Lexicomp®

Drug Information Handbook *for Dentistry*

Including Oral Medicine for Medically Compromised Patients & Specific Oral Conditions

26th Edition

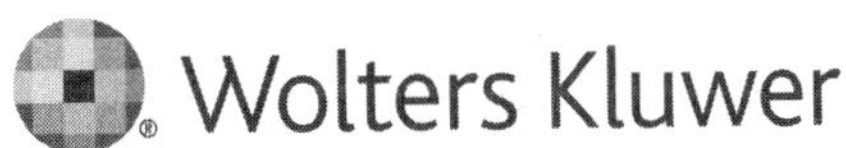

Lexicomp®

Drug Information Handbook *for Dentistry*

Including Oral Medicine for Medically Compromised Patients & Specific Oral Conditions

Richard L. Wynn, BSPharm, PhD
Professor of Pharmacology
Baltimore College of Dental Surgery
Dental School
University of Maryland Baltimore
Baltimore, Maryland

Timothy F. Meiller, DDS, PhD
Professor
Oncology and Diagnostic Sciences
Baltimore College of Dental Surgery
Professor of Oncology
Marlene and Stewart Greenebaum Cancer Center
University of Maryland Medical System
Baltimore, Maryland

Harold L. Crossley, DDS, MS, PhD
Professor Emeritus
Baltimore College of Dental Surgery
Dental School
University of Maryland Baltimore
Baltimore, Maryland

Lexicomp®

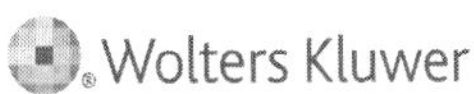
Wolters Kluwer

NOTICE

This data is intended to serve the user as a handy reference and not as a complete drug information resource. It does not include information on every therapeutic agent available. The publication covers over 1,600 commonly used drugs. In addition, it does not include all potentially relevant information about any particular drug. Instead, it is intended to present important aspects of drug data in a more concise and accessible format than is typically found in medical literature or product material supplied by manufacturers.

The nature of drug information is that it is constantly evolving because of ongoing research and clinical experience and is often subject to interpretation. UpToDate, Inc. ("UpToDate") publishes summary drug information in this reference resource for use by healthcare professionals in the course of their professional practice. The content in this resource is intended only to supplement – not substitute for or replace – the knowledge and judgment of physicians, nurses, pharmacists and other healthcare professionals regarding drug therapy and patient-specific health conditions.

The content is published based upon publicly available sources generally viewed as reliable in the healthcare community, including specifically pharmaceutical manufacturer labeling, information published by regulatory agencies and primary medical literature. UpToDate does not engage in any independent review, testing or study of any medication, medical device, condition, illness, injury, test, procedure, treatment, or therapy in connection with the publication of the content. The content is not intended to explicitly or implicitly endorse any particular medication as safe or effective for treating any particular patient or health condition. Certain of UpToDate's authors, editors, reviewers, and contributors have written portions of this book in their individual capacities. The inclusion of content is not intended to indicate that it has been reviewed or endorsed by any federal or state agency, pharmaceutical company, or regulatory body.

UpToDate assumes no responsibility or liability for errors or omissions of any kind in the content. UpToDate expressly disclaims any liability for any loss or damage claimed to have resulted from the use of the content. Users of the content shall hold UpToDate harmless from any such claims and shall indemnify UpToDate for any expenses incurred if such claims are made. In no event shall UpToDate nor any of its authors, editors, reviewers, contributors or publishers be liable to any user or any third-party, including specifically any customer or patient of a user, for direct, special, indirect, incidental, or consequential damages. UpToDate disclaims all warranties of any kind or nature, whether expressed or implied, including any warranty as to the quality, accuracy, comprehensiveness, currency, suitability, availability, compatibility, merchantability, and fitness for a particular purpose of the content.

If you have any suggestions or questions regarding any information presented in this data, please contact our drug information pharmacists at (855) 633-0577. Book revisions are available at our website at http://www.wolterskluwercdi.com/clinical-notices/revisions/.

This manual was produced using LIMS — a publishing service of UpToDate, Inc.

Lexicomp®

ISBN 978-1-59195-382-1

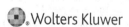

TABLE OF CONTENTS

TABLE OF CONTENTS

ABOUT THE EDITORS

Richard L. Wynn, BSPharm, PhD

Richard L. Wynn, PhD, is Professor of Pharmacology at the Baltimore College of Dental Surgery, Dental School, University of Maryland Baltimore. Dr Wynn has served as a dental educator, researcher, and teacher of dental pharmacology and dental hygiene pharmacology for his entire professional career. He holds a BS in Pharmacy, an MS (physiology), and a PhD (pharmacology) from the University of Maryland. He was a practicing pharmacist for 10 years in the Baltimore area. Dr Wynn chaired the Department of Pharmacology at the University of Maryland Dental School from 1980 to 1995. From 1990 to 1995 he was also the appointed Chair of the Department of Biochemistry at the Dental School. Previously, he chaired the Department of Oral Biology at the University of Kentucky College of Dentistry, for six years.

Dr Wynn has to his credit over 400 publications, including original research articles in scientific journals, textbooks, textbook chapters, monographs, and articles in continuing education journals. He has given over 600 continuing education seminars to dental professionals in the US, Canada, and Europe. Dr Wynn has been a consultant to the drug industry for over 30 years and his research laboratories have contributed to the development of new analgesics and anesthetics. He is a former consultant to the Academy of General Dentistry, the American Dental Association, and a former consultant to the Council on Dental Education, Commission on Accreditation. One of his primary interests continues to be keeping dental professionals informed on all aspects of drug use in dental practice.

Timothy F. Meiller, DDS, PhD

Dr Meiller is Professor of Oncology and Diagnostic Sciences at the University of Maryland Dental School and Professor of Oncology at the Marlene and Stewart Greenebaum Comprehensive Cancer Center, University of Maryland Medical System in Baltimore. He is Director of the Oral Medicine Program in the dental school and the cancer center. He has held his position at the Dental School for 43 years.

Dr Meiller is a Diplomate of the American Board of Oral Medicine and a graduate of Johns Hopkins University and the University of Maryland Dental and Graduate Schools, holding a DDS and a PhD in Immunology/Virology. He has over 200 publications to his credit, maintains an active general dental practice, and is a consultant to the National Institutes of Health and the Veterans Administration. He is currently engaged in ongoing investigations into cellular immune dysfunction in premalignant oral lesions, oral diseases associated with AIDS, in patients receiving therapies for cancer and in other medically-compromised patients.

Harold L. Crossley, DDS, MS, PhD

Dr Crossley is Professor Emeritus at the University of Maryland Dental School. A native of Rhode Island, Dr Crossley received a Bachelor of Science degree in Pharmacy from the University of Rhode Island in 1964. He later was awarded the Master of Science (1970) and Doctorate degrees (1972) in Pharmacology. The University of Maryland Dental School in Baltimore awarded Dr Crossley the DDS degree in 1980. The liaison between the classroom and his dental practice, which he maintained on a part-time basis in the Dental School Intramural Faculty Practice, produced a practical approach to understanding the pharmacology of drugs used in the dental office.

Dr Crossley has coauthored a number of articles and four books dealing with a variety of topics within the field of pharmacology. Other areas of expertise include the pharmacology of street drugs and chemical dependency. He serves on the Maryland State Dental Association's Well-Being Committee. He is an active member of Phi Kappa Phi, Omicron Kappa Upsilon Honorary Dental Society, the American College of Dentists, International College of Dentists, and an honorary member of the Thomas B. Hinman Dental Society. He was the recipient of the 2008 Gordon Christensen Lecturer Recognition award presented by the Chicago Dental Society, and the recipient of the 2012 Award of Distinction presented by the Academy of Dentistry International for his efforts in continuing dental education. He has been a consultant for the United States Drug Enforcement Administration and other law enforcement agencies since 1974. Drawing on this unique background, Dr Crossley has become nationally and internationally recognized as an expert on street drugs and chemical dependency as well as the clinical pharmacology of dental drugs.

DRUG INTERACTIONS EDITORIAL ADVISORY PANEL

Nina Bemben, PharmD, BCPS
Senior Clinical Content Specialist
Wolters Kluwer

Melody Berg, PharmD, MPH, BCPS-AQ ID, AAHIVP
Senior Clinical Content Specialist
Wolters Kluwer

Kay Burke, PharmD
Senior Clinical Content Specialist
Wolters Kluwer

Nadia Haque, PharmD, MHSA, BCPS, FASHP
Senior Clinical Content Specialist
Wolters Kluwer

Jamie Hoffman, PharmD, BCPS
Senior Clinical Content Specialist
Wolters Kluwer

Carrie Nemerovski, PharmD, BCPS-AQ Cardiology
Senior Clinical Content Specialist
Wolters Kluwer

Kandace M. Schuft, PharmD
Senior Clinical Content Specialist
Wolters Kluwer

Steve Sklar, PharmD
Senior Clinical Manager
Wolters Kluwer

Stephen Marc Stout, PharmD, MS, BCPS
Director, Clinical Content
Wolters Kluwer

Daniel S. Streetman, PharmD, MS, RPh
Clinical Manager, Metabolism, Interactions, & Genomics Group
Wolters Kluwer

Sarah Warren, PharmD
Senior Clinical Content Specialist, Clinical Decision Support Pharmacogenomics Content
Wolters Kluwer

David M. Weinstein, PhD, RPh
Senior Director, Clinical Content
Wolters Kluwer

EDITORIAL ADVISORY PANEL

Christine M. Cohn, PharmD, BCPS
Senior Clinical Content Specialist
Wolters Kluwer

Justin W. Cole, PharmD, BCPS
Chair of Pharmacy Practice, Director,
Center for Pharmacy Innovation
Cedarville University School of Pharmacy

Michelle Condren, PharmD, BCPPS, AE-C, CDE, FPPAG
Professor and Director of Pediatric Research
University of Oklahoma
School of Community Medicine,
Department of Pediatrics

Jessica Connell, RN, BSN
Pharmacotherapy Contributor
Tifton, Georgia

Kim Connell, PharmD
Pharmacotherapy Contributor
Thomasville, Georgia

Elizabeth V. Connor, MD
Gynecologic Oncologist
Billings Clinic

Ann P. Conrad, ANP-BC, RN, ACRN
Advanced Practice Nurse
Community Hospitalists

James Coons, PharmD, FCCP, BCCP
Clinical Pharmacist, Cardiology
University of Pittsburgh School of Pharmacy

Marilyn Cortell, RDH, MS, FAADH
Associate Professor
New York City College of Technology,
City University of New York

Jessica Cottreau, PharmD, BCPS
Infectious Diseases Clinical Pharmacist
Northwestern Memorial Hospital

Harold L. Crossley, DDS, MS, PhD
Professor Emeritus
Baltimore College of Dental Surgery,
University of Maryland

Erica Lee Breden Crouse, PharmD, BCPP, BCGP, FASCP, FASHP
Clinical Pharmacy Specialist, Psychiatry
Virginia Commonwealth University Health

Melanie W. Cucchi, BS, PharmD, RPh
Clinical Manager, Pediatric & Neonatal Content
Wolters Kluwer

Judy Cvetinovich, RPh
Clinical Manager,
Clinical Decision Support Dosing Content
Wolters Kluwer

Martha Dagen, MT (ASCP), SBB
Laboratory Assistant Director
Williamson Medical Center

Mitchell J. Daley, PharmD, FCCM, BCPS
Clinical Pharmacy Specialist – Critical Care
University Medical Center Brackenridge

Kathryn E. Dane, PharmD, BCPS
Clinical Pharmacy Specialist,
Inpatient Anticoagulation and Hematology
The Johns Hopkins Hospital

Emily E. Davies, PharmD, CPE
Clinical Pharmacist
University Hospital Home Health

Christine Tisdale Davis, PharmD
Clinical Pharmacy Specialist
St. Boniface Hospital (Canada)

Joseph M. Davis, PharmD, BCPS
Clinical Nephrology/Decentralized Medicine Pharmacist
Vidant Medical Center

Lacey Davis, PharmD, BCPS
Clinical Pharmacist, Hospice, Palliative Care, and
Post-Acute Care
Aultman Hospital

Beth Deen, PharmD, BDNSP
Senior Pediatric Clinical Pharmacy Specialist
Cook Children's Medical Center

Renee K. Dixon, MD
Pulmonary Attending/Pulmonologist
Christiana Care Hospital

Elisabeth Donahey, PharmD, BCPS, BCCCP
Senior Clinical Content Specialist
Wolters Kluwer

Heather M. Draper, PharmD, BCPS
Clinical Pharmacist, Emergency Medicine
Mercy Health Saint Mary's

Kim S. Dufner, PharmD
Clinical Content Specialist
Wolters Kluwer

Steven Patrick Dunn, PharmD, FAHA, FCCP, BCPS-AQ Cardiology, BCCP
Pharmacy Clinical Coordinator
University of Virginia Health System

Emily A. Durr, PharmD, BCCCP
Clinical Pharmacy Specialist, Surgical Critical Care
Grady Health System

Ijeoma Julie Eche, MSN, FNP-BC, AOCNP, CPHON, BMT-CN
Family Nurse Practitioner, Staff Nurse
Beth Israel Deaconess Medical Center,
Boston Children's Hospital

Megan Jo Ehret, PharmD, MS, BCPP
Associate Professor
University of Maryland, School of Pharmacy

Vicki L. Ellingrod, PharmD, BCPP
Head, Clinical Pharmacogenomics
Laboratory and *Associate Professor*
Department of Psychiatry,
Colleges of Pharmacy and Medicine,
University of Michigan

Jacqueline Ellis, RN, MSN
Pharmacotherapy Contributor
Twinsburg, Ohio

Kelley K. Engle, BSPharm
Pharmacotherapy Contributor
Stow, Ohio

Christopher Ensor, PharmD, BCPS-AQ Cardiology, FAST, FCCP
Pharmacotherapy Specialist, Thoracic Transplantation and Clinical Coordinator
Florida Hospital

Gregory A. Eschenauer, PharmD, BCPS-AQ ID
Infectious Diseases Clinical Pharmacist
Michigan Medicine

Kirk Evoy, PharmD, BCACP, BC-ADM, CTTS
Ambulatory Clinical Pharmacist
Southeast Clinic, University Health System

Nicole L. Eye, PharmD
Pain Clinical Specialist Pharmacist
Avera McKennan Hospital

Erin Fabian, PharmD, RPh, BCPS
Senior Clinical Content Specialist
Wolters Kluwer

Michael Fahey, BSc, MSc, PhD, MRPharmS
Director
Alignment Consulting

Jessica F. Farrell, PharmD
Associate Professor
Albany College of Pharmacy and Health Sciences

Elizabeth A. Farrington, PharmD, FCCP, FCCM, FPPAG, BCPS
Pharmacist III - Pediatrics
New Hanover Regional Medical Center

Salia Farrokh, PharmD, BCPS, BCCP
Neuro ICU Clinical Pharmacist Specialist
The John Hopkins Hospital

J. Emanuel Finet, MD
Staff, Section of Heart Failure and Transplantation Medicine
Cleveland Clinic

Christine Fitzgerald, PharmD, BCPS
Pharmacotherapy Contributor
Valleio, California

David Frame, PharmD
Hematology/Oncology/BMT Clinical Specialist
Michigan Medicine

Kristina M. Frangella, PharmD, BCPS, CDE, BCACP
Clinical Pharmacy Specialist, Ambulatory Care
Louis Stokes
Cleveland Department of Veteran Affairs
Medical Center

Michelle A. Fravel, PharmD, BCPS
Clinical Pharmacy Specialist
University of Iowa Health Care

Carole W. Fuseck, MSN, RN, ACCNS-AG, VA-BC
Clinical Nurse Specialist, Critical Care
Louis Stokes
Cleveland Department of Veteran Affairs
Medical Center

Jennifer Gatsos-Walter, PharmD
Senior Clinical Content Specialist, Clinical Decision Support Dosing Content
Wolters Kluwer

Charles Gaudet, BSN, RN, CCRN
Staff Nurse
Tufts Medical Center

Laura Gaudet, BDN, RN-BC
Staff Nurse
Massachusetts General Hospital

Bruce Gaynes, BS, OD, MS, PharmD
Staff Optometrist
Edward Hines, Jr. VA Hospital,
Department of Veterans Affairs Medical Center

Joyce Generali, RPh, MS, FASHP
Senior Clinical Manager, In-depth Content
Wolters Kluwer

Angela G. German, PharmD, BCOP
Clinical Pharmacy Specialist
Henry Ford Hospital

Jennifer Gibbons, PT, DPT
Early Intervention Physical Therapist
Cuyahoga County Board of Developmental Disabilities

Angela M. Gibson, PharmD, RPh
Staff Pharmacist
Floyd Memorial Hospital and
Health Services/Baptist Health Floyd

Vi Gilmore, PharmD, BCPS
Clinical Pharmacy Specialist, Internal Medicine
The Johns Hopkins Hospital

Heather L. Girand, PharmD
Professor of Pharmacy, Pediatrics
Pharmacy Practice, Ferris State University
College of Pharmacy

Meredith D. Girard, MD, FACP
Medical Staff
Department of Internal Medicine, Summa Health Systems

Jennifer Ellis Girotto, PharmD, BCPPS, BCIDP
Infectious Diseases Clinical Pharmacist
Connecticut Children's Medical Center

Jeffrey P. Gonzales, PharmD, BCPS
Senior Clinical Content Specialist
Wolters Kluwer

John D. Grabenstein, RPh, PhD
Vaccinologist
Easton, Maryland

Kelley Graham, RN
Home Health Nurse
Bayada Home Health

Tania H. Gregorian, PharmD
Clinical Pharmacist, Ambulatory Care
Cedars-Sinai Medical Care Foundation

Shellee A. Grim, PharmD, MS-CTS, BCPS, BCIDP
Senior Clinical Content Specialist
Wolters Kluwer

Alison Gambill Grisso, PharmD, BCPPS
Pediatrics Clinical Pharmacist
Vanderbilt Children's Hospital

Kelly Gruver, RDH, EFDA, MHHS
Preceptor and Clinical Coordinator
Cuyahoga Community College

Mitra Habibi, PharmD
Clinical Pharmacist
University of Illinois
Hospital and Health Sciences System

Tracy Hagemann, PharmD
Associate Dean and *Professor of Clinical Pharmacy*
University of Tennessee College of Pharmacy

Kat Hall, MPharm, IPresc, PGCertClinEd, PGDipGPP, MFRPSII, MRPharmS, FHEA
Director of Centre for Inter-Professional Postgraduate Education and Training
University of Reading

Nadia Haque, PharmD, MHSA, BCPS, FASHP
Senior Clinical Content Specialist
Wolters Kluwer

Jacqueline Harris, MSN, RN
Nurse Manager
Louis Stokes Cleveland VA Medical Center

Steve Hart, MD
Director, Clinical Decision Support Precautions Team
Wolters Kluwer

Kristin L. Harter, PharmD, BCPS
Clinical Pharmacist
San Francisco General Hospital

Emily L. Heil, PharmD, BCIDP, BCPS-AQ ID, AAHIVP
Infectious Diseases Clinical Pharmacy Specialist
University of Maryland Medical Center

Sarrah Hein, PharmD, BCPPS
Pediatric Clinical Coordinator
Akron Children's Hospital

Eric Henry, PharmD
Clinical Content Specialist, Drug Files
Wolters Kluwer

Alicia M. Hernandez, MPH, RN, BSN
Family Nurse Practitioner
MetroHealth Medical System

Carla Hernandez, RN, BSN
Clinical Research Nurse
University Hospitals Cleveland Medical Center

Michael Heung, MD, MS
Associate Chief for Clinical Affairs and Service Chief, Division of Nephrology
University of Michigan Medical School

Tara A. Higgins, PharmD, BCPPS
Clinical Pharmacy Specialist, Pediatric Hematology/Oncology/BMT
UF Health Shands Hospital

Jacob Hirsekorn, PharmD
Clinical Content Specialist
Wolters Kluwer

Jamie Hoffman, PharmD, BCPS
Senior Clinical Content Specialist
Wolters Kluwer

Mark T. Holdsworth, PharmD
Associate Professor of Pharmacy & Pediatrics and *Pharmacy Practice Area Head*
College of Pharmacy, The University of New Mexico

Christine Holman, PharmD, BCGP, BCPS
Clinical Pharmacy Specialist
Kaiser Permanente Springfield Medical Center

Amy P. Holmes, PharmD, BCPPS
Neonatal Intensive Care Clinical Specialist
Novant Health Forsyth Medical Center

Edward Horn, PharmD, BCPS
Clinical Specialist, Transplant/Cardiothoracic Surgery
Allegheny General Hospital

Collin A. Hovinga, PharmD, MS, FCCP
Director of Research Support Services
Seton Healthcare Family, Dell Children's Medical Center

Joanna Hudson, PharmD, BCPS, FASN, FCCP, FNKF
Clinical Pharmacist, Nephrology
Methodist University Hospital

Robert W. Hutchison Jr, PharmD, BCACP
Clinical Associate Professor of Pharmacy Practice
Texas A&M Irma Lerma Rangel College of Pharmacy

Lauren Hynicka, PharmD, BCPS
Clinical Pharmacy Specialist
University of Maryland Medical Center

Makiko Iwasawa, PharmD, BCPS
Chief Pharmacist, Drug Information Center
National Cerebral and Cardiovascular Center

Adam B. Jackson, PharmD, BCPS
Clinical Pharmacy Specialist in Infectious Diseases
Kaiser Permanente

Anna M. Wodlinger Jackson, PharmD, BCPS-AQ Cardiology
Pharmacotherapy Contributor
Fort Lauderdale, Florida

Annette Jenkins, RPh
Clinical Content Specialist
Wolters Kluwer

Tamika Johnson, BSN, RN, CCM
Ambulatory Oncology Nurse Case Manager
Children's National Medical Center

Beth Outland Jones, RPh
Clinical Content Specialist, Clinical Decision Support Precautions Team
Wolters Kluwer

Jeffrey D. Lewis, PharmD, MACM
Dean and Professor
Lloyd L. Gregory School of Pharmacy,
Palm Beach Atlantic University

John Lindsley, PharmD, BCPS
Cardiology Clinical Pharmacy Specialist
The Johns Hopkins Hospital

Nicholas A. Link, PharmD, BCOP
Clinical Specialist, Oncology
Cleveland Clinic Hillcrest Hospital

Lisa K. Lohr, PharmD
Oncology Pharmacy Specialist
Masonic Cancer Clinic

Julie Lothamer, RPh
Clinical Content Specialist,
Clinical Decision Support Dosing Content
Wolters Kluwer

Jennifer Loucks, PharmD, BCPS
Solid Organ Transplant Clinical Pharmacist
The University of Kansas Hospital

Jennifer Fisher Lowe, PharmD, BCOP
Clinical Oncology Pharmacist
IU Health Simon Cancer Center

Sherry Luedtke, PharmD
Associate Professor
Department of Pharmacy Practice,
Texas Tech University HSC School of Pharmacy

Viki Lui, BPharm, MPH, MSHP
Lead Education Pharmacist for Pharmacy Department
The Royal Melbourne Hospital

Jordan D. Lundberg, PharmD, BCOP
Clinical Specialist Pharmacist, Hematology
The James Cancer Hospital and
Solove Research Institute

Scott Lundy, MD, PhD
Resident Physician
Cleveland Clinic Foundation

Melissa Makii, PharmD, BCPS
Clinical Pharmacy Specialist, Pediatric Oncology
Rainbow Babies & Children's Hospital

Karen Falck Marlowe, PharmD, BCPS, CPE
Assistant Dean, Associate Department Head
Auburn University, Harrison School of Pharmacy

Patricia L. Marshik, PharmD
Associate Professor of Pharmacy with Tenure
University of New Mexico Health Sciences Center,
College of Pharmacy

Marketa Marvanova, PharmD, PhD, BCGP, BCPP, FASCP
Dean and *Professor*
University of Montana

Kelly Matatics, BSN, RN-BC, OCN
Clinical Nurse Research Specialist
University Hospitals Cleveland Medical Center

Vincent F. Mauro, BS, PharmD, FCCP
Professor of Clinical Pharmacy and
Adjunct Professor of Medicine
Colleges of Pharmacy and Medicine,
The University of Toledo

Rebecca Ann Maxson, PharmD, BCPS
Assistant Clinical Professor
Auburn University, Harrison School of Pharmacy

Joseph Mazur, BScPharm, PharmD, BCPS
Clinical Specialist – MICU/Pulmonary
Medical University of South Carolina

Shawn Mazur, PharmD
Clinical Pharmacy Manager, Infectious Diseases
New York-Presbyterian/Weill Cornell Medical Center

Jamie L. McConaha, PharmD, NCTTP, BCACP, CDE
Associate Professor of Pharmacy Practice
Duquesne University Mylan School of Pharmacy

Joseph McGraw, PharmD, MPH, PhD, BCPS
Assistant Professor of Pharmaceutical Science and
Metabolism Laboratory Director
Concordia University Wisconsin, School of Pharmacy

Shawn McKinney, RPh
Clinical Manager, Drug Files
Wolters Kluwer

Ann Marie McMullin, MD
Associate Staff
Emergency Services Institute, Cleveland Clinic

Christopher McPherson, PharmD
Clinical Pharmacy Practice Manager
Neonatal Intensive Care Unit, St. Louis Children's Hospital

Calvin J. Meaney, PharmD, BCPS
Clinical Assistant Professor
University at Buffalo School of Pharmacy and
Pharmaceutical Sciences

Varsha Mehta, PharmD, MS, FCCP
Clinical Pharmacist
Michigan Medicine

Timothy F. Meiller, DDS, PhD
Professor
Oncology and Diagnostic Sciences,
Baltimore College of Dental Surgery

Micheline Meiners, MSc, PhD
Pharmacotherapy Contributor
Lago Norte, Brazil

Cathy A. Meives, PharmD
Clinical Manager, Core Pharmacology
Wolters Kluwer

Megan Menon, PharmD, BCOP
Clinical Pharmacy Specialist
Roswell Park Cancer Institute

Jenna Meredith, APRN, MSN, NNP-BC
Neonatal Nurse Practitioner
MetroHealth Medical Center

Jessica Beth Michaud, PharmD, BCPS
Clinical Pharmacist
Froedtert & the Medical College of Wisconsin

Ji Hyun Park, PharmD, RPh
Clinical Pharmacist
KEPCO Medical Center, Hanjeon Hospital, KMC

Susie H. Park, PharmD, BCPP
Assistant Professor of Clinical Pharmacy
University of Southern Califormia

Mary Herring Parker, PharmD, FASHP, FCCP, BCPS, BCCP
Clinical Pharmacist Specialist
Durham VA HealthCare System

Nicole Passerrello, PharmD, BCPPS, BCPS
Senior Clinical Content Specialist
Wolters Kluwer

Neha Patel, PharmD, BCPS
Clinical Specialist, Solid Organ Transplant, Adjunct Facility
Medical University of South Carolina

Nisha K. Patel, PharmD, MBA, BCPS
Clinical Pharmacy Specialist
The Johns Hopkins Hospital

Brent Pettijohn Sr., RPh
Clinical Content Specialist, Drug Files
Wolters Kluwer

Rebecca Pettit, PharmD, MBA, BCPS
Pediatric Pulmonary Clinical Pharmacy Specialist
Riley Hospital for Children,
Indiana University Health,
Department of Pharmacy

Hanna Phan, PharmD, FCCP
Clinical Pharmacy Specialist,
Pediatric Pulmonology and Sleep
Banner University Medical Center, Tucson

Cameron Phillips, BPharm, MClin Pharm
Academic Affiliate
College of Medicine and Public Health,
Flinders University

Kristie Phillips, psy.APRN.CNS-BC
Research Nurse
Louis Stokes VA Medical Center

Julie Pingel, PharmD, BCPPS
Pediatric Critical Care Clinical Pharmacy Specialist
Monroe Carell Jr. Children's Hospital at Vanderbilt

Jennifer L. Placencia, PharmD
Neonatal Clinical Pharmacy Specialist
Texas Children's Hospital

Karen Post, RPh
Clinical Manager, Drug Files
Wolters Kluwer

Ted Post, MD
Editor-in-Chief
Wolters Kluwer

Amy L. Potts, PharmD, BCPS
Program Director, Quality, Safety, and Education
Monroe Carell Jr. Children's Hospital at Vanderbilt

Erin Powell, PharmD
Clinical Content Specialist, Drug Files
Wolters Kluwer

Jessica Price, PharmD
Clinical Pharmacy Specialist
Children's Hospital of the King's Daughter

Mary Quigley, BSN, RN
Clinical Nurse Manager
Barnes Jewish Hospital

Saira Rab, PharmD, BCPS-AQ ID, AAHIVP
Infectious Diseases/HIV Clinical Pharmacist Specialist
Grady Health System

Sally Rafie, PharmD, BCPS
Medical Safety Pharmacist
UC San Diego Health System

Esta Razavi, PharmD, MBA
Clinical Content Specialist,
Clinical Decision Support Precautions Team
Wolters Kluwer

Brent Reed, BS, PharmD, BCPS-AQ Cardiology, FAHA
Clinical Pharmacy Specialist, Heart Transplantation Clinic
University of Maryland Heart Center

James Reissig, PharmD, BCPS
Pharmacy Specialist, Residency Program Director
UH Parma Medical Center

Neil Reynolds, BPharm, MSc
Senior Pharmacist
Fiona Stanley Hospital

Vanitra Richards, PharmD
Clinical Content Specialist,
Clinical Decision Support Precautions Teams
Wolters Kluwer

Linda Riski-Lindorff, RPh
Senior Clinical Content Specialist, Drug Files
Wolters Kluwer

Darren Roberts, BPharm, MBBS, PhD, FRACP
Staff Specialist, Clinical Pharmacology and Toxicology
St. Vincent's Hospital (Australia)

Jason A. Roberts, PhD, BPharm (Hons), B App Sc, FSHP
Clinical Pharmacist
Royal Brisbane and Women's Hospital

Melissa E. Rotz, PharmD, BCPS
Staff Pharmacist
Cooper University Hospital

Lisa Ryan, MD
General Pediatrician
BJC Medical Group

Amy Rybarczyk, PharmD, BCPS
Pharmacy Clinical Manager
Wooster Community Hospital

Rikki L. Rychel, PharmD, BCPS, CDE
Clinical Pharmacy Specialist, Ambulatory Care
Louis Stokes Cleveland Department of Veterans Affairs Medical Center

Shannon Saldana, PharmD, MS, BCPP
Psychiatry Advanced Clinical Pharmacist
Primary Children's Hospital

Alexandra L. Thompson, RN
Staff RN, Inpatient Pediatrics
Newton Wellesley Hospital

Kathryn Timberlake, PharmD, FCSHP
Clinical Pharmacy Specialist, Infectious Diseases
The Hospital for Sick Children

Sandra R. Tolbert, PharmD, BCGP
Pharmacotherapy Contributor
North Royalton, Ohio

Lindsey Toman, PharmD, BCPS
Clinical Pharmacy Specialist, Solid Organ Transplantation
The Johns Hopkins Hospital

Elizabeth A. Tomsik, PharmD, BCPS
Senior Clinical Director, Drug Content
Wolters Kluwer

Van L. Tran, PharmD, BCPS, BCPPS, MBA
Clinical Pharmacy Specialist
INOVA Children's Hospital

Dana Travis, RPh
Clinical Content Specialist
Wolters Kluwer

Heidi Trinkman, PharmD
Pediatric Hematology/Oncology
Clinical Pharmacy Specialist
Cook Children's Medical Center

Tanya Uritsky, PharmD, BCPS
Clinical Pharmacy Specialist in Pain and Palliative Care
Hospital of the University of Pennsylvania

Amy M. VandenBerg, PharmD, BCPP
Clinical Pharmacy Specialist, Psychiatry and Neurology
Michigan Medicine

Andriette van Jaarsveld, BPharm, MScMed
Clinical Pharmacy Specialist
Mediclinic Southern Africa (Stellenbosch)

Amy Van Orman, PharmD, BCPS
Senior Clinical Content Specialist
Wolters Kluwer

Craig Vargo, PharmD, BCOP
Specialty Practice Pharmacist, Breast Oncology
The James Cancer Hospital and Solove Research Institute

Carlos Vidotti
Pharmacotherapy Contributor
Brasilia DF, Brazil

A. Mary Vilay, PharmD
Associate Professor
University of New Mexico

Polly Waggoner, RPh
Clinical Director, Drug Files
Wolters Kluwer

Robert Wahler Jr, PharmD
Director, Clinical Pharmacy Services
Niagara Hospice Inc

Sarah Warren, PharmD
Senior Clinical Content Specialist
Wolters Kluwer

Kristin Watson, PharmD, BCPS
Clinical Pharmacy Specialist, Heart Failure Clinic
Veterans Affairs Medical Center

Lori D. Wazny, PharmD, BSc (Pharm), EPPH
Clinical Pharmacist
Manitoba Renal Program, Health Sciences Centre

Kyle A. Weant, PharmD, BCPS, BCCCP, FCCP
Clinical Pharmacist Specialist, Emergency Medicine
Medical University of South Carolina

JoEllen L. Weilnau, PharmD
Clinical Coordinator
Department of Hematology/Oncology/Bone Marrow Transplant, Akron Children's Hospital

David M. Weinstein, PhD, RPh
Senior Director, Clinical Content
Wolters Kluwer

Paula Welker, RPh
Clinical Content Specialist
Wolters Kluwer

Cindy Wethington, RPh
Clinical Content Specialist,
Clinical Decision Support Dosing Content
Wolters Kluwer

Regine L. White, PharmD, RPh
Senior Clinical Content Specialist
Wolters Kluwer

Ashley Whitley, APRN, FNP-C
Family Nurse Practitioner
USAF GUARD

Greg Wiggers, PharmD, PhD
Clinical Content Specialist
Wolters Kluwer

Barbara S. Wiggins, PharmD, MBA, BCPS, BCCP, BCCCP, CLS, FNLA, FAHA, FCCP, FACC
Clinical Pharmacy Specialist, Cardiology
Medical University of South Carolina

Sheilia M. Wilhelm, PharmD, FCCP, BCPS
Associate Professor (Clinical),
Department of Pharmacy Practice
Wayne State University,
Eugene Applebaum College of Pharmacy

Andrea Williams, RPh
Pharmacotherapy Contributor
St. Louis, MO

Nathan Wirick, PharmD, BCPS
Clinical Specialist in Infectious Diseases and
Antibiotic Management
Cleveland Clinic Hillcrest Hospital

G. Christopher Wood, PharmD, BCCCP, BCPS-AQ ID
Clinical Pharmacist
Regional One Health Medical Center,
University of Tennessee Health Science Center

Lisa A. Wood, PharmD, BCPS, BCPPS
Clinical Pharmacist, Critical Care
Ann & Robert H. Lurie Children's Hospital of Chicago

PREFACE TO THE TWENTY-SIXTH EDITION

The editors of the 26th edition of the *Drug Information Handbook for Dentistry* are extremely proud that the book remains as popular and as successful as its readers have affirmed. We thank each practitioner and student who has made the previous editions so widely accepted in the field of dentistry. In this new 26th edition, we have responded to all of the comments and creative suggestions that come from our readership each year. We know that our text remains the premier companion to the daily practice of dentistry and that it complements Oral Medicine and medical reference libraries that every clinician has available in their office.

The latest Guidelines for Antimicrobial Stewardship endorsed by the ADA have been added, including the guideline effects on the management of patients at risk of endocarditis or those with joint prostheses. In addition, the new recommendations for antibiotic use in odontogenic infections by the American Association of Endodontists have been included.

The chapter related to the dentist's involvement with the cancer patient now has an expanded section for salivary testing for HPV and HPV vaccines as well as addresses diagnostic testing in the dental office. Stand-alone sections have been updated for the crucial topics of Antiplatelet and Anticoagulation Considerations in Dentistry, adding information on the newly approved reversal agent for one of the novel anticoagulation drugs. Medication related osteonecrosis of the jaw (MRONJ) information has been updated. Recommended readings have been edited for chapter subsections. Sections have been expanded and added related to prescribing medications with NSAIDs including their risk association with MI and stroke, acetaminophen, and sarcoidosis. Prescribing information options are outlined and are available for easy cross-referencing for the busy dental practitioner.

As in each previous edition, the Oral Medicine chapters have been updated offering a clearly highlighted selection of common dental office prescription choices and Rx examples for management of common oral conditions often encountered during patient care. These example prescriptions have been updated and are presented in a stand alone section for quicker reference.

There have been expanded discussions inserted of how opioid prescribing guidelines and non-narcotic alternative medication choices can be prudently evaluated by dentists to manage acute and chronic oral pain.

The monographs now include over 1,600 drugs and these have been updated in the 26th edition with the fields expanded in common monographs to make them easier to read and identify for all of the drugs. The fields most important to practicing dentists have been enhanced. The drugs most commonly used in dentistry have the added fields regarding specific use considerations in dentistry. Medical drugs also include dosing and dose formulation information. In addition, the adverse reaction section and the important uses and effects on dental treatment for all drugs have been updated throughout the text, now categorizing common oral adverse events as frequent, infrequent, or rare.

In addition to the extensive information presented, we are confident that the dental practitioners and dental hygienists who utilize the text will find the size and format to be easy to navigate. The drug information section of the handbook, in which all drugs are listed alphabetically, includes extensive cross-referencing by US brand names and index terms, making the text the true complete drug reference guide for dental practice.

We hope that the active general dentist, the specialist, the dental hygienist, and the advanced student of dentistry remain better prepared for patient care while using this new 26th edition of the DIHD.

Richard L. Wynn

Timothy F. Meiller

Harold L. Crossley

DESCRIPTION OF SECTIONS AND FIELDS USED IN THIS HANDBOOK

The *Drug Information Handbook for Dentistry, 26th Edition* is organized into six sections: Introductory text; sample prescriptions, alphabetical listing of drug monographs; natural products; oral medicine topics; appendix; and a Pharmacologic Category Index which lists all drugs in this handbook in their unique pharmacologic class.

INTRODUCTORY TEXT

Helpful guides to understanding the organization and format of the information in this handbook.

SAMPLE PRESCRIPTIONS

Examples provided for prototype drugs and popular prescriptions. Prescriptions included for the following uses: Prevention of endocarditis and to reduce the risk of late infections of joint prostheses, oral pain, bacterial infections and periodontal diseases, sinus infection treatment, antimicrobial oral rinse, fungal infections, viral infections, ulcerative and erosive disorders, sedation (prior to dental treatment).

DRUG MONOGRAPHS

This alphabetical listing of drugs contains comprehensive monographs for medications commonly prescribed in dentistry and concise monographs for other popular drugs which dental patients may be taking. Extensive cross-referencing is provided by US brand names and index terms. Monographs may contain the following fields:

Generic Name	US adopted name
Pronunciation	Phonetic pronunciation guide
Related Information	Cross-reference(s) to pertinent information in other sections of this handbook
Related Sample Prescriptions	Cross-reference(s) to sample prescriptions.
Brand Names: US	Trade names found in the United States (manufacturer-specific). The symbol [DSC] appears after trade names that have been recently discontinued.
Brand Names: Canada	Trade names found in Canada.
Generic Availability (US)	Indicates availability of generic products in the United States
Pharmacologic Category	Indicates one or more systematic classifications of the drug
Dental Use	Information in the **Dental Use** field indicates when a drug has an established use specific to dentistry and/or oral medicine. In some cases, these uses are considered to be unlabeled, as they are not included in the FDA-approved product labeling (see Description of Dental Use).
Use	Statements under the **Use** field reflect the approved labeling by the FDA based on accepted clinical evaluation on safety and efficacy of the drug as submitted in the New Drug Application (NDA). The "gold standard" of clinical testing of a new drug requires a randomly selected cohort of subjects, using a double-blind and placebo controlled protocol and an acceptable method of assessment to test differences between test compound and placebo. It is assumed that by their approval of the labeling, the FDA considers the new drug "safe and effective" for treating a particular condition in a given patient population.
Local Anesthetic/Vasoconstrictor Precautions	Specific information for the dental health professional to prevent potential drug interactions related to anesthesia
Effects on Dental Treatment	Includes significant side effects of drug therapy which may directly or indirectly affect dental treatment or diagnosis; may also contain suggested management approaches and patient handling or care.
Effects on Bleeding	How the product affects bleeding during dental procedures
Adverse Reactions	Side effects are grouped by percentage of incidence (if known) and/or body system; in the interest of saving space, <1% effects are grouped only by percentage. Adverse drug reactions and incidences are derived from product labeling unless otherwise specified within this field.
Dental Usual Dosage	The amount of the drug to be typically given or taken during dental treatment for children and adults

Dosing	The amount of drug to be typically given or taken during therapy; may include the following:
Adult	The recommended amount of drug to be given to adult patients
Adult & Geriatric	This combined field is only used to indicate that no specific adjustments for elderly patients were identified. However, other issues should be considered (eg, renal or hepatic impairment).
Geriatric	A suggested amount of drug to be given to elderly patients; may include adjustments from adult dosing (lack of information in the monograph may imply that the drug is not used in the elderly patient or no specific adjustments could be identified)
Renal Impairment: Adult	Suggested dosage adjustments for adults based on compromised renal function; may include dosing instructions for patients on dialysis
Hepatic Impairment: Adult	Suggested dosage adjustments for adults based on compromised liver function
Obesity: Adult	Dosing adjustment or dosing considerations for the obese adult patient. Obesity is defined as a BMI ≥30 kg/m^2 (based on the World Health Organization [WHO]).
Adjustment for Toxicity: Adult	Suggested adult dosage adjustments in the event specific toxicities related to therapy are noted, such as hematologic toxicities related to cancer chemotherapy
Pediatric	The amount of the drug to be typically administered during therapy; may include dosing information for infants, children, and adolescents (up through 18 years of age) and other suggested dosing adjustments for toxicity or concomitant medication(s). Dosing information not from product labeling will be preceded with "Limited data available" and have a citation. When both fixed-doses and weight-directed doses (eg, milligram per kilogram [mg/kg]) are listed, the preferred method is the weight-directed. When weight-directed dosing (eg, mg/kg) and maximum doses are provided, use the weight-directed (mg/kg) dose to calculate the milligram dose for the patient, but do not exceed the maximum dose listed, unless otherwise noted. Do not exceed adult maximum dosage for a given indication, unless otherwise noted. If using fixed dosing based upon age, special care and lower doses should be considered in pediatric patients who have a low weight for their age. When ranges of doses are provided, initiate therapy at the lower end of the range and titrate the dose accordingly, unless otherwise indicated. The following age group definitions are utilized to characterize age-related dosing, unless otherwise specified in the monograph: Neonate (0 to 28 days of age), infant (>28 days to 1 year of age), children (1 to 12 years of age), and adolescent (13 to 18 years of age).
Renal Impairment: Pediatric	Suggested dosage adjustments for pediatric patients based on compromised renal function; may include dosing instructions for patients on dialysis
Hepatic Impairment: Pediatric	Suggested dosage adjustments for pediatric patients based on compromised liver function
Mechanism of Action	How the drug works in the body to elicit a response
Contraindications	Information pertaining to inappropriate use of the drug as dictated by approved labeling
Warnings/Precautions	Precautionary considerations, hazardous conditions related to use of the drug, and disease states or patient populations in which the drug should be cautiously used. Boxed warnings, when present, are clearly identified and are adapted from the FDA approved labeling. Consult the product labeling for the exact black box warning through the manufacturer's or the FDA website.
Warnings: Additional Pediatric Considerations	Provides further details for precautionary considerations that are specific to pediatric and neonatal patients

Drug Interactions	
Metabolism/Transport Effects	If a drug has demonstrated involvement with cytochrome P450 enzymes, or other metabolism or transport proteins, this field will identify the drug as an inhibitor, inducer, or substrate of the specific enzyme(s) (eg, CYP1A2 or UGT1A1). CYP450 isoenzymes are identified as substrates (minor or major), inhibitors (weak, moderate, or strong), and inducers (weak or strong).
Avoid Concomitant Use	Designates drug combinations which should not be used concomitantly, due to an unacceptable risk:benefit assessment. Frequently, the concurrent use of the agents is explicitly prohibited or contraindicated by the product labeling.
Increased Effect/Toxicity	Drug combinations that result in an increased or toxic therapeutic effect between the drug listed in the monograph and other drugs or drug classes.
Decreased Effect	Drug combinations that result in a decreased therapeutic effect between the drug listed in the monograph and other drugs or drug classes.
Food Interactions	Possible important interactions between the drug listed in the monograph and food, alcohol, or other beverages.
Dietary Considerations	Specific dietary modifications and/or restrictions (eg, information about sodium content)
Pharmacodynamics/Kinetics	
Onset of Action	The time after drug administration when therapeutic effect is observed; may also include time for peak therapeutic effect.
Duration of Action	Length of therapeutic effect.
Half-life Elimination	The reported half-life of elimination for the parent or metabolites of the drug
Time to Peak	Describes the relative time after ingestion when concentration achieves the highest serum concentration
Reproductive Considerations	A summary of human information pertinent to or associated with use of the drug related to pregnancy testing, contraception, and infertility in females and males.
Pregnancy Risk Factor	Five categories established by the FDA to indicate the potential of a systemically absorbed drug for causing risk to the fetus; the FDA is replacing this category system with scientific data and other information specific to the use of the drug in pregnant women as new drugs and product labeling on existing drugs are approved
Pregnancy Considerations	A summary of human and/or animal information pertinent to or associated with the use of the drug as it relates to clinical effects on the fetus, newborn, or pregnant women.
Breastfeeding Considerations	Information pertinent to or associated with the human use of the drug as it relates to clinical effects on the breastfeeding infant or postpartum woman.
Product Availability	Provides availability information on products that have been approved by the FDA but are not yet available for use. Estimates for when a product may be available are included, when this information is known. May also provide any unique or critical drug availability issues.
Controlled Substance	Contains controlled substance schedule information as assigned by the United States Drug Enforcement Administration (DEA) or Canada's Controlled Drugs and Substance Act (CDSA). CDSA information is only provided for drugs available in Canada and not available in the US.
Prescribing and Access Restrictions	Provides information on any special requirements regarding the prescribing, obtaining, or dispensing of drugs, including any unique access restrictions

Dosage Forms Considerations	More specific information regarding product concentrations, ingredients, package sizes, amount of doses per container, and other important details pertaining to various formulations of medications
Dosage Forms: US	Information with regard to form, strength, and availability of the drug in the United States. **Note:** Additional formulation information (eg, excipients, preservatives) is included when available. Please consult product labeling for further information.
Dosage Forms: Canada	Information with regard to form, strength, and availability of the drug in Canada. The symbol [DSC] appears after trade names that have been recently discontinued.
Dental Health Professional Considerations	Pharmacology-related comments and considerations relevant to the dental professional

NATURAL PRODUCTS: HERBAL AND DIETARY SUPPLEMENTS

The natural product content is adapted from *The Review of Natural Products* a Facts & Comparisons online database. This section consists of a clinical overview that summarizes the uses, dosing, contraindications, pregnancy/lactation, interactions, adverse reactions, and toxicology information for each natural product. The dental-specific information is also included to further assist the dental professional in patient care.

ORAL MEDICINE TOPICS

This section is divided into two major parts and contains text on Oral Medicine topics. In each subsection, the systemic condition or the oral disease state is described briefly, followed by the pharmacologic considerations with which the dentist must be familiar.

I. **Dental Management and Therapeutic Considerations in Medically Compromised Patients:** Focuses on common medical conditions and their associated drug therapies with which the dentist must be familiar. Patient profiles with commonly associated drug regimens are described.

II. **Dental Management and Therapeutic Considerations in Patients With Specific Oral Conditions:** Focuses on therapies the dentist may choose to prescribe for patients suffering from oral disease or who are in need of special care. Some overlap between these sections has resulted from systemic conditions that have oral manifestations and vice-versa. Cross-references to the descriptions and the monographs for individual drugs described elsewhere in this handbook allow for easy retrieval of information. Example prescriptions for drugs commonly used in the treatment of each condition are presented so that the clinician can evaluate alternate approaches to treatment. Seldom is there a single drug of choice.
Note: Prescriptions listed represent prototype drugs and popular prescriptions and are examples only. The pharmacologic category index is available for cross-referencing if alternatives or additional drugs are sought.

APPENDIX

The appendix is broken down into various sections for easy use and offers a compilation of tables and guidelines which can often be helpful when considering patient care.

INDEX

This section includes a pharmacologic category index with an easy-to-use classification system in alphabetical order.

DESCRIPTION OF DENTAL USE

Unlabeled Use and Routes of Administration in Dentistry and Oral Medicine

The off-label use of a medication may involve differences in either the intended purpose or the route of administration of a particular medication. In dentistry, there are some situations which are common (clindamycin for endocarditis prophylaxis), and uncommon (application of Oralone paste to the oral mucosa) which may be termed "unlabeled use". Depending on the degree of familiarity, the prescription of a drug for an off-label purpose may create concern on the part of healthcare professionals who are less familiar with the dental use of these medications. For example, a pharmacist may note the statement "for external use only" on the label of a tube of topical cream and question whether the drug should be applied to the oral mucosa. Usually, reinforcement of the use of a drug as well as an analysis of the likely systemic exposure/toxicity, can address these concerns.

The dentist who prescribes a drug bears the responsibility for deciding on the purpose of the prescription and the detail of the dosing regimen. These professional decisions are based on information from a variety of sources, including (but not limited to) the official labeling, sound scientific evidence, expert medical judgment, or published literature. In selected situations, these sources may justify the use of a drug in an off-label manner. Accepted professional standards indicate off-label use of a drug must be initiated in good faith, serve the best interest of the patient, and must be undertaken without fraudulent intent. Healthcare providers should recognize that the approved labeling is not intended to limit the practitioners in the exercise of his or her best professional judgment in serving the interest of patients. However, it should be noted that a practitioner may be accountable for the negligent use in a civil action regardless of whether the FDA has approved the use of the drug in question. Based on these assertions, at least one medical organization (the American Academy of Pediatrics) has published in an official policy statement that the practice of medicine may actually require a practitioner to use drugs in an off-label manner in order to provide the most appropriate treatment for a given patient. Off-label use in dentistry and oral medicine is a frequently encountered issue. A discussion of the off-label use of drugs in dentistry appears in the *ADA/PDR Guide to Dental Therapeutics*, 5th Edition, edited by Sebastian G. Ciancio, DDS in cooperation with the ADA Division of Legal Affairs.

CONTROLLED SUBSTANCES

Schedule I = C-I

The drugs and other substances in this schedule have no legal medical uses except research. They have a **high** potential for abuse. They include selected opiates such as heroin, opium derivatives, and hallucinogens.

Schedule II = C-II

The drugs and other substances in this schedule have legal medical uses and a **high** abuse potential which may lead to severe dependence. They include former "Class A" opioids, amphetamines, barbiturates, and other drugs.

Schedule III = C-III

The drugs and other substances in this schedule have legal medical uses and a **lesser** degree of abuse potential which may lead to **moderate** dependence. They include former "Class B" opioids and other drugs.

Schedule IV = C-IV

The drugs and other substances in this schedule have legal medial uses and **low** abuse potential which may lead to **moderate** dependence. They include barbiturates, benzodiazepines, propoxyphenes, and other drugs.

Schedule V = C-V

The drugs and other substances in this schedule have legal medical uses and **low** abuse potential which may lead to **moderate** dependence. They include opioids cough preparations, diarrhea preparations, and other drugs.

Note: These are federal classifications. Your individual state may place a substance into a more restricted category. When this occurs, the more restricted category applies. Consult your state law.

PREGNANCY CATEGORIES

Pregnancy Categories (sometimes referred to as pregnancy risk factors) are a letter system presented under the *Teratogenic Effects* subsection of the product labeling. The system was initiated in 1979. The categories were required to be part of the package insert for prescription drugs that are systemically absorbed. The Food and Drug Administration (FDA) has updated prescribing labeling requirements and as of June 2015, the pregnancy categories will no longer be part of new product labeling. Prescription products which currently have a pregnancy category letter will be phasing this out of their product information.

The categories are defined as follows:

A	Adequate and well-controlled studies in pregnant women have not shown that the drug increases the risk of fetal abnormalities.
B	Animal reproduction studies show no evidence of impaired fertility or harm to the fetus; however, no adequate and well-controlled studies have been conducted in pregnant women. **or** Animal reproduction studies have shown adverse events; however, studies in pregnant women have not shown that the drug increases the risk of abnormalities.
C	Animal reproduction studies have shown an adverse effect on the fetus. There are no adequate and well-controlled studies in humans and the benefits from the use of the drug in pregnant women may be acceptable, despite its potential risks. **or** Animal reproduction studies have not been conducted.
D	Based on human data, the drug can cause fetal harm when administered to pregnant women, but the potential benefits from the use of the drug may be acceptable, despite its potential risks.
X	Studies in animals or humans have demonstrated fetal abnormalities (or there is positive evidence of fetal risk based on reports and/or marketing experience) and the risk of using the drug in pregnant women clearly outweighs any possible benefit (for example, safer drugs or other forms of therapy are available).

In 2008, the Food and Drug Administration (FDA) proposed new labeling requirements which would eliminate the use of the pregnancy category system and replace it with scientific data and other information specific to the use of the drug in pregnant women. These proposed changes were suggested because the current category system may be misleading. For instance, some practitioners may believe that risk increases from category A to B to C to D to X, which is not the intent. In addition, practitioners may not be aware that some medications are categorized based on animal data, while others are based on human data. The new labeling requirements will contain pregnancy and lactation subsections, each describing a risk summary, clinical considerations, and section for specific data.

For full descriptions of the final rule, refer to the following website: http://www.fda.gov/Drugs/DevelopmentApprovalProcess/DevelopmentResources/Labeling/ucm093307.htm

PRESCRIPTION WRITING

Doctor's Name
Address
Phone Number

Patient's Name/Date

Patient's Address/Age

Rx

Drug Name/Dosage Size
Disp: Number of tablets, capsules, ounces to be dispensed (roman numerals added as precaution for abused drugs)
Sig: Direction on how drug is to be taken

Doctor's signature
State license number
DEA number (if required)

PRESCRIPTION REQUIREMENTS

1. Date
2. Full name and address of patient
3. Name and address of prescriber
4. Signature of prescriber

If Class II drug, Drug Enforcement Agency (DEA) number necessary.

If Class II and Class III opioid, a triplicate prescription form (in the state of California) is necessary and it must be handwritten by the prescriber.

Please turn to appropriate oral medicine chapters for examples of prescriptions.

PREVENTING PRESCRIBING ERRORS

Prescribing errors account for the majority of reported medication errors and have prompted health care professionals to focus on the development of steps to make the prescribing process safer. Prescription legibility has been attributed to a portion of these errors and legislation has been enacted in several states to address prescription legibility. However, eliminating handwritten prescriptions and ordering medications through the use of technology [eg, computerized prescriber order entry (CPOE)] has been the primary recommendation. Whether a prescription is electronic, typed, or hand-printed, additional safe practices should be considered for implementation to maximize the safety of the prescribing process. Listed below are suggestions for safer prescribing:

- Ensure correct patient by using at least 2 patient identifiers on the prescription (eg, full name, birth date, or address). Review prescription with the patient or patient's caregiver.
- If pediatric patient, document patient's birth date or age and most recent weight. If geriatric patient, document patient's birth date or age.
- Prevent drug name confusion: For more information, see http://www.ismp.org/tools/confuseddrugnames.pdf.
  - Use TALLman lettering (eg, buPROPion, busPIRone, predniSONE, prednisoLONE). For more information, see http://www.fda.gov/drugs/drugsafety/medicationerrors/default.htm.
  - Avoid abbreviated drug names (eg, MSO_4, $MgSO_4$, MS, HCT, 6MP, MTX), as they may be misinterpreted and cause error.
  - Avoid investigational names for drugs with FDA approval (eg, FK-506, CBDCA).
  - Avoid chemical names such as 6-mercaptopurine or 6-thioguanine, as sixfold overdoses have been given when these were not recognized as chemical names. The proper names of these drugs are mercaptopurine or thioguanine.
  - Use care when prescribing drugs that look or sound similar (eg, look- alike, sound-alike drugs). Common examples include: CeleBREX vs CeleXA, hydrOXYzine vs hydrALAZINE, ZyPREXA vs ZyrTEC.
- Avoid dangerous, error-prone abbreviations (eg, regardless of letter-case: U, IU, QD, QOD, µg, cc, @). Do not use apothecary system or symbols. Additionally, text messaging abbreviations (eg, "2Day") should never be used.
  - For more information, see http://www.ismp.org/tools/errorproneabbreviations.pdf.
- Always use a leading zero for numbers <1 (0.5 mg is correct and .5 mg is **incorrect**) and never use a trailing zero for whole numbers (2 mg is correct and 2.0 mg is **incorrect**).
- Always use a space between a number and its units as it is easier to read. There should be no periods after the abbreviations mg or mL (10 mg is correct and 10mg is **incorrect**).
- For doses that are ≥1,000 dosing units, use properly placed commas to prevent 10-fold errors (100,000 units is correct and 100000 units is **incorrect**).
- Do not prescribe drug dosage by the type of container in which the drug is available (eg, do not prescribe "1 amp", "2 vials", etc).
- Do not write vague or ambiguous orders which have the potential for misinterpretation by other health care providers. Examples of vague orders to avoid: "Resume pre-op medications," "give drug per protocol," or "continue home medications."
- Review each prescription with patient (or patient's caregiver) including the medication name, indication, and directions for use.
- Take extra precautions when prescribing *high alert drugs* (drugs that can cause significant patient harm when prescribed in error). Common examples of these drugs include: Anticoagulants, chemotherapy, insulins, opioids, and sedatives.
  - For more information, see http://www.ismp.org/tools/institutionalhighalert.asp.

To Err Is Human: Building a Safer Health System, Kohn LT, Corrigan JM, Donaldson MS, eds. Washington, D.C.: National Academy Press. 2000.

A Complete Outpatient Prescription[1]

A complete outpatient prescription can prevent the prescriber, the pharmacist, and/or the patient from making a mistake and can eliminate the need for further clarification. The complete outpatient prescription should contain:

- Patient's full name
- Medication indication
- Allergies
- Prescriber name and telephone or pager number
- For pediatric patients: Their birth date or age and current weight
- For geriatric patients: Their birth date or age
- Drug name, dosage form and strength
- For pediatric patients: Intended daily weight-based dose so that calculations can be checked by the pharmacist (ie, mg/kg/day or units/kg/day)
- Number or amount to be dispensed
- Complete instructions for the patient or caregiver, including the purpose of the medication, directions for use (including dose), dosing frequency, route of administration, duration of therapy, and number of refills.
- Dose should be expressed in convenient units of measure.
- When there are recognized contraindications for a prescribed drug, the prescriber should indicate knowledge of this fact to the pharmacist (ie, when prescribing a potassium salt for a patient receiving an ACE inhibitor, the prescriber should write "K serum leveling being monitored").

Upon dispensing of the final product, the pharmacist should ensure that the patient or caregiver can effectively demonstrate the appropriate administration technique. An appropriate measuring device should be provided or recommended. Household teaspoons and tablespoons should not be used to measure liquid medications due to their variability and inaccuracies in measurement; oral medication syringes are recommended.

[1]Levine SR, Cohen MR, Blanchard NR, et al. Guidelines for preventing medication errors in pediatrics. *J Pediatr Pharmacol Ther.* 2001;6:426-442.

SAMPLE PRESCRIPTIONS

Drug prescriptions shown in this section represent prototype drugs and popular prescriptions and are examples only. The pharmacologic category index is available for cross-referencing if alternatives and additional drugs are sought. See the Oral Medicine Chapters for a complete description of Diagnosis and Management considerations.

TABLE OF CONTENTS

ORAL PAIN - SAMPLE PRESCRIPTIONS

The patient with existing acute or chronic oral pain requires appropriate treatment and sensitivity on the part of the dentist, all for the purpose of achieving relief from the oral source of pain. Pain can be divided into mild, moderate, and severe levels and requires a subjective assessment by the dentist based on knowledge of the dental procedures to be performed, the presenting signs and symptoms of the patient, and the realization that most dental procedures are invasive often leading to pain once the patient has left the dental office. The practitioner must be aware that the treatment of the source of the pain is usually the best management. ***Opioid analgesics can be used on a short-term basis or intermittently in combination with nonopioid therapy in the chronic pain patient. Judicious prescribing, monitoring, and maintenance by the practitioner are imperative, particularly whenever considering the use of an opioid analgesic due to the abuse and addiction liabilities.*** For all prescribers of extended release and long-acting opioid analgesics, patient information as noted below is required. The CDC has released guidelines for opioid prescriptions. Numerous states have adopted prescription monitoring programs particularly targeting opioids and benzodiazapines; refer to your home state guidelines for specific regulations and reporting requirements. In general opioids should not be the first-line therapy choice for chronic pain except for active cancer, palliative therapy, or end of life care. Please visit www.cdc.gov/drugoverdose/prescribing/guideline.html for more specific details. The FDA also has a required Opioid Analgesic Risk Evaluation and Mitigation Strategy (REMS) for opioid analgesic drug products used in the outpatient setting, see www.opioidanalgesicrems.com.

DOs and DON'Ts of Extended Release/Long-Acting Opioid Analgesics

DO:

- Read the **Medication Guide**.
- Take your medicine exactly as prescribed.
- Store your medicine away from children and in a safe place.
- Check with pharmacy about disposal of unused medicine.
- Call your health care provider for medical advice about side effects. You may report side effects to the FDA at (800) FDA-1088.

Call 911 or your local emergency service right away if:

- You take too much medicine.
- You have trouble breathing or shortness of breath.
- A child has taken this medicine.

Talk to your health care provider:

- If the dose you are taking does not control your pain.
- About any side effects you may be having.
- About all the medicines you take, including over-the-counter medicines, vitamins, and dietary supplements.

DON'T:

- **Do not** give your medicine to others.
- **Do not** take medicine unless it was prescribed for you.
- **Do not** stop taking your medicine without talking to your health care provider.
- **Do not** break, chew, crush, dissolve, or inject your medicine. If you cannot swallow your medicine whole, talk to your health care provider.
- **Do not** drink alcohol while taking this medicine.

MILD/MODERATE ORAL PAIN

General Prescription Comments

The FDA has formally requested manufacturers to limit the amount of acetaminophen in prescription combination products (eg, Vicodin, Lortab) to no more than 325 mg per dosage unit. The FDA is also requiring manufacturers to update labeling of all prescription combination acetaminophen products to warn of the potential risk for severe liver injury (see Oral Pain on page 1734 for more information). Most manufacturers have already reduced acetaminophen amounts to 300 to 325 mg per tablet in combination prescription products.

Note: Numerous brand name products for infants and children that contain ibuprofen or acetaminophen have been voluntarily recalled by manufacturers due to investigation by the FDA.

Closely monitor and reevaluate response at least every 2 weeks. If response is inadequate, reevaluate diagnosis, medication choice, and dosage.

Note: The following sample prescriptions are for **adults.**

Sample Prescriptions

For additional information, see Acetaminophen on page 59, Diflunisal on page 495, Ibuprofen on page 786, Naproxen on page 1080

Rx:

Acetaminophen 325 mg tablets
Disp: To be determined by practitioner
Sig: Take 2 tablets every 4 hours

Note: Products include Tylenol and others.

Note: Acetaminophen can be given if patient has allergies, bleeding problems, or stomach upset secondary to aspirin or NSAIDs.

Rx:

Ibuprofen 200 mg tablets
Disp: To be determined by practitioner
Sig: Take 1 to 2 tablets every 4 hours

Note: Ibuprofen is an available OTC as Advil, Motrin IB, and many store brand generic names. NSAIDs should not be combined with aspirin. NSAIDs may increase post-treatment bleeding. Use with caution in patients receiving anticoagulants or antiplatelet drugs.

Rx:

Naproxen sodium 220 mg tablets
Disp: To be determined by practitioner
Sig: Take 1 to 2 tablets every 8 hours

Note: Naproxen sodium is an available OTC as Aleve and many store brand generic names.

Rx:

Ibuprofen 400 mg tablets
Disp: 20 tablets
Sig: Take 1 tablet every 4 to 6 hours as needed for pain

Note: Prescription strength ibuprofen is available as the brand name Motrin.

Rx:

Dolobid 500 mg tablets
Disp: 16 tablets
Sig: Take 2 tablets initially, then 1 tablet every 12 hours as needed for pain

Ingredient: Diflunisal

MODERATE/MODERATELY SEVERE ORAL PAIN

General Prescription Comments

Closely monitor and reevaluate response at least every 2 weeks. If response is inadequate, reevaluate diagnosis, medication choice, and dosage.
Note: The following sample prescriptions are for **adults.**

Sample Prescriptions

For additional information, see Acetaminophen and Codeine on page 65, Acetaminophen and Tramadol on page 71, Hydrocodone and Acetaminophen on page 764, Hydrocodone and Ibuprofen on page 769, Ibuprofen on page 786, Naproxen on page 1080, TraMADol on page 1468

Rx:

Ibuprofen 800 mg tablets
Disp: 16 tablets
Sig: Take 1 tablet 3 times/day as needed for pain

Note: For severe pain can be given up to 4 times/day. Also available as 600 mg tablets.

Rx:
TraMADol 50 mg tablets
Disp: 36 tablets
Sig: Take 1 to 2 tablets every 4 to 6 hours as needed for pain (maximum: 400 mg/day)

Note: Also available as the brand name Ultram.
Important notification regarding TraMADol: Effective August 18, 2014, Tramadol was classified as a Schedule IV controlled dangerous substance (CDS) under federal regulation. If you dispense Tramadol to your patients, you are required to report this to the Prescription Drug Monitoring Program (PDMP). If you write a prescription for Tramadol, but do **not** dispense this medication, you are not required to report to the PDMP. The Division of Drug Control (DDC) has posted the following information on its website: USDOJ/DEA, 21 CFR (Federal Register) Part 1308: Schedules of Controlled Dangerous Substances: Placement of Tramadol Into Schedule IV (Final Rule). DEA (CFR Final Rule) Tramadol Schedule IV Placement (Effective: 8/18/14).

Rx:
Ultracet tablets
Disp: 36 tablets
Sig: Take 2 tablets every 4 to 6 hours as needed for pain, not to exceed 8 tablets in 24 hours

Ingredients: Acetaminophen 325 mg and Tramadol 37.5 mg

Rx:
Vicoprofen tablets
Disp: 16 tablets
Sig: Take 1 to 2 tablets every 4 to 6 hours as needed for pain (maximum: 5 tablets/day)

Note: Restrictions: C-II; no refills
Ingredients: Hydrocodone 7.5 mg and ibuprofen 200 mg; available as generic equivalent

Rx:
Vicodin ES tablets 7.5 mg hydrocodone/300 mg acetaminophen (per tablet)
Disp: 16 tablets
Sig: Take 1 tablet every 4 to 6 hours as needed for pain (maximum: 5 tablets/day)

Note: Restrictions: C-II; no refills
Ingredients: Hydrocodone bitartrate 7.5 mg and acetaminophen 300 mg; available as generic equivalent.

Rx:
Norco 10 mg
Disp: 16 tablets
Sig: Take 1 or 2 tablets every 4 hours as needed for pain; not to exceed 8 tablets in 24 hours

Note: Restrictions: C-II; no refills
Ingredients: Hydrocodone 10 mg and acetaminophen 325 mg; available as generic equivalent

Rx:
Tylenol #3
Disp: 16 tablets
Sig: Take 1 tablet every 4 hours as needed for pain

Note: Restrictions: C-III; no refills
Ingredients: Codeine 30 mg and acetaminophen 300 mg; available as generic equivalent

Rx:
Naproxen 275 mg tablets
Disp: 16 tablets
Sig: Take 2 tablets initially, then one tablet 3 times/day as needed for pain

SEVERE ORAL PAIN

General Prescription Comments

Closely monitor and reevaluate response at least every 2 weeks. If response is inadequate, reevaluate diagnosis, medication choice, and dosage.

Liquid volumes are suggested for a typical 2-week course. Check with pharmacist for available sizes.

Cream and ointment tube sizes may vary based on availability. Refer to individual monograph or check with pharmacist for available sizes.
Note: The following sample prescriptions are for **adults.**

Sample Prescriptions

For additional information, see Oxycodone and Acetaminophen on page 1164 and Oxycodone and Ibuprofen

Rx:

Percocet tablets
Disp: 16 tablets
Sig: Take 1 tablet every 6 hours as needed for pain

Note: Restrictions: C-II; no refills
Ingredients: Oxycodone 5 mg and acetaminophen 325 mg; available as generic equivalent; triplicate prescription required in some states

Rx:

Oxycodone and Ibuprofen tablets
Disp: 16 tablets
Sig: Take 1 tablet every 6 hours as needed for pain

Note: Restrictions: C-II; no refills
Ingredients: Oxycodone 5 mg and ibuprofen 400 mg; triplicate prescription required in some states

ANTIMICROBIAL ORAL RINSE - SAMPLE PRESCRIPTIONS

General Prescription Comments

Closely monitor and reevaluate response at least every 2 weeks. If response is inadequate, reevaluate diagnosis, medication choice, and dosage.

Liquid volumes for antimicrobial rinses are suggested for a typical 1 month course. Check with pharmacist for available sizes.

Sample Prescriptions

For additional information, see Chlorhexidine Gluconate (Oral) on page 334, Mouthwash (Antiseptic) on page 1062.

Rx:

Chlorhexidine gluconate 0.12% oral rinse
Disp: 16 oz bottle
Sig: Rinse vigorously twice daily with 15 mL for 30 seconds and expectorate

Note: Chlorhexidine gluconate available as the following brands: Peridex Oral Rinse, PerioGard, GUM Paroex, ORO-Clense, Perichlor; it is also available in an alcohol-free formulation in most pharmaceutical locations. Advise patient of risk of reversible tooth staining. Some brands are available in various volumes.

Rx:

Listerine antiseptic mouthwash [OTC]
Disp: Various size bottles
Sig: Rinse vigorously twice daily with 15 to 20 mL for 30 seconds and expectorate

Note: Various formulations, such as Cool Mint, are also available in an alcohol-free formulation.

BACTERIAL INFECTIONS AND PERIODONTAL DISEASES - SAMPLE PRESCRIPTIONS

General Prescription Comments

For the use of all antibiotic medications, prescribers should review the guidelines related to antimicrobial stewardship endorsed by the ADA that is cited in Bacterial Infections on page 1739. Sample prescription dosing is for adults. Closely monitor and reevaluate response at least every 2 weeks. If response is inadequate, reevaluate diagnosis, medication choice, and dosage.

Sample Prescriptions

For additional information, see Bacterial Infections on page 1739, Amoxicillin on page 124, Amoxicillin and Clavulanate on page 130, Azithromycin (Systemic) on page 203, Cephalexin on page 322, Clindamycin (Systemic) on page 368, Doxycycline on page 522, Erythromycin (Systemic) on page 588, LevoFLOXacin (Systemic) on page 898, MetroNIDAZOLE (Systemic) on page 1011, Minocycline (Systemic) on page 1032, Penicillin V Potassium on page 1211.

PLEASE NOTE: Citing concerns over risk of pseudomembranous colitis the American Association of Endodontists has recently altered their recommendations for use of antibiotics to now recommend azithromycin as the alternative to penicillin in allergic individuals and also as a better choice in cases where response to penicillin is inadequate.

Rx:

Penicillin V potassium 500 mg
Disp: 40 tablets
Sig: Take 1 tablet 4 times/day for 7 to 10 days (consider a loading dose of 1 g for acute infection). Reevaluate 48 to 72 hours after initiating antibiotics, if minimal or no response, consider changing to another class.

Rx:

Clindamycin (Systemic) 150 mg
Disp: 40 capsules
Sig: Take 1 capsule 4 times/day for 7 to 10 days

Note: Prescription usually selected for patients allergic to penicillin; may be prescribed for 3 or 4 times/day. Recommend to be taken after food to reduce GI concerns.

Rx:

Clindamycin (Systemic) 300 mg
Disp: 40 capsules
Sig: Take 1 capsule 4 times/day for 7 to 10 days

Note: Prescription usually selected for patients allergic to penicillin; may be prescribed for 3 or 4 times/day. Recommend to be taken after food to reduce GI concerns.

Rx:

Azithromycin (Systemic) 250 mg
Disp: 1 Z-Pak
Sig: 2 tablets day 1, then 1 tablet/day until gone

Note: This option has been cited as an alternative in penicillin allergic patients by the Association of Endodontists due to concerns over pseudomembranous colitis.

OTHER ANTIBIOTICS:

Rx:

Amoxicillin 250 mg
Disp: 30 capsules
Sig: Take 1 capsule 3 times/day for 7 to 10 days

Rx:

Amoxicillin 500 mg
Disp: 30 capsules or tablets
Sig: Take 1 capsule or tablet 3 times/day for 7 to 10 days

Rx:

Amoxicillin 875 mg
Disp: 20 tablets
Sig: Take 1 tablet twice daily

Rx:

Augmentin 250 mg
Disp: 30 tablets
Sig: Take 1 tablet 3 times/day for 7 to 10 days

Rx:
Augmentin 500 mg
Disp: 30 tablets
Sig: Take 1 tablet 3 times/day for 7 to 10 days

Rx:
Augmentin 875 mg
Disp: 20 tablets
Sig: Take 1 tablet twice daily for 7 to 10 days

Rx:
Augmentin XR 1,000 mg
Disp: 20 tablets
Sig: Take 1 tablet twice daily for 7 to 10 days; not the same as taking two 500 mg tablets

Rx:
Cephalexin 250 mg
Disp: 40 capsules
Sig: Take 1 capsule 4 times/day for 7 to 10 days

Rx:
MetroNIDAZOLE (Systemic) 500 mg
Disp: 40 tablets
Sig: Take 1 tablet 3 or 4 times/day for 7 to 10 days

Note: For acute periodontal infections or as therapy in osteonecrosis of the jaw, usually used in combination with amoxicillin or amoxicillin plus clavulanic acid; may be prescribed for 3 or 4 times/day. When prescribed at 500 mg tid the patient can take both medications together enhancing compliance.

Rx:
Erythromycin (Systemic) 250 mg
Disp: 40 tablets
Sig: Take 1 tablet 4 times/day for 7 to 10 days

Note: Prescription for patients allergic to penicillin, however, is seldom prescribed due to concern over general efficacy and considerable GI effects.

Rx:
Zithromax TRI-PAK 500 mg
Disp: 1 PAK
Sig: Follow package insert directions until gone

Ingredient: Azithromycin (Systemic)

Rx:
Levaquin 500 mg
Disp: 10 tablets
Sig: Take 1 tablet/day until gone

Ingredient: LevoFLOXacin, available as 250, 500, and 750 mg tablets

Note: Not the ideal drug for general dental and/or periodontal infections; however, levofloxacin is approved for treatment of acute bacterial rhinosinusitis.

PERIODONTAL DISEASE

Note: Sample prescriptions based on dosing suggestions from the American Academy of Periodontology

Rx:
Azithromycin (Systemic) 500 mg tablets
Disp: Dispense a dose pack
Sig: Take 1 tablet daily for 4 to 7 days as directed

Rx:
Clindamycin (Systemic) 300 mg tablets
Disp: 24 tablets
Sig: Take 1 tablet 3 times/day for 8 days

Rx:
Doxycycline or Minocycline 100 to 200 mg tablets
Disp: 21 tablets of selected dose
Sig: Take 1 tablet daily for 21 days

Rx:
Doxycycline 100 mg tablets
Disp: 42 tablets
Sig: Take 1 tablet twice daily for 21 days

Note: Prescription used for Lyme disease: Early stage (erythema migrans)

Rx:
MetroNIDAZOLE (Systemic) 500 mg
Disp: 24 tablets
Sig: Take 1 tablet 3 times/day for 8 days

Note: Metronidazole is often used in acute periodontal infections and in the early management of infected osteonecrosis of the jaw in combination with amoxicillin, or amoxicillin plus clavulanic acid.

Rx:
MetroNIDAZOLE (Systemic) and Amoxicillin 250 mg or 500 mg tablets
Disp: 24 tablets of each drug
Sig: Take 1 tablet of each drug 3 times/day for 8 days

FUNGAL INFECTIONS - SAMPLE PRESCRIPTIONS

FUNGAL INFECTIONS REQUIRING TOPICAL THERAPY

General Prescription Comments

Closely monitor and reevaluate response at least every 2 weeks. If response is inadequate, reevaluate diagnosis, medication choice, and dosage.

Liquid volumes are suggested for a typical 2-week course. Check with pharmacist for available sizes.

Cream and ointment tube may vary from 5 g, 15 g, 30 g, 45 g, or 60 g sizes, based on availability. Refer to individual monograph or check with pharmacist for available sizes.

Sample Prescriptions

For additional information, see Fungal Infections on page 1752, Clotrimazole (Oral) on page 396, Nystatin (Oral) on page 1121, Nystatin (Topical) on page 1122

Rx:

Nystatin (Oral) 100,000 units/mL oral suspension
Disp: 300 mL
Sig: Rinse with 1 teaspoon (5 mL) for 2 minutes 4 to 5 times/day and expectorate

Rx:

Nystatin (Topical) ointment
Disp: 15 g tube
Sig: Apply locally as directed with a thin coat to inner surface of denture and the affected area 4 to 5 times/day

Rx:

Mycelex 10 mg troches
Disp: 70 troches
Sig: Dissolve 1 troche in mouth 4 to 5 times/day until gone; leave any prosthesis out during treatment and soak prosthesis in nystatin liquid suspension overnight

Ingredient: Clotrimazole (Oral)

FUNGAL INFECTIONS REQUIRING SYSTEMIC THERAPY

General Prescription Comments

Note: Decision to use systemic antifungals should be based on diagnostic culture results or positive smear.

Closely monitor and reevaluate response at least every 2 weeks. If response is inadequate, reevaluate diagnosis, medication choice, and dosage.

Sample Prescriptions

For additional information, see Fluconazole on page 674, Itraconazole on page 849, Posaconazole on page 1248, Voriconazole on page 1552

Rx:

Diflucan 100 mg tablets
Disp: 14 tablets
Sig: Take 2 tablets on day 1, then take 1 tablet/day until gone

Note: Sometimes a shorter course is adequate. However, oral infections are more commonly difficult to eradicate and often a 21-day course, or even a second course, may be necessary.

Ingredient: Fluconazole

Rx:

Sporanox oral solution 10 mg/mL
Disp: 300 mL
Sig: Take 200 mg (4 teaspoonfuls) once daily for 14 days

Ingredient: Itraconazole

Rx:

Noxafil oral suspension 40 mg/mL
Disp: 210 mL
Sig: Take 400 mg (2 teaspoonfuls) twice daily for 3 days, then 400 mg (2 teaspoonfuls) once daily for 14 days

Ingredient: Posaconazole

Note: For use in patients refractory to itraconazole or fluconazole

Rx:

Voriconazole 200 mg tablets
Disp: 28 tablets
Sig: Take 1 tablet twice daily for 14 days

ANGULAR CHEILITIS

General Prescription Comments

Closely monitor and reevaluate response at least every 2 weeks. If response is inadequate, reevaluate diagnosis, medication choice, and dosage. Other associated etiologies for angular cheilitis must also be considered, such as loss of vertical dimension, trauma, and vitamin deficiencies.

Cream and ointment tube may vary from 15 g, 30 g, or 45 g sizes, based on availability. Refer to individual monograph or check with pharmacist for available sizes.

Sample Prescriptions

For additional information, see Iodoquinol and Hydrocortisone on page 836, Nystatin and Triamcinolone on page 1123

Rx:

Nystatin and Triamcinolone acetonide ointment
Disp: 30 g tube
Sig: Dry affected area of angular cheilitis, apply locally as directed to affected area 4 times/day for 10 to 14 days and then reevaluate

Rx:

Iodoquinol and Hydrocortisone cream
Disp: 45 g tube
Sig: Dry affected area of angular cheilitis, apply locally as directed 3 to 4 times/day for 10 days to 2 weeks and then reevaluate

PREVENTION OF ENDOCARDITIS AND TO REDUCE THE RISK OF LATE INFECTIONS OF JOINT PROSTHESES - SAMPLE PRESCRIPTIONS

General Prescription Comments

For any patients requiring preprocedural antibiotics for prevention of infective endocarditis or to reduce the risk of late infections in joint prostheses, the dental team must be aware of significant changes in the practice guidelines endorsed by the American Dental Association, the American Heart Association, and the American Association of Orthopedic Surgeons. The American Association of Orthopedic Surgeons (AAOS) has developed Appropriate Use Criteria (AUC) for thirteen selected situations encountered by orthopedists, including, "Management of patients with orthopedic implants undergoing dental procedures". This was added as of November 2016. Please review the chapter on preprocedural antibiotics for the complete discussion.

Regarding antibiotic selection, when after consultation preprocedural antibiotics are deemed necessary, one important change occurred. In the latest release from the AAOS, clindamycin is no longer recommended as the suggested alternative in patients allergic to penicillins. The AAOS now recommends, in allergic patients still able to take oral medication, 2 g cephalexin, or 500 mg of azithromycin or clarithromycin, in that order of selection. Since this release the ADA and the AHA have not taken any steps to alter their endocarditis recommendations. Terico AT, Gallagher JC. Beta-lactam hypersensitivity and cross-reactivity. *J Pharm Pract.* 2014;27(6):530-544 is cited as the reference for considerations of cross-allergenicity of cephalosporins and penicillins.

Preprocedural antibiotics are only recommended in very specific medical circumstances relative to endocarditis and they are generally not recommended for patients with joint prostheses. The dentist is encouraged as always to record a thorough medical history to determine risks and to consult with the appropriate physician in order to make the final decision to prescribe antibiotic prophylaxis or not. See Antibiotic Prophylaxis on page 1715 for additional information regarding high-risk patients and the goals of consultation.

Prescriptions dispense amounts are for three visits. These numbers can be adjusted for each patient treatment plan.

Sample Prescriptions

For additional information, see Amoxicillin on page 124, Azithromycin (Systemic) on page 203, Cephalexin on page 322, Clarithromycin on page 361, Clindamycin (Systemic) on page 368

Rx:

Amoxicillin 500 mg
Disp: 12 tablets
Sig: 4 tablets (2 g) 30 to 60 minutes prior to dental visit and repeat at each appointment

Rx:

Clindamycin (Systemic) 150 mg
Disp: 12 capsules
Sig: 4 capsules (600 mg) 30 to 60 minutes prior to dental visit and repeat at each appointment

Rx:

Cephalexin 500 mg
Disp: 12 tablets
Sig: 4 tablets (2 g) 30 to 60 minutes prior to dental visit and repeat at each appointment

Note: Clindamycin is no longer recommended in the AAOS guidelines but is still an alternative in the AHA and ADA guidelines.

Rx:

Azithromycin (Systemic) 500 mg
Disp: 3 tablets
Sig: 1 tablet 30 to 60 minutes prior to dental visit and repeat at each appointment

Rx:

Clarithromycin 500 mg
Disp: 3 tablets
Sig: 1 tablet 30 to 60 minutes prior to dental visit and repeat at each appointment

SINUS INFECTION TREATMENT - SAMPLE PRESCRIPTIONS

General Prescription Comments

Please review the guidelines related to antimicrobial stewardship endorsed by the ADA that is cited in Bacterial Infections on page 1739. Closely monitor and reevaluate response at least every 2 weeks. If response is inadequate, reevaluate diagnosis, medication choice, and dosage.

Sinus infections represent a common condition which may present with confounding dental complaints. Treatment is sometimes instituted by the dentist, but due to the often chronic and recurrent nature of sinus infections, early involvement of an otolaryngologist is advised. These infections may require antibiotics of varying spectrum, as well as requiring the management of sinus congestion. Although amoxicillin is usually adequate, many otolaryngologists initially prescribe Augmentin. Second generation cephalosporins, azithromycin, and clarithromycin are sometimes used depending on the chronicity of the problem. Although not the ideal drug for general dental and/or periodontal infections, levofloxacin (Levoquin) is approved for treatment of acute bacterial rhinosinusitis.

Sample Prescriptions

For additional information, see Amoxicillin on page 124, Amoxicillin and Clavulanate on page 130, Azithromycin (Systemic) on page 203, Chlorpheniramine on page 340, LevoFLOXacin on page 898, Oxymetazoline (Nasal) on page 1173, Pseudoephedrine on page 1291

Rx:
Afrin nasal spray [OTC]
Disp: 15 mg
Sig: Spray once in each nostril every 6 to 8 hours for no more than 3 days

Ingredient: Oxymetazoline (Nasal)

Rx:
Sudafed 60 mg tablets [OTC]
Disp: 30 tablets
Sig: Take 1 tablet every 4 to 6 hours as needed for congestion

Note: Some reports have suggested alterations in blood pressure with pseudoephedrine which can range from minor to significant. This should be considered prior to prescribing.
Ingredient: Pseudoephedrine

Rx:
Chlor-Trimeton 4 mg [OTC]
Disp: 14 tablets
Sig: Take 1 tablet twice daily

Ingredient: Chlorpheniramine

ANTIBIOTICS:

Note: Antibiotics are not always required but may be useful in acute management of infection.

Rx:
Azithromycin (Systemic) 250 mg
Disp: 1 Z-Pak
Sig: 2 tablets day 1, then 1 tablet/day until gone

Rx:
Amoxicillin 250 mg
Disp: 30 capsules
Sig: Take 1 capsule 3 times/day for 7 to 10 days

Rx:
Amoxicillin 500 mg
Disp: 30 capsules or tablets
Sig: Take 1 capsule or tablet 3 times/day for 7 to 10 days

Rx:
Amoxicillin 875 mg
Disp: 20 tablets
Sig: Take 1 tablet twice daily

Rx:
Augmentin 250 mg
Disp: 30 tablets
Sig: Take 1 tablet 3 times/day for 7 to 10 days

Rx:
Augmentin 500 mg
Disp: 30 tablets
Sig: Take 1 tablet 3 times/day for 7 to 10 days

Rx:
Augmentin 875 mg
Disp: 20 tablets
Sig: Take 1 tablet twice daily for 7 to 10 days

Rx:
Augmentin XR 1,000 mg
Disp: 20 tablets
Sig: Take 2 tablets twice daily for 7 to 10 days

Rx:
LevoFLOXacin
Disp: Either five 750 mg tablets or seven or fourteen 500 mg tablets
Sig: Depending on the reference therapy you are following, select 1 tablet/day from the dosage and durations above

Note: For Acute Bacterial Rhinosinusitis, available as 500 mg or 750 mg tablets. Not generally recommended for dental or periodontal infections.

VIRAL INFECTIONS - SAMPLE PRESCRIPTIONS

HERPES SIMPLEX (INITIAL or PRIMARY)

General Prescription Comments

Closely monitor and reevaluate response. If response is inadequate, reevaluate diagnosis, medication choice, and dosage.

Sample Prescriptions

For additional information, see Acyclovir (Systemic) on page 75, Acyclovir (Topical) on page 82, Famciclovir on page 635, ValACYclovir on page 1512

Rx:
Zovirax 200 mg capsules
Disp: 35 to 60 capsules depending on regimen selected
Sig: Take 1 capsule 5 times/day or 2 capsules 3 times/day for 7 to 10 days
Ingredient: Acyclovir (Systemic)

Note: Regimens for HSV initial infections using valacyclovir or famciclovir are considered Off-Label Use (ie, not approved by the FDA).

Rx:
Famciclovir 500 mg tablets
Disp: 14 tablets
Sig: Take 1 tablet every 12 hours for 7 days

Rx:
Valacyclovir 1 g tablet
Disp: 14 tablets
Sig: Take 1 tablet every 12 hours for 7 days

Rx:
Zovirax cream 5%
Disp: 5 g tube
Sig: Apply thin layer to lesions 5 times/day for the duration of the external lesions

Ingredient: Acyclovir (Topical)

HERPES SIMPLEX (RECURRENT)

General Prescription Comments

Therapy should be initiated at the first sign of any prodrome such as tingling, burning, or itching.

Cream and ointment tube sizes may vary based on availability. Refer to individual monograph or check with pharmacist for available sizes.

Sample Prescriptions

For additional information, see Acyclovir (Topical) on page 82, Docosanol on page 508, Famciclovir on page 635, Penciclovir on page 1207, ValACYclovir on page 1512

Rx:
Denavir topical cream 1%
Disp: 1.5 g tube
Sig: Apply locally as directed to lesion every 2 hours during waking hours (begin when prodromal symptoms first occur)

Ingredient: Penciclovir

Rx:
Famciclovir 500 mg tablets
Disp: 3 tablets
Sig: Take 3 tablets (1,500 mg) as a single dose; therapy should be initiated at the first sign of any prodrome such as tingling, burning, or itching

Note: Dispense in multiples of 3 so that patient has drug on hand for any recurrences; available as generic equivalent

Rx:
ValACYclovir 500 mg
Disp: 8 caplets
Sig: 4 caplets twice daily for 1 day (separate doses by 12 hours); therapy should be initiated at the first sign of any prodrome such as tingling, burning, or itching

Rx:

Abreva cream [OTC]
Disp: 2 g tube
Sig: Apply to lesion 5 times/day during waking hours for the duration of the external lesions (begin when prodrome/ symptoms first occur)

Ingredient: Docosanol

Rx:

Zovirax cream 5%
Disp: 2 g tube; 5 g tube
Sig: Apply 5 times/day for the duration of the external lesions

Ingredient: Acyclovir (Topical)

SHINGLES (VARICELLA-ZOSTER VIRUS)

General Prescription Comments

Closely monitor and reevaluate response. If response is inadequate, reevaluate diagnosis, medication choice, and dosage.

Sample Prescriptions

For additional information, see Acyclovir (Systemic) on page 75, Famciclovir on page 635, ValACYclovir on page 1512

Rx:

Zovirax 200 mg capsules
Disp: 200 capsules
Sig: Take 4 capsules 4 times/day for 5 days

Ingredient: Acyclovir (Systemic)

Rx:

ValACYclovir 500 mg
Disp: 42 caplets
Sig: Take 2 caplets 3 times/day for 7 days

Rx:

Famciclovir 500 mg
Disp: 21 tablets
Sig: 1 tablet 3 times/day for 7 days

SEDATION (PRIOR TO DENTAL TREATMENT) - SAMPLE PRESCRIPTIONS

General Prescription Comments

Sample prescription doses are for healthy adults. Use of these drugs and/or dosage may not be appropriate for children, elderly, and/or debilitated patients. Dental sedation should be used cautiously in these patients. Patients receiving sedative agents must be advised that they will need to have someone drive them to and from their appointment.

Sample Prescriptions for Adults

For additional information, see ALPRAZolam on page 106, DiazePAM on page 477, HydrOXYzine on page 780, LORazepam on page 931, Triazolam on page 1493

Rx:

Valium 5 mg
Disp: 1 tablet
Sig: Take 1 tablet 1 hour before appointment

Note: Also available as 2 mg and 10 mg
Ingredient: DiazePAM

Rx:

Ativan 1 mg
Disp: 2 tablets
Sig: Take 2 tablets 1 hour before appointment

Note: Also available as 0.5 mg and 2 mg
Ingredient: LORazepam

Rx:

Xanax 0.5 mg
Disp: 1 tablet
Sig: Take 1 tablet 1 hour before appointment

Ingredient: ALPRAZolam

Rx:

Vistaril 25 mg
Disp: 2 capsules
Sig: Take 2 capsules 1 hour before appointment

Ingredient: HydrOXYzine

Rx:

Halcion 0.25 mg
Disp: 1 tablet
Sig: Take 1 tablet 1 hour before appointment

Ingredient: Triazolam

ULCERATIVE AND EROSIVE DISORDERS - SAMPLE PRESCRIPTIONS

RECURRENT APHTHOUS STOMATITIS

General Prescription Comments

Some intraoral uses are off-label. Write directions as "use locally as directed" and closely monitor and reevaluate response at least every 2 weeks. If response is inadequate, reevaluate diagnosis, medication choice, and dosage.

Liquid volumes are suggested for a typical 2-week course. Check with pharmacist for available sizes.

Cream, gel, and ointment tube sizes may vary based on availability. Refer to individual monograph or check with pharmacist for available sizes. Ointments, creams, and gels work well when the lesions are few in number and/or localized to the anterior areas of the oral cavity. When the lesions are more extensive or in the posterior areas of the mouth, steroid rinses and/or systemic steroids or other medications that suppress inflammation may be necessary.

Sample Prescriptions

For additional information, see Betamethasone (Topical) on page 237, Clobetasol on page 377, Dexamethasone (Systemic) on page 463, DiphenhydrAMINE (Systemic) on page 502, Fluocinonide on page 691, Triamcinolone (Topical) on page 1490

Palliative

Rx:

Orabase Protective Barrier [OTC]
Disp: 1 package
Sig: Apply locally as directed, every 6 hours as needed

Rx:

Benadryl liquid 12.5 mg per 5 mL (mix 50/50) with Kaopectate
Disp: 8 oz total
Sig: Rinse with 1 to 2 teaspoonfuls every 2 hours and expectorate

Note: Maalox can be used in place of Kaopectate if constipation is a problem. Benadryl is available as a generic DiphenhydrAMINE liquid.

Rx:

Benadryl liquid 12.5 mg per 5 mL / Kaopectate / Lidocaine viscous (mix 1/3, 1/3, 1/3)
Disp: 8 oz total
Sig: Rinse with 1 to 2 teaspoonfuls every 2 hours and expectorate

Note: Maalox can be used in place of Kaopectate if constipation is a problem. Benadryl is available as a generic DiphenhydrAMINE liquid. Lidocaine viscous is available as a prescription only. Combinations of medications like these are often called MAGIC MOUTHWASH and are not a direct treatment for the oral ulcerations but may provide some relief as the ulcers are present.

Rx:

Benadryl liquid 12.5 mg per 5 mL
Disp: 4 oz bottle
Sig: Rinse with 1 to 2 teaspoonfuls every 2 hours and expectorate

Note: Benadryl is available as a generic DiphenhydrAMINE liquid.

Therapy-Based (Contain Steroids)

Rx:

Oralone 0.1%
Disp: 5 g tube
Sig: Apply locally as directed to the lesion after each meal and at bedtime

Ingredient: Triamcinolone (Topical)

Rx:

Fluocinonide 0.05% gel
Disp: 45 g tube
Sig: Apply locally as directed to lesion 4 times/day

Rx:

Temovate 0.05%
Disp: 45 g tube
Sig: Apply locally as directed a small quantity with a Q-tip to affected area 3 to 4 times/day

Ingredient: Clobetasol propionate

Note: Pharmacies can be asked to compound drugs with higher potency, such as clobetasol with Orabase to achieve bioadhesive properties to help deliver the steroid effects.

Rx:

Betamethasone 0.1% ointment
Disp: 45 g tube
Sig: Apply a small quantity with a Q-tip locally as directed to affected area 3 to 4 times/day

Rx:

Decadron elixir 0.5 mg per 5 mL
Disp: 500 mL
Sig: Rinse with 1 teaspoon for 4 to 5 minutes 3 to 4 times/day and expectorate at the conclusion of each rinse

Ingredient: Dexamethasone (Systemic)

Note: Depending on severity of ulceration, instructions can be tailored to include swallowing initial doses and then tapering to every other dose eventually over 4 to 7 days to no swallowing. See Erosive Lichen Planus, Other Biopsy-Proven Desquamative Oral Diseases, and Major Aphthae for more examples.

MILD LICHEN PLANUS

General Prescription Comments

Some intraoral uses are off-label. Write directions as "use locally as directed" and closely monitor and reevaluate response at least every 2 weeks. If response is inadequate, reevaluate diagnosis, medication choice, and dosage.

Cream and ointment tube sizes may vary based on availability. Refer to individual monograph or check with pharmacist for available sizes.

Sample Prescriptions

For additional information, see Betamethasone (Topical) on page 237, Clobetasol on page 377, Dexamethasone (Systemic) on page 463, Fluocinonide on page 691, Triamcinolone (Topical) on page 1490

Rx:

Oralone 0.1%
Disp: 5 g tube
Sig: Apply locally as directed by coating the lesion with a thin film after each meal and at bedtime

Ingredient: Triamcinolone (Topical) 0.1%

Rx:

Fluocinonide 0.05% gel
Disp: 45 g tube
Sig: Apply locally as directed to lesion 4 times/day

Rx:

Temovate 0.05%
Disp: 45 g tube
Sig: Apply a small quantity with a Q-tip locally as directed to affected area 3 to 4 times/day

Ingredient: Clobetasol

Note: The pharmacist can compound potent steroids, such as clobetasol with Orabase, to enhance adherence to oral tissues.

Rx:

Betamethasone 0.1% ointment
Disp: 45 g tube
Sig: Apply a small quantity with a Q-tip locally as directed to affected area 3 to 4 times/day

Rx:

Decadron elixir 0.5 mg per 5 mL
Disp: 500 mL
Sig: Rinse with 1 teaspoon for 4 to 5 minutes 3 to 4 times/day and expectorate at the conclusion of each rinse

Ingredient: Dexamethasone (Systemic)

Note: Depending on severity of ulceration, instructions can be tailored to include swallowing initial doses and then tapering to every other dose eventually over 4 to 7 days to no swallowing. See Erosive Lichen Planus, Other Biopsy-Proven Desquamative Oral Diseases, and Major Aphthae for more examples.

EROSIVE LICHEN PLANUS, OTHER BIOPSY-PROVEN DESQUAMATIVE ORAL DISEASES (ie, PEMPHIGOID, PEMPHIGUS), AND MAJOR APHTHAE

General Prescription Comments

Some intraoral uses are off-label. Write directions as "use locally as directed" and closely monitor and reevaluate response at least every 2 weeks. If response is inadequate, reevaluate diagnosis, medication choice, and dosage.

Liquid volumes are suggested for a typical 2-week course. Check with pharmacist for available sizes.

Cream, gel, and ointment formulations should only be selected if the sites of the oral lesions are localized and are accessible for applications.

Cream, gel, and ointment tube sizes may vary based on availability. Refer to individual monograph or check with pharmacist for available sizes.

Note: Soft, thin, vacuum-formed trays can be made (similar to bleaching trays but extending slightly onto the gingiva) to deliver steroid ointments or creams to any gingival lesions. Also, the pharmacist can compound potent steroids, such as clobetasol with Orabase, to enhance adherence to oral tissues. For chronically recurring lesions, prednisone can be prescribed at 40 mg/day for week 1, 30 mg/day for week 2, continue tapering dose each week to 0. Occasionally, the clinician needs to tailor the regimen by using alternating doses every other day, such as 20 mg day 1, 10 mg day 2, then back to 20 mg. It is important to assess patient compliance when such a regimen is considered.

Sample Prescriptions

For additional information, see Clobetasol on page 377, Dexamethasone (Systemic) on page 463, MethylPREDNISolone on page 999, PredniSONE on page 1260

If a combination topical and systemic treatment is considered and the pill form followed by a rinse regimen is not preferred:

Rx:

Decadron 0.5 mg per 5 mL elixir
Disp: 500 mL bottle
Sig: For 3 days, rinse with 1 tablespoonful (15 mL) 4 times/day and swallow; then for 3 days, rinse with 1 teaspoonful (5 mL) 4 times/day and swallow; then for 3 days, rinse with 1 teaspoonful (5 mL) 4 times/day and swallow every other time. Then for 3 days rinse with 1 teaspoonful (5 mL) 4 times/day and expectorate. Continue the rinse and expectorate mode for 2 minutes but discontinue medication when mouth becomes completely comfortable.

Ingredient: Dexamethasone (Systemic); the practitioner can tailor this rinse, hold expectorate and/or swallow prescription to the severity and lesion location for each individual patient.

Rx:

Temovate 0.05% cream
Disp: 15 g tube
Sig: Apply locally as directed 4 to 5 times/day

Ingredient: Clobetasol; high potency topical steroid

Rx:

PredniSONE 5 mg tablets
Disp: 40 tablets
Sig: Take 5 tablets in the morning for 5 days, then 5 tablets in the morning every other day until gone

Rx:

PredniSONE 10 mg tablets
Disp: 50 tablets
Sig: Take 4 tablets in the morning for 5 days, then decrease by 1 tablet on each successive series of 5 days.

Note: Longer durations of a regimen (eg, 7 to 10 days) can be tailored to the severity of the oral condition.

Rx:

Medrol Dose Pak
Disp: 1 Pack
Sig: Follow package insert directions until gone

Ingredient: MethylPREDNISolone

Rx:

Protopic ointment (available in 0.03% and 0.1% strengths)
Disp: Available in 30 g, 60 g, and 100 g tubes
Sig: Apply locally as directed 2 times/day

Ingredient: Tacrolimus (Calcineurin Inhibitor; Immunosuppressant Agent)

ALPHABETICAL LISTING OF DRUGS

- ◆ **14115700** *see* Aclidinium *on page 74*
- ◆ **A-25 [OTC]** *see* Vitamin A *on page 1549*
- ◆ **A-200 Lice Treatment Kit [OTC]** *see* Pyrethrins and Piperonyl Butoxide *on page 1293*
- ◆ **A-200 Maximum Strength [OTC]** *see* Pyrethrins and Piperonyl Butoxide *on page 1293*
- ◆ **A771726** *see* Teriflunomide *on page 1423*

Abacavir (a BAK a veer)

Related Information

HIV Infection and AIDS *on page 1690*

Brand Names: US Ziagen

Brand Names: Canada APO-Abacavir; MINT-Abacavir; Ziagen

Pharmacologic Category Antiretroviral, Reverse Transcriptase Inhibitor, Nucleoside (Anti-HIV)

Use HIV-1 infection: Treatment of HIV-1 infection in combination with other antiretroviral agents

Local Anesthetic/Vasoconstrictor Precautions No information available to require special precautions

Effects on Dental Treatment No significant effects or complications reported

Effects on Bleeding No information available to require special precautions relative to altered hemostasis

Adverse Reactions Rates of adverse reactions were defined during combination therapy with other antiretrovirals.

>10%:

Central nervous system: Headache (adults: ≤13%; infants, children, & adolescents: 1%), fatigue (≤12%), malaise (≤12%)

Gastrointestinal: Nausea (7% to 19%)

1% to 10%:

Central nervous system: Abnormal dreams (≤10%), sleep disorder (≤10%), chills (≤9%), migraine (≤7%), depression (6%), dizziness (6%), anxiety (5%)

Dermatologic: Skin rash (5% to 7%)

Endocrine & metabolic: Hypertriglyceridemia (grades 3/4: 2% to 6%)

Gastrointestinal: Nausea and vomiting (9% to 10%), diarrhea (7%), abdominal pain (≤6%), gastritis (≤6%), gastrointestinal signs and symptoms (≤6%), increased serum amylase (grades 3/4: 2% to 4%), vomiting (2%)

Hematologic & oncologic: Neutropenia (grades 3/4: 2% to 5%), thrombocytopenia (grades 3/4: 1%)

Hepatic: Increased serum alanine aminotransferase (grades 3/4: 6%), increased serum aspartate aminotransferase (grades 3/4: 6%)

Hypersensitivity: Drug-induced hypersensitivity (9%), hypersensitivity reaction (including anaphylaxis and multiorgan failure; 8%; excluding subjects carrying the HLA-B*5701 allele: 1%)

Neuromuscular & skeletal: Increased creatine phosphokinase (grades 3/4: 7% to 8%), musculoskeletal pain (5% to 6%)

Respiratory: ENT infection (5%), viral respiratory tract infection (5%), bronchitis (4%), pneumonia (infants, children, & adolescents: 4%)

Miscellaneous: Fever (≤9%)

Frequency not defined:

Endocrine & metabolic: Increased gamma-glutamyl transferase

Gastrointestinal: Pancreatitis

<1%, postmarketing, and/or case reports: Anemia, autoimmune disease, erythema multiforme, Graves disease, Guillain-Barre syndrome, hepatomegaly, hyperglycemia, immune reconstitution syndrome, lactic acidosis, leukopenia, lipotrophy, liver steatosis, myocardial infarction, pain, polymyositis, redistribution of body fat, renal function abnormality, Stevens-Johnson syndrome, toxic epidermal necrolysis

Mechanism of Action Nucleoside reverse transcriptase inhibitor. Abacavir is a guanosine analogue which is phosphorylated to carbovir triphosphate which interferes with HIV viral RNA-dependent DNA polymerase resulting in inhibition of viral replication.

Pharmacodynamics/Kinetics

Half-life Elimination

Serum:

Pediatric patients ≥3 months to ≤13 years: 1 to 1.5 hours (Hughes 1999; Kline 1999)

Adults: 1.54 ± 0.63 hours

Hepatic impairment (mild): Increases half-life by 58%

Intracellular: 12 to 26 hours

Time to Peak Pediatric patients ≥3 months to ≤13 years: Within 1.5 hours (Hughes 1999); Adults: 0.7 to 1.7 hours

Reproductive Considerations

The Health and Human Services (HHS) perinatal HIV guidelines consider abacavir a preferred nucleoside reverse transcriptase inhibitor for females living with HIV who are not yet pregnant but are trying to conceive.

For males and females living with HIV and planning a pregnancy, maximum viral suppression below the limits of detection with antiretroviral therapy (ART), modification of therapy (if needed), optimization of the woman's health, and a discussion of the potential risks and benefits of ART therapy during pregnancy is recommended prior to conception (HHS [perinatal] 2019).

Pregnancy Considerations

Abacavir has a high level of transfer across the human placenta.

No increased risk of overall birth defects has been observed following first trimester exposure according to data collected by the antiretroviral pregnancy registry. Maternal antiretroviral therapy (ART) may be associated with adverse pregnancy outcomes including preterm delivery, stillbirth, low birth weight, and small for gestational age infants. Actual risks may be influenced by maternal factors, such as disease severity, gestational age at initiation of therapy, and specific ART regimen, therefore close fetal monitoring is recommended. Because there is clear benefit to appropriate treatment, maternal ART should not be withheld due to concerns for adverse neonatal outcomes. Long-term follow-up is recommended for all infants exposed to antiretroviral medications; children without HIV but who were exposed to ART in utero and develop significant organ system abnormalities of unknown etiology (particularly of the CNS or heart) should be evaluated for potential mitochondrial dysfunction. Cases of lactic acidosis and hepatic steatosis have been reported in pregnant women with use of nucleoside reverse transcriptase inhibitors (NRTIs).

The Health and Human Services (HHS) perinatal HIV guidelines consider abacavir a preferred NRTI for pregnant females living with HIV who are antiretroviral-naive, who have had ART therapy in the past but are restarting, or who require a new ART regimen (due to poor tolerance or poor virologic response of current regimen). In addition, females who become pregnant while taking abacavir may continue if viral suppression is effective and the regimen is well tolerated. The pharmacokinetics of abacavir are not significantly changed by pregnancy and dose adjustment is not needed for pregnant females.

The HHS perinatal HIV guidelines consider abacavir in combination with lamivudine to be a preferred NRTI backbone for initial therapy in antiretroviral-naive pregnant females (do not use in females who are positive for the HLA-B*5701 allele). This backbone is not recommended with atazanavir/ritonavir or efavirenz if pretreatment HIV RNA is >100,000 copies/mL. In addition, the HHS perinatal HIV guidelines consider abacavir in combination with lamivudine and dolutegravir to be a preferred integrase strand transfer inhibitor regimen for initial therapy in antiretroviral-naive pregnant females.

In general, ART is recommended for all pregnant females living with HIV to keep the viral load below the limit of detection and reduce the risk of perinatal transmission. Therapy should be individualized following a discussion of the potential risks and benefits of treatment during pregnancy. Monitoring of pregnant females is more frequent than in nonpregnant adults. ART should be continued postpartum for all females living with HIV and can be modified after delivery.

Health care providers are encouraged to enroll pregnant females exposed to antiretroviral medications as early in pregnancy as possible in the Antiretroviral Pregnancy Registry (1-800-258-4263 or http://www.APRegistry.com). Health care providers caring for pregnant females living with HIV and their infants may contact the National Perinatal HIV Hotline (888-448-8765) for clinical consultation (HHS [perinatal] 2019).

Abacavir and Lamivudine

(a BAK a veer & la MI vyoo deen)

Related Information

Abacavir *on page 50*

LamiVUDine *on page 872*

Brand Names: US Epzicom

Brand Names: Canada APO-Abacavir-Lamivudine; Auro-Abacavir/Lamivudine; Kivexa; MYLAN-Abacavir/Lamivudine; PMS-Abacavir-Lamivudine; TEVA-Abacavir/Lamivudine

Pharmacologic Category Antiretroviral, Reverse Transcriptase Inhibitor, Nucleoside (Anti-HIV)

Use HIV-1 infection, treatment: Treatment of HIV-1 infection in combination with other antiretroviral agents.

Local Anesthetic/Vasoconstrictor Precautions No information available to require special precautions

Effects on Dental Treatment No significant effects or complications reported

Effects on Bleeding No information available to require special precautions relative to altered hemostasis

Adverse Reactions See individual agents as well as other combination products for additional information. Rates of adverse reactions were defined during combination therapy with other antiretrovirals.

1% to 10%:

Central nervous system: Abnormal dreams, anxiety, depression, dizziness, fatigue, headache, insomnia, malaise, migraine, vertigo

Dermatologic: Skin rash

Gastrointestinal: Abdominal pain, diarrhea, gastritis

Hypersensitivity: Hypersensitivity (including multiorgan failure and anaphylaxis; ≤9%; higher incidence in subjects carrying the HLA-B*5701 allele)

Miscellaneous: Fever

<1%, postmarketing, and/or case reports: Abnormal breath sounds, alopecia, anemia (including pure red cell aplasia and severe anemias progressing on therapy), aplastic anemia, erythema multiforme, exacerbation of hepatitis B, hepatitis, hyperglycemia, immune reconstitution syndrome, increased creatine phosphokinase, lactic acidosis, liver steatosis, lymphadenopathy, myasthenia, paresthesia, peripheral neuropathy, redistribution of body fat, rhabdomyolysis, seizure, splenomegaly, Stevens-Johnson syndrome, stomatitis, weakness, wheezing

Mechanism of Action Nucleoside reverse transcriptase inhibitor combination.

Abacavir is a guanosine analogue which is phosphorylated to carbovir triphosphate which interferes with HIV viral RNA-dependent DNA polymerase resulting in inhibition of viral replication.

Lamivudine is a cytosine analog. After lamivudine is triphosphorylated, the principle mode of action is inhibition of HIV reverse transcription via viral DNA chain termination; inhibits RNA-dependent DNA polymerase activities of reverse transcriptase.

Reproductive Considerations

The Health and Human Services (HHS) perinatal HIV guidelines consider abacavir in combination with lamivudine to be a preferred nucleoside reverse transcriptase inhibitor combination for females living with HIV who are not yet pregnant but are trying to conceive (HHS [perinatal] 2019).

Refer to individual monographs for additional information.

Pregnancy Considerations

The Health and Human Services (HHS) perinatal HIV guidelines consider abacavir in combination with lamivudine to be a preferred nucleoside reverse transcriptase inhibitor combination for pregnant females living with HIV who are antiretroviral-naive, who have had antiretroviral therapy (ART) in the past but are restarting, or who require a new ART regimen (due to poor tolerance or poor virologic response of current regimen). In addition, females who become pregnant while taking abacavir/lamivudine may continue if viral suppression is effective and the regimen is well tolerated. Do not use in females who are positive for the HLA-B*5701 allele. This backbone is not recommended with atazanavir/ritonavir or efavirenz if pretreatment HIV RNA is >100,000 copies/mL (HHS [perinatal] 2019).

Refer to individual monographs for additional information.

Abacavir, Dolutegravir, and Lamivudine

(a BAK a veer, doe loo TEG ra vir, & la MI vyoo deen)

Brand Names: US Triumeq

Brand Names: Canada Triumeq

Pharmacologic Category Antiretroviral, Integrase Inhibitor (Anti-HIV); Antiretroviral, Reverse Transcriptase Inhibitor, Nucleoside (Anti-HIV)

Use

HIV infection, treatment: Treatment of HIV-1 infection in adult and pediatric patients weighing ≥40 kg.

Limitations of use: Not recommended for use in patients with known or clinically suspected integrase strand transfer inhibitor resistance because the dose of dolutegravir is insufficient in these subpopulations.

Local Anesthetic/Vasoconstrictor Precautions No information available to require special precautions

Effects on Dental Treatment No significant effects or complications reported

Effects on Bleeding No information available to require special precautions

Adverse Reactions See individual agents as well as other combination products for additional information.

>10%:

Endocrine & metabolic: Hyperglycemia (≥126 mg/dL)

Gastrointestinal: Increased serum lipase (>1.5 x ULN)

Neuromuscular & skeletal: Increased creatine phosphokinase (≥6.0 x ULN)

1% to 10%:

Central nervous system: Drowsiness (<2%), lethargy (<2%), nightmares (<2%), sleep disorder (<2%), suicidal ideation (<2%), depression, fatigue, headache, insomnia

Dermatologic: Pruritus (<2%)

Endocrine & metabolic: Hypertriglyceridemia (<2%)

Gastrointestinal: Abdominal distention (<2%), abdominal distress (<2%), abdominal pain (<2%), anorexia (<2%), dyspepsia (<2%), flatulence (<2%), gastroesophageal reflux disease (<2%), upper abdominal pain (<2%), vomiting (<2%)

Hematologic & oncologic: Decreased neutrophils

Hepatic: Hepatitis (<2%), increased serum ALT (>2.5 x ULN), increased serum AST (>2.5 x ULN)

Neuromuscular & skeletal: Arthralgia (<2%), myositis (<2%)

Renal: Renal insufficiency (<2%)

Miscellaneous: Fever (<2%)

<1%, postmarketing, and/or case reports: Abnormal dreams, diarrhea, dizziness, hypersensitivity reaction, immune reconstitution syndrome, nausea, skin rash

Mechanism of Action Dolutegravir inhibits HIV integrase by binding to the integrase active site and blocking the strand transfer step of retroviral DNA integration. Abacavir is converted by cellular enzymes to the active metabolite, carbovir triphosphate (CBV-TP), an analogue of deoxyguanosine-5′-triphosphate (dGTP). CBV-TP inhibits the activity of HIV-1 reverse transcriptase (RT) both by competing with the natural substrate dGTP and by its incorporation into viral DNA. Intracellularly, lamivudine is phosphorylated to its active 5′-triphosphate metabolite, lamivudine triphosphate (3TC-TP). The principal mode of action of 3TC-TP is inhibition of reverse transcriptase via DNA chain termination after incorporation of the nucleotide analogue.

Reproductive Considerations

The Health and Human Services (HHS) perinatal HIV guidelines consider this fixed-dose combination an alternative regimen for women living with HIV who are not yet pregnant but are trying to conceive (HHS [perinatal] 2019).

Refer to individual monographs for additional information.

Pregnancy Considerations

The Health and Human Services (HHS) perinatal HIV guidelines consider this fixed-dose combination a preferred regimen in pregnant females living with HIV who are antiretroviral naive, who have had antiretroviral therapy (ART) in the past but are restarting, and who require a new ART regimen (due to poor tolerance or poor virologic response of current regimen). In addition, females who become pregnant while taking this regimen may continue if viral suppression is effective and the regimen is well tolerated (HHS [perinatal] 2019).

Refer to individual monographs for additional information.

◆ **Abacavir/Dolutegravir/Lamivudine** *see* Abacavir, Dolutegravir, and Lamivudine *on page 51*

Abacavir, Lamivudine, and Zidovudine

(a BAK a veer, la MI vyoo deen, & zye DOE vyoo deen)

Related Information

Abacavir *on page 50*

HIV Infection and AIDS *on page 1690*

LamiVUDine *on page 872*

Zidovudine *on page 1569*

Brand Names: US Trizivir

Brand Names: Canada APO-Abacavir-Lamivud-Zidovud; Trizivir [DSC]

Pharmacologic Category Antiretroviral, Reverse Transcriptase Inhibitor, Nucleoside (Anti-HIV)

Use

HIV infection: Treatment of HIV-1 infection in combination with other antiretroviral agents.

Local Anesthetic/Vasoconstrictor Precautions No information available to require special precautions

Effects on Dental Treatment No significant effects or complications reported

Effects on Bleeding No information available to require special precautions relative to altered hemostasis

Adverse Reactions See individual agents as well as other combination products for additional information. Frequency not always defined.

Central nervous system: Headache (13%), fatigue (12%), malaise (12%), depression (6%), anxiety (5%)

Dermatologic: Skin rash (5%)

Endocrine & metabolic: Increased amylase (2%), increased serum triglycerides (grade 3-4: 2%), increased gamma-glutamyl transferase, redistribution of body fat

Gastrointestinal: Nausea (19%), nausea and vomiting (10%), diarrhea (7%), pancreatitis

Hematologic & oncologic: Neutropenia (5%)

Hepatic: Increased serum ALT (6%)

Hypersensitivity: Hypersensitivity (1% to 9%; based on abacavir component; higher risk in carriers of the HLA-B*5701 allele)

Immunologic: Immune reconstitution syndrome

Infection: Viral infection (5%)

Miscellaneous: Fever and chills (6%)

Neuromuscular & skeletal: Increased creatine phosphokinase (7%)

Respiratory: ENT infection (5%)

<1%, postmarketing, and/or case reports: Abdominal pain, abnormal breath sounds, allergic sensitization (including anaphylaxis), alopecia, anemia, anorexia, aplastic anemia, arthralgia, cardiomyopathy, decreased appetite, dizziness, dyspepsia, erythema multiforme, exacerbation of hepatitis B (posttreatment), gynecomastia, increased serum bilirubin, increased serum transaminases, insomnia, lactic acidosis, liver steatosis, lymphadenopathy, myalgia, myasthenia, oral mucosa hyperpigmentation, paresthesia, peripheral neuropathy, rhabdomyolysis, seizure, sleep disorder, splenomegaly, Stevens-Johnson syndrome, stomatitis, thrombocytopenia, urticaria, vasculitis, weakness, wheezing

Mechanism of Action The combination of abacavir, lamivudine, and zidovudine is believed to act synergistically to inhibit reverse transcriptase via DNA chain termination after incorporation of the nucleoside analogue as well as to delay the emergence of mutations conferring resistance.

Reproductive Considerations

The Health and Human Services (HHS) perinatal HIV guidelines do not recommend use of this fixed-dose combination regimen in females who are not yet pregnant but are trying to conceive (HHS [perinatal] 2019).

Refer to individual monographs for additional information.

Pregnancy Considerations

The Health and Human Services (HHS) perinatal HIV guidelines do not recommend use of this fixed-dose combination regimen in pregnancy. Women who become pregnant while taking this combination should be changed to a recommended regimen (HHS [perinatal] 2019).

Refer to individual monographs for additional information.

- **Abacavir/Lamivudine/Zidovudine** *see* Abacavir, Lamivudine, and Zidovudine *on page 52*
- **Abacavir Sulfate** *see* Abacavir *on page 50*
- **Abacavir Sulfate and Lamivudine** *see* Abacavir and Lamivudine *on page 51*
- **Abacavir Sulfate, Dolutegravir, and Lamivudine** *see* Abacavir, Dolutegravir, and Lamivudine *on page 51*

Abaloparatide (a bal oh PAR a tide)

Brand Names: US Tymlos

Pharmacologic Category Parathyroid Hormone Analog

Use Osteoporosis: Treatment of postmenopausal females with osteoporosis at high risk for fracture (defined as a history of osteoporotic fracture or multiple risk factors for fracture). May also be used in patients who have failed or are intolerant to other available osteoporosis therapy.

Limitations of use: Cumulative lifetime duration of abaloparatide and any other parathyroid hormone therapy (eg, teriparatide) should not exceed 2 years.

Local Anesthetic/Vasoconstrictor Precautions
No information available to require special precautions

Effects on Dental Treatment No significant effects or complications reported

Effects on Bleeding No information available to require special precautions

Adverse Reactions

>10%:

Endocrine & metabolic: Increased uric acid (25%)

Genitourinary: Hypercalciuria (11% to 20%)

Immunologic: Antibody development (49%; neutralizing antibodies: 68%; antibody formation was not found to have any clinical significance)

Local: Erythema at injection site (58%)

1% to 10%:

Cardiovascular: Palpitations (5%), orthostatic hypotension (1% to 4%), sinus tachycardia (≤2%), tachycardia (≤2%)

Central nervous system: Dizziness (10%), headache (8%), fatigue (3%)

Endocrine & metabolic: Hypercalcemia (3%)

Gastrointestinal: Nausea (8%), upper abdominal pain (3%)

Local: Swelling at injection site (10%), pain at injection site (9%)

Mechanism of Action Abaloparatide is an analog of human parathyroid hormone related peptide (PTHrP [1-34]), which acts as an agonist at the PTH1 receptor (PTH1R). This results in stimulation of osteoblast function and increased bone mass (Harslof 2016; Leder 2017).

Pharmacodynamics/Kinetics

Half-life Elimination 1.7 hours

Time to Peak 0.51 hours (range: 0.25 to 0.52 hours)

Pregnancy Considerations Abaloparatide is not indicated for use in women of reproductive potential. Animal reproduction studies have not been conducted.

Abatacept (ab a TA sept)

Related Information

Rheumatoid Arthritis, Osteoarthritis, and Osteoporosis *on page 1697*

Brand Names: US Orencia; Orencia ClickJect

Brand Names: Canada Orencia

Pharmacologic Category Antirheumatic, Disease Modifying; Selective T-Cell Costimulation Blocker

Use

Juvenile idiopathic arthritis: Treatment of moderately to severely active polyarticular juvenile idiopathic arthritis in patients ≥2 years of age; may be used as monotherapy or in combination with methotrexate.

Psoriatic arthritis: Treatment of active psoriatic arthritis in adults.

Rheumatoid arthritis: Treatment of moderately to severely active adult rheumatoid arthritis; may be used as monotherapy or in combination with other disease-modifying antirheumatic drugs (DMARDs).

Note: Abatacept should **not** be used in combination with other potent immunosuppressants (eg, biologic DMARDs, Janus kinase inhibitors).

Local Anesthetic/Vasoconstrictor Precautions
No information available to require special precautions

Effects on Dental Treatment Key adverse event(s) related to dental treatment: Abatacept belongs to the class of disease-modifying antirheumatic drugs and, as such, has immunosuppressive properties. Consider a medical consult prior to any invasive treatment for patients under active treatment with abatacept. Delayed wound healing due to the immunosuppressive effects and increased potential for postsurgical infection may be of concern.

Effects on Bleeding No information available to require special precautions

Adverse Reactions COPD patients experienced a higher frequency of COPD-related adverse reactions (COPD exacerbation, cough, dyspnea, pneumonia, rhonchi).

>10%:

Central nervous system: Headache (18%)

Gastrointestinal: Nausea (≥10%)

Immunologic: Antibody development (2% to 41%)

Infection: Infection (54%), influenza (5% to 13%)

Respiratory: Bronchitis (5% to 13%), sinusitis (5% to 13%), upper respiratory tract infection (5% to 13%), nasopharyngitis (12%)

1% to 10%:

Cardiovascular: Hypertension (7%)

Central nervous system: Dizziness (9%)

Dermatologic: Skin rash (4%)

Gastrointestinal: Dyspepsia (6%)

Genitourinary: Urinary tract infection (6%)

Immunologic: Immunogenicity (1% to 2%)
Infection: Herpes simplex infection (<5%)
Local: Injection site reaction (3% to 4%)
Neuromuscular & skeletal: Back pain (7%), limb pain (3%)
Respiratory: Cough (8%), pneumonia (<5%), rhinitis (<5%)
Miscellaneous: Infusion-related reaction (≤9%)

<1% and/or case reports: Anaphylaxis, cellulitis, diverticulitis of the gastrointestinal tract, dyspnea, flushing, hypersensitivity reaction, hypotension, malignant lymphoma, malignant neoplasm of lung, nonimmune anaphylaxis, pruritus, pyelonephritis, sepsis, urticaria, wheezing

Frequency not defined:
Genitourinary: Malignant neoplasm of cervix
Hematologic & oncologic: Endometrial carcinoma, malignant melanoma, malignant neoplasm of the bile duct, malignant neoplasm of bladder, malignant neoplasm of breast, malignant neoplasm of kidney, malignant neoplasm of ovary, malignant neoplasm of prostate, malignant neoplasm of skin, malignant neoplasm of thyroid, malignant neoplasm of uterus, myelodysplastic syndrome
Respiratory: Exacerbation of chronic obstructive pulmonary disease, rhonchi

Postmarketing: Exacerbation of psoriasis, hypersensitivity angiitis, psoriasis, vasculitis

Mechanism of Action Selective costimulation modulator; inhibits T-cell (T-lymphocyte) activation by binding to CD80 and CD86 on antigen presenting cells (APC), thus blocking the required CD28 interaction between APCs and T cells. Activated T lymphocytes are found in the synovium of rheumatoid arthritis patients.

Pharmacodynamics/Kinetics

Half-life Elimination

Rheumatoid arthritis (RA): IV: 13.1 days (range: 8 to 25 days).

Clearance: **Note:** Clearance increases with increasing body weight.

Children 6 to 17 years: Juvenile idiopathic arthritis: 0.4 mL/hour/kg (0.2 to 1.12 mL/hour/kg).

Adults: RA: 0.22 mL/hour/kg (0.13 to 0.47 mL/hour/kg).

Reproductive Considerations

Until additional data are available related to use in pregnancy, it is recommended to discontinue use and switch to a safer medication prior to conception unless no other pregnancy compatible medication is able to control maternal disease (Götestam Skorpen 2016).

Pregnancy Considerations

Information related to the use of abatacept in pregnancy is limited (Kumar 2015).

A pregnancy registry has been established to monitor outcomes of women exposed to abatacept during pregnancy (1-877-311-8972).

◆ **Abbott-43818** *see* Leuprolide *on page 890*

◆ **ABC** *see* Abacavir *on page 50*

◆ **ABCD** *see* Amphotericin B Cholesteryl Sulfate Complex *on page 137*

◆ **ABDEK [OTC]** *see* Vitamins (Multiple/Oral) *on page 1550*

◆ **Abelcet** *see* Amphotericin B (Lipid Complex) *on page 138*

◆ **ABI-007** *see* PACLitaxel (Protein Bound) *on page 1179*

◆ **Abilify** *see* ARIPiprazole *on page 164*

◆ **Abilify Maintena** *see* ARIPiprazole *on page 164*

◆ **Abilify MyCite** *see* ARIPiprazole *on page 164*

◆ **Abiraterone** *see* Abiraterone Acetate *on page 54*

Abiraterone Acetate (a bir A ter one AS e tate)

Brand Names: US Yonsa; Zytiga

Brand Names: Canada Zytiga

Pharmacologic Category Antiandrogen; Antineoplastic Agent, Antiandrogen

Use

Prostate cancer, metastatic:

Treatment of metastatic, castration-resistant prostate cancer (in combination with prednisone [Zytiga] or methylprednisolone [Yonsa])

Treatment of metastatic, high-risk castration-sensitive prostate cancer (in combination with prednisone [Zytiga])

Local Anesthetic/Vasoconstrictor Precautions No information available to require special precautions

Effects on Dental Treatment No significant effects or complications reported

Effects on Bleeding No information available to require special precautions

Adverse Reactions Adverse reactions reported for use in combination with a corticosteroid.

>10%:
Cardiovascular: Hypertension (9% to 37%), edema (25% to 27%)
Central nervous system: Fatigue (39%), insomnia (14%)
Endocrine & metabolic: Hypertriglyceridemia (63%), hyperglycemia (57%), hypernatremia (33%), hypokalemia (17% to 30%), hypophosphatemia (24%), hot flash (15% to 22%)
Gastrointestinal: Constipation (23%), diarrhea (18% to 22%), dyspepsia (6% to 11%)
Genitourinary: Urinary tract infection (7% to 12%)
Hematologic & oncologic: Lymphocytopenia (20% to 38%; grades 3/4: 4% to 9%), bruise (13%)
Hepatic: Increased serum alanine aminotransferase (11% to 46%), increased serum aspartate aminotransferase (15% to 37%), increased serum bilirubin (7% to 16%)
Neuromuscular & skeletal: Arthralgia (≤30%), joint swelling (≤30%), myalgia (26%)
Respiratory: Cough (7% to 17%), upper respiratory infection (5% to 13%), dyspnea (12%), nasopharyngitis (11%)

1% to 10%:
Cardiovascular: Cardiac arrhythmia (7%), chest discomfort (≤4%), chest pain (≤4%), cardiac failure (2%)
Central nervous system: Headache (8%), falling (6%)
Dermatologic: Skin rash (8%)
Genitourinary: Hematuria (10%), groin pain (7%), urinary frequency (7%), nocturia (6%)
Neuromuscular & skeletal: Bone fracture (6%)
Miscellaneous: Fever (9%)

<1%, postmarketing, and/or case reports: Acute hepatic failure, adrenocortical insufficiency, fulminant hepatitis, myopathy, pneumonitis, rhabdomyolysis

Mechanism of Action Abiraterone selectively and irreversibly inhibits CYP17 (17 alpha-hydroxylase/C17,20-lyase), an enzyme required for androgen biosynthesis which is expressed in testicular, adrenal, and prostatic tumor tissues. Inhibits the formation of the testosterone precursors dehydroepiandrosterone (DHEA) and androstenedione.

Pharmacodynamics/Kinetics

Half-life Elimination 14.4 to 16.5 hours (Acharya 2012)

Time to Peak 2 hours (Acharya 2012)

Reproductive Considerations

Male patients with female partners of reproductive potential should use effective contraception during treatment and for 3 weeks after the last abiraterone dose.

Abiraterone is available in uncoated and film-coated tablets and in micronized tablets; the manufacturer recommends females who may become pregnant wear gloves if handling uncoated tablets, micronized tablets, or tablets that are broken, crushed, or damaged. NIOSH recommends single gloving for administration of hazardous intact oral tablets (NIOSH 2016).

Pregnancy Considerations

Based on the mechanism of action and adverse effects observed in animal reproduction studies, abiraterone may cause fetal harm or fetal loss if administered during pregnancy. Abiraterone is not indicated for use in females.

Abiraterone is available in uncoated and film-coated tablets and in micronized tablets; the manufacturer recommends females who are pregnant wear gloves if handling uncoated tablets, micronized tablets, or tablets that are broken, crushed, or damaged. NIOSH recommends single gloving for administration of hazardous intact oral tablets (NIOSH 2016).

◆ **Abiraterone Acetate Fine Particle (Yonsa)** *see* Abiraterone Acetate *on page 54*

◆ **Abiraterone Acetate Micronized (Yonsa)** *see* Abiraterone Acetate *on page 54*

◆ **Abiraterone Acetate Originator (Zytiga)** *see* Abiraterone Acetate *on page 54*

◆ **ABLC** *see* Amphotericin B (Lipid Complex) *on page 138*

AbobotulinumtoxinA

(aye bo BOT yoo lin num TOKS in aye)

Brand Names: US Dysport

Brand Names: Canada Dysport Aesthetic; Dysport Therapeutic

Pharmacologic Category Neuromuscular Blocker Agent, Toxin

Use

Cervical dystonia: Treatment of adults with cervical dystonia.

Glabellar lines: Temporary improvement in the appearance of moderate to severe glabellar lines associated with corrugator and procerus muscle activity in adults <65 years of age.

Spasticity: Treatment of spasticity in patients ≥2 years of age.

Local Anesthetic/Vasoconstrictor Precautions No information available to require special precautions

Effects on Dental Treatment Key adverse event(s) related to dental treatment: Xerostomia (normal salivary flow resumes upon discontinuation) and facial paresis.

Effects on Bleeding No information available to require special precautions

Adverse Reactions

Cervical dystonia:

>10%:

Gastrointestinal: Dysphagia (15% to 39%), xerostomia (13% to 39%)

Local: Discomfort at injection site (13% to 22%)

Nervous system: Voice disorder (6% to 28%), fatigue (12%), headache (11%), facial paresis (5% to 11%)

Neuromuscular & skeletal: Myasthenia (11% to 56%)

Ophthalmic: Eye disease (6% to 17%)

1% to 10%:

Immunologic: Antibody development (binding or neutralizing; 3%)

Local: Pain at injection site (5%)

Nervous system: Dizziness (4%)

Neuromuscular & skeletal: Musculoskeletal pain (7%), amyotrophy (1%)

Respiratory: Dyspnea (3%; onset: ~1 week; duration: ~3 weeks)

Frequency not defined:

Cardiovascular: Decreased heart rate

Endocrine & metabolic: Increased serum glucose

Glabellar lines:

1% to 10%:

Dermatologic: Contact dermatitis (2% to 3%)

Gastrointestinal: Nausea (2%)

Genitourinary: Hematuria (2%)

Infection: Influenza (2% to 3%)

Local: Pain at injection site (3%), discomfort at injection site (2% to 3%), injection site reaction (2% to 3%), swelling at injection site (2% to 3%)

Nervous system: Headache (9%)

Ophthalmic: Blepharoptosis (2%), eyelid edema (2%)

Respiratory: Nasopharyngitis (10%), upper respiratory tract infection (3%), bronchitis (2% to 3%), cough (2% to 3%), pharyngolaryngeal pain (2% to 3%), sinusitis (2%)

Upper limb spasticity:

>10%: Respiratory: Upper respiratory tract infection (children and adolescents: 9% to 11%)

1% to 10%:

Cardiovascular: Hypertension (adults: 1% to 2%), syncope (adults: 1% to 2%)

Dermatologic: Eczema (children and adolescents: <3%; injection site), rash at injection site (children and adolescents: <3%)

Endocrine & metabolic: Increased serum triglycerides (adults: 1% to 2%)

Gastrointestinal: Nausea (children and adolescents: 1% to 3%), constipation (adults: 2%), diarrhea (adults: 1% to 2%)

Hematologic & oncologic: Bruise (adults: 1% to 2%)

Immunologic: Antibody development (4% to 7%; neutralizing: ≤4%)

Infection: Influenza (1% to 3%), infection (adults: 2%)

Local: Bruising at injection site (children and adolescents: <3%), pain at injection site (children and adolescents: <3%), swelling at injection site (children and adolescents: <3%)

Nervous system: Headache (children and adolescents: 3% to 6%; adults: 2%), myasthenia (2% to 6%), epilepsy (2% to 4%), falling (adults: 3%), fatigue (<3%), depression (adults: 2% to 3%), hypoesthesia (adults: 2%), seizure (adults: 2%)

Neuromuscular & skeletal: Limb pain (children and adolescents: <3%), myalgia (children and adolescents: <3%), back pain (adults: 2%), asthenia (adults: 1% to 2%)

Respiratory: Pharyngitis (children and adolescents: 6% to 10%), flu-like symptoms (children and adolescents: <3%), cough (adults: 2%)
Miscellaneous: Accidental injury (adults: 2%)
Frequency not defined: Local: Injection site reaction

Lower limb spasticity:
>10%:
Respiratory: Nasopharyngitis (children and adolescents: 9% to 16%), cough (children and adolescents: 7% to 14%)
Miscellaneous: Fever (children and adolescents: 7% to 12%)
1% to 10%:
Cardiovascular: Peripheral edema (adults: 2%)
Gastrointestinal: Constipation (adults: 2%)
Hepatic: Increased serum alanine aminotransferase (adults: 2%)
Immunologic: Antibody development (4%; neutralizing: ≤2%)
Nervous system: Falling (adults: 6% to 9%), epilepsy (children and adolescents: ≤7%), seizure (children and adolescents: ≤7%), myasthenia (adults: 7%), fatigue (adults: 1% to 4%), headache (adults: 3%), depression (adults: 2% to 3%), insomnia (adults: 2%)
Neuromuscular & skeletal: Limb pain (6% to 7%), arthralgia (adults: 2% to 4%)
Respiratory: Bronchitis (children and adolescents: 7% to 8%), flu-like symptoms (adults: 2%)

Any indication: <1%, postmarketing and/or case reports: Abnormal gait, amyotrophy, anaphylaxis, antibody development, blurred vision, burning sensation, connective tissue disease (excessive granulation tissue), corneal disease, decreased lacrimation, diplopia, disturbance in attention, dry eye syndrome, dysarthria, dysphagia, dyspnea, edema (soft tissue), erythema of skin, facial paresis, feeling abnormal, feeling of heaviness, flu-like symptoms, hypersensitivity reaction, hypertonia, hypoesthesia, photophobia, reduced blinking, respiratory failure, serum sickness, severe dyspnea, urinary incontinence, urticaria, vertigo

Mechanism of Action AbobotulinumtoxinA (previously known as botulinum toxin type A) is a neurotoxin produced by *Clostridium botulinum*, spore-forming anaerobic bacillus, which appears to affect only the presynaptic membrane of the neuromuscular junction in humans, where it prevents calcium-dependent release of acetylcholine and produces a state of denervation. Muscle inactivation persists until new fibrils grow from the nerve and form junction plates on new areas of the muscle-cell walls.

Pharmacodynamics/Kinetics

Onset of Action Peak effect: Cervical dystonia: 2 to 4 weeks; Upper limb spasticity: 1 week

Duration of Action Cervical dystonia, glabellar lines: ≥4 months; Lower limb spasticity: ≥5 ½ months; Upper limb spasticity: ≥5 months

Pregnancy Considerations Adverse events have been observed in animal reproduction studies.

- **Abraxane** *see* PACLitaxel (Protein Bound) *on page 1179*
- **Abreva [OTC]** *see* Docosanol *on page 508*
- **Abrilada** *see* Adalimumab *on page 83*
- **Absorbable Collagen Hemostat** *see* Collagen Hemostat *on page 410*
- **Absorbable Cotton** *see* Cellulose (Oxidized/Regenerated) *on page 320*
- **Absorbable Gelatin Sponge** *see* Gelatin (Absorbable) *on page 731*
- **Absorica** *see* ISOtretinoin (Systemic) *on page 846*
- **Absorica LD** *see* ISOtretinoin (Systemic) *on page 846*
- **Abstral** *see* FentaNYL *on page 642*
- **ABT-0199** *see* Venetoclax *on page 1538*
- **ABT-335** *see* Fenofibrate and Derivatives *on page 640*
- **ABT-493 and ABT-530** *see* Glecaprevir and Pibrentasvir *on page 738*
- **ABT-620** *see* Elagolix *on page 547*
- **ABX-EGF** *see* Panitumumab *on page 1187*
- **AC 2993** *see* Exenatide *on page 633*

Acalabrutinib (a KAL a broo ti nib)

Brand Names: US Calquence
Brand Names: Canada Calquence
Pharmacologic Category Antineoplastic Agent; Antineoplastic Agent, Bruton Tyrosine Kinase Inhibitor; Antineoplastic Agent, Tyrosine Kinase Inhibitor

Use

Chronic lymphocytic leukemia or small lymphocytic lymphoma: Treatment of chronic lymphocytic leukemia or small lymphocytic lymphoma in adults.

Mantle cell lymphoma (previously treated): Treatment of mantle cell lymphoma in adults who have received at least 1 prior therapy.

Local Anesthetic/Vasoconstrictor Precautions No information available to require special precautions

Effects on Dental Treatment No significant effects or complications reported

Effects on Bleeding Chemotherapy may result in significant myelosuppression, potentially including significant reduction in platelet counts (thrombocytopenia grades 3 or 4: 8%), neutropenia (grade 3 or 4: 23%) and altered hemostasis. Hematoma ~8% and hemorrhage ~8% of patients. In patients who are under active treatment with these agents, medical consult is suggested.

Adverse Reactions
>10%:
Central nervous system: Headache (39%), fatigue (28%)
Dermatologic: Skin rash (18%)
Gastrointestinal: Diarrhea (31%), nausea (19%), abdominal pain (15%), constipation (15%), vomiting (13%)
Hematologic & oncologic: Neutropenia (grade 3 or 4: 23%), bruise (21%; grade 1: 19%), anemia (grade 3 or 4: 11%), malignant neoplasm (11%)
Neuromuscular & skeletal: Myalgia (21%)
1% to 10%:
Cardiovascular: Atrial fibrillation (≤3%), atrial flutter (≤3%)
Hematologic & oncologic: Thrombocytopenia (grade 3 or 4: 8%), hematoma (≤8%; grade ≥3: ≤1%), hemorrhage (≤8%; grade ≥3: ≤1%), skin carcinoma (7%)
Renal: Increased serum creatinine (grade 2: 5%)
Respiratory: Epistaxis (6%)
Frequency not defined:
Central nervous system: Progressive multifocal leukoencephalopathy
Infection: Opportunistic infection, reactivation of HBV, serious infection
Respiratory: Pneumonia

Mechanism of Action Acalabrutinib is a selective and irreversible second-generation Bruton's tyrosine kinase (BTK) inhibitor (Byrd 2016). Acalabrutinib and the active metabolite (ACP-5862) form a bond (covalent) with a cysteine residue in the active BTK site to inhibit BTK enzyme activity. BTK is an integral component of the B-cell receptor (BCR) and cytokine receptor pathways. BTK signals activation of the pathways necessary for B-cell proliferation, trafficking, chemotaxis and adhesion. BTK inhibition results in decreased malignant B-cell proliferation and tumor growth.

Pharmacodynamics/Kinetics

Half-life Elimination Acalabrutinib: 1 hour; ACP-5862 (active metabolite): 3.5 hours.

Time to Peak Acalabrutinib: 0.9 hours (range: 0.5 to 1.9 hours); ACP-5862: 1.6 hours (range: 0.9 to 2.7 hours).

Reproductive Considerations

Evaluate pregnancy status prior to use in females of reproductive potential. Females of reproductive potential should use effective contraception during therapy and for at least 1 week after the last acalabrutinib dose.

Pregnancy Considerations

Based on data from animal reproduction studies, in utero exposure to acalabrutinib may cause fetal harm.

Prescribing and Access Restrictions

Available through specialty pharmacy distributors. Information regarding distribution is available from the manufacturer at www.calquence.com.

Acamprosate (a kam PROE sate)

Brand Names: Canada Campral

Pharmacologic Category GABA Agonist/Glutamate Antagonist

Use

Alcohol use disorder: Maintenance of abstinence from alcohol in patients with alcohol use disorder who are abstinent at treatment initiation, as part of a comprehensive management program

Limitations of use: Efficacy has not been demonstrated in subjects who have not undergone detoxification and not achieved alcohol abstinence prior to beginning treatment. Efficacy in promoting abstinence from alcohol in polysubstance abusers has not been adequately assessed.

Local Anesthetic/Vasoconstrictor Precautions No information available to require special precautions

Effects on Dental Treatment Key adverse event(s) related to dental treatment: Xerostomia and changes in salivation (normal salivary flow resumes upon discontinuation) and taste perversion.

Effects on Bleeding No information available to require special precautions

Adverse Reactions Many adverse effects associated with treatment may be related to alcohol abstinence; reported frequency range may overlap with placebo.

>10%: Gastrointestinal: Diarrhea (10% to 17%)

1% to 10%:

Cardiovascular: Chest pain, hypertension, palpitations, peripheral edema, syncope, vasodilation

Central nervous system: Insomnia (6% to 9%), anxiety (5% to 8%), depression (4% to 8%), dizziness (3% to 4%), pain (2% to 4%), paresthesia (2% to 3%), abnormality in thinking, amnesia, attempted suicide, chills, drowsiness, headache

Dermatologic: Pruritus (3% to 4%), diaphoresis (2% to 3%), skin rash

Endocrine & metabolic: Decreased libido, weight gain

Gastrointestinal: Anorexia (2% to 5%), nausea (3% to 4%), flatulence (1% to 4%), xerostomia (1% to 3%), abdominal pain, constipation, dysgeusia, dyspepsia, increased appetite, vomiting

Genitourinary: Impotence

Infection: Infection

Neuromuscular & skeletal: Weakness (5% to 7%), arthralgia, back pain, myalgia, tremor

Ophthalmic: Visual disturbance

Respiratory: Bronchitis, dyspnea, flu-like symptoms, increased cough, pharyngitis, rhinitis

<1%, postmarketing, and/or case reports: Abnormal hepatic function tests, agitation, alopecia, anemia, angina pectoris, asthma, brain disease, colitis, confusion, deafness, diabetes mellitus, duodenal ulcer, eosinophilia, epistaxis, exfoliative dermatitis, fever, gastrointestinal hemorrhage, gout, hallucination, hemorrhage, hepatic cirrhosis, hepatitis, hostility, hyperbilirubinemia, hyperesthesia, hyperglycemia, hypersensitivity reaction, hyperuricemia, hyponatremia, hypotension, hypothyroidism, increased serum creatinine, increased serum transaminases, leukopenia, lymphadenopathy, lymphocytosis, myocardial infarction, nephrolithiasis, neuralgia, ophthalmic inflammation, orthostatic hypotension, pancreatitis, pneumonia, psychoneurosis, psychosis, pulmonary embolism, rectal hemorrhage, renal failure, seizure, skin photosensitivity, suicidal ideation, tachycardia, thrombocytopenia, urticaria, withdrawal syndrome

Mechanism of Action Mechanism not fully defined. Structurally similar to gamma-amino butyric acid (GABA), acamprosate appears to increase the activity of the GABA-ergic system, and decreases activity of glutamate within the CNS, including a decrease in activity at N-methyl D-aspartate (NMDA) receptors; may also affect CNS calcium channels. Restores balance to GABA and glutamate activities which appear to be disrupted in alcohol use disorder. During therapeutic use, reduces alcohol intake, but does not cause a disulfiram-like reaction following alcohol ingestion. Insignificant CNS activity, outside its effect on alcohol use disorder, was observed including no anxiolytic, anticonvulsant, or antidepressant activity.

Pharmacodynamics/Kinetics

Half-life Elimination 20 to 33 hours

Time to Peak Plasma: 3 to 8 hours

Pregnancy Risk Factor C

Pregnancy Considerations Adverse events were observed in animal reproduction studies.

Pharmacological agents should not be used for the treatment of alcohol use disorder in pregnant women unless needed for the treatment of acute alcohol withdrawal or a coexisting disorder; agents other than acamprosate are recommended for acute alcohol withdrawal (APA [Reus 2018]).

◆ **Acamprosate Calcium** *see* Acamprosate *on page 57*

◆ **Acanya** *see* Clindamycin and Benzoyl Peroxide *on page 375*

Acarbose (AY car bose)

Related Information

Endocrine Disorders and Pregnancy *on page 1684*

Brand Names: US Precose

Brand Names: Canada Glucobay; MAR-Acarbose

Pharmacologic Category Antidiabetic Agent, Alpha-Glucosidase Inhibitor

Use Diabetes mellitus, type 2: Adjunct to diet and exercise to improve glycemic control in adults with type 2 diabetes mellitus

Local Anesthetic/Vasoconstrictor Precautions No information available to require special precautions.

Effects on Dental Treatment No significant effects or complications reported.

Effects on Bleeding No information available to require special precautions.

Adverse Reactions

>10%: Gastrointestinal: Frequency and intensity of flatulence (74%) tend to abate with time; diarrhea (31%) and abdominal pain (19%) tend to return to pretreatment levels over time

1% to 10%: Hepatic: Increased serum transaminases (≤4%)

<1%, postmarketing, and/or case reports: Edema, erythema, hepatic injury, hepatitis, intestinal obstruction, jaundice, pneumatosis cystoides intestinalis, skin rash, thrombocytopenia, urticaria

Mechanism of Action Competitive inhibitor of pancreatic α-amylase and intestinal brush border α-glucosidases, resulting in delayed hydrolysis of ingested complex carbohydrates and disaccharides and absorption of glucose; dose-dependent reduction in postprandial serum insulin and glucose peaks; inhibits the metabolism of sucrose to glucose and fructose

Pharmacodynamics/Kinetics

Half-life Elimination ~2 hours

Time to Peak Active drug: ~1 hour

Pregnancy Risk Factor B

Pregnancy Considerations

Information related to the use of acarbose in pregnancy is limited (Bertini 2005; Narayanan 2016). Less than 2% of an oral dose of acarbose is absorbed systemically, which should limit fetal exposure.

Poorly controlled diabetes during pregnancy can be associated with an increased risk of adverse maternal and fetal outcomes, including diabetic ketoacidosis, preeclampsia, spontaneous abortion, preterm delivery, delivery complications, major birth defects, stillbirth, and macrosomia (ACOG 201 2018). To prevent adverse outcomes, prior to conception and throughout pregnancy, maternal blood glucose and HbA_{1c} should be kept as close to target goals as possible but without causing significant hypoglycemia (ADA 2020; Blumer 2013).

Agents other than acarbose are currently recommended to treat diabetes mellitus in pregnancy (ADA 2020).

- **A-Caro-25 [OTC]** *see* Beta-Carotene *on page* 233
- **Accolate** *see* Zafirlukast *on page* 1565
- **Accrufer** *see* Ferric Maltol *on page* 663
- **AccuNeb** *see* Albuterol *on page* 90
- **Accupril** *see* Quinapril *on page* 1298
- **Accutane** *see* ISOtretinoin (Systemic) *on page* 846

Acebutolol (a se BYOO toe lole)

Related Information

Cardiovascular Diseases *on page* 1654

Brand Names: US Sectral [DSC]

Brand Names: Canada APO-Acebutolol, MYLAN-Acebutolol [DSC]; SANDOZ Acebutolol [DSC]; Sectral 200 [DSC]; Sectral [DSC]; TEVA-Acebutolol

Pharmacologic Category Antiarrhythmic Agent, Class II; Antihypertensive; Beta-Blocker With Intrinsic Sympathomimetic Activity

Use

Hypertension: Management of hypertension. **Note:** Beta-blockers are **not** recommended as first-line therapy (ACC/AHA [Whelton 2017]).

Ventricular premature beats: Management of ventricular premature beats

Local Anesthetic/Vasoconstrictor Precautions No information available to require special precautions. Local anesthetic with vasoconstrictor can be safely used in patients medicated with acebutolol.

Effects on Dental Treatment Acebutolol is a cardioselective beta-blocker. Local anesthetic with vasoconstrictor can be safely used in patients medicated with acebutolol. Nonselective beta-blockers (ie, propranolol, nadolol) enhance the pressor response to epinephrine, or levonordefrin resulting in hypertension and bradycardia; this has not been reported for acebutolol. Many nonsteroidal anti-inflammatory drugs, such as ibuprofen and indomethacin, can reduce the hypotensive effect of beta-blockers after 3 or more weeks of therapy with the NSAID. Short-term NSAID use (ie, 3 days) requires no special precautions in patients taking beta-blockers.

Effects on Bleeding No information available to require special precautions

Adverse Reactions

>10%: Central nervous system: Fatigue (11%)

1% to 10%:

Cardiovascular: Chest pain (2%), edema (2%), bradycardia (≤2%), cardiac failure (≤2%), hypotension (≤2%)

Central nervous system: Dizziness (6%), headache (6%), insomnia (3%), abnormal dreams (2%), depression (2%), anxiety (≤2%), hyperesthesia (≤2%), hypoesthesia (≤2%)

Dermatologic: Skin rash (2%), pruritus (≤2%)

Gastrointestinal: Constipation (4%), diarrhea (4%), dyspepsia (4%), nausea (4%), flatulence (3%), abdominal pain (≤2%), vomiting (≤2%)

Genitourinary: Urinary frequency (3%), dysuria (≤2%), impotence (≤2%), nocturia (≤2%)

Hepatic: Hepatic abnormality (≤2%)

Neuromuscular & skeletal: Myalgia (2%), arthralgia (≤2%), back pain (≤2%)

Ophthalmic: Visual disturbance (2%), conjunctivitis (≤2%), dry eye syndrome (≤2%), eye pain (≤2%)

Respiratory: Dyspnea (4%), rhinitis (2%), cough (1%), pharyngitis (≤2%), wheezing (≤2%)

<1%, postmarketing, and/or case reports: Increased ANA titer, systemic lupus erythematosus

Mechanism of Action Competitively blocks $beta_1$-adrenergic receptors with little or no effect on $beta_2$-receptors except at high doses; exhibits membrane stabilizing and intrinsic sympathomimetic activity

Pharmacodynamics/Kinetics

Onset of Action 1 to 2 hours

Duration of Action 12 to 24 hours

Half-life Elimination Parent drug: 3 to 4 hours; Metabolite: 8 to 13 hours

Time to Peak 2 to 4 hours

Pregnancy Risk Factor B

Pregnancy Considerations

Acebutolol and diacetolol (active metabolite) cross the placenta.

Decreases in birth weight, blood pressure, and heart rate have been observed in neonates following maternal use of acebutolol during pregnancy. If maternal use of a beta-blocker is needed, fetal growth should be monitored during pregnancy and the newborn should be monitored for 48 hours after delivery for bradycardia, hypoglycemia, and respiratory depression (ESC [Regitz-Zagrosek 2018]).

Chronic maternal hypertension is also associated with adverse events in the fetus/infant. Chronic maternal hypertension may increase the risk of birth defects, low birth weight, premature delivery, stillbirth, and neonatal death. Actual fetal/neonatal risks may be related to duration and severity of maternal hypertension. Untreated chronic hypertension may also increase the risks of adverse maternal outcomes, including gestational diabetes, preeclampsia, delivery complications, stroke and myocardial infarction (ACOG 203 2019).

The plasma elimination half-life of acebutolol is longer in pregnant women at term (Bianchetti 1981a; Boutroy 1982). When treatment of chronic hypertension in pregnancy is indicated, agents other than acebutolol are preferred (ACOG 203 2019; ESC [Regitz-Zagrosek 2018]; Magee 2014). Females with preexisting hypertension may continue their medication during pregnancy unless contraindications exist (ESC [Regitz-Zagrosek 2018])

◆ **Acebutolol HCl** *see* Acebutolol *on page 58*

◆ **Acebutolol Hydrochloride** *see* Acebutolol *on page 58*

◆ **Aceon [DSC]** *see* Perindopril *on page 1218*

◆ **Acephen [OTC]** *see* Acetaminophen *on page 59*

Acetaminophen (a seet a MIN oh fen)

Related Information

Oral Pain *on page 1734*

Related Sample Prescriptions

Oral Pain - Sample Prescriptions *on page 30*

Brand Names: US Acephen [OTC]; Aspirin Free Anacin Extra Strength [OTC]; Cetafen Extra [OTC]; Cetafen [OTC]; FeverAll Adult [OTC]; FeverAll Children's [OTC]; FeverAll Infants' [OTC]; FeverAll Junior Strength [OTC]; GoodSense Pain Relief; GoodSense Pain Relief Extra Strength [OTC]; Little Fevers [OTC]; Mapap Arthritis Pain [OTC]; Mapap Children's [OTC]; Mapap Extra Strength [OTC]; Mapap [OTC]; Midol Long Lasting Relief [OTC]; Non-Aspirin Pain Reliever [OTC]; Nortemp Children's [OTC]; Ofirmev; Pain & Fever Children's [OTC]; Pain Eze [OTC]; Pain Relief Extra Strength [OTC]; Pharbetol Extra Strength [OTC]; Pharbetol [OTC]; Q-Pap Children's [OTC] [DSC]; Q-Pap Extra Strength [OTC] [DSC]; Q-Pap Infants' [OTC] [DSC]; Q-Pap [OTC] [DSC]; Silapap Children's [OTC]; Triaminic Children's Fever Reducer Pain Reliever [OTC]; Tylenol 8 HR Arthritis Pain [OTC]; Tylenol 8 HR [OTC] [DSC]; Tylenol Children's [OTC]; Tylenol Extra Strength [OTC]; Tylenol Infants' [OTC]; Tylenol [OTC]; Valorin Extra [OTC]; Valorin [OTC]

Brand Names: Canada Abenol; Apo-Acetaminophen; Atasol; Novo-Gesic; Pediatrix; Tempra; Tylenol

Generic Availability (US) Yes: Excludes extended release products; injectable formulation

Pharmacologic Category Analgesic, Nonopioid

Dental Use Treatment of postoperative pain

Use

Fever: Temporary reduction of fever.

Pain:

Injection: Management of mild to moderate pain in patients ≥2 years of age; management of moderate to severe pain when combined with opioid analgesia in patients ≥2 years.

Oral, Rectal: Temporary relief of minor aches, pains, and headache.

Local Anesthetic/Vasoconstrictor Precautions No information available to require special precautions

Effects on Dental Treatment No significant effects or complications reported (see Dental Health Professional Considerations)

Effects on Bleeding As a single agent, acetaminophen does not appear to affect bleeding or platelet aggregation. Acetaminophen may prolong the INR and increase bleeding in patients taking warfarin (Coumadin). For patients taking warfarin, single acetaminophen doses or acetaminophen therapy of short duration should be safe, but if large (>1.3 g/day) doses are administered for longer than 10 to 14 days, then the INR should be monitored (see Dental Health Professional Considerations).

Adverse Reactions

Oral, Rectal: Frequency not defined:

Dermatologic: Skin rash

Endocrine & metabolic: Decreased serum bicarbonate, decreased serum calcium, decreased serum sodium, hyperchloremia, hyperuricemia, increased serum glucose

Genitourinary: Nephrotoxicity (with chronic overdose)

Hematologic & oncologic: Anemia, leukopenia, neutropenia, pancytopenia

Hepatic: Increased serum alkaline phosphatase, increased serum bilirubin

Hypersensitivity: Hypersensitivity reaction (rare)

Renal: Hyperammonemia, renal disease (analgesic)

IV:

>10%: Gastrointestinal: Nausea (adults: 34%; neonates, infants, children, and adolescents: ≥5%), vomiting (adults: 15%; neonates, infants, children, and adolescents: ≥5%)

1% to 10%:

Cardiovascular: Hypertension (≥1%), hypotension (≥1%), peripheral edema (adults: ≥1%), tachycardia

Central nervous system: Headache (adults: 10%; neonates, infants, children, and adolescents: ≥1%), insomnia (adults: 7%), agitation (neonates, infants, children, and adolescents: ≥1%), anxiety (adults: ≥1%), fatigue (adults: ≥1%), trismus (adults: ≥1%)

Dermatologic: Pruritus (neonates, infants, children, and adolescents: ≥5%), skin rash

Endocrine & metabolic: Hypoalbuminemia (neonates, infants, children, and adolescents: ≥1%), hypokalemia (≥1%), hypomagnesemia (neonates, infants, children, and adolescents: ≥1%), hypophosphatemia (neonates, infants, children, and adolescents: ≥1%), hypervolemia

Gastrointestinal: Constipation (neonates, infants, children, and adolescents: ≥5%), diarrhea (neonates, infants, children, and adolescents: ≥1%), abdominal pain

Genitourinary: Oliguria (neonates, infants, children, and adolescents: ≥1%)

Hematologic & oncologic: Anemia (≥1%)

Hepatic: Increased serum transaminases

Local: Pain at injection site (≥1%)

Neuromuscular & skeletal: Limb pain, muscle spasm (≥1%)
Ophthalmic: Periorbital edema
Respiratory: Abnormal breath sounds (adults: ≥1%), atelectasis (neonates, infants, children, and adolescents: ≥1%), dyspnea (adults: ≥1%), hypoxia, pleural effusion (neonates, infants, children, and adolescents: ≥1%), pulmonary edema (neonates, infants, children, and adolescents: ≥1%), stridor (adults: ≥1%), wheezing (adults: ≥1%)
Miscellaneous: Fever (neonates, infants, children, and adolescents: ≥1%)

All formulations: <1%, postmarketing, and/or case reports: Anaphylaxis, hypersensitivity reaction

Dental Usual Dosage Postoperative pain: Oral, rectal:
Children <12 years: 10 to 15 mg/kg/dose every 4 to 6 hours as needed; do **not** exceed 5 doses (2.6 g) in 24 hours
Adults: 325 to 650 mg every 4 to 6 hours or 1000 mg 3 to 4 times/day; do **not** exceed 4 g/day

Dosing

Adult Note: Safety: Acetaminophen-induced hepatotoxicity, which can be life threatening, has been associated with doses >4 g/day. Although doses up to 4 g/day are generally well tolerated (Dart 2007; Krenzelok 2012; Larson 2007; Temple 2006; Whitcomb 1994), hepatotoxicity has been reported rarely at this dose limit (Amar 2007). Due to this risk, some experts recommend a lower maximum dose of 3 g/day in adults with normal liver function, particularly when used for longer durations (eg, >7 days) for pain (Chou 2019). Heavy alcohol use, malnutrition, fasting, low body weight, advanced age, febrile illness, select liver disease, and use of drugs that interact with acetaminophen metabolism may increase risk of hepatotoxicity; a lower total daily dose (eg, 2 g/day) or avoidance may be preferred (Hamilton 2019b; Hayward 2016; Larson 2007). When calculating total daily dose, confirm that all sources (eg, prescription, OTCs, combinations) are included.

Pain (mild to moderate) and/or fever (monotherapy or as an adjunct):

Oral: 325 to 650 mg every 4 to 6 hours as needed **or** 1 g every 6 hours as needed; maximum dose: 4 g/day (Amar 2007; APS 2016). See **"Note: Safety"** above regarding maximum dose.

OTC labeling (patient-guided therapy): **Note:** Dosage recommendations, including maximum doses, vary among OTC manufacturers.
Immediate release:
Regular strength (325 mg/tablet): 2 tablets (650 mg) every 4 to 6 hours as needed; maximum daily dose: 10 tablets/day (3.25 g/day).
Extra strength (500 mg/tablet): 2 tablets (1 g) every 6 hours as needed; maximum daily dose: 6 tablets/day (3 g/day).
Extended release (650 mg/tablet): 2 tablets (1.3 g) every 8 hours as needed; maximum daily dose: 6 tablets/day (3.9 g/day).

IV:
≥50 kg: 650 mg every 4 hours **or** 1 g every 6 hours; maximum single dose: 1 g/dose; maximum daily dose: 4 g/day.
<50 kg: 12.5 mg/kg every 4 hours **or** 15 mg/kg every 6 hours; maximum single dose: 15 mg/kg/dose (≤750 mg/dose); maximum daily dose: 75 mg/kg/day (≤3.75 g/day). **Note:** Some experts recommend this reduced dosing if used in patients with chronic alcoholism, malnutrition, or dehydration regardless of weight (Mariano 2019).

Rectal: 325 to 650 mg every 4 to 6 hours as needed (Pandharipande 2019); maximum daily dose: 3.9 g/day. **Note:** Absorption is irregular; bioavailability may be reduced by ~10% to 20% relative to oral administration (Bannwarth 2003).

Geriatric

Pain (acute) or fever: Oral, IV: Refer to adult dosing.
Persistent pain (off-label): Adults ≥75 years: Oral:
Initial: 325 to 500 mg every 4 hours **or** 500 to 1,000 mg every 6 hours
Maximum: ≤4,000 mg/day. In older adults with hepatic impairment or history of alcohol abuse being treated for persistent pain, do not exceed a maximum of 2,000 to 3,000 mg/day (AGS 2009)

Renal Impairment: Adult

The renal dosing recommendations are based upon the best available evidence and clinical expertise. Senior Editorial Team: Bruce Mueller, PharmD, FCCP, FASN, FNKF; Jason Roberts, PhD, BPharm (Hons), B App Sc, FSHP, FISAC; Michael Heung, MD, MS.

IV, Oral, Rectal:
Mild to severe impairment: No dosage adjustment likely to be necessary. The manufacturer's labeling for IV acetaminophen states that longer dosing intervals and a reduced total daily dose may be warranted in patients with severe kidney impairment (CrCl ≤30 mL/minute); however, acetaminophen concentrations and half-life are increased but similar to those in patients with normal renal function (Berg 1990; Forrest 1982; Martin 1991; Prescott 1989). Glucuronide and sulfate conjugate metabolites accumulate in renal impairment, but the clinical effects are unknown (Martin 1991).
Hemodialysis, intermittent (thrice weekly): Acetaminophen and its conjugates are readily dialyzable (Øie 1975): No dosage adjustment necessary (Davison 2014; Martin 1993).
Peritoneal dialysis: Not dialyzed (Lee 1996): No dosage adjustment necessary (Davison 2014).
CRRT: Dialyzed (Scoville 2018): No dosage adjustment necessary (expert opinion).
PIRRT (eg, sustained, low-efficiency diafiltration): No dosage adjustment necessary (Böhler 1999, expert opinion).

Hepatic Impairment: Adult

Oral: Use with caution and consider dosage adjustment or avoiding use, depending on degree of hepatic impairment and other patient-specific factors. Although limited data exist, low-dose therapy (maximum: ≤2 to 3 g/day) is usually well tolerated in patients with chronic liver disease or cirrhosis, provided patients are not actively drinking alcohol; however, the presence of other factors increasing the risk of acetaminophen-induced hepatotoxicity (eg, malnutrition, fasting, low body weight, advanced age, febrile illness, concurrent use of drugs that interact with acetaminophen metabolism) must also be taken into consideration (Bosilkovska 2012; Chandok 2010; Dwyer 2014; Hayward 2016; Imani 2014). Some experts would limit the maximum dose to ≤2 g/day in any patient with advanced chronic liver disease or cirrhosis (provided the patient is not actively drinking alcohol) and would avoid use in any patient with severe alcoholic hepatitis or acute liver injury. Avoiding use is also recommended by some experts in patients with advanced chronic liver disease or cirrhosis who are actively drinking alcohol, malnourished, not eating, or receiving a concomitant interacting medication. For short-term or one-time use, a maximum of ≤4 g/day may be considered in lower risk patients with chronic liver disease or early-stage compensated cirrhosis who are **not** actively drinking alcohol (Hamilton 2019b).

IV:

Mild to moderate impairment: There are no dosage adjustments provided in the manufacturer's labeling. Use with caution; a reduced total daily dosage may be warranted.

Severe impairment: Use is contraindicated.

Pediatric Note: Oral liquids are available in multiple concentrations (eg, 160 mg/5 mL, 500 mg/5 mL, 500 mg/15 mL); precautions should be taken to verify and avoid confusion between the different concentrations; dose should be clearly presented as "mg."

Pain (mild to moderate) or fever: Note: All sources of acetaminophen (eg, prescription, OTC, combination products) should be considered when evaluating a patient's maximum daily dose. To lower the risk for hepatotoxicity, limit daily dose to ≤75 mg/kg/**day** (maximum of 5 daily doses), not to exceed 4,000 mg/**day**; while recommended doses are generally considered safe, hepatotoxicity has been reported (rarely) even with doses below recommendations (AAP [Sullivan 2011]; Heard 2014; Lavonas 2010).

Oral:

Weight-directed dosing: Infants, Children, and Adolescents: 10 to 15 mg/kg/dose every 4 to 6 hours as needed (American Pain Society 2008; Kliegman 2011; AAP [Sullivan 2011]); do not exceed 5 doses in 24 hours; maximum daily dose: 75 mg/kg/**day** not to exceed 4,000 mg/**day**.

Fixed dosing:

Oral suspension, chewable tablets: Infants and Children <12 years: Consult specific product formulations for appropriate age groups. See table; use of weight to select dose is preferred; if weight is not available, then use age; doses may be repeated every 4 hours; maximum: 5 doses/day.

Acetaminophen Dosing (Oral)

Weight (preferred)[A]		Age	Dosage (mg)
kg	lbs		
2.7 to 5.3	6 to 11	0 to 3 mo	40
5.4 to 8.1	12 to 17	4 to 11 mo	80
8.2 to 10.8	18 to 23	1 to 2 y	120
10.9 to 16.3	24 to 35	2 to 3 y	160
16.4 to 21.7	36 to 47	4 to 5 y	240
21.8 to 27.2	48 to 59	6 to 8 y	320 to 325
27.3 to 32.6	60 to 71	9 to 10 y	325 to 400
32.7 to 43.2	72 to 95	11 y	480 to 500

[A]Manufacturer's recommendations are based on weight in pounds (OTC labeling); weight in kg listed here is derived from pounds and rounded; kg weight listed also is adjusted to allow for continuous weight ranges in kg. OTC labeling instructs consumer to consult with physician for dosing instructions in infants and children under 2 years of age.

Immediate-release solid dosage formulations: **Note:** Actual OTC dosing recommendations may vary by product and/or manufacturer:

Children 6 to 11 years: 325 mg every 4 to 6 hours; maximum daily dose: 1,625 mg/**day**; **Note:** Do not use more than 5 days unless directed by a physician.

Children ≥12 years and Adolescents:

Regular strength: 650 mg every 4 to 6 hours; maximum daily dose: 3,250 mg/**day** unless directed by a physician; under physician supervision daily doses ≤4,000 mg may be used.

Extra strength: 1,000 mg every 6 hours; maximum daily dose: 3,000 mg/**day** unless directed by a physician; under physician supervision daily doses ≤4,000 mg may be used.

Extended release: Children ≥12 years and Adolescents: 1,300 mg every 8 hours; maximum daily dose: 3,900 mg/**day**.

IV:

Infants and Children <2 years:

Manufacturer's labeling: Fever: 15 mg/kg/dose every 6 hours; maximum daily dose: 60 mg/kg/**day**.

Alternate dosing: Limited data available: Pain and fever: 7.5 to 15 mg/kg/dose every 6 hours; maximum daily dose: 60 mg/kg/**day** (Wilson-Smith 2009).

Children ≥2 years (Shastri 2015; Zuppa 2011):

<50 kg: 15 mg/kg/dose every 6 hours **or** 12.5 mg/kg/dose every 4 hours; maximum single dose: 15 mg/kg up to 750 mg; maximum daily dose: 75 mg/kg/**day** not to exceed 3,750 mg/**day**.

≥50 kg: 15 mg/kg/dose every 6 hours **or** 12.5 mg/kg/dose every 4 hours; maximum single dose: 15 mg/kg up to 1,000 mg; maximum daily dose: 75 mg/kg/**day** not to exceed 4,000 mg/**day**.

Adolescents:

<50 kg: 15 mg/kg/dose every 6 hours or 12.5 mg/kg/dose every 4 hours; maximum single dose: 15 mg/kg up to 750 mg; maximum daily dose: 75 mg/kg/**day** not to exceed 3,750 mg/**day**.

≥50 kg: 1,000 mg every 6 hours **or** 650 mg every 4 hours; maximum single dose: 1,000 mg; maximum daily dose: 4,000 mg/**day**.

Rectal:

Weight-directed dosing: Limited data available: Infants and Children <12 years: 10 to 20 mg/kg/dose every 4 to 6 hours as needed; **do not exceed 5 doses in 24 hours** (Kliegman 2011; Vernon 1979); maximum daily dose: 75 mg/kg/**day**.

Fixed dosing:

Infants 6 to 11 months: 80 mg every 6 hours; maximum daily dose: 320 mg/**day**.

Infants and Children 12 to 36 months: 80 mg every 4 to 6 hours; maximum daily dose: 400 mg/**day**.

Children >3 to 6 years: 120 mg every 4 to 6 hours; maximum daily dose: 600 mg/**day**.

Children >6 up to 12 years: 325 mg every 4 to 6 hours; maximum daily dose: 1,625 mg/**day**.

Children ≥12 years and Adolescents: 650 mg every 4 to 6 hours; maximum daily dose: 3,900 mg/**day**.

Pain; peri-/postoperative management; adjunct to opioid therapy:

IV:

Infants and Children <2 years: Limited data available: 7.5 to 15 mg/kg/dose every 6 hours; maximum daily dose: 60 mg/kg/**day** (Wilson-Smith 2009).

Children ≥2 years (Shastri 2015; Zuppa 2011):

<50 kg: 15 mg/kg/dose every 6 hours **or** 12.5 mg/kg/dose every 4 hours; maximum single dose: 15 mg/kg up to 750 mg; maximum daily dose: 75 mg/kg/**day** not to exceed 3,750 mg/**day**.

≥50 kg: 15 mg/kg/dose every 6 hours **or** 12.5 mg/kg/dose every 4 hours; maximum single dose: 15 mg/kg up to 1,000 mg; maximum daily dose: 75 mg/kg/**day** not to exceed 4,000 mg/**day**.

Adolescents:

<50 kg: 15 mg/kg/dose every 6 hours **or** 12.5 mg/kg/dose every 4 hours; maximum single dose: 15 mg/kg up to 750 mg; maximum daily dose: 75 mg/kg/**day** not to exceed 3,750 mg/**day**.

≥50 kg: 1,000 mg every 6 hours or 650 mg every 4 hours; maximum single dose: 1,000 mg; maximum daily dose: 4,000 mg/**day**.

Rectal: Limited data available: Children and Adolescents:

Loading dose: 40 mg/kg for 1 dose, in most trials, the dose was administered postoperatively (Birmingham 2001; Capici 2008; Hahn 2000; Mireskandari 2011; Prins 2008; Riad 2007; Viitanen 2003); a maximum dose of 1,000 mg was most frequently reported. However, in one trial evaluating 24 older pediatric patients (all patients ≥25 kg; mean age: ~13 years), the data suggested that a dose of 1,000 mg does not produce therapeutic serum concentrations (target for study: >10 mcg/mL) compared to a 40 mg/kg dose (up to ~2,000 mg); the resultant C_{max} was: 7.8 mcg/mL (1,000 mg dose group) vs 15.9 mcg/mL (40 mg/kg dose group). **Note:** Therapeutic serum concentrations for analgesia have not been well-established (Howell 2003).

Maintenance dose: 20 to 25 mg/kg/dose every 6 hours as needed for 2 to 3 days has been suggested if further pain control is needed postoperatively; maximum daily dose: 100 mg/kg/**day**; therapy longer than 5 days has not been evaluated (Birmingham 2001; Hahn 2000; Prins 2008).

Note: In the majority of trials, suppositories were not divided due to unequal distribution of drug within suppository; doses were rounded to the nearest mg amount using 1 or 2 suppositories of available product strengths.

Renal Impairment: Pediatric

IV: Children ≥2 years and Adolescents:

CrCl >30 mL/minute: No dosage adjustment necessary.

CrCl ≤30 mL/minute: Use with caution; consider decreasing daily dose and extending dosing interval.

Oral: Infants, Children, and Adolescents: There are no dosage adjustments provided in the manufacturer's labeling.

Hemodialysis: Readily dialyzable (Øie 1975).

Hepatic Impairment: Pediatric Use with caution. Limited, low-dose therapy is usually well-tolerated in hepatic disease/cirrhosis; however, cases of hepatotoxicity at daily acetaminophen dosages <4,000 mg/day have been reported. Avoid chronic use in hepatic impairment.

Mechanism of Action Although not fully elucidated, the analgesic effects are believed to be due to activation of descending serotonergic inhibitory pathways in the CNS. Interactions with other nociceptive systems may be involved as well (Smith 2009). Antipyresis is produced from inhibition of the hypothalamic heat-regulating center.

Contraindications

Injection: Hypersensitivity to acetaminophen or any component of the formulation; severe hepatic impairment or severe active liver disease

OTC labeling: When used for self-medication, do not use with other drug products containing acetaminophen or if allergic to acetaminophen or any of the inactive ingredients

Warnings/Precautions [Injection: US Boxed Warning]: Acetaminophen has been associated with acute liver failure, at times resulting in liver transplant and death. Hepatotoxicity is usually associated with excessive acetaminophen intake and often involves more than one product that contains acetaminophen. Do not exceed the maximum recommended daily dose (>4 g daily in adults). In addition, chronic daily dosing may also result in liver damage in some patients. Limit acetaminophen dose from all sources (prescription, OTC, combination products) and all routes of administration (IV, oral, rectal) to ≤4 g/day (adults). Use with caution in patients with alcoholic liver disease; consuming ≥3 alcoholic drinks/day may increase the risk of liver damage. Use caution in patients with hepatic impairment or active liver disease; use of IV formulation is contraindicated in patients with severe hepatic impairment or severe active liver disease.

[Injection: US Boxed Warning]: Take care to avoid dosing errors with acetaminophen injection, which could result in accidental overdose and death; ensure that the dose in mg is not confused with mL, dosing in patients <50 kg is based on body weight, infusion pumps are properly programmed, and total daily dose of acetaminophen from all sources does not exceed the maximum daily limits.

Hypersensitivity and anaphylactic reactions have been reported including life-threatening anaphylaxis; discontinue immediately if symptoms occur. Serious and potentially fatal skin reactions, including acute generalized exanthematous pustulosis (AGEP), Stevens-Johnson syndrome (SJS), and toxic epidermal necrolysis (TEN), have occurred rarely with acetaminophen use. Discontinue therapy at the first appearance of skin rash.

Benzyl alcohol and derivatives: Some dosage forms may contain benzyl alcohol and/or sodium benzoate/benzoic acid; benzoic acid (benzoate) is a metabolite of benzyl alcohol; large amounts of benzyl alcohol (≥99 mg/kg/day) have been associated with a potentially fatal toxicity ("gasping syndrome") in neonates; the "gasping syndrome" consists of metabolic acidosis, respiratory distress, gasping respirations, CNS dysfunction (including convulsions, intracranial hemorrhage), hypotension and cardiovascular collapse (AAP ["Inactive" 1997]; CDC, 1982); some data suggests that benzoate displaces bilirubin from protein binding sites (Ahlfors, 2001); avoid or use dosage forms containing benzyl alcohol and/or benzyl alcohol derivative with caution in neonates. See manufacturer's labeling.

Polysorbate 80: Some dosage forms may contain polysorbate 80 (also known as Tweens). Hypersensitivity reactions, usually a delayed reaction, have been reported following exposure to pharmaceutical products containing polysorbate 80 in certain individuals (Isaksson, 2002; Lucente 2000; Shelley, 1995).

Thrombocytopenia, ascites, pulmonary deterioration, and renal and hepatic failure have been reported in premature neonates after receiving parenteral products containing polysorbate 80 (Alade, 1986; CDC, 1984). See manufacturer's labeling. Some products may contain aspartame which is metabolized to phenylalanine and must be avoided (or used with caution) in patients with phenylketonuria.

Propylene glycol: Some dosage forms may contain propylene glycol; large amounts are potentially toxic and have been associated hyperosmolality, lactic acidosis, seizures, and respiratory depression; use caution (AAP ["Inactive" 1997]; Zar, 2007).

When used for self-medication, patients should be instructed to contact health care provider if symptoms get worse or new symptoms appear, redness or swelling is present in the painful area, fever lasts >3 days (all ages), or pain (excluding sore throat) lasts longer than: Children ≥12 years, Adolescents, and Adults: 10 days; Infants and Children <12 years: 5 days. When treating children with sore throat, if sore throat is severe, persists for >2 days, or is followed by fever, rash, headache, nausea, or vomiting, consult health care provider immediately.

Use with caution in patients with chronic malnutrition; use intravenous formulation with caution in patients with severe hypovolemia. Use with caution in patients with known G6PD deficiency.

Warnings: Additional Pediatric Considerations Prophylactic use of acetaminophen to reduce fever and discomfort associated vaccination is not recommended by the Advisory Committee on Immunization Practices (ACIP). Additionally, the ACIP does not recommend prophylactic acetaminophen to reduce risk of febrile seizure in infants and children with or without a history of febrile seizures. Antipyretics have not been shown to prevent febrile seizures (NCIRD/ACIP 2011). One study reported that routine prophylactic administration of acetaminophen to prevent fever prior to vaccination decreased the immune response of some vaccines; in the trial evaluating 459 infants (including 226 who received acetaminophen), antibody geometric mean concentrations (GMCs) for targeted vaccine immune response markers were lower in significantly more infants in the acetaminophen group compared with control. Before the booster dose, children who received prophylactic acetaminophen had lower antibody GMCs for all vaccine serotypes than children in the control group; this effect persisted after boosting even in the absence of additional acetaminophen doses. The clinical significance of this reduction in immune response has not been established (Prymula 2009). Antipyretics may be used to treat fever or discomfort following vaccination (NCIRD/ACIP 2011).

Hepatoxicity has been reported in patients using acetaminophen. In pediatric patients, this is most commonly associated with supratherapeutic dosing, more frequent administration than recommended, and use of multiple acetaminophen-containing products; however, hepatotoxicity has been rarely reported with recommended dosages (AAP [Sullivan 2011]; Heard 2014). All sources of acetaminophen (eg, prescription, OTC, combination) should be considered when evaluating a patient's maximum daily dose. To lower the risk for hepatotoxicity, the maximum daily acetaminophen dose should be limited to ≤75 mg/kg/day (maximum of 5 daily doses), not to exceed 4,000 mg/day (AAP [Sullivan 2011]; Heard 2014; Krenzelok 2012; Lavonas 2010). Acetaminophen avoidance or a lower total daily dose (2,000 to 3,000 mg/day) has been suggested for adults with increased risk for acetaminophen hepatotoxicity (eg, malnutrition, certain liver diseases, use of drugs that interact with acetaminophen metabolism); similar data are unavailable in pediatric patients (Hayward 2016; Larson 2007; Worriax 2007).

Some dosage forms may contain propylene glycol; in neonates, large amounts of propylene glycol delivered orally, intravenously (eg, >3,000 mg/day), or topically have been associated with potentially fatal toxicities which can include metabolic acidosis, seizures, renal failure, and CNS depression; toxicities have also been reported in children and adults including hyperosmolality, lactic acidosis, seizures, and respiratory depression; use caution (AAP 1997; Shehab 2009).

Drug Interactions

Metabolism/Transport Effects **Substrate** of CYP1A2 (minor), CYP2A6 (minor), CYP2C9 (minor), CYP2D6 (minor), CYP2E1 (major), CYP3A4 (minor); **Note:** Assignment of Major/Minor substrate status based on clinically relevant drug interaction potential

Avoid Concomitant Use There are no known interactions where it is recommended to avoid concomitant use.

Increased Effect/Toxicity

Acetaminophen may increase the levels/effects of: Busulfan; Dasatinib; Imatinib; Local Anesthetics; Mipomersen; Phenylephrine (Systemic); Prilocaine; Sodium Nitrite; SORAfenib; Vitamin K Antagonists

The levels/effects of Acetaminophen may be increased by: Alcohol (Ethyl); Dapsone (Topical); Dasatinib; Flucloxacillin; Isoniazid; MetyraPONE; Nitric Oxide; Probenecid; SORAfenib

Decreased Effect

Acetaminophen may decrease the levels/effects of: LamoTRIgine

The levels/effects of Acetaminophen may be decreased by: Barbiturates; CarBAMazepine; Fosphenytoin-Phenytoin; Isoniazid; Lorlatinib

Food Interactions Rate of absorption may be decreased when given with food. Management: Administer without regard to food.

Dietary Considerations Some products may contain phenylalanine and/or sodium.

Pharmacodynamics/Kinetics

Onset of Action

Oral: <1 hour

IV: Analgesia: 5 to 10 minutes; Antipyretic: Within 30 minutes

Peak effect: IV: Analgesic: 1 hour

Duration of Action

IV, Oral: Analgesia: 4 to 6 hours

IV: Antipyretic: ≥6 hours

Half-life Elimination Prolonged following toxic doses

Neonates: 7 hours (range: 4 to 10 hours)

Infants: ~4 hours (range: 1 to 7 hours)

Children: 3 hours (range: 2 to 5 hours)

Adolescents: ~3 hours (range: 2 to 4 hours)

Adults: ~2 hours (range: 2 to 3 hours); may be slightly prolonged in severe renal insufficiency (CrCl <30 mL/minute): 2 to 5.3 hours

Time to Peak Serum: Oral: Immediate release: 10 to 60 minutes (may be delayed in acute overdoses); IV: 15 minutes

Pregnancy Considerations

Acetaminophen crosses the placenta (Naga Rani 1989).

Based on epidemiological data, an increased risk of major congenital malformations has not been observed following maternal use of acetaminophen during pregnancy. Although not considered a major birth defect, an association between maternal acetaminophen use and cryptorchidism (undescended testis) has been observed (Fisher 2016; Jensen 2010; Kristensen 2011; Snijder 2012). The use of acetaminophen in normal doses during pregnancy is not associated with an increased risk of miscarriage or still birth; however, an increase in fetal death or spontaneous abortion may be seen following maternal overdose if treatment is delayed (Li 2003; Rebordosa 2009; Riggs 1989). Prenatal constriction of the ductus arteriosus has been noted in case reports following maternal use during the third trimester (Allegaert 2019); although this association was not confirmed in a large observational study (Dathe 2019), acetaminophen has been evaluated for the treatment of a persistent patent ductus arteriosus in preterm neonates (Terrin 2016). Additional adverse events such as wheezing and asthma in early childhood and adverse neurodevelopmental effects such as ADHD following in utero acetaminophen exposure have been evaluated in multiple studies; outcome information is inconclusive, and a causal association has not been established (Cheelo 2014; Fan 2017; Lourido-Cebreiro 2017; Scialli 2010; SMFM 2017). It should be noted that maternal fever is also associated with adverse fetal outcomes, including neural tube defects, oral clefts, and congenital heart defects. Treatment of maternal fever with an antipyretic may reduce these risks (Drier 2014).

Due to pregnancy-induced physiologic changes, some pharmacokinetic properties of acetaminophen may be altered. Dose adjustments are not recommended (Kulo 2014). Acetaminophen is considered appropriate for the treatment of pain and fever in pregnancy (SMFM 2017). Acetaminophen may be used as part of a multimodal approach to pain relief following cesarean delivery (ACOG 209 2019), for the treatment of acute migraine in pregnant patients (Burch 2019; Hamilton 2019a; Marmura 2015) and is recommended for the treatment of fever in pregnant women diagnosed with influenza (ACOG 753 2018). Acetaminophen is recommended to be used at the lowest effective dose for the shortest duration of time to effectively treat the mother and protect the health of the fetus (Kilcoyne 2017).

Breastfeeding Considerations Acetaminophen is present in breast milk (Notarianni 1987).

The relative infant dose (RID) of acetaminophen is 3.98% when calculated using the highest breast milk concentration located and compared to an infant therapeutic dose of 60 mg/kg/day.

In general, breastfeeding is considered acceptable when the RID is <10% (Anderson 2016; Ito 2000).

The RID of acetaminophen was calculated using a milk concentration of 15.9 mcg/mL providing an estimated daily infant dose via breast milk of 2.385 mg/kg/day. This milk concentration was obtained following a single maternal dose of oral acetaminophen 1,000 mg given to 11 women, 3 to 9 days' postpartum (Hurden 1980).

Following a single oral maternal dose of acetaminophen 650 mg, the half-life of acetaminophen is 1.35 to 3.5 hours in breast milk (Berlin 1980). Acetaminophen can be detected in the urine of breastfeeding infants (Notarianni 1987). Except for a single case report of a rash (Matheson 1985), adverse reactions have generally not been observed in breastfeeding infants (Ito 1993).

Nonopioid analgesics are preferred for breastfeeding females who require pain control peripartum or for surgery outside of the postpartum period (ABM [Martin 2018]; ABM [Reece-Stremtan 2017]; Sachs 2013). Acetaminophen is one of the preferred non-narcotic agents (Sachs 2013) and is considered compatible with breastfeeding when used in usual recommended doses (WHO 2002).

Dosage Forms: US

Caplet, oral: 500 mg
- Cetafen Extra [OTC]: 500 mg
- Mapap Extra Strength [OTC]: 500 mg
- Pain Eze [OTC]: 650 mg
- Tylenol [OTC]: 325 mg
- Tylenol Extra Strength [OTC]: 500 mg

Caplet, extended release, oral:
- Mapap Arthritis Pain [OTC]: 650 mg
- Midol Long Lasting Relief [OTC]: 650 mg
- Tylenol 8 HR Arthritis Pain [OTC]: 650 mg

Capsule, oral:
- Mapap Extra Strength [OTC]: 500 mg
- Tylenol [OTC]: 325 mg
- Tylenol Extra Strength [OTC]: 500 mg

Injection, solution [preservative free]:
- Ofirmev: 10 mg/mL (100 mL)

Liquid, oral: 160 mg/5 mL (120 mL, 473 mL)
- Silapap Children's [OTC]: 160 mg/5 mL (118 mL, 237 mL, 473 mL)

Solution, oral: 160 mg/5 mL (5 mL, 10 mL, 20 mL, 118 mL, 473 mL); 325 mg/10.15 mL (10.15 mL); 650 mg/20.3 mL (20.3 mL)

Suppository, rectal: 120 mg (12s, 50s, 100s); 325 mg (12s); 650 mg (12s, 50s, 100s)
- Acephen [OTC]: 120 mg (12s, 50s, 100s); 325 mg (6s, 12s, 50s, 100s); 650 mg (12s, 50s, 100s)
- Feverall [OTC]: 80 mg (6s, 50s); 120 mg (6s, 50s); 325 mg (6s, 50s); 650 mg (50s)

Suspension, oral: 160 mg/5 mL (5 mL, 10 mL, 10.15 mL, 20 mL, 20.3 mL)
- Mapap Children's [OTC]: 160 mg/5 mL (118 mL)
- Nortemp Children's [OTC]: 160 mg/5 mL (118 mL)
- Pain & Fever Children's [OTC]: 160 mg/5 mL (60 mL)
- Tylenol Children's [OTC]: 160 mg/5 mL (60 mL, 120 mL)
- Tylenol Infants' [OTC]: 160 mg/5 mL (60 mL)

Syrup, oral:
- Triaminic Children's Fever Reducer Pain Reliever [OTC]: 160 mg/5 mL (118 mL)

Tablet, oral: 325 mg, 500 mg
- Aspirin Free Anacin Extra Strength [OTC]: 500 mg
- Cetafen [OTC]: 325 mg
- GoodSense Pain Relief [OTC]: 325 mg
- GoodSense Pain Relief Extra Strength [OTC]: 500 mg
- Mapap [OTC]: 325 mg
- Mapap Extra Strength [OTC]: 500 mg
- Non-Aspirin Pain Reliever [OTC]: 325 mg
- Pain Relief Extra Strength [OTC]: 500 mg
- Pharbetol [OTC]: 325 mg
- Pharbetol Extra Strength [OTC]: 500 mg
- Tylenol [OTC]: 325 mg
- Tylenol Extra Strength [OTC]: 500 mg
- Valorin [OTC]: 325 mg
- Valorin Extra [OTC]: 500 mg

Tablet, chewable, oral: 80 mg, 160 mg
Mapap Children's [OTC]: 80 mg
Tablet, dispersible, oral: 80 mg, 160 mg
Mapap Children's [OTC]: 80 mg
Tablet, extended release, oral: 650 mg

Dental Health Professional Considerations

Although the ***OTC product labeling*** for acetaminophen products state to limit the maximum dose to 3,000 mg daily (for extra strength) or 3,250 mg (for regular strength) (see this site for details: http://www.-tylenolprofessional.com/products-and-dosages.html), it is still appropriate for patients to take up to 4,000 mg daily "under the direction of a health care provider" (http://www.tylenolprofessional.com/dosage.html).

The acetaminophen component requires use with caution in patients who use alcohol, with preexisting liver disease, and those receiving more than one source of acetaminophen-containing medication.

Hepatotoxicity caused by acetaminophen is potentiated by chronic alcohol consumption. People who are taking acetaminophen, even at therapeutic doses, and consume alcohol are at risk of developing hepatotoxicity.

Acetaminophen may increase the levels and enhance the anticoagulant effects of vitamin K antagonists acenocoumarol and warfarin (Coumadin). Studies have reported that acetaminophen has increased the INR in warfarin-treated patients with daily acetaminophen doses as low as 2 g, particularly when taking acetaminophen for >1 week (Gebauer 2003; Hylek 1998). In addition, case reports of bleeding as a result of increased INR have been published (Bagheri 1999). There is no known mechanism of the interaction; furthermore, some studies have failed to demonstrate this interaction (Gadisseur 2003; Kwan 1995; van den Bemt 2002). In terms of risk, the data suggest that acetaminophen and warfarin could interact in some clinically significant manner but that the benefits of concomitant use of acetaminophen for pain control in dental patients taking warfarin usually outweigh the risks. An appropriate monitoring plan should be in place to identify potential negative effects and dosage adjustments may be necessary in a minority of patients. The interaction may be more likely to occur with daily acetaminophen doses of >1.3 g for >1 week. In a review of seven random controlled trials comparing acetaminophen versus placebo in warfarin-treated patients (Caldeira 2015), acetaminophen was associated with a mean 0.62 INR increase compared to placebo. Specifically, there was 0.17 mean increase of the INR per each daily gram of acetaminophen. Statistically, this was significant; however, the clinical relevance was questionable since the reviewed studies did not report any major bleeding event.

There are no reports of acetaminophen interacting with antiplatelet drugs such as aspirin, clopidogrel (Plavix), ticagrelor (Brilinta), or prasugrel (Effient). Also, there are no reports of acetaminophen in combination with hydrocodone, codeine, or oxycodone interacting with warfarin (Coumadin).

◆ **Acetaminophen and Benzhydrocodone** *see* Benzhydrocodone and Acetaminophen *on page 228*

Acetaminophen and Codeine

(a seet a MIN oh fen & KOE deen)

Related Information

Acetaminophen *on page 59*
Codeine *on page 404*

Related Sample Prescriptions

Oral Pain - Sample Prescriptions *on page 30*

Brand Names: US Capital/Codeine [DSC]; Tylenol with Codeine #3 [DSC]; Tylenol with Codeine #4 [DSC]

Brand Names: Canada Acet Codeine 30 [DSC]; Acet Codeine 60 [DSC]; PMS-Acetaminophen/Codeine; Procet-30 [DSC]; TEVA-Emtec-30; TEVA-Lenoltec No 4; Triatec-30; Tylenol #4

Generic Availability (US) May be product dependent

Pharmacologic Category Analgesic Combination (Opioid); Analgesic, Opioid

Dental Use Treatment of postoperative pain

Use

Pain management: Management of mild to moderate pain where treatment with an opioid is appropriate and for which alternative treatments are inadequate.

Limitations of use: Reserve for use in patients for whom alternative treatment options (eg, nonopioid analgesics) are ineffective, not tolerated, or would be otherwise inadequate.

Local Anesthetic/Vasoconstrictor Precautions No information available to require special precautions

Effects on Dental Treatment No significant effects or complications reported (see Dental Health Professional Considerations)

Effects on Bleeding As a single agent, acetaminophen does not appear to affect bleeding or platelet aggregation. Acetaminophen may prolong the INR and increase bleeding in patients taking warfarin (Coumadin). For patients taking warfarin, single acetaminophen doses or acetaminophen therapy of short duration should be safe, but if large (>1.3 g/day) doses are administered for longer than 10-14 days, then the INR should be monitored (see Dental Health Professional Considerations).

Adverse Reactions Also see individual agents.

Frequency not defined:

Central nervous system: Dizziness, drowsiness, dysphoria, euphoria, sedation, serotonin syndrome
Dermatologic: Pruritus, skin rash
Endocrine & metabolic: Adrenocortical insufficiency
Gastrointestinal: Abdominal pain, constipation, nausea, vomiting
Hematologic & oncologic: Agranulocytosis, thrombocytopenia
Hypersensitivity: Hypersensitivity reaction
Respiratory: Dyspnea

<1%, postmarketing, and/or case reports: Hypogonadism (Brennan 2013; Debono 2011), respiratory depression

Dental Usual Dosage Postoperative pain: Adults: Analgesic: Based on codeine (30-60 mg/dose) every 4-6 hours (maximum: 4000 mg/24 hours based on acetaminophen component)

Dosing

Adult Note: Adult doses ≥60 mg codeine fail to give commensurate relief of pain but merely prolong analgesia and are associated with an appreciably increased incidence of side effects.

Pain management: Oral:

Solution or suspension:

Acetaminophen 120 mg/codeine 12 mg per 5 mL: 15 mL every 4 hours as needed; adjust dose according to severity of pain and response of patient (maximum: acetaminophen 4,000 mg per 24 hours).

Acetaminophen 160 mg/codeine 8 mg per 5 mL [Canadian product]: 10 to 20 mL every 4 hours as needed; adjust dose according to severity of pain and response of patient (maximum: 100 mL per 24 hours)

Tablets: Acetaminophen (300 to 1,000 mg/dose)/codeine (15 to 60 mg/dose) every 4 hours as needed; adjust dose according to severity of pain and response of patient (maximum: acetaminophen 4,000 mg/codeine 360 mg per 24 hours).

Discontinuation of therapy: When discontinuing chronic opioid therapy, the dose should be gradually tapered down. An optimal universal tapering schedule for all patients has not been established (CDC [Dowell 2016]). Proposed schedules range from slow (eg, 10% reductions per week) to rapid (eg, 25% to 50% reduction every few days) (CDC 2015). Tapering schedules should be individualized to minimize opioid withdrawal while considering patient-specific goals and concerns as well as the pharmacokinetics of the opioid being tapered. An even slower taper may be appropriate in patients who have been receiving opioids for a long duration (eg, years), particularly in the final stage of tapering, whereas more rapid tapers may be appropriate in patients experiencing severe adverse events (CDC [Dowell 2016]). Monitor carefully for signs/symptoms of withdrawal. If the patient displays withdrawal symptoms, consider slowing the taper schedule; alterations may include increasing the interval between dose reductions, decreasing amount of daily dose reduction, pausing the taper and restarting when the patient is ready, and/or coadministration of an $alpha_2$ agonist (eg, clonidine) to blunt withdrawal symptoms (Berna 2015; CDC [Dowell 2016]). Continue to offer nonopioid analgesics as needed for pain management during the taper; consider nonopioid adjunctive treatments for withdrawal symptoms (eg, GI complaints, muscle spasm) as needed (Berna 2015; Sevarino 2018).

Geriatric Refer to adult dosing. Use with caution and consider initiation at the low end of the dosing range; titrate slowly.

Renal Impairment: Adult There are no specific dosage adjustments provided in the manufacturer's labeling; use with caution. Also see individual agents.

Hepatic Impairment: Adult There are no specific dosage adjustments provided in the manufacturer's labeling; use with caution. Also see individual agents.

Pediatric Note: Doses should be titrated to appropriate analgesic effect. All sources of acetaminophen (eg, prescription, OTC, combination products) should be considered when evaluating a patient's maximum daily dose. To lower the risk for hepatotoxicity, limit daily dose to ≤75 mg/kg/**day** (maximum of 5 daily doses), not to exceed 4,000 mg/**day**; while recommended doses are generally considered safe, hepatotoxicity has been reported (rarely) even with doses below recommendations (AAP [Sullivan 2011]; Heard 2014; Lavonas 2010).

Pain management, mild to moderate:

Note: Use is contraindicated in pediatric patients <12 years of age and for postoperative management in pediatric patients 12 to 18 years of age who have undergone tonsillectomy and/or adenoidectomy. Avoid codeine use in all pediatric patient populations in which it is contraindicated and in pediatric patients 12 to 18 years of age who have other risk factors that increase risk for respiratory depression associated with codeine (eg, conditions associated with hypoventilation like postoperative status, obstructive sleep apnea, obesity, severe pulmonary disease, neuromuscular disease, use of other medications known to depress respiratory drive); in rare cases in which codeine-containing product is the only option, consider genotype testing prior to use; use extra precaution; monitor closely for adverse effects. Codeine has been associated with reports of life-threatening or fatal respiratory depression in children and adolescents; multifactorial causes have been identified; of primary concern are unrecognized ultrarapid metabolizers of CYP2D6 who may have extensive conversion of codeine (prodrug) to morphine and thus increased opioid-mediated effects (AAP [Tobias 2016]; Dancel 2017; Gammal 2016; Goldschneider 2017; Poonai 2015).

Children and Adolescents: Limited data available in ages <12 years and in postoperative tonsillectomy and/or adenoidectomy patients: Not a preferred agent; use only when determined codeine is only option

Weight-directed dosing: Dosage for individual components:

Codeine: Oral: 0.5 to 1 mg/kg/dose every 4 to 6 hours; maximum dose: 60 mg/dose (APS 2016). **Note:** Do not use for postoperative tonsillectomy and/or adenoidectomy pain management

Acetaminophen: Oral: 10 to 15 mg/kg/dose every 4 to 6 hours; do **not** exceed 5 doses in 24 hours; maximum daily dose: 75 mg/kg/**day** not to exceed 4,000 mg/**day**

Acetaminophen 160 mg/codeine 8 mg per 5 mL [Canadian product]: Children ≥12 years and Adolescents: Oral: 10 to 20 mL every 4 to 6 hours as needed; adjust dose according to severity of pain and response of patient; maximum daily dose: 100 mL/24 hours

Renal Impairment: Pediatric Children and Adolescents: There are no specific dosage adjustments provided in the manufacturer's labeling; however, clearance may be reduced; active metabolites may accumulate. Use with caution; initiate at lower doses or longer dosing intervals followed by careful titration. See individual monographs for specific adjustments.

Hepatic Impairment: Pediatric Children and Adolescents: There are no dosage adjustments provided in the manufacturer's labeling; however, product contains acetaminophen; use with caution. Cases of hepatotoxicity at daily acetaminophen dosages <4 g/day have been reported. See individual monographs.

Mechanism of Action

Acetaminophen: Although not fully elucidated, the analgesic effects are believed to be due to activation of descending serotonergic inhibitory pathways in the CNS. Interactions with other nociceptive systems may be involved as well (Smith 2009). Antipyresis is produced from inhibition of the hypothalamic heat-regulating center.

Codeine: Binds to opiate receptors in the CNS, causing inhibition of ascending pain pathways, altering the perception of and response to pain; causes cough suppression by direct central action in the medulla; produces generalized CNS depression.

Contraindications

Hypersensitivity (eg, anaphylaxis) to acetaminophen, codeine, or any component of the formulation; pediatric patients <12 years of age; postoperative management in pediatric patients <18 years of age who have undergone tonsillectomy and/or adenoidectomy; significant respiratory depression; acute or severe bronchial asthma in an unmonitored setting or in the absence of resuscitative equipment; GI obstruction, including paralytic ileus (known or suspected); concurrent use with or within 14 days following monoamine oxidase inhibitors (MAOIs) therapy.

Canadian labeling: Additional contraindications (not in US labeling): Hypersensitivity to other opioid analgesics; mechanical GI obstruction (eg, bowel obstruction, strictures) or any disease/condition that affects bowel transit (known or suspected); suspected surgical abdomen (eg, acute appendicitis, pancreatitis); mild pain that can be managed with other pain medications; severe hepatic or renal impairment; acute or severe bronchial asthma, chronic obstructive airway disease; status asthmaticus; hypercapnia; cor pulmonale; acute alcoholism; delirium tremens; seizure disorder; severe CNS depression; increased cerebrospinal or intracranial pressure; head injury; pregnancy; use during labor and delivery; CYP2D6 ultra-rapid metabolizers. Some products may contraindicate use in patients <18 years (refer to specific product labeling).

Documentation of allergenic cross-reactivity for opioids is limited. However, because of similarities in chemical structure and/or pharmacologic actions, the possibility of cross-sensitivity cannot be ruled out with certainty.

Warnings/Precautions **[US Boxed Warning]: Life-threatening respiratory depression and death have occurred in children who received codeine. Most of the reported cases occurred following tonsillectomy and/or adenoidectomy, and many of the children had evidence of being ultrarapid metabolizers of codeine due to a CYP2D6 polymorphism. Acetaminophen/codeine is contraindicated in pediatric patients <12 years of age and pediatric patients <18 years of age following tonsillectomy and/or adenoidectomy. Avoid the use of acetaminophen/codeine in pediatric patients 12 to 18 years of age who have other risk factors that may increase their sensitivity to the respiratory depressant effects of codeine.** Risk factors include conditions associated with hypoventilation, such as postoperative status, obstructive sleep apnea, obesity, severe pulmonary disease, neuromuscular disease, and concomitant use of other medications that cause respiratory depression. Deaths have also occurred in breastfeeding infants after being exposed to high concentrations of morphine because the mothers were ultrarapid metabolizers. **[US Boxed Warning]: Prolonged use during pregnancy can cause neonatal opioid withdrawal syndrome, which may be life-threatening if not recognized and treated according to protocols developed by neonatology experts. If opioid use is required for a prolonged period in a pregnant woman, advise the patient of the risk of neonatal opioid withdrawal syndrome and ensure that appropriate treatment will be available.** Signs and symptoms include irritability, hyperactivity and abnormal sleep pattern, high pitched cry, tremor, vomiting, diarrhea, and failure to gain weight. Onset, duration, and severity depend on the drug used, duration of use, maternal dose, and rate of drug elimination by the newborn.

Avoid use of codeine in patients with impaired consciousness or coma as these patients are susceptible to intracranial effects of CO_2 retention. Some products may contain metabisulfite, which may cause allergic reactions. Use caution in patients with ≥2 copies of the variant CYP2D6*2 allele; may have extensive conversion to morphine and thus increased opioid-mediated effects. Avoid the use of codeine in these patients; consider alternative analgesics such as morphine or a nonopioid agent (Crews 2012). The occurrence of this phenotype is seen in 0.5% to 1% of Chinese and Japanese, 0.5% to 1% of Hispanics, 1% to 10% of Caucasians, 3% of African-Americans, and 16% to 28% of North Africans, Ethiopians, and Arabs.

Serious and potentially fatal skin reactions, including acute generalized exanthematous pustulosis, Stevens-Johnson syndrome, and toxic epidermal necrolysis have occurred rarely with acetaminophen use. Discontinue therapy at the first appearance of skin rash or any other sign of hypersensitivity. Limit acetaminophen dose from all sources (prescription, OTC, combination products) to <4 g/day in adults. Do not use acetaminophen/codeine concomitantly with other acetaminophen-containing products.

[US Boxed Warning]: Acetaminophen has been associated with cases of acute liver failure, at times resulting in liver transplant and death. Most of the cases of liver injury are associated with the use of acetaminophen at dosages that exceed 4 g/day, and often involve more than one acetaminophen-containing product. Risk is increased with alcohol use, preexisting liver disease, and intake of more than one source of acetaminophen-containing medications. Chronic daily dosing in adults has also resulted in liver damage in some patients. Hypersensitivity and anaphylactic reactions have been reported with acetaminophen use; discontinue immediately if symptoms of allergic or hypersensitivity reactions occur. Use with caution in patients with hypersensitivity reactions to other phenanthrene-derivative opioid agonists (hydrocodone, hydromorphone, levorphanol, oxycodone, oxymorphone). Use acetaminophen with caution in patients with known G6PD deficiency. Use with caution in patients with alcoholic liver disease; consuming ≥3 alcoholic drinks/day may increase the risk of liver damage.

May cause CNS depression, which may impair physical or mental abilities; patients must be cautioned about performing tasks that require mental alertness (eg, operating machinery or driving). **[US Boxed Warning]: Use exposes patients and other users to the risks of opioid addiction, abuse, and misuse, which can lead to overdose and death. Assess each patient's risk prior to prescribing acetaminophen/codeine, and monitor all patients regularly for the development of these behaviors or conditions.** Use with caution in patients with a history of drug abuse or acute alcoholism; potential for drug dependency exists. Other factors associated with increased risk for misuse include younger age, concomitant depression (major), and psychotropic medication use. Consider offering naloxone prescriptions in patients with factors associated with an increased risk for overdose, such as history of overdose or substance use disorder, higher opioid dosages (≥50 morphine milligram equivalents

[MME]/day orally), and concomitant benzodiazepine use (Dowell [CDC 2016]). Abuse or misuse of ER tablets by crushing, chewing, snorting, or injecting the dissolved product will result in the uncontrolled delivery of the oxycodone and can result in overdose and death.

Chronic pain (outside of end-of-life or palliative care, active cancer treatment, sickle cell disease, or medication-assisted treatment for opioid use disorder) in outpatient setting in adults: Opioids should **not** be used as first-line therapy for chronic pain management (pain >3-month duration or beyond time of normal tissue healing) due to limited short-term benefits, undetermined long-term benefits, and association with serious risks (eg, overdose, myocardial infarction [MI], auto accidents, risk of developing opioid use disorder). Preferred management includes nonpharmacologic therapy and nonopioid therapy (eg, NSAIDs, acetaminophen, certain anticonvulsants and antidepressants). If opioid therapy is initiated, it should be combined with nonpharmacologic and nonopioid therapy, as appropriate. Prior to initiation, known risks of opioid therapy should be discussed and realistic treatment goals for pain/function should be established, including consideration for discontinuation if benefits do not outweigh risks. Therapy should be continued only if clinically meaningful improvement in pain/function outweighs risks. Therapy should be initiated at the lowest effective dosage using immediate-release opioids (instead of extended-release/long-acting opioids). Risk associated with use increases with higher opioid dosages. Risks and benefits should be re-evaluated when increasing dosage to ≥50 MME/day orally; dosages ≥90 MME/day orally should be avoided unless carefully justified (Dowell [CDC 2016]).

Abrupt discontinuation in patients who are physically dependent on opioids has been associated with serious withdrawal symptoms, uncontrolled pain, attempts to find other opioids (including illicit), and suicide. Use a collaborative, patient-specific taper schedule that minimizes the risk of withdrawal, considering factors such as current opioid dose, duration of use, type of pain, and physical and psychological factors. Monitor pain control, withdrawal symptoms, mood changes, suicidal ideation, and for use of other substances; provide care as needed. Concurrent use of mixed agonist/antagonist (eg, pentazocine, nalbuphine, butorphanol) or partial agonist (eg, buprenorphine) analgesics may also precipitate withdrawal symptoms and/or reduced analgesic efficacy in patients following prolonged therapy with mu opioid agonists. Potentially significant drug-drug interactions may exist, requiring dose or frequency adjustment, additional monitoring, and/or selection of alternative therapy. **[US Boxed Warning]: Concomitant use of opioids with benzodiazepines or other CNS depressants, including alcohol, may result in profound sedation, respiratory depression, coma, and death. Reserve concomitant prescribing of acetaminophen/codeine and benzodiazepines or other CNS depressants for use in patients for whom alternative treatment options are inadequate. Limit dosages and durations to the minimum required. Follow patients for signs and symptoms of respiratory depression and sedation. [US Boxed Warning]: The effects of concomitant use or discontinuation of CYP-450 3A4 inducers, 3A4 inhibitors, or 2D6 inhibitors with codeine are complex. Use of CYP-450 3A4 inducers, 3A4 inhibitors, or 2D6 inhibitors with acetaminophen/codeine requires careful consideration of the effects on the parent drug, codeine, and the active metabolite, morphine.**

Use with caution in cachectic or debilitated patients, or in morbidly obese patients; adrenal insufficiency (including Addison disease); biliary tract impairment (including acute pancreatitis); renal or severe hepatic impairment; toxic psychosis; delirium tremens; thyroid disorders; prostatic hyperplasia and/or urethral stricture; seizure disorder; head injury, intracranial lesions or increased intracranial pressure. May cause or aggravate constipation; chronic use may result in obstructive bowel disease, particularly in those with underlying intestinal motility disorders. May also be problematic in patients with unstable angina and patients post-MI. Consider preventive measures (eg, stool softener, increased fiber) to reduce the potential for constipation. **[US Boxed Warning]: Serious, life-threatening, or fatal respiratory depression may occur with use. Monitor for respiratory depression, especially during initiation of therapy or following a dose increase.** Carbon dioxide retention from opioid-induced respiratory depression can exacerbate the sedating effects of opioids. Use with caution and monitor for respiratory depression in patients with significant chronic obstructive pulmonary disease or cor pulmonale, and those with a substantially decreased respiratory reserve, hypoxia, hypercapnia, or preexisting respiratory depression, particularly when initiating and titrating therapy; critical respiratory depression may occur, even at therapeutic dosages. Consider the use of alternative nonopioid analgesics in these patients. May obscure diagnosis or clinical course of patients with acute abdominal conditions. Use with caution in the elderly; may be more sensitive to adverse effects, such as respiratory depression. Use opioids for chronic pain with caution in this age group; monitor closely due to an increased potential for risks, including certain risks such as falls/fracture, cognitive impairment, and constipation. Clearance may also be reduced in older adults (with or without renal impairment) resulting in a narrow therapeutic window and increasing the risk for respiratory depression or overdose (Dowell [CDC 2016]).

[US Boxed Warning]: Accidental ingestion of acetaminophen/codeine, especially by children, can result in a fatal overdose of codeine. [US Boxed Warning]: Ensure accuracy when prescribing, dispensing, and administering acetaminophen/codeine oral solution or suspension. Dosing errors due to confusion between mg and mL and other codeine containing oral products of different concentrations can result in accidental overdose and death. May cause severe hypotension (including orthostatic hypotension and syncope); use with caution in patients with hypovolemia, cardiovascular disease (including acute MI), or drugs that may exaggerate hypotensive effects (including phenothiazines or general anesthetics). Monitor for symptoms of hypotension following initiation or dose titration. Avoid use in patients with circulatory shock. Use opioids with caution for chronic pain in patients with mental health conditions (eg, depression, anxiety disorders, post-traumatic stress disorder) due to increased risk for opioid use disorder and overdose; more frequent monitoring is recommended (Dowell [CDC 2016]). Opioid use increases the risk for sleep-related disorders (eg, central sleep apnea [CSA], hypoxemia) in a dose-dependent fashion. Use with caution for chronic pain and titrate dosage cautiously in patients with risk factors for sleep-disordered breathing (eg, heart failure, obesity). Consider dose reduction in patients presenting with CSA. Avoid opioids in patients with moderate to severe sleep-disordered breathing (Dowell [CDC 2016]). An opioid-containing analgesic regimen should be tailored to each patient's needs and based upon the type of pain being treated (acute versus chronic), the route of administration, degree of tolerance for opioids (naive versus chronic user), age, weight, and medical condition. The optimal analgesic dose varies widely among patients; doses should be titrated to pain relief/prevention. Opioids decrease bowel motility; monitor for decreased bowel motility in postop patients receiving opioids. Use with caution in the perioperative setting; individualize treatment when transitioning from parenteral to oral analgesics.

[US Boxed Warning]: To ensure that the benefits of opioid analgesics outweigh the risks of addiction, abuse, and misuse, the FDA has required a Risk Evaluation and Mitigation Strategy (REMS) for these products. Under the requirements of the REMS, drug companies with approved opioid analgesic products must make REMS-compliant education programs available to health care providers. Health care providers are strongly encouraged to complete a REMS-compliant education program; counsel patients and/or their caregivers, with every prescription, on safe use, serious risks, storage, and disposal of these products; emphasize to patients and their caregivers the importance of reading the Medication Guide every time it is provided by their pharmacist; and consider other tools to improve patient, household, and community safety.

Some dosage forms may contain propylene glycol; large amounts are potentially toxic and have been associated hyperosmolality, lactic acidosis, seizures and respiratory depression; use caution (AAP ["Inactive" 1997]; Zar 2007).

Some dosage forms may contain sodium benzoate/ benzoic acid; benzoic acid (benzoate) is a metabolite of benzyl alcohol; large amounts of benzyl alcohol (≥99 mg/kg/day) have been associated with a potentially fatal toxicity ("gasping syndrome") in neonates; the "gasping syndrome" consists of metabolic acidosis, respiratory distress, gasping respirations, CNS dysfunction (including convulsions, intracranial hemorrhage), hypotension, and cardiovascular collapse (AAP ["Inactive" 1997]; CDC 1982); some data suggests that benzoate displaces bilirubin from protein binding sites (Ahlfors 2001); avoid or use dosage forms containing benzyl alcohol derivative with caution in neonates. See manufacturer's labeling.

Warnings: Additional Pediatric Considerations

Use is contraindicated in pediatric patients <12 years of age and for postoperative management in pediatric patients 12 to 18 years of age who have undergone tonsillectomy and/or adenoidectomy. Avoid codeine use in all pediatric patient populations in which it is contraindicated and in pediatric patients 12 to 18 years of age who have other risk factors that increase risk for respiratory depression associated with codeine (eg, conditions associated with hypoventilation like postoperative status, obstructive sleep apnea, obesity, severe pulmonary disease, neuromuscular disease, use of other medications known to depress respiratory drive); in rare cases in which codeine-containing product is the only option, consider genotype testing prior to use; use extra precaution; monitor closely for adverse effects. Prior to 2017, acetaminophen/codeine was approved for use in children as young as 3 years of age. Codeine has also been removed from the WHO List of Essential Medications in Children since 2011. Codeine has been associated with reports of life-threatening or fatal respiratory depression in children and adolescents; a review of FDA adverse events data and the literature includes reports of at least 21 deaths in infants or children (1965-2015). Multifactorial causes for the respiratory depression have been identified; of primary concern are unrecognized ultrarapid metabolizers of CYP2D6 who may have extensive conversion of codeine (prodrug) to morphine and thus increased opioid-mediated effects (ie, respiratory depression). Other oral opioid and nonopioid analgesics are alternate options depending upon severity of pain and other patient specific factors (eg, age, route of administration, etc); however, each also has unique therapeutic challenges and concerns; refer to individual monographs for detailed information (AAP [Tobias 2016]; Dancel 2017; Gammal 2016; Goldschneider 2017; Poonai 2015).

Hepatoxicity has been reported in patients using acetaminophen. In pediatric patients, this is most commonly associated with supratherapeutic dosing, more frequent administration than recommended, and use of multiple acetaminophen-containing products; however, hepatotoxicity has been rarely reported with recommended dosages (AAP [Sullivan 2011]; Heard 2014). All sources of acetaminophen (eg, prescription, OTC, combination) should be considered when evaluating a patient's maximum daily dose. To lower the risk for hepatotoxicity, the maximum daily acetaminophen dose should be limited to ≤75 mg/kg/day (maximum of 5 daily doses), not to exceed 4,000 mg/day (AAP [Sullivan 2011]; Heard 2014; Krenzelok 2012; Lavonas 2010). Acetaminophen avoidance or a lower total daily dose (2,000 to 3,000 mg/day) has been suggested for adults with increased risk for acetaminophen hepatotoxicity (eg, malnutrition, certain liver diseases, use of drugs that interact with acetaminophen metabolism); similar data are unavailable in pediatric patients (Hayward 2016; Larson 2007; Worriax 2007).

Some dosage forms may contain propylene glycol; in neonates large amounts of propylene glycol delivered orally, intravenously (eg, >3,000 mg/day), or topically have been associated with potentially fatal toxicities which can include metabolic acidosis, seizures, renal failure, and CNS depression; toxicities have also been reported in children and adults including hyperosmolality, lactic acidosis, seizures, and respiratory depression; use caution (AAP 1997; Shehab 2009).

Drug Interactions

Metabolism/Transport Effects Refer to individual components.

Avoid Concomitant Use

Avoid concomitant use of Acetaminophen and Codeine with any of the following: Azelastine (Nasal); Bromperidol; Eluxadoline; Monoamine Oxidase Inhibitors; Opioids (Mixed Agonist / Antagonist); Orphenadrine; Oxomemazine; Paraldehyde; Thalidomide

Increased Effect/Toxicity

Acetaminophen and Codeine may increase the levels/ effects of: Alvimopan; Azelastine (Nasal); Blonanserin; Busulfan; Dasatinib; Desmopressin; Diuretics; Eluxadoline; Flunitrazepam; Imatinib; Local Anesthetics; Methotrimeprazine; MetyroSINE; Mipomersen; Opioid Agonists; Orphenadrine; OxyCODONE; Paraldehyde; Phenylephrine (Systemic); Piribedil; Pramipexole; Prilocaine; Ramosetron; ROPINIRole; Rotigotine;

Serotonergic Agents (High Risk); Sodium Nitrite; SORAfenib; Suvorexant; Thalidomide; Vitamin K Antagonists; Zolpidem

The levels/effects of Acetaminophen and Codeine may be increased by: Ajmaline; Alizapride; Amphetamines; Anticholinergic Agents; Brimonidine (Topical); Bromopride; Bromperidol; Cannabidiol; Cannabis; Chlormethiazole; Chlorphenesin Carbamate; CNS Depressants; Cobicistat; CYP3A4 Inhibitors (Moderate); CYP3A4 Inhibitors (Strong); Dapsone (Topical); Dasatinib; Dimethindene (Topical); Dronabinol; Droperidol; Flucloxacillin; Isoniazid; Kava Kava; Lemborexant; Lisuride; Lofexidine; Lumefantrine; Magnesium Sulfate; Methotrimeprazine; Metoclopramide; MetyraPONE; Minocycline (Systemic); Monoamine Oxidase Inhibitors; Nabilone; Nitric Oxide; Oxomemazine; Peginterferon Alfa-2b; Perampanel; PHENobarbital; Primidone; Probenecid; Rufinamide; Sodium Oxybate; Somatostatin Analogs; SORAfenib; Succinylcholine; Tetrahydrocannabinol; Tetrahydrocannabinol and Cannabidiol

Decreased Effect

Acetaminophen and Codeine may decrease the levels/effects of: Diuretics; Gastrointestinal Agents (Prokinetic); Pegvisomant; Sincalide

The levels/effects of Acetaminophen and Codeine may be decreased by: CarBAMazepine; CYP2D6 Inhibitors (Moderate); CYP2D6 Inhibitors (Strong); CYP3A4 Inducers (Moderate); CYP3A4 Inducers (Strong); Fosphenytoin-Phenytoin; Isoniazid; Lorlatinib; Nalmefene; Naltrexone; Opioids (Mixed Agonist / Antagonist); Peginterferon Alfa-2b; PHENobarbital; Primidone

Reproductive Considerations Long-term opioid use may cause secondary hypogonadism, which may lead to sexual dysfunction and infertility (Brennan 2013).

Pregnancy Considerations

[US Boxed Warning]: Prolonged use during pregnancy can result in neonatal opioid withdrawal syndrome, which may be life-threatening if not recognized and treated, and requires management according to protocols developed by neonatology experts. If opioid use is required for a prolonged period in a pregnant woman, advise the patient of the risk of neonatal opioid withdrawal syndrome and ensure that appropriate treatment will be available.

Refer to individual monographs for additional information.

Breastfeeding Considerations

Acetaminophen and codeine are present in breast milk. Due to the potential for serious adverse reactions in the breastfed infant, breastfeeding is not recommended by the manufacturer.

Refer to individual monographs for additional information.

Controlled Substance Liquid products: C-V; Tablet: C-III

Dosage Forms: US

Solution, Oral:

Generic: Acetaminophen 120 mg and codeine phosphate 12 mg per 5 mL (5 mL, 12.5 mL, 118 mL, 473 mL)

Tablet, Oral:

Generic: Acetaminophen 300 mg and codeine phosphate 15 mg, Acetaminophen 300 mg and codeine phosphate 30 mg, Acetaminophen 300 mg and codeine phosphate 60 mg

Dosage Forms: Canada

Elixir, Oral:

Generic: Acetaminophen 160 mg and codeine 8 mg per 5 mL (100 mL, 500 mL)

Tablet, Oral:

Triatec-30: Acetaminophen 300 mg and codeine phosphate 30 mg

Tylenol #4: Acetaminophen 300 mg and codeine phosphate 60 mg

Generic: Acetaminophen 300 mg and codeine phosphate 30 mg, Acetaminophen 300 mg and codeine phosphate 60 mg

Dental Health Professional Considerations

Although the ***OTC product labeling*** for acetaminophen products state to limit the maximum dose to 3,000 mg daily (for extra strength) or 3,250 mg (for regular strength) (see this site for details: http://www.tylenolprofessional.com/products-and-dosages.html), it is still appropriate for patients to take up to 4,000 mg daily "under the direction of a health care provider" (http://www.tylenolprofessional.com/dosage.html).

The acetaminophen component requires use with caution in patients who use alcohol, with preexisting liver disease, and those receiving more than one source of acetaminophen-containing medication.

Hepatotoxicity caused by acetaminophen is potentiated by chronic alcohol consumption. People who are taking acetaminophen, even at therapeutic doses, and consume alcohol are at risk of developing hepatotoxicity.

Acetaminophen may increase the levels and enhance the anticoagulant effects of vitamin K antagonists acenocoumarol and warfarin (Coumadin). Studies have reported that acetaminophen has increased the INR in warfarin treated patients with daily acetaminophen doses as low as 2 g, particularly when taking acetaminophen for >1 week (Antlitz, 1968; Boeijinga, 1982; Gebauer, 2003; Hylek, 1998; Rubin, 1984). In addition, case reports of bleeding as a result of increased INR have been published (Bagheri, 1999; Bartle, 1991). There is no known mechanism of the interaction; furthermore, some studies have failed to demonstrate this interaction (Gadisseur, 2003; Kwan, 1995; van den Bemt, 2002). In terms of risk, the data suggest that acetaminophen and warfarin could interact in some clinically significant manner but that the benefits of concomitant use of acetaminophen for pain control in dental patients taking warfarin usually outweigh the risks. An appropriate monitoring plan should be in place to identify potential negative effects and dosage adjustments may be necessary in a minority of patients. The interaction may be more likely to occur with daily acetaminophen doses of >1.3 g for >1 week.

There are no reports of acetaminophen interacting with antiplatelet drugs such as aspirin, clopidogrel (Plavix), ticagrelor (Brilinta), or prasugrel (Effient). Also, there are no reports of acetaminophen in combination with hydrocodone, codeine, or oxycodone interacting with warfarin (Coumadin).

◆ **Acetaminophen and Hydrocodone** *see* Hydrocodone and Acetaminophen *on page 761*

◆ **Acetaminophen and Oxycodone** *see* Oxycodone and Acetaminophen *on page 1164*

Acetaminophen and Tramadol

(a seet a MIN oh fen & TRA ma dole)

Related Information

Acetaminophen *on page 59*
Oral Pain *on page 1734*
TraMADol *on page 1468*

Related Sample Prescriptions

Oral Pain - Sample Prescriptions *on page 30*

Brand Names: US Ultracet

Brand Names: Canada ACT Tramadol/Acet [DSC]; APO-Tramadol/Acet; Auro-Tramadol/Acetaminophen; JAMP-Acet-Tramadol; Mar-Tramadol/Acet; MINT-Tramadol/Acet; MYLAN-Tramadol/Acet [DSC]; NRA-Tramadol/Acet [DSC]; PMS-Tramadol-Acet; Priva-Tramadol/Acet; TARO-Tramadol/Acet; TEVA-Tramadol/Acetaminophen; Tramacet; Tramadol-Acet [DSC]; Tramadol/Acet

Generic Availability (US) Yes

Pharmacologic Category Analgesic Combination (Opioid); Analgesic, Opioid

Dental Use Treatment of postoperative pain (≤5 days)

Use

Pain management: Short-term (≤5 days) management of acute pain severe enough to require an opioid analgesic and for which alternative treatments are inadequate.

Limitations of use: Reserve tramadol/acetaminophen for use in patients for whom alternative treatment options (eg, nonopioid analgesics) are ineffective, not tolerated, or would be otherwise inadequate to provide sufficient management of pain.

Local Anesthetic/Vasoconstrictor Precautions No information available to require special precautions

Effects on Dental Treatment Key adverse event(s) related to dental treatment: Xerostomia and changes in salivation (normal salivary flow resumes upon discontinuation) (see Dental Health Professional Considerations).

Effects on Bleeding As a single agent, acetaminophen does not appear to affect bleeding or platelet aggregation. Acetaminophen may prolong the INR and increase bleeding in patients taking warfarin (Coumadin). For patients taking warfarin, single acetaminophen doses or acetaminophen therapy of short duration should be safe, but if large (>1.3 g/day) doses are administered for longer than 10-14 days, then the INR should be monitored (see Dental Health Professional Considerations).

Adverse Reactions Also see individual agents.

1% to 10%:

Central nervous system: Drowsiness (6%), dizziness (3%), insomnia (2%), anxiety, confusion, euphoria, fatigue, headache, nervousness

Dermatologic: Diaphoresis (4%), pruritus (2%), skin rash

Endocrine & metabolic: Hot flash

Gastrointestinal: Constipation (6%), anorexia (3%), diarrhea (3%), nausea (3%), xerostomia (2%), abdominal pain, dyspepsia, flatulence, vomiting

Genitourinary: Prostatic disease (2%)

Neuromuscular & skeletal: Tremor, weakness

<1%, postmarketing, and/or case reports: Abnormality in thinking, albuminuria, amnesia, anemia, ataxia, cardiac arrhythmia, changes in liver function, chest pain, convulsions, depersonalization, depression, drug abuse, dysphagia, dyspnea, emotional lability, exacerbation of migraine headache, exacerbation of hypertension, hallucination, hypertension, hypertonia, hypotension, impotence, melena, migraine, muscle spasm, nightmares, oliguria, palpitations, paresthesia, rigors, stupor, syncope, tachycardia, tinnitus, tongue edema, urinary retention, urination disorder, vertigo, visual disturbance, weight loss, withdrawal syndrome (with abrupt discontinuation; includes anxiety, diarrhea, hallucinations [rare], nausea, pain, piloerection, rigors, sweating, and tremor; uncommon discontinuation symptoms may include severe anxiety, panic attacks, or paresthesia)

Dental Usual Dosage Acute postoperative pain (≤5 days): Adults: Oral: Two tablets every 4-6 hours as needed for pain relief (maximum: 8 tablets/day); treatment should not exceed 5 days

Dosing

Adult

Pain management: Oral: Acetaminophen 325 mg/tramadol 37.5 mg: Two tablets every 4 to 6 hours as needed for pain relief (maximum: 8 tablets/day [acetaminophen 2,600 mg/tramadol 300 mg per day]); do not exceed 5 days of therapy

Discontinuation of therapy: If discontinuing in a physically dependent patient, decrease the dose by no more than 10% to 25% and use a gradual downward titration. If patient displays withdrawal symptoms, temporarily interrupt the taper or increase dose to previous dose and then reduce dose more slowly by increasing interval between dose reductions, decreasing amount of daily dose reduction, or both.

Geriatric Refer to adult dosing. Use with caution.

Renal Impairment: Adult

CrCl ≥30 mL/minute: No dosage adjustment necessary.

CrCl <30 mL/minute: Maximum: Two tablets every 12 hours

Hepatic Impairment: Adult Use is not recommended (acetaminophen and tramadol undergo extensive hepatic metabolism).

Mechanism of Action

Acetaminophen: Although not fully elucidated, the analgesic effects are believed to be due to activation of descending serotonergic inhibitory pathways in the CNS. Interactions with other nociceptive systems may be involved as well (Smith 2009). Antipyresis is produced from inhibition of the hypothalamic heat-regulating center.

Tramadol: Binds to μ-opiate receptors in the CNS causing inhibition of ascending pain pathways, altering the perception of and response to pain; also inhibits the reuptake of norepinephrine and serotonin, which also modifies the ascending pain pathway

Contraindications

Hypersensitivity to acetaminophen, tramadol, or any component of the formulation; pediatric patients <12 years; postoperative management in pediatric patients <18 years who have undergone tonsillectomy and/or adenoidectomy; significant respiratory depression; acute or severe bronchial asthma in an unmonitored setting or in the absence of resuscitative equipment; GI obstruction, including paralytic ileus (known or suspected); concomitant use with or within 14 days following MAO inhibitor therapy.

Documentation of allergenic cross-reactivity for opioids is limited. However, because of similarities in chemical structure and/or pharmacologic actions, the possibility of cross-sensitivity cannot be ruled out with certainty.

Canadian labeling: Additional contraindications (not in US labeling): Known or suspected mechanical GI obstruction (eg, bowel obstruction, strictures) or any disease/condition that affects bowel transit; suspected surgical abdomen (eg, acute appendicitis, pancreatitis); severe renal impairment (creatinine clearance <30 mL/minute); severe hepatic impairment (Child-Pugh class C); mild pain that can be managed with other pain medications; acute or severe bronchial asthma, chronic obstructive airway, or status asthmaticus; acute respiratory depression, hypercapnia, or cor pulmonale; acute alcoholism, delirium tremens, or seizure disorder; severe CNS depression, increased cerebrospinal or intracranial pressure, or head injury; any situation where opioids are contraindicated (eg, acute intoxication with alcohol, hypnotics, centrally acting analgesics, opioids or psychotropic drugs); breastfeeding; pregnancy; use during labor and delivery.

Warnings/Precautions See individual agents.

Drug Interactions

Metabolism/Transport Effects Refer to individual components.

Avoid Concomitant Use

Avoid concomitant use of Acetaminophen and Tramadol with any of the following: Azelastine (Nasal); Bromperidol; CarBAMazepine; Dapoxetine; Eluxadoline; Iobenguane Radiopharmaceutical Products; Monoamine Oxidase Inhibitors (Antidepressant); Monoamine Oxidase Inhibitors (Type B); Opioids (Mixed Agonist / Antagonist); Orphenadrine; Oxomemazine; Paraldehyde; Thalidomide

Increased Effect/Toxicity

Acetaminophen and Tramadol may increase the levels/effects of: Alvimopan; Amifampridine; Azelastine (Nasal); Blonanserin; Busulfan; CarBAMazepine; Dasatinib; Desmopressin; Diuretics; Eluxadoline; Flunitrazepam; Hypoglycemia-Associated Agents; Imatinib; Iohexol; Iomeprol; Iopamidol; Local Anesthetics; Methotrimeprazine; MetyroSINE; Mipomersen; Monoamine Oxidase Inhibitors (Type B); Orphenadrine; Oxitriptan; OxyCODONE; Paraldehyde; Phenylephrine (Systemic); Piribedil; Pramipexole; Prilocaine; Ramosetron; ROPINIRole; Rotigotine; Selective Serotonin Reuptake Inhibitors; Serotonergic Agents (High Risk, Miscellaneous); Sodium Nitrite; SORAfenib; Suvorexant; Thalidomide; Tricyclic Antidepressants; Vitamin K Antagonists; Zolpidem

The levels/effects of Acetaminophen and Tramadol may be increased by: Ajmaline; Alizapride; Almotriptan; Amphetamines; Androgens; Anticholinergic Agents; Antidiabetic Agents; Antiemetics (5HT3 Antagonists); Brimonidine (Topical); Bromopride; Bromperidol; BuPROPion; BusPIRone; Cannabidiol; Cannabis; Chlormethiazole; Chlorphenesin Carbamate; CNS Depressants; Cobicistat; CYP2D6 Inhibitors (Moderate); CYP2D6 Inhibitors (Strong); CYP3A4 Inhibitors (Strong); Dapoxetine; Dapsone (Topical); Dasatinib; Dexmethylphenidate-Methylphenidate; Dextromethorphan; Dimethindene (Topical); Dronabinol; Droperidol; DULoxetine; Eletriptan; Ergot Derivatives; Flucloxacillin; Herbs (Hypoglycemic Properties); Isoniazid; Kava Kava; Lemborexant; Linezolid; Lisuride; Lofexidine; Lorcaserin (Withdrawn From US Market); Lumefantrine; Magnesium Sulfate; Maitake; Methotrimeprazine; Methylene Blue; Metoclopramide; MetyraPONE; Minocycline (Systemic); Monoamine Oxidase Inhibitors (Antidepressant); Nabilone; Nefazodone; Nitric Oxide; Ondansetron; Oxomemazine; Ozanimod; Peginterferon Alfa-2b; Pegvisomant; Perampanel; PHENobarbital; Primidone; Probenecid; Prothionamide; Quinolones; Ritonavir; Rufinamide; Salicylates; Selective Serotonin Reuptake Inhibitors (Strong CYP2D6 Inhibitors); Serotonergic Non-Opioid CNS Depressants; Serotonergic Opioids (High Risk); Serotonin 5-HT1D Receptor Agonists (Triptans); Serotonin/Norepinephrine Reuptake Inhibitors; Sodium Oxybate; SORAfenib; St John's Wort; Succinylcholine; Syrian Rue; Tetrahydrocannabinol; Tetrahydrocannabinol and Cannabidiol; Tricyclic Antidepressants

Decreased Effect

Acetaminophen and Tramadol may decrease the levels/effects of: CarBAMazepine; Diuretics; Gastrointestinal Agents (Prokinetic); Iobenguane Radiopharmaceutical Products; Pegvisomant; Sincalide

The levels/effects of Acetaminophen and Tramadol may be decreased by: CarBAMazepine; CYP2D6 Inhibitors (Moderate); CYP2D6 Inhibitors (Strong); CYP3A4 Inducers (Moderate); CYP3A4 Inducers (Strong); Dabrafenib; Deferasirox; DULoxetine; Enzalutamide; Erdafitinib; Fosphenytoin-Phenytoin; Isoniazid; Ivosidenib; Lorlatinib; Mitotane; Nalmefene; Naltrexone; Ondansetron; Opioids (Mixed Agonist / Antagonist); Peginterferon Alfa-2b; PHENobarbital; Primidone; Quinolones; Ritonavir; Sarilumab; Selective Serotonin Reuptake Inhibitors (Strong CYP2D6 Inhibitors); Siltuximab; St John's Wort; Tocilizumab

Food Interactions Food may delay time to peak plasma levels, however, the extent of absorption is not affected. Management: Administer without regard to meals.

Reproductive Considerations

Chronic use of opioids may decrease fertility in females and males of reproductive potential.

Pregnancy Considerations

Acetaminophen and tramadol cross the placenta.

[US Boxed Warning]: Prolonged use of opioids during pregnancy can cause neonatal withdrawal syndrome, which may be life-threatening if not recognized and treated according to protocols developed by neonatology experts. If opioid use is required for a prolonged period in a pregnant woman, advise the patient of the risk of neonatal opioid withdrawal syndrome and ensure that appropriate treatment will be available.

Refer to individual monographs for additional information.

Breastfeeding Considerations

Acetaminophen and tramadol are present in breast milk. Due to the potential for serious adverse reactions in the breastfed infant, breastfeeding is not recommended by the manufacturer. Refer to individual monographs.

Controlled Substance C-IV

Dosage Forms: US

Tablet, Oral:

Ultracet: Acetaminophen 325 mg and tramadol hydrochloride 37.5 mg

Generic: Acetaminophen 325 mg and tramadol hydrochloride 37.5 mg

Dosage Forms: Canada

Tablet, Oral:

Tramacet: Acetaminophen 325 mg and tramadol hydrochloride 37.5 mg

Generic: Acetaminophen 325 mg and tramadol hydrochloride 37.5 mg

Dental Health Professional Considerations Although the ***OTC product labeling*** for acetaminophen products state to limit the maximum dose to 3,000 mg daily (for extra strength) or 3,250 mg (for regular strength) (see this site for details: http://www.-tylenolprofessional.com/products-and-dosages.html), it is still appropriate for patients to take up to 4,000 mg daily "under the direction of a health care provider" (http://www.tylenolprofessional.com/dosage.html).

The acetaminophen component requires use with caution in patients who use alcohol, with preexisting liver disease, and those receiving more than one source of acetaminophen-containing medication.

Hepatotoxicity caused by acetaminophen is potentiated by chronic alcohol consumption. People who are taking acetaminophen, even at therapeutic doses, and consume alcohol are at risk of developing hepatotoxicity.

Acetaminophen may increase the levels and enhance the anticoagulant effects of vitamin K antagonists acenocoumarol and warfarin (Coumadin®). Studies have reported that acetaminophen has increased the INR in warfarin treated patients with daily acetaminophen doses as low as 2 g, particularly when taking acetaminophen for >1 week (Antlitz, 1968; Boeijinga, 1982; Gebauer, 2003; Hylek, 1998; Rubin, 1984). In addition, case reports of bleeding as a result of increased INR have been published (Bagheri, 1999; Bartle, 1991). There is no known mechanism of the interaction; furthermore, some studies have failed to demonstrate this interaction (Gadisseur, 2003; Kwan, 1995; van den Bemt, 2002). In terms of risk, the data suggest that acetaminophen and warfarin could interact in some clinically significant manner but that the benefits of concomitant use of acetaminophen for pain control in dental patients taking warfarin usually outweigh the risks. An appropriate monitoring plan should be in place to identify potential negative effects and dosage adjustments may be necessary in a minority of patients. The interaction may be more likely to occur with daily acetaminophen doses of >1.3 g for >1 week.

There are no reports of acetaminophen interacting with antiplatelet drugs such as aspirin, clopidogrel (Plavix®), or prasugrel (Effient™). Also, there are no reports of acetaminophen in combination with hydrocodone, codeine, or oxycodone interacting with warfarin (Coumadin®).

◆ **Acetaminophen/Benzhydrocodone** *see* Benzhydrocodone and Acetaminophen *on page 228*

◆ **Acetaminophen/Butalbital/Caffeine/Codeine** *see* Butalbital, Acetaminophen, Caffeine, and Codeine *on page 274*

◆ **Acetaminophen, Caffeine, Codeine, and Butalbital** *see* Butalbital, Acetaminophen, Caffeine, and Codeine *on page 274*

◆ **Acetaminophen/Codeine** *see* Acetaminophen and Codeine *on page 65*

◆ **Acetaminophen/Hydrocodone** *see* Hydrocodone and Acetaminophen *on page 764*

AcetaZOLAMIDE (a set a ZOLE a mide)

Brand Names: US Diamox Sequels [DSC]

Pharmacologic Category Anticonvulsant, Miscellaneous; Carbonic Anhydrase Inhibitor; Diuretic, Carbonic Anhydrase Inhibitor; Ophthalmic Agent, Antiglaucoma

Use

Altitude illness: Prevention or amelioration of symptoms associated with acute mountain sickness (immediate and extended release dosage forms)

Edema: Adjunctive treatment of drug-induced edema or edema due to congestive heart failure (IV and immediate release dosage forms)

Elevated intraocular pressure: Treatment of elevated intraocular pressure (IOP) in patients with chronic open-angle glaucoma or acute angle-closure glaucoma prior to surgery or as part of a 4-drug medical management regimen when a patient cannot be seen by an ophthalmologist for ≥1 hour

Epilepsy: Adjunctive treatment of centrencephalic epilepsies (IV and immediate release dosage forms)

Local Anesthetic/Vasoconstrictor Precautions No information available to require special precautions

Effects on Dental Treatment Key adverse event(s) related to dental treatment: Metallic taste (resolves upon discontinuation)

Effects on Bleeding No information available to require special precautions

Adverse Reactions Frequency not defined.

Cardiovascular: Flushing

Central nervous system: Ataxia, confusion, convulsions, depression, dizziness, drowsiness, excitement, fatigue, flaccid paralysis, headache, malaise, paresthesia

Dermatologic: Allergic skin reaction, skin photosensitivity, Stevens-Johnson syndrome, toxic epidermal necrolysis, urticaria

Endocrine & metabolic: Electrolyte imbalance, growth retardation (children), hyperglycemia, hypoglycemia, hypokalemia, hyponatremia, metabolic acidosis

Gastrointestinal: Decreased appetite, diarrhea, dysgeusia, glycosuria, melena, nausea, vomiting

Genitourinary: Crystalluria, hematuria

Hematologic and oncologic: Agranulocytosis, aplastic anemia, leukopenia, thrombocytopenia, thrombocytopenic purpura

Hepatic: Abnormal hepatic function tests, cholestatic jaundice, fulminant hepatic necrosis, hepatic insufficiency

Hypersensitivity: Anaphylaxis

Local: Pain at injection site

Ophthalmic: Myopia

Otic: Auditory disturbance, tinnitus

Renal: Polyuria, renal failure

Miscellaneous: Fever

Mechanism of Action Reversible inhibition of the enzyme carbonic anhydrase resulting in reduction of hydrogen ion secretion at renal tubule and an increased renal excretion of sodium, potassium, bicarbonate, and water. Decreases production of aqueous humor and inhibits carbonic anhydrase in central nervous system to retard abnormal and excessive discharge from CNS neurons.

Pharmacodynamics/Kinetics

Onset of Action

Capsule (extended release): 2 hours; Tablet (immediate release): 1 to 1.5 hours; IV: 2 to 10 minutes

Peak effect: Capsule (extended release): 8 to 18 hours; IV: 15 minutes; Tablet: 2 to 4 hours

Duration of Action Inhibition of aqueous humor secretion: Capsule (extended release): 18 to 24 hours; IV: 4 to 5 hours; Tablet: 8 to 12 hours

Half-life Elimination 2.4 to 5.8 hours

Time to Peak Plasma: Capsule (extended release): 3 to 6 hours; Tablet: 1 to 4 hours; IV: 15 minutes

Pregnancy Considerations

Limited data is available following the use of acetazolamide in pregnant women for the treatment of idiopathic intracranial hypertension (Falardeau 2013; Kesler 2013).

Pregnant women exposed to acetazolamide during pregnancy for the treatment of seizure disorders are encouraged to enroll themselves into the AED Pregnancy Registry by calling 1-888-233-2334. Additional information is available at aedpregnancyregistry.org

- ◆ **Acetoxymethylprogesterone** *see* MedroxyPROGESTERone *on page 953*
- ◆ **Acetylsalicylic Acid** *see* Aspirin *on page 177*
- ◆ **Achromycin** *see* Tetracycline (Systemic) *on page 1431*
- ◆ **Aciclovir** *see* Acyclovir (Systemic) *on page 75*
- ◆ **Aciclovir** *see* Acyclovir (Topical) *on page 82*
- ◆ **Acid Controller Max St [OTC]** *see* Famotidine *on page 635*
- ◆ **Acid Controller Original Str [OTC]** *see* Famotidine *on page 635*
- ◆ **Acidophilus/Bulgaricus** *see Lactobacillus on page 869*
- ◆ **Acidoph/L.Bulg/Bif.B/S.Thermop** *see Lactobacillus on page 869*
- ◆ **Acid Reducer [OTC]** *see* Famotidine *on page 635*
- ◆ **Acid Reducer Maximum Strength [OTC]** *see* Famotidine *on page 635*
- ◆ **Acidulated Phosphate Fluoride** *see* Fluoride *on page 693*
- ◆ **Aciphex** *see* RABEprazole *on page 1302*
- ◆ **AcipHex Sprinkle** *see* RABEprazole *on page 1302*

Aclidinium (a kli DIN ee um)

Related Information

Respiratory Diseases *on page 1680*

Brand Names: US Tudorza Pressair

Brand Names: Canada Tudorza Genuair

Pharmacologic Category Anticholinergic Agent; Anticholinergic Agent, Long-Acting

Use Chronic obstructive pulmonary disease: Maintenance treatment of patients with chronic obstructive pulmonary disease (COPD).

Local Anesthetic/Vasoconstrictor Precautions No information available to require special precautions

Effects on Dental Treatment Key adverse event(s) related to dental treatment: Cough, nasopharyngitis, rhinitis, sinusitis, and toothache have been reported.

Effects on Bleeding No information available to require special precautions

Adverse Reactions

1% to 10%:

Central nervous system: Headache (7%), falling (1%)

Gastrointestinal: Diarrhea (3%), toothache (1%), vomiting (1%)

Respiratory: Nasopharyngitis (6%), cough (3%), rhinitis (2%), sinusitis (2%)

<1%, postmarketing, and/or case reports: Anaphylaxis, angioedema, blurred vision, bronchospasm, cardiac failure, diabetes mellitus, first-degree atrioventricular block, nausea, osteoarthritis, pruritus, skin rash, stomatitis, tachycardia, type 1 hypersensitivity reaction, urinary retention, urticaria, voice disorder, xerostomia

Mechanism of Action Competitively and reversibly inhibits the action of acetylcholine at type 3 muscarinic (M_3) receptors in bronchial smooth muscle causing bronchodilation

Pharmacodynamics/Kinetics

Half-life Elimination 5 to 8 hours (following inhalation)

Time to Peak Plasma: Within 10 minutes (steady state, following inhalation)

Pregnancy Considerations Adverse events have been observed in animal reproduction studies.

- ◆ **Aclidinium Bromide** *see* Aclidinium *on page 74*
- ◆ **Aclovate [DSC]** *see* Alclometasone *on page 91*
- ◆ **ACP-103** *see* Pimavanserin *on page 1232*
- ◆ **ACP-196** *see* Acalabrutinib *on page 56*
- ◆ **Act [OTC]** *see* Fluoride *on page 693*
- ◆ **ACT-D** *see* DACTINomycin *on page 430*
- ◆ **ACT-064992** *see* Macitentan *on page 945*
- ◆ **ACT-293987** *see* Selexipag *on page 1364*
- ◆ **ActD** *see* DACTINomycin *on page 430*
- ◆ **Actemra** *see* Tocilizumab *on page 1457*
- ◆ **Actemra ACTPen** *see* Tocilizumab *on page 1457*
- ◆ **ACTH** *see* Corticotropin *on page 412*
- ◆ **Acthar** *see* Corticotropin *on page 412*
- ◆ **Acthrel** *see* Corticorelin *on page 411*
- ◆ **Acticlate** *see* Doxycycline *on page 522*
- ◆ **Actifoam Collagen Sponge** *see* Collagen Hemostat *on page 410*
- ◆ **Actimmune** *see* Interferon Gamma-1b *on page 836*
- ◆ **Actinomycin** *see* DACTINomycin *on page 430*
- ◆ **Actinomycin D** *see* DACTINomycin *on page 430*
- ◆ **Actinomycin CI** *see* DACTINomycin *on page 430*
- ◆ **Actiq** *see* FentaNYL *on page 642*
- ◆ **Activase** *see* Alteplase *on page 111*
- ◆ **Activated Ergosterol** *see* Ergocalciferol *on page 582*
- ◆ **Activated PCC** *see* Anti-inhibitor Coagulant Complex (Human) *on page 156*
- ◆ **Active Injection D** *see* DexAMETHasone (Systemic) *on page 463*
- ◆ **Activella** *see* Estradiol and Norethindrone *on page 598*
- ◆ **Act Kids [OTC]** *see* Fluoride *on page 693*
- ◆ **Actonel** *see* Risedronate *on page 1331*
- ◆ **Actoplus Met** *see* Pioglitazone and Metformin *on page 1236*
- ◆ **Actoplus Met XR [DSC]** *see* Pioglitazone and Metformin *on page 1236*
- ◆ **Actos** *see* Pioglitazone *on page 1234*
- ◆ **Act Restoring [OTC]** *see* Fluoride *on page 693*
- ◆ **Act Total Care [OTC]** *see* Fluoride *on page 693*
- ◆ **Act Total Care Dry Mouth [OTC]** *see* Fluoride *on page 693*
- ◆ **Act Total Care Sensitive [OTC]** *see* Fluoride *on page 693*
- ◆ **ACV** *see* Acyclovir (Systemic) *on page 75*
- ◆ **ACV** *see* Acyclovir (Topical) *on page 82*
- ◆ **Acycloguanosine** *see* Acyclovir (Systemic) *on page 75*
- ◆ **Acycloguanosine** *see* Acyclovir (Topical) *on page 82*

Acyclovir (Systemic) (ay SYE kloe veer)

Related Information

Systemic Viral Diseases *on page 1709*
ValACYclovir *on page 1512*
Viral Infections *on page 1754*

Related Sample Prescriptions

Viral Infections - Sample Prescriptions *on page 43*

Brand Names: US Zovirax

Brand Names: Canada APO-Acyclovir; MYLAN-Acyclovir; RATIO-Acyclovir [DSC]; TEVA-Acyclovir; Zovirax

Generic Availability (US) Yes

Pharmacologic Category Antiviral Agent

Dental Use Treatment of initial and prophylaxis of recurrent mucosal and cutaneous herpes simplex (HSV-1 and HSV-2) infections in immunocompromised patients

Use

Oral:

Herpes simplex virus (HSV), genital: Treatment of initial episodes and the management of recurrent episodes of genital herpes.

Herpes zoster (shingles): Acute treatment of herpes zoster (shingles).

Varicella (chickenpox): Treatment of varicella (chickenpox).

Injection:

Herpes simplex encephalitis: Treatment of herpes simplex encephalitis.

Herpes simplex virus (HSV), genital infection (severe): Treatment of severe initial clinical episodes of genital herpes in immunocompetent patients.

Herpes simplex virus (HSV), mucocutaneous infection in immunocompromised patients: Treatment of initial and recurrent mucosal and cutaneous herpes simplex (HSV-1 and HSV-2) in immunocompromised patients.

Herpes simplex virus (HSV), neonatal: Treatment of neonatal herpes infections.

Herpes zoster (shingles) in immunocompromised patients: Treatment of herpes zoster (shingles) in immunocompromised patients.

Local Anesthetic/Vasoconstrictor Precautions No information available to require special precautions

Effects on Dental Treatment No significant effects or complications reported (see Dental Health Professional Considerations)

Effects on Bleeding No information available to require special precautions

Adverse Reactions As reported with IV administration, unless otherwise noted.

>10%:

Central nervous system: Malaise (oral: 12%)

Hematologic & oncologic: Decrease in absolute neutrophil count (neonates: 3% to 16%), decreased hemoglobin (neonates: 13%)

1% to 10%:

Central nervous system: Headache (oral: ≤2%)

Dermatologic: Pruritus (2%), skin rash (2%), urticaria (2%)

Gastrointestinal: Nausea (oral and IV: ≤7%), vomiting (oral and IV: ≤7%), diarrhea (oral: 2% to 3%; IV: <1%)

Hematologic & oncologic: Thrombocytopenia (neonates: 5% to 10%; children, adolescents, and adults: <1%)

Hepatic: Increased serum bilirubin (neonates, grades 3/4: 4%), increased serum transaminases (1% to 2%)

Local: Inflammation at injection site (≤9%), injection site phlebitis (≤9%)

Renal: Increased blood urea nitrogen (5% to 10%), increased serum creatinine (5% to 10%)

<1%, postmarketing, and/or case reports (all routes): Abdominal pain, aggressive behavior, agitation, alopecia, anaphylaxis, anemia, angioedema, anorexia, ataxia, coma, confusion, delirium, disseminated intravascular coagulation, dizziness, drowsiness, dysarthria, encephalopathy, erythema multiforme, fatigue, fever, gastrointestinal distress, hallucination, hematuria, hemolysis, hepatitis, hyperbilirubinemia, hypersensitivity angiitis, hypotension, impaired consciousness, increased liver enzymes, jaundice, leukocytosis, leukopenia, lymphadenopathy, myalgia, neutropenia, neutrophilia, obtundation, pain, paresthesia, peripheral edema, psychosis, renal failure syndrome, renal pain, seizure, skin photosensitivity, Stevens-Johnson syndrome, thrombocythemia, toxic epidermal necrolysis, tremor, visual disturbance

Dental Usual Dosage

Mucocutaneous HSV: Adults:

Immunocompromised (off-label use): Oral: 400 mg 5 times a day for 7-14 days

Chronic suppression of recurrent herpes labialis (cold sores) (off-label use): Immunocompetent adults: oral: 400 mg twice daily (Rooney 1993)

Dosing

Adult

Bell palsy, new onset (adjunctive therapy) (alternative agent) (off-label use): Oral: 400 mg 5 times daily for 10 days in combination with corticosteroids; begin within 3 days of symptom onset. **Note:** Antiviral therapy alone is **not** recommended (AAN [Gronseth 2012]; AAO-HNSF [Baugh 2013]; Ronthal 2020); some experts only recommend addition of an antiviral to steroid therapy in patients with severe Bell palsy (de Almeida 2014).

Cytomegalovirus, prevention in low-risk allogeneic hematopoietic cell transplant recipients (alternative agent) (off-label use): Note: Begin at engraftment and continue to day 100; requires close monitoring for cytomegalovirus (CMV) reactivation (due to weak activity); not for use in patients at high risk for CMV disease (ASBMT/IDSA [Tomblyn 2009]):

IV: 500 mg/m^2/dose every 8 hours for up to 4 weeks or until hospital discharge, followed by oral therapy (ASBMT/IDSA [Tomblyn 2009]; Boeckh 2009; Ljungman 2002)

Oral: Following initial IV therapy: 800 mg 4 times daily (ASBMT/IDSA [Tomblyn 2009]; Boeckh 2009; Ljungman 2002)

Herpes simplex virus, central nervous system infection (encephalitis or meningitis): IV: 10 mg/kg/dose every 8 hours. Duration for encephalitis is 14 to 21 days and for meningitis is 10 to 14 days; treatment of encephalitis requires IV therapy while treatment of meningitis may include step-down oral antiviral therapy. **Note:** Empiric herpes simplex virus (HSV) therapy should be initiated in all patients with suspected encephalitis (AST-IDCOP [Lee 2019]; IDSA [Tunkel 2008]; Tunkel 2020).

Herpes simplex virus, mucocutaneous infection:

Esophagitis (off-label use):

Immunocompetent patients: **Oral:** 400 mg 3 times daily **or** 200 mg 5 times daily for 7 to 10 days (Bonis 2020; Canalejo Castrillero 2010)

Immunocompromised patients: **Oral:** 400 mg 5 times daily for 14 to 21 days (Bonis 2020)

Patients with severe odynophagia or dysphagia: **IV:** 5 mg/kg/dose every 8 hours; patients who rapidly improve can be switched to an oral antiviral to complete a total of 7 to 14 days of therapy (Bonis 2020; Canalejo Castrillero 2010).

Genital:

Immunocompetent patients:

Treatment, initial episode:

Oral: 400 mg 3 times daily **or** 200 mg 5 times daily for 7 to 10 days; extend duration if lesions have not healed completely after 10 days (CDC [Workowski 2015]).

IV (for severe disease): 5 to 10 mg/kg/dose every 8 hours for 2 to 7 days, followed by oral acyclovir (or similar antiviral) to complete ≥10 days of therapy total (CDC [Workowski 2015])

Treatment, recurrent episode: **Oral:** 400 mg 3 times daily for 5 days **or** 800 mg twice daily for 5 days **or** 800 mg 3 times daily for 2 days. **Note**: Treatment is most effective when initiated during the prodrome or within 1 day of lesion onset (CDC [Workowski 2015]).

Suppressive therapy (eg, for severe and/or frequent recurrences): **Oral:** 400 mg twice daily. **Note:** Reassess need periodically (eg, annually) (CDC [Workowski 2015]).

Immunocompromised patients (including patients with HIV):

Treatment, initial ***or*** *recurrent episode*:

Oral: 400 mg 3 times daily for 5 to 10 days; extend treatment duration if lesions have not healed completely after 10 days (AST-IDCOP [Lee 2019]; CDC [Workowski 2015]; HHS [OI adult 2020]).

IV (for severe disease): 5 to 10 mg/kg/dose every 8 hours for 2 to 7 days, followed by oral acyclovir (or similar antiviral) once lesions begin to regress and continue for ≥10 days of therapy and until complete resolution (CDC [Workowski 2015]; HHS [OI adult 2020]).

Suppressive therapy (eg, for severe and/or frequent recurrences): **Oral:** 400 to 800 mg 2 to 3 times daily. **Note:** Reassess need periodically (eg, annually) (CDC [Workowski 2015]; HHS [OI adult 2020]).

Pregnant females:

Treatment, initial episode: **Oral:** 400 mg 3 times daily for 7 to 10 days; extend treatment duration if lesion has not healed completely after 10 days (ACOG 2007).

Treatment, recurrent episode (symptomatic): **Oral:** 400 mg 3 times daily **or** 800 mg twice daily for 5 days (ACOG 2007). **Note:** Some experts reserve treatment of recurrent episodes for patients with severe and/or frequent symptoms (Riley 2020).

Suppressive therapy, for patients with a genital HSV lesion anytime during pregnancy: **Oral:** 400 mg 3 times daily, beginning at 36 weeks' gestation and continued until the onset of labor (ACOG 2007; CDC [Workowski 2015]; Riley 2020). **Note:** Some experts offer suppressive therapy earlier than 36 weeks' gestation for women who have a first-episode lesion during the third trimester (Riley 2020).

Orolabial: **Note:** Initiate therapy at earliest symptom.

Immunocompetent and immunocompromised patients (including patients with HIV):

Treatment, initial ***or*** *recurrent episode*:

Oral: 400 mg 3 times daily for 5 to 10 days and until complete lesion resolution in immunocompromised patients (AST-IDCOP [Lee 2019]; HHS [OI adult 2020]; Klein 2020)

IV (for severe disease in immunocompromised patients): 5 mg/kg/dose every 8 hours; switch to oral acyclovir (or similar antiviral) once lesions begin to regress and continue until complete resolution (AST-IDCOP [Lee 2019]; HHS [OI adult 2020]).

Suppressive therapy (eg, for severe and/or frequent recurrences): **Oral:** 400 mg twice daily (HHS [OI adult 2020]; Rooney 1993). **Note:** Reassess need periodically (eg, annually) (HHS [OI adult 2020]).

Herpes simplex virus, prevention in immunocompromised patients (off-label use):

Seropositive hematopoietic cell transplant recipients (allogeneic or autologous) or seropositive patients undergoing leukemia induction chemotherapy:

IV: 250 mg/m^2/dose every 12 hours (ASBMT/IDSA [Tomblyn 2009])

Oral: 400 to 800 mg twice daily (ASBMT/IDSA [Tomblyn 2009])

Note: Initiate with the chemotherapeutic or conditioning regimen and continue until recovery of WBC count and resolution of mucositis; duration may be extended in patients with frequent recurrences or graft-vs-host disease (ASBMT/IDSA [Tomblyn 2009]; ASCO/IDSA [Taplitz 2018]).

Solid organ transplant recipients (HSV-seropositive patients who do **not** require CMV prophylaxis): **Oral:** 400 to 800 mg twice daily for ≥1 month (AST-IDCOP [Lee 2019]); some experts recommend continuing for 3 to 6 months after transplantation and during periods of lymphodepletion associated with treatment of rejection (Fishman 2020).

Herpes zoster (shingles), treatment:

Immunocompetent patients: **Oral:** 800 mg 5 times daily for 7 days (Pott Junior 2018; Shafran 2004). Initiate at earliest sign or symptom; treatment is most effective when initiated ≤72 hours after rash onset, but may initiate treatment >72 hours after rash onset if new lesions are continuing to appear (Cohen 1999).

Immunocompromised patients (including patients with HIV):

Acute localized dermatomal: **Oral:** 800 mg 5 times daily for 7 to 10 days; consider longer duration if lesions resolve slowly (AST-IDCOP [Pergam 2019]; HHS [OI adult 2020]).

Extensive cutaneous lesions or visceral involvement: **IV:** 10 mg/kg/dose every 8 hours (AST-IDCOP [Pergam 2019]; HHS [OI adult 2020]). When formation of new lesions has ceased and signs/symptoms of visceral infection are improving, switch to an oral antiviral to complete a total of 10 to 14 days of therapy (HHS [OI adult 2020]).

Herpes zoster ophthalmicus (off-label use): Immunocompromised patients or patients who require hospitalization for sight-threatening disease: **IV:** 10 mg/kg/dose every 8 hours for 7 days (Albrecht 2020a)

Varicella (chickenpox), treatment: Ideally initiate therapy within 24 hours of symptom onset, but may start later if the patient still has active lesions:

Immunocompetent patients with uncomplicated infection: **Oral:** 800 mg 5 times daily for ≥5 to 7 days and until all lesions have crusted (Albrecht 2020b; Arvin 1996; Wallace 1992)

Immunocompromised patients (including patients with HIV):

Severe or complicated infection: **IV:** 10 mg/kg/dose every 8 hours for 7 to 10 days (AST-IDCOP [Pergam 2019]; HHS [OI adult 2020]). May switch to oral antiviral after defervescence if no evidence of visceral involvement; continue until all lesions have crusted (AST-IDCOP [Pergam 2019]; HHS [OI adult 2020]).

Uncomplicated infection: **Oral:** 800 mg 5 times daily for 5 to 7 days (HHS [OI adult 2020]); some experts recommend a minimum duration of 7 days, extending the course until all lesions have crusted (AST-IDCOP [Pergam 2019]).

Varicella zoster virus, acute retinal necrosis (off-label use): IV: 10 mg/kg/dose every 8 hours for 10 to 14 days, followed by ~6 weeks of valacyclovir (Albrecht 2020a; HHS [OI adult 2020]); in patients with HIV, intravitreal ganciclovir should be added (HHS [OI adult 2020]).

Varicella zoster virus, encephalitis (off-label use): IV: 10 to 15 mg/kg/dose every 8 hours for 10 to 14 days (IDSA [Tunkel 2008])

Varicella zoster virus, prevention in immunocompromised patients (off-label use):

Seropositive hematopoietic cell transplant recipients (allogeneic and autologous): **Oral:** 800 mg twice daily (ASBMT/IDSA [Tomblyn 2009]; Boeckh 2006). **Note:** Initiate with the chemotherapeutic or conditioning regimen and continue for 1 year; may extend duration in patients requiring ongoing immunosuppression (some experts continue prophylaxis in these patients until 6 months after discontinuation of all systemic immunosuppression) (ASBMT/IDSA [Tomblyn 2009]).

Solid organ transplant recipients (VZV-seropositive patients who do **not** require CMV prophylaxis): **Oral:** 200 mg 3 to 5 times daily for 3 to 6 months after transplantation and during periods of lymphodepletion associated with treatment of rejection (AST-IDCOP [Pergam 2019]; Fishman 2020).

Geriatric Refer to adult dosing; use with caution.

Renal Impairment: Adult Note: Monitor closely for neurotoxicity (Chowdhury 2016)

Note: The manufacturer's labeling dosing adjustments are reported as mL/minute/1.73 m^2 based on data using CrCl adjusted for BSA (Blum 1982; de Miranda 1983).

Oral:

CrCl >25 mL/minute/1.73 m^2: No dosage adjustment necessary.

CrCl 10 to 25 mL/minute/1.73 m^2: If the usual recommended dose is 800 mg 5 times daily: Administer 800 mg every 8 hours

CrCl <10 mL/minute/1.73 m^2:

If the usual recommended dose is 200 mg 5 times daily or 400 mg every 12 hours: Administer 200 mg every 12 hours

If the usual recommended dose is 800 mg 5 times daily: Administer 200 mg every 12 hours (IDSA [Gupta 2005])

Intermittent hemodialysis (IHD): Dialyzable (60% reduction following a 6-hour session):

Note: Dosing dependent on the assumption of 3-times-weekly, complete IHD sessions. Administer after hemodialysis on dialysis days.

If the usual recommended dose is 200 mg 5 times daily or 400 mg every 12 hours: Administer 200 mg every 12 hours

If the usual recommended dose is 800 mg 5 times daily: Administer a loading dose of 400 mg and a maintenance dose of 200 mg twice daily plus a single 400 mg dose after each dialysis (Almond 1995). **Note:** Dose based on pharmacokinetic data and computer modeling.

Continuous ambulatory peritoneal dialysis (CAPD): 600 to 800 mg daily (Stathoulopoulou 1996)

IV:

If the usual recommended dose is 10 mg/kg/dose every 8 hours:

CrCl >50 mL/minute/1.73 m^2: No dosage adjustment necessary.

CrCl 25 to 50 mL/minute/1.73 m^2: 10 mg/kg/dose every 12 hours

CrCl 10 to <25 mL/minute/1.73 m^2: 10 mg/kg/dose every 24 hours

CrCl <10 mL/minute/1.73 m^2: 5 mg/kg/dose every 24 hours

If the usual recommended dose is 5 mg/kg/dose every 8 hours:

CrCl >50 mL/minute/1.73 m^2: No dosage adjustment necessary.

CrCl 25 to 50 mL/minute/1.73 m^2: 5 mg/kg/dose every 12 hours

CrCl 10 to <25 mL/minute/1.73 m^2: 5 mg/kg/dose every 24 hours

CrCl <10 mL/minute/1.73 m^2: 2.5 mg/kg/dose every 24 hours

Intermittent hemodialysis (IHD): Dialyzable (60% reduction following a 6-hour session): 2.5 to 5 mg/kg/dose every 24 hours (Heintz 2009). **Note:** Use higher end of dosing range for viral meningoencephalitis and varicella-zoster infections. Dosing dependent on the assumption of 3-times-weekly, complete IHD sessions. Administer after hemodialysis on dialysis days

Peritoneal dialysis (PD): 2.5 to 5 mg/kg/dose every 24 hours; no supplemental dose needed (Aronoff 2007). **Note:** Use higher end of dosing range for viral meningoencephalitis and varicella-zoster infections.

Continuous renal replacement therapy (CRRT) (Heintz 2009): Drug clearance is highly dependent on the method of renal replacement, filter type, and flow rate. Appropriate dosing requires close monitoring of pharmacologic response, signs of adverse reactions due to drug accumulation, as well as drug concentrations in relation to target trough (if appropriate). The following are general recommendations only (based on dialysate flow/ultrafiltration rates of 1 to 2 L/hour and minimal residual renal function) and should not supersede clinical judgment:

CVVH: 5 to 10 mg/kg/dose every 24 hours

CVVHD/CVVHDF: 5 to 10 mg/kg/dose every 12 to 24 hours

Note: The higher end of dosage range is recommended for viral meningoencephalitis and varicella-zoster virus infections.

Hepatic Impairment: Adult Oral, IV: There are no dosage adjustments provided in the manufacturer's labeling; use caution in patients with severe impairment.

Obesity: Adult IV: In obese patients, acyclovir IV has been dosed using ideal body weight (IBW) to avoid overdosing and subsequent toxicity. However, in a pharmacokinetic study using a single acyclovir IV dose, morbidly obese patients (BMI ≥40 kg/m^2) dosed using IBW had lower systemic exposures compared to normal weight subjects dosed using actual body weight (exposure based on AUC, C_{max}, and T > IC_{50} [time the drug concentration remains above the 50% inhibitory concentration]) (Turner 2016). Therefore, to avoid potentially underdosing obese patients who are severely ill (eg, HSV encephalitis), some clinicians use adjusted body weight (AjBW) to determine the IV dose (AjBW=IBW + [0.4 x (actual body weight-IBW)]) (Wong 2017), although this approach has not been evaluated in clinical studies.

Pediatric Note: Obese patients should be dosed using ideal body weight. Parenteral IV doses >15 mg/kg/dose or 500 mg/**m^2** may be associated with an increased risk of nephrotoxicity; close monitoring of renal function is recommended (Rao 2015).

Cytomegalovirus (CMV) prophylaxis: Low-risk allogeneic hematopoietic stem cell transplant (HSCT) in seropositive recipient. **Note:** Begin at engraftment and continue to day 100; requires close monitoring for CMV reactivation (due to weak activity); not for use in patients at high risk for CMV disease (Tomblyn 2009):

Oral:

Infants, Children, and Adolescents <40 kg: 600 mg/**m^2**/dose 4 times daily; maximum dose: 800 mg/dose.

Children and Adolescents ≥40 kg: 800 mg 4 times daily.

IV: Infants, Children, and Adolescents: 500 mg/**m^2**/dose every 8 hours.

Varicella zoster virus, acute retinal necrosis, treatment (HIV-exposed/-infected):

Initial treatment: **Note:** Follow up IV therapy with oral valacyclovir or acyclovir therapy (valacyclovir preferred) (HHS [OI adult 2020]; HHS [OI pediatric 2019]).

Infants and Children: IV: 10 to 15 mg/kg/dose every 8 hours for 10 to 14 days (HHS [OI pediatric 2019]).

Adolescents: IV: 10 mg/kg/dose every 8 hours for 10 to 14 days; recommended to be used in combination with 1 to 2 doses of intravitreal ganciclovir (HHS [OI adult 2020]).

Maintenance treatment (alternative to valacyclovir): Infants and Children: Oral: 20 mg/kg/dose 4 times daily for 4 to 6 weeks to begin after 10- to 14-day course of IV acyclovir (HHS [OI pediatric 2019]).

Herpes zoster (shingles), treatment:

Immunocompetent host:

Ambulatory therapy: Children ≥12 years and Adolescents: Oral: 800 mg every 4 hours (5 doses per day) for 5 to 7 days (*Red Book* [AAP 2018]).

Hospitalized patient:

Infants and Children <2 years: IV: 10 mg/kg/dose every 8 hours for 7 to 10 days (*Red Book* [AAP 2018]).

Children ≥2 years and Adolescents: IV: 500 mg/**m^2**/dose every 8 hours for 7 to 10 days; some experts recommend 10 mg/kg/dose every 8 hours (*Red Book* [AAP 2018]).

Immunocompromised host (non-HIV-exposed/-infected): IV: Infants, Children, and Adolescents: 10 mg/kg/dose every 8 hours for 7 to 10 days (*Red Book* [AAP 2018]).

HIV-exposed/-infected:

Mild, uncomplicated disease and no or moderate immune suppression:

Infants and Children: Oral: 20 mg/kg/dose 4 times daily for 7 to 10 days; maximum dose: 800 mg/dose; consider longer course if resolution of lesions is slow (HHS [OI pediatric 2019]).

Adolescents (alternative therapy): Oral: 800 mg 5 times daily for 7 to 10 days, longer if lesions resolve slowly (HHS [OI adult 2020]).

Severe immune suppression or complicated disease; trigeminal nerve involvement, extensive multidermatomal zoster or extensive cutaneous lesions or visceral involvement:

Infants: IV: 10 mg/kg/dose every 8 hours until resolution of cutaneous lesions and visceral disease clearly begins, then convert to oral therapy to complete a 10- to 14-day total course of therapy (HHS [OI pediatric 2019]).

Children: IV: 10 mg/kg/dose **or** 500 mg/**m^2**/dose every 8 hours until resolution of cutaneous lesions and visceral disease clearly begins, then convert to oral therapy to complete a 10- to 14-day total course of therapy (HHS [OI pediatric 2019]).

Adolescents: IV: 10 mg/kg/dose every 8 hours until clinical improvement is evident, then convert to oral therapy to complete a 10- to 14-day total course of therapy (HHS [OI adult 2020]).

Herpes simplex virus (HSV) neonatal infection, treatment and suppressive therapy in very young infants (independent of HIV status):

Treatment (disseminated, CNS, or skin, eye, or mouth disease): Infants 1 to 3 months: IV: 20 mg/kg/dose every 8 hours; treatment duration: For cutaneous and mucous membrane infections (skin, eye, or mouth): 14 days; for CNS or disseminated infection: 21 days (AAP [Kimberlin 2013]; Bradley 2019; CDC [Workowski 2015]; HHS [OI pediatric 2019]; *Red Book* [AAP 2018]).

Chronic suppressive therapy following any neonatal HSV infection: Infants: Oral: 300 mg/**m^2**/dose every 8 hours for 6 months; begin after completion of a 14- to 21-day-course of IV therapy dependent upon type of infection (AAP [Kimberlin 2013]; Bradley 2019; Kimberlin 2011; *Red Book* [AAP 2018]).

HSV encephalitis, treatment:

Independent of HIV status:

Infants and Children 3 months to <12 years: IV: 10 to 15 mg/kg/dose every 8 hours for 14 to 21 days. **Note:** Due to increased risk of neurotoxicity and nephrotoxicity, higher doses (20 mg/kg) are not routinely recommended (Bradley 2019; HHS [OI pediatric 2019]; *Red Book* [AAP 2018]).

Children ≥12 years and Adolescents: IV: 10 mg/kg/dose every 8 hours for 14 to 21 days (HHS [OI pediatric 2019]; *Red Book* [AAP 2018]).

HSV genital infection:

First infection, mild to moderate:

Non-HIV-exposed/-infected:

Children <12 years: Oral: 40 to 80 mg/kg/**day** divided in 3 to 4 doses per day for 7 to 10 days; maximum daily dose: 1,200 mg/**day** (Bradley 2019; *Red Book* [AAP 2018]).

Children and Adolescents ≥12 years: Oral: 200 mg every 4 hours while awake (5 times daily) **or** 400 mg 3 times daily for 7 to 10 days; treatment can be extended beyond 10 days if healing is not complete (CDC [Workowski 2015]; *Red Book* [AAP 2018]).

HIV-exposed/-infected:

Children: Oral: 20 mg/kg/dose 3 times daily for 7 to 10 days; maximum dose: 400 mg/dose (HHS [OI pediatric 2019]).

Adolescents: Oral: 400 mg 3 times daily for 5 to 10 days (HHS [OI adult 2020]).

First infection, severe (independent of HIV status): IV: Children and Adolescents ≥12 years: 5 mg/kg/dose every 8 hours for 5 to 7 days **or** 5 to 10 mg/kg/dose every 8 hours for 2 to 7 days, followed with oral therapy to complete at least 10 days of therapy (CDC [Workowski 2015]; *Red Book* [AAP 2018]).

Recurrent infection:

Children <12 years (independent of HIV status): Oral: 20 mg/kg/dose 3 times daily for 5 days; maximum dose: 400 mg/dose (Bradley 2019; HHS [OI pediatric 2019]).

Children and Adolescents ≥12 years:

Non-HIV-exposed/-infected: Oral: 200 mg every 4 hours while awake (5 times daily) for 5 days, **or** 400 mg 3 times daily for 5 days, **or** 800 mg twice daily for 5 days **or** 800 mg 3 times daily for 2 days (CDC [Workowski 2015]; *Red Book* [AAP 2018]).

HIV-exposed/-positive: Adolescents: Oral: 400 mg 3 times daily for 5 to 10 days (HHS [OI adult 2020]).

Suppression, chronic:

Non-HIV-exposed/-infected:

Children <12 years: Limited data available: Oral: 20 mg/kg/dose twice daily; maximum dose: 400 mg/dose (Bradley 2019).

Children and Adolescents ≥12 years: Oral: 400 mg twice daily; reassess therapy after 12 months (Bradley 2019; CDC [Workowski 2015]; *Red Book* [AAP 2018]).

HIV-exposed/-infected:

Infants and Children: Oral: 20 mg/kg/dose twice daily; maximum dose: 800 mg/dose (HHS [OI pediatric 2019]).

Adolescents: Oral: 400 mg twice daily (HHS [OI adult 2020]).

HSV orolabial disease (ie, gingivostomatitis, herpes labialis):

Non-HIV-exposed/-infected: Primary infection: Infants, Children, and Adolescents: Oral: 20 mg/kg/dose 4 times daily for 5 to 7 days; usual maximum dose: 800 mg/dose (Bradley 2019; Cernik 2008; *Red Book* [AAP 2018]).

HIV-exposed/-infected (HHS [OI pediatric 2019]):

Mild, symptomatic:

Infants and Children: Oral: 20 mg/kg/dose 4 times daily for 7 to 10 days; maximum dose: 400 mg/dose.

Adolescents: Oral: 400 mg 3 times daily for 5 to 10 days (HHS [OI adult 2020]).

Moderate to severe, symptomatic: **Note:** Switch to oral therapy once lesions begin to regress and continue oral therapy until lesions completely healed.

Infants and Children: IV: 5 to 10 mg/kg/dose every 8 hours.

Adolescents: IV: 5 mg/kg/dose every 8 hours.

HSV mucocutaneous infection:

Immunocompetent host: Infants, Children, and Adolescents:

Treatment:

IV: 5 mg/kg/dose every 8 hours (Bradley 2019).

Oral: 20 mg/kg/dose 4 times daily for 5 to 7 days; maximum dose: 800 mg/dose (Bradley 2019; *Red Book* [AAP 2018]).

Suppression, chronic: Limited data available; no pediatric data; some experts recommend oral 20 mg/kg/dose 2 to 3 times daily for 6 to 12 months, then reevaluate need; maximum dose: 400 mg/dose (Bradley 2019).

Immunocompromised host:

Treatment:

IV:

Infants and Children: IV: 10 mg/kg/dose every 8 hours for 7 to 14 days (*Red Book* [AAP 2018]).

Adolescents: IV: 5 to 10 mg/kg/dose every 8 hours; change to oral therapy after lesions begin to regress (HHS [OI adult 2020]; *Red Book* [AAP 2018]).

Oral: Children ≥2 years and Adolescents: 1,000 mg/**day** in 3 to 5 divided doses for 7 to 14 days (*Red Book* [AAP 2018]).

Suppression, chronic (cutaneous, ocular) episodes:

Non-HIV-exposed/-infected:

Children ≥12 years and Adolescents: Oral: 400 mg twice daily; reassess at 12 months (*Red Book* [AAP 2018]).

HIV-exposed/-infected:

Infants and Children: Oral: 20 mg/kg/dose twice daily; maximum dose: 800 mg/dose; reassess after 12 months (HHS [OI pediatric 2019]).

Adolescents: Oral: 400 mg twice daily; reassess at 12 months (HHS [OI adult 2020]).

HSV progressive or disseminated infection, treatment (immunocompromised host):

Non-HIV-exposed/-infected: Infants, Children, and Adolescents: IV: 10 mg/kg/dose every 8 hours for 7 to 14 days (*Red Book* [AAP 2018]).

HIV-exposed/-infected: Infants, Children, and Adolescents: IV: 10 mg/kg/dose every 8 hours for 21 days; higher doses (up to 20 mg/kg/dose) may be used in children <12 years of age (HHS [OI pediatric 2019]; *Red Book* [AAP 2018]).

HSV, acute retinal necrosis, treatment (HIV-exposed/-infected): Infants and Children (HHS [OI pediatric 2019]):

Initial treatment: IV: 10 to 15 mg/kg/dose every 8 hours for 10 to 14 days. **Note:** Follow up IV therapy with oral acyclovir or valacyclovir maintenance therapy.

Maintenance treatment (alternative to valacyclovir): Begin after 10- to 14-day course of IV acyclovir: Oral: 20 mg/kg/dose 4 times daily for 4 to 6 weeks.

HSV prophylaxis; immunocompromised hosts, seropositive:

HSCT in seropositive recipient (Tomblyn 2009):

Prevention of early reactivation: **Note:** Begin at conditioning and continue until engraftment or resolution of mucositis; whichever is longer (~30 days post-HSCT)

Infants, Children, and Adolescents <40 kg:

IV: 250 mg/$\mathbf{m^2}$/dose every 8 hours **or** 125 mg/$\mathbf{m^2}$/dose every 6 hours; maximum daily dose: 80 mg/kg/**day**

Oral: 60 to 90 mg/kg/**day** in 2 to 3 divided doses; maximum dose: 800 mg/dose twice daily

Children and Adolescents ≥40 kg:
IV: 250 mg/**m²**/dose every 12 hours
Oral: 400 to 800 mg twice daily
Prevention of late reactivation: **Note:** Treatment during first year after HSCT.
Infants, Children, and Adolescents <40 kg: Oral: 60 to 90 mg/kg/**day** in 2 to 3 divided doses; maximum daily dose: 800 mg twice daily
Children and Adolescents ≥40 kg: Oral: 800 mg twice daily
Other immunocompromised hosts who are HSV seropositive:
IV: Infants, Children, and Adolescents: 5 mg/kg/dose every 8 hours during period of risk (*Red Book* [AAP 2018]).
Oral: Children ≥2 years and Adolescents: 200 mg every 4 hours while awake (5 doses daily) **or** 200 mg every 8 hours; administer during periods of risk (*Red Book* [AAP 2018]).

Varicella (chickenpox) or Herpes zoster (shingles), prophylaxis
HSCT: Prophylaxis of disease reactivation: **Note:** Continue therapy for 1 year after HSCT (Tomblyn 2009):
Infants, Children, and Adolescents <40 kg: Oral: 60 to 80 mg/kg/day in 2 to 3 divided doses
Children and Adolescents ≥40 kg: Oral: 800 mg twice daily
HIV-exposed/-infected: Limited data available: **Note:** Consider use if >96 hours postexposure or if VZV-immune globulin is not available; begin therapy 7 to 10 days after exposure; some experts begin therapy at first appearance of rash (HHS [OI pediatric 2019]).
Infants and Children: Oral: 20 mg/kg/dose 4 times daily for 7 days; maximum dose: 800 mg/dose (HHS [OI pediatric 2019]).
Adolescents: Oral: 800 mg 5 times daily for 5 to 7 days (HHS [OI adult 2020]).
Other immunocompromised hosts: Infants, Children, and Adolescents: Oral: 20 mg/kg/dose 4 times daily for 7 days; maximum dose: 800 mg/dose. **Note:** Consider use if VZV-immune globulin or IVIG is not available; begin therapy 7 to 10 days after exposure (*Red Book* [AAP 2018]).

Varicella (chickenpox), treatment: Begin treatment within the first 24 hours of rash onset:
Immunocompetent host:
Ambulatory therapy: Oral: Infants, Children, and Adolescents: 20 mg/kg/dose 4 times daily for 5 days; maximum daily dose: 3,200 mg/**day** (Bradley 2019; *Red Book* [AAP 2018]).
Hospitalized patient: IV: Infants, Children, and Adolescents: 10 mg/kg/dose **or** 500 mg/**m²**/dose every 8 hours for 7 to 14 days (Bradley 2019; *Red Book* [AAP 2018]); some experts recommend 15 to 20 mg/kg/dose for severe disseminated or CNS infection (Bradley 2019).
Immunocompromised host (non-HIV-exposed/-infected):
Infants and Children <2 years: IV: 10 mg/kg/dose every 8 hours; duration dependent upon clinical response, typically 7 to 14 days (Bradley 2019; *Red Book* [AAP 2018]).
Children ≥2 years and Adolescents: IV: 500 mg/**m²**/dose every 8 hours duration dependent upon clinical response, typically 7 to 14 days; some experts recommend 10 mg/kg/dose every 8 hours (Bradley 2019; *Red Book* [AAP 2018]).
HIV-exposed/-infected:
Mild, uncomplicated disease and no or moderate immune suppression:
Infants and Children: Oral: 20 mg/kg/dose 4 times daily for 7 to 10 days and until no new lesions for 48 hours; maximum dose: 800 mg/dose (HHS [OI pediatric 2019]).
Adolescents (alternative therapy): Oral: 800 mg 5 times daily for 5 to 7 days (HHS [OI adult 2020]).
Severe, complicated disease or severe immune suppression:
Infants: IV: 10 mg/kg/dose every 8 hours for 7 to 10 days and until no new lesions for 48 hours (HHS [OI pediatric 2019]).
Children: IV: 10 mg/kg/dose or 500 mg/m²/dose every 8 hours for 7 to 10 days or until no new lesions for 48 hours (HHS [OI pediatric 2019]).
Adolescents: IV: 10 mg/kg/dose every 8 hours for 7 to 10 days; may convert to oral therapy after defervescence and if no evidence of visceral involvement is evident (HHS [OI adult 2020]).

Renal Impairment: Pediatric
Monitor closely for neurotoxicity (Chowdhury 2016).
Infants, Children and Adolescents: IV:
CrCl >50 mL/minute/1.73 m²: No dosage adjustment necessary
CrCl 25 to 50 mL/minute/1.73 m²: Administer the usual recommended dose every 12 hours
CrCl 10 to <25 mL/minute/1.73 m²: Administer the usual recommended dose every 24 hours
CrCl <10 mL/minute/1.73 m²: Administer 50% of the usual recommended dose every 24 hours (eg, if the usual recommended dose is 10 mg/kg/dose every 8 hours, then administer 5 mg/kg/dose every 24 hours)
Intermittent hemodialysis (IHD): Dialyzable (60% reduction following a 6-hour session): 5 mg/kg/dose every 24 hours; administer after hemodialysis on dialysis days (Aronoff 2007)
Peritoneal dialysis (PD): 5 mg/kg/dose every 24 hours; no supplemental dose needed (Aronoff 2007)
Continuous renal replacement therapy (CRRT): 10 mg/kg/dose every 12 hours (Aronoff 2007)

Hepatic Impairment: Pediatric There are no dosage adjustments provided in the manufacturer's labeling.

Mechanism of Action Acyclovir is converted to acyclovir monophosphate by virus-specific thymidine kinase then further converted to acyclovir triphosphate by other cellular enzymes. Acyclovir triphosphate inhibits DNA synthesis and viral replication by competing with deoxyguanosine triphosphate for viral DNA polymerase and being incorporated into viral DNA.

Contraindications Hypersensitivity to acyclovir, valacyclovir, or any component of the formulation

Warnings/Precautions Neurotoxicity (eg, tremor/myoclonus, confusion, agitation, lethargy, hallucination, impaired consciousness) has been reported; risk may be increased with higher doses and in patients with renal failure. Monitor patients for signs/symptoms of neurotoxicity; ensure appropriate dosage reductions in patients with renal impairment (Chowdhury 2016). Use with caution in immunocompromised patients; thrombotic microangiopathy has been reported. Use caution in the elderly or preexisting renal disease (may require dosage modification). Renal failure (sometimes fatal) has been reported. Maintain adequate hydration during oral or IV therapy. Use IV preparation with caution in patients with underlying neurologic abnormalities, serious hepatic or electrolyte abnormalities, or substantial hypoxia. Encephalopathic changes characterized by lethargy, obtundation, confusion, hallucination, tremors, agitation, seizure, or coma have been observed in patients receiving IV acyclovir. Acyclovir IV is an irritant (depending on concentration); avoid extravasation. Potentially significant drug-drug interactions may exist, requiring dose or frequency adjustment, additional monitoring, and/or selection of alternative therapy.

Varicella: For maximum benefit, treatment should begin within 24 hours of appearance of rash; oral route not recommended for routine use in otherwise healthy children with varicella but may be effective in patients at increased risk of moderate to severe infection (>12 years of age, chronic cutaneous or pulmonary disorders, long-term salicylate therapy, corticosteroid therapy).

Warnings: Additional Pediatric Considerations Acyclovir can cause intrarenal obstructive nephropathy, interstitial nephritis, and tubular necrosis resulting in significant renal insufficiency. In one study, 35% (131/373 courses) in 371 pediatric patients treated with IV acyclovir mostly for meningoencephalitis were observed to have renal dysfunction. Renal dysfunction typically occurred within 48 hours of initiation and was reversible in most cases after dosage reduction or discontinuation, although in some instances, return to baseline was not observed. Analysis of the degree of dysfunction based on percent reduction of estimated GFR (eGFR) showed that of the 373 acyclovir courses, 22% (81/373) had an eGFR reduction of 25% to 49%, renal injury (defined as a 50% to 75% reduction in eGFR) in 9.7% (36/373), and renal failure (eGFR reduction >75%) in 3.8% (14/373). Doses >500 mg/m^2 were significantly associated with all levels of nephrotoxicity and acyclovir doses >15 mg/kg were significantly associated with a 25% to 49% reduction in eGFR. Statistically significant risk factors for renal failure identified through univariate analysis were age >8 years, weight >20 kg, BMI >19 kg/m^2, and concurrent ceftriaxone with or without gadolinium. Associations of other antibiotics and contrast agents were not statistically significant. Monitor renal function during therapy, particularly for high doses and in older pediatric patients (>8 years). Outside of the neonatal period, reduced dosing or use of mg/m^2 dosing in larger children may need to be considered; further studies are necessary (Rao 2015).

Drug Interactions

Metabolism/Transport Effects **Inhibits** CYP1A2 (weak)

Avoid Concomitant Use

Avoid concomitant use of Acyclovir (Systemic) with any of the following: Cladribine; Foscarnet; Varicella Virus Vaccine; Zoster Vaccine (Live/Attenuated)

Increased Effect/Toxicity

Acyclovir (Systemic) may increase the levels/effects of: CloZAPine; Mycophenolate; Tenofovir Products; Theophylline Derivatives; TiZANidine; Zidovudine

The levels/effects of Acyclovir (Systemic) may be increased by: Foscarnet; Mycophenolate; Tenofovir Products

Decreased Effect

Acyclovir (Systemic) may decrease the levels/effects of: Cladribine; Talimogene Laherparepvec; Varicella Virus Vaccine; Zoster Vaccine (Live/Attenuated)

Dietary Considerations Some products may contain sodium.

Pharmacodynamics/Kinetics

Half-life Elimination Half-life elimination: Terminal: Neonates and Infants ≤3 months: 3.8 ± 1.19 hours; Infants >3 months to Children ≤12 years: 2.36 ± 0.97 hours; Adults: ~2.5 hours (with normal renal function); 20 hours (ESRD) (Gorlitsky 2017); Hemodialysis: ~5 hours

Pregnancy Considerations Acyclovir has been shown to cross the human placenta (Henderson 1992).

Results from a pregnancy registry, established in 1984 and closed in 1999, did not find an increase in the number of birth defects with exposure to acyclovir when compared to those expected in the general population. However, due to the small size of the registry and lack of long-term data, the manufacturer recommends using during pregnancy with caution and only when clearly needed. Acyclovir is recommended for the treatment of genital herpes in pregnant patients (ACOG 2007; CDC [Workowski 2015]).

Breastfeeding Considerations Acyclovir is present in breast milk.

The relative infant dose (RID) of acyclovir is 1.83% to 3.65% when calculated using the highest breast milk concentration located and compared to an IV infant therapeutic dose of 30 to 60 mg/kg/day.

In general, breastfeeding is considered acceptable when the RID of a medication is <10% (Anderson 2016; Ito 2000).

The RID of acyclovir was calculated using a milk concentration of 7.3 mcg/mL, providing an estimated daily infant dose via breast milk of 1.095 mg/kg/day. This milk concentration was obtained following maternal administration acyclovir 900 mg IV daily for 5 days (Bork 1995). The mean half-life of acyclovir in breast milk was 3.2 hours in one study (Lau 1987); acyclovir was measurable in breast milk for up to 88 hours after the last maternal dose in another (Bork 1995). Acyclovir has been detected in the urine of a breastfeeding infant (Lau 1987).

In one case report, the mother reported no adverse events in her exclusively breastfed infant following a maternal dose of acyclovir 800 mg orally 5 times daily for 7 days (Taddio 1994).

Acyclovir is considered compatible with breastfeeding (WHO 2002). Acyclovir may be used for the treatment of genital herpes in breastfeeding women (ACOG 2007; CDC [Workowski 2015]). The manufacturer recommends that caution be exercised when administering acyclovir to breastfeeding women. Breastfeeding mothers with herpetic lesions near or on the breast should avoid breastfeeding (Gartner 2005); precautions should be taken to prevent infant contact with active lesions (ACOG 2007).

Dosage Forms: US

Capsule, Oral:

Generic: 200 mg

Solution, Intravenous:

Generic: 50 mg/mL (20 mL)

Solution, Intravenous [preservative free]:

Generic: 50 mg/mL (10 mL, 20 mL)

Suspension, Oral:

Zovirax: 200 mg/5 mL (473 mL)

Generic: 200 mg/5 mL (473 mL)

Tablet, Oral:

Generic: 400 mg, 800 mg

Dosage Forms: Canada

Solution, Intravenous:

Generic: 25 mg/mL (20 mL); 50 mg/mL (10 mL, 20 mL)

Suspension, Oral:

Zovirax: 200 mg/5 mL (125 mL)

Tablet, Oral:

Generic: 200 mg, 400 mg, 800 mg

Dental Health Professional Considerations

Although some conflicting data, dental treatment may be a risk factor for asymptomatic viral shedding of herpes simplex virus type-1 (HSV-1) into human saliva in patients with previous exposure to the virus (Hyland 2007).

It is recommended to reappoint the patient if an active lesion is present. If the lesion is already "crusted" over, treatment will not induce spread of the virus but treatment is aimed at patient comfort during the procedure relating to the wound healing on their lip.

Acyclovir (Topical) (ay SYE kloe veer)

Related Information

Systemic Viral Diseases *on page 1709*

Viral Infections *on page 1754*

Related Sample Prescriptions

Viral Infections - Sample Prescriptions *on page 43*

Brand Names: US Sitavig; Zovirax

Brand Names: Canada APO-Acyclovir; Zovirax

Generic Availability (US) May be product dependent

Pharmacologic Category Antiviral Agent, Topical

Dental Use Treatment of initial and prophylaxis of recurrent mucosal and cutaneous herpes simplex (HSV-1 and HSV-2) infections in immunocompromised patients

Use Herpes virus:

Buccal tablet: Treatment of recurrent herpes labialis (cold sores) in immunocompetent adults

Cream: Treatment of recurrent herpes labialis (cold sores) in immunocompetent children ≥12 years of age, adolescents, and adults

Ointment: Management of limited non-life-threatening mucocutaneous herpes simplex virus infections in immunocompromised patients

Local Anesthetic/Vasoconstrictor Precautions No information available to require special precautions

Effects on Dental Treatment Key adverse event(s) related to dental treatment: Topical (Zovirax cream): Dry/cracked lips and dry/flaky skin were reported in fewer than 1 in 100 patients in clinical studies.

Effects on Bleeding No information available to require special precautions

Adverse Reactions

>10%: Dermatologic: Local pain (ointment 30%; mild; includes transient burning and stinging)

1% to 10%:

Central nervous system: Lethargy (buccal tablet 1%)

Dermatologic: Erythema (buccal tablet 1%), skin rash (buccal tablet 1%)

Gastrointestinal: Aphthous stomatitis (buccal tablet 1%), gingival pain (buccal tablet 1%)

Local: Application site reaction (cream 5%; including dry lips, desquamation, dryness of skin, cracked lips, burning skin, pruritus, flakiness of skin, and stinging on skin); application site irritation (buccal tablet 1%)

<1%, postmarketing, and/or case reports: Anaphylaxis, angioedema, contact dermatitis, eczema, localized edema, local pruritus, pruritus

Dental Usual Dosage

Herpes labialis (cold sores): Children ≥12 years and Adults: Topical: Cream: Apply 5 times/day for 4 days

Mucocutaneous HSV: Adults: Nonlife-threatening, immunocompromised: Topical: Ointment: 1/2" ribbon of ointment for a 4" square surface area every 3 hours (6 times/day) for 7 days

Dosing

Adult & Geriatric

Herpes labialis (cold sores), recurrent:

Topical cream: Apply 5 times daily for 4 days

Buccal tablet: Apply one 50 mg tablet as a single dose to the upper gum region (canine fossa)

HSV, mucocutaneous (non-life-threatening, immunocompromised): Topical ointment: 1/2" ribbon of ointment for a 4" square surface area every 3 hours (6 times daily) for 7 days

Renal Impairment: Adult There are no dosage adjustments provided in the manufacturer's labeling. However, dosage adjustment is unlikely due to low systemic absorption.

Hepatic Impairment: Adult There are no dosage adjustments provided in the manufacturer's labeling. However, dosage adjustment is unlikely due to low systemic absorption.

Pediatric Herpes labialis (cold sores): Topical cream: Children ≥12 years and Adolescents: Apply 5 times/day for 4 days

Renal Impairment: Pediatric There are no dosage adjustments provided in the manufacturer's labeling; however, dosage adjustment is unlikely due to low systemic absorption.

Hepatic Impairment: Pediatric There are no dosage adjustments provided in the manufacturer's labeling; however, dosage adjustment is unlikely due to low systemic absorption.

Mechanism of Action Acyclovir is converted to acyclovir monophosphate by virus-specific thymidine kinase then further converted to acyclovir triphosphate by other cellular enzymes. Acyclovir triphosphate inhibits DNA synthesis and viral replication by competing with deoxyguanosine triphosphate for viral DNA polymerase and being incorporated into viral DNA.

Contraindications

Hypersensitivity to acyclovir, valacyclovir, or any component of the formulation

Buccal tablet: Additional contraindications: Hypersensitivity to milk protein concentrate

Warnings/Precautions Genital herpes: Physical contact should be avoided when lesions are present; transmission may also occur in the absence of symptoms. Treatment should begin with the first signs or symptoms. There are no data to support the use of acyclovir ointment to prevent transmission of infection to other persons or prevent recurrent infections if no signs or symptoms are present.

Herpes labialis: Treatment should begin with the first signs or symptoms. Cream is for external use only to the lips and face; do not apply to eye or inside the mouth or nose, or any mucous membranes. Ointment should also not be used in the eye and be used with caution in immunocompromised patients. Cream may be irritating and cause contact sensitization. Buccal tablets are applied to the area of the upper gum above the incisor tooth on the same side as the symptoms; do not apply to the inside of the lip or cheek. Some products may contain milk protein concentrate.

Warnings: Additional Pediatric Considerations Some dosage forms may contain propylene glycol; in neonates large amounts of propylene glycol delivered orally, intravenously (eg, >3,000 mg/day), or topically have been associated with potentially fatal toxicities which can include metabolic acidosis, seizures, renal failure, and CNS depression; toxicities have also been reported in children and adults including hyperosmolality, lactic acidosis, seizures, and respiratory depression; use caution (AAP 1997; Shehab 2009).

Drug Interactions

Metabolism/Transport Effects None known.

Avoid Concomitant Use There are no known interactions where it is recommended to avoid concomitant use.

Increased Effect/Toxicity There are no known significant interactions involving an increase in effect.

Decreased Effect

Acyclovir (Topical) may decrease the levels/effects of: Talimogene Laherparepvec

Pregnancy Considerations

When administered orally, acyclovir crosses the placenta. The amount of acyclovir available systemically following topical application of the cream, buccal tablet, or ointment is significantly less in comparison to oral doses.

Refer to the Acyclovir (Systemic) monograph for details.

Breastfeeding Considerations

When administered orally, acyclovir is present in breast milk.

The amount of acyclovir available systemically following topical application of the cream, buccal tablet, or ointment is significantly less in comparison to oral doses. According to the manufacturer, the decision to continue or discontinue breastfeeding during therapy should consider the risk of infant exposure, the benefits of breastfeeding to the infant, and the benefits of treatment to the mother. Women with herpetic lesions near or on the breast should avoid breastfeeding.

Refer to the Acyclovir (Systemic) monograph for details.

Dosage Forms: US

Cream, External:

Zovirax: 5% (5 g)

Generic: 5% (5 g)

Ointment, External:

Zovirax: 5% (30 g)

Generic: 5% (5 g, 15 g, 30 g)

Tablet, Buccal:

Sitavig: 50 mg

Dosage Forms: Canada

Cream, External:

Zovirax: 5% (5 g)

Ointment, External:

Zovirax: 5% (4 g, 15 g, 30 g)

Generic: 5% (4 g, 5 g, 15 g, 30 g)

Dental Health Professional Considerations

Although some conflicting data, dental treatment may be a risk factor for asymptomatic viral shedding of herpes simplex virus type-1 (HSV-1) into human saliva in patients with previous exposure to the virus (Hyland 2007).

It is recommended to reappoint the patient if an active lesion is present. If the lesion is already "crusted" over, treatment will not induce spread of the virus but treatment is aimed at patient comfort during the procedure relating to the wound healing on their lip.

◆ **Acyclovir Sodium** *see* Acyclovir (Systemic) *on page 75*

◆ **Aczone** *see* Dapsone (Topical) *on page 437*

◆ **AD32** *see* Valrubicin *on page 1520*

◆ **aDabi-Fab** *see* IdaruCIZUmab *on page 795*

◆ **Adakveo** *see* Crizanlizumab *on page 414*

◆ **Adalat CC [DSC]** *see* NIFEdipine *on page 1104*

Adalimumab (a da LIM yoo mab)

Related Information

Rheumatoid Arthritis, Osteoarthritis, and Osteoporosis *on page 1697*

Brand Names: US Humira; Humira Pediatric Crohns Start; Humira Pen; Humira Pen-CD/UC/HS Starter; Humira Pen-Ps/UV/Adol HS Start

Brand Names: Canada Humira

Pharmacologic Category Antirheumatic, Disease Modifying; Gastrointestinal Agent, Miscellaneous; Monoclonal Antibody; Tumor Necrosis Factor (TNF) Blocking Agent

Use

Ankylosing spondylitis: Treatment (to reduce signs/symptoms) of active ankylosing spondylitis in adults.

Crohn disease: Treatment (to reduce signs/symptoms and to induce and maintain clinical remission) of active Crohn disease (moderate to severe) in adults and pediatric patients ≥6 years of age (Humira only) with an inadequate response to conventional therapy or who have lost response to or are intolerant to infliximab.

Hidradenitis suppurativa (Humira only): Treatment of moderate to severe hidradenitis suppurativa in adults and children ≥12 years of age.

Juvenile idiopathic arthritis: Treatment (to reduce signs/symptoms) of active polyarticular juvenile idiopathic arthritis (moderate to severe) in pediatric patients ≥2 years of age (Humira) or ≥4 years of age (Amjevita; Cyltezo); may be used alone or in combination with methotrexate.

Plaque psoriasis: Treatment of chronic plaque psoriasis (moderate to severe) in adults who are candidates for systemic therapy or phototherapy, and when other systemic therapies are less appropriate (with close monitoring and regular follow-up).

Psoriatic arthritis: Treatment (to reduce signs/symptoms, inhibit progression of structural damage, and improve physical function) of active psoriatic arthritis in adults; may be used alone or in combination with nonbiologic disease-modifying antirheumatic drugs (DMARDs).

Rheumatoid arthritis: Treatment (to reduce signs/symptoms, induce major clinical response, inhibit progression of structural damage, and improve physical function) of active rheumatoid arthritis (moderate to severe) in adults; may be used alone or in combination with methotrexate or other nonbiologic DMARDs.

Ulcerative colitis: Treatment (to induce and sustain clinical remission) of active ulcerative colitis (moderate to severe) in adults who have had an inadequate response to conventional therapy (**Note:** Efficacy in patients that are intolerant to or no longer responsive to other TNF blockers has not been established).

Uveitis (Humira only): Treatment of non-infectious intermediate, posterior, and panuveitis in adults and children ≥2 years of age.

Local Anesthetic/Vasoconstrictor Precautions

No information available to require special precautions

Effects on Dental Treatment Key adverse event(s) related to dental treatment: Adalimumab belongs to the class of disease-modifying antirheumatic drugs and, as such, has immunosuppressive properties. Consider a medical consult prior to any invasive treatment for patients under active treatment with adalimumab. Delayed wound healing due to the immunosuppressive effects and increased potential for postsurgical infection may be of concern.

Effects on Bleeding Rare reports of pancytopenia (including aplastic anemia), as well as medically significant thrombocytopenia, have been reported with tumor necrosis factor-alpha therapy; in patients undergoing active treatment, a medical consult is recommended

Adverse Reactions

>10%:

Central nervous system: Headache (12%)

Dermatologic: Skin rash (6% to 12%)

Hematologic & oncologic: Positive ANA titer (12%)

Immunologic: Antibody development (3% to 26%)

Infection: Infection (children and adolescents: 45%)

Local: Injection site reaction (5% to 20%)

Neuromuscular & skeletal: Increased creatine phosphokinase (15%)

Respiratory: Upper respiratory tract infection (17%), sinusitis (11%)

1% to 10%:

Cardiovascular: Hypertension (5%), atrial fibrillation (<5%), cardiac arrhythmia (<5%), chest pain (<5%), coronary artery disease (<5%), deep vein thrombosis (<5%), hypertensive encephalopathy (<5%), myocardial infarction (<5%), palpitations (<5%), pericardial effusion (<5%), pericarditis (<5%), peripheral edema (<5%), subdural hematoma (<5%), syncope (<5%), tachycardia (<5%)

Central nervous system: Confusion (<5%), myasthenia (<5%), paresthesia (<5%), torso pain (<5%)

Dermatologic: Cellulitis, erysipelas

Endocrine & metabolic: Hyperlipidemia (7%), hypercholesterolemia (6%), dehydration (<5%), ketosis (<5%), menstrual disease (<5%), parathyroid disease (<5%)

Gastrointestinal: Nausea (9%), abdominal pain (7%), cholecystitis (<5%), cholelithiasis (<5%), esophagitis (<5%), gastrointestinal hemorrhage (<5%), vomiting (<5%), diverticulitis of the gastrointestinal tract

Genitourinary: Urinary tract infection (≤8%), hematuria (5%), cystitis (<5%), pelvic pain (<5%)

Hematologic & oncologic: Adenoma (<5%), agranulocytosis (<5%), paraproteinemia (<5%), polycythemia (<5%), carcinoma (including breast, gastrointestinal, skin, urogenital), malignant lymphoma, malignant melanoma

Hepatic: Increased serum alkaline phosphatase (5%), hepatic necrosis (<5%)

Hypersensitivity: Hypersensitivity reaction (children 5% to 6%; adults 1%)

Infection: Serious infection (4%), herpes simplex infection (≤4%), herpes zoster infection (≤4%), sepsis

Neuromuscular & skeletal: Back pain (6%), arthritis (<5%), arthropathy (<5%), bone disease (<5%), bone fracture (<5%), limb pain (<5%), muscle cramps (<5%), myasthenia (<5%), osteonecrosis (<5%), septic arthritis (<5%), synovitis (<5%), tendon disease (<5%), tremor (<5%), arthralgia (3%; plaque psoriasis)

Ophthalmic: Cataract (<5%)

Renal: Nephrolithiasis (<5%), pyelonephritis

Respiratory: Flu-like symptoms (7%), asthma (<5%), bronchospasm (<5%), dyspnea (<5%), pleural effusion (<5%), respiratory depression (<5%), pharyngitis (juvenile idiopathic arthritis: ≤4%), pneumonia (≤4%), tuberculosis (including reactivation of latent infection; disseminated, miliary, lymphatic, peritoneal, and pulmonary)

Miscellaneous: Accidental injury (10%), abnormal healing (<5%), postoperative complication (infection)

<1%, postmarketing, and/or case reports: Abscess (limb, perianal), alopecia, anal fissure, anaphylactoid shock, anaphylaxis, anemia, angioedema, aplastic anemia, appendicitis, asthenia, bacterial infection, basal cell carcinoma, blepharitis, bronchitis, cardiac failure, cerebrovascular accident, cervical dysplasia, circulatory shock, clonus, cytopenia, dermal ulcer, diarrhea, diplopia, endometrial hyperplasia, eosinophilia, erythema multiforme, fever, fixed drug eruption, fulminant necrotizing fasciitis, fungal infection, Guillain-Barré syndrome, hepatic failure, hepatitis B (reactivation), hepatosplenic T-cell lymphomas (children, adolescents, and young adults), hepatotoxicity (idiosyncratic) (Chalasani 2014), histoplasmosis, hyperreflexia, hypersensitivity angiitis, increased serum transaminases, interstitial pulmonary disease (including pulmonary fibrosis), intestinal obstruction, intestinal perforation, leukemia, leukopenia, lichenoid eruption, liver metastases, lupus-like syndrome, lymphadenopathy, lymphocytosis, malignant neoplasm of ovary, meningitis (viral), Merkel cell carcinoma, multiple sclerosis, musculoskeletal chest pain, mycobacterium avium complex, myositis (children and adolescents), neutropenia, nocturia, optic neuritis, pancreatitis, pancytopenia, protozoal infection, psoriasis (including new onset, palmoplantar, pustular, or exacerbation), pulmonary embolism, respiratory failure, sarcoidosis, septic shock, skin granuloma (annulare; children and adolescents), Stevens-Johnson syndrome, streptococcal pharyngitis (children and adolescents), supraventricular cardiac arrhythmia, swelling of eye, systemic lupus erythematosus, testicular neoplasm, thrombocytopenia, urticaria, vascular disease, vasculitis (systemic), viral infection

Mechanism of Action Adalimumab is a recombinant monoclonal antibody that binds to human tumor necrosis factor alpha (TNF-alpha), thereby interfering with binding to TNFα receptor sites and subsequent cytokine-driven inflammatory processes. Elevated TNF levels in the synovial fluid are involved in the pathologic pain and joint destruction in immune-mediated arthritis. Adalimumab decreases signs and symptoms of psoriatic arthritis, rheumatoid arthritis, and ankylosing spondylitis. It inhibits progression of structural damage of rheumatoid and psoriatic arthritis. Reduces signs and symptoms and maintains clinical remission in Crohn disease and ulcerative colitis; reduces epidermal thickness and inflammatory cell infiltration in plaque psoriasis.

Pharmacodynamics/Kinetics

Half-life Elimination Terminal: ~2 weeks (range: 10 to 20 days)

Time to Peak Serum: SubQ: 131 ± 56 hours

Reproductive Considerations

The American Academy of Dermatology considers tumor necrosis factor (TNF) blocking agents for the treatment of psoriasis to be compatible for use in male patients planning to father a child (AAD-NPF [Menter 2019]). Women with psoriasis planning a pregnancy may continue treatment with adalimumab. Women with well-controlled psoriasis who wish to avoid fetal exposure can consider discontinuing adalimumab 10 weeks prior to attempting pregnancy (Rademaker 2018).

Treatment algorithms are available for use of biologics in female patients with Crohn disease who are planning a pregnancy (Weizman 2019).

Pregnancy Considerations Adalimumab crosses the placenta.

Adalimumab is a humanized monoclonal antibody (IgG_1). Placental transfer of human IgG is dependent upon the IgG subclass, maternal serum concentrations, birth weight, and gestational age, generally increasing as pregnancy progresses. The lowest exposure would be expected during the period of organogenesis (Palmeira 2012; Pentsuk 2009).

Following administration to pregnant patients with inflammatory bowel disease, cord blood and newborn serum concentrations of adalimumab are greater than maternal serum at delivery (Julsgaard 2016; Mahadevan 2013). The mean time to adalimumab clearance was 4 months (range: 2.9 to 5 months) in a study in 36 infants exposed in utero. The estimated mean half-life of adalimumab in these infants was 26 days (Julsgaard 2016). One case report notes adalimumab was detectable in the infant serum for 19 months following in utero exposure (Labetoulle 2018).

Outcome data from a pregnancy registry are available. Included were women with rheumatoid arthritis treated with adalimumab at least during the first trimester (n=74), women with RA not treated with adalimumab (n=80), and healthy pregnant women without RA (n=219). The incidence of major birth defects was not significantly different between the treatment groups. No pattern of specific defects was noted. There were no adverse pregnancy outcomes associated with therapy (Burmester 2017). Information related to this class of medications is emerging, but based on available data, tumor necrosis factor alpha (TNFα) blocking agents are considered to have low to moderate risk when used in pregnancy (ACOG 776 2019).

The risk of immunosuppression may be increased following third trimester maternal use of TNFα blocking agents; the fetus, neonate/infant should be considered immunosuppressed for 1 to 3 months following in utero exposure (AAD-NPF [Menter 2019]). Vaccination with live vaccines (eg, rotavirus vaccine) should be avoided for the first 6 months of life if exposure to a biologic agent occurs during the third trimester of pregnancy (eg, >27 weeks' gestation) (Mahadevan 2019).

Maternal adalimumab serum concentrations were found to remain stable during pregnancy in a study of nine women with Crohn disease (Seow 2017).

Inflammatory bowel disease is associated with adverse pregnancy outcomes including an increased risk of miscarriage, premature delivery, delivery of a low birth weight infant, and poor maternal weight gain. Management of maternal disease should be optimized prior to pregnancy. Treatment decreases disease flares, disease activity, and the incidence of adverse pregnancy outcomes (Mahadevan 2019).

Use of immune modulating therapies in pregnancy should be individualized to optimize maternal disease and pregnancy outcomes (ACOG 776 2019). The American Academy of Dermatology considers TNFα blocking agents for the treatment of psoriasis to be compatible with pregnancy (AAD-NPF [Menter 2019]). When treatment for inflammatory bowel disease is needed in pregnant women, appropriate biologic therapy can be continued without interruption. Serum levels should be evaluated prior to conception and optimized to avoid subtherapeutic concentrations or high levels which may increase placental transfer. Dosing can be adjusted so delivery occurs at the lowest serum concentration. For adalimumab, the final injection can be given 2 to 3 weeks prior to the estimated date of delivery (1 to 2 weeks if weekly dosing), then continued 48 hours postpartum (Mahadevan 2019).

Data collection to monitor pregnancy and infant outcomes following exposure to adalimumab is ongoing. Women exposed to adalimumab during pregnancy for the treatment of an autoimmune disease (eg, inflammatory bowel disease) may contact the OTIS Autoimmune Diseases Study at 877-311-8972.

Product Availability

Abrilada (adalimumab-afzb): FDA approved November 2019; availability anticipated in 2023. Information pertaining to this product within the monograph is pending revision. Consult the prescribing information for additional information.

Amjevita (adalimumab-atto): FDA approved September 2016; anticipated availability is currently unknown. Amjevita is approved as biosimilar to Humira. Consult the prescribing information for additional information.

Cyltezo (adalimumab-adbm): FDA approved August 2017; anticipated availability is currently unknown. Cyltezo is approved as biosimilar to Humira. Information pertaining to this product within the monograph is pending revision. Consult the prescribing information for additional information.

Hadlima (adalimumab-bwwd): FDA approved July 2019; anticipated availability is currently unknown. Hadlima is approved as biosimilar to Humira. Consult the prescribing information for additional information.

Hulio (adalimumab-fkjp): FDA approved July 2020; availability anticipated July 2023. Hulio is approved as a biosimilar to Humira.

◆ **Adalimumab-adbm** *see* Adalimumab *on page 83*

◆ **Adalimumab-afzb** *see* Adalimumab *on page 83*

◆ **Adalimumab-atto** *see* Adalimumab *on page 83*

◆ **Adamantanamine Hydrochloride** *see* Amantadine *on page 112*

Adapalene (a DAP a leen)

Brand Names: US Differin; Differin [OTC]

Brand Names: Canada Differin; Differin XP

Pharmacologic Category Acne Products; Retinoic Acid Derivative; Topical Skin Product, Acne

Use Acne vulgaris: Treatment of acne vulgaris.

Local Anesthetic/Vasoconstrictor Precautions No information available to require special precautions

Effects on Dental Treatment No significant effects or complications reported

Effects on Bleeding No information available to require special precautions

Adverse Reactions

>10%: Dermatologic: Xeroderma (≤45%), exfoliation of skin (≤44%), erythema (≤38%), burning sensation of skin (≤29%), stinging of the skin (≤29%)

1% to 10%: Dermatologic: Skin abnormalities (1% to 6%; discomfort), desquamation (2%), pruritus (≤2%), skin irritation (1% to 2%), sunburn (1% to 2%)

≤1%, postmarketing, and/or case reports: Acne flare, angioedema (gel), application site pain (gel), conjunctivitis, contact dermatitis, dermatitis, eczema, eyelid edema, facial edema (gel), skin discoloration, skin rash (cream/gel), swelling of lips (gel)

Mechanism of Action Retinoid-like compound which is a modulator of cellular differentiation, keratinization, and inflammatory processes, all of which represent important features in the pathology of acne vulgaris

Pharmacodynamics/Kinetics

Onset of Action 8 to 12 weeks

Half-life Elimination Terminal: 7 to 51 hours (gel)

Reproductive Considerations In clinical trials, women of childbearing potential were required to have a negative pregnancy test prior to therapy.

Pregnancy Risk Factor C

Pregnancy Considerations

Inadvertent exposure to a limited number of pregnant women occurred during premarketing studies. Published information related to adapalene exposure in pregnancy is limited (Autret 1997).

In general, topical products are recommended for the treatment of acne in pregnancy due to lower systemic exposure. However, because adapalene may share the characteristic of teratogenicity with other retinoids, agents other than adapalene are preferred. Avoid applying large amounts over prolonged periods of time to decrease the potential for systemic absorption (Akhavan 2003; Kong 2013; Leechman 2006).

- ◆ **Adasuve** *see* Loxapine *on page 940*
- ◆ **ADC DS-8201a** *see* Fam-Trastuzumab Deruxtecan *on page 636*
- ◆ **Adcirca** *see* Tadalafil *on page 1401*
- ◆ **ADD 234037** *see* Lacosamide *on page 868*
- ◆ **Addaprin [OTC]** *see* Ibuprofen *on page 786*
- ◆ **Adderall** *see* Dextroamphetamine and Amphetamine *on page 475*
- ◆ **Adderall XR** *see* Dextroamphetamine and Amphetamine *on page 475*

Adefovir (a DEF o veer)

Related Information

HIV Infection and AIDS *on page 1690*

Systemic Viral Diseases *on page 1709*

Brand Names: US Hepsera

Brand Names: Canada APO-Adefovir; Hepsera

Pharmacologic Category Antihepadnaviral, Reverse Transcriptase Inhibitor, Nucleotide (Anti-HBV)

Use Treatment of chronic hepatitis B with evidence of active viral replication (based on persistent elevation of ALT/AST or histologic evidence)

Local Anesthetic/Vasoconstrictor Precautions No information available to require special precautions

Effects on Dental Treatment No significant effects or complications reported

Effects on Bleeding No information available to require special precautions

Adverse Reactions In liver transplant patients with baseline renal dysfunction, frequency of increased serum creatinine has been observed to be as high as 32% to 51% at 48 and 96 weeks post-transplantation, respectively; considering the concomitant use of other potentially nephrotoxic medications, baseline renal insufficiency, and predisposing comorbidities, the role of adefovir in these changes could not be established.

>10%:

Central nervous system: Headache (24% to 25%)

Gastrointestinal: Abdominal pain (15%), diarrhea (≤13%)

Genitourinary: Hematuria (grade ≥3: 11%)

Hepatic: Hepatitis (exacerbation; ≤25% within 12 weeks of adefovir discontinuation)

Neuromuscular & skeletal: Weakness (≤25%)

1% to 10%:

Dermatologic: Pruritus, skin rash

Endocrine & metabolic: Hypophosphatemia (<2 mg/dL: 1% and 3% in pre-/post-liver transplant patients, respectively)

Gastrointestinal: Flatulence (≤8%), dyspepsia (5% to 9%), nausea, vomiting

Neuromuscular & skeletal: Back pain (≤10%)

Renal: Increased serum creatinine (≥0.5 mg/dL: 2% to 3% in compensated liver disease; incidence may be higher in patients with decompensated cirrhosis or in liver transplant recipients), renal failure

Respiratory: Cough (6% to 8%), rhinitis (≤5%)

<1%, postmarketing, and/or case reports: Fanconi's syndrome, hepatitis, myopathy, nephrotoxicity, osteomalacia, pancreatitis, proximal tubular nephropathy

Mechanism of Action Acyclic nucleotide reverse transcriptase inhibitor (adenosine analog) which interferes with HBV viral RNA-dependent DNA polymerase resulting in inhibition of viral replication.

Pharmacodynamics/Kinetics

Half-life Elimination 7.5 hours; prolonged in renal impairment

Time to Peak Median: 1.75 hours (range: 0.58 to 4 hours)

Pregnancy Considerations Information related to the use of adefovir in pregnancy is limited (Yi 2012); use of other agents is recommended (AASLD [Terrault 2016]).

Health care providers are encouraged to enroll women exposed to adefovir during pregnancy in the Hepsera pregnancy registry (800-258-4263).

- ◆ **Adefovir Dipivoxil** *see* Adefovir *on page 86*
- ◆ **ADH** *see* Vasopressin *on page 1535*
- ◆ **Adhansia XR** *see* Methylphenidate *on page 997*
- ◆ **Adipex-P** *see* Phentermine *on page 1224*
- ◆ **ADL-2698** *see* Alvimopan *on page 112*
- ◆ **Adlyxin** *see* Lixisenatide *on page 925*
- ◆ **Adlyxin Starter Pack** *see* Lixisenatide *on page 925*
- ◆ **Admelog** *see* Insulin Lispro *on page 824*
- ◆ **Admelog SoloStar** *see* Insulin Lispro *on page 824*
- ◆ **Ado Trastuzumab** *see* Ado-Trastuzumab Emtansine *on page 86*

Ado-Trastuzumab Emtansine
(a do tras TU zoo mab em TAN seen)

Brand Names: US Kadcyla

Brand Names: Canada Kadcyla

Pharmacologic Category Antineoplastic Agent, Anti-HER2; Antineoplastic Agent, Antibody Drug Conjugate; Antineoplastic Agent, Antimicrotubular; Antineoplastic Agent, Monoclonal Antibody

Use

Breast cancer, early: Treatment (single agent) of human epidermal growth factor receptor 2 (HER2)-positive early breast cancer in patients with residual invasive disease following neoadjuvant taxane and trastuzumab-based treatment.

Breast cancer, metastatic: Treatment (single agent) of HER2-positive, metastatic breast cancer in patients who previously received trastuzumab and a taxane, separately or in combination, and have either received prior therapy for metastatic disease or developed disease recurrence during or within 6 months of completing adjuvant therapy.

Limitations of use: Patients should be selected for therapy based on an approved companion diagnostic test for HER2 protein overexpression or HER2 gene amplification in tumor specimens.

Local Anesthetic/Vasoconstrictor Precautions No information available to require special precautions

Effects on Dental Treatment Key adverse event(s) related to dental treatment: Abnormal taste, oral discomfort, xerostomia and changes in salivation (normal salivary flow resumes upon discontinuation)

Effects on Bleeding Chemotherapy may result in significant myelosuppression, thrombocytopenia (31%; grades 3/4: 15%; Asians grades 3/4: 45%), anemia (14%; grades 3/4: 4%), neutropenia (7%; grades 3/4: 2%). In patients who are under active treatment with these agents, medical consult is suggested.

Adverse Reactions

>10%:

Central nervous system: Fatigue (36% to 50%), headache (28%), peripheral neuropathy (21% to 28%; grades 3/4: 2%), insomnia (12% to 14%)

Dermatologic: Skin rash (1% to 12%)

Gastrointestinal: Nausea (40% to 42%), constipation (17% to 27%), diarrhea (12% to 24%), vomiting (15% to 19%), abdominal pain (11% to 19%), xerostomia (14% to 17%), stomatitis (14% to 15%; grades 3/4: <1%)

Hematologic & oncologic: Hemorrhage (29% to 32%; grades 3/4: ≤2%), thrombocytopenia (29% to 31%; grades 3/4: 6% to 15%; Asian patients, grades 3/4: 19% to 45%), anemia (10% to 14%; grades 3/4: 1% to 4%)

Hepatic: Increased serum aspartate aminotransferase (79% to 98%), increased serum alanine aminotransferase (55% to 82%), increased serum transaminases (29% to 32%), increased serum bilirubin (7% to 17%)

Neuromuscular & skeletal: Musculoskeletal pain (30% to 36%), arthralgia (19% to 26%), asthenia (≤18%), myalgia (14% to 15%)

Respiratory: Epistaxis (22% to 23%), cough (14% to 18%), dyspnea (8% to 12%)

Miscellaneous: Fever (10% to 19%)

1% to 10%:

Cardiovascular: Peripheral edema (4% to 7%), hypertension (5% to 6%), left ventricular dysfunction (2% to 3%)

Central nervous system: Dizziness (10%), chills (5% to 8%)

Dermatologic: Pruritus (6% to 7%)

Endocrine & metabolic: Hypokalemia (7% to 10%)

Gastrointestinal: Dyspepsia (4% to 9%), dysgeusia (8%)

Genitourinary: Urinary tract infection (9% to 10%)

Hematologic & oncologic: Neutropenia (7% to 8%; grades 3/4: 2%)

Hepatic: Increased serum alkaline phosphatase (5% to 8%)

Hypersensitivity: Hypersensitivity reaction (2% to 3%)

Immunologic: Antibody development (4% to 6%; neutralizing: 1% to 3%)

Ophthalmic: Increased lacrimation (3% to 6%), blurred vision (4% to 5%), dry eye syndrome (4% to 5%), conjunctivitis (4%)

Respiratory: Radiation pneumonitis (2%), pneumonitis (≤1%)

Miscellaneous: Infusion related reaction (1% to 2%)

Frequency not defined:

Cardiovascular: Decreased left ventricular ejection fraction

Hepatic: Hepatic encephalopathy, hepatic failure, hepatotoxicity

Respiratory: Acute respiratory distress syndrome, interstitial pulmonary disease

<1%: Nonimmune anaphylaxis, portal hypertension (including nodular regenerative hyperplasia), tumor lysis syndrome

Mechanism of Action Ado-trastuzumab emtansine is a HER2-antibody drug conjugate which incorporates the HER2 targeted actions of trastuzumab with the microtubule inhibitor DM1 (a maytansine derivative). The conjugate, which is linked via a stable thioether linker, allows for selective delivery into HER2 overexpressing cells, resulting in cell cycle arrest and apoptosis.

Pharmacodynamics/Kinetics

Half-life Elimination ~4 days

Time to Peak Near the end of the infusion

Reproductive Considerations

[US Boxed Warning]: Exposure to ado-trastuzumab emtansine during pregnancy can result in embryo-fetal harm. Advise patients of these risks and the need for effective contraception.

Evaluate pregnancy status prior to treatment in females of reproductive potential; effective contraception should be used during therapy and for 7 months after the last dose of ado-trastuzumab emtansine. Males with female partners of reproductive potential should use effective contraception during therapy and for 4 months after the last dose.

Pregnancy Considerations

[US Boxed Warning]: Exposure to ado-trastuzumab emtansine during pregnancy can result in embryo-fetal harm. Advise patients of these risks.

Oligohydramnios and oligohydramnios sequence (manifested as pulmonary hypoplasia, skeletal malformations, and neonatal death) were observed following trastuzumab exposure during pregnancy (trastuzumab is the antibody component of ado-trastuzumab emtansine). Monitor for oligohydramnios if trastuzumab exposure occurs during pregnancy or within 7 months prior to conception; conduct appropriate fetal testing if oligohydramnios occurs. Based on the mechanism of action, the DM1 component of the ado-trastuzumab emtansine formulation may also cause fetal harm if administered during pregnancy.

European Society for Medical Oncology guidelines for cancer during pregnancy recommend delaying treatment with HER-2 targeted agents until after delivery in pregnant patients with HER-2 positive disease (Peccatori 2013).

Data collection to monitor pregnancy and infant outcomes following exposure to ado-trastuzumab emtansine is ongoing. If ado-trastuzumab emtansine exposure occurs during pregnancy or within 7 months prior to conception, healthcare providers should report the exposure to the Genentech (888-835-2555).

◆ **Adoxa [DSC]** *see* Doxycycline *on page* 522

Afamelanotide (A fa me LAN oh tide)

Brand Names: US Scenesse

Pharmacologic Category Alpha-Melanocyte Stimulating Hormone Analog, Synthetic

Use Erythropoietic protoporphyria: To increase pain free light exposure in adult patients with a history of phototoxic reactions from erythropoietic protoporphyria.

Local Anesthetic/Vasoconstrictor Precautions No information available to require special precautions

Effects on Dental Treatment No significant effects or complications reported

Effects on Bleeding No information available to require special precautions

Adverse Reactions

>10%:

Gastrointestinal: Nausea (19%)

Local: Application site reaction (21%)

1% to 10%:

Central nervous system: Fatigue (6%), dizziness (4%), drowsiness (2%)

Dermatologic: Melanocytic nevus (4%), skin hyperpigmentation (4%), skin irritation (2%)

Endocrine & metabolic: Porphyria (2%)

Local: Local skin discoloration (10%)

Respiratory: Oropharyngeal pain (7%), cough (6%), respiratory tract infection (4%)

Mechanism of Action Afamelanotide is a melanocortin receptor agonist that binds predominantly to MC1-R; increases production of eumelanin in the skin independently of exposure to sunlight or artificial UV light sources.

Pharmacodynamics/Kinetics

Half-life Elimination ~15 hours.

Time to Peak 36 hours.

Pregnancy Considerations Adverse events were not observed in animal reproduction studies.

- ◆ **Afrin NoDrip Sinus [OTC]** *see* Oxymetazoline (Nasal) *on page 1173*
- ◆ **Afrin Sinus [OTC]** *see* Oxymetazoline (Nasal) *on page 1173*
- ◆ **Afstyla** *see* Antihemophilic Factor (Recombinant) *on page 153*
- ◆ **Aftertest Topical Pain Relief [OTC]** *see* Benzocaine *on page 228*
- ◆ **AG-120** *see* Ivosidenib *on page 851*
- ◆ **AG-221** *see* Enasidenib *on page 562*
- ◆ **AG-013736** *see* Axitinib *on page 197*
- ◆ **Aggrastat** *see* Tirofiban *on page 1453*
- ◆ **Aggrenox** *see* Aspirin and Dipyridamole *on page 185*
- ◆ **AGN 1135** *see* Rasagiline *on page 1311*
- ◆ **$AgNO_3$** *see* Silver Nitrate *on page 1371*
- ◆ **AgonEaze** *see* Lidocaine and Prilocaine *on page 911*
- ◆ **Agrylin** *see* Anagrelide *on page 148*
- ◆ **AHF (Human)** *see* Antihemophilic Factor (Human) *on page 152*
- ◆ **AHF (Human)** *see* Antihemophilic Factor/von Willebrand Factor Complex (Human) *on page 154*
- ◆ **AHF (Recombinant [Fc Fusion Protein])** *see* Antihemophilic Factor (Recombinant [Fc Fusion Protein]) *on page 154*
- ◆ **AHF (Recombinant)** *see* Antihemophilic Factor (Recombinant) *on page 153*
- ◆ **A-hydroCort** *see* Hydrocortisone (Systemic) *on page 773*
- ◆ **A-hydroCort** *see* Hydrocortisone (Topical) *on page 775*
- ◆ **AICC** *see* Anti-inhibitor Coagulant Complex (Human) *on page 156*
- ◆ **Aimovig** *see* Erenumab *on page 581*
- ◆ **Aimovig (140 MG Dose) [DSC]** *see* Erenumab *on page 581*
- ◆ **AIN457** *see* Secukinumab *on page 1361*
- ◆ **AirDuo Digihaler** *see* Fluticasone and Salmeterol *on page 705*
- ◆ **AirDuo RespiClick** *see* Fluticasone and Salmeterol *on page 705*
- ◆ **Aklief** *see* Trifarotene *on page 1496*
- ◆ **Akovaz** *see* EPHEDrine (Systemic) *on page 568*
- ◆ **Akynzeo** *see* Fosnetupitant and Palonosetron *on page 717*
- ◆ **Akynzeo** *see* Netupitant and Palonosetron *on page 1095*
- ◆ **ALA** *see* Aminolevulinic Acid (Topical) *on page 117*
- ◆ **5-ALA** *see* Aminolevulinic Acid (Topical) *on page 117*
- ◆ **Ala-Cort** *see* Hydrocortisone (Topical) *on page 775*
- ◆ **Ala Scalp** *see* Hydrocortisone (Topical) *on page 775*
- ◆ **Alavert [OTC]** *see* Loratadine *on page 930*
- ◆ **Alavert Allergy and Sinus [OTC]** *see* Loratadine and Pseudoephedrine *on page 931*

Albiglutide (al bi GLOO tide)

Brand Names: US Tanzeum [DSC]

Pharmacologic Category Antidiabetic Agent, Glucagon-Like Peptide-1 (GLP-1) Receptor Agonist

Use Diabetes mellitus, type 2: Adjunct to diet and exercise to improve glycemic control in the treatment of type 2 diabetes mellitus

Local Anesthetic/Vasoconstrictor Precautions No information available to require special precautions

Effects on Dental Treatment Key adverse event(s) related to dental treatment: Schedule type 1 and type 2 diabetic patients for dental treatment in the morning in order to minimize chance of stress-induced hypoglycemia.

Effects on Bleeding No information available to require special precautions

Adverse Reactions Reactions reported from monotherapy and combination therapy.

>10%:

Endocrine & metabolic: Hypoglycemia (combination therapy; 3% to 17%)

Gastrointestinal: Diarrhea (13%), nausea (11%)

Local: Injection site reaction (11% to 18%, including erythema at injection site [2%], hypersensitivity reaction at injection site [1%], rash at injection site [1%], itching at injection site)

Respiratory: Upper respiratory tract infection (14%)

1% to 10%:

Cardiovascular: Atrial fibrillation (1%)

Endocrine & metabolic: Increased gamma-glutamyl transferase (2%)

Gastrointestinal: Gastroesophageal reflux disease (4%), vomiting (4%)

Immunologic: Antibody development (non-neutralizing; 6%)

Infection: Influenza (5%)

Neuromuscular & skeletal: Arthralgia (7%), back pain (7%)

Respiratory: Cough (7%), pneumonia (2%)

<1%: Angioedema, appendicitis, atrial flutter, constipation, hypersensitivity reaction, increased heart rate (1-2 bpm), increased serum ALT, increased serum bilirubin, pancreatitis

Mechanism of Action Albiglutide is an agonist of human glucagon-like peptide-1 (GLP-1) receptor and augments glucose-dependent insulin secretion and slows gastric emptying.

Pharmacodynamics/Kinetics

Half-life Elimination ~5 days

Time to Peak 3 to 5 days

Reproductive Considerations

Because of the long washout period, consider stopping albiglutide at least 1 month before a planned pregnancy.

Pregnancy Risk Factor C

Pregnancy Considerations

Adverse events have been observed in some animal reproduction studies.

Poorly controlled diabetes during pregnancy can be associated with an increased risk of adverse maternal and fetal outcomes, including diabetic ketoacidosis, preeclampsia, spontaneous abortion, preterm delivery, delivery complications, major birth defects, stillbirth, and macrosomia (ACOG 201 2018). To prevent adverse outcomes, prior to conception and throughout pregnancy, maternal blood glucose and HbA_{1c} should be kept as close to target goals as possible but without causing significant hypoglycemia (ADA 2020; Blumer 2013).

Agents other than albiglutide are currently recommended to treat diabetes mellitus in pregnancy (ADA 2020).

Product Availability Tanzeum has been discontinued in the US for >1 year.

◆ **Albumin-Bound Paclitaxel** *see* PACLitaxel (Protein Bound) *on page 1179*

◆ **Albumin-Stabilized Nanoparticle Paclitaxel** *see* PACLitaxel (Protein Bound) *on page 1179*

Albuterol (al BYOO ter ole)

Related Information

Respiratory Diseases *on page 1680*

Brand Names: US ProAir Digihaler; ProAir HFA; ProAir RespiClick; Proventil HFA; Ventolin HFA; VoSpire ER [DSC]

Brand Names: Canada Airomir; APO-Salbutamol HFA; APO-Salvent; APO-Salvent Sterules; DOM-Salbutamol; PHL-Salbutamol Respirator [DSC]; PHL-Salbutamol [DSC]; PMS-Salbutamol; RATIO-Salbutamol [DSC]; SANDOZ Salbutamol [DSC]; TEVA-Salbutamol; TEVA-Salbutamol HFA; Ventolin; Ventolin Diskus; Ventolin HFA; Ventolin PF

Pharmacologic Category $Beta_2$ Agonist

Use

Bronchospasm: Treatment or prevention of bronchospasm in patients with reversible obstructive airway disease (eg, asthma).

Exercise-induced bronchospasm: Prevention of exercise-induced bronchospasm.

Local Anesthetic/Vasoconstrictor Precautions No information available to require special precautions

Effects on Dental Treatment Key adverse event(s) related to dental treatment: Infrequent occurrence of unpleasant taste, glossitis, sinusitis, and xerostomia (normal salivary flow resumes upon discontinuation) have been reported. Rare occurrence of dysgeusia and tongue ulcers have also been reported.

Effects on Bleeding No information available to require special precautions

Adverse Reactions Incidence of adverse effects is dependent upon age of patient, dose, and route of administration. Frequency not always defined.

>10%:

Central nervous system: Excitement (children and adolescents 2 to 14 years: 20%), nervousness (4% to 15%)

Neuromuscular & skeletal: Tremor (≥5% to 38%; frequency increases with age)

Respiratory: Upper respiratory tract infection (≥5% to 21%), rhinitis (5% to 16%), bronchospasm (8% to 15%; exacerbation of underlying pulmonary disease), pharyngitis (14%), exacerbation of asthma (11% to 13%)

1% to 10%:

Cardiovascular: Tachycardia (≤7%), hypertension (1% to 3%), chest pain (<3%), edema (<3%), extrasystoles (<3%), chest discomfort, flushing, palpitations

Central nervous system: Shakiness (children and adolescents 6 to 14 years: 9%), headache (3% to 7%), dizziness (<7%), insomnia (1% to 3%), anxiety (<3%), ataxia (<3%), depression (<3%), drowsiness (<3%), rigors (<3%), voice disorder (<3%), hyperactive behavior (children and adolescents 6 to 14 years: 2%), malaise (2%), pain (2%), migraine (≤2%), emotional lability (1%), fatigue (1%), restlessness, vertigo

Dermatologic: Diaphoresis (<3%), skin rash (<3%), urticaria (≤2%), pallor (children 2 to 6 years: 1%)

Endocrine & metabolic: Increased serum glucose (10%), diabetes mellitus (<3%)

Gastrointestinal: Nausea (2% to 10%), vomiting (3% to 7%), unpleasant taste (inhalation site, 4%), gastroenteritis (3%), increased appetite (children and adolescents 6 to 14 years: 3%), viral gastroenteritis (1% to 3%), diarrhea (<3%), eructation (<3%), flatulence (<3%), glossitis (<3%), xerostomia (<3%), gastrointestinal signs and symptoms (children 2 to 6 years: 2%), dyspepsia (1% to 2%), anorexia (children 2 to 6 years: 1%)

Genitourinary: Urinary tract infection (≤3%), difficulty in micturition

Hematologic & oncologic: Decreased hematocrit (7%), decreased hemoglobin (7%), decreased white blood cell count (4%), lymphadenopathy (3%)

Hepatic: Increased serum ALT (5%), increased serum AST (4%)

Hypersensitivity: Hypersensitivity reaction (3% to 6%)

Infection: Cold symptoms (3%), infection (<3%; skin/appendage: ≤2%)

Local: Application site reaction (HFA inhaler: 6%)

Neuromuscular & skeletal: Muscle cramps (1% to 7%; frequency increases with age), musculoskeletal pain (3% to 5%), back pain (2% to 4%), hyperkinesia (≤4%), leg cramps (<3%)

Ophthalmic: Conjunctivitis (children 2 to 6 years: 1%)

Otic: Otitis media (≤4%), ear disease (<3%), otalgia (<3%), tinnitus (<3%)

Respiratory: Throat irritation (10%), viral upper respiratory tract infection (7%), respiratory tract disease (6%), nasopharyngitis (≥5%; children: 2%), oropharyngeal pain (≥5%; children: 2%), sinusitis (≥5%), upper respiratory tract inflammation (5%), cough (≥3%), flu-like symptoms (3%), dyspnea (<3%), laryngitis (<3%), oropharyngeal edema (<3%), pulmonary disease (<3%), bronchitis (≥2%), increased bronchial secretions (2%), wheezing (1% to 2%), epistaxis (children and adolescents 6 to 14 years: 1%), nasal congestion (1%), sinus headache (1%)

Miscellaneous: Fever (≥5% to 6%), accidental injury (<3%)

<1%, postmarketing, and/or case reports: Anaphylaxis, angina pectoris, angioedema, atrial fibrillation, dysgeusia, exacerbation of diabetes mellitus, gag reflex, hoarseness, hyperglycemia, hypokalemia, hypotension, irritability, ketoacidosis, lactic acidosis, metabolic acidosis, muscle spasm (children and adolescents 6 to 14 years), mydriasis (children and adolescents 6 to 14 years), oropharyngeal irritation, paradoxical bronchospasm, peripheral vasodilation, stomach pain (children and adolescents 6 to 14 years), supraventricular tachycardia, tongue ulcer, weakness

Mechanism of Action Relaxes bronchial smooth muscle by action on $beta_2$-receptors with little effect on heart rate.

Pharmacodynamics/Kinetics

Onset of Action Nebulization solution: ≤5 minutes; Oral inhalation: DPI: 5.7 minutes (median), MDI: 5.4 to 8.2 minutes (median); Oral: Immediate release: ≤30 minutes.

Duration of Action Nebulization solution: 3 to 6 hours; Oral inhalation: DPI: ~2 hours (median), MDI: ~4 to 6 hours; Oral: Immediate release: 6 to 8 hours, Extended release: Up to 12 hours.

Half-life Elimination Oral inhalation: 3.8 to ~5 hours; Oral: Immediate release: 5 to 6 hours, Extended release: 9.3 hours.

Time to Peak

Time to peak, serum:

Nebulization solution: 30 minutes; Oral inhalation: DPI: 30 minutes, MDI: 25 minutes (mean); Oral: Immediate release: ≤2 hours, Extended release: 6 hours.

Time to peak, FEV_1:

Nebulization solution: ~1 to 2 hours; Oral inhalation: DPI: Within 30 minutes, MDI: 47 minutes; Oral: Immediate release: 2 to 3 hours.

Pregnancy Considerations Albuterol crosses the placenta (Boulton 1997).

Maternal use of beta-2 agonists are not associated with an increased risk of fetal malformations (GINA 2020). Systemic use may be associated with hypoglycemia and tachycardia in the mother and fetus (ERS/TSANZ [Middleton 2020]). Uncontrolled asthma is associated with adverse events on pregnancy (increased risk of perinatal mortality, preeclampsia, preterm birth, low-birth-weight infants, cesarean delivery, and the development of gestational diabetes). Poorly controlled asthma or asthma exacerbations may have a greater fetal/maternal risk than what is associated with appropriately used asthma medications. Maternal treatment improves pregnancy outcomes by reducing the risk of some adverse events (eg, preterm birth and gestational diabetes) (ERS/TSANZ [Middleton 2020]; GINA 2020).

Short-acting beta-2 agonists (SABA) should be used to treat acute asthma exacerbations in pregnant women (GINA 2020). SABA are preferred over long-acting agents when treatment for asthma is needed during pregnancy; maternal asthma symptoms should be monitored monthly during pregnancy (ERS/TSANZ [Middleton 2020]). If high doses are required during labor and delivery, monitoring of glucose concentrations in the newborn for 24 hours is recommended, especially in preterm infants (GINA 2020).

Albuterol may affect uterine contractility. Maternal pulmonary edema and other adverse events have been reported when albuterol was used for tocolysis. Albuterol is not approved for use as a tocolytic; use caution when needed to treat bronchospasm in pregnant women.

Data collection to monitor pregnancy and infant outcomes associated with asthma and the medications used to treat asthma in pregnancy is ongoing. Healthcare providers are encouraged to enroll exposed pregnant females in the MotherToBaby Pregnancy Studies conducted by the Organization of Teratology Information Specialists (1-877-311-8972 or https://mothertobaby.org). Patients may also enroll themselves.

◆ **Albuterol and Ipratropium** *see* Ipratropium and Albuterol *on page 839*

◆ **Albuterol/Ipratropium** *see* Ipratropium and Albuterol *on page 839*

◆ **Albuterol Sulfate** *see* Albuterol *on page 90*

◆ **Alcaine** *see* Proparacaine *on page 1286*

Alclometasone (al kloe MET a sone)

Brand Names: US Aclovate [DSC]

Pharmacologic Category Corticosteroid, Topical

Use Steroid-responsive dermatosis: Treatment of inflammation and pruritic manifestations of corticosteroid-responsive dermatosis in adults and pediatric patients ≥1 year.

Local Anesthetic/Vasoconstrictor Precautions No information available to require special precautions

Effects on Dental Treatment No significant effects or complications reported

Effects on Bleeding No information available to require special precautions

Adverse Reactions Frequency not always defined.

Central nervous system: Localized burning (1% to 2%)

Dermatologic: Local dryness (2%), papular rash (2%), erythema (1% to 2%), pruritus (1% to 2%), acne vulgaris, allergic dermatitis, atrophic striae, folliculitis, hypopigmentation, miliaria, perioral dermatitis, skin atrophy

Endocrine & metabolic: Cushing's syndrome, growth suppression, HPA-axis suppression

Infection: Secondary infection

Local: Local irritation (2%)

Mechanism of Action Topical corticosteroids have anti-inflammatory, antipruritic, and vasoconstrictive properties. May depress the formation, release, and activity of endogenous chemical mediators of inflammation (kinins, histamine, liposomal enzymes, prostaglandins) through the induction of phospholipase A_2 inhibitory proteins (lipocortins) and sequential inhibition of the release of arachidonic acid. Alclometasone has low range potency.

Pharmacodynamics/Kinetics

Onset of Action Initial response (Ruthven 1988): Eczema: 5.3 days; Psoriasis: 6.7 days

Time to Peak Peak response (Ruthven 1988): Eczema: 13.9 days; Psoriasis: 14.8 days

Pregnancy Risk Factor C

Pregnancy Considerations

Adverse events have been observed with corticosteroids following topical application in animal reproduction studies.

Systemic bioavailability of topical corticosteroids is variable (integrity of skin, use of occlusion, etc) and may be further influenced by trimester of pregnancy (Chi 2017). In general, the use of topical corticosteroids is not associated with a significant risk of adverse pregnancy outcomes. However, there may be an increased risk of low birth weight infants following maternal use of potent or very potent topical products, especially in high doses. Use of mild to moderate potency topical corticosteroids is preferred in pregnant women and the use of large amounts or use for prolonged periods of time should be avoided (Chi 2016; Chi 2017; Murase 2014). Also avoid areas of high percutaneous absorption (Chi 2017). The risk of stretch marks may be increased with use of topical corticosteroids (Murase 2014).

◆ **Alclometasone Dipropionate** *see* Alclometasone *on page 91*

◆ **Alcortin A** *see* Iodoquinol and Hydrocortisone *on page 836*

◆ **Aldactone** *see* Spironolactone *on page 1386*

◆ **Aldara** *see* Imiquimod *on page 802*

Aldesleukin (al des LOO kin)

Brand Names: US Proleukin

Brand Names: Canada Proleukin

Pharmacologic Category Antineoplastic Agent, Biological Response Modulator; Antineoplastic Agent, Miscellaneous

Use

Melanoma, metastatic: Treatment of metastatic melanoma in adults.

Renal cell cancer, metastatic: Treatment of metastatic renal cell cancer in adults.

Limitations of use: Careful patient selection is necessary. Assess performance status (PS); patients with a more favorable PS (Eastern Cooperative Oncology Group [ECOG] PS 0) at treatment initiation respond better to aldesleukin (higher response rate and lower toxicity). Experience in patients with ECOG PS >1 is limited.

Local Anesthetic/Vasoconstrictor Precautions No information available to require special precautions

Effects on Dental Treatment Key adverse event(s) related to dental treatment: Stomatitis

Effects on Bleeding Chemotherapy may result in significant myelosuppression, including thrombocytopenia. In patients who are under active treatment, a medical consult is suggested.

Adverse Reactions

>10%:

Cardiovascular: Hypotension (71%, grade 4: 3%), peripheral edema (28%), tachycardia (23%), edema (15%), vasodilation (13%), supraventricular tachycardia (12%, grade 4: 1%), cardiac disease (11%; includes blood pressure changes, HF and ECG changes)

Central nervous system: Chills (52%), confusion (34%, grade 4: 1%), malaise (27%), drowsiness (22%), anxiety (12%), pain (12%), dizziness (11%)

Dermatologic: Skin rash (42%), pruritus (24%), exfoliative dermatitis (18%)

Endocrine & metabolic: Weight gain (16%), acidosis (12%, grade 4: 1%), hypomagnesemia (12%), hypocalcemia (11%)

Gastrointestinal: Diarrhea (67%, grade 4: 2%), vomiting (19% to 50%, grade 4: 1%), nausea (19% to 35%), stomatitis (22%), anorexia (20%), abdominal pain (11%)

Genitourinary: Oliguria (63%, grade 4: 6%)

Hematologic & oncologic: Thrombocytopenia (37%, grade 4: 1%), anemia (29%), leukopenia (16%)

Hepatic: Hyperbilirubinemia (40%, grade 4: 2%), increased serum AST (23%, grade 4: 1%)

Immunologic: Antibody development (66% to 74%)

Infection: Infection (13%, grade 4: 1%)

Neuromuscular & skeletal: Weakness (23%)

Renal: Increased serum creatinine (33%, grade 4: 1%)

Respiratory: Dyspnea (43%, grade 4: 1%), pulmonary disease (24%; includes pulmonary congestion, rales, rhonchi), cough (11%), respiratory tract disease (11%; includes acute respiratory distress syndrome, pulmonary infiltrates, and pulmonary changes)

Miscellaneous: Fever (29%, grade 4: 1%)

1% to 10%:

Cardiovascular: Cardiac arrhythmia (10%), cardiac arrest (grade 4: 1%), myocardial infarction (grade 4: 1%), ventricular tachycardia (grade 4: 1%)

Central nervous system: Coma (grade 4: 2%), psychosis (grade 4: 1%), stupor (grade 4: 1%)

Gastrointestinal: Enlargement of abdomen (10%)

Genitourinary: Anuria (grade 4: 5%)

Hematologic & oncologic: Blood coagulation disorder (grade 4: 1%; includes intravascular coagulopathy)

Hepatic: Increased serum alkaline phosphatase (10%)

Infection: Sepsis (grade 4: 1%)

Renal: Acute renal failure (grade 4: 1%)

Respiratory: Rhinitis (10%), apnea (grade 4: 1%)

<1%, postmarketing, and/or case reports: Agitation, allergic interstitial nephritis, anaphylaxis, angioedema, asthma, atrial arrhythmia, atrioventricular block, blindness (transient or permanent), bowel infarction, bradycardia, brain disease, bullous pemphigoid, capillary leak syndrome, cardiomyopathy, cellulitis, cerebral edema, cerebral lesion, cerebral vasculitis, cerebrovascular accident, cholecystitis, colitis, delirium, depression (severe; leading to suicide), diabetes mellitus, duodenal ulcer, endocarditis, eosinophilia, exacerbation of Crohn's disease, extrapyramidal reaction, gastritis, hematemesis, hemoptysis, hemorrhage (including cerebral, gastrointestinal, retroperitoneal, subarachnoid, subdural), hepatic failure, hepatitis, hepatosplenomegaly, hypertension, hyperthyroidism, hyperuricemia, hyperventilation, hypothermia, hypoventilation, hypoxia, IgA glomerulonephritis (crescentic), increased blood urea nitrogen, increased nonprotein nitrogen, inflammatory arthritis, insomnia, intestinal necrosis, intestinal obstruction, intestinal perforation, ischemic heart disease, leukocytosis, lymphocytopenia, malignant hyperthermia, meningitis, myasthenia gravis (oculo-bulbar), mydriasis, myocarditis, myopathy, myositis, neuralgia, neuritis, neuropathy, neutropenia, optic neuritis, pancreatitis, paranoia, pericardial effusion, pericarditis, peripheral gangrene, phlebitis, pneumonia, pneumothorax, pulmonary edema, pulmonary embolism, renal tubular necrosis, respiratory acidosis, respiratory arrest, respiratory failure, restricted systemic blood flow, rhabdomyolysis, scleroderma, seizure, shock, Stevens-Johnson syndrome, syncope, thrombosis, thyroiditis, tissue necrosis at injection site, tracheoesophageal fistula, transient ischemic attacks, urticaria, ventricular premature contractions

Mechanism of Action Aldesleukin is a human recombinant interleukin-2 product which promotes proliferation, differentiation, and recruitment of T and B cells, natural killer (NK) cells, and thymocytes; causes cytolytic activity in a subset of lymphocytes and subsequent interactions between the immune system and malignant cells; can stimulate lymphokine-activated killer (LAK) cells and tumor-infiltrating lymphocytes (TIL) cells.

Pharmacodynamics/Kinetics

Half-life Elimination

IV:

Children: Distribution: 14 ± 6 minutes; Elimination: 51 ± 11 minutes

Adults: Distribution: 13 minutes; Terminal: 85 minutes

Reproductive Considerations

Effective contraception is recommended for males and/or females of reproductive potential using this medication.

Pregnancy Risk Factor C

Pregnancy Considerations

Adverse events were observed in animal reproduction studies.

- ◆ **Aldomet** *see* Methyldopa *on page 995*
- ◆ **Aldurazyme** *see* Laronidase *on page 878*
- ◆ **Alecensa** *see* Alectinib *on page 92*

Alectinib (al EK ti nib)

Brand Names: US Alecensa

Brand Names: Canada Alecensaro

Pharmacologic Category Antineoplastic Agent, Anaplastic Lymphoma Kinase Inhibitor; Antineoplastic Agent, Tyrosine Kinase Inhibitor

Use Non-small cell lung cancer, metastatic: Treatment of anaplastic lymphoma kinase (ALK)-positive, metastatic non-small cell lung cancer (NSCLC) as detected by an approved test.

Local Anesthetic/Vasoconstrictor Precautions No information available to require special precautions

Effects on Dental Treatment No significant effects or complications reported

Effects on Bleeding No reports of bleeding or thrombocytopenia.

Adverse Reactions

>10%:

Cardiovascular: Edema (30%), bradycardia (8% to 18%)

Central nervous system: Fatigue (≤41%), headache (17%)

Dermatologic: Skin rash (18%)

Endocrine & metabolic: Hyperglycemia (36%), hypocalcemia (32%), hypokalemia (29%), hypophosphatemia (21%), hyponatremia (20%), weight gain (11%)

Gastrointestinal: Constipation (34%), nausea (18%), diarrhea (16%), vomiting (12%)

Hematologic & oncologic: Anemia (56%, grades 3/4: 2%), lymphocytopenia (22%, grades 3/4: 5%)

Hepatic: Increased serum AST (51%), increased serum alkaline phosphatase (47%), hyperbilirubinemia (39%), increased serum ALT (34%)

Neuromuscular & skeletal: Increased creatine phosphokinase (43%), weakness (≤41%), musculoskeletal pain (≤29%), myalgia (≤29%), back pain (12%)

Renal: Increased serum creatinine (28%)

Respiratory: Cough (19%), dyspnea (16%)

1% to 10%:

Cardiovascular: Pulmonary embolism (1%)

Dermatologic: Skin photosensitivity (10%)

Ophthalmic: Visual disturbances (10%)

Renal: Renal insufficiency (8%)

<1%, postmarketing, and/or case reports: Interstitial pulmonary disease, pneumonitis

Mechanism of Action Alectinib is a tyrosine kinase receptor inhibitor which inhibits anaplastic lymphoma kinase (ALK) and RET (with similar potency to ALK; Ou 2016). ALK gene abnormalities due to mutations or translocations may result in expression of oncogenic fusion proteins (eg, ALK fusion protein) which alter signaling and expression and result in increased cellular proliferation and survival in tumors which express these fusion proteins. Inhibition of ALK phosphorylation and ALK-mediated activation of downstream signaling results in decreased tumor cell viability. Alectinib is more potent than crizotinib against ALK, and can inhibit most of the clinically observed acquired ALK resistance mutations to crizotinib (Ou 2016).

Pharmacodynamics/Kinetics

Half-life Elimination Parent drug: 33 hours; M4: 31 hours

Time to Peak 4 hours

Reproductive Considerations

Females of reproductive potential should use effective contraception during therapy and for 1 week after the final dose. Males with female partners of reproductive potential should use effective contraception during therapy and for 3 months after the last dose.

Pregnancy Considerations

Based on data from animal reproduction studies and its mechanism of action, alectinib may be expected to cause fetal harm if administered during pregnancy.

Prescribing and Access Restrictions Available through specialty pharmacies and distributors. Further information may be obtained from the manufacturer, Genentech, at 1-888-249-4918 or at https://www.alecensa.com/.

◆ **Alectinib Hydrochloride** *see* Alectinib *on page* 92

Alemtuzumab (ay lem TU zoo mab)

Brand Names: US Campath; Lemtrada

Brand Names: Canada Lemtrada; MabCampath

Pharmacologic Category Antineoplastic Agent, Anti-CD52; Antineoplastic Agent, Monoclonal Antibody; Monoclonal Antibody

Use

B-cell chronic lymphocytic leukemia: Campath or MabCampath [Canadian product]: Treatment (as a single agent) of B-cell chronic lymphocytic leukemia.

Multiple sclerosis, relapsing: Lemtrada: Treatment of relapsing-remitting and active secondary progressive multiple sclerosis (MS); generally reserved for patients who have had an inadequate response to ≥2 medications indicated for the treatment of MS.

Limitations of use: Alemtuzumab is not recommended for use in patients with clinically isolated syndrome due to its safety profile.

Local Anesthetic/Vasoconstrictor Precautions No information available to require special precautions

Effects on Dental Treatment Key adverse event(s) related to dental treatment: Frequent occurrence of oral candidiasis, oropharyngeal pain; occurrence of stomatitis, distortion of the sense of taste, oral herpes simplex infection, tooth infection

Effects on Bleeding Chemotherapy may result in significant myelosuppression, including thrombocytopenia. In patients who are under active treatment, a medical consult is suggested.

Adverse Reactions

Multiple sclerosis:

>10%:

Central nervous system: Headache (52%), fatigue (18%), insomnia (16%), paresthesia (10%)

Dermatologic: Skin rash (53%), urticaria (16%), pruritus (14%)

Endocrine & metabolic: Thyroid disease (13% to 37%)

Gastrointestinal: Nausea (21%), diarrhea (12%)

Genitourinary: Urinary tract infection (19%)

Hematologic & oncologic: Lymphocytopenia (100%)

Immunologic: Antibody development (neutralizing: 5% to 94%; anti-alemtuzumab: 2% to 83%; no effect on drug efficacy)

Infection: Infection (71%), herpes virus infection (16%), fungal infection (12% to 13%; including oral candidiasis, vulvovaginal candidiasis)

Local: Infusion-related reaction (92%)

Neuromuscular & skeletal: Arthralgia (12%), back pain (12%), limb pain (12%)

Respiratory: Nasopharyngitis (25%), upper respiratory tract infection (16%), oropharyngeal pain (11%), sinusitis (11%)

Miscellaneous: Fever (29%)

1% to 10%:

Cardiovascular: Flushing (10%), tachycardia (8%), chest discomfort (7%), peripheral edema (5%), atrial fibrillation (≤3%), bradycardia (≤3%), chest pain (≤3%), hypertension (≤3%), hypotension (≤3%)

Central nervous system: Dizziness (10%), chills (9%), anxiety (7%), neurological signs and symptoms (≤3%; transient)

Dermatologic: Dermatitis (8%), erythema of skin (5%)

Gastrointestinal: Abdominal pain (10%), vomiting (10%), oral herpes simplex infection (9%), dysgeusia (8%), dyspepsia (8%), appendicitis (≤3%), gastroenteritis (≤3%), tooth infection (≤3%)

Genitourinary: Microscopic hematuria (8%), uterine hemorrhage (5%), genital herpes simplex (1%)

Hematologic & oncologic: Decreased CD-4 cell count (6%), decreased CD-8 cell counts (6%), decreased T cell lymphocytes (5%), immune thrombocytopenia (2%), hematoma (1%), petechia (1%)

Hypersensitivity: Angioedema (≤3%)

Infection: Influenza (8%), herpes zoster infection (4%), herpes simplex infection (2%), human papilloma virus infection (2%)

Neuromuscular & skeletal: Myasthenia (7%), muscle spasm (6%), myalgia (6%), neck pain (5%), asthenia (5%)

Ophthalmic: Graves' ophthalmopathy (1%)

Respiratory: Cough (9%), dyspnea (8%), bronchitis (7%), epistaxis (5%), bronchospasm (≤3%), pneumonia (≤3%)

Frequency not defined:

Central nervous system: Pain

Respiratory: Hypersensitivity pneumonitis, pneumonitis (with fibrosis), pulmonary infiltrates

B-cell chronic lymphocytic leukemia:

>10%:

Cardiovascular: Hypotension (16%), cardiac arrhythmia (14%), hypertension (14%)

Central nervous system: Chills (53%), headache (14%)

Dermatologic: Urticaria (16%), skin rash (13%)

Hematologic & oncologic: Lymphocytopenia (97%; grades 3/4: 97%), neutropenia (77%; grades 3/4: 42% to 64%), anemia (76%; grades 3/4: 12% to 38%), thrombocytopenia (71%; grades 3/4: 13% to 52%)

Infection: Infection (50% to 74%), CMV viremia (55%), cytomegalovirus disease (6% to 16%)

Respiratory: Dyspnea (14%)

Miscellaneous: Fever (69%)

1% to 10%:

Cardiovascular: Tachycardia (10%)

Central nervous system: Insomnia (10%), anxiety (8%), dysesthesia (>5%), fatigue (>5%)

Dermatologic: Erythema of skin (4%)

Gastrointestinal: Diarrhea (10%), anorexia (>5%), nausea (>5%), stomatitis (>5%), vomiting (>5%)

Hematologic & oncologic: Febrile neutropenia (grades ≥3: 5% to 10%), autoimmune thrombocytopenia (2%)

Immunologic: Antibody development (2% to 8%; neutralizing: 2%)

Infection: Sepsis (grades ≥3: 3% to 10%)

Neuromuscular & skeletal: Musculoskeletal pain (>5%), tremor (3%)

Respiratory: Bronchospasm (>5%)

<1%, postmarketing, and/or case reports (any indication): Anaphylactic shock, anaphylaxis, anemia, anti-GBM disease, aplastic anemia, autoimmune hemolytic anemia, autoimmune hepatitis, bone marrow aplasia, bone marrow depression, cardiac failure, cardiomyopathy, cerebrovascular accident, cholecystitis, chronic inflammatory demyelinating polyneuropathy, connective tissue disease (undifferentiated), Epstein-Barr-associated lymphoproliferative disorder, Epstein-Barr infection, goiter, Goodpasture's syndrome, graft versus host disease (transfusion associated), Graves' disease, Guillain-Barre syndrome, hemolytic anemia, hemophilia A (acquired [anti-Factor VIII antibodies]), hemorrhagic stroke, hyperthyroidism, hypothyroidism, immunological signs and symptoms (hemophagocytic lymphohistiocytosis), ischemic stroke, listeriosis (including gastroenteritis, encephalitis, sepsis), lymphoproliferative disorder, malignant lymphoma, malignant melanoma, malignant neoplasm of thyroid, membranous glomerulonephritis, meningitis due to listeria monocytogenes, meningitis (herpes), neutropenia, opportunistic infection, optic neuropathy, pancytopenia, pneumonitis, progressive multifocal leukoencephalopathy, pulmonary alveolar hemorrhage, pure red cell aplasia, reactivation of disease, reduced ejection fraction, retinal pigment changes (epitheliopathy), rheumatoid arthritis, serum sickness, suicidal ideation, suicidal tendencies, syncope, thyroiditis, tuberculosis, tumor lysis syndrome, type 1 diabetes mellitus, vasculitis, vitiligo

Mechanism of Action Alemtuzumab binds to CD52, a nonmodulating antigen present on the surface of B and T lymphocytes, a majority of monocytes, macrophages, NK cells, and a subpopulation of granulocytes. After binding to $CD52^+$ cells, an antibody-dependent lysis of malignant cells occurs. In multiple sclerosis, alemtuzumab immunomodulatory effects may include alteration in the number, proportions, and properties of some lymphocyte subsets following treatment.

Pharmacodynamics/Kinetics

Half-life Elimination IV: Campath: 11 hours (following first 30 mg dose; range: 2 to 32 hours); 6 days (following the last 30 mg dose; range: 1 to 14 days); Lemtrada: ~2 weeks

Reproductive Considerations

Females and males of reproductive potential should use effective contraception during therapy and for at least 6 months after the last dose of Campath. Females of reproductive potential should use effective contraception during therapy and for 4 months after the last dose of Lemtrada.

In general, disease-modifying therapies for multiple sclerosis are stopped prior to a planned pregnancy except in females at high risk of multiple sclerosis activity (AAN [Rae-Grant 2018]). Consider use of agents other than alemtuzumab for females at high risk of disease reactivation who are planning a pregnancy. Delaying pregnancy is recommended for females with persistent high disease activity; however, use of alemtuzumab may be an alternative option in these patients if the last infusion is at least 4 months prior to conception (ECTRIMS/EAN [Montalban 2018]).

Pregnancy Considerations

Alemtuzumab is a humanized monoclonal antibody (IgG_1). Potential placental transfer of human IgG is dependent upon the IgG subclass and gestational age, generally increasing as pregnancy progresses. The lowest exposure would be expected during the period of organogenesis (Palmeira 2012; Pentsuk

2009). Based on animal studies, alemtuzumab may cause fetal B- and T-lymphocyte depletion.

Information related to the use of alemtuzumab in pregnant females with multiple sclerosis is limited (Alroughani 2016; Tuohy 2015). Alemtuzumab induces persistent thyroid disorders which may cause adverse maternal and fetal events. In a patient who developed Graves disease during alemtuzumab therapy, neonatal Graves disease with thyroid storm developed in her infant exposed in utero 1 year following maternal treatment.

In general, disease-modifying therapies for multiple sclerosis are not initiated during pregnancy, except in females at high risk of multiple sclerosis activity (AAN [Rae-Grant 2018]).

Data collection to monitor pregnancy and infant outcomes following exposure to alemtuzumab is ongoing. Health care providers are encouraged to enroll females exposed to alemtuzumab during pregnancy in the pregnancy exposure registry (1-866-758-2990).

Prescribing and Access Restrictions As of September 4, 2012, alemtuzumab (Campath) is no longer commercially available in the United States (or Europe); a restricted distribution program will allow access (free of charge) for appropriate patients. Information on necessary documentation and requirements is available at Campath Distribution Program (1-877-422-6728) or Genzyme Medical Information (1-800-745-4447, option 2).

Alendronate (a LEN droe nate)

Related Information

Osteonecrosis of the Jaw *on page 1699*

Rheumatoid Arthritis, Osteoarthritis, and Osteoporosis *on page 1697*

Brand Names: US Binosto; Fosamax

Brand Names: Canada ACCEL-Alendronate [DSC]; ACH-Alendronate; ACT Alendronate [DSC]; Alendronate-70; APO-Alendronate; Auro-Alendronate; DOM-Alendronate; DOM-Alendronate-FC; Fosamax; GEN-Alendronate; JAMP-Alendronate; MINT-Alendronate; MYLAN-Alendronate [DSC]; PHL-Alendronate [DSC]; PMS-Alendronate; PMS-Alendronate-FC; RAN-Alendronate; RIVA-Alendronate; SANDOZ Alendronate; TEVA-Alendronate; VAN-Alendronate [DSC]

Generic Availability (US) May be product dependent

Pharmacologic Category Bisphosphonate Derivative

Use

Osteoporosis:

Binosto: Treatment of osteoporosis in postmenopausal females and to increase bone mass in males with osteoporosis

Fosamax: Treatment and prevention of osteoporosis in postmenopausal females; treatment to increase bone mass in males with osteoporosis; treatment of glucocorticoid-induced osteoporosis in males and females with low bone mineral density who are receiving a prednisone dosage of ≥7.5 mg/day (or equivalent)

Paget disease: *Fosamax:* Treatment of Paget disease of the bone in patients (males and females) who are symptomatic, at risk for future complications, or with alkaline phosphatase ≥2 times the upper limit of normal

Local Anesthetic/Vasoconstrictor Precautions No information available to require special precautions

Effects on Dental Treatment Osteonecrosis of the jaw (ONJ), generally associated with local infection and/or tooth extraction and often with delayed healing, has been reported in patients taking bisphosphonates. Symptoms included nonhealing extraction socket or an exposed jawbone. Most reported cases of bisphosphonate-associated osteonecrosis have been in cancer patients treated with intravenous bisphosphonates. However, some have occurred in patients with postmenopausal osteoporosis taking oral bisphosphonates. The risk of developing ONJ in patients taking oral bisphosphonates remains low with an estimated prevalence of 0.1% (one out of every 1000 cases of patients exposed to oral bisphosphonates). The benefits of using the oral bisphosphonates to prevent osteoporosis significantly outweighs the small risk of developing bisphosphonate-associated ONJ. Also, at the present time, there are no validated diagnostic techniques to determine which patients are at increased risk of developing ONJ. ONJ in patients taking these drugs can occur spontaneously. In addition, the risk of ONJ increases with specific procedures that increase bone trauma, particularly tooth extractions. Other factors that increase risk of ONJ in patients taking these drugs are age (>65 years of age), periodontitis, use of bisphosphonates for >2 years, smoking, wearing dentures, and diabetes. Patients who develop ONJ while on bisphosphonate therapy should receive care by an oral surgeon. See Dental Health Professional Considerations.

Effects on Bleeding No information available to require special precautions

Adverse Reactions Note: Incidence of adverse effects (mostly GI) increases significantly in patients treated for Paget disease at 40 mg/day.

>10%: Endocrine & metabolic: Decreased serum calcium (18%; transient, mild)

1% to 10%:

Central nervous system: Headache (3%)

Endocrine & metabolic: Decreased serum phosphate (10%; transient, mild)

Gastrointestinal: Abdominal pain (2% to 7%), acid regurgitation (1% to 5%), flatulence (≤4%), gastroesophageal reflux disease (3%), constipation (≤3%), diarrhea (≤3%), dyspepsia (1% to 3%), nausea (1% to 3%), esophageal ulcer (2%), dysphagia (1%), melena (1%), abdominal distension (≤1%), gastric ulcer (≤1%; may be severe with complications), gastritis (≤1%)

Neuromuscular & skeletal: Musculoskeletal pain (≤6%; includes bone pain, joint pain, and muscle pain), muscle cramps (≤1%)

<1%, postmarketing, and/or case reports: Alopecia, conjunctivitis, dizziness, duodenal ulcer (may be severe with complications), dysgeusia, episcleritis, erythema, erosive esophagitis, esophageal perforation, esophageal stenosis, esophageal ulcer, esophagitis, exacerbation of asthma, femur fracture (low-energy fractures, including subtrochanteric and diaphyseal), fever, hypersensitivity reaction (includes angioedema and urticaria), hypocalcemia (symptomatic), joint swelling, malaise, oropharyngeal ulcer; osteonecrosis of the jaw, peripheral edema, pruritus, scleritis, skin rash (occasionally with photosensitivity), Stevens-Johnson syndrome, toxic epidermal necrolysis, uveitis, vertigo, weakness

Dosing

Adult & Geriatric Note: In order for alendronate to be sufficiently absorbed, it needs to be administered in the morning ≥30 minutes before the first food, beverage (except plain water), or other medications. Patients with swallowing difficulties, esophageal motility disorders, or the inability to stand or sit upright for ≥30 minutes should not receive oral bisphosphate therapy. Patients should receive supplemental calcium and vitamin D if dietary intake is inadequate. Calcium and other supplements/medications containing polyvalent cations (eg, aluminum, iron, magnesium, zinc) can cause bisphosphonates to be insufficiently absorbed; accordingly, wait ≥30 to 60 minutes after taking alendronate to take calcium or other medications and supplements that interfere with the absorption of alendronate (Gertz 1999; Rosen 2019).

Androgen deprivation therapy-associated osteoporosis, prevention (alternative agent) (off-label use): Note: For use in men with prostate cancer **without** bone metastases treated long term with androgen deprivation therapy who are at elevated risk of osteoporotic fractures. Due to uncertain efficacy relative to preferred agents, some experts recommend against the use of alendronate for this indication unless preferred agents are unavailable or inappropriate (Smith 2019).

Oral: 70 mg once weekly (Bruder 2006; Greenspan 2007; Klotz 2013).

Osteoporosis, prevention of fractures (males and postmenopausal females): Note: Prior to use, evaluate and treat any potential causes of secondary osteoporosis (eg, hypogonadism in males) (ES [Watts 2012]).

High fracture risk patients include those with a history of fragility fracture, as well as males ≥50 years of age and postmenopausal females with a T-score ≤−2.5, or a T-score between −1 and −2.5 at high fracture risk according to an assessment (Finkelstein 2019; NOF [Cosman 2014]):

Treatment: Oral: 70 mg once weekly **or** 10 mg once daily.

Patients with T-scores between −1 and −2.5 and **not** at high fracture risk according to an assessment but who desire pharmacologic therapy for prevention of bone loss and/or fracture (Lewiecki 2019):

Prevention: Oral: 35 mg once weekly **or** 5 mg once daily.

Duration of therapy: The optimal duration of therapy has not been established. If fracture risk remains high (eg, fragility fracture before or during therapy) after the initial 5 years, consider extending therapy for up to 10 years or switching to alternative therapy (AACE/ACE [Camacho 2016]; Adler 2016; ES [Eastell 2019]; Watts 2010). Alternatively, if bone mineral density (BMD) is stable, there have been no previous fragility fractures, and short-term fracture risk is low, consider discontinuation (ie, drug holiday) after the initial 5 years. The optimal length of a drug holiday has not been established, although it is usually for a period of up to 5 years for oral bisphosphonates (ES [Eastell 2019]). The decision to resume therapy following a drug holiday is based on multiple factors, including decline in BMD, duration of discontinuation, and risk factors for fracture (ES [Eastell 2019]; Rosen 2019).

Osteoporosis, glucocorticoid-induced: Note: Recommended for use in males ≥50 years of age and postmenopausal females with low BMD (T-scores between −1 and −2.5 in either group) and expected to receive systemic glucocorticoid therapy for at least 3 months at a prednisone dose of ≥7.5 mg/day (or its equivalent); or in any patient whose baseline risk of fracture is high and is receiving a glucocorticoid at any dose or duration. In younger males and premenopausal females, patient selection must be individualized (Rosen 2019). Avoid use in females who are pregnant, who plan on becoming pregnant, or who are not using effective birth control (ACR [Buckley 2017]).

Prevention (off-label use) or treatment: Oral: 70 mg once weekly (Stoch 2009; Yeap 2008) **or** 10 mg once daily (de Nijs 2006; Tee 2012).

Paget disease, treatment (alternative agent): Note: For symptomatic patients with active disease and select patients with asymptomatic disease (eg, abnormal biochemical marker, prior to planned surgery at an active pagetic site) (Charles 2019; ES [Singer 2014]).

Initial: Oral: 40 mg once daily for 6 months (ES [Singer 2014]; manufacturer's labeling).

Re-treatment: A second course (ie, 40 mg orally once daily for 6 months) may be considered following a 6-month posttreatment evaluation period in patients whose serum alkaline phosphatase normalized during initial treatment but then subsequently rose above normal after discontinuation **or** if serum alkaline phosphatase failed to normalize during the initial course (Charles 2019; manufacturer's labeling).

Missed doses (once weekly): If a once-weekly dose is missed, administer the next morning after remembered; then return to the original scheduled day of the week on the once-weekly schedule; however, do not administer 2 doses on the same day.

Renal Impairment: Adult

CrCl ≥35 mL/minute: No dosage adjustment necessary.

CrCl <35 mL/minute: Use not recommended.

Hepatic Impairment: Adult No dosage adjustment necessary.

Pediatric Note: Patients should receive supplemental calcium and vitamin D if dietary intake is inadequate.

Osteogenesis imperfecta: Limited data available, dosing regimens and efficacy results variable (Akcay 2008; Pizones 2005; Seikaly 2005; Ward 2011): Children ≥2 years and Adolescents:

≤30 kg: Oral: 5 mg once daily

30 to <40 kg: 5 or 10 mg once daily

≥40 kg: Oral: 10 mg once daily

Dosing based on several prospective and retrospective trials; most smaller studies reported increased bone mineral density (BMD), decreased frequency of fractures, alleviation of chronic pain, and in some patients increased mobility (Akcay 2008; Pizones 2005; Seikaly2005; Unal 2005; Vyskocil 2005). The largest trial, a multicenter, randomized, placebo-controlled trial (n=109 in treatment group, n=83 completed 2-year follow-up) reported significant increases in lumbar spine BMD; however, other efficacy markers including long-bone fracture rate and pediatric disability score were no different than placebo (Ward 2011).

Osteopenia associated with cystic fibrosis (CF): Limited data available: Children ≥5 years and Adolescents: Oral:

≤25 kg: 5 mg once daily

>25 kg: 10 mg once daily

Dosing based on a randomized, placebo-controlled trial of CF patients (n=128, treatment group: n=65) with low apparent BMD age and inadequate response to calcium and calcifediol treatment; results showed a significant increase in BMD (16.3% vs 3.1% from baseline); evaluation of effect on fracture rate not possible due to sample size and duration (trial duration: 2 years); alendronate appeared to be well-tolerated with no notable difference in adverse effects reported (Bianchi 2013)

Osteopenia, nonambulatory patients (eg, cerebral palsy, muscular dystrophy): Limited data available, efficacy results variable: **Note**: Due to added complexity of administration requirements (eg, remaining in an upright position for an extended time) weekly dosing is preferred in these patients.

Fixed dosing (Apkon 2008; Houston 2014; Sholas 2005): Children ≥6 years and Adolescents: Oral: Usual reported dose: 35 mg once **weekly.** Dosing based on experience in 42 patients (age range: 6 to 16 years) from two case series and a retrospective trial. In the retrospective cohort study (n=29 mean age: 12 years), treatment showed a non-statistically significant trend in Z-score stabilization (Houston 2014). A case series of 10 patients (age range: 6 to 16 years) reported fewer fractures after treatment started compared to the prior year; alendronate was reported as being well tolerated; one patient discontinued therapy for hematemesis (also receiving high-dose ibuprofen therapy) (Sholas 2005).

Weight-directed dosing: Children ≥3 years and Adolescents: Oral: 1 mg/kg/dose once **weekly** (Paksu 2012); if using a solid dosage form, consider dose rounding to the nearest 10 mg (up or down as appropriate) (Lethaby 2007). Dosing based on a prospective trial of 26 patients (age range: 3 to 17 years); results showed after one year of treatment, increased BMD and decreased alkaline phosphatase.

Osteopenia/Osteoporosis, rheumatology patients (eg, JIA, SLE, dermatomyositis): Limited data available: Children ≥4 years and Adolescents:

≤20 kg: Oral: 5 mg once daily

>20 kg to 30 kg: Oral: 5 or 10 mg once daily

>30 kg: Oral: 10 mg once daily

Dosing based on a prospective trial (multicenter and single center) (Bianchi 2000; Cimaz 2002; Unal 2006); results from trials showed bone mineral density (BMD) was significantly increased (to normal values in some patients) after alendronate therapy; in some cases, bone turnover markers were reduced without a reduction of inflammatory activity (underlying rheumatologic disease process)

Renal Impairment: Pediatric There are no pediatric-specific recommendations provided in the manufacturer's labeling; based on experience in adult patients, use is not recommended in patients with a CrCl of <35 mL/minute.

Hepatic Impairment: Pediatric There are no pediatric-specific recommendations provided in the manufacturer's labeling; based on experience in adult patients, no adjustment required.

Mechanism of Action A bisphosphonate which inhibits bone resorption via actions on osteoclasts or on osteoclast precursors; decreases the rate of bone resorption, leading to an indirect increase in bone mineral density. In Paget disease, characterized by disordered resorption and formation of bone, inhibition of resorption leads to an indirect decrease in bone formation; but the newly-formed bone has a more normal architecture.

Contraindications

Hypersensitivity to alendronate or any component of the formulation; hypocalcemia; abnormalities of the esophagus (eg, stricture, achalasia) which delay esophageal emptying; inability to stand or sit upright for at least 30 minutes; increased risk of aspiration (effervescent tablets; oral solution)

Canadian labeling: Additional contraindications (not in the US labeling): Renal insufficiency with CrCl <35 mL/minute

Documentation of allergenic cross-reactivity for bisphosphonates is limited. However, because of similarities in chemical structure and/or pharmacologic actions, the possibility of cross-sensitivity cannot be ruled out with certainty.

Warnings/Precautions Use caution in patients with renal impairment (not recommended for use in patients with CrCl <35 mL/minute); hypocalcemia must be corrected before therapy initiation; ensure adequate calcium and vitamin D intake. May cause irritation to upper GI mucosa. Esophagitis, dysphagia, esophageal ulcers, esophageal erosions, and esophageal stricture (rare) have been reported; risk increases in patients unable to comply with dosing instructions. Use with caution in patients with dysphagia, esophageal disease, gastritis, duodenitis, or ulcers (may worsen underlying condition). Discontinue use if new or worsening symptoms develop.

Osteonecrosis of the jaw (ONJ), also referred to as medication-related osteonecrosis of the jaw (MRONJ), has been reported in patients receiving bisphosphonates. Known risk factors for MRONJ include invasive dental procedures (eg, tooth extraction, dental implants, boney surgery), cancer diagnosis, concomitant therapy (eg, chemotherapy, corticosteroids, angiogenesis inhibitors), poor oral hygiene, ill-fitting dentures, and comorbid disorders (anemia, coagulopathy, infection, preexisting dental or periodontal disease). Risk may increase with increased duration of bisphosphonate use. According to a position paper by the American Association of Maxillofacial Surgeons (AAOMS), MRONJ has been associated with bisphosphonate and other antiresorptive agents (denosumab), and antiangiogenic agents (eg, bevacizumab, sunitinib) used for the treatment of osteoporosis or malignancy; risk of MRONJ is significantly higher in cancer patients receiving antiresorptive therapy compared to patients receiving osteoporosis treatment (regardless of medication used or dosing schedule). MRONJ risk is also increased with intravenous antiresorptive use compared to the minimal risk associated with oral bisphosphonate use, although risk appears to increase with oral bisphosphonates when duration of therapy exceeds 4 years (AAOMS [Ruggiero 2014]). The manufacturer's labeling states that in patients requiring invasive dental procedures, discontinuing bisphosphonates may reduce the risk of ONJ and clinical judgment should guide the decision. However, the AAOMS suggests there is currently no evidence that interrupting oral bisphosphonate therapy alters the risk of ONJ following tooth extraction, and that in patients receiving oral bisphosphonates for <4 years who have no clinical risk factors, no alternations or delay in any procedure common to oral/maxillofacial surgeons, periodontists, and other dental providers is necessary (special considerations apply to patients receiving dental implants). Conversely, in patients receiving oral bisphosphonates for >4 years **or** in patients receiving oral bisphosphonates for <4 years who have also taken corticosteroids or antiangiogenic medications concomitantly, the AAOMS recommends considering a 2-month, drug-free period prior to invasive dental procedures (recommendation based on a theoretical benefit). Patients developing ONJ during therapy should receive care by an oral surgeon (AAOMS [Ruggiero 2014]). According to the manufacturer, discontinuation of the bisphosphonate therapy should be considered (based on risk/benefit evaluation) in patients who develop ONJ. Avoid oral bisphosphates after bariatric surgery; inadequate oral absorption and potential anastomotic ulceration may occur. If therapy is indicated, IV administered bisphosphonates are recommended.

Atypical femur fractures (AFF) have been reported in patients receiving bisphosphonates. The fractures include subtrochanteric femur (bone just below the hip joint) and diaphyseal femur (long segment of the thigh bone). Some patients experience prodromal pain weeks or months before the fracture occurs. It is unclear if bisphosphonate therapy is the cause for these fractures; AFFs have also been reported in patients not taking bisphosphonates, and in patients receiving glucocorticoids. Patients receiving long-term (>3 to 5 years) bisphosphonate therapy may be at an increased risk (Adler 2016; NOF [Cosman 2014]); however, benefits of therapy (when used for osteoporosis) generally outweigh absolute risk of AFF within the first 5 years of treatment, especially in patients with high fracture risk (Adler 2016; ES [Eastell 2019]). Patients presenting with thigh or groin pain with a history of receiving bisphosphonates should be evaluated for femur fracture. Consider interrupting bisphosphonate therapy in patients who develop a femoral shaft fracture; assess for fracture in the contralateral limb.

Severe (and occasionally debilitating) bone, joint, and/or muscle pain have been reported during bisphosphonate treatment. The onset of pain ranged from a single day to several months. Consider discontinuing therapy in patients who experience severe symptoms; symptoms usually resolve upon discontinuation. Some patients experienced recurrence when rechallenged with the same drug or another bisphosphonate; avoid use in patients with a history of these symptoms in association with bisphosphonate therapy.

Survivors of adult cancers with nonmetastatic disease who have osteoporosis (T score of -2.5 or lower in femoral neck, total hip, or lumbar spine) or who are at increased risk of osteoporotic fractures, should be offered bone modifying agents (utilizing the osteoporosis-indicated dose) to reduce the risk of fracture. For patients without hormonal responsive cancers, when clinically appropriate, estrogens may be administered along with other bone modifying agents (ASCO [Shapiro 2019]). The choice of bone modifying agent (eg, oral or IV bisphosphonates or subQ denosumab) should be based on several factors (eg, patient preference, potential adverse effects, quality of life considerations, availability, adherence, cost). Adequate calcium and vitamin D intake, exercise (using a combination of exercise types), as well as lifestyle modifications (if indicated), should also be encouraged.

Conjunctivitis, uveitis, episcleritis, and scleritis have been reported with alendronate; patients presenting with signs of ocular inflammation may require further ophthalmologic evaluation. Potentially significant drug-drug interactions may exist, requiring dose or frequency adjustment, additional monitoring, and/or selection of alternative therapy. Each effervescent tablet contains 650 mg of sodium (NaCl 1,650 mg); use with caution in patients following a sodium-restricted diet.

Warnings: Additional Pediatric Considerations The potential adverse effects of bisphosphonate therapy on the immature bones of growing children are concerning and data to fully describe are insufficient. Animal data has shown alendronate (high-dose) inhibits longitudinal bone growth (Rauch 2004); pediatric patients with osteogenesis imperfecta (OI) treated with pamidronate for 4 years showed increased height z scores (Zeitlin 2003); pediatric growth effects with other bisphosphonates is lacking. Possible decreased bone remodeling affecting growth or fracture healing may occur with bisphosphonate therapy; a case-report in an adolescent treated with high-dose pamidronate described abnormal long-bone modeling (Rauch 2004); a large, placebo-controlled OI trial (n=109, age range: 4 to 19 years) reported that alendronate did not interfere with fracture healing (Ward 2011). Rapid and in some cases significant weight gain has been reported with pamidronate therapy in pediatric patients which may negatively affect rehabilitation in patients with OI (Zeitlin 2003). Monitor patients closely.

Drug Interactions

Metabolism/Transport Effects None known.

Avoid Concomitant Use

Avoid concomitant use of Alendronate with any of the following: Parathyroid Hormone

Increased Effect/Toxicity

Alendronate may increase the levels/effects of: Deferasirox

The levels/effects of Alendronate may be increased by: Aminoglycosides; Angiogenesis Inhibitors (Systemic); Aspirin; Nonsteroidal Anti-Inflammatory Agents

Decreased Effect

Alendronate may decrease the levels/effects of: Parathyroid Hormone

The levels/effects of Alendronate may be decreased by: Polyvalent Cation Containing Products; Proton Pump Inhibitors

Food Interactions All food and beverages interfere with absorption. Coadministration with dairy products may decrease alendronate absorption. Beverages (especially orange juice, coffee, and mineral water) and food may reduce the absorption of alendronate as much as 60%. Management: Alendronate must be taken first thing in the morning and ≥30 minutes before the first food, beverage (except plain water), or other medication of the day.

Dietary Considerations Ensure adequate calcium and vitamin D intake; if dietary intake is inadequate, dietary supplementation is recommended. Males and females should consume:

Calcium: 1,000 mg/day (men: 50 to 70 years) **or** 1,200 mg/day (females ≥51 years and males ≥71 years) (IOM 2011; NOF [Cosman 2014]).

Vitamin D: 800 to 1,000 int. units/day (males and females ≥50 years) (NOF [Cosman 2014]). Recommended Dietary Allowance (RDA): 600 int. units daily (males and females ≤70 years) **or** 800 int. units/day (males and females ≥71 years) (IOM 2011).

Pharmacodynamics/Kinetics

Half-life Elimination Exceeds 10 years

Reproductive Considerations

Underlying causes of osteoporosis should be evaluated and treated prior to considering bisphosphonate therapy in premenopausal women; effective contraception is recommended when bisphosphonate therapy is required (Pepe 2020). Bisphosphonates are incorporated into the bone matrix and gradually released over time. Because exposure prior to pregnancy may theoretically increase the risk of fetal harm, most sources recommend discontinuing bisphosphonate therapy in females of reproductive potential as early as possible prior to a planned pregnancy. Use in premenopausal females should be reserved for special circumstances when rapid bone loss is occurring; a bisphosphonate with the shortest half-life should then be used (Bhalla 2010; Pereira 2012; Stathopoulos 2011).

Oral bisphosphonates can be considered for the prevention of glucocorticoid-induced osteoporosis in premenopausal females with moderate to high risk of fracture who do not plan to become pregnant during the treatment period and who are using effective birth control (or are not sexually active); intravenous therapy should be reserved for high risk patients only (Buckley [ACR 2017]).

Pregnancy Considerations

It is not known if bisphosphonates cross the placenta, but based on their lower molecular weight, fetal exposure is expected (Djokanovic 2008; Stathopoulos 2011).

Information related to the use of alendronate in pregnancy is available from case reports and small retrospective studies (Gerin 2016; Green 2014; Levy 2009; Ornoy 2006; Sokal 2019; Stathopoulos 2011).

Bisphosphonates are incorporated into the bone matrix and gradually released over time. The amount available in the systemic circulation varies by drug, dose, and duration of therapy. Theoretically, there may be a risk of fetal harm when pregnancy follows the completion of therapy (hypocalcemia, low birth weight, and decreased gestation have been observed in some case reports); however, available data have not shown that exposure to bisphosphonates during pregnancy significantly increases the risk of adverse fetal events (Djokanovic 2008; Green 2014; Levy 2009; Machairiotis 2019; Sokal 2019; Stathopoulos 2011). Exposed infants should be monitored for hypocalcemia after birth (Djokanovic 2008; Stathopoulos 2011).

Breastfeeding Considerations

It is not known if alendronate is present in breast milk.

According to the manufacturer, the decision to breastfeed during therapy should consider the risk of infant exposure, the benefits of breastfeeding to the infant, and the benefits of treatment to the mother.

Dosage Forms: US

Solution, Oral:

Generic: 70 mg/75 mL (75 mL)

Tablet, Oral:

Fosamax: 70 mg

Generic: 5 mg, 10 mg, 35 mg, 70 mg

Tablet Effervescent, Oral:

Binosto: 70 mg

Dosage Forms: Canada

Tablet, Oral:

Fosamax: 70 mg

Generic: 5 mg, 10 mg, 40 mg, 70 mg

Dental Health Professional Considerations

A review of 2,408 published cases of bisphosphonate-associated osteonecrosis of the jaw bone (BP-associated ONJ) was done by Filleul 2010. BP therapy was associated with 89% of the cases to treat malignancies and 11% of the cases to treat nonmalignant conditions. Information on the specific bisphosphonate used was available for 1,694 of the patients. Intravenous therapy (primarily zoledronic acid) was received by 88% of the patients and 12% received oral treatment (primarily alendronate). Of all the cases of BP-associated ONJ, 67% were preceded by tooth extraction and for 26% of patients, there was no predisposing factor identified.

A 2010 retrospective case review reported the prevalence of BP-associated ONJ in patients using alendronate-type drugs was one out of 952 patients or ~0.1% (Lo 2010). Of the 8,572 respondents, nine cases of ONJ were identified; five had developed ONJ spontaneously and four developed ONJ after tooth extraction. When extrapolated to patient-years of bisphosphonate exposure, this prevalence rate of 0.1% equates to a frequency of 28 cases per 100,000 person-years of oral bisphosphonate treatment. An Australian group (Mavrokokki 2007), identified the frequency of BP-associated ONJ in osteoporotic patients, mainly taking weekly oral alendronate, was 1 in 8,470 to 1 in 2,260 (0.01% to 0.04%) patients. If extractions were carried out, the calculated frequency was 1 in 1,130 to 1 in 296 (0.09% to 0.34%) patients. The median time to onset of ONJ in alendronate patients was 24 months.

According to the 2011 report by the American Dental Association (ADA), the incidence of BP-associated ONJ remains low and the benefits of using oral bisphosphonates significantly outweighs the risk of developing BP-associated ONJ for treatment and prevention of osteoporosis and cancer treatment (Hellstein 2011). The full 47-page report can be accessed at http://www.-ada.org/~/media/ADA/Member%20Center/FIles/topics_ARONJ_report.ashx.

The ADA review of 2011 stated the incidence of oral BP-associated ONJ was one case for every 1,000 individuals exposed to oral bisphosphonates (0.1%) (Hellstein 2011).

The most comprehensive review to date on osteonecrosis of the jaw bone (ONJ) has been published in the *Journal of Bone and Mineral Research* (Khan 2015), and written by an International Task Force of authors, totaling 34, from academe; industry; clinical medical and dental practice; oral and maxillofacial surgery; bone and mineral research; epidemiology; medical and dental oncology; orthopedic surgery; osteoporosis research; muscle and bone research; endocrinology and diagnostic sciences. The work provides a systematic review of the literature and international consensus on the classification, incidence, pathophysiology, diagnosis, and management of ONJ in both oncology and osteoporosis patient populations. This review of the literature from January 2003 to April 2014, with 299 references, offers recommendations for management of ONJ based on multidisciplinary international consensus.

Prevalence and incidence of ONJ in osteoporosis patients from the Task Force report:

Prevalence – the percent of osteoporotic population affected with ONJ

After reviewing all literature reports on this subject, the Task Force concluded that the prevalence of ONJ in patients prescribed oral BPs for the treatment of osteoporosis ranges from 0% to 0.04% with the majority being below 0.001%. However, the Task Force does cite the study of (Lo et al) that evaluated the Kaiser Permanente database and found the prevalence of ONJ in those receiving BPs for more than 2 years to range from 0.05% to 0.21% and appeared to be related to duration of exposure. As mentioned above, the American Dental Association has previously reported that the prevalence of ONJ in osteoporosis patients using oral BPs to be 1 out of 1,000 or 0.1% (Hellstein 2011).

Incidence - the rate at which ONJ occurs or the number of times it happens

From currently available data, the incidence of ONJ in the osteoporosis patient population appears to be low ranging from 0.15% to less than 0.001% person-years drug exposure. In terms of the osteoporosis patient population taking oral BPs, the incidence ranges from 1.04 to 69 per 100,000 patient years of drug exposure.

Alendronate and Cholecalciferol

(a LEN droe nate & kole e kal SI fer ole)

Related Information

Alendronate *on page 95*

Cholecalciferol *on page 344*

Brand Names: US Fosamax Plus D

Brand Names: Canada APO-Alendronate/Vitamin D3; Fosavance; SANDOZ Alendronate/Cholecalcif; TEVA-Alendronate/Cholecal

Pharmacologic Category Bisphosphonate Derivative; Vitamin D Analog

Use

Osteoporosis: Treatment of osteoporosis in postmenopausal females; treatment to increase bone mass in males with osteoporosis.

Limitations of use: Not for use in the treatment of vitamin D deficiency.

Local Anesthetic/Vasoconstrictor Precautions No information available to require special precautions

Effects on Dental Treatment Osteonecrosis of the jaw (ONJ), generally associated with local infection and/or tooth extraction and often with delayed healing, has been reported in patients taking bisphosphonates. Symptoms included nonhealing extraction socket or an exposed jawbone. Most reported cases of bisphosphonate-associated osteonecrosis have been in cancer patients treated with intravenous bisphosphonates. However, some have occurred in patients with postmenopausal osteoporosis taking oral bisphosphonates. The risk of developing ONJ in patients taking oral bisphosphonates remains low with an estimated prevalence of 0.1% (one out of every 1000 cases of patients exposed to oral bisphosphonates). The benefits of using the oral bisphosphonates to prevent osteoporosis significantly outweighs the small risk of developing bisphosphonate-associated ONJ. Also, at the present time, there are no validated diagnostic techniques to determine which patients are at increased risk of developing ONJ. ONJ in patients taking these drugs can occur spontaneously. In addition, the risk of ONJ increases with specific procedures that increase bone trauma, particularly tooth extractions. Other factors that increase risk of ONJ in patients taking these drugs are age (>65 years of age), periodontitis, use of bisphosphonates for >2 years, smoking, wearing dentures, and diabetes. Patients who develop ONJ while on bisphosphonate therapy should receive care by an oral surgeon. See Dental Health Professional Considerations.

Effects on Bleeding No information available to require special precautions

Adverse Reactions See individual agents.

Mechanism of Action See individual agents.

Pregnancy Considerations Refer to individual monographs.

Dental Health Professional Considerations See Alendronate monograph.

◆ **Alendronate Sodium** *see* Alendronate *on page 95*

◆ **Alendronate Sodium and Cholecalciferol** *see* Alendronate and Cholecalciferol *on page 100*

◆ **Alendronic Acid Monosodium Salt Trihydrate** *see* Alendronate *on page 95*

◆ **Aler-Dryl [OTC]** *see* DiphenhydrAMINE (Systemic) *on page 502*

◆ **Alevazol [OTC]** *see* Clotrimazole (Topical) *on page 397*

◆ **Aleve [OTC]** *see* Naproxen *on page 1080*

Alfentanil (al FEN ta nil)

Pharmacologic Category Analgesic, Opioid; Anilidopiperidine Opioid

Use

Analgesia: Analgesic adjunct for the maintenance of anesthesia with barbiturate/nitrous oxide/oxygen; analgesic with nitrous oxide/oxygen in the maintenance of general anesthesia; analgesic component for monitored anesthesia care.

Anesthetic: Primary anesthetic for induction of anesthesia in general surgery when endotracheal intubation and mechanical ventilation are required.

Local Anesthetic/Vasoconstrictor Precautions No information available to require special precautions

Effects on Dental Treatment Key adverse event(s) related to dental treatment: Patients may experience orthostatic hypotension as they stand up after treatment; especially if lying in dental chair for extended periods of time. Use caution with sudden changes in position during and after dental treatment.

Erythromycin inhibits the liver metabolism of alfentanil resulting in increased sedation and prolonged respiratory depression. Clarithromycin may act similarly.

Effects on Bleeding No information available to require special precautions

Adverse Reactions

>10%:

Cardiovascular: Hypertension (18%), chest wall rigidity (17%), bradycardia (14%), tachycardia (12%)

Gastrointestinal: Nausea (28%), vomiting (18%)

1% to 10%:

Cardiovascular: Hypotension (10%), cardiac arrhythmia (1% to 3%)

Central nervous system: Dizziness (3% to 9%), drowsiness (≤3%), sedation (≤3%; postoperative)

Neuromuscular & skeletal: Muscle movements (3% to 9%; skeletal)

Ophthalmic: Blurred vision (1% to 3%)

Respiratory: Apnea (3% to 9%), respiratory depression (1% to 3%; postoperative)

Frequency not defined:

Cardiovascular: Peripheral vasodilation

Gastrointestinal: Constipation

Ophthalmic: Miosis

<1%, postmarketing, and/or case reports: Anaphylaxis, bronchospasm, confusion (postoperative), drug dependence, euphoria (postoperative), headache, hypercapnia, laryngospasm, muscle rigidity (neck and extremities), myoclonus, pruritus, shivering, urticaria

Mechanism of Action Binds with stereospecific receptors at many sites within the CNS, increases pain threshold, alters pain perception, inhibits ascending pain pathways; is an ultra short-acting opioid

Pharmacodynamics/Kinetics

Onset of Action Rapid, within 5 minutes

Duration of Action Dose dependent: 30 to 60 minutes

Half-life Elimination

Newborns (premature): 5.33 to 9 hours (Davis 1988; Marlow 1990)

Children: 40 to 63 minutes (Davis 1988; Meistelman 1987; Roure 1987)

Adults: 90 to 111 minutes

Reproductive Considerations

Long-term opioid use may cause secondary hypogonadism, which may lead to sexual dysfunction or infertility (Brennan 2013).

Pregnancy Considerations

Alfentanil crosses the placenta (Cartwright 1989; Gepts 1986).

Prolonged use of opioids during pregnancy can cause neonatal withdrawal syndrome, which may be life-threatening if not recognized and treated according to protocols developed by neonatology experts. If opioid use is required for a prolonged period in a pregnant woman, advise the patient of the risk of neonatal opioid withdrawal syndrome and ensure that appropriate treatment will be available. Opioids may cause respiratory depression and psychophysiologic effects in the neonate; newborns of mothers receiving opioids during labor should be monitored.

The pharmacokinetic properties of alfentanil are not influenced by pregnancy when administered prior to delivery (Gepts 1986). Alfentanil has been evaluated for use in obstetrical analgesia (Mattingly 2003); other agents are more commonly used (ACOG 209 2019).

The ACOG recommends that pregnant women should not be denied medically necessary surgery, regardless of trimester. If the procedure is elective, it should be delayed until after delivery (ACOG 775 2019).

Controlled Substance C-II

◆ **Alfentanil Hydrochloride** *see* Alfentanil *on page 100*

◆ **Alfentanyl** *see* Alfentanil *on page 100*

◆ **Alferon N** *see* Interferon Alfa-n3 *on page 833*

Alfuzosin (al FYOO zoe sin)

Related Information

Clinical Risk Related to Drugs Prolonging QT Interval *on page 1675*

Brand Names: US Uroxatral

Brand Names: Canada APO-Alvuzosin; Auro-Alfuzosin; SANDOZ Alfuzosin; TEVA-Alfuzosin PR [DSC]; Xatral

Pharmacologic Category Alpha$_1$ Blocker

Use Benign prostatic hyperplasia: Treatment of signs and symptoms of benign prostatic hyperplasia (BPH)

Local Anesthetic/Vasoconstrictor Precautions

Alfuzosin is one of the drugs confirmed to prolong the QT interval and is accepted as having a risk of causing torsade de pointes. The risk of drug-induced torsade de pointes is extremely low when a single QT interval prolonging drug is prescribed. In terms of epinephrine, it is not known what effect vasoconstrictors in the local anesthetic regimen will have in patients with a known history of congenital prolonged QT interval or in patients taking any medication that prolongs the QT interval. Until more information is obtained, it is suggested that the clinician consult with the physician prior to the use of a vasoconstrictor in suspected patients, and that the vasoconstrictor (epinephrine, mepivacaine and levonordefrin [Carbocaine® 2% with Neo-Cobefrin®]) be used with caution.

Effects on Dental Treatment No significant effects or complications reported

Effects on Bleeding No information available to require special precautions

Adverse Reactions

1% to 10%:

Central nervous system: Dizziness (6%), fatigue (3%), headache (3%), pain (1% to 2%)

Gastrointestinal: Abdominal pain (1% to 2%), constipation (1% to 2%), dyspepsia (1% to 2%), nausea (1% to 2%)

Genitourinary: Impotence (1% to 2%)

Respiratory: Upper respiratory tract infection (3%), bronchitis (1% to 2%), pharyngitis (1% to 2%), sinusitis (1% to 2%)

<1%, postmarketing, and/or case reports: Angina pectoris (preexisting CAD), angioedema, atrial fibrillation, chest pain, diarrhea, edema, flushing, hepatic injury (including cholestatic), hypotension, intraoperative floppy iris syndrome (with cataract surgery), jaundice, orthostatic hypotension, priapism, pruritus, rhinitis, skin rash, syncope, systolic hypotension, tachycardia, thrombocytopenia, toxic epidermal necrolysis, urticaria, vomiting

Mechanism of Action An antagonist of alpha$_1$-adrenoreceptors in the lower urinary tract. Smooth muscle tone is mediated by the sympathetic nervous stimulation of alpha$_1$-adrenoreceptors, which are abundant in the prostate, prostatic capsule, prostatic urethra, and bladder neck. Blockade of these adrenoreceptors can cause smooth muscles in the bladder neck and prostate to relax, resulting in an improvement in urine flow rate and a reduction in BPH symptoms.

Pharmacodynamics/Kinetics

Half-life Elimination 10 hours

Time to Peak Plasma: 8 hours following a meal

Pregnancy Considerations Adverse events have not been observed in animal reproduction studies.

Dental Health Professional Considerations See Local Anesthetic/Vasoconstrictor Precautions

◆ **Alfuzosin HCl** *see* Alfuzosin *on page 101*

◆ **Alfuzosin Hydrochloride** *see* Alfuzosin *on page 101*

◆ **Alimta** *see* PEMEtrexed *on page 1206*

Alirocumab (al i ROK ue mab)

Brand Names: US Praluent

Brand Names: Canada Praluent

Pharmacologic Category Antilipemic Agent, PCSK9 Inhibitor; Monoclonal Antibody

Use

Hyperlipidemia, primary: Adjunct to diet, alone or in combination with other lipid-lowering therapies (eg, statins, ezetimibe) for the treatment of adults with primary hyperlipidemia (including heterozygous familial hypercholesterolemia [HeFH]) to reduce low-density lipoprotein cholesterol (LDL-C).

Secondary prevention of cardiovascular events: To reduce the risk of MI, stroke, and unstable angina requiring hospitalization in adults with established cardiovascular disease (Schwartz 2018).

Local Anesthetic/Vasoconstrictor Precautions

No information available to require special precautions

Effects on Dental Treatment No significant effects or complications reported

Effects on Bleeding No information available to require special precautions

Adverse Reactions

>10%: Local: Injection site reaction (4% to 17%)

1% to 10%:

Gastrointestinal: Diarrhea (5%)

Hematologic & oncologic: Bruise (2%)

Hepatic: Liver enzyme disorder (3%), increased serum transaminases (>3 x ULN: 2%)

Hypersensitivity: Hypersensitivity reaction (9%)

Immunologic: Antibody development (6%; neutralizing: <1%)

Infection: Influenza (6%)

Neuromuscular & skeletal: Myalgia (4% to 6%), muscle spasm (3%)

Respiratory: Cough (3%)

Frequency not defined:

Cardiovascular: Hypersensitivity angiitis

Endocrine & metabolic: Decreased LDL cholesterol (<25 mg/dL)

<1%, postmarketing, and/or case reports: Angioedema, flu-like symptoms

Mechanism of Action Alirocumab is a human monoclonal antibody (IgG1isotype) that binds to proprotein convertase subtilisin kexin type 9 (PCSK9). PCSK9 binds to the low-density lipoprotein receptors (LDLR) on hepatocyte surfaces to promote LDLR degradation within the liver. LDLR is the primary receptor that clears circulating LDL; therefore, the decrease in LDLR levels by PCSK9 results in higher blood levels of LDL-C. By inhibiting the binding of PCSK9 to LDLR, alirocumab increases the number of LDLRs available to clear LDL, thereby lowering LDL-C levels.

Pharmacodynamics/Kinetics

Onset of Action Peak effect: Proprotein convertase subtilisin kexin type 9 (PCSK9) suppression: 4 to 8 hours

Half-life Elimination SubQ: Steady-state: 17 to 20 days; reduced to 12 days when administered with a statin

Time to Peak SubQ: 3 to 7 days

Pregnancy Considerations

Alirocumab is a humanized monoclonal antibody (IgG_1). Potential placental transfer of human IgG is dependent upon the IgG subclass and gestational age, generally increasing as pregnancy progresses. The lowest exposure would be expected during the period of organogenesis (Palmeira 2012; Pentsuk 2009).

Health care providers are encouraged to enroll women exposed to alirocumab during pregnancy in the MotherToBaby Pregnancy Studies by contacting the Organization of Teratology Information Specialists (OTIS) (877-311-8972) or https://mothertobaby.org/ongoing-study/praluent/alirocumab/.

Prescribing and Access Restrictions Only available via specialty pharmacies. Call 844-772-5836 or visit https://www.praluenthcp.com/support for additional information.

Aliskiren (a lis KYE ren)

Related Information

Cardiovascular Diseases *on page 1654*

Brand Names: US Tekturna

Brand Names: Canada Rasilez

Pharmacologic Category Renin Inhibitor

Use

Hypertension: Management of hypertension in adults and pediatric patients ≥50 kg and ≥6 years of age.

Note: Not recommended for the initial treatment of hypertension (ACC/AHA [Whelton 2017]).

Local Anesthetic/Vasoconstrictor Precautions No information available to require special precautions

Effects on Dental Treatment No significant effects or complications required

Effects on Bleeding No information available to require special precautions

Adverse Reactions

1% to 10%:

Dermatologic: Skin rash (1%)

Gastrointestinal: Diarrhea (2%)

Neuromuscular & skeletal: Increased creatine phosphokinase (>300% increase: 1%)

Renal: Increased blood urea nitrogen (≤7%), increased serum creatinine (≤7%)

Respiratory: Cough (1%)

<1%, postmarketing, and/or case reports: Abdominal pain, anaphylaxis, anemia, angioedema, decreased hematocrit, decreased hemoglobin, dyspepsia, erythema, gastroesophageal reflux disease, gout, hepatic insufficiency, hyperkalemia, hyponatremia, increased liver enzymes, increased uric acid, myositis, nausea, nephrolithiasis, periorbital edema, peripheral edema, pruritus, rhabdomyolysis, seizure, severe hypotension, Stevens-Johnson syndrome, tonic-clonic seizures, toxic epidermal necrolysis, urticaria, vomiting

Mechanism of Action Decreases plasma renin activity and inhibits conversion of angiotensinogen to angiotensin I.

Pharmacodynamics/Kinetics

Onset of Action Maximum antihypertensive effect: Within 2 weeks

Half-life Elimination ~24 hours (range: 16 to 32 hours)

Time to Peak 1 to 3 hours

Pregnancy Considerations [US Boxed Warning]: Drugs that act on the renin-angiotensin system can cause injury and death to the developing fetus. Discontinue as soon as possible once pregnancy is detected. The use of drugs which act on the renin-angiotensin system are associated with oligohydramnios. Oligohydramnios, due to decreased fetal renal function, may lead to fetal lung hypoplasia and skeletal malformations. Use is also associated with anuria, hypotension, renal failure, skull hypoplasia, and death in the fetus/neonate. The exposed fetus should be monitored for fetal growth, amniotic fluid volume, and organ formation. Infants exposed *in utero* should be monitored for hyperkalemia, hypotension, and oliguria.

◆ **Aliskiren Hemifumarate** *see* Aliskiren *on page 102*

Alitretinoin (Topical) (a li TRET i noyn)

Brand Names: US Panretin

Pharmacologic Category Antineoplastic Agent, Retinoic Acid Derivative

Use

Kaposi sarcoma: Topical treatment of cutaneous lesions in AIDS-related Kaposi sarcoma.

Limitations of use: Alitretinoin is not indicated when systemic therapy is necessary (eg, >10 new Kaposi sarcoma lesions in previous month, symptomatic visceral involvement, symptomatic pulmonary Kaposi sarcoma, symptomatic lymphedema). There is no experience in using alitretinoin (topical) in combination with systemic treatment for Kaposi sarcoma.

Local Anesthetic/Vasoconstrictor Precautions No information available to require special precautions

Effects on Dental Treatment No significant effects or complications reported

Effects on Bleeding No information available to require special precautions

Adverse Reactions

>10%:

Central nervous system: Pain (≤34%), paresthesia (3% to 22%)

Dermatologic: Skin rash (25% to 77%), pruritus (8% to 11%)

1% to 10%:

Cardiovascular: Edema (3% to 8%)

Dermatologic: Exfoliative dermatitis (3% to 9%), dermatological disease (≤8%)

Mechanism of Action Alitretinoin is a naturally occurring endogenous retinoid that binds to and activates intracellular retinoid receptors (RAR and RXR subtypes); this results in altered expression of the genes controlling cellular differentiation and proliferation in normal and neoplastic cells, inhibiting the growth of Kaposi sarcoma

Reproductive Considerations

Females of reproductive potential should avoid becoming pregnant during treatment with topical alitretinoin.

Pregnancy Considerations

Alitretinoin may cause fetal harm if significant absorption occurs in a female who is pregnant.

- **Alkeran** *see* Melphalan *on page 961*
- **All Day Allergy [OTC]** *see* Cetirizine (Systemic) *on page 328*
- **All Day Allergy Childrens [OTC] [DSC]** *see* Cetirizine (Systemic) *on page 328*
- **All Day Pain Relief [OTC]** *see* Naproxen *on page 1080*
- **All Day Relief [OTC]** *see* Naproxen *on page 1080*
- **Allegra Allergy [OTC]** *see* Fexofenadine *on page 666*
- **Allegra Allergy Childrens [OTC]** *see* Fexofenadine *on page 666*
- **Aller-Chlor [OTC]** *see* Chlorpheniramine *on page 340*
- **Allerest** *see* Chlorpheniramine and Pseudoephedrine *on page 341*
- **Allergy [OTC]** *see* Chlorpheniramine *on page 340*
- **Allergy [OTC] [DSC]** *see* Loratadine *on page 930*
- **Allergy 24-HR [OTC]** *see* Fexofenadine *on page 666*
- **Allergy Childrens [OTC]** *see* DiphenhydrAMINE (Systemic) *on page 502*
- **Allergy Non-Drowsy [OTC] [DSC]** *see* Loratadine *on page 930*
- **Allergy Relief [OTC]** *see* Cetirizine (Systemic) *on page 328*
- **Allergy Relief [OTC]** *see* Chlorpheniramine *on page 340*
- **Allergy Relief [OTC]** *see* DiphenhydrAMINE (Systemic) *on page 502*
- **Allergy Relief [OTC]** *see* Fexofenadine *on page 666*
- **Allergy Relief [OTC]** *see* Loratadine *on page 930*
- **Allergy Relief-D [OTC]** *see* Loratadine and Pseudoephedrine *on page 931*
- **Allergy Relief Cetirizine [OTC]** *see* Cetirizine (Systemic) *on page 328*
- **Allergy Relief Childrens [OTC]** *see* Cetirizine (Systemic) *on page 328*
- **Allergy Relief Childrens [OTC]** *see* DiphenhydrAMINE (Systemic) *on page 502*
- **Allergy Relief/Indoor/Outdoor [OTC]** *see* Cetirizine (Systemic) *on page 328*
- **Allergy Relief/Indoor/Outdoor [OTC]** *see* Fexofenadine *on page 666*
- **Allergy Relief Loratadine [OTC]** *see* Loratadine *on page 930*
- **Allergy-Time [OTC]** *see* Chlorpheniramine *on page 340*
- **Allevacaine [OTC]** *see* Benzocaine *on page 228*
- **Allevess [OTC]** *see* Capsaicin *on page 284*
- **Alli [OTC]** *see* Orlistat *on page 1145*

Allopurinol (al oh PURE i nole)

Brand Names: US Aloprim; Zyloprim

Brand Names: Canada AG-Allopurinol; APO-Allopurinol; GEN-Allopurinol; JAMP-Allopurinol; Mar-Allopurinol; Zyloprim

Pharmacologic Category Antigout Agent; Xanthine Oxidase Inhibitor

Use

Oral:

Gout, treatment: Management of primary or secondary gout (acute attack, tophi, joint destruction, uric acid lithiasis, and/or nephropathy)

Guideline recommendations: EULAR guidelines: Urate-lowering therapy (ULT) (eg, allopurinol) is indicated in all patients with recurrent flares, tophi, urate arthropathy, and/or renal stones. ULT initiation is recommended close in time to first diagnosis in patients presenting at a young age (<40 years of age) or with very high serum uric acid levels (>8 mg/dL) and/or comorbidities (eg, renal impairment, hypertension, ischemic heart disease, heart failure) (EULAR [Richette 2017]).

Nephrolithiasis, prevention of recurrent calcium stones: Management in patients with hyperuricosuria (uric acid excretion >800 mg/day in men and >750 mg/day in women)

Tumor lysis syndrome, prevention: Management of hyperuricemia associated with cancer treatment for leukemia, lymphoma, and other malignancies

Limitations of use: Allopurinol is not recommended for the treatment of asymptomatic hyperuricemia. Allopurinol reduces serum and urinary uric acid concentrations; its use should be individualized for each patient and requires an understanding of its mode of action and pharmacokinetics.

IV:

Tumor lysis syndrome, prevention : Management of hyperuricemia associated with cancer treatment for leukemia, lymphoma, or solid tumor malignancies in patients who cannot tolerate oral therapy.

Local Anesthetic/Vasoconstrictor Precautions No information available to require special precautions

Effects on Dental Treatment No significant effects or complications reported

Effects on Bleeding No information available to require special precautions

Adverse Reactions

1% to 10%:

Dermatologic: Maculopapular rash (≤3%; pruritic), skin rash (≤2%)

Endocrine & metabolic: Gout (≤6%; acute)
Gastrointestinal: Nausea (1%), vomiting (≤1%)
Renal: Renal failure syndrome (≤1%), renal insufficiency (≤1%)

Frequency not defined:
Gastrointestinal: Diarrhea
Hepatic: Increased serum alanine aminotransferase, increased serum alkaline phosphatase, increased serum aspartate aminotransferase

<1%, postmarketing, and/or case reports: Abdominal pain, acute respiratory distress syndrome, ageusia, agitation, agranulocytosis, albuminuria, alopecia, amblyopia, amnesia, anemia, anorexia, aplastic anemia, apnea, arthralgia, asthenia, asthma, bone marrow aplasia, bone marrow suppression, bradycardia, bronchospasm, cardiac disorder, cardiac failure, cataract, cellulitis, cerebral infarction, cerebrovascular accident, chills, cholestatic jaundice, chronic myelocytic leukemia (blast crisis), coma, confusion, conjunctivitis, constipation, decreased libido, depression, diaphoresis, disseminated intravascular coagulation, dizziness, drowsiness, dysgeusia, dyspepsia, dystonia, ecchymoses, ECG abnormality, eczema, edema, electrolyte disorder, enlargement of abdomen, enlargement of salivary glands, eosinophilia, eosinophilic fibrohistiocytic bone marrow lesion, epistaxis, exfoliative dermatitis, facial edema, fever, flatulence, flushing, foot-drop, furunculosis, gastritis, gastrointestinal hemorrhage, glycosuria, granulomatous hepatitis, gynecomastia, headache, hematuria, hemolytic anemia, hemorrhage, hemorrhagic pancreatitis, hepatic failure, hepatic necrosis, hepatomegaly, hepatotoxicity, hyperbilirubinemia, hypercalcemia, hyperglycemia, hyperkalemia, hyperlipidemia, hypernatremia, hyperphosphatemia, hypersensitivity angiitis, hypersensitivity reaction, hypertension, hyperuricemia, hypervolemia, hypocalcemia, hypokalemia, hypomagnesemia, hyponatremia, hypoprothrombinemia, hypotension, hypotonia, impotence, increased serum creatinine, infection, injection site reaction, insomnia, intestinal obstruction, iritis, jaundice, lactic acidosis, leukocytosis, leukopenia, lichen planus, low cardiac output, lymphadenopathy, lymphocytosis, macular retinitis, malaise, male infertility, mental status changes, metabolic acidosis, mucositis, myalgia, myoclonus, myopathy, necrotizing angiitis, nephritis, neuritis, neutropenia, oliguria, onycholysis, optic neuritis, pain, pancytopenia, paralysis, paresthesia, pericarditis, peripheral neuropathy, peripheral vascular disease, pharyngitis, proctitis, pruritus, pulmonary embolism, purpuric rash, respiratory failure, respiratory insufficiency, reticulocytosis, rhinitis, seizure, sepsis, septic shock, skin edema, splenomegaly, status epilepticus, Stevens-Johnson syndrome, stomatitis, tachypnea, thrombocytopenia, thrombophlebitis, tinnitus, tongue edema, toxic epidermal necrolysis, tremor, tumor lysis syndrome, twitching, uremia, urinary tract infection, urticaria, vasculitis, vasodilation, ventricular fibrillation, vertigo, vesicobullous dermatitis, water intoxication

Mechanism of Action Allopurinol inhibits xanthine oxidase, the enzyme responsible for the conversion of hypoxanthine to xanthine to uric acid. Allopurinol is metabolized to oxypurinol which is also an inhibitor of xanthine oxidase; allopurinol acts on purine catabolism, reducing the production of uric acid without disrupting the biosynthesis of vital purines.

Pharmacodynamics/Kinetics

Onset of Action

Gout: Decrease in serum and urine uric acid: 2 to 3 days; peak effect: 1 week or longer; normal serum urate levels achieved typically within 1 to 3 weeks

Cancer therapy-induced hyperuricemia: Median time to plasma uric acid control: 27 hours (Cortes 2010)

Half-life Elimination Parent drug: ~1 to 2 hours; Oxypurinol: ~15 hours

Time to Peak Plasma: Oral: Allopurinol: 1.5 hours; Oxypurinol: 4.5 hours

Pregnancy Considerations Allopurinol crosses the placenta (Torrance 2009).

Information related to allopurinol in pregnancy is limited. Based on available information, an increased risk of adverse fetal events has not been observed (Hoeltzenbein 2013).

- **Allopurinol and Lesinurad** *see* Lesinurad and Allopurinol *on page 887*
- **Allopurinol Sodium** *see* Allopurinol *on page 103*
- **All trans Retinoic Acid** *see* Tretinoin (Systemic) *on page 1483*
- **All-trans Vitamin A Acid** *see* Tretinoin (Systemic) *on page 1483*

Almotriptan (al moh TRIP tan)

Related Information

Temporomandibular Dysfunction (TMD), Chronic Pain, and Fibromyalgia *on page 1773*

Brand Names: US Axert [DSC]

Brand Names: Canada APO-Almotriptan; Axert [DSC]; MYLAN-Almotriptan; SANDOZ Almotriptan; TEVA-Almotriptan

Pharmacologic Category Antimigraine Agent; Serotonin 5-$HT_{1B,\ 1D}$ Receptor Agonist

Use Acute treatment of migraine with or without aura in adults (with a history of migraine) and adolescents (with a history of migraine lasting ≥4 hours when left untreated)

Local Anesthetic/Vasoconstrictor Precautions No information available to require special precautions

Effects on Dental Treatment Key adverse effect(s) related to dental treatment: Xerostomia (normal salivary flow resumes upon discontinuation)

Effects on Bleeding No information available to require special precautions

Adverse Reactions

1% to 10%:
Central nervous system: Drowsiness (≤5%), dizziness (≤4%), headache (≤2%)
Gastrointestinal: Nausea (1% to 3%), vomiting (≤2%), xerostomia (1%)
Neuromuscular & skeletal: Paresthesia (≤1%)

<1%, postmarketing, and/or case reports: Abdominal cramps, abdominal discomfort, abdominal pain, abnormal dreams, altered sense of smell, anaphylactic shock, anaphylaxis, angina pectoris, angioedema, anxiety, arthralgia, arthritis, ataxia, back pain, blepharospasm, blurred vision, bronchitis, central nervous system stimulation, chest pain, chills, cold extremities, colitis, confusion, conjunctivitis, coronary artery vasospasm, decreased visual acuity, depression, dermatitis, diaphoresis, diarrhea, diplopia, dry eye syndrome, dysgeusia, dysmenorrhea, dyspepsia, dyspnea, epistaxis, erythema, euphoria, eye irritation, eye pain, fatigue, fever, gastritis, gastroenteritis,

gastroesophageal reflux disease, hemiplegia, hyperacusis, hypercholesterolemia, hyperglycemia, hyperhidrosis, hyperreflexia, hypersensitivity reaction, hypertension, hypertonia, hyperventilation, hypoesthesia, increased creatine phosphokinase, increased gamma-glutamyl transferase, increased thirst, insomnia, ischemic heart disease, lack of concentration, laryngismus, laryngitis, limb pain, malaise, mastalgia, myalgia, myasthenia, myocardial infarction, myopathy, neck pain, neck stiffness, nervousness, neuropathy, nightmares, nystagmus, otalgia, otitis media, palpitations, pharyngitis, pruritus, restlessness, rhinitis, scotoma, seizure, shakiness, sialorrhea, sinusitis, skin photosensitivity, skin rash, sneezing, syncope, tachycardia, tinnitus, tremor, vasodilation, ventricular fibrillation, ventricular tachycardia, vertigo, weakness

Mechanism of Action Selective agonist for serotonin ($5\text{-}HT_{1B}$ and $5\text{-}HT_{1D}$ receptors) in cranial arteries; causes vasoconstriction and reduces sterile inflammation associated with antidromic neuronal transmission correlating with relief of migraine

Pharmacodynamics/Kinetics

Half-life Elimination Mean: 3 to 5 hours (Baldwin 2004; McEnroe 2005)

Time to Peak Plasma: 1 to 3 hours

Pregnancy Risk Factor C

Pregnancy Considerations Adverse events were observed in animal reproduction studies. Information related to almotriptan use in pregnancy is limited (Källén, 2011; Nezvalová-Henriksen, 2010; Nezvalová-Henriksen, 2012). Until additional information is available, other agents are preferred for the initial treatment of migraine in pregnancy (Da Silva, 2012; MacGregor, 2012; Williams, 2012).

- ◆ **Almotriptan Malate** *see* Almotriptan *on page 104*
- ◆ **Alocane Emergency Burn Max Str [OTC]** *see* Lidocaine (Topical) *on page 902*
- ◆ **Aloclair** *see* Polyvinylpyrrolidone and Sodium Hyaluronate *on page 1244*
- ◆ **Alocril** *see* Nedocromil (Ophthalmic) *on page 1090*
- ◆ **Aloe Vesta Antifungal [OTC]** *see* Miconazole (Topical) *on page 1019*
- ◆ **Aloe Vesta Clear Antifungal [OTC]** *see* Miconazole (Topical) *on page 1019*

Alogliptin (al oh GLIP tin)

Brand Names: US Nesina

Brand Names: Canada Nesina

Pharmacologic Category Antidiabetic Agent, Dipeptidyl Peptidase 4 (DPP-4) Inhibitor

Use Diabetes mellitus, type 2, treatment: As an adjunct to diet and exercise to improve glycemic control in adults with type 2 diabetes mellitus as monotherapy or combination therapy.

Local Anesthetic/Vasoconstrictor Precautions No information available to require special precautions

Effects on Dental Treatment Alogliptin-dependent patients with diabetes (noninsulin dependent, type 2) should be appointed for dental treatment in morning in order to minimize chance of stress-induced hypoglycemia.

Effects on Bleeding No information available to require special precautions

Adverse Reactions

1% to 10%:

Central nervous system: Headache (4%)

Renal: Renal function abnormality (3%), decreased creatinine clearance (2%)

Respiratory: Nasopharyngitis (5%), upper respiratory tract infection (5%)

<1%, postmarketing, and/or case reports: Acute pancreatitis, anaphylaxis, angioedema, bullous pemphigoid, constipation, diarrhea, hepatic failure, hypersensitivity reaction, increased liver enzymes, intestinal obstruction, nausea, rhabdomyolysis, severe arthralgia, severe dermatological reaction, skin rash, Stevens-Johnson syndrome, urticaria

Mechanism of Action Alogliptin inhibits dipeptidyl peptidase 4 (DPP-4) enzyme resulting in prolonged active incretin levels. Incretin hormones (eg, glucagon-like peptide-1 [GLP-1] and glucose-dependent insulinotropic polypeptide [GIP]) regulate glucose homeostasis by increasing insulin synthesis and release from pancreatic beta cells and decreasing glucagon secretion from pancreatic alpha cells. Decreased glucagon secretion results in decreased hepatic glucose production. Under normal physiologic circumstances, incretin hormones are released by the intestine throughout the day and levels are increased in response to a meal; incretin hormones are rapidly inactivated by the DPP-4 enzyme.

Pharmacodynamics/Kinetics

Half-life Elimination ~21 hours

Time to Peak ~1 to 2 hours

Pregnancy Considerations

Poorly controlled diabetes during pregnancy can be associated with an increased risk of adverse maternal and fetal outcomes, including diabetic ketoacidosis, preeclampsia, spontaneous abortion, preterm delivery, delivery complications, major birth defects, stillbirth, and macrosomia (ACOG 201 2018). To prevent adverse outcomes, prior to conception and throughout pregnancy, maternal blood glucose and HbA_{1c} should be kept as close to target goals as possible but without causing significant hypoglycemia (ADA 2020; Blumer 2013).

Agents other than alogliptin are currently recommended to treat diabetes mellitus in pregnancy (ADA 2020).

- ◆ **Alogliptin Benzoate** *see* Alogliptin *on page 105*
- ◆ **Alomide** *see* Lodoxamide *on page 926*
- ◆ **Aloprim** *see* Allopurinol *on page 103*
- ◆ **Alora** *see* Estradiol (Systemic) *on page 596*

Alosetron (a LOE se tron)

Brand Names: US Lotronex

Pharmacologic Category Selective $5\text{-}HT_3$ Receptor Antagonist

Use Irritable bowel syndrome: Treatment of women with severe diarrhea-predominant irritable bowel syndrome (IBS) who have chronic IBS symptoms (generally lasting 6 months or longer), have had anatomic or biochemical abnormalities of the GI tract excluded, and who have not responded adequately to conventional therapy.

Local Anesthetic/Vasoconstrictor Precautions No information available to require special precautions

Effects on Dental Treatment No significant effects or complications reported

Effects on Bleeding No information available to require special precautions

Adverse Reactions

>10%: Gastrointestinal: Constipation (9% to 29%; dose related)

1% to 10%:

Central nervous system: Fatigue (≥3%), headache (≥3%)

Gastrointestinal: Abdominal distress (≤1% to 7%), abdominal pain (≤1% to 7%), nausea (6%), gastrointestinal distress (≤5%), gastrointestinal pain (≤5%), gastroenteritis (≥3%), vomiting (≥3%), diarrhea (2% to 3%), flatulence (1% to 3%), hemorrhoids (1% to 3%), abdominal distention (2%), acid regurgitation (≤2%), gastroesophageal reflux disease (≤2%)

Genitourinary: Urinary tract infection (≥3%)

Neuromuscular & skeletal: Muscle spasm (≥3%)

Respiratory: Cough (≥3%), nasopharyngitis (≥3%), upper respiratory tract infection (≥3%)

<1%, postmarketing, and/or case reports: Abnormal bilirubin levels, abnormal erythrocytes, active gastrointestinal lesion, allergic skin reaction, alopecia, anxiety, cardiac arrhythmia, cholecystitis, cognitive dysfunction, colitis, confusion, cystitis, decreased gastrointestinal motility, depression, dermatitis, diaphoresis, disruption of body temperature regulation, disturbance in fluid balance, diverticulitis, drowsiness, dyspepsia, extrasystoles, fecal impaction, gastrointestinal obstruction, gastrointestinal perforation, gastrointestinal spasm, gastrointestinal ulcer, hematoma, hemoglobinopathy, hemorrhage, hepatitis, hyperacidity, hyperglycemia, hypertension, hypoesthesia, hypoglycemia, hypothalamic disease, intestinal obstruction, intussusception, ischemic colitis, memory impairment, mesenteric ischemia (small bowel), muscle cramps, muscle rigidity, myalgia, occult blood in stools, ostealgia, pain, pituitary insufficiency, proctitis, respiratory tract disease, sedation, sexual disorder, skeletal pain, skin rash, tachyarrhythmia, tremor, ulcerative colitis, urinary frequency, urticaria

Mechanism of Action Alosetron is a potent and selective antagonist of a subtype of the serotonin 5-HT_3 receptor. 5-HT_3 receptors are ligand-gated ion channels extensively distributed on enteric neurons in the human gastrointestinal tract, as well as other peripheral and central locations. Activation of these channels affect the regulation of visceral pain, colonic transit, and gastrointestinal secretions. In patients with irritable bowel syndrome, blockade of these channels may reduce pain, abdominal discomfort, urgency, and diarrhea.

Pharmacodynamics/Kinetics

Half-life Elimination 1.5 hours

Time to Peak 1 hour

Pregnancy Considerations Adverse events have not been observed in animal reproduction studies.

◆ **Alosetron HCl** *see* Alosetron *on page 105*

◆ **Aloxi** *see* Palonosetron *on page 1184*

◆ **1α-Hydroxyergocalciferol** *see* Doxercalciferol *on page 519*

◆ **α-2-interferon** *see* Interferon Alfa-2b *on page 831*

◆ **Alphanate/VWF Complex/Human** *see* Antihemophilic Factor/von Willebrand Factor Complex (Human) *on page 154*

◆ **AlphaTrex [DSC]** *see* Betamethasone (Topical) *on page 237*

◆ **Alph-E [OTC]** *see* Vitamin E (Systemic) *on page 1549*

◆ **Alph-E-Mixed [OTC]** *see* Vitamin E (Systemic) *on page 1549*

◆ **Alph-E-Mixed 1000 [OTC]** *see* Vitamin E (Systemic) *on page 1549*

ALPRAZolam (al PRAY zoe lam)

Related Information

Dentin Hypersensitivity, Acid Erosion, High Caries Index, Management of Alveolar Osteitis, and Xerostomia *on page 1762*

Management of the Patient With Anxiety or Depression *on page 1778*

Temporomandibular Dysfunction (TMD), Chronic Pain, and Fibromyalgia *on page 1773*

Related Sample Prescriptions

Sedation (Prior to Dental Treatment) - Sample Prescriptions *on page 45*

Brand Names: US ALPRAZolam Intensol; ALPRAZolam XR; Xanax; Xanax XR

Brand Names: Canada ALPRAZolam TS; ALPRAZolam-1; APO-Alpraz; APO-Alpraz TS; JAMP-Alprazolam [DSC]; MYLAN-ALPRAZolam [DSC]; NAT-ALPRAZolam [DSC]; RIVA-ALPRAZolam [DSC]; TEVA-Alprazolam; Xanax; Xanax TS

Generic Availability (US) May be product dependent

Pharmacologic Category Benzodiazepine

Dental Use Preoperative anxiety

Use Anxiety disorders: Treatment of generalized anxiety disorder, short-term anxiety, and anxiety associated with depression (IR tablet, oral concentrate, orally disintegrating tablets); treatment of panic disorder with or without agoraphobia (IR tablet, ER tablet, oral concentrate, orally disintegrating tablets).

Local Anesthetic/Vasoconstrictor Precautions No information available to require special precautions

Effects on Dental Treatment Key adverse event(s) related to dental treatment: Significant xerostomia and changes in salivation (normal salivary flow resumes upon discontinuation)

Effects on Bleeding No information available to require special precautions

Adverse Reactions

>10%:

Central nervous system: Drowsiness (immediate-release: 41% to 77%; extended-release: 23%), fatigue (immediate-release: 49%; extended-release: 14%), sedation (extended-release: 45%), ataxia (immediate-release: 40%; extended-release: 7% to 9%), memory impairment (immediate-release: 33%; extended-release: 15%), irritability (immediate-release: 33%; extended-release: ≥1%), cognitive dysfunction (immediate-release: 29%), dysarthria (immediate-release: 23%; extended-release: 11%), dizziness (immediate-release: 2% to 21%; extended-release: ≥1%), depression (extended-release: 1% to 12%)

Dermatologic: Skin rash (immediate-release: 11%; extended-release: <1%)

Endocrine & metabolic: Weight gain (immediate-release: 27%; extended-release: 5%), weight loss (immediate-release: 23%), decreased libido (6% to 14%)

Gastrointestinal: Increased appetite (immediate-release: 33%; extended-release: 7%), decreased appetite (immediate release: 28%), constipation (immediate-release: 26%; extended-release: 8%), xerostomia (immediate-release: 15%)

Genitourinary: Difficulty in micturition (immediate-release: 12%; extended-release: ≥1%)

1% to 10%:

Cardiovascular: Hypotension (immediate-release: 5%; extended-release: <1%), chest pain (extended-release: ≥1%), palpitations (extended-release: ≥1%)

Central nervous system: Confusion (immediate-release: 10%; extended-release: 2%), altered mental status (extended-release: 7%), disinhibition (immediate-release: 3%), disturbance in attention (extended-release: 3%), equilibrium disturbance (extended-release: 3%), akathisia (immediate-release: 2%), disorientation (extended-release: 2%), lethargy (extended-release: 2%), talkativeness (immediate-release: 2%), derealization (≥1% to 2%), agitation (extended-release: ≥1%), depersonalization (extended-release: ≥1%), headache (extended-release: ≥1%), insomnia (extended-release: ≥1%), malaise (extended-release: ≥1%), nervousness (extended-release: ≥1%), nightmares (extended-release: ≥1%), restlessness (≥1%), vertigo (extended-release: ≥1%), anxiety (extended-release: 1%), feeling hot (immediate-release: 1%; extended-release: <1%), hypersomnia (extended-release: 1%), hypoesthesia (extended-release: 1%), dystonia

Dermatologic: Allergic skin reaction (≤4%), dermatitis (immediate-release: ≤4%), diaphoresis (extended-release: ≥1%), pruritus (extended-release: 1%)

Endocrine & metabolic: Menstrual disease (immediate-release: 10%; extended-release: 2%), increased libido (immediate-release: 8%; extended-release: ≥1%), change in libido (immediate-release: 7%), hot flash (extended-release: 2%)

Gastrointestinal: Nausea (extended-release: 6%), sialorrhea (immediate-release: 4% to 6%; extended-release: ≥1%), anorexia (extended-release: 2%), abdominal pain (extended-release: ≥1%), diarrhea (extended-release: ≥1%), dyspepsia (extended-release: ≥1%), vomiting (extended-release: ≥1%)

Genitourinary: Sexual disorder (immediate-release: 7%; extended-release: 2%), dysmenorrhea (extended-release: 4%), urinary incontinence (immediate-release: 2%; extended-release: <1%)

Neuromuscular & skeletal: Arthralgia (extended-release: 2%), dyskinesia (extended-release: 2%), myalgia (extended-release: 2%), back pain (extended-release: ≥1%), muscle cramps (extended-release: ≥1%), muscle twitching (extended-release: ≥1%), tremor (extended-release: ≥1%), weakness (extended-release: ≥1%), limb pain (extended-release: 1%)

Ophthalmic: Blurred vision (extended-release: ≥1%)

Respiratory: Dyspnea (extended-release: 2%), hyperventilation (extended-release: ≥1%), nasal congestion (extended-release: ≥1%), allergic rhinitis (extended-release: 1%)

Frequency not defined:

Central nervous system: Drug dependence, drug withdrawal

<1%, postmarketing, and/or case reports: Abnormal dreams, aggressive behavior, amnesia, angioedema, apathy, chest tightness, choking sensation, clumsiness, cold and clammy skin, diplopia, dysgeusia, dysphagia, edema, emotional lability, epistaxis, euphoria, falling, fever, galactorrhea, gastrointestinal disease, gynecomastia, hallucination, hangover effect, hepatic failure, hepatitis, homicidal ideation, hyperprolactinemia, hypomania, hypotonia, impaired consciousness, impulse control disorder, increased energy, increased liver enzymes, increased serum bilirubin, increased thirst, intoxicated feeling, jaundice, jitteriness, mania, mydriasis, otalgia, outbursts of anger, paraplegia, peripheral edema, photophobia, psychomotor retardation, relaxation, rhinorrhea, rigors, seizure, sensation of cold, sinus tachycardia, skin photosensitivity, sleep apnea, sleep talking, Stevens-Johnson syndrome, stupor, suicidal ideation, syncope, tinnitus, urinary frequency, urticaria, voice disorder

Dental Usual Dosage Preoperative anxiety (off-label use) Adults: Oral: 0.5 mg 60-90 minutes before procedure (De Witte, 2002)

Dosing

Adult Note: Reduce dose or avoid use in patients receiving opioids, with significant chronic disease (eg, respiratory compromise), or at increased risk for accumulation (eg, advanced cirrhosis). Generally, avoid use in patients with, or at risk for, substance use disorders; if used, closely supervise.

Anxiety:

Anxiety disorders (adjunctive therapy or monotherapy) (alternative agent):

Note: Generally used short term for symptom relief until concurrent therapy is effective (eg, ≤12 weeks). Long-term, low-dose therapy (eg, 2 mg/day) may be considered for select patients when other treatments are ineffective or poorly tolerated (Craske 2020; Katzman 2014; WFSBP [Bandelow 2012]). Use with caution in patients with posttraumatic stress disorder; benzodiazepines may worsen symptoms (VA/DoD 2017).

Immediate release: **Oral:** Initial: 0.25 mg 3 to 4 times daily; may increase dose based on response and tolerability in increments ≤1 mg/day at intervals ≥3 days up to a usual dose of 2 to 6 mg/day in 3 to 4 divided doses. Some patients may require up to 8 mg/day for optimal response; manufacturer's labeling maximum: 10 mg/day. With doses >4 mg/day, increase more gradually to minimize adverse effects; periodically reassess and consider dosage reduction (APA [Stein 2009]; WFSBP [Bandelow 2012]; manufacturer's labeling).

Extended release (panic disorder labeled use): **Oral:** Initial: 0.5 to 1 mg once daily; may increase dose based on response and tolerability in increments ≤1 mg/day at intervals ≥3 days up to a usual dose of 2 to 6 mg/day. Some patients may require up to 8 mg/day for optimal response; manufacturer's labeling maximum: 10 mg/day. With doses >4 mg/day, increase more gradually to minimize adverse effects; periodically reassess and consider dosage reduction. Administration in 2 divided doses may be considered to maximize efficacy (APA [Stein 2009]; WFSBP [Bandelow 2012]; manufacturer's labeling).

Procedural anxiety (premedication) (off-label use):

Immediate release: **Oral, Sublingual:** 0.5 mg 30 to 90 minutes before procedure; if needed due to incomplete response and/or duration of procedure, may repeat the dose (usually at 50% of the initial dose) after 30 to 60 minutes (Choy 2020; De Witte 2002; Shavakhi 2014).

Vertigo, acute episodes, treatment (alternative agent) (off-label use):

Note: Reserve use for episodes lasting several hours to days. Dosing based on expert opinion.

Immediate release: **Oral:** Initial: 0.5 mg every 8 hours as needed with a usual duration of 24 to 48 hours (Furman 2020).

Dosing conversions: Immediate release to extended release: ER tablet may be substituted for the IR tablet on a mg-per-mg basis, administering the ER tablet once daily. Administration of the ER formulation in 2 divided doses may be considered to maximize efficacy (APA [Stein 2009]).

Discontinuation of therapy: In patients receiving extended or higher-dose benzodiazepine therapy, unless safety concerns require a more rapid withdrawal, gradually withdraw to detect reemerging symptoms and minimize rebound and withdrawal symptoms. Taper total daily dose by 10% to 25% every 1 to 2 weeks based on response and tolerability. The optimal taper rate and duration will vary; durations up to 6 months may be necessary for some patients (Bystritsky 2020; Lader 2011; VA/DoD 2015). For patients on high doses, taper more rapidly in the beginning and slow the reduction rate as the taper progresses. For example, reduce the dose weekly by 25% until half of the dose remains. Thereafter, continue to reduce by ~12% every 4 to 7 days. For benzodiazepines with half-lives significantly less than 24 hours, including alprazolam, consider substituting an equivalent dose of a long-acting benzodiazepine to allow for a more gradual reduction in drug serum concentrations (VA/DoD 2015).

Dosage adjustment for concomitant therapy: Significant drug interactions exist, requiring dose/frequency adjustment or avoidance. Consult drug interactions database for more information.

Geriatric

Immediate release: **Oral:** Use lower initial doses of 0.25 mg 2 to 3 times daily and titrate slowly; refer to adult dosing.

Extended release: **Oral:** Use lower initial doses of 0.5 mg once daily and titrate slowly; refer to adult dosing.

Dosing conversions: Refer to adult dosing.

Discontinuation of therapy: Refer to adult dosing.

Renal Impairment: Adult There are no dosage adjustments provided in the manufacturer's labeling; use caution.

Hepatic Impairment: Adult

Advanced liver disease:

IR tablet, oral concentrate, orally disintegrating tablet: 0.25 mg 2 to 3 times daily.

Extended release: 0.5 mg once daily

Pediatric Note: Titrate dose to effect; use lowest effective dose. The usefulness of this medication should be periodically reassessed.

Anxiety:

Children ≥7 years and Adolescents <18 years: Limited data available: Oral: Immediate release: Initial: 0.005 to 0.02 mg/kg/dose 3 times daily (Kliegman 2007); dosing based on a trial in patients 7 to 16 years of age (n=13), initial doses of 0.005 mg/kg or 0.125 mg/dose were given 3 times/day for situational anxiety and increments of 0.125 to 0.25 mg/dose were used to increase doses to maximum of 0.02 mg/kg/dose or 0.06 mg/kg/**day**; a range of 0.375 to 3 mg/**day** was needed (Pfefferbaum 1987). Another study in 17 children (8 to 17 years of age) with overanxious disorder or avoidant disorders used initial daily doses of 0.25 mg for children <40 kg and 0.5 mg for those >40 kg. The dose was titrated at 2-day intervals to a maximum of 0.04 mg/kg/**day**. Required doses ranged from 0.5 to 3.5 mg/day with a mean of 1.6 mg/day. Based on clinical global ratings, alprazolam appeared to be better than placebo; however, this difference was **not** statistically significant (Simeon 1992).

Adolescents ≥18 years: Oral: Immediate release: Initial: 0.25 to 0.5 mg 3 times daily; titrate dose upward as needed every 3 to 4 days; usual maximum daily dose: 4 mg/**day**. Patients requiring doses >4 mg/**day** should be increased cautiously. Periodic reassessment and consideration of dosage reduction is recommended.

Panic disorder: Adolescents ≥18 years: Oral:

Immediate release: Initial: 0.5 mg 3 times daily; titrate dose upward as needed every 3 to 4 days in increments ≤1 mg/day; mean dose used in controlled trials: 5 to 6 mg/**day**; maximum daily dose: 10 mg/**day** (rarely required)

Extended release: Initial: 0.5 to 1 mg once daily; titrate dose upward as needed every 3 to 4 days in increments ≤1 mg/day; usual dose: 3 to 6 mg/**day**; maximum daily dose: 10 mg/**day** (rarely required)

Switching from immediate release to extended release: Administer the same total daily dose, but give once daily; if effect is not adequate, titrate dose as above.

Premenstrual dysphoric disorder: Limited data available: Adolescents: Oral: Initial dose: 0.25 mg 3 times daily; titrate as needed. Usual daily dose: 1.25 to 2.25 mg/**day** (Kliegman 2011)

Discontinuation of therapy: Abrupt discontinuation should be avoided. Daily dose must be gradually decreased no more frequently than every 3 days; however, some patients may require a slower reduction. If withdrawal symptoms occur, resume previous dose and discontinue on a less rapid schedule.

Renal Impairment: Pediatric There are no dosage adjustments provided in the manufacturer's labeling.

Mechanism of Action Binds to stereospecific benzodiazepine receptors on the postsynaptic GABA neuron at several sites within the central nervous system, including the limbic system, reticular formation. Enhancement of the inhibitory effect of GABA on neuronal excitability results by increased neuronal membrane permeability to chloride ions. This shift in chloride ions results in hyperpolarization (a less excitable state) and stabilization. Benzodiazepine receptors and effects appear to be linked to the GABA-A receptors. Benzodiazepines do not bind to GABA-B receptors.

Contraindications Hypersensitivity to alprazolam or any component of the formulation (cross-sensitivity with other benzodiazepines may exist); acute narrow-angle glaucoma; concurrent use with ketoconazole, itraconazole, or other potent CYP3A4 inhibitors.

Canadian labeling: Additional contraindications (not in US labeling): Myasthenia gravis; severe hepatic insufficiency; severe respiratory insufficiency; sleep apnea.

Warnings/Precautions [US Boxed warning]: Concomitant use of benzodiazepines and opioids may result in profound sedation, respiratory depression, coma, and death. Reserve concomitant prescribing of these drugs for use in patients for whom alternative treatment options are inadequate. Limit dosages and durations to the minimum required. Follow patients for signs and symptoms of respiratory depression and sedation.

Rebound or withdrawal symptoms, including seizures, may occur following abrupt discontinuation or large decreases in dose (more common in adult patients receiving >4 mg/day or prolonged treatment); the risk of seizures appears to be greatest 24 to 72 hours following discontinuation of therapy. Breakthrough anxiety may occur at the end of dosing interval. Use with caution in patients receiving concurrent CYP3A4 inhibitors, moderate or strong CYP3A4 inducers, and major CYP3A4 substrates; consider alternative agents that avoid or lessen the potential for CYP-mediated interactions. Use with caution in renal impairment or predisposition to urate nephropathy; has weak uricosuric properties. Use with caution in or debilitated patients (use lower starting dose), patients with hepatic disease (including alcoholics) or respiratory disease, or obese patients. Cigarette smoking may decrease alprazolam concentrations up to 50%. Elderly patients may be at an increased risk of death with use; risk has been found highest within the first 4 months of use in elderly dementia patients (Jennum 2015; Saarelainen 2018).

Causes CNS depression (dose related) which may impair physical and mental capabilities. Patients must be cautioned about performing tasks that require mental alertness (eg, operating machinery or driving). Effects with other sedative drugs or ethanol may be potentiated. Benzodiazepines have been associated with falls and traumatic injury and should be used with extreme caution in patients who are at risk of these events (Nelson 1999). Hazardous sleep-related activities such as sleep-driving, cooking and eating food, and making phone calls while asleep have been noted with benzodiazepines (Dolder 2008).

Use caution in patients with depression, particularly if suicidal risk may be present. Episodes of mania or hypomania have occurred in depressed patients treated with alprazolam. May cause physical or psychological dependence. Acute withdrawal may be precipitated in patients after administration of flumazenil. Tolerance does not develop to the anxiolytic effects (Vinkers 2012). Chronic use of this agent may increase the perioperative benzodiazepine dose needed to achieve desired effect.

Benzodiazepines have been associated with anterograde amnesia (Nelson 1999). Paradoxical reactions, including hyperactive or aggressive behavior, have been reported with benzodiazepines; risk may be increased in adolescent/pediatric patients, geriatric patients, or patients with a history of alcohol use disorder or psychiatric/personality disorders (Mancuso 2004). Does not have analgesic, antidepressant, or antipsychotic properties.

Drug Interactions

Metabolism/Transport Effects **Substrate** of CYP3A4 (major); **Note:** Assignment of Major/Minor substrate status based on clinically relevant drug interaction potential; **Inhibits** CYP3A4 (weak)

Avoid Concomitant Use

Avoid concomitant use of ALPRAZolam with any of the following: Abametapir; Azelastine (Nasal); Bromperidol; Conivaptan; Fusidic Acid (Systemic); Idelalisib; Indinavir; Itraconazole; Ketoconazole (Systemic); OLANZapine; Orphenadrine; Oxomemazine; Paraldehyde; Pimozide; Sodium Oxybate; Thalidomide

Increased Effect/Toxicity

ALPRAZolam may increase the levels/effects of: Alcohol (Ethyl); Azelastine (Nasal); Blonanserin; Brexanolone; Buprenorphine; CloZAPine; CNS Depressants; Dofetilide; Flibanserin; Flunitrazepam; Lemborexant; Lomitapide; Methadone; Methotrimeprazine; MetyroSINE; NiMODipine; Opioid Agonists; Orphenadrine; OxyCODONE; Paraldehyde; Pimozide; Piribedil; Pramipexole; ROPINIRole; Rotigotine; Sodium Oxybate; Suvorexant; Thalidomide; Triazolam; Ubrogepant; Zolpidem

The levels/effects of ALPRAZolam may be increased by: Abametapir; Alizapride; Aprepitant; Brimonidine (Topical); Bromopride; Bromperidol; Cannabidiol; Cannabis; Chlormethiazole; Chlorphenesin Carbamate; Clofazimine; Conivaptan; CYP3A4 Inhibitors (Moderate); CYP3A4 Inhibitors (Strong); Dimethindene (Topical); Doxylamine; Dronabinol; Droperidol; Duvelisib; Erdafitinib; Erythromycin (Systemic); Esketamine; FluvoxaMINE; Fosaprepitant; Fosnetupitant; Fusidic Acid (Systemic); HydrOXYzine; Idelalisib; Indinavir; Itraconazole; Kava Kava; Ketoconazole (Systemic); Larotrectinib; Lemborexant; Lisuride; Lofexidine; Magnesium Sulfate; Melatonin; Methotrimeprazine; Metoclopramide; MiFEPRIStone; Minocycline (Systemic); Nabilone; Netupitant; OLANZapine; Ombitasvir, Paritaprevir, and Ritonavir; Ombitasvir, Paritaprevir, Ritonavir, and Dasabuvir; Oxomemazine; Palbociclib; Perampanel; Rufinamide; Simeprevir; Stiripentol; Teduglutide; Tetrahydrocannabinol; Tetrahydrocannabinol and Cannabidiol; Trimeprazine

Decreased Effect

The levels/effects of ALPRAZolam may be decreased by: CYP3A4 Inducers (Moderate); CYP3A4 Inducers (Strong); Dabrafenib; Deferasirox; Enzalutamide; Erdafitinib; Ivosidenib; Mitotane; Sarilumab; Siltuximab; Theophylline Derivatives; Tocilizumab; Yohimbine

Food Interactions The C_{max} of the extended release formulation is increased by 25% when a high-fat meal is given 2 hours before dosing. T_{max} is decreased 33% when food is given immediately prior to dose and increased by 33% when food is given ≥1 hour after dose. Management: Administer without regard to food.

Dietary Considerations Orally-disintegrating tablets may contain phenylalanine.

Pharmacodynamics/Kinetics

Half-life Elimination

Adults: Mean: 11.2 hours (Immediate release range: 6.3 to 26.9 hours; Extended release range: 10.7 to 15.8 hours); Orally-disintegrating tablet: Mean: 12.5 hours (range: 7.9 to 19.2 hours)

Alcoholic liver disease: 19.7 hours (range: 5.8 to 65.3 hours)

Obesity: 21.8 hours (range: 9.9 to 40.4 hours)

Elderly: 16.3 hours (range: 9 to 26.9 hours)

Time to Peak

Immediate release: 1 to 2 hours

Extended release: Adolescents and Adults: ~9 hours, relatively steady from 4 to 12 hours (Glue 2006); decreased by 1 hour when administered at bedtime (as compared to morning administration); decreased by 33% when administered with a high-fat meal; increased by 33% when administered ≥1 hour after a high-fat meal

Orally-disintegrating tablet: 1.5 to 2 hours; occurs ~15 minutes earlier when administered with water; increased to ~4 hours when administered with a high-fat meal

Pregnancy Risk Factor D

Pregnancy Considerations Benzodiazepines have the potential to cause harm to the fetus. Alprazolam and its metabolites cross the human placenta. Teratogenic effects have been observed with some benzodiazepines; however, additional studies are needed. The incidence of premature birth and low birth weights may be increased following maternal use of benzodiazepines; hypoglycemia and respiratory problems in the neonate may occur following exposure late in pregnancy. Neonatal withdrawal symptoms may occur within days to weeks after birth and "floppy infant syndrome" (which also includes withdrawal symptoms) has been reported with some benzodiazepines (Bergman 1992; Iqbal 2002; Wikner 2007). When treating pregnant females with panic disorder, psychosocial interventions should be considered prior to pharmacotherapy (APA [Stein 2009]). If a benzodiazepine is needed in pregnancy, agents other than alprazolam are preferred (Larsen 2015).

Breastfeeding Considerations Alprazolam is present in breast milk.

The relative infant dose (RID) of alprazolam is 7.9% when calculated using a mean breast milk concentration and compared to a weight-adjusted maternal dose of 0.5 mg.

In general, breastfeeding is considered acceptable when an RID of a medication is <10% (Anderson 2016; Ito 2000). However, some sources note breastfeeding should only be considered if the RID is <5% for psychotropic agents (Larsen 2015).

The RID of alprazolam was calculated using a mean maximum milk concentration of 3.7 ng/mL, providing an estimated daily infant dose via breast milk of 0.555 mcg/kg/day. This milk concentration was obtained following administration of a single oral dose of alprazolam 0.5 mg to eight postpartum females. Peak breast milk concentrations of alprazolam occurred at ~1 hour and the half-life was ~14 hours; metabolites were not detected (Oo 1995).

Case reports have noted drowsiness (Ito 1993) or CNS depression (Kelly 2012) in infants exposed to alprazolam while breastfeeding. Symptoms of withdrawal were described in an infant following alprazolam exposure in utero and via breast milk (Anderson 1989).

Breastfeeding is not recommended by the manufacturer. If a benzodiazepine is needed in breastfeeding females, use of shorter acting agents is preferred (Larsen 2015; WHO 2002).

Controlled Substance C-IV

Dosage Forms: US

Concentrate, Oral:
ALPRAZolam Intensol: 1 mg/mL (30 mL)

Tablet, Oral:
Xanax: 0.25 mg, 0.5 mg, 1 mg, 2 mg
Generic: 0.25 mg, 0.5 mg, 1 mg, 2 mg

Tablet Disintegrating, Oral:
Generic: 0.25 mg, 0.5 mg, 1 mg, 2 mg

Tablet Extended Release 24 Hour, Oral:
ALPRAZolam XR: 0.5 mg, 1 mg, 2 mg, 3 mg
Xanax XR: 0.5 mg, 1 mg, 2 mg, 3 mg
Generic: 0.5 mg, 1 mg, 2 mg, 3 mg

Dosage Forms: Canada

Tablet, Oral:
Xanax: 0.25 mg, 0.5 mg, 1 mg
Xanax TS: 2 mg
Generic: 0.25 mg, 0.5 mg, 1 mg, 2 mg

Dental Health Professional Considerations
Patient should not drive themselves to and from the dental office. It is recommended an adult companion accompany the patient to their appointment.

◆ **ALPRAZolam Intensol** *see* ALPRAZolam *on page 106*

◆ **ALPRAZolam XR** *see* ALPRAZolam *on page 106*

Alprostadil (al PROS ta dill)

Brand Names: US Caverject; Caverject Impulse; Edex; Muse; Prostin VR

Brand Names: Canada Caverject; Muse; Prostin VR

Pharmacologic Category Prostaglandin; Vasodilator

Use

Patent ductus arteriosus (Prostin VR Pediatric): Temporary maintenance of patency of ductus arteriosus in neonates with ductal-dependent congenital heart disease until surgery can be performed. These defects include cyanotic (eg, pulmonary atresia, pulmonary stenosis, tricuspid atresia, Fallot's tetralogy, transposition of the great vessels) and acyanotic (eg, interruption of aortic arch, coarctation of aorta, hypoplastic left ventricle) heart disease.

Erectile dysfunction:

Caverject, Edex, Caverject Impulse: Treatment of erectile dysfunction due to vasculogenic, psychogenic, neurogenic, or mixed etiology; Caverject may be a useful adjunct to other diagnostic tests in the diagnosis of erectile dysfunction

Muse: Treatment of erectile dysfunction

Local Anesthetic/Vasoconstrictor Precautions
No information available to require special precautions

Effects on Dental Treatment No significant effects or complications reported

Effects on Bleeding No information available to require special precautions

Adverse Reactions

Intraurethral:

>10%: Genitourinary: Penile pain, urethral burning

2% to 10%:
Central nervous system: Dizziness, headache, pain
Genitourinary: Testicular pain, urethral bleeding (minor), vulvovaginal pruritus (female partner)

<2%: Leg pain, perineal pain, tachycardia

Intracavernosal injection:

>10%: Genitourinary: Penile pain

1% to 10%:
Cardiovascular: Hypertension
Central nervous system: Dizziness, headache
Genitourinary: Prolonged erection (>4 hours, 4%), penile disease, penile rash, penile swelling, Peyronie's disease
Local: Bruising at injection site, hematoma at injection site

<1%: Balanitis, injection site hemorrhage, priapism (0.4%)

Intravenous:

>10%:
Cardiovascular: Flushing
Respiratory: Apnea
Miscellaneous: Fever

1% to 10%:
Cardiovascular: Bradycardia, cardiac arrest, edema, hypertension, hypotension, tachycardia
Central nervous system: Dizziness, headache, seizure
Endocrine & metabolic: Hypokalemia
Gastrointestinal: Diarrhea
Hematologic & oncologic: Disseminated intravascular coagulation
Infection: Sepsis
Local: Local pain (in structures other than the injection site)
Neuromuscular & skeletal: Back pain
Respiratory: Cough, flu-like symptoms, nasal congestion, sinusitis, upper respiratory tract infection

<1%: Anemia, anuria, bradypnea, cardiac failure, cerebral hemorrhage, gastroesophageal reflux disease, hematuria, hemorrhage, hyperbilirubinemia, hyperemia, hyperirritability, hyperkalemia, hypoglycemia, hypothermia, jitteriness, lethargy, neck hyperextension, peritonitis, second degree atrioventricular block, shock, stiffness, supraventricular tachycardia, thrombocytopenia, ventricular fibrillation, wheezing (bronchial)

Mechanism of Action Causes vasodilation by means of direct effect on vascular and ductus arteriosus smooth muscle; relaxes trabecular smooth muscle by dilation of cavernosal arteries when injected along the penile shaft, allowing blood flow to and entrapment in the lacunar spaces of the penis (ie, corporeal veno-occlusive mechanism)

Pharmacodynamics/Kinetics

Onset of Action Erectile dysfunction: 5 to 20 minutes

Duration of Action Ductus arteriosus will begin to close within 1 to 2 hours after drug is stopped; Erectile dysfunction: Intended duration <1 hour

Half-life Elimination 30 seconds to 10 minutes

Time to Peak

Acyanotic congenital heart disease: Usual: 1.5 to 3 hours; Range: 15 minutes to 11 hours

Cyanotic congenital heart disease: Usual: ~30 minutes

Erectile dysfunction: Intracavernosal: 30 to 60 minutes; Transurethral: ~16 minutes

Reproductive Considerations

Muse is contraindicated in males having sexual intercourse with a pregnant woman unless a condom barrier is being used.

Pregnancy Considerations Alprostadil is not indicated for use in women.

◆ **Alprostadil Alfadex** *see* Alprostadil *on page 110*

◆ **Altabax** *see* Retapamulin *on page 1318*

◆ **Altace** *see* Ramipril *on page 1307*

◆ **Altavera** *see* Ethinyl Estradiol and Levonorgestrel *on page 612*

Alteplase (AL te plase)

Related Information

Cardiovascular Diseases *on page 1654*

Brand Names: US Activase; Cathflo Activase

Brand Names: Canada Activase RT-PA; Alteplase RT-PA; Cathflo

Pharmacologic Category Thrombolytic Agent

Use

Activase:

Acute ischemic stroke: Treatment of acute ischemic stroke (AIS) as soon as possible but within 3 hours of symptom onset.

Pulmonary embolism: Management of acute massive pulmonary embolism (PE)

ST-elevation myocardial infarction: Management of ST-elevation myocardial infarction (STEMI) for the lysis of thrombi in coronary arteries.

Limitations of use: The risk of stroke may outweigh the benefit produced by thrombolytic therapy in patients whose acute myocardial infarction (MI) puts them at low risk for death or heart failure.

Recommended criteria for treatment:

STEMI (ACCF/AHA [O'Gara 2013]): Ischemic symptoms within 12 hours of treatment or evidence of ongoing ischemia 12 to 24 hours after symptom onset with a large area of myocardium at risk or hemodynamic instability.

STEMI ECG definition: New ST-segment elevation at the J point in at least 2 contiguous leads of ≥2 mm (0.2 mV) in men or ≥1.5 mm (0.15 mV) in women in leads V_2-V_3 and/or of ≥1 mm (0.1 mV) in other contiguous precordial leads or limb leads. New or presumably new left bundle branch block (LBBB) may interfere with ST-elevation analysis and should not be considered diagnostic in isolation.

At non-PCI-capable hospitals, the ACCF/AHA recommends thrombolytic therapy administration when the anticipated first medical contact (FMC)-to-device time at a PCI-capable hospital is >120 minutes due to unavoidable delays.

AIS: Onset of stroke symptoms within 3 hours of treatment

Pulmonary embolism (PE), acute (hemodynamically unstable/massive): Acute PE in patients with sustained hypotension (SBP <90 mm Hg for 15 minutes) or with signs/symptoms of shock and without a high bleeding risk (Kearon 2012; Kearon 2016).

Cathflo Activase: Restoration of function to central venous access device

Local Anesthetic/Vasoconstrictor Precautions No information available to require special precautions

Effects on Dental Treatment Key adverse event(s) related to dental treatment: As with all drugs which may affect hemostasis, bleeding is the major adverse effect associated with alteplase. Hemorrhage may occur at virtually any site; risk is dependent on multiple variables, including the dosage administered, concurrent use of multiple agents which alter hemostasis, and patient predisposition. Rapid lysis of coronary artery thrombi by thrombolytic agents may be associated with reperfusion-related atrial and/or ventricular arrhythmias. See Effects on Bleeding.

Effects on Bleeding Bleeding is the major adverse effect associated with thrombolytic agents, such as alteplase. It is unlikely that ambulatory patients presenting for dental treatment will be taking parenteral thrombolytic therapy.

Adverse Reactions

>10%: Cardiovascular: Intracranial hemorrhage (CVA: Within 90 days: 15%, within 36 hours: 6%; AMI: <1%)

1% to 10%:

Cerebrovascular accident (new ischemic stroke in CVA: 6%)

Dermatologic: Ecchymosis (AMI: 1%)

Gastrointestinal: Gastrointestinal hemorrhage (AMI: 5%)

Genitourinary: Genitourinary tract hemorrhage (AMI: 4%)

Frequency not defined:

Hematologic & oncologic: Arterial embolism, major hemorrhage, pulmonary embolism

Infection: Sepsis

1%, postmarketing, and/or case reports: Anaphylaxis, angioedema, atrioventricular block, atrioventricular dissociation, cardiac arrhythmia, cardiac failure, cardiac tamponade, cardiogenic shock, cerebral edema, cerebral herniation, deep vein thrombosis, embolism, epistaxis, fever, gingival hemorrhage, hypersensitivity reaction, hypotension, ischemia (recurrent), laryngeal edema, mitral valve insufficiency, myocardial reinfarction, myocardial rupture, nausea, pericardial effusion, pericarditis, pleural effusion, pulmonary edema, retroperitoneal hemorrhage, seizure, skin rash, thromboembolism, urticaria, vomiting

Mechanism of Action Initiates local fibrinolysis by binding to fibrin in a thrombus (clot) and converts entrapped plasminogen to plasmin

Pharmacodynamics/Kinetics

Duration of Action >50% present in plasma cleared ~5 minutes after infusion terminated, ~80% cleared within 10 minutes; fibrinolytic activity persists for up to 1 hour after infusion terminated (Semba 2000)

Half-life Elimination Initial: 5 minutes

Pregnancy Considerations

Based on the molecular weight, alteplase is not expected to cross the placenta (Pacheco 2019).

Bleeding may occur with alteplase therapy and the risk of bleeding may be increased by pregnancy.

Case reports describe the use of alteplase in pregnant women primarily for acute ischemic stroke (Khan 2017; Landais 2018; Rodrigues 2019; Ryman 2019; Sousa Gomes 2019; Watanabe 2019). Use of alteplase may be appropriate for the treatment of moderate or severe acute stroke in pregnant women. Close monitoring for uterine bleeding is recommended (AHA/ASA [Powers 2019]; Leffert 2016; Pacheco 2019).

Use of alteplase in pregnant patients with pulmonary embolism (ESC [Konstantinides 2020]; Rodriguez 2020) and mechanical prosthetic valve thrombosis (Sousa Gomes 2019) has also been reported. Information related to early postpartum use is limited (Akazawa 2017).

- **Alteplase Recombinant** *see* Alteplase *on page 111*
- **Alteplase, Tissue Plasminogen Activator, Recombinant** *see* Alteplase *on page 111*
- **Altoprev** *see* Lovastatin *on page 940*
- **Altreno** *see* Tretinoin (Topical) *on page 1484*
- **Aluminum Potassium Sulfate and Epinephrine (Racemic) (Dental)** *see* Epinephrine (Racemic) and Aluminum Potassium Sulfate *on page 575*
- **Aluminum Sucrose Sulfate, Basic** *see* Sucralfate *on page 1389*
- **Alunbrig** *see* Brigatinib *on page 250*
- **Alupent** *see* Metaproterenol *on page 982*
- **Alvesco** *see* Ciclesonide (Oral Inhalation) *on page 346*

Alvimopan (al VI moe pan)

Brand Names: US Entereg

Pharmacologic Category Gastrointestinal Agent, Miscellaneous; Opioid Antagonist, Peripherally-Acting

Use Postoperative ileus: To accelerate the time to upper and lower GI recovery following surgeries including partial bowel resection with primary anastomosis

Local Anesthetic/Vasoconstrictor Precautions No information available to require special precautions

Effects on Dental Treatment No significant effects or complications reported

Effects on Bleeding No information available to require special precautions

Adverse Reactions Note: Incidence reported limited to bowel resection patients only.

1% to 10%:

Endocrine & metabolic: Hypokalemia (10%)
Gastrointestinal: Dyspepsia (2% to 7%)
Genitourinary: Urinary retention (3%)
Hematologic and oncologic: Anemia (5%)
Neuromuscular & skeletal: Back pain (3%)

Frequency not defined:

Cardiovascular: Myocardial infarction

Mechanism of Action An opioid receptor antagonist which blocks opioid binding at the mu receptor; alvimopan has restricted ability to cross the blood-brain barrier at therapeutic doses. It selectively and competitively binds to the GI tract mu opioid receptors and antagonizes the peripheral effects of opioids on gastrointestinal motility and secretion. Does not affect opioid analgesic effects or induce opioid withdrawal symptoms.

Pharmacodynamics/Kinetics

Half-life Elimination 10 to 17 hours

Time to Peak Plasma: Parent drug: ~2 hours; Metabolite: 36 hours

Pregnancy Considerations Adverse events have not been observed in animal reproduction studies.

- **ALX-0600** *see* Teduglutide *on page 1410*
- **ALXN 1210** *see* Ravulizumab *on page 1313*
- **Alyacen 1/35** *see* Ethinyl Estradiol and Norethindrone *on page 614*
- **Alyacen 7/7/7** *see* Ethinyl Estradiol and Norethindrone *on page 614*
- **Alyq** *see* Tadalafil *on page 1401*
- **Amabelz** *see* Estradiol and Norethindrone *on page 598*

Amantadine (a MAN ta deen)

Related Information

Systemic Viral Diseases *on page 1709*

Brand Names: US Gocovri; Osmolex ER

Brand Names: Canada DOM-Amantadine HCl [DSC]; PDP-Amantadine; PHL-Amantadine [DSC]

Pharmacologic Category Anti-Parkinson Agent, Dopamine Agonist; Antiviral Agent; Antiviral Agent, Adamantane

Use

Drug-induced extrapyramidal symptoms (IR and ER tablet only): Treatment of drug-induced extrapyramidal symptoms.

Parkinson disease, dyskinesias (adjunctive therapy) or mild motor symptoms (monotherapy):

Extended release:

Capsule: Treatment of dyskinesias in patients with Parkinson disease receiving levodopa-based therapy, with or without concomitant dopaminergic medications.

Tablet: Treatment of Parkinson disease.

Immediate release: Treatment of idiopathic Parkinson disease (paralysis agitans), postencephalitic parkinsonism, parkinsonism in association with cerebral arteriosclerosis, and symptomatic parkinsonism, which may follow injury to the nervous system by carbon monoxide intoxication.

Local Anesthetic/Vasoconstrictor Precautions No information available to require special precautions

Effects on Dental Treatment Key adverse event(s) related to dental treatment: Xerostomia (prolonged use may cause significant xerostomia; normal salivary flow resumes upon discontinuation); Patients may experience orthostatic hypotension as they stand up after treatment; especially if lying in dental chair for extended periods of time. Use caution with sudden changes in position during and after dental treatment.

Effects on Bleeding No information available to require special precautions

Adverse Reactions

>10%:

Cardiovascular: Orthostatic hypotension (≤29%; may be more common in men), presyncope (≤29%), syncope (≤29%), peripheral edema (1% to 16%)

Central nervous system: Dizziness (≤29%), delusions (≤25%), hallucination (≤25%), illusion (≤25%), paranoia (≤25%), falling (13%)

Gastrointestinal: Xerostomia (1% to 16%; may be more common in women), constipation (1% to 13%)

1% to 10%:

Cardiovascular: Livedo reticularis (1% to 6%; may be more common in women)

Central nervous system: Insomnia (5% to 10%), anxiety (1% to 7%), depression (1% to 6%), headache (1% to 6%), abnormal dreams (1% to 5%; may be more common in women), agitation (1% to 5%), ataxia (1% to 5%; may be more common in men and adults ≥65 years old), confusion (1% to 5%), drowsiness (1% to 5%), fatigue (1% to 5%), irritability (1% to 5%), nervousness (1% to 5%), dyschromia (3%), dystonia (3%), apathy (2%), suicidal ideation (≤2%)

Gastrointestinal: Nausea (5% to 10%; may be more common in women), decreased appetite (6%), anorexia (1% to 5%), diarrhea (1% to 5%), vomiting (3%)

Genitourinary: Urinary tract infection (10%), benign prostatic hypertrophy (6%)

Hematologic & oncologic: Bruise (6%)

Neuromuscular & skeletal: Joint swelling (3%), muscle spasm (3%)

Ophthalmic: Blurred vision (4%), cataract (3%; may be more common in women), xerophthalmia (3%)

Respiratory: Dry nose (1% to 5%), cough (3%)

<1%, postmarketing, and/or case reports: Abnormal gait, abnormality in thinking, acute respiratory tract failure, aggressive behavior, agranulocytosis, amnesia, anaphylaxis, cardiac arrhythmia (including malignant arrhythmias), cardiac failure, coma, corneal edema, decreased libido, decreased visual acuity, delirium, diaphoresis, dysphagia, dyspnea, eczema, edema, EEG pattern changes, euphoria, fever, hyperkinesia, hypersensitivity reaction, hypertension, hypertonia, hypokinesia, hypotension, impulse control disorder, increased blood urea nitrogen, increased creatine phosphokinase, increased gamma-glutamyl transferase, increased lactate dehydrogenase, increased libido, increased serum alkaline phosphatase, increased serum ALT, increased serum AST, increased serum bilirubin, increased serum creatinine, keratitis, leukocytosis, leukopenia, mania, mydriasis, neuroleptic malignant syndrome (associated with dosage reduction or abrupt withdrawal of amantadine), neutropenia, oculogyric crisis, optic nerve palsy, paresthesia, pathological gambling, pruritus, psychosis, pulmonary edema, seizure, skin photosensitivity, skin rash, slurred speech, stupor, tachycardia, tachypnea, tremor, urinary retention, visual disturbance (including punctate subepithelial or other corneal opacity), weakness

Mechanism of Action

Antiviral:

Amantadine is no longer recommended as an antiviral (CDC 2018; IDSA [Uyeki 2019]). The mechanism of amantadine's antiviral activity has not been fully elucidated. It appears to primarily prevent the release of infectious viral nucleic acid into the host cell by interfering with the transmembrane domain of the viral M2 protein. Amantadine is also known to prevent viral assembly during replication. Amantadine inhibits the replication of influenza A virus isolates from each of the subtypes (ie, H1N1, H2N2, and H3N2), but has very little or no activity against influenza B virus isolates.

Parkinson disease:

The exact mechanism of amantadine in the treatment of Parkinson disease and drug-induced extrapyramidal symptoms is not known. Data from early animal studies suggest that amantadine may have direct and indirect effects on dopamine neurons; however, recent studies have demonstrated that amantadine is a weak, noncompetitive NMDA receptor antagonist. Although amantadine has not been shown to possess direct anticholinergic activity, clinically, it exhibits anticholinergic-like side effects (dry mouth, urinary retention, and constipation).

Pharmacodynamics/Kinetics

Onset of Action Antidyskinetic: Within 48 hours

Half-life Elimination Normal renal function: 16 ± 6 hours (9 to 31 hours); Healthy, older (≥60 years) males: 29 hours (range: 20 to 41 hours) (Aoki 1988); End-stage renal disease: 8 days

Time to Peak Plasma: Extended-release capsule: 12 hours (mean; range: 6 to 20 hours); extended-release tablet: 7.5 hours (median; range: 5.5 to 12 hours); immediate release: 2 to 4 hours

Pregnancy Risk Factor C

Pregnancy Considerations

Adverse events have been observed in animal reproduction studies, and teratogenic events have been observed in humans (case reports) (Seier 2017).

When treatment for Parkinson disease is needed, agents other than amantadine are recommended in pregnant women (Seier 2017).

◆ **Amantadine Hydrochloride** *see* Amantadine *on page 112*

◆ **Amaryl** *see* Glimepiride *on page 740*

◆ **Ambien** *see* Zolpidem *on page 1582*

◆ **Ambien CR** *see* Zolpidem *on page 1582*

◆ **AmBisome** *see* Amphotericin B (Liposomal) *on page 138*

Ambrisentan (am bri SEN tan)

Brand Names: US Letairis

Brand Names: Canada APO-Ambrisentan; Volibris

Pharmacologic Category Endothelin Receptor Antagonist; Vasodilator

Use Pulmonary arterial hypertension: Treatment of pulmonary artery hypertension (PAH) (World Health Organization [WHO] Group I) to improve exercise ability and delay clinical worsening; in combination with tadalafil to reduce the risks of disease progression and hospitalization for worsening PAH, and to improve exercise ability. Studies establishing effectiveness included predominantly patients with WHO Functional Class II to III symptoms and etiologies of idiopathic or heritable PAH (60%) or PAH associated with connective tissue diseases (34%).

Local Anesthetic/Vasoconstrictor Precautions No information available to require special precautions

Effects on Dental Treatment Key adverse event(s) related to dental treatment: Endothelin antagonists have caused bleeding gums; there have been no specific reports for ambrisentan

Effects on Bleeding No information available to require special precautions

Adverse Reactions Frequency not always defined.

Cardiovascular: Peripheral edema (14% to 38%), flushing (4%)

Central nervous system: Headache (34%)

Gastrointestinal: Dyspepsia (3%)

Genitourinary: Oligospermia

Hematologic & oncologic: Decreased hemoglobin (7% to 10%; dose-dependent), anemia (7%), decreased hematocrit

Respiratory: Nasal congestion (6% to 16%), cough (13%), bronchitis (4%), sinusitis (3%)

<1%, postmarketing, and/or case reports: Cardiac failure, dizziness, fatigue, fluid retention, hypersensitivity, hypotension, increased liver enzymes, nausea, vomiting, weakness

Mechanism of Action Blocks endothelin receptor subtypes ET_A and ET_B on vascular endothelium and smooth muscle. Stimulation of ET_A receptors, located primarily in pulmonary vascular smooth muscle cells is associated with vasoconstriction and cellular proliferation. Stimulation of ET_B receptors, located in both pulmonary vascular endothelial cells and smooth muscle cells is associated with vasodilation, antiproliferative effects, and endothelin clearance. Although ambrisentan blocks both ET_A and ET_B receptors, the affinity is greater for the ET_A receptor (>4,000-fold higher affinity).

Pharmacodynamics/Kinetics

Half-life Elimination ~9 hours

Time to Peak ~2 hours

Reproductive Considerations

[US Boxed Warning]: Exclude pregnancy before the initiation of treatment with ambrisentan. Females of reproductive potential must have a negative pregnancy test prior to initiation of therapy.

[US Boxed Warning]: Females of reproductive potential must use acceptable methods of contraception during treatment and for 1 month after treatment. Obtain monthly pregnancy tests during treatment and 1 month after discontinuation of treatment. One highly effective form of contraception (intrauterine device, contraceptive implant, or tubal sterilization) or a combination of contraceptive methods (hormone contraceptive with a barrier method or 2 barrier methods) may be used. If the partner has had a vasectomy, a hormone or barrier method must also be used. A missed menses or suspected pregnancy should be reported to a health care provider and prompt immediate pregnancy testing.

Sperm counts may be reduced in men during treatment (as observed with bosentan).

Pregnancy Considerations Ambrisentan is contraindicated in pregnancy.

[US Boxed Warning]: Do not administer ambrisentan to a pregnant female because it may cause fetal harm. Ambrisentan is very likely to produce serious birth defects if used by pregnant females because this effect has been seen consistently when it is administered to animals.

Females with pulmonary arterial hypertension are encouraged to avoid pregnancy (McLaughlin 2009; Taichman 2014).

- **AMD3100** *see* Plerixafor *on page 1241*
- **Amdinocillin Pivoxil** *see* Pivmecillinam *on page 1240*
- **Ameluz** *see* Aminolevulinic Acid (Topical) *on page 117*
- **Amerge** *see* Naratriptan *on page 1085*
- **Americaine Hemorrhoidal Ointment** *see* Benzocaine *on page 228*
- **Ameseal™** *see* Polyvinylpyrrolidone and Sodium Hyaluronate *on page 1244*
- **A-Methapred** *see* MethylPREDNISolone *on page 999*
- **Amethia** *see* Ethinyl Estradiol and Levonorgestrel *on page 612*
- **Amethia Lo** *see* Ethinyl Estradiol and Levonorgestrel *on page 612*
- **Amethocaine Hydrochloride** *see* Tetracaine (Systemic) *on page 1427*
- **Amethocaine Hydrochloride** *see* Tetracaine (Topical) *on page 1428*
- **Amethopterin** *see* Methotrexate *on page 990*
- **Amethyst** *see* Ethinyl Estradiol and Levonorgestrel *on page 612*
- **Amfepramone** *see* Diethylpropion *on page 494*
- **AMG145** *see* Evolocumab *on page 631*
- **AMG-162** *see* Denosumab *on page 453*
- **Amicar** *see* Aminocaproic Acid *on page 116*

Amifampridine (AM i fam pri deen)

Brand Names: US Firdapse; Ruzurgi

Pharmacologic Category Cholinergic Agonist; Potassium Channel Blocker

Use Lambert-Eaton myasthenic syndrome: Treatment of Lambert-Eaton myasthenic syndrome (LEMS) in adults (Firdapse) and pediatric patients 6 to <17 years (Ruzurgi).

Local Anesthetic/Vasoconstrictor Precautions Amifampridine causes increases in blood pressure. Consider monitoring blood pressure prior to using local anesthetic with a vasoconstrictor.

Effects on Dental Treatment No significant effects or complications reported

Effects on Bleeding No information available to require special precautions

Adverse Reactions

>10%:

Cardiovascular: Hypertension (12%)

Central nervous system: Paresthesia (62%), headache (14%), muscle spasm (12%)

Gastrointestinal: Abdominal pain (14%), diarrhea (14%), nausea (14%)

Hepatic: Increased liver enzymes (14%)

Neuromuscular & skeletal: Back pain (14%)

Respiratory: Upper respiratory tract infection (33%)

1% to 10%:

Cardiovascular: Peripheral edema (≥5%)

Central nervous system: Dizziness (10%), myasthenia (10%), falling (7%), depression (≥5%), insomnia (≥5%), seizure (2%)

Dermatologic: Erythema (≥5%)

Endocrine & metabolic: Hypercholesterolemia (≥5%)

Gastrointestinal: Constipation (7%), gastroesophageal reflux disease (≥5%)

Genitourinary: Urinary tract infection (≥5%)

Hematologic: Lymphadenopathy (7%)

Infection: Influenza (≥5%), viral infection (≥5%)

Neuromuscular & skeletal: Asthenia (10%), limb pain (10%), increased creatine phosphokinase in blood specimen (≥5%)

Ophthalmic: Cataract (10%)
Respiratory: Bronchitis (7%), dyspnea (≥5%)
Miscellaneous: Fever (≥5%)

Mechanism of Action Increases acetylcholine release in nerve terminals via potassium channel blockade (Wirtz 2010).

Pharmacodynamics/Kinetics

Half-life Elimination Firdapse: 1.8 to 2.5 hours; Ruzurgi: 3.6 to 4.2 hours

Time to Peak Firdapse: 20 minutes to 1 hour; Ruzurgi: Median: 0.5 hour; increased with high fat meal (1 hour)

Pregnancy Considerations

Information related to the use of amifampridine in pregnancy is limited (Pelufo-Pellicer 2006).

◆ **Amifampridine Phosphate** *see* Amifampridine *on page 114*

Amikacin (Systemic) (am i KAY sin)

Brand Names: Canada Erfa-Amikacin

Pharmacologic Category Antibiotic, Aminoglycoside

Use Serious infections: Treatment of serious infections (eg, bone infections, respiratory tract infections, endocarditis, septicemia) due to gram-negative organisms, including *Pseudomonas*, *Escherichia coli*, *Proteus*, *Providencia*, *Klebsiella*, *Enterobacter*, *Serratia*, and *Acinetobacter*

Local Anesthetic/Vasoconstrictor Precautions

No information available to require special precautions

Effects on Dental Treatment No significant effects or complications reported

Effects on Bleeding No information available to require special precautions

Adverse Reactions

1% to 10%:

Central nervous system: Neurotoxicity
Genitourinary: Nephrotoxicity
Otic: Auditory ototoxicity, vestibular ototoxicity

<1%, postmarketing, and/or case reports: Arthralgia, drowsiness, drug fever, dyspnea, eosinophilia, headache, hypersensitivity reaction, hypotension, nausea, paresthesia, skin rash, tremor, vomiting, weakness

Mechanism of Action Inhibits protein synthesis in susceptible bacteria by binding to 30S ribosomal subunits

Pharmacodynamics/Kinetics

Half-life Elimination Renal function and age dependent:

Infants: Low birth weight (1 to 3 days): 7 to 9 hours; Full-term >7 days: 4 to 5 hours (Howard 1975)
Children: 1.6 to 2.5 hours
Adolescents: 1.5 ± 1 hour
Adults: Normal renal function: ~2 hours; Anuria/end-stage renal disease: 17 to 150 hours (Aronoff 2007)

Time to Peak Serum: IM: 60 minutes; IV: Within 30 minutes following a 30-minute infusion; **Note:** Distribution is prolonged after larger doses (≥60 minutes after 30 minute-infusion of 20 mg/kg [Tod 1998]; ≥90 minutes after 60-minute infusion of a high-dose aminoglycoside [gentamicin 7 mg/kg] [Demczar 1997]).

Pregnancy Risk Factor D

Pregnancy Considerations Amikacin crosses the placenta.

Aminoglycosides may cause fetal harm if administered to a pregnant woman. There are several reports of total irreversible bilateral congenital deafness in children whose mothers received a different aminoglycoside (streptomycin) during pregnancy. Although serious side effects to the fetus/infant have not been reported following maternal use of all aminoglycosides, a potential for harm exists.

Due to pregnancy-induced physiologic changes, some pharmacokinetic parameters of intravenous amikacin may be altered (Bernard 1977).

Amikacin may be one of the preferred antibiotics when an aminoglycoside is needed for multidrug resistant TB in pregnancy (HHS [OI] 2018). Amikacin is recommended as part of a multiantibiotic treatment regimen of *Mycobacterium avium* complex (MAC) in patients with cystic fibrosis in certain situations (Floto 2016); use of the IV route should be reserved for life-threatening infections in pregnant females (Panchaud 2016).

Amikacin (Oral Inhalation) (am i KAY sin)

Brand Names: US Arikayce

Pharmacologic Category Antibiotic, Aminoglycoside

Use

***Mycobacterium avium* complex:** Treatment of *Mycobacterium avium* complex (MAC) lung disease in adults who have limited or no alternative treatment options, as part of a combination antibacterial drug regimen in patients who do not achieve negative sputum cultures after a minimum of 6 consecutive months of a multidrug background regimen therapy.

Limitation of use: Amikacin oral inhalation has only been studied in patients with refractory MAC lung disease defined as patients who did not achieve negative sputum cultures after a minimum of 6 consecutive months of a multidrug background regimen therapy. The use of amikacin is not recommended for patients with non-refractory MAC lung disease.

Local Anesthetic/Vasoconstrictor Precautions

No information available to require special precautions

Effects on Dental Treatment Key adverse event(s) related to dental treatment: Occurrence of oral candidiasis, altered sense of taste, xerostomia (normal salivary flow resumes upon discontinuance)

Effects on Bleeding No information available to require special precautions

Adverse Reactions

>10%:

Gastrointestinal: Diarrhea (13%), nausea (12%)
Nervous system: Fatigue (≤16%), voice disorder (47%)
Neuromuscular & skeletal: Asthenia (≤16%), musculoskeletal pain (17%)
Otic: Ototoxicity (17%)
Respiratory: Bronchospasm (29%), cough (39%), exacerbation of pulmonary symptoms (15%; including chronic obstructive pulmonary disease and bronchiectasis), hemoptysis (18%), pneumonia (10%), upper respiratory system symptoms (17%; including irritation, pain, inflammation, edema)

1% to 10%:

Cardiovascular: Chest discomfort (5%)
Dermatologic: Skin rash (6%)
Endocrine & metabolic: Weight loss (6%)
Gastrointestinal: Dysgeusia (3%), oral candidiasis (4%), vomiting (7%), xerostomia (2%)
Nervous system: Anxiety (5%), balance impairment (1%), dizziness (6%), headache (10%)
Neuromuscular & skeletal: Neuromuscular symptoms (2%; including myasthenia, peripheral neuropathy)
Otic: Tinnitus (8%)

Respiratory: Bronchitis (4%), change in bronchial secretions (5%), epistaxis (3%), hypersensitivity pneumonitis (3% to 4%), pneumothorax (2%), respiratory failure (3%)

Miscellaneous: Decreased exercise tolerance (1%), fever (7%)

Frequency not defined: Genitourinary: Nephrotoxicity

Postmarketing: Hypersensitivity: Anaphylaxis, hypersensitivity reaction

Mechanism of Action Inhibits protein synthesis in susceptible bacteria by binding to 30S ribosomal subunits

Pharmacodynamics/Kinetics

Half-life Elimination ~5.9 to 19.5 hours

Pregnancy Considerations

Aminoglycosides may cause fetal harm if administered to a pregnant woman. Systemic absorption of amikacin following oral inhalation is expected to be low compared to intravenous administration; however, systemic exposure was associated with total irreversible bilateral congenital deafness in children whose mothers received a different aminoglycoside during pregnancy.

Refer to the Amikacin (Systemic) monograph for details.

◆ **Amikacin Sulfate** *see* Amikacin (Oral Inhalation) *on page 115*

◆ **Amikacin Sulfate** *see* Amikacin (Systemic) *on page 115*

AMILoride (a MIL oh ride)

Related Information

Cardiovascular Diseases *on page 1654*

Brand Names: Canada Midamor

Pharmacologic Category Antihypertensive; Diuretic, Potassium-Sparing

Use

Heart failure or hypertension: Counteracts potassium loss induced by other diuretics in the treatment of hypertension or heart failure; usually used in conjunction with more potent diuretics such as thiazides or loop diuretics.

Note: Potassium-sparing diuretics are **not** recommended for the initial treatment of hypertension (ACC/AHA [Whelton 2018]).

Local Anesthetic/Vasoconstrictor Precautions No information available to require special precautions

Effects on Dental Treatment No significant effects or complications reported

Effects on Bleeding No information available to require special precautions

Adverse Reactions

1% to 10%:

Central nervous system: Dizziness, fatigue, headache

Endocrine & metabolic: Hyperkalemia (up to 10%; risk reduced in patients receiving kaliuretic diuretics), dehydration, gynecomastia, hyperchloremic metabolic acidosis, hyponatremia

Gastrointestinal: Abdominal pain, change in appetite, constipation, diarrhea, gas pain, nausea, vomiting

Genitourinary: Impotence

Neuromuscular & skeletal: Muscle cramps, weakness

Respiratory: Cough, dyspnea

<1%, postmarketing, and/or case reports: Alopecia, bladder spasm, cardiac arrhythmia, chest pain, dysuria, gastrointestinal hemorrhage, increased intraocular pressure, jaundice, orthostatic hypotension, palpitations, polyuria

Mechanism of Action Blocks epithelial sodium channels in the late distal convoluted tubule (DCT), and collecting duct which inhibits sodium reabsorption from the lumen. This effectively reduces intracellular sodium, decreasing the function of Na+/K+ATPase, leading to potassium retention and decreased calcium, magnesium, and hydrogen excretion. As sodium uptake capacity in the DCT/collecting duct is limited, the natriuretic, diuretic, and antihypertensive effects are generally considered weak.

Pharmacodynamics/Kinetics

Onset of Action Within 2 hours; Peak effect: 6 to 10 hours

Duration of Action ~24 hours

Half-life Elimination Normal renal function: 6 to 9 hours; renal impairment (CrCl <50 mL/minute): 21 to 144 hours (George 1980)

Time to Peak Serum:3 to 4 hours

Pregnancy Risk Factor B

Pregnancy Considerations Adverse events were not observed in animal reproduction studies.

◆ **Amiloride HCl** *see* AMILoride *on page 116*

◆ **Amiloride Hydrochloride** *see* AMILoride *on page 116*

◆ **2-Amino-6-Mercaptopurine** *see* Thioguanine *on page 1438*

◆ **2-Amino-6-Methoxypurine Arabinoside** *see* Nelarabine *on page 1091*

◆ **2-Amino-6-Trifluoromethoxy-benzothiazole** *see* Riluzole *on page 1328*

◆ **Aminobenzylpenicillin** *see* Ampicillin *on page 140*

Aminocaproic Acid (a mee noe ka PROE ik AS id)

Related Information

Antiplatelet and Anticoagulation Considerations in Dentistry *on page 1666*

Brand Names: US Amicar

Pharmacologic Category Antifibrinolytic Agent; Antihemophilic Agent; Hemostatic Agent; Lysine Analog

Use To enhance hemostasis when fibrinolysis contributes to bleeding (causes may include cardiac surgery, hematologic disorders, neoplastic disorders, abruptio placentae, hepatic cirrhosis, and urinary fibrinolysis)

Local Anesthetic/Vasoconstrictor Precautions No information available to require special precautions

Effects on Dental Treatment No significant effects or complications reported (see Effects on Bleeding)

Effects on Bleeding Used as an off-label indication to prevent or treat dental bleeding in patients with Hemophilia A; may cause thrombocytopenia

Adverse Reactions Frequency not defined.

Cardiovascular: Arrhythmia, bradycardia, edema, hypotension, intracranial hypertension, peripheral ischemia, syncope, thrombosis

Central nervous system: Confusion, delirium, dizziness, fatigue, hallucinations, headache, malaise, seizure, stroke

Dermatologic: Rash, pruritus

Gastrointestinal: Abdominal pain, anorexia, cramps, diarrhea, GI irritation, nausea, vomiting

Genitourinary: Dry ejaculation

Hematologic: Agranulocytosis, bleeding time increased, leukopenia, thrombocytopenia

Local: Injection site necrosis, injection site pain, injection site reactions

Neuromuscular & skeletal: CPK increased, myalgia, myositis, myopathy, rhabdomyolysis (rare), weakness
Ophthalmic: Vision decreased, watery eyes
Otic: Tinnitus
Renal: BUN increased, intrarenal obstruction (glomerular capillary thrombosis), myoglobinuria (rare), renal failure (rare)
Respiratory: Dyspnea, nasal congestion, pulmonary embolism
Miscellaneous: Allergic reaction, anaphylactoid reaction, anaphylaxis
Postmarketing and/or case reports: Hepatic lesion, hyperkalemia, myocardial lesion

Mechanism of Action Binds competitively to plasminogen; blocking the binding of plasminogen to fibrin and the subsequent conversion to plasmin, resulting in inhibition of fibrin degradation (fibrinolysis).

Pharmacodynamics/Kinetics

Onset of Action ~1 to 72 hours

Half-life Elimination 1 to 2 hours

Time to Peak Oral: 1.2 ± 0.45 hours

Pregnancy Risk Factor C

Pregnancy Considerations Animal reproduction studies have not been conducted.

◆ **Amino Levulinic Acid** *see* Aminolevulinic Acid (Topical) *on page 117*

◆ **5-Aminolevulinic Acid** *see* Aminolevulinic Acid (Topical) *on page 117*

Aminolevulinic Acid (Topical)

(a MEE noh lev yoo lin ik AS id)

Brand Names: US Ameluz; Levulan Kerastick

Brand Names: Canada Levulan Kerastick

Pharmacologic Category Photosensitizing Agent, Topical; Topical Skin Product

Use

Actinic keratoses:

Gel (Ameluz): Lesion-directed and field-directed topical treatment of mild to moderate actinic keratosis of the face and scalp; to be used in conjunction with photodynamic therapy with narrowband red light illumination (using BF-RhodoLED lamp).

Solution (Levulan Kerastick): Topical treatment of minimally to moderately thick actinic keratoses of the face, scalp, or upper extremities; to be used in conjunction with photodynamic therapy with blue light illumination (using BLU-U blue light).

Local Anesthetic/Vasoconstrictor Precautions No information available to require special precautions

Effects on Dental Treatment Key adverse event(s) related to dental treatment: Bleeding/hemorrhage (limited to application/treatment site).

Effects on Bleeding Bleeding/hemorrhage at application or treatment site.

Adverse Reactions

>10%:

Central nervous system: Localized burning (≤92%; severe: ≤73%)
Dermatologic: Stinging of the skin (severe: ≤73%), crusted skin (≤71%; severe: ≤5%), desquamation (≤71%; severe: ≤22%), local dryness (≤65%; severe: ≤22%), hyperpigmentation (≤64%), hypopigmentation (≤36%), localized vesiculation (≤36%), exfoliation of skin (≤19%), skin erosion (≤14%; may be severe), dermatological disease (5% to 12%)
Local: Application site reaction (100%), application site erythema (65% to 99%), local pain (≤92%; severe: ≤30%), application site irritation (72%), localized edema (1% to 51%; may be severe), application site discharge (≤36%), application site pruritus (8% to 34%; severe: 1% to 7%), application site induration (12%)

1% to 10%:

Central nervous system: Paresthesia (9%), hyperalgesia (6%), local discomfort (3%), dysesthesia (≤2%), pain (≤1%), chills, headache
Dermatologic: Urticaria (1% to 7%; may be severe), pustules (1% to 4%), dermal ulcer (≤4%), excoriation (≤2%), pruritic rash (perilesional: <2%), skin blister (<2%)
Hematologic & oncologic: Squamous cell carcinoma (2% to <10%), squamous cell carcinoma of skin (2% to <10%), hemorrhage (≤4%)
Local: Localized tenderness (1% to 2%)
Ophthalmic: Eyelid edema
Respiratory: Sinusitis (2% to <10%)

<1%, postmarketing, and/or case reports: Blurred vision, diplopia, eye irritation, fatigue, feeling hot, fever, local inflammation, local swelling, nervousness, ocular hyperemia, petechia, photophobia, pruritus, pustular rash, skin discoloration, skin photosensitivity, temporary amnesia

Mechanism of Action Aminolevulinic acid is a metabolic precursor of the photosensitizer protoporphyrin IX (PpIX). Photosensitization following local/topical application of aminolevulinic acid occurs through the metabolic conversion to PpIX. When exposed to light of appropriate wavelength and energy, accumulated PpIX produces a photodynamic reaction resulting in local cytotoxicity. Precancerous and cancerous cells exhibit a higher rate of porphyrin induction compared to normal cells.

Pharmacodynamics/Kinetics

Onset of Action Peak fluorescence intensity of protoporphyrin IX (PpIX): Actinic keratosis: Solution: 11 hours ± 1 hour; Perilesional skin: 12 hours ± 1 hour

Half-life Elimination Mean fluorescence clearance half-life of PpIX for lesions: Solution: 30 ± 10 hours

Time to Peak Gel: 3 hours

Pregnancy Considerations Animal reproduction studies have not been conducted. Systemic absorption following topical application is negligible.

◆ **Aminolevulinic Acid HCl** *see* Aminolevulinic Acid (Topical) *on page 117*

◆ **Aminolevulinic Acid Hydrochloride** *see* Aminolevulinic Acid (Topical) *on page 117*

Aminophylline (am in OFF i lin)

Related Information

Respiratory Diseases *on page 1680*
Theophylline *on page 1437*

Pharmacologic Category Phosphodiesterase Enzyme Inhibitor, Nonselective

Use

Reversible airflow obstruction: Treatment of acute exacerbations of symptoms and reversible airflow obstruction due to asthma or other chronic lung diseases (eg, emphysema, chronic bronchitis) as an adjunct to inhaled beta-2 selective agonists and systemically administered corticosteroids.

Guideline recommendations:

Asthma: The 2007 National Heart, Lung, and Blood Institute Asthma Guidelines and the 2020 Global Initiative for Asthma Guidelines recommend against aminophylline for the treatment of asthma exacerbations because of poor efficacy and safety concerns (GINA 2020; NAEPP 2007).

Chronic obstructive pulmonary disease: The 2019 Global Initiative for Chronic Obstructive Lung Disease Guidelines recommends against aminophylline for the treatment of chronic obstructive pulmonary disease exacerbations because of significant adverse effects (GOLD 2019).

Local Anesthetic/Vasoconstrictor Precautions No information available to require special precautions

Effects on Dental Treatment Prescribe erythromycin products with caution to patients taking theophylline products. Erythromycin will delay the normal metabolic inactivation of theophyllines leading to increased blood levels; this has resulted in nausea, vomiting, and CNS restlessness.

Effects on Bleeding No information available to require special precautions

Adverse Reactions Frequency not defined. Adverse events observed at therapeutic serum levels:

Central nervous system: Headache, insomnia, irritability, restlessness, seizure

Dermatologic: Allergic skin reaction, exfoliative dermatitis

Gastrointestinal: Diarrhea, nausea, vomiting

Genitourinary: Diuresis (transient)

Neuromuscular & skeletal: Tremor

Mechanism of Action Theophylline has two distinct actions; smooth muscle relaxation (ie, bronchodilation) and suppression of the response of the airways to stimuli (ie, non-bronchodilator prophylactic effects). Bronchodilation is mediated by inhibition of two isoenzymes, phosphodiesterase (PDE III and, to a lesser extent, PDE IV) while non-bronchodilation effects are mediated through other molecular mechanisms. Theophylline increases the force of contraction of diaphragmatic muscles through enhancement of calcium uptake through adenosine-mediated channels.

Pharmacodynamics/Kinetics

Half-life Elimination Theophylline: Highly variable and dependent upon age, hepatic function, cardiac function, lung disease, and smoking history

Premature infants, postnatal age 3 to 15 days: 30 hours (range: 17 to 43 hours)

Premature infants, postnatal age 25 to 57 days: 20 hours (range: 9.4 to 30.6 hours)

Term infants, postnatal age 1 to 2 days: 25.7 hours (range: 25 to 26.5 hours)

Term infants, postnatal age 3 to 30 weeks: 11 hours (range: 6 to 29 hours)

Children 1 to 4 years: 3.4 hours (range: 1.2 to 5.6 hours)

Children and Adolescents 6 to 17 years: 3.7 hours (range: 1.5 to 5.9 hours)

Adults ≥18 years to ≤60 years (asthma, nonsmoking, otherwise healthy): 8.7 hours (range: 6.1 to 12.8 hours)

Elderly >60 years (nonsmoking, healthy): 9.8 hours (range: 1.6 to 18 hours)

Time to Peak Serum: Theophylline: Within 30 minutes

Pregnancy Considerations

Aminophylline is a complex of theophylline and ethylenediamine. Theophylline crosses the placenta. Refer to Theophylline monograph for additional information.

◆ **4-aminopyridine** *see* Dalfampridine *on page 431*

◆ **Aminosalicylate Calcium** *see* Aminosalicylic Acid *on page 118*

◆ **Aminosalicylate Sodium** *see* Aminosalicylic Acid *on page 118*

Aminosalicylic Acid (a mee noe sal i SIL ik AS id)

Brand Names: US Paser

Pharmacologic Category Antitubercular Agent

Use Adjunctive treatment of tuberculosis used in combination with other antitubercular agents

Local Anesthetic/Vasoconstrictor Precautions No information available to require special precautions

Effects on Dental Treatment NSAID formulations are known to reversibly decrease platelet aggregation via mechanisms different than observed with aspirin. The dentist should be aware of the potential of abnormal coagulation. Caution should also be exercised in the use of NSAIDs in patients already on anticoagulant therapy with drugs such as warfarin (Coumadin®).

Effects on Bleeding No information available to require special precautions

Adverse Reactions Frequency not defined.

Cardiovascular: Pericarditis, vasculitis

Central nervous system: Brain disease

Dermatologic: Skin rash (including exfoliative dermatitis)

Endocrine & metabolic: Goiter (with or without myxedema), hypoglycemia, hypothyroidism

Gastrointestinal: Abdominal pain, diarrhea, nausea, vomiting

Hematologic & oncologic: Agranulocytosis, hemolytic anemia, leukopenia, thrombocytopenia

Hepatic: Hepatitis, jaundice

Miscellaneous: Fever

Ophthalmic: Optic neuritis

Respiratory: Eosinophilic pneumonitis

Mechanism of Action Aminosalicylic acid (PAS) is a highly-specific bacteriostatic agent active against *M. tuberculosis*. Structurally related to para-aminobenzoic acid (PABA) and its mechanism of action is thought to be similar to the sulfonamides, a competitive antagonism with PABA; disrupts plate biosynthesis in sensitive organisms.

Pharmacodynamics/Kinetics

Half-life Elimination Reduced with renal impairment

Time to Peak Serum: 6 hours

Pregnancy Risk Factor C

Pregnancy Considerations Teratogenic effects have been reported in animal reproduction studies. Salicylates have been noted to cross the placenta and enter fetal circulation. Aminosalicylic acid has been used safely during pregnancy; however, it should only be used if there are no alternatives for the treatment of multidrug-resistant tuberculosis (*MMWR*, 2003).

◆ **4-Aminosalicylic Acid** *see* Aminosalicylic Acid *on page 118*

◆ **5-Aminosalicylic Acid** *see* Mesalamine *on page 980*

Amiodarone (a MEE oh da rone)

Related Information

Cardiovascular Diseases *on page 1654*

Clinical Risk Related to Drugs Prolonging QT Interval *on page 1675*

Brand Names: US Nexterone; Pacerone

Brand Names: Canada APO-Amiodarone; DOM-Amiodarone; MYLAN-Amiodarone [DSC]; PMS-Amiodarone; PRO-Amiodarone-200; RIVA-Amiodarone; SANDOZ Amiodarone; TEVA-Amiodarone

Pharmacologic Category Antiarrhythmic Agent, Class III

Use Ventricular arrhythmias: Management of life-threatening recurrent ventricular fibrillation (VF) or recurrent hemodynamically unstable ventricular tachycardia (VT) refractory to other antiarrhythmic agents or in patients intolerant of other agents used for these conditions

Local Anesthetic/Vasoconstrictor Precautions Consider consult with patient's cardiologist prior to use of a vasonconstrictor. Closely monitor for additive/synergistic pharmacologic effects, and consider electrocardiographic monitoring, when a local anesthetic is used in a ptient receiving amiodarone. Amiodarone prolongs the QT interval and may cause torsade de pointes. The risk of drug-induced torsade de pointes may be small when a single QT interval prolonging drug is prescribed. In terms of epinephrine, it is not known what effect vasoconstrictors in the local anesthetic regimen will have in patients with a known history of congenital prolonged QT interval or in patients taking any medication that prolongs the QT interval.

Effects on Dental Treatment Key adverse event(s) related to dental treatment: Distortion of the sense of taste along with abnormal salivation; rare occurrence of xerostomia (normal salivary flow resumes upon discontinuation).

Effects on Bleeding No information available to require special precautions

Adverse Reactions

>10%:

Cardiovascular: Hypotension (intravenous: 20%; oral: <1%; refractory in rare cases)

Endocrine & metabolic: Phospholipidemia (pulmonary phospholipidosis; oral: 50%; intravenous: <1%)

Gastrointestinal: Nausea (oral: 10% to 33%; intravenous: 4%), vomiting (10% to 33%; intravenous: <2%)

Ophthalmic: Epithelial keratopathy (98% to 99%; vortex; Raizman 2016)

Respiratory: Pulmonary toxicity (oral: 2% to 17%; intravenous: <1%)

1% to 10%:

Cardiovascular: Bradycardia (2% to 6%), atrioventricular block (≤5%), sinus bradycardia (≤5%), exacerbation of cardiac arrhythmia (oral: 2% to 5%), cardiac failure (2% to 3%), cardiac arrhythmia (1% to 3%), edema (oral: 1% to 3%; intravenous: <1%), flushing (oral: 1% to 3% intravenous: <1%), sinus node dysfunction (≤3%), ventricular tachycardia (2%), atrial fibrillation (intravenous: <2%), cardiogenic shock (intravenous: <2%), nodal arrhythmia (intravenous: <2%), prolonged QT interval on ECG (<2%; associated with worsening arrhythmia), torsades de pointes (<2%), ventricular fibrillation (<2%)

Dermatologic: Skin photosensitivity (10%), solar dermatitis (oral: ≤9%), Stevens-Johnson syndrome (<2%)

Endocrine & metabolic: Hypothyroidism (1% to 10%), decreased libido (oral: 1% to 3%), hyperthyroidism (2%)

Gastrointestinal: Anorexia (oral: 4% to 9%), constipation (oral: 4% to 9%), altered salivation (oral: 1% to 3%), dysgeusia (oral: 1% to 3%), abdominal pain (oral: 1% to 3%), diarrhea (intravenous: <2%)

Hematologic & oncologic: Disorder of hemostatic components of blood (oral: 1% to 3%), thrombocytopenia (<2%)

Hepatic: Abnormal hepatic function tests (4%), hepatic disease (oral: 1% to 3%), increased serum alanine aminotransferase (<2%), increased serum aspartate aminotransferase (<2%)

Nervous system: Abnormal gait (oral: ≤9%), ataxia (oral: ≤9%), fatigue (oral: ≤9%), involuntary body movements (oral: ≤9%), malaise (oral: ≤9%), dizziness (oral: 4% to 9%; intravenous: <1%), paresthesia (oral: 4% to 9%), altered sense of smell (oral: 1% to 3%), headache (oral: 1% to 3%), insomnia (oral: 1% to 3%), sleep disorder (oral: 1% to 3%)

Neuromuscular & skeletal: Tremor (oral: ≤9%)

Ophthalmic: Blurred vision (oral: ≤10%; intravenous: <1%), visual halos around lights (oral: ≤10%), visual disturbance (oral: 4% to 9%), optic neuritis (1%)

Renal: Renal insufficiency (<2%)

Respiratory: Pneumonitis (oral: ≤9%), pulmonary fibrosis (oral: ≤9%; intravenous: <1%), acute respiratory distress syndrome (≤2%), pulmonary edema (intravenous: <2%)

Miscellaneous: Fever (intravenous: 3%; oral: <1%)

Frequency not defined:

Cardiovascular: Asystole

Nervous system: Peripheral neuropathy

Ophthalmic: Dry eye syndrome, photophobia

Respiratory: Hypersensitivity pneumonitis, pneumonitis (alveolar)

<1%, postmarketing, and/or case reports: Acute pancreatitis, acute renal failure, agranulocytosis, alopecia, anaphylactic shock, anaphylaxis, angioedema, aplastic anemia, back pain, blue-gray skin pigmentation, bronchiolitis obliterans organizing pneumonia, bronchospasm, bullous dermatitis, cardiac conduction disturbance (including bundle branch block, infra-HIS block, and antegrade conduction via an accessory pathway), cholestasis, cholestatic hepatitis, confusion, cough, delirium, demyelinating disease (polyneuropathy), disorientation, drug-induced Parkinson's disease, drug reaction with eosinophilia and systemic symptoms, dyspnea, eczema, eosinophilic pneumonitis, epididymitis, erythema multiforme, exfoliative dermatitis, granulocytosis, hallucination, hemolytic anemia, hemoptysis, hepatic cirrhosis, hepatic failure, hepatitis, hepatotoxicity (idiosyncratic) (Chalasani 2014), hypoesthesia, hypoxia, idiopathic intracranial hypertension, impotence, increased intracranial pressure, increased lactate dehydrogenase, increased serum alkaline phosphatase, increased serum creatinine, infusion site reaction (including cellulitis, edema, erythema, extravasation possibly leading to venous/infusion site necrosis, granuloma, hypoesthesia, induration, inflammation, intravascular amiodarone deposition/mass, pain, phlebitis, pigment changes, pruritus, skin sloughing, thrombophlebitis, thrombosis, urticaria), interstitial pneumonitis, intracranial hypertension (Tan 2019), jaundice, lupus-like syndrome, malignant neoplasm of skin, malignant neoplasm of thyroid, mass (pulmonary), muscle spasm, myasthenia, myopathy, myxedema (including myxedema coma), neutropenia, nonimmune anaphylaxis, optic neuropathy, pancytopenia, pleural effusion, pleurisy, pruritus, pulmonary alveolar hemorrhage, pulmonary infiltrates, respiratory failure, rhabdomyolysis, SIADH, sinoatrial arrest, skin carcinoma, skin granuloma, skin rash, spontaneous ecchymoses, thyroid nodule, thyrotoxicosis, toxic epidermal necrolysis,

urticaria, vasculitis, ventricular premature contractions, visual field defect, wheezing, xerostomia

Mechanism of Action Class III antiarrhythmic agent which inhibits adrenergic stimulation (alpha- and beta-blocking properties), affects sodium, potassium, and calcium channels, prolongs the action potential and refractory period in myocardial tissue; decreases AV conduction and sinus node function

Pharmacodynamics/Kinetics

Onset of Action Oral: 2 days to 3 weeks; IV: (electrophysiologic effects) within hours; antiarrhythmic effects: 2 to 3 days to 1 to 3 weeks; mean onset of effect may be shorter in children vs adults and in patients receiving IV loading doses; Peak effect: 1 week to 5 months

Duration of Action

After discontinuing therapy: Variable, 2 weeks to months: Children: Less than a few weeks; Adults: Several months

Note: Duration after discontinuation may be shorter in children than adults

Half-life Elimination Note: Half-life is shortened in children vs adults

Amiodarone:

Single dose: 58 days (range: 15 to 142 days)

Oral chronic therapy: Mean range: 40 to 55 days (range: 26 to 107 days)

IV single dose: Mean range: 9 to 36 days

N-desethylamiodarone (active metabolite): Prolonged in severe left ventricular dysfunction

Single dose: 36 days (range: 14 to 75 days)

Oral chronic therapy: 61 days

IV single dose: Mean range: 9 to 30 days

Time to Peak Oral: Serum: 3 to 7 hours

Pregnancy Considerations

Amiodarone and the active metabolite, N-desethylamiodarone, cross the placenta (Plomp 1992).

In utero exposure may cause fetal harm. Reported risks include neonatal bradycardia, QT prolongation, and periodic ventricular extrasystoles; neonatal hypothyroidism (with or without goiter); neonatal hyperthyroxinemia; neurodevelopmental abnormalities independent of thyroid function; jerk nystagmus with synchronous head titubation; fetal growth retardation; and/or premature birth.

Oral or IV amiodarone should be used in pregnancy only to treat arrhythmias refractory to other treatments or when other treatments are contraindicated (ACC/AHA/HRS [Page 2015]).

Amiodarone (administered either maternally or directly to the fetus) may be considered for the in utero management of fetal atrial flutter and in life-threatening cases of sustained fetal supraventricular tachycardia refractory to first and second line agents, but because of potential toxicity, risks and benefits should be assessed (AHA [Donofrio 2014]; Kang 2015).

If in utero exposure occurs, newborns should be monitored for thyroid disorders and cardiac arrhythmias.

Dental Health Professional Considerations Amiodarone is one of the drugs confirmed to prolong the QT interval. See Local Anesthetic/Vasoconstrictor Precautions

◆ **Amiodarone HCl** *see* Amiodarone *on page 118*

◆ **Amiodarone Hydrochloride** *see* Amiodarone *on page 118*

◆ **Amitiza** *see* Lubiprostone *on page 941*

Amitriptyline (a mee TRIP ti leen)

Related Information

Dentin Hypersensitivity, Acid Erosion, High Caries Index, Management of Alveolar Osteitis, and Xerostomia *on page 1762*

Temporomandibular Dysfunction (TMD), Chronic Pain, and Fibromyalgia *on page 1773*

Vasoconstrictor Interactions With Antidepressants *on page 1821*

Brand Names: US Elavil [DSC]

Brand Names: Canada AG-Amitriptyline; Amitriptyline-10; Amitriptyline-25; APO-Amitriptyline; BIO-Amitriptyline; Elavil; JAMP-Amitriptyline; Levate; Mar-Amitriptyline; NOVO-Triptyn [DSC]; PMS-Amitriptyline; PRIVA-Amitriptyline; TEVA-Amitriptyline

Pharmacologic Category Antidepressant, Tricyclic (Tertiary Amine)

Use Major depressive disorder (unipolar): Treatment of unipolar major depressive disorder

Local Anesthetic/Vasoconstrictor Precautions Amitriptyline is one of the drugs confirmed to prolong the QT interval and is accepted as having a risk of causing torsade de pointes. In terms of epinephrine, it is not known what effect vasoconstrictors in the local anesthetic regimen will have in patients with a known history of congenital prolonged QT interval or in patients taking any medication that prolongs the QT interval. Until more information is obtained, it is suggested that the clinician consult with the physician prior to the use of a vasoconstrictor in suspected patients, and that the vasoconstrictor (epinephrine, mepivacaine and levonordefrin [Carbocaine® 2% with Neo-Cobefrin®]) be used with caution.

Effects on Dental Treatment Key adverse event(s) related to dental treatment: Frequent occurrence of xerostomia and changes in salivation (normal salivary flow resumes upon discontinuation); stomatitis, peculiar taste, orthostatic hypotension, and black tongue have also been reported. Infrequent occurrences of facial edema, tongue edema, parotid gland enlargement, and ageusia have also been reported. Use caution with sudden changes in position during and after dental treatment. Amitriptyline is the most anticholinergic and sedating of the antidepressants; has pronounced effects on the cardiovascular system. Long-term treatment with tricyclic antidepressants (TCAs), such as amitriptyline, increases the risk of caries by reducing salivation and salivary buffer capacity. In a study by Rundergren, et al, pathological alterations were observed in the oral mucosa of 72% of 58 patients; 55% had new carious lesions after taking TCAs for a median of 5½ years. Current research is investigating the use of the salivary stimulant pilocarpine (Salagen) to overcome the xerostomia from amitriptyline.

Effects on Bleeding May cause thrombocytopenia

Adverse Reactions Anticholinergic effects may be pronounced; moderate to marked sedation can occur (tolerance to these effects usually occurs).

Frequency not defined:

Cardiovascular: Acute myocardial infarction, atrioventricular conduction disturbance, cardiac arrhythmia, cardiomyopathy (rare) (Briec 2006), cerebrovascular accident, ECG changes (nonspecific), edema, facial edema, heart block, hypertension, orthostatic hypotension, palpitations, sinus tachycardia, syncope

Dermatologic: Allergic skin rash, alopecia, diaphoresis, skin photosensitivity, urticaria

Endocrine & metabolic: Altered serum glucose, decreased libido, galactorrhea not associated with childbirth, gynecomastia, increased libido, SIADH, weight gain, weight loss

Gastrointestinal: Ageusia, anorexia, constipation, melanoglossia, nausea, paralytic ileus, parotid gland enlargement, stomatitis, unpleasant taste, vomiting, xerostomia

Genitourinary: Breast hypertrophy, impotence, testicular swelling, urinary frequency, urinary retention, urinary tract dilation

Hematologic & oncologic: Bone marrow depression (including agranulocytosis, leukopenia, and thrombocytopenia), eosinophilia, purpuric disease

Hepatic: Hepatic failure, hepatitis (rare; including altered liver function and jaundice)

Hypersensitivity: Tongue edema

Nervous system: Anxiety, ataxia, cognitive dysfunction, coma, confusion, delusion, disorientation, dizziness, drowsiness, dysarthria, EEG pattern changes, excitement, extrapyramidal reaction (including abnormal involuntary movements and tardive dyskinesia), fatigue, hallucination, headache, hyperpyrexia, insomnia, lack of concentration, nightmares, numbness, paresthesia, peripheral neuropathy, restlessness, sedated state, seizure, tingling of extremities, withdrawal syndrome (nausea, headache, malaise, irritability, restlessness, dream and sleep disturbance, mania [rare], and hypomania [rare]) (Davison 1993; Dilsaver 1984)

Neuromuscular & skeletal: Asthenia, lupus-like syndrome, tremor

Ophthalmic: Accommodation disturbance, blurred vision, increased intraocular pressure, mydriasis

Otic: Tinnitus

Postmarketing:

Nervous system: Neuroleptic malignant syndrome (rare) (Corrigan 1988; Janati 2012; Stevens 2008), serotonin syndrome (rare) (Dougherty 2002; Perry 2000)

Ophthalmic: Angle-closure glaucoma (Lowe 1966)

Mechanism of Action Increases the synaptic concentration of serotonin and/or norepinephrine in the central nervous system by inhibition of their reuptake by the presynaptic neuronal membrane pump.

Pharmacodynamics/Kinetics

Onset of Action Depression: Initial effects may be observed within 1 to 2 weeks of treatment with continued improvements through 4 to 6 weeks (Papakostas 2006; Posternak 2005; Szegedi 2009).

Half-life Elimination ~13 to 36 hours (Schulz 1985)

Time to Peak Serum: ~2 to 5 hours (Schulz 1985)

Pregnancy Risk Factor C

Pregnancy Considerations

Amitriptyline crosses the human placenta; CNS effects, limb deformities, and developmental delay have been noted in case reports (causal relationship not established). Tricyclic antidepressants may be associated with irritability, jitteriness, and convulsions (rare) in the neonate (Yonkers 2009). Crying, constipation, problems with urinating, and nausea may also occur in neonates exposed during pregnancy (Larsen 2015).

The ACOG recommends that therapy for depression during pregnancy be individualized; treatment should incorporate the clinical expertise of the mental health clinician, obstetrician, primary health care provider, and pediatrician (ACOG 2008). According to the American Psychiatric Association (APA), the risks of medication treatment should be weighed against other treatment options and untreated depression. For women who discontinue antidepressant medications during pregnancy and who may be at high risk for postpartum depression, the medications can be restarted following delivery (APA 2010). Treatment algorithms have been developed by the ACOG and the APA for the management of depression in women prior to conception and during pregnancy (Yonkers 2009). Tricyclic antidepressants are not the preferred therapy for depression in pregnant women but may be helpful when agitation is also present. If a TCA is needed, amitriptyline is one of the preferred agents. Maternal serum concentrations should be monitored during pregnancy (Larsen 2015; Yonkers 2009). Migraine prophylaxis should be avoided during pregnancy; if needed, amitriptyline may be used if other agents are ineffective or contraindicated (Pringsheim 2012).

Pregnant women exposed to antidepressants during pregnancy are encouraged to enroll in the National Pregnancy Registry for Antidepressants (NPRAD). Women 18 to 45 years of age or their health care providers may contact the registry by calling 844-405-6185. Enrollment should be done as early in pregnancy as possible.

Dental Health Professional Considerations See Local Anesthetic/Vasoconstrictor Precautions

- **Amitriptyline Hydrochloride** *see* Amitriptyline *on page 120*
- **AMJ 9701** *see* Palifermin *on page 1181*
- **Amjevita** *see* Adalimumab *on page 83*

AmLODIPine (am LOE di peen)

Related Information

Calcium Channel Blockers and Gingival Hyperplasia *on page 1816*

Cardiovascular Diseases *on page 1654*

Brand Names: US Katerzia; Norvasc

Brand Names: Canada ACCEL-AmLODIPine [DSC]; ACT AmLODIPine; AG-AmLODIPine; APO-AmLODIPine; Auro-AmLODIPine; BIO-AmLODIPine; DOM-AmLODIPine; GD-AmLODIPine [DSC]; JAMP-AmLODIPine; M-Amlodipine; Mar-AmLODIPine; MINT-AmLODIPine; MYLAN-AmLODIPine; Norvasc; NRA-Amlodipine; PDP-Amlodipine; PHARMA-AmLODIPine; PMS-AmLODIPine; Priva-AmLODIPine; RAN-AmLODIPine; RIVA-AmLODIPine; SANDOZ AmLODIPine; SANDOZ-AmLODIPine; Septa-AmLODIPine; TEVA-AmLODIPine; VAN-AmLODIPine [DSC]

Pharmacologic Category Antianginal Agent; Antihypertensive; Calcium Channel Blocker; Calcium Channel Blocker, Dihydropyridine

Use

Angina: Treatment of symptomatic chronic stable angina; treatment of confirmed or suspected vasospastic angina (previously referred to as Prinzmetal or variant angina). May be used alone or in combination with other antianginal agents.

Hypertension: Management of hypertension in adults and children ≥6 years of age.

Local Anesthetic/Vasoconstrictor Precautions No information available to require special precautions

Effects on Dental Treatment Key adverse event(s) related to dental treatment: Rare occurrence of gingival hyperplasia with amlodipine than with other calcium channel blockers (usually resolves upon discontinuation); consultation with physician is suggested if gingival hyperplasia is observed. Rare occurrences of xerostomia, orthostatic hypotension, and erythema multiforme (severe oral ulcerations that respond well to systemic steroid therapy).

Effects on Bleeding No information available to require special precautions

Adverse Reactions

>10%: Cardiovascular: Peripheral edema (2% to 11% [placebo 1%], dose related; females: 15% [placebo 5%]; males: 6% [placebo 1%])

1% to 10%:

Cardiovascular: Flushing (≤3%, dose related, more frequent in females), palpitations (≤5%, dose related, more frequent in females)

Dermatologic: Pruritus (≤2%), skin rash (≤2%)

Gastrointestinal: Abdominal pain (2%), nausea (3%)

Nervous system: Dizziness (3%, doses ≥5 mg/day), drowsiness (2%, females), fatigue (5%), male sexual disorder (≤2%)

Neuromuscular & skeletal: Asthenia (≤2%), muscle cramps (≤2%)

Respiratory: Dyspnea (≤2%)

<1%:

Cardiovascular: Peripheral ischemia, sinus tachycardia, syncope, vasculitis

Dermatologic: Diaphoresis, erythema multiforme

Endocrine & metabolic: Hot flash, hyperglycemia, weight gain, weight loss

Gastrointestinal: Anorexia, constipation, dysphagia, flatulence, gingival hyperplasia, pancreatitis, vomiting, xerostomia

Genitourinary: Difficulty in micturition, nocturia, urinary frequency

Hematologic & oncologic: Leukopenia, purpuric disease, thrombocytopenia (Cvetković 2013)

Hypersensitivity: Angioedema, hypersensitivity reaction

Nervous system: Abnormal dreams, anxiety, depersonalization, depression, female sexual disorder, hypoesthesia, insomnia, malaise, pain, paresthesia, peripheral neuropathy, rigors, vertigo

Neuromuscular & skeletal: Arthralgia, back pain, myalgia, osteoarthritis, tremor

Ophthalmic: Conjunctivitis, diplopia, eye pain

Otic: Tinnitus

Respiratory: Epistaxis

Postmarketing:

Dermatologic: Dermatologic disorder (Schamberg's disease) (Schetz 2015), toxic epidermal necrolysis (Baetz 2011)

Endocrine & metabolic: Gynecomastia (Cornes 2001)

Hepatic: Cholestatic hepatitis (Egbuonu 2019; Zinsser 2004), hepatotoxicity (Demirci 2013; Hammerstrom 2015), increased liver enzymes (Lafuente 2000; Zinsser 2004), jaundice (Lafuente 2000)

Renal: Acute interstitial nephritis (Ejaz 2000)

Mechanism of Action Inhibits calcium ion from entering the "slow channels" or select voltage-sensitive areas of vascular smooth muscle and myocardium during depolarization, producing a relaxation of coronary vascular smooth muscle and coronary vasodilation; increases myocardial oxygen delivery in patients with vasospastic angina. Amlodipine directly acts on vascular smooth muscle to produce peripheral arterial vasodilation reducing peripheral vascular resistance and blood pressure.

Pharmacodynamics/Kinetics

Onset of Action Antihypertensive effect: Significant reductions in blood pressure at 24 to 48 hours after first dose; slight increase in heart rate within 10 hours of administration may reflect some vasodilating activity (Donnelly 1993)

Duration of Action Antihypertensive effect: At least 24 hours (Donnelly 1993); has been shown to extend to at least 72 hours when discontinued after 6 to 7 weeks of therapy (Biston 1999)

Half-life Elimination Terminal (biphasic): 30 to 50 hours; increased with hepatic dysfunction

Time to Peak Plasma: 6 to 12 hours

Pregnancy Considerations

Amlodipine crosses the placenta. Cord blood concentrations were ~40% of maternal serum at delivery, and concentrations in the newborn were below the limit of quantification (<0.1 ng/mL) when measured in eight infants within 48 hours of delivery (Morgan 2017; Morgan 2018).

Due to pregnancy-induced pharmacologic changes, amlodipine pharmacokinetics may be altered immediately postpartum (Morgan 2018; Naito 2015b).

Chronic maternal hypertension may increase the risk of birth defects, low birth weight, preterm delivery, stillbirth, and neonatal death. Actual fetal/neonatal risks may be related to duration and severity of maternal hypertension. Untreated hypertension may also increase the risks of adverse maternal outcomes, including gestational diabetes, myocardial infarction, preeclampsia, stroke, and delivery complications (ACOG 203 2019).

Calcium channel blockers may be used to treat hypertension in pregnant women; however, agents other than amlodipine are more commonly used (ACOG 203 2019; ESC [Regitz-Zagrosek 2018]). Females with preexisting hypertension may continue their medication during pregnancy unless contraindications exist (ESC [Regitz-Zagrosek 2018]).

Amlodipine and Olmesartan

(am LOE di peen & olme SAR tan)

Related Information

AmLODIPine *on page 121*

Olmesartan *on page 1131*

Brand Names: US Azor

Pharmacologic Category Angiotensin II Receptor Blocker; Antianginal Agent; Antihypertensive; Calcium Channel Blocker; Calcium Channel Blocker, Dihydropyridine

Use Hypertension: Management of hypertension (monotherapy or with other antihypertensive agents).

Local Anesthetic/Vasoconstrictor Precautions No information available to require special precautions

Effects on Dental Treatment Key adverse event(s) related to dental treatment: Patients may experience orthostatic hypotension as they stand up after treatment; especially if lying in dental chair for extended periods of time. Use caution with sudden changes in position during and after dental treatment.

Fewer reports of gingival hyperplasia with amlodipine than with other CCBs (usually resolves upon discontinuation); consultation with physician is suggested.

Effects on Bleeding No information available to require special precautions

Adverse Reactions Reactions/percentages reported with combination product; also see individual agents

>10%: Cardiovascular: Peripheral edema (dose related: 18% to 26%)

Frequency not defined (limited to important or life-threatening): Anaphylaxis, hypotension, nocturia, orthostatic hypotension, palpitations, pruritus, skin rash, urinary frequency

Mechanism of Action

Amlodipine: Directly acts on vascular smooth muscle to produce peripheral arterial vasodilation reducing peripheral vascular resistance and blood pressure.

Olmesartan: Blocks the vasoconstrictor and aldosterone-secreting effects of angiotensin II.

Pregnancy Risk Factor D

Pregnancy Considerations [US Boxed Warning]: Drugs that act on the renin-angiotensin system can cause injury and death to the developing fetus. Discontinue as soon as possible once pregnancy is detected. See individual agents.

- **Amlodipine and Telmisartan** *see* Telmisartan and Amlodipine *on page 1414*
- **Amlodipine Benzoate** *see* AmLODIPine *on page 121*
- **Amlodipine Besylate** *see* AmLODIPine *on page 121*
- **Amlodipine Besylate and Olmesartan Medoxomil** *see* Amlodipine and Olmesartan *on page 122*
- **Amlodipine Besylate and Telmisartan** *see* Telmisartan and Amlodipine *on page 1414*
- **Ammonapse** *see* Sodium Phenylbutyrate *on page 1378*
- **AMN107** *see* Nilotinib *on page 1105*
- **Amnesteem** *see* ISOtretinoin (Systemic) *on page 846*

Amoxapine (a MOKS a peen)

Related Information

Dentin Hypersensitivity, Acid Erosion, High Caries Index, Management of Alveolar Osteitis, and Xerostomia *on page 1762*

Vasoconstrictor Interactions With Antidepressants *on page 1821*

Pharmacologic Category Antidepressant, Tricyclic (Secondary Amine)

Use Major depressive disorder (unipolar): Treatment of unipolar major depression, including depression with psychotic features

Local Anesthetic/Vasoconstrictor Precautions Use with caution; epinephrine and levonordefrin have been shown to have an increased pressor response in combination with TCAs. Amoxapine is one of the drugs confirmed to prolong the QT interval and is accepted as having a risk of causing torsade de pointes. The risk of drug-induced torsade de pointes is extremely low when a single QT interval prolonging drug is prescribed. In terms of epinephrine, it is not known what effect vasoconstrictors in the local anesthetic regimen will have in patients with a known history of congenital prolonged QT interval or in patients taking any medication that prolongs the QT interval. Until more information is obtained, it is suggested that the clinician consult with the physician prior to the use of a vasoconstrictor in suspected patients, and that the vasoconstrictor (epinephrine, mepivacaine and levonordefrin [Carbocaine® 2% with Neo-Cobefrin®]) be used with caution.

Effects on Dental Treatment Key adverse event(s) related to dental treatment: Xerostomia and changes in salivation (normal salivary flow resumes upon discontinuation). Long-term treatment with TCAs, such as amoxapine, increases the risk of caries by reducing salivation and salivary buffer capacity.

Effects on Bleeding May cause thrombocytopenia

Adverse Reactions

>10%:

Central nervous system: Drowsiness (14%)

Gastrointestinal: Xerostomia (14%), constipation (12%)

1% to 10%:

Cardiovascular: Edema, palpitations

Central nervous system: Anxiety, ataxia, confusion, dizziness, EEG pattern changes, excitement, fatigue, headache, insomnia, nervousness, nightmares, restlessness

Dermatologic: Diaphoresis, skin rash

Endocrine & metabolic: Increased serum prolactin

Gastrointestinal: Increased appetite, nausea

Neuromuscular & skeletal: Tremor, weakness

Ophthalmic: Blurred vision (7%)

<1% (Limited to important or life-threatening): Abdominal pain, accommodation disturbance, agranulocytosis, alopecia, altered serum glucose, angle-closure glaucoma, anorexia, atrial arrhythmia, atrial fibrillation, breast hypertrophy, decreased libido, delayed micturition, diarrhea, disorientation, eosinophilia, epigastric distress, extrapyramidal reaction, fever, flatulence, galactorrhea, hallucination, heart block, hepatic insufficiency, hepatitis, hypersensitivity reaction, hypertension, hyperthermia, hypomania, hypotension, impotence, increased intraocular pressure, increased libido, jaundice, lack of concentration, lacrimation, leukopenia, menstrual disease, mydriasis, myocardial infarction, nasal congestion, neuroleptic malignant syndrome, numbness, painful ejaculation, pancreatitis, paralytic ileus, paresthesia, parotid swelling, petechia, pruritus, purpura, seizure, SIADH, skin photosensitivity, syncope, tachycardia, tardive dyskinesia, testicular swelling, thrombocytopenia, tingling sensation, tinnitus, unusual taste, urinary frequency, urinary retention, urticaria, vasculitis, vomiting, weight gain, weight loss

Mechanism of Action Reduces the reuptake of serotonin and norepinephrine. The metabolite, 7-OH-amoxapine has significant dopamine receptor blocking activity similar to antipsychotic agents.

Pharmacodynamics/Kinetics

Onset of Action Depression: Initial effects may be observed within 1 to 2 weeks of treatment, with continued improvements through 4 to 6 weeks (Papakostas 2006; Posternak 2005; Szegedi 2009).

Half-life Elimination 8 hours; 8-hydroxyamoxapine metabolite: 30 hours

Time to Peak Serum: ~90 minutes

Pregnancy Risk Factor C

Pregnancy Considerations Adverse events were observed in some animal reproduction studies. Tricyclic antidepressants may be associated with irritability, jitteriness, and convulsions (rare) in the neonate (Yonkers, 2009).

The ACOG recommends that therapy for depression during pregnancy be individualized; treatment should incorporate the clinical expertise of the mental health clinician, obstetrician, primary healthcare provider, and pediatrician (ACOG, 2008). According to the American Psychiatric Association (APA), the risks of medication treatment should be weighed against other treatment options and untreated depression. For women who discontinue antidepressant medications during pregnancy and who may be at high risk for postpartum depression, the medications can be restarted following delivery (APA, 2010). Treatment algorithms have been developed by the ACOG and the APA for the management of depression in women prior to conception and during pregnancy (Yonkers, 2009).

Pregnant women exposed to antidepressants during pregnancy are encouraged to enroll in the National Pregnancy Registry for Antidepressants (NPRAD). Women 18 to 45 years of age or their health care providers may contact the registry by calling 844-405-6185. Enrollment should be done as early in pregnancy as possible.

Dental Health Professional Considerations See Local Anesthetic/Vasoconstrictor Precautions

Amoxicillin (a moks i SIL in)

Related Information

Antibiotic Prophylaxis *on page 1715*
Bacterial Infections *on page 1739*
Gastrointestinal Disorders *on page 1678*
Osteonecrosis of the Jaw *on page 1699*
Periodontal Diseases *on page 1748*

Related Sample Prescriptions

Bacterial Infections and Periodontal Diseases - Sample Prescriptions *on page 35*
Prevention of Endocarditis and to Reduce the Risk of Late Infections of Joint Prostheses - Sample Prescriptions *on page 40*
Sinus Infection Treatment - Sample Prescriptions *on page 41*

Brand Names: US Moxatag [DSC]

Brand Names: Canada AG-Amoxicillin; APO-Amoxi; APO-Amoxi Sugar Free; Auro-Amoxicillin; DOM-Amoxicillin; JAMP-Amoxicillin; Moxilean 50 [DSC]; MYLAN-Amoxicillin [DSC]; Novamoxin; PMS-Amoxicillin; Polymox; PRO Amox-500; PRO-Amox-250

Generic Availability (US) Yes

Pharmacologic Category Antibiotic, Penicillin

Dental Use Antibiotic for standard prophylactic regimen for dental patients who are at risk for infective endocarditis; prophylaxis in total joint replacement patients undergoing dental procedures; antibiotic used to treat orofacial infections. Useful (as amoxicillin or amoxicillin/clavulanic acid) in combination with metronidazole in addition to scaling and root planing in the treatment of periodontitis associated with the presence of *Actinobacillus actinomycetemcomitans* (AA).

Use

Ear, nose, and throat infections (pharyngitis/tonsillitis, otitis media):

Immediate release: Treatment of infections due to beta-lactamase-negative *Streptococcus* spp. (alpha- and beta-hemolytic isolates only), *Streptococcus pneumoniae*, *Staphylococcus* spp., or *Haemophilus influenzae*.

Extended release: Treatment of tonsillitis and/or pharyngitis due to *Streptococcus pyogenes* in adults and pediatric patients ≥12 years of age.

Genitourinary tract infections: Immediate release: Treatment of infections of the genitourinary tract due to beta-lactamase-negative *Escherichia coli*, *Proteus mirabilis*, or *Enterococcus faecalis*.

***Helicobacter pylori* eradication:** Immediate release: Eradication of *H. pylori* to reduce the risk of duodenal ulcer recurrence as a component of combination therapy in patients with active or 1-year history of duodenal ulcer disease.

Lower respiratory tract infections (including pneumonia): Immediate release: Treatment of infections of the lower respiratory tract due to beta-lactamase-negative *Streptococcus* spp. (alpha- and beta-hemolytic strains only), *S. pneumoniae*, *Staphylococcus* spp., or *H. influenzae*.

Rhinosinusitis, acute bacterial: Immediate release: Treatment of infections due to beta-lactamase-negative *Streptococcus* spp. (alpha- and beta-hemolytic isolates only), *S. pneumoniae*, *Staphylococcus* spp., or *H. influenzae*.

Skin and skin structure infections: Immediate release: Treatment of infections of the skin and skin structure due to beta-lactamase-negative *Streptococcus* spp. (alpha- and beta-hemolytic strains only), *Staphylococcus* spp., or *E. coli*.

Local Anesthetic/Vasoconstrictor Precautions No information available to require special precautions

Effects on Dental Treatment Prolonged use of penicillins may lead to development of oral candidiasis

Effects on Bleeding No information available to require special precautions

Adverse Reactions

1% to 10%:

- Central nervous system: Headache (1%)
- Gastrointestinal: Diarrhea (2%), nausea (1%), vomiting (1%)
- Genitourinary: Vulvovaginal infection (2%)

Frequency not defined:

- Cardiovascular: Hypersensitivity angiitis
- Central nervous system: Agitation, anxiety, behavioral changes, confusion, dizziness, insomnia, reversible hyperactivity, seizure
- Dermatologic: Acute generalized exanthematous pustulosis, erythematous maculopapular rash, erythema multiforme, exfoliative dermatitis, skin rash, Stevens-Johnson syndrome, toxic epidermal necrolysis, urticaria
- Gastrointestinal: *Clostridioides difficile* associated diarrhea, *Clostridioides difficile* colitis, hemorrhagic colitis, melanoglossia, mucocutaneous candidiasis, staining of tooth
- Genitourinary: Crystalluria
- Hematologic & oncologic: Agranulocytosis, anemia, eosinophilia, hemolytic anemia, immune thrombocytopenia, leukopenia, thrombocytopenia
- Hepatic: Cholestatic hepatitis, cholestatic jaundice, hepatitis (acute cytolytic), increased serum alanine aminotransferase, increased serum aspartate aminotransferase
- Hypersensitivity: Anaphylaxis
- Immunologic: Serum sickness-like reaction

<1%, postmarketing, and/or case reports: Abdominal pain

Dental Usual Dosage Oral:

Children >3 months and <40 kg: Prophylaxis against infective endocarditis: 50 mg/kg 30-60 minutes before procedure. **Note:** American Heart Association (AHA) guidelines now recommend prophylaxis only in patients undergoing invasive procedures and in whom underlying cardiac conditions may predispose to a higher risk of adverse outcomes should infection occur.

Adults:

Periodontitis (aggressive) (in combination with metronidazole) associated with presence of *Actinobacillus actinomycetemcomitans* (AA): 500 mg every 8 hours for 10 days used in addition to scaling and root planing (Varela 2011). In aggressive periodontitis, greatest benefit is seen after 3 months of therapy. No benefit was seen after 6 months of therapy (Varela 2011).

Prophylaxis against infective endocarditis: 2 g 30-60 minutes before procedure. **Note:** American Heart Association (AHA) guidelines now recommend prophylaxis only in patients undergoing invasive procedures and in whom underlying cardiac conditions may predispose to a higher risk of adverse outcomes should infection occur.

Orofacial infection: 250-500 mg every 8 hours or 500-875 mg twice daily

Prophylaxis in total joint replacement patients undergoing dental procedures which produce bacteremia: 2 g 1 hour prior to procedure

Note: In general, patients with prosthetic joint implants do not require prophylactic antibiotics prior to dental procedures. In planning an invasive oral procedure, dental consultation with the patient's orthopedic surgeon may be advised to review the risks of infection.

Dosing

Adult & Geriatric Note: Amoxicillin 775 mg ER tablets (brand and generic) have been discontinued in the United States for >1 year.

Note: Unless otherwise specified, all dosing recommendations based on immediate-release product formulations.

Usual dosage range:

Immediate release: **Oral:** 500 mg to 1 g every 8 to 12 hours.

Extended release: 775 mg once daily.

Actinomycosis (off-label use):

Note: For initial therapy of mild infection or step-down therapy following parenteral treatment of severe infection.

Oral: 500 mg 3 to 4 times daily **or** 1 g 3 times daily (Brook 2020; Martin 1984; Paulo 2018); higher doses of 4 to 6 g/day in divided doses have been utilized in case reports (Moghimi 2013; Valour 2014). Duration of therapy is 2 to 6 months for mild infection and 6 to 12 months (including 4 to 6 weeks of parenteral therapy) for severe or extensive infection (Brook 2020).

Anthrax (alternative agent for penicillin-susceptible strains) (off-label use):

Note: Consult public health officials for event-specific recommendations. A high index of suspicion for emergent beta-lactam resistance during therapy is warranted (Wilson 2019).

Inhalational exposure postexposure prophylaxis (PEP): **Oral:** 1 g every 8 hours for 42 to 60 days.

Note: Anthrax vaccine should also be administered to exposed individuals (CDC [Bower 2019]; CDC [Hendricks 2014]). **Duration of therapy:** If the PEP anthrax vaccine series is administered on schedule (for all regimens), antibiotics may be discontinued in immunocompetent adults 18 to 65 years of age at 42 days after initiation of vaccine or 2 weeks after the last dose of the vaccine (whichever comes last and not to exceed 60 days); if the vaccination series cannot be completed, antibiotics should continue for 60 days (CDC [Bower 2019]). In addition, adults with immunocompromising conditions or receiving immunosuppressive therapy, patients >65 years of age, and patients who are pregnant or breastfeeding should receive antibiotics for 60 days (CDC [Bower 2019]).

Cutaneous, without systemic involvement: **Oral:** 1 g every 8 hours; duration is 60 days following biological weapon-related event and 7 to 10 days after naturally acquired infection. **Note:** Patients with cutaneous lesions of the head or neck or extensive edema should be treated with a parenteral regimen recommended for systemic involvement (CDC [Hendricks 2014]).

Asplenia, prophylaxis against bacterial infection in select high-risk patients (off-label use): Oral: Based on expert opinion: 500 mg twice daily. Duration varies based on patient-specific factors (Pasternack 2018).

Bronchiectasis (off-label use):

Treatment of pulmonary exacerbations in patients ***without*** *beta-lactamase-positive Haemophilus influenzae or Pseudomonas aeruginosa:* **Oral:** 500 mg 3 times daily (Barker 2018; Finegold 1981) **or** 1 g 3 times daily (Prigogine 1988) for up to 14 days (Barker 2018; ERS [Polverino 2017]).

Prevention of pulmonary exacerbations: **Oral:** 500 mg twice daily; dosing based on expert opinion (Barker 2018). **Note:** Recommended for patients with ≥3 exacerbations per year who are **not** colonized with *P. aeruginosa* and not candidates for long-term macrolide therapy (Barker 2018; ERS [Polverino 2017]).

Endocarditis, prophylaxis (dental or invasive respiratory tract procedures) (off-label use): Oral: 2 g 30 to 60 minutes before procedure. **Note:** Only recommended for patients with cardiac conditions associated with the highest risk of an adverse outcome from endocarditis **and** who are undergoing a procedure likely to result in bacteremia with an organism that has the potential ability to cause endocarditis (AHA [Wilson 2007]).

Helicobacter pylori **eradication: Oral:**

Clarithromycin triple regimen: Amoxicillin 1 g twice daily in combination with clarithromycin 500 mg twice daily, plus a standard-dose or double-dose proton pump inhibitor; continue regimen for 14 days. **Note:** Avoid use in patients with risk factors for macrolide resistance (eg, prior macrolide exposure or local clarithromycin resistance rates ≥15%, which is assumed in the United States) (ACG [Chey 2017]; Fallone 2016).

Concomitant regimen: Amoxicillin 1 g twice daily in combination with clarithromycin 500 mg twice daily, either metronidazole or tinidazole 500 mg twice daily, plus a standard-dose proton pump inhibitor twice daily; continue regimen for 10 to 14 days (ACG [Chey 2017]).

Sequential regimen (alternative regimen): Amoxicillin 1 g twice daily plus a standard-dose proton pump inhibitor twice daily for 5 to 7 days; followed by clarithromycin 500 mg twice daily, either metronidazole or tinidazole 500 mg twice daily, plus a standard-dose proton pump inhibitor twice daily for 5 to 7 days; some experts prefer the 10-day regimen due to the lack of data showing superiority of the 14-day sequential regimen in North America (ACG [Chey 2017]; Crowe 2020).

Hybrid regimen (alternative regimen): Amoxicillin 1 g twice daily, plus a standard-dose proton pump inhibitor twice daily for 7 days; followed by amoxicillin 1 g twice daily, clarithromycin 500 mg twice daily, either metronidazole or tinidazole 500 mg twice daily, plus a standard-dose proton pump inhibitor twice daily for 7 days (ACG [Chey 2017]).

Levofloxacin triple regimen (salvage regimen): Amoxicillin 1 g twice daily in combination with a standard-dose proton pump inhibitor twice daily plus levofloxacin 500 mg once daily; continue regimen for 10 to 14 days (ACG [Chey 2017]).

High-dose dual therapy (salvage regimen): Amoxicillin 750 mg 4 times daily **or** 1 g 3 times daily; in combination with a standard-dose or double-dose proton pump inhibitor 3 to 4 times daily for 14 days (ACG [Chey 2017]).

Lyme disease (*Borrelia* spp. infection) (off-label use):

Early localized (eg, erythema migrans): **Oral:** 500 mg 3 times daily for 14 to 21 days (IDSA [Wormser 2006]).

Early disseminated, carditis (initial therapy for mild disease [first-degree atrioventricular block with PR interval <300 msec] or step-down therapy after initial parenteral treatment for more severe disease once PR interval <300 msec): **Oral:** 500 mg 3 times daily for 14 to 21 days (Hu 2018; IDSA [Wormser 2006]); for step-down therapy, some experts prefer a total antibiotic duration of 21 to 28 days (Hu 2018).

Early disseminated, mild neurologic involvement (isolated facial nerve palsy [no evidence of meningitis]) (alternative agent): **Oral:** 500 mg 3 times daily for 14 to 21 days (IDSA [Wormser 2006]).

Late disease, arthritis without neurologic involvement: **Oral:** 500 mg 3 times daily for 28 days (IDSA [Wormser 2006]).

Otitis media, acute (alternative agent): Limited data: **Oral:** 500 mg every 8 hours **or** 875 mg every 12 hours (WHO 2001; manufacturer's labeling). Some experts use 1 g every 8 hours for patients at high risk of severe infection or resistant *Streptococcus pneumoniae*. Duration is 5 to 7 days for mild to moderate infection and 10 days for severe infection (Limb 2019).

Note: Some experts recommend amoxicillin/clavulanate over amoxicillin alone because of concern for decreased penicillin susceptibility in *Streptococcus pneumoniae* and other otopathogens (Limb 2019).

Periodontitis, severe (off-label use): Oral: 500 mg every 8 hours in combination with metronidazole for 7 to 14 days; used in addition to periodontal debridement (Caton 2018; Chow 2019; Silva-Senem 2013; Wilder 2020).

Pneumonia, community acquired, outpatient empiric therapy (patients without comorbidities or risk factors for antibiotic resistant pathogens): **Oral:** 1 g 3 times daily (ATS/IDSA [Metlay 2019]); some experts prefer use of amoxicillin in combination with an antibiotic that targets atypical pathogens (File 2020). Duration is for a minimum of 5 days; patients should be clinically stable with normal vital signs before therapy is discontinued (ATS/IDSA [Metlay 2019]).

Prosthetic joint infection (off-label use):

Note: For chronic antimicrobial suppression of prosthetic joint infection caused by beta-hemolytic streptococci, penicillin-susceptible *Enterococcus* spp., or *Cutibacterium* spp. (following pathogen-specific IV therapy in patients undergoing 1-stage exchange or debridement with retention of prosthesis).

Oral: 500 mg 3 times daily (IDSA [Osmon 2013]; Siqueria 2015); duration depends on patient-specific factors (Berbari 2019).

Rhinosinusitis, acute bacterial:

Note: For initial therapy of nonsevere infection in patients without risk factors for pneumococcal resistance or poor outcome (eg, age ≥65 years, recent hospitalization or antibiotic use, immunocompromising condition, residence in a region with high rates of resistance) (Patel 2018).

Oral: 500 mg every 8 hours **or** 875 mg every 12 hours for 5 to 7 days (AAO-HNS [Rosenfeld 2015]; Garbutt 2012; Lindbaek 1996; Patel 2018). In uncomplicated acute bacterial rhinosinusitis, initial observation and symptom management without antibiotic therapy is appropriate in most patients (AAO-HNS [Rosenfeld 2015]; ACG/CDC [Harris 2016]).

Skin and soft tissue infection:

Erysipelas, mild: **Oral:** 500 mg 3 times daily **or** 875 mg twice daily for 5 days, with extension to 14 days for slow response, severe infection, or immunosuppression (Spelman 2019; manufacturer's labeling).

Erysipeloid, localized cutaneous: **Oral:** 500 mg 3 times daily for 7 to 10 days (IDSA [Stevens 2014]).

Streptococcal pharyngitis (group A): Oral: 500 mg twice daily **or** 1 g once daily for 10 days (AHA [Gerber 2009]; IDSA [Shulman 2012]).

Extended release: 775 mg once daily for 10 days.

Urinary tract infection:

Note: Not recommended for empiric therapy given decreased efficacy compared to first-line agents and high prevalence of resistance (IDSA/ESCMID [Gupta 2011]).

Acute uncomplicated or simple cystitis (infection limited to the bladder and no signs/symptoms of upper tract or systemic infection) due to Enterococcus spp.: **Oral:** 500 mg every 8 hours **or** 875 mg every 12 hours for 5 days (Cole 2015; Hooton 2019a; Hooton 2019b; Murray 2020; Swaminathan 2010).

Asymptomatic group B Streptococcus bacteriuria (≥10^5 CFU per mL) in pregnancy: **Oral:** 500 mg every 8 hours **or** 875 mg every 12 hours for 4 to 7 days (ACOG 782 2019; Hooton 2019c; IDSA [Nicolle 2019]).

Renal Impairment: Adult

The renal dosing recommendations are based upon the best available evidence and clinical expertise. Senior Editorial Team: Bruce Mueller, PharmD, FCCP, FASN, FNKF; Jason Roberts, PhD, BPharm (Hons), B App Sc, FSHP, FISAC; Michael Heung, MD, MS.

Altered kidney function:

Oral: Immediate release:

Amoxicillin Dose Adjustments in Kidney Impairment

GFR (mL/minute)	If the normal recommended dose is 250 to 500 mg every 8 hours[a]	If the normal recommended dose is 875 mg to 1 g every 12 hours[b]	If the normal recommended dose is 1 g every 8 hours[b,c]
≥30	No dosage adjustment necessary	No dosage adjustment necessary	No dosage adjustment necessary
10 to 30	250 to 500 mg every 12 hours	500 mg every 12 hours	1 g every 12 hours
<10	250 to 500 mg every 12 to 24 hours	500 mg every 12 to 24 hours	500 mg every 12 hours
Hemodialysis, intermittent (thrice weekly)[d]	250 to 500 mg every 12 to 24 hours	500 mg every 12 to 24 hours	500 mg every 12 hours
Peritoneal dialysis	250 to 500 mg every 12 hours	500 mg every 12 hours	500 mg every 12 hours

[a]Golightly 2013; Szeto 2017; manufacturer's labeling; expert opinion

[b]Expert opinion

[c]Keller 2015

[d]Dialyzable (30% to 47% with low flux filters [Davies 1988; Francke 1979]). If utilizing a 24-hour dosing interval, administer dose after dialysis or give an additional dose after dialysis on dialysis days.

Oral: Extended release:

CrCl ≥30 mL/minute: There are no dosage adjustments provided in the manufacturer's labeling (has not been studied).

CrCl <30 mL/minute: Not recommended.

Hemodialysis, intermittent (thrice weekly): Not recommended.

Hepatic Impairment: Adult There are no dosage adjustments provided in the manufacturer's labeling.

Pediatric Note: Unless otherwise specified, all pediatric dosing recommendations based on immediate-release product formulations (oral suspension, chewable tablet, tablet, and capsule). Amoxicillin 775 mg ER tablets (brand [Moxatag] and generic) have been discontinued in the US for >1 year.

General dosing, susceptible infection:

Mild to moderate infection:

Infants ≤3 months: Oral: 25 to 50 mg/kg/day in divided doses every 8 hours (*Red Book* [AAP 2015]). **Note:** Manufacturer's labeling recommends a maximum daily dose of 30 mg/kg/**day** divided into 2 doses per day for this age group.

Infants >3 months, Children, and Adolescents:

AAP recommendations (*Red Book* [AAP 2015]): Oral: 25 to 50 mg/kg/day in divided doses every 8 hours; maximum dose: 500 mg/dose.

Manufacturer's labeling: Oral: 20 to 40 mg/kg/day in divided doses every 8 hours (maximum dose: 500 mg/dose) **or** 25 to 45 mg/kg/day in divided doses every 12 hours (maximum dose: 875 mg/dose).

Severe infection (as step-down therapy): Infants, Children, and Adolescents: Oral: 80 to 100 mg/kg/day in divided doses every 8 hours; maximum dose: 500 mg/dose for most indications (*Red Book* [AAP 2015]).

Anthrax:

Cutaneous, without systemic involvement: Infants, Children, and Adolescents: Oral: 75 mg/kg/day in 3 divided doses. Maximum dose: 1,000 mg/dose. Duration of therapy: 7 to 10 days for naturally acquired infection, up to 60 days for biological weapon-related exposure (AAP [Bradley 2014]).

Inhalational, postexposure prophylaxis: Infants, Children, and Adolescents: Oral: 75 mg/kg/day in divided doses every 8 hours for 60 days after exposure; maximum dose: 1,000 mg/dose (AAP [Bradley 2014]).

Catheter (peritoneal dialysis), exit-site or tunnel infection: Infants, Children, and Adolescents: Oral: 10 to 20 mg/kg once daily; maximum dose: 1,000 mg/dose (ISPD [Warady 2012]).

Endocarditis, prophylaxis: Note: AHA guidelines (Baltimore 2015) limit the use of prophylactic antibiotics to patients at the highest risk for infective endocarditis (IE) or adverse outcomes (eg, prosthetic heart valves, patients with previous IE, unrepaired cyanotic congenital heart disease, repaired congenital heart disease with prosthetic material or device during first 6 months after procedure, repaired congenital heart disease with residual defects at the site or adjacent to site of prosthetic patch or device, heart transplant recipients with cardiac valvulopathy):

Dental or oral procedures or respiratory tract procedures (eg, tonsillectomy, adenoidectomy): Infants, Children, and Adolescents: Oral: 50 mg/kg 30 to 60 minutes before procedure; maximum dose: 2,000 mg/dose (AHA [Wilson 2007]).

***H. pylori* eradication:** Children and Adolescents: Oral: 50 mg/kg/day in 2 divided doses for 10 to 14 days. **Note:** Duration dependent on regimen used; maximum daily dose: 2,000 mg/**day**. Administer in combination with a proton pump inhibitor or bismuth subsalicylate and at least one other antibiotic (clarithromycin and/or metronidazole) (NASPGHAN/ESPGHAN [Koletzko 2011]).

Lyme disease: Infants, Children, and Adolescents: Oral: 50 mg/kg/day in divided doses every 8 hours; maximum dose: 500 mg/dose (Halperin 2007; IDSA [Wormser 2006]).

Otitis media, acute (AOM): Infants ≥2 months and Children: Oral: 80 to 90 mg/kg/day in divided doses every 12 hours; variable duration of therapy, if <2 years of age or severe symptoms (any age): 10-day course; if 2 to 5 years of age with mild to moderate symptoms: 7-day course; ≥6 years of age with mild to moderate symptoms: 5- to 7-day course; some experts recommend initiating with 90 mg/kg/day (AAP [Lieberthal 2013]; *Red Book* [AAP 2015]); a maximum dose is not provided in the Guidelines for The Diagnosis and Management of Acute Otitis Media (AAP [Lieberthal 2013]); however, some experts suggest a maximum daily dose of 4,000 mg/**day** for high-dose amoxicillin therapy (Bradley 2015).

Peritonitis (peritoneal dialysis), prophylaxis for patients requiring invasive dental procedures: Infants, Children, and Adolescents: Oral: 50 mg/kg administered 30 to 60 minutes before dental procedure; maximum dose: 2,000 mg/dose (ISPD [Warady 2012]).

Pneumonia, community-acquired: Infants ≥3 months, Children, and Adolescents:

Empiric therapy for presumed bacterial pneumonia: Oral: 90 mg/kg/day in divided doses every 12 hours; maximum daily dose: 4,000 mg/**day** (IDSA [Bradley 2011]).

Group A *Streptococcus,* mild infection or step-down therapy: Oral: 50 to 75 mg/kg/day in divided doses every 12 hours; maximum daily dose: 4,000 mg/**day** (IDSA [Bradley 2011]).

Haemophilus influenzae, mild infection or step-down therapy: Oral: 75 to 100 mg/kg/day in divided doses every 8 hours; maximum daily dose: 4,000 mg/**day** (IDSA [Bradley 2011]).

Streptococcus pneumonia, mild infection or step-down therapy (penicillin MIC ≤2 mcg/mL): Oral: 90 mg/kg/day in divided doses every 12 hours **or** 45 mg/kg/day in divided doses every 8 hours; maximum daily dose: 4,000 mg/**day** (IDSA [Bradley 2011]).

Streptococcus pneumonia, relatively resistant (penicillin MIC = 2 mcg/mL): Oral: 90 to 100 mg/kg/day in divided doses every 8 hours; dosing based on pharmacokinetic modeling; Monte Carlo simulations show that this dose provides optimal lung exposures to increase efficacy (Bradley 2010; IDSA [Bradley 2011]).

Pneumococcal infection prophylaxis for anatomic or functional asplenia [eg, sickle cell disease (SCD)] (Price 2007; *Red Book* [AAP 2015]):

Before 2 months of age (or as soon as SCD is diagnosed or asplenia occurs) through 5 years of age: Oral: 20 mg/kg/day in divided doses every 12 hours; maximum dose: 250 mg/dose.

Children ≥6 years and Adolescents: Oral: 250 mg every 12 hours; **Note:** The decision to discontinue penicillin prophylaxis after 5 years of age in children who have not experienced invasive pneumococcal infection and have received recommended pneumococcal immunizations is patient and clinician dependent.

Rhinosinusitis, acute bacterial; uncomplicated: Note: AAP guidelines recommend amoxicillin as first-line empiric therapy for pediatric patients 1 to 18 years with uncomplicated cases and where resistance is not suspected; however, the IDSA guidelines consider amoxicillin/clavulanate as the preferred therapy (IDSA [Chow 2012]; AAP [Wald 2013]):

Low dose: Children ≥2 years and Adolescents: Oral: 45 mg/kg/day in divided doses every 12 hours; **Note:** Only use for uncomplicated, mild to moderate infections in children who do not attend daycare and who have not received antibiotics within the last month (AAP [Wald 2013]).

High dose (use reserved for select patients; see **Note**): Children ≥2 years and Adolescents: Oral: 80 to 90 mg/kg/day in divided doses every 12 hours; maximum dose: 2,000 mg/dose; **Note:** Should only use for mild to moderate infections in children who do not attend daycare and who have not received antibiotics within the last month and live in communities with a high prevalence of non-susceptible *S. pneumoniae* resistance (AAP [Wald 2013]).

Tonsillopharyngitis; Group A streptococcal infection, treatment and primary prevention of rheumatic fever:

Immediate release (oral suspension, chewable tablets, tablets, capsules): Children and Adolescents 3 to 18 years: Oral: 50 mg/kg once daily **or** 25 mg/kg twice daily for 10 days; maximum daily dose: 1,000 mg/**day** (AHA [Gerber 2009]; IDSA [Shulman 2012]).

Extended-release tablets: Children ≥12 years and Adolescents: Oral: 775 mg once daily for 10 days; **Note:** Patient must be able to swallow tablet whole.

UTI, prophylaxis (hydronephrosis, vesicoureteral reflux): Infants ≤2 months: Oral: 10 to 15 mg/kg once daily; some suggest administration in the evening (drug resides in bladder longer); **Note:** Due to resistance, amoxicillin should not be used for prophylaxis after 2 months of age (Belarmino 2006; Greenbaum 2006; Mattoo 2007).

Renal Impairment: Pediatric

There are no dosage adjustments provided in the manufacturer's labeling; however, the following guidelines have been used by some clinicians (Aronoff 2007): Oral:

Immediate release: Infants, Children, and Adolescents:

Mild to moderate infection: Dosing based on 25 to 50 mg/kg/day divided every 8 hours:

GFR >30 mL/minute/1.73 m^2: No adjustment required

GFR 10 to 29 mL/minute/1.73 m^2: 8 to 20 mg/kg/dose every 12 hours

GFR <10 mL/minute/1.73 m^2: 8 to 20 mg/kg/dose every 24 hours

Hemodialysis: Moderately dialyzable (20% to 50%); ~30% removed by 3-hour hemodialysis: 8 to 20 mg/kg/dose every 24 hours; give after dialysis

Peritoneal dialysis: 8 to 20 mg/kg/dose every 24 hours

Severe infection (high dose): Dosing based on 80 to 90 mg/kg/day divided every 12 hours:

GFR >30 mL/minute/1.73 m^2: No adjustment required

GFR 10 to 29 mL/minute/1.73 m^2: 20 mg/kg/dose every 12 hours; do not use the 875 mg tablet

GFR <10 mL/minute/1.73 m^2: 20 mg/kg/dose every 24 hours; do not use the 875 mg tablet

Hemodialysis: Moderately dialyzable (20% to 50%); ~30% removed by 3-hour hemodialysis: 20 mg/kg/dose every 24 hours; give after dialysis

Peritoneal dialysis: 20 mg/kg/dose every 24 hours

Extended release: Children ≥12 years and Adolescents: CrCl <30 mL/minute: Not recommended

Hepatic Impairment: Pediatric There are no dosage adjustments provided in the manufacturer's labeling.

Mechanism of Action Inhibits bacterial cell wall synthesis by binding to one or more of the penicillin-binding proteins (PBPs) which in turn inhibits the final transpeptidation step of peptidoglycan synthesis in bacterial cell walls, thus inhibiting cell wall biosynthesis. Bacteria eventually lyse due to ongoing activity of cell wall autolytic enzymes (autolysins and murein hydrolases) while cell wall assembly is arrested.

Contraindications

Serious hypersensitivity to amoxicillin (eg, anaphylaxis, Stevens-Johnson syndrome) or to other beta-lactams, or any component of the formulation

Canadian labeling: Additional contraindications (not in US labeling): Infectious mononucleosis (suspected or confirmed)

Warnings/Precautions In patients with renal impairment, doses and/or frequency of administration should be modified in response to the degree of renal impairment; dosage adjustment recommended in patients with GFR <30 mL/minute. Avoid extended release 775 mg tablet and immediate release 875 mg tablet in patients with GFR <30 mL/minute or patients requiring hemodialysis. A high percentage of patients with infectious mononucleosis develop an erythematous rash during amoxicillin therapy; avoid use in these patients. Serious and occasionally severe or fatal hypersensitivity (anaphylactic) reactions have been reported in patients on penicillin therapy, including amoxicillin, especially with a history of beta-lactam hypersensitivity (including severe reactions with cephalosporins) and/or a history of sensitivity to multiple allergens. Prolonged use may result in fungal or bacterial superinfection, including *C. difficile*-associated diarrhea (CDAD) and pseudomembranous colitis; CDAD has been observed >2 months postantibiotic treatment. Potentially significant interactions may exist, requiring dose or frequency adjustment, additional monitoring, and/or selection of alternative therapy.

Chewable tablets may contain phenylalanine; see manufacturer's labeling.

Benzyl alcohol and derivatives: Some dosage forms may contain sodium benzoate/benzoic acid; benzoic acid (benzoate) is a metabolite of benzyl alcohol; large amounts of benzyl alcohol (≥99 mg/kg/day) have been associated with a potentially fatal toxicity ("gasping syndrome") in neonates; the "gasping syndrome" consists of metabolic acidosis, respiratory distress, gasping respirations, CNS dysfunction (including convulsions, intracranial hemorrhage), hypotension, and cardiovascular collapse (AAP ["Inactive" 1997]; CDC 1982); some data suggests that benzoate displaces bilirubin from protein binding sites (Ahlfors 2001); avoid or use dosage forms containing benzyl alcohol derivative with caution in neonates. See manufacturer's labeling.

Warnings: Additional Pediatric Considerations Epstein-Barr virus infection (infectious mononucleosis), acute lymphocytic leukemia, or cytomegalovirus infection increases risk for amoxicillin-induced maculopapular rash. Appearance of a rash should be carefully evaluated to differentiate a nonallergic amoxicillin rash from a hypersensitivity reaction. Amoxicillin rash occurs in 5% to 10% of children receiving amoxicillin and is a generalized dull, red, maculopapular rash, generally appearing 3 to 14 days after the start of therapy. It normally begins on the trunk and spreads over most of the body. It may be most intense at pressure areas, elbows, and knees. A high percentage (43% to 100%) of patients with infectious mononucleosis have developed rash during therapy; amoxicillin-class antibiotics are not recommended in these patients.

In a meta-analysis of pediatric acute otitis media trials, high-dose amoxicillin regimens were associated with a higher incidence of adverse effects compared to standard-dose; the incidence of diarrhea was 18.9% with high-dose amoxicillin/clavulanate, 13.8% with high-dose amoxicillin, and 8.7% with standard-dose amoxicillin; the incidence of generalized rash was 6.5% with high-dose amoxicillin, 4.9% with high-dose amoxicillin/clavulanate, and 2.9% with standard-dose amoxicillin; however, significant heterogeneity was observed (Hum 2019).

Drug Interactions

Metabolism/Transport Effects None known.

Avoid Concomitant Use

Avoid concomitant use of Amoxicillin with any of the following: BCG (Intravesical); Cholera Vaccine

Increased Effect/Toxicity

Amoxicillin may increase the levels/effects of: Dichlorphenamide; Methotrexate; Vitamin K Antagonists

The levels/effects of Amoxicillin may be increased by: Acemetacin; Allopurinol; Probenecid

Decreased Effect

Amoxicillin may decrease the levels/effects of: Aminoglycosides; BCG (Intravesical); BCG Vaccine (Immunization); Cholera Vaccine; Lactobacillus and Estriol; Mycophenolate; Sodium Picosulfate; Typhoid Vaccine

The levels/effects of Amoxicillin may be decreased by: Tetracyclines

Dietary Considerations Some products may contain phenylalanine.

Pharmacodynamics/Kinetics

Half-life Elimination Adults: Immediate-release: 61.3 minutes; Extended-release: 90 minutes

Time to Peak Capsule; oral suspension: 1 to 2 hours; Chewable tablet: 1 hour; Extended-release tablet: 3.1 hours

Pregnancy Risk Factor B

Pregnancy Considerations Amoxicillin crosses the placenta (Muller 2009).

Due to pregnancy-induced physiologic changes, some pharmacokinetic parameters of amoxicillin may be altered (Andrew 2007). Oral ampicillin-class antibiotics are poorly absorbed during labor.

Amoxicillin may be used for the management of *Bacillus anthracis* in pregnant women when penicillin susceptibility is documented (Meaney-Delman 2014). Amoxicillin is an alternative antibiotic for the treatment of chlamydial infections in pregnancy (CDC [Workowski 2015]). Amoxicillin can also be used in the management of preterm prelabor rupture of membranes (PROM) and in certain situations prior to vaginal delivery in women at high risk for endocarditis (ACOG 188 2019; ACOG 199 2018).

Breastfeeding Considerations Amoxicillin is present in breast milk (Kafetzis 1981).

The relative infant dose (RID) of amoxicillin is 0.15% to 0.54% when calculated using the highest average breast milk concentration located and compared to an infant therapeutic dose of 25 to 90 mg/kg/day.

In general, breastfeeding is considered acceptable when the RID is <10% (Anderson 2016; Ito 2000).

The RID of amoxicillin was calculated using a milk concentration of 0.9 mcg/mL, providing an estimated daily infant dose via breast milk of 0.135 mg/kg/day. This milk concentration was obtained following maternal administration of a single oral dose of amoxicillin 1,000 mg (Kafetzis 1981).

Self-limiting diarrhea, rash, and somnolence have been reported in nursing infants exposed to amoxicillin (Benyamini 2005; Goldstein 2009; Ito 1993); the manufacturer warns of the potential for allergic sensitization in the infant. In general, antibiotics that are present in breast milk may cause non-dose-related modification of bowel flora. Monitor infants for GI disturbances, such as thrush or diarrhea (WHO 2002).

Although the manufacturer recommends that caution be exercised when administering amoxicillin to breastfeeding women, amoxicillin is considered compatible with breastfeeding when used in usual recommended doses (WHO 2002). Amoxicillin has been recommended to treat mastitis in breastfeeding women when penicillin susceptibility is documented (WHO 2000) and also for the management of *Bacillus anthracis* (Meaney-Delman 2014).

Product Availability

Amoxicillin 775 mg ER tablets (brand and generic) have been discontinued in the United States for >1 year.

Dosage Forms: US

Capsule, Oral:

Generic: 250 mg, 500 mg

Suspension Reconstituted, Oral:

Generic: 125 mg/5 mL (80 mL, 100 mL, 150 mL); 200 mg/5 mL (50 mL, 75 mL, 100 mL); 250 mg/5 mL (80 mL, 100 mL, 150 mL); 400 mg/5 mL (50 mL, 75 mL, 100 mL)

Tablet, Oral:

Generic: 500 mg, 875 mg

Tablet Chewable, Oral:

Generic: 125 mg, 250 mg

Dosage Forms: Canada

Capsule, Oral:

Polymox: 250 mg, 500 mg

Generic: 250 mg, 500 mg

Suspension Reconstituted, Oral:

Polymox: 125 mg/5 mL (150 mL); 250 mg/5 mL (150 mL)

Generic: 125 mg/5 mL (15 mL, 75 mL, 100 mL, 150 mL); 250 mg/5 mL (15 mL, 75 mL, 100 mL, 150 mL)

Tablet Chewable, Oral:

Generic: 125 mg, 250 mg

Amoxicillin and Clavulanate

(a moks i SIL in & klav yoo LAN ate)

Related Information

Amoxicillin *on page 124*

Bacterial Infections *on page 1739*

Related Sample Prescriptions

Bacterial Infections and Periodontal Diseases - Sample Prescriptions *on page 35*

Sinus Infection Treatment - Sample Prescriptions *on page 41*

Brand Names: US Augmentin; Augmentin ES-600; Augmentin XR [DSC]

Brand Names: Canada Amoxi-Clav [DSC]; APO-Amoxi Clav; Clavulin; Clavulin-125F; Clavulin-250F; Clavulin-500F; RATIO-Aclavulanate 250F [DSC]; RATIO-Aclavulanate [DSC]; RATIO-Aclavulanate-125F [DSC]; SANDOZ Amoxi-Clav

Generic Availability (US) Yes

Pharmacologic Category Antibiotic, Penicillin

Dental Use Treatment of orofacial infections when beta-lactamase-producing staphylococci and beta-lactamase-producing *Bacteroides* are present

Use

Oral:

Otitis media, acute:

IR tablets, chewable tablets, oral suspension (400/57 mg per 5 mL, 250/62.5 mg per 5 mL, 200/28.5 mg per 5 mL, and 125/31.25 mg per 5 mL only): Treatment of otitis media caused by beta-lactamase-producing strains of *Haemophilus influenzae* and *Moraxella catarrhalis*.

Oral suspension (600/42.9 mg per 5 mL concentration): Treatment of acute otitis media, recurrent or persistent, caused by *Streptococcus pneumoniae* (penicillin MIC = 2 mcg/mL or less), *H. influenzae* (including beta-lactamase-producing strains), and *M. catarrhalis* (including beta-lactamase-producing strains) in pediatric patients with a history of antibiotic exposure for acute otitis media in the preceding 3 months and who are either ≤2 years of age or attend day care.

Pneumonia:

ER tablets only: Treatment of patients with community-acquired pneumonia (CAP) caused by confirmed or suspected beta-lactamase-producing pathogens (ie, *H. influenzae*, *M. catarrhalis*, *Haemophilus parainfluenzae*, *Klebsiella pneumoniae*, methicillin-susceptible *Staphylococcus aureus*) and *S. pneumoniae* with reduced susceptibility to penicillin (penicillin minimum inhibitory concentration [MIC] = 2 mcg/mL).

Limitations of use: Augmentin XR is not indicated for the treatment of infections caused by *S. pneumoniae* with penicillin MIC of ≥4 mcg/mL (limited data).

IR tablets, chewable tablets, oral suspension (400/57 mg per 5 mL, 250/62.5 mg per 5 mL, 200/28.5 mg per 5 mL, and 125/31.25 mg per 5 mL only): Treatment of lower respiratory tract infection caused by beta-lactamase-producing strains of *H. influenzae* and *M. catarrhalis*.

Rhinosinusitis, acute bacterial:

ER tablets: Treatment of patients with acute bacterial sinusitis caused by confirmed or suspected beta-lactamase-producing pathogens (ie, *H. influenzae*, *M. catarrhalis*, *H. parainfluenzae*, *K. pneumoniae*, methicillin-susceptible *S. aureus*) and *S. pneumoniae* with reduced susceptibility to penicillin (penicillin MIC = 2 mcg/mL).

Limitations of use: Augmentin XR is not indicated for the treatment of infections caused by *S. pneumoniae* with penicillin MIC of ≥4 mcg/mL (limited data).

IR tablets, chewable tablets, oral suspension (400/57 mg per 5 mL, 250/62.5 mg per 5 mL, 200/28.5 mg per 5 mL, and 125/31.25 mg per 5 mL only): Treatment of sinusitis caused by beta-lactamase-producing strains of *H. influenzae* and *M. catarrhalis*.

Skin and skin structure infections: IR tablets, chewable tablets, oral suspension (400/57 mg per 5 mL, 250/62.5 mg per 5 mL, 200/28.5 mg per 5 mL, and 125/31.25 mg per 5 mL only): Treatment of skin and skin structure infections caused by beta-lactamase-producing strains of *S. aureus*, *Escherichia coli*, and *Klebsiella* spp.

Urinary tract infections: IR tablets, chewable tablets, oral suspension (400/57 mg per 5 mL, 250/62.5 mg per 5 mL, 200/28.5 mg per 5 mL, and 125/31.25 mg per 5 mL only): Treatment of urinary tract infections caused by beta-lactamase-producing strains of *E. coli*, *Klebsiella* spp, and *Enterobacter* spp.

IV [Canadian product]: Treatment of severe upper respiratory infections, chronic bronchitis (acute exacerbation), CAP, cystitis, pyelonephritis, skin and soft tissue infections, osteomyelitis, intra-abdominal infections, and female genital infections caused by susceptible organisms in adults and pediatric patients; surgical prophylaxis in procedures involving the GI tract, pelvic cavity, head and neck, or biliary tract in adults.

Local Anesthetic/Vasoconstrictor Precautions No information available to require special precautions

Effects on Dental Treatment Prolonged use of penicillins may lead to development of oral candidiasis (see Dental Health Professional Considerations)

Effects on Bleeding No information available to require special precautions

Adverse Reactions

>10%: Gastrointestinal: Diarrhea (3% to 34%; incidence varies upon dose and regimen used)

1% to 10%:

Dermatologic: Diaper rash, skin rash, urticaria

Gastrointestinal: Abdominal distress, loose stools, nausea, vomiting

Genitourinary: Vaginitis

Infection: Candidiasis, vaginal mycosis

<1%, postmarketing, and/or case reports: Cholestatic jaundice, flatulence, headache, hepatic insufficiency, hepatitis, hepatotoxicity (idiosyncratic) (Chalasani 2014), increased liver enzymes, increased serum alkaline phosphatase, prolonged prothrombin time, thrombocythemia, vasculitis (hypersensitivity)

Additional adverse reactions seen with **ampicillin-class antibiotics:** Acute generalized exanthematous pustulosis, agitation, agranulocytosis, anaphylaxis, anemia, angioedema, anxiety, behavioral changes, confusion, convulsions, crystalluria, dental discoloration, dizziness, dyspepsia, enterocolitis, eosinophilia, erythema multiforme, exfoliative dermatitis, gastritis, glossitis, hematuria, hemolytic anemia, hemorrhagic colitis, hyperactivity, immune thrombocytopenia, increased serum bilirubin, increased serum transaminases, insomnia, interstitial nephritis, leukopenia, melanoglossia, mucocutaneous candidiasis, pruritus, pseudomembranous colitis, serum sickness-like reaction, Stevens-Johnson syndrome, stomatitis, thrombocytopenia, toxic epidermal necrolysis

Dental Usual Dosage Orofacial infections: Children >40 kg and Adults: Oral: 250-500 mg every 8 hours or 875 mg every 12 hours

Dosing

Adult & Geriatric Note: Dose is based on the amoxicillin component. Dose and frequency are product specific; not all products are interchangeable. For adults who have difficulty swallowing the tablets, the 125 mg/5 mL or 250 mg/5 mL suspension (in appropriate amounts) may be given in place of the 500 mg tablet; the 200 mg/5 mL or 400 mg/5 mL suspension (in appropriate amounts) may be given in place of the 875 mg tablet.

Usual dosing range:

Oral: Immediate release: 500 mg every 8 to 12 hours **or** 875 mg every 12 hours; Extended release: 2 g every 12 hours.

IV [Canadian product]: 1 g every 8 hours or 2 g every 8 to 12 hours; surgical prophylaxis: 1 to 2 g at induction of anesthesia for procedures <1 hour (for procedures >1 hour may administer up to 2 additional doses in 24 hours).

Bite wound, prophylaxis or treatment (animal or human bite) (off-label use): Oral: Immediate release: 875 mg every 12 hours (IDSA [Stevens 2014]). **Note:** For prophylaxis, duration is 3 to 5 days (IDSA [Stevens 2014]); for treatment of established infection, duration is typically 5 to 14 days and varies based on clinical response and patient-specific factors (Baddour 2019a; Baddour 2019b).

Chronic obstructive pulmonary disease, acute exacerbation (off-label use): Note: Some experts reserve for patients with risk factors for poor outcomes (eg, age ≥65 years, FEV_1 <50% predicted, frequent exacerbations, major comorbidities), but low risk of *Pseudomonas* infection (Sethi 2020).

Oral: Immediate release: 500 mg every 8 hours **or** 875 mg every 12 hours for 3 to 7 days (GOLD 2020; Llor 2012; Sethi 2020; Wilson 2012).

Diabetic foot infection (off-label use): Note: May be used alone for mild infections or after clinical response to parenteral therapy in patients without risk factors or concern for infection caused by *Pseudomonas aeruginosa* (IDSA [Lipsky 2012]; Weintrob 2018).

Oral: Immediate release: 875 mg every 12 hours (IDSA [Lipsky 2012]; Lipsky 2004; Weintrob 2018). Duration of therapy should be tailored to individual clinical circumstances; most patients with infection limited to skin and soft tissue respond to 1 to 2 weeks of therapy (IDSA [Lipsky 2012]; Weintrob 2018).

Intra-abdominal infection (off-label use):

Diverticulitis, acute (for uncomplicated infection that meets criteria for outpatient therapy or as step-down therapy after clinical improvement on initial parenteral therapy): Oral:

Immediate release: 875 mg every 8 hours (Biondo 2014; Mora Lopez 2013).

Extended release: 2 g every 12 hours (Pemberton 2020).

Other intra-abdominal infection, step-down therapy (when clinically improved and able to tolerate oral therapy): Oral: Immediate release: 875 mg 2 to 3 times daily (Barshak 2018; Lucasti 2008; SIS [Mazuski 2017]; SIS/IDSA [Solomkin 2010]).

Duration of therapy is for 4 to 7 days following adequate source control (SIS/IDSA [Solomkin 2010]); for uncomplicated appendicitis and diverticulitis managed nonoperatively, a longer duration is necessary (Barshak 2018; Pemberton 2020).

Neutropenic fever, low-risk cancer patients (empiric therapy) (off-label use): Oral: Immediate release: 500 mg every 8 hours (Freifeld 1999; Kern 1999) **or** 875 mg every 12 hours (Kern 2013). Combine either dosing regimen with oral ciprofloxacin; continue until resolution of fever and neutropenia. **Note:** Avoid in patients who have received fluoroquinolone prophylaxis. Administer first dose in the health care setting (after blood cultures are drawn); observe patient for ≥4 hours before discharge (ASCO/IDSA [Taplitz 2018]; IDSA [Freifeld 2011]).

Odontogenic infection (initial therapy for mild infection or step-down therapy after parenteral treatment) (off-label use): Oral: Immediate release: 875 mg twice daily (Tancawan 2015); continue to complete a total of 7 to 14 days of therapy (Chow 2019).

Otitis media, acute: Oral:

Immediate release: 875 mg twice daily (Mira 2001) **or** 500 mg every 8 hours (WHO 2001).

Extended release: 1 or 2 g twice daily, based on weight and severity of infection; some experts prefer the extended release formulation for patients at high risk of severe infection or resistant *S. pneumoniae* (Limb 2019).

Duration: 5 to 7 days for mild to moderate infection and 10 days for severe infection (Limb 2019).

Peritonsillar cellulitis or abscess (off-label-use): Note: For step-down therapy after parenteral treatment. Limited data available; dosing based on expert opinion. Reserve for use in regions where *Staphylococcus aureus* remains susceptible to methicillin or based upon susceptibility results of isolated pathogens, if available. Oral: Immediate release: 875 mg every 12 hours to complete a total of 14 days of therapy (Wald 2018).

Pneumonia:

Aspiration pneumonia (community acquired [mild]): Oral:

Immediate release: 875 mg twice daily (Bartlett 2019).

Extended release: 2 g twice daily (Bartlett 2019).

Duration of therapy: Generally 7 days (Bartlett 2019).

Community acquired, outpatient empiric therapy (patients with comorbidities): Oral:

Immediate release: 500 mg 3 times daily **or** 875 mg twice daily as part of an appropriate combination regimen (ATS/IDSA [Metlay 2019]).

Extended release: 2 g twice daily as part of an appropriate combination regimen (ATS/IDSA [Metlay 2019]).

Duration of therapy: Minimum of 5 days; patients should be clinically stable with normal vital signs before therapy is discontinued (ATS/IDSA [Metlay 2019]).

Rhinosinusitis, acute bacterial: Note: In uncomplicated acute bacterial rhinosinusitis, initial observation and symptom management without antibiotic therapy is appropriate in most patients (AAO-HNS [Rosenfeld 2015]; Harris 2016).

Standard dose: Oral: Immediate release: 500 mg every 8 hours **or** 875 mg every 12 hours for 5 to 7 days (IDSA [Chow 2012])

High dose: Oral: Extended release: 2 g every 12 hours. **Note:** Recommended for patients at risk for poor outcome or pneumococcal resistance based on the following features: age ≥65 years, recent hospitalization, antibiotic use within the past month, immunocompromise, residence in a region with high rates of penicillin-resistant *S. pneumoniae*, or failure to respond to initial treatment (AAO-HNS [Rosenfeld 2015]; IDSA [Chow 2012]). For initial therapy, the duration is 5 to 7 days; for patients who have failed initial therapy and require re-treatment, the duration is 7 to 10 days (Patel 2018).

Streptococcus (group A), chronic carriage (off-label use): Oral: Immediate release: 40 mg/kg/day in divided doses (eg, 875 mg every 12 hours) (maximum: 2 g/day) for 10 days (IDSA [Shulman 2012]; Mahakit 2006). **Note:** Most individuals with chronic carriage do not require antibiotics (IDSA [Shulman 2012]).

Urinary tract infection (UTI) (alternative agent): Note: Although evidence is limited, some experts recommend the use of amoxicillin/clavulanate in this setting. Use with caution and only when first-line agents cannot be used (due to decreased efficacy of oral beta-lactams compared to other agents) (ESCMID/IDSA [Gupta 2011]; Hooton 2018a). Closely monitor patient.

Acute uncomplicated cystitis or acute simple cystitis (infection limited to bladder and no signs/symptoms of upper tract or systemic infection): Oral: Immediate release: 500 mg twice daily (Hooton 2005) for 5 to 7 days (ESCMID/IDSA [Gupta 2011]; Hooton 2018a).

Complicated UTI (including pyelonephritis): Oral: Immediate release: 875 mg twice daily for 10 to 14 days (ESCMID/IDSA [Gupta 2011]; Johnson 2018). **Note:** Oral therapy should follow appropriate parenteral therapy. For outpatient treatment of mild infection, a single dose of a long-acting parenteral agent is acceptable; for outpatients who are more ill or are at risk for more severe illness, consider continuing parenteral therapy until culture and susceptibility results are available (ESCMID/IDSA [Gupta 2011]; Hooton 2018b).

Renal Impairment: Adult

The renal dosing recommendations are based upon the best available evidence and clinical expertise. Senior Editorial Team: Bruce Mueller, PharmD, FCCP, FASN, FNKF; Jason Roberts, PhD, BPharm (Hons), B App Sc, FSHP, FISAC; Michael Heung, MD, MS.

Oral:

Note: Renally adjusted dose recommendations are based on the amoxicillin 250 mg/clavulanate 125 mg and amoxicillin 500 mg/clavulanate 125 mg tablets. Avoid IR 875 mg tablet or ER tablets in patients with CrCl <30 mL/minute.

Altered kidney function:

GFR ≥30 mL/minute: No dosage adjustment necessary.

GFR 10 to 30 mL/minute: 250 to 500 mg every 12 hours.

GFR <10 mL/minute: 250 to 500 mg every 12 to 24 hours (expert opinion; manufacturer's labeling).

Hemodialysis, intermittent (thrice weekly): Dialyzable (30% to 47% [amoxicillin component], 34% [clavulanic acid] with low-flux filters [Davies 1988; Francke 1979]): 250 to 500 mg every 12 to 24 hours (Hui 2017; manufacturer's labeling). If utilizing a 24-hour dosing interval, administer dose after dialysis or give an additional dose after dialysis on dialysis days.

Peritoneal dialysis: 250 to 500 mg every 12 hours (expert opinion).

IV [Canadian product]: **Note:** Dose based on amoxicillin component.

Altered kidney function:

CrCl ≥30 mL/minute: No dosage adjustment necessary.

CrCl 10 to 30 mL/minute: Initial: 1 g followed by 500 mg every 12 hours.

CrCl <10 mL/minute: Initial: 1 g followed by 500 mg every 12 to 24 hours (expert opinion).

Hemodialysis, intermittent (thrice weekly): Dialyzable (30% to 47% [amoxicillin component] with low-flux filters [Davies 1988; Francke 1979]): Initial: 1 g followed by 500 mg every 12 to 24 hours. If utilizing a 24-hour dosing interval, administer dose after dialysis or give an additional 500 mg dose after dialysis on dialysis days (expert opinion; manufacturer's labeling).

Peritoneal dialysis: Initial: 1 g followed by 500 mg every 12 hours (expert opinion).

Hepatic Impairment: Adult Oral, IV [Canadian product]: There are no dosage adjustments provided in the manufacturer's labeling; use with caution. Use contraindicated in patients with a history of amoxicillin and clavulanate-associated hepatic dysfunction.

Pediatric Note: Dosing based on amoxicillin component; dose and frequency are product specific; not all products are interchangeable; using a product with the incorrect amoxicillin:clavulanate ratio could result in subtherapeutic clavulanic acid concentrations or severe diarrhea.

Frequency of dosing generally based on ratio of amoxicillin to clavulanate:

- 2:1 formulations are dosed 3 times daily (amoxicillin 250 mg/clavulanate 125 mg). **Note:** Per the manufacturer, the amoxicillin 250 mg/clavulanate 125 mg tablet should only be used in patients ≥40 kg due to the amoxicillin to clavulanate ratio.

- 4:1 formulations are dosed 3 times daily (amoxicillin 125 mg/clavulanate 31.25 mg; amoxicillin 250 mg/clavulanate 62.5 mg; amoxicillin 500 mg/clavulanate 125 mg).
- 7:1 formulations are dosed 2 times daily (amoxicillin 200 mg/clavulanate 28.5 mg; amoxicillin 400 mg/clavulanate 57 mg; amoxicillin 875 mg/clavulanate 125 mg).
- 14:1 formulations are dosed 2 times daily (amoxicillin 600 mg/clavulanate 42.9 mg).
- 16:1 formulations (extended release) are dosed 2 times daily (amoxicillin 1,000 mg/clavulanate 62.5 mg).

General dosing, susceptible infection: Note: Dosing determined by formulations amoxicillin:clavulanate ratio:

Immediate-release formulations (*Red Book* [AAP 2018]): Infants, Children, and Adolescents: Oral:

4:1 formulation: 20 to 40 mg amoxicillin/kg/day in divided doses 3 times daily; maximum daily dose: 1,500 mg/**day**.

7:1 formulation: 25 to 45 mg amoxicillin/kg/day in divided doses twice daily; maximum daily dose: 1,750 mg/**day**.

14:1 formulation: 90 mg amoxicillin/kg/day in divided doses twice daily; maximum daily dose: 4,000 mg/**day**.

Extended-release formulation (16:1): Children and Adolescents >40 kg: Oral: 2,000 mg amoxicillin every 12 hours.

Impetigo: Infants, Children, and Adolescents: Oral: 25 mg amoxicillin/kg/day in divided doses twice daily; maximum dose: 875 mg amoxicillin/dose (IDSA [Stevens 2014]).

Otitis media, acute: Infants ≥3 months and Children: Oral suspension (600 mg/5 mL): Oral: 90 mg amoxicillin/kg/day divided every 12 hours for up to 10 days; recommended for use in children with severe illness, who have received amoxicillin in the past 30 days, who have treatment failure at 48 to 72 hours on first-line therapy, and when coverage for beta-lactamase positive *H. influenzae* and *M. catarrhalis* is needed. Variable duration of therapy; the manufacturer suggests 10-day course in all patients; however, new data suggests a shorter course in some cases: If <2 years of age or severe symptoms (any age): 10-day course; if 2 to 5 years of age with mild to moderate symptoms: 7-day course; if ≥6 years of age with mild to moderate symptoms: 5- to 7-day course (AAP [Lieberthal 2013]).

Pneumonia, community-acquired (IDSA/PIDS [Bradley 2011]): Infants ≥3 months, Children, and Adolescents:

Empiric therapy: Oral: 90 mg amoxicillin/kg/day in divided doses twice daily; maximum daily dose: 4,000 mg/**day**.

H. influenzae, beta-lactamase positive strains, mild infection, or step-down therapy: Oral:

Standard dose: 45 mg amoxicillin/kg/day in divided doses 3 times daily.

High dose: 90 mg amoxicillin/kg/day in divided doses twice daily.

Rhinosinusitis, acute bacterial:

Infants ≥3 months: Oral: 45 mg amoxicillin/kg/day divided every 12 hours **or** 40 mg/kg/day divided every 8 hours.

Children and Adolescents: Oral:

Standard dose: 45 mg amoxicillin/kg/day divided every 12 hours for 10 to 14 days; usual adult dose: 875 mg amoxicillin/dose (IDSA [Chow 2012]).

High dose: 80 to 90 mg amoxicillin/kg/day divided every 12 hours; maximum dose: 2,000 mg/dose (AAP [Wald 2013]; IDSA [Chow 2012]); treatment duration variable: 10 to 28 days, some have suggested discontinuation of therapy 7 days after resolution of signs and symptoms of infection (AAP [Wald 2013]); some experts recommend a duration of 10 to 14 days (IDSA [Chow 2012]). **Note:** Recommended for patients who live in areas with high endemic rates of penicillin-non-susceptible *S. pneumonia*, patients with moderate to severe infections, daycare attendance, age <2 years, recent hospitalization, antibiotic use within the past month, patients who are immunocompromised or if initial therapy fails (second-line therapy) (AAP [Wald 2013]; IDSA [Chow 2012]).

Streptococci, group A; chronic carrier treatment: Children and Adolescents: Oral: 40 mg amoxicillin/kg/day in divided doses every 8 hours for 10 days; maximum daily dose: 2,000 mg amoxicillin/**day** (IDSA [Shulman 2012]).

Urinary tract infections: Infants ≥2 months and Children ≤2 years: Oral: 20 to 40 mg amoxicillin/kg/day in divided doses 3 times daily (AAP 2011).

Renal Impairment: Pediatric

Infants, Children, and Adolescents: There are no dosage adjustments provided in the manufacturer's labeling; however, the following guidelines have been used by some clinicians (Aronoff 2007): Oral:

Mild to moderate infection: Dosing based on 20 to 40 mg amoxicillin/kg/day divided every 8 hours or 25 to 45 mg amoxicillin/kg/day divided every 12 hours:

GFR >30 mL/minute/1.73 m^2: No adjustment required

GFR 10 to 29 mL/minute/1.73 m^2: 8 to 20 mg amoxicillin/kg/dose every 12 hours

GFR <10 mL/minute/1.73 m^2: 8 to 20 mg amoxicillin/kg/dose every 24 hours

Hemodialysis: 8 to 20 mg amoxicillin/kg/dose every 24 hours; give after dialysis

Peritoneal dialysis: 8 to 20 mg amoxicillin/kg/dose every 24 hours

Severe infection (high dose): Dosing based on 80 to 90 mg amoxicillin/kg/day divided every 12 hours:

CrCl >30 mL/minute/1.73 m^2: No adjustment required

CrCl 10 to 29 mL/minute/1.73 m^2: 20 mg amoxicillin/kg/dose every 12 hours; do not use the 875 mg tablet

CrCl <10 mL/minute/1.73 m^2: 20 mg amoxicillin/kg/dose every 24 hours; do not use the 875 mg tablet

Hemodialysis: 20 mg amoxicillin/kg/dose every 24 hours; give after dialysis; do not use the 875 mg tablet

Peritoneal dialysis: 20 mg amoxicillin/kg/dose every 24 hours; do not use the 875 mg tablet

Hepatic Impairment: Pediatric There are no dosage adjustments provided in the manufacturer's labeling; use with caution. Use contraindicated in patients with a history of amoxicillin and clavulanate-associated hepatic dysfunction.

Mechanism of Action Clavulanic acid binds and inhibits beta-lactamases that inactivate amoxicillin resulting in amoxicillin having an expanded spectrum of activity. Amoxicillin inhibits bacterial cell wall synthesis by binding to one or more of the penicillin-binding proteins (PBPs) which in turn inhibits the final transpeptidation step of peptidoglycan synthesis in bacterial cell walls, thus inhibiting cell wall biosynthesis. Bacteria eventually lyse due to ongoing activity of cell wall autolytic enzymes (autolysins and murein hydrolases) while cell wall assembly is arrested.

Contraindications

Hypersensitivity to amoxicillin, clavulanic acid, other beta-lactam antibacterial drugs (eg, penicillins, cephalosporins), or any component of the formulation; history of cholestatic jaundice or hepatic dysfunction with amoxicillin/clavulanate potassium therapy.

Augmentin XR: Additional contraindications: Severe renal impairment (CrCl <30 mL/minute) and hemodialysis patients.

Canadian labeling: Additional contraindications (not in the US labeling): Oral: Suspected or confirmed mononucleosis.

Warnings/Precautions Hypersensitivity reactions, including anaphylaxis (some fatal), have been reported. Prolonged use may result in fungal or bacterial superinfection, including *C. difficile*-associated diarrhea (CDAD) and pseudomembranous colitis; CDAD has been observed >2 months postantibiotic treatment. Although rarely fatal, hepatic dysfunction (eg, cholestatic jaundice, hepatitis) has been reported. Patients at highest risk include those with serious underlying disease or concomitant medications. Hepatic toxicity is usually reversible. Monitor LFTs at regular intervals in patients with hepatic impairment. High percentage of patients with infectious mononucleosis have developed rash during therapy; ampicillin class antibiotics not recommended in these patients. Incidence of diarrhea is higher than with amoxicillin alone. Due to differing content of clavulanic acid, not all formulations are interchangeable; use of an inappropriate product for a specific dosage could result in either diarrhea (which may be severe) or subtherapeutic clavulanic acid concentrations leading to decreased clinical efficacy. Low incidence of cross-allergy with cephalosporins exists. Monitor renal, hepatic, and hematopoietic function if therapy extends beyond approved duration times. Dosage adjustment recommended in patients with CrCl ≤30 mL/minute. Some products contain phenylalanine. Potentially significant drug-drug interactions may exist, requiring dose or frequency adjustment, additional monitoring, and/or selection of alternative therapy.

Warnings: Additional Pediatric Considerations Epstein-Barr virus infection (infectious mononucleosis), acute lymphocytic leukemia, or cytomegalovirus infection increase risk for penicillin-induced maculopapular rash. Appearance of a rash should be carefully evaluated to differentiate a nonallergic ampicillin rash from a hypersensitivity reaction; rash occurs in 5% to 10% of children and is a generalized dull red, maculopapular rash, generally appearing 3 to 14 days after the start of therapy. It normally begins on the trunk and spreads over most of the body. It may be most intense at pressure areas, elbows, and knees. A high percentage (43% to 100%) of patients with infectious mononucleosis have developed rash during therapy; ampicillin-class antibiotics are not recommended in these patients.

In a meta-analysis of pediatric acute otitis media trials, high-dose amoxicillin regimens were associated with a higher incidence of adverse effects compared to standard-dose; the incidence of diarrhea was 18.9% with high-dose amoxicillin/clavulanate, 13.8% with high-dose amoxicillin, and 8.7% with standard-dose amoxicillin; the incidence of generalized rash was 6.5% with high-dose amoxicillin, 4.9% with high-dose amoxicillin/clavulanate, and 2.9% with standard-dose amoxicillin; however, significant heterogeneity was observed (Hum 2019).

Drug Interactions

Metabolism/Transport Effects None known.

Avoid Concomitant Use

Avoid concomitant use of Amoxicillin and Clavulanate with any of the following: BCG (Intravesical); Cholera Vaccine

Increased Effect/Toxicity

Amoxicillin and Clavulanate may increase the levels/effects of: Dichlorphenamide; Methotrexate; Vitamin K Antagonists

The levels/effects of Amoxicillin and Clavulanate may be increased by: Acemetacin; Allopurinol; Probenecid

Decreased Effect

Amoxicillin and Clavulanate may decrease the levels/effects of: Aminoglycosides; BCG (Intravesical); BCG Vaccine (Immunization); Cholera Vaccine; Lactobacillus and Estriol; Mycophenolate; Sodium Picosulfate; Typhoid Vaccine

The levels/effects of Amoxicillin and Clavulanate may be decreased by: Tetracyclines

Dietary Considerations May be taken with meals or on an empty stomach; take with meals to increase absorption and decrease GI upset; may mix with milk, formula, or juice. Extended release tablets should be taken with food. Some products may contain sodium. Some products contain phenylalanine. All dosage forms contain potassium.

Pharmacodynamics/Kinetics

Half-life Elimination Clavulanic acid: 1 hour

Time to Peak Clavulanic acid: Serum: 1.5 hours

Pregnancy Risk Factor B

Pregnancy Considerations Both amoxicillin and clavulanic acid cross the placenta (Weber 1984). Oral ampicillin-class antibiotics are poorly absorbed during labor.

Breastfeeding Considerations

Amoxicillin is present in breast milk following administration amoxicillin/clavulanate (Weber 1984).

The relative infant dose (RID) of amoxicillin following administration of amoxicillin/clavulanate is 0.02% to 0.07% when calculated using the highest average breast milk concentration located and compared to an infant therapeutic dose of 25 to 90 mg/kg/day. In general, breastfeeding is considered acceptable when the RID is <10% (Anderson 2016; Ito 2000).

Using the highest average milk concentration (0.12 mcg/mL), the estimated daily infant dose via breast milk is 0.018 mg/kg/day. This milk concentration was obtained 4 to 6 hours following maternal administration of oral amoxicillin/clavulanate 250 mg/125 mg (Takase 1982).

Constipation, diarrhea, restlessness, and rash have been reported in breastfeeding infants exposed to amoxicillin and clavulanate; reversible elevations in AST and ALT have been noted in one infant (Benyamini 2005). The manufacturer warns of the potential for allergic sensitization in the infant. In general, antibiotics that are present in breast milk may cause non-dose-related modification of bowel flora. Monitor infants for GI disturbances, such as thrush and diarrhea (WHO 2002).

Although the manufacturer recommends that caution be exercised when administering amoxicillin and clavulanate to breastfeeding women, amoxicillin/clavulanate is considered compatible with breastfeeding when used in usual recommended doses (WHO 2002).

Dosage Forms Considerations

IV [Canadian product]: 500 mg, 1 g, and 2 g vials contain 31.4 mg (1.4 mmoL), 62.9 mg (2.7 mmoL), and 125.9 mg (5.5 mmoL) of sodium and 19.6 (0.5 mmoL), 39.3 mg (1 mmoL) and 39.3 mg (1 mmoL) of potassium, respectively.

Dosage Forms: US

Suspension Reconstituted, Oral:

Augmentin: Amoxicillin 250 mg and clavulanate potassium 62.5 mg per 5 mL (75 mL, 100 mL, 150 mL); Amoxicillin 125 mg and clavulanate potassium 31.25 mg per 5 mL (75 mL, 100 mL, 150 mL)

Augmentin ES-600: Amoxicillin 600 mg and clavulanate potassium 42.9 mg per 5 mL (75 mL, 125 mL, 200 mL)

Generic: Amoxicillin 200 mg and clavulanate potassium 28.5 mg per 5 mL (50 mL, 75 mL, 100 mL); Amoxicillin 250 mg and clavulanate potassium 62.5 mg per 5 mL (75 mL, 100 mL, 150 mL); Amoxicillin 400 mg and clavulanate potassium 57 mg per 5 mL (50 mL, 75 mL, 100 mL); Amoxicillin 600 mg and clavulanate potassium 42.9 mg per 5 mL (75 mL, 125 mL, 200 mL)

Tablet, Oral:

Augmentin: Amoxicillin 500 mg and clavulanate potassium 125 mg

Generic: Amoxicillin 250 mg and clavulanate potassium 125 mg, Amoxicillin 500 mg and clavulanate potassium 125 mg, Amoxicillin 875 mg and clavulanate potassium 125 mg

Tablet Chewable, Oral:

Generic: Amoxicillin 200 mg and clavulanate potassium 28.5 mg, Amoxicillin 400 mg and clavulanate potassium 57 mg

Tablet Extended Release 12 Hour, Oral:

Generic: Amoxicillin 1000 mg and clavulanate potassium 62.5 mg

Dosage Forms: Canada

Solution Reconstituted, Intravenous:

Generic: Amoxicillin 1000 mg and clavulanate potassium 200 mg (1 ea); Amoxicillin 2000 mg and clavulanate potassium 200 mg (1 ea); Amoxicillin 500 mg and clavulanate potassium 100 mg (1 ea)

Suspension Reconstituted, Oral:

Clavulin: Amoxicillin 400 mg and clavulanate potassium 57 mg per 5 mL (70 mL); Amoxicillin 200 mg and clavulanate potassium 28.5 mg per 5 mL (70 mL)

Clavulin-125F: Amoxicillin 125 mg and clavulanate potassium 31.25 mg per 5 mL (100 mL, 150 mL)

Clavulin-250F: Amoxicillin 250 mg and clavulanate potassium 62.5 mg per 5 mL (100 mL, 150 mL)

Generic: Amoxicillin 125 mg and clavulanate potassium 31.25 mg per 5 mL (100 mL, 150 mL); Amoxicillin 250 mg and clavulanate potassium 62.5 mg per 5 mL (100 mL, 150 mL); Amoxicillin 400 mg and clavulanate potassium 57 mg per 5 mL (70 mL)

Tablet, Oral:

Clavulin: Amoxicillin 875 mg and clavulanate potassium 125 mg

Clavulin-500F: Amoxicillin 500 mg and clavulanate potassium 125 mg

Generic: Amoxicillin 250 mg and clavulanate potassium 125 mg, Amoxicillin 500 mg and clavulanate potassium 125 mg, Amoxicillin 875 mg and clavulanate potassium 125 mg

Dental Health Professional Considerations In maxillary sinus, anterior nasal cavity, and deep neck infections, beta-lactamase-producing staphylococci and beta-lactamase-producing *Bacteroides* usually are present. In these situations, antibiotics that resist the beta-lactamase enzyme are indicated. Amoxicillin and clavulanic acid is administered orally for moderate infections. Ampicillin sodium and sulbactam sodium (Unasyn®) is administered parenterally for more severe infections.

- ◆ **Amoxicillin and Clavulanate Potassium** *see* Amoxicillin and Clavulanate *on page 130*
- ◆ **Amoxicillin and Clavulanic Acid** *see* Amoxicillin and Clavulanate *on page 130*
- ◆ **Amoxicillin, Clarithromycin, and Lansoprazole** *see* Lansoprazole, Amoxicillin, and Clarithromycin *on page 877*
- ◆ **Amoxicillin, Clarithromycin, and Omeprazole** *see* Omeprazole, Clarithromycin, and Amoxicillin *on page 1140*
- ◆ **Amoxicillin-Clavulanate** *see* Amoxicillin and Clavulanate *on page 130*
- ◆ **Amoxicillin/Clavulanate K** *see* Amoxicillin and Clavulanate *on page 130*
- ◆ **Amoxicillin, Omeprazole, and Rifabutin** *see* Omeprazole, Amoxicillin, and Rifabutin *on page 1140*
- ◆ **Amoxicillin/Potassium Clav** *see* Amoxicillin and Clavulanate *on page 130*
- ◆ **Amoxicillin Trihydrate** *see* Amoxicillin *on page 124*
- ◆ **Amoxil** *see* Amoxicillin *on page 124*
- ◆ **Amoxycillin** *see* Amoxicillin *on page 124*
- ◆ **Amoxycillin and Clavulanate Potassium** *see* Amoxicillin and Clavulanate *on page 130*
- ◆ **Amoxycillin and Clavulanic Acid** *see* Amoxicillin and Clavulanate *on page 130*

Amphetamine (am FET a meen)

Related Information

Dentin Hypersensitivity, Acid Erosion, High Caries Index, Management of Alveolar Osteitis, and Xerostomia *on page 1762*

Management of the Chemically Dependent Patient *on page 1724*

Brand Names: US Adzenys ER; Adzenys XR-ODT; Dyanavel XR; Evekeo; Evekeo ODT

Pharmacologic Category Central Nervous System Stimulant

Use

Attention-deficit/hyperactivity disorder: Treatment of ADHD

Exogenous obesity (immediate-release tablet only): Short-term treatment of exogenous obesity as an adjunct to caloric restriction for patients refractory to alternative therapy (eg, repeated diets, group programs, other drugs)

Narcolepsy (immediate-release tablet only): Treatment of narcolepsy

Local Anesthetic/Vasoconstrictor Precautions Use vasoconstrictor with caution in patients taking amphetamine. Amphetamines enhance the sympathomimetic response of epinephrine and norepinephrine leading to potential hypertension and cardiotoxicity.

Effects on Dental Treatment Key adverse event(s) related to dental treatment: Amphetamines cause tachycardia, increases in blood pressure, and palpitations. Consider monitoring blood pressure prior to using local anesthetic with a vasoconstrictor. Symptoms associated with bruxism have been observed in some patients.

Effects on Bleeding No information available to require special precautions

Adverse Reactions

1% to 10%:

Central nervous system: Insomnia (children: 4%), emotional lability (children: 3%)

Gastrointestinal: Decreased appetite (children: 4%), upper abdominal pain (children: 4%), abdominal pain (children: 3%)

Respiratory: Allergic rhinitis (children: 4%), epistaxis (children: 4%)

Miscellaneous: Accidental injury (children: 3%)

Frequency not defined:

Central nervous system: Drug abuse, drug dependence

Gastrointestinal: Diarrhea

<1%, postmarketing, and/or case reports: Acute myocardial infarction, aggressive behavior, alopecia, anaphylaxis, angioedema, anorexia, blurred vision, bruxism, cardiomyopathy, change in libido, constipation, dermatillomania, dizziness, dysgeusia, dyskinesia, dysphoria, euphoria, exacerbation of Gilles de la Tourette syndrome, fatigue, frequent erections, gastrointestinal disease, headache, hypersensitivity reaction, impotence, increased blood pressure, irritability, mydriasis, nausea, outbursts of anger, overstimulation, palpitations, paresthesia, peripheral vascular disease, prolonged erection, psychosis, Raynaud's disease, restlessness, rhabdomyolysis, skin rash, Stevens-Johnson syndrome, tachycardia, talkativeness, tic disorder (including exacerbation), toxic epidermal necrolysis, tremor, unpleasant taste, urticaria, vocal tics (including exacerbation), weight loss, xerostomia

Mechanism of Action Amphetamines are noncatecholamine sympathomimetic amines that promote release of catecholamines (primarily dopamine and norepinephrine) from their storage sites in the presynaptic nerve terminals. A less significant mechanism may include their ability to block the reuptake of catecholamines by competitive inhibition. The anorexigenic effect is probably secondary to the CNS-stimulating effect; the site of action is probably the hypothalamic feeding center.

Pharmacodynamics/Kinetics

Duration of Action Oral:

Immediate-release tablet: Evekeo: 4 to 6 hours (Jain 2017)

Extended-release orally-disintegrating tablet: Adzenys XR-ODT: 10 to 12 hours

Half-life Elimination Oral:

Immediate-release tablet: 12 hours (de la Torre 2004)

Immediate-release orally-disintegrating tablet: Evekeo ODT: Adults: d-amphetamine 10 hours and l-amphetamine 11.7 hours

Extended-release orally-disintegrating tablet: Adzenys XR-ODT:

Children 6 to 12 years: d-amphetamine 9 to 10 hours and l-amphetamine 10 to 11 hours

Adults: d-amphetamine 11 hours and l-amphetamine 14 hours

Extended-release suspension:

Adzenys ER:

Children 6 to 12 years: d-amphetamine 12.7 hours (mean) and l-amphetamine 15.3 hours

Adults: d-amphetamine 11.4 hours and l-amphetamine 14.1 hours

Dyanavel XR:

Children: d-amphetamine 10.43 ± 2.01 hours and l-amphetamine 12.14 ± 3.15 hours

Adults: d-amphetamine 12.36 ± 2.95 hours and l-amphetamine 15.12 ± 4.4 hours

Time to Peak Oral:

Immediate-release tablet: Within 4 hours (de la Torre 2004)

Immediate-release orally-disintegrating tablet: Evekeo ODT: Median time d-amphetamine and l-amphetamine 3.5 hours (with water) and 3 hours (without water); increased with food in adults

Extended-release orally-disintegrating tablet: Adzenys XR-ODT: Median time d-amphetamine 5 hours (7 hours with food) and l-amphetamine ~5.25 hours (7.75 hours with food)

Extended-release suspension:

Adzenys ER suspension: d-amphetamine and l-amphetamine: 5 hours (median) with or without food

Dyanavel XR suspension:

Children: Median time d-amphetamine 3.9 hours and l-amphetamine 4.5 hours

Adults: 4 (2 to 7) hours

Pregnancy Considerations

Information related to use of amphetamine in pregnancy is limited (Maurovich-Horvat 2013). The majority of human data are based on illicit amphetamine/methamphetamine exposure and not from therapeutic maternal use (Golub 2005). Use of amphetamines during pregnancy may lead to an increased risk of premature birth and low birth weight; newborns may experience symptoms of withdrawal. Behavioral problems may also occur later in childhood (LaGasse 2012). Newborns should be monitored for agitation, irritability, excessive drowsiness, or feeding difficulties

Data collection to monitor pregnancy outcomes following exposure to amphetamine is ongoing. Healthcare providers are encouraged to enroll females exposed to amphetamine during pregnancy in the National Pregnancy Registry for Psychostimulants (1-866-961-2388 and/or https://womensmentalhealth.org/clinical-and-research-programs/pregnancyregistry/othermedications/).

Controlled Substance C-II

◆ **Amphetamine and Dextroamphetamine** *see* Dextroamphetamine and Amphetamine *on page 475*

◆ **Amphetamine Sulfate** *see* Amphetamine *on page 135*

◆ **Amphet Asp/Amphet/D-Amphet** *see* Dextroamphetamine and Amphetamine *on page 475*

Amphotericin B Cholesteryl Sulfate Complex

(am foe TER i sin bee kole LES te ril SUL fate KOM plecks)

Pharmacologic Category Antifungal Agent, Parenteral

Use Treatment of invasive aspergillosis in patients who have failed amphotericin B deoxycholate treatment, or who have renal impairment or experience unacceptable toxicity which precludes treatment with amphotericin B deoxycholate in effective doses.

Local Anesthetic/Vasoconstrictor Precautions No information available to require special precautions

Effects on Dental Treatment No significant effects or complications reported

Effects on Bleeding No information available to require special precautions

Adverse Reactions Amphotericin B colloidal dispersion has an improved therapeutic index compared to conventional amphotericin B, and has been used safely in patients with amphotericin B-related nephrotoxicity; however, continued decline of renal function has occurred in some patients.

>10%:

Cardiovascular: Hypotension, tachycardia
Central nervous system: Chills
Endocrine & metabolic: Hypokalemia
Gastrointestinal: Vomiting
Hepatic: Hyperbilirubinemia
Renal: Increased serum creatinine
Miscellaneous: Fever

5% to 10%:

Cardiovascular: Chest pain, facial edema, hypertension
Central nervous system: Abnormality in thinking, drowsiness, headache, insomnia
Dermatologic: Diaphoresis, pruritus, skin rash
Endocrine & metabolic: Hyperglycemia, hypocalcemia, hypomagnesemia, hypophosphatemia
Gastrointestinal: Abdominal pain, diarrhea, enlargement of abdomen, hematemesis, nausea, stomatitis, xerostomia
Hematologic & oncologic: Anemia, hemorrhage, thrombocytopenia
Hepatic: Abnormal hepatic function tests, increased serum alkaline phosphatase, jaundice
Neuromuscular & skeletal: Back pain, muscle rigidity, tremor
Respiratory: Dyspnea, epistaxis, hypoxia, increased cough, rhinitis

<5%, postmarketing, and/or case reports: Acidosis, atrial arrhythmia, cardiac arrest, cardiac failure, gastrointestinal hemorrhage, hepatic failure, injection site reaction, oliguria, pain at injection site, pleural effusion, renal failure, seizure, syncope, ventricular arrhythmia

Mechanism of Action Binds to ergosterol altering cell membrane permeability in susceptible fungi and causing leakage of cell components with subsequent cell death. Proposed mechanism suggests that amphotericin causes an oxidation-dependent stimulation of macrophages (Lyman, 1992).

Pharmacodynamics/Kinetics

Half-life Elimination ~28 hours; prolonged with higher doses

Pregnancy Risk Factor B

Pregnancy Considerations Amphotericin crosses the placenta and enters the fetal circulation. Amphotericin B is recommended for the treatment of serious systemic fungal diseases in pregnant women; refer to current guidelines (IDSA [Pappas 2016]; King 1998; Pilmis 2015).

Product Availability Amphotec has been discontinued in the US for more than 1 year.

◆ **Amphotericin B Colloidal Dispersion** *see* Amphotericin B Cholesteryl Sulfate Complex *on page 137*

Amphotericin B (Conventional)

(am foe TER i sin bee con VEN sha nal)

Related Information

Fungal Infections *on page 1752*

Brand Names: Canada Fungizone IV

Pharmacologic Category Antifungal Agent, Parenteral

Use

Life-threatening fungal infections: Treatment of patients with progressive, potentially life-threatening fungal infections: Aspergillosis, cryptococcosis (torulosis), North American blastomycosis, systemic candidiasis, coccidioidomycosis, histoplasmosis, zygomycosis (including mucormycosis due to susceptible species of the genera *Absidia, Mucor,* and *Rhizopus*), and infections due to related susceptible species of *Conidiobolus, Basidiobolus,* and sporotrichosis.

Leishmaniasis: Alternative treatment in patients with American (New World) mucocutaneous leishmaniasis

Local Anesthetic/Vasoconstrictor Precautions No information available to require special precautions

Effects on Dental Treatment No significant effects or complications reported

Effects on Bleeding No information available to require special precautions

Adverse Reactions

Systemic:

>10%:

Cardiovascular: Hypotension
Central nervous system: Chills, headache (less frequent with I.T.), malaise, pain (less frequent with I.T.)
Endocrine & metabolic: Hypokalemia, hypomagnesemia
Gastrointestinal: Anorexia, diarrhea, epigastric pain, heartburn, nausea (less frequent with I.T.), stomach cramps, vomiting (less frequent with I.T.)
Hematologic & oncologic: Anemia (normochromic-normocytic)
Local: Pain at injection site (with or without phlebitis or thrombophlebitis [incidence may increase with peripheral infusion of admixtures])
Renal: Renal function abnormality (including azotemia, renal tubular acidosis, nephrocalcinosis [>0.1 mg/mL]), renal insufficiency
Respiratory: Tachypnea
Miscellaneous: Fever

1% to 10%:

Cardiovascular: Flushing, hypertension
Central nervous system: Arachnoiditis, delirium, neuralgia (lumbar; especially with intrathecal therapy), paresthesia (especially with intrathecal therapy)
Genitourinary: Urinary retention
Hematologic & oncologic: Leukocytosis

<1% (Limited to important or life-threatening): Acute hepatic failure, agranulocytosis, anuria, blood coagulation disorder, bone marrow depression, bronchospasm, cardiac arrest, cardiac arrhythmia, cardiac failure, convulsions, diplopia, dyspnea, eosinophilia,

exfoliation of skin, hearing loss, hemorrhagic gastroenteritis, hepatitis, hypersensitivity pneumonitis, increased liver enzymes, jaundice, leukoencephalopathy, leukopenia, maculopapular rash, melena, nephrogenic diabetes insipidus, oliguria, peripheral neuropathy, pruritus, pulmonary edema, renal failure, renal tubular acidosis, shock, Stevens-Johnson syndrome, thrombocytopenia, tinnitus, toxic epidermal necrolysis, ventricular fibrillation, vertigo (transient), visual disturbance, wheezing

Mechanism of Action Binds to ergosterol altering cell membrane permeability in susceptible fungi and causing leakage of cell components with subsequent cell death. Proposed mechanism suggests that amphotericin causes an oxidation-dependent stimulation of macrophages (Lyman 1992).

Pharmacodynamics/Kinetics

Half-life Elimination

Premature neonates (GA: 27.4 ± 5 weeks): 14.8 hours (range: 5 to 82 hours) (Baley 1990)

Infants and Children (4 months to 14 years): 18.1 ± 6.6 hours (range: 11.9 to 40.3 hours) (Benson 1989)

Adults: Biphasic: Initial: 15 to 48 hours; Terminal: 15 days

Time to Peak Within 1 hour following a 4- to 6-hour dose

Pregnancy Risk Factor B

Pregnancy Considerations

Amphotericin crosses the placenta and enters the fetal circulation. Amphotericin B is recommended for the treatment of serious systemic fungal diseases in pregnant women. Refer to current guidelines (IDSA [Pappas 2016]; King 1998; Pilmis 2015).

◆ **Amphotericin B Deoxycholate** *see* Amphotericin B (Conventional) *on page 137*

◆ **Amphotericin B Desoxycholate** *see* Amphotericin B (Conventional) *on page 137*

Amphotericin B (Lipid Complex)

(am foe TER i sin bee LIP id KOM pleks)

Brand Names: US Abelcet

Brand Names: Canada Abelcet

Pharmacologic Category Antifungal Agent, Parenteral

Use Fungal infection (invasive): Treatment of invasive fungal infection in patients who are refractory to or intolerant of conventional amphotericin B (amphotericin B deoxycholate) therapy

Local Anesthetic/Vasoconstrictor Precautions No information available to require special precautions

Effects on Dental Treatment No significant effects or complications reported

Effects on Bleeding No information available to require special precautions

Adverse Reactions Nephrotoxicity and infusion-related hyperpyrexia, rigor, and chilling are reduced relative to amphotericin deoxycholate.

>10%:

Central nervous system: Chills (18%)

Renal: Increased serum creatinine (11%)

Miscellaneous: Fever (14%), multi-organ failure (11%)

1% to 10%:

Cardiovascular: Hypotension (8%), cardiac arrest (6%), hypertension (5%), chest pain (3%)

Central nervous system: Headache (6%), pain (5%)

Dermatologic: Skin rash (4%)

Endocrine & metabolic: Hypokalemia (5%)

Gastrointestinal: Nausea (9%), vomiting (8%), diarrhea (6%), abdominal pain (4%), gastrointestinal hemorrhage (4%)

Hematologic & oncologic: Thrombocytopenia (5%), anemia (4%), leukopenia (4%)

Hepatic: Hyperbilirubinemia (4%)

Infection: Sepsis (7%), infection (5%)

Renal: Renal failure (5%)

Respiratory: Respiratory failure (8%), dyspnea (6%), respiratory tract disease (4%)

<1%, postmarketing, and/or case reports: Acute hepatic failure, anaphylactoid reaction, anuria, asthma, blood coagulation disorder, brain disease, bronchospasm, cardiac arrhythmia, cardiomyopathy, cerebrovascular accident, cholangitis, cholecystitis, deafness, dysuria, eosinophilia, erythema multiforme, exfoliative dermatitis, extrapyramidal reaction, hearing loss, hematologic disease, hemoptysis, hepatic sinusoidal obstruction syndrome (formerly known as hepatic veno-occlusive disease), hepatitis, hepatomegaly, hepatotoxicity, hypercalcemia, hyperkalemia, hypersensitivity reaction, hypocalcemia, hypomagnesemia, increased blood urea nitrogen, increased serum transaminases, injection site reaction, jaundice, leukocytosis, myasthenia, myocardial infarction, oliguria, peripheral neuropathy, pleural effusion, pulmonary edema, pulmonary embolism, renal insufficiency, renal tubular acidosis, seizure, shock, tachycardia, thrombophlebitis, ventricular fibrillation, vertigo (transient), visual impairment

Mechanism of Action Binds to ergosterol altering cell membrane permeability in susceptible fungi and causing leakage of cell components with subsequent cell death. Proposed mechanism suggests that amphotericin causes an oxidation-dependent stimulation of macrophages.

Pharmacodynamics/Kinetics

Half-life Elimination 173 hours following multiple doses

Pregnancy Risk Factor B

Pregnancy Considerations

Amphotericin crosses the placenta and enters the fetal circulation. Amphotericin B is recommended for the treatment of serious, systemic fungal diseases in pregnant women, refer to current guidelines (IDSA [Pappas 2016]; King 1998; Pilmus 2015).

Amphotericin B (Liposomal)

(am foe TER i sin bee lye po SO mal)

Brand Names: US AmBisome

Brand Names: Canada AmBisome

Pharmacologic Category Antifungal Agent, Parenteral

Use

Cryptococcal meningitis in patients with HIV: Treatment of cryptococcal meningitis in patients with HIV.

Fungal infections, empiric therapy: Empiric treatment in febrile neutropenic patients with presumed fungal infection.

Fungal infections, systemic therapy: Treatment of systemic infections caused by *Aspergillus* sp, *Candida* sp, and/or *Cryptococcus* sp in patients refractory to conventional amphotericin B deoxycholate therapy or when renal impairment or unacceptable toxicity precludes the use of the deoxycholate formulation.

Leishmaniasis (visceral): Treatment of visceral leishmaniasis.

Local Anesthetic/Vasoconstrictor Precautions No information available to require special precautions

Effects on Dental Treatment Key adverse event(s) related to dental treatment: Facial swelling, mucositis, stomatitis, and ulcerative stomatitis; Patients may experience orthostatic hypotension as they stand up after treatment; especially if lying in dental chair for extended periods of time. Use caution with sudden changes in position during and after dental treatment (see Dental Health Professional Considerations).

Effects on Bleeding No information available to require special precautions

Adverse Reactions Percentage of adverse reactions is dependent upon population studied and may vary with respect to premedications and underlying illness. Incidence of decreased renal function and infusion-related events are lower than rates observed with amphotericin B deoxycholate.

>10%:

Cardiovascular: Hypertension (8% to 20%), tachycardia (9% to 19%), peripheral edema (15%), edema (12% to 14%), hypotension (7% to 14%), chest pain (8% to 12%), localized phlebitis (9% to 11%)

Central nervous system: Chills (29% to 48%), insomnia (17% to 22%), headache (9% to 20%), pain (14%), anxiety (7% to 14%), confusion (9% to 13%)

Dermatologic: Skin rash (5% to 25%), pruritus (11%)

Endocrine & metabolic: Hypokalemia (31% to 51%), hypomagnesemia (15% to 50%), hyperglycemia (8% to 23%), hypocalcemia (5% to 18%), hyponatremia (9% to 12%), hypervolemia (8% to 12%)

Gastrointestinal: Nausea (16% to 40%), vomiting (11% to 32%), diarrhea (11% to 30%), abdominal pain (7% to 20%), constipation (15%), anorexia (10% to 14%)

Genitourinary: Nephrotoxicity (14% to 47%), hematuria (14%)

Hematologic & oncologic: Anemia (27% to 48%), leukopenia (15% to 17%), thrombocytopenia (6% to 13%)

Hepatic: Increased serum alkaline phosphatase (7% to 22%), hyperbilirubinemia (≤18%), increased serum ALT (15%), increased serum AST (13%), abnormal hepatic function tests (not specified) (4% to 13%)

Hypersensitivity: Transfusion reaction (9% to 18%)

Infection: Sepsis (7% to 14%), infection (11% to 13%)

Neuromuscular & skeletal: Weakness (6% to 13%), back pain (12%)

Renal: Increased serum creatinine (18% to 40%), increased blood urea nitrogen (7% to 21%)

Respiratory: Dyspnea (18% to 23%), pulmonary disease (14% to 18%), cough (2% to 18%), epistaxis (9% to 15%), pleural effusion (13%), rhinitis (11%)

Miscellaneous: Infusion related reactions (4% to 21%; fever [7% to 24%], chills [6% to 24%], vomiting [4% to 16%], nausea [8% to 14%], dyspnea [5% to 10%], tachycardia [2% to 10%], hypertension [2% to 9%], vasodilation [5%], hypotension [4%], hyperventilation [1%], hypoxia [≤1%])

2% to 10%:

Cardiovascular: Atrial fibrillation, bradycardia, cardiac arrest, cardiac arrhythmia, cardiomegaly, facial edema, flushing, heart valve disease, orthostatic hypotension, vascular disorder, vasodilation

Central nervous system: Dizziness (7% to 9%), abnormality in thinking, agitation, coma, depression, drowsiness, dysesthesia, dystonia, hallucination, malaise, nervousness, paresthesia, rigors, seizure

Dermatologic: Diaphoresis (7%), alopecia, cellulitis, dermal ulcer, dermatological reaction, maculopapular rash, skin discoloration, urticaria, vesiculobullous dermatitis, xeroderma

Endocrine & metabolic: Hypernatremia (4%), acidosis, hyperchloremia, hyperkalemia, hypermagnesemia, hyperphosphatemia, hypophosphatemia, increased lactate dehydrogenase, increased nonprotein nitrogen

Gastrointestinal: Gastrointestinal hemorrhage (10%), aphthous stomatitis, dyspepsia, dysphagia, enlargement of abdomen, eructation, fecal incontinence, flatulence, gingival hemorrhage, hematemesis, hemorrhoids, hiccups, increased serum amylase, intestinal obstruction, mucositis, rectal disease, stomatitis, xerostomia

Genitourinary: Dysuria, toxic nephrosis, urinary incontence, vaginal hemorrhage

Hematologic & oncologic: Blood coagulation disorder, bruise, decreased prothrombin time, hemophthalmos, hemorrhage, hypoproteinemia, increased prothrombin time, oral hemorrhage, petechia, purpura

Hepatic: Hepatic injury, hepatic sinusoidal obstruction syndrome (formerly known as hepatic veno-occlusive disease), hepatomegaly

Hypersensitivity: Delayed hypersensitivity, hypersensitivity reaction

Immunologic: Graft versus host disease

Infection: Herpes simplex infection

Local: Inflammation at injection site

Neuromuscular & skeletal: Arthralgia, myalgia, neck pain, ostealgia, tremor

Ophthalmic: Conjunctivitis, dry eyes

Renal: Acute renal failure, renal failure, renal function abnormality

Respiratory: Hypoxia (6% to 8%), asthma, atelectasis, dry nose, flu-like symptoms, hemoptysis, hyperventilation, pharyngitis, pneumonia, pulmonary edema, respiratory alkalosis, respiratory failure, respiratory insufficiency, sinusitis

Miscellaneous: Procedural complication (8% to 10%)

Postmarketing and/or case reports: Agranulocytosis, angioedema, bronchospasm, cyanosis, erythema, hemorrhagic cystitis, hypoventilation, rhabdomyolysis

Mechanism of Action Binds to ergosterol altering cell membrane permeability in susceptible fungi and causing leakage of cell components with subsequent cell death. Proposed mechanism suggests that amphotericin causes an oxidation-dependent stimulation of macrophages (Lyman 1992).

Pharmacodynamics/Kinetics

Half-life Elimination 7 to 10 hours (following a single 24-hour dosing interval); Terminal half-life: 100 to 153 hours (following multiple dosing up to 49 days)

Pregnancy Considerations

Amphotericin crosses the placenta and enters the fetal circulation. Amphotericin B is recommended for the treatment of serious systemic fungal diseases in pregnant women; refer to current guidelines (IDSA [Pappas 2016]; King 1998; Pilmis 2015).

Dental Health Professional Considerations

Amphotericin B, liposomal is a true single bilayer liposomal drug delivery system. Liposomes are closed, spherical vesicles created by mixing specific proportions of amphophilic substances such as phospholipids and cholesterol so that they arrange themselves into multiple concentric bilayer membranes when hydrated in aqueous solutions. Single bilayer liposomes are then formed by microemulsification of multilamellar vesicles using a homogenizer. Amphotericin B, liposomal consists of these unilamellar bilayer liposomes with amphotericin B intercalated within the membrane. Due to the nature and quantity of amphophilic substances used, and the lipophilic moiety in the amphotericin B molecule, the drug is an integral part of the overall structure of the amphotericin B liposomes. Amphotericin B, liposomal contains true liposomes that are <100 nm in diameter.

◆ **Amphotericin B Liposome** *see* Amphotericin B (Liposomal) *on page 138*

Ampicillin (am pi SIL in)

Related Information

Antibiotic Prophylaxis *on page 1715*

Brand Names: Canada APO-Ampi [DSC]; NOVO-Ampicillin

Generic Availability (US) Yes

Pharmacologic Category Antibiotic, Penicillin

Dental Use IV or IM administration for the prevention of infective endocarditis in patients not allergic to penicillin and unable to take oral amoxicillin; IV or IM administration for prophylaxis in total joint replacement patients (hip replacement, knee replacement) not allergic to penicillin and unable to take oral medications undergoing dental procedures

Use

Oral:

GI tract infections: Treatment of GI tract infections caused by *Shigella*, *Salmonella typhosa* and other *Salmonella*, *Escherichia coli*, *Proteus mirabilis*, and enterococci. **Note:** Ampicillin is **not** recommended as a first-line agent for shigellosis, salmonellosis (nontyphoid), or *Salmonella enterica* species (typhoid fever) due to development of resistance (CDC 2014).

GU tract infections: Treatment of GU tract infections caused by *E. coli*, *P. mirabilis*, enterococci, *Shigella*, *S. typhosa* and other *Salmonella*, and nonpenicillinase-producing *Neisseria gonorrhoeae*. **Note:** Ampicillin is **not** recommended by the CDC as a first-line agent in the treatment of gonorrhea (CDC 2010).

Respiratory tract infections: Treatment of respiratory tract infections caused by nonpenicillinase-producing *Haemophilus influenzae* and staphylococci, and streptococci, including *Streptococcus pneumoniae*.

Injection:

Bloodstream infection: Treatment of bloodstream infection caused by susceptible gram-positive organisms, including *Streptococcus* species, penicillin G-susceptible staphylococci, and enterococci; gram-negative bloodstream infection caused by *E. coli*, *P. mirabilis*, and *Salmonella* species.

Endocarditis, treatment: Treatment of endocarditis caused by susceptible gram-positive organisms, including *Streptococcus* species, penicillin G-susceptible staphylococci, and enterococci.

GI infections: Treatment of GI infections caused by *S. typhi* (typhoid fever), other *Salmonella* species, and *Shigella* species (dysentery). **Note:** Ampicillin is **not** recommended as a first-line agent for shigellosis, salmonellosis (nontyphoid), or *S. enterica* species (typhoid fever) due to development of resistance (CDC 2014).

Meningitis, bacterial: Treatment of bacterial meningitis caused by *E. coli*, group B streptococci, and other gram-negative bacteria (*Neisseria meningitidis*).

Respiratory tract infections: Treatment of respiratory tract infections caused by *S. pneumoniae*, *Staphylococcus aureus* (penicillinase and nonpenicillinase producing), *H. influenzae*, and group A beta-hemolytic streptococci.

Urinary tract infections: Treatment of urinary tract infections caused by *E. coli* and *P. mirabilis*.

Local Anesthetic/Vasoconstrictor Precautions No information available to require special precautions

Effects on Dental Treatment Key adverse event(s) related to dental treatment: Infrequent occurrences of oral candidiasis, dysgeusia, glossitis, sore mouth, and stomatitis.

Effects on Bleeding No information available to require special precautions

Adverse Reactions Frequency not defined.

Central nervous system: Brain disease (penicillin-induced), glossalgia, seizure, sore mouth

Dermatologic: Erythema multiforme, exfoliative dermatitis, skin rash, urticaria

Note: Appearance of a rash should be carefully evaluated to differentiate (if possible) nonallergic ampicillin rash from hypersensitivity reaction. Incidence is higher in patients with viral infection, *Salmonella* infection, lymphocytic leukemia, or patients that have hyperuricemia.

Gastrointestinal: Diarrhea, enterocolitis, glossitis, melanoglossia, nausea, oral candidiasis, pseudomembranous colitis, stomatitis, vomiting

Hematologic & oncologic: Agranulocytosis, anemia, eosinophilia, hemolytic anemia, immune thrombocytopenia, leukopenia

Hepatic: Increased serum AST

Hypersensitivity: Anaphylaxis

Immunologic: Serum sickness-like reaction

Renal: Interstitial nephritis (rare)

Respiratory: Stridor

Miscellaneous: Fever

<1%, postmarketing, and/or case reports: Dysgeusia (Syed 2016)

Dental Usual Dosage

Infective endocarditis prophylaxis: IM, IV: Dental, oral, or respiratory tract procedures:

Infants and Children: 50 mg/kg within 30 to 60 minutes prior to procedure in patients not allergic to penicillin and unable to take oral amoxicillin.

Adults: 2 g within 30 to 60 minutes prior to procedure in patients not allergic to penicillin and unable to take oral amoxicillin.

Note: Intramuscular injections should be avoided in patients who are receiving anticoagulant therapy. In these circumstances, orally administered regimens should be given whenever possible. Intravenously administered antibiotics should be used for patients who are unable to tolerate or absorb oral medications.

Note: American Heart Association (AHA) guidelines now recommend prophylaxis only in patients undergoing invasive procedures and in whom underlying cardiac conditions may predispose to a higher risk of adverse outcomes should infection occur.

Prophylaxis in total joint replacement patient: Adults: IM, IV: 2 g 1 hour prior to the procedure

Note: In general, patients with prosthetic joint implants do not require prophylactic antibiotics prior to dental procedures. In planning an invasive oral procedure, dental consultation with the patient's orthopedic surgeon may be advised to review the risks of infection.

Dosing

Adult & Geriatric Note: For oral therapy, including oral step-down therapy after IV ampicillin, oral amoxicillin is usually preferred over oral ampicillin due to improved bioavailability and absorption (bioavailability 77% *versus* 39% to 54%, respectively) (Arancibia 1980; Bolme 1976). For ease of outpatient IV ampicillin administration, the total daily dose may be administered as a 24-hour continuous infusion (IDSA [Berbari 2015]; IDSA [Osmon 2013]; Lewis 2018; Ogawa 2014).

Bloodstream infection:

Pathogen-directed therapy for Enterococcus spp.: IV: 2 g every 4 hours; use as part of an appropriate combination regimen in the setting of suspected endocarditis or critical illness (Graninger 1992; IDSA [Mermel 2009]; Murray 2019). Duration of therapy is 7 to 14 days for uncomplicated infection (ie, fever resolution within 72 hours **and** absence of metastatic focus of infection or endovascular hardware) (IDSA [Mermel 2009]). Some experts recommend a duration of 5 to 7 days for uncomplicated infection with rapid blood culture clearance (within 24 hours) **and** in the absence of metastatic infection (Murray 2019).

Pathogen-directed therapy for Listeria monocytogenes: IV: 2 g every 4 hours; use in combination with gentamicin for nonpregnant patients. Duration should be individualized based on patient factors, source and extent of infection, and clinical response, but ampicillin is usually continued for at least 14 to 21 days (Charlier 2017; Gelfand 2020; Hof 1997).

Endocarditis, prophylaxis (dental or invasive respiratory tract procedures) (alternative agent for patients unable to take oral therapy) (off-label use): IM, IV: 2 g as a single dose 30 to 60 minutes before procedure. **Note:** Only recommended for patients with cardiac conditions associated with the highest risk of an adverse outcome from endocarditis **and** who are undergoing a procedure likely to result in bacteremia with an organism that has the potential ability to cause endocarditis (AHA [Wilson 2007]).

Endocarditis, treatment:

Enterococcus faecalis, native or prosthetic valve (penicillin-susceptible): IV: 2 g every 4 hours as part of an appropriate combination regimen (eg, with ceftriaxone or gentamicin). Duration is usually 6 weeks; for patients with native valve endocarditis and symptoms <3 months, the combination of ampicillin and gentamicin can be given for 4 weeks. **Note:** Ampicillin plus ceftriaxone is the preferred regimen in patients with or at risk of renal insufficiency or with gentamicin resistance (AHA [Baddour 2015]; Fernández-Hidalgo 2013; Sexton 2019), and some experts favor this combination for all patients with native valve endocarditis (Sexton 2019).

HACEK organisms, native or prosthetic valve (ampicillin-susceptible) (off-label use): IV: 2 g every 4 hours for 4 weeks (native valve) or 6 weeks (prosthetic valve) (AHA [Baddour 2015]). **Note**: In vitro susceptibility should be confirmed prior to use.

Viridans group streptococci and Streptococcus gallolyticus (Streptococcus bovis) (alternative agent):

Native valve: Highly penicillin-susceptible (minimum inhibitory concentration [MIC] ≤0.12 mcg/mL): IV: 2 g every 4 hours for 4 weeks (AHA [Baddour 2015]).

Native valve: Relatively penicillin-resistant (MIC >0.12 to <0.5 mcg/mL): IV: 2 g every 4 hours for 4 weeks in combination with gentamicin for the first 2 weeks (AHA [Baddour 2015]).

Native valve: Penicillin-resistant (MIC ≥0.5 mcg/mL): IV: 2 g every 4 hours in combination with gentamicin. The duration of this regimen is not well established; infectious diseases consultation recommended (AHA [Baddour 2015]).

Prosthetic valve: Highly penicillin-susceptible (MIC ≤0.12 mcg/mL): IV: 2 g every 4 hours for 6 weeks (with or without concomitant gentamicin for the first 2 weeks) (AHA [Baddour 2015]).

Prosthetic valve: Relatively penicillin-resistant (MIC >0.12 to <0.5 mcg/mL) or fully penicillin-resistant (MIC ≥0.5 mcg/mL): IV: 2 g every 4 hours in combination with gentamicin for 6 weeks (AHA [Baddour 2015]). For relatively resistant strains, some experts prefer a shorter duration of the gentamicin component (≥2 weeks) (Karchmer 2019).

Intra-abdominal infection (off-label use): *Empiric or pathogen-directed therapy for Enterococcus spp. in high-risk patients (eg, postoperative infection or healthcare-associated infection in patients with prior use of antibiotics that select for Enterococcus, immunocompromising condition, valvular heart disease, or prosthetic intravascular material)*:

IV: 2 g every 4 hours as part of an appropriate combination regimen (Barshak 2019; SIS [Mazuski 2017]). Total duration of therapy (which may include oral step-down therapy) is 4 to 7 days following adequate source control (SIS [Mazuski 2017]; SIS/IDSA [Solomkin 2010]); for infections managed without surgical or percutaneous intervention, a longer duration may be necessary (Barshak 2019).

Meningitis, bacterial: *As a component of empiric therapy (community-acquired infections in immunocompetent patients >50 years of age and immunocompromised patients) or pathogen-directed therapy (eg, Haemophilus influenzae [beta-lactamase negative], L. monocytogenes, Neisseria meningitidis [penicillin MIC <0.1 mcg/mL], Streptococcus agalactiae, Streptococcus pneumoniae [penicillin MIC ≤0.06 mcg/mL], Enterococcus spp. [ampicillin-susceptible])*:

IV: 2 g every 4 hours; for empiric therapy and for directed therapy for *Enterococcus* or *Listeria*, use as part of an appropriate combination regimen. Treatment duration is 7 to 21 days, depending on causative pathogen(s) and clinical response (IDSA [Tunkel 2004]; IDSA [Tunkel 2017]).

Osteomyelitis and/or discitis, treatment (off-label use): *Pathogen-directed therapy for penicillin-susceptible Enterococcus or Streptococcus spp.*: IV: 2 g every 4 hours **or** 12 g as a continuous infusion every 24 hours, generally for ≥6 weeks. Shorter courses are appropriate if the affected bone is completely resected (eg, by amputation) (IDSA [Berbari 2015]; Osmon 2019). For *Enterococcus*, some experts use with ceftriaxone in the setting of retained hardware (Osmon 2019).

Pelvic infections (off -label use):

Intra-amniotic infection (chorioamnionitis): IV: 2 g every 6 hours in combination with gentamicin. In females undergoing cesarean delivery, an anti-anaerobic agent should also be added. Continue regimen until vaginal delivery or for 1 dose after cesarean delivery (ACOG 2017). **Note:** Some experts recommend 1 additional dose after vaginal delivery and extension of antibiotics after cesarean delivery until patient is afebrile and asymptomatic ≥48 hours (Tita 2019).

Postpartum endometritis: **Note:** For patients known to be colonized with GBS (Chen 2019).

IV: 2 g every 6 hours in combination with clindamycin **and** gentamicin; treat until patient is clinically improved (no fundal tenderness) and afebrile for 24 to 48 hours (Brumfield 2000; Chen 2019).

Tubo-ovarian abscess: IV: 2 g every 6 hours in combination with clindamycin **and** gentamicin (Beigi 2019). After 24 to 48 hours of sustained clinical improvement, may transition to oral therapy to complete ≥14 days of treatment (CDC [Workowski 2015]).

Peritonitis, treatment (peritoneal dialysis patients) (off-label use): Note: Intraperitoneal administration is preferred to IV administration (ISPD [Li 2016]). Consider a 25% dose increase in patients with significant residual renal function (urine output >100 mL/day) (ISPD [Li 2010]; ISPD [Li 2016]; Mancini 2018; Szeto 2018).

Pathogen-directed therapy (eg, Enterococcus spp., Streptococcus spp.): Continuous (with every exchange): Intraperitoneal: 125 mg/L of dialysate with each exchange (ISPD [Li 2016]). Duration of therapy is ≥2 weeks for patients with adequate clinical response (Burkart 2019; ISPD [Li 2016]).

Prosthetic joint infection (off-label use): *Pathogen-directed therapy (eg, penicillin-susceptible Enterococcus spp. or Streptococcus spp.)*: IV: 2 g every 4 hours **or** 12 g continuous infusion every 24 hours. Duration varies, but is generally 4 to 6 weeks; for enterococcal infections, some experts use with ceftriaxone in the setting of retained hardware (Berbari 2019; IDSA [Osmon 2013]).

Streptococcus (group B), maternal prophylaxis for prevention of neonatal disease (alternative agent) (off-label use): Note: Prophylaxis is reserved for pregnant women with a positive group B *Streptococcus* (GBS) vaginal or rectal screen in late gestation; GBS bacteriuria during the current pregnancy; history of birth of an infant with early-onset GBS disease; and unknown GBS culture status with any of the following: birth <37 0/7 weeks' gestation, intrapartum fever, prolonged rupture of membranes, known GBS positive in a previous pregnancy, or intrapartum nucleic acid amplification testing positive for GBS (ACOG 2019).

IV: 2 g as a single dose at onset of labor or prelabor rupture of membranes, then 1 g every 4 hours until delivery (ACOG 2019).

Urinary tract infection: Note: Uncomplicated urinary tract infection (UTI) has traditionally been defined as infection in an otherwise healthy nonpregnant female with a normal urinary tract; UTI in other patient populations has been considered complicated. Some experts instead categorize UTI as either acute simple cystitis (mild infection limited to the bladder with no signs/symptoms of upper tract or systemic infection in a nonpregnant adult) or complicated UTI (pyelonephritis or cystitis symptoms with other signs/symptoms of systemic infection) (Hooton 2019a; Hooton 2019b; Hooton 2019c). Ampicillin is not recommended for empiric therapy given decreased efficacy compared to first-line agents and high prevalence of resistance (IDSA/ESCMID [Gupta 2011]).

Acute uncomplicated or simple cystitis due to Enterococcus spp.: Oral: 500 mg every 6 hours for 5 to 7 days (Hooton 2019a; Hooton 2019b; IDSA/ESCMID [Gupta 2011]; Shah 2018).

Acute pyelonephritis or other complicated urinary tract infection due to Enterococcus spp. (off label): IV: 1 to 2 g every 4 to 6 hours; can give with an aminoglycoside for critical illness (Cole 2015; Heintz 2010; IDSA/ESCMID [Gupta 2011]). Switch to an appropriate oral regimen once patient has improvement in symptoms. Duration of therapy depends on the antimicrobial chosen to complete the regimen and ranges from 5 to 14 days (Hooton 2019c).

Renal Impairment: Adult

There are no dosage adjustments provided in the manufacturer's labeling; however, the following adjustments have been recommended (Aronoff 2007):

CrCl >50 mL/minute: Administer every 6 hours.

CrCl 10 to 50 mL/minute: Administer every 6 to 12 hours.

CrCl <10 mL/minute: Administer every 12 to 24 hours.

End-stage renal disease on intermittent hemodialysis (IHD) (administer after hemodialysis on dialysis days): Dialyzable (20% to 50%): IV: 1 to 2 g every 12 to 24 hours (administer after hemodialysis on dialysis days) (Heintz 2009). **Note:** Dosing dependent on the assumption of 3 times/week, complete IHD sessions.

Peritoneal dialysis: Not dialyzable: IV: 1 to 2 g every 12 to 24 hours (Blackwell 1990; Ruedy 1966).

Continuous renal replacement therapy (Heintz 2009): Drug clearance is highly dependent on the method of renal replacement, filter type, and flow rate. Appropriate dosing requires close monitoring of pharmacologic response, signs of adverse reactions due to drug accumulation, as well as drug concentrations in relation to target trough (if appropriate). The following are general recommendations only (based on dialysate flow/ultrafiltration rates of 1 to 2 L/hour and minimal residual renal function) and should not supersede clinical judgment: IV:

CVVH: Loading dose of 2 g followed by 1 to 2 g every 8 to 12 hours.

CVVHD: Loading dose of 2 g followed by 1 to 2 g every 8 hours.

CVVHDF: Loading dose of 2 g followed by 1 to 2 g every 6 to 8 hours.

Hepatic Impairment: Adult There are no dosage adjustments provided in the manufacturer's labeling.

Pediatric

General dosing, susceptible infection (Bradley 2019; *Red Book* [AAP 2018]): Infants, Children, and Adolescents:

Mild to moderate infection:

Oral: 50 to 100 mg/kg/**day** divided every 6 hours; maximum daily dose: 2,000 mg/**day**.

IM, IV: 50 to 200 mg/kg/**day** divided every 6 hours; maximum daily dose: 8 **g/day**.

Severe infection (eg, meningitis, endocarditis): IM, IV: 300 to 400 mg/kg/**day** divided every 4 to 6 hours; maximum daily dose: 12 **g/day**.

Community-acquired pneumonia (CAP) (IDSA/PIDS [Bradley 2011]): Infants >3 months, Children, and Adolescents: **Note:** May consider addition of vancomycin or clindamycin to empiric therapy if community-acquired MRSA suspected. In children

≥5 years, a macrolide antibiotic should be added if atypical pneumonia cannot be ruled out.

Empiric treatment or *S. pneumoniae* (MICs for penicillin ≤2 mcg/mL) or *H. influenzae* (beta-lactamase negative) in fully immunized patients: IV: 150 to 200 mg/kg/**day** divided every 6 hours.

Group A *Streptococcus*: IV: 200 mg/kg/**day** divided every 6 hours.

S. pneumoniae (MICs for penicillin ≥4 mcg/mL): IV: 300 to 400 mg/kg/**day** divided every 6 hours.

Endocarditis:

Treatment: Children and Adolescents: IV: 200 to 300 mg/kg/day divided every 4 to 6 hours; maximum daily dose: 12 g/**day**; use in combination with other antibiotics for at least 4 weeks; some organisms may require longer duration (AHA [Baltimore 2015]).

Prophylaxis: **Note:** AHA guidelines (Baltimore 2015) limit the use of prophylactic antibiotics to patients at the highest risk for infective endocarditis (IE) or adverse outcomes (eg, prosthetic heart valves, patients with previous IE, unrepaired cyanotic congenital heart disease, repaired congenital heart disease with prosthetic material or device during first 6 months after procedure, repaired congenital heart disease with residual defects at the site or adjacent to site of prosthetic patch or device, and heart transplant recipients with cardiac valvulopathy):

Dental or oral procedures or respiratory tract procedures (eg, tonsillectomy, adenoidectomy): Infants, Children, and Adolescents: IV, IM: 50 mg/kg within 30 to 60 minutes before procedure; maximum dose: 2,000 mg/dose. Intramuscular (IM) injections should be avoided in patients who are receiving anticoagulant therapy. In these circumstances, orally administered regimens should be used whenever possible. Intravenously (IV) administered antibiotics should be used for patients who are unable to tolerate or absorb oral medications (Wilson 2007).

Intra-abdominal infection, complicated: Infants, Children, and Adolescents: IV: 200 mg/kg/**day** divided every 6 hours; maximum single dose: 2,000 mg; maximize doses if undrained abdominal abscesses (IDSA [Solomkin 2010]).

Meningitis (including health care-associated meningitis and ventriculitis): Infants, Children, and Adolescents: IV: 300 to 400 mg/kg/**day** divided every 4 to 6 hours; maximum daily dose: 12 **g/day** (Bradley 2019; IDSA [Tunkel 2004]; IDSA [Tunkel 2017]; *Red Book* [AAP 2018]).

Peritonitis (CAPD) Limited data available: Infants, Children, and Adolescents: Intraperitoneal: 125 mg per liter of dialysate for 2 weeks (ISPD [Warady 2012]).

Surgical prophylaxis: Infants, Children, and Adolescents: IV: 50 mg/kg within 60 minutes prior to surgical incision; may repeat in 2 hours if lengthy procedure or excessive blood loss; maximum dose: 2,000 mg/dose (ASHP/IDSA [Bratzler 2013]; *Red Book* [AAP 2018]).

Renal Impairment: Pediatric

Infants, Children, and Adolescents: There are no dosage adjustments provided in the manufacturer's labeling; however, the following adjustments have been recommended (Aronoff 2007). **Note:** Renally adjusted dose recommendations are based on IM, IV doses of 100 to 200 mg/kg/day divided every 6 hours: IM, IV:

GFR 30 to 50 mL/minute/1.73 m^2: 35 to 50 mg/kg/dose every 6 hours

GFR 10 to 29 mL/minute/1.73 m^2: 35 to 50 mg/kg/dose every 8 to 12 hours

GFR <10 mL/minute/1.73 m^2: 35 to 50 mg/kg/dose every 12 hours

Intermittent hemodialysis: 35 to 50 mg/kg/dose every 12 hours

Peritoneal dialysis (PD): 35 to 50 mg/kg/dose every 12 hours

Continuous renal replacement therapy (CRRT): 35 to 50 mg/kg/dose every 6 hours

Hepatic Impairment: Pediatric There are no dosage adjustments provided in the manufacturer's labeling.

Mechanism of Action Inhibits bacterial cell wall synthesis by binding to one or more of the penicillin-binding proteins (PBPs) which in turn inhibits the final transpeptidation step of peptidoglycan synthesis in bacterial cell walls, thus inhibiting cell wall biosynthesis. Bacteria eventually lyse due to ongoing activity of cell wall autolytic enzymes (autolysins and murein hydrolases) while cell wall assembly is arrested.

Contraindications Hypersensitivity (eg, anaphylaxis) to ampicillin, any component of the formulation, or other penicillins; infections caused by penicillinase-producing organisms

Warnings/Precautions Dosage adjustment may be necessary in patients with renal impairment. Serious and occasionally severe or fatal hypersensitivity (anaphylactoid) reactions have been reported in patients on penicillin therapy, especially with a history of beta-lactam hypersensitivity, history of sensitivity to multiple allergens, or previous IgE-mediated reactions (eg, anaphylaxis, angioedema, urticaria). Serious anaphylactoid reactions require emergency treatment and airway management. Appropriate treatments must be readily available. Use with caution in asthmatic patients. Appearance of any rash should be carefully evaluated to differentiate a nonallergic ampicillin rash from a hypersensitivity reaction. High percentage of patients with infectious mononucleosis have developed rash during therapy with ampicillin; ampicillin-class antibiotics not recommended in these patients This rash (generalized maculopapular and pruritic) usually appears 7 to 10 days after initiation and usually resolves within a week of discontinuation. It is not known whether these patients are truly allergic to ampicillin. Ampicillin rash occurs in 5% to 10% of children receiving ampicillin and is a generalized dull red, maculopapular rash, generally appearing 3 to 14 days after the start of therapy. It normally begins on the trunk and spreads over most of the body. It may be most intense at pressure areas, elbows, and knees. Prolonged use may result in fungal or bacterial superinfection, including *Clostridium difficile*-associated diarrhea (CDAD) and pseudomembranous colitis; CDAD has been observed >2 months postantibiotic treatment.

Warnings: Additional Pediatric Considerations Ampicillin has been shown to prolong the bleeding time in neonates in 2 prospective studies. The first study found a prolonged bleeding time by an average of 60 seconds longer than baseline in neonates (n=15; GA: 33 to 41 weeks; weight: 1,760 to 3,835 g) after receiving the third and fourth doses of ampicillin (50 to 100 mg/kg/dose every 12 hours) (Sheffield 2010). The second study evaluated the effect on bleeding time in very low birth weight patients (n=20; GA: 23 to 33 weeks; weight: 400 to 1,410 g); results showed that patients receiving ampicillin for ≥10 days had a prolonged bleeding time compared to baseline; on average bleeding time was 2 minutes longer (p=0.001) (Sheffield 2011). The clinical significance of ampicillin's effect on bleeding time is unknown, but probably depends on the patient's clinical status and risk of hemorrhage.

Drug Interactions

Metabolism/Transport Effects None known.

Avoid Concomitant Use

Avoid concomitant use of Ampicillin with any of the following: BCG (Intravesical); Cholera Vaccine

Increased Effect/Toxicity

Ampicillin may increase the levels/effects of: Dichlorphenamide; Methotrexate; Vitamin K Antagonists

The levels/effects of Ampicillin may be increased by: Acemetacin; Allopurinol; Probenecid

Decreased Effect

Ampicillin may decrease the levels/effects of: Aminoglycosides; Atenolol; BCG (Intravesical); BCG Vaccine (Immunization); Cholera Vaccine; Lactobacillus and Estriol; Mycophenolate; Sodium Picosulfate; Typhoid Vaccine

The levels/effects of Ampicillin may be decreased by: Chloroquine; Lanthanum; Tetracyclines

Food Interactions Food decreases ampicillin absorption rate; may decrease ampicillin serum concentration. Management: Take at equal intervals around-the-clock, preferably on an empty stomach (30 minutes before or 2 hours after meals). Maintain adequate hydration, unless instructed to restrict fluid intake.

Dietary Considerations Take on an empty stomach 30 minutes before or 2 hours after meals. Some products may contain sodium.

Pharmacodynamics/Kinetics

Half-life Elimination

Neonates:

PNA 2 to 7 days: 4 hours

PNA 8 to 14 days: 2.8 hours

PNA 15 to 30 days: 1.7 hours

Children and Adults: 1 to 1.8 hours (Bergan 1978)

Anuric patients: 8 to 20 hours

Time to Peak Serum concentration: Oral: Within 1 to 2 hours

Pregnancy Risk Factor B

Pregnancy Considerations

Ampicillin crosses the placenta, providing detectable concentrations in the cord serum and amniotic fluid (Bolognese 1968; Fisher 1967; MacAulay 1966).

Due to pregnancy induced physiologic changes, the pharmacokinetics of IV and oral ampicillin may be altered. In addition, oral ampicillin is poorly absorbed during labor (Philipson 1977; Philipson 1978; Wasz-Hockert 1970).

Ampicillin is recommended for use in pregnant women for the management of preterm prelabor rupture of membranes (PROM) and is an option for the prevention of early-onset group B streptococcal (GBS) disease in newborns. Ampicillin may also be used in certain situations prior to vaginal delivery in women at high risk for endocarditis (ACOG 188 2018; ACOG 199 2018; ACOG 797 2020).

Breastfeeding Considerations Ampicillin is present in breast milk.

In general, antibiotics that are present in breast milk may cause nondose-related modification of bowel flora. Monitor infants for GI disturbances, such as thrush or diarrhea (WHO 2002).

Although the manufacturer recommends that caution be exercised when administering ampicillin to breastfeeding women, ampicillin is considered compatible with breastfeeding when used in usual recommended doses (WHO 2002).

Dosage Forms: US

Capsule, Oral:

Generic: 500 mg

Solution Reconstituted, Injection [preservative free]:

Generic: 125 mg (1 ea); 250 mg (1 ea); 500 mg (1 ea); 1 g (1 ea); 2 g (1 ea)

Solution Reconstituted, Intravenous [preservative free]:

Generic: 1 g (1 ea); 2 g (1 ea); 10 g (1 ea)

Dosage Forms: Canada

Capsule, Oral:

Generic: 250 mg, 500 mg

Solution Reconstituted, Injection:

Generic: 250 mg (1 ea); 500 mg (1 ea); 1 g (1 ea); 2 g (1 ea)

Ampicillin and Sulbactam

(am pi SIL in & SUL bak tam)

Related Information

Ampicillin *on page* 140

Brand Names: US Unasyn

Generic Availability (US) Yes

Pharmacologic Category Antibiotic, Penicillin

Dental Use Parenteral beta-lactamase-resistant antibiotic combination to treat more severe orofacial infections where beta-lactamase-producing staphylococci and beta-lactamase-producing *Bacteroides* are present

Use Bacterial infections: Treatment of skin and skin structure, intra-abdominal, and gynecological infections caused by susceptible bacteria; spectrum is that of ampicillin plus organisms producing beta-lactamases such as *Staphylococcus aureus*, *Haemophilus influenzae*, *Escherichia coli*, *Klebsiella*, *Acinetobacter*, *Enterobacter*, and anaerobes.

Local Anesthetic/Vasoconstrictor Precautions No information available to require special precautions

Effects on Dental Treatment Key adverse event(s) related to dental treatment: Rare occurrences of candidiasis, erythema multiforme, facial swelling, glossitis, stomatitis, Stevens-Johnson syndrome, and hairy tongue have been reported.

Effects on Bleeding No information available to require special precautions

Adverse Reactions Also see Ampicillin.

>10%: Local: Pain at injection site (IM; 16%)

1% to 10%:

Cardiovascular: Thrombophlebitis (3%), phlebitis (1%)

Dermatologic: Skin rash (<2%)

Gastrointestinal: Diarrhea (3%)

Local: Pain at injection site (IV; 3%)

<1%, postmarketing, and/or case reports: Abdominal distention, abdominal pain, acute generalized exanthematous pustulosis, agranulocytosis, anaphylactic shock, anaphylaxis, anemia, angioedema, basophilia, candidiasis, casts in urine (hyaline), chest pain, chills, cholestasis, cholestatic hepatitis, cholestatic jaundice, *Clostridioides* (formerly *Clostridium*) *difficile*-associated diarrhea, constriction of the pharynx, convulsions, decreased hematocrit, decreased hemoglobin, decreased neutrophils, decreased red blood cells, decreased serum albumin, decreased serum total protein, dermatitis, dizziness, drowsiness, dyspepsia, dyspnea, dysuria, edema, eosinophilia, epistaxis, erythema, erythema multiforme, erythrocyturia, exfoliative dermatitis, facial swelling, fatigue, flatulence, gastritis, glossitis, hairy tongue, headache, hemolytic anemia, hepatic insufficiency, hepatitis, hyperbilirubinemia, hypersensitivity reaction, immune thrombocytopenia, increased blood urea nitrogen, increased lactate dehydrogenase, increased liver enzymes, increased monocytes, increased serum alkaline phosphatase, increased serum ALT, increased serum AST, increased serum creatinine, injection site reaction, interstitial nephritis, jaundice, leukopenia, lymphocytopenia, lymphocytosis (abnormal), malaise, melena, mucous membrane bleeding, nausea, positive direct Coombs test, pruritus, pseudomembranous colitis, sedation, Stevens-Johnson syndrome, stomatitis, substernal pain, thrombocythemia, thrombocytopenia, toxic epidermal necrolysis, urinary retention, urticaria, vomiting

Dental Usual Dosage Severe orofacial infections: Adults: IM, IV: 1000 to 2000 mg ampicillin (1500 to 3000 mg Unasyn) every 6 hours (maximum: 8 g ampicillin/day, 12 g Unasyn)

Dosing

Adult & Geriatric Note: Ampicillin/sulbactam is a combination product formulated in a 2:1 ratio. Adult dosage recommendations are expressed as total grams of ampicillin/sulbactam.

Usual dosage range: IM, IV: 1.5 to 3 g every 6 hours (maximum: ampicillin/sulbactam 12 g daily) (manufacturer's labeling); for the treatment of infections caused by *Acinetobacter* spp., higher doses have been described (Assimakopoulos 2019; Gilad 2008; Levin 2003; Makris 2018; Mosaed 2018).

Bite wound infection, treatment (animal or human bite) (off-label use): IV: 1.5 to 3 g every 6 hours (IDSA [Stevens 2014]); some experts prefer 3 g every 6 hours (Baddour 2019a; Baddour 2019b). Duration of treatment for established infection is typically 5 to 14 days (including oral step-down therapy) (Baddour 2019a; Baddour 2019b; IDSA [Stevens 2014]).

Bloodstream infection (off-label use): *For pathogen-directed therapy of susceptible organisms:*

IV: 3 g every 6 hours (IDSA [Mermel 2009]; Jellison 2001; Murray 2019); for infections caused by *Acinetobacter* spp., higher doses (eg, 3 g every 4 hours) have been described (Gilad 2008; Levin 2003). Usual duration is 7 to 14 days; individualize depending on organism, source of infection, and clinical response. A 7-day duration is recommended for patients with uncomplicated Enterobacteriaceae infection who respond appropriately to antibiotic therapy (Kanafani 2019; Moehring 2019; Yahav 2018).

Diabetic foot infection, moderate to severe: IV: 3 g every 6 hours (Harkless 2005). Usual duration of therapy (including oral step-down therapy) is 2 to 4 weeks (in the absence of osteomyelitis) (Harkless 2005; IDSA [Lipsky 2012]; Weintrob 2019).

Endocarditis, treatment (off-label use): *Enterococcus (native or prosthetic valve; beta-lactamase-producing strains susceptible to aminoglycosides):*

IV: 3 g every 6 hours in combination with gentamicin for 6 weeks (AHA [Baddour 2015]).

Odontogenic infection, pyogenic (off-label use): IV: 3 g every 6 hours; duration is 7 to 14 days (including oral step-down therapy) (Chow 2019).

Pelvic infections (alternative agent):

Intra-amniotic infection (chorioamnionitis): IV: 3 g every 6 hours. Continue until vaginal delivery or for 1 dose after cesarean delivery (ACOG 2017). **Note:** Some experts recommend 1 additional dose after vaginal delivery and extension of antibiotics after cesarean delivery until patient is afebrile and asymptomatic ≥48 hours (Tita 2019).

Pelvic inflammatory disease (including tubo-ovarian abscess): IV: 3 g every 6 hours in combination with doxycycline. After 24 to 48 hours of sustained clinical improvement, may transition to oral therapy to complete ≥14 days of treatment (CDC [Workowski 2015). **Note:** Some experts include this combination as a preferred regimen for tubo-ovarian abscess (Beigi 2019).

Postpartum endometritis: IV: 3 g every 6 hours; treat until patient is clinically improved (no fundal tenderness) and afebrile for 24 to 48 hours (Chen 2019; Gall 1996).

Peritonitis, treatment (peritoneal dialysis patients): Pathogen-directed therapy for susceptible organisms. **Note:** Intraperitoneal administration is preferred to IV administration. Duration of therapy is ≥2 weeks for patients with adequate clinical response (Burkart 2019; ISPD [Li 2016]). Consider a 25% dose increase in patients with significant residual renal function (urine output >100 mL/day) (ISPD [Li 2010]; ISPD [Li 2016]; Mancini 2018; Szeto 2018).

Intermittent (preferred): Intraperitoneal: 3 g per exchange every 12 hours; allow to dwell for ≥6 hours (Blackwell 1990; ISPD [Li 2016]).

Continuous (with every exchange) (dose is per liter of dialysate): Intraperitoneal: Loading dose: 750 mg/**L** to 1 g/**L** of dialysate with first exchange of dialysate; maintenance dose: 100 mg/**L** of dialysate with each subsequent exchange (ISPD [Li 2016]; Lam 2008).

Pneumonia (off-label use):

Aspiration pneumonia : IV: 1.5 to 3 g every 6 hours, generally for 7 days (Bartlett 2019).

Community-acquired pneumonia: Inpatients without risk factors for *P. aeruginosa:* IV: 3 g every 6 hours in combination with other agent(s) when appropriate. Total duration (including oral step-down therapy) is a minimum of 5 days; patients should be clinically stable with normal vital signs prior to discontinuation (ATS/IDSA [Metlay 2019]; Majcher-Peszynska 2014; Rossoff 1995).

Hospital-acquired or ventilator-associated pneumonia: Targeted therapy for susceptible pathogens: IV: 3 g every 6 hours, in combination with other agent(s) when appropriate, typically for 7 days and individualized based on response to therapy (Chan 2010; IDSA/ATS [Kalil 2016]; Ye 2016; Zalts 2016). **Note:** For infections caused by *Acinetobacter* spp., higher doses (eg, 3 g every 4 hours) have been described (Assimakopoulos 2019; Gilad 2008; Levin 2003; Makris 2018; Mosaed 2018).

Surgical prophylaxis (off-label use): IV: 3 g within 60 minutes prior to surgical incision. Doses may be repeated in 2 hours if procedure is lengthy or if there is excessive blood loss. **Note:** Consider local susceptibility patterns prior to use (Anderson 2019; ASHP/IDSA/SIS/SHEA [Bratzler 2013]). In cases in which extension of prophylaxis is warranted postoperatively, total duration should be ≤24 hours (Anderson 2019). Postoperative prophylaxis is not recommended in clean and clean-contaminated surgeries (CDC [Berríos-Torres 2017]).

Surgical site infections (eg, intestinal, GU tract, abdominal wall) (off-label use): IV: 3 g every 6 hours. Duration depends on extent and severity of infection as well as response to therapy; may switch to oral treatment when clinically improved. **Note:** Consult local susceptibility patterns prior to empiric use (IDSA [Stevens 2014]; Mancino 2020).

Renal Impairment: Adult

The renal dosing recommendations are based upon the best available evidence and clinical expertise. Senior Editorial Team: Bruce Mueller, PharmD, FCCP, FASN, FNKF; Jason Roberts, PhD, BPharm (Hons), B App Sc, FSHP, FISAC; Michael Heung, MD, MS.

Note: Renally adjusted dose recommendations are based on a usual recommended dose of 1.5 to 3 g every 6 hours.

Altered kidney function: IV:

Note: Estimation of renal function for the purpose of drug dosing should be done using the Cockcroft-Gault formula. Dosage recommendations are expressed as grams of **ampicillin/sulbactam** combination (Wright 1983; manufacturer's labeling):

CrCl ≥30 mL/minute: No dosage adjustment necessary.

CrCl 15 to 29 mL/minute: 1.5 to 3 g every 12 hours.

CrCl 5 to 14 mL/minute: 1.5 to 3 g every 24 hours.

Augmented renal clearance (measured urinary CrCl ≥130 mL/minute/1.73 m^2): Augmented renal clearance (ARC) is a condition that occurs in certain critically-ill patients without organ dysfunction and with normal serum creatinine concentrations. Young patients (<55 years of age) admitted post trauma or major surgery are at highest risk for ARC, as well as those with sepsis, burns, or hematologic malignancies. An 8- to 24-hour measured urinary CrCl is necessary to identify these patients (Bilbao-Meseguer 2018; Udy 2010).

IV: 1.5 to 3 g every 4 to 6 hours (expert opinion).

Hemodialysis, intermittent (thrice weekly): Dialyzable (39% to 63% [Jusko 1973]):

IV: 1.5 to 3 g every 12 to 24 hours; administer after dialysis when scheduled dose falls on dialysis days (Heintz 2009).

Peritoneal dialysis: IV: 1.5 g every 12 hours or 3 g every 24 hours (Blackwell 1990; expert opinion).

CRRT: Drug clearance is dependent on the effluent flow rate, filter type, and method of renal replacement. Recommendations are based on high-flux dialyzers and effluent flow rates of 20 to 25 mL/kg/hour (or ~1,500 to 3,000 mL/hour) unless otherwise noted. Appropriate dosing requires consideration of adequate drug concentrations (eg, site of infection) and consideration of initial loading doses. Close monitoring of response and adverse reactions (eg, neurotoxicity) due to drug accumulation is important.

CVVH/CVVHD/CVVHDF: **IV:** 3 g every 8 to 12 hours (Heintz 2009; expert opinion).

PIRRT (eg, sustained, low-efficiency diafiltration): Drug clearance is dependent on the effluent flow rate, filter type, and method of renal replacement. Appropriate dosing requires consideration of adequate drug concentrations (eg, site of infection) and consideration of initial loading doses. Close monitoring of response and adverse reactions (eg, neurotoxicity) due to drug accumulation is important.

IV: Initial: 3 g followed by 1.5 to 3 g every 8 to 12 hours. Where possible, give one dose after PIRRT session (Lorenzen 2012; expert opinion).

Hepatic Impairment: Adult There is no dosage adjustment provided in the manufacturer's labeling.

Pediatric Note: Unasyn (ampicillin/sulbactam) is a combination product formulated in a 2:1 ratio (eg, each 3 g vial contains 2 g of ampicillin and 1 g of sulbactam); review dosing units carefully. Dosage recommendations are expressed as either mg of the **ampicillin** component or as total grams of the **ampicillin/sulbactam combination** within the dosing field; review dosing units in each indication carefully.

General dosing, susceptible infection: Infants, Children, and Adolescents:

Mild to moderate infection: IV: 100 to 200 mg ampicillin/kg/day divided every 6 hours; maximum dose: 2,000 mg ampicillin/dose (*Red Book* [AAP 2018]); may also be administered IM (Bradley 2018)

Severe infection (eg, meningitis, resistant *Streptococcus pneumonia*): IV: 200 to 400 mg ampicillin/kg/day divided every 6 hours; maximum dose: 2,000 mg ampicillin/dose (Bradley 2018; *Red Book* [AAP 2018]); may also be administered IM (Bradley 2018)

Endocarditis, treatment: Children and Adolescents: IV: 200 to 300 mg ampicillin/kg/day divided every 4 to 6 hours; maximum dose: 2,000 mg ampicillin/dose; may use in combination with gentamicin, vancomycin, and/or rifampin (optional; dependent upon organism) for at least 4 to 6 weeks; some organisms may require longer duration (AHA [Baltimore 2015])

Intra-abdominal infection, complicated: Infants, Children, and Adolescents: IV: 200 mg ampicillin/kg/day divided every 6 hours; **Note:** Due to high rates of *E. coli* resistance, not recommended for the treatment of community-acquired intra-abdominal infections (IDSA [Solomkin 2010])

Pelvic inflammatory disease: Adolescents: IV: 3 **g** ampicillin/sulbactam every 6 hours with doxycycline (CDC [Workowski 2015])

Rhinosinusitis, severe infection requiring hospitalization: Children and Adolescents: IV: 200 to 400 mg ampicillin/kg/day divided every 6 hours for 10 to 14 days; maximum dose: 2,000 mg ampicillin/dose (IDSA [Chow 2012])

Skin and skin structure infection: Children and Adolescents: IV: 200 mg ampicillin/kg/day divided every 6 hours for up to 14 days; maximum dose: 2,000 mg ampicillin/dose

Surgical prophylaxis: Children and Adolescents: IV: 50 mg ampicillin/kg/dose within 60 minutes prior to procedure; may repeat in 2 hours if lengthy procedure or excessive blood loss; maximum dose: 2,000 mg ampicillin/dose (Bratzler 2013)

Renal Impairment: Pediatric

Children and Adolescents: IV:

CrCl ≥30 mL/minute/1.73 m^2: No dosage adjustment required.

CrCl 15 to 29 mL/minute/1.73 m^2: Administer every 12 hours.

CrCl 5 to 14 mL/minute/1.73 m^2: Administer every 24 hours.

Hepatic Impairment: Pediatric There are no dosage adjustments provided in the manufacturer's labeling.

Mechanism of Action Inhibits bacterial cell wall synthesis by binding to one or more of the penicillin-binding proteins (PBPs) which in turn inhibits the final transpeptidation step of peptidoglycan synthesis in bacterial cell walls, thus inhibiting cell wall biosynthesis. Bacteria eventually lyse due to ongoing activity of cell wall autolytic enzymes (autolysins and murein hydrolases) while cell wall assembly is arrested. The addition of sulbactam, a beta-lactamase inhibitor, to ampicillin extends the spectrum of ampicillin to include some beta-lactamase-producing organisms.

Contraindications Hypersensitivity (eg, anaphylaxis or Stevens-Johnson syndrome) to ampicillin, sulbactam, or to other beta-lactam antibacterial drugs (eg, penicillins, cephalosporins), or any component of the formulations; history of cholestatic jaundice or hepatic dysfunction associated with ampicillin/sulbactam

Warnings/Precautions Dosage adjustment may be necessary in patients with renal impairment. Serious and occasionally severe or fatal hypersensitivity (anaphylactic) reactions have been reported in patients on penicillin therapy, especially with a history of beta-lactam hypersensitivity, history of sensitivity to multiple allergens. Patients with a history of penicillin hypersensitivity have experienced severe reactions when treated with cephalosporins. Before initiating therapy, carefully investigate previous penicillin, cephalosporin, or other allergen hypersensitivity. If an allergic reaction occurs, discontinue and institute appropriate therapy. Hepatitis and cholestatic jaundice have been reported (including fatalities). Toxicity is usually reversible. Monitor hepatic function at regular intervals in patients with hepatic impairment. High percentage of patients with infectious mononucleosis have developed rash during therapy with ampicillin; ampicillin-class antibacterials are not recommended in these patients. Appearance of a rash should be carefully evaluated to differentiate a nonallergic ampicillin rash from a hypersensitivity reaction. Prolonged use may result in fungal or bacterial superinfection, including *C. difficile*-associated diarrhea (CDAD) and pseudomembranous colitis; CDAD has been observed >2 months postantibiotic treatment.

Drug Interactions

Metabolism/Transport Effects None known.

Avoid Concomitant Use

Avoid concomitant use of Ampicillin and Sulbactam with any of the following: BCG (Intravesical); Cholera Vaccine

Increased Effect/Toxicity

Ampicillin and Sulbactam may increase the levels/effects of: Dichlorphenamide; Methotrexate; Vitamin K Antagonists

The levels/effects of Ampicillin and Sulbactam may be increased by: Acemetacin; Allopurinol; Probenecid

Decreased Effect

Ampicillin and Sulbactam may decrease the levels/effects of: Aminoglycosides; Atenolol; BCG (Intravesical); BCG Vaccine (Immunization); Cholera Vaccine; Lactobacillus and Estriol; Mycophenolate; Sodium Picosulfate; Typhoid Vaccine

The levels/effects of Ampicillin and Sulbactam may be decreased by: Chloroquine; Lanthanum; Tetracyclines

Dietary Considerations Some products may contain sodium.

Pharmacodynamics/Kinetics

Half-life Elimination Sulbactam: Children 1 to 12 years (normal renal function): Mean range: ~0.7 to 0.9 hours (Nahata 1999); Adults (normal renal function): 1 to 1.3 hours; **Note:** Elimination kinetics of both ampicillin and sulbactam are similarly affected in patients with renal impairment, therefore, the blood concentration ratio is expected to remain constant regardless of renal function.

Pregnancy Considerations Both ampicillin and sulbactam cross the placenta.

Due to pregnancy-induced physiologic changes, some pharmacokinetic properties of ampicillin/sulbactam may be altered (Chamberlain 1993). Ampicillin/sulbactam may be considered for prophylactic use prior to cesarean delivery (consult current recommendations) (ACOG 199 2018).

Breastfeeding Considerations Ampicillin and sulbactam are present in breast milk.

A review article notes the exposure of ampicillin and sulbactam to a breastfeeding infant would be ~1% to 2% of a typical adult dose (Foulds 1986).

The manufacturer recommends that caution be used if administering to breastfeeding women. Ampicillin is considered compatible with breastfeeding when used in usual recommended doses. In general, antibiotics that are present in breast milk may cause nondose-related modification of bowel flora. Monitor infants for GI disturbances (WHO 2002).

Also refer to the Ampicillin monograph.

Dosage Forms: US

Solution Reconstituted, Injection [preservative free]:

Unasyn: 3 g: Ampicillin 2 g and sulbactam 1 g (1 ea); 1.5 g: Ampicillin 1 g and sulbactam 0.5 g (1 ea)

Generic: 1.5 g: Ampicillin 1 g and sulbactam 0.5 g (1 ea); 3 g: Ampicillin 2 g and sulbactam 1 g (1 ea)

Solution Reconstituted, Intravenous [preservative free]:

Unasyn: 15 g: Ampicillin 10 g and sulbactam 5 g (1 ea)

Generic: 1.5 g: Ampicillin 1 g and sulbactam 0.5 g (1 ea); 15 g: Ampicillin 10 g and sulbactam 5 g (1 ea); 3 g: Ampicillin 2 g and sulbactam 1 g (1 ea)

Dental Health Professional Considerations In maxillary sinus, anterior nasal cavity, and deep neck infections, beta-lactamase-producing staphylococci and beta-lactamase-producing *Bacteroides* usually are present. In these situations, antibiotics that resist the beta-lactamase enzyme should be administered. Amoxicillin and clavulanic acid is administered orally for moderate infections. Ampicillin sodium and sulbactam sodium (Unasyn) is administered parenterally for more severe infections.

- ◆ **Ampicillin Sodium** *see* Ampicillin *on page 140*
- ◆ **Ampicillin Sodium/Sulbactam Na** *see* Ampicillin and Sulbactam *on page 144*
- ◆ **Ampicillin Trihydrate** *see* Ampicillin *on page 140*
- ◆ **Ampyra** *see* Dalfampridine *on page 431*
- ◆ **AMR101** *see* Omega-3 Fatty Acids *on page 1137*
- ◆ **Amrix** *see* Cyclobenzaprine *on page 418*
- ◆ **Amvisc** *see* Hyaluronate and Derivatives *on page 761*
- ◆ **Amvisc Plus** *see* Hyaluronate and Derivatives *on page 761*

Amyl Nitrite (AM il NYE trite)

Pharmacologic Category Antianginal Agent; Antidote; Vasodilator

Local Anesthetic/Vasoconstrictor Precautions No information available to require special precautions

Effects on Dental Treatment Key adverse event(s) related to dental treatment: Patients may experience orthostatic hypotension as they stand up after treatment; especially if lying in dental chair for extended periods of time. Use caution with sudden changes in position during and after dental treatment.

Effects on Bleeding No information available to require special precautions

Adverse Reactions Frequency not defined.

Cardiovascular: Cerebral ischemia, facial flushing, hypotension, orthostatic hypotension, shock, syncope, tachycardia, vasodilation

Central nervous system: Dizziness, headache, increased intracranial pressure, restlessness

Dermatologic: Dermatitis, diaphoresis, pallor, skin irritation

Gastrointestinal: Fecal incontinence, nausea, vomiting

Genitourinary: Urinary incontinence

Hematologic & oncologic: Hemolytic anemia, methemoglobinemia

Neuromuscular & skeletal: Weakness

Ophthalmic: Eye irritation, increased intraocular pressure

Mechanism of Action Relaxes vascular smooth muscle; decreases venous ratios and arterial blood pressure; reduces left ventricular work; decreases myocardial O_2 consumption. When used for cyanide poisoning, amyl nitrite promotes the formation of methemoglobin which competes with cytochrome oxidase for the cyanide ion. Cyanide combines with methemoglobin to form cyanomethemoglobin, thereby freeing the cytochrome oxidase and allowing aerobic metabolism to continue.

Pharmacodynamics/Kinetics

Onset of Action Angina: Within 30 seconds.

Duration of Action Angina: 3-15 minutes; Pharmacologic provocation of latent left ventricular outflow tract (LVOT) gradient in hypertrophic cardiomyopathy (HCM): ~30 seconds (Wesley Reagan 2005).

Half-life Elimination Amyl nitrite: <1 hour; Methemoglobin: 1 hour.

Pregnancy Risk Factor C

Pregnancy Considerations Animal reproduction studies have not been conducted. Because amyl nitrite significantly decreases systemic blood pressure and therefore blood flow to the fetus, use is contraindicated in pregnancy (per manufacturer). In addition, fetal hemoglobin may be more susceptible methemoglobin conversion (Valenzuela, 1986).

- **Amzeeq** *see* Minocycline (Topical) *on page* 1036
- **AN100226** *see* Natalizumab *on page* 1086
- **Anacaine** *see* Benzocaine *on page* 228
- **Anadrol-50** *see* Oxymetholone *on page* 1175
- **Anafranil** *see* ClomiPRAMINE *on page* 383

Anagrelide (an AG gre lide)

Brand Names: US Agrylin

Brand Names: Canada Agry-Gen; Agrylin; DOM-Anagrelide; PMS-Anagrelide; SANDOZ Anagrelide

Pharmacologic Category Antiplatelet Agent; Phosphodiesterase-3 Enzyme Inhibitor

Use

Essential thrombocythemia: Treatment of thrombocythemia secondary to myeloproliferative neoplasms to reduce elevated platelets and the risk of thrombosis and to reduce associated symptoms (including thrombo-hemorrhagic events).

Note: The use of hydroxyurea and low-dose aspirin may be preferred over anagrelide for the initial treatment of essential thrombocythemia; however, anagrelide may be appropriate in patients who are resistant or intolerant to hydroxyurea (ESMO [Vannucchi 2015]).

Local Anesthetic/Vasoconstrictor Precautions No information available to require special precautions

Effects on Dental Treatment Key adverse event(s) related to dental treatment: Patients may experience orthostatic hypotension as they stand up after treatment; especially if lying in dental chair for extended periods of time. Use caution with sudden changes in position during and after dental treatment.

Effects on Bleeding Anagrelide causes dose-related reduction in platelet production and could affect normal clotting; hemorrhage has been reported. Medical consult is suggested for patients under active treatment with anagrelide.

Adverse Reactions Reactions similar in adult and pediatric patients unless otherwise noted.

>10%:

Cardiovascular: Edema (21%), palpitations (26%)

Gastrointestinal: Abdominal pain (16%), diarrhea (26%), nausea (17%)

Nervous system: Dizziness (15%), headache (44%), pain (15%)

Neuromuscular & skeletal: Asthenia (23%)

1% to 10%:

Cardiovascular: Angina pectoris (1% to <5%), cardiac arrhythmia (1% to <5%), cardiac failure (1% to <5%), chest pain (8%), hypertension (1% to <5%), orthostatic hypotension (1% to <5%), peripheral edema (9%), syncope (1% to <5%), tachycardia (8%), vasodilation (1% to <5%)

Dermatologic: Alopecia (1% to <5%), ecchymoses (1% to <5%), pruritus (6%), skin rash (8%)

Gastrointestinal: Anorexia (8%), constipation (1% to <5%), dyspepsia (5%), flatulence (10%), gastritis (1% to <5%), gastrointestinal hemorrhage (1% to <5%), vomiting (10%)

Hematologic & oncologic: Anemia (1% to <5%), hemorrhage (1% to <5%), thrombocytopenia (1% to <5%)

Hepatic: Increased liver enzymes (1% to <5%)

Nervous system: Amnesia (1% to <5%), chills (1% to <5%), confusion (1% to <5%), depression (1% to <5%), drowsiness (1% to <5%), insomnia (1% to <5%), malaise (6%), migraine (1% to <5%), nervousness (1% to <5%), paresthesia (6%)

Neuromuscular & skeletal: Arthralgia (1% to <5%), back pain (6%), myalgia (1% to <5%)

Ophthalmic: Diplopia (1% to <5%), visual disturbance (1% to <5%)

Otic: Tinnitus (1% to <5%)

Renal: Hematuria (1% to <5%), renal failure syndrome (1% to <5%)

Respiratory: Cough (6%), dyspnea (12%), epistaxis (1% to <5%), flu-like symptoms (1% to <5%), pleural effusion, pneumonia (1% to <5%)

Miscellaneous: Fever (9%)

<1%:

Cardiovascular: Supraventricular tachycardia, ventricular tachycardia

Nervous system: Hypoesthesia

Frequency not defined:

Cardiovascular: Acute myocardial infarction, atrial fibrillation, cardiomegaly, cardiomyopathy, cerebrovascular accident, complete atrioventricular block, decreased diastolic pressure (pediatric patients), increased pulse (pediatric patients), pericardial effusion, prolonged QT interval on ECG, systolic hypotension (pediatric patients)

Gastrointestinal: Pancreatitis

Nervous system: Fatigue (pediatric patients)

Neuromuscular & skeletal: Muscle cramps (pediatric patients)

Respiratory: Pulmonary fibrosis, pulmonary hypertension, pulmonary infiltrates

Postmarketing:

Cardiovascular: Prinzmetal angina, torsades de pointes

Dermatologic: Skin photosensitivity (pediatric patients)

Hematologic & oncologic: Leukocytosis

Hepatic: Hepatotoxicity (including increased serum alanine aminotransferase [>3 x ULN], increased serum aspartate aminotransferase [>3 x ULN])

Renal: Interstitial nephritis

Respiratory: Interstitial pulmonary disease (including eosinophilic pneumonitis, hypersensitivity pneumonitis, interstitial pneumonitis)

Mechanism of Action Anagrelide appears to inhibit cyclic nucleotide phosphodiesterase and the release of arachidonic acid from phospholipase, possibly by inhibiting phospholipase A_2. Anagrelide also causes a dose-related reduction in platelet production, which results from decreased megakaryocyte hypermaturation (disrupts the postmitotic phase of maturation).

Pharmacodynamics/Kinetics

Onset of Action Initial: Within 7 to 14 days; complete response (platelets ≤600,000/mm^3): 4 to 12 weeks

Duration of Action Platelet rebound: Variable; upon discontinuation, platelet count begins to rise within 4 days and returns to baseline in 1 to 2 weeks (may rebound above baseline)

Half-life Elimination Anagrelide: ~1.5 hours, similar data reported in pediatric patients 7 to 14 years of age; 3-hydroxy anagrelide: ~2.5 hours

Time to Peak Serum: ~1 hour (in fasted state), similar data reported in pediatric patients 7 to 14 years of age

Pregnancy Considerations

Data regarding use of anagrelide during pregnancy is limited (Alkindi 2005; Birgegård 2018; Cornet 2017; Doubek 2004; Sobas 2009; Wright 2001).

Thrombocythemia is associated with an increased risk for adverse pregnancy outcomes including miscarriage, stillbirth, and preeclampsia. When treatment for essential thrombocythemia is needed during pregnancy, other agents are currently preferred (Tefferi 2018).

◆ **Anagrelide Hydrochloride** *see* Anagrelide *on page 148*

Anakinra (an a KIN ra)

Related Information

Rheumatoid Arthritis, Osteoarthritis, and Osteoporosis *on page 1697*

Brand Names: US Kineret

Brand Names: Canada Kineret

Pharmacologic Category Antirheumatic, Disease Modifying; Interleukin-1 Receptor Antagonist

Use

Neonatal-onset multisystem inflammatory disease: Treatment of neonatal-onset multisystem inflammatory disease (NOMID).

Rheumatoid arthritis: Reduction in signs and symptoms and slowing the progression of structural damage of moderately to severely active rheumatoid arthritis (RA) in patients 18 years and older who have failed 1 or more disease-modifying antirheumatic drugs (DMARDs).

Local Anesthetic/Vasoconstrictor Precautions No information available to require special precautions

Effects on Dental Treatment Key adverse event(s) related to dental treatment: Anakinra belongs to the class of disease-modifying antirheumatic drugs and, as such, has immunosuppressive properties. Consider a medical consult prior to any invasive treatment for patients under active treatment with anakinra. Delayed wound healing due to the immunosuppressive effects and increased potential for postsurgical infection may be of concern.

Effects on Bleeding No information available to require special precautions

Adverse Reactions

>10%:

Central nervous system: Headache (12% to 14%)

Gastrointestinal: Vomiting (NOMID: 14%)

Immunologic: Antibody development (RA: 49%; neutralizing: 2%; no correlation of antibody development and adverse effects)

Infection: Infection (RA: 39%; serious infection: 2% to 3%; including cellulitis, pneumonia, and bone and joint infections)

Local: Injection site reaction (RA: 71%; mild: 73%; moderate: 24%; severe: 2% to 3%; NOMID: 16%; mild: 76%; moderate: 24%)

Neuromuscular & skeletal: Arthralgia (NOMID: 12%)

Respiratory: Nasopharyngitis (NOMID: 12%)

Miscellaneous: Fever (NOMID: 12%)

1% to 10%:

Gastrointestinal: Nausea (RA: 8%), diarrhea (RA: 7%)

Hematologic & oncologic: Eosinophilia (RA: 9%), decreased white blood cell count (RA: 8%), change in platelet count (RA; decreased: 2%

Frequency not defined:

Dermatologic: Skin rash (NOMID)

Endocrine & metabolic: Hypercholesterolemia (RA)

Respiratory: Upper respiratory tract infection (NOMID)

<1%, postmarketing, and/or case reports: Hepatitis (noninfectious), hypersensitivity reaction (including anaphylaxis, angioedema, pruritus, skin rash, urticaria), increased serum transaminases, metastases (malignant lymphoma, malignant melanoma), opportunistic infection, thrombocytopenia (including severe)

Mechanism of Action Antagonist of the interleukin-1 (IL-1) receptor. Endogenous IL-1 is induced by inflammatory stimuli and mediates a variety of immunological responses, including degradation of cartilage (loss of proteoglycans) and stimulation of bone resorption.

Pharmacodynamics/Kinetics

Half-life Elimination Terminal: 4 to 6 hours; Severe renal impairment (CrCl <30 mL/minute): ~7 hours; ESRD: 9.7 hours (Yang 2003)

Time to Peak SubQ: 3 to 7 hours

Reproductive Considerations

Based on limited information, use of anakinra may be continued through conception in women with rheumatic and musculoskeletal diseases who are planning a pregnancy and not able to use alternative therapies; use should be discontinued once pregnancy is confirmed. Conception should be planned during a period of quiescent/low disease activity (ACR [Sammaritano 2020]).

Based on limited information, use of anakinra may be continued in males with rheumatic and musculoskeletal diseases who are planning to father a child (ACR [Sammaritano 2020]).

Pregnancy Considerations Information related to the use of anakinra during pregnancy is limited (Berger 2009; Chang 2014; Duman 2019; İlgen 2017; Ozdogan 2019; Smith 2018; Youngstein 2017).

Until additional information is available, anakinra is not currently recommended for the treatment of rheumatic and musculoskeletal diseases during pregnancy. Anakinra should be discontinued once pregnancy is confirmed (ACR [Sammaritano 2020]).

Women exposed to anakinra during pregnancy may contact the Organization of Teratology Information Services (OTIS), Rheumatoid Arthritis and Pregnancy Study at 1-877-311-8972.

Prescribing and Access Restrictions For patient self-administration, product may be obtained via the Kineret On Track program. Further information is available at https://www.kineretrx.com/hcp/kineret-on-track.php or 1-866-547-0644.

◆ **Anaprox DS [DSC]** *see* Naproxen *on page 1080*

◆ **Anastia [DSC]** *see* Lidocaine (Topical) *on page 902*

Anastrozole (an AS troe zole)

Brand Names: US Arimidex

Brand Names: Canada ACH-Anastrozole; APO-Anastrozole; Arimidex; BIO-Anastrozole; CCP-Anastrozole; JAMP-Anastrozole; Mar-Anastrozole; MED-Anastrozole; MINT-Anastrozole; MYLAN-Anastrozole [DSC]; NAT-Anastrozole; PMS-Anastrozole; RAN-Anastrozole; RIVA-Anastrozole; SANDOZ Anastrozole; TARO-Anastrozole; TEVA-Anastrozole; VAN-Anastrozole [DSC]; Zinda-Anastrozole

Pharmacologic Category Antineoplastic Agent, Aromatase Inhibitor

Use Breast cancer:

First-line treatment of locally-advanced or metastatic breast cancer (hormone receptor-positive or unknown) in postmenopausal women

Adjuvant treatment of early hormone receptor-positive breast cancer in postmenopausal women

Treatment of advanced breast cancer in postmenopausal women with disease progression following tamoxifen therapy

Local Anesthetic/Vasoconstrictor Precautions No information available to require special precautions

Effects on Dental Treatment Key adverse event(s) related to dental treatment: Xerostomia (normal salivary flow resumes upon discontinuation).

Effects on Bleeding No information available to require special precautions

Adverse Reactions Comparator: Tamoxifen

>10%:

Cardiovascular: Angina pectoris (2% [comparator: 1.6%]; 12% [comparator: 5.2%] in patients with preexisting ischemic heart disease), hypertension (5% to 13%), ischemic heart disease (4% [comparator: 3%]; 17% [comparator: 10%] in patients with preexisting ischemic heart disease), vasodilation (25% to 36%)

Dermatologic: Skin rash (6% to 11%)

Endocrine & metabolic: Hot flash (12% to 36%)

Gastrointestinal: Gastrointestinal distress (29% to 34%), nausea (11% to 19%), vomiting (≤13%)

Nervous system: Depression (5% to 13%), fatigue (≤19%), headache (9% to 13%), mood disorder (19%), pain (11% to 17%)

Neuromuscular & skeletal: Arthralgia (15% [comparator: 11%]), arthritis (17% [comparator: 14%]), asthenia (≤19%), back pain (10% to 12% [comparator: 10% to 13%]), ostealgia (7% to 11% [comparator: 6% to 10%]), osteoporosis (11% [comparator: 7%])

Respiratory: Increased cough (8% to 11%), pharyngitis (6% to 14%)

1% to 10%:

Cardiovascular: Acute myocardial infarction (1% [comparator: 1.1%]; 1% [comparator: 3.2%] in patients with preexisting ischemic heart disease), cerebral ischemia (2%), chest pain (5% to 7%), deep vein thrombosis (2%), edema (7%), peripheral edema (5% to 10%), thromboembolic disease (3% to 4%), thrombophlebitis (2% to 5%), venous thrombosis (3%)

Dermatologic: Alopecia (2% to 5%), diaphoresis (2% to 5%), pruritus (2% to 5%)

Endocrine & metabolic: Hypercholesterolemia (9%), increased gamma-glutamyl transferase (2% to 5%), weight gain (2% to 9%), weight loss (2% to 5%)

Gastrointestinal: Abdominal pain (7% to 9%), anorexia (5% to 7%), constipation (7% to 9%), diarrhea (8% to 9%), dyspepsia (7%), gastrointestinal disease (7%), xerostomia (4% to 6%)

Genitourinary: Leukorrhea (2% to 3%), mastalgia (8%), pelvic pain (5%), urinary tract infection (8%), vaginal discharge (4%), vaginal dryness (2%), vaginal hemorrhage (1% to 5%), vaginitis (4%), vulvovaginitis (6%)

Hematologic & oncologic: Anemia (4%), leukopenia (2% to 5%), lymphedema (10%), neoplasm (5%), tumor flare (3%)

Hepatic: Increased serum alanine aminotransferase (2% to 5%), increased serum alkaline phosphatase (2% to 5%), increased serum aminotransferase (2% to 5%)

Infection: Infection (9%)

Nervous system: Anxiety (6%), carpal tunnel syndrome (3% [comparator: 0.7%]), confusion (2% to 5%), dizziness (6% to 8%), drowsiness (2% to 5%), hypertonia (3%), insomnia (6% to 10%), lethargy (1%), malaise (2% to 5%), nervousness (2% to 5%), paresthesia (5% to 7%)

Neuromuscular & skeletal: Arthropathy (6% to 7% [comparator: 5%]), bone fracture (1% to 10% [comparator: 1% to 7%]), myalgia (6% [comparator: 5%]), neck pain (2% to 5%), pathological fracture (2% to 5%)

Ophthalmic: Cataract (6%)

Respiratory: Bronchitis (5%), dyspnea (8% to 10%), flu-like symptoms (6% to 7%), rhinitis (2% to 5%), sinusitis (6%)

Miscellaneous: Accidental injury (10%), cyst (5%), fever (2% to 5%)

<1%:

Dermatologic: Dermal ulcer, skin blister

Hematologic & oncologic: Endometrial carcinoma

Hepatic: Abnormal hepatic function tests, hepatitis, hepatomegaly, jaundice

Frequency not defined:
Cardiovascular: Cerebral infarction (Sagara 2010), pulmonary embolism (Lycette 2006), retinal thrombosis (Eisner 2008)
Neuromuscular & skeletal: Decreased bone mineral density (Eastell 2008; Markopoulos 2010)
Postmarketing:
Dermatologic: Dermatitis (Kim 2020), dermatologic disorder (lichen sclerosus) (Agrawal 2017; Potter 2013), erythema multiforme (Cozzani 2018; Wollina 2018), hypersensitivity angiitis (Shoda 2005), pruritic rash (Bremec 2009; Tanaka 2019), Stevens-Johnson syndrome, urticaria (Bock 2014), xeroderma (Cristofanilli 2010)
Endocrine & metabolic: Hypercalcemia (Järhult 2014; Yu 2016), hyperparathyroidism (Järhult 2014)
Hematologic & oncologic: Polycythemia (Kapoor 2019; Yeruva 2015)
Hepatic: Increased serum bilirubin, liver steatosis (Lacey 2014)
Hypersensitivity: Anaphylaxis, angioedema
Infection: Pulmonary cryptococcosis (Wei 2020)
Nervous system: Tardive dyskinesia (Manjunatha 2013)
Neuromuscular & skeletal: Subacute cutaneous lupus erythematosus (Fisher 2016), tendon disease (Martens 2007), tenosynovitis (stenosing)
Ophthalmic: Vitreous traction (Eisner 2008)

Mechanism of Action Anastrozole is a potent and selective nonsteroidal aromatase inhibitor. By inhibiting aromatase, the conversion of androstenedione to estrone, and testosterone to estradiol, is prevented, thereby decreasing tumor mass or delaying progression in patients with tumors responsive to hormones. Anastrozole causes an 85% decrease in estrone sulfate levels.

Pharmacodynamics/Kinetics

Onset of Action Onset of estradiol reduction: 70% reduction after 24 hours; 80% after 2 weeks of therapy

Duration of Action Duration of estradiol reduction: 6 days

Half-life Elimination ~50 hours

Time to Peak Plasma: ~2 hours without food; 5 hours with food

Reproductive Considerations Evaluate pregnancy status prior to therapy. Females of reproductive potential should use effective contraception during therapy and for at least 3 weeks after the last anastrozole dose.

Pregnancy Considerations
Based on the mechanism of action and information from animal reproduction studies, anastrozole may cause fetal harm if exposure occurs during pregnancy.

◆ **Anbesol [OTC]** *see* Benzocaine *on page* 228

◆ **Anbesol Cold Sore Therapy [OTC]** *see* Benzocaine *on page* 228

◆ **Anbesol JR [OTC] [DSC]** *see* Benzocaine *on page* 228

◆ **Anbesol Maximum Strength [OTC]** *see* Benzocaine *on page* 228

◆ **Ancef** *see* CeFAZolin *on page* 301

◆ **Ancobon** *see* Flucytosine *on page* 682

Andexanet Alfa (an DEX a net AL fa)

Brand Names: US Andexxa

Pharmacologic Category Antidote

Use Life-threatening bleeding associated with apixaban or rivaroxaban: Reversal of anticoagulation in patients treated with apixaban or rivaroxaban experiencing life-threatening or uncontrolled bleeding.

Local Anesthetic/Vasoconstrictor Precautions
No information available to require special precautions

Effects on Dental Treatment No significant effects or complications reported

Effects on Bleeding **FDA has issued a black box warning on the possibility of andexanet alfa inducing thromboembolic events as a reversal agent to apixaban (Eliquis) and rivaroxaban (Xarelto). It is anticipated its use will be in a medical emergency and not in the dental setting.**

Adverse Reactions
>10%:
Immunologic: Antibody development (6% to 17%)
Miscellaneous: Infusion related reaction (18%)
1% to 10%:
Cardiovascular: Deep vein thrombosis (6%), ischemic stroke (5%), acute myocardial infarction (3%), pulmonary embolism (3%), cardiogenic shock (2%), cardiac failure (1%)
Genitourinary: Urinary tract infection (≥5%)
Respiratory: Pneumonia (≥5%), acute respiratory failure (1%)
Frequency not defined: Cardiovascular: Arterial thromboembolism, venous thromboembolism
<1%, postmarketing, and/or case reports: Coronary thrombosis, intracardiac thrombus, nonsustained ventricular tachycardia

Mechanism of Action Andexanet alfa binds and sequesters the factor Xa inhibitors rivaroxaban and apixaban. In addition, andexanet alfa inhibits the activity of Tissue Factor Pathway Inhibitor, increasing tissue factor-initiated thrombin generation.

Pharmacodynamics/Kinetics

Onset of Action Rapid (Lu 2013)

Half-life Elimination Note: Clinical trials have shown that when andexanet alfa is administered to patients taking apixaban or rivaroxaban, anti-factor Xa activity increases to placebo levels ~2 hours after completion of the infusion (Connolly 2016; Siegel 2015). However, elevation of tissue factor-initiated thrombin generation above pretreatment baseline occurs within 2 minutes after administration and is sustained above placebo for at least 22 hours after administration.
Pharmacokinetic half-life:
Generation 1 product: Low dose: 4.3 (range: 3.3 to 11.9) hours; High dose: 4 (range: 2 to 5.7) hours
Generation 2 product: Low dose: 3.3 (range: 2.3 to 4) hours; High dose: 2.7 (range: 1.9 to 3.4) hours
Pharmacodynamic half-life: ~1 hour (Siegal 2015).

Pregnancy Considerations Animal reproduction studies have not been conducted.

◆ **Andexxa** *see* Andexanet Alfa *on page* 151

◆ **Androderm** *see* Testosterone *on page* 1425

◆ **AndroGel** *see* Testosterone *on page* 1425

◆ **AndroGel Pump** *see* Testosterone *on page* 1425

◆ **Android [DSC]** *see* MethylTESTOSTERone *on page* 1006

◆ **Androvite [OTC]** *see* Vitamins (Multiple/Oral) *on page* 1550

◆ **Androxy** *see* Fluoxymesterone *on page* 699

◆ **Androxy [DSC]** *see* Fluoxymesterone *on page* 699

◆ **AneCream [OTC]** *see* Lidocaine (Topical) *on page* 902

- **AneCream5 [OTC]** *see* Lidocaine (Topical) *on page 902*
- **Angeliq** *see* Drospirenone and Estradiol *on page 534*
- **Angiomax** *see* Bivalirudin *on page 246*

Anidulafungin (ay nid yoo la FUN jin)

Related Information
Fungal Infections *on page 1752*
Brand Names: US Eraxis
Brand Names: Canada Eraxis
Pharmacologic Category Antifungal Agent, Parenteral; Echinocandin
Use Treatment of candidemia, esophageal candidiasis, and other forms of *Candida* infections (intra-abdominal abscess and peritonitis)
Local Anesthetic/Vasoconstrictor Precautions Post marketing or case reports have reported rare occurrences of ECG changes, including prolongation of QT interval associated with anidulafungin. Until more information is obtained, and the patient is not taking any additional medication which prolongs QT interval, there is no reason to require special precautions with the use of vasoconstrictor.
Effects on Dental Treatment Key adverse event(s) related to dental treatment: Occurrence of oral candidiasis
Effects on Bleeding Thrombocytopenia and prolonged prothrombin time has been reported; medical consult suggested.
Adverse Reactions
>10%:
Cardiovascular: Hypotension (15%), hypertension (12%), peripheral edema (11%)
Central nervous system: Insomnia (15%)
Endocrine & metabolic: Hypokalemia (≤25%), hypomagnesemia (12%)
Gastrointestinal: Nausea (7% to 24%), diarrhea (9% to 18%), vomiting (7% to 18%)
Genitourinary: Urinary tract infection (15%)
Hepatic: Increased serum alkaline phosphatase (12%)
Infection: Bacteremia (18%)
Respiratory: Dyspnea (12%)
Miscellaneous: Fever (9% to 18%)
2% to 10%:
Cardiovascular: Deep vein thrombosis (10%), chest pain (5%)
Central nervous system: Confusion (8%), headache (8%), depression (6%)
Dermatologic: Decubitus ulcer (5%)
Endocrine & metabolic: Hypoglycemia (7%), dehydration (6%), hyperglycemia (6%), hyperkalemia (6%)
Gastrointestinal: Constipation (8%), dyspepsia (7%), abdominal pain (6%), oral candidiasis (5%)
Hematologic & oncologic: Anemia (8% to 9%), leukocytosis (5% to 8%), thrombocythemia (6%)
Hepatic: Increased serum transaminases (≤5%)
Infection: Sepsis (7%)
Neuromuscular & skeletal: Back pain (5%)
Renal: Increased serum creatinine (5%)
Respiratory: Pleural effusion (10%), cough (7%), pneumonia (6%), respiratory distress (6%)
<2%, postmarketing, and/or case reports: Anaphylactic shock, anaphylaxis, angioedema, atrial fibrillation, blood coagulation disorder, blurred vision, bronchospasm, cholestasis, clostridium infection, diaphoresis, dizziness, ECG abnormality (including ECG changes – prolonged QT interval), erythema, eye pain, flushing, hepatic insufficiency, hepatic necrosis, hepatitis, hot flash, increased amylase, increased blood urea nitrogen, increased creatine phosphokinase, increased gamma-glutamyl transferase, increased serum bilirubin, increased serum lipase, infusion related reaction, prolonged prothrombin time, pruritus, right bundle branch block, rigors, seizure, sinus arrhythmia, skin rash, thrombocytopenia, thrombophlebitis, urticaria, ventricular premature contractions, visual disturbance
Mechanism of Action Noncompetitive inhibitor of 1,3-beta-D-glucan synthase resulting in reduced formation of 1,3-beta-D-glucan, an essential polysaccharide comprising 30% to 60% of *Candida* cell walls (absent in mammalian cells); decreased glucan content leads to osmotic instability and cellular lysis
Pharmacodynamics/Kinetics
Half-life Elimination Terminal: 40-50 hours
Pregnancy Considerations Adverse effects were observed in animal reproduction studies. Other agents are currently preferred for the treatment of *Candida* infections in pregnant women (IDSA [Pappas 2016]).

- **Anjeso** *see* Meloxicam *on page 957*
- **Annovera** *see* Segesterone Acetate and Ethinyl Estradiol *on page 1362*
- **Anodyne LPT** *see* Lidocaine and Prilocaine *on page 911*
- **Anoro Ellipta** *see* Umeclidinium and Vilanterol *on page 1508*
- **Ansamycin** *see* Rifabutin *on page 1323*
- **Antabuse** *see* Disulfiram *on page 505*
- **Antara** *see* Fenofibrate and Derivatives *on page 640*
- **Anti-4 Alpha Integrin** *see* Natalizumab *on page 1086*
- **Anti-CD19/CD28/CD3zeta CAR Gammaretroviral Vector-transduced Autologous T Lymphocytes KTE-C19** *see* Axicabtagene Ciloleucel *on page 196*
- **Anti-CD20 Monoclonal Antibody** *see* RiTUXimab *on page 1336*
- **Anti-CD20 Monoclonal Antibody** *see* Rituximab and Hyaluronidase *on page 1338*
- **Anti-CD22 Immunotoxin CAT-8015** *see* Moxetumomab Pasudotox *on page 1063*
- **Anti-CD38 monoclonal antibody SAR650984** *see* Isatuximab *on page 842*
- **Anti-CD52 Monoclonal Antibody** *see* Alemtuzumab *on page 93*
- **anti-c-erB-2** *see* Trastuzumab *on page 1479*
- **Anti-Diarrheal [OTC]** *see* Loperamide *on page 928*
- **Antidiuretic Hormone** *see* Vasopressin *on page 1535*
- **Anti-EGFR Monoclonal Antibody IMC-11F8** *see* Necitumumab *on page 1089*
- **anti-ERB-2** *see* Trastuzumab *on page 1479*
- **Antifungal [OTC]** *see* Miconazole (Topical) *on page 1019*
- **Anti-Fungal [OTC]** *see* Tolnaftate *on page 1462*

Antihemophilic Factor (Human)
(an tee hee moe FIL ik FAK tor HYU man)

Brand Names: US Hemofil M; Koate; Koate-DVI; Monoclate-P [DSC]
Pharmacologic Category Antihemophilic Agent; Blood Product Derivative

Use

Hemophilia A: Control and prevention of bleeding episodes in patients with hemophilia A (classic hemophilia); perioperative management of hemophilia A.

Limitations of use: Not indicated for the treatment of von Willebrand disease.

Local Anesthetic/Vasoconstrictor Precautions No information available to require special precautions

Effects on Dental Treatment No significant effects or complications reported

Effects on Bleeding Following large doses, an increased bleeding tendency has rarely been reported. Mild thrombocytopenia has been reported. Due to underlying hemophilia and complications of thrombotic events, a medical consultation is warranted.

Adverse Reactions

1% to 10%:

Hematologic & oncologic: Increased Factor VIII inhibitors (6%)

Local: Inflammation at injection site (2%)

<1%: Chest tightness, dizziness, dysgeusia, fever, headache

Frequency not defined: Hypersensitivity: Hypersensitivity reaction

Postmarketing: Abdominal pain, anaphylaxis, bradycardia, bronchospasm, chest pain, chills, cough, cyanosis, diarrhea, dyspnea, edema, facial edema, fatigue, flushing, hyperhidrosis, hyperventilation, hypotension, irritability, musculoskeletal pain, nausea, ocular hyperemia, pruritus, skin rash, tachycardia, urticaria, visual impairment, vomiting

Mechanism of Action Protein (factor VIII) in normal plasma which is necessary for clot formation and maintenance of hemostasis; activates factor X in conjunction with activated factor IX; activated factor X converts prothrombin to thrombin, which converts fibrinogen to fibrin, and with factor XIII forms a stable clot

Pharmacodynamics/Kinetics

Half-life Elimination Mean: 14.8 to 17.5 hours

Pregnancy Considerations Pregnant hemophilia A carriers may have an increased bleeding risk following abortion, invasive procedures, miscarriage, and delivery; close surveillance is recommended. Factor VIII levels should be monitored at the first antenatal visit, once or twice during the third trimester, prior to surgical or invasive procedures, and at delivery. Although factor VIII concentrations increase in pregnant patients, factor VIII replacement is recommended if concentrations are <0.5 IU/mL and any of the following occur: need for invasive procedures (including delivery), spontaneous miscarriage, insertion and removal of epidural catheters, or active bleeding. Hemostatic factor VIII concentrations should be maintained for at least 3 to 5 days following invasive procedures or postpartum. If a replacement product is indicated, a recombinant product is preferred (NHF 2017; RCOG [Pavord 2017]; WFH [Srivastava 2013]).

Antihemophilic Factor (Recombinant)

(an tee hee moe FIL ik FAK tor ree KOM be nant)

Brand Names: US Advate; Afstyla; Helixate FS [DSC]; Kogenate FS; Kogenate FS Bio-Set [DSC]; Kovaltry; Novoeight; Nuwiq; Recombinate; Xyntha; Xyntha Solofuse

Brand Names: Canada Advate; Kovaltry; Nuwiq; Xyntha; Xyntha Solofuse; Zonovate

Pharmacologic Category Antihemophilic Agent

Use

Hemophilia A:

Control and prevention of bleeding episodes: Prevention and control of bleeding episodes in adults and children with hemophilia A.

Perioperative management: Surgical prophylaxis in adults and children with hemophilia A.

Routine prophylaxis to prevent or reduce the frequency of bleeding: Routine prophylactic treatment to prevent or reduce the frequency of bleeding episodes in adults and children with hemophilia A.

Routine prophylaxis to prevent bleeding episodes and joint damage (Helixate FS, Kogenate FS): Routine prophylactic treatment to reduce the frequency of bleeding episodes and the risk of joint damage in children without preexisting joint damage.

Limitations of use: Not indicated for the treatment of von Willebrand disease.

Local Anesthetic/Vasoconstrictor Precautions No information available to require special precautions

Effects on Dental Treatment Key adverse event(s) related to dental treatment: Taste perversion.

Effects on Bleeding Following large doses, an increased bleeding tendency has rarely been reported. Mild thrombocytopenia has been reported. Due to underlying hemophilia and complications of thrombotic events, a medical consultation is warranted.

Adverse Reactions Actual frequency may vary by product.

>10%:

Dermatologic: Pruritus (≤16%), skin rash (≤16%), urticaria (≤16%)

Hematologic & oncologic: Increased factor VIII inhibitors (≤52%)

Local: Catheter infection (18% to 19%)

Nervous system: Headache (7% to 24%)

Neuromuscular & skeletal: Arthralgia (8% to 23%)

Respiratory: Cough (12% to 13%), nasopharyngitis (12%)

Miscellaneous: Fever (≤23%)

1% to 10%:

Cardiovascular: Chest discomfort (1%), palpitations (1%), sinus tachycardia (1%)

Dermatologic: Allergic dermatitis (1%)

Gastrointestinal: Abdominal distress (2%), abdominal pain (2%), diarrhea (6% to 8%), dyspepsia (2%), vomiting (7% to 8%)

Hematologic & oncologic: Lymphadenopathy (1%)

Hypersensitivity: Hypersensitivity reaction (2%)

Local: Infusion site reaction (4% to 7%), injection site reaction (1% to 3%)

Nervous system: Chills (≤1%), dizziness (≤1%), insomnia (3%), procedural pain (5%)

Neuromuscular & skeletal: Asthenia (6%), back pain (≤3%; more common in children)

Otic: Otic infection (≤5%)

Respiratory: Nasal congestion (6%), pharyngolaryngeal pain (5%), upper respiratory tract infection (7%)

Miscellaneous: Limb injury (6%)

<1%:

Cardiovascular: Cold extremity, facial flushing, flushing, hypotension

Dermatologic: Erythema of skin, hyperhidrosis, maculopapular rash, pallor

Gastrointestinal: Dysgeusia, nausea, xerostomia

Hematologic & oncologic: Hematoma

Local: Inflammation at injection site, pain at injection site

Nervous system: Fatigue, feeling hot, vertigo

Neuromuscular & skeletal: Limb pain, paresthesia, tremor

Respiratory: Epistaxis

Frequency not defined: Endocrine & metabolic: Hot flash

Postmarketing:

Cardiovascular: Chest pain, facial edema, tachycardia

Hypersensitivity: Anaphylaxis, angioedema

Nervous system: Loss of consciousness, malaise, restlessness

Respiratory: Cyanosis, dyspnea, laryngeal edema

Mechanism of Action Factor VIII replacement, necessary for clot formation and maintenance of hemostasis. It activates factor X in conjunction with activated factor IX; activated factor X converts prothrombin to thrombin, which converts fibrinogen to fibrin, and with factor XIII forms a stable clot.

Pharmacodynamics/Kinetics

Half-life Elimination

Advate: Children <12 years: 8.7 to 11.2 hours; Adolescents and Adults: 12 hours

Afstyla: Children <12 years: 10.2 to 10.4 hours; Children ≥12 years and Adolescents: 14.3 hours; Adults: 14.2 hours

Helixate FS, Kogenate FS: Children: 10.7 hours; Adults: 13.7 to 14.6 hours

Kovaltry: Children <12 years: ~12 hours; Children ≥12 years, Adolescents, and Adults: ~14 hours

Novoeight: Children <12 years: 7.7 to 10 hours; Adolescents and Adults: 11 to 12 hours

Nuwiq: Children ≤12 years: 11.9 to 13.1 hours; Adolescents and Adults: 17.1 hours

Recombinate: Adults: 14.6 ± 4.9 hours

Xyntha, Xyntha Solofuse: Children and Adolescents: 6.9 to 8.3 hours; Adults: 11 to 17 hours

Pregnancy Considerations Pregnant hemophilia A carriers may have an increased bleeding risk following abortion, invasive procedures, miscarriage, and delivery; close surveillance is recommended. Factor VIII levels should be monitored at the first antenatal visit, once or twice during the third trimester, prior to surgical or invasive procedures, and at delivery. Although factor VIII concentrations increase in pregnant patients, factor VIII replacement is recommended if concentrations are <0.5 IU/mL and any of the following occur: need for invasive procedures (including delivery), spontaneous miscarriage, insertion and removal of epidural catheters, or active bleeding. Hemostatic factor VIII concentrations should be maintained for at least 3 to 5 days following invasive procedures or postpartum. If a replacement product is indicated, a recombinant product is preferred (NHF 2017; RCOG [Pavord 2017]; WFH [Srivastava 2013]).

Antihemophilic Factor (Recombinant [Fc Fusion Protein])

(an tee hee moe FIL ik FAK tor ree KOM be nant eff see FYOO zhun PRO teen)

Brand Names: US Eloctate

Brand Names: Canada Eloctate

Pharmacologic Category Antihemophilic Agent

Use Hemophilia A:

Control and prevention of bleeding episodes: For the prevention and control of bleeding episodes in adults and children with hemophilia A.

Perioperative management: For surgical prophylaxis in adults and children with hemophilia A.

Routine prophylaxis to prevent or reduce the frequency of bleeding: For routine prophylactic treatment to prevent or reduce the frequency of bleeding episodes in adults and children with hemophilia A.

Limitation of use: Not indicated for the treatment of von Willebrand disease.

Local Anesthetic/Vasoconstrictor Precautions No information available to require special precautions

Effects on Dental Treatment No significant effects or complications reported

Effects on Bleeding Following large doses, an increased bleeding tendency has rarely been reported. Mild thrombocytopenia has been reported. Due to underlying hemophilia and complications of thrombotic events, a medical consultation is warranted.

Adverse Reactions

<1%, postmarketing, and/or case reports: Antibody development (neutralizing), arthralgia, back pain, bradycardia, chest pain, cough, dizziness, dysgeusia, feeling hot, headache, hot flash, hypersensitivity reaction, hypertension, joint swelling, lower abdominal pain, malaise, myalgia, procedural hypotension, sensation of cold, skin rash, venous pain (postinjection)

Mechanism of Action Factor VIII replacement, necessary for clot formation and maintenance of hemostasis. It activates factor X in conjunction with activated factor IX; activated factor X converts prothrombin to thrombin, which converts fibrinogen to fibrin, and with factor XIII forms a stable clot.

Pharmacodynamics/Kinetics

Half-life Elimination Children <12 years: 12.7 to 14.9 hours; Children ≥12 years, Adolescents, and Adults: 16.4 to 19.7 hours

Pregnancy Considerations Pregnant hemophilia A carriers may have an increased bleeding risk following abortion, invasive procedures, miscarriage, and delivery; close surveillance is recommended. Factor VIII levels should be monitored at the first antenatal visit, once or twice during the third trimester, prior to surgical or invasive procedures, and at delivery. Although factor VIII concentrations increase in pregnant patients, factor VIII replacement is recommended if concentrations are <0.5 IU/mL and any of the following occur: need for invasive procedures (including delivery), spontaneous miscarriage, insertion and removal of epidural catheters, or active bleeding. Hemostatic factor VIII concentrations should be maintained for at least 3 to 5 days following invasive procedures or postpartum. If a replacement product is indicated, a recombinant product is preferred (NHF 2017; RCOG [Pavord 2017]; WFH [Srivastava 2013]).

◆ **Antihemophilic Factor (Recombinant), Single Chain** *see* Antihemophilic Factor (Recombinant) *on page 153*

Antihemophilic Factor/von Willebrand Factor Complex (Human)

(an tee hee moe FIL ik FAK tor von WILL le brand FAK tor KOM plex HYU man)

Brand Names: US Alphanate/VWF Complex/Human; Humate-P; Wilate

Brand Names: Canada Humate-P; Wilate

Pharmacologic Category Antihemophilic Agent; Blood Product Derivative

Use

Hemophilia A:

Alphanate: Treatment and prevention of bleeding in adult and pediatric patients with factor VIII deficiency due to hemophilia A (classical hemophilia).

Humate-P: Treatment and prevention of bleeding in adults with hemophilia A (classical hemophilia).

Wilate: Treatment and prevention of bleeding in adults and pediatric patients ≥12 years of age with hemophilia A (classical hemophilia).

von Willebrand disease:

Alphanate: Surgical and/or invasive procedures in adult and pediatric patients with von Willebrand disease when desmopressin is either ineffective or contraindicated

Limitations of use: Not indicated for patients with severe von Willebrand disease (type 3) undergoing major surgery.

Humate-P: Treatment of spontaneous or trauma-induced bleeding, as well as prevention of excessive bleeding during and after surgery in adult and pediatric patients with severe von Willebrand disease, including mild or moderate von Willebrand disease where use of desmopressin is known or suspected to be inadequate.

Limitations of use: Safety and efficacy of prophylactic dosing to prevent spontaneous bleeding have not been conducted in patients with von Willebrand disease.

Wilate: On demand treatment and control of bleeding episodes, and perioperative management of bleeding in adult and pediatric patients with von Willebrand disease.

Local Anesthetic/Vasoconstrictor Precautions No information available to require special precautions

Effects on Dental Treatment No significant effects or complications reported

Effects on Bleeding Following large doses, an increased bleeding tendency has rarely been reported. Mild thrombocytopenia has been reported. Due to underlying hemophilia and complications of thrombotic events, a medical consultation is warranted.

Adverse Reactions

>10%:

Gastrointestinal: Nausea (24%; postoperative)

Hematologic & oncologic: Hemorrhage (30%; postoperative)

Miscellaneous: Postoperative pain (17%)

1% to 10%:

Cardiovascular: Chest tightness (>5%), edema (>5%), facial edema (>1%), peripheral edema (1%), vasodilation (1%)

Central nervous system: Chills (>1%), headache (>1%), pain (>1%), paresthesia (>1%), dizziness (≥1%)

Dermatologic: Pruritus (>1%), skin rash (>1%), urticaria (>1%)

Hematologic & oncologic: Thrombocythemia (4%; exacerbation)

Hypersensitivity: Hypersensitivity reaction (2%)

Infection: Parvovirus B19 seroconversion (3%; not accompanied by clinical signs of disease)

Neuromuscular & skeletal: Back pain (>1%), limb pain (1%)

Respiratory: Respiratory distress (>1%)

Miscellaneous: Fever (≥1%)

Frequency not defined:

Cardiovascular: Orthostatic hypotension, phlebitis, pulmonary embolism, subdural hematoma, thrombophlebitis

Central nervous system: Cerebral hemorrhage

Endocrine & metabolic: Heavy menstrual bleeding

Gastrointestinal: Gastrointestinal hemorrhage, vomiting

Hematologic & oncologic: Decreased hematocrit (moderate), increased factor VIII inhibitors

Hepatic: Increased serum alanine aminotransferase

Hypersensitivity: Anaphylaxis, angioedema

Infection: Infection, sepsis

Renal: Pyelonephritis

Postmarketing and/or case reports: Abdominal pain, antibody development (neutralizing), arthralgia, bleeding tendency disorder, chest discomfort, cough, dyspnea, fatigue, hemolysis, hemolytic anemia, hypertension, hypervolemia, infusion-site pain, lethargy, shock, sleep disorder, thromboembolic complications

Mechanism of Action Factor VIII and von Willebrand factor (VWF), obtained from pooled human plasma, are used to replace endogenous factor VIII and VWF in patients with hemophilia or von Willebrand disease. Factor VIII in conjunction with activated factor IX, activates factor X which converts prothrombin to thrombin and fibrinogen to fibrin. VWF promotes platelet aggregation and adhesion to damaged vascular endothelium and acts as a stabilizing carrier protein for factor VIII. (Circulating levels of functional VWF are measured as ristocetin cofactor activity [VWF:RCo]).

Pharmacodynamics/Kinetics

Onset of Action Shortening of bleeding time: Immediate; maximum effect: 1 to 2 hours.

Duration of Action von Willebrand disease: Shortening of bleeding time: <6 hours postinfusion; presence of VWF multimers detected in the plasma: ≥24 hours (Alphanate).

Half-life Elimination

Factor VIII coagulant activity (FVIII:C): Range (in patients with hemophilia A): Alphanate: 8 to 28 hours; Humate: 8 to 17 hours; Wilate: Adult: 6 to 15 hours; pediatric: 9 to 15 hours.

VWF:RCo: Range (in patients with von Willebrand disease): Alphanate: 4 to 16 hours; Humate: 3 to 34 hours; Wilate: 6 to 49 hours.

Pregnancy Considerations Pregnant hemophilia A carriers and those with von Willebrand disease may have an increased bleeding risk following abortion, invasive procedures, miscarriage, and delivery; close surveillance is recommended. Factor VIII concentrations may increase in pregnant patients; changes in von Willebrand factor levels may vary during pregnancy depending on type. Patients should be monitored at the first antenatal visit, once or twice during the third trimester, prior to surgical or invasive procedures, and at delivery. Replacement is recommended if concentrations are <0.5 IU/mL and any of the following occur: need for invasive procedures (including delivery), spontaneous miscarriage, insertion and removal of epidural catheters, or active bleeding. Hemostatic concentrations should be maintained for at least 3 to 5 days following invasive procedures or postpartum. When VWF replacement therapy is needed, a recombinant product or a product made from a safe plasma source with viral testing that contains both factor VIII and von Willebrand factor is recommended. A recombinant product is one of the preferred agents if prophylaxis or treatment is needed for hemophilia A during pregnancy (NHF 2017; RCOG [Pavord 2017]; WFH [Srivastava 2013]).

◆ **Antihemophilic Factor/Vwf** *see* Antihemophilic Factor/von Willebrand Factor Complex (Human) *on page 154*

◆ **Anti-HER2 ADC DS-8201a** *see* Fam-Trastuzumab Deruxtecan *on page 636*

- **Anti-HER2 Antibody Drug Conjugate DS-8201a** *see* Fam-Trastuzumab Deruxtecan *on page 636*
- **Anti-Hist Allergy [OTC]** *see* DiphenhydrAMINE (Systemic) *on page 502*

Anti-inhibitor Coagulant Complex (Human)

(an TEE in HI bi tor coe AG yoo lant KOM pleks HYU man)

Brand Names: US FEIBA

Brand Names: Canada Feiba NF

Pharmacologic Category Activated Prothrombin Complex Concentrate (aPCC); Antihemophilic Agent; Blood Product Derivative

Use

Hemorrhage in patients with hemophilia: Control and prevention of bleeding episodes in patients with hemophilia A and B with inhibitors.

Perioperative bleeding management in patients with hemophilia: Perioperative bleeding management in patients with hemophilia A and B with inhibitors.

Routine prophylaxis of bleeding events in patients with hemophilia: Routine prophylaxis to prevent or reduce the frequency of bleeding episodes in patients with hemophilia A and B with inhibitors.

Local Anesthetic/Vasoconstrictor Precautions No information available to require special precautions

Effects on Dental Treatment No significant effects or complications reported

Effects on Bleeding Due to underlying hemophilia and complications of thrombotic events, a medical consultation is warranted.

Adverse Reactions Frequency not defined.

Cardiovascular: Cerebrovascular accident (embolic/thrombotic stroke), chest discomfort, chest pain, decreased blood pressure, flushing, hypertension, hypotension, myocardial infarction, pulmonary embolism, tachycardia, thromboembolism, thrombosis (arterial thrombosis, venous thrombosis)

Central nervous system: Chills, dizziness, drowsiness, headache, hypoesthesia (including facial), malaise, paresthesia

Dermatologic: Pruritus, skin rash, urticaria

Gastrointestinal: Abdominal distress, diarrhea, dysgeusia, nausea, vomiting

Hematologic & oncologic: Disseminated intravascular coagulation

Hypersensitivity: Angioedema, hypersensitivity reaction (including anaphylaxis)

Immunologic: Antibody development (anamnestic response)

Local: Pain at injection site

Respiratory: Bronchospasm, cough, dyspnea, wheezing

Miscellaneous: Fever

Mechanism of Action Multiple interactions of the components in anti-inhibitor coagulant complex restore the impaired thrombin generation of hemophilia patients with inhibitors. In vitro, anti-inhibitor coagulant complex shortens the activated partial thromboplastin time of plasma containing factor VIII inhibitor.

Pharmacodynamics/Kinetics

Onset of Action Peak thrombin generation: Within 15 to 30 minutes (Varadi 2003)

Duration of Action 8 to 12 hours (based on thrombin generation) (Varadi 2003)

Half-life Elimination 4 to 7 hours (based on thrombin generation) (Varadi 2003)

Pregnancy Considerations

Limited outcome information is available from a pregnancy registry following use of anti-inhibitor coagulant complex (human) in pregnant women with acquired hemophilia A (Tengborn 2012). Other products are preferred for the routine prophylaxis of bleeding events in pregnant patients with known hemophilia (NHF 2017; WFH [Srivastava 2013]; RCOG [Pavord 2017]). However, the use of anti-inhibitor coagulant complex (human) may be considered in select patients with bleeding associated with postpartum acquired hemophilia A (a recombinant product may be preferred) (Huth-Kuhne 2009; Kruse-Jarres 2017; Windyga 2019).

- **Anti-Itch [OTC]** *see* DiphenhydrAMINE (Topical) *on page 503*
- **Anti-Itch Maximum Strength [OTC] [DSC]** *see* DiphenhydrAMINE (Topical) *on page 503*
- **Anti-Itch Maximum Strength [OTC]** *see* Hydrocortisone (Topical) *on page 775*
- **Anti-nectin 4 ADC ASG-22CE** *see* Enfortumab Vedotin *on page 564*
- **Anti-PD-1 Human Monoclonal Antibody MDX-1106** *see* Nivolumab *on page 1114*
- **Anti-PD-1 Monoclonal Antibody MK-3475** *see* Pembrolizumab *on page 1204*
- **Anti-PD-1 Monoclonal Antibody REGN2810** *see* Cemiplimab *on page 320*
- **Anti-PDGFR Alpha Monoclonal Antibody IMC-3G3** *see* Olaratumab *on page 1131*
- **Anti-PD-L1 Monoclonal Antibody MSB0010718C** *see* Avelumab *on page 195*
- **Antiseptic Mouthwash** *see* Mouthwash (Antiseptic) *on page 1062*
- **Antiseptic Oral Rinse [OTC] [DSC]** *see* Cetylpyridinium *on page 330*
- **Antiseptic Skin Cleanser [OTC] [DSC]** *see* Chlorhexidine Gluconate (Topical) *on page 335*
- **Anti-Tac Monoclonal Antibody** *see* Daclizumab *on page 428*

Antithrombin (an tee THROM bin)

Brand Names: US Thrombate III

Pharmacologic Category Anticoagulant; Blood Product Derivative

Use Hereditary antithrombin deficiency: Thrombate III: Treatment and prevention of thromboembolism and prevention of perioperative and peripartum thromboembolism in patients with hereditary antithrombin deficiency.

Local Anesthetic/Vasoconstrictor Precautions No information available to require special precautions

Effects on Dental Treatment No significant effects or complications reported

Effects on Bleeding As with all anticoagulant drugs, bleeding is a potential adverse effect of antithrombin during dental surgery; risk is dependent on multiple variables, including the intensity of anticoagulation and patient susceptibility. Medical consult is suggested. It is unlikely that ambulatory patients presenting for dental treatment will be taking intravenous anticoagulant therapy such as antithrombin.

Adverse Reactions

1% to 10%:

Cardiovascular: Chest pain (≤2%)

Central nervous system: Dizziness (2%)

Gastrointestinal: Liver enzyme abnormalities (≤2%)
Genitourinary: Hematuria (≤2%)
Hematologic & oncologic: Hemorrhage (≥5%), hematoma (≤2%)
Local: Infusion site reaction (≥5%)
Neuromuscular & skeletal: Hemarthrosis (≤2%)

<1%, postmarketing, and/or case reports: Blurred vision, chest tightness, chills, dizziness, dyspnea, fever, gastrointestinal fullness, muscle cramps, nausea, unpleasant taste, urticaria

Mechanism of Action Antithrombin is the primary physiologic inhibitor of *in vivo* coagulation. It is an alpha$_2$-globulin. Its principal actions are the inactivation of thrombin, plasmin, and other active serine proteases of coagulation, including factors IXa, Xa, XIa, and XIIa. The inactivation of proteases is a major step in the normal clotting process. The strong activation of clotting enzymes at the site of every bleeding injury facilitates fibrin formation and maintains normal hemostasis. Thrombosis in the circulation would be caused by active serine proteases if they were not inhibited by antithrombin after the localized clotting process (Schwartz, 1989).

In patients with hereditary antithrombin (AT) deficiency, spontaneous thrombosis may occur due to decreased AT concentrations; therapy with human or recombinant AT restores functional AT activity.

Pharmacodynamics/Kinetics

Half-life Elimination

Plasma derived (Thrombate III): Biologic: 2.5 days (immunologic assay); 3.8 days (functional AT assay). Half-life may be decreased following surgery, with hemorrhage, acute thrombosis, and/or during heparin administration.

Pregnancy Considerations

The risk of thromboembolic events such as venous thromboembolism (VTE) is increased in patients with hereditary antithrombin (AT) deficiency. Pregnancy-induced physiologic changes also increase this risk; risk is dependent upon maternal antithrombin levels and personal or family history of thromboembolism (ACOG 197 2018). Thrombate III is approved for use in pregnant women with hereditary AT deficiency to replace endogenous antithrombin and reduce the risk of peripartum thromboembolism. Antithrombin replacement can be used in pregnant patients with hereditary AT deficiency in high-risk settings (eg, childbirth, miscarriage, surgery) when other anticoagulant therapy (eg, low molecular weight heparin [LMWH]) is withheld or as adjunctive therapy to LMWH in pregnant women at high risk for VTE (Bauer 2016; Ilonczai 2015; James 2017; Rogenhofer 2014).

◆ **Antithrombin III** *see* Antithrombin *on page* *156*

◆ **Antithrombin Alfa** *see* Antithrombin *on page* *156*

Antithymocyte Globulin (Equine)

(an te THY moe site GLOB yu lin, E kwine)

Brand Names: US Atgam

Brand Names: Canada Atgam

Pharmacologic Category Immune Globulin; Immunosuppressant Agent; Polyclonal Antibody

Use

Aplastic anemia: Treatment of moderate-to-severe aplastic anemia in patients not considered suitable candidates for bone marrow transplantation

Limitations of use: The usefulness of antithymocyte globulin (equine) has not been demonstrated in patients with aplastic anemia who are suitable candidates for transplantation, or in aplastic anemia secondary to neoplastic disease, storage disease, myelofibrosis, Fanconi syndrome, or in patients with known prior treatment with myelotoxic agents or radiation therapy

Local Anesthetic/Vasoconstrictor Precautions No information available to require special precautions

Effects on Dental Treatment Key adverse event(s) related to dental treatment: Stomatitis

Effects on Bleeding No information available to require special precautions

Adverse Reactions

>10%:

Central nervous system: Chills, headache
Dermatologic: Dermatological reaction (wheal/flare), pruritus, skin rash, urticaria
Hematologic & oncologic: Leukopenia, thrombocytopenia
Neuromuscular & skeletal: Arthralgia
Miscellaneous: Fever

1% to 10%:

Cardiovascular: Bradycardia, cardiac disease, cardiac failure, chest pain, edema, hypertension, hypotension, myocarditis, phlebitis, thrombophlebitis
Central nervous system: Agitation, brain disease (viral), burning sensation (burning of soles and burning of palms), dizziness, encephalitis, generalized ache, lethargy, seizure
Dermatologic: Diaphoresis, night sweats
Gastrointestinal: Diarrhea, nausea, stomatitis, vomiting
Genitourinary: Proteinuria
Hematologic & oncologic: Lymphadenopathy
Hepatic: Abnormal hepatic function tests, hepatosplenomegaly
Hypersensitivity: Anaphylaxis, serum sickness
Infection: Viral infection
Local: Injection site reaction (pain, redness, swelling)
Neuromuscular & skeletal: Back pain, joint stiffness, myalgia
Ophthalmic: Periorbital edema
Renal: Renal function test abnormality
Respiratory: Dyspnea, pleural effusion, respiratory distress

<1%, postmarketing, and/or case reports: Abdominal pain, acute renal failure, anaphylactoid reaction, anemia, apnea, confusion, cough, deep vein thrombosis, disorientation, dizziness, eosinophilia, epigastric pain, epistaxis, erythema, flank pain, gastrointestinal hemorrhage, gastrointestinal perforation, granulocytopenia, hemolysis, hemolytic anemia, herpes simplex infection (reactivation), hiccups, hyperglycemia, infection, involuntary body movements, laryngospasm, malaise, muscle rigidity, neutropenia, pancytopenia, paresthesia, pulmonary edema, pure red cell aplasia, renal artery thrombosis, sore mouth, sore throat, tachycardia, thrombosis of vein (iliac), toxic epidermal necrolysis, tremor, vasculitis, viral hepatitis, weakness, wound dehiscence

Mechanism of Action Immunosuppressant involved in the elimination of antigen-reactive T lymphocytes (killer cells) in peripheral blood or alteration in the function of T-lymphocytes, which are involved in humoral immunity and partly in cell-mediated immunity; induces complete or partial hematologic response in aplastic anemia

Pharmacodynamics/Kinetics

Half-life Elimination 5.7 ± 3 days

Pregnancy Considerations

Antithymocyte globulin (equine) is a purified immunoglobulin G. Placental transfer of human IgG is dependent upon the IgG subclass, maternal serum concentrations, newborn birth weight, and gestational age, generally increasing as pregnancy progresses. The lowest exposure would be expected during the period of organogenesis (Palmeira 2012; Pentsuk 2009).

Information related to the use of antithymocyte globulin (equine) in pregnancy is limited (Aitchison 1989; Miller 1995; Pajor 1992). Antithymocyte globulin (equine) is not recommended for the treatment of aplastic anemia in pregnancy (Killick 2016).

The Transplant Pregnancy Registry International (TPR) is a registry that follows pregnancies that occur in maternal transplant recipients or those fathered by male transplant recipients. The TPR encourages reporting of pregnancies following solid organ transplant by contacting them at 1-877-955-6877 or https://www.transplantpregnancyregistry.org.

- **Anti-Thymocyte Globulin (Equine)** *see* Antithymocyte Globulin (Equine) *on page 157*
- **Antithymocyte Immunoglobulin** *see* Antithymocyte Globulin (Equine) *on page 157*
- **Anti-TROP-2 Antigen Antibody-drug Conjugate IMMU-132** *see* Sacituzumab Govitecan *on page 1352*
- **Antitumor Necrosis Factor Alpha (Human)** *see* Adalimumab *on page 83*
- **Anti-VEGF Monoclonal Antibody** *see* Bevacizumab *on page 242*
- **Anti-VEGF rhuMAb** *see* Bevacizumab *on page 242*
- **Antivert** *see* Meclizine *on page 952*
- **Antizol** *see* Fomepizole *on page 710*
- **Anucort-HC** *see* Hydrocortisone (Topical) *on page 775*
- **Anu-Med [OTC] [DSC]** *see* Phenylephrine (Topical) *on page 1227*
- **Anusol-HC** *see* Hydrocortisone (Topical) *on page 775*
- **Anzemet** *see* Dolasetron *on page 510*
- **4-AP** *see* Dalfampridine *on page 431*
- **AP24534** *see* PONATinib *on page 1246*
- **AP26113** *see* Brigatinib *on page 250*
- **Apadaz** *see* Benzhydrocodone and Acetaminophen *on page 228*

Apalutamide (a pa LOO ta mide)

Brand Names: US Erleada

Brand Names: Canada Erleada

Pharmacologic Category Antineoplastic Agent, Antiandrogen

Use

Prostate cancer:

Treatment of metastatic, castration-sensitive prostate cancer.

Treatment of nonmetastatic, castration-resistant prostate cancer.

Local Anesthetic/Vasoconstrictor Precautions

No information available to require special precautions

Effects on Dental Treatment No significant effects or complications reported

Effects on Bleeding Chemotherapy with apalutamide may result in significant myelosuppression, including anemia (70%; grades 3/4: <1%), leukopenia (47%; grades 3/4: <1%), and lymphocytopenia (41%; grades 3/4: 2%). In patients who are under active treatment with apalutamide, medical consult is suggested.

Adverse Reactions

>10%:

Cardiovascular: Hypertension (18% to 25%), peripheral edema (11%)

Central nervous system: Fatigue (26% to 39%), falling (16%)

Dermatologic: Skin rash (25% to 28%), pruritus (6% to 11%)

Endocrine & metabolic: Hypercholesterolemia (76%), hyperglycemia (70%), hypertriglyceridemia (17% to 67%), hyperkalemia (32%), increased thyroid stimulating hormone level (25%), hot flash (14% to 23%), weight loss (16%)

Gastrointestinal: Diarrhea (9% to 20%), nausea (18%), decreased appetite (12%)

Hematologic & oncologic: Anemia (70%; grades 3/4: <1%), leukopenia (47%; grades 3/4: <1%), lymphocytopenia (41%; grades 3/4: 2%)

Neuromuscular & skeletal: Arthralgia (16% to 17%), bone fracture (9% to 12%)

1% to 10%:

Cardiovascular: Ischemic heart disease (4%), cardiac failure (2%)

Endocrine & metabolic: Hypothyroidism (4% to 8%)

Gastrointestinal: Dysgeusia (3%)

Neuromuscular & skeletal: Muscle spasm (3%)

<1%, postmarketing, and/or case reports: Seizure

Mechanism of Action Apalutamide is a nonsteroidal androgen receptor inhibitor; apalutamide binds directly to the androgen receptor ligand-binding domain to prevent androgen-receptor translocation, DNA binding, and receptor-mediated transcription (Smith 2018). Androgen receptor inhibition results in decreased proliferation of tumor cells and increased apoptosis, leading to a decrease in tumor volume.

Pharmacodynamics/Kinetics

Half-life Elimination ~3 days

Time to Peak 2 hours (range: 1 to 5 hours)

Reproductive Considerations

Males with female partners of reproductive potential should use effective contraception during therapy and for 3 months after the last apalutamide dose.

Pregnancy Considerations

Based on the mechanism of action, in utero exposure to apalutamide may cause fetal harm and potential fetal loss.

Prescribing and Access Restrictions Apalutamide is available through a specialty pharmacy network. Refer to https://www.janssencarepath.com/hcp/erleada or call 877-227-3728 for more information.

- **APAP (abbreviation is not recommended)** *see* Acetaminophen *on page 59*
- **APC8015** *see* Sipuleucel-T *on page 1374*
- **aPCC** *see* Anti-inhibitor Coagulant Complex (Human) *on page 156*
- **ApexiCon E** *see* Diflorasone *on page 494*
- **Apidra** *see* Insulin Glulisine *on page 823*
- **Apidra SoloStar** *see* Insulin Glulisine *on page 823*

Apixaban (a PIX a ban)

Related Information

Antiplatelet and Anticoagulation Considerations in Dentistry *on page 1666*

Brand Names: US Eliquis; Eliquis DVT/PE Starter Pack

Brand Names: Canada Eliquis

Pharmacologic Category Anticoagulant; Anticoagulant, Factor Xa Inhibitor; Direct Oral Anticoagulant (DOAC)

Use

Deep vein thrombosis: Treatment of deep vein thrombosis (DVT); to reduce the risk of recurrent DVT following initial therapy

Nonvalvular atrial fibrillation: To reduce the risk of stroke and systemic embolism in patients with nonvalvular atrial fibrillation (AF)

Postoperative venous thromboprophylaxis following hip or knee replacement surgery: Prophylaxis of DVT, which may lead to pulmonary embolism (PE), in patients who have undergone hip or knee replacement surgery

Pulmonary embolism: Treatment of PE; to reduce the risk of recurrent PE following initial therapy

Local Anesthetic/Vasoconstrictor Precautions No information available to require special precautions

Effects on Dental Treatment Key adverse event(s) related to dental treatment: Surgical site bleeding may occur. See Effects on Bleeding.

Effects on Bleeding Apixaban inhibits platelet activation and fibrin clot formation via direct, selective, and reversible inhibition of factor Xa. As with all anticoagulants, bleeding is the major adverse effect of apixaban. Hemorrhage may occur at virtually any site; risk is dependent on multiple variables including the intensity of anticoagulation and patient susceptibility. Medical consult is suggested.

Adverse Reactions

>10%: Hematologic & oncologic: Hemorrhage (≤15%; major hemorrhage: ≤2%; clinically relevant nonmajor: 4%)

1% to 10%:

Endocrine & metabolic: Heavy menstrual bleeding (1%)

Gastrointestinal: Gingival hemorrhage (≤1%), nausea (3%)

Genitourinary: Hematuria (≤2%)

Hematologic & oncologic: Anemia (3%), bruise (1% to 2%), hematoma (1% to 2%), rectal hemorrhage (≤1%)

Respiratory: Epistaxis (≤4%), hemoptysis (≤1%)

<1%:

Cardiovascular: Perioperative blood loss, syncope

Dermatologic: Dermal hemorrhage, skin rash, wound secretion

Endocrine & metabolic: Increased gamma-glutamyl transferase

Gastrointestinal: Gastrointestinal hemorrhage, hematemesis, hematochezia, hemorrhoidal bleeding, melena

Genitourinary: Abnormal uterine bleeding, genital bleeding

Hematologic & oncologic: Hemophthalmos, periorbital hematoma, petechia, postoperative hematoma (incision site), postprocedural hemorrhage, puncture site bleeding, thrombocytopenia, wound hemorrhage

Hepatic: Increased serum alkaline phosphatase, increased serum bilirubin, increased serum transaminases

Hypersensitivity: Allergic angioedema, anaphylaxis

Local: Hematoma at injection site, incision site hemorrhage

Nervous system: Intracranial hemorrhage

Neuromuscular & skeletal: Muscle hemorrhage

Ophthalmic: Conjunctival hemorrhage, retinal hemorrhage

Postmarketing:

Cardiovascular: Thrombosis (with premature discontinuation) (Garcia 2014; Granger 2015)

Hematologic & oncologic: Spinal hematoma (El Alayli 2020; Ardebol 2019)

Nervous system: Epidural intracranial hemorrhage (El Alayli 2020; Ardebol 2019)

Ophthalmic: Periorbital edema (Ahmad 2018)

Mechanism of Action Inhibits platelet activation and fibrin clot formation via direct, selective and reversible inhibition of free and clot-bound factor Xa (FXa). FXa, as part of the prothrombinase complex consisting also of factor Va, calcium ions, and phospholipid, catalyzes the conversion of prothrombin to thrombin. Thrombin both activates platelets and catalyzes the conversion of fibrinogen to fibrin.

Pharmacodynamics/Kinetics

Onset of Action 3 to 4 hours

Half-life Elimination ~12 hours (8 to 15 hours) (AHA [Raval 2017])

Time to Peak 3 to 4 hours

Reproductive Considerations

Information related to the use of direct acting oral anticoagulants in pregnancy is limited; until safety data are available, adequate contraception is recommended during therapy for females of childbearing potential. Females planning a pregnancy should be switched to alternative anticoagulants prior to conception (Cohen 2016).

Pregnancy Considerations

Based on placenta perfusion studies, apixaban is expected to cross the placenta (Bapat 2016).

Information specific to the use of apixaban in pregnancy is limited (Beyer-Westendorf 2016; Königsbrügge 2014; Lameijer 2018). Use of direct acting oral anticoagulants increases the risk of bleeding in all patients. When used in pregnancy, there is also the potential for fetal bleeding or subclinical placental bleeding which may increase the risk of miscarriage, preterm delivery, fetal compromise, or stillbirth (Cohen 2016).

Data are insufficient to evaluate the safety of direct acting oral anticoagulants during pregnancy (Bates 2012) and use in pregnant females is not recommended (Regitz-Zagrosek [ESC 2018]). Agents other than apixaban are preferred for the treatment of AF, PE, or VTE in pregnant patients (Howard 2018; Kearon 2016; Lip 2018; Regitz-Zagrosek [ESC 2018]). Patients should be switched to an alternative anticoagulant if pregnancy occurs during therapy. Fetal monitoring that includes evaluations for fetal bleeding and assessments for risk of preterm delivery are recommended if the direct acting oral anticoagulant is continued (Cohen 2016).

Dental Health Professional Considerations At this time there are no coagulation parameters for apixaban to predict the extent of bleeding. Increased bleeding may occur during invasive dental procedures in patients taking apixaban. Medical consult is suggested prior to dental invasive procedures. Routine coagulation testing (INR) is not required, or necessary, for Direct-Acting Oral Anticoagulants (DOAC).

◆ **Aplenzin** *see* BuPROPion *on page 271*

◆ **Aplicare Povidone-Iodine [OTC]** *see* Povidone-Iodine (Topical) *on page 1249*

◆ **Aplicare Povidone-Iodine Scrub [OTC]** *see* Povidone-Iodine (Topical) *on page 1249*

◆ **Aplisol** *see* Tuberculin Tests *on page 1503*

◆ **Aplonidine** *see* Apraclonidine *on page 161*

◆ **Apokyn** *see* Apomorphine *on page 160*

Apomorphine (a poe MOR feen)

Brand Names: US Apokyn; Kynmobi; Kynmobi Titration Kit

Brand Names: Canada Movapo

Pharmacologic Category Anti-Parkinson Agent, Dopamine Agonist

Use

Parkinson disease:

Sublingual film: Treatment of acute, intermittent "off" episodes in patients with Parkinson disease.

SubQ: Treatment of hypomobility "off" episodes in patients with advanced Parkinson disease.

Local Anesthetic/Vasoconstrictor Precautions Apomorphine is one of the drugs confirmed to prolong the QT interval and is accepted as having a risk of causing torsade de pointes. The risk of drug-induced torsade de pointes is extremely low when a single QT interval prolonging drug is prescribed. In terms of epinephrine, it is not known what effect vasoconstrictors in the local anesthetic regimen will have in patients with a known history of congenital prolonged QT interval or in patients taking any medication that prolongs the QT interval. Until more information is obtained, it is suggested that the clinician consult with the physician prior to the use of a vasoconstrictor in suspected patients, and that the vasoconstrictor (epinephrine, mepivacaine and levonordefrin [Carbocaine® 2% with Neo-Cobefrin®]) be used with caution.

Effects on Dental Treatment Key adverse event(s) related to dental treatment: Patients may experience orthostatic hypotension as they stand up after treatment; especially if lying in dental chair for extended periods of time. Use caution with sudden changes in position during and after dental treatment.

Effects on Bleeding No information available to require special precautions

Adverse Reactions

>10%:

Cardiovascular: Angina pectoris (≤15%), chest pain (≤15%), chest pressure (≤15%), hypotension (≤11%), orthostatic hypotension (diastolic or systolic: ≤43%; can be severe), syncope (≤11%)

Gastrointestinal: Nausea (≤30%; can be severe nausea; can occur with antiemetic pretreatment), oral paresthesia (sublingual film: ≤13%), vomiting (≤30%; can be severe vomiting; can occur with antiemetic pretreatment)

Local: Injection site reaction (5% to 26%; bruising at injection site [16%], injection site granuloma [4%], injection site pruritus [2%])

Nervous system: Dizziness (≤20%), drowsiness (11% to 35%), falling (4% to 30%), hallucination (≤14%), yawning (40%)

Neuromuscular & skeletal: Dyskinesia (24% to 35%)

Respiratory: Oropharyngeal edema (sublingual film: 1% to 15%), oropharyngeal pain (sublingual film: ≤13%), rhinorrhea (6% to 20%)

1% to 10%:

Cardiovascular: Acute myocardial infarction (≤4%), cardiac failure (≥5%), edema (≤10%), presyncope (≤4%)

Dermatologic: Diaphoresis (≥5%), ecchymoses (≥5%), facial swelling (≤6%), hyperhidrosis (6%), urticaria (≤6%)

Endocrine & metabolic: Dehydration (≥5%)

Gastrointestinal: Constipation (≥5%), diarrhea (≥5%), oral mucosal erythema (sublingual film: 7%), oral mucosa ulcer (sublingual film: ≤7%), stomatitis (sublingual film: ≤7%), xerostomia (sublingual film: 1% to 6%)

Genitourinary: Urinary tract infection (≥5%)

Hypersensitivity: Hypersensitivity reaction (≤6%)

Nervous system: Anxiety (≥5%), confusion (≤10%), delusion (≤6%), depression (≥5%), disorientation (≤6%), exacerbation of Parkinson's disease (≥5%), fatigue (3% to 7%), headache (5% to 8%), insomnia (≥5%)

Neuromuscular & skeletal: Arthralgia (≥5%), asthenia (≥5%), back pain (≥5%), limb pain (≥5%), swelling of extremities (≤10%)

Respiratory: Dyspnea (≥5%), pneumonia (≥5%)

Miscellaneous: Laceration (sublingual film: 1% to 6%)

<1%: Genitourinary: Priapism

Postmarketing:

Cardiovascular: Prolonged QT interval on ECG (dose related)

Hematologic & oncologic: Hemolytic anemia (combination therapy) (Colosimo 1994; Frankel 1990)

Nervous system: Aggressive behavior, agitation, behavioral changes, impulse control disorder (including pathological gambling, increased libido), mental status changes, paranoid ideation, psychosis (acute), sudden onset of sleep

Mechanism of Action Stimulates postsynaptic D2-type receptors within the caudate putamen in the brain.

Pharmacodynamics/Kinetics

Onset of Action SubQ: Rapid

Half-life Elimination Terminal: Sublingual: ~1.7 hours (range: 0.8 to 3 hours); SubQ: ~40 minutes.

Time to Peak Plasma: Sublingual: 0.5 to 1 hour; SubQ: 10 to 60 minutes.

Pregnancy Considerations Adverse events have been observed in animal reproduction studies.

Product Availability Kynmobi sublingual film: FDA approved May 2020; availability anticipated September 2020.

Prescribing and Access Restrictions Apokyn is only available through specialty pharmacies and cannot be obtained through a retail pharmacy. For more information, contact 1-877-7APOKYN (1-877-727-6596).

Dental Health Professional Considerations See Local Anesthetic/Vasoconstrictor Precautions

◆ **Apomorphine Hydrochloride** *see* Apomorphine *on page 160*

◆ **Apomorphine Hydrochloride Hemihydrate** *see* Apomorphine *on page 160*

◆ **APPG** *see* Penicillin G Procaine *on page 1210*

Apraclonidine (a pra KLOE ni deen)

Brand Names: US Iopidine
Brand Names: Canada Iopidine
Pharmacologic Category $Alpha_2$ Agonist, Ophthalmic
Use
Elevated intraocular pressure:
0.5% solution: Short-term, adjunctive therapy in patients who require additional reduction of intraocular pressure (IOP)
1% solution: Prevention and treatment of postsurgical IOP elevation following argon laser trabeculoplasty, argon laser iridotomy or Nd:YAG posterior capsulotomy (manufacturer's labeling) or as part of a 4-drug medical management regimen in acute angle-closure glaucoma when the patient cannot be seen by an ophthalmologist for ≥1 hour (off-label use) (Krawitz 1990; Pokhrel 2007).
Local Anesthetic/Vasoconstrictor Precautions No information available to require special precautions
Effects on Dental Treatment Key adverse event(s) related to dental treatment: Xerostomia (normal salivary flow resumes upon discontinuation)
Effects on Bleeding No information available to require special precautions
Adverse Reactions Frequency not always defined.
5% to 15%:
Gastrointestinal: Xerostomia (10%)
Ophthalmic: Eye discomfort, eye pruritus, ocular hyperemia
1% to 5%:
Cardiovascular: Cardiac arrhythmia (<3%), chest pain (<3%), facial edema (<3%), peripheral edema (<3%), localized blanching
Central nervous system: Altered sense of smell (<3%), ataxia (<3%), depression (<3%), dizziness (<3%), drowsiness (<3%), headache (<3%), insomnia (<3%), malaise (<3%), nervousness (<3%), paresthesia (<3%)
Dermatologic: Contact dermatitis (<3%), dermatitis (<3%)
Gastrointestinal: Constipation (<3%), dysgeusia (<3%), nausea (<3%)
Neuromuscular & skeletal: Myalgia (<3%), weakness (<3%)
Ophthalmic: Blurred vision, conjunctivitis, dry eye syndrome, eyelid edema, eye discharge, foreign body sensation of eye, lacrimation
Respiratory: Asthma (<3%), dry nose (<3%), dyspnea (<3%), pharyngitis (<3%), rhinitis (<3%)
<1%, postmarketing, and/or case reports: Blepharitis, blepharoconjunctivitis, bradycardia, conjunctival edema, corneal erosion, corneal infiltrates, corneal staining, crusting of eyelid, epithelial keratopathy, erythema of eyelid, eyelid disease, eyelid retraction, eye irritation, eye pain, follicular conjunctivitis, hypersensitivity reaction, keratitis, ocular edema, photophobia, scaling of eyelid, visual disturbance
Mechanism of Action Apraclonidine is a potent alpha-adrenergic agent similar to clonidine; relatively selective for $alpha_2$-receptors but does retain some binding to $alpha_1$-receptors; appears to result in reduction of aqueous humor formation; its penetration through the blood-brain barrier is more polar than clonidine which reduces its penetration through the blood-brain barrier and suggests that its pharmacological profile is characterized by peripheral rather than central effects.
Pharmacodynamics/Kinetics
Onset of Action 1 hour; Peak effect: Decreased intraocular pressure: 3 to 5 hours
Half-life Elimination Systemic: 0.5% solution: 8 hours
Pregnancy Considerations
Adverse events have been observed in animal reproduction studies. If ophthalmic agents are needed during pregnancy, the minimum effective dose should be used in combination with punctal occlusion to decrease potential exposure to the fetus (Samples 1988).

◆ **Apraclonidine HCl** *see* Apraclonidine *on page 161*

◆ **Apraclonidine Hydrochloride** *see* Apraclonidine *on page 161*

Apremilast (a PRE mi last)

Brand Names: US Otezla
Brand Names: Canada Otezla
Pharmacologic Category Phosphodiesterase-4 Enzyme Inhibitor
Use
Behçet disease: Treatment of oral ulcers associated with Behçet disease.
Psoriasis: Treatment of patients with moderate to severe plaque psoriasis who are candidates for phototherapy or systemic therapy.
Psoriatic arthritis: Treatment of patients with active psoriatic arthritis.
Local Anesthetic/Vasoconstrictor Precautions No information available to require special precautions
Effects on Dental Treatment No significant effects or complications reported
Effects on Bleeding No information available to require special precautions
Adverse Reactions Frequency not always defined.
Central nervous system: Tension headache (7%), headache (6%), fatigue (3%), depression (2%), insomnia (2%), migraine (2%), paresthesia (<2%)
Dermatologic: Skin rash (<2%), folliculitis (1%)
Endocrine & metabolic: Weight loss (5% to 10% of body weight: 10% to 12%; ≥10% of body weight: 2%)
Gastrointestinal: Diarrhea (18%), nausea (17%), vomiting (4%), decreased appetite (3%), dyspepsia (3%), abdominal distress (2%), abdominal pain (2%), frequent bowel movements (2%), upper abdominal pain (2%), abdominal distention (<2%), gastroesophageal reflux disease (<2%)
Hypersensitivity: Hypersensitivity reaction (<2%)
Infection: Influenza (<2%), tooth abscess (1%)
Neuromuscular & skeletal: Back pain (2%), arthralgia (<2%), muscle spasm (<2%), myalgia (<2%)
Respiratory: Upper respiratory tract infection (8%), nasopharyngitis (7%), sinusitis (2%), bronchitis (<2%), cough (<2%), pharyngitis (<2%), rhinitis (<2%), sinus headache (<2%)
<1%: Atrial fibrillation, exacerbation of psoriasis (rebound following discontinuation), severe diarrhea, suicidal ideation, tachyarrhythmia
Mechanism of Action Apremilast inhibits phosphodiesterase 4 (PDE4) specific for cyclic adenosine monophosphate (cAMP) which results in increased intracellular cAMP levels and regulation of numerous inflammatory mediators (eg, decreased expression of nitric oxide synthase, TNF-α, and interleukin [IL]-23, as well as increased IL-10) (Schafer, 2012).

Pharmacodynamics/Kinetics

Half-life Elimination ~6 to 9 hours

Time to Peak ~2.5 hours

Reproductive Considerations

Due to potential toxicity, discontinue use ≥2 days prior to a planned pregnancy (Rademaker 2018).

Pregnancy Considerations

Due to potential toxicity and limited information related to use in pregnancy, use is not currently recommended in pregnant females (Rademaker 2018).

A registry is available for women exposed to apremilast during pregnancy (877-311-8972).

Aprepitant (ap RE pi tant)

Brand Names: US Cinvanti; Emend; Emend Tri-Pack

Brand Names: Canada Emend; Emend Tri-Pack

Pharmacologic Category Antiemetic; Substance P/ Neurokinin 1 Receptor Antagonist

Use

IV (Cinvanti):

Prevention of chemotherapy-induced nausea and vomiting:

Prevention of acute and delayed nausea and vomiting associated with initial and repeat courses of **highly** emetogenic chemotherapy, including high-dose cisplatin, as single-dose aprepitant regimen (in combination with other antiemetics) in adults.

Prevention of delayed nausea and vomiting associated with initial and repeat courses of **moderately** emetogenic chemotherapy as a single-dose aprepitant regimen (in combination with other antiemetics) in adults.

Prevention of nausea and vomiting associated with initial and repeat courses of **moderately** emetogenic chemotherapy as a 3-day aprepitant regimen (in combination with other antiemetics) in adults.

Oral (Emend oral):

Prevention of chemotherapy-induced nausea and vomiting:

Prevention of acute and delayed nausea and vomiting associated with **highly** emetogenic chemotherapy (initial and repeat courses; in combination with other antiemetics) in patients ≥12 years (capsules) and in patients ≥6 months (oral suspension).

Prevention of nausea and vomiting associated with **moderately** emetogenic chemotherapy (initial and repeat courses; in combination with other antiemetics) in patients ≥12 years (capsules) and in patients ≥6 months (oral suspension).

Note: Generic aprepitant capsules are only approved for use in adults.

Postoperative nausea and vomiting (generic capsules): Prevention of postoperative nausea and vomiting (PONV) in adults. **Note:** The PONV indication was removed from the Emend capsule US prescribing information (in September 2019); however, it remains in the labeling for generic aprepitant capsules.

Limitations of use: Aprepitant has not been studied for the management of existing nausea and vomiting. Chronic, continuous administration is not recommended (has not been studied and chronic use may alter aprepitant's drug interaction profile).

Local Anesthetic/Vasoconstrictor Precautions No information available to require special precautions

Effects on Dental Treatment Key adverse event(s) related to dental treatment: Hiccups, stomatitis, and mucous membrane disorder.

Effects on Bleeding No information available to require special precautions

Adverse Reactions Adverse reactions may be reported in combination with other antiemetic agents. As reported for highly emetogenic cancer chemotherapy or moderately emetogenic cancer chemotherapy, unless otherwise noted as reported for postoperative nausea and vomiting (PONV).

>10%:

Central nervous system: Fatigue (adults: 1% to 13%; children & adolescents: 5%)

Hematologic & oncologic: Neutropenia (children & adolescents: 13%; adults: <3%)

1% to 10%:

Cardiovascular: Hypotension (PONV: 6%), bradycardia (PONV: <3%), flushing (<3%), palpitations (<3%), peripheral edema (<3%), syncope (PONV: <3%)

Central nervous system: Headache (children & adolescents: 9%), dizziness (<3% to 5%), anxiety (<3%), hypoesthesia (PONV: <3%), hypothermia (PONV: <3%), malaise (<3%), peripheral neuropathy (<3%), abnormal behavior (children & adolescents: 2%), agitation (children & adolescents: 2%)

Dermatologic: Pruritus (3%), alopecia (<3%), hyperhidrosis (<3%), skin rash (<3%), urticaria (<3%)

Endocrine & metabolic: Dehydration (≤3%), decreased serum albumin (PONV: <3%), decreased serum potassium (PONV: <3%), decreased serum sodium (<3%), hot flash (<3), hypokalemia (<3%), hypovolemia (PONV: <3%), increased serum glucose (PONV: <3%), weight loss (<3%)

Gastrointestinal: Constipation (PONV: ≤9%), diarrhea (6% to 9%), dyspepsia (≤7%), abdominal pain (≤6%), hiccups (4% to 5%), decreased appetite (<3% to 5%), dysgeusia (<3%), eructation (<3%), flatulence (<3%), gastritis (<3%), gastroesophageal reflux disease (<3%), nausea (<3%), vomiting (<3%), xerostomia (<3%)

Genitourinary: Proteinuria (<3%)

Hematologic & oncologic: Decreased hemoglobin (children & adolescents: 5%), decreased white blood cell count (≤4%), anemia (<3%), febrile neutropenia (<3%), hematoma (PONV: <3%), thrombocytopenia (<3%)

Hepatic: Increased serum alanine aminotransferase (3%), increased serum alkaline phosphatase (<3%), increased serum aspartate aminotransferase (<3%), increased serum bilirubin (PONV: <3%)

Infection: Candidiasis (<3%), postoperative infection (PONV: <3%)

Local: Induration at injection site (3%), inflammation at injection site (3%), infusion site reaction (3%)

Neuromuscular & skeletal: Asthenia (≤7%), musculoskeletal pain (<3%)

Renal: Increased blood urea nitrogen (<3%)

Respiratory: Cough (<3% to 5%), dyspnea (<3%), hypoxia (PONV: <3%), oropharyngeal pain (<3%), pharyngitis (<3%), respiratory depression (PONV: <3%)

Miscellaneous: Wound dehiscence (PONV: <3%)

<1%, postmarketing, and/or case reports: Abdominal distention, abnormal dreams, abnormal gait, acne vulgaris, anaphylaxis, angioedema, anxiety, cardiac disease, chest discomfort, chills, cognitive dysfunction, conjunctivitis, decreased neutrophils, disorientation, drowsiness, dysfunction, dysuria, edema, epigastric distress, euphoria, hematuria,

hyperglycemia, hypersensitivity reaction, hyponatremia, increased thirst, lethargy, muscle cramps, myalgia, neutropenic enterocolitis, oily skin, perforated duodenal ulcer, pollakiuria, polyuria, polydipsia, post nasal drip, skin lesion, skin photosensitivity, sneezing, staphylococcal infection, Stevens-Johnson syndrome, stomatitis, throat irritation, tinnitus, toxic epidermal necrolysis, weight gain

Mechanism of Action Aprepitant prevents acute and delayed vomiting by inhibiting the substance P/neurokinin 1 (NK_1) receptor; augments the antiemetic activity of 5-HT_3 receptor antagonists and corticosteroids to inhibit acute and delayed phases of chemotherapy-induced emesis.

Pharmacodynamics/Kinetics

Half-life Elimination Terminal: IV, Oral: ~9 to 13 hours

Time to Peak Plasma: Pediatric: Capsule: ~4 hours; Suspension ~6 hours; Adults: 40 mg: ~3 hours; 125 mg followed by 80 mg for 2 days: ~4 hours

Reproductive Considerations

Efficacy of hormonal contraceptive may be reduced during and for 28 days following the last aprepitant dose; alternative or additional effective methods of contraception should be used both during treatment with aprepitant and for at least 1 month following the last aprepitant dose.

Pregnancy Considerations

The injection formulation contains ethanol; use should be avoided in females who are pregnant.

- **Apri** *see* Ethinyl Estradiol and Desogestrel *on page 609*
- **Apriso** *see* Mesalamine *on page 980*
- **Aptensio XR** *see* Methylphenidate *on page 997*
- **Aptiom** *see* Eslicarbazepine *on page 592*
- **Aptivus** *see* Tipranavir *on page 1452*
- **Aquanil HC [OTC]** *see* Hydrocortisone (Topical) *on page 775*
- **Aquasol A** *see* Vitamin A *on page 1549*
- **Aqueous Crystalline Penicillin G** *see* Penicillin G (Parenteral/Aqueous) *on page 1209*
- **Aqueous Procaine Penicillin G** *see* Penicillin G Procaine *on page 1210*
- **Aqueous Vitamin D [OTC]** *see* Cholecalciferol *on page 344*
- **Aqueous Vitamin E [OTC]** *see* Vitamin E (Systemic) *on page 1549*
- **Aquoral** *see* Saliva Substitute *on page 1354*
- **Ara-C** *see* Cytarabine (Conventional) *on page 424*
- **Arabinosylcytosine** *see* Cytarabine (Conventional) *on page 424*
- **Arakoda** *see* Tafenoquine *on page 1402*
- **Aranelle** *see* Ethinyl Estradiol and Norethindrone *on page 614*
- **Aranesp (Albumin Free)** *see* Darbepoetin Alfa *on page 440*
- **Arava** *see* Leflunomide *on page 882*
- **Arazlo** *see* Tazarotene *on page 1408*
- **Arbinoxa [DSC]** *see* Carbinoxamine *on page 292*
- **Arcapta Neohaler** *see* Indacaterol *on page 807*
- **Arestin** *see* Minocycline Hydrochloride (Periodontal) *on page 1036*

Arformoterol (ar for MOE ter ol)

Related Information

Respiratory Diseases *on page 1680*

Brand Names: US Brovana

Pharmacologic Category $Beta_2$-Adrenergic Agonist; $Beta_2$-Adrenergic Agonist, Long-Acting

Use Chronic obstructive pulmonary disease: Long-term maintenance treatment of bronchoconstriction in patients with chronic obstructive pulmonary disease (COPD), including chronic bronchitis and emphysema

Local Anesthetic/Vasoconstrictor Precautions

Arformoterol is one of the drugs confirmed to prolong the QT interval and is accepted as having a risk of causing torsade de pointes. The risk of drug-induced torsade de pointes is extremely low when a single QT interval prolonging drug is prescribed. In terms of epinephrine, it is not known what effect vasoconstrictors in the local anesthetic regimen will have in patients with a known history of congenital prolonged QT interval or in patients taking any medication that prolongs the QT interval. Until more information is obtained, it is suggested that the clinician consult with the physician prior to the use of a vasoconstrictor in suspected patients, and that the vasoconstrictor (epinephrine, mepivacaine and levonordefrin [Carbocaine 2% with Neo-Cobefrin]) be used with caution.

Effects on Dental Treatment Key adverse event(s) related to dental treatment: Occurrence of oral candidiasis

Effects on Bleeding No information available to require special precautions

Adverse Reactions

2% to 10%:

Cardiovascular: Chest pain (7%), peripheral edema (3%)

Central nervous system: Pain (8%)

Dermatologic: Skin rash (4%)

Gastrointestinal: Diarrhea (6%)

Neuromuscular & skeletal: Back pain (6%), leg cramps (4%)

Respiratory: Dyspnea (4%), sinusitis (5%), flu-like symptoms (3%), respiratory congestion (2%)

<2%: Abscess, agitation, arteriosclerosis, arthralgia, arthritis, atrial flutter, atrioventricular block, bone disease, calcium crystalluria, cardiac failure, cerebral infarction, constipation, cystitis, decreased glucose tolerance, dehydration, digitalis intoxication, drowsiness, ECG changes, edema, fever, gastritis, glaucoma, glycosuria, gout, heart block, hematuria, hernia, hyperglycemia, hyperlipidemia, hypersensitivity reaction, hypoglycemia, hypokalemia, hypokinesia, inversion T wave on ECG, lung carcinoma, melena, myocardial infarction, neck stiffness, neoplasm, nephrolithiasis, nocturia, oral candidiasis, paradoxical bronchospasm, paralysis, paresthesia (circumoral), pelvic pain, periodontal abscess, prolonged QT interval on ECG, prostate specific antigen increase, pyuria, rectal hemorrhage, retroperitoneal hemorrhage, rheumatoid arthritis, skin discoloration, skin hypertrophy, supraventricular tachycardia, tendinous contracture, tremor, urinary tract abnormality, urine abnormality, viral infection, visual disturbance, voice disorder, xeroderma

Mechanism of Action Arformoterol, the (R,R)-enantiomer of the racemic formoterol, is a long-acting $beta_2$-agonist that relaxes bronchial smooth muscle by selective action on $beta_2$-receptors with little effect on cardiovascular system.

Pharmacodynamics/Kinetics

Onset of Action 7-20 minutes; Peak effect: 1-3 hours

Half-life Elimination 26 hours

Time to Peak 0.5-3 hours

Pregnancy Considerations

Beta-agonists may interfere with uterine contractility if administered during labor.

Arformoterol in an enantiomer of formoterol. Refer to the Formoterol monograph for information.

- **Arformoterol Tartrate** *see* Arformoterol *on page 163*

Argatroban (ar GA troh ban)

Related Information

Cardiovascular Diseases *on page 1654*

Pharmacologic Category Anticoagulant; Anticoagulant, Direct Thrombin Inhibitor

Use

Heparin-induced thrombocytopenia: Prophylaxis or treatment of thrombosis in adults with heparin-induced thrombocytopenia (HIT).

Percutaneous coronary intervention: As an anticoagulant for percutaneous coronary intervention (PCI) in adults who have or are at risk of developing HIT.

Local Anesthetic/Vasoconstrictor Precautions No information available to require special precautions

Effects on Dental Treatment Key adverse event(s) related to dental treatment: Bleeding is a potential adverse effect of argatroban during dental surgery; it is unlikely that ambulatory patients presenting for dental treatment will be taking intravenous anticoagulant therapy. See Effects on Bleeding.

Effects on Bleeding As with all anticoagulants, bleeding is a potential adverse effect of argatroban during dental surgery; risk is dependent on multiple variables, including the intensity of anticoagulation and patient susceptibility. Medical consult is suggested. It is unlikely that ambulatory patients presenting for dental treatment will be taking intravenous anticoagulant therapy such as argatroban.

Adverse Reactions As with all anticoagulants, bleeding is the major adverse effect of argatroban. Hemorrhage may occur at virtually any site. Risk is dependent on multiple variables, including the intensity of anticoagulation and patient susceptibility.

>10%:

Cardiovascular: Chest pain (PCI related: <1% to 15%), hypotension (7% to 11%)

Genitourinary: Genitourinary tract hemorrhage (including hematuria; major: <1%; minor: 2% to 12%)

1% to 10%:

Cardiovascular: Vasodilation (1% to 10%), cardiac arrest (6%), bradycardia (5%), ventricular tachycardia (5%), myocardial infarction (PCI: 4%), angina pectoris (2%), coronary occlusion (2%), ischemic heart disease (2%), thrombosis (<1% to 2%)

Central nervous system: Headache (5%), pain (5%), intracranial hemorrhage (1% to 4%)

Dermatologic: Dermatological reaction (bullous eruption, rash; 1% to <10%)

Gastrointestinal: Nausea (5% to 7%), diarrhea (6%), vomiting (4% to 6%), abdominal pain (3% to 4%), gastrointestinal hemorrhage (major: <1% to 3%; minor: 3%)

Hematologic & oncologic: Decreased hematocrit (minor: ≤10%; major: <1%), decreased hemoglobin (minor: ≤10%; major: <1%; ≥2 g/dL), groin bleeding (5%), brachial bleeding (2%), minor hemorrhage (CABG related: 2%)

Neuromuscular & skeletal: Back pain (PCI related: 8%)

Respiratory: Dyspnea (10%), cough (3% to 10%), hemoptysis (minor: ≤1% to 3%)

Miscellaneous: Fever (<1% to 7%)

<1% (Limited to important or life-threatening): Aortic valve stenosis, bleeding at injection site (or access site; minor), cerebrovascular disease, gastroesophageal reflux disease, hypersensitivity reaction, local hemorrhage (limb and below-the-knee stump), pulmonary edema, retroperitoneal bleeding

Mechanism of Action A direct, highly-selective thrombin inhibitor. Reversibly binds to the active thrombin site of free and clot-associated thrombin. Inhibits fibrin formation; activation of coagulation factors V, VIII, and XIII; activation of protein C; and platelet aggregation.

Pharmacodynamics/Kinetics

Onset of Action Immediate

Half-life Elimination 39 to 51 minutes; Hepatic impairment: 181 minutes

Time to Peak Steady-state: 1 to 3 hours

Pregnancy Considerations Information related to argatroban in pregnancy is limited. Use of parenteral direct thrombin inhibitors in pregnancy should be limited to those women who have severe allergic reactions to heparin, including heparin-induced thrombocytopenia, and who cannot receive danaparoid (Guyatt 2012).

- **Arginine Vasopressin** *see* Vasopressin *on page 1535*
- **8-Arginine Vasopressin** *see* Vasopressin *on page 1535*
- **Aricept** *see* Donepezil *on page 512*
- **Arikayce** *see* Amikacin (Oral Inhalation) *on page 115*
- **Arimidex** *see* Anastrozole *on page 150*

ARIPiprazole (ay ri PIP ray zole)

Brand Names: US Abilify; Abilify Maintena; Abilify MyCite

Brand Names: Canada Abilify; Abilify Maintena; APO-ARIPiprazole; Auro-ARIPiprazole; MINT-Aripiprazole; PMS-ARIPiprazole; RIVA-ARIPiprazole; SANDOZ ARIPiprazole; TEVA-ARIPiprazole

Pharmacologic Category Second Generation (Atypical) Antipsychotic

Use

Oral:

Bipolar disorder: As monotherapy or as an adjunct to lithium or valproate for acute treatment of manic or mixed episodes associated with bipolar disorder and maintenance treatment (tablet with sensor only) of bipolar disorder.

Irritability associated with autistic disorder: Treatment of irritability associated with autistic disorder (tablet, orally disintegrating tablet, and oral solution only) in children and adolescents.

Major depressive disorder (unipolar), treatment resistant: Adjunctive treatment of unipolar major depressive disorder in patients with an inadequate response to prior antidepressant therapy.

Schizophrenia: Treatment of schizophrenia.

Tourette disorder: Treatment of Tourette disorder (tablet, orally disintegrating tablet, and oral solution only) in children and adolescents.

Injection: Extended release:

Bipolar disorder: Maintenance monotherapy treatment of bipolar disorder.

Schizophrenia: Treatment of schizophrenia.

Local Anesthetic/Vasoconstrictor Precautions No information available to require special precautions

Effects on Dental Treatment Key adverse event(s) related to dental treatment: Infrequent occurrence of toothache, xerostomia, and changes in salivation including drooling (normal salivary flow resumes upon discontinuation) have been reported. Rare occurrence of bruxism, dysgeusia, dystonia (oromandibular), tongue tremors, and trismus have also been reported. For additional rare considerations, see Dental Health Professional Considerations.

Effects on Bleeding No information available to require special precautions

Adverse Reactions Unless otherwise noted, frequency of adverse reactions is shown as reported for adult patients receiving aripiprazole monotherapy. Spectrum and incidence of adverse effects similar in children; exceptions noted when incidence is much higher in children.

IM:

>10%:

Endocrine & metabolic: Decreased HDL cholesterol (14%), increased LDL cholesterol (10% to 14%), increased serum cholesterol (4% to 22%), increased serum triglycerides (7% to 27%), weight gain (17% to 22%)

Nervous system: Akathisia (dose-related; 2% to 12%), headache (12%)

1% to 10%:

Cardiovascular: Orthostatic hypotension (3%), tachycardia (≤2%)

Endocrine & metabolic: Increased serum glucose (8%), weight loss (4%)

Gastrointestinal: Abdominal distress (2%), constipation (10%), diarrhea (3%), nausea (9%), vomiting (3%), xerostomia (4%)

Hematologic & oncologic: Neutropenia (6%)

Local: Injection site reaction (≤1%; including erythema, induration, inflammation, hemorrhage, pruritus, rash, swelling), pain at injection site (5%)

Nervous system: Anxiety (≥1%), dizziness (4% to 8%), drowsiness (7% to 9%), dystonia (2%), extrapyramidal reaction (10%), fatigue (dose-related; 1% to 2%), insomnia (≥1%), sedated state (3% to 5%), restlessness (≥1%)

Neuromuscular & skeletal: Arthralgia (4%), back pain (4%), musculoskeletal pain (3%), myalgia (4%), tremor (dose-related; 3%)

Respiratory: Nasal congestion (2%), upper respiratory tract infection (4%)

<1%:

Cardiovascular: Abnormal T waves on ECG, bradycardia, chest discomfort, hypertension, increased blood pressure, presyncope, prolonged QT interval on ECG, sinus tachycardia

Endocrine & metabolic: Decreased serum cholesterol, decreased serum triglycerides, glycosuria, hyperprolactinemia, increased libido, obesity

Gastrointestinal: Bruxism, decreased appetite, dysgeusia, dyspepsia, hyperinsulinism, swollen tongue, upper abdominal pain

Genitourinary: Pollakiuria, urinary incontinence

Hematologic & oncologic: Thrombocytopenia

Hepatic: Abnormal hepatic function tests, hepatotoxicity

Hypersensitivity: Hypersensitivity reaction

Nervous system: Abnormal gait, aggressive behavior, agitation, delayed ejaculation, dystonia (oromandibular), hypersomnia, irritability, lethargy, memory impairment, panic attack, psychotic reaction, seizure, suicidal ideation, syncope, trismus

Neuromuscular & skeletal: Bradykinesia, increased creatinine phosphokinase in blood specimen, joint stiffness, muscle twitching, rhabdomyolysis

Ophthalmic: Blurred vision, oculogyric crisis

Respiratory: Nasopharyngitis

Miscellaneous: Fever

Oral:

>10%:

Endocrine & metabolic: Increased serum glucose (adults: 18%; children and adolescents: 3% to 5%), weight gain (children and adolescents: 3% to 26%; adults: 2% to 8%)

Gastrointestinal: Constipation (adults: 11%; children and adolescents: 2%), nausea (8% to 15%), vomiting (8% to 14%)

Local: Application site rash (Mycite patch: 12%)

Nervous system: Agitation (19%), akathisia (dose-related; 2% to 13%), anxiety (17%), drowsiness (dose-related; children and adolescents: 10% to 26%; adults: 5% to 13%), extrapyramidal reaction (dose-related; children and adolescents: 6% to 27%; adults: 5% to 16%), fatigue (dose-related; children and adolescents: 4% to 22%; adults: 6%), headache (adults: 27%; children and adolescents: 10% to 12%), sedated state (dose-related; children and adolescents: 9% to 21%; adults: 3% to 11%), insomnia (18%)

Neuromuscular & skeletal: Tremor (dose-related; 5% to 12%)

1% to 10%:

Cardiovascular: Orthostatic hypotension (≤4%)

Dermatologic: Skin rash (children and adolescents: ≤2%)

Endocrine & metabolic: Decreased HDL cholesterol (children and adolescents: 4%), increased serum cholesterol (children and adolescents: 1%), increased serum triglycerides (5% to 10%), weight loss (≥1%)

Gastrointestinal: Abdominal distress (2% to 3%), anorexia, decreased appetite (children and adolescents: 5% to 7%), diarrhea (children and adolescents: 4%), dyspepsia (9%), increased appetite (children and adolescents: 7%), sialorrhea (dose-related; children and adolescents; 4% to 8%), stomach discomfort (3%), upper abdominal pain (children and adolescents: 3%), xerostomia (5%)

Genitourinary: Urinary incontinence (≥1%)

Nervous system: Dizziness (3% to 10%), drooling (children and adolescents: 3% to 9%), dystonia (2%), irritability (children and adolescents: 2%), lethargy (adults: 5%; children and adolescents: 3% to 5%), pain (3%), restlessness (5% to 6%)

Neuromuscular & skeletal: Asthenia (≥1%), limb pain (4%), muscle rigidity (children and adolescents: 2%), muscle spasm (2%), myalgia (2%), stiffness (2% to 4%)

Ophthalmic: Blurred vision (3% to 8%)

Respiratory: Cough (3%), epistaxis (children and adolescents: 2%), nasopharyngitis (children and adolescents: 6% to 9%), pharyngolaryngeal pain (3%)

Miscellaneous: Fever (children and adolescents: 4% to 9%)

<1%:

Cardiovascular: Acute myocardial infarction, angina pectoris, atrial fibrillation, atrial flutter, atrioventricular block, bradycardia, chest pain, choreoathetosis, facial edema, hypertension, hypotension, ischemic heart disease, palpitations, peripheral edema, prolonged QT interval on ECG

Dermatologic: Alopecia, hyperhidrosis, pruritus, skin photosensitivity, urticaria

Endocrine & metabolic: Amenorrhea, change in libido, gynecomastia, hirsutism (children and adolescents), hypoglycemia, hypokalemia, hyponatremia, increased gamma-glutamyl transferase, increased lactate dehydrogenase, increased serum prolactin, menstrual disease

Gastrointestinal: Gastroesophageal reflux disease, tongue spasm (children and adolescents)

Genitourinary: Erectile dysfunction, mastalgia, nocturia, priapism, urinary retention

Hematologic & oncologic: Elevated glycosylated hemoglobin, thrombocytopenia

Hepatic: Hepatitis, increased liver enzymes, increased serum bilirubin, jaundice

Hypersensitivity: Hypersensitivity reaction

Nervous system: Aggressive behavior, anorgasmia, ataxia, catatonia, cogwheel rigidity, delirium, hypertonia, impaired mobility, memory impairment, myasthenia, myoclonus, parkinsonism, seizure, sleep talking (children and adolescents), somnambulism, speech disturbance, tic disorder

Neuromuscular & skeletal: Akinesia, bradykinesia, hypokinesia, rhabdomyolysis

Ophthalmic: Diplopia, oculogyric crisis, photophobia

Renal: Increased blood urea nitrogen, increased creatinine clearance

Respiratory: Dyspnea, nasal congestion

Postmarketing (any indication):

Cardiovascular: Cerebrovascular accident, transient ischemic attacks

Endocrine & metabolic: Diabetic ketoacidosis, hyperglycemia

Gastrointestinal: Dysphagia

Hematologic & oncologic: Agranulocytosis, leukopenia, neutropenia

Hypersensitivity: Anaphylaxis, angioedema

Immunologic: Drug reaction with eosinophilia and systemic symptoms

Nervous system: Impulse control disorder (including pathological gambling, hypersexuality, increased shopping or eating), neuroleptic malignant syndrome, sleep apnea (obstructive) (Health Canada, August 16, 2016; Shirani 2011), suicidal ideation, suicidal tendencies, syncope, tardive dyskinesia

Mechanism of Action Aripiprazole is a quinolinone antipsychotic which exhibits high affinity for D_2, D_3, 5-HT_{1A}, and 5-HT_{2A} receptors; moderate affinity for D_4, 5-HT_{2C}, 5-HT_7, $alpha_1$ adrenergic, and H_1 receptors. It also possesses moderate affinity for the serotonin reuptake transporter; has no affinity for muscarinic (cholinergic) receptors. Aripiprazole functions as a partial agonist at the D_2 and 5-HT_{1A} receptors, and as an antagonist at the 5-HT_{2A} receptor (de Bartolomeis 2015).

Pharmacodynamics/Kinetics

Onset of Action Initial: 1 to 3 weeks

Half-life Elimination

Aripiprazole: 75 hours; dehydro-aripiprazole: 94 hours; IM, extended release (terminal): ~30 to 47 days (dose-dependent)

CYP2D6 poor metabolizers: Aripiprazole: 146 hours

Time to Peak Plasma:

IM: Extended release (after multiple doses): 4 days (deltoid administration); 5 to 7 days (gluteal administration).

Tablet: 3 to 5 hours; high-fat meals delay time to peak by 3 hours for aripiprazole and 12 hours for dehydro-aripiprazole.

Reproductive Considerations

If treatment is needed in a woman planning a pregnancy, use of an agent other than aripiprazole is preferred (Larsen 2015).

Pregnancy Considerations

Aripiprazole crosses the placenta; aripiprazole and dehydro-aripiprazole can be detected in the cord blood at delivery (Nguyen 2011; Watanabe 2011).

Antipsychotic use during the third trimester of pregnancy has a risk for abnormal muscle movements (extrapyramidal symptoms [EPS]) and/or withdrawal symptoms in newborns following delivery. Symptoms in the newborn may include agitation, feeding disorder, hypertonia, hypotonia, respiratory distress, somnolence, and tremor; these effects may be self-limiting or require hospitalization.

Treatment algorithms have been developed by the ACOG and the APA for the management of depression in women prior to conception and during pregnancy (Yonkers 2009). The ACOG recommends that therapy during pregnancy be individualized; treatment with psychiatric medications during pregnancy should incorporate the clinical expertise of the mental health clinician, obstetrician, primary health care provider, and pediatrician. Safety data related to atypical antipsychotics during pregnancy is limited, as such, routine use is not recommended. However, if a woman is inadvertently exposed to an atypical antipsychotic while pregnant, continuing therapy may be preferable to switching to an agent that the fetus has not yet been exposed to; consider risk:benefit (ACOG 2008). If treatment is initiated during pregnancy, use of an agent other than aripiprazole is preferred (Larsen 2015).

Health care providers are encouraged to enroll women exposed to aripiprazole during pregnancy in the National Pregnancy Registry for Atypical Antipsychotics (866-961-2388 or http://www.womensmentalhealth.org/clinical-and-research-programs/pregnancyregistry/).

Product Availability

Abilify immediate-release injection (9.75 mg/1.3 mL) has been discontinued in the US for more than 1 year.

Dental Health Professional Considerations Aripiprazole works differently from the classic antipsychotics, such as chlorpromazine, in that it does not appear to block central dopaminergic receptors, but rather seems to be a stabilizer of dopamine-serotonin central systems. The risk of extrapyramidal reactions such as pseudoparkinsonism, acute dystonic reactions, akathisia, and tardive dyskinesia are low and the frequencies reported are similar to placebo. Aripiprazole may be associated with neuroleptic malignant syndrome (NMS).

ARIPiprazole Lauroxil (ay ri PIP ray zole lawr OX il)

Brand Names: US Aristada; Aristada Initio

Pharmacologic Category Second Generation (Atypical) Antipsychotic

Use

Schizophrenia: Treatment of schizophrenia in adults.

Limitations of use: The **675 mg** strength aripiprazole lauroxil nanocrystal dispersion (Aristada Initio) is only to be used as a single dose in combination with oral aripiprazole for initiation of long-term treatment with aripiprazole lauroxil (Aristada) or as a single dose to reinitiate treatment after a missed dose of aripiprazole lauroxil (Aristada). It is not intended for repeat dosing.

Local Anesthetic/Vasoconstrictor Precautions No information available to require special precautions.

Effects on Dental Treatment Key adverse event(s) related to dental treatment: Infrequent occurrence of headache, xerostomia, and changes in salivation including drooling (normal salivary flow resumes upon discontinuation) have been reported. Rare occurrence of bruxism, dysgeusia, dystonia (oromandibular), tongue tremors, trismus, and Parkinson-like syndrome/restlessness have also been reported. Patients on higher doses may experience orthostatic hypotension as they stand up after treatment; especially if lying in dental chair for extended periods of time. Use caution with sudden changes in position during and after dental treatment. For additional rare considerations, see Dental Health Professional Considerations.

Effects on Bleeding No information available to require special precautions

Adverse Reactions

>10%: Central nervous system: Akathisia (11%)

1% to 10%:

- Central nervous system: Headache (5%), parkinsonian-like syndrome (4%), insomnia (3% to 4%), restlessness (3%), dystonia (2%)
- Endocrine & metabolic: Weight gain (2%; ≥7% increase: 9% to 10%)
- Local: Pain at injection site (3% to 4%)
- Neuromuscular & skeletal: Increased creatine phosphokinase (1% to 2%)

Frequency not defined:

- Cardiovascular: Angina pectoris, palpitations, tachycardia
- Central nervous system: Anxiety, dizziness, myasthenia
- Gastrointestinal: Constipation, xerostomia
- Neuromuscular & skeletal: Asthenia

<1%, postmarketing, and/or case reports: Erythema at injection site, impulse control disorder (including compulsive shopping, intense gambling urges, binge eating, and hypersexuality), induration at injection site, orthostatic hypotension (patient taking 882 mg aripiprazole lauroxil), swelling at injection site

Mechanism of Action Aripiprazole lauroxil is a prodrug of aripiprazole. Following intramuscular injection, aripiprazole lauroxil is likely converted by enzyme-mediated hydrolysis to N-hydroxymethyl aripiprazole, which is then hydrolyzed to aripiprazole. Aripiprazole is a quinolinone antipsychotic that exhibits high affinity for D_2, D_3, 5-HT_{1A}, and 5-HT_{2A} receptors; moderate affinity for D_4, 5-HT_{2C}, 5-HT_7, $alpha_1$ adrenergic, and H_1 receptors. It also possesses moderate affinity for the serotonin reuptake transporter; has no affinity for muscarinic (cholinergic) receptors. Aripiprazole functions as a partial agonist at the D_2 and 5-HT_{1A} receptors, and as an antagonist at the 5-HT_{2A} receptor (de Bartolomeis 2015).

Pharmacodynamics/Kinetics

Onset of Action

Aristada: 5 to 6 days following injection; within 4 days following injection when administered concomitantly with oral aripiprazole.

Aristada Initio (675 mg strength nanocrystal dispersion): Reaches systemic circulation on day of injection; reaches clinically relevant serum concentrations 4 days following injection when administered concomitantly with oral aripiprazole 30 mg.

Duration of Action Aristada: 36 days following appearance in the systemic circulation.

Half-life Elimination

Aristada: 53.9 to 57.2 days.

Aristada Initio (675 mg strength nanocrystal dispersion): 15 to 18 days.

Time to Peak Serum: Aristada Initio (675 mg strength nanocrystal dispersion): 16 to 35 days (median 27 days).

Pregnancy Considerations

Aripiprazole crosses the placenta; aripiprazole and dehydro-aripiprazole can be detected in the cord blood at delivery (Nguyen 2011; Watanabe 2011).

Antipsychotic use during the third trimester of pregnancy has a risk for abnormal muscle movements (extrapyramidal symptoms [EPS]) and/or withdrawal symptoms in newborns following delivery. Symptoms in the newborn may include agitation, feeding disorder, hypertonia, hypotonia, respiratory distress, somnolence, and tremor; these effects may be self-limiting or require hospitalization.

Data collection to monitor pregnancy and infant outcomes following exposure to aripiprazole lauroxil is ongoing. Health care providers are encouraged to enroll women exposed to aripiprazole lauroxil during pregnancy in the National Pregnancy Registry for Atypical Antipsychotics at 1-866-961-2388 or visit http://womensmentalhealth.org/clinical-and-research-programs/pregnancyregistry.

Dental Health Professional Considerations Aripiprazole Lauroxil works differently from the classic antipsychotics, such as chlorpromazine, in that it does not appear to block central dopaminergic receptors, but rather seems to be a stabilizer of dopamine-serotonin central systems. The risk of extrapyramidal reactions such as pseudoparkinsonism, acute dystonic reactions, akathisia, and tardive dyskinesia are low and the frequencies reported are similar to placebo. Aripiprazole may be associated with neuroleptic malignant syndrome (NMS).

- ◆ **Aristada** *see* ARIPiprazole Lauroxil *on page 167*
- ◆ **Aristada Initio** *see* ARIPiprazole Lauroxil *on page 167*
- ◆ **Arixtra** *see* Fondaparinux *on page 710*

Armodafinil (ar moe DAF i nil)

Brand Names: US Nuvigil

Pharmacologic Category Central Nervous System Stimulant

Use

Narcolepsy: To improve wakefulness in patients with excessive sleepiness associated with narcolepsy.

Obstructive sleep apnea: To improve wakefulness in patients with excessive sleepiness associated with obstructive sleep apnea (OSA).

Limitations of use: In OSA, armodafinil is indicated to treat excessive sleepiness and not as treatment for the underlying obstruction. If continuous positive airway pressure (CPAP) is the treatment of choice for a patient, a maximal effort to treat with CPAP for an adequate period of time should be made prior to initiating armodafinil for excessive sleepiness.

Shift-work disorder: To improve wakefulness in patients with excessive sleepiness associated with shift-work disorder.

Local Anesthetic/Vasoconstrictor Precautions Use vasoconstrictor with caution. Patients may experience heart palpitations and increased heart rate when taking armodafinil.

Effects on Dental Treatment Key adverse event(s) related to dental treatment: Armodafinil causes tachycardia, increases in blood pressure, and palpitations. Consider monitoring blood pressure prior to using local anesthetic with a vasoconstrictor. Symptoms associated with bruxism have been observed in some patients.

Effects on Bleeding No information available to require special precautions

Adverse Reactions

>10%: Central nervous system: Headache (14% to 23%; dose related)

1% to 10%:

Cardiovascular: Palpitations (2%), increased heart rate (1%)

Central nervous system: Insomnia (4% to 6%; dose related), dizziness (5%), anxiety (4%), depression (1% to 3%; dose related), fatigue (2%), agitation (1%), depressed mood (1%), lack of concentration (1%), migraine (1%), nervousness (1%), pain (1%), paresthesia (1%)

Dermatologic: Skin rash (1% to 4%; dose related), contact dermatitis (1%), diaphoresis (1%)

Endocrine & metabolic: Increased gamma-glutamyl transferase (1%), increased thirst (1%)

Gastrointestinal: Nausea (6% to 9%; dose related), xerostomia (2% to 7%; dose related), diarrhea (4%), dyspepsia (2%), upper abdominal pain (2%), anorexia (1%), constipation (1%), decreased appetite (1%), loose stools (1%), vomiting (1%)

Hypersensitivity: Seasonal allergy (1%)

Neuromuscular & skeletal: Tremor (1%)

Renal: Polyuria (1%)

Respiratory: Dyspnea (1%), flu-like symptoms (1%)

Miscellaneous: Fever (1%)

<1%, postmarketing, and/or case reports: Anaphylaxis, angioedema, DRESS syndrome, hypersensitivity reaction (including bronchospasm, dysphagia), hypouricemia, increased liver enzymes, increased serum alkaline phosphatase, irritability, multi-organ hypersensitivity, oral mucosa changes (including blistering, sores, ulceration), pancytopenia, skin changes (including blistering, sores, ulceration), Stevens-Johnson syndrome, suicidal ideation, systolic hypertension, toxic epidermal necrolysis

Mechanism of Action The exact mechanism of action of armodafinil is unknown. It is the R-enantiomer of modafinil. Armodafinil binds to the dopamine transporter and inhibits dopamine reuptake, which may result in increased extracellular dopamine levels in the brain. However, it does not appear to be a dopamine receptor agonist and also does not appear to bind to or inhibit the most common receptors or enzymes that are relevant for sleep/wake regulation.

Pharmacodynamics/Kinetics

Half-life Elimination ~15 hours

Time to Peak 2 hours (fasted)

Reproductive Considerations Efficacy of steroidal contraceptives (including depot and implantable contraceptives) may be decreased; alternate means of effective contraception or the addition of a barrier method should be considered during armodafinil therapy and for 1 month after armodafinil is discontinued.

Pregnancy Considerations

Preliminary data from the Nuvigil/Provigil pregnancy registry suggest an increased risk of major fetal congenital malformations, including congenital cardiac anomalies (Alertec Canadian product monograph 2019). Intrauterine growth restriction and spontaneous abortion have been reported in association with armodafinil.

A pregnancy registry has been established for patients exposed to armodafinil; healthcare providers are encouraged to register pregnant patients or pregnant females may register themselves by calling 1-866-404-4106.

Controlled Substance C-IV

- **ArmonAir Digihaler** *see* Fluticasone (Oral Inhalation) *on page 703*
- **ArmonAir RespiClick** *see* Fluticasone (Oral Inhalation) *on page 703*
- **ArmonAir RespiClick 55 [DSC]** *see* Fluticasone (Oral Inhalation) *on page 703*
- **ArmonAir RespiClick 113 [DSC]** *see* Fluticasone (Oral Inhalation) *on page 703*
- **ArmonAir RespiClick 232 [DSC]** *see* Fluticasone (Oral Inhalation) *on page 703*
- **Armour Thyroid** *see* Thyroid, Desiccated *on page 1442*
- **ARN-509** *see* Apalutamide *on page 158*
- **Arnuity Ellipta** *see* Fluticasone (Oral Inhalation) *on page 703*
- **Aromasin** *see* Exemestane *on page 632*
- **Arranon** *see* Nelarabine *on page 1091*
- **ARRY-162** *see* Binimetinib *on page 244*
- **ARRY-380** *see* Tucatinib *on page 1503*
- **ARRY-142886** *see* Selumetinib *on page 1365*
- **ARRY-438162** *see* Binimetinib *on page 244*
- **Artane** *see* Trihexyphenidyl *on page 1498*
- **Artemether and Benflumetol** *see* Artemether and Lumefantrine *on page 168*

Artemether and Lumefantrine

(ar TEM e ther & loo me FAN treen)

Related Information

Clinical Risk Related to Drugs Prolonging QT Interval *on page 1675*

Brand Names: US Coartem

Pharmacologic Category Antimalarial Agent

Use Malaria, treatment: Treatment of acute, uncomplicated malaria infections due to *Plasmodium falciparum*, including geographical regions where chloroquine resistance has been reported. **Note:** CDC guidelines also recommend artemether/lumefantrine as an alternative agent for chloroquine-sensitive *Plasmodium* species, for chloroquine-resistant *Plasmodium vivax* or *Plasmodium ovale*, and as oral treatment for severe malaria after completion of IV therapy or as interim therapy pending IV therapy (CDC 2020).

Local Anesthetic/Vasoconstrictor Precautions Artemether and lumefantrine is one of the drugs confirmed to prolong the QT interval and is accepted as having a risk of causing torsade de pointes. The risk of drug-induced torsade de pointes is extremely low when a single QT interval prolonging drug is prescribed. In terms of epinephrine, it is not known what effect vasoconstrictors in the local anesthetic regimen will have in patients with a known history of congenital prolonged QT interval or in patients taking any medication that prolongs the QT interval. Until more information is obtained, it is suggested that the clinician consult with the physician prior to the use of a vasoconstrictor in suspected patients, and that the vasoconstrictor (epinephrine, mepivacaine and levonordefrin [Carbocaine® 2% with Neo-Cobefrin®]) be used with caution.

Effects on Dental Treatment No significant effects or complications reported

Effects on Bleeding No information available to require special precautions

Adverse Reactions

>10%:

Cardiovascular: Palpitation (adults: 18%)

Central nervous system: Headache (adults 56%; children 13%), dizziness (adults 39%; children 4%), fever (25% to 29%), chills (adults 23%; children 5%), sleep disorder (adults: 22%), fatigue (adults 17%; children 3%)

Gastrointestinal: Anorexia (adults 40%; children 13%), nausea (adults 26%; children 5%), vomiting (17% to 18%), abdominal pain (8% to 17%)

Infection: Plasmodium falciparum (exacerbation: children: 17%)

Neuromuscular & skeletal: Weakness (adults 38%; children 5%), arthralgia (adults 34%; children 3%), myalgia (adults 32%; children 3%)

Respiratory: Cough (adults 6%; children 23%)

Miscellaneous: Fever (25% to 29%)

3% to 10%:

Central nervous system: Insomnia (adults: 5%), malaise (adults: 3%), vertigo (adults: 3%)

Dermatologic: Pruritus (adults: 4%), skin rash (3%)

Gastrointestinal: Diarrhea (7% to 8%)

Hematologic & oncologic: Anemia (4% to 9%)

Hepatic: Hepatomegaly (6% to 9%), increased serum AST (≤4%)

Infection: Malaria (≤3%)

Respiratory: Rhinitis (4%), nasopharyngitis (≤3%)

<3%, postmarketing, and/or case reports: Abnormal gait, abnormal lymphocytes, abscess, agitation, anaphylaxis, angioedema, asthma, ataxia, back pain, bronchitis, bullous dermatitis, change in platelet count (increased), clonus, conjunctivitis, constipation, decreased hematocrit, decreased platelet count, decreased white blood cell count, dermatitis (hands and feet), dyspepsia, dysphagia, emotional lability, eosinophilia, fine motor control disorder, gastroenteritis, helminthiasis, hematuria, hemolytic anemia (delayed), hookworm infection, hyper-reflexia, hypoesthesia, hypokalemia, impetigo, increased serum ALT, influenza, leukocytosis, leukopenia, lower respiratory tract infection, nystagmus, oral herpes, otic infection, peptic ulcer, pharyngolaryngeal pain, pneumonia, proteinuria, respiratory tract infection, subcutaneous abscess, tinnitus, tremor, upper respiratory tract infection, urinary tract infection, urticaria

Mechanism of Action A coformulation of artemether and lumefantrine with activity against *Plasmodium falciparum*. Artemether and major metabolite dihydroartemisinin (DHA) are rapid schizontocides with activity attributed to the endoperoxide moiety common to each substance. Artemether inhibits an essential calcium adenosine triphosphatase. The exact mechanism of lumefantrine is unknown, but it may inhibit the formation of β-hematin by complexing with hemin. Both artemether and lumefantrine inhibit nucleic acid and protein synthesis. Artemether rapidly reduces parasite biomass and lumefantrine eliminates residual parasites.

Pharmacodynamics/Kinetics

Half-life Elimination Artemether: 1-2 hours; DHA: 2 hours; Lumefantrine: 72-144 hours

Time to Peak Plasma: Artemether: ~2 hours; Lumefantrine: ~6-8 hours

Reproductive Considerations

Artemether may reduce the effectiveness of hormonal contraceptives. An additional nonhormonal method of birth control should be used during therapy.

Pregnancy Considerations

A meta-analysis of observational pregnancy studies, which included 500 pregnant women exposed to artemether/lumefantrine in their first trimester, and data from observational and open-label studies of >1,200 pregnant women exposed to artemether/lumefantrine in their second or third trimesters have not shown an increased risk of major birth defects, miscarriage, or adverse maternal/fetal outcomes.

Malaria infection in pregnant women may be more severe than in nonpregnant women and has a high risk of maternal and perinatal morbidity and mortality. Malaria infection during pregnancy can lead to miscarriage, premature delivery, low birth weight, congenital infection, and/or perinatal death. Therefore, pregnant women and women who are likely to become pregnant are advised to avoid travel to malaria-risk areas. When travel is unavoidable, pregnant women should take precautions to avoid mosquito bites and use effective prophylactic medications (CDC 2020; CDC Yellow Book 2020).

Artemether/lumefantrine may be used to treat chloroquine resistant uncomplicated malaria during the second and third trimesters. Artemether/lumefantrine also may be used as an alternative treatment during the first trimester when preferred agents are not available. In pregnant patients with severe malaria, artemether/lumefantrine is the preferred interim oral therapy when the preferred IV agent is not readily available (discontinue once IV treatment is initiated). Dosing is the same as nonpregnant patients (Ballard [CDC 2018]; CDC 2020).

Dental Health Professional Considerations See Local Anesthetic/Vasoconstrictor Precautions

◆ **Artemether/Lumefantrine** *see* Artemether and Lumefantrine *on page 168*

◆ **Artemisinin Derivative** *see* Artesunate *on page 169*

Artesunate (ar TES oo nate)

Pharmacologic Category Antimalarial Agent; Artemisinin Derivative

Use

Malaria (severe), treatment: Initial treatment of severe malaria in adult and pediatric patients.

Limitations of use: Artesunate for injection does not treat the hypnozoite liver stage forms of *Plasmodium* and will therefore not prevent relapses of malaria due to *Plasmodium vivax* or *Plasmodium ovale*. Concomitant therapy with an antimalarial agent such as an 8-aminoquinoline drug is necessary for the treatment of severe malaria due to *P. vivax* or *P. ovale*.

Local Anesthetic/Vasoconstrictor Precautions No information available to require special precautions

Effects on Dental Treatment Key adverse event(s) related to dental treatment: Metallic taste has been reported

Effects on Bleeding No information available to require special precautions

Adverse Reactions

1% to 10%:

Genitourinary: Hemoglobinuria (7%)

Hepatic: Jaundice (2%)

Nervous system: Neurological signs and symptoms (1%)

Renal: Acute renal failure (9%)

Frequency not defined:

Nervous system: Ataxia, balance impairment, confusion, paresis, restlessness

Neuromuscular & skeletal: Asthenia, tremor

Postmarketing:

Hematologic & oncologic: Autoimmune hemolytic anemia, hemolysis, hemolytic anemia

Hypersensitivity: Anaphylaxis, hypersensitivity reaction

Mechanism of Action Artesunate, a semisynthetic derivative of artemisinin, is a prodrug that is rapidly metabolized to the active metabolite, dihydroartemisinin (DHA). Artesunate and DHA contain an endoperoxide bridge that is activated by heme iron binding, resulting in oxidative stress, inhibition of protein and nucleic acid synthesis, ultrastructural changes, and a decrease in parasite growth and survival. Both are active against the blood-stage asexual parasites and gametocytes of *Plasmodium* species (including chloroquine-resistant strains) but **not** active against the hypnozoite liver stage forms of *P. vivax* and *P. ovale*.

Pharmacodynamics/Kinetics

Half-life Elimination Artesunate: 0.3 hours; dihydroartemisinin (DHA): 1.3 hours.

Time to Peak Dihydroartemisinin (DHA): Adults infected with severe malaria: Within 15 minutes (Newton 2006).

Pregnancy Considerations An increased risk of adverse pregnancy outcomes has not been observed following maternal use of artesunate.

Malaria infection in pregnant women may be more severe than in nonpregnant women and has a high risk of maternal and perinatal morbidity and mortality. Malaria infection during pregnancy can lead to miscarriage, premature delivery, low birth weight, congenital infection, and/or perinatal death. Therefore, pregnant women and women who are likely to become pregnant are advised to avoid travel to malaria-risk areas. When travel is unavoidable, pregnant women should take precautions to avoid mosquito bites and use effective prophylactic medications (CDC 2020; CDC Yellow Book 2020).

Artesunate is recommended for the treatment of severe malaria during pregnancy (CDC 2020; WHO 2015). Severe malaria is life threatening to the mother and fetus; when otherwise indicated, treatment should not be withheld because of fears of teratogenicity.

Data collection to monitor pregnancy and infant outcomes following exposure to artesunate is ongoing. Health care providers are encouraged to enroll females exposed to artesunate during pregnancy in the pregnancy safety study (1-855-526-4827).

Product Availability Artesunate: FDA approved May 2020; anticipated availability currently unknown. Until product is available through the hospital supply chain, health care professionals seeking artesunate for treatment of patients with severe malaria should contact the CDC for information on product ordering from CDC quarantine stations. CDC malaria hotline: (770) 488-7788 or (855) 856-4713 (toll free) Monday to Friday 9am to 5pm EST or (770) 488-7100 after hours, weekends, and holidays.

◆ **Artesunic Acid** *see* Artesunate *on page 169*

◆ **Arthrotec** *see* Diclofenac and Misoprostol *on page 490*

◆ **Articadent** *see* Articaine and Epinephrine *on page 170*

Articaine and Epinephrine

(AR ti kane & ep i NEF rin)

Related Information

EPINEPHrine (Systemic) *on page 569*

Oral Pain *on page 1734*

Brand Names: US Articadent; Orabloc; Septocaine with Epinephrine 1:100,000; Septocaine with Epinephrine 1:200,000; Zorcaine

Brand Names: Canada Astracaine with Epinephrine 1:200,000; Astracaine with Epinephrine forte 1:100,000; Karticaine; Karticaine Forte; Orabloc 1:100,000; Orabloc 1:200,000; Posicaine N; Posicaine SP; Septanest N; Septanest SP; Ultracaine DS; Ultracaine DS Forte; Zorcaine

Generic Availability (US) No

Pharmacologic Category Local Anesthetic

Dental Use Local, infiltrative, or conductive anesthesia in both simple and complex dental and periodontal procedures

Use Dental anesthesia: Local, infiltrative, or conductive anesthesia in both simple and complex dental procedures

Local Anesthetic/Vasoconstrictor Precautions No information available to require special precautions (see Dental Health Professional Considerations)

Effects on Dental Treatment No significant effects or complications reported

Effects on Bleeding No information available to require special precautions

Adverse Reactions Frequency not always defined.

Adverse reactions are characteristic of those associated with other amide-type local anesthetics; adverse reactions to this group of drugs may also result from excessive plasma levels which may be due to overdosage, unintentional intravascular injection, or slow metabolic degradation.

Cardiovascular: Facial edema (1%), cardiac arrhythmia, cardiac insufficiency

Central nervous system: Pain (13%), headache (4%), paresthesia (1%), seizure

Gastrointestinal: Gingivitis (1%)

Hypersensitivity: Hypersensitivity reaction

Local: Injection site reaction

Respiratory: Asthma

Miscellaneous: Tissue necrosis

<1%, postmarketing, and/or case reports: Abdominal pain, accidental injury, arthralgia, back pain, constipation, dermatological disease, diarrhea, dizziness, drowsiness, dysgeusia, dysmenorrhea, dyspepsia, ecchymoses, edema, facial paralysis, gingival hemorrhage, glossitis, hemorrhage, hyperesthesia, increased thirst, lymphadenopathy, malaise, methemoglobinemia, migraine, myalgia, nausea, neck pain, nervousness, neuropathy, oral mucosa ulcer, osteomyelitis, otalgia, pharyngitis, pruritus, rhinitis, sialorrhea, stomatitis, syncope, tachycardia, tongue edema, vomiting, weakness, xerostomia

Dental Usual Dosage Adults:

Infiltration: Injection volume of 4% solution: 0.5-2.5 mL; total dose: 20-100 mg

Nerve block: Injection volume of 4% solution: 0.5-3.4 mL; total dose: 20-136 mg

Oral surgery: Injection volume of 4% solution: 1-5.1 mL; total dose: 40-204 mg

Note: These dosages are guides only; other dosages may be used; however, do not exceed maximum recommended dose

Special populations: The clinician is reminded that these doses serve only as a guide to the amount of anesthetic required for most routine procedures. The actual volumes to be used depend upon a number of factors, such as type and extent of surgical procedure, depth of anesthesia, degree of muscular relaxation, and condition of the patient. In all cases, the smallest dose that will produce the desired result should be given. Dosages should be reduced for pediatric patients, elderly patients, and patients with cardiac and/or liver disease.

Dosing

Adult

Dental anesthesia: Submucosal infiltration and/or nerve block: Articaine 4%/epinephrine: **Note:** These dosages are guides only; other dosages may be used; however, do not exceed maximum recommended dose. The actual volumes to be used depend upon a number of factors, such as type and extent of surgical procedure, depth of anesthesia, degree of muscular relaxation, and condition of the patient. In all cases, the smallest dose that will produce the desired result should be given. For most routine dental procedures, epinephrine 1:200,000 is preferred; when more pronounced hemostasis or improved visualization of the surgical field are required, epinephrine 1:100,000 may be used. Dosages should be reduced for patients with cardiac disease and acutely ill and/or debilitated patients:

Infiltration: 0.5 to 2.5 mL; total dose of articaine: 20 to 100 mg; maximum dose of articaine: 7 mg/kg (0.175 mL/kg).

Nerve block: 0.5 to 3.4 mL; total dose of articaine: 20 to 136 mg; maximum dose of articaine: 7 mg/kg (0.175 mL/kg).

Oral surgery: 1 to 5.1 mL; total dose of articaine: 40 to 204 mg; maximum dose of articaine: 7 mg/kg (0.175 mL/kg).

Geriatric

Dental anesthesia: Submucosal infiltration and/or nerve block: Articaine 4%/epinephrine: **Note:** These dosages are guides only; other dosages may be used; however, do not exceed maximum recommended dose. The actual volumes to be used depend upon a number of factors, such as type and extent of surgical procedure, depth of anesthesia, degree of muscular relaxation, and condition of the patient. In all cases, the smallest dose that will produce the desired result should be given. For most routine dental procedures, epinephrine 1:200,000 is preferred; when more pronounced hemostasis or improved visualization of the surgical field are required, epinephrine 1:100,000 may be used. Dosages should be reduced for patients with cardiac disease and acutely ill and/or debilitated patients:

65 to 75 years:

Simple procedures: 0.43 to 4.76 mg/kg of articaine.

Complex procedures: 1.05 to 4.27 mg/kg of articaine.

≥75 years:

Simple procedures: 0.78 to 4.76 mg/kg of articaine.

Complex procedures: 1.12 to 2.17 mg/kg of articaine.

Renal Impairment: Adult There are no dosage adjustments provided in the manufacturer's labeling (has not been studied).

Hepatic Impairment: Adult There are no dosage adjustments provided in the manufacturer's labeling (has not been studied). Use with caution in patients with severe hepatic disease.

Pediatric

Dental anesthesia: Note: The provided dosages are guides only; other dosages may be necessary; however, do not exceed maximum recommended dose. The actual volumes to be used depend upon a number of factors, such as type and extent of surgical procedure, depth of anesthesia, degree of muscular relaxation, and condition of the patient. In all cases, the smallest dose that will produce the desired result should be used. Two concentrations of epinephrine (1:100,000 or 1:200,00) with 4% articaine are available; when more pronounced hemostasis or improved visualization of the surgical field are required, epinephrine 1:100,000 may be used; in clinical trials of pediatric patients 4 to 16 years of age, the 1:100,000 was also used; in adults, the manufacturer recommends epinephrine 1:200,000 for most routine dental procedures. Dosages should be reduced for patients with cardiac disease and acutely ill and/or debilitated patients. Dosing presented in variable unit (mg/kg, mg, mL/kg, and mL); use extra precaution to verify dosing units.

Children ≥4 years and Adolescents ≤16 years: Submucosal infiltration and/or nerve block: Articaine 4%/epinephrine: Injection:

Simple procedures: Reported range: 0.76 to 5.65 mg/kg of articaine; maximum articaine dose: 7 mg/kg (0.175 mL/kg of 4% solution)

Complex procedures: 0.37 to 7 mg/kg of articaine; maximum articaine dose: 7 mg/kg (0.175 mL/kg of 4% solution)

Adolescents ≥17 years: Submucosal infiltration and/or nerve block: Articaine 4%/epinephrine: Injection:

Infiltration: 0.5 to 2.5 mL (total articaine dose: 20 to 100 mg); not to exceed 7 mg/kg (0.175 mL/kg of 4% solution) of articaine

Nerve block: 0.5 to 3.4 mL (total articaine dose: 20 to 136 mg); not to exceed 7 mg/kg (0.175 mL/kg of 4% solution) of articaine

Oral surgery: 1 to 5.1 mL (total articaine dose: 40 to 204 mg); not to exceed 7 mg/kg (0.175 mL/kg of 4% solution) of articaine

Renal Impairment: Pediatric There are no dosage adjustments provided in the manufacturer's labeling (has not been studied).

Hepatic Impairment: Pediatric There are no dosage adjustments provided in the manufacturer's labeling (has not been studied). Use with caution in patients with severe hepatic disease.

Mechanism of Action

Articaine: Blocks both the initiation and conduction of nerve impulses by increasing the threshold for electrical excitation in the nerve, slowing the propagation of the nerve impulse, and reducing the rate of rise of the action potential.

Epinephrine: Increases the duration of action of articaine by causing vasoconstriction (via alpha effects) which slows the vascular absorption of articaine.

Contraindications Sulfite hypersensitivity.

Documentation of allergenic cross-reactivity for local anesthetics is limited. However, because of similarities in chemical structure and/or pharmacologic actions, the possibility of cross-sensitivity cannot be ruled out with certainty.

Canadian labeling: Additional contraindications (not in US labeling): Hypersensitivity to articaine, epinephrine, or any component of the formulation; allergies to dental anesthetics; patients with inflammation and/or sepsis near the proposed injection site, severe shock, paroxysmal tachycardia, frequent arrhythmia, neurological disease, severe hypertension; children <4 years of age; anesthesia of fingers, toes, tip of nose, ears, and penis; narrow-angle glaucoma; severe heart disease, heart block, or known arrhythmias; recent (3 to 6 months) myocardial infarction; recent (3 months) coronary artery bypass surgery; concurrent use of non-cardioselective beta-blockers, tricyclic antidepressants, MAO inhibitors, ergot derivatives, and halothane (or other similar inhalation type drugs); pheochromocytoma; thyrotoxicosis; severe hepatic/renal insufficiency; bronchial asthma; intravascular use.

Warnings/Precautions Systemic toxicity may occur. Systemic absorption of local anesthetics may produce cardiovascular and/or CNS effects. Toxic blood concentrations of local anesthetics depress cardiac conduction and excitability, which may lead to AV block, ventricular arrhythmias, and cardiac arrest (sometimes resulting in death). In addition, myocardial contractility is depressed and peripheral vasodilation occurs, leading to decreased cardiac output and arterial blood pressure. Restlessness, anxiety, tinnitus, dizziness, blurred vision, tremors, depression, or drowsiness may be early warning signs of CNS toxicity. Small doses of local anesthetics injected into dental blocks may produce adverse reactions similar to systemic toxicity, including confusion, convulsions, respiratory depression and/or respiratory arrest, and cardiovascular stimulation or depression; these reactions may be due to intra-arterial injection of the local anesthetic with retrograde flow to the cerebral circulation. Constantly monitor cardiovascular and respiratory vital signs and patient's state of consciousness carefully following each injection. Epinephrine may cause local toxicity, including ischemic injury or necrosis. Methemoglobinemia has been reported with local anesthetics; clinically significant methemoglobinemia requires immediate treatment along with discontinuation of the anesthetic and other oxidizing agents. Onset may be immediate or delayed (hours) after anesthetic exposure. Patients with glucose-6-phosphate dehydrogenase deficiency, congenital or idiopathic methemoglobinemia, cardiac or pulmonary compromise, exposure to oxidizing agents or their metabolites, or infants <6 months of age are more susceptible and should be closely monitored for signs and symptoms of methemoglobinemia (eg, cyanosis, headache, rapid pulse, shortness of breath, lightheadedness, fatigue). Use with caution in patients with impaired cardiovascular function, including patients with heart block. Use local anesthetics containing a vasoconstrictor with caution in patients with vascular disease; patients with peripheral vascular disease or hypertensive vascular disease may exhibit exaggerated vasoconstrictor response, possibly resulting in ischemic injury or necrosis. Dosages should be reduced for patients with cardiac disease. Use with caution in patients with severe hepatic disease (has not been studied).

Administer reduced dosages, commensurate with age and physical condition to pediatric, elderly, debilitated and/or acutely-ill patients. Avoid intravascular injection; accidental intravascular injection may be associated with convulsions, followed by CNS or cardiorespiratory depression and coma, progressing ultimately to respiratory arrest. Aspiration should be performed prior to administration; the needle must be repositioned until no return of blood can be elicited by aspiration; however, absence of blood in the syringe does not guarantee that intravascular injection has been avoided. To avoid serious adverse effects and high plasma levels, use the lowest dosage resulting in effective anesthesia. Repeated doses may cause significant increases in blood levels due to the possibility of accumulation of the drug or its metabolites. Dosage recommendations should not be exceeded. Health care providers should be well trained in diagnosis and management of emergencies that may arise from the use of these agents. Resuscitative equipment, oxygen, and other resuscitative drugs should be available for immediate use. May contain sodium metabisulfite, which may cause allergic-type reactions (including anaphylactic symptoms, and life-threatening or less severe asthmatic episodes) in certain susceptible patients. The overall prevalence of the sulfite sensitivity in the general population is unknown, and is seen more frequently in asthmatic than in nonasthmatic persons. Potentially significant interactions may exist, requiring dose or frequency adjustment, additional monitoring, and/or selection of alternative therapy.

Drug Interactions

Metabolism/Transport Effects Refer to individual components.

Avoid Concomitant Use

Avoid concomitant use of Articaine and Epinephrine with any of the following: Blonanserin; Bromperidol; Bupivacaine (Liposomal); Ergot Derivatives; Lurasidone

Increased Effect/Toxicity

Articaine and Epinephrine may increase the levels/effects of: Bupivacaine (Liposomal); Doxofylline; Lurasidone; Neuromuscular-Blocking Agents; Solriamfetol; Sympathomimetics

The levels/effects of Articaine and Epinephrine may be increased by: AtoMOXetine; Beta-Blockers (Nonselective); Bretylium; Cannabinoid-Containing

Products; Chloroprocaine; Cocaine (Topical); COMT Inhibitors; Ergot Derivatives; Guanethidine; Hyaluronidase; Inhalational Anesthetics; Linezolid; Methemoglobinemia Associated Agents; Monoamine Oxidase Inhibitors; Ozanimod; Procarbazine; Serotonin/Norepinephrine Reuptake Inhibitors; Tedizolid; Tricyclic Antidepressants

Decreased Effect

Articaine and Epinephrine may decrease the levels/effects of: Antidiabetic Agents; Benzylpenicilloyl Polylysine; Technetium Tc 99m Tilmanocept

The levels/effects of Articaine and Epinephrine may be decreased by: Alpha1-Blockers; Benperidol; Beta-Blockers (Beta1 Selective); Beta-Blockers (with Alpha-Blocking Properties); Blonanserin; Bromperidol; CloZAPine; Haloperidol; Promethazine; Spironolactone

Pharmacodynamics/Kinetics

Onset of Action 1 to 9 minutes

Duration of Action Complete anesthesia: ~1 hour (infiltration); ~2 hours (nerve block)

Half-life Elimination Articaine/epinephrine: 43.8 to 44.4 minutes

Time to Peak Articaine: ~25 minutes (single dose); 48 minutes (3 doses)

Pregnancy Risk Factor C

Pregnancy Considerations Adverse events have been observed in some animal reproduction studies using this combination. Articaine crosses the placenta (Strasser 1977).

Breastfeeding Considerations It is not known if articaine or epinephrine are excreted in breast milk. The manufacturer recommends that caution be exercised when administering articaine/epinephrine to breastfeeding women; consideration may be given to pumping and discarding milk for 4 hours after the last dose. In general, women administered single dose local anesthesia for dental procedures may resume breastfeeding once they are awake and stable (Montgomery 2012).

Dosage Forms: US

Injection, solution [for dental use]:

Articadent: Articaine hydrochloride 4% [40 mg/mL] and epinephrine 1:100,000 (1.7 mL)

Articadent: Articaine hydrochloride 4% [40 mg/mL] and epinephrine 1:200,000 (1.7 mL)

Orabloc: Articaine hydrochloride 4% [40 mg/mL] and epinephrine 1:100,000 (1.8 mL)

Orabloc: Articaine hydrochloride 4% [40 mg/mL] and epinephrine 1:200,000 (1.8 mL)

Septocaine with epinephrine 1:100,000: Articaine 4% [40 mg/mL] and epinephrine 1:100,000 (1.7 mL)

Septocaine with epinephrine 1:200,000: Articaine 4% [40 mg/mL] and epinephrine 1:200,000 (1.7 mL)

Zorcaine: Articaine 4% [40 mg/mL] and epinephrine 1:100,000 (1.7 mL)

Dosage Forms: Canada

Injection, solution [for dental use]:

Astracaine with epinephrine 1:200,000: Articaine 4% and epinephrine 1:200,000 (1.8 mL)

Astracaine Forte with epinephrine forte 1:100,000: Articaine 4% and epinephrine 1:100,000 (1.8 mL)

Septanest N: Articaine 4% and epinephrine 1:200,000 (1.7 mL)

Septanest SP: Articaine 4% and epinephrine 1:100,000 (1.7 mL)

Ultracaine DS: Articaine 4% and epinephrine 1:200,000 (1.7 mL)

Ultracaine DS Forte: Articaine 4% and epinephrine 1:100,000 (1.7 mL)

Dental Health Professional Considerations Septocaine (articaine hydrochloride 4% and epinephrine 1:100,000) is the first FDA approval in 30 years of a new local dental anesthetic providing complete pulpal anesthesia for approximately 1 hour. Chemically, articaine contains both an amide linkage and an ester linkage, making it chemically unique in the class of local anesthetics. Since it contains the ester linkage, articaine HCl is rapidly metabolized by plasma carboxyesterase to its primary metabolite, articainic acid, which is an inactive product of this metabolism. According to the manufacturer, *in vitro* studies show that the human liver microsomal P450 isoenzyme system metabolizes approximately 5% to 10% of available articaine with nearly quantitative conversion to articainic acid. The elimination half-life of articaine is about 1.8 hours, and that of articainic acid is about 1.5 hours. Articaine is excreted primarily through urine with 53% to 57% of the administered dose eliminated in the first 24 hours following submucosal administration. Articainic acid is the primary metabolite in urine. A minor metabolite, articainic acid glucuronide, is also excreted in the urine. Articaine constitutes only 2% of the total dose excreted in urine.

The anesthetic efficacy of the articaine 4% with 1:200,000 epinephrine (A/200) was compared to that of articaine 4% with 1:100,000 (A/100) using electric pulp tester to assess anesthesia using 63 subjects after either maxillary infiltration (Moore, 2006) or inferior alveolar block (Hersh, 2006).

After maxillary infiltration of 1 mL of each formula, the onset times to anesthesia were 3.1 ± 2.3 minutes for articaine 4% and 1:200,000 epinephrine (A/200), 3 ± 2.1 minutes for articaine 4% and 1:100,000 epinephrine (A/100), 3 ± 2 minutes for articaine 4% with no epinephrine (A/no). These three mean times of onset were not statistically different. Durations of anesthesia were 41.6 ± 21.1 minutes A/200, 45 ± 23.6 minutes A/100, 13.3 ± 6.8 minutes for A/no. There was no statistically significant difference between the durations elicited by the A/200 and A/100 formulations (Moore, 2006). In the second trial of the study, also using 63 subjects, the investigators administered an inferior alveolar nerve block injection of one cartridge (1.7 mL) using a standard intra-oral injection technique for inferior alveolar block anesthesia. Pulpal anesthesia was measured again using the pulp tester.

The onset times to anesthesia were 4.7 ± 2.6 minutes A/200, 4.2 ± 2.8 minutes A/100, and 4.3 ± 2.5 minutes for A/no. There were no statistically significant differences in these times to onset. Durations of anesthesia were 51.2 ± 55.9 minutes A/200, 61.8 ± 59 minutes A/100, and 49.7 ± 44.6 minutes for A/no. There were no statistically significant differences in the duration between A/200, A/100, and A/no formulations (Hersh, 2006).

Oral paresthesia: The occurrence of oral paresthesia associated with 4% solutions of prilocaine or articaine, although rare, continue to be slightly more frequent than other local anesthetics. From 1999-2008, there were 182 cases of nonsurgical paresthesia (Gaffen, 2009). Of the cases, 172 involved mandibular block injection only. Another eight cases involved mandibular block combined with at least one other type of anesthetic injection. A single case involved infiltration around tooth number 35 (European numbering system; tooth number 20 for Universal numbering system) and the final case involved infiltration and intraligamentary injection in the maxillary anterior region.

A 2010 report, reviewed adverse events submitted voluntarily over a 10-year period involving the dental local anesthetics articaine, bupivacaine, lidocaine, mepivacaine, and prilocaine in the United States. Articaine reported incidence: One case per 4,159,848 cartridges sold. The reported incidence of paresthesia was one case for 13,800,970 cartridges of all local anesthetics sold in the U.S. (Garisto, 2010).

- **Artificial Saliva** *see* Saliva Substitute *on page 1354*
- **Artiss** *see* Fibrin Sealant *on page 667*
- **Arymo ER** *see* Morphine (Systemic) *on page 1050*
- **Arze-Ject-A [DSC]** *see* Triamcinolone (Systemic) *on page 1485*
- **Arzerra** *see* Ofatumumab *on page 1126*
- **ASA** *see* Aspirin *on page 177*
- **5-ASA** *see* Mesalamine *on page 980*
- **Asacol** *see* Mesalamine *on page 980*
- **Asacol HD** *see* Mesalamine *on page 980*
- **Asceniv** *see* Immune Globulin *on page 803*
- **Ascriptin Maximum Strength [OTC]** *see* Aspirin *on page 177*
- **Ascriptin Regular Strength [OTC]** *see* Aspirin *on page 177*

Asenapine (a SEN a peen)

Related Information

Clinical Risk Related to Drugs Prolonging QT Interval *on page 1675*

Brand Names: US Saphris; Secuado

Brand Names: Canada Saphris

Pharmacologic Category Antimanic Agent; Second Generation (Atypical) Antipsychotic

Use

Bipolar disorder (sublingual tablet only): Treatment of acute manic or mixed episodes associated with bipolar I disorder (as monotherapy in adult and pediatric patients ≥10 years of age or adjunctive treatment with lithium or valproate in adults) and maintenance treatment in adults (as monotherapy).

Schizophrenia (transdermal patch, sublingual tablet): Treatment of adults with schizophrenia.

Local Anesthetic/Vasoconstrictor Precautions Asenapine is one of the drugs confirmed to prolong the QT interval and is accepted as having a risk of causing torsade de pointes. The risk of drug-induced torsade de pointes is extremely low when a single QT interval prolonging drug is prescribed. In terms of epinephrine, it is not known what effect vasoconstrictors in the local anesthetic regimen will have in patients with a known history of congenital prolonged QT interval or in patients taking any medication that prolongs the QT interval. Until more information is obtained, it is suggested that the clinician consult with the physician prior to the use of a vasoconstrictor in suspected patients, and that the vasoconstrictor (epinephrine, mepivacaine and levonordefrin [Carbocaine® 2% with Neo-Cobefrin®]) be used with caution.

Effects on Dental Treatment Key adverse event(s) related to dental treatment: Xerostomia and increase in salivation (normal salivary flow resumes upon discontinuation). Abnormal taste, toothache, and edema of the tongue have been reported. Patients may experience orthostatic hypotension as they stand up after treatment; especially if lying in dental chair for extended periods of time. Use caution with sudden changes in position during and after dental treatment. Asenapine may cause extrapyramidal symptoms including tardive dyskinesia; risk may be greater with increased doses.

Effects on Bleeding No information available to require special precautions

Adverse Reactions Actual frequency may be dependent upon dose and/or indication.

>10%:

Central nervous system: Drowsiness (children and adolescents: 46% to 53%; adults: 3% to 26%;), insomnia (adults: 15% to 16%; children and adolescents: 4%), akathisia (adults: 4% to 15%; children and adolescents: 1% to 2%), fatigue (4% to 14%), extrapyramidal reaction (adults: 8% to 13%; children and adolescents: 1% to 2%), headache (8% to 11%)

Endocrine & metabolic: Weight gain (adults: 1% to 22%; children and adolescents: 2% to 12%), increased serum triglycerides (adults: 3% to 18%; children and adolescents: 2% to 4%), increased serum glucose (adults: 3% to 16%; children and adolescents: 2%), decreased HDL cholesterol (6% to 15%), increased serum cholesterol (adults: 2% to 14%)

Gastrointestinal: Oral hypoesthesia (5% to 30%)

Local: Application site reaction (transdermal: 14% to 15%)

Neuromuscular & skeletal: Increased creatine phosphokinase in blood specimen (adults: 11%)

1% to 10%:

Cardiovascular: Hypertension (adults: 2% to 3%), tachycardia (1% to 3%), orthostatic hypotension (2%), syncope (≤1%)

Central nervous system: Dizziness (5% to 10%), bipolar mood disorder (exacerbation; adults: ≤8%), mania (adults: ≤8%), agitation (adults: 3% to 4%), suicidal ideation (children and adolescents: 3% to 4%), anxiety (adults: 3%), dystonia (1% to 3%), outbursts of anger (children and adolescents: 2%), drug-induced Parkinson's disease (children and adolescents: 1% to 2%), irritability (1% to 2%), disruption of body temperature regulation (≤1%)

Dermatologic: Skin rash (children and adolescents: 2%)

Endocrine & metabolic: Increased serum prolactin (2% to 3%), dehydration (children and adolescents: 2%), increased LDL cholesterol (1%)

Gastrointestinal: Increased appetite (2% to 10%), abdominal pain (children and adolescents: 9%; adults: 2% to 3%), dysgeusia (3% to 9%), constipation (adults: 3% to 7%), vomiting (3% to 7%), nausea (4% to 6%), sialorrhea (adults: ≤4%), diarrhea (3%), dyspepsia (adults: 3%), stomach discomfort (adults: 2% to 3%), toothache (adults: 2% to 3%), xerostomia (adults: 2% to 3%), hyperinsulinism (children and adolescents: 1% to 3%), glossalgia (children and adolescents: 2%)

Genitourinary: Dysmenorrhea (≤2%), galactorrhea not associated with childbirth (≤2%)

Hepatic: Increased serum transaminases (adults: 2% to 3%), increased serum alanine aminotransferase (1% to 3%), increased liver enzymes (2%), increased serum aspartate aminotransferase (children and adolescents: 2%)

Local: Application site erythema (transdermal: 9% to 10%), application-site pruritus (transdermal: 4% to 5%)

Neuromuscular & skeletal: Arthralgia (adults: 2%), muscle strain (children and adolescents: 2%), myalgia (1% to 2%), asthenia (<2%)

Respiratory: Nasopharyngitis (adults: 3% to 5%), oropharyngeal pain (children and adolescents: 3%), upper respiratory tract infection (3%), dyspnea (children and adolescents: 2%), nasal congestion (children and adolescents: 2%)

Miscellaneous: Fever (≤1%)

Frequency not defined:

Cardiovascular: Prolonged QT interval on ECG

Central nervous system: Altered mental status, falling, neuroleptic malignant syndrome, tardive dyskinesia

Gastrointestinal: Oral paresthesia, swollen tongue

<1%, postmarketing, and/or case reports: Accommodation disturbance, anaphylaxis, anemia, angioedema, application site irritation, blurred vision, bundle branch block (temporary), choking sensation, diabetes mellitus, diplopia, dysarthria, dyslipidemia, dysphagia, exfoliation of skin (sublingual: oral mucosal), gastroesophageal reflux disease, hyperpigmentation, hypersensitivity reaction, hyponatremia, hypotension, leukopenia, neutropenia, oral inflammation (sublingual), oral mucosal ulcer (sublingual), oropharyngeal blister (sublingual), seizure, skin photosensitivity, thrombocytopenia, urinary incontinence, wheezing

Mechanism of Action Asenapine is a dibenzo-oxepino pyrrole atypical antipsychotic with mixed serotonin-dopamine antagonist activity. It exhibits high affinity for 5-HT_{1A}, 5-HT_{1B}, 5-HT_{2A}, 5-HT_{2B}, 5-HT_{2C}, 5-HT_{5-7}, D_{1-4}, H_1 and, alpha$_1$- and alpha$_2$-adrenergic receptors; moderate affinity for H_2 receptors. Asenapine has no significant affinity for muscarinic receptors. The binding affinity to the D_2 receptor is 19 times lower than the 5-HT_{2A} affinity (Weber 2009). The addition of serotonin antagonism to dopamine antagonism (classic neuroleptic mechanism) is thought to improve negative symptoms of psychoses and reduce the incidence of extrapyramidal side effects as compared to typical antipsychotics (Huttunen 1995).

Pharmacodynamics/Kinetics

Half-life Elimination Sublingual: Terminal: ~24 hours; Transdermal: ~30 hours.

Time to Peak Sublingual: 0.5 to 1.5 hours; Transdermal: 12 to 24 hours.

Reproductive Considerations

Asenapine may cause hyperprolactinemia, which may decrease reproductive function in both males and females.

If treatment is needed in a woman planning a pregnancy, use of an agent other than asenapine is preferred (Larsen 2015).

Pregnancy Considerations

Antipsychotic use during the third trimester of pregnancy has a risk for abnormal muscle movements (extrapyramidal symptoms) and/or withdrawal symptoms in newborns following delivery. Symptoms in the newborn may include agitation, feeding disorder, hypertonia, hypotonia, respiratory distress, somnolence, and tremor; these effects may be self-limiting or require hospitalization; monitoring of the neonate is recommended.

The American College of Obstetricians and Gynecologists (ACOG) recommends that therapy during pregnancy be individualized; treatment with psychiatric medications during pregnancy should incorporate the clinical expertise of the mental health clinician, obstetrician, primary health care provider, and pediatrician. Safety data related to atypical antipsychotics during pregnancy are limited and routine use is not recommended. However, if a woman is inadvertently exposed to an atypical antipsychotic while pregnant, continuing therapy may be preferable to switching to a typical antipsychotic that the fetus has not yet been exposed to; consider risk:benefit (ACOG 92 2008). If treatment is initiated during pregnancy, use of an agent other than asenapine is preferred (Larsen 2015).

Health care providers are encouraged to enroll women 18 to 45 years of age exposed to asenapine during pregnancy in the Atypical Antipsychotics Pregnancy Registry (1-866-961-2388 or http://www.womensmentalhealth.org/pregnancyregistry).

Dental Health Professional Considerations See Local Anesthetic/Vasoconstrictor Precautions

- **Asenapine Maleate** *see* Asenapine *on page 174*
- **Asendin [DSC]** *see* Amoxapine *on page 123*
- **ASG-22CE** *see* Enfortumab Vedotin *on page 564*
- **Ashlyna** *see* Ethinyl Estradiol and Levonorgestrel *on page 612*
- **Asmanex (7 Metered Doses)** *see* Mometasone (Oral Inhalation) *on page 1046*
- **Asmanex (14 Metered Doses)** *see* Mometasone (Oral Inhalation) *on page 1046*
- **Asmanex (30 Metered Doses)** *see* Mometasone (Oral Inhalation) *on page 1046*
- **Asmanex (60 Metered Doses)** *see* Mometasone (Oral Inhalation) *on page 1046*
- **Asmanex (120 Metered Doses)** *see* Mometasone (Oral Inhalation) *on page 1046*
- **Asmanex HFA** *see* Mometasone (Oral Inhalation) *on page 1046*
- **ASNase** *see* Asparaginase (*E. coli*) *on page 175*
- **ASP2215** *see* Gilteritinib *on page 736*
- **Asparaginase** *see* Asparaginase (*E. coli*) *on page 175*

Asparaginase (*E. coli*) (a SPEAR a ji nase e ko lye)

Brand Names: Canada Kidrolase

Pharmacologic Category Antineoplastic Agent, Enzyme; Antineoplastic Agent, Miscellaneous

Use Acute lymphoblastic leukemia: Treatment (remission induction) of acute lymphoblastic leukemia (in combination with other chemotherapy).

Local Anesthetic/Vasoconstrictor Precautions No information available to require special precautions

Effects on Dental Treatment Key adverse event(s) related to dental treatment: Stomatitis

Effects on Bleeding Thrombotic and hemorrhagic events have been reported with asparaginase (*E. coli*). A medical consult is recommended.

Adverse Reactions Frequency not defined:

Cardiovascular: Acute myocardial infarction, arterial thrombosis, cerebral thrombosis, cerebrovascular accident (Morgan 2011), embolism, facial edema, flushing, hypertension, hypotension, peripheral edema, thrombosis, venous thrombosis

Dermatologic: Erythema of skin, pruritus, urticaria

Endocrine & metabolic: Amenorrhea, decreased glucose tolerance, diabetic ketoacidosis, hyperammonemia (with clinical signs of metabolic encephalopathy), hypercholesterolemia, hyperglycemia, hypertriglyceridemia, hypoalbuminemia, hypocholesterolemia, increased serum amylase, increased uric acid, weight loss

Gastrointestinal: Abdominal pain, acute pancreatitis, cholestasis, diarrhea, hemorrhagic pancreatitis, intestinal perforation (rare), nausea (frequent, but rarely severe; may be secondary to increased blood urea nitrogen and increased uric acid), necrotizing pancreatitis, swelling of lips, vomiting (frequent, but rarely severe; may be secondary to increased blood urea nitrogen and increased uric acid)

Genitourinary: Azoospermia

Hematologic & oncologic: Anemia, antithrombin III deficiency, bone marrow depression, decreased clotting factors (factors VII, VIII, IX, and X), disorder of hemostatic components of blood (change in hemostatic function; decrease in plasminogen), febrile neutropenia, hemorrhage, hypofibrinogenemia, leukopenia, neutropenia, prolonged partial thromboplastin time, prolonged prothrombin time, thrombocytopenia

Hepatic: Cholestatic hepatitis, hepatic failure, hepatic injury, hepatitis, hepatomegaly, hepatotoxicity, increased serum alanine aminotransferase, increased serum alkaline phosphatase, increased serum aspartate aminotransferase, increased serum bilirubin, jaundice, liver steatosis

Hypersensitivity: Anaphylactic shock, anaphylaxis, hypersensitivity reaction, type I hypersensitivity reaction

Immunologic: Antibody development (including neutralizing), increased serum globulins (beta and gamma)

Infection: Bacterial infection, fungal infection, opportunistic infection, sepsis, viral infection

Local: Injection site reaction

Nervous system: Cerebrovascular hemorrhage (Morgan 2011), chills, confusion, delusion, disorientation, fatigue, malaise, mild depression, pain, parkinsonism, personality disorder, reversible posterior leukoencephalopathy syndrome, seizure

Renal: Increased blood urea nitrogen, renal failure syndrome

Respiratory: Bronchospasm, dyspnea, laryngeal edema, respiratory distress (with retrosternal pressure)

Miscellaneous: Fever

Mechanism of Action In leukemic cells, asparaginase hydrolyzes L-asparagine to ammonia and L-aspartic acid, leading to depletion of asparagine. Leukemia cells, especially lymphoblasts, require exogenous asparagine; normal cells can synthesize asparagine. Asparagine depletion in leukemic cells leads to inhibition of protein synthesis and apoptosis. Asparaginase is cycle-specific for the G_1 phase.

Pharmacodynamics/Kinetics

Half-life Elimination IM: 34 to 49 hours; IV: 8 to 30 hours

Time to Peak IM: 14 to 24 hours

Reproductive Considerations

Per the manufacturer, females of reproductive potential should avoid pregnancy during chemotherapy, and males should not father a child during chemotherapy and for a period of time after the last dose of asparaginase (*E. coli*).

Pregnancy Considerations

Based on data from animal reproduction studies, in utero exposure to asparaginase (*E. coli*) may cause fetal harm.

Asparaginase (*Erwinia*)

(a SPEAR a ji nase er WIN i ah)

Brand Names: US Erwinaze

Pharmacologic Category Antineoplastic Agent, Enzyme; Antineoplastic Agent, Miscellaneous

Use Acute lymphoblastic leukemia: Treatment (in combination with other chemotherapy) of acute lymphoblastic leukemia (ALL) in patients with hypersensitivity to *E. coli*-derived asparaginase

Local Anesthetic/Vasoconstrictor Precautions No information available to require special precautions

Effects on Dental Treatment No significant effects or complications reported

Effects on Bleeding Thrombotic and hemorrhagic events have been reported with asparaginase *(Erwinia)*. A medical consult is recommended.

Adverse Reactions

>10%:

Endocrine & metabolic: Hyperglycemia

Gastrointestinal: Nausea, vomiting

Hepatic: Increased serum transaminases

Hypersensitivity: Hypersensitivity reaction

Immunologic: Antibody development

1% to 10%:

Cardiovascular: Thrombosis

Endocrine & metabolic: Decreased glucose tolerance

Gastrointestinal: Abdominal distress, abdominal pain, diarrhea, pancreatitis, stomatitis

Hematologic & oncologic: Hemorrhage

Hepatic: Hyperbilirubinemia

Hypersensitivity: Local hypersensitivity reaction

Miscellaneous: Fever

<1%: Anaphylaxis, hyperammonemia

Frequency not defined: Cardiovascular: Cerebrovascular accident

Postmarketing: Pulmonary embolism, sagittal sinus thrombosis

Mechanism of Action Asparaginase catalyzes the deamidation of asparagine to aspartic acid and ammonia, reducing circulating levels of asparagine. Leukemia cells lack asparagine synthetase and are unable to synthesize asparagine. Asparaginase reduces the exogenous asparagine source for the leukemic cells, resulting in cytotoxicity specific to leukemic cells.

Pharmacodynamics/Kinetics

Half-life Elimination IM: ~16 hours (Asselin 1993; Avramis 2005); IV: ~7.5 hours

Reproductive Considerations Evaluate pregnancy status prior to use in females of reproductive potential. Females of reproductive potential should use effective contraception during therapy and for 3 months after the last dose of asparaginase (*Erwinia*); use of oral contraceptives is not recommended.

Pregnancy Considerations

Based on data from animal reproduction studies, in utero exposure to asparaginase (*Erwinia*) may cause fetal harm.

Prescribing and Access Restrictions For order information contact 877-625-2566 or visit http://erwinaze.com/healthcare-professionals/order-erwinaze/

- **Asparaginase *Erwinia chrysanthemi*** *see* Asparaginase (*Erwinia*) *on page 176*
- **Asparlas** *see* Calaspargase Pegol *on page 278*
- **Aspart Insulin** *see* Insulin Aspart *on page 817*

◆ **Aspart Insulin and Insulin Aspart Protamine** *see* Insulin Aspart Protamine and Insulin Aspart *on page 818*

◆ **Aspercin [OTC]** *see* Aspirin *on page 177*

◆ **Asperflex Max St [OTC]** *see* Lidocaine (Topical) *on page 902*

Aspirin (AS pir in)

Related Information

Antiplatelet and Anticoagulation Considerations in Dentistry *on page 1666*

Cardiovascular Diseases *on page 1654*

Oral Pain *on page 1734*

Rheumatoid Arthritis, Osteoarthritis, and Osteoporosis *on page 1697*

Brand Names: US Ascriptin Maximum Strength [OTC]; Ascriptin Regular Strength [OTC]; Aspercin [OTC]; Aspir-low [OTC]; Aspirin Adult Low Dose [OTC]; Aspirin Adult Low Strength [OTC]; Aspirin EC Low Strength [OTC]; Aspirtab [OTC]; Bayer Aspirin EC Low Dose [OTC]; Bayer Aspirin Extra Strength [OTC]; Bayer Aspirin Regimen Adult Low Strength [OTC]; Bayer Aspirin Regimen Children's [OTC]; Bayer Aspirin Regimen Regular Strength [OTC]; Bayer Aspirin [OTC]; Bayer Genuine Aspirin [OTC]; Bayer Plus Extra Strength [OTC]; Bayer Women's Low Dose Aspirin [OTC]; Buffasal [OTC]; Bufferin Extra Strength [OTC]; Bufferin [OTC]; Buffinol [OTC]; Durlaza; Ecotrin Arthritis Strength [OTC]; Ecotrin Low Strength [OTC]; Ecotrin [OTC]; GoodSense Low Dose [OTC]; Halfprin [OTC] [DSC]; St Joseph Adult Aspirin [OTC]; Tri-Buffered Aspirin [OTC]

Brand Names: Canada Asaphen; Asaphen E.C.; Entrophen; Novasen; Praxis ASA EC 81 Mg Daily Dose; Pro-AAS EC-80

Generic Availability (US) May be product dependent

Pharmacologic Category Analgesic, Nonopioid; Antiplatelet Agent; Nonsteroidal Anti-inflammatory Drug (NSAID), Oral; Salicylate

Dental Use Treatment of postoperative pain

Use

Immediate release:

Analgesic, antipyretic, and anti-inflammatory: For the temporary relief of headache, pain, and fever caused by colds, muscle aches and pains, menstrual pain, toothache pain, and minor aches and pains of arthritis.

Revascularization procedures: For use in patients who have undergone revascularization procedures (ie, coronary artery bypass graft, percutaneous transluminal coronary angioplasty, or carotid endarterectomy).

Vascular indications, including ischemic stroke, transient ischemic attack, acute coronary syndromes (ST-elevation myocardial infarction or non-ST-elevation acute coronary syndromes [non-ST-elevation myocardial infarction or unstable angina]), secondary prevention after acute coronary syndromes, and management of stable ischemic heart disease: To reduce the combined risk of death and nonfatal stroke in patients who have had ischemic stroke or transient ischemia of the brain due to fibrin platelet emboli; to reduce the risk of vascular mortality in patients with a suspected acute myocardial infarction (MI); to reduce the combined risk of death and nonfatal MI in patients with a previous MI or unstable angina; to reduce the combined risk of MI and sudden death in patients with stable ischemic heart disease.

ER capsules:

Ischemic stroke or transient ischemic attack: To reduce the risk of death and recurrent stroke in patients who have had an ischemic stroke or transient ischemic attack.

Stable ischemic heart disease: To reduce the risk of death and MI in patients with stable ischemic heart disease.

Limitations of use: Do not use ER capsules in situations for which a rapid onset of action is required (such as acute treatment of MI or before percutaneous coronary intervention); use IR formulations instead.

Local Anesthetic/Vasoconstrictor Precautions No information available to require special precautions

Effects on Dental Treatment Key adverse event(s) related to dental treatment: As with all drugs which may affect hemostasis, bleeding is associated with aspirin. Hemorrhage may occur at virtually any site; risk is dependent on multiple variables including dosage, concurrent use of multiple agents which alter hemostasis, and patient susceptibility. Many adverse effects of aspirin are dose related, and are rare at low dosages. Other serious reactions are idiosyncratic, related to allergy or individual sensitivity (see Dental Health Professional Considerations).

Aspirin as sole antiplatelet agent: Patients taking aspirin for ischemic stroke prevention are safe to continue it during dental procedures (Armstrong, 2013).

Concurrent aspirin use with other antiplatelet agents: Aspirin in combination with clopidogrel (Plavix), prasugrel (Effient), or ticagrelor (Brilinta) is the primary prevention strategy against stent thrombosis after placement of drug-eluting metal stents in coronary patients. Premature discontinuation of combination antiplatelet therapy (ie, dual antiplatelet therapy) strongly increases the risk of a catastrophic event of stent thrombosis leading to myocardial infarction and/or death, so says a science advisory issued in January 2007 from the American Heart Association in collaboration with the American Dental Association and other professional healthcare organizations. The advisory stresses a 12-month therapy of dual antiplatelet therapy after placement of a drug-eluting stent in order to prevent thrombosis at the stent site. Any elective surgery should be postponed for 1 year after stent implantation, and if surgery must be performed, consideration should be given to continuing the antiplatelet therapy during the perioperative period in high-risk patients with drug-eluting stents.

This advisory was issued from a science panel made up of representatives from the American Heart Association (AHA), the American College of Cardiology, the Society for Cardiovascular Angiography and Interventions, the American College of Surgeons, the American Dental Association (ADA), and the American College of Physicians (Grines, 2007).

Effects on Bleeding Aspirin irreversibly inhibits platelet aggregation which can prolong bleeding. Upon discontinuation, normal platelet function returns only when new platelets are released (~7 to 10 days). However, in the case of dental surgery, there is no scientific evidence to support discontinuation of aspirin. This was recently supported by the American Academy of Neurology in patients with ischemic cerebrovascular disease (Armstrong, 2013). A recent study compared blood loss after a single tooth extraction in coronary artery disease patients who were either on aspirin (100 mg daily) or off aspirin for the extraction. The mean volume of bleeding was not statistically different between the groups. Local hemostatic measures were sufficient to control bleeding and there were no reported episodes of hemorrhaging intra- or postoperatively (Medeiros, 2011).

Adverse Reactions As with all drugs which may affect hemostasis, bleeding is associated with aspirin. Hemorrhage may occur at virtually any site. Risk is dependent on multiple variables including dosage, concurrent use of multiple agents which alter hemostasis, and patient susceptibility. Many adverse effects of aspirin are dose related, and are rare at low dosages. Other serious reactions are idiosyncratic, related to allergy or individual sensitivity. Accurate estimation of frequencies is not possible. The reactions listed below have been reported for aspirin.

Cardiovascular: Cardiac arrhythmia, edema, hypotension, tachycardia

Central nervous system: Agitation, cerebral edema, coma, confusion, dizziness, fatigue, headache, hyperthermia, insomnia, lethargy, nervousness, Reye's syndrome

Dermatologic: Skin rash, urticaria

Endocrine & metabolic: Acidosis, dehydration, hyperglycemia, hyperkalemia, hypernatremia (buffered forms), hypoglycemia (children)

Gastrointestinal: Gastrointestinal ulcer (6% to 31%), duodenal ulcer, dyspepsia, epigastric distress, gastritis, gastrointestinal erosion, heartburn, nausea, stomach pain, vomiting

Genitourinary: Postpartum hemorrhage, prolonged gestation, prolonged labor, proteinuria, stillborn infant

Hematologic & oncologic: Anemia, blood coagulation disorder, disseminated intravascular coagulation, hemolytic anemia, hemorrhage, iron deficiency anemia, prolonged prothrombin time, thrombocytopenia

Hepatic: Hepatitis (reversible), hepatotoxicity, increased serum transaminases

Hypersensitivity: Anaphylaxis, angioedema

Neuromuscular & skeletal: Acetabular bone destruction, rhabdomyolysis, weakness

Otic: Hearing loss, tinnitus

Renal: Increased blood urea nitrogen, increased serum creatinine, interstitial nephritis, renal failure (including cases caused by rhabdomyolysis), renal insufficiency, renal papillary necrosis

Respiratory: Asthma, bronchospasm, dyspnea, hyperventilation, laryngeal edema, noncardiogenic pulmonary edema, respiratory alkalosis, tachypnea

Miscellaneous: Low birth weight

Postmarketing and/or case reports: Anorectal stenosis (suppository), atrial fibrillation (toxicity), cardiac conduction disturbance (toxicity), cerebral infarction (ischemic), cholestatic jaundice, colitis, colonic ulceration, coronary artery vasospasm, delirium, esophageal obstruction, esophagitis (with esophageal ulcer), hematoma (esophageal), macular degeneration (age-related) (Li 2015), periorbital edema, rhinosinusitis

Dental Usual Dosage Postoperative pain:

Analgesic and antipyretic: Oral, rectal:

Children: 10 to 15 mg/kg/dose every 4 to 6 hours, up to a total of 4 g/day

Adults: 325 to 650 mg every 4 to 6 hours up to 4 g/day

Anti-inflammatory: Oral: Initial:

Children: 60 to 90 mg/kg/day in divided doses; usual maintenance: 80 to 100 mg/kg/day divided every 6 to 8 hours; monitor serum concentrations

Adults: 2.4 to 3.6 g/day in divided doses; usual maintenance: 3.6 to 5.4 g/day; monitor serum concentrations

Dosing

Adult & Geriatric Note: Ibuprofen, naproxen, and possibly other nonselective nonsteroidal anti-inflammatory drugs (NSAIDs) may reduce the cardioprotective effects of aspirin (Capone 2005; Catella-Lawson 2001; MacDonald 2003). Avoid regular or frequent use of NSAIDs in patients receiving aspirin for cardiovascular protection. An ER formulation exists (162.5 mg capsule); however, it should not be used in situations when a rapid onset of action is necessary (eg, ST-elevation myocardial infarction [MI]); dosing information provided is based on the IR formulations.

Analgesic and antipyretic: Immediate release: Oral: 325 mg to 1 g every 4 to 6 hours as needed; usual maximum daily dose: 4 g/day (Abramson 2019).

Note: If patient cannot take orally, rectal suppositories (300 or 600 mg) are available.

Anti-inflammatory for arthritis associated with rheumatic disease: Immediate release: Oral: 4 to 8 g/day in 4 to 5 divided doses as needed; titrate dose based on response and tolerability. Continue treatment until symptoms resolve (typically 1 to 2 weeks, but potentially up to 8 weeks). Use of aspirin at these high doses (4 to 8 g/day) may be limited by adverse effects (tinnitus, diminished auditory acuity, GI intolerance) (Abramson 2019; Carapetis 2012; Steer 2019).

Atherosclerotic cardiovascular disease:

Acute coronary syndrome:

Note: For rapid onset, non-enteric-coated IR tablet(s) should be chewed and swallowed upon identification of clinical and ECG findings suggesting an acute coronary syndrome. Enteric-coated aspirin is not preferred, since onset of action may be delayed. If it is the only product available, enteric-coated IR tablet(s) may be chewed and swallowed (ACCP [Eikelboom 2012]; Sai 2011). For maintenance therapy, any oral formulation is acceptable for use.

Non-ST-elevation acute coronary syndromes or ST-elevation myocardial infarction:

Note: For initial therapy, administer aspirin in combination with an IV anticoagulant and a P2Y12 inhibitor (ACC/AHA [Amsterdam 2014]; ACCF/AHA [O'Gara 2013]).

Initial:

Immediate release (non-enteric-coated): Oral: 162 to 325 mg administered once (chew and swallow) at the time of diagnosis (ACC/AHA [Amsterdam 2014]; ACCF/AHA [O'Gara 2013]).

Rectal (alternative route): 600 mg administered once at the time of diagnosis if an IR oral formulation is unavailable or oral route is not feasible (Maalouf 2009).

Maintenance (secondary prevention):

Immediate release: Oral: 75 to 100 mg once daily (ACC/AHA [Levine 2016]; Hennekens 2019; Mehta 2001).

Duration of therapy: Aspirin plus a P2Y12 inhibitor (dual antiplatelet therapy [DAPT]) should be continued for ≥12 months, unless bleeding risk is a concern. If there have been no major bleeding complications after 12 months, continuation of DAPT may be considered. Reevaluate the need for DAPT at regular intervals based on bleeding and thrombotic risks. When DAPT is complete, discontinue the P2Y12 inhibitor and continue aspirin indefinitely (ACC/AHA [Levine 2016]; Bonaca 2015; Cutlip 2019a; Lincoff 2019; Mauri 2014; Mehta 2001; Wallentin 2009; Wiviott 2007; Yusuf 2001).

Percutaneous coronary intervention for stable ischemic heart disease (off-label use):

Initial:

Note: For initial therapy, non-enteric-coated IR tablet(s) should be administered. Enteric-coated aspirin is not preferred since onset of action is delayed. For patients who receive a coronary stent during percutaneous coronary intervention, administer aspirin in combination with an IV anticoagulant and clopidogrel (ACCF/AHA/SCAI [Levine 2011]).

Patients chronically taking aspirin ≥325 mg/day prior to percutaneous coronary intervention: **Immediate release (non-enteric-coated): Oral:** 75 to 100 mg prior to the procedure (Cutlip 2020); some experts recommend doses up to 325 mg (ACCF/AHA/SCAI [Levine 2011]).

Patients** not **chronically taking aspirin or chronically taking aspirin <325 mg/day prior to percutaneous coronary intervention: **Immediate release (non-enteric-coated): Oral:** 300 to 325 mg given ≥2 hours (preferably 24 hours) before the procedure (ACCF/AHA/SCAI [Levine 2011]; Cutlip 2020).

Maintenance:

Immediate release: Oral: 75 to 100 mg once daily in combination with clopidogrel (DAPT); upon completion of the recommended duration of DAPT, continue aspirin indefinitely (ACC/AHA [Levine 2016]; Cutlip 2019c). Refer to Clopidogrel monograph for information on duration of DAPT.

Atherosclerotic cardiovascular disease, primary prevention (off-label use):

Note: Use should be a shared decision between health care professionals and patients after weighing the cardiovascular disease risk versus benefits (ACC/AHA [Arnett 2019]).

Immediate release: Oral: 75 to 100 mg once daily (ACC/AHA [Arnett 2019]).

Atherosclerotic cardiovascular disease, secondary prevention:

Carotid artery atherosclerosis, asymptomatic or symptomatic (off-label use): Immediate release: Oral: 75 to 325 mg once daily (ACCP [Alonso-Coello 2012]; Walker 1995).

Coronary artery bypass graft surgery: Immediate release: Oral: 75 to 81 mg once daily beginning preoperatively; continue indefinitely following surgery (AHA [Kulik 2015]; Aranki 2019).

Off-pump coronary artery bypass graft surgery: Following surgery, consider adding clopidogrel in combination with aspirin for 12 months then discontinue clopidogrel and continue aspirin indefinitely (AHA [Kulik 2015]).

Patients with acute coronary syndrome followed by coronary artery bypass graft surgery: Administer aspirin in combination with a P2Y12 inhibitor for 12 months then continue aspirin indefinitely (AHA [Kulik 2015]). Some experts do not use P2Y12 inhibitors postoperatively in these patients (Aranki 2019).

Ischemic stroke/Transient ischemic attack:

Cardioembolic stroke (alternative agent):

Note: Oral anticoagulation is preferred. For patients who cannot take an oral anticoagulant, may consider aspirin as an alternative (AHA/ASA [Kernan 2014]).

Immediate release: Oral: 75 to 100 mg once daily (AHA/ASA [Kernan 2014]).

Intracranial atherosclerosis (50% to 99% stenosis of a major intracranial artery), secondary prevention: **Immediate release: Oral:** 325 mg once daily; for patients with recent stroke or transient ischemic attack (within 30 days) may consider short-term use of clopidogrel (for 21 or 90 days depending on degree of stenosis) in combination with aspirin (AHA/ASA [Kernan 2014]; Chimowitz 2011) followed by single-agent antiplatelet therapy with aspirin, clopidogrel, or aspirin/ER dipyridamole indefinitely (ACCP [Lansberg 2012]; AHA/ASA [Kernan 2014]; Cucchiara 2019).

Noncardioembolic ischemic stroke/transient ischemic attack:

Note: For patients with a minor stroke (National Institutes of Health Stroke Scale score ≤3) or high-risk transient ischemic attack ($ABCD^2$ score ≥4), may consider short-term use of clopidogrel (for 21 days) in combination with aspirin (AHA/ASA [Kernan 2014]; AHA/ASA [Powers 2018]) followed by single-agent antiplatelet therapy with aspirin, clopidogrel, or aspirin/ER dipyridamole indefinitely (ACCP [Lansberg 2012]; AHA/ASA [Kernan 2014]; Cucchiara 2019).

Initial:

Immediate release: Oral: 162 to 325 mg administered once at the time of diagnosis; in patients who receive IV alteplase, antiplatelet therapy is generally delayed for ≥24 hours, but administered as soon as possible thereafter (AHA/ASA [Kernan 2014]; AHA/ASA [Powers 2018]; Filho 2019).

Rectal (alternative route): 300 mg administered once at the time of diagnosis if oral route is not feasible (IST 1997; Sandercock 2014).

Maintenance (alternative agent):

Note: Some experts prefer clopidogrel over aspirin or combination aspirin/ER dipyridamole over aspirin alone for long-term secondary prevention (ACCP [Lansberg 2012]; Cucchiara 2019).

Immediate release: Oral: 50 to 100 mg once daily (ACCP [Lansberg 2012]; AHA/ASA [Kernan 2014]; Cucchiara 2019).

Peripheral atherosclerotic disease (upper or lower extremity; with or without a revascularization procedure) (off-label use): Immediate release: Oral: 75 to 100 mg once daily (ACCP [Alonso-Coello 2012]; AHA/ACC [Gerhard-Herman 2017]).

Stable ischemic heart disease: Immediate release: Oral: 75 to 100 mg once daily (ACCF/AHA [Fihn 2012]; Kannam 2019).

Carotid artery stenting (off-label use):

Initial:

***Initiation ≥48 hours before procedure*:** **Immediate release: Oral:** 325 to 650 mg once daily in combination with clopidogrel (Brott 2010; Fairman 2019a).

Initiation <48 hours before procedure: **Immediate release: Oral:** 650 mg once ≥4 hours before procedure in combination with clopidogrel (Brott 2010; Fairman 2019a).

Maintenance:

Immediate release: Oral: 325 mg once daily in combination with clopidogrel for 6 weeks, then discontinue clopidogrel and continue aspirin 325 mg once daily indefinitely thereafter. In patients with history of neck irradiation, some experts recommend continuing aspirin plus clopidogrel indefinitely (Brott 2010; Fairman 2019a).

Carotid endarterectomy: Immediate release: Oral: 75 to 325 mg once daily starting prior to surgery and continued indefinitely (ACCP [Alonso-Coello 2012]; Fairman 2019b).

Colorectal cancer risk reduction, primary prevention (off-label use):

Note: The optimal dose and duration of therapy for colorectal cancer risk reduction are unknown. Utilization should be a shared decision between health care professionals and patients that weighs the risk versus benefits of treatment (Chan 2020).

Immediate release: Oral: 75 to 325 mg once daily (Chan 2020; Rothwell 2010; Ye 2013).

Migraine, acute (off-label use):

Note: For mild to moderate attacks not associated with vomiting or severe nausea (Smith 2020).

Immediate release: Oral: 900 mg or 1 g once as needed (Lipton 2005; MacGregor 2002).

Pericarditis, acute or recurrent (treatment) (off-label use):

Note: Preferred over other NSAIDs in patients with ischemic heart disease since aspirin is required. If pericarditis occurs after an MI, avoid anti-inflammatory doses for 7 to 10 days unless symptoms require acute treatment (LeWinter 2019).

Immediate release: Oral: Initial: 650 mg to 1 g every 8 hours until resolution of symptoms; gradually taper off over several weeks by decreasing the dose by 250 to 500 mg every 1 to 2 weeks (ESC [Adler 2015]; Imazio 2020). Use in combination with colchicine. In patients at risk of NSAID-related GI toxicity, prophylaxis (generally with a proton pump inhibitor) is recommended (Adler 2019; ESC [Adler 2015]; Imazio 2020).

Polycythemia vera, prevention of thrombosis (off-label use):

Note: Avoid use in patients with concurrent acquired von Willebrand syndrome (Tefferi 2019).

Immediate release: Oral: 75 to 100 mg once or twice daily (Barbui 2006; Landolfi 2004; McMullin 2005; Pascale 2012; Tefferi 2017).

Preeclampsia prevention (off-label use):

Note: Consider for use in pregnant women with ≥2 moderate risk factors or ≥1 high risk factor for preeclampsia (ACOG 743 2018).

Immediate release: Oral: 81 to 162 mg once daily, ideally beginning between 12 to 16 weeks' gestation but may be started up to 28 weeks' gestation; continue therapy until delivery (ACOG 743 2018; Rolnik 2017).

Valvular heart disease:

Surgical prosthetic heart valve replacement, thromboprophylaxis:

Bioprosthetic aortic or mitral heart valve replacement (off-label use): Immediate release: Oral: 75 to 100 mg once daily; use in combination with warfarin for the first 3 to 6 months after surgery; continue aspirin indefinitely (ACC [Otto 2017]; AHA/ACC [Nishimura 2014]; AHA/ACC [Nishimura 2017]).

Mechanical aortic or mitral heart valve replacement (off-label use): Immediate release: Oral: 75 to 100 mg once daily in combination with warfarin (AHA/ACC [Nishimura 2014]; AHA/ACC [Nishimura 2017]).

Transcatheter *aortic* valve replacement, thromboprophylaxis (off-label use):

Note: Refer to institutional policies and procedures on use of antiplatelet therapy for patients who require therapeutic anticoagulation for a different indication.

Immediate release: Oral: 75 to 100 mg once daily; in combination with clopidogrel for 3 to 6 months after transcatheter aortic valve replacement, depending on type of valve implanted; continue aspirin indefinitely (AHA/ACC [Nishimura 2014]; AHA/ACC [Nishimura 2017]). To minimize risk of bleeding complications, may give aspirin **or** clopidogrel alone and reserve dual antiplatelet therapy during the first 3 to 6 months for patients at high risk of a thrombotic event (Kuno 2019).

Transcatheter *mitral* valve repair with MitraClip device, thromboprophylaxis (off-label use):

Note: Patients are generally treated with antithrombotic therapy (antiplatelet or anticoagulant if there is a concurrent indication) for at least 6 months following the procedure.

Immediate release: Oral:

Loading dose: 325 mg once immediately following MitraClip insertion or within 24 hours prior to the procedure; use in combination with clopidogrel (Stone 2018).

Maintenance: 81 mg once daily for at least 6 months; may use as monotherapy or in combination with clopidogrel (Stone 2018).

Venous thromboembolism prevention, indefinite therapy (off-label use):

Note: For use in select patients to prevent recurrent venous thromboembolism (VTE) if unable to take an anticoagulant. In patients who have completed ≥6 months of anticoagulation and in whom indefinite therapeutic anticoagulation is indicated, aspirin is not recommended since it is less effective (Lip 2019).

Immediate release: Oral: 100 mg once daily after completion of a conventional treatment course with therapeutic anticoagulation (Becattini 2012; Brighton 2012; Lip 2019; Simes 2014).

Venous thromboembolism prophylaxis for total hip or total knee arthroplasty (off-label use):

Note: This is a hybrid strategy using rivaroxaban followed by aspirin. Limit this strategy to low-risk patients who undergo elective unilateral total hip arthroplasty (THA) or total knee arthroplasty (TKA), ambulate within 24 hours after surgery, and do not have additional risk factors for VTE, indications for long-term anticoagulation, lower limb or hip fracture in the previous 3 months, or expected major surgery in the upcoming 3 months (Pai 2020).

Immediate release: Oral: After a 5-day course of postoperative rivaroxaban prophylaxis, initiate aspirin 81 mg once daily on postoperative day 6 and continue for 9 days for TKA (total duration: 14 days) or 30 days for THA (total duration: 35 days) (Anderson 2018).

Renal Impairment: Adult

Analgesia or anti-inflammatory uses: The manufacturer recommends avoiding in patients with CrCl <10 mL/minute. However, may use with caution and monitor renal function or consider the use of an alternative analgesic/anti-inflammatory agent (NKF [Henrich 1996]; Whelton 2000).

Antiplatelet uses: The manufacturer recommends avoiding in patients with CrCl <10 mL/minute. However, in general, the benefit of low-dose aspirin outweighs any risk associated with nephropathy or other adverse effects even in the setting of severe renal impairment; the recommended aspirin dose should not be reduced in any patient with suspected or documented cardiovascular disease, or other antithrombotic indication (Fernandez 2001; Harter 1979; Summaria 2015). In patients with diabetes and chronic kidney disease or in dialysis patients, the National Kidney Foundation recommends the use of antithrombotic doses of aspirin (ie, 75 to 162 mg daily) for prevention and management of ischemic heart disease or primary prevention of atherosclerotic disease (KDOQI 2005; KDOQI 2007).

Hemodialysis: Dialyzable (concentration dependent; higher salicylate concentrations are more readily dialyzable: 50% to 60%) (Juurlink 2015; Rosenberg 1981); consider administration after hemodialysis on dialysis days (Aronoff 2007).

Hepatic Impairment: Adult Avoid use in severe liver disease.

Pediatric Note: All pediatric dosing for immediate-release formulations unless otherwise specified. Doses are typically rounded to a convenient amount (eg, 1/4 of 81 mg tablet).

Analgesic: Oral, rectal: **Note:** Do not use aspirin in pediatric patients <18 years who have or who are recovering from chickenpox or flu symptoms (eg, viral illness) due to the association with Reye syndrome (APS 2016):

Infants, Children, and Adolescents weighing <50 kg: Limited data available: 10 to 15 mg/kg/dose every 4 to 6 hours; maximum daily dose: 90 mg/kg/**day** or 4,000 mg/**day** whichever is less (APS 2016).

Children ≥12 years and Adolescents weighing ≥50 kg: 325 to 650 mg every 4 to 6 hours; maximum daily dose: 4,000 mg/**day**.

Anti-inflammatory: Limited data available: Infants, Children, and Adolescents: Oral: Initial: 60 to 90 mg/kg/**day** in divided doses; usual maintenance: 80 to 100 mg/kg/**day** divided every 6 to 8 hours; monitor serum concentrations (Levy 1978).

Antiplatelet effects: Limited data available: Infants, Children, and Adolescents: Oral: Adequate pediatric studies have not been performed; pediatric dosage is derived from adult studies. Usual adult maximum daily dose for antiplatelet effects is 325 mg/**day**.

Acute ischemic stroke (AIS):

Noncardioembolic: 1 to 5 mg/kg/dose once daily for ≥2 years; patients with recurrent AIS or TIAs should be transitioned to clopidogrel, LMWH, or warfarin (ACCP [Monagle 2012]).

Secondary to Moyamoya and non-Moyamoya vasculopathy: 1 to 5 mg/kg/dose once daily; **Note:** In non-Moyamoya vasculopathy, continue aspirin for 3 months, with subsequent use guided by repeat cerebrovascular imaging (ACCP [Monagle 2012]).

Prosthetic heart valve:

Bioprosthetic aortic valve (with normal sinus rhythm): 1 to 5 mg/kg/dose once daily for 3 months (AHA [Giglia 2013]; ACCP [Guyatt 2012]; ACCP [Monagle 2012]).

Mechanical aortic and/or mitral valve: 1 to 5 mg/kg/dose once daily combined with vitamin K antagonist (eg, warfarin) is recommended as first-line antithrombotic therapy (ACCP [Guyatt 2012]; ACCP [Monagle 2012]). Alternative regimens: 6 to 20 mg/kg/dose once daily in combination with dipyridamole (Bradley 1985; el Makhlouf 1987; LeBlanc 1993; Serra 1987; Solymar 1991).

Shunts: Blalock-Taussig; Glenn; postoperative; primary prophylaxis: 1 to 5 mg/kg/dose once daily (ACCP [Monagle 2012]; AHA [Giglia 2013]).

Norwood, Fontan surgery, postoperative; primary prophylaxis: 1 to 5 mg/kg/dose once daily (ACCP [Monagle 2012]; AHA [Giglia 2013]).

Transcatheter Atrial Septal Defect (ASD) or Ventricular Septal Defect (VSD) devices, postprocedure prophylaxis: 1 to 5 mg/kg/dose once daily starting one to several days prior to implantation and continued for at least 6 months. For older children and adolescents, after device closure of ASD, an additional anticoagulant may be given with aspirin for 3 to 6 months, but the aspirin should continue for at least 6 months (AHA [Giglia 2013]).

Ventricular assist device (VAD) placement: 1 to 5 mg/kg/dose once daily initiated within 72 hours of VAD placement; should be used with heparin (initiated between 8 to 48 hours following implantation) and with or without dipyridamole (ACCP [Monagle 2012]).

Kawasaki disease: Limited data available; optimal dose not established: **Note:** Patients with Kawasaki disease and presenting with influenza or viral illness should not receive aspirin; acetaminophen is suggested as an antipyretic in these patients and an alternate antiplatelet agent suggested for a minimum of 2 weeks (AHA [McCrindle 2017]).

Infants, Children, and Adolescents: Oral:

Initial therapy (acute phase): Recommended dosing regimens vary. Use in combination with IV immune globulin (within first 10 days of symptom onset) and corticosteroids in some cases.

High dose: 80 to 100 mg/kg/**day** divided every 6 hours for up to 14 days until fever resolves for at least 48 to 72 hours (AAP [*Red Book* 2015]; ACCP [Monagle 2012]; AHA [Giglia 2013]; AHA [McCrindle 2017]).

Moderate dose: 30 to 50 mg/kg/**day** divided every 6 hours for up to 14 days until fever resolves for at least 48 to 72 hours (AHA [McCrindle 2017]).

Subsequent therapy (low-dose; antiplatelet effects): 3 to 5 mg/kg/**day** once daily; reported dosing range: 1 to 5 mg/kg/day; initiate after fever resolves for at least 48 to 72 hours (or after 14 days). In patients without coronary artery abnormalities, administer the lower dose for 6 to 8 weeks. In patients with coronary artery abnormalities, low-dose aspirin should be continued indefinitely (in addition to therapy with warfarin) (AAP [*Red Book* 2015]; ACCP [Monagle 2012]; AHA [Giglia 2013]; AHA [McCrindle 2017]).

Rheumatic fever: Limited data available: Infants, Children, and Adolescents: Oral: Initial: 100 mg/kg/**day** divided into 4 to 5 doses; if response inadequate, may increase dose to 125 mg/kg/**day**; continue for 2 weeks; then decrease dose to 60 to 70 mg/kg/**day** in divided doses for an additional 3 to 6 weeks (WHO Guidelines 2004).

Migratory polyarthritis, with carditis without cardiomegaly or congestive heart failure: Oral: Initial: 50 to 70 mg/kg/**day** in 4 divided doses for 3 to 5 days, followed by 50 mg/kg/**day** in 4 divided doses for 2 to 3 weeks, followed by 25 mg/kg/**day** in 4 divided doses for 2 to 4 weeks (Kliegman 2020); escalation to doses up to 80 to 100 mg/kg/**day** in 4 or 5 divided doses has been described for arthritis management (RHD Australia 2020).

Carditis and more than minimal cardiomegaly or congestive heart failure: **Note:** Aspirin should be initiated at the beginning of prednisone taper regimen to prevent rebound inflammation: Oral: 50 mg/kg/**day** in 4 divided doses for 6 weeks (Kliegman 2020).

Renal Impairment: Pediatric

Infants, Children, and Adolescents: There are no recommendations in the manufacturer's labeling; however, the following adjustments have been recommended (Aronoff 2007):

GFR ≥10 mL/minute/1.73 m^2: No dosage adjustment necessary.

GFR <10 mL/minute/1.73 m^2: Avoid use.

Intermittent hemodialysis: Dialyzable: 50% to 100% (concentration dependent; higher salicylate concentrations are more readily dialyzable) (Juurlink 2015; Rosenberg 1981); administer daily dose after dialysis session on dialysis days (Aronoff 2007).

Peritoneal dialysis: Avoid use.

CRRT: No dosage adjustment necessary; monitor serum concentrations.

Hepatic Impairment: Pediatric All ages: Avoid use in severe liver disease.

Mechanism of Action Irreversibly inhibits cyclooxygenase-1 and 2 (COX-1 and 2) enzymes, via acetylation, which results in decreased formation of prostaglandin precursors; irreversibly inhibits formation of prostaglandin derivative, thromboxane A_2, via acetylation of platelet cyclooxygenase, thus inhibiting platelet aggregation; has antipyretic, analgesic, and anti-inflammatory properties

Contraindications

Hypersensitivity to NSAIDs; patients with asthma, rhinitis, and nasal polyps; use in children or teenagers for viral infections, with or without fever.

Documentation of allergenic cross-reactivity for salicylates is limited. However, because of similarities in chemical structure and/or pharmacologic actions, the possibility of cross-sensitivity cannot be ruled out with certainty.

Warnings/Precautions Clinical or population-based data regarding the risks of nonsteroidal anti-inflammatory drugs (NSAIDs) in the setting of coronavirus disease 2019 (COVID-19) are limited (FDA Safety Communication 2020; Kim 2020). Some experts recommend the use of acetaminophen as the preferred antipyretic agent, when possible, and if NSAIDs are needed, to use the lowest effective dose and shortest duration (EMA 2020; Kim 2020). In general, for patients already taking an NSAID for a comorbid condition, it is recommended to continue the NSAID as directed by their health care provider (EMA 2020; NIH 2020; WHO 2020).

Use with caution in patients with platelet and bleeding disorders, renal dysfunction, dehydration, or erosive gastritis. Avoid use in patients with active peptic ulcer disease. Heavy ethanol use (>3 drinks/day) can increase bleeding risks. When using high dosages (eg, analgesic or anti-inflammatory uses), use with caution and monitor renal function or consider the use of an alternative analgesic/anti-inflammatory agent (NKF [Henrich 1996]; Whelton 2000). Low-dose aspirin (eg, 75 to 162 mg daily) may be safely used in patients with any degree of renal impairment (KDOQI 2005; KDOQI 2007). Avoid use in severe hepatic failure. Low-dose aspirin for cardioprotective effects is associated with a two- to fourfold increase in UGI events (eg, symptomatic or complicated ulcers); risks of these events increase with increasing aspirin dose; during the chronic phase of aspirin dosing, doses >81 mg are not recommended unless indicated (Bhatt 2008).

Discontinue use if tinnitus or impaired hearing occurs. Caution in mild-to-moderate renal failure (only at high dosages). Patients with sensitivity to tartrazine dyes, nasal polyps, and asthma may have an increased risk of salicylate sensitivity. In the treatment of acute ischemic stroke, avoid aspirin for 24 hours following administration of alteplase; administration within 24 hours increases the risk of hemorrhagic transformation (Jauch 2013). Concurrent use of aspirin and clopidogrel is not recommended for secondary prevention of ischemic stroke or TIA in patients unable to take oral anticoagulants due to hemorrhagic risk (Furie 2011). Aspirin should be avoided (if possible) in surgical patients for 1 to 2 weeks prior to elective surgery, to reduce the risk of excessive bleeding. Patients who have recently undergone percutaneous coronary intervention with stenting or balloon angioplasty should continue antiplatelet therapy until it is safe to temporarily hold treatment. Elective surgery for these patients should be delayed. Patient specific situations should be discussed with cardiologist (ACC/AHA [Fleisher 2014]; ACC/AHA [Levine 2016]; AHA/ACC/SCAI/ACS/ADA [Grines 2007]).

An individualized and multidisciplinary approach should be used to manage patients with an acute lower GI bleed (LGIB) who are on antiplatelet medications. Aspirin for primary prevention of cardiovascular events should be avoided in most patients with LGIB who do not have high risk factors for cardiovascular events. However, aspirin for secondary cardiovascular prevention should generally *not* be discontinued in patients with established cardiovascular disease and a history of lower GI bleeding (Strate 2016).

When used for self-medication (OTC labeling): Children and teenagers who have or are recovering from chickenpox or flu-like symptoms should not use this product. Changes in behavior (along with nausea and vomiting) may be an early sign of Reye's syndrome; patients should be instructed to contact their healthcare provider if these occur.

Some dosage forms may contain polysorbate 80 (also known as Tweens). Hypersensitivity reactions, usually a delayed reaction, have been reported following exposure to pharmaceutical products containing polysorbate 80 in certain individuals (Isaksson 2002; Lucente 2000; Shelley 1995). Thrombocytopenia, ascites, pulmonary deterioration, and renal and hepatic failure have been reported in premature neonates after receiving parenteral products containing polysorbate 80 (Alade 1986; CDC 1984). See manufacturer's labeling.

Aspirin resistance is defined as measurable, persistent platelet activation that occurs in patients prescribed a therapeutic dose of aspirin. Clinical aspirin resistance, the recurrence of some vascular event despite a regular therapeutic dose of aspirin, is considered aspirin treatment failure. Estimates of biochemical aspirin resistance range from 5.5% to 60% depending on the population studied and the assays used (Gasparyan 2008). Patients with aspirin resistance may have a higher risk of cardiovascular events compared to those who are aspirin sensitive (Gum 2003). Evaluate the risk vs benefit of aspirin after bariatric surgery in patients. If aspirin therapy is continued (eg, cardiovascular indications), use the lowest possible dose with coadministration of proton pump inhibitor.

Warnings: Additional Pediatric Considerations Do not use aspirin in pediatric patients <18 years of age (APS 2016) who have or who are recovering from chickenpox or flu symptoms (due to the association with Reye syndrome); when using aspirin, changes in behavior (along with nausea and vomiting) may be an early sign of Reye syndrome; instruct patients and caregivers to contact their health care provider if these symptoms occur; patients should be kept current on their influenza and varicella immunizations. Although Reye syndrome has been observed in patients receiving prolonged, high-dose aspirin therapy after Kawasaki disease presentation; it has not been observed in pediatric patients receiving low (antiplatelet) dosing regimens. Patients with Kawasaki disease and presenting with influenza or viral illness should not receive aspirin; acetaminophen is suggested as an antipyretic in these patients, and an alternate antiplatelet agent is suggested for a minimum of 2 weeks (AHA [McCrindle 2017]).

Drug Interactions

Metabolism/Transport Effects **Substrate** of CYP2C9 (minor); **Note:** Assignment of Major/Minor substrate status based on clinically relevant drug interaction potential

Avoid Concomitant Use

Avoid concomitant use of Aspirin with any of the following: Dexibuprofen; Dexketoprofen; Floctafenine; Influenza Virus Vaccine (Live/Attenuated); Ketorolac (Nasal); Ketorolac (Systemic); Macimorelin; Omacetaxine; Sulfinpyrazone; Urokinase; Varicella Virus-Containing Vaccines

Increased Effect/Toxicity

Aspirin may increase the levels/effects of: Agents with Antiplatelet Properties; Agents with Blood Glucose Lowering Effects; Ajmaline; Alendronate; Angiotensin-Converting Enzyme Inhibitors; Anticoagulants; Apixaban; Bemiparin; Carbonic Anhydrase Inhibitors; Carisoprodol; Cephalothin; Collagenase (Systemic); Corticosteroids (Systemic); Dabigatran Etexilate; Deoxycholic Acid; Dexibuprofen; Dexketoprofen; Edoxaban; Enoxaparin; Gold Sodium Thiomalate; Heparin; Ibritumomab Tiuxetan; Methotrexate; Nicorandil; Nonsteroidal Anti-Inflammatory Agents (COX-2 Selective); Obinutuzumab; Omacetaxine; PRALAtrexate; Rivaroxaban; Salicylates; Talniflumate; Thiopental; Thrombolytic Agents; Ticagrelor; Urokinase; Valproate Products; Varicella Virus-Containing Vaccines; Vitamin K Antagonists

The levels/effects of Aspirin may be increased by: Acalabrutinib; Agents with Antiplatelet Properties; Alcohol (Ethyl); Ammonium Chloride; Calcium Channel Blockers (Nondihydropyridine); Dasatinib; Fat Emulsion (Fish Oil Based); Felbinac; Floctafenine; Ginkgo Biloba; Glucosamine; Herbs (Anticoagulant/Antiplatelet Properties); Ibrutinib; Influenza Virus Vaccine (Live/Attenuated); Inotersen; Ketorolac (Nasal); Ketorolac (Systemic); Limaprost; Loop Diuretics; Multivitamins/Fluoride (with ADE); Multivitamins/Minerals (with ADEK, Folate, Iron); Multivitamins/Minerals (with AE, No Iron); Nonsteroidal Anti-Inflammatory Agents (Nonselective); Omega-3 Fatty Acids; Pentosan Polysulfate Sodium; Pentoxifylline; Potassium Phosphate; Prostacyclin Analogues; Selective Serotonin Reuptake Inhibitors; Selumetinib; Serotonin/Norepinephrine Reuptake Inhibitors; Tipranavir; Tricyclic Antidepressants (Tertiary Amine); Vitamin E (Systemic); Zanubrutinib

Decreased Effect

Aspirin may decrease the levels/effects of: Angiotensin-Converting Enzyme Inhibitors; Benzbromarone; Carisoprodol; Dexketoprofen; Hyaluronidase; Lesinurad; Loop Diuretics; Macimorelin; Multivitamins/Fluoride (with ADE); Multivitamins/Minerals (with ADEK, Folate, Iron); Multivitamins/Minerals (with AE, No Iron); Nonsteroidal Anti-Inflammatory Agents (Nonselective); Probenecid; Sincalide; Spironolactone; Sulfinpyrazone; Ticagrelor; Tiludronate

The levels/effects of Aspirin may be decreased by: Alcohol (Ethyl); Corticosteroids (Systemic); Dexibuprofen; Dexketoprofen; Floctafenine; Ketorolac (Nasal); Ketorolac (Systemic); Nonsteroidal Anti-Inflammatory Agents (Nonselective); Sucroferric Oxyhydroxide

Food Interactions Food may decrease the rate but not the extent of oral absorption. Benedictine liqueur, prunes, raisins, tea, and gherkins have a potential to cause salicylate accumulation. Fresh fruits containing vitamin C may displace drug from binding sites, resulting in increased urinary excretion of aspirin. Curry powder, paprika, licorice; may cause salicylate accumulation. These foods contain 6 mg salicylate/100 g. An ordinary American diet contains 10-200 mg/day of salicylate. Management: Administer with food or large volume of water or milk to minimize GI upset. Limit curry powder, paprika, licorice.

Pharmacodynamics/Kinetics

Onset of Action Immediate release: Platelet inhibition: Nonenteric-coated: <1 hour; enteric-coated: 3 to 4 hours (Eikelboom 2012). **Note:** Chewing nonenteric-coated or enteric-coated tablets results in inhibition of platelet aggregation within 20 minutes (Eikelboom 2012; Feldman 1999; Sai 2011).

Duration of Action Immediate release: 4 to 6 hours; however, platelet inhibitory effects last the lifetime of the platelet (~10 days) due to its irreversible inhibition of platelet COX-1 (Eikelboom, 2012).

Half-life Elimination Parent drug: Plasma concentration: 15 to 20 minutes; Salicylates (dose dependent): 3 hours at lower doses (300 to 600 mg), 5 to 6 hours (after 1 g), 10 hours with higher doses

Time to Peak Serum: Immediate release: ~1 to 2 hours (nonenteric-coated), 3 to 4 hours (enteric-coated) (Eikelboom, 2012); Extended-release capsule: ~2 hours. **Note:** Chewing nonenteric-coated tablets results in a time to peak concentration of 20 minutes (Feldman, 1999). Chewing enteric-coated tablets results in a time to peak concentration of 2 hours (Sai, 2011).

Pregnancy Considerations

Salicylate is present in umbilical cord and newborn serum following maternal use of aspirin prior to delivery (Garrettson 1975; Levy 1975; Palmisano 1960). Salicylic acid and other metabolites can also be detected in the newborn urine following in utero exposure (Garrettson 1975).

Fetal outcomes are influenced by maternal dose; low dose aspirin (≤150 mg/day) is not associated with the same risks as higher doses and has a positive effect on some pregnancy outcomes (ACOG 743 2018; Turner 2019). Adverse effects reported in the fetus following maternal use of high dose aspirin include mortality, intrauterine growth retardation, salicylate intoxication, bleeding abnormalities, and neonatal acidosis. Use of aspirin close to delivery may cause premature closure of the ductus arteriosus. Adverse effects reported in the mother include anemia, hemorrhage, prolonged gestation, and prolonged labor (Corby 1978; Østensen 1998).

Due to pregnancy-induced physiologic changes, some pharmacokinetic properties of aspirin may be altered (Rymark 1994; Shanmugalingam 2019).

Low-dose aspirin may be used to prevent preeclampsia in women at high risk (history of preeclampsia, multifetal gestation, chronic hypertension, type 1 or type 2 diabetes mellitus, renal disease, autoimmune disease [systemic lupus erythematosus, antiphospholipid syndrome]) (ACOG 203 2019; ACOG 743 2018; ESC [Regitz-Zagrosek 2018]; EULAR [Andreoli 2017]). Use of low-dose aspirin may be considered to prevent preeclampsia in women with moderate risk factors (including but not limited to BMI >30, family history of preeclampsia, maternal age ≥35 years) (ACOG 743 2018). Treatment is started between 12 and 28 weeks' gestation (optimally before 16 weeks' gestation) (ACCP [Bates 2012]; ACOG 743 2018; LeFevre 2014). Low-dose aspirin to prevent thrombosis may also be used during the second and third trimesters in women with prosthetic valves (mechanical or bioprosthetic). The use of warfarin is recommended throughout pregnancy, along with low-dose aspirin during second and third trimesters, in patients with mechanical prosthetic valves (AHA/ACC [Nishimura 2014]). Low-dose aspirin may also be used after the first trimester in women with low-risk conditions requiring antiplatelet therapy (AHA/ASA [Kernan 2014]). When needed in doses required for the management of pain, agents other than aspirin are preferred in pregnant women and use in the third trimester is not recommended (Källén 2016; Shah 2015).

Breastfeeding Considerations

Salicylic acid is present in breast milk following maternal use of aspirin (Bailey 1982; Findlay 1981; Jamali 1981).

Actual breast milk concentrations of salicylic acid vary by maternal dose. In a study of six breastfeeding women, 1 to 8 months' postpartum, the highest breast milk concentration of salicylic acid was 0.0001654 mcg/mL in six women, following a maternal dose of aspirin 81 mg/day (duration of treatment not presented). Authors of this study calculated the RID of aspirin to be <1% of the weight-adjusted maternal dose (Datta 2017). In general, breastfeeding is considered acceptable when the RID is <10% (Anderson 2016; Ito 2000). Significantly higher breast milk concentrations (48.1 mcg/mL) were reported following maternal administration of aspirin 1,500 mg as a single dose (Jamali 1981).

The reported time to peak milk concentration of salicylic acid is variable (2 to 9 hours), milk concentrations decline slowly, and do not correlate strongly to maternal serum concentration (Bailey 1982; Bar-Oz 2003; Datta 2017; Findlay 1981; Jamali 1981). Salicylate is measurable in the serum (Unsworth 1987) and urine (Clark 1981) of breastfed infants following maternal use of oral aspirin. Higher salicylate concentrations may be present in breast milk following multiple maternal doses. In addition, salicylate concentrations may be higher than reported as metabolite concentrations of salicylic acid were not evaluated in most studies; the longer elimination half-life in infants compared to adults should also be considered (Bar-Oz 2003; Spigset 2000).

Metabolic acidosis was reported in a 16-day old breastfed full-term infant following maternal doses of aspirin 3.9 g/day (Clark 1981). Thrombocytopenic purpura was also reported in one infant following salicylate exposure via breast milk (maternal dose not specified) (Spigset 2000; Terrangna 1967). There were no cases of diarrhea, drowsiness, or irritability noted in breastfed infants in the study which included 15 mother-infant pairs following aspirin exposure (dose, duration, and relationship to breastfeeding not provided) (Ito 1993).

Nonopioid analgesics are preferred for breastfeeding females who require pain control peripartum or for surgery outside of the postpartum period. Low doses of aspirin (75 to 162 mg/day) may be used; however, other agents are preferred if higher doses are needed (ABM [Martin 2018]; ABM [Reece-Stremtan 2017]; Sachs 2013). When used for vascular indications, breastfeeding may be continued during low-dose aspirin therapy (ACCP [Bates 2012]; AHA/ASA [Kernan 2014]; ESC [Regitz-Zagrosek 2018]; WHO 2002). The WHO considers occasional doses of aspirin to be compatible with breastfeeding but recommends avoiding long-term therapy and consider monitoring the infant for adverse effects (hemolysis, prolonged bleeding, metabolic acidosis) (WHO 2002). Other sources also suggest avoiding high doses of aspirin while breastfeeding due to the theoretical risk of Reye syndrome (Bar-Oz 2003; Spigset 2000).

Dosage Forms: US

Caplet, oral: 500 mg

Ascriptin Maximum Strength [OTC]: 500 mg
Bayer Aspirin Extra Strength [OTC]: 500 mg
Bayer Genuine Aspirin [OTC]: 325 mg
Bayer Plus Extra Strength [OTC]: 500 mg
Bayer Women's Low Dose Aspirin [OTC]: 81 mg

Caplet, enteric coated, oral:

Bayer Aspirin Regimen Regular Strength [OTC]: 325 mg

Capsule Extended Release, oral:

Durlaza: 162.5 mg

Suppository, rectal: 300 mg (12s); 600 mg (12s)

Tablet, oral: 325 mg
Ascriptin Regular Strength [OTC]: 325 mg
Aspercin [OTC]: 325 mg
Aspirtab [OTC]: 325 mg
Bayer Genuine Aspirin [OTC]: 325 mg
Buffasal [OTC]: 325 mg
Bufferin [OTC]: 325 mg
Bufferin Extra Strength [OTC]: 500 mg
Buffinol [OTC]: 324 mg
Tri-Buffered Aspirin [OTC]: 325 mg
Tablet, chewable, oral: 81 mg
Bayer Aspirin Regimen Children's [OTC]: 81 mg
St Joseph Adult Aspirin [OTC]: 81 mg
Tablet, delayed release, oral: 81 mg
Aspirin Adult Low Dose: 81 mg
Aspirin Adult Low Strength: 81 mg
Aspirin EC Low Strength: 81 mg
Bayer Aspirin: 325 mg
GoodSense Low Dose [OTC]: 81 mg
Tablet, enteric coated, oral: 81 mg, 325 mg, 650 mg
Aspir-low [OTC]: 81 mg
Bayer Aspirin Regimen Adult Low Strength [OTC]: 81 mg
Ecotrin [OTC]: 325 mg
Ecotrin Arthritis Strength [OTC]: 500 mg
Ecotrin Low Strength [OTC]: 81 mg
St Joseph Adult Aspirin [OTC]: 81 mg

Dental Health Professional Considerations The Food and Drug Administration (FDA), has issued a letter updating information and considerations regarding the use of ibuprofen (400 mg doses) in patients who are taking low dose aspirin (81 mg, immediate release; not enteric coated) for cardioprotection and stroke prevention. Ibuprofen, at these doses, may interfere with aspirin's antiplatelet effect depending upon when it is administered. Patients initiated on aspirin first (for ~1 week) then ibuprofen (400 mg 3 times/day for 10 days) seem to maintain aspirin's platelet effect (Cryer, 2005). Ibuprofen has the greatest impact on aspirin if administered less than 8 hours before aspirin (Catella-Lawson, 2001).

Patients may require counseling about the appropriate timing of ibuprofen dosing in relationship to aspirin therapy. With occasional use of ibuprofen, a clinically-significant interaction with aspirin in unlikely. To avoid interference during chronic dosing, a single dose of ibuprofen should be taken 30 to 120 minutes after aspirin ingestion or at least 8 hours should elapse after ibuprofen dosing before giving aspirin (Catella-Lawson, 2001; FDA, 2006).

The clinical implications of the interaction are unclear. There have not been any clinical endpoint studies conducted at this time. Avoidance of this interaction is potentially important because aspirin's vascular protection could be decreased or negated.

Other nonselective NSAIDs may have potential for a similar interaction with aspirin. Such has been described with naproxen (Capone, 2005). Acetaminophen does not appear to interfere with the antiplatelet effect of aspirin. Other clinical scenarios (use of smaller ibuprofen doses, other aspirin products, other doses of aspirin) have not been evaluated.

Additional information is available at: http://www.fda.gov/Drugs/DrugSafety/PostmarketDrugSafetyInformationforPatientsandProviders/ucm125222.htm

◆ **Aspirin Adult Low Dose [OTC]** *see* Aspirin *on page 177*

◆ **Aspirin Adult Low Strength [OTC]** *see* Aspirin *on page 177*

Aspirin and Dipyridamole

(AS pir in & dye peer ID a mole)

Related Information
Aspirin *on page 177*
Dipyridamole *on page 503*

Brand Names: US Aggrenox

Brand Names: Canada Aggrenox [DSC]; TARO-Dipyridamole w/ ASA

Pharmacologic Category Antiplatelet Agent

Use Stroke prevention: Reduction in the risk of stroke in patients who have had transient ischemia of the brain or complete ischemic stroke due to thrombosis.

Local Anesthetic/Vasoconstrictor Precautions No information available to require special precautions

Effects on Dental Treatment Key adverse event(s) related to dental treatment: As with all drugs which may affect hemostasis, bleeding is associated with aspirin. Hemorrhage may occur at virtually any site; risk is dependent on multiple variables including dosage, concurrent use of multiple agents which alter hemostasis, and patient susceptibility. Many adverse effects of aspirin are dose related, and are rare at low dosages. Other serious reactions are idiosyncratic, related to allergy or individual sensitivity (see Dental Health Professional Considerations).

Aspirin as sole antiplatelet agent: Patients taking aspirin for ischemic stroke prevention are safe to continue it during dental procedures (Armstrong 2013).

Concurrent aspirin use with other antiplatelet agents: Aspirin in combination with clopidogrel (Plavix), prasugrel (Effient), or ticagrelor (Brilinta™) is the primary prevention strategy against stent thrombosis after placement of drug-eluting metal stents in coronary patients. Premature discontinuation of combination antiplatelet therapy (ie, dual antiplatelet therapy) strongly increases the risk of a catastrophic event of stent thrombosis leading to myocardial infarction and/or death, so says a science advisory issued in January 2007 from the American Heart Association in collaboration with the American Dental Association and other professional healthcare organizations. The advisory stresses a 12-month therapy of dual antiplatelet therapy after placement of a drug-eluting stent in order to prevent thrombosis at the stent site. Any elective surgery should be postponed for 1 year after stent implantation, and if surgery must be performed, consideration should be given to continuing the antiplatelet therapy during the perioperative period in high-risk patients with drug-eluting stents.

This advisory was issued from a science panel made up of representatives from the American Heart Association (AHA), the American College of Cardiology, the Society for Cardiovascular Angiography and Interventions, the American College of Surgeons, the American Dental Association (ADA), and the American College of Physicians (Grines 2007).

Effects on Bleeding Aspirin irreversibly inhibits platelet aggregation which can prolong bleeding. Upon discontinuation, normal platelet function returns only when new platelets are released (~7-10 days). However, in the case of dental surgery, there is no scientific evidence to support discontinuation of aspirin. This was recently supported by the American Academy of Neurology in patients with ischemic cerebrovascular disease (Armstrong 2013). A recent study compared blood loss after a single tooth extraction in coronary artery disease patients who were either on aspirin (100 mg daily) or off aspirin for the extraction. The mean volume of bleeding was not statistically different between the groups. Local hemostatic measures were sufficient to control bleeding and there were no reported episodes of hemorrhaging intra- or postoperatively (Medeiros 2011).

Adverse Reactions

>10%:

Central nervous system: Headache (39%; tolerance usually develops)

Gastrointestinal: Abdominal pain (18%), dyspepsia (18%), nausea (16%), diarrhea (13%)

1% to 10%:

Gastrointestinal: Vomiting (8%), gastrointestinal hemorrhage (3%)

Hematologic & oncologic: Hemorrhage (3%)

<1%, postmarketing, and/or case reports: Agitation, alopecia, anaphylaxis, angina pectoris, angioedema, anorexia, aplastic anemia, bronchospasm, bruise, cardiac arrhythmia, cerebral edema, cerebral hemorrhage, chest pain, cholelithiasis, confusion, dehydration, disorder of hemostatic components of blood, disseminated intravascular coagulation, dizziness, dyspnea, ecchymoses, flushing, gastritis, gastrointestinal perforation, gastrointestinal ulcer, gingival hemorrhage, hearing loss, hematemesis, hematoma, hematuria, hemoptysis, hepatic failure, hepatic insufficiency, hepatitis, hyperkalemia, hypersensitivity angiitis, hypersensitivity reaction, hypoglycemia, hypokalemia, hypotension, hypothermia, interstitial nephritis, intracranial hemorrhage, jaundice, laryngeal edema, melena, metabolic acidosis, migraine, myalgia, nonthrombocytopenic purpura, palpitations, pancreatitis, pancytopenia, prolonged prothrombin time, proteinuria, pruritus, rectal hemorrhage, renal failure syndrome, renal insufficiency, renal papillary necrosis, respiratory alkalosis, Reye's syndrome, rhabdomyolysis, skin rash, Stevens-Johnson syndrome, subarachnoid hemorrhage, supraventricular tachycardia, syncope, tachycardia, tachypnea, thrombocythemia, thrombocytopenia, urticaria

Mechanism of Action The antithrombotic action results from additive antiplatelet effects. Dipyridamole inhibits the uptake of adenosine into platelets, endothelial cells, and erythrocytes. Aspirin inhibits platelet aggregation by irreversible inhibition of platelet cyclooxygenase and thus inhibits the generation of thromboxane A_2.

Pregnancy Considerations Refer to individual monographs

Dental Health Professional Considerations The Food and Drug Administration (FDA), has issued a letter updating information and considerations regarding the use of ibuprofen (400 mg doses) in patients who are taking low dose aspirin (81 mg, immediate release; not enteric coated) for cardioprotection and stroke prevention. Ibuprofen, at these doses, may interfere with aspirin's antiplatelet effect depending upon when it is administered. Patients initiated on aspirin first (for ~1 week) then ibuprofen (400 mg 3 times/day for 10 days) seem to maintain aspirin's platelet effect (Cryer 2005). Ibuprofen has the greatest impact on aspirin if administered less than 8 hours before aspirin (Catella-Lawson 2001).

Patients may require counseling about the appropriate timing of ibuprofen dosing in relationship to aspirin therapy. With occasional use of ibuprofen, a clinically-significant interaction with aspirin in unlikely. To avoid interference during chronic dosing, a single dose of ibuprofen should be taken 30-120 minutes after aspirin ingestion or at least 8 hours should elapse after ibuprofen dosing before giving aspirin (Catella-Lawson 2001; FDA 2006).

The clinical implications of the interaction are unclear. There have not been any clinical endpoint studies conducted at this time. Avoidance of this interaction is potentially important because aspirin's vascular protection could be decreased or negated.

Other nonselective NSAIDs may have potential for a similar interaction with aspirin. Such has been described with naproxen (Capone 2005). Acetaminophen does not appear to interfere with the antiplatelet effect of aspirin. Other clinical scenarios (use of smaller ibuprofen doses, other aspirin products, other doses of aspirin) have not been evaluated.

Additional information is available at: http://www.fda.gov/Drugs/DrugSafety/PostmarketDrugSafetyInformationforPatientsandProviders/ucm125222.htm

◆ **Aspirin and Extended-Release Dipyridamole** *see* Aspirin and Dipyridamole *on page* 185

◆ **Aspirin, Caffeine, and Orphenadrine** *see* Orphenadrine, Aspirin, and Caffeine *on page* 1146

◆ **Aspirin/Dipyridamole** *see* Aspirin and Dipyridamole *on page* 185

◆ **Aspirin EC Low Strength [OTC]** *see* Aspirin *on page* 177

◆ **Aspirin Free Anacin Extra Strength [OTC]** *see* Acetaminophen *on page* 59

◆ **Aspirin, Orphenadrine, and Caffeine** *see* Orphenadrine, Aspirin, and Caffeine *on page* 1146

◆ **Aspir-low [OTC]** *see* Aspirin *on page* 177

◆ **Aspirtab [OTC]** *see* Aspirin *on page* 177

◆ **Astagraf XL** *see* Tacrolimus (Systemic) *on page* 1398

◆ **Astelin** *see* Azelastine (Nasal) *on page* 201

◆ **Astepro** *see* Azelastine (Nasal) *on page* 201

◆ **Astero** *see* Lidocaine (Topical) *on page* 902

◆ **Asthmanefrin Refill [OTC]** *see* EPINEPHrine (Oral Inhalation) *on page* 573

◆ **ASTX727** *see* Decitabine and Cedazuridine *on page* 448

◆ **AT** *see* Antithrombin *on page* 156

◆ **AT-III** *see* Antithrombin *on page* 156

◆ **AT1001** *see* Migalastat *on page* 1030

◆ **Atacand** *see* Candesartan *on page* 282

Atazanavir (at a za NA veer)

Related Information

HIV Infection and AIDS *on page* 1690

Brand Names: US Reyataz

Brand Names: Canada MYLAN-Atazanavir; Reyataz; TEVA-Atazanavir

Pharmacologic Category Antiretroviral, Protease Inhibitor (Anti-HIV)

Use HIV-1 infection, treatment:

Treatment of HIV-1 infection in combination with other antiretroviral agents in patients ≥3 months of age weighing ≥5 kg.

Limitations of use:

Not recommended for use in pediatric patients <3 months of age due to the risk of kernicterus.

Use in treatment-experienced patients should be guided by the number of baseline primary protease inhibitor resistance substitutions.

Local Anesthetic/Vasoconstrictor Precautions No information available to require special precautions

Effects on Dental Treatment No significant effects or complications reported

Effects on Bleeding Increased bleeding has been noted with protease inhibitors, such as atazanavir, in patients with hemophilia A or B. Thrombocytopenia has been reported. No other information is available to require special precautions in other patients.

Adverse Reactions Includes data from both treatment-naive and treatment-experienced patients. Unless otherwise noted, frequency of adverse events is as reported in adults receiving combination antiretroviral therapy.

>10%:

Dermatologic: Skin rash (adults 3% to 21%; median onset: 7 weeks; children 14%)

Endocrine & metabolic: Increased serum cholesterol (≥240 mg/dL: 6% to 25%), increased amylase (adults: >2 x ULN: ≤14%)

Gastrointestinal: Nausea (3% to 14%)

Hepatic: Increased serum bilirubin (≥2.6 x ULN: adults 35% to 49%; children 16%), jaundice (children 13% to 15%; adults 5% to 9%)

Neuromuscular & skeletal: Increased creatine phosphokinase (>5 times ULN: 6% to 11%)

Respiratory: Cough (children 21%)

Miscellaneous: Fever (children 18% to 19%; adults 2%)

1% to 10%:

Cardiovascular: Peripheral edema (children 7%), first degree atrioventricular block (6%), second degree atrioventricular block (children ≤2%; adults [rare])

Central nervous system: Headache (adults 1% to 6%; children 7% to 8%), peripheral neuropathy (<1% to 4%), insomnia (<1% to 3%), depression (2%), dizziness (<1% to 2%)

Endocrine & metabolic: Increased serum triglycerides (≥751 mg/dL: <1% to 8%), hyperglycemia (≥251 mg/dL: 5%), hypoglycemia (children: grades 3/4: 4%)

Gastrointestinal: Vomiting (children 8% to 12%; adults 3% to 4%), diarrhea (children 8% to 9%; adults 1% to 3%), increased serum lipase (adults: >2 x ULN: ≤5%), abdominal pain (4%)

Hematologic & oncologic: Decreased neutrophils (<750 cells/mm^3: 3% to 7%), decreased hemoglobin (<8.0 g/dL: <1% to 5%), decreased platelet count (<50,000 cells/mm^3: 2%)

Hepatic: Increased serum ALT (adults and children: >5 x ULN: 3% to 9%; 10% to 25% in adult patients co-infected with hepatitis B and/or C), increased serum AST (>5 times ULN: 2% to 7%; 9% to 10% in patients co-infected with hepatitis B and/or C)

Neuromuscular & skeletal: Myalgia (4%), limb pain (children 6%)

Respiratory: Nasal congestion (children 6%), oropharyngeal pain (children 6%), rhinorrhea (children 6%), wheezing (children 6%)

Postmarketing and/or case reports: Alopecia, angioedema, arthralgia, cholecystitis, cholelithiasis, cholestasis, chronic renal failure, complete atrioventricular block (rare), diabetes mellitus, DRESS syndrome, edema, erythema multiforme, granulomatous interstitial nephritis, hepatic abnormality, immune reconstitution syndrome, interstitial nephritis, left bundle branch block, maculopapular rash, nephrolithiasis, pancreatitis, prolongation P-R interval on ECG, prolonged QT interval on ECG, pruritus, Stevens-Johnson syndrome, torsades de pointes

Mechanism of Action Binds to the site of HIV-1 protease activity and inhibits cleavage of viral Gag-Pol polyprotein precursors into individual functional proteins required for infectious HIV. This results in the formation of immature, noninfectious viral particles.

Pharmacodynamics/Kinetics

Half-life Elimination Unboosted therapy: 7 to 8 hours; Boosted therapy (with ritonavir): 9 to 18 hours; 12 hours in patients with hepatic impairment

Time to Peak Plasma: 2 to 3 hours

Reproductive Considerations

The Health and Human Services (HHS) perinatal HIV guidelines consider atazanavir (when combined with low-dose ritonavir boosting) a preferred protease inhibitor for females living with HIV who are not yet pregnant but are trying to conceive. Atazanavir (when combined with low-dose cobicistat boosting) is not recommended for in women who are planning a pregnancy.

Females living with HIV not planning a pregnancy may use any available type of contraception, considering possible drug interactions and contraindications of the specific method. Consult drug interactions database for more detailed information specific to use of atazanavir and combination oral contraceptives.

For males and females living with HIV and planning a pregnancy, maximum viral suppression below the limits of detection with antiretroviral therapy (ART), modification of therapy (if needed), optimization of the woman's health, and a discussion of the potential risks and benefits of ART therapy during pregnancy is recommended prior to conception (HHS [perinatal] 2019).

Pregnancy Considerations

Atazanavir has a low level of transfer across the human placenta with cord blood concentrations reported as 13% to 21% of maternal serum concentrations at delivery.

An increased risk of teratogenic effects has not been observed based on information collected by the antiretroviral pregnancy registry. Maternal antiretroviral therapy (ART) may be associated with adverse pregnancy outcomes including preterm delivery, stillbirth, low birth weight, and small for gestational age infants. Actual risks may be influenced by maternal factors such as disease severity, gestational age at initiation of therapy, and specific ART regimen, therefore close fetal monitoring is recommended. Because there is clear benefit to appropriate treatment, maternal ART should not be withheld due to concerns for adverse neonatal outcomes. Long-term follow-up is recommended for all infants exposed to antiretroviral medications; children without HIV but who were exposed to ART in utero and develop significant organ system abnormalities of unknown etiology (particularly of the CNS or heart) should be evaluated for potential mitochondrial dysfunction. Hyperbilirubinemia or hypoglycemia may occur in neonates following in utero exposure to atazanavir, although data are conflicting (monitor). Hyperglycemia, new onset of diabetes mellitus, or diabetic ketoacidosis have been reported with protease inhibitors; it is not clear if pregnancy increases this risk. Consider performing the standard glucose screening test earlier in pregnancy in women who initiated protease inhibitor therapy prior to conception.

Use of unboosted atazanavir is not recommended during pregnancy. The Health and Human Services (HHS) perinatal HIV guidelines consider atazanavir (when combined with low-dose ritonavir boosting) a preferred protease inhibitor for pregnant females living with HIV who are antiretroviral-naive (initial therapy), who have had ART therapy in the past but are restarting, or who require a new ART regimen (due to poor tolerance or poor virologic response of current regimen). In addition, females who become pregnant while taking atazanavir may continue if viral suppression is effective and the regimen is well tolerated. Atazanavir (when combined with low-dose cobicistat boosting) is not recommended for use during pregnancy. If pregnancy occurs during therapy, consideration should be given to changing to a more effective regimen. If continued, close monitoring, including more frequent therapeutic drug monitoring if available, is recommended.

Atazanavir is not recommended in treatment-experienced pregnant females taking both H_2-receptor blockers and tenofovir disoproxil fumarate. Pharmacokinetic studies suggest that standard dosing during pregnancy may provide decreased plasma concentrations and some experts recommend increased doses during the second and third trimesters. However, the manufacturer notes that dose adjustment is not required unless using concomitant H_2-receptor blockers or tenofovir disoproxil fumarate in antiretroviral-experienced pregnant females. Therapeutic drug monitoring may be useful.

In general, ART is recommended for all pregnant females living with HIV to keep the viral load below the limit of detection and reduce the risk of perinatal transmission. Therapy should be individualized following a discussion of the potential risks and benefits of treatment during pregnancy. Monitoring of pregnant females is more frequent than in non-pregnant adults. ART should be continued postpartum for all females living with HIV and can be modified after delivery.

Health care providers are encouraged to enroll pregnant females exposed to antiretroviral medications as early in pregnancy as possible in the Antiretroviral Pregnancy Registry (1-800-258-4263 or http://www.APRegistry.com). Health care providers caring for pregnant females living with HIV and their infants may contact the National Perinatal HIV Hotline (888-448-8765) for clinical consultation (HHS [perinatal] 2019).

Atazanavir and Cobicistat

(at a za NA veer & koe BIK i stat)

Brand Names: US Evotaz

Brand Names: Canada Evotaz [DSC]

Pharmacologic Category Antiretroviral, Protease Inhibitor (Anti-HIV); Cytochrome P-450 Inhibitor

Use

HIV-1 infection, treatment: Treatment of HIV-1 infection in adults and pediatric patients weighing ≥35 kg in combination with other antiretroviral agents.

Limitations of use: Use in treatment-experienced patients should be guided by the number of baseline primary protease inhibitor resistance substitutions

Local Anesthetic/Vasoconstrictor Precautions No information available to require special precautions

Effects on Dental Treatment No significant effects or complications reported

Effects on Bleeding Increased bleeding has been noted with protease inhibitors, such as atazanavir, in patients with hemophilia A or B. Thrombocytopenia has been reported. No other information is available to require special precautions in other patients.

Adverse Reactions All adverse reactions are from trials using cobicistat coadministered with atazanavir, emtricitabine + tenofovir. Also see individual agents.

>10%: Hepatic: Increased serum bilirubin (grades 3/4: 73%)

1% to 10%:

Central nervous system: Headache (2%), abnormal dreams (<2%), depression (<2%), fatigue (<2%), insomnia (<2%)

Dermatologic: Skin rash (5%)

Endocrine & metabolic: Increased gamma-glutamyl transferase (grades 3/4: 4%), glycosuria (grades 3/4: 3%), increased serum glucose (grades 3/4: 2%), Fanconi syndrome (<2%)

Gastrointestinal: Increased serum amylase (grades 3/4: 4%), diarrhea (2%), nausea (2%), upper abdominal pain (<2%), vomiting (<2%)

Genitourinary: Hematuria (grades 3/4: 6%)

Hematologic & oncologic: Decreased neutrophils (grades 3/4: 3%)

Hepatic: Increased serum ALT (grades 3/4: 6%), jaundice (6%), increased serum AST (grades 3/4: 4%)

Neuromuscular & skeletal: Increased creatine phosphokinase (grades 3/4: 8%), rhabdomyolysis (<2%)

Ophthalmic: Scleral icterus (4%)

Renal: Nephrolithiasis (<2%), renal disease (<2%)

Frequency not defined: Endocrine & metabolic: Increased HDL cholesterol, increased LDL cholesterol, increased serum glucose, increased serum triglycerides

Mechanism of Action

Atazanavir binds to the site of HIV-1 protease activity and inhibits cleavage of viral Gag-Pol polyprotein precursors into individual functional proteins required for infectious HIV. This results in the formation of immature, noninfectious viral particles.

Cobicistat is a mechanism-based inhibitor of cytochrome P450 3A (CYP3A). Inhibition of CYP3A-mediated metabolism by cobicistat and increases the systemic exposure of CYP3A substrates (eg, atazanavir).

Reproductive Considerations

The Health and Human Services perinatal HIV guidelines do not recommend this fixed-dose combination for females living with HIV who are not yet pregnant but are trying to conceive (HHS [perinatal] 2019).

Females living with HIV not planning a pregnancy may use any available type of contraception, considering possible drug interactions and contraindications of the specific method. Consult drug interactions database for more detailed information specific to use of atazanavir/cobicistat and combination oral contraceptives. The manufacturer recommends considering use of nonhormonal contraceptives.

Refer to individual monographs for additional information.

Pregnancy Considerations
The Health and Human Services (HHS) perinatal HIV guidelines do not recommend this fixed-dose combination for pregnant females living with HIV who are antiretroviral-naive, who have had antiretroviral therapy (ART) in the past but are restarting, or who require a new ART regimen (due to poor tolerance or poor virologic response of current regimen). For females who become pregnant while taking this combination, consider altering the regimen, or continue with frequent monitoring if viral suppression is effective and the regimen is well tolerated. Trough concentrations of atazanavir may be significantly reduced during the second and third trimesters when used in combination with cobicistat (HHS [perinatal] 2019).

Refer to individual monographs for additional information.

◆ **Atazanavir Sulfate** *see* Atazanavir *on page 186*

◆ **Atazanavir Sulfate/Cobicistat** *see* Atazanavir and Cobicistat *on page 188*

◆ **Atelvia** *see* Risedronate *on page 1331*

Atenolol (a TEN oh lole)

Related Information
Cardiovascular Diseases *on page 1654*

Brand Names: US Tenormin

Brand Names: Canada ACT Atenolol; AG-Atenolol; APO-Atenol; BIO-Atenolol; DOM-Atenolol; GMD-Atenolol; JAMP-Atenolol; Mar-Atenolol; MINT-Atenol; MYLAN-Atenolol [DSC]; PMS-Atenolol; RIVA-Atenolol; SANDOZ Atenolol [DSC]; Septa-Atenolol; TARO-Atenolol; Tenormin; TEVA-Atenolol; TRIA-Atenolol

Pharmacologic Category Antianginal Agent; Antihypertensive; Beta-Blocker, Beta-1 Selective

Use

Acute MI: Management of hemodynamically stable patients with definite or suspected acute MI to reduce cardiovascular mortality.

Guideline recommendations: According to the American College of Cardiology Foundation/American Heart Association (ACC/AHA) guidelines for the management of ST-elevation myocardial infarction (STEMI) and the ACC/AHA guidelines for the management of non-ST-elevation ACS (NSTE-ACS), oral beta-blockers should be initiated within the first 24 hours unless the patient has signs of heart failure, evidence of a low-output state, an increased risk for cardiogenic shock, or other contraindications. However, recommendations do not specify any particular beta-blocking agent for optimal treatment of NSTE-ACS. Thus, clinicians must use practical experience to determine proper therapy in managing patients (ACC/AHA [Amsterdam 2014]; ACC/AHA [O'Gara 2013]).

Angina pectoris caused by coronary atherosclerosis: Long-term management of patients with angina pectoris.

Hypertension: Management of hypertension. **Note:** Beta-blockers are **not** recommended as first-line therapy (ACC/AHA [Whelton 2017]).

Local Anesthetic/Vasoconstrictor Precautions No information available to require special precautions

Effects on Dental Treatment Atenolol is a cardioselective beta-blocker. Local anesthetic with vasoconstrictor can be safely used in patients medicated with atenolol. Nonselective beta-blockers (ie, propranolol, nadolol) enhance the pressor response to epinephrine, resulting in hypertension and bradycardia; this has not been reported for atenolol. Many nonsteroidal anti-inflammatory drugs, such as ibuprofen and indomethacin, can reduce the hypotensive effect of beta-blockers after 3 or more weeks of therapy with the NSAID. Short-term NSAID use (ie, 3 days) requires no special precautions in patients taking beta-blockers.

Effects on Bleeding No information available to require special precautions

Adverse Reactions Incidence rates are from studies in hypertensive patients unless otherwise noted.

>10%:

Cardiovascular: Hypotension (acute myocardial infarction: 25%), cardiac failure (acute myocardial infarction: 19%), bradycardia (acute myocardial infarction: 18%; 3%), ventricular tachycardia (acute myocardial infarction: 16%), cold extremities (12%), supraventricular tachycardia (acute myocardial infarction: 12%)

Central nervous system: Fatigue (≤26%), dizziness (1% to 13%), depression (≤12%)

1% to 10%:

Cardiovascular: Bundle branch block (acute myocardial infarction: 7%), atrial fibrillation (acute myocardial infarction: 5%), heart block (acute myocardial infarction: 5%), atrial flutter (acute myocardial infarction: 2%), orthostatic hypotension (2%), pulmonary embolism (acute myocardial infarction: 1%)

Central nervous system: Abnormal dreams (3%), lethargy (1% to 3%), vertigo (2%), drowsiness (≤2%)

Gastrointestinal: Nausea (3% to 4%), diarrhea (2% to 3%)

Neuromuscular & skeletal: Limb pain (3%)

Respiratory: Bronchospasm (acute myocardial infarction: 1%)

<1%, postmarketing, and/or case reports: Antibody development, cardiogenic shock, exacerbation of psoriasis, hallucination, headache, impotence, increased liver enzymes, increased serum bilirubin, lupus-like syndrome, nonthrombocytopenic purpura, Peyronie disease, psoriasiform eruption, psychosis, Raynaud disease, renal failure syndrome, sick sinus syndrome, thrombocytopenia, transient alopecia, visual disturbance, xerostomia

Mechanism of Action Competitively blocks response to beta-adrenergic stimulation, selectively blocks $beta_1$-receptors with little or no effect on $beta_2$-receptors except at high doses

Pharmacodynamics/Kinetics

Onset of Action Oral: ≤1 hour; Peak effect: Oral: 2 to 4 hours

Duration of Action Normal renal function: Beta-blocking effect: 12 to 24 hours; Antihypertensive effect: Oral: 24 hours

Half-life Elimination Beta:

Newborns (<24 hours of age) born to mothers receiving atenolol: Mean: 16 hours; up to 35 hours (Rubin 1983)

Children and Adolescents 5 to 16 years of age: Mean: 4.6 hours; range: 3.5 to 7 hours; Patients >10 years of age may have longer half-life (>5 hours) compared to children 5 to 10 years of age (<5 hours) (Buck 1989)

Adults: Normal renal function: 6 to 7 hours, prolonged with renal impairment; End-stage renal disease (ESRD): 15 to 35 hours

Time to Peak Plasma: Oral: 2 to 4 hours

Pregnancy Risk Factor D

Pregnancy Considerations

Atenolol crosses the placenta and is found in cord blood.

Maternal use of atenolol may cause harm to the fetus. Adverse events, such as bradycardia, hypoglycemia and reduced birth weight, have been observed following in utero exposure to atenolol. If maternal use of a beta-blocker is needed, fetal growth should be monitored during pregnancy and the newborn should be monitored for 48 hours after delivery for bradycardia, hypoglycemia, and respiratory depression (ESC [Regitz-Zagrosek 2018]).

Chronic maternal hypertension is also associated with adverse events in the fetus/infant. Chronic maternal hypertension may increase the risk of birth defects, low birth weight, premature delivery, stillbirth, and neonatal death. Actual fetal/neonatal risks may be related to duration and severity of maternal hypertension. Untreated chronic hypertension may also increase the risks of adverse maternal outcomes, including gestational diabetes, preeclampsia, delivery complications, stroke, and myocardial infarction (ACOG 203 2019).

The maternal pharmacokinetic parameters of atenolol during the second and third trimesters are within the ranges reported in nonpregnant patients (Hebert 2005). When treatment of chronic hypertension in pregnancy is indicated, atenolol is not recommended due to adverse fetal/neonatal events (ACOG 203 2019; ESC [Regitz-Zagrosek 2018]; Magee 2014). If atenolol is used in women with preexisting hypertension, it should be discontinued as soon as pregnancy is diagnosed (Magee 2014). Atenolol is also not recommended for the treatment of atrial fibrillation or supraventricular tachycardia during pregnancy; consult current guidelines for specific recommendations (ESC [Regitz-Zagrosek 2018]).

Atenolol and Chlorthalidone

(a TEN oh lole & klor THAL i done)

Related Information

Atenolol *on page 189*

Chlorthalidone *on page 343*

Brand Names: US Tenoretic

Brand Names: Canada Tenoretic

Pharmacologic Category Antihypertensive; Beta-Blocker, Beta-1 Selective; Diuretic, Thiazide

Use Hypertension: Management of hypertension

Local Anesthetic/Vasoconstrictor Precautions No information available to require special precautions

Effects on Dental Treatment Atenolol is a cardioselective beta-blocker. Local anesthetic with vasoconstrictor can be safely used in patients medicated with atenolol. Nonselective beta-blockers (ie, propranolol, nadolol) enhance the pressor response to epinephrine, resulting in hypertension and bradycardia; this has not been reported for atenolol. Many nonsteroidal anti-inflammatory drugs, such as ibuprofen and indomethacin, can reduce the hypotensive effect of beta-blockers after 3 or more weeks of therapy with the NSAID. Short-term NSAID use (ie, 3 days) requires no special precautions in patients taking beta-blockers.

Effects on Bleeding No information available to require special precautions

Adverse Reactions See individual agents.

Pregnancy Risk Factor D

Pregnancy Considerations Atenolol and chlorthalidone cross the placenta.

Refer to individual monographs for additional information.

- **Atenolol/Chlorthalidone** *see* Atenolol and Chlorthalidone *on page 190*
- **Atenolol+SyrSpend SF PH4** *see* Atenolol *on page 189*
- **ATG** *see* Antithymocyte Globulin (Equine) *on page 157*
- **Atgam** *see* Antithymocyte Globulin (Equine) *on page 157*
- **Athletes Foot Spray [OTC]** *see* Tolnaftate *on page 1462*
- **ATIII** *see* Antithrombin *on page 156*
- **Ativan** *see* LORazepam *on page 931*
- **Atlizumab** *see* Tocilizumab *on page 1457*

AtoMOXetine (AT oh mox e teen)

Related Information

Dentin Hypersensitivity, Acid Erosion, High Caries Index, Management of Alveolar Osteitis, and Xerostomia *on page 1762*

Brand Names: US Strattera

Brand Names: Canada APO-Atomoxetine; AURO-Atomoxetine; DOM-Atomoxetine; MYLAN-Atomoxetine [DSC]; PMS-Atomoxetine; RIVA-Atomoxetine; SANDOZ Atomoxetine; Strattera; TEVA-Atomoxetine

Pharmacologic Category Norepinephrine Reuptake Inhibitor, Selective

Use Attention-deficit/hyperactivity disorder: Treatment of attention-deficit/hyperactivity disorder (ADHD)

Local Anesthetic/Vasoconstrictor Precautions Use vasoconstrictor with caution. Atomoxetine may increase heart rate or blood pressure in the presence of pressor agents. Pressor agents include the vasoconstrictors epinephrine or mepivacaine and levonordefrin (Carbocaine® 2% with Neo-Cobefrin®)

Effects on Dental Treatment Key adverse event(s) related to dental treatment: Xerostomia (normal salivary flow resumes upon discontinuation)

Effects on Bleeding No information available to require special precautions

Adverse Reactions Percentages as reported in children and adults; some adverse reactions may be increased in "poor metabolizers" (CYP2D6). Frequency not always defined.

>10%:

Central nervous system: Headache (19%; children and adolescents), insomnia (1% to 19%), drowsiness (8% to 11%)

Dermatologic: Hyperhidrosis (4% to 15%)

Gastrointestinal: Xerostomia (17% to 35%), nausea (7% to 26%), decreased appetite (15% to 23%), abdominal pain (7% to 18%), vomiting (4% to 11%), constipation (1% to 11%)

Genitourinary: Erectile dysfunction (8% to 21%)

1% to 10%:

Cardiovascular: Increased diastolic blood pressure (5% to 9%; ≥15 mm Hg), systolic hypertension (4% to 5%), palpitations (3%), cold extremities (1% to 3%), syncope (≤3%), flushing (≥2%), orthostatic hypotension (≤2%), tachycardia (≤2%), prolonged QT interval on ECG

Central nervous system: Fatigue (6% to 10%), dizziness (5% to 8%), depression (4% to 7%), disturbed sleep (3% to 7%), irritability (5% to 6%), jitteriness (2% to 5%), abnormal dreams (4%), chills (3%), paresthesia (adults 3%; postmarketing observation in children), anxiety (≥2%), hostility (children and adolescents 2%), emotional lability (1% to 2%), agitation, restlessness, sensation of cold

Dermatologic: Excoriation (2% to 4%), skin rash (2%), pruritus, urticaria

Endocrine & metabolic: Weight loss (2% to 7%), decreased libido (3%), hot flash (3%), increased thirst (2%), menstrual disease

Gastrointestinal: Dyspepsia (4%), anorexia (3%), dysgeusia, flatulence

Genitourinary: Ejaculatory disorder (2% to 6%), urinary retention (1% to 6%), dysmenorrhea (3%), dysuria (2%), orgasm abnormal, pollakiuria, prostatitis, testicular pain, urinary frequency

Neuromuscular & skeletal: Tremor (1% to 5%), muscle spasm, weakness

Ophthalmic: Blurred vision (1% to 4%), conjunctivitis (1% to 3%), mydriasis

Respiratory: Pharyngolaryngeal pain

Miscellaneous: Therapeutic response unexpected (2%)

<1%, postmarketing, and/or case reports: Aggressive behavior, akathisia, alopecia, anaphylaxis, angioedema, cerebrovascular accident, change in libido, delusions, growth suppression (children), hallucination, hepatotoxicity, hypersensitivity reaction, hypoesthesia, hypomania, impulsivity, jaundice, lethargy, mania, myocardial infarction, panic attack, pelvic pain, priapism, Raynaud's phenomenon, rhabdomyolysis, seizure (including patients with no prior history or known risk factors for seizure), severe hepatic disease, suicidal ideation, tics

Mechanism of Action Selectively inhibits the reuptake of norepinephrine (Ki 4.5 nM) with little to no activity at the other neuronal reuptake pumps or receptor sites.

Pharmacodynamics/Kinetics

Duration of Action Up to 24 hours (Jain 2017)

Half-life Elimination Atomoxetine: 5 hours (up to 24 hours in poor metabolizers); Active metabolites: 4-hydroxyatomoxetine: 6-8 hours; N-desmethylatomoxetine: 6-8 hours (34-40 hours in poor metabolizers)

Time to Peak Plasma: 1-2 hours; delayed 3 hours by high-fat meal

Reproductive Considerations Appropriate contraception is recommended for sexually active women of childbearing potential (Heiligenstein 2003). An agent other than atomoxetine is preferred for the treatment of attention-deficit/hyperactivity disorder (ADHD) in women planning a pregnancy (Larsen 2015).

Pregnancy Considerations

In comparison to other agents used for the treatment of attention-deficit/hyperactivity disorder (ADHD), information related to atomoxetine use in pregnancy is limited (Bro 2015; Haervig 2014; Heiligenstein 2003; Ornoy 2018).

If medication is needed for the treatment of ADHD during pregnancy, an agent other than atomoxetine is preferred. Consider discontinuing or changing treatment in women who become pregnant during atomoxetine therapy (Larsen 2015).

Data collection to monitor pregnancy and infant outcomes following exposure to atomoxetine is ongoing. Health care providers are encouraged to enroll females exposed to atomoxetine during pregnancy in the National Pregnancy Registry for ADHD medications at 1-866-961-2388.

◆ **Atomoxetine Hydrochloride** *see* AtoMOXetine *on page 190*

AtorvaSTATin (a TORE va sta tin)

Related Information

Cardiovascular Diseases *on page 1654*

Brand Names: US Lipitor

Brand Names: Canada ACH-Atorvastatin Calcium; AG-Atorvastatin; APO-Atorvastatin; Atorvastatin-10; Atorvastatin-20; Atorvastatin-40; Atorvastatin-80; Auro-Atorvastatin; BIO-Atorvastatin; DOM-Atorvastatin; GD-Atorvastatin [DSC]; JAMP-Atorvastatin; Lipitor; M-Atorvastatin; Mar-Atorvastatin; MINT-Atorvastatin; MYLAN-Atorvastatin; NRA-Atorvastatin; PMS-Atorvastatin; PRIVA-Atorvastatin; RATIO-Atorvastatin [DSC]; REDDY-Atorvastatin; RIVA-Atorvastatin; SANDOZ Atorvastatin; TARO-Atorvastatin; TEVA-Atorvastatin

Pharmacologic Category Antilipemic Agent, HMG-CoA Reductase Inhibitor

Use

Heterozygous familial hypercholesterolemia: To reduce elevated total cholesterol (total-C), LDL cholesterol (LDL-C), apolipoprotein B (apo B), and triglyceride levels, and to increase HDL cholesterol in patients with primary hypercholesterolemia.

Heterozygous familial hypercholesterolemia (pediatrics): To reduce total-C, LDL-C, and apo B levels in pediatric patients 10 to 17 years of age with heterozygous familial hypercholesterolemia with LDL-C ≥190 mg/dL, LDL-C ≥160 mg/dL with positive family history of premature cardiovascular disease (CVD), or LDL-C ≥160 mg/dL with 2 or more other CVD risk factors.

Homozygous familial hypercholesterolemia: To reduce total-C and LDL-C in patients with homozygous familial hypercholesterolemia as an adjunct to other lipid-lowering treatments (eg, LDL apheresis) or if such treatments are unavailable.

Prevention of atherosclerotic cardiovascular disease:

Primary prevention of atherosclerotic cardiovascular disease (ASCVD): To reduce the risk of myocardial infarction (MI), stroke, revascularization procedures, and angina in adult patients without a history of coronary heart disease (CHD) but who have multiple CHD risk factors.

Secondary prevention in patients with established ASCVD: To reduce the risk of MI, stroke, revascularization procedures, and angina in patients with a history of CHD.

Local Anesthetic/Vasoconstrictor Precautions No information available to require special precautions

Effects on Dental Treatment Key adverse event(s) related to dental treatment: Assess unusual presentations of muscle weakness or myopathy resulting from lipid therapy such as patient having a difficult time brushing teeth or weakness with chewing. Refer patient back to their physician for evaluation and adjustment of lipid therapy.

Effects on Bleeding No information available to require special precautions

Adverse Reactions

>10%:

Gastrointestinal: Diarrhea (7% to 14%)

Neuromuscular & skeletal: Arthralgia (9% to 12%)

Respiratory: Nasopharyngitis (13%)

1% to 10%:

Cardiovascular: Hemorrhagic stroke (2%)

Central nervous system: Insomnia (5%), malaise (<2%), nightmares (<2%)

Dermatologic: Urticaria (<2%)

Endocrine & metabolic: Diabetes mellitus (6%), hyperglycemia (<2%)

Gastrointestinal: Nausea (7%), dyspepsia (6%), abdominal distress (<2%), cholestasis (<2%), eructation (<2%), flatulence (<2%)

Genitourinary: Urinary tract infection (7% to 8%), urine abnormality (white blood cells positive in urine: <2%)

Hepatic: Increased serum transaminases (≤2%), abnormal hepatic function tests (<2%), hepatitis (<2%), increased serum alkaline phosphatase (<2%)

Neuromuscular & skeletal: Limb pain (9%), myalgia (4% to 8%), musculoskeletal pain (5%), muscle spasm (4% to 5%), increased creatine phosphokinase (<2%), joint swelling (<2%), muscle fatigue (<2%), neck pain (<2%)

Ophthalmic: Blurred vision (<2%)

Otic: Tinnitus (<2%)

Respiratory: Pharyngolaryngeal pain (3% to 4%), epistaxis (<2%)

Miscellaneous: Fever (<2%)

Frequency not defined: Central nervous system: Myasthenia

<1%, postmarketing, and/or case reports: Abdominal pain, alopecia, amnesia (reversible), anaphylaxis, anemia, angioedema, anorexia, back pain, bullous rash, chest pain, cognitive dysfunction (reversible), confusion (reversible), cystitis (interstitial; Huang 2015), depression, dizziness, dysgeusia, elevated glycosylated hemoglobin (HbA_{1c}), erythema multiforme, fatigue, gynecomastia, hepatic failure, hypoesthesia, increased serum glucose, interstitial pulmonary disease, jaundice, memory impairment (reversible), myopathy, myositis, pancreatitis, paresthesia, peripheral edema, peripheral neuropathy, pruritus, rhabdomyolysis, rupture of tendon, Stevens-Johnson syndrome, thrombocytopenia, toxic epidermal necrolysis, vomiting, weight gain

Mechanism of Action Inhibitor of 3-hydroxy-3-methylglutaryl coenzyme A (HMG-CoA) reductase, the rate-limiting enzyme in cholesterol synthesis (reduces the production of mevalonic acid from HMG-CoA); this then results in a compensatory increase in the expression of LDL receptors on hepatocyte membranes and a stimulation of LDL catabolism. In addition to the ability of HMG-CoA reductase inhibitors to decrease levels of high-sensitivity C-reactive protein (hsCRP), they also possess pleiotropic properties including improved endothelial function, reduced inflammation at the site of the coronary plaque, inhibition of platelet aggregation, and anticoagulant effects (de Denus 2002; Ray 2005).

Pharmacodynamics/Kinetics

Onset of Action Initial changes: 3 to 5 days; Maximal reduction in plasma cholesterol and triglycerides: 2 to 4 weeks; LDL reduction: 10 mg/day: 39% (for each doubling of this dose, LDL is lowered approximately 6%)

Half-life Elimination Parent drug: ~14 hours; Equipotent metabolites: 20 to 30 hours

Time to Peak Serum: 1 to 2 hours

Reproductive Considerations

Atorvastatin is contraindicated in females who may become pregnant.

Adequate contraception is recommended if an HMG-CoA reductase inhibitor is required in females of reproductive potential. Females planning a pregnancy should discontinue the HMG-CoA reductase inhibitor 1 to 2 months prior to attempting to conceive (AHA/ACC [Grundy 2019]).

Pregnancy Considerations Atorvastatin is contraindicated in pregnant females.

There are reports of congenital anomalies following maternal use of HMG-CoA reductase inhibitors in pregnancy; however, maternal disease, differences in specific agents used, and the low rates of exposure limit the interpretation of the available data (Godfrey 2012; Lecarpentier 2012). Cholesterol biosynthesis may be important in fetal development; serum cholesterol and triglycerides increase normally during pregnancy. The discontinuation of lipid-lowering medications temporarily during pregnancy is not expected to have significant impact on the long-term outcomes of primary hypercholesterolemia treatment.

Atorvastatin should be discontinued immediately if an unplanned pregnancy occurs during treatment.

◆ **Atorvastatin Calcium** *see* AtorvaSTATin *on page 191*

Atovaquone (a TOE va kwone)

Related Information

Systemic Viral Diseases *on page 1709*

Brand Names: US Mepron

Brand Names: Canada Mepron

Pharmacologic Category Antiprotozoal

Use

Pneumocystis jirovecii pneumonia (PCP), prophylaxis: Prevention of PCP in adults and adolescents 13 years and older who are intolerant to trimethoprim-sulfamethoxazole (TMP-SMZ)

Pneumocystis jirovecii pneumonia (PCP), treatment: Acute oral treatment of mild to moderate PCP in adults and adolescents 13 years and older who are intolerant to TMP-SMZ

Local Anesthetic/Vasoconstrictor Precautions No information available to require special precautions

Effects on Dental Treatment Key adverse event(s) related to dental treatment: Occurrence of oral *Candida* infection, altered sense of taste; frequent occurrence of cough, rhinitis, sinusitis

Effects on Bleeding No information available to require special precautions

Adverse Reactions Frequency not always defined. Adverse reaction statistics have been compiled from studies including patients with advanced HIV disease. Consequently, it is difficult to distinguish reactions attributed to atovaquone from those caused by the underlying disease or a combination thereof.

>10%:

Central nervous system: Headache (16% to 31%), insomnia (10% to 19%), depression, pain

Dermatologic: Skin rash (22% to 46%), pruritus (5% to ≥10%), diaphoresis

Gastrointestinal: Diarrhea (19% to 42%), nausea (21% to 32%), vomiting (14% to 22%), abdominal pain (4% to 21%)

Infection: Infection (18% to 22%)

Neuromuscular & skeletal: Weakness (8% to 31%), myalgia

Respiratory: Cough (14% to 25%), rhinitis (5% to 24%), dyspnea (15% to 21%), sinusitis (7% to ≥10%), flu-like symptoms

Miscellaneous: Fever (14% to 40%)

1% to 10%:

Cardiovascular: Hypotension (≤1%)

Central nervous system: Dizziness (3% to 8%), anxiety (≤7%)

Endocrine & metabolic: Hyponatremia (7% to 10%), hyperglycemia (≤9%), increased amylase (7% to 8%), hypoglycemia (≤1%)

Gastrointestinal: Oral candidiasis (5% to 10%), anorexia (≤7%), dyspepsia (≤5%), constipation (≤3%), dysgeusia (≤3%)

Hematologic & oncologic: Anemia (4% to 6%), neutropenia (3% to 5%)

Hepatic: Increased liver enzymes (4% to 8%)

Renal: Increased blood urea nitrogen (≤1%), increased serum creatinine (≤1%)

Respiratory: Bronchospasm (2% to 4%)

<1%, postmarketing, and/or case reports: Acute renal failure, angioedema, constriction of the pharynx, corneal disease (vortex keratopathy), desquamation, erythema multiforme, hepatic failure (rare), hepatitis (rare), hypersensitivity reaction, methemoglobinemia, pancreatitis, Stevens-Johnson syndrome, thrombocytopenia, urticaria

Mechanism of Action Inhibits electron transport in mitochondria resulting in the inhibition of key metabolic enzymes responsible for the synthesis of nucleic acids and ATP

Pharmacodynamics/Kinetics

Half-life Elimination Range: 67 ± 33.4 hours to 77.6 ± 23.1 hours

Pregnancy Considerations

Information specific to the use of atovaquone in pregnancy is limited.

Diagnosis and treatment of *Pneumocystis jirovecii* pneumonia (PCP) in pregnant women is the same as in nonpregnant women. Atovaquone may be used as an alternative agent for PCP and *Toxoplasma gondii* infections when needed in pregnancy (HHS [OI adult 2020]).

Atovaquone and Proguanil

(a TOE va kwone & pro GWA nil)

Related Information

Atovaquone *on page 192*

Brand Names: US Malarone

Brand Names: Canada Malarone; Malarone Pediatric

Pharmacologic Category Antimalarial Agent

Use

Malaria, prophylaxis: Prophylaxis of *Plasmodium falciparum* malaria, including areas where chloroquine resistance has been reported. **Note:** CDC also recommends atovaquone/proguanil as prophylaxis for other *Plasmodium* species (CDC Yellow Book 2020).

Malaria, treatment: Treatment of acute, uncomplicated *P. falciparum* malaria. **Note:** CDC guidelines also recommend atovaquone/proguanil as an alternative agent for chloroquine-sensitive *Plasmodium* species, for chloroquine-resistant *Plasmodium vivax or Plasmodium ovale*, and as alternative oral treatment for severe malaria after completion of IV therapy or as interim therapy pending IV therapy (CDC 2020).

Local Anesthetic/Vasoconstrictor Precautions No information available to require special precautions

Effects on Dental Treatment No significant effects or complications reported

Effects on Bleeding No information available to require special precautions

Adverse Reactions The following adverse reactions were reported in patients being treated for malaria. When used for prophylaxis, reactions are similar to those seen with placebo.

>10%:

Gastrointestinal: Abdominal pain (17%), nausea (12%), vomiting (children: 10% to 13%; adults: 12%)

Hepatic: Increased serum ALT (27%; increased liver function test values typically normalized after ~4 weeks), increased serum AST (17%; increased liver function test values typically normalized after ~4 weeks)

1% to 10%:

Central nervous system: Headache (10%), dizziness (5%)

Dermatologic: Pruritus (children: 6%)

Gastrointestinal: Diarrhea (children: 6%; adults: 8%), anorexia (5%)

Neuromuscular & skeletal: Weakness (8%)

<1%, postmarketing, and/or case reports: Anaphylaxis (rare), anemia (rare), angioedema, cholestasis, erythema multiforme (rare), hallucination, hepatic failure (case report), hepatitis (rare), neutropenia, pancytopenia (with severe renal impairment), psychotic reaction (rare), seizure (rare), skin photosensitivity, skin rash, Stevens-Johnson syndrome (rare), stomatitis, urticaria, vasculitis (rare)

Mechanism of Action

Atovaquone: Selectively inhibits parasite mitochondrial electron transport.

Proguanil: The metabolite cycloguanil inhibits dihydrofolate reductase, disrupting deoxythymidylate synthesis. Together, atovaquone/cycloguanil affect the erythrocytic and exoerythrocytic stages of development.

Pharmacodynamics/Kinetics

Half-life Elimination

Atovaquone: 2-3 days (adults), 1-2 days (children)

Proguanil: 12-21 hours

Pregnancy Considerations

Outcome information following maternal use of atovaquone and proguanil in pregnancy is limited (Andrejko 2019; Mayer 2018; Pasternak 2011).

The pharmacokinetics of atovaquone and proguanil may be altered during pregnancy (Burger 2016).

Malaria infection in pregnant women may be more severe than in nonpregnant women and has a high risk of maternal and perinatal morbidity and mortality. Malaria infection during pregnancy can lead to miscarriage, premature delivery, low birth weight, congenital infection, and/or perinatal death. Therefore, pregnant women and women who are likely to become pregnant are advised to avoid travel to malaria-risk areas. When travel is unavoidable, pregnant women should take precautions to avoid mosquito bites and use effective prophylactic medications (CDC 2020; CDC Yellow Book 2020).

Due to limited information, atovaquone/proguanil is not preferred for use during pregnancy. However, atovaquone/proguanil may be used as an alternative treatment of malaria in pregnant women when other treatment options are not available or not being tolerated; consult current CDC guidelines (CDC 2020).

- **Atovaquone and Proguanil Hydrochloride** *see* Atovaquone and Proguanil *on page 193*
- **Atovaquone/Proguanil HCl** *see* Atovaquone and Proguanil *on page 193*
- **ATRA** *see* Tretinoin (Systemic) *on page 1483*
- **Atralin** *see* Tretinoin (Topical) *on page 1484*
- **Atripla** *see* Efavirenz, Emtricitabine, and Tenofovir Disoproxil Fumarate *on page 545*
- **Atropine and Diphenoxylate** *see* Diphenoxylate and Atropine *on page 503*
- **Atrovent HFA** *see* Ipratropium (Oral Inhalation) *on page 838*
- **ATV** *see* Atazanavir *on page 186*
- **Aubagio** *see* Teriflunomide *on page 1423*
- **Aubra** *see* Ethinyl Estradiol and Levonorgestrel *on page 612*
- **Aubra EQ** *see* Ethinyl Estradiol and Levonorgestrel *on page 612*
- **Audenz** *see* Influenza A Virus Vaccine (H5N1) *on page 811*
- **Augmentin** *see* Amoxicillin and Clavulanate *on page 130*
- **Augmentin ES-600** *see* Amoxicillin and Clavulanate *on page 130*
- **Augmentin XR [DSC]** *see* Amoxicillin and Clavulanate *on page 130*
- **Auraphene-B [OTC]** *see* Carbamide Peroxide *on page 289*
- **Aurodryl Allergy Childrens [OTC]** *see* DiphenhydrAMINE (Systemic) *on page 502*
- **Aurovela 1.5/30** *see* Ethinyl Estradiol and Norethindrone *on page 614*
- **Aurovela 1/20** *see* Ethinyl Estradiol and Norethindrone *on page 614*
- **Aurovela 24 FE** *see* Ethinyl Estradiol and Norethindrone *on page 614*
- **Aurovela Fe 1.5/30** *see* Ethinyl Estradiol and Norethindrone *on page 614*
- **Aurovela FE 1/20** *see* Ethinyl Estradiol and Norethindrone *on page 614*
- **Autologous Anti-CD19 CAR-positive T lymphocytes KTE-C19** *see* Axicabtagene Ciloleucel *on page 196*
- **Autologous CART-19 TCR:4-1BB cells** *see* Tisagenlecleucel *on page 1454*
- **Auvi-Q** *see* EPINEPHrine (Systemic) *on page 569*
- **Avage [DSC]** *see* Tazarotene *on page 1408*
- **Avakine** *see* InFLIXimab *on page 809*

Avanafil (a VAN a fil)

Brand Names: US Stendra

Pharmacologic Category Phosphodiesterase-5 Enzyme Inhibitor

Use Erectile dysfunction: Treatment of erectile dysfunction

Local Anesthetic/Vasoconstrictor Precautions No information available to require special precautions

Effects on Dental Treatment No significant effects or complications reported

Effects on Bleeding No information available to require special precautions

Adverse Reactions

>10%: Central nervous system: Headache (1% to 12%)

2% to 10%:

Cardiovascular: Flushing (3% to 10%), ECG abnormality (1% to 3%)

Central nervous system: Dizziness (1% to 2%)

Gastrointestinal: Viral gastroenteritis (≤2%)

Neuromuscular & skeletal: Back pain (1% to 3%)

Respiratory: Nasopharyngitis (1% to 5%), nasal congestion (1% to 3%), upper respiratory tract infection (1% to 3%)

<2%, postmarketing, and/or case reports: Abdominal distress, angina pectoris, anterior ischemic optic neuropathy (nonarteritic), arthralgia, balanitis, bronchitis, constipation, cough, deep vein thrombosis, depression, diarrhea, drowsiness, dyspepsia, dyspnea on exertion, epistaxis, fatigue, gastritis, gastroesophageal reflux disease, hearing loss, hematuria, hyperglycemia, hypertension, hypoglycemia, hypotension, increased serum ALT, influenza, insomnia, limb pain, muscle spasm, musculoskeletal pain, myalgia, nausea, nephrolithiasis, oropharyngeal pain, palpitations, peripheral edema, pollakiuria, priapism, pruritus, sinus congestion, sinusitis, skin rash, tinnitus, urinary tract infection, vertigo, vision color changes, vision loss (temporary or permanent), vomiting, wheezing

Mechanism of Action Does not directly cause penile erections, but affects the response to sexual stimulation. The physiologic mechanism of erection of the penis involves release of nitric oxide (NO) in the corpus cavernosum during sexual stimulation. NO then activates the enzyme guanylate cyclase, which results in increased levels of cyclic guanosine monophosphate (cGMP), producing smooth muscle relaxation and inflow of blood to the corpus cavernosum. Avanafil enhances the effect of NO by inhibiting phosphodiesterase type 5 (PDE-5), which is responsible for degradation of cGMP in the corpus cavernosum; when sexual stimulation causes local release of NO, inhibition of PDE-5 by avanafil causes increased levels of cGMP in the corpus cavernosum, resulting in smooth muscle relaxation and inflow of blood to the corpus cavernosum; at recommended doses, it has no effect in the absence of sexual stimulation.

Pharmacodynamics/Kinetics

Half-life Elimination Terminal: ~5 hours

Time to Peak Plasma: 30 to 45 minutes (fasting); 1.12 to 1.25 hours (high-fat meal)

Pregnancy Considerations Adverse events were not observed in animal reproduction studies. This product is not indicated for use in females.

- **Avandia** *see* Rosiglitazone *on page 1347*

Avapritinib (A va PRI ti nib)

Brand Names: US Ayvakit

Pharmacologic Category Antineoplastic Agent, PDGFR-alpha Blocker; Antineoplastic Agent, Tyrosine Kinase Inhibitor

Use Gastrointestinal stromal tumor, unresectable or metastatic: Treatment of unresectable or metastatic gastrointestinal stromal tumor harboring a PDGFRA exon 18 mutation, including PDGFRA D842V mutations in adults.

Local Anesthetic/Vasoconstrictor Precautions No information available to require special precautions.

Effects on Dental Treatment Key adverse event(s) related to dental treatment: Frequent occurrence of loss of taste, altered taste.

Effects on Bleeding Chemotherapy may result in significant myelosuppression, potentially including significant reduction in platelet counts (thrombocytopenia grades 27%; grades ≥3: <1%) and altered hemostasis. In patients who are under active treatment with these agents, medical consult is suggested.

Adverse Reactions Incidence of adverse reactions include unapproved dosing regimens.

>10%:

Cardiovascular: Edema (72%)

Central nervous system: Fatigue (≤61%), central nervous system toxicity (58%), cognitive dysfunction (41% to 48%), dizziness (20% to 22%), headache (17%), sleep disorder (15% to 16%), mood disorder (13%)

Dermatologic: Skin rash (23%), hair discoloration (21%), alopecia (13%)

Endocrine & metabolic: Decreased serum phosphate (49%), decreased serum potassium (34%), decreased serum albumin (31%), decreased serum magnesium (29%), decreased serum sodium (28%), ageusia (≤15%), dysgeusia (≤15%), weight loss (13%)

Gastrointestinal: Nausea (64%), decreased appetite (38%), vomiting (38%), diarrhea (37%), abdominal pain (31%), constipation (23%), dyspepsia (16%)

Hematologic & oncologic: Leukopenia (62%; grade ≥3: 5%), decreased neutrophils (43%; grades ≥3: 6%), thrombocytopenia (27%; grades ≥3: <1%), increased INR (24%; grades ≥3: <1%), prolonged partial thromboplastin time (13%)

Hepatic: Increased serum bilirubin (69%), increased serum aspartate aminotransferase (51%), increased serum alanine aminotransferase (19%), increased serum alkaline phosphatase (14%)

Neuromuscular & skeletal: Asthenia (≤61%)

Ophthalmic: Increased lacrimation (33%)

Renal: Increased serum creatinine (29%)

Respiratory: Dyspnea (17%), pleural effusion (12%)

Miscellaneous: Fever (14%)

1% to 10%:

Cardiovascular: Hypertension (8%)

Central nervous system: Speech disturbance (6%), intracranial hemorrhage (3%), hallucination (2%)

Dermatologic: Palmar-plantar erythrodysesthesia (1%)

Endocrine & metabolic: Hyperthyroidism (≤3%), hypothyroidism (≤3%), thyroid disease (3%)

Gastrointestinal: Severe abdominal pain (3%), gastrointestinal hemorrhage (2%), severe vomiting (2%)

Hematologic & oncologic: Anemia (9%), tumor hemorrhage (1%)

Infection: Sepsis (3%)

Renal: Acute renal failure (2%)

Respiratory: Pneumonia (1%)

Frequency not defined:

Cardiovascular: Facial edema, peripheral edema, subdural hematoma

Central nervous system: Agitation, amnesia, anxiety, cerebral hemorrhage, dementia, disturbance in attention, drowsiness, dysphoria, encephalopathy, irritability, personality changes, retrograde amnesia, suicidal ideation

Genitourinary: Testicular swelling

Hepatic: Hyperbilirubinemia

Ophthalmic: Ocular edema, periorbital edema

Respiratory: Pharyngeal edema

Mechanism of Action Avapritinib is a potent tyrosine kinase inhibitor that blocks PDGFRA; it targets PDGFRA and PDGFR D842 mutants, as well as KIT exon 11, 11/17, and 17 mutants. Certain PDGFRA and KIT mutations may result in autophosphorylation and constitutive activation of these receptors, which may contribute to tumor cell proliferation. Avapritinib inhibits autophosphorylation of KIT D816V and PDGFRA D842V, which are mutants associated with resistance to approved kinase inhibitors.

Pharmacodynamics/Kinetics

Half-life Elimination 32 to 57 hours.

Time to Peak 2 to 4.1 hours.

Reproductive Considerations

Evaluate pregnancy status prior to use in females of reproductive potential. Females of reproductive potential and males with female partners of reproductive potential should use effective contraception during therapy and for 6 weeks after the last dose of avapritinib.

Pregnancy Considerations

Based on the mechanism of action and data from animal reproduction studies, in utero exposure to avapritinib may cause fetal harm.

Prescribing and Access Restrictions

Avapritinib is available through a select network of specialty pharmacies. For more information, refer to https://ayvakit.com/hcp/.

- ◆ **Avapro** *see* Irbesartan *on page 840*
- ◆ **Avastin** *see* Bevacizumab *on page 242*
- ◆ **AVE0010** *see* Lixisenatide *on page 925*
- ◆ **Aveed** *see* Testosterone *on page 1425*
- ◆ **Avelox [DSC]** *see* Moxifloxacin (Systemic) *on page 1064*
- ◆ **Avelox ABC Pack [DSC]** *see* Moxifloxacin (Systemic) *on page 1064*

Avelumab (a VEL ue mab)

Brand Names: US Bavencio

Brand Names: Canada Bavencio

Pharmacologic Category Antineoplastic Agent, Anti-PD-L1 Monoclonal Antibody; Antineoplastic Agent, Monoclonal Antibody

Use

Merkel cell carcinoma, metastatic: Treatment of metastatic Merkel cell carcinoma in adults and children ≥12 years of age.

Renal cell carcinoma, advanced: First-line treatment of advanced renal cell carcinoma (in combination with axitinib).

Urothelial carcinoma, locally advanced or metastatic:

First-line maintenance treatment of locally advanced or metastatic urothelial carcinoma that has not progressed with first-line platinum-containing chemotherapy.

Treatment of locally advanced or metastatic urothelial carcinoma in previously treated patients who have disease progression during or following platinum-containing chemotherapy or have disease progression within 12 months of neoadjuvant or adjuvant treatment with platinum-containing chemotherapy.

Local Anesthetic/Vasoconstrictor Precautions

No information available to require special precautions

Effects on Dental Treatment No significant effects or complications reported

Effects on Bleeding **Chemotherapy may result in significant myelosuppression, potentially including significant reduction in platelet counts (thrombocytopenia 27%; grades 3/4:1%) and altered hemostasis. In patients who are under active treatment with these agents, medical consult is suggested.**

Adverse Reactions

>10%:

Cardiovascular: Peripheral edema (17% to 20%), hypertension (10% to 13%)

Central nervous system: Fatigue (41% to 50%), dizziness (14%)

Dermatologic: Skin rash (15% to 22%)

Endocrine & metabolic: Weight loss (15% to 19%), hyponatremia (grades 3/4: 16%), increased gamma-glutamyl transferase (grades 3/4: 12%)

Gastrointestinal: Nausea (22% to 24%), diarrhea (18% to 23%), decreased appetite (20% to 21%), abdominal pain (16% to 19%), constipation (17% to 18%), increased serum lipase (14%), vomiting (13% to 14%)

Genitourinary: Urinary tract infection (21%)

Hematologic & oncologic: Lymphocytopenia (49%; grades 3/4: 11% to 19%), anemia (35%; grades 3/4: 6% to 9%), thrombocytopenia (27%; grades 3/4: 1%)

Hepatic: Increased serum aspartate aminotransferase (34%), increased serum alanine aminotransferase (20%)

Neuromuscular & skeletal: Musculoskeletal pain (25% to 32%), arthralgia (16%)

Renal: Increased serum creatinine (≤16%), renal failure syndrome (≤16%)

Respiratory: Cough (14% to 18%), dyspnea (11% to 17%)

Miscellaneous: Infusion-related reaction (14% to 30%), fever (16%)

1% to 10%:

Central nervous system: Headache (10%)

Dermatologic: Pruritus (10%), cellulitis (>1%)

Endocrine & metabolic: Hyperglycemia (grades 3/4: 3% to 9%), increased amylase (8%), hypothyroidism (5%)

Gastrointestinal: Colitis (2%), intestinal obstruction (≥2%)

Hematologic & oncologic: Neutropenia (6%; grades 3/4: 1%)

Hepatic: Increased serum alkaline phosphatase (grades 3/4: 7%), increased serum bilirubin (6%)

Immunologic: Antibody development (4%)

Neuromuscular & skeletal: Asthenia (>1%)

Renal: Acute renal failure (>1%)

Respiratory: Pneumonitis (1%)

Frequency not defined: Cardiovascular: Pericardial effusion

<1%, postmarketing, and/or case reports: Adrenocortical insufficiency, arthritis, erythema multiforme, exfoliative dermatitis, Guillain-Barré syndrome, hepatitis, hyperthyroidism, myocarditis, myositis, nephritis, pemphigoid, pituitary insufficiency, psoriasis, sepsis (systemic inflammatory response), thyroiditis, type 1 diabetes mellitus, uveitis

Mechanism of Action Avelumab is a fully human monoclonal antibody that binds to programmed death ligand 1 (PD-L1) to selectively prevent the interaction between the programmed cell death-1 (PD-1) and B7.1 receptors, while still allowing interaction between PD-L2 and PD-1 (Kaufman 2016). PD-L1 is an immune check point protein expressed on tumor cells and tumor infiltrating cells and down regulates anti-tumor t-cell function by binding to PD-1 and B7.1; blocking PD-1 and B7.1 interactions restores antitumor t-cell function (Fehrenbacher 2016; Rosenberg 2016).

Pharmacodynamics/Kinetics

Half-life Elimination 6.1 days

Reproductive Considerations

Females of reproductive potential should use effective contraception during therapy and for at least 1 month after the last avelumab dose.

Pregnancy Considerations

Immunoglobulins are known to cross the placenta and fetal exposure to avelumab is expected. Based on the mechanism of action, avelumab may cause fetal harm. Immune-mediated fetal rejection causing increased abortion or stillbirth was observed in animal reproduction studies.

- ◆ **Aviane** *see* Ethinyl Estradiol and Levonorgestrel *on page 612*
- ◆ **Avian Influenza Virus Vaccine** *see* Influenza A Virus Vaccine (H5N1) *on page 811*
- ◆ **Avibactam and Ceftazidime** *see* Ceftazidime and Avibactam *on page 314*
- ◆ **Avidoxy** *see* Doxycycline *on page 522*
- ◆ **Avita** *see* Tretinoin (Topical) *on page 1484*
- ◆ **Avitene** *see* Collagen Hemostat *on page 410*
- ◆ **Avitene Flour** *see* Collagen Hemostat *on page 410*
- ◆ **Avodart** *see* Dutasteride *on page 539*
- ◆ **Avonex** *see* Interferon Beta-1a *on page 833*
- ◆ **Avonex Pen** *see* Interferon Beta-1a *on page 833*
- ◆ **AVP** *see* Vasopressin *on page 1535*
- ◆ **Avsola** *see* InFLIXimab *on page 809*
- ◆ **Avycaz** *see* Ceftazidime and Avibactam *on page 314*
- ◆ **Axert [DSC]** *see* Almotriptan *on page 104*

Axicabtagene Ciloleucel

(ax i CAB tay jeen sye LO loo sel)

Brand Names: US Yescarta

Pharmacologic Category Antineoplastic Agent, Anti-CD19; Antineoplastic Agent, CAR-T Immunotherapy; CAR-T Cell Immunotherapy; Cellular Immunotherapy, Autologous; Chimeric Antigen Receptor T-Cell Immunotherapy

Use

Large B-cell lymphoma, relapsed or refractory: Treatment of relapsed or refractory large B-cell lymphoma after 2 or more lines of systemic therapy, including diffuse large B-cell lymphoma (DLBCL) not otherwise specified, primary mediastinal large B-cell lymphoma, high grade B-cell lymphoma, and DLBCL arising from follicular lymphoma

Limitations of use: Not indicated for the treatment of patients with primary CNS lymphoma

Local Anesthetic/Vasoconstrictor Precautions

No information available to require special precautions

Effects on Dental Treatment Xerostomia, normal salivary flow with discontinuation

Effects on Bleeding No information available to require special precautions

Adverse Reactions

>10%:

Cardiovascular: Hypotension (57%), tachycardia (57%), cardiac arrhythmia (23%), edema (19%), hypertension (15%), thrombosis (10%), cardiac failure (6%), capillary leak syndrome (3%)

Central nervous system: Brain disease (57%; lasted up to 173 days), fatigue (46%), headache (44% to 45%), chills (40%), dizziness (21%), motor dysfunction (19%), aphasia (18%), delirium (17%)

Endocrine & metabolic: Hypophosphatemia (grade 3 or 4: 50%), hyponatremia (grade 3 or 4: 19%), weight loss (16%), increased uric acid (grade 3 or 4: 13%), dehydration (11%)

Gastrointestinal: Decreased appetite (44%), diarrhea (38%), nausea (34%), vomiting (26%), constipation (23%), abdominal pain (14%), xerostomia (11%)

Hematologic & oncologic: Lymphocytopenia (grade 3 or 4: 100%), leukopenia (grade 3 or 4: 96%), neutropenia (grade 3 or 4: 93%), anemia (grade 3 or 4: 66%), thrombocytopenia (grade 3 or 4: 58%), febrile neutropenia (36%), hypogammaglobulinemia (15%)

Hepatic: Increased direct serum bilirubin (grade 3 or 4: 13%)

Hypersensitivity: Cytokine release syndrome (94%)

Infection: Infection (26%), viral infection (16%), bacterial infection (13%)

Neuromuscular & skeletal: Tremor (31%), limb pain (17%), back pain (15%), myalgia (14%)

Renal: Renal insufficiency (12%)

Respiratory: Hypoxia (32%), cough (30%), dyspnea (19%), pleural effusion (13%)

Miscellaneous: Fever (86%)

1% to 10%:

Central nervous system: Anxiety (9%), insomnia (9%), ataxia (6%), seizure (4%), cognitive dysfunction (comprehending mathematics: 2%), myoclonus (2%)

Dermatologic: Skin rash (9%)

Endocrine & metabolic: Hypokalemia (grade 3 or 4: 10%)

Genitourinary: Urinary tract infection (>2%)

Hematologic & oncologic: Blood coagulation disorder (2%), natural killer cell count increased (hemophagocytic lymphohistiocytosis/macrophage activation syndrome: 1%)

Hepatic: Increased serum ALT (grade 3 or 4: 10%)

Hypersensitivity: Hypersensitivity reaction (1%)

Infection: Fungal infection (5%), clostridium infection (>2%)

Neuromuscular & skeletal: Arthralgia (10%)

Respiratory: Pulmonary edema (9%), pulmonary infection (>2%)

Frequency not defined: Central nervous system: Cerebral edema, leukoencephalopathy, seizure

Mechanism of Action Axicabtagene ciloleucel is a CD19-directed genetically modified autologous T cell immunotherapy in which a patient's T cells are reprogrammed with a transgene encoding a chimeric antigen receptor (CAR) to identify and eliminate CD19-expressing malignant and normal cells. The CAR is comprised of a murine single-chain antibody fragment which recognizes CD19 and is fused to CD28 and CD3 zeta. CD3 zeta is a critical component for initiating T-cell activation and antitumor activity. After binding to CD19-expressing cells, the CD28 and CD3-zeta co-stimulatory domains activate downstream signaling cascades, which results in T cell activation, proliferation, acquisition of effector functions, and secretion of inflammatory cytokines and chemokines, leading to destruction of CD19-expressing cells. Axicabtagene ciloleucel is prepared from the patient's peripheral blood cells obtained via leukapheresis.

Pharmacodynamics/Kinetics

Onset of Action Median time to response: 1 month (range: 0.8 to 6 months) (Neelapu 2017)

Duration of Action Anti-CD19 CAR T cells displayed an initial rapid expansion followed by a decline to near baseline levels by 3 months post axicabtagene ciloleucel infusion

Time to Peak Peak levels of anti-CD19 CAR T cells occurred within the first 7 to 14 days after infusion

Reproductive Considerations

Evaluate pregnancy status prior to therapy in females of reproductive potential; pregnancy testing is recommended prior to therapy in sexually active women of reproductive potential. Refer to the cyclophosphamide and fludarabine monographs for information related to use of effective contraception in patients using these medications for lymphodepleting chemotherapy. The duration of contraception needed following axicabtagene ciloleucel administration is not known. Potential pregnancies (following treatment) should be discussed with the prescriber.

Pregnancy Considerations

Treatment with axicabtagene ciloleucel is not recommended during pregnancy. If placental transfer were to occur, fetal toxicity, including B-cell lymphocytopenia, may occur.

Potential pregnancies (following treatment) should be discussed with the prescriber.

◆ **Axi-Cel** *see* Axicabtagene Ciloleucel *on page 196*

◆ **Axiron [DSC]** *see* Testosterone *on page 1425*

Axitinib (ax I ti nib)

Brand Names: US Inlyta

Brand Names: Canada Inlyta

Pharmacologic Category Antineoplastic Agent, Tyrosine Kinase Inhibitor; Antineoplastic Agent, Vascular Endothelial Growth Factor (VEGF) Inhibitor

Use

Renal cell carcinoma, advanced:

First-line treatment (in combination with avelumab **or** pembrolizumab) of advanced renal cell carcinoma.

Treatment (as a single-agent) of advanced renal cell carcinoma after failure of 1 prior systemic therapy.

Local Anesthetic/Vasoconstrictor Precautions

Significant hypertension can occur with the use of this drug; monitor for hypertension prior to using local anesthetic with vasoconstrictor; medical consult if necessary

Effects on Dental Treatment Key adverse event(s) related to dental treatment: Oral mucosal inflammation, stomatitis, and taste alteration have been reported

Effects on Bleeding Chemotherapy may result in significant myelosuppression, potentially including significant reduction in platelet counts and altered hemostasis. Hemorrhagic events have been reported. In patients who are under active treatment with axitinib, medical consult is suggested.

Adverse Reactions

>10%:

Cardiovascular: Hypertension (40%)

Dermatologic: Palmar-plantar erythrodysesthesia (27%), skin rash (13%)

Endocrine & metabolic: Decreased serum bicarbonate (44%), hyperglycemia (28%), hyperkalemia (15%), hypernatremia (17%), hypoalbuminemia (15%), hypocalcemia (39%), hypoglycemia (11%), hyponatremia (13%), hypophosphatemia (13%), hypothyroidism (19%), weight loss (25%)

Gastrointestinal: Abdominal pain (14%), constipation (20%), decreased appetite (34%), diarrhea (55%), dysgeusia (11%), increased serum amylase (25%), increased serum lipase (3% to 27%), mucosal swelling (15%), nausea (32%), stomatitis (15%; grades 3/4: 1%), vomiting (24%)
Genitourinary: Proteinuria (11%)
Hematologic & oncologic: Decreased absolute lymphocyte count (33%; grades 3/4: 3%), decreased platelet count (15%; grades 3/4: <1%), decreased white blood cell count (11%), hemorrhage (16%; grades 3/4: 1%)
Hepatic: Increased serum alanine aminotransferase (22%), increased serum alkaline phosphatase (30%), increased serum aspartate aminotransferase (20%)
Nervous system: Fatigue (39%), headache (14%), voice disorder (31%)
Neuromuscular & skeletal: Arthralgia (15%), asthenia (21%), limb pain (13%)
Renal: Increased serum creatinine (55%)
Respiratory: Cough (15%), dyspnea (15%)

1% to 10%:
Cardiovascular: Arterial thrombosis (2%), cardiac failure (2%), deep vein thrombosis (1%), pulmonary embolism (2%), retinal thrombosis (≤1%), transient ischemic attacks (1%), venous thrombosis (3%)
Dermatologic: Alopecia (4%), erythema of skin (2%), pruritus (7%), xeroderma (10%)
Endocrine & metabolic: Dehydration (6%), hypercalcemia (6%), hyperthyroidism (1%)
Gastrointestinal: Dyspepsia (10%), gastrointestinal fistula (1%), gastrointestinal perforation (≤1%), glossalgia (3%), hemorrhoids (4%), upper abdominal pain (8%)
Genitourinary: Hematuria (3%)
Hematologic & oncologic: Anemia (4%), increased hemoglobin (9%), polycythemia (1%), rectal hemorrhage (2%)
Nervous system: Dizziness (9%)
Neuromuscular & skeletal: Myalgia (7%)
Ophthalmic: Retinal vein occlusion (≤1%)
Otic: Tinnitus (3%)
Respiratory: Epistaxis (6%), hemoptysis (2%)

<1%:
Cardiovascular: Cerebrovascular accident, hypertensive crisis
Nervous system: Reversible posterior leukoencephalopathy syndrome

Frequency not defined:
Cardiovascular: Acute myocardial infarction
Gastrointestinal: Gastrointestinal hemorrhage, melena
Nervous system: Cerebral hemorrhage
Ophthalmic: Retinal artery occlusion

Mechanism of Action Axitinib is a selective second-generation tyrosine kinase inhibitor which blocks angiogenesis and tumor growth by inhibiting vascular endothelial growth factor receptors (VEGFR-1, VEGFR-2, and VEGFR-3).

Pharmacodynamics/Kinetics

Half-life Elimination 2.5 to 6.1 hours

Time to Peak 2.5 to 4 hours

Reproductive Considerations

Females of reproductive potential should have a pregnancy test prior to therapy; effective contraception should be used during axitinib therapy and for 1 week after the final axitinib dose.

Males with female partners of reproductive potential should also use effective contraception during axitinib therapy and for 1 week after the final axitinib dose.

Pregnancy Considerations

Based on its mechanism of action and findings from animal reproduction studies, adverse effects on pregnancy would be expected.

Prescribing and Access Restrictions Available from select specialty pharmacies. Further information may be obtained at 877-744-5675 or www.inlytahcp.com.

- **AY-25650** *see* Triptorelin *on page 1500*
- **Aygestin** *see* Norethindrone *on page 1117*
- **Ayuna** *see* Ethinyl Estradiol and Levonorgestrel *on page 612*
- **Ayvakit** *see* Avapritinib *on page 194*
- **5-Aza-2'-deoxycytidine** *see* Decitabine *on page 447*

AzaCITIDine (ay za SYE ti deen)

Brand Names: US Vidaza

Brand Names: Canada NAT-AzaCITIDine; REDDY-Azacitidine; Vidaza

Pharmacologic Category Antineoplastic Agent, Antimetabolite; Antineoplastic Agent, DNA Methylation Inhibitor

Use Myelodysplastic syndromes: Treatment of myelodysplastic syndromes (MDS) in patients with the following French-American-British (FAB) classification subtypes: Refractory anemia or refractory anemia with ringed sideroblasts (if accompanied by neutropenia or thrombocytopenia or requiring transfusions), refractory anemia with excess blasts, refractory anemia with excess blasts in transformation, and chronic myelomonocytic leukemia.

Local Anesthetic/Vasoconstrictor Precautions No information available to require special precautions

Effects on Dental Treatment Key adverse event(s) related to dental treatment: Mucositis, gingival bleeding, oral mucosal petechiae, stomatitis, oral hemorrhage, and tongue ulceration.

Effects on Bleeding Gingival bleeding is reported in 10% of patients. Thrombocytopenia is reported in 66% to 70% of patients receiving azacitidine subcutaneously.

Adverse Reactions

>10%:
Cardiovascular: Chest pain (16%)
Dermatologic: Ecchymoses (31%), erythema (7% to 17%), pruritus (12%), skin rash (10% to 14%)
Gastrointestinal: Abdominal pain (13%), abdominal tenderness (12%), anorexia (21%), constipation (34% to 50%), diarrhea (36%), nausea (48% to 71%), vomiting (27% to 54%)
Hematologic & oncologic: Anemia (51% to 70%; grades 3/4: 14%), febrile neutropenia (14% to 16%; grades 3/4: 13%), leukopenia (18% to 48%; grades 3/4: 15%), neutropenia (32% to 66%; grades 3/4: 61%), petechia (11% to 24%; more common with IV administration), thrombocytopenia (66% to 70%; grades 3/4: 58%)
Local: Bruising at injection site (5% to 14%), erythema at injection site (35% to 43%), injection site reaction (14% to 29%), pain at injection site (19% to 23%)
Nervous system: Anxiety (5% to 13%), dizziness (19%), fatigue (24%), headache (22%), insomnia (9% to 11%), malaise (11%)
Neuromuscular & skeletal: Arthralgia (22%), myalgia (16%)
Respiratory: Dyspnea (5% to 29%), nasopharyngitis (15%), pneumonia (11%), upper respiratory infection (9% to 13%)

Miscellaneous: Fever (30% to 52%)

1% to 10%:

Cardiovascular: Atrial fibrillation (<5%), cardiac failure (<5%), chest wall pain (5%), congestive cardiomyopathy (<5%), hypertension (9%), hypotension (7%), orthostatic hypotension (<5%), septic shock (<5%)

Dermatologic: Cellulitis (<5%), pruritic rash (<5%), pyoderma gangrenosum (<5%), rash at injection site (6%), skin nodules (5%), skin sclerosis (<5%), urticaria (6%), xeroderma (5%)

Endocrine & metabolic: Dehydration (<5%), hypokalemia (6%; more common with IV administration), weight loss (8%)

Gastrointestinal: Cholecystectomy (<5%), cholecystitis (<5%), diverticulitis of the gastrointestinal tract (<5%), dyspepsia (6%), gastrointestinal hemorrhage (<5%), gingival hemorrhage (10%), loose stools (6%), melena (<5%), stomatitis (8%)

Genitourinary: Abscess of rectum and/or peri-rectal area (<5%), hematuria (6%), urinary tract infection (9%)

Hematologic & oncologic: Agranulocytosis (<5%), bone marrow failure (<5%), hematoma (9%), leukemia cutis (<5%), oral hemorrhage (5%), pancytopenia (<5%), postprocedural hemorrhage (6%), splenomegaly (<5%)

Hypersensitivity: Anaphylactic shock (<5%), hypersensitivity reaction (<5%)

Infection: Bacterial infection (<5%), blastomycosis (<5%), limb abscess (<5%), neutropenic sepsis (<5%), sepsis (<5%, including *Klebsiella* sepsis), staphylococcal bacteremia (<5%), staphylococcal infection (<5%), systemic inflammatory response syndrome (<5%), toxoplasmosis (<5%)

Local: Catheter site hemorrhage (<5%), hematoma at injection site (6%), induration at injection site (5%), injection site granuloma (5%), injection site infection (<5%), itching at injection site (7%), skin discoloration at injection site (5%), swelling at injection site (5%)

Nervous system: Aggravated bone pain (<5%), cerebral hemorrhage (<5%), flank pain (<5%), intracranial hemorrhage (<5%), lethargy (7% to 8%), myasthenia (<5%), seizure (<5%)

Neuromuscular & skeletal: Neck pain (<5%)

Ophthalmic: Subconjunctival hemorrhage (<5%)

Renal: Renal failure syndrome (<5%)

Respiratory: Hemoptysis (<5%), *Klebsiella pneumoniae* infection (<5%), pharyngolaryngeal pain (6%), pneumonitis (<5%), pulmonary infiltrates (<5%), respiratory distress (<5%), rhinitis (6%), streptococcal pharyngitis (<5%)

Miscellaneous: Physical health deterioration (<5%)

Frequency not defined:

Hepatic: Hepatic coma

Nervous system: Rigors (more common with IV administration)

Neuromuscular & skeletal: Asthenia (more common with IV administration)

Postmarketing:

Dermatologic: Sweet's syndrome

Hematologic & oncologic: Differentiation syndrome, tumor lysis syndrome

Infection: Necrotizing fasciitis

Local: Tissue necrosis at injection site

Respiratory: Interstitial pulmonary disease

Mechanism of Action Antineoplastic effects may be a result of azacitidine's ability to promote hypomethylation of DNA, restoring normal gene differentiation and proliferation. Azacitidine also exerts direct toxicity to abnormal hematopoietic cells in the bone marrow.

Pharmacodynamics/Kinetics

Half-life Elimination IV, SubQ: ~4 hours

Time to Peak SubQ: 30 minutes

Reproductive Considerations

Evaluate pregnancy status prior to therapy. Women of childbearing potential should be advised to avoid pregnancy during treatment. Males with female partners of reproductive potential should not father a child and should use effective contraception during therapy.

Pregnancy Considerations

Based on its mechanism of action, azacitidine may cause fetal harm if administered during pregnancy.

- **AZA-CR** *see* AzaCITIDine *on page 198*
- **Azactam** *see* Aztreonam (Systemic) *on page 211*
- **Azactam in Dextrose [DSC]** *see* Aztreonam (Systemic) *on page 211*
- **Azacytidine** *see* AzaCITIDine *on page 198*
- **5-Azacytidine** *see* AzaCITIDine *on page 198*
- **5-Aza-dCyd** *see* Decitabine *on page 447*
- **Azaepothilone B** *see* Ixabepilone *on page 852*
- **Azasan** *see* AzaTHIOprine *on page 199*

AzaTHIOprine (ay za THYE oh preen)

Brand Names: US Azasan; Imuran

Brand Names: Canada APO-AzaTHIOprine; Aza-THIOprine-50; Imuran; MYLAN-AzaTHIOprine [DSC]; NU-AzaTHIOprine [DSC]; TEVA-AzaTHIOprine

Pharmacologic Category Immunosuppressant Agent

Use

Kidney transplantation: Adjunctive therapy in prevention of rejection of kidney transplants

Guideline recommendations: While azathioprine is FDA approved for adjunctive therapy in prevention of rejection after kidney transplantation, it is no longer recommended as a first-line agent. The KDIGO clinical practice guidelines for care of kidney transplant recipients recommend a combination of maintenance immunosuppressive medications as maintenance therapy, including a calcineurin inhibitor and an antiproliferative agent (mycophenolate preferred) with or without corticosteroids. Azathioprine is recommended as a second-line antiproliferative agent for prevention of acute rejection (KDIGO [Kasiske 2010]).

Rheumatoid arthritis: Treatment of active rheumatoid arthritis (RA), to reduce signs and symptoms.

Appropriate use: While azathioprine is FDA approved for the treatment of active arthritis, the 2012 and 2015 guideline updates from the American College of Rheumatology for the treatment of rheumatoid arthritis do not include azathioprine due to infrequent use in rheumatoid arthritis and a lack of new data (ACR [Singh 2012]; ACR [Singh 2016]). However, azathioprine may be acceptable in certain situations where methotrexate is contraindicated and other alternatives are unable to be used (Cohen 2019).

Local Anesthetic/Vasoconstrictor Precautions

No information available to require special precautions

Effects on Dental Treatment No significant effects or complications reported

Effects on Bleeding Thrombocytopenia and bleeding may occur.

Adverse Reactions Frequency not always defined; dependent upon dose, duration, indication, and concomitant therapy.

Central nervous system: Malaise

Gastrointestinal: Nausea and vomiting (rheumatoid arthritis: 12%), diarrhea

Hematologic & oncologic: Leukopenia (renal transplant: >50%; rheumatoid arthritis: 28%), neoplasia (renal transplant 3% [other than lymphoma], 0.5% [lymphoma]), thrombocytopenia

Hepatic: Hepatotoxicity, increased serum alkaline phosphatase, increased serum bilirubin, increased serum transaminases

Infection: Increased susceptibility to infection (renal transplant 20%; rheumatoid arthritis <1%; includes bacterial, fungal, protozoal, viral, opportunistic, and reactivation of latent infections)

Neuromuscular & skeletal: Myalgia

Miscellaneous: Fever

<1%, postmarketing and/or case reports: Abdominal pain, acute myelocytic leukemia, alopecia, anemia, arthralgia, bone marrow depression, hemorrhage, hepatic sinusoidal obstruction syndrome (formerly known as hepatic veno-occlusive disease), hepatosplenic T-cell lymphomas, hepatotoxicity (idiosyncratic) (Chalasani, 2014), hypersensitivity, hypotension, interstitial pneumonitis (reversible), JC virus infection, macrocytic anemia, malignant lymphoma, malignant neoplasm of skin, negative nitrogen balance, pancreatitis, pancytopenia, progressive multifocal leukoencephalopathy, skin rash, steatorrhea, Sweet's syndrome (acute febrile neutrophilic dermatosis)

Mechanism of Action Azathioprine is an imidazolyl derivative of mercaptopurine; metabolites are incorporated into replicating DNA and halt replication; also block the pathway for purine synthesis (Taylor 2005). The 6-thioguanine nucleotide metabolites appear to mediate the majority of azathioprine's immunosuppressive and toxic effects.

Pharmacodynamics/Kinetics

Onset of Action Immune thrombocytopenia (oral): Initial response: 30 to 90 days; Peak response: 30 to 120 days (Neunert 2011)

Half-life Elimination Azathioprine and mercaptopurine: Variable: ~2 hours (Taylor 2005)

Time to Peak Oral: 1 to 2 hours (including metabolites)

Reproductive Considerations

The manufacturer recommends that females of reproductive potential avoid becoming pregnant during treatment. However, additional recommendations are available for use in females and males on azathioprine who are planning a pregnancy.

Azathioprine is an acceptable immunosuppressant for use in kidney transplant recipients planning a pregnancy (EBPG 2002; KDIGO 2009; López 2014). Azathioprine should be substituted for mycophenolate 6 weeks prior to conception. Conception may be considered for females on a stable/low maintenance dose for ≥1 year following transplant (EBPG 2002; López 2014).

Azathioprine is also acceptable for use in females with rheumatoid arthritis (BSR/BHPR [Flint 2016]) and other rheumatic and musculoskeletal diseases who are planning a pregnancy. Conception should be planned during a period of quiescent/low disease activity (ACR [Sammaritano 2020]). Females treated with azathioprine for lupus nephritis should continue treatment while planning a pregnancy; conception may be considered after 6 months of inactive disease (EULAR/ERA-EDTA [Bertsias 2012]).

Females with autoimmune hepatitis who are planning pregnancy should continue use of azathioprine prior to conception to decrease the risk of flare and hepatic decompensation; biological remission is recommended for 1 year prior to conception (AASLD [Mack 2019]).

Information related to paternal use of azathioprine is limited. However, available data have not shown azathioprine adversely impacting male fertility or increasing the risk of adverse pregnancy outcomes when used within 3 months prior to conception (Bermas 2019; Mouyis 2019). Azathioprine is acceptable for use in males with rheumatoid arthritis (Flint 2016) and other rheumatic and musculoskeletal diseases (ACR [Sammaritano 2020]) who are planning to father a child.

Pregnancy Risk Factor D

Pregnancy Considerations Azathioprine crosses the placenta.

Adverse events, including congenital anomalies, immunosuppression, hematologic toxicities (lymphopenia, pancytopenia), and intrauterine growth retardation have been observed in case reports following maternal use in kidney allograft recipients. Some of these adverse outcomes may be dose-related or a result of maternal disease (ACR [Sammaritano 2020]; EBPG 2002). Adverse pregnancy outcomes may also be associated with a kidney transplant, including preterm delivery and low birth weight in the infant and hypertension and preeclampsia in the mother. Appropriate maternal use of lower risk immunosuppressants may help decrease these risks (KDIGO 2009).

Azathioprine can be continued and should be substituted for mycophenolate in patients who become pregnant following a kidney transplant (EBPG 2002; KDIGO 2009; López 2014). Azathioprine may also be used in some pregnant patients who have had a liver (AASLD [Lucey 2013]), heart (ISHLT [Costanzo 2010]) or uterine (Jones 2019 [limited data]) transplant.

Available guidelines suggest that use of azathioprine is acceptable for the treatment of rheumatoid arthritis in pregnant females (BSR/BHPR [Flint 2016]), although use for this indication is contraindicated by the manufacturer. Azathioprine may also be used in the treatment of lupus nephritis (ACR [Hahn 2012]; EULAR/ERA-EDTA [Bertsias 2012]) and other rheumatic and musculoskeletal diseases (ACR [Sammaritano 2020]) during pregnancy.

Females with inflammatory bowel disease who are on maintenance therapy with azathioprine monotherapy may continue treatment during pregnancy; initiating treatment during pregnancy is not recommended. Combination therapy with azathioprine should be avoided due to increased risk of newborn infection (AGA [Mahadevan 2019]).

Treatment with azathioprine for autoimmune hepatitis should be continued during pregnancy. Because pregnancy may increase the risk of a flare, monitor closely for 6 months' postpartum (AASLD [Mack 2019]). Azathioprine may also be useful for the treatment of immune thrombocytopenia in a pregnant female refractory to preferred agents (Provan 2010). Azathioprine is considered acceptable for the treatment of myasthenia gravis in pregnant patients who are not controlled with or unable to tolerate corticosteroids (Sanders 2016).

The Transplant Pregnancy Registry International (TPR) is a registry that follows pregnancies that occur in maternal transplant recipients or those fathered by male transplant recipients. The TPR encourages reporting of pregnancies following solid organ transplant by contacting them at 1-877-955-6877 or https://www.transplantpregnancyregistry.org.

◆ **Azathioprine Sodium** *see* AzaTHIOprine *on page 199*
◆ **5-AZC** *see* AzaCITIDine *on page 198*
◆ **AZD2281** *see* Olaparib *on page 1130*
◆ **AZD6140** *see* Ticagrelor *on page 1444*
◆ **AZD-6244** *see* Selumetinib *on page 1365*
◆ **AZD6474** *see* Vandetanib *on page 1531*
◆ **AZD9291** *see* Osimertinib *on page 1149*

Azelastine (Nasal) (a ZEL as teen)

Brand Names: US Astepro

Pharmacologic Category Histamine H_1 Antagonist; Histamine H_1 Antagonist, Second Generation

Use

Perennial allergic rhinitis (Astepro 0.1% and 0.15% solution only): Relief of symptoms of perennial allergic rhinitis in adults and pediatric patients ≥6 months.

Seasonal allergic rhinitis: Relief of symptoms of seasonal allergic rhinitis in adults and pediatric patients ≥2 years (Astepro 0.1% and 0.15% solution) and ≥5 years (azelastine [generic] 0.1% solution).

Vasomotor rhinitis (azelastine [generic] 0.1% solution): Relief of symptoms of vasomotor rhinitis in adults and adolescents ≥12 years.

Local Anesthetic/Vasoconstrictor Precautions No information available to require special precautions

Effects on Dental Treatment Key adverse event(s) related to dental treatment: Bitter taste, xerostomia (normal salivary flow resumes upon discontinuation), aphthous stomatitis, glossitis, and burning sensation in throat. Chronic use of antihistamines will inhibit salivary flow, particularly in elderly patients. May contribute to periodontal disease and oral discomfort.

Effects on Bleeding No information available to require special precautions

Adverse Reactions Adverse reactions may be dose-, indication-, or product-dependent:

>10%:

Central nervous system: Bitter taste (4% to 20%), headache (1% to 15%), drowsiness (≤12%)

Infection: Cold symptoms (children ≤17%)

Respiratory: Rhinitis (exacerbation; ≤17%), cough (children: 11%; infants and children: ≥2%)

2% to 10%:

Central nervous system: Dysesthesia (8%), dizziness (2%), fatigue (2%)

Dermatologic: Contact dermatitis

Endocrine & metabolic: Weight gain (2%)

Gastrointestinal: Dysgeusia (children: 2% to 4%), nausea (3%), xerostomia (3%), vomiting

Infection: Upper respiratory tract infection (children: ≥2% to 3%)

Neuromuscular & skeletal: Myalgia (≤2%)

Ophthalmic: Conjunctivitis (<2% to 5%)

Otic: Otitis media (infants & children: ≥2%)

Respiratory: Epistaxis (2% to 7%), asthma (5%), sinusitis (3% to >5%), burning sensation of the nose (4%), pharyngitis (4%), nasal discomfort (≤4%), sneezing (1% to 3%), sore nose (infants and children: ≥2%), nasal mucosa ulcer (≤2%), pharyngolaryngeal pain

Miscellaneous: Fever

<2%:

Cardiovascular: Flushing, hypertension, tachycardia

Central nervous system: Abnormality in thinking, anxiety, depersonalization, depression, hypoesthesia, malaise, nervousness, sleep disorder, vertigo

Dermatologic: Eczema, folliculitis, furunculosis

Endocrine & metabolic: Albuminuria, amenorrhea

Gastrointestinal: Abdominal pain, ageusia, aphthous stomatitis, constipation, diarrhea, gastroenteritis, glossitis, increased appetite, toothache

Genitourinary: Hematuria, mastalgia

Hepatic: Increased serum ALT

Hypersensitivity: Hypersensitivity reaction

Infection: Herpes simplex infection, viral infection

Neuromuscular & skeletal: Back pain, dislocation of temporomandibular joint, hyperkinesia, limb pain, rheumatoid arthritis

Ophthalmic: Eye pain, watery eyes

Renal: Polyuria

Respiratory: Bronchitis, bronchospasm, laryngitis, nasal congestion, paranasal sinus hypersecretion, paroxysmal nocturnal dyspnea, postnasal drip, sore throat

Miscellaneous: Laceration

<1%, postmarketing, and/or case reports: Altered sense of smell, anaphylactoid reaction, anosmia, application site irritation, atrial fibrillation, blurred vision, chest pain, confusion, drug tolerance, dyspnea, facial edema, increased serum transaminases, insomnia, muscle spasm, nasal sores, palpitations, paresthesia, pruritus, skin rash, urinary retention, visual disturbance, xerophthalmia

Mechanism of Action Competes with histamine for H_1-receptor sites on effector cells and inhibits the release of histamine and other mediators involved in the allergic response; when used intranasally, reduces hyper-reactivity of the airways; increases the motility of bronchial epithelial cilia, improving mucociliary transport

Pharmacodynamics/Kinetics

Onset of Action 30 minutes (Wallace 2008); maximum effect: 3 hours

Duration of Action 12 hours

Half-life Elimination Azelastine: 22 hours (0.1% solution), 25 hours (0.15% solution); Desmethylazelastine: 52 hours (0.1% solution), 57 hours (0.15% solution)

Time to Peak 2 to 3 hours (Azelastine [generic] 0.1% solution); 3 to 4 hours (Astepro)

Pregnancy Considerations

An increased risk of adverse pregnancy outcomes has not been observed; however, information related to the use of nasal azelastine in pregnancy is limited. Use of other agents for the treatment of allergic rhinitis in pregnant women may be preferred (BSACI [Scadding 2017]).

- **Azelastine HCl** *see* Azelastine (Nasal) *on page 201*
- **Azelastine Hydrochloride** *see* Azelastine (Nasal) *on page 201*
- **Azidothymidine** *see* Zidovudine *on page 1569*
- **Azidothymidine, Abacavir, and Lamivudine** *see* Abacavir, Lamivudine, and Zidovudine *on page 52*
- **Azilect** *see* Rasagiline *on page 1311*

Azilsartan (ay zil SAR tan)

Related Information

Cardiovascular Diseases *on page 1654*

Brand Names: US Edarbi

Brand Names: Canada Edarbi

Pharmacologic Category Angiotensin II Receptor Blocker; Antihypertensive

Use

Hypertension: Management of hypertension

Guideline recommendations:

The 2017 Guideline for the Prevention, Detection, Evaluation, and Management of High Blood Pressure in Adults recommends if monotherapy is warranted, in the absence of comorbidities (eg, cerebrovascular disease, chronic kidney disease, diabetes, heart failure, ischemic heart disease, etc.), that thiazide-like diuretics or dihydropyridine calcium channel blockers may be preferred options due to improved cardiovascular endpoints (eg, prevention of heart failure and stroke). ACE inhibitors and ARBs are also acceptable for monotherapy. Combination therapy may be required to achieve blood pressure goals and is initially preferred in patients at high risk (stage 2 hypertension or atherosclerotic cardiovascular disease [ASCVD] risk ≥10%) (ACC/AHA [Whelton 2017]).

Local Anesthetic/Vasoconstrictor Precautions No information available to require special precautions

Effects on Dental Treatment Key adverse event(s) related to dental treatment: Patients may experience orthostatic hypotension as they stand up after treatment; especially if lying in dental chair for extended periods of time. Use caution with sudden changes in position during and after dental treatment.

Effects on Bleeding No information available to require special precautions

Adverse Reactions

1% to 10%: Gastrointestinal: Diarrhea (≤2%)

Frequency not defined:

Cardiovascular: Hypotension, orthostatic hypotension

Central nervous system: Dizziness, fatigue, orthostatic dizziness

Gastrointestinal: Nausea

Neuromuscular & skeletal: Asthenia, muscle spasm

Renal: Increased serum creatinine

Respiratory: Cough

<1%, postmarketing, and/or case reports: Angioedema, decreased hematocrit, decreased hemoglobin, decreased red blood cells, leukocytosis, pruritus, skin rash, thrombocytopenia

Mechanism of Action Angiotensin II (which is formed by enzymatic conversion from angiotensin I) is the primary pressor agent of the renin-angiotensin system. Effects of angiotensin II include vasoconstriction, stimulation of aldosterone synthesis/release, cardiac stimulation, and renal sodium reabsorption. Azilsartan inhibits angiotensin II's vasoconstrictor and aldosterone-secreting effects by selectively blocking the binding of angiotensin II to the AT_1 receptor in vascular smooth muscle and adrenal gland tissues (azilsartan has a stronger affinity for the AT_1 receptor than the AT_2 receptor). The action is independent of the angiotensin II synthesis pathways. Azilsartan does not inhibit ACE (kininase II), therefore it does not affect the response to bradykinin (the clinical relevance of this is unknown) and does not bind to or inhibit other receptors or ion channels of importance in cardiovascular regulation.

Pharmacodynamics/Kinetics

Half-life Elimination ~11 hours

Time to Peak Serum: 1.5-3 hours

Reproductive Considerations

The use of angiotensin II receptor blockers should generally be avoided in women planning a pregnancy (ACOG 203 2019).

Pregnancy Considerations

[US Boxed Warning]: Drugs that act on the renin-angiotensin system can cause injury and death to the developing fetus. When pregnancy is detected, discontinue as soon as possible. The use of drugs which act on the renin-angiotensin system are associated with oligohydramnios. Oligohydramnios, due to decreased fetal renal function, may lead to fetal lung hypoplasia and skeletal malformations. Oligohydramnios may not appear until after irreversible fetal injury has occurred. Use in pregnancy is also associated with anuria, hypotension, renal failure, skull hypoplasia, and death in the fetus/neonate. The exposed fetus should be monitored for fetal growth, amniotic fluid volume, and organ formation. Infants exposed in utero should be monitored for hyperkalemia, hypotension, and oliguria (exchange transfusions or dialysis may be needed). These adverse events are generally associated with maternal use in the second and third trimesters.

Chronic maternal hypertension itself is also associated with adverse events in the fetus/infant. The risk of birth defects, low birth weight, premature delivery, stillbirth, and neonatal death may be increased with chronic hypertension in pregnancy. Actual risks may be related to duration and severity of maternal hypertension (ACOG 203 2019).

The use of angiotensin II receptor blockers is generally not recommended to treat chronic hypertension in pregnant women (ACOG 203 2019).

- **Azilsartan Medoxomil** *see* Azilsartan *on page 202*

Azithromycin (Systemic) (az ith roe MYE sin)

Related Information

Antibiotic Prophylaxis *on page 1715*
Bacterial Infections *on page 1739*
Clinical Risk Related to Drugs Prolonging QT Interval *on page 1675*
Periodontal Diseases *on page 1748*
Sexually-Transmitted Diseases *on page 1707*

Related Sample Prescriptions

Bacterial Infections and Periodontal Diseases - Sample Prescriptions *on page 35*
Prevention of Endocarditis and to Reduce the Risk of Late Infections of Joint Prostheses - Sample Prescriptions *on page 40*
Sinus Infection Treatment - Sample Prescriptions *on page 41*

Brand Names: US Zithromax; Zithromax Tri-Pak; Zithromax Z-Pak; Zmax [DSC]

Brand Names: Canada ACT Azithromycin [DSC]; AG-Azithromycin; APO-Azithromycin; APO-Azithromycin Z; AURO-Azithromycin; DOM-Azithromycin; GD-Azithromycin [DSC]; GEN-Azithromycin; JAMP-Azithromycin; Mar-Azithromycin; MYLAN-Azithromycin [DSC]; Novo-Azithromycin Pediatric [DSC]; NRA-Azithromycin; PHL-Azithromycin [DSC]; PMS-Azithromycin; PRO-Azithromycin; RATIO-Azithromycin; RIVA-Azithromycin; SANDOZ Azithromycin; TEVA-Azithromycin; Zithromax

Generic Availability (US) Yes

Pharmacologic Category Antibiotic, Macrolide

Dental Use Alternate oral antibiotic for prevention of infective endocarditis in individuals allergic to penicillins or ampicillin, when amoxicillin cannot be used; alternate antibiotic in the treatment of common orofacial infections caused by aerobic gram-positive cocci and susceptible anaerobes

Use

Oral, IV:

Chancroid: Treatment of genital ulcer disease (in men) due to *Haemophilus ducreyi* (chancroid)

Chronic obstructive pulmonary disease, acute exacerbation: Treatment of acute bacterial exacerbations of chronic obstructive pulmonary disease (COPD) due to *Haemophilus influenzae, Moraxella catarrhalis*, or *Streptococcus pneumoniae*

***Mycobacterium avium* complex:** Prevention of *Mycobacterium avium* complex (MAC) in patients with advanced HIV infection; treatment of disseminated MAC (in combination with ethambutol) in patients with advanced HIV infection

Otitis media, acute: Treatment of acute otitis media due to *H. influenzae, M. catarrhalis*, or *S. pneumoniae*

Pneumonia, community-acquired: Treatment of community-acquired pneumonia (CAP) due to *Chlamydophila pneumoniae, H. influenzae, Legionella pneumophila, M. catarrhalis, Mycoplasma pneumoniae,* or *S. pneumoniae*

Skin and skin structure infection, uncomplicated: Treatment of uncomplicated skin and skin structure infections due to *Staphylococcus aureus, Streptococcus pyogenes*, or *Streptococcus agalactiae*

Streptococcal pharyngitis (group A): Treatment of pharyngitis/tonsillitis due to *S. pyogenes* as an alternative to first-line therapy

Urethritis/cervicitis: Treatment of urethritis and cervicitis due to *Chlamydia trachomatis* or *Neisseria gonorrhoeae*

Local Anesthetic/Vasoconstrictor Precautions Consider consult with patient's cardiologist prior to use of a vasoconstrictor. Closely monitor for additive/synergistic pharmacologic effects, and consider electrocardiographic monitoring when a local anesthetic is used in a patient receiving azithromycin. Azithromycin prolongs the QT interval and may cause torsade de pointes. The risk of drug-induced torsade de pointes is extremely low when a single QT interval prolonging drug is prescribed. In terms of epinephrine, it is not known what effect vasoconstrictors in the local anesthetic regimen will have in patients with a known history of congenital prolonged QT interval or in patients taking any medication that prolongs the QT interval.

Effects on Dental Treatment Key adverse event(s) related to dental treatment: Rare occurrences of mucositis, oral candidiasis, and tongue discoloration

Effects on Bleeding No information available to require special precautions

Adverse Reactions

>10%: Gastrointestinal: Diarrhea (≤14%; high single-dose regimens tend to be associated with increased incidence), nausea (≤7%; high single-dose regimens: 5% to 18%), vomiting (adults: ≤2%; adults, single 2 g dose: 2% to 7%; children, single-dose regimens tend to be associated with increased incidence: 1% to 6%)

1% to 10%:

Cardiovascular: Chest pain (≤1%), facial edema (children: ≤1%), palpitations (adults: ≤1%)

Dermatologic: Diaphoresis (children: ≤1%), eczema (children: ≤1%), fungal dermatitis (children: ≤1%), pruritus (≤2%), skin photosensitivity (adults: ≤1%), skin rash (≤2%; single-dose regimens tend to be associated with increased incidence), urticaria (≤1%), vesiculobullous dermatitis (children: ≤1%)

Endocrine & metabolic: Decreased serum glucose (adults: >1%), increased gamma-glutamyl transferase (1% to 2%), increased lactate dehydrogenase (1% to 3%), increased serum glucose (adults: >1%), increased serum potassium (1% to 2%)

Gastrointestinal: Abdominal pain (1% to 7%; single-dose regimens tend to be associated with increased incidence), anorexia (≤2%), constipation (≤1%), dysgeusia (adults: ≤1%), dyspepsia (≤1%), enteritis (children: ≤1%), flatulence (≤1%), gastritis (≤1%), melena (adults: ≤1%), oral candidiasis (≤1%), stomatitis (≤1%)

Genitourinary: Genital candidiasis (adults: ≤1%), vaginitis (adults: ≤3%)

Hematologic & oncologic: Anemia (≤1%), eosinophilia (≥1%), increased neutrophils (adults: >1%), leukopenia (≤1%), lymphocytopenia (>1%), lymphocytosis (>1%), thrombocythemia (>1%), monocytosis (adults: ≤1%)

Hepatic: Cholestatic jaundice (≤1%), increased serum alanine aminotransferase (≤6%), increased serum aspartate aminotransferase (≤6%), increased serum bilirubin (≤3%), jaundice (children: ≤1%)

Hypersensitivity: Angioedema (≤1%), hypersensitivity reaction (≤1%)

Infection: Fungal infection (children: ≤1%)

Local: Local inflammation (adults, IV: 3%), pain at injection site (adults, IV: 7%)

Nervous system: Agitation (≤1%), dizziness (≤1%), drowsiness (≤1%), fatigue (≤1%), headache (≤1%), insomnia (children: ≤1%), malaise (children: ≤1%), nervousness (children: ≤1%), pain (children: ≤1%), vertigo (≤1%)

Neuromuscular & skeletal: Hyperkinetic muscle activity (children: ≤1%), increased creatine phosphokinase in blood specimen (1% to 2%)
Renal: Increased blood urea nitrogen (≤3%), increased serum creatinine (≤6%), nephritis (adults: ≤1%)
Respiratory: Bronchospasm (≤1%), cough (children: ≤1%), pleural effusion (children: ≤1%)
Miscellaneous: Fever (children: ≤1%)

<1%:
Endocrine & metabolic: Increased serum bicarbonate, increased serum phosphate, decreased serum potassium, decreased serum sodium
Hematologic & oncologic: Basophilia, neutropenia
Hepatic: Increased serum alkaline phosphatase

Postmarketing:
Cardiovascular: Cardiac arrhythmia, edema, hypotension, prolonged QT interval on ECG, syncope, torsades de pointes, ventricular tachycardia
Dermatologic: Acute generalized exanthematous pustulosis, erythema multiforme, Stevens-Johnson syndrome, toxic epidermal necrolysis
Gastrointestinal: Ageusia, *Clostridioides difficile* associated diarrhea, *Clostridioides difficile* colitis, pancreatitis, pyloric stenosis (infantile hypertrophic), tongue discoloration
Hematologic & oncologic: Thrombocytopenia
Hepatic: Hepatic failure, hepatic insufficiency, hepatic necrosis, hepatitis, hepatotoxicity (idiosyncratic) (Chalasani 2014)
Hypersensitivity: Anaphylaxis
Immunologic: Drug reaction with eosinophilia and systemic symptoms
Nervous system: Aggressive behavior, altered sense of smell, anosmia, anxiety, asthenia, exacerbation of myasthenia gravis, hyperactive behavior, paresthesia, seizure
Neuromuscular & skeletal: Arthralgia
Otic: Deafness, hearing loss, tinnitus
Renal: Acute renal failure, interstitial nephritis

Dental Usual Dosage

Prophylaxis against infective endocarditis (off-label use): Oral:
Children: 15 mg/kg 30-60 minutes before procedure (maximum: 500 mg). **Note:** American Heart Association (AHA) guidelines now recommend prophylaxis only in patients undergoing invasive procedures and in whom underlying cardiac conditions may predispose to a higher risk of adverse outcomes should infection occur. As of April 2007, routine prophylaxis for GI/GU procedures is no longer recommended by the AHA.
Adolescents ≥16 years and Adults: 500 mg 30-60 minutes prior to the procedure. **Note:** American Heart Association (AHA) guidelines now recommend prophylaxis only in patients undergoing invasive procedures and in whom underlying cardiac conditions may predispose to a higher risk of adverse outcomes should infection occur. As of April 2007, routine prophylaxis for GI/GU procedures is no longer recommended by the AHA.

Bacterial sinusitis: Oral:
Children ≥6 months: 10 mg/kg once daily for 3 days (maximum: 500 mg/day)
Adolescents ≥16 years and Adults: 500 mg/day for a total of 3 days
Extended release suspension (Zmax): 2 g as a single dose

Orofacial infections: Adolescents ≥16 years and Adults: Oral: 500 mg/day, then 250 mg days 2-5
Treatment of periodontal disease: 500 mg once daily for 4-7 days

Dosing

Adult & Geriatric

Coronavirus disease 2019 (COVID-19): Azithromycin, in combination with hydroxychloroquine, is under investigation for use in the treatment of COVID-19 (see ClinicalTrials.gov) and should **only** be given as part of a clinical trial (HHS 2020; IDSA [Bhimraj 2020]).

Note: Zmax suspension has been discontinued in the United States for >1 year.

Note: ER suspension (Zmax) is not interchangeable with IR formulations. Use should be limited to approved indications. All doses are expressed as IR azithromycin unless otherwise specified.

Acne vulgaris, inflammatory (moderate to severe) (off-label use):
Note: Use as an adjunct to topical acne therapy (AAD [Zaenglein 2016]).
Oral: Dosing regimens used in clinical trials have varied greatly. All trials used pulse-dosing regimens; regimens included: 500 mg once daily for 4 consecutive days per month for 3 consecutive months (Babaeinejad 2011; Parsad 2001) **or** 500 mg once daily for 3 days in the first week, followed by 500 mg once weekly until week 10 (Maleszka 2011) **or** 500 mg once daily for 3 consecutive days each week in month 1, followed by 500 mg once daily for 2 consecutive days each week in month 2, then 500 mg once daily for 1 day each week in month 3 (Kus 2005). The shortest possible duration should be used to minimize development of bacterial resistance; reevaluate at 3 to 4 months (AAD [Zaenglein 2016]).

Babesiosis (off-label use):
Mild to moderate disease: **Oral:** 500 mg on day 1, followed by 250 mg once daily in combination with atovaquone for 7 to 10 days in immunocompetent patients (IDSA [Wormser 2006]; Krause 2000; Vannier 2020); higher doses of azithromycin may be used in immunocompromised patients (600 mg to 1 g daily) (IDSA [Wormser 2006]; Weiss 2001; Wormser 2010).
Severe disease: **IV:** 500 mg daily in combination with atovaquone for 7 to 10 days (Kletsova 2017; Sanchez 2016); a longer duration is needed for those at high risk for relapse (Krause 2008; Sanchez 2016; Vannier 2020). **Note:** May switch to oral azithromycin (at the same dose) following improvement on IV therapy (Sanchez 2016); when switching to oral treatment in immunocompromised patients, a higher dose (600 mg to 1 g daily) has been used (IDSA [Wormser 2006]; Sanchez 2016; Weiss 2001).

Bronchiectasis (noncystic fibrosis), prevention of pulmonary exacerbations (off-label use): Oral: 500 mg 3 times weekly (Wong 2012) or 250 mg once daily (Altenburg 2013). **Note:** Recommended for patients with ≥2 (Barker 2020) or ≥3 (ERS [Polverino 2017]) exacerbations per year; for those who do not have *Pseudomonas aeruginosa* infection, have *P. aeruginosa* but cannot take an inhaled antibiotic, or continue to have exacerbations despite an inhaled antibiotic. Patients should be screened for nontuberculous mycobacterial infection prior to treatment, and azithromycin should not be given if present (ERS [Polverino 2017]).

Bronchiolitis obliterans syndrome in lung transplant recipients, treatment (off-label use): Oral: 250 mg daily for 5 days, followed by 250 mg 3 times weekly for at least a 3-month trial (ISHLT/ATS/ERS [Meyer 2014]); some experts continue indefinitely, regardless of response to therapy (Pilewski 2019). **Note:** When studied to prevent bronchiolitis obliterans syndrome in patients with hematologic malignancy who underwent allogeneic hematopoietic cell transplantation, rates of cancer relapse and mortality were increased among patients receiving long-term azithromycin, leading to early trial termination (Bergeron 2017; FDA Drug Safety Communication 2018).

Cat scratch disease (lymphadenitis) (off-label use): Oral: 500 mg as a single dose, then 250 mg once daily for 4 additional days (Bass 1998; IDSA [Stevens 2014]; Psarros 2012).

Cesarean delivery (intrapartum or after rupture of membranes), preoperative prophylaxis (off-label use): IV: 500 mg as a single dose 1 hour prior to surgical incision; use in combination with standard preoperative antibiotics (ACOG 199 2018; Tita 2016).

Chronic obstructive pulmonary disease, acute exacerbation:

Acute exacerbation, treatment: **Note:** Avoid use in patients with risk factors for *Pseudomonas* infection or poor outcomes (eg, ≥65 years of age with major comorbidities, FEV_1 <50% predicted, frequent exacerbations) (Sethi 2020).

Oral: 500 mg in a single loading dose on day 1, followed by 250 mg once daily on days 2 to 5 (Castaldo 2003) **or** 500 mg once daily for 3 days (Swanson 2005).

Prevention of exacerbations (off- label use): **Oral:** 250 to 500 mg 3 times weekly (Berkhof 2013; GOLD 2019; Uzun 2014) **or** 250 mg once daily (Albert 2011; GOLD 2019).

Cystic fibrosis, anti-inflammatory (off-label use): Oral: 250 mg (<40 kg) or 500 mg (≥40 kg) 3 times weekly (Saiman 2003) **or** 250 mg once daily (Wolter 2002). **Note:** Patients should be screened for nontuberculous mycobacterial infection prior to treatment and azithromycin should not be given if present (Mogayzel 2013; Saiman 2003).

Diarrhea, infectious (off-label use):

Campylobacter gastroenteritis: Oral: 1 g as a single dose **or** 500 mg once daily for 3 days (ACG [Riddle 2016]; Tribble 2007). If symptoms have not resolved after 24 hours following single-dose therapy, continue with 500 mg once daily for 2 more days (ACG [Riddle 2016]). For HIV-infected patients, 500 mg once daily for 5 days is recommended (HHS [OI adult] 2020). **Note:** Increased nausea may occur with the 1 g single-dose regimen (Tribble 2007), which may be reduced by administering azithromycin as 2 divided doses on the same day (CDC 2018; Riddle 2017).

Cholera (alternative agent): **Oral:** 1 g as a single dose (Saha 2006).

Shigella gastroenteritis: **Note:** Confirm susceptibility if possible (Agha 2018; HHS [OI adult] 2020; WHO 2005). Oral: 500 mg once daily for 3 days (ACG [Riddle 2016]); 5 days of therapy should be given for *Shigella dysenteriae* type 1 infection or for patients with HIV coinfection (Agha 2018; HHS [OI adult] 2020).

Travelers' diarrhea , empiric treatment: **Oral:** 1 g as a single dose **or** 500 mg once daily for 3 days (ACG [Riddle 2016]; CDC 2018; Riddle 2017; Tribble 2007). If symptoms have not resolved after 24 hours following single-dose therapy, continue with 500 mg once daily for 2 more days. A 3-day course of 500 mg once daily is the preferred regimen for dysentery or febrile diarrhea (ACG [Riddle 2016]). **Note:** Most cases are self-limited and may not warrant antimicrobial therapy. Increased nausea may occur with the 1 g single-dose regimen (Tribble 2007), which may be reduced by administering azithromycin as 2 divided doses on the same day (CDC 2018; Riddle 2017).

Endocarditis prophylaxis, dental or invasive respiratory tract procedure (alternative agent for penicillin-allergic patients) (off-label use): Oral: 500 mg 30 to 60 minutes prior to procedure. **Note:** Only recommended for patients with cardiac conditions associated with the highest risk of an adverse outcome from endocarditis and who are undergoing a procedure likely to result in bacteremia with an organism that has the potential to cause endocarditis. (AHA [Wilson 2007]).

Lyme disease (erythema migrans or borrelial lymphocytoma) (alternative agent) (off-label use): Oral: 500 mg once daily for 7 to 10 days. **Note:** Use with caution and only when recommended agents cannot be used (due to decreased efficacy compared to other agents) (IDSA [Wormser 2006]).

Mycobacterial (nontuberculous) infection:

Mycobacterium avium complex (MAC) infection:

Disseminated disease in patients with HIV:

Treatment: Oral: 500 to 600 mg daily as part of a combination therapy regimen (HHS [OI adult] 2020).

Primary prophylaxis (patients with CD4 count <50 cells/mm^3 who are **not** initiated on fully suppressive antiretroviral therapy [ART]): **Oral:** 1.2 g once weekly (preferred) **or** 600 mg twice weekly; may discontinue prophylaxis when patient is initiated on effective ART (HHS [OI adult] 2020; IAS-USA [Saag 2018]).

Secondary prophylaxis: **Oral:** 500 to 600 mg daily as part of an appropriate combination regimen; may discontinue when patient has completed ≥12 months of therapy, has no signs/symptoms of MAC disease, and has sustained (>6 months) CD4 count >100 cells/mm^3 in response to ART (HHS [OI adult] 2020).

Pulmonary disease (nodular/bronchiectatic disease) (off-label use): **Oral:** 500 to 600 mg 3 times weekly as part of an appropriate combination regimen; continue treatment until patient is culture negative on therapy for ≥1 year (ATS/IDSA [Griffith 2007]); some experts prefer 500 mg 3 times weekly due to improved tolerability (BTS [Haworth 2017]).

Pulmonary disease (severe nodular/bronchiectatic or cavitary disease) (off-label use): **Oral:** 250 to 500 mg once daily as part of an appropriate combination regimen (ATS/IDSA [Griffith 2007]; BTS [Haworth 2017]; Deshpande 2016; van Ingen 2012); continue treatment until patient is culture negative on therapy for ≥1 year (ATS/IDSA [Griffith 2007]; BTS [Haworth 2017]). Preliminary data suggest a relationship between peak concentration and clinical outcome among patients receiving daily therapy for pulmonary MAC (Jeong 2016); as such, some experts recommend checking levels and/or using higher doses of azithromycin (Kasperbauer 2019).

Pulmonary disease in patients with cystic fibrosis (off-label use): **Oral:** 250 to 500 mg once daily as part of an appropriate combination regimen; continue treatment until patient is culture negative on therapy for ≥1 year. **Note:** Intermittent dosing (3 times weekly) is not recommended for patients with cystic fibrosis (CFF/ECFS [Floto 2016]).

Mycobacterium abscessus infection (off-label use):

Note: Presence of inducible *erm* gene can result in decreased susceptibility even with a "susceptible" MIC result; perform susceptibility testing before and after ≥14 days of clarithromycin incubation to evaluate for the presence of an active *erm* gene, which may preclude use of azithromycin (CFF/ECFS [Floto 2016]; Griffith 2019).

Pulmonary, skin, soft tissue, or bone infection: **Oral:** 250 to 500 mg once daily as part of an appropriate combination regimen and continued for ≥6 to 12 months for pulmonary and bone infections, and ≥4 months for skin/soft tissue infections (ATS/IDSA [Griffith 2007]; CFF/ECFS [Floto 2016]; Griffith 2019). **Note:** Patients should be under the care of a clinician with expertise in managing mycobacterial infection.

Pertussis (off-label use): Oral: 500 mg on day 1, followed by 250 mg once daily on days 2 to 5 (CDC [Tiwari 2005]).

Pneumonia, community acquired:

Outpatient: **Oral:** 500 mg on day 1, followed by 250 mg once daily for 4 days **or** 500 mg once daily for 3 days (Amsden 1999; ATS/IDSA [Metlay 2019]; Schönwald 1991). **Note:** May use as monotherapy (alternative agent) for outpatients without comorbidities or risk factors for antibiotic-resistant pathogens only if local pneumococcal resistance is <25%. Must be used as part of an appropriate combination regimen in outpatients with comorbidities (ATS/IDSA [Metlay 2019]); some experts prefer to use as part of an appropriate combination regimen in all outpatients, regardless of comorbidities (File 2020).

Inpatient: **Oral, IV:** 500 mg once daily for a minimum of 3 days, as part of an appropriate combination regimen (ATS/IDSA [Metlay 2019]; File 2020).

Sexually transmitted infections:

Cervicitis, empiric therapy: **Oral:** 1 g as a single dose, preferably under direct observation; give in combination with ceftriaxone if the patient is at high risk for gonorrhea, if follow-up is a concern, or if the local prevalence of gonorrhea is high (eg, >5%) (CDC [Workowski 2015]; Hsu 2019).

Chancroid (due to Haemophilus ducreyi): **Oral:** 1 g as a single dose. **Note:** Data are limited concerning efficacy in HIV infected patients (CDC [Workowski 2015]).

Chlamydia trachomatis infection of the cervix, urethra, or pharynx (off-label use [pharynx]): **Oral:** 1 g as a single dose, preferably under direct observation (CDC [Workowski 2015]).

Chlamydia trachomatis infection, expedited partner therapy (off-label use): **Oral:** 1 g as a single dose, preferably under direct observation. **Note:** Clinical evaluation and presumptive treatment is preferred for sexual partners of patients with chlamydia. Alternatively, expedited partner therapy for chlamydia can be used for heterosexual partners if the provider is concerned that the partner will otherwise not be promptly evaluated and treated; state laws regarding expedited partner therapy vary (CDC [Workowski 2015]).

Empiric treatment following sexual assault (off-label use): **Oral:** 1 g as a single dose in combination with ceftriaxone (plus metronidazole or tinidazole) (CDC [Workowski 2015]).

Gonococcal infection, disseminated (arthritis, arthritis-dermatitis) (off-label use): **Oral:** 1 g as a single dose in combination with ceftriaxone, preferably under direct observation (CDC [Workowski 2015]).

Gonococcal infection, expedited partner therapy (off-label use): **Oral:** 1 g as a single dose in combination with cefixime. **Note:** Clinical evaluation and presumptive treatment is preferred for sexual partners of patients with gonorrhea. Alternatively, expedited partner therapy for gonorrhea can be used for heterosexual partners if the provider is concerned that the partner will otherwise not be promptly evaluated and treated; state laws regarding expedited partner therapy vary (CDC [Workowski 2015]).

Gonococcal infection, uncomplicated (infection of the cervix, urethra, rectum, or pharynx; conjunctivitis): **Oral:**

Dual-therapy regimen (off-label): 1 g as a single dose in combination with ceftriaxone (CDC [Workowski 2015]).

Patients with severe cephalosporin allergy (off-label): 2 g as a single dose in combination with gemifloxacin (not available in the US) or gentamicin IM (CDC [Workowski 2015]). **Note:** Patients with pharyngeal infection treated with an alternative regimen should have a test-of-cure performed. Consult an infectious diseases specialist when treatment failure is suspected and report failures to the CDC through state and local health departments within 24 hours of diagnosis (CDC [Workowski 2015]).

Granuloma inguinale (donovanosis) (off-label use): **Oral:** 1 g once weekly **or** 500 mg once daily for ≥3 weeks and until lesions have healed. **Note:** If symptoms do not improve within the first few days of therapy, the addition of gentamicin may be considered (CDC [Workowski 2015]).

Mycoplasma genitalium (off-label use): Oral:

Note: Azithromycin resistance is rapidly emerging; consider alternative therapy. Azithromycin is not recommended for persistent infection when included in the initial regimen (CDC [Workowski 2015]; Martin 2019).

Initial treatment: 500 mg on day 1, followed by 250 mg once daily on days 2 through 5 (CDC [Workowski 2015]; Falk 2015); some experts favor high dose (1 g on day 1 followed by 500 mg once daily on days 2 through 4 with a test of cure 3 to 4 weeks after initiation) (Durukan 2019; Martin 2019; Read 2019).

Syphilis, primary and secondary (alternative agent for penicillin-allergic patients) (off-label use): **Oral:** 2 g as a single dose. **Note:** Limited data support the use of alternatives to penicillin; close serologic and clinical follow-up is warranted. Use only if no other options are available due to the potential for rapid emergence of macrolide resistance in *Treponema pallidum* and treatment failure; do not use to treat syphilis in patients with HIV, pregnant women, or the men who have sex with men (MSM) population (CDC [Workowski 2015]).

Urethritis, empiric therapy: **Oral:** 1 g as a single dose, preferably under direct observation; give in combination with ceftriaxone if there is microscopic evidence of gonococcal urethritis or if there is high clinical suspicion for gonococcal infection (Bachmann 2020; CDC [Workowski 2015]).

Streptococcal pharyngitis (group A) (alternative agent for severely penicillin-allergic patients): Oral: 500 mg on day 1, followed by 250 mg once daily on days 2 through 5 (IDSA [Shulman 2012]) **or** 500 mg once daily for 3 days (Casey 2005).

Surgical prophylaxis, uterine evacuation (induced abortion or pregnancy loss) (alternative agent) (off-label use): Oral: 500 mg as a single dose 1 hour before the procedure; may be administered up to 24 hours before the procedure (Shih 2020). **Note:** The optimal dosing regimen has not been established; various protocols are in use (RCOG 2015; White 2018; White 2019).

Renal Impairment: Adult The renal dosing recommendations are based upon the best available evidence and clinical expertise. Senior Editorial Team: Bruce Mueller, PharmD, FCCP, FASN, FNKF; Jason Roberts, PhD, BPharm (Hons), B App Sc, FSHP, FISAC; Michael Heung, MD, MS.

Oral, IV:

Mild to severe impairment: No dosage adjustment necessary (Höffler 1995).

Hemodialysis: No dosage adjustment or supplemental dose necessary (Aronoff 2007; Heintz 2009).

Peritoneal dialysis: Minimally dialyzed (Kent 2001): No dosage adjustment or supplemental dose necessary (Ma 2014).

CRRT: No dosage adjustment or supplemental dose necessary (Aronoff 2007; Heintz 2009).

Hepatic Impairment: Adult Azithromycin is predominantly hepatically eliminated; however, there is no dosage adjustment provided in the manufacturer's labeling. Use with caution due to potential for hepatotoxicity (rare); discontinue immediately for signs or symptoms of hepatitis.

Pediatric Note: Extended-release suspension (Zmax) is not interchangeable with immediate-release formulations. All doses are expressed as immediate-release azithromycin unless otherwise specified. Zmax 2 g extended-release oral suspension has been discontinued in the US for >1 year.

General dosing, susceptible infection (*Red Book* [AAP 2018]): Infants, Children, and Adolescents:

Oral: 5 to 12 mg/kg/dose; typically administered as 10 to 12 mg/kg/dose on day 1 (usual maximum dose: 500 mg/dose) followed by 5 to 6 mg/kg once daily (usual maximum dose: 250 mg/dose) for remainder of treatment duration.

IV: 10 mg/kg once daily; maximum dose: 500 mg/dose.

Babesiosis: Limited data available: Infants, Children, and Adolescents: Oral: 10 mg/kg once on day 1 (maximum dose: 500 mg/dose), then 5 mg/kg/dose once daily (maximum dose: 250 mg/dose) in combination with atovaquone for a total duration of 7 to 10 days; longer duration may be necessary in some patients with severe or persistent symptoms until parasitemia is cleared; in immunocompromised patients, higher doses (eg, adults: 600 to 1,000 mg daily) have been used (IDSA [Wormser 2006]; *Red Book* [AAP 2018]).

Cat scratch disease (*Bartonella henselae*) (lymphadenitis) (IDSA [Stevens 2014]): Limited data available:

Infants, Children, and Adolescents weighing ≤45 kg: Oral: 10 mg/kg once on day 1 (maximum dose: 500 mg/dose), then 5 mg/kg/dose once daily for 4 additional days (maximum dose: 250 mg/dose).

Children and Adolescents weighing >45 kg: Oral: 500 mg as a single dose on day 1, then 250 mg once daily for 4 additional days.

Cervicitis or urethritis, empiric treatment: Limited data available:

Infants and Children <45 kg: Optimal dose uncertain: Oral: 60 mg/kg as a single dose in combination with ceftriaxone; maximum dose: 1,000 mg/dose (*Red Book* [AAP 2018]).

Children ≥45 kg and Adolescents: Oral: 1,000 mg as a single dose in combination with ceftriaxone (CDC [Workowski 2015]; *Red Book* [AAP 2018]).

Chancroid *(Haemophilus ducreyi)* (CDC [Workowski 2015]; *Red Book* [AAP 2018]): Limited data available:

Infants and Children <45 kg: Oral: 20 mg/kg as a single dose; maximum dose: 1,000 mg/dose.

Children ≥45 kg and Adolescents: Oral: 1,000 mg as a single dose.

***Chlamydia trachomatis* infection:**

Urogenital/anogenital tract or oropharyngeal infection (eg, cervicitis, urethritis): Oral: Children <8 years weighing ≥45 kg **or** Children ≥8 years and Adolescents: Oral: 1,000 mg as a single dose (CDC [Workowski 2015]; *Red Book* [AAP 2018]).

Pneumonia: Infants: Oral, IV: 20 mg/kg/dose once daily for 3 days (CDC [Workowski 2015]; *Red Book* [AAP 2018]).

Cystic fibrosis; improve lung function, reduce exacerbation frequency: Limited data available; dosing regimen variable (Mogayzel 2013; Saiman 2003; Saiman 2010):

Children ≥6 years and Adolescents: Oral:

18 to 35.9 kg: 250 mg three times weekly (Monday, Wednesday, Friday).

≥36 kg: 500 mg three times weekly (Monday, Wednesday, Friday).

Diarrhea, infectious:

Campylobacter infection:

Non-HIV-exposed/-infected: Infants, Children, and Adolescents: Oral: 10 mg/kg/dose once daily for 3 days (*Red Book* [AAP 2018]); maximum dose: 500 mg/dose (Riddle 2017).

HIV-exposed/-infected: Adolescents: Oral: 500 mg once daily for 5 days (HHS [adult OI 2020].

Shigellosis:

Non-HIV-exposed/-infected: Infants, Children, and Adolescents: Oral: 10 mg/kg/dose once daily for 3 days (Dupont 2009; Mackell 2005); maximum dose: 500 mg/dose (Riddle 2017); WHO Guidelines recommend up to 20 mg/kg/dose (usual adult dose: 1,000 to 1,500 mg/dose) and in some cases, a wider range of duration of therapy (eg, 1 to 5 days) (WHO 2005).

HIV-exposed/-infected: Adolescents: Oral: 500 mg once daily for 5 days (HHS [adult OI 2020].

Endocarditis; prophylaxis: Infants, Children, and Adolescents: Oral: 15 mg/kg/dose 30 to 60 minutes before procedure; maximum dose: 500 mg/dose (AHA [Wilson 2007]).

Gonococcal infection:

Uncomplicated (infection of the cervix, urethra, rectum, or pharynx; conjunctivitis) (CDC [Workowski 2015]); *Red Book* [AAP 2018]): Limited data available: Children >45 kg and Adolescents: Oral: 1,000 mg as a single dose in combination with ceftriaxone; for patients with a severe cephalosporin allergy use azithromycin 2,000 mg orally as a single dose in combination with IM gentamicin or gemifloxacin (not available in the US).

Disseminated (arthritis, arthritis-dermatitis, meningitis, endocarditis): Limited data available: Children >45 kg and Adolescents: Oral: 1,000 mg as a single dose in combination with daily ceftriaxone (CDC [Workowski 2015]); *Red Book* [AAP 2018]).

Group A streptococcal infection; treatment of streptococcal tonsillopharyngitis (alternative agent for severely penicillin-allergic patients) (IDSA [Shulman 2012]):

Manufacturer's labeling and AHA recommendations: Infants, Children, and Adolescents: Oral: 12 mg/kg/dose once daily for 5 days; maximum dose: 500 mg/dose (AHA [Gerber 2009]).

Alternate dosing:

IDSA recommendations: Infants, Children, and Adolescents: Oral: 12 mg/kg (maximum: 500 mg/dose) on day 1 followed by 6 mg/kg/dose (maximum: 250 mg/dose) once daily on days 2 through 5 (IDSA [Shulman 2012]).

Three-day regimen: Limited data available: Children and Adolescents: Oral: 20 mg/kg/dose once daily for 3 days; maximum dose: 1,000 mg/dose (Cohen 2004; O'Doherty 1996).

Meningococcal disease, chemoprophylaxis of high-risk contacts: Infants, Children, and Adolescents: Oral: 10 mg/kg as a single dose; maximum dose: 500 mg/dose; **Note:** Not routinely recommended; may consider if fluoroquinolone resistance detected (*Red Book* [AAP 2018]).

***Mycobacterium avium* complex (MAC) infection (HIV-exposed/-infected):**

Infants and Children (HHS [pediatric OI 2019]):

Primary prophylaxis (patients who meet age-specific CD4 count thresholds): Oral: 20 mg/kg once **weekly** (maximum dose: 1,200 mg/dose) (preferred regimen) **or** alternatively, 5 mg/kg/dose once daily (maximum dose: 250 mg/dose); may be discontinued in children ≥2 years of age receiving stable antiretroviral therapy (ART) for ≥6 months and experiencing sustained (>3 months) CD4 count recovery well above age-specific targets.

Treatment (alternative to clarithromycin): Oral: 10 to 12 mg/kg/dose once daily as part of an appropriate combination regimen; maximum dose: 500 mg/dose; continue therapy for at least 12 months; following completion of treatment, initiate long-term suppression (secondary prophylaxis).

Long-term suppression (secondary prophylaxis) (alternative to clarithromycin): Oral: 5 mg/kg/dose once daily as part of an appropriate combination regimen; consideration can be given to discontinuation of therapy in children ≥2 years when patient has completed ≥12 months of therapy, has no signs/symptoms of MAC disease, and has sustained (≥6 months) CD4 count recovery meeting age-specific thresholds in response to stable ART.

Adolescents (HHS [adult OI 2020]):

Primary prophylaxis (patients with CD4 count <50 cells/mm^3 who are not initiated on fully suppressive ART): Oral: 1,200 mg once weekly (preferred) **or** 600 mg twice weekly; may discontinue prophylaxis when patient is initiated on effective ART.

Treatment and long-term suppression (secondary prophylaxis): Oral: 500 to 600 mg daily as part of an appropriate combination regimen; may discontinue when patient has completed ≥12 months of therapy, has no signs or symptoms of MAC disease, and has sustained (≥6 months) CD4 count >100 cells/mm^3 in response to ART.

Otitis media, acute (AOM): Infants ≥6 months, Children, and Adolescents: Oral: **Note:** Due to increased *S. pneumonia* and *H. influenzae* resistance, azithromycin is not routinely recommended as a treatment option (AAP [Lieberthal 2013]).

Single-dose regimen: 30 mg/kg as a single dose; maximum dose: 1,500 mg/dose; if patient vomits within 30 minutes of dose, repeat dosing has been administered although limited data available on safety.

Three-day regimen: 10 mg/kg once daily for 3 days; maximum dose: 500 mg/dose.

Five-day regimen: 10 mg/kg once on day 1 (maximum dose: 500 mg/dose), followed by 5 mg/kg (maximum dose: 250 mg/dose) once daily on days 2 to 5.

Peritonitis (peritoneal dialysis), prophylaxis for patients receiving peritoneal dialysis who require dental procedures:

Infants, Children, and Adolescents: Oral: 15 mg/kg administered 30 to 60 minutes before dental procedure; maximum dose: 500 mg/dose (Warady [ISPD 2012]).

Pertussis (CDC 2005; *Red Book* [AAP 2018]): Oral, IV:

Infants 1 to 5 months: 10 mg/kg/dose once daily for 5 days.

Infants ≥6 months, Children, and Adolescents: 10 mg/kg once on day 1 (maximum dose: 500 mg/dose), followed by 5 mg/kg once daily on days 2 to 5 (maximum dose: 250 mg/dose).

Pneumonia, community-acquired (presumed atypical pneumonia or proven *Chlamydia* or *Mycoplasma* infection) (IDSA/PIDS [Bradley 2011]):

Mild infection or step-down therapy: Infants >3 months, Children, and Adolescents: Oral: 10 mg/kg once on day 1 (maximum dose: 500 mg/dose), followed by 5 mg/kg/dose (maximum dose: 250 mg/dose) once daily on days 2 to 5 (IDSA/PIDS [Bradley 2011]).

Severe infection: Infants >3 months, Children, and Adolescents: IV: 10 mg/kg/dose once daily for at least 2 days (maximum dose: 500 mg/dose); when able transition to the oral route with a single daily dose of 5 mg/kg/dose (maximum dose: 250 mg/dose) to complete a 5-day course of therapy (IDSA/PIDS [Bradley 2011]).

Recurrent asthma-like symptoms, reduction in duration: Limited data available: Children ≤3 years: Oral: 10 mg/kg/dose once daily for 3 days; dosing based on a randomized placebo-controlled trial (n=72; episodes of recurrent asthma-like symptoms analyzed=148; mean age: 2 ± 0.6 years); patients were diagnosed with recurrent troublesome lung symptoms (asthma-like episodes) and included in the study if they had ≥5 episodes in 6 months, persistent symptoms for ≥4 weeks, or previously experienced a severe acute episode requiring an oral steroid or hospital admission, patients presenting with ≥3 days of consecutive symptoms were randomized to azithromycin or placebo. Patients received a beta-2 agonist, with the potential to receive inhaled corticosteroids (82%), montelukast (60%), and/or oral prednisolone as well. Children who received azithromycin experienced fewer days of symptoms (3.4 days) as compared to those who received placebo (7.7 days; $p<0.0001$); the biggest impact was noted when azithromycin was given before day 6 of symptoms (Stokholm 2016).

Rhinosinusitis, bacterial: Infants ≥6 months, Children, and Adolescents: Oral: 10 mg/kg/dose once daily for 3 days; maximum dose: 500 mg/dose; **Note:** Although FDA approved, macrolides are not recommended for empiric therapy due to high rates of resistance (AAP [Wald 2013]); IDSA [Chow 2012]).

Sexual victimization, prophylaxis: Note: Consider administering hepatitis B or human papillomavirus vaccines if needed based on patient's immunization status (CDC [Workowski 2015]; *Red Book* [AAP 2018]).

Adolescents: Oral: 1,000 mg as a single dose in combination with ceftriaxone and either metronidazole or tinidazole (CDC [Workowski 2015]; *Red Book* [AAP 2018]).

Renal Impairment: Pediatric

Altered kidney function: Infants, Children, and Adolescents: Oral, IV:

Mild to severe impairment: There are no dosage adjustments provided in the manufacturer's labeling; however, some experts suggest that no dosage adjustment is necessary (Aronoff 2007).

Hemodialysis: There are no dosage adjustments provided in the manufacturer's labeling; however, some experts suggest no dosage adjustment or supplemental doses are necessary (Aronoff 2007).

Peritoneal dialysis: There are no dosage adjustments provided in the manufacturer's labeling; however, some experts suggest no dosage adjustment or supplemental doses are necessary (Aronoff 2007). Based on adult information, azithromycin is not removed with continuous ambulatory peritoneal dialysis (Kent 2001).

Continuous renal replacement therapy (CRRT): There are no dosage adjustments provided in the manufacturer's labeling; however, some experts suggest no dosage adjustment or supplemental doses are necessary (Aronoff 2007).

Hepatic Impairment: Pediatric Azithromycin is predominantly hepatically eliminated; however, there is no dosage adjustment provided in the manufacturer's labeling. Use with caution due to potential for hepatotoxicity (rare); discontinue immediately for signs or symptoms of hepatitis.

Mechanism of Action Inhibits RNA-dependent protein synthesis at the chain elongation step; binds to the 50S ribosomal subunit resulting in blockage of transpeptidation

Contraindications

Hypersensitivity to azithromycin, erythromycin, other macrolide (eg, azalide or ketolide) antibiotics, or any component of the formulation; history of cholestatic jaundice/hepatic dysfunction associated with prior azithromycin use

Note: The manufacturer does not list concurrent use of pimozide as a contraindication; however, azithromycin is listed as a contraindication in the manufacturer's labeling for pimozide.

Warnings/Precautions Use with caution in patients with preexisting liver disease; hepatocellular and/or cholestatic hepatitis (with or without jaundice), hepatic necrosis, failure and death have occurred. Discontinue immediately if symptoms of hepatitis occur (malaise, nausea, vomiting, abdominal colic, fever). Allergic (hypersensitivity) reactions (eg, angioedema, anaphylaxis, Stevens-Johnson syndrome, toxic epidermal necrolysis and drug reaction with eosinophilia and systemic symptoms [DRESS]) have been reported (rare), including fatalities; reappearance of allergic reaction may occur shortly after discontinuation without further azithromycin exposure. When studied to prevent bronchiolitis obliterans syndrome in patients with hematologic malignancy who underwent allogeneic hematopoietic cell transplantation, rates of cancer relapse and mortality were increased among patients receiving long-term azithromycin, leading to early trial termination (Bergeron 2017; FDA Drug Safety Communication 2018). May mask or delay symptoms of incubating gonorrhea or syphilis, so appropriate culture and susceptibility tests should be performed prior to initiating a treatment regimen. Prolonged use may result in fungal or bacterial superinfection, including *C. difficile*-associated diarrhea (CDAD); CDAD has been observed >2 months postantibiotic treatment. Use caution with renal dysfunction. Macrolides (especially erythromycin) have been associated with rare QT_c prolongation and ventricular arrhythmias, including torsades de pointes; consider avoiding use in patients with prolonged QT interval, congenital long QT syndrome, history of torsades de pointes, bradyarrhythmias, uncorrected hypokalemia or hypomagnesemia, clinically significant bradycardia, uncompensated heart failure, or concurrent use of Class IA (eg, quinidine, procainamide) or Class III (eg, amiodarone, dofetilide, sotalol) antiarrhythmic agents or other drugs known to prolong the QT interval. Use with caution in patients with myasthenia gravis. Use of azithromycin in neonates and infants <6 weeks of age has been associated with infantile hypertrophic pyloric stenosis (IHPS); the strongest association occurred with exposure during the first 2 weeks of life; observe for nonbilious vomiting or irritability with feeding (Eberly 2015). The risks and benefits of azithromycin use should be carefully considered in neonates; some experts recommend avoidance except for in the treatment of pertussis or *C. trachomatis* pneumonia; specific risk-benefit ratio should be considered before use for *Ureaplasma* spp. eradication (Meyers 2020).

Oral suspensions (immediate release and extended release) are not interchangeable.

Drug Interactions

Metabolism/Transport Effects **Substrate** of CYP3A4 (minor); **Note:** Assignment of Major/Minor substrate status based on clinically relevant drug interaction potential; **Inhibits** P-glycoprotein/ABCB1

Avoid Concomitant Use

Avoid concomitant use of Azithromycin (Systemic) with any of the following: BCG (Intravesical); Bilastine; Cholera Vaccine; DOXOrubicin (Conventional); Fexinidazole [INT]; Mizolastine; PAZOPanib; Pimozide; QT-prolonging Strong CYP3A4 Inhibitors (Moderate Risk); Rimegepant; Topotecan; VinCRIStine (Liposomal)

Increased Effect/Toxicity

Azithromycin (Systemic) may increase the levels/effects of: Afatinib; Aliskiren; AtorvaSTATin; Betrixaban; Bilastine; Cardiac Glycosides; Celiprolol; Chloroquine; Clofazimine; Colchicine; CycloSPORINE (Systemic); Dabigatran Etexilate; Domperidone; DOXOrubicin (Conventional); Edoxaban; Etoposide; Etoposide Phosphate; Everolimus; Gadobenate Dimeglumine; Glecaprevir and Pibrentasvir; Halofantrine; Haloperidol; Inotuzumab Ozogamicin; Lapatinib; Larotrectinib; Lefamulin; Lofexidine; Lovastatin; Midostaurin; Mizolastine; Morphine (Systemic); Nadolol; Naldemedine; Naloxegol; Ondansetron; PAZOPanib; Pentamidine (Systemic); P-glycoprotein/ABCB1 Substrates; Piperaquine; Probucol; QT-prolonging Antipsychotics (Moderate Risk); QT-prolonging Class IC Antiarrhythmics (Moderate Risk); QT-prolonging Quinolone Antibiotics (Moderate Risk); Ranolazine; RifAXIMin; Rimegepant; RisperiDONE; RomiDEPsin; Silodosin; Simvastatin; Sirolimus; Sodium Stibogluconate; Tacrolimus (Systemic); Tacrolimus (Topical); Talazoparib; Tegaserod; Teniposide; Tolvaptan; Topotecan; Toremifene; Ubrogepant; VinCRIStine (Liposomal); Vitamin K Antagonists

The levels/effects of Azithromycin (Systemic) may be increased by: Amisulpride (Oral); Fexinidazole [INT]; Nelfinavir; Pimozide; QT-prolonging Agents (Highest Risk); QT-prolonging Antidepressants (Moderate Risk); QT-prolonging Kinase Inhibitors (Moderate Risk); QT-prolonging Moderate CYP3A4 Inhibitors (Moderate Risk); QT-prolonging Strong CYP3A4 Inhibitors (Moderate Risk)

Decreased Effect

Azithromycin (Systemic) may decrease the levels/effects of: BCG (Intravesical); BCG Vaccine (Immunization); Cholera Vaccine; Lactobacillus and Estriol; Sincalide; Sodium Picosulfate; Typhoid Vaccine

Food Interactions Rate and extent of GI absorption may be altered depending upon the formulation. Azithromycin suspension, not tablet form, has significantly increased absorption (46%) with food. Management: Immediate release suspension and tablet may be taken without regard to food; extended release suspension should be taken on an empty stomach (at least 1 hour before or 2 hours following a meal).

Dietary Considerations

Some products may contain sodium and/or sucrose.

Oral suspension, immediate release, may be administered with or without food.

Oral suspension, extended release, should be taken on an empty stomach (at least 1 hour before or 2 hours following a meal).

Tablet may be administered with food to decrease GI effects.

Pharmacodynamics/Kinetics

Half-life Elimination Terminal: Oral, IV: Infants and Children 4 months to 15 years: 54.5 hours; Adults: Immediate release: 68 to 72 hours; Extended release: 59 hours

Time to Peak Oral: Serum: Immediate release: ~2 to 3 hours; Extended release: 3 to 5 hours

Pregnancy Considerations

Azithromycin crosses the placenta (Ramsey 2003)

The maternal serum half-life of azithromycin is unchanged in early pregnancy and decreased at term; however, high concentrations of azithromycin are sustained in the myometrium and adipose tissue (Fischer 2012; Ramsey 2003).

Azithromycin may be used as an alternative or adjunctive prophylactic antibiotic in females undergoing unplanned cesarean delivery (ACOG 199 2018). Azithromycin is recommended for the treatment of several infections, including chlamydia, gonococcal infections, and *Mycobacterium avium* complex in pregnant patients (consult current guidelines) (CDC [Workowski 2015]; HHS [OI adult 2020]). Azithromycin may also be used in certain situations prior to vaginal delivery in females at high risk for endocarditis (ACOG 199 2018).

Azithromycin is under investigation for use in the treatment of coronavirus disease 2019 (COVID-19) (see ClinicalTrials.gov) and should **only** be given as part of a clinical trial for this indication (HHS 2020). The American College of Obstetricians and Gynecologists and the Society for Maternal-Fetal Medicine have developed an algorithm to aid practitioners in assessing and managing pregnant women with suspected or confirmed COVID-19 (https://www.acog.org/topics/covid-19; https://www.smfm.org/covid19). Interim guidance is also available from the Centers for Disease Control and Prevention for pregnant women who are diagnosed with COVID-19 (https://www.cdc.gov/coronavirus/2019-ncov/hcp/inpatient-obstetric-healthcare-guidance.html).

Data collection to monitor maternal and infant outcomes following exposure to COVID-19 during pregnancy is ongoing. Health care providers are encouraged to enroll females exposed to COVID-19 during pregnancy in the Organization of Teratology Information Specialists pregnancy registry (1-877-311-8972; https://mothertobaby.org/join-study/) or PRIORITY (Pregnancy Coronavirus Outcomes Registry) (1-415-754-3729; https://priority.ucsf.edu/).

Breastfeeding Considerations Azithromycin is present in breast milk.

Following administration of oral azithromycin 2 g as a single dose to 20 women during labor, azithromycin was measurable in breast milk for up to 28 days; adverse events were not observed in the breastfed infants (Salman 2015). In a different study, a woman was given oral azithromycin as a 1 g loading dose followed in 48 hours by azithromycin 500 mg for 3 days; milk concentrations increased over time and reached a peak 30 hours after the last oral dose (Kelsey 1994). In a third study, the median half-life in breast milk was 15.6 hours (Sutton 2015).

Decreased appetite, diarrhea, rash, and somnolence have been reported in nursing infants exposed to macrolide antibiotics (Goldstein 2009). In general, antibiotics that are present in breast milk may cause non-dose-related modification of bowel flora. Monitor infants for GI disturbances (WHO 2002). In addition, an increased risk for infantile hypertrophic pyloric stenosis (IHPS) may be present in infants who are exposed to macrolides via breast milk, especially during the first 2 weeks of life (Lund 2014); however, data are conflicting (Goldstein 2009). According to the manufacturer, the decision to breastfeed during therapy should consider the risk of infant exposure, the benefits of breastfeeding to the infant, and benefits of treatment to the mother.

The Centers for Disease Control and Prevention's (CDC's) Sexually Transmitted Diseases Treatment Guidelines state that azithromycin is one of the recommended agents for the treatment of granuloma inguinale in lactating women. For lymphogranuloma venereum, azithromycin may be considered as an alternative agent in this patient population (CDC [Workowski 2015]).

Azithromycin is under investigation for use in the treatment of coronavirus disease 2019 (COVID-19) (see ClinicalTrials.gov) and should **only** be given as part of a clinical trial for this indication (HHS 2020). Interim guidance is available from the CDC for lactating women who are diagnosed with COVID-19 (https://www.cdc.gov/coronavirus/2019-ncov/hcp/inpatient-obstetric-healthcare-guidance.html). Information related to COVID-19 and breastfeeding is also available from the World Health Organization (https://www.who.int/docs/default-source/maternal-health/faqs-breastfeeding-and-covid-19.pdf?sfvrsn=d839e6c0_1).

Product Availability Zmax suspension has been discontinued in the US for more than 1 year.

Dosage Forms: US

Packet, Oral:
Zithromax: 1 g (3 ea, 10 ea)
Generic: 1 g (3 ea, 10 ea)

Solution Reconstituted, Intravenous [preservative free]:
Zithromax: 500 mg (1 ea)
Generic: 500 mg (1 ea)

Suspension Reconstituted, Oral:
Zithromax: 100 mg/5 mL (15 mL); 200 mg/5 mL (15 mL, 22.5 mL, 30 mL)
Generic: 100 mg/5 mL (15 mL); 200 mg/5 mL (15 mL, 22.5 mL, 30 mL)

Tablet, Oral:
Zithromax: 250 mg, 500 mg
Zithromax Tri-Pak: 500 mg
Zithromax Z-Pak: 250 mg
Generic: 250 mg, 500 mg, 600 mg

Dosage Forms: Canada

Solution Reconstituted, Intravenous:
Zithromax: 500 mg (5 mL)
Generic: 500 mg (1 ea)

Suspension Reconstituted, Oral:
Zithromax: 100 mg/5 mL (15 mL); 200 mg/5 mL (15 mL, 22.5 mL)
Generic: 100 mg/5 mL (15 mL, 22.5 mL); 200 mg/5 mL (15 mL, 22.5 mL, 37.5 mL)

Tablet, Oral:
Zithromax: 250 mg, 600 mg
Generic: 250 mg, 600 mg

Dental Health Professional Considerations There is evidence that azithromycin is proarrhythmic (see Local Anesthetic/Vasoconstrictor Precautions)

A recent large retrospective review of the cardiovascular risks of azithromycin was published. Researchers reviewed a Tennessee Medicaid cohort of patients to evaluate cardiovascular mortality in patients taking azithromycin, amoxicillin, ciprofloxacin, levofloxacin, or no antibiotic. The cohort included patients who took azithromycin (347,795 prescriptions); propensity-score-matched persons who took no antibiotics (1,391,180 control periods); and patients who took amoxicillin (1,348,672 prescriptions), ciprofloxacin (264,626 prescriptions), or levofloxacin (193,906 prescriptions). The risk of cardiovascular death was greater with azithromycin than with ciprofloxacin, but similar to levofloxacin. Amoxicillin showed no increase in risk of cardiovascular death. The estimated risk for azithromycin was 47 additional cardiovascular deaths per million courses of treatment (Ray 2012).

- **Azithromycin Dihydrate** *see* Azithromycin (Systemic) *on page 203*
- **Azithromycin Monohydrate** *see* Azithromycin (Systemic) *on page 203*
- **AZL-M** *see* Azilsartan *on page 202*
- **Azolen Tincture [OTC]** *see* Miconazole (Topical) *on page 1019*
- **Azor** *see* Amlodipine and Olmesartan *on page 122*
- **AZO Urinary Pain Relief [OTC]** *see* Phenazopyridine *on page 1222*
- **AZT + 3TC (error-prone abbreviation)** *see* Lamivudine and Zidovudine *on page 874*
- **AZT, Abacavir, and Lamivudine** *see* Abacavir, Lamivudine, and Zidovudine *on page 52*
- **AZT (error-prone abbreviation)** *see* Zidovudine *on page 1569*
- **Azthreonam** *see* Aztreonam (Systemic) *on page 211*
- **Aztreonam** *see* Aztreonam (Oral Inhalation) *on page 212*

Aztreonam (Systemic) (AZ tree oh nam)

Brand Names: US Azactam; Azactam in Dextrose [DSC]

Pharmacologic Category Antibiotic, Monobactam

Use Treatment of patients with urinary tract infections, lower respiratory tract infections, septicemia, skin/skin structure infections, intra-abdominal infections, and gynecological infections caused by susceptible gram-negative bacilli

Local Anesthetic/Vasoconstrictor Precautions No information available to require special precautions

Effects on Dental Treatment No significant effects or complications reported

Effects on Bleeding No information available to require special precautions

Adverse Reactions

>10%:

Hematologic & oncologic: Neutropenia (children 3% to 11%; adults <1%)

Hepatic: Increased serum transaminases (children, high dose: >3 times ULN: 15% to 20%; children, standard dose: increased serum AST 4%, increased serum ALT 7%)

Local: Pain at injection site (children 12%, adults 2%)

1% to 10%:

Cardiovascular: Phlebitis (intravenous: ≤2%), thrombophlebitis (intravenous: ≤2%)

Dermatologic: Skin rash (children 4%, adults ≤1%)

Gastrointestinal: Diarrhea (≤1%), nausea (≤1%), vomiting (≤1%)

Hematologic & oncologic: Eosinophilia (children 6%, adults <1%), thrombocythemia (children 4%, adults <1%)

Local: Erythema at injection site (intravenous: Children 3%, adults <1%), discomfort at injection site (intramuscular: ≤2%), swelling at injection site (intramuscular: ≤2%)

Renal: Increased serum creatinine (children 6%)

Miscellaneous: Fever (≤1%)

<1%, postmarketing, and/or case reports: Abdominal cramps, anaphylaxis, anemia, angioedema, breast tenderness, bronchospasm, chest pain, *Clostridioides* (formerly *Clostridium*) *difficile*-associated diarrhea, confusion, diaphoresis, diplopia, dizziness, dysgeusia, dyspnea, erythema multiforme, exfoliative dermatitis, flushing, gastrointestinal hemorrhage, halitosis, headache, hepatitis, hepatobiliary disease, hypotension, increased serum alkaline phosphatase, increased serum ALT (adults), increased serum AST (adults), induration at injection site, insomnia, jaundice,

leukocytosis, malaise, myalgia, nasal congestion, numbness of tongue, oral mucosa ulcer, pancytopenia, paresthesia, petechia, positive direct Coombs test, prolonged partial thromboplastin time, prolonged prothrombin time, pruritus, pseudomembranous colitis, purpura, seizure, sneezing, thrombocytopenia, tinnitus, toxic epidermal necrolysis, urticaria, vaginitis, ventricular bigeminy (transient), ventricular premature contractions (transient), vertigo, vulvovaginal candidiasis, weakness, wheezing

Mechanism of Action Inhibits bacterial cell wall synthesis by binding to one or more of the penicillin-binding proteins (PBPs) which in turn inhibits the final transpeptidation step of peptidoglycan synthesis in bacterial cell walls, thus inhibiting cell wall biosynthesis. Bacteria eventually lyse due to ongoing activity of cell wall autolytic enzymes (autolysins and murein hydrolases) while cell wall assembly is arrested. Monobactam structure makes cross-allergenicity with beta-lactams unlikely.

Pharmacodynamics/Kinetics

Half-life Elimination

Neonates: <7 days, ≤2.5 kg: 5.5 to 9.9 hours; <7 days, >2.5 kg: 2.6 hours; 1 week to 1 month: 2.4 hours

Children 2 months to 12 years: 1.7 hours

Children with cystic fibrosis: 1.3 hours

Adults: Normal renal function: 1.5 to 2 hours

End-stage renal disease: 6 to 8.4 hours (Brogden 1986)

Time to Peak IM: Within 60 minutes (Mattie 1988)

Pregnancy Risk Factor B

Pregnancy Considerations

Aztreonam crosses the placenta and can be detected in the fetus.

Information related to aztreonam for the treatment of urinary tract infections in pregnancy is limited. Use may be considered in pregnant patients allergic to preferred antibiotics (Glaser 2015; Jolley 2010).

Aztreonam (Oral Inhalation) (AZ tree oh nam)

Brand Names: US Cayston

Brand Names: Canada Cayston

Pharmacologic Category Antibiotic, Monobactam

Use Cystic fibrosis: Improve respiratory symptoms in cystic fibrosis (CF) patients with pulmonary *Pseudomonas aeruginosa* infections.

Local Anesthetic/Vasoconstrictor Precautions

No information available to require special precautions

Effects on Dental Treatment No significant effects or complications reported

Effects on Bleeding No information available to require special precautions

Adverse Reactions

>10%:

Gastrointestinal: Pharyngolaryngeal pain (12%)

Respiratory: Cough (54%), nasal congestion (16%), wheezing (16%)

Miscellaneous: Fever (13%; more common in children)

1% to 10%:

Cardiovascular: Chest discomfort (8%)

Dermatologic: Skin rash (2%)

Gastrointestinal: Abdominal pain (7%), vomiting (6%)

Respiratory: Bronchospasm (3%; patients experienced ≥15% reduction in FEV_1)

<1%, postmarketing, and/or case reports: Arthralgia, facial rash, facial swelling, hypersensitivity reaction, joint swelling, pharyngeal edema

Mechanism of Action Inhibits bacterial cell wall synthesis by binding to one or more of the penicillin-binding proteins (PBPs), which in turn inhibits the final transpeptidation step of peptidoglycan synthesis in bacterial cell walls, thus inhibiting cell wall biosynthesis. Bacteria eventually lyse due to ongoing activity of cell wall autolytic enzymes (autolysins and murein hydrolases), while cell wall assembly is arrested. Monobactam structure makes cross-allergenicity with beta-lactams unlikely.

Pharmacodynamics/Kinetics

Half-life Elimination Adults: 2.1 hours.

Time to Peak ~1 hour (plasma).

Pregnancy Considerations

Aztreonam crosses the placenta and reaches the fetal circulation following IV administration; however, peak plasma concentrations following inhalation of aztreonam are significantly less than those observed following aztreonam IV.

Due to its poor systemic absorption, use of aztreonam inhalation is likely acceptable for the management of cystic fibrosis in pregnant patients with *Pseudomonas aeruginosa* (Kroon 2018; Middleton 2019). When required, use may continue during pregnancy (Middleton 2019).

Prescribing and Access Restrictions Cayston (aztreonam inhalation solution) is only available through a select group of specialty pharmacies and cannot be obtained through a retail pharmacy. Because Cayston may only be used with the Altera Nebulizer System, it can only be obtained from the following specialty pharmacies; IV Solutions/Maxor; Foundation Care; Pharmaceutical Specialties Inc; TLCRx/ModernHEALTH; and Walgreens Specialty Pharmacy. This network of specialty pharmacies ensures proper access to both the drug and device. To obtain the medication and proper nebulizer, contact the Cayston Access Program at 1-877-7CAYSTON (1-877-722-9786) or at www.cayston.com. In Canada, Cayston is distributed by Innomar Solutions specialty pharmacy; Canadian healthcare providers and patients may obtain additional information at http://cayston.ca/

- **Azulfidine** *see* SulfaSALAzine *on page 1392*
- **Azulfidine EN-tabs** *see* SulfaSALAzine *on page 1392*
- **Azuphen MB [DSC]** *see* Methenamine, Sodium Phosphate Monobasic, Phenyl Salicylate, Methylene Blue, and Hyoscyamine *on page 987*
- **Azurette** *see* Ethinyl Estradiol and Desogestrel *on page 609*
- **B-2-400 [OTC]** *see* Riboflavin *on page 1323*
- **B6** *see* Pyridoxine *on page 1294*
- **B-12 Compliance Injection** *see* Cyanocobalamin *on page 417*
- **B1939** *see* EriBULin *on page 584*
- **Baby Anbesol [OTC]** *see* Benzocaine *on page 228*
- **Baby Aspirin** *see* Aspirin *on page 177*

Bacitracin (Topical) (bas i TRAY sin)

Pharmacologic Category Antibiotic, Topical

Use Topical infection prevention: Prevention of infection in minor cuts, scrapes, or burns.

Local Anesthetic/Vasoconstrictor Precautions

No information available to require special precautions

Effects on Dental Treatment No significant effects or complications reported

Effects on Bleeding No information available to require special precautions

Adverse Reactions Postmarketing and/or case reports: Anaphylaxis (Elsner, 1990; Farley, 1995)

Mechanism of Action Inhibits bacterial cell wall synthesis by preventing transfer of mucopeptides into the growing cell wall

Pregnancy Considerations Although large studies have not been conducted, absorption is limited following topical application; use during pregnancy has not been associated with an increased risk of adverse fetal events (Leachman, 2006; Murase, 2014).

Baclofen (BAK loe fen)

Brand Names: US Gablofen; Lioresal; Ozobax

Brand Names: Canada APO-Baclofen; Baclofen-10; Baclofen-20; DOM-Baclofen; Lioresal DS [DSC]; Lioresal Intrathecal; Lioresal [DSC]; MYLAN-Baclofen; PMS-Baclofen; RATIO-Baclofen [DSC]; RIVA-Baclofen

Pharmacologic Category Skeletal Muscle Relaxant

Use

Spasticity:

Oral: Management of reversible spasticity associated with multiple sclerosis or spinal cord lesions.

Intrathecal: Management of severe spasticity of spinal cord origin (eg, spinal cord injury, multiple sclerosis) or cerebral origin (eg, cerebral palsy, traumatic brain injury) in patients ≥4 years of age; may be considered as an alternative to destructive neurosurgical procedures.

Limitations of use: Patients should first respond to a screening dose of intrathecal baclofen prior to consideration for long-term infusion via an implantable pump. For spasticity of spinal cord origin, chronic infusion via an implantable pump should be reserved for patients unresponsive to oral baclofen therapy, or those who experience intolerable CNS adverse effects at effective doses. Patients with spasticity due to traumatic brain injury should wait at least 1 year after the injury before consideration of long-term intrathecal baclofen therapy.

Local Anesthetic/Vasoconstrictor Precautions No information available to require special precautions

Effects on Dental Treatment Key adverse event(s) related to dental treatment: Infrequent occurrence of xerostomia (normal salivary flow resumes upon discontinuation) has been reported. Rare occurrence of dysgeusia and tongue irritations have also been reported.

Effects on Bleeding No information available to require special precautions

Adverse Reactions

>10%:

Central nervous system: Hypotonia (2% to 35%), drowsiness (6% to 21%), confusion (1% to 11%), headache (2% to 11%)

Gastrointestinal: Nausea (1% to 12%), vomiting (2% to 11%)

1% to 10%:

Cardiovascular: Hypotension (≤9%), peripheral edema (≤3%)

Central nervous system: Seizure (≤10%), dizziness (2% to 8%), insomnia (≤7%), paresthesia (≤7%), hypertonia (≤6%), pain (≤4%), speech disturbance (≤4%), depression (2%), coma (≤2%), abnormality in thinking (≤1%), agitation (≤1%), chills (≤1%)

Dermatologic: Pruritus (4%), urticaria (≤1%)

Gastrointestinal: Constipation (≤6%), sialorrhea (≤3%), xerostomia (≤3%), diarrhea (≤2%)

Genitourinary: Urinary retention (≤8%), urinary frequency (≤6%), difficulty in micturition (2%), impotence (≤2%), urinary incontinence (≤2%)

Neuromuscular & skeletal: Asthenia (≤2%), back pain (≤2%), tremor (≤1%)

Ophthalmic: Amblyopia (≤2%)

Respiratory: Hypoventilation (≤4%), pneumonia (≤2%), dyspnea (≤1%)

Miscellaneous: Accidental injury (≤4%)

<1%, postmarketing, and/or case reports: Abdominal pain, accommodation disturbance, akathisia, albuminuria, alopecia, amnesia, ankle edema, anorexia, anxiety, apnea, ataxia, blurred vision, bradycardia, carcinoma, chest pain, contact dermatitis, decreased libido, deep vein thrombophlebitis, dehydration, dermal ulcer, diaphoresis, diplopia, dysarthria, dysautonomia, dysgeusia, dysphagia, dystonia, dysuria, epilepsy, erectile dysfunction, euphoria, excitement, facial edema, fecal incontinence, fever, gastrointestinal hemorrhage, hallucination, hematuria, hyperglycemia, hyperhidrosis, hypertension, hyperventilation, hypothermia, hysteria, inhibited ejaculation, intestinal obstruction, leukocytosis, loss of postural reflex, malaise, miosis, muscle rigidity, myalgia, mydriasis, nasal congestion, nephrolithiasis, nocturia, nystagmus disorder, occult blood in stools, oliguria, opisthotonus, orgasm disturbance, pallor, palpitations, paranoid ideation, personality disorder, petechial rash, priapism, pulmonary embolism, scoliosis, scoliosis progression, sedated state, sexual disorder, skin rash, slurred speech, strabismus, suicidal ideation, syncope, taste disorder, tinnitus, tongue irritation, vaginitis, vasodilation, weight gain, weight loss

Mechanism of Action Inhibits the transmission of both monosynaptic and polysynaptic reflexes at the spinal cord level, possibly by hyperpolarization of primary afferent fiber terminals, with resultant relief of muscle spasticity

Pharmacodynamics/Kinetics

Onset of Action

Intrathecal bolus: 30 minutes to 1 hour; Continuous infusion: 6 to 8 hours after infusion initiation

Peak effect: Intrathecal bolus: 4 hours (effects may last 4 to 8 hours); Continuous infusion: 24 to 48 hours

Half-life Elimination

Oral:

Pediatric patients with cerebral palsy (age range: 2 to 17 years): 4.5 hours (He 2014)

Adults: Solution: 5.7 hours; Tablets: 3.75 ± 0.96 hours (Brunton 2011)

Intrathecal: CSF elimination half-life: 1.5 hours over the first 4 hours

Time to Peak Serum: Oral: 1 hour (0.5 to 4 hours) (Brunton 2011)

Pregnancy Considerations

Late-onset neonatal withdrawal may occur following in utero exposure. Feeding difficulties, high-pitched cry, hyperthermia, hypertonicity, loose stools, tremors, and seizures have been reported in newborns following maternal use of oral baclofen throughout pregnancy (Duncan 2013; Freeman 2016; Ratnayaka 2001). Use of intrathecal baclofen in pregnant females has been described (Dalton 2008; Hara 2018; Méndez-Lucena 2016; Tandon 2010). Maternal plasma concentrations following administration of intrathecal baclofen are significantly less than those with oral doses; exposure to the fetus is expected to be limited and adverse neonatal events have not been noted in available reports (Morton 2009).

◆ **Bactrim** *see* Sulfamethoxazole and Trimethoprim *on page 1391*

◆ **Bactrim DS** *see* Sulfamethoxazole and Trimethoprim *on page 1391*

◆ **Bactroban [DSC]** *see* Mupirocin *on page 1066*

◆ **Bactroban Nasal [DSC]** *see* Mupirocin *on page 1066*

◆ **Bafiertam** *see* Monomethyl Fumarate *on page 1048*

◆ **BAL8557** *see* Isavuconazonium Sulfate *on page 843*

◆ **Balcoltra** *see* Ethinyl Estradiol and Levonorgestrel *on page 612*

Baloxavir Marboxil (ba LOX A veer mar BOX el)

Brand Names: US Xofluza (40 MG Dose); Xofluza (80 MG Dose)

Pharmacologic Category Antiviral Agent; Endonuclease Inhibitor

Use

Influenza, seasonal, treatment: Treatment of acute uncomplicated influenza (A or B) infection in patients ≥12 years of age who have been symptomatic for no more than 48 hours and who are otherwise healthy or at high risk of developing influenza-related complications.

Limitations of use: Influenza viruses change over time, and factors such as the virus type or subtype, emergence of resistance, or changes in viral virulence may diminish the clinical benefit of antiviral drugs. Consider available information on influenza drug susceptibility patterns and treatment effects when deciding whether to use baloxavir marboxil.

Local Anesthetic/Vasoconstrictor Precautions No information available to require special precautions

Effects on Dental Treatment Key adverse event(s) related to dental treatment: Nasopharyngitis has been reported

Effects on Bleeding No information available to require special precautions

Adverse Reactions

1% to 10%: Gastrointestinal: Diarrhea (2% [Hayden 2018])

Postmarketing:

Dermatologic: Erythema multiforme, facial swelling, skin rash, urticaria

Gastrointestinal: Bloody diarrhea, colitis, melena, swollen tongue, vomiting

Hypersensitivity: Anaphylactic shock, anaphylaxis, angioedema, hypersensitivity reaction, nonimmune anaphylaxis

Nervous system: Abnormal behavior, delirium, hallucination, voice disorder

Ophthalmic: Eyelid edema

Mechanism of Action Baloxavir marboxil is an oral prodrug that is converted to baloxavir, an inhibitor of the endonuclease activity of a selective polymerase acidic (PA) protein, which is required for viral gene transcription, resulting in inhibition of influenza virus replication. Baloxavir has demonstrated antiviral activity against influenza A and B viruses, including strains resistant to standard current antiviral agents (Hayden 2018).

Pharmacodynamics/Kinetics

Half-life Elimination 79.1 hour

Time to Peak 4 hours

Pregnancy Considerations

Adverse events were not observed in animal reproduction studies.

Untreated influenza infection is associated with an increased risk of adverse events to the fetus and an increased risk of complications or death to the mother. Other agents are currently recommended for the treatment of influenza in pregnant females and females up to 2 weeks postpartum (ACOG 2018; CDC [Fiore] 2011).

Balsalazide (bal SAL a zide)

Brand Names: US Colazal; Giazo [DSC]

Pharmacologic Category 5-Aminosalicylic Acid Derivative; Anti-inflammatory Agent

Use

Ulcerative colitis: Treatment of mildly- to moderately-active ulcerative colitis

Limitations of use: Efficacy of Giazo has not been demonstrated in females.

Local Anesthetic/Vasoconstrictor Precautions No information available to require special precautions

Effects on Dental Treatment No significant effects or complications reported

Effects on Bleeding No information available to require special precautions

Adverse Reactions

>10%:

Central nervous system: Headache (children: 15%; adults: 8%)

Gastrointestinal: Abdominal pain (children: 12% to 13%; adults: ≤6%)

1% to 10%:

Central nervous system: Fatigue (children: 4%; adults: ≤2%), insomnia (adults: 2%)

Gastrointestinal: Vomiting (children: 10%; adults: ≤4%), diarrhea (children: 9%; adults: ≤5%), exacerbation of ulcerative colitis (children: 6%; adults: 1%), nausea (adults: 5%; children: 4%), hematochezia (children: 4%), stomatitis (children: 3%), anorexia (adults: 2%), dyspepsia (adults: 2%), flatulence (adults: ≤2%), abdominal cramps (adults: 1%), constipation (adults: ≤1%), xerostomia (adults: ≤1%)

Genitourinary: Urinary tract infection (adults: 1% to 4%), dysmenorrhea (children: 3%)

Hematologic & oncologic: Anemia (4%)

Neuromuscular & skeletal: Arthralgia (adults: ≤4%), musculoskeletal pain (adults: 2%), myalgia (adults: ≤1%)

Respiratory: Pharyngitis (children: 6%; adults: 2%), flu-like symptoms (children: 4%; adults: 1%), respiratory infection (adults: ≤4%), cough (children: 3%; adults: 2%), pharyngolaryngeal pain (adults: 4%, children: 3%), rhinitis (adults: 2%)

Miscellaneous: Fever (children: 6%; adults: 2%)

<1%, postmarketing, and/or case reports: Alopecia, back pain, bowel urgency, bronchopneumonia, cholestatic jaundice, dizziness, dyspnea, edema, erythema nodosum, facial edema, fecal impaction, gastroenteritis, gastroesophageal reflux disease, hepatic cirrhosis, hepatic failure, hepatic injury, hepatic necrosis, hepatotoxicity, hyperbilirubinemia, hypersensitivity reaction, increased blood pressure, increased heart rate, increased liver enzymes, increased serum AST, interstitial nephritis, jaundice, Kawasaki-like syndrome, lethargy, malaise, myocarditis, pain, pancreatitis, pericarditis, pleural effusion,

pneumonia (with and without eosinophilia), pruritus, renal failure, skin rash, vasculitis

Mechanism of Action Balsalazide is a prodrug, converted by bacterial azoreduction to 5-aminosalicylic acid (mesalamine, active), 4-aminobenzoyl-β-alanine (inert), and their metabolites. 5-aminosalicylic acid may decrease inflammation by blocking the production of arachidonic acid metabolites topically in the colon mucosa.

Pharmacodynamics/Kinetics

Half-life Elimination Primary effect is topical (colonic mucosa); therapeutic effect appears not to be influenced by the systemic half-life of balsalazide (1.9 hours) or its metabolites (5-ASA [9.5 hours], N-Ac-5-ASA [10.4 hours])

Time to Peak Balsalazide: Capsule: 1 to 2 hours; Tablet: 0.5 hours

Pregnancy Considerations Mesalamine (5-aminosalicylic acid) is the active metabolite of balsalazide; mesalamine is known to cross the placenta. Refer to the mesalamine monograph for additional information.

Product Availability Giazo has been discontinued in the United States for more than 1 year.

- ◆ **Balsalazide Disodium** *see* Balsalazide *on page 214*
- ◆ **Balziva** *see* Ethinyl Estradiol and Norethindrone *on page 614*
- ◆ **Banophen [OTC]** *see* DiphenhydrAMINE (Systemic) *on page 502*
- ◆ **Banophen [OTC]** *see* DiphenhydrAMINE (Topical) *on page 503*
- ◆ **Banzel** *see* Rufinamide *on page 1350*
- ◆ **Baraclude** *see* Entecavir *on page 567*

Baricitinib (bar i SYE ti nib)

Brand Names: US Olumiant

Brand Names: Canada Olumiant

Pharmacologic Category Antirheumatic Miscellaneous; Antirheumatic, Disease Modifying; Janus Associated Kinase Inhibitor

Use

Rheumatoid arthritis: Treatment of adult patients with moderately to severely active rheumatoid arthritis who have had an inadequate response to one or more tumor necrosis factor antagonist therapies.

Limitation of use: Use of baricitinib in combination with other JAK inhibitors, biologic DMARDs, or with potent immunosuppressants such as azathioprine and cyclosporine is not recommended.

Local Anesthetic/Vasoconstrictor Precautions Prolongation of the EKG QT interval has been reported as a rare occurrence associated with other Janus kinase inhibitors (see ruxolitinib). Assuming the patient has no history of arrhythmia or not taking any medications which are associated with prolongation of the QT interval, there is nothing to suggest that baricitinib will increase the risk of an arrhythmia.

Effects on Dental Treatment Key adverse event(s) related to dental treatment: Opportunistic infections are possible; rare occurrence of esophageal candidiasis and fungal infections have been reported. Although there are no specific reports, patients may be at risk for candida albicans infections in the oral cavity.

Effects on Bleeding Active therapy with immunosuppressants such as baricitinib may result in myelosuppression; medical consult suggested. Baricitinib labeling reports the occurrence of anemia and lymphocytopenia; rare occurrence of deep vein thrombosis.

Adverse Reactions

>10%:

Infection: Infection (29%; serious infection: 1%)

Respiratory: Upper respiratory tract infection (16%)

1% to 10%:

Gastrointestinal: Nausea (3%)

Hepatic: Increased serum alanine aminotransferase (≥3 x ULN) (2%), increased serum aspartate aminotransferase (≥3 x ULN) (1%)

Infection: Herpes zoster infection (1%)

<1%:

Cardiovascular: Arterial thrombosis

Dermatologic: Acne vulgaris

Hematologic & oncologic: Malignant lymphoma, malignant neoplasm, neutropenia

Frequency not defined:

Cardiovascular: Venous thrombosis (including deep vein thrombosis and pulmonary embolism)

Endocrine & metabolic: Increased HDL cholesterol, increased LDL cholesterol, increased serum cholesterol, increased serum triglycerides

Gastrointestinal: Esophageal candidiasis, gastrointestinal perforation

Genitourinary: Urinary tract infection

Hematologic & oncologic: Anemia, lymphocytopenia

Hepatic: Increased liver enzymes

Infection: Bacterial infection, BK virus, candidiasis, cryptococcosis, cytomegalovirus disease, fungal infection, histoplasmosis, mycobacterium infection, viral infection

Neuromuscular & skeletal: Increased creatine phosphokinase in blood specimen

Renal: Increased serum creatinine

Respiratory: Infection due to an organism in genus *Pneumocystis*

Postmarketing:

Dermatologic: Facial swelling, skin rash, urticaria

Hematologic & oncologic: Skin carcinoma

Mechanism of Action Baricitinib inhibits Janus kinase (JAK) enzymes, which are intracellular enzymes involved in stimulating hematopoiesis and immune cell function through a signaling pathway. In response to extracellular cytokine or growth factor signaling, JAKs activate signal transducers and activators of transcription (STATs), which regulate gene expression and intracellular activity. Inhibition of JAKs prevents the activation of STATs and reduces serum IgG, IgM, IgA, and C-reactive protein.

Pharmacodynamics/Kinetics

Half-life Elimination ~12 hours

Time to Peak ~1 hour

Reproductive Considerations

Recommendations for use of baricitinib to treat rheumatic and musculoskeletal diseases in women who are planning a pregnancy or males who are planning to father a child are not available due to lack of data (ACR [Sammaritano 2020]). Consider discontinuing use 1 month prior to conception (Costanzo 2020).

Pregnancy Considerations

Information related to use of baricitinib in pregnancy is limited (Costanzo 2020).

Recommendations for use of baricitinib in pregnant women with rheumatic and musculoskeletal diseases are not available due to lack of data. Placental transfer may be expected based on molecular weight (ACR [Sammaritano 2020]).

Dental Health Professional Considerations The actions of baricitinib in treating rheumatoid arthritis is due to its ability to inhibit cytokines, including some in the interleukin family, from attaching to receptors that exacerbate arthritic symptoms. The receptors rely on the Janus kinase family of enzymes for receptor activations. These activations occur because the kinases phosphorylate receptor components (definition of kinases is enzymes that phosphorylate substrates). Janus kinases are members of the larger family of tyrosine kinases. Janus kinases, sometimes referred to as JAKs, due to the phosphorylation, recruit signal transducers and activators of transcription (STATs) which regulate intracellular activity. Drugs, such as baricitinib, that inhibit the activity of the Janus kinases block the receptor activations. Unfortunately, one undesired result is suppression of immune responses, leading to increased risk of infections. A US Boxed Warning reminds the clinician of the increased risk of serious infections in patients receiving baricitinib. Infections can often develop in patients receiving concomitant immunosuppressive agents, such as corticosteroids or methotrexate. It is suggested to closely monitor patients for the development of signs/symptoms of infection during and after baricitinib treatment.

◆ **Baridium [OTC] [DSC]** *see* Phenazopyridine *on page 1222*

◆ **Basaglar KwikPen** *see* Insulin Glargine *on page 822*

Basiliximab (ba si LIK si mab)

Brand Names: US Simulect

Brand Names: Canada Simulect

Pharmacologic Category Immunosuppressant Agent; Interleukin-2 Inhibitor; Monoclonal Antibody

Use

Renal transplant (prophylaxis of acute rejection): Prophylaxis of acute organ rejection in renal transplantation in combination with cyclosporine (modified) and corticosteroids

Guideline recommendations: While basiliximab is FDA-approved for prophylaxis of acute organ rejection in renal transplantation in combination with cyclosporine (modified) and corticosteroids, cyclosporine is no longer recommended as the first line agent of choice. The Kidney Disease: Improving Global Outcomes (KDIGO) clinical practice guidelines for care of kidney transplant recipients recommend induction as part of the initial immunosuppressive regimen for all kidney transplants to reduce the risk of acute rejection. KDIGO recommends an interleukin 2 receptor antagonist (eg, basiliximab) as the first line induction agent for acute rejection prophylaxis except in those patients at high immunologic risk. (KDIGO [Kasiske 2009]).

Local Anesthetic/Vasoconstrictor Precautions No information available to require special precautions

Effects on Dental Treatment Key adverse event(s) related to dental treatment: Facial edema and ulcerative stomatitis. Causes gingival hypertrophy (GH) similar to that caused by cyclosporine; early reports indicate that frequency/incidence of basiliximab-induced GH not as high as cyclosporine-induced GH.

Effects on Bleeding No information available to require special precautions

Adverse Reactions Frequency not defined. Administration of basiliximab did not appear to increase the incidence or severity of adverse effects in clinical trials. Adverse events were reported in 96% of both the placebo and basiliximab groups.

>10%:

Cardiovascular: Hypertension, peripheral edema

Central nervous system: Headache, insomnia, pain

Dermatologic: Acne vulgaris

Endocrine & metabolic: Hypercholesterolemia, hyperglycemia, hyperkalemia, hyperuricemia, hypokalemia, hypophosphatemia

Gastrointestinal: Abdominal pain, constipation, diarrhea, dyspepsia, nausea, vomiting

Genitourinary: Urinary tract infection

Hematologic & oncologic: Anemia

Infection: Viral infection

Neuromuscular & skeletal: Tremor

Respiratory: Dyspnea, upper respiratory infection

Miscellaneous: Fever, postoperative wound complication

3% to 10%:

Cardiovascular: Abnormal heart sounds, angina pectoris, atrial fibrillation, cardiac arrhythmia, cardiac failure, chest pain, hypotension, tachycardia, thrombosis

Central nervous system: Agitation, anxiety, depression, dizziness, fatigue, hypoesthesia, malaise, rigors

Dermatologic: Dermal ulcer, dermatological disease, hypertrichosis, pruritus, skin rash

Endocrine & metabolic: Acidosis, albuminuria, anasarca, dehydration, diabetes mellitus, hypercalcemia, hyperlipidemia, hypertriglyceridemia, hypervolemia, hypocalcemia, hypoglycemia, hypomagnesemia, hyponatremia, increased nonprotein nitrogen, increased serum glucocorticoids, weight gain

Gastrointestinal: Enlargement of abdomen, esophagitis, flatulence, gastroenteritis, gastrointestinal hemorrhage, GI moniliasis, gingival hyperplasia, hernia, melena, stomatitis (including ulcerative)

Genitourinary: Bladder dysfunction, dysuria, genital edema (male), hematuria, impotence, oliguria, ureteral disease, urinary frequency, urinary retention

Hematologic & oncologic: Hematoma, hemorrhage, hypoproteinemia, leukopenia, polycythemia, purpura, thrombocytopenia

Infection: Cytomegalovirus disease, herpes virus infection (simplex and zoster), infection, sepsis

Neuromuscular & skeletal: Arthralgia, arthropathy, back pain, bone fracture, leg pain, muscle cramps, myalgia, neuropathy, paresthesia, weakness

Ophthalmic: Cataract, conjunctivitis, visual disturbance

Renal: Renal insufficiency, renal tubular necrosis

Respiratory: Bronchitis, bronchospasm, cough, pharyngitis, pneumonia, pulmonary edema, rhinitis, sinusitis

Miscellaneous: Accidental injury, cyst

<1%, postmarketing, and/or case reports: Anaphylaxis, capillary leak syndrome, cytokine release syndrome, diabetes (new onset), hypersensitivity reaction (includes bronchospasm, cardiac failure, dyspnea, hypotension, pruritus, pulmonary edema, respiratory failure, skin rash, sneezing, tachycardia, urticaria), impaired glucose tolerance, increase in fasting plasma glucose, lymphoproliferative disorder

Mechanism of Action Basiliximab is a chimeric (murine/human) immunosuppressant monoclonal antibody which blocks the alpha-chain of the interleukin-2 (IL-2) receptor complex; this receptor is expressed on activated T lymphocytes and is a critical pathway for activating cell-mediated allograft rejection

Pharmacodynamics/Kinetics

Duration of Action Mean: 36 ± 14 days (determined by IL-2R alpha saturation in patients also on cyclosporine and corticosteroids)

Half-life Elimination Children 1 to 11 years: 9.5 ± 4.5 days; Adolescents 12 to 16 years: 9.1 ± 3.9 days; Adults: Mean: 7.2 ± 3.2 days

Reproductive Considerations

Women of childbearing potential should use effective contraceptive measures before beginning treatment, during, and for 4 months after completion of basiliximab treatment.

Pregnancy Considerations

Basiliximab is a monoclonal IgG antibody which targets IL-2 receptors. IgG is known to cross the placenta; IL-2 receptors play an important role in the development of the immune system.

The Transplant Pregnancy Registry International (TPR) is a registry that follows pregnancies that occur in maternal transplant recipients or those fathered by male transplant recipients. The TPR encourages reporting of pregnancies following solid organ transplant by contacting them at 1-877-955-6877 or https://www.transplantpregnancyregistry.org.

- **Bavencio** *see* Avelumab *on page 195*
- **Baxdela** *see* Delafloxacin *on page 451*
- **BAY 43-9006** *see* SORAfenib *on page 1383*
- **BAY 59-7939** *see* Rivaroxaban *on page 1340*
- **BAY 73-4506** *see* Regorafenib *on page 1314*
- **Bayer Aspirin [OTC]** *see* Aspirin *on page 177*
- **Bayer Aspirin EC Low Dose [OTC]** *see* Aspirin *on page 177*
- **Bayer Aspirin Extra Strength [OTC]** *see* Aspirin *on page 177*
- **Bayer Aspirin Regimen Adult Low Strength [OTC]** *see* Aspirin *on page 177*
- **Bayer Aspirin Regimen Children's [OTC]** *see* Aspirin *on page 177*
- **Bayer Aspirin Regimen Regular Strength [OTC]** *see* Aspirin *on page 177*
- **Bayer Genuine Aspirin [OTC]** *see* Aspirin *on page 177*
- **Bayer Plus Extra Strength [OTC]** *see* Aspirin *on page 177*
- **Bayer Women's Low Dose Aspirin [OTC]** *see* Aspirin *on page 177*
- **Baza Antifungal [OTC] [DSC]** *see* Miconazole (Topical) *on page 1019*
- **Bazedoxifene and Estrogens (Conjugated/Equine)** *see* Estrogens (Conjugated/Equine) and Bazedoxifene *on page 603*
- **Bazedoxifene and Oestrogens** *see* Estrogens (Conjugated/Equine) and Bazedoxifene *on page 603*
- **BC-3781** *see* Lefamulin *on page 881*
- **B-Caro-T [OTC]** *see* Beta-Carotene *on page 233*
- **BCL-2 Inhibitor GDC-0199** *see* Venetoclax *on page 1538*
- **B Complex Combinations** *see* Vitamin B Complex Combinations *on page 1549*
- **BCX-1812** *see* Peramivir *on page 1216*
- **BCX 2600** *see* Stiripentol *on page 1388*

Becaplermin (be KAP ler min)

Brand Names: US Regranex

Pharmacologic Category Growth Factor, Platelet-Derived; Topical Skin Product

Use Diabetic ulcers: Adjunctive treatment of lower extremity diabetic neuropathic ulcers that extend into the subcutaneous tissue or beyond and have an adequate blood supply.

Limitations of use: Efficacy has not been established for pressure and venous stasis ulcers; has not been evaluated for diabetic neuropathic ulcers that do not extend through the dermis into subcutaneous tissue (stage I or II, International Association of Enterostomal Therapy [IAET] staging classification) or ischemic diabetic ulcers.

Local Anesthetic/Vasoconstrictor Precautions No information available to require special precautions

Effects on Dental Treatment No significant effects or complications reported

Effects on Bleeding No information available to require special precautions

Adverse Reactions

1% to 10%: Dermatologic: Erythematous rash (2%)

<1%, postmarketing, and/or case reports: Connective tissue disorder (excessive granulation tissue), dermal ulcer (with or without tunneling), erythema (with purulent discharge), local pain

Mechanism of Action Recombinant B-isoform homodimer of human platelet-derived growth factor (rPDGF-BB) which enhances formation of new granulation tissue, induces fibroblast proliferation and differentiation to promote wound healing; also promotes angiogenesis.

Pregnancy Considerations Animal reproduction studies have not been conducted.

Beclomethasone (Nasal) (be kloe METH a sone)

Brand Names: US Beconase AQ; Qnasl; Qnasl Childrens

Brand Names: Canada APO-Beclomethasone AQ; MYLAN-Beclo AQ; Rivanase AQ

Pharmacologic Category Corticosteroid, Nasal

Use

Nasal polyps, postsurgical prophylaxis (Beconase AQ only): Prevention of recurrence of nasal polyps following surgical removal in adults and children 6 years and older.

Rhinitis, allergic:

Beconase AQ: Relief of symptoms of seasonal or perennial allergic rhinitis in adults and children 6 years and older.

Qnasl: Treatment of the nasal symptoms associated with seasonal or perennial allergic rhinitis in adults and children 4 years and older.

Rhinitis, nonallergic (vasomotor): Beconase AQ: Relief of symptoms of nonallergic (vasomotor) rhinitis in adults and children 6 years and older.

Local Anesthetic/Vasoconstrictor Precautions No information available to require special precautions

Effects on Dental Treatment Key adverse event(s) related to dental treatment: Occurrence of oral, nasal, or pharyngeal candidiasis; rare occurrence of unpleasant taste, loss of taste

Effects on Bleeding Frequent occurrence of nose bleed

Adverse Reactions Frequency not always defined.

>10%: Respiratory: Nasopharyngitis (≤24%; children: 2%), epistaxis (2% to 11%)

1% to 10%:

Central nervous system: Dizziness (≤5%), headache (≤5%)

Endocrine & metabolic: Adrenal suppression (at high doses or in susceptible individuals), hypercorticoidism (at high doses or in susceptible individuals)

Gastrointestinal: Nausea (≤5%), oral candidiasis (rare; more likely with aqueous solution)

Immunologic: Immunosuppression

Neuromuscular & skeletal: Decreased linear skeletal growth rate

Ophthalmic: Intraocular pressure increased (5%), lacrimation (≤3%)

Respiratory: Sneezing (4%), upper respiratory tract infection (children: 3%), nasal congestion (≤3%), rhinorrhea (≤3%), nasal mucosa irritation (erosion) (≤1%), nasal candidiasis (rare; more likely with aqueous solution), pharyngeal candidiasis (rare; more likely with aqueous solution)

Miscellaneous: Fever (children: 3%), wound healing impairment

<1%, postmarketing, and/or case reports: Ageusia, altered sense of smell, anaphylactoid reaction, anaphylaxis, angioedema, anosmia, blurred vision, bronchospasm, burning sensation, cataract, chorioretinitis, dry nose, glaucoma, hypersensitivity reaction, nasal mucosa ulcer, nasal septum perforation, skin rash, unpleasant taste, urticaria, wheezing

Mechanism of Action Controls the rate of protein synthesis; depresses the migration of polymorphonuclear leukocytes, fibroblasts; reverses capillary permeability and lysosomal stabilization at the cellular level to prevent or control inflammation

Pharmacodynamics/Kinetics

Onset of Action Within a few days up to 2 weeks

Half-life Elimination BDP: 0.5 hours; 17-BMP: 2.7 hours

Pregnancy Considerations

Intranasal corticosteroids may be acceptable for the treatment of rhinitis during pregnancy when used at recommended doses (Lal 2016).

Pregnant females adequately controlled on beclomethasone may continue therapy; if initiating treatment during pregnancy, use of an agent with more data in pregnant females and less systemic absorption may be preferred (Alhussien 2018; Namazy 2016).

Beclomethasone (Oral Inhalation)

(be kloe METH a sone)

Related Information

Respiratory Diseases *on page 1680*

Brand Names: US Qvar RediHaler; Qvar [DSC]

Brand Names: Canada Qvar

Generic Availability (US) No

Pharmacologic Category Corticosteroid, Inhalant (Oral)

Use

Asthma: Maintenance and prophylactic treatment of asthma in patients ≥5 years of age (QVAR) or ≥4 years of age (QVAR RediHaler).

Limitations of use: Not for relief of acute bronchospasm.

Local Anesthetic/Vasoconstrictor Precautions No information available to require special precautions

Effects on Dental Treatment Key adverse event(s) related to dental treatment: Oral candidiasis, xerostomia (normal salivary flow resumes upon discontinuation), nasal dryness, and dry throat. Localized infections with *Candida albicans* or *Aspergillus niger* occur frequently in the mouth and pharynx with repetitive use of an oral inhaler; may require treatment with appropriate antifungal therapy or discontinuance of inhaler use. Occurrence of oropharyngeal pain; rare occurrence of altered sense of taste.

Effects on Bleeding No information available to require special precautions

Adverse Reactions

>10%:

Central nervous system: Headache (1% to 25%)

Respiratory: Pharyngitis (3% to 27%)

1% to 10%:

Central nervous system: Pain (1% to 5%), voice disorder (4%)

Gastrointestinal: Oral candidiasis (1% to 8%), vomiting (children: 3%), diarrhea (children: 1% to 3%), nausea (1% to 3%)

Genitourinary: Dysmenorrhea (1% to 3%), viral gastroenteritis (children: 1% to 3%)

Infection: Influenza (children: 1% to 3%)

Neuromuscular & skeletal: Back pain (1% to 4%), myalgia (children: 1% to 3%)

Otic: Otitis (children: 1% to 3%)

Respiratory: Nasopharyngitis (2% to 9%), upper respiratory tract infection (3% to 8%), cough (1% to 7%), viral upper respiratory tract infection (2% to 4%), oropharyngeal pain (1% to 4%), sinusitis (3%), allergic rhinitis (≤3%)

Miscellaneous: Fever (children: 3%)

<1%, postmarketing, and/or case reports: Aggressive behavior, blurred vision, depression, dysgeusia (Tuccori 2011), psychomotor agitation, retinopathy, sleep disorder, suicidal ideation

Dosing

Adult & Geriatric Note: Titrate to the lowest effective dose once asthma is controlled.

Asthma: Oral inhalation: **Note:** To decrease the severity or duration of an asthma exacerbation, may consider temporarily quadrupling the dose (early in the course of illness) in patients with mild to moderate asthma with a mild flare in symptoms. Reserve this approach for patients with no prior history of life-threatening asthma exacerbations, and in those with good self-management skills; return to baseline dose after normalization of symptoms or at a maximum of 14 days of the quadrupled dose (GINA 2020; McKeever 2018).

US labeling: Metered-dose inhaler:

QVAR/QVAR RediHaler: **Note:** Dosing based on previous asthma therapy and asthma severity. May increase dose after 2 weeks of therapy in patients who are not adequately controlled.

Patients not currently on inhaled corticosteroids: Initial: 40 to 80 mcg twice daily; maximum dose: 320 mcg twice daily

Patients previously on inhaled corticosteroids: Initial: 40 to 320 mcg twice daily; maximum dose: 320 mcg twice daily

Canadian labeling: Metered-dose inhaler:

Mild asthma: 50 to 100 mcg twice daily; maximum dose: 100 mcg twice daily

Moderate asthma: 100 to 250 mcg twice daily; maximum dose: 250 mcg twice daily

Severe asthma: 300 to 400 mcg twice daily; maximum dose: 400 mcg twice daily

Asthma Guidelines:

Global Initiative for Asthma and National Asthma Education and Prevention Program guidelines (GINA 2020; NAEPP 2007): Metered-dose inhaler: **Note:** Administer in 1 to 4 inhalations/day depending on strength of inhaler.

Low-dose therapy: 80 to 200 mcg/day

Medium-dose therapy: >200 to 400 mcg/day

High-dose therapy: >400 mcg/day

Chronic obstructive pulmonary disease (stable) (off-label use): Oral inhalation: 50 to 400 mcg daily as a component of dual or triple combination therapy (GOLD 2014; GOLD 2019).

Renal Impairment: Adult There are no dosage adjustments provided in the manufacturer's labeling (has not been studied).

Hepatic Impairment: Adult There are no dosage adjustments provided in the manufacturer's labeling (has not been studied).

Pediatric Note: Doses should be titrated to the lowest effective dose once asthma is controlled.

Asthma:

Maintenance therapy:

Manufacturer's labeling: Qvar RediHaler: Oral inhalation: **Note:** Twice daily doses should be administered approximately 12 hours apart.

Children 4 to 11 years: Initial: 40 mcg twice daily; maximum dose: 80 mcg twice daily.

Children ≥12 years and Adolescents:

No previous inhaled corticosteroids: Initial: 40 to 80 mcg twice daily; maximum dose: 320 mcg twice daily.

Previous inhaled corticosteroid use: Initial: 40 to 160 mcg twice daily; maximum dose: 320 mcg twice daily.

Note: Therapeutic ratio between Qvar Redihaler and other beclomethasone inhalers (eg, CFC formulations; however, none are currently available in US) has not been established.

National Asthma Education and Prevention Program Guidelines (NAEPP 2007): HFA formulation (Qvar RediHaler): Oral inhalation:

Children 5 to 11 years: Administer in divided doses:

"Low" dose: 80 to 160 mcg/day (40 mcg/puff: 2 to 4 puffs/day or 80 mcg/puff: 1 to 2 puffs/day).

"Medium" dose: >160 to 320 mcg/day (40 mcg/puff: 4 to 8 puffs/day or 80 mcg/puff: 2 to 4 puffs/day).

"High" dose: >320 mcg/day (40 mcg/puff: >8 puffs/day or 80 mcg/puff: >4 puff/day).

Children ≥12 years and Adolescents:

"Low" dose: 80 to 240 mcg/day (40 mcg/puff: 2 to 6 puffs/day or 80 mcg/puff: 1 to 3 puffs/day).

"Medium" dose: >240 to 480 mcg/day (40 mcg/puff: 6 to 12 puffs/day or 80 mcg/puff: 3 to 6 puffs/day).

"High" dose: >480 mcg/day (40 mcg/puff: >12 puffs/day or 80 mcg/puff: 6 puffs/day).

Mild flare, exacerbation: Limited data available:

Children ≥12 years and Adolescents with mild to moderate asthma, no prior history of life-threatening asthma exacerbations, and with good self-management skills:

It is recommended to temporarily quadruple the inhaled corticosteroid dose early in the course of a mild flare to decrease the severity of an asthma exacerbation. After symptoms stabilize or after a maximum of 14 days of quadrupled dose, whichever occurs first, patients should be returned to their baseline dose (GINA 2019). Quadrupling the inhaled corticosteroid dose has been shown to decrease the severity of an asthma exacerbation in select patients. In a randomized trial of adolescents ≥16 years and adults (n=1,871), temporarily quadrupling the inhaled corticosteroid dose when asthma control began to deteriorate resulted in fewer severe asthma exacerbations (ie, less treatment with systemic glucocorticoids or unscheduled appointments for asthma) compared to patients who maintained their inhaled corticosteroid dose (McKeever 2018). No data for quadrupling the dose in patients <16 years of age has been published. Quintupling the dose of inhaled corticosteroids (fluticasone) in children 5 to 11 years of age was not shown to reduce the rate of severe exacerbations and may have been associated adverse effects (decreased linear growth, particularly in patients <8 years of age) (GINA 2019; Jackson 2018).

Conversion from oral systemic corticosteroid to orally-inhaled corticosteroid: Initiation of oral inhalation therapy in patients on oral corticosteroids (OCS) should include a gradual dose reduction of OCS. If adrenal insufficiency occurs, temporarily increase the OCS dose and follow with a more gradual withdrawal. **Note:** When transitioning from systemic to inhaled corticosteroids, supplemental systemic corticosteroid therapy may be necessary during periods of stress or during severe asthma attacks.

Canadian labeling: Maintenance therapy: Metered-dose inhaler: Oral inhalation:

Children 5 to 11 years: Initial: 50 mcg twice daily; maximum dose: 100 mcg twice daily.

Children ≥12 years of age and Adolescents:

Mild asthma: 50 to 100 mcg twice daily; maximum dose: 100 mcg twice daily.

Moderate asthma: 100 to 250 mcg twice daily; maximum dose: 250 mcg twice daily.

Severe asthma: 300 to 400 mcg twice daily; maximum dose: 400 mcg twice daily.

Renal Impairment: Pediatric There are no dosage adjustments provided in the manufacturer's labeling.

Hepatic Impairment: Pediatric There are no dosage adjustments provided in the manufacturer's labeling.

Mechanism of Action Controls the rate of protein synthesis; depresses the migration of polymorphonuclear leukocytes, fibroblasts; reverses capillary permeability and lysosomal stabilization at the cellular level to prevent or control inflammation

Contraindications

Hypersensitivity to beclomethasone or any component of the formulation; status asthmaticus, or other acute asthma episodes requiring intensive measures

Documentation of allergenic cross-reactivity for corticosteroids is limited. However, because of similarities in chemical structure and/or pharmacologic actions, the possibility of cross-sensitivity cannot be ruled out with certainty.

Canadian labeling: Additional contraindications (not in US labeling): Moderate to severe bronchiectasis requiring intensive measures; untreated fungal, bacterial, or tubercular infections of the respiratory tract

Warnings/Precautions May cause hypercortisolism or suppression of hypothalamic-pituitary-adrenal (HPA) axis, particularly in younger children or in patients receiving high doses for prolonged periods. HPA axis suppression may lead to adrenal crisis. Withdrawal and discontinuation of a corticosteroid should be done slowly and carefully. Particular care is required when patients are transferred from systemic corticosteroids to inhaled products due to possible adrenal insufficiency or withdrawal from steroids, including an increase in allergic symptoms. Adult patients receiving ≥20 mg per day of prednisone (or equivalent) may be most susceptible. Fatalities have occurred due to adrenal insufficiency in asthmatic patients during and after transfer from systemic corticosteroids to aerosol steroids; aerosol steroids do **not** provide the systemic steroid needed to treat patients having trauma, surgery, or infections (particularly gastroenteritis), or other conditions with severe electrolyte loss. Select surgical patients on long-term, high-dose, inhaled corticosteroid should be given stress doses of hydrocortisone intravenously during the surgical period and the dose reduced rapidly within 24 hours after surgery (NAEPP 2007).

Paradoxical bronchospasm that may be life-threatening may occur with use of inhaled bronchodilating agents; reaction should be distinguished from inadequate response. If paradoxical bronchospasm occurs, discontinue beclomethasone and institute alternative therapy. Supplemental steroids (oral or parenteral) may be needed during stress or severe asthma attacks. Use is contraindicated in status asthmaticus or during other acute asthma episodes requiring intensive measures. Hypersensitivity reactions (eg, angioedema, bronchospasm, rash, and urticaria) may occur; discontinue use if reaction occurs. Prolonged use of corticosteroids may increase the incidence of secondary infection, mask acute infection (including fungal infections), prolong or exacerbate viral infections, or limit response to vaccines. Avoid use, if possible, in patients with ocular herpes, active or quiescent respiratory or untreated viral, fungal, parasitic or bacterial systemic infections. Exposure to chickenpox and measles should be avoided; if the patient is exposed, prophylaxis with varicella zoster immune globulin or pooled intramuscular immunoglobulin, respectively, may be indicated; if chickenpox develops, treatment with antiviral agents may be considered. Local oropharyngeal *Candida albicans* infections have been reported; if this occurs, treat appropriately while continuing therapy. Patients should be instructed to rinse mouth with water without swallowing after each use.

Use with caution in patients with major risk factors for decreased bone mineral count. Use with caution in patients with cataracts and/or glaucoma; blurred vision, increased intraocular pressure, glaucoma, and cataracts have occurred with prolonged use. Consider routine eye exams in chronic users. Because of the risk of adverse effects, systemic corticosteroids should be used cautiously in elderly patients in the smallest possible effective dose for the shortest duration.

Orally inhaled corticosteroids may cause a reduction in growth velocity in pediatric patients (~1 centimeter per year [range: 0.3 to 1.8 cm per year] and related to dose and duration of exposure). To minimize the systemic effects of orally inhaled corticosteroids, each patient should be titrated to the lowest effective dose. Growth should be routinely monitored in pediatric patients. A gradual tapering of dose may be required prior to discontinuing therapy; there have been reports of systemic corticosteroid withdrawal symptoms (eg, joint/muscle pain, lassitude, depression) when withdrawing oral inhalation therapy. When transferring to oral inhalation therapy from systemic corticosteroid therapy, previously suppressed allergic conditions (rhinitis, conjunctivitis, eczema, arthritis, and eosinophilic conditions) may be unmasked. Withdraw systemic corticosteroid therapy by gradually tapering the dose. Monitor lung function, beta-agonist use, asthma symptoms, and for signs and symptoms of adrenal insufficiency (eg, fatigue, lassitude, weakness, nausea/vomiting, hypotension) during withdrawal.

Potentially significant drug-drug interactions may exist, requiring dose or frequency adjustment, additional monitoring, and/or selection of alternative therapy.

Warnings: Additional Pediatric Considerations Reduction in growth velocity may occur when corticosteroids are administered to pediatric patients, even at recommended doses via inhaled route; reduction in growth velocity is related to dose and duration of exposure; monitor growth. With beclomethasone-HFA (Qvar), the mean reduction in growth velocity was 0.5 cm/year less than that with the previous beclomethasone CFC inhaler formulation. Use of Qvar with a spacer device is not recommended in children <5 years of age due to the decreased amount of medication that is delivered with increasing wait times; patients should be instructed to inhale immediately if using a spacer device.

Although recommended in children ≥12 years and adolescents, using higher doses (quintupled) in children <12 years of age has not shown efficacy and may be associated with a higher risk of adverse effects. A study in children 5 to 11 years of age with mild to moderate persistent asthma evaluated quintupling the dose of the inhaled corticosteroid (fluticasone) following the early signs of decreased asthma control; results showed that quintupled fluticasone dosages did not reduce the rate of severe exacerbations and may have been associated adverse effects (decreased linear growth, particularly in patients <8 years of age) (Jackson 2018).

Drug Interactions

Metabolism/Transport Effects None known.

Avoid Concomitant Use

Avoid concomitant use of Beclomethasone (Oral Inhalation) with any of the following: Aldesleukin; BCG (Intravesical); Cladribine; Desmopressin; Loxapine; Natalizumab; Pimecrolimus; Tacrolimus (Topical)

Increased Effect/Toxicity

Beclomethasone (Oral Inhalation) may increase the levels/effects of: Amphotericin B; Baricitinib; Deferasirox; Desmopressin; Fingolimod; Leflunomide; Loop Diuretics; Loxapine; Natalizumab; Ozanimod; Ritodrine; Siponimod; Thiazide and Thiazide-Like Diuretics; Tofacitinib

The levels/effects of Beclomethasone (Oral Inhalation) may be increased by: Cladribine; Denosumab; Inebilizumab; Ocrelizumab; Pimecrolimus; Tacrolimus (Topical); Trastuzumab

Decreased Effect

Beclomethasone (Oral Inhalation) may decrease the levels/effects of: Aldesleukin; BCG (Intravesical); Coccidioides immitis Skin Test; Corticorelin; Cosyntropin; Hyaluronidase; Nivolumab; Pidotimod; Sipuleucel-T; Smallpox and Monkeypox Vaccine (Live); Tertomotide; Vaccines (Inactivated)

The levels/effects of Beclomethasone (Oral Inhalation) may be decreased by: Echinacea; Tobacco (Smoked)

Pharmacodynamics/Kinetics

Onset of Action Within 1 to 2 days in some patients; usually within 1 to 2 weeks; Maximum effect: 3 to 4 weeks

Half-life Elimination

QVAR: BDP: 0.5 hours; 17-BMP: 2.8 hours

RediHaler:; BDP: 2 minutes; 17-BMP: 4 hours

Time to Peak

Plasma: Inhalation:

QVAR: BDP: 0.5 hours; 17-BMP: 0.7 hours

RediHaler: BDP: 2 minutes; 17-BMP: 10 minutes

Pregnancy Considerations Maternal use of inhaled corticosteroids (ICS) in usual doses is not associated with an increased risk of fetal malformations; a small risk of malformations was observed in one study following maternal doses of beclomethasone >1,000 mcg/day. Uncontrolled asthma is associated with adverse events on pregnancy (increased risk of perinatal mortality, preeclampsia, preterm birth, low-birth-weight infants, cesarean delivery, and the development of gestational diabetes). Poorly controlled asthma or asthma exacerbations may have a greater fetal/maternal risk than what is associated with appropriately used asthma medications. Maternal treatment improves pregnancy outcomes by reducing the risk of some adverse events (eg, preterm birth and gestational diabetes) (ERS/TSANZ [Middleton 2020]; GINA 2020).

Inhaled corticosteroids are recommended for the treatment of asthma during pregnancy (GINA 2020). Beclomethasone is one of the preferred agents. The lowest dose that maintains asthma control should be used. Maternal asthma symptoms should be monitored monthly during pregnancy (ERS/TSANZ [Middleton 2020])

Data collection to monitor pregnancy and infant outcomes associated with asthma and the medications used to treat asthma in pregnancy is ongoing. Health care providers are encouraged to enroll exposed pregnant females in the MotherToBaby Pregnancy Studies conducted by the Organization of Teratology Information Specialists (OTIS) (877-311-8972 or https://mothertobaby.org). Patients may also enroll themselves.

Breastfeeding Considerations

It is not known if beclomethasone is present in breast milk following oral inhalation; however, other corticosteroids are present in breast milk.

According to the manufacturer, the decision to continue or discontinue breastfeeding during therapy should consider the risk of infant exposure, the benefits of breastfeeding to the infant, and benefits of treatment to the mother. However, females with asthma should be encouraged to breastfeed (GINA 2020). Beclomethasone oral inhalation is considered compatible with breastfeeding (ERS/TSANZ [Middleton 2020]).

Dosage Forms Considerations Qvar 8.7 g and Qvar Redihaler 10.6 g canisters contain 120 inhalations.

Dosage Forms: US

Aerosol Breath Activated, Inhalation:

Qvar RediHaler: 40 mcg/actuation (10.6 g); 80 mcg/actuation (10.6 g)

Dosage Forms: Canada

Aerosol Solution, Inhalation:

Qvar: 50 mcg/actuation (6.5 g, 12.4 g); 100 mcg/actuation (6.5 g, 12.4 g)

◆ **Beclomethasone Dipropionate** *see* Beclomethasone (Nasal) *on page 217*

◆ **Beconase AQ** *see* Beclomethasone (Nasal) *on page 217*

◆ **Behenyl Alcohol** *see* Docosanol *on page 508*

◆ **Bekyree** *see* Ethinyl Estradiol and Desogestrel *on page 609*

Belatacept (bel AT a sept)

Brand Names: US Nulojix

Pharmacologic Category Selective T-Cell Costimulation Blocker

Use

Kidney transplant (de novo use): Prophylaxis of organ rejection concomitantly with basiliximab induction, mycophenolate, and corticosteroids in adult Epstein-Barr virus (EBV) seropositive kidney transplant recipients

Limitations of use: Use only in EBV seropositive patients; use for prophylaxis of organ rejection in transplanted organs other than the kidney has not been established.

Local Anesthetic/Vasoconstrictor Precautions

No information available to require special precautions

Effects on Dental Treatment Key adverse event(s) related to dental treatment: Stomatitis has been reported

Effects on Bleeding No information available to require special precautions

Adverse Reactions Incidences reported as part of a combination therapy regimen.

>10%:

Cardiovascular: Peripheral edema (34%), hypertension (32%), hypotension (18%)

Central nervous system: Headache (21%), insomnia (15%)

Endocrine & metabolic: Hypokalemia (21%), hyperkalemia (20%), hypophosphatemia (19%), lipid metabolism disorder (19%), hyperglycemia (16%), hypocalcemia (13%), hypercholesterolemia (11%)

Gastrointestinal: Diarrhea (39%), constipation (33%), nausea (24%), vomiting (22%), abdominal pain (19%)

Genitourinary: Urinary tract infection (37%), dysuria (11%)

Hematologic & oncologic: Anemia (45%), leukopenia (20%)

Infection: Infection (72% to 82%, serious infection 24% to 36%), fungal infection (18%), herpes virus infection (7% to 14%), cytomegalovirus disease (11% to 13%), influenza (11%)

Neuromuscular & skeletal: Arthralgia (17%), back pain (13%)

Renal: Proteinuria (16%; up to 33% 2+ proteinuria at 1 month post-transplant), graft complications (renal: 25%), hematuria (16%), increased serum creatinine (15%)

Respiratory: Cough (24%), upper respiratory tract infection (15%), nasopharyngitis (13%), dyspnea (12%)

Miscellaneous: Fever (28%)

1% to 10%:

Cardiovascular: Arteriovenous fistula site complication (thrombosis, <10%), atrial fibrillation (<10%)

Central nervous system: Anxiety (10%), Guillain-Barré syndrome (<10%), dizziness (9%)

Dermatologic: Alopecia (<10%), hyperhidrosis (<10%), acne vulgaris (8%)

Endocrine & metabolic: Diabetes mellitus (new onset, 5% to 8%), hypomagnesemia (7%), hyperuricemia (5%)
Gastrointestinal: Stomatitis (<10%; including aphthous stomatitis), upper abdominal pain (9%)
Genitourinary: Urinary incontinence (<10%)
Hematologic & oncologic: Hematoma (<10%), lymphocele (<10%), neutropenia (<10%), malignant neoplasm (4%), malignant neoplasm of skin (nonmelanoma, 2%)
Immunologic: Antibody development (2%)
Infection: Polyoma virus infection (3% to 4%)
Neuromuscular & skeletal: Musculoskeletal pain (<10%), tremor (8%)
Renal: Acute renal failure (<10%), hydronephrosis (<10%), kidney transplant dysfunction (chronic allograft nephropathy: <10%), renal disease (renal artery stenosis: <10%), renal insufficiency (<10%), renal tubular necrosis (9%)
Respiratory: Bronchitis (10%), tuberculosis (1% to 2%)
Miscellaneous: Infusion related reaction (5%)

<1%, postmarketing, and/or case reports: Anaphylaxis, aspergillosis (cerebral; higher dosing regimen), encephalitis (Chagas, West Nile; higher dosing regimen), graft rejection (renal), lymphoproliferative disorder (post transplant; incidence is 9-fold higher in non-EBV seropositive patients), meningitis (cryptococcal), nephropathy (polyoma virus-associated mainly BK), progressive multifocal leukoencephalopathy (higher dosing regimen)

Mechanism of Action Fusion protein which acts as a selective T-cell (lymphocyte) costimulation blocker by binding to CD80 and CD86 receptors on antigen presenting cells (APC), blocking the required CD28 mediated interaction between APCs and T cells needed to activate T lymphocytes. T-cell stimulation results in cytokine production and proliferation, mediators in immunologic rejection associated with kidney transplantation.

Pharmacodynamics/Kinetics

Half-life Elimination ~10 days (healthy patients and kidney transplant patients)

Pregnancy Considerations

Adverse events have been observed in animal reproduction studies.

The Transplant Pregnancy Registry International (TPR) is a registry that follows pregnancies that occur in maternal transplant recipients or those fathered by male transplant recipients. The TPR encourages reporting of pregnancies following solid organ transplant by contacting them at 1-877-955-6877 or www.transplantpregnancyregistry.org.

Prescribing and Access Restrictions

Patients (new and existing) must be registered in the Nulojix Distribution Program. Additional information is available by calling (855) 511-6180 or at http://www.-nulojixhcp.bmscustomerconnect.com/index.

◆ **Belbuca** *see* Buprenorphine *on page 260*

◆ **Beleodaq** *see* Belinostat *on page 223*

Belimumab (be LIM yoo mab)

Brand Names: US Benlysta
Brand Names: Canada Benlysta
Pharmacologic Category Monoclonal Antibody

Use

Systemic lupus erythematosus: Treatment of adults and children ≥5 years of age with active, autoantibody-positive systemic lupus erythematosus (SLE) who are receiving standard therapy.

Limitations of use: Use is not recommended in patients with severe active lupus nephritis, severe active CNS lupus, or in combination with other biologics, including B-cell targeted therapies or IV cyclophosphamide.

Local Anesthetic/Vasoconstrictor Precautions No information available to require special precautions

Effects on Dental Treatment No significant effects or complications reported

Effects on Bleeding No information available to require special precautions

Adverse Reactions

>10%:
Gastrointestinal: Diarrhea (12%), nausea (15%)
Hypersensitivity: Hypersensitivity reaction (13%)
Infection: Infection (IV: 71%, SubQ: 55%)
Nervous system: Psychiatric disturbance (16%; serious: 1%)
Miscellaneous: Infusion related reaction (17%)

1% to 10%:
Dermatologic: Dermatological reaction (≥3%)
Gastrointestinal: Viral gastroenteritis (3%)
Genitourinary: Cystitis (4%), urinary tract infection (>5%)
Hematologic & oncologic: Leukopenia (4%)
Immunologic: Antibody development (≤5%)
Infection: Influenza (>5%), serious infection (6%)
Local: Injection site reaction (6%)
Nervous system: Anxiety (4%), depression (5% to 6%), headache (≥3%), insomnia (6% to 7%), migraine (5%), suicidal behavior (≤1%), suicidal ideation (≤1%)
Neuromuscular & skeletal: Limb pain (6%)
Respiratory: Bronchitis (9%), nasopharyngitis (9%), pharyngitis (5%), sinusitis (>5%), upper respiratory tract infection (>5%)
Miscellaneous: Fever (10%)

Frequency not defined:
Dermatologic: Cellulitis
Respiratory: Pneumonia

<1%:
Cardiovascular: Bradycardia
Neuromuscular & skeletal: Myalgia

Postmarketing:
Hypersensitivity: Anaphylaxis, angioedema
Nervous system: Progressive multifocal leukoencephalopathy

Mechanism of Action Belimumab is an IgG1-lambda monoclonal antibody that prevents the survival of B lymphocytes by blocking the binding of soluble human B lymphocyte stimulator protein (BLyS) to receptors on B lymphocytes. This reduces the activity of B-cell mediated immunity and the autoimmune response.

Pharmacodynamics/Kinetics

Onset of Action B cells: 8 weeks; Clinical improvement (SLE Responder Index and flare reduction): 16 weeks (Navarra 2011)

Half-life Elimination Terminal: IV: 19.4 days; SubQ: 18.3 days

Time to Peak SubQ: 2.6 days

Reproductive Considerations

Females of reproductive potential should use effective contraception during therapy and for at least 4 months after the last belimumab dose.

Based on limited information, use of belimumab may be continued through conception in women with rheumatic and musculoskeletal diseases who are planning a pregnancy and not able to use alternative therapies; use should be discontinued once pregnancy is confirmed. Conception should be planned during a period of quiescent/low disease activity (ACR [Sammaritano 2020]).

Recommendations for use of belimumab to treat rheumatic and musculoskeletal diseases in males who are planning to father a child are not available due to limited data (ACR [Sammaritano 2020]).

Pregnancy Considerations

Belimumab is a humanized monoclonal antibody (IgG_1). Potential placental transfer of human IgG is dependent upon the IgG subclass and gestational age, generally increasing as pregnancy progresses. The lowest exposure would be expected during the period of organogenesis (Palmeira 2012; Pentsuk 2009).

Information related to use of belimumab in pregnancy is limited (Bitter 2018; Danve 2014; Emmi 2016; Kumthekar 2017). If exposure occurs during pregnancy, the manufacturer recommends monitoring the newborn for B-cell reduction and other immune dysfunction.

Until additional information is available, belimumab is not currently recommended for the treatment of rheumatic and musculoskeletal diseases during pregnancy. Belimumab should be discontinued once pregnancy is confirmed (ACR [Sammaritano 2020]).

Health care providers are encouraged to enroll women exposed to belimumab during pregnancy in a pregnancy registry (877-681-6296); patients may also enroll themselves.

Belinostat (be LIN oh stat)

Brand Names: US Beleodaq

Pharmacologic Category Antineoplastic Agent, Histone Deacetylase (HDAC) Inhibitor

Use Peripheral T-cell lymphoma, relapsed or refractory: Treatment of relapsed or refractory peripheral T-cell lymphoma (PTCL).

Local Anesthetic/Vasoconstrictor Precautions Belinostat is one of the drugs confirmed to prolong the QT interval and is accepted as having a risk of causing torsade de pointes. The risk of drug-induced torsade de pointes is extremely low when a single QT interval prolonging drug is prescribed. In terms of epinephrine, it is not known what effect vasoconstrictors in the local anesthetic regimen will have in patients with a known history of congenital prolonged QT interval or in patients taking any medication that prolongs the QT interval. Until more information is obtained, it is suggested that the clinician consult with the physician prior to the use of a vasoconstrictor in suspected patients, and that the vasoconstrictor (epinephrine, mepivacaine and levonordefrin [Carbocaine® 2% with Neo-Cobefrin®]) be used with caution.

Effects on Dental Treatment Key adverse event(s) related to dental treatment: Hypotension reported (10% incidence); monitor patient for dizziness when arising from dental chair

Effects on Bleeding Chemotherapy may result in significant myelosuppression, potentially including significant reduction in platelet counts (thrombocytopenia grades 3/4: 7%) and altered hemostasis. In patients who are under active treatment with these agents, medical consult is suggested.

Adverse Reactions

>10%:

- Cardiovascular: Peripheral edema (20%), prolonged QT interval on ECG (11%; grades 3/4: 4%)
- Central nervous system: Fatigue (37%; grades 3/4: 5%), chills (16%; grades 3/4: 1%), headache (15%)
- Dermatologic: Skin rash (20%; grades 3/4: 1%), pruritus (16%; grades 3/4: 3%)
- Endocrine & metabolic: Increased lactate dehydrogenase (16%; grades 3/4: 2%), hypokalemia (12%; grades 3/4: 4%)
- Gastrointestinal: Nausea (42%; grades 3/4: 1%), vomiting (29%; grades 3/4: 1%), constipation (23%; grades 3/4: 1%), diarrhea (23%; grades 3/4: 2%), decreased appetite (15%; grades 3/4: 2%), abdominal pain (11%; grades 3/4: 1%)
- Hematologic & oncologic: Anemia (32%; grades 3/4: 11%), thrombocytopenia (16%; grades 3/4: 7%)
- Local: Pain at injection site (14%)
- Respiratory: Dyspnea (22%; grades 3/4: 6%), cough (19%)
- Miscellaneous: Fever (35%; grades 3/4: 2%)

1% to 10%:

- Cardiovascular: Hypotension (10%; grades 3/4: 3%), phlebitis (10%; grades 3/4: 1%)
- Central nervous system: Dizziness (10%)
- Infection: Infection (>2%)
- Renal: Increased serum creatinine (>2%)
- Respiratory: Pneumonia (>2%)
- Miscellaneous: Multi-organ failure (>2%)

<1%, postmarketing, and/or case reports: Abnormal hepatic function tests, febrile neutropenia, hepatic failure, hepatotoxicity, leukopenia, sepsis, tumor lysis syndrome, ventricular fibrillation

Mechanism of Action Belinostat is a histone deacetylase (HDAC) inhibitor which catalyzes acetyl group removal from protein lysine residues (of histone and some nonhistone proteins). Inhibition of histone deacetylase results in accumulation of acetyl groups, leading to cell cycle arrest and apoptosis. Belinostat has preferential cytotoxicity toward tumor cells versus normal cells.

Pharmacodynamics/Kinetics

Half-life Elimination 1.1 hours

Time to Peak At end of infusion (Steele 2011)

Reproductive Considerations

Evaluate pregnancy status prior to use in females of reproductive potential. Females of reproductive potential should use effective contraception during therapy and for 6 months after the last belinostat dose. Males with female partners of reproductive potential should use effective contraception during therapy and for 3 months after the last dose of belinostat.

Pregnancy Considerations

Based on the mechanism of action and findings of genotoxicity, in utero exposure to belinostat may cause fetal harm.

Dental Health Professional Considerations This drug is known to prolong the QT interval (see Local Anesthetic/Vasocontrictor Precautions)

◆ **Belrapzo** *see* Bendamustine *on page* 226

◆ **Belsomra** *see* Suvorexant *on page* 1397

Bempedoic Acid (BEM pe DOE ik AS id)

Brand Names: US Nexletol

Pharmacologic Category Antilipemic Agent, Adenosine Triphosphate-Citrate Lyase (ACL) Inhibitor

Use

Atherosclerotic cardiovascular disease, established: Treatment of established atherosclerotic cardiovascular disease, as an adjunct to diet and maximally tolerated statin therapy, in adult patients who require additional lowering of low-density lipoprotein cholesterol (LDL-C).

Heterozygous familial hypercholesterolemia: Treatment of heterozygous familial hypercholesterolemia, as an adjunct to diet and maximally tolerated statin therapy, in adult patients who require additional lowering of LDL-C.

Limitations of use: The effect of bempedoic acid on cardiovascular morbidity and mortality has not been determined.

Local Anesthetic/Vasoconstrictor Precautions No information available to require special precautions.

Effects on Dental Treatment No significant effects or complications reported.

Effects on Bleeding No information available to require special precautions.

Adverse Reactions

>10%: Endocrine & metabolic: Gout (2% [placebo: 0.4%]; with prior gout history: 11% [placebo: 2%]), hyperuricemia (4% to 26% [placebo: 1% to 10%])

1% to 10%:

Cardiovascular: Atrial fibrillation (2%), increased serum creatine kinase (1%)

Gastrointestinal: Abdominal distress (≤3%), abdominal pain (≤3%)

Genitourinary: Benign prostatic hyperplasia (1%)

Hematologic & oncologic: Anemia (3%), leukopenia (9%), thrombocythemia (10%)

Hepatic: Increased liver enzymes (2%), increased serum aspartate aminotransferase (1%)

Neuromuscular & skeletal: Back pain (3%), limb pain (3%), muscle spasm (4%)

Renal: Increased blood urea nitrogen (4%), increased serum creatinine (2%)

Respiratory: Upper respiratory tract infection (5%)

<1%: Neuromuscular & skeletal: Rupture of tendon (placebo: 0%)

Mechanism of Action Bempedoic acid is an adenosine triphosphate-citrate lyase (ACL) inhibitor that lowers low-density lipoprotein cholesterol (LDL-C) by inhibiting cholesterol synthesis in the liver. ACL is an enzyme upstream of 3-hydroxy-3-methyl-glutaryl-coenzyme A reductase in the cholesterol biosynthesis pathway. Bempedoic acid and its active metabolite, ESP15228, require coenzyme A (CoA) activation by very long-chain acyl-CoA synthetase 1 (ACSVL1) to ETC-1002-CoA and ESP15228-CoA, respectively. ACSVL1 is expressed primarily in the liver. Inhibition of ACL by ETC-1002-CoA results in decreased cholesterol synthesis in the liver and lowers LDL-C in blood via upregulation of LDL receptors.

Pharmacodynamics/Kinetics

Half-life Elimination 21 ± 11 hours.

Time to Peak 3.5 hours.

Pregnancy Considerations

Based on the mechanism of action, in utero exposure to bempedoic acid may cause fetal harm. In general, bempedoic acid should be discontinued if pregnancy occurs.

Other agents may be preferred if treatment is needed in a pregnant woman (AACE [Jellinger 2017]; NLA [Jacobson 2015]).

Bempedoic Acid and Ezetimibe

(BEM pe DOE ik AS id & ez ET i mibe)

Brand Names: US Nexlizet

Pharmacologic Category Antilipemic Agent, 2-Azetidinone; Antilipemic Agent, Adenosine Triphosphate-Citrate Lyase (ACL) Inhibitor

Use

Atherosclerotic cardiovascular disease, established: Treatment of established atherosclerotic cardiovascular disease, as an adjunct to diet and maximally tolerated statin therapy, in adult patients who require additional lowering of LDL-C.

Heterozygous familial hypercholesterolemia: Treatment of heterozygous familial hypercholesterolemia, as an adjunct to diet and maximally tolerated statin therapy, in adult patients who require additional lowering of LDL-C.

Limitations of use: The effect of bempedoic acid/ezetimibe on cardiovascular morbidity and mortality has not been determined.

Local Anesthetic/Vasoconstrictor Precautions No information available to require special precautions.

Effects on Dental Treatment Key adverse event(s) related to dental treatment: Occurrence of nasopharyngitis.

Effects on Bleeding No information available to require special precautions.

Adverse Reactions Also see individual agents.

1% to 10%:

Gastrointestinal: Constipation (5%)

Genitourinary: Urinary tract infection (6%)

Respiratory: Nasopharyngitis (5%)

Frequency not defined: Gastrointestinal: Oral discomfort

Mechanism of Action

Bempedoic acid: An adenosine triphosphate-citrate lyase (ACL) inhibitor that lowers LDL-C by inhibiting cholesterol synthesis in the liver. ACL is an enzyme upstream of 3-hydroxy-3-methyl-glutaryl-coenzyme A reductase in the cholesterol biosynthesis pathway. Bempedoic acid and its active metabolite, ESP15228, require coenzyme A (CoA) activation by very long-chain acyl-CoA synthetase 1 (ACSVL1) to ETC-1002-CoA and ESP15228-CoA, respectively. ACSVL1 is expressed primarily in the liver. Inhibition of ACL by ETC-1002-CoA results in decreased cholesterol synthesis in the liver and lowers LDL-C in blood via upregulation of low-density lipoprotein receptors.

Ezetimibe: Inhibits absorption of cholesterol at the brush border of the small intestine via the sterol transporter, Niemann-Pick C1-Like1. This leads to a decreased delivery of cholesterol to the liver, reduction of hepatic cholesterol stores, and an increased clearance of cholesterol from the blood; decreases total C, LDL-C, ApoB, and triglycerides while increasing HDL-cholesterol.

Pregnancy Considerations

Based on the mechanism of action, in utero exposure may cause fetal harm. In general, use should be discontinued once pregnancy is recognized.

Refer to individual monographs for additional information.

- **Benadryl** *see* DiphenhydrAMINE (Systemic) *on page 502*
- **Benadryl Allergy [OTC]** *see* DiphenhydrAMINE (Systemic) *on page 502*
- **Benadryl Allergy Childrens [OTC]** *see* DiphenhydrAMINE (Systemic) *on page 502*
- **Benadryl Itch Stopping [OTC]** *see* DiphenhydrAMINE (Topical) *on page 503*

Benazepril (ben AY ze pril)

Related Information

Cardiovascular Diseases *on page 1654*

Brand Names: US Lotensin

Brand Names: Canada Lotensin [DSC]; PMS-Benazepril [DSC]

Pharmacologic Category Angiotensin-Converting Enzyme (ACE) Inhibitor; Antihypertensive

Use

Hypertension: Management of hypertension

Guideline recommendations: The 2017 Guideline for the Prevention, Detection, Evaluation, and Management of High Blood Pressure in Adults recommends if monotherapy is warranted, in the absence of comorbidities (eg, cerebrovascular disease, chronic kidney disease, diabetes, heart failure, ischemic heart disease, etc.), that thiazide-like diuretics or dihydropyridine calcium channel blockers may be preferred options due to improved cardiovascular endpoints (eg, prevention of heart failure and stroke). ACE inhibitors and ARBs are also acceptable for monotherapy. Combination therapy may be required to achieve blood pressure goals and is initially preferred in patients at high risk (stage 2 hypertension or atherosclerotic cardiovascular disease [ASCVD] risk ≥10%) (ACC/AHA [Whelton 2017]).

Local Anesthetic/Vasoconstrictor Precautions No information available to require special precautions

Effects on Dental Treatment Key adverse event(s) related to dental treatment: Patients may experience orthostatic hypotension as they stand up after treatment; especially if lying in dental chair for extended periods of time. Use caution with sudden changes in position during and after dental treatment.

An angiotensin-converting enzyme (ACE) Inhibitor cough is a dry, hacking, nonproductive cough that can potentially interfere with longer dental procedures if patient has this side effect.

Effects on Bleeding No information available to require special precautions

Adverse Reactions

1% to 10%:

Cardiovascular: Hypotension

Central nervous system: Headache (6%), dizziness (4%), drowsiness (2%), orthostatic dizziness (2%)

<1%, postmarketing, and/or case reports: Alopecia, angioedema, anxiety, arthralgia, arthritis, asthma, bronchitis, constipation, decreased libido, dermatitis, diaphoresis, dyspnea, ECG changes, eosinophilia, fatigue, flushing, gastritis, hemolytic anemia, hypersensitivity, hypertonia, hyponatremia, impotence, increased liver enzymes, increased serum bilirubin, increased serum glucose, increased uric acid, infection, insomnia, melena, myalgia, nausea, nervousness, pancreatitis, paresthesia, pemphigus, proteinuria, pruritus, sinusitis, skin photosensitivity, skin rash, Stevens-Johnson syndrome, thrombocytopenia, urinary frequency, urinary tract infection, vomiting, weakness

Mechanism of Action Competitive inhibition of angiotensin I being converted to angiotensin II, a potent vasoconstrictor, through the angiotensin I-converting enzyme (ACE) activity, with resultant lower levels of angiotensin II which causes an increase in plasma renin activity and a reduction in aldosterone secretion

Pharmacodynamics/Kinetics

Onset of Action

Reduction in plasma angiotensin-converting enzyme (ACE) activity: Peak effect: 1 to 2 hours after 2 to 20 mg dose (Nussberger 1987; Nussberger 1989)

Reduction in blood pressure: Peak effect: Single dose: 2 to 4 hours; Continuous therapy: 2 weeks (Fogari 1990)

Duration of Action Reduction in plasma angiotensin-converting enzyme (ACE) activity: >90% inhibition for 24 hours after 5 to 20 mg dose (Balfour 1991)

Half-life Elimination Benazeprilat: Effective: 10 to 11 hours; Terminal: Children: 5 hours, Adults: 22 hours

Time to Peak

Parent drug: 0.5 to 1 hour

Active metabolite (benazeprilat): Fasting: 1 to 2 hours; Nonfasting: 2 to 4 hours

Reproductive Considerations

Angiotensin-converting enzyme (ACE) inhibitors should be avoided in sexually active females of reproductive potential not using effective contraception (ADA 2020).

ACE inhibitors should generally be avoided for the treatment of hypertension in women planning a pregnancy; use should only be considered for cases of hypertension refractory to other medications (ACOG 203 2019).

Pregnancy Considerations Benazepril crosses the placenta.

Exposure to an angiotensin-converting enzyme (ACE) inhibitor during the first trimester of pregnancy may be associated with an increased risk of fetal malformations (ACOG 203 2019; ESC [Regitz-Zagrosek 2018]); however, outcomes observed may also be influenced by maternal disease (ACC/AHA [Whelton 2018]).

[US Boxed Warning]: Drugs that act on the renin-angiotensin system can cause injury and death to the developing fetus. Discontinue as soon as possible once pregnancy is detected.

Drugs that act on the renin-angiotensin system are associated with oligohydramnios. Oligohydramnios, due to decreased fetal renal function, may lead to fetal lung hypoplasia and skeletal malformations. Their use in pregnancy is also associated with anuria, hypotension, renal failure, skull hypoplasia, and death in the fetus/neonate.

Infants exposed to an ACE inhibitor in utero should be monitored for hyperkalemia, hypotension, and oliguria. Oligohydramnios may not appear until after irreversible fetal injury has occurred. Exchange transfusions or dialysis may be required to reverse hypotension or improve renal function.

Chronic maternal hypertension is also associated with adverse events in the fetus/infant. Chronic maternal hypertension may increase the risk of birth defects, low birth weight, premature delivery, stillbirth, and neonatal death. Actual fetal/neonatal risks may be related to duration and severity of maternal hypertension. Untreated chronic hypertension may also increase the risks of adverse maternal outcomes, including gestational diabetes, preeclampsia, delivery complications, stroke, and myocardial infarction (ACOG 203 2019).

When treatment of hypertension in pregnancy is indicated, ACE inhibitors should generally be avoided due to their adverse fetal events; use in pregnant women should only be considered for cases of hypertension refractory to other medications (ACOG 203 2019). ACE inhibitors are not recommended for the treatment of heart failure in pregnancy (Regitz-Zagrosek [ESC 2018]).

◆ **Benazepril HCl** *see* Benazepril *on page* 225

◆ **Benazepril Hydrochloride** *see* Benazepril *on page* 225

Bendamustine (ben da MUS teen)

Brand Names: US Belrapzo; Bendeka; Treanda

Brand Names: Canada Treanda

Pharmacologic Category Antineoplastic Agent, Alkylating Agent; Antineoplastic Agent, Alkylating Agent (Nitrogen Mustard)

Use

Chronic lymphocytic leukemia: Treatment of chronic lymphocytic leukemia (CLL).

Non-Hodgkin lymphoma, indolent (refractory): Treatment of indolent B-cell non-Hodgkin lymphoma (NHL) which has progressed during or within 6 months of rituximab treatment or a rituximab-containing regimen.

Local Anesthetic/Vasoconstrictor Precautions No information available to require special precautions

Effects on Dental Treatment Key adverse event(s) related to dental treatment: Frequent occurrence of stomatitis and xerostomia (normal salivary flow resumes upon discontinuation) have been reported. Occurrence of altered taste, oral candidiasis, and mucositis (frequency not defined) have also been reported.

Effects on Bleeding Thrombocytopenia has been reported in 77% to 86% (grade 3/4: 11% to 25%) of patients.

Adverse Reactions

>10%:

Cardiovascular: Peripheral edema (13%)

Central nervous system: Fatigue (9% to 57%), headache (21%), dizziness (14%), chills (6% to 14%), insomnia (13%)

Dermatologic: Skin rash (8% to 16%)

Endocrine & metabolic: Weight loss (7% to 18%), dehydration (14%)

Gastrointestinal: Nausea (20% to 75%), vomiting (16% to 40%), diarrhea (9% to 37%), constipation (29%), anorexia (23%), stomatitis (15%; grades 3/4: <1%), abdominal pain (13%), decreased appetite (13%), dyspepsia (11%)

Hematologic & oncologic: Lymphocytopenia (68% to 99%; grades 3/4: 47% to 94%), bone marrow depression (grades 3/4: 98%; nadir in week 3), leukopenia (61% to 94%; grades 3/4: 28% to 56%), decreased hemoglobin (88% to 89%; grades 3/4: 11% to 13%), decreased neutrophils (75% to 86%; grades 3/4: 43% to 60%), thrombocytopenia (77% to 86%; grades 3/4: 11% to 25%)

Hepatic: Increased serum bilirubin (34%)

Neuromuscular & skeletal: Back pain (14%), asthenia (8% to 11%)

Respiratory: Cough (4% to 22%), dyspnea (16%)

Miscellaneous: Fever (24% to 34%)

1% to 10%:

Cardiovascular: Tachycardia (7%), chest pain (6%), hypotension (6%), exacerbation of hypertension (3%)

Central nervous system: Anxiety (8%), depression (6%), pain (6%)

Dermatologic: Pruritus (5% to 6%), hyperhidrosis (5%), night sweats (5%), xeroderma (5%)

Endocrine & metabolic: Hypokalemia (9%), hyperuricemia (7%), hyperglycemia (grades 3/4: 3%), hypocalcemia (grades 3/4: 2%), hyponatremia (grades 3/4: 2%)

Gastrointestinal: Gastroesophageal reflux disease (10%), xerostomia (9%), dysgeusia (7%), oral candidiasis (6%), abdominal distention (5%), upper abdominal pain (5%)

Genitourinary: Urinary tract infection (10%)

Hematologic & oncologic: Febrile neutropenia (grades 3/4: 6%)

Hepatic: Increased serum alanine aminotransferase (grades 3/4: 3%), increased serum aspartate transaminase (grades 3/4: 1%)

Hypersensitivity: Hypersensitivity reaction (5%)

Infection: Herpes zoster infection (10%), infection (6%), herpes simplex infection (3%)

Local: Infusion site pain (6%), catheter pain (5%)

Neuromuscular & skeletal: Arthralgia (6%), limb pain (5%), ostealgia (5%)

Renal: Increased serum creatinine (grades 3/4: 2%)

Respiratory: Upper respiratory tract infection (10%), sinusitis (9%), pharyngolaryngeal pain (8%), pneumonia (8%), nasopharyngitis (6% to 7%), nasal congestion (5%), wheezing (5%)

Frequency not defined:

Central nervous system: Drowsiness, malaise

Dermatologic: Dermatitis, skin necrosis

Gastrointestinal: Mucositis

Hematologic & oncologic: Hemolysis

<1%, postmarketing, and/or case reports: Acute renal failure, anaphylactoid shock, anaphylaxis, atrial fibrillation, bronchogenic carcinoma, bullous rash, cardiac failure, dermatological reaction (toxic), DRESS syndrome, erythema, extravasation injury, hepatitis, hepatotoxicity, injection site reaction, myelodysplastic syndrome, myeloid leukemia (acute), myocardial infarction, neutropenic sepsis, palpitations, pancytopenia, pneumonia due to *Pneumocystis jirovecii*, pneumonitis, pulmonary alveolar hemorrhage (with grade 3 thrombocytopenia), pulmonary fibrosis, reactivation of disease (including, but not limited to hepatitis B, cytomegalovirus, *Mycobacterium tuberculosis*, herpes zoster), sepsis, septic shock, Stevens-Johnson syndrome, toxic epidermal necrolysis, tumor lysis syndrome

Mechanism of Action Bendamustine is an alkylating agent (nitrogen mustard derivative) with a benzimidazole ring (purine analog) which demonstrates only partial cross-resistance (*in vitro*) with other alkylating agents. It leads to cell death via single and double strand DNA cross-linking. Bendamustine is active against quiescent and dividing cells. The primary cytotoxic activity is due to bendamustine (as compared to metabolites).

Pharmacodynamics/Kinetics

Half-life Elimination Bendamustine: ~40 minutes; M3: ~3 hours; M4: ~30 minutes

Time to Peak Typically at end of infusion

Reproductive Considerations

Evaluate pregnancy status prior to use in females of reproductive potential. Females of reproductive potential should use effective contraception during therapy and for at least 6 months after the last dose. Males with female partners of reproductive potential should use effective contraception during therapy and for at least 3 months after the last dose of bendamustine.

Adverse effects to male fertility have been observed in clinical studies. Effects include impaired spermatogenesis, azoospermia, and total germinal aplasia. Risks are increased with combination therapy. Spermatogenesis may return in some patients following remission and may occur several years after therapy has been discontinued.

Pregnancy Considerations

Based on the mechanism of action and data from animal reproduction studies, in utero exposure to bendamustine may cause fetal harm. The European Society for Medical Oncology has published guidelines for diagnosis, treatment, and follow-up of cancer during pregnancy; the guidelines recommend referral to a facility with expertise in cancer during pregnancy and encourage a multidisciplinary team (obstetrician, neonatologist, oncology team). In general, if chemotherapy is indicated, it should be avoided in the first trimester and there should be a 3-week time period between the last chemotherapy dose and anticipated delivery, and chemotherapy should not be administered beyond week 33 of gestation (Peccatori 2013).

A pregnancy registry is available for all cancers diagnosed during pregnancy at Cooper Health (877-635-4499).

- ◆ **Bendamustine HCl** *see* Bendamustine *on page 226*
- ◆ **Bendamustine Hydrochloride** *see* Bendamustine *on page 226*
- ◆ **Bendeka** *see* Bendamustine *on page 226*
- ◆ **Benemid [DSC]** *see* Probenecid *on page 1277*
- ◆ **Benflumetol and Artemether** *see* Artemether and Lumefantrine *on page 168*
- ◆ **Benicar** *see* Olmesartan *on page 1131*
- ◆ **Benlysta** *see* Belimumab *on page 222*

Benralizumab (ben ra LIZ ue mab)

Brand Names: US Fasenra; Fasenra Pen

Brand Names: Canada Fasenra

Pharmacologic Category Interleukin-5 Receptor Antagonist; Monoclonal Antibody, Anti-Asthmatic

Use

Asthma, severe: Add-on maintenance treatment of severe asthma in adults and children ≥12 years of age with an eosinophilic phenotype

Limitations of use: Not indicated for treatment of other eosinophilic conditions or for the relief of acute bronchospasm or status asthmaticus

Local Anesthetic/Vasoconstrictor Precautions

No information available to require special precautions

Effects on Dental Treatment Key adverse event(s) related to dental treatment: Pharyngitis has been reported.

Effects on Bleeding No information available to require special precautions

Adverse Reactions

>10%: Immunologic: Antibody development (13%; neutralizing: 12%)

1% to 10%:

Central nervous system: Headache (8%)

Respiratory: Pharyngitis (5%)

Miscellaneous: Fever (3%)

Postmarketing: Anaphylaxis, angioedema, hypersensitivity reaction

Mechanism of Action Benralizumab, a humanized afucosylated, monoclonal antibody (IgG1, kappa) that binds to the alpha subunit of the interleukin-5 receptor. IL-5 is the major cytokine responsible for the growth and differentiation, recruitment, activation, and survival of eosinophils (a cell type associated with inflammation and an important component in the pathogenesis of asthma). Benralizumab, by inhibiting IL-5 signaling, reduces the production and survival of eosinophils and basophils through antibody dependent cell-mediated cytotoxicity; however, the mechanism of benralizumab action in asthma has not been definitively established.

Pharmacodynamics/Kinetics

Half-life Elimination ~15.5 days

Pregnancy Considerations

Benralizumab is a humanized monoclonal antibody (IgG_1). Placental transfer of human IgG is dependent upon the IgG subclass, maternal serum concentrations, newborn birth weight, and gestational age, generally increasing as pregnancy progresses. The lowest exposure would be expected during the period of organogenesis (Palmeira 2012; Pentsuk 2009).

Uncontrolled asthma is associated with adverse events on pregnancy (increased risk of perinatal mortality, preeclampsia, preterm birth, low-birth-weight infants, cesarean delivery, and the development of gestational diabetes). Poorly controlled asthma or asthma exacerbations may have a greater fetal/maternal risk than what is associated with appropriately used asthma medications. Maternal treatment improves pregnancy outcomes by reducing the risk of some adverse events (eg, preterm birth, gestational diabetes). Maternal asthma symptoms should be monitored monthly during pregnancy (ERS/TSANZ [Middleton 2020]; GINA 2020).

Use of monoclonal antibodies for the treatment of asthma in pregnancy may be considered when conventional therapies are insufficient; use of an agent other than benralizumab may be preferred (ERS/TSANZ [Middleton 2020]).

Data collection to monitor pregnancy and infant outcomes following exposure to benralizumab is ongoing. Health care providers are encouraged to enroll exposed pregnant females in the MotherToBaby Pregnancy Studies conducted by the Organization of Teratology Information Specialists (OTIS) (877-311-8972 or https://mothertobaby.org). Patients may also enroll themselves.

- ◆ **Bentyl** *see* Dicyclomine *on page 492*

◆ **BenzaClin** *see* Clindamycin and Benzoyl Peroxide *on page 375*

◆ **BenzaClin with Pump** *see* Clindamycin and Benzoyl Peroxide *on page 375*

◆ **Benzathine Benzylpenicillin** *see* Penicillin G Benzathine *on page 1208*

◆ **Benzathine Penicillin G** *see* Penicillin G Benzathine *on page 1208*

◆ **Benzatropine** *see* Benztropine *on page 231*

◆ **Benzhexol Hydrochloride** *see* Trihexyphenidyl *on page 1498*

Benzhydrocodone and Acetaminophen

(benz hye droe KOE done & a seet a MIN oh fen)

Brand Names: US Apadaz

Pharmacologic Category Analgesic Combination (Opioid); Analgesic, Opioid

Use

Pain management: Short-term (≤14 days) management of acute pain severe enough to require an opioid analgesic and for which alternative treatments are inadequate.

Limitations of use: Reserve for use in patients for whom alternative treatment options (eg, nonopioid analgesics) are ineffective, not tolerated, or would be otherwise inadequate to provide sufficient management of pain.

Local Anesthetic/Vasoconstrictor Precautions No information available to require special precautions

Effects on Dental Treatment No significant effects or complications reported

Effects on Bleeding As a single agent, acetaminophen does not appear to affect bleeding or platelet aggregation. Acetaminophen may prolong the INR and increase bleeding in patients taking warfarin (Coumadin). For patients taking warfarin, single acetaminophen doses or acetaminophen therapy of short duration should be safe, but if large (>1.3 g/day) doses are administered for longer than 10 to 14 days, then the INR should be monitored.

Adverse Reactions Also see acetaminophen and hydrocodone.

>10%:

Central nervous system: Drowsiness (19%)

Dermatologic: Pruritus (12%)

Gastrointestinal: Nausea (22%), vomiting (13%), constipation (12%)

1% to 10%:

Cardiovascular: Hypotension (1% to 5%), presyncope (1% to 5%)

Central nervous system: Dizziness (8%), headache (6%)

Endocrine & metabolic: Hot flash (1% to 5%)

Gastrointestinal: Abdominal distention (1% to 5%), abdominal pain (1% to 5%), flatulence (1% to 5%)

Neuromuscular & skeletal: Tremor (1% to 5%), weakness (1% to 5%)

Respiratory: Dyspnea (1% to 5%)

<1%, postmarketing, and/or case reports: Agitation, chest discomfort, diarrhea, euphoria, eye pruritus, gastroesophageal reflux disease, hematemesis, hypoesthesia, nightmares, rhinitis, syncope

Mechanism of Action

Benzhydrocodone: Prodrug of hydrocodone; binds to opiate receptors in the CNS, altering the perception of and response to pain; suppresses cough in medullary center; produces generalized CNS depression.

Acetaminophen: Although not fully elucidated, the analgesic effects are believed to be due to activation of descending serotonergic inhibitory pathways in the central nervous system. Interactions with other nociceptive systems may be involved as well (Smith 2009). Antipyresis is produced from inhibition of the hypothalamic heat-regulating center.

Reproductive Considerations

Long-term opioid use may cause secondary hypogonadism, which may lead to sexual dysfunction and infertility (Brennan 2013).

Pregnancy Considerations

[US Boxed Warning]: Prolonged use of opioids during pregnancy can cause neonatal withdrawal syndrome, which may be life-threatening if not recognized and treated according to protocols developed by neonatology experts. If opioid use is required for a prolonged period in a pregnant woman, advise the patient of the risk of neonatal opioid withdrawal syndrome and ensure that appropriate treatment will be available.

Also refer to the individual Acetaminophen monograph.

Product Availability Apadaz: FDA approved February 2018; anticipated availability unknown

Controlled Substance C-II

◆ **Benzmethyzin** *see* Procarbazine *on page 1278*

Benzocaine (BEN zoe kane)

Related Information

Oral Pain *on page 1734*

Related Sample Prescriptions

Ulcerative and Erosive Disorders - Sample Prescriptions *on page 46*

Brand Names: US Aftertest Topical Pain Relief [OTC]; Allevacaine [OTC]; Anacaine; Anbesol Cold Sore Therapy [OTC]; Anbesol JR [OTC] [DSC]; Anbesol Maximum Strength [OTC]; Anbesol [OTC]; Baby Anbesol [OTC]; Benz-O-Sthetic [OTC]; Bi-Zets/Benzotroches [OTC]; Cepacol INSTAMAX [OTC]; Cepacol [OTC]; Chiggerex [OTC] [DSC]; Chiggertox [OTC] [DSC]; Dent-O-Kain/20 [OTC]; Dentapaine [OTC]; Dermoplast [OTC] [DSC]; Foille [OTC] [DSC]; GoodSense Oral Pain Relief [OTC]; HurriCaine One [OTC]; Hurricaine [OTC]; HurriPak Starter Kit [OTC]; Ivy-Rid [OTC]; Kank-A Mouth Pain [OTC] [DSC]; Ora-film [OTC]; Sore Throat Relief [OTC] [DSC]; Topex Topical Anesthetic; Trocaine Throat [OTC] [DSC]; Zilactin Baby [OTC]

Generic Availability (US) May be product dependent

Pharmacologic Category Analgesic, Topical; Local Anesthetic

Dental Use Ester-type topical local anesthetic for temporary relief of pain associated with toothache, minor sore throat pain, and canker sore

Use Note: Approved ages and uses for products may vary; consult product labeling for specific information:

Topical, external:

Dermal irritation: Ointment 5%, spray 5% and 20%: Temporary relief of pain and itching associated with minor skin irritations, cuts, scrapes, minor burns, sunburn, and insect bites; prevention of infection in minor cuts, scrapes and burns.

Hemorrhoids: Ointment 20%: Temporary relief of hemorrhoid symptoms.

Poison ivy/sumac: Spray 5% (Ivy-Rid only): Temporary relief of pain and itching associated with poison ivy/oak/sumac.

Topical, oral:

Mouth and gum irritation:

Ointment 20%: Temporary relief of pain associated with fever blisters and cold sores.

Gel 10% and 20%, lozenge, spray 5%, liquid 10% and 20%: Temporary relief of pain associated with toothache, sore gums, sore throat, canker sores, braces, minor dental procedures, or minor injury of the mouth and gum caused by dentures or orthodontic appliances. **Note:** Although product is available in a gel formulation for relief of pain associated with teething in infants ≥4 months, the FDA, AAP, and American Academy of Pediatric Dentistry do not recommend use due to safety concerns related to increased methemoglobinemia risk in infants and children <2 years of age (AAP 2011; FDA 2018).

Sore throat/mouth, gag reflex suppression: Spray 20%: Topical anesthetic for oral or mucosal areas; temporary relief of occasional minor irritation and pain associated with sore mouth and throat; temporary suppression of gag reflex.

Topical anesthetic: Gel or liquid 20% (Topex only): Topical anesthetic for use on oral mucosa prior to local anesthetic injections, scaling and prophylaxis; to relieve discomfort associated with taking impressions and intraoral radiographs.

Local Anesthetic/Vasoconstrictor Precautions No information available to require special precautions

Effects on Dental Treatment A patient history of allergy to ester-type local anesthetics contraindicates the use of this product.

Effects on Bleeding No information available to require special precautions

Adverse Reactions Frequency not defined.

Central nervous system: Localized burning, stinging sensation

Dermatologic: Contact dermatitis, localized erythema, localized rash, urticaria

Hematologic & oncologic: Methemoglobinemia

Hypersensitivity: Hypersensitivity

Local: Local pruritus, localized edema, localized tenderness

Dental Usual Dosage Relief of pain (toothache, minor sore throat pain, and canker sore): Children ≥2 years and Adults: Topical (oral): 10% to 20%: Apply thin layer to affected area up to 4 times daily

Dosing

Adult & Geriatric Note: General dosing guidelines provided; refer to specific product labeling for dosing instructions.

Dermal irritation: Topical (external): Spray 5% and 20%, ointment 5%: Apply to affected area or use 1 spray up to 4 times daily as needed. In cases of bee stings, remove stinger before treatment.

Hemorrhoids: Topical (rectal, external): Ointment 20%: Apply to affected area up to 6 times daily.

Mouth and gum irritation: Topical (oral): Gel 10% or 20%, liquid 10% or 20%, ointment 20%, spray 5%: Apply thin layer to affected area or use 1 spray up to 4 times daily as needed.

Poison ivy/sumac: Topical (external): Spray 5% (Ivy-Rid only): Spray affected area until wet.

Sore throat/mouth, gag reflex suppression: Topical (oral):

Lozenge: Allow 1 lozenge to dissolve slowly in mouth; may repeat every 2 hours as needed.

Spray 20%:

Benz-O-Sthetic: Spray 2 to 3 times or as needed. Repeat if needed for larger areas.

Hurricaine: Spray on affected area or throat up to 4 times daily.

Topical anesthetic: Topical (oral): Gel or liquid 20% (Topex only): Apply a small amount to mucosa to achieve topical anesthesia.

Renal Impairment: Adult There are no dosage adjustments provided in the manufacturer's labeling.

Hepatic Impairment: Adult There are no dosage adjustments provided in the manufacturer's labeling.

Pediatric Note: General dosing recommendations provided; refer to specific product labeling for dosing instructions. Due to risk of methemoglobinemia, AAP, FDA, and the American Academy of Pediatric Dentistry do **NOT** recommend use for teething and mouth pain in infants and children <2 years (AAP 2011; AAPD 2012; FDA Safety Announcement 2018).

Dermal irritation (insect bites, minor cuts, scrapes, minor burns, sunburn): Topical: 20% spray, 5% ointment: Children ≥2 years and Adolescents: Apply to affected area 3 to 4 times daily as needed.

Mouth and gum irritation (including fever blisters and cold sores): Topical:

Oral 10% or 20% gel/liquid: Children ≥2 years and Adolescents: Apply thin layer to affected area up to 4 times daily as needed.

Oral 5% spray: Children ≥6 years and Adolescents: Use 1 spray to affected area up to 4 times daily.

Sore throat/mouth, gag reflex suppression:

Oral: Oral lozenge: Children ≥5 years and Adolescents: Allow 1 lozenge to dissolve slowly in mouth; may repeat every 2 hours as needed.

Topical: **Note:** Consult product labeling for specific dose recommendations.

Oral spray 5%: Children ≥6 years and Adolescents: Use 1 spray to affected area or throat up to 4 times daily.

Oral spray 20%: Children ≥2 years and Adolescents: Spray on affected area or throat up to 4 times daily.

Renal Impairment: Pediatric There are no dosage adjustments provided in the manufacturer's labeling.

Hepatic Impairment: Pediatric There are no dosage adjustments provided in the manufacturer's labeling.

Mechanism of Action Blocks both the initiation and conduction of nerve impulses by decreasing the neuronal membrane's permeability to sodium ions, which results in inhibition of depolarization with resultant blockade of conduction

Contraindications

Hypersensitivity to benzocaine, para-aminobenzoic acid (PABA), or any component of the formulation

OTC labeling: When used for self-medication, do not use if you have allergy to local anesthetics (procaine, butacaine, benzocaine, or other "caine" anesthetics). Do not use over deep or puncture wounds, infections, serious burns, or lacerations.

Warnings/Precautions Methemoglobinemia has been reported following topical use, particularly with higher concentration (14% to 20%) spray formulations applied to the mouth or mucous membranes. When applied as a spray to the mouth or throat, multiple sprays (or sprays of longer than indicated duration) are not recommended. Use caution with breathing problems (asthma, bronchitis, emphysema, in smokers), inflamed/damaged mucosa, heart disease, children <6 months of age, and hemoglobin or enzyme abnormalities (glucose-6-phosphate dehydrogenase deficiency, hemoglobin-M disease, NADH-methemoglobin reductase deficiency, pyruvate-kinase deficiency). Alternatives to benzocaine sprays, such as topical lidocaine preparations, should be considered for patients at higher risk of this reaction. The classical clinical finding of methemoglobinemia is chocolate brown-colored arterial blood. However, suspected cases should be confirmed by co-oximetry, which yields a direct and accurate measure of methemoglobin levels. Standard pulse oximetry readings or arterial blood gas values are not reliable. Clinically significant methemoglobinemia requires immediate treatment (Anderson 1988; Cooper 1997; Moore 2004). Due to risk of methemoglobinemia, AAP, FDA, and the American Academy of Pediatric Dentistry do **NOT** recommend use for teething and mouth pain in infants and children <2 years of age (AAP 2011; AAPD 2012; FDA 2018).

Some dosage forms may contain benzyl alcohol; large amounts of benzyl alcohol (≥99 mg/kg/day) have been associated with a potentially fatal toxicity ("gasping syndrome") in neonates; the "gasping syndrome" consists of metabolic acidosis, respiratory distress, gasping respirations, CNS dysfunction (including convulsions, intracranial hemorrhage), hypotension and cardiovascular collapse (AAP ["Inactive" 1997]; CDC 1982); some data suggests that benzoate displaces bilirubin from protein binding sites (Ahlfors 2001); avoid or use dosage forms containing benzyl alcohol with caution in neonates. See manufacturer's labeling. Some dosage forms may contain propylene glycol; large amounts are potentially toxic and have been associated hyperosmolality, lactic acidosis, seizures and respiratory depression; use caution (AAP 1997 Zar 2007). See manufacturer's labeling. For external use only; do not insert into rectum using fingers or any mechanical device or applicator.

When used for self-medication, notify healthcare provider if condition worsens, or does not improve within 7 days; clears up and occurs again within a few days; or if accompanied by additional symptoms (eg, swelling, rash, headache, nausea, vomiting, or fever). Do not use topical products on open wounds; avoid contact with the eyes. Do not use for a prolonged time and/or on large portions of the body. When topical anesthetics are used prior to cosmetic or medical procedures, the lowest amount of anesthetic necessary for pain relief should be applied. High systemic levels and toxic effects (eg, methemoglobinemia, irregular heartbeats, respiratory depression, seizures, death) have been reported in patients who (without supervision of a trained professional) have applied topical anesthetics in large amounts (or to large areas of the skin), left these products on for prolonged periods of time, or have used wraps/dressings to cover the skin following application.

Warnings: Additional Pediatric Considerations

There is a significant safety risk of methemoglobinemia with benzocaine use. The majority of cases of methemoglobinemia associated with benzocaine use have been in infants and children <2 years of age for treatment of teething and mouth pain; also at greater risk for development are patients with asthma, bronchitis, emphysema, mucosal damage, or inflammation at the application site, heart disease, and malnutrition. The FDA has strengthened their warning against using topical OTC benzocaine for teething pain and are urging manufacturers to stop marketing OTC oral benzocaine products for treatment of teething in infants and children <2 years of age and to add contraindications to use in teething and treatment in infants and children <2 years (FDA Safety Announcement 2018). The use of OTC topical anesthetics (eg, benzocaine) for teething pain is also discouraged by AAP and The American Academy of Pediatric Dentistry (AAP 2011; AAPD 2012). The AAP recommends managing teething pain with a chilled (not frozen) teething ring or gently rubbing/massaging with the caregiver's finger.

Some dosage forms may contain propylene glycol; in neonates large amounts of propylene glycol delivered orally, intravenously (eg, >3,000 mg/day), or topically have been associated with potentially fatal toxicities which can include metabolic acidosis, seizures, renal failure, and CNS depression; toxicities have also been reported in children and adults including hyperosmolality, lactic acidosis, seizures and respiratory depression; use caution (AAP 1997; Shehab 2009).

Drug Interactions

Metabolism/Transport Effects None known.

Avoid Concomitant Use There are no known interactions where it is recommended to avoid concomitant use.

Increased Effect/Toxicity

Benzocaine may increase the levels/effects of: Local Anesthetics; Prilocaine; Sodium Nitrite

The levels/effects of Benzocaine may be increased by: Dapsone (Topical); Methemoglobinemia Associated Agents; Nitric Oxide

Decreased Effect There are no known significant interactions involving a decrease in effect.

Pharmacodynamics/Kinetics

Onset of Action Anesthetic effect: Spray: 15 to 30 seconds.

Dosage Forms: US

Aerosol, External:

Ivy-Rid [OTC]: 2% (85 g)

Aerosol, Mouth/Throat:

Hurricaine [OTC]: 20% (57 g)
Topex Topical Anesthetic: 20% (57 g)

Gel, Mouth/Throat:

Anbesol [OTC]: 10% (9 g)
Anbesol Maximum Strength [OTC]: 20% (9 g)
Baby Anbesol [OTC]: 7.5% (9 g)
Benz-O-Sthetic [OTC]: 20% (15 g, 29 g)
Dentapaine [OTC]: 20% (11 g)
GoodSense Oral Pain Relief [OTC]: 20% (14 g)
Hurricaine [OTC]: 20% (5.25 g, 30 g)
Zilactin Baby [OTC]: 10% (9.4 g)

Kit, Mouth/Throat:

HurriPak Starter Kit [OTC]: 20%

Liquid, Mouth/Throat:

Anbesol [OTC]: 10% (12 mL)
Anbesol Maximum Strength [OTC]: 20% (12 mL)
Benz-O-Sthetic [OTC]: 20% (56 g)
Dent-O-Kain/20 [OTC]: 20% (9 mL)
Hurricaine [OTC]: 20% (30 mL)

Lozenge, Mouth/Throat:

Bi-Zets/Benzotroches [OTC]: 15 mg (10 ea)
Cepacol [OTC]: Benzocaine 15 mg and menthol 2.3 mg (16 ea)
Cepacol INSTAMAX [OTC]: Benzocaine 15 mg and menthol 20 mg (16 ea)

Ointment, External:
Anacaine: 10% (30 g)
Anbesol Cold Sore Therapy [OTC]: (9 g)
Solution, Mouth/Throat:
Allevacaine [OTC]: 20% (1 ea, 25 ea)
Benz-O-Sthetic [OTC]: 20% (30 mL)
Hurricaine [OTC]: 20% (30 mL)
HurriCaine One [OTC]: 20% (2 ea, 25 ea)
Stick, External:
Aftertest Topical Pain Relief [OTC]: 10% (4 mL)
Strip, Mouth/Throat:
Ora-film [OTC]: 6% (12 ea)
Swab, Mouth/Throat:
Benz-O-Sthetic [OTC]: 20% (2 ea)

Dental Health Professional Considerations Health Canada has issued a reminder to healthcare professionals that benzocaine sprays must be used judiciously to minimize the risk of methemoglobinemia. Almost all reported cases have been associated with higher concentration (14% to 20% benzocaine) spray products used in the mouth and on other mucous membranes. Alternatives to benzocaine sprays, such as topical lidocaine preparations, should be considered for patients at higher risk of this reaction.

◆ **Benzoic Acid, Hyoscyamine, Methenamine, Methylene Blue, and Phenyl Salicylate** *see* Methenamine, Phenyl Salicylate, Methylene Blue, Benzoic Acid, and Hyoscyamine *on page 987*

◆ **Benzoic Acid, Methenamine, Methylene Blue, Phenyl Salicylate, and Hyoscyamine** *see* Methenamine, Phenyl Salicylate, Methylene Blue, Benzoic Acid, and Hyoscyamine *on page 987*

Benzonatate (ben ZOE na tate)

Related Information
Perioral Premalignant Lesions and Management of Patients Undergoing Cancer Therapy *on page 1781*

Brand Names: US Tessalon Perles

Pharmacologic Category Antitussive

Use Cough: Symptomatic relief of cough

Local Anesthetic/Vasoconstrictor Precautions
No information available to require special precautions

Effects on Dental Treatment No significant effects or complications reported

Effects on Bleeding No information available to require special precautions

Adverse Reactions Frequency not defined.
Cardiovascular: Chest numbness
Central nervous system: Chills, confusion, dizziness, hallucination, headache, sedation
Dermatologic: Pruritus, skin rash
Gastrointestinal: Constipation, gastrointestinal distress, nausea
Hypersensitivity: Hypersensitivity reaction (bronchospasm, laryngospasm, cardiovascular collapse)
Ophthalmic: Burning sensation of eyes
Respiratory: Nasal congestion

Mechanism of Action Tetracaine congener with antitussive properties; suppresses cough by topical anesthetic action on the respiratory stretch receptors

Pharmacodynamics/Kinetics
Onset of Action Therapeutic: 15 to 20 minutes
Duration of Action 3 to 8 hours

Pregnancy Risk Factor C

Pregnancy Considerations Animal reproduction studies have not been conducted. Information related to use in pregnancy is limited (Heinonen 1977).

◆ **Benz-O-Sthetic [OTC]** *see* Benzocaine *on page 228*

◆ **Benzoyl Metronidazole** *see* MetroNIDAZOLE (Systemic) *on page 1011*

◆ **Benzoyl Peroxide and Clindamycin** *see* Clindamycin and Benzoyl Peroxide *on page 375*

Benztropine (BENZ troe peen)

Related Information
Dentin Hypersensitivity, Acid Erosion, High Caries Index, Management of Alveolar Osteitis, and Xerostomia *on page 1762*

Brand Names: US Cogentin

Brand Names: Canada Benztropine Omega; PDP-Benztropine; PMS-Benztropine; VPI-Benztropine

Pharmacologic Category Anti-Parkinson Agent, Anticholinergic; Anticholinergic Agent

Use
Drug-induced extrapyramidal symptoms, acute treatment: Acute treatment drug-induced extrapyramidal symptoms (excluding tardive dyskinesia).
Parkinsonism: Adjunctive therapy of all forms of parkinsonism.

Local Anesthetic/Vasoconstrictor Precautions
No information available to require special precautions

Effects on Dental Treatment Key adverse event(s) related to dental treatment: Xerostomia and changes in salivation (normal salivary flow resumes upon discontinuation), dry throat, and nasal dryness (very prevalent).

Effects on Bleeding No information available to require special precautions

Adverse Reactions Frequency not defined.
Cardiovascular: Tachycardia
Central nervous system: Confusion, depression, disorientation, heatstroke, hyperthermia, lethargy, memory impairment, nervousness, numbness of fingers, psychotic symptoms (exacerbation of preexisting symptoms), toxic psychosis, visual hallucination
Dermatologic: Skin rash
Gastrointestinal: Constipation, nausea, paralytic ileus, vomiting, xerostomia
Genitourinary: Dysuria, urinary retention
Ophthalmic: Blurred vision, mydriasis

Mechanism of Action Possesses both anticholinergic and antihistaminic effects. *In vitro* anticholinergic activity approximates that of atropine; *in vivo* it is only about half as active as atropine. Animal data suggest its antihistaminic activity and duration of action approach that of pyrilamine maleate.

Pharmacodynamics/Kinetics
Onset of Action
IM, IV: Within a few minutes; there is no significant difference between onset of effect after intravenous or intramuscular injection
Oral: Within 1 hour
Time to Peak Plasma: Oral: 7 hours (Brocks 1999)

Pregnancy Considerations
Paralytic ileus (which resolved rapidly) was reported in two newborns exposed to a combination of benztropine and chlorpromazine during the second and third trimesters and the last 6 weeks of pregnancy, respectively (Falterman 1980).

◆ **Benztropine Mesylate** *see* Benztropine *on page 231*

◆ **Benzylpenicillin Benzathine** *see* Penicillin G Benzathine *on page 1208*

◆ **Benzylpenicillin Potassium** *see* Penicillin G (Parenteral/Aqueous) *on page 1209*

◆ **Benzylpenicillin Sodium** *see* Penicillin G (Parenteral/Aqueous) *on page 1209*

◆ **Beovu** *see* Brolucizumab *on page 251*

Bepotastine (be poe TAS teen)

Brand Names: US Bepreve

Brand Names: Canada Bepreve

Pharmacologic Category Histamine H_1 Antagonist; Histamine H_1 Antagonist, Second Generation; Mast Cell Stabilizer

Use Allergic conjunctivitis: Treatment of itching associated with allergic conjunctivitis

Local Anesthetic/Vasoconstrictor Precautions No information available to require special precautions

Effects on Dental Treatment Key adverse event(s) related to dental treatment: Taste abnormalities reported in ≤25% of patients

Effects on Bleeding No information available to require special precautions

Adverse Reactions

>10%: Gastrointestinal: Dysgeusia (25%)

1% to 10%:

Central nervous system: Headache (2% to 5%)

Ophthalmic: Eye irritation (2% to 5%)

Respiratory: Nasopharyngitis (2% to 5%)

<1%, postmarketing, and/or case reports: Hypersensitivity reaction, pharyngeal edema, pruritus, skin rash, swelling of lips, swollen tongue

Mechanism of Action Direct H_1-receptor antagonist and inhibits release of histamine from mast cells

Pharmacodynamics/Kinetics

Onset of Action Within 3 minutes (Macejko 2010)

Duration of Action Up to 16 hours (Williams 2011)

Time to Peak Serum: 1 to 2 hours

Pregnancy Considerations

Plasma concentrations are below the limits of detection 24 hours after ophthalmic use. If ophthalmic agents are needed during pregnancy, the minimum effective dose should be used in combination with punctal occlusion to decrease potential exposure to the fetus (Samples 1988).

◆ **Bepotastine Besilate** *see* Bepotastine *on page 232*

◆ **Bepreve** *see* Bepotastine *on page 232*

Beractant (ber AKT ant)

Brand Names: US Survanta

Brand Names: Canada Survanta

Pharmacologic Category Lung Surfactant

Use Respiratory distress syndrome: Prevention of respiratory distress syndrome (RDS) in premature neonates with birth weight <1,250 g or with evidence of surfactant deficiency (administer within 15 minutes of birth); treatment of RDS in neonates with x-ray confirmation of RDS and requiring mechanical ventilation (administer within 8 hours of birth).

Local Anesthetic/Vasoconstrictor Precautions No information available to require special precautions

Effects on Dental Treatment No significant effects or complications reported

Effects on Bleeding No information available to require special precautions

Adverse Reactions Frequency not defined. The following occurred during the dosing procedure:

>10%: Cardiovascular: Bradycardia (transient)

1% to 10%: Respiratory: Oxygen desaturation

<1%, postmarketing, and/or case reports: Apnea, emphysema (pulmonary interstitial), hypercapnia, hypertension, hypotension, increased susceptibility to infection (post-treatment nosocomial sepsis), low blood CO2, obstruction of endotracheal tube, pallor, pneumothorax (including pneumopericardium), vasoconstriction

Mechanism of Action Replaces deficient or ineffective endogenous lung surfactant in neonates with respiratory distress syndrome (RDS) or in neonates at risk of developing RDS. Surfactant prevents the alveoli from collapsing during expiration by lowering surface tension between air and alveolar surfaces.

Pharmacodynamics/Kinetics

Onset of Action Improved oxygenation: Within minutes

Pregnancy Considerations Beractant is only indicated for use in premature neonates

Besifloxacin (be si FLOX a sin)

Brand Names: US Besivance

Brand Names: Canada Besivance

Pharmacologic Category Antibiotic, Fluoroquinolone; Antibiotic, Ophthalmic

Use Bacterial conjunctivitis: Treatment of bacterial conjunctivitis caused by susceptible isolates of the following bacteria: *Aerococcus viridans*, CDC coryneform group G, *Haemophilus influenzae*, *Staphylococcus aureus*, *Staphylococcus epidermidis*, *Streptococcus mitis* group, *Streptococcus oralis*, *Streptococcus pneumoniae*, *Corynebacterium pseudodiphtheriticum*, *Corynebacterium striatum*, *Moraxella lacunata*, *Moraxella catarrhalis*, *Pseudomonas aeruginosa*, *Staphylococcus hominis*, *Staphylococcus lugdunensis*, *Staphylococcus warneri*, *Streptococcus salivarius*.

Local Anesthetic/Vasoconstrictor Precautions No information available to require special precautions

Effects on Dental Treatment No significant effects or complications reported

Effects on Bleeding No information available to require special precautions

Adverse Reactions Frequency not always defined.

1% to 2%:

Central nervous system: Headache

Ophthalmic: Conjunctival erythema (2%), blurred vision, eye irritation, eye pain, eye pruritus

Mechanism of Action Inhibits both DNA gyrase and topoisomerase IV. DNA gyrase is an essential bacterial enzyme required for DNA replication, transcription, and repair. Topoisomerase IV is an essential bacterial enzyme required for decatenation during cell division. Inhibition effect is bactericidal.

Pharmacodynamics/Kinetics

Half-life Elimination ~7 hours

Pregnancy Considerations

Systemic concentrations of besifloxacin following ophthalmic administration are low. If ophthalmic agents are needed during pregnancy, the minimum effective dose should be used in combination with punctal occlusion for 3 to 5 minutes after application to decrease potential exposure to the fetus (Samples 1988).

◆ **Besifloxacin HCl** *see* Besifloxacin *on page 232*

- **Besifloxacin Hydrochloride** *see* Besifloxacin *on page 232*
- **Besivance** *see* Besifloxacin *on page 232*
- **β Carotene** *see* Beta-Carotene *on page 233*

Beta-Carotene (BAY ta KARE oh teen)

Brand Names: US A-Caro-25 [OTC]; B-Caro-T [OTC]; Caroguard [OTC]

Pharmacologic Category Vitamin, Fat Soluble

Use Dietary supplement: Use as a dietary supplement to increase vitamin A when dietary intake is inadequate

Local Anesthetic/Vasoconstrictor Precautions No information available to require special precautions

Effects on Dental Treatment No significant effects or complications reported

Effects on Bleeding No information available to require special precautions

Adverse Reactions Frequency not defined.

Central nervous system: Dizziness

Dermatologic: Skin discoloration (yellowing of palms, hands, or soles of feet, and to a lesser extent the face)

Mechanism of Action The exact mechanism of action in erythropoietic protoporphyria has not as yet been elucidated; although patient must become carotenemic before effects are observed, there appears to be more than a simple internal light screen responsible for the drug's action. A protective effect was achieved when beta-carotene was added to blood samples. The concentrations of solutions used were similar to those achieved in treated patients. Topically applied beta-carotene is considerably less effective than systemic therapy.

Pregnancy Considerations Maternal intake of beta-carotene influences cord blood concentrations (Scaife 2006).

- **Betadine [OTC]** *see* Povidone-Iodine (Topical) *on page 1249*
- **Betadine Skin Cleanser [OTC] [DSC]** *see* Povidone-Iodine (Topical) *on page 1249*
- **Betadine Surgical Scrub [OTC]** *see* Povidone-Iodine (Topical) *on page 1249*
- **Betadine Swab Aid [OTC] [DSC]** *see* Povidone-Iodine (Topical) *on page 1249*
- **Betadine Swabsticks [OTC]** *see* Povidone-Iodine (Topical) *on page 1249*
- **17-beta E2** *see* Estradiol (Systemic) *on page 596*
- **17-beta estradiol** *see* Estradiol (Systemic) *on page 596*
- **Beta HC [OTC]** *see* Hydrocortisone (Topical) *on page 775*
- **Betamet Acet/Betamet Na pH** *see* Betamethasone (Systemic) *on page 233*

Betamethasone (Systemic)

(bay ta METH a sone)

Related Information

Respiratory Diseases *on page 1680*

Brand Names: US Celestone Soluspan; Pod-Care 100C; ReadySharp Betamethasone

Brand Names: Canada Betaject [DSC]; Celestone Soluspan

Generic Availability (US) Yes

Pharmacologic Category Corticosteroid, Systemic

Dental Use Treatment of a variety of oral diseases of allergic, inflammatory, or autoimmune origin

Use

Intramuscular:

Allergic states: Control of severe or incapacitating allergic conditions intractable to adequate trials of conventional treatment in asthma, atopic dermatitis, contact dermatitis, drug hypersensitivity reactions, perennial or seasonal allergic rhinitis, serum sickness, transfusion reactions

Dermatologic diseases: Bullous dermatitis herpetiformis, exfoliative erythroderma, mycosis fungoides, pemphigus, severe erythema multiforme (Stevens-Johnson syndrome)

Endocrine disorders: Congenital adrenal hyperplasia, hypercalcemia associated with cancer, nonsuppurative thyroiditis. **Note:** Hydrocortisone or cortisone is the drug of choice in primary or secondary adrenocortical insufficiency. Synthetic analogs may be used in conjunction with mineralocorticoids where applicable; in infancy mineralocorticoid supplementation is of particular importance

Gastrointestinal diseases: During acute episodes in regional enteritis and ulcerative colitis

Hematologic disorders: Acquired (autoimmune) hemolytic anemia, Diamond-Blackfan anemia, pure red cell aplasia, selected cases of secondary thrombocytopenia

Neoplastic diseases: Palliative management of leukemias and lymphomas

Nervous system: Acute exacerbations of multiple sclerosis; cerebral edema associated with primary or metastatic brain tumor or craniotomy. **Note**: Treatment guidelines recommend the use of high-dose IV or oral methylprednisolone for acute exacerbations of multiple sclerosis (AAN [Scott 2011]; NICE 2014).

Ophthalmic diseases: Sympathetic ophthalmia, temporal arteritis, uveitis and ocular inflammatory conditions unresponsive to topical corticosteroids

Renal diseases: To induce diuresis or remission of proteinuria in idiopathic nephrotic syndrome or that due to lupus erythematosus

Respiratory diseases: Berylliosis, fulminating or disseminated pulmonary tuberculosis when used concurrently with appropriate antituberculous chemotherapy, idiopathic eosinophilic pneumonias, symptomatic sarcoidosis

Rheumatic disorders: Adjunctive therapy for short-term administration in acute gout flares; acute rheumatic carditis; ankylosing spondylitis; psoriatic arthritis; rheumatoid arthritis, including juvenile rheumatoid arthritis (selected cases may require low-dose maintenance therapy); treatment of dermatomyositis, polymyositis, and systemic lupus erythematosus.

Miscellaneous: Trichinosis with neurologic or myocardial involvement, tuberculous meningitis with subarachnoid block or impending block when used with appropriate antituberculous chemotherapy

Intra-articular or soft tissue administration:

Adjunctive therapy for short-term administration in acute gout flares, acute and subacute bursitis, acute nonspecific tenosynovitis, epicondylitis, rheumatoid arthritis, synovitis of osteoarthritis

Intralesional:
Treatment of alopecia areata; discoid lupus erythematosus; keloids; localized hypertrophic, infiltrated, inflammatory lesions of granuloma annulare, lichen planus, lichen simplex chronicus (neurodermatitis), and psoriatic plaques; necrobiosis lipoidica diabeticorum

Local Anesthetic/Vasoconstrictor Precautions No information available to require special precautions

Effects on Dental Treatment No significant effects or complications reported

Effects on Bleeding Variable effects on anticoagulant therapy are observed with glucocorticoids such as betamethasone.

Adverse Reactions Frequency not defined:

Cardiovascular: Bradycardia, cardiac arrhythmia, cardiomegaly, circulatory shock, edema, embolism (fat), hypertension, hypertrophic cardiomyopathy, myocardial rupture (following recent MI), syncope, tachycardia, thromboembolism, thrombophlebitis, vasculitis

Central nervous system: Abnormal sensory symptoms, arachnoiditis, depression, emotional lability, euphoria, headache, increased intracranial pressure, insomnia, malaise, meningitis, myasthenia, neuritis, neuropathy, paraplegia, paresthesia, personality changes, pseudotumor cerebri, psychic disorder, seizure, spinal cord compression, vertigo

Dermatologic: Acne vulgaris, allergic dermatitis, atrophic striae, diaphoresis, ecchymoses, erythema, exfoliation of skin, fragile skin, hyperpigmentation, hypertrichosis, hypopigmentation, skin atrophy, skin rash, subcutaneous atrophy, suppression of skin test reaction, thinning hair, urticaria, xeroderma

Endocrine & metabolic: Amenorrhea, calcinosis, cushingoid state, decreased glucose tolerance, decreased serum potassium, fluid retention, glycosuria, growth suppression (pediatric), hirsutism, HPA-axis suppression, hypokalemic alkalosis, impaired glucose tolerance/prediabetes, insulin resistance (increased requirements for insulin or oral hyperglycemic agents), moon face, negative nitrogen balance, protein catabolism, sodium retention, weight gain

Gastrointestinal: Abdominal distention, change in bowel habits, hiccups, increased appetite, intestinal perforation, nausea, pancreatitis, peptic ulcer, ulcerative esophagitis

Genitourinary: Bladder dysfunction, spermatozoa disorder (decreased motility and number)

Hematologic & oncologic: Petechia

Hepatic: Hepatomegaly, increased liver enzymes

Hypersensitivity: Anaphylactoid reaction, anaphylaxis, angioedema

Infection: Infection (decreased resistance), sterile abscess

Local: Injection site reaction (intra-articular use). post-injection flare (intra-articular use)

Neuromuscular & skeletal: Amyotrophy, aseptic necrosis of femoral head, aseptic necrosis of humeral head, bone fracture, Charcot arthropathy, lipotrophy, myopathy, osteoporosis, rupture of tendon, steroid myopathy

Ophthalmic: Blindness, blurred vision, cataract, exophthalmos, glaucoma, increased intraocular pressure, papilledema

Respiratory: Pulmonary edema

Miscellaneous: Wound healing impairment

Dosing

Adult Note: Dosages expressed as combined amount of betamethasone sodium phosphate and betamethasone acetate; 1 mg is equivalent to betamethasone sodium phosphate 0.5 mg and betamethasone acetate 0.5 mg.

Usual dosage range: IM: Initial: 0.25 to 9 mg/day (based on severity of disease and patient response).

Indication-specific dosing:

Antenatal fetal maturation (off-label use): IM: 12 mg every 24 hours for a total of 2 doses (ACOG 171 2016). A single course of betamethasone is recommended for women between 24 and 34 weeks of gestation, including those with ruptured membranes or multiple gestations, who are at risk of delivering within 7 days. A single course may be appropriate in some women beginning at 23 weeks gestation or late preterm (between 34 0/7 weeks and 36 6/7 weeks gestation). A single repeat course may be considered in some women with pregnancies less than 34 weeks gestation at risk for delivery within 7 days and who had a course of antenatal corticosteroids >14 days prior (ACOG 171 2016; ACOG 217 2020; ACOG 713 2017).

Bursitis (other than of foot): Intra-articular: 3 to 6 mg (0.5 to 1 mL) for one dose; additional injections may be required for acute exacerbations or chronic conditions; generally, injections should be separated by a minimum of 4 to 6 weeks and limited to ≤4 injections per year. If symptoms are not improved after 1 or 2 injections, additional injections are unlikely to provide benefit (Cardone 2002); following resolution of acute episodes, reduced doses may be warranted for chronic conditions.

Dermatologic conditions: Intradermal: 1.2 mg/cm^2 (0.2 mL/cm^2) into lesion for one dose (maximum: 6 mg [1 mL] weekly).

Foot disorders: Intra-articular: 1.5 mg to 6 mg (0.25 to 1 mL) per dose. Dose is based upon condition; additional injections (when required) should generally be separated by a minimum of 4 to 6 weeks and limited to ≤4 injections per year. If symptoms are not improved after 1 or 2 injections, additional injections are unlikely to provide benefit (Cardone 2002):

Bursitis: 1.5 mg to 3 mg (0.25 to 0.5 mL).

Tenosynovitis: 3 mg (0.5 mL).

Acute gouty arthritis: 3 mg to 6 mg (0.5 to 1 mL).

Multiple sclerosis: Note: Treatment guidelines recommend the use of high-dose IV or oral methylprednisolone for acute exacerbations of multiple sclerosis (AAN [Scott 2011]; NICE 2014).

IM: 30 mg daily for 1 week, followed by 12 mg every other day for 4 weeks.

Rheumatoid and osteoarthritis: Intra-articular: 3 mg to 12 mg (0.5 to 2 mL) for one dose. Dose is based upon the joint size:

Very large (eg, hip): 6 to 12 mg (1 to 2 mL).

Large (eg, knee, ankle, shoulder): 6 mg (1 mL).

Medium (eg, elbow, wrist): 3 mg to 6 mg (0.5 to 1 mL).

Small (eg, inter- or metacarpophalangeal, sternoclavicular): 1.5 mg to 3 mg (0.25 to 0.5 mL).

Tenosynovitis (other than of foot), peritendinitis: Intra-articular: 1.5 to 6 mg (0.25 to 1 mL) depending on joint size for one dose (Cardone 2002; Churgay 2009; Waryasz 2017; manufacturer labeling); additional injections (when required) should generally be separated by a minimum of 4 to 6 weeks and limited to ≤4 injections per year. If symptoms are not improved after 1 or 2 injections, additional injections are unlikely to provide benefit (Cardone 2002; Waryasz 2017).

Geriatric Refer to adult dosing. Use the lowest effective dose.

Renal Impairment: Adult There are no dosage adjustments provided in the manufacturer's labeling.

Hepatic Impairment: Adult There are no dosage adjustments provided in the manufacturer's labeling.

Pediatric Note: Dosages expressed as combined amount of betamethasone sodium phosphate and betamethasone acetate; 1 mg is equivalent to betamethasone sodium phosphate 0.5 mg and betamethasone acetate 0.5 mg. Dosage should be based on severity of disease and patient response; use lowest effective dose for shortest period of time to avoid HPA axis suppression

General dosing, treatment of inflammatory and allergic conditions: Infants, Children, and Adolescents: IM: Initial: 0.02 to 0.3 mg/kg/day (0.6 to 9 mg/m^2/day) in 3 or 4 divided doses

Infantile hemangioma, severe: Limited data available: Infants and Children: Intralesional: Dosage dependent upon size of lesion: Commonly reported: 6 mg administered as a 6 mg/mL (in combination with triamcinolone injection) divided into multiple injections along the lesion perimeter; reported range: 1.5 to 18 mg/dose; doses usually administered every 8 to 14 weeks; reported range: 6 to 25 weeks (Buckmiller, 2008; Chowdri, 1994; Kushner, 1985; Praseyono, 2011). Dosing based on small trials and case-series, mostly reported in infants and children ≤4 years of age. The largest experience (n=70, age range: 2 months to 12 years) prospectively used a betamethasone/triamcinolone combination injection (1.5 to 18 mg betamethasone acetate) and showed that 89.23% of lesions with an initial volume <20 cc^3 regressed by more than 50%, but only 22.2% of lesions with an initial volume >20 cc^3 displayed a good or excellent response (Chowdri, 1994). Another trial (n=25, age range: 7 weeks to 2 years) used lower doses of 3 to 12 mg (in combination with triamcinolone); 16 patients experienced a marked response (Kushner, 1985).

Renal Impairment: Pediatric There are no dosage adjustments provided in the manufacturer's labeling.

Hepatic Impairment: Pediatric There are no dosage adjustments provided in the manufacturer's labeling.

Mechanism of Action Controls the rate of protein synthesis; depresses the migration of polymorphonuclear leukocytes, fibroblasts; reverses capillary permeability and lysosomal stabilization at the cellular level to prevent or control inflammation

Contraindications

Hypersensitivity to any component of the formulation; IM administration contraindicated in immune thrombocytopenia (formerly known as idiopathic thrombocytopenic purpura).

Canadian labeling: Additional contraindications (not in US labeling): Herpes simplex of the eye; systemic fungal infections; vaccinia; cerebral malaria; use in areas with local infection.

Documentation of allergenic cross-reactivity for glucocorticoids is limited. However, because of similarities in chemical structure and/or pharmacologic actions, the possibility of cross-sensitivity cannot be ruled out with certainty.

Warnings/Precautions Avoid concurrent use of other corticosteroids.

May cause hypercortisolism or suppression of hypothalamic-pituitary-adrenal (HPA) axis, particularly in younger children or in patients receiving high doses for prolonged periods. HPA axis suppression may lead to adrenal crisis. Withdrawal and discontinuation of a corticosteroid should be done slowly and carefully. Particular care is required when patients are transferred from systemic corticosteroids to inhaled products due to possible adrenal insufficiency or withdrawal from steroids, including an increase in allergic symptoms. Adult patients receiving >20 mg per day of prednisone (or equivalent) may be most susceptible. Fatalities have occurred due to adrenal insufficiency in asthmatic patients during and after transfer from systemic corticosteroids to aerosol steroids; aerosol steroids do not provide the systemic steroid needed to treat patients having trauma, surgery, or infections. In stressful situations, HPA axis-suppressed patients should receive adequate supplementation with natural glucocorticoids (hydrocortisone or cortisone) rather than betamethasone (due to lack of mineralocorticoid activity).

Acute myopathy has been reported with high-dose corticosteroids, usually in patients with neuromuscular transmission disorders; may involve ocular and/or respiratory muscles; monitor creatine kinase; recovery may be delayed. Corticosteroid use may cause psychiatric disturbances, including depression, euphoria, insomnia, mood swings, and personality changes. Preexisting psychiatric conditions may be exacerbated by corticosteroid use. Prolonged use of corticosteroids may also increase the incidence of secondary infection, mask acute infection (including fungal infections), prolong or exacerbate viral infections, or limit response to killed or inactivated vaccines. Special pathogens (*Amoeba*, *Candida*, *Cryptococcus*, *Mycobacterium*, *Nocardia*, *Pneumocystis*, *Strongyloides*, or *Toxoplasma*) may be activated or an infection exacerbation may occur (may be fatal). Amebiasis or *Strongyloides* infections should be particularly ruled out. Exposure to varicella zoster (chickenpox) should be avoided; corticosteroids should not be used to treat ocular herpes simplex. Corticosteroids should not be used for cerebral malaria or viral hepatitis. Close observation is required in patients with latent tuberculosis and/or TB reactivity; restrict use in active TB (only in conjunction with antituberculosis treatment). Prolonged treatment with corticosteroids has been associated with the development of Kaposi sarcoma (case reports); if noted, discontinuation of therapy should be considered. High-dose corticosteroids should not be used to manage acute head injury. Rare cases of anaphylactoid reactions have been observed in patients receiving corticosteroids.

Use with caution in patients with thyroid disease, hepatic impairment, renal impairment, cardiovascular disease, diabetes, glaucoma, cataracts, myasthenia gravis, patients at risk for osteoporosis, patients at risk for seizures, or GI diseases (diverticulitis, fresh intestinal anastomoses, peptic ulcer, ulcerative colitis) due to perforation risk. Use caution following acute MI (corticosteroids have been associated with myocardial rupture). Use with caution in patients with HF and/or hypertension; long-term use has been associated with fluid retention and electrolyte disturbances. Dietary modifications may be necessary. Use with caution in patients with a recent history of myocardial infarction (MI); left ventricular free wall rupture has been reported after the use of corticosteroids. Use with caution in patients with renal impairment; fluid and sodium retention and increased potassium and calcium excretion may occur. Dietary modifications may be necessary. Not recommended for the treatment of optic neuritis; may increase frequency of new episodes. Intra-articular injection may result in joint tissue damage. Injection into an infected site should be avoided. Injection into a previously infected join is usually not recommended. If infection is suspected, joint fluid examination is recommended. If septic arthritis occurs after injection, institute appropriate antimicrobial therapy. Suspension for injection is for intramuscular, intra-articular or intralesional use only, do not administer intravenously. Corticosteroids are not approved for epidural injection. Serious neurologic events (eg, spinal cord infarction, paraplegia, quadriplegia, cortical blindness, stroke), some resulting in death, have been reported with epidural injection of corticosteroids, with and without use of fluoroscopy. Intra-articular injected corticosteroids may be systemically absorbed. May produce systemic as well as local effects. Appropriate examination of any joint fluid present is necessary to exclude a septic process. Avoid injection into an infected site. Do not inject into unstable joints. Intra-articular injection may result in damage to joint tissues. Potentially significant drug-drug interactions may exist, requiring dose or frequency adjustment, additional monitoring, and/or selection of alternative therapy. Because of the risk of adverse effects, systemic corticosteroids should be used cautiously in the elderly in the smallest possible effective dose for the shortest duration. Withdraw therapy with gradual tapering of dose.

Use with caution in patients with systemic sclerosis; an increase in scleroderma renal crisis incidence has been observed with corticosteroid use. Monitor BP and renal function in patients with systemic sclerosis treated with corticosteroids (EULAR [Kowal-Bielecka 2017]).

Prolonged use in children may affect growth velocity; growth should be routinely monitored in pediatric patients.

Warnings: Additional Pediatric Considerations

Adrenal suppression with failure to thrive has been reported in infants after receiving intralesional corticosteroid injections for treatment of hemangioma (Goyal, 2004). May cause osteoporosis (at any age) or inhibition of bone growth in pediatric patients. Use with caution in patients with osteoporosis. In a population-based study of children, risk of fracture was shown to be increased with >4 courses of corticosteroids; underlying clinical condition may also impact bone health and osteoporotic effect of corticosteroids (Leonard, 2007).

Drug Interactions

Metabolism/Transport Effects None known.

Avoid Concomitant Use

Avoid concomitant use of Betamethasone (Systemic) with any of the following: Aldesleukin; BCG (Intravesical); Cladribine; Desmopressin; Fexinidazole [INT]; Indium 111 Capromab Pendetide; Macimorelin; Mifamurtide; MiFEPRIStone; Natalizumab; Pimecrolimus; Tacrolimus (Topical)

Increased Effect/Toxicity

Betamethasone (Systemic) may increase the levels/effects of: Acetylcholinesterase Inhibitors; Amphotericin B; Androgens; Baricitinib; Deferasirox; Desirudin; Desmopressin; Fexinidazole [INT]; Fingolimod; Leflunomide; Loop Diuretics; Natalizumab; Nicorandil; Nonsteroidal Anti-Inflammatory Agents (COX-2 Selective); Nonsteroidal Anti-Inflammatory Agents (Nonselective); Ozanimod; Quinolones; Ritodrine; Sargramostim; Siponimod; Thiazide and Thiazide-Like Diuretics; Tofacitinib; Upadacitinib; Vaccines (Live); Vitamin K Antagonists

The levels/effects of Betamethasone (Systemic) may be increased by: Aprepitant; Cladribine; CYP3A4 Inhibitors (Strong); Denosumab; DilTIAZem; Estrogen Derivatives; Fosaprepitant; Indacaterol; Inebilizumab; MiFEPRIStone; Neuromuscular-Blocking Agents (Nondepolarizing); Ocrelizumab; Pimecrolimus; Roflumilast; Salicylates; Tacrolimus (Topical); Trastuzumab

Decreased Effect

Betamethasone (Systemic) may decrease the levels/effects of: Aldesleukin; Antidiabetic Agents; Axicabtagene Ciloleucel; BCG (Intravesical); Calcitriol (Systemic); Coccidioides immitis Skin Test; Corticorelin; Cosyntropin; Hyaluronidase; Indium 111 Capromab Pendetide; Isoniazid; Macimorelin; Mifamurtide; Nivolumab; Pidotimod; Salicylates; Sipuleucel-T; Somatropin; Tacrolimus (Systemic); Tertomotide; Tisagenlecleucel; Urea Cycle Disorder Agents; Vaccines (Inactivated); Vaccines (Live)

The levels/effects of Betamethasone (Systemic) may be decreased by: CYP3A4 Inducers (Strong); Echinacea; MiFEPRIStone; Mitotane

Pharmacodynamics/Kinetics

Half-life Elimination 6.5 hours (Peterson 1983)

Time to Peak Serum: IV: 10 to 36 minutes (Peterson 1983)

Pregnancy Considerations

Betamethasone crosses the placenta (Brownfoot 2013) and is partially metabolized by placental enzymes to an inactive metabolite (Murphy 2007).

Some studies have shown an association between first trimester systemic corticosteroid use and oral clefts or decreased birth weight; however, information is conflicting and may be influenced by maternal dose/indication for use (Lunghi 2010; Park-Wyllie 2000; Pradat 2003). Hypoadrenalism may occur in newborns following maternal use of corticosteroids during pregnancy; monitor.

Betamethasone is classified as a fluorinated corticosteroid. When systemic corticosteroids are needed in pregnancy for rheumatic disorders, nonfluorinated corticosteroids (eg, prednisone) are preferred. Chronic high doses should be avoided (ACR [Sammaritano 2020]).

Antenatal corticosteroid administration promotes fetal lung maturity and is associated with the reduction of intraventricular hemorrhage, necrotizing enterocolitis, neonatal mortality, and respiratory distress syndrome. A single course of betamethasone is recommended for women between 24 0/7 and 33 6/7 weeks' gestation who are at risk of delivering within 7 days. This recommendation includes those with ruptured membranes or multiple gestations. A single course of betamethasone may be considered for women beginning at 23 0/7 weeks' gestation who are at risk of delivering within 7 days, in consultation with the family regarding resuscitation. In addition, a single course of betamethasone may be given to women between 34 0/7 weeks and 36 6/7 weeks who are at risk of preterm delivery within 7 days and who have not previously received corticosteroids if induction or delivery will proceed ≥24 hours and ≤7 days; delivery should not be delayed for administration of antenatal corticosteroids. Use of concomitant tocolytics is not currently recommended and administration of late preterm corticosteroids has not been evaluated in women with intrauterine infection, multiple gestations, pregestational diabetes, or women who delivered previously by cesarean section at term. Multiple repeat courses are not recommended.

However, in women with pregnancies less than 34 weeks' gestation at risk for delivery within 7 days and who had a course of antenatal corticosteroids >14 days prior, a single repeat course may be considered; use of a repeat course in women with preterm prelabor rupture of membranes is controversial (ACOG 171 2016; ACOG 217 2020; ACOG 713 2017). Modifications are not required in pregnant patients diagnosed with coronavirus disease 2019 (COVID-19) (ACOG FAQ 2020).

The American College of Obstetricians and Gynecologists (ACOG) and the Society for Maternal-Fetal Medicine (SMFM) have developed an algorithm to aid practitioners in assessing and managing pregnant women with suspected or confirmed COVID-19 (https://www.acog.org/topics/covid-19; https://www.smfm.org/covid19). Interim guidance is also available from the CDC for pregnant women who are diagnosed with COVID-19 (https://www.cdc.gov/coronavirus/2019-ncov/hcp/inpatient-obstetric-healthcare-guidance.html).

Breastfeeding Considerations Corticosteroids are present in breast milk.

The onset of milk secretion after birth may be delayed and the volume of milk produced may be decreased by antenatal betamethasone therapy; this affect was seen when delivery occurred 3 to 9 days after the betamethasone dose in women between 28 and 34 weeks gestation. Antenatal betamethasone therapy did not affect milk production when birth occurred <3 days or >10 days of treatment (Henderson 2008).

The manufacturer notes that when used systemically, maternal use of corticosteroids have the potential to cause adverse events in a breastfed infant (eg, growth suppression, interfere with endogenous corticosteroid production) and therefore, recommends that caution be exercised when administering betamethasone to breastfeeding women. Corticosteroids are generally considered compatible with breastfeeding when used in usual doses; however, monitoring of the breastfeeding infant for adverse reactions is recommended (WHO 2002). Betamethasone is classified as a fluorinated corticosteroid. When systemic corticosteroids are needed in a lactating woman for rheumatic disorders, low doses of nonfluorinated corticosteroids (eg, prednisone) are preferred (ACR [Sammaritano 2020]).

Dosage Forms: US

Kit, Injection:

Pod-Care 100C: Betamethasone sodium phosphate 3 mg and betamethasone acetate 3 mg per 1 mL

ReadySharp Betamethasone: Betamethasone sodium phosphate 3 mg and betamethasone acetate 3 mg per 1 mL

Suspension, Injection:

Celestone Soluspan: Betamethasone sodium phosphate 3 mg and betamethasone acetate 3 mg per 1 mL (5 mL)

Generic: Betamethasone sodium phosphate 3 mg and betamethasone acetate 3 mg per 1 mL (5 mL)

Dosage Forms: Canada

Suspension, Injection:

Celestone Soluspan: Betamethasone sodium phosphate 3 mg and betamethasone acetate 3 mg per 1 mL (1 mL, 5 mL)

Betamethasone (Topical) (bay ta METH a sone)

Related Sample Prescriptions

Ulcerative and Erosive Disorders - Sample Prescriptions *on page 46*

Brand Names: US AlphaTrex [DSC]; Diprolene; Diprolene AF; Luxiq; Sernivo

Brand Names: Canada Betaderm; Beteflam; Celestoderm V; Celestoderm V/2; Diprolene; Diprosone; Luxiq [DSC]; Prevex B [DSC]; Rivasone Scalp; Rolene; Rosone; TARO-Sone; TEVA-Ectosone; TEVA-Topilene; TEVA-Topisone; Valisone Scalp

Generic Availability (US) May be product dependent

Pharmacologic Category Corticosteroid, Topical

Dental Use Treatment of a variety of oral diseases of allergic, inflammatory, or autoimmune origin

Use

Dermatoses: Relief of inflammatory and pruritic manifestations of corticosteroid-responsive dermatoses.

Dermatoses of the scalp (foam): Relief of inflammatory and pruritic manifestations of corticosteroid-responsive dermatoses of the scalp.

Plaque psoriasis (spray; patch [Canadian product]): Treatment of mild to moderate plaque psoriasis in patients 18 years and older.

Local Anesthetic/Vasoconstrictor Precautions No information available to require special precautions

Effects on Dental Treatment No significant effects or complications reported

Effects on Bleeding Variable effects on anticoagulant therapy are observed with glucocorticoids such as betamethasone.

Adverse Reactions

>10%:

Endocrine & metabolic: HPA axis suppression

Local: Application site reaction (≤54%; includes application site burning, stinging of the skin, and application-site pruritus; most reactions were mild)

1% to 10%:

Dermatologic: Acne vulgaris (2%), alopecia (2%)

Nervous system: Paresthesia (2%)

Ophthalmic: Conjunctivitis (2%)

<1%, postmarketing, and/or case reports: Bullous dermatitis, cataract, contact dermatitis, dermatitis, dysgeusia, erythema, erythematous rash, folliculitis, glaucoma, hyperglycemia, hypersensitivity reaction, increased intraocular pressure, localized vesiculation, retinopathy (central serous), skin discoloration, skin rash, telangiectasia

Dental Usual Dosage Allergic or inflammatory diseases: Topical: Gel: Apply small quantity with cotton swab to affected area 3-4 times/day

Dosing

Adult Note: Base dosage on severity of disease and patient response. Use lowest dose possible for shortest period of time to avoid HPA axis suppression. Therapy should be discontinued when control is achieved.

Corticosteroid-responsive dermatoses: Topical:

Cream, augmented formulation: Betamethasone dipropionate 0.05%: Apply once or twice daily (maximum: 50 g weekly).

Cream, unaugmented formulation:

Betamethasone dipropionate 0.05%: Apply once daily; may increase to twice daily if needed

Betamethasone valerate 0.1%: Apply 1 to 3 times daily. **Note:** Once- or twice-daily applications are usually effective.

Foam: Apply to the scalp twice daily, once in the morning and once at night. **Note:** Reassess if no improvement after 2 weeks of treatment.

Gel, augmented formulation: Apply once or twice daily; rub in gently (maximum: 50 g weekly). **Note:** Reassess if no improvement after 2 weeks of treatment.

Lotion, augmented formulation: Betamethasone dipropionate 0.05%: Apply a few drops once or twice daily (maximum: 50 mL weekly). **Note:** Reassess if no improvement after 2 weeks of treatment.

Lotion, unaugmented formulation:

Betamethasone dipropionate 0.05%: Apply a few drops twice daily

Betamethasone valerate 0.1%: Apply a few drops twice daily; may consider increasing dose for resistant cases. Following improvement, may apply once daily.

Ointment, augmented formulation: Betamethasone dipropionate 0.05%: Apply once or twice daily (maximum: 50 g weekly). **Note:** Reassess if no improvement after 2 weeks of treatment.

Ointment, unaugmented formulation:

Betamethasone dipropionate 0.05%: Apply once daily; may increase to twice daily if needed

Betamethasone valerate 0.1%: Apply 1 to 3 times daily. **Note:** Once- or twice-daily applications are usually effective.

Plaque psoriasis: Topical:

Patch [Canadian product]: Betamethasone valerate: Apply 1 patch (2.25 mg) to each affected area once daily [up to 5 patches (11.25 mg) may be applied daily]; maximum duration of therapy: 30 days.

Spray, unaugmented formulation: Betamethasone dipropionate 0.05%: Apply twice daily for up to 4 weeks

Geriatric Refer to adult dosing. Use the lowest effective dose.

Renal Impairment: Adult There are no dosage adjustments provided in the manufacturer's labeling.

Hepatic Impairment: Adult There are no dosage adjustments provided in the manufacturer's labeling.

Pediatric Note: Dosage should be based on severity of disease and patient response; use smallest amount for shortest period of time to avoid HPA axis suppression. Therapy should be discontinued when control is achieved.

Dermatoses (corticosteroid-responsive):

Betamethasone valerate:

Cream 0.1%, ointment 0.1%: Children and Adolescents: Topical: Apply a thin film to the affected area once to 3 times daily; usually once- or twice-daily application is effective.

Lotion 0.1%: Children and Adolescents: Topical: Apply a few drops to the affected area twice daily in the morning and at night; in some cases, more frequent application may be necessary; following improvement reduce to once-daily application.

Betamethasone dipropionate (augmented formulation):

Cream 0.05%, ointment 0.05%: Adolescents: Topical: Apply a thin film to affected area once or twice daily; maximum dose: 50 g/week; evaluate continuation of therapy if no improvement within 2 weeks of treatment.

Gel 0.05%: Children ≥12 years and Adolescents: Topical: Apply a thin layer to the affected area once or twice daily; rub in gently; maximum dose: 50 g/week; not recommended for use longer than 2 weeks.

Lotion 0.05%: Adolescents: Topical: Apply a few drops to the affected area once or twice daily; rub in gently; maximum dose: 50 mL/week; not recommended for use for longer than 2 weeks.

Psoriasis (plaque), treatment: Adolescents ≥18 years of age: *Betamethasone dipropionate spray 0.05%*: Topical: Apply spray to affected area twice daily and rub in gently for up to 4 weeks.

Renal Impairment: Pediatric There are no dosage adjustments provided in the manufacturer's labeling.

Hepatic Impairment: Pediatric There are no dosage adjustments provided in the manufacturer's labeling.

Mechanism of Action Topical corticosteroids have anti-inflammatory, antipruritic, and vasoconstrictive properties. May depress the formation, release, and activity of endogenous chemical mediators of inflammation (kinins, histamine, liposomal enzymes, prostaglandins) through the induction of phospholipase A_2 inhibitory proteins (lipocortins) and sequential inhibition of the release of arachidonic acid. Betamethasone has intermediate to very high range potency (dosage-form dependent).

Contraindications

Hypersensitivity to betamethasone, other corticosteroids, or any component of the formulation

Cream, Lotion: Untreated bacterial, tubercular, and fungal skin infections; viral diseases (eg, herpes simplex, chicken pox, vaccinia)

Canadian labeling: Additional contraindications (not in US labeling): Treatment of rosacea, acne vulgaris, perioral dermatitis, or pruritus without inflammation (foam); skin manifestations relating to tuberculosis or syphilis, eruptions following vaccinations; application to eyes (foam); <18 years of age (patch). **Note:** Product labels may vary (refer also to product labels).

Warnings/Precautions Very high potency topical products are not for treatment of rosacea, perioral dermatitis; not for use on face, groin, or axillae; not for use in a diapered area. Avoid concurrent use of other corticosteroids.

May cause hypercortisolism or suppression of hypothalamic-pituitary-adrenal (HPA) axis, particularly in younger children or in patients receiving high doses for prolonged periods. HPA axis suppression may lead to adrenal crisis.

Topical corticosteroids, including betamethasone, may increase the risk of posterior subcapsular cataracts and glaucoma. Monitor for ocular symptoms. Avoid contact with eyes.

Topical corticosteroids may be absorbed percutaneously. Absorption of topical corticosteroids may cause manifestations of Cushing syndrome (rare), hyperglycemia, or glycosuria. Absorption is increased by the use of occlusive dressings, application to denuded skin, application to large surface areas, or prolonged use. Potentially significant interactions may exist, requiring dose or frequency adjustment, additional monitoring, and/or selection of alternative therapy.

Discontinue if skin irritation or contact dermatitis should occur; do not use in patients with decreased skin circulation. Withdraw therapy with gradual tapering of dose by reducing the frequency of application or substitution of a less potent steroid. Allergic contact dermatitis can occur and is usually diagnosed by failure to heal rather than clinical exacerbation; discontinue use if irritation occurs and treat appropriately.

For topical use only; avoid contact with eyes. Not for oral, ophthalmic, or intravaginal use. Augmented (eg, very high potency) product use in patients <13 years of age is not recommended. Not for treatment of rosacea, perioral dermatitis, or if skin atrophy is present at treatment site; not for facial, groin, axillary, oral, ophthalmic, or intravaginal use. Children may absorb proportionally larger amounts after topical application and may be more prone to systemic effects. HPA axis suppression, intracranial hypertension, and Cushing syndrome have been reported in children receiving topical corticosteroids. Prolonged use may affect growth velocity; growth should be routinely monitored in pediatric patients. Use lowest dose possible for shortest period of time to avoid HPA axis suppression. Foam contains flammable propellants. Avoid fire, flame, and smoking during and immediately following administration. Patch [Canadian product] has not been studied in psoriasis of the face, scalp or intertriginous areas; contains methyl and propyl parahydroxybenzoate, which may cause hypersensitivity (sometimes delayed).

Warnings: Additional Pediatric Considerations

The extent of percutaneous absorption is dependent on several factors, including epidermal integrity (intact vs abraded skin), formulation, age of the patient, prolonged duration of use, and the use of occlusive dressings. Percutaneous absorption of topical steroids is increased in neonates (especially preterm neonates), infants, and young children. Infants and small children may be more susceptible to HPA axis suppression, intracranial hypertension, Cushing syndrome, or other systemic toxicities due to larger skin surface area to body mass ratio. HPA axis suppression was observed in 32% of infants and children (age range: 3 months to 12 years) being treated with betamethasone dipropionate cream (0.05%) for atopic dermatitis in an open-label trial (n=60); the incidence was greater younger patients vs older children (mean reported incidence for age ranges: ≤1 year: 50%; 2 to 8 years: 32% to 38%; 9 to 12 years: 17%).

Some dosage forms may contain propylene glycol; in neonates large amounts of propylene glycol delivered orally, intravenously (eg, >3,000 mg/day), or topically have been associated with potentially fatal toxicities which can include metabolic acidosis, seizures, renal failure, and CNS depression; toxicities have also been reported in children and adults including hyperosmolality, lactic acidosis, seizures and respiratory depression; use caution (AAP 1997; Shehab 2009).

Drug Interactions

Metabolism/Transport Effects None known.

Avoid Concomitant Use

Avoid concomitant use of Betamethasone (Topical) with any of the following: Aldesleukin

Increased Effect/Toxicity

Betamethasone (Topical) may increase the levels/effects of: Deferasirox; Ritodrine

Decreased Effect

Betamethasone (Topical) may decrease the levels/effects of: Aldesleukin; Corticorelin; Hyaluronidase

Pregnancy Considerations

Systemic bioavailability of topical corticosteroids is variable (eg, integrity of skin, use of occlusion) and may be further influenced by trimester of pregnancy (Chi 2017). In general, the use of topical corticosteroids is not associated with a significant risk of adverse pregnancy outcomes. However, there may be an increased risk of low birth weight infants following maternal use of potent or very potent topical products, especially in high doses. Use of mild to moderate potency topical corticosteroids is preferred in pregnant females, and the use of large amounts or use for prolonged periods of time should be avoided (Chi 2016; Chi 2017; Murase 2014). Also avoid areas of high percutaneous absorption (Chi 2017). The risk of stretch marks may be increased with use of topical corticosteroids (Murase 2014).

Breastfeeding Considerations

It is not known if systemic absorption following topical administration results in detectable quantities of betamethasone in breast milk.

Systemic corticosteroids are present in breast milk. According to the manufacturer, the decision to breastfeed during therapy should consider the risk of infant exposure, the benefits of breastfeeding to the infant, and benefits of treatment to the mother. However, topical corticosteroids are generally considered acceptable for use (Butler 2014; WHO 2002).

Do not apply topical corticosteroids to breast until breastfeeding ceases (Leachman 2006); hypertension was noted in a breastfed infant when a high potency topical corticosteroid was applied to the nipple (Butler 2014; Leachman 2006).

Dosage Forms: US

Cream, External:
Diprolene AF: 0.05% (15 g, 50 g)
Generic: 0.05% (15 g, 45 g, 50 g); 0.1% (15 g, 45 g)

Emulsion, External:
Sernivo: 0.05% (120 mL)

Foam, External:
Luxiq: 0.12% (50 g, 100 g)
Generic: 0.12% (50 g, 100 g)

Gel, External:
Generic: 0.05% (15 g, 50 g)

Lotion, External:
Generic: 0.05% (30 mL, 60 mL); 0.1% (60 mL)

Ointment, External:
Diprolene: 0.05% (15 g, 50 g)
Generic: 0.05% (15 g, 45 g, 50 g); 0.1% (15 g, 45 g)

Dosage Forms: Canada

Cream, External:
Betaderm: 0.05% (15 g, 454 g); 0.1% (15 g, 454 g)
Celestoderm V/2: 0.05% (450 g)
Celestoderm V: 0.1% (450 g)
Diprosone: 0.05% (15 g, 50 g)
TARO-Sone: 0.05% (15 g, 50 g, 450 g)
Generic: 0.05% (15 g, 50 g, 450 g); 0.1% (15 g, 450 g)

Lotion, External:
Betaderm: 0.1% (30 mL, 75 mL)
Diprosone: 0.05% (75 mL)
TARO-Sone: 0.05% (30 mL, 75 mL)
Valisone Scalp: 0.1% (30 mL, 75 mL)
Generic: 0.05% (30 mL, 60 mL, 75 mL); 0.1% (30 mL, 60 mL, 75 mL)

Ointment, External:
Betaderm: 0.05% (15 g, 454 g); 0.1% (15 g, 454 g)
Celestoderm V/2: 0.05% (450 g)
Celestoderm V: 0.1% (450 g)
Diprolene: 0.05% (15 g, 50 g)
Diprosone: 0.05% (15 g, 50 g)
Generic: 0.05% (15 g, 50 g, 450 g)

Patch 24 Hour, External:
Beteflam: 2.25 mg (4 ea, 8 ea, 16 ea)

◆ **Betamethasone Acetate** *see* Betamethasone (Systemic) *on page* 233

◆ **Betamethasone Dipropionate** *see* Betamethasone (Topical) *on page* 237

- ◆ **Betamethasone Dipropionate, Augmented** *see* Betamethasone (Topical) *on page 237*
- ◆ **Betamethasone/Propylene Glyc** *see* Betamethasone (Topical) *on page 237*
- ◆ **Betamethasone Sodium Phosphate** *see* Betamethasone (Systemic) *on page 233*
- ◆ **Betamethasone Sod Phos/Acetate** *see* Betamethasone (Systemic) *on page 233*
- ◆ **Betamethasone Valerate** *see* Betamethasone (Topical) *on page 237*
- ◆ **Betapace** *see* Sotalol *on page 1384*
- ◆ **Betapace AF** *see* Sotalol *on page 1384*
- ◆ **Betaquik [OTC]** *see* Medium Chain Triglycerides *on page 953*
- ◆ **Betasept Surgical Scrub [OTC]** *see* Chlorhexidine Gluconate (Topical) *on page 335*
- ◆ **Betaseron** *see* Interferon Beta-1b *on page 835*

Betaxolol (Systemic) (be TAKS oh lol)

Related Information

Cardiovascular Diseases *on page 1654*

Pharmacologic Category Antihypertensive; Beta-Blocker, Beta-1 Selective

Use

Hypertension: Management of hypertension. **Note:** Beta-blockers are **not** recommended as first-line therapy (ACC/AHA [Whelton 2017]).

Local Anesthetic/Vasoconstrictor Precautions No information available to require special precautions

Effects on Dental Treatment Betaxolol is a cardioselective beta-blocker. Local anesthetic with vasoconstrictor can be safely used in patients medicated with betaxolol. Nonselective beta-blockers (ie, propranolol, nadolol) enhance the pressor response to epinephrine or levonordefrin, resulting in hypertension and bradycardia; this has not been reported for betaxolol. Many nonsteroidal anti-inflammatory drugs, such as ibuprofen and indomethacin, can reduce the hypotensive effect of beta-blockers after 3 or more weeks of therapy with the NSAID. Short-term NSAID use (ie, 3 days) requires no special precautions in patients taking beta-blockers.

Effects on Bleeding No information available to require special precautions

Adverse Reactions

2% to 10%:

Cardiovascular: Bradycardia (6% to 8%; symptomatic bradycardia: ≤2%; dose-dependent), chest pain (2% to 7%), cold extremities (2%), palpitations (2%), edema (≤2%; similar to placebo)

Central nervous system: Fatigue (3% to 10%), insomnia (1% to 5%), lethargy (3%), paresthesia (2%)

Gastrointestinal: Nausea (2% to 6%), dyspepsia (4% to 5%), diarrhea (2%)

Hematologic & oncologic: Positive ANA titer (5%)

Neuromuscular & skeletal: Arthralgia (3% to 5%)

Respiratory: Dyspnea (2%), pharyngitis (2%)

<2%, postmarketing, and/or case reports: Abnormal dreams, abnormality in thinking, acidosis, alopecia, amnesia, anemia, angina pectoris, anorexia, arthropathy, ataxia, atrioventricular block, blepharitis, breast fibroadenosis, bronchitis, bronchospasm, cardiac arrhythmia, cardiac failure, cataract, cerebrovascular disease, conjunctivitis, constipation, cough, cystitis, deafness, decreased libido, depression, diabetes mellitus, diaphoresis, dysgeusia, dysphagia, dysuria, emotional lability, epistaxis, erythematous rash, exacerbation of psoriasis, fever, flushing, hallucination, hemophthalmos, hypercholesterolemia, hyperglycemia, hyperkalemia, hyperlipidemia, hypersensitivity reaction, hypertension, hypertrichosis, hyperuricemia, hypoglycemia, hypokalemia, hypotension, impotence, increased lactate dehydrogenase, increased serum ALT, increased serum AST, influenza, intermittent claudication, iritis, labyrinth disease, leukocytosis, lymphadenopathy, malaise, menstrual disease, muscle cramps, myocardial infarction, nervousness, neuralgia, neuropathy, numbness, oliguria, peripheral ischemia, Peyronie's disease, pneumonia, prostatitis, proteinuria, pruritus, purpura, renal insufficiency, rhinitis, rigors, scotoma, sinusitis, skin rash, stupor, syncope, tendonitis, thrombocytopenia, thrombophlebitis, thrombosis, tinnitus, tremor, twitching, visual disturbance, vomiting, weight gain, weight loss, xerostomia

Mechanism of Action Competitively blocks $beta_1$-receptors, with little or no effect on $beta_2$-receptors

Pharmacodynamics/Kinetics

Onset of Action 1 to 1.5 hours

Half-life Elimination 14 to 22 hours; prolonged in hepatic disease and/or chronic renal failure. In patients with chronic renal failure undergoing dialysis, the half-life and AUC are approximately doubled.

Time to Peak 1.5 to 6 hours

Pregnancy Risk Factor C

Pregnancy Considerations

Betaxolol crosses the placenta (Morselli 1990).

Following maternal use of betaxolol, the beta-blocker effects may persist in the neonate for several days after birth. The risk of cardiac and pulmonary complications is increased in the neonate. Bradycardia, hypoglycemia, and respiratory distress have been reported and monitoring of the neonate for 3 to 5 days after birth is recommended.

Chronic maternal hypertension is also associated with adverse events in the fetus/infant. Chronic maternal hypertension may increase the risk of birth defects, low birth weight, premature delivery, stillbirth, and neonatal death. Actual fetal/neonatal risks may be related to duration and severity of maternal hypertension. Untreated chronic hypertension may also increase the risks of adverse maternal outcomes, including gestational diabetes, preeclampsia, delivery complications, stroke, and myocardial infarction (ACOG 203 2019).

The maternal half-life and serum concentration of betaxolol immediately postpartum are not significantly different than what is observed in nonpregnant women (Boutroy 1990; Morselli 1990). When treatment of chronic hypertension in pregnancy is indicated, agents other than betaxolol are preferred (ACOG 203 2019; ESC [Regitz-Zagrosek 2018]; Magee 2014). Females with preexisting hypertension may continue their medication during pregnancy unless contraindications exist (ESC [Regitz-Zagrosek 2018]).

- ◆ **Betaxolol HCl** *see* Betaxolol (Systemic) *on page 240*
- ◆ **Betaxolol Hydrochloride** *see* Betaxolol (Systemic) *on page 240*

Bethanechol (be THAN e kole)

Brand Names: US Urecholine [DSC]

Brand Names: Canada Duvoid; PHL-Bethanechol Chloride [DSC]; PMS-Bethanechol Chloride

Pharmacologic Category Cholinergic Agonist

Use

Neurogenic bladder: Treatment of neurogenic atony of the urinary bladder with retention

Urinary retention: Treatment of acute postoperative and postpartum nonobstructive (functional) urinary retention

Local Anesthetic/Vasoconstrictor Precautions No information available to require special precautions

Effects on Dental Treatment This is a cholinergic agent similar to pilocarpine; expect to see salivation and sweating in patients.

Effects on Bleeding No information available to require special precautions

Adverse Reactions Frequency not defined.

Cardiovascular: Flushing, hypotension, tachycardia

Central nervous system: Colic, headache, malaise, seizure

Dermatologic: Diaphoresis

Gastrointestinal: Abdominal cramps, borborygmi, diarrhea, eructation, nausea, salivation, vomiting

Genitourinary: Urinary urgency

Ophthalmic: Lacrimation, miosis

Respiratory: Asthma, bronchoconstriction

Mechanism of Action Due to stimulation of the parasympathetic nervous system, bethanechol increases bladder muscle tone causing contractions which initiate urination. Bethanechol also stimulates gastric motility, increases gastric tone and may restore peristalsis.

Pharmacodynamics/Kinetics

Onset of Action 30 minutes; Peak effect: ~60 to 90 minutes

Duration of Action ~1 hour (with therapeutic doses); up to 6 hours with large doses (300 to 400 mg)

Pregnancy Risk Factor C

Pregnancy Considerations Animal reproduction studies have not been conducted.

◆ **Bethanechol Chloride** *see* Bethanechol *on page 240*

◆ **Bethkis** *see* Tobramycin (Oral Inhalation) *on page 1456*

Betrixaban (be TRIX a ban)

Related Information

Antiplatelet and Anticoagulation Considerations in Dentistry *on page 1666*

Brand Names: US Bevyxxa [DSC]

Pharmacologic Category Anticoagulant; Anticoagulant, Factor Xa Inhibitor; Direct Oral Anticoagulant (DOAC)

Use

VTE (prophylaxis): Prophylaxis of VTE in adults hospitalized for an acute medical illness who are at risk for thromboembolic complications due to moderate or severe restricted mobility and other risk factors for VTE.

Limitations of use: Safety and effectiveness have not been established in patients with prosthetic heart valves (has not been studied).

Local Anesthetic/Vasoconstrictor Precautions No information available to require special precautions

Effects on Dental Treatment Key adverse event(s) related to dental treatment: Surgical site bleeding may occur; see Effects on Bleeding

Effects on Bleeding Betrixaban inhibits platelet activation and fibrin clot formation via direct, selective, and reversible inhibition of factor Xa. As with all anticoagulants, bleeding is the major adverse effect of betrixaban. Hemorrhage may occur at virtually any site; risk is dependent on multiple variables including the intensity of anticoagulation and patient susceptibility. Medical consult is suggested.

Adverse Reactions

1% to 10%:

Cardiovascular: Hypertension (2%)

Central nervous system: Headache (2%)

Endocrine & metabolic: Hypokalemia (3%)

Gastrointestinal: Constipation (3%), diarrhea (2%), nausea (2%)

Genitourinary: Urinary tract infection (3%), hematuria (2%)

Hematologic & oncologic: Hemorrhage (2%; clinically relevant non-major bleeding)

Respiratory: Epistaxis (2%)

<1%, postmarketing, and/or case reports: Hypersensitivity reaction, major hemorrhage (including gastrointestinal bleeding, intracranial hemorrhage, and intraocular bleeding)

Mechanism of Action Inhibits fibrin clot formation via direct and selective inhibition of factor Xa (FXa). FXa, as part of the prothrombinase complex consisting also of factor Va, calcium ions, and phospholipid, catalyzes the conversion of prothrombin to thrombin. Thrombin both activates platelets and catalyzes the conversion of fibrinogen to fibrin.

Pharmacodynamics/Kinetics

Onset of Action Peak effect: 3 to 4 hours

Duration of Action ≥72 hours

Half-life Elimination 19 to 27 hours

Time to Peak 3 to 4 hours

Reproductive Considerations

Information related to use of direct acting oral anticoagulants in pregnancy is limited; until safety data are available, adequate contraception is recommended during therapy for females of childbearing potential. Females planning a pregnancy should be switched to alternative anticoagulants prior to conception (Cohen 2016b).

Pregnancy Considerations

Information related to the use of direct acting oral anticoagulants during pregnancy is limited and information specific to betrixaban has not been reported (Beyer-Westendorf 2016; Lameijer 2018). Use of direct acting oral anticoagulants increases the risk of bleeding in all patients. When used in pregnancy, there is also the potential for fetal bleeding or subclinical placental bleeding which may increase the risk of miscarriage, preterm delivery, fetal compromise, or stillbirth (Cohen 2016b).

Data are insufficient to evaluate the safety of direct acting oral anticoagulants during pregnancy (Bates 2012) and use in pregnant females is not recommended (ESC [Regitz-Zagrosek 2018]). Agents other than betrixaban are preferred for VTE prophylaxis in pregnant patients (ESC [Regitz-Zagrosek 2018]). Patients should be switched to an alternative anticoagulant if pregnancy occurs during therapy. Fetal monitoring that includes evaluations for fetal bleeding and assessments for risk of preterm delivery are recommended if the direct acting oral anticoagulant is continued (Cohen 2016b).

Product Availability Bevyxxa is no longer available in the United States.

Dental Health Professional Considerations Routine coagulation testing (INR) is not required, or necessary, for Direct-Acting Oral Anticoagulants (DOAC).

◆ **Betrixaban Maleate** *see* Betrixaban *on page 241*

Bevacizumab (be vuh SIZ uh mab)

Related Information

Osteonecrosis of the Jaw *on page 1699*

Brand Names: US Avastin; Mvasi; Zirabev

Brand Names: Canada Avastin; Mvasi; Zirabev

Pharmacologic Category Antineoplastic Agent, Monoclonal Antibody; Antineoplastic Agent, Vascular Endothelial Growth Factor (VEGF) Inhibitor; Vascular Endothelial Growth Factor (VEGF) Inhibitor

Use

Cervical cancer, persistent/recurrent/metastatic (Avastin and bevacizumab biosimilars): Treatment of persistent, recurrent, or metastatic cervical cancer (in combination with paclitaxel and either cisplatin or topotecan).

Colorectal cancer, metastatic (Avastin and bevacizumab biosimilars): First- or second-line treatment of metastatic colorectal cancer (CRC) (in combination with fluorouracil-based chemotherapy); second-line treatment of metastatic CRC (in combination with fluoropyrimidine-irinotecan- or fluoropyrimidine-oxaliplatin-based chemotherapy) after progression on a first-line treatment containing bevacizumab.

Limitations of use: Not indicated for the adjuvant treatment of colon cancer.

Glioblastoma, recurrent (Avastin and bevacizumab biosimilars): Treatment of recurrent glioblastoma in adults.

Hepatocellular carcinoma, unresectable or metastatic (Avastin only): Treatment of unresectable or metastatic hepatocellular carcinoma (in combination with atezolizumab) in patients who have not received prior systemic therapy.

Non-small cell lung cancer, nonsquamous (Avastin and bevacizumab biosimilars): First-line treatment of unresectable, locally advanced, recurrent or metastatic nonsquamous non-small cell lung cancer (in combination with carboplatin and paclitaxel).

Ovarian (epithelial), fallopian tube, or primary peritoneal cancer (Avastin only):

Stage III or IV disease, following initial surgical resection: Treatment of stage III or IV epithelial ovarian, fallopian tube, or primary peritoneal cancer following initial surgical resection (in combination with carboplatin and paclitaxel, followed by single-agent bevacizumab).

Platinum-resistant recurrent: Treatment of platinum-resistant recurrent epithelial ovarian, fallopian tube, or primary peritoneal cancer (in combination with paclitaxel, doxorubicin [liposomal], or topotecan) in patients who received no more than 2 prior chemotherapy regimens.

Platinum-sensitive recurrent: Treatment of platinum-sensitive recurrent epithelial ovarian, fallopian tube, or primary peritoneal cancer (in combination with carboplatin and paclitaxel or with carboplatin and gemcitabine and then followed by single-agent bevacizumab).

Renal cell carcinoma, metastatic (Avastin and bevacizumab biosimilars): Treatment of metastatic renal cell carcinoma (in combination with interferon alfa).

Note: Mvasi (bevacizumab-awwb) and Zirabev (bevacizumab-bvzr) are approved as biosimilars to Avastin (bevacizumab).

Local Anesthetic/Vasoconstrictor Precautions No information available to require special precautions

Effects on Dental Treatment Key adverse event(s) related to dental treatment: Xerostomia (normal salivary flow resumes upon discontinuation), stomatitis, taste disorder, and gingival bleeding.

Cases of osteonecrosis of the jaw (ONJ) have been associated with bevacizumab exposure. ONJ presents clinically as exposed necrotic bone of at least 8 weeks duration with or without the presence of pain, infection, or previous trauma in a patient who has not received radiation to the jaw. Since ONJ is also associated with bisphosphonate exposure and bisphosphonates are known to have antiangiogenic properties, inhibition of angiogenesis may play a role in ONJ associated with these two classes of drugs. Patients developing ONJ while on bevacizumab therapy should receive care by an oral surgeon. See Dental Health Professional Considerations.

Effects on Bleeding Minor gum bleeding has been reported in 2% to 4% of patients. Thrombocytopenia has been reported. A medical consult is suggested.

Adverse Reactions Percentages reported as monotherapy and as part of combination chemotherapy regimens. Some studies only reported hematologic toxicities grades ≥4 and nonhematologic toxicities grades ≥3.

>10%:

Cardiovascular: Hypertension (24% to 42%), peripheral edema (15%), venous thromboembolism (grades 3/4: 5% to 11%)

Dermatologic: Exfoliative dermatitis, xeroderma

Endocrine & metabolic: Hyperglycemia (26%), hypoalbuminemia (16%), hypomagnesemia (24%), hyponatremia (19%), ovarian failure (34%), weight loss (20% to 21%)

Gastrointestinal: Abdominal pain (grade 3/4: 8% to 12%), decreased appetite (34% to 36%), diarrhea (21% to 40%), dysgeusia, nausea (53% to 72%), stomatitis (15% to 25%)

Genitourinary: Pelvic pain (14%), proteinuria (5% to 20%), urinary tract infection (22%)

Hematologic & oncologic: Bruise (17%), leukopenia (grades 3/4: 37% to 53%), lymphocytopenia (12%; grades 3/4: 6%), neutropenia (12%; grades 3/4: 8% to 21%), pulmonary hemorrhage (4% to 31%), thrombocytopenia (58%; grade 3/4: 20% to 40%)

Nervous system: Anxiety (17%), dizziness (23%), dysarthria (8% to 12%), fatigue (33% to 82%), headache (22% to 49%), insomnia (21%), myasthenia (13% to 15%), voice disorder (5% to 13%)

Neuromuscular & skeletal: Arthralgia (28% to 41%), back pain (12% to 21%), limb pain (19% to 25%), myalgia (19%)

Ophthalmic: Disease of the lacrimal apparatus

Renal: Increased serum creatinine (16%)

Respiratory: Cough (26%), dyspnea (26% to 30%), epistaxis (17% to 55%), oropharyngeal pain (16%), sinusitis (15%)

Miscellaneous: Postoperative wound complication (5% to 15%)

1% to 10%:

Cardiovascular: Arterial thrombosis (grades ≥3: 5%), decreased left ventricular ejection fraction (10%), deep vein thrombosis (grades 3/4: 9%), intra-abdominal venous thrombosis (grades 3/4: 3%), left ventricular dysfunction (grades 3/4: 1%), pulmonary embolism (1%), syncope (grades 3/4: 3%), thrombosis (10%)

Dermatologic: Acne vulgaris (1%), cellulitis (grades 3/4: 3%)

Endocrine & metabolic: Dehydration (grades 3/4: 4%), hypokalemia (grades 3/4: 7%)
Gastrointestinal: Constipation (grades 3/4: 4%), fistula of bile duct (≤2%), gastritis (1%), gastroesophageal reflux disease (2%), gastrointestinal fistula (≤2%), gastrointestinal perforation (≤3%), gingival hemorrhage (4% to 7%), gingival pain (1%), gingivitis (2%), hemorrhoids (8%), oral mucosa ulcer (2%), rectal fistula (6%), rectal pain (6%), tracheoesophageal fistula (≤2%)
Genitourinary: Bladder fistula (≤2%), vaginal fistula (≤2%)
Hematologic & oncologic: Hemorrhage (grades ≥3: ≤7%; including major hemorrhage)
Infection: Infection (10%), tooth abscess (2%)
Nervous system: Pain (grades 3/4: 8%)
Neuromuscular & skeletal: Asthenia (grades 3/4: 10%)
Ophthalmic: Blurred vision (2%)
Otic: Deafness (1%), tinnitus (2%)
Renal: Renal fistula (≤2%)
Respiratory: Bronchopleural fistula (≤2%), nasal congestion (8%), nasal signs and symptoms (7% to 10%), rhinitis (≥3%), rhinorrhea (10%)
Miscellaneous: Fistula (≤2%), infusion related reaction (<3%; severe infusion related reaction: <1%, including hypertensive crisis)

<1%:
Genitourinary: Nephrotic syndrome
Immunologic: Antibody development
Nervous system: Reversible posterior leukoencephalopathy syndrome

Frequency not defined:
Cardiovascular: Acute myocardial infarction, angina pectoris, cerebral infarction, transient ischemic attacks
Gastrointestinal: Gastrointestinal hemorrhage, hematemesis
Genitourinary: Vaginal hemorrhage
Hypersensitivity reaction: Hypersensitivity reaction
Nervous system: Intracranial hemorrhage
Respiratory: Hemoptysis

Postmarketing:
Cardiovascular: Mesenteric thrombosis
Gastrointestinal: Gallbladder perforation, gastrointestinal anastomotic ulcer, gastrointestinal ulcer, intestinal necrosis
Hematologic & oncologic: Pancytopenia
Neuromuscular & skeletal: Fulminant necrotizing fasciitis, osteonecrosis of the jaw, polyserositis
Ophthalmic: Inflammation of anterior segment of eye (toxic anterior segment syndrome) (Sato 2010)
Renal: Renal thrombotic microangiopathy
Respiratory: Nasal septum perforation, pulmonary hypertension

Mechanism of Action Bevacizumab is a recombinant, humanized monoclonal antibody which binds to, and neutralizes, vascular endothelial growth factor (VEGF), preventing its association with endothelial receptors, Flt-1 and KDR. VEGF binding initiates angiogenesis (endothelial proliferation and the formation of new blood vessels). The inhibition of microvascular growth is believed to retard the growth of all tissues (including metastatic tissue).

Pharmacodynamics/Kinetics

Half-life Elimination

IV:
Pediatric patients (age: 1 to 21 years): Median: 11.8 days (range: 4.4 to 14.6 days) (Glade Bender 2008)
Adults: ~20 days (range: 11 to 50 days)
Intravitreal: ~5 to 10 days (Bakri 2007; Krohne 2008)

Reproductive Considerations

Evaluate pregnancy status prior to use in females of reproductive potential. Women of reproductive potential should use effective contraception during therapy and for 6 months following the last bevacizumab dose.

In premenopausal women with solid tumors receiving adjuvant therapy, the incidence of ovarian failure was 34% for bevacizumab with chemotherapy versus 2% for chemotherapy alone. Recovery of ovarian function (resumption of menses, positive serum β-HCG pregnancy test, or follicle-stimulating hormone level <30 mIU/mL) at all time points in the post-treatment period after bevacizumab discontinuation was demonstrated in approximately 22% of females who received bevacizumab. The long-term effects of bevacizumab on fertility are unknown. Females of reproductive potential should be informed of the potential risk of ovarian failure prior to bevacizumab initiation.

Pregnancy Considerations

Bevacizumab is a vascular endothelial growth factor (VEGF) inhibitor; VEGF is required to achieve and maintain normal pregnancies (Peracha 2016). Based on findings in animal reproduction studies and on the mechanism of action, bevacizumab may cause fetal harm if administered to a pregnant woman. Information from postmarketing reports following systemic exposure in pregnancy is limited.

Information following intravitreal bevacizumab use in pregnancy is also limited (Introini 2012; Kianersi 2016; Petrou 2010; Polizzi 2015a; Polizzi 2015b; Sarmad 2016; Sullivan 2014; Tarantola 2010; Wu 2010). Based on studies in nonpregnant adults, VEGF inhibitors can alter systemic concentrations of VEGF and placental growth factor following intravitreal administration (Peracha 2016; Zehetner 2015). Until additional information is available, intravitreal use during the first trimester should be avoided and use later in pregnancy should be based on patient specific risks versus benefits (Peracha 2016; Polizzi 2015b).

Systemic administration of bevacizumab was found to cause a preeclampsia-like syndrome in nonpregnant females (Cross 2012). Preeclampsia was reported in a pregnant female following intravitreal administration; however, this case also had a significant obstetric history which may have contributed to this finding (Sullivan 2014).

Dental Health Professional Considerations Three case reports describe the development of ONJ in association with bevacizumab therapy. All three cases were cancer patients treated with bevacizumab 10 mg/kg every 2 weeks and 15 mg/kg every 3 weeks (Estilo 2009; Greuter 2008). Another report showed that a combination of bisphosphonates and antiangiogenic factors (primarily bevacizumab) induces ONJ more frequently than bisphosphonates alone. Of the 25 patients receiving concurrent treatment with bisphosphonates and the antiangiogenic drug bevacizumab, four developed ONJ (16%). Of the 91 patients receiving bisphosphonates without antiangiogenic factors, one developed ONJ (1.1%), a significant statistical difference (Christodoulou 2009).

◆ **Bevacizumab-awwb** *see* Bevacizumab *on page 242*
◆ **Bevacizumab-bvzr** *see* Bevacizumab *on page 242*
◆ **Bevacizumab, inj** *see* Bevacizumab *on page 242*
◆ **Bevespi Aerosphere** *see* Glycopyrrolate and Formoterol *on page 743*
◆ **Bevyxxa [DSC]** *see* Betrixaban *on page 241*

- **Bexsero** *see* Meningococcal Group B Vaccine *on page 963*
- **Beyaz** *see* Ethinyl Estradiol, Drospirenone, and Levomefolate *on page 618*
- **BG-12** *see* Dimethyl Fumarate *on page 501*
- **BGB-3111** *see* Zanubrutinib *on page 1568*
- **BI 397** *see* Dalbavancin *on page 430*
- **BI-1356** *see* LinaGLIPtin *on page 917*
- **BI10773** *see* Empagliflozin *on page 555*
- **Biaxin [DSC]** *see* Clarithromycin *on page 361*
- **BIBF1120** *see* Nintedanib *on page 1108*
- **Bicillin L-A** *see* Penicillin G Benzathine *on page 1208*
- **Bicillin C-R** *see* Penicillin G Benzathine and Penicillin G Procaine *on page 1209*
- **Bicillin C-R 900/300** *see* Penicillin G Benzathine and Penicillin G Procaine *on page 1209*

Binimetinib (bin i ME ti nib)

Brand Names: US Mektovi

Pharmacologic Category Antineoplastic Agent, MEK Inhibitor

Use Melanoma, unresectable or metastatic: Treatment of unresectable or metastatic melanoma with a BRAF V600E or V600K mutation (in combination with encorafenib) as detected by an approved test.

Local Anesthetic/Vasoconstrictor Precautions No information available to require special precautions

Effects on Dental Treatment Key adverse event(s) related to dental treatment: Hypertension reported (>10%); consider monitoring blood pressure prior to using local anesthetic with a vasoconstrictor

Effects on Bleeding Frequent hemorrhagic events reported which were gastrointestinal in nature, although none involving the oral cavity

Adverse Reactions Incidences of adverse reactions were defined during combination therapy with encorafenib.

>10%:

Cardiovascular: Peripheral edema (13%), hypertension (11%)

Central nervous system: Fatigue (43%), dizziness (15%)

Dermatologic: Skin rash (22%)

Endocrine & metabolic: Increased gamma-glutamyl transferase (45%), hyponatremia (18%)

Gastrointestinal: Nausea (41%), diarrhea (36%), vomiting (30%), abdominal pain (28%), constipation (22%)

Hematologic & oncologic: Anemia (36%, grades 3/4: 4%), hemorrhage (19%; grades 3/4:3%), leukopenia (13%), lymphocytopenia (13%, grades 3/4: 2%), neutropenia (13%, grades 3/4: 3%)

Hepatic: Increased serum alanine aminotransferase (29%), increased serum aspartate aminotransferase (27%), increased serum alkaline phosphatase (21%)

Neuromuscular & skeletal: Increased creatine phosphokinase in blood specimen (58%)

Ophthalmic: Visual impairment (20%), retinal pigment changes (≤20%, retinal pigment epithelial dystrophy), retinopathy (≤20%, serous including 8% retinal detachment and 6% macular edema)

Renal: Increased serum creatinine (93%)

Miscellaneous: Fever (18%)

1% to 10%:

Cardiovascular: Decreased left ventricular ejection fraction (7%), venous thromboembolism (6%), pulmonary embolism (3%)

Gastrointestinal: Colitis (<10%), hematochezia (3%), hemorrhoidal bleeding (1%)

Hematologic & oncologic: Rectal hemorrhage (4%)

Hypersensitivity: Hypersensitivity (<10%)

Neuromuscular & skeletal: Panniculitis (<10%)

Ophthalmic: Uveitis (4%)

Frequency not defined:

Cardiovascular: Left ventricular dysfunction

Central nervous system: Headache

<1%, postmarketing, and/or case reports: Interstitial pulmonary disease, pneumonitis, retinal vein occlusion, rhabdomyolysis

Mechanism of Action Binimetinib reversibly inhibits mitogen-activated extracellular kinase (MEK) 1 and 2 activation and kinase activity. MEK proteins are upstream regulators of the extracellular signal-related kinase (ERK) pathway. Binimetinib inhibits ERK phosphorylation and viability and MEK-dependent phosphorylation of the protein kinase B-raf (BRAF) mutant cell lines. The combination of binimetinib and encorafenib allows for greater antitumor activity in BRAF V600 mutant cell lines; in animal studies, the combination also delayed the emergence of resistance in BRAF V600E mutant cells compared to either drug alone.

Pharmacodynamics/Kinetics

Half-life Elimination 3.5 hours

Time to Peak 1.6 hours

Reproductive Considerations Verify pregnancy status in females of reproductive potential prior to initiating binimetinib therapy. Females of reproductive potential should use a highly effective contraceptive during therapy and for at least 30 days after the final binimetinib dose.

Pregnancy Considerations

Based on its mechanism of action and on findings in animal reproduction studies, binimetinib may cause fetal harm if administered during pregnancy.

Prescribing and Access Restrictions Binimetinib is available through a network of select specialty pharmacies. Refer to https://www.braftovimektovi.com/hcp/ for more information.

- **Binosto** *see* Alendronate *on page 95*
- **Bio-D-Mulsion [OTC] [DSC]** *see* Cholecalciferol *on page 344*
- **Bio-D-Mulsion Forte [OTC] [DSC]** *see* Cholecalciferol *on page 344*
- **Bionect** *see* Hyaluronate and Derivatives *on page 761*
- **Biorphen** *see* Phenylephrine (Systemic) *on page 1227*
- **Bio-Statin** *see* Nystatin (Oral) *on page 1121*
- **Biotene Dry Mouth Gentle [OTC]** *see* Saliva Substitute *on page 1354*
- **Biotene Moisturizing Mouth Spray [OTC]** *see* Saliva Substitute *on page 1354*
- **Biotene Oral Balance [OTC]** *see* Saliva Substitute *on page 1354*
- **Bird Flu Vaccine** *see* Influenza A Virus Vaccine (H5N1) *on page 811*
- **Bismuth/Metronid/Tetracycline** *see* Bismuth Subcitrate, Metronidazole, and Tetracycline *on page 245*

Bismuth Subcitrate, Metronidazole, and Tetracycline

(BIZ muth sub CIT rate, me troe NI da zole, & tet ra SYE kleen)

Brand Names: US Pylera

Pharmacologic Category Antibiotic, Miscellaneous; Antibiotic, Tetracycline Derivative; Antidiarrheal

Use Duodenal ulcer associated with *Helicobacter pylori* infection: In combination with omeprazole for the treatment of patients with *H. pylori* infection and duodenal ulcer disease (active or history of within the past 5 years) to eradicate *H. pylori*.

Local Anesthetic/Vasoconstrictor Precautions No information available to require special precautions

Effects on Dental Treatment Tetracyclines are not recommended for use during pregnancy since they can cause enamel hypoplasia and permanent teeth discoloration; long-term use associated with oral candidiasis; taste perversion has been reported.

Effects on Bleeding No information available to require special precautions

Adverse Reactions Also see individual agents. Adverse reactions are associated with concomitant administration of omeprazole.

>10%: Gastrointestinal: Abnormal stools (16%)

1% to 10%:

Central nervous system: Headache (5%), dizziness (3%)

Dermatologic: Maculopapular rash (1%)

Gastrointestinal: Nausea (8%), diarrhea (7%), abdominal pain (5%), dysgeusia (4%), dyspepsia (3%), constipation (1%), xerostomia (1%)

Genitourinary: Vaginitis (3%), urine abnormality (1%)

Hepatic: Increased serum ALT (1%), increased serum AST (1%)

Neuromuscular & skeletal: Weakness (3%)

Miscellaneous: Laboratory test abnormality (2%)

<1%, postmarketing, and/or case reports: Abdominal distention, anxiety, back pain, candidiasis, chest discomfort, chest pain, drowsiness, duodenal ulcer, eructation, fatigue, flatulence, gastritis, gastroenteritis, increased appetite, increased creatine phosphokinase, malaise, myalgia, skin rash, tachycardia, tongue discoloration (darkening), visual disturbance, vomiting, weight gain

Mechanism of Action

Bismuth: Has both antisecretory and antimicrobial action; may provide some anti-inflammatory action as well.

Metronidazole: After diffusing into the organism, interacts with DNA to cause a loss of helical DNA structure and strand breakage resulting in inhibition of protein synthesis and cell death in susceptible organisms.

Tetracycline: Inhibits bacterial protein synthesis by binding with the 30S and possibly the 50S ribosomal subunit(s) of susceptible bacteria; may also cause alterations in the cytoplasmic membrane.

Bismuth, metronidazole, and tetracycline individually have demonstrated *in vitro* activity against most susceptible strains of *H. pylori* isolated from patients with duodenal ulcers.

Pregnancy Considerations

This combination is contraindicated in women who are pregnant. Metronidazole and tetracycline both cross the human placenta and may have adverse effects to the fetus. See individual monographs for additional information.

◆ **Bismuth Subcitrate Potassium, Tetracycline, and Metronidazole** *see* Bismuth Subcitrate, Metronidazole, and Tetracycline *on page 245*

◆ **Bismuth Subsalicylate, Metronidazole, and Tetracycline** *see* Tetracycline, Bismuth Subsalicylate, and Metronidazole *on page 1433*

◆ **Bismuth Subsalicylate, Metronidazole, and Tetracycline Hydrochloride** *see* Tetracycline, Bismuth Subsalicylate, and Metronidazole *on page 1433*

◆ **Bismuth Subsalicylate, Tetracycline, and Metronidazole** *see* Tetracycline, Bismuth Subsalicylate, and Metronidazole *on page 1433*

Bisoprolol (bis OH proe lol)

Related Information

Cardiovascular Diseases *on page 1654*

Brand Names: US Zebeta [DSC]

Brand Names: Canada APO-Bisoprolol; MINT-Bisoprolol; MYLAN-Bisoprolol [DSC]; PMS-Bisoprolol; PRO-Bisoprolol-10; PRO-Bisoprolol-5; RIVA-Bisoprolol; SANDOZ Bisoprolol; TEVA-Bisoprolol

Pharmacologic Category Antihypertensive; Beta-Blocker, Beta-1 Selective

Use Hypertension: Management of hypertension. **Note:** Beta-blockers are **not** recommended as first-line therapy (ACC/AHA [Whelton 2017]).

Local Anesthetic/Vasoconstrictor Precautions No information available to require special precautions

Effects on Dental Treatment Bisoprolol is a cardioselective beta-blocker. Local anesthetic with vasoconstrictor can be safely used in patients medicated with bisoprolol. Nonselective beta-blockers (ie, propranolol, nadolol) enhance the pressor response to epinephrine, resulting in hypertension and bradycardia; this has not been reported for bisoprolol. Many nonsteroidal anti-inflammatory drugs, such as ibuprofen and indomethacin, can reduce the hypotensive effect of beta-blockers after 3 or more weeks of therapy with the NSAID. Short-term NSAID use (ie, 3 days) requires no special precautions in patients taking beta-blockers.

Effects on Bleeding No information available to require special precautions

Adverse Reactions

1% to 10%:

Cardiovascular: Chest pain (1%)

Central nervous system: Fatigue (7%), hypoesthesia (1%)

Gastrointestinal: Diarrhea (3%), vomiting (1%)

Hepatic: Increased serum alanine aminotransferase (≤4%), increased serum aspartate aminotransferase (≤4%)

Respiratory: Upper respiratory tract infection (5%), dyspnea (1%)

Frequency not defined:

Cardiovascular: Cardiac arrhythmia, cardiac failure, claudication, cold extremities, edema, flushing, hypersensitivity angiitis, hypotension, orthostatic hypotension, palpitations

Central nervous system: Anxiety, depression, dizziness, drowsiness, headache, hyperesthesia, insomnia, lack of concentration, malaise, memory impairment, paresthesia, restlessness, sensation of eye pressure, twitching, vertigo, vivid dream

Dermatologic: Acne vulgaris, alopecia, diaphoresis, eczema, pruritus, skin irritation, skin rash

Endocrine & metabolic: Decreased libido, gout, increased serum glucose, increased serum phosphate, increased serum potassium, increased serum triglycerides, increased uric acid, weight gain
Gastrointestinal: Abdominal pain, constipation, dysgeusia, dyspepsia, epigastric pain, gastric pain, gastritis, nausea, peptic ulcer, xerostomia
Genitourinary: Cystitis, impotence
Hematologic & oncologic: Decreased white blood cell count, positive ANA titer, purpuric rash, thrombocytopenia
Neuromuscular & skeletal: Back pain, muscle cramps, myalgia, neck pain, tremor
Ophthalmic: Abnormal lacrimation, eye pain, visual disturbance
Otic: Otalgia, tinnitus
Renal: increased blood urea nitrogen, increased serum creatinine, polyuria, renal colic
Respiratory: Asthma, bronchitis, bronchospasm, cough, dyspnea on exertion, pharyngitis, rhinitis, sinusitis

<1%, postmarketing, and/or case reports: Angioedema, arthralgia, asthenia, auditory impairment, bradycardia, dermatitis, exfoliative dermatitis, Peyronie disease, psoriasis, sleep disturbance, syncope, unsteadiness

Mechanism of Action Selective inhibitor of $beta_1$-adrenergic receptors; competitively blocks $beta_1$-receptors, with little or no effect on $beta_2$-receptors at doses ≤20 mg

Pharmacodynamics/Kinetics

Onset of Action 1 to 2 hours

Half-life Elimination Normal renal function: 9 to 12 hours; CrCl <40 mL/minute: 27 to 36 hours; Hepatic cirrhosis: 8 to 22 hours

Time to Peak 2 to 4 hours

Pregnancy Risk Factor C

Pregnancy Considerations

Exposure to beta-blockers during pregnancy may increase the risk for adverse events in the neonate. If maternal use of a beta-blocker is needed, fetal growth should be monitored during pregnancy and the newborn should be monitored for 48 hours after delivery for bradycardia, hypoglycemia, and respiratory depression (ESC [Regitz-Zagrosek 2018]).

Chronic maternal hypertension is also associated with adverse events in the fetus/infant. Chronic maternal hypertension may increase the risk of birth defects, low birth weight, premature delivery, stillbirth, and neonatal death. Actual fetal/neonatal risks may be related to duration and severity of maternal hypertension. Untreated chronic hypertension may also increase the risks of adverse maternal outcomes, including gestational diabetes, preeclampsia, delivery complications, stroke, and myocardial infarction (ACOG 203 2019).

When treatment of chronic hypertension in pregnancy is indicated, agents other than bisoprolol are preferred (ACOG 203 2019; ESC [Regitz-Zagrosek 2018]; Magee 2014). Females with preexisting hypertension may continue their medication during pregnancy unless contraindications exist (ESC [Regitz-Zagrosek 2018]).

◆ **Bisoprolol Fumarate** *see* Bisoprolol *on page 245*

◆ **Bis-POM PMEA** *see* Adefovir *on page 86*

◆ **Bistropamide** *see* Tropicamide *on page 1502*

◆ **Bivalent Human Papillomavirus Vaccine** *see* Papillomavirus (Types 16, 18) Vaccine (Human, Recombinant) *on page 1191*

Bivalirudin (bye VAL i roo din)

Related Information

Cardiovascular Diseases *on page 1654*

Brand Names: US Angiomax

Brand Names: Canada Angiomax

Pharmacologic Category Anticoagulant; Anticoagulant, Direct Thrombin Inhibitor

Use Percutaneous coronary intervention: Anticoagulant for use in patients undergoing percutaneous coronary intervention (PCI) including patients with heparin-induced thrombocytopenia (HIT) and heparin-induced thrombocytopenia/thrombosis syndrome (HIT/TS)

Local Anesthetic/Vasoconstrictor Precautions No information available to require special precautions

Effects on Dental Treatment Key adverse event(s) related to dental treatment: Bleeding is the major adverse effect of bivalirudin. Additional adverse effects are often related to idiosyncratic reactions, the frequency is difficult to estimate. Adverse reactions reported were generally less than those seen with heparin. See Effects on Bleeding.

Effects on Bleeding As with all anticoagulants, bleeding is a potential adverse effect of bivalirudin during dental surgery; risk is dependent on multiple variables, including the intensity of anticoagulation and patient susceptibility. Medical consult is suggested. It is unlikely that ambulatory patients presenting for dental treatment will be taking intravenous anticoagulant therapy such as bivalirudin.

Adverse Reactions As with all anticoagulants, bleeding is the major adverse effect of bivalirudin. Hemorrhage may occur at virtually any site. Risk is dependent on multiple variables, including the intensity of anticoagulation, concurrent use of a glycoprotein IIb/IIIa inhibitor, and patient susceptibility. Additional adverse effects are often related to idiosyncratic reactions, and the frequency is difficult to estimate. Adverse reactions reported were generally less than those seen with heparin.

>10%:
Cardiovascular: Hypotension (≤12%)
Central nervous system: Pain (≤15%), headache (≤12%)
Gastrointestinal: Nausea (≤15%)
Hematologic & oncologic: Minor hemorrhage (Protocol defined: 14%; heparin 26%; TIMI defined: 1%; heparin 3% [Lincoff, 2003])
Neuromuscular & skeletal: Back pain (9% to 42%)

1% to 10%:
Cardiovascular: Hypertension (6%), bradycardia (5%), angina pectoris (≤5%), thrombosis (1%; <4 hours, in patients with STEMI undergoing primary PCI)
Central nervous system: Insomnia (7%), anxiety (6%), nervousness (5%)
Gastrointestinal: Vomiting (≤6%), abdominal pain (5%), dyspepsia (5%)
Genitourinary: Pelvic pain (6%), urinary retention (4%)
Hematologic & oncologic: Major hemorrhage (Protocol defined: 2% to 4%; heparin 4% to 9%; TIMI defined: 0.6%; heparin 0.9%; transfusion required: 1% to 2%; heparin 2% to 6% [Lincoff, 2003])
Local: Pain at injection site (≤8%)
Miscellaneous: Fever (5%)

<1%, postmarketing, and/or case reports: Cardiac tamponade, cerebral ischemia, confusion, facial paralysis, hemorrhage, hypersensitivity reaction (including anaphylaxis), increased INR, increased susceptibility to infection, intracranial hemorrhage, oliguria, pulmonary

edema, pulmonary hemorrhage, renal failure, retroperitoneal hemorrhage, sepsis, syncope, thrombocytopenia, vascular disease, venous thrombosis (during PCI, including intracoronary brachytherapy), ventricular fibrillation

Mechanism of Action Bivalirudin acts as a specific and reversible direct thrombin inhibitor; it binds to the catalytic and anionic exosite of both circulating and clot-bound thrombin. Catalytic binding site occupation functionally inhibits coagulant effects by preventing thrombin-mediated cleavage of fibrinogen to fibrin monomers, and activation of factors V, VIII, and XIII. Shows linear dose- and concentration-dependent prolongation of ACT, aPTT, PT, and TT.

Pharmacodynamics/Kinetics

Onset of Action Immediate

Duration of Action Coagulation times return to baseline ~1 hour following discontinuation of infusion

Half-life Elimination

Normal renal function and mild renal impairment: 25 minutes

Moderate renal impairment: 34 minutes

Severe renal impairment: 57 minutes

Dialysis: 3.5 hours

Pregnancy Considerations Bivalirudin is used in conjunction with aspirin, which may lead to maternal or fetal adverse effects, especially during the third trimester. Use of parenteral direct thrombin inhibitors in pregnancy should be limited to those women who have severe allergic reactions to heparin, including heparin-induced thrombocytopenia, and who cannot receive danaparoid (Guyatt 2012).

- ◆ **Bivigam** *see* Immune Globulin *on page 803*
- ◆ **Bi-Zets/Benzotroches [OTC]** *see* Benzocaine *on page 228*
- ◆ **BL4162A** *see* Anagrelide *on page 148*
- ◆ **Blenoxane** *see* Bleomycin *on page 247*
- ◆ **Bleo** *see* Bleomycin *on page 247*

Bleomycin (blee oh MYE sin)

Pharmacologic Category Antineoplastic Agent, Antibiotic

Use

Head and neck cancers: Treatment of squamous cell carcinomas of the head and neck

Hodgkin lymphoma: Treatment of Hodgkin lymphoma

Malignant pleural effusion: Sclerosing agent for malignant pleural effusion

Testicular cancer: Treatment of testicular cancer

Local Anesthetic/Vasoconstrictor Precautions

No information available to require special precautions

Effects on Dental Treatment Key adverse event(s) related to dental treatment: Stomatitis and mucositis.

Effects on Bleeding No information available to require special precautions

Adverse Reactions Frequency not always defined. The pathogenesis of respiratory adverse effects is not certain, but may be due to damage of pulmonary, vascular, or connective tissue. Response to steroid therapy is variable and somewhat controversial.

>10%:

Cardiovascular: Phlebitis

Central nervous system: Tumor pain

Dermatologic: Hyperpigmentation (50%), atrophic striae (≤50%), erythema (≤50%), exfoliation of the skin (≤50%; particularly on the palmar and plantar surfaces of the hands and feet), hyperkeratosis (≤50%), localized vesiculation (≤50%), skin rash (≤50%), skin sclerosis (≤50%), alopecia (may be dose-related and reversible with discontinuation), nailbed changes (may be dose-related and reversible with discontinuation)

Endocrine & metabolic: Weight loss

Gastrointestinal: Stomatitis (≤30%), mucositis (≤30%), anorexia

Miscellaneous: Febrile reaction (25% to 50%; acute)

1% to 10%:

Dermatologic: Onycholysis, pruritus, thickening of skin

Hypersensitivity: Anaphylactoid reaction (including chills, confusion, fever, hypotension, wheezing; onset may be immediate or delayed for several hours; includes idiosyncratic reaction in 1% of lymphoma patients)

Neuromuscular & skeletal: Scleroderma (diffuse)

Respiratory: Tachypnea (≤5% to 10%), rales (≤5% to 10%), interstitial pneumonitis (acute or chronic: ≤5% to 10%), pulmonary fibrosis (≤5% to 10%), hypoxia (1%)

<1%, postmarketing, and/or case reports: Angioedema, bone marrow depression (rare), cerebrovascular accident, cerebral arteritis, chest pain, coronary artery disease, hepatotoxicity, hyperpigmentation (flagellate), ischemic heart disease, malaise, myocardial infarction, nausea, nephrotoxicity, pericarditis, Raynaud's phenomenon, scleroderma (scleroderma-like skin changes), Stevens-Johnson syndrome, thrombotic thrombocytopenic purpura, toxic epidermal necrolysis, vomiting

Mechanism of Action Bleomycin inhibits synthesis of DNA; binds to DNA leading to single- and double-strand breaks; also inhibits (to a lesser degree) RNA and protein synthesis

Pharmacodynamics/Kinetics

Half-life Elimination Terminal: IV: 2 hours

Time to Peak Serum: IM, SubQ, Intrapleural: 30 to 60 minutes

Reproductive Considerations

According to the manufacturer, women of childbearing potential should avoid becoming pregnant during bleomycin treatment.

Pregnancy Risk Factor D

Pregnancy Considerations

Adverse effects were observed in animal reproduction studies. The European Society for Medical Oncology has published guidelines for diagnosis, treatment, and follow-up of cancer during pregnancy; the guidelines recommend referral to a facility with expertise in cancer during pregnancy and encourage a multidisciplinary team (obstetrician, neonatologist, oncology team). In general, if chemotherapy is indicated, it should be avoided in the first trimester and there should be a 3-week time period between the last chemotherapy dose and anticipated delivery, and chemotherapy should not be administered beyond week 33 of gestation (Peccatori 2013). When multiagent therapy is needed to treat Hodgkin lymphoma during pregnancy, bleomycin (as a component of the ABVD [doxorubicin, bleomycin, vinblastine, and dacarbazine] regimen) may be used, starting with the second trimester (Follows 2014; Peccatori 2013).

- ◆ **Bleomycin Sulfate** *see* Bleomycin *on page 247*
- ◆ **Blisovi 24 Fe** *see* Ethinyl Estradiol and Norethindrone *on page 614*
- ◆ **Blisovi Fe 1.5/30** *see* Ethinyl Estradiol and Norethindrone *on page 614*

◆ **Blisovi FE 1/20** *see* Ethinyl Estradiol and Norethindrone *on page 614*
◆ **BLM** *see* Bleomycin *on page 247*
◆ **BLU-285** *see* Avapritinib *on page 194*
◆ **Blue Tube/ Aloe [OTC]** *see* Lidocaine (Topical) *on page 902*
◆ **BMN 673** *see* Talazoparib *on page 1402*
◆ **BMS-188667** *see* Abatacept *on page 53*
◆ **BMS 201038** *see* Lomitapide *on page 927*
◆ **BMS-224818** *see* Belatacept *on page 221*
◆ **BMS-232632** *see* Atazanavir *on page 186*
◆ **BMS-247550** *see* Ixabepilone *on page 852*
◆ **BMS 337039** *see* ARIPiprazole *on page 164*
◆ **BMS-354825** *see* Dasatinib *on page 443*
◆ **BMS-477118** *see* SAXagliptin *on page 1360*
◆ **BMS-512148** *see* Dapagliflozin *on page 435*
◆ **BMS-901608** *see* Elotuzumab *on page 550*
◆ **BMS-936558** *see* Nivolumab *on page 1114*
◆ **BocaSal** *see* Saliva Substitute *on page 1354*
◆ **BOL-303224-A** *see* Besifloxacin *on page 232*
◆ **Bondronate** *see* Ibandronate *on page 782*
◆ **Bonine [OTC]** *see* Meclizine *on page 952*
◆ **Boniva** *see* Ibandronate *on page 782*
◆ **Bontril PDM** *see* Phendimetrazine *on page 1223*

Bortezomib (bore TEZ oh mib)

Brand Names: US Velcade

Brand Names: Canada ACT Bortezomib; PMS-Bortezomib; Velcade

Pharmacologic Category Antineoplastic Agent, Proteasome Inhibitor

Use

Mantle cell lymphoma: Treatment of mantle cell lymphoma in adults.

Multiple myeloma: Treatment of multiple myeloma in adults.

Local Anesthetic/Vasoconstrictor Precautions Bortezomib is one of the drugs confirmed to prolong the QT interval and is accepted as having a risk of causing torsades de pointes. The risk of drug-induced torsades de pointes is extremely low when a single QT interval prolonging drug is prescribed. In terms of epinephrine, it is not known what effect vasoconstrictors in the local anesthetic regimen will have in patients with a known history of congenital prolonged QT interval or in patients taking any medication that prolongs the QT interval. Until more information is obtained, it is suggested that the clinician consult with the physician prior to the use of a vasoconstrictor in suspected patients and that the vasoconstrictor (epinephrine, mepivacaine, and levonordefrin [Carbocaine 2% with Neo-Cobefrin]) be used with caution.

Effects on Dental Treatment Key adverse event(s) related to dental treatment: Rare occurrence of abnormal taste has been reported. Oral candidiasis and stomatitis have also been reported; frequency not defined.

Effects on Bleeding Dose-related thrombocytopenia (~35%; nadir: day 11; recovery: by day 21) is most common hematological event with platelet counts usually returning to baseline following active therapy each cycle. A medical consult is suggested.

Adverse Reactions

>10%:

Central nervous system: Peripheral neuropathy (IV: 35% to 54%; SubQ: 37%; grade ≥2: 24% to 39%; grade ≥3: IV: 7% to 15%; SubQ: 5% to 6%; grade 4: <1%), fatigue (7% to 52%), neuralgia (23%), headache (10% to 19%), paresthesia (7% to 19%), dizziness (10% to 18%; excludes vertigo)

Dermatologic: Skin rash (12% to 23%)

Gastrointestinal: Diarrhea (19% to 52%), nausea (14% to 52%), constipation (24% to 34%), vomiting (9% to 29%), anorexia (14% to 21%), abdominal pain (11%), decreased appetite (11%)

Hematologic & oncologic: Thrombocytopenia (16% to 52%; grade 3: 5% to 24%; grade 4: 3% to 7%; nadir: Day 11; recovery: By day 21), neutropenia (5% to 27%; grade 3: 8% to 18%; grade 4: 2% to 4%; nadir: Day 11; recovery: By day 21), anemia (12% to 23%; grade 3: 4% to 6%; grade 4: <1%), leukopenia (18% to 20%; grade 3: 5%; grade 4: ≤1%)

Infection: Herpes zoster infection (reactivation; 6% to 11%)

Neuromuscular & skeletal: Asthenia (7% to 16%)

Respiratory: Dyspnea (11%)

Miscellaneous: Fever (8% to 23%)

1% to 10%:

Cardiovascular: Hypotension (8% to 9%), cardiac disease (treatment emergent; 8%), acute pulmonary edema (≤1%), cardiac failure (≤1%), cardiogenic shock (≤1%), pulmonary edema (≤1%)

Endocrine & metabolic: Dehydration (2%)

Hematologic & oncologic: Hemorrhage (≥ grade 3: 2%)

Infection: Herpes simplex infection (1% to 3%), herpes zoster (1% to 2%)

Local: Injection site reaction (mostly redness; SubQ: 6%), irritation at injection site (IV: 5%)

Respiratory: Pneumonia (1% to 3%)

Frequency not defined:

Cardiovascular: Aggravated atrial fibrillation, angina pectoris, atrial flutter, atrioventricular block, bradycardia, cerebrovascular accident, deep vein thrombosis, edema, embolism (peripheral), facial edema, hemorrhagic stroke, hypersensitivity angiitis, hypertension, ischemic heart disease, myocardial infarction, pericardial effusion, pericarditis, peripheral edema, phlebitis, portal vein thrombosis, pulmonary embolism, septic shock, sinoatrial arrest, subdural hematoma, torsades de pointes, transient ischemic attacks, ventricular tachycardia

Central nervous system: Agitation, anxiety, ataxia, brain disease, cerebral hemorrhage, chills, coma, confusion, cranial nerve palsy, dysarthria, dysautonomia, dysesthesia, insomnia, malaise, mental status changes, motor dysfunction, paralysis, psychosis, seizure, spinal cord compression, suicidal ideation, vertigo

Dermatologic: Pruritus, urticaria

Endocrine & metabolic: Amyloid heart disease, hyperglycemia (diabetic patients), hyperkalemia, hypernatremia, hyperuricemia, hypocalcemia, hypoglycemia (diabetic patients), hypokalemia, hyponatremia, weight loss

Gastrointestinal: Cholestasis, duodenitis (hemorrhagic), dysphagia, fecal impaction, gastritis (hemorrhagic), gastroenteritis, gastroesophageal reflux disease, hematemesis, intestinal obstruction, intestinal perforation, melena, oral candidiasis, pancreatitis, paralytic ileus, peritonitis, stomatitis

Genitourinary: Bladder spasm, hematuria, hemorrhagic cystitis, urinary incontinence, urinary retention, urinary tract infection

Hematologic & oncologic: Disseminated intravascular coagulation, febrile neutropenia, lymphocytopenia, oral mucosal petechiae

Hepatic: Ascites, hepatic failure, hepatic hemorrhage, hepatitis, hyperbilirubinemia

Hypersensitivity: Anaphylaxis, angioedema, hypersensitivity reaction

Infection: Aspergillosis, bacteremia, listeriosis, toxoplasmosis

Local: Catheter infection

Neuromuscular & skeletal: Arthralgia, back pain, bone fracture, limb pain, myalgia, ostealgia

Ophthalmic: Blurred vision, conjunctival infection, conjunctival irritation, diplopia

Otic: Auditory impairment

Renal: Bilateral hydronephrosis, nephrolithiasis, proliferative glomerulonephritis, renal failure

Respiratory: Acute respiratory distress syndrome, aspiration pneumonia, atelectasis, bronchitis, chronic obstructive pulmonary disease (exacerbation), cough, epistaxis, hemoptysis, hypoxia, laryngeal edema, nasopharyngitis, pleural effusion, pneumonitis, pulmonary hypertension, pulmonary infiltrates (including diffuse), respiratory tract infection, sinusitis

<1%, postmarketing, and/or case reports: Amyloidosis, blepharitis, blindness, cardiac tamponade, chalazion (Fraunfelder 2016), deafness (bilateral), decreased left ventricular ejection fraction, dysgeusia, dyspepsia, hemolytic-uremic syndrome, herpes meningoencephalitis, increased serum transaminases, interstitial pneumonitis, intestinal obstruction, ischemic colitis, ocular herpes simplex, optic neuritis, optic neuropathy, progressive multifocal leukoencephalopathy, prolonged QT interval on ECG, pulmonary disease, respiratory insufficiency, reversible posterior leukoencephalopathy syndrome, sepsis, Stevens-Johnson syndrome, Sweet syndrome, syncope, thrombotic microangiopathy, thrombotic thrombocytopenic purpura, toxic epidermal necrolysis, tumor lysis syndrome

Mechanism of Action Bortezomib inhibits proteasomes, enzyme complexes which regulate protein homeostasis within the cell. Specifically, it reversibly inhibits chymotrypsin-like activity at the 26S proteasome, leading to activation of signaling cascades, cell-cycle arrest, and apoptosis.

Pharmacodynamics/Kinetics

Half-life Elimination Single dose: IV: 9 to 15 hours; Multiple dosing: 1 mg/m^2: 40 to 193 hours; 1.3 mg/m^2: 76 to 108 hour

Reproductive Considerations

Evaluate pregnancy status in women of reproductive potential prior to initiating therapy; women of reproductive potential should avoid becoming pregnant during bortezomib treatment. Females of reproductive potential should use effective contraception during therapy and for 7 months following bortezomib treatment. Males with female partners of reproductive potential should use effective contraception during and for 4 months following bortezomib treatment.

Bortezomib may potentially affect male or female fertility (based on the mechanism of action).

Pregnancy Considerations

Based on the mechanism of action and on findings in animal reproduction studies, bortezomib may cause fetal harm if administered during pregnancy.

Bosentan (boe SEN tan)

Brand Names: US Tracleer

Brand Names: Canada ACT Bosentan [DSC]; APO-Bosentan; BIO-Bosentan; MYLAN-Bosentan [DSC]; NAT-Bosentan; PMS-Bosentan; SANDOZ Bosentan; TARO-Bosentan; TEVA-Bosentan; Tracleer

Pharmacologic Category Endothelin Receptor Antagonist; Vasodilator

Use Pulmonary arterial hypertension: Treatment of pulmonary artery hypertension (PAH) (WHO Group I) in adults with WHO-FC II, III, or IV symptoms to improve exercise ability and to decrease clinical deterioration; treatment of PAH (WHO Group 1) in pediatric patients ≥3 years with idiopathic or congenital PAH to improve pulmonary vascular resistance (PVR), resulting in an improvement in exercise ability.

Local Anesthetic/Vasoconstrictor Precautions No information available to require special precautions

Effects on Dental Treatment Key adverse event(s) related to dental treatment: Endothelin antagonists have caused bleeding gums; there have been no specific reports for bosentan

Effects on Bleeding No information available to require special precautions

Adverse Reactions

>10%:

Cardiovascular: Edema (≤11%)

Central nervous system: Headache (15%)

Hepatic: Increased serum ALT (≥3 times ULN: ≤12%; 8 times ULN: ≤2%; dose-related), increased serum AST (≥3 times ULN: ≤12%; 8 times ULN: ≤2%; dose-related)

Respiratory: Respiratory tract infection (22%)

1% to 10%:

Cardiovascular: Chest pain (5%), syncope (5%), flushing (4%), hypotension (4%), palpitations (4%)

Endocrine & metabolic: Fluid retention (≤2%)

Hematologic & oncologic: Anemia (3%)

Neuromuscular & skeletal: Arthralgia (4%)

Respiratory: Sinusitis (4%)

<1%, postmarketing, and/or case reports: Anaphylaxis, angioedema, DRESS syndrome, hepatic cirrhosis (prolonged therapy), hepatic failure (rare), hypersensitivity reaction, jaundice, leukopenia, nasal congestion, neutropenia, peripheral edema, severe anemia, skin rash, thrombocytopenia

Mechanism of Action Endothelin receptor antagonist that blocks endothelin receptors on endothelium and vascular smooth muscle (stimulation of these receptors is associated with vasoconstriction). Bosentan blocks both ET_A and ET_B receptors, with a slightly higher affinity for the A subtype.

Pharmacodynamics/Kinetics

Half-life Elimination ~5 hours; prolonged with heart failure, possibly with PAH

Time to Peak Plasma: 3 to 5 hours

Reproductive Considerations

Bosentan is contraindicated in females who may become pregnant.

[US Boxed Warning]: Pregnancy must be excluded before the start of treatment with bosentan. Throughout treatment and for 1 month after stopping bosentan, women of childbearing potential

must use two reliable methods of contraception unless the patient has an intrauterine device (IUD) or tubal sterilization in which case no other contraception is needed. Hormonal contraceptives, including oral, injectable, transdermal, and implantable contraceptives, should not be used as the sole means of contraception because these may not be effective in patients receiving bosentan. Obtain monthly pregnancy tests. When a hormonal or barrier contraceptive is used, one additional method of contraception is still needed if a male partner has had a vasectomy. A missed menses or suspected pregnancy should be reported to a health care provider and prompt immediate pregnancy testing.

Decreased sperm counts and adverse effects on spermatogenesis have been observed in men during treatment; fertility may be impaired. It is not known if effects on fertility are reversible.

Pregnancy Considerations

Bosentan is contraindicated in females who are pregnant.

[US Boxed Warning]: Bosentan is likely to cause major birth defects if used by pregnant women based on animal data.

Women with pulmonary arterial hypertension (PAH) are encouraged to avoid pregnancy (McLaughlin 2009; Taichman 2014).

◆ **Botox** *see* OnabotulinumtoxinA *on page 1140*

◆ **Botox Cosmetic** *see* OnabotulinumtoxinA *on page 1140*

◆ **Botulinum Toxin Type A** *see* AbobotulinumtoxinA *on page 55*

◆ **Botulinum Toxin Type A** *see* IncobotulinumtoxinA *on page 806*

◆ **Botulinum Toxin Type A** *see* OnabotulinumtoxinA *on page 1140*

◆ **Botulinum Toxin Type B** *see* RimabotulinumtoxinB *on page 1328*

◆ **Bovine Lung Surfactant** *see* Beractant *on page 232*

◆ **BProtected Pedia D-Vite [OTC]** *see* Cholecalciferol *on page 344*

◆ **BProtected Pedia Iron [OTC]** *see* Ferrous Sulfate *on page 664*

◆ **Braftovi** *see* Encorafenib *on page 563*

◆ **BRAF(V600E) Kinase Inhibitor RO5185426** *see* Vemurafenib *on page 1537*

◆ **Bravelle [DSC]** *see* Urofollitropin *on page 1509*

◆ **Breath Rx [OTC] [DSC]** *see* Cetylpyridinium *on page 330*

◆ **Breo Ellipta** *see* Fluticasone and Vilanterol *on page 706*

◆ **Brethaire** *see* Terbutaline *on page 1422*

◆ **Brethine** *see* Terbutaline *on page 1422*

◆ **Brevibloc** *see* Esmolol *on page 593*

◆ **Brevibloc in NaCl** *see* Esmolol *on page 593*

◆ **Brevibloc Premixed** *see* Esmolol *on page 593*

◆ **Brevibloc Premixed DS** *see* Esmolol *on page 593*

◆ **Brevicon (28) [DSC]** *see* Ethinyl Estradiol and Norethindrone *on page 614*

◆ **Brevital Sodium** *see* Methohexital *on page 989*

◆ **Bricanyl** *see* Terbutaline *on page 1422*

◆ **Briellyn** *see* Ethinyl Estradiol and Norethindrone *on page 614*

Brigatinib (bri GA ti nib)

Brand Names: US Alunbrig

Brand Names: Canada Alunbrig

Pharmacologic Category Antineoplastic Agent, Anaplastic Lymphoma Kinase Inhibitor; Antineoplastic Agent, Tyrosine Kinase Inhibitor

Use Non-small cell lung cancer, metastatic: Treatment of anaplastic lymphoma kinase (ALK)-positive (as detected by an approved test) metastatic non-small cell lung cancer (NSCLC) in adults.

Local Anesthetic/Vasoconstrictor Precautions No information available to require special precautions

Effects on Dental Treatment Key adverse event(s) related to dental treatment: Hypertension has been reported in approximately 10% to 20% of patients receiving brigatinib. Monitoring of blood pressure prior to dental treatment is advised.

Effects on Bleeding No information available to require special precautions

Adverse Reactions

>10%:

Cardiovascular: Hypertension (11% to 21%)

Central nervous system: Fatigue (29% to 36%), headache (27% to 28%), peripheral neuropathy (13%, grades 3/4: ≤2%), insomnia (7% to 11%)

Dermatologic: Skin rash (15% to 24%)

Endocrine & metabolic: Increased serum AST (38% to 65%), hyperglycemia (38% to 49%; including exacerbations), increased serum ALT (34% to 40%), increased amylase (27% to 39%)

Gastrointestinal: Increased serum lipase (21% to 45%), nausea (33% to 40%), diarrhea (19% to 38%), vomiting (23% to 24%), decreased appetite (15% to 22%), constipation (15% to 19%), abdominal pain (10% to 17%)

Hematologic & oncologic: Anemia (23% to 40%; grades 3/4: <1%), lymphocytopenia (19% to 27%; grades 3/4: 3% to 5%), abnormal phosphorus levels (decreased; 15% to 23%; grades 3/4: <1%), prolonged partial thromboplastin time (20% to 22%; grades 3/4: ≤2%)

Hepatic: Increased serum alkaline phosphatase (15% to 29%)

Neuromuscular & skeletal: Increased creatine phosphokinase (27% to 48%), muscle spasm (12% to 17%), back pain (10% to 15%), myalgia (9% to 15%), arthralgia (14%), limb pain (4% to 11%)

Respiratory: Cough (18% to 34%), dyspnea (21% to 27%)

Miscellaneous: Fever (6% to 14%)

1% to 10%:

Cardiovascular: Bradycardia (6% to 8%)

Ophthalmic: Visual disturbance (7% to 10%; including blurred vision, diplopia, and reduced visual acuity)

Respiratory: Interstitial pneumonitis (≤9%), pneumonitis (≤9%), hypoxia (≤3%), pneumonia (5% to 10%)

Mechanism of Action Brigatinib is a broad spectrum multikinase inhibitor with activity against anaplastic lymphoma kinase (ALK), ROS1, insulin-like growth factor-1 receptor (IGF-1R), and FLT-3, as well as EGFR deletion and point mutations. ALK autophosphorylation and ALK-mediated phosphorylation of downstream signaling proteins STAT3, AKT, ERK1/2, and S6 are inhibited by brigatinib. In vitro, brigatinib also inhibited proliferation of cell lines expressing EML4-ALK and

NPM-ALK fusion proteins. Brigatinib has activity against cells expressing EML4-ALK and 17 mutant forms associated with ALK inhibitor resistance, as well as EGFR-Del (E746-A750), ROS1-L2026M, FLT3-F691L, and FLT3-D835Y. Clinically, brigatinib showed anti-tumor activity against EML4-ALK mutant forms (including G1202R and L1196M) which were identified in NSCLC cells in patients who progressed on crizotinib.

Pharmacodynamics/Kinetics

Half-life Elimination 25 hours.

Time to Peak 1 to 4 hours.

Reproductive Considerations Evaluate pregnancy status in females of reproductive potential prior to therapy initiation. Females of reproductive potential should use an effective nonhormonal contraceptive during therapy and for at least 4 months after the last brigatinib dose. Males with female partners of reproductive potential should use effective contraception during therapy and for at least 3 months after the last dose.

Pregnancy Considerations

Based on the mechanism of action and adverse events observed in animal reproduction studies, brigatinib may be expected to cause fetal harm if used during pregnancy.

◆ **Brilinta** *see* Ticagrelor *on page* 1444

◆ **Brisdelle** *see* PARoxetine *on page* 1194

Brivaracetam (briv a RA se tam)

Brand Names: US Briviact

Brand Names: Canada Brivlera

Pharmacologic Category Anticonvulsant, Miscellaneous

Use Partial-onset seizures: Treatment of partial-onset seizures in patients with epilepsy as monotherapy or adjunctive therapy.

Local Anesthetic/Vasoconstrictor Precautions No information available to require special precautions

Effects on Dental Treatment Key adverse event(s) related to dental treatment: Incidence of sedation and equilibrium disturbances in patients taking brivaracetam reported; monitor for symptoms, particularly for equilibrium problems, as patient arises from dental chair, and assist as necessary.

Effects on Bleeding No information available to require special precautions

Adverse Reactions

>10%:

Central nervous system: Drowsiness (≤27%), fatigue (≤27%), hypersomnia (≤27%), lethargy (≤27%), malaise (≤27%), sedation (≤27%), abnormal gait (≤16%), ataxia (≤16%), dizziness (≤16%), equilibrium disturbance (≤16%), vertigo (≤16%), psychiatric disturbance (13%; includes psychotic and nonpsychotic)

Neuromuscular & skeletal: Asthenia (≤27%)

Ophthalmic: Nystagmus (≤16%)

1% to 10%:

Central nervous system: Euphoria (IV: ≥3%), infusion site pain (IV: ≥3%), intoxicated feeling (IV: ≥3%), irritability (3%)

Gastrointestinal: Nausea (≤5%), vomiting (≤5%), dysgeusia (IV: ≥3%), constipation (2%)

Hematologic & oncologic: Decreased white blood cell count (2%)

Frequency not defined:

Central nervous system: Suicidal ideation

Hypersensitivity: Hypersensitivity reaction

<1%, postmarketing, and/or case reports: Angioedema, bronchospasm, decreased neutrophils

Mechanism of Action The precise mechanism by which brivaracetam exerts its antiepileptic activity is unknown. Brivaracetam displays a high and selective affinity for synaptic vesicle protein 2A (SV2A) in the brain, which may contribute to the antiepileptic effect.

Pharmacodynamics/Kinetics

Half-life Elimination ~9 hours

Time to Peak Oral: 1 hour (fasting, range: 0.25 to 3 hours).

Pregnancy Considerations

Adverse events have been observed in animal reproduction studies.

Females exposed to brivaracetam during pregnancy are encouraged to enroll themselves into the North American Antiepileptic Drug (NAAED) Pregnancy Registry by calling 1-888-233-2334. Additional information is available at http://www.aedpregnancyregistry.org.

Controlled Substance C-V

◆ **Briviact** *see* Brivaracetam *on page* 251

◆ **BRL 43694** *see* Granisetron *on page* 748

Brolucizumab (BROE lue SIZ ue mab)

Brand Names: US Beovu

Brand Names: Canada Beovu

Pharmacologic Category Ophthalmic Agent; Vascular Endothelial Growth Factor (VEGF) Inhibitor

Use Neovascular (wet) age-related macular degeneration: Treatment of neovascular (wet) age-related macular degeneration.

Local Anesthetic/Vasoconstrictor Precautions No information available to require special precautions

Effects on Dental Treatment No significant effects or complications reported

Effects on Bleeding No information available to require special precautions

Adverse Reactions

>10%: Immunologic: Antibody development (53% to 67%)

1% to 10%:

Cardiovascular: Arterial thromboembolism (5%)

Hypersensitivity: Hypersensitivity reaction (2%)

Ophthalmic: Abnormal sensation in eyes (1%), blindness (1%), blurred vision (10%), cataract (7%), conjunctival hemorrhage (6%), conjunctival hyperemia (1%), conjunctivitis (3%), corneal abrasion (2%), endophthalmitis (1%), eye pain (5%), increased intraocular pressure (4%), increased lacrimation (1%), intraocular inflammation (4% to 6%), punctate keratitis (1%), retinal artery occlusion (1%), retinal detachment (1%), retinal hemorrhage (4%), retinal hole without detachment (1%), retinal pigment epithelium detachment (1%), retinal pigment epithelium tear (3%), vitreous detachment (4%), vitreous opacity (5%)

Postmarketing: Ophthalmic: Retinal vein occlusion

Mechanism of Action Brolucizumab is a recombinant humanized monoclonal antibody vascular endothelial growth factor (VEGF) inhibitor that binds to the 3 major isoforms of VEGF-A, thereby suppressing endothelial cell proliferation, neovascularization, and vascular permeability to slow vision loss.

Pharmacodynamics/Kinetics

Half-life Elimination 4.4 ± 2 days.

Time to Peak Serum: 24 hours (free brolucizumab).

Reproductive Considerations Evaluate pregnancy status prior to use in females of reproductive potential. Females of reproductive potential should use highly effective contraception (methods with pregnancy rates <1%) during therapy and for ≥1 month following the last brolucizumab dose.

Pregnancy Considerations

Brolucizumab is a vascular endothelial growth factor (VEGF) inhibitor; VEGF is required to achieve and maintain normal pregnancies (Peracha 2016). Based on findings in animal reproduction studies and on the mechanism of action, brolucizumab may cause fetal harm if administered to a pregnant female.

- **Brolucizumab-dbll** *see* Brolucizumab *on page 251*

Brompheniramine (brome fen IR a meen)

Brand Names: US Respa-BR [DSC]

Pharmacologic Category Alkylamine Derivative; Histamine H_1 Antagonist; Histamine H_1 Antagonist, First Generation

Use **Upper respiratory allergies:** Temporary relief of sneezing; itchy, watery eyes; itchy nose or throat; and runny nose caused by hay fever (allergic rhinitis) or other upper respiratory allergies.

Local Anesthetic/Vasoconstrictor Precautions

No information available to require special precautions

Effects on Dental Treatment Key adverse event(s) related to dental treatment: Xerostomia (normal salivary flow resumes upon discontinuation). Chronic use of antihistamines will inhibit salivary flow, particularly in elderly patients; this may contribute to periodontal disease and oral discomfort.

Effects on Bleeding No information available to require special precautions

Adverse Reactions Frequency not defined.

Cardiovascular: Angina pectoris, chest tightness, circulatory shock, extrasystoles, hypotension, increased blood pressure, palpitations, tachycardia

Central nervous system: Anxiety, ataxia, central nervous system stimulation, chills, confusion, dizziness, drowsiness, euphoria, excitement, fatigue, headache, hysteria, insomnia, irritability, nervousness, neuritis, paresthesia, restlessness, sedation, seizure, tension, vertigo

Dermatologic: Diaphoresis, skin photosensitivity, skin rash, urticaria

Gastrointestinal: Abdominal cramps, anorexia, constipation, diarrhea, epigastric distress, heartburn, nausea, vomiting, xerostomia

Genitourinary: Dysuria, early menses, urinary retention

Hematologic & oncologic: Agranulocytosis, hemolytic anemia, hypoplastic anemia, thrombocytopenia

Hypersensitivity: Anaphylactic shock

Neuromuscular & skeletal: Tremor, weakness

Ophthalmic: Blurred vision, diplopia, mydriasis

Otic: Acute labyrinthitis, tinnitus

Renal: Polyuria

Respiratory: Dry nose, dry throat, nasal congestion, thickening of bronchial secretions, wheezing

Mechanism of Action Competes with histamine for H_1-receptor sites on effector cells

Pharmacodynamics/Kinetics

Half-life Elimination Children: ~12 hours (Simons, 1999); Adults: ~25 hours (Simons, 1982)

Time to Peak Serum: Children: 3-3.5 hours (Simons, 1999); Adults: 2-4 hours (Simons, 1982)

Pregnancy Considerations

Maternal first-generation antihistamine use has generally not resulted in an increased risk of birth defects (Babalola 2013; Murase 2014); however, information specific to brompheniramine is limited (Heinonen 1977; Seto 1993).

Brompheniramine is not the preferred antihistamine for the treatment of rhinitis or urticaria in pregnant women (BSACI [Scadding 2017]; Zuberbier 2018).

- **Brompheniramine Maleate** *see* Brompheniramine *on page 252*
- **Brompheniramine Tannate** *see* Brompheniramine *on page 252*
- **Brovana** *see* Arformoterol *on page 163*
- **Brukinsa** *see* Zanubrutinib *on page 1568*
- **BSF208075** *see* Ambrisentan *on page 113*
- **BTK-InhB** *see* Zanubrutinib *on page 1568*
- **BTK Inhibitor ACP-196** *see* Acalabrutinib *on page 56*
- **BTK Inhibitor PCI-32765** *see* Ibrutinib *on page 785*
- **BTX-A** *see* OnabotulinumtoxinA *on page 1140*
- **B-type Natriuretic Peptide (Human)** *see* Nesiritide *on page 1094*
- **Buckleys Cough [OTC]** *see* Dextromethorphan *on page 476*
- **Budeprion SR** *see* BuPROPion *on page 271*

Budesonide (Systemic) (byoo DES oh nide)

Brand Names: US Entocort EC; Ortikos; Uceris

Brand Names: Canada Cortiment; Entocort

Pharmacologic Category Corticosteroid, Systemic

Use

Crohn disease, mild to moderate (capsules): Treatment of active Crohn disease (mild to moderate) involving the ileum and/or the ascending colon in patients ≥8 years of age; maintenance of clinical remission (for up to 3 months) of Crohn disease (mild to moderate) involving the ileum and/or the ascending colon in adults

Ulcerative colitis (tablets): Induction of remission in patients with active ulcerative colitis (mild to moderate)

Local Anesthetic/Vasoconstrictor Precautions

No information available to require special precautions

Effects on Dental Treatment Key adverse event(s) related to dental treatment: Occurrence of glossitis, oral candidiasis, and swelling of the tongue has been reported.

Effects on Bleeding No information available to require special precautions

Adverse Reactions

>10%:

Central nervous system: Headache (15% to 21%)

Dermatologic: Acne vulgaris (15%)

Endocrine & metabolic: Decreased cortisol (foam 17%; tablets 2% to 4%), bruise (15%), moon face (11%)

Gastrointestinal: Nausea (2% to 11%)

Respiratory: Respiratory tract infection (11%)

1% to 10%:

Cardiovascular: Chest pain (<5%), edema (<5%), facial edema (<5%), flushing (<5%), hypertension (<5%), palpitations (<5%), tachycardia (<5%)

Central nervous system: Dizziness (<5% to 7%), fatigue (3% to 5%), agitation (<5%), amnesia (<5%), confusion (<5%), drowsiness (<5%), insomnia (<5%), malaise (<5%), nervousness (<5%), paresthesia (<5%), sleep disorder (<5%), vertigo (<5%)
Dermatologic: Alopecia (<5%), dermatitis (<5%), dermatological disease (<5%), diaphoresis (<5%), eczema (<5%)
Endocrine & metabolic: Hirsutism (≤5%), hypokalemia (1% to <5%), intermenstrual bleeding (<5%), menstrual disease (<5%), weight gain (<5%), adrenocortical insufficiency (foam 4%; capsules >1%), redistribution of body fat (1%)
Gastrointestinal: Diarrhea (10%), dyspepsia (6%), anal disease (<5%), enteritis (<5%), epigastric pain (<5%), exacerbation of Crohn's disease (<5%), gastrointestinal fistula (<5%), glossitis (<5%), hemorrhoids (<5%), increased appetite (<5%), intestinal obstruction (<5%), oral candidiasis (<5%), upper abdominal pain (3% to 4%), flatulence (3%), abdominal distention (2%), constipation (2%)
Genitourinary: Urinary tract infection (2% to <5%), dysuria (<5%), nocturia (<5%), urinary frequency (<5%), hematuria (≥1%), pyuria (≥1%)
Hematologic & oncologic: C-reactive protein increased (1% to <5%), leukocytosis (1% to <5%), purpura (<5%), abnormal neutrophils (≥1%), anemia (≥1%), increased erythrocyte sedimentation rate (≥1%)
Hepatic: Increased serum alkaline phosphatase (≥1%)
Hypersensitivity: Tongue edema (<5%)
Infection: Viral infection (6%), abscess (<5%)
Neuromuscular & skeletal: Ankle edema (7%), arthralgia (5%), arthritis (≤5%), hyperkinesia (<5%), muscle cramps (<5%), myalgia (<5%), tremor (<5%), weakness (<5%)
Ophthalmic: Eye disease (<5%), visual disturbance (<5%)
Otic: Otic infection (<5%)
Respiratory: Sinusitis (8%), bronchitis (<5%), dyspnea (<5%), flu-like symptoms (<5%), pharyngeal disease (<5%), rhinitis (<5%)
Miscellaneous: Fever (<5%)

<1%, postmarketing, and/or case reports: Allergic dermatitis, anaphylaxis, emotional lability, hyperglycemia, maculopapular rash, pancreatitis, peripheral edema, pruritus, pseudotumor cerebri, rectal bleeding, skin rash

Mechanism of Action Budesonide, a glucocorticoid with high topical potency and limited systemic effects, depresses the activity of endogenous chemical mediators of inflammation (eg, kinins, prostaglandins). Oral budesonide formulations allow for targeted, pH-dependent budesonide release in the treatment of IBD (eg, Crohn disease, ulcerative colitis). The controlled release capsule contains enteric coated granules that dissolve at a pH ≥5.5, delivering budesonide to the ileum and ascending colon. The multimatrix enteric coated tablet dissolves at a pH ≥7, delivering budesonide to the entire colon (Abdalla 2016; Iborra 2014).

Pharmacodynamics/Kinetics

Half-life Elimination

Children ≥9 years of age and adolescents ≤14 years: IV: 1.9 hours.

Adults: IV: 2 to 3.6 hours; Capsule: 6.3 ± 1.6 hours (range: 2 to 8 hours).

Time to Peak Capsule: Children ≥9 years and Adolescents ≤14 years: Median: 5 hours; Adults: 0.5 to 10 hours; Tablet (extended release): 13.3 ± 5.9 hours

Reproductive Considerations Fertility may be decreased in females with active inflammatory bowel disease. Corticosteroids used for the management of inflammatory bowel disease are not expected to decrease female fertility (AGA [Mahadevan 2019]).

Pregnancy Considerations

Some studies have shown an association between first trimester systemic corticosteroid use and oral clefts (Park-Wyllie 2000; Pradat 2003). Systemic corticosteroids may also influence fetal growth (decreased birth weight); however, information is conflicting (Lunghi 2010). Hypoadrenalism may occur in newborns following maternal use of corticosteroids in pregnancy (monitor).

Because systemic corticosteroids may increase the risk of gestational diabetes and other adverse pregnancy outcomes, use for maintenance therapy in pregnant women with inflammatory bowel disease is not recommended. However, corticosteroids may be used to treat disease flares in pregnant patients (AGA [Mahadevan 2019]).

Product Availability Ortikos (budesonide extended-release capsules): FDA approval June 2019; anticipated availability is currently unknown. Consult the prescribing information for additional information.

Budesonide (Nasal) (byoo DES oh nide)

Brand Names: US Rhinocort Allergy [OTC]; Rhinocort Aqua [DSC]

Brand Names: Canada MYLAN-Budesonide AQ; Rhinocort Aqua; Rhinocort Turbuhaler [DSC]

Pharmacologic Category Corticosteroid, Nasal

Use

US labeling:

Rx: Allergic rhinitis: Management of symptoms of seasonal or perennial allergic rhinitis in adults and children ≥6 years.

OTC: Upper respiratory symptoms: Relief of symptoms of hay fever or other upper respiratory allergies (eg, nasal congestion, runny nose, itchy nose, sneezing) in adults and children ≥6 years.

Canadian labeling:

Nasal polyps: Treatment of nasal polyps; prevention of nasal polyps after polypectomy.

Rhinitis: Management of symptoms of seasonal allergic, perennial, and vasomotor rhinitis unresponsive to conventional therapy.

Local Anesthetic/Vasoconstrictor Precautions
No information available to require special precautions

Effects on Dental Treatment No significant effects or complications reported

Effects on Bleeding No information available to require special precautions

Adverse Reactions

1% to 10%: Respiratory: Epistaxis (8%), pharyngitis (4%), bronchospasm (2%), cough (2%), nasal mucosa irritation (2%)

<1%, postmarketing, and/or case reports: Anosmia, cataract, crusting of nose, dizziness, fatigue, glaucoma, growth suppression, headache, hypersensitivity reaction, increased intraocular pressure, mucous membrane ulceration, nasal septum perforation, nausea, pharyngeal disease (irritation, itchy throat, throat pain), wheezing

Mechanism of Action Controls the rate of protein synthesis; depresses the migration of polymorphonuclear leukocytes, fibroblasts; reverses capillary permeability and lysosomal stabilization at the cellular level to prevent or control inflammation. Has potent glucocorticoid activity and weak mineralocorticoid activity.

Pharmacodynamics/Kinetics

Onset of Action Rhinocort Aqua: Within 10 hours; Peak effect: Up to 2 weeks

Half-life Elimination 2 to 3 hours

Time to Peak Plasma: Nasal: 30 minutes

Pregnancy Considerations Maternal use of intranasal corticosteroids (INCS) in usual doses are not associated with an increased risk of fetal malformations or preterm birth (ERS/TSANZ [Middleton 2020]). Although an agent with less systemic absorption may be considered, budesonide is one of the INCS that may be used during pregnancy (Alhussien 2018; BSACI [Scadding 2017]; ERS/TSANZ [Middleton 2020]).

Budesonide (Oral Inhalation)

(byoo DES oh nide)

Brand Names: US Pulmicort; Pulmicort Flexhaler

Brand Names: Canada Pulmicort Nebuamp; Pulmicort Turbuhaler; TEVA-Budesonide

Pharmacologic Category Corticosteroid, Inhalant (Oral)

Use

Asthma: Maintenance and prophylactic treatment of asthma in patients ≥6 years of age (dry powder inhaler) or 12 months to 8 years of age (nebulization suspension).

Limitations of use: Not for relief of acute bronchospasm.

Local Anesthetic/Vasoconstrictor Precautions No information available to require special precautions

Effects on Dental Treatment Key adverse event(s) related to dental treatment: Xerostomia (normal salivary flow resumes upon discontinuation), dry throat, abnormal taste, and herpes simplex. Localized infections with *Candida albicans* or *Aspergillus niger* have occurred frequently in the mouth and pharynx with repetitive use of oral inhaler of corticosteroids. These infections may require treatment with appropriate antifungal therapy or discontinuance of treatment with corticosteroid inhaler.

Effects on Bleeding Variable effects on anticoagulant therapy are observed with glucocorticoids such as budesonide (systemic, oral inhalation).

Adverse Reactions

Frequencies are for both formulations unless otherwise indicated.

>10%:

Otic: Otitis media (suspension: 12%; powder: 1%)

Respiratory: Respiratory infection (suspension: 38%; powder: ≥3%), rhinitis (5% to 12%)

1% to 10%:

Cardiovascular: Syncope (powder: 1% to 3%), chest pain (suspension: 1% to <3%)

Central nervous system: Headache (powder: ≥3%; suspension: <1%), pain (powder: ≥3%), hypertonia (powder: 1% to 3%), insomnia (powder: 1% to 3%), voice disorder (powder: 1% to 3%), emotional lability (suspension: 1% to <3%), fatigue (suspension: 1% to <3%)

Dermatologic: Skin rash (suspension: 4%; powder: <1%), contact dermatitis (suspension: 1% to <3%), eczema (suspension: 1% to <3%), pruritus (suspension: 1% to <3%), pustular rash (suspension: 1% to <3%)

Endocrine & metabolic: Weight gain (1% to 3%)

Gastrointestinal: Dyspepsia (≥5%), nausea (2% to ≥5%), gastroenteritis (suspension: 5%), diarrhea (suspension: 4%), vomiting (1% to 4%), abdominal pain (1% to 3%), dysgeusia (powder: 1% to 3%), xerostomia (powder: 1% to 3%), anorexia (suspension: 1% to <3%), viral gastroenteritis (powder: 2%), oral candidiasis (powder: 1%)

Hematologic & oncologic: Ecchymosis (powder: 1% to 3%), cervical lymphadenopathy (suspension: 1% to <3%), purpura (suspension: 1% to <3%)

Hypersensitivity: Hypersensitivity reaction (1% to <3%)

Infection: Candidiasis (suspension: 4% to 5%), viral infection (suspension: 4% to 5%), infection (1% to 3%), herpes simplex infection (suspension: 1% to <3%)

Neuromuscular & skeletal: Arthralgia (≥5%), weakness (≥5%), back pain (powder: ≥3%), bone fracture (1% to 3%), myalgia (1% to 3%), neck pain (powder: 1% to 3%), hyperkinesia (suspension: 1% to <3%)

Ophthalmic: Conjunctivitis (suspension: 4%), eye infection (suspension: 1% to <3%)

Otic: Otic infection (suspension: 5%), otalgia (suspension: 1% to <3%), otitis externa (suspension: 1% to <3%)

Respiratory: Nasopharyngitis (powder: 9%), cough (5% to 9%), epistaxis (suspension: 2% to 4%), respiratory tract infection (powder: ≥3%), sinusitis (powder: ≥3%; suspension: <1%), nasal congestion (powder: 3%), pharyngitis (powder: 3%; suspension: <1%), flu-like symptoms (suspension: 1% to <3%), stridor (suspension: 1% to <3%), allergic rhinitis (powder: 2%), viral upper respiratory tract infection (powder: 2%)

Miscellaneous: Fever (≥3%)

Postmarketing and/or case reports: Adrenocortical insufficiency, aggressive behavior, anxiety, avascular necrosis of femoral head, bronchitis, bruise, cataract, depression, glaucoma, growth suppression, hypercorticoidism, increased intraocular pressure, irritability, nervousness, osteoporosis, pain, psychosis, restlessness, skin irritation (facial), throat irritation, wheezing

Mechanism of Action Controls the rate of protein synthesis; depresses the migration of polymorphonuclear leukocytes, fibroblasts; reverses capillary permeability and lysosomal stabilization at the cellular level to prevent or control inflammation. Has potent glucocorticoid activity and weak mineralocorticoid activity.

Pharmacodynamics/Kinetics

Onset of Action Nebulization: 2 to 8 days; Inhalation: 24 hours

Peak effect: Nebulization: 4 to 6 weeks; Inhalation: 1 to 2 weeks

Half-life Elimination

Children 4 to 6 years: 2.3 hours (after nebulization)

Children and Adolescents 10 to 14 years: 1.5 hours

Adults: 2 to 3.6 hours

Time to Peak

Nebulization: Pulmicort Respules: Children: 20 minutes

Oral inhalation: Pulmicort Flexhaler:

Children and Adolescents: 15 to 30 minutes

Adults: 10 minutes

Pregnancy Considerations

Studies of pregnant women using inhaled budesonide have not demonstrated an increased risk of congenital abnormalities.

Maternal use of inhaled corticosteroids (ICS) in usual doses is not associated with an increased risk of fetal malformations; a small risk of malformations was observed in one study following high maternal doses of an alternative inhaled corticosteroid. Uncontrolled asthma is associated with adverse events on pregnancy (increased risk of perinatal mortality, preeclampsia, preterm birth, low-birth-weight infants, cesarean delivery, and the development of gestational diabetes). Poorly controlled asthma or asthma exacerbations may have a greater fetal/maternal risk than what is associated with appropriately used asthma medications. Maternal treatment improves pregnancy outcomes by reducing the risk of some adverse events (eg, preterm birth, gestational diabetes) (ERS/TSANZ [Middleton 2020]; GINA 2020).

ICS are recommended for the treatment of asthma during pregnancy (GINA 2020). Budesonide is one of the preferred agents. The lowest dose that maintains asthma control should be used. Maternal asthma symptoms should be monitored monthly during pregnancy (ERS/TSANZ [Middleton 2020]).

Data collection to monitor pregnancy and infant outcomes associated with asthma and the medications used to treat asthma in pregnancy is ongoing. Health care providers are encouraged to enroll exposed pregnant females in the MotherToBaby Pregnancy Studies conducted by the Organization of Teratology Information Specialists (OTIS) (877-311-8972 or https://mothertobaby.org). Patients may also enroll themselves.

Budesonide (Topical) (byoo DES oh nide)

Brand Names: US Uceris
Brand Names: Canada Entocort
Pharmacologic Category Corticosteroid, Rectal
Use

Ulcerative colitis: Remission induction in patients with active mild to moderate distal ulcerative colitis extending up to 40 cm from the anal verge

Entocort Enema [Canadian product]: Management of distal ulcerative colitis (rectum, sigmoid, and descending colon)

Local Anesthetic/Vasoconstrictor Precautions No information available to require special precautions

Effects on Dental Treatment No significant effects or complications reported

Effects on Bleeding No information available to require special precautions

Adverse Reactions Frequency not always defined.

>10%: Endocrine & metabolic: Decreased plasma cortisol (17%)

1% to 10%:

Endocrine & metabolic: Adrenocortical insufficiency (4%), hpa-axis suppression, hypercortisolism

Gastrointestinal: Nausea (2%)

<1%, postmarketing, and/or case reports: Acne vulgaris, adrenal cortex hypofunction, agitation, allergic dermatitis, anaphylaxis, anxiety, depression, diarrhea, dizziness, drowsiness, dysphoria, emotional lability, exacerbation of diabetes mellitus, fever, flatulence, hyperacidity (peptic ulcer), hyperglycemia, hypertension, insomnia, maculopapular rash, pancreatitis, peripheral edema, pruritus, pseudotumor cerebri, skin rash, sleep disorder, urticaria

Mechanism of Action Controls the rate of protein synthesis; depresses the migration of polymorphonuclear leukocytes, fibroblasts; reverses capillary permeability and lysosomal stabilization at the cellular level to prevent or control inflammation. Has potent glucocorticoid activity and weak mineralocorticoid activity.

Pharmacodynamics/Kinetics

Half-life Elimination Rectal enema [Canadian product]: 2 to 3 hours

Time to Peak Rectal enema [Canadian product]: 1.5 hours

Reproductive Considerations Fertility may be decreased in females with active inflammatory bowel disease. Corticosteroids used for the management of inflammatory bowel disease are not expected to decrease female fertility (AGA [Mahadevan 2019]).

Pregnancy Considerations

Hypoadrenalism may occur in newborns following maternal use of corticosteroids in pregnancy; monitor.

Because systemic corticosteroids may increase the risk of gestational diabetes and other adverse pregnancy outcomes, use for maintenance therapy in pregnant women with inflammatory bowel disease is not recommended. However, corticosteroids may be used to treat disease flares in pregnant patients (AGA [Mahadevan 2019]).

◆ **Budesonide and Eformoterol** *see* Budesonide and Formoterol *on page 255*

Budesonide and Formoterol

(byoo DES oh nide & for MOH te rol)

Related Information

Budesonide (Oral Inhalation) *on page 254*

Formoterol *on page 711*

Brand Names: US Symbicort
Brand Names: Canada Symbicort 100 Turbuhaler; Symbicort 200 Turbuhaler; Symbicort Forte Turbuhaler
Pharmacologic Category $Beta_2$ Agonist; $Beta_2$-Adrenergic Agonist, Long-Acting; Corticosteroid, Inhalant (Oral)
Use

Asthma (controller/maintenance): Treatment of asthma in patients ≥6 years of age.

Chronic obstructive pulmonary disease: Maintenance treatment of airflow obstruction in patients with chronic obstructive pulmonary disease (COPD), including chronic bronchitis and/or emphysema; to reduce COPD exacerbations.

Local Anesthetic/Vasoconstrictor Precautions No information available to require special precautions

Effects on Dental Treatment Key adverse event(s) related to dental treatment: Formoterol: Xerostomia (normal salivary flow resumes upon discontinuation). Localized infections with *Candida albicans* or *Aspergillus niger* have occurred frequently in the mouth and pharynx with repetitive use of oral inhaler of corticosteroids. These infections may require treatment with appropriate antifungal therapy or discontinuance of treatment with corticosteroid inhaler.

Effects on Bleeding No information available to require special precautions

Adverse Reactions Reported incidences are for adolescents and adults unless specified otherwise. Also see individual agents.

>10%:

Central nervous system: Headache (7% to 11%; children: ≥3%)

Respiratory: Nasopharyngitis (7% to 11%), upper respiratory tract infection (4% to 11%; children: ≥3%)

1% to 10%:

Gastrointestinal: Abdominal distress (1% to 7%), oral candidiasis (1% to 6%), vomiting (1% to 3%)

Infection: Influenza (2% to 3%)

Neuromuscular & skeletal: Back pain (2% to 3%)

Respiratory: Pharyngolaryngeal pain (6% to 9%), pulmonary infection (7% to 8%), lower respiratory tract infection (3% to 8%), sinusitis (4% to 6%), bronchitis (5%), nasal congestion (3%), pharyngitis (children: ≥3%), rhinitis (children: ≥3%)

<1%, postmarketing, and/or case reports: Agitation, anaphylaxis, angina pectoris, angioedema, atrial arrhythmia, behavioral changes, bronchospasm, bruise, cataract, cough, decreased linear skeletal growth rate (pediatric patients), depression, dermatitis, dizziness, extrasystoles, glaucoma, hypercorticoidism signs and symptoms, hyperglycemia, hypersensitivity reaction, hypertension, hypokalemia, hypotension, immunosuppression, increased intraocular pressure, insomnia, muscle cramps, nausea, nervousness, palpitations, pruritus, restlessness, skin rash, tachycardia, throat irritation, tremor, urticaria, ventricular arrhythmia, voice disorder

Mechanism of Action

Formoterol: Relaxes bronchial smooth muscle by selective action on beta$_2$ receptors with little effect on heart rate; formoterol has a long-acting effect.

Budesonide: A corticosteroid which controls the rate of protein synthesis, depresses the migration of polymorphonuclear leukocytes/fibroblasts, and reverses capillary permeability and lysosomal stabilization at the cellular level to prevent or control inflammation.

Pregnancy Considerations Adverse events were observed in animal reproduction studies using this combination. Refer to individual agents.

- ◆ **Budesonide Foam** *see* Budesonide (Topical) *on page 255*
- ◆ **Buffasal [OTC]** *see* Aspirin *on page 177*
- ◆ **Bufferin [OTC]** *see* Aspirin *on page 177*
- ◆ **Bufferin Extra Strength [OTC]** *see* Aspirin *on page 177*
- ◆ **Buffinol [OTC]** *see* Aspirin *on page 177*

Bumetanide (byoo MET a nide)

Related Information

Cardiovascular Diseases *on page 1654*

Brand Names: US Bumex

Brand Names: Canada Burinex

Pharmacologic Category Antihypertensive; Diuretic, Loop

Use Edema: Management of edema secondary to heart failure or hepatic or renal disease (including nephrotic syndrome).

Local Anesthetic/Vasoconstrictor Precautions No information available to require special precautions

Effects on Dental Treatment No significant effects or complications reported

Effects on Bleeding No information available to require special precautions

Adverse Reactions

>10%:

Endocrine & metabolic: Hyperuricemia (18%), hypochloremia (15%), hypokalemia (15%)

Genitourinary: Azotemia (11%)

1% to 10%:

Central nervous system: Dizziness (1%)

Endocrine & metabolic: Hyponatremia (9%), hyperglycemia (7%), phosphorus change (5%), variations in bicarbonate (3%), abnormal serum calcium (2%), abnormal lactate dehydrogenase (1%)

Neuromuscular & skeletal: Muscle cramps (1%)

Renal: Increased serum creatinine (7%)

Respiratory: Variations in CO_2 content (4%)

<1%, postmarketing, and/or case reports: Abdominal pain, abnormal alkaline phosphatase, abnormal bilirubin levels, abnormal hematocrit, abnormal hemoglobin level, abnormal transaminase, arthritic pain, asterixis, auditory impairment, blood cholesterol abnormal, brain disease (in patients with preexisting liver disease), change in creatinine clearance, change in prothrombin time, change in WBC count, chest pain, dehydration, diaphoresis, diarrhea, dyspepsia, ECG changes, erectile dysfunction, fatigue, glycosuria, headache, hyperventilation, hypotension, musculoskeletal pain, nausea, nipple tenderness, orthostatic hypotension, otalgia, ototoxicity, premature ejaculation, proteinuria, pruritus, renal failure, skin rash, Stevens-Johnson syndrome, thrombocytopenia, toxic epidermal necrolysis, urticaria, vertigo, vomiting, weakness, xerostomia

Mechanism of Action Inhibits reabsorption of sodium and chloride in the ascending loop of Henle and proximal renal tubule, interfering with the chloride-binding cotransport system, thus causing increased excretion of water, sodium, chloride, magnesium, phosphate, and calcium; it does not appear to act on the distal tubule

Pharmacodynamics/Kinetics

Onset of Action Oral: 0.5 to 1 hour; IV: 2 to 3 minutes.

Peak effect: Oral: 1 to 2 hours; IV: 15 to 30 minutes.

Duration of Action Oral: 4 to 6 hours; IV: 2 to 3 hours

Half-life Elimination

Premature and full term neonates: 6 hours (range up to 15 hours)

Infants <2 months: 2.5 hours

Infants 2 to 6 months: 1.5 hours

Adults: 1 to 1.5 hours

Pregnancy Considerations Adverse events have been observed in some animal reproduction studies.

- ◆ **Bumex** *see* Bumetanide *on page 256*
- ◆ **Bunavail** *see* Buprenorphine and Naloxone *on page 270*
- ◆ **Buphenyl** *see* Sodium Phenylbutyrate *on page 1378*

Bupivacaine (byoo PIV a kane)

Related Information

Oral Pain *on page 1734*

Brand Names: US Bupivacaine Fisiopharma; Bupivacaine Spinal; Marcaine; Marcaine Preservative Free; Marcaine Spinal; P-Care M; ReadySharp Bupivacaine [DSC]; Sensorcaine; Sensorcaine-MPF; Sensorcaine-MPF Spinal [DSC]

Brand Names: Canada Marcaine; Marcaine Spinal; Sensorcaine

Pharmacologic Category Local Anesthetic

Use Local or regional anesthesia; spinal anesthesia (0.75% in dextrose 8.25% injection); diagnostic and therapeutic procedures; obstetrical procedures (only 0.25% and 0.5% concentrations)

0.25%: Local infiltration, peripheral nerve block, sympathetic block, caudal or epidural block

0.5%: Peripheral nerve block, caudal and epidural block

0.75% **(not for obstetrical anesthesia)**: Retrobulbar block, epidural block. **Note:** Reserve for surgical procedures where a high degree of muscle relaxation and prolonged effect are necessary

Local Anesthetic/Vasoconstrictor Precautions No information available to require special precautions

Effects on Dental Treatment No significant effects or complications reported

Effects on Bleeding No information available to require special precautions

Adverse Reactions Frequency not defined. Reactions listed are based on reports for other agents in this same pharmacologic class and may not be specifically reported for bupivacaine.

Cardiovascular: Bradycardia, cardiac insufficiency, circulatory shock, heart block, hypotension, ventricular arrhythmia

Central nervous system: Anxiety, arachnoiditis, central nervous system depression, central nervous system stimulation, chills, cranial nerve palsy, dizziness, headache, localized numbness (perineal), meningism, paralysis, paraplegia, paresthesia, persistent anesthesia, restlessness, seizure, shivering

Gastrointestinal: Fecal incontinence, loss of anal sphincter control, nausea, vomiting

Genitourinary: Prolonged labor, sexual disorder (loss of function), urinary incontinence, urinary retention

Hematologic & oncologic: Methemoglobinemia

Hypersensitivity: Hypersensitivity reaction

Infection: Septic meningitis

Neuromuscular & skeletal: Asthenia, back pain, lower extremity weakness, tremor

Ophthalmic: Blurred vision, miosis

Otic: Tinnitus

Respiratory: Apnea, hypoventilation (usually associated with unintentional subarachnoid injection during high spinal anesthesia), respiratory paralysis

Mechanism of Action Blocks both the initiation and conduction of nerve impulses by decreasing the neuronal membrane's permeability to sodium ions, which results in inhibition of depolarization with resultant blockade of conduction

Pharmacodynamics/Kinetics

Onset of Action Anesthesia (route and dose dependent):

Epidural: Up to 17 minutes to spread to T6 dermatome (Scott 1980)

Infiltration: Fast (Barash 2009); Dental injection: 2 to 10 minutes

Spinal: Within 1 minute; maximum dermatome level achieved within 15 minutes in most cases

Duration of Action Route and dose dependent:

Epidural: 2 to 7.7 hours (Barash 2009)

Infiltration: 2 to 8 hours (Barash 2009); Dental injection: Up to 7 hours

Spinal: 1.5 to 2.5 hours (Tsai 2007)

Half-life Elimination Age dependent: Neonates: 8.1 hours; Adults: 2.7 hours

Time to Peak Plasma: Caudal, epidural, or peripheral nerve block: 30 to 45 minutes

Pregnancy Considerations

Bupivacaine crosses the placenta. Bupivacaine is approved for use at term in obstetrical anesthesia or analgesia. **[US Boxed Warning]: The 0.75% is not recommended for obstetrical anesthesia.** Bupivacaine 0.75% solutions have been associated with cardiac arrest following epidural anesthesia in obstetrical patients and use of this concentration is not recommended for this purpose. Use in obstetrical paracervical block anesthesia is contraindicated.

Bupivacaine and Epinephrine

(byoo PIV a kane & ep i NEF rin)

Related Information

Bupivacaine *on page 256*

EPINEPHrine (Systemic) *on page 569*

Oral Pain *on page 1734*

Brand Names: US Marcaine/Epinephrine; Marcaine/Epinephrine PF; Sensorcaine-MPF/EPINEPHrine; Sensorcaine/EPINEPHrine

Brand Names: Canada Marcaine; Marcaine E; Sensorcaine/Epinephrine; Vivacaine

Generic Availability (US) Yes

Pharmacologic Category Local Anesthetic

Dental Use Local anesthesia

Use Anesthesia/analgesia: Local or regional anesthesia or analgesia for surgery, dental and oral procedures, diagnostic and therapeutic procedures, and obstetrical procedure

0.25%: Local infiltration, peripheral nerve block, sympathetic block, lumbar epidural, or caudal

0.5%: Peripheral nerve block, lumbar epidural, caudal, epidural test dose, or dental blocks

0.75% **(not for obstetrical anesthesia)**: Retrobulbar block or lumbar epidural; **Note:** Reserve for surgical procedures where a high degree of muscle relaxation and prolonged effect are necessary.

Local Anesthetic/Vasoconstrictor Precautions No information available to require special precautions

Effects on Dental Treatment It is common to misinterpret psychogenic responses to local anesthetic injection as an allergic reaction. Intraoral injections are perceived by many patients as a stressful procedure in dentistry. Common symptoms to this stress are diaphoresis, palpitations, and hyperventilation. Patients may exhibit hypersensitivity to bisulfites contained in local anesthetic solution to prevent oxidation of epinephrine. In general, patients reacting to bisulfites have a history of asthma and their airways are hyper-reactive to asthmatic syndrome.

Degree of adverse effects in the CNS and cardiovascular system is directly related to the blood levels of bupivacaine: Bradycardia, hypersensitivity reactions (rare; may be manifest as dermatologic reactions and edema at injection site), asthmatic syndromes.

High blood levels: Anxiety, restlessness, disorientation, confusion, dizziness, tremors, seizures, CNS depression (resulting in somnolence, unconsciousness and possible respiratory arrest), nausea, and vomiting.

Effects on Bleeding No information available to require special precautions

Adverse Reactions See individual agents.

Dental Usual Dosage

Infiltration and nerve block in maxillary and mandibular area: Children >12 years and Adults: 9 mg (1.8 mL) of bupivacaine as a 0.5% solution with epinephrine 1:200,000 per injection site. A second dose may be administered if necessary to produce adequate anesthesia after allowing up to 10 minutes for onset. Up to a maximum of 90 mg of bupivacaine hydrochloride per dental appointment. The effective anesthetic dose varies with procedure, intensity of anesthesia needed, duration of anesthesia required, and physical condition of the patient; always use the lowest effective dose along with careful aspiration.

The following numbers of dental carpules (1.8 mL) provide the indicated amounts of bupivacaine hydrochloride 0.5% and vasoconstrictor (epinephrine 1:200,000). See table.

# of Cartridges (1.8 mL)	mg Bupivacaine (0.5%)	mg Vasoconstrictor (Epinephrine 1:200,000)
1	9	0.009
2	18	0.018
3	27	0.027
4	36	0.036
5	45	0.045
6	54	0.054
7	63	0.063
8	72	0.072
9	81	0.081
10	90	0.090

Note: Adult and children doses of bupivacaine hydrochloride with epinephrine cited from USP Dispensing Information (USP DI), 17th ed, The United States Pharmacopeial Convention, Inc, Rockville, MD, 1997, 134.

Dosing

Adult & Geriatric Dose varies with procedure, depth of anesthesia, vascularity of tissues, duration of anesthesia, and condition of patient. Do not use solutions containing preservatives for caudal or epidural block. Doses may be repeated up to once every 3 hours (maximum: 400 mg/day of bupivacaine).

Caudal and lumbar epidural block test dose (preservative free): 2 to 3 mL of 0.5% (maximum: 15 mg/dose of bupivacaine or 15 mcg/dose of epinephrine)

Caudal block (preservative free): 15 to 30 mL of 0.25% or 0.5% (maximum: 75 mg/dose of 0.25% bupivacaine or 150 mg/dose of 0.5% bupivacaine)

Epidural block (other than caudal block, preservative free): 10 to 20 mL of 0.25% or 0.5% (maximum: 50 mg/dose of 0.25% bupivacaine or 100 mg/dose of 0.5% bupivacaine). Administer in 3 to 5 mL increments, allowing sufficient time to detect toxic manifestations of inadvertent IV or intrathecal administration.

Surgical procedures requiring a high degree of muscle relaxation and prolonged effects only: 10 to 20 mL of 0.75%; **Note:** Not to be used in obstetrical cases (maximum: 150 mg/dose of bupivacaine)

Local anesthesia: Infiltration: 0.25% infiltrated locally (maximum: 400 mg/day of bupivacaine)

Peripheral nerve block: 5 mL of 0.25% or 0.5% (maximum: 400 mg/day of bupivacaine)

Retrobulbar anesthesia: 2 to 4 mL of 0.75% (maximum: 30 mg/dose of bupivacaine)

Sympathetic nerve block: 20 to 50 mL of 0.25% (maximum: 125 mg/dose of bupivacaine)

Dental block: 1.8 mL (9 mg) of bupivacaine as a 0.5% solution with epinephrine 1:200,000 per injection site. A second dose may be administered if necessary to produce adequate anesthesia after allowing up to 10 minutes for onset. Up to a maximum of 90 mg of bupivacaine per dental appointment. The effective anesthetic dose varies with procedure, intensity of anesthesia needed, duration of anesthesia required, and physical condition of the patient; always use the lowest effective dose along with careful aspiration.

Renal Impairment: Adult There are no dosage adjustments provided in the manufacturer's labeling; use with caution.

Hepatic Impairment: Adult There are no dosage adjustments provided in the manufacturer's labeling; use with caution.

Pediatric Children >12 years and Adolescents: Refer to adult dosing.

Renal Impairment: Pediatric There are no dosage adjustments provided in manufacturer's labeling; use with caution.

Hepatic Impairment: Pediatric There are no dosage adjustments provided in manufacturer's labeling; use with caution.

Mechanism of Action Local anesthetics bind selectively to the intracellular surface of sodium channels to block influx of sodium into the axon. As a result, depolarization necessary for action potential propagation and subsequent nerve function is prevented. The block at the sodium channel is reversible. When drug diffuses away from the axon, sodium channel function is restored and nerve propagation returns.

Epinephrine prolongs the duration of the anesthetic actions of bupivacaine by causing vasoconstriction (alpha-adrenergic receptor agonist) of the vasculature surrounding the nerve axons. This prevents the diffusion of bupivacaine away from the nerves resulting in a longer retention in the axon

Contraindications

Hypersensitivity to bupivacaine, epinephrine, amide-type local anesthetics, or any component of the formulation; obstetrical paracervical block anesthesia

Canadian labeling: Additional contraindications (not in US labeling): IV regional anesthesia (Bier block)

Warnings/Precautions Some commercially available formulations contain sodium metabisulfite, which may cause allergic-type reactions. Do not use solutions containing preservatives for caudal or epidural block. Intravascular injections should be avoided. Local anesthetics have been associated with rare occurrences of sudden respiratory arrest. Convulsions due to systemic toxicity leading to cardiac arrest have also been reported, presumably following unintentional intravascular injection. **[US Boxed Warning]: The 0.75% is not recommended for obstetrical anesthesia.** A test dose is recommended prior to epidural administration and all reinforcing doses with continuous catheter technique. Use caution with cardiovascular dysfunction, hepatic impairment, or patients with compromised blood supply. Bupivacaine-containing products have been associated with rare occurrences of arrhythmias, cardiac arrest, and death. Use caution in debilitated, elderly, or acutely ill patients; dose reduction may be required. Dental practitioners and/or clinicians using local anesthetic agents should be well trained in diagnosis and management of emergencies that may arise from the use of these agents. Resuscitative equipment, oxygen, and other resuscitative drugs should be available for immediate use. Not recommended for use in children <12 years of age.

Methemoglobinemia has been reported with local anesthetics; clinically significant methemoglobinemia requires immediate treatment along with discontinuation of the anesthetic and other oxidizing agents. Onset may be immediate or delayed (hours) after anesthetic exposure. Patients with glucose-6-phosphate dehydrogenase deficiency, congenital or idiopathic methemoglobinemia, cardiac or pulmonary compromise, exposure to oxidizing agents or their metabolites, or infants <6 months of age are more susceptible and should be closely monitored for signs and symptoms of methemoglobinemia (eg, cyanosis, headache, rapid pulse, shortness of breath, lightheadedness, fatigue).

Continuous intra-articular infusion of local anesthetics after arthroscopic or other surgical procedures is **not** an approved use; chondrolysis (primarily shoulder joint) has occurred following infusion, with some requiring arthroplasty or shoulder replacement.

Drug Interactions

Metabolism/Transport Effects Refer to individual components.

Avoid Concomitant Use

Avoid concomitant use of Bupivacaine and Epinephrine with any of the following: Blonanserin; Bromperidol; Ergot Derivatives; Lurasidone

Increased Effect/Toxicity

Bupivacaine and Epinephrine may increase the levels/effects of: Amifostine; Antipsychotic Agents (Second Generation [Atypical]); Bupivacaine (Liposomal); Doxofylline; Hypotension-Associated Agents; Levodopa-Containing Products; Lurasidone; Neuromuscular-Blocking Agents; Nitroprusside; Pholcodine; Solriamfetol; Sympathomimetics

The levels/effects of Bupivacaine and Epinephrine may be increased by: Alfuzosin; Amisulpride (Oral); AtoMOXetine; Barbiturates; Beta-Blockers; Beta-Blockers (Nonselective); Blood Pressure Lowering Agents; Bretylium; Brimonidine (Topical); Cannabinoid-Containing Products; Chloroprocaine; Cocaine (Topical); COMT Inhibitors; Diazoxide; Ergot Derivatives; Guanethidine; Herbs (Hypotensive Properties); Hyaluronidase; Inhalational Anesthetics; Linezolid; Lormetazepam; Methemoglobinemia Associated Agents; Molsidomine; Monoamine Oxidase Inhibitors; Naftopidil; Nicergoline; Nicorandil; Obinutuzumab; Ozanimod; Pentoxifylline; Phosphodiesterase 5 Inhibitors; Procarbazine; Prostacyclin Analogues; Quinagolide; Serotonin/Norepinephrine Reuptake Inhibitors; Tedizolid; Tricyclic Antidepressants

Decreased Effect

Bupivacaine and Epinephrine may decrease the levels/effects of: Antidiabetic Agents; Benzylpenicilloyl Polylysine; Technetium Tc 99m Tilmanocept

The levels/effects of Bupivacaine and Epinephrine may be decreased by: Alpha1-Blockers; Benperidol; Beta-Blockers (Beta1 Selective); Beta-Blockers (with Alpha-Blocking Properties); Blonanserin; Bromperidol; CloZAPine; Haloperidol; Promethazine; Spironolactone

Pregnancy Risk Factor C

Pregnancy Considerations See individual agents.

Dosage Forms: US

Solution, Injection:

Marcaine/Epinephrine: Bupivacaine hydrochloride 0.5% and epinephrine 1:200,000 (50 mL); Bupivacaine hydrochloride 0.25% and epinephrine 1:200,000 (50 mL)

Sensorcaine/EPINEPHrine: Bupivacaine hydrochloride 0.5% and epinephrine 1:200,000 (50 mL); Bupivacaine hydrochloride 0.25% and epinephrine 1:200,000 (50 mL)

Generic: Bupivacaine hydrochloride 0.25% and epinephrine 1:200,000 (50 mL); Bupivacaine hydrochloride 0.5% and epinephrine 1:200,000 (50 mL)

Solution, Injection [preservative free]:

Marcaine/Epinephrine PF: Bupivacaine hydrochloride 0.5% and epinephrine 1:200,000 (10 mL, 30 mL); Bupivacaine hydrochloride 0.25% and epinephrine 1:200,000 (10 mL, 30 mL)

Sensorcaine-MPF/EPINEPHrine: Bupivacaine hydrochloride 0.5% and epinephrine 1:200,000 (10 mL, 30 mL); Bupivacaine hydrochloride 0.25% and epinephrine 1:200,000 (10 mL, 30 mL); Bupivacaine hydrochloride 0.75% and epinephrine 1:200,000 (30 mL)

Generic: Bupivacaine hydrochloride 0.25% and epinephrine 1:200,000 (10 mL, 30 mL); Bupivacaine hydrochloride 0.5% and epinephrine 1:200,000 (1.8 mL, 10 mL, 30 mL)

Dosage Forms: Canada

Solution, Injection:

Marcaine: Bupivacaine hydrochloride 0.5% and epinephrine 1:200,000 (1.8 mL)

Marcaine E: Bupivacaine hydrochloride 0.5% and epinephrine 1:200,000 (3 mL, 20 mL); Bupivacaine hydrochloride 0.25% and epinephrine 1:200,000 (20 mL)

Sensorcaine/Epinephrine: Bupivacaine hydrochloride 0.5% and epinephrine 1:200,000 (20 mL); Bupivacaine hydrochloride 0.25% and epinephrine 1:200,000 (20 mL)

Vivacaine: Bupivacaine hydrochloride 0.5% and epinephrine 1:200,000 (1.8 mL)

Generic: Bupivacaine hydrochloride 0.5% and epinephrine 1:200,000 (1.8 mL)

Dental Health Professional Considerations A 2010 report, reviewed adverse events submitted voluntarily over a 10-year period involving the dental local anesthetics articaine, bupivacaine, lidocaine, mepivacaine, and prilocaine in the United States. Bupivacaine reported incidence: One case per 124,286,050 cartridges sold. The reported incidence of paresthesia was one case for 13,800,970 cartridges of all local anesthetics sold in the U.S. (Garisto, 2010).

- **Bupivacaine/Epinephrine** *see* Bupivacaine and Epinephrine *on page 257*
- **Bupivacaine Fisiopharma** *see* Bupivacaine *on page 256*
- **Bupivacaine HCl** *see* Bupivacaine *on page 256*
- **Bupivacaine HCl/Epinephrine** *see* Bupivacaine and Epinephrine *on page 257*
- **Bupivacaine Hydrochloride** *see* Bupivacaine *on page 256*

Bupivacaine (Liposomal)

(byoo PIV a kane lye po SO mal)

Brand Names: US Exparel

Pharmacologic Category Local Anesthetic

Use Analgesia, postsurgical: Single-dose infiltration in adults to produce postsurgical local analgesia and as an interscalene brachial plexus nerve block to produce postsurgical regional analgesia.

Local Anesthetic/Vasoconstrictor Precautions No information available to require special precautions

Effects on Dental Treatment No significant effects or complications reported

Effects on Bleeding No information available to require special precautions

Adverse Reactions

>10%:

Central nervous system: Motor dysfunction (12% to 21%)

Gastrointestinal: Nausea (<40%), vomiting (28%), constipation (2% to 22%)

Miscellaneous: Fever (2% to 23%)

1% to 10%:

Cardiovascular: Hypertension (<10%; includes procedural hypertension), hypotension (7%), procedural hypotension (4%), tachycardia (4%), peripheral edema (2% to 3%), sinus tachycardia (2% to 3%), atrial fibrillation (<2%), bradycardia (<2%), bundle branch block (<2%), cardiac arrhythmia (<2%), deep vein thrombosis (<2%), edema (<2%), first degree atrioventricular block (<2%), oxygen saturation decreased (<2%), orthostatic hypotension (<2%), palpitations (<2%), presyncope (<2%), prolonged QT interval on ECG (<2%), sinus bradycardia (<2%), supraventricular extrasystole (<2%), syncope (2%), ventricular premature contractions (<2%), ventricular tachycardia (<2%)

Central nervous system: Insomnia (2% to <10%), procedural pain (2% to <10%), headache (4% to 8%), dizziness (≤6%; includes postural dizziness), confusion (5%), fatigue (5%), drowsiness (2% to 5%), hypoesthesia (2% to 4%), anxiety (3%), sensation of cold (3%), falling (2% to 3%), feeling hot (2%), mobility disorder (decreased: 2%), sensation disorder (sensory loss: 2%), agitation (<2%), chills (<2%), delirium (<2%), depression (<2%), hyperthermia (<2%), myasthenia (<2%), pain (<2%), paresthesia (<2%), restlessness (<2%), sedation (<2%), lethargy (1%)

Dermatologic: Hyperhidrosis (5%), pruritus (3%), cellulitis (<2%), diaphoresis (<2%), erythema (<2%), increased wound secretion (<2%), pallor (<2%), pruritic rash (<2%), skin blister (<2%), skin rash (<2%), urticaria (<2%)

Gastrointestinal: Dysgeusia (7%), oral hypoesthesia (3% to 4%), hiccups (1% to 2%)

Genitourinary: Urinary retention (8%), dysuria (<2%), urinary incontinence (<2%)

Hematologic & oncologic: Acute posthemorrhagic anemia (2% to <10%; postoperative), anemia (6%), bruise (≤2%), hematoma (<2%), leukocytosis (<2%), postoperative hematoma (≤2%)

Hepatic: Increased liver enzymes (4%), increased serum aspartate aminotransferase (3%), increased serum alanine aminotransferase (1%)

Hypersensitivity: Fixed drug eruption (<2%), hypersensitivity reaction (<2%)

Infection: Fungal infection (2%)

Local: Localized edema (incision site: <2%)

Neuromuscular & skeletal: Back pain (<10%), muscle spasm (<10%), muscle twitching (8%), arthralgia (<2%), asthenia (<2%), joint swelling (<2%), laryngospasm (<2%), musculoskeletal pain (<2%), neck pain (<2%), tremor (<2%)

Ophthalmic: Blurred vision (<2%), decreased visual acuity (<2%)

Otic: Auditory impairment (<2%), tinnitus (<2%)

Renal: Increased serum creatinine (2%)

Respiratory: Hypoxia (1% to 2%), apnea (<2%), atelectasis (<2%), cough (<2%), dyspnea (<2%), pulmonary infiltrates (<2%), pneumonia (<2%), pulmonary infection (<2%), respiratory depression (<2%), respiratory failure (<2%)

Miscellaneous: Procedural complications (postprocedural swelling: 2%), dehiscence (<2%)

<1%, postmarketing, and/or case reports: Paralysis, seizure

Mechanism of Action Blocks both the initiation and conduction of nerve impulses by decreasing the neuronal membrane's permeability to sodium ions, which results in inhibition of depolarization with resultant blockade of conduction.

Pharmacodynamics/Kinetics

Onset of Action Rapid (Hu 2013)

Duration of Action Local: Up to 72 hours (Hu 2013); Systemic: Plasma levels can persist for 96 hours after local administration and 120 hours after interscalene brachial plexus nerve block.

Half-life Elimination 13 to 34 hours (Hu 2013)

Time to Peak Within 1 hour (initial peak); 12 to 36 hours (second peak) (Hu 2013)

Pregnancy Considerations

Bupivacaine crosses the placenta. Not recommended for use in pregnancy. Use in obstetrical paracervical block anesthesia is contraindicated; may cause fetal bradycardia and death.

- ◆ **Bupivacaine Liposome** *see* Bupivacaine (Liposomal) *on page 259*
- ◆ **Bupivacaine Liposome/Pf** *see* Bupivacaine (Liposomal) *on page 259*
- ◆ **Bupivacaine Spinal** *see* Bupivacaine *on page 256*
- ◆ **Buprenex** *see* Buprenorphine *on page 260*

Buprenorphine (byoo pre NOR feen)

Brand Names: US Belbuca; Buprenex; Butrans; Probuphine Implant Kit; Sublocade

Brand Names: Canada Belbuca [DSC]; BuTrans 10; BuTrans 15; BuTrans 20; BuTrans 5; Probuphine; Sublocade; Subutex

Generic Availability (US) May be product dependent

Pharmacologic Category Analgesic, Opioid; Analgesic, Opioid Partial Agonist

Use

Opioid use disorder:

Extended-release injection: Maintenance treatment of moderate to severe opioid use disorder in patients who have initiated treatment with 8 to 24 mg of a transmucosal buprenorphine-containing product, followed by dose adjustment for a minimum of 7 days.

Subdermal implant: Maintenance treatment of opioid use disorder in patients who have achieved and sustained prolonged clinical stability on low to moderate doses (≤8 mg/day) of a transmucosal buprenorphine-containing product for 3 months or longer with no need for supplemental dosing or adjustments

Sublingual tablet: Medically supervised withdrawal and maintenance treatment of opioid use disorder.

Limitations of use: Buprenorphine should be used as part of a complete treatment program to include counseling and psychosocial support.

Pain management:

Buccal film, transdermal patch: Management of pain severe enough to require around-the-clock, long-term opioid treatment and for which alternative treatment options are inadequate

Immediate-release injection: Management of pain severe enough to require an opioid analgesic and for which treatments are inadequate

Limitations of use: Reserve buprenorphine for use in patients for whom alternative treatment options (eg, nonopioid analgesics, opioid combination products, immediate-release opioids) are ineffective, not tolerated, or would be otherwise inadequate to provide sufficient management of pain. Buprenorphine buccal film and transdermal patch are not indicated as an as needed analgesic.

Local Anesthetic/Vasoconstrictor Precautions No information available to require special precautions

Effects on Dental Treatment No significant effects or complications reported

Effects on Bleeding No information available to require special precautions

Adverse Reactions

Buccal film:

1% to 10%:

Cardiovascular: Hypertension (1% to <5%), peripheral edema (1% to <5%)

Central nervous system: Fatigue (≥5%), headache (4% to ≥5%), dizziness (2% to ≥5%), drowsiness (1% to ≥5%), anxiety (1% to <5%), depression (1% to <5%), falling (1% to <5%), insomnia (1% to <5%), opioid withdrawal syndrome (1% to <5%)

Dermatologic: Hyperhidrosis (1% to <5%), pruritus (1% to <5%), skin rash (1% to <5%)

Endocrine & metabolic: Hot flash (1% to <5%)

Gastrointestinal: Nausea (9% to 10%), diarrhea (≥5%), xerostomia (≥5%), vomiting (4% to ≥5%), constipation (3% to ≥5%), abdominal pain (1% to <5%), decreased appetite (1% to <5%), gastroenteritis (1% to <5%)

Genitourinary: Urinary tract infection (1% to <5%)

Hematologic & oncologic: Anemia (1% to <5%), bruise (1% to <5%)

Neuromuscular & skeletal: Back pain (1% to <5%), muscle spasm (1% to <5%)

Respiratory: Upper respiratory tract infection (≥5%), bronchitis (1% to <5%), nasopharyngitis (1% to <5%), oropharyngeal pain (1% to <5%), paranasal sinus congestion (1% to <5%), sinusitis (1% to <5%)

Miscellaneous: Fever (1% to <5%)

Implant:

>10%:

Central nervous system: Headache (13%)

Local: Local pain (13%; at implant site), local pruritus (12%; at implant site)

1% to 10%:

Cardiovascular: Chest pain (1%)

Central nervous system: Depression (6%), dizziness (4%), pain (4%), drowsiness (3%), fatigue (3%), chills (2%), migraine (2%), paresthesia (1%), sedation (1%), sensation of cold (1%)

Dermatologic: Localized erythema (10%; at implant site), skin rash (2%), excoriation (1% to 2%; including scratch), skin lesion (1%)

Gastrointestinal: Constipation (6%), nausea (6%), vomiting (6%), toothache (5%), upper abdominal pain (3%), flatulence (1%)

Hematologic & oncologic: Local hemorrhage (7%; at implant site)

Local: Localized edema (5%; at implant site), local swelling (1%)

Neuromuscular & skeletal: Back pain (6%), limb pain (3%), asthenia (2%)

Respiratory: Oropharyngeal pain (5%), cough (3%), dyspnea (1%)

Miscellaneous: Fever (3%), laceration (3%)

Injection:

>10%: Central nervous system: Sedation (≤66%)

1% to 10%:

Cardiovascular: Hypotension (1% to 5%)

Central nervous system: Vertigo (5% to 10%), dizziness (2% to 10%), headache (1% to 9%), fatigue (4% to 6%), drowsiness (2% to 5%)

Dermatologic: Injection site pruritus (6% to 10%), diaphoresis (1% to 5%)

Endocrine & metabolic: Increased gamma-glutamyl transferase (3% to 4%)

Gastrointestinal: Nausea (5% to 10%), constipation (8% to 9%), vomiting (1% to 9%)

Hepatic: Increased serum aspartate aminotransferase (3% to 5%), increased serum alanine aminotransferase (1% to 5%)

Local: Pain at injection site (5% to 6%), erythema at injection site (3% to 4%), bruising at injection site (1%), induration at injection site (1%), swelling at injection site (≤1%)

Neuromuscular & skeletal: Increased creatine phosphokinase (3% to 5%)

Ophthalmic: Miosis (1% to 5%)

Respiratory: Hypoventilation (1% to 5%)

Sublingual tablet:

>10%:

Central nervous system: Headache (29%), insomnia (21%)

Dermatologic: Diaphoresis (13%)

Gastrointestinal: Nausea (14%), abdominal pain (12%)

Infection: Infection (12%)

1% to 10%: Gastrointestinal: Constipation (8%), vomiting (8%)

Transdermal patch:

>10%:

Central nervous system: Dizziness (2% to 15%), headache (3% to 14%), drowsiness (2% to 13%)

Gastrointestinal: Nausea (6% to 21%), constipation (3% to 13%)

Local: Application-site pruritus (5% to 15%)

1% to 10%:

Cardiovascular: Chest pain (<5%), hypertension (<5%), peripheral edema (1% to <5%)

Central nervous system: Fatigue (≤5%), insomnia (<5%), anxiety (1% to <5%), depression (1% to <5%), falling (1% to <5%), hypoesthesia (1% to <5%), migraine (1% to <5%), pain (1% to <5%), paresthesia (1% to <5%)

Dermatologic: Pruritus (1% to 5%), hyperhidrosis (1% to <5%), skin rash (1% to <5%)

Gastrointestinal: Vomiting (≤9%), xerostomia (≥5% to 6%), anorexia (1% to <5%), diarrhea (1% to <5%), dyspepsia (1% to <5%), upper abdominal pain (1% to <5%), stomach discomfort (2%)

Genitourinary: Urinary tract infection (1% to <5%)

Infection: Influenza (1% to <5%)

Local: Application site erythema (5% to 10%), application site rash (5% to 8%), application site irritation (1% to 6%)

Neuromuscular & skeletal: Arthralgia (1% to <5%), asthenia (1% to <5%), back pain (1% to <5%), joint swelling (1% to <5%), limb pain (1% to <5%), muscle spasm (1% to <5%), musculoskeletal pain (1% to <5%), myalgia (1% to <5%), neck pain (1% to <5%), tremor (1% to <5%)

Respiratory: Bronchitis (1% to <5%), cough (1% to <5%), dyspnea (1% to <5%), nasopharyngitis (1% to <5%), pharyngolaryngeal pain (1% to <5%), sinusitis (1% to <5%), upper respiratory tract infection (1% to <5%)

Miscellaneous: Fever (1% to <5%)

<1%, postmarketing, and/or case reports: Abdominal distention, abdominal distress, abdominal pain, abnormal dreams, abnormal gait, abnormal hepatic function tests, accidental injury, acute sinusitis, agitation, amblyopia, anaphylactic shock, angina pectoris, angioedema, apathy, apnea, application site burning, application site dermatitis, application site discharge, application site reaction, application site vesicles, asthenia, ataxia, atrial fibrillation, blurred vision, bone fracture, bradycardia, bronchospasm, cellulitis, cellulitis at injection site, cerebrovascular accident, changes in respiration, chest pain, chills, cholecystitis, coma, confusion, conjunctivitis, contact dermatitis, coronary artery disease, cough, cyanosis, decreased libido, decreased mental acuity, decreased plasma testosterone, dehydration, depersonalization, depressed mood, depression, diarrhea, diplopia, disorientation, disturbance in attention, diverticulitis of the gastrointestinal tract, drug dependence (physical dependence), dysarthria, dysgeusia, dyspepsia, dysphagia, dysphoria, dyspnea, emotional lability, euphoria, exacerbation of asthma, excoriation, facial edema, flatulence, flushing, gallbladder disease (intracholedochal pressure), glossalgia, glossitis, hallucination, hepatic encephalopathy, hepatic failure, hepatic necrosis, hepatitis (including cytolytic), hepatorenal syndrome, hiccups, hot flash, hypersensitivity reaction, hyperventilation, hypoesthesia, hypogonadism (Brennan 2013; Debono 2011), hypotension, hypoventilation, increased blood pressure, increased serum alanine aminotransferase, increased serum aspartate aminotransferase, increased serum transaminases, injection site reaction, intestinal obstruction, jaundice, laceration, lethargy, local discomfort, localized warm feeling, loss of consciousness, malaise, memory impairment, mental status changes, migraine, miosis, musculoskeletal pain, myasthenia, nasal congestion, neck pain, nervousness, nightmares, noncardiac chest pain, opioid withdrawal syndrome, oral hypoesthesia, oral mucosa erythema, orthostatic hypotension, osteoarthritis, pallor, palpitations, pneumonia, prolonged QT interval on ECG, pruritus, psychosis, respiratory depression, respiratory distress, respiratory failure, restlessness, rhinitis, rhinorrhea, sedation, seizure, sensation of cold, sexual disorder, skin rash, slurred speech, stomatitis, syncope, tachycardia, tinnitus, tooth abscess, toothache, transient ischemic attacks, tremor, urinary hesitancy, urinary incontinence, urinary retention, urticaria, vasodilation, vertigo, visual disturbance, weight loss, Wenckebach period on ECG, wheezing, xeroderma, xerophthalmia, xerostomia

Dosing

Adult

Note: Buprenorphine 8 mg sublingual tablet = buprenorphine/naloxone 8 mg/2 mg sublingual film = buprenorphine/naloxone 4.2 mg/0.7 mg buccal film = buprenorphine/naloxone 5.7 mg/1.4 mg sublingual tablet.

Acute pain (moderate to severe): Note: Long-term use is not recommended. The following recommendations are guidelines and do not represent the maximum doses that may be required in all patients. Doses should be titrated to pain relief/prevention.

Immediate-release injection:

IM: Initial: 0.3 mg every 6 to 8 hours as needed; initial dose (up to 0.3 mg) may be repeated once in 30 to 60 minutes after the initial dose if needed.

Slow IV: Initial: 0.3 mg every 6 to 8 hours as needed; initial dose (up to 0.3 mg) may be repeated once in 30 to 60 minutes after the initial dose if needed.

Chronic pain (moderate to severe):

Buccal film: **Note:** Buprenorphine buccal film doses of 600, 750, and 900 mcg are only for use following titration from lower doses (maximum dose: 900 mcg every 12 hours).

Opioid-naive patients and opioid-non-tolerant patients: Initial: 75 mcg once daily or, if tolerated, every 12 hours for ≥4 days, then increase to 150 mcg every 12 hours.

Opioid-experienced patients (conversion from other opioids to buprenorphine): Discontinue all other around-the-clock opioids when buprenorphine is initiated. Taper patient's current opioid to no more than 30 mg oral morphine sulfate equivalents daily before initiating buprenorphine. Following analgesic taper, base the initial buprenorphine dose on the patient's daily opioid dose prior to taper. Patients may require additional short-acting analgesics during the taper period.

Patients who were receiving daily dose of <30 mg of oral morphine equivalents: Initial: 75 mcg once daily or every 12 hours.

Patients who were receiving daily dose of 30 to 89 mg of oral morphine equivalents: Initial: 150 mcg every 12 hours.

Patients who were receiving daily dose of 90 to 160 mg of oral morphine equivalents: Initial: 300 mcg every 12 hours.

Patients who were receiving daily dose of >160 mg of oral morphine equivalents: Buprenorphine buccal film may not provide adequate analgesia; **consider the use of an alternate analgesic.**

Conversion from methadone: Close monitoring is required when converting methadone to another opioid. Ratio between methadone and other opioid agonists varies widely according to previous dose exposure. Methadone has a long half-life and can accumulate in the plasma.

Dose titration (opioid-naive or opioid-experienced patients): Individually titrate in increments of 150 mcg every 12 hours, no more frequently than every 4 days, to a dose that provides adequate analgesia and minimizes adverse reactions (maximum dose: 900 mcg every 12 hours; doses up to 450 mcg every 12 hours were studied in opioid naive patients). Patients may require additional short-acting analgesics during titration.

Discontinuation of therapy: When discontinuing buccal film, use a gradual downward titration, such as decreasing the dose by no more than 10% to 25% in a physically dependent patient and continue downward titration every 2 to 4 weeks. If patient displays withdrawal symptoms, temporarily interrupt the taper or increase dose to previous level and then reduce dose more slowly by increasing interval between dose reductions, decreasing amount of daily dose reduction, or both.

Patients with oral mucositis: Reduce the starting dose and titration incremental dose by 50%.

Transdermal patch:

Opioid-naive patients: Initial: 5 **mcg**/hour applied once every 7 days.

Opioid-experienced patients (conversion from other opioids to buprenorphine): Discontinue all other around-the-clock opioid drugs when buprenorphine therapy is initiated. Short-acting analgesics as needed may be continued until analgesia with transdermal buprenorphine is attained. There is a potential for buprenorphine to precipitate withdrawal in patients already receiving opioids.

Patients who were receiving daily dose of <30 mg of oral morphine equivalents: Initial: 5 **mcg**/hour applied once every 7 days.

Patients who were receiving daily dose of 30 to 80 mg of oral morphine equivalents: Taper the current around-the-clock opioid for up to 7 days to ≤30 mg/day of oral morphine or equivalent before initiating therapy. Initial: 10 **mcg**/hour applied once every 7 days.

Patients who were receiving daily dose of >80 mg of oral morphine equivalents: Buprenorphine transdermal patch, even at the maximum dose of 20 **mcg**/hour applied once every 7 days, may not provide adequate analgesia; **consider the use of an alternate analgesic.**

Dose titration (opioid-naive or opioid-experienced patients): May increase dose in 5 mcg/hour, 7.5 mcg/hour, or 10 mcg/hour increments (using no more than two patches), based on patient's supplemental short-acting analgesic requirements, with a minimum titration interval of 72 hours (maximum dose: 20 mcg/hour applied once every 7 days; risk for QTc prolongation increases with doses >20 mcg/hour patch).

Discontinuation of therapy: When discontinuing transdermal patch, use a gradual downward titration, such as decreasing the dose by no more than 10% to 25% in a physically dependent patient and continue downward titration every 2 to 4 weeks. If patient displays withdrawal symptoms, temporarily interrupt the taper or increase dose to previous level and then reduce dose more slowly by increasing interval between dose reductions, decreasing amount of daily dose reduction, or both.

Opioid use disorder:

Extended-release injection: SubQ: Initial: 300 mg monthly for the first 2 months, after treatment has been inducted and adjusted with 8 to 24 mg of a transmucosal buprenorphine-containing product for a minimum of 7 days. Maintenance: 100 mg monthly, increasing to 300 mg monthly for patients who tolerate the 100 mg dose but do not demonstrate a satisfactory clinical response (as evidenced by self-reported illicit opioid use or urine drug screens positive for illicit opioid use). **Note**: Administer doses ≥26 days apart.

Extended interval dosing (only for use in select instances such as extended travel): Patients established on a maintenance dose of 100 mg monthly may receive a single 300 mg dose to cover a 2-month period followed by resumption of the 100 mg monthly dose. Patients should be cautioned about sedation and other buprenorphine-related effects due to higher peak levels following the 300 mg dose.

Subdermal implant: Insert 4 implants subdermally in the inner side of the upper arm 12 to 24 hours after last dose of transmucosal buprenorphine-containing product (SAMHSA 2018). Remove no later than 6 months after the date of insertion; if continued treatment is desired, insert 4 new implants subdermally in the inner side of the contralateral arm. After one insertion in each arm, discontinue treatment with subdermal implants.

Converting back to sublingual tablet: On day of implant removal, resume buprenorphine treatment at previous sublingual dose.

Sublingual tablet:

Induction: 2 to 4 mg; if no signs of precipitated withdrawal after 60 to 90 minutes, may increase in increments of 2 to 4 mg. Consider an initial dose of 1 mg in patients with a history of opioid use disorder with a high risk of relapse but not currently dependent on opioids; titration in these patients should occur much more slowly than tolerant patients to avoid oversedation/overdose (SAMHSA 2018). Once initial dose is tolerated, may increase to a dose that is clinically effective and provides 24 hours of stabilization. Buprenorphine treatment initiation should begin after mild to moderate opioid withdrawal signs appear (to avoid precipitated withdrawal), which is generally ≥6 to 12 hours after last use of short-acting opioids (eg, heroin, oxycodone) and 24 to 72 hours after last use of long-acting opioids (methadone) (Kampman [ASAM 2015]). Patients on methadone should have their methadone maintenance dose reduced to the minimum tolerable dose and remain on that dose for ≥7 days. Waiting ≥36 hours after last use of methadone and initiating at lower doses (buprenorphine 2 mg) decreases risk of precipitated methadone withdrawal (SAMHSA 2018).

After induction and titration, daily dose usually ≥8 mg/day. In patients continuing to use opioids, consider increasing the dose by 4 to 8 mg to a daily dose of ≥12 to 16 mg/day (Kampman [ASAM 2015]).

Manufacturer's labeling: Dosing in the prescribing information may not reflect current clinical practice.

Induction: Day 1: 8 mg; Day 2 and subsequent induction days: Induction usually accomplished over 3 to 4 days. Dosing on the first day may be given in 2 to 4 mg increments.

Maintenance: Target dose: 16 mg/day; doses >24 mg/day have not been demonstrated to provide any clinical advantage.

Discontinuation of therapy: When discontinuing sublingual buprenorphine for long-term treatment of opioid use disorder, use a gradual downward titration of the dose to prevent withdrawal; do not abruptly discontinue (SAMHSA 2018).

Opioid withdrawal in heroin-dependent hospitalized patients (off-label use): Immediate-release injection: IV infusion: 0.3 to 0.9 mg (diluted in 50 to 100 mL of NS) over 20 to 30 minutes every 6 to 12 hours (Welsh 2002).

Perineural anesthesia (off-label use): Immediate-release perineural injection: 200 to 300 mcg added to local anesthetic (eg, bupivacaine, mepivacaine, tetracaine) with or without epinephrine and administered as a single injection (Kosel 2015; Krishnan 2016).

Geriatric

Acute pain (moderate to severe): Immediate-release injection: IM, slow IV: Refer to adult dosing; use with caution.

Chronic pain (moderate to severe): Buccal film, transdermal patch: No specific dosage adjustments required; use caution and titrate slowly due to potential for increased risk of adverse events.

Opioid use disorder: Extended-release injection, subdermal implant: No specific dosage adjustments required; use caution due to potential for increased risk of adverse events and inability to adjust dosage.

Renal Impairment: Adult There are no dosage adjustments provided in the manufacturer's labeling (has not been adequately studied); use with caution. In pharmacokinetic studies, renal impairment (including administration pre- or post-hemodialysis) was not associated with increased buprenorphine plasma concentrations.

Hepatic Impairment: Adult

Buccal film:

Mild impairment (Child-Pugh class A): No dosage adjustment necessary.

Moderate impairment (Child-Pugh class B): No dosage adjustment necessary; use caution and monitor for signs and symptoms of toxicity or overdose.

Severe impairment (Child-Pugh class C): Reduce starting dose and reduce titration dose by 50% (ie, from 150 mcg to 75 mcg).

Extended-release injection (SubQ):

Mild impairment: There are no dosage adjustments provided in the manufacturer's labeling.

Moderate to severe impairment: Use is not recommended. If signs and symptoms of hepatic impairment occur within 2 weeks of injection, removal of depot may be required. Monitor for signs and symptoms of toxicity or overdose.

Immediate-release injection (IM, IV):

Mild or moderate impairment: There are no dosage adjustments provided in the manufacturer's labeling; however, need for dosage adjustment is unlikely as systemic exposure following IV buprenorphine in these patients was similar to healthy subjects.

Severe impairment: There are no dosage adjustments provided in the manufacturer's labeling; use with caution.

Subdermal implant:

Mild impairment: There are no dosage adjustments provided in the manufacturer's labeling (has not been studied).

Moderate or severe impairment: Use is not recommended.

Sublingual:

Mild impairment: No dosage adjustment necessary.

Moderate impairment: No dosage adjustment necessary; use caution and monitor for signs and symptoms of toxicity or overdose.

Severe impairment: Consider reducing initial and titration incremental dose by 50%; monitor for signs and symptoms of toxicity or overdose.

Transdermal patch:

Mild or moderate impairment: There are no dosage adjustments provided in the manufacturer's labeling; however, need for dosage adjustment is unlikely as systemic exposure following IV buprenorphine in these patients was similar to that observed in healthy subjects.

Severe impairment: There are no dosage adjustments provided in the manufacturer's labeling (has not been studied); consider alternative therapy with more flexibility for dosing adjustments.

Pediatric

Acute pain (moderate to severe): Dose should be titrated to appropriate effect. The following recommendations are guidelines and do not represent the maximum doses that may be required in all patients.

Children 2 to 12 years: IM, slow IV injection: Initial: Opioid-naive: 2 to 6 **mcg**/kg/dose every 4 to 6 hours (APS 2016); **Note:** Not all children have faster clearance rates than adults; some children may require dosing intervals of every 6 to 8 hours; observe clinical effects to establish the proper dosing interval.

Adolescents: IM, slow IV injection: Initial: Opioid-naive: 0.3 mg every 6 to 8 hours as needed; initial dose may be repeated once in 30 to 60 minutes if clinically needed

Chronic pain (moderate to severe): Adolescents ≥18 years: Transdermal patch:

Opioid-naive patients: Initial: 5 **mcg**/hour applied once every 7 days

Opioid-experienced patients (conversion from other opioids to buprenorphine patch): Discontinue all other around-the-clock opioid drugs when buprenorphine therapy is initiated. Short-acting analgesics as needed may be continued until analgesia with transdermal buprenorphine is attained. There is a potential for buprenorphine to precipitate withdrawal in patients already receiving opioids.

Patients who were receiving daily dose of <30 mg of oral morphine equivalents: Initial: 5 **mcg**/hour applied once every 7 days

Patients who were receiving daily dose of 30 to 80 mg of oral morphine equivalents: Taper the current around-the-clock opioid for up to 7 days to ≤30 mg/day of oral morphine or equivalent before initiating therapy. Initial: 10 **mcg**/hour applied once every 7 days.

Patients who were receiving daily dose of >80 mg of oral morphine equivalents: Buprenorphine transdermal patch, even at the maximum dose of 20 **mcg**/hour applied once every 7 days, may not provide adequate analgesia; consider the use of an alternate analgesic.

Dose titration (opioid-naive or opioid-experienced patients): May increase dose in 5 **mcg**/hour, 7.5 **mcg**/hour, or 10 **mcg**/hour increments (using no more than two 5 **mcg**/hour patches); titrate no more frequently than every 72 hours; maximum dose: 20 **mcg**/hour applied once every 7 days due to risk of QTc prolongation associated with higher doses.

Discontinuation of therapy: Taper dose gradually every 7 days to prevent withdrawal in the physically dependent patient; consider initiating immediate-release opioids, if needed for signs and symptoms of withdrawal.

Opioid dependence: Note: Do not start induction with buprenorphine until objective and clear signs of withdrawal are apparent (otherwise withdrawal may be precipitated).

Sublingual tablet: **Note**: The combination product, buprenorphine and naloxone, is preferred therapy over buprenorphine monotherapy for induction treatment (and stabilization/maintenance treatment) for short-acting opioid dependence (US Department of Health and Human Services 2005)

American Society of Addiction Medicine Guidelines (Kampman [ASAM 2015]): Limited data available:

Adolescents: Sublingual tablet:

Note: Buprenorphine treatment initiation should begin after mild to moderate opioid withdrawal signs appear (to avoid precipitated withdrawal), which is generally at least 6 to 12 hours after last use of short-acting opioids (eg, heroin, oxycodone) and 24 to 72 hours after last use of long-acting opioids (methadone).

Induction: Initial: 2 to 4 mg; if no signs of precipitated withdrawal after 60 to 90 minutes, may increase in increments of 2 to 4 mg. Once initial dose is tolerated, may increase to a dose that is clinically effective and provides 24 hours of stabilization.

After induction and titration, daily dose usually ≥8 mg/day are necessary. In patients continuing to use opioids, consider increasing the dose by 4 to 8 mg to a daily dose of ≥12 to 16 mg/day. Maximum daily dose 24 mg/**day.**

Manufacturer's labeling: Adolescents ≥16 years:

Induction: Day 1: 8 mg/day divided in 2 to 4 mg increments; day 2 and subsequent induction days dose dependent upon patient response. In 1 study, patients received 8 mg on day 1, followed by 16 mg on day 2; induction usually accomplished over 3 to 4 days. Treatment should begin only when objective and clear signs of moderate opioid withdrawal appear, and not less than 4 hours after last use of heroin or other short-acting opioids or not less than 24 hours after last use of methadone or other long-acting opioids. Titrating dose to clinical effectiveness should be done as rapidly as possible to prevent undue withdrawal symptoms and patient dropout during the induction period.

Maintenance: Target dose: 16 mg/day; reported range: 4 to 24 mg/day; doses higher than 24 mg/day have not been demonstrated to provide any clinical advantage; patients should be switched to the buprenorphine/naloxone combination product for maintenance and unsupervised therapy

Subdermal implant: Adolescents ≥16 years: Insert 4 implants subdermally in the inner side of the upper arm. Remove no later than 6 months after the date of insertion; if continued treatment is desired, insert 4 new implants subdermally in the inner side of the contralateral arm. After 1 insertion in each arm, discontinue treatment with subdermal implants.

To convert back to sublingual tablet: On day of implant removal, resume buprenorphine treatment at previous sublingual dose

Renal Impairment: Pediatric There are no dosage adjustments provided in manufacturer's labeling (has not been studied); use with caution. In pharmacokinetic studies, renal impairment (including administration pre- or posthemodialysis) was not associated with increased buprenorphine plasma concentrations.

Hepatic Impairment: Pediatric

Injection (immediate release): Children ≥2 years and Adolescents: Use caution due to extensive hepatic metabolism; dosage adjustments may be necessary.

Subdermal implant: Adolescents ≥16 years:

Mild impairment: There are no dosage adjustments provided in the manufacturer's labeling (has not been studied).

Moderate or severe impairment: Use is not recommended.

Mechanism of Action Buprenorphine exerts its analgesic effect via high-affinity binding to mu opiate receptors in the CNS; displays partial mu agonist and weak kappa antagonist activity. Due to it being a partial mu agonist, its analgesic effects plateau at higher doses and it then behaves like an antagonist. The extended-release formulation is injected subcutaneously as a liquid; subsequent precipitation following injection results in a solid depot which will gradually release buprenorphine via diffusion and biodegradation of the depot.

Contraindications

Hypersensitivity (eg, anaphylaxis) to buprenorphine or any component of the formulation.

Buccal film, IR injection, transdermal patch: Additional contraindications: Significant respiratory depression; acute or severe asthma in an unmonitored setting or in the absence of resuscitative equipment; GI obstruction, including paralytic ileus (known or suspected).

Documentation of allergenic cross-reactivity for opioids is limited. However, because of similarities in chemical structure and/or pharmacologic actions, the possibility of cross-sensitivity cannot be ruled out with certainty.

Canadian labeling: Additional contraindications (not in US labeling): Acute respiratory depression; hypercapnia; cor pulmonale; acute alcoholism or current physiological alcohol dependence; delirium tremens; convulsive disorders; severe CNS depression; increased cerebrospinal or intracranial pressure; head injury; severe hepatic insufficiency.

Buccal film, transdermal patch: Additional contraindications: Hypersensitivity to other opioids; suspected surgical abdomen (eg, acute appendicitis or pancreatitis); mild, intermittent or short duration pain that can otherwise be managed; management of acute pain, including use in outpatient or day surgeries; management of perioperative pain relief, or in other situations characterized by rapidly varying analgesic requirements; obstructive airway (other than asthma); status asthmaticus; concurrent use or use within 14 days of monoamine oxidase inhibitors (MAOIs); myasthenia gravis; patients with opioid use disorder and for opioid withdrawal treatment; pregnancy or during labor and delivery; breastfeeding; known or suspected oral mucositis (buccal film only).

ER injection: Additional contraindications: Suspected surgical abdomen (eg, acute appendicitis or pancreatitis); obstructive airway (other than asthma); status asthmaticus; concurrent use with or within 14 days of MAOIs; known or suspected GI obstruction (bowel obstruction or stricture) or any condition affecting bowel transit (ileus of any type); congenital long QT syndrome or QTc prolongation at baseline; uncorrected hypokalemia, hypomagnesemia, hypocalcemia.

Subdermal implant: Additional contraindications: Severe respiratory insufficiency, opioid-naive patients, known or suspected GI obstruction or any condition affecting bowel transit, congenital long QT prolongation or QTc prolongation at baseline, uncorrected hypokalemia, hypomagnesemia, hypocalcemia.

Warnings/Precautions An opioid-containing analgesic regimen should be tailored to each patient's needs and based upon the type of pain being treated (acute versus chronic), the route of administration, degree of tolerance for opioids (naive versus chronic user), age, weight, and medical condition. The optimal analgesic dose varies widely among patients. Doses should be titrated to pain relief/prevention. When switching patients from buprenorphine to naltrexone, do not initiate naltrexone until 7 to 14 days after buprenorphine discontinuation. No time delay is required when switching patients from buprenorphine to methadone (Kampman [ASAM 2015]).

[US Boxed Warning]: To ensure that the benefits of opioid analgesics outweigh the risks of addiction, abuse, and misuse, a REMS is required. Drug companies with approved opioid analgesic products must make REMS-compliant education programs available to health care providers. Health care providers are encouraged to complete a REMS-compliant education program; counsel patients and/or their caregivers, with every prescription, on safe use, serious risks, storage, and disposal of these products; emphasize to patients and their caregivers the importance of reading the Medication Guide every time it is provided by their pharmacist; and consider other tools to improve patient, household, and community safety.

May cause CNS depression, which may impair physical or mental abilities; patients must be cautioned about performing tasks that require mental alertness (eg, operating machinery, driving). **[US Boxed Warning]: Serious, life-threatening, or fatal respiratory depression may occur. Monitor closely for respiratory depression, especially during initiation or dose escalation. Misuse or abuse by chewing, swallowing, snorting, or injecting buprenorphine extracted from the buccal film or transdermal system will result in the uncontrolled delivery of buprenorphine and pose a significant risk of overdose and death.** Misuse by self-injection of buprenorphine or the concomitant use of buprenorphine and benzodiazepines (or other CNS depressants, including alcohol) may result in coma or death. Carbon dioxide retention from opioid-induced respiratory depression can exacerbate the sedating effects of opioids. If the extended release injection is discontinued due to respiratory depression, monitor the patient for ongoing respiratory depression for several months due to its extended release characteristics. Use with caution in patients with compromised respiratory function (eg, chronic obstructive pulmonary disease, cor pulmonale, decreased respiratory reserve, hypoxia, hypercapnia, or preexisting respiratory depression). Accidental exposure to even one dose, especially in children, can result in a fatal overdose. Use with caution and monitor for respiratory depression in patients with significant chronic obstructive pulmonary disease or cor pulmonale and those with a substantially decreased respiratory reserve, hypoxia, hypercapnia, or preexisting respiratory depression, particularly when initiating and titrating therapy; critical respiratory depression may occur, even at therapeutic dosages. Consider the use of alternative nonopioid analgesics in these patients. Opioid use increases the risk for sleep-related disorders (eg, central sleep apnea [CSA], hypoxemia) in a dose-dependent fashion. Use with caution for chronic pain and titrate dosage cautiously in patients with risk factors for sleep-disordered breathing (eg, heart failure, obesity). Consider dose reduction in patients presenting with CSA (Dowell [CDC 2016]). When using buprenorphine for treatment of opioid use disorder, treat acute pain with nonopioid analgesics whenever possible. If treatment with a high-affinity full opioid analgesic is required, monitor closely for respiratory depression, as high doses may be necessary to achieve pain relief. Use with caution in elderly patients; may be more sensitive to adverse effects (eg, life-threatening respiratory depression). In chronic pain, monitor opioid use closely in this age group due to an increased potential for risks, including certain risks such as falls/fracture, cognitive impairment, and constipation (Dowell [CDC 2016]). Consider the use of alternative nonopioid analgesics in these patients. Also use with caution in debilitated or cachectic patients; there is a greater potential for life-threatening respiratory depression, even at therapeutic dosages. Consider the use of alternative nonopioid analgesics in these patients.

Hypersensitivity reactions, including bronchospasm, angioneurotic edema, and anaphylactic shock, have been reported. The most common symptoms include rash, hives, and pruritus.

Hepatitis has been reported; hepatic events ranged from transient, asymptomatic transaminase elevations to hepatic failure; in many cases, patients had preexisting hepatic impairment. Monitor liver function tests in patients at increased risk for hepatotoxicity (eg, history of alcohol or IV drug abuse, preexisting hepatic dysfunction) prior to and during therapy. Remove buprenorphine subdermal implant if signs and symptoms of buprenorphine toxicity develop concurrent with hepatic impairment. If signs and symptoms of toxicity or overdose occur within 2 weeks of extended-release injection, removal of the depot may be required. Use buccal film and sublingual tablet with caution in patients with moderate hepatic impairment; dosage adjustment recommended in severe hepatic impairment. Use immediate-release injection with caution in patients with severe impairment. Subdermal implants should not be used in patients with preexisting moderate to severe hepatic impairment. Transdermal patch should not be used in patients with severe hepatic impairment; consider alternative therapy with more flexibility for dosing adjustments. Patients with preexisting moderate or severe hepatic impairment are not candidates for the extended-release injection. If moderate or severe impairment develops during treatment with the extended-release injection, continue with caution and monitor for toxicity for several months.

Avoid use in patients with CNS depression or coma as these patients are susceptible to intracranial effects of CO_2 retention. Use with extreme caution in patients with head injury, intracranial lesions, or elevated intracranial pressure (ICP); exaggerated elevation of ICP may occur. Buprenorphine can produce miosis and changes in the level of consciousness that may interfere with patient evaluation. May cause severe hypotension, including orthostatic hypotension and syncope; use with caution in patients with hypovolemia, cardiovascular disease (including acute MI), or drugs that may exaggerate hypotensive effects (including phenothiazines or general anesthetics). Monitor for symptoms of hypotension following initiation or dose titration. Avoid use in patients with circulatory shock. May obscure diagnosis or clinical course of patients with acute abdominal conditions. Use with caution in patients with a history of ileus or bowel obstruction; buccal film, immediate-release injection, and transdermal patch are contraindicated in patients with known or suspected GI obstruction, including paralytic ileus. Use with caution in patients with biliary tract dysfunction, including acute pancreatitis; may cause constriction of sphincter of Oddi. Use with caution in patients with a history of seizure disorders; may cause or exacerbate preexisting seizures. Use with caution in patients with adrenal insufficiency, including Addison disease. Long-term opioid use may cause adrenal insufficiency (nausea, vomiting, anorexia, fatigue, weakness, dizziness, and low BP) or secondary hypogonadism, which may lead to mood disorders and osteoporosis (Brennan 2013). Use with caution in patients with renal impairment, morbid obesity, toxic psychosis, thyroid dysfunction, or prostatic hyperplasia and/or urinary stricture. Potentially significant drug-drug interactions may exist, requiring dose or frequency adjustment, additional monitoring, and/or selection of alternative therapy. **[US Boxed Warning]: Buccal film, extended-release and immediate-release injection, transdermal patch: Concomitant use of benzodiazepines or other CNS depressants, including alcohol and opioids, may result in profound sedation, respiratory depression, coma, and death. Reserve concomitant prescribing of opioids and benzodiazepines or other CNS depressants for use in patients for whom alternative treatment options are inadequate. Limit dosages and durations to the minimum required. Follow patients for signs and symptoms of respiratory depression and sedation.** Prohibiting medication-assisted treatment of opioid use disorder may increase the risk of morbidity and mortality, therefore patients should be educated on the risks of concomitant use with benzodiazepines, sedatives, opioid analgesics, and alcohol. Strategies should be developed to manage use of prescribed or illicit benzodiazepines or other CNS depressants at initiation of or during treatment with buprenorphine; adjustments to induction procedures and additional monitoring may be required. If appropriate, delay or omit buprenorphine dose if a patient is sedated at time of buprenorphine dosing. Discontinuation of benzodiazepines or other CNS depressants is preferred; gradual tapering of benzodiazepine or other CNS depressant, decreasing to lowest effective dose, or monitoring in a higher level of care for taper may be appropriate. Benzodiazepines are not the treatment of choice for anxiety or insomnia for patients in buprenorphine treatment; make sure patients are appropriately diagnosed and consider alternative medications for anxiety and insomnia prior to co-administration of benzodiazepines and buprenorphine.

[US Boxed Warning]: Use exposes patients and other users to the risks of addiction, abuse, and misuse, potentially leading to overdose and death. Assess each patient's risk before prescribing; monitor all patients regularly for development of these behaviors or conditions. Use with caution in patients with a history of substance use disorder; potential for opioid use disorder exists. Other factors associated with increased risk for misuse include younger age and psychotropic medication use. Consider offering naloxone prescriptions in patients with factors associated with an increased risk for overdose, such as history of overdose or substance use disorder, higher opioid dosages (≥50 morphine milligram equivalents/day orally), and concomitant benzodiazepine use (Dowell [CDC 2016]). The misuse of buccal film by swallowing or of transdermal patch by placing it in the mouth, chewing it, swallowing it, or using it in ways other than indicated may cause choking, overdose, and death. Use with caution in patients with delirium tremens. Buccal film and transdermal patch are indicated for the management of pain severe enough to require daily, around-the-clock, long-term opioid treatment; should not be used for as-needed pain relief. Therapy with the buccal film, immediate-release injection, or transdermal patch is not appropriate for use in the management of opioid use disorder. Handle removed depots or implants with adequate security, accountability, and proper disposal, per facility procedure for a Schedule III drug product, and per applicable federal, state, and local regulations. To properly dispose of transdermal patch, fold it over on itself and flush down the toilet immediately (if a drug take-back option is not readily available); alternatively, seal the used patch in the provided Patch-Disposal Unit and dispose of in the trash. When used for chronic pain (outside of end-of-life or palliative care, active cancer treatment, sickle cell disease, or medication-assisted treatment for opioid use disorder) in outpatient setting in adults, opioids should not be used as first-line therapy for chronic pain management (pain >3-month duration or beyond time of normal tissue healing) due to limited short-term benefits, undetermined long-term benefits, and association with serious risks (eg, overdose, MI, auto accidents, risk of developing opioid use disorder). Preferred management includes nonpharmacologic therapy and nonopioid therapy (eg, NSAIDs, acetaminophen, certain anticonvulsants and antidepressants). If opioid therapy is initiated, it should be combined with nonpharmacologic and nonopioid therapy, as appropriate. Prior to initiation, known risks of opioid therapy should be discussed and realistic treatment goals for pain/function should be established, including consideration for discontinuation if benefits do not outweigh risks. Therapy should be continued only if clinically meaningful improvement in pain/function outweighs risks. Therapy should be initiated at the lowest effective dosage using immediate-release opioids (instead of extended-release/long-acting opioids). Risk associated with use increases with higher opioid dosages. Risks and benefits should be re-evaluated when increasing dosage to ≥50 morphine milligram equivalents (MME)/day orally; dosages ≥90 MME/day orally should be avoided unless carefully justified (Dowell [CDC 2016]).

Buprenorphine has been observed to cause QTc prolongation. Do not exceed a dose of 900 mcg every 12 hours buccal film or one 20 **mcg**/hour transdermal patch. Avoid using in patients with a personal or family history of long QT syndrome or in patients taking concurrent class IA or III antiarrhythmics or other medications that prolong the QT interval. Use with caution in patients with hypokalemia, hypomagnesemia, or clinically unstable cardiac disease, including unstable heart failure, unstable atrial fibrillation, symptomatic bradycardia, or active MI. Avoid exposure of transdermal patch application site and surrounding area to direct external heat sources (eg, heating pads, electric blankets, heat or tanning lamps, hot baths/saunas, hot water bottles, or direct sunlight). Buprenorphine release from the patch is temperature-dependent and may result in overdose. Patients who experience fever or increase in core temperature should be monitored closely and adjust dose if signs or respiratory depression or CNS depression occur. Application-site reactions, including rare cases of severe reactions (eg, vesicles, discharge, "burns"), have been observed with transdermal patch use; onset varies from days to months after initiation; patients should be instructed to report severe reactions promptly and discontinue therapy. Oral mucositis may result in more rapid absorption and higher buprenorphine plasma levels in patients using buccal film; reduce dose in patients with oral mucositis and monitor closely for signs and symptoms of toxicity or overdose. **[US Boxed Warning]: Prolonged use during pregnancy can cause neonatal withdrawal syndrome, which may be life-threatening if not recognized and treated according to according to protocols developed by neonatology experts. If opioid use is required for a prolonged period in a pregnant woman, advise the patient of the risk of neonatal withdrawal syndrome and ensure that appropriate treatment will be available.** Signs and symptoms include irritability, hyperactivity and abnormal sleep pattern, high-pitched cry, tremor, vomiting, diarrhea, and failure to gain weight. Onset, duration, and severity depend on the drug used, duration of use, maternal dose, and rate of drug elimination by the newborn.

Reversal of partial opioid agonists or mixed opioid agonist/antagonists (eg, buprenorphine, pentazocine) may be incomplete and large doses of naloxone may be required. Abrupt discontinuation in patients who are physically dependent to opioids has been associated with serious withdrawal symptoms, uncontrolled pain, attempts to find other opioids (including illicit), and suicide. Use a collaborative, patient-specific taper schedule that minimizes the risk of withdrawal, considering factors such as current opioid dose, duration of use, type of pain, and physical and psychological factors. Monitor pain control, withdrawal symptoms, mood changes, suicidal ideation, and for use of other substances and provide care as needed. Concurrent use of opioid agonist/antagonist analgesics may also precipitate withdrawal symptoms and/or reduced analgesic efficacy in patients following prolonged therapy with mu opioid agonists. Withdrawal signs and symptoms will be delayed in patients who discontinue the ER injection or have it removed; transmucosal buprenorphine may be needed to treat withdrawal in these patients.

Tablets, which are used for induction treatment of opioid use disorder, should not be started until objective and clear signs of moderate withdrawal are evident. If subdermal implants are not immediately replaced in contralateral arm after removal, maintain patients on their previous dosage of sublingual buprenorphine.

[US Boxed Warning]: Serious harm or death could result if extended-release injection is administered IV. The injection forms a solid mass upon contact with body fluids and may cause occlusion, local tissue damage, and thromboembolic events, including life-threatening pulmonary emboli if administered IV. Because of the risk of serious harm or death that could result from IV self-administration, buprenorphine extended-release injection is only available through a restricted program called the Sublocade REMS Program. Health care settings and pharmacies that order and dispense buprenorphine extended-release injection must be certified in this program and comply with the REMS requirements. Administer via subcutaneous route only. Do not administer IM or IV.

There is no maximum recommended duration for the use of buprenorphine sublingual tablets in the maintenance treatment of opioid use disorder; patients may require treatment indefinitely. Advise patients of the potential to relapse to illicit drug use following discontinuation of opioid agonist/partial agonist medication-assisted treatment. If the extended-release injection is discontinued or the depot is removed, monitor the patient for several months for signs and symptoms of withdrawal. After steady-state has been achieved (4 to 6 months), patients discontinuing extended-release injections may have detectable plasma levels of buprenorphine for 12 months or longer.

In patients undergoing elective surgery (excluding caesarean section), discontinuation of buprenorphine 24 to 36 hours before anticipated need for surgical anesthesia may be considered. Short-acting opioids may be given during and/or after surgery. In patients unable to abruptly discontinue buprenorphine prior to surgery, full opioid agonists may be added to the buprenorphine to maintain proper anesthesia; however, increased doses may be required to overcome buprenorphine receptor blockade. If opioid therapy is required as part of anesthesia, patients should be continuously monitored in an anesthesia care setting by persons not involved in in the conduct of the surgical or diagnostic procedure. This guidance applies to anyone who has been treated with extended release buprenorphine injection within the past 6 months. The decision whether to discontinue buprenorphine prior to elective surgery should be made in consultation with the surgeon and anesthesiologist (Kampman [ASAM 2015]).

[US Boxed Warning]: Insertion and removal of implant are associated with the risk of implant migration, protrusion, and expulsion. Rare but serious complications including nerve damage and migration resulting in embolism and death may result from improper insertion in the upper arm. Additional complications may include local migration, protrusion, and expulsion. Incomplete insertions or infections may lead to protrusion or expulsion. Because of the risks associated with insertion and removal, buprenorphine implant is available only through a restricted program. All health care providers must successfully complete a live training program on the insertion and removal procedures and become certified, prior to performing insertions or prescribing buprenorphine implants. Patients must be monitored to ensure that the implant is removed by a health care provider certified to perform insertions. Infection may occur at site of insertion or removal, with excessive palpation shortly after insertion and improper removal increasing the risk. Examine the insertion site one week following insertion for signs of infection or problems with wound healing. Use subdermal implants with caution in patients with a history of keloid formation, connective tissue disease (ie, scleroderma) or history of recurrent MRSA infections. Subdermal implant is not appropriate for patients who are new to treatment or have not sustained prolonged clinical stability on buprenorphine ≤8 mg/day.

Drug Interactions

Metabolism/Transport Effects

Substrate of CYP3A4 (major); **Note:** Assignment of Major/Minor substrate status based on clinically relevant drug interaction potential

Avoid Concomitant Use

Avoid concomitant use of Buprenorphine with any of the following: Abametapir; Atazanavir; Azelastine (Nasal); Bromperidol; Conivaptan; Eluxadoline; Fusidic Acid (Systemic); Idelalisib; Monoamine Oxidase Inhibitors; Opioid Agonists; Opioids (Mixed Agonist / Antagonist); Orphenadrine; Oxomemazine; Paraldehyde; Thalidomide

Increased Effect/Toxicity

Buprenorphine may increase the levels/effects of: Alvimopan; Azelastine (Nasal); Blonanserin; Desmopressin; Diuretics; Eluxadoline; Flunitrazepam; Methotrimeprazine; MetyroSINE; Monoamine Oxidase Inhibitors; Orphenadrine; Paraldehyde; Piribedil; Pramipexole; QT-prolonging Agents (Highest Risk); Ramosetron; ROPINIRole; Rotigotine; Serotonergic Agents (High Risk); Suvorexant; Thalidomide; Zolpidem

The levels/effects of Buprenorphine may be increased by: Abametapir; Alcohol (Ethyl); Alizapride; Amphetamines; Anticholinergic Agents; Aprepitant; Atazanavir; Brimonidine (Topical); Bromopride; Bromperidol; Cannabidiol; Cannabis; Chlormethiazole;

Chlorphenesin Carbamate; Clofazimine; CNS Depressants; Cobicistat; Conivaptan; CYP3A4 Inhibitors (Moderate); CYP3A4 Inhibitors (Strong); Daclatasvir; Dimethindene (Topical); Dronabinol; Droperidol; Duvelisib; Erdafitinib; Fosaprepitant; Fosnetupitant; Fusidic Acid (Systemic); Idelalisib; Kava Kava; Larotrectinib; Lemborexant; Lisuride; Lofexidine; Magnesium Sulfate; Methotrimeprazine; Metoclopramide; MiFEPRIStone; Minocycline (Systemic); Nabilone; Netupitant; Ombitasvir, Paritaprevir, and Ritonavir; Ombitasvir, Paritaprevir, Ritonavir, and Dasabuvir; Oxomemazine; Palbociclib; Perampanel; PHENobarbital; Primidone; Rufinamide; Simeprevir; Sodium Oxybate; Stiripentol; Succinylcholine; Tetrahydrocannabinol; Tetrahydrocannabinol and Cannabidiol

Decreased Effect

Buprenorphine may decrease the levels/effects of: Atazanavir; Diuretics; Gastrointestinal Agents (Prokinetic); Opioid Agonists; Pegvisomant; Sincalide

The levels/effects of Buprenorphine may be decreased by: CYP3A4 Inducers (Moderate); CYP3A4 Inducers (Strong); Dabrafenib; Deferasirox; Efavirenz; Enzalutamide; Erdafitinib; Etravirine; Ivosidenib; Mitotane; Nalmefene; Naltrexone; Opioids (Mixed Agonist / Antagonist); PHENobarbital; Primidone; Rifabutin; Sarilumab; Siltuximab; Tocilizumab

Pharmacodynamics/Kinetics

Onset of Action Analgesic: Immediate-release IM: ≥15 minutes; Peak effect: Immediate-release IM: ~1 hour

Duration of Action Immediate-release IM: ≥6 hours; Extended-release SubQ: 28 days

Half-life Elimination

Premature neonates (GA: 27 to 32 weeks): Immediate-release IV: 20 ± 8 hours (Barrett 1993)

Children 4 to 7 years: Immediate-release IV: ~1 hour (Olkkola 1989)

Adults: Immediate-release IV: 2.2 to 3 hours; Buccal film: 27.6 ± 11.2 hours; Apparent terminal half-life: Sublingual tablet: ~37 hours; Transdermal patch: ~26 hours. **Note:** Extended elimination half-life for sublingual administration may be due to depot effect (Kuhlman 1996)

Time to Peak Plasma: Buccal film: 2.5 to 3 hours; Extended-release SubQ: 24 hours, with steady state achieved after 4 to 6 months; Subdermal implant: 12 hours after insertion, with steady state achieved by week 4; Sublingual: 30 minutes to 1 hour (Kuhlman 1996); Transdermal patch: Steady state achieved by day 3

Reproductive Considerations

Pregnancy testing is recommended prior to initiating therapy for opioid use disorders (SAMHSA 2018). Long-term opioid use may cause infertility in males and females of reproductive potential. Amenorrhea may develop secondary to substance abuse. Initiation of buprenorphine maintenance treatment may improve fertility resulting in unplanned pregnancy. Contraception counseling is recommended (Dow 2012).

Pregnancy Considerations

Buprenorphine crosses the placenta; buprenorphine and norbuprenorphine can be detected in newborn serum, urine, hair, and meconium following in utero exposure (Di Trana 2019).

According to some studies, maternal use of opioids may be associated with birth defects (including neural tube defects, congenital heart defects, and gastroschisis), poor fetal growth, stillbirth, and preterm delivery (CDC [Dowell 2016]). Opioids used as part of obstetric analgesia/anesthesia during labor and delivery may temporarily affect the fetal heart rate (ACOG 209 2019). **[US Boxed Warning]: Prolonged use of opioids during pregnancy can result in neonatal opioid withdrawal syndrome, which may be life-threatening if not recognized and treated and requires management according to protocols developed by neonatology experts. If opioid use is required for a prolonged period in a pregnant woman, advise the patient of the risk of neonatal opioid withdrawal syndrome and ensure appropriate treatment will be available.** Symptoms of neonatal abstinence syndrome (NAS) following opioid exposure may be autonomic (eg, fever, temperature instability), gastrointestinal (eg, diarrhea, vomiting, poor feeding/weight gain), or neurologic (eg, high-pitched crying, hyperactivity, increased muscle tone, increased wakefulness/abnormal sleep pattern, irritability, sneezing, seizure, tremor, yawning) (Dow 2012; Hudak 2012). The onset and duration of neonatal withdrawal symptoms are dependent upon the specific opioid used, maternal dosing, and rate of elimination by the newborn. NAS associated with buprenorphine may correlate to concentrations of norbuprenorphine in the cord blood (Shah 2016). Opioids may cause respiratory depression and psycho-physiologic effects in the neonate; newborns of mothers receiving opioids during pregnancy and/or labor should be monitored.

Opioid agonist pharmacotherapy is recommended for pregnant women with an opioid use disorder. Transmucosal buprenorphine is a recommended treatment option (ACOG 711 2017; SAMHSA 2018). Due to pregnancy-induced physiologic changes, some pharmacokinetic properties of sublingual buprenorphine may be altered (Bastian 2017; Caritis 2017; Zhang 2018). Use of the subcutaneous implant is not currently recommended in pregnant women (SAMHSA 2018). Maintenance doses of buprenorphine will not provide adequate pain relief during labor. Women receiving buprenorphine for the treatment of opioid use disorder should be maintained on their daily dose of buprenorphine in addition to receiving the same pain management options during labor and delivery as opioid-naive women; Opioid agonist-antagonists should be avoided for the treatment of labor pain in women maintained on buprenorphine due to the risk of precipitating acute withdrawal (ACOG 711 2017; SAMHSA 2018). Use of a multimodal approach to pain relief which can maximize non-opioid interventions is recommended. Monitor for maternal over sedation and somnolence (Krans 2019).

Breastfeeding Considerations

Buprenorphine is present in breast milk.

Product labeling notes the relative infant dose (RID) of buprenorphine to be <1% when calculated using median breast milk concentrations and compared to weight-adjusted maternal doses following sublingual dosing. In general, breastfeeding is considered acceptable when the RID of a medication is <10% (Anderson 2016; Ito 2000).

The RID of buprenorphine is available from two published studies. One is based on data from six women taking a median sublingual dose of buprenorphine 0.29 mg/kg/day (range: 0.06 to 0.41 mg/kg/day), 5 to 8 days' postpartum. The RID of buprenorphine and the norbuprenorphine metabolite were 0.2% (range: 0.03% to 0.31%) and 0.12% (range: 0.04% to 0.18%) of the weight-adjusted maternal dose, respectively. Breast milk concentrations varied in parallel to the maternal plasma concentrations (Lindemalm

2009). A second study used data from seven women taking an average sublingual dose of buprenorphine 7 mg/day (range: 2.4 to 24 mg/day), ~1 month postpartum. The mean RID of buprenorphine was calculated to be 0.38% (range: 0.04% to 0.63%) of the weight-adjusted maternal dose, using a mean milk concentration of 3.65 mcg/L (range: 0.83 to 8.27 mcg/L), providing an estimated daily infant dose via breast milk of 0.55 mcg/kg/day (range: 0.12 to 1.24 mcg/kg/day). The mean RID of norbuprenorphine was calculated to be 0.18% (range: 0.03% to 0.31%) of the weight-adjusted maternal dose, using a mean milk concentration of 1.94 mcg/L (range: 0.45 to 4.96 mcg/L), providing an estimated daily infant dose via breast milk of 0.29 mcg/kg/day (range: 0.07 to 0.74 mcg/kg/day) (Ilett 2012). Higher breast milk concentrations of buprenorphine have also been reported following chronic maternal use (Jansson 2016). Buprenorphine and norbuprenorphine were detected in the urine and serum of breasted infants (Jansson 2016; Lindemalm 2009); adverse events were not observed (Ilett 2012; Lindemalm 2009).

Nonopioid analgesics are preferred for breastfeeding females who require pain control peripartum or for surgery outside of the postpartum period (ABM [Martin 2018]; ABM [Reece-Stremtan 2017]). However, when a narcotic is needed to treat maternal pain following surgery in a breastfeeding woman, use of buprenorphine can be considered. The lowest effective dose for the shortest duration of time should be used to limit adverse events in the mother and breastfeeding infant (ABM [Reece-Stremtan 2017]).

When buprenorphine is used to treat opioid use disorder in breastfeeding women, most guidelines allow breastfeeding as long as the infant is tolerant to the dose and other contraindications, such as HIV infection or other illicit drug use do not exist (AAP 2012; ABM [Reece-Stremtan 2015]; ACOG 711 2017; SAMHSA 2018). Breastfeeding can be encouraged regardless of maternal buprenorphine dose (ABM [Reece-Stremtan 2015]). If additional illicit substances are being abused, women treated with buprenorphine should pump and discard breast milk until sobriety is established (Dow 2012).

The decision to breastfeed during therapy should consider the risk of infant exposure, the benefits of breastfeeding to the infant, and the benefits of treatment to the mother. Breastfeeding women using opioids for postpartum pain or for the treatment of chronic maternal pain should monitor their infants for drowsiness, sedation, feeding difficulties, or limpness (ACOG 209 2019). Withdrawal symptoms may occur when maternal use is discontinued, or breastfeeding is stopped.

Controlled Substance C-III

Prescribing and Access Restrictions

Extended-release injection: Prescribing of the extended release injection is limited to healthcare providers who meet qualifying requirements, have notified the Secretary of Health and Human Services (HHS) of their intent to prescribe this product for the treatment of opioid dependence and have been assigned a unique identification number to include on every prescription.

Subdermal implant: Prescribing of implants and inserting or removing implants are limited to healthcare providers who have completed a live training program. Additionally, inserting or removing implants is limited to healthcare providers who have demonstrated procedural competency. As a prerequisite for participating in the live training program, the healthcare provider must have performed at least one qualifying surgical procedure in the last 3 months. Qualifying procedures are those performed under local anesthesia using aseptic technique and include, at a minimum, making skin incisions or placing sutures. Buprenorphine subdermal implant will only be distributed to certified prescribers through a restricted distribution program. Information concerning the insertion and removal procedures can be obtained by calling 1-844-859-6341.

Sublingual tablet: Prescribing of tablets for opioid dependence is limited to physicians who have met the qualification criteria and have received a DEA number specific to prescribing this product. Tablets will be available through pharmacies and wholesalers which normally provide controlled substances.

Dosage Forms Considerations Note: Subdermal implant and subcutaneous implant both refer to Probuphine.

Dosage Forms: US

Film, Buccal:

Belbuca: 75 mcg (1 ea, 60 ea); 150 mcg (1 ea, 60 ea); 300 mcg (1 ea, 60 ea); 450 mcg (1 ea, 60 ea); 600 mcg (1 ea, 60 ea); 750 mcg (1 ea, 60 ea); 900 mcg (1 ea, 60 ea)

Implant, Subcutaneous:

Probuphine Implant Kit: 74.2 mg (4 ea)

Patch Weekly, Transdermal:

Butrans: 5 mcg/hr (4 ea); 7.5 mcg/hr (4 ea); 10 mcg/hr (4 ea); 15 mcg/hr (4 ea); 20 mcg/hr (4 ea)

Generic: 5 mcg/hr (1 ea, 4 ea); 7.5 mcg/hr (4 ea); 10 mcg/hr (1 ea, 4 ea); 15 mcg/hr (1 ea, 4 ea); 20 mcg/hr (1 ea, 4 ea)

Solution, Injection:

Buprenex: 0.3 mg/mL (1 mL)

Generic: 0.3 mg/mL (1 mL)

Solution, Injection [preservative free]:

Generic: 0.3 mg/mL (1 mL)

Solution Prefilled Syringe, Subcutaneous [preservative free]:

Sublocade: 100 mg/0.5 mL (0.5 mL); 300 mg/1.5 mL (1.5 mL)

Tablet Sublingual, Sublingual:

Generic: 2 mg, 8 mg

Dosage Forms: Canada

Implant, Subcutaneous:

Probuphine: 74.2 mg (4 ea)

Patch Weekly, Transdermal:

BuTrans 5: 5 mcg/hr (4 ea)

BuTrans 10: 10 mcg/hr (4 ea)

BuTrans 15: 15 mcg/hr (4 ea)

BuTrans 20: 20 mcg/hr (4 ea)

Solution Prefilled Syringe, Subcutaneous:

Sublocade: 100 mg/0.5 mL (0.5 mL); 300 mg/1.5 mL (1.5 mL)

Tablet Sublingual, Sublingual:

Subutex: 2 mg, 8 mg

Buprenorphine and Naloxone

(byoo pre NOR feen & nal OKS one)

Related Information

Buprenorphine *on page 260*

Naloxone *on page 1074*

Brand Names: US Bunavail; Suboxone; Zubsolv

Brand Names: Canada ACT Buprenorphine/Naloxone; MYLAN-Buprenorphine/Naloxone [DSC]; PMS-Buprenorphine-Naloxone; Suboxone

Pharmacologic Category Analgesic, Opioid; Analgesic, Opioid Partial Agonist

Use

Opioid use disorder: Treatment of opioid use disorder.

General information: Buprenorphine/naloxone should be used as part of a complete treatment plan to include counseling and psychosocial support.

Local Anesthetic/Vasoconstrictor Precautions No information available to require special precautions

Effects on Dental Treatment No significant effects or complications reported

Effects on Bleeding No information available to require special precautions

Adverse Reactions Also see individual agents.

>10%:

Central nervous system: Headache (7% to 37%), pain (22%)

Dermatologic: Diaphoresis (>1% to 14%)

Gastrointestinal: Nausea (sublingual tablet: 5% to 15%), constipation (>1% to 12%), abdominal pain (11%)

1% to 10%:

Cardiovascular: Vasodilation (9%), palpitations (sublingual film: >1%)

Central nervous system: Disturbance in attention (sublingual film: >1%), insomnia (>1%), intoxicated feeling (sublingual film: >1%), withdrawal syndrome (>1%)

Gastrointestinal: Vomiting (5% to 8%), glossalgia (sublingual film: >1%), oral hypoesthesia (sublingual film: >1%), oral mucosa erythema (sublingual film: >1%)

Ophthalmic: Blurred vision (sublingual film: >1%)

Frequency not defined:

Central nervous system: Anxiety, irritability, restlessness

Dermatologic: Piloerection

Gastrointestinal: Stomach discomfort

Neuromuscular & skeletal: Arthralgia

Ophthalmic: Increased lacrimation

Respiratory: Rhinorrhea

<1%, postmarketing, and/or case reports: Glossitis, oral bullae, oral mucosa ulcer, peripheral edema, stomatitis

Mechanism of Action

Buprenorphine: Buprenorphine exerts its analgesic effect via high affinity binding to mu opiate receptors in the CNS; displays partial mu agonist and weak kappa antagonist activity

Naloxone: Pure opioid antagonist that competes and displaces opioids at opioid receptor sites

Pharmacodynamics/Kinetics

Half-life Elimination Suboxone: Buprenorphine 24 to 42 hours; Naloxone 2 to 12 hours; Bunavail: Buprenorphine 16.4 to 27.5 hours; Naloxone 1.9 to 2.4 hours; Cassipa: Buprenorphine 35 to 37 hours; Naloxone 5.6 to 6.6 hours

Reproductive Considerations

Pregnancy testing is recommended prior to initiating therapy for opioid use disorders (SAMHSA 2018). Long-term opioid use may cause infertility in males and females of reproductive potential. Amenorrhea may develop secondary to substance abuse. Initiation of buprenorphine maintenance treatment may improve fertility resulting in unplanned pregnancy. Contraception counseling is recommended (Dow 2012).

Pregnancy Considerations

Buprenorphine and naloxone can be detected in cord blood following maternal use of sublingual tablets; cord blood concentrations of buprenorphine and naloxone correlate with maternal serum levels (Weigand 2016).

Prolonged use of opioids during pregnancy can result in neonatal opioid withdrawal syndrome, which may be life-threatening if not recognized and treated and requires management according to protocols developed by neonatology experts. If opioid use is required for a prolonged period in a pregnant woman, advise the patient of the risk of neonatal opioid withdrawal syndrome and ensure appropriate treatment will be available.

Opioid agonist pharmacotherapy is recommended when treating opioid use disorder in pregnancy; however, use of buprenorphine monotherapy is currently preferred due to limited safety data with the buprenorphine/naloxone combination product (ACOG 711 2017; SAMHSA 2018). Treatment with the combination product should not be initiated during pregnancy (SAMHSA 2018).

Refer to individual monographs for additional information.

Product Availability Cassipa (buprenorphine 16 mg and naloxone 4 mg) sublingual film: FDA approved September 2018; anticipated availability is currently unknown. Information pertaining to this product within the monograph is pending revision. Consult the prescribing information for additional information.

Controlled Substance C-III

Prescribing and Access Restrictions In the US prescribing of tablets for opioid dependence is limited to physicians who have met the qualification criteria and have received a DEA number specific to prescribing this product. Tablets will be available through pharmacies and wholesalers which normally provide controlled substances.

◆ **Buprenorphine HCl** *see* Buprenorphine *on page 260*

◆ **Buprenorphine HCl/Naloxone HCl** *see* Buprenorphine and Naloxone *on page 270*

◆ **Buprenorphine Hydrochloride** *see* Buprenorphine *on page 260*

◆ **Buprenorphine Hydrochloride and Naloxone Hydrochloride Dihydrate** *see* Buprenorphine and Naloxone *on page 270*

BuPROPion (byoo PROE pee on)

Related Information

Cardiovascular Diseases *on page 1654*

Dentin Hypersensitivity, Acid Erosion, High Caries Index, Management of Alveolar Osteitis, and Xerostomia *on page 1762*

Vasoconstrictor Interactions With Antidepressants *on page 1821*

Brand Names: US Aplenzin; Forfivo XL; Wellbutrin SR; Wellbutrin XL; Zyban [DSC]

Brand Names: Canada MYLAN-BuPROPion XL; PMS-BuPROPion SR; RATIO-BuPROPion SR [DSC]; SANDOZ BuPROPion; TARO-Bupropion XL; TEVA-Bupropion XL; Wellbutrin SR; Wellbutrin XL; Zyban

Pharmacologic Category Antidepressant, Dopamine/Norepinephrine-Reuptake Inhibitor; Smoking Cessation Aid

Use

Major depressive disorder (unipolar [excluding Zyban]): Treatment of major depressive disorder (MDD)

Seasonal affective disorder (24-hour extended release [Aplenzin, Wellbutrin XL]): Prevention of seasonal major depressive episodes in patients with a diagnosis of seasonal affective disorder (SAD)

Smoking cessation (12-hour extended release [sustained release; Zyban]): As an aid to smoking cessation treatment

Local Anesthetic/Vasoconstrictor Precautions Part of the mechanism of bupropion is to block reuptake of norepinephrine along with dopamine. Because of the potential for norepinephrine elevation within CNS synapses, it is suggested that vasoconstrictor be administered with caution and to monitor vital signs in dental patients taking antidepressants that affect norepinephrine in this way.

Effects on Dental Treatment Key adverse event(s) related to dental treatment: Significant xerostomia (normal salivary flow resumes with discontinuation); infrequent occurrence of abnormal taste, oral mucosal ulcers; rare occurrence of stomatitis, tongue edema, gingivitis, glossitis.

Effects on Bleeding Rare occurrences of thrombocytopenia and gingival hemorrhage.

Adverse Reactions

>10%:

Cardiovascular: Tachycardia (≤11%)

Central nervous system: Insomnia (11% to 40%), headache (25% to 34%), agitation (2% to 32%), dizziness (6% to 22%)

Dermatologic: Diaphoresis (5% to 22%)

Endocrine & metabolic: Weight loss (14% to 23%)

Gastrointestinal: Xerostomia (10% to 28%), constipation (8% to 26%), nausea and vomiting (23%), nausea (1% to 18%)

Neuromuscular & skeletal: Tremor (1% to 21%)

Ophthalmic: Blurred vision (3% to 15%)

Respiratory: Nasopharyngitis (13%), pharyngitis (3% to 13%), rhinitis (12%)

1% to 10%:

Cardiovascular: Palpitations (2% to 6%), cardiac arrhythmia (5%), chest pain (≤4%), flushing (≤4%), hypertension (1% to 4%; may be severe), hypotension (3%)

Central nervous system: Lack of concentration (9%), confusion (≤8%), anxiety (3% to 8%), hostility (≤6%), nervousness (4% to 5%), abnormal dreams (3% to 5%), abnormal sensory symptoms (4%), sleep disorder (4%), migraine (≤4%), irritability (3%), memory impairment (≤3%), drowsiness (2% to 3%), pain (3%), akathisia (≤2%), central nervous system stimulation (≤2%), paresthesia (≤2%), twitching (≤2%), dystonia (≥1%), abnormality in thinking (1%), depression

Dermatologic: Skin rash (1% to 8%), pruritus (2% to 4%), xeroderma (2%), urticaria (1% to 2%)

Endocrine & metabolic: Weight gain (9%), menstrual disease (2% to 5%), decreased libido (≤3%), hot flash (1% to 3%)

Gastrointestinal: Abdominal pain (2% to 9%), diarrhea (4% to 7%), flatulence (6%), anorexia (1% to 5%), dysgeusia (2% to 4%), increased appetite (2% to 4%), vomiting (≥1% to 4%), dyspepsia (3%), oral mucosa ulcer (2%), dysphagia (≤2%)

Genitourinary: Urinary frequency (≥1% to 5%), urinary urgency (≤2%), vaginal hemorrhage (≤2%), urinary tract infection (≤1%)

Hypersensitivity: Hypersensitivity reaction (1%)

Infection: Infection (8% to 9%)

Neuromuscular & skeletal: Myalgia (2% to 6%), arthralgia (4% to 5%), asthenia (4%), neck pain (2%), arthritis (≤2%), dyskinesia (≥1%)

Ophthalmic: Diplopia (≤3%)

Otic: Tinnitus (1% to 6%), auditory disturbance (5%)

Renal: Polyuria (≤1%)

Respiratory: Upper respiratory infection (9%), sinusitis (2% to 5%), cough (2% to 4%), increased cough (2% to 3%), epistaxis (2%), bronchitis (≤2%)

Miscellaneous: Accidental injury (2%), fever (1% to 2%)

<1%, postmarketing, and/or case reports: Abnormal stools, accommodation disturbance, acute myocardial infarction, aggressive behavior, akinesia, alopecia, amnesia, anaphylactic shock, anaphylaxis, anemia, angioedema, angle-closure glaucoma, aphasia, ataxia, atrioventricular block, bronchospasm, bruxism, cerebrovascular accident, change in prothrombin time, chills, colitis, coma, complete atrioventricular block, cutaneous lupus erythematosus (Hannah 2018), cystitis, deafness, delirium, delusion, depersonalization, derealization, drug-induced Parkinson disease, dry eye syndrome, dysarthria, dyspareunia, dysphoria, dysuria, ecchymoses, edema, EEG pattern changes, ejaculatory disorder, emotional lability, erythema multiforme, esophagitis, euphoria, exfoliative dermatitis, extrapyramidal reaction, extrasystoles, facial edema, gastric ulcer, gastroesophageal reflux disease, gastrointestinal hemorrhage, gingival hemorrhage, gingivitis, glossitis, glycosuria, gynecomastia, hallucination, hepatic injury, hepatic insufficiency, hepatitis, hirsutism, homicidal ideation, hyperglycemia, hyperkinetic muscle activity, hypertonia, hypoesthesia, hypoglycemia, hypokinesia, hypomania, hyponatremia, impotence, increased intraocular pressure, increased libido, increased thirst, inguinal hernia, intestinal perforation, jaundice, leukocytosis, leukopenia, lower limb cramp, lymphadenopathy, maculopapular rash, malaise, manic behavior, menopause, muscle rigidity, musculoskeletal chest pain, myasthenia, mydriasis, myoclonus, neuralgia, neuropathy, nonimmune anaphylaxis, orthostatic hypotension, painful erection, pancreatitis, pancytopenia, panic, paranoid ideation, peripheral edema, phlebitis, pneumonia, prostatic disease, psychiatric signs and symptoms, psychosis, pulmonary embolism, restlessness, rhabdomyolysis, salpingitis, sciatica, seizure (dose-related), serum sickness-like reaction, SIADH, sialorrhea, skin photosensitivity, Stevens-Johnson syndrome, stomatitis, subacute cutaneous lupus erythematosus (Hannah 2018), suicidal ideation, syncope, tardive dyskinesia, thrombocytopenia, tongue edema, type IV hypersensitivity reaction, urinary incontinence, urinary retention, vaginitis, vasodilation, vertigo

Mechanism of Action Aminoketone antidepressant structurally different from all other marketed antidepressants; like other antidepressants the mechanism of bupropion's activity is not fully understood. Bupropion is a relatively weak inhibitor of the neuronal uptake of norepinephrine and dopamine, and does not inhibit monoamine oxidase or the reuptake of serotonin. Metabolite inhibits the reuptake of norepinephrine. The primary mechanism of action is thought to be dopaminergic and/or noradrenergic.

Pharmacodynamics/Kinetics

Onset of Action Depression: Initial effects may be observed within 1 to 2 weeks of treatment, with continued improvements through 4 to 6 weeks (Papakostas 2006; Posternak 2005; Szegedi 2009).

Duration of Action 1 to 2 days

Half-life Elimination
Distribution: 3 to 4 hours
Elimination:
Hydrochloride salt: ~21 hours after chronic dosing (± 9 hours); Metabolites (after a single dose): Hydroxybupropion: 20 ± 5 hours; Erythrohydrobupropion: 33 ± 10 hours; Threohydrobupropion: 37 ± 13 hours
Hydrobromide salt: 21 ± 7 hours; Metabolites: Hydroxybupropion: 24 ± 5 hours; Erythrohydrobupropion: 31 ± 8 hours; Threohydrobupropion: 51 ± 9 hours

Time to Peak
Bupropion: Immediate release: Within 2 hours; 12-hour extended release (sustained release): Within 3 hours; 24-hour extended release: ~5 hours; 12 hours (fed)
Metabolite: Hydroxybupropion: Immediate release: ~3 hours; Extended release: ~6 to 7 hours

Pregnancy Considerations
Bupropion and its metabolites cross the placenta (Fokina 2016).

An increased risk of congenital malformations has not been observed following maternal use of bupropion during pregnancy; however, data specific to cardiovascular malformations is inconsistent. The long-term effects on development and behavior have not been studied.

Therapy with antidepressants during pregnancy should be individualized (ACOG 2008). Psychotherapy or other nonmedication therapies may be considered for some women; however, antidepressant medication should be considered for pregnant women with moderate to severe major depressive disorder (APA 2010). If treatment for MDD is initiated for the first time during pregnancy, agents other than bupropion are preferred (MacQueen 2016). Treatment algorithms have been developed by the ACOG and the APA for the management of depression in women prior to conception and during pregnancy (ACOG 2008; APA 2010; Yonkers 2009).

There is insufficient information related to the use of bupropion to recommend use for smoking cessation during pregnancy (ACOG 721 2017).

Pregnant women exposed to antidepressants during pregnancy are encouraged to enroll in the National Pregnancy Registry for Antidepressants (NPRAD). Women 18 to 45 years of age or their health care providers may contact the registry by calling 844-405-6185. Enrollment should be done as early in pregnancy as possible.

◆ **Bupropion and Naltrexone** *see* Naltrexone and Bupropion *on page 1078*

◆ **Bupropion HCl** *see* BuPROPion *on page 271*

◆ **Bupropion Hydrobromide** *see* BuPROPion *on page 271*

◆ **Bupropion Hydrochloride** *see* BuPROPion *on page 271*

◆ **Bupropion Hydrochloride and Naltrexone Hydrochloride** *see* Naltrexone and Bupropion *on page 1078*

◆ **BuSpar** *see* BusPIRone *on page 273*

BusPIRone (byoo SPYE rone)

Related Information
Management of the Patient With Anxiety or Depression *on page 1778*

Brand Names: Canada APO-BusPIRone; CO BusPIRone; DOM-BusPIRone; GMD-Buspirione; NU-BusPIRone [DSC]; PMS-BusPIRone; RIVA-BusPIRone [DSC]; TEVA-BusPIRone

Pharmacologic Category Antianxiety Agent, Miscellaneous

Use Generalized anxiety disorder: Management of generalized anxiety disorder or the short-term relief of the symptoms of anxiety

Local Anesthetic/Vasoconstrictor Precautions
No information available to require special precautions

Effects on Dental Treatment Key adverse event(s) related to dental treatment: Xerostomia (normal salivary flow resumes upon discontinuation).

Effects on Bleeding No information available to require special precautions

Adverse Reactions
>10%: Central nervous system: Dizziness (3% to 12%)
1% to 10%:
Cardiovascular: Chest pain (≥1%)
Central nervous system: Drowsiness (10%), headache (6%), nervousness (5%), confusion (2%), excitement (2%), numbness (2%), outbursts of anger (2%), abnormal dreams (≥1%), ataxia (1%) paresthesia (1%)
Dermatologic: Diaphoresis (1%), skin rash (1%)
Gastrointestinal: Nausea (8%), diarrhea (2%), sore throat (≥1%)
Neuromuscular & skeletal: Weakness (2%), musculoskeletal pain (1%), tremor (1%)
Ophthalmic: Blurred vision (2%)
Otic: Tinnitus (≥1%)
Respiratory: Nasal congestion (≥1%)
<1%, postmarketing, and/or case reports: Acne vulgaris, akathisia, alcohol abuse, alopecia, altered sense of smell, amenorrhea, angioedema, anorexia, apathy, arthralgia, bradycardia, bruise, cardiac failure, cardiomyopathy, cerebrovascular accident, change in libido, claustrophobia, cogwheel rigidity, cold intolerance, conjunctivitis, delayed ejaculation, depersonalization, dissociative reaction, dysgeusia, dyskinesia, dysphoria, dyspnea, dystonia, dysuria, edema, emotional lability, eosinophilia, epistaxis, euphoria, extrapyramidal reaction, eye pain, facial edema, fear, fever, flatulence, flushing, galactorrhea, glossopyrosis, hallucination, hemorrhagic diathesis, hiccups, hyperacusis, hypersensitivity reaction, hypertension, hyperventilation, hypotension, impotence, increased appetite, increased intraocular pressure, increased serum ALT, increased serum AST, increased serum transaminases, inner ear disturbance, involuntary muscle movements, irritable bowel syndrome, laryngitis, leukopenia, malaise, memory impairment, menstrual disease, muscle cramps, muscle spasm, myocardial infarction, nocturia, parkinsonian-like syndrome, pelvic inflammatory disease, personality disorder, photophobia, pruritus, psychosis, rectal hemorrhage, restless leg syndrome, restlessness, roaring sensation in head, salivation, seizure, serotonin syndrome, skin blister, slowed reaction time, slurred speech, stiffness, stupor, suicidal ideation, syncope, thinning of nails, thrombocytopenia, thyroid disease, urinary frequency, urinary hesitancy, urinary incontinence, urinary retention, urticaria, vertigo,

visual disturbance (tunnel vision), weight gain, weight loss, xeroderma

Mechanism of Action The mechanism of action of buspirone is unknown. Buspirone has a high affinity for serotonin 5-HT_{1A} and 5-HT_2 receptors, without affecting benzodiazepine-GABA receptors. Buspirone has moderate affinity for dopamine D_2 receptors.

Pharmacodynamics/Kinetics

Half-life Elimination 2 to 3 hours; increased with renal or hepatic impairment

Time to Peak Serum: 40 to 90 minutes

Pregnancy Risk Factor B

Pregnancy Considerations Adverse events have not been observed in animal reproduction studies.

◆ **Buspirone Hydrochloride** *see* BusPIRone *on page 273*

◆ **Butalbit/Acetamin/Caff/Codeine** *see* Butalbital, Acetaminophen, Caffeine, and Codeine *on page 274*

Butalbital, Acetaminophen, Caffeine, and Codeine

(byoo TAL bi tal, a seet a MIN oh fen, KAF een, & KOE deen)

Related Information

Acetaminophen *on page 59*

Caffeine *on page 277*

Codeine *on page 404*

Brand Names: US Fioricet/Codeine

Pharmacologic Category Analgesic Combination (Opioid); Analgesic, Opioid; Barbiturate

Use

Tension or muscle contraction headache: Management of the symptom complex of tension (muscle contraction) headache when nonopioid analgesic and alternative treatments are inadequate.

Limitations of use: Reserve for use in patients for whom alternative treatment options (eg, nonopioid, non-barbiturate analgesics) are ineffective, not tolerated, or would be otherwise inadequate to provide sufficient management of pain.

Local Anesthetic/Vasoconstrictor Precautions No information available to require special precautions

Effects on Dental Treatment No significant effects or complications reported (see Dental Health Professional Considerations)

Effects on Bleeding As a single agent, acetaminophen does not appear to affect bleeding or platelet aggregation. Acetaminophen may prolong the INR and increase bleeding in patients taking warfarin (Coumadin). For patients taking warfarin, single acetaminophen doses or acetaminophen therapy of short duration should be safe, but if large (>1.3 g/day) doses are administered for longer than 10-14 days, then the INR should be monitored (see Dental Health Professional Considerations).

Adverse Reactions Frequency not defined.

Cardiovascular: Syncope, tachycardia

Central nervous system: Agitation, confusion, depression, dizziness, drowsiness, euphoria, excitement, fatigue, headache, increased energy, intoxicated feeling, lethargy, numbness, paresthesia, sedation, seizure, shakiness

Dermatologic: Hyperhidrosis, pruritus

Endocrine & metabolic: Hot flash

Gastrointestinal: Abdominal pain, constipation, dysphagia, flatulence, heartburn, nausea, vomiting, xerostomia

Genitourinary: Diuresis

Hypersensitivity: Hypersensitivity reaction

Neuromuscular & skeletal: Leg pain, muscle fatigue

Otic: Otalgia, tinnitus

Respiratory: Dyspnea, nasal congestion

Miscellaneous: Fever, heavy eyelids

Postmarketing and/or case reports: Hypogonadism (Brennan 2013; Debono 2011)

Note: Potential reactions associated with components of Fioricet with Codeine include agranulocytosis, cardiac stimulation, dependence, erythema multiforme, hyperglycemia, irritability, nephrotoxicity, rash, thrombocytopenia, toxic epidermal necrolysis, tremor

Mechanism of Action

Acetaminophen: Although not fully elucidated, the analgesic effects are believed to be due to activation of descending serotonergic inhibitory pathways in the CNS. Interactions with other nociceptive systems may be involved as well (Smith 2009). Antipyresis is produced from inhibition of the hypothalamic heat-regulating center.

Butalbital: Short- to intermediate-acting barbiturate; depresses the sensory cortex, decreases motor activity, alters cerebellar function, and produces drowsiness, sedation, hypnosis, and dose-dependent respiratory depression.

Caffeine: CNS stimulant; use with acetaminophen and dihydrocodeine increases the level of analgesia provided by each agent.

Codeine: Binds to opiate receptors in the CNS, causing inhibition of ascending pain pathways, altering the perception of and response to pain; produces generalized CNS depression.

Reproductive Considerations

Long-term opioid use may cause secondary hypogonadism, which may lead to sexual dysfunction and infertility (Brennan 2013).

Pregnancy Considerations

[US Boxed Warning]: Prolonged use of opioids during pregnancy can cause neonatal withdrawal syndrome, which may be life-threatening if not recognized and treated according to protocols developed by neonatology experts. If opioid use is required for a prolonged period in a pregnant woman, advise the patient of the risk of neonatal opioid withdrawal syndrome and ensure that appropriate treatment will be available. Refer to the acetaminophen/butalbital, caffeine, or codeine monographs for additional information.

Controlled Substance C-III

Dental Health Professional Considerations

Although the ***OTC product labeling*** for acetaminophen products state to limit the maximum dose to 3,000 mg daily (for extra strength) or 3,250 mg (for regular strength) (see this site for details: http://www.-tylenolprofessional.com/products-and-dosages.html), it is still appropriate for patients to take up to 4,000 mg daily "under the direction of a health care provider" (http://www.tylenolprofessional.com/dosage.html).

The acetaminophen component requires use with caution in patients who use alcohol, with preexisting liver disease, and those receiving more than one source of acetaminophen-containing medication.

Hepatotoxicity caused by acetaminophen is potentiated by chronic alcohol consumption. People who are taking acetaminophen, even at therapeutic doses, and consume alcohol are at risk of developing hepatotoxicity.

Acetaminophen may increase the levels and enhance the anticoagulant effects of vitamin K antagonists acenocoumarol and warfarin (Coumadin). Studies have reported that acetaminophen has increased the INR in warfarin treated patients with daily acetaminophen doses as low as 2 g, particularly when taking acetaminophen for >1 week (Antlitz, 1968; Boeijinga, 1982; Gebauer, 2003; Hylek, 1998; Rubin, 1984). In addition, case reports of bleeding as a result of increased INR have been published (Bagheri, 1999; Bartle, 1991). There is no known mechanism of the interaction; furthermore, some studies have failed to demonstrate this interaction (Gadisseur, 2003; Kwan, 1995; van den Bemt, 2002). In terms of risk, the data suggest that acetaminophen and warfarin could interact in some clinically significant manner but that the benefits of concomitant use of acetaminophen for pain control in dental patients taking warfarin usually outweigh the risks. An appropriate monitoring plan should be in place to identify potential negative effects and dosage adjustments may be necessary in a minority of patients. The interaction may be more likely to occur with daily acetaminophen doses of >1.3 g for >1 week.

There are no reports of acetaminophen interacting with antiplatelet drugs such as aspirin, clopidogrel (Plavix), or prasugrel (Effient). Also, there are no reports of acetaminophen in combination with hydrocodone, codeine, or oxycodone interacting with warfarin (Coumadin).

Butoconazole (byoo toe KOE na zole)

Brand Names: US Gynazole-1

Pharmacologic Category Antifungal Agent, Imidazole Derivative; Antifungal Agent, Vaginal

Use **Vulvovaginal candidiasis:** Local treatment of vulvovaginal candidiasis due to *Candida albicans*

Local Anesthetic/Vasoconstrictor Precautions No information available to require special precautions

Effects on Dental Treatment No significant effects or complications reported

Effects on Bleeding No information available to require special precautions

Adverse Reactions Frequency not defined.

Gastrointestinal: Abdominal cramps, abdominal pain

Genitourinary: Pelvic pain, vulvovaginal burning, vulvovaginal disease (soreness), vulvovaginal pruritus

Local: Local swelling

Mechanism of Action Inhibits biosynthesis of ergosterol, damaging the fungal cell wall membrane, which increases permeability in susceptible fungi (*Candida*), causing leaking of nutrients

Pharmacodynamics/Kinetics

Time to Peak Plasma: 12 to 24 hours

Reproductive Considerations

This product may weaken latex or rubber condoms or diaphragms (CDC [Workowski 2015]).

Pregnancy Risk Factor C

Pregnancy Considerations

Adverse events have been observed in some animal reproduction studies. Following vaginal administration, small amounts are absorbed systemically. Single dose, topical azole regimens are not recommended for the treatment of vulvovaginal candidiasis; only topical azole therapies with 7 day regimens are recommended in pregnant women with vulvovaginal candidiasis (CDC [Workowski 2015]).

◆ **Butoconazole Nitrate** *see* Butoconazole *on page* 275

Butorphanol (byoo TOR fa nole)

Brand Names: Canada PMS-Butorphanol [DSC]

Pharmacologic Category Analgesic, Opioid; Analgesic, Opioid Partial Agonist

Use

Pain management: Management of pain severe enough to require an opioid analgesic and for which alternative treatments are inadequate

Limitations of use: Reserve for use in patients for whom alternative treatment options (eg, nonopioid analgesics, opioid combination products) are ineffective, not tolerated, or would be otherwise inadequate to provide sufficient management of pain.

Pain during labor (injection only): Management of pain during labor.

Preoperative medication (injection only): Preoperative or preanesthetic medication

Supplement to balanced anesthesia (injection only): Supplement to balanced anesthesia

Local Anesthetic/Vasoconstrictor Precautions No information available to require special precautions

Effects on Dental Treatment Key adverse event(s) related to dental treatment: Xerostomia (normal salivary flow resumes upon discontinuation) and unpleasant aftertaste.

Effects on Bleeding No information available to require special precautions

Adverse Reactions

>10%:

Central nervous system: Drowsiness (43%), dizziness (19%), insomnia (nasal spray 11%)

Gastrointestinal: Nausea and vomiting (13%)

Respiratory: Nasal congestion (nasal spray 13%)

1% to 10%:

Cardiovascular: Palpitations, vasodilation

Central nervous system: Anxiety, burning sensation, confusion, euphoria, floating feeling, headache, lethargy, nervousness, paresthesia

Dermatologic: Cold and clammy skin, diaphoresis, pruritus

Gastrointestinal: Anorexia, constipation, stomach pain, unpleasant taste, xerostomia

Neuromuscular & skeletal: Tremor, weakness

Ophthalmic: Blurred vision

Otic: Otalgia, tinnitus

Respiratory: Bronchitis, cough, dyspnea, epistaxis, nasal discomfort, pharyngitis, rhinitis, sinus congestion, sinusitis, upper respiratory tract infection

<1%, postmarketing, and/or case reports: Abnormal dreams, agitation, apnea, chest pain, convulsions, delusions, depression, drug dependence, dysphoria, edema, hallucination, hostility, hypertension, hypogonadism (Brennan, 2013; Debono, 2011), hypotension, respiratory depression, seizure, shallow respiration, skin rash, speech disturbance, syncope, tachycardia, urination disorder, urticaria, vertigo, withdrawal syndrome

Mechanism of Action Agonist of kappa opiate receptors and partial agonist of mu opiate receptors in the CNS, causing inhibition of ascending pain pathways, altering the perception of and response to pain; produces analgesia, respiratory depression, and sedation similar to opioids

Pharmacodynamics/Kinetics

Onset of Action IM, Nasal: ≤15 minutes; IV: Within a few minutes

Peak effect: IM, IV: 0.5 to 1 hour; Nasal: 1 to 2 hours

Duration of Action IM, IV: 3 to 4 hours; Nasal: 4 to 5 hours

Half-life Elimination

IV, nasal: ~2 to 9 hours; Hydroxybutorphanol: ~18 hours

Elderly: IV, nasal: ~3 to 9 hours

Renal impairment (CrCl <30 mL/minute): ~10.5 hours

Hepatic impairment: ~16.8 hours

Time to Peak Plasma: IM: 20 to 40 minutes; Nasal: 30 to 60 minutes

Reproductive Considerations

Long-term opioid use may cause secondary hypogonadism, which may lead to sexual dysfunction or infertility in men and women (Brennan 2013).

Pregnancy Risk Factor C

Pregnancy Considerations Butorphanol crosses the placenta

Butorphanol can be detected in neonatal serum following maternal IM injection prior to delivery (Pittman 1980).

According to some studies, maternal use of opioids may be associated with birth defects (including neural tube defects, congenital heart defects, and gastroschisis), poor fetal growth, stillbirth, and preterm delivery (CDC [Dowell 2016]). Opioids used as part of obstetric analgesia/anesthesia during labor and delivery may temporarily affect the fetal heart rate (ACOG 209 2019).

[US Boxed Warning]: Prolonged use of butorphanol during pregnancy can result in neonatal opioid withdrawal syndrome, which may be life-threatening if not recognized and treated, and requires management according to protocols developed by neonatology experts. If opioid use is required for a prolonged period in a pregnant woman, advise the patient of the risk of neonatal opioid withdrawal syndrome and ensure that appropriate treatment will be available. If chronic opioid exposure occurs in pregnancy, adverse events in the newborn (including withdrawal) may occur (Chou 2009). Symptoms of neonatal abstinence syndrome (NAS) following opioid exposure may be autonomic (eg, fever, temperature instability), gastrointestinal (eg, diarrhea, vomiting, poor feeding/weight gain), or neurologic (eg, high-pitched crying, hyperactivity, increased muscle tone, increased wakefulness/abnormal sleep pattern, irritability, sneezing, seizure, tremor, yawning) (Dow 2012; Hudak 2012). Mothers who are physically dependent on opioids may give birth to infants who are also physically dependent. Opioids may cause respiratory depression and psychophysiologic effects in the neonate; newborns of mothers receiving opioids during labor should be monitored.

Butorphanol injection is approved for the management of pain during labor; apnea or respiratory distress in the newborn may occur. Opioids used as part of obstetric analgesia/anesthesia during labor and delivery may temporarily affect the fetal heart rate (ACOG 209 2019). The manufacturer recommends that caution be used if abnormal fetal heart rate patterns are present.

The ACOG recommends that pregnant women should not be denied medically necessary surgery, regardless of trimester. If the procedure is elective, it should be delayed until after delivery (ACOG 775 2019).

Controlled Substance C-IV

- ◆ **Butorphanol Tartrate** *see* Butorphanol *on page 275*
- ◆ **Butrans** *see* Buprenorphine *on page 260*
- ◆ **B Vitamin Combinations** *see* Vitamin B Complex Combinations *on page 1549*
- ◆ **BW-430C** *see* LamoTRIgine *on page 874*
- ◆ **BW524W91** *see* Emtricitabine *on page 556*
- ◆ **Bydureon** *see* Exenatide *on page 633*
- ◆ **Bydureon BCise** *see* Exenatide *on page 633*
- ◆ **Byetta 5 MCG Pen** *see* Exenatide *on page 633*
- ◆ **Byetta 10 MCG Pen** *see* Exenatide *on page 633*
- ◆ **Byfavo** *see* Remimazolam *on page 1316*
- ◆ **Bystolic** *see* Nebivolol *on page 1088*
- ◆ **Byvalson [DSC]** *see* Nebivolol and Valsartan *on page 1089*
- ◆ **C2B8 Monoclonal Antibody** *see* RiTUXimab *on page 1336*
- ◆ **2C4 Antibody** *see* Pertuzumab *on page 1220*
- ◆ **311C90** *see* ZOLMitriptan *on page 1581*
- ◆ **C225** *see* Cetuximab *on page 329*

Cabergoline (ca BER goe leen)

Brand Names: Canada ACT Cabergoline; APO-Cabergoline; Dostinex

Pharmacologic Category Ergot Derivative

Use

Hyperprolactinemic disorders: Treatment of hyperprolactinemic disorders, either idiopathic or caused by pituitary adenomas.

Limitations of use: Not indicated for inhibition or suppression of physiologic lactation.

Canadian labeling: Additional use (not in US labeling): Prevention of the onset of physiological lactation in the puerperium when clinically indicated (eg, still born baby or neonatal death, conditions that interfere with suckling, severe acute or chronic mental illness, maternal disease which may be transmitted to the baby that require medications which are excreted in the milk).

Limitations of use: Not indicated for suppression of already established postpartum lactation.

Local Anesthetic/Vasoconstrictor Precautions

Cabergoline is a semisynthetic ergot alkaloid derivative; there is a possibility that it has vasoconstricting effects; use vasoconstrictor with caution

Effects on Dental Treatment Key adverse event(s) related to dental treatment: Xerostomia (normal salivary flow resumes upon discontinuation), throat irritation, and toothache.

Effects on Bleeding No information available to require special precautions

Adverse Reactions

>10%:

Gastrointestinal: Nausea (27% to 29%)

Nervous system: Headache (26%), dizziness (15% to 17%)

1% to 10%:

Cardiovascular: Orthostatic hypotension (4%), peripheral edema (1%), hypotension (≤1%), palpitations (≤1%), syncope (≤1%)

Dermatologic: Acne vulgaris (≤1%), pruritus (≤1%)

Endocrine & metabolic: Hot flash (3%), dependent edema (1%)

Gastrointestinal: Constipation (7% to 10%), abdominal pain (5%), dyspepsia (2% to 5%), vomiting (2% to 4%), diarrhea (≤2%), flatulence (≤2%), xerostomia (≤2%), toothache (1%), anorexia (≤1%)

Genitourinary: Mastalgia (1% to 2%), dysmenorrhea (≤1%)
Nervous system: Fatigue (5% to 7%), vertigo (1% to 4%), depression (3%), pain (2%), drowsiness (≤2%), nervousness (≤2%), paresthesia (≤2%), lack of concentration (1%), anxiety (≤1%), insomnia (≤1%), malaise (≤1%)
Neuromuscular & skeletal: Asthenia (6%), arthralgia (1%)
Ophthalmic: Periorbital edema (1%), visual disturbance (≤1%)
Respiratory: Rhinitis (1%), throat irritation (1%), flu-like symptoms (≤1%)

<1%, postmarketing, and/or case reports: Aggressive behavior, alopecia, epistaxis, facial edema, heart valve disease, impulse control disorder, increased libido (including hypersexuality), pathological gambling, pericardial effusion, pleural effusion, psychosis, pulmonary fibrosis, retroperitoneal fibrosis, weight gain, weight loss

Mechanism of Action Cabergoline is a long acting dopamine receptor agonist with a high affinity for D_2 receptors; prolactin secretion by the anterior pituitary is predominantly under hypothalamic inhibitory control exerted through the release of dopamine. It is a potent 5-HT_{2B}-receptor agonist, which may contribute to observed fibrotic/valvulopathic events.

Pharmacodynamics/Kinetics

Half-life Elimination 63 to 69 hours

Time to Peak Plasma: 2 to 3 hours

Reproductive Considerations Dose-related decreases in prolactin occur with cabergoline therapy. Treatment may restore fertility in previously infertile women.

Pregnancy Considerations

Information related to the use of cabergoline for the treatment of hyperprolactinemia in pregnancy is available but limited compared to the use of other agents (Almistehi 2018; Auriemma 2013; Colao 2008; Lebbe 2010; Moltich 2015; Ricci 2002; Robert 1996; Stalldecker 2010). Although available evidence suggests cabergoline use early in pregnancy does not cause harm to the fetus, it is recommended that therapy be discontinued once pregnancy is discovered.

If treatment of hyperprolactinemia during pregnancy is required, cabergoline may be used, but other agents are preferred. Monitoring of prolactin levels should be suspended during pregnancy (Endocrine Society [Melmed 2011]). If treatment for acromegaly (off-label use) is required during pregnancy for worsening symptoms (such as headache) or evidence of tumor growth, use of cabergoline may be considered. Monitoring of insulin-like growth factor 1 and/or growth hormone (GH) are not recommended during pregnancy as an active placental GH variant present in maternal blood limits the usefulness of the results (Endocrine Society [Katznelson 2014]). Information related to cabergoline for the treatment of Cushing Syndrome (off-label use) during pregnancy is limited; agents other than cabergoline are recommended (Nakhleh 2016; Nieman 2015; Sek 2017).

Cabergoline is contraindicated in patients with uncontrolled hypertension; use is not recommended by the manufacturer in women with pregnancy-induced hypertension (eg, preeclampsia, eclampsia, postpartum hypertension) unless benefit outweighs potential risk.

◆ **Cafcit** *see* Caffeine *on page 277*

◆ **CAFdA** *see* Clofarabine *on page 381*

◆ **Cafergot** *see* Ergotamine and Caffeine *on page 583*

Caffeine (KAF een)

Brand Names: US Cafcit; Keep Alert [OTC]; No Doz Maximum Strength [OTC] [DSC]; Stay Awake Maximum Strength [OTC]; Stay Awake [OTC]; Vivarin [OTC]

Brand Names: Canada Diurex; Extra Strength Pep-Back; Pep-Back; Peyona; Therma Pro; Wake Ups

Pharmacologic Category Central Nervous System Stimulant; Phosphodiesterase Enzyme Inhibitor, Nonselective

Use

Caffeine citrate: Treatment of idiopathic apnea of prematurity

Caffeine [OTC labeling]: Restore mental alertness or wakefulness when experiencing fatigue

Local Anesthetic/Vasoconstrictor Precautions No information available to require special precautions

Effects on Dental Treatment Key adverse event(s) related to dental treatment: Caffeine causes tachycardia, increases in blood pressure, and palpitations. Consider monitoring blood pressure prior to using local anesthetic with a vasoconstrictor. Symptoms associated with bruxism have been observed in some patients.

Effects on Bleeding No information available to require special precautions

Adverse Reactions

1% to 10%:
Dermatologic: Skin rash (9%), epidermal thinning (2%), xeroderma (2%)
Endocrine & metabolic: Acidosis (2%)
Gastrointestinal: Gastritis (2%), gastrointestinal hemorrhage (2%)
Hematologic & oncologic: Disseminated intravascular coagulation (2%), hemorrhage (2%)
Infection: Sepsis (4%)
Nervous system: Cerebral hemorrhage (2%)
Ophthalmic: Retinopathy of prematurity (2%)
Renal: Renal failure syndrome (2%)
Respiratory: Dyspnea (2%), pulmonary edema (2%)
Miscellaneous: Reduced intake of food/liquids (9%, feeding intolerance), abnormal healing (2%), accidental injury (2%)

Frequency not defined: Gastrointestinal: Necrotizing enterocolitis

Postmarketing: Cardiac disorder (including increased left ventricular output, increased stroke volume), central nervous system stimulation, gastrointestinal disease (including gastric aspirate), hyperglycemia, hypoglycemia, increased creatinine clearance, increased heart rate, increased urinary sodium, increased urine calcium excretion, increased urine output, irritability, jitteriness, restlessness, tachycardia

Mechanism of Action Increases levels of 3'5' cyclic AMP by inhibiting phosphodiesterase; CNS stimulant which increases medullary respiratory center sensitivity to carbon dioxide, stimulates central inspiratory drive, and improves skeletal muscle contraction (diaphragmatic contractility); prevention of apnea may occur by competitive inhibition of adenosine

Pharmacodynamics/Kinetics

Half-life Elimination

Neonates: 72 to 96 hours.

Infants ≥9 months, Children, Adolescents, and Adults: 5 hours.

Time to Peak Serum: Preterm neonates: Oral: 30 minutes to 2 hours.

Pregnancy Considerations

Caffeine crosses the placenta; serum concentrations in the fetus are similar to those in the mother (Grosso 2005).

Based on current studies, usual dietary exposure to caffeine is unlikely to cause congenital malformations (Brent 2011). However, available data show conflicting results related to maternal caffeine use and the risk of other adverse events, such as spontaneous abortion or growth retardation (Brent 2011; Jahanfar 2013; Nehlig 1994). Chronic maternal consumption of high amounts of caffeine during pregnancy may lead to neonatal withdrawal at delivery (eg, apnea, irritability, jitteriness, vomiting) (Martin 2007).

The half-life of caffeine is prolonged during the second and third trimesters of pregnancy and maternal and fetal exposure is also influenced by maternal tobacco or alcohol consumption (Brent 2011; Koren 2000). Current guidelines recommend limiting caffeine intake from all sources to ≤200 mg/day during pregnancy (ACOG 2010).

◆ **Caffeine, Acetaminophen, Butalbital, and Codeine** *see* Butalbital, Acetaminophen, Caffeine, and Codeine *on page 274*

◆ **Caffeine and Ergotamine** *see* Ergotamine and Caffeine *on page 583*

◆ **Caffeine and Sodium Benzoate** *see* Caffeine *on page 277*

◆ **Caffeine Citrate** *see* Caffeine *on page 277*

◆ **Caffeine, Orphenadrine, and Aspirin** *see* Orphenadrine, Aspirin, and Caffeine *on page 1146*

◆ **Caffeine Sodium Benzoate** *see* Caffeine *on page 277*

◆ **CAL-101** *see* Idelalisib *on page 795*

◆ **Calaclear [OTC]** *see* Pramoxine *on page 1252*

◆ **Caladryl Clear [OTC]** *see* Pramoxine *on page 1252*

◆ **Calan [DSC]** *see* Verapamil *on page 1540*

◆ **Calan SR** *see* Verapamil *on page 1540*

Calaspargase Pegol (kal AS par jase PEG ol)

Brand Names: US Asparlas

Pharmacologic Category Antineoplastic Agent, Enzyme; Antineoplastic Agent, Miscellaneous

Use Acute lymphoblastic leukemia: Treatment of acute lymphoblastic leukemia (ALL) (as part of a combination chemotherapy regimen) in children and adults age 1 month to 21 years.

Local Anesthetic/Vasoconstrictor Precautions
No information available to require special precautions

Effects on Dental Treatment Key adverse event(s) related to dental treatment: Decreased blood pressure associated with the use of calaspargase pegol-mknl; patients may experience orthostatic hypotension as they stand up after treatment, especially if lying in dental chair for extended periods of time. Use caution with sudden changes in position during and after dental treatment.

Effects on Bleeding Hemorrhage: Hemorrhage associated with increased prothrombin time (PT), increased partial thromboplastin time (PTT), and hypofibrinogenemia have been reported in patients receiving calaspargase pegol-mknl.

Adverse Reactions

>10%:

- Cardiovascular: Decreased blood pressure
- Gastrointestinal: Pancreatitis (12% to 16%)
- Hematologic & oncologic: Disorder of hemostatic components of blood (grades 3/4: 14%)
- Hepatic: Increased serum transaminases (grades 3/4: 52%), increased serum bilirubin (grades 3/4: 20%)
- Hypersensitivity: Hypersensitivity (grades 3/4: 7% to 21%), angioedema
- Ophthalmic: Swelling of eye
- Respiratory: Bronchospasm

1% to 10%:

- Cardiovascular: Embolism (grades 3/4: ≤8%), thrombosis (grades 3/4: ≤8%), cardiac arrhythmia (grades 3/4: 2%), cardiac failure (grades 3/4: 2%)
- Gastrointestinal: Diarrhea (grades 3/4: 9%)
- Hematologic & oncologic: Hemorrhage (grades 3/4: 4%)
- Infection: Sepsis (grades 3/4: 5%), fungal infection (grades 3/4: 3%)
- Respiratory: Dyspnea (grades 3/4: 4%), pneumonia (grades 3/4: 3%)

Frequency not defined:

- Hematologic & oncologic: Hypofibrinogenemia, prolonged partial thromboplastin time, prolonged prothrombin time
- Hypersensitivity: Anaphylaxis

Mechanism of Action Calaspargase pegol contains an *E. coli*-derived asparagine-specific enzyme, as a conjugate of L-asparaginase and monomethoxypolyethylene glycol (mPEG) with a succinimidyl carbonate linker which produces a stable bond between the mPEG component and the L-asparaginase lysine groups. L-asparaginase is an enzyme which catalyzes the deamidation of asparagine to aspartic acid and ammonia, reducing circulating levels of asparagine. Leukemic cells with low asparagine synthetase expression have a reduced ability to synthesize L-asparagine. L-asparaginase reduces the exogenous asparagine source for the leukemic cells, resulting in cytotoxicity specific to leukemic cells.

Pharmacodynamics/Kinetics

Half-life Elimination 16.1 days

Time to Peak 1.17 hours

Reproductive Considerations Evaluate pregnancy status prior to use in females of reproductive potential. Effective nonhormonal contraception should be used during therapy and for at least 3 months after the last calaspargase pegol dose. Hormonal contraceptives may not be effective and are not recommended as a form of contraception.

Pregnancy Considerations

Based on animal reproduction studies conducted with L-asparaginase, adverse effects to the fetus may be expected if exposure occurs during pregnancy.

Product Availability Asparlas: FDA approved December 2018; anticipated availability is currently undetermined

◆ **Calaspargase Pegol-mknl** *see* Calaspargase Pegol *on page 278*

◆ **Calcet Petites [OTC]** *see* Calcium and Vitamin D *on page 280*

◆ **Calcidiol** *see* Calcifediol *on page 279*

◆ **Calcidol [OTC]** *see* Ergocalciferol *on page 582*

Calcifediol (kal si fe DYE ole)

Brand Names: US Rayaldee

Pharmacologic Category Vitamin D Analog

Use

Secondary hyperparathyroidism: Treatment of secondary hyperparathyroidism in adults with stage 3 or 4 chronic kidney disease and serum total 25-hydroxyvitamin D levels less than 30 ng/mL.

Limitations of use: Not indicated for the treatment of secondary hyperparathyroidism in patients with stage 5 chronic kidney disease or in patients with end-stage renal disease (ESRD) on dialysis.

Local Anesthetic/Vasoconstrictor Precautions No information available to require special precautions

Effects on Dental Treatment Key adverse event(s) related to dental treatment: Nasopharyngitis has been reported

Effects on Bleeding No information available to require special precautions

Adverse Reactions

>10%: Hematologic & oncologic: Abnormal phosphorus levels (increased: 45%; hyperphosphatemia: <1%)

1% to 10%:

Cardiovascular: Cardiac failure (4%)

Endocrine & metabolic: Hypercalcemia (4%; patients requiring dose reduction for hypercalcemia: 2%), hyperkalemia (3%), hyperuricemia (2%)

Hematologic & oncologic: Anemia (5%), bruise (2%)

Neuromuscular & skeletal: Osteoarthritis (2%)

Renal: Increased serum creatinine (5%)

Respiratory: Nasopharyngitis (5%), cough (4%), dyspnea (4%), bronchitis (3%), chronic obstructive pulmonary disease (1%), pneumonia (1%)

Mechanism of Action Calcifediol, a prohormone of the active form of vitamin D_3, calcitriol (1,25 dihydroxyvitamin D_3), is catalyzed to calcitriol by the 1-alpha-hydroxylase enzyme, CYP27B1, primarily in the kidney. Calcitriol binds to vitamin D receptors in target tissues activating vitamin D responsive pathways resulting in increased intestinal absorption of calcium and phosphorus and reduced parathyroid hormone synthesis.

Pharmacodynamics/Kinetics

Onset of Action ~2 weeks; maximum effect: ~3 months

Half-life Elimination Healthy adults: ~11 days; Stage 3 and 4 CKD: ~25 days

Pregnancy Considerations Endogenous calcifediol crosses the placenta in concentrations generally lower than those in the maternal plasma; supplementation increases cord blood 25OHD concentrations (IOM 2011).

◆ **Calciferol [OTC]** *see* Ergocalciferol *on page 582*

◆ **CalciFol** *see* Vitamins (Multiple/Oral) *on page 1550*

◆ **CalciFolic-D** *see* Vitamins (Multiple/Oral) *on page 1550*

◆ **Calcitrate [OTC]** *see* Calcium and Vitamin D *on page 280*

Calcitriol (Systemic) (kal si TRYE ole)

Brand Names: US Rocaltrol

Brand Names: Canada Calcijex [DSC]; Calcitriol-Odan; Rocaltrol; TARO-Calcitriol

Pharmacologic Category Vitamin D Analog

Use

Hypoparathyroidism/pseudohypoparathyroidism: Management of hypocalcemia in patients with hypoparathyroidism or pseudohypoparathyroidism (oral)

Secondary hyperparathyroidism in patients with chronic kidney disease: Management of secondary hyperparathyroidism in patients with moderate to severe chronic kidney disease (CKD) not on dialysis (oral) or in patients on dialysis (oral or IV). **Note:** Although the manufacturer's labeling states that calcitriol may be used specifically to treat hypocalcemia in dialysis patients, due to the risk of hypercalcemia, use should generally be reserved for patients with severe and progressive hyperparathyroidism (KDIGO 2017).

Local Anesthetic/Vasoconstrictor Precautions No information available to require special precautions

Effects on Dental Treatment Key adverse event(s) related to dental treatment: Metallic taste and xerostomia (normal salivary flow resumes upon discontinuation).

Effects on Bleeding No information available to require special precautions

Adverse Reactions

>10%: Endocrine & metabolic: Hypercalcemia

1% to 10%:

Central nervous system: Headache

Dermatologic: Skin rash

Endocrine & metabolic: Polydipsia

Gastrointestinal: Abdominal pain, nausea

Genitourinary: Urinary tract infection

Frequency not defined:

Cardiovascular: Cardiac arrhythmia, hypertension

Central nervous system: Apathy, drowsiness, hyperthermia, metallic taste, psychosis, sensory disturbance

Dermatologic: Erythema, erythema multiforme, pruritus, urticaria

Endocrine & metabolic: Albuminuria, calcinosis, decreased libido, dehydration, growth suppression, hypercholesterolemia, weight loss

Gastrointestinal: Anorexia, constipation, pancreatitis, stomach pain, vomiting, xerostomia

Genitourinary: Hypercalciuria, nocturia

Hepatic: Increased serum ALT, increased serum AST

Hypersensitivity: Hypersensitivity reaction

Local: Pain at injection site (mild)

Neuromuscular & skeletal: Dystrophy, myalgia, ostealgia, weakness

Ophthalmic: Conjunctivitis, photophobia

Renal: Calcium nephrolithiasis, increased blood urea nitrogen, increased serum creatinine, polyuria

Respiratory: Rhinorrhea

<1%, postmarketing and/or case reports: Agitation, anaphylaxis, apprehension, hypermagnesemia, hyperphosphatemia, hypervitaminosis D, increased hematocrit, increased hemoglobin, increased neutrophils, increased serum alkaline phosphatase, insomnia, limb pain, lymphocytosis

Mechanism of Action Calcitriol, the active form of vitamin D (1,25 hydroxyvitamin D_3), binds to and activates the vitamin D receptor in kidney, parathyroid gland, intestine, and bone, stimulating intestinal calcium transport and absorption. It reduces parathyroid hormone (PTH) levels and improves calcium and phosphate homeostasis by stimulating bone resorption of calcium and increasing renal tubular reabsorption of calcium. Decreased renal conversion of vitamin D to its primary active metabolite (1,25 hydroxyvitamin D) in chronic renal failure leads to reduced activation of vitamin D receptor, which subsequently removes inhibitory suppression of parathyroid hormone (PTH) release; increased serum PTH (secondary hyperparathyroidism) reduces calcium excretion and enhances bone resorption.

Pharmacodynamics/Kinetics

Onset of Action Oral: 2 hours; maximum effect: 10 hours

Duration of Action Oral, IV: 3 to 5 days

Half-life Elimination Children 1.8 to 16 years undergoing peritoneal dialysis: 27.4 hours; Healthy adults: 5 to 8 hours; Hemodialysis: 16 to 22 hours

Time to Peak Serum: Oral: 3 to 6 hours; Hemodialysis: 8 to 12 hours

Pregnancy Risk Factor C

Pregnancy Considerations

Maternal calcitriol may be detected in the fetal circulation. Mild hypercalcemia has been reported in a newborn following maternal use of calcitriol during pregnancy. Adverse effects on fetal development were not observed with use of calcitriol during pregnancy in women (N=9) with pseudovitamin D-dependent rickets. Doses were adjusted every 4 weeks to keep calcium concentrations within normal limits (Edouard 2011). If calcitriol is used for the management of hypoparathyroidism in pregnancy, dose adjustments may be needed as pregnancy progresses and again following delivery. Vitamin D and calcium levels should be monitored closely and kept in the lower normal range (Callies 1998).

Calcitriol (Topical) (kal si TRYE ole)

Brand Names: US Vectical

Brand Names: Canada Silkis

Pharmacologic Category Vitamin D Analog

Use Plaque psoriasis: Management of mild to moderate plaque psoriasis in adults and pediatric patients ≥2 years of age.

Local Anesthetic/Vasoconstrictor Precautions
No information available to require special precautions

Effects on Dental Treatment Key adverse event(s) related to dental treatment: Metallic taste and xerostomia (normal salivary flow resumes upon discontinuation).

Effects on Bleeding No information available to require special precautions

Adverse Reactions

>10%: Endocrine: Hypercalcemia (24%)

1% to 10%:

Dermatologic: Psoriasis (4%), pruritus (1% to 3%), skin discomfort

Genitourinary: Urine abnormality (4%), hypercalciuria (3%)

<1%, postmarketing, and/or case reports: Burning sensation of skin, dermatitis (acute; blistering), eczema (including extensive flare up), erythema, nephrolithiasis, skin atrophy

Mechanism of Action The mechanism by which calcitriol is beneficial in the treatment of psoriasis has not been established.

Pharmacodynamics/Kinetics

Duration of Action Oral, IV: 3 to 5 days

Half-life Elimination Children 1.8 to 16 years undergoing peritoneal dialysis: 27.4 hours; Healthy adults: 5 to 8 hours; Hemodialysis: 16 to 22 hours

Time to Peak Oral: 3 to 6 hours; Hemodialysis: 8 to 12 hours

Pregnancy Considerations Topical agents are recommended for the treatment of psoriasis in pregnancy; however, agents with information specific to use in pregnant patients is preferred (Babalola 2013; Bae 2012).

- **Calcium Acetylhomotaurinate** *see* Acamprosate *on page 57*

Calcium and Vitamin D
(KAL see um & VYE ta min dee)

Brand Names: US Calcet Petites [OTC]; Calcitrate [OTC]; Caltrate 600+D [OTC] [DSC]; Caltrate 600+D3 Soft [OTC]; Caltrate 600+D3 [OTC]; Caltrate 600+Soy [OTC]; Caltrate ColonHealth [OTC]; Caltrate Gummy Bites [OTC]; Citracal Maximum [OTC]; Citracal Petites [OTC]; Citracal Regular [OTC]; Os-Cal Calcium + D3 [OTC]; Os-Cal Extra D3 [OTC]; Os-Cal [OTC]; Oysco 500+D [OTC]; Oysco D [OTC] [DSC]

Pharmacologic Category Calcium Salt; Electrolyte Supplement, Oral; Vitamin, Fat Soluble

Use Dietary supplement: Use as a dietary supplement when calcium intake may be inadequate

Local Anesthetic/Vasoconstrictor Precautions
No information available to require special precautions

Effects on Dental Treatment No significant effects or complications reported

Effects on Bleeding No information available to require special precautions

Adverse Reactions Frequency not defined; also see individual agents

Central nervous system: Headache

Endocrine & metabolic: Hypercalcemia

Gastrointestinal: Gastrointestinal distress

Genitourinary: Hypercalciuria

- **Calcium Carb & Cit/Vitamin D3** *see* Calcium and Vitamin D *on page 280*
- **Calcium Carbonate and Etidronate Disodium** *see* Etidronate and Calcium Carbonate *on page 621*
- **Calcium Carbonate/Vitamin D2** *see* Calcium and Vitamin D *on page 280*
- **Calcium Carbonate/Vitamin D3** *see* Calcium and Vitamin D *on page 280*
- **Calcium Citrate and Vitamin D** *see* Calcium and Vitamin D *on page 280*
- **Calcium Citrate/Vitamin D2** *see* Calcium and Vitamin D *on page 280*
- **Calcium Citrate/Vitamin D3** *see* Calcium and Vitamin D *on page 280*
- **Calcium Folinate** *see* Leucovorin Calcium *on page 889*
- **Calcium Leucovorin** *see* Leucovorin Calcium *on page 889*
- **Calcium Levoleucovorin** *see* LEVOleucovorin *on page 899*
- **Calcium Paraaminosalicylate** *see* Aminosalicylic Acid *on page 118*
- **Calcium Phosphate and Vitamin D** *see* Calcium and Vitamin D *on page 280*
- **Calcium/Vitamin D** *see* Calcium and Vitamin D *on page 280*
- **Caldolor** *see* Ibuprofen *on page 786*
- **Caldyphen Clear [OTC]** *see* Pramoxine *on page 1252*
- **Callergy Clear [OTC]** *see* Pramoxine *on page 1252*

- ◆ **CaloMist** *see* Cyanocobalamin *on page 417*
- ◆ **Calquence** *see* Acalabrutinib *on page 56*
- ◆ **Caltrate 600+D [OTC] [DSC]** *see* Calcium and Vitamin D *on page 280*
- ◆ **Caltrate 600+D3 [OTC]** *see* Calcium and Vitamin D *on page 280*
- ◆ **Caltrate 600+D3 Soft [OTC]** *see* Calcium and Vitamin D *on page 280*
- ◆ **Caltrate 600+Soy [OTC]** *see* Calcium and Vitamin D *on page 280*
- ◆ **Caltrate ColonHealth [OTC]** *see* Calcium and Vitamin D *on page 280*
- ◆ **Caltrate Gummy Bites [OTC]** *see* Calcium and Vitamin D *on page 280*
- ◆ **Cambia** *see* Diclofenac (Systemic) *on page 484*
- ◆ **Camila** *see* Norethindrone *on page 1117*
- ◆ **Campath** *see* Alemtuzumab *on page 93*
- ◆ **Campath-1H** *see* Alemtuzumab *on page 93*
- ◆ **Camphorated Tincture of Opium (error-prone synonym)** *see* Paregoric *on page 1192*
- ◆ **Campral** *see* Acamprosate *on page 57*
- ◆ **Camptosar** *see* Irinotecan (Conventional) *on page 841*
- ◆ **Camptothecin-11** *see* Irinotecan (Conventional) *on page 841*
- ◆ **Camrese** *see* Ethinyl Estradiol and Levonorgestrel *on page 612*
- ◆ **Camrese Lo** *see* Ethinyl Estradiol and Levonorgestrel *on page 612*

Canagliflozin (kan a gli FLOE zin)

Brand Names: US Invokana

Brand Names: Canada Invokana

Pharmacologic Category Antidiabetic Agent, Sodium-Glucose Cotransporter 2 (SGLT2) Inhibitor; Sodium-Glucose Cotransporter 2 (SGLT2) Inhibitor

Use Diabetes mellitus, type 2, treatment: As an adjunct to diet and exercise to improve glycemic control in adults with type 2 diabetes mellitus; risk reduction of major cardiovascular events (cardiovascular death, nonfatal myocardial infarction, and nonfatal stroke) in adults with type 2 diabetes mellitus and established cardiovascular disease; risk reduction of end-stage kidney disease, doubling of serum creatinine, cardiovascular death, and hospitalization for heart failure in adults with type 2 diabetes mellitus and diabetic nephropathy with urinary albumin excretion >300 mg/day.

Local Anesthetic/Vasoconstrictor Precautions No information available to require special precautions

Effects on Dental Treatment Key adverse event(s) related to dental treatment: Hypoglycemia reported; patients should be appointed for dental treatment in the morning in order to minimize chance of stress-induced hypoglycemia. Dizziness and syncope have been reported; patients may experience orthostatic hypotension as they stand up after treatment; especially if lying in dental chair for extended periods of time. Use caution with sudden changes in position during and after dental treatment.

Canagliflozin-dependent patients with diabetes (non-insulin dependent, type 2) should be questioned by the dental professional at each dental visit to assess their risk for stress-induced hypoglycemia. The dental professional should inquire about the patient's routine (ie, work, sleep schedule, eating patterns), history of hypoglycemia, time of last medication dose, last meal, and most recent blood sugar assessment. Keep a supply of glucose tablets and other carbohydrates in the office to prepare for a hypoglycemic event. Seek medical attention when necessary (American Diabetes Association 2016).

Effects on Bleeding No information available to require special precautions

Adverse Reactions

>10%: Infection: Genitourinary fungal infection (females: 11% to 12%; males: 4%; patients who developed infections were more likely to experience recurrence)

1% to 10%:

Cardiovascular: Hypotension (3%)

Central nervous system: Falling (2%), fatigue (2%)

Endocrine & metabolic: Hypoglycemia (4%), hypovolemia (2% to 3%), increased thirst (2% to 3%), increased serum potassium (eGFR 45 to 60 mL/minute: >5.4 mEq/mL: 9%; ≥6.5% mEQ/mL: 1%)

Gastrointestinal: Abdominal pain (2%), constipation (2%), nausea (2%)

Genitourinary: Urinary tract infection (6%), increased urine output (5%), vulvovaginal pruritus (2% to 3%)

Hematologic & oncologic: Increased hemoglobin (3% to 4%)

Hypersensitivity: Hypersensitivity reaction (4%)

Neuromuscular & skeletal: Asthenia (≤1%)

Miscellaneous: Limb injury (toe, foot, lower limb amputations: 2% to 4%)

Frequency not defined:

Endocrine & metabolic: Increased LDL cholesterol, increased serum cholesterol (non-HDL)

Neuromuscular & skeletal: Bone fracture, decreased bone mineral density

Renal: Decreased estimated GFR (eGFR), increased serum creatinine

<1%, postmarketing, and/or case reports: Acute renal failure, anaphylaxis, angioedema, ketoacidosis, necrotizing fasciitis (perineum), pancreatitis, phimosis, pyelonephritis, skin photosensitivity, urinary tract infection with sepsis

Mechanism of Action By inhibiting sodium-glucose cotransporter 2 (SGLT2) in the proximal renal tubules, canagliflozin reduces reabsorption of filtered glucose from the tubular lumen and lowers the renal threshold for glucose (RT_G). SGLT2 is the main site of filtered glucose reabsorption; reduction of filtered glucose reabsorption and lowering of RT_G result in increased urinary excretion of glucose, thereby reducing plasma glucose concentrations.

Pharmacodynamics/Kinetics

Onset of Action Within 24 hours (dose-dependent)

Duration of Action Suppression of the renal threshold for glucose (RT_G) occurs throughout the 24-hour dosing interval; maximal RT_G suppression occurred with the 300 mg dose (RT_G decreased from baseline of ~240 mg/dL to a mean of 70 to 90 mg/dL over 24 hours).

Half-life Elimination Apparent terminal half-life: 100 mg dose: 10.6 hours; 300 mg dose: 13.1 hours

Time to Peak Plasma: 1 to 2 hours

Pregnancy Considerations

Due to adverse effects on renal development observed in animal studies, the manufacturer does not recommend use of canagliflozin during the second and third trimesters of pregnancy.

Poorly controlled diabetes during pregnancy can be associated with an increased risk of adverse maternal and fetal outcomes, including diabetic ketoacidosis, preeclampsia, spontaneous abortion, preterm delivery, delivery complications, major birth defects, stillbirth, and macrosomia. To prevent adverse outcomes, prior to conception and throughout pregnancy, maternal blood glucose and HbA_{1c} should be kept as close to target goals as possible but without causing significant hypoglycemia (ADA 2020; Blumer 2013).

Agents other than canagliflozin are currently recommended to treat diabetes mellitus in pregnancy (ADA 2020).

◆ **Canasa** *see* Mesalamine *on page 980*

◆ **Cancidas** *see* Caspofungin *on page 296*

Candesartan (kan de SAR tan)

Related Information

Cardiovascular Diseases *on page 1654*

Brand Names: US Atacand

Brand Names: Canada ACCEL-Candesartan [DSC]; ACH-Candesartan; ACT Candesartan [DSC]; AG-Candesartan; APO-Candesartan; Atacand; Auro-Candesartan; DOM-Candesartan [DSC]; JAMP-Candesartan; MINT-Candesartan; MYLAN-Candesartan [DSC]; PMS-Candesartan; RIVA-Candesartan [DSC]; SANDOZ Candesartan; TARO-Candesartan; TEVA-Candesartan

Pharmacologic Category Angiotensin II Receptor Blocker; Antihypertensive

Use

Heart failure with reduced ejection fraction: Treatment of heart failure (NYHA class II to IV) in adults with left ventricular systolic dysfunction (ejection fraction <40%) to reduce cardiovascular death and heart failure hospitalization.

Hypertension: Management of hypertension in adults and children ≥1 year of age.

Local Anesthetic/Vasoconstrictor Precautions No information available to require special precautions

Effects on Dental Treatment Key adverse event(s) related to dental treatment: Patients may experience orthostatic hypotension as they stand up after treatment; especially if lying in dental chair for extended periods of time. Use caution with sudden changes in position during and after dental treatment.

Effects on Bleeding No information available to require special precautions

Adverse Reactions

>10%:

Cardiovascular: Hypotension (19%)

Renal: Renal function abnormality (13%)

1% to 10%:

Central nervous system: Dizziness (4%)

Endocrine & metabolic: Hyperkalemia (6%)

Neuromuscular & skeletal: Back pain (3%)

Respiratory: Upper respiratory tract infection (6%), pharyngitis (2%), rhinitis (2%)

Frequency not defined:

Central nervous system: Headache

Renal: Exacerbation of renal disease (children & adolescents), increased serum creatinine

<1%, postmarketing, and/or case reports: Abnormal hepatic function tests, agranulocytosis, angioedema, cough, hepatitis, hyponatremia, leukopenia, neutropenia, pruritus, skin rash, urticaria

Mechanism of Action Candesartan is an angiotensin receptor antagonist. Angiotensin II acts as a vasoconstrictor. In addition to causing direct vasoconstriction, angiotensin II also stimulates the release of aldosterone. Once aldosterone is released, sodium as well as water are reabsorbed. The end result is an elevation in blood pressure. Candesartan binds to the AT1 angiotensin II receptor. This binding prevents angiotensin II from binding to the receptor thereby blocking the vasoconstriction and the aldosterone secreting effects of angiotensin II.

Pharmacodynamics/Kinetics

Onset of Action

2 to 3 hours; antihypertensive effect: Within 2 weeks

Peak effect: 6 to 8 hours; maximum antihypertensive effect: 4 to 6 weeks

Duration of Action >24 hours

Half-life Elimination Dose dependent: 5 to 9 hours

Time to Peak Children (1 to 17 years); Adults: 3 to 4 hours

Reproductive Considerations

The use of angiotensin II receptor blockers should generally be avoided in women planning a pregnancy (ACOG 203 2019). When treatment is needed in females of reproductive potential with diabetic nephropathy, candesartan should be discontinued at the first positive pregnancy test (Cabiddu 2016; Porta 2011).

Pregnancy Considerations

[US Boxed Warning]: Drugs that act on the renin-angiotensin system can cause injury and death to the developing fetus. When pregnancy is detected, discontinue as soon as possible. The use of drugs which act on the renin-angiotensin system are associated with oligohydramnios. Oligohydramnios, due to decreased fetal renal function, may lead to fetal lung hypoplasia and skeletal malformations. Oligohydramnios may not appear until after irreversible fetal injury has occurred. Use in pregnancy is also associated with anuria, hypotension, renal failure, skull hypoplasia, and death in the fetus/neonate. The exposed fetus should be monitored for fetal growth, amniotic fluid volume, and organ formation. Infants exposed in utero should be monitored for hyperkalemia, hypotension, and oliguria (exchange transfusions or dialysis may be needed). These adverse events are generally associated with maternal use in the second and third trimesters.

Chronic maternal hypertension itself is also associated with adverse events in the fetus/infant. The risk of birth defects, low birth weight, premature delivery, stillbirth, and neonatal death may be increased with chronic hypertension in pregnancy. Actual risks may be related to duration and severity of maternal hypertension (ACOG 203 2019).

The use of angiotensin II receptor blockers is generally not recommended to treat chronic hypertension in pregnant women (ACOG 203 2019). When treatment is needed in females of reproductive potential with diabetic nephropathy, candesartan should be discontinued at the first positive pregnancy test (Cabiddu 2016; Porta 2011).

◆ **Candesartan Cilexetil** *see* Candesartan *on page 282*

Cangrelor (KAN grel or)

Brand Names: US Kengreal

Pharmacologic Category Antiplatelet Agent; Antiplatelet Agent, Non-thienopyridine; P2Y12 Antagonist

Use Percutaneous coronary intervention (PCI): Adjunct to PCI to reduce the risk of periprocedural myocardial infarction, repeat coronary revascularization, and stent thrombosis in patients who have not been treated with a $P2Y_{12}$ platelet inhibitor and are not being given a glycoprotein IIb/IIIa inhibitor.

Local Anesthetic/Vasoconstrictor Precautions No information available to require special precautions

Effects on Dental Treatment No significant effects or complications reported

Effects on Bleeding Cangrelor increases the risk of bleeding. However, it is indicated as an intravenous infusion prior to and during percutaneous coronary intervention and has a short elimination half-life. No antiplatelet effect is observed an hour after discontinuation. There is no information to require any special precautions for dental procedures in patients previously exposed to Cangrelor.

Adverse Reactions

Hematologic & oncologic: Hemorrhage (GUSTO: 16%; TIMI: <1%)

Renal: Renal insufficiency (3%; severe; creatinine clearance <30 mL/minute)

Respiratory: Dyspnea (1%)

<1%, postmarketing, and/or case reports: Hypersensitivity reaction

Mechanism of Action Cangrelor, a nonthienopyridine adenosine triphosphate analogue, is a direct $P2Y_{12}$ platelet receptor inhibitor that blocks adenosine diphosphate (ADP)-induced platelet activation and aggregation. Cangrelor binds selectively and reversibly to the $P2Y_{12}$ receptor, preventing further signaling and platelet activation.

Pharmacodynamics/Kinetics

Onset of Action Platelet inhibition occurs within 2 minutes

Duration of Action Antiplatelet effect is maintained throughout duration of infusion. After discontinuation, platelet function returns to normal within 1 hour

Half-life Elimination ~3 to 6 minutes

Time to Peak Within 2 minutes

Pregnancy Risk Factor C

Pregnancy Considerations Adverse events were observed in some animal reproduction studies.

◆ **Cangrelor Tetrasodium** *see* Cangrelor *on page* 282

Cannabidiol (kan a bi DYE ol)

Brand Names: US Epidiolex

Pharmacologic Category Anticonvulsant; Cannabinoid

Use Seizure disorders: Treatment of seizures associated with Lennox-Gastaut syndrome, Dravet syndrome, or tuberous sclerosis complex in patients ≥1 year of age.

Local Anesthetic/Vasoconstrictor Precautions No information available to require special precautions

Effects on Dental Treatment Key adverse event(s) related to dental treatment: Sedation is most common early in treatment and may resolve with continued use. Excessive salivation has been reported.

Effects on Bleeding No information available to require special precautions

Adverse Reactions

>10%:

Central nervous system: Drowsiness (≤32%), lethargy (≤32%), sedation (≤32%), fatigue (≤12%), malaise (≤12%), insomnia (≤11%), sleep disorder (≤11%), sleep disturbance (≤11%)

Dermatologic: Skin rash (7% to 13%)

Endocrine & metabolic: Weight loss (3% to 18%)

Gastrointestinal: Decreased appetite (16% to 22%), diarrhea (9% to 20%)

Hematologic & oncologic: Anemia (30%)

Hepatic: Increased serum alanine aminotransferase (>3x ULN: 13% to 17%), increased serum transaminases (8% to 16%)

Infection: Infection (25% to 41%), viral infection (7% to 11%)

Neuromuscular & skeletal: Asthenia (≤12%)

1% to 10%:

Central nervous system: Agitation (≤9%), irritability (≤9%), aggressive behavior (≤5%), outbursts of anger (≤5%), drooling (≤4%), abnormal gait (2% to 3%)

Gastrointestinal: Gastroenteritis (4%), sialorrhea (≤4%), abdominal distress (≤3%), abdominal pain (≤3%)

Infection: Fungal infection (1% to 3%)

Respiratory: Pneumonia (5% to 8%), hypoxia (≤3%), respiratory failure (≤3%)

Frequency not defined:

Hematologic & oncologic: Decreased hematocrit, decreased hemoglobin

Hepatic: Increased serum aspartate aminotransferase, increased serum transaminases (>20x ULN)

Hypersensitivity: Hypersensitivity reaction

Renal: Increased serum creatinine

<1%, postmarketing, and/or case reports: Angioedema, erythema, pruritus

Mechanism of Action The exact antiepileptic mechanism of action of cannabidiol is unknown; however, it does not appear to involve its effects on cannabinoid receptors.

Pharmacodynamics/Kinetics

Onset of Action Within 4 weeks

Half-life Elimination 56 to 61 hours

Time to Peak 2.5 to 5 hours at steady state

Pregnancy Considerations

Cannabidiol can be detected in the umbilical cord serum and meconium following maternal use of inhaled, non-medicinal cannabis during pregnancy (Kim 2018).

Patients exposed to cannabidiol during pregnancy are encouraged to enroll in the North American Antiepileptic Drug (NAAED) Pregnancy Registry by calling 1-888-233-2334. Additional information is available at www.aedpregnancyregistry.org.

Controlled Substance

Descheduled April 2020

◆ **Cannabidiol and Tetrahydrocannabinol** *see* Tetrahydrocannabinol and Cannabidiol *on page* 1434

◆ **Capex** *see* Fluocinolone (Topical) *on page* 689

◆ **Caphosol** *see* Saliva Substitute *on page* 1354

◆ **Capital/Codeine [DSC]** *see* Acetaminophen and Codeine *on page* 65

◆ **Caplyta** *see* Lumateperone *on page* 942

Capmatinib (kap MA ti nib)

Brand Names: US Tabrecta

Pharmacologic Category Antineoplastic Agent, MET Inhibitor; Antineoplastic Agent, Tyrosine Kinase Inhibitor

Use Non-small cell lung cancer, metastatic: Treatment of metastatic non-small cell lung cancer (NSCLC) in adults whose tumors have a mutation that leads to mesenchymal-epithelial transition (MET) exon 14 skipping as detected by an approved test.

Local Anesthetic/Vasoconstrictor Precautions No information available to require special precautions.

Effects on Dental Treatment No significant effects or complications reported.

Effects on Bleeding No information available to require special precautions.

Adverse Reactions

>10%:

Cardiovascular: Peripheral edema (52%)

Endocrine & metabolic: Decreased serum albumin (68%), decreased serum glucose (21%), decreased serum phosphate (23%), decreased serum sodium (23%), increased gamma-glutamyl transferase (29%), increased serum potassium (23%)

Gastrointestinal: Constipation (18%), decreased appetite (21%), diarrhea (18%), increased serum amylase (31%), increased serum lipase (26%), nausea (44%; severe nausea: 2%), vomiting (28%; severe vomiting: 2%)

Hematologic & oncologic: Decreased hemoglobin (24%, grades 3/4: 3%), leukopenia (23%, grades 3/4: <1%), lymphocytopenia (44%, grades 3/4: 14%)

Hepatic: Increased serum alanine aminotransferase (37%), increased serum alkaline phosphatase (32%), increased serum aspartate aminotransferase (25%)

Nervous system: Fatigue (32%), noncardiac chest pain (15%)

Neuromuscular & skeletal: Back pain (14%)

Renal: Increased serum creatinine (62%)

Respiratory: Cough (16%), dyspnea (24%)

Miscellaneous: Fever (14%)

1% to 10%:

Dermatologic: Cellulitis (<10%), pruritus (<10%), urticaria (<10%)

Endocrine & metabolic: Weight loss (10%)

Gastrointestinal: Acute pancreatitis (<10%)

Renal: Acute renal failure (<10%, including renal failure syndrome)

Respiratory: Interstitial pulmonary disease (≤5%), pleural effusion (4%), pneumonia (5%), pneumonitis (≤5%)

Frequency not defined: Hepatic: Hepatotoxicity

Mechanism of Action Capmatinib is a potent and highly-selective inhibitor of mesenchymal-epithelial transition (MET), including the mutant variant produced by exon 14 skipping. MET exon 14 skipping results in increased downstream MET signaling. Through MET inhibition, capmatinib decreases cancer cell growth. Capmatinib inhibits MET phosphorylation triggered by binding of c-MET (also known as hepatocyte growth factor) or by MET amplification, as well as MET-mediated phosphorylation of downstream signaling proteins.

Pharmacodynamics/Kinetics

Half-life Elimination 6.5 hours.

Time to Peak ~1 to 2 hours.

Reproductive Considerations

Evaluate pregnancy status prior to use in females of reproductive potential.

Females of reproductive potential should use effective contraception during therapy and for 1 week after the last capmatinib dose. Males with female partners of reproductive potential should use effective contraception during therapy and for 1 week after the last capmatinib dose.

Pregnancy Considerations

Based on the mechanism of action and data from animal reproduction studies, in utero exposure to capmatinib may cause fetal harm.

◆ **Capmatinib Hydrochloride** *see* Capmatinib *on page 283*

◆ **Capoten** *see* Captopril *on page 286*

◆ **Caprelsa** *see* Vandetanib *on page 1531*

Capsaicin (kap SAY sin)

Related Information

Capsicum Peppers *on page 1601*

Brand Names: US Allevess [OTC]; Captracin [DSC]; Capzasin-HP [OTC]; Capzasin-P [OTC]; Capzix [OTC]; DiabetAid Pain and Tingling Relief [OTC]; Flexin; Levatio; MaC Patch [DSC]; MenCaps [OTC]; Neuvaxin [DSC]; Qutenza; Releevia MC [DSC]; Releevia [DSC]; Renovo; Salonpas Gel-Patch Hot [OTC]; Salonpas Hot [OTC] [DSC]; Sinelee [DSC]; Sure Result SR Relief [OTC]; Trixaicin HP [OTC]; Trixaicin [OTC] [DSC]; Zostrix HP [OTC]; Zostrix Natural Pain Relief [OTC]

Brand Names: Canada Zostrix; Zostrix H.P.

Generic Availability (US) Yes: Cream

Pharmacologic Category Analgesic, Topical; Topical Skin Product; Transient Receptor Potential Vanilloid 1 (TRPV1) Agonist

Dental Use Potential use as topical agent in burning mouth syndrome and oral mucositis

Use

Muscle/Joint pain: Temporary relief of minor aches and pains of muscles and joints associated with simple backache, muscle strains, sprains, arthritis, bruises, or cramps.

Neuropathic pain (8% patch): Management of neuropathic pain associated with postherpetic neuralgia and diabetic peripheral neuropathy of the feet in adults.

Local Anesthetic/Vasoconstrictor Precautions No information available to require special precautions

Effects on Dental Treatment No significant effects or complications reported

Effects on Bleeding No information available to require special precautions

Adverse Reactions The following adverse events occurred with topical patch administration.

>10%: Local: Application site erythema (63%), application site pain (42%)

1% to 10%:

Cardiovascular: Hypertension (2%)

Dermatologic: Papule of skin (6%), local dryness of skin (2%), pruritus (2%)

Gastrointestinal: Nausea (5%), vomiting (3%)

Local: Application site edema (2% to 4%), application site pruritus (6%)

Respiratory: Nasopharyngitis (4%), sinusitis (3%), bronchitis (2%)

<1%:

Cardiovascular: Peripheral edema

Dermatologic: Abnormal skin odor

Gastrointestinal: Dysgeusia

Local: Application site reaction (includes anesthesia, bruise, dermatitis, excoriation, exfoliation, hyperesthesia, inflammation, irritation, paresthesia, urticaria, vesicles, warmth)

Nervous system: Burning sensation, dizziness, headache, hyperesthesia, hypoesthesia, peripheral sensory neuropathy
Ophthalmic: Eye irritation, eye pain
Respiratory: Cough, throat irritation
Postmarketing: Accidental injury, burn (second degree), cicatrix of skin

Dental Usual Dosage Topical: Apply cream or gel to affected area 3-4 times/day

Dosing

Adult & Geriatric

Diabetic neuropathy: Topical:

Cream (0.075%) (off-label use): Apply 4 times/day (Bril 2011).

Patch (Qutenza): Apply patch to most painful areas of the feet for 30 minutes. Up to 4 patches may be applied in a single application. Treatment may be repeated ≥3 months as needed for return of pain (do not apply more frequently than every 3 months). Area should be pretreated with a topical anesthetic prior to patch application.

Muscle/Joint pain: Topical:

Cream, gel, liquid, lotion: Apply thin film to affected areas 3 to 4 times daily.

Patch: 0.025%, 0.03%, 0.0375%: Apply 1 patch to affected area for up to 8 hours (maximum: 4 patches/day); do not use for >5 consecutive days (product specific).

Neuropathic pain: Topical: Patch (Qutenza): Apply patch to most painful area for 60 minutes. Up to 4 patches may be applied in a single application. Treatment may be repeated ≥3 months as needed for return of pain (do not apply more frequently than every 3 months). Area should be pretreated with a topical anesthetic prior to patch application.

Renal Impairment: Adult There are no dosage adjustments provided in the manufacturer's labeling.

Hepatic Impairment: Adult There are no dosage adjustments provided in the manufacturer's labeling.

Pediatric

Muscle ache and joint pain, minor: Topical:

Lotion 0.025% (DiabetAid Tingling and Pain Relief) Children ≥2 years and Adolescents: Topical: Apply to affected area not more than 3 to 4 times/day

Patch: **Note:** With OTC products, approved ages and uses may vary; consult product specific labeling.

Product strength <0.05%: Adolescents ≥12 years: Topical:

Flexin (0.0375%): Apply 1 patch to affected area; may change 2 to 3 times/day; maximum daily dose: 3 patches/**day**

Levatio (0.03%): Apply 1 patch to affected area for up to 8 hours; change patch 1 to 2 times daily; maximum daily dose: 4 patches/**day**; do not use for >5 consecutive days

MaC (0.0375%): Apply 1 patch to affected area for up to 8 hours; change patch 2 to 3 times/day; maximum daily dose: 4 patches/24 hours

MenCaps (0.0225%): Apply 1 patch to affected area for up to 8 hours; may change patch up to 3 times daily

Releevia MC (0.0375%), Renovo (0.0375%): Apply 1 patch to affected area; may change patch 1 to 2 times daily; maximum daily dose: 3 patches/**day**

Salonpas Pain Relieving Hot Patch (0.025%): Apply 1 patch to affected area for up to 8 hours; may change patch up to 3 to 4 times daily

Product strength 0.05%: Adolescents ≥16 years: Topical: Allevess patch: Apply 1 patch to affected area; may change patch 1 to 2 times daily

Renal Impairment: Pediatric There are no dosage adjustments provided in the manufacturer's labeling.

Hepatic Impairment: Pediatric There are no dosage adjustments provided in the manufacturer's labeling.

Mechanism of Action Capsaicin, a transient receptor potential vanilloid 1 receptor (TRPV1) agonist, activates TRPV1 ligand-gated cation channels on nociceptive nerve fibers, resulting in depolarization, initiation of action potential, and pain signal transmission to the spinal cord; capsaicin exposure results in subsequent desensitization of the sensory axons and inhibition of pain transmission initiation. In arthritis, capsaicin induces release of substance P, the principal chemomediator of pain impulses from the periphery to the CNS, from peripheral sensory neurons; after repeated application, capsaicin depletes the neuron of substance P and prevents reaccumulation. The functional link between substance P and the capsaicin receptor, TRPV1, is not well understood.

Contraindications

Hypersensitivity to capsaicin, menthol, or any component of the formulation.

OTC labeling: When used for self-medication, do not use on wounds, damaged, broken, irritated skin, or into skin folds; do not cover with bandage; do not apply within 1 hour before or after bath, shower, hot tub, or sauna; do not use in combination with external heat source (eg, heating pad); do not use concurrently with other topical analgesics.

Warnings/Precautions May cause serious burns (eg, first- to third-degree chemical burns) at the application site. In some cases, hospitalization has been required. Discontinue use and seek medical attention if signs of skin injury (eg, pain, swelling, or blistering) occur following application (FDA Drug Safety Communication 2012). May cause CNS depression, which may impair physical or mental abilities; patients must be cautioned about performing tasks that require mental alertness (eg, operating machinery, driving). Use the 8% patch with caution in patients with uncontrolled hypertension, or a history of cardiovascular or cerebrovascular events; transient increases in BP due to treatment-related pain have occurred during and after application of RX patch. Monitor BP periodically during and following treatment.

8% patch: Severe irritation to the eyes, mucous membranes, respiratory tract, or skin may occur due to unintended capsaicin exposure. If irritation of the eyes or mucous membranes occurs, remove the individual from the area of the capsaicin patch and flush eyes and mucous membranes with cool water. If respiratory tract irritation (eg, coughing, sneezing) occurs, remove the individual from the area of the capsaicin patch and provide supportive care if shortness of breath develops. If skin not intended to be treated is exposed to the patch, apply cleansing gel for 1 minute and remove with dry gauze; after cleansing gel has been removed, wash the area with soap and water; postapplication pain should be treated with local cooling methods (ice pack) and/or analgesics. Clean all areas that had contact with capsaicin. Decreased sensory function, including to thermal and other harmful stimuli, has been reported; effects are usually minor and temporary. Patients with preexisting sensory deficits should be assessed for sensory deterioration or loss prior to each patch application. Continued use should be reevaluated for new onset or worsening of existing sensory deficits.

For external use only; avoid contact with eyes, mouth, genitals, or any or other mucous membranes. Do not use immediately before or after activities such as bathing, swimming, showering, sunbathing, strenuous exercise, steam bath, sauna, or other heat or sunlight exposure to the treated area. Stop use and consult a health care provider if excessive redness, blistering, burning, or irritation develops, symptoms get worse, symptoms persist for >7 days, symptoms resolve and then recur, or if difficulty breathing or swallowing occurs. Do not handle contact lenses for 1 hour after handling, applying, or removing capsaicin (product specific).

RX labeling: Do not cover with bandage or compression. Use only on intact skin; do not use on wounds, damaged, broken, infected, sensitive, or inflamed skin. Do not apply to face or scalp. Do not use concurrently with other external pain-relieving products.

OTC labeling: Transient burning may occur and generally disappears after several days.

Patch (8%): Avoid inhaling airborne material from dried residue. Remove patches gently and slowly to decrease risk of aerosolization; inhalation of airborne capsaicin may result in coughing or sneezing.

Benzyl alcohol and derivatives: Some dosage forms may contain benzyl alcohol; large amounts of benzyl alcohol (≥99 mg/kg/day) have been associated with a potentially fatal toxicity ("gasping syndrome") in neonates; the "gasping syndrome" consists of metabolic acidosis, respiratory distress, gasping respirations, CNS dysfunction (including convulsions, intracranial hemorrhage), hypotension, and cardiovascular collapse (AAP ["Inactive" 1997]; CDC 1982); some data suggest that benzoate displaces bilirubin from protein binding sites (Ahlfors 2001); avoid or use dosage forms containing benzyl alcohol with caution in neonates. See manufacturer's labeling.

Drug Interactions

Metabolism/Transport Effects Substrate of CYP2E1 (minor); **Note:** Assignment of Major/Minor substrate status based on clinically relevant drug interaction potential

Avoid Concomitant Use There are no known interactions where it is recommended to avoid concomitant use.

Increased Effect/Toxicity There are no known significant interactions involving an increase in effect.

Decreased Effect There are no known significant interactions involving a decrease in effect.

Pharmacodynamics/Kinetics

Onset of Action OTC products (capsaicin 0.025% to 0.1%): 2 to 4 weeks of continuous therapy; Qutenza patch: 1 week after application

Half-life Elimination Topical patch (capsaicin 8%): 1.64 hours (Babbar 2009)

Pregnancy Considerations Systemic absorption is limited following topical administration of the patch, and fetal exposure is not expected following maternal use; plasma concentrations are below the limit of detection 3 to 6 hours after the patch is removed.

Breastfeeding Considerations

Systemic absorption is limited following topical administration of the 8% patch, and exposure via breast milk is not expected following maternal use.

According to the manufacturer, the decision to breastfeed during therapy should consider the risk of infant exposure, the benefits of breastfeeding to the infant, and the benefits of treatment to the mother. To minimize potential exposure to a breastfed infant, avoid application to the nipple and surrounding area.

Dosage Forms: US

Cream, topical:

Capzasin-HP [OTC]: 0.1% (42.5 g)
Capzasin-P [OTC]: 0.035% (42.5 g)
Capzix [OTC]: 0.1% (56.6 g)
Sure Result SR Relief [OTC]: 0.025% (118 mL)
Trixaicin HP [OTC]: 0.075% (60 g)
Zostrix HP [OTC]: 0.1% (60 g)
Zostrix Natural Pain Relief [OTC]: 0.033% (56.6 g)
Generic: 0.025% (25 g, 50 g, 60 g, 120 g); 0.1% (42.5 g)

Gel, topical:

Capzasin-P [OTC]: 0.025% (42.5 g) [contains menthol]

Liquid, topical:

Capzasin-P [OTC]: 0.15% (29.5 mL)

Lotion, topical:

DiabetAid Pain and Tingling Relief [OTC]: 0.025% (120 mL)

Patch, topical:

Allevess [OTC]: 0.05% (15s) [contains menthol 5%]
Flexin: 0.0375% (15s) [contains menthol 5%]
Levatio: 0.03% (15s) [contains menthol 5%]
MenCaps [OTC]: 0.0225% (15s) [contains menthol 4.5%]
Qutenza: 8% (1s, 2s)
Renovo: 0.0375% (15s) [contains menthol 5%]
Salonpas Gel-Patch Hot [OTC]: 0.025% (3s, 6s)

◆ **Capsaicin/Menthol** *see* Capsaicin *on page 284*

Captopril (KAP toe pril)

Related Information

Cardiovascular Diseases *on page 1654*

Brand Names: Canada APO-Capto; BCI Captopril [DSC]; CO Captopril; DOM-Captopril [DSC]; MYLAN-Captopril [DSC]; PMS-Captopril; TEVA-Captopril; TRIA-Captopril [DSC]

Pharmacologic Category Angiotensin-Converting Enzyme (ACE) Inhibitor; Antihypertensive

Use

Diabetic nephropathy: Treatment of diabetic nephropathy (proteinuria >500 mg/day) in patients with type 1 insulin-dependent diabetes mellitus and retinopathy.

Heart failure with reduced ejection fraction: Treatment of heart failure.

Hypertension: Management of hypertension.

Myocardial infarction with left ventricular dysfunction: To improve survival following myocardial infarction (MI) (eg, ST-elevation MI or non-ST-elevation MI) in clinically stable patients with left ventricular dysfunction manifested as an ejection fraction of ≤40%, and to reduce the incidence of overt heart failure and subsequent hospitalizations for heart failure in these patients.

Local Anesthetic/Vasoconstrictor Precautions No information available to require special precautions

Effects on Dental Treatment Key adverse event(s) related to dental treatment: Loss or diminished perception of taste; Patients may experience orthostatic hypotension as they stand up after treatment; especially if lying in dental chair for extended periods of time. Use caution with sudden changes in position during and after dental treatment.

An angiotensin-converting enzyme (ACE) Inhibitor cough is a dry, hacking, nonproductive cough that can potentially interfere with longer dental procedures if patient has this side effect.

Effects on Bleeding No information available to require special precautions

Adverse Reactions

Frequency not defined:

Cardiovascular: Angina pectoris, cardiac arrest, cardiac arrhythmia, cardiac failure, flushing, myocardial infarction, orthostatic hypotension, Raynaud's phenomenon, syncope

Central nervous system: Ataxia, cerebrovascular insufficiency, confusion, depression, drowsiness, myasthenia, nervousness

Dermatologic: Bullous pemphigoid, erythema multiforme, exfoliative dermatitis, pallor, Stevens-Johnson syndrome

Endocrine & metabolic: Gynecomastia, hyponatremia (symptomatic)

Gastrointestinal: Cholestasis, dyspepsia, glossitis, pancreatitis

Genitourinary: Impotence, nephrotic syndrome, oliguria, urinary frequency

Hematologic & oncologic: Agranulocytosis, anemia, pancytopenia, thrombocytopenia

Hepatic: Hepatic necrosis (rare), hepatitis, increased serum alkaline phosphatase, increased serum bilirubin, increased serum transaminases, jaundice

Hypersensitivity: Anaphylactoid reaction, angioedema

Neuromuscular & skeletal: Myalgia, weakness

Ophthalmic: Blurred vision

Renal: Polyuria, renal failure, renal insufficiency

Respiratory: Bronchospasm, eosinophilic pneumonitis, rhinitis

1% to 10%:

Cardiovascular: Hypotension (1% to 3%), chest pain (1%), palpitations (1%), tachycardia (1%)

Dermatologic: Skin rash (maculopapular or urticarial [4% to 7%]; in patients with rash, a positive ANA and/or eosinophilia has been noted in 7% to 10%), pruritus (2%)

Endocrine & metabolic: Hyperkalemia (1% to 11%)

Gastrointestinal: Dysgeusia (2% to 4%; loss of taste or diminished perception)

Genitourinary: Proteinuria (1%)

Hematologic & oncologic: Neutropenia (≤4%; in patients with renal insufficiency or collagen-vascular disease)

Hypersensitivity: Hypersensitivity reaction (rash, pruritus, fever, arthralgia, and eosinophilia: 4% to 7%; depending on dose and renal function)

Renal: Increased serum creatinine, renal insufficiency (worsening; may occur in patients with bilateral renal artery stenosis or hypovolemia)

Respiratory: Cough (<1% to 2%)

Miscellaneous: Hypersensitivity reactions (rash, pruritus, fever, arthralgia, and eosinophilia) have occurred in 4% to 7% of patients (depending on dose and renal function); dysgeusia - loss of taste or diminished perception (2% to 4%)

<1%, postmarketing, and/or case reports: Abdominal pain, alopecia, angina pectoris, anorexia, aphthous stomatitis, aplastic anemia, arthralgia, cholestatic jaundice, constipation, diarrhea, dizziness, dyspnea, eosinophilia, fatigue, fever, gastric irritation, glomerulonephritis, Guillain-Barre syndrome, headache, hemolytic anemia, Huntington's chorea (exacerbation), hyperthermia, increased erythrocyte sedimentation rate, insomnia, interstitial nephritis, Kaposi's sarcoma, malaise, myalgia, nausea, paresthesia, peptic ulcer, pericarditis, psoriasis, seizure (in premature infants), systemic lupus erythematosus, vasculitis, visual hallucination (Doane, 2013), vomiting, xerostomia

Mechanism of Action Competitive inhibitor of angiotensin-converting enzyme (ACE); prevents conversion of angiotensin I to angiotensin II, a potent vasoconstrictor; results in lower levels of angiotensin II which causes an increase in plasma renin activity and a reduction in aldosterone secretion.

Pharmacodynamics/Kinetics

Onset of Action Within 15 minutes; Peak effect: Blood pressure reduction: 1 to 1.5 hours after dose; Maximum effect: Antihypertensive: 60 to 90 minutes; may require several weeks of therapy before full hypotensive effect is seen

Duration of Action Dose related, may require several weeks of therapy before full hypotensive effect

Half-life Elimination

Infants with CHF: 3.3 hours; range: 1.2 to 12.4 hours (Pereira 1991)

Children: 1.5 hours; range: 0.98 to 2.3 hours (Levy 1991)

Adults: Healthy volunteers: ~1.7 hours (Duchin 1982). In 2 studies, patients with chronic renal failure demonstrated ~2-fold longer half-lives as compared to normal subjects (Giudicelli 1984; Onoyama 1981). Half-life was up to 21 hours in patients with severe renal impairment and up to 32 hours in patients on chronic hemodialysis in another study (Duchin 1984)

Time to Peak Within 1 to 2 hours

Reproductive Considerations

Angiotensin-converting enzyme (ACE) inhibitors should be avoided in sexually active females of reproductive potential not using effective contraception (ADA 2020).

ACE inhibitors should generally be avoided for the treatment of hypertension in women planning a pregnancy; use should only be considered for cases of hypertension refractory to other medications (ACOG 203 2019).

When treatment is needed in females of reproductive potential with diabetic nephropathy, the ACE inhibitor should be discontinued at the first positive pregnancy test (Cabiddu 2016; Spotti 2018).

Pregnancy Risk Factor D

Pregnancy Considerations

Captopril crosses the placenta (Hurault de Ligny 1987).

Exposure to an angiotensin-converting enzyme (ACE) inhibitor during the first trimester of pregnancy may be associated with an increased risk of fetal malformations (ACOG 203 2019; ESC [Regitz-Zagrosek 2018]); however, outcomes observed may also be influenced by maternal disease (ACC/AHA [Whelton 2018]).

[US Boxed Warning]: Drugs that act on the renin-angiotensin system can cause injury and death to the developing fetus. Discontinue as soon as possible once pregnancy is detected. Drugs that act on the renin-angiotensin system are associated with oligohydramnios. Oligohydramnios, due to decreased fetal renal function, may lead to fetal lung hypoplasia and skeletal malformations. Their use in pregnancy is also associated with anuria, hypotension, renal failure, skull hypoplasia, and death in the fetus/neonate. Infants exposed to an ACE inhibitor in utero should be monitored for hyperkalemia, hypotension, and oliguria. Oligohydramnios may not appear until after irreversible fetal injury has occurred. Exchange transfusions or dialysis may be required to reverse hypotension or improve renal function, although data related to the effectiveness in neonates is limited.

Chronic maternal hypertension is also associated with adverse events in the fetus/infant. Chronic maternal hypertension may increase the risk of birth defects, low birth weight, premature delivery, stillbirth, and neonatal death. Actual fetal/neonatal risks may be related to duration and severity of maternal hypertension. Untreated chronic hypertension may also increase the risks of adverse maternal outcomes, including gestational diabetes, preeclampsia, delivery complications, stroke and myocardial infarction (ACOG 203 2019).

When treatment of hypertension in pregnancy is indicated, ACE inhibitors should generally be avoided due to their adverse fetal events; use in pregnant women should only be considered for cases of hypertension refractory to other medications (ACOG 203 2019). ACE inhibitors are not recommended for the treatment of heart failure in pregnancy (Regitz-Zagrosek [ESC 2018]).

When treatment is needed in females of reproductive potential with diabetic nephropathy, the ACE inhibitor should be discontinued at the first positive pregnancy test (Cabiddu 2016; Spotti 2018).

◆ **Captracin [DSC]** *see* Capsaicin *on page 284*
◆ **Capzasin-HP [OTC]** *see* Capsaicin *on page 284*
◆ **Capzasin-P [OTC]** *see* Capsaicin *on page 284*
◆ **Capzix [OTC]** *see* Capsaicin *on page 284*
◆ **Carafate** *see* Sucralfate *on page 1389*

CarBAMazepine (kar ba MAZ e peen)

Related Information

Temporomandibular Dysfunction (TMD), Chronic Pain, and Fibromyalgia *on page 1773*

Brand Names: US Carbatrol; Epitol; Equetro; TEGretol; TEGretol-XR

Brand Names: Canada APO-CarBAMazepine; DOM-CarBAMazepine; DOM-CarBAMazepine CR; Mazepine; MYLAN-CarBAMazepine [DSC]; PMS-CarBAMazepine; PMS-CarBAMazepine CR; PMS-CarBAMazepine-CR; SANDOZ CarBAMazepine CR; SANDOZ CarBAMazepine [DSC]; TARO-CarBAMazepine; TEGretol; TEGretol CR; TEVA-Carbamazepine

Pharmacologic Category Anticonvulsant, Miscellaneous

Use

Bipolar disorder: Monotherapy in the acute treatment of hypomania and mild to moderate manic or mixed episodes associated with bipolar disorder

Focal (partial) onset seizures and generalized onset seizures: Monotherapy and adjunctive therapy in the treatment of patients with focal onset seizures and generalized onset seizures

Limitations of use: Carbamazepine is not indicated for the treatment of nonmotor (absence) seizures; it has been associated with increased frequency of generalized convulsions in these patients.

Neuropathic pain: Treatment of trigeminal or glossopharyngeal neuralgia

Local Anesthetic/Vasoconstrictor Precautions No information available to require special precautions

Effects on Dental Treatment Key adverse event(s) related to dental treatment: Xerostomia (normal salivary flow resumes upon discontinuation). Rare occurrence of taste alteration, lip edema, laryngeal edema; glossitis and stomatitis has been reported but frequency not defined. Both hypertension and hypotension has been reported. Blood pressure monitoring is essential prior to dental treatment. Hypotension could predispose the patient to orthostatic hypotension.

Effects on Bleeding A spectrum of hematologic effects has been reported including agranulocytosis, aplastic anemia, neutropenia and thrombocytopenia; detection of hematologic change to include symptoms of fever, sore throat, mouth ulcers and easy bruising would necessitate a medical consult prior to dental treatment.

Adverse Reactions

>10%:

Central nervous system: Dizziness (44%), drowsiness (32%), ataxia (15%)

Gastrointestinal: Nausea (29%), vomiting (18%)

1% to 10%:

Cardiovascular: Hypertension (3%)

Central nervous system: Speech disturbance (6%), abnormality in thinking (2%), paresthesia (2%), twitching (2%), vertigo (2%)

Dermatologic: Pruritus (8%), skin rash (7%)

Gastrointestinal: Constipation (10%), xerostomia (8%)

Neuromuscular & skeletal: Weakness (8%), tremor (3%)

Ophthalmic: Blurred vision (5% to 6%)

Frequency not defined:

Cardiovascular: Arterial insufficiency (cerebral artery), atrioventricular block, cardiac arrhythmia, cardiac failure, collapse, coronary artery disease (aggravation), edema, exacerbation of hypertension, hypotension, pulmonary embolism, syncope, thromboembolism, thrombophlebitis

Central nervous system: Agitation, chills, confusion, depression, fatigue, headache, hyperacusis, involuntary body movements, neuroleptic malignant syndrome, peripheral neuritis, talkativeness, unsteadiness, visual hallucination

Dermatologic: Acute generalized exanthematous pustulosis, alopecia, diaphoresis, dyschromia, erythema multiforme, erythema nodosum, erythematous rash, exfoliative dermatitis, maculopapular rash, onychomadesis, pruritic rash, skin photosensitivity, Stevens-Johnson syndrome, toxic epidermal necrolysis, urticaria

Endocrine & metabolic: Acute porphyria, albuminuria, decreased serum calcium, glycosuria, hirsutism, hyponatremia, porphyria cutanea tarda, porphyria (variegate), SIADH

Gastrointestinal: Abdominal pain, anorexia, diarrhea, gastric distress, glossitis, pancreatitis, stomatitis

Genitourinary: Acute urinary retention, azotemia, defective spermatogenesis, impotence, microscopic urine deposits, oliguria, reduced fertility (male), urinary frequency

Hematologic & oncologic: Adenopathy, agranulocytosis, aplastic anemia, bone marrow depression, eosinophilia, hypogammaglobulinemia, leukocytosis, leukopenia, lymphadenopathy, pancytopenia, purpura, thrombocytopenia

Hepatic: Abnormal hepatic function tests, cholestatic jaundice, hepatic failure, hepatitis, hepatocellular jaundice, increased liver enzymes

Hypersensitivity: Hypersensitivity reaction

Immunologic: DRESS syndrome

Neuromuscular & skeletal: Arthralgia, exacerbation of systemic lupus erythematosus, leg cramps, lupus-like syndrome, myalgia, osteoporosis

Ophthalmic: Conjunctivitis, diplopia, increased intraocular pressure, punctate cataract, nystagmus, oculomotor disturbance

Otic: Tinnitus

Renal: Increased blood urea nitrogen, renal failure

Respiratory: Dry throat, pulmonary hypersensitivity

Miscellaneous: Fever

<1%, postmarketing, and/or case reports: Anaphylaxis, angioedema, aseptic meningitis, decreased thyroid hormones, dysgeusia (Syed 2016), eyelid edema, glottis edema, hepatotoxicity (idiosyncratic: Chalasani 2014), intrahepatic cholestasis (vanishing bile duct syndrome), laryngeal edema, lip edema, suicidal tendencies

Mechanism of Action In addition to anticonvulsant effects, carbamazepine has anticholinergic, antineuralgic, antidiuretic, muscle relaxant, antimanic, antidepressive, and antiarrhythmic properties; may depress activity in the nucleus ventralis of the thalamus or decrease synaptic transmission or decrease summation of temporal stimulation leading to neural discharge by limiting influx of sodium ions across cell membrane or other unknown mechanisms; stimulates the release of ADH and potentiates its action in promoting reabsorption of water; chemically related to tricyclic antidepressants

Pharmacodynamics/Kinetics

Half-life Elimination Half-life is variable because of autoinduction which is usually complete 3 to 5 weeks after initiation of a fixed carbamazepine regimen.

Carbamazepine: Initial: 25 to 65 hours; Extended release: 35 to 40 hours; Multiple doses: Children and Adolescents: Mean range: 3.1 to 20.8 hours (Battino 1995); Adults: 12 to 17 hours

Epoxide metabolite: Initial: 34 ± 9 hours

Time to Peak Unpredictable:

Immediate release: Suspension: Multiple doses: 1.5 hour; tablet: 4 to 5 hours

Extended release: Carbatrol, Equetro: 12 to 26 hours (single dose), 4 to 8 hours (multiple doses); Tegretol®-XR: 3 to 12 hours

Reproductive Considerations

Carbamazepine may decrease plasma concentrations of hormonal contraceptives; alternate or back-up methods of contraception should be considered. Carbamazepine may interfere with some pregnancy tests.

Pregnancy Considerations

Carbamazepine and its active metabolite cross the placenta; concentrations are variable but correlate with maternal serum concentrations (Kacirova 2016).

Carbamazepine may be associated with teratogenic effects, including spina bifida, craniofacial defects, and cardiovascular malformations. Data from the International Registry of Antiepileptic Drugs and Pregnancy (EURAP) and the UK and Ireland Epilepsy Pregnancy Registers (UKEPR) note the risk of congenital malformations increases with higher doses (Campbell 2014; Tomson 2011). The risk of teratogenic effects is higher with anticonvulsant polytherapy than monotherapy. Developmental delays have also been observed following in utero exposure to carbamazepine (per manufacturer).

Due to pregnancy-induced physiologic changes, some pharmacokinetic properties of carbamazepine may be altered; however, available studies have slightly conflicting results (Deligiannidis 2014; Tomson 2013). Therapeutic drug monitoring of carbamazepine is recommended in pregnant women (Harden 2009; Hiemke 2018).

Carbamazepine is not recommended for the treatment of bipolar disorder in pregnancy (Larsen 2015).

Patients exposed to carbamazepine during pregnancy are encouraged to enroll themselves into the North American Antiepileptic Drug (NAAED) Pregnancy Registry by calling 1-888-233-2334. Additional information is available at www.aedpregnancyregistry.org.

Carbamide Peroxide (KAR ba mide per OKS ide)

Brand Names: US Auraphene-B [OTC]; Clearcanal Earwax Softener [OTC]; E-R-O Ear Drops [OTC] [DSC]; E-R-O Ear Wax Removal System [OTC] [DSC]; Ear Drops Earwax Aid [OTC]; Ear Drops [OTC]; Earwax Treatment Drops [OTC] [DSC]; Gly-Oxide [OTC]; GoodSense Ear Wax Kit [OTC]; GoodSense Ear Wax Removal [OTC]

Pharmacologic Category Anti-inflammatory, Locally Applied; Otic Agent, Cerumenolytic

Use

Oral: Temporary use in cleansing of canker sore and minor wounds or gum inflammation due to minor dental procedures, dentures, orthodontic appliances, accidental injury, or other irritations of mouth and gums; aids in removal of phlegm, mucus, or other secretions associated with occasional sore mouth.

Otic: Aid to soften, loosen, and remove excessive earwax.

Local Anesthetic/Vasoconstrictor Precautions No information available to require special precautions

Effects on Dental Treatment No significant effects or complications reported (see Dental Health Professional Considerations)

Effects on Bleeding No information available to require special precautions

Adverse Reactions Frequency not defined.

Dermatologic: Localized erythema, skin rash

Infection: Superinfection

Local: Local irritation, redness

Mechanism of Action Carbamide peroxide releases hydrogen peroxide which serves as a source of nascent oxygen upon contact with catalase; deodorant action is probably due to inhibition of odor-causing bacteria; softens impacted cerumen due to its foaming action

Pharmacodynamics/Kinetics

Onset of Action ~24 hours

Dental Health Professional Considerations When used as tooth whitening product, most common side effect is tooth sensitivity.

◆ **Carbatrol** *see* CarBAMazepine *on page 288*

Carbidopa (kar bi DOE pa)

Brand Names: US Lodosyn

Pharmacologic Category Anti-Parkinson Agent, Decarboxylase Inhibitor

Use

Parkinsonism: Given with carbidopa/levodopa in the treatment of idiopathic Parkinson disease, postencephalitic parkinsonism, and symptomatic parkinsonism, which may follow injury to the nervous system by carbon monoxide and/or manganese intoxication.

Note: Administration of carbidopa allows use of a lower dosage of levodopa, more rapid titration, and a decrease in nausea and vomiting associated with levodopa; use with carbidopa/levodopa in patients requiring additional carbidopa; has no effect without levodopa.

Local Anesthetic/Vasoconstrictor Precautions No information available to require special precautions

Effects on Dental Treatment Key adverse event(s) related to dental treatment: Dopaminergic therapy in Parkinson's disease includes the use of carbidopa in combination with levodopa. Carbidopa/levodopa combination is associated with orthostatic hypotension. Patients may experience orthostatic hypotension as they stand up after treatment; especially if lying in dental chair for extended periods of time. Use caution with sudden changes in position during and after dental treatment.

Effects on Bleeding No information available to require special precautions

Adverse Reactions Adverse reactions are associated with concomitant administration with levodopa.

Cardiovascular: Cardiac arrhythmia, chest pain, edema, flushing, hypertension, hypotension, myocardial infarction, orthostatic hypotension, palpitation, phlebitis, syncope

Central nervous system: Abnormal dreams, abnormal gait, agitation, anxiety, ataxia, confusion, decreased mental acuity, delusions, dementia, depression (with or without suicidal tendencies), disorientation, dizziness, drowsiness, euphoria, extrapyramidal reaction, falling, fatigue, glossopyrosis, hallucination, headache, Horner's syndrome, impulse control disorder, insomnia, malaise, memory impairment, nervousness, neuroleptic malignant syndrome, nightmares, numbness, on-off phenomenon, paranoia, paresthesia, pathological gambling, peripheral neuropathy, psychosis, seizure (causal relationship not established), trismus

Dermatologic: Alopecia, bulla, diaphoresis, discoloration of sweat, skin rash

Endocrine & metabolic: Abnormal lactate dehydrogenase, glycosuria, hot flash, hyperglycemia, hypokalemia, increased libido (including hypersexuality), increased uric acid, weight changes

Gastrointestinal: Abdominal distress, abdominal pain, anorexia, bruxism, constipation, diarrhea, discoloration of saliva, duodenal ulcer, dysgeusia, dyspepsia, dysphagia, flatulence, gastrointestinal hemorrhage, heartburn, hiccups, nausea, sialorrhea, sore throat, vomiting, xerostomia

Genitourinary: Priapism, proteinuria, urinary frequency, urinary incontinence, urinary retention, urinary tract infection, urine discoloration

Hematologic & oncologic: Abnormal Coombs' test, agranulocytosis, anemia, decreased hematocrit, decreased hemoglobin, hemolytic anemia, leukopenia, malignant melanoma, thrombocytopenia

Hepatic: Abnormal alanine aminotransferase, abnormal alkaline phosphatase, abnormal aspartate transaminase, abnormal bilirubin levels, abnormal lactate dehydrogenase

Hypersensitivity: Angioedema, hypersensitivity reaction (bulla, IgA vasculitis, pruritus, urticaria)

Neuromuscular & skeletal: Back pain, dyskinesia (including choreiform, dystonic, and other involuntary movements), leg pain, muscle cramps, muscle twitching, shoulder pain, tremor, weakness

Ophthalmic: Blepharospasm, blurred vision, diplopia, mydriasis, oculogyric crisis (may be associated with acute dystonic reactions)

Renal: Increased blood urea nitrogen, increased serum creatinine

Respiratory: Cough, dyspnea, hoarseness, upper respiratory tract infection

Mechanism of Action Carbidopa is a peripheral decarboxylase inhibitor with little or no pharmacological activity when given alone in usual doses. It inhibits the peripheral decarboxylation of levodopa to dopamine; and as it does not cross the blood-brain barrier, unlike levodopa, effective brain concentrations of dopamine are produced with lower doses of levodopa. At the same time, reduced peripheral formation of dopamine reduces peripheral side-effects, notably nausea and vomiting, and cardiac arrhythmias, although the dyskinesias and adverse mental effects associated with levodopa therapy tend to develop earlier.

Pregnancy Considerations

Carbidopa can be detected in the umbilical cord but absorption in fetal tissue is minimal (Merchant 1995). The incidence of Parkinson disease in pregnancy is relatively rare and information related to the use of carbidopa in pregnant women is limited to use with other agents. Refer to the carbidopa and levodopa monograph for additional information.

Carbidopa and Levodopa

(kar bi DOE pa & lee voe DOE pa)

Related Information

Carbidopa *on page 289*

Brand Names: US Duopa; Rytary; Sinemet; Sinemet CR [DSC]

Brand Names: Canada AA-Levocarb CR; APO-Levocarb; APO-Levocarb 100/25; APO-Levocarb 250/25; DOM-Levo-Carbidopa; Duodopa; MINT-Levocarb; PMS-Levocarb CR; Pro-Lecarb; PRO-Levocarb-100/25; Sinemet 100/10 [DSC]; Sinemet 100/25; Sinemet 250/25; Sinemet CR 200/50 [DSC]; Sinemet CR [DSC]; TEVA-Levocarbidopa

Pharmacologic Category Anti-Parkinson Agent, Decarboxylase Inhibitor; Anti-Parkinson Agent, Dopamine Precursor

Use Parkinson disease: Treatment of Parkinson disease, postencephalitic parkinsonism, and symptomatic parkinsonism that may follow carbon monoxide and/or manganese intoxication; treatment of motor fluctuations in advanced Parkinson disease (intestinal suspension [Duopa] only).

Local Anesthetic/Vasoconstrictor Precautions No information available to require special precautions

Effects on Dental Treatment Key adverse event(s) related to dental treatment: Xerostomia (normal salivary flow resumes upon discontinuation) and taste alterations; Dopaminergic therapy in Parkinson's disease (ie, treatment with levodopa and carbidopa combination) is associated with orthostatic hypotension. Patients may experience orthostatic hypotension as they stand up after treatment; especially if lying in dental chair for extended periods of time. Use caution with sudden changes in position during and after dental treatment.

Effects on Bleeding No information available to require special precautions

Adverse Reactions

>10%:

Cardiovascular: Orthostatic hypotension (enteral suspension: 70% to 73%; oral: 1% to 5%)

Central nervous system: Dizziness (2% to 19%), headache (oral: 1% to 17%), depression (enteral suspension: 11%; oral: 1% to 2%)
Gastrointestinal: Nausea (enteral suspension: 30%; oral: 3% to 20%), constipation (enteral suspension: 22%; oral: ≤6%)
Neuromuscular & skeletal: Dyskinesia (2% to 17%), increased creatine phosphokinase (enteral suspension: ≤17%)
Renal: Increased blood urea nitrogen (enteral suspension: ≤13%)

1% to 10%:
Cardiovascular: Hypertension (enteral suspension: 8%), peripheral edema (enteral suspension: 8%), ischemia (oral: ≤2%), chest pain (oral: ≤1%)
Central nervous system: Insomnia (oral: 1% to 9%), anxiety (2% to 8%), confusion (2% to 8%), abnormal dreams (oral: ≤6%), polyneuropathy (enteral suspension: 5%), sleep disorder (enteral suspension: 5%), hallucination (≤5%), psychosis (≤5%), dystonia (oral: ≤2%), on-off phenomenon (oral: 1% to 2%), paresthesia (oral: ≤1%)
Dermatologic: Skin rash (enteral suspension: 5%)
Endocrine & metabolic: Increased serum glucose (≥1%)
Gastrointestinal: Xerostomia (oral: 1% to 7%), diarrhea (≤5%), dyspepsia (≤5%), vomiting (oral: 2% to 5%), anorexia (oral: 1%)
Genitourinary: Bacteriuria (enteral suspension: 5%; oral: ≥1%), urinary tract infection (oral: 2%), hematuria (oral: ≥1%), urinary frequency (oral: ≤1%)
Hematologic & oncologic: Leukocyturia (enteral suspension: 5%; oral: ≥1%), decreased hematocrit (oral: ≥1%), decreased hemoglobin (oral: ≥1%)
Neuromuscular & skeletal: Back pain (oral: ≤2%), muscle cramps (oral: ≤1%), shoulder pain (oral: ≤1%)
Respiratory: Atelectasis (enteral suspension: 8%), oropharyngeal pain (enteral suspension: 8%), upper respiratory tract infection (enteral suspension: 8%; oral: 1% to 2%), dyspnea (oral: ≤2%)
Miscellaneous: Fever (enteral suspension: 5%)

<1%, postmarketing, and/or case reports: Abdominal distress, abdominal pain, abnormal behavior, abnormal gait, abnormality in thinking, agitation, agranulocytosis, alopecia, anemia, angioedema, asthenia, ataxia, blepharospasm, blurred vision, bruxism, bullous rash (including pemphigus-like reactions), cardiac arrhythmia, common cold, cough, decreased mental acuity, decreased serum potassium, delirium, delusions, dementia, diaphoresis, diplopia, discoloration of saliva, discoloration of sweat, disorientation, drowsiness, duodenal ulcer, dysgeusia, dysphagia, edema, euphoria, extrapyramidal reaction, falling, fatigue, flatulence, flushing, gastrointestinal hemorrhage, glossopyrosis, glycosuria, heartburn, hemolytic anemia, Henoch-Schonlein purpura, hiccups, hoarseness, Horner syndrome (reactivation), hot flash, hypotension, impulse control disorder, increased lactate dehydrogenase, increased libido (including hypersexuality), increased serum alanine aminotransferase, increased serum alkaline phosphatase, increased serum aspartate transaminase, increased serum bilirubin, increased tremors, increased uric acid, leukopenia, lower extremity pain, malaise, malignant melanoma, memory impairment, muscle twitching, mydriasis, myocardial infarction, narcolepsy, nervousness, neuroleptic malignant syndrome, nightmares, numbness, oculogyric crisis, palpitations, paranoia, pathological gambling, peripheral neuropathy, phlebitis, positive direct Coombs test, priapism, proteinuria, pruritus, seizure, sense of stimulation, sialorrhea, suicidal ideation, suicidal tendencies, syncope, thrombocytopenia, trismus, urinary incontinence, urinary retention, urine discoloration, urticaria, weight gain, weight loss

Mechanism of Action Parkinson disease symptoms are due to a lack of striatal dopamine; levodopa circulates in the plasma to the blood-brain-barrier (BBB), where it crosses, to be converted by striatal enzymes to dopamine; carbidopa inhibits the peripheral plasma breakdown of levodopa by inhibiting its decarboxylation, and thereby increases available levodopa at the BBB

Pharmacodynamics/Kinetics

Half-life Elimination Levodopa (in presence of carbidopa): Immediate release: 1.5 hours; controlled release: 1.6 hours; extended release: 1.9 hours (Hsu 2015; manufacturer's labeling).

Time to Peak Levodopa component: Immediate release: 0.5 to 1 hour; controlled release: 1.5 to 2 hours; extended release: 1 to 4.5 hours (Hsu 2015; manufacturer's labeling). Intestinal gel [Canadian product]: 2.9 hours with therapeutic plasma levels reached 10 to 30 minutes following morning bolus dose; intestinal suspension: 2.5 hours.

Pregnancy Considerations

Carbidopa can be detected in the umbilical cord, but absorption in fetal tissue is minimal. Levodopa crosses the placenta and can be metabolized by the fetus and detected in fetal tissue (Merchant 1995).

The incidence of Parkinson disease in pregnancy is relatively rare, and although information related to the use of carbidopa/levodopa in pregnant women is limited (Ball 1995; Cook 1985; Golbe 1987; Serikawa 2011; Shulman 2000; Tüfekçioğlu 2018; Zlotnik 2014), this combination has the most outcome information available for the treatment of pregnant women (Seier 2017). Current guidelines note that the available information is insufficient to make a recommendation for the treatment of restless legs syndrome in pregnant women (Aurora 2012).

Prescribing and Access Restrictions Duodopa intestinal gel [Canadian product]: In Canada, the Duodopa Education Program is a risk mitigation program established to provide safe and effective use of Duodopa in advanced Parkinson patients. The program involves:

- Education of prescribing neurologists and other health care providers on suitable candidates for treatment, surgical procedures (PEG tube placement), and follow-up care including infusion device education.
- Distribution of educational materials to patients and caregivers describing Duodopa intestinal gel and its proper use, PEG tube placement, and complications associated with the mode of administration and/or PEG tube placement.

◆ **Carbidopa, Entacapone, and Levodopa** *see* Levodopa, Carbidopa, and Entacapone *on page 897*

◆ **Carbidopa/Levodopa** *see* Carbidopa and Levodopa *on page 290*

◆ **Carbidopa, Levodopa, and Entacapone** *see* Levodopa, Carbidopa, and Entacapone *on page 897*

◆ **Carbidopa/Levodopa/Entacapone** *see* Levodopa, Carbidopa, and Entacapone *on page 897*

Carbinoxamine (kar bi NOKS a meen)

Brand Names: US Arbinoxa [DSC]; Karbinal ER; RyVent

Pharmacologic Category Ethanolamine Derivative; Histamine H_1 Antagonist; Histamine H_1 Antagonist, First Generation

Use Allergies: For the symptomatic treatment of seasonal and perennial allergic rhinitis; vasomotor rhinitis; allergic conjunctivitis caused by inhalant allergens and foods; mild, uncomplicated allergic skin manifestations of urticaria and angioedema; dermatographism; as therapy for anaphylactic reactions adjunctive to epinephrine and other standard measures after the acute manifestations have been controlled; amelioration of the severity of allergic reactions to blood or plasma.

Local Anesthetic/Vasoconstrictor Precautions No information available to require special precautions

Effects on Dental Treatment Key adverse event(s) related to dental treatment: Xerostomia (normal salivary flow resumes upon discontinuation).

Effects on Bleeding No information available to require special precautions

Adverse Reactions Frequency not defined.

Cardiovascular: Chest tightness, extrasystoles, hypotension, palpitations, tachycardia

Central nervous system: Ataxia (most frequent), chills, confusion, dizziness (most frequent), drowsiness (most frequent), euphoria, excitability, fatigue, headache, hysteria, insomnia, irritability, nervousness, neuritis, paresthesia, restlessness, sedation (most frequent), seizure, vertigo

Dermatologic: Diaphoresis, skin photosensitivity, skin rash, urticaria

Endocrine & metabolic: Increased uric acid

Gastrointestinal: Anorexia, constipation, diarrhea, epigastric distress (most frequent), nausea, vomiting, xerostomia

Genitourinary: Difficulty in micturition, early menses, urinary frequency, urinary retention

Hematologic & oncologic: Agranulocytosis, hemolytic anemia, thrombocytopenia

Hypersensitivity: Anaphylactic shock, hypersensitivity reaction

Neuromuscular & skeletal: Tremor

Ophthalmic: Blurred vision, diplopia

Otic: Labyrinthitis, tinnitus

Respiratory: Dry nose, dry throat, nasal congestion, thickening of bronchial secretions (most frequent), wheezing

Mechanism of Action Carbinoxamine competes with histamine for H_1-receptor sites on effector cells in the gastrointestinal tract, blood vessels, and respiratory tract.

Pharmacodynamics/Kinetics

Duration of Action ~4 hours (immediate release)

Half-life Elimination 17 hours (extended release)

Time to Peak Serum: 1.5 to 5 hours

Pregnancy Risk Factor C

Pregnancy Considerations Animal reproduction studies have not been conducted. Maternal antihistamine use has generally not resulted in an increased risk of birth defects; however, information specific for the use of carbinoxamine during pregnancy has not been located. Although antihistamines are recommended for some indications in pregnant women, the use of other agents with specific pregnancy data may be preferred.

- ◆ **Carbinoxamine Maleate** *see* Carbinoxamine *on page 292*
- ◆ **Carbocaine** *see* Mepivacaine *on page 972*
- ◆ **Carbocaine 2% with Neo-Cobefrin** *see* Mepivacaine and Levonordefrin *on page 975*
- ◆ **Carbocaine Preservative-Free** *see* Mepivacaine *on page 972*

CARBOplatin (KAR boe pla tin)

Brand Names: US Paraplatin

Pharmacologic Category Antineoplastic Agent, Alkylating Agent; Antineoplastic Agent, Platinum Analog

Use Ovarian cancer, advanced: Initial treatment of advanced ovarian cancer in combination with other established chemotherapy agents; palliative treatment of recurrent ovarian cancer after prior chemotherapy, including cisplatin-based treatment

Local Anesthetic/Vasoconstrictor Precautions No information available to require special precautions

Effects on Dental Treatment Key adverse event(s) related to dental treatment: Stomatitis, mucositis, and taste dysgeusia.

Effects on Bleeding Hemorrhagic complication (ie, bleeding) has been reported in 5% of patients. Thrombocytopenia is one of the dose-limiting complications of carboplatin's myelosuppression. A medical consult is suggested.

Adverse Reactions Percentages reported with single-agent therapy.

>10%:

Central nervous system: Pain (23%)

Endocrine & metabolic: Hyponatremia (29% to 47%), hypomagnesemia (29% to 43%), hypocalcemia (22% to 31%), hypokalemia (20% to 28%)

Gastrointestinal: Vomiting (65% to 81%), abdominal pain (17%), nausea (without vomiting: 10% to 15%)

Hematologic & oncologic: Bone marrow depression (dose related and dose limiting; nadir at ~21 days with single-agent therapy), anemia (71% to 90%; grades 3/4: 21%), leukopenia (85%; grades 3/4: 15% to 26%), neutropenia (67%; grades 3/4: 16% to 21%), thrombocytopenia (62%; grades 3/4: 25% to 35%)

Hepatic: Increased serum alkaline phosphatase (24% to 37%), increased serum AST (15% to 19%)

Hypersensitivity: Hypersensitivity (2% to 16%)

Neuromuscular & skeletal: Weakness (11%)

Renal: Decreased creatinine clearance (27%), increased blood urea nitrogen (14% to 22%)

1% to 10%:

Central nervous system: Peripheral neuropathy (4% to 6%), neurotoxicity (5%)

Dermatologic: Alopecia (2% to 3%)

Gastrointestinal: Constipation (6%), diarrhea (6%), dysgeusia (1%), mucositis (≤1%), stomatitis (≤1%)

Hematologic & oncologic: Bleeding complications (5%), hemorrhage (5%)

Hepatic: Increased serum bilirubin (5%)

Infection: Infection (5%)

Ophthalmic: Visual disturbance (1%)

Otic: Ototoxicity (1%)

Renal: Increased serum creatinine (6% to 10%)

<1%, postmarketing, and/or case reports (Limited to important or life-threatening): Anaphylaxis, anorexia, bronchospasm, cardiac failure, cerebrovascular accident, dehydration, embolism, erythema, febrile neutropenia, hemolytic anemia (acute), hemolytic-uremic syndrome, hypertension, hypotension, injection site reaction (pain, redness, swelling), limb ischemia (acute), malaise, metastases, pruritus, skin rash, tissue necrosis (associated with extravasation), urticaria, vision loss

Mechanism of Action Carboplatin is a platinum compound alkylating agent which covalently binds to DNA; interferes with the function of DNA by producing interstrand DNA cross-links. Carboplatin is apparently not cell-cycle specific.

Pharmacodynamics/Kinetics

Half-life Elimination CrCl >60 mL/minute: Carboplatin: 2.6 to 5.9 hours (based on a dose of 300 to 500 mg/m^2); Platinum (from carboplatin): ≥5 days

Reproductive Considerations

Women of childbearing potential should avoid becoming pregnant during treatment

Pregnancy Considerations

Carboplatin may cause fetal harm if administered during pregnancy.

- ◆ **Cardene** *see* NiCARdipine *on page 1100*
- ◆ **Cardene IV** *see* NiCARdipine *on page 1100*
- ◆ **Cardizem** *see* DilTIAZem *on page 499*
- ◆ **Cardizem CD** *see* DilTIAZem *on page 499*
- ◆ **Cardizem LA** *see* DilTIAZem *on page 499*
- ◆ **Cardura** *see* Doxazosin *on page 517*
- ◆ **Cardura XL** *see* Doxazosin *on page 517*
- ◆ **Carimune NF** *see* Immune Globulin *on page 803*

Cariprazine (kar IP ra zeen)

Brand Names: US Vraylar

Pharmacologic Category Second Generation (Atypical) Antipsychotic

Use

Bipolar disorder: Acute treatment of manic or mixed episodes and major depression associated with bipolar I disorder

Schizophrenia: Treatment of schizophrenia

Local Anesthetic/Vasoconstrictor Precautions

No information available to require special precautions

Effects on Dental Treatment Key adverse event(s) related to dental treatment: Toothache and xerostomia has been reported

Effects on Bleeding No information available to require special precautions

Adverse Reactions

>10%:

Central nervous system: Drug-induced extrapyramidal reaction (15% to 41%), Parkinsonian-like syndrome (13% to 21%), akathisia (9% to 20%), headache (14%), insomnia (9% to 13%)

Gastrointestinal: Nausea (7% to 13%)

1% to 10%:

Cardiovascular: Hypertension (2% to 5%), tachycardia (2%)

Central nervous system: Drowsiness (7% to 8%), restlessness (4% to 7%), dizziness (3% to 7%), anxiety (5% to 6%), agitation (5%), dystonia (2% to 5%), fatigue (3% to 4%), suicidal ideation

Dermatologic: Hyperhidrosis

Endocrine & metabolic: Weight gain (2% to 8%), hyponatremia

Gastrointestinal: Vomiting (4% to 10%), constipation (6% to 7%), dyspepsia (5% to 7%), abdominal pain (6%), diarrhea (4%), toothache (4%), decreased appetite (3%), xerostomia (3%)

Genitourinary: Pollakiuria

Hepatic: Increased serum transaminases (≥3x ULN; 2% to 4%), increased liver enzymes (1%)

Neuromuscular & skeletal: Increased creatine phosphokinase (2% to 6%), limb pain (4%), back pain (3%), muscle rigidity (2% to 3%), arthralgia (2%)

Ophthalmic: Blurred vision (4%)

<1%, postmarketing, and/or case reports: Cerebrovascular accident, dysphagia, gastritis, gastroesophageal reflux disease, hepatitis, leukopenia, neutropenia, rhabdomyolysis, Stevens-Johnson syndrome

Mechanism of Action Cariprazine is a second generation antipsychotic which displays partial agonist activity at dopamine D_2 and serotonin 5-HT_{1A} receptors and antagonist activity at serotonin 5-HT_{2A} receptors. It exhibits high affinity for dopamine (D_2 and D_3) and serotonin (5-HT_{1A}) receptors and has low affinity for serotonin 5-HT_{2C} and alpha$_{1A}$-adrenergic receptors. Cariprazine functions as an antagonist for 5-HT_{2B} (high affinity) and 5-HT_{2A} receptors (moderate affinity), binds to histamine H_1 receptors, and has no affinity for muscarinic (cholinergic) receptors.

Pharmacodynamics/Kinetics

Half-life Elimination Cariprazine: 2 to 4 days; DCAR: 1 to 2 days; DDCAR: 1 to 3 weeks

Time to Peak Plasma: Cariprazine: 3 to 6 hours

Pregnancy Considerations Antipsychotic use during the third trimester of pregnancy has a risk for abnormal muscle movements (extrapyramidal symptoms [EPS]) and/or withdrawal symptoms in newborns following delivery. Symptoms in the newborn may include agitation, feeding disorder, hypertonia, hypotonia, respiratory distress, somnolence, and tremor; these effects may be self-limiting or require hospitalization.

The ACOG recommends that therapy during pregnancy be individualized; treatment with psychiatric medications during pregnancy should incorporate the clinical expertise of the mental health clinician, obstetrician, primary health care provider, and pediatrician. Safety data related to atypical antipsychotics during pregnancy are limited and routine use is not recommended. However, if a woman is inadvertently exposed to an atypical antipsychotic while pregnant, continuing therapy may be preferable to switching to a typical antipsychotic that the fetus has not yet been exposed to; consider risk: benefit (ACOG 2008).

Health care providers are encouraged to enroll women exposed to cariprazine during pregnancy in the National Pregnancy Registry for Atypical Antipsychotics (866-961-2388 or http://www.womensmentalhealth.org/clinical-and-research-programs/pregnancyregistry/).

- ◆ **Cariprazine Hydrochloride** *see* Cariprazine *on page 293*
- ◆ **Carisoprodate** *see* Carisoprodol *on page 293*

Carisoprodol (kar eye soe PROE dole)

Brand Names: US Soma; Vanadom

Pharmacologic Category Skeletal Muscle Relaxant

Use

Musculoskeletal conditions: Short-term (2 to 3 weeks) treatment of discomfort associated with acute painful musculoskeletal conditions.

Limitations of use: Carisoprodol should only be used for short periods (up to 2 or 3 weeks); adequate evidence of effectiveness for more prolonged use has not been established and acute, painful musculoskeletal conditions are generally of short duration.

Local Anesthetic/Vasoconstrictor Precautions No information available to require special precautions

Effects on Dental Treatment No significant effects or complications reported

Effects on Bleeding No information available to require special precautions

Adverse Reactions

>10%: Central nervous system: Drowsiness (13% to 17%)

1% to 10%: Central nervous system: Dizziness (7% to 8%), headache (3% to 5%)

Postmarketing and/or case reports: Abdominal cramps, agitation, allergic dermatitis, anaphylaxis, angioedema, ataxia, burning sensation of eyes, depression, drug dependence, dyspnea, epigastric pain, eosinophilia, erythema multiforme, exacerbation of asthma, fixed drug eruption, hallucination, headache, hiccups, hypersensitivity reaction, idiosyncratic reaction (symptoms may include agitation, ataxia, confusion, diplopia, disorientation, dysarthria, euphoria, extreme weakness, muscle twitching, mydriasis, temporary vision loss, and/or transient quadriplegia); insomnia, irritability, leukopenia, nausea, orthostatic hypotension, pancytopenia, paradoxical central nervous system stimulation, pruritus, psychosis, seizure, skin rash, syncope, tachycardia, transient flushing of face, tremor, urticaria, vertigo, vomiting, weakness, withdrawal syndrome (abdominal cramps, headache, insomnia, nausea, seizure)

Mechanism of Action Precise mechanism is not yet clear, but many effects have been ascribed to its central depressant actions. In animals, carisoprodol blocks interneuronal activity and depresses polysynaptic neuron transmission in the spinal cord and reticular formation of the brain. It is also metabolized to meprobamate, which has anxiolytic and sedative effects.

Pharmacodynamics/Kinetics

Onset of Action Rapid

Duration of Action 4 to 6 hours

Half-life Elimination Carisoprodol: ~2 hours; Meprobamate: ~10 hours

Time to Peak Plasma: 1.5 to 2 hours

Pregnancy Considerations Postmarketing data with meprobamate (the active metabolite) do not show a consistent association between maternal use and an increased risk or pattern of major congenital malformations. In one study, maternal use did not adversely affect mental or motor development, or IQ scores in children exposed in utero.

Controlled Substance C-IV

◆ **Carnitine** *see* LevOCARNitine *on page 896*

◆ **Carnitor** *see* LevOCARNitine *on page 896*

◆ **Carnitor SF** *see* LevOCARNitine *on page 896*

◆ **Caroguard [OTC]** *see* Beta-Carotene *on page 233*

◆ **CaroSpir** *see* Spironolactone *on page 1386*

◆ **Carrington Antifungal [OTC]** *see* Miconazole (Topical) *on page 1019*

◆ **Cartia XT** *see* DilTIAZem *on page 499*

Carvedilol (KAR ve dil ole)

Related Information

Cardiovascular Diseases *on page 1654*

Brand Names: US Coreg; Coreg CR

Brand Names: Canada APO-Carvedilol; Auro-Carvedilol; DOM-Carvedilol; JAMP-Carvedilol; MYLAN-Carvedilol [DSC]; NU-Carvedilol [DSC]; PMS-Carvedilol; RAN-Carvedilol; TEVA-Carvedilol

Pharmacologic Category Antihypertensive; Beta-Blocker With Alpha-Blocking Activity

Use

Heart failure with reduced ejection fraction, including left ventricular dysfunction following myocardial infarction: Treatment of mild to severe chronic heart failure of ischemic or cardiomyopathic origin or left ventricular dysfunction following myocardial infarction (clinically stable with left ventricular ejection fraction ≤40%).

Hypertension: Management of hypertension. **Note:** Beta-blockers are **not** recommended as first-line therapy (ACC/AHA [Whelton 2018]).

Local Anesthetic/Vasoconstrictor Precautions Carvedilol is a nonselective beta-blocker, but also has alpha-adrenergic blocking actions. No intrinsic sympathomimetic activity has been documented for carvedilol. Unlike other nonselective beta-blockers such as propranolol, with which epinephrine has interacted with to result in initial hypertensive episode followed by tachycardia, any interaction with carvedilol and vasoconstrictor to result in hypertensive episode would not be expected. There is no information available to require special precautions.

Effects on Dental Treatment Key adverse event(s) related to dental treatment: Frequent occurrence of orthostatic hypotension has been reported (use caution with sudden changes in position during and after dental treatment). Infrequent occurrence of periodontitis and xerostomia (normal salivary flow resumes upon discontinuation) have been reported. Rare occurrence of erythema multiforme and Stevens-Johnson syndrome have also been reported.

Note: Many nonsteroidal anti-inflammatory drugs, such as ibuprofen and indomethacin, can reduce the hypotensive effect of beta-blockers after 3 or more weeks of therapy with the NSAID. Short-term NSAID use (ie, 3 days) requires no special precautions in patients taking beta-blockers.

Effects on Bleeding No information available to require special precautions

Adverse Reactions

>10%:

Cardiovascular: Hypotension (≤20%), orthostatic hypotension (≤20%)

Central nervous system: Dizziness (2% to 32%), fatigue (24%)

Endocrine & metabolic: Weight gain (10% to 12%), hyperglycemia (5% to 12%)

Gastrointestinal: Diarrhea (1% to 12%)

Neuromuscular & skeletal: Asthenia (11%)

1% to 10%:

Cardiovascular: Bradycardia (≤10%), syncope (≤8%), peripheral edema (1% to 7%), angina pectoris (6%), edema (5% to 6%), atrioventricular block (>1% to ≤3%), cerebrovascular accident (>1% to ≤3%), exacerbation of angina pectoris (>1% to ≤3%), hypertension (>1% to ≤3%), lower extremity edema (>1% to ≤3%), palpitations (>1% to ≤3%), peripheral vascular disease (>1% to ≤3%), peripheral ischemia (≤1%), tachycardia (≤1%)

Central nervous system: Headache (5% to 8%), depression (>1% to ≤3%), drowsiness (>1% to ≤3%), hypoesthesia (>1% to ≤3%), hypotonia (>1% to ≤3%), malaise (>1% to ≤3%), vertigo (>1% to ≤3%), paresthesia (1% to ≤3%), insomnia (1% to 2%), abnormality in thinking (≤1%), emotional lability (≤1%), exacerbation of depression (≤1%), lack of concentration (≤1%), nervousness (≤1%), nightmares (≤1%), sleep disorder (≤1%)

Dermatologic: Diaphoresis (≤1%), erythematous rash (≤1%), maculopapular rash (≤1%), pruritus (≤1%), psoriasiform eruption (≤1%), skin photosensitivity (≤1%)

Endocrine & metabolic: Increased nonprotein nitrogen (6%), dependent edema (4%), hypercholesterolemia (4%), albuminuria (>1% to ≤3%), diabetes mellitus (>1% to ≤3%), glycosuria (>1% to ≤3%), gout (>1% to ≤3%), hyperkalemia (>1% to ≤3%), hyperuricemia (>1% to ≤3%), hypervolemia (>1% to ≤3%), hypoglycemia (>1% to ≤3%), hyponatremia (>1% to ≤3%), hypovolemia (>1% to ≤3%), impotence (>1% to ≤3%), increased gamma-glutamyl transferase (>1% to ≤3%), weight loss (>1% to ≤3%), decreased libido (≤1%), hypertriglyceridemia (≤1%), hypokalemia (≤1%)

Gastrointestinal: Nausea (2% to 9%), vomiting (6%), melena (>1% to ≤3%), periodontitis (>1% to ≤3%), gastrointestinal pain (1% to ≤3%), xerostomia (≤1%)

Genitourinary: Hematuria (>1% to ≤3%), urinary frequency (≤1%)

Hematologic & oncologic: Hypoprothrombinemia (>1% to ≤3%), nonthrombocytopenic purpura (>1% to ≤3%), thrombocytopenia (1% to ≤3%), leukopenia (≤1%)

Hepatic: Increased serum alanine aminotransferase (>1% to ≤3%), increased serum alkaline phosphatase (>1% to ≤3%), increased serum aspartate aminotransferase (>1% to ≤3%), hyperbilirubinemia (≤1%), increased liver enzymes (≤1%)

Hypersensitivity: Hypersensitivity reaction (>1% to ≤3%)

Neuromuscular & skeletal: Arthralgia (6%), arthritis (>1% to ≤3%), muscle cramps (>1% to ≤3%), hypokinesia (≤1%)

Ophthalmic: Visual disturbance (5%), blurred vision (>1% to ≤3%)

Otic: Tinnitus (≤1%)

Renal: Increased blood urea nitrogen (≤6%), increased serum creatinine (>1% to ≤3%), renal insufficiency (>1% to ≤3%)

Respiratory: Increased cough (5%), nasopharyngitis (4%), rales (4%), dyspnea (>3%), flu-like symptoms (>1% to ≤3%), nasal congestion (1%), paranasal sinus congestion (1%), asthma (≤1%)

Miscellaneous: Fever (>1% to ≤3%)

Frequency not defined:

Hematologic & oncologic: Anemia

Respiratory: Pulmonary edema

<1%, postmarketing, and/or case reports: Abnormal lymphocytes, alopecia, anaphylactoid shock, anaphylaxis, angioedema, aplastic anemia, amnesia, auditory impairment, bronchospasm, bundle branch block, cerebrovascular disease, complete atrioventricular block, decreased HDL cholesterol, erythema multiforme, exfoliative dermatitis, gastrointestinal hemorrhage, interstitial pneumonitis, ischemic heart disease, migraine, neuralgia, pancytopenia, paresis, respiratory alkalosis, seizure, Stevens-Johnson syndrome, toxic epidermal necrolysis, urinary incontinence

Mechanism of Action As a racemic mixture, carvedilol has nonselective beta-adrenoreceptor and alpha-adrenergic blocking activity. No intrinsic sympathomimetic activity has been documented. Associated effects in hypertensive patients include reduction of cardiac output, exercise- or beta-agonist-induced tachycardia, reduction of reflex orthostatic tachycardia, vasodilation, decreased peripheral vascular resistance (especially in standing position), decreased renal vascular resistance, reduced plasma renin activity, and increased levels of atrial natriuretic peptide. In CHF, associated effects include decreased pulmonary capillary wedge pressure, decreased pulmonary artery pressure, decreased heart rate, decreased systemic vascular resistance, increased stroke volume index, and decreased right atrial pressure (RAP).

Pharmacodynamics/Kinetics

Onset of Action Antihypertensive effect: Alpha-blockade: Within 30 minutes; Beta-blockade: Within 1 hour. Peak antihypertensive effect: ~1 to 2 hours

Half-life Elimination

Infants and Children 6 weeks to 3.5 years (n=8): 2.2 hours (Läer 2002)

Children and Adolescents 5.5 to 19 years (n=7): 3.6 hours (Läer 2002)

Adults 7 to 10 hours; some have reported lower values: Adults 24 to 37 years (n=9): 5.2 hours (Läer 2002)

R(+)-carvedilol: 5 to 9 hours

S(-)-carvedilol: 7 to 11 hours

Time to Peak Extended release: ~5 hours

Pregnancy Considerations

Exposure to beta-blockers during pregnancy may increase the risk for adverse events in the neonate. If maternal use of a beta-blocker is needed, fetal growth should be monitored during pregnancy and the newborn should be monitored for 48 hours after delivery for bradycardia, hypoglycemia, and respiratory depression (ESC [Regitz-Zagrosek 2018]).

Chronic maternal hypertension is also associated with adverse events in the fetus/infant. Chronic maternal hypertension may increase the risk of birth defects, low birth weight, premature delivery, stillbirth, and neonatal death. Actual fetal/neonatal risks may be related to duration and severity of maternal hypertension. Untreated chronic hypertension may also increase the risks of adverse maternal outcomes, including gestational diabetes, preeclampsia, delivery complications, stroke, and myocardial infarction (ACOG 203 2019).

When treatment of chronic hypertension in pregnancy is indicated, agents other than carvedilol are preferred (ACOG 203 2019; ESC [Regitz-Zagrosek 2018]; Magee 2014). Females with preexisting hypertension may continue their medication during pregnancy unless contraindications exist (ESC [Regitz-Zagrosek 2018]). Carvedilol may be considered for use in pregnant patients with heart failure (ESC [Regitz-Zagrosek 2018]).

◆ **CAS 1403254-99-8** *see* Tazemetostat *on page 1408*

Caspofungin (kas poe FUN jin)

Related Information

Fungal Infections *on page 1752*

Brand Names: US Cancidas

Brand Names: Canada Cancidas

Pharmacologic Category Antifungal Agent, Parenteral; Echinocandin

Use

Aspergillosis, invasive: Treatment of invasive aspergillosis in patients ≥3 months of age who are refractory to or intolerant of other therapies (eg, amphotericin B, lipid formulations of amphotericin B, itraconazole).

Limitations of use: Has not been studied as initial therapy for invasive aspergillosis.

Candidemia and other *Candida* infections: Treatment of candidemia and the following *Candida* infections in patients ≥3 months of age: Intra-abdominal abscesses, peritonitis, and pleural space infections.

Limitations of use: Has not been studied in endocarditis, osteomyelitis, and meningitis due to *Candida*.

Candidiasis, esophageal: Treatment of esophageal candidiasis in patients ≥3 months of age.

Limitations of use: Not approved for the treatment of oropharyngeal candidiasis (OPC).

Fungal infections, empiric therapy (neutropenic patients): Empiric therapy for presumed fungal infections in febrile, neutropenic patients ≥3 months of age.

Local Anesthetic/Vasoconstrictor Precautions

No information available to require special precautions

Effects on Dental Treatment No significant effects or complications reported

Effects on Bleeding No information available to require special precautions

Adverse Reactions

>10%:

Cardiovascular: Hypotension (adults: 3% to 20%; infants, children, and adolescents: 9%), peripheral edema (adults: 6% to 11%), tachycardia (7% to 11%)

Central nervous system: Chills (adults: 9% to 23%; infants, children, and adolescents: 13%), headache (9% to 15%)

Dermatologic: Skin rash (4% to 23%)

Gastrointestinal: Diarrhea (adults: 6% to 27%; infants, children, and adolescents: 7%), vomiting (6% to 17%), nausea (adults: 5% to 15%; infants, children, and adolescents: 4%)

Hematologic & oncologic: Decreased hemoglobin (adults: 18% to 21%), decreased hematocrit (adults: 13% to 18%), decreased white blood cell count (adults: 12%), anemia (adults: 11%)

Hepatic: Increased serum alkaline phosphatase (adults: 9% to 22%), increased serum ALT (adults: 4% to 18%; infants, children, and adolescents: 5%), increased serum AST (adults: 6% to 16%; infants, children, and adolescents: 2%), increased serum bilirubin (adults: 5% to 13%)

Local: Localized phlebitis (adults: 18%)

Renal: Increased serum creatinine (adults: 3% to 11%)

Respiratory: Respiratory failure (adults: 2% to 20%), cough (adults: 6% to 11%), pneumonia (adults: 4% to 11%)

Miscellaneous: Infusion related reaction (20% to 35%), fever (6% to 30%), septic shock (adults: 11% to 14%)

1% to 10%:

Cardiovascular: Hypertension (5% to 9%), atrial fibrillation (<5%), bradycardia (<5%), cardiac arrhythmia (<5%), edema (<5%), flushing (<5%), myocardial infarction (<5%)

Central nervous system: Anxiety (<5%), confusion (<5%), depression (<5%), dizziness (<5%), drowsiness (<5%), fatigue (<5%), insomnia (<5%), seizure (<5%)

Dermatologic: Erythema (5% to 9%), pruritus (infants, children, and adolescents: 6%), skin lesion (<5%), urticaria (<5%), decubitus ulcer (adults: 3% to 5%)

Endocrine & metabolic: Hypomagnesemia (adults: 7%), hyperglycemia (adults: 6%), hypokalemia (5% to 6%), hypercalcemia (<5%), hypervolemia (<5%)

Gastrointestinal: Abdominal pain (4% to 9%), mucosal inflammation (4% to 6%), abdominal distention (<5%), anorexia (<5%), constipation (<5%), decreased appetite (<5%), dyspepsia (<5%), upper abdominal pain (<5%)

Genitourinary: Urinary tract infection (<5%), nephrotoxicity (adults: 3%; serum creatinine ≥2 x baseline value or ≥1 mg/dL in patients with serum creatinine above ULN range)

Hematologic & oncologic: Blood coagulation disorder (<5%), febrile neutropenia (<5%), neutropenia (<5%), petechia (<5%), thrombocytopenia (<5%)

Hepatic: Decreased serum albumin (adults: 7%), hepatic failure (<5%), hepatomegaly (<5%), hepatotoxicity (<5%), hyperbilirubinemia (<5%), jaundice (<5%)

Infection: Sepsis (adults: 5% to 7%), bacteremia (<5%)

Local: Catheter infection (infants, children, and adolescents: 9%), infusion site reaction (<5%; pain/pruritus/swelling)

Neuromuscular & skeletal: Arthralgia (<5%), back pain (<5%), limb pain (<5%), tremor (<5%), weakness (<5%)

Renal: Hematuria (adults: 10%), increased blood urea nitrogen (adults: 4% to 9%), renal failure (<5%)

Respiratory: Dyspnea (adults: 9%), pleural effusion (adults: 9%), respiratory distress (adults: ≤8%), rales (adults: 7%), epistaxis (<5%), hypoxia (<5%), tachypnea (<5%)

<1%, postmarketing, and/or case reports: Anaphylaxis, erythema multiforme, exfoliation of skin, hepatic necrosis, hepatitis, histamine release (including facial swelling, bronchospasm, sensation of warmth), increased gamma-glutamyl transferase, pancreatitis, renal insufficiency, Stevens-Johnson syndrome, swelling, toxic epidermal necrolysis

Mechanism of Action Inhibits synthesis of β(1,3)-D-glucan, an essential component of the cell wall of susceptible fungi. Highest activity is in regions of active cell growth. Mammalian cells do not require β(1,3)-D-glucan, limiting potential toxicity.

Pharmacodynamics/Kinetics

Half-life Elimination Beta (distribution): 9 to 11 hours (~8 hours in children <12 years); Terminal: 40 to 50 hours; beta phase half-life is 32% to 43% lower in pediatric patients than in adult patients

Pregnancy Considerations

Based on animal data, in utero exposure to caspofungin may cause fetal harm.

When treatment of invasive *Aspergillus* or *Candida* infections is needed during pregnancy, other agents are preferred (HHS [OI adult 2020]; IDSA [Pappas 2016]).

Cefaclor (SEF a klor)

Related Information

Antibiotic Prophylaxis *on page 1715*
Bacterial Infections *on page 1739*

Brand Names: Canada APO-Cefaclor [DSC]; CO Cefaclor; DOM-Cefaclor; NOVO-Cefaclor [DSC]; PMS-Cefaclor 125 [DSC]; PMS-Cefaclor 250 [DSC]; PMS-Cefaclor BID [DSC]; PMS-Cefaclor [DSC]

Generic Availability (US) Yes

Pharmacologic Category Antibiotic, Cephalosporin (Second Generation)

Dental Use Alternative antibiotic for treatment of orofacial infections in patients allergic to penicillins; susceptible bacteria including aerobic gram-positive bacteria and anaerobes

Use

Acute bacterial exacerbations of chronic bronchitis (extended-release tablets only): Treatment of acute bacterial exacerbations of chronic bronchitis due to *Haemophilus influenzae* (excluding beta-lactamase-negative, ampicillin-resistant strains only), *Moraxella catarrhalis*, or *Streptococcus pneumoniae*.

Lower respiratory tract infections (capsules and oral suspension only): Treatment of lower respiratory tract infections, including pneumonia, caused by *S. pneumoniae*, *H. influenzae*, and *Streptococcus pyogenes*.

Otitis media (capsules and oral suspension only): Treatment of otitis media caused by *S. pneumoniae*, *H. influenzae*, staphylococci, and *S. pyogenes*.

Pharyngitis and tonsillitis: Treatment of pharyngitis and tonsillitis due to *S. pyogenes*.

Secondary bacterial infections of acute bronchitis (extended-release tablets only): Treatment of secondary bacterial infections of acute bronchitis due to *H. influenzae* (excluding beta-lactamase negative, ampicillin-resistant strains), *M. catarrhalis*, or *S. pneumoniae*.

Skin and skin structure infections, uncomplicated: Treatment of uncomplicated skin and skin structure infections due to *Staphylococcus aureus* (methicillin-susceptible) or *S. pyogenes* (capsules and oral suspension only).

Urinary tract infections (capsules and oral suspension only): Treatment of urinary tract infections, including pyelonephritis and cystitis, caused by *Escherichia coli*, *Proteus mirabilis*, *Klebsiella* spp, and coagulase-negative staphylococci.

Local Anesthetic/Vasoconstrictor Precautions No information available to require special precautions

Effects on Dental Treatment No significant effects or complications reported (see Dental Health Professional Considerations)

Effects on Bleeding No information available to require special precautions

Adverse Reactions

1% to 10%:

Dermatologic: Rash (1% to 2%; includes erythematous rash, maculopapular rash, or morbilliform rash)

Gastrointestinal: Diarrhea (3%)

Genitourinary: Vaginitis (2%), vulvovaginal candidiasis (2%)

Hematologic & oncologic: Eosinophilia (2%)

Hepatic: Increased serum transaminases (3%)

<1%, postmarketing, and/or case reports: Agitation, agranulocytosis, anaphylaxis, angioedema, aplastic anemia, arthralgia, cholestatic jaundice, confusion, dizziness, drowsiness, hallucination, hemolytic

anemia, hepatitis, hyperactivity, insomnia, interstitial nephritis, irritability, nausea, nervousness, neutropenia, paresthesia, prolonged prothrombin time, pruritus, pseudomembranous colitis, seizure, serum sickness, Stevens-Johnson syndrome, thrombocytopenia, toxic epidermal necrolysis, urticaria, vomiting

Dental Usual Dosage Orofacial infections: Adults: Oral: Dosing range: 250-500 mg every 8 hours

Dosing

Adult & Geriatric

Treatment of susceptible infections: Oral:
Immediate-release: 250 to 500 mg every 8 hours
Extended-release: 500 mg every 12 hours

Indication-specific dosing: Note: An extended-release tablet dose of 500 mg twice daily is clinically equivalent to an immediate-release capsule dose of 250 mg 3 times daily; an extended-release tablet dose of 500 mg twice daily is **NOT** clinically equivalent to 500 mg 3 times daily of other cefaclor formulations.

Acute bacterial exacerbations of chronic bronchitis: Oral: Extended-release: 500 mg every 12 hours for 7 days

Secondary bacterial infection of acute bronchitis: Oral: Extended-release: 500 mg every 12 hours for 7 days

Renal Impairment: Adult

Manufacturer's labeling:

Oral, immediate-release: There are no dosage adjustments provided in the manufacturer's labeling; however, half-life is increased in anuric patients; use with caution.

Oral, extended-release: There are no dosage adjustments provided in the manufacturer's labeling.

Dialysis: Moderately dialyzable (20% to 50%)

Alternative recommendations (off-label dosing) (Aronoff 2007):

Oral, immediate-release:

Mild to severe impairment: No dosage adjustment necessary.

End-stage renal disease (ESRD) on intermittent hemodialysis (IHD) (administer after hemodialysis on dialysis days): Supplement with 250 to 500 mg after dialysis.

Peritoneal dialysis: Administer 250 to 500 mg every 8 hours.

Hepatic Impairment: Adult There are no dosage adjustments provided in the manufacturer's labeling.

Pediatric

General dosing, susceptible infection: Mild to moderate infection: Infants, Children, and Adolescents: Oral, immediate release: 20 to 40 mg/kg/day divided every 8 to 12 hours. Maximum daily dose: 1,500 mg/**day** (*Red Book* [AAP 2015])

Bronchitis: Adolescents ≥16 years: Extended release tablet: **Note:** An extended release tablet dose of 500 mg twice daily is clinically equivalent to an immediate release capsule dose of 250 mg 3 times daily; an extended release tablet dose of 500 mg twice daily is **NOT** clinically equivalent to 500 mg 3 times daily of other cefaclor formulations.

Acute bacterial exacerbations of chronic bronchitis: Oral: Extended release: 500 mg every 12 hours for 7 days

Secondary bacterial infection of acute bronchitis: Oral: Extended release: 500 mg every 12 hours for 7 days

Lower respiratory tract infections: Infants, Children, and Adolescents: Oral immediate release: 20 to 40 mg/kg/day divided every 8 hours; maximum daily dose: 1,000 mg/**day**. If beta-hemolytic streptococcus/*S. pyogenes* suspected, treat for at least 10 days.

Otitis media: Infants, Children, and Adolescents: Oral immediate release: 40 mg/kg/day divided every 8 to 12 hours (oral suspension) or every 8 hours (capsule); maximum daily dose: 1,000 mg/**day**. If beta-hemolytic streptococcus/*S. pyogenes* suspected, treat for at least 10 days. **Note:** Cefaclor is not a recommended treatment option in the AAP guidelines (Lieberthal 2013).

Pharyngitis/tonsillitis: Infants, Children, and Adolescents: Oral immediate release: 20 mg/kg/day divided every 8 to 12 hours (oral suspension) or every 8 hours (capsule); maximum daily dose: 1,000 mg/**day**. If beta-hemolytic streptococcus/*S. pyogenes* confirmed, treat for at least 10 days. **Note:** Cefaclor is not a recommended treatment option in the IDSA guidelines and is not considered preferred by the AHA due to its broad spectrum (AHA [Gerber 2009], IDSA [Shulman 2012]).

Skin and skin structure infections, uncomplicated: Infants, Children, and Adolescents: Oral: Immediate release: 20 to 40 mg/kg/day divided every 8 hours; maximum daily dose: 1,000 mg/**day**. If due to beta-hemolytic streptococcus/*S. pyogenes*, treat for at least 10 days.

Urinary tract infections: Infants, Children, and Adolescents: Oral: Immediate release: 20 to 40 mg/kg/day divided every 8 hours; maximum daily dose: 1,000 mg/**day**

Renal Impairment: Pediatric

Manufacturer's labeling:

Oral, immediate release: Infants, Children, and Adolescents: There are no dosage adjustments provided in the manufacturer's labeling; however, half-life is increased in anuric patients; use with caution.

Oral, extended release: There are no dosage adjustments provided in the manufacturer's labeling.

Alternative recommendations (Aronoff 2007): Dosing based on usual dose of 20 to 40 mg/kg/day in divided doses every 8 to 12 hours

Infants, Children, and Adolescents: Oral, immediate release:

GFR ≥10 mL/minute/1.73 m^2: No dosage adjustment necessary.

GFR <10 mL/minute/1.73 m^2: Administer 50% of the recommended dose.

End-stage renal disease (ERD) on intermittent hemodialysis (IHD) (supplemental dose posthemodialysis needed): Administer 50% of the recommended dose.

Peritoneal dialysis: Administer 50% of the recommended dose.

Hemodialysis: Hemodialysis shortens half-life by 25% to 35%

Moderately dialyzable (20% to 50%) (Aronoff 2007)

Hepatic Impairment: Pediatric There are no dosage adjustments provided in the manufacturer's labeling.

Mechanism of Action Inhibits bacterial cell wall synthesis by binding to one or more of the penicillin-binding proteins (PBPs), which in turn inhibits the final transpeptidation step of peptidoglycan synthesis in bacterial cell walls, thus inhibiting cell wall biosynthesis. Bacteria eventually lyse due to ongoing activity of cell wall autolytic enzymes (autolysins and murein hydrolases) while cell wall assembly is arrested.

Contraindications Hypersensitivity to cefaclor, any component of the formulation, or other cephalosporins

Warnings/Precautions Anaphylactic reactions have occurred. If a serious hypersensitivity reaction occurs, discontinue and institute emergency supportive measures, including airway management and treatment (eg, epinephrine, antihistamines and/or corticosteroids). Use with caution in patients with a history of gastrointestinal disease, particularly colitis. Use with caution in patients with renal impairment. Prolonged use may result in fungal or bacterial superinfection, including *C. difficile*-associated diarrhea (CDAD) and pseudomembranous colitis; CDAD has been observed >2 months postantibiotic treatment. Use with caution in patients with a history of penicillin allergy. An extended-release tablet dose of 500 mg twice daily is clinically equivalent to an immediate-release capsule dose of 250 mg 3 times daily; an extended-release tablet dose of 500 mg twice daily is **NOT** clinically equivalent to 500 mg 3 times daily of other cefaclor formulations. Potentially significant interactions may exist, requiring dose or frequency adjustment, additional monitoring, and/or selection of alternative therapy.

Benzyl alcohol and derivatives: Some dosage forms may contain sodium benzoate/benzoic acid; benzoic acid (benzoate) is a metabolite of benzyl alcohol; large amounts of benzyl alcohol (≥99 mg/kg/day) have been associated with a potentially fatal toxicity ("gasping syndrome") in neonates; the "gasping syndrome" consists of metabolic acidosis, respiratory distress, gasping respirations, CNS dysfunction (including convulsions, intracranial hemorrhage), hypotension, and cardiovascular collapse (AAP ["Inactive" 1997]; CDC, 1982); some data suggests that benzoate displaces bilirubin from protein binding sites (Ahlfors, 2001); avoid or use dosage forms containing benzyl alcohol derivative with caution in neonates. See manufacturer's labeling.

Warnings: Additional Pediatric Considerations May cause serum sickness-like reaction (estimated incidence ranges from 0.024% to 0.2% per drug course); majority of reactions have occurred in children <5 years of age with symptoms of fever, rash, erythema multiforme, and arthralgia, often occurring during the second or third exposure.

Drug Interactions

Metabolism/Transport Effects **Substrate** of OAT1/3

Avoid Concomitant Use

Avoid concomitant use of Cefaclor with any of the following: BCG (Intravesical); Cholera Vaccine

Increased Effect/Toxicity

Cefaclor may increase the levels/effects of: Aminoglycosides; Vitamin K Antagonists

The levels/effects of Cefaclor may be increased by: Nitisinone; Pretomanid; Probenecid; Teriflunomide; Tolvaptan

Decreased Effect

Cefaclor may decrease the levels/effects of: Aminoglycosides; BCG (Intravesical); BCG Vaccine (Immunization); Cholera Vaccine; Lactobacillus and Estriol; Sodium Picosulfate; Typhoid Vaccine

Food Interactions The bioavailability of cefaclor extended-release tablets is decreased 23% and the maximum concentration is decreased 67% when taken on an empty stomach. Management: Administer with food.

Dietary Considerations Extended release tablets should be taken with or within 1 hour of food.

Pharmacodynamics/Kinetics

Half-life Elimination 0.6 to 0.9 hours; prolonged with renal impairment (2.3 to 2.8 hours in anuria)

Time to Peak Capsules, oral suspension: 30 to 60 minutes; Extended-release tablets: 2.5 hours

Pregnancy Risk Factor B

Pregnancy Considerations

An increased risk of teratogenic effects has not been observed following maternal use of cefaclor.

Breastfeeding Considerations Small amounts of cefaclor are excreted in breast milk. The manufacturer recommends that caution be exercised when administering cefaclor to nursing women. Nondose-related effects could include modification of bowel flora.

Dosage Forms: US

Capsule, Oral:

Generic: 250 mg, 500 mg

Suspension Reconstituted, Oral:

Generic: 125 mg/5 mL (150 mL); 250 mg/5 mL (150 mL); 375 mg/5 mL (100 mL)

Tablet Extended Release 12 Hour, Oral:

Generic: 500 mg

Dosage Forms: Canada

Capsule, Oral:

Generic: 250 mg, 500 mg

Dental Health Professional Considerations Cefaclor is effective against anaerobic bacteria, but the sensitivity of alpha-hemolytic Streptococcus vary; approximately 10% of strains are resistant. Nearly 70% are intermediately sensitive. Patients allergic to penicillins can use a cephalosporin; the incidence of cross-reactivity between penicillins and cephalosporins is 1% to 5% when the allergic reaction to penicillin is delayed. If the patient has a history of anaphylaxis to penicillin, cephalosporins are contraindicated in these patients.

Cefadroxil (sef a DROKS il)

Related Information

Antibiotic Prophylaxis *on page 1715*

Bacterial Infections *on page 1739*

Brand Names: Canada APO-Cefadroxil; PRO-Cefadroxil-500; TEVA-Cefadroxil

Generic Availability (US) Yes

Pharmacologic Category Antibiotic, Cephalosporin (First Generation)

Dental Use Alternative antibiotic for treatment of orofacial infections in patients allergic to penicillins; susceptible bacteria including aerobic gram-positive bacteria and anaerobes

Use

Pharyngitis and/or tonsillitis: Treatment of pharyngitis and/or tonsillitis caused by *Streptococcus pyogenes* (group A beta-hemolytic streptococci).

Skin and skin structure infections: Treatment of skin and skin structure infections caused by staphylococci and/or streptococci.

Urinary tract infection: Treatment of urinary tract infections caused by *Escherichia coli*, *Proteus mirabilis*, and *Klebsiella* species.

Local Anesthetic/Vasoconstrictor Precautions No information available to require special precautions

Effects on Dental Treatment No significant effects or complications reported

Effects on Bleeding No information available to require special precautions

Adverse Reactions

1% to 10%: Gastrointestinal: Diarrhea

<1%: postmarketing, and/or case reports: Abdominal pain, agranulocytosis, anaphylaxis, angioedema, arthralgia, cholestasis, *Clostridioides* (formerly *Clostridium*) *difficile*-associated diarrhea, dyspepsia, erythema multiforme, erythematous rash, fever, genital candidiasis, hepatic failure, increased serum transaminases, maculopapular rash, nausea, neutropenia, pruritus, pseudomembranous colitis, serum sickness, Stevens-Johnson syndrome, thrombocytopenia, urticaria, vaginitis, vomiting

Dental Usual Dosage Orofacial infections: Oral: Adults: Dosage range: 250-500 mg every 8 hours

Dosing

Adult & Geriatric

Prosthetic joint infection, staphylococci (oxacillin-susceptible), chronic oral antimicrobial suppression (off-label use): 500 mg every 12 hours (Osmon 2013)

Skin and skin structure infections: Oral: 1 g daily in a single or 2 divided doses

Streptococcal pharyngitis (group A) (alternative agent for mild [non-anaphylactic] penicillin allergy): Oral: 1 g once daily for 10 days (IDSA [Shulman 2012]; Pichichero 2018; manufacturer's labeling)

Manufacturer's labeling: Dosing in the prescribing information may not reflect current clinical practice. 500 mg twice daily

Urinary tract infection (UTI) (alternative agent):

Note: Use with caution and only when recommended agents cannot be used (due to decreased efficacy of oral beta-lactams compared to other agents) (Hooton 2018a; ESMID/IDSA [Gupta 2011]; Greenberg 1986; Sandberg 1990).

Cystitis, acute uncomplicated: Oral: 500 mg twice daily (Greenberg 1986; Hooton 1995) for 5 to 7 days (Greenberg 1986; Hooton 2018a)

UTI, complicated (including pyelonephritis): Oral: 1 g twice daily (Sandberg 1990) for 10 to 14 days (Hooton 2018b; Sandberg 1990). **Note:** Oral therapy should follow appropriate parenteral therapy. For outpatient treatment of mild infection, a single dose of a long-acting parenteral agent is acceptable; for outpatients who are more ill or are at risk for more severe illness, consider continuing parenteral therapy until culture and susceptibility results are available (ESMID/IDSA [Gupta 2011]; Hooton 2018b).

Renal Impairment: Adult

Initial: 1 g as a single dose.

Maintenance:

CrCl >50 mL/minute: No dosage adjustment necessary.

CrCl 25 to 50 mL/minute: 500 mg every 12 hours.

CrCl 10 to 25 mL/minute: 500 mg every 24 hours.

CrCl <10 mL/minute: 500 mg every 36 hours.

Hepatic Impairment: Adult There are no dosage adjustments provided in the manufacturer's labeling.

Pediatric

General dosing, susceptible infection: Mild to moderate infection: Infants, Children, and Adolescents: Oral: 15 mg/kg/dose twice daily; maximum daily dose: 2,000 mg/**day** (*Red Book* [AAP 2015])

Impetigo: Children and Adolescents: Oral: 30 mg/kg/day in a single dose or divided every 12 hours; maximum daily dose: 1,000 mg/**day**

Pharyngitis/tonsillitis: Children and Adolescents: Oral: 30 mg/kg/day in a single dose or divided every 12 hours for 10 days; maximum daily dose: 1,000 mg/**day**

Skin and skin structure infections: Children and Adolescents: Oral: 15 mg/kg/dose every 12 hours; maximum daily dose: 1,000 mg/**day**

Urinary tract infections: Children and Adolescents: Oral: 15 mg/kg/dose every 12 hours; maximum daily dose: 2,000 mg/**day**

Renal Impairment: Pediatric

Infants, Children, and Adolescents: There are no dosage adjustments provided in the manufacturer's labeling for this age group; however, the following have been used by some clinicians (Aronoff 2007): Dosing based on a usual dose of 30 mg/kg/day in divided doses every 12 hours:

CrCl ≥30 mL/minute/1.73 m^2: No dosage adjustment necessary

CrCl 10 to 29 mL/minute/1.73 m^2: 15 mg/kg/dose every 24 hours

CrCl <10 mL/minute/1.73 m^2: 15 mg/kg/dose every 36 hours

Hemodialysis, intermittent: 15 mg/kg/dose every 24 hours

Peritoneal dialysis: 15 mg/kg/dose every 36 hours

Hepatic Impairment: Pediatric There are no dosage adjustments provided in the manufacturer's labeling.

Mechanism of Action Inhibits bacterial cell wall synthesis by binding to one or more of the penicillin-binding proteins (PBPs) which in turn inhibits the final transpeptidation step of peptidoglycan synthesis in bacterial cell walls, thus inhibiting cell wall biosynthesis. Bacteria eventually lyse due to ongoing activity of cell wall autolytic enzymes (autolysins and murein hydrolases) while cell wall assembly is arrested.

Contraindications Hypersensitivity to cefadroxil, any component of the formulation, or other cephalosporins

Warnings/Precautions Use with caution in patients with renal impairment (CrCl <50 mL/minute/1.73 m^2); dosage adjustment may be needed. Hypersensitivity reactions, including anaphylaxis, may occur. If an allergic reaction occurs, discontinue treatment and institute appropriate supportive measures. Use with caution in patients with a history of penicillin allergy. Use with caution in patients with a history of gastrointestinal disease, particularly colitis. Prolonged use may result in fungal or bacterial superinfection, including *C. difficile*-associated diarrhea (CDAD) and pseudomembranous colitis; CDAD has been observed >2 months postantibiotic treatment. Only IM penicillin has been shown to be effective in the prophylaxis of rheumatic fever. Cefadroxil is generally effective in the eradication of streptococci from the oropharynx; efficacy data for cefadroxil in the prophylaxis of subsequent rheumatic fever episodes are not available. Potentially significant drug-drug interactions may exist, requiring dose or frequency adjustment, additional monitoring, and/or selection of alternative therapy.

Suspension may contain sulfur dioxide (sulfite); hypersensitivity reactions, including anaphylaxis and/or asthmatic exacerbations, may occur (may be life threatening).

Dosage form specific issues: Some dosage forms may contain sodium benzoate/benzoic acid; benzoic acid (benzoate) is a metabolite of benzyl alcohol; large amounts of benzyl alcohol (≥99 mg/kg/day) have been associated with a potentially fatal toxicity ("gasping syndrome") in neonates; the "gasping syndrome" consists of metabolic acidosis, respiratory distress, gasping respirations, CNS dysfunction (including convulsions, intracranial hemorrhage), hypotension, and cardiovascular collapse (AAP ["Inactive" 1997]; CDC 1982); some data suggests that benzoate displaces bilirubin from protein binding sites (Ahlfors, 2001); avoid or use dosage forms containing benzyl alcohol derivative with caution in neonates. Some dosage forms may contain propylene glycol; large amounts are potentially toxic and have been associated with hyperosmolality, lactic acidosis, seizures, and respiratory depression; use caution (AAP 1997; Zar 2007). See manufacturer's labeling.

Warnings: Additional Pediatric Considerations Some dosage forms may contain propylene glycol; in neonates large amounts of propylene glycol delivered orally, intravenously (eg, >3,000 mg/day), or topically have been associated with potentially fatal toxicities which can include metabolic acidosis, seizures, renal failure, and CNS depression; toxicities have also been reported in children and adults including hyperosmolality, lactic acidosis, seizures, and respiratory depression; use caution (AAP 1997; Shehab 2009).

Drug Interactions

Metabolism/Transport Effects None known.

Avoid Concomitant Use

Avoid concomitant use of Cefadroxil with any of the following: BCG (Intravesical); Cholera Vaccine

Increased Effect/Toxicity

Cefadroxil may increase the levels/effects of: Aminoglycosides; Vitamin K Antagonists

The levels/effects of Cefadroxil may be increased by: Probenecid

Decreased Effect

Cefadroxil may decrease the levels/effects of: Aminoglycosides; BCG (Intravesical); BCG Vaccine (Immunization); Cholera Vaccine; Lactobacillus and Estriol; Sodium Picosulfate; Typhoid Vaccine

Pharmacodynamics/Kinetics

Half-life Elimination 1 to 2 hours; 20 to 24 hours in renal failure

Time to Peak

Serum: Within 70 to 90 minutes

Pregnancy Risk Factor B

Pregnancy Considerations

Cefadroxil crosses the placenta. Limited data are available concerning the use of cefadroxil in pregnancy; however, adverse fetal effects were not noted in a small clinical trial.

Breastfeeding Considerations Very small amounts of cefadroxil are excreted in breast milk. The manufacturer recommends that caution be exercised when administering cefadroxil to nursing women. Nondose-related effects could include modification of bowel flora.

Dosage Forms: US

Capsule, Oral:

Generic: 500 mg

Suspension Reconstituted, Oral:

Generic: 250 mg/5 mL (50 mL, 100 mL); 500 mg/5 mL (75 mL, 100 mL)

Tablet, Oral:

Generic: 1 g

Dosage Forms: Canada

Capsule, Oral:

Generic: 500 mg

◆ **Cefadroxil Monohydrate** *see* Cefadroxil *on page 299*

CeFAZolin (sef A zoe lin)

Related Information

Antibiotic Prophylaxis *on page 1715*

Generic Availability (US) Yes

Pharmacologic Category Antibiotic, Cephalosporin (First Generation)

Dental Use Alternative antibiotic for prevention of infective endocarditis when parenteral administration is needed. Individuals allergic to amoxicillin (penicillins) may receive cefazolin provided they have not had an immediate, local, or systemic IgE-mediated anaphylactic allergic reaction to penicillin.

Use

Biliary tract infection: Treatment of biliary tract infections due to *Escherichia coli*, various strains of streptococci, *Proteus mirabilis*, *Klebsiella* species, and *Staphylococcus aureus*.

Bloodstream infection: Treatment of bloodstream infection due to methicillin-susceptible staphylococci, *E. coli* , *P. mirabilis*, and *Klebsiella* species.

Bone and joint infection: Treatment of bone and joint infections due to *S. aureus*.

Endocarditis, treatment: Treatment of endocarditis due to methicillin-susceptible staphylococci and group A beta-hemolytic streptococci (*Streptococcus pyogenes*).

Genital infection: Treatment of genital infections (ie, prostatitis, epididymitis) due to *E. coli*, *P. mirabilis*, and *Klebsiella* species.

Respiratory tract infection: Treatment of respiratory tract infections due to *Streptococcus pneumoniae*, *Klebsiella* species, *Haemophilus influenzae*, methicillin-susceptible *S. aureus*, and group A beta-hemolytic streptococci.

Skin and soft tissue infection: Treatment of skin and soft tissue infections due to methicillin-susceptible *S. aureus*, group A beta-hemolytic streptococci, and other strains of streptococci.

Surgical prophylaxis: To reduce the incidence of certain postoperative infections in patients undergoing surgical procedures.

Urinary tract infection: Treatment of urinary tract infections due to *E. coli*, *P. mirabilis*, *Klebsiella* species, and some strains of *Enterobacter*.

Local Anesthetic/Vasoconstrictor Precautions No information available to require special precautions

Effects on Dental Treatment Key adverse event(s) related to dental treatment: Rare occurrence of oral candidiasis

Effects on Bleeding May potentiate the anticoagulant effects of vitamin K anticoagulants (ie, warfarin)

Adverse Reactions Frequency not defined.

Cardiovascular: Localized phlebitis

Central nervous system: Seizure

Dermatologic: Pruritus, skin rash, Stevens-Johnson syndrome

Gastrointestinal: Abdominal cramps, anorexia, diarrhea, nausea, oral candidiasis, pseudomembranous colitis, vomiting

Genitourinary: Vaginitis

Hepatic: Hepatitis, increased serum transaminases

Hematologic: Eosinophilia, leukopenia, neutropenia, thrombocythemia, thrombocytopenia

Hypersensitivity: Anaphylaxis

Local: Pain at injection site

Renal: Increased blood urea nitrogen, increased serum creatinine, renal failure

Miscellaneous: Fever

Dental Usual Dosage

Infective endocarditis prophylaxis (off-label use): IM, IV:

Infants and Children: 50 mg/kg 30 to 60 minutes before procedure; maximum dose: 1 g

Adults: 1 g 30 to 60 minutes before procedure.

Note: Intramuscular injections should be avoided in patients who are receiving anticoagulant therapy. In these circumstances, orally administered regimens should be given whenever possible. Intravenously administered antibiotics should be used for patients who are unable to tolerate or absorb oral medications.

Note: American Heart Association (AHA) guidelines now recommend prophylaxis only in patients undergoing invasive procedures and in whom underlying cardiac conditions may predispose to a higher risk of adverse outcomes should infection occur. As of April 2007, routine prophylaxis for GI/GU procedures is no longer recommended by the AHA.

Dosing

Adult & Geriatric

Bloodstream infection:

Pathogen-directed therapy for methicillin-susceptible staphylococci (alternative agent):

IV: 2 g every 8 hours (Fowler 2019; IDSA [Mermel 2009]); treat uncomplicated *Staphylococcus aureus* bacteremia for ≥14 days starting from day of first negative blood culture, with longer courses warranted for endocarditis or metastatic sites of infection (IDSA [Mermel 2009]).

Pathogen-directed therapy for susceptible Enterobacteriaceae:

IV: 2 g every 8 hours (Hsieh 2016; Turnidge 2011). Usual duration is 7 to 14 days; individualize depending on source and extent of infection as well as clinical response. A 7-day duration is recommended for patients with uncomplicated Enterobacteriaceae infection who respond appropriately to antibiotic therapy (Moehring 2019; Yahav 2018).

Antibiotic lock technique (catheter-salvage strategy):

Note: For infections caused by susceptible organisms when the catheter cannot be removed; use in addition to systemic antibiotics. Catheter salvage is **not** recommended for *S. aureus*.

Intracatheter: Prepare lock solution to final concentration of cefazolin 5 to 10 mg/mL (may be combined with heparin). Instill into each lumen of the catheter access port using a volume sufficient to fill the catheter (2 to 5 mL), with a dwell time of up to 72 hours depending on frequency of catheter use and solution stability. Withdraw lock solution prior to catheter use; replace with fresh cefazolin lock solution after catheter use. Antibiotic lock therapy is given for the same duration as systemic antibiotics (Bookstaver 2009; Girand 2020; IDSA [Mermel 2009]).

Endocarditis, prophylaxis (dental or invasive respiratory tract procedures) (alternative agent for patients with nonsevere, non-IgE-mediated penicillin allergy who cannot take oral therapy) (off-label use):

IM, IV: 1 g as a single dose 30 to 60 minutes before procedure. **Note:** Only recommended for patients with cardiac conditions associated with the highest risk of adverse outcome from endocarditis **and** who are undergoing a procedure likely to result in bacteremia with an organism that has the potential ability to cause endocarditis (AHA [Wilson 2007]).

Endocarditis, treatment:

Note: Cefazolin should not be used in patients with concomitant CNS infections (eg, brain abscess) (AHA [Baddour 2015]).

Pathogen-directed therapy for methicillin-susceptible staphylococci (alternative agent for patients with nonsevere, non-IgE-mediated penicillin allergy):

Native valve: **IV:** 2 g every 8 hours for 6 weeks (AHA [Baddour 2015]).

Prosthetic valve: **IV:** 2 g every 8 hours for ≥6 weeks (combine with rifampin for entire duration of therapy and gentamicin for the first 2 weeks) (AHA [Baddour 2015]).

Intra-abdominal infection, community-acquired (mild to moderate infection in low-risk patients):

Note: Reserve for patients with low risk for resistant pathogens (eg, local Enterobacteriaceae resistance rate to cefazolin <10% and no recent antibiotic exposure) (Barshak 2019).

Cholecystitis, acute: **IV:** 1 to 2 g every 8 hours; continue for 1 day after gallbladder removal or until clinical resolution in patients managed nonoperatively (IDSA/SIS [Solomkin 2010]; Vollmer 2019). **Note:** The addition of anaerobic therapy is recommended if biliary-enteric anastomosis is present (IDSA/SIS [Solomkin 2010]).

Other intra-abdominal infections (eg, perforated appendix, appendiceal abscess, diverticulitis) (off-label use): **IV:** 1 to 2 g every 8 hours in combination with metronidazole. Total duration of therapy (which may include oral step-down therapy) is 4 to 7 days following adequate source control (IDSA/SIS [Solomkin 2010]); for uncomplicated appendicitis managed nonoperatively, a longer duration may be necessary (Barshak 2019; Pemberton 2020; Salminen 2015).

Osteomyelitis and/or discitis:

Treatment, pathogen-directed therapy for methicillin-susceptible S. aureus:

IV: 2 g every 8 hours for ≥6 weeks depending on extent of infection, debridement, and clinical response (IDSA [Berbari 2015]; Osmon 2019).

Prevention, following open fractures:

IV: 2 g for patients <120 kg or 3 g for patients ≥120 kg every 8 hours; ideally administer within 6 hours of injury. For type I or II fractures (no more than moderate comminution or contamination, no or minimal periosteal stripping, adequate soft tissue coverage), discontinue 24 hours following wound closure. For type III fractures (severe contamination or comminution), use as part of an appropriate combination regimen and continue for 72 hours after injury or up to 24 hours after wound closure (EAST [Hoff 2011]; Schmitt 2020). **Note:** For patients with risk for methicillin-resistant *S. aureus* (MRSA), potential water exposure, or fecal or clostridial contamination, alternative or additional antibiotics are recommended (Schmitt 2020).

Peritonitis, treatment (peritoneal dialysis patients) (off-label use):

Note: As a component of empiric therapy in patients at low risk for MRSA or as pathogen-directed therapy. Intraperitoneal administration is preferred to IV administration. Duration of therapy is ≥2 to 3 weeks, depending on organism, for patients with adequate clinical response (Burkart 2019; ISPD [Li 2016]). Consider a 25% dose increase in patients with significant residual renal function (urine output

>100 mL/day) (ISPD [Li 2010]; ISPD [Li 2016]; Mancini 2018; Szeto 2018).

Intermittent: **Intraperitoneal:** 15 to 20 mg/kg added to one exchange of dialysis solution once daily (allow to dwell for ≥6 hours). For patients on continuous ambulatory peritoneal dialysis, add cefazolin to the overnight dwell. **Note:** Some experts recommend adding cefazolin to each exchange in patients on automated peritoneal dialysis as nighttime intraperitoneal levels of cefazolin may fall below the minimum inhibitory concentration of most organisms (ISPD [Li 2016]).

Continuous (with every exchange) (dose is per liter of dialysate): **Intraperitoneal:** Loading dose: 500 mg/L of dialysate added to first exchange of dialysate; maintenance dose: 125 mg/L of dialysate with each subsequent exchange of dialysate (ISPD [Li 2016]).

Pneumonia: *Pathogen-directed therapy for methicillin-susceptible S. aureus:* IV: 2 g every 8 hours (Klompas 2019; Miller 2018). Minimum duration is 5 to 7 days; patients should be clinically stable with normal vital signs before therapy is discontinued (IDSA/ATS [Kalil 2016]; IDSA/ATS [Metlay 2019]).

Prostatitis, acute bacterial: *Pathogen-directed therapy for susceptible organisms:* **IV:** 1 g every 8 hours; may switch to oral therapy 24 to 48 hours after improvement in fever and clinical symptoms. Total duration of therapy is 4 to 6 weeks (Meyrier 2019).

Prosthetic joint infection: *Pathogen-directed therapy for methicillin-susceptible S. aureus:* **IV:** 2 g every 8 hours. Duration ranges from 2 to 6 weeks depending on prosthesis management, use of rifampin, and other patient-specific factors. **Note:** In select cases (eg, debridement and retention of prosthesis or one-stage arthroplasty), combine with oral rifampin and give oral suppressive antibiotic therapy following completion of IV treatment (Berbari 2019; IDSA [Osmon 2013]).

Septic arthritis, without prosthetic material: *Pathogen-directed therapy for methicillin-susceptible S. aureus:* **IV:** 2 g every 8 hours. Duration is 3 to 4 weeks (in the absence of osteomyelitis), including oral step-down therapy (Goldenberg 2019; Ross 2017). Some experts recommend 4 weeks of parenteral therapy for patients with concomitant bacteremia (Goldenberg 2019).

Skin and soft tissue infection:

Erysipelas or nonpurulent cellulitis in patients without risk for methicillin-resistant S. aureus: **IV:** 1 to 2 g every 8 hours. Total duration of therapy ≥5 days (including oral step-down therapy); may extend to 14 days depending on severity and clinical response (IDSA [Stevens 2014]; Spelman 2019).

Pathogen-directed therapy for methicillin-susceptible S. aureus: **IV:** 1 to 2 g every 8 hours. Total duration of therapy is 5 to 14 days (including oral step-down therapy) depending on severity of infection, need for debridement, and clinical response (IDSA [Stevens 2014]; Spelman 2019). **Note:** For necrotizing infections, antibiotic therapy must be used in conjunction with early and aggressive surgical exploration and debridement of necrotic tissue; continue until further debridement is not necessary and the patient has clinically improved and is afebrile for 48 to 72 hours (IDSA [Stevens 2014]).

Surgical site incisional infection (trunk or extremity surgery, not involving axilla or perineum): **IV:** 1 g every 8 hours; duration is dependent upon severity, need for debridement, and clinical response (IDSA [Stevens 2014]).

Streptococcus (group B), maternal prophylaxis for prevention of neonatal disease (alternative agent) (off-label use):

Note: Prophylaxis is reserved for pregnant women with a positive group B streptococcus (GBS) vaginal or rectal screening in late gestation or GBS bacteriuria during the current pregnancy, history of birth of an infant with early-onset GBS disease, and unknown GBS culture status with any of the following: birth <37 0/7 weeks gestation, intrapartum fever, prolonged rupture of membranes, known GBS positive in a previous pregnancy, or intrapartum nucleic acid amplification testing positive for GBS (ACOG 782 2019).

IV: 2 g as a single dose at onset of labor or prelabor rupture of membranes, then 1 g every 8 hours until delivery (ACOG 782 2019). **Note:** Use of cefazolin should be reserved for penicillin-allergic patients at **low** risk for anaphylaxis (eg, rash without urticaria and no systemic symptoms, family history of penicillin allergy but no personal history, patients who report penicillin allergy but have no recollection of symptoms or treatment) (ACOG 782 2019).

Surgical prophylaxis: IV: 2 g for patients <120 kg or 3 g for patients ≥120 kg; administer within 60 minutes of surgical incision. Use in combination with metronidazole for procedures requiring anaerobic coverage (eg, colorectal and clean-contaminated head and neck procedures). May repeat dose intraoperatively in 4 hours if procedure is lengthy or if there is excessive blood loss (ASHP/IDSA/SIS/SHEA [Bratzler 2013]); maximum dose: 12 g/day (manufacturer's labeling). In cases where an extension of prophylaxis is warranted postoperatively, total duration should be ≤24 hours (Anderson 2014). Postoperative prophylaxis is not recommended in clean and clean-contaminated surgeries (CDC [Berríos-Torres 2017]).

Toxic shock syndrome (off-label use): *Pathogen-directed therapy for group A streptococcus or methicillin-susceptible S. aureus (alternative agent for patients with nonsevere, non-IgE-mediated penicillin allergy) (off-label use):* **IV:** 2 g every 8 hours in combination with clindamycin. In the absence of bacteremia, treat for a total of ≥10 days, including oral step-down therapy (Chu 2019; Stevens 2019).

Urinary tract infection, complicated (including pyelonephritis): *Pathogen-directed therapy for susceptible organisms*: **IV:** 1 g every 8 hours (Millar 1995; Wing 1998). Switch to an appropriate oral regimen once patient has improvement in symptoms if culture and susceptibility results allow. Duration of therapy depends on the antimicrobial chosen to complete the regimen and ranges from 5 to 14 days (IDSA [Gupta 2011]; IDSA [Hooton 2010]).

Renal Impairment: Adult

CrCl ≥55 mL/minute: No dosage adjustment necessary

CrCl 35 to 54 mL/minute: Administer full dose in intervals of ≥8 hours

CrCl 11 to 34 mL/minute: Administer 50% of usual dose every 12 hours

CrCl ≤10 mL/minute: Administer 50% of usual dose every 18 to 24 hours

Intermittent hemodialysis (IHD) (administer after hemodialysis on dialysis days): Dialyzable (20% to 50%): 500 mg to 1 g every 24 hours **or** use 1 to 2 g every 48 to 72 hours (Heintz 2009) **or** 15 to 20 mg/kg (maximum dose: 2 g) after dialysis 3 times weekly (Ahern 2003; Sowinski 2001) **or** 2 g after dialysis if next dialysis expected in 48 hours or 3 g after dialysis if next dialysis is expected in 72 hours (Stryjewski 2007).

Note: Dosing dependent on the assumption of 3 times weekly, complete IHD sessions.

Peritoneal dialysis (PD): IV: 500 mg every 12 hours

Continuous renal replacement therapy (CRRT) (Heintz 2009; Trotman 2005): Drug clearance is highly dependent on the method of renal replacement, filter type, and flow rate. Appropriate dosing requires close monitoring of pharmacologic response, signs of adverse reactions due to drug accumulation, as well as drug concentrations in relation to target trough (if appropriate). The following are general recommendations only (based on dialysate flow/ultrafiltration rates of 1 to 2 L/hour and minimal residual renal function) and should not supersede clinical judgment:

CVVH: Loading dose of 2 g followed by 1 to 2 g every 12 hours

CVVHD/CVVHDF: Loading dose of 2 g followed by either 1 g every 8 hours **or** 2 g every 12 hours. **Note:** Dosage of 1 g every 8 hours results in similar steady-state concentrations as 2 g every 12 hours and is more cost effective (Heintz 2009).

Hepatic Impairment: Adult There are no dosage adjustments provided in the manufacturer's labeling.

Obesity: Adult Refer to indication-specific dosing for obesity-related information (may not be available for all indications).

Pediatric

General dosing, susceptible infection (Bradley 2019; *Red Book* [AAP 2018]): Infants, Children, and Adolescents: IM, IV:

Mild to moderate infections: 25 to 100 mg/kg/day divided every 8 hours; maximum daily dose: 6 **g/day**

Severe infections (eg, bone/joint infections): 100 to 150 mg/kg/day divided every 6 to 8 hours; maximum daily dose: 12 **g/day**

Endocarditis, bacterial:

Prophylaxis for dental and upper respiratory procedures: Infants, Children, and Adolescents: IM, IV: 50 mg/kg 30 to 60 minutes before procedure; maximum dose: 1,000 mg/dose (AHA [Wilson 2007]). **Note**: AHA guidelines (Baltimore 2015) limit the use of prophylactic antibiotics to patients at the highest risk for infective endocarditis (IE) or adverse outcomes (eg, prosthetic heart valves, patients with previous IE, unrepaired cyanotic congenital heart disease, repaired congenital heart disease with prosthetic material or device during first 6 months after procedure, repaired congenital heart disease with residual defects at the site or adjacent to site of prosthetic patch or device, and heart transplant recipients with cardiac valvulopathy).

Treatment: Children and Adolescents: IV: 100 mg/kg/day in divided doses every 8 hours; usual adult dose: 2,000 mg/dose; maximum daily dose: 12 **g/day**; treat for at least 4 weeks; longer durations may be necessary; may use with or without gentamicin (AHA [Baltimore 2015])

Peritonitis (peritoneal dialysis) (ISPD [Warady 2012]): Limited data available: Infants, Children, and Adolescents:

Prophylaxis:

Touch contamination of PD line: Intraperitoneal: 125 mg per liter

Invasive dental procedures: IV: 25 mg/kg administered 30 to 60 minutes before procedure; maximum dose: 1,000 mg/dose

Gastrointestinal or genitourinary procedures: IV: 25 mg/kg administered 60 minutes before procedure; maximum dose: 2,000 mg/dose

Treatment: Intraperitoneal:

Intermittent: 20 mg/kg every 24 hours in the long dwell

Continuous: Loading dose: 500 mg per liter of dialysate; maintenance: 125 mg per liter of dialysate

Pneumonia, community-acquired pneumonia (CAP), *S. aureus*, methicillin susceptible: Infants >3 months, Children, and Adolescents: IV: 50 mg/kg/dose every 8 hours (Bradley 2011); usual maximum dose for severe infections: 12 **g/day** (*Red Book* [AAP 2018])

Skin and soft tissue infections, *S. aureus*, methicillin susceptible (mild to moderate): (IDSA [Stevens 2014]): Infants, Children, and Adolescents:

S. aureus, methicillin susceptible skin and soft tissue infections including pyomyositis: IV: 50 mg/kg/day divided every 8 hours; maximum dose: 1,000 mg/dose; higher doses may be required in severe cases; duration of therapy at least 5 days, but longer may be necessary in some cases, eg, febrile and neutropenic patients: 7 to 14 days; pyomyositis: 14 to 21 days

S. aureus, methicillin susceptible necrotizing infection of skin, fascia, or muscle: IV: 100 mg/kg/day divided every 8 hours; maximum dose: 1,000 mg/dose; continue therapy until surgical debridement no longer necessary, clinical improvement and afebrile for 48 to 72 hours

Streptococcal, nonpurulent skin infection (cellulitis): IV: 100 mg/kg/day divided every 8 hours; maximum dose: 1,000 mg/dose; duration of therapy at least 5 days, but longer may be necessary in some cases

Surgical prophylaxis: Infants, Children, and Adolescents: IV: 30 mg/kg within 60 minutes prior to procedure, may repeat in 4 hours for prolonged procedure or excessive blood loss (eg, >1,500 mL in adults); maximum dose dependent upon patient weight: Weight <120 kg: 2,000 mg/dose; weight ≥120 kg: 3,000 mg/dose (ASHP/IDSA [Bratzler 2013]; *Red Book* [AAP 2018])

Renal Impairment: Pediatric

IM, IV:

Infants >1 month, Children, and Adolescents: After initial loading dose is administered, modify dose based on the degree of renal impairment:

CrCl >70 mL/minute: No dosage adjustment required

CrCl 40 to 70 mL/minute: Administer 60% of the usual daily dose divided every 12 hours

CrCl 20 to 40 mL/minute: Administer 25% of the usual daily dose divided every 12 hours

CrCl 5 to 20 mL/minute: Administer 10% of the usual daily dose given every 24 hours

Hemodialysis: 25 mg/kg/dose every 24 hours (Aronoff 2007)

Peritoneal dialysis: 25 mg/kg/dose every 24 hours (Aronoff 2007)

Continuous renal replacement therapy: 25 mg/kg/dose every 8 hours (Aronoff 2007)

Hepatic Impairment: Pediatric There are no dosage adjustments provided in the manufacturer's labeling.

Mechanism of Action Inhibits bacterial cell wall synthesis by binding to one or more of the penicillin-binding proteins (PBPs) which in turn inhibits the final transpeptidation step of peptidoglycan synthesis in bacterial cell walls, thus inhibiting cell wall biosynthesis. Bacteria eventually lyse due to ongoing activity of cell wall autolytic enzymes (autolysins and murein hydrolases) while cell wall assembly is arrested.

Contraindications Hypersensitivity to cefazolin, other cephalosporin antibiotics, penicillins, other beta-lactams, or any component of the formulation.

Warnings/Precautions Hypersensitivity reactions, including anaphylaxis, may occur. If an allergic reaction occurs, discontinue treatment and institute appropriate supportive measures. Use with caution in patients with a history of penicillin allergy. Use with caution in patients with renal impairment; dosage adjustment required. Prolonged use may result in fungal or bacterial superinfection, including *Clostridioides* (formerly *Clostridium*) *difficile*-associated diarrhea (CDAD) and pseudomembranous colitis; CDAD has been observed >2 months postantibiotic treatment. May be associated with increased INR, especially in nutritionally-deficient patients, prolonged treatment, hepatic or renal disease. Use with caution in patients with a history of seizure disorder; high levels, particularly in the presence of renal impairment, may increase risk of seizures. Potentially significant drug-drug interactions may exist, requiring dose or frequency adjustment, additional monitoring, and/or selection of alternative therapy.

Drug Interactions

Metabolism/Transport Effects None known.

Avoid Concomitant Use

Avoid concomitant use of CeFAZolin with any of the following: BCG (Intravesical); Cholera Vaccine

Increased Effect/Toxicity

CeFAZolin may increase the levels/effects of: Aminoglycosides; Fosphenytoin; Phenytoin; RifAMPin; Vitamin K Antagonists

The levels/effects of CeFAZolin may be increased by: Probenecid

Decreased Effect

CeFAZolin may decrease the levels/effects of: Aminoglycosides; BCG (Intravesical); BCG Vaccine (Immunization); Cholera Vaccine; Lactobacillus and Estriol; Sodium Picosulfate; Typhoid Vaccine

Dietary Considerations Some products may contain sodium.

Pharmacodynamics/Kinetics

Half-life Elimination IM or IV: Neonates: 3 to 5 hours; Adults: 1.8 hours (IV); ~2 hours (IM) (prolonged with renal impairment)

Time to Peak Serum: IM: 0.5 to 2 hours; IV: Within 5 minutes

Pregnancy Risk Factor B

Pregnancy Considerations Cefazolin crosses the placenta.

Adverse events have not been reported in the fetus following administration of cefazolin prior to cesarean delivery.

Due to pregnancy-induced physiologic changes, some pharmacokinetic parameters of cefazolin may be altered (Allegaert 2009; Elkomy 2014; Philipson 1987). In addition to pregnancy, obesity has been found to influence the pharmacokinetics of cefazolin (Pevzner 2011; Stitely 2013; Young 2015). Dose adjustments may be required in pregnant women who are obese (ACOG 199 2018).

Cefazolin is recommended for group B streptococcus prophylaxis in pregnant patients with a nonanaphylactic penicillin allergy. It is also one of the antibiotics recommended for prophylactic use prior to cesarean delivery and may be used in certain situations prior to vaginal delivery in women at high risk for endocarditis (ACOG 199 2018; ACOG 782 2019).

Breastfeeding Considerations Cefazolin is present in breast milk.

Based on limited information, the relative infant dose (RID) of cefazolin is <1% following a single maternal dose of 2 g (Yoshioka 1979).

In general, breastfeeding is considered acceptable when the RID of a medication is <10% (Anderson 2016; Ito 2000).

The RID of cefazolin was calculated using a milk concentration of 1.51 mcg/mL, providing an estimated daily infant dose via breast milk of 0.2265 mcg/kg/day. This milk concentration was obtained 3 hours following maternal administration cefazolin 2 g IV to 20 postpartum women (Yoshioka 1979).

The manufacturer recommends that caution be exercised when administering cefazolin to breastfeeding women. In general, antibiotics that are present in breast milk may cause non-dose-related modification of bowel flora (WHO 2002).

Dosage Forms: US

Solution, Intravenous [preservative free]:

Generic: 1 g/50 mL in Dextrose 4% (50 mL); 2 g/100 mL in Dextrose 4% (100 mL)

Solution Reconstituted, Injection:

Generic: 10 g (1 ea)

Solution Reconstituted, Injection [preservative free]:

Generic: 500 mg (1 ea); 1 g (1 ea); 10 g (1 ea); 100 g (1 ea); 300 g (1 ea)

Solution Reconstituted, Intravenous [preservative free]:

Generic: 1 g (1 ea); 1 g and Dextrose 4% (1 ea); 2 g and Dextrose 3% (1 ea)

Dosage Forms: Canada

Solution Reconstituted, Injection:

Generic: 500 mg (1 ea); 1 g (1 ea); 10 g (1 ea); 20 g (1 ea); 100 g (1 ea)

◆ **Cefazolin Sodium** *see* CeFAZolin *on page 301*

Cefdinir (SEF di ner)

Brand Names: Canada Omnicef

Pharmacologic Category Antibiotic, Cephalosporin (Third Generation)

Use

Chronic obstructive pulmonary disease, acute exacerbation: Treatment of acute exacerbations of chronic bronchitis in adults and adolescents caused by *Haemophilus influenzae* (including beta-lactamase-producing strains), *Haemophilus parainfluenzae* (including beta-lactamase-producing strains), *Streptococcus pneumoniae* (penicillin-susceptible strains only), and *Moraxella catarrhalis* (including beta-lactamase-producing strains)

Otitis media, acute: Treatment of acute bacterial otitis media in pediatric patients caused by *H. influenzae* (including beta-lactamase-producing strains), *S. pneumoniae* (penicillin-susceptible strains only), and *M. catarrhalis* (including beta-lactamase-producing strains)

Pneumonia, community-acquired: Treatment of community-acquired pneumonia in adults and adolescents caused by *H. influenzae* (including beta-lactamase-producing strains), *H. parainfluenzae* (including beta-lactamase-producing strains), *S. pneumoniae* (penicillin-susceptible strains only), and *M. catarrhalis* (including beta-lactamase-producing strains)

Sinusitis, acute: Treatment of acute maxillary sinusitis in adults and adolescents caused by *H. influenzae* (including beta-lactamase-producing strains), *S. pneumoniae* (penicillin-susceptible strains only), and *M. catarrhalis* (including beta-lactamase-producing strains). **Note:** Limitations of use: According to the IDSA guidelines for acute bacterial rhinosinusitis, cefdinir is no longer recommended as monotherapy for initial empiric treatment (IDSA [Chow 2012]).

Skin and skin structure infections, uncomplicated: Treatment of uncomplicated skin and skin structure infections in adults, adolescents, and pediatric patients caused by *Staphylococcus aureus* (including beta-lactamase-producing strains) and *Streptococcus pyogenes*

Streptococcal pharyngitis (group A): Treatment of pharyngitis/tonsillitis in adults, adolescents, and pediatric patients caused by *S. pyogenes*

Local Anesthetic/Vasoconstrictor Precautions No information available to require special precautions

Effects on Dental Treatment Key adverse event(s) related to dental treatment: Rare occurrences of stomatitis, candidiasis, erythema multiforme, Stevens-Johnson syndrome, facial edema, and xerostomia have been reported.

Effects on Bleeding No information available to require special precautions

Adverse Reactions

>10%: Gastrointestinal: Diarrhea (8% to 15%)

1% to 10%:

Central nervous system: Headache (2%)

Dermatologic: Skin rash (≤3%)

Endocrine & metabolic: Decreased serum bicarbonate (≤1%), glycosuria (≤1%), hyperglycemia (≤1%), hyperphosphatemia (≤1%), increased gamma-glutamyl transferase (≤1%), increased lactate dehydrogenase (≤1%)

Gastrointestinal: Nausea (≤3%), abdominal pain (≤1%), vomiting (≤1%)

Genitourinary: Vulvovaginal candidiasis (≤4%), urine abnormality (increased leukocytes: ≤2%), proteinuria (1% to 2%), occult blood in urine (≤1%), vaginitis (≤1%)

Hematologic & oncologic: Lymphocytosis (≤2%), eosinophilia (1%), lymphocytopenia (1%), abnormal neutrophils (functional disorder of polymorphonuclear neutrophils: ≤1%), thrombocythemia (≤1%), change in WBC count (≤1%)

Hepatic: Increased serum alkaline phosphatase (≤1%), increased serum ALT (≤1%)

Renal: Increased urine pH (≤1%), increased urine specific gravity (≤1%)

<1%, postmarketing, and/or case reports: Abnormal stools, anaphylaxis, anorexia, asthma, blood coagulation disorder, bloody diarrhea, candidiasis, cardiac failure, chest pain, cholestasis, conjunctivitis, constipation, cutaneous candidiasis, decreased hemoglobin, decreased urine specific gravity, disseminated intravascular coagulation, dizziness, drowsiness, dyspepsia, enterocolitis (acute), eosinophilic pneumonitis, erythema multiforme, erythema nodosum, exfoliative dermatitis, facial edema, fever, flatulence, fulminant hepatitis, granulocytopenia, hemolytic anemia, hemorrhagic colitis, hemorrhagic diathesis, hepatic failure, hepatitis (acute), hyperkalemia, hyperkinesia, hypersensitivity angiitis, hypertension, hypocalcemia, hypophosphatemia, immune thrombocytopenia, increased amylase, increased blood urea nitrogen, increased monocytes, increased serum AST, increased serum bilirubin, insomnia, interstitial pneumonitis (idiopathic), intestinal obstruction, involuntary body movements, jaundice, laryngeal edema, leukopenia, leukorrhea, loss of consciousness, maculopapular rash, melena, myocardial infarction, pancytopenia, peptic ulcer, pneumonia (drug-induced), pruritus, pseudomembranous colitis, renal disease, renal failure (acute), respiratory failure (acute), rhabdomyolysis, serum sickness, shock, Stevens-Johnson syndrome, stomatitis, thrombocytopenia, toxic epidermal necrolysis, upper gastrointestinal hemorrhage, weakness, xerostomia

Mechanism of Action Inhibits bacterial cell wall synthesis by binding to one or more of the penicillin-binding proteins (PBPs) which in turn inhibits the final transpeptidation step of peptidoglycan synthesis in bacterial cell walls, thus inhibiting cell wall biosynthesis. Bacteria eventually lyse due to ongoing activity of cell wall autolytic enzymes (autolysins and murein hydrolases) while cell wall assembly is arrested.

Pharmacodynamics/Kinetics

Half-life Elimination 1.7 (± 0.6) hours with normal renal function

Time to Peak 2 to 4 hours

Pregnancy Risk Factor B

Pregnancy Considerations

An increase in most types of birth defects was not found following first trimester exposure to cephalosporins.

Cefditoren (sef de TOR en)

Related Information

Bacterial Infections *on page* 1739

Brand Names: US Spectracef

Pharmacologic Category Antibiotic, Cephalosporin (Third Generation)

Use Treatment of acute bacterial exacerbation of chronic bronchitis or community-acquired pneumonia (due to susceptible organisms including *Haemophilus influenzae, Haemophilus parainfluenzae, Streptococcus pneumoniae*-penicillin susceptible only, *Moraxella catarrhalis*); pharyngitis or tonsillitis (*Streptococcus pyogenes*); and uncomplicated skin and skin-structure infections (*Staphylococcus aureus* - not MRSA, *Streptococcus pyogenes*)

Local Anesthetic/Vasoconstrictor Precautions No information available to require special precautions

Effects on Dental Treatment No significant effects or complications reported

Effects on Bleeding No information available to require special precautions

Adverse Reactions

>10%: Gastrointestinal: Diarrhea (11% to 15%)

1% to 10%:

Endocrine & metabolic: Increased serum glucose (1% to 2%)

Gastrointestinal: Nausea (4% to 6%), abdominal pain (2%), dyspepsia (1% to 2%), vomiting (1%)
Genitourinary: Vulvovaginal candidiasis (3% to 6%), hematuria (3%), urine abnormality (increased leukocytes: 2%)
Hematologic & oncologic: Decreased hematocrit (2%)
Nervous system: Headache (2% to 3%)

<1%, postmarketing, and/or case reports: Abnormal dreams, acute renal failure, decreased serum albumin, anorexia, arthralgia, asthma, change in WBC count (decrease or increase), coagulation time increased, constipation, decreased hemoglobin, decreased neutrophils, decreased serum calcium, decreased serum sodium, diaphoresis, dizziness, drowsiness, dysgeusia, eosinophilic pneumonitis, eosinophilia, eructation, erythema multiforme, facial edema, fever, flatulence, fungal infection, gastritis, gastrointestinal disease, hyperglycemia, hypersensitivity reaction, hypochloremia, hypoglycemia (Kennedy 2019), hypophosphatemia, increased appetite, increased blood urea nitrogen, increased serum ALT, increased serum AST, increased serum cholesterol, increased serum potassium, increased thirst, insomnia, interstitial pneumonitis, leukopenia, leukorrhea, lymphocytosis, myalgia, nervousness, oral candidiasis, oral mucosa ulcer, pain, peripheral edema, pharyngitis, positive direct Coombs test, pseudomembranous colitis, proteinuria, pruritus, rhinitis, sinusitis, skin rash, Stevens-Johnson syndrome, stomatitis, thrombocythemia, thrombocytopenia, toxic epidermal necrolysis, urinary frequency, urticaria, vaginitis, weakness, weight loss, xerostomia

Mechanism of Action Inhibits bacterial cell wall synthesis by binding to one or more of the penicillin-binding proteins (PBPs) which in turn inhibits the final transpeptidation step of peptidoglycan synthesis in bacterial cell walls, thus inhibiting cell wall biosynthesis. Bacteria eventually lyse due to ongoing activity of cell wall autolytic enzymes (autolysins and murein hydrolases) while cell wall assembly is arrested.

Pharmacodynamics/Kinetics

Half-life Elimination 1.6 ± 0.4 hours; increased with moderate (2.7 hours) and severe (4.7 hours) renal impairment

Time to Peak 1.5 to 3 hours

Pregnancy Risk Factor B

Pregnancy Considerations

An increase in most types of birth defects was not found following first trimester exposure to cephalosporins.

◆ **Cefditoren Pivoxil** *see* Cefditoren *on page 306*

Cefepime (SEF e pim)

Brand Names: US Maxipime [DSC]

Brand Names: Canada APO-Cefepime

Pharmacologic Category Antibiotic, Cephalosporin (Fourth Generation)

Use

Intra-abdominal infection: Treatment, in combination with metronidazole, of complicated intra-abdominal infections caused by *Escherichia coli*, viridans group streptococci, *Pseudomonas aeruginosa*, *Klebsiella pneumoniae*, *Enterobacter* species, or *Bacteroides fragilis*.

Neutropenic fever: Empiric treatment of febrile neutropenic patients.

Pneumonia (moderate to severe): Treatment of moderate to severe pneumonia caused by *Streptococcus pneumoniae*, including cases associated with concurrent bacteremia, *P. aeruginosa*, *K. pneumoniae*, or *Enterobacter* species.

Skin and soft tissue infection: Treatment of moderate to severe skin and soft tissue infections caused by *Staphylococcus aureus* (methicillin-susceptible isolates only) or *Streptococcus pyogenes*.

Urinary tract infection, including pyelonephritis: Treatment of urinary tract infections, including pyelonephritis, caused by *E. coli*, *K. pneumoniae*, or *Proteus mirabilis*, including cases associated with concurrent bacteremia with these microorganisms.

Local Anesthetic/Vasoconstrictor Precautions No information available to require special precautions

Effects on Dental Treatment Key adverse event(s) related to dental treatment: Rare occurrence of oral candidiasis.

Effects on Bleeding No information available to require special precautions

Adverse Reactions

>10%: Hematologic & oncologic: Positive direct Coombs test (without hemolysis; 16%)

1% to 10%:
Cardiovascular: Localized phlebitis (1%)
Central nervous system: Headache (≤1%)
Dermatologic: Skin rash (1% to 4%), pruritus (≤1%)
Endocrine & metabolic: Hypophosphatemia (3%)
Gastrointestinal: Diarrhea (≤3%), nausea (≤2%), vomiting (≤1%)
Hematologic & oncologic: Eosinophilia (2%)
Hepatic: Increased serum ALT (3%), abnormal partial thromboplastin time (2%), increased serum AST (2%), abnormal prothrombin time (1%)
Hypersensitivity: Hypersensitivity (in patients with a history of penicillin allergy: ≤10%)
Miscellaneous: Fever (≤1%)

<1%, postmarketing, and/or case reports: Agranulocytosis, anaphylactic shock, anaphylaxis, anemia, aphasia, brain disease, *Clostridioides* (formerly *Clostridium*) *difficile*-associated diarrhea, colitis, coma, confusion, decreased hematocrit, erythema, hallucination, hypercalcemia, hyperkalemia, hyperphosphatemia, hypocalcemia, increased blood urea nitrogen, increased serum alkaline phosphatase, increased serum bilirubin, increased serum creatinine, leukopenia, local inflammation, local pain, myoclonus, neurotoxicity, neutropenia, oral candidiasis, pseudomembranous colitis, seizure, status epilepticus (nonconvulsive), stupor, thrombocytopenia, urticaria, vaginitis

Mechanism of Action Inhibits bacterial cell wall synthesis by binding to one or more of the penicillin-binding proteins (PBPs) which in turn inhibits the final transpeptidation step of peptidoglycan synthesis in bacterial cell walls, thus inhibiting cell wall biosynthesis. Bacteria eventually lyse due to ongoing activity of cell wall autolytic enzymes (autolysis and murein hydrolases) while cell wall assembly is arrested.

Pharmacodynamics/Kinetics

Half-life Elimination
Neonates: 4 to 5 hours (Lima-Rogel 2008)
Children 2 months to 6 years: 1.77 to 1.96 hours
Adults: 2 hours
Hemodialysis: 13.5 hours
Continuous peritoneal dialysis: 19 hours

Time to Peak IM: 1 to 2 hours; IV: 0.5 hours

Pregnancy Considerations Cefepime crosses the placenta (Ozyuncu 2010).

An increased risk of major birth defects or other adverse fetal or maternal outcomes has generally not been observed following use of cephalosporin antibiotics during pregnancy.

When an antibiotic is needed for the treatment of maternal infection, cefepime can be considered. However, other, more well-studied cephalosporins are preferred for use in pregnancy (Betschart 2020; ERS/TSANZ [Middleton 2020]; Panchaud 2016).

◆ **Cefepime HCl** *see* Cefepime *on page 307*
◆ **Cefepime HCl/D5W** *see* Cefepime *on page 307*
◆ **Cefepime Hydrochloride** *see* Cefepime *on page 307*

Cefiderocol (SEF i DER oh kol)

Brand Names: US Fetroja

Pharmacologic Category Antibiotic, Cephalosporin

Use Urinary tract infection, complicated (including pyelonephritis): Treatment of complicated urinary tract infections, including pyelonephritis, caused by the following susceptible gram-negative microorganisms: *Escherichia coli, Klebsiella pneumoniae, Proteus mirabilis, Pseudomonas aeruginosa*, and *Enterobacter cloacae* complex, in patients ≥18 years of age who have limited or no alternative treatment options.

Local Anesthetic/Vasoconstrictor Precautions No information available to require special precautions

Effects on Dental Treatment Key adverse event(s) related to dental treatment: Occurrence of taste alteration, stomatitis, candidiasis, xerostomia

Effects on Bleeding Increased INR (prolonged prothrombin times), thrombocythemia have been reported

Adverse Reactions

1% to 10%:

Cardiovascular: Atrial fibrillation (<2%), bradycardia (<2%), cardiac failure (<2%), peripheral edema (<2%)

Central nervous system: Headache (2%), insomnia (<2%), restlessness (<2%), seizure (<2%)

Dermatologic: Skin rash (3%), pruritus (<2%)

Endocrine & metabolic: Hypokalemia (2%), hypervolemia (<2%), hypocalcemia (<2%)

Gastrointestinal: Diarrhea (4%), constipation (3%), nausea (2%), vomiting (2%), abdominal pain (<2%), biliary colic (<2%), cholecystitis (<2%), cholelithiasis (<2%), *Clostridioides difficile* associated diarrhea (<2%), decreased appetite (<2%), dysgeusia (<2%), stomatitis (<2%), xerostomia (<2%)

Genitourinary: Finding of blood in urine (<2%)

Hematologic & oncologic: Increased INR (<2%), prolonged prothrombin time (<2%), thrombocythemia (<2%)

Hepatic: Increased liver enzymes (2%)

Hypersensitivity: Drug-induced hypersensitivity reaction (<2%)

Infection: Candidiasis (2%)

Local: Infusion site reaction (4%)

Neuromuscular & skeletal: Increased creatine phosphokinase in blood specimen (<2%)

Respiratory: Cough (2%), dyspnea (<2%), pleural effusion (<2%)

Miscellaneous: Fever (<2%)

Mechanism of Action Cefiderocol is a siderophore cephalosporin. A catechol side chain promotes formation of chelated complexes with ferric iron, allowing use of iron transport systems to deliver cefiderocol across the outer membrane of gram-negative bacilli. The cephalosporin moiety binds to penicillin-binding proteins which in turn inhibits the final transpeptidation step of peptidoglycan synthesis in bacterial cell walls, thus inhibiting cell wall biosynthesis.

Pharmacodynamics/Kinetics

Half-life Elimination 2 to 3 hours.

Pregnancy Considerations

In general, an increase in most types of birth defects or adverse maternal or fetal outcomes was not found following exposure to cephalosporins.

◆ **Cefiderocol Sulfate Tosylate** *see* Cefiderocol *on page 308*

Cefixime (sef IKS eem)

Related Information

Sexually-Transmitted Diseases *on page 1707*

Brand Names: US Suprax

Brand Names: Canada Auro-Cefixime; Suprax

Pharmacologic Category Antibiotic, Cephalosporin (Third Generation)

Use

Treatment of uncomplicated urinary tract infections (due to *Escherichia coli* and *Proteus mirabilis*), otitis media (due to *Haemophilus influenzae, Moraxella catarrhalis,* and *Streptococcus pyogenes*), pharyngitis and tonsillitis (due to *Streptococcus pyogenes*), acute exacerbations of chronic bronchitis (due to *Streptococcus pneumoniae* and *Haemophilus influenzae*); uncomplicated cervical/urethral gonorrhea (due to *N. gonorrhoeae* [penicillinase- and nonpenicillinase-producing])

Note: Due to concerns of resistance, the CDC no longer recommends use of cefixime as a first-line regimen in the treatment of uncomplicated gonorrhea in the US; ceftriaxone is the preferred cephalosporin in combination with azithromycin (CDC 2012; CDC [Workowski 2015]).

Local Anesthetic/Vasoconstrictor Precautions No information available to require special precautions

Effects on Dental Treatment No significant effects or complications reported

Effects on Bleeding No information available to require special precautions

Adverse Reactions

>10%: Gastrointestinal: Diarrhea (16%)

2% to 10%: Gastrointestinal: Abdominal pain, nausea, dyspepsia, flatulence, loose stools

<2%: Acute renal failure, anaphylactoid reaction, anaphylaxis, angioedema, candidiasis, dizziness, drug fever, eosinophilia, erythema multiforme, facial edema, fever, headache, hepatitis, hyperbilirubinemia, increased blood urea nitrogen, increased serum creatinine, increased serum transaminases, jaundice, leukopenia, neutropenia, prolonged prothrombin time, pruritus, pseudomembranous colitis, seizure, serum sickness-like reaction, skin rash, Stevens-Johnson syndrome, thrombocytopenia, toxic epidermal necrolysis, urticaria, vaginitis, vomiting

Mechanism of Action Inhibits bacterial cell wall synthesis by binding to one or more of the penicillin-binding proteins (PBPs); which in turn inhibits the final transpeptidation step of peptidoglycan synthesis in bacterial cell walls, thus inhibiting cell wall biosynthesis. Bacteria eventually lyse due to ongoing activity of cell wall autolytic enzymes (autolysins and murein hydrolases) while cell wall assembly is arrested.

Pharmacodynamics/Kinetics

Half-life Elimination Normal renal function: 3 to 4 hours; Moderate impairment (CrCl 20 to 40 mL/minute): 6.4 hours; Renal failure: Up to 11.5 hours

Time to Peak Serum: Suspension: 2 to 6 hours; Capsule: 3 to 8 hours; Delayed with food

Pregnancy Considerations

Cefixime crosses the placenta and can be detected in the amniotic fluid (Ozyüncü 2010).

An increased risk of major birth defects or other adverse fetal or maternal outcomes has generally not been observed following use of cephalosporin antibiotics.

◆ **Cefixime Trihydrate** *see* Cefixime *on page 308*

◆ **Cefotan** *see* CefoTEtan *on page 310*

Cefotaxime (sef oh TAKS eem)

Brand Names: US Claforan [DSC]

Brand Names: Canada Claforan [DSC]

Pharmacologic Category Antibiotic, Cephalosporin (Third Generation)

Use

Bacteremia/Septicemia: Treatment of bacteremia/septicemia caused by *Escherichia coli*, *Klebsiella* species, and *Serratia marcescens*, *Staphylococcus aureus* and *Streptococcus* species (including *Streptococcus pneumoniae*).

Bone or joint infections: Treatment of bone or joint infections caused by *S. aureus* (penicillinase and nonpenicillinase producing strains), *Streptococcus* species (including *Streptococcus pyogenes*), and *Proteus mirabilis*.

CNS infections: Treatment of CNS infections (eg, meningitis, ventriculitis) caused by *Neisseria meningitidis*, *Haemophilus influenzae*, *S. pneumoniae*, *Klebsiella pneumoniae*, and *E. coli*.

Genitourinary infections: Treatment of genitourinary infections, including urinary tract infections (UTIs), caused by *Staphylococcus epidermidis*, *S. aureus* (penicillinase and nonpenicillinase producing), *Citrobacter* species, *Enterobacter* species, *E. coli*, *Klebsiella* species, *P. mirabilis*, *Proteus vulgaris*, *Providencia stuartii*, *Morganella morganii*, *Providencia rettgeri*, and *S. marcescens*

Gynecologic infections: Treatment of gynecologic infections, including pelvic inflammatory disease, endometritis, and pelvic cellulitis, caused by *S. epidermidis*, *Streptococcus* species, *Enterobacter* species, *Klebsiella* species, *E. coli*, *P. mirabilis*, *Bacteroides* species (including *Bacteroides fragilis*), *Clostridium* species, and anaerobic cocci (including *Peptostreptococcus* and *Peptococcus* species) and *Fusobacterium* species (including *Fusobacterium nucleatum*).

Intraabdominal infections: Treatment of intraabdominal infections, including peritonitis caused by *Streptococcus* species, *E. coli*, *Klebsiella* species, *Bacteroides* species, and anaerobic cocci (including *Peptostreptococcus* species and *Peptococcus* species), *P. mirabilis*, and *Clostridium* species.

Lower respiratory tract infections: Treatment of lower respiratory tract infections, including pneumonia, caused by *S. pneumoniae*, *S. pyogenes* (group A streptococci) and other streptococci (excluding enterococci, [eg, *Enterococcus faecalis*]), *S. aureus* (penicillinase and nonpenicillinase producing), *E. coli*, *Klebsiella* species, *H. influenzae* (including ampicillin-resistant strains), *H. parainfluenzae*, *P. mirabilis*, *S. marcescens*, *Enterobacter* species, and indole-positive *Proteus*

Skin and skin structure infections: Treatment of skin and skin structure infections caused by *S. aureus* (penicillinase and nonpenicillinase producing), *S. epidermidis*, *S. pyogenes* (group A streptococci) and other streptococci, *Acinetobacter* species, *E. coli*, *Citrobacter* species (including *Citrobacter freundii*), *Enterobacter* species, *Klebsiella* species, *P. mirabilis*, *P. vulgaris*, *M. morganii*, *P. rettgeri*, *S. marcescens*, *Bacteroides* species, and anaerobic cocci (including *Peptostreptococcus* species and *Peptococcus* species).

Surgical prophylaxis: Reduce the incidence of certain infections in patients undergoing surgical procedures (eg, abdominal or vaginal hysterectomy, GI and GU tract surgery) that may be classified as contaminated or potentially contaminated; reduce the incidence of certain postoperative infections in patients undergoing cesarean section.

Local Anesthetic/Vasoconstrictor Precautions

No information available to require special precautions

Effects on Dental Treatment No significant effects or complications reported

Effects on Bleeding No information available to require special precautions

Adverse Reactions

1% to 10%:

Dermatologic: Pruritus (≤2%), skin rash (≤2%)

Gastrointestinal: Colitis (≤1%), diarrhea (≤1%), nausea (≤1%), vomiting (≤1%)

Hematologic & oncologic: Eosinophilia (≤2%)

Local: Induration at injection site (IM ≤4%), inflammation at injection site (IV ≤4%), pain at injection site (IM ≤4%), tenderness at injection site (IM ≤4%)

Miscellaneous: Fever (≤2%)

<1%, postmarketing and/or case reports: Acute generalized exanthematous pustulosis, acute renal failure, agranulocytosis, anaphylaxis, bone marrow failure, brain disease, candidiasis, cardiac arrhythmia (after rapid IV injection via central catheter), cholestasis, *Clostridioides* (formerly *Clostridium*) *difficile*-associated diarrhea, dizziness, erythema multiforme, granulocytopenia, headache, hemolytic anemia, hepatitis, increased blood urea nitrogen, increased gamma-glutamyl transferase, increased lactate dehydrogenase, increased serum alkaline phosphatase, increased serum ALT, increased serum AST, increased serum bilirubin, increased serum creatinine, injection site phlebitis, interstitial nephritis, jaundice, leukopenia, local irritation, neutropenia, pancytopenia, positive direct Coombs test, pseudomembranous colitis, Stevens-Johnson syndrome, thrombocytopenia, toxic epidermal necrolysis, urticaria, vaginitis

Mechanism of Action Inhibits bacterial cell wall synthesis by binding to one or more of the penicillin-binding proteins (PBPs) which in turn inhibits the final transpeptidation step of peptidoglycan synthesis in bacterial cell walls, thus inhibiting cell wall biosynthesis. Bacteria eventually lyse due to ongoing activity of cell wall autolytic enzymes (autolysins and murein hydrolases) while cell wall assembly is arrested. Cefotaxime has activity in the presence of some beta-lactamases, both penicillinases and cephalosporinases, of gram-negative and gram-positive bacteria. *Enterococcus* species may be intrinsically resistant to cefotaxime. Most extended-spectrum beta-lactamase (ESBL)-producing and carbapenemase-producing isolates are resistant to cefotaxime.

Pharmacodynamics/Kinetics

Half-life Elimination

Cefotaxime: Infants ≤1500 g: 4.6 hours; Infants >1500 g: 3.4 hours; Children: 1.5 hours; Adults: 1 to 1.5 hours; prolonged with renal and/or hepatic impairment

Desacetylcefotaxime: 1.3 to 1.9 hours; prolonged with renal impairment (Ings 1982)

Time to Peak Serum: IM: Within 30 minutes

Pregnancy Risk Factor B

Pregnancy Considerations Cefotaxime crosses the human placenta.

Cefotaxime is approved for use in women undergoing cesarean section (consult current guidelines for appropriate use).

◆ **Cefotaxime Sodium** *see* Cefotaxime *on page 309*

CefoTEtan (SEF oh tee tan)

Brand Names: US Cefotan

Pharmacologic Category Antibiotic, Cephalosporin (Second Generation)

Use

Bone and joint infections: Treatment of bone and joint infections caused by *Staphylococcus aureus*.

Gynecologic infections: Treatment of gynecologic infections caused by *S. aureus*, (including penicillinase- and non-penicillinase-producing strains), *Staphylococcus epidermidis, Streptococcus* spp. (excluding enterococci), *Streptococcus agalactiae, Escherichia coli, Proteus mirabilis, Neisseria gonorrhoeae, Bacteroides* spp. (excluding *Bacteroides distasonis, Bacteroides ovatus, Bacteroides thetaiotaomicron*), *Fusobacterium* spp., and gram-positive anaerobic cocci (including *Peptococcus* and *Peptostreptococcus* spp.).

Limitations of use: Cefotetan has no activity against *Chlamydia (Chlamydophila) trachomatis*. When treating pelvic inflammatory disease, add appropriate antichlamydial coverage.

Lower respiratory tract infections: Treatment of lower respiratory tract infections caused by *Streptococcus pneumoniae, S. aureus* (penicillinase- and non-penicillinase-producing strains), *Haemophilus influenzae* (including ampicillin-resistant strains), *Klebsiella* spp. (including *K. pneumoniae*), *E. coli, P. mirabilis*, and *Serratia marcescens*.

Serious infections: Treatment of confirmed or suspected gram-positive or gram-negative sepsis or in patients with other serious infections (often administered with concomitant aminoglycosides).

Skin and skin structure infections: Treatment of skin and skin structure infections due to *S. aureus* (penicillinase- and non-penicillinase-producing strains), *Staphylococcus epidermidis, Streptococcus pyogenes, Streptococcus* spp. (excluding enterococci), *E. coli, K. pneumoniae, Peptococcus niger, Peptostreptococcus* spp.

Surgical (perioperative) prophylaxis: Preoperative administration in surgical procedures that are classified as clean contaminated or potentially contaminated (eg, cesarean section, abdominal or vaginal hysterectomy, transurethral surgery, biliary tract surgery, GI surgery).

Urinary tract infections: Treatment of urinary tract infections caused by *E. coli, Klebsiella* spp. (including *K. pneumoniae*), *P. mirabilis* and *Proteus* spp. (which may include the organisms now called *Proteus vulgaris, Providencia rettgeri*, and *Morganella morganii*).

Local Anesthetic/Vasoconstrictor Precautions No information available to require special precautions

Effects on Dental Treatment No significant effects or complications reported

Effects on Bleeding May potentiate the anticoagulant effects of vitamin K anticoagulants (ie, warfarin) due to alterations of gut flora. Cefotetan may have additional hypoprothrombinemic activity.

Adverse Reactions

1% to 10%:

Gastrointestinal: Diarrhea (1%)

Hepatic: Increased serum transaminases (1%)

Hypersensitivity: Hypersensitivity reaction (1%)

<1%, postmarketing, and/or case reports: Agranulocytosis, anaphylaxis, eosinophilia, fever, hemolytic anemia, hemorrhage, increased blood urea nitrogen, increased serum creatinine, leukopenia, nausea, nephrotoxicity, phlebitis, prolonged prothrombin time, pruritus, pseudomembranous colitis, skin rash, thrombocythemia, thrombocytopenia, urticaria, vomiting

Mechanism of Action Inhibits bacterial cell wall synthesis by binding to one or more of the penicillin-binding proteins (PBPs) which in turn inhibits the final transpeptidation step of peptidoglycan synthesis in bacterial cell walls, thus inhibiting cell wall biosynthesis. Bacteria eventually lyse due to ongoing activity of cell wall autolytic enzymes (autolysins and murein hydrolases) while cell wall assembly is arrested.

Pharmacodynamics/Kinetics

Half-life Elimination 3 to 4.6 hours, prolonged in patients with moderately impaired renal function (up to 10 hours)

Time to Peak Serum: IM: 1 to 3 hours

Pregnancy Risk Factor B

Pregnancy Considerations

Cefotetan crosses the placenta and produces therapeutic concentrations in the amniotic fluid and cord serum. Cefotetan is one of the antibiotics recommended for prophylactic use prior to cesarean delivery.

◆ **Cefotetan Disodium** *see* CefoTEtan *on page 310*

CefOXitin (se FOKS i tin)

Pharmacologic Category Antibiotic, Cephalosporin (Second Generation)

Use

Bacteremia/sepsis: Treatment of bacteremia/sepsis caused by *Streptococcus pneumoniae, Staphylococcus aureus* (including penicillinase-producing strains), *Escherichia coli, Klebsiella* species, and *Bacteroides* species including *B. fragilis*.

Bone and joint infections: Treatment of bone and joint infections caused by *S. aureus* (including penicillinase-producing strains).

Gynecological infections: Treatment of endometritis, pelvic cellulitis, and pelvic inflammatory disease caused by *E. coli, Neisseria gonorrhoeae* (including penicillinase-producing strains), *Bacteroides* species including *Bacteroides fragilis, Clostridium* species, *P. niger, Peptostreptococcus* species, and *Streptococcus agalactiae*.

Limitations of use: Cefoxitin does not have activity against *Chlamydia trachomatis*. When cefoxitin is used to treat pelvic inflammatory disease, add appropriate antichlamydial coverage.

Lower respiratory tract infections: Treatment of pneumonia and lung abscess, caused by *S. pneumoniae*, other streptococci (excluding enterococci; eg, *Enterococcus faecalis* [formerly *Streptococcus faecalis*]), *S. aureus* (including penicillinase-producing strains), *E. coli*, *Klebsiella* species, *Haemophilus influenzae*, and *Bacteroides* species.

Septicemia: Treatment of septicemia caused by *S. pneumoniae*, *S. aureus* (including penicillinase-producing strains), *E. coli*, *Klebsiella* species, and *Bacteroides* species including *B. fragilis*.

Skin and skin structure infections: Treatment of skin and skin structure infections caused by *S. aureus* (including penicillinase-producing strains), *Staphylococcus epidermidis*, *Streptococcus pyogenes* and other streptococci (excluding enterococci [eg, *E. faecalis*] [formerly *S. faecalis*]), *E. coli*, *Proteus mirabilis*, *Klebsiella* species, *Bacteroides* species including *B. fragilis*, *Clostridium* species, *P. niger*, and *Peptostreptococcus* species.

Urinary tract infections: Treatment of UTIs caused by *E. coli*, *Klebsiella* species, *P. mirabilis*, *Morganella morganii*, *Proteus vulgaris*, and *Providencia* species (including *Providencia rettgeri*).

Local Anesthetic/Vasoconstrictor Precautions No information available to require special precautions

Effects on Dental Treatment No significant effects or complications reported

Effects on Bleeding May potentiate the anticoagulant effects of vitamin K anticoagulants (ie, warfarin) due to alterations of gut flora.

Adverse Reactions

1% to 10%: Gastrointestinal: Diarrhea

<1%: Anaphylaxis, angioedema, bone marrow depression, dyspnea, eosinophilia, exacerbation of myasthenia gravis, exfoliative dermatitis, fever, hemolytic anemia, hypotension, increased blood urea nitrogen, increased serum creatinine, increased serum transaminases, interstitial nephritis, jaundice, leukopenia, nausea, nephrotoxicity (increased; with aminoglycosides), phlebitis, prolonged prothrombin time, pruritus, pseudomembranous colitis, skin rash, thrombocytopenia, thrombophlebitis, toxic epidermal necrolysis, urticaria, vomiting

Mechanism of Action Inhibits bacterial cell wall synthesis by binding to one or more of the penicillin-binding proteins (PBPs) which in turn inhibits the final transpeptidation step of peptidoglycan synthesis in bacterial cell walls, thus inhibiting cell wall biosynthesis. Bacteria eventually lyse due to ongoing activity of cell wall autolytic enzymes (autolysins and murein hydrolases) while cell wall assembly is arrested.

Pharmacodynamics/Kinetics

Half-life Elimination Neonates and Infants (PNA: 10-53 days): 1.4 hours (Regazzi 1983); Adults: 41-59 minutes; prolonged with renal impairment

Time to Peak Serum: IM: Within 20-30 minutes

Pregnancy Considerations

Cefoxitin crosses the placenta and reaches the cord serum and amniotic fluid.

An increased risk of major birth defects or other adverse fetal or maternal outcomes has generally not been observed following use of cephalosporin antibiotics, including cefoxitin, during pregnancy.

Cefoxitin is one of the antibiotics recommended for prophylactic use prior to cesarean delivery (ACOG 199 2018).

◆ **Cefoxitin Sodium** *see* CefOXitin *on page 310*

◆ **Cefoxitin Sodium/D5W** *see* CefOXitin *on page 310*

Cefpodoxime (sef pode OKS eem)

Pharmacologic Category Antibiotic, Cephalosporin (Third Generation)

Use

Chronic obstructive pulmonary disease, acute exacerbation: Treatment of acute bacterial exacerbation of chronic obstructive pulmonary disease caused by *Streptococcus pneumoniae*, *Haemophilus influenzae* (non-beta-lactamase-producing strains only), or *Moraxella catarrhalis*.

Cystitis, acute uncomplicated: Treatment of acute uncomplicated cystitis caused by *Escherichia coli*, *Klebsiella pneumoniae*, *Proteus mirabilis*, or *Staphylococcus saprophyticus*.

Otitis media, acute: Treatment of acute otitis media caused by *S. pneumoniae* (excluding penicillin-resistant strains), *Streptococcus pyogenes*, *H. influenzae* (including beta-lactamase-producing strains), or *M. catarrhalis* (including beta-lactamase-producing strains).

Pneumonia, community-acquired: Treatment of community-acquired pneumonia caused by *S. pneumoniae* or *H. influenzae* (including beta-lactamase-producing strains).

Rhinosinusitis, acute bacterial: Treatment of acute bacterial rhinosinusitis caused by *H. influenzae* (including beta-lactamase-producing strains), *S. pneumoniae*, and *M. catarrhalis*. **Note:** According to the Infectious Diseases Society of America guidelines for acute bacterial rhinosinusitis, cefpodoxime is recommended in combination with clindamycin due to concern for pneumococcal resistance (IDSA [Chow 2012]).

Skin and soft tissue infection: Treatment of uncomplicated skin and soft tissue infection caused by *Staphylococcus aureus* (including penicillinase-producing strains) or *S. pyogenes*.

Streptococcal pharyngitis (group A) : Treatment of pharyngitis or tonsillitis caused by *S. pyogenes*.

Local Anesthetic/Vasoconstrictor Precautions No information available to require special precautions

Effects on Dental Treatment No significant effects or complications reported

Effects on Bleeding No information available to require special precautions

Adverse Reactions

>10%:

Dermatologic: Diaper rash (12%)

Gastrointestinal: Diarrhea (infants and toddlers 15%)

1% to 10%:

Central nervous system: Headache (1%)

Dermatologic: Skin rash (1%)

Gastrointestinal: Diarrhea (7%), nausea (4%), abdominal pain (2%), vomiting (1% to 2%)

Genitourinary: Vaginal infection (3%)

<1%: Anaphylaxis, anxiety, chest pain, cough, decreased appetite, dizziness, dysgeusia, epistaxis, eye pruritus, fatigue, fever, flatulence, flushing, fungal skin infection, hypotension, insomnia, malaise, nightmares, pruritus, pseudomembranous colitis, purpuric nephritis, tinnitus, vulvovaginal candidiasis, weakness, xerostomia

Mechanism of Action Inhibits bacterial cell wall synthesis by binding to one or more of the penicillin-binding proteins (PBPs) which in turn inhibits the final transpeptidation step of peptidoglycan synthesis in bacterial cell walls, thus inhibiting cell wall biosynthesis. Bacteria eventually lyse due to ongoing activity of cell wall autolytic enzymes (autolysins and murein hydrolases) while cell wall assembly is arrested.

Pharmacodynamics/Kinetics

Half-life Elimination ~2 to 3 hours; prolonged with renal impairment (~10 hours for CrCl <30 mL/minute)

Time to Peak Tablets: Within 2 to 3 hours; Oral suspension: Slower in presence of food, 48% increase in T_{max}

Pregnancy Risk Factor B

Pregnancy Considerations

Adverse events were not observed in animal reproduction studies.

◆ **Cefpodoxime Proxetil** *see* Cefpodoxime *on page 311*

Cefprozil (sef PROE zil)

Related Information

Antibiotic Prophylaxis *on page 1715*

Brand Names: Canada APO-Cefprozil; Auro-Cefprozil; Cefzil [DSC]; SANDOZ Cefprozil; TARO-Cefprozil

Pharmacologic Category Antibiotic, Cephalosporin (Second Generation)

Use

Acute bacterial exacerbation of chronic bronchitis: Treatment of mild to moderate acute bacterial exacerbations of chronic bronchitis caused by *S. pneumoniae*, *H. influenzae* (including beta-lactamase-producing strains), and *M. catarrhalis* (including beta-lactamase-producing strains).

Otitis media: Treatment of mild to moderate otitis media caused by *S. pneumoniae*, *Haemophilus influenzae* (including beta-lactamase-producing strains), and *Moraxella (Branhamella) catarrhalis* (including beta-lactamase-producing strains).

Pharyngitis/tonsillitis: Treatment of mild to moderate pharyngitis/tonsillitis caused by *Streptococcus pyogenes*.

Limitations of use: Cefprozil is generally effective in the eradication of *S. pyogenes* from the nasopharynx; however, substantial data establishing the efficacy of cefprozil in the subsequent prevention of rheumatic fever are not available at present.

Skin and skin-structure infections, uncomplicated: Treatment of mild to moderate uncomplicated skin and skin-structure infections caused by *Staphylococcus aureus* (including penicillinase-producing strains) and *S. pyogenes*.

Local Anesthetic/Vasoconstrictor Precautions No information available to require special precautions

Effects on Dental Treatment No significant effects or complications reported

Effects on Bleeding No information available to require special precautions

Adverse Reactions Frequency not always defined.

1% to 10%:

Central nervous system: Dizziness (1%)

Dermatologic: Diaper rash (2%), genital pruritus (2%)

Gastrointestinal: Nausea (4%), diarrhea (3%), abdominal pain (1%), vomiting (1%)

Genitourinary: Vaginitis

Hepatic: Increased serum transaminases (2%)

Infection: Superinfection

<1%, postmarketing, and/or case reports: Anaphylaxis, angioedema, arthralgia, cholestatic jaundice, confusion, drowsiness, eosinophilia, erythema multiforme, fever, headache, hyperactivity, increased blood urea nitrogen, increased serum creatinine, insomnia, leukopenia, pseudomembranous colitis, serum sickness, skin rash, Stevens-Johnson syndrome, thrombocytopenia, urticaria

Mechanism of Action Inhibits bacterial cell wall synthesis by binding to one or more of the penicillin-binding proteins (PBPs) which in turn inhibits the final transpeptidation step of peptidoglycan synthesis in bacterial cell walls, thus inhibiting cell wall biosynthesis. Bacteria eventually lyse due to ongoing activity of cell wall autolytic enzymes (autolysins and murein hydrolases) while cell wall assembly is arrested.

Pharmacodynamics/Kinetics

Half-life Elimination

Infants ≥6 months and Children: 1.5 hours.

Adults:

Normal: 1.3 hours.

Kidney impairment: Up to 5.2 hours (dependent upon degree of kidney impairment).

Kidney failure: Up to 5.9 hours.

Hepatic impairment: ~2 hours.

Time to Peak

Serum:

Infants ≥6 months and Children: 1 to 2 hours.

Adult: Fasting: 1.5 hours.

Pregnancy Risk Factor B

Pregnancy Considerations Adverse events were not observed in animal reproduction studies.

Ceftaroline Fosamil (sef TAR oh leen FOS a mil)

Brand Names: US Teflaro

Pharmacologic Category Antibiotic, Cephalosporin (Fifth Generation)

Use

Pneumonia, community-acquired: Treatment of community-acquired bacterial pneumonia in adults and pediatric patients ≥2 months of age caused by *Streptococcus pneumoniae* (including cases with concurrent bacteremia), *Staphylococcus aureus* (methicillin-susceptible isolates only), *Haemophilus influenzae*, *Klebsiella pneumoniae*, *Klebsiella oxytoca*, and *Escherichia coli*.

Skin and skin structure infections: Treatment of acute bacterial skin and skin structure infections in adults and pediatric patients (≥34 weeks gestational age and 12 days postnatal age) caused by *S. aureus* (including methicillin-susceptible and methicillin-resistant isolates), *Streptococcus pyogenes*, *Streptococcus agalactiae*, *E. coli*, *K. pneumoniae*, and *K. oxytoca*.

Local Anesthetic/Vasoconstrictor Precautions No information available to require special precautions

Effects on Dental Treatment No significant effects or complications reported

Effects on Bleeding No information available to require special precautions

Adverse Reactions

>10%: Hematologic & oncologic: Positive direct Coombs test (10% to 18%; no evidence of hemolysis)

1% to 10%:

Cardiovascular: Phlebitis (adults: 2%), bradycardia (adults: <2%), palpitations (adults: <2%)

Central nervous system: Headache (infants, children, and adolescents: <3%), dizziness (adults: <2%), seizure (adults: <2%)

Dermatologic: Skin rash (3% to 7%), pruritus (infants, children, and adolescents: <3%), urticaria (adults: <2%)
Endocrine & metabolic: Hypokalemia (adults: 2%), hyperglycemia (adults: <2%), hyperkalemia (adults: <2%)
Gastrointestinal: Diarrhea (5% to 8%), vomiting (2% to 5%), nausea (3% to 4%), constipation (adults: 2%), abdominal pain (adults: <2%), *Clostridioides difficile* colitis (adults: <2%)
Hematologic & oncologic: Anemia (adults: <2%), eosinophilia (adults: <2%), neutropenia (adults: <2%), thrombocytopenia (adults: <2%)
Hepatic: Increased serum alanine aminotransferase (infants, children, and adolescents: <3%), increased serum aspartate aminotransferase (infants, children, and adolescents: <3%), increased serum transaminases (adults: 2%), hepatitis (adults: <2%)
Hypersensitivity: Anaphylaxis (adults: <2%), hypersensitivity reaction (adults: <2%)
Renal: Renal failure syndrome (adults: <2%)
Miscellaneous: Fever (≤3%)
Postmarketing: Agranulocytosis, *Clostridioides difficile* associated diarrhea, eosinophilic pneumonia, leukopenia

Mechanism of Action Inhibits bacterial cell wall synthesis by binding to penicillin-binding proteins (PBPs) 1 through 3. This action blocks the final transpeptidation step of peptidoglycan synthesis in bacterial cell walls and inhibits cell wall biosynthesis. Bacteria eventually lyse due to ongoing activity of cell wall autolytic enzymes (autolysis and murein hydrolases) while cell wall assembly is arrested. Ceftaroline has a strong affinity for PBP2a, a modified PBP in MRSA, and PBP2x in *S. pneumoniae*, contributing to its spectrum of activity against these bacteria.

Pharmacodynamics/Kinetics

Half-life Elimination 1.6 ± 0.38 hours (single dose); 2.66 ± 0.4 hours (multiple dose)

Time to Peak ~1 hour

Pregnancy Considerations Adverse events have been observed in some animal reproduction studies.

◆ **Ceftaroline Fosamil Acetate** *see* Ceftaroline Fosamil *on page 312*

CefTAZidime (SEF tay zi deem)

Brand Names: US Fortaz; Fortaz in D5W [DSC]; Tazicef

Brand Names: Canada Fortaz

Pharmacologic Category Antibiotic, Cephalosporin (Third Generation)

Use

Bloodstream infection (gram-negative bacteremia): Treatment of bloodstream infection caused by *Pseudomonas aeruginosa*, *Klebsiella* spp., *Haemophilus influenzae*, *Escherichia coli*, *Serratia* spp., *Streptococcus pneumoniae*, and *Staphylococcus aureus* (methicillin-susceptible strains).

Bone and joint infections: Treatment of bone and joint infections caused by *P. aeruginosa*, *Klebsiella* spp., *Enterobacter* spp., and *S. aureus* (methicillin-susceptible strains).

CNS infections: Treatment of CNS infections, including meningitis, caused by *H. influenzae* and *Neisseria meningitidis*. Ceftazidime has also been used successfully in cases of meningitis due to *P. aeruginosa* and *S. pneumoniae*.

Empiric therapy in immunocompromised patients: Empiric treatment of infections in immunocompromised patients.

Gynecologic infections: Treatment of endometritis, pelvic cellulitis, and other infections of the female genital tract caused by *E. coli*.

Intra-abdominal infections: Treatment of peritonitis caused by *E. coli*, *Klebsiella* spp., and *S. aureus* (methicillin-susceptible strains) and polymicrobial intra-abdominal infections caused by aerobic and anaerobic organisms and some *Bacteroides* spp. (many isolates of *Bacteroides fragilis* are resistant).

Lower respiratory tract infections: Treatment of lower respiratory tract infections, including pneumonia, caused by *P. aeruginosa* and other *Pseudomonas* spp.; *H. influenzae*, including ampicillin-resistant isolates; *Klebsiella* spp.; *Enterobacter* spp.; *Proteus mirabilis*; *E. coli*; *Serratia* spp.; *Citrobacter* spp.; *S. pneumoniae*; and *S. aureus* (methicillin-susceptible strains).

Skin and soft tissue infections: Treatment of skin and soft tissue infections caused by *P. aeruginosa*; *Klebsiella* spp.; *E. coli*; *Proteus* spp., including *P. mirabilis* and indole-positive *Proteus*; *Enterobacter* spp.; *Serratia* spp.; *S. aureus* (methicillin-susceptible strains); and *Streptococcus pyogenes* (group A beta-hemolytic streptococci).

Urinary tract infections: Treatment of complicated and uncomplicated urinary tract infections caused by *P. aeruginosa*; *Enterobacter* spp.; *Proteus* spp., including *P. mirabilis* and indole-positive *Proteus*; *Klebsiella* spp.; and *E. coli*.

Local Anesthetic/Vasoconstrictor Precautions No information available to require special precautions

Effects on Dental Treatment No significant effects or complications reported

Effects on Bleeding No information available to require special precautions

Adverse Reactions

1% to 10%:
Dermatologic: Pruritus (<2%), skin rash (<2%)
Endocrine & metabolic: Increased lactate dehydrogenase (6%), increased gamma-glutamyl transferase (5%)
Gastrointestinal: Diarrhea (1%)
Hematologic & oncologic: Eosinophilia (8%), positive direct Coombs test (4%; without hemolysis), thrombocythemia (2%)
Hepatic: Increased serum ALT (7%), increased serum AST (6%), increased serum alkaline phosphatase (4%)
Hypersensitivity: Hypersensitivity reactions (2%)
Local: Inflammation at injection site (1%), injection site phlebitis (1%)
Miscellaneous: Fever (<2%)

Frequency not defined:
Central nervous system: Seizure
Hematologic & oncologic: Agranulocytosis, leukopenia, lymphocytosis, neutropenia, thrombocytopenia
Renal: Increased blood urea nitrogen, increased serum creatinine

<1%, postmarketing, and/or case reports: Abdominal pain, anaphylaxis (severe in rare instances, including cardiopulmonary arrest), angioedema, candidiasis, *Clostridioides* (formerly *Clostridium*) *difficile*-associated diarrhea, dizziness, erythema multiforme, headache, hemolytic anemia, hyperbilirubinemia, jaundice, nausea, pain at injection site, paresthesia, renal insufficiency, Stevens-Johnson syndrome, toxic epidermal necrolysis, urticaria, vaginitis, vomiting

Mechanism of Action Inhibits bacterial cell wall synthesis by binding to one or more of the penicillin-binding proteins (PBPs), which in turn inhibits the final transpeptidation step of peptidoglycan synthesis in bacterial cell walls, thus inhibiting cell wall biosynthesis. Bacteria eventually lyse due to ongoing activity of cell wall autolytic enzymes (autolysins and murein hydrolases) while cell wall assembly is arrested.

Pharmacodynamics/Kinetics

Half-life Elimination

Preterm neonates <32 weeks GA (van den Anker 1995):

PNA 3 days: 8.7 ± 2.8 hours.

PNA 10 days: 5 ± 0.9 hours.

Adult: 1 to 2 hours, significantly prolonged with renal impairment.

Time to Peak Serum: IM: ~1 hour

Pregnancy Risk Factor B

Pregnancy Considerations

Ceftazidime crosses the placenta (Jørgensen 1987).

Due to pregnancy-induced physiologic changes, some pharmacokinetic parameters of ceftazidime may be altered (Giamarellou 1983; Jørgensen 1987; Nathorst-Böös 1995).

Ceftazidime and Avibactam

(SEF tay zi deem & a vi BAK tam)

Brand Names: US Avycaz

Pharmacologic Category Cephalosporin Combination

Use

Intra-abdominal infections, complicated: Treatment of complicated intra-abdominal infections (cIAI) in adult and pediatric patients ≥3 months of age, in combination with metronidazole, caused by *Citrobacter freundii* complex, *Enterobacter cloacae*, *Escherichia coli*, *Klebsiella oxytoca*, *Klebsiella pneumoniae*, *Proteus mirabilis*, and *Pseudomonas aeruginosa*.

Pneumonia, hospital-acquired and ventilator-associated: Treatment of hospital-acquired bacterial pneumonia and ventilator-associated (HAP/VAP) bacterial pneumonia in adult patients caused by ceftazidime/avibactam-susceptible *K. pneumoniae*, *E. cloacae*, *E. coli*, *Serratia marcescens*, *P. mirabilis*, *P. aeruginosa*, and *Haemophilus influenzae*.

Urinary tract infections, complicated (including pyelonephritis): Treatment of complicated urinary tract infections (cUTI) (including pyelonephritis) in adult and pediatric patients ≥3 months of age, caused by *C. freundii* complex, *E. cloacae*, *E. coli*, *K. pneumoniae*, *P. mirabilis*, and *P. aeruginosa*.

Local Anesthetic/Vasoconstrictor Precautions No information available to require special precautions

Effects on Dental Treatment No significant effects or complications reported

Effects on Bleeding No information available to require special precautions

Adverse Reactions Also see ceftazidime monograph.

>10%: Hematologic & oncologic: Positive direct coombs test (3% to 21%)

1% to 10%:

Dermatologic: Injection site phlebitis (children and adolescents: >3%; adults: <1%), skin rash (children and adolescents: >3%; adults: <1%), pruritus (2%)

Gastrointestinal: Vomiting (>3%), diarrhea (≥3%), nausea (3%), constipation (2%), upper abdominal pain (1%)

<1%, postmarketing, and/or case reports: Acute renal failure, anxiety, candidiasis, *Clostridioides difficile*-associated diarrhea, dysgeusia, hypokalemia, increased gamma-glutamyl transferase, increased serum alanine aminotransferase, increased serum aspartate aminotransferase, leukopenia, maculopapular rash, nephrolithiasis, renal insufficiency, thrombocythemia, thrombocytopenia, urticaria

Mechanism of Action

Ceftazidime inhibits bacterial cell wall synthesis by binding to one or more of the penicillin-binding proteins (PBPs) which in turn inhibits the final transpeptidation step of peptidoglycan synthesis in bacterial cell walls, thus inhibiting cell wall biosynthesis. Bacteria eventually lyse due to ongoing activity of cell wall autolytic enzymes (autolysins and murein hydrolases) while cell wall assembly is arrested.

Avibactam inactivates some beta-lactamases and protects ceftazidime from degradation.

Pharmacodynamics/Kinetics

Half-life Elimination

Single dose:

Ceftazidime:

Children ≥6 years to <12 years: Median: 1.6 hours (0.9 to 1.8 hours) (Bradley 2016)

Children ≥12 years and Adolescents: Median: 1.7 hours (0.9 to 2.8 hours) (Bradley 2016)

Adults: Mean: 3.27 hours

Avibactam:

Children ≥6 years to <12 years: Median: 1.7 hours (0.9 to 2 hours) (Bradley 2016)

Children ≥12 years and Adolescents: Median: 1.6 hours (0.9 to 2.8 hours) (Bradley 2016)

Adults: Mean: 2.22 hours

Multiple dose: Adults: Mean: Ceftazidime: 2.76 hours; Avibactam: 2.71 hours

Pregnancy Considerations Adverse events have not been observed in animal reproduction studies conducted with ceftazidime; adverse events have been observed in some animal reproduction studies conducted with avibactam.

◆ **Ceftazidime/Avibactam** *see* Ceftazidime and Avibactam *on page* 314

Ceftibuten (sef TYE byoo ten)

Related Information

Bacterial Infections *on page* 1739

Brand Names: US Cedax [DSC]

Pharmacologic Category Antibiotic, Cephalosporin (Third Generation)

Use

Acute bacterial exacerbations of chronic bronchitis: Treatment of mild to moderate acute bacterial exacerbations of chronic bronchitis due to *Haemophilus influenzae* (including beta-lactamase-producing strains), *Moraxella catarrhalis* (including beta-lactamase-producing strains), or *Streptococcus pneumoniae* (penicillin-susceptible strains only).

Limitations of use: In acute bacterial exacerbations of chronic bronchitis clinical trials where *M. catarrhalis* was isolated from infected sputum at baseline, ceftibuten clinical efficacy was 22% less than control.

Acute bacterial otitis media: Treatment of mild to moderate acute bacterial otitis media due to *H. influenzae* (including beta-lactamase-producing strains), *M. catarrhalis* (including beta-lactamase-producing strains), or *Streptococcus pyogenes*.

Limitations of use: Although ceftibuten used empirically was equivalent to comparators in the treatment of clinically and/or microbiologically documented acute otitis media, the efficacy against *S. pneumoniae* was 23% less than control. Therefore, ceftibuten should be given empirically only when adequate antimicrobial coverage against *S. pneumoniae* has been previously administered.

Pharyngitis/tonsillitis: Treatment of mild to moderate pharyngitis and tonsillitis due to *S. pyogenes*.

Local Anesthetic/Vasoconstrictor Precautions No information available to require special precautions

Effects on Dental Treatment No significant effects or complications reported

Effects on Bleeding No information available to require special precautions

Adverse Reactions

1% to 10%:

Central nervous system: Headache (≤3%), dizziness (≤1%)

Gastrointestinal: Nausea (≤4%), diarrhea (3% to 4%), dyspepsia (≤2%), loose stools (≤2%), abdominal pain (1% to 2%), vomiting (1% to 2%)

Hematologic & oncologic: Eosinophilia (3%), decreased hemoglobin (1% to 2%), change in platelet count (increase: ≤1%)

Hepatic: Increased serum ALT (≤1%), increased serum bilirubin (≤1%)

Renal: Increased blood urea nitrogen (2% to 4%)

<1%, postmarketing, and/or case reports: Agitation, anorexia, aphasia, candidiasis, constipation, dehydration, diaper rash, drowsiness, dysgeusia, dyspnea, dysuria, eructation, fatigue, fever, flatulence, hematuria, hyperkinesia, increased serum alkaline phosphatase, increased serum AST, increased serum creatinine, insomnia, irritability, jaundice, leukopenia, melena, nasal congestion, paresthesia, pruritus, pseudomembranous colitis, psychosis, rigors, serum sickness, skin rash, Stevens-Johnson syndrome, stridor, thrombocytopenia, toxic epidermal necrolysis, urticaria, vaginitis, xerostomia

Mechanism of Action Inhibits bacterial cell wall synthesis by binding to one or more of the penicillin-binding proteins (PBPs) which in turn inhibits the final transpeptidation step of peptidoglycan synthesis in bacterial cell walls, thus inhibiting cell wall biosynthesis. Bacteria eventually lyse due to ongoing activity of cell wall autolytic enzymes (autolysins and murein hydrolases) while cell wall assembly is arrested.

Pharmacodynamics/Kinetics

Half-life Elimination Children: 2 hours; Adults: 2.4 hours; CrCl 30 to 49 mL/minute: 7.1 hours; CrCl 5 to 29 mL/minute: 13.4 hours; CrCl <5 mL/minute: 22.3 hours

Time to Peak 2 to 2.6 hours

Pregnancy Risk Factor B

Pregnancy Considerations Adverse events have not been observed in animal reproduction studies. An increase in most types of birth defects was not found following first trimester exposure to cephalosporins (Crider 2009).

Product Availability All ceftibuten formulations (brand and generic) have been discontinued in the US for more than 1 year.

◆ **Ceftin [DSC]** *see* Cefuroxime *on page 317*

Ceftolozane and Tazobactam

(sef TOL oh zane & taz oh BAK tam)

Brand Names: US Zerbaxa

Brand Names: Canada Zerbaxa

Pharmacologic Category Cephalosporin Combination

Use

Intra-abdominal infection: Treatment of complicated intra-abdominal infection in patients ≥18 years, in combination with metronidazole, caused by *Enterobacter cloacae, Escherichia coli, Klebsiella oxytoca, Klebsiella pneumoniae, Proteus mirabilis, Pseudomonas aeruginosa, Bacteroides fragilis, Streptococcus anginosus, Streptococcus constellatus*, and *Streptococcus salivarius*.

Pneumonia, (hospital-acquired or ventilator-associated): Treatment of hospital-acquired pneumonia and ventilator-associated bacterial pneumonia in patients ≥18 years, caused by *E. cloacae, E. coli, Haemophilus influenzae, K. oxytoca, K. pneumoniae, P. mirabilis, P. aeruginosa*, and *Serratia marcescens*.

Urinary tract infection: Treatment of complicated urinary tract infection, including pyelonephritis, in patients ≥18 years caused by *E. coli, K. pneumoniae, P. mirabilis*, and *P. aeruginosa*.

Local Anesthetic/Vasoconstrictor Precautions No information available to require special precautions

Effects on Dental Treatment No significant effects or complications reported

Effects on Bleeding No information available to require special precautions

Adverse Reactions

>10%:

Hematologic & oncologic: Positive direct Coombs test (hospital-acquired bacterial pneumonia [HAP] and ventilator-associated bacterial pneumonia [VAP]: 31%; complicated intra-abdominal infections and UTIs: <1%)

Hepatic: Increased serum transaminases (HAP and VAP: 12%)

1% to 10%:

Cardiovascular: Hypotension (≤2%), atrial fibrillation (≤1%)

Central nervous system: Headache (3% to 6%), intracranial hemorrhage (HAP and VAP: 4%), insomnia (1% to 4%), anxiety (≤2%), dizziness (≤1%)

Dermatologic: Skin rash (≤2%)

Endocrine & metabolic: Hypokalemia (≤3%), increased gamma-glutamyl transferase (<2%)

Gastrointestinal: Nausea (3% to 8%), diarrhea (2% to 6%), constipation (2% to 4%), *Clostridioides difficile* associated diarrhea (3%), vomiting (1% to 3%), abdominal pain (≤1%)

Hematologic & oncologic: Anemia (≤2%), thrombocythemia (≤2%)

Hepatic: Increased serum alanine aminotransferase (2%), increased serum alkaline phosphatase (<2%), increased serum aspartate aminotransferase (1% to 2%)

Renal: Renal failure syndrome (HAP and VAP: ≤9%; complicated intra-abdominal infections and UTIs: <1%), renal insufficiency (HAP and VAP: ≤9%; complicated intra-abdominal infections and UTIs: <1%)

Miscellaneous: Fever (2% to 6%)

<1%, postmarketing, and/or case reports: Abdominal distention, angina pectoris, candidiasis, dyspepsia, dyspnea, flatulence, fungal urinary tract infection, gastritis, hyperglycemia, hypomagnesemia,

hypophosphatemia, infusion site reaction, ischemic stroke, oropharyngeal candidiasis, paralytic ileus, tachycardia, urticaria, venous thrombosis, vulvovaginal candidiasis

Mechanism of Action Ceftolozane inhibits bacterial cell wall synthesis by binding to one or more of the penicillin-binding proteins (PBPs); which in turn inhibits the final transpeptidation step of peptidoglycan synthesis in bacterial cell walls, thus inhibiting cell wall biosynthesis. Ceftolozane is an inhibitor of PBPs of *Pseudomonas aeruginosa* (eg, PBP1b, PBP1c, and PBP3) and *Escherichia coli* (eg, PBP3). Tazobactam irreversibly inhibits some beta-lactamases (eg, certain penicillinases and cephalosporinases), and can covalently bind to some plasmid-mediated and chromosomal bacterial beta-lactamases.

Pharmacodynamics/Kinetics

Half-life Elimination Ceftolozane: ~3 to 4 hours; Tazobactam: ~2 to 3 hours

Pregnancy Considerations

Tazobactam crosses the placenta (Bourget 1998).

In general, an increased risk of major birth defects or other adverse fetal or maternal outcomes has not been observed following maternal use of cephalosporin antibiotics

◆ **Ceftolozane/Tazobactam** *see* Ceftolozane and Tazobactam *on page 315*

CefTRIAXone (sef trye AKS one)

Related Information

Antibiotic Prophylaxis *on page 1715*

Sexually-Transmitted Diseases *on page 1707*

Brand Names: Canada SANDOZ CefTRIAXone [DSC]

Pharmacologic Category Antibiotic, Cephalosporin (Third Generation)

Use

Bloodstream infection: Caused by *Staphylococcus aureus*, *Streptococcus pneumoniae*, *Escherichia coli*, *Haemophilus influenzae*, or *Klebsiella pneumoniae*.

Bone and joint infections (osteomyelitis and/or discitis, prosthetic joint infection, septic arthritis): Caused by *S. aureus*, *S. pneumoniae*, *E. coli*, *Proteus mirabilis*, *K. pneumoniae*, or *Enterobacter* spp.

Gonococcal infection, uncomplicated (cervical/urethral, rectal, and pharyngeal): Caused by *Neisseria gonorrhoeae*, including both penicillinase- and nonpenicillinase-producing strains, and pharyngeal gonorrhea caused by nonpenicillinase-producing strains of *N. gonorrhoeae*.

Intra-abdominal infection, community-acquired (mild to moderate infection in low-risk patients): Caused by *E. coli*, *K. pneumoniae*, *Bacteroides fragilis*, *Clostridium* spp. (**Note:** Most strains of *C. difficile* are resistant), or *Peptostreptococcus* spp.

Lower respiratory tract infections (pneumonia, community-acquired): Caused by *S. pneumoniae*, *S. aureus*, *H. influenzae*, *Haemophilus parainfluenzae*, *K. pneumoniae*, *E. coli*, *Enterobacter aerogenes*, *P. mirabilis*, or *Serratia marcescens*.

Meningitis, bacterial: Caused by *H. influenzae*, *Neisseria meningitidis*, or *S. pneumoniae*. Ceftriaxone has also been used successfully in a limited number of cases of meningitis and shunt infection caused by *Staphylococcus epidermidis* and *E. coli* (efficacy for these 2 organisms in this organ system was studied in fewer than 10 infections).

Otitis media, acute: Caused by *S. pneumoniae*, *H. influenzae* (including beta-lactamase-producing strains), or *Moraxella catarrhalis* (including beta-lactamase-producing strains).

Pelvic inflammatory disease (mild to moderate): Caused by *N. gonorrhoeae*. Ceftriaxone, like other cephalosporins, has no activity against *Chlamydia trachomatis*; therefore, when cephalosporins are used in the treatment of patients with pelvic inflammatory disease and *C. trachomatis* is one of the suspected pathogens, appropriate antichlamydial coverage should be added.

Skin and soft tissue infections: Caused by *S. aureus*, *S. epidermidis*, *Streptococcus pyogenes*, viridans group streptococci, *E. coli*, *Enterobacter cloacae*, *Klebsiella oxytoca*, *K. pneumoniae*, *P. mirabilis*, *Morganella morganii* (efficacy for this organism in this organ system was studied in fewer than 10 infections), *S. marcescens*, *Acinetobacter calcoaceticus*, *B. fragilis* (efficacy for this organism in this organ system was studied in fewer than 10 infections), or *Peptostreptococcus* spp.

Surgical prophylaxis, colorectal: To reduce the incidence of postoperative infections in patients undergoing surgical procedures classified as contaminated or potentially contaminated.

Urinary tract infection, complicated (including pyelonephritis): Caused by *E. coli*, *P. mirabilis*, *Proteus vulgaris*, *M. morganii*, or *K. pneumoniae*.

Local Anesthetic/Vasoconstrictor Precautions No information available to require special precautions

Effects on Dental Treatment No significant effects or complications reported

Effects on Bleeding May potentiate the anticoagulant effects of vitamin K anticoagulants (ie, warfarin) due to alterations of gut flora.

Adverse Reactions

>10%:

Dermatologic: Skin tightness (IM: ≤5% to ≤17%; local)

Local: Induration at injection site (≤5% to ≤17%; incidence higher with IM), warm sensation at injection site (IM: ≤5% to ≤17%)

1% to 10%:

Dermatologic: Skin rash (2%)

Gastrointestinal: Diarrhea (3%)

Hematologic & oncologic: Eosinophilia (6%), leukopenia (2%), thrombocythemia (5%)

Hepatic: Increased serum transaminases (3%)

Local: Pain at injection site (≤1%), tenderness at injection site (≤1%)

Renal: Increased blood urea nitrogen (1%)

<1%:

Cardiovascular: Flushing, palpitations, phlebitis

Dermatologic: Diaphoresis, pruritus

Endocrine & metabolic: Glycosuria

Gastrointestinal: Abdominal pain, choledocholithiasis, cholelithiasis, *Clostridioides difficile* colitis, dysgeusia, dyspepsia, flatulence, gallbladder sludge, nausea, pancreatitis, vomiting

Genitourinary: Casts in urine, hematuria, vaginitis

Hematologic & oncologic: Agranulocytosis, anemia, basophilia, decreased prothrombin time, disorder of hemostatic components of blood, granulocytopenia, hemolytic anemia, lymphocytopenia, lymphocytosis, monocytosis, neutropenia, prolonged prothrombin time, thrombocytopenia

Hepatic: Increased serum alkaline phosphatase, increased serum bilirubin, jaundice

Hypersensitivity: Anaphylaxis, serum sickness

Infection: Candidiasis, genitourinary fungal infection

Nervous system: Chills, dizziness, headache, seizure
Renal: Increased serum creatinine, nephrolithiasis
Respiratory: Bronchospasm, epistaxis, hypersensitivity pneumonitis

Postmarketing:

Dermatologic: Acute generalized exanthematous pustulosis (Salman 2019), allergic dermatitis, erythema multiforme, Stevens-Johnson syndrome (Liberopoulos 2003), toxic epidermal necrolysis (Atanaskovic-Markovic 2013; Lam 2008), urticaria
Gastrointestinal: *Clostridioides difficile* associated diarrhea, glossitis, kernicterus, stomatitis
Genitourinary: Oliguria (Shen 2014), ureteral obstruction (Lu 2012), urolithiasis (Shen 2014)
Immunologic: Drug reaction with eosinophilia and systemic symptoms (Hansel 2017)
Renal: Acute renal failure (post-renal) (Li 2014; Shen 2014); hypercalciuria (Zeng 2020)

Mechanism of Action Inhibits bacterial cell wall synthesis by binding to one or more of the penicillin-binding proteins (PBPs) which in turn inhibits the final transpeptidation step of peptidoglycan synthesis in bacterial cell walls, thus inhibiting cell wall biosynthesis. Bacteria eventually lyse due to ongoing activity of cell wall autolytic enzymes (autolysins and murein hydrolases) while cell wall assembly is arrested.

Pharmacodynamics/Kinetics

Half-life Elimination

Neonates (Martin 1984): 1 to 4 days: 16 hours; 9 to 30 days: 9 hours
Infants and Children: 4 to 6.6 hours (Richards 1984)
Adults: Normal renal and hepatic function: ~5 to 9 hours
Adults: Renal impairment (mild-to-severe): ~12 to 16 hours

Time to Peak Serum: IM: 2 to 3 hours

Pregnancy Risk Factor B

Pregnancy Considerations Ceftriaxone crosses the placenta.

Pregnancy was found to influence the single dose pharmacokinetics of ceftriaxone when administered prior to delivery (Popović 2007). The pharmacokinetics of ceftriaxone following multiple doses in the third trimester are similar to those of nonpregnant patients (Bourget 1993). Ceftriaxone is recommended for use in pregnant women for the treatment of gonococcal infections, Lyme disease, and may be used in certain situations prior to vaginal delivery in women at high risk for endocarditis (consult current guidelines) (ACOG 199 2018; CDC [Workowski 2015]; Wormser 2006).

◆ **Ceftriaxone Sodium** *see* CefTRIAXone *on page 316*

Cefuroxime (se fyoor OKS eem)

Related Information

Antibiotic Prophylaxis *on page 1715*
Bacterial Infections *on page 1739*

Brand Names: US Ceftin [DSC]; Zinacef in Sterile Water [DSC]; Zinacef [DSC]

Brand Names: Canada APO-Cefuroxime; Auro-Cefuroxime; Ceftin; PRO-Cefuroxime-500; RATIO-Cefuroxime [DSC]

Pharmacologic Category Antibiotic, Cephalosporin (Second Generation)

Use

Bone and joint infections (injection only): Treatment of bone and joint infections caused by *Staphylococcus aureus* (penicillinase- and non-penicillinase-producing strains).

Chronic obstructive pulmonary disease, acute exacerbation (tablets only): Treatment of mild to moderate acute bacterial exacerbations of chronic bronchitis in adults and adolescents ≥13 years of age caused by *Streptococcus pneumoniae, Haemophilus influenzae* (beta-lactamase negative strains), or *Haemophilus parainfluenzae* (beta-lactamase negative strains).

Lower respiratory tract infections (injection only): Treatment of lower respiratory tract infections, including pneumonia, caused by *S. pneumoniae*, *H. influenzae* (including ampicillin-resistant strains), *Klebsiella* spp., *S. aureus* (penicillinase- and non-penicillinase-producing strains), *Streptococcus pyogenes,* and *Escherichia coli.*

Lyme disease (early) (tablets only): Treatment of adults and adolescents ≥13 years of age with early Lyme disease caused by *Borrelia burgdorferi.*

Otitis media, acute (tablets and oral suspension only): Treatment of pediatric patients ≥3 months of age with acute bacterial otitis media caused by *S. pneumoniae*, *H. influenzae* (including beta-lactamase-producing strains), *Moraxella catarrhalis* (including beta-lactamase-producing strains), or *S. pyogenes.*

Pharyngitis/tonsillitis (tablets and oral suspension only): Treatment of mild to moderate pharyngitis/tonsillitis caused by *S. pyogenes* in adults and pediatric patients ≥3 months of age.

Limitations of use: Efficacy in the prevention of rheumatic fever has not been established in clinical trials. Efficacy in the treatment of penicillin-resistant strains of *S. pyogenes* has not been demonstrated.

Septicemia (injection only): Treatment of septicemia caused by *S. aureus* (penicillinase- and non-penicillinase-producing strains), *S. pneumoniae*, *E. coli*, *H. influenzae* (including ampicillin-resistant strains), and *Klebsiella* spp.

Sinusitis, acute bacterial (tablets and oral suspension only): Treatment of mild to moderate acute bacterial maxillary sinusitis caused by *S. pneumoniae* or *H. influenzae* (non-beta-lactamase-producing strains only).

Limitations of use: Effectiveness for sinus infections caused by beta-lactamase-producing *H. influenzae* or *M. catarrhalis* in patients with acute bacterial maxillary sinusitis has not been established. **Note**: According to the IDSA guidelines for acute bacterial rhinosinusitis, cefuroxime is no longer recommended as monotherapy for initial empiric treatment (IDSA [Chow 2012]).

Skin and skin-structure infections (impetigo) (oral suspension only): Treatment of pediatric patients 3 months to 12 years of age with skin or skin-structure infections (impetigo) caused by *S. aureus* (including beta-lactamase-producing strains) or *S. pyogenes.*

Skin and skin-structure infections (injection; tablets [uncomplicated infections only]): Treatment of adults and pediatric patients >3 months of age with skin and skin-structure infections (including impetigo) caused by *S. aureus* (penicillinase- and non-penicillinase-producing strains), *S. pyogenes*, *E. coli*, *Klebsiella* spp., and *Enterobacter* spp.

Surgical prophylaxis (injection only): Prophylaxis of infection in patients undergoing surgical procedures that are classified as clean-contaminated or potentially contaminated procedures.

Urinary tract infections (tablets and injection only): Treatment of adults and pediatric patients >3 months of age with urinary tract infections caused by *E. coli* and *Klebsiella* spp.

Local Anesthetic/Vasoconstrictor Precautions No information available to require special precautions

Effects on Dental Treatment Rare occurrence of candidiasis, glossitis, oral mucosal ulcers and trismus.

Effects on Bleeding No information available to require special precautions

Adverse Reactions

>10%: Gastrointestinal: Diarrhea (4% to 11%, duration dependent)

1% to 10%:

Cardiovascular: Local thrombophlebitis (2%)

Dermatologic: Diaper rash (children 3%)

Endocrine & metabolic: Increased lactate dehydrogenase (1%)

Gastrointestinal: Nausea and vomiting (3% to 7%), unpleasant taste (children 5%)

Genitourinary: Vaginitis (≤5%)

Hematologic & oncologic: Decreased hematocrit (≤10%), decreased hemoglobin (≤10%), eosinophilia (1% to 7%)

Hepatic: Increased serum transaminases (2% to 4%), increased serum alkaline phosphatase (2%)

Immunologic: Jarisch-Herxheimer reaction (6%)

<1%, postmarketing, and/or case reports (Limited to important or life-threatening): Abdominal pain, anaphylaxis, angioedema, anorexia, arthralgia, brain disease, candidiasis, chest pain, chest tightness, chills, cholestasis, *Clostridioides* (formerly *Clostridium*) *difficile*-associated diarrhea, colitis, cough, decreased creatinine clearance, dizziness, drowsiness, drug fever, dyspepsia, dyspnea, dysuria, erythema, erythema multiforme, fever, flatulence, gastrointestinal hemorrhage, gastrointestinal infection, glossitis, headache, hearing loss, hemolytic anemia, hepatitis, hyperactivity, hyperbilirubinemia, hypersensitivity, hypersensitivity angiitis, increased blood urea nitrogen, increased liver enzymes, increased serum creatinine, increased thirst, interstitial nephritis, irritability, jaundice, joint swelling, leukopenia, muscle cramps, muscle rigidity, muscle spasm (neck), neutropenia, oral mucosa ulcer, pancytopenia, positive direct Coombs test, prolonged prothrombin time, pruritus, pseudomembranous colitis, renal insufficiency, renal pain, seizure, serum sickness-like reaction, sialorrhea, sinusitis, skin rash, Stevens-Johnson syndrome, stomach cramps, tachycardia, thrombocytopenia (rare), toxic epidermal necrolysis, trismus, upper respiratory tract infection, urethral bleeding, urethral pain, urinary tract infection, urticaria, vaginal discharge, vaginal irritation, viral infection, vulvovaginal candidiasis, vulvovaginal pruritus

Mechanism of Action Inhibits bacterial cell wall synthesis by binding to one or more of the penicillin-binding proteins (PBPs) which in turn inhibits the final transpeptidation step of peptidoglycan synthesis in bacterial cell walls, thus inhibiting cell wall biosynthesis. Bacteria eventually lyse due to ongoing activity of cell wall autolytic enzymes (autolysins and murein hydrolases) while cell wall assembly is arrested.

Pharmacodynamics/Kinetics

Half-life Elimination

Premature neonates:

PNA ≤3 days: Median: 5.8 hours (de Louvois 1982)

PNA ≥8 days: Median: 1.6 to 3.8 hours (de Louvois 1982)

Children and Adolescents: 1.4 to 1.9 hours

Adults: ~1 to 2 hours; prolonged with renal impairment

Time to Peak Serum: IM: ~15 to 60 minutes; IV: 2 to 3 minutes; Oral: Children: ~3 to 4 hours; Adults: ~2 to 3 hours

Pregnancy Considerations

Cefuroxime crosses the placenta (Dallmann 2017; Lalic-Popovic 2016).

An increased risk of major birth defects or other adverse fetal or maternal outcomes has generally not been observed following maternal use of cephalosporin antibiotics, including cefuroxime.

Due to pregnancy-induced physiologic changes, some pharmacokinetic properties of cefuroxime may be altered (Dallmann 2017; Lalic-Popovic 2016).

Cefuroxime is one of the antibiotics effective for prophylactic use prior to cesarean delivery (ACOG 199 2018).

Product Availability Ceftin oral suspension has been discontinued in the US for more than 1 year.

◆ **Cefuroxime Axetil** *see* Cefuroxime *on page 317*

◆ **Cefuroxime Sodium** *see* Cefuroxime *on page 317*

◆ **Cefzil** *see* Cefprozil *on page 312*

◆ **CeleBREX** *see* Celecoxib *on page 318*

Celecoxib (se le KOKS ib)

Related Information

Oral Pain *on page 1734*

Rheumatoid Arthritis, Osteoarthritis, and Osteoporosis *on page 1697*

Brand Names: US CeleBREX

Brand Names: Canada ACCEL-Celecoxib [DSC]; ACT Celecoxib; AG-Celecoxib; APO-Celecoxib; Auro-Celecoxib; BIO-Celecoxib; CeleBREX; GD-Celecoxib [DSC]; JAMP-Celecoxib; Mar-Celecoxib; MINT-Celecoxib; MYLAN-Celecoxib [DSC]; NRA-Celecoxib; PMS-Celecoxib; Priva-Celecoxib; RAN-Celecoxib; RIVA-Celecox; SANDOZ Celecoxib [DSC]; SDZ Celecoxib; TEVA-Celecoxib [DSC]

Pharmacologic Category Analgesic, Nonopioid; Nonsteroidal Anti-inflammatory Drug (NSAID), COX-2 Selective

Use

Acute pain: Management of acute pain.

Ankylosing spondylitis: Relief of the signs/symptoms of ankylosing spondylitis.

Juvenile idiopathic arthritis: Relief of the signs/symptoms of juvenile idiopathic arthritis (JIA) in patients 2 years and older.

Osteoarthritis: Relief of the signs/symptoms of osteoarthritis.

Primary dysmenorrhea: Treatment of primary dysmenorrhea.

Rheumatoid arthritis: Relief of the signs/symptoms of rheumatoid arthritis.

Local Anesthetic/Vasoconstrictor Precautions No information available to require special precautions

Effects on Dental Treatment Key adverse event(s) related to dental treatment: Stomatitis, abnormal taste, and xerostomia (normal salivary flow resumes upon discontinuation).

Effects on Bleeding No effects on bleeding or platelet function have been reported. See Dental Health Professional Considerations.

Adverse Reactions

≥2%:

Cardiovascular: Peripheral edema (2%)

Gastrointestinal: Diarrhea (6%), dyspepsia (9%), abdominal pain (4%), flatulence (2%), gastroesophageal reflux disease, vomiting

Hepatic: Increased liver enzymes (<3x ULN: ≤6%)

Renal: Nephrolithiasis (3%)

Respiratory: Upper respiratory tract infection (8%), sinusitis (5%), pharyngitis (2%), rhinitis (2%), dyspnea

Miscellaneous: Accidental injury (3%)

Frequency not defined:

Dermatologic: Acute generalized exanthematous pustulosis, exfoliative dermatitis

Gastrointestinal: Gastrointestinal perforation, gastrointestinal ulcer, GI inflammation, intestinal perforation

Hypersensitivity: Anaphylaxis

Immunologic: DRESS syndrome

Respiratory: Local alveolar osteitis (post oral surgery patients)

<2%, postmarketing, and/or case reports: Acute renal failure, ageusia, agranulocytosis, albuminuria, alopecia, anaphylactoid reaction, anemia, angina pectoris, angioedema, anorexia, anosmia, anxiety, aplastic anemia, arthralgia, aseptic meningitis, ataxia, bronchitis, bronchospasm, bronchospasm (aggravated), cellulitis, cerebrovascular accident, chest pain, cholelithiasis, colitis (with bleeding), constipation, contact dermatitis, coronary artery disease, cough, cyst, cyst (NOS), cystitis, deafness, decreased hemoglobin, deep vein thrombosis, depression, dermatitis, diaphoresis, diverticulitis, drowsiness, dysphagia, dysuria, ecchymoses, edema, epistaxis, eructation, erythema multiforme, erythematous rash, esophageal perforation, esophagitis, exacerbation of hypertension, facial edema, fatigue, fever, flu-like symptoms, gangrene of skin or other tissue, gastritis, gastroenteritis, gastroesophageal reflux disease, gastrointestinal hemorrhage, hematuria, hemorrhoids, hepatic failure, hepatic necrosis, hepatitis, hiatal hernia, hot flash, hypercholesterolemia, hyperglycemia, hypersensitivity exacerbation, hypersensitivity reaction, hypertonia, hypoesthesia, hypoglycemia, hypokalemia, hyponatremia, increased appetite, increased blood urea nitrogen, increased creatine phosphokinase, increased nonprotein nitrogen, increased serum alkaline phosphatase, interstitial nephritis, intestinal obstruction, intracranial hemorrhage, jaundice, laryngitis, leg cramps, leukopenia, maculopapular rash, melena, migraine, myalgia, myocardial infarction, nervousness, osteoarthritis, pain, palpitations, pancreatitis, pancytopenia, paresthesia, peripheral pain, pneumonia, pruritus, pulmonary embolism, skin changes, skin photosensitivity, Stevens-Johnson syndrome, stomatitis, syncope, synovitis, tachycardia, tendonitis, tenesmus, thrombocythemia, thrombocytopenia, thrombophlebitis, tinnitus, toxic epidermal necrolysis, urinary frequency, urticaria, vasculitis, ventricular fibrillation, vertigo, weight gain, xeroderma, xerostomia

Mechanism of Action Inhibits prostaglandin synthesis by decreasing the activity of the enzyme, cyclooxygenase-2 (COX-2), which results in decreased formation of prostaglandin precursors; has antipyretic, analgesic, and anti-inflammatory properties. Celecoxib does not inhibit cyclooxygenase-1 (COX-1) at therapeutic concentrations.

Pharmacodynamics/Kinetics

Half-life Elimination Children and Adolescents ~7-16 years (steady-state): 6 ± 2.7 hours (range: 3-10 hours) (Stempak 2002); Adults: ~11 hours (fasted)

Time to Peak Children: Median: 3 hours (range: 1-5.8 hours) (Stempak 2002); Adults: ~3 hours

Reproductive Considerations

The chronic use of NSAIDs in women of reproductive age may be associated with infertility that is reversible upon discontinuation of the medication. Consider discontinuing use in women having difficulty conceiving or those undergoing investigation of fertility. The use of NSAIDs close to conception may be associated with an increased risk of miscarriage (Bermas 2014; Bloor 2013).

Pregnancy Risk Factor C (prior to 30 weeks' gestation)/D (≥30 weeks' gestation)

Pregnancy Considerations

Birth defects have been observed following in utero NSAID exposure in some studies, however data is conflicting (Bloor 2013). Nonteratogenic effects, including prenatal constriction of the ductus arteriosus, persistent pulmonary hypertension of the newborn, oligohydramnios, necrotizing enterocolitis, renal dysfunction or failure, and intracranial hemorrhage have been observed in the fetus/neonate following in utero NSAID exposure. In addition, nonclosure of the ductus arteriosus postnatally may occur and be resistant to medical management (Bermas 2014; Bloor 2013). Because NSAIDs may cause premature closure of the ductus arteriosus, product labeling for celecoxib specifically states use should be avoided starting at 30 weeks' gestation.

Use of NSAIDs can be considered for the treatment of mild rheumatoid arthritis flares in pregnant women, however use should be minimized or avoided early and late in pregnancy (Bermas 2014; Saavedra Salinas 2015). Some guidelines recommend avoiding use of selective Cox-2 inhibitors completely during pregnancy due to limited data (Flint 2016).

Product Availability Elyxyb (celecoxib 25 mg/mL oral solution): FDA approved May 2020; anticipated availability currently unknown. Elyxyb is indicated for the acute treatment of migraine with or without aura in adults. Information pertaining to this product within the monograph is pending revision. Consult the prescribing information for additional information.

Dental Health Professional Considerations The product labeling for **all** prescription nonsteroidal anti-inflammatory agents (NSAIDs) now include boxed warnings regarding an increased risk of cardiovascular (CV) events and gastrointestinal (GI) bleeding associated with their use and a contraindication for use in patients who have recently undergone coronary artery bypass graft (CABG) surgery. Medication guides are also now required for these products. Manufacturers of over-the-counter products are to include warnings about potential skin reactions, which are already included in prescription labeling.

The FDA encourages physicians to consider this information in risk-to-benefit evaluations while considering the use of the COX-2 selective celecoxib (CeleBREX®) in patients. Similar COX-2 selective drugs, including rofecoxib (Vioxx®) and valdecoxib (Bextra®), were pulled from the market due to increased risks of adverse CV events associated with their use. In addition, the FDA advises an evaluation of alternative therapy. If physicians determine that continued use is appropriate for individual patients, the lowest effective dose of celecoxib should be prescribed.

The association between selective COX-2 inhibitors and increased cardiovascular risk has been noted previously and prompted by publication of a meta-analysis entitled "Risk of Cardiovascular Events Associated With Selective COX-2 Inhibitors" in the August 22, 2001, edition of the *Journal of the American Medical Association (JAMA)*. The researchers re-evaluated four previously published trials, assessing cardiovascular events in patients receiving either celecoxib or rofecoxib. They found an association between the use of COX-2 inhibitors and cardiovascular events (including MI and ischemic stroke). The annualized MI rate was found to be significantly higher in patients receiving celecoxib or rofecoxib than in the control (placebo) group from a recent meta-analysis of primary prevention trials. Although cause and effect cannot be established (these trials were originally designed to assess GI effects, not cardiovascular ones), the authors believe the available data raise a cautionary flag concerning the risk of cardiovascular events with the use of COX-2 inhibitors.

Cross-reactivity, including bronchospasm, is a concern with aspirin and other NSAIDs, in aspirin-sensitive patients. The manufacturer suggests that celecoxib should not be administered to patients with this type of aspirin sensitivity and should be used with caution in patients with preexisting asthma.

The manufacturer studied the effect of celecoxib on the anticoagulant effect of warfarin and found no alteration of anticoagulant effect, as determined by prothrombin time, in patients taking 2-5 mg daily. However, the manufacturer has issued a caution when using celecoxib with warfarin since those patients are at increased risk of bleeding complications.

◆ **Celestone Soluspan** *see* Betamethasone (Systemic) *on page 233*

◆ **CeleXA** *see* Citalopram *on page 353*

◆ **CellCept** *see* Mycophenolate *on page 1067*

◆ **CellCept Intravenous** *see* Mycophenolate *on page 1067*

◆ **Cell Culture Inactivated Influenza Vaccine, Quadrivalent [Flucelvax Quadrivalent]** *see* Influenza Virus Vaccine (Inactivated) *on page 812*

Cellulose (Oxidized/Regenerated)

(SEL yoo lose, OKS i dyzed re JEN er aye ted)

Related Information

Antiplatelet and Anticoagulation Considerations in Dentistry *on page 1666*

Brand Names: US Interceed; Surgicel SNoW 1"x2" [DSC]; Surgicel SNoW 2"x4" [DSC]; Surgicel SNoW 4"x4" [DSC]

Pharmacologic Category Hemostatic Agent

Use Hemostasis: Adjunctive use in surgical procedures to control capillary, venous, or small arterial hemorrhage when ligation or other conventional methods of control are impractical or ineffective.

Local Anesthetic/Vasoconstrictor Precautions No information available to require special precautions

Effects on Dental Treatment No significant effects or complications reported

Effects on Bleeding No information available to require special precautions

Adverse Reactions <1%, postmarketing, and/or case reports: Application site burning, application site edema (encapsulation), blindness (when placed in anterior cranial fossa), difficulty in micturition (after prostatectomy), foreign body reaction, headache, neurotoxicity, paralysis, postoperative complication (adhesions; prolonged drainage after cholecystectomy), sneezing (epistaxis and rhinological procedures), stinging sensation, ureteral obstruction (after kidney resection), vascular insufficiency (stenosis when applied as a wrap)

Mechanism of Action Cellulose, oxidized regenerated is saturated with blood at the bleeding site and swells into a brownish or black gelatinous mass which aids in the formation of a clot. When used in small amounts, it is absorbed from the sites of implantation with little or no tissue reaction. In addition to providing hemostasis, oxidized regenerated cellulose also has been shown *in vitro* to have bactericidal properties. Its hemostatic effect is not enhanced by the addition of thrombin.

Pregnancy Considerations Has been evaluated for use in gynecologic surgeries (Ahmad 2015; Sharma 2003; Sharma 2006).

◆ **Celontin** *see* Methsuximide *on page 994*

Cemiplimab (SEM ip LI mab)

Brand Names: US Libtayo

Brand Names: Canada Libtayo

Pharmacologic Category Antineoplastic Agent, Anti-PD-1 Monoclonal Antibody; Antineoplastic Agent, Immune Checkpoint Inhibitor; Antineoplastic Agent, Monoclonal Antibody

Use Cutaneous squamous cell carcinoma, metastatic or locally advanced: Treatment of metastatic cutaneous squamous cell carcinoma (CSCC) or locally advanced CSCC in patients who are not candidates for curative surgery or curative radiation.

Local Anesthetic/Vasoconstrictor Precautions No information available to require special precautions

Effects on Dental Treatment No significant effects or complications reported

Effects on Bleeding Therapy with immune checkpoint inhibitors may result in significant myelosuppression, including thrombocytopenia. In patients under active treatment a medical consult is suggested.

Adverse Reactions

>10%:

Central nervous system: Fatigue (29%)

Dermatologic: Skin rash (25%), dermatologic disorders (≤2%; with drug reinitiation: 22%), pruritus (15%)

Gastrointestinal: Diarrhea (22%), nausea (19%), constipation (12%)

Neuromuscular & skeletal: Musculoskeletal pain (17%)

1% to 10%:

Cardiovascular: Hypertension (grades 3/4: ≥2%)

Dermatologic: Cellulitis (grades 3/4: ≥2%), skin infection (grades 3/4: ≥2%), erythema multiforme (≤2%), pemphigoid (≤2%)

Endocrine & metabolic: Hypothyroidism (6%), hypophosphatemia (grades 3/4: 4%), hyponatremia (grades 3/4: 3%), hyperthyroidism (2%), hypercalcemia (grades 3/4: 1%), hypoalbuminemia (grades 3/4: 1%)

Gastrointestinal: Decreased appetite (10%)

Genitourinary: Urinary tract infection (grades 3/4: ≥2%)

Hematologic & oncologic: Lymphocytopenia (grades 3/4: 7%), anemia (grades 3/4: 2%), increased INR (grades 3/4: 2%)
Hepatic: Increased serum aspartate aminotransferase (grades 3/4: 3%), hepatitis (2%)
Immunologic: Antibody development (1%)
Infection: Sepsis (grades 3/4: ≥2%)
Respiratory: Pneumonia (grades 3/4: ≥2%), pneumonitis (≥2%)

Frequency not defined: Dermatologic: Stevens-Johnson syndrome, toxic epidermal necrolysis

<1%, postmarketing, and/or case reports: Adrenocortical insufficiency, aplastic anemia, arthritis, blindness, colitis, demyelinating disease, diabetes mellitus, duodenitis, encephalitis, gastritis, Guillain-Barre syndrome, hematologic disease (hemophagocytic lymphohistiocytosis), hemolytic anemia, hypophysitis, immune thrombocytopenia, increased serum amylase, increased serum lipase, infusion related reaction, iritis, lymphadenitis (Kikuchi), meningitis, myasthenia, myasthenia gravis, myelitis, myocarditis, myositis, nephritis, neuropathy (autoimmune), ophthalmic inflammation, organ transplant rejection, pancreatitis, paresis (nerve), pericarditis, polymyalgia rheumatica, renal failure syndrome, retinal detachment, rhabdomyolysis, sarcoidosis, systemic inflammatory response syndrome, uveitis, vasculitis, visual impairment, Vogt-Koyanagi-Harada syndrome

Mechanism of Action Cemiplimab is a recombinant human IgG4 monoclonal antibody that inhibits programmed death-1 (PD-1) activity by binding to PD-1 and blocking the interactions with the ligands PD-L1 and PD-L2, releasing PD-1 pathway-mediated inhibition of immune response, including anti-tumor response. PD-1 ligand upregulation may occur in some tumors and signaling through this pathway can contribute to inhibition of active T-cell immune surveillance of tumors. Blocking PD-1 activity has resulted in decreased tumor growth.

Pharmacodynamics/Kinetics

Half-life Elimination 19 days

Reproductive Considerations

Evaluate pregnancy status prior to therapy. Females of reproductive potential should use effective contraception during therapy and for at least 4 months after the last cemiplimab dose.

Pregnancy Considerations

Cemiplimab is a recombinant human immunoglobulin (IgG4) monoclonal antibody; human IgG4 is known to cross the placenta. Based on the mechanism of action and information from animal reproduction studies, use of cemiplimab during pregnancy may cause fetal harm.

◆ **Cemiplimab-rwlc** *see* Cemiplimab *on page 320*

Cenegermin (sen EH jer men)

Brand Names: US Oxervate

Pharmacologic Category Recombinant Human Nerve Growth Factor

Use Neurotrophic keratitis: Treatment of neurotrophic keratitis

Local Anesthetic/Vasoconstrictor Precautions No information available to require special precautions

Effects on Dental Treatment No significant effects or complications reported

Effects on Bleeding No information available to require special precautions

Adverse Reactions

>10%: Ophthalmic: Eye pain (16%)

1% to 10%:
Central nervous system: Foreign body sensation
Ophthalmic: Corneal deposits, lacrimation, ocular hyperemia, ophthalmic inflammation

Mechanism of Action Nerve growth factor is an endogenous protein involved in the differentiation and maintenance of neurons, which acts through specific high-affinity (ie, TrkA) and low-affinity (ie, p75NTR) nerve growth factor receptors in the anterior segment of the eye to support corneal innervation and integrity.

Pregnancy Considerations Adverse events were not observed in animal reproduction studies.

◆ **Cenegermin-bkbj** *see* Cenegermin *on page 321*

Cenobamate (SEN oh BAM ate)

Brand Names: US Xcopri; Xcopri (250 MG Daily Dose); Xcopri (350 MG Daily Dose)

Pharmacologic Category Anticonvulsant, Miscellaneous

Use Focal (partial) onset seizures: Treatment of focal (partial) onset seizures in adult patients.

Local Anesthetic/Vasoconstrictor Precautions Frequent occurrence of ECG abnormality identified as shortening of the QT interval. In terms of epinephrine, it is not known what effect vasoconstrictors in the local anesthetic regimen will have in patients with a known history of familial short QT interval or in patients taking any medication that shortens the QT interval. Until more information is obtained, it is suggested that the clinician consult with the physician prior to the use of a vasoconstrictor in suspected patients, and that the vasoconstrictor (epinephrine, levonordefrin [Neo-Cobefrin]) be used with caution.

Effects on Dental Treatment Key adverse event(s) related to dental treatment: Taste alteration; nasopharyngitis.

Effects on Bleeding No information available to require special precautions.

Adverse Reactions

>10%:
Cardiovascular: ECG abnormality (QT shortening: 31% to 66%)
Central nervous system: Hypersomnia (≤57%), lethargy (≤57%), malaise (≤57%), drowsiness (19% to 37%), dizziness (18% to 33%), fatigue (12% to 24%), headache (10% to 12%)
Endocrine & metabolic: Increased serum potassium (8% to 17%)
Ophthalmic: Visual disturbance (9% to 18%), diplopia (6% to 15%)

1% to 10%:
Cardiovascular: Palpitations (2%)
Central nervous system: Amnesia (≤9%), disorientation (≤9%), disturbance in attention (≤9%), psychomotor impairment (≤9%), voice disorder (≤9%), balance impairment (3% to 9%), abnormal gait (3% to 8%), dysarthria (1% to 7%), ataxia (3% to 6%), vertigo (6%), aphasia (1% to 4%), confusion (2% to 3%), euphoria (2%), migraine (2%), irritability (1% to 2%), memory impairment (1% to 2%), sedated state (1% to 2%), suicidal ideation (1% to 2%)
Dermatologic: Pustular rash (2%), pruritus (1% to 2%)
Endocrine & metabolic: Weight loss (1% to 2%)
Gastrointestinal: Nausea (6% to 9%), constipation (2% to 8%), decreased appetite (3% to 5%), vomiting (2% to 5%), diarrhea (1% to 5%), xerostomia (1% to 3%), dysgeusia (2%), dyspepsia (2%), abdominal pain (1% to 2%), hiccups (1%)

Genitourinary: Urinary tract infection (5%), dysmenorrhea (1% to 2%), pollakiuria (1%)

Hepatic: Increased serum alanine aminotransferase (1% to 4%; >3 x ULN: ≤3%), increased serum aspartate aminotransferase (1% to 3%)

Neuromuscular & skeletal: Back pain (4% to 5%), asthenia (3%), tremor (3%), musculoskeletal chest pain (1% to 2%)

Ophthalmic: Nystagmus disorder (3% to 7%), blurred vision (2% to 4%)

Respiratory: Nasopharyngitis (4% to 5%), dyspnea (3%), pharyngitis (1% to 2%)

Miscellaneous: Head trauma (1% to 2%)

Frequency not defined:

Gastrointestinal: Appendicitis

Immunologic: Drug reaction with eosinophilia and systemic symptoms

Mechanism of Action Cenobamate inhibits voltage-gated sodium channels, reducing repetitive neuronal firing. Cenobamate also acts as a positive allosteric modulator of $GABA_A$ ion channels.

Pharmacodynamics/Kinetics

Half-life Elimination Terminal: 50 to 60 hours.

Time to Peak 1 to 4 hours.

Reproductive Considerations Cenobamate may decrease the efficacy of oral contraceptives. Females of childbearing potential should use additional or alternative nonhormonal contraceptive measures during treatment with cenobamate.

Pregnancy Considerations

Adverse events were observed in some animal reproduction studies.

Data collection to monitor pregnancy and infant outcomes following exposure to cenobamate is ongoing. Health care providers are encouraged to enroll females exposed to cenobamate during pregnancy in the North American Antiepileptic Drug Pregnancy Registry (1-888-233-2334 or http://www.aedpregnancyregistry.org/).

Controlled Substance C-V

- **Centamin [OTC]** *see* Vitamins (Multiple/Oral) *on page 1550*
- **Centany** *see* Mupirocin *on page 1066*
- **Centany AT** *see* Mupirocin *on page 1066*
- **Centrum [OTC]** *see* Vitamins (Multiple/Oral) *on page 1550*
- **Centrum Cardio [OTC]** *see* Vitamins (Multiple/Oral) *on page 1550*
- **Centrum Flavor Burst [OTC]** *see* Vitamins (Multiple/Oral) *on page 1550*
- **Centrum MultiGummies [OTC]** *see* Vitamins (Multiple/Oral) *on page 1550*
- **Centrum Performance [OTC]** *see* Vitamins (Multiple/Oral) *on page 1550*
- **Centrum Silver [OTC]** *see* Vitamins (Multiple/Oral) *on page 1550*
- **Centrum Silver Ultra Men's [OTC]** *see* Vitamins (Multiple/Oral) *on page 1550*
- **Centrum Silver Ultra Women's [OTC]** *see* Vitamins (Multiple/Oral) *on page 1550*
- **Centrum Ultra Men's [OTC]** *see* Vitamins (Multiple/Oral) *on page 1550*
- **Centrum Ultra Women's [OTC]** *see* Vitamins (Multiple/Oral) *on page 1550*
- **Cepacol [OTC]** *see* Benzocaine *on page 228*
- **Cepacol Antibacterial [OTC]** *see* Cetylpyridinium *on page 330*
- **Cepacol INSTAMAX [OTC]** *see* Benzocaine *on page 228*

Cephalexin (sef a LEKS in)

Related Information

Antibiotic Prophylaxis *on page 1715*

Bacterial Infections *on page 1739*

Related Sample Prescriptions

Bacterial Infections and Periodontal Diseases - Sample Prescriptions *on page 35*

Prevention of Endocarditis and to Reduce the Risk of Late Infections of Joint Prostheses - Sample Prescriptions *on page 40*

Brand Names: US Daxbia [DSC]; Keflex

Brand Names: Canada APO-Cephalex; AURO-Cephalexin; DOM-Cephalexin [DSC]; Keflex; LUPIN-Cephalexin; PMS-Cephalexin; TEVA-Cephalexin; TEVA-Cephalexin 125; TEVA-Cephalexin 250

Generic Availability (US) Yes

Pharmacologic Category Antibiotic, Cephalosporin (First Generation)

Dental Use Prophylaxis in total joint replacement patients undergoing dental procedures; alternative oral antibiotic for prevention of infective endocarditis in individuals allergic to penicillins or ampicillin

Note: Individuals allergic to amoxicillin (penicillins) may receive cephalexin provided they have not had an immediate, local, or systemic IgE-mediated anaphylactic allergic reaction to penicillin.

Use

Bone infections: Treatment of bone infections caused by *Staphylococcus aureus* and/or *Proteus mirabilis*.

Genitourinary tract infections: Treatment of genitourinary tract infections, including acute prostatitis, caused by *Escherichia coli*, *P. mirabilis*, and *Klebsiella pneumoniae*.

Otitis media: Treatment of otitis media caused by *Streptococcus pneumoniae*, *Haemophilus influenzae*, *S. aureus*, *Streptococcus pyogenes*, and *Moraxella catarrhalis*.

Respiratory tract infections: Treatment of respiratory tract infections (including pharyngitis) caused by *S. pneumoniae* and *S. pyogenes*.

Skin and skin structure infections: Treatment of skin and skin structure infections caused by *S. aureus* and/or *S. pyogenes*.

Local Anesthetic/Vasoconstrictor Precautions No information available to require special precautions

Effects on Dental Treatment No significant effects or complications reported (see Dental Health Professional Considerations)

Effects on Bleeding No information available to require special precautions

Adverse Reactions Frequency not defined.

Central nervous system: Agitation, confusion, dizziness, fatigue, hallucination, headache

Dermatologic: Erythema multiforme (rare), genital pruritus, skin rash, Stevens-Johnson syndrome (rare), toxic epidermal necrolysis (rare), urticaria

Gastrointestinal: Abdominal pain, diarrhea, dyspepsia, gastritis, nausea (rare), pseudomembranous colitis, vomiting (rare)

Genitourinary: Genital candidiasis, vaginal discharge, vaginitis

Hematologic & oncologic: Eosinophilia, hemolytic anemia, neutropenia, thrombocytopenia

Hepatic: Cholestatic jaundice (rare), hepatitis (transient, rare), increased serum ALT, increased serum AST

Hypersensitivity: Anaphylaxis, angioedema, hypersensitivity reaction

Neuromuscular & skeletal: Arthralgia, arthritis, arthropathy

Renal: Interstitial nephritis (rare)

Dental Usual Dosage

Prophylaxis against infective endocarditis (dental, oral, or respiratory tract procedures): Oral:

Children >1 year: 50 mg/kg 30 to 60 minutes prior to procedure; maximum: 2 g

Children >15 years and Adults: 2 g 30 to 60 minutes prior to procedure

Note: American Heart Association (AHA) guidelines now recommend prophylaxis only in patients undergoing invasive procedures and in whom underlying cardiac conditions may predispose to a higher risk of adverse outcomes should infection occur.

Prophylaxis in total joint replacement patients undergoing dental procedures which produce bacteremia: Oral: Adults: 2 g 1 hour prior to procedure

Note: In general, patients with prosthetic joint implants do not require prophylactic antibiotics prior to dental procedures. In planning an invasive oral procedure, dental consultation with the patient's orthopedic surgeon may be advised to review the risks of infection.

Dosing

Adult & Geriatric

Usual dosage range: Oral: 250 to 1,000 mg every 6 hours or 500 mg every 12 hours (maximum: 4 g/day).

Indication-specific dosing:

Cellulitis (nonpurulent)/erysipelas, mild (alternative agent): Oral: 500 mg 4 times daily for at least 5 days (duration should be extended if not resolved/slow response) (IDSA [Stevens 2014]).

Endocarditis, prophylaxis (dental or invasive respiratory tract procedures) (alternative agent) (off-label use): Oral: 2 g 30 to 60 minutes prior to procedure. **Note:** AHA guidelines recommend prophylaxis only in patients undergoing invasive procedures and in whom underlying cardiac conditions may predispose to a higher risk of adverse outcomes should infection occur (AHA [Wilson 2007]).

Impetigo or ecthyma: Oral: 250 to 500 mg 4 times daily for 7 days. **Note:** Not an appropriate agent if MRSA is suspected or confirmed (Baddour 2019; IDSA [Stevens 2014]).

Prosthetic joint infection (off-label use): Oral: Treatment (following pathogen-specific IV therapy in patients undergoing 1-stage exchange or debridement with retention of prosthesis). **Note:** Duration ranges from a minimum of 3 months to indefinitely, depending on patient-specific factors (Berbari 2019):

Staphylococci (methicillin-susceptible): 500 mg every 6 to 8 hours **or** 1 g every 8 to 12 hours. For the first 3 to 6 months of therapy, combine with rifampin (Berbari 2019; IDSA [Osmon 2013]).

Streptococci, beta-hemolytic (alternative agent): 500 mg every 6 to 8 hours (Berbari 2019; IDSA [Osmon 2013]).

Cutibacterium spp (alternative agent): 500 mg every 6 to 8 hours (IDSA [Osmon 2013]; Kanafani 2019).

Streptococcal pharyngitis (group A) (alternative agent for mild [non-anaphylactic] penicillin allergy): Oral: 500 mg every 12 hours for 10 days (IDSA [Shulman 2012]; Pichichero 2020; manufacturer's labeling).

Urinary tract infection:

Acute uncomplicated or simple cystitis, treatment (alternative agent): Oral: 250 to 500 mg every 6 hours for 5 to 7 days (Bolding 1978; Hooton 2019a; Hooton 2019b; Johnson 1972; Menday 2000).

Bacteriuria (≥10^5 CFU per mL), asymptomatic, in pregnancy: Oral: 250 to 500 mg every 6 hours for 4 to 7 days (ACOG 782 2019; Hooton 2019c; IDSA [Nicolle 2019]; Pedler 1985).

Cystitis, uncomplicated, prophylaxis for recurrent infection (off-label use):

Note: Prophylaxis may be considered in nonpregnant women with bothersome, recurrent uncomplicated cystitis despite nonantimicrobial preventative measures. The optimal duration of prophylaxis has not been established; duration ranges from 3 to 12 months, with periodic assessment and monitoring (AUA/CUA/SUFU [Anger 2019]; Hooton 2019d).

Continuous prophylaxis: Oral: 125 to 250 mg once daily (AUA/CUA/SUFU [Anger 2019]; Gower 1975).

Postcoital prophylaxis: Females with cystitis temporally related to sexual intercourse: Oral: 250 mg as a single dose immediately before or after sexual intercourse (AUA/CUA/SUFU [Anger 2019]; Pfau 1992).

Renal Impairment: Adult

CrCl ≥60 mL/minute: No dosage adjustment necessary.

CrCl 30 to 59 mL/minute: There are no specific dosage adjustments provided in the manufacturer's labeling; maximum recommended daily dose: 1,000 mg/day.

CrCl 15 to 29 mL/minute: 250 mg every 8 to 12 hours

CrCl 5 to 14 mL/minute (not yet on dialysis): 250 every 24 hours

CrCl 1 to 4 mL/minute (not yet on dialysis): 250 mg every 48 to 60 hours

End-stage renal disease (on intermittent hemodialysis: There are no dosage adjustments provided in the manufacturer's labeling; however, the following guidelines have been used by some clinicians (Aronoff 2007): Oral: 250 to 500 mg every 12 to 24 hours; moderately dialyzable (20% to 50%); give dose after dialysis session.

Peritoneal dialysis: There are no dosage adjustments provided in the manufacturer's labeling; however, the following guidelines have been used by some clinicians (Aronoff 2007): Oral: 250 to 500 mg every 12 to 24 hours.

Hepatic Impairment: Adult

There are no dosage adjustments provided in the manufacturer's labeling.

Pediatric

General dosing, susceptible infection (Bradley 2019; *Red Book* [AAP 2018]): Infants, Children, and Adolescents:

Mild to moderate infection: Oral: 25 to 50 mg/kg/day divided every 6 or 12 hours; maximum daily dose: 2,000 mg/**day**.

Severe infection (eg, bone and joint infections): Oral: 75 to 100 mg/kg/day divided every 6 to 8 hours; maximum daily dose: 4,000 mg/**day**.

Catheter (peritoneal dialysis); exit-site or tunnel infection: Limited data available: Infants, Children, and Adolescents: Oral: 10 to 20 mg/kg/day once daily or divided into 2 doses; maximum dose: 1,000 mg/dose (ISPD [Warady 2012]).

Pharyngitis/tonsillitis (group A streptococcal): Note: Use is reserved for patients with penicillin allergy (non-anaphylactic) (IDSA [Shulman 2012]).

Infants, Children, and Adolescents: Oral: 40 mg/kg/day divided every 12 hours for 10 days, maximum dose: 500 mg/dose (IDSA [Shulman 2012]).

Impetigo (*staphylococcus* or *streptococcus*): Note: Do not use if MRSA is suspected or confirmed.

Infants, Children, and Adolescents: Oral: 25 to 50 mg/kg/day divided every 6 or 8 hours; some experts suggest up to 75 mg/kg/day divided every 8 hours may be necessary in some cases; maximum daily dose: 1,000 mg/**day**; continue for at least 7 days, full duration dependent upon clinical response (Bradley 2019; IDSA [Stevens 2014]).

Otitis media, acute (AOM): Note: Cephalexin is not routinely recommended as an empiric treatment option (AAP [Lieberthal 2013]).

Children >1 year and Adolescents <15 years: Oral: 75 to 100 mg/kg/day divided every 6 hours; maximum dose not established for AOM; usual maximum adult dose for mild to moderate infections: 500 mg/dose and for severe infections: 1,000 mg/dose.

Skin and skin structure infections (eg, cellulitis, erysipelas): Infants, Children, and Adolescents: Oral: 25 to 50 mg/kg/day divided every 6 hours; maximum dose: 500 mg/dose; continue for at least 5 days or longer depending upon clinical response (IDSA [Stevens 2014]).

Endocarditis prophylaxis: Note: AHA guidelines (Baltimore 2015) limit the use of prophylactic antibiotics to patients at the highest risk for infective endocarditis (IE) or adverse outcomes (eg, prosthetic heart valves, patients with previous IE, unrepaired cyanotic congenital heart disease, repaired congenital heart disease with prosthetic material or device during first 6 months after procedure, repaired congenital heart disease with residual defects at the site or adjacent to site of prosthetic patch or device, and heart transplant recipients with cardiac valvulopathy):

Dental or oral procedures, or respiratory tract procedures (eg, tonsillectomy, adenoidectomy): **Note:** Recommended for use in patients with penicillin allergy (non-anaphylactic):

Infants, Children, and Adolescents: Oral: 50 mg/kg administered 30 to 60 minutes prior to procedure; maximum dose: 2,000 mg/dose (AHA [Wilson 2007]).

Pneumonia, community-acquired: *S. aureus* (methicillin-susceptible), mild infection or step-down therapy: Infants >3 months, Children, and Adolescents: Oral: 75 to 100 mg/kg/day in 3 to 4 divided doses (IDSA/PIDS [Bradley 2011]); maximum daily dose: 4,000 mg/**day** (*Red Book* [AAP 2018]).

Urinary tract infection:

Empiric therapy in febrile patients: Infants ≥2 months and Children <24 months: Oral: 50 to 100 mg/kg/day divided every 6 hours for 7 to 14 days (AAP 2011).

Treatment:

Children and Adolescents <15 years: Oral: 25 to 50 mg/kg/day divided every 6 to 12 hours for 7 to 14 days, maximum dose: 500 mg/dose; for severe infections, 50 to 100 mg/kg/day divided every 6 to 12 hours may be necessary; maximum daily dose: 4,000 mg/**day**.

Adolescents ≥15 years: Oral: 250 mg every 6 hours or 500 mg every 12 hours for 7 to 14 days; higher doses may be necessary for severe infections; maximum daily dose: 4,000 mg/**day**.

Osteoarticular infection (eg, septic arthritis, osteomyelitis); step-down therapy: Infants, Children, and Adolescents: Oral: 100 mg/kg/day divided every 6 to 8 hours; maximum daily dose: 4,000 mg/**day**; duration of therapy variable, dependent upon clinical response and typically extensive (weeks of therapy); compliance should be monitored (Bradley 2019; *Red Book* [AAP 2018]); a small (n=11) prospective, open-label pharmacokinetic study reported a median dose of 40 mg/kg/dose every 8 hours (mean age: 7 years; range: 1 to 16 years; dose range: 19 to 51 mg/kg/dose every 8 hours) maintained serum concentrations long enough to meet the pharmacokinetic/pharmacodynamic target for efficacy (T>MIC ≥40%) (Autmizguine 2013).

Renal Impairment: Pediatric

Weight-based dosing: Infants, Children, and Adolescents: There are no recommendations in the manufacturer's labeling; the following adjustments have been recommended (Aronoff 2007). **Note:** Renally-adjusted dose recommendations are based on doses of 25 to 50 mg/kg/day divided every 6 hours: Oral:

CrCl >50 mL/minute/1.73 m^2: No adjustment necessary.

CrCl 30 to 50 mL/minute/1.73 m^2: 5 to 10 mg/kg/dose every 8 hours (maximum dose: 500 mg/dose).

CrCl 10 to 29 mL/minute/1.73 m^2: 5 to 10 mg/kg/dose every 12 hours (maximum dose: 500 mg/dose).

CrCl <10 mL/minute/1.73 m^2: 5 to 10 mg/kg/dose every 24 hours (maximum dose: 500 mg/dose).

Intermittent hemodialysis: 5 to 10 mg/kg/dose every 24 hours after dialysis (maximum dose: 500 mg/dose).

Peritoneal dialysis: 5 to 10 mg/kg/dose every 24 hours (maximum dose: 500 mg/dose).

Fixed dosing: Adolescents ≥15 years: Oral:

CrCl ≥60 mL/minute: No dosage adjustment necessary.

CrCl 30 to 59 mL/minute: No adjustment necessary; maximum recommended daily dose: 1,000 mg/**day**.

CrCl 15 to 29 mL/minute: 250 mg every 8 to 12 hours.

CrCl 5 to 14 mL/minute (not yet on dialysis): 250 every 24 hours.

CrCl 1 to 4 mL/minute (not yet on dialysis): 250 mg every 48 to 60 hours.

Hepatic Impairment: Pediatric There are no dosing adjustments provided in the manufacturer's labeling.

Mechanism of Action Inhibits bacterial cell wall synthesis by binding to one or more of the penicillin-binding proteins (PBPs) which in turn inhibits the final transpeptidation step of peptidoglycan synthesis in bacterial cell walls, thus inhibiting cell wall biosynthesis. Bacteria eventually lyse due to ongoing activity of cell wall autolytic enzymes (autolysins and murein hydrolases) while cell wall assembly is arrested.

Contraindications Hypersensitivity to cephalexin, other cephalosporins, or any component of the formulation

Warnings/Precautions Allergic reactions (eg, rash, urticaria, angioedema, anaphylaxis, erythema multiforme, Stevens-Johnson syndrome, toxic epidermal necrolysis [TEN]) have been reported. If an allergic reaction occurs, discontinue immediately and institute appropriate treatment. Use with caution in patients with a history of seizure disorder; high levels, particularly in the presence of renal impairment, may increase risk of seizures. Modify dosage in patients with severe renal impairment. Use with caution in patients with a history of penicillin allergy, especially IgE-mediated reactions (eg, anaphylaxis, urticaria). Positive direct Coombs tests and acute intravascular hemolysis has been reported. If anemia develops during or after therapy, discontinue use and work up for drug-induced hemolytic anemia. Prolonged use may result in fungal or bacterial superinfection, including *C. difficile*-associated diarrhea (CDAD) and pseudomembranous colitis; CDAD has been observed >2 months post antibiotic treatment. May be associated with increased INR, especially in nutritionally-deficient patients, prolonged treatment, hepatic or renal disease. Potentially significant interactions may exist, requiring dose or frequency adjustment, additional monitoring, and/or selection of alternative therapy.

Drug Interactions

Metabolism/Transport Effects None known.

Avoid Concomitant Use

Avoid concomitant use of Cephalexin with any of the following: BCG (Intravesical); Cholera Vaccine

Increased Effect/Toxicity

Cephalexin may increase the levels/effects of: Aminoglycosides; MetFORMIN; Vitamin K Antagonists

The levels/effects of Cephalexin may be increased by: Probenecid

Decreased Effect

Cephalexin may decrease the levels/effects of: Aminoglycosides; BCG (Intravesical); BCG Vaccine (Immunization); Cholera Vaccine; Lactobacillus and Estriol; Sodium Picosulfate; Typhoid Vaccine

The levels/effects of Cephalexin may be decreased by: Multivitamins/Minerals (with ADEK, Folate, Iron); Multivitamins/Minerals (with AE, No Iron); Sucroferric Oxyhydroxide; Zinc Salts

Food Interactions Peak antibiotic serum concentration is lowered and delayed, but total drug absorbed is not affected. Cephalexin serum levels may be decreased if taken with food. Management: Administer without regard to food.

Pharmacodynamics/Kinetics

Half-life Elimination Neonates: 5 hours; Children 3 to 12 months: 2.5 hours; Adults: 0.5 to 1.2 hours (prolonged with renal impairment)

Time to Peak Serum: ~1 hour

Pregnancy Considerations

Cephalexin crosses the placenta and produces therapeutic concentrations in the fetal circulation and amniotic fluid (Creatsas 1980).

An increased risk of major birth defects or other adverse fetal or maternal outcomes has generally not been observed following use of cephalosporin antibiotics, including cephalexin, during pregnancy.

Peak concentrations in pregnant patients are similar to those in nonpregnant patients. Prolonged labor may decrease oral absorption (Griffith 1983; Paterson 1972). Cephalexin may be used in certain situations prior to vaginal delivery in females at high risk for endocarditis, and use may be considered for postcesarean delivery prophylaxis in obese females (ACOG 199 2018). Use of cephalexin may also be considered for the treatment of asymptomatic bacteriuria in pregnant women (Nicolle [IDSA 2019]).

Breastfeeding Considerations Cephalexin is present in breast milk.

The relative infant dose (RID) of cephalexin is 0.13% to 0.52% when compared to an infant therapeutic dose of 25 to 100 mg/kg/day.

In general, breastfeeding is considered acceptable when the relative infant dose is <10% (Anderson 2016; Ito 2000).

The RID of cephalexin was calculated using a milk concentration of 0.85 mcg/mL, providing an estimated daily infant dose via breast milk of 0.13 mg/kg/day. This milk concentration was obtained following a single maternal dose of cephalexin 1,000 mg orally on the third postpartum day. The mean peak milk concentration occurred 4 to 5 hours after the dose (Kafetzis 1981). Slightly higher concentrations of cephalexin were detected in the breast milk of a breastfeeding woman also administered probenecid and cephalexin for ≥16 days (Ilett 2006).

Diarrhea has been reported in breastfeeding infants (Ilett 2006; Ito 1993). In general, antibiotics that are present in breast milk may cause non-dose-related modification of bowel flora. Monitor infants for GI disturbances (WHO 2002).

When an antibiotic is needed, cephalexin may be used to treat mastitis in breastfeeding women allergic to preferred agents (Amir 2014; Berens 2015). According to the manufacturer, the decision to breastfeed during therapy should consider the risk of infant exposure, the benefits of breastfeeding to the infant, and benefits of treatment to the mother

Dosage Forms: US

Capsule, Oral:

Keflex: 250 mg, 500 mg, 750 mg

Generic: 250 mg, 500 mg, 750 mg

Suspension Reconstituted, Oral:

Generic: 125 mg/5 mL (100 mL, 200 mL); 250 mg/5 mL (100 mL, 200 mL)

Tablet, Oral:

Generic: 250 mg, 500 mg

Dosage Forms: Canada

Capsule, Oral:

Generic: 250 mg, 500 mg

Suspension Reconstituted, Oral:

Keflex: 125 mg/5 mL (100 mL, 200 mL); 250 mg/5 mL (200 mL)

Generic: 125 mg/5 mL (100 mL, 150 mL, 200 mL); 250 mg/5 mL (100 mL, 120 mL, 150 mL, 200 mL)

Tablet, Oral:

Keflex: 250 mg, 500 mg

Generic: 250 mg, 500 mg

Dental Health Professional Considerations Cephalexin is effective against anaerobic bacteria, but the sensitivity of alpha-hemolytic Streptococcus vary; approximately 10% of strains are resistant. Nearly 70% are intermediately sensitive. Patients allergic to penicillins can use a cephalosporin; the incidence of cross-reactivity between penicillins and cephalosporins is 1% to 5% when the allergic reaction to penicillin is delayed. If the patient has a history of anaphylaxis to penicillin, cephalosporins are contraindicated in these patients.

◆ **Cephalexin Monohydrate** *see* Cephalexin *on page 322*

◆ **Cequa** *see* CycloSPORINE (Ophthalmic) *on page 423*

◆ **CERA** *see* Methoxy Polyethylene Glycol-Epoetin Beta *on page 993*

◆ **CeraVe Itch Relief [OTC] [DSC]** *see* Pramoxine *on page 1252*

◆ **Cerdelga** *see* Eliglustat *on page 549*

◆ **Cerebyx** *see* Fosphenytoin *on page 717*

Ceritinib (se RI ti nib)

Brand Names: US Zykadia

Brand Names: Canada Zykadia

Pharmacologic Category Antineoplastic Agent, Anaplastic Lymphoma Kinase Inhibitor; Antineoplastic Agent, Tyrosine Kinase Inhibitor

Use Non-small cell lung cancer, metastatic: Treatment of anaplastic lymphoma kinase (ALK)-positive (as detected by an approved test) metastatic non-small cell lung cancer (NSCLC).

Local Anesthetic/Vasoconstrictor Precautions Ceritinib is one of the drugs confirmed to prolong the QT interval and is accepted as having a risk of causing torsade de pointes. The risk of drug-induced torsade de pointes is extremely low when a single QT interval prolonging drug is prescribed. In terms of epinephrine, it is not known what effect vasoconstrictors in the local anesthetic regimen will have in patients with a known history of congenital prolonged QT interval or in patients taking any medication that prolongs the QT interval. Until more information is obtained, it is suggested that the clinician consult with the physician prior to the use of a vasoconstrictor in suspected patients, and that the vasoconstrictor (epinephrine, mepivacaine and levonordefrin [Carbocaine® 2% with Neo-Cobefrin®]) be used with caution.

Effects on Dental Treatment No significant effects or complications reported

Effects on Bleeding No information available to require special precautions

Adverse Reactions

>10%:

Cardiovascular: Prolonged QT interval on ECG (4% to 12%)

Central nervous system: Fatigue (45% to 52%), noncardiac chest pain (21%), headache (19%), neuropathy (17%), dizziness (12%)

Dermatologic: Skin rash (16% to 21%), pruritus (11%)

Endocrine & metabolic: Increased gamma-glutamyl transferase (84%), hyperglycemia (49% to 53%), decreased serum phosphate (36% to 38%), weight loss (24%)

Gastrointestinal: Diarrhea (56% to 86%), nausea (45% to 80%), vomiting (35% to 67%), abdominal pain (40% to 54%), increased serum amylase (37%), decreased appetite (34%), constipation (20% to 29%), increased serum lipase (13% to 28%), dyspepsia (≤16%), dysphagia (≤16%), gastroesophageal reflux disease (≤16%)

Hematologic & oncologic: Anemia (67% to 84%; grades 3/4: 4% to 5%), neutropenia (27%; grades 3/4: 2%), thrombocytopenia (16%; grades 3/4: 1%)

Hepatic: Increased serum ALT (80% to 91%; >5x ULN: 28%), increased serum AST (75% to 86%; >5x ULN: 16%), increased serum alkaline phosphatase (81%), increased serum bilirubin (15%)

Neuromuscular & skeletal: Back pain (19%), limb pain (13%), musculoskeletal pain (11%)

Renal: Increased serum creatinine (58% to 77%)

Respiratory: Cough (25%)

Miscellaneous: Fever (19%)

1% to 10%:

Cardiovascular: Pericarditis (4%), bradycardia (1% to 4%) pericardial effusion (≥2%), sinus bradycardia (1%)

Central nervous system: Seizure (≥2%)

Endocrine & metabolic: Dehydration (≥2%)

Hepatic: Hepatotoxicity (2%)

Ophthalmic: Visual disturbance (4% to 9%)

Renal: Renal failure (2%)

Respiratory: Pleural effusion (4%), pneumonia (4%), interstitial pulmonary disease (2% to 4%), pulmonary infection (≥2%), severe dyspnea (≥2%)

<1%, postmarketing and/or case reports: Pancreatitis

Mechanism of Action Ceritinib is a potent inhibitor of anaplastic lymphoma kinase (ALK), a tyrosine kinase involved in the pathogenesis of non-small cell lung cancer. ALK gene abnormalities due to mutations or translocations may result in expression of oncogenic fusion proteins (eg, ALK fusion protein) which alter signaling and expression and result in increased cellular proliferation and survival in tumors which express these fusion proteins. ALK inhibition reduces proliferation of cells expressing the genetic alteration. Ceritinib also inhibits insulin-like growth factor 1 receptor (IGF-1R), insulin receptor (InsR), and ROS1. Ceritinib has demonstrated activity in crizotinib-resistant tumors in NSCLC xenograft models.

Pharmacodynamics/Kinetics

Half-life Elimination 41 hours (following a single 750 mg fasted dose)

Time to Peak ~4 to 6 hours

Reproductive Considerations

Women of reproductive potential should use effective contraception during treatment and for 6 months following therapy discontinuation. Based on the potential for genotoxicity, males with female partners of reproductive potential should use condoms during treatment and for 3 months following completion of therapy.

Pregnancy Considerations

Based on findings in animal reproduction studies and its mechanism of action, ceritinib may cause fetal harm if administered to a pregnant woman.

Dental Health Professional Considerations See Local Anesthetic/Vasoconstrictor Precautions

Certolizumab Pegol (cer to LIZ u mab PEG ol)

Related Information

Rheumatoid Arthritis, Osteoarthritis, and Osteoporosis *on page 1697*

Brand Names: US Cimzia; Cimzia Prefilled; Cimzia Starter Kit

Brand Names: Canada Cimzia

Pharmacologic Category Antirheumatic, Disease Modifying; Gastrointestinal Agent, Miscellaneous; Tumor Necrosis Factor (TNF) Blocking Agent

Use

Ankylosing spondylitis: Treatment of adults with active ankylosing spondylitis (AS)

Axial spondyloarthritis, nonradiographic: Treatment of adults with nonradiographic axial spondyloarthritis (nr-axSpA) with objective signs of inflammation.

Crohn disease: Treatment of moderately to severely active Crohn disease in patients who have inadequate response to conventional therapy

Plaque psoriasis: Treatment of moderate to severe plaque psoriasis in adults who are candidates for systemic therapy or phototherapy

Psoriatic arthritis: Treatment of adult patients with active psoriatic arthritis

Rheumatoid arthritis: Treatment of adults with moderately to severely active rheumatoid arthritis (RA) (as monotherapy or in combination with nonbiological disease-modifying antirheumatic drugs [DMARDS])

Local Anesthetic/Vasoconstrictor Precautions No information available to require special precautions

Effects on Dental Treatment Key adverse event(s) related to dental treatment: Certolizumab pegol belongs to the class of disease-modifying antirheumatic drugs and, as such, has immunosuppressive properties. Consider a medical consult prior to any invasive treatment for patients under active treatment with certolizumab pegol. Delayed wound healing due to the immunosuppressive effects and increased potential for postsurgical infection may be of concern.

Effects on Bleeding No information available to require special precautions

Adverse Reactions

>10%:

- Gastrointestinal: Nausea (≤11% [Schreiber 2005])
- Immunologic: Antibody development (7% to 23%; neutralizing: 3% to 8%)
- Infection: Infection (38%)
- Respiratory: Upper respiratory tract infection (18% to 22%)

1% to 10%:

- Central nervous system: Headache (4%)
- Dermatologic: Skin rash (9%)
- Genitourinary: Urinary tract infection (7% to 8%)
- Hematologic & oncologic: Positive ANA titer (4%)
- Hepatic: Increased serum transaminases (≤4%)
- Infection: Herpes virus infections (2%)
- Local: Injection site reaction (2% to 3%)
- Neuromuscular & skeletal: Arthralgia (6%)
- Respiratory: Cough (3%)

Frequency not defined:

- Dermatologic: Cellulitis
- Gastrointestinal: Diarrhea, intestinal obstruction
- Hematologic & oncologic: Hematoma, leukopenia, pancytopenia
- Infection: Abscess (abdominal), aspergillosis, blastomycosis, candidiasis, coccidioidomycosis, fungal infection, histoplasmosis, listeriosis, opportunistic infection, sepsis, serious infection, tuberculosis
- Renal: Pyelonephritis
- Respiratory: Infection due to an organism in genus Pneumocystis, lower respiratory tract infection, pneumonia

<1%, postmarketing, and/or case reports: Abdominal pain, allergic dermatitis, anaphylaxis, angioedema, aplastic anemia, autoimmune hepatitis (Shelton 2015), cardiac failure, cytopenia, dyspnea, erythema at injection site, erythema nodosum, hepatosplenic T-cell lymphomas, hepatotoxicity (idiosyncratic) (Chalasani 2014), Hodgkin lymphoma, hot flash, hypersensitivity reaction, hypotension, lichenoid eruption, limb pain, lupus-like syndrome, malaise, malignant lymphoma, malignant melanoma, malignant neoplasm, Merkel cell carcinoma, non-Hodgkin lymphoma, optic neuritis, orthostatic dizziness, pain at injection site, peripheral edema, peripheral neuropathy, psoriasis (including new onset, palmoplantar, pustular, or exacerbation), reactivation of HBV, sarcoidosis, seizure, serum sickness, syncope, thrombocytopenia, urticaria, viral infection

Mechanism of Action Certolizumab is a pegylated humanized antibody Fab' fragment of tumor necrosis factor alpha (TNF-alpha) monoclonal antibody. Certolizumab binds to and selectively neutralizes human TNF-alpha activity. (Elevated levels of TNF-alpha have a role in the inflammatory process associated with Crohn disease and in joint destruction associated with rheumatoid arthritis.) Since it is not a complete antibody (lacks Fc region), it does not induce complement activation, antibody-dependent cell-mediated cytotoxicity, or apoptosis. Pegylation of certolizumab allows for delayed elimination and therefore an extended half-life.

Pharmacodynamics/Kinetics

Half-life Elimination ~14 days

Time to Peak Plasma: 54 to 171 hours

Reproductive Considerations

The American Academy of Dermatology considers tumor necrosis factor alpha (TNFα) blocking agents for the treatment of psoriasis to be compatible for use in male patients planning to father a child (AAD-NPF [Menter 2019]). Women with psoriasis planning a pregnancy may continue treatment with certolizumab pegol. Women with well-controlled psoriasis who wish to avoid fetal exposure can consider discontinuing certolizumab pegol 10 weeks prior to attempting pregnancy (Rademaker 2018).

Treatment algorithms are available for use of biologics in female patients with Crohn disease who are planning a pregnancy (Weizman 2019).

Pregnancy Considerations

Placental transfer of certolizumab pegol is minimal (Förger 2016; Mariette 2018).

Certolizumab pegol is a humanized Fab-fragment conjugated to polyethylene glycol (PEG). Placental transfer of Fab-fragments is expected to be low to absent (Pentsuk 2009).

Serum concentrations of certolizumab pegol in 12 infants of 10 mothers were ≥75% lower than the maternal serum at delivery (last maternal dose of 400 mg given 5 to 42 days prior to birth; median: 19 days). PEG was not present in infant plasma or cord blood. Although placental transfer of certolizumab pegol was low, based on the rate certolizumab pegol decline in one case, infants may have a slower rate of elimination than adults (Mahadevan 2013). In a study with information from 11 infants, certolizumab pegol cord concentrations were below the limit of detection (n=8) to 1 mcg/mL (n=3). In comparison, median maternal serum levels were 32.97 mcg/mL following administration of certolizumab 200 mg every 2 weeks (Förger 2016). Information is also available from a multicenter study which included 16 mothers on various certolizumab doses during pregnancy. All mothers in the study had therapeutic drug concentrations. The median time between the last maternal dose and delivery was 11 days (range: 1 to 27 days). Certolizumab pegol was measurable in the cord blood in one of 14 infants; concentrations were 0.09% of the maternal plasma levels. Certolizumab pegol was not present in infant serum 4 and 8 weeks after birth. In addition, 14 of 15 umbilical cord samples did not have detectable concentrations of PEG (Mariette 2018).

Pregnancy outcome data from the UCB Pharma safety database collected through March 6, 2017 has been published. Among 528 prospective pregnancies with

538 known outcomes (10 twin pregnancies), 85.3% resulted in live births; among these, 81.2% had at least first trimester exposure. Other outcomes reported were miscarriage (8.7%), elective abortions (5%), major congenital malformations (1.7%), and stillbirths (0.9%). There were no patterns of birth defects among the eight infants with congenital malformations and the rate of birth defects was not greater than that observed in the general population. Pregnancy outcomes were not known for 411 cases reported to the database; 198 additional pregnancies were ongoing at the time of the report (Clowse 2018). Information related to this class of medications is emerging, but based on available data, tumor necrosis factor alpha (TNFα) blocking agents are considered to have low to moderate risk when used in pregnancy (ACOG 776 2019).

Inflammatory bowel disease is associated with adverse pregnancy outcomes including an increased risk of miscarriage, premature delivery, delivery of a low birth weight infant, and poor maternal weight gain. Management of maternal disease should be optimized prior to pregnancy. Treatment decreases disease flares, disease activity, and the incidence of adverse pregnancy outcomes (Mahadevan 2019).

Use of immune modulating therapies in pregnancy should be individualized to optimize maternal disease and pregnancy outcomes (ACOG 776 2019). The American Academy of Dermatology considers TNFα blocking agents for the treatment of psoriasis to be compatible with pregnancy (AAD-NPF [Menter 2019]). When treatment for inflammatory bowel disease is needed in pregnant women, certolizumab pegol can be continued without interruption. Serum levels should be evaluated prior to conception and optimized to avoid subtherapeutic concentrations or high levels which may increase placental transfer (Mahadevan 2019).

Data collection to monitor pregnancy and infant outcomes following exposure to certolizumab pegol is ongoing. Health care providers are encouraged to enroll women exposed to certolizumab pegol during pregnancy in the MotherToBaby Pregnancy Studies by contacting the Organization of Teratology Information Specialists (OTIS) (877-311-8972) or http://mothertobaby.org/pregnancy-studies/.

◆ **Cerubidine** *see* DAUNOrubicin (Conventional) *on page 445*

◆ **C.E.S.** *see* Estrogens (Conjugated/Equine, Systemic) *on page 601*

◆ **C.E.S.** *see* Estrogens (Conjugated/Equine, Topical) *on page 602*

◆ **Cetafen [OTC]** *see* Acetaminophen *on page 59*

◆ **Cetafen Extra [OTC]** *see* Acetaminophen *on page 59*

Cetirizine (Systemic) (se TI ra zeen)

Brand Names: US All Day Allergy Childrens [OTC] [DSC]; All Day Allergy [OTC]; Allergy Relief Cetirizine [OTC]; Allergy Relief Childrens [OTC]; Allergy Relief [OTC]; Allergy Relief/Indoor/Outdoor [OTC]; Cetirizine HCl Allergy Child [OTC]; Cetirizine HCl Childrens Alrgy [OTC]; Cetirizine HCl Childrens [OTC]; Cetirizine HCl Hives Relief [OTC]; GoodSense All Day Allergy [OTC]; Quzyttir; ZyrTEC Allergy Childrens [OTC]; ZyrTEC Allergy [OTC]; ZyrTEC Childrens Allergy [OTC]

Brand Names: Canada APO-Cetirizine; JAMP-Cetirizine; Mar-Cetirizine; MINT-Cetirizine; PMS-Cetirizine; Priva-Cetirizine; Reactine

Pharmacologic Category Histamine H_1 Antagonist; Histamine H_1 Antagonist, Second Generation; Piperazine Derivative

Use

Oral:

Allergic rhinitis: Relief of symptoms associated with allergic rhinitis.

Urticaria, chronic spontaneous: Treatment of uncomplicated skin manifestations of chronic spontaneous urticaria.

Injection:

Urticaria, acute: Treatment of acute urticaria.

Local Anesthetic/Vasoconstrictor Precautions No information available to require special precautions

Effects on Dental Treatment Key adverse event(s) related to dental treatment: Xerostomia and decreased salivation (normal salivary flow resumes upon discontinuation). Rare occurrence of aphthous stomatitis, altered taste, orofacial dyskinesia, stomatitis, tongue edema, tongue discoloration.

Effects on Bleeding No information available to require special precautions

Adverse Reactions

>10%: Nervous system: Drowsiness (adolescents and adults: 11% to 14%; children: 2% to 4%), headache (children: 14%; adults: <1%)

1% to 10%:

Cardiovascular: Cardiac failure (<2%), chest pain (<2%), edema (<2%), facial edema (<2%), flushing (<2%), hypertension (<2%), lower extremity edema (<2%), palpitations (<2%), peripheral edema (<2%), syncope (<2%), tachycardia (<2%)

Dermatologic: Acne vulgaris (<2%), alopecia (<2%), bullous rash (<2%), cutaneous nodule (<2%), dermatitis (<2%), diaphoresis (<2%), eczema (<2%), erythematous rash (<2%), furunculosis (<2%), hyperkeratosis (<2%), hypertrichosis (<2%), maculopapular rash (<2%), pallor (<2%), pruritus (<2%), seborrhea (<2%), skin photosensitivity (<2%), skin rash (<2%), urticaria (<2%), xeroderma (<2%)

Endocrine & metabolic: Decreased libido (<2%), dehydration (<2%), diabetes mellitus (<2%), heavy menstrual bleeding (<2%), hot flash (<2%), increased thirst (<2%), intermenstrual bleeding (<2%), weight gain (<2%)

Gastrointestinal: Abdominal pain (children: 4% to 6%), xerostomia (adolescents and adults: 5%), nausea (children: 3%), diarrhea (children: 2% to 3%), vomiting (children: 2% to 3%), ageusia (<2%), anorexia (<2%), aphthous stomatitis (<2%), constipation (<2%), dental caries (<2%), dysgeusia (<2%), dyspepsia (<2%), enlargement of abdomen (<2%), eructation (<2%), flatulence (<2%), gastritis (<2%), hemorrhoids (<2%), increased appetite (<2%), melena (<2%), sialorrhea (<2%), stomatitis (<2%), tongue discoloration (<2%)

Genitourinary: Cystitis (<2%), dysmenorrhea (<2%), dysuria (<2%), hematuria (<2%), leukorrhea (<2%), mastalgia (<2%), urinary frequency (<2%), urinary incontinence (<2%), urinary retention (<2%), urinary tract infection (<2%), vaginitis (<2%)

Hematologic & oncologic: Hemophthalmos (<2%), lymphadenopathy (<2%), purpuric disease (<2%), rectal hemorrhage (<2%)

Hepatic: Hepatic insufficiency (<2%)

Hypersensitivity: Angioedema (<2%), tongue edema (<2%)

Nervous system: Insomnia (≤9%), fatigue (4% to 6%), malaise (≤4%), dizziness (adolescents and adults: 2%), abnormality in thinking (<2%), agitation (<2%), altered sense of smell (<2%), amnesia (<2%), anxiety (<2%), ataxia (<2%), confusion (<2%), depersonalization (<2%), depression (<2%), emotional lability (<2%), euphoria (<2%), hyperesthesia (<2%), hypertonia (<2%), hypoesthesia (<2%), impaired concentration (<2%), migraine (<2%), myasthenia (<2%), nervousness (<2%), nightmares (<2%), pain (<2%), paralysis (<2%), paresthesia (<2%), rigors (<2%), sleep disorder (<2%), twitching (<2%), vertigo (<2%), voice disorder (<2%)

Neuromuscular & skeletal: Arthralgia (<2%), arthritis (<2%), asthenia (<2%), back pain (<2%), hyperkinetic muscle activity (<2%), lower limb cramp (<2%), myalgia (<2%), myelitis (<2%), osteoarthrosis (<2%), tremor (<2%)

Ophthalmic: Accommodation disturbance (<2%), blepharoptosis (<2%), blindness (<2%), conjunctivitis (<2%), eye pain (<2%), glaucoma (<2%), periorbital edema (<2%), visual field defect (<2%), xerophthalmia (<2%)

Otic: Deafness (<2%), otalgia (<2%), ototoxicity (<2%), tinnitus (<2%)

Renal: Polyuria (<2%)

Respiratory: Pharyngitis (children: 6%), epistaxis (children: 4%), bronchospasm (children: 3%), bronchitis (<2%), dyspnea (<2%), hyperventilation (<2%), increased bronchial secretions (<2%), nasal polyposis (<2%), pneumonia (<2%), respiratory system disorder (<2%), rhinitis (<2%), sinusitis (<2%), upper respiratory tract infection (<2%)

Miscellaneous: Fever (<2%)

<1%: Feeling hot, hyperhidrosis, presyncope

Frequency not defined:

Hepatic: Increased serum transaminases

Nervous system: Irritability

Miscellaneous: Fussiness in an infant or toddler

Postmarketing: Aggressive behavior, anaphylaxis, cholestasis, glomerulonephritis, hallucination, hemolytic anemia, hepatitis, increased serum bilirubin, orofacial dyskinesia, sedated state, seizure, severe hypotension, suicidal ideation, suicidal tendencies, thrombocytopenia

Mechanism of Action Competes with histamine for H_1-receptor sites on effector cells in the gastrointestinal tract, blood vessels, and respiratory tract

Pharmacodynamics/Kinetics

Onset of Action Suppression of skin wheal and flare: Oral: 20 to 60 minutes.

Duration of Action Suppression of skin wheal and flare: Oral: ≥24 hours.

Half-life Elimination Children: 6.2 hours; Adults: 8 hours

Time to Peak Serum: Oral: 1 hour; IV: 108 seconds.

Pregnancy Considerations

Guidelines for the use of antihistamines in the treatment of allergic rhinitis or urticaria in pregnancy are generally the same as in nonpregnant females. Cetirizine may be used when a second generation antihistamine is needed. The lowest effective dose should be used (Powell 2015; Scadding 2017; Wallace 2008; Zuberbier 2018).

◆ **Cetirizine HCl Allergy Child [OTC]** *see* Cetirizine (Systemic) *on page 328*

◆ **Cetirizine HCl Childrens [OTC]** *see* Cetirizine (Systemic) *on page 328*

◆ **Cetirizine HCl Childrens Alrgy [OTC]** *see* Cetirizine (Systemic) *on page 328*

◆ **Cetirizine HCl Hives Relief [OTC]** *see* Cetirizine (Systemic) *on page 328*

◆ **Cetirizine Hydrochloride** *see* Cetirizine (Systemic) *on page 328*

Cetuximab (se TUK see mab)

Brand Names: US Erbitux

Brand Names: Canada Erbitux

Pharmacologic Category Antineoplastic Agent, Epidermal Growth Factor Receptor (EGFR) Inhibitor; Antineoplastic Agent, Monoclonal Antibody

Use

Colorectal cancer, metastatic: Treatment of *KRAS* wild-type (without mutation), epidermal growth factor receptor (EGFR)-expressing metastatic colorectal cancer as determined by an approved test (in combination with FOLFIRI [irinotecan, fluorouracil, and leucovorin] as first-line treatment, in combination with irinotecan [in patients refractory to irinotecan-based chemotherapy], or as a single agent in patients who have failed irinotecan- and oxaliplatin-based chemotherapy or who are intolerant to irinotecan).

Limitation of use: Cetuximab is not indicated for the treatment of *RAS*-mutant colorectal cancer or when results of the *RAS* mutation tests are unknown.

Head and neck cancer, squamous cell: Treatment of squamous cell cancer of the head and neck (as a single agent for recurrent or metastatic disease after platinum-based chemotherapy failure; in combination with radiation therapy as initial treatment of locally or regionally advanced disease; in combination with platinum and fluorouracil-based chemotherapy as first-line treatment of locoregional or metastatic disease).

Local Anesthetic/Vasoconstrictor Precautions No information available to require special precautions

Effects on Dental Treatment No significant effects or complications reported

Effects on Bleeding No information available to require special precautions

Adverse Reactions

>10%:

Cardiovascular: Cardiac disorder (6% to 11%)

Central nervous system: Fatigue (91%), malaise (≤73%), pain (59%), peripheral sensory neuropathy (45%; grades 3/4: 1%), headache (19% to 38%), insomnia (27%), confusion (18%), chills (≤16%), rigors (≤16%), anxiety (14%), depression (14%)

Dermatologic: Desquamation (95%), acneiform eruption (15% to 88%), radiodermatitis (86%), xeroderma (14% to 57%), pruritus (14% to 47%), skin rash (28% to 44%), changes in nails (31%), acne vulgaris (14% to 22%), paronychia (20%), palmar-plantar erythrodysesthesia (19%), skin fissure (19%), alopecia (12%)

Endocrine & metabolic: Weight loss (15% to 84%), hypomagnesemia (6% to 55%), dehydration (13% to 25%), hypocalcemia (12%), hypokalemia (12%)

Gastrointestinal: Diarrhea (19% to 72%), nausea (49% to 64%), abdominal pain (59%), constipation (53%), vomiting (29% to 40%), stomatitis (31% to 32%; grades 3/4: 1% to 3%), anorexia (25% to 30%), dyspepsia (14% to 16%), xerostomia (12%)

Hematologic & oncologic: Neutropenia (49%; grades 3/4: 31%), leukopenia (grades 3/4: 17%)

Hepatic: Increased serum alanine aminotransferase (43%), increased serum aspartate aminotransferase (38%), increased serum alkaline phosphatase (33%)
Infection: Infection (13% to 44%), infection without neutropenia (38%)
Local: Application site reaction (18%)
Neuromuscular & skeletal: Asthenia (≤73%), ostealgia (15%), arthralgia (14%)
Ophthalmic: Conjunctivitis (10% to 18%)
Respiratory: Dyspnea (49%), cough (30%), pharyngitis (26%)
Miscellaneous: Fever (22% to 29%), infusion related reaction (8% to 18%)

1% to 10%:
Cardiovascular: Pulmonary embolism (4%), ischemic heart disease (2%)
Gastrointestinal: Dysgeusia (10%)
Immunologic: Antibody development (<5%)
Infection: Sepsis (1% to 4%)
Renal: Renal failure syndrome (1%: colorectal cancer patients; frequency not defined in other populations)

Frequency not defined:
Dermatologic: Hypertrichosis
Endocrine & metabolic: Electrolyte disorder

<1%, postmarketing, and/or case reports: Abscess, acute myocardial infarction, aseptic meningitis, blepharitis, bullous pemphigoid, cardiac arrhythmia, cellulitis, cheilitis, corneal ulcer, interstitial pulmonary disease, keratitis, skin infection, Stevens-Johnson syndrome, toxic epidermal necrolysis

Mechanism of Action Cetuximab is a recombinant human/mouse chimeric monoclonal antibody which binds specifically to the epidermal growth factor receptor (EGFR, HER1, c-ErbB-1) and competitively inhibits the binding of epidermal growth factor (EGF) and other ligands. Binding to the EGFR blocks phosphorylation and activation of receptor-associated kinases, resulting in inhibition of cell growth, induction of apoptosis, and decreased matrix metalloproteinase and vascular endothelial growth factor production. EGFR signal transduction results in *RAS* wild-type activation; cells with *RAS* mutations appear to be unaffected by EGFR inhibition.

Pharmacodynamics/Kinetics

Half-life Elimination ~112 hours (range: 63 to 230 hours)

Reproductive Considerations

Verify pregnancy status in females of reproductive potential prior to treatment initiation. The manufacturer recommends that females of reproductive potential use effective contraception during therapy and for 2 months following the last dose of cetuximab.

Pregnancy Considerations

Based on animal data and the mechanism of action, cetuximab may be expected to cause fetal harm if administered during pregnancy.

Cetylpyridinium (SEE til peer i DI nee um)

Brand Names: US Antiseptic Oral Rinse [OTC] [DSC]; Breath Rx [OTC] [DSC]; Cepacol Antibacterial [OTC]; Clean Zing [OTC]; GoodSense Oral Rinse [OTC]; Larynex [OTC]

Pharmacologic Category Antiseptic, Oral Mouthwash

Use Antiseptic to aid in the prevention and reduction of plaque and gingivitis, and to freshen breath

Local Anesthetic/Vasoconstrictor Precautions No information available to require special precautions

Effects on Dental Treatment Key adverse event(s) related to dental treatment: Tooth and tongue staining and oral irritation.

Effects on Bleeding No information available to require special precautions

Adverse Reactions Frequency not defined. Gastrointestinal: Dental discoloration, mouth irritation, tongue discoloration

Pregnancy Considerations Cetylpyridinium chloride mouthwash (alcohol free) has been associated with a reduction in preterm births in pregnant women with periodontal disease (Jeffcoat, 2011).

Dental Health Professional Considerations Numerous mouthwashes contain cetylpyridinium, review product labeling for additional information.

◆ **Cetylpyridinium Chloride** *see* Cetylpyridinium *on page 330*

Cevimeline (se vi ME leen)

Related Information

Dentin Hypersensitivity, Acid Erosion, High Caries Index, Management of Alveolar Osteitis, and Xerostomia *on page 1762*

Perioral Premalignant Lesions and Management of Patients Undergoing Cancer Therapy *on page 1781*

Brand Names: US Evoxac

Generic Availability (US) Yes

Pharmacologic Category Cholinergic Agonist

Dental Use Treatment of symptoms of dry mouth in patients with Sjögren's syndrome

Use Xerostomia (associated with Sjögren's syndrome): Treatment of symptoms of dry mouth in patients with Sjögren's syndrome.

Local Anesthetic/Vasoconstrictor Precautions No information available to require special precautions

Effects on Dental Treatment Key adverse event(s) related to dental treatment: Excessive salivation, salivary gland pain

Effects on Bleeding No information available to require special precautions

Adverse Reactions Frequency not always defined.

>10%:
Dermatologic: Diaphoresis (19%)
Gastrointestinal: Nausea (14%)
Respiratory: Sinusitis (12%), rhinitis (11%), upper respiratory tract infection (11%)

1% to 10%:
Cardiovascular: Chest pain, edema, palpitations, peripheral edema
Central nervous system: Fatigue (3%), insomnia (2%), depression, hypertonia, hypoesthesia, hyporeflexia, migraine, vertigo
Dermatologic: Dermatological disease, erythematous rash, pruritus
Endocrine & metabolic: Hot flash (2%), increased amylase
Gastrointestinal: Abdominal pain (8%), vomiting (5%), sialorrhea (2%), anorexia, aphthous stomatitis, constipation, eructation, flatulence, gastroesophageal reflux disease, hiccups, salivary gland pain, sialadenitis, toothache, xerostomia
Genitourinary: Urinary tract infection (6%), cystitis, vaginitis
Hematologic & oncologic: Anemia
Hypersensitivity: Hypersensitivity reaction
Infection: Abscess, candidiasis, fungal infection, infection

Neuromuscular & skeletal: Back pain (5%), arthralgia (4%), skeletal pain (3%), weakness (1%), leg cramps, myalgia, tremor
Ophthalmic: Eye disease, eye infection, eye pain, visual disturbance, xerophthalmia
Otic: Otalgia, otitis media
Respiratory: Cough (6%), bronchitis (4%), epistaxis, flu-like symptoms, pneumonia
Miscellaneous: Accidental injury (5%), fever

<1%, postmarketing, and/or case reports: acute exacerbations of multiple sclerosis, aggressive behavior, alopecia, angina pectoris, anterior chamber eye hemorrhage, aphasia, apnea, arthropathy, avascular necrosis of femoral head, bronchospasm, bullous rash, bundle branch block, cardiac arrhythmia, cardiac disease, cholecystitis, cholelithiasis, cholinergic syndrome, deafness, dehydration, delirium, dementia, depersonalization, diabetes mellitus, dyskinesia, ECG abnormality, emotional lability, eosinophilia, esophageal stenosis, esophagitis, extrasystoles, facial edema, gastric ulcer, gastrointestinal hemorrhage, gingival hyperplasia, glaucoma, granulocytopenia, hallucination, hematoma, hematuria, hepatic insufficiency, hyperglycemia, hyperkalemia, hypertension, hypoglycemia, hypotension, hypothyroidism, immune thrombocytopenia, impotence, increased liver enzymes, intestinal obstruction, inversion T wave on ECG, irritable bowel syndrome, leukopenia, lymphocytosis, manic reaction, menstrual disease, myocardial infarction, nephrolithiasis, neuropathy, paralysis, paranoia, paresthesia, peptic ulcer, pericarditis, peripheral ischemia, skin photosensitivity reaction, pleural effusion, pulmonary embolism, pulmonary fibrosis, rectal disease, renal insufficiency, seizure, sepsis, supraventricular tachycardia, syncope, systemic lupus erythematosus, tachycardia, tenosynovitis, thrombocytopenia, thrombophlebitis, ulcerative colitis, urinary retention, urination disorder, vasculitis

Dental Usual Dosage Dry mouth (in Sjögren's syndrome): Adults: Oral: 30 mg 3 times/day

Dosing

Adult & Geriatric Xerostomia (associated with Sjögren's syndrome): Oral: 30 mg 3 times/day

Renal Impairment: Adult There are no dosage adjustment provided in the manufacturer's labeling.

Hepatic Impairment: Adult There are no dosage adjustment provided in the manufacturer's labeling.

Mechanism of Action Binds to muscarinic (cholinergic) receptors, causing an increase in secretion of exocrine glands (such as salivary and sweat glands) and increase tone of smooth muscle in gastrointestinal and urinary tracts

Contraindications Hypersensitivity to cevimeline or any component of the formulation; uncontrolled asthma; when miosis is undesirable (eg, narrow-angle glaucoma, acute iritis)

Warnings/Precautions May alter cardiac conduction and/or heart rate; use caution in patients with significant cardiovascular disease, including angina, or myocardial infarction. Cevimeline has the potential to increase bronchial smooth muscle tone, airway resistance, and bronchial secretions; use with caution in patients with controlled asthma, COPD, or chronic bronchitis. May cause blurred vision, decreased visual acuity (particularly at night and in patients with central lens changes) and impaired depth perception. Patients should be cautioned about driving at night or performing hazardous activities in reduced lighting. Use with caution in patients with a history of cholelithiasis; may induce contractions of the gallbladder or biliary smooth muscle, precipitating complications such as cholangitis, cholecystitis, or biliary obstruction.

Use with caution in patients with a history of cholelithiasis; may induce contractions of the gallbladder or biliary smooth muscle, precipitating complications such as cholangitis, cholecystitis, or biliary obstruction. Use with caution in patients with a history of nephrolithiasis; may induce smooth muscle spasms, precipitating renal colic or ureteral reflux in patients with nephrolithiasis. Patients with a known or suspected deficiency of CYP2D6 may be at higher risk of adverse effects.

Drug Interactions

Metabolism/Transport Effects Substrate of CYP2D6 (minor), CYP3A4 (minor); **Note:** Assignment of Major/Minor substrate status based on clinically relevant drug interaction potential

Avoid Concomitant Use There are no known interactions where it is recommended to avoid concomitant use.

Increased Effect/Toxicity

The levels/effects of Cevimeline may be increased by: Acetylcholinesterase Inhibitors; Beta-Blockers

Decreased Effect

Cevimeline may decrease the levels/effects of: Cimetropium; Sincalide

Pharmacodynamics/Kinetics

Half-life Elimination 5 ± 1 hours

Time to Peak 1.5 to 2 hours

Pregnancy Considerations Adverse effects were observed in animal reproduction studies.

Breastfeeding Considerations It is not known if cevimeline is excreted in breast milk. Due to the potential for serious adverse reactions in the nursing infant, the manufacturer recommends a decision be made whether to discontinue nursing or to discontinue the drug, taking into account the importance of treatment to the mother.

Dosage Forms: US

Capsule, Oral:

Evoxac: 30 mg
Generic: 30 mg

Dental Health Professional Considerations Patient may experience sweating and/or facial flushing when beginning treatment.

- ◆ **Chateal** *see* Ethinyl Estradiol and Levonorgestrel *on page 612*
- ◆ **Chateal EQ** *see* Ethinyl Estradiol and Levonorgestrel *on page 612*
- ◆ **CHG** *see* Chlorhexidine Gluconate (Topical) *on page 335*
- ◆ **Chickenpox vaccine** *see* Measles, Mumps, Rubella, and Varicella Virus Vaccine *on page 950*
- ◆ **Chiggerex [OTC] [DSC]** *see* Benzocaine *on page 228*
- ◆ **Chiggertox [OTC] [DSC]** *see* Benzocaine *on page 228*
- ◆ **Childrens Advil [OTC]** *see* Ibuprofen *on page 786*
- ◆ **Childrens Loratadine [OTC]** *see* Loratadine *on page 930*
- ◆ **Childrens Motrin [OTC]** *see* Ibuprofen *on page 786*
- ◆ **Childrens Silfedrine [OTC]** *see* Pseudoephedrine *on page 1291*
- ◆ **Chloditan** *see* Mitotane *on page 1041*
- ◆ **Chlodithane** *see* Mitotane *on page 1041*

Chlophedianol, Dexbrompheniramine, and Pseudoephedrine

(kloe fe DYE a nol deks brom fen EER a meen & soo doe e FED rin)

Brand Names: US Chlo Tuss [OTC]

Pharmacologic Category Alkylamine Derivative; Alpha/Beta Agonist; Antitussive; Decongestant; Histamine H_1 Antagonist; Histamine H_1 Antagonist, First Generation

Use Common cold/upper respiratory allergies : Temporary relief of symptoms due to the common cold, hay fever (allergic rhinitis), or other upper respiratory allergies (eg, runny nose, itchy watery eyes, itching of the nose or throat, sneezing, nasal congestion).

Local Anesthetic/Vasoconstrictor Precautions Pseudoephedrine - Use with caution since pseudoephedrine is a sympathomimetic amine which could interact with epinephrine to cause a pressor response.

Effects on Dental Treatment Key adverse event(s) related to dental treatment: Pseudoephedrine - Xerostomia (normal salivary flow resumes upon discontinuation).

Effects on Bleeding No information available to require special precautions.

Adverse Reactions Also see Pseudoephedrine.

Frequency not defined:

Nervous system: Dizziness, drowsiness, excitability, insomnia, nervousness

Mechanism of Action

Chlophedianol is an antitussive.

Dexbrompheniramine is an antihistamine; competitively antagonizes histamine at histamine-1 receptor sites.

Pseudoephedrine is a sympathomimetic amine and isomer of ephedrine; acts as a decongestant in respiratory tract mucous membranes with less vasoconstrictor action than ephedrine in normotensive individuals.

- ◆ **Chlophedianol, Pseudoephedrine, and Dexbrompheniramine** *see* Chlophedianol, Dexbrompheniramine, and Pseudoephedrine *on page 332*

Chlorambucil (klor AM byoo sil)

Brand Names: US Leukeran

Brand Names: Canada Leukeran

Pharmacologic Category Antineoplastic Agent, Alkylating Agent; Antineoplastic Agent, Alkylating Agent (Nitrogen Mustard)

Use

Chronic lymphocytic leukemia: Management of chronic lymphocytic leukemia

Hodgkin lymphoma: Management of Hodgkin lymphoma

Non-Hodgkin lymphoma: Management of non-Hodgkin lymphomas

Local Anesthetic/Vasoconstrictor Precautions No information available to require special precautions

Effects on Dental Treatment Key adverse event(s) related to dental treatment: Stomatitis.

Effects on Bleeding Thrombocytopenia has been reported to occur 1-2 weeks after a short course of therapy and persist for up to 4 weeks.

Adverse Reactions Frequency not defined.

Central nervous system: Drug fever, peripheral neuropathy

Dermatologic: Allergic skin reaction, skin rash, urticaria

Endocrine & metabolic: Amenorrhea

Gastrointestinal: Diarrhea (infrequent), nausea (infrequent), oral mucosa ulcer (infrequent), vomiting (infrequent)

Genitourinary: Azoospermia, cystitis (sterile), infertility

Hematologic & oncologic: Anemia, bone marrow depression, bone marrow failure (irreversible), leukemia (secondary), leukopenia, lymphocytopenia, malignant neoplasm (secondary), neutropenia (onset: 3 weeks; recovery: 10 days after last dose), pancytopenia, thrombocytopenia

Hepatic: Hepatotoxicity, jaundice

Hypersensitivity: Angioedema, hypersensitivity reaction

Respiratory: Interstitial pneumonitis, pulmonary fibrosis

Miscellaneous: Fever

1%, postmarketing, and/or case reports: Agitation, ataxia, confusion, erythema multiforme, flaccid paralysis, seizure (focal/generalized), hallucination, muscle twitching, myoclonus, SIADH (syndrome of inappropriate antidiuretic hormone secretion), Stevens-Johnson syndrome, toxic epidermal necrolysis, tremor

Mechanism of Action Chlorambucil is an alkylating agent that interferes with DNA replication and RNA transcription by alkylation and cross-linking the strands of DNA, inducing cellular apoptosis.

Pharmacodynamics/Kinetics

Half-life Elimination Chlorambucil: ~1.5 hours; Phenylacetic acid mustard: 1.8 ± 0.4 hours

Time to Peak Chlorambucil: Within 1 hour; Phenylacetic acid mustard: 1.9 ± 0.7 hours

Reproductive Considerations

[US Boxed Warning]: Chlorambucil produces human infertility. Chromosomal damage has been documented. Reversible and irreversible sterility (when administered to prepubertal and pubertal males), azoospermia (in adult males), and amenorrhea (in females) have been observed. Fibrosis, vasculitis, and depletion of primordial follicles have been noted on autopsy of the ovaries.

Women of childbearing potential should avoid becoming pregnant while receiving treatment.

Pregnancy Risk Factor D

Pregnancy Considerations
Following exposure during the first trimester, case reports have noted adverse renal effects (unilateral agenesis) in the newborn.

[US Boxed Warning]: Chlorambucil is probably mutagenic and teratogenic in humans.

◆ **Chlorambucilum** *see* Chlorambucil *on page 332*

◆ **Chloraminophene** *see* Chlorambucil *on page 332*

Chloramphenicol (Systemic)
(klor am FEN i kole)

Brand Names: Canada Chloromycetin Succinate

Pharmacologic Category Antibiotic, Miscellaneous

Use

Serious infections: Treatment of serious infections, including cystic fibrosis exacerbations, bacterial meningitis, and bacteremia, caused by *Chlamydiaceae*, *Haemophilus influenzae*, *Rickettsia*, *Salmonella* spp. (acute infections), and other organisms when other less toxic agents are ineffective or contraindicated.

Guideline recommendations: Chloramphenicol may be considered for use as an alternative agent to doxycycline in the treatment of tickborne rickettsial diseases (eg, Rocky Mountain spotted fever [RMSF]); however, epidemiologic studies suggest that chloramphenicol-treated patients with RMSF are at a higher risk of death compared to tetracycline-treated patients. In addition, chloramphenicol is *not* effective in the treatment of human ehrlichiosis or anaplasmosis, therefore, use with caution in the *empiric* treatment of tickborne rickettsial diseases (CDC [Biggs 2016]).

Local Anesthetic/Vasoconstrictor Precautions
No information available to require special precautions

Effects on Dental Treatment Key adverse event(s) related to dental treatment: Glossitis and stomatitis.

Effects on Bleeding Thrombocytopenia has been reported with short or long courses of therapy due to bone marrow suppression.

Adverse Reactions Frequency not defined.

Central nervous system: Confusion, delirium, depression, headache

Dermatologic: Skin rash, urticaria

Gastrointestinal: Diarrhea, enterocolitis, glossitis, nausea, stomatitis, vomiting

Hematologic & oncologic: Aplastic anemia, bone marrow depression, granulocytopenia, hypoplastic anemia, pancytopenia, thrombocytopenia

Hypersensitivity: Anaphylaxis, angioedema, hypersensitivity reaction

Ophthalmic: Optic neuritis

Miscellaneous: Drug toxicity (Gray syndrome), fever

Mechanism of Action Reversibly binds to 50S ribosomal subunits of susceptible organisms preventing amino acids from being transferred to growing peptide chains thus inhibiting protein synthesis

Pharmacodynamics/Kinetics

Half-life Elimination

Neonates: 1 to 2 days: 24 hours; 10 to 16 days: 10 hours

Chloramphenicol: Infants: Significantly prolonged (Powell 1982); Children 4 to 6 hours; Adults: ~4 hours (Ambrose 1984)

Hepatic disease: Prolonged (Ambrose 1984)

Pregnancy Risk Factor C

Pregnancy Considerations
Chloramphenicol crosses the placenta producing cord concentrations approaching maternal serum concentrations. An increased risk of teratogenic effects has not been associated with the use of chloramphenicol in pregnancy (Czeizel 2000; Heinonen 1977). "Gray Syndrome" has occurred in premature infants and newborns receiving chloramphenicol. Chloramphenicol may be used as an alternative agent for the treatment of Rocky Mountain spotted fever in pregnant women although caution should be used when administration occurs during the third trimester (CDC [Biggs 2016]).

◆ **ChloraPrep One Step [OTC] [DSC]** *see* Chlorhexidine Gluconate (Topical) *on page 335*

◆ **Chlorbutinum** *see* Chlorambucil *on page 332*

ChlordiazePOXIDE (klor dye az e POKS ide)

Related Information
Dentin Hypersensitivity, Acid Erosion, High Caries Index, Management of Alveolar Osteitis, and Xerostomia *on page 1762*

Pharmacologic Category Benzodiazepine

Use

Alcohol withdrawal syndrome: Management of acute alcohol withdrawal symptoms.

Anxiety disorders: Management of anxiety disorders or short-term relief of anxiety symptoms.

Local Anesthetic/Vasoconstrictor Precautions
No information available to require special precautions

Effects on Dental Treatment Key adverse event(s) related to dental treatment: Xerostomia (normal salivary flow resumes upon discontinuation).

Effects on Bleeding No information available to require special precautions

Adverse Reactions Frequency not defined

Cardiovascular: Edema, syncope

Central nervous system: Abnormal electroencephalogram, ataxia, confusion, drowsiness, drug-induced extrapyramidal reaction

Dermatologic: Skin rash

Endocrine & metabolic: Change in libido, menstrual disease

Gastrointestinal: Constipation, nausea

Hematologic & oncologic: Agranulocytosis, bone marrow depression

Hepatic: Hepatic insufficiency, jaundice

Miscellaneous: Paradoxical reaction

Mechanism of Action Binds to stereospecific benzodiazepine receptors on the postsynaptic GABA neuron at several sites within the CNS, including the limbic system, reticular formation. Enhancement of the inhibitory effect of GABA on neuronal excitability results by increased neuronal membrane permeability to chloride ions. This shift in chloride ions results in hyperpolarization (a less excitable state) and stabilization. Benzodiazepine receptors and effects appear to be linked to the GABA-A receptors. Benzodiazepines do not bind to GABA-B receptors (Vinkers 2012).

Pharmacodynamics/Kinetics

Half-life Elimination Parent: 24 to 48 hours; demoxepam 14 to 95 hours (Schwartz 1971)

Time to Peak Serum: 0.5 to 2 hours (Baskin 1982)

Pregnancy Considerations
Chlordiazepoxide crosses the human placenta and fetal serum concentrations are similar to those in the mother. Teratogenic effects have been observed with some benzodiazepines (including chlordiazepoxide);

however, additional studies are needed. The incidence of premature birth and low birth weights may be increased following maternal use of benzodiazepines; hypoglycemia and respiratory problems in the neonate may occur following exposure late in pregnancy. Neonatal withdrawal symptoms may occur within days to weeks after birth and "floppy infant syndrome" (which also includes withdrawal symptoms) has been reported with some benzodiazepines (Bergman 1992; Iqbal 2002; Wikner 2007).

Controlled Substance C-IV

◆ **Chlordiazepoxide Hydrochloride** *see* ChlordiazePOXIDE *on page 333*

Chlorhexidine Gluconate (Oral)

(klor HEKS i deen GLOO koe nate)

Brand Names: US Paroex; Peridex; Periogard

Brand Names: Canada APO-Chlorhexidine; Chlorhexidine Alcohol Free; DentiCare Rinse; GUM Paroex Oral Rinse; Oro Clear; Oro-Clense; Perichlor; Peridex; Periogard; X-Pur Chlorhexidine

Generic Availability (US) Yes

Pharmacologic Category Antibiotic, Oral Rinse

Dental Use

Antibacterial dental rinse; chlorhexidine is active against gram-positive and gram-negative organisms, facultative anaerobes, aerobes, and yeast

Chip, for periodontal pocket insertion: Indicated as an adjunct to scaling and root planing procedures for reduction of pocket depth in patients with adult periodontitis; may be used as part of a periodontal maintenance program

Use

Gingivitis: Oral rinse: Antimicrobial dental rinse for gingivitis treatment

Periodontitis: Periodontal chip: Adjunctive therapy to scaling and root planning procedures to reduce pocket depth in patients with periodontitis

Local Anesthetic/Vasoconstrictor Precautions
No information available to require special precautions

Effects on Dental Treatment Key adverse event(s) related to dental treatment: Increased tartar on teeth, altered taste perception, staining of oral surfaces (mucosa, teeth, dorsum of tongue), and oral/tongue irritation. Staining may be visible as soon as 1 week after therapy begins and is more pronounced when there is a heavy accumulation of unremoved plaque and when teeth fillings have rough surfaces. Stain does not have a clinically adverse effect but because removal may not be possible, patient with anterior restorations should be advised of the potential permanency of the stain.

Effects on Bleeding No information available to require special precautions

Adverse Reactions

>10%:

Gastrointestinal: Toothache (51%)

Respiratory: Upper respiratory tract infection (28%), sinusitis (14%)

1% to 10%:

Gastrointestinal: Gingival hyperplasia (4%), aphthous stomatitis (2%)

Neuromuscular & skeletal: Arthritis (3%), tendonitis (2%)

Respiratory: Bronchitis (6%), pharyngitis (4%)

Frequency not defined:

Dermatologic: Cellulitis

Gastrointestinal: Dental discoloration (with oral rinse), dental discomfort, increased tartar formation, mouth discoloration

Infection: Abscess

<1%, postmarketing, and/or case reports: Coated tongue, desquamation, dysgeusia, erythema, geographic tongue, gingivitis, glossitis, hyperkeratosis, hypersensitivity reaction, hypoesthesia, mouth irritation, oral lesion, oral mucosa ulcer, paresthesia, parotid gland enlargement, sialadenitis, stomatitis, tongue changes (short frenum), tongue edema, tongue irritation, trauma, xerostomia

Dental Usual Dosage Adults:

Oral rinse (Peridex, PerioGard):

Floss and brush teeth, completely rinse toothpaste from mouth and swish 15 mL (one capful) undiluted oral rinse around in mouth for 30 seconds, then expectorate. Caution patient not to swallow the medicine and instruct not to eat for 2-3 hours after treatment (cap on bottle measures 15 mL).

Treatment of gingivitis: Oral prophylaxis: Swish for 30 seconds with 15 mL chlorhexidine, then expectorate; repeat twice daily (morning and evening). Patient should have a re-evaluation followed by a dental prophylaxis every 6 months.

Periodontal chip: One chip is inserted into a periodontal pocket with a probing pocket depth ≥5 mm. Up to 8 chips may be inserted in a single visit. Treatment is recommended every 3 months in pockets with a remaining depth ≥5 mm. If dislodgment occurs 7 days or more after placement, the subject is considered to have had the full course of treatment. If dislodgment occurs within 48 hours, a new chip should be inserted. The chip biodegrades completely and does not need to be removed. Patients should avoid dental floss at the site of periochip® insertion for 10 days after placement because flossing might dislodge the chip.

Insertion of periodontal chip: Pocket should be isolated and surrounding area dried prior to chip insertion. The chip should be grasped using forceps with the rounded edges away from the forceps. The chip should be inserted into the periodontal pocket to its maximum depth. It may be maneuvered into position using the tips of the forceps or a flat instrument.

Dosing

Adult & Geriatric

Gingivitis: Oral rinse: Swish for 30 seconds with 15 mL (one capful) of undiluted oral rinse after toothbrushing, then expectorate; repeat twice daily (morning and evening). Therapy should be initiated immediately following a dental prophylaxis. Patient should be reevaluated and given a dental prophylaxis at intervals no longer than every 6 months.

Periodontitis: Periodontal chip: One chip is inserted into a periodontal pocket with a probing pocket depth ≥5 mm. Up to 8 chips may be inserted in a single visit. Treatment is recommended every 3 months in pockets with a remaining depth ≥5 mm. If dislodgment occurs 7 days or more after placement, the subject is considered to have had the full course of treatment. If dislodgment occurs within 48 hours, a new chip should be inserted.

Oropharyngeal decontamination (to reduce the risk of hospital-acquired or ventilator-associated pneumonia) (off-label use): Oral rinse:

Cardiac surgical patients: 15 mL swished and gargled **or** applied to intubated patients by swabbing the oral cavity (buccal, pharyngeal, gingival, tongue, and tooth surfaces) for 30 seconds twice daily. Initiate preoperatively and continue postoperatively for 10 days or until extubation. Avoid food or drink for 30 minutes after rinsing (DeRiso 1996; Houston 2002).

Mechanically-ventilated patients: No specific dosing recommended due to the heterogeneous nature of the studies and paucity of conclusive data.

Renal Impairment: Adult There are no dosage adjustments provided in the manufacturer's labeling.

Hepatic Impairment: Adult There are no dosage adjustments provided in the manufacturer's labeling.

Pediatric Gingivitis: Limited data available: Children ≥8 years and Adolescents: Oral: Oral rinse (0.12%): Swish 15 mL (one capful) for 30 seconds after toothbrushing, then expectorate; repeat twice daily (morning and evening) (de la Rosa 1998)

Renal Impairment: Pediatric There are no dosage adjustments provided in the manufacturer's labeling.

Hepatic Impairment: Pediatric There are no dosage adjustments provided in the manufacturer's labeling.

Mechanism of Action Chlorhexidine has activity against gram-positive and gram-negative organisms, facultative anaerobes, aerobes, and yeast; it is both bacteriostatic and bactericidal, depending on its concentration. The bactericidal effect of chlorhexidine is a result of the binding of this cationic molecule to negatively charged bacterial cell walls and extramicrobial complexes. At low concentrations, this causes an alteration of bacterial cell osmotic equilibrium and leakage of potassium and phosphorous resulting in a bacteriostatic effect. At high concentrations of chlorhexidine, the cytoplasmic contents of the bacterial cell precipitate and result in cell death.

Contraindications Hypersensitivity to chlorhexidine or any component of the formulation

Warnings/Precautions Serious allergic reactions, including anaphylaxis, have been reported with use.

Oral rinse: Staining of oral surfaces (teeth, tooth restorations, dorsum of tongue) may occur; patients exhibited a measurable increase of staining in the facial anterior after six months of therapy that is more pronounced when there is a heavy accumulation of unremoved plaque. Stain does not adversely affect health of the gingivae or other oral tissues, and most stain can be removed from most tooth surfaces by dental prophylaxis. Because removal may not be possible, patients with anterior facial restorations with rough surfaces or margins should be advised of the potential permanency of the stain. An increase in supragingival calculus has been observed with use; it is not known if the incidence of subgingival calculus is increased. Dental prophylaxis to remove calculus deposits should be performed at least every 6 months. May alter taste perception during use; has rarely been associated with permanent taste alteration.

Effect on periodontitis has not been determined; has not been tested in patients with acute necrotizing ulcerative gingivitis.

Periodontal chip: Infectious events (eg, abscesses, cellulitis) have been observed rarely with adjunctive chip placement post scaling and root planing; use with caution in patients with periodontal disease and concomitant diseases potentially decreasing immune status (eg, diabetes, cancer). Use in acute periodontal abscess pocket is not recommended.

Warnings: Additional Pediatric Considerations Some dosage forms may contain propylene glycol; in neonates large amounts of propylene glycol delivered orally, intravenously (eg, >3,000 mg/day), or topically have been associated with potentially fatal toxicities which can include metabolic acidosis, seizures, renal failure, and CNS depression; toxicities have also been reported in children and adults including hyperosmolality, lactic acidosis, seizures, and respiratory depression; use caution (AAP 1997; Shehab 2009).

Drug Interactions

Metabolism/Transport Effects None known.

Avoid Concomitant Use There are no known interactions where it is recommended to avoid concomitant use.

Increased Effect/Toxicity There are no known significant interactions involving an increase in effect.

Decreased Effect There are no known significant interactions involving a decrease in effect.

Pharmacodynamics/Kinetics

Duration of Action Serum concentrations: Detectable levels are not present in the plasma 12 hours after administration

Pregnancy Risk Factor B/C (manufacturer specific)

Pregnancy Considerations Adverse events have not been observed in animal reproduction studies following use of the oral rinse; use of periodontal chip has not been studied. Chlorhexidine oral rinse is poorly absorbed from the GI tract.

Breastfeeding Considerations It is not known if chlorhexidine is excreted in breast milk. The manufacturer recommends that caution be exercised when administering chlorhexidine oral rinse to nursing women. However, oral rinse is not intended for ingestion; patient should expectorate after rinsing.

Dosage Forms: US

Solution, Mouth/Throat:

Paroex: 0.12% (473 mL)

Peridex: 0.12% (118 mL, 473 mL, 1893 mL)

Periogard: 0.12% (473 mL)

Generic: 0.12% (15 mL, 118 mL, 473 mL)

Dosage Forms: Canada

Solution, Mouth/Throat:

DentiCare Rinse: 0.12% (500 mL)

GUM Paroex Oral Rinse: 0.12% (473 mL)

Oro Clear: 0.12% (500 mL, 4000 mL)

Perichlor: 0.12% (475 mL)

Peridex: 0.12% (475 mL)

Periogard: 0.12% (15 mL, 473 mL)

Generic: 0.12% (15 mL, 250 mL, 473 mL, 475 mL, 480 mL, 500 mL, 4000 mL)

Chlorhexidine Gluconate (Topical)

(klor HEKS i deen GLOO koe nate)

Brand Names: US Antiseptic Skin Cleanser [OTC] [DSC]; Betasept Surgical Scrub [OTC]; ChloraPrep One Step [OTC] [DSC]; Dyna-Hex 2 [OTC]; Dyna-Hex 4 [OTC]; Hibiclens [OTC]; Tegaderm CHG Dressing [OTC]

Generic Availability (US) May be product dependent

Pharmacologic Category Antibiotic, Topical

Dental Use External surgical antiseptic scrub; not to be used as an oral rinse, see Chlorhexidine Gluconate (Oral)

Use Antiseptic: Skin cleanser for preoperative skin preparation, skin wound and general skin cleanser for patients; surgical scrub and antiseptic hand rinse for healthcare personnel

Local Anesthetic/Vasoconstrictor Precautions No information available to require special precautions

Effects on Dental Treatment No significant effects or complications reported

Effects on Bleeding No information available to require special precautions

Adverse Reactions

Dermatologic: Allergic sensitization, erythema, hypersensitivity reaction, rough skin, xeroderma

<1%, postmarketing, and/or case reports: Anaphylaxis (Health Canada May 2016), dyspnea, facial edema, nasal congestion

Dosing

Adult & Geriatric Note: General dosing guidelines provided; refer to specific product labeling for dosing instructions.

Antiseptic: Topical:

Surgical scrub: Scrub hands and forearms with ~5 mL for 3 minutes paying close attention to nails, cuticles, and interdigital spaces, and rinse thoroughly, wash for an additional 3 minutes with 5 mL, rinse, and dry thoroughly.

Health care personnel hand antiseptic: Liquid or solution: Wash with ~5 mL for 15 seconds; rinse thoroughly with water and dry

Preoperative skin preparation:

Solution: Apply liberally to surgical site and swab for at least 2 minutes. Dry with sterile towel. Repeat procedure (swab for additional 2 minutes and dry with sterile towel).

Applicator (ChloraPrep One-Step):

Dry surgical sites (eg, abdomen, arm): Completely wet treatment area; use gentle back and forth strokes for ~30 seconds. Allow solution to air dry for ~30 seconds. If using an ignition source (eg, electrocautery), allow solution to completely dry for a minimum of 3 minutes for hairless skin and up to 1 hour in hair; do not blot or wipe away. **Note:** Prior to use with electrocautery procedures, consult specific product labeling to determine if the ChloraPrep product may be used near an ignition source.

Moist surgical sites (eg, inguinal area): Completely wet treatment area; use gentle back and forth strokes for ~2 minutes. Allow solution to air dry for ~1 minute. If using an ignition source (eg, electrocautery), allow solution to completely dry for a minimum of 3 minutes for hairless skin and up to 1 hour in hair; do not blot or wipe away. **Note:** Prior to use with electrocautery procedures, consult specific product labeling to determine if the ChloraPrep product may be used near an ignition source.

Wound care and general skin cleansing: Rinse area with water, then apply minimum amount necessary to cover skin or wound area and wash gently. Rinse again thoroughly.

Renal Impairment: Adult There are no dosage adjustments provided in the manufacturer's labeling.

Hepatic Impairment: Adult There are no dosage adjustments provided in the manufacturer's labeling.

Pediatric

Skin cleanser for preoperative skin preparation, skin wound and general skin cleanser for patients: Topical:

Infants <2 months: **Note:** It is recommended to use with care in this population due to potential risk of dermal irritation or chemical burns. Expert suggestions are variable depending upon site and clinical scenario. Not all products may be appropriate for use in this population; refer to product specific labeling. Some experience in neonatal patients applicable to this patient population (Garland 2009; Tamma 2010).

Preoperative skin preparation: Solution: Apply liberally to surgical site and swab for at least 2 minutes. Dry with sterile towel. Repeat procedure (swab for additional 2 minutes and dry with sterile towel).

Wound care and general skin cleansing: Rinse area with water, then apply the minimum amount of chlorhexidine necessary to cover skin or wound area and wash gently. Rinse again thoroughly.

Infants ≥2 months, Children, and Adolescents: Topical solution:

Preoperative skin preparation: Solution: Apply liberally to surgical site and swab for at least 2 minutes. Dry with sterile towel. Repeat procedure (swab for additional 2 minutes and dry with sterile towel).

Wound care and general skin cleansing: Rinse area with water, then apply the minimum amount of chlorhexidine necessary to cover skin or wound area and wash gently. Rinse again thoroughly.

Renal Impairment: Pediatric There are no dosage adjustments provided in the manufacturer's labeling.

Hepatic Impairment: Pediatric There are no dosage adjustments provided in the manufacturer's labeling.

Mechanism of Action Chlorhexidine has activity against gram-positive and gram-negative organisms, facultative anaerobes, aerobes, and yeast; it is both bacteriostatic and bactericidal, depending on its concentration. The bactericidal effect of chlorhexidine is a result of the binding of this cationic molecule to negatively charged bacterial cell walls and extramicrobial complexes. At low concentrations, this causes an alteration of bacterial cell osmotic equilibrium and leakage of potassium and phosphorous resulting in a bacteriostatic effect. At high concentrations of chlorhexidine, the cytoplasmic contents of the bacterial cell precipitate and result in cell death.

Contraindications Hypersensitivity to chlorhexidine or any component of the formulation

Warnings/Precautions Serious allergic reactions, including anaphylaxis, have been reported with use. For topical use only. Keep out of eyes, ears, and the mouth; if contact occurs, rinse with cold water immediately; permanent eye injury may result if agent enters and remains in the eye. Deafness has been reported following instillation in the middle ear through perforated ear drums. Avoid applying to wounds that involve more than the superficial skin layers. Avoid repeated use as general skin cleansing of large surfaces (unless necessary for condition). Not for preoperative preparation of face or head; avoid contact with meninges (do not use on lumbar puncture sites). Avoid applying to genital areas; generalized allergic reactions, irritation, and sensitivity have been reported. Solutions may be flammable (products may contain alcohol); avoid exposure to open flame and/or ignition source (eg, electrocautery) until completely dry; avoid application to hairy areas which may significantly delay drying time. Use with caution in children <2 months of age due to potential for increased absorption, and risk of irritation or chemical burns. May cause staining of fabrics (brown stain) due to a chemical reaction between chlorhexidine gluconate bound to fabric and chlorine (if sufficient chlorine is present from certain laundry detergents used during laundering process). When used as a topical antiseptic, improper use may lead to product contamination. Although infrequent, product contamination has been associated with reports of localized and systemic infections. To reduce the risk of infection, ensure antiseptic products are used according to the labeled instructions; avoid diluting products after opening; and apply single-use containers only one time to one patient and discard any unused solution (FDA Drug Safety Communication, 2013).

Warnings: Additional Pediatric Considerations Although topical chlorhexidine is widely used in many NICUs as a skin cleanser prior to procedures (eg, central venous line placement/care) (Tamma 2010), data is lacking to support use in premature infants. Manufacturer's labeling recommends using with caution in premature neonates and infants <2 months of age as chlorhexidine-containing products may cause irritation or chemical burns. A survey of US NICU chlorhexidine use reports dermal burns occurring more frequently in neonates with birth weight <1,500 g (Tamma 2010). If used for neonatal dermal site cleansing, some suggest using sterile water or normal saline to remove excess disinfectant after procedures may help avoid chemical burns (Eichenwald 2017; Nuntnarumit 2013). Several studies have noted detectable serum concentrations in neonates after chlorhexidine exposure; no correlation between serum concentration and GA, birth weight, or PNA was identified; the clinical significance is undetermined (Chapman 2013; Garland 2009).

Drug Interactions

Metabolism/Transport Effects None known.

Avoid Concomitant Use There are no known interactions where it is recommended to avoid concomitant use.

Increased Effect/Toxicity There are no known significant interactions involving an increase in effect.

Decreased Effect There are no known significant interactions involving a decrease in effect.

Pregnancy Considerations No reports of adverse effects in newborns have been reported, even though chlorhexidine is commonly used during labor and in the neonate. Moreover, only very small amounts of disinfectant reach the maternal circulation and the fetus.

Breastfeeding Considerations It is not known if chlorhexidine is excreted in breast milk.

Dosage Forms: US

Liquid, External:

Betasept Surgical Scrub [OTC]: 4% (118 mL, 237 mL, 473 mL, 946 mL)

Hibiclens [OTC]: 4% (15 mL, 118 mL, 236 mL, 473 mL, 946 mL, 3790 mL)

Generic: 2% (118 mL); 4% (118 mL, 237 mL, 473 mL, 946 mL, 3800 mL)

Miscellaneous, External:

Tegaderm CHG Dressing [OTC]: (Dressing) (1 ea)

Pad, External:

Generic: 2% (2 ea, 6 ea)

Solution, External:

Dyna-Hex 2 [OTC]: 2% (473 mL)

Dyna-Hex 4 [OTC]: 4% (118 mL, 473 mL)

◆ **Chlormeprazine** *see* Prochlorperazine *on page 1279*

◆ **2-Chlorodeoxyadenosine** *see* Cladribine *on page 359*

Chloroprocaine (klor oh PROE kane)

Related Information

Oral Pain *on page 1734*

Brand Names: US Clorotekal; Nesacaine; Nesacaine-MPF

Pharmacologic Category Local Anesthetic

Use

Local anesthesia:

Chloroprocaine (with preservatives):

Production of local anesthesia by infiltration and peripheral nerve block.

Chloroprocaine (without preservatives):

Production of local anesthesia by infiltration and peripheral nerve block, as well as epidural and caudal administration; production of local anesthesia by subarachnoid block (spinal anesthesia) in adults (Clorotekal only).

Note: Due to chloroprocaine's fast onset and short duration of action, it is most often used to establish adequate epidural anesthesia (eg, in a parturient prior to delivery) or possibly, for peripheral nerve block in a patient undergoing short (<60 minutes) ambulatory surgery that is not anticipated to produce significant postoperative pain (Alley 2014; Miller 2010).

Limitations of use: Nesacaine, Nesacaine-MPF: The manufacturer recommends against using either formulation (ie, with or without preservatives) for subarachnoid administration (ie, spinal anesthesia); however, the use of chloroprocaine without preservatives (Nesacaine-MPF) has been safely used off-label for spinal anesthesia (Goldblum 2013; Miller 2010; Yoos 2005). Do not use chloroprocaine with preservatives (Nesacaine) for epidural or spinal anesthesia.

Local Anesthetic/Vasoconstrictor Precautions No information available to require special precautions

Effects on Dental Treatment No significant effects or complications reported

Effects on Bleeding No information available to require special precautions

Adverse Reactions

>10%: Central nervous system: Procedural pain (16%)

1% to 10%:

Cardiovascular: Hypotension (5%)

Central nervous system: Headache (<2%)

Endocrine & metabolic: Hyperglycemia (<2%)

Gastrointestinal: Nausea (<2%)

Local: Injection site pain (4%)

Frequency not defined.

Cardiovascular: Syncope, ventricular arrhythmia

Central nervous system: Central nervous system depression, central nervous system stimulation, increased body temperature

Dermatologic: Diaphoresis, erythema

Gastrointestinal: Loss of anal sphincter control

Hypersensitivity: Anaphylactoid reaction, angioedema

Respiratory: Laryngeal edema, respiratory arrest, sneezing

<1%, postmarketing, and/or case reports: Akathisia, anaphylaxis, anxiety, arachnoiditis, auditory impairment, back pain, blurred vision, bradycardia, burning sensation, cardiac arrest, cardiac arrhythmia, cardiac insufficiency, cauda equine syndrome, chondrolysis of articular cartilage, diplopia, dizziness, drowsiness, dysesthesia, dyspnea, erythema multiforme, fecal incontinence, feeling hot, groin pain, hypersensitivity reaction, hypertension, hypoesthesia, limb pain, localized numbness (perineal; causing sexual dysfunction), loss of consciousness, malaise, motor dysfunction, myoclonus, oral hypoesthesia, oral paresthesia, paresthesia, peripheral neuropathy, photophobia, presyncope, prolonged emergency from anesthesia, pruritus, respiratory arrest, respiratory depression, restlessness, seizure, sexual disorder, speech disturbance, spinal cord injury, tachycardia, tinnitus, tremor, urinary

incontinence, urinary retention, urticaria, visual disturbance, vomiting

Mechanism of Action Chloroprocaine is an ester-type local anesthetic, which stabilizes the neuronal membranes and prevents initiation and transmission of nerve impulses thereby affecting local anesthetic actions. Chloroprocaine reversibly prevents generation and conduction of electrical impulses in neurons by decreasing the transient increase in permeability to sodium. The differential sensitivity generally depends on the size of the fiber; small fibers are more sensitive than larger fibers and require a longer period for recovery. Sensory pain fibers are usually blocked first, followed by fibers that transmit sensations of temperature, touch, and deep pressure. High concentrations block sympathetic somatic sensory and somatic motor fibers. The spread of anesthesia depends upon the distribution of the solution. This is primarily dependent on the volume of drug injected.

Pharmacodynamics/Kinetics

Onset of Action 6 to 12 minutes

Duration of Action Up to 60 minutes (patient, type of block, concentration, and method of anesthesia dependent)

Half-life Elimination In vitro, plasma: Neonates: 43 ± 2 seconds; Adults: 21 ± 2 seconds (males), 25 ± 1 second (females)

Pregnancy Risk Factor C

Pregnancy Considerations Animal reproduction studies have not been conducted. Local anesthetics rapidly cross the placenta and may cause varying degrees of maternal, fetal, and neonatal toxicity. Close maternal and fetal monitoring (heart rate and electronic fetal monitoring advised) are required during obstetrical use. Maternal hypotension has resulted from regional anesthesia. Positioning the patient on her left side and elevating the legs may help. Epidural, paracervical, or pudendal anesthesia may alter the forces of parturition through changes in uterine contractility or maternal expulsive efforts. The use of some local anesthetic drugs during labor and delivery may diminish muscle strength and tone for the first day or two of life. Administration as a paracervical block is not recommended with toxemia of pregnancy, fetal distress, or prematurity. Administration of a paracervical block early in pregnancy has resulted in maternal seizures and cardiovascular collapse. Fetal bradycardia and acidosis also have been reported. Fetal depression has occurred following unintended fetal intracranial injection while administering a paracervical and/or pudendal block.

◆ **Chloroprocaine Hydrochloride** *see* Chloroprocaine *on page 337*

Chloroquine (KLOR oh kwin)

Related Information

Clinical Risk Related to Drugs Prolonging QT Interval *on page 1675*

Brand Names: Canada TEVA-Chloroquine

Pharmacologic Category Aminoquinoline (Antimalarial); Antimalarial Agent

Use

Malaria: Treatment of uncomplicated malaria due to susceptible strains of *Plasmodium vivax, Plasmodium malariae, Plasmodium ovale,* and *Plasmodium falciparum*; prophylaxis of malaria (in geographic areas where chloroquine resistance is not present). **Note:** The CDC guidelines also recommend chloroquine for chloroquine-sensitive *Plasmodium knowlesi* malaria (CDC 2020).

Limitations of use: Chloroquine alone does not prevent relapses in patients with *P. vivax* or *P. ovale* malaria (not effective against exoerythrocytic forms). Do not use for the treatment of complicated malaria (high-grade parasitemia and/or complications [eg, cerebral malaria, acute renal failure]) or for malaria prophylaxis in areas where chloroquine resistance occurs (resistance to chloroquine is widespread in *P. falciparum* and reported in *P. vivax*).

Extraintestinal amebiasis: Treatment of extraintestinal amebiasis.

Local Anesthetic/Vasoconstrictor Precautions Chloroquine is one of the drugs confirmed to prolong the QT interval and is accepted as having a risk of causing torsade de pointes. The risk of drug-induced torsade de pointes is extremely low when a single QT interval prolonging drug is prescribed. In terms of epinephrine, it is not known what effect vasoconstrictors in the local anesthetic regimen will have in patients with a known history of congenital prolonged QT interval or in patients taking any medication that prolongs the QT interval. Until more information is obtained, it is suggested that the clinician consult with the physician prior to the use of a vasoconstrictor in suspected patients, and that the vasoconstrictor (epinephrine, mepivacaine and levonordefrin [Carbocaine® 2% with Neo-Cobefrin®]) be used with caution.

Effects on Dental Treatment Key adverse event(s) related to dental treatment: Stomatitis.

Effects on Bleeding Thrombocytopenia has been reported.

Adverse Reactions

Frequency not defined:

Cardiovascular: Atrioventricular block, bundle branch block, cardiac arrhythmia, cardiac failure, cardiomyopathy, ECG changes (including flattened T wave on ECG, inversion T wave on ECG, prolonged QT interval on ECG, widened QRS complex on ECG), hypotension, torsades de pointes, ventricular fibrillation, ventricular tachycardia

Dermatologic: Alopecia, bleaching of hair, blue-gray skin pigmentation (oral mucosa and hard palate, nails, and skin [Gallo 2009; Horta-Bass 2018; Manger 2017]), erythema multiforme, exacerbation of psoriasis, exfoliative dermatitis, lichen planus, pleomorphic rash, pruritus, skin photosensitivity, Stevens-Johnson syndrome, toxic epidermal necrolysis, urticaria

Endocrine & metabolic: Exacerbation of porphyria, severe hypoglycemia

Gastrointestinal: Abdominal cramps, anorexia, diarrhea, nausea, vomiting

Hematologic & oncologic: Agranulocytosis (reversible), aplastic anemia, hemolytic anemia (in G6PD-deficient patients), neutropenia, pancytopenia, thrombocytopenia

Hepatic: Hepatitis, increased liver enzymes

Hypersensitivity: Anaphylaxis, angioedema

Immunologic: Drug reaction with eosinophilia and systemic symptoms

Nervous system: Agitation, anxiety, confusion, decreased deep tendon reflex, delirium, depression, extrapyramidal reaction (dystonia, dyskinesia, protrusion of the tongue, torticollis), hallucination, headache, insomnia, personality changes, polyneuropathy, psychosis, seizure, sensorimotor neuropathy, sensorineural hearing loss, suicidal tendencies

Neuromuscular & skeletal: Asthenia, myopathy, neuromuscular disease, proximal myopathy

Ophthalmic: Accommodation disturbances, blurred vision, corneal opacity (reversible), macular degeneration (may be irreversible), maculopathy (may be irreversible), night blindness, retinal pigment changes (bull's eye appearance), retinopathy (including irreversible changes in long-term or high-dose therapy), transient scotomata, visual field defect (paracentral scotomas)

Otic: Hearing loss (risk increased in patients with preexisting auditory damage), tinnitus

Postmarketing:

Hepatic: Hepatic impairment (FDA Safety Alert, April 1, 2020)

Renal: Renal insufficiency (FDA Safety Alert, April 1, 2020)

Mechanism of Action

Antimalarial: Binds to and inhibits DNA and RNA polymerase; interferes with metabolism and hemoglobin utilization by parasites; inhibits prostaglandin effects; chloroquine concentrates within parasite acid vesicles and raises internal pH resulting in inhibition of parasite growth; may involve aggregates of ferriprotoporphyrin IX acting as chloroquine receptors causing membrane damage; may also interfere with nucleoprotein synthesis.

Antiviral (coronavirus disease 2019 [COVID-19]): Not fully understood; however, it may change the pH at the cell membrane surface and inhibit viral fusion. It may also inhibit glycosylation of viral proteins (Wang 2020).

Pharmacodynamics/Kinetics

Half-life Elimination

Healthy subjects: 74.7 ± 30.1 hours (Salako 1984).

Chronic renal insufficiency: 191.4 ± 69.1 hours (range: 103.5 to 309.9 hours) (Salako 1984).

Time to Peak Serum: Oral: Within 1-2 hours

Pregnancy Considerations

Chloroquine and its metabolites cross the placenta and can be detected in the cord blood and urine of the newborn infant (Akintonwa 1988; Essien 1982; Law 2008). In one study, chloroquine and its metabolites were measurable in the cord blood 89 days (mean) after the last maternal dose (Law 2008).

Chloroquine has not been found to increase the risk of adverse fetal events when used in recommended doses for malaria prophylaxis (CDC Yellow Book 2020). Retinal toxicity is a known risk following long-term use or high doses of chloroquine. Although animal reproduction studies have shown accumulation of chloroquine in fetal ocular tissues, an association between chloroquine and fetal ocular toxicity has not been confirmed in available human studies (Gaffar 2019; Osadchy 2011).

Malaria infection in pregnant women may be more severe than in nonpregnant women and has a high risk of maternal and perinatal morbidity and mortality. Malaria infection during pregnancy can lead to miscarriage, premature delivery, low birth weight, congenital infection, and/or perinatal death. Therefore, pregnant women and women who are likely to become pregnant are advised to avoid travel to malaria-risk areas. When travel is unavoidable, pregnant women should take precautions to avoid mosquito bites and use effective prophylactic medications.

Indications and dosing for chloroquine treatment and prophylaxis of uncomplicated malaria are the same in pregnant and nonpregnant adults. Chloroquine may be used in all trimesters of pregnancy (CDC 2020; CDC Yellow Book 2020).

Due to pregnancy-induced physiologic changes, some pharmacokinetic properties of chloroquine may be altered (Chukwuani 2004; Fakeye 2002; Karunajeewa 2010; Lee 2008; Massele 1997; Olafuyi 2019; Salman 2017; Wilby 2011). Available studies suggest dose adjustments could be needed, but data are not sufficient to determine what an appropriate dosing change is when chloroquine is used for the treatment or prophylaxis of malaria during pregnancy (Karunajeewa 2010; Salman 2017). Pregnant patients should be closely monitored for response to treatment, especially when chloroquine is used during the second and third trimesters (WHO 2015).

Chloroquine has been under evaluation for the management of coronavirus disease 2019 (COVID-19). An emergency use authorization (EUA) was issued by the FDA in April 2020 authorizing use of chloroquine for hospitalized patients. It was revoked in June 2020 amid concerns for safety and lack of efficacy. Chloroquine should only be given as part of a clinical trial (FDA 2020; HHS 2020).

Data collection to monitor maternal and infant outcomes following exposure to COVID-19 during pregnancy is ongoing. Health care providers are encouraged to enroll females exposed to COVID-19 during pregnancy in the Organization of Teratology Information Specialists (OTIS) pregnancy registry (877-311-8972; https://mothertobaby.org/join-study/) or the PRIORITY (**Preg**nancy **C**o**R**onav**I**rus **O**utcomes **R**eg**I**s**T**r**Y**) (415-754-3729, https://priority.ucsf.edu/).

Dental Health Professional Considerations See Local Anesthetic/Vasoconstrictor Precautions

◆ **Chloroquine Phosphate** *see* Chloroquine *on page 338*

Chlorothiazide (klor oh THYE a zide)

Related Information

Cardiovascular Diseases *on page 1654*

Brand Names: US Diuril; Sodium Diuril

Pharmacologic Category Antihypertensive; Diuretic, Thiazide

Use

Edema: Adjunctive treatment of edema

Hypertension: Management of hypertension

Guideline recommendations: The 2017 Guideline for the Prevention, Detection, Evaluation, and Management of High Blood Pressure in Adults recommends if monotherapy is warranted, in the absence of comorbidities (eg, cerebrovascular disease, chronic kidney disease, diabetes, heart failure, ischemic heart disease, etc), that thiazide-like diuretics or dihydropyridine calcium channel blockers may be preferred options due to improved cardiovascular endpoints (eg, prevention of heart failure and stroke). ACE inhibitors and ARBs are also acceptable for monotherapy. Combination therapy may be required to achieve blood pressure goals and is initially preferred in patients at high risk (stage 2 hypertension or atherosclerotic cardiovascular disease [ASCVD] risk ≥10%) (ACC/AHA [Whelton 2017]).

Local Anesthetic/Vasoconstrictor Precautions

No information available to require special precautions

Effects on Dental Treatment Key adverse event(s) related to dental treatment: Patients may experience orthostatic hypotension as they stand up after treatment; especially if lying in dental chair for extended periods of time. Use caution with sudden changes in position during and after dental treatment.

Effects on Bleeding No information available to require special precautions

Adverse Reactions Frequency not defined.

Cardiovascular: Hypotension, necrotizing angiitis, orthostatic hypotension

Central nervous system: Dizziness, headache, paresthesia, restlessness, vertigo

Dermatologic: Alopecia, erythema multiforme, exfoliative dermatitis, skin photosensitivity, skin rash, Stevens-Johnson syndrome, toxic epidermal necrolysis, urticaria

Endocrine & metabolic: Glycosuria, hypercalcemia, hyperglycemia, hyperuricemia, hypochloremic alkalosis, hypokalemia, hypomagnesemia, hyponatremia, increased serum cholesterol, increased serum triglycerides

Gastrointestinal: Abdominal cramps, anorexia, constipation, diarrhea, gastric irritation, nausea, pancreatitis, sialadenitis, vomiting

Genitourinary: Hematuria (IV), impotence

Hematologic & oncologic: Agranulocytosis, aplastic anemia, hemolytic anemia, leukopenia, purpura, thrombocytopenia

Hepatic: Jaundice

Hypersensitivity: Anaphylaxis

Neuromuscular & skeletal: Muscle spasm, systemic lupus erythematosus, weakness

Ophthalmic: Blurred vision, xanthopsia

Renal: Interstitial nephritis, renal failure, renal insufficiency

Respiratory: Pneumonitis, pulmonary edema, respiratory distress

Miscellaneous: Fever

Mechanism of Action Inhibits sodium and chloride reabsorption in the distal tubules causing increased excretion of sodium, chloride, and water resulting in diuresis. Loss of potassium, hydrogen ions, magnesium, phosphate, and bicarbonate also occurs.

Pharmacodynamics/Kinetics

Onset of Action Diuresis: Oral: Within 2 hours; IV: 15 minutes; Peak effect: Oral: ~4 hours; IV: 30 minutes

Duration of Action Diuretic action: Oral: ~6 to 12 hours; IV: 2 hours

Half-life Elimination 45 to 120 minutes

Pregnancy Considerations

Chlorothiazide crosses the placenta and is found in cord blood. Maternal use may cause may cause fetal or neonatal jaundice, thrombocytopenia, or other adverse events observed in adults.

Use of thiazide diuretics to treat edema during normal pregnancies is not appropriate; use may be considered when edema is due to pathologic causes (as in the nonpregnant patient); monitor.

Chronic maternal hypertension is associated with adverse events in the fetus/infant. The risk of birth defects, low birth weight, premature delivery, stillbirth, and neonatal death may be increased with chronic hypertension in pregnancy. Actual risks may be related to duration and severity of maternal hypertension. Diuretics are considered second-line therapy for treating chronic hypertension in pregnancy (ACOG 203 2019).

The treatment of edema associated with chronic heart failure during pregnancy is similar to that of nonpregnant patients. Use of thiazide diuretics may be considered but use with caution due to the potential reduction in placental blood flow. Patients diagnosed after delivery can be treated according to heart failure guidelines (ESC [Bauersachs 2016]; ESC [Regitz-Zagrosek 2018]).

- **Chlorothiazide Sodium** *see* Chlorothiazide *on page 339*
- **Chlorphenamine** *see* Chlorpheniramine *on page 340*

Chlorpheniramine (klor fen IR a meen)

Related Information

Bacterial Infections *on page 1739*

Brand Names: US Aller-Chlor [OTC]; Allergy Relief [OTC]; Allergy [OTC]; Allergy-Time [OTC]; Chlor-Trimeton Allergy [OTC]; Chlor-Trimeton [OTC]; Ed Chlorped Jr [OTC]; Ed ChlorPed [OTC] [DSC]; Ed-Chlortan [OTC] [DSC]; Pharbechlor [OTC]

Pharmacologic Category Alkylamine Derivative; Histamine H_1 Antagonist; Histamine H_1 Antagonist, First Generation

Use Allergic symptoms, allergic rhinitis, urticaria, pruritus: Perennial and seasonal allergic rhinitis and other allergic symptoms including urticaria, pruritus

Local Anesthetic/Vasoconstrictor Precautions No information available to require special precautions

Effects on Dental Treatment Key adverse event(s) related to dental treatment: Xerostomia (normal salivary flow resumes upon discontinuation). Chronic use of antihistamines will inhibit salivary flow, particularly in elderly patients; this may contribute to periodontal disease, tooth decay, and oral discomfort.

Effects on Bleeding No information available to require special precautions

Adverse Reactions

>10%:

Central nervous system: Drowsiness (slight to moderate)

Respiratory: Thickening of bronchial secretions

1% to 10%:

Central nervous system: Dizziness, excitability, fatigue, headache, nervousness

Endocrine & metabolic: Weight gain

Gastrointestinal: Abdominal pain, diarrhea, increased appetite, nausea, xerostomia

Genitourinary: Urinary retention

Neuromuscular & skeletal: Arthralgia, weakness

Ophthalmic: Diplopia

Renal: Polyuria

Respiratory: Pharyngitis

Mechanism of Action Competes with histamine for H_1-receptor sites on effector cells in the gastrointestinal tract, blood vessels, and respiratory tract

Pharmacodynamics/Kinetics

Half-life Elimination Serum: Children and Adolescents 6 to 16 years: 13.1 ± 6.6 hours (range: 6.3 to 23.1 hours) (Simons 1982); Adults: 14-24 hours (Paton 1985)

Time to Peak Children and Adolescents 6 to 16 years: Oral: 2.5 ± 1.5 hours (range: 1 to 6 hours) (Simons 1982); Adults: 2-3 hours (Sharma 2003)

Pregnancy Considerations

Maternal chlorpheniramine use has generally not resulted in an increased risk of birth defects (Aselton 1985; Gilboa 2009; Heinonen 1977; Jick 1981).

Antihistamines may be used for the treatment of rhinitis, urticaria, and pruritus with rash in pregnant women (although second generation antihistamines may be preferred) (Angier 2010; Murase 2014; Wallace 2008; Zuberbier 2014). Antihistamines are not recommended for treatment of pruritus associated with intrahepatic cholestasis in pregnancy (Ambros-Rudolph 2011; Kremer 2011).

◆ **Chlorpheniramine and Codeine** *see* Codeine and Chlorpheniramine *on page 404*

Chlorpheniramine and Pseudoephedrine

(klor fen IR a meen & soo doe e FED rin)

Related Information

Chlorpheniramine *on page 340*

Pseudoephedrine *on page 1291*

Brand Names: US LoHist-D [OTC]; Maxichlor PSE [OTC]; Neutrahist Pediatric [OTC] [DSC]; SudoGest Sinus & Allergy [OTC]

Brand Names: Canada Triaminic Cold & Allergy

Pharmacologic Category Alkylamine Derivative; Alpha/Beta Agonist; Decongestant; Histamine H_1 Antagonist; Histamine H_1 Antagonist, First Generation

Use Upper respiratory tract conditions: Temporary relief of symptoms (nasal congestion; sinus congestion/pressure, runny nose; sneezing; itching of the eyes, nose, or throat) associated with the common cold, allergic rhinitis, and other upper respiratory tract conditions.

Local Anesthetic/Vasoconstrictor Precautions Use with caution since pseudoephedrine is a sympathomimetic amine which could interact with epinephrine to cause a pressor response

Effects on Dental Treatment Key adverse event(s) related to dental treatment:

Chlorpheniramine: Prolonged use will cause significant xerostomia (normal salivary flow resumes upon discontinuation).

Pseudoephedrine: Xerostomia (prolonged use worsens; normal salivary flow resumes upon discontinuation).

Effects on Bleeding No information available to require special precautions

Adverse Reactions See individual agents.

Mechanism of Action

Chlorpheniramine competes with histamine for H_1-receptor sites on effector cells in the gastrointestinal tract, blood vessels, and respiratory tract.

Pseudoephedrine is a sympathomimetic amine and isomer of ephedrine; acts as a decongestant in respiratory tract mucous membranes with less vasoconstrictor action than ephedrine in normotensive individuals.

Pregnancy Risk Factor C

Pregnancy Considerations

Reproduction studies have not been conducted with this combination product. See individual agents.

◆ **Chlorpheniramine Maleate** *see* Chlorpheniramine *on page 340*

◆ **Chlorpheniramine Maleate and Pseudoephedrine Hydrochloride** *see* Chlorpheniramine and Pseudoephedrine *on page 341*

Chlorpheniramine, Pseudoephedrine, and Codeine

(klor fen IR a meen, soo doe e FED rin, & KOE deen)

Related Information

Chlorpheniramine *on page 340*

Codeine *on page 404*

Pseudoephedrine *on page 1291*

Brand Names: US Phenylhistine DH [OTC] [DSC]; Tricode AR [DSC]

Pharmacologic Category Alkylamine Derivative; Alpha/Beta Agonist; Analgesic, Opioid; Antitussive; Decongestant; Histamine H_1 Antagonist; Histamine H_1 Antagonist, First Generation

Use Cough and upper respiratory allergy symptoms: Temporary relief of symptoms (runny nose, sneezing, itching of nose or throat, itchy/watery eyes, cough due to minor throat and bronchial irritation, nasal congestion, reduces swelling of nasal passages) associated with the common cold, allergic rhinitis, or other upper respiratory allergies.

Local Anesthetic/Vasoconstrictor Precautions Use with caution since pseudoephedrine is a sympathomimetic amine which could interact with epinephrine to cause a pressor response

Effects on Dental Treatment Key adverse event(s) related to dental treatment:

Chlorpheniramine: Significant xerostomia with prolonged use (normal salivary flow resumes upon discontinuation).

Pseudoephedrine: Xerostomia (normal salivary flow resumes upon discontinuation).

Effects on Bleeding No information available to require special precautions

Adverse Reactions Also see individual agents.

<1%, postmarketing, and/or case reports: Hypogonadism (Brennan 2013; Debono 2011)

Mechanism of Action

Codeine: Binds to opioid receptors in the CNS, causing inhibition of ascending pain pathways, altering the perception of and response to pain; causes cough suppression by direct central action in the medulla; produces generalized CNS depression.

Chlorpheniramine: A propylamine derivative antihistamine drug (H_1 receptor antagonist) that also possesses anticholinergic and sedative activity. It prevents released histamine from dilating capillaries and causing edema of the respiratory mucosa.

Pseudoephedrine: Directly stimulates alpha-adrenergic receptors of respiratory mucosa causing vasoconstriction; directly stimulates beta-adrenergic receptors causing bronchial relaxation.

Controlled Substance C-V

◆ **Chlorpheniramine Tannate and Pseudoephedrine Tannate** *see* Chlorpheniramine and Pseudoephedrine *on page 341*

◆ **Chlorphen/Pseudoephed/Codeine** *see* Chlorpheniramine, Pseudoephedrine, and Codeine *on page 341*

ChlorproMAZINE (klor PROE ma zeen)

Related Information

Clinical Risk Related to Drugs Prolonging QT Interval *on page 1675*

Brand Names: Canada TEVA-ChlorproMAZINE

Pharmacologic Category Antimanic Agent; First Generation (Typical) Antipsychotic; Phenothiazine Derivative

Use

Agitation/aggression (severe, acute) associated with psychiatric disorders (eg, schizophrenia, bipolar disorder): Treatment of agitation and aggression related to bipolar disorder, schizophrenia, and other psychotic disorders.

Behavioral problems: Treatment of severe behavioral problems in children 1 to 12 years of age marked by combativeness and/or explosive hyperexcitable behavior (out of proportion to immediate provocations).

Bipolar disorder: Treatment of manic episodes associated with bipolar disorder.

Hiccups, prolonged or intractable: Treatment of intractable hiccups.

Hyperactivity: Short-term treatment of hyperactive children who show excessive motor activity with accompanying conduct disorders consisting of some or all of the following symptoms: impulsivity, difficulty sustaining attention, aggressiveness, mood lability, and poor frustration tolerance.

Nausea and vomiting, acute self-limiting: Management of nausea and vomiting. Also used off label as an alternative agent for refractory nausea and vomiting of pregnancy (ACOG 2018).

Schizophrenia: Treatment of schizophrenia and psychotic disorders.

Tetanus: Adjunctive therapy in the treatment of tetanus.

Limitation of use: Generally not a first- or second-line agent due to availability of safer, equally effective alternatives for most indications (Jibson 2020).

Local Anesthetic/Vasoconstrictor Precautions Chlorpromazine is one of the drugs confirmed to prolong the QT interval and is accepted as having a risk of causing torsade de pointes. The risk of drug-induced torsade de pointes is extremely low when a single QT interval prolonging drug is prescribed. In terms of epinephrine, it is not known what effect vasoconstrictors in the local anesthetic regimen will have in patients with a known history of congenital prolonged QT interval or in patients taking any medication that prolongs the QT interval. Until more information is obtained, it is suggested that the clinician consult with the physician prior to the use of a vasoconstrictor in suspected patients, and that the vasoconstrictor (epinephrine, mepivacaine and levonordefrin [Carbocaine® 2% with Neo-Cobefrin®]) be used with caution.

Effects on Dental Treatment Key adverse event(s) related to dental treatment:

Xerostomia (normal salivary flow resumes upon discontinuation).

Significant hypotension may occur, especially when the drug is administered parenterally. Patients may experience orthostatic hypotension as they stand up after treatment; especially if lying in dental chair for extended periods of time. Use caution with sudden changes in position during and after dental treatment. Orthostatic hypotension is due to alpha-receptor blockade; elderly are at greater risk.

Tardive dyskinesia: Prevalence rate may be 40% in elderly; development of the syndrome and the irreversible nature are proportional to duration and total cumulative dose over time. Extrapyramidal reactions are more common in elderly with up to 50% developing these reactions after 60 years of age. Drug-induced Parkinson's syndrome occurs often; akathisia is the most common extrapyramidal reaction in elderly.

Increased confusion, memory loss, psychotic behavior, and agitation frequently occur as a consequence of anticholinergic effects. Antipsychotic-associated sedation in nonpsychotic patients is extremely unpleasant due to feelings of depersonalization, derealization, and dysphoria.

Effects on Bleeding No information available to require special precautions

Adverse Reactions

Frequency not defined.

Cardiovascular: ECG abnormality (nonspecific QT changes), orthostatic hypotension, syncope, tachycardia

Central nervous system: Brain edema, catatonic-like state, dizziness, drowsiness, dystonia, extrapyramidal reaction, hyperpyrexia, neuroleptic malignant syndrome, parkinsonism, psychotic symptoms, restlessness, tardive dyskinesia, tardive dystonia

Dermatologic: Contact dermatitis, cutaneous lupus erythematosus (Pavlidakey 1985), skin photosensitivity, skin pigmentation (slate gray)

Endocrine & metabolic: Weight gain

Gastrointestinal: Atony of colon, constipation, increased appetite, nausea, obstipation, paralytic ileus, xerostomia

Genitourinary: Breast engorgement, ejaculatory disorder, false positive pregnancy test, impotence, lactation, priapism, urinary retention

Hematologic & oncologic: Agranulocytosis, aplastic anemia, eosinophilia, hemolytic anemia, immune thrombocytopenia, leukopenia

Hepatic: Jaundice

Hypersensitivity: Nonimmune anaphylaxis

Neuromuscular & skeletal: Lupus-like syndrome (Pavlidakey 1985)

Ophthalmic: Corneal deposits, lens disease (deposits), miosis, mydriasis, star-shaped cataract, visual impairment

Respiratory: Nasal congestion

Miscellaneous: Low fever

Postmarketing: Abnormal proteins in cerebrospinal fluid, amenorrhea, angioedema, asthma, epithelial keratopathy, exfoliative dermatitis, glycosuria, gynecomastia, hyperglycemia, hypoglycemia, laryngeal edema, pancytopenia, peripheral edema, retinitis pigmentosa, seizure

Mechanism of Action Chlorpromazine is an aliphatic phenothiazine antipsychotic which blocks postsynaptic mesolimbic dopaminergic receptors in the brain; exhibits a strong alpha-adrenergic blocking effect and depresses the release of hypothalamic and hypophyseal hormones; believed to depress the reticular activating system, thus affecting basal metabolism, body temperature, wakefulness, vasomotor tone, and emesis

Pharmacodynamics/Kinetics

Onset of Action IM: 15 minutes; Oral: 30 to 60 minutes; Antipsychotic effects: Gradual, may take up to several weeks; Maximum antipsychotic effect: 6 weeks to 6 months

Duration of Action Oral: 4 to 6 hours

Half-life Elimination Biphasic: Initial: Children: 1.1 hours; Adults: ~2 hours; Terminal: Children: 7.7 hours; Adults: ~30 hours

Pregnancy Considerations

Jaundice or hyper- or hyporeflexia have been reported in newborn infants following maternal use of phenothiazines. Antipsychotic use during the third trimester of pregnancy has a risk for abnormal muscle movements (extrapyramidal symptoms [EPS]) and withdrawal symptoms in newborns following delivery. Symptoms in the newborn may include agitation, feeding disorder, hypertonia, hypotonia, respiratory distress, somnolence, and tremor; these effects may be self-limiting or require hospitalization.

Chlorpromazine may be considered for the adjunctive treatment of nausea and vomiting in pregnant women. Use is reserved for women with dehydration when symptoms persist following preferred pharmacologic therapies (ACOG 189 2018).

Dental Health Professional Considerations See Local Anesthetic/Vasoconstrictor Precautions

- **Chlorpromazine HCl** *see* ChlorproMAZINE *on page 341*
- **Chlorpromazine Hydrochloride** *see* ChlorproMAZINE *on page 341*

ChlorproPAMIDE (klor PROE pa mide)

Related Information

Endocrine Disorders and Pregnancy *on page 1684*

Brand Names: Canada APO-ChlorproPAMIDE

Pharmacologic Category Antidiabetic Agent, Sulfonylurea

Use Diabetes mellitus, type 2: As an adjunct to diet and exercise to improve glycemic control in adults with type 2 diabetes mellitus

Guideline recommendations: First-generation sulfonylureas (eg, chlorpropamide) are not recommended treatment options for type 2 diabetes; later generation sulfonylureas with lower hypoglycemic risks (eg, glipizide) are preferred (ADA 2020).

Local Anesthetic/Vasoconstrictor Precautions No information available to require special precautions

Effects on Dental Treatment Key adverse event(s) related to dental treatment: Patients with diabetes should be questioned by the dental professional at each dental visit to assess their risk for stress-induced hypoglycemia. The dental professional should inquire about the patient's routine (ie, work, sleep schedule, eating patterns), history of hypoglycemia, time of last medication dose, last meal, and most recent blood sugar assessment. Keep a supply of glucose tablets and other carbohydrates in the office to prepare for a hypoglycemic event. Seek medical attention when necessary (American Diabetes Association, 2018).

Effects on Bleeding No information available to require special precautions

Adverse Reactions Frequency not always defined.

Central nervous system: Disulfiram-like reaction, dizziness, headache

Dermatologic: Pruritus (<3%), maculopapular rash (≤1%), urticaria (≤1%), erythema multiforme, exfoliative dermatitis, skin photosensitivity

Endocrine & metabolic: Hepatic porphyria, hypoglycemia, porphyria cutanea tarda, SIADH (syndrome of inappropriate antidiuretic hormone secretion), weight gain

Gastrointestinal: Nausea (<5%), anorexia (<2%), diarrhea (<2%), hunger (<2%), vomiting (<2%)

Hematologic & oncologic: Agranulocytosis, aplastic anemia, eosinophilia, hemolytic anemia, leukopenia, pancytopenia, thrombocytopenia

Hepatic: Cholestatic jaundice, hepatic failure, hepatitis

<1%, postmarketing, and/or case reports: Proctocolitis

Mechanism of Action Stimulates insulin release from the pancreatic beta cells; reduces glucose output from the liver; insulin sensitivity is increased at peripheral target sites

Pharmacodynamics/Kinetics

Onset of Action 1 hour; Peak effect: 3-6 hours

Duration of Action 24 hours

Half-life Elimination ~36 hours, prolonged in elderly or with renal impairment; End-stage renal disease: 50-200 hours

Time to Peak Serum: 2-4 hours

Pregnancy Considerations Chlorpropamide crosses the placenta.

Severe hypoglycemia lasting 4 to 10 days has been noted in infants born to mothers taking a sulfonylurea (including chlorpropamide) at the time of delivery; additional adverse events have also been reported and may be influenced by maternal glycemic control (Jackson 1962; Kemball 1970; Uhrig 1983; Zucker 1968). The manufacturer recommends if chlorpropamide is used during pregnancy, it should be discontinued at least 1 month before the expected delivery date.

Poorly controlled diabetes during pregnancy can be associated with an increased risk of adverse maternal and fetal outcomes, including diabetic ketoacidosis, preeclampsia, spontaneous abortion, preterm delivery, delivery complications, major birth defects, stillbirth, and macrosomia (ACOG 201 2018). To prevent adverse outcomes, prior to conception and throughout pregnancy, maternal blood glucose and HbA_{1c} should be kept as close to target goals as possible but without causing significant hypoglycemia (ADA 2020; Blumer 2013).

Agents other than chlorpropamide are currently recommended to treat diabetes mellitus in pregnancy (ADA 2020).

Chlorthalidone (klor THAL i done)

Related Information

Cardiovascular Diseases *on page 1654*

Brand Names: Canada APO-Chlorthalidone [DSC]

Pharmacologic Category Antihypertensive; Diuretic, Thiazide-Related

Use

Edema, refractory: Adjunctive treatment (eg, added to loop diuretics) of edema associated with heart failure, renal impairment, hepatic cirrhosis, or corticosteroid and estrogen therapy.

Hypertension: Management of hypertension.

Local Anesthetic/Vasoconstrictor Precautions No information available to require special precautions

Effects on Dental Treatment No significant effects or complications reported

Effects on Bleeding No information available to require special precautions

Adverse Reactions

Frequency not defined:

Cardiovascular: Necrotizing angiitis, orthostatic hypotension, vasculitis

Central nervous system: Dizziness, headache, paresthesia, restlessness, vertigo

Dermatologic: Skin photosensitivity, skin rash, toxic epidermal necrolysis, urticaria

Endocrine & metabolic: Glycosuria, hyperglycemia, hyperuricemia, hypochloremic alkalosis, hypokalemia, hyponatremia

Gastrointestinal: Abdominal cramps, anorexia, constipation, diarrhea, gastric irritation, nausea, pancreatitis, vomiting

Genitourinary: Impotence

Hematologic & oncologic: Agranulocytosis, aplastic anemia, hypersensitivity angiitis, leukopenia, nonthrombocytopenic purpura, thrombocytopenia
Hepatic: Intrahepatic cholestatic jaundice
Neuromuscular & skeletal: Asthenia, muscle spasm
Ophthalmic: Xanthopsia

Mechanism of Action Sulfonamide-derived diuretic that inhibits sodium and chloride reabsorption in the distal convoluted tubule (Gamba 2005; Moes 2014; Rose 1991).

Pharmacodynamics/Kinetics

Onset of Action ~2.6 hours; Peak effect: 2 to 6 hours (Carter 2004)

Duration of Action Single dose: 24 to 48 hours; Long-term dosing: 48 to 72 hours (Carter 2004)

Half-life Elimination Single dose: 40 hours; Long-term dosing: 45 to 60 hours (Carter 2004); may be prolonged with renal impairment

Pregnancy Considerations

Chlorthalidone crosses the placenta and can be detected in cord blood (Mulley 1978).

Maternal use may cause fetal or neonatal jaundice, thrombocytopenia, hypoglycemia, and electrolyte abnormalities.

Chronic maternal hypertension is associated with adverse events in the fetus/infant. The risk of birth defects, low birth weight, premature delivery, stillbirth, and neonatal death may be increased with chronic hypertension in pregnancy. Actual risks may be related to duration and severity of maternal hypertension. Diuretics are considered second-line therapy for treating chronic hypertension in pregnancy (ACOG 203 2019).

The treatment of edema associated with chronic heart failure during pregnancy is similar to that of nonpregnant patients. Use of thiazide diuretics may be considered but use with caution due to the potential reduction in placental blood flow. Patients diagnosed after delivery can be treated according to heart failure guidelines (ESC [Bauersachs 2016]; ESC [Regitz-Zagrosek 2018]).

◆ **Chlorthalidone and Atenolol** *see* Atenolol and Chlorthalidone *on page 190*

◆ **Chlor-Trimeton [OTC]** *see* Chlorpheniramine *on page 340*

◆ **Chlor-Trimeton Allergy [OTC]** *see* Chlorpheniramine *on page 340*

Chlorzoxazone (klor ZOKS a zone)

Related Information

Temporomandibular Dysfunction (TMD), Chronic Pain, and Fibromyalgia *on page 1773*

Brand Names: US Lorzone; Parafon Forte DSC [DSC]

Pharmacologic Category Skeletal Muscle Relaxant

Use Musculoskeletal conditions: Adjunct to rest, physical therapy, and other measures for the relief of discomfort associated with acute, painful musculoskeletal conditions

Local Anesthetic/Vasoconstrictor Precautions No information available to require special precautions

Effects on Dental Treatment No significant effects or complications reported

Effects on Bleeding No information available to require special precautions

Adverse Reactions Frequency not defined.

Central nervous system: Dizziness, drowsiness, malaise, paradoxical central nervous system stimulation
Genitourinary: Urine discoloration
<1%, postmarketing, and/or case reports: Allergic skin rash, anaphylaxis (very rare), angioedema (very rare), ecchymoses, gastrointestinal hemorrhage, hepatotoxicity, petechia

Mechanism of Action Centrally acting agent; acts on the spinal cord and subcortical areas of the brain to inhibit polysynaptic reflex arcs involved in causing and maintaining skeletal muscle spasms

Pharmacodynamics/Kinetics

Onset of Action Within 1 hour (Desiraju 1983)

Duration of Action Up to 6 hours (Desiraju 1983)

Half-life Elimination ~1 hour (Desiraju 1983)

Time to Peak ~1 to 2 hours

Pregnancy Considerations

Animal reproduction studies have not been conducted.

◆ **Chlo Tuss [OTC]** *see* Chlophedianol, Dexbrompheniramine, and Pseudoephedrine *on page 332*

Cholecalciferol (kole e kal SI fer ole)

Brand Names: US Aqueous Vitamin D [OTC]; Bio-D-Mulsion Forte [OTC] [DSC]; Bio-D-Mulsion [OTC] [DSC]; BProtected Pedia D-Vite [OTC]; D-3-5 [OTC]; D-Vi-Sol [OTC]; D-Vita [OTC] [DSC]; D-Vite Pediatric [OTC]; D3 Vitamin [OTC] [DSC]; D3-50 [OTC]; Decara [OTC]; Delta D3 [OTC]; Dialyvite Vitamin D 5000 [OTC]; Dialyvite Vitamin D3 Max [OTC]; Pronutrients Vitamin D3 [OTC]; Vitamin D3 Super Strength [OTC]; Vitamin D3 Ultra Potency [OTC]; Weekly-D [OTC]

Brand Names: Canada D-Tabs; EURO D 10000; EURO-D; JAMP-Vitamin D; Luxa-D; ViDextra

Pharmacologic Category Vitamin D Analog

Use Dietary supplement: As a vitamin D dietary supplement

Local Anesthetic/Vasoconstrictor Precautions No information available to require special precautions

Effects on Dental Treatment Key adverse event(s) related to dental treatment: Metallic taste and xerostomia (normal salivary flow resumes upon discontinuation).

Effects on Bleeding No information available to require special precautions

Adverse Reactions No adverse reactions listed in the manufacturer's labeling.

Mechanism of Action Cholecalciferol (vitamin D_3) is a provitamin. The active metabolite, 1,25-dihydroxyvitamin D (calcitriol), stimulates calcium and phosphate absorption from the small intestine, promotes secretion of calcium from bone to blood; promotes renal tubule phosphate resorption (IOM 2011)

Pharmacodynamics/Kinetics

Half-life Elimination Circulating: 25(OH)D: 2 to 3 weeks; 1,25-dihydroxyvitamin D: ~4 hours

Pregnancy Considerations

The cholecalciferol metabolite, 25(OH)D, crosses the placenta; maternal serum concentrations correlate with fetal concentrations at birth (Misra 2008; Wagner 2008).

Adequate maternal vitamin D is required for fetal growth and development (Misra 2008). Vitamin D deficiency in a pregnant woman may lead to a vitamin D deficiency in the neonate (Misra 2008; Wagner 2008). Serum 25(OH) D concentrations should be measured in pregnant women considered to be at increased risk of deficiency

(ACOG 2011). The amount of vitamin D contained in prenatal vitamins may not be adequate to treat a deficiency during pregnancy; although larger doses may be needed, current guidelines recommend a total of 1,000 to 2,000 units/day until more safety data is available (ACOG 2011). In women not at risk for deficiency, doses larger than the RDA should be avoided during pregnancy (ACOG 2011; IOM 2011).

◆ **Cholecalciferol and Alendronate** *see* Alendronate and Cholecalciferol *on page 100*

Cholestyramine Resin

(koe LES teer a meen REZ in)

Related Information

Cardiovascular Diseases *on page 1654*

Brand Names: US Prevalite; Questran; Questran Light

Brand Names: Canada Cholestyramine-ODAN; DOM-Cholestyramine; JAMP-Cholestyramine Sugar Free; Olestyr; Olestyr Light

Pharmacologic Category Antilipemic Agent, Bile Acid Sequestrant

Use

Dyslipidemia: Adjunct in the management of primary hypercholesterolemia; regression of arteriolosclerosis

Pruritus associated with cholestasis: Treatment of pruritus associated with partial biliary obstruction

Local Anesthetic/Vasoconstrictor Precautions No information available to require special precautions

Effects on Dental Treatment No significant effects or complications reported

Effects on Bleeding No information available to require special precautions

Adverse Reactions Frequency not defined.

Cardiovascular: Edema, syncope

Central nervous system: Anxiety, dizziness, drowsiness, fatigue, headache, neuralgia, paresthesia, vertigo

Dermatologic: Perianal skin irritation, skin irritation, skin rash, urticaria

Endocrine & metabolic: Hyperchloremic metabolic acidosis (children), increased libido, weight gain, weight loss

Gastrointestinal: Abdominal pain, anorexia, biliary colic, constipation, dental bleeding, dental caries, dental discoloration, diarrhea, diverticulitis, duodenal ulcer with hemorrhage, dysgeusia, dysphagia, eructation, flatulence, gallbladder calcification, gastric ulcer, gastrointestinal hemorrhage, hemorrhoidal bleeding, hiccups, intestinal obstruction (rare), melena, nausea, pancreatitis, rectal pain, steatorrhea, tongue irritation, tooth enamel damage (dental erosion), vomiting

Genitourinary: Diuresis, dysuria, hematuria

Hematologic & oncologic: Adenopathy, anemia, bruise, hemorrhage, hypoprothrombinemia, prolonged prothrombin time, rectal hemorrhage

Hepatic: Abnormal hepatic function tests

Neuromuscular & skeletal: Arthralgia, arthritis, back pain, myalgia, osteoporosis

Ophthalmic: Nocturnal amblyopia (rare), uveitis

Otic: Tinnitus

Respiratory: Asthma, dyspnea, wheezing

Mechanism of Action Forms a nonabsorbable complex with bile acids in the intestine, releasing chloride ions in the process; inhibits enterohepatic reuptake of intestinal bile salts and thereby increases the fecal loss of bile salt-bound low density lipoprotein cholesterol

Pharmacodynamics/Kinetics

Onset of Action Peak effect: 21 days

Pregnancy Considerations

Lipid concentrations increase during pregnancy as required for normal fetal development. When increases are greater than expected, supervised dietary intervention should be initiated. Bile acid sequestrants are recommended when treatment is needed (Avis 2009; Jacobson 2015).

Cholestyramine is not absorbed systemically, but may interfere with maternal vitamin absorption; therefore, regular prenatal supplementation may not be adequate.

◆ **Choline Fenofibrate** *see* Fenofibrate and Derivatives *on page 640*

◆ **CI-1008** *see* Pregabalin *on page 1268*

◆ **Cialis** *see* Tadalafil *on page 1401*

Ciclesonide (Nasal) (sye KLES oh nide)

Brand Names: US Omnaris; Zetonna

Brand Names: Canada APO-Ciclesonide; Omnaris; Omnaris HFA [DSC]

Pharmacologic Category Corticosteroid, Nasal

Use Seasonal and perennial allergic rhinitis: Management of seasonal and perennial allergic rhinitis.

Local Anesthetic/Vasoconstrictor Precautions No information available to require special precautions

Effects on Dental Treatment No significant effects or complications reported

Effects on Bleeding No information available to require special precautions

Adverse Reactions

>10%:

Respiratory: Epistaxis (≤11%)

1% to 10%:

Central nervous system: Headache (3% to 7%)

Gastrointestinal: Nausea (≥2%)

Genitourinary: Urinary tract infection (≥2%)

Infection: Influenza (≥2%)

Neuromuscular & skeletal: Back pain (≥2%), strain (≥2%)

Otic: Otalgia (2%)

Respiratory: Nasopharyngitis (2% to 7%), nasal discomfort (3% to 6%), pharyngolaryngeal pain (≥3%), bronchitis (≥2%), cough (≥2%; may be dose-responsive), nasal septum disorder (≥2%; may be dose-responsive), oropharyngeal pain (≥2%), sinusitis (≥2%), streptococcal pharyngitis (≥2%), viral upper respiratory tract infection (≥2%), upper respiratory infection (≤2%)

<1%, postmarketing, and/or case reports: Angioedema (with angioedema of the lips, angioedema of the oropharynx, and angioedema of the tongue), dizziness, dysgeusia, dyspepsia, leukocytosis, nasal candidiasis, nasal congestion, nasal mucosa ulcer, pharyngeal candidiasis, rhinorrhea, throat irritation, xerostomia

Pharmacodynamics/Kinetics

Onset of Action 24-48 hours; further improvement observed over 1-2 weeks in seasonal allergic rhinitis or 5 weeks in perennial allergic rhinitis

Pregnancy Considerations

Information related to the use of ciclesonide in pregnancy has not been located (Alhussien 2018).

Maternal use of intranasal corticosteroids in usual doses are not associated with an increased risk of fetal malformations or preterm birth (ERS/TSANZ [Middleton 2020]). Although use of intranasal ciclesonide is likely acceptable, other agents may be preferred for the treatment of allergic rhinitis during pregnancy (Alhussien 2018; BSACI [Scadding 2017]; ERS/TSANZ [Middleton 2020]).

Ciclesonide (Oral Inhalation)

(sye KLES oh nide)

Related Information

Respiratory Diseases *on page 1680*

Brand Names: US Alvesco

Brand Names: Canada Alvesco

Pharmacologic Category Corticosteroid, Inhalant (Oral)

Use

Asthma: Maintenance treatment of asthma as prophylactic therapy in patients ≥12 years of age.

Limitations of use: Not indicated for relief of acute bronchospasm.

Local Anesthetic/Vasoconstrictor Precautions No information available to require special precautions

Effects on Dental Treatment Key adverse event(s) related to dental treatment: Dysphonia has been reported with use of this medication. Localized infections with *Candida albicans* or *Aspergillus niger* occur frequently in the mouth and pharynx with repetitive use of an oral inhaler; may require treatment with appropriate antifungal therapy or discontinuance of inhaler use.

Effects on Bleeding No information available to require special precautions

Adverse Reactions

>10%:

Central nervous system: Headache (≤11%)

Respiratory: Nasopharyngitis (≤11%)

1% to 10%:

Cardiovascular: Facial edema (≥3%)

Central nervous system: Dizziness (≥3%), fatigue (≥3%), voice disorder (1%)

Dermatologic: Urticaria (≥3%)

Gastrointestinal: Gastroenteritis (≥3%), oral candidiasis (≥3%)

Infection: Influenza (≥3%)

Neuromuscular & skeletal: Arthralgia (≥3%), back pain (≥3%), limb pain (≥3%), musculoskeletal chest pain (≥3%)

Ophthalmic: Conjunctivitis (≥3%)

Otic: Otalgia (2%)

Respiratory: Upper respiratory tract infection (≤9%), nasal congestion (≤6%), pharyngolaryngeal pain (≤5%), hoarseness (≥3%), pneumonia (≥3%), sinusitis (≥3%), paradoxical bronchospasm (2%)

<1%, postmarketing, and/or case reports: Angioedema (with swelling of lip/pharynx/tongue), cataract, chest discomfort, increased gamma-glutamyl transferase, increased intraocular pressure, increased serum ALT, nausea, palpitations, pharyngeal candidiasis, skin rash, weight gain, xerostomia

Mechanism of Action Ciclesonide is a nonhalogenated, glucocorticoid prodrug that is hydrolyzed to the pharmacologically active metabolite des-ciclesonide following administration. Des-ciclesonide has a high affinity for the glucocorticoid receptor and exhibits anti-inflammatory activity. The mechanism of action for corticosteroids is believed to be a combination of three important properties – anti-inflammatory activity, immunosuppressive properties, and antiproliferative actions.

Pharmacodynamics/Kinetics

Onset of Action >4 weeks for maximum benefit

Half-life Elimination Ciclesonide: 0.7 hours; des-ciclesonide: 6 to 7 hours

Time to Peak ~1 hour (des-ciclesonide)

Pregnancy Risk Factor C

Pregnancy Considerations

Maternal use of inhaled corticosteroids in usual doses are not associated with an increased risk of fetal malformations; a small risk of malformations was observed in one study following high maternal doses of an alternative inhaled corticosteroid (ERS/TSANZ [Middleton 2020]; GINA 2020). Hypoadrenalism may occur in infants born to mothers receiving corticosteroids during pregnancy.

Uncontrolled asthma is associated with adverse events on pregnancy (increased risk of perinatal mortality, preeclampsia, preterm birth, low birth weight infants, cesarean delivery, and the development of gestational diabetes). Poorly controlled asthma or asthma exacerbations may have a greater fetal/maternal risk than what is associated with appropriately used asthma medications. Maternal treatment improves pregnancy outcomes by reducing the risk of some adverse events (eg, preterm birth, gestational diabetes) (ERS/TSANZ [Middleton 2020]; GINA 2020).

Inhaled corticosteroids are recommended for the treatment of asthma during pregnancy (GINA 2020). Ciclesonide oral inhalation is considered probably acceptable for use during pregnancy. Pregnant females adequately controlled on ciclesonide for asthma may continue therapy; if initiating treatment during pregnancy, use of an agent with more data in pregnant females may be preferred. The lowest dose that maintains asthma control should be used. Maternal asthma symptoms should be monitored monthly during pregnancy (ERS/TSANZ [Middleton 2020]).

Data collection to monitor pregnancy and infant outcomes associated with asthma and the medications used to treat asthma in pregnancy is ongoing. Health care providers are encouraged to enroll exposed pregnant females in the MotherToBaby Pregnancy Studies conducted by the Organization of Teratology Information Specialists (877-311-8972 or https://mothertobaby.org). Patients may also enroll themselves.

◆ **Ciclodan** *see* Ciclopirox *on page 346*

◆ **Ciclodan Cream [DSC]** *see* Ciclopirox *on page 346*

◆ **Ciclodan Solution [DSC]** *see* Ciclopirox *on page 346*

Ciclopirox

(sye kloe PEER oks)

Brand Names: US Ciclodan; Ciclodan Cream [DSC]; Ciclodan Solution [DSC]; Ciclopirox Treatment; CNL8 Nail [DSC]; Loprox; Penlac [DSC]

Brand Names: Canada APO-Ciclopirox; Loprox; Penlac Nail Lacquer; PMS-Ciclopirox; Stieprox; TARO-Ciclopirox

Pharmacologic Category Antifungal Agent, Topical

Use

Dermatologic conditions (infectious and seborrheal):

Cream, suspension: Topical treatment of tinea pedis, tinea cruris, and tinea corporis due to *Trichophyton rubrum*, *Trichophyton mentagrophytes*, *Epidermophyton floccosum*, and *Microsporum canis*; candidiasis (moniliasis) due to *Candida albicans*; tinea (pityriasis) versicolor due to *Malassezia furfur*.

Gel: Topical treatment of interdigital tinea pedis and tinea corporis due to *T. rubrum*, *T. mentagrophytes*, or *E. floccosum*; seborrheic dermatitis of the scalp.

Nail lacquer topical solution: Topical treatment of immunocompetent patients with mild to moderate onychomycosis of fingernails and toenails, without lunula involvement, due to *Trichophyton rubrum*, as a component of a comprehensive management program.

Shampoo: Topical treatment of seborrheic dermatitis of the scalp in adults.

Local Anesthetic/Vasoconstrictor Precautions No information available to require special precautions

Effects on Dental Treatment No significant effects or complications reported

Effects on Bleeding No information available to require special precautions

Adverse Reactions Frequency not always defined.

Cardiovascular: Facial edema, ventricular tachycardia (shampoo)

Central nervous system: Headache

Dermatologic: Acne vulgaris, alopecia, contact dermatitis, erythema, hair discoloration (rare; shampoo formulation in light-haired individuals), localized erythema, nail disease (shape or color change with lacquer), pruritus, skin rash, xeroderma

Local: Application site burning (gel: 7% to 34%; other dose forms: ≤1%), local irritation, local pain

Ophthalmic: Eye pain

Mechanism of Action Inhibiting transport of essential elements in the fungal cell disrupting the synthesis of DNA, RNA, and protein

Pharmacodynamics/Kinetics

Half-life Elimination Biologic: Cream, suspension: 1.7 hours; Elimination: Gel: 5.5 hours

Pregnancy Risk Factor B

Pregnancy Considerations Adverse events were not observed in animal reproduction studies.

◆ **Ciclopirox Olamine** *see* Ciclopirox *on page 346*

◆ **Ciclopirox Treatment** *see* Ciclopirox *on page 346*

◆ **Ciclosporin** *see* CycloSPORINE (Ophthalmic) *on page 423*

◆ **Ciclosporin** *see* CycloSPORINE (Systemic) *on page 421*

◆ **CidalEaze [DSC]** *see* Lidocaine (Topical) *on page 902*

◆ **Cidecin** *see* DAPTOmycin *on page 437*

Cidofovir (si DOF o veer)

Related Information

Systemic Viral Diseases *on page 1709*

Brand Names: Canada Mar-Cidofovir

Pharmacologic Category Antiviral Agent

Use

Cytomegalovirus retinitis: Treatment of cytomegalovirus (CMV) retinitis in patients with AIDS.

Limitations of use: Safety and efficacy have not been established for treatment of other CMV infections (eg, pneumonitis, gastroenteritis), congenital or neonatal CMV disease, or CMV disease in non-HIV infected individuals.

Local Anesthetic/Vasoconstrictor Precautions No information available to require special precautions

Effects on Dental Treatment Key adverse event(s) related to dental treatment: Stomatitis and abnormal taste.

Effects on Bleeding No reports of bleeding or thrombocytopenia with cidofovir alone.

Adverse Reactions

Frequency not defined. *Incidence not specifically defined, but reported in the range of >10%. **Incidence not specifically defined, but reported in the range of 1% to 10%.

Cardiovascular: Cardiac disease, cardiac failure, cardiomyopathy, edema, orthostatic hypotension, shock, syncope, tachycardia

Central nervous system: Chills,* headache,* pain,* agitation, amnesia, anxiety, confusion, convulsions, dizziness, hallucination, insomnia, malaise, vertigo

Dermatologic: Alopecia,* skin rash,* skin discoloration, skin photosensitivity, urticaria

Endocrine & metabolic: Decreased serum bicarbonate,* Fanconi's syndrome,** adrenocortical insufficiency

Gastrointestinal: Anorexia,* diarrhea,* nausea,* oral candidiasis,* vomiting,* abdominal pain, aphthous stomatitis, colitis, constipation, dysphagia, fecal incontinence, gastritis, gastrointestinal hemorrhage, gingivitis, melena, proctitis, stomatitis, tongue discoloration

Genitourinary: Nephrotoxicity,* proteinuria,* urinary incontinence

Hematologic & oncologic: Anemia,* neutropenia,* hypochromic anemia, immune thrombocytopenia, leukocytosis, leukopenia, lymphadenopathy, pancytopenia, pseudolymphoma, splenomegaly, thrombocytopenia

Hepatic: Abnormal liver function tests, hepatic disease, hepatic necrosis, hepatomegaly, hepatosplenomegaly, jaundice

Hypersensitivity: Hypersensitivity reaction

Infection: Infection,* sepsis

Local: Injection site reaction

Neuromuscular & skeletal: Weakness,* tremor

Ophthalmic: Decreased intraocular pressure,* iritis,* uveitis,* amblyopia, blindness, cataract, conjunctivitis, corneal lesion, diplopia, visual disturbance

Otic: Hearing loss

Renal: Increased serum creatinine*

Respiratory: Cough,* dyspnea,* pneumonia**

Miscellaneous: Fever*

<1%, postmarketing, and/or case reports: Hepatic failure, metabolic acidosis, pancreatitis

Mechanism of Action Cidofovir is converted to cidofovir diphosphate (the active intracellular metabolite); cidofovir diphosphate suppresses CMV replication by selective inhibition of viral DNA synthesis. Incorporation of cidofovir diphosphate into growing viral DNA chain results in viral DNA synthesis rate reduction.

Pharmacodynamics/Kinetics

Half-life Elimination Plasma: ~2.6 hours; intracellular elimination half-lives of metabolites are longer (range: 24 to 87 hours) (Lea, 1996)

Reproductive Considerations

[US Boxed Warning]: In animal studies, cidofovir caused hypospermia.

Women of childbearing potential should use effective contraception during therapy and for 1 month following treatment. Males should use a barrier contraceptive during therapy and for 3 months following treatment.

Pregnancy Risk Factor C

Pregnancy Considerations

[US Boxed Warning]: In animal studies, cidofovir was teratogenic.

The indications for treating CMV retinitis during pregnancy are the same as in nonpregnant HIV infected woman; however, systemic therapy should be avoided during the first trimester when possible. When therapy is needed to treat maternal infection, use of cidofovir is not recommended (HHS [Adult OI 2020]).

- **Cilastatin and Imipenem** *see* Imipenem and Cilastatin *on page 799*
- **Cilastatin, Imipenem, and Relebactam** *see* Imipenem, Cilastatin, and Relebactam *on page 800*
- **Cilastatin, Relebactam, and Imipenem** *see* Imipenem, Cilastatin, and Relebactam *on page 800*
- **Cilastatin Sodium, Imipenem Monohydrate, and Relebactam Monohydrate** *see* Imipenem, Cilastatin, and Relebactam *on page 800*

Cilazapril (sye LAY za pril)

Brand Names: Canada APO-Cilazapril; CO Cilazapril [DSC]; Inhibace; MYLAN-Cilazapril; PMS-Cilazapril; TEVA-Cilazapril [DSC]

Pharmacologic Category Angiotensin-Converting Enzyme (ACE) Inhibitor; Antihypertensive

Use Note: Not approved in the US

Heart failure: Adjunctive treatment of heart failure

Guideline recommendations: The American College of Cardiology/American Heart Association (ACC/AHA) 2013 Heart Failure Guidelines recommend the use of ACE inhibitors, along with other guideline-directed medical therapies, to prevent progression of HF and reduced ejection fraction in asymptomatic patients with or without a history of myocardial infarction (Stage B HF), or to treat those with symptomatic heart failure and reduced ejection fraction to reduce morbidity and mortality (Stage C HFrEF).

Hypertension: Management of hypertension

Guideline recommendations: The 2017 Guideline for the Prevention, Detection, Evaluation, and Management of High Blood Pressure in Adults recommends if monotherapy is warranted, in the absence of comorbidities (eg, cerebrovascular disease, chronic kidney disease, diabetes, heart failure, ischemic heart disease, etc.), that thiazide-like diuretics or dihydropyridine calcium channel blockers may be preferred options due to improved cardiovascular endpoints (eg, prevention of heart failure and stroke). ACE inhibitors and ARBs are also acceptable for monotherapy. Combination therapy may be required to achieve blood pressure goals and is initially preferred in patients at high risk (stage 2 hypertension or atherosclerotic cardiovascular disease [ASCVD] risk ≥10%) (ACC/AHA [Whelton 2017]).

Local Anesthetic/Vasoconstrictor Precautions No information available to require special precautions

Effects on Dental Treatment Key adverse event(s) related to dental treatment: Patients may experience orthostatic hypotension as they stand up after treatment; especially if lying in dental chair for extended periods of time. Use caution with sudden changes in position during and after dental treatment.

An angiotensin-converting enzyme (ACE) Inhibitor cough is a dry, hacking, nonproductive cough that can potentially interfere with longer dental procedures if patient has this side effect.

Effects on Bleeding No information available to require special precautions

Adverse Reactions Frequency not always defined.

1% to 10%:

Cardiovascular: Orthostatic hypotension (2%), palpitations (≤1%), symptomatic hypotension (heart failure patients: ≤1%)

Central nervous system: Dizziness (3% to 8%), headache (3% to 5%), fatigue (2% to 3%)

Gastrointestinal: Nausea (1% to 3%)

Neuromuscular & skeletal: Weakness (≤2%)

Renal: Increased serum creatinine

Respiratory: Cough (hypertension patients: 2%; heart failure patients: ≤8%; sometimes severe)

1%, postmarketing, and/or case reports: Abdominal pain, agranulocytosis (rare), alopecia, anaphylaxis (rare), anemia, angina pectoris, angioedema (including facial edema), anorexia, anxiety, arthralgia, ataxia, atrial fibrillation, atrioventricular block, bradycardia, bronchitis, bronchospasm, bullous dermatitis (rare), cardiac arrhythmia, cardiac decompensation, cardiac failure, cerebrovascular accident (rare), chest pain, confusion, conjunctivitis, constipation, decreased libido, depression, dermatitis, diarrhea, diaphoresis, drowsiness, dysgeusia, dyspepsia, dyspnea, dysuria, epistaxis, erythema multiforme (rare), exacerbation of psoriasis (rare), exfoliative dermatitis (rare), extrasystoles, fatigue, flatulence, flushing, gastrointestinal hemorrhage, gout, hemolytic anemia, hyperbilirubinemia, hyperglycemia, hyperkalemia (more common in renal patients), hypoesthesia, immune thrombocytopenia (rare), impotence, increased liver enzymes (rare), increased serum transaminases, insomnia, leg cramps, leukopenia, lichen planus (rare), lupus-like syndrome (rare), malaise, migraine, myalgia, myocardial infarction (rare), nausea, nervousness, neutropenia (rare), pancreatitis (rare), paresthesia, pemphigus, pharyngitis, photophobia, polyuria, proteinuria, pruritus, psoriasiform eruption (rare), purpura (rare), rectal hemorrhage, renal failure (rare), respiratory tract infection, rhinitis, rigors, sinusitis, skin rash (rare; including erythematous rash and maculopapular rash), Stevens-Johnson syndrome (rare), syncope, tachycardia, tinnitus, toxic epidermal necrolysis, transient ischemic attacks (rare), tremor, uremia, urinary frequency, urticaria (rare), vertigo, visual disturbance, visual hallucination (Doane 2013), voice disorder, vomiting, xerostomia

Mechanism of Action Cilazapril is a prodrug that is rapidly converted to cilazaprilat (active metabolite), a competitive inhibitor of angiotensin-converting enzyme (ACE); prevents conversion of angiotensin I to angiotensin II, a potent vasoconstrictor; results in lower levels of angiotensin II which causes an increase in plasma renin activity and a reduction in aldosterone secretion.

Pharmacodynamics/Kinetics

Onset of Action ~1 to 2 hours; Peak effect: Antihypertensive effect: 3 to 7 hours; Heart failure (reduction of systemic vascular resistance and pulmonary capillary wedge pressure): 2 to 4 hours

Duration of Action Therapeutic effect: Up to 24 hours

Half-life Elimination Cilazaprilat: Terminal: Single dose: 36 to 49 hours; Multidose: ~54 hours

Time to Peak Cilazaprilat: Within 2 hours

Reproductive Considerations
Use is contraindicated in females who intend to become pregnant or who are of childbearing potential and are not using adequate contraception.

[Canadian Boxed Warning]: Patients planning pregnancy should be changed to alternative antihypertensive treatments which have an established safety profile for use in pregnancy.

Pregnancy Considerations
[Canadian Boxed Warning]: When used in pregnancy, angiotensin converting enzyme (ACE) inhibitors can cause injury or even death of the developing fetus. Drugs that act on the renin-angiotensin system are associated with oligohydramnios. Oligohydramnios, due to decreased fetal renal function, may lead to fetal lung hypoplasia and skeletal malformations. Their use in pregnancy is also associated with anuria, hypotension, renal failure, skull hypoplasia, and death in the fetus/neonate. Infants exposed to an ACE inhibitor in utero should be monitored for hyperkalemia, hypotension, and oliguria. Oligohydramnios may not appear until after irreversible fetal injury has occurred. Exchange transfusions or dialysis may be required to reverse hypotension or improve renal function, although data related to the effectiveness in neonates are limited.

Chronic maternal hypertension may increase the risk of birth defects, low birth weight, preterm delivery, stillbirth, and neonatal death. Actual fetal/neonatal risks may be related to duration and severity of maternal hypertension. Untreated hypertension may also increase the risks of adverse maternal outcomes, including gestational diabetes, myocardial infarction, preeclampsia, stroke, and delivery complications (ACOG 203 2019).

[Canadian Boxed Warning]: Use of cilazapril is contraindicated during pregnancy. Pregnant women should be informed of the potential hazards to the fetus and must not take cilazapril during pregnancy. When pregnancy is detected, cilazapril should be discontinued as soon as possible and, if appropriate, alternative therapy should be started.

Product Availability Not available in the US

◆ **Cilazapril Monohydrate** *see* Cilazapril *on page 348*

Cilostazol (sil OH sta zol)

Related Information

Antiplatelet and Anticoagulation Considerations in Dentistry *on page 1666*
Cardiovascular Diseases *on page 1654*

Pharmacologic Category Antiplatelet Agent; Phosphodiesterase-3 Enzyme Inhibitor; Vasodilator

Use Intermittent claudication: Reduction of symptoms of intermittent claudication, as indicated by an increased walking distance.

Local Anesthetic/Vasoconstrictor Precautions
No information available to require special precautions

Effects on Dental Treatment No significant effects or complications reported

Effects on Bleeding Cilostazol causes reversible inhibition of platelet aggregation. To restore platelet function, cilostazol should be discontinued for 96 hours (4 days). A medical consult is recommended to determine the benefit:risk of continuing or discontinuing cilostazol for invasive dental procedures.

Adverse Reactions
>10%:
Central nervous system: Headache (27% to 34%)
Gastrointestinal: Diarrhea (12% to 19%), abnormal stools (12% to 15%)
Infection: Infection (10% to 14%)
Respiratory: Rhinitis (7% to 12%)

1% to 10%:
Cardiovascular: Palpitations (5% to 10%), peripheral edema (7% to 9%), tachycardia (4%), atrial fibrillation (<2%), atrial flutter (<2%), cardiac arrest (<2%), cardiac failure (<2%), cerebral infarction (<2%), edema (<2%), facial edema (<2%), hypotension (<2%), myocardial infarction (<2%), nodal arrhythmia (<2%), orthostatic hypotension (<2%), supraventricular tachycardia (<2%), syncope (<2%), varicose veins (<2%), ventricular premature contractions (<2%), ventricular tachycardia (<2%)
Central nervous system: Dizziness (9% to 10%), vertigo (3%), anxiety (<2%), chills (<2%), insomnia (<2%), malaise (<2%), neuralgia (<2%)
Dermatologic: Ecchymoses (<2%), furunculosis (eye: <2%), skin hypertrophy (<2%), urticaria (<2%), xeroderma (<2%)
Endocrine & metabolic: Albuminuria (<2%), diabetes mellitus (<2%), gout (<2%), hyperlipidemia (<2%), hyperuricemia (<2%), increased gamma-glutamyl transferase (<2%)
Gastrointestinal: Nausea (7%), dyspepsia (6%), abdominal pain (4% to 5%), flatulence (3%), anorexia (<2%), cholelithiasis (<2%), colitis (<2%), duodenal ulcer (<2%), duodenitis (<2%), esophageal hemorrhage (<2%), esophagitis (<2%), gastric ulcer (<2%), gastritis (<2%), gastroenteritis (<2%), gingival hemorrhage (<2%), hematemesis (<2%), melena (<2%), peptic ulcer (<2%), periodontal abscess (<2%)
Genitourinary: Cystitis (<2%), pelvic pain (<2%), urinary frequency (<2%), vaginal hemorrhage (<2%), vaginitis (<2%)
Hematologic & oncologic: Anemia (<2%), hemorrhage (<2%), hemorrhage (eye, <2%), iron deficiency anemia (<2%), polycythemia (<2%), purpura (<2%), rectal hemorrhage (<2%), retroperitoneal hemorrhage (<2%)
Hypersensitivity: Tongue edema (<2%)
Neuromuscular & skeletal: Back pain (7%), myalgia (3%), arthralgia (<2%), bursitis (<2%), neck stiffness (<2%), ostealgia (<2%)
Ophthalmic: Amblyopia (<2%), blindness (<2%), conjunctivitis (<2%), diplopia (<2%), retinal hemorrhage (<2%)
Otic: Otalgia (<2%), tinnitus (<2%)
Renal: Increased serum creatinine (<2%)
Respiratory: Pharyngitis (10%), cough (3% to 4%), asthma (<2%), epistaxis (<2%), hemoptysis (<2%), pneumonia (<2%), sinusitis (<2%)
Miscellaneous: Fever (<2%)

Postmarketing and/or case reports: Abnormal hepatic function tests, agranulocytosis, anaphylaxis, angina pectoris, angioedema, aplastic anemia, cerebrovascular accident, cerebral hemorrhage, chest pain, coronary thrombosis (stent), fixed drug eruption, gastrointestinal hemorrhage, granulocytopenia, hematoma (extradural), hematuria, hemorrhagic diathesis, hepatic insufficiency, hot flash, hyperglycemia, hypersensitivity, hypertension, increased blood pressure, increased blood urea nitrogen, interstitial pneumonitis, intracranial hemorrhage, jaundice, left ventricular dysfunction (outflow tract obstruction; in patients with sigmoid-shaped interventricular septum), leukopenia, pain, pancytopenia, pulmonary hemorrhage, pruritus, prolonged QT interval on ECG, skin rash, Stevens-Johnson syndrome, subcutaneous hemorrhage, subdural hematoma, thrombocytopenia, thrombosis, torsades de pointes, vasodilation, vomiting

Mechanism of Action Cilostazol and its metabolites are inhibitors of phosphodiesterase III. As a result, cyclic AMP is increased leading to reversible inhibition of platelet aggregation, vasodilation, and inhibition of vascular smooth muscle cell proliferation.

Pharmacodynamics/Kinetics

Onset of Action Effect on walking distance: 2 to 4 weeks; may require up to 12 weeks

Half-life Elimination ~11 to 13 hours

Pregnancy Risk Factor C

Pregnancy Considerations Adverse events have been observed in animal reproduction studies.

- **Cimduo** *see* Lamivudine and Tenofovir Disoproxil Fumarate *on page 873*
- **Cimzia** *see* Certolizumab Pegol *on page 326*
- **Cimzia Prefilled** *see* Certolizumab Pegol *on page 326*
- **Cimzia Starter Kit** *see* Certolizumab Pegol *on page 326*
- **Cinqair** *see* Reslizumab *on page 1317*
- **Cinvanti** *see* Aprepitant *on page 162*
- **Cipro** *see* Ciprofloxacin (Systemic) *on page 350*

Ciprofloxacin (Systemic) (sip roe FLOKS a sin)

Related Information

Periodontal Diseases *on page 1748*

Brand Names: US Cipro; Cipro in D5W [DSC]; Cipro XR [DSC]

Brand Names: Canada ACT Ciprofloxacin; AG-Ciprofloxacin; APO-Ciproflox; Auro-Ciprofloxacin; BIO-Ciprofloxacin; Cipro; Cipro XL; DOM-Ciprofloxacin; GEN-Ciprofloxacin; GMD-Ciprofloxacin; JAMP-Ciprofloxacin; Mar-Ciprofloxacin; MINT-Ciproflox; MINT-Ciprofloxacin [DSC]; MYLAN-Ciprofloxacin [DSC]; NU-Ciprofloxacin [DSC]; PMS-Ciprofloxacin; PMS-Ciprofloxacin XL; Priva-Ciprofloxacin; PRO-Ciprofloxacin; RATIO-Ciprofloxacin; RIVA-Ciprofloxacin; SANDOZ Ciprofloxacin; Septa-Ciprofloxacin; TARO-Ciproflox; TARO-Ciprofloxacin; TEVA-Ciprofloxacin [DSC]; VAN-Ciprofloxacin [DSC]

Pharmacologic Category Antibiotic, Fluoroquinolone

Use

Children and Adolescents: Treatment of complicated urinary tract infections and pyelonephritis due to *E. coli*. **Note:** Although effective, ciprofloxacin is not the drug of first choice in children.

Infants, Children, Adolescents, and Adults: Prophylaxis to reduce incidence or progression of disease following inhalation exposure to *Bacillus anthracis*; prophylaxis and treatment of plague (*Yersinia pestis*).

Adults: Treatment of the following infections when caused by susceptible bacteria: Urinary tract infections; acute uncomplicated cystitis in females, chronic bacterial prostatitis, bone and joint infections, complicated intra-abdominal infections (in combination with metronidazole), infectious diarrhea, typhoid fever (*Salmonella typhi*), hospital-acquired (nosocomial) pneumonia.

Limitations of use: Because fluoroquinolones have been associated with disabling and potentially irreversible serious adverse reactions (eg, tendinitis and tendon rupture, peripheral neuropathy, CNS effects), reserve ciprofloxacin for use in patients who have no alternative treatment options for acute uncomplicated cystitis.

Local Anesthetic/Vasoconstrictor Precautions No information available to require special precautions

Effects on Dental Treatment No significant effects or complications reported

Effects on Bleeding No information available to require special precautions

Adverse Reactions

>10%: Neuromuscular & skeletal: Musculoskeletal signs and symptoms (children: 9% to 22%)

1% to 10%:

Dermatologic: Skin rash (1% to 2%)

Gastrointestinal: Abdominal pain (children: 3%; adults: <1%), diarrhea (2% to 5%), dyspepsia (1% to 3%), nausea (3% to 4%), vomiting (1% to 5%)

Genitourinary: Vulvovaginal candidiasis (2%)

Hepatic: Abnormal hepatic function tests (1%)

Local: Injection site reactions (IV: >1%)

Nervous system: Dizziness (oral: 2%; IV: <1%; may be more common in elderly) (Mattappalil 2014), drowsiness, headache (oral: 1% to 3%; IV: >1%), insomnia, nervousness, neurological signs and symptoms (IV: children: 3%), restlessness (IV: >1%; oral: <1%)

Respiratory: Asthma (children: 2%)

Miscellaneous: Fever (children: 2%; adults: <1%)

<1%:

Cardiovascular: Acute myocardial infarction, angina pectoris, bradycardia, flushing, hypertension, hypotension, syncope, tachycardia, thrombophlebitis, vasculitis, vasodilation

Dermatologic: Diaphoresis, erythema multiforme, erythema nodosum, exfoliative dermatitis, maculopapular rash, phototoxicity, pruritus, skin photosensitivity, Stevens-Johnson syndrome (Hallgren 2003), toxic epidermal necrolysis, urticaria, vesicobullous dermatitis, xeroderma

Endocrine & metabolic: Albuminuria, gynecomastia, hyperglycemia (Chou 2013), hypoglycemia (Berhe 2019; Chou 2013), increased thirst

Gastrointestinal: Abdominal distress, anorexia, *Clostridioides difficile* colitis (Cain 1990), constipation, dysgeusia, flatulence, gastrointestinal hemorrhage, intestinal obstruction, intestinal perforation, oral mucosa ulcer, pancreatitis, xerostomia

Genitourinary: Casts in urine, crystalluria, dysmenorrhea, hematuria, hemorrhagic cystitis, urinary frequency, vaginitis

Hematologic & oncologic: Agranulocytosis, petechia, prolonged prothrombin time, purpuric disease

Hepatic: Cholestatic jaundice, hepatic necrosis

Hypersensitivity: Anaphylactic shock, anaphylaxis, angioedema, hypersensitivity reaction

Nervous system: Abnormal dreams, abnormal gait, anosmia, ataxia, burning sensation, confusion, depersonalization, depression, hallucination, hypertonia, irritability, malaise, manic reaction, migraine, myasthenia, nightmares, pain, paranoid ideation, paresthesia, phobia, seizure, status epilepticus, suicidal ideation, suicidal tendencies, taste disorder, toxic psychosis, unresponsive to stimuli, vertigo

Neuromuscular & skeletal: Arthralgia, asthenia, joint stiffness, tremor

Ophthalmic: Blurred vision, chromatopsia, decreased visual acuity, diplopia, nystagmus disorder, photopsia
Otic: Hearing loss, tinnitus
Renal: Acute renal failure, interstitial nephritis (Farid 2018; Lim 2003), nephrolithiasis, renal insufficiency
Respiratory: Bronchospasm, dyspnea, hemoptysis, laryngeal edema

Postmarketing:
Cardiovascular: Aortic aneurysm (Meng 2018), aortic dissection (Meng 2018), prolonged QT interval on ECG, torsades de pointes (Teng 2019), ventricular arrhythmia
Dermatologic: Acute generalized exanthematous pustulosis (Foti 2017; Hauserman 2005)
Gastrointestinal: Ageusia, *Clostridioides difficile* associated diarrhea
Hematologic & oncologic: Anemia, eosinophilia, hemolytic anemia, leukopenia, lymphocytosis, methemoglobinemia, monocytosis, pancytopenia, thrombocythemia, thrombocytopenia (Sim 2018)
Hepatic: Hepatic failure, hepatotoxicity (Alshammari 2014; Orman 2011; Radovanovic 2018), increased serum alkaline phosphatase, increased serum bilirubin, jaundice
Hypersensitivity: Fixed drug eruption (Illiyas 2019; Mollica 2019; Nair 2015), nonimmune anaphylaxis (Ouni 2019)
Immunologic: Drug reaction with eosinophilia and systemic symptoms (Alkhateeb 2013), serum sickness-like reaction (Slama 1990)
Infection: Candidiasis
Nervous system: Agitation, anxiety, delirium, disturbance in attention, exacerbation of myasthenia gravis (Jones 2011), Guillain-Barré syndrome (Ali 2014), hyperesthesia, hypoesthesia, idiopathic intracranial hypertension (Milanlioglu 2011), increased intracranial pressure, intracranial hypertension (Tan 2019), memory impairment, myoclonus, peripheral neuropathy (Ali 2014; Francis 2014; Popescu 2018), polyneuropathy, twitching
Neuromuscular & skeletal: Myalgia, rupture of tendon (Arabyat 2015; Yu 2019), tendonitis
Ophthalmic: Retinal detachment (inconsistent data) (Shin 2018)
Respiratory: Pneumonitis

Mechanism of Action Inhibits DNA-gyrase in susceptible organisms; inhibits relaxation of supercoiled DNA and promotes breakage of double-stranded DNA

Pharmacodynamics/Kinetics

Half-life Elimination Children: 4 to 5 hours; Adults: Normal renal function: 4 to 6 hours

Time to Peak Oral:
Immediate release tablet: 0.5 to 2 hours
Extended release tablet: Cipro XR: 1 to 2.5 hours

Pregnancy Considerations

Ciprofloxacin crosses the placenta and produces measurable concentrations in the amniotic fluid and cord serum (Ludlam 1997).

Based on available data, an increased risk of major birth defects, miscarriage, or other adverse fetal and maternal outcomes have not been observed following ciprofloxacin use during pregnancy.

Due to pregnancy-induced physiologic changes, some pharmacokinetic properties of ciprofloxacin may be altered. Serum concentrations of ciprofloxacin may be lower during pregnancy than in nonpregnant patients (Giamarellou 1989).

Ciprofloxacin is recommended for prophylaxis and treatment of pregnant women exposed to anthrax (Meaney-Delman 2014). Alternative antibiotics are recommended in pregnant women for indications such as chancroid (CDC [Workowski 2015]), meningococcal disease (CDC [Bilukha 2005]), or perianal disease and pouchitis in women with inflammatory bowel disease (AGA [Mahadevan 2019]).

Ciprofloxacin and Fluocinolone

(sip roe FLOKS a sin & floo oh SIN oh lone)

Brand Names: US Otovel

Brand Names: Canada Otixal Single Use

Pharmacologic Category Antibiotic, Fluoroquinolone; Antibiotic, Otic; Antibiotic/Corticosteroid, Otic; Corticosteroid, Otic

Use Acute otitis media: Treatment of acute otitis media with tympanostomy tubes (AOMT) due to susceptible isolates of *Staphylococcus aureus, Streptococcus pneumoniae, Haemophilus influenza, Moraxella catarrhalis,* and *Pseudomonas aeruginosa* in pediatric patients 6 months and older.

Local Anesthetic/Vasoconstrictor Precautions No information available to require special precautions

Effects on Dental Treatment No significant effects or complications reported

Effects on Bleeding No information available to require special precautions

Adverse Reactions

1% to 10%:
Dermatologic: Connective tissue disorder (excessive granulation tissue; 1%)
Local: Application site discharge (otorrhea: 5%)

Frequency not defined: Infection: Bacterial superinfection

<1%, postmarketing, and/or case reports: Auricular edema, candidiasis, dizziness, dysgeusia, equilibrium disturbance, eustachian tube congestion, exfoliation of skin, flushing, headache, hypersensitivity reaction, hypoacusis, otalgia, otic infection, paresthesia, pruritus of ear, tinnitus, tympanic membrane disease, tympanostomy tube blockage (device occlusion)

Mechanism of Action

Ciprofloxacin: Inhibits DNA-gyrase in susceptible organisms; inhibits relaxation of supercoiled DNA and promotes breakage of double-stranded DNA.

Fluocinolone: Topical corticosteroids have anti-inflammatory, antipruritic, and vasoconstrictive properties. May depress the formation, release, and activity of endogenous chemical mediators of inflammation (kinins, histamine, liposomal enzymes, prostaglandins) through the induction of phospholipase A_2 inhibitory proteins (lipocortins) and sequential inhibition of the release of arachidonic acid.

Pregnancy Considerations

Due to limited systemic absorption, exposure of ciprofloxacin or fluocinolone to the fetus is not expected following maternal otic administration.

- ◆ **Ciprofloxacin and Fluocinolone Acetonide** *see* Ciprofloxacin and Fluocinolone *on page* 351
- ◆ **Ciprofloxacin HCl** *see* Ciprofloxacin (Systemic) *on page* 350
- ◆ **Ciprofloxacin Hydrochloride** *see* Ciprofloxacin (Systemic) *on page* 350
- ◆ **Cipro in D5W [DSC]** *see* Ciprofloxacin (Systemic) *on page* 350

- ◆ **Cipro XR [DSC]** *see* Ciprofloxacin (Systemic) *on page 350*

Cisapride (SIS a pride)

Brand Names: US Propulsid®

Pharmacologic Category Gastrointestinal Agent, Prokinetic

Use Treatment of nocturnal symptoms of gastroesophageal reflux disease (GERD); has demonstrated effectiveness for gastroparesis, refractory constipation, and nonulcer dyspepsia

Local Anesthetic/Vasoconstrictor Precautions Cisapride is one of the drugs confirmed to prolong the QT interval and is accepted as having a risk of causing torsade de pointes. The risk of drug-induced torsade de pointes is extremely low when a single QT interval prolonging drug is prescribed. In terms of epinephrine, it is not known what effect vasoconstrictors in the local anesthetic regimen will have in patients with a known history of congenital prolonged QT interval or in patients taking any medication that prolongs the QT interval. Until more information is obtained, it is suggested that the clinician consult with the physician prior to the use of a vasoconstrictor in suspected patients, and that the vasoconstrictor (epinephrine, mepivacaine and levonordefrin [Carbocaine® 2% with Neo-Cobefrin®]) be used with caution.

Effects on Dental Treatment Key adverse event(s) related to dental treatment: Xerostomia (normal salivary flow resumes upon discontinuation).

Effects on Bleeding No information available to require special precautions

Adverse Reactions Frequency not defined.

>5%:

Central nervous system: Headache

Dermatologic: Skin rash

Gastrointestinal: Abdominal cramps, diarrhea, dyspepsia, flatulence, nausea, xerostomia

Respiratory: Rhinitis

<5%:

Cardiovascular: Tachycardia

Central nervous system: Anxiety, drowsiness, extrapyramidal reaction, fatigue, insomnia, seizure

Hematologic & oncologic: Aplastic anemia, granulocytopenia, leukopenia, pancytopenia, thrombocytopenia

Hepatic: Increased liver enzymes

Infection: Viral infection (increased incidence)

Respiratory: Cough, sinusitis, upper respiratory tract infection

<1%, postmarketing, and/or case reports: Apnea, bronchospasm, gynecomastia, hyperprolactinemia, methemoglobinemia, psychiatric disturbance, skin photosensitivity

Mechanism of Action Enhances the release of acetylcholine at the myenteric plexus. *In vitro* studies have shown cisapride to have serotonin-4 receptor agonistic properties which may increase gastrointestinal motility and cardiac rate; increases lower esophageal sphincter pressure and lower esophageal peristalsis; accelerates gastric emptying of both liquids and solids.

Pharmacodynamics/Kinetics

Onset of Action 0.5-1 hour

Half-life Elimination 6-12 hours

Pregnancy Risk Factor C

Pregnancy Considerations Adverse events were observed in animal reproduction studies.

Prescribing and Access Restrictions In U.S., available via limited-access protocol only. Call 877-795-4247 for more information.

Dental Health Professional Considerations See Local Anesthetic/Vasoconstrictor Precautions

- ◆ **cis-DDP** *see* CISplatin *on page 352*
- ◆ **cis-Diamminedichloroplatinum** *see* CISplatin *on page 352*

CISplatin (SIS pla tin)

Pharmacologic Category Antineoplastic Agent, Alkylating Agent; Antineoplastic Agent, Platinum Analog

Use

Bladder cancer, advanced: Treatment of advanced bladder cancer

Ovarian cancer, advanced: Treatment of advanced ovarian cancer

Testicular cancer, advanced: Treatment of advanced testicular cancer

Local Anesthetic/Vasoconstrictor Precautions No information available to require special precautions

Effects on Dental Treatment No significant effects or complications reported

Effects on Bleeding Cisplatin causes relatively less bone marrow suppression than many other antineoplastic agents. Thrombocytopenia may occur 18-23 days following treatment.

Adverse Reactions

>10%:

Central nervous system: Neurotoxicity (peripheral neuropathy is dose and duration dependent)

Gastrointestinal: Nausea and vomiting (76% to 100%)

Genitourinary: Nephrotoxicity (28% to 36%; acute renal failure and chronic renal insufficiency)

Hematologic & oncologic: Anemia (≤40%), leukopenia (25% to 30%; nadir: Day 18 to 23; recovery: By day 39; dose related), thrombocytopenia (25% to 30%; nadir: Day 18 to 23; recovery: By day 39; dose related)

Hepatic: Increased liver enzymes

Otic: Ototoxicity (children 40% to 60%; adults 10% to 31%; as tinnitus, high frequency hearing loss)

1% to 10%: Local: Local irritation

<1%, postmarketing, and/or case reports: Alopecia (mild), ageusia, anaphylaxis, autonomic neuropathy, bradycardia (Schlumbrecht 2015), bronchoconstriction, cardiac arrhythmia, cardiac failure, cerebral arteritis, cerebrovascular accident, dehydration, diarrhea, dysgeusia (Rehwaldt 2009), extravasation, heart block, hemolytic anemia (acute), hemolytic-uremic syndrome, hiccups, hypercholesterolemia, hyperuricemia, hypocalcemia, hypokalemia, hypomagnesemia, hyponatremia, hypophosphatemia, hypotension, increased serum amylase, ischemic heart disease, leukoencephalopathy, Lhermitte's sign, mesenteric ischemia (acute; Morgan 2011), myocardial infarction, neutropenic enterocolitis (Furonaka 2005), optic neuritis, pancreatitis (Trivedi 2005), papilledema, peripheral ischemia (acute), phlebitis (Tokuda 2015), reversible posterior leukoencephalopathy syndrome, seizure, SIADH, skin rash, tachycardia, tetany, thrombosis (aortic; Fernandes 2011), thrombotic thrombocytopenic purpura, vasospasm (acute arterial; Morgan 2011), vision color changes, vision loss

Mechanism of Action Cisplatin inhibits DNA synthesis by the formation of DNA cross-links; denatures the double helix; covalently binds to DNA bases and disrupts DNA function; may also bind to proteins; the *cis*-isomer is 14 times more cytotoxic than the *trans*-isomer; both forms cross-link DNA but cis-platinum is less easily recognized by cell enzymes and, therefore, not repaired. Cisplatin can also bind two adjacent guanines on the same strand of DNA producing intrastrand cross-linking and breakage.

Pharmacodynamics/Kinetics

Half-life Elimination

Children: Free drug: 1.3 hours; Total platinum: 44 hours

Adults: Cisplatin: 20 to 30 minutes; Platinum: ≥5 days

Reproductive Considerations

Verify pregnancy status prior to treatment initiation in females of reproductive potential. Females of reproductive potential should use effective contraception during treatment and for 14 months after the last cisplatin dose. Male patients with female partners of reproductive potential should use effective contraception during treatment and for 11 months after the last cisplatin dose.

Cisplatin has been associated with cumulative dose-dependent ovarian failure, premature menopause, impairment of spermatogenesis (oligospermia, azoospermia; possibly irreversible), and reduced female and male fertility.

Pregnancy Considerations

Cisplatin has been reported to cross the human placenta.

Cisplatin may cause fetal harm if administered to a pregnant female. Adverse events associated with cisplatin containing regimens include oligohydramnios, intrauterine growth restriction and preterm birth; acute respiratory distress syndrome, cytopenias, and hearing loss have been reported in the neonate.

- **cis-platinum** *see* CISplatin *on page 352*
- ***Cis*-Retinoic Acid** *see* ISOtretinoin (Systemic) *on page 846*
- **9-cis-retinoic acid** *see* Alitretinoin (Topical) *on page 102*
- **13-*cis*-Retinoic Acid** *see* ISOtretinoin (Systemic) *on page 846*
- **13-*cis*-Vitamin A Acid** *see* ISOtretinoin (Systemic) *on page 846*

Citalopram (sye TAL oh pram)

Related Information

Clinical Risk Related to Drugs Prolonging QT Interval *on page 1675*

Escitalopram *on page 590*

Vasoconstrictor Interactions With Antidepressants *on page 1821*

Brand Names: US CeleXA

Brand Names: Canada ACCEL-Citalopram [DSC]; ACT Citalopram; AG-Citalopram; APO-Citalopram; Auro-Citalopram; BIO-Citalopram; CCP-Citalopram; CeleXA; Citalopram-10; Citalopram-20; Citalopram-40; CTP 30; DOM-Citalopram; ECL-Citalopram [DSC]; JAMP-Citalopram; Mar-Citalopram; MINT-Citalopram; MYLAN-Citalopram [DSC]; NAT-Citalopram; NRA-Citalopram; NU-Citalopram [DSC]; PMS-Citalopram; Priva-Citalopram; RAN-Citalo; RIVA-Citalopram; SANDOZ Citalopram; SEPTA-Citalopram; TEVA-Citalopram; VAN-Citalopram [DSC]

Generic Availability (US) Yes

Pharmacologic Category Antidepressant, Selective Serotonin Reuptake Inhibitor

Use Major depressive disorder (unipolar): Treatment of unipolar major depressive disorder

Local Anesthetic/Vasoconstrictor Precautions Although caution should be used in patients taking tricyclic antidepressants, no interactions have been reported with vasoconstrictors and citalopram, a nontricyclic antidepressant which acts to increase serotonin; no precautions appear to be needed

Citalopram is one of the drugs confirmed to prolong the QT interval and is accepted as having a risk of causing torsade de pointes. The risk of drug-induced torsade de pointes is extremely low when a single QT interval prolonging drug is prescribed. In terms of epinephrine, it is not known what effect vasoconstrictors in the local anesthetic regimen will have in patients with a known history of congenital prolonged QT interval or in patients taking any medication that prolongs the QT interval. Until more information is obtained, it is suggested that the clinician consult with the physician prior to the use of a vasoconstrictor in suspected patients, and that the vasoconstrictor (epinephrine, mepivacaine and levonordefrin [Carbocaine® 2% with Neo-Cobefrin®]) be used with caution.

Effects on Dental Treatment Key adverse event(s) related to dental treatment: Xerostomia (normal salivary flow resumes upon discontinuation). Premarketing trials reported abnormal taste. See Effects on Bleeding and Dental Health Professional Considerations.

Effects on Bleeding Selective serotonin reuptake inhibitors, such as citalopram, may impair platelet aggregation due to platelet serotonin depletion, possibly increasing the risk of a bleeding complication. The risk of a bleeding complication can be increased by coadministration of other antiplatelet agents, such as NSAIDs and aspirin.

Adverse Reactions

>10%:

Dermatologic: Diaphoresis (11%; dose related)

Gastrointestinal: Nausea (21%), xerostomia (20%)

Nervous system: Drowsiness (18%; dose related; literature suggests incidence occurs less frequently in children and adolescents compared to adults [Safer 2006]), insomnia (15%; dose related)

1% to 10%:

Cardiovascular: Bradycardia (1%), hypotension (≥1%), orthostatic hypotension (≥1%), prolonged QT interval on ECG (2% [placebo: 1%]) (Hasnain 2014), tachycardia (≥1%)

Dermatologic: Pruritus (≥1%), skin rash (≥1%)

Endocrine & metabolic: Amenorrhea (≥1%), decreased libido (1% to 4% [placebo: <1%]), weight gain (≥1%), weight loss (≥1%)

Gastrointestinal: Abdominal pain (3%), anorexia (4%), diarrhea (8%), dysgeusia (≥1%), dyspepsia (5%), flatulence (≥1%), increased appetite (≥1%), sialorrhea (≥1%), vomiting (4%; literature suggests incidence is higher in adolescents compared to adults, and is two- to threefold higher in children compared to adults [Safer 2006])

Genitourinary: Dysmenorrhea (3%), ejaculatory disorder (6% [placebo: 1%]), impotence (3%; dose related [placebo: <1%])

Nervous system: Agitation (3%), amnesia (≥1%), anxiety (4%), apathy (≥1%), confusion (≥1%), depression (≥1%), fatigue (5%; dose related), lack of concentration (≥1%), migraine (≥1%), paresthesia (≥1%), yawning (2%; dose related)
Neuromuscular & skeletal: Arthralgia (2%), myalgia (2%), tremor (8%)
Ophthalmic: Accommodation disturbance (≥1%)
Renal: Polyuria (≥1%)
Respiratory: Cough (≥1%), rhinitis (5%), sinusitis (3%), upper respiratory tract infection (5%)
Miscellaneous: Fever (2%)

<1%:

Cardiovascular: Acute myocardial infarction, angina pectoris, atrial fibrillation, bundle branch block, cardiac failure, cerebrovascular accident, extrasystoles, facial edema, flushing, hypertension, ischemic heart disease, peripheral edema, phlebitis, pulmonary embolism, syncope, transient ischemic attacks
Dermatologic: Acne vulgaris, alopecia, cellulitis, dermatitis, eczema, hypertrichosis, hypohidrosis, psoriasis, skin discoloration, skin photosensitivity, urticaria, xeroderma
Endocrine & metabolic: Altered serum glucose, dehydration, galactorrhea not associated with childbirth, goiter, gynecomastia, hot flash, hypoglycemia, hypokalemia, hyponatremia (Flores 2014; Odeh 2011), hypothyroidism, increased libido, increased thirst, obesity
Gastrointestinal: Bruxism, cholecystitis, cholelithiasis, colitis, diverticulitis of the gastrointestinal tract, duodenal ulcer, dysphagia, eructation, esophagitis, gastric ulcer, gastritis, gastroenteritis, gastroesophageal reflux disease, gingival hemorrhage, gingivitis, glossitis, hemorrhoids, hiccups, melanosis, pruritus ani, stomatitis
Genitourinary: Breast hypertrophy, dysuria, hematuria, mastalgia, oliguria, urinary incontinence, urinary retention, vaginal hemorrhage (Durmaz 2015)
Hematologic & oncologic: Anemia, disorder of hemostatic components of blood, hypochromic anemia, leukocytosis, leukopenia, lymphadenopathy, lymphocytopenia, lymphocytosis, purpuric disease
Hepatic: Hepatitis, hyperbilirubinemia, increased liver enzymes, increased serum alkaline phosphatase, jaundice
Nervous system: Abnormal gait, aggressive behavior, ataxia, catatonia, delusion, depersonalization, drug dependence, dystonia (Moosavi 2014), emotional lability, euphoria, extrapyramidal reaction, hallucination, hyperesthesia, hypertonia, hypoesthesia, involuntary muscle movements, myasthenia, neuralgia, nightmares, panic attack, paranoid ideation, psychosis, rigors, seizure, serotonin syndrome (Tseng 2014), stupor, vertigo
Neuromuscular & skeletal: Arthritis, bursitis, hyperkinetic muscle activity, hypokinesia, lower limb cramp, osteoporosis, skeletal pain
Ophthalmic: Abnormal lacrimation, blepharoptosis, cataract, conjunctivitis, diplopia, dry eye syndrome, eye pain, keratitis, mydriasis, photophobia
Otic: Tinnitus
Renal: Nephrolithiasis, pyelonephritis, renal pain
Respiratory: Asthma, bronchitis, bronchospasm, dyspnea, epistaxis, flu-like symptoms, laryngitis, pneumonia, pneumonitis, seasonal allergic rhinitis

Frequency not defined: Nervous system: Suicidal ideation (Coughlin 2016), suicidal tendencies (Zisook 2009)

Postmarketing:

Cardiovascular: Chest pain, Raynaud's disease (Khouri 2016; Peiró 2007), thrombosis, torsades de pointes (de Gregorio 2011), ventricular arrhythmia
Dermatologic: Ecchymoses, erythema multiforme, toxic epidermal necrolysis
Endocrine & metabolic: Increased serum prolactin, orgasm abnormal (Montejo 2001), SIADH (Odeh 2011)
Gastrointestinal: Gastrointestinal hemorrhage, pancreatitis
Genitourinary: Erectile dysfunction (Montejo 2001), priapism (including clitoral priapism) (Berk 1997; Berk 1997; Reisman 2017), sexual difficulty (decreased genital sensation) (Csoka 2008), sexual disorder (persistent post-SSRI) (Csoka 2008)
Hematologic & oncologic: Hemolytic anemia, hypoprothrombinemia, thrombocytopenia (Andersohn 2009)
Hepatic: Hepatic necrosis
Hypersensitivity: Anaphylaxis, angioedema, hypersensitivity reaction
Nervous system: Akathisia, anorgasmia (Clayton 2015), choreoathetosis, delirium, hyperactive behavior (agitation, hyperactivation, hyperkinesis, restlessness occurring in children at a two- to threefold higher incidence compared to adolescents [Safer 2006]), mania (Pravin 2004), myoclonus, neuroleptic malignant syndrome (Stevens 2008), withdrawal syndrome
Neuromuscular & skeletal: Dyskinesia (Gaanderse 2016), rhabdomyolysis
Ophthalmic: Acute angle-closure glaucoma (Croos 2005; Massaoutis 2007), nystagmus disorder
Renal: Acute renal failure

Dosing

Adult Note: Maximum daily dose: Due to the risk of QT prolongation, the maximum recommended daily dose for all indications is 40 mg. A lower maximum daily dose of 20 mg is recommended in patients >60 years of age, those with significant hepatic impairment, and patients who are concurrently receiving medications that significantly increase citalopram levels (eg, cimetidine, omeprazole) or known poor metabolizers of CYP2C19 substrates. **Initial dose and titration:** In patients sensitive to side effects, some experts suggest a lower starting dose of 10 mg daily and gradual titration in increments of no more than 10 mg, particularly in patients with anxiety who are generally more sensitive to overstimulation effects (eg, anxiety, insomnia) with antidepressants (Hirsch 2018c; WFSBP [Bandelow 2012]).

Aggressive or agitated behavior associated with dementia (off-label use): Oral: Initial: 10 mg once daily; increase to 20 mg once daily after ≥3 days. In adults ≤60 years, may further increase dose based on response and tolerability up to 30 mg/day (Pollock 2002; Pollock 2007; Porsteinsson 2014); for adults >60 years, do not exceed the maximum dose of 20 mg/day.

Binge eating disorder (off-label use): Oral: Initial: 20 mg once daily. In adults ≤60 years of age, may gradually increase dose based on response and tolerability at intervals ≥1 week to 40 mg once daily. Although doses up to 60 mg/day have been studied, due to safety considerations the recommended maximum dose is 40 mg/day for adults ≤60 years of age and 20 mg/day for adults >60 years (McElroy 2003).

Generalized anxiety disorder (off-label use): Oral: Initial: 10 mg once daily; may gradually increase dose based on response and tolerability in 10 mg increments at intervals ≥1 week to a maximum dose of 40 mg/day for adults ≤60 years and 20 mg/day for adults >60 years of age (Blank 2006; Varia 2002).

Major depressive disorder (unipolar): Oral: Initial: 20 mg once daily. In adults ≤60 years of age, may gradually increase dose based on response and tolerability at intervals ≥1 week to a maximum dose of 40 mg/day; for adults >60 years of age, do not exceed the maximum dose of 20 mg/day. Daily doses that exceeded these limits have been studied but are not recommended due to safety considerations.

Obsessive-compulsive disorder (off-label use): Oral: Initial: 20 mg once daily. In adults ≤60 years of age, may gradually increase dose based on response and tolerability in 10 to 20 mg increments at intervals ≥1 week to a maximum dose of 40 mg/day; for adults >60 years of age, do not exceed the maximum dose of 20 mg/day. Daily doses that exceeded these limits have been studied but are not recommended due to safety considerations (APA [Koran 2007]; Montgomery 2001). **Note:** An adequate trial for assessment of effect in obsessive-compulsive disorder is considered to be ≥6 weeks at maximum tolerated dose (Issari 2016).

Panic disorder (off-label use): Oral: Initial: 10 mg once daily for 3 to 7 days, then 20 mg once daily. In adults ≤60 years, may gradually increase dose based on response and tolerability in 10 to 20 mg increments at intervals ≥1 week to a maximum of 40 mg/day; for adults >60 years of age, do not exceed the maximum dose of 20 mg/day. Daily doses that exceeded these limits have been studied but are not recommended due to safety considerations (APA 2009b; Leinonen 2000; Perna 2001; Seedat 2003; Stahl 2003; Wade 1997).

Posttraumatic stress disorder (off-label use): Oral: Initial: 20 mg once daily. In adults ≤60 years of age, may gradually increase dose based on response and tolerability in 10 to 20 mg increments at intervals ≥1 week to a maximum dose of 40 mg once daily; for adults >60 years of age, do not exceed the maximum dose of 20 mg/day. Daily doses that exceeded these limits have been studied but are not recommended due to safety considerations (English 2006; Tucker 2003).

Premature ejaculation (off-label use): Oral: Initial: 20 mg once daily. In adults ≤60 years of age, may gradually increase dose based on response and tolerability at intervals of ≥1 week (some experts suggest 3- to 4-week titration intervals [Khera 2020]) up to a maximum of 40 mg/day (Althof 2014; Atmaca 2002a; Safarinejad 2006); for adults >60 years of age, do not exceed the maximum dose of 20 mg/day.

Premenstrual dysphoric disorder (PMDD) (off-label use):

Continuous daily dosing regimen: Oral: Initial: 10 mg once daily; over the first month increase to usual effective dose of 20 mg once daily; in subsequent menstrual cycles, further dose increases (eg, in 10 mg increments per menstrual cycle) up to 40 mg/day may be necessary in some patients for optimal response (Casper 2020; Freeman 2002; Wikander 1998).

Intermittent regimens:

Luteal phase dosing regimen: Oral: Initial: 10 mg once daily during the luteal phase of menstrual cycle only (ie, beginning therapy 14 days before anticipated onset of menstruation and continued to the onset of menses); over the first month increase to usual effective dose of 20 mg once daily during the luteal phase; in a subsequent menstrual cycle, a further increase to 30 mg/day during the luteal phase may be necessary in some patients for optimal response (Casper 2020; Freeman 2002; Wikander 1998).

Symptom-onset dosing regimen: Oral: Initial: 10 mg once daily from the day of symptom onset until a few days after the start of menses; over the first month increase to usual effective dose of 20 mg once daily; in a subsequent menstrual cycle a further increase to 30 mg/day may be necessary in some patients for optimal response (Casper 2020; Ravindran 2007).

Social anxiety disorder (off-label use): Oral: Initial: 10 to 20 mg once daily. In adults ≤60 years of age, after ~6 weeks may gradually increase dose based on response and tolerability in 10 to 20 mg increments at intervals ≥1 week up to maximum of 40 mg/day; for adults >60 years of age, do not exceed the maximum dose of 20 mg/day. Daily doses that exceeded these limits have been studied but are not recommended due to safety considerations (Atmaca 2002b; Furmark 2005; Stein 2019; WFSBP [Bandelow 2012]).

Vasomotor symptoms associated with menopause (alternative agent) (off-label use): Oral: Initial: 10 mg once daily; may increase dose to 20 mg once daily after 1 week. In adults ≤60 years of age, doses as high as 40 mg/day have been studied; however, doses >20 mg/day have demonstrated little additional benefit and greater adverse effects (Barton 2010; Kalay 2007; NAMS 2015). For adults >60 years of age, do not exceed the maximum dose of 20 mg/day.

Dosage adjustments: For concomitant therapy with moderate to strong CYP2C19 inhibitors or other drugs that significantly increase citalopram levels (eg, cimetidine, omeprazole, voriconazole) and in persons who are known to be poor metabolizers of CYP2C19: Maximum dose: 20 mg/day.

Discontinuation of therapy:When discontinuing antidepressant treatment that has lasted for >3 weeks, gradually taper the dose (eg, over 2 to 4 weeks) to minimize withdrawal symptoms and detect reemerging symptoms (APA 2010; WFSBP [Bauer 2015]). Reasons for a slower taper (eg, over 4 weeks) include use of a drug with a half-life <24 hours (eg, paroxetine, venlafaxine), prior history of antidepressant withdrawal symptoms, or high doses of antidepressants (APA 2010; Hirsch 2019). If intolerable withdrawal symptoms occur, resume the previously prescribed dose and/or decrease dose at a more gradual rate (Shelton 2001). Select patients (eg, those with a history of discontinuation syndrome) on long-term treatment (>6 months) may benefit from tapering over >3 months (WFSBP [Bauer 2015]). Evidence supporting ideal taper rates is limited (Shelton 2001; WFSBP [Bauer 2015]).

Switching antidepressants: Evidence for ideal antidepressant switching strategies is limited; strategies include cross-titration (gradually discontinuing the first antidepressant while at the same time gradually increasing the new antidepressant) and direct switch (abruptly discontinuing the first antidepressant and then starting the new antidepressant at an equivalent dose or lower dose and increasing it gradually). Cross-titration (eg, over 1 to 4 weeks depending upon sensitivity to discontinuation symptoms and adverse effects) is standard for most switches, but is contraindicated when switching to or from an MAOI. A direct switch may be an appropriate approach when switching to another agent in the same or similar class (eg, when switching between two SSRIs), when the antidepressant to be discontinued has been used for <1 week, or when the discontinuation is for adverse effects. When choosing the switch strategy, consider the risk of discontinuation symptoms, potential for drug interactions, other antidepressant properties (eg, half-life, adverse effects, pharmacodynamics), and the degree of symptom control desired (Hirsch 2018b; Ogle 2013; WFSBP [Bauer 2013]).

Switching to or from an MAOI:

Allow 14 days to elapse between discontinuing an MAOI and initiation of citalopram.

Allow 14 days to elapse between discontinuing citalopram and initiation of an MAOI.

Geriatric Note: For patients >60 years of age, the maximum recommended dose is 20 mg/day due to the risk of QT prolongation.

Generalized anxiety disorder (off-label use): Oral: Initial: 10 mg once daily; may increase dose based on response and tolerability in 10 mg increments at intervals ≥1 week up to 20 mg/day. Doses up to 40 mg/day have been studied; however, according to the manufacturer, dosing should not exceed 20 mg/day (Blank 2006; Crocco 2017; Lenze 2005).

Major depressive disorder (unipolar): Adults >60 years: Oral: Initial: 10 to 20 mg once daily (Marano 2015; VA/DoD 2016); maximum dose: 20 mg/day due to increased exposure and the risk of QT prolongation.

Discontinuation of therapy: Refer to adult dosing.

Switching antidepressants: Refer to adult dosing.

Renal Impairment: Adult

Mild to moderate impairment: No dosage adjustment necessary.

Severe impairment: CrCl <20 mL/minute: No dosage adjustment provided in manufacturer's labeling (has not been studied); use caution.

Hepatic Impairment: Adult Maximum recommended dose: 20 mg daily due to decreased clearance and the risk of QT prolongation

Pediatric Note: Slower titration of dose every 2 to 4 weeks may minimize risk of SSRI associated behavioral activation, which has been shown to increase risk of suicidal behavior. Doses >40 mg are not recommended due to risk of QTc prolongation.

Depression: Limited data available; efficacy results variable: One randomized, placebo-controlled trial has shown citalopram to be effective for the treatment of depression in pediatric patients (Wagner 2004); other controlled pediatric trials have **not** shown benefit (Sharp 2006; von Knorring 2006; Wagner 2005). Some experts recommend the following doses (Dopheide 2006): Oral:

Children 7 to ≤11 years: Initial: 10 mg/day given once daily; increase dose slowly by 5 mg/day every 2 weeks as clinically needed; dosage range: 20 to 40 mg/day

Children and Adolescents ≥12 years: Initial: 20 mg/day given once daily; increase dose slowly by 10 mg/day every 2 weeks as clinically needed; dosage range: 20 to 40 mg/day

Obsessive-compulsive disorder: Limited data available: Several open label trials have been published (Mukaddes 2003; Thomsen 1997; Thomsen 2001). Some experts recommend the following doses: Oral:

Children 7 to ≤11 years: Initial: 5 to 10 mg/day given once daily; increase dose slowly by 5 mg/day every 2 weeks as clinically needed; dosage range: 10 to 40 mg/day

Children and Adolescents ≥12 years: Initial: 10 to 20 mg/day given once daily; increase dose slowly by 10 mg/day every 2 weeks as clinically needed; dosage range: 10 to 40 mg/day

Note: Higher mg/kg doses are needed in children compared to adolescents.

Discontinuation of therapy: Consider planning antidepressant discontinuation for lower-stress times, recognizing non-illness-related factors could cause stress or anxiety and be misattributed to antidepressant discontinuation (Hathaway 2018). Upon discontinuation of antidepressant therapy, gradually taper the dose to minimize the incidence of discontinuation syndromes (withdrawal) and allow for the detection of reemerging disease state symptoms (eg, relapse). Evidence supporting ideal taper rates after illness remission is limited. APA and NICE guidelines suggest tapering therapy over at least several weeks with consideration to the half-life of the antidepressant; antidepressants with a shorter half-life may need to be tapered more conservatively. After long-term (years) antidepressant treatment, WFSBP guidelines recommend tapering over 4 to 6 months, with close monitoring during and for 6 months after discontinuation. If intolerable discontinuation symptoms occur following a dose reduction, consider resuming the previously prescribed dose and/or decrease dose at a more gradual rate (APA 2010; Bauer 2002; Fenske 2009; Haddad 2001; NCCMH 2010; Schatzberg 2006; Shelton 2001; Warner 2006).

MAO inhibitor recommendations:

Switching to or from an MAO inhibitor intended to treat psychiatric disorders:

Allow 14 days to elapse between discontinuing an MAO inhibitor intended to treat psychiatric disorders and initiation of citalopram.

Allow 14 days to elapse between discontinuing citalopram and initiation of an MAO inhibitor intended to treat psychiatric disorders.

Renal Impairment: Pediatric Specific recommendations in pediatric patients are not available; based on experience in adult patients, in mild to moderate impairment, no adjustment needed, and in severe impairment, use with caution (has not been studied).

Hepatic Impairment: Pediatric Specific recommendations in pediatric patients are not available; based on experience in adult patients, consider reduced daily doses due to increased serum concentrations and the risk of QT prolongation.

Mechanism of Action A racemic bicyclic phthalane derivative, citalopram selectively inhibits serotonin reuptake in the presynaptic neurons and has minimal effects on norepinephrine or dopamine. Uptake inhibition of serotonin is primarily due to the *S*-enantiomer of citalopram. Displays little to no affinity for serotonin, dopamine, adrenergic, histamine, GABA, or muscarinic receptor subtypes.

Contraindications

Hypersensitivity to citalopram or any component of the formulation; use of MAO inhibitors intended to treat psychiatric disorders (concurrently or within 14 days of discontinuing either citalopram or the MAO inhibitor); initiation of citalopram in a patient receiving linezolid or intravenous methylene blue; concomitant use with pimozide

Canadian labeling: Additional contraindications (not in US labeling): Known QT interval prolongation or congenital long QT syndrome

Warnings/Precautions [US Boxed Warning]: Antidepressants increase the risk of suicidal thinking and behavior in children, adolescents, and young adults (18 to 24 years of age) with major depressive disorder (MDD) and other psychiatric disorders; consider risk prior to prescribing. Short-term studies did not show an increased risk in patients >24 years of age and showed a decreased risk in patients ≥65 years. Closely monitor patients for clinical worsening, suicidality, or unusual changes in behavior, particularly during the initial 1 to 2 months of therapy or during periods of dosage adjustments (increases or decreases); the patient's family or caregiver should be instructed to closely observe the patient and communicate condition with health care provider. A medication guide concerning the use of antidepressants should be dispensed with each prescription. **Citalopram is not FDA approved for use in children.**

The possibility of a suicide attempt is inherent in major depression and may persist until remission occurs. Use caution in high-risk patients. Worsening depression and severe abrupt suicidality that are not part of the presenting symptoms may require discontinuation or modification of drug therapy.

May precipitate a shift to mania or hypomania in patients with bipolar disorder. Monotherapy in patients with bipolar disorder should be avoided. Combination therapy with an antidepressant and a mood stabilizer may be effective for acute treatment of bipolar major depressive episodes, but should be avoided in acute mania or mixed episodes, as well as maintenance treatment in bipolar disorder due to the mood-destabilizing effects of antidepressants (CANMAT [Yatham 2018]; WFSBP [Grunze 2018]). Patients presenting with depressive symptoms should be screened for bipolar disorder **Citalopram is not FDA approved for the treatment of bipolar depression.**

Potentially life-threatening serotonin syndrome (SS) has occurred with serotonergic agents (eg, SSRIs, SNRIs), particularly when used in combination with other serotonergic agents (eg, triptans, TCAs, fentanyl, lithium, tramadol, buspirone, St John's wort, tryptophan) or agents that impair metabolism of serotonin (eg, MAO inhibitors intended to treat psychiatric disorders, other MAO inhibitors [ie, linezolid and intravenous methylene blue]). Discontinue treatment (and any concomitant serotonergic agent) immediately if signs/symptoms arise. May increase the risks associated with electroconvulsive therapy. Has a low potential to impair cognitive or motor performance; caution operating hazardous machinery or driving. Bone fractures have been associated with antidepressant treatment. Consider the possibility of a fragility fracture if an antidepressant-treated patient presents with unexplained bone pain, point tenderness, swelling, or bruising (Rabenda 2013; Rizzoli 2012).

Citalopram causes dose-dependent QTc prolongation; torsades de pointes, ventricular tachycardia, and sudden death have been reported. Use is not recommended in patients with congenital long QT syndrome, bradycardia, recent MI, uncompensated heart failure, hypokalemia, and/or hypomagnesemia, or patients receiving concomitant medications which prolong the QT interval; if use is essential and cannot be avoided in these patients, ECG monitoring is recommended. Discontinue therapy in any patient with persistent QTc measurements >500 msec. Serum electrolytes, particularly potassium and magnesium, should be monitored prior to initiation and periodically during therapy in any patient at increased risk for significant electrolyte disturbances; hypokalemia and/or hypomagnesemia should be corrected prior to use. Due to the QT prolongation risk, doses >40 mg/day are not recommended. In a scientific statement from the American Heart Association, citalopram has been determined to be an agent that may exacerbate underlying myocardial dysfunction (magnitude: major) (AHA [Page 2016]). Additionally, the maximum daily dose should not exceed 20 mg/day in certain populations (eg, CYP2C19 poor metabolizers, patients with hepatic impairment, elderly patients). Potentially significant drug-drug interactions may exist, requiring dose or frequency adjustment, additional monitoring, and/or selection of alternative therapy.

Use with caution in patients with a previous seizure disorder or condition predisposing to seizures such as brain damage or alcoholism. Pharmacokinetics are altered in patients >60 years of age; a lower maximum dose of 20 mg/day is recommended in this population because of the risk of QT prolongation. May cause mild pupillary dilation, which in susceptible individuals can lead to an episode of narrow-angle glaucoma. Consider evaluating patients who have not had an iridectomy for narrow-angle glaucoma risk factors. Citalopram is not FDA-approved for use in children; however, if used, monitor weight and growth regularly during therapy due to the potential for decreased appetite and weight loss with SSRI use.

Abrupt discontinuation or interruption of antidepressant therapy has been associated with a discontinuation syndrome. Symptoms arising may vary with antidepressant however commonly include nausea, vomiting, diarrhea, headaches, light-headedness, dizziness, diminished appetite, sweating, chills, tremors, paresthesias, fatigue, somnolence, and sleep disturbances (eg, vivid dreams, insomnia). Greater risks for developing a discontinuation syndrome have been associated with antidepressants with shorter half-lives, longer durations of treatment, and abrupt discontinuation. For antidepressants of short or intermediate half-lives, symptoms may emerge within 2 to 5 days after treatment discontinuation and last 7 to 14 days (APA 2010; Fava 2006; Haddad 2001; Shelton 2001; Warner 2006).

Warnings: Additional Pediatric Considerations

Selective serotonin reuptake inhibitor (SSRI)-associated behavioral activation (ie, restlessness, hyperkinesis, hyperactivity, agitation) is two- to threefold more prevalent in children compared to adolescents; it is more prevalent in adolescents compared to adults. Somnolence (including sedation and drowsiness) is more common in adults compared to children and adolescents (Safer, 2006). SSRI-associated vomiting is two- to threefold more prevalent in children compared to adolescents and is more prevalent in adolescents compared to adults (Safer, 2006).

Drug Interactions

Metabolism/Transport Effects **Substrate** of CYP2C19 (major), CYP2D6 (minor), CYP3A4 (major); **Note:** Assignment of Major/Minor substrate status based on clinically relevant drug interaction potential; **Inhibits** CYP2D6 (weak)

Avoid Concomitant Use

Avoid concomitant use of Citalopram with any of the following: Bromopride; Dapoxetine; Escitalopram; Fexinidazole [INT]; Linezolid; Methylene Blue; Monoamine Oxidase Inhibitors (Antidepressant); Pimozide; QT-prolonging Agents (Highest Risk); Rasagiline; Selegiline; Urokinase

Increased Effect/Toxicity

Citalopram may increase the levels/effects of: Agents with Antiplatelet Properties; Agents with Blood Glucose Lowering Effects; Anticoagulants; Antipsychotic Agents; Apixaban; Aspirin; Bemiparin; Brexanolone; Cephalothin; Collagenase (Systemic); Dabigatran Etexilate; Deoxycholic Acid; Desmopressin; Domperidone; Doxepin-Containing Products; DULoxetine; Edoxaban; Enoxaparin; Escitalopram; FLUoxetine; FluvoxaMINE; Gilteritinib; Haloperidol; Heparin; Hydroxychloroquine; Ibritumomab Tiuxetan; Lofexidine; Methylene Blue; Monoamine Oxidase Inhibitors (Antidepressant); Nonsteroidal Anti-Inflammatory Agents (COX-2 Selective); Nonsteroidal Anti-Inflammatory Agents (Nonselective); Obinutuzumab; Oxitriptan; Perhexiline; QT-prolonging Kinase Inhibitors (Moderate Risk); QT-prolonging Miscellaneous Agents (Moderate Risk); QT-prolonging Moderate CYP3A4 Inhibitors (Moderate Risk); QT-prolonging Strong CYP3A4 Inhibitors (Moderate Risk); Rasagiline; Rivaroxaban; Salicylates; Selective Serotonin Reuptake Inhibitors; Selegiline; Serotonergic Non-Opioid CNS Depressants; Serotonin/Norepinephrine Reuptake Inhibitors; Thiazide and Thiazide-Like Diuretics; Thrombolytic Agents; Tricyclic Antidepressants; Urokinase; Vitamin K Antagonists; Voriconazole

The levels/effects of Citalopram may be increased by: Acalabrutinib; Alcohol (Ethyl); Almotriptan; Alosetron; Amisulpride (Oral); Amphetamines; Antiemetics (5HT3 Antagonists); Antipsychotic Agents; Bromopride; BuPROPion; BusPIRone; Cimetidine; Cyclobenzaprine; CYP2C19 Inhibitors (Moderate); Dapoxetine; Dexmethylphenidate-Methylphenidate; Dextromethorphan; Eletriptan; Ergot Derivatives; Escitalopram; Esomeprazole; Fat Emulsion (Fish Oil Based); Fenfluramine; Fexinidazole [INT]; Fluconazole; FLUoxetine; FluvoxaMINE; Glucosamine; Herbs (Anticoagulant/Antiplatelet Properties); Hydroxychloroquine; Ibrutinib; Inotersen; Lasmiditan; Limaprost; Linezolid; Lofexidine; Lorcaserin (Withdrawn From US Market); Metaxalone; MetyroSINE; Multivitamins/Fluoride (with ADE); Multivitamins/Minerals (with ADEK, Folate, Iron); Multivitamins/Minerals (with AE, No Iron); Nefazodone; Nonsteroidal Anti-Inflammatory Agents (Topical); Omega-3 Fatty Acids; Omeprazole; Ondansetron; Opioid Agonists; Ozanimod; Pentamidine (Systemic); Pentosan Polysulfate Sodium; Pentoxifylline; Pimozide; Prostacyclin Analogues; QT-prolonging Agents (Highest Risk); QT-prolonging Antipsychotics (Moderate Risk); QT-prolonging Class IC Antiarrhythmics (Moderate Risk); QT-prolonging Moderate CYP3A4 Inhibitors (Moderate Risk); QT-prolonging Quinolone Antibiotics (Moderate Risk); QT-prolonging Strong CYP3A4 Inhibitors (Moderate Risk); Ramosetron; Safinamide; Selumetinib; Serotonergic Agents (High Risk, Miscellaneous); Serotonergic Opioids (High Risk); Serotonin 5-HT1D Receptor Agonists (Triptans); St John's Wort; Syrian Rue; Tipranavir; TraMADol; Tricyclic Antidepressants; Vitamin E (Systemic); Voriconazole; Zanubrutinib

Decreased Effect

Citalopram may decrease the levels/effects of: Ioflupane I 123; Thyroid Products

The levels/effects of Citalopram may be decreased by: CarBAMazepine; CYP3A4 Inducers (Moderate); CYP3A4 Inducers (Strong); Cyproheptadine; Dabrafenib; Deferasirox; Enzalutamide; Erdafitinib; Gilteritinib; Lumacaftor and Ivacaftor; Mitotane; Nonsteroidal Anti-Inflammatory Agents (COX-2 Selective); Nonsteroidal Anti-Inflammatory Agents (Nonselective); RifAMPin; Sarilumab; Siltuximab; St John's Wort; Tocilizumab

Dietary Considerations May be taken without regard to food.

Pharmacodynamics/Kinetics

Onset of Action

Anxiety disorders (generalized anxiety, obsessive-compulsive, panic, and posttraumatic stress disorder): Initial effects may be observed within 2 weeks of treatment, with continued improvements through 4 to 6 weeks (Issari 2016; Varigonda 2016; WFSBP [Bandelow 2012]); some experts suggest up to 12 weeks of treatment may be necessary for response, particularly in patients with obsessive-compulsive disorder and posttraumatic stress disorder (BAP [Baldwin 2014]; Katzman 2014; WFSBP [Bandelow 2012]).

Depression: Initial effects may be observed within 1 to 2 weeks of treatment, with continued improvements through 4 to 6 weeks (Papakostas 2006; Posternak 2005; Szegedi 2009; Taylor 2006).

Premenstrual dysphoric disorder: Initial effects may be observed within the first few days of treatment, with response at the first menstrual cycle of treatment (ISPMD [Nevatte 2013]).

Duration of Action 1 to 2 days

Half-life Elimination 24 to 48 hours (average: 35 hours); doubled with hepatic impairment and increased by 30% (following multiple doses) to 50% (following single dose) in elderly patients (≥60 years)

Time to Peak Serum: 1 to 6 hours, average within 4 hours

Reproductive Considerations Citalopram may cause or exacerbate sexual dysfunction. Decreased libido and anorgasmia have been reported in females. Abnormal ejaculation, decreased libido, and impotence have been reported in males.

Pregnancy Risk Factor C

Pregnancy Considerations

Citalopram and its metabolites cross the human placenta (Heikkinen, Ekblad, Kero 2002). An increased risk of teratogenic effects, including cardiovascular defects, may be associated with maternal use of citalopram or other SSRIs; however, available information is conflicting. Nonteratogenic effects in the newborn following SSRI/SNRI exposure late in the third trimester include respiratory distress, cyanosis, apnea, seizures, temperature instability, feeding difficulty, vomiting, hypoglycemia, hypo- or hypertonia, hyper-reflexia, jitteriness, irritability, constant crying, and tremor. Symptoms may be due to the toxicity of the SSRIs/SNRIs or a discontinuation syndrome and may be consistent with serotonin syndrome associated with SSRI treatment. Persistent pulmonary hypertension of the newborn (PPHN) has also been reported with SSRI exposure. The long-term effects of in utero SSRI exposure on infant development and behavior are not known.

Due to pregnancy-induced physiologic changes, women who are pregnant may require adjusted doses of citalopram to achieve euthymia (Heikkinen, Ekblad, Kero 2002). The ACOG recommends that therapy with SSRIs or SNRIs during pregnancy be individualized; treatment of depression during pregnancy should incorporate the clinical expertise of the mental health clinician, obstetrician, primary health care provider, and pediatrician. According to the American Psychiatric Association (APA), the risks of medication treatment should be weighed against other treatment options and untreated depression. For women who discontinue antidepressant medications during pregnancy and who may be at high risk for postpartum depression, the medications can be restarted following delivery. Treatment algorithms have been developed by the ACOG and the APA for the management of depression in women prior to conception and during pregnancy (ACOG 2008; APA 2010; Yonkers 2009).

Pregnant women exposed to antidepressants during pregnancy are encouraged to enroll in the National Pregnancy Registry for Antidepressants (NPRAD). Women 18 to 45 years of age or their health care providers may contact the registry by calling 844-405-6185. Enrollment should be done as early in pregnancy as possible.

Breastfeeding Considerations

Citalopram and its active metabolites are present in breast milk.

The relative infant dose (RID) of citalopram has been evaluated in numerous studies; the reported RID of citalopram ranges from 3% to 10% of the weight-adjusted maternal dose (maternal dose not stated; Berle 2011), and may be higher (Berle 2011; Sriraman 2015).

In general, breastfeeding is considered acceptable when the RID is <10% (Anderson 2016; Ito 2000); however, some sources note breastfeeding should only be considered if the RID is <5% for psychotropic agents (Larsen 2015). Active metabolites of citalopram can also be detected in breast milk. Peak milk concentrations of citalopram and desmethylcitalopram occur 4 and 6 hours, respectively, after the maternal dose in women on chronic therapy (Rampono 2000). However, avoiding breastfeeding during the expected peak concentrations will generally not decrease infant exposure significantly for antidepressants with long half-lives (Berle 2011). Although the absolute infant plasma concentrations are generally negligible, in some cases the infant plasma concentration of citalopram was up to 10% of the maternal concentration (Berle 2011).

Excessive somnolence, decreased feeding, and weight loss have been noted in infants exposed to citalopram from breast milk. Infants of mothers using psychotropic medications should be monitored daily for changes in sleep, feeding patterns, and behavior (Bauer 2013) as well as infant growth and neurodevelopment (Sachs 2013; Sriraman 2015). Maternal use of an SSRI during pregnancy may cause delayed lactogenesis (Marshall 2010).

When first initiating an antidepressant in a breastfeeding woman, agents other than citalopram are preferred. Women successfully treated with citalopram during pregnancy may continue use while breastfeeding if there are no other contraindications (Berle 2011; Sriraman 2015). According to the manufacturer, the decision to continue or discontinue breastfeeding during therapy should take into account the risk of infant exposure, the benefits of breastfeeding to the infant, and benefits of treatment to the mother.

Dosage Forms: US

Solution, Oral:

Generic: 10 mg/5 mL (10 mL, 240 mL)

Tablet, Oral:

CeleXA: 10 mg, 20 mg, 40 mg

Generic: 10 mg, 20 mg, 40 mg

Dosage Forms: Canada

Tablet, Oral:

CeleXA: 20 mg, 40 mg

CTP 30: 30 mg

Generic: 10 mg, 20 mg, 40 mg

Dental Health Professional Considerations Problems with SSRI-induced bruxism have been reported and may preclude their use; clinicians attempting to evaluate any patient with bruxism or involuntary muscle movement, who is simultaneously being treated with an SSRI drug, should be aware of the potential association.

Also see Local Anesthetic/Vasoconstrictor Precautions

- ◆ **Citalopram Hydrobromide** *see* Citalopram *on page 353*
- ◆ **Citanest Plain Dental** *see* Prilocaine *on page 1274*
- ◆ **Citracal Maximum [OTC]** *see* Calcium and Vitamin D *on page 280*
- ◆ **Citracal Petites [OTC]** *see* Calcium and Vitamin D *on page 280*
- ◆ **Citracal Regular [OTC]** *see* Calcium and Vitamin D *on page 280*
- ◆ **Citrovorum Factor** *see* Leucovorin Calcium *on page 889*
- ◆ **CL-118,532** *see* Triptorelin *on page 1500*
- ◆ **CI-719** *see* Gemfibrozil *on page 733*
- ◆ **CL-184116** *see* Porfimer *on page 1247*
- ◆ **CL-232315** *see* MitoXANTRONE *on page 1042*

Cladribine (KLA dri been)

Brand Names: US Mavenclad (10 Tabs); Mavenclad (4 Tabs); Mavenclad (5 Tabs); Mavenclad (6 Tabs); Mavenclad (7 Tabs); Mavenclad (8 Tabs); Mavenclad (9 Tabs)

Brand Names: Canada Mavenclad

Pharmacologic Category Antineoplastic Agent, Antimetabolite; Antineoplastic Agent, Antimetabolite (Purine Analog); Immunosuppressant Agent

Use

Hairy cell leukemia (injection only): Treatment of active hairy cell leukemia as defined by clinically significant anemia, neutropenia, thrombocytopenia, or disease-related symptoms.

Multiple sclerosis, relapsing (oral tablet only): Treatment of relapsing forms of multiple sclerosis (MS), including relapsing-remitting (RRMS) and active secondary progressive disease in adults who have had inadequate response or are intolerant to other therapies for multiple sclerosis.

Limitations of use: Not recommended for patients with clinically isolated syndrome.

Local Anesthetic/Vasoconstrictor Precautions No information available to require special precautions

Effects on Dental Treatment No significant effects or complications reported

Effects on Bleeding The major dose-limiting adverse effect of cladribine is bone marrow suppression including severe (grade 4) thrombocytopenia in ~12% of patients receiving repeated courses of therapy; recovery is usually by day 12.

Adverse Reactions

IV:

>10%:

Hematologic & oncologic: Bone marrow depression (34%, may be delayed onset), febrile neutropenia (47%), severe anemia (37%), severe neutropenia (70%), thrombocytopenia (12%)

Infection: Bacterial infection (12%), infection (28%; serious infection: 6%)

Miscellaneous: Fever (69%; high fever: 11%)

1% to 10%: Infection: Fungal infection (6%), herpes zoster infection (4%), viral infection (6%)

Frequency not defined:

Cardiovascular: Edema, peripheral edema, phlebitis, tachycardia

Dermatologic: Ecchymosis, hyperhidrosis, pruritus, skin rash

Gastrointestinal: Abdominal pain, constipation, decreased appetite, diarrhea, flatulence, nausea, vomiting

Hematologic & oncologic: Bruise, decreased CD-4 cell count (nadir occurred 4 to 6 months following treatment and may continue to be depressed >15 months), petechia, purpuric disease

Infection: Bacteremia, localized infection, septicemia

Local: Bleeding at injection site, injection site reaction, localized edema

Nervous system: Anxiety, chills, dizziness, fatigue, headache, insomnia, malaise, myasthenia, pain, severe neurotoxicity

Neuromuscular & skeletal: Arthralgia, asthenia, myalgia

Respiratory: Abnormal breath sounds, cough, dyspnea, rales

Postmarketing:

Dermatologic: Stevens-Johnson syndrome, toxic epidermal necrolysis, viral skin infection

Hematologic & oncologic: Tumor lysis syndrome

Nervous system: Progressive multifocal leukoencephalopathy

Respiratory: Pneumonia, respiratory tract infection

Oral:

>10%:

Hematologic & oncologic: Decreased hemoglobin (26%), decreased platelet count (11%), lymphocytopenia (24% to 87%)

Hypersensitivity: Hypersensitivity reaction (11%; severe hypersensitivity reaction: <1%)

Infection: Infection (49%)

Nervous system: Headache (25%)

Respiratory: Upper respiratory tract infection (38%)

1% to 10%:

Cardiovascular: Hypertension (5%)

Dermatologic: Alopecia (3%)

Gastrointestinal: Nausea (10%), oral herpes simplex infection (3%)

Hematologic & oncologic: Neutropenia (4%)

Infection: Herpes virus infection (6%), herpes zoster infection (2%)

Nervous system: Depression (5%), insomnia (6%)

Neuromuscular & skeletal: Arthralgia (≤7%), arthritis (≤7%), back pain (8%)

Respiratory: Bronchitis (5%)

Miscellaneous: Fever (5%)

<1%:

Cardiovascular: Cardiac failure, myocarditis

Hepatic: Hepatic injury

Nervous system: Seizure (tonic clonic), status epilepticus

Respiratory: Tuberculosis

Frequency not defined:

Dermatologic: Skin rash

Hematologic & oncologic: Malignant melanoma, malignant neoplasm, malignant neoplasm of ovary, pancreatic adenocarcinoma

Infection: Coccidioidomycosis, fungal infection

Renal: Pyelonephritis

Mechanism of Action Cladribine is a purine nucleoside analogue; it is a prodrug which is activated by phosphorylation and converted into the active moiety, Cd-ATP. This active form incorporates into DNA to result in the breakage of DNA strand and shutdown of DNA synthesis and repair. This also results in a depletion of nicotinamide adenine dinucleotide and adenosine triphosphate (ATP). Cladribine is cell-cycle nonspecific. The mechanism of cladribine in treating multiple sclerosis (MS) is unknown, but may involve cytotoxic effects on B and T lymphocytes that result from the shutdown of DNA synthesis, leading to a depletion of lymphocytes.

Pharmacodynamics/Kinetics

Half-life Elimination Children 8 months to 18 years: IV: 19.7 ± 3.4 hours (Kearns 1994); Adults: After a 2-hour infusion (with normal renal function): 5.4 hours; Oral: ~24 hours

Time to Peak Oral: Median 0.5 hour (range 0.5 to 1.5 hours) (fasting); 1.5 hours (range 1 to 3 hours) (with high-fat meal)

Reproductive Considerations

Females of reproductive potential should use highly effective contraception during therapy regardless of the route of administration/indication for treatment.

[US Boxed Warning]: Oral tablet: Cladribine is contraindicated for use in women and men of reproductive potential who do not plan to use effective contraception because of the potential for fetal harm. Exclude pregnancy before the start of treatment with cladribine in females of reproductive potential. Advise females and males of reproductive potential to use effective contraception during cladribine dosing and for 6 months after the last dose in each treatment course. Pregnancy should be excluded in females of reproductive potential prior to each course of cladribine. The effect of cladribine on hormonal contraceptives is not known, use of a barrier method is recommended in addition to systemic hormonal contraceptives during therapy and for 4 weeks after the last cladribine dose.

In general, disease-modifying therapies for multiple sclerosis are stopped prior to a planned pregnancy except in females at high risk of multiple sclerosis activity (AAN [Rae-Grant 2018]). Consider use of agents other than cladribine for females at high risk of disease reactivation who are planning a pregnancy. Delaying pregnancy is recommended for females with persistent high disease activity; when disease-modifying therapy is needed in these patients, other agents are preferred (ECTRIMS/EAN [Montalban 2018]).

Pregnancy Considerations

Based on the mechanism of action and data from animal reproduction studies, in utero exposure to cladribine is expected to cause fetal harm.

[US Boxed Warning]: Oral tablet: Cladribine is contraindicated for use in pregnant women because of the potential for fetal harm. Malformations and embryolethality occurred in animals. Stop cladribine if the patient becomes pregnant.

In general, disease-modifying therapies for multiple sclerosis are not initiated during pregnancy, except in females at high risk of multiple sclerosis activity (AAN [Rae-Grant 2018]).

Information related to the use of cladribine for the treatment of hairy cell leukemia in pregnancy is limited (Daver 2013).

A pregnancy registry is available for all cancers diagnosed during pregnancy at Cooper Health (877-635-4499).

- ◆ **Claforan [DSC]** *see* Cefotaxime *on page 309*
- ◆ **Claravis** *see* ISOtretinoin (Systemic) *on page 846*
- ◆ **Clarinex** *see* Desloratadine *on page 459*
- ◆ **ClariSpray** *see* Fluticasone (Nasal) *on page 703*

Clarithromycin (kla RITH roe mye sin)

Related Information

Antibiotic Prophylaxis *on page 1715*
Bacterial Infections *on page 1739*
Clinical Risk Related to Drugs Prolonging QT Interval *on page 1675*
Gastrointestinal Disorders *on page 1678*

Brand Names: US Biaxin [DSC]

Brand Names: Canada ACT Clarithromycin XL; APO-Clarithromycin; APO-Clarithromycin XL; Biaxin; Biaxin XL; DOM-Clarithromycin; GEN-Clarithromycin; M-Clarithromycin; MYLAN-Clarithromycin [DSC]; PMS-Clarithromycin; RAN-Clarithromycin; RIVA-Clarithromycin; SANDOZ Clarithromycin; TARO-Clarithromycin; TEVA-Clarithromycin

Generic Availability (US) Yes

Pharmacologic Category Antibiotic, Macrolide

Dental Use Alternate oral antibiotic for prevention of infective endocarditis in individuals allergic to penicillins or ampicillin, when amoxicillin cannot be used

Use

Chronic obstructive pulmonary disease, acute exacerbation: Treatment of acute bacterial exacerbation of chronic bronchitis in adults due to susceptible *Haemophilus influenzae*, *Haemophilus parainfluenzae*, *Moraxella catarrhalis*, or *Streptococcus pneumoniae*.

Helicobacter pylori **eradication:** Eradication of *Helicobacter pylori* to reduce the risk of duodenal ulcer recurrence as a component of combination therapy (triple therapy) in adults with *H. pylori* infection and duodenal ulcer disease (active or 5-year history of duodenal ulcer).

Limitations of use: Regimens that contain clarithromycin as the single antibacterial agent are more likely to be associated with the development of clarithromycin resistance. Clarithromycin-containing regimens should not be used in patients with known or suspected clarithromycin-resistant isolates (efficacy is reduced).

Mycobacterial (nontuberculous) infection: Prophylaxis and treatment of disseminated mycobacterial infections due to *Mycobacterium avium* complex (MAC) in patients with advanced HIV infection.

Otitis media: Treatment of acute otitis media in pediatric patients due to susceptible *H. influenzae*, *M. catarrhalis*, or *S. pneumoniae*.

Pneumonia, community-acquired: Treatment of community-acquired pneumonia due to susceptible *Mycoplasma pneumoniae*, *S. pneumoniae*, or *Chlamydophila pneumoniae* (adult and pediatric patients) and *H. influenzae, H. parainfluenzae,* or *M. catarrhalis* (adults).

Skin/skin structure infection: Treatment of uncomplicated skin/skin structure infection due to susceptible *Staphylococcus aureus* or *Streptococcus pyogenes*.

Streptococcal pharyngitis: Treatment of pharyngitis/tonsillitis due to susceptible *S. pyogenes* (alternative agent for patients with severe penicillin allergy).

Local Anesthetic/Vasoconstrictor Precautions Clarithromycin is one of the drugs confirmed to prolong the QT interval and is accepted as having a risk of causing torsade de pointes. In terms of epinephrine, it is not known what effect vasoconstrictors in the local anesthetic regimen will have in patients with a known history of congenital prolonged QT interval or in patients taking any medication that prolongs the QT interval. Until more information is obtained, it is suggested that the clinician consult with the physician prior to the use of a vasoconstrictor in suspected patients, and that the vasoconstrictor (epinephrine, mepivacaine and levonordefrin [Carbocaine® 2% with Neo-Cobefrin®]) be used with caution. See Dental Health Professional Considerations.

Effects on Dental Treatment Key adverse event(s) related to dental treatment: Abnormal taste.

Effects on Bleeding No information available to require special precautions

Adverse Reactions

1% to 10%:

Central nervous system: Headache (2%), insomnia

Dermatologic: Skin rash (children 3%)

Gastrointestinal: Dysgeusia (adults 3% to 7%), vomiting (children 6%), diarrhea (3% to 6%), nausea (adults 3%), abdominal pain (2% to 3%), dyspepsia (adults 2%)

Hematologic & oncologic: Prolonged prothrombin time (adults 1%)

Hepatic: Abnormal hepatic function tests

Hypersensitivity: Anaphylactoid reaction

Infection: Candidiasis (including oral)

Renal: Increased blood urea nitrogen (4%)

<1%, postmarketing, and/or case reports: Abdominal distension, abnormal albumin-globulin ratio, acne vulgaris, acute generalized exanthematous pustulosis, ageusia, agranulocytosis, altered sense of smell, anaphylaxis, angioedema, anorexia, anosmia, anxiety, asthma, atrial fibrillation, behavioral changes, bullous dermatitis, cellulitis, chest pain, chills, cholestasis, cholestatic hepatitis, *Clostridioides* (formerly *Clostridium*) *difficile*-associated diarrhea, *Clostridioides* (formerly *Clostridium*) *difficile* (colitis), confusion, constipation, dark urine (abnormal urine color associated with liver injury), decreased appetite, decreased white blood cell count, dental discoloration (reversible with dental cleaning), depersonalization, depression, disorientation, dizziness, DRESS syndrome, drowsiness, dyskinesia, eosinophilia, epistaxis, eructation, esophagitis, extrasystoles, fatigue, fever, flatulence, gastritis, gastroenteritis, gastroesophageal reflux disease, glossitis, hallucination, hearing loss (reversible), hemorrhage, hepatic failure, hepatic insufficiency, hepatitis, hepatotoxicity (idiosyncratic) (Chalasani 2014), hyperhidrosis, hypersensitivity reaction,

hypoglycemia, IgA vasculitis, increased gamma-glutamyl transferase, increased INR, increased lactate dehydrogenase, increased serum alkaline phosphatase, increased serum ALT, increased serum AST, increased serum bilirubin, increased serum creatinine, infection, interstitial nephritis, jaundice, leukopenia, loss of consciousness, maculopapular rash, malaise, manic behavior, muscle spasm, myalgia, myopathy, neck stiffness, nervousness, neutropenia, nightmares, palpitations, pancreatitis, parasomnias, paresthesia, prolonged QT interval on ECG, pruritus, pseudomembranous colitis, psychosis, pulmonary embolism, rectal pain, renal failure, rhabdomyolysis, seizure, Stevens-Johnson syndrome, stomatitis, thrombocytopenia, tinnitus, tongue discoloration, torsades de pointes, toxic epidermal necrolysis, tremor, urticaria, vaginal infection, ventricular arrhythmia, ventricular tachycardia, vertigo, weakness, xerostomia

Dental Usual Dosage Prophylaxis against infective endocarditis (off-label use): Oral:

Children: 15 mg/kg 30-60 minutes before procedure

Adults: 500 mg 30-60 minutes prior to procedure

Dosing

Adult & Geriatric General dosing note: IR and ER formulations are available; 500 mg every 12 hours of immediate release is equivalent to 1 g of extended release (two 500 mg ER tablets) once daily.

Bartonella spp. infection (off-label use):

Bacillary angiomatosis, peliosis hepatitis, bacteremia, or osteomyelitis in patients with HIV:

Note: Not to be used for endocarditis or CNS infections (HHS [OI adult] 2019).

Primary treatment (alternative agent): **Oral:** Immediate release: 500 mg twice daily for at least 3 to 4 months (HHS [OI adult] 2019).

Long-term suppression for patients with relapse after ≥3 months of primary treatment: **Oral:** Immediate release: 500 mg twice daily; may discontinue if completed 3 to 4 months of therapy and CD4 >200 cells/mm^3 for ≥6 months. **Note:** Some experts discontinue only if *Bartonella* titers have also decreased 4-fold (HHS [OI adult] 2019).

Cat scratch disease, lymphadenitis (alternative agent): **Oral:** Immediate release: 500 mg twice daily for 7 to 10 days (Spach 2020).

Bronchiolitis obliterans, including diffuse panbronchiolitis and symptomatic cryptogenic bronchiolitis obliterans (off-label use): Oral: Immediate release: 250 to 500 mg once daily (Kadota 2003; King 2020). After a 3- to 6-month trial, long-term therapy may be continued based on response (King 2020).

Chronic obstructive pulmonary disease, acute exacerbation: Note: Avoid use in patients with risk factors for *Pseudomonas* infection or poor outcomes (eg, ≥65 years of age with major comorbidities, FEV_1 <50% predicted, frequent exacerbations) (Sethi 2020).

Oral: Immediate release: 500 mg every 12 hours for 3 to 7 days (Falagas 2008; GOLD 2019; Hunter 2001; Sethi 2020).

Endocarditis prophylaxis, dental or invasive respiratory tract procedure (alternative agent for patients with penicillin allergy) (off-label use): Oral: Immediate release: 500 mg administered 30 to 60 minutes prior to procedure. **Note:** Reserve for select situations (cardiac condition with the highest risk of adverse endocarditis outcomes and procedure likely to result in bacteremia with an organism that can cause endocarditis) (AHA [Wilson 2007]).

***Helicobacter pylori* eradication: Note:** Avoid clarithromycin-based therapy in patients with risk factors for macrolide resistance (eg, prior macrolide exposure, local clarithromycin resistance rates ≥15% [which is assumed in the United States] or eradication rates with clarithromycin triple therapy ≤85%) (ACG [Chey 2017]; Crowe 2020; Fallone 2016).

Oral: Immediate release: 500 mg twice daily for 7 to 14 days as part of an appropriate combination regimen (ACG [Chey 2017]; Crowe 2020; Fallone 2016; McNicholl 2020).

Mycobacterial (nontuberculous) infection:

Mycobacterium avium complex infection:

Disseminated disease in patients with HIV:

Treatment: **Oral:** Immediate release: 500 mg twice daily as part of an appropriate combination regimen for a minimum of 12 months; subsequently may discontinue once there are no signs/symptoms of *Mycobacterium avium* complex disease and the CD4 count has exceeded 100 cells/mm^3 for >6 months in response to antiretroviral therapy (ART) (HHS [OI adult] 2019).

Primary prophylaxis: **Note:** Not routinely recommended; reserve for patients with CD4 count <50 cells/mm^3 who are **not** initiated on fully suppressive ART.

Oral: Immediate release: 500 mg twice daily; may discontinue prophylaxis when patient is initiated on effective ART (HHS [OI adult] 2019; IAS-USA [Saag 2018]).

Pulmonary disease, nonsevere noncavitary nodular/bronchiectatic disease in patients without cystic fibrosis (off-label use): **Oral:** Immediate release: 500 mg twice daily 3 times weekly as part of an appropriate combination regimen; continue treatment until patient is culture negative on therapy for ≥1 year (ATS/IDSA [Griffith 2007]; BTS [Haworth 2017]).

Pulmonary disease, severe nodular/bronchiectatic disease, cavitary disease, or disease in patients with cystic fibrosis (off-label use): **Oral:** Immediate release: 500 mg twice daily as part of an appropriate combination regimen; 250 mg twice daily can be used in patients without cystic fibrosis who are <50 kg or >70 years of age to avoid GI intolerance. Continue treatment until patient is culture negative on therapy for ≥1 year (ATS/IDSA [Griffith 2007]; BTS [Haworth 2017]; CFF/ECFS [Floto 2016]).

Mycobacterium abscessus infection (off-label use): **Note:** Perform susceptibility testing before and after ≥14 days of clarithromycin incubation to evaluate for the presence of an inducible *erm* gene, which can result in decreased macrolide susceptibility even with a "susceptible" MIC result and may preclude use of clarithromycin (CFF/ECFS [Floto 2016]; Griffith 2020).

Pulmonary, skin, soft tissue, or bone infection: **Oral:** Immediate release: 500 mg twice daily as part of an appropriate combination regimen and continued for ≥6 to 12 months (ATS/IDSA [Griffith 2007]; CFF/ECFS [Floto 2016]; Griffith 2020). **Note:** Patients should be under the care of a clinician with expertise in managing mycobacterial infection.

Pertussis (off-label use):

Treatment: **Note:** Treatment should be initiated within 21 days of cough onset. After this interval, some experts reserve treatment for pregnant women, patients >65 years of age, and those with asthma, chronic obstructive pulmonary disease, or immunocompromising conditions (Cornia 2020).

Oral: Immediate release: 500 mg twice daily for 7 days (CDC [Tiwari 2005]).

Postexposure prophylaxis: **Note:** Postexposure prophylaxis should be administered, regardless of vaccination history, to close contacts of persons with pertussis during the first 21 days of cough.

Oral: Immediate release: 500 mg twice daily for 7 days (CDC [Tiwari 2005]).

Pneumonia, community-acquired:

Inpatient: Oral: Immediate release: 500 mg twice daily as part of an appropriate combination regimen (ATS/IDSA [Metlay 2019]).

Outpatient: **Oral:** 500 mg (immediate release) twice daily (ATS/IDSA [Metlay 2019]) or 1 g (two 500 mg ER tablets) once daily. **Note:** Use as part of an appropriate combination regimen; if local pneumococcal macrolide resistance is <25%, monotherapy is an alternative approach for outpatients without comorbidities or risk factors for antibiotic-resistant pathogens (ATS/IDSA [Metlay 2019]).

Duration of therapy: Minimum of 5 days; patients should be clinically stable with normal vital signs before therapy is discontinued (ATS/IDSA [Metlay 2019]).

Q fever (*Coxiella burnetii*), acute symptomatic (alternative agent) (off-label use): Note: Reserved for nonpregnant patients who are not at risk for complications (eg, no endocarditis or underlying valvular disease) (Raoult 2020). Treatment is most effective if given within the first 3 days of symptoms (CDC [Anderson 2013]).

Oral: Immediate release: 500 mg twice daily for 14 days (Gikas 2001; Raoult 2020).

Streptococcal pharyngitis (group A) (alternative agent for patients with severe penicillin allergy): Oral: Immediate release: 250 mg every 12 hours for 10 days (IDSA [Shulman 2012]).

Renal Impairment: Adult

CrCl ≥30 mL/minute: No dosage adjustment necessary.

CrCl <30 mL/minute: Decrease clarithromycin dose by 50%

Hemodialysis: Administer after HD session is completed (Aronoff 2007).

In combination with atazanavir or ritonavir:

CrCl 30 to 60 mL/minute: Decrease clarithromycin dose by 50%.

CrCl <30 mL/minute: Decrease clarithromycin dose by 75%.

Hepatic Impairment: Adult No dosage adjustment necessary if renal function is normal; however, in patients with hepatic impairment and concomitant severe renal impairment, a dosage reduction or prolonged dosing intervals may be appropriate.

Pediatric

Note: All pediatric dosing recommendations based on immediate release product formulations (tablet and oral suspension):

General dosing, susceptible infection, mild to moderate infection: Infants, Children, and Adolescents: Oral: 15 mg/kg/day divided every 12 hours; maximum single dose: 500 mg (*Red Book* [AAP 2012])

Bartonellosis, treatment and secondary prophylaxis in HIV-exposed/-positive patients (excluding CNS infections and endocarditis): Limited data available: Oral:

Infants and Children: 15 mg/kg/day divided every 12 hours for at least 3 months; maximum single dose: 500 mg (CDC 2009)

Adolescents: 500 mg twice daily administered for at least 3 months (DHHS [adult] 2013)

Endocarditis, prophylaxis: Note: AHA guidelines (Baltimore 2015) limit the use of prophylactic antibiotics to patients at the highest risk for infective endocarditis (IE) or adverse outcomes (eg, prosthetic heart valves, patients with previous IE, unrepaired cyanotic congenital heart disease, repaired congenital heart disease with prosthetic material or device during first 6 months after procedure, repaired congenital heart disease with residual defects at the site or adjacent to site of prosthetic patch or device, heart transplant recipients with cardiac valvulopathy):

Dental procedures in patients allergic to penicillins: Limited data available: Infants, Children, and Adolescents: Oral: 15 mg/kg; maximum single dose: 500 mg; administer 30 to 60 minutes before procedure (AHA [Wilson 2007]).

Group A streptococcal infection; rheumatic fever, primary prevention and treatment of streptococcal tonsillopharyngitis: Infants, Children, and Adolescents: Oral: 15 mg/kg/day divided every 12 hours for 10 days; maximum single dose: 250 mg (Gerber 2009; IDSA [Shulman 2012])

***Helicobacter pylori* eradication:** Children and Adolescents: Oral: 20 mg/kg/day divided every 12 hours for 7 to 14 days. **Note:** Duration dependent on regimen used; maximum single dose: 500 mg. Administer as part of triple or quadruple combination regimens with amoxicillin and proton pump inhibitor with or without metronidazole (Koletzko 2011)

Lyme disease: Limited data available: Infants, Children, and Adolescents: Oral: 7.5 mg/kg twice daily for 14 to 21 days; maximum single dose: 500 mg (IDSA [Wormser 2006])

Mycobacterium avium complex infection (MAC) (HIV-exposed/-positive):

Infants and Children (DHHS [pediatric] 2013):

Prophylaxis:

Primary prophylaxis: Oral: 15 mg/kg/day divided every 12 hours; maximum single dose: 500 mg; to prevent first episode begin therapy at the following $CD4^+$ T-lymphocyte counts (see below):

Infants <12 months: <750 cells/mm^3

Children 1 to <2 years: <500 cells/mm^3

Children 2 to 5 years: <75 cells/mm^3

Children ≥6 years: <50 cells/mm^3

Secondary prophylaxis: Oral: 15 mg/kg/day divided every 12 hours; maximum single dose: 500 mg; use in combination with ethambutol with or without rifabutin

Treatment: Oral: 15 to 30 mg/kg/day divided every 12 hours; maximum single dose: 500 mg; use in combination with ethambutol and if severe infection, rifabutin; follow with chronic suppressive therapy

Adolescents (DHHS [adult] 2013):

Prophylaxis:

Primary prophylaxis: Oral: 500 mg twice daily

Secondary prophylaxis: Oral: 500 mg twice daily plus ethambutol; consider additional agents (eg, rifabutin, aminoglycoside, fluoroquinolone) for CD4 <50 cells/mm^3, high mycobacterial load, or ineffective antiretroviral therapy.

Treatment: Oral: 500 mg twice daily in combination with ethambutol: Consider additional agents (eg, rifabutin, aminoglycoside, fluoroquinolone) for CD4 <50 cells/mm^3, high mycobacterial load, or ineffective antiretroviral therapy.

Otitis media, acute (AOM): Infants ≥6 months and Children: Oral: 15 mg/kg/day divided every 12 hours for 10 days; maximum single dose: 500 mg; **Note:** Due to increased *S. pneumoniae* and *H. influenzae* resistance, clarithromycin is not routinely recommended as a treatment option (AAP [Lieberthal 2013])

Peritonitis (peritoneal dialysis), prophylaxis for patients requiring invasive dental procedures: Infants, Children, and Adolescents: Oral: 15 mg/kg 30 to 60 minutes before dental procedure; maximum single dose: 500 mg (Warady [ISPD 2012])

Pertussis: Infants, Children, and Adolescents: Oral: 15 mg/kg/day divided every 12 hours for 7 days; maximum single dose: 500 mg (CDC [Tiwari 2005])

Pneumonia, community-acquired (CAP); presumed atypical pneumonia (*M. pneumoniae, C. pneumoniae, C. trachomatis*); mild infection or step-down therapy: Infants >3 months, Children, and Adolescents: Oral: 15 mg/kg/day every 12 hours for 10 days; shorter courses may be appropriate for mild disease; maximum single dose: 500 mg; **Note:** A beta-lactam antibiotic should be added if typical bacterial pneumonia cannot be ruled out (Bradley 2011).

Renal Impairment: Pediatric

Infants, Children, and Adolescents: The following adjustments have been recommended (Aronoff 2007). **Note:** Renally adjusted dose recommendations are based on a dose 15 mg/kg/day divided twice daily.

GFR ≥30 mL/minute/1.73 m^2: No dosage adjustment necessary

GFR 10 to 29 mL/minute/1.73 m^2: 4 mg/kg/dose every 12 hours

GFR <10 mL/minute/1.73 m^2: 4 mg/kg/dose once daily

Hemodialysis: Administer after HD session is completed: 4 mg/kg/dose once daily

Peritoneal dialysis: 4 mg/kg/dose once daily

Hepatic Impairment: Pediatric Infants, Children, and Adolescents: No dosage adjustment necessary if renal function is normal; however, in patients with hepatic impairment and concomitant severe renal impairment, a dosage reduction or prolonged dosing intervals may be appropriate.

Mechanism of Action Exerts its antibacterial action by binding to 50S ribosomal subunit resulting in inhibition of protein synthesis. The 14-OH metabolite of clarithromycin is twice as active as the parent compound against certain organisms.

Contraindications

Hypersensitivity to clarithromycin, erythromycin, any of the macrolide antibiotics, or any component of the formulation; history of cholestatic jaundice/hepatic dysfunction associated with prior use of clarithromycin; concomitant use with cisapride, pimozide, ergot alkaloids (eg, ergotamine, dihydroergotamine), lomitapide, or HMG-CoA reductase inhibitors extensively metabolized by CYP3A4 (eg, lovastatin, simvastatin); concomitant use with colchicine in patients with renal or hepatic impairment

Canadian labeling: Additional contraindications (not in US labeling): Severe hepatic failure in combination with renal impairment; history of QT prolongation (congenital or documented acquired QT prolongation or ventricular cardiac arrhythmia, including torsades de pointes; hypokalemia; concomitant use with saquinavir, midazolam (oral), colchicine (regardless of hepatic/renal impairment), ticagrelor; concomitant use with astemizole, domperidone, terfenadine, or ranolazine (not available in Canada)

Warnings/Precautions Use has been associated with QT prolongation and infrequent cases of arrhythmias, including torsade de pointes (may be fatal). Use with caution in elderly patients; may be at increased risk of torsades de pointes. Avoid use in patients with known prolongation of the QT interval, ventricular cardiac arrhythmia (including torsades de pointes), uncorrected hypokalemia or hypomagnesemia, clinically significant bradycardia, and patients receiving Class IA (eg, quinidine, procainamide) or Class III (eg, amiodarone, dofetilide, sotalol) antiarrhythmic agents or other drugs known to prolong the QT interval. Use caution in patients with coronary artery disease. A clinical trial in patients with CAD demonstrated an increase in risk of all-cause mortality ≥1 year after the end of treatment in patients randomized to receive clarithromycin. Other epidemiologic studies evaluating this risk have variable results.

Elevated liver function tests and hepatitis (hepatocellular and/or cholestatic with or without jaundice) have been reported; usually reversible after discontinuation of clarithromycin. May lead to hepatic failure or death (rarely), especially in the presence of preexisting diseases and/or concomitant use of medications. Discontinue immediately if symptoms of hepatitis (eg, anorexia, jaundice, abdominal tenderness, pruritus, dark urine) occur. Use with caution in patients with myasthenia gravis; exacerbation of symptoms and new onset of symptoms has occurred. Use with caution in severe renal impairment; dosage adjustment required.

Potentially significant drug-drug interactions may exist, requiring dose or frequency adjustment, additional monitoring, and/or selection of alternative therapy. Prolonged use may result in fungal or bacterial superinfection, including *C. difficile*-associated diarrhea (CDAD) and pseudomembranous colitis; CDAD has been observed >2 months postantibiotic treatment. Decreased *H. pylori* eradication rates have been observed with short-term (≤7 days) combination therapy. Current guidelines recommend 10 to 14 days of therapy (triple or quadruple) for eradication of *H. pylori* in pediatric and adult patients (Chey 2007; NASPHGAN [Koletzko 2011]). Decreased survival has been observed in patients with HIV with *Mycobacterium avium* complex (MAC) receiving clarithromycin doses above the maximum recommended dose; maximum recommended dosing should not be exceeded in this population. Development of resistance to clarithromycin has been observed when used as prophylaxis and treatment of MAC infection (Biaxin Canadian product labeling).

Severe acute reactions have (rarely) been reported, including anaphylaxis, Stevens-Johnson syndrome (SJS), toxic epidermal necrolysis (TEN), drug rash with eosinophilia and systemic symptoms (DRESS), Henoch-Schönlein purpura (IgA vasculitis), and acute generalized exanthematous pustulosis; discontinue therapy and initiate treatment immediately for severe acute hypersensitivity reactions. The presence of ER tablets in the stool has been reported, particularly in patients with anatomic (eg, ileostomy, colostomy) or functional GI disorders with decreased transit times. Consider alternative dosage forms (eg, suspension) or an alternative antimicrobial for patients with tablet residue in the stool and no signs of clinical improvement. Some dosage forms may contain propylene glycol. Large amounts are potentially toxic and have been associated hyperosmolality, lactic acidosis, seizures, and respiratory depression; use caution (AAP 1997; Zar 2007).

Drug Interactions

Metabolism/Transport Effects **Substrate** of CYP3A4 (major); **Note:** Assignment of Major/Minor substrate status based on clinically relevant drug interaction potential; **Inhibits** CYP3A4 (strong), OATP1B1/1B3 (SLCO1B1/1B3), P-glycoprotein/ABCB1

Avoid Concomitant Use

Avoid concomitant use of Clarithromycin with any of the following: Abametapir; Acalabrutinib; Ado-Trastuzumab Emtansine; Alfuzosin; Aprepitant; Astemizole; Asunaprevir; Avanafil; Avapritinib; Barnidipine; BCG (Intravesical); Bilastine; Blonanserin; Bosutinib; Bromocriptine; Budesonide (Systemic); Cholera Vaccine; Cisapride; Cobimetinib; Conivaptan; Dabrafenib; Dapoxetine; Dihydroergotamine; Domperidone; DOXOrubicin (Conventional); Dronedarone; Elagolix; Elagolix, Estradiol, and Norethindrone; Eletriptan; Entrectinib; Eplerenone; Ergot Derivatives; Ergotamine; Everolimus; Fexinidazole [INT]; Flibanserin; Fluticasone (Nasal); Fosaprepitant; Fusidic Acid (Systemic); Grazoprevir; Halofantrine; Ibrutinib; Idelalisib; Irinotecan Products; Isavuconazonium Sulfate; Ivabradine; Lefamulin; Lemborexant; Lercanidipine; Lomitapide; Lopinavir; Lovastatin; Lumateperone; Lurasidone; Lurbinectedin; Macitentan; Mizolastine; Naloxegol; Neratinib; NiMODipine; Nisoldipine; PAZOPanib; Pimozide; Posaconazole; QT-prolonging Agents (Highest Risk); QT-prolonging Miscellaneous Agents (Moderate Risk); Radotinib; Ranolazine; Red Yeast Rice; Regorafenib; Revefenacin; Rimegepant; Rupatadine; Salmeterol; Saquinavir; Silodosin; Simeprevir; Simvastatin; Sonidegib; Suvorexant; Tamsulosin; Tazemetostat; Terfenadine; Ticagrelor; Tolvaptan; Topotecan; Trabectedin; Triazolam; Ubrogepant; Udenafil; Ulipristal; VinCRIStine (Liposomal); Vinflunine; Vorapaxar; Voxilaprevir

Increased Effect/Toxicity

Clarithromycin may increase the levels/effects of: Abemaciclib; Acalabrutinib; Ado-Trastuzumab Emtansine; Afatinib; Alfuzosin; Aliskiren; Alitretinoin (Systemic); Almotriptan; Alosetron; ALPRAZolam; Antineoplastic Agents (Vinca Alkaloids); Apixaban; Aprepitant; ARIPiprazole; ARIPiprazole Lauroxil; Astemizole; Asunaprevir; AtorvaSTATin; Avanafil; Avapritinib; Axitinib; Barnidipine; Benperidol; Benzhydrocodone; Betamethasone (Ophthalmic); Betrixaban; Bictegravir; Bilastine; Blonanserin; Bortezomib; Bosentan; Bosutinib; Brentuximab Vedotin; Brexpiprazole; Brigatinib; Brinzolamide; Bromocriptine; Budesonide (Nasal); Budesonide (Oral Inhalation); Budesonide (Systemic); Budesonide (Topical); Buprenorphine; BusPIRone; Cabazitaxel; Cabergoline; Cabozantinib; Calcifediol; Calcium Channel Blockers; Cannabidiol; Cannabis; Capmatinib; CarBAMazepine; Cardiac Glycosides; Cariprazine; Celiprolol; Ceritinib; Cilostazol; Cinacalcet; Cisapride; Citalopram; Cobicistat; Cobimetinib; Codeine; Colchicine; Conivaptan; Copanlisib; Corticosteroids (Orally Inhaled); Corticosteroids (Systemic); Crizotinib; CycloSPORINE (Systemic); CYP3A4 Inducers (Strong); CYP3A4 Substrates (High risk with Inhibitors); Dabigatran Etexilate; Dabrafenib; Daclatasvir; Dapoxetine; Darifenacin; Darolutamide; Dasatinib; Deflazacort; DexAMETHasone (Ophthalmic); Dienogest; Dihydroergotamine; DOCEtaxel; Domperidone; DOXOrubicin (Conventional); Dronabinol; Dronedarone; Drospirenone; Dutasteride; Duvelisib; Edoxaban; Elagolix; Elagolix, Estradiol, and Norethindrone; Eletriptan; Elexacaftor, Tezacaftor, and Ivacaftor; Eliglustat; Eluxadoline; Encorafenib; Enfortumab Vedotin; Entrectinib; Eplerenone; Erdafitinib; Ergot Derivatives; Ergotamine; Erlotinib; Estrogen Derivatives; Eszopiclone; Etizolam; Etoposide; Etoposide Phosphate; Everolimus; Evogliptin; Fedratinib; FentaNYL; Fesoterodine; Flibanserin; FLUoxetine; Fluticasone (Nasal); Fluticasone (Oral Inhalation); Fosaprepitant; Fostamatinib; Galantamine; Gefitinib; Gilteritinib; Glasdegib; Glecaprevir and Pibrentasvir; GlipiZIDE; GlyBURIDE; Grazoprevir; GuanFACINE; Halofantrine; HYDROcodone; Ibrutinib; Iloperidone; Imatinib; Imidafenacin; Irinotecan Products; Isavuconazonium Sulfate; Istradefylline; Ivabradine; Ivacaftor; Ixabepilone; Lapatinib; Larotrectinib; Lefamulin; Lemborexant; Lercanidipine; Levobupivacaine; Levomilnacipran; Lomitapide; Lopinavir; Lorlatinib; Lovastatin; Lumateperone; Lumefantrine; Lurasidone; Lurbinectedin; Macitentan; Manidipine; Maraviroc; MedroxyPROGESTERone; Meperidine; MethylPREDNISolone; Midazolam; Midostaurin; MiFEPRIStone; Mirodenafil; Mirtazapine; Mizolastine; Morphine (Systemic); Nadolol; Naldemedine; Nalfurafine; Naloxegol; Neratinib; Nilotinib; NiMODipine; Nintedanib; Nisoldipine; Olaparib; Ondansetron; Osilodrostat; Ospemifene; Oxybutynin; Palbociclib; Panobinostat; Parecoxib; Paricalcitol; PARoxetine; PAZOPanib; Pemigatinib; Pexidartinib; P-glycoprotein/ABCB1 Substrates; Pimavanserin; Pimecrolimus; Pimozide; Piperaquine; Pitavastatin; Polatuzumab Vedotin; PONATinib; Pranlukast; Pravastatin; Praziquantel; PrednisoLONE (Systemic); PredniSONE; QT-prolonging Antidepressants (Moderate Risk); QT-prolonging Miscellaneous Agents (Moderate Risk); QUEtiapine; Radotinib; Ramelteon; Ranolazine; Red Yeast Rice; Regorafenib; Repaglinide; Retapamulin; Revefenacin; Ribociclib; RifAXIMin; Rilpivirine; Rimegepant; Riociguat; Ripretinib; RisperiDONE; Rivaroxaban; RomiDEPsin; Rupatadine; Ruxolitinib; Salmeterol; Saquinavir; SAXagliptin; Selumetinib; Sibutramine; Sildenafil; Silodosin; Simeprevir; Simvastatin; Sirolimus; Solifenacin; Sonidegib; SORAfenib; SUFentanil; SUNItinib; Suvorexant; Tacrolimus (Systemic); Tacrolimus (Topical); Tadalafil; Talazoparib; Tamsulosin; Tasimelteon; Tazemetostat; Tegaserod; Temsirolimus; Terfenadine; Tetrahydrocannabinol; Tetrahydrocannabinol and Cannabidiol; Tezacaftor and Ivacaftor; Theophylline Derivatives; Thiotepa; Ticagrelor; Tofacitinib; Tolterodine; Tolvaptan; Topotecan; Toremifene; Trabectedin; TraMADol; TraZODone; Triazolam; Ubrogepant; Udenafil; Ulipristal; Upadacitinib; Valbenazine; Vardenafil; Vemurafenib; Venetoclax; Vilazodone; VinCRIStine

(Liposomal); Vinflunine; Vitamin K Antagonists; Vorapaxar; Voriconazole; Voxelotor; Voxilaprevir; Zanubrutinib; Zidovudine; Zopiclone

The levels/effects of Clarithromycin may be increased by: Abametapir; Amisulpride (Oral); Antihepaciviral Combination Products; Atazanavir; Bosentan; CarBAMazepine; Ceritinib; Citalopram; Cobicistat; Conivaptan; Crizotinib; CYP3A4 Inducers (Moderate); CYP3A4 Inducers (Strong); CYP3A4 Inhibitors (Moderate); CYP3A4 Inhibitors (Strong); Dasatinib; Efavirenz; Encorafenib; Entrectinib; Erythromycin (Systemic); Fexinidazole [INT]; Fluconazole; FLUoxetine; Fosnetupitant; Fusidic Acid (Systemic); Idelalisib; Lefamulin; Lopinavir; MiFEPRIStone; Netupitant; Nilotinib; Osimertinib; Pentamidine (Systemic); Pimozide; Posaconazole; QT-prolonging Agents (Highest Risk); QT-prolonging Antipsychotics (Moderate Risk); QT-prolonging Class IC Antiarrhythmics (Moderate Risk); QT-prolonging Quinolone Antibiotics (Moderate Risk); QUEtiapine; Ribociclib; Ritonavir; Saquinavir; Stiripentol; Toremifene; Vemurafenib; Vilanterol; Voriconazole

Decreased Effect

Clarithromycin may decrease the levels/effects of: BCG (Intravesical); BCG Vaccine (Immunization); Cholera Vaccine; Doxercalciferol; Ifosfamide; Lactobacillus and Estriol; Sincalide; Sodium Picosulfate; Thiotepa; Ticagrelor; Typhoid Vaccine; Zidovudine

The levels/effects of Clarithromycin may be decreased by: Atazanavir; Bosentan; CarBAMazepine; CYP3A4 Inducers (Moderate); CYP3A4 Inducers (Strong); Deferasirox; Efavirenz; Enzalutamide; Lopinavir; Mitotane; Ritonavir; Sarilumab; Siltuximab; Tocilizumab

Food Interactions Immediate release: Food delays rate, but not extent of absorption; Extended release: Food increases clarithromycin AUC by ~30% relative to fasting conditions. Management: Administer immediate release products without regard to meals. Administer extended release products with food.

Pharmacodynamics/Kinetics

Half-life Elimination Immediate release: Clarithromycin: 3-7 hours; 14-OH-clarithromycin: 5-9 hours

Time to Peak Immediate release: 2-3 hours; Extended release: 5-8 hours

Pregnancy Considerations Clarithromycin crosses the placenta (Witt 2003).

The manufacturer recommends that clarithromycin not be used in a pregnant woman unless there are no alternative therapies. Clarithromycin is not recommended as a first-line agent for the treatment or prophylaxis of *Mycobacterium avium* complex or for treatment of bacterial respiratory disease in HIV-infected pregnant patients (HHS [OI adult] 2019]).

Breastfeeding Considerations

Clarithromycin and its active metabolite (14-hydroxy clarithromycin) are present in breast milk.

The relative infant dose (RID) of clarithromycin is ≤1% when calculated using the highest mean breast milk concentration located and compared to an infant therapeutic dose of 15 mg/kg/day.

In general, breastfeeding is considered acceptable when the RID is <10% (Anderson 2016; Ito 2000).

Using the highest mean milk concentrations (clarithromycin: 0.85 mg/L; 14-hydroxy clarithromycin: 0.63 mg/L), the estimated daily infant dose via breast milk was calculated to be 136 mcg/kg/day. This milk concentration was obtained following maternal administration of oral clarithromycin 250 mg twice daily; the half-lives of clarithromycin and 14-hydroxy clarithromycin in breast milk were 4.3 ± 0.3 hours and 9 ± 1.2 hours, respectively (Sedlmayr 1993).

Decreased appetite, diarrhea, rash, and somnolence have been reported in breastfed infants exposed to macrolide antibiotics (Goldstein 2009). In general, antibiotics that are present in breast milk may cause non-dose-related modification of bowel flora. Monitor infants for GI disturbances, such as thrush and diarrhea (WHO 2002). In addition, an increased risk for infantile hypertrophic pyloric stenosis (IHPS) may be present in infants who are exposed to macrolides via breast milk, especially during the first two weeks of life (Lund 2014); however, data are conflicting (Goldstein 2009). According to the manufacturer, the decision to breastfeed during therapy should consider the risk of infant exposure, the benefits of breastfeeding to the infant, and benefits of treatment to the mother.

Dosage Forms: US

Suspension Reconstituted, Oral:

Generic: 125 mg/5 mL (50 mL, 100 mL); 250 mg/5 mL (50 mL, 100 mL)

Tablet, Oral:

Generic: 250 mg, 500 mg

Tablet Extended Release 24 Hour, Oral:

Generic: 500 mg

Dosage Forms: Canada

Suspension Reconstituted, Oral:

Biaxin: 125 mg/5 mL (55 mL, 105 mL); 250 mg/5 mL (105 mL)

Generic: 125 mg/5 mL (55 mL, 105 mL, 150 mL); 250 mg/5 mL (55 mL, 105 mL, 150 mL)

Tablet, Oral:

Biaxin: 250 mg, 500 mg

Generic: 250 mg, 500 mg

Tablet Extended Release 24 Hour, Oral:

Biaxin XL: 500 mg

Generic: 500 mg

Dental Health Professional Considerations The FDA issued a special alert in December 2005 stating that short-term therapy with clarithromycin in patients with stable coronary artery disease may cause significantly higher cardiovascular mortality. The use of 500 mg clarithromycin daily for 14 days in patients with the above condition resulted in significantly higher all-cause mortality compared to patients taking placebo. This information is provided to the dental practitioner on the possible association between short-term use of clarithromycin for infections and increases in mortality in patients with a history of stable coronary artery disease.

Also see Local Anesthetic/Vasoconstrictor Precautions

- ◆ **Clarithromycin, Amoxicillin, and Omeprazole** *see* Omeprazole, Clarithromycin, and Amoxicillin *on page 1140*
- ◆ **Clarithromycin, Lansoprazole, and Amoxicillin** *see* Lansoprazole, Amoxicillin, and Clarithromycin *on page 877*
- ◆ **Claritin [OTC]** *see* Loratadine *on page 930*
- ◆ **Claritin-D 12 Hour Allergy & Congestion [OTC]** *see* Loratadine and Pseudoephedrine *on page 931*
- ◆ **Claritin-D 24 Hour Allergy & Congestion [OTC]** *see* Loratadine and Pseudoephedrine *on page 931*
- ◆ **Claritin Allergy Childrens [OTC]** *see* Loratadine *on page 930*
- ◆ **Claritin Childrens [OTC]** *see* Loratadine *on page 930*
- ◆ **Claritin Reditabs [OTC]** *see* Loratadine *on page 930*

◆ **Clavulanic Acid and Amoxicillin** *see* Amoxicillin and Clavulanate *on page 130*

◆ **Clavulanic Acid and Amoxycillin** *see* Amoxicillin and Clavulanate *on page 130*

◆ **Clean Zing [OTC]** *see* Cetylpyridinium *on page 330*

◆ **Clearcanal Earwax Softener [OTC]** *see* Carbamide Peroxide *on page 289*

Clemastine (KLEM as teen)

Brand Names: US Dayhist Allergy 12 Hour Relief [OTC]; Tavist Allergy [OTC] [DSC]

Pharmacologic Category Ethanolamine Derivative; Histamine H_1 Antagonist; Histamine H_1 Antagonist, First Generation

Use

Allergic rhinitis: Relief of symptoms associated with allergic rhinitis or other upper respiratory allergies (eg, sneezing, rhinorrhea, pruritus, and lacrimation) in children ≥12 years of age and adults (tablets and syrup) and in children 6 to 12 years (syrup only)

Urticaria/angioedema: Relief of mild, uncomplicated allergic skin manifestations of urticaria and angioedema in children ≥12 years of age and adults (tablets and syrup) and in children 6 to 12 years (syrup only)

OTC Labeling: **Common cold/hay fever/upper respiratory allergies:** Relief of symptoms associated with the common cold (eg, rhinorrhea, sneezing, throat/nose pruritus, lacrimation) in children ≥12 years of age and adults

Local Anesthetic/Vasoconstrictor Precautions No information available to require special precautions

Effects on Dental Treatment Key adverse event(s) related to dental treatment: Xerostomia (normal salivary flow resumes upon discontinuation).

Effects on Bleeding No information available to require special precautions

Adverse Reactions Frequency not defined.

Cardiovascular: Hypotension, palpitations, tachycardia

Central nervous system: Ataxia, confusion, dizziness, drowsiness (slight to moderate), fatigue, headache, insomnia, irritability, nervousness, restlessness, sedation

Dermatologic: Skin photosensitivity, skin rash

Gastrointestinal: Constipation, diarrhea, epigastric distress, nausea, vomiting, xerostomia

Genitourinary: Difficulty in micturition, urinary frequency, urinary retention

Hematologic & oncologic: Agranulocytosis, hemolytic anemia, thrombocytopenia

Hypersensitivity: Anaphylaxis

Ophthalmic: Blurred vision

Otic: Tinnitus

Respiratory: Thickening of bronchial secretions

Mechanism of Action Competes with histamine for H_1-receptor sites on effector cells in the gastrointestinal tract, blood vessels, and respiratory tract; anticholinergic and sedative effects are also seen.

Pharmacodynamics/Kinetics

Onset of Action 2 hours after administration; Peak effect: Therapeutic: 5 to 7 hours

Duration of Action 10 to 12 hours; may persist for up to 24 hours

Half-life Elimination ~21 hours (range: 10 to 33 hours) (Sharma 2003)

Time to Peak 2 to 4 hours

Pregnancy Risk Factor B

Pregnancy Considerations Maternal clemastine use has generally not resulted in an increased risk of birth defects. Antihistamines are recommended for the treatment of rhinitis, urticaria, and pruritus with rash in pregnant women (although second generation antihistamines may be preferred). Antihistamines are not recommended for treatment of pruritus associated with intrahepatic cholestasis in pregnancy.

◆ **Clemastine Fumarate** *see* Clemastine *on page 367*

◆ **Cleocin** *see* Clindamycin (Systemic) *on page 368*

◆ **Cleocin** *see* Clindamycin (Topical) *on page 375*

◆ **Cleocin in D5W [DSC]** *see* Clindamycin (Systemic) *on page 368*

◆ **Cleocin Phosphate** *see* Clindamycin (Systemic) *on page 368*

◆ **Cleocin-T** *see* Clindamycin (Topical) *on page 375*

Clevidipine (klev ID i peen)

Related Information

Calcium Channel Blockers and Gingival Hyperplasia *on page 1816*

Brand Names: US Cleviprex

Pharmacologic Category Antihypertensive; Calcium Channel Blocker; Calcium Channel Blocker, Dihydropyridine

Use Hypertension: Management of hypertension when oral therapy is not feasible or not desirable.

Local Anesthetic/Vasoconstrictor Precautions No information available to require special precautions

Effects on Dental Treatment Key adverse event(s) related to dental treatment: Although other calcium channel blockers (eg, nifedipine, diltiazem) have been associated with gingival hyperplasia, there are no reports that clevidipine has caused this adverse effect.

Effects on Bleeding No information available to require special precautions

Adverse Reactions

>10%:

Cardiovascular: Atrial fibrillation (21%)

Central nervous system: Insomnia (12%)

Gastrointestinal: Nausea (5% to 21%)

Miscellaneous: Fever (19%)

1% to 10%:

Central nervous system: Headache (6%)

Gastrointestinal: Vomiting (3%)

Hematologic & oncologic: Postprocedural hemorrhage (3%)

Renal: Acute renal failure (9%)

Respiratory: Pneumonia (3%), respiratory failure (3%)

<1%, postmarketing, and/or case reports: Dyspnea, hypersensitivity reaction, hypotension, increased serum triglycerides, intestinal obstruction, myocardial infarction, oxygen saturation decreased, syncope, tachycardia (reflex), thrombophlebitis

Mechanism of Action Dihydropyridine calcium channel blocker with potent arterial vasodilating activity. Inhibits calcium ion influx through the L-type calcium channels during depolarization in arterial smooth muscle, producing a decrease in mean arterial pressure (MAP) by reducing systemic vascular resistance.

Pharmacodynamics/Kinetics

Onset of Action 2 to 4 minutes after start of infusion

Duration of Action IV: 5 to 15 minutes

Half-life Elimination Biphasic: Initial: 1 minute (predominant); Terminal: ~15 minutes

Pregnancy Risk Factor C

Pregnancy Considerations
Adverse events have been observed in animal reproduction studies.

Chronic maternal hypertension may increase the risk of birth defects, low birth weight, preterm delivery, stillbirth, and neonatal death. Actual fetal/neonatal risks may be related to duration and severity of maternal hypertension. Untreated hypertension may also increase the risks of adverse maternal outcomes, including gestational diabetes, myocardial infarction, preeclampsia, stroke, and delivery complications (ACOG 203 2019).

Calcium channel blockers may be used to treat hypertension in pregnant women; however, clevidipine is only available as an IV infusion. If a patient needs IV therapy for hypertension during pregnancy, other agents are more commonly utilized (ACOG 203 2019; ESC [Regitz-Zagrosek 2018]). Females with preexisting hypertension may continue their medication during pregnancy unless contraindications exist (ESC [Regitz-Zagrosek 2018]).

◆ **Clevidipine Butyrate** *see* Clevidipine *on page* 367
◆ **Cleviprex** *see* Clevidipine *on page* 367
◆ **Climara** *see* Estradiol (Systemic) *on page* 596
◆ **Climara Pro** *see* Estradiol and Levonorgestrel *on page* 598
◆ **Clindacin ETZ** *see* Clindamycin (Topical) *on page* 375
◆ **Clindacin-P** *see* Clindamycin (Topical) *on page* 375
◆ **Clindacin Pac** *see* Clindamycin (Topical) *on page* 375
◆ **Clindagel** *see* Clindamycin (Topical) *on page* 375

Clindamycin (Systemic) (klin da MYE sin)

Related Information
Antibiotic Prophylaxis *on page* 1715
Bacterial Infections *on page* 1739
Osteonecrosis of the Jaw *on page* 1699
Periodontal Diseases *on page* 1748

Related Sample Prescriptions
Bacterial Infections and Periodontal Diseases - Sample Prescriptions *on page* 35
Prevention of Endocarditis and to Reduce the Risk of Late Infections of Joint Prostheses - Sample Prescriptions *on page* 40

Brand Names: US Cleocin; Cleocin in D5W [DSC]; Cleocin Phosphate; CLIN Single Use [DSC]

Brand Names: Canada AG-Clindamycin; APO-Clindamycin; Auro-Clindamycin; Clindamycine-150 [DSC]; Clindamycine-300 [DSC]; Dalacin C; Dalacin C Palmitate; Dalacin C Phosphate; JAMP Clindamycin; M-Clindamycin; MYLAN-Clindamycin [DSC]; PMS-Clindamycin [DSC]; RIVA-Clindamycin; TEVA-Clindamycin

Generic Availability (US) May be product dependent

Pharmacologic Category Antibiotic, Lincosamide

Dental Use Alternate oral antibiotic for prevention of infective endocarditis in individuals allergic to penicillins or ampicillin, when amoxicillin cannot be used; alternate IM or IV antibiotic for prevention of infective endocarditis in patients allergic to penicillins or ampicillin and unable to take oral medication; alternate oral antibiotic for prophylaxis for dental patients with total joint replacement who are allergic to penicillin; alternate IV antibiotic for prophylaxis for dental patients with total joint replacement who are allergic to penicillin and unable to take oral medications; alternate antibiotic in the treatment of common orofacial infections caused by aerobic gram-positive cocci and susceptible anaerobes; treatment of periodontal disease

Use

Bone and joint infections: Treatment of bone and joint infections, including acute hematogenous osteomyelitis caused by *Staphylococcus aureus* and as adjunctive therapy in the surgical treatment of chronic bone and joint infections caused by susceptible organisms.

Gynecological infections: Treatment of gynecologic infections, including endometritis, nongonococcal tubo-ovarian abscess, pelvic cellulitis, and postsurgical vaginal cuff infection caused by susceptible anaerobes.

Intraabdominal infections: Treatment of intraabdominal infections, including peritonitis and intraabdominal abscess caused by susceptible anaerobic organisms.

Lower respiratory tract infections: Treatment of lower respiratory tract infections, including pneumonia, empyema, and lung abscess caused by susceptible anaerobes, *Streptococcus pneumoniae*, other streptococci (except *Enterococcus faecalis*), and *S. aureus*.

Septicemia: Treatment of septicemia caused by *S. aureus*, streptococci (except *E. faecalis*), and susceptible anaerobes.

Skin and soft tissue infection: Treatment of skin and soft tissue infection caused by *Streptococcus pyogenes*, *S. aureus*, and susceptible anaerobes.

Local Anesthetic/Vasoconstrictor Precautions No information available to require special precautions

Effects on Dental Treatment No significant effects or complications reported (See Dental Health Professional Considerations)

Effects on Bleeding No information available to require special precautions

Adverse Reactions Frequency not defined.

Cardiovascular: Hypotension (rare; IV administration), thrombophlebitis (IV)
Central nervous system: Metallic taste (IV)
Dermatologic: Acute generalized exanthematous pustulosis, erythema multiforme (rare), exfoliative dermatitis (rare), maculopapular rash, pruritus, skin rash, Stevens-Johnson syndrome (rare), toxic epidermal necrolysis, urticaria, vesiculobullous dermatitis
Gastrointestinal: Abdominal pain, antibiotic-associated colitis, *Clostridioides* (formerly *Clostridium*) *difficile*-associated diarrhea, diarrhea, esophageal ulcer, esophagitis, nausea, pseudomembranous colitis, unpleasant taste (IV), vomiting
Genitourinary: Azotemia, oliguria, proteinuria, vaginitis
Hematologic & oncologic: Agranulocytosis, eosinophilia (transient), neutropenia (transient), thrombocytopenia
Hepatic: Abnormal hepatic function tests, jaundice
Hypersensitivity: Anaphylactic shock, anaphylactoid reaction (rare), anaphylaxis, angioedema, hypersensitivity reaction
Immunologic: DRESS syndrome
Local: Abscess at injection site (IM), induration at injection site (IM), irritation at injection site (IM), pain at injection site (IM)
Neuromuscular & skeletal: Polyarthritis (rare)
Renal: Renal insufficiency (rare)

Dental Usual Dosage
Orofacial infection:
Children:
Oral: 10-20 mg/kg/day in 3-4 equally divided doses
IV: 15-25 mg/kg/day in 3-4 equally divided doses

Adults:
Oral: 150-450 mg/dose for 7 days; maximum dose: 1.8 g/day
IV: 600-900 mg every 8 hours
Treatment of periodontal disease: Oral: 300 mg every 8 hours for 8 days
Infective endocarditis prophylaxis:
Children:
Oral: 20 mg/kg 30-60 minutes before procedure
IM, IV: 20 mg/kg 30-60 minutes before procedure. **Note:** Intramuscular injections should be avoided in patients who are receiving anticoagulant therapy. In these circumstances, orally administered regimens should be given whenever possible. Intravenously administered antibiotics should be used for patients who are unable to tolerate or absorb oral medications.
Adults:
Oral: 600 mg 30-60 minutes before procedure
IM, IV: 600 mg 30-60 minutes before procedure. **Note:** Intramuscular injections should be avoided in patients who are receiving anticoagulant therapy. In these circumstances, orally administered regimens should be given whenever possible. Intravenously administered antibiotics should be used for patients who are unable to tolerate or absorb oral medications.
Prophylaxis in total joint replacement patients undergoing dental procedures which produce bacteremia:
Adults:
Oral: 600 mg 1 hour prior to procedure
IV: 600 mg 1 hour prior to procedure (for patients unable to take oral medication)
Note: In general, patients with prosthetic joint implants do not require prophylactic antibiotics prior to dental procedures. In planning an invasive oral procedure, dental consultation with the patient's orthopedic surgeon may be advised to review the risks of infection.

Dosing

Adult & Geriatric

Usual dose:
Oral: 600 to 1,800 mg/day in 2 to 4 divided doses; up to 2,400 mg/day in 4 divided doses may be given for severe infections.
IM, IV: 600 to 2,700 mg/day in 2 to 4 divided doses; according to the manufacturer, up to 4,800 mg/day IV (in divided doses) has been used in life-threatening infections; however, data supporting this dose are lacking; maximum: 600 mg/dose IM.

Anthrax (off-label use): Note: Consult public health officials for event-specific recommendations.
Inhalational exposure postexposure prophylaxis (PEP) (alternative agent): **Oral:** 600 mg every 8 hours for 42 to 60 days.
Note: Anthrax vaccine should also be administered to exposed individuals (CDC [Bower 2019]; CDC [Hendricks 2014]). **Duration of therapy:** If the PEP anthrax vaccine series is administered on schedule (for all regimens), antibiotics may be discontinued in immunocompetent adults 18 to 65 years of age at 42 days after initiation of vaccine or 2 weeks after the last dose of the vaccine (whichever comes last and not to exceed 60 days); if the vaccination series cannot be completed, antibiotics should continue for 60 days (CDC [Bower 2019]). In addition, adults with immunocompromising conditions or receiving immunosuppressive therapy, patients >65 years of age, and patients who are pregnant or breastfeeding should receive antibiotics for 60 days (CDC [Bower 2019]).
Cutaneous, without systemic involvement, empiric therapy (alternative agent): **Oral:** 600 mg every 8 hours for 60 days following biological weapon-related event; duration is 7 to 10 days after naturally acquired infection. **Note**: Patients with cutaneous lesions of the head or neck or extensive edema should be treated for systemic involvement (CDC [Hendricks 2014]).
Systemic, meningitis excluded: **IV:** 900 mg every 8 hours in combination with other appropriate agents for at least 2 weeks or until clinically stable, whichever is longer (CDC [Hendricks 2014]).
Meningitis (alternative agent): **IV:** 900 mg every 8 hours in combination with other appropriate agents for at least 2 to 3 weeks or until clinically stable, whichever is longer (CDC [Hendricks 2014]).
Note: Antitoxin should also be administered for systemic anthrax. Following the course of IV combination therapy for systemic anthrax infection (including meningitis), patients exposed to aerosolized spores require oral monotherapy to complete a total antimicrobial course of 60 days (CDC [Hendricks 2014]).

Babesiosis (off-label use):
Mild to moderate disease: **Oral:** 600 mg every 8 hours in combination with quinine for 7 to 10 days (IDSA [Wormser 2006]).
Severe disease: **IV:** 600 mg every 6 hours for 7 to 10 days in combination with quinine (IDSA [Wormser 2006]; Krause 2019); a longer duration is needed for those at high risk for relapse (Krause 2008; Sanchez 2016; Vannier 2020). Clindamycin can be given orally once symptoms have abated and parasitemia is reduced (Krause 2019; Sanchez 2016).

Bacterial vaginosis (alternative agent) (off-label use): Oral: 300 mg twice daily for 7 days (CDC [Workowski 2015]).

Bite wound, prophylaxis or treatment, animal or human bite (alternative agent) (off-label use): **Note:** For animal bite, use in combination with an appropriate agent for *Pasteurella multocida*. For human bite, use in combination with an appropriate agent for *Eikenella corrodens* (IDSA [Stevens 2014]).
Oral: 300 to 450 mg 3 times daily (Baddour 2019a; Baddour 2019b; IDSA [Stevens 2014]).
IV: 600 mg every 6 to 8 hours (IDSA [Stevens 2014]). **Note:** In selected patients with high-risk wounds, some experts recommend parenteral therapy be given initially until infection is resolving, followed by oral therapy (Baddour 2019a; Baddour 2019b).
Note: For prophylaxis, duration is 3 to 5 days (IDSA [Stevens 2014]); for treatment of established infection, duration is typically 5 to 14 days and varies based on patient-specific factors, including clinical response (Baddour 2019a; Baddour 2019b).

Diabetic foot infection, mild to moderate (alternative agent) (off-label use): Oral: 300 to 450 mg every 6 to 8 hours (Bader 2008; IDSA [Lipsky 2012]; Lipsky 1990; Weintrob 2018). **Note:** May be used alone for empiric therapy of mild infections; if there are risk factors for gram-negative bacilli, must be used in combination with other appropriate agents. Duration of therapy should be tailored to individual clinical circumstances; most patients respond to 1 to 2 weeks of therapy (IDSA [Lipsky 2012]; Weintrob 2018).

Endocarditis, prophylaxis (dental or invasive respiratory tract procedures) (alternative agent for penicillin-allergic patients) (off-label use):

Oral: 600 mg as a single dose 30 to 60 minutes prior to procedure (AHA [Wilson 2007]).

IM, IV: 600 mg as a single dose 30 to 60 minutes before procedure (only if unable to tolerate or absorb oral therapy) (AHA [Wilson 2007]).

Note: Only recommended for patients with cardiac conditions associated with the highest risk of an adverse outcome from endocarditis **and** who are undergoing a procedure likely to result in bacteremia with an organism that has the potential ability to cause endocarditis (AHA [Wilson 2007]).

Hidradenitis suppurativa (off-label use): Oral: 300 mg twice daily in combination with rifampin for 10 to 12 weeks (Dessinioti 2016; Gener 2009; Gulliver 2016; Zouboulis 2015).

Malaria, treatment (alternative agent) (off-label use): Oral: 20 mg/kg/**day** in divided doses every 8 hours for 7 days in combination with quinine sulfate (quinine sulfate duration is region specific). **Note:** If used for *P. vivax* or *P. ovale*, use in combination with primaquine. If used for severe malaria (after completion of IV therapy), use full 7-day schedule of clindamycin. (CDC 2020).

Neutropenic fever, empiric therapy for low-risk cancer patients (alternative agent for penicillin-allergic patients) (off-label use): Oral: 600 mg every 8 hours (Rubenstein 1993); some experts recommend 300 mg every 6 hours (Bow 2018) (data on appropriate dose are limited). Use in combination with oral ciprofloxacin; continue until afebrile and neutropenia has resolved. **Note:** Avoid in patients who have received fluoroquinolone prophylaxis. Administer first dose in the health care setting (after blood cultures are drawn); observe patient for ≥4 hours before discharge (ASCO/IDSA [Taplitz 2018]; IDSA [Freifeld 2011]).

Odontogenic infection (alternative agent for penicillin-allergic patients) (off-label use):

IV: 600 mg every 8 hours until improved, then transition to oral clindamycin (Bhagania 2018; Chow 2018).

Oral (initial therapy for mild infection or step-down after parenteral treatment): 450 mg every 8 hours to complete a 7- to 14-day course (Chow 2018); doses in the literature varied from 150 mg every 6 hours (Tancawan 2015) to 300 mg every 6 hours (Cachovan 2011) to 600 mg every 8 hours (Bhagania 2018).

Osteomyelitis:

Osteomyelitis due to methicillin-resistant Staphylococcus aureus (MRSA) (alternative agent): **IV, Oral:** 600 mg 3 times daily for a minimum of 8 weeks; some experts combine with rifampin (IDSA [Liu 2011]).

Osteomyelitis, native vertebral due to staphylococci, methicillin-susceptible (alternative agent):

IV: 600 to 900 mg every 8 hours for 6 weeks (IDSA [Berbari 2015]).

Oral: 300 to 450 mg 4 times daily (IDSA [Berbari 2015]) or 600 mg 3 times daily (IDSA [Liu 2011]) for 6 weeks (IDSA [Berbari 2015]). **Note:** Clindamycin may also be used as suppressive therapy in selected patients (Osmon 2019).

Osteomyelitis, native vertebral due to Cutibacterium acnes (alternative agent): **IV:** 600 to 900 mg every 8 hours for 6 weeks (IDSA [Berbari 2015]).

Pelvic inflammatory disease, severe: IV: 900 mg every 8 hours with gentamicin; after 24 to 48 hours of sustained clinical improvement, transition to clindamycin 450 mg orally 4 times daily (or oral doxycycline) to complete 14 days of therapy. **Note:** If tubo-ovarian abscess is present, oral clindamycin should be given in combination with doxycycline to complete at least 14 days of therapy rather than giving doxycycline alone (CDC [Workowski 2015]).

***Pneumocystis jirovecii* pneumonia (PCP), treatment (alternative agent) (off-label use):**

Mild to moderate disease: **Oral:** 450 mg every 6 hours or 600 mg every 8 hours with primaquine for 21 days (HHS [OI adult 2020]).

Severe disease: **IV:** 600 mg every 6 hours or 900 mg every 8 hours with primaquine for 21 days; following clinical improvement, clindamycin can be given orally at 450 mg every 6 hours or 600 mg every 8 hours (HHS [OI adult 2020]; Thomas 2018).

Note: Patients with moderate or severe infection (PaO_2 <70 mm Hg at room air or alveolar-arterial oxygen gradient ≥35 mm Hg) should receive adjunctive glucocorticoids (HHS [OI adult 2020]).

Pneumonia due to MRSA (alternative agent) (off-label use): Oral, IV: 600 mg 3 times daily; duration is for a minimum of 7 days and varies based on disease severity and response to therapy (IDSA [Liu 2011]).

Postpartum endometritis: IV: 900 mg every 8 hours plus gentamicin; treat until the patient is clinically improved (no fundal tenderness) and afebrile for 24 to 48 hours (Chen 2018; Gall 1996).

Prosthetic joint infection (off-label use):

Cutibacterium acnes, treatment (alternative agent for penicillin allergy):

IV: 600 to 900 mg every 8 hours for 4 to 6 weeks (IDSA [Osmon 2013]).

Oral: 300 to 450 mg every 6 hours (IDSA [Osmon 2013]), following at least 2 weeks of parenteral therapy (Kanafani 2018).

Methicillin-resistant staphylococci, treatment (chronic suppression): **Oral:** 600 mg every 8 hours (Berbari 2019).

Rhinosinusitis, acute bacterial (alternative agent for penicillin-allergic patients able to tolerate cephalosporins with concern for pneumococcal resistance) (off-label use): Oral: 300 mg every 6 to 8 hours in combination with a third-generation cephalosporin (eg, cefixime or cefpodoxime) for 5 to 7 days (IDSA [Chow 2012]; Patel 2018; Rosenfeld 2016). **Note:** In uncomplicated acute bacterial rhinosinusitis, initial observation and symptom management without antibiotic therapy is appropriate in most patients (AAO-HNS [Rosenfeld 2015]; Harris 2016).

Septic arthritis due to *Staphylococcus aureus* (including MRSA) (alternative agent): Oral, IV: 600 mg 3 times daily for 3 to 4 weeks (Goldenberg 2018; IDSA [Liu 2011]). **Note:** A longer course of parenteral therapy (4 weeks) may be required for patients with concomitant bacteremia (in the absence of endocarditis) (Goldenberg 2019).

Skin and soft tissue infection:

Impetigo or ecthyma if MRSA is suspected or confirmed (alternative agent): Oral: 300 mg 4 times daily or 450 mg 3 times daily for 7 days (Baddour 2020; IDSA [Stevens 2014]).

Nonpurulent cellulitis or erysipelas due to beta-hemolytic streptococci or Staphylococcus aureus (including MRSA), empiric or pathogen-directed therapy (alternative agent):

Oral: 300 mg 4 times daily or 450 mg 3 times daily.

IV: 600 mg to 900 mg every 8 hours.

Note: Transition to oral therapy once improving; treat for at least 5 days but may extend to 14 days depending on severity and clinical response (IDSA [Stevens 2014]; Spelman 2020).

Purulent cellulitis or abscess due to S. aureus (including MRSA) or beta-hemolytic streptococci (alternative agent):

Oral: 300 mg 4 times daily or 450 mg 3 times daily. Treat for 5 to 14 days depending on severity and clinical response.

Note: Systemic antibiotics only indicated for certain instances (eg, immunocompromised patients, signs of systemic infection, large or multiple abscess, indwelling device, high risk for adverse outcome with endocarditis). If at risk for gram-negative bacilli, use in combination with an appropriate agent (IDSA [Stevens 2014]; Spelman 2020).

Necrotizing soft tissue infection (alternative agent): **IV:** 600 to 900 mg every 8 hours as part of an appropriate combination regimen. **Note:** Antibiotic therapy must be used in conjunction with early and aggressive surgical exploration and debridement of necrotic tissue (IDSA [Stevens 2014]; Stevens 2018).

Streptococcus (group A):

Bloodstream infection: **IV:** 900 mg every 8 hours in combination with IV penicillin G; duration is individualized, but clindamycin may be discontinued within 48 hours for patients without septic shock, organ failure, or necrotizing infection. Continue penicillin G to complete ≥14 days of therapy (Stevens 2019).

Pharyngitis (alternative agent for penicillin-allergic patients) (off-label use): **Oral:** 300 mg 3 times daily for 10 days (IDSA [Shulman 2012]).

Chronic carriage (off-label use): **Oral:** 300 mg 3 times daily for 10 days. **Note:** Most individuals with chronic carriage do not require antimicrobial treatment (IDSA [Shulman 2012]).

Streptococcus (group B), maternal prophylaxis for prevention of neonatal disease (alternative agent) (off-label use):

Note: Prophylaxis is reserved for pregnant women with a positive group B streptococci (GBS) vaginal or rectal screening in late gestation or GBS bacteriuria during the current pregnancy, history of birth of an infant with early-onset GBS disease, and unknown GBS culture status with any of the following: birth <37 0/7 weeks gestation, intrapartum fever, prolonged rupture of membranes, known GBS positive in a previous pregnancy, or intrapartum nucleic acid amplification testing positive for GBS (ACOG 2019).

IV: 900 mg at onset of labor or prelabor rupture of membranes, then every 8 hours until delivery. **Note:** Clindamycin should be reserved for penicillin-allergic patients at high risk for anaphylaxis (ACOG 2019).

Surgical prophylaxis (in combination with other appropriate agents when coverage for MRSA is indicated or for gram-positive coverage in patients unable to tolerate cephalosporins) (off-label use): IV: 900 mg started within 60 minutes prior to initial surgical incision. Clindamycin doses may be repeated intraoperatively at 6-hour intervals if procedure is lengthy or if there is excessive blood loss (ASHP/IDSA/SIS/SHEA [Bratzler 2013]). In cases where an extension of prophylaxis is warranted postoperatively, total duration should be ≤24 hours (Anderson 2014; ASHP/IDSA/SIS/SHEA [Bratzler 2013]). For clean and clean-contaminated procedures, continued prophylactic antibiotics beyond surgical incision closure is not recommended, even in the presence of a drain (CDC [Berríos-Torres 2017]).

Toxic shock syndrome, toxin production suppression (empiric therapy): IV: 900 mg every 8 hours as part of an appropriate combination regimen (Lappin 2009; Wong 2013). Duration is until clinically and hemodynamically stable for at least 48 to 72 hours; then discontinue clindamycin and give monotherapy with an appropriate agent (Chu 2019; Stevens 2019).

***Toxoplasma gondii* encephalitis and pneumonitis (alternative agent) (off-label use):**

Initial treatment: **Oral, IV:** 600 mg every 6 hours in combination with pyrimethamine and leucovorin. Continue therapy for at least 6 weeks; longer duration may be required if incomplete response or extensive disease; after completion of acute therapy, all patients should receive long-term maintenance therapy (HHS [OI adult 2020]; Schwartz 2013).

Long-term maintenance therapy: **Oral:** 600 mg every 8 hours in combination with pyrimethamine and leucovorin (HHS [OI adult 2020]; Schwartz 2013); in patients with HIV, may discontinue when asymptomatic with a CD4 count >200 cells/mm^3 and an undetectable HIV viral load for >6 months in response to ART (HHS [OI adult 2020]).

Renal Impairment: Adult

The renal dosing recommendations are based upon the best available evidence and clinical expertise. Senior Editorial Team: Bruce Mueller, PharmD, FCCP, FASN, FNKF; Jason Roberts, PhD, BPharm (Hons), B App Sc, FSHP, FISAC; Michael Heung, MD, MS.

IV, Oral:

Mild to severe impairment: No dosage adjustment necessary.

Hemodialysis, intermittent (thrice weekly): Poorly dialyzed; no supplemental dose or dosage adjustment necessary (Cimino 1969).

Peritoneal dialysis: Poorly dialyzed; no dosage adjustment necessary (Malacoff 1975).

CRRT: No dosage adjustment necessary (Heintz 2009).

PIRRT (eg, sustained, low-efficiency diafiltration): No dosage adjustment necessary (expert opinion).

Hepatic Impairment: Adult

Mild impairment: There are no dosage adjustments provided in the manufacturer's labeling.

Moderate to severe impairment: There are no dosage adjustments provided in the manufacturer's labeling. In studies of patients with moderate or severe liver disease, half-life is prolonged; however, when administered on an every-8-hour schedule, accumulation should rarely occur. In severe liver disease, use caution and monitor liver enzymes periodically during therapy.

Pediatric Note: Dosage should be based on total body weight for obese children ≥2 years of age and adolescents (Smith 2017; manufacturer's labeling).

General dosing, susceptible infection:
IM, IV:
Manufacturer's labeling: Infants, Children, and Adolescents 1 month to 16 years:
Weight-directed dosing: 20 to 40 mg/kg/day divided every 6 to 8 hours.
BSA-directed dosing: 350 to 450 mg/m^2/day divided every 6 to 8 hours.
Alternate dosing (*Red Book* [AAP] 2012): Infants, Children, and Adolescents:
Mild to moderate infections: 20 mg/kg/day divided every 8 hours; maximum daily dose: 1,800 mg/**day**.
Severe infections: 40 mg/kg/day divided every 6 to 8 hours; maximum daily dose: 2,700 mg/**day**.
Oral:
Manufacturer's labeling: Infants, Children, and Adolescents:
Hydrochloride salt (capsule): 8 to 20 mg/kg/day divided every 6 to 8 hours.
Palmitate salt (solution): 8 to 25 mg/kg/day divided every 6 to 8 hours; minimum dose: 37.5 mg 3 times daily.
Alternate dosing (*Red Book* [AAP]; 2012): Infants, Children, and Adolescents:
Mild to moderate infections: 10 to 25 mg/kg/day divided every 8 hours; maximum daily dose: 1,800 mg/**day**.
Severe infections: 30 to 40 mg/kg/day divided every 6 to 8 hours; maximum daily dose: 1,800 mg/**day**.

Babesiosis: Infants, Children, and Adolescents: Oral: 20 to 40 mg/kg/day divided every 8 hours for 7 to 10 days plus quinine; maximum single dose: 600 mg (*Red Book* [AAP] 2012).

Bacterial endocarditis prophylaxis for dental and upper respiratory procedures in penicillin-allergic patients (*Red Book* [AAP] 2012; Wilson 2007): Infants, Children, and Adolescents:
IM, IV: 20 mg/kg 30 minutes before procedure; maximum single dose: 600 mg.
Oral: 20 mg/kg 1 hour before procedure; maximum single dose: 600 mg.
Note: American Heart Association (AHA) guidelines now recommend prophylaxis only in patients undergoing invasive procedures and in whom underlying cardiac conditions may predispose to a higher risk of adverse outcomes should infection occur. As of April 2007, routine prophylaxis for GI/GU procedures is no longer recommended by the AHA.

Catheter (peritoneal dialysis); exit-site or tunnel infection: Infant, Children, and Adolescents: Oral: 10 mg/kg/dose 3 times daily; maximum dose: 600 mg/dose (Warady [ISPD 2012]).

Intra-abdominal infection, complicated: Infants, Children, and Adolescents: IV: **Note:** Not recommended for community-acquired infections due to increasing *Bacteroides fragilis* resistance: 20 to 40 mg/kg/day divided every 6 to 8 hours in combination with gentamicin or tobramycin (Solomkin 2010).

Malaria, treatment: Infants, Children, and Adolescents:
Uncomplicated: Oral: 20 mg/kg/day divided every 8 hours for 7 days plus quinine (CDC 2011; *Red Book* [AAP] 2012).
Severe: IV: Loading dose: 10 mg/kg once followed by 15 mg/kg/day divided every 8 hours plus IV quinidine gluconate; switch to oral therapy (clindamycin and quinine, see above) when able for total treatment duration of 7 days. **Note:** Quinine duration is region specific; consult CDC for current recommendations (CDC 2011).

Osteomyelitis, septic arthritis, due to MRSA: Infants, Children, and Adolescents: IV, Oral: 40 mg/kg/day divided every 6 to 8 hours for at least 4 to 6 weeks (osteomyelitis) or 3 to 4 weeks (septic arthritis) (IDSA [Liu 2011]).

Otitis media, acute: Infants ≥6 months, Children, and Adolescents: Oral: 30 to 40 mg/kg/day divided every 8 hours; administer with or without a third generation cephalosporin (AAP [Lieberthal 2013]).

Peritonitis (peritoneal dialysis):
Prophylaxis (Warady [ISPD 2012]):
Invasive dental procedures: Oral: 20 mg/kg administered 30 to 60 minutes before procedure; maximum dose: 600 mg.
Gastrointestinal or genitourinary procedures: IV: 10 mg/kg administered 30 to 60 minutes before procedure; maximum dose: 600 mg.
Treatment: Intraperitoneal, continuous: Loading dose: 300 mg per liter of dialysate; maintenance dose: 150 mg per liter; **Note:** 125 mg/liter has also been recommended as a maintenance dose (Aronoff 2007; Warady [ISPD 2012]).

Pharyngitis:
AHA guidelines (Gerber 2009): Children and Adolescents: Oral: 20 mg/kg/day in divided doses 3 times daily for 10 days; maximum single dose: 600 mg.
IDSA guidelines (Shulman, 2012): Children and Adolescents: Oral:
Treatment and primary prevention of rheumatic fever: 21 mg/kg/day in divided doses 3 times daily for 10 days; maximum single dose: 300 mg.
Treatment of chronic carriers: 20 to 30 mg/kg/day in divided doses 3 times daily for 10 days; maximum single dose: 300 mg.

Pneumococcal disease, invasive: Infants, Children, and Adolescents: IV: 25 to 40 mg/kg/day divided every 6 to 8 hours (*Red Book* [AAP] 2012).

***Pneumocystis jirovecii* (formerly *carnii*) pneumonia (PCP):**
Non HIV-exposed/-positive (*Red Book* [AAP] 2012): Infants, Children, and Adolescents:
Mild to moderate disease: Oral: 10 mg/kg 3 to 4 times daily for 21 days; in combination with other agents; maximum single dose: 450 mg.
Moderate to severe disease: IV: 15 to 25 mg/kg 3 to 4 times daily for 21 days; give with pentamidine or primaquine; maximum single dose: 600 mg. May switch to oral dose after clinical improvement.
HIV-exposed/-positive: Adolescents (DHHS [adult] 2013):
Mild to moderate disease: Oral: 300 mg every 6 hours **or** 450 mg every 8 hours with primaquine for 21 days.
Moderate to severe disease:
Oral: 300 mg every 6 hours **or** 450 mg every 8 hours with primaquine for 21 days.
IV: 600 mg every 6 hours **or** 900 mg every 8 hours with primaquine for 21 days.

Pneumonia:
Community-acquired pneumonia (CAP) (IDSA/PIDS [Bradley 2011]): Infants ≥3 months, Children, and Adolescents: **Note:** In children ≥5 years, a macrolide antibiotic should be added if atypical pneumonia cannot be ruled out.
Moderate to severe infection: IV: 40 mg/kg/day divided every 6 to 8 hours.

Mild infection, step-down therapy: Oral: 30 to 40 mg/kg/day divided every 6 to 8 hours.

MRSA pneumonia: IV: 40 mg/kg/day divided every 6 to 8 hours for 7 to 21 days (IDSA [Liu 2011]).

Rhinosinusitis, acute bacterial: Children and Adolescents: Oral: 30 to 40 mg/kg/day divided every 8 hours with concomitant cefixime or cefpodoxime for 10 to 14 days. **Note:** Recommended in patients with nontype I penicillin allergy, after failure to initial therapy, or in patients at risk for antibiotic resistance (eg, daycare attendance, age <2 years, recent hospitalization, antibiotic use within the past month) (Chow 2012).

Skin and soft tissue infection: Infants, Children, and Adolescents:

Impetigo: Oral: 20 mg/kg/day in divided doses 3 times daily for 7 days; maximum dose: 400 mg/dose (IDSA [Stevens 2014]).

MRSA infection: **Note:** Treatment duration based on clinical response, usually 7 to 14 days for complicated skin and soft tissue infection and 5 to 10 days for outpatient cellulitis (nonpurulent or purulent) (IDSA [Liu 2011]).

IV: 25 to 40 mg/kg/day in divided doses 3 times daily (IDSA [Stevens 2014]) or 40 mg/kg/day in divided doses every 6 to 8 hours (IDSA [Liu 2011]); maximum dose: 600 mg/dose.

Oral: 30 to 40 mg/kg/day in divided doses 3 times daily (IDSA [Stevens 2014]) or 30 to 40 mg/kg/day in divided doses every 6 to 8 hours (IDSA [Liu 2011]); maximum dose: 450 mg/dose.

MSSA infection (IDSA [Stevens 2014]): Duration of treatment dependent upon site and severity of infection; cellulitis and abscesses that have been drained typically require 5 to 10 days of therapy.

IV: 25 to 40 mg/kg/day in divided doses 3 times daily; maximum dose: 600 mg/dose.

Oral: 25 to 30 mg/kg/day in divided doses 3 times daily; maximum dose: 450 mg/dose.

Necrotizing infections: IV: 10 to 13 mg/kg/**dose** every 8 hours; maximum dose: 900 mg/dose; may use in combination with other antibiotics based on organism. Continue until further debridement is not necessary, patient has clinically improved, and patient is afebrile for 48 to 72 hours (IDSA [Stevens 2014]).

Surgical prophylaxis: Children and Adolescents: IV: 10 mg/kg 30 to 60 minutes prior to the procedure; may repeat in 6 hours; maximum single dose: 900 mg (Bratzler 2013).

Toxoplasmosis (HIV-exposed/positive or hematopoietic cell transplantation recipients):

Infants and Children (CDC 2009; *Red Book* [AAP] 2012; Tomblyn 2009):

Treatment, HIV-exposed/-positive: IV, Oral: 5 to 7.5 mg/kg/dose 4 times daily with pyrimethamine and leucovorin; maximum single dose: 600 mg.

Secondary prevention:

HIV-exposed/-positive: Oral: 7 to 10 mg/kg/dose every 8 hours and pyrimethamine plus leucovorin; maximum single dose: 600 mg (DHHS [pediatric] 2013).

Hematopoietic cell transplantation recipients: Oral: 5 to 7.5 mg/kg/dose every 6 hours and pyrimethamine plus leucovorin; maximum single dose: 450 mg.

Adolescents (DHHS [adult] 2013; *Red Book* [AAP] 2012; Tomblyn 2009):

Treatment: Oral, IV: 600 mg every 6 hours with pyrimethamine and leucovorin for at least 6 weeks; longer if clinical or radiologic disease is extensive or response is incomplete.

Secondary prevention:

HIV-exposed/-positive: Oral: 600 mg every 8 hours with pyrimethamine and leucovorin.

Hematopoietic cell transplantation recipients: Oral: 300 to 450 mg every 6 to 8 hours with pyrimethamine and leucovorin.

Renal Impairment: Pediatric

Altered kidney function: Infants, Children, and Adolescents: IV, Oral:

Mild to severe impairment: No dosage adjustment necessary.

Hemodialysis, intermittent (thrice weekly): Poorly dialyzed; based on adult information, no supplemental dose or dosage adjustment necessary (Cimino 1969).

Peritoneal dialysis: Poorly dialyzed; based on adult information, no dosage adjustment necessary (Malacoff 1975).

Continuous renal replacement therapy (CRRT): Based on adult information, no dosage adjustment necessary (Heintz 2009).

Hepatic Impairment: Pediatric No adjustment required. Use caution with severe hepatic impairment.

Mechanism of Action Reversibly binds to 50S ribosomal subunits preventing peptide bond formation thus inhibiting bacterial protein synthesis; bacteriostatic or bactericidal depending on drug concentration, infection site, and organism

Contraindications

Hypersensitivity to clindamycin, lincomycin, or any component of the formulation.

Canadian labeling: Additional contraindications (not in US labeling): Oral clindamycin: Infants <30 days of age.

Warnings/Precautions Dosage adjustment may be necessary in patients with severe hepatic dysfunction. **[US Boxed Warning]: Can cause severe and possibly fatal colitis. Should be reserved for serious infections where less toxic antimicrobial agents are inappropriate. It should not be used in patients with nonbacterial infections such as most upper respiratory tract infections. Hypertoxin-producing strains of *C. difficile* cause increased morbidity and mortality, as these infections can be refractory to antimicrobial therapy and may require colectomy. *C. difficile* -associated diarrhea (CDAD) must be considered in all patients who present with diarrhea following antibiotic use. CDAD has been observed >2 months postantibiotic treatment. If CDAD is suspected or confirmed, ongoing antibiotic use not directed against *C. difficile* may need to be discontinued. Institute appropriate fluid and electrolyte management, protein supplementation, antibiotic treatment of C. difficile, and surgical evaluation as clinically indicated.** Use with caution in patients with a history of gastrointestinal disease, particularly colitis. Use may result in overgrowth of nonsusceptible organisms, particularly yeast. Should superinfection occur, appropriate measures should be taken as indicated by the clinical situation. Severe hypersensitivity reactions, including severe skin reactions (eg, drug reaction with eosinophilia and systemic symptoms [DRESS], Stevens-Johnson syndrome [SJS], and toxic epidermal necrolysis [TEN]), some fatal, and anaphylactic reactions, including anaphylactic shock, have been reported. Permanently discontinue treatment and institute appropriate therapy if these reactions occur. Some products may contain tartrazine (FD&C yellow no. 5), which may cause allergic reactions in certain individuals. Allergy is frequently seen in patients who also have an aspirin hypersensitivity. Use caution in atopic patients. A subgroup of older patients with associated severe illness may tolerate diarrhea less well. Monitor carefully for changes in bowel frequency. Not appropriate for use in the treatment of meningitis due to inadequate penetration into the CSF. Do not inject IV undiluted as a bolus. Product should be diluted in compatible fluid and infused over 10 to 60 minutes. Potentially significant interactions may exist, requiring dose or frequency adjustment, additional monitoring, and/or selection of alternative therapy.

Benzyl alcohol and derivatives: Some dosage forms may contain benzyl alcohol; large amounts of benzyl alcohol (≥99 mg/kg/day) have been associated with a potentially fatal toxicity ("gasping syndrome") in neonates; the "gasping syndrome" consists of metabolic acidosis, respiratory distress, gasping respirations, CNS dysfunction (including convulsions, intracranial hemorrhage), hypotension and cardiovascular collapse (AAP ["Inactive" 1997]; CDC 1982); some data suggests that benzoate displaces bilirubin from protein binding sites (Ahlfors 2001); avoid or use dosage forms containing benzyl alcohol with caution in neonates. See manufacturer's labeling.

Drug Interactions

Metabolism/Transport Effects **Substrate** of CYP3A4 (minor); **Note:** Assignment of Major/Minor substrate status based on clinically relevant drug interaction potential

Avoid Concomitant Use

Avoid concomitant use of Clindamycin (Systemic) with any of the following: BCG (Intravesical); Cholera Vaccine; Mecamylamine

Increased Effect/Toxicity

Clindamycin (Systemic) may increase the levels/effects of: Mecamylamine; Neuromuscular-Blocking Agents

Decreased Effect

Clindamycin (Systemic) may decrease the levels/effects of: BCG (Intravesical); BCG Vaccine (Immunization); Cholera Vaccine; Lactobacillus and Estriol; Sodium Picosulfate; Typhoid Vaccine

The levels/effects of Clindamycin (Systemic) may be decreased by: CYP3A4 Inducers (Strong); Kaolin

Pharmacodynamics/Kinetics

Half-life Elimination

Neonates (Gonzalez 2016):

PMA ≤28 weeks: Median: 5.89 hours (range: 2.42 to 12.9 hours).

PMA >28 to 32 weeks: Median: 5.25 hours (range: 2.34 to 8.87 hours).

PMA >32 to 40 weeks: Median: 3.96 hours (range: 1.3 to 8.83 hours).

Neonates and Infants ≤5 months (Gonzalez 2016):

PMA >40 to 60 weeks: Median: 2.35 hours (range: 0.94 to 6.44 hours).

Infants >5 months to 1 year (Gonzalez 2016): Median: 2.05 hours (range: 1.26 to 3.47 hours).

Children ≥2 years and Adolescents (Smith 2017):

Non-obese: Median range: 2.15 to 2.84 hours.

Obese: Median range: 2.15 to 3.55 hours.

Adults: 3 hours.

Elderly (oral) ~4 hours (range: 3.4 to 5.1 hours).

Time to Peak Serum: Oral: Within 60 minutes; IM: 1 to 3 hours

Pregnancy Considerations

Clindamycin crosses the placenta and can be detected in the cord blood and fetal tissue (Philipson 1973; Weinstein 1976). Clindamycin injection contains benzyl alcohol, which may also cross the placenta.

Clindamycin pharmacokinetics are not affected by pregnancy (Philipson 1976; Weinstein 1976).

Clindamycin is recommended for use in pregnant women for the prophylaxis of group B streptococcal disease in newborns (alternative option for patients at high risk for anaphylaxis to penicillin [or whose risk is unknown], and who have GBS susceptible to clindamycin) (ACOG 797 2020); prophylaxis and treatment of *Toxoplasma gondii* encephalitis (alternative therapy), or treatment of *Pneumocystis pneumonia* (PCP) (alternative therapy) (HHS [OI adult 2020]); bacterial vaginosis (CDC [Workowski 2015]); anthrax (Meaney-Delman 2014); or malaria (CDC 2020). Clindamycin is also one of the antibiotics recommended for prophylactic use prior to cesarean delivery and may be used in certain situations prior to vaginal delivery in women at high risk for endocarditis (ACOG 199 2018).

Breastfeeding Considerations Clindamycin is present in breast milk.

The relative infant dose (RID) of clindamycin is 1.2% to 4.7% when calculated using the highest verifiable breast milk concentration located and compared to an infant therapeutic dose of 10 to 40 mg/kg/day.

In general, breastfeeding is considered acceptable when the RID is <10% (Anderson 2016; Ito 2000).

Using the highest verifiable milk concentration (3.1 mcg/mL), the estimated daily infant dose via breast milk is 0.465 mg/kg/day. This milk concentration was obtained following maternal administration of oral clindamycin 150 mg three times daily for at least 1 week (Stéen 1982). The manufacturer reports that clindamycin breast milk concentrations range from <0.5 to 3.8 mcg/mL following doses of 150 mg orally to 600 mg IV.

One case of bloody stools in an infant occurred after a mother received clindamycin while breastfeeding; however, a causal relationship was not confirmed (Mann 1980). In general, antibiotics that are present in breast milk may cause non-dose-related modification of bowel flora.

According to the manufacturer, the decision to continue or discontinue breastfeeding during therapy should take into account the risk of infant exposure, the benefits of breastfeeding to the infant, and benefits of treatment to the mother; alternate therapies may be preferred. Additional guidelines recommend to avoid clindamycin in breastfeeding women if possible; monitor breastfeeding infants for GI disturbances, diarrhea, and bloody stools if maternal treatment is required (WHO 2002).

Dosage Forms: US

Capsule, Oral:

Cleocin: 75 mg, 150 mg, 300 mg

Generic: 75 mg, 150 mg, 300 mg

Solution, Injection:

Cleocin Phosphate: 300 mg/2 mL (2 mL); 600 mg/4 mL (4 mL); 900 mg/6 mL (6 mL); 9 g/60 mL (60 mL)

Generic: 300 mg/2 mL (2 mL); 600 mg/4 mL (4 mL); 900 mg/6 mL (6 mL); 9000 mg/60 mL (60 mL); 9 g/60 mL (60 mL)

Solution, Intravenous:
Generic: 600 mg/50 mL (50 mL); 900 mg/50 mL (50 mL); 900 mg/6 mL (6 mL)
Solution, Intravenous [preservative free]:
Generic: 300 mg/50 mL (50 mL); 600 mg/50 mL (50 mL); 900 mg/50 mL (50 mL); 300 mg/50 mL in NaCl 0.9% (50 mL); 600 mg/50 mL in NaCl 0.9% (50 mL); 900 mg/50 mL in NaCl 0.9% (50 mL)
Solution Reconstituted, Oral:
Cleocin: 75 mg/5 mL (100 mL)
Generic: 75 mg/5 mL (100 mL)

Dosage Forms: Canada
Capsule, Oral:
Dalacin C: 150 mg, 300 mg
Generic: 150 mg, 300 mg
Solution, Injection:
Dalacin C Phosphate: 150 mg/mL (2 mL, 4 mL, 6 mL, 60 mL)
Generic: 150 mg/mL (2 mL, 4 mL, 6 mL, 60 mL, 120 mL)
Solution, Intravenous:
Generic: 300 mg/50 mL (50 mL); 600 mg/50 mL (50 mL); 900 mg/50 mL (50 mL)
Solution Reconstituted, Oral:
Dalacin C Palmitate: 75 mg/5 mL (100 mL)

Dental Health Professional Considerations About 1% of clindamycin users develop pseudomembranous colitis. Symptoms may occur 2 to 9 days after initiation of therapy; however, it has never occurred with the 1-dose regimen of clindamycin used to prevent bacterial endocarditis.

Clindamycin (Topical) (klin da MYE sin)

Brand Names: US Cleocin; Cleocin-T; Clindacin ETZ; Clindacin Pac; Clindacin-P; Clindagel; Clindesse; Evoclin

Brand Names: Canada Clinda-T; Clindets [DSC]; Dalacin T; Dalacin Vaginal; TARO-Clindamycin

Pharmacologic Category Antibiotic, Lincosamide; Topical Skin Product, Acne

Use
Acne vulgaris: Treatment of acne vulgaris (topical gel, topical lotion, topical solution)
Bacterial vaginosis: Treatment of bacterial vaginosis (vaginal cream, vaginal suppository)

Local Anesthetic/Vasoconstrictor Precautions No information available to require special precautions

Effects on Dental Treatment No significant effects or complications reported

Effects on Bleeding No information available to require special precautions

Adverse Reactions
Topical: >10%: Dermatologic: Xeroderma (18% to 23%; gel, lotion, solution), oily skin (gel, lotion: 10% to 18%; solution: 1%), erythema (7% to 16%; gel, lotion, solution), burning sensation of skin (10% to 11%; gel, lotion, solution), exfoliation of skin (7% to 11%; lotion, solution), pruritus (7% to 11%; gel, lotion, solution)

Vaginal:
>10%: Genitourinary: Vaginal moniliasis (≤13%)
1% to 10%:
Dermatologic: Pruritus (≤1% nonapplication site; <1% application site)
Genitourinary: Vulvovaginal disease (3% to 9%), vulvovaginitis (≤7%), vaginal pain (2%), trichomonal vaginitis (≤1%)
Infection: Fungal infection (≤1%)

<1%, postmarketing, and/or case reports (all routes): Abdominal cramps, abdominal pain, application site pain, bacterial infection, bloody diarrhea, colitis, constipation, contact dermatitis, diarrhea (hemorrhagic or severe), dizziness, dysgeusia, dyspepsia, dysuria, edema, endometriosis, epistaxis, erythema, eye pain, fever, flank pain, flatulence, folliculitis, folliculitis (gram-negative infection), gastrointestinal disease, gastrointestinal distress, halitosis, headache, hypersensitivity reaction, hyperthyroidism, maculopapular rash, menstrual disease, nausea, pain, pseudomembranous colitis, pyelonephritis, severe colitis, skin rash, upper respiratory infection, urinary tract infection, urticaria, uterine hemorrhage, vaginal discharge, vertigo, vomiting, vulvovaginal pruritus

Mechanism of Action Reversibly binds to 50S ribosomal subunits preventing peptide bond formation thus inhibiting bacterial protein synthesis; bacteriostatic or bactericidal depending on drug concentration, infection site, and organism

Pharmacodynamics/Kinetics
Half-life Elimination Vaginal cream: 1.5 to 2.6 hours following repeated dosing; Vaginal suppository: 11 hours (range: 4 to 35 hours, limited by absorption rate)
Time to Peak Vaginal cream: ~10 to 14 hours (range: 4 to 24 hours); Vaginal suppository: ~5 hours (range: 1 to 10 hours)

Reproductive Considerations
Some vaginal products contain mineral oil which may weaken condoms or contraceptive diaphragms. Therefore, use of these products are not recommended for birth control during therapy or for 3 to 5 days (depending on the product) following treatment.

Pregnancy Considerations
Clindamycin crosses the placenta following oral and parenteral dosing (Philipson 1973; Weinstein 1976). The amount of clindamycin available systemically is less following topical and vaginal application than with IV or oral administration.

Various clindamycin vaginal products are available for the treatment of bacterial vaginosis. Recommendations for use in pregnant woman vary by product labeling. Current guidelines note that the same oral or vaginal regimens used in nonpregnant women may be used during pregnancy, including oral or vaginal clindamycin (CDC [Workowski 2015]).

If treatment for acne is needed during pregnancy, topical clindamycin may be considered if an antibiotic is needed. To decrease systemic exposure, pregnant women should avoid application to inflamed skin for long periods of time, or to large body surface areas (Kong 2013).

Clindamycin and Benzoyl Peroxide
(klin da MYE sin & BEN zoe il peer OKS ide)

Related Information
Clindamycin (Topical) *on page 375*

Brand Names: US Acanya; BenzaClin; BenzaClin with Pump; Duac [DSC]; Neuac; Onexton

Brand Names: Canada BenzaClin; Clindoxyl; Clindoxyl ADV; TARO-Benzoyl/Clindamycin Kit; TARO-Clindamycin/Benzoyl Perox

Pharmacologic Category Acne Products; Topical Skin Product; Topical Skin Product, Acne

Use Acne: Topical treatment of acne vulgaris

Local Anesthetic/Vasoconstrictor Precautions No information available to require special precautions

Effects on Dental Treatment No significant effects or complications reported

Effects on Bleeding No information available to require special precautions

Adverse Reactions Also see individual agents.

>10%:

Dermatologic: Application site scaling (≤21%), local dryness (≤16%)

Local: Application site erythema (<31%), local desquamation (2% to 19%), application site itching (≤17%)

1% to 10%:

Dermatologic: Stinging of the skin (application site: ≤7%), sunburn (local; 1%)

Local: Application site burning (≤10%), application site reaction (3%)

<1%, postmarketing, and/or case reports: Anaphylaxis, application site irritation, application site pain, contact dermatitis, hypersensitivity reaction, local discoloration, local skin exfoliation, skin rash, urticaria

Mechanism of Action

Benzoyl peroxide: Releases free-radical oxygen, which oxidizes bacterial proteins in the sebaceous follicles, decreasing the number of anaerobic bacteria and decreasing irritating-type free fatty acids.

Clindamycin: Reversibly binds to 50S ribosomal subunits preventing peptide bond formation thus inhibiting bacterial protein synthesis; bacteriostatic or bactericidal depending on drug concentration, infection site, and organism.

Pregnancy Considerations

Topical therapy is preferred for the treatment of acne during pregnancy. The combination of topical clindamycin with benzoyl peroxide is recommended for mild to moderate inflammatory acne in pregnant women (Chien 2016).

Refer to individual monographs for additional information.

- ◆ **Clindamycin HCl** *see* Clindamycin (Systemic) *on page* 368
- ◆ **Clindamycin Hydrochloride** *see* Clindamycin (Systemic) *on page* 368
- ◆ **Clindamycin Palmitate** *see* Clindamycin (Systemic) *on page* 368
- ◆ **Clindamycin Palmitate HCl** *see* Clindamycin (Systemic) *on page* 368
- ◆ **Clindamycin Phos/Benzoyl Perox** *see* Clindamycin and Benzoyl Peroxide *on page* 375
- ◆ **Clindamycin Phosphate** *see* Clindamycin (Topical) *on page* 375
- ◆ **Clindamycin Phosphate and Benzoyl Peroxide** *see* Clindamycin and Benzoyl Peroxide *on page* 375
- ◆ **Clindesse** *see* Clindamycin (Topical) *on page* 375
- ◆ **Clinoril** *see* Sulindac *on page* 1394
- ◆ **Clinpro 5000** *see* Fluoride *on page* 693
- ◆ **CLIN Single Use [DSC]** *see* Clindamycin (Systemic) *on page* 368

CloBAZam (KLOE ba zam)

Brand Names: US Onfi; Sympazan

Brand Names: Canada APO-Clobazam; Clobazam-10 [DSC]; DOM-Clobazam [DSC]; Frisium [DSC]; PMS-Clobazam; TEVA-Clobazam

Pharmacologic Category Anticonvulsant, Benzodiazepine; Benzodiazepine

Use

Lennox-Gastaut syndrome: Adjunctive treatment of seizures associated with Lennox-Gastaut syndrome in patients ≥2 years

Local Anesthetic/Vasoconstrictor Precautions No information available to require special precautions

Effects on Dental Treatment Key adverse event(s) related to dental treatment: Xerostomia (normal salivary flow resumes upon discontinuation). Paradoxical reactions (including excitation, agitation, hallucinations, and psychosis) are known to occur with benzodiazepines.

Effects on Bleeding No information available to require special precautions

Adverse Reactions

>10%:

Central nervous system: Drowsiness (16% to 25%), lethargy (10% to 15%), drooling (13% to 14%), aggressive behavior (8% to 14%), irritability (11%)

Respiratory: Upper respiratory tract infection (13% to 14%)

Miscellaneous: Fever (10% to 17%)

1% to 10%:

Central nervous system: Ataxia (10%), sedation (9%), insomnia (5% to 7%), psychomotor agitation (5%), fatigue (3% to 5%), dysarthria (2% to 5%)

Gastrointestinal: Constipation (2% to 10%), vomiting (7% to 9%), decreased appetite (7%), increased appetite (2% to 5%), dysphagia (5%)

Genitourinary: Urinary tract infection (2% to 5%)

Respiratory: Cough (3% to 7%), pneumonia (3% to 7%), bronchitis (2% to 5%)

Postmarketing and/or case reports: Abdominal distention, agitation, anemia, angioedema, anxiety, apathy, behavioral changes, blurred vision, confusion, delirium, delusions, depression, diplopia, eosinophilia, facial edema, hallucination, hypothermia, increased liver enzymes, leukopenia, lip edema, mood changes, muscle spasm, pulmonary aspiration, respiratory depression, skin rash, Stevens-Johnson syndrome, suicidal ideation, suicidal tendencies, thrombocytopenia, toxic epidermal necrolysis, urinary retention, urticaria, withdrawal syndrome

Mechanism of Action Clobazam is a 1,5 benzodiazepine which binds to stereospecific benzodiazepine receptors on the postsynaptic GABA neuron at several sites within the central nervous system, including the limbic system, reticular formation. Enhancement of the inhibitory effect of GABA on neuronal excitability results by increased neuronal membrane permeability to chloride ions. This shift in chloride ions results in hyperpolarization (a less excitable state) and stabilization. Benzodiazepine receptors and effects appear to be linked to the GABA-A receptors. Benzodiazepines do not bind to GABA-B receptors (Vinkers 2012).

Pharmacodynamics/Kinetics

Onset of Action Maximum effect: 5 to 9 days

Half-life Elimination Children: Clobazam: 16 hours (Ng 2007); Adults: Clobazam: 36 to 42 hours; N-desmethyl (active): 71 to 82 hours

Time to Peak Oral film: 0.33 to 4 hours; Tablet: 0.5 to 4 hours; Oral suspension: 0.5 to 2 hours

Pregnancy Considerations Clobazam crosses the placenta.

An increased risk of fetal malformations may be associated with first trimester benzodiazepine exposure (data not consistent). Exposure to benzodiazepines immediately prior to or during birth may result in hypothermia, hypotonia, respiratory depression, and difficulty feeding in the neonate; neonates exposed to benzodiazepines late in pregnancy may develop dependence and withdrawal. The incidence of premature birth and low birth weights may be increased following maternal use of benzodiazepines; hypoglycemia and respiratory problems in the neonate may occur following exposure late in pregnancy. Neonatal withdrawal symptoms may occur within days to weeks after birth and "floppy infant syndrome" (which also includes withdrawal symptoms) has been reported with some benzodiazepines (Bergman 1992; Iqbal 2002; Wikner 2007). A combination of factors influences the potential teratogenicity of anticonvulsant therapy. When treating women with epilepsy, monotherapy with the lowest effective dose and avoidance medications known to have a high incidence of teratogenic effects is recommended (Harden 2009; Wlodarczyk 2012).

Patients exposed to clobazam during pregnancy are encouraged to enroll themselves into the North American Antiepileptic Drug (NAAED) Pregnancy Registry by calling 1-888-233-2334. Additional information is available at www.aedpregnancyregistry.org.

Controlled Substance C-IV

Clobetasol (kloe BAY ta sol)

Related Information

Ulcerative, Erosive, and Painful Oral Mucosal Disorders *on page 1758*

Related Sample Prescriptions

Ulcerative and Erosive Disorders - Sample Prescriptions *on page 46*

Brand Names: US Clobetasol Propionate E; Clobex; Clobex Spray; Clodan; Cormax Scalp Application [DSC]; Impoyz; Olux; Olux-E; Tasoprol; Temovate; Temovate E [DSC]; Tovet

Brand Names: Canada APO-Clobetasol; Clobex; Clobex Spray; Dermovate; MYLAN-Clobetasol; NOVO-Clobetasol [DSC]; ODAN Clobetasol; Olux-E [DSC]; PMS-Clobetasol; Sandoz Clobetasol; TARO-Clobetasol; TARO-Clobetasol Topical; TEVA-Clobetasol

Generic Availability (US) May be product dependent

Pharmacologic Category Corticosteroid, Topical

Dental Use Short-term relief of oral mucosal inflammation

Use **Steroid-responsive dermatoses:** Short-term relief of inflammation and pruritic manifestations of moderate to severe corticosteroid-responsive dermatoses

Local Anesthetic/Vasoconstrictor Precautions No information available to require special precautions

Effects on Dental Treatment No significant effects or complications reported

Effects on Bleeding No information available to require special precautions

Adverse Reactions Frequency may depend upon formulation used, length of application, surface area covered, and the use of occlusive dressings.

>10%: Endocrine & metabolic: HPA-axis suppression (13% to 56%)

1% to 10%:

Central nervous system: Localized burning (≤10%), headache (≤2%), numbness of fingers (<2%), local discomfort (1%)

Dermatologic: Skin atrophy (≤4%), telangiectasia (≤3%), eczema (pruritus hiemalis: 2%), xeroderma (≤2%), erythema (<2%), folliculitis (<2%), pruritus (<2%), skin fissure (<2%), stinging of skin (<2%), hypopigmentation (1% to 2%)

Local: Application site reaction (2% to 4%), local irritation (<2%)

Respiratory: Upper respiratory tract infection (8%), nasopharyngitis (5%), streptococcal pharyngitis (1%)

Frequency not defined:

Dermatologic: Local acneiform eruptions, urticaria

Local: Application site edema

<1%, postmarketing, and/or case reports: Alopecia, application site induration, atrophic striae, cataract, contact dermatitis, Cushing syndrome, dermatitis, desquamation, exacerbation of psoriasis, excoriation, exfoliation of skin, eye irritation, glaucoma, hypertrichosis, increased intraocular pressure, indurated plaques of the skin, lichenoid eruption, miliaria, papule, perioral dermatitis, retinopathy (central serous), scalp pustules, scalp tightness, secondary infection, skin pain, skin rash, skin tenderness (scalp), tingling of skin (scalp)

Dental Usual Dosage Oral mucosal inflammation: Children ≥12 years and Adults: Cream: Apply twice daily for up to 2 weeks (maximum dose: 50 g/week); discontinue application when control is achieved; if no improvement is seen, reassessment of diagnosis may be necessary

Dosing

Adult & Geriatric Note: Discontinue when control achieved; if improvement not seen within 2 weeks, reassessment of diagnosis may be necessary.

Mild to moderate plaque-type psoriasis of nonscalp areas: Topical: *Foam:* Apply twice daily for up to 2 weeks (maximum dose: 50 g/week).

Moderate to severe plaque-type psoriasis: Topical:

Cream (0.025%), emollient cream, lotion: Apply twice daily for up to 2 weeks (cream) or up to 4 weeks if needed (emollient cream, lotion) when application is <10% of body surface area (maximum dose: 50 g/week or 50 mL/week). Treatment with lotion beyond 2 weeks should be limited to localized lesions (<10% body surface area) that have not improved sufficiently.

Spray: Apply by spraying directly onto affected area twice daily and gently rub into skin. Limit treatment to 4 consecutive weeks; treatment beyond 2 weeks should be limited to localized lesions that have not improved sufficiently. Maximum total dose: 50 g/week or 59 mL/week. Do not use more than 26 sprays per application or 52 sprays per day.

Oral mucosal inflammation (off-label use): Topical: *Cream:* Apply twice daily for up to 2 weeks (maximum dose: 50 g/week); discontinue application when control is achieved; if no improvement is seen, reassessment of diagnosis may be necessary.

Scalp psoriasis, moderate to severe: Topical:

Foam: Apply twice daily for up to 2 weeks (maximum dose: 50 g/week).

Shampoo: Apply thin film to dry scalp once daily (maximum dose: 50 g/week or 50 mL/week); leave in place for 15 minutes, then add water, lather, and rinse thoroughly. Limit treatment to 4 consecutive weeks.

Steroid-responsive dermatoses: Topical: *Cream (0.05%), emollient cream, emollient foam, foam, gel, lotion, ointment, solution:* Apply twice daily for up to 2 weeks (maximum dose: 50 g/week or 50 mL/week).

Renal Impairment: Adult There are no dosage adjustments provided in the manufacturer's labeling.

Hepatic Impairment: Adult There are no dosage adjustments provided in the manufacturer's labeling.

Pediatric Note: Dosage should be based on severity of disease and patient response; use the smallest amount for the shortest period of time to avoid HPA axis suppression; discontinue therapy when control is achieved; reassess diagnosis if no improvement is seen within 2 weeks. Due to the high incidence of adrenal suppression noted in clinical studies, clobetasol lotion, shampoo, and spray are not recommended for use in patients <18 years of age.

Dermatoses (steroid-responsive):

Cream 0.05%, emollient cream, gel, ointment: Children ≥12 years and Adolescents: Topical: Apply sparingly to affected area twice daily for up to 2 weeks; maximum weekly dose: 50 g/**week**.

Emollient foam: Children ≥12 years and Adolescents: Topical: Apply a thin layer to affected area twice daily in the morning and evening for up to 2 weeks; maximum weekly dose: 50 g/**week**.

Lotion: Adolescents ≥18 years: Topical: Apply twice daily for up to 2 weeks; maximum weekly dose: 50 g/**week** or 50 mL/**week**.

Solution: Children ≥12 years and Adolescents: Topical: Apply sparingly to affected area of scalp twice daily for up to 2 weeks; maximum weekly dose: 50 mL/**week**.

Plaque-type psoriasis of nonscalp areas, mild to moderate: Children ≥12 years and Adolescents: Foam: Topical: Apply thin layer to affected area twice daily for up to 2 weeks; maximum weekly dose: 50 g/**week** or 21 capfuls/**week**.

Plaque-type psoriasis, moderate to severe:

Cream 0.025%: Adolescents ≥18 years: Topical: Apply thin layer twice daily for up to 2 weeks; maximum weekly dose: 50 g/**week**.

Emollient cream: Adolescents ≥16 years: Topical: Apply sparingly twice daily for up to 2 weeks; if response is not adequate, may be used for up to 2 more weeks if application is <10% of BSA; use with caution; maximum weekly dose: 50 g/**week**.

Lotion: Adolescents ≥18 years: Topical: Apply twice daily for up to 2 weeks; may extend treatment for an additional 2 weeks for localized lesions <10% of BSA; maximum weekly dose: 50 g/**week** or 50 mL/**week**.

Spray: Adolescents ≥18 years: Apply by spraying directly onto affected area twice daily and gently rub into skin for up to 4 weeks; treatment beyond 2 weeks should be limited to localized lesions which have not improved sufficiently. Maximum weekly dose: 50 g/**week** or 59 mL/**week**. Do not use more than 26 sprays per application or 52 sprays per day.

Scalp psoriasis, moderate to severe:

Foam: Children ≥12 years and Adolescents: Topical: Apply thin layer twice daily for up to 2 weeks; maximum weekly dose: 50 g/**week** or 21 capfuls/**week**.

Shampoo: Adolescents ≥18 years: Topical: Apply thin film to affected area of dry scalp once daily for up to 4 weeks; maximum weekly dose: 50 g/**week** or 50 mL/**week**.

Renal Impairment: Pediatric There are no dosage adjustments provided in manufacturer's labeling.

Hepatic Impairment: Pediatric There are no dosage adjustments provided in manufacturer's labeling.

Mechanism of Action Topical corticosteroids have anti-inflammatory, antipruritic, and vasoconstrictive properties. May depress the formation, release, and activity of endogenous chemical mediators of inflammation (kinins, histamine, liposomal enzymes, prostaglandins) through the induction of phospholipase A_2 inhibitory proteins (lipocortins) and sequential inhibition of the release of arachidonic acid. Clobetasol has very high range potency.

Contraindications

Hypersensitivity to clobetasol, other corticosteroids, or any component of the formulation; primary infections of the scalp (scalp solution only)

Canadian labeling: Additional contraindications (not in US labeling): Treatment of rosacea, acne vulgaris, perioral dermatitis, or perianal and genital pruritus; viral (eg, herpes or varicella) lesions of the skin, bacterial or fungal skin infections, parasitic infections, skin manifestations relating to tuberculosis or syphilis, eruptions following vaccinations; ulcerous wounds; application to eyes or eyelids; children <2 years of age (shampoo); children <1 year of age (cream, ointment, scalp application). **Note:** Product labels may vary (refer also to product labels).

Warnings/Precautions Systemic absorption of topical corticosteroids may cause hypothalamic-pituitary-adrenal (HPA) axis suppression particularly in younger children. HPA axis suppression may lead to adrenal crisis. Allergic contact dermatitis may occur; it is usually diagnosed by failure to heal rather than clinical exacerbation. Prolonged treatment with corticosteroids has been associated with the development of Kaposi sarcoma (case reports); if noted, discontinuation of therapy should be considered. Local effects may occur, including folliculitis, acneiform eruptions, hypopigmentation, perioral dermatitis, allergic contact dermatitis, secondary infection, striae, miliaria, skin atrophy and telangiectasia; may be irreversible. Topical corticosteroids, including clobetasol, may increase the risk of posterior subcapsular cataracts and glaucoma. Monitor for ocular changes. Avoid contact with eyes. Concomitant skin infections may be present or develop during therapy; discontinue if dermatological infection persists despite appropriate antimicrobial therapy. Adverse systemic effects including Cushing syndrome, hyperglycemia, glycosuria, and HPA suppression may occur when used on large surface areas, denuded skin, or with an occlusive dressing. Use in children <12 years of age is not recommended. Children may absorb proportionally larger amounts after topical application and may be more prone to systemic effects. Prolonged use may affect growth velocity; growth should be routinely monitored in pediatric patients. Clobex lotion, Clobex shampoo, Clobex spray, and Clodan shampoo are not recommended for use in pediatric patients ≤17 years.

Do not use on the face, axillae, or groin or for the treatment of acne vulgaris, rosacea or perioral dermatitis. Emollient cream contains imidurea; may cause allergic sensitization or irritation upon skin contact with the skin. Foam and spray are flammable; do not use near open flame.

Warnings: Additional Pediatric Considerations The extent of percutaneous absorption is dependent on several factors, including epidermal integrity (intact vs abraded skin), formulation, age of the patient, prolonged duration of use, and the use of occlusive dressings. Percutaneous absorption of topical steroids is increased in neonates (especially preterm neonates), infants, and young children. Infants and small children may be more susceptible to HPA axis suppression, intracranial hypertension, Cushing syndrome, or other systemic toxicities due to larger skin surface area to body mass ratio. Due to the high incidence of adrenal suppression noted in clinical studies, clobetasol lotion, shampoo, and spray are not recommended for use in patients <18 years of age. In a study of patients with moderate to severe atopic dermatitis (involving ≥20% BSA) receiving Clobex 0.05% lotion twice daily for 2 weeks, 9 of the14 pediatric patients (12 to 17 years of age) included developed adrenal suppression, compared to 2 of the 10 pediatric patients receiving the cream. In a study of patients receiving Clobex 0.05% shampoo, 5 of 12 pediatric patients (12 to 17 years of age) developed HPA axis suppression.

Some dosage forms may contain propylene glycol; in neonates, large amounts of propylene glycol delivered orally, intravenously (eg, >3,000 mg/day), or topically have been associated with potentially fatal toxicities which can include metabolic acidosis, seizures, renal failure, and CNS depression; toxicities have also been reported in children and adults including hyperosmolality, lactic acidosis, seizures, and respiratory depression; use caution (AAP 1997; Shehab 2009).

Drug Interactions

Metabolism/Transport Effects None known.

Avoid Concomitant Use

Avoid concomitant use of Clobetasol with any of the following: Aldesleukin

Increased Effect/Toxicity

Clobetasol may increase the levels/effects of: Deferasirox; Ritodrine

Decreased Effect

Clobetasol may decrease the levels/effects of: Aldesleukin; Corticorelin; Hyaluronidase

Pregnancy Considerations

Information related to the use of clobetasol in pregnancy is limited (Westermann 2012).

Systemic bioavailability of topical corticosteroids is variable (integrity of skin, use of occlusion, etc.) and may be further influenced by trimester of pregnancy (Chi 2017). In general, the use of topical corticosteroids is not associated with a significant risk of adverse pregnancy outcomes. However, there may be an increased risk of low birth weight infants following maternal use of potent or very potent topical products, especially in high doses. Use of mild to moderate potency topical corticosteroids is preferred in pregnant females and the use of large amounts or use for prolonged periods of time should be avoided (Chi 2016; Chi 2017; Murase 2014). Also avoid areas of high percutaneous absorption (Chi 2017). The risk of stretch marks may be increased with use of topical corticosteroids (Murase 2014).

The treatment of psoriasis in pregnancy is initiated with conservative treatment as in nonpregnant females. When a topical steroid is needed, low to moderate potency corticosteroids are preferred initially. High potency topical steroids should be used only when clearly needed and after the first trimester (Bae 2012).

Breastfeeding Considerations

Systemic corticosteroids are present in human milk. It is not known if topical application of clobetasol will result in detectable quantities in breast milk.

Information related to the use of clobetasol and breastfeeding is limited (Carrillo Dde 2006). According to the manufacturer, the decision to breastfeed during therapy should consider the risk of infant exposure, the benefits of breastfeeding to the infant, and benefits of treatment to the mother. Low to moderate potency topical corticosteroids are preferred for initial treatment of psoriasis in breastfeeding females (Bae 2012). Do not apply topical corticosteroids to breast until breastfeeding ceases (Leachman 2006); hypertension was noted in a breastfed infant when a high potency topical corticosteroid was applied to the nipple (Butler 2014; Leachman 2006).

Product Availability Impeklo 0.05% lotion: FDA approved May 2020; anticipated availability currently unknown. Information pertaining to this product within the monograph is pending revision. Impeklo is indicated for the relief of the inflammatory and pruritic manifestations of corticosteroid-responsive dermatoses.

Dosage Forms: US

Cream, External:
Clobetasol Propionate E: 0.05% (15 g, 30 g, 60 g)
Impoyz: 0.025% (100 g)
Temovate: 0.05% (30 g, 60 g)
Generic: 0.05% (15 g, 30 g, 45 g, 60 g)

Foam, External:
Olux: 0.05% (50 g, 100 g)
Olux-E: 0.05% (50 g, 100 g)
Tovet: 0.05% (100 g)
Generic: 0.05% (50 g, 100 g)

Gel, External:
Generic: 0.05% (15 g, 30 g, 60 g)

Kit, External:
Clodan: 0.05%
Tasoprol: 0.05%
Tovet: 0.05%

Liquid, External:
Clobex Spray: 0.05% (59 mL, 125 mL)
Generic: 0.05% (59 mL, 125 mL)

Lotion, External:
Clobex: 0.05% (59 mL, 118 mL)
Generic: 0.05% (59 mL, 118 mL)

Ointment, External:
Temovate: 0.05% (15 g, 30 g)
Generic: 0.05% (15 g, 30 g, 45 g, 60 g)

Shampoo, External:
Clobex: 0.05% (118 mL)
Clodan: 0.05% (118 mL)
Generic: 0.05% (118 mL)

Solution, External:
Generic: 0.05% (25 mL, 50 mL)

Dosage Forms: Canada

Cream, External:
Dermovate: 0.05% (15 g, 50 g)
Generic: 0.05% (15 g, 30 g, 50 g, 450 g, 454 g)

Liquid, External:
Clobex Spray: 0.05% (59 mL, 125 mL)
Generic: 0.05% (59 mL)

Ointment, External:
Dermovate: 0.05% (15 g, 50 g)
Generic: 0.05% (15 g, 50 g, 450 g, 454 g)

Shampoo, External:
Clobex: 0.05% (15 mL, 118 mL)

Solution, External:
Dermovate: 0.05% (20 mL, 60 mL)
Generic: 0.05% (20 mL, 59 mL, 60 mL, 90 mL)

◆ **Clobetasol Propionate** *see* Clobetasol *on page 377*

◆ **Clobetasol Propionate E** *see* Clobetasol *on page 377*

◆ **Clobex** *see* Clobetasol *on page 377*

◆ **Clobex Spray** *see* Clobetasol *on page 377*

◆ **Clodan** *see* Clobetasol *on page 377*

Clodronate (KLOE droh nate)

Related Information

Osteonecrosis of the Jaw *on page 1699*

Brand Names: Canada Bonefos [DSC]; Clasteon

Pharmacologic Category Bisphosphonate Derivative

Use Note: Not approved in the US

Hypercalcemia of malignancy: Management of hypercalcemia of malignancy

Osteolytic bone metastases: Adjunct in the management of osteolysis due to bone metastases of malignant tumors

Local Anesthetic/Vasoconstrictor Precautions
No information available to require special precautions

Effects on Dental Treatment Osteonecrosis of the jaw (ONJ), generally associated with local infection and/or tooth extraction and often with delayed healing, has been reported in patients taking bisphosphonates. Symptoms included nonhealing extraction socket or an exposed jawbone. Most reported cases of bisphosphonate-associated osteonecrosis have been in cancer patients treated with intravenous bisphosphonates. However, some have occurred in patients with postmenopausal osteoporosis taking oral bisphosphonates. Dental surgery, particularly tooth extraction, may increase the risk for ONJ. Patients who develop ONJ while on bisphosphonate therapy should receive care by an oral surgeon. See Dental Health Professional Considerations.

Effects on Bleeding No information available to require special precautions

Adverse Reactions

>10%: Hepatic: Increased serum transaminases (postmenopausal osteopenic women: 18%; >2 x ULN: 2%)

1% to 10%:

Cardiovascular: Cardiac failure (1%)

Endocrine & metabolic: Hypocalcemia (2% to 3%)

Gastrointestinal: Gastrointestinal disease (≤10%; includes stomach pain), nausea (3%), diarrhea (2%), anorexia (1%)

Neuromuscular & skeletal: Bone fracture (1%)

Renal: Increased serum creatinine (1%)

Respiratory: Pneumonia (1%)

<1%, postmarketing, and/or case reports: Arthralgia (severe), bronchospasm (patients with aspirin-sensitive asthma), conjunctivitis, dysphagia, erythematous rash, femur fracture (atypical subtrochanteric and diaphyseal), hypersensitivity reactions (angioedema, dyspnea [in patients with aspirin-sensitive asthma], pruritus, respiratory disorder, skin rash, urticaria), hypophosphatemia (transient), increased liver enzymes, increased parathyroid hormone, leukemia (rare), maculopapular rash, mouth irritation, myalgia (severe), myelodysplasia (rare), oropharyngeal ulcer, ostealgia (severe), osteonecrosis (jaw or external auditory canal), proteinuria, renal failure, renal insufficiency, uveitis

Mechanism of Action A bisphosphonate that lowers serum calcium by inhibition of bone resorption via actions on osteoclasts or on osteoclast precursors; may also have indirect inhibitory effects through osteoblastic cells, which control recruitment and activity of osteoclasts.

Pharmacodynamics/Kinetics

Onset of Action Calcium-lowering effects: IV: Within 48 hours

Duration of Action Calcium-lowering effects: 5 days to 3 weeks following discontinuation

Half-life Elimination Terminal: Oral: ~6 hours; IV: 13 hours (serum); prolonged in bone tissue

Time to Peak Plasma: Oral: 30 minutes

Reproductive Considerations
Bisphosphonates are incorporated into the bone matrix and gradually released over time. Because exposure prior to pregnancy may theoretically increase the risk of fetal harm, most sources recommend discontinuing bisphosphonate therapy in females of reproductive potential as early as possible prior to a planned pregnancy. Use in premenopausal females should be reserved for special circumstances when rapid bone loss is occurring; a bisphosphonate with the shortest half-life should then be used (Bhalla 2010; Pereira 2012; Stathopoulos 2011).

Pregnancy Considerations Use is contraindicated during pregnancy.

It is not known if bisphosphonates cross the placenta, but based on their lower molecular weight, fetal exposure is expected (Djokanovic 2008; Stathopoulos 2011).

Bisphosphonates are incorporated into the bone matrix and gradually released over time. The amount available in the systemic circulation varies by drug, dose, and duration of therapy. Theoretically, there may be a risk of fetal harm when pregnancy follows the completion of therapy (hypocalcemia, low birth weight, and decreased gestation have been observed in some case reports); however, available data have not shown that exposure to bisphosphonates during pregnancy significantly increases the risk of adverse fetal events (Djokanovic 2008; Green 2014; Levy 2009; Machairiotis 2019; Sokal 2019; Stathopoulos 2011). Exposed infants should be monitored for hypocalcemia after birth (Djokanovic 2008; Stathopoulos 2011).

Product Availability Not available in the US

Dental Health Professional Considerations A review of 2,408 published cases of bisphosphonate-associated osteonecrosis of the jaw bone (BP-associated ONJ) was done by Filleul 2010. BP therapy was associated with 89% of the cases to treat malignancies and 11% of the cases to treat nonmalignant conditions. Information on the specific bisphosphonate used was available for 1,694 of the patients. Intravenous therapy (primarily zoledronic acid) was received by 88% of the patients and 12% received oral treatment (primarily alendronate). Of all the cases of BP-associated ONJ, 67% were preceded by tooth extraction and for 26% of patients, there was no predisposing factor identified.

A 2010 retrospective case review reported the prevalence of BP-associated ONJ in patients using alendronate-type drugs was 1 out of 952 patients or ~0.1% (Lo 2010). Of the 8,572 respondents, nine cases of ONJ were identified; five had developed ONJ spontaneously and four developed ONJ after tooth extraction. When extrapolated to patient-years of bisphosphonate exposure, this prevalence rate of 0.1% equates to a frequency of 28 cases per 100,000 person-years of oral bisphosphonate treatment. An Australian group (Mavrokokki 2007), identified the frequency of BP-associated ONJ in osteoporotic patients, mainly taking weekly oral alendronate, was 1 in 8,470 to 1 in 2,260 (0.01% to 0.04%) patients. If extractions were carried out, the calculated frequency was 1 in 1,130 to 1 in 296 (0.09% to 0.34%) patients. The median time to onset of ONJ in alendronate patients was 24 months.

According to the 2011 report by the American Dental Association (ADA), the incidence of BP-associated ONJ remains low and the benefits of using oral bisphosphonates significantly outweighs the risk of developing BP-associated ONJ for treatment and prevention of osteoporosis and cancer treatment (Hellstein 2011). The full 47-page report can be accessed at http://www.ada.org/~/media/ADA/Member%20Center/FIles/topics_ARONJ_report.ashx.

The ADA review of 2011 stated the incidence of oral BP-associated ONJ was one case for every 1,000 individuals exposed to oral bisphosphonates (0.1%) (Hellstein 2011).

The most comprehensive review to date on osteonecrosis of the jaw bone (ONJ) has been published in the *Journal of Bone and Mineral Research* (Khan 2015), and written by an International Task Force of authors, totaling 34, from academe; industry; clinical medical and dental practice; oral and maxillofacial surgery; bone and mineral research; epidemiology; medical and dental oncology; orthopedic surgery; osteoporosis research; muscle and bone research; endocrinology and diagnostic sciences. The work provides a systematic review of the literature and international consensus on the classification, incidence, pathophysiology, diagnosis, and management of ONJ in both oncology and osteoporosis patient populations. This review of the literature from January 2003 to April 2014, with 299 references, offers recommendations for management of ONJ based on multidisciplinary international consensus.

Prevalence and incidence of ONJ in osteoporosis patients from the Task Force report:

Prevalence – the percent of osteoporotic population affected with ONJ

After reviewing all literature reports on this subject, the Task Force concluded that the prevalence of ONJ in patients prescribed oral BPs for the treatment of osteoporosis ranges from 0% to 0.04% with the majority being below 0.001%. However, the Task Force does cite the study of (Lo et al) that evaluated the Kaiser Permanente database and found the prevalence of ONJ in those receiving BPs for more than 2 years to range from 0.05% to 0.21% and appeared to be related to duration of exposure. As mentioned above, the American Dental Association has previously reported that the prevalence of ONJ in osteoporosis patients using oral BPs to be 1 out of 1,000 or 0.1% (Hellstein 2011).

Incidence - the rate at which ONJ occurs or the number of times it happens

From currently available data, the incidence of ONJ in the osteoporosis patient population appears to be low ranging from 0.15% to less than 0.001% person-years drug exposure. In terms of the osteoporosis patient population taking oral BPs, the incidence ranges from 1.04 to 69 per 100,000 patient years of drug exposure.

◆ **Clodronate Disodium** *see* Clodronate *on page* 380

Clofarabine (klo FARE a been)

Brand Names: US Clolar
Brand Names: Canada Clolar
Pharmacologic Category Antineoplastic Agent, Antimetabolite; Antineoplastic Agent, Antimetabolite (Purine Analog)

Use Acute lymphoblastic leukemia, relapsed or refractory: Treatment of relapsed or refractory acute lymphoblastic leukemia (ALL) in patients 1 to 21 years of age (after at least 2 prior regimens)

Local Anesthetic/Vasoconstrictor Precautions No information available to require special precautions

Effects on Dental Treatment Key adverse event(s) related to dental treatment: Mucosal inflammation and gingival bleeding.

Effects on Bleeding Chemotherapy may result in significant myelosuppression, potentially including significant reduction in platelet counts and altered hemostasis. In patients who are under active treatment with these agents, medical consult is suggested.

Due to the thrombocytopenic effects of clofarabine, an increased risk of bleeding may be seen in patients receiving concomitant NSAIDs (including aspirin).

Adverse Reactions Incidences include off-label use in the treatment of AML.

>10%:

- Cardiovascular: Tachycardia (35%), hypotension (29%), flushing (19%), hypertension (13%), edema (12%)
- Central nervous system: Headache (43%), chills (34%), fatigue (34%), anxiety (21%), pain (15%)
- Dermatologic: Pruritus (43%), skin rash (38%), palmar-plantar erythrodysesthesia (16%), erythema (11%)
- Gastrointestinal: Vomiting (78%), nausea (73%), diarrhea (56%), abdominal pain (35%), anorexia (30%), gingival bleeding (17%), mucosal inflammation (16%), oral candidiasis (11%)
- Genitourinary: Hematuria (13%)
- Hematologic & oncologic: Leukopenia (88%; grades 3/4: 88%), anemia (83%; grades 3/4: 75%), lymphocytopenia (82%; grades 3/4: 82%), thrombocytopenia (81%; grades 3/4: 80%), neutropenia (10% to 64%; grades 3/4: 64%; grade 4: 7%), febrile neutropenia (55%; grade 3: 51%; grade 4: 3%), petechia (26%; grade 3: 6%)
- Hepatic: Increased serum ALT (81%), increased serum AST (74%), increased bilirubin (45%)
- Infection: Infection (83%; includes bacterial, fungal, and viral), sepsis (including septic shock; 17%)
- Local: Catheter infection (12%)
- Neuromuscular & skeletal: Limb pain (30%), myalgia (14%)
- Renal: Increased serum creatinine (50%)
- Respiratory: Epistaxis (27%), dyspnea (13%), pleural effusion (12%)
- Miscellaneous: Fever (39%)

1% to 10%:

- Cardiovascular: Pericardial effusion (8%), capillary leak syndrome (4%)
- Central nervous system: Drowsiness (10%), irritability (10%), lethargy (10%), agitation (5%), mental status changes (1% to 4%)
- Dermatologic: Cellulitis (8%), pruritic rash (8%)
- Gastrointestinal: Rectal pain (8%), upper abdominal pain (8%), pseudomembranous colitis (7%), stomatitis (7%), pancreatitis (1% to 4%), typhlitis (1% to 4%)
- Hematologic & oncologic: Tumor lysis syndrome (6%; grade 3: 6%), oral mucosal petechiae (5%; grade 3: 4%)
- Hepatic: Jaundice (8%), hyperbilirubinemia (1% to 4%), hepatic sinusoidal obstruction syndrome (formerly known as hepatic veno-occlusive disease: 2%)
- Hypersensitivity: Hypersensitivity (1% to 4%)

Infection: Herpes simplex infection (10%), bacteremia (9%), candidiasis (7%), herpes zoster (7%), staphylococcal bacteremia (6%), staphylococcal sepsis (5%), influenza (1% to 4%), sepsis syndrome (2%)

Neuromuscular & skeletal: Back pain (10%), ostealgia (10%), weakness (10%), arthralgia (9%)

Renal: Acute renal failure

Respiratory: Pneumonia (10%), respiratory distress (10%), tachypnea (9%), upper respiratory tract infection (5%), pulmonary edema (1% to 4%), sinusitis (1% to 4%)

<1%, postmarketing, and/or case reports: Enterocolitis (occurs more frequently within 30 days of treatment and with combination chemotherapy), exfoliative dermatitis, gastrointestinal hemorrhage, hallucination (Jeha 2006), hepatic failure, hepatitis, hepatomegaly (Jeha 2006), hypokalemia (Jeha 2006), hyponatremia, hypophosphatemia, increased right ventricular pressure (Jeha 2006), left ventricular systolic dysfunction (Jeha 2006), major hemorrhage (including cerebral and pulmonary; majority of cases associated with thrombocytopenia), Stevens-Johnson syndrome, toxic epidermal necrolysis

Mechanism of Action Clofarabine, a purine (deoxyadenosine) nucleoside analog, is metabolized to clofarabine 5'-triphosphate. Clofarabine 5'-triphosphate decreases cell replication and repair as well as causing cell death. To decrease cell replication and repair, clofarabine 5'-triphosphate competes with deoxyadenosine triphosphate for the enzymes ribonucleotide reductase and DNA polymerase. Cell replication is decreased when clofarabine 5'-triphosphate inhibits ribonucleotide reductase from reacting with deoxyadenosine triphosphate to produce deoxynucleotide triphosphate which is needed for DNA synthesis. Cell replication is also decreased when clofarabine 5'-triphosphate competes with DNA polymerase for incorporation into the DNA chain; when done during the repair process, cell repair is affected. To cause cell death, clofarabine 5'-triphosphate alters the mitochondrial membrane by releasing proteins, an inducing factor and cytochrome C.

Pharmacodynamics/Kinetics

Half-life Elimination Children and Adolescents 2 to 19 years: 5.2 hours; Children and Adults: 7 hours; may be prolonged in in the elderly and in patients with renal impairment (Bonate, 2011)

Reproductive Considerations

Evaluate pregnancy status prior to use in females of reproductive potential. Females of reproductive potential should use effective contraception during therapy and for ≥6 months after the last clofarabine dose. Males with female partners of reproductive potential should use effective contraception during therapy and for ≥3 months after the last dose of clofarabine.

Pregnancy Considerations

Based on the mechanism of action and data from animal reproduction studies, in utero exposure to clofarabine may cause fetal harm.

◆ **Clofarex** *see* Clofarabine *on page* 381

◆ **Clolar** *see* Clofarabine *on page* 381

◆ **Clomid** *see* ClomiPHENE *on page* 382

ClomiPHENE (KLOE mi feen)

Brand Names: Canada Clomid [DSC]; Serophene [DSC]

Pharmacologic Category Ovulation Stimulator; Selective Estrogen Receptor Modulator (SERM)

Use Treatment of ovulatory dysfunction: Treatment of ovulatory dysfunction in women desiring pregnancy

Local Anesthetic/Vasoconstrictor Precautions No information available to require special precautions

Effects on Dental Treatment No significant effects or complications reported

Effects on Bleeding No information available to require special precautions

Adverse Reactions

>10%: Endocrine & metabolic: Ovary enlargement (14%)

1% to 10%:

Central nervous system: Headache (1%)

Endocrine & metabolic: Hot flash (10%)

Gastrointestinal: Abdominal distention (≤6%), abdominal distress (≤6%), bloating (≤6%), nausea (≤2%), vomiting (≤2%)

Genitourinary: Breast disease (discomfort: 2%), abnormal uterine bleeding (1%)

Ophthalmic: Visual disturbance (2%)

<1%, postmarketing/case reports: Accommodation disturbance, acne vulgaris, alopecia, anxiety, arthralgia, back pain, cardiac arrhythmia, cataract, cerebrovascular accident, chest pain, constipation, depression, dermatitis, diarrhea, dizziness, dry hair, dyspnea, ectopic pregnancy, edema, endometriosis, endometrium disease (reduced thickness), erythema, erythema multiforme, erythema nodosum, eye pain, fatigue, fever, hepatitis, hypersensitivity reaction, hypertension, hypertrichosis, hypertriglyceridemia, increased appetite, increased serum transaminases, increased urine output, insomnia, irritability, leukocytosis, macular edema, migraine, mood changes, myalgia, neoplasm, nervousness, optic neuritis, ovarian cyst, ovarian hemorrhage, ovarian hyperstimulation syndrome, palpitations, pancreatitis, paresthesia, phlebitis, photopsia, pruritus, psychosis, pulmonary embolism, retinal hemorrhage, retinal thrombosis, retinal vascular spasm, seizure, severe abdominal pain, skin rash, syncope, tachycardia, thrombophlebitis, thyroid disease, tinnitus, urinary frequency, urticaria, uterine hemorrhage, vaginal dryness, vertigo, vision loss (temporary/prolonged), vitreous detachment (posterior), weakness, weight gain, weight loss

Mechanism of Action Clomiphene is a racemic mixture consisting of zuclomiphene (~38%) and enclomiphene (~62%), each with distinct pharmacologic properties. Clomiphene acts at the level of the hypothalamus, occupying cell surface and intracellular estrogen receptors (ERs) for longer durations than estrogen. This interferes with receptor recycling, effectively depleting hypothalamic ERs and inhibiting normal estrogenic negative feedback. Impairment of the feedback signal results in increased pulsatile GnRH secretion from the hypothalamus and subsequent pituitary gonadotropin (FSH, LH) release, causing growth of the ovarian follicle, followed by follicular rupture (ASRM 2013; Dickey 1996).

Pharmacodynamics/Kinetics

Onset of Action Ovulation: 5 to 10 days following course of treatment

Duration of Action Effects are cumulative; ovulation may occur in the cycle following the last treatment (Dickey 1996)

Half-life Elimination ~5 days (Goldstein 2000)

Time to Peak ~6 hours (Goldstein 2000)

Pregnancy Considerations
Use is contraindicated in females who are already pregnant.

The incidence of adverse fetal effects following maternal use of clomiphene for ovulation induction is similar to those seen in the general population.

◆ **Clomiphene Citrate** *see* ClomiPHENE *on page 382*

ClomiPRAMINE (kloe MI pra meen)

Related Information
Dentin Hypersensitivity, Acid Erosion, High Caries Index, Management of Alveolar Osteitis, and Xerostomia *on page 1762*
Vasoconstrictor Interactions With Antidepressants *on page 1821*

Brand Names: US Anafranil

Brand Names: Canada Anafranil; DOM-ClomiPRAMINE [DSC]; MED ClomiPRAMINE; PMS-Clomipramine [DSC]; TARO-Clomipramine

Pharmacologic Category Antidepressant, Tricyclic (Tertiary Amine)

Use Obsessive-compulsive disorder: Treatment of obsessive-compulsive disorder

Local Anesthetic/Vasoconstrictor Precautions Use with caution; epinephrine and levonordefrin have been shown to have an increased pressor response in combination with TCAs. Clomipramine is one of the drugs confirmed to prolong the QT interval and is accepted as having a risk of causing torsade de pointes. The risk of drug-induced torsade de pointes is extremely low when a single QT interval prolonging drug is prescribed. In terms of epinephrine, it is not known what effect vasoconstrictors in the local anesthetic regimen will have in patients with a known history of congenital prolonged QT interval or in patients taking any medication that prolongs the QT interval. Until more information is obtained, it is suggested that the clinician consult with the physician prior to the use of a vasoconstrictor in suspected patients, and that the vasoconstrictor (epinephrine, mepivacaine and levonordefrin [Carbocaine® 2% with Neo-Cobefrin®]) be used with caution.

Effects on Dental Treatment Key adverse event(s) related to dental treatment: Xerostomia and changes in salivation (normal salivary flow resumes upon discontinuation). Long-term treatment with TCAs, such as clomipramine, increases the risk of caries by reducing salivation and salivary buffer capacity.

Effects on Bleeding No information available to require special precautions

Adverse Reactions

>10%:

Central nervous system: Dizziness (adults: 54%; children and adolescents: 41%), drowsiness (46% to 54%), headache (adults: 52%), fatigue (35% to 39%), insomnia (adults: 25%; children and adolescents: 11%), nervousness (adults: 18%; children and adolescents: 4%), myoclonus (adults: 13%; children and adolescents: 2%)

Dermatologic: Diaphoresis (adults: 29%; children and adolescents: 9%)

Endocrine & metabolic: Change in libido (adults: 21%), weight gain (adults: 18%; children and adolescents: 2%)

Gastrointestinal: Xerostomia (adults: 84%, children and adolescents: 63%), constipation (adults: 47%; children and adolescents: 22%), nausea (adults: 33%), dyspepsia (13% to 22%), anorexia (12% to 22%), diarrhea (7% to 13%), abdominal pain (adults: 11%), increased appetite (adults: 11%)

Genitourinary: Ejaculation failure (adults: 42%, children and adolescents: 6%), impotence (adults: 20%), difficulty in micturition (adults: 14%; children and adolescents: 4%)

Neuromuscular & skeletal: Tremor (adults: 54%; children and adolescents: 33%), myalgia (adults: 13%)

Ophthalmic: Visual disturbance (adults: 18%; children and adolescents: 7%)

Respiratory: Pharyngitis (adults: 14%), rhinitis (adults: 12%)

1% to 10%:

Cardiovascular: Flushing (7% to 8%), chest pain (children and adolescents: 7%), orthostatic hypotension (children, adolescents, and adults: 4% to 6%), palpitations (4%), tachycardia (children, adolescents, and adults: 2% to 4%), ECG abnormality (2%), syncope (children and adolescents: 2%)

Central nervous system: Anxiety (adults: 9%; children and adolescents: 2%), paresthesia (adults: 9%), memory impairment (7% to 9%), sleep disorder (4% to 9%), twitching (adults: 7%), depression (adults: 5%), lack of concentration (adults: 5%), pain (3% to 4%), hypertonia (2% to 4%), abnormal dreams (adults: 3%), agitation (adults: 3%), migraine (adults: 3%), psychosomatic disorder (adults: 3%), speech disturbance (adults: 3%), yawning (adults: 3%), confusion (2% to 3%), aggressive behavior (children and adolescents: 2%), chills (adults: 2%), depersonalization (2%), emotional lability (adults: 2%), irritability (children and adolescents: 2%), paresis (children and adolescents: 2%), myasthenia (1% to 2%), panic attack (1% to 2%), abnormality in thinking (≥1%), vertigo (≥1%), seizure (≤1%)

Dermatologic: Skin rash (4% to 8%), pruritus (adults: 6%), body odor (children and adolescents: 2%), dermatitis (adults: 2%), xeroderma (adults: 2%), urticaria (adults: 1%)

Endocrine & metabolic: Weight loss (children and adolescents: 7%), hot flash (2% to 5%), menstrual disease (adults: 4%), amenorrhea (adults: 1%)

Gastrointestinal: Dysgeusia (4% to 8%), vomiting (7%), flatulence (adults: 6%), aphthous stomatitis (children and adolescents: 2%), dysphagia (adults: 2%), gastrointestinal disease (adults: 2%), halitosis (children and adolescents: 2%), esophagitis (adults: 1%)

Genitourinary: Urinary retention (children and adolescents: 7%; adults: 2%), urinary tract infection (adults: 6%), urinary frequency (adults: 5%), lactation (nonpuerperal; adults: 4%), breast hypertrophy (adults: 2%), cystitis (adults: 2%), leukorrhea (adults: 2%), vaginitis (adults: 2%), mastalgia (adults: 1%)

Hematologic & oncologic: Purpuric disease (adults: 3%)

Hepatic: Increased serum alanine aminotransferase (>3 x ULN: 3%), increased serum aspartate aminotransferase (>3 x ULN: 1%)

Hypersensitivity: Hypersensitivity reaction (children and adolescents: 7%)

Neuromuscular & skeletal: Asthenia (1% to 2%)

Ophthalmic: Abnormal lacrimation (adults: 3%), anisocoria (children and adolescents: 2%), blepharospasm (children and adolescents: 2%), mydriasis (adults: 2%), ocular allergy (children and adolescents: 2%), conjunctivitis (adults: 1%)

Otic: Tinnitus (4% to 6%)

Respiratory: Bronchospasm (children and adolescents: 7%; adults: 2%), sinusitis (adults: 6%), dyspnea (children and adolescents: 2%), epistaxis (adults: 2%), laryngitis (children and adolescents: 2%)

Miscellaneous: Fever (adults: 4%)

<1%, postmarketing, and/or case reports: Abnormal electroencephalogram, abnormal sensory symptoms, accommodation disturbance, acute myocardial infarction, agranulocytosis, albuminuria, alopecia, altered sense of smell, anemia, aneurysm, angle-closure glaucoma, anticholinergic syndrome, apathy, aphasia, apraxia, ataxia, atrial flutter, blepharitis, blood in stool, bone marrow depression, bradycardia, brain disease, breast fibroadenosis, bronchitis, bundle branch block, cardiac arrhythmia, cardiac failure, catatonic-like state, cellulitis, cerebral hemorrhage, cervical dysplasia, cheilitis, chloasma, cholinergic syndrome, choreoathetosis, chromatopsia, chronic enteritis, colitis, coma, conjunctival hemorrhage, cyanosis, deafness, dehydration, delirium, delusions, dental caries, dermal ulcer, diabetes mellitus, diplopia, drug reaction with eosinophilia and systemic symptoms, duodenitis, dyskinesia, dystonia, eczema, edema, edema (oral), endometrial hyperplasia, endometriosis, enlargement of salivary glands, epididymitis, erythematous rash, exophthalmos, exostosis, extrapyramidal reaction, extrasystoles, gastric dilation, gastric ulcer, gastroesophageal reflux disease, glycosuria, goiter, gout, gynecomastia, hallucination, heart block, hematuria, hemiparesis, hemoptysis, hepatic injury (severe), hepatitis, hostility, hyperacusis, hypercholesterolemia, hyperesthesia, hyperglycemia, hyperkinetic muscle activity, hyperreflexia, hyperthermia, hyperthyroidism, hyperuricemia, hyperventilation, hypnogenic hallucinations, hypoesthesia, hypokalemia, hypokinesia, hyponatremia, hypothyroidism, hypoventilation, intestinal obstruction, irritable bowel syndrome, ischemic heart disease, keratitis, laryngismus, leukemoid reaction, leukopenia, local inflammation (uterine), lupus erythematous-like rash, lymphadenopathy, maculopapular rash, manic reaction, muscle spasm, mutism, myopathy, myositis, nephrolithiasis, neuralgia, neuropathy, nocturnal amblyopia, oculogyric crisis, oculomotor nerve paralysis, ovarian cyst, pancytopenia, paralytic ileus, paranoid ideation, peptic ulcer, periarteritis nodosa, peripheral ischemia, pharyngeal edema, phobia, photophobia, pneumonia, premature ejaculation, pseudolymphoma, psoriasis, psychosis, pyelonephritis, pyuria, rectal hemorrhage, renal cyst, schizophreniform disorder, scleritis, serotonin syndrome, SIADH, skin hypertrophy, skin photosensitivity, somnambulism, strabismus, stupor, suicidal ideation, suicidal tendencies, teeth clenching, thrombocytopenia, thrombophlebitis, tongue ulcer, torticollis, urinary incontinence, uterine hemorrhage, vaginal hemorrhage, vasospasm, ventricular tachycardia, visual field defect, voice disorder, withdrawal syndrome

Mechanism of Action Clomipramine appears to affect serotonin uptake while its active metabolite, desmethylclomipramine, affects norepinephrine uptake

Pharmacodynamics/Kinetics

Onset of Action

Anxiety disorders (obsessive-compulsive, panic disorder): Initial effects may be observed within 2 weeks of treatment, with continued improvements through 4 to 6 weeks (Varigonda 2016; WFSBP [Bandelow 2012]); some experts suggest up to 12 weeks of treatment may be necessary for response, particularly in patients with obsessive-compulsive disorder (BAP [Baldwin 2014]; Katzman 2014; WFSBP [Bandelow 2012]).

Depression: Initial effects may be observed within 1 to 2 weeks of treatment, with continued improvements through 4 to 6 weeks (Papakostas 2006; Posternak 2005; Szegedi 2009).

Duration of Action 1 to 2 days

Half-life Elimination Adults (following a 150 mg dose): Clomipramine 19 to 37 hours (mean: 32 hours); DMI: 54 to 77 hours (mean: 69 hours)

Time to Peak 2 to 6 hours

Pregnancy Risk Factor C

Pregnancy Considerations

Clomipramine and its metabolite desmethylclomipramine cross the placenta and can be detected in cord blood and neonatal serum at birth (Loughhead 2006; ter Horst 2012). Data from five newborns found the half-life for clomipramine in the neonate to be 42 ± 16 hours following in utero exposure. Serum concentrations were not found to correlate to withdrawal symptoms (ter Horst 2012). Withdrawal symptoms (including jitteriness, tremor, and seizures) have been observed in neonates whose mothers took clomipramine up to delivery.

The ACOG recommends that therapy for depression during pregnancy be individualized; treatment should incorporate the clinical expertise of the mental health clinician, obstetrician, primary health care provider, and pediatrician (ACOG 2008). According to the American Psychiatric Association (APA), the risks of medication treatment should be weighed against other treatment options and untreated depression. For women who discontinue antidepressant medications during pregnancy and who may be at high risk for postpartum depression, the medications can be restarted following delivery (APA 2010). Treatment algorithms have been developed by the ACOG and the APA for the management of depression in women prior to conception and during pregnancy (Yonkers 2009).

Data collection to monitor pregnancy and infant outcomes following exposure to clomipramine is ongoing. Pregnant women exposed to antidepressants during pregnancy are encouraged to enroll in the National Pregnancy Registry for Antidepressants (NPRAD). Women 18 to 45 years of age or their health care providers may contact the registry by calling 844-405-6185. Enrollment should be done as early in pregnancy as possible.

Dental Health Professional Considerations See Local Anesthetic/Vasoconstrictor Precautions

◆ **Clomipramine HCl** *see* ClomiPRAMINE *on page 383*

◆ **Clomipramine Hydrochloride** *see* ClomiPRAMINE *on page 383*

ClonazePAM (kloe NA ze pam)

Related Information

Dentin Hypersensitivity, Acid Erosion, High Caries Index, Management of Alveolar Osteitis, and Xerostomia *on page 1762*

Brand Names: US KlonoPIN

Brand Names: Canada APO-ClonazePAM; Clonapam; CO ClonazePAM [DSC]; DOM-ClonazePAM [DSC]; DOM-ClonazePAM-R [DSC]; MYLAN-ClonazePAM [DSC]; PMS-ClonazePAM; PMS-ClonazePAM-R; PRO-ClonazePAM; RIVA-ClonazePAM; Rivotril; SANDOZ ClonazePAM [DSC]; TEVA-ClonazePAM

Generic Availability (US) Yes

Pharmacologic Category Anticonvulsant, Benzodiazepine; Benzodiazepine

Dental Use Burning mouth syndrome

Use

Panic disorder: Treatment of panic disorder, with or without agoraphobia.

Seizure disorders: Monotherapy or adjunctive therapy in the treatment of the Lennox-Gastaut syndrome (petit mal variant), akinetic, and myoclonic seizures; absence seizures (petit mal) unresponsive to succinimides.

Local Anesthetic/Vasoconstrictor Precautions No information available to require special precautions

Effects on Dental Treatment Key adverse event(s) related to dental treatment: Infrequent occurrence of sinusitis, gingival pain, and xerostomia (normal salivary flow resumes upon discontinuance) have been reported. Rare occurrence of candidiasis, toothache, jaw pain, fungal infections, tongue swelling, herpes simplex infection, and orthostatic hypotension have also been reported.

Effects on Bleeding No information available to require special precautions

Adverse Reactions Reactions reported in patients with seizure disorder, unless otherwise noted. Frequency not always defined.

>10%: Central nervous system: Drowsiness (seizure disorder: ~50%; panic disorder: 26% to 50%), ataxia (seizure disorder: ~30%; panic disorder: 1% to 9%), behavioral problems (seizure disorder: ~25%), dizziness (panic disorder: 5% to 12%)

1% to 10%:

Central nervous system: Fatigue (panic disorder: 6% to 9%), depression (panic disorder: 6% to 8%), memory impairment (panic disorder: 4% to 5%), nervousness (panic disorder: 3% to 4%), dysarthria (panic disorder: ≤4%), reduced intellectual ability (panic disorder: ≤4%), emotional lability (panic disorder: 2%), confusion (panic disorder: ≤2%), delayed ejaculation (panic disorder ≤2%)

Endocrine & metabolic: Decreased libido (panic disorder: ≤3%)

Gastrointestinal: Constipation (panic disorder: 3% to 5%), decreased appetite (panic disorder: 3%), abdominal pain (panic disorder: 2%)

Genitourinary: Dysmenorrhea (panic disorder: 3% to 6%), vaginitis (panic disorder: 2% to 4%), impotence (panic disorder: ≤3%), urinary tract infection (panic disorder: ≤2%), urinary frequency (panic disorder: 1% to 2%)

Hypersensitivity: Hypersensitivity (panic disorder: 2% to 4%)

Neuromuscular & skeletal: Myalgia (panic disorder: 2% to 4%)

Ophthalmic: Blurred vision (panic disorder: 2% to 3%)

Respiratory: Upper respiratory tract infection (panic disorder: 6% to 10%), sinusitis (panic disorder: 4% to 8%), influenza (panic disorder: 4% to 5%), cough (panic disorder: ≤4%), rhinitis (panic disorder: 2% to 4%), pharyngitis (panic disorder: 2% to 3%), bronchitis (panic disorder: 2%)

Frequency not defined:

Cardiovascular: Edema (ankle or facial), palpitations

Central nervous system: Amnesia, aphonia, choreiform movements, coma, glassy-eyed appearance, hallucination, headache, hemiparesis, hypotonia, hysteria, insomnia, myasthenia, psychosis, slurred speech, vertigo

Dermatologic: Alopecia, skin rash

Endocrine & metabolic: Dehydration, hirsutism, increased libido, weight gain, weight loss

Gastrointestinal: Anorexia, coated tongue, diarrhea, encopresis, gastritis, gingival pain, increased appetite, nausea, xerostomia

Genitourinary: Dysuria, nocturia, urinary incontinence, urinary retention

Hematologic & oncologic: Anemia, eosinophilia, leukopenia, lymphadenopathy, thrombocytopenia

Hepatic: Hepatomegaly, increased serum alkaline phosphatase (transient), increased serum transaminases (transient)

Neuromuscular & skeletal: Dysdiadochokinesia, tremor

Ophthalmic: Abnormal eye movements, diplopia, nystagmus

Respiratory: Chest congestion, dyspnea, respiratory depression, rhinorrhea, upper respiratory complaint (hypersecretion)

Miscellaneous: Fever, paradoxical reactions (including aggressive behavior, agitation, anxiety excitability, hostility, irritability, nervousness, nightmares, sleep disturbance, vivid dreams), physical health deterioration

<1%, postmarketing, and/or case reports (any indication): Abdominal distress, abnormal behavior (increased oppositional behavior), accidental injury, acne flare, ageusia, aggressive behavior, alcohol intoxication, anxiety, apathy, arthralgia, back pain, bladder dysfunction, bone fracture, burn, burning sensation of skin, candidiasis, cellulitis, chest pain, contact dermatitis, cystitis, depersonalization, dermal hemorrhage, dermatological reaction, disinhibition (organic), dyspepsia, ejaculatory disorder, epistaxis, exacerbation of asthma, excitement, excoriation, eye irritation, falling, flatulence, flushing, foot pain, frequent bowel movements, fungal infection, gastric distress, gout, heartburn, heavy headedness, hemorrhoids, herpes simplex infection, hoarseness, hordeolum, hyperactivity, hypertonia, hypoesthesia, hunger, illusion, increased dream activity, increased thirst, infectious mononucleosis, irregular menses, irritability, jaw pain, knee effusion, knee pain, lack of concentration, leg pain, leg thrombophlebitis, local inflammation, lower back pain, malaise, mastalgia, migraine, motion sickness, orthostatic hypotension, otalgia, otitis, pain, paresis, paresthesia, pedal edema, pelvic pain, periorbital edema, pleurisy, pneumonia, polyuria, pruritus, pustular rash, shivering, shoulder pain, sialorrhea, sleep disorder, slowed reaction time, sneezing, sprain, strain, streptococcal infection, suicidal ideation, suicidal tendencies, tendonitis, tongue edema, toothache, twitching, twitching of eye, urinary tract hemorrhage, urine discoloration, viral infection, visual disturbance, visual field defect, withdrawal syndrome, xeroderma, xerophthalmia, yawning

Dental Usual Dosage Burning mouth syndrome (off-label use): Adults: Oral: 0.25-3 mg/day in 2 divided doses, in morning and evening

Dosing

Adult Note: Reduce dose or avoid use in patients receiving opioids, with significant chronic disease (eg, respiratory compromise), or at increased risk for accumulation (eg, hepatic impairment). Generally, avoid use in patients with, or at risk for, substance use disorders; if prescribed, closely supervise use.

Anxiety:

Anxiety and agitation, acute (adjunctive therapy or monotherapy) (off-label use):

Oral: Initial: 0.5 mg/day in 2 divided doses; may be given as needed or scheduled (Fang 2012; Marder 2020; Mojtabai 2020; manufacturer's labeling). May increase dose based on response and tolerability up to 4 mg/day in 2 to 4 divided doses (Roy-Byrne 2020b; manufacturer's labeling). In severe agitation due to psychosis, some experts consider further increasing dose, if needed and tolerated, up to a reported maximum of 8 mg/day in divided doses (Fang 2012).

Anxiety disorder (adjunctive therapy or monotherapy) (alternative agent):

Note: While FDA-approved for panic disorder, clinical trials also support use in other anxiety disorders (Pollack 2014; Wang 2016). Generally used short-term for symptom relief until concurrent therapy is effective (eg, ≤12 weeks). Long-term, low-dose therapy may be used for select patients when other treatments are ineffective or poorly tolerated (Katzman 2014; WFSBP [Bandelow 2012]). Use with caution in patients with posttraumatic stress disorder; benzodiazepines may worsen symptoms (VA/DoD 2017).

Oral: Initial: 0.25 to 1 mg/day in 1 to 2 divided doses; may be given as needed or scheduled. If needed, may increase daily dose based on response and tolerability in increments of 0.25 to 0.5 mg every few days (eg, ≥3 days); usual target range: 1 to 3 mg/day; maximum: 4 mg/day in 1 to 4 divided doses. To minimize daytime motor impairment and drowsiness, may be taken as a single dose at bedtime (Bystritsky 2020; Roy-Byrne 2020a; Roy-Byrne 2020b; Stein 2020; manufacturer's labeling).

Myoclonus (monotherapy or adjunctive therapy) (off-label use):

Oral: Initial: 0.5 mg/day in 2 divided doses; may gradually increase daily dose based on response and tolerability to a usual dose of 1.5 to 3 mg/day in 3 divided doses (Caviness 2020; Jankovic 1986; Obeso 1989; Tijssen 1997).

Rapid eye movement sleep behavior disorder (monotherapy or adjunctive therapy) (off-label use):

Oral: Initial: 0.25 to 0.5 mg within 30 minutes of bedtime; usual dose range: 0.25 to 2 mg before bedtime (AASM [Aurora 2010]; Howell 2020). In most patients, 0.5 to 1 mg before bedtime is sufficient and better tolerated than doses >1 mg (Howell 2020).

Note: In patients with dementia, gait disorders, or obstructive sleep apnea, avoid use or reduce dose (eg, initial dose: 0.125 to 0.25 mg before bedtime) (AASM [Aurora 2010]; Fernández-Arcos 2016; Li 2016).

Seizure disorders, refractory (adjunctive therapy or monotherapy) (alternative agent):

Note: FDA-approved for Lennox-Gastaut syndrome and resistant absence seizures; however, also used off label as adjunctive or bridge therapy in other seizure types, including myoclonic and atonic seizures and drug-resistant epilepsy syndromes (Bank 2017; Schachter 2020).

Oral:

Monotherapy: Initial: 0.5 to 1.5 mg/day in 1 to 3 divided doses (Brodie 1997; manufacturer's labeling).

Adjunctive therapy: Initial: 0.5 to 1 mg/day in 1 to 3 divided doses (Schachter 2020).

Dosage adjustment: May increase dose based on response and tolerability in increments of 0.5 to 1 mg every 3 to 7 days to usual maintenance dose of 2 to 8 mg/day in 1 to 2 divided doses; maximum dose: 20 mg/day (Brodie 1997; Schachter 2020; manufacturer's labeling).

Tardive dyskinesia (alternative agent) (off-label use):

Note: For reduction of dyskinesia and anxiety in milder forms of tardive dyskinesia in conjunction with appropriate therapy modification(s) such as tapering/discontinuing offending drug (Liang 2020).

Oral: Initial: 0.5 mg/day; increase daily dose based on response and tolerability by 0.5 mg every 5 days up to 4 mg/day (Liang 2020; Thaker 1990).

Vertigo, acute episodes, treatment (alternative agent) (off-label use):

Note: Reserve use for episodes lasting several hours to days.

Oral: 0.25 to 0.5 mg every 8 to 12 hours as needed for 24 to 48 hours (Furman 2020; Ganança 2002).

Discontinuation of therapy: In patients receiving extended or higher-dose benzodiazepine therapy, unless safety concerns require a more rapid withdrawal, gradually withdraw to detect reemerging symptoms and minimize rebound and withdrawal symptoms. Taper total daily dose by ~10% to 25% every 1 to 2 weeks based on response and tolerability. The optimal taper rate and duration will vary; durations up to 6 months may be necessary for some patients (Bystritsky 2020; Lader 2011; VA/DoD 2015). For patients on high doses, taper more rapidly in the beginning and slow the reduction rate as the taper progresses. For example, reduce the dose weekly by 25% until half of the dose remains. Thereafter, continue to reduce by ~12% every 4 to 7 days (VA/DoD 2015).

Geriatric Refer to adult dosing. Initiate with low doses and observe closely.

Renal Impairment: Adult There are no dosage adjustments provided in the manufacturer's labeling; use with caution. Clonazepam metabolites may accumulate in patients with renal impairment.

Hepatic Impairment: Adult There are no dosage adjustments provided in the manufacturer's labeling; use with caution. Clonazepam undergoes hepatic metabolism. Contraindicated in patients with significant hepatic impairment.

Pediatric Note: If necessary to discontinue clonazepam therapy, drug should be withdrawn gradually.

Neuroirritability, agitation (palliative care): Limited data available: Infants, Children, and Adolescents: Oral:

Patient weight:

<30 kg: Initial: 0.01 to 0.03 mg/kg/day in divided doses up to 3 to 4 times daily; increase dose to desired effect up to a maximum daily dose: 0.2 mg/kg/**day** in 3 divided doses (Kliegman 2017; Wustoff 2007)

≥30 kg: Initial: ≤0.25 mg/dose 3 times daily; may increase by 0.5 to 1 mg/day every 3 days up to maintenance dose range: 0.05 to 0.2 mg/kg/day up to maximum daily dose: 20 mg/**day** (Kliegman 2017)

Seizure disorders:

Infants and Children <10 years or ≤30 kg: Oral:

Initial: 0.01 to 0.03 mg/kg/day in 2 to 3 divided doses; maximum initial daily dose: 0.05 mg/kg/**day**; increase by ≤0.25 to 0.5 mg every third day until seizures are controlled or adverse effects observed

Maintenance dose: 0.1 to 0.2 mg/kg/day in 3 divided doses; maximum daily dose: 0.2 mg/kg/**day**

Children ≥10 years or >30 kg and Adolescents: Oral:

Initial: 0.01 to 0.05 mg/kg/day in 2 or 3 divided doses; maximum initial dose: 0.5 mg/dose 3 times daily; may increase dose by 25% or by 0.5 to 1 mg every 3 to 7 days until seizures are controlled or adverse effects observed (Kliegman 2017)

Maintenance dose range: 0.05 to 0.2 mg/kg/day in 2 to 3 divided doses; maximum daily dose: 20 mg/**day** (Kliegman 2017)

Panic disorder: Adolescents ≥18 years: Oral: Initial: 0.25 mg twice daily; increase in increments of 0.125 to 0.25 mg twice daily every 3 days; target dose: 1 mg/day in divided doses; some patients may require higher doses up to a maximum daily dose: 4 mg/**day.** To discontinue, treatment should be withdrawn gradually; decrease dose by 0.125 mg twice daily every 3 days until medication is completely withdrawn.

Renal Impairment: Pediatric There are no dosage adjustments provided in the manufacturer's labeling; use with caution. Clonazepam metabolites may accumulate in patients with renal impairment.

Hepatic Impairment: Pediatric There are no dosage adjustments provided in the manufacturer's labeling; use with caution. Clonazepam undergoes hepatic metabolism. Contraindicated in patients with significant hepatic impairment.

Mechanism of Action The exact mechanism is unknown, but believed to be related to its ability to enhance the activity of GABA; suppresses the spike-and-wave discharge in absence seizures by depressing nerve transmission in the motor cortex.

Contraindications

Hypersensitivity to clonazepam, other benzodiazepines, or any component of the formulation; significant liver disease; acute narrow-angle glaucoma

Canadian labeling: Additional contraindications (not in US labeling): Severe respiratory insufficiency; sleep apnea syndrome; myasthenia gravis

Warnings/Precautions Pooled analysis of trials involving various antiepileptics (regardless of indication) showed an increased risk of suicidal thoughts/behavior (incidence rate: 0.43% treated patients compared to 0.24% of patients receiving placebo); risk observed as early as 1 week after initiation and continued through duration of trials (most trials ≤24 weeks). Monitor all patients for notable changes in behavior that might indicate suicidal thoughts or depression; notify health care provider immediately if symptoms occur. Use caution in patients with depression, particularly if suicidal risk may be present.

Benzodiazepines have been associated with anterograde amnesia (Nelson 1999). May cause CNS depression, which may impair physical or mental abilities; patients must be cautioned about performing tasks which require mental alertness (eg, operating machinery or driving); increased risk may occur with the use of multiple anticonvulsants. Paradoxical reactions, including hyperactive or aggressive behavior, have been reported with benzodiazepines; risk may be increased in adolescent/pediatric patients, geriatric patients, or patients with a history of alcohol use disorder or psychiatric/personality disorders (Mancuso 2004). Clonazepam may cause respiratory depression and may produce an increase in salivation; use with caution in patients with compromised respiratory function (eg, chronic obstructive pulmonary disease, sleep apnea) and in patients who have difficulty handling secretions. May be used in patients with open angle glaucoma who are receiving appropriate therapy; contraindicated in acute narrow angle glaucoma. Use with caution in patients with a history of drug abuse or acute alcoholism; potential for drug dependency exists. Tolerance, psychological and physical dependence may occur with prolonged use. Use with caution in patients with hepatic impairment; accumulation likely to occur. Contraindicated in patients with significant hepatic impairment. Use with caution in patients with renal impairment; clonazepam metabolites are renally eliminated. Use with caution in debilitated patients. Elderly patients may be at an increased risk of death with use; risk has been found highest within the first 4 months of use in elderly dementia patients (Jennum 2015; Saarelainen 2018). Use with extreme caution in patients who are at risk of falls; benzodiazepines have been associated with falls and traumatic injury (Nelson 1999). Use with caution in patients with porphyria; may have a porphyrogenic effect. Hazardous sleep-related activities such as sleep-driving, cooking and eating food, and making phone calls while asleep have been noted with benzodiazepines (Dolder 2008).

Does not have analgesic, antidepressant, or antipsychotic properties. Worsening of seizures may occur when added to patients with multiple seizure types. Loss of anticonvulsant activity may occur (typically within 3 months of initiation); dose adjustment may be necessary. Periodically reevaluate the long-term usefulness of clonazepam for the individual patient. Clonazepam is a long half-life benzodiazepine. Duration of action after a single dose is determined by redistribution rather than metabolism. Tolerance develops to the anticonvulsant effects. It does not develop to the anxiolytic effects (Vinkers 2012). Chronic use of this agent may increase the perioperative benzodiazepine dose needed to achieve desired effect. Rebound or withdrawal symptoms may occur following abrupt discontinuation or large decreases in dose. Use caution when reducing dose or withdrawing therapy; decrease slowly and monitor for withdrawal symptoms. Flumazenil may cause withdrawal in patients receiving long-term benzodiazepine therapy (Brogden 1988). Potentially significant drug-drug interactions may exist, requiring dose or frequency adjustment, additional monitoring, and/or selection of alternative therapy. **[US Boxed Warning]: Concomitant use of benzodiazepines and opioids may result in profound sedation, respiratory depression, coma, and death. Reserve concomitant prescribing of these drugs for use in patients for whom alternative treatment options are inadequate. Limit dosages to the minimum required. Follow patients for signs and symptoms of respiratory depression and sedation.**

Drug Interactions

Metabolism/Transport Effects **Substrate** of CYP3A4 (major); **Note:** Assignment of Major/Minor substrate status based on clinically relevant drug interaction potential

Avoid Concomitant Use

Avoid concomitant use of ClonazePAM with any of the following: Abametapir; Azelastine (Nasal); Bromperidol; Conivaptan; Fusidic Acid (Systemic); Idelalisib; OLANZapine; Orphenadrine; Oxomemazine; Paraldehyde; Sodium Oxybate; Thalidomide

Increased Effect/Toxicity

ClonazePAM may increase the levels/effects of: Alcohol (Ethyl); Azelastine (Nasal); Blonanserin; Brexanolone; Buprenorphine; CloZAPine; CNS Depressants; Flunitrazepam; Methadone; Methotrimeprazine; MetyroSINE; Opioid Agonists; Orphenadrine; OxyCODONE; Paraldehyde; Piribedil; Pramipexole; ROPINIRole; Rotigotine; Sodium Oxybate; Suvorexant; Thalidomide; Zolpidem

The levels/effects of ClonazePAM may be increased by: Abametapir; Alizapride; Aprepitant; Brimonidine (Topical); Bromopride; Bromperidol; Cannabidiol; Cannabis; Chlormethiazole; Chlorphenesin Carbamate; Clofazimine; Cobicistat; Conivaptan; Cosyntropin; CYP3A4 Inhibitors (Moderate); CYP3A4 Inhibitors (Strong); Dimethindene (Topical); Doxylamine; Dronabinol; Droperidol; Duvelisib; Erdafitinib; Esketamine; Fosaprepitant; Fosnetupitant; Fusidic Acid (Systemic); HydrOXYzine; Idelalisib; Kava Kava; Larotrectinib; Lemborexant; Lisuride; Lofexidine; Magnesium Sulfate; Melatonin; Methotrimeprazine; Metoclopramide; MiFEPRIStone; Minocycline (Systemic); Nabilone; Netupitant; OLANZapine; Oxomemazine; Palbociclib; Perampanel; Rufinamide; Simeprevir; Stiripentol; Teduglutide; Tetrahydrocannabinol; Tetrahydrocannabinol and Cannabidiol; Trimeprazine; Vigabatrin

Decreased Effect

The levels/effects of ClonazePAM may be decreased by: CYP3A4 Inducers (Moderate); CYP3A4 Inducers (Strong); Dabrafenib; Deferasirox; Enzalutamide; Erdafitinib; Fosphenytoin; Ivosidenib; Mitotane; Phenytoin; Sarilumab; Siltuximab; Theophylline Derivatives; Tocilizumab; Yohimbine

Pharmacodynamics/Kinetics

Onset of Action ~20 to 40 minutes (Hanson 1972)

Duration of Action Infants and young children: 6 to 8 hours (Hanson 1972); Adults: ≤12 hours (Hanson 1972)

Half-life Elimination Neonates: 22 to 81 hours (Patsalos 2018); Children: 22 to 33 hours (Walson 1996); Adults: 17 to 60 hours (Walson 1996).

Time to Peak Serum: 1 to 4 hours

Pregnancy Considerations

Clonazepam crosses the placenta. Teratogenic effects have been observed with some benzodiazepines; however, additional studies are needed. The incidence of premature birth and low birth weights may be increased following maternal use of benzodiazepines; hypoglycemia and respiratory problems in the neonate may occur following exposure late in pregnancy. Neonatal withdrawal symptoms may occur within days to weeks after birth and "floppy infant syndrome" (which also includes withdrawal symptoms) has been reported with some benzodiazepines, including clonazepam (Bergman 1992; Iqbal 2002; Wikner 2007). A combination of factors influences the potential teratogenicity of anticonvulsant therapy. When treating pregnant females with epilepsy, monotherapy with the lowest effective dose and avoidance medications known to have a high incidence of teratogenic effects is recommended (Harden 2009; Wlodarczyk 2012). When treating pregnant females with panic disorder, psychosocial interventions should be considered prior to pharmacotherapy (APA 2009).

Patients exposed to clonazepam during pregnancy are encouraged to enroll themselves into the AED Pregnancy Registry by calling 1-888-233-2334. Additional information is available at www.aedpregnancyregistry.org.

Breastfeeding Considerations Clonazepam is present in breast milk.

The relative infant dose (RID) of clonazepam is 2.8% when calculated using the highest breast milk concentration from a case report and compared to a weight-adjusted maternal dose of 4 mg/day.

In general, breastfeeding is considered acceptable when an RID of a medication is <10% (Anderson 2016; Ito 2000). However, some sources note breastfeeding should only be considered if the RID is <5% for psychotropic agents (Larsen 2015).

The RID of clonazepam was calculated using a milk concentration of 0.0107 mcg/mL, providing an estimated daily infant dose via breast milk of 1.6 mcg/kg/day. This milk concentration was obtained following maternal administration of clonazepam 2 mg twice daily during pregnancy and after delivery; milk samples were obtained on days 2 to 4 postpartum (Söderman 1988). Slightly higher milk concentrations (0.013 mcg/mL) were noted in a second report. The mother was taking clonazepam throughout pregnancy (dose not specified); milk sampling began 72 hours after delivery (Fisher 1985). Clonazepam was detected in the serum of the breastfeeding infants (Fisher 1985; Söderman 1988) and concentrations may have been influenced not only by breast milk but also by in utero exposure.

Apnea, CNS depression, hypotonia, and somnolence have been reported in infants exposed to clonazepam via breast milk (Fisher 1985; Kelly 2012; Soussan 2014). In a review of females taking various doses of clonazepam (range: 0.5 to 2 mg/day) during pregnancy and postpartum (n=10) or only postpartum (n=1), clonazepam was measurable in the serum of two infants; however, adverse events were not reported (Birnbaum 1999).

Clonazepam has a long half-life and may accumulate in the breastfed infant, especially preterm infants or those exposed to chronic maternal doses (Davanzo 2013). A single maternal dose may be compatible with breastfeeding (WHO 2002). If chronic use of a benzodiazepine is needed in breastfeeding females, use of shorter acting agents is preferred (Davanzo 2013; Veiby 2015; WHO 2002). Infants of females using medications for seizure disorders should be monitored for drowsiness, decreased feeding, and poor weight gain (Veiby 2015).

According to the manufacturer, the decision to breastfeed during therapy should consider the risk of infant exposure, the benefits of breastfeeding to the infant, and benefits of treatment to the mother.

Controlled Substance C-IV

Dosage Forms: US

Tablet, Oral:

KlonoPIN: 0.5 mg, 1 mg, 2 mg

Generic: 0.5 mg, 1 mg, 2 mg

Tablet Disintegrating, Oral:

Generic: 0.125 mg, 0.25 mg, 0.5 mg, 1 mg, 2 mg

Dosage Forms: Canada

Tablet, Oral:

Rivotril: 0.5 mg, 2 mg

Generic: 0.25 mg, 0.5 mg, 1 mg, 2 mg

CloNIDine (KLON i deen)

Related Information

Cardiovascular Diseases *on page 1654*

Dentin Hypersensitivity, Acid Erosion, High Caries Index, Management of Alveolar Osteitis, and Xerostomia *on page 1762*

Brand Names: US Catapres; Catapres-TTS-1; Catapres-TTS-2; Catapres-TTS-3; Duraclon; Kapvay

Brand Names: Canada APO-CloNIDine; Catapres [DSC]; Dixarit [DSC]; DOM-CloNIDine; MINT-CloNIDine; TEVA-CloNIDine

Pharmacologic Category Alpha$_2$-Adrenergic Agonist; Antihypertensive

Use

Attention-deficit/hyperactivity disorder (extended-release tablet): Treatment of attention-deficit/hyperactivity disorder (monotherapy or as adjunctive therapy)

Hypertension (immediate-release tablet and transdermal patch): Management of hypertension. **Note: Not** recommended for the initial treatment of hypertension (ACC/AHA [Whelton 2018]). Clonidine should be avoided for the treatment of hypertension in patients with heart failure with reduced ejection fraction of ischemic origin (AHA/ACC/ASH [Rosendorff 2015]).

Vasomotor symptoms associated with menopause (0.025 mg tablet [Canadian product]): Relief of menopausal flushing in patients for whom hormonal replacement therapy is unnecessary or not desirable.

Local Anesthetic/Vasoconstrictor Precautions Clonidine is one of the drugs confirmed to prolong the QT interval and is accepted as having a risk of causing torsade de pointes. The risk of drug-induced torsade de pointes is extremely low when a single QT interval prolonging drug is prescribed. In terms of epinephrine, it is not known what effect vasoconstrictors in the local anesthetic regimen will have in patients with a known history of congenital prolonged QT interval or in patients taking any medication that prolongs the QT interval. Until more information is obtained, it is suggested that the clinician consult with the physician prior to the use of a vasoconstrictor in suspected patients and that the vasoconstrictor (epinephrine, mepivacaine and levonordefrin [Carbocaine 2% with Neo-Cobefrin]) be used with caution.

Effects on Dental Treatment Key adverse event(s) related to dental treatment: Significant xerostomia (normal salivary flow resumes upon discontinuation), headache, and abnormal taste; patients may experience orthostatic hypotension as they stand up after treatment, especially if lying in dental chair for extended periods of time. Use caution with sudden changes in position during and after dental treatment.

Effects on Bleeding No information available to require special precautions

Adverse Reactions Frequency not always defined.

Oral, Transdermal: Incidence of adverse events may be less with transdermal compared to oral due to the lower peak/trough ratio.

>10%:

Central nervous system: Drowsiness (2% to 38%), headache (1% to 29%), fatigue (4% to 16%), dizziness (2% to 16%)

Dermatologic: Transient skin rash (localized; characterized by pruritus and erythema; transdermal 15% to 50%), contact dermatitis (transdermal 8% to 34%)

Gastrointestinal: Xerostomia (≤40%), upper abdominal pain (15%)

1% to 10%:

Cardiovascular: Bradycardia (≤4%), edema (3%), localized blanching (transdermal 1%), palpitations (1%), tachycardia (≤3%), atrioventricular block, cardiac arrhythmia, cardiac failure, cerebrovascular accident, chest pain, ECG abnormality, flushing, orthostatic hypotension, prolonged QT Interval on ECG, Raynaud's phenomenon, syncope

Central nervous system: Sedation (3% to 10%), irritability (5% to 9%), nightmares (4% to 9%), insomnia (≤6%), emotional disturbance (4%), lethargy (3%), nervousness (1% to 3%), depression (1%), throbbing (transdermal 1%), withdrawal syndrome (1%), aggressive behavior, agitation, anxiety, behavioral changes, delirium, delusions, hallucination (visual and auditory), malaise, numbness (localized; transdermal), paresthesia, parotid pain (oral), restlessness, vivid dream

Dermatologic: Localized vesiculation (transdermal 7%), allergic contact sensitivity (transdermal 5%), hyperpigmentation (transdermal 5%), burning sensation of skin (transdermal 3%), excoriation (transdermal 3%), macular eruption (1%), papule (transdermal 1%), alopecia, hypopigmentation (localized; transdermal), pallor, skin rash, urticaria

Endocrine & metabolic: Gynecomastia (1%), weight gain (<1%), decreased libido, hyperglycemia (transient; oral), increased thirst

Gastrointestinal: Constipation (1% to 10%), viral gastrointestinal infection (5%), anorexia (1%), abdominal pain (oral), diarrhea, gastrointestinal pseudo-obstruction (oral), nausea, parotitis (oral), sore throat, vomiting

Genitourinary: Urinary incontinence (4%), sexual disorder (3%), erectile dysfunction (2% to 3%), nocturia (1%), pollakiuria, urinary retention

Hematologic & oncologic: Thrombocytopenia (oral)

Hepatic: Abnormal hepatic function tests (mild transient abnormalities; <1%), hepatitis

Hypersensitivity: Angioedema

Neuromuscular & skeletal: Weakness (10%), tremor (1% to 4%), arthralgia (1%), myalgia (1%), leg cramps (<1%), increased creatine phosphokinase (transient; oral), limb pain

Ophthalmic: Accommodation disturbance, blurred vision, burning sensation of eyes, decreased lacrimation, dry eye syndrome, increased lacrimation

Otic: Otitis media (≤3%), otalgia

Respiratory: Asthma, dry nose, epistaxis, flu-like symptoms, nasal congestion, nasopharyngitis, respiratory tract infection, rhinorrhea

Miscellaneous: Crying (1% to 3%), fever

Epidural: Note: The following adverse events occurred more often than placebo in cancer patients with intractable pain being treated with concurrent epidural morphine.

>10%:

Cardiovascular: Hypotension (45%), orthostatic hypotension (32%)

Central nervous system: Confusion (13%), dizziness (13%)

Gastrointestinal: Xerostomia (13%)

1% to 10%:

Cardiovascular: Chest pain (5%)

Central nervous system: Hallucination (5%)

Dermatologic: Diaphoresis (5%)

Gastrointestinal: Nausea and vomiting (8%)

Otic: Tinnitus (5%)

Mechanism of Action Stimulates alpha-2 adrenoceptors in the brain stem, thus activating an inhibitory neuron, resulting in reduced sympathetic outflow from the CNS, producing a decrease in peripheral resistance, renal vascular resistance, heart rate, and blood pressure; epidural clonidine may produce pain relief at spinal presynaptic and postjunctional alpha-2 adrenoceptors by preventing pain signal transmission; pain relief occurs only for the body regions innervated by the spinal segments where analgesic concentrations of clonidine exist. For the treatment of ADHD, the mechanism of action is unknown; it has been proposed that postsynaptic alpha-2 agonist stimulation regulates subcortical activity in the prefrontal cortex, the area of the brain responsible for emotions, attentions, and behaviors and causes reduced hyperactivity, impulsiveness, and distractibility. Epidurally administered clonidine produces dose-dependent analgesia not antagonized by opiate antagonists. The analgesia is limited to the body regions innervated by the spinal segments where analgesic concentrations of clonidine are present. Clonidine is thought to produce analgesia at presynaptic and postjunctional alpha-2 adrenoceptors in the spinal cord by preventing pain signal transmission to the brain.

Pharmacodynamics/Kinetics

Onset of Action

Antihypertensive effect: Oral: Immediate release: 0.5 to 1 hour (maximum reduction in blood pressure: 2 to 4 hours); Transdermal: Initial application: 2 to 3 days; Transdermal: Steady state reached in ~3 days

Attention-deficit/hyperactivity disorder: Oral: Extended release (Kapvay): Onset of action: 1 to 2 weeks (AAP [Wolraich 2011])

Half-life Elimination

Children: 6.13 ± 1.33 hours (Lonnqvist 1993)

Adults: Normal renal function: 12 to 16 hours; Renal impairment: ≤41 hours

Epidural administration: CSF half-life elimination: 1.3 ± 0.5 hours; plasma half-life elimination: 22 ± 15 hours

Transdermal: Half-life elimination (after patch removal): ~20 hours (due to skin depot effect; increase in plasma clonidine concentrations may occur after patch removal [MacGregor 1985])

Time to Peak Plasma: Oral: Immediate release: 1 to 3 hours; Extended release (Kapvay): 7 to 8 hours

Pregnancy Considerations

Clonidine crosses the placenta; concentrations in the umbilical cord plasma are similar to those in the maternal serum and concentrations in the amniotic fluid may be 4 times those in the maternal serum.

The pharmacokinetics of clonidine may be altered during pregnancy due to an increase in nonrenal clearance, possibly regulated by maternal CYP2D6 genotype (Buchanan 2009; Claessens 2010).

Chronic maternal hypertension may increase the risk of birth defects, low birth weight, preterm delivery, stillbirth, and neonatal death. Actual fetal/neonatal risks may be related to duration and severity of maternal hypertension. Untreated hypertension may also increase the risks of adverse maternal outcomes, including gestational diabetes, myocardial infarction, preeclampsia, stroke, and delivery complications (ACOG 203 2019). Agents other than clonidine are more commonly used to treat hypertension in pregnancy (ACOG 203 2019; ESC [Regitz-Zagrosek 2018]); use of clonidine should be considered in consult with subspecialists (ACOG 203 2019). Females with preexisting hypertension may continue their medication during pregnancy unless contraindications exist (ESC [Regitz-Zagrosek 2018]).

If treatment for attention-deficit/hyperactivity disorder (ADHD) in pregnancy is needed, other agents are preferred (Ornoy 2018). Data collection to monitor pregnancy and infant outcomes following exposure to ADHD medications is ongoing. Health care providers are encouraged to enroll females exposed to Kapvay during pregnancy in the National Pregnancy Registry for ADHD Medications (866-961-2388).

[US Boxed Warning]: Epidural clonidine is not recommended for obstetrical or postpartum pain due to risk of hemodynamic instability. However, in a rare obstetrical, or postpartum patient, potential benefits may outweigh the possible risks. Severe maternal hypotension may occur following epidural use which may result in decreased placental perfusion. Clonidine has been evaluated for use as an adjunctive agent for epidural labor analgesia (Allen 2018; Kumari 2018; Landau 2002; Roelants 2015; Zhang 2015) including patients who are opioid dependent (Hoyt 2018).

◆ **Clonidine HCl** *see* CloNIDine *on page* 389

◆ **Clonidine Hydrochloride** *see* CloNIDine *on page* 389

Clopidogrel (kloh PID oh grel)

Related Information

Antiplatelet and Anticoagulation Considerations in Dentistry *on page* 1666

Cardiovascular Diseases *on page* 1654

Brand Names: US Plavix

Brand Names: Canada ACT Clopidogrel; APO-Clopidogrel; Auro-Clopidogrel; BIO-Clopidogrel; DOM-Clopidogrel; JAMP-Clopidogrel; Mar-Clopidogrel; MINT-Clopidogrel [DSC]; MYLAN-Clopidogrel [DSC]; NRA-Clopidogrel; Plavix; PMS-Clopidogrel; RIVA-Clopidogrel; SANDOZ Clopidogrel; TARO-Clopidogrel; TEVA-Clopidogrel

Generic Availability (US) Yes

Pharmacologic Category Antiplatelet Agent; Antiplatelet Agent, Thienopyridine; P2Y12 Antagonist

Use

Acute coronary syndrome:

ST-segment elevation myocardial infarction: To reduce the rate of myocardial infarction (MI) and stroke in conjunction with aspirin in patients with acute ST-elevation MI who are to be managed medically.

Non-ST-segment elevation acute coronary syndromes: To decrease the rate of MI and stroke in conjunction with aspirin in patients with non-ST-segment elevation acute coronary syndromes (unstable angina/non-ST-elevation MI), including patients who are to be managed medically and those who are to be managed with coronary revascularization.

Myocardial infarction, ischemic stroke, or peripheral atherosclerotic disease: To reduce the rate of MI and stroke in patients with a history of recent MI, recent stroke, or established peripheral atherosclerotic disease.

Local Anesthetic/Vasoconstrictor Precautions No information available to require special precautions

Effects on Dental Treatment Key adverse event(s) related to dental treatment: Rare occurrence of loss of taste, taste disorder, lichen planus, and stomatitis have been reported.

Effects on Bleeding Clopidogrel irreversibly inhibits platelet aggregation which persists for the life of the platelet (7-10 days) and until new platelets are released. Clopidogrel should **not** be discontinued in patients with cardiac stents that have not completed their full course of dual antiplatelet therapy (eg, aspirin and clopidogrel [prasugrel or ticagrelor]); patient-specific situations need to be discussed with cardiologist. If normal platelet function is desired, clopidogrel should be discontinued for at least 5 days. A medical consult is recommended to determine the benefit:risk of continuing or discontinuing clopidogrel therapy for invasive dental procedures.

Adverse Reactions As with all drugs that may affect hemostasis, bleeding is associated with clopidogrel. Hemorrhage may occur at virtually any site. Risk is dependent on multiple variables, including the concurrent use of multiple agents that alter hemostasis and patient susceptibility.

1% to 10%:

Hematologic & oncologic: Minor hemorrhage (4% to 5%), major hemorrhage (4%)

Frequency not defined:

Hematologic & oncologic: Bruise, hematoma

Respiratory: Epistaxis

<1%, postmarketing, and/or case reports: Abnormal hepatic function tests, acute generalized exanthematous pustulosis, acute hepatic failure, ageusia, agranulocytosis, angioedema, aplastic anemia, arthralgia, arthritis, bronchospasm, bullous rash, colitis (including ulcerative or lymphocytic), confusion, diarrhea, drug-induced hypersensitivity reaction, drug reaction with eosinophilia and systemic symptoms, duodenal ulcer, eczema, eosinophilic pneumonitis, erythema multiforme, erythematous rash, exfoliative dermatitis, fever, gastric ulcer, hallucination, headache, hemophilia A (acquired), hepatitis (noninfectious), hypersensitivity reaction, hypotension, increased serum creatinine, insulin autoimmune syndrome, interstitial pneumonitis, intracranial hemorrhage, lichen planus, maculopapular rash, myalgia, nonimmune anaphylaxis, pancreatitis, pancytopenia, pruritus, serum sickness, Stevens-Johnson syndrome, stomatitis, taste disorder, thrombotic thrombocytopenic purpura, toxic epidermal necrolysis, urticaria, vasculitis

Dosing

Adult & Geriatric

Acute coronary syndrome:

Note: Routine platelet-function testing or genetic testing for CYP2C19 polymorphisms is not recommended (ACC/AHA [Levine 2016]; Scott 2013; Sibbing 2019).

ST-segment elevation myocardial infarction:

Note: Regardless of the reperfusion strategy, administer clopidogrel in combination with a parenteral anticoagulant and aspirin (ACCF/AHA [O'Gara 2013]).

If using fibrinolytic therapy for reperfusion:

Age ≤75 years: **Oral:** Initial loading dose: 300 mg once at the time of diagnosis; followed by 75 mg once daily (ACCF/AHA [O'Gara 2013]; Sabatine 2005a).

Age >75 years: **Oral:** 75 mg once daily (ACCF/AHA [O'Gara 2013]).

Patient requires percutaneous coronary intervention following fibrinolytic therapy:

Fibrinolytic administered **with** a loading dose of clopidogrel: **Oral:** Continue 75 mg once daily (do not administer an additional loading dose) (ACCF/AHA [O'Gara 2013]).

Fibrinolytic administered **≤24 hours ago without** a loading dose of clopidogrel: **Oral:** Initial: 300 mg once prior to percutaneous coronary intervention (PCI); followed by 75 mg once daily after PCI (ACCF/AHA [O'Gara 2013]).

Fibrinolytic administered **>24 hours ago without** a loading dose of clopidogrel: **Oral:** Initial: 600 mg once prior to PCI; followed by 75 mg once daily after PCI (ACCF/AHA [O'Gara 2013]).

If using percutaneous coronary intervention for reperfusion (alternative agent) (off-label use):

Note: Some experts prefer ticagrelor or prasugrel over clopidogrel unless there is high risk for bleeding (Lincoff 2019; Wallentin 2009; Wiviott 2007).

Oral: Initial: 600 mg once as early as possible before PCI; followed by 75 mg once daily after PCI (ACCF/AHA [O'Gara 2013]; Dangas 2009; Mehta 2010).

If no planned reperfusion strategy (alternative agent):

Note: Some experts prefer ticagrelor over clopidogrel (Lincoff 2019).

Oral: Initial: 300 mg once at the time of diagnosis; followed by 75 mg once daily (Lincoff 2019).

Duration of therapy: Clopidogrel plus aspirin (dual antiplatelet therapy [DAPT]) should be continued for ≥12 months unless bleeding is a concern. If there have been no major bleeding complications after 12 months, continuation of DAPT may be considered. Reevaluate the need for DAPT at regular intervals based on bleeding and thrombotic risks. When DAPT is complete, discontinue clopidogrel and continue aspirin indefinitely (ACC/AHA [Levine 2016]; ACCF/AHA [O'Gara 2013]; Lincoff 2019; Mauri 2014).

Non-ST-segment elevation acute coronary syndromes:

Note: Regardless of the management strategy, administer clopidogrel in combination with a parenteral anticoagulant and aspirin (ACC/AHA [Amsterdam 2014]).

If using an ischemia-guided approach (medical management) (alternative agent):

Note: Some experts prefer ticagrelor over clopidogrel (Cutlip 2019a).

Oral: Initial: 300 or 600 mg once at the time of diagnosis; followed by 75 mg once daily (ACC/AHA [Amsterdam 2014]). Some experts prefer an initial dose of 600 mg unless there is high risk for bleeding, in which case, an initial dose of 300 mg is also appropriate (Cutlip 2019a).

If using an invasive approach (reperfusion using percutaneous coronary intervention) (alternative agent):

Note: Some experts prefer ticagrelor or prasugrel over clopidogrel unless there is high risk for bleeding (Cutlip 2019a; Wallentin 2009; Wiviott 2007).

Oral: Initial: 600 mg once as early as possible before PCI; followed by 75 mg once daily after PCI (ACC/AHA [Amsterdam 2014]).

Duration of therapy: Clopidogrel plus aspirin (DAPT) should be continued for ≥12 months unless bleeding is a concern. If there have been no major bleeding complications after 12 months, continuation of DAPT may be considered. Reevaluate the need for DAPT at regular intervals based on bleeding and thrombotic risks. When DAPT is complete, discontinue clopidogrel and continue aspirin indefinitely (ACC/AHA [Amsterdam 2014]; ACC/AHA [Levine 2016]; Cutlip 2019a; Mauri 2014; Mehta 2001; Yusuf 2001).

Percutaneous coronary intervention for stable ischemic heart disease (off-label use):

Note: Administer clopidogrel in combination with a parenteral anticoagulant and aspirin for patients who undergo PCI with stenting (ACCF/AHA/SCAI [Levine 2011]).

Oral: Initial: 600 mg once, administered ≥2 hours before PCI, ideally ≥24 hours before PCI; followed by 75 mg once daily (ACCF/AHA/SCAI [Levine 2011]; Cutlip 2020).

Duration of therapy: Upon completion of the recommended duration of DAPT (clopidogrel plus aspirin), discontinue clopidogrel and continue aspirin indefinitely (ACC/AHA [Levine 2016]; Cutlip 2019c):

- Bare metal stent implantation: DAPT for a minimum of 1 month (ACC/AHA [Levine 2016]). Some experts recommend at least 6 months and up to 12 months; in patients at high bleeding risk, shorter duration may be considered. After 6 to 12 months, assess bleeding and ischemic risks to determine if patient should receive longer therapy (eg, for an additional 18 to 24 months) (Cutlip 2019c).
- Drug eluting stent implantation: DAPT for at least 6 months and up to 12 months; if bleeding occurs or patient is at high risk of bleeding, may stop after 3 months (ACC/AHA [Levine 2016]). After 6 to 12 months, assess bleeding and ischemic risks to determine if patient should receive longer therapy (eg, for an additional 18 to 24 months) (Cutlip 2019c).

Carotid artery atherosclerosis, symptomatic (alternative agent) (off-label use):

Note: For patients who are intolerant of aspirin.

Oral: 75 mg once daily (ACCP [Alonso-Coello 2012]; Cucchiara 2019).

Carotid artery stenting (off-label use):

Initial:

Initiation ≥48 hours before procedure: **Oral:** 75 mg **twice daily** in combination with aspirin (Brott 2010; Fairman 2019).

Initiation <48 hours of procedure: **Oral:** 450 mg once ≥4 hours before procedure in combination with aspirin (Brott 2010; Fairman 2019).

Maintenance: **Oral:** 75 mg **once daily** in combination with aspirin for ≥6 weeks; after 6 weeks of DAPT with clopidogrel and aspirin, assess bleeding and ischemic risks to determine total duration of therapy; upon completion of DAPT, discontinue clopidogrel and continue aspirin indefinitely. In patients with history of neck irradiation, some experts recommend continuing clopidogrel plus aspirin indefinitely (Brott 2010; Fairman 2019).

Coronary artery bypass graft surgery (off-label use):

Aspirin-allergic or aspirin-intolerant patients: **Oral:** 75 mg once daily; continue indefinitely (AHA [Kulik 2015]).

Following off-pump coronary artery bypass graft surgery: Oral: 75 mg once daily in combination with aspirin for 1 year, then discontinue clopidogrel and continue aspirin indefinitely (AHA [Kulik 2015]; Deo 2013; Mannacio 2012).

Patients with acute coronary syndrome followed by coronary artery bypass graft surgery: Oral: 75 mg once daily in combination with aspirin for 1 year, then discontinue clopidogrel and continue aspirin indefinitely (AHA [Kulik 2015]). Some experts do not use clopidogrel postoperatively in these patients (Aranki 2020).

Peripheral atherosclerotic disease (upper or lower extremity; with or without revascularization): **Oral:** 75 mg once daily (ACCP [Alonso-Coello 2012]; AHA/ACC [Gerhard-Herman 2017]; CAPRIE 1996).

Stable ischemic heart disease (alternative agent) (off-label use):

Note: Aspirin is preferred; clopidogrel is an alternative for patients who have a history of GI bleeding or are allergic to aspirin (ACCF/AHA [Fihn 2012]).

Oral: 75 mg once daily (ACCF/AHA [Fihn 2012]; ACCP [Vandvik 2012]; CAPRIE 1996).

Stroke/Transient ischemic attack:

Intracranial atherosclerosis (50% to 99% stenosis of a major intracranial artery), secondary prevention:

Note: Aspirin is recommended for all patients; may consider clopidogrel (in combination with aspirin) for short-term use in patients with recent stroke or transient ischemic attack (within 30 days) (AHA/ASA [Kernan 2014]; Ehtisham 2019). For long-term stroke prevention, indefinite use of clopidogrel monotherapy is an alternative to aspirin (AHA/ASA [Kernan 2014]).

Oral: 75 mg once daily in combination with aspirin; duration of clopidogrel depends on degree of stenosis.

Stenosis of 50% to 69%: Clopidogrel may be added to aspirin for 21 days; after 21 days, discontinue clopidogrel and continue aspirin indefinitely (Ehtisham 2019).

Stenosis of 70% to 99%: Clopidogrel may be added to aspirin for 90 days; after 90 days, discontinue clopidogrel and continue aspirin indefinitely (AHA/ASA [Kernan 2014]; Derdeyn 2014; Ehtisham 2019).

Ischemic stroke or transient ischemic attack, noncardioembolic, secondary prevention:

Note: Single-agent antiplatelet therapy is recommended for long-term secondary prevention. Aspirin, clopidogrel, or aspirin/ER dipyridamole are all reasonable options depending on patient-specific factors. Some experts, however, prefer clopidogrel or aspirin/ER dipyridamole (ACCP [Lansberg 2012]; AHA/ASA [Kernan 2014]; Cucchiara 2019).

Oral: 75 mg once daily indefinitely; in patients who receive IV alteplase, antiplatelet therapy is generally delayed for ≥24 hours, but administered as soon as possible thereafter (AHA/ASA [Kernan 2014]; AHA/ASA [Powers 2018]).

Minor ischemic stroke (NIHSS score ≤3) or high-risk transient ischemic attack (ABCD^2 score ≥4):

Note: Short-term use of clopidogrel in combination with aspirin may be considered in patients who meet this criteria. Initiate antiplatelet therapy as soon as possible and within 24 hours of stroke onset. If an IV thrombolytic was administered, delay starting antiplatelet therapy for ≥24 hours but administer as soon as possible thereafter (AHA/ASA [Kernan 2014]; AHA/ASA [Powers 2018]; Johnston 2018; Wang 2013).

Oral: Initial: 300 to 600 mg in combination with aspirin; followed by 75 mg once daily in combination with aspirin for 21 days. After 21 days, transition to single-agent antiplatelet therapy with aspirin, clopidogrel, or aspirin/ER dipyridamole and continue indefinitely. If clopidogrel is used, continue to administer 75 mg once daily (ACCP [Lansberg 2012]; AHA/ASA [Kernan 2014]; AHA/ASA [Powers 2018]; Johnston 2018; Wang 2013).

Transcatheter *aortic* valve replacement, thromboprophylaxis (off-label use):

Note: Refer to institutional policies and procedures on use of antiplatelet therapy for patients who require therapeutic anticoagulation for a different indication.

Oral: 300 mg once prior to valve implantation in combination with aspirin; followed by 75 mg once daily for 3 to 6 months depending on the type of valve implanted; after completion of clopidogrel, continue aspirin indefinitely (ACC [Otto 2017]; AHA/ACC [Nishimura 2014], AHA/ACC [Nishimura 2017]; Kalich 2018). To minimize risk of bleeding complications, may give aspirin **or** clopidogrel alone and reserve dual antiplatelet therapy during the first 3 to 6 months for patients at high risk of a thrombotic event; for either strategy, continue aspirin indefinitely (Kuno 2019).

Transcatheter *mitral* valve repair with MitraClip device, thromboprophylaxis (off-label use):

Note: Patients are generally treated with antithrombotic therapy (antiplatelet or anticoagulant if there is a concurrent indication) for at least 6 months following the procedure (Stone 2018).

Oral:

Loading dose: 300 mg once immediately following MitraClip insertion or within 24 hours prior to the procedure; may use as monotherapy or in combination with aspirin (Stone 2018).

Maintenance: 75 mg once daily for at least 6 months; may use as monotherapy or in combination with aspirin (Stone 2018).

Transitioning between P2Y$_{12}$ inhibitors: Note: This provides general guidance on transitioning between P2Y12 inhibitors.

Transitioning from another P2Y$_{12}$ inhibitor to clopidogrel:

Transitioning from prasugrel:

Patient received prasugrel for ≤5 days: Give a clopidogrel 300 mg loading dose 24 hours after the last dose of prasugrel, followed by 75 mg once daily; some experts do not administer a loading dose (Lincoff 2019).

Patient received prasugrel for >5 days: Give clopidogrel 75 mg once daily, starting 24 hours after the last dose of prasugrel (Kerneis 2013; Lincoff 2019).

Transitioning from ticagrelor: Give a clopidogrel 600 mg loading dose 12 hours after the last dose of ticagrelor, followed by 75 mg once daily (Franchi 2018).

Renal Impairment: Adult

No dosage adjustment necessary (Basra 2011). **Note:** Chronic kidney disease stage 5 (ie, end-stage renal disease or an eGFR <15 mL/minute) is associated with higher residual platelet reactivity with maintenance dosing (Muller 2012).

Hemodialysis: Not dialyzable (NCS/SCCM [Frontera 2016])

Hepatic Impairment: Adult No dosage adjustment necessary.

Pediatric

Antiplatelet effect: Limited data available:

Infants and Children ≤24 months: In the PICOLO trial, a dose of 0.2 mg/kg/dose once daily was found to achieve a mean inhibition of platelet aggregation similar to adults receiving the adult recommended dose; **Note:** This study included pediatric patients with a systemic-to-pulmonary artery shunt, intracardiac or intravascular stent, Kawasaki disease, or arterial graft; 79% of patients received concomitant aspirin (ACCP [Monagle 2012]; Li 2008).

Children >2 years and Adolescents: Initial dose: 1 mg/kg once daily; in general, do not exceed adult dose (ACCP [Monagle 2012]; Finkelstein 2005; Soman 2006).

CYP2C19 poor metabolizers (ie, CYP2C19*2 or *3 carriers): Specific pediatric recommendations are lacking; based on experience in adult patients, routine genetic testing is not recommended in patients treated with clopidogrel undergoing percutaneous coronary intervention, testing may be considered to identify poor metabolizers who would be at risk for poor response while receiving clopidogrel; if identified, these patients may be considered for an alternative P2Y12 inhibitor (AHA [Levine 2011]).

Renal Impairment: Pediatric There are no pediatric-specific dosage adjustments provided in the manufacturer's labeling; use with caution. Based on adult data, no dosage adjustment is required; in adults, GFR stage 5 (ie, end-stage renal disease or an eGFR <15 mL/minute) is associated with higher residual platelet reactivity with maintenance dosing (Muller 2012).

Hepatic Impairment: Pediatric There are no pediatric-specific dosage adjustments provided in the manufacturer's labeling; in adults, no dosage adjustment is necessary.

Mechanism of Action Clopidogrel requires *in vivo* biotransformation to an active thiol metabolite. The active metabolite irreversibly blocks the $P2Y_{12}$ component of ADP receptors on the platelet surface, which prevents activation of the GPIIb/IIIa receptor complex, thereby reducing platelet aggregation. Platelets blocked by clopidogrel are affected for the remainder of their lifespan (~7 to 10 days).

Contraindications

Hypersensitivity (eg, anaphylaxis) to clopidogrel or any component of the formulation; active pathological bleeding (eg, peptic ulcer, intracranial hemorrhage).

Canadian labeling: Additional contraindications (not in US labeling): Significant liver impairment or cholestatic jaundice; concomitant use of repaglinide.

Warnings/Precautions [US Boxed Warning]: Effectiveness of clopidogrel results from its antiplatelet activity, which is dependent on its conversion to an active metabolite by the CYP-450 system, principally CYP2C19. In patients who are homozygous for nonfunctional alleles of the CYP2C19 genes (termed "CYP2C19 poor metabolizers"), clopidogrel at recommended doses forms less of the active metabolite and has a reduced effect on platelet activity. Tests are available to identify patients who are CYP2C19 poor metabolizers. Consider use of another platelet $P2Y_{12}$ inhibitor in patients identified as CYP2C19 poor metabolizers. Routine platelet function testing or genetic testing for CYP2C19 polymorphisms is not recommended (ACC/AHA [Levine 2016]; Scott 2013; Sibbing 2019). An individualized and multidisciplinary approach should be utilized to determine therapy discontinuation and management in patients with acute lower GI bleed (LGIB) who are on antiplatelet medications; risk of ongoing bleeding should be weighed with risk of thromboembolic events. If antiplatelet agents are discontinued, they should generally be resumed as soon as possible and at least within 7 days taking into account control of bleeding and cardiovascular risk. Aspirin should generally *not* be discontinued. Dual antiplatelet therapy (DAPT) should generally *not* be discontinued in the 90 days post-acute coronary syndrome or 30 days post-coronary stenting (Strate 2016).

In patients with coronary stents, premature interruption of therapy may result in stent thrombosis with subsequent fatal and nonfatal myocardial infarction. Duration of therapy, in general, is determined by the type of stent placed (bare metal or drug eluting) and whether an acute coronary syndrome event was ongoing at the time of placement (ACC/AHA [Levine 2016]; AHA/ACC/SCAI/ACS/ADA [Grines 2007]). In patients undergoing elective surgery, consider discontinuing 5 days before surgery (except in patients with cardiac stents that have not completed their full course of DAPT; patient-specific situations need to be discussed with cardiologist; AHA/ACC/SCAI/ACS/ADA Science Advisory provides recommendations) (Grines 2007). Elective noncardiac surgery should not be performed in patients in whom DAPT will need to be discontinued perioperatively within 30 days following bare metal stent (BMS) placement or within 12 months after drug-eluting stent (DES) placement. In patients undergoing urgent non-cardiac surgery during the first 4 to 6 weeks after BMS or DES placement, DAPT may be continued. In patients with stents undergoing surgery that requires discontinuation of the $P2Y_{12}$ inhibitor, continue aspirin and re-start the $P2Y_{12}$ inhibitor as soon as possible after surgery (ACC/AHA [Fleisher 2014]). In patients undergoing elective CABG, discontinue clopidogrel at least 5 days before procedure; when urgent CABG is necessary, the ACC/AHA CABG guidelines recommend discontinuation for at least 24 hours prior to surgery (ACC/AHA [Hillis 2011]). The ACC/AHA STEMI guidelines recommend discontinuation for at least 24 hours prior to *on-pump* CABG if possible; *off-pump* CABG may be performed within 24 hours of clopidogrel administration if the benefits of prompt revascularization outweigh the risks of bleeding (ACCF/AHA [O'Gara 2013]).

Because of structural similarities, cross-reactivity has been reported among the thienopyridines (clopidogrel, prasugrel, and ticlopidine); use with caution or avoid in patients with hypersensitivity or hematologic reactions to previous thienopyridine use. Use of clopidogrel is contraindicated in patients with hypersensitivity to clopidogrel. Although desensitization may be considered for mild to moderate hypersensitivity, do not desensitize patients with prior life-threatening allergic reactions to clopidogrel (eg, toxic epidermal necrolysis, exfoliative dermatitis, Stevens-Johnson syndrome, thrombotic thrombocytopenic purpura [TTP]) (Lokhandwala 2011). Use with caution in patients with moderate to severe renal impairment (experience is limited).

Clopidogrel increases the risk of bleeding. Use is contraindicated in patients with active pathological bleeding (eg, peptic ulcer, intracranial hemorrhage). Additional risk factors for bleeding include age ≥75 years, propensity to bleed (eg, recent trauma or surgery, recent or recurrent GI bleeding, active peptic ulcer disease, severe hepatic impairment), body weight <60 kg, CABG or other surgical procedure, concomitant use of medications that increase risk of bleeding (eg, warfarin, nonsteroidal anti-inflammatory drugs). Use with caution in patients with platelet disorders, bleeding disorders, and/or at increased risk for bleeding. Bleeding should be suspected if patient becomes hypotensive, even if overt signs of bleeding do not exist. It may be possible to restore hemostasis by administering exogenous platelets; however, platelet transfusions within 4 hours of the clopidogrel loading dose or 2 hours of the maintenance dose may be less effective. Cases of TTP (usually occurring within the first 2 weeks of therapy), resulting in some fatalities, have been reported; urgent plasmapheresis is required. In patients with recent lacunar stroke (within 180 days), the use of clopidogrel in addition to aspirin did not significantly reduce the incidence of the primary outcome of stroke recurrence (any ischemic stroke or intracranial hemorrhage) compared to aspirin alone; the use of clopidogrel in addition to aspirin did however increase the risk of major hemorrhage and the rate of all-cause mortality (SPS3 Investigators 2012). Potentially significant interactions may exist, requiring dose or frequency adjustment, additional monitoring, and/or selection of alternative therapy.

Drug Interactions

Metabolism/Transport Effects Substrate of CYP2C19 (major), CYP3A4 (minor); **Note:** Assignment of Major/Minor substrate status based on clinically relevant drug interaction potential; **Inhibits** BCRP/ABCG2, CYP2B6 (weak), CYP2C8 (moderate)

Avoid Concomitant Use

Avoid concomitant use of Clopidogrel with any of the following: Amodiaquine; Ozanimod; PAZOPanib; Rimegepant; Topotecan; Urokinase

Increased Effect/Toxicity

Clopidogrel may increase the levels/effects of: Agents with Antiplatelet Properties; Alpelisib; Amodiaquine; Anticoagulants; Apixaban; Bemiparin; BuPROPion;

Cephalothin; Cladribine; Collagenase (Systemic); Dabigatran Etexilate; Dabrafenib; Dasabuvir; Deoxycholic Acid; Desloratadine; Edoxaban; Enoxaparin; Enzalutamide; Heparin; Ibritumomab Tiuxetan; Obinutuzumab; Ombitasvir, Paritaprevir, Ritonavir, and Dasabuvir; Ozanimod; PACLitaxel (Conventional); PACLitaxel (Protein Bound); PAZOPanib; Pioglitazone; Repaglinide; Rimegepant; Rivaroxaban; Rosuvastatin; Salicylates; Selexipag; Sibutramine; Talazoparib; Thrombolytic Agents; Topotecan; Treprostinil; Tucatinib; Ubrogepant; Urokinase; Warfarin

The levels/effects of Clopidogrel may be increased by: Acalabrutinib; CYP2C19 Inducers (Strong); Dasatinib; Fat Emulsion (Fish Oil Based); Glucosamine; Herbs (Anticoagulant/Antiplatelet Properties); Ibrutinib; Inotersen; Limaprost; Multivitamins/Fluoride (with ADE); Multivitamins/Minerals (with ADEK, Folate, Iron); Multivitamins/Minerals (with AE, No Iron); Omega-3 Fatty Acids; Pentosan Polysulfate Sodium; Pentoxifylline; Prostacyclin Analogues; Selumetinib; Tipranavir; Vitamin E (Systemic); Zanubrutinib

Decreased Effect

The levels/effects of Clopidogrel may be decreased by: Amiodarone; Calcium Channel Blockers; Cangrelor; CYP2C19 Inhibitors (Moderate); CYP2C19 Inhibitors (Strong); Erythromycin (Systemic); Esomeprazole; Etravirine; FentaNYL; Grapefruit Juice; Lansoprazole; Morphine (Systemic); Omeprazole; Pantoprazole; Ritonavir; Sodium Zirconium Cyclosilicate

Food Interactions Consumption of three 200 mL glasses of grapefruit juice a day may substantially reduce clopidogrel antiplatelet effects. Management: Avoid or minimize the consumption of grapefruit or grapefruit juice (Holmberg 2013).

Dietary Considerations Avoid or minimize the consumption of grapefruit juice (Holmberg 2013).

Pharmacodynamics/Kinetics

Onset of Action

Onset of action: Inhibition of platelet aggregation (IPA): Dose-dependent:
- 300 to 600 mg loading dose: Detected within 2 hours
- 50 to 100 mg/day: Detected by the second day of treatment

Peak effect: Time to maximal IPA: Dose-dependent: **Note:** Degree of IPA based on adenosine diphosphate (ADP) concentration used during light aggregometry:
- 300 to 600 mg loading dose:
  - ADP 5 micromole/L: 20% to 30% IPA at 6 hours post administration (Montelescot 2006)
  - ADP 20 micromole/L: 30% to 37% IPA at 6 hours post administration (Montelescot 2006)
- 50 to 100 mg/day: ADP 5 micromole/L: 50% to 60% IPA at 5 to 7 days (Herbert 1993)

Duration of Action Platelet aggregation and bleeding time gradually return to baseline after ~5 days after discontinuation.

Half-life Elimination Parent drug: ~6 hours; Thiol derivative (active metabolite) ~30 minutes; carboxylic acid derivative (inactive; main circulating metabolite): ~8 hours; **Note:** A clopidogrel radiolabeled study has shown that covalent binding to platelets accounts for 2% of radiolabel and has a half-life of 11 days.

Time to Peak Serum: ~0.75 hours

Pregnancy Considerations

Information related to use during pregnancy is limited (Bauer 2012; De Santis 2011; Myers 2011). Based on available data, an increased risk of major birth defects, miscarriage, or adverse fetal outcomes has not been associated with maternal use of clopidogrel. According to the manufacturer, use should not be withheld if needed for emergent treatment of stroke or myocardial infarction during pregnancy. Discontinue use 5 to 7 days prior to labor, delivery, or neuraxial blockade if possible due to increased risk of maternal bleeding and hemorrhage.

Available guidelines recommend using clopidogrel only when strictly needed and for the shortest duration possible until additional fetal safety data are available (ESC [Regitz-Zagrosek 2018]).

Breastfeeding Considerations It is not known if clopidogrel is present in breast milk.

Adverse events have not been reported in breastfed infants (limited data). According to the manufacturer, the decision to breastfeed during therapy should consider the risk of infant exposure, the benefits of breastfeeding to the infant, and benefits of treatment to the mother.

Dosage Forms: US

Tablet, Oral:

Plavix: 75 mg

Generic: 75 mg, 300 mg

Dosage Forms: Canada

Tablet, Oral:

Plavix: 75 mg, 300 mg

Generic: 75 mg, 300 mg

Dental Health Professional Considerations

Aspirin in combination with clopidogrel (Plavix), prasugrel (Effient), or ticagrelor (Brilinta) is the primary prevention strategy against stent thrombosis after placement of drug-eluting metal stents in coronary patients. Premature discontinuation of combination antiplatelet therapy (ie, dual antiplatelet therapy) strongly increases the risk of a catastrophic event of stent thrombosis leading to myocardial infarction and/or death, according to a science advisory issued in January 2007 from the American Heart Association in collaboration with the American Dental Association and other professional health care organizations. The advisory stresses a 12-month therapy of dual antiplatelet therapy after placement of a drug-eluting stent in order to prevent thrombosis at the stent site. Any elective surgery should be postponed for 1 year after stent implantation and if surgery must be performed, consideration should be given to continue the antiplatelet therapy during the perioperative period in high-risk patients with drug-eluting stents.

This was issued from a science panel made up of representatives from the American Heart Association, the American College of Cardiology, the Society for Cardiovascular Angiography and Interventions, the American College of Surgeons, the American Dental Association, and the American College of Physicians (Grines 2007).

- **Clopidogrel Bisulfate** *see* Clopidogrel *on page 390*
- **Clopidogrel Hydrogen Sulfate** *see* Clopidogrel *on page 390*

Clorazepate (klor AZ e pate)

Related Information

Dentin Hypersensitivity, Acid Erosion, High Caries Index, Management of Alveolar Osteitis, and Xerostomia *on page 1762*

Brand Names: US Tranxene-T

Pharmacologic Category Anticonvulsant, Benzodiazepine; Benzodiazepine

Use

Alcohol withdrawal: Symptomatic relief of acute alcohol withdrawal.

Anxiety disorders: Management of anxiety disorders and short-term relief of the symptoms of anxiety.

Partial seizures: Adjunct therapy in the management of partial seizures.

Local Anesthetic/Vasoconstrictor Precautions No information available to require special precautions

Effects on Dental Treatment Key adverse event(s) related to dental treatment: Xerostomia (normal salivary flow resumes upon discontinuation); drowsiness; Patients may experience orthostatic hypotension as they stand up after treatment; especially if lying in dental chair for extended periods of time. Use caution with sudden changes in position during and after dental treatment. It is suggested that opioid analgesics not be given for pain control to patients taking clorazepate due to enhanced sedation.

Effects on Bleeding No information available to require special precautions

Adverse Reactions Frequency not defined.

Cardiovascular: Hypotension

Central nervous system: Anxiety, ataxia, confusion, depression, dizziness, drowsiness, dysarthria, fatigue, headache, insomnia, irritability, memory impairment, nervousness, slurred speech

Dermatologic: Skin rash

Endocrine & metabolic: Decreased libido

Gastrointestinal: Constipation, decreased appetite, diarrhea, increased appetite, nausea, vomiting, xerostomia

Hepatic: Increased serum transaminases, jaundice

Neuromuscular & skeletal: Tremor

Ophthalmic: Blurred vision, diplopia

Mechanism of Action Binds to stereospecific benzodiazepine receptors on the postsynaptic GABA neuron at several sites within the central nervous system, including the limbic system and reticular formation. Enhancement of the inhibitory effect of GABA on neuronal excitability results by increased neuronal membrane permeability to chloride ions. This shift in chloride ions results in hyperpolarization (a less excitable state) and stabilization. Benzodiazepine receptors and effects appear to be linked to the GABA-A receptors. Benzodiazepines do not bind to GABA-B receptors (Nelson 1999).

Pharmacodynamics/Kinetics

Half-life Elimination Nordiazepam: 20 to 160 hours; Oxazepam: 6 to 24 hours (Riss, 2008)

Time to Peak Serum: ~0.5 to 2 hour (Carrigan, 1977; Riss, 2008)

Pregnancy Considerations Nordiazepam, the active metabolite of clorazepate, crosses the placenta and is measurable in cord blood and amniotic fluid. Teratogenic effects have been observed with some benzodiazepines (including clorazepate); however, additional studies are needed. The incidence of premature birth and low birth weights may be increased following maternal use of benzodiazepines; hypoglycemia and respiratory problems in the neonate may occur following exposure late in pregnancy. Neonatal withdrawal symptoms may occur within days to weeks after birth and "floppy infant syndrome" (which also includes withdrawal symptoms) has been reported with some benzodiazepines (Bergman 1992; Iqbal 2002; Patel 1980; Rey 1979; Wikner 2007). A combination of factors influences the potential teratogenicity of anticonvulsant therapy. When treating women with epilepsy, monotherapy with the lowest effective dose and avoidance of medications known to have a high incidence of teratogenic effects is recommended (Harden 2009; Wlodarczyk 2012).

Patients exposed to clorazepate during pregnancy are encouraged to enroll themselves into the AED Pregnancy Registry by calling 1-888-233-2334. Additional information is available at www.aedpregnancyregistry.org.

Controlled Substance C-IV

- **Clorazepate Dipotassium** *see* Clorazepate *on page 395*
- **Cloroteka1** *see* Chloroprocaine *on page 337*
- **Clorox Nasal Antiseptic [OTC] [DSC]** *see* Povidone-Iodine (Topical) *on page 1249*
- **Clotrimazole 3 Day [OTC]** *see* Clotrimazole (Topical) *on page 397*

Clotrimazole (Oral) (kloe TRIM a zole)

Related Information

Fungal Infections *on page 1752*

Related Sample Prescriptions

Fungal Infections - Sample Prescriptions *on page 38*

Generic Availability (US) Yes

Pharmacologic Category Antifungal Agent, Imidazole Derivative; Antifungal Agent, Oral Nonabsorbed

Dental Use Treatment of susceptible fungal infections, including oropharyngeal candidiasis; limited data suggest that clotrimazole troches may be effective for prophylaxis against oropharyngeal candidiasis in neutropenic patients

Use

Oropharyngeal candidiasis (treatment): Local treatment of oropharyngeal candidiasis.

Oropharyngeal candidiasis (prophylaxis): To reduce the incidence of oropharyngeal candidiasis in immunocompromised patients undergoing chemotherapy, radiotherapy, or steroid therapy utilized in the treatment of leukemia, solid tumors, or renal transplantation.

Local Anesthetic/Vasoconstrictor Precautions No information available to require special precautions

Effects on Dental Treatment No significant effects or complications reported

Effects on Bleeding No information available to require special precautions

Adverse Reactions

>10%: Hepatic: Abnormal liver function tests

Frequency not defined:

Dermatologic: Pruritus

Gastrointestinal: Nausea, vomiting

Dental Usual Dosage Oropharyngeal candidiasis: Children >3 years and Adults: Oral:

Prophylaxis: 10 mg troche dissolved 3 times/day for the duration of chemotherapy or until steroids are reduced to maintenance levels

Treatment: 10 mg troche dissolved slowly 5 times/day for 14 consecutive days

Dosing

Adult & Geriatric

Oropharyngeal candidiasis, prophylaxis: Oral: 10 mg dissolved slowly 3 times daily for the duration of chemotherapy or until steroids are reduced to maintenance levels.

Oropharyngeal candidiasis, treatment (mild disease): Oral: 10 mg dissolved slowly 5 times daily for 7 to 14 consecutive days (AST-IDCOP [Aslam 2019]; HHS [OI adult 2020]; IDSA [Pappas 2016]).

Renal Impairment: Adult There are no dosage adjustments provided in the manufacturer's labeling.

Hepatic Impairment: Adult There are no dosage adjustments provided in the manufacturer's labeling.

Pediatric Candidiasis, oropharyngeal; treatment: Children ≥3 years and Adolescents: Oral: 10 mg troche dissolved slowly 5 times daily for 14 consecutive days. **Note:** When used for initial treatment in patients with HIV, duration of therapy is 7 to 14 days (HHS [OI adult 2016]; HHS [OI pediatric 2016]).

Renal Impairment: Pediatric There are no dosage adjustments provided in the manufacturer's labeling.

Hepatic Impairment: Pediatric There are no dosage adjustments provided in the manufacturer's labeling.

Mechanism of Action Binds to phospholipids in the fungal cell membrane altering cell wall permeability resulting in loss of essential intracellular elements

Contraindications

Hypersensitivity to clotrimazole or any component of the formulation

Documentation of allergenic cross-reactivity for antifungals is limited. However, because of similarities in chemical structure and/or pharmacologic actions, the possibility of cross-sensitivity can not be ruled out with certainty.

Warnings/Precautions Clotrimazole should not be used for treatment of systemic fungal infection. Abnormal LFTs have been reported, including abnormal aspartate aminotransferase (AST). Elevations are usually minimal. Monitor LFTs periodically, especially in patients with preexisting hepatic impairment. Clotrimazole must be slowly dissolved in the mouth for maximum efficacy. Potentially significant drug-drug interactions may exist, requiring dose or frequency adjustment, additional monitoring, and/or selection of alternative therapy.

Drug Interactions

Metabolism/Transport Effects Inhibits CYP3A4 (weak)

Avoid Concomitant Use

Avoid concomitant use of Clotrimazole (Oral) with any of the following: Pimozide

Increased Effect/Toxicity

Clotrimazole (Oral) may increase the levels/effects of: Dofetilide; Flibanserin; Lemborexant; Lomitapide; NiMODipine; Pimozide; Tacrolimus (Systemic); Triazolam; Ubrogepant

Decreased Effect There are no known significant interactions involving a decrease in effect.

Pregnancy Risk Factor C

Pregnancy Considerations

Adverse events have been observed in animal reproduction studies.

Breastfeeding Considerations It is not known if clotrimazole is excreted in breast milk following oral (troche) administration (data not located); however, systemic absorption is low (Sawyer 1975).

Dosage Forms: US

Troche, Mouth/Throat:

Generic: 10 mg

Clotrimazole (Topical) (kloe TRIM a zole)

Brand Names: US 3 Day Vaginal [OTC]; Alevazol [OTC]; Clotrimazole 3 Day [OTC]; Clotrimazole Anti-Fungal [OTC]; Clotrimazole GRx [OTC]; Desenex [OTC]; Gyne-Lotrimin 3 [OTC]; Gyne-Lotrimin [OTC]; Lotrimin AF For Her [OTC]; Lotrimin AF [OTC] [DSC]; Pro-Ex Antifungal [OTC]; Shopko Athletes Foot [OTC]

Generic Availability (US) Yes

Pharmacologic Category Antifungal Agent, Imidazole Derivative; Antifungal Agent, Oral Nonabsorbed/Partially Absorbed; Antifungal Agent, Topical; Antifungal Agent, Vaginal

Use

Topical cream and solution: Topical treatment of candidiasis due to *Candida albicans* and tinea versicolor caused by *Malassezia furfur*

OTC labeling: Topical treatment of tinea pedis, tinea cruris, and tinea corporis

Topical ointment: *OTC labeling:* Topical treatment of tinea cruris, *C. albicans*, tinea corporis, and tinea pedis

Vaginal cream: Treatment of vaginal yeast infections and relief of associated external vulvar itching and irritation

Vaginal tablet [Canadian product]: Treatment of vaginal candidiasis

Local Anesthetic/Vasoconstrictor Precautions No information available to require special precautions

Effects on Dental Treatment No significant effects or complications reported

Effects on Bleeding No information available to require special precautions

Adverse Reactions Vaginal:

1% to 10%: Genitourinary: Vulvovaginal burning

<1% (Limited to important or life-threatening): Burning sensation of the penis (of sexual partner), polyuria, pruritus vulvae, vaginal discharge, vulvar pain, vulvar swelling

Dental Usual Dosage Cutaneous candidiasis: Children >3 years and Adults: Topical (cream, solution): Apply twice daily; if no improvement occurs after 4 weeks of therapy, re-evaluate diagnosis.

Dosing

Adult & Geriatric

Cutaneous candidiasis: Topical:

Cream, solution: Apply to affected area twice daily; if no improvement occurs after 4 weeks of therapy, re-evaluate diagnosis.

Ointment (OTC labeling): Apply to affected area twice daily for 2 weeks.

Otomycosis (off-label use): Topical: Solution: Instill 4 to 5 drops into the affected ear(s) twice daily for 10 to 14 days (Chander 1996; de la Paz Cota 2018; Goguen 2019); application should begin after thorough cleansing of the ear canal by the provider. Reassess after completion of therapy; if fungal elements are still present, repeat cleansing of the ear canal followed by another 10- to 14-day course of clotrimazole and reassessment. Several cycles of ear cleansing followed by topical therapy and reassessment may be required; persistent otomycosis should be managed by an otolaryngologist (Goguen 2019).

Tinea corporis, tinea cruris, tinea pedis (OTC labeling): Topical: Cream, ointment, solution: Apply to affected area twice daily for 2 weeks (tinea cruris) or 4 weeks (tinea corporis, tinea pedis).

Tinea versicolor: Topical: Cream, solution: Apply to affected area twice daily; if no improvement occurs after 4 weeks of therapy, re-evaluate diagnosis.

Vulvovaginal candidiasis: Intravaginal: **Note:** A longer duration may be necessary in patients with complicated infection (ie, recurrent or severe infection, infection with non-*albicans Candida*, or infection in an immunocompromised host) (CDC [Workowski 2015]; HHS [OI adult 2020]).

Cream (1%): Insert 1 applicatorful of 1% vaginal cream daily (at bedtime) for 7 consecutive days. **Note:** Guidelines recommend a duration of 7 to 14 days (CDC [Workowski 2015]). May also apply externally twice daily for 7 days as needed for itching and irritation.

Canesten 6 day intravaginal cream (1%) [Canadian product]: Insert 1 applicatorful of 1% vaginal cream daily (preferably at bedtime) for 6 consecutive days.

Cream (2%): Insert 1 applicatorful of 2% vaginal cream daily (preferably at bedtime) for 3 consecutive days. May also apply externally twice daily for 7 days as needed for itching and irritation.

Cream (10%) [Canadian product]: Insert 1 applicatorful of 10% vaginal cream as a single dose (preferably at bedtime)

Tablet [Canadian product]:

500 mg tablet: Insert 1 vaginal tablet as a single dose (preferably at bedtime)

200 mg tablet: Insert 1 vaginal tablet once daily for 3 consecutive days (preferably at bedtime)

Note: When tablets are used in conjunction with an external cream, apply cream over the irritated area 1 to 2 times/day as needed for up to 7 consecutive days

Renal Impairment: Adult There are no dosage adjustments provided in the manufacturer's labeling; however, dosage adjustment unlikely due to low systemic absorption.

Hepatic Impairment: Adult There are no dosage adjustments provided in the manufacturer's labeling; however, dosage adjustment unlikely due to low systemic absorption.

Pediatric

Cutaneous candidiasis: Topical ointment: Children ≥2 years and Adolescents: Topical: Apply twice daily (morning and night) for 2 weeks.

Tinea corporis, tinea cruris, and tinea pedis: Topical cream, ointment, or solution: Children ≥2 years and Adolescents: Topical: Apply twice daily (morning and night). Duration: 2 weeks for tinea cruris; 4 weeks for tinea corporis and tinea pedis

Vulvovaginal candidiasis: Children ≥12 years and Adolescents: Intravaginal:

Cream (1%): Insert 1 applicatorful of 1% vaginal cream daily (preferably at bedtime) for 7 consecutive days; some patients may require 14 days (CDC [Workowski 2015]). May also apply externally twice daily for 7 days as needed for itching and irritation.

Cream (2%): Insert 1 applicatorful of 2% vaginal cream daily (preferably at bedtime) for 3 consecutive days. May also apply externally twice daily for 7 days as needed for itching and irritation.

Renal Impairment: Pediatric There are no dosage adjustments provided in the manufacturer's labeling; however, dosage adjustment unlikely needed due to low systemic absorption.

Hepatic Impairment: Pediatric There are no dosage adjustments provided in the manufacturer's labeling; however, dosage adjustment unlikely needed due to low systemic absorption.

Mechanism of Action Binds to phospholipids in the fungal cell membrane altering cell wall permeability resulting in loss of essential intracellular elements

Contraindications

Hypersensitivity to clotrimazole or any component of the formulation.

OTC labeling: When used for self-medication, do not use vaginal cream if you have never had a vaginal yeast infection diagnosed by a doctor.

Documentation of allergenic cross-reactivity for imidazole antifungals is limited. However, because of similarities in chemical structure and/or pharmacologic actions, the possibility of cross-sensitivity cannot be ruled out with certainty.

Warnings/Precautions Topical formulations are for external use only; avoid contact with the eyes. Not effective for treatment of scalp or nails. When used for self-medication, discontinue use and contact a healthcare provider if there is no improvement in 2 weeks (jock itch) or 4 weeks (athlete's foot, ringworm). If irritation/sensitivity develops, discontinue therapy and institute appropriate alternative therapy. When vaginal formulations are used for self-medication (OTC), consult a health care provider before use if experiencing vaginal itching and discomfort for the first time, frequent vaginal yeast infections (eg, monthly, 3 in 6 months), or exposure to HIV. A mild increase in vaginal itching, burning, or irritation may occur with use; a health care provider should be consulted before switching to another agent if patient does not experience complete relief. Discontinue use and contact a health care provider if symptoms do not improve in 3 days or last more than 7 days, or if symptoms of a more serious condition occur (eg, abdominal pain, back/shoulder pain, fever, chills, nausea, vomiting, foul-smelling vaginal discharge). For vaginal use only; do not use tampons, douches, spermicides, or other vaginal products or have vaginal intercourse during treatment.

Benzyl alcohol and derivatives: Some dosage forms may contain benzyl alcohol; large amounts of benzyl alcohol (≥99 mg/kg/day) have been associated with a potentially fatal toxicity ("gasping syndrome") in neonates; the "gasping syndrome" consists of metabolic acidosis, respiratory distress, gasping respirations, CNS dysfunction (including convulsions, intracranial hemorrhage), hypotension and cardiovascular collapse (AAP ["Inactive" 1997]; CDC 1982); some data suggests that benzoate displaces bilirubin from protein binding sites (Ahlfors 2001); avoid or use dosage forms containing benzyl alcohol with caution in neonates. See manufacturer's labeling.

Drug Interactions

Metabolism/Transport Effects None known.

Avoid Concomitant Use

Avoid concomitant use of Clotrimazole (Topical) with any of the following: Progesterone

Increased Effect/Toxicity

Clotrimazole (Topical) may increase the levels/effects of: Sirolimus; Tacrolimus (Systemic)

Decreased Effect

Clotrimazole (Topical) may decrease the levels/effects of: Progesterone

Pharmacodynamics/Kinetics

Time to Peak Serum: Vaginal cream: ~24 hours

Reproductive Considerations
Vaginal products may weaken latex condoms and diaphragms (CDC [Workowski 2015]) and may not be effective in preventing pregnancy or sexually transmitted diseases.

Pregnancy Considerations
Following topical and vaginal administration, small amounts of imidazoles are absorbed systemically (Duhm 1974). Vaginal topical azole products (7-day therapies only) are the preferred treatment of vulvovaginal candidiasis in pregnant women.

Breastfeeding Considerations
It is not known if clotrimazole is present in breast milk. The manufacturer recommends that caution be exercised when administering clotrimazole to breastfeeding women.

Dosage Forms: US

Cream, External:
Clotrimazole Anti-Fungal [OTC]: 1% (45 g)
Clotrimazole GRx [OTC]: 1% (14 g)
Desenex [OTC]: 1% (30 g)
Lotrimin AF For Her [OTC]: 1% (24 g)
Pro-Ex Antifungal [OTC]: 1% (42 g)
Shopko Athletes Foot [OTC]: 1% (28.4 g)
Generic: 1% (15 g, 28 g, 30 g, 45 g)

Cream, Vaginal:
3 Day Vaginal [OTC]: 2% (21 g)
Clotrimazole 3 Day [OTC]: 2% (22.2 g)
Gyne-Lotrimin [OTC]: 1% (45 g)
Gyne-Lotrimin 3 [OTC]: 2% (21 g)
Generic: 1% (45 g)

Ointment, External:
Alevazol [OTC]: 1% (56.7 g)

Solution, External:
Generic: 1% (10 mL, 29.57 mL, 30 mL)

- **Clotrimazole Anti-Fungal [OTC]** *see* Clotrimazole (Topical) *on page 397*
- **Clotrimazole GRx [OTC]** *see* Clotrimazole (Topical) *on page 397*

Cloxacillin (kloks a SIL in)

Brand Names: Canada APO-Cloxi; TEVA-Cloxacillin
Pharmacologic Category Antibiotic, Penicillin
Use Note: Not approved in the US

Bacterial infections: Treatment of bacterial infections including endocarditis, pneumonia, bone and joint infections, skin and soft-tissue infections, and sepsis that are caused by susceptible strains of penicillinase-producing staphylococci.

Limitations of use: Exhibits good activity against *Staphylococcus aureus*; has activity against many streptococci, but is less active than penicillin and is generally not used in clinical practice to treat streptococcal infections. Not effective against methicillin-resistant staphylococci.

Local Anesthetic/Vasoconstrictor Precautions
No information available to require special precautions

Effects on Dental Treatment Key adverse event(s) related to dental treatment: Prolonged use of penicillins may lead to development of oral candidiasis.

Effects on Bleeding No information available to require special precautions

Adverse Reactions Frequency not defined. Adverse effects may be reported as class effects rather than specific to cloxacillin.
Cardiovascular: Hypotension, thrombophlebitis
Central nervous system: Confusion, lethargy, myoclonus, seizure (high doses and/or renal failure), twitching
Dermatologic: Pruritus, skin rash, urticaria
Gastrointestinal: Abdominal pain, diarrhea, epigastric distress, flatulence, hairy tongue, loose stools, melanoglossia, nausea, oral candidiasis, pseudomembranous colitis, stomatitis, vomiting
Genitourinary: Hematuria, proteinuria
Hematologic & oncologic: Agranulocytosis, anemia, bone marrow depression, eosinophilia, granulocytopenia, hemolytic anemia, immune thrombocytopenia, leukopenia, neutropenia, thrombocytopenia
Hepatic: Increased serum alkaline phosphatase, increased serum ALT, increased serum AST, hepatotoxicity
Hypersensitivity: Anaphylaxis, angioedema, hypersensitivity reaction (immediate and delayed)
Immunologic: Serum sickness-like reaction
Neuromuscular & skeletal: Laryngospasm
Renal: Interstitial nephritis, renal insufficiency, renal tubular disease
Respiratory: Bronchospasm, laryngeal edema, sneezing, wheezing
Miscellaneous: Fever

Mechanism of Action Inhibits bacterial cell wall synthesis by binding to one or more of the penicillin-binding proteins (PBPs) which in turn inhibit the final transpeptidation step of peptidoglycan synthesis in bacterial cell walls, thus inhibiting cell wall biosynthesis. Bacteria eventually lyse due to ongoing activity of cell wall autolytic enzymes (autolysins and murein hydrolases) while cell wall assembly is arrested.

Pharmacodynamics/Kinetics
Half-life Elimination 0.5 to 1.5 hours; prolonged with renal impairment and in neonates
Time to Peak Oral: Serum: ~1 hour

Pregnancy Considerations
Penicillin class antibiotics cross the placenta in varying degrees. Cloxacillin is highly protein bound which may influence fetal exposure (Nau 1987).

As a class, penicillin antibiotics are widely used in pregnant women. Based on available data, penicillin antibiotics are generally considered compatible for use during pregnancy (Ailes 2016; Bookstaver 2015; Crider 2009; Damkier 2019; Lamont 2014; Muanda 2017a; Muanda 2017b).

Product Availability Not available in the US

- **Cloxacillin Sodium** *see* Cloxacillin *on page 399*

CloZAPine (KLOE za peen)

Brand Names: US Clozaril; FazaClo [DSC]; Versacloz
Brand Names: Canada AA-Clozapine; Clozaril; GEN-Clozapine
Pharmacologic Category Second Generation (Atypical) Antipsychotic

Use

Schizophrenia, treatment resistant: Treatment of severely ill patients with schizophrenia who fail to respond adequately to antipsychotic treatment.

Suicidal behavior in schizophrenia or schizoaffective disorder: To reduce the risk of suicidal behavior in patients with schizophrenia or schizoaffective disorder who are judged to be at chronic risk for reexperiencing suicidal behavior, based on history and recent clinical state.

Local Anesthetic/Vasoconstrictor Precautions Most pharmacology textbooks state that in presence of phenothiazines, systemic doses of epinephrine paradoxically decrease the blood pressure. This is the so called "epinephrine reversal" phenomenon. This has never been observed when epinephrine is given by infiltration as part of the local anesthesia procedure.

Effects on Dental Treatment Key adverse event(s) related to dental treatment: Sialorrhea and xerostomia (normal salivary flow resumes upon discontinuation); Patients may experience orthostatic hypotension as they stand up after treatment; especially if lying in dental chair for extended periods of time. Use caution with sudden changes in position during and after dental treatment. Do not use atropine-like drugs for xerostomia in patients taking clozapine due to significant potentiation.

Effects on Bleeding No information available to require special precautions

Adverse Reactions

>10%:

Cardiovascular: Hypertension (4% to 12%), hypotension (9% to 13%), tachycardia (17% to 25%)

Gastrointestinal: Constipation (14% to 25%), dyspepsia (14%), nausea (≤3% to 17%), sialorrhea (13% to 48%), vomiting (≤3% to 17%), weight gain (4% to 31%)

Nervous system: Dizziness (14% to 27%), drowsiness (≤39% to 46%), insomnia (2% to 20%), sedated state (≤39%), vertigo (≤19%)

Miscellaneous: Fever (5% to 13%)

1% to 10%:

Cardiovascular: Syncope (6%)

Dermatologic: Diaphoresis (6%), skin rash (2%)

Gastrointestinal: Abdominal distress (≤4%), diarrhea (2%), heartburn (≤4%), xerostomia (5% to 6%)

Genitourinary: Urine abnormality (2%)

Hematologic & oncologic: Eosinophilia (1%), leukopenia (≤3%), neutropenia (≤3%)

Nervous system: Agitation (4%), akathisia (3%), akinesia (≤4%), confusion (3%), disturbed sleep (≤4%), fatigue (2%), headache (7% to 10%), nightmares (≤4%), restlessness (4%), seizure (3%; dose related)

Neuromuscular & skeletal: Hypokinesia (≤4%), muscle rigidity (3%), tremor (6%)

Ophthalmic: Visual disturbance (5%)

<1%, postmarketing, and/or case reports: Abnormal electroencephalogram, acute myocardial infarction, agranulocytosis, angioedema, angle-closure glaucoma, atrial fibrillation, bradycardia, cardiac failure, cardiomyopathy, cataplexy, cerebrovascular accident, cholestasis, colitis, decreased gastrointestinal motility, deep vein thrombosis, delirium, diabetes mellitus, diabetes mellitus with hyperosmolar coma, drug reaction with eosinophilia and systemic symptoms, dyschromia, dysphagia, enlargement of salivary glands, erythema multiforme, fecal impaction, gastrointestinal infarction, granulocytopenia, hepatic cirrhosis, hepatic failure, hepatic fibrosis, hepatic necrosis, hepatitis, hepatotoxicity, hyperglycemia, hypersensitivity angiitis, hypersensitivity reaction, hyperuricemia, hyponatremia, increased creatine phosphokinase in blood specimen, increased erythrocyte sedimentation rate, increased hematocrit, increased hemoglobin, increased serum cholesterol, increased serum triglycerides, interstitial nephritis (acute), intestinal obstruction, ischemia (intestinal), jaundice, ketoacidosis, liver injury, liver steatosis, lower respiratory tract infection, mitral valve insufficiency, myasthenia, myocarditis, myoclonus, neuroleptic malignant syndrome, nocturnal enuresis, non-Hirschsprung megacolon, obsessive compulsive disorder, obstructive sleep apnea syndrome (Shirani 2011), orthostatic hypotension, palpitations, pancreatitis (acute), paralytic ileus, paresthesia, periorbital edema, pheochromocytoma (pseudo), pleural effusion, pneumonia, priapism, prolonged QT interval on ECG, psychosis (exacerbated), pulmonary aspiration, pulmonary embolism, renal failure, retrograde ejaculation, rhabdomyolysis, sepsis, sialadenitis, skin photosensitivity, status epilepticus, Stevens-Johnson syndrome, syncope, systemic lupus erythematosus, tardive dyskinesia, thrombocytopenia, thrombocytosis, torsades de pointes, transient ischemic attacks, vasculitis, ventricular fibrillation, ventricular tachycardia, weight loss

Mechanism of Action The therapeutic efficacy of clozapine (dibenzodiazepine antipsychotic) is proposed to be mediated through antagonism of the dopamine type 2 (D_2) and serotonin type 2A (5-HT_{2A}) receptors. In addition, it acts as an antagonist at alpha-adrenergic, histamine H_1, cholinergic, and other dopaminergic and serotonergic receptors.

Pharmacodynamics/Kinetics

Onset of Action Within 1 week for sedation, improvement in sleep; 6 to 12 weeks for antipsychotic effects; Adequate trial: 6 to 12 weeks at a therapeutic dose and blood level; Maximum effect: 6 to 12 months; improvement may continue 6 to 12 months after clozapine initiation (Meltzer 2003).

Duration of Action Variable

Half-life Elimination Steady state: 12 hours (range: 4 to 66 hours)

Time to Peak Suspension: 2.2 hours (range: 1 to 3.5 hours); Tablets: 2.5 hours (range: 1 to 6 hours); Dispersible tablets: 2.3 hours (range: 1 to 6 hours)

Pregnancy Considerations

Clozapine crosses the placenta and can be detected in the fetal blood and amniotic fluid (Barnas 1994; Imaz 2018).

Outcome information following maternal use of clozapine during pregnancy is limited (Beex-Oosterhuis 2020; Larsen 2015; Mehta 2017; Nguyen 2020). Antipsychotic use during the third trimester of pregnancy has a risk for abnormal muscle movements (extrapyramidal symptoms) and/or withdrawal symptoms in newborns following delivery. Symptoms in the newborn may include agitation, feeding disorder, hypertonia, hypotonia, respiratory distress, somnolence, and tremor; these effects may be self-limiting or require hospitalization.

The American College of Obstetricians and Gynecologists (ACOG) recommends that therapy during pregnancy be individualized; treatment with psychiatric medications during pregnancy should incorporate the clinical expertise of the mental health clinician, obstetrician, primary healthcare provider, and pediatrician. Safety data related to atypical antipsychotics during pregnancy is limited and routine use is not recommended. However, if a woman is inadvertently exposed to an atypical antipsychotic while pregnant, continuing therapy may be preferable to switching to an agent that the fetus has not yet been exposed to; consider risk: benefit (ACOG 2008). An increased risk of exacerbation of psychosis should be considered when discontinuing or changing treatment during pregnancy and postpartum. In general, other agents are preferred for use in pregnancy; however, clozapine may be used in women who cannot be switched to recommended antipsychotics (Larsen 2015).

Health care providers are encouraged to enroll women 18 to 45 years of age exposed to clozapine during pregnancy in the Atypical Antipsychotics Pregnancy Registry (1-866-961-2388 or http://www.womensmentalhealth.org/pregnancyregistry).

Prescribing and Access Restrictions Canada: Currently, there are multiple manufacturers that distribute clozapine and each manufacturer has its own registry and distribution system. Patients must be registered in a database that includes their location, prescribing physician, testing laboratory, and dispensing pharmacist before using clozapine. Patients may not be switched from one brand of clozapine to another without completion of a new registry-specific patient registration form by signed by the prescribing physician. Information specific to each monitoring program is available from the individual manufacturers.

- **Clozaril** *see* CloZAPine *on page* 399
- **CMA-676** *see* Gemtuzumab Ozogamicin *on page* 734
- **4CMenB** *see* Meningococcal Group B Vaccine *on page* 963
- **C-Met/Hepatocyte Growth Factor Receptor Tyrosine Kinase Inhibitor PF-02341066** *see* Crizotinib *on page* 415
- **C-Met/HGFR Tyrosine Kinase Inhibitor PF-02341066** *see* Crizotinib *on page* 415
- **C-MET Inhibitor INCB028060** *see* Capmatinib *on page* 283
- **CNJ-016** *see* Vaccinia Immune Globulin (Intravenous) *on page* 1511
- **CNL8 Nail [DSC]** *see* Ciclopirox *on page* 346
- **CNTO-148** *see* Golimumab *on page* 744
- **CNTO 328** *see* Siltuximab *on page* 1371
- **CNTO 1275** *see* Ustekinumab *on page* 1510
- **CNTO 1959** *see* Guselkumab *on page* 750
- **Coagulant Complex Inhibitor** *see* Anti-inhibitor Coagulant Complex (Human) *on page* 156
- **Coagulation Factor I** *see* Fibrinogen Concentrate (Human) *on page* 666
- **Coagulation Factor Xa (Recombinant), Inactivated zhzo** *see* Andexanet Alfa *on page* 151
- **Co-Amoxiclav** *see* Amoxicillin and Clavulanate *on page* 130
- **Coartem** *see* Artemether and Lumefantrine *on page* 168

Cobicistat (koe BIK i stat)

Brand Names: US Tybost

Brand Names: Canada Tybost

Pharmacologic Category Cytochrome P-450 Inhibitor

Use

HIV-1 infection, treatment: Treatment of HIV-1 infection in adults to increase systemic exposure of atazanavir or darunavir (once-daily dosing regimen) in combination with other antiretroviral agents; treatment of HIV-1 infection to increase systemic exposure of atazanavir or darunavir (once-daily regimen) in pediatric patients weighing ≥35 kg or ≥40 kg, respectively, in combination with other antiretroviral agents.

Limitations of use: Cobicistat is **not** interchangeable with ritonavir to increase systemic exposure of darunavir 600 mg twice daily, fosamprenavir, saquinavir, or tipranavir due to lack of exposure data. The use of cobicistat is not recommended with darunavir 600 mg twice daily, fosamprenavir, saquinavir, or tipranavir.

Local Anesthetic/Vasoconstrictor Precautions No information available to require special precautions

Effects on Dental Treatment No significant effects or complications reported

Effects on Bleeding No information available to require special precautions

Adverse Reactions All adverse reactions are from trials using cobicistat coadministered with atazanavir, emtricitabine + tenofovir unless otherwise noted.

>10%: Hepatic: Hyperbilirubinemia (grades 3/4: 73%)

1% to 10%:

Cardiovascular: Increased serum creatine kinase (grades 3/4: 8%)

Central nervous system: Headache (2%), abnormal dreams (<2%), depression (<2%), fatigue (<2%), insomnia (<2%)

Dermatologic: Skin rash (5%)

Endocrine & metabolic: Increased gamma-glutamyl transferase (grades 3/4: 4%), glycosuria (grades 3/4: 3%), hyperglycemia (grades 3/4: 2%), Fanconi's syndrome (<2%)

Gastrointestinal: Increased serum lipase (grades 3/4: 7%), increased serum amylase (grades 3/4: 4%), diarrhea (2%), nausea (2%), upper abdominal pain (<2%), vomiting (<2%)

Genitourinary: Hematuria (grades 3/4: 6%), proximal tubular nephropathy (2%)

Hematologic & oncologic: Decreased neutrophils (grades 3/4: 3%)

Hepatic: Increased serum alanine aminotransferase (grades 3/4: 6%), jaundice (6%), increased serum aspartate aminotransferase (grades 3/4: 4%)

Neuromuscular & skeletal: Rhabdomyolysis (<2%)

Ophthalmic: Scleral icterus (4%)

Renal: Nephrolithiasis (<2%), renal disease (<2%)

Frequency not defined:

Endocrine & metabolic: Increased HDL cholesterol, increased LDL cholesterol, increased serum cholesterol, increased serum triglycerides

Renal: Decreased creatinine clearance (no effect on renal glomerular function in patients with normal renal function), increased serum creatinine, renal insufficiency

Mechanism of Action Cobicistat is a mechanism-based inhibitor of cytochrome P450 3A (CYP3A). Inhibition of CYP3A-mediated metabolism by cobicistat and increases the systemic exposure of CYP3A substrates atazanavir and darunavir.

Pharmacodynamics/Kinetics

Half-life Elimination Terminal: ~3 to 4 hours

Time to Peak ~3.5 hours

Reproductive Considerations

The Health and Human Services (HHS) perinatal HIV guidelines do not recommend cobicistat for females living with HIV who are not yet pregnant but are trying to conceive.

For males and females living with HIV and planning a pregnancy, maximum viral suppression below the limits of detection with antiretroviral therapy (ART), modification of therapy (if needed), optimization of the woman's health, and a discussion of the potential risks and benefits of ART therapy during pregnancy is recommended prior to conception (HHS [perinatal] 2019).

Pregnancy Considerations Cobicistat has low placental transfer.

An increased risk of teratogenic effects has not been observed based on information collected by the antiretroviral pregnancy registry. Maternal antiretroviral therapy (ART) may be associated with adverse pregnancy outcomes including preterm delivery, stillbirth, low birth weight, and small for gestational age infants. Actual risks may be influenced by maternal factors, such as disease severity, gestational age at initiation of therapy, and specific ART regimen, therefore close fetal monitoring is recommended. Because there is clear benefit to appropriate treatment, maternal ART should not be withheld due to concerns for adverse neonatal outcomes. Long-term follow-up is recommended for all infants exposed to antiretroviral medications; children without HIV but who were exposed to ART in utero and develop significant organ system abnormalities of unknown etiology (particularly of the CNS or heart) should be evaluated for potential mitochondrial dysfunction.

The Health and Human Services (HHS) perinatal HIV guidelines do not recommend cobicistat for use in pregnant females living with HIV who are antiretroviral-naive, who have had ART therapy in the past but are restarting, or who require a new ART regimen (due to poor tolerance or poor virologic response of current regimen). Cobicistat exposure is decreased in pregnancy. Use of cobicistat boosted atazanavir, darunavir, or elvitegravir in pregnancy is **not recommended;** patients who become pregnant during therapy should consider changing to a more effective, recommended regimen. If cobicistat is continued in a pregnant patient who is virally suppressed, monitor the viral load more frequently (eg, monthly during the second and third trimesters).

In general, ART is recommended for all pregnant females living with HIV to keep the viral load below the limit of detection and reduce the risk of perinatal transmission. Therapy should be individualized following a discussion of the potential risks and benefits of treatment during pregnancy. Monitoring of pregnant females is more frequent than in nonpregnant adults. ART should be continued postpartum for all females living with HIV and can be modified after delivery.

Health care providers are encouraged to enroll pregnant females exposed to antiretroviral medications as early in pregnancy as possible in the Antiretroviral Pregnancy Registry (800-258-4263 or http://www.-APRegistry.com). Health care providers caring for pregnant females living with HIV and their infants may contact the National Perinatal HIV Hotline (888-448-8765) for clinical consultation (HHS [perinatal] 2019).

- ◆ **Cobicistat and Atazanavir** *see* Atazanavir and Cobicistat *on page 188*
- ◆ **Cobicistat, Emtricitabine, Tenofovir Alafenamide, and Darunavir,** *see* Darunavir, Cobicistat, Emtricitabine, and Tenofovir Alafenamide *on page 442*
- ◆ **Cobicistat, Emtricitabine, Tenofovir Alafenamide, and Elvitegravir** *see* Elvitegravir, Cobicistat, Emtricitabine, and Tenofovir Alafenamide *on page 553*
- ◆ **Cobicistat, Emtricitabine, Tenofovir Disoproxil Fumarate, and Elvitegravir** *see* Elvitegravir, Cobicistat, Emtricitabine, and Tenofovir Disoproxil Fumarate *on page 553*

Cobimetinib (koe bi ME ti nib)

Brand Names: US Cotellic
Brand Names: Canada Cotellic

Pharmacologic Category Antineoplastic Agent, MEK Inhibitor

Use Melanoma, unresectable or metastatic: Treatment of unresectable or metastatic melanoma in patients with a BRAF V600E or V600K mutation (in combination with vemurafenib)

Local Anesthetic/Vasoconstrictor Precautions Hypertension can occur with the use of this drug. Monitor for hypertension prior to using local anesthetic with vasoconstrictor; medical consult if necessary.

Effects on Dental Treatment Key adverse event(s) related to dental treatment: Stomatitis (14%; includes aphthous stomatitis, mucositis, and oral mucosa ulcer) has been observed

Effects on Bleeding Hemorrhage may occur with cobimetinib; Grade 3 to 4 bleeding has occurred. In patients who are under active treatment with these agents, medical consult is suggested.

Adverse Reactions Percentages reported as part of combination chemotherapy regimens.

>10%:

Cardiovascular: Decreased left ventricular ejection fraction (grades 2/3: 26%), hypertension (15%)

Dermatologic: Skin photosensitivity (46% to 47%, grades 3/4: 4%; includes solar dermatitis and sunburn), acneiform eruption (16%, grades 3/4: 2%)

Endocrine & metabolic: Hypophosphatemia (68%), increased gamma-glutamyl transferase (65%; grades 3/4: 21%), hypoalbuminemia (42%), hyponatremia (38%), hyperkalemia (26%), hypokalemia (25%), hypocalcemia (24%)

Gastrointestinal: Diarrhea (60%), nausea (41%), vomiting (24%), stomatitis (14%; includes aphthous stomatitis, mucositis, and oral mucosa ulcer)

Hematologic & oncologic: Lymphocytopenia (73%, grades 3/4: 10%), anemia (69%; grades 3/4: 3%), thrombocytopenia (18%), hemorrhage (13%, grades 3/4: 1%; includes bruise, ecchymoses, epistaxis, gingival hemorrhage, hematemesis, hematochezia, hemoptysis, hemorrhoidal bleeding, hypermenorrhea, melena, menometrorrhagia, nail bed bleeding, pulmonary hemorrhage, purpura, rectal hemorrhage, rupture of ovarian cyst, subarachnoid hemorrhage, subgaleal hematoma, traumatic hematoma, uterine hemorrhage, and vaginal hemorrhage)

Hepatic: Increased serum AST (73%, grades 3/4: 7% to 8%), increased serum alkaline phosphatase (71%, grades 3/4: 7%), increased serum ALT (68%, grades 3/4: 11%)

Neuromuscular & skeletal: Increased creatine phosphokinase (79%, grades 3/4: 12% to 14%)

Ophthalmic: Visual impairment (15%, grades 3/4: <1%; includes blurred vision, decreased visual acuity), chorioretinopathy (13%, grades 3/4: <1%), retinal detachment (12%, grades 3/4: 2%; includes detachment of macular retinal pigment epithelium and retinal pigment epithelium detachment)

Renal: Increased serum creatinine (100%; grades 3/4: 3%)

Miscellaneous: Fever (28%)

1% to 10%:

Central nervous system: Chills (10%)

Dermatologic: Skin rash (grades 3/4: 16%; grade 4: 2%; rash resulting in hospitalization: 3%)

Gastrointestinal: Gastrointestinal hemorrhage (4%)

Genitourinary: Genitourinary tract hemorrhage (2%), hematuria (2%)

Hematologic & oncologic: Keratoacanthoma (≤6%), squamous cell carcinoma of skin (≤6%), basal cell carcinoma (5%)

Hepatic: Abnormal bilirubin levels (grades 3/4: 2%)

<1%, postmarketing, and/or case reports: Cerebral hemorrhage, malignant melanoma (second primary), malignant neoplasm (noncutaneous)

Mechanism of Action Cobimetinib is a potent and selective inhibitor of the mitogen-activated extracellular kinase (MEK) pathway (Larkin 2014); it reversibly inhibits MEK1 and MEK2, which are upstream regulators of the extracellular signal-related kinase (ERK) pathway. The ERK pathway promotes cellular proliferation. MEK1 and MEK2 are part of the BRAF pathway, which is activated by BRAF V600E and K mutations. Vemurafenib targets a different kinase in the RAS/RAF/MEK/ERK pathway; when cobimetinib and vemurafenib are used in combination, increased apoptosis and reduced tumor growth occurs.

Pharmacodynamics/Kinetics

Half-life Elimination Mean: 44 hours (range: 23 to 70 hours)

Time to Peak Median: 2.4 hours (range: 1 to 24 hours)

Reproductive Considerations

Women of reproductive potential should use effective contraception during therapy and for 2 weeks after the final dose.

Pregnancy Considerations

Based on the mechanism of action and data from animal reproduction studies, cobimetinib would be expected to cause fetal harm.

Prescribing and Access Restrictions Available through specialty pharmacies. Further information may be obtained from the manufacturer, Genentech, at 1-888-249-4918, or at http://www.cotellic.com.

◆ **Cobimetinib Fumarate** *see* Cobimetinib *on page 402*

◆ **Cocaine Hydrochloride** *see* Cocaine (Topical) *on page 403*

Cocaine (Topical) (koe KANE)

Related Information

Management of the Chemically Dependent Patient *on page 1724*

Brand Names: US C-Topical; Goprelto; Numbrino

Brand Names: Canada PMS-Cocaine HCl

Pharmacologic Category Local Anesthetic

Use

Anesthesia:

Generic topical solution: Topical anesthesia (and vasoconstriction) for mucous membranes of the oral, laryngeal, or nasal cavities.

Goprelto, Numbrino: Topical anesthesia for mucous membranes when performing diagnostic procedures and surgeries on or through nasal cavities.

Local Anesthetic/Vasoconstrictor Precautions Although plain local anesthetic is not contraindicated, vasoconstrictor is absolutely contraindicated in any patient under the influence of or within 2 hours of cocaine use

Effects on Dental Treatment Key adverse event(s) related to dental treatment: Loss of taste perception. See Dental Health Professional Considerations.

Effects on Bleeding No information available to require special precautions

Adverse Reactions Note: Use of the topical solution may produce systemic reactions from excessive and rapid absorption.

>10%: Cardiovascular: Hypertension (78%)

1% to 10%:

Cardiovascular: Prolonged QT interval on ECG (3%), sinus tachycardia (2%), tachycardia (5%)

Nervous system: Headache (3%)

Respiratory: Epistaxis (1%)

Frequency not defined:

Cardiovascular: Acute myocardial infarction (Lenders 2013; Makaryus 2006), increased blood pressure, increased heart rate

Nervous system: Drug abuse, drug dependence, nervousness, tonic clonic epilepsy

Neuromuscular & skeletal: Tremor

Ophthalmic: Corneal changes (epithelium sloughing), corneal ulcer

Postmarketing: Anxiety, atrial arrhythmia, ischemic heart disease, ventricular arrhythmia (Lenders 2013)

Mechanism of Action Ester local anesthetic blocks both the initiation and conduction of nerve impulses by decreasing the neuronal membrane's permeability to sodium ions, which results in inhibition of depolarization with resultant blockade of conduction; interferes with the uptake of norepinephrine by adrenergic nerve terminals producing vasoconstriction

Pharmacodynamics/Kinetics

Onset of Action ~1 minute; Peak effect: ~5 minutes

Duration of Action Dose dependent: ≥30 minutes.

Half-life Elimination 1 to 1.7 hours

Pregnancy Considerations Cocaine rapidly crosses the placenta in concentrations equal to those in the mother. Adverse events occur in the fetus (eg, congenital malformations, growth restriction), infant (neonatal abstinence syndrome), and mother (eg, preterm labor, placental abruption) following maternal abuse (Fajemirokun-Odudeyi 2004).

Controlled Substance C-II

Dental Health Professional Considerations The cocaine user, regardless of how the cocaine was administered, presents a potential life-threatening situation in the dental operatory. A patient under the influence of cocaine could be compared to a car going 100 mph. Blood pressure is elevated, heart rate is likely increased, and the use of a local anesthetic with epinephrine may result in a medical emergency. Such patients can be identified by their jitteriness, irritability, talkativeness, tremors, and short, abrupt speech patterns. These same signs and symptoms may also be seen in a normal dental patient with preoperative dental anxiety; therefore, the dentist must be particularly alert in order to identify the potential cocaine abuser. If cocaine use is suspected, the patient should never be given a local anesthetic with vasoconstrictor, for fear of exacerbating the cocaine-induced sympathetic response. Life-threatening episodes of cardiac arrhythmias and hypertensive crises have been reported when local anesthetic with vasoconstrictor was administered to a patient under the influence of cocaine. No local anesthetic, used by any dentist, can interfere with, nor test positive by cocaine in any urine testing screen. Therefore, the dentist does not need to be concerned with any false drug-use accusations associated with dental anesthesia.

Codeine (KOE deen)

Related Information

Oral Pain *on page 1734*

Brand Names: Canada Codeine 15; Codeine 30; Codeine Contin; Linctus Codeine Blanc; PMS-Codeine [DSC]; RATIO-Codeine [DSC]; TEVA-Codeine

Pharmacologic Category Analgesic, Opioid; Antitussive

Use

Pain management: Management of mild- to moderately-severe pain

Limitations of use: Reserve codeine for use in patients for whom alternative treatment options (eg, nonopioid analgesics, opioid combination products) are ineffective, not tolerated, or would be otherwise inadequate.

Local Anesthetic/Vasoconstrictor Precautions No information available to require special precautions

Effects on Dental Treatment No significant effects or complications reported (see Dental Health Professional Considerations)

Effects on Bleeding No information available to require special precautions

Adverse Reactions Frequency not defined.

Cardiovascular: Bradycardia, cardiac arrest, circulatory depression, flushing, hypertension, hypotension, palpitations, shock, syncope, tachycardia

Central nervous system: Abnormal dreams, agitation, anxiety, apprehension, ataxia, chills, depression, disorientation, dizziness, drowsiness, dysphoria, euphoria, fatigue, hallucination, headache, increased intracranial pressure, insomnia, nervousness, paresthesia, sedation, shakiness, taste disorder, vertigo

Dermatologic: Diaphoresis, pruritus, skin rash, urticaria

Gastrointestinal: Abdominal cramps, abdominal pain, anorexia, biliary tract spasm, constipation, diarrhea, nausea, pancreatitis, vomiting, xerostomia

Genitourinary: Urinary hesitancy, urinary retention

Hypersensitivity: Hypersensitivity reaction

Neuromuscular & skeletal: Laryngospasm, muscle rigidity, tremor, weakness

Ophthalmic: Blurred vision, diplopia, miosis, nystagmus, visual disturbance

Respiratory: Bronchospasm, dyspnea, respiratory arrest, respiratory depression

<1%, postmarketing, and/or case reports: Hypogonadism (Brennan 2013; Debono 2011)

Mechanism of Action Binds to opioid receptors in the CNS, causing inhibition of ascending pain pathways, altering the perception of and response to pain; causes cough suppression by direct central action in the medulla; produces generalized CNS depression

Pharmacodynamics/Kinetics

Onset of Action

Oral: Immediate release: 0.5 to 1 hour; Injection [Canadian product]: 10 to 30 minutes

Peak effect: Oral: Immediate release: 1 to 1.5 hours; Injection [Canadian product]: 30 to 60 minutes

Duration of Action Oral: Immediate release: 4 to 6 hours; Injection [Canadian product]: 4 to 6 hours

Half-life Elimination ~3 hours

Time to Peak Plasma: Immediate release: 1 hour; Controlled release [Canadian product]: 3.3 hours

Reproductive Considerations

Long-term opioid use may cause secondary hypogonadism, which may lead to sexual dysfunction or infertility in men and women (Brennan 2013).

Pregnancy Considerations Opioids cross the placenta.

According to some studies, maternal use of opioids may be associated with birth defects (including neural tube defects, congenital heart defects, and gastroschisis), poor fetal growth, stillbirth, and preterm delivery (CDC [Dowell 2016]).

[US Boxed Warning]: Prolonged use of codeine during pregnancy can result in neonatal opioid withdrawal syndrome, which may be life-threatening if not recognized and treated, and requires management according to protocols developed by neonatology experts. If opioid use is required for a prolonged period in a pregnant woman, advise the patient of the risk of neonatal opioid withdrawal syndrome and ensure that appropriate treatment will be available. If chronic opioid exposure occurs in pregnancy, adverse events in the newborn (including withdrawal) may occur (Chou 2009). Symptoms of neonatal abstinence syndrome (NAS) following opioid exposure may be autonomic (eg, fever, temperature instability), gastrointestinal (eg, diarrhea, vomiting, poor feeding/weight gain), or neurologic (eg, high-pitched crying, hyperactivity, increased muscle tone, increased wakefulness/abnormal sleep pattern, irritability, sneezing, seizure, tremor, yawning) (Dow 2012; Hudak 2012). Mothers who are physically dependent on opioids may give birth to infants who are also physically dependent. Opioids may cause respiratory depression and psychophysiologic effects in the neonate; newborns of mothers receiving opioids during labor should be monitored.

Codeine is not commonly used to treat pain during labor and immediately postpartum (ACOG 209 2019) or chronic noncancer pain in pregnant women or those who may become pregnant (CDC [Dowell 2016]; Chou 2009).

Controlled Substance C-II

Dental Health Professional Considerations It is recommended that codeine not be used as the sole entity for analgesia because of moderate efficacy along with relatively high incidence of nausea, sedation, and constipation. In addition, codeine has some opioid addiction liability. Codeine in combination with acetaminophen or aspirin is recommended. Maximum effective analgesic dose of codeine is 60 mg (1 grain). Beyond 60 mg increases respiratory depression only.

◆ **Codeine, Acetaminophen, Butalbital, and Caffeine** *see* Butalbital, Acetaminophen, Caffeine, and Codeine *on page 274*

◆ **Codeine and Acetaminophen** *see* Acetaminophen and Codeine *on page 65*

Codeine and Chlorpheniramine

(KOE deen & klor fen IR a meen)

Brand Names: US Tuxarin ER; Tuzistra XR; Z-Tuss AC [OTC]

Pharmacologic Category Analgesic, Opioid; Antitussive; Histamine H_1 Antagonist; Histamine H_1 Antagonist, First Generation

Use Cough and upper respiratory symptoms: Temporary relief of cough and upper respiratory symptoms (runny nose; sneezing; nose, throat, or eye itching; cough) associated with allergies or a common cold in adults ≥18 years of age.

Local Anesthetic/Vasoconstrictor Precautions No information available to require special precautions

Effects on Dental Treatment Key adverse event(s) related to dental treatment: Xerostomia (normal salivary flow resumes upon discontinuation).

Effects on Bleeding No information available to require special precautions

Adverse Reactions Frequency not defined; reactions reported with combination product and/or individual agents. Also see individual agents.

Cardiovascular: Chest pain, chest tightness, decreased heart rate, facial flushing, hypertension, hypotension, orthostatic hypotension, palpitations, peripheral edema, prolonged QT interval on ECG, shock, syncope, tachycardia

Central nervous system: Agitation, anxiety, ataxia, coma, confusion, decreased mental acuity, depression, dizziness, drowsiness, drug abuse, drug dependence, dysphoria, euphoria, excitability, falling, false sense of well-being, fatigue, fear, hallucination, headache, increased intracranial pressure, insomnia, irritability, lethargy, malaise, migraine, nervousness, opioid withdrawal syndrome, relaxation, restlessness, sedated state, seizure, vertigo

Dermatologic: Dermatitis, diaphoresis, erythema of skin, facial swelling, hyperhidrosis, pruritus, skin rash, urticaria

Endocrine & metabolic: Altered serum glucose (change in glucose utilization), glycosuria, gynecomastia, hot flash, hypoglycemia, increased libido, pheochromocytoma crisis

Gastrointestinal: Abdominal distention, abdominal pain, acute pancreatitis, anorexia, biliary tract spasm, constipation, decreased appetite, decreased gastrointestinal motility, diarrhea, dyspepsia, dysphagia, epigastric distress, gastroesophageal reflux disease, hiccups, increased appetite, increased serum amylase, intestinal obstruction, nausea, paralytic ileus, spasm of sphincter of Oddi, vomiting, xerostomia

Genitourinary: Dysuria, early menses, hypogonadism, infertility, irritable bladder, lactation insufficiency, ureteral spasm, urinary frequency, urinary hesitancy, urinary retention, urinary tract infection

Hematologic & oncologic: Agranulocytosis, aplastic anemia, thrombocytopenia

Hypersensitivity: Anaphylaxis

Neuromuscular & skeletal: Arthralgia, asthenia, back pain, dyskinesia, facial dyskinesia, laryngospasm (allergic), muscle spasm, tremor, vesicle sphincter spasm

Ophthalmic: Blurred vision, diplopia, hypermetropia, increased lacrimation, miosis, mydriasis, photophobia, visual disturbance

Otic: Labyrinthitis, tinnitus

Respiratory: Allergic bronchospastic disease, atelectasis, bronchitis, cough, dry nose, dry throat, dyspnea, laryngismus, nasal congestion, nasopharyngitis, respiratory depression, respiratory distress, sinusitis, thickening of bronchial secretions, upper respiratory tract infection, wheezing

Miscellaneous: Impaired physical performance

Mechanism of Action

Codeine: Binds to opioid receptors in the CNS, causing inhibition of ascending pain pathways, altering the perception of and response to pain; causes cough suppression by direct central action in the medulla; produces generalized CNS depression.

Chlorpheniramine: H_1 receptor antagonist that also possesses anticholinergic and sedative activity. It prevents released histamine from dilating capillaries and causing edema of the respiratory mucosa.

Reproductive Considerations

Long-term opioid use may cause secondary hypogonadism, which may lead to sexual dysfunction and infertility (Brennan 2013).

Pregnancy Considerations

[US Boxed Warning]: Use is not recommended in pregnant women. Prolonged use of opioids during pregnancy can cause neonatal withdrawal syndrome, which may be life-threatening if not recognized and treated according to protocols developed by neonatology experts. If opioid use is required for a prolonged period in a pregnant woman, advise the patient of the risk of neonatal opioid withdrawal syndrome and ensure that appropriate treatment will be available.

See individual agents for additional information.

Controlled Substance Extended Release Suspension: C-III; Liquid products: C-V

- ◆ **Codeine and Promethazine** *see* Promethazine and Codeine *on page* 1283
- ◆ **Codeine, Chlorpheniramine, and Pseudoephedrine** *see* Chlorpheniramine, Pseudoephedrine, and Codeine *on page* 341
- ◆ **Codeine Phos/Acetaminophen** *see* Acetaminophen and Codeine *on page* 65
- ◆ **Codeine Phosphate** *see* Codeine *on page* 404
- ◆ **Codeine Sulfate** *see* Codeine *on page* 404
- ◆ **Cogentin** *see* Benztropine *on page* 231
- ◆ **Colace [OTC]** *see* Docusate *on page* 509
- ◆ **Colace Clear [OTC] [DSC]** *see* Docusate *on page* 509
- ◆ **Colazal** *see* Balsalazide *on page* 214
- ◆ **ColBenemid** *see* Colchicine and Probenecid *on page* 406

Colchicine (KOL chi seen)

Brand Names: US Colcrys; Gloperba; Mitigare

Brand Names: Canada EURO-Colchicine; JAMP-Colchicine; PMS-Colchicine; SANDOZ Colchicine

Pharmacologic Category Antigout Agent

Use

Familial Mediterranean fever (tablet [eg, Colcrys] only): Treatment of familial Mediterranean fever in adults and children 4 years and older.

Gout flares: Prophylaxis and treatment of acute gout flares when taken at the first sign of a flare.

Limitations of use: Gloperba and Mitigare are only approved for prophylaxis of gout flares; use for acute treatment during gout flares has not been studied.

Local Anesthetic/Vasoconstrictor Precautions No information available to require special precautions

Effects on Dental Treatment No significant effects or complications reported

Effects on Bleeding No information available to require special precautions

Adverse Reactions Frequency not always defined.

>10%: Gastrointestinal: Gastrointestinal disease (26% to 77%), diarrhea (23% to 77%), vomiting (17%), nausea (4% to 17%)

1% to 10%:

Central nervous system: Fatigue (1% to 4%), headache (1% to 2%)

Endocrine & metabolic: Gout (4%)

Gastrointestinal: Abdominal cramps, abdominal pain

Respiratory: Pharyngolaryngeal pain (2% to 3%)

<1%, postmarketing, and/or case reports: Alopecia, aplastic anemia, azoospermia, bone marrow depression, dermatitis, disseminated intravascular coagulation, dysgeusia (Syed 2016), granulocytopenia, hepatotoxicity, hypersensitivity reaction, increased creatine phosphokinase in blood specimen, increased serum alanine aminotransferase, increased serum aspartate aminotransferase, lactose intolerance, leukopenia, maculopapular rash, myalgia, myasthenia, myopathy, myotonia, neuropathy, oligospermia, pancytopenia, peripheral neuritis, nonthrombocytopenic purpura, rhabdomyolysis, skin rash, thrombocytopenia, toxic neuromuscular disease

Mechanism of Action Disrupts cytoskeletal functions by inhibiting β-tubulin polymerization into microtubules, preventing activation, degranulation, and migration of neutrophils associated with mediating some gout symptoms. In familial Mediterranean fever, may interfere with intracellular assembly of the inflammasome complex present in neutrophils and monocytes that mediate activation of interleukin-1β.

Pharmacodynamics/Kinetics

Onset of Action Oral: Pain relief: ~18 to 24 hours

Half-life Elimination 27 to 31 hours (multiple oral doses; young, healthy volunteers)

Time to Peak Serum: Oral: 0.5 to 3 hours

Reproductive Considerations

Colchicine should not be discontinued in females with familial Mediterranean fever who are planning a pregnancy (EULAR [Ozen 2016]). Conception in females with rheumatic and musculoskeletal diseases should be planned during a period of quiescent/low disease activity (ACR [Sammaritano 2020]).

Continuation of colchicine therapy is strongly recommended for use in males with rheumatic and musculoskeletal diseases who are planning to father a child (ACR [Sammaritano 2020]). Use in males may rarely be associated with reversible infertility. A temporary dose reduction or discontinuation may be needed if azoospermia or oligospermia is related to use; however, men generally do not need to discontinue colchicine prior to conception (EULAR [Ozen 2016]).

Pregnancy Considerations Colchicine crosses the placenta.

Based on available information, an increased risk of major birth defects or pregnancy loss has not been observed following maternal use of colchicine for the treatment of rheumatic diseases, such as familial Mediterranean fever (FMF) (EULAR [Ozen 2016]; Indraratna 2018). However, untreated FMF is associated with adverse pregnancy outcomes including abortion, miscarriage, and exacerbations of FMF attacks (EULAR [Ozen 2016]).

Colchicine can be continued during pregnancy in females with rheumatic and musculoskeletal diseases (ACR [Sammaritano 2020]). Available guidelines recommend continuing colchicine during pregnancy for the treatment of conditions such as FMF when there are no acceptable alternatives and discontinuation of treatment may lead to uncontrolled disease and adverse pregnancy outcomes. Increased monitoring during pregnancy is recommended; amniocentesis is not warranted (ACR [Sammaritano 2020]; EULAR [Ozen 2016]).

Colchicine and Probenecid

(KOL chi seen & proe BEN e sid)

Related Information

Colchicine *on page 405*
Probenecid *on page 1277*

Pharmacologic Category Anti-inflammatory Agent; Antigout Agent; Uricosuric Agent

Use Treatment of chronic gouty arthritis when complicated by frequent, recurrent acute attacks of gout

Local Anesthetic/Vasoconstrictor Precautions No information available to require special precautions

Effects on Dental Treatment No significant effects or complications reported

Effects on Bleeding No information available to require special precautions

Adverse Reactions See individual agents.

Pregnancy Considerations See individual agents.

◆ **Colcrys** *see* Colchicine *on page 405*

Colesevelam (koh le SEV a lam)

Related Information

Cardiovascular Diseases *on page 1654*

Brand Names: US Welchol

Brand Names: Canada APO-Colesevelam; Lodalis

Generic Availability (US) Yes

Pharmacologic Category Antilipemic Agent, Bile Acid Sequestrant

Use

Diabetes mellitus, type 2: Improve glycemic control in adults with type 2 diabetes mellitus in conjunction with diet and exercise

Guideline recommendations: Colesevelam is not generally used in patients with type 2 diabetes but may be tried in specific situations (ADA 2020).

Hyperlipidemia (primary):

Management of elevated LDL-C in adults with primary hyperlipidemia in conjunction with diet and exercise.

Management of heterozygous familial hypercholesterolemia (heFH) in adolescent patients (males and postmenarcheal females 10 to 17 years of age) who are unable to reach LDL-C target levels despite an adequate trial of dietary therapy and lifestyle modification.

Local Anesthetic/Vasoconstrictor Precautions No information available to require special precautions

Effects on Dental Treatment No significant effects or complications reported

Effects on Bleeding No information available to require special precautions

Adverse Reactions Actual frequency may be dependent upon indication. Unless otherwise noted, frequency of adverse effects is reported for adult patients.

>10%: Gastrointestinal: Constipation (3% to 11%)

1% to 10%:

Cardiovascular: Cardiovascular toxicity (2%, including myocardial infarction, aortic stenosis, bradycardia), hypertension (2% to 3%)

Central nervous system: Headache (children and adults 4% to 8%), fatigue (children 4%)

Endocrine & metabolic: Hypertriglyceridemia (4% to 5%; >500 mg/dL: <1%; >1,000 mg/dL: <1%), hyperglycemia (3%), hypoglycemia (3%)

Gastrointestinal: Dyspepsia (3% to 8%), diarrhea (4%), nausea (children and adults 3% to 4%), gastroesophageal reflux disease (2%), periodontal abscess (2%), vomiting (children 2%)

Hematologic & oncologic: C-reactive protein increased (3%)

Infection: Influenza (children and adolescents 4%)

Neuromuscular & skeletal: Weakness (4%), back pain (2%), increased creatine phosphokinase (children and adults 2%), myalgia (2%)

Respiratory: Nasopharyngitis (children 5% to 6%), upper respiratory tract infection (children and adults 3% to 5%), flu-like symptoms (children 4%), pharyngitis (3%), rhinitis (children 2%)

<1%, postmarketing, and/or case reports: Abdominal distension, dysphagia, esophageal obstruction, fecal impaction, flatulence, worsening of hemorrhoids, increased serum transaminases, infection, intestinal obstruction, pancreatitis, unstable angina pectoris

Dosing

Adult & Geriatric

Diarrhea associated with bile acid malabsorption (off-label use): Oral: 3.75 g/day in 1 or 2 divided doses (Beigel 2014; Wilcox 2014)

Hyperlipidemia (primary), diabetes mellitus (type 2): Oral: 3.75 g/day in 1 or 2 divided doses

Note: Use may be considered in patients with fasting triglyceride level ≤300 mg/dL who do not meet cholesterol treatment goals with dietary modification and other lipid lowering therapies (eg, maximally tolerated statin and ezetimibe) (AHA/ACC [Grundy 2018]).

Renal Impairment: Adult No dosage adjustments necessary; not absorbed from the gastrointestinal tract.

Hepatic Impairment: Adult No dosage adjustments necessary; not absorbed from the gastrointestinal tract.

Pediatric Note: Due to large tablet size, the manufacturer recommends packets of oral suspension for pediatric patients. Overall with dyslipidemia management, lifestyle changes are recommended to be implemented for at least 6 to 12 months before beginning pharmacotherapy (AACE [Jellinger 2017]). Bile acid sequestrant therapy may be considered for LDL/apo B reduction and mild HDL increases but should not be used in pediatric patients with hypertriglyceridemia. Multivitamin supplementation recommended due to potential folic acid and cholecalciferol malabsorption (AACE [Jellinger 2017]).

Heterozygous familial hypercholesterolemia: Children ≥10 years and Adolescents: Oral: 3.75 g once daily or in divided doses twice daily.

Renal Impairment: Pediatric Children ≥10 years and Adolescents: No adjustment necessary; not absorbed from the GI tract.

Hepatic Impairment: Pediatric Children ≥10 years and Adolescents: No dosage adjustment necessary; not absorbed from the GI tract.

Mechanism of Action Cholesterol is the major precursor of bile acid. Colesevelam binds with bile acids in the intestine to form an insoluble complex that is eliminated in feces. This increased excretion of bile acids results in an increased oxidation of cholesterol to bile acid and a lowering of the serum cholesterol.

Contraindications

History of bowel obstruction; serum TG concentrations of more than 500 mg/dL; history of hypertriglyceridemia-induced pancreatitis.

Canadian labeling: Additional contraindications (not in US labeling): Hypersensitivity to colesevelam or any component of the formulation; biliary obstruction

Warnings/Precautions Bile acid sequestrants can increase serum triglyceride concentrations; severely elevated triglycerides can cause acute pancreatitis. The manufacturer contraindicates use if triglycerides exceed 500 mg/dL and in patients with a history of hypertriglyceridemia-induced pancreatitis. The American College of Cardiology/American Heart Association recommends avoiding use in patients with baseline fasting triglyceride levels ≥300 mg/dL (ACC/AHA [Grundy 2018]). Use with caution in patients using insulin, thiazolidinediones, or sulfonylureas (may cause increased triglyceride concentrations) or in patients susceptible to fat-soluble vitamin deficiencies. Discontinue if symptoms of acute pancreatitis occur (eg, severe abdominal pain with or without nausea and vomiting). Use is not recommended in patients with gastroparesis, other severe GI motility disorders, or a history of major GI tract surgery or patients at risk for bowel obstruction. Use tablets with caution in patients with dysphagia or swallowing disorders; use the oral suspension form of colesevelam due to large tablet size and risk for esophageal obstruction. Discontinue if symptoms of bowel obstruction occur (eg, severe abdominal pain, severe constipation).

Minimal effects are seen on HDL-C and triglyceride levels. Secondary causes of hypercholesterolemia should be excluded before initiation. Colesevelam has not been studied in Fredrickson Type I, III, IV, or V dyslipidemias. Colesevelam is not indicated for the management of type 1 diabetes, particularly in the acute management (eg, DKA). It is also not indicated in type 2 diabetes mellitus as monotherapy and must be used as an adjunct to diet, exercise, and glycemic control with insulin or oral antidiabetic agents. The use of colesevelam in pediatric patients with type 2 diabetes has not been evaluated. Combination with dipeptidyl peptidase 4 inhibitors or thiazolidinediones has not been studied extensively. There is no evidence of macrovascular disease risk reduction with colesevelam.

Use with caution in patients susceptible to fat-soluble vitamin deficiencies. Absorption of fat soluble vitamins A, D, E, and K may be decreased; patients should take vitamins ≥4 hours before colesevelam. Potentially significant drug-drug interactions may exist, requiring dose or frequency adjustment, additional monitoring, and/or selection of alternative therapy. Some products may contain phenylalanine; use with caution. Not for use in patients with diabetic ketoacidosis (DKA) or patients with type 1 diabetes mellitus.

Drug Interactions

Metabolism/Transport Effects None known.

Avoid Concomitant Use

Avoid concomitant use of Colesevelam with any of the following: Mycophenolate

Increased Effect/Toxicity There are no known significant interactions involving an increase in effect.

Decreased Effect

Colesevelam may decrease the levels/effects of: Amiodarone; Chenodiol; Cholic Acid; Corticosteroids (Oral); CycloSPORINE (Systemic); Deferasirox; Estrogen Derivatives (Contraceptive); Ethinyl Estradiol; Ezetimibe; Glimepiride; GlipiZIDE; GlyBURIDE; Leflunomide; Lomitapide; Loop Diuretics; Methotrexate; Multivitamins/Fluoride (with ADE); Multivitamins/Minerals (with ADEK, Folate, Iron); Multivitamins/Minerals (with AE, No Iron); Mycophenolate; Niacin; Nonsteroidal Anti-Inflammatory Agents; Norethindrone; Obeticholic Acid; Olmesartan; Phenytoin; Pravastatin;

Progestins (Contraceptive); Propranolol; Raloxifene; Teriflunomide; Tetracyclines; Thiazide and Thiazide-Like Diuretics; Thyroid Products; Ursodiol; Vancomycin; Vitamin D Analogs; Warfarin

Dietary Considerations Some products may contain phenylalanine.

Pharmacodynamics/Kinetics

Onset of Action

Lipid lowering: Therapeutic: ~2 weeks

Reduction of hemoglobin A_{1C} (Type II diabetes): 4-6 weeks initial onset; 12-18 weeks maximal effect

Reproductive Considerations

Colesevelam may reduce the efficacy of oral contraception; consult drug interactions database for detailed information.

Pregnancy Considerations

Colesevelam is not absorbed systemically following oral administration and maternal use is not expected to result in fetal exposure to the drug.

Lipid concentrations increase during pregnancy as required for normal fetal development. When increases are greater than expected, supervised dietary intervention should be initiated. Bile acid sequestrants are recommended when treatment is needed, and therapy with colesevelam is preferred (Avis 2009; Jacobson 2015).

Colesevelam may interfere with maternal vitamin absorption; therefore, regular supplementation may not be adequate.

Breastfeeding Considerations

Due to lack of systemic absorption, colesevelam is not expected to be present in breast milk.

When treatment for hypercholesterolemia in breastfeeding women is needed, therapy with bile acid sequestrants may be considered, and therapy with colesevelam is preferred (Jacobson 2015; NICE 2008).

Dosage Forms Considerations Welchol contains phenylalanine 27 mg per 3.75 gram packet

Dosage Forms: US

Packet, Oral:

Welchol: 3.75 g (30 ea)

Generic: 3.75 g (30 ea)

Tablet, Oral:

Welchol: 625 mg

Generic: 625 mg

Dosage Forms: Canada

Packet, Oral:

Lodalis: 3.75 g (30 ea)

Tablet, Oral:

Lodalis: 625 mg

Generic: 625 mg

Colistimethate (koe lis ti METH ate)

Brand Names: US Coly-Mycin M

Brand Names: Canada Coly-Mycin M

Pharmacologic Category Antibiotic, Miscellaneous

Use Treatment of acute or chronic infections due to sensitive strains of certain gram-negative bacilli (particularly *Pseudomonas aeruginosa*) which are resistant to other antibacterials or in patients allergic to other antibacterials

Local Anesthetic/Vasoconstrictor Precautions No information available to require special precautions

Effects on Dental Treatment No significant effects or complications reported

Effects on Bleeding No information available to require special precautions

Adverse Reactions

>10%:

Genitourinary: Nephrotoxicity (18% to 26% [Dalfino 2012; Oliveira 2009])

Renal: Acute renal failure (33% to 60% [Akajagbor 2013; Deryke 2010])

1% to 10%:

Central nervous system: Neurotoxicity (7%; higher incidence with high-dose IV use in cystic fibrosis [Bosso 1991; Koch-Weser 1970])

Frequency not defined:

Central nervous system: Dizziness, oral paresthesia, paresthesia, peripheral paresthesia, seizures, slurred speech, vertigo

Dermatologic: Pruritus, skin rash, urticaria

Gastrointestinal: *Clostridioides* (formerly *Clostridium*) *difficile*-associated diarrhea, gastric distress

Genitourinary: Decreased urine output

Hypersensitivity: Anaphylaxis

Renal: Decreased creatinine clearance, increased blood urea nitrogen, increased serum creatinine

Respiratory: Apnea, respiratory distress

Miscellaneous: Fever

Mechanism of Action Colistimethate (or the sodium salt [colistimethate sodium]) is the inactive prodrug that is hydrolyzed to colistin, which acts as a cationic detergent and damages the bacterial cytoplasmic membrane causing leaking of intracellular substances and cell death

Pharmacodynamics/Kinetics

Half-life Elimination IM, IV: Colistimethate: 2 to 3 hours

Critically ill: Infants (including premature infants), Children, Adolescents, and Adults: IV: Colistimethate: 2.3 hours; Colistin: 14.4 hours (Plachouras 2009)

Cystic fibrosis: IV: Colistin: ~3.5 hours (Li 2003)

ESRD patients receiving CAPD: IV: Colistin: 13.2 hours (Koomanachai 2014)

Time to Peak

Healthy volunteers: IV: Colistin: 2 hours (range: 1 to 4 hours) (Couet 2011)

Critically ill: IV: Colistin: ~7 hours (Plachouras 2009)

Pregnancy Risk Factor C

Pregnancy Considerations Adverse events have been observed in animal reproduction studies. Colistimethate crosses the placenta in humans.

◆ **Colistimethate Sodium** *see* Colistimethate *on page 408*

◆ **Colistin Methanesulfonate** *see* Colistimethate *on page 408*

◆ **Colistin Methanesulphonate** *see* Colistimethate *on page 408*

◆ **Colistin Sulfomethate** *see* Colistimethate *on page 408*

◆ **CollaCote** *see* Collagen (Absorbable) *on page 408*

◆ **Collagen** *see* Collagen Hemostat *on page 410*

Collagen (Absorbable) (KOL la jen, ab SORB able)

Related Information

Antiplatelet and Anticoagulation Considerations in Dentistry *on page 1666*

Brand Names: US CollaCote; CollaPatch; CollaPlug; HeliCote; HeliPlug; HeliTape

Pharmacologic Category Hemostatic Agent

Use Hemostatic

Local Anesthetic/Vasoconstrictor Precautions No information available to require special precautions

Effects on Dental Treatment No significant effects or complications reported

Effects on Bleeding No information available to require special precautions

Adverse Reactions Frequency not defined. Reactions listed are based on reports for other agents in this same pharmacologic class and may not be specifically reported for collagen (adsorbable/dental).

Hypersensitivity: Hypersensitivity reaction

Miscellaneous: Foreign body reaction

<1%, postmarketing, and/or case reports: Seroma (subgaleal)

Mechanism of Action The highly porous sponge structure absorbs blood and wound exudate. The collagen component causes aggregation of platelets which bind to collagen fibrils. The aggregated platelets degranulate, releasing coagulation factors that promote the formation of fibrin.

◆ **Collagen Absorbable Hemostat** *see* Collagen Hemostat *on page 410*

Collagenase (Systemic) (KOL la je nase)

Brand Names: US Xiaflex

Brand Names: Canada Xiaflex [DSC]

Pharmacologic Category Enzyme

Use

Dupuytren contracture: Treatment of adults with Dupuytren contracture with a palpable cord

Peyronie disease: Treatment of adult men with Peyronie disease with a palpable plaque and curvature deformity of at least 30 degrees at the start of therapy

Adverse Reactions

Dupuytren's contracture:

>10%:

Cardiovascular: Peripheral edema (primarily as swelling of injected hand: 73% to 77%)

Dermatologic: Pruritus (4% to 15%), hemorrhagic blister (12%)

Hematologic & oncologic: Bruise (59% to 70%), lymphadenopathy (13%)

Immunologic: Antibody development (≥86%; neutralizing antibodies: AUX-I: 10%; AUX-II: 21%)

Local: Bleeding at injection site (6% to 38%), injection site reaction (35%; includes erythema, inflammation, irritation), swelling at injection site (5% to 24%), tenderness at injection site (24%), pain at injection site (14%)

Neuromuscular & skeletal: Limb pain (35% to 51%)

Miscellaneous: Laceration (9% to 22%)

1% to 10%:

Central nervous system: Lymph node pain (8%), axillary pain (6% to 7%)

Dermatologic: Erythema (6%), ecchymoses (5%)

Local: Hematoma at injection site (8%)

<1%, postmarketing, and/or case reports: Anaphylaxis, antibody development (IgE; increased with successive injections), causalgia, ligament disorder, pulley rupture, rupture of tendon, sensory disturbance, vasodepressor syncope

Peyronie disease:

>10%:

Genitourinary: Penile hematoma (66%; severe: 4% to 6%), penile swelling (55%), penile pain (45%), penile ecchymoses (15%), penile popping sensation (13%)

Immunologic: Antibody development (55% to >99%; neutralizing antibodies: AUX-I: 60%; AUX-II: 52%; no correlation to clinical response or adverse reaction)

1% to 10%:

Central nervous system: Procedural pain (2%), suprapubic pain (1%)

Dermatologic: Hemorrhagic blister (5%), genital pruritus (3%), skin discoloration (2%), localized vesiculation (injection site, 1%)

Genitourinary: Blisters on penis (3%), painful erection (3%), erectile dysfunction (2%), dyspareunia (1%)

Local: Itching at injection site (1% to 4%), localized edema (1%)

Miscellaneous: Nodule (1%)

<1%, postmarketing, and/or case reports: Penile fracture, sudden penile detumescence

Mechanism of Action Collagenase clostridium histolyticum contains two forms of microbial collagenase (Collagenase AUX-I and Collagenase AUX-II) isolated and purified from the fermentation of *Clostridium histolyticum* bacteria; collagenase lyses collagen, leading to enzymatic disruption of contracted Dupuytren cord or Peyronie plaque (both comprised primarily of collagen).

Pregnancy Risk Factor B

Pregnancy Considerations

Pharmacokinetic studies in humans did not show quantifiable systemic levels following intralesional injection into a Dupuytren cord; however, low levels were quantifiable in the plasma following administration into the penile plaque. IgE-anti-drug antibodies commonly develop in treated patients; effects to the fetus are unknown.

Product Availability Qwo: FDA approved July 2020; availability anticipated Spring 2021. Information pertaining to this product within the monograph is pending revision. Qwo is indicated for the treatment of moderate to severe cellulite in the buttocks of adult women. Consult the prescribing information for additional information.

Collagenase (Topical) (KOL la je nase)

Brand Names: US Santyl

Brand Names: Canada Santyl

Pharmacologic Category Enzyme, Topical Debridement

Use Dermal ulcers: Debriding chronic dermal ulcers and severely burned areas.

Local Anesthetic/Vasoconstrictor Precautions No information available to require special precautions

Effects on Dental Treatment No significant effects or complications reported

Effects on Bleeding No information available to require special precautions

Adverse Reactions Frequency not defined.

Local: Application site burning, application site irritation, application site pain

<1%, postmarketing and/or case reports: Hypersensitivity reaction

Mechanism of Action Collagenase is an enzyme derived from the fermentation by *Clostridium histolyticum* and differs from other proteolytic enzymes in that its enzymatic action has a high specificity for native and denatured collagen in necrotic tissue; collagenase will not attack collagen in healthy tissue or newly formed granulation tissue. Therefore, collagenase is effective for the removal of detritus, formation of granulation tissue, and subsequent epithelization of dermal ulcers and severely burned areas.

Pregnancy Considerations It is not known if collagenase is absorbed systemically following topical application.

- **Collagenase Clostridium Histolyticum** *see* Collagenase (Systemic) *on page* *409*

Collagen Hemostat (KOL la jen HEE moe stat)

Related Information

Antiplatelet and Anticoagulation Considerations in Dentistry *on page* *1666*

Brand Names: US Actifoam Collagen Sponge; Avitene; Avitene Flour; Endo Avitene; Syringe Avitene; Ultrafoam Sponge 2x6.25x7CM; Ultrafoam Sponge 8x12.5x1CM; Ultrafoam Sponge 8x12.5x3CM; Ultrafoam Sponge 8x25x1CM; Ultrafoam Sponge 8x6.25x1CM

Pharmacologic Category Hemostatic Agent

Use Hemostasis: Adjunct to hemostasis in surgical procedures when control of bleeding by ligature or conventional procedures is ineffective or impractical.

Local Anesthetic/Vasoconstrictor Precautions No information available to require special precautions

Effects on Dental Treatment No significant effects or complications reported

Effects on Bleeding Used in surgical procedures as an adjunct to hemostasis when control of bleeding by ligature or conventional procedures is ineffective or impractical.

Adverse Reactions Frequency not defined.

Miscellaneous: Adhesion formation, allergic reaction, edema, foreign body reaction, hematoma, inflammation, potentiation of infection

Postmarketing and/or case reports: Numbness, pain, paralysis, subgaleal seroma; alveolalgia and transient laryngospasm with dental use

Mechanism of Action Collagen hemostat is an absorbable topical hemostatic agent prepared from purified bovine corium collagen and shredded into fibrils. Physically, microfibrillar collagen hemostat yields a large surface area. Chemically, it is collagen with hydrochloric acid noncovalently bound to some of the available amino groups in the collagen molecules. When in contact with a bleeding surface, collagen hemostat attracts platelets which adhere to its fibrils and undergo the release phenomenon. This triggers aggregation of the platelets into thrombi in the interstices of the fibrous mass, initiating the formation of a physiologic platelet plug.

Pharmacodynamics/Kinetics

Onset of Action Hemostasis: 2 to 5 minutes

- **CollaPatch** *see* Collagen (Absorbable) *on page* *408*
- **CollaPlug** *see* Collagen (Absorbable) *on page* *408*
- **Colocort [DSC]** *see* Hydrocortisone (Topical) *on page* *775*
- **Coly-Mycin M** *see* Colistimethate *on page* *408*
- **CombiPatch** *see* Estradiol and Norethindrone *on page* *598*
- **Combivent Respimat** *see* Ipratropium and Albuterol *on page* *839*
- **Combivir** *see* Lamivudine and Zidovudine *on page* *874*
- **Compazine** *see* Prochlorperazine *on page* *1279*
- **Complement C5 Inhibitor ALXN1210** *see* Ravulizumab *on page* *1313*
- **Complera** *see* Emtricitabine, Rilpivirine, and Tenofovir Disoproxil Fumarate *on page* *559*
- **Complete Allergy Medication [OTC] [DSC]** *see* DiphenhydrAMINE (Systemic) *on page* *502*
- **Complete Allergy Relief [OTC]** *see* DiphenhydrAMINE (Systemic) *on page* *502*
- **Compound E** *see* Cortisone *on page* *413*
- **Compound F** *see* Hydrocortisone (Systemic) *on page* *773*
- **Compound F** *see* Hydrocortisone (Topical) *on page* *775*
- **Compound S** *see* Zidovudine *on page* *1569*
- **Compound S, Abacavir, and Lamivudine** *see* Abacavir, Lamivudine, and Zidovudine *on page* *52*
- **Compro** *see* Prochlorperazine *on page* *1279*
- **Comtan** *see* Entacapone *on page* *567*
- **Concerta** *see* Methylphenidate *on page* *997*
- **Conjugated Estrogen** *see* Estrogens (Conjugated/Equine, Systemic) *on page* *601*
- **Conjugated Estrogen** *see* Estrogens (Conjugated/Equine, Topical) *on page* *602*
- **Conjupri** *see* Levamlodipine *on page* *893*
- **Continuous Erythropoietin Receptor Activator** *see* Methoxy Polyethylene Glycol-Epoetin Beta *on page* *993*
- **Contrave** *see* Naltrexone and Bupropion *on page* *1078*
- **Conventional Amphotericin B** *see* Amphotericin B (Conventional) *on page* *137*
- **Conventional Cytarabine** *see* Cytarabine (Conventional) *on page* *424*
- **Conventional Daunomycin** *see* DAUNOrubicin (Conventional) *on page* *445*
- **Conventional Doxorubicin** *see* DOXOrubicin (Conventional) *on page* *520*
- **Conventional Irinotecan** *see* Irinotecan (Conventional) *on page* *841*
- **Conventional Paclitaxel** *see* PACLitaxel (Conventional) *on page* *1178*
- **Conventional Trastuzumab** *see* Trastuzumab *on page* *1479*
- **Conventional Vincristine** *see* VinCRIStine *on page* *1546*
- **ConZip** *see* TraMADol *on page* *1468*
- **Copegus [DSC]** *see* Ribavirin (Systemic) *on page* *1320*
- **Copiktra** *see* Duvelisib *on page* *540*
- **Copper Intrauterine Device** *see* Copper IUD *on page* *410*

Copper IUD (KOP er eye uh dee)

Brand Names: US Paragard Intrauterine Copper

Pharmacologic Category Contraceptive

Use Contraception: For prevention of pregnancy, intrauterine device (IUD) may be in place for up to 10 years

Local Anesthetic/Vasoconstrictor Precautions No information available to require special precautions

Effects on Dental Treatment No significant effects or complications reported

Effects on Bleeding No information available to require special precautions

Adverse Reactions

Frequency not defined:

Endocrine & metabolic: Heavy menstrual bleeding, spotty menstruation

Genitourinary: Abnormal vaginal hemorrhage, cervical perforation, dysmenorrhea, dyspareunia, ectopic pregnancy, embedment of intrauterine system in the myometrium, endometriosis (may be asymptomatic), pelvic cramps, pelvic inflammatory disease (may be asymptomatic), pelvic pain, spontaneous migration of the IUD, uterine perforation, vaginitis

Hematologic & oncologic: Anemia

Infection: Sepsis (including Group A streptococcal sepsis), infection (including severe and actinomycosis)

Neuromuscular & skeletal: Back pain

Miscellaneous: Female birth control device expulsion from genital tract

Postmarketing: Abdominal distention, amenorrhea, breakage of IUD, dizziness, fever, hypersensitivity reaction (including metal allergy), muscle spasm, nausea, pelvic region infection (uterus), Stevens-Johnson syndrome

Mechanism of Action The mechanism of action is not well defined but may involve interfering with sperm transport, fertilization, and prevention of implantation. A copper IUD may prevent fertilization by interfering with the ability of sperm to reach the fallopian tube, or decrease the sperm's ability to fertilize by causing a foreign body reaction and chemical changes that may be toxic. Implantation can rarely occur with a copper IUD; however, the number of fertilized ova is decreased when compared to sexually active women not using a contraceptive. When fertilized ova are present, they do not develop normally (Rivera, 1999). The number of women with a copper IUD who have an unintended pregnancy within the first year of insertion following typical use and perfect use is <1%.

Reproductive Considerations

In a study evaluating use for emergency contraception (off-label indication), eligible females were required to have ≥1 spontaneous normal cycle(s) following discontinued hormonal contraception, or a recent delivery, miscarriage, or induced abortion, plus a negative urine pregnancy test in addition to the usual contraindications to intrauterine device insertion (Wu 2010).

Pregnancy Considerations Use during pregnancy is contraindicated.

Septic abortion with septicemia, septic shock, and death may occur if pregnancy occurs with the intrauterine device (IUD) in place. The risk of miscarriage, premature labor, premature delivery, and sepsis are increased if an intrauterine pregnancy occurs and continues with the IUD in place. If pregnancy occurs, the device should be removed if the strings are visible (pregnancy loss may occur). If the strings are not visible but it is determined that the device is still in place, the female should be informed of the risks if pregnancy is continued.

- **Cordran** *see* Flurandrenolide *on page 700*
- **Coreg** *see* Carvedilol *on page 294*
- **Coreg CR** *see* Carvedilol *on page 294*
- **CoreMino** *see* Minocycline (Systemic) *on page 1032*
- **Corgard** *see* Nadolol *on page 1070*
- **Corlanor** *see* Ivabradine *on page 850*
- **Corlopam** *see* Fenoldopam *on page 641*
- **Cormax Scalp Application [DSC]** *see* Clobetasol *on page 377*
- **Coronavirus** *see* Azithromycin (Systemic) *on page 203*
- **Coronavirus** *see* Chloroquine *on page 338*
- **Coronavirus** *see* Hydroxychloroquine *on page 778*
- **Coronavirus** *see* Lopinavir and Ritonavir *on page 929*
- **Coronavirus** *see* Sarilumab *on page 1359*
- **Coronavirus** *see* Tocilizumab *on page 1457*
- **Cortaid Maximum Strength [OTC]** *see* Hydrocortisone (Topical) *on page 775*
- **Cortef** *see* Hydrocortisone (Systemic) *on page 773*
- **Cortenema** *see* Hydrocortisone (Topical) *on page 775*
- **Corticool [OTC] [DSC]** *see* Hydrocortisone (Topical) *on page 775*

Corticorelin (kor ti koe REL in)

Brand Names: US Acthrel

Pharmacologic Category Diagnostic Agent

Use Cushing syndrome, differential diagnosis: Used as a diagnostic aid to differentiate between pituitary and ectopic production of ACTH in patients with ACTH-dependent disease

Local Anesthetic/Vasoconstrictor Precautions

No information available to require special precautions

Effects on Dental Treatment No significant effects or complications reported

Effects on Bleeding No information available to require special precautions

Adverse Reactions Frequency not always defined. Incidence of adverse effects is dependent upon dose.

Cardiovascular: Decreased blood pressure (7%), asystole, flushing (face, neck, and upper chest), palpitations (Corticorelin 2004)

Central nervous system: Tonic-clonic seizures (1%), dizziness, (Corticorelin 2004), metallic taste (Corticorelin 2004)

Gastrointestinal: Vomiting (Corticorelin 2004), xerostomia (Corticorelin 2004)

Respiratory: Dyspnea (urge to inspire)

<1%, postmarketing, and/or case reports: Angioedema, chest tightness, hypotension (severe), increased heart rate, loss of consciousness, tachycardia (severe), wheezing

Mechanism of Action Corticorelin ovine, a peptide of ovine corticotropin-releasing hormone (oCRH) and an analogue of human CRH (hCRH), stimulates adrenocorticotropic hormone (ACTH) release from the anterior pituitary. ACTH stimulates the adrenal cortex to produce cortisol. Depending on the plasma ACTH and cortisol response following the corticorelin stimulation test, the results aid the clinician in the differentiation between the source of ACTH-dependent hypercortisolism (pituitary vs ectopic).

Pharmacodynamics/Kinetics

Onset of Action IV:

Plasma ACTH concentration: Increases 2 minutes after injection

Plasma cortisol concentration: Increases within 10 minutes after injection

Peak effect: Response to injection is biphasic with a second lower peak 2 to 3 hours postinjection; basal and peak response levels vary depending on AM or PM administration. In general, baseline ACTH and cortisol concentrations are higher in the AM.

Plasma ACTH concentration: Initial peak: 15 to 60 minutes after injection

Plasma cortisol concentration: Initial peak at 30 to 120 minutes after injection

Duration of Action IV: Plasma ACTH and cortisol concentrations remain elevated for up to 2 hours after injection.

Half-life Elimination $t_{1/2}$: Exhibits biexponential decay; Fast component: 11.6 ± 1.5 minutes; slow component: 73 ± 8 minutes

Pregnancy Considerations Animal reproduction studies have not been conducted.

◆ **Corticorelin Ovine Triflutate** *see* Corticorelin *on page 411*

Corticotropin (kor ti koe TROE pin)

Brand Names: US Acthar

Brand Names: Canada ACTH 40

Pharmacologic Category Adrenocorticotropin Stimulating Hormone

Use

Diuresis in nephrotic syndrome: To induce a diuresis or remission of proteinuria in patients with nephrotic syndrome without uremia of the idiopathic type or due to lupus erythematosus. **Note:** Based on the 2012 KDIGO clinical practice guidelines for glomerulonephritis, recommendations cannot be made for the use of corticotropin for initial therapy or relapses of idiopathic membranous nephropathy until more randomized, controlled trials are conducted. The KDIGO guidelines do not include recommendations for use of corticotropin in the treatment of proteinuria due to lupus nephritis (KDIGO 2012).

Infantile spasms: Treatment of infantile spasms in infants and children younger than 2 years. **Note:** Corticotropin is the preferred treatment in most patients (AAN [Go 2012])

Multiple sclerosis: Treatment of acute exacerbations of multiple sclerosis in adults. **Note**: Treatment guidelines recommend the use of high dose IV or oral methylprednisolone for acute exacerbations of multiple sclerosis (AAN [Scott 2011]; NICE 2014). Corticotropin may be an alternative therapy if IV corticosteroids cannot be administered or are not tolerated (Simsarian 2011).

Ophthalmic diseases: Treatment of severe acute and chronic allergic and inflammatory processes involving the eye and its adnexa (eg, keratitis, iritis, iridocyclitis, diffuse posterior uveitis, choroiditis, optic neuritis, chorioretinitis, anterior segment inflammation). **Note:** FDA approved use; however, available data to support use in these conditions is limited.

Symptomatic sarcoidosis: Treatment of symptomatic sarcoidosis. **Note:** FDA approved use; however, available data to support use in this condition is limited. Glucocorticoids (eg, prednisone) are generally recommended as first-line treatment for sarcoidosis (Soto-Gomez 2016).

Local Anesthetic/Vasoconstrictor Precautions No information available to require special precautions

Effects on Dental Treatment No significant effects or complications reported

Effects on Bleeding No information available to require special precautions

Adverse Reactions Adverse events associated with infantile spasm treatment unless otherwise indicated. Other adverse events associated with corticosteroids may also occur.

>10%:

Cardiovascular: Hypertension (11%)

Central nervous system: Convulsions (12%)

Infection: Infection (20%)

1% to 10%:

Cardiovascular: Cardiac abnormality (3%)

Central nervous system: Irritability (7%)

Endocrine & metabolic: Cushingoid state (3%)

Gastrointestinal: Decreased appetite (3%), diarrhea (3%), vomiting (3%), weight gain (1%)

Infection: Candidiasis (≥2%)

Otic: Otitis media (≥2%)

Respiratory: Pneumonia (≥2%), upper respiratory tract infection (≥2%), nasal congestion (1%)

Miscellaneous: Fever (5%)

Frequency not defined:

Cardiovascular: Increased blood pressure (associated with cortisol elevation)

Central nervous system: Behavioral changes (associated with cortisol elevation), mood changes (associated with cortisol elevation)

Endocrine & metabolic: Decreased glucose tolerance (associated with cortisol elevation), fluid retention (associated with cortisol elevation)

Gastrointestinal: Increased appetite (associated with cortisol elevation), weight gain (associated with cortisol elevation)

<1%, postmarketing and/or case reports: Abdominal distention, carbohydrate intolerance (infants), cardiac failure, diaphoresis (adults), dizziness, epidermal thinning (adults), facial erythema, headache (adults), hirsutism (adults), hypersensitivity reaction, hypokalemic alkalosis (infants), impaired intestinal carbohydrate absorption, injection site reaction, intracranial hemorrhage (adults), myasthenia, nausea, necrotizing angiitis (adults), pancreatitis (adults), reversible cerebral atrophy (infants; usually secondary to hypertension), shock (adults), subdural hematoma, ulcerative esophagitis, vertebral compression fracture (infants), vertigo (adults)

Mechanism of Action Stimulates the adrenal cortex to secrete adrenal steroids (including cortisol), weakly androgenic substances, and aldosterone. Prolonged administration of large doses induces hyperplasia and hypertrophy of the adrenal cortex and continuous high output of cortisol, corticosterone, and weak androgens. Trophic effects on the adrenal cortex appear to be mediated by cyclic adenosine monophosphate. Also reported to bind to melanocortin receptors.

Pharmacodynamics/Kinetics

Onset of Action Maximum effect: Cortisol serum concentration: IM, SubQ: 3-12 hours

Duration of Action Repository: 10-25 hours, up to 3 days

Half-life Elimination ACTH: 15 minutes

Pregnancy Risk Factor C

Pregnancy Considerations

Endogenous corticotropin concentrations are increased near delivery (Smith, 2007).

Some studies have shown an association between first trimester systemic corticosteroid use and oral clefts (Park-Wyllie 2000; Prada, 2003). Systemic corticosteroids may also influence fetal growth (decreased birth weight); however, information is conflicting (Lunghi 2010). When systemic corticosteroids are needed in pregnancy, it is generally recommended to use the lowest effective dose for the shortest duration of time, avoiding high doses during the first trimester (Leachman 2006; Lunghi 2010; Makol 2011; Østensen 2009).

Prescribing and Access Restrictions Acthar Gel is only available through specialty pharmacy distribution and not through traditional distribution sources (eg, wholesalers, retail pharmacies). Hospitals wishing to acquire Acthar Gel should contact CuraScript Specialty Distribution (1-877-599-7748).

After treatment is initiated, discharge or outpatient prescriptions should be submitted to the Acthar Support and Access Program (A.S.A.P.) in order to ensure an uninterrupted supply of the medication. The Acthar Referral/Prescription form is available online at http://www.acthar.com/files/Acthar-Prescription-Referral-Form.pdf.

Additional information is available for the A.S.A.P. at http://www.acthar.com/healthcare-professionals/physician-patient-referrals or by calling 1-888-435-2284.

◆ **Corticotropin, Repository** *see* Corticotropin *on page 412*
◆ **Cortifoam** *see* Hydrocortisone (Topical) *on page 775*
◆ **Cortisol** *see* Hydrocortisone (Systemic) *on page 773*
◆ **Cortisol** *see* Hydrocortisone (Topical) *on page 775*

Cortisone (KOR ti sone)

Related Information

Respiratory Diseases *on page 1680*
Triamcinolone (Systemic) *on page 1485*

Pharmacologic Category Corticosteroid, Systemic

Use

Allergic states: Control of severe or incapacitating allergic conditions intractable to adequate trials of conventional treatment of atopic dermatitis, bronchial asthma, contact dermatitis, drug hypersensitivity reactions, seasonal or perennial allergic rhinitis, and serum sickness.

Dermatologic diseases: Bullous dermatitis herpetiformis, exfoliative dermatitis, mycosis fungoides, pemphigus, severe erythema multiforme (Stevens-Johnson syndrome), severe psoriasis, severe seborrheic dermatitis.

Endocrine disorders: Congenital adrenal hyperplasia, hypercalcemia associated with cancer, nonsuppurative thyroiditis, primary or secondary adrenocortical insufficiency (hydrocortisone or cortisone is the first choice; synthetic analogs may be used in conjunction with mineralocorticoids when applicable; in infancy, mineralocorticoid supplementation is of particular importance).

Gastrointestinal diseases: To tide the patient over a critical period of the disease in regional enteritis and ulcerative colitis.

Hematologic disorders: Acquired (autoimmune) hemolytic anemia, congenital (erythroid) hypoplastic anemia, erythroblastopenia (red blood cell [RBC] anemia), immune thrombocytopenia (formerly known as idiopathic thrombocytopenic purpura) in adults, secondary thrombocytopenia in adults.

Neoplastic diseases: Palliative management of leukemias and lymphomas in adults; acute leukemia of childhood.

Ophthalmic diseases: Severe acute and chronic allergic and inflammatory processes involving the eye and its adnexa (eg, allergic conjunctivitis, allergic corneal marginal ulcers, anterior segment inflammation, chorioretinitis, diffuse posterior uveitis and choroiditis, keratitis, herpes zoster ophthalmicus, iritis and iridocyclitis, optic neuritis, sympathetic ophthalmia).

Renal diseases: To induce diuresis or remission of proteinuria in nephrotic syndrome, without uremia, of the idiopathic type or that is caused by lupus erythematosus.

Respiratory diseases: Aspiration pneumonitis, berylliosis, fulminating or disseminated pulmonary tuberculosis when used concurrently with appropriate antituberculosis chemotherapy, Loeffler syndrome not manageable by other means, symptomatic sarcoidosis.

Rheumatic disorders: Adjunctive therapy for short-term administration (to tide the patient over an acute episode or exacerbation) in acute and subacute bursitis; acute gouty arthritis; acute nonspecific tenosynovitis; ankylosing spondylitis; epicondylitis; posttraumatic osteoarthritis; psoriatic arthritis; rheumatoid arthritis (RA), including juvenile RA (select cases may require low-dose maintenance therapy); and synovitis of osteoarthritis. During an exacerbation or as maintenance therapy in select cases of acute rheumatic carditis, systemic dermatomyositis (polymyositis), and systemic lupus erythematosus.

Miscellaneous: Tuberculous meningitis with subarachnoid block or impending block when used concurrently with appropriate antituberculous chemotherapy; trichinosis with neurologic or myocardial involvement.

Local Anesthetic/Vasoconstrictor Precautions No information available to require special precautions

Effects on Dental Treatment A compromised immune response may occur if patient has been taking systemic cortisone. The need for corticosteroid coverage in these patients should be considered before any dental treatment; consult with physician.

Effects on Bleeding Variable effects on anticoagulant therapy are observed with glucocorticoids, such as cortisone.

Adverse Reactions Frequency not defined.

>10%:
- Central nervous system: Insomnia, nervousness
- Gastrointestinal: Dyspepsia, increased appetite

1% to 10%:
- Endocrine & metabolic: Diabetes mellitus, hirsutism
- Neuromuscular & skeletal: Arthralgia
- Ophthalmic: Cataract, glaucoma
- Respiratory: Epistaxis

<1%, postmarketing, and/or case reports: Abdominal distention, acne vulgaris, alkalosis, amenorrhea, amyotrophy, bone fracture, bruise, Cushing's syndrome, decreased glucose tolerance, delirium, edema, emotional lability, euphoria, fluid retention, growth suppression, hallucination, headache, HPA-axis suppression, hyperglycemia, hyperpigmentation, hypersensitivity reaction, hypertension, hypokalemia, myalgia, nausea, osteoporosis, pancreatitis, peptic ulcer, pseudotumor cerebri, psychosis, seizure, skin atrophy, sodium retention, ulcerative esophagitis, vertigo, vomiting

Mechanism of Action Decreases inflammation by suppression of migration of polymorphonuclear leukocytes and reversal of increased capillary permeability

Pharmacodynamics/Kinetics

Half-life Elimination ~0.5 hours

Time to Peak ~2 hours

Pregnancy Considerations

Cortisone crosses the placenta (Migeon 1957). Some studies have shown an association between first trimester systemic corticosteroid use and oral clefts (Park-Wyllie 2000; Pradat 2003). Systemic corticosteroids may also influence fetal growth (decreased birth weight); however, information is conflicting (Lunghi

2010). Hypoadrenalism may occur in newborns following maternal use of corticosteroids in pregnancy (monitor). When systemic corticosteroids are needed in pregnancy, it is generally recommended to use the lowest effective dose for the shortest duration of time, avoiding high doses during the first trimester (Leachman 2006; Lunghi 2010; Makol 2011; Østensen 2009). Cortisone may be used (alternative agent) to treat primary adrenal insufficiency (PAI) in pregnant women. Pregnant women with PAI should be monitored at least once each trimester (Bornstein 2016).

- ◆ **Cortisone Acetate** *see* Cortisone *on page 413*
- ◆ **Corvert** *see* Ibutilide *on page 794*
- ◆ **Corvite 150** *see* Vitamins (Multiple/Oral) *on page 1550*
- ◆ **Cosentyx** *see* Secukinumab *on page 1361*
- ◆ **Cosentyx (300 MG Dose)** *see* Secukinumab *on page 1361*
- ◆ **Cosentyx Sensoready (300 MG)** *see* Secukinumab *on page 1361*
- ◆ **Cosentyx Sensoready Pen** *see* Secukinumab *on page 1361*
- ◆ **Cosmegen** *see* DACTINomycin *on page 430*
- ◆ **Cosopt** *see* Dorzolamide and Timolol *on page 516*
- ◆ **Cosopt PF** *see* Dorzolamide and Timolol *on page 516*
- ◆ **Cotellic** *see* Cobimetinib *on page 402*
- ◆ **Cotempla XR-ODT** *see* Methylphenidate *on page 997*
- ◆ **Cotrimoxazole** *see* Sulfamethoxazole and Trimethoprim *on page 1391*
- ◆ **Cough DM [OTC]** *see* Dextromethorphan *on page 476*
- ◆ **Coumadin [DSC]** *see* Warfarin *on page 1557*
- ◆ **Covaryx** *see* Estrogens (Esterified) and Methyltestosterone *on page 605*
- ◆ **Covaryx H.S.** *see* Estrogens (Esterified) and Methyltestosterone *on page 605*
- ◆ **COVID-19** *see* Azithromycin (Systemic) *on page 203*
- ◆ **COVID-19** *see* Chloroquine *on page 338*
- ◆ **COVID-19** *see* Hydroxychloroquine *on page 778*
- ◆ **COVID-19** *see* Lopinavir and Ritonavir *on page 929*
- ◆ **COVID-19** *see* Sarilumab *on page 1359*
- ◆ **COVID-19** *see* Tocilizumab *on page 1457*
- ◆ **Coviracil** *see* Emtricitabine *on page 556*
- ◆ **Cozaar** *see* Losartan *on page 938*
- ◆ **CP-690, 550** *see* Tofacitinib *on page 1459*
- ◆ **CP358774** *see* Erlotinib *on page 584*
- ◆ **CPC** *see* Cetylpyridinium *on page 330*
- ◆ **CPM** *see* Cyclophosphamide *on page 420*
- ◆ **CPT-11** *see* Irinotecan (Conventional) *on page 841*
- ◆ **CPX-351** *see* Daunorubicin and Cytarabine (Liposomal) *on page 445*
- ◆ **CPZ** *see* ChlorproMAZINE *on page 341*
- ◆ **13-CRA** *see* ISOtretinoin (Systemic) *on page 846*
- ◆ **CRA-032765** *see* Ibrutinib *on page 785*
- ◆ **Creomulsion Adult [OTC] [DSC]** *see* Dextromethorphan *on page 476*
- ◆ **Creomulsion for Children [OTC] [DSC]** *see* Dextromethorphan *on page 476*
- ◆ **Cresemba** *see* Isavuconazonium Sulfate *on page 843*
- ◆ **Crestor** *see* Rosuvastatin *on page 1348*
- ◆ **Crest Scope [OTC]** *see* Mouthwash (Antiseptic) *on page 1062*
- ◆ **Crest Scope Outlast [OTC]** *see* Mouthwash (Antiseptic) *on page 1062*
- ◆ **Crinone** *see* Progesterone *on page 1280*
- ◆ **Crisantaspase** *see* Asparaginase (*Erwinia*) *on page 176*
- ◆ **Critic-Aid Clear AF [OTC] [DSC]** *see* Miconazole (Topical) *on page 1019*
- ◆ **Crixivan** *see* Indinavir *on page 807*

Crizanlizumab (KRIZ an LIZ ue mab)

Brand Names: US Adakveo

Pharmacologic Category Monoclonal Antibody; Monoclonal Antibody, Anti-P-Selectin

Use Sickle cell disease: To reduce the frequency of vaso-occlusive crises in adults and pediatric patients ≥16 years of age with sickle cell disease.

Local Anesthetic/Vasoconstrictor Precautions No information available to require special precautions

Effects on Dental Treatment Key adverse event(s) related to dental treatment: Frequent occurrence of oropharyngeal pain

Effects on Bleeding Decreased platelet aggregation

Adverse Reactions

>10%:

Gastrointestinal: Nausea (18%)

Neuromuscular & skeletal: Arthralgia (18%), back pain (15%)

Miscellaneous: Fever (11%)

1% to 10%:

Dermatologic: Pruritus (<10%)

Gastrointestinal: Abdominal distress (<10%), abdominal pain (<10%), diarrhea (<10%), vomiting (<10%)

Genitourinary: Vulvovaginal pruritus (<10%)

Immunologic: Antibody development (2%)

Local: Infusion site pain (<10%), infusion site reaction (<10%), injection site extravasation (<10%), swelling at injection site (<10%)

Neuromuscular & skeletal: Musculoskeletal chest pain (<10%), myalgia (<10%)

Respiratory: Oropharyngeal pain (<10%)

Miscellaneous: Infusion related reaction (3% to 10%)

Frequency not defined: Hematologic & oncologic: Abnormal platelet aggregation

Mechanism of Action Crizanlizumab is a humanized IgG_2 kappa monoclonal antibody which binds to P-selectin and blocks interaction with ligands, including P-selectin glycoprotein ligand 1. Translocation of P-selectin to the activated endothelial cell surface results in adhesion of sickle erythrocytes to vessels and the development of vascular occlusion (Ataga 2017). By binding to P-selectin, crizanlizumab inhibits interactions between endothelial cells, platelets, red blood cells, and leukocytes, which may result in decreased platelet aggregation, maintenance of blood flow, and minimized sickle cell-related pain crises.

Pharmacodynamics/Kinetics

Half-life Elimination 7.6 days in patients with sickle cell disease; 10.6 days in healthy volunteers.

Pregnancy Considerations

Based on data from animal reproduction studies, in utero exposure to crizanlizumab may cause fetal harm.

Crizanlizumab is a humanized monoclonal antibody (IgG_2). Placental transfer of human IgG is dependent upon the IgG subclass, maternal serum concentrations, birth weight, and gestational age, generally increasing as pregnancy progresses. The lowest exposure would be expected during the period of organogenesis (Palmeira 2012; Pentsuk 2009).

Sickle cell disease increases the risk of adverse maternal and fetal outcomes, including an increased risk for vaso-occlusive crises, preeclampsia, eclampsia, intrauterine growth restriction, preterm delivery, low birth weight, and maternal and perinatal mortality.

◆ **Crizanlizumab-tmca** *see* Crizanlizumab *on page 414*

Crizotinib (kriz OH ti nib)

Related Information

Clinical Risk Related to Drugs Prolonging QT Interval *on page 1675*

Brand Names: US Xalkori

Brand Names: Canada Xalkori

Pharmacologic Category Antineoplastic Agent, Anaplastic Lymphoma Kinase Inhibitor; Antineoplastic Agent, Tyrosine Kinase Inhibitor

Use Non-small cell lung cancer, metastatic: Treatment of metastatic non-small cell lung cancer (NSCLC) in patients whose tumors are anaplastic lymphoma kinase (ALK)-positive or are ROS1-positive (as detected by an approved test)

Local Anesthetic/Vasoconstrictor Precautions Crizotinib is one of the drugs confirmed to prolong the QT interval and is accepted as having a risk of causing torsade de pointes. The risk of drug-induced torsade de pointes is extremely low when a single QT interval prolonging drug is prescribed. In terms of epinephrine, it is not known what effect vasoconstrictors in the local anesthetic regimen will have in patients with a known history of congenital prolonged QT interval or in patients taking any medication that prolongs the QT interval. Until more information is obtained, it is suggested that the clinician consult with the physician prior to the use of a vasoconstrictor in suspected patients, and that the vasoconstrictor (epinephrine, mepivacaine, and levonordefrin [Carbocaine® 2% with Neo-Cobefrin®]) be used with caution.

Effects on Dental Treatment Key adverse event(s) related to dental treatment: Stomatitis and taste alteration have been reported

Effects on Bleeding No reports of bleeding or thrombocytopenia

Adverse Reactions

>10%:

Cardiovascular: Edema (31% to 49%), bradycardia (5% to 14%)

Central nervous system: Fatigue (27% to 29%), neuropathy (19% to 25%), headache (22%), dizziness (18% to 22%)

Dermatologic: Skin rash (9% to 11%)

Endocrine & metabolic: Hypophosphatemia (28% to 32%), hypokalemia (18%)

Gastrointestinal: Diarrhea (60% to 61%), nausea (55% to 56%), vomiting (46% to 47%), constipation (42% to 43%), decreased appetite (30%), abdominal pain (26%), dysgeusia (26%), dyspepsia (8% to 14%)

Genitourinary: Decreased estimated GFR (eGFR) (<90 mL/min/1.73 m^2: 76%; <60 mL/min/1.73 m^2: 38%; <30 mL/min/1.73 m^2: 4%)

Hematologic & oncologic: Neutropenia (49% to 52%; grades 3/4: 11% to 12%), lymphocytopenia (48% to 51%; grades 3/4: 7% to 9%)

Hepatic: Increased serum alanine aminotransferase (76% to 79%), increased serum aspartate aminotransferase (61% to 66%)

Neuromuscular & skeletal: Limb pain (16%)

Ophthalmic: Visual disturbance (60% to 71%; onset: <2 weeks)

Respiratory: Upper respiratory tract infection (26% to 32%)

Miscellaneous: Fever (19%)

1% to 10%:

Cardiovascular: Pulmonary embolism (6%), prolonged QT interval on ECG (5% to 6%), syncope (1% to 3%)

Endocrine & metabolic: Weight loss (10%), weight gain (8%), diabetic ketoacidosis (≤2%), decreased plasma testosterone (1%; hypogonadism)

Gastrointestinal: Dysphagia (10%), esophagitis (2% to 6%)

Hepatic: Hepatic failure (1%)

Infection: Sepsis (≤5%)

Neuromuscular & skeletal: Muscle spasm (8%)

Renal: Renal cyst (3% to 5%)

Respiratory: Acute respiratory distress syndrome (≤5%), interstitial pulmonary disease (≤5%; includes acute respiratory distress syndrome, pneumonitis), pneumonia (≤5%), respiratory failure (≤5%), dyspnea (2%)

Frequency not defined:

Cardiovascular: Cardiac arrhythmia, septic shock

Central nervous system: Abnormal gait, dysesthesia, hypoesthesia, myasthenia, neuralgia, peripheral neuropathy

Dermatologic: Burning sensation of skin

Ophthalmic: Blurred vision, decreased visual acuity, diplopia, photophobia, photopsia, visual field defect, visual impairment, vitreous opacity

<1%, postmarketing, and/or case reports: Hepatotoxicity, increased creatine phosphokinase in blood specimen, vision loss

Mechanism of Action Crizotinib is a tyrosine kinase receptor inhibitor which inhibits anaplastic lymphoma kinase (ALK), Hepatocyte Growth Factor Receptor (HGFR, c-MET), ROS1 (c-ros), and Recepteur d'Origine Nantais (RON). ALK gene abnormalities due to mutations or translocations may result in expression of oncogenic fusion proteins (eg, ALK fusion protein) which alter signaling and expression and result in increased cellular proliferation and survival in tumors which express these fusion proteins. Approximately 2% to 7% of patients with NSCLC have the abnormal echinoderm microtubule-associated protein-like 4, or EML4-ALK gene (which has a higher prevalence in never smokers or light smokers and in patients with adenocarcinoma). Inhibition of ALK, ROS1, and c-Met phosphorylation is concentration-dependent. Crizotinib selectively inhibits ALK tyrosine kinase, which reduces proliferation of cells expressing the genetic alteration.

Pharmacodynamics/Kinetics

Half-life Elimination Terminal: 42 hours

Time to Peak 4 to 6 hours

Reproductive Considerations

Evaluate pregnancy status prior to use in females of reproductive potential. Females of reproductive potential should use adequate contraception during treatment and for at least 45 days after the last crizotinib dose; males with female partners of reproductive potential should use condoms during treatment and for at least 90 days after the final crizotinib dose.

Pregnancy Considerations
Based on the mechanism of action and data from animal reproduction studies, crizotinib may cause fetal harm if administered during pregnancy.

Prescribing and Access Restrictions Available through specialty pharmacies. Further information may be obtained from the manufacturer, Pfizer, at 1-877-744-5675, or at http://www.pfizerpro.com

Dental Health Professional Considerations See Local Anesthetic/Vasoconstrictor Precautions

- **Cromoglicate** *see* Cromolyn (Oral Inhalation) *on page 416*
- **Cromoglicate** *see* Cromolyn (Systemic) *on page 416*
- **Cromoglycic Acid** *see* Cromolyn (Oral Inhalation) *on page 416*
- **Cromoglycic Acid** *see* Cromolyn (Systemic) *on page 416*

Cromolyn (Systemic) (KROE moe lin)

Brand Names: US Gastrocrom

Pharmacologic Category Mast Cell Stabilizer

Use

Food allergy: Nalcrom [Canadian product]: Treatment of food allergy in conjunction with restriction of main causative allergens

Systemic mastocytosis: Management of systemic mastocytosis

Local Anesthetic/Vasoconstrictor Precautions
No information available to require special precautions

Effects on Dental Treatment Key adverse event(s) related to dental treatment:
Systemic: Glossitis, stomatitis, and unpleasant taste.

Effects on Bleeding No information available to require special precautions

Adverse Reactions
Cardiovascular: Chest pain, edema, flushing, palpitations, tachycardia, ventricular premature contractions
Central nervous system: Headache (5%), irritability (2%), malaise (1%), anxiety, behavioral changes, burning sensation, convulsions, depression, dizziness, dizziness (postprandial), fatigue, hallucination, hypoesthesia, insomnia, lethargy, migraine, nervousness, paresthesia, psychosis
Dermatologic: Pruritus (3%), skin rash (2%), erythema, skin photosensitivity, urticaria
Gastrointestinal: Diarrhea (5%), nausea (3%), abdominal pain (2%), constipation, dyspepsia, dysphagia, esophageal spasm, flatulence, glossitis, stomatitis, unpleasant taste, vomiting
Genitourinary: Dysuria, urinary frequency
Hematologic & oncologic: Neutropenia, pancytopenia, polycythemia, purpura
Hepatic: Abnormal hepatic function tests
Hypersensitivity: Anaphylaxis, angioedema
Neuromuscular & skeletal: Myalgia (3%), arthralgia, lower extremity weakness, lupus erythematosus, stiffness of legs
Otic: Tinnitus
Respiratory: Dyspnea, pharyngitis

Mechanism of Action Prevents the mast cell release of histamine, leukotrienes, and slow-reacting substance of anaphylaxis by inhibiting degranulation after contact with antigens

Pharmacodynamics/Kinetics

Onset of Action Response to treatment: Oral: May occur within 2 to 6 weeks

Half-life Elimination 80 to 90 minutes

Pregnancy Considerations Adverse events were not observed in animal reproduction studies. Systemic absorption following oral administration is <1%.

Cromolyn (Oral Inhalation) (KROE moe lin)

Brand Names: Canada DOM-Sodium Cromoglycate [DSC]; PMS-Sodium Cromoglycate

Pharmacologic Category Mast Cell Stabilizer

Use Note: Current expert recommendations do not recommend cromolyn for routine use for asthma, due to lower efficacy relative to other therapies (GINA 2019). Cromolyn may be considered for exercise-induced bronchospasm; however, regular controller therapy with inhaled corticosteroids or combination as-needed short-acting beta agonist and corticosteroids is preferred (GINA 2019).

Asthma: Maintenance and prophylactic therapy for asthma.

Exercise- or allergen-induced bronchospasm, prevention: Prevention of exercise- or allergen-induced bronchospasm.

Local Anesthetic/Vasoconstrictor Precautions
No information available to require special precautions

Effects on Dental Treatment Key adverse event(s) related to dental treatment:
Inhalation: Unpleasant taste.

Effects on Bleeding No information available to require special precautions

Adverse Reactions Frequency not always defined.
Central nervous system: Drowsiness
Dermatologic: Burning sensation of the nose, pruritus of nose
Gastrointestinal: Nausea, stomach pain
Hypersensitivity: Serum sickness
Respiratory: Cough (20%; transient), wheezing (4%; mild), epistaxis, nasal congestion, sneezing
<1%, postmarketing, and/or case reports: Anaphylaxis, anemia, angioedema, arthralgia, bronchospasm, dizziness, dysuria, exfoliative dermatitis, headache, hemoptysis, hoarseness, joint swelling, lacrimation, laryngeal edema, nephrosis, myalgia, parotid gland enlargement, pericarditis, peripheral neuritis, photodermatitis, polymyositis, pulmonary infiltrates (with eosinophilia), skin rash, urinary frequency, urticaria, vasculitis (periarteritis), vertigo

Mechanism of Action Prevents the mast cell release of histamine, leukotrienes, and slow-reacting substance of anaphylaxis by inhibiting degranulation after contact with antigens

Pharmacodynamics/Kinetics

Half-life Elimination 80 to 90 minutes

Time to Peak Serum: Inhalation: ~15 minutes

Pregnancy Risk Factor B

Pregnancy Considerations
Limited data suggest little or no placental transfer (Brogden 1974).

Uncontrolled asthma is associated with adverse events on pregnancy (increased risk of perinatal mortality, preeclampsia, preterm birth, low birth weight infants, cesarean delivery, and the development of gestational diabetes). Poorly controlled asthma or asthma exacerbations may have a greater fetal/maternal risk than what is associated with appropriately used asthma medications. Maternal treatment improves pregnancy outcomes by reducing the risk of some adverse events (eg, preterm birth, gestational diabetes). Maternal asthma symptoms should be monitored monthly during pregnancy (ERS/TSANZ [Middleton 2020]; GINA 2020).

Other agents are preferred for the control of asthma in pregnancy (GINA 2020).

Data collection to monitor pregnancy and infant outcomes associated with asthma and the medications used to treat asthma in pregnancy is ongoing. Health care providers are encouraged to enroll exposed pregnant females in the MotherToBaby Pregnancy Studies conducted by the Organization of Teratology Information Specialists (877-311-8972 or https://mothertobaby.org). Patients may also enroll themselves.

- ◆ **Cromolyn Sodium** *see* Cromolyn (Oral Inhalation) *on page 416*
- ◆ **Cromolyn Sodium** *see* Cromolyn (Systemic) *on page 416*
- ◆ **Cruex Prescription Strength [OTC]** *see* Miconazole (Topical) *on page 1019*
- ◆ **Cryselle-28** *see* Ethinyl Estradiol and Norgestrel *on page 617*
- ◆ **Crystalline Penicillin** *see* Penicillin G (Parenteral/Aqueous) *on page 1209*
- ◆ **CS-747** *see* Prasugrel *on page 1252*
- ◆ **CsA** *see* CycloSPORINE (Ophthalmic) *on page 423*
- ◆ **CsA** *see* CycloSPORINE (Systemic) *on page 421*
- ◆ **CTL019** *see* Tisagenlecleucel *on page 1454*
- ◆ **CTLA-4Ig** *see* Abatacept *on page 53*
- ◆ **CTM** *see* Chlorpheniramine *on page 340*
- ◆ **C-Topical** *see* Cocaine (Topical) *on page 403*
- ◆ **CTX** *see* Cyclophosphamide *on page 420*
- ◆ **Cubicin** *see* DAPTOmycin *on page 437*
- ◆ **Cubicin RF** *see* DAPTOmycin *on page 437*
- ◆ **Cu-IUD** *see* Copper IUD *on page 410*
- ◆ **Culturelle [OTC]** *see Lactobacillus on page 869*
- ◆ **Culturelle Baby [OTC]** *see Lactobacillus on page 869*
- ◆ **Curad Hydrocortisone [OTC]** *see* Hydrocortisone (Topical) *on page 775*
- ◆ **Curosurf** *see* Poractant Alfa *on page 1247*
- ◆ **CuT380A** *see* Copper IUD *on page 410*
- ◆ **Cutaquig** *see* Immune Globulin *on page 803*
- ◆ **Cuvitru** *see* Immune Globulin *on page 803*
- ◆ **Cuvposa** *see* Glycopyrrolate (Systemic) *on page 742*
- ◆ **CXA 201** *see* Ceftolozane and Tazobactam *on page 315*
- ◆ **CyA** *see* CycloSPORINE (Ophthalmic) *on page 423*
- ◆ **CyA** *see* CycloSPORINE (Systemic) *on page 421*

Cyanocobalamin (sye an oh koe BAL a min)

Brand Names: US B-12 Compliance Injection; Nascobal; Physicians EZ Use B-12; Vitamin Deficiency System-B12

Brand Names: Canada Cobex; Cyano Vit B12; JAMP-Cyanocobalamin

Pharmacologic Category Vitamin, Water Soluble

Use Vitamin B_{12} deficiency: Treatment of pernicious anemia, vitamin B_{12} deficiency due to dietary deficiencies, gastrointestinal malabsorption, folic acid deficiency, parasitic infestation, inadequate secretion of intrinsic factor, and inadequate utilization of B_{12} (eg, during neoplastic treatment); treatment of increased B_{12} requirements due to pregnancy, thyrotoxicosis, hemorrhage, malignancy, liver or kidney disease

Local Anesthetic/Vasoconstrictor Precautions No information available to require special precautions

Effects on Dental Treatment No significant effects or complications reported

Effects on Bleeding No information available to require special precautions

Adverse Reactions

>10%:

Central nervous system: Headache (IM: 20%; intranasal: 4%)

Infection: Infection (12% to 13%)

Neuromuscular & skeletal: Asthenia (IM: 16%; intranasal: 4%)

1% to 10%:

Central nervous system: Paresthesia (4%)

Gastrointestinal: Glossitis (nasal: 4%), nausea (4%)

Respiratory: Rhinitis (4% to 8%)

Frequency not defined:

Cardiovascular: Cardiac failure, thrombosis (peripheral)

Dermatologic: Pruritus, skin rash (transient)

Endocrine & metabolic: Hypokalemia

Gastrointestinal: Diarrhea

Hematologic & oncologic: Polycythemia vera, thrombocythemia

Hypersensitivity: Anaphylactic shock (IM/SubQ)

Respiratory: Pulmonary edema

Miscellaneous: Swelling

Mechanism of Action Coenzyme for various metabolic functions, including fat and carbohydrate metabolism and protein synthesis, used in cell replication and hematopoiesis

Pharmacodynamics/Kinetics

Onset of Action

Megaloblastic anemia: IM:

Conversion of megaloblastic to normoblastic erythroid hyperplasia within bone marrow: 8 hours

Increased reticulocytes: 2 to 5 days

Complicated vitamin B_{12} deficiency: IM, SubQ: Resolution of:

Psychiatric sequelae: 24 hours

Thrombocytopenia: 10 days

Granulocytopenia: 2 weeks

Time to Peak Serum: IM, SubQ: 30 minutes to 2 hours; Intranasal: 1.25 ± 1.9 hours

Pregnancy Considerations

Water soluble vitamins cross the placenta. Absorption of vitamin B_{12} may increase during pregnancy. Vitamin B_{12} requirements may be increased in pregnant women compared to nonpregnant women. Serum concentrations of vitamin B_{12} are higher in the neonate at birth than the mother (IOM 1998).

- ◆ **Cyanokit** *see* Hydroxocobalamin *on page 778*
- ◆ **Cyclafem 1/35** *see* Ethinyl Estradiol and Norethindrone *on page 614*
- ◆ **Cyclafem 7/7/7** *see* Ethinyl Estradiol and Norethindrone *on page 614*
- ◆ **Cyclessa [DSC]** *see* Ethinyl Estradiol and Desogestrel *on page 609*

Cyclobenzaprine (sye kloe BEN za preen)

Related Information

Dentin Hypersensitivity, Acid Erosion, High Caries Index, Management of Alveolar Osteitis, and Xerostomia *on page 1762*

Temporomandibular Dysfunction (TMD), Chronic Pain, and Fibromyalgia *on page 1773*

Brand Names: US Amrix; Fexmid

Brand Names: Canada AG-Cyclobenzaprine; APO-Cyclobenzaprine; Auro-Cyclobenzaprine; DOM-Cyclobenzaprine; Flexeril; JAMP-Cyclobenzaprine; MYLAN-Cyclobenzaprine [DSC]; PMS-Cyclobenzaprine; RIVA-Cyclobenzaprine; TEVA-Cyclobenzaprine

Generic Availability (US) Yes

Pharmacologic Category Skeletal Muscle Relaxant

Dental Use Treatment of muscle spasm associated with acute temporomandibular joint pain (TMJ)

Use Muscle spasm: As an adjunct to rest and physical therapy for short-term (2 to 3 weeks) relief of muscle spasm associated with acute, painful musculoskeletal conditions.

Local Anesthetic/Vasoconstrictor Precautions No information available to require special precautions

Effects on Dental Treatment Key adverse event(s) related to dental treatment: Xerostomia and changes in salivation (normal salivary flow resumes upon discontinuation). Occurrence of unpleasant taste. Rare occurrence of loss of taste (ageusia); rare occurrence of facial edema and tongue edema.

Effects on Bleeding No information available to require special precautions

Adverse Reactions

>10%:

Central nervous system: Drowsiness (1% to 39%), dizziness (1% to 11%)

Gastrointestinal: Xerostomia (6% to 32%)

1% to 10%:

Central nervous system: Fatigue (1% to 6%), headache (1% to 5%), confusion (1% to 3%), decreased mental acuity (1% to 3%), irritability (1% to 3%), nervousness (1% to 3%)

Gastrointestinal: Dyspepsia (≤4%), abdominal pain (1% to 3%), acid regurgitation (1% to 3%), constipation (1% to 3%), diarrhea (1% to 3%), nausea (1% to 3%), unpleasant taste (1% to 3%)

Neuromuscular & skeletal: Weakness (1% to 3%)

Ophthalmic: Blurred vision (1% to 3%)

Respiratory: Pharyngitis (1% to 3%), upper respiratory tract infection (1% to 3%)

<1%, postmarketing, and/or case reports: Abnormal dreams, abnormal hepatic function tests, abnormality in thinking, ageusia, agitation, anaphylaxis, angioedema, anorexia, anxiety, ataxia, cardiac arrhythmia, cholestasis, convulsions, depression, diaphoresis, diplopia, disorientation, dysarthria, excitement (paradoxical, children), facial edema, flatulence, gastritis, gastrointestinal pain, hallucination, hepatitis (rare), hypertonia, hypotension, increased thirst, insomnia, jaundice, malaise, muscle twitching, palpitations, paresthesia, pruritus, psychosis, seizure, serotonin syndrome, skin rash, syncope, tachycardia, tinnitus, tongue edema, tremor, urinary frequency, urinary retention, urticaria, vasodilation, vertigo, vomiting

Dental Usual Dosage Treatment of muscle spasm associated with acute TMJ pain (Burket 2008) (**Note:** Do not use longer than 2-3 weeks): Oral:

Adults: Initial: 5 mg 3 times/day; may increase to 7.5-10 mg 3 times/day if needed

Elderly: 5 mg 3 times/day; plasma concentration and incidence of adverse effects are increased in the elderly; dose should be titrated slowly

Dosing

Adult

Note: Patients more sensitive to sedating and other CNS adverse effects (eg, those who are older, debilitated patients, those with organ impairment) may better tolerate a reduced dose, less frequent administration, and/or more gradual titration (Chou 2019).

Fibromyalgia (alternative agent) (off-label use):

Note: For mild to moderate symptoms, particularly with sleep disturbance (EULAR [Macfarlane 2017]; Goldenberg 2020; Tofferi 2004).

Oral: Immediate release: Initial: 5 to 10 mg once daily before bedtime; may gradually titrate as needed and tolerated up to 10 to 40 mg daily in 1 to 3 divided doses (Calandre 2015; EULAR [Macfarlane 2017]; Goldenberg 2020; Tofferi 2004). If excessive sedation occurs, may divide dose so larger portion is taken at bedtime (eg, 5 mg in morning and 10 or 15 mg at bedtime) (Goldenberg 2020; Tofferi 2004).

Muscle spasm and/or musculoskeletal pain (adjunctive therapy):

Note: For skeletal muscle spasm and/or pain (eg, low back pain, neck pain) with muscle spasm, usually in combination with a nonsteroidal anti-inflammatory drug (NSAID) and/or acetaminophen (ACP [Chou 2017]; Borenstein 2003; van Tulder 2003). In general, muscle relaxants should be used temporarily (eg, for a few days or intermittently for a few days when needed) (APS 2016).

Oral: Immediate release: Initial: 5 mg 3 times daily scheduled or as needed with one of the doses administered at bedtime (Chou 2019). May increase dose based on response and tolerability up to 10 mg 3 times daily as needed. Once-daily use at bedtime (with daytime NSAID and/or acetaminophen) may be better tolerated (Knight 2020).

Oral: Extended release: Usual: 15 mg once daily; some patients may require up to 30 mg once daily.

Temporomandibular disorder, acute (adjunctive therapy) (off-label use):

Note: Adjunct to an NSAID in select patients with pain on palpation of the lower jaw muscle (Alencar 2014; Herman 2002; Mehta 2019).

Oral: Immediate release: Usual: 10 mg once daily at bedtime for 10 to 14 days (Alencar 2014; Herman 2002; Mehta 2019).

Geriatric Avoid use (Beers Criteria [AGS 2019]).

Renal Impairment: Adult There are no dosage adjustments provided in the manufacturer's labeling.

Hepatic Impairment: Adult

Extended release: Mild to severe impairment: Use not recommended.

Immediate release:

Mild impairment: Initial: 5 mg; use with caution; titrate slowly and consider less frequent dosing.

Moderate to severe impairment: Use not recommended.

Pediatric Muscle spasm, treatment: Adolescents ≥15 years: Oral: Immediate release tablet: Initial: 5 mg 3 times daily; may increase up to 10 mg 3 times daily if needed. Do not use longer than 2 to 3 weeks.

Renal Impairment: Pediatric There are no dosage adjustments provided in the manufacturer's labeling.

Hepatic Impairment: Pediatric

Immediate release tablet: Adolescents ≥15 years:

Mild impairment: Initial: 5 mg; use with caution; titrate slowly and consider less frequent dosing

Moderate to severe impairment: Use not recommended

Mechanism of Action Centrally-acting skeletal muscle relaxant pharmacologically related to tricyclic antidepressants; reduces tonic somatic motor activity influencing both alpha and gamma motor neurons

Contraindications Hypersensitivity to cyclobenzaprine or any component of the formulation; during or within 14 days of MAO inhibitors; hyperthyroidism; heart failure; arrhythmias; heart block or conduction disturbances; acute recovery phase of MI

Warnings/Precautions May cause CNS depression, which may impair physical or mental abilities; ethanol and/or other CNS depressants may enhance these effects. Patients must be cautioned about performing tasks which require mental alertness (eg, operating machinery or driving). Cyclobenzaprine shares the toxic potentials of the tricyclic antidepressants (including arrhythmias, tachycardia, and conduction time prolongation) and the usual precautions of tricyclic antidepressant therapy should be observed; use with caution in patients with urinary hesitancy or retention, angle-closure glaucoma or increased intraocular pressure, hepatic impairment, or in the elderly.

Potentially life-threatening serotonin syndrome has occurred with cyclobenzaprine when used in combination with other serotonergic agents (eg, SSRIs, SNRIs, TCAs, meperidine, tramadol, buspirone, MAO inhibitors), bupropion, and verapamil. Monitor patients closely especially during initiation/dose titration for signs/symptoms of serotonin syndrome such as mental status changes (eg, agitation, hallucinations); autonomic instability (eg, tachycardia, labile blood pressure, diaphoresis); neuromuscular changes (eg, tremor, rigidity, myoclonus); GI symptoms (eg, nausea, vomiting, diarrhea); and/or seizures. Discontinue cyclobenzaprine and any concomitant serotonergic agent immediately if signs/symptoms arise. Concomitant use or use within 14 days of discontinuing an MAO inhibitor is contraindicated.

Extended release capsules not recommended for use in mild-to-severe hepatic impairment or in the elderly. Potentially significant drug-drug interactions may exist, requiring dose or frequency adjustment, additional monitoring, and/or selection of alternative therapy. Effects may be potentiated when used with other CNS depressants or ethanol.

Warnings: Additional Pediatric Considerations Not effective in the treatment of spasticity due to cerebral or spinal cord disease or in children with cerebral palsy.

Drug Interactions

Metabolism/Transport Effects **Substrate** of CYP1A2 (minor), CYP2D6 (minor), CYP3A4 (minor); **Note:** Assignment of Major/Minor substrate status based on clinically relevant drug interaction potential

Avoid Concomitant Use

Avoid concomitant use of Cyclobenzaprine with any of the following: Aclidinium; Azelastine (Nasal); Bromperidol; Cimetropium; Eluxadoline; Glycopyrrolate (Oral Inhalation); Glycopyrronium (Topical); Ipratropium (Oral Inhalation); Levosulpiride; Monoamine Oxidase Inhibitors; Orphenadrine; Oxatomide; Oxomemazine; Paraldehyde; Potassium Chloride; Potassium Citrate; Pramlintide; Revefenacin; Thalidomide; Tiotropium; Umeclidinium

Increased Effect/Toxicity

Cyclobenzaprine may increase the levels/effects of: Alcohol (Ethyl); Anticholinergic Agents; Azelastine (Nasal); Blonanserin; Botulinum Toxin-Containing Products; Brexanolone; Buprenorphine; Cimetropium; CloZAPine; CNS Depressants; Eluxadoline; Flunitrazepam; Glucagon; Glycopyrrolate (Oral Inhalation); Methotrimeprazine; MetyroSINE; Mirabegron; Monoamine Oxidase Inhibitors; Opioid Agonists; Orphenadrine; OxyCODONE; Paraldehyde; Piribedil; Potassium Chloride; Potassium Citrate; Pramipexole; Ramosetron; Revefenacin; ROPINIRole; Rotigotine; Serotonergic Agents (High Risk); Suvorexant; Thalidomide; Thiazide and Thiazide-Like Diuretics; Tiotropium; Topiramate; Zolpidem

The levels/effects of Cyclobenzaprine may be increased by: Aclidinium; Alizapride; Amantadine; Botulinum Toxin-Containing Products; Brimonidine (Topical); Bromopride; Bromperidol; Cannabidiol; Cannabis; Chloral Betaine; Chlormethiazole; Chlorphenesin Carbamate; Dimethindene (Topical); Doxylamine; Dronabinol; Droperidol; Esketamine; Glycopyrronium (Topical); HydrOXYzine; Ipratropium (Oral Inhalation); Kava Kava; Lemborexant; Lisuride; Lofexidine; Magnesium Sulfate; Methotrimeprazine; Metoclopramide; Mianserin; Minocycline (Systemic); Nabilone; Oxatomide; Oxomemazine; Perampanel; Pramlintide; Rufinamide; Sodium Oxybate; Tetrahydrocannabinol; Tetrahydrocannabinol and Cannabidiol; Tolperisone; Trimeprazine; Umeclidinium

Decreased Effect

Cyclobenzaprine may decrease the levels/effects of: Acetylcholinesterase Inhibitors; Gastrointestinal Agents (Prokinetic); Itopride; Levosulpiride; Nitroglycerin; Secretin

The levels/effects of Cyclobenzaprine may be decreased by: Acetylcholinesterase Inhibitors; Ombitasvir, Paritaprevir, and Ritonavir; Ombitasvir, Paritaprevir, Ritonavir, and Dasabuvir

Food Interactions Food increases bioavailability (peak plasma concentrations increased by 35% and area under the curve by 20%) of the extended release capsule. Management: Monitor for increased effects if taken with food.

Pharmacodynamics/Kinetics

Onset of Action Immediate release: Within 1 hour

Duration of Action Immediate release: 12 to 24 hours

Half-life Elimination Normal hepatic function: Range: 8 to 37 hours; Immediate release: 18 hours; Extended release: 32 hours; Impaired hepatic function: 46.2 hours (range: 22.4 to 188 hours) (Winchell 2002)

Time to Peak Immediate release: ~4 hours (Winchell 2002); Extended release: 7 to 8 hours

Pregnancy Considerations Published information related to cyclobenzaprine use in pregnancy is limited (Flannery 1989; Moreira 2014).

Breastfeeding Considerations

Cyclobenzaprine is present in breast milk (Burra 2019).

The relative infant dose (RID) of cyclobenzaprine is 1.4% when calculated using the highest breast milk concentration located, compared to a weight-adjusted maternal dose of 10 mg twice daily.

In general, breastfeeding is considered acceptable when the RID of a medication is <10% (Anderson 2016; Ito 2000).

The RID of cyclobenzaprine was calculated using a milk concentration of 24.5 ng/mL, providing an estimated daily infant dose via breast milk of 0.004 mg/kg/day. This milk concentration was obtained following maternal administration of cyclobenzaprine 10 mg twice daily for 3 years following delivery. This same study also sampled breast milk of a mother taking cyclobenzaprine 5 mg once daily for 3 months following delivery. Authors of the study calculated the RID of cyclobenzaprine in both cases to be 0.5% using average breast milk concentrations and actual maternal weight. Adverse events were not observed in the breastfed infants. Until additional information is available, assessment of the infant for adverse events is recommended (Burra 2019). According to the manufacturer, the decision to breastfeed during therapy should consider the risk of infant exposure, the benefits of breastfeeding to the infant, and benefits of treatment to the mother.

Dosage Forms: US

Capsule Extended Release 24 Hour, Oral:
Amrix: 15 mg, 30 mg
Generic: 15 mg, 30 mg

Tablet, Oral:
Fexmid: 7.5 mg
Generic: 5 mg, 7.5 mg, 10 mg

Dosage Forms: Canada

Tablet, Oral:
Flexeril: 10 mg
Generic: 10 mg

◆ **Cyclobenzaprine HCl** *see* Cyclobenzaprine *on page 418*

◆ **Cyclobenzaprine Hydrochloride** *see* Cyclobenzaprine *on page 418*

Cyclophosphamide (sye kloe FOS fa mide)

Brand Names: Canada Procytox

Pharmacologic Category Antineoplastic Agent, Alkylating Agent; Antineoplastic Agent, Alkylating Agent (Nitrogen Mustard); Antirheumatic Miscellaneous; Immunosuppressant Agent

Use

Oncology uses: Treatment of acute lymphoblastic leukemia (ALL), acute myelocytic leukemia (AML), breast cancer, chronic lymphocytic leukemia (CLL), chronic myeloid leukemia (CML), Hodgkin lymphoma, mycosis fungoides, multiple myeloma, neuroblastoma, non-Hodgkin lymphomas (including Burkitt lymphoma), ovarian adenocarcinoma, and retinoblastoma

Limitations of use: Although potentially effective as a single-agent in susceptible malignancies, cyclophosphamide is more frequently used in combination with other chemotherapy drugs

Nononcology uses: Nephrotic syndrome: Treatment of minimal change nephrotic syndrome (biopsy proven) in children who are unresponsive or intolerant to corticosteroid therapy

Limitations of use: The safety and efficacy for the treatment of nephrotic syndrome in adults or in other renal diseases has not been established.

Local Anesthetic/Vasoconstrictor Precautions No information available to require special precautions

Effects on Dental Treatment Key adverse event(s) related to dental treatment: Mucositis and stomatitis.

Effects on Bleeding Hematologic toxicities including thrombocytopenia are among the important dose-limiting effects of cyclophosphamide. A medical consult is recommended.

Adverse Reactions Frequency not defined.

Dermatologic: Alopecia (reversible; onset: 3 to 6 weeks after start of treatment)

Endocrine & metabolic: Altered hormone level (increased gonadotropin secretion), amenorrhea

Gastrointestinal: Abdominal pain, anorexia, diarrhea, mucositis, nausea and vomiting (dose-related), stomatitis

Genitourinary: Azoospermia, defective oogenesis, hemorrhagic cystitis, oligospermia, sterility

Hematologic & oncologic: Anemia, bone marrow depression, febrile neutropenia, leukopenia (dose-related; recovery: 7 to 10 days after cessation), neutropenia, thrombocytopenia

Infection: Infection

<1%, postmarketing, and/or case reports: Acute respiratory distress, anaphylaxis, auditory disturbance, blurred vision, cardiac arrhythmia (with high-dose [HSCT] therapy), cardiac failure (with high-dose [HSCT] therapy), cardiac tamponade (with high-dose [HSCT] therapy), cardiotoxicity, confusion, C-reactive protein increased, dizziness, dyschromia (skin/fingernails), dyspnea, erythema multiforme, gastrointestinal hemorrhage, heart block, hematuria, hemopericardium, hemorrhagic colitis, hemorrhagic myocarditis (with high-dose [HSCT] therapy), hemorrhagic ureteritis, hepatic sinusoidal obstruction syndrome (formerly known as hepatic veno-occlusive disease), hepatitis, hepatotoxicity, hypersensitivity reaction, hyperuricemia, hypokalemia, hyponatremia, increased lactate dehydrogenase, interstitial pneumonitis, jaundice, malaise, mesenteric ischemia (acute), metastases, methemoglobinemia (with high-dose [HSCT] therapy), multi-organ failure, myocardial necrosis (with high-dose [HSCT] therapy), neurotoxicity, neutrophilic eccrine hidradenitis, ovarian fibrosis, pancreatitis, pericarditis, pneumonia, pulmonary hypertension, pulmonary infiltrates, pulmonary interstitial fibrosis (with high doses), pulmonary veno-occlusive disease, pyelonephritis, radiation recall phenomenon, reactivation of disease, reduced ejection fraction, renal tubular necrosis, reversible posterior leukoencephalopathy syndrome, rhabdomyolysis, sepsis, septic shock, SIADH, skin rash, Stevens-Johnson syndrome, testicular atrophy, thrombocytopenia (immune-mediated), thrombosis (arterial and venous), toxic epidermal necrolysis, toxic megacolon, tumor lysis syndrome, urinary fibrosis, weakness, wound healing impairment

Mechanism of Action Cyclophosphamide is an alkylating agent that prevents cell division by cross-linking DNA strands and decreasing DNA synthesis. It is a cell cycle phase nonspecific agent. Cyclophosphamide also possesses potent immunosuppressive activity. Cyclophosphamide is a prodrug that must be metabolized to active metabolites in the liver.

Pharmacodynamics/Kinetics

Half-life Elimination IV: 3 to 12 hours; Children: 4 hours; Adults: 6 to 8 hours

Time to Peak Oral: ~1 hour; IV: Metabolites: 2 to 3 hours

Reproductive Considerations

Evaluate pregnancy status prior to use in females of reproductive potential.

Females of reproductive potential should use effective contraception while receiving cyclophosphamide and for up to 1 year after completion of cyclophosphamide treatment. Males with female partners who are or may become pregnant should use a condom during and for at least 4 months after cyclophosphamide treatment.

Cyclophosphamide is used off label in the management of lupus nephritis in nonpregnant adults (Hahn 2012). Females treated for rheumatic and musculoskeletal diseases should consider discontinuing cyclophosphamide 3 to 6 months prior to attempted pregnancy to allow for disease monitoring and potential change to another immunosuppressant. Cyclophosphamide should also be discontinued 12 weeks prior to attempted conception in males with rheumatic and musculoskeletal diseases who are planning to father a child (ACR [Sammaritano 2020]).

Cyclophosphamide may cause ovarian insufficiency in females, and infertility and long-term gonadal damage in males. Dose-related sterility (which may be irreversible) may occur in both males and females. Recommendations are available for fertility preservation of male and female adult patients treated with anticancer agents (ASCO [Oktay 2018]). Recommendations for preserving fertility in females and males treated with cyclophosphamide for autoimmune and systemic inflammatory diseases are available (ACR [Sammaritano 2020]).

Pregnancy Considerations

Cyclophosphamide crosses the placenta and can be detected in amniotic fluid (D'Incalci 1982).

Birth defects (including malformations of the skeleton, palate, limbs, and eyes), miscarriage, fetal growth retardation, and fetotoxic effects in the newborn (including anemia, gastroenteritis leukopenia, pancytopenia, and severe bone marrow hypoplasia) have been reported.

Cyclophosphamide, if indicated, may be administered to pregnant women with breast cancer as part of some combination chemotherapy regimens; chemotherapy should not be administered during the first trimester, after 35 weeks' gestation, or within 3 weeks of planned delivery (Amant 2010; Loibl 2015; Shachar 2017). Use of regimens containing cyclophosphamide are generally avoided for the treatment of Hodgkin or non-Hodgkin lymphoma in pregnancy. However, use of cyclophosphamide may be considered as part of some regimens to treat patients diagnosed with aggressive non-Hodgkin lymphomas during the second or third trimester (Lishner 2016; Moshe 2017). The European Society for Medical Oncology has published guidelines for diagnosis, treatment, and follow-up of cancer during pregnancy. The guidelines recommend referral to a facility with expertise in cancer during pregnancy and encourage a multidisciplinary team (obstetrician, neonatologist, oncology team). In general, if chemotherapy is indicated, it should be avoided during in the first trimester, there should be a 3-week time period between the last chemotherapy dose and anticipated delivery, and chemotherapy should not be administered beyond week 33 of gestation (ESMO [Peccatori 2013]).

Cyclophosphamide is used off label in the management of lupus nephritis in nonpregnant adults (Hahn 2012). In patients with life- or organ-threatening maternal disease, cyclophosphamide may be used in the second or third trimesters only when an alternative therapy is not available (ACR [Sammaritano 2020]).

Cyclophosphamide is used off label as second-line therapy for the management of refractory immune thrombocytopenia (ITP) in nonpregnant adults; however, cyclophosphamide is not recommended for the treatment of ITP during pregnancy (ASH [Neunert 2019]; Provan 2019).

A pregnancy registry is available for all cancers diagnosed during pregnancy at Cooper Health (1-877-635-4499).

CycloSERINE (sye kloe SER een)

Pharmacologic Category Antibiotic, Miscellaneous; Antitubercular Agent

Use

Tuberculosis: Treatment of active pulmonary or extrapulmonary tuberculosis, in combination with other agents, when treatment with primary tuberculosis therapy has proved inadequate

Urinary tract infections: May be effective in treatment of acute urinary tract infections caused by susceptible strains of gram-positive and gram-negative bacteria, especially *Enterobacter* spp. and *Escherichia coli.* **Note:** Should be considered only when more conventional therapy has failed and when the organism has been demonstrated to be susceptible to the drug.

Local Anesthetic/Vasoconstrictor Precautions

No information available to require special precautions

Effects on Dental Treatment No significant effects or complications reported

Effects on Bleeding No information available to require special precautions

Adverse Reactions Frequency not defined.

Cardiovascular: Cardiac arrhythmia, cardiac failure

Central nervous system: Coma, confusion, dizziness, drowsiness, dysarthria, headache, hyperreflexia, paresis, paresthesia, psychosis, restlessness, seizure, vertigo

Dermatologic: Skin rash

Endocrine & metabolic: Cyanocobalamin deficiency, folate deficiency

Hepatic: Increased liver enzymes

Hypersensitivity: Hypersensitivity reaction

Neuromuscular & skeletal: Tremor

Mechanism of Action Inhibits bacterial cell wall synthesis by competing with amino acid (D-alanine) for incorporation into the bacterial cell wall; bacteriostatic or bactericidal

Pharmacodynamics/Kinetics

Half-life Elimination Normal renal function: 12 hours

Time to Peak Serum: 4 to 8 hours

Pregnancy Risk Factor C

Pregnancy Considerations

Cycloserine crosses the placenta and can be detected in the fetal blood and amniotic fluid. The American Thoracic Society recommends use in pregnant women only if there are no alternatives (CDC 2003).

◆ **Cyclosporin A** *see* CycloSPORINE (Ophthalmic) *on page 423*

◆ **Cyclosporin A** *see* CycloSPORINE (Systemic) *on page 421*

CycloSPORINE (Systemic) (SYE kloe spor een)

Brand Names: US Gengraf; Neoral; SandIMMUNE

Brand Names: Canada APO-CycloSPORINE; Neoral; SandIMMUNE IV; SANDOZ CycloSPORINE

Pharmacologic Category Calcineurin Inhibitor; Immunosuppressant Agent

Use

Cyclosporine modified:

Transplant rejection prophylaxis: Prophylaxis of organ rejection in kidney, liver, and heart transplants (commonly used in combination with an antiproliferative immunosuppressive agent and corticosteroid).

Rheumatoid arthritis: Treatment of severe, active rheumatoid arthritis (RA) not responsive to methotrexate alone

Psoriasis: Treatment of severe, recalcitrant plaque psoriasis in non-immunocompromised adults unresponsive to or unable to tolerate other systemic therapy

Cyclosporine non-modified:

Transplant rejection (prophylaxis): Prophylaxis of organ rejection in kidney, liver, and heart transplants (commonly used in combination with an antiproliferative agent and a corticosteroid)

Transplant rejection, chronic (treatment): May be used for the treatment of chronic rejection (kidney, liver, and heart) in patients previously treated with other immunosuppressive agents. **Note:** While approved for the treatment of chronic organ rejection, other therapies are clinically preferred in this setting.

Local Anesthetic/Vasoconstrictor Precautions No information available to require special precautions

Effects on Dental Treatment Key adverse event(s) related to dental treatment: Mouth sores, swallowing difficulty, gingivitis, gum hyperplasia, xerostomia (normal salivary flow resumes upon discontinuation), abnormal taste, tongue disorder, and gingival bleeding (see Dental Health Professional Considerations)

Effects on Bleeding No information available to require special precautions

Adverse Reactions Adverse reactions reported with systemic use, including rheumatoid arthritis, psoriasis, and transplantation (kidney, liver, and heart). Percentages noted include the highest frequency regardless of indication/dosage. Frequencies may vary for specific conditions or formulation.

>10%:

Cardiovascular: Hypertension (8% to 53%), edema (5% to 14%)

Central nervous system: Headache (2% to 25%), paresthesia (1% to 11%)

Dermatologic: Hypertrichosis (5% to 19%)

Endocrine & metabolic: Hirsutism (21% to 45%), increased serum triglycerides (15%), female genital tract disease (9% to 11%)

Gastrointestinal: Nausea (2% to 23%), diarrhea (3% to 13%), gingival hyperplasia (2% to 16%), abdominal distress (<1% to 15%), dyspepsia (2% to 12%)

Genitourinary: Urinary tract infection (kidney transplant: 21%)

Infection: Increased susceptibility to infection (3% to 25%), viral infection (kidney transplant: 16%)

Neuromuscular & skeletal: Tremor (7% to 55%), leg cramps (2% to 12%)

Renal: Increased serum creatinine (16% to ≥50%), renal insufficiency (10% to 38%)

Respiratory: Upper respiratory tract infection (1% to 14%)

Kidney, liver, and heart transplant only (≤2% unless otherwise noted):

Cardiovascular: Chest pain (≤4%), flushing (<1% to 4%), glomerular capillary thrombosis, myocardial infarction

Central nervous system: Convulsions (1% to 5%), anxiety, confusion, lethargy, tingling sensation

Dermatologic: Skin infection (7%), acne vulgaris (1% to 6%), nail disease (brittle fingernails), hair breakage, night sweats, pruritus

Endocrine & metabolic: Gynecomastia (<1% to 4%), hyperglycemia, hypomagnesemia, weight loss

Gastrointestinal: Vomiting (2% to 10%), anorexia, aphthous stomatitis, constipation, dysphagia, gastritis, hiccups, pancreatitis

Genitourinary: Hematuria

Hematologic & oncologic: Leukopenia (<1% to 6%), lymphoma (<1% to 6%), anemia, thrombocytopenia, upper gastrointestinal hemorrhage

Hepatic: Hepatotoxicity (<1% to 7%)

Infection: Localized fungal infection (8%), cytomegalovirus disease (5%), septicemia (5%), abscess (4%), fungal infection (systemic: 2%)

Neuromuscular & skeletal: Arthralgia, myalgia, weakness

Ophthalmic: Conjunctivitis, visual disturbance

Otic: Hearing loss, tinnitus

Respiratory: Sinusitis (<1% to 7%), pneumonia (6%)

Miscellaneous: Fever

Rheumatoid arthritis only (1% to <3% unless otherwise noted):

Cardiovascular: Chest pain (4%), cardiac arrhythmia (2%), abnormal heart sounds, cardiac failure, myocardial infarction, peripheral ischemia

Central nervous system: Dizziness (8%), pain (6%), insomnia (4%), depression (3%), migraine (2% to 3%), anxiety, drowsiness, emotional lability, hypoesthesia, lack of concentration, malaise, neuropathy, nervousness, paranoia, vertigo

Dermatologic: Cellulitis, dermatological reaction, dermatitis, diaphoresis, dyschromia, eczema, enanthema, folliculitis, nail disease, pruritus, urticaria, xeroderma

Endocrine & metabolic: Menstrual disease (3%), decreased libido, diabetes mellitus, goiter, hot flash, hyperkalemia, hyperuricemia, hypoglycemia, increased libido, weight gain, weight loss

Gastrointestinal: Vomiting (9%), flatulence (5%), gingivitis (4%), constipation, dysgeusia, dysphagia, enlargement of salivary glands, eructation, esophagitis, gastric ulcer, gastritis, gastroenteritis, gingival hemorrhage, glossitis, peptic ulcer, tongue disease, xerostomia

Genitourinary: Leukorrhea (1%), breast fibroadenosis, hematuria, mastalgia, nocturia, urine abnormality, urinary incontinence, urinary urgency, uterine hemorrhage

Hematologic & oncologic: Purpura (3% to 4%), anemia, carcinoma, leukopenia, lymphadenopathy

Hepatic: Hyperbilirubinemia

Infection: Abscess (including renal), bacterial infection, candidiasis, fungal infection, herpes simplex infection, herpes zoster, viral infection

Neuromuscular & skeletal: Arthralgia, bone fracture, dislocation, myalgia, stiffness, synovial cyst, tendon disease, weakness

Ophthalmic: Cataract, conjunctivitis, eye pain, visual disturbance

Otic: Tinnitus, deafness, vestibular disturbance

Renal: Abscess (renal), increased blood urea nitrogen, polyuria, pyelonephritis

Respiratory: Cough (5%), dyspnea (5%), sinusitis (4%), abnormal breath sounds, bronchospasm, epistaxis, tonsillitis

Psoriasis only (1% to <3% unless otherwise noted):
- Cardiovascular: Chest pain, flushing
- Central nervous system: Psychiatric disturbance (4% to 5%), pain (3% to 4%), dizziness, insomnia, nervousness, vertigo
- Dermatologic: Acne vulgaris, folliculitis, hyperkeratosis, pruritus, skin rash, xeroderma
- Endocrine & metabolic: Hot flash
- Gastrointestinal: Abdominal distention, constipation, gingival hemorrhage, increased appetite
- Genitourinary: Urinary frequency
- Hematologic & oncologic: Abnormal erythrocytes, altered platelet function, blood coagulation disorder, carcinoma, hemorrhagic diathesis
- Hepatic: Hyperbilirubinemia
- Neuromuscular & skeletal: Arthralgia (1% to 6%)
- Ophthalmic: Visual disturbance
- Respiratory: Flu-like symptoms (8% to 10%), bronchospasm (5%), cough (5%), dyspnea (5%), rhinitis (5%), respiratory tract infection
- Miscellaneous: Fever

Postmarketing and/or case reports (any indication): Anaphylaxis/anaphylactoid reaction (possibly associated with Cremophor EL vehicle in injection formulation), brain disease, central nervous system toxicity, cholestasis, cholesterol increased, exacerbation of psoriasis (transformation to erythrodermic or pustular psoriasis), fatigue, gout, haemolytic uremic syndrome, hepatic insufficiency, hepatitis, hyperbilirubinemia, hyperkalemia, hyperlipidemia, hypertrichosis, hyperuricemia, hypomagnesemia, impaired consciousness, increased susceptibility to infection (including JC virus and BK virus), jaundice, leg pain (possibly a manifestation of Calcineurin-Inhibitor Induced Pain Syndrome), malignant lymphoma, migraine, myalgia, myopathy, myositis, papilledema, progressive multifocal leukoencephalopathy, pseudotumor cerebri, pulmonary edema (noncardiogenic), renal disease (polyoma virus-associated), reversible posterior leukoencephalopathy syndrome, rhabdomyolysis, thrombotic microangiopathy

Mechanism of Action Inhibition of production and release of interleukin II and inhibits interleukin II-induced activation of resting T-lymphocytes.

Pharmacodynamics/Kinetics

Half-life Elimination Oral: May be prolonged with hepatic impairment and shorter in pediatric patients due to the higher metabolism rate

Cyclosporine (non-modified): Biphasic: Alpha: 1.4 hours; Terminal: 19 hours (range: 10-27 hours)

Cyclosporine (modified): Biphasic: Terminal: 8.4 hours (range: 5-18 hours)

Time to Peak Serum: Oral:

Cyclosporine (non-modified): 2-6 hours; some patients have a second peak at 5-6 hours

Cyclosporine (modified): Renal transplant: 1.5-2 hours

Pregnancy Considerations

Cyclosporine crosses the placenta; maternal concentrations do not correlate with those found in the umbilical cord. Cyclosporine may be detected in the serum of newborns for several days after birth (Claris 1993). Based on clinical use, premature births and low birth weight were consistently observed in pregnant transplant patients (additional pregnancy complications also present). Formulations may contain alcohol; the alcohol content should be taken into consideration in pregnant women.

The pharmacokinetics of cyclosporine may be influenced by pregnancy (Grimer 2007). Cyclosporine may be used in pregnant renal, liver, or heart transplant patients (Cowan 2012; EBPG Expert Group on Renal Transplantation 2002; McGuire 2009; Parhar 2012). If therapy is needed for psoriasis, other agents are preferred; however, cyclosporine may be used as an alternative agent along with close clinical monitoring; use should be avoided during the first trimester if possible (Bae 2012). If treatment is needed for lupus nephritis, other agents are recommended to be used in pregnant women (Hahn 2012).

The Transplant Pregnancy Registry International (TPR) is a registry that follows pregnancies that occur in maternal transplant recipients or those fathered by male transplant recipients. The TPR encourages reporting of pregnancies following solid organ transplant by contacting them at 1-877-955-6877 or https://www.transplantpregnancyregistry.org.

Dental Health Professional Considerations Consider a medical consultation prior to any invasive dental procedure in patients who have received an organ transplant; delayed wound healing due to the immunosuppressive effects and an increased potential for postoperative infection may be of concern.

CycloSPORINE (Ophthalmic)

(SYE kloe spor een)

Brand Names: US Cequa; Restasis; Restasis MultiDose

Brand Names: Canada Restasis; Restasis MultiDose; TEVA-CycloSPORINE; Verkazia

Pharmacologic Category Calcineurin Inhibitor; Immunosuppressant Agent

Use Keratoconjunctivitis sicca: Increase tear production when suppressed tear production is presumed to be due to keratoconjunctivitis sicca-associated ocular inflammation (in patients not already using topical anti-inflammatory drugs or punctal plugs)

Local Anesthetic/Vasoconstrictor Precautions No information available to require special precautions

Effects on Dental Treatment No significant effects or complications reported

Effects on Bleeding No information available to require special precautions

Adverse Reactions

>10%: Ophthalmic: Eye pain (1% to 22%), burning sensation of eyes (17%)

1% to 10%:
- Central nervous system: Foreign body sensation of eye (1% to 5%), headache (1% to 5%)
- Genitourinary: Urinary tract infection (1% to 5%)
- Ophthalmic: Conjunctival hyperemia (1% to 6%), blepharitis (1% to 5%), blurred vision (1% to 5%), epiphora (1% to 5%), eye discharge (1% to 5%), eye irritation (1% to 5%), eye pruritus (1% to 5%), stinging of eyes (1% to 5%), visual disturbance (1% to 5%)

<1%, postmarketing and/or case reports: Hypersensitivity reaction

Pregnancy Considerations

Serum concentrations are below the limit of detection (<0.1 ng/mL) following ophthalmic use; fetal exposure following ophthalmic administration is not expected.

- ◆ **CyFolex** *see* Vitamins (Multiple/Oral) *on page* 1550
- ◆ **Cyklokapron** *see* Tranexamic Acid *on page* 1478
- ◆ **Cyltezo** *see* Adalimumab *on page* 83
- ◆ **Cymbalta** *see* DULoxetine *on page* 536

Cyproheptadine (si proe HEP ta deen)

Pharmacologic Category Histamine H_1 Antagonist; Histamine H_1 Antagonist, First Generation; Piperidine Derivative

Use Allergic conditions: Perennial and seasonal allergic rhinitis; vasomotor rhinitis; allergic conjunctivitis caused by inhalant allergens and foods; mild, uncomplicated allergic skin manifestations of urticaria and angioedema; amelioration of allergic reactions to blood or plasma; cold urticaria; dermatographism; adjunctive anaphylactic therapy.

Local Anesthetic/Vasoconstrictor Precautions No information available to require special precautions

Effects on Dental Treatment Key adverse event(s) related to dental treatment: Xerostomia (normal salivary flow resumes upon discontinuation)

Effects on Bleeding No information available to require special precautions

Adverse Reactions Frequency not defined.

Cardiovascular: Extrasystoles, hypotension, palpitations, tachycardia

Central nervous system: Ataxia, chills, confusion, dizziness, drowsiness, euphoria, excitement, fatigue, hallucination, headache, hysteria, insomnia, irritability, nervousness, neuritis, paresthesia, restlessness, sedation, seizure, vertigo

Dermatologic: Diaphoresis, skin photosensitivity, skin rash, urticaria

Gastrointestinal: Abdominal pain, anorexia, cholestasis, constipation, diarrhea, increased appetite, nausea, vomiting, xerostomia

Genitourinary: Difficulty in micturition, urinary frequency, urinary retention

Hematologic & oncologic: Agranulocytosis, hemolytic anemia, leukopenia, thrombocytopenia

Hepatic: Hepatic failure, hepatitis, jaundice

Hypersensitivity: Anaphylactic shock, angioedema, hypersensitivity reaction

Neuromuscular & skeletal: Tremor

Ophthalmic: Blurred vision, diplopia

Otic: Labyrinthitis (acute), tinnitus

Respiratory: Nasal congestion, pharyngitis, thickening of bronchial secretions

Mechanism of Action A potent antihistamine and serotonin antagonist with anticholinergic effects; competes with histamine for H_1-receptor sites on effector cells in the gastrointestinal tract, blood vessels, and respiratory tract (Paton 1985).

Pharmacodynamics/Kinetics

Half-life Elimination Metabolites: ~16 hours (Paton 1985)

Time to Peak Plasma: Metabolites: 6 to 9 hours (Paton 1985)

Pregnancy Risk Factor B

Pregnancy Considerations

Per the product labeling, an increased risk of congenital abnormalities was not observed following maternal use of cyproheptadine during the first, second, or third trimesters in two studies of pregnant women; however the possibility of harm cannot be ruled out. Although cyproheptadine is approved for the treatment of allergic conditions such as rhinitis and uritcaria, other agents are preferred for use in pregnant women (Scadding 2008; Wallace 2008; Zuberbier 2014). Antihistamines are not recommended for treatment of pruritus associated with intrahepatic cholestasis in pregnancy (Ambros-Rudolph 2011; Kremer 2014).

◆ **Cyproheptadine HCl** *see* Cyproheptadine *on page 424*

◆ **Cyproheptadine Hydrochloride** *see* Cyproheptadine *on page 424*

◆ **Cyramza** *see* Ramucirumab *on page 1308*

◆ **Cyred** *see* Ethinyl Estradiol and Desogestrel *on page 609*

◆ **Cyred EQ** *see* Ethinyl Estradiol and Desogestrel *on page 609*

◆ **CYT** *see* Cyclophosphamide *on page 420*

◆ **Cytarabine** *see* Cytarabine (Conventional) *on page 424*

Cytarabine (Conventional)

(sye TARE a been con VEN sha nal)

Brand Names: Canada Cytosar; PMS-Cytarabine

Pharmacologic Category Antineoplastic Agent, Antimetabolite; Antineoplastic Agent, Antimetabolite (Pyrimidine Analog)

Use

Acute lymphoblastic leukemia: Treatment of acute lymphoblastic leukemia.

Acute myeloid leukemia: Remission induction (in combination with other chemotherapy medications) in acute myeloid leukemia in adult and pediatric patients.

Chronic myeloid leukemia: Treatment of chronic myeloid leukemia in blast phase.

Meningeal leukemia: Prophylaxis and treatment of meningeal leukemia.

Local Anesthetic/Vasoconstrictor Precautions No information available to require special precautions

Effects on Dental Treatment Key adverse event(s) related to dental treatment: Mucositis

Effects on Bleeding Hematologic effects depend on dose and schedule of treatment. Platelets are one of the primary cell lines affected. Patients will develop thrombocytopenia on approximately day 7 which resolves about day 21-28. A medical consult is recommended.

Adverse Reactions Frequency not always defined. CNS, gastrointestinal, ophthalmic, and pulmonary toxicities are more common with high-dose regimens.

Cardiovascular: Angina pectoris, chest pain, local thrombophlebitis, pericarditis

Central nervous system: Aseptic meningitis, cerebral dysfunction, dizziness, headache, neuritis, neurotoxicity, paralysis (intrathecal and IV combination therapy), reversible posterior leukoencephalopathy syndrome

Dermatologic: Acute generalized exanthematous pustulosis, alopecia, dermal ulcer, ephelis, pruritus, skin rash, urticaria

Endocrine & metabolic: Hyperuricemia

Gastrointestinal: Abdominal pain, anal fissure, anorexia, diarrhea, esophageal ulcer, esophagitis, increased serum amylase, increased serum lipase, intestinal necrosis, mucositis, nausea, pancreatitis, sore throat, toxic megacolon, vomiting

Genitourinary: Urinary retention

Hematologic & oncologic: Anemia, bone marrow depression, hemorrhage, leukopenia, megaloblastic anemia, neutropenia (onset: 1 to 7 days; nadir [biphasic]: 7 to 9 days and at 15 to 24 days; recovery [biphasic]: 9 to 12 days and at 24 to 34 days), reticulocytopenia, thrombocytopenia (onset: 5 days; nadir: 12 to 15 days; recovery 15 to 25 days)

Hepatic: Hepatic insufficiency, hepatic sinusoidal obstruction syndrome (formerly known as hepatic veno-occlusive disease), increased serum transaminases (acute), jaundice
Hypersensitivity: Allergic edema, anaphylaxis
Infection: Sepsis
Local: Cellulitis at injection site, inflammation at injection site (SC injection), local inflammation (anus), pain at injection site (SC injection)
Neuromuscular & skeletal: Rhabdomyolysis
Ophthalmic: Conjunctivitis
Renal: Renal insufficiency
Respiratory: Acute respiratory distress, dyspnea, interstitial pneumonitis
Miscellaneous: Drug toxicity (cytarabine syndrome; chest pain, conjunctivitis, fever, maculopapular rash, malaise, myalgia, ostealgia), fever

Adverse events associated with high-dose cytarabine

Cardiovascular: Cardiomegaly, cardiomyopathy (in combination with cyclophosphamide)
Central nervous system: Neurotoxicity (patients with renal impairment: ≤55%), coma, drowsiness, neurocerebellar toxicity, peripheral neuropathy (motor and sensory), personality changes
Dermatologic: Alopecia (complete), desquamation, skin rash (severe)
Gastrointestinal: Gastrointestinal ulcer, necrotizing enterocolitis, pancreatitis, peritonitis, pneumatosis cystoides intestinalis
Hepatic: Hepatic abscess, hepatic injury, hyperbilirubinemia
Infection: Sepsis
Ophthalmic: Corneal toxicity, hemorrhagic conjunctivitis
Respiratory: Acute respiratory distress, pulmonary edema

Adverse events associated with intrathecal cytarabine administration

Central nervous system: Aphonia, leukoencephalopathy (necrotizing; with concurrent cranial irradiation, intrathecal methotrexate, and intrathecal hydrocortisone), nerve palsy (accessory nerve), neurotoxicity, paraplegia
Gastrointestinal: Dysphagia, nausea, vomiting
Ophthalmic: Blindness (with concurrent systemic chemotherapy and cranial irradiation), diplopia
Respiratory: Cough, hoarseness
Miscellaneous: Fever

Mechanism of Action Cytarabine inhibits DNA synthesis. Cytarabine gains entry into cells by a carrier process, and then must be converted to its active compound, aracytidine triphosphate. Cytarabine is a pyrimidine analog and is incorporated into DNA; however, the primary action is inhibition of DNA polymerase resulting in decreased DNA synthesis and repair. The degree of cytotoxicity correlates linearly with incorporation into DNA; therefore, incorporation into the DNA is responsible for drug activity and toxicity. Cytarabine is specific for the S phase of the cell cycle (blocks progression from the G_1 to the S phase).

Pharmacodynamics/Kinetics

Half-life Elimination IV: Initial: 7 to 20 minutes; Terminal: 1 to 3 hours; Intrathecal: 2 to 6 hours

Time to Peak IM, SubQ: 20 to 60 minutes

Reproductive Considerations

Females of reproductive potential should avoid becoming pregnant during treatment and be advised of the potential risks if exposure during pregnancy would occur.

Pregnancy Considerations

Based on the mechanism of action and findings from animal reproduction studies, fetal harm may occur if cytarabine is administered during pregnancy. Limb and ear defects have been noted in case reports of cytarabine exposure during the first trimester of pregnancy. The following have also been noted in the neonate: Pancytopenia, WBC depression, electrolyte abnormalities, prematurity, low birth weight, decreased hematocrit or platelets. Risk to the fetus is decreased if treatment can be avoided during the first trimester.

- **Cytarabine and Daunorubicin (Liposomal)** *see* Daunorubicin and Cytarabine (Liposomal) *on page 445*
- **Cytarabine Hydrochloride** *see* Cytarabine (Conventional) *on page 424*
- **Cytarabine Lipid Complex** *see* Cytarabine (Liposomal) *on page 425*

Cytarabine (Liposomal)

(sye TARE a been lye po SO mal)

Brand Names: US DepoCyt [DSC]

Brand Names: Canada Depocyt [DSC]

Pharmacologic Category Antineoplastic Agent, Antimetabolite; Antineoplastic Agent, Antimetabolite (Pyrimidine Analog)

Use Lymphomatous meningitis: Intrathecal treatment of lymphomatous meningitis

Local Anesthetic/Vasoconstrictor Precautions No information available to require special precautions

Effects on Dental Treatment No significant effects or complications reported

Effects on Bleeding Hematologic effects depend on dose and schedule of treatment. Platelets are one of the primary cell lines affected. Patients will develop thrombocytopenia on approximately day 7 which resolves about day 21-28. A medical consult is recommended.

Adverse Reactions

>10%:

Cardiovascular: Peripheral edema (11%)
Central nervous system: Chemical arachnoiditis (without dexamethasone premedication: 100%; with dexamethasone premedication: 33% to 42%; grade 4: 19% to 30%; onset: ≤5 days), headache (56%), confusion (33%), fatigue (25%), abnormal gait (23%), seizure (20% to 22%), dizziness (18%), lethargy (16%), insomnia (14%), memory impairment (14%), pain (14%)
Endocrine & metabolic: Dehydration (13%)
Gastrointestinal: Nausea (46%), vomiting (44%), constipation (25%), diarrhea (12%), decreased appetite (11%)
Genitourinary: Urinary tract infection (14%)
Hematologic & oncologic: Anemia (12%), thrombocytopenia (3% to 11%)
Neuromuscular & skeletal: Weakness (40%), back pain (24%), limb pain (15%), neck pain (14%), arthralgia (11%), neck stiffness (11%)
Ophthalmic: Blurred vision (11%)
Miscellaneous: Fever (32%)

1% to 10%:

Cardiovascular: Tachycardia (9%), hypotension (8%), hypertension (6%), syncope (3%), edema (2%)

Central nervous system: Agitation (10%), hypoesthesia (10%), myasthenia (10%), depression (8%), anxiety (7%), peripheral neuropathy (3% to 4%), abnormal reflexes (3%), sensorimotor neuropathy (3%)
Dermatologic: Diaphoresis (2%), pruritus (2%)
Endocrine & metabolic: Hypokalemia (7%), hyponatremia (7%), hyperglycemia (6%)
Gastrointestinal: Abdominal pain (9%), dysphagia (8%), anorexia (5%), hemorrhoids (3%), mucosal inflammation (3%)
Genitourinary: Urinary incontinence (7%), urinary retention (5%)
Hematologic & oncologic: Neutropenia (10%), bruise (2%)
Neuromuscular & skeletal: Tremor (9%)
Otic: Hypoacusis (6%)
Respiratory: Dyspnea (10%), cough (7%), pneumonia (6%)

<1%, postmarketing, and/or case reports: Anaphylaxis, bladder disease (bladder control impaired), blindness, brain disease, cauda equina syndrome, cranial nerve palsy, deafness, drowsiness, fecal incontinence, hemiplegia, hydrocephalus, increased intracranial pressure, leukocytosis (in CSF), meningitis (infectious), myelopathy, nervous system disease (neurologic deficit), numbness, papilledema, visual disturbance

Mechanism of Action Cytarabine liposomal is a sustained-release formulation of the active ingredient cytarabine, an antimetabolite which acts through inhibition of DNA synthesis and is cell cycle-specific for the S phase of cell division. Cytarabine is converted intracellularly to its active metabolite cytarabine-5'-triphosphate (ara-CTP). Ara-CTP also appears to be incorporated into DNA and RNA; however, the primary action is inhibition of DNA polymerase, resulting in decreased DNA synthesis and repair. The liposomal formulation allows for gradual release, resulting in prolonged exposure.

Pharmacodynamics/Kinetics

Half-life Elimination Cerebrospinal fluid: ~6 to 82 hours.

Time to Peak Cerebrospinal fluid: Intrathecal: Within 1 hour.

Reproductive Considerations

Systemic exposure following intrathecal administration of cytarabine liposomal is negligible; however, women of childbearing potential should avoid becoming pregnant during treatment.

Pregnancy Considerations

Adverse effects were observed in animal reproductive studies with conventional cytarabine. Conventional cytarabine has been associated with fetal malformations when given as a component of systemic combination chemotherapy during the first trimester. Systemic exposure following intrathecal administration of cytarabine liposomal is negligible.

Product Availability DepoCyt is no longer available in the US.

- ◆ **Cytarabine (Liposomal) and Daunorubicin (Liposomal)** *see* Daunorubicin and Cytarabine (Liposomal) *on page 445*
- ◆ **Cytarabine Liposome** *see* Cytarabine (Liposomal) *on page 425*
- ◆ **Cytarabine Liposome and Daunorubicin Liposome** *see* Daunorubicin and Cytarabine (Liposomal) *on page 445*
- ◆ **Cytarabine Liposome Injection** *see* Cytarabine (Liposomal) *on page 425*
- ◆ **Cytomel** *see* Liothyronine *on page 919*
- ◆ **Cytosar-U** *see* Cytarabine (Conventional) *on page 424*
- ◆ **Cytosine Arabinosine Hydrochloride** *see* Cytarabine (Conventional) *on page 424*
- ◆ **Cytostasan** *see* Bendamustine *on page 226*
- ◆ **Cytotec** *see* MiSOPROStol *on page 1040*
- ◆ **Cytovene** *see* Ganciclovir (Systemic) *on page 728*
- ◆ **Cytoxan** *see* Cyclophosphamide *on page 420*
- ◆ **D2** *see* Ergocalciferol *on page 582*
- ◆ **D2E7** *see* Adalimumab *on page 83*
- ◆ **D3** *see* Cholecalciferol *on page 344*
- ◆ **D-3-5 [OTC]** *see* Cholecalciferol *on page 344*
- ◆ **D3-50 [OTC]** *see* Cholecalciferol *on page 344*
- ◆ **D3 Vitamin [OTC] [DSC]** *see* Cholecalciferol *on page 344*
- ◆ **d4T** *see* Stavudine *on page 1387*
- ◆ **DA-7157** *see* Tedizolid *on page 1409*
- ◆ **DA-7158** *see* Tedizolid *on page 1409*
- ◆ **DA-7218** *see* Tedizolid *on page 1409*

Dabigatran Etexilate (da BIG a tran ett EX ill ate)

Related Information

Antiplatelet and Anticoagulation Considerations in Dentistry *on page 1666*
Cardiovascular Diseases *on page 1654*

Brand Names: US Pradaxa

Brand Names: Canada APO-Dabigatran; Pradaxa

Pharmacologic Category Anticoagulant; Anticoagulant, Direct Thrombin Inhibitor; Direct Oral Anticoagulant (DOAC)

Use

Deep venous thrombosis and pulmonary embolism treatment and prevention: Treatment of deep venous thrombosis (DVT) and pulmonary embolism (PE) in patients who have been treated with a parenteral anticoagulant for 5 to 10 days; to reduce the risk of recurrence of DVT and PE in patients who have been previously treated.

Nonvalvular atrial fibrillation: Prevention of stroke and systemic embolism in patients with nonvalvular atrial fibrillation.

Venous thromboembolism prophylaxis in total hip arthroplasty: Prophylaxis of DVT and PE in patients who have undergone total hip arthroplasty.

Local Anesthetic/Vasoconstrictor Precautions No information available to require special precautions

Effects on Dental Treatment Dabigatran etexilate is converted *in vivo* to the active dabigatran, a specific, reversible, direct thrombin inhibitor. It causes bleeding by preventing thrombin-mediated effects, and by inhibiting thrombin-induced platelet aggregation. Patients taking dabigatran etexilate are at increased risk of bleeding. See Effects on Bleeding.

Effects on Bleeding Dabigatran etexilate inhibits clot formation via direct inhibition of thrombin (factor IIa). Dabigatran increases the risk of bleeding and can cause significant and sometimes fatal bleeding. Hemorrhage may occur at virtually any site; risk is dependent on multiple variables, including the intensity of anticoagulation and patient susceptibility. Medical consult is suggested.

Adverse Reactions

>10%:

Gastrointestinal: Gastrointestinal signs and symptoms (25% to 40%)

Hematologic & oncologic: Hemorrhage (10% to 19%), major hemorrhage (≤6%)

1% to 10%: Gastrointestinal: Abdominal discomfort (≤8%), abdominal pain (≤8%), dyspepsia (4% to 8%), epigastric discomfort (≤8%), esophagitis (≤3%), gastroesophageal reflux disease (≤3%), gastritis (≤3%), gastrointestinal hemorrhage (≤7%; major: ≤3%), hemorrhagic gastritis (≤3%), upper abdominal pain (≤8%)

<1%:

Cardiovascular: Acute myocardial infarction, hemorrhagic stroke, subarachnoid hemorrhage, subdural hematoma

Genitourinary: Genitourinary tract hemorrhage (major)

Hematologic & oncologic: Retroperitoneal hemorrhage (major), spinal hematoma (with spinal puncture or spinal/epidural anesthesia)

Hypersensitivity: Allergic angioedema, anaphylactic shock, anaphylaxis, hypersensitivity reaction

Nervous system: Epidural intracranial hemorrhage (with spinal puncture or spinal/epidural anesthesia), intracranial hemorrhage

Neuromuscular & skeletal: Hemarthrosis (major), muscle hemorrhage (major)

Frequency not defined: Gastrointestinal: Gastrointestinal ulcer

Postmarketing:

Dermatologic: Alopecia

Gastrointestinal: Esophageal ulcer

Hematologic & oncologic: Thrombocytopenia

Mechanism of Action Prodrug lacking anticoagulant activity that is converted in vivo to the active dabigatran, a specific, reversible, direct thrombin inhibitor that inhibits both free and fibrin-bound thrombin. Inhibits coagulation by preventing thrombin-mediated effects, including cleavage of fibrinogen to fibrin monomers, activation of factors V, VIII, XI, and XIII, and inhibition of thrombin-induced platelet aggregation.

Pharmacodynamics/Kinetics

Half-life Elimination 12 to 17 hours; Elderly: 14 to 17 hours; Mild-to-moderate renal impairment: 15 to 18 hours; Severe renal impairment: 28 hours (Stangier 2010)

Time to Peak Plasma: Dabigatran: 1 hour; delayed 2 hours by food (no effect on bioavailability)

Reproductive Considerations

Information related to the use of direct acting oral anticoagulants in pregnancy is limited; until safety data are available, adequate contraception is recommended during therapy for females of childbearing potential. Females planning a pregnancy should be switched to alternative anticoagulants prior to conception (Cohen 2016).

Pregnancy Considerations

An ex vivo human placenta dual perfusion model illustrated that dabigatran crossed the placenta at term; dabigatran etexilate mesylate (prodrug) had limited placental transfer (Bapat 2014). Use of direct acting oral anticoagulants increases the risk of bleeding in all patients. When used in pregnancy, there is also the potential for fetal bleeding or subclinical placental bleeding which may increase the risk of miscarriage, preterm delivery, fetal compromise, or stillbirth (Cohen 2016).

Information related to the use of dabigatran etexilate in pregnancy is limited (Beyer-Westendorf 2016; Lameijer 2018). Data are insufficient to evaluate the safety of direct acting oral anticoagulants during pregnancy (Guyatt 2012) and use in pregnant females is not recommended (Regitz-Zagrosek [ESC 2018]). Agents other than dabigatran etexilate are preferred for the treatment of AF or VTE in pregnant patients (Kearon 2016; Lip 2018; Regitz-Zagrosek [ESC 2018]). Patients should be switched to an alternative anticoagulant if pregnancy occurs during therapy. Fetal monitoring that includes evaluations for fetal bleeding and assessments for risk of preterm delivery are recommended if the direct acting oral anticoagulant is continued (Cohen 2016).

Dental Health Professional Considerations At recommended therapeutic doses, dabigatran etexilate prolongs the activated partial thromboplastin time (aPTT). With an oral dose of 150 mg twice daily, the median peak aPTT is approximately twice that of control values. Twelve hours after the last dose, the median aPTT is 1.5 x control. The INR test is relatively insensitive to the activity of dabigatran etexilate and may not be elevated in patients on dabigatran etexilate. Medical consult is suggested. Routine coagulation testing (INR) is not required, or necessary, for Direct-Acting Oral Anticoagulants (DOAC).

◆ **Dabigatran Etexilate Mesylate** *see* Dabigatran Etexilate *on page 426*

Dacarbazine (da KAR ba zeen)

Pharmacologic Category Antineoplastic Agent, Alkylating Agent (Triazene)

Use

Hodgkin lymphoma: Treatment of Hodgkin lymphoma (in combination with other chemotherapy agents)

Melanoma, metastatic malignant: Treatment of metastatic malignant melanoma

Local Anesthetic/Vasoconstrictor Precautions No information available to require special precautions

Effects on Dental Treatment Key adverse event(s) related to dental treatment: Metallic taste.

Effects on Bleeding Hematopoietic suppression (including platelets) is the most common toxicity of dacarbazine. Risk of thrombocytopenia, which can be life-threatening, reaches a nadir at 7-10 days. A medical consult is recommended.

Adverse Reactions Frequency not always defined.

Central nervous system: Infusion-site pain

Dermatologic: Alopecia

Gastrointestinal: Nausea and vomiting (>90%), anorexia

Hematologic & oncologic: Bone marrow depression (onset: 5 to 7 days; nadir: 7 to 10 days; recovery: 21 to 28 days), leukopenia, thrombocytopenia

<1%, postmarketing, and/or case reports: Anaphylaxis, anemia, diarrhea, dysgeusia, eosinophilia, erythema, facial flushing, facial paresthesia, flu-like symptoms (fever, myalgia, malaise), hepatic necrosis, increased liver enzymes (transient), paresthesia, renal function test abnormality, skin photosensitivity, skin rash, urticaria, venous obstruction (hepatic vein)

Mechanism of Action Dacarbazine is an alkylating agent which is converted to the active alkylating metabolite MTIC [(methyl-triazene-1-yl)-imidazole-4-carboxamide] via the cytochrome P450 system. The cytotoxic effects of MTIC are manifested through alkylation (methylation) of DNA at the O^6, N^7 guanine positions which lead to DNA double strand breaks and apoptosis. Dacarbazine is non-cell cycle specific (Marchesi 2007).

Pharmacodynamics/Kinetics

Half-life Elimination Biphasic: Initial: 19 minutes, 55 minutes (renal and hepatic dysfunction); Terminal: 5 hours, 7.2 hours (renal and hepatic dysfunction)

Pregnancy Risk Factor C

Pregnancy Considerations

[US Boxed Warning]: Studies have demonstrated this agent to be carcinogenic and/or teratogenic when used in animals.

The European Society for Medical Oncology has published guidelines for diagnosis, treatment, and follow-up of cancer during pregnancy. The guidelines recommend referral to a facility with expertise in cancer during pregnancy and encourage a multidisciplinary team (obstetrician, neonatologist, oncology team). In general, if chemotherapy is indicated, it should be avoided during in the first trimester, there should be a 3-week time period between the last chemotherapy dose and anticipated delivery, and chemotherapy should not be administered beyond week 33 of gestation (Peccatori 2013). An international consensus panel has published guidelines for hematologic malignancies during pregnancy. Dacarbazine is a component of the ABVD regimen, which is used for the treatment of Hodgkin lymphoma. If treatment cannot be deferred until after delivery in patients with early stage Hodgkin lymphoma, ABVD may be administered safely and effectively in the latter phase of pregnancy (based on limited data); for patients with advanced-stage disease, ABVD can be administered in the second and third trimesters (Lishner 2016).

Daclatasvir (dak LAT as vir)

Brand Names: US Daklinza [DSC]

Brand Names: Canada Daklinza [DSC]

Pharmacologic Category Antihepaciviral, NS5A Inhibitor; NS5A Inhibitor

Use

Chronic hepatitis C: Treatment of chronic hepatitis C virus (HCV) genotype 1 or genotype 3 infection in combination with sofosbuvir, with or without ribavirin

Limitations of use: Sustained virologic response rates are reduced in HCV genotype 3-infected patients with cirrhosis receiving daclatasvir in combination with sofosbuvir for 12 weeks.

Local Anesthetic/Vasoconstrictor Precautions No information available to require special precautions

Effects on Dental Treatment No significant effects or complications reported

Effects on Bleeding No information available to require special precautions

Adverse Reactions All adverse drug reactions are from combination therapy trials with sofosbuvir.

>10%:

- Central nervous system: Fatigue (14% to 15%), headache (12% to 14%)
- Gastrointestinal: Nausea (8% to 15%)
- Hematologic & Oncologic: Anemia (20%)

1% to 10%:

- Central nervous system: Drowsiness (5%), insomnia (3%)
- Dermatologic: Skin rash (8%)
- Gastrointestinal: Diarrhea (3% to 5%), increased serum lipase (>3x ULN, transient)

<1%, postmarketing, and/or case reports: Reactivation of HBV (FDA Safety Alert Dec. 8, 2016)

Mechanism of Action Daclatasvir binds to the N-terminus within Domain 1 of HCV nonstructural protein 5A (NS5A) and inhibits viral RNA replication and virion assembly.

Pharmacodynamics/Kinetics

Half-life Elimination ~12 to 15 hours

Time to Peak Plasma: ≤2 hours

Reproductive Considerations

If used in combination with ribavirin, all warnings related to the use of ribavirin and contraception should be followed.

HCV-infected females of childbearing potential should consider postponing pregnancy until therapy is complete to reduce the risk of HCV transmission (AASLD/IDSA 2018).

Pregnancy Considerations

Daclatasvir must not be used as monotherapy. If used in combination with ribavirin, use is contraindicated in pregnant females and males whose female partners are pregnant. All warnings related to the use of ribavirin and pregnancy should be followed.

Treatment of hepatitis C is not currently recommended to treat maternal infection or to decrease the risk of mother-to-child transmission during pregnancy (Tran 2016). When HCV infection is detected during pregnancy, treatment should be deferred until after delivery. Direct-acting antiviral medications should not be used in pregnant females outside of clinical trials until safety and efficacy information is available (SMFM [Hughes 2017]).

Product Availability The manufacturer of Daklinza, Bristol Myers Squibb, plans to cease distribution of the 90 mg tablets as of December 2018 and the 30 mg and 60 mg tablets as of June 2019.

◆ **Daclatasvir Dihydrochloride** *see* Daclatasvir *on page 428*

◆ **Dacliximab** *see* Daclizumab *on page 428*

Daclizumab (dac KLYE zue mab)

Brand Names: US Zinbryta [DSC]

Brand Names: Canada Zinbryta

Pharmacologic Category Immunosuppressant Agent; Interleukin-2 Inhibitor; Monoclonal Antibody

Use Multiple sclerosis, relapsing: Treatment of relapsing forms of multiple sclerosis (MS) in adults. Daclizumab should generally be reserved for patients who have had an inadequate response to 2 or more medications indicated for the treatment of MS.

Local Anesthetic/Vasoconstrictor Precautions No information available to require special precautions

Effects on Dental Treatment Key adverse event(s) related to dental treatment: Oropharyngeal pain, bronchitis, pharyngitis, rhinitis, tonsillitis have been reported

Effects on Bleeding No information available to require special precautions

Adverse Reactions

>10%:

- Dermatologic: Allergic skin reaction (18% to 37%), skin rash (7% to 11%)
- Immunologic: Autoimmune disease (13% to 32%)
- Infection: Infection (50% to 65%)
- Respiratory: Nasopharyngitis (25%), upper respiratory tract infection (9% to 17%)

1% to 10%:

- Central nervous system: Depression (7% to 10%), seizure (1%)

Dermatologic: Dermatitis (3% to 9%), eczema (5%), acne vulgaris (3%)
Hematologic & oncologic: Lymphadenopathy (5%), anemia (3%)
Hepatic: Increased serum ALT (5% to 6%), increased serum AST (3% to 6%), hepatic injury (≤1%)
Infection: Influenza (9%)
Respiratory: Oropharyngeal pain (8%), bronchitis (7%), pharyngitis (6%), rhinitis (4%), tonsillitis (4%)
Miscellaneous: Fever (3%)

Frequency not defined:
Dermatologic: Desquamation, erythema, folliculitis, pruritus, psoriasis, skin photosensitivity, skin rash (toxic), xeroderma
Gastrointestinal: Diarrhea
Hematologic & oncologic: Decreased absolute lymphocyte count, lymphadenitis
Hepatic: Abnormal hepatic function tests, increased liver enzymes
Hypersensitivity: Hypersensitivity reaction (including anaphylaxis, angioedema, and urticaria)
Infection: Cytomegalovirus disease, viral infection
Respiratory: Laryngitis, pneumonia, respiratory tract infection

<1%, postmarketing, and/or case reports: Autoimmune hepatitis, colitis (serious; noninfectious), increased serum alkaline phosphatase (<2 x ULN), increased serum bilirubin (≥2 x ULN), increased serum transaminases (≥3 x ULN), malignant neoplasm of breast (more common in women), suicidal ideation

Mechanism of Action Daclizumab is a humanized monoclonal antibody which binds to the CD25 subunit of the high-affinity interleukin-2 (IL-2) receptor to prevent signaling at the high-affinity IL-2 receptor while allowing increased IL-2 availability for signaling at the intermediate-affinity IL-2 receptor (Gold 2013, Kappos 2015). Because IL-2 has a role in activating and regulating the immune system; CD25 antagonism may result in therapeutic benefit in multiple sclerosis (Gold 2013).

Pharmacodynamics/Kinetics

Half-life Elimination SubQ: 21 days

Time to Peak SubQ: 5 to 7 days

Reproductive Considerations In general, disease-modifying therapies for multiple sclerosis are stopped prior to a planned pregnancy except in females at high risk of multiple sclerosis activity (AAN [Rae-Grant 2018]). Consider use of agents other than daclizumab for females at high risk of disease reactivation who are planning a pregnancy. Delaying pregnancy is recommended for females with persistent high disease activity; when disease-modifying therapy is needed in these patients, other agents are preferred (ECTRIMS/EAN [Montalban 2018]).

Pregnancy Considerations

Information related to the use of daclizumab in pregnancy is limited (Gold 2016).

In general, disease-modifying therapies for multiple sclerosis are not initiated during pregnancy, except in females at high risk of multiple sclerosis activity (AAN [Rae-Grant 2018]). When disease-modifying therapy is needed in these patients, other agents are preferred (ECTRIMS/EAN [Montalban 2018]).

Product Availability

As of March 2, 2018, Biogen and AbbVie have announced the voluntary worldwide withdrawal of Zinbryta (daclizumab) for the treatment of adult patients with relapsing forms of multiple sclerosis. The drug will be available in the United States and Canada for patients as needed until April 30, 2018.

More information may be found at http://media.biogen.com/press-release/autoimmune-diseases/biogen%C2%A0and-abbvie-announce%C2%A0-voluntary%C2%A0worldwide-withdrawal-marketi or https://www.-fda.gov/Drugs/DrugSafety/ucm600999.htm?utm_campaign=FDA%20working%20with%20manufacturers%20to%20withdraw%20Zinbryta%20from%20the%20market%20in&utm_medium=email&utm_source=Eloqua or http://healthycanadians.gc.ca/recall-alert-rappel-avis/hc-sc/2018/66214a-eng.php.

◆ **Daclizumab beta [Canadian generic name]** *see* Daclizumab *on page 428*

◆ **Daclizumab High Yield Process** *see* Daclizumab *on page 428*

◆ **Daclizumab HYP** *see* Daclizumab *on page 428*

◆ **Dacogen** *see* Decitabine *on page 447*

Dacomitinib (DAK oh MI ti nib)

Brand Names: US Vizimpro

Brand Names: Canada Vizimpro

Pharmacologic Category Antineoplastic Agent, Epidermal Growth Factor Receptor (EGFR) Inhibitor; Antineoplastic Agent, Tyrosine Kinase Inhibitor

Use Non-small cell lung cancer, metastatic: First-line treatment of metastatic non-small cell lung cancer (NSCLC) in patients with epidermal growth factor receptor (EGFR) exon 19 deletion or exon 21 L858R substitution mutations as detected by an approved test.

Local Anesthetic/Vasoconstrictor Precautions
No information available to require special precautions

Effects on Dental Treatment Key adverse event(s) related to dental treatment: Frequent occurrence of stomatitis, oral mucosa ulcers

Effects on Bleeding No information available to require special precautions

Adverse Reactions

>10%:
Cardiovascular: Chest pain (10%)
Central nervous system: Insomnia (11%)
Dermatologic: Skin rash (69% to 78%), paronychia (64%), xeroderma (30%), alopecia (23%), pruritus (21%), palmar-plantar erythrodysesthesia (15%), dermatitis (11%)
Endocrine & metabolic: Hypoalbuminemia (44%), hyperglycemia (36%), hypocalcemia (33%), hypokalemia (29%), hyponatremia (26%), weight loss (26%), hypomagnesemia (22%)
Gastrointestinal: Diarrhea (87%), stomatitis (45%; grades 3/4: 4%), decreased appetite (31%), nausea (19%), constipation (13%), oral mucosa ulcer (12%)
Hematologic & oncologic: Anemia (44%; grades 3/4: <1%), lymphocytopenia (42%; grades 3/4: 6%)
Hepatic: Increased serum alanine aminotransferase (40%), increased serum aspartate aminotransferase (35%), increased serum alkaline phosphatase (22%), hyperbilirubinemia (16%)
Neuromuscular & skeletal: Limb pain (14%), asthenia (13%), musculoskeletal pain (12%)
Ophthalmic: Conjunctivitis (19%)
Renal: Increased creatinine clearance (24%)
Respiratory: Cough (21%), nasal signs and symptoms (19%), dyspnea (13%), upper respiratory tract infection (12%)

1% to 10%:
Central nervous system: Fatigue (9%)

Dermatologic: Skin fissure (9%), exfoliation of skin (4% to 7%), hypertrichosis (1%)
Endocrine & metabolic: Dehydration (1%)
Gastrointestinal: Vomiting (9%), dysgeusia (7%)
Ophthalmic: Keratitis (2%)
Respiratory: Interstitial pulmonary disease (3%)
<1%, postmarketing, and/or case reports: Pneumonitis

Mechanism of Action Dacomitinib is an irreversible epidermal growth factor receptor (EGFR) tyrosine kinase inhibitor which has activity against EGFR/HER1, HER2, and HER4, as well as some EGFR-activating mutations (exon 19 deletion or exon 21 L858R substitution mutation). Dacomitinib also has activity against DDR1, EPHA6, LCK, DDR2, and MNK1 (in vitro).

Pharmacodynamics/Kinetics

Half-life Elimination 70 hours

Time to Peak ~6 hours (range: 2 to 24 hours)

Reproductive Considerations

Verify pregnancy status in females of reproductive potential prior to initiating dacomitinib. Females of reproductive potential should use effective contraception during therapy and for at least 17 days after the last dacomitinib dose.

Pregnancy Considerations

Based on data from animal reproduction studies and the mechanism of action, dacomitinib use during pregnancy may cause fetal harm.

◆ **DACT** *see* DACTINomycin *on page* 430

DACTINomycin (dak ti noe MYE sin)

Brand Names: US Cosmegen

Brand Names: Canada Cosmegen

Pharmacologic Category Antineoplastic Agent, Antibiotic

Use

Ewing sarcoma: Treatment of Ewing sarcoma (as part of a multi-phase, combination chemotherapy regimen)

Gestational trophoblastic neoplasia: Treatment of gestational trophoblastic neoplasia in post-menarchal patients (as a single agent or as part of a combination chemotherapy regimen)

Rhabdomyosarcoma: Treatment of rhabdomyosarcoma (as part of a multi-phase, combination chemotherapy regimen)

Solid tumors: Palliative and/or adjunctive treatment of locally recurrent or locoregional solid malignancies (as a component of regional perfusion) in adult patients

Wilms tumor: Treatment of Wilms tumor (as part of a multi-phase, combination chemotherapy regimen)

Local Anesthetic/Vasoconstrictor Precautions
No information available to require special precautions

Effects on Dental Treatment Key adverse event(s) related to dental treatment: Stomatitis and mucositis

Effects on Bleeding Onset of thrombocytopenia, which can be severe, occurs at 7 days with the nadir at 14-21 days. A medical consult is recommended.

Adverse Reactions

Frequency not defined:
Cardiovascular: Thrombophlebitis
Central nervous system: Fatigue, malaise, peripheral neuropathy
Dermatologic: Acne vulgaris, alopecia, cheilitis, dermatitis, erythema multiforme, skin rash, Stevens-Johnson syndrome, toxic epidermal necrolysis
Endocrine & metabolic: Growth suppression, hypocalcemia
Gastrointestinal: Abdominal pain, anorexia, aphthous stomatitis, constipation, diarrhea, dysphagia, esophagitis, gastrointestinal ulcer, mucositis, nausea, proctitis, vomiting
Hematologic & oncologic: Anemia, bone marrow depression, disseminated intravascular coagulation, febrile neutropenia, hemorrhage, leukopenia, neutropenia (nadir: 14 to 21 days), pancytopenia, reticulocytopenia, second primary malignant neoplasm (including leukemia), thrombocytopenia, tumor lysis syndrome
Hepatic: Abnormal hepatic function tests, ascites, hepatic failure, hepatic sinusoidal obstruction syndrome, hepatitis, hepatomegaly, hepatotoxicity, severe hepatic disease (hepatopathy-thrombocytopenia syndrome, Farruggia 2011)
Hypersensitivity: Hypersensitivity reaction
Infection: Infection, sepsis
Neuromuscular & skeletal: Myalgia
Ophthalmic: Optic neuropathy
Renal: Renal function abnormality, renal failure syndrome, renal insufficiency
Respiratory: Pneumonitis, pneumothorax
Miscellaneous: Fever, radiation recall phenomenon

Mechanism of Action Dactinomycin binds to the guanine portion of DNA intercalating between guanine and cytosine base pairs inhibiting DNA and RNA synthesis and protein synthesis

Pharmacodynamics/Kinetics

Half-life Elimination 30 to 40 hours (Perry 2012); Children: Range: 14 to 43 hours (Veal 2005)

Reproductive Considerations

Verify pregnancy status of females of reproductive potential prior to initiating dactinomycin therapy; effective contraception should be used during therapy and for at least 6 months after the last dactinomycin dose.

When used for gestational trophoblastic neoplasm, unfavorable outcomes have been reported when subsequent pregnancies occur within 6 months of treatment. It is recommended to use effective contraception for 6 months to 1 year after therapy (Matsui 2004; Seckl 2013).

Males with female partners of reproductive potential should use effective contraception during therapy and for 3 months after the last dactinomycin dose.

Pregnancy Considerations

Based on data from animal reproduction studies and its mechanism of action, dactinomycin may cause fetal harm if administered to a pregnant female.

When used for gestational trophoblastic neoplasm, unfavorable outcomes have been reported when subsequent pregnancies occur within 6 months of treatment (Matsui 2004; Seckl 2013).

◆ **Daklinza [DSC]** *see* Daclatasvir *on page* 428

Dalbavancin (dal ba VAN sin)

Brand Names: US Dalvance

Pharmacologic Category Glycopeptide

Use Acute bacterial skin and skin structure infections: Treatment of adult patients with acute bacterial skin and skin structure infections (ABSSSI) caused by susceptible isolates of the following gram-positive microorganisms: *Staphylococcus aureus* (including methicillin-susceptible and methicillin-resistant strains), *Streptococcus pyogenes*, *Streptococcus agalactiae*, *S. dysgalactiae*, *Streptococcus anginosus* group (including *S. anginosus*, *S. intermedius*, *S. constellatus*), and *Enterococcus faecalis* (vancomycin-susceptible strains)

Local Anesthetic/Vasoconstrictor Precautions No information available to require special precautions

Effects on Dental Treatment Key adverse event(s) related to dental treatment: Use may result in fungal superinfection including *Candida albicans* in the oral cavity.

Effects on Bleeding Dalbavancin may affect bleeding times including spontaneous hematoma and wound hemorrhage; may interfere with test used to monitor coagulation such as INR.

Adverse Reactions

1% to 10%:

Cardiovascular: Flushing (<2%), phlebitis (<2%)

Central nervous system: Headache (5%), dizziness (<2%)

Dermatologic: Skin rash (3%), pruritus (2%), urticaria (<2%)

Endocrine & metabolic: Hypoglycemia (<2%), increased gamma-glutamyl transferase (<2%), increased lactate dehydrogenase (<2%)

Gastrointestinal: Nausea (6%), diarrhea (4%), vomiting (3%), abdominal pain (<2%), *Clostridioides* (formerly *Clostridium*) *difficile* colitis (<2%), gastrointestinal hemorrhage (<2%), hematochezia (<2%), melena (<2%), oral candidiasis (<2%)

Hematologic & oncologic: Acute posthemorrhagic anemia (<2%), anemia (<2%), eosinophilia (<2%), hematoma (spontaneous; <2%), increased INR (<2%), leukopenia (<2%), neutropenia (<2%), petechia (<2%), thrombocythemia (<2%), thrombocytopenia (<2%), wound hemorrhage (<2%)

Hepatic: Hepatotoxicity (<2%), increased serum alkaline phosphatase (<2%), increased serum transaminases (<2%)

Hypersensitivity: Anaphylactoid reaction (<2%)

Infection: Vulvovaginal infection (mycotic; <2%)

Respiratory: Bronchospasm (<2%)

Miscellaneous: Infusion related reaction (<2%; including red man syndrome)

<1%, postmarketing, and/or case reports: Anaphylaxis, back pain, *Clostridioides* (formerly *Clostridium*) *difficile*-associated diarrhea, hypersensitivity reaction, increased serum alanine aminotransferase

Mechanism of Action Dalbavancin is a lipoglycopeptide which binds to the D-alanyl-D-alanine terminus of the stem pentapeptide in nascent cell wall peptidoglycan, preventing cross-linking and interfering with cell wall synthesis. It is bactericidal in vitro against *Staphylococcus aureus* and *Streptococcus pyogenes*

Pharmacodynamics/Kinetics

Half-life Elimination 346 hours

Pregnancy Considerations Adverse events have been observed in animal reproduction studies. The long half-life of dalbavancin should be considered when evaluating potential exposure to the fetus.

◆ **Dalbavancin HCl** *see* Dalbavancin *on page 430*

Dalfampridine (dal FAM pri deen)

Brand Names: US Ampyra

Brand Names: Canada Fampyra

Pharmacologic Category Potassium Channel Blocker

Use Treatment to improve walking in patients with multiple sclerosis (MS)

Local Anesthetic/Vasoconstrictor Precautions No information available to require special precautions

Effects on Dental Treatment No significant effects or complications reported

Effects on Bleeding No information available to require special precautions

Adverse Reactions

>10%: Genitourinary: Urinary tract infection (12%)

1% to 10%:

Central nervous system: Insomnia (9%), dizziness (7%), headache (7%), equilibrium disturbance (5%), paresthesia (4%)

Gastrointestinal: Nausea (7%), constipation (3%), dyspepsia (2%)

Neuromuscular & skeletal: Weakness (7%), back pain (5%), acute exacerbations of multiple sclerosis (4%)

Respiratory: Nasopharyngitis (4%), pharyngolaryngeal pain (2%)

<1%, postmarketing and/or case reports: Hypersensitivity reaction, seizure, vomiting

Mechanism of Action Nonspecific potassium channel blocker which improves conduction in focally demyelinated axons by delaying repolarization and prolonging the duration of action potentials. Enhanced neuronal conduction is thought to strengthen skeletal muscle fiber twitch activity, thereby, improving peripheral motor neurologic function.

Pharmacodynamics/Kinetics

Half-life Elimination 5.2-6.5 hours; prolonged in severe renal impairment (~3 times longer)

Time to Peak Plasma: 3-4 hours

Pregnancy Considerations Information related to the use of dalfampridine in pregnancy is limited (Maillart 2016).

◆ **Dalfopristin and Quinupristin** *see* Quinupristin and Dalfopristin *on page 1301*

◆ **Daliresp** *see* Roflumilast *on page 1343*

◆ ***d*-Alpha Tocopherol** *see* Vitamin E (Systemic) *on page 1549*

Dalteparin (dal TE pa rin)

Related Information

Cardiovascular Diseases *on page 1654*

Brand Names: US Fragmin

Brand Names: Canada Fragmin

Pharmacologic Category Anticoagulant; Anticoagulant, Low Molecular Weight Heparin

Use

Anticoagulant for hemodialysis and hemofiltration (Fragmin [Canadian product only]): Prevention of clotting in the extracorporeal system during hemodialysis and hemofiltration in connection with acute renal failure or chronic renal insufficiency

Non-ST elevation acute coronary syndromes: Prevention of ischemic complications in patients with unstable angina or non-Q-wave myocardial infarction on concurrent aspirin therapy.

Venous thromboembolism prophylaxis: Prevention of DVT which may lead to PE, in patients requiring abdominal surgery who are at risk for thromboembolism complications (eg, >40 years, obesity, malignancy, history of DVT or PE, surgical procedures requiring general anesthesia lasting >30 minutes); patients undergoing total hip arthroplasty; or in patients who are at risk for thromboembolism complications due to severe immobility during an acute illness.

Venous thromboembolism treatment in patients with active cancer: Extended treatment (6 months) of acute symptomatic VTE (ie, DVT and/or PE) to reduce the recurrence of VTE in cancer patients.

Venous thromboembolism treatment in pediatric patients: Treatment of symptomatic VTE (ie, DVT and/or PE) to reduce the recurrence of VTE in infants ≥1 month of age, children, and adolescents.

Local Anesthetic/Vasoconstrictor Precautions No information available to require special precautions

Effects on Dental Treatment Key adverse event(s) related to dental treatment: Bleeding is the major adverse effect of dalteparin. Adverse reactions reported were generally less than those seen with heparin. See Effects on Bleeding.

Effects on Bleeding The risk of bleeding and thrombocytopenia is high with low molecular weight heparin anticoagulants such as dalteparin. The use of NSAIDs and aspirin should be avoided. A medical consult is recommended.

Adverse Reactions

>10%:

Hematologic & oncologic: Thrombocytopenia (infants, children, and adolescents: 21% to 37%; adults: 11% to 14%; grades 3/4: ≤7%), hemorrhage (3% to 14%), bruise (infants, children, and adolescents: 12%)

Local: Bruising at injection site (infants, children, and adolescents: 30%)

1% to 10%:

Hematologic & oncologic: Major hemorrhage (1% to 4%), wound hematoma (≤3%)

Hepatic: Increased serum alanine aminotransferase (4% to 10%), increased serum aspartate aminotransferase (5% to 9%)

Local: Pain at injection site (5% to 12%), hematoma at injection site (≤6%)

Respiratory: Epistaxis (infants, children, and adolescents: 10%)

Miscellaneous: Re-operation due to bleeding (≤1%)

<1%: Gastrointestinal hemorrhage, hemoptysis, skin necrosis

Frequency not defined:

Cardiovascular: Spinal hematoma

Central nervous system: Epidural intracranial hemorrhage

Postmarketing: Alopecia, hypersensitivity reaction, nonimmune anaphylaxis, osteoporosis, postoperative wound bleeding

Mechanism of Action Low molecular weight heparin analog with a molecular weight of 4,000 to 6,000 daltons; the commercial product contains 3% to 15% heparin with a molecular weight <3,000 daltons, 65% to 78% with a molecular weight of 3,000 to 8,000 daltons and 14% to 26% with a molecular weight >8,000 daltons; while dalteparin has been shown to inhibit both factor Xa and factor IIa (thrombin), the antithrombotic effect of dalteparin is characterized by a higher ratio of anti-Factor Xa to anti-Factor IIa activity (ratio = 4)

Pharmacodynamics/Kinetics

Onset of Action Anti-Factor Xa activity: Within 1 to 2 hours.

Duration of Action >12 hours.

Half-life Elimination

Route dependent:

IV: Mean terminal half-life: 2.1 ± 0.3 hours (40 unit/kg/dose) to 2.3 ± 0.4 hours (60 unit/kg/dose); mean terminal half-life (anti-Factor Xa activity): 5.7 ± 2.0 hours (5,000 unit dose in chronic renal impairment requiring hemodialysis).

SubQ:

Pediatric: Age-dependent changes were observed.

3 to <8 weeks: 2.25 ± 0.173 hours.

≥8 weeks to <2 years: 3.02 ± 0.688 hours.

≥2 years to <8 years: 4.27 ± 1.05 hours.

≥8 years to <12 years: 5.11 ± 0.509 hours.

≥12 years to <20 years: 6.28 ± 0.937 hours.

Adult: Mean terminal half-life: 3 to 5 hours.

Time to Peak Serum: SubQ: Anti-Factor Xa activity: ~4 hours.

Reproductive Considerations

For women who require long-term anticoagulation with warfarin and who are considering pregnancy, LMWH substitution should be done prior to conception when possible. When choosing therapy, fetal outcomes (ie, pregnancy loss, malformations), maternal outcomes (ie, VTE, hemorrhage), burden of therapy, and maternal preference should be considered (ACCP [Guyatt 2012]).

Pregnancy Considerations

Low molecular weight heparin (LMWH) does not cross the placenta; increased risks of fetal bleeding or teratogenic effects have not been reported (ACCP [Bates 2012]).

LMWH is recommended over unfractionated heparin for the treatment of acute VTE in pregnant women. LMWH is also recommended over unfractionated heparin for VTE prophylaxis in pregnant women with certain risk factors. LMWH should be discontinued at least 24 hours prior to induction of labor or a planned cesarean delivery. For women undergoing cesarean section and who have additional risk factors for developing VTE, the prophylactic use of LMWH may be considered (ACCP [Guyatt 2012]). LMWH may also be used in women with mechanical heart valves (consult current guidelines for details) (ACC/AHA [Nishimura 2014]; ACCP [Bates 2012]).

Multiple-dose vials contain benzyl alcohol (avoid in pregnant women due to association with gasping syndrome in premature infants); use of preservative-free formulation is recommended.

◆ **Dalteparin Sodium** *see* Dalteparin *on page 431*

◆ **Dalvance** *see* Dalbavancin *on page 430*

Danaparoid (da NAP a roid)

Brand Names: Canada Orgaran

Pharmacologic Category Anticoagulant

Use Note: Not approved in the US

Catheter patency: Intermittent flushing to maintain patency of catheters/IV lines and/or access ports

Deep vein thrombosis: Prevention of postoperative deep vein thrombosis (DVT) following orthopedic or major abdominal and thoracic surgery; prevention of DVT in patients with confirmed diagnosis of non-hemorrhagic stroke

Heparin-induced thrombocytopenia: Management of heparin-induced thrombocytopenia (HIT)

Local Anesthetic/Vasoconstrictor Precautions No information available to require special precautions

Effects on Dental Treatment Key adverse event(s) related to dental treatment: Bleeding is the major adverse effect of danaparoid. See Effects on Bleeding.

Effects on Bleeding As with all anticoagulants, bleeding is the major adverse effect of danaparoid. Hemorrhage may occur at virtually any site; risk is dependent on multiple variables including the intensity of anticoagulation and patient susceptibility. At the recommended doses, LMWHs do not significantly influence platelet aggregation or affect global clotting time (ie, PT or aPTT). Medical consult is suggested.

Adverse Reactions Frequency not always defined. As with all anticoagulants, bleeding is the major adverse effect of danaparoid. Hemorrhage may occur at virtually any site. Risk is dependent on multiple variables.

1% to 10%:

- Central nervous system: Pain (5%)
- Dermatologic: Skin rash (1%)
- Gastrointestinal: Nausea (3%), constipation (2%)
- Genitourinary: Urinary retention (1%)
- Hematologic & oncologic: Leukocytosis (1%)
- Infection: Infection (2%)
- Local: Hematoma at injection site (≤5%)
- Respiratory: Pneumonia (1%)
- Miscellaneous: Fever (2% to 5%)

Frequency not defined:

- Cardiovascular: Atrial fibrillation, cerebral infarction, decreased blood pressure (arterial), deep vein thrombosis, hypotension, peripheral edema
- Central nervous system: Cerebral hemorrhage, confusion, fatigue, hemiparesis, insomnia, loss of consciousness, restlessness
- Genitourinary: Hematuria, urinary incontinence, urinary tract hemorrhage (including microscopic), urine abnormality
- Hematologic & oncologic: Bruise, hematoma, hemorrhage (dose-related), thrombocytopenia
- Hypersensitivity: Hypersensitivity reaction
- Infection: Sepsis
- Neuromuscular & skeletal: Muscle spasm, tremor
- Respiratory: Apnea, asthma

<1%, postmarketing, and/or case reports: Increased serum alkaline phosphatase, increased serum ALT (transient), increased serum AST (transient)

Mechanism of Action Inhibits factor Xa and IIa (anti-Xa effects >20 times anti-IIa effects). Prevents fibrin formation in the coagulation pathway via thrombin generation inhibition.

Pharmacodynamics/Kinetics

Onset of Action Peak effect: SubQ: Maximum anti-factor Xa activities occur in 4-5 hours

Half-life Elimination Anti-Xa activity: ~25 hours (renal impairment: 29-35 hours); Thrombin generation inhibition activity: ~7 hours

Pregnancy Considerations

The manufacturer labeling states that incidental observations in pregnant women during the last trimesters, gave no indication that use during pregnancy results in fetal abnormalities or exacerbation of bleeding in the mother or infant during delivery. Use in pregnant women however is generally not recommended unless deemed medically necessary and alternative therapy is unavailable. Danaparoid does not cross the placenta and is the preferred anticoagulant in pregnant women with HIT (Guyatt 2012).

Product Availability Not available in the US

◆ **Danaparoid Sodium** *see* Danaparoid *on page 432*

Danazol (DA na zole)

Brand Names: Canada Cyclomen

Pharmacologic Category Androgen

Use

Endometriosis: Treatment of endometriosis amenable to hormonal management.

Hereditary angioedema (HAE), prophylaxis: Prevention of attacks of angioedema of all types (cutaneous, abdominal, laryngeal) in males and females.

Guideline recommendations: Danazol may be considered for short-term pre-procedural and long-term HAE prophylaxis as an alternative to CI inhibitor (human). Danazol is **not** recommended for treatment of acute HAE attacks (WAO/EAACI [Maurer 2018]).

Local Anesthetic/Vasoconstrictor Precautions No information available to require special precautions

Effects on Dental Treatment No significant effects or complications reported

Effects on Bleeding Thrombocytopenia and thrombotic events have been reported.

Adverse Reactions

Frequency not defined:

- Cardiovascular: Acute myocardial infarction, edema, flushing, hypertension, palpitations, syncope, tachycardia
- Dermatologic: Acne vulgaris, alopecia, diaphoresis, maculopapular rash, papular rash, pruritus, seborrhea, urticaria, vesicular eruption
- Endocrine & metabolic: Amenorrhea (may continue post-therapy), change in libido, decreased glucose tolerance (and glucagon changes), decreased HDL cholesterol, decreased thyroxine binding globulin, hirsutism (mild), increased LDL cholesterol, increased thyroxine binding globulin, menstrual disease (altered timing of cycle, spotting), weight gain
- Gastrointestinal: Constipation, gastroenteritis, nausea, vomiting
- Genitourinary: Asthenospermia, breast atrophy, decreased ejaculate volume, hematuria, inhibition of spermatogenesis, spermatozoa disorder (changes in sperm count and semen viscosity), vaginal dryness, vaginal irritation
- Hematologic & oncologic: Abnormal erythrocytes (increased), decreased sex hormone binding globulin, eosinophilia, increased sex hormone-binding globulin, leukocytosis, leukopenia, malignant neoplasm (after prolonged use), petechial rash, polycythemia, purpuric rash, thrombocythemia, thrombocytopenia
- Hepatic: Cholestatic jaundice, hepatic adenoma, hepatic neoplasm (malignant; after prolonged use), increased liver enzymes, jaundice, peliosis hepatitis
- Nervous system: Depression, dizziness, emotional lability, fatigue, headache, nervousness, paresthesia, sleep disorder, voice disorder (deepening of the voice, hoarseness, instability, sore throat)
- Neuromuscular & skeletal: Ankylosing spondylitis, arthralgia, asthenia, back pain, increased creatine phosphokinase in blood specimen, joint swelling, limb pain, muscle cramps, muscle spasm, neck pain, tremor
- Ophthalmic: Visual disturbance
- Respiratory: Interstitial pneumonitis

<1%, postmarketing, and/or case reports: Anxiety, carpal tunnel syndrome, cataract, change in appetite, chills, clitoromegaly, erythema multiforme, fever, gingival hemorrhage, Guillain-Barre syndrome, hepatotoxicity (idiosyncratic) (Chalasani 2014), intracranial hypertension (Tan 2019), nasal congestion, nipple discharge, pancreatitis, pelvic pain, pseudotumor cerebri, purpuric disease (splenic peliosis), seizure, skin photosensitivity, Stevens-Johnson syndrome

Mechanism of Action Suppresses pituitary output of follicle-stimulating hormone (FSH) and luteinizing hormone (LH), resulting in regression and atrophy of normal and ectopic endometrial tissue; decreases rate ▶

of growth of abnormal breast tissue; reduces attacks associated with hereditary angioedema by increasing levels of C4 component of complement

Pharmacodynamics/Kinetics

Onset of Action Immune thrombocytopenia (off-label use): Initial response: 14 to 90 days; Peak response: 28 to 180 days (Neunert 2011)

Half-life Elimination 9.7 ± 3.29 hours (variable; up to 24 hours following long-term use for endometriosis)

Time to Peak Serum: 4 hours (range: 2 to 8 hours)

Reproductive Considerations

[US Boxed Warning]: A sensitive test (eg, beta subunit test, if available) capable of determining early pregnancy is recommended immediately prior to start of therapy. Additionally, a nonhormonal method of contraception should be used during therapy.

Pregnancy Considerations

Use of danazol in pregnancy is contraindicated. If a patient becomes pregnant while taking danazol, administration of the drug should be discontinued and the patient should be apprised of the potential risk to the fetus. Exposure to danazol in utero may result in androgenic effects on the female fetus; reports of clitoral hypertrophy, labial fusion, urogenital sinus defect, vaginal atresia, and ambiguous genitalia have been received.

The use of danazol for the management of hereditary angioedema (HAE) in pregnancy that is not responsive to preferred therapy has been described in case reports (Altman 2006; Boulos 1994; González-Quevedo 2016; Milingos 2009). However, danazol is contraindicated during pregnancy; current guidelines recommend use of other agents in pregnant females (WAO/EAACI [Maurer 2018]).

◆ **Danocrine** *see* Danazol *on page* 433

◆ **Dantrium** *see* Dantrolene *on page* 434

Dantrolene (DAN troe leen)

Brand Names: US Dantrium; Revonto; Ryanodex

Brand Names: Canada Dantrium

Pharmacologic Category Skeletal Muscle Relaxant

Use

Chronic spasticity: Oral: Treatment of spasticity associated with upper motor neuron disorders (eg, spinal cord injury, stroke, cerebral palsy, or multiple sclerosis).

Malignant hyperthermia:

IV: Management of malignant hyperthermia (MH) crisis.

Oral, IV: Following a malignant hyperthermic crisis to prevent recurrence.

Note: Dantrolene is not recommended for preoperative prophylaxis of MH, even in susceptible patients, provided non-triggering anesthetic agents are used.

Local Anesthetic/Vasoconstrictor Precautions No information available to require special precautions

Effects on Dental Treatment No significant effects or complications reported

Effects on Bleeding No information available to require special precautions

Adverse Reactions Frequency not always defined.

Cardiovascular: Flushing (intravenous: 27%), atrioventricular block (intravenous: 3%), tachycardia (3%), cardiac failure, phlebitis, variable blood pressure

Central nervous system: Drowsiness (17%; drowsiness may persist for 48 hours post dose), voice disorder (intravenous: 13%), feeling abnormal (intravenous: 10%), dizziness (3%), headache (3%), myasthenia (3%), chills, choking sensation, confusion, depression, fatigue, insomnia, malaise, nervousness, seizure, speech disturbance

Dermatologic: Acneiform eruption (capsules), diaphoresis, eczematous rash, erythema (intravenous), hair disease (abnormal growth), pruritus, urticaria

Gastrointestinal: Dysphagia (10%; use caution at meal time on day of administration as swallowing may be difficult), nausea (10%), vomiting (3%), abdominal cramps, anorexia, constipation, diarrhea, dysgeusia, gastric irritation, gastrointestinal hemorrhage, sialorrhea

Genitourinary: Crystalluria, difficulty in micturition, erectile dysfunction, hematuria, nocturia, urinary frequency, urinary incontinence, urinary retention

Hematologic & oncologic: Anemia, aplastic anemia, leukopenia, lymphocytic lymphoma, thrombocytopenia

Hepatic: Hepatitis

Hypersensitivity: Anaphylaxis

Local: Injection site reaction (intravenous: 3%; pain, erythema, swelling), local tissue necrosis (with extravasation due to high product pH)

Neuromuscular & skeletal: Limb pain (intravenous: 3%), back pain, myalgia

Ophthalmic: Blurred vision (intravenous: 3%), diplopia, epiphora, visual disturbance

Respiratory: Dyspnea (intravenous), pleural effusion (with pericarditis), pulmonary edema (rare), respiratory depression

Miscellaneous: Fever

<1%, postmarketing, and/or case reports: Decrease in forced vital capacity (intravenous), dyspnea (intravenous), hepatic disease, hepatotoxicity (oral), increased liver enzymes (oral), respiratory muscle failure (intravenous)

Mechanism of Action Acts directly on skeletal muscle by interfering with release of calcium ion from the sarcoplasmic reticulum; prevents or reduces the increase in myoplasmic calcium ion concentration that activates the acute catabolic processes associated with malignant hyperthermia

Pharmacodynamics/Kinetics

Half-life Elimination

Neonates (at birth): ~20 hours (Shime 1988)

Children 2 to 7 years: 10 hours (range: 8.1 to 14.8 hours) (Lerman 1989)

Adults: 4 to 11 hours

Pregnancy Risk Factor C

Pregnancy Considerations

Dantrolene crosses the human placenta. Cord blood concentrations are similar to those in the maternal plasma at term. and dantrolene can be detected in the newborn serum at delivery. Adverse events were not observed in the newborn following maternal doses of 100 mg/day administered orally prior to delivery (Shime 1988). Uterine atony has been reported following dantrolene injection after delivery; however, this may be due in part to the mannitol contained in the IV preparation (Shin 1995; Weingarten 1987). Prophylactic use of dantrolene is not routinely recommended in pregnant women susceptible to MH prior to obstetric surgery, if use is needed, close monitoring of the mother and newborn is recommended (Krause 2004; Norman 1995).

◆ **Dantrolene Sodium** *see* Dantrolene *on page 434*

Dapagliflozin (dap a gli FLOE zin)

Brand Names: US Farxiga

Brand Names: Canada Forxiga

Pharmacologic Category Antidiabetic Agent, Sodium-Glucose Cotransporter 2 (SGLT2) Inhibitor; Sodium-Glucose Cotransporter 2 (SGLT2) Inhibitor

Use

Diabetes mellitus, type 2, treatment: As an adjunct to diet and exercise to improve glycemic control in adults with type 2 diabetes mellitus; risk reduction of hospitalization for heart failure in patients with type 2 diabetes mellitus and established cardiovascular disease or multiple cardiovascular risk factors.

Heart failure with reduced ejection fraction: To reduce the risk of cardiovascular death and hospitalization for heart failure in adults with heart failure with reduced ejection fraction (NYHA class II to IV).

Local Anesthetic/Vasoconstrictor Precautions No information available to require special precautions

Effects on Dental Treatment Key adverse event(s) related to dental treatment: Dizziness and syncope have been reported; patients may experience orthostatic hypotension as they stand up after treatment; especially if lying in dental chair for extended periods of time. Use caution with sudden changes in position during and after dental treatment.

Dapagliflozin-dependent patients with diabetes (non-insulin dependent, type 2) should be questioned by the dental professional at each dental visit to assess their risk for stress-induced hypoglycemia. The dental professional should inquire about the patient's routine (ie, work, sleep schedule, eating patterns), history of hypoglycemia, time of last medication dose, last meal, and most recent blood sugar assessment. Keep a supply of glucose tablets and other carbohydrates in the office to prepare for a hypoglycemic event. Seek medical attention when necessary (American Diabetes Association 2016).

Effects on Bleeding No information available to require special precautions

Adverse Reactions Incidences may include dapagliflozin used as add-on therapy.

1% to 10%:

Endocrine & metabolic: Dyslipidemia (3%), hypovolemia (1% to 3%)

Gastrointestinal: Nausea (3%)

Genitourinary: Dysuria (2%), increased urine output (3% to 4%), urinary tract infection (6%)

Hematologic & oncologic: Increased hematocrit (1%)

Infection: Genitourinary fungal infection (3% to 8%), influenza (3%)

Neuromuscular & skeletal: Back pain (4%), limb pain (2%)

Respiratory: Nasopharyngitis (7%)

Frequency not defined:

Genitourinary: Decreased estimated GFR (eGFR)

Hypersensitivity: Hypersensitivity reaction

Neuromuscular & skeletal: Bone fracture

Renal: Increased serum creatinine

<1%, postmarketing, and/or case reports: Acute renal failure, anaphylaxis (severe), angioedema, increased LDL cholesterol, ketoacidosis, necrotizing fasciitis (perineum), pyelonephritis, severe dermatological reaction, skin rash, urinary tract infection with sepsis

Mechanism of Action By inhibiting sodium-glucose cotransporter 2 (SGLT2) in the proximal renal tubules, dapagliflozin reduces reabsorption of filtered glucose from the tubular lumen and lowers the renal threshold for glucose (RT_G). SGLT2 is the main site of filtered glucose reabsorption; reduction of filtered glucose reabsorption and lowering of RT_G result in increased urinary excretion of glucose, thereby reducing plasma glucose concentrations. Dapagliflozin also reduces sodium reabsorption and increases sodium delivery to the distal tubule, which may decrease cardiac preload/afterload and downregulate sympathetic activity.

Pharmacodynamics/Kinetics

Duration of Action Following discontinuation, urinary glucose excretion returns to baseline within ~3 days for the 10 mg dose.

Half-life Elimination ~12.9 hours

Time to Peak 2 hours

Pregnancy Considerations

Due to adverse effects on renal development observed in animal studies, the manufacturer does not recommend use of dapagliflozin during the second and third trimesters of pregnancy

Poorly controlled diabetes during pregnancy can be associated with an increased risk of adverse maternal and fetal outcomes, including diabetic ketoacidosis, preeclampsia, spontaneous abortion, preterm delivery, delivery complications, major birth defects, stillbirth, and macrosomia. To prevent adverse outcomes, prior to conception and throughout pregnancy, maternal blood glucose and HbA_{1c} should be kept as close to target goals as possible but without causing significant hypoglycemia (ADA 2020; Blumer 2013).

Agents other than dapagliflozin are currently recommended to treat diabetes mellitus in pregnancy (ADA 2020).

Dapagliflozin and Metformin

(dap a gli FLOE zin & met FOR min)

Brand Names: US Xigduo XR

Brand Names: Canada Xigduo

Pharmacologic Category Antidiabetic Agent, Biguanide; Antidiabetic Agent, Sodium-Glucose Cotransporter 2 (SGLT2) Inhibitor; Sodium-Glucose Cotransporter 2 (SGLT2) Inhibitor

Use Diabetes mellitus, type 2, treatment: Adjunct to diet and exercise to improve glycemic control in adults with type 2 diabetes mellitus. **Note:** Dapagliflozin is also indicated for risk reduction of hospitalization for heart failure in patients with type 2 diabetes mellitus and established cardiovascular disease or multiple cardiovascular risk factors.

Local Anesthetic/Vasoconstrictor Precautions No information available to require special precautions

Effects on Dental Treatment Key adverse event(s) related to dental treatment: Dizziness and syncope have been reported; patients may experience orthostatic hypotension as they stand up after treatment; especially if lying in dental chair for extended periods of time. Use caution with sudden changes in position during and after dental treatment.

Dapagliflozin-dependent patients with diabetes (non-insulin dependent, type 2) should be questioned by the dental professional at each dental visit to assess their risk for stress-induced hypoglycemia. The dental professional should inquire about the patient's routine (ie, work, sleep schedule, eating patterns), history of hypoglycemia, time of last medication dose, last meal, and most recent blood sugar assessment. Keep a supply of glucose tablets and other carbohydrates in the office to prepare for a hypoglycemic event. Seek medical attention when necessary (American Diabetes Association 2016).

Effects on Bleeding No information available to require special precautions

Adverse Reactions See individual monographs for additional adverse effects reported with each agent

1% to 10%:

Central nervous system: Headache (5%), dizziness (3%)

Endocrine & metabolic: Dyslipidemia (2% to 3%)

Infection: Genitourinary fungal infection (female: 9%, includes bacterial vaginosis, female genital tract infection, genital abscess, vaginal infection, vulvovaginal candidiasis; male: 4%, includes balanitis, balanitis [candida], balanoposthitis, posthitis), influenza (3% to 4%)

Gastrointestinal: Nausea (3% to 4%), constipation (3%)

Genitourinary: Urinary tract infection (6%), increased urine output (2% to 3%), dysuria (2%)

Respiratory: Cough (3%), pharyngitis (2% to 3%)

<1%, postmarketing, and/or case reports: Ketoacidosis (FDA Safety Communication, December 4, 2015), pyelonephritis (FDA Safety Communication, December 4, 2015), urosepsis (FDA Safety Communication, December 4, 2015)

Mechanism of Action

Dapagliflozin: By inhibiting sodium-glucose cotransporter 2 (SGLT2) in the proximal renal tubules, dapagliflozin reduces reabsorption of filtered glucose from the tubular lumen and lowers the renal threshold for glucose (RTG). SGLT2 is the main site of filtered glucose reabsorption; reduction of filtered glucose reabsorption and lowering of RTG result in increased urinary excretion of glucose, thereby reducing plasma glucose concentrations. Dapagliflozin also reduces sodium reabsorption and increases sodium delivery to the distal tubule, which may decrease cardiac preload/afterload and downregulate sympathetic activity.

Metformin: Decreases hepatic glucose production, decreases intestinal absorption of glucose, improves insulin sensitivity by increasing peripheral glucose uptake and utilization.

Pregnancy Considerations Metformin crosses the placenta (ADA 2020).

Refer to individual monographs for additional information.

◆ **Dapagliflozin/Metformin HCl** *see* Dapagliflozin and Metformin *on page 435*

◆ **Dapagliflozin Propanediol** *see* Dapagliflozin *on page 435*

Dapagliflozin, Saxagliptin, and Metformin

(dap a gli FLOE zin, sax a GLIP tin, & met FOR min)

Pharmacologic Category Antidiabetic Agent, Biguanide; Antidiabetic Agent, Dipeptidyl Peptidase 4 (DPP-4) Inhibitor; Sodium-Glucose Cotransporter 2 (SGLT2) Inhibitor

Use Diabetes mellitus, type 2, treatment: Adjunct to diet and exercise to improve glycemic control in adults with type 2 diabetes mellitus.

Local Anesthetic/Vasoconstrictor Precautions No information available to require special precautions

Effects on Dental Treatment Key adverse event(s) related to dental treatment:

Dapagliflozin: Dizziness and syncope have been reported; patients may experience orthostatic hypotension as they stand up after treatment, especially if lying in dental chair for extended periods of time. Use caution with sudden changes in position during and after dental treatment.

Dapagliflozin, saxagliptin, metformin-dependent patients with diabetes (noninsulin dependent, type 2) should be questioned by the dental professional at each dental visit to assess their risk for stress-induced hypoglycemia. The dental professional should inquire about the patient's routine (ie, work, sleep schedule, eating patterns), history of hypoglycemia, time of last medication dose, last meal, and most recent blood sugar assessment. Keep a supply of glucose tablets and other carbohydrates in the office to prepare for a hypoglycemic event. Seek medical attention when necessary (American Diabetes Association 2016).

Effects on Bleeding No information available to require special precautions

Adverse Reactions See individual agents.

Mechanism of Action See individual agents.

Pregnancy Considerations

The manufacturer does not recommend use of this combination during the second or third trimesters of pregnancy.

Refer to individual monographs for additional information.

Product Availability Qternmet XR: FDA approved May 2019; anticipated availability is currently unknown.

◆ **Dapagliflozin, Saxagliptin, and Metformin Hydrochloride** *see* Dapagliflozin, Saxagliptin, and Metformin *on page 436*

◆ **Dapcin** *see* DAPTOmycin *on page 437*

Dapsone (Systemic) (DAP sone)

Related Information

HIV Infection and AIDS *on page 1690*

Brand Names: Canada MAR-Dapsone; RIVA-Dapsone

Pharmacologic Category Antibiotic, Miscellaneous

Use Treatment of leprosy (due to susceptible strains of *Mycobacterium leprae*) and dermatitis herpetiformis

Local Anesthetic/Vasoconstrictor Precautions No information available to require special precautions

Effects on Dental Treatment No significant effects or complications reported

Effects on Bleeding No information available to require special precautions

Adverse Reactions Frequency not always defined.

>10%: Hematologic: Reticulocyte increase (2% to 12%), hemolysis (>10%; dose related; seen in patients with and without G6PD deficiency), hemoglobin decrease (>10%; 1-2 g/dL; almost all patients), methemoglobinemia (>10%), red cell life span shortened (>10%), Agranulocytosis, anemia, leukopenia, pure red cell aplasia (case report)

Cardiovascular: Tachycardia

Central nervous system: Fever, headache, insomnia, psychosis, vertigo

Dermatologic: Bullous and exfoliative dermatitis, erythema nodosum, exfoliative dermatitis, morbilliform and scarlatiniform reactions, phototoxicity, Stevens-Johnson syndrome, toxic epidermal necrolysis, urticaria
Endocrine & metabolic: Hypoalbuminemia (without proteinuria), male infertility
Gastrointestinal: Abdominal pain, nausea, pancreatitis, vomiting
Hepatic: Cholestatic jaundice, hepatitis
Neuromuscular & skeletal: Lower motor neuron toxicity (prolonged therapy), lupus-like syndrome, peripheral neuropathy (rare, nonleprosy patients)
Ophthalmic: Blurred vision
Otic: Tinnitus
Renal: Albuminuria, nephrotic syndrome, renal papillary necrosis
Respiratory: Interstitial pneumonitis, pulmonary eosinophilia
Miscellaneous: Infectious mononucleosis-like syndrome (rash, fever, lymphadenopathy, hepatic dysfunction)

Mechanism of Action Competitive antagonist of para-aminobenzoic acid (PABA) and prevents normal bacterial utilization of PABA for the synthesis of folic acid

Pharmacodynamics/Kinetics

Half-life Elimination Children: 15.1 hours (Mirochnick 1993); Adults: 28 hours (range: 10 to 50 hours)

Time to Peak 4 to 8 hours

Pregnancy Risk Factor C

Pregnancy Considerations Dapsone crosses the placenta (Brabin 2004). Per the manufacturer, dapsone has not shown an increased risk of congenital anomalies when given during all trimesters of pregnancy. Several reports have described adverse effects in the newborn after in utero exposure to dapsone, including neonatal hemolytic disease, methemoglobinemia, and hyperbilirubinemia (Hocking 1968; Kabra 1998; Thornton 1989). Dapsone may be used in pregnant women requiring maintenance therapy of either leprosy or dermatitis herpetiformis. Dapsone may be used as an alternative agent for management of *Pneumocystis jirovecii* pneumonia (PCP) or *T. gondii* encephalitis in pregnant patients with HIV (HHS [OI Adult 2020]). Because of the theoretical increased risk for hyperbilirubinemia and kernicterus, neonatal care providers should be informed if maternal dapsone is used near term (HHS [OI Adult 2020]).

Dapsone (Topical) (DAP sone)

Brand Names: US Aczone

Brand Names: Canada Aczone

Pharmacologic Category Topical Skin Product, Acne

Use Acne vulgaris: Topical treatment of acne vulgaris in patients ≥9 years of age (7.5% gel) or patients ≥12 years of age (5% gel).

Guideline recommendations: American Academy of Dermatology (AAD) acne guidelines recommend dapsone 5% topical gel for inflammatory acne, particularly in adult females with acne (AAD [Zaenglein 2016]).

Local Anesthetic/Vasoconstrictor Precautions No information available to require special precautions

Effects on Dental Treatment No significant effects or complications reported

Effects on Bleeding No information available to require special precautions

Adverse Reactions

1% to 10%:
Respiratory: Sinusitis (2%)

Frequency not defined:
Central nervous system: Attempted suicide, tonic-clonic movements
Gastrointestinal: Abdominal pain, pancreatitis, severe vomiting
Respiratory: Pharyngitis

<1%, postmarketing, and/or case reports: Application site rash, depression, erythema, erythematous rash, facial edema, lip edema, methemoglobinemia, periorbital swelling, psychosis, skin rash

Pregnancy Considerations

The amount of topical dapsone available systemically is minimal compared to oral administration.

Topical products are recommended as initial therapy for the treatment of acne vulgaris in pregnant females; however, information specific to dapsone is lacking (Kong 2013). Agents other than topical dapsone are preferred (Chien 2016).

DAPTOmycin (DAP toe mye sin)

Brand Names: US Cubicin; Cubicin RF

Brand Names: Canada Cubicin; Cubicin RF

Pharmacologic Category Antibiotic, Cyclic Lipopeptide

Use

Bloodstream infection: Treatment of bloodstream infection caused by *Staphylococcus aureus* (methicillin-susceptible and methicillin-resistant isolates) in adults, including those with right-sided infective endocarditis; treatment of bloodstream infection due to *S. aureus* in pediatric patients 1 to 17 years of age.

Skin and skin structure infections, complicated: Treatment of complicated skin and skin structure infections caused by *S. aureus* (including methicillin-resistant isolates), *Streptococcus pyogenes*, *Streptococcus agalactiae*, *Streptococcus dysgalactiae* subspecies *equisimilis*, and *Enterococcus faecalis* (vancomycin-susceptible isolates only) in adult and pediatric patients 1 to 17 years of age.

Limitations of use: Not indicated for the treatment of pneumonia.

Local Anesthetic/Vasoconstrictor Precautions No information available to require special precautions

Effects on Dental Treatment No significant effects or complications reported

Effects on Bleeding No information available to require special precautions

Adverse Reactions

1% to 10%:
Cardiovascular: Chest pain (adults: 7%), edema (adults: 7%), hypertension (adults: 6%), hypotension (adults: 2%)
Central nervous system: Insomnia (adults: 9%), headache (3% to 5%), dizziness (adults: 2%)
Dermatologic: Pruritus (3% to 6%), diaphoresis (adults: 5%), skin rash (adults: 4%)
Gastrointestinal: Diarrhea (5% to 7%), abdominal pain (adults: 6%; children and adolescents: 2%), vomiting (children and adolescents: 3% to 11%; adults: <1%)
Genitourinary: Urinary tract infection (adults: 2%)
Hepatic: Abnormal hepatic function tests (adults: 3%), increased serum alkaline phosphatase (adults: 2%)
Infection: Gram-negative organism infection (adults: 8%), bacteremia (adults: 5%), sepsis (adults: 5%)
Neuromuscular & skeletal: Increased creatine phosphokinase (3% to 9%)
Respiratory: Pharyngolaryngeal pain (adults: 8%), dyspnea (adults: 2%)

Miscellaneous: Fever (≤4%)
Frequency not defined:
Cardiovascular: Atrial fibrillation, atrial flutter
Central nervous system: Hallucination, hypoesthesia (including oral)
Endocrine & metabolic: Increased serum phosphate
Gastrointestinal: Decreased appetite, epigastric distress, gingival pain, oral candidiasis, xerostomia
Genitourinary: Fungal urinary tract infection, proteinuria, vulvovaginal candidiasis
Hematologic & oncologic: Lymphadenopathy
Hepatic: Increased serum ALT, increased serum AST
Infection: Candidiasis, fungal septicemia
Neuromuscular & skeletal: Dyskinesia
Ophthalmic: Blurred vision
Otic: Tinnitus
Renal: Renal insufficiency

<1%, postmarketing, and/or case reports: Abdominal distension, acute generalized exanthematous pustulosis, acute renal failure, anaphylaxis, anemia, arthralgia, bronchiolitis obliterans organizing pneumonia, *Clostridioides* (formerly *Clostridium*) *difficile*-associated diarrhea, cough, decreased appetite, dysgeusia, eczema, electrolyte disturbance, eosinophilia, eosinophilic pneumonitis, eye irritation, fatigue, flushing, hypomagnesemia, hypersensitivity reaction (including angioedema, drug rash with eosinophilia and systemic symptoms [DRESS], dysphagia, hives, pulmonary eosinophilia, truncal erythema), increased lactate dehydrogenase, increased myoglobin, increased serum bicarbonate, jaundice, leukocytosis, mental status changes, muscle cramps, myalgia, myasthenia, myopathy, nausea, neutropenia (Knoll 2013), paresthesia, peripheral neuropathy, renal failure, rhabdomyolysis, rigors, Stevens-Johnson syndrome, stomatitis, supraventricular cardiac arrhythmia, thrombocythemia, thrombocytopenia, vertigo, vesiculobullous dermatitis, visual disturbance, weakness

Mechanism of Action Daptomycin binds to components of the cell membrane of susceptible organisms and causes rapid depolarization, inhibiting intracellular synthesis of DNA, RNA, and protein. Daptomycin is bactericidal in a concentration-dependent manner.

Pharmacodynamics/Kinetics

Half-life Elimination

Neonates and Infants <3 months: Median: 6.2 hours (range: 3.7 to 9 hours) (Cohen-Wolkowiez 2012)
Children 2 to 6 years: Mean range: 5.3 to 5.7 hours (Abdel-Rahman 2008; Abdel-Rahman 2011)
Children 7 to 11 years: 5.6 ± 2.2 hours (Abdel-Rahman 2008)
Children 12 to 17 years: 6.7 ± 2.2 hours (Abdel-Rahman 2008)
Adults: 8 to 9 hours (up to 28 hours in renal impairment)

Pregnancy Considerations Adverse events were not observed in animal reproduction studies. Successful use of daptomycin during the second and third trimesters of pregnancy has been described; however, only limited information is available from case reports.

◆ **Daraprim** *see* Pyrimethamine *on page 1294*

◆ **Dara/rHuPH20** *see* Daratumumab and Hyaluronidase *on page 439*

Daratumumab (dar a TOOM ue mab)

Brand Names: US Darzalex
Brand Names: Canada Darzalex

Pharmacologic Category Antineoplastic Agent, Anti-CD38; Antineoplastic Agent, Monoclonal Antibody

Use

Multiple myeloma (newly diagnosed):

Treatment of newly diagnosed multiple myeloma (in combination with bortezomib, thalidomide, and dexamethasone) in adults who are eligible for autologous stem cell transplant.

Treatment of newly diagnosed multiple myeloma (in combination with bortezomib, melphalan, and prednisone) in adults who are ineligible for autologous stem cell transplant.

Treatment of newly diagnosed multiple myeloma (in combination with lenalidomide and dexamethasone) in adults who are ineligible for autologous stem cell transplant.

Multiple myeloma (relapsed/refractory):

Treatment of multiple myeloma (in combination with dexamethasone and lenalidomide) in adults who have received at least 1 prior therapy.

Treatment of multiple myeloma (in combination with dexamethasone and bortezomib) in adults who have received at least 1 prior therapy.

Treatment of multiple myeloma (in combination with dexamethasone and pomalidomide) in adults who have received at least 2 prior therapies, including lenalidomide and a proteasome inhibitor.

Treatment of multiple myeloma (as monotherapy) in adults who have received at least 3 prior lines of therapy, including a proteasome inhibitor and an immunomodulatory agent or who are double refractory to a proteasome inhibitor and an immunomodulatory agent.

Local Anesthetic/Vasoconstrictor Precautions No information available to require special precautions

Effects on Dental Treatment No significant effects or complications reported

Effects on Bleeding Chemotherapy may result in significant myelosuppression, including thrombocytopenia. In patients under active treatment a medical consult is suggested.

Adverse Reactions

>10%:
Gastrointestinal: Constipation (15%), decreased appetite (15%), diarrhea (16%), nausea (27%), vomiting (14%)
Hematologic & oncologic: Anemia (45%; grade 3: 19%), lymphocytopenia (72%; grade 3: 30%; grade 4: 10%), neutropenia (60%; grade 3: 17%; grade 4: 3%), thrombocytopenia (48%; grade 3: 10%; grade 4: 8%)
Nervous system: Fatigue (39%), headache (12%)
Neuromuscular & skeletal: Arthralgia (17%), back pain (23%), limb pain (15%), musculoskeletal chest pain (12%)
Respiratory: Cough (21%), dyspnea (15%), nasal congestion (17%), nasopharyngitis (15%), pneumonia (11%), upper respiratory tract infection (20%)
Miscellaneous: Fever (21%), infusion related reaction (48%)

1% to 10%:
Cardiovascular: Hypertension (10%)
Infection: Herpes zoster infection (3%)
Nervous system: Chills (10%)
Miscellaneous: Physical health deterioration (3%)

<1%:
Immunologic: Antibody development
Infection: Reactivation of HBV

Frequency not defined: Hematologic & oncologic: Positive indirect Coombs test

Postmarketing:
Gastrointestinal: Pancreatitis
Hypersensitivity: Anaphylaxis

Mechanism of Action Daratumumab is an IgG1κ human monoclonal antibody directed against CD38. CD38 is a cell surface glycoprotein which is highly expressed on myeloma cells, yet is expressed at low levels on normal lymphoid and myeloid cells (Lokhorst 2015). By binding to CD38, daratumumab inhibits the growth of CD38 expressing tumor cells by inducing apoptosis directly through Fc mediated cross linking as well as by immune-mediated tumor cell lysis through complement dependent cytotoxicity, antibody dependent cell mediated cytotoxicity, and antibody dependent cellular phagocytosis.

Pharmacodynamics/Kinetics

Half-life Elimination 18 ± 9 days

Reproductive Considerations Females of reproductive potential should use effective contraception during therapy and for 3 months after the last daratumumab dose.

Pregnancy Considerations

Daratumumab is a humanized monoclonal antibody (IgG_1). Potential placental transfer of human IgG is dependent upon the IgG subclass and gestational age, generally increasing as pregnancy progresses. The lowest exposure would be expected during the period of organogenesis (Palmeira 2012; Pentsuk 2009).

Based on the mechanism of action, daratumumab may cause myeloid or lymphoid cell depletion and decreased bone density in the fetus. The administration of live vaccines should be deferred for neonates and infants exposed to daratumumab in utero until a hematology evaluation can be completed. When using in combination regimens, also refer to individual monographs for additional information.

Daratumumab and Hyaluronidase

(DAR a TOOM ue mab & HYE al ure ON i dase)

Brand Names: US Darzalex Faspro

Pharmacologic Category Antineoplastic Agent, Anti-CD38; Antineoplastic Agent, Monoclonal Antibody

Use

Multiple myeloma (newly diagnosed):

Treatment of newly diagnosed multiple myeloma (in combination with bortezomib, melphalan, and prednisone) in adults who are ineligible for autologous stem cell transplant.

Treatment of newly diagnosed multiple myeloma (in combination with lenalidomide and dexamethasone) in adults who are ineligible for autologous stem cell transplant.

Multiple myeloma (relapsed/refractory):

Treatment of relapsed or refractory multiple myeloma (in combination with lenalidomide and dexamethasone) in adults who have received at least 1 prior therapy.

Treatment of relapsed or refractory multiple myeloma (in combination with bortezomib and dexamethasone) in adults who have received at least 1 prior therapy.

Treatment of relapsed or refractory multiple myeloma (as monotherapy) in adults who have received at least 3 prior lines of therapy, which included a proteasome inhibitor and an immunomodulatory agent, or who are double refractory to a proteasome inhibitor and an immunomodulatory agent.

Local Anesthetic/Vasoconstrictor Precautions No information available to require special precautions.

Effects on Dental Treatment No significant effects or complications reported.

Effects on Bleeding Chemotherapy may result in significant myelosuppression, including thrombocytopenia. In patients under active treatment a medical consult is suggested.

Adverse Reactions Also see individual agents.

>10%:
Gastrointestinal: Diarrhea (15%)
Hematologic & oncologic: Decreased hemoglobin (42%; grades 3/4: 14%), decreased neutrophils (55%; grades 3/4: 19%), decreased platelet count (43%; grades 3/4: 16%), leukopenia (65%; grades 3/4: 19%), lymphocytopenia (59%; grades 3/4: 36%)
Hypersensitivity: Hypersensitivity reaction (11%, including severe hypersensitivity reactions)
Nervous system: Fatigue (15%)
Respiratory: Upper respiratory tract infection (24%)
Miscellaneous: Fever (13%), infusion related reaction (13%)

1% to 10%:
Cardiovascular: Atrial fibrillation (<10%), hypertension (<10%), hypotension (<10%), peripheral edema (<10%)
Dermatologic: Pruritus (<10%), skin rash (<10%)
Endocrine & metabolic: Dehydration (<10%), hyperglycemia (<10%), hypocalcemia (<10%)
Gastrointestinal: Abdominal pain (<10%), constipation (<10%), decreased appetite (<10%), nausea (8%), vomiting (<10%)
Genitourinary: Urinary tract infection (<10%)
Immunologic: Antibody development (8%; neutralizing: 0%)
Infection: Herpes zoster infection (<10%), influenza (<10%), reactivation of HBV (<10%), sepsis (<10%)
Local: Erythema at injection site (>1%), injection site reaction (8%)
Nervous system: Chills (6%), dizziness (<10%), insomnia (<10%), paresthesia (<10%), peripheral sensory neuropathy (<10%)
Neuromuscular & skeletal: Arthralgia (<10%), back pain (10%), muscle spasm (<10%), musculoskeletal chest pain (<10%)
Respiratory: Bronchitis (<10%), cough (9%), dyspnea (6%), pneumonia (8%), pulmonary edema (<10%)

Frequency not defined:
Hematologic & oncologic: Positive indirect Coombs test
Hypersensitivity: Anaphylaxis

Mechanism of Action Daratumumab is an IgG1κ human monoclonal antibody directed against CD38. CD38 is a cell surface glycoprotein which is highly expressed on myeloma cells. By binding to CD38, daratumumab inhibits the growth of CD38-expressing tumor cells by inducing apoptosis directly through Fc mediated cross linking as well as by immune-mediated tumor cell lysis through complement dependent cytotoxicity, antibody dependent cell mediated cytotoxicity, and antibody dependent cellular phagocytosis. Hyaluronidase increases permeability of the subcutaneous tissue by depolymerizing hyaluronan. At the recommended dose, hyaluronidase acts locally and the effects are reversible; permeability of subcutaneous tissue is restored within 24 to 48 hours.

Pharmacodynamics/Kinetics

Half-life Elimination SubQ: 20 days.

Time to Peak SubQ: ~3 days.

Reproductive Considerations

Evaluate pregnancy status prior to use in females of reproductive potential.

Females of reproductive potential should use effective contraception during therapy and for 3 months after the last daratumumab/hyaluronidase dose. If daratumumab/hyaluronidase is used in combination with lenalidomide, pregnancy testing and contraception requirements for lenalidomide should also be followed.

Daratumumab/hyaluronidase may be used as monotherapy or in combination with other agents (eg, bortezomib, lenalidomide, melphalan); refer to the Daratumumab, Hyaluronidase, and other individual monographs for additional information.

Pregnancy Considerations

Based on the mechanism of action, in utero exposure to daratumumab/hyaluronidase may cause fetal harm.

Daratumumab/hyaluronidase in combination with lenalidomide is contraindicated for use during pregnancy.

Daratumumab/hyaluronidase may be used as monotherapy or in combination with other agents (eg, bortezomib, lenalidomide, melphalan); refer to the Daratumumab, Hyaluronidase, and other individual monographs for additional information.

◆ **Daratumumab and hyaluronidase-fihj** *see* Daratumumab and Hyaluronidase *on page 439*

◆ **Daratumumab plus rHuPH20** *see* Daratumumab and Hyaluronidase *on page 439*

◆ **Daratumumab-rHuPH20** *see* Daratumumab and Hyaluronidase *on page 439*

◆ **Daratumumab with rHuPH20** *see* Daratumumab and Hyaluronidase *on page 439*

Darbepoetin Alfa (dar be POE e tin AL fa)

Brand Names: US Aranesp (Albumin Free)
Brand Names: Canada Aranesp
Pharmacologic Category Colony Stimulating Factor; Erythropoiesis-Stimulating Agent (ESA); Hematopoietic Agent

Use

Anemia due to chemotherapy in patients with cancer: Treatment of anemia in patients with nonmyeloid malignancies when anemia is due to the effect of concomitant myelosuppressive chemotherapy, and upon initiation, there is a minimum of 2 additional months of planned chemotherapy.

Anemia due to chronic kidney disease: Treatment of anemia due to chronic kidney disease, including patients on dialysis and patients not on dialysis.

Limitations of use: Darbepoetin alfa has not demonstrated improved quality of life, fatigue, or well-being. Darbepoetin alfa is **not** indicated for use under the following conditions:

- Cancer patients receiving hormonal therapy, therapeutic biologic products, or radiation therapy unless also receiving concurrent myelosuppressive chemotherapy
- Cancer patients receiving myelosuppressive chemotherapy when the expected outcome is curative
- Cancer patients receiving myelosuppressive chemotherapy when anemia can be managed by transfusion
- As a substitute for red blood cell (RBC) transfusion in patients requiring immediate correction of anemia

Local Anesthetic/Vasoconstrictor Precautions
No information available to require special precautions

Effects on Dental Treatment No significant effects or complications reported

Effects on Bleeding Erythropoiesis-stimulating agents have been associated with thromboembolic events.

Adverse Reactions Adverse reactions occurred in adults with chronic kidney disease unless otherwise specified.

>10%:

Cardiovascular: Hypertension (31%; children and adolescents: frequency not defined), peripheral edema (17%), edema (cancer patients: 13%)

Gastrointestinal: Abdominal pain (cancer patients: 13%)

Respiratory: Dyspnea (17%), cough (12%)

1% to 10%:

Cardiovascular: Procedural hypotension (10%), angina pectoris (8%), thrombosis (cancer patients: 5%), thrombosis of vascular graft (arteriovenous: 5%), thromboembolism (cancer patients, venous: 4%), pulmonary embolism (cancer patients: 2%), arterial thromboembolism (cancer patients: 1%)

Dermatologic: Erythema of skin (≤5%), skin rash (≤5%)

Endocrine & metabolic: Hypervolemia (7%)

Immunologic: Antibody development (children & adolescents: 4% to 6%, adults: <1%)

Frequency not defined:

Cardiovascular: Myocardial infarction, significant cardiovascular event

Central nervous system: Cerebrovascular disease

Local: Pain at injection site

<1%, postmarketing, and/or case reports: Anaphylaxis, angioedema, bronchospasm, cardiac failure, cerebrovascular accident, erythema multiforme, exfoliation of skin, hypertensive encephalopathy, pure red cell aplasia (occurs following development of antibodies to erythropoietin), seizure, severe dermatological reaction, severe hypersensitivity reaction, skin blister, Stevens-Johnson syndrome, toxic epidermal necrolysis, urticaria

Mechanism of Action Darbepoetin alfa induces erythropoiesis by stimulating the division and differentiation of committed erythroid progenitor cells; induces the release of reticulocytes from the bone marrow into the bloodstream, where they mature to erythrocytes. There is a dose-response relationship with this effect. This results in an increase in reticulocyte counts followed by a rise in hematocrit and hemoglobin levels. When administered SubQ or IV, darbepoetin alfa's half-life is ~3 times that of epoetin alfa concentrations.

Pharmacodynamics/Kinetics

Onset of Action Increased hemoglobin levels not generally observed until 2 to 6 weeks after initiating treatment

Half-life Elimination Note: Darbepoetin alfa half-life is approximately 3-fold longer than epoetin alfa following IV administration

CKD:

Children and Adolescents: (Lerner 2002):

IV: Terminal: 22.1 ± 4.8 hours

SubQ: Terminal: 42.8 ± 23 hours

Adults:

IV: 21 hours

SubQ: Nondialysis patients: 70 hours (range: 35 to 139 hours), Dialysis patients: 46 hours (range: 12 to 89 hours)

Cancer:

Children and Adolescents: SubQ: 49.4 ± 32 hours (Blumer 2007)

Adults: SubQ: 74 hours (range: 24 to 144 hours)

Time to Peak SubQ:

CKD:

Children and Adolescents: 36.2 ± 14.1 hours (Lerner 2002)

Adults: 48 hours (range: 12 to 72 hours; independent of dialysis)

Cancer:

Children and Adolescents: 87.5 ± 53 hours (Blumer 2007)

Adults: 71 hours (range: 28 to 120 hours)

Pregnancy Considerations Use of darbepoetin alfa in pregnancy has been described in case reports (Ghosh 2007; Goshorn 2005; Macciò 2009; Sobiło-Jarek 2006).

◆ **Darbepoetin Alfa Polysorbate** *see* Darbepoetin Alfa *on page 440*

Darifenacin (dar i FEN a sin)

Brand Names: US Enablex

Brand Names: Canada Enablex

Pharmacologic Category Anticholinergic Agent

Use Overactive bladder: Treatment of overactive bladder with symptoms of urinary frequency, urgency, or urge incontinence.

Local Anesthetic/Vasoconstrictor Precautions No information available to require special precautions

Effects on Dental Treatment Key adverse event(s) related to dental treatment: Xerostomia (normal salivary flow resumes upon discontinuation). Prolonged xerostomia may contribute to discomfort and dental disease (eg, caries, periodontal disease, and oral candidiasis).

Effects on Bleeding No information available to require special precautions

Adverse Reactions

>10%: Gastrointestinal: Xerostomia (19% to 35%), constipation (15% to 21%)

1% to 10%:

Cardiovascular: Hypertension (≥1%), peripheral edema (≥1%)

Central nervous system: Headache (7%), dizziness (<2%), pain (≥1%)

Dermatological: Pruritus (≥1%), skin rash (≥1%), xeroderma (≥1%)

Endocrine & metabolic: Weight gain (≥1%)

Gastrointestinal: Dyspepsia (3% to 8%), abdominal pain (2% to 4%), nausea (2% to 4%), vomiting (≥1%)

Genitourinary: Urinary tract infection (4% to 5%), vaginitis (≥1%), urinary retention (acute)

Neuromuscular & skeletal: Weakness (<3%), arthralgia (≥1%), back pain (≥1%)

Ophthalmic: Dry eye syndrome (2%), visual disturbance (≥1%)

Respiratory: Flu-like symptoms (1% to 3%), bronchitis (≥1%), pharyngitis (≥1%), rhinitis (≥1%), sinusitis (≥1%)

Postmarketing and/or case reports: Anaphylaxis, angioedema, confusion, erythema multiforme, granuloma (annulare), hallucination, hypersensitivity reaction, palpitations

Mechanism of Action Selective antagonist of the M3 muscarinic (cholinergic) receptor subtype. Blockade of the receptor limits bladder contractions, reducing the symptoms of bladder irritability/overactivity (urge incontinence, urgency and frequency).

Pharmacodynamics/Kinetics

Half-life Elimination ~13 to 19 hours

Time to Peak Plasma: ~7 hours

Pregnancy Risk Factor C

Pregnancy Considerations Adverse events have been observed in animal reproduction studies.

◆ **Darifenacin Hydrobromide** *see* Darifenacin *on page 441*

Darunavir (dar OO na veer)

Related Information

HIV Infection and AIDS *on page 1690*

Brand Names: US Prezista

Brand Names: Canada APO-Darunavir; AURO-Darunavir; Prezista

Pharmacologic Category Antiretroviral, Protease Inhibitor (Anti-HIV)

Use HIV-1 infection, treatment: Treatment of HIV-1 infection, coadministered with ritonavir and other antiretroviral agents, in adults and pediatric patients 3 years and older

Local Anesthetic/Vasoconstrictor Precautions No information available to require special precautions

Effects on Dental Treatment No significant effects or complications reported

Effects on Bleeding Increased bleeding has been noted with protease inhibitors, such as darunavir, in patients with hemophilia A or B. No other information is available to require special precautions in other patients.

Adverse Reactions Frequency of adverse events is reported for darunavir/ritonavir in both treatment-naive and experienced patients. Frequency, type, and severity of adverse events in pediatric patients are comparable to adult patients unless otherwise noted. See also Ritonavir monograph.

>10%:

Dermatologic: Skin rash (children: 5% to 19%; adults: 6% to 7%)

Endocrine & metabolic: Increased serum cholesterol (adults: 1% to 25%; children & adolescents: grade 3: 1%), increased LDL cholesterol (adults: 8% to 14%; children & adolescents: grade 3: 3%), increased serum glucose (≤11%)

Gastrointestinal: Vomiting (children & adolescents: 13% to 33%; adults: 2% to 5%), nausea (children: 4% to 25%; adults: 4% to 7%), diarrhea (children & adolescents: 11% to 24%; adults: 9% to 14%)

1% to 10%:

Central nervous system: Headache (3% to 9%), fatigue (≤3%), abnormal dreams (<2%)

Dermatologic: Pruritus (children & adolescents: 8%; adults: <2%), Stevens-Johnson syndrome (<2%), urticaria (<2%)

Endocrine & metabolic: Increased serum triglycerides (1% to 10%), increased amylase (≤7%), diabetes mellitus (≤2%)

Gastrointestinal: Abdominal pain (5% to 10%), decreased appetite (children & adolescents: 8%), anorexia (2% to 5%), increased serum lipase (adults: ≤3%; children & adolescents: grade 3: 1%), abdominal distention (2%), dyspepsia (≤2%), flatulence (<2%), acute pancreatitis (<2%)

Hepatic: Increased serum ALT (adults: ≤9%; children: 1% to 3%), increased serum AST (adults: 1% to 7%; children & adolescents: grade 3: 1%), hepatitis (<2%; includes acute and cytolytic), increased serum alkaline phosphatase (≤1%)
Hypersensitivity: Angioedema (<2%), hypersensitivity reaction (<2%)
Immunologic: Immune reconstitution syndrome (<2%)
Neuromuscular & skeletal: Weakness (≤3%), myalgia (<2%), osteonecrosis (<2%)

<1%, postmarketing, and/or case reports: Acute generalized exanthematous pustulosis, dermatological reaction, DRESS syndrome, erythema multiforme (DHHS 2011), hepatic disease, hepatotoxicity, hyperbilirubinemia, hyperglycemia, hypercholesterolemia (DHHS 2011), hypertriglyceridemia, redistribution of body fat, toxic epidermal necrolysis

Mechanism of Action Binds to the site of HIV-1 protease activity and inhibits cleavage of viral Gag-Pol polyprotein precursors into individual functional proteins required for infectious HIV. This results in the formation of immature, noninfectious viral particles.

Pharmacodynamics/Kinetics

Half-life Elimination ~15 hours

Reproductive Considerations

The Health and Human Services (HHS) perinatal HIV guidelines consider darunavir (when combined with low-dose ritonavir boosting) a preferred protease inhibitor for females living with HIV who are not yet pregnant but are trying to conceive. Darunavir (when combined with low-dose cobicistat boosting) is not recommended for use in women who are planning a pregnancy.

Females living with HIV not planning a pregnancy may use any available type of contraception, considering possible drug interactions and contraindications of the specific method. Consult drug interactions database for more detailed information specific to use of darunavir and specific contraceptives.

For males and females living with HIV and planning a pregnancy, maximum viral suppression below the limits of detection with antiretroviral therapy (ART), modification of therapy (if needed), optimization of the woman's health, and a discussion of the potential risks and benefits of ART therapy during pregnancy is recommended prior to conception (HHS [perinatal] 2019).

Pregnancy Considerations

Darunavir has a low level of transfer across the human placenta.

No increased risk of overall birth defects has been observed following first trimester exposure according to data collected by the antiretroviral pregnancy registry. Maternal antiretroviral therapy (ART) may be associated with adverse pregnancy outcomes including preterm delivery, stillbirth, low birth weight, and small for gestational age infants. Actual risks may be influenced by maternal factors, such as disease severity, gestational age at initiation of therapy, and specific ART regimen, therefore close fetal monitoring is recommended. Because there is clear benefit to appropriate treatment, maternal ART should not be withheld due to concerns for adverse neonatal outcomes. Long-term follow-up is recommended for all infants exposed to antiretroviral medications; children without HIV but who were exposed to ART in utero and develop significant organ system abnormalities of unknown etiology (particularly of the CNS or heart) should be evaluated for potential mitochondrial dysfunction. Hyperglycemia, new onset of diabetes mellitus, or diabetic ketoacidosis have been reported with protease inhibitors; it is not clear if pregnancy increases this risk. Consider performing the standard glucose screening test earlier in pregnancy in women who initiated protease inhibitor therapy prior to conception.

The Health and Human Services (HHS) perinatal HIV guidelines consider darunavir (when combined with low-dose ritonavir boosting) a preferred protease inhibitor for pregnant females living with HIV who are antiretroviral-naive (initial therapy), who have had ART therapy in the past but are restarting, or who require a new ART regimen (due to poor tolerance or poor virologic response of current regimen). In addition, females who become pregnant while taking darunavir may continue if viral suppression is effective and the regimen is well tolerated. Darunavir (when combined with low-dose cobicistat boosting) is not recommended for use during pregnancy. If pregnancy occurs during therapy, consideration should be given to changing to a more effective regimen. If continued, close monitoring, including more frequent therapeutic drug monitoring if available, is recommended.

Serum concentrations are decreased during pregnancy; therefore, ritonavir-boosted twice-daily dosing should be used. Exposure to darunavir is decreased in pregnant women when combined with cobicistat. Product labeling provides guidance for use of once daily darunavir dosing in pregnant women, however, the current HHS perinatal guidelines do not recommend once daily dosing during pregnancy.

In general, ART is recommended for all pregnant females living with HIV to keep the viral load below the limit of detection and reduce the risk of perinatal transmission. Therapy should be individualized following a discussion of the potential risks and benefits of treatment during pregnancy. Monitoring of pregnant females is more frequent than in nonpregnant adults. ART should be continued postpartum for all females living with HIV and can be modified after delivery.

Health care providers are encouraged to enroll pregnant females exposed to antiretroviral medications as early in pregnancy as possible in the Antiretroviral Pregnancy Registry (1-800-258-4263 or http://www.APRegistry.com). Health care providers caring for pregnant females living with HIV and their infants may contact the National Perinatal HIV Hotline (888-448-8765) for clinical consultation (HHS [perinatal] 2019).

Darunavir, Cobicistat, Emtricitabine, and Tenofovir Alafenamide

(dar UE na vir, koe BIK i stat, EM trye SYE ta been, and ten OF oh vir AL a FEN a mide)

Brand Names: US Symtuza

Brand Names: Canada Symtuza

Pharmacologic Category Antiretroviral, Protease Inhibitor (Anti-HIV); Antiretroviral, Reverse Transcriptase Inhibitor, Nucleoside (Anti-HIV); Antiretroviral, Reverse Transcriptase Inhibitor, Nucleotide (Anti-HIV); Cytochrome P-450 Inhibitor

Use HIV-1 infection, treatment: Treatment of HIV-1 infection in adults and pediatric patients ≥40 kg who have no prior antiretroviral treatment history or who are virologically suppressed (HIV-1 RNA <50 copies per mL) on a stable antiretroviral regimen for ≥6 months and have no known substitutions associated with resistance to darunavir or tenofovir.

Local Anesthetic/Vasoconstrictor Precautions No information available to require special precautions

Effects on Dental Treatment No significant effects or complications reported

Effects on Bleeding No information available to require special precautions

Adverse Reactions

>10%:

Dermatologic: Skin rash (8% to 15%)

Endocrine & metabolic: Increased serum cholesterol (2% to 17%)

Neuromuscular & skeletal: Decreased bone mineral density (16%)

1% to 10%:

Central nervous system: Fatigue (4%), headache (3%), abnormal dreams (<2%)

Dermatologic: Pruritus (<2%), Stevens-Johnson syndrome (<2%)

Endocrine & metabolic: Increased LDL cholesterol (5% to 9%), increased serum triglycerides (≤7%), increased serum glucose (≤6%), diabetes mellitus (<2%), gynecomastia (<2%), lipodystrophy (<2%)

Gastrointestinal: Diarrhea (9%), nausea (6%), abdominal distress (2%), flatulence (2%), acute pancreatitis (<2%), anorexia (<2%), dyspepsia (<2%), vomiting (<2%)

Hepatic: Increased serum alanine aminotransferase (2%), increased serum aspartate aminotransferase (2%), hepatitis (<2%)

Hypersensitivity: Angioedema (<2%), hypersensitivity (<2%)

Immunologic: Immune reconstitution syndrome (<2%)

Neuromuscular & skeletal: Myalgia (<2%), osteonecrosis (<2%)

Renal: Increased serum creatinine (≤4%)

Mechanism of Action Darunavir binds to the site of HIV-1 protease activity and inhibits cleavage of viral Gag-Pol polyprotein precursors into individual functional proteins required for infectious HIV. This results in the formation of immature, noninfectious viral particles. Cobicistat is a mechanism-based inhibitor of cytochrome P450 3A (CYP3A). Inhibition of CYP3A-mediated metabolism by cobicistat increases the systemic exposure of CYP3A substrates (eg, darunavir). Emtricitabine is a cytosine analogue and tenofovir alafenamide is converted intracellularly to tenofovir (adenosine nucleotide analog) and subsequently phosphorylated by cellular kinases to the active moiety, tenofovir diphosphate. Emtricitabine and tenofovir alafenamide interfere with HIV viral RNA-dependent DNA polymerase activities resulting in inhibition of viral replication.

Reproductive Considerations

The Health and Human Services (HHS) perinatal HIV guidelines do not recommend this fixed-dose combination for females living with HIV who are not yet pregnant but are trying to conceive (HHS [perinatal] 2019).

Refer to individual monographs for additional information.

Pregnancy Considerations

The Health and Human Services (HHS) perinatal HIV guidelines do not recommend this fixed-dose combination for pregnant females living with HIV who are antiretroviral-naive, who have had antiretroviral therapy (ART) in the past but are restarting, or who require a new ART regimen (due to poor tolerance or poor virologic response of current regimen). For females who become pregnant while taking this combination, consider altering the regimen, or continue with frequent monitoring if viral suppression is effective and the regimen is well tolerated (HHS [perinatal] 2019).

Refer to individual monographs for additional information.

- **Darunavir, Emtricitabine, Tenofovir Alafenamide, and Cobicistat** *see* Darunavir, Cobicistat, Emtricitabine, and Tenofovir Alafenamide *on page 442*
- **Darunavir Ethanolate** *see* Darunavir *on page 441*
- **Darzalex** *see* Daratumumab *on page 438*
- **Darzalex Faspro** *see* Daratumumab and Hyaluronidase *on page 439*
- **Darzalex/rHuPH20** *see* Daratumumab and Hyaluronidase *on page 439*
- **Dasabuvir, Ombitasvir, Paritaprevir, and Ritonavir** *see* Ombitasvir, Paritaprevir, Ritonavir, and Dasabuvir *on page 1136*

Dasatinib (da SA ti nib)

Brand Names: US Sprycel

Brand Names: Canada APO-Dasatinib; Sprycel

Pharmacologic Category Antineoplastic Agent, BCR-ABL Tyrosine Kinase Inhibitor; Antineoplastic Agent, Tyrosine Kinase Inhibitor

Use

Acute lymphoblastic leukemia:

Adult: Treatment of Philadelphia chromosome-positive (Ph+) acute lymphoblastic leukemia (ALL) in adult patients with resistance or intolerance to prior therapy.

Pediatric: Treatment of newly diagnosed Ph+ ALL (in combination with chemotherapy) in pediatric patients ≥1 year of age.

Chronic myeloid leukemia:

Adult: Treatment of newly diagnosed Ph+ chronic myeloid leukemia (CML) in chronic phase; treatment of chronic, accelerated, or myeloid or lymphoid blast phase Ph+ CML with resistance or intolerance to prior therapy, including imatinib.

Pediatric: Treatment of Ph+ CML in chronic phase in pediatric patients ≥1 year of age.

Local Anesthetic/Vasoconstrictor Precautions Dasatinib is one of the drugs confirmed to prolong the QT interval and is accepted as having a risk of causing torsade de pointes. The risk of drug-induced torsade de pointes is extremely low when a single QT interval prolonging drug is prescribed. In terms of epinephrine, it is not known what effect vasoconstrictors in the local anesthetic regimen will have in patients with a known history of congenital prolonged QT interval or in patients taking any medication that prolongs the QT interval. Until more information is obtained, it is suggested that the clinician consult with the physician prior to the use of a vasoconstrictor in suspected patients, and that the vasoconstrictor (epinephrine, mepivacaine and levonordefrin [Carbocaine® 2% with Neo-Cobefrin®]) be used with caution.

Effects on Dental Treatment Key adverse event(s) related to dental treatment: Mucositis/stomatitis, taste perversion.

Effects on Bleeding Bleeding was experienced in ≤9% of patients with ≤7% severe. Thrombocytopenia is prevalent. A medical consult is recommended.

Adverse Reactions Adverse reactions occurred in adults unless otherwise indicated.

≥10%:

Cardiovascular: Facial edema, peripheral edema

Central nervous system: Headache (adults and children: 12% to 33%), fatigue (adults: 8% to 26%; children: 10%), pain (11%)
Dermatologic: Skin rash (adults and children: 11% to 21%), pruritus (12%)
Endocrine & metabolic: Fluid retention (adults: 19% to 48%; children: 10%; cardiac-related: 9%)
Gastrointestinal: Diarrhea (adults: 17% to 31%; children: 21%), nausea (adults and children: 8% to 24%), vomiting (adults and children: 5% to 16%), abdominal pain (adults and children: 7% to 16%)
Hematologic & oncologic: Thrombocytopenia (grades 3/4: 22% to 85%), neutropenia (grades 3/4: 29% to 79%), anemia (grades 3/4: 13% to 74%), hemorrhage (8% to 26%; grades 3/4: 1% to 9%), febrile neutropenia (4% to 12%; grades 3/4: 4% to 12%)
Infection: Infection (9% to 14%)
Local: Localized edema (3% to 22%; superficial)
Neuromuscular & skeletal: Musculoskeletal pain (<22%), limb pain (children: 19%), myalgia (7% to 13%), arthralgia (adults and children: ≤13%)
Respiratory: Pleural effusion (5% to 28%), dyspnea (3% to 24%)
Miscellaneous: Fever (6% to 18%)

1% to <10%:
Cardiovascular: Cardiac conduction disturbance (7%), ischemic heart disease (4%), cardiac disorder (≤4%), edema (≤4%), pericardial effusion (≤4%), prolonged QT interval on ECG (≤1%), cardiac arrhythmia, chest pain, flushing, hypertension, palpitations, tachycardia
Central nervous system: Intracranial hemorrhage (≤3%), chills, depression, dizziness, drowsiness, insomnia, myasthenia, neuropathy, peripheral neuropathy
Dermatologic: Acne vulgaris, alopecia, dermatitis, eczema, hyperhidrosis, urticaria, xeroderma
Endocrine & metabolic: Growth suppression, hyperuricemia, weight gain, weight loss
Gastrointestinal: Constipation (10%), gastrointestinal hemorrhage (2% to 9%), abdominal distention, change in appetite, colitis (including neutropenic colitis), dysgeusia, dyspepsia, enterocolitis, gastritis, mucositis, stomatitis
Hematologic & oncologic: Bruise
Hepatic: Increased serum bilirubin (grades 3/4: ≤6%), increased serum alanine aminotransferase (grades 3/4: ≤5%), increased serum aspartate aminotransferase (grades 3/4: ≤4%), ascites (≤1%)
Infection: Herpes virus infection, sepsis
Neuromuscular & skeletal: Muscle spasm (5%), abnormal bone growth (children; epiphyses delayed fusion), asthenia, stiffness
Ophthalmic: Blurred vision, decreased visual acuity, dry eye syndrome, visual disturbance
Otic: Tinnitus
Renal: Increased serum creatinine (grades 3/4: ≤8%)
Respiratory: Pulmonary hypertension (≤5%), pulmonary edema (≤4%), cough, pneumonia, pneumonitis, pulmonary infiltrates, upper respiratory tract infection
Miscellaneous: Soft tissue injury (oral)

<1%, postmarketing, and/or case reports: Abnormal gait, abnormal platelet aggregation, abnormal T waves on ECG, acute coronary syndrome, acute pancreatitis, acute respiratory distress, amnesia, anal fissure, angina pectoris, anxiety, arthritis, asthma, ataxia, atrial fibrillation, atrial flutter, bronchospasm, bullous skin disease, cardiomegaly, cerebrovascular accident, cholecystitis, cholestasis, confusion, conjunctivitis, coronary artery disease, cor pulmonale, cranial nerve palsy (facial), decreased libido, deep vein thrombosis, dehydration, dementia, dermal ulcer, diabetes mellitus, dyschromia, dysphagia, embolism, emotional lability, epistaxis, equilibrium disturbance, erythema nodosum, esophagitis, fibrosis (dermal), fistula (anal), gastroesophageal reflux disease, gastrointestinal disease (protein wasting), gingival hemorrhage, gynecomastia (adults and children), hearing loss, hematoma, hematuria, hemoptysis, hemorrhage (ocular), hepatitis, hypercholesterolemia, hypersensitivity reaction, hypersensitivity angiitis, hyperthyroidism, hypoalbuminemia, hypotension, hypothyroidism, increased creatine phosphokinase, increased gamma-glutamyl transferase, increased lacrimation, increased pulmonary artery pressure, increased troponin, inflammation (panniculitis), interstitial pulmonary disease, intestinal obstruction, livedo reticularis, lymphadenopathy, lymphocytopenia, malaise, menstrual disease, myocarditis, nail disease, nephrotic syndrome, optic neuritis, osteonecrosis, osteopenia (children), ototoxicity (hemorrhage), palmar-plantar erythrodysesthesia, pancreatitis, pericarditis, petechia, photophobia, pleuropericarditis, prolongation P-R interval on ECG, proteinuria, pulmonary embolism, pure red cell aplasia, reactivation of HBV, renal failure syndrome, renal insufficiency, rhabdomyolysis, seizure, skin photosensitivity, Stevens-Johnson syndrome, Sweet's syndrome, syncope, tendonitis, thrombophlebitis, thrombosis, thrombotic microangiopathy, thyroiditis, transient ischemic attacks, tremor, tumor lysis syndrome, upper gastrointestinal tract ulcer, urinary frequency, uterine hemorrhage, vaginal hemorrhage, ventricular arrhythmia, ventricular tachycardia, vertigo, voice disorder

Mechanism of Action Dasatinib is a BCR-ABL tyrosine kinase inhibitor that targets most imatinib-resistant BCR-ABL mutations (except the T315I and F317V mutants) by distinctly binding to active and inactive ABL-kinase. Kinase inhibition halts proliferation of leukemia cells. It also inhibits SRC family (including SRC, LKC, YES, FYN); c-KIT, EPHA2 and platelet derived growth factor receptor (PDGFRβ).

Pharmacodynamics/Kinetics

Half-life Elimination Terminal: 3 to 5 hours (adults); 2 to 5 hours (pediatrics)

Time to Peak 0.5 to 6 hours

Reproductive Considerations

Females of reproductive potential should use effective contraception during treatment and for 30 days after the final dasatinib dose.

Pregnancy Considerations

Dasatinib crosses the placenta, with fetal plasma and amniotic concentrations comparable to maternal concentrations. Adverse effects, including hydrops fetalis and fetal leukopenia and thrombocytopenia have been reported following maternal exposure to dasatinib. Pregnant females are advised to avoid exposure to crushed or broken tablets.

Dental Health Professional Considerations See Local Anesthetic/Vasoconstrictor Precautions

◆ **Dasetta 1/35** *see* Ethinyl Estradiol and Norethindrone *on page 614*

◆ **Dasetta 7/7/7** *see* Ethinyl Estradiol and Norethindrone *on page 614*

◆ **Daunomycin** *see* DAUNOrubicin (Conventional) *on page 445*

◆ **Daunorubicin and Cytarabine Liposome** *see* Daunorubicin and Cytarabine (Liposomal) *on page 445*

◆ **DAUNOrubicin Citrate** *see* DAUNOrubicin (Liposomal) *on page 446*

◆ **DAUNOrubicin Citrate (Liposomal)** *see* DAUNOrubicin (Liposomal) *on page 446*

◆ **DAUNOrubicin Citrate Liposome** *see* DAUNOrubicin (Liposomal) *on page 446*

DAUNOrubicin (Conventional)

(daw noe ROO bi sin con VEN sha nal)

Brand Names: Canada Cerubidine

Pharmacologic Category Antineoplastic Agent, Anthracycline; Antineoplastic Agent, Topoisomerase II Inhibitor

Use

Acute lymphocytic leukemia: Treatment (remission induction) of acute lymphocytic leukemia (ALL) in children and adults (in combination with other chemotherapy)

Acute myeloid leukemia: Treatment (remission induction) of acute myeloid leukemia (AML) in adults (in combination with other chemotherapy)

Local Anesthetic/Vasoconstrictor Precautions No information available to require special precautions

Effects on Dental Treatment Key adverse event(s) related to dental treatment: Stomatitis and discoloration of saliva.

Effects on Bleeding Thrombocytopenia occurs with the nadir in 10-14 days and recovery in 21-28 days. A medical consult is suggested.

Adverse Reactions Frequency not defined.

>10%:

Cardiovascular: Cardiac failure (dose-related, may be delayed for 7 to 8 years after treatment), ECG abnormality (transient, generally asymptomatic and self-limiting; includes atrial premature contractions, ST segment changes on ECG, supraventricular tachycardia, ventricular premature contractions)

Dermatologic: Alopecia (reversible)

Gastrointestinal: Nausea (mild), stomatitis, vomiting (mild)

Genitourinary: Red urine discoloration

Hematologic & oncologic: Bone marrow depression (onset: 7 days; nadir: 10 to 14 days; recovery: 21 to 28 days; primarily leukopenia; anemia, thrombocytopenia)

Miscellaneous: Radiation recall phenomenon

1% to 10%:

Dermatologic: Discoloration of sweat

Endocrine & metabolic: Hyperuricemia

Gastrointestinal: Abdominal pain, diarrhea, discoloration of saliva, gastrointestinal ulcer

Local: Post-injection flare

Ophthalmic: Discoloration of tears

<1%, postmarketing, and/or case reports: Anaphylactoid reaction, cardiac arrhythmia, cardiomyopathy, hepatitis, hypersensitivity reaction (systemic; includes angioedema, dysphagia, dyspnea, pruritus, urticaria), increased serum bilirubin, increased serum transaminases, infertility, injection site reaction (includes injection site cellulitis, local thrombophlebitis, pain at injection site), leukemia (secondary), myocardial infarction, myocarditis, nail bed changes (pigmentation), nail disease (banding), onycholysis, pericarditis, skin rash, sterility, typhlitis (neutropenic)

Mechanism of Action Daunorubicin inhibits DNA and RNA synthesis by intercalation between DNA base pairs and by steric obstruction. Daunomycin intercalates at points of local uncoiling of the double helix. Although the exact mechanism is unclear, it appears that direct binding to DNA (intercalation) and inhibition of DNA repair (topoisomerase II inhibition) result in blockade of DNA and RNA synthesis and fragmentation of DNA.

Pharmacodynamics/Kinetics

Half-life Elimination Initial: 45 minutes; Terminal: 18.5 hours; Daunorubicinol plasma half-life: ~27 hours

Reproductive Considerations

Women of reproductive potential should avoid pregnancy.

Pregnancy Considerations

Daunorubicin crosses the placenta. Based on data from animal reproduction studies, in utero exposure to daunorubicin may cause fetal harm.

Daunorubicin and Cytarabine (Liposomal)

(daw noe ROO bi sin & sye TARE a been lye po SO mal)

Brand Names: US Vyxeos

Pharmacologic Category Antineoplastic Agent, Anthracycline; Antineoplastic Agent, Antimetabolite; Antineoplastic Agent, Antimetabolite (Pyrimidine Analog); Antineoplastic Agent, Topoisomerase II Inhibitor

Use Acute myeloid leukemia: Treatment of adults with newly-diagnosed therapy-related acute myeloid leukemia (t-AML) or AML with myelodysplasia-related changes (AML-MRC)

Local Anesthetic/Vasoconstrictor Precautions No information available to require special precautions

Effects on Dental Treatment No significant effects or complications reported

Effects on Bleeding Thrombocytopenia

Adverse Reactions

>10%:

Cardiovascular: Edema (51%), cardiac arrhythmia (30%), cardiotoxicity (20%), hypotension (20%), hypertension (18%), chest pain (17%)

Central nervous system: Headache (33%), fatigue (32%), sleep disorder (25%), chills (23%), dizziness (18%), delirium (16%), anxiety (14%)

Dermatologic: Skin rash (54%), pruritus (15%)

Endocrine & metabolic: Hyponatremia (grades 3/4: 6% to 14%)

Gastrointestinal: Diarrhea (≤66%), nausea (47%), colitis (≤45%), mucositis (44%), constipation (40%), abdominal pain (33%), decreased appetite (29%), vomiting (24%), hemorrhoids (11%)

Hematologic & oncologic: Anemia (100%), neutropenia (100%; grade 4 [prolonged]: 10% to 17%), thrombocytopenia (100%; grade 3 [prolonged]: 25% to 28%), hemorrhage (70%; grades 3 to 5: 10%), febrile neutropenia (68%; grades 3 to 5: 66%), petechia (11%)

Hypersensitivity: Transfusion reaction (11%)

Infection: Bacteremia (24%), fungal infection (18%), sepsis (11%)

Local: Injection site reaction (16%; includes catheter and device site)

Neuromuscular & skeletal: Musculoskeletal pain (38%)

Ophthalmic: Visual impairment (11%)

Renal: Renal insufficiency (11%)

Respiratory: Cough (33%), dyspnea (32%), pneumonia (26%), hypoxia (18%), upper respiratory tract infection (18%), pleural effusion (16%)

Miscellaneous: Fever (17%)

1% to 10%:

Central nervous system: Hallucination (<10%)

Endocrine & metabolic: Hypokalemia (grades 3/4: 6% to 9%), hypoalbuminemia (grades 3/4: 2% to 7%), abnormal alanine aminotransferase (grades 3/4: ≤5%)

Gastrointestinal: Dyspepsia (<10%)

Hepatic: Hyperbilirubinemia (grades 3/4: 2% to 6%)

Ophthalmic: Conjunctivitis (<10%), dry eye syndrome (<10%), eye irritation (<10%), eye pain (<10%), injected sclera (<10%), ocular hyperemia (<10%), periorbital edema (<10%), swelling of eye (<10%)

Otic: Deafness (<10%)

Respiratory: Pneumonitis (<10%)

Mechanism of Action

Daunorubicin and cytarabine (liposomal) is a combination product with a fixed 1:5 (daunorubicin:cytarabine) molar ratio; this ratio has been shown to have synergistic effects in killing leukemia cells in vitro and in animal models.

Daunorubicin (conventional) inhibits DNA and RNA synthesis by intercalation between DNA base pairs and by steric obstruction. Daunomycin intercalates at points of local uncoiling of the double helix. Although the exact mechanism is unclear, it appears that direct binding to DNA (intercalation) and inhibition of DNA repair (topoisomerase II inhibition) result in blockade of DNA and RNA synthesis and fragmentation of DNA. Cytarabine (conventional) is a pyrimidine analog and is incorporated into DNA; however, the primary action is inhibition of DNA polymerase resulting in decreased DNA synthesis and repair. The degree of cytotoxicity correlates linearly with incorporation into DNA; therefore, incorporation into the DNA is responsible for drug activity and toxicity. Cytarabine is specific for the S phase of the cell cycle (blocks progression from the G1 to the S phase).

Per animal data, liposomes are taken up intact by bone marrow cells (to a greater degree in leukemia cells versus normal bone marrow cells) and are degraded following cellular internalization, thus releasing cytarabine and daunorubicin within the cells.

Pharmacodynamics/Kinetics

Half-life Elimination 31.5 hours (daunorubicin); 40.4 hours (cytarabine) with >99% of drug(s) remaining encapsulated in the liposomes

Reproductive Considerations

Evaluate pregnancy status prior to use in women of reproductive potential; effective contraception should be used during therapy and for at least 6 months after the last dose. Male patients with female partners of reproductive potential should also use effective contraception during therapy and for at least 6 months after the last dose.

Pregnancy Considerations

Based on the mechanism of action, anecdotal data of cytarabine use in pregnant women, and data from animal reproduction studies, use of daunorubicin and cytarabine (liposomal) in pregnancy may cause fetal harm.

Also refer to individual monographs for additional information.

◆ **DAUNOrubicin Hydrochloride** *see* DAUNOrubicin (Conventional) *on page* 445

DAUNOrubicin (Liposomal)

(daw noe ROO bi sin lye po SO mal)

Pharmacologic Category Antineoplastic Agent, Anthracycline; Antineoplastic Agent, Topoisomerase II Inhibitor

Use

Kaposi sarcoma: First-line treatment of advanced HIV-associated Kaposi sarcoma

Limitation of use: Daunorubicin (liposomal) is not recommended in HIV-related Kaposi sarcoma which is less than advanced.

Local Anesthetic/Vasoconstrictor Precautions No information available to require special precautions

Effects on Dental Treatment Key adverse event(s) related to dental treatment: Stomatitis.

Effects on Bleeding Thrombocytopenia occurs with the nadir in 14 days and recovery in 21 days. A medical consult is recommended.

Adverse Reactions Frequency not always defined.

Cardiovascular: Edema (11%), chest pain (10%), angina pectoris (≤5%), atrial fibrillation (≤5%), cardiac arrest (≤5%), cardiac tamponade (≤5%), hypertension (≤5%), myocardial infarction (≤5%), palpitations (≤5%), pericardial effusion (≤5%), pulmonary hypertension (≤5%), sinus tachycardia (≤5%), supraventricular tachycardia (≤5%), syncope (≤5%), tachycardia (≤5%), ventricular premature contractions (≤5%), decreased left ventricular ejection fraction (3%; reduction of 20% to 25%), cardiomyopathy (cumulative, dose-related; total dose above 300 mg/m^2)

Central nervous system: Fatigue (49%), headache (25%), rigors (19%), neuropathy (13%), depression (10%), malaise (10%), dizziness (8%), insomnia (6%), abnormality in thinking (≤5%), amnesia (≤5%), anxiety (≤5%), ataxia (≤5%), confusion (≤5%), drowsiness (≤5%), emotional lability (≤5%), hallucination (≤5%), hypertonia (≤5%), meningitis (≤5%), seizure (≤5%)

Dermatologic: Diaphoresis (14%), alopecia (8%), pruritus (7%), folliculitis (≤5%), seborrhea (≤5%), xeroderma (≤5%)

Endocrine & metabolic: Dehydration (≤5%), hot flash (≤5%), increased thirst (≤5%)

Gastrointestinal: Nausea (54%), diarrhea (38%), abdominal pain (23%), anorexia (23%), vomiting (23%), stomatitis (10%), constipation (7%), tenesmus (5%), dental caries (≤5%), dysgeusia (≤5%), dysphagia (≤5%), gastritis (≤5%), gastrointestinal hemorrhage (≤5%), gingival hemorrhage (≤5%), hemorrhoids (≤5%), hiccups (≤5%), increased appetite (≤5%), melena (≤5%), xerostomia (≤5%)

Genitourinary: Dysuria (≤5%), nocturia (≤5%)

Hematologic & oncologic: Neutropenia (<1,000 cells/mm^3: 36%; grade 4: 15%), lymphadenopathy (≤5%), splenomegaly (≤5%), bone marrow depression (especially granulocytes; platelets and erythrocytes less effected), severe granulocytopenia (may be associated with fever and result in infection)

Hepatic: Hepatomegaly (≤5%)

Hypersensitivity: Hypersensitivity reaction (24%)

Infection: Opportunistic infection (40%; median time to first infection/illness: 214 days)

Local: Inflammation at injection site (≤5%)

Neuromuscular & skeletal: Back pain (16%), arthralgia (7%), myalgia (7%), abnormal gait (≤5%), hyperkinesia (≤5%), tremor (≤5%)

Ophthalmic: Visual disturbance (5%), conjunctivitis (≤5%), eye pain (≤5%)

Otic: Deafness (≤5%), otalgia (≤5%), tinnitus (≤5%)
Renal: Polyuria (≤5%)
Respiratory: Cough (28%), dyspnea (26%), rhinitis (12%), sinusitis (8%), flu-like symptoms (5%), hemoptysis (≤5%), increased bronchial secretions (≤5%), pulmonary infiltrates (≤5%)
Miscellaneous: Fever (47%), infusion-related reaction (14%; includes back pain, flushing, chest tightness)

Mechanism of Action Liposomal preparation of daunorubicin; liposomes have been shown to penetrate solid tumors more effectively, possibly because of their small size and longer circulation time. Once in tissues, daunorubicin is released (over time). Daunorubicin inhibits DNA and RNA synthesis by intercalation between DNA base pairs and by steric obstruction; and intercalates at points of local uncoiling of the double helix. Although the exact mechanism is unclear, it appears that direct binding to DNA (intercalation) and inhibition of DNA repair (topoisomerase II inhibition) result in blockade of DNA and RNA synthesis and fragmentation of DNA.

Pharmacodynamics/Kinetics

Half-life Elimination Distribution: 4.4 hours

Pregnancy Risk Factor D

Pregnancy Considerations Adverse events were observed in animal reproduction studies.

Product Availability DaunoXome has been discontinued in the US for more than 1 year.

- ◆ **Daunorubicin (Liposomal) and Cytarabine (Liposomal)** *see* Daunorubicin and Cytarabine (Liposomal) *on page 445*
- ◆ **Daurismo** *see* Glasdegib *on page 737*
- ◆ **Daxbia [DSC]** *see* Cephalexin *on page 322*
- ◆ **Dayhist Allergy 12 Hour Relief [OTC]** *see* Clemastine *on page 367*
- ◆ **Daypro** *see* Oxaprozin *on page 1152*
- ◆ **Daysee** *see* Ethinyl Estradiol and Levonorgestrel *on page 612*
- ◆ **Daytrana** *see* Methylphenidate *on page 997*
- ◆ **3 Day Vaginal [OTC]** *see* Clotrimazole (Topical) *on page 397*
- ◆ **Dayvigo** *see* Lemborexant *on page 883*
- ◆ **DayVigo** *see* Lemborexant *on page 883*
- ◆ **D-Care 100X** *see* Lidocaine and Epinephrine *on page 908*
- ◆ **D-Care DM2 [DSC]** *see* MetFORMIN *on page 983*
- ◆ **DCC-2618** *see* Ripretinib *on page 1330*
- ◆ **2′-DCF** *see* Pentostatin *on page 1214*
- ◆ **dCF** *see* Pentostatin *on page 1214*
- ◆ **DDAVP** *see* Desmopressin *on page 460*
- ◆ **DDAVP Rhinal Tube** *see* Desmopressin *on page 460*
- ◆ **ddI** *see* Didanosine *on page 492*
- ◆ **DDP** *see* CISplatin *on page 352*
- ◆ **1-Deamino-8-D-Arginine Vasopressin** *see* Desmopressin *on page 460*
- ◆ **Deblitane** *see* Norethindrone *on page 1117*
- ◆ **Decadron** *see* DexAMETHasone (Systemic) *on page 463*
- ◆ **Decapinol** *see* Delmopinol *on page 452*
- ◆ **Decara [OTC]** *see* Cholecalciferol *on page 344*

Decitabine (de SYE ta been)

Brand Names: US Dacogen

Pharmacologic Category Antineoplastic Agent, Antimetabolite; Antineoplastic Agent, DNA Methylation Inhibitor

Use Myelodysplastic syndromes: Treatment of myelodysplastic syndromes (MDS), including previously treated and untreated, de novo and secondary MDS of all French-American-British (FAB) subtypes (refractory anemia, refractory anemia with ringed sideroblasts, refractory anemia with excess blasts, refractory anemia with excess blasts in transformation, and chronic myelomonocytic leukemia) and intermediate-1, intermediate-2, and high-risk International Prognostic Scoring System (IPSS) groups

Local Anesthetic/Vasoconstrictor Precautions No information available to require special precautions

Effects on Dental Treatment Key adverse event(s) related to dental treatment: Oral mucosal petechiae, stomatitis, gingival bleeding, tongue ulceration, oral candidiasis, lip ulceration, mucosal inflammation, gingival pain have been reported.

Effects on Bleeding Gingival bleeding and oral mucosal petechiae have been reported with decitabine therapy as well as a high incidence (27% to 89%) of thrombocytopenia. A medical consult is recommended.

Adverse Reactions

>10%:

Cardiovascular: Edema (5% to 18%), heart murmur (16%), hypotension (6% to 11%), peripheral edema (25% to 27%)
Dermatologic: Cellulitis (9% to 12%), ecchymoses (9% to 22%), erythema of skin (5% to 14%), pallor (23%), pruritus (9% to 11%), skin lesion (5% to 11%), skin rash (11% to 19%)
Endocrine & metabolic: Hyperglycemia (6% to 33%), hyperkalemia (13%), hypoalbuminemia (24%), hypokalemia (12% to 22%), hypomagnesemia (5% to 24%), hyponatremia (19%)
Gastrointestinal: Abdominal pain (14%), anorexia (16% to 23%), constipation (30% to 35%), decreased appetite (8% to 16%), diarrhea (28% to 34%), dyspepsia (10% to 12%), nausea (40% to 42%), stomatitis (11% to 12%), vomiting (16% to 25%)
Hematologic & oncologic: Anemia (31% to 82%), febrile neutropenia (20% to 29%; grades 3/4: 23%), leukopenia (6% to 28%), lymphadenopathy (12%), neutropenia (38% to 90%; grades 3/4: 87%), oral mucosal petechiae (13%), petechia (12% to 39%), thrombocytopenia (27% to 89%; grades 3/4: 85%)
Hepatic: Hyperbilirubinemia (14%), increased serum alkaline phosphatase (11%)
Local: Localized tenderness (11%)
Nervous system: Anxiety (9% to 11%), chills (16%), confusion (8% to 12%), dizziness (18% to 21%), fatigue (46%), headache (23% to 28%), hypoesthesia (11%), insomnia (14% to 28%), lethargy (12%), pain (5% to 13%), rigors (22%)
Neuromuscular & skeletal: Arthralgia (17% to 20%), asthenia (15%), back pain (17% to 18%), limb pain (18% to 19%)
Respiratory: Cough (27% to 40%), dyspnea (29%), epistaxis (13%), pharyngitis (16%), pneumonia (20% to 22%), rales (8% to 14%)
Miscellaneous: Fever (6% to 53%)

1% to 10%:

Cardiovascular: Acute cardiorespiratory failure (<5%), acute myocardial infarction (<5%), atrial fibrillation (<5%), cardiac failure (5%), cardiomyopathy (<5%), chest discomfort (7%), chest pain (≤6%), chest wall pain (7%), hypertension (6%), pulmonary embolism (<5%), supraventricular tachycardia (<5%), tachycardia (8%)

Dermatologic: Alopecia (8%), catheter-site erythema (5%), excoriation of skin (5%), facial swelling (6%), night sweats (5%), urticaria (6%), xeroderma (8%)

Endocrine & metabolic: Decreased serum bicarbonate (5%), decreased serum total protein (5%), dehydration (6% to 8%), hypochloremia (6%), increased lactate dehydrogenase (8%), increased serum bicarbonate (6%), weight loss (9%)

Gastrointestinal: Abdominal distention (5%), cholecystitis (<5%), dysphagia (5% to 6%), gastroesophageal reflux disease (5%), gingival hemorrhage (8%), gingival pain (<5%), glossalgia (5%), hemorrhoids (8%), loose stools (7%), mucosal swelling (9%), oral candidiasis (6%), oral changes (soft tissue: 6%), oral mucosa ulcer (lip: 5%), tongue ulcer (7%), toothache (6%), upper abdominal pain (5% to 6%)

Genitourinary: Dysuria (6%), urethral bleeding (<5%), urinary frequency (5%), urinary tract infection (7%)

Hematologic & oncologic: Bone marrow depression (<5%), hematoma (5%), pancytopenia (5%), postprocedural hemorrhage (<5%), splenomegaly (<5%), thrombocythemia (5%), upper gastrointestinal hemorrhage (<5%)

Hepatic: Ascites (10%), decreased serum bilirubin (5%), increased serum aspartate aminotransferase (10%)

Hypersensitivity: Anaphylaxis (<5%), hypersensitivity reaction (<5%), transfusion reaction (7%)

Infection: Abscess (peridiverticular, <5%), bacteremia (5%), candidiasis (10%), fungal infection (<5%), sepsis (<5%), staphylococcal bacteremia (8%), staphylococcal infection (7%), tooth abscess (5%)

Local: Catheter infection (8%), catheter pain (5%), catheter site hemorrhage (<5%), swelling at injection site (5%)

Nervous system: Depression (9%), falling (8%), intracranial hemorrhage (<5%), malaise (5%), mental status changes (<5%), mouth pain (5%), myasthenia (5%)

Neuromuscular & skeletal: Muscle spasm (7%), musculoskeletal pain (≤6%; includes discomfort), myalgia (5% to 9%), ostealgia (6%)

Ophthalmic: Blurred vision (6%)

Otic: Otalgia (6%)

Renal: Acute renal failure (<5%), increased blood urea nitrogen (10%)

Respiratory: Abnormal breath sounds (5% to 10%), hemoptysis (<5%), hypoxia (10%), mycobacterium avium complex (<5%), paranasal sinus congestion (5%), pharyngolaryngeal pain (8%), pleural effusion (5%), post nasal drip (5%), pulmonary aspergillosis (<5%), pulmonary edema (6%), pulmonary infection (pseudomonas: <5%), pulmonary infiltrates (<5%), pulmonary signs and symptoms (crepitations: 5%), respiratory tract infection (<5%), sinusitis (5% to 6%), upper respiratory tract infection (10%)

Miscellaneous: Mass (pulmonary, <5%), postoperative pain (<5%)

Frequency not defined: Hepatic: Abnormal hepatic function tests

Postmarketing:

Dermatologic: Sweet's syndrome (acute febrile neutrophilic dermatosis)

Hematologic & oncologic: Differentiation syndrome

Mechanism of Action Decitabine is a hypomethylating agent. After phosphorylation, decitabine is incorporated into DNA and inhibits DNA methyltransferase causing hypomethylation and subsequent cell death (within the S-phase of the cell cycle).

Pharmacodynamics/Kinetics

Half-life Elimination ~0.5 to 0.6 hours

Reproductive Considerations

Evaluate pregnancy status prior to therapy. Females of reproductive potential should use effective contraception during treatment and for 6 months after the last decitabine dose. Males with female partners of reproductive potential should use effective contraception during treatment and for 3 months after the last decitabine dose.

Pregnancy Considerations

Based on the mechanism of action and information from animal reproduction studies, decitabine may cause fetal harm if exposure occurs during pregnancy. Information related to the use of decitabine in pregnancy is limited.

Decitabine and Cedazuridine

(de SYE ta been & SED az URE i deen)

Brand Names: US Inqovi

Pharmacologic Category Antineoplastic Agent, Antimetabolite; Antineoplastic Agent, DNA Methylation Inhibitor; Cytidine Deaminase Inhibitor

Use Myelodysplastic syndromes: Treatment of myelodysplastic syndromes (MDS), including previously treated and untreated, de novo and secondary MDS with the following French-American-British subtypes (refractory anemia, refractory anemia with ringed sideroblasts, refractory anemia with excess blasts, and chronic myelomonocytic leukemia [CMML]) and intermediate-1, intermediate-2, and high-risk International Prognostic Scoring System groups, in adults.

Local Anesthetic/Vasoconstrictor Precautions No information available to require special precautions.

Effects on Dental Treatment No significant effects or complications reported.

Effects on Bleeding Bone marrow suppression: Fatal and serious myelosuppression can occur with decitabine and cedazuridine. New or worsening thrombocytopenia (including grades 3 or 4) occurred commonly. A medical consult is recommended for patients under active treatment with this drug.

Mechanism of Action

Decitabine is a hypomethylating agent. After phosphorylation, decitabine is incorporated into DNA and inhibits DNA methyltransferase causing hypomethylation and subsequent cell death (within the S-phase of the cell cycle). Hypomethylation in cancer cells may restore normal function to genes that are necessary for control of cellular differentiation and proliferation.

Cedazuridine is a cytidine deaminase (CDA) inhibitor. CDA is an enzyme that catalyzes the degradation of cytidine, including the cytidine analog decitabine; high CDA levels in the GI tract and liver degrade decitabine and limit its oral bioavailability. The combination of cedazuridine with decitabine increases systemic decitabine exposure.

Pharmacodynamics/Kinetics

Half-life Elimination Decitabine: 1.5 hours; Cedazuridine: 6.7 hours.

Time to Peak Decitabine: 1 hour (range: 0.3 to 3 hours); Cedazuridine: 3 hours (range: 1.5 to 6.1 hours).

Reproductive Considerations

Evaluate pregnancy status prior to use in females of reproductive potential.

Females of reproductive potential should use effective contraception during therapy and for 6 months after the last dose of decitabine/cedazuridine. Males with female partners of reproductive potential should use effective contraception during therapy and for 3 months after the last decitabine/cedazuridine dose.

Pregnancy Considerations Based on the mechanism of action, data from animal reproduction studies, as well as limited human data, in utero exposure to decitabine/cedazuridine may cause fetal harm.

Product Availability Inqovi: FDA approved July 2020; anticipated availability currently unknown.

- **Decitabine/Cedazuridine** *see* Decitabine and Cedazuridine *on page 448*
- **Decongestant 12Hour Max St [OTC]** *see* Pseudoephedrine *on page 1291*

Defibrotide (DE fib ro tide)

Brand Names: US Defitelio

Brand Names: Canada Defitelio

Pharmacologic Category Antiplatelet Agent; Thrombolytic Agent

Use Hepatic sinusoidal obstruction syndrome (treatment): Treatment of hepatic sinusoidal obstruction syndrome (SOS; formerly called veno-occlusive disease [VOD]) with renal or pulmonary dysfunction following hematopoietic stem cell transplant (HSCT).

Local Anesthetic/Vasoconstrictor Precautions No information available to require special precautions

Effects on Dental Treatment Key adverse event(s) related to dental treatment: Increased bleeding with invasive procedures (see Effects on Bleeding)

Effects on Bleeding Defibrotide has antiplatelet and fibrinolytic properties; expect increased bleeding with invasive dental procedures; medical consult is recommended

Adverse Reactions

>10%:

Cardiovascular: Hypotension (11% to 37%)
Gastrointestinal: Diarrhea (24%), vomiting (18%), nausea (16%)
Hematologic & oncologic: Hemorrhage (59%; any type)
Respiratory: Epistaxis (14%)

1% to 10%:

Central nervous system: Intracranial hemorrhage (3%), cerebral hemorrhage (2%)
Endocrine & metabolic: Hyperuricemia (2%)
Gastrointestinal: Gastrointestinal hemorrhage (9%)
Hematologic & oncologic: Pulmonary hemorrhage (4%)
Hypersensitivity: Hypersensitivity reaction (<2%)
Immunologic: Graft versus host disease (6%)
Infection: Sepsis (7%), infection (3%)
Respiratory: Pulmonary alveolar hemorrhage (7% to 9%), pulmonary infiltrates (6%), pneumonia (5%)

Frequency not defined:

Cardiovascular: Thrombophlebitis
Endocrine & metabolic: Hot flash
Gastrointestinal: Abdominal cramps, abdominal pain, bloody diarrhea, hematemesis
Genitourinary: Hematuria
Hematologic & oncologic: Oral hemorrhage
Renal: Renal failure
Miscellaneous: Fever

Mechanism of Action Defibrotide augments plasmin enzymatic activity to hydrolyze fibrin clots. It reduces endothelial cell (EC) activation and increases EC-mediated fibrinolysis by increasing tissue plasminogen activator and thrombomodulin expression, as well as by decreasing von Willebrand factor and plasminogen activator inhibitor-1 expression.

Pharmacodynamics/Kinetics

Half-life Elimination <2 hours

Pregnancy Considerations Adverse effects have been observed in animal reproduction studies.

- **Defibrotide Sodium** *see* Defibrotide *on page 449*
- **Defitelio** *see* Defibrotide *on page 449*

Deflazacort (de FLAZE a kort)

Brand Names: US Emflaza

Pharmacologic Category Corticosteroid, Systemic

Use Duchenne muscular dystrophy: Treatment of Duchenne muscular dystrophy (DMD) in patients ≥2 years of age.

Local Anesthetic/Vasoconstrictor Precautions No information available to require special precautions

Effects on Dental Treatment No significant effects or complications reported

Effects on Bleeding No information available to require special precautions

Adverse Reactions

>10%:

Dermatologic: Erythema (8% to 28%)
Endocrine & metabolic: Cushingoid appearance (33% to 60%), hirsutism (10% to 35%), weight gain (20% to 28%), obesity (central, 10% to 25%)
Gastrointestinal: Abdominal pain (including upper abdominal pain: 18%), increased appetite (14%)
Genitourinary: Pollakiuria (12% to 15%)
Respiratory: Cough (12%), upper respiratory tract infection (12%)

1% to 10%:

Cardiovascular: Cardiac arrhythmia (≥1%)
Central nervous system: Irritability (8% to 10%), abnormal behavior (9%), psychomotor agitation (6%), aggressive behavior (≥1%), depression (≥1%), dizziness (≥1%), emotional disturbance (≥1%), emotional lability (≥1%), heat exhaustion (≥1%), hypertonia (≥1%, hypertonic bladder), insomnia (≥1%), mood changes (≥1%), sleep disorder (≥1%)
Dermatologic: Skin rash (7%), atrophic striae (6%), acneiform eruption (≥1%), acne vulgaris (≥1%), alopecia (≥1%), impetigo (≥1%)
Endocrine & metabolic: Glycosuria (≥1%), hot flash (≥1%), increased thirst (≥1%)
Gastrointestinal: Constipation (10%), abdominal distress (6%), nausea (6%), dyspepsia (≥1%), gastrointestinal disease (≥1%)
Genitourinary: Dysuria (≥1%), testicular pain (≥1%), urinary tract infection (≥1%), urine discoloration (≥1%)
Hematologic & oncologic: Bruise (6%)
Infection: Influenza (≥1%), tooth abscess (≥1%), viral infection (≥1%)
Neuromuscular & skeletal: Back pain (7%), back injury (≥1%), limb pain (≥1%), muscle spasm (≥1%), myalgia (≥1%), neck pain (≥1%)

Ophthalmic: Hordeolum (≥1%), increased lacrimation (≥1%)
Otic: Otitis externa (≥1%)
Respiratory: Nasopharyngitis (10%), rhinorrhea (8%), epistaxis (6%), hypoventilation (≥1%), pharyngitis (≥1%)
Miscellaneous: Fever (9%), accidental injury (≥1%, face), mass (≥1%, neck)

Frequency not defined.
Central nervous system: Myasthenia (associated with long-term use)
Neuromuscular & skeletal: Bone fracture (long bones including the fibula as well as greenstick fractures), decreased bone mineral density, osteopenia (associated with long-term use), tendon disease (associated with long-term use)

<1%, postmarketing, and/or case reports: Abnormal serum calcium (negative calcium balance), acute pancreatitis (especially in children), acute peptic ulcer with hemorrhage and perforation, amyotrophy, anaphylaxis, anxiety, avascular necrosis of bones, carbohydrate intolerance, change in serum protein (negative protein balance), chorioretinitis, cognitive dysfunction (including confusion, amnesia, delusions, hallucinations, mania, or suicidal thoughts), corneal thinning, decreased serum potassium, edema, exacerbation of epilepsy, hemorrhage, hypersensitivity, hypokalemic alkalosis, increased intracranial pressure (with papilledema in children), leukocytosis, negative nitrogen balance, peptic ulcer, pseudotumor cerebri, scleral thinning, thromboembolism (especially in patients with underlying conditions associated with increased thrombotic tendency), toxic epidermal necrolysis, vertebral compression fracture, vertigo, wound healing impairment

Mechanism of Action Deflazacort is a corticosteroid prodrug; its active metabolite, 21-desDFZ, acts on the glucocorticoid receptor to exert anti-inflammatory and immunosuppressive effects. The precise mechanism by which deflazacort exerts its therapeutic effects in patients with Duchenne muscular dystrophy is unknown.

Pharmacodynamics/Kinetics

Time to Peak 1 hour (range: 0.25 to 2 hours); delayed by 1 hour with a high-fat meal

Pregnancy Considerations Deflazacort crosses the placenta. Orofacial clefts, intrauterine growth restriction, and decreased birth weight have been reported following maternal use. Hypoadrenalism may occur in newborns following maternal use of corticosteroids in pregnancy; monitor.

◆ **Deflazacorte** *see* Deflazacort *on page* 449

Degarelix (deg a REL ix)

Brand Names: US Firmagon; Firmagon (240 MG Dose)

Brand Names: Canada Firmagon

Pharmacologic Category Antineoplastic Agent, Gonadotropin-Releasing Hormone Antagonist; Gonadotropin Releasing Hormone Antagonist

Use Prostate cancer, advanced: Treatment of advanced prostate cancer

Local Anesthetic/Vasoconstrictor Precautions Degarelix may prolong QT interval; it is suggested that the clinician consult with the physician prior to use of vasoconstrictor in suspected patients; use vasoconstrictor (epinephrine, mepivacaine and levonordefrin [Carbocaine® 2% with Neo-Cobefrin®]) with caution.

Effects on Dental Treatment No significant effects or complications reported

Effects on Bleeding No information available to require special precautions

Adverse Reactions

>10%:
Endocrine & metabolic: Hot flash (26%), increased gamma-glutamyl transferase (≥10%)
Hepatic: Increased serum transaminases (≥10%)
Local: Injection site reaction (35%; including erythema at injection site [17%], induration at injection site [4%], injection site nodule [3%], pain at injection site [28%], swelling at injection site [6%])

1% to 10%:
Cardiovascular: Hypertension (6%)
Dermatologic: Diaphoresis (≥1%)
Endocrine & metabolic: Gynecomastia (≥1%), weight gain (9%)
Gastrointestinal: Constipation (5%), diarrhea, (≥1%), nausea (1% to <5%)
Genitourinary: Erectile dysfunction (≥1%), testicular atrophy (≥1%), urinary tract infection (5%)
Immunologic: Antibody development (antidegarelix: 10%)
Nervous system: Chills (5%), dizziness (1% to <5%), fatigue (1% to <5%), headache (1% to <5%), insomnia (1% to <5%)
Neuromuscular & skeletal: Arthralgia (5%), asthenia (1% to <5%), back pain (6%)
Miscellaneous: Fever (1% to <5%), night sweats (1% to <5%)

<1%: Cardiovascular: Prolonged QT interval on ECG

Frequency not defined: Hepatic: Abnormal liver function tests

Postmarketing: Hypersensitivity: Hypersensitivity reaction (including anaphylaxis, urticaria, and angioedema)

Mechanism of Action Gonadotropin-releasing hormone (GnRH) antagonist which reversibly binds to GnRH receptors in the anterior pituitary gland, blocking the receptor and decreasing secretion of luteinizing hormone (LH) and follicle stimulation hormone (FSH), resulting in rapid androgen deprivation by decreasing testosterone production, thereby decreasing testosterone levels. Testosterone levels do not exhibit an initial surge, or flare, as is typical with GnRH agonists (Crawford 2011).

Pharmacodynamics/Kinetics

Onset of Action Rapid; ~96% of patients had testosterone levels ≤50 ng/dL within 3 days (Klotz 2008)

Half-life Elimination Loading dose: SubQ: ~53 days; Maintenance dose: SubQ: ~31 days (Canadian labeling)

Time to Peak Plasma: Loading dose: SubQ: Within 2 days

Reproductive Considerations Degarelix may impair fertility in males and females (based on the mechanism of action). Use of degarelix for ovarian suppression is under study (Dellapasqua 2019; Papanikolaou 2018).

Pregnancy Considerations Based on the mechanism of action and data from animal reproduction studies, in utero exposure to degarelix may cause fetal harm.

Dental Health Professional Considerations See Local Anesthetic/Vasoconstrictor Precautions

◆ **Degarelix Acetate** *see* Degarelix *on page* 450
◆ **Degludec Insulin** *see* Insulin Degludec *on page* 819
◆ **Degludec Insulin and Liraglutide** *see* Insulin Degludec and Liraglutide *on page* 820

◆ **Dehydrobenzperidol** *see* Droperidol *on page 534*

Delafloxacin (del a FLOKS a sin)

Brand Names: US Baxdela

Pharmacologic Category Antibiotic, Fluoroquinolone

Use

Pneumonia, community-acquired: Treatment of adults with community-acquired bacterial pneumonia caused by the following susceptible microorganisms: *Streptococcus pneumoniae, Staphylococcus aureus* (methicillin-susceptible isolates), *Klebsiella pneumoniae, Escherichia coli, Pseudomonas aeruginosa, Haemophilus influenzae, Haemophilus parainfluenzae, Legionella pneumophila, Mycoplasma pneumoniae,* and *Chlamydophila pneumoniae.*

Skin and skin structure infection: Treatment of acute bacterial skin and skin structure infection caused by susceptible isolates of *S. aureus* (including methicillin-resistant and methicillin-susceptible isolates), *Staphylococcus haemolyticus, Staphylococcus lugdunensis, Streptococcus agalactiae, Streptococcus anginosus* group (including *Streptococcus anginosus, Streptococcus intermedius,* and *Streptococcus constellatus*), *Streptococcus pyogenes, Enterococcus faecalis, E. coli, Enterobacter cloacae, K. pneumoniae,* and *P. aeruginosa.*

Local Anesthetic/Vasoconstrictor Precautions No information available to require special precautions

Effects on Dental Treatment Key adverse event(s) related to dental treatment: Oral candidiasis has been reported, particularly with prolonged use of delafloxacin

Effects on Bleeding No information available to require special precautions

Adverse Reactions

1% to 10%:

Cardiovascular: Bradycardia (<2%), flushing (<2%), hypertension (<2%), hypotension (<2%), palpitations (<2%), presyncope (<2%), sinus tachycardia (<2%), syncope (<2%), ventricular premature contractions (<2%)

Central nervous system: Headache (3%), abnormal dreams (<2%), agitation (<2%), anxiety (<2%), confusion (<2%), dizziness (<2%), hypoesthesia (<2%), insomnia (<2%), paresthesia (<2%), vertigo (<2%)

Dermatologic: Dermatitis (<2%), pruritus (<2%), skin rash (<2%), urticaria (<2%)

Endocrine & metabolic: Hyperglycemia (<2%), hypoglycemia (<2%)

Gastrointestinal: Nausea (8%), diarrhea (5% to 8%), vomiting (2%), abdominal pain (<2%), *Clostridioides difficile* associated diarrhea (<2%), dysgeusia (<2%), dyspepsia (<2%), oral candidiasis (<2%)

Genitourinary: Vulvovaginal candidiasis (<2%)

Hematologic & oncologic: Agranulocytosis (<2%), anemia (<2%), leukopenia (<2%), neutropenia (<2%), pancytopenia (<2%)

Hepatic: Increased serum transaminases (3% to 5%), increased serum alkaline phosphatase (<2%)

Hypersensitivity: Hypersensitivity reaction (<2%)

Infection: Fungal infection (<2%)

Neuromuscular & skeletal: Increased creatine phosphokinase in blood specimen (<2%), myalgia (<2%)

Ophthalmic: Blurred vision (<2%)

Otic: Tinnitus (<2%), vestibular disturbance (<2%)

Renal: Increased serum creatinine (<2%), renal failure syndrome (<2%), renal insufficiency (<2%)

Miscellaneous: Infusion related reaction (<2%)

Frequency not defined:

Central nervous system: Central nervous system disease, exacerbation of myasthenia gravis, peripheral neuropathy

Neuromuscular & skeletal: Rupture of tendon, tendonitis

Mechanism of Action Delafloxacin inhibits DNA gyrase (topoisomerase II) and topoisomerase IV enzymes, which are required for bacterial DNA replication, transcription, repair, and recombination.

Pharmacodynamics/Kinetics

Half-life Elimination IV: 3.7 hours (single dose); Oral: 4.2 to 8.5 hours (multiple dose)

Time to Peak ~1 hour

Pregnancy Considerations Adverse events were observed in some animal reproduction studies.

◆ **Delafloxacin Meglumine** *see* Delafloxacin *on page 451*

◆ **Delatestryl** *see* Testosterone *on page 1425*

Delavirdine (de la VIR deen)

Related Information

HIV Infection and AIDS *on page 1690*

Brand Names: US Rescriptor [DSC]

Brand Names: Canada Rescriptor [DSC]

Pharmacologic Category Antiretroviral, Reverse Transcriptase Inhibitor, Non-nucleoside (Anti-HIV)

Use HIV-1 infection: Treatment of HIV-1 infection in combination with at least two additional antiretroviral agents. **Note:** Delavirdine is no longer recommended for use in the treatment of HIV (HHS [adult] 2019).

Local Anesthetic/Vasoconstrictor Precautions No information available to require special precautions

Effects on Dental Treatment No significant effects or complications reported

Effects on Bleeding No reports of bleeding or thrombocytopenia.

Adverse Reactions Frequency not always defined. Frequency of adverse reactions reported from occurrence in clinical trials with delavirdine when used as part of combination antiretroviral therapy.

Cardiovascular: Cardiac arrhythmia, cardiac insufficiency, cardiac rate disturbance, cardiomyopathy, hypersensitivity angiitis, hypertension, orthostatic hypotension, peripheral vascular disease

Central nervous system: Headache (19% to 20%), depression (10% to 15%), anxiety (6% to 8%), cognitive dysfunction, confusion, emotional lability, hallucination, paralysis, vertigo

Dermatologic: Skin rash (16% to 32%), desquamation, erythema multiforme, fungal dermatitis, Stevens-Johnson syndrome

Endocrine & metabolic: Increased serum transaminases (2% to 5%), increased amylase (3%), increased serum bilirubin (2%), hyperglycemia, hyperkalemia, hypertriglyceridemia, hyperuricemia, hypocalcemia, hyponatremia, hypophosphatemia, increased gamma-glutamyl transferase, menstrual disease, redistribution of body fat

Gastrointestinal: Nausea (20% to 25%), vomiting (3% to 11%), abdominal pain (4% to 6%), anorexia, bloody stools, colitis, diarrhea, diverticulitis, fecal incontinence, gastroenteritis, gastrointestinal hemorrhage, gingival hemorrhage, increased serum lipase, pancreatitis, vomiting

Genitourinary: Hematuria, urinary tract infection

Hematologic & oncologic: Decreased hemoglobin (1% to 3%), prolonged prothrombin time (2%), adenopathy, bruise, eosinophilia, granulocytosis, leukopenia, pancytopenia, purpura, spleen disease, thrombocytopenia
Hepatic: Hepatomegaly, increased serum alkaline phosphatase, jaundice
Hypersensitivity: Angioedema, hypersensitivity reaction
Infection: Abscess, candidiasis (oral/vaginal), infection
Neuromuscular & skeletal: Ostealgia, tetany
Ophthalmic: Conjunctivitis
Renal: Increased serum creatinine, nephrolithiasis, renal pain
Respiratory: Bronchitis (6% to 8%), chest congestion, dyspnea, pneumonia
Miscellaneous: Fever (4% to 12%)
<1%, postmarketing and/or case reports: Acute renal failure, hemolytic anemia, hepatic failure, immune reconstitution syndrome, rhabdomyolysis

Mechanism of Action Delavirdine binds directly to reverse transcriptase, blocking RNA-dependent and DNA-dependent DNA polymerase activities

Pharmacodynamics/Kinetics

Half-life Elimination 5.8 hours (range: 2 to 11 hours)

Time to Peak Plasma: 1 hour

Reproductive Considerations

Based on the Health and Humans Services (HHS) perinatal HIV guidelines, delavirdine is not one of the recommended antiretroviral agents for use in females who are trying to conceive.

For males and females living with HIV and planning a pregnancy, maximum viral suppression below the limits of detection with antiretroviral therapy (ART), modification of therapy (if needed), optimization of the woman's health, and a discussion of the potential risks and benefits of ART therapy during pregnancy is recommended prior to conception (HHS [perinatal] 2019).

Pregnancy Considerations

Outcome information specific to delavirdine use in pregnancy is no longer being reviewed and updated in the Health and Humans Services (HHS) perinatal guidelines. Maternal antiretroviral therapy (ART) may be associated with adverse pregnancy outcomes including preterm delivery, stillbirth, low birth weight, and small for gestational age infants. Actual risks may be influenced by maternal factors such as disease severity, gestational age at initiation of therapy, and specific ART regimen, therefore close fetal monitoring is recommended. Because there is clear benefit to appropriate treatment, maternal ART should not be withheld due to concerns for adverse neonatal outcomes. Long-term follow-up is recommended for all infants exposed to antiretroviral medications; children without HIV but who were exposed to ART in utero and develop significant organ system abnormalities of unknown etiology (particularly of the CNS or heart) should be evaluated for potential mitochondrial dysfunction. Hypersensitivity reactions (including hepatic toxicity and rash) are more common in women on non-nucleoside reverse transcriptase inhibitor therapy; it is not known if pregnancy increases this risk.

Based on the HHS perinatal HIV guidelines, delavirdine is not one of the recommended antiretroviral agents for use during pregnancy.

In general, ART is recommended for all pregnant females living with HIV to keep the viral load below the limit of detection and reduce the risk of perinatal transmission. Therapy should be individualized following a discussion of the potential risks and benefits of treatment during pregnancy. Monitoring of pregnant females is more frequent than in nonpregnant adults. ART should be continued postpartum for all females living with HIV and can be modified after delivery.

Health care providers are encouraged to enroll pregnant females exposed to antiretroviral medications as early in pregnancy as possible in the Antiretroviral Pregnancy Registry (1-800-258-4263 or http://www.-APRegistry.com). Health care providers caring for pregnant females living with HIV and their infants may contact the National Perinatal HIV Hotline (888-448-8765) for clinical consultation (HHS [perinatal] 2019).

◆ **Delestrogen** *see* Estradiol (Systemic) *on page 596*

Delmopinol (del MOE pi nol)

Brand Names: US Decapinol

Pharmacologic Category Antibacterial, Oral Rinse

Local Anesthetic/Vasoconstrictor Precautions
No information available to require special precautions

Effects on Dental Treatment No significant effects or complications reported

Mechanism of Action Reduces adhesion of plaque-causing bacteria, reducing the formation of new plaque and promoting the removal of deposits with normal mechanical disruption (brushing and flossing). Ultimately causes a reduction in both plaque and gingivitis. Decapinol® is regulated as a medical device because the primary mode of action is to serve as a physical barrier without chemical activity.

Pregnancy Risk Factor The manufacturer does not recommend use in pregnant women.

◆ **Delmopinol Hydrochloride** *see* Delmopinol *on page 452*

◆ **Delstrigo** *see* Doravirine, Lamivudine, and Tenofovir Disoproxil Fumarate *on page 514*

◆ **Delsym [OTC]** *see* Dextromethorphan *on page 476*

◆ **Delsym Cough Childrens [OTC]** *see* Dextromethorphan *on page 476*

◆ **Delta-9-tetrahydro-cannabinol** *see* Dronabinol *on page 532*

◆ **Delta-9-Tetrahydrocannabinol and Cannabinol** *see* Tetrahydrocannabinol and Cannabidiol *on page 1434*

◆ **Delta-9 THC** *see* Dronabinol *on page 532*

◆ **Delta- Aminolevulinic Acid Hydrochloride** *see* Aminolevulinic Acid (Topical) *on page 117*

◆ **Deltacortisone** *see* PredniSONE *on page 1260*

◆ **Delta D3 [OTC]** *see* Cholecalciferol *on page 344*

◆ **Deltadehydrocortisone** *see* PredniSONE *on page 1260*

◆ **Deltasone** *see* PredniSONE *on page 1260*

◆ **Delyla** *see* Ethinyl Estradiol and Levonorgestrel *on page 612*

◆ **Delzicol** *see* Mesalamine *on page 980*

◆ **Demadex** *see* Torsemide *on page 1467*

◆ **Demadex [DSC]** *see* Torsemide *on page 1467*

◆ **Demerol** *see* Meperidine *on page 966*

◆ **Demulen** *see* Ethinyl Estradiol and Ethynodiol Diacetate *on page 611*

◆ **Denavir** *see* Penciclovir *on page 1207*

Denosumab (den OH sue mab)

Related Information

Osteonecrosis of the Jaw *on page 1699*

Brand Names: US Prolia; Xgeva

Brand Names: Canada Prolia; Xgeva

Generic Availability (US) No

Pharmacologic Category Bone-Modifying Agent; Monoclonal Antibody

Use

Bone metastases from solid tumors (Xgeva): Prevention of skeletal-related events in patients with bone metastases from solid tumors.

Giant cell tumor of bone (Xgeva): Treatment of giant cell tumor of bone (in adults and skeletally mature adolescents) that is unresectable or where surgical resection is likely to result in severe morbidity.

Hypercalcemia of malignancy (Xgeva): Treatment of hypercalcemia of malignancy refractory to bisphosphonate therapy.

Multiple myeloma (Xgeva): Prevention of skeletal-related events in patients with multiple myeloma.

Osteoporosis/bone loss (Prolia): Treatment of osteoporosis in postmenopausal females at high risk of fracture; treatment of osteoporosis (to increase bone mass) in males at high risk of fracture; treatment of bone loss (to increase bone mass) in males receiving androgen-deprivation therapy for nonmetastatic prostate cancer; treatment of bone loss (to increase bone mass) in females receiving aromatase inhibitor therapy for breast cancer; treatment of glucocorticoid-induced osteoporosis in patients at high risk of fracture who are initiating or continuing systemic glucocorticoids at a daily dose equivalent to ≥7.5 mg of prednisone for an anticipated duration of at least 6 months (high risk defined as osteoporotic fracture history, multiple risk factors for fracture, or failure of or intolerance to other available osteoporosis therapy).

Local Anesthetic/Vasoconstrictor Precautions No information available to require special precautions

Effects on Dental Treatment Cases of osteonecrosis of the jaw bone (ONJ) have been associated with denosumab exposure. ONJ presents clinically as exposed necrotic bone of at least 8 weeks duration with or without the presence of pain, infection, or previous trauma in a patient who has not received radiation to the jaws. Since ONJ is also associated with bisphosphonate exposure, and osteoclasts are the common targets of bisphosphonates and denosumab, osteoclastic inhibition may play a central role in ONJ associated with these two classes of drugs. Patients developing ONJ while on denosumab therapy should receive care by an oral surgeon. See Warnings/Precautions and Dental Health Professional Considerations.

Effects on Bleeding No information available to require special precautions

Adverse Reactions Percentages noted with Prolia (60 mg every 6 months) or Xgeva (120 mg every 4 weeks).

>10%:

Cardiovascular: Peripheral edema (Xgeva: 17% to 24%; Prolia: 5%), hypertension (Prolia: 4%)

Central nervous system: Fatigue (Xgeva: ≤45%), headache (Xgeva: 11% to 24%; Prolia: 4%)

Dermatologic: Skin rash (≤14%), dermatitis (Prolia: ≤11%), eczema (Prolia: ≤11%)

Endocrine & metabolic: Hypophosphatemia (Xgeva: 32%; severe: 10% to 21%), hypocalcemia (Xgeva: 3% to 18%; Prolia: 2%)

Gastrointestinal: Diarrhea (Xgeva: 20% to 34%), nausea (Xgeva: 30% to 32%), decreased appetite (Xgeva: 24%), vomiting (Xgeva: 24%; Prolia 2%), constipation (Xgeva: 21%; Prolia: 3%)

Hematologic & oncologic: Anemia (Xgeva: 21% to 22%), thrombocytopenia (Xgeva: 19%)

Neuromuscular & skeletal: Asthenia (Xgeva: ≤45%), back pain (Xgeva: 21%; Prolia: 5% to 12%), arthralgia (7% to 14%), limb pain (Prolia: 10% to 12%)

Respiratory: Dyspnea (Xgeva: 21% to 27%), cough (Xgeva: 15%), upper respiratory tract infection (Xgeva: 15%; Prolia: 5%)

1% to 10%:

Cardiovascular: Angina pectoris (Prolia: 3%)

Central nervous system: Sciatica (Prolia: 5%)

Endocrine & metabolic: Hypercholesterolemia (Prolia: 7%), hypokalemia (Xgeva: grade 3: 3%); hypomagnesemia (Xgeva: grade 3: 3%), severe hypocalcemia (symptomatic; Xgeva: 2% to 3%; Prolia: <1%)

Gastrointestinal: Upper abdominal pain (Prolia: 3%), flatulence (Prolia: 2%)

Genitourinary: Urinary tract infection (Prolia: 3%)

Hematologic & oncologic: Malignant neoplasm (Prolia: new; 3% to 5%)

Infection: Serious infection (Prolia: 4%)

Neuromuscular & skeletal: Musculoskeletal pain (Prolia: 6%), ostealgia (Prolia: 4%), myalgia (Prolia: 3%), osteonecrosis of the jaw (Xgeva ≤4%; Prolia: <1%), polymyalgia rheumatic (Prolia: 2%)

Ophthalmic: Cataract (Prolia: 5%)

Respiratory: Pneumonia (Xgeva: 8%), nasopharyngitis (Prolia: 7%), bronchitis (Prolia: 4%)

<1%, postmarketing, and/or case reports: Alopecia, anaphylaxis, antibody development, endocarditis, erythema of skin, facial swelling, femur fracture (diaphyseal, subtrochanteric), hypercalcemia (Xgeva, following discontinuation), hypersensitivity reaction, lichenoid eruption, osteomyelitis, pancreatitis, increased parathyroid hormone, urticaria

Dosing

Adult & Geriatric Note: Correct hypocalcemia prior to initiation of therapy. Administer calcium and vitamin D as necessary to prevent or treat hypocalcemia during therapy.

Bone metastases from solid tumors (prevention of skeletal-related events; Xgeva): SubQ: 120 mg every 4 weeks (Fizazi 2011; Henry 2011; Stopeck 2010).

Giant cell tumor of bone (Xgeva): SubQ: 120 mg once every 4 weeks; during the first month, give an additional 120 mg on days 8 and 15 (Blay 2011; Thomas 2010).

Hypercalcemia of malignancy (Xgeva): SubQ: 120 mg every 4 weeks; during the first month, give an additional 120 mg on days 8 and 15 (Hu 2014).

Multiple myeloma (prevention of skeletal-related events; Xgeva): SubQ: 120 mg every 4 weeks (Raje 2018). Denosumab has a reversible mechanism of action and therefore should not be discontinued abruptly (ASCO [Anderson 2018]).

Osteoporosis/bone loss (Prolia):

Androgen deprivation therapy-induced bone loss in males with prostate cancer, treatment: SubQ: 60 mg as a single dose, once every 6 months (Smith 2009).

Aromatase inhibitor-induced bone loss in females with breast cancer, treatment: SubQ: 60 mg as a single dose, once every 6 months (Ellis 2008).

Osteoporosis, glucocorticoid-induced (males and females): SubQ: 60 mg as a single dose, once every 6 months (Saag 2018).

Osteoporosis, treatment (males and postmenopausal females): Note: Alternative initial agent if bisphosphonate therapy is not suitable (ES [Eastell 2019]). Prior to use, evaluate and treat any potential causes of secondary osteoporosis (eg, hypogonadism in males) (ES [Watts 2012]).

SubQ: 60 mg as a single dose, once every 6 months.

Discontinuation/interruption of therapy: Bone mineral density (BMD) returns to baseline within 18 to 24 months following discontinuation; bone turnover markers increase within 3 to 6 months and then return to baseline within 24 months following discontinuation. Therefore, a drug holiday is not recommended (Bone 2011; ES [Eastell 2019]). If continued osteoporosis therapy is necessary, discontinuation or interruption of denosumab should not occur without subsequent antiresorptive therapy (eg, bisphosphonate or alternative) to prevent a rebound in bone turnover and to decrease rapid BMD loss and risk of fracture (ES [Eastell 2019]).

Duration of therapy: If fracture risk remains high after initial 5 to 10 years, consider extending therapy or switching to alternative therapy; there are no data on use beyond 10 years (ES [Eastell 2019]).

Missed dose: If a dose is missed, administer as soon as possible, then continue dosing every 6 months from the date of the last injection.

Bone destruction caused by rheumatoid arthritis (off-label use; based on limited data): SubQ: 60 mg or 180 mg as a single one time dose and repeated at 6 months (in combination with continued methotrexate); a total of 2 doses was administered in the study (Cohen 2008).

Renal Impairment: Adult

The renal dosing recommendations are based upon the best available evidence and clinical expertise. Senior Editorial Team: Bruce Mueller, PharmD, FCCP, FASN, FNKF; Jason Roberts, PhD, BPharm (Hons), B App Sc, FSHP, FISAC; Michael Heung, MD, MS.

Note: Monitor patients with severe impairment (CrCl <30 mL/minute or on dialysis) closely, as significant and prolonged hypocalcemia (incidence of 29% and potentially lasting weeks to months) and marked elevations of serum parathyroid hormone are serious risks in this population (Bhanot 2019; Jalleh 2018; Marlow 2018; Ueki 2015; manufacturer's labeling). Ensure adequate calcium and vitamin D intake/supplementation.

Altered kidney function:

CrCl ≥30 mL/minute: No dosage adjustment necessary.

CrCl <30 mL/minute:

Prolia: No dosage adjustment necessary; use in conjunction with guidance from patient's nephrology team, as osteoporosis is difficult to distinguish from chronic kidney disease mineral and bone disorder (expert opinion). The risk of Prolia administration must be weighed against the accuracy of the diagnosis of the underlying bone disease (KDIGO 2017).

Xgeva: There are no specific dosage adjustments recommended. Guidelines suggest dosage adjustment is not necessary; close monitoring for hypocalcemia is recommended (ASCO [Anderson 2018]; ASCO/CCO [Van Poznak 2017]; Grávalos 2016).

Hemodialysis, intermittent (thrice weekly): Unlikely to be removed by hemodialysis (Bailie 2020); dose as for patients with CrCl <30 mL/minute; use with caution and monitor calcium levels closely, with appropriate adjustment in dialysate calcium concentration in addition to adequate calcium and active vitamin D supplementation (Thongprayoon 2018).

Peritoneal dialysis: Unlikely to be removed by peritoneal dialysis (Bailie 2020); dose as for patients with CrCl <30 mL/minute; use with caution and monitor calcium levels closely.

Hepatic Impairment: Adult There are no dosage adjustments provided in the manufacturer's labeling (has not been studied).

Pediatric Note: Administer calcium and vitamin D as necessary to prevent or treat hypocalcemia.

Giant cell tumor of the bone, treatment: Xgeva: Adolescents (skeletally mature) weighing ≥45 kg: SubQ: 120 mg once every 4 weeks; during the first month, give an additional dose of 120 mg on days 8 and 15 (Chawla 2013; Thomas 2010).

Renal Impairment: Pediatric

Monitor patients with severe impairment (CrCl <30 mL/minute or on dialysis) due to increased risk of hypocalcemia.

Xgeva: There are no dosage adjustments provided in the manufacturer's labeling; however, in studies of patients with varying degrees of renal impairment, the degree of renal impairment had no effect on denosumab pharmacokinetics or pharmacodynamics.

Hepatic Impairment: Pediatric There are no dosage adjustments provided in manufacturer's labeling (has not been studied).

Mechanism of Action Denosumab is a monoclonal antibody with affinity for nuclear factor-kappa ligand (RANKL). Osteoblasts secrete RANKL; RANKL activates osteoclast precursors and subsequent osteolysis which promotes release of bone-derived growth factors, such as insulin-like growth factor-1 (IGF1) and transforming growth factor-beta (TGF-beta), and increases serum calcium levels. Denosumab binds to RANKL, blocks the interaction between RANKL and RANK (a receptor located on osteoclast surfaces), and prevents osteoclast formation, leading to decreased bone resorption and increased bone mass in osteoporosis. In solid tumors with bony metastases, RANKL inhibition decreases osteoclastic activity leading to decreased skeletal related events and tumor-induced bone destruction. In giant cell tumors of the bone (which express RANK and RANKL), denosumab inhibits tumor growth by preventing RANKL from activating its receptor (RANK) on the osteoclast surface, osteoclast precursors, and osteoclast-like giant cells.

Contraindications

Prolia: Hypersensitivity (systemic) to denosumab or any component of the formulation; preexisting hypocalcemia; pregnancy

Xgeva: Known clinically significant hypersensitivity to denosumab or any component of the formulation; preexisting hypocalcemia

Warnings/Precautions Clinically significant hypersensitivity (including anaphylaxis) has been reported. May include throat tightness, facial edema, upper airway edema, lip swelling, dyspnea, pruritus, rash, urticaria, and hypotension. If anaphylaxis or clinically significant hypersensitivity occurs, initiate appropriate management and permanently discontinue. Denosumab may cause or exacerbate hypocalcemia; severe symptomatic cases (including fatalities) have been reported. An increased risk has been observed with increasing renal dysfunction, most commonly severe dysfunction (CrCl <30 mL/minute and/or on dialysis), and with inadequate/no calcium supplementation. Monitor calcium levels; correct preexisting hypocalcemia prior to therapy. Monitor levels more frequently when denosumab is administered with other drugs that can also lower calcium levels. Use caution in patients with a history of hypoparathyroidism, thyroid surgery, parathyroid surgery, malabsorption syndromes, excision of small intestine, severe renal impairment/dialysis, treatment with other calcium-lowering agents, or other conditions which would predispose the patient to hypocalcemia; monitor calcium, phosphorus, and magnesium closely during therapy (the manufacturer recommends monitoring within 14 days of injection [Prolia] or during the first weeks of therapy initiation [Xgeva]). Concomitant use of calcimimetic medications may worsen hypocalcemia. Hypocalcemia lasting weeks to months (and requiring frequent monitoring) has been reported in postmarketing analyses. Administer calcium, vitamin D, and magnesium as necessary. Patients with severe renal impairment (CrCl <30 mL/minute) or those on dialysis may also develop marked elevations of serum parathyroid hormone (PTH). Hypercalcemia (clinically significant requiring hospitalization and complicated by acute renal injury) may occur in patients with giant cell tumor of bone and patients with growing skeletons weeks to months following discontinuation of denosumab therapy. Monitor for signs/symptoms of hypercalcemia (eg, nausea, vomiting, headache, decreased alertness), assess serum calcium periodically, and treat accordingly. Incidence of infections may be increased, including serious skin infections, abdominal, urinary, ear, or periodontal infections. Endocarditis has also been reported following use. Patients should be advised to contact their healthcare provider if signs or symptoms of severe infection or cellulitis develop. Use with caution in patients with impaired immune systems or using concomitant immunosuppressive therapy; may be at increased risk for serious infections. Evaluate the need for continued treatment with serious infection.

Atypical femur fractures have been reported in patients receiving denosumab. The fractures may occur anywhere along the femoral shaft (may be bilateral) and commonly occur with minimal to no trauma to the area. Some patients experience prodromal pain weeks or months before the fracture occurs. Because these fractures also occur in osteoporosis patients not treated with denosumab, it is unclear if denosumab therapy is the cause for the fractures; concomitant glucocorticoids may contribute to fracture risk. Advise patients to report new/unusual hip, thigh, or groin pain; and if so, evaluate for atypical/incomplete fracture. Contralateral limb should be assessed if atypical fracture occurs. Consider interrupting therapy in patients who develop an atypical femoral fracture. Following treatment discontinuation, the fracture risk increases, including risk of multiple vertebral fractures; patients with a history of prior fractures or osteoporosis are at higher risk. Vertebral fractures occurred as early as 7 months (average: 19 months) after the last dose of denosumab. Evaluate benefit/risk before initiating denosumab treatment for osteoporosis, especially in patients with prior vertebral fracture. If denosumab is discontinued, evaluate risk for vertebral fracture and consider transitioning to an alternative osteoporosis therapy. Because denosumab is associated with a severe bone turnover rebound following discontinuation, post-denosumab antiresorptive therapy (eg, bisphosphonate therapy or alternative) is suggested to mitigate decline in bone mineral density (ES [Eastell 2019]; Tsourdi 2017). Bisphosphonate therapy following denosumab discontinuation may reduce/prevent bone turnover rebound (Lamy 2017).

Osteonecrosis of the jaw (ONJ), also referred to as medication-related osteonecrosis of the jaw (MRONJ), has been reported in patients receiving denosumab. ONJ may manifest as jaw pain, osteomyelitis, osteitis, bone erosion, tooth/periodontal infection, toothache, gingival ulceration/erosion. Risk factors include invasive dental procedures (eg, tooth extraction, dental implants, oral surgery), cancer diagnosis, immunosuppressive therapy, angiogenesis inhibitor therapy, chemotherapy, systemic corticosteroids, poor oral hygiene, use of a dental appliance, ill-fitting dentures, periodontal and/or other preexisting dental disease, diabetes and gingival infections, local infection with delayed healing, anemia, and/or coagulopathy. In studies of patients with cancer, a longer duration of denosumab exposure was associated with a higher incidence of ONJ, although a majority of patients had predisposing factors, including a history of poor oral hygiene, tooth extraction, or the use of a dental appliance. Patients should maintain good oral hygiene during treatment. A dental exam and appropriate preventive dentistry should be performed prior to therapy. The manufacturer's labeling recommends avoiding invasive dental procedures in patients with bone metastases receiving denosumab for prevention of skeletal-related events and to consider temporary discontinuation of therapy in these patients if invasive dental procedure is required. According to a position paper by the American Association of Maxillofacial Surgeons (AAOMS), MRONJ has been associated with bisphosphonates and other antiresorptive agents (denosumab), and antiangiogenic agents (eg, bevacizumab, sunitinib) used for the treatment of osteoporosis or malignancy; risk is significantly higher in cancer patients receiving antiresorptive therapy compared to patients receiving osteoporosis treatment (regardless of medication used or dosing schedule). MRONJ risk is increased with intravenous antiresorptive therapy compared to the minimal risk associated with oral bisphosphonate use, although risk appears to increase with oral bisphosphonates when duration of therapy exceeds 4 years. The AAOMS suggests that if medically permissible, initiation of denosumab for cancer therapy should be delayed until optimal dental health is attained (if extractions are required, antiresorptive therapy should delayed until the extraction site has mucosalized or until after adequate osseous healing). Once denosumab is initiated for oncologic disease, procedures that involve direct osseous injury and placement of dental implants should be avoided. Patients developing ONJ during therapy should receive care by an oral surgeon (AAOMS [Ruggiero 2014]). According to the manufacturer, discontinuation of denosumab should be considered (based on risk/benefit evaluation) in patients who develop ONJ.

Postmenopausal osteoporosis: For use in females at high risk for fracture which is defined as a history of osteoporotic fracture or multiple risk factors for fracture.

May also be used in females who failed or did not tolerate other therapies.

The American Society of Clinical Oncology (ASCO) has updated guidelines on the role of bone-modifying agents (BMAs) in multiple myeloma (ASCO [Anderson 2018]). The update now includes denosumab as an alternate to zoledronic acid or pamidronate in patients with lytic disease, and as an additional option in adjunctive pain control in patients with pain due to osteolytic disease and patients receiving other interventions for fractures or impending fractures. Denosumab may also be preferred (to zoledronic acid) in patients with renal impairment. The ASCO guidelines recommend continuing the BMA for up to 2 years in multiple myeloma patients; BMAs may then be resumed upon relapse with new onset skeletal-related events. Denosumab has a reversible mechanism of action and therefore should not be discontinued abruptly (refer to Bone fractures [above] for further information).

Breast cancer: The American Society of Clinical Oncology (ASCO) /Cancer Care Ontario (CCO) updated guidelines on the role of BMAs for metastatic breast cancer patients (ASCO/CCO [Van Poznak 2017]). The guidelines recommend initiating a BMA (denosumab, pamidronate, zoledronic acid) in patients with metastatic breast cancer to the bone. One BMA is not recommended over another (evidence supporting one BMA over another is insufficient). The optimal duration of BMA therapy is not defined; however, the guidelines recommend continuing BMA therapy indefinitely. The analgesic effect of BMAs are modest and BMAs should not be used alone for pain management; supportive care, analgesics, adjunctive therapies, radiation therapy, surgery, and/or systemic anticancer therapy should be utilized.

Survivors of adult cancers with nonmetastatic disease who have osteoporosis (T score of -2.5 or lower in femoral neck, total hip, or lumbar spine) or who are at increased risk of osteoporotic fractures, should be offered bone modifying agents (utilizing the osteoporosis-indicated dose) to reduce the risk of fracture. For patients without hormonal responsive cancers, when clinically appropriate, estrogens may be administered along with other bone modifying agents (ASCO [Shapiro 2019]). The choice of bone modifying agent (eg, oral or IV bisphosphonates or subQ denosumab) should be based on several factors (eg, patient preference, potential adverse effects, quality of life considerations, availability, adherence, cost). Adequate calcium and vitamin D intake, exercise (using a combination of exercise types), as well as lifestyle modifications (if indicated), should also be encouraged.

Denosumab therapy results in significant suppression of bone turnover; the long term effects of treatment are not known but may contribute to adverse outcomes such as ONJ, atypical fractures, or delayed fracture healing; monitor. Use with caution in patients with renal impairment (CrCl <30 mL/minute) or patients on dialysis; risk of hypocalcemia is increased. Dose adjustment is not needed when administered at 60 mg every 6 months (Prolia); once-monthly dosing has not been evaluated in patients with renal impairment (Xgeva). Dermatitis, eczema, and rash (which are not necessarily specific to the injection site) have been reported; consider discontinuing if severe symptoms occur. Packaging may contain natural latex rubber. May impair bone growth in children with open growth plates or inhibit eruption of dentition. In pediatrics, indicated only for the treatment of giant cell tumor of bone in adolescents who are skeletally mature. Do not administer Prolia and Xgeva to the same patient for different indications. Potentially significant interactions may exist, requiring dose or frequency adjustment, additional monitoring, and/or selection of alternative therapy.

Drug Interactions

Metabolism/Transport Effects None known.

Avoid Concomitant Use There are no known interactions where it is recommended to avoid concomitant use.

Increased Effect/Toxicity

Denosumab may increase the levels/effects of: Calcimimetic Agents; Immunosuppressants

Decreased Effect There are no known significant interactions involving a decrease in effect.

Dietary Considerations Ensure adequate calcium and vitamin D intake to prevent or treat hypocalcemia. Calcium 1,000 mg/day and vitamin D ≥400 units/day is recommended in product labeling (Prolia). If dietary intake is inadequate, dietary supplementation is recommended. Females and males should consume:

Calcium: 1,000 mg/day (males: 50 to 70 years) **or** 1,200 mg/day (females ≥51 years and males ≥71 years) (IOM 2011; NOF 2014).

Vitamin D: 800 to 1,000 units/day (males and females ≥50 years) (NOF 2014). Recommended Dietary Allowance (RDA): 600 units/day (males and females ≤70 years) **or** 800 units/day (males and females ≥71 years) (IOM 2011).

Pharmacodynamics/Kinetics

Onset of Action Decreases markers of bone resorption by ~85% within 3 days; maximal reductions observed within 1 month

Hypercalcemia of malignancy: Time to response (median): 9 days; Time to complete response (median): 23 days (Hu 2014)

Duration of Action Markers of bone resorption return to baseline within 12 months of discontinuing therapy

Hypercalcemia of malignancy: Duration of response (median): 104 days; Duration of complete response (median): 34 days (Hu 2014)

Half-life Elimination ~25 to 28 days

Time to Peak Serum: 10 days (range: 3 to 21 days)

Reproductive Considerations

Evaluate pregnancy status prior to use in females of reproductive potential. Females of reproductive potential should be advised to use effective contraception during denosumab treatment and for at least 5 months following the last denosumab dose. Studies of denosumab following a single 60 mcg subcutaneous dose in healthy men demonstrated that denosumab is present in the semen in low concentrations (~2% of serum exposure) and therefore unlikely that a female partner or fetus would be exposed during unprotected sex to pharmacologically relevant denosumab concentrations via seminal fluid (Sohn 2016).

Pregnancy Considerations

Based on the mechanism of action and data from animal reproduction studies, in utero exposure to denosumab may cause fetal harm. Denosumab is a humanized monoclonal antibody (IgG_2). Potential placental transfer of human IgG is dependent upon the IgG subclass and gestational age, generally increasing as pregnancy progresses. The lowest exposure would be expected during the period of organogenesis (Palmeira 2012; Pentsuk 2009). Use of Prolia is contraindicated during pregnancy.

Data collection to monitor pregnancy and infant outcomes following exposure to denosumab is ongoing. Health care providers are encouraged to enroll females exposed to denosumab during pregnancy in the Amgen Pregnancy Surveillance Program (1-800-772-6436).

Breastfeeding Considerations It is not known if denosumab is present in breast milk.

According to the manufacturer, the decision to breastfeed during therapy should consider the risk of infant exposure, the benefits of breastfeeding to the infant, and benefits of treatment to the mother.

Dosage Forms Considerations Prolia prefilled syringe gray needle cap contains dry natural rubber (a derivative of latex).

Dosage Forms: US

Solution, Subcutaneous [preservative free]:

Xgeva: 120 mg/1.7 mL (1.7 mL)

Solution Prefilled Syringe, Subcutaneous [preservative free]:

Prolia: 60 mg/mL (1 mL)

Dosage Forms: Canada

Solution, Subcutaneous:

Xgeva: 120 mg/1.7 mL (1.7 mL)

Solution Prefilled Syringe, Subcutaneous:

Prolia: 60 mg/mL (1 mL)

Dental Health Professional Considerations In head-to-head comparison trials of denosumab and zoledronate (a bisphosphonate) for the treatment of bone metastasis in patients with cancer, 20 cases of ONJ were detected out of a total of 1026 subjects (2.0%) exposed to denosumab. There were 14 cases of ONJ observed out of a total of 1020 subjects (1.4%) exposed to zoledronate (Kyrgidis, 2010). The case of a 60-year old male cancer patient who developed ONJ after treatment with denosumab has been published (Taylor, 2010). In that report, the patient participated in a trial for a phase 3 study of denosumab. The patient had never been prescribed a bisphosphonate medication before treatment with denosumab. Clinical and radiological features of the lesion were diagnostic of probable ONJ. After discontinuation of the denosumab, the patient was treated with antibiotics and chlorhexidine rinses for a week. The necrotic bone sequestered 12 months later, and 15 months after initial presentation, the mucosa had healed with no further symptoms. Another case reported the development of ONJ in a 65-year old women being treated for giant cell tumor with denosumab. Although the patient was medically compromised and on multiple medications, the authors proposed that a common thread in ONJ development is inhibition of osteoclastic activity, mediated in this case by denosumab.

◆ **Denovo [OTC]** *see* Methylfolate *on page 996*

◆ **Denta 5000 Plus** *see* Fluoride *on page 693*

◆ **DentaGel** *see* Fluoride *on page 693*

◆ **Dentapaine [OTC]** *see* Benzocaine *on page 228*

◆ **Dent-O-Kain/20 [OTC]** *see* Benzocaine *on page 228*

◆ **Deoxyazacytidine** *see* Decitabine *on page 447*

◆ **Deoxycoformycin** *see* Pentostatin *on page 1214*

◆ **2'-Deoxycoformycin** *see* Pentostatin *on page 1214*

◆ **Depacon [DSC]** *see* Valproic Acid and Derivatives *on page 1518*

◆ **Depakene [DSC]** *see* Valproic Acid and Derivatives *on page 1518*

◆ **Depakote** *see* Valproic Acid and Derivatives *on page 1518*

◆ **Depakote ER** *see* Valproic Acid and Derivatives *on page 1518*

◆ **Depakote Sprinkles** *see* Valproic Acid and Derivatives *on page 1518*

◆ **Deplin 7.5** *see* Methylfolate *on page 996*

◆ **Deplin 15** *see* Methylfolate *on page 996*

◆ **DepoCyt [DSC]** *see* Cytarabine (Liposomal) *on page 425*

◆ **Depo-Estradiol** *see* Estradiol (Systemic) *on page 596*

◆ **DepoFoam Bupivacaine** *see* Bupivacaine (Liposomal) *on page 259*

◆ **DepoFoam-Encapsulated Cytarabine** *see* Cytarabine (Liposomal) *on page 425*

◆ **DEPO-Medrol** *see* MethylPREDNISolone *on page 999*

◆ **Depo-Provera** *see* MedroxyPROGESTERone *on page 953*

◆ **Depo-SubQ Provera 104** *see* MedroxyPROGESTERone *on page 953*

◆ **Depo-Testosterone** *see* Testosterone *on page 1425*

◆ **Deprenyl** *see* Selegiline *on page 1363*

◆ **Depsipeptide** *see* RomiDEPsin *on page 1343*

◆ **DermacinRx Empricaine** *see* Lidocaine and Prilocaine *on page 911*

◆ **DermacinRx Prizopak** *see* Lidocaine and Prilocaine *on page 911*

◆ **DermaFungal [OTC]** *see* Miconazole (Topical) *on page 1019*

◆ **Derma-Smoothe/FS Body** *see* Fluocinolone (Topical) *on page 689*

◆ **Derma-Smoothe/FS Scalp** *see* Fluocinolone (Topical) *on page 689*

◆ **Dermasorb HC [DSC]** *see* Hydrocortisone (Topical) *on page 775*

◆ **Dermasorb TA [DSC]** *see* Triamcinolone (Topical) *on page 1490*

◆ **Dermatop [DSC]** *see* Prednicarbate *on page 1255*

◆ **Dermazene** *see* Iodoquinol and Hydrocortisone *on page 836*

◆ **Dermazone [DSC]** *see* Triamcinolone (Topical) *on page 1490*

◆ **Dermoplast [OTC] [DSC]** *see* Benzocaine *on page 228*

◆ **Descovy** *see* Emtricitabine and Tenofovir Alafenamide *on page 557*

◆ **Desenex [OTC]** *see* Clotrimazole (Topical) *on page 397*

◆ **Desenex [OTC]** *see* Miconazole (Topical) *on page 1019*

◆ **Desenex Jock Itch [OTC]** *see* Miconazole (Topical) *on page 1019*

◆ **Desiccated Thyroid** *see* Thyroid, Desiccated *on page 1442*

Desipramine (des IP ra meen)

Related Information

Dentin Hypersensitivity, Acid Erosion, High Caries Index, Management of Alveolar Osteitis, and Xerostomia *on page 1762*

Vasoconstrictor Interactions With Antidepressants *on page 1821*

Brand Names: US Norpramin

Brand Names: Canada DOM-Desipramine; NOVO-Desipramine FC [DSC]; NOVO-Desipramine SC [DSC]; NOVO-Desipramine [DSC]; NU-Desipramine [DSC]; PMS-Desipramine; PMS-Desipramine Hydro

Pharmacologic Category Antidepressant, Tricyclic (Secondary Amine)

Use Depression: Treatment of depression

Local Anesthetic/Vasoconstrictor Precautions Use with caution; epinephrine and levonordefrin have been shown to have an increased pressor response in combination with TCAs. Desipramine is one of the drugs confirmed to prolong the QT interval and is accepted as having a risk of causing torsade de pointes. The risk of drug-induced torsade de pointes is extremely low when a single QT interval prolonging drug is prescribed. In terms of epinephrine, it is not known what effect vasoconstrictors in the local anesthetic regimen will have in patients with a known history of congenital prolonged QT interval or in patients taking any medication that prolongs the QT interval. Until more information is obtained, it is suggested that the clinician consult with the physician prior to the use of a vasoconstrictor in suspected patients, and that the vasoconstrictor (epinephrine, mepivacaine and levonordefrin [Carbocaine® 2% with Neo-Cobefrin®]) be used with caution.

Effects on Dental Treatment Key adverse event(s) related to dental treatment: Xerostomia and changes in salivation (normal salivary flow resumes upon discontinuation), unpleasant taste, stomatitis, and black tongue. Long-term treatment with TCAs increases the risk of caries by reducing salivation and salivary buffer capacity.

Effects on Bleeding Thrombocytopenia has been reported.

Adverse Reactions Frequency not defined. Some reactions listed are based on reports for other agents in this same pharmacologic class, and may not be specifically reported for desipramine.

Cardiovascular: Cardiac arrhythmia, cerebrovascular accident, edema, flushing, heart block, hypertension, hypotension, myocardial infarction, palpitations, premature ventricular contractions, tachycardia, ventricular fibrillation, ventricular tachycardia

Central nervous system: Agitation, anxiety, ataxia, confusion, delusions, disorientation, dizziness, drowsiness, drug fever, EEG pattern changes, extrapyramidal reaction, falling, fatigue, hallucination, headache, hypomania, insomnia, neuroleptic malignant syndrome, nightmares, numbness, peripheral neuropathy, psychosis (exacerbation), restlessness, seizure, tingling of extremities, tingling sensation, withdrawal syndrome

Dermatologic: Alopecia, diaphoresis (excessive), pruritus, skin photosensitivity, skin rash, urticaria

Endocrine & metabolic: Decreased libido, decreased serum glucose, galactorrhea, gynecomastia, increased libido, increased serum glucose, SIADH, weight gain, weight loss

Gastrointestinal: Abdominal cramps, anorexia, constipation, diarrhea, epigastric distress, increased pancreatic enzymes, melanoglossia, nausea, paralytic ileus, parotid gland enlargement, stomatitis, sublingual adenitis, unpleasant taste, vomiting, xerostomia

Genitourinary: Breast hypertrophy, impotence, nocturia, painful ejaculation, testicular swelling, urinary hesitancy, urinary retention, urinary tract dilation

Hematologic & oncologic: Agranulocytosis, eosinophilia, petechia, purpura, thrombocytopenia

Hepatic: Abnormal hepatic function tests, cholestatic jaundice, hepatitis, increased liver enzymes, increased serum alkaline phosphatase

Neuromuscular & skeletal: Tremor, weakness

Ophthalmic: Accommodation disturbance, blurred vision, increased intraocular pressure, mydriasis

Otic: Tinnitus

Renal: Polyuria

Miscellaneous: Fever

Postmarketing and/or case reports: Angle-closure glaucoma, serotonin syndrome, suicidal ideation, suicidal tendencies

Mechanism of Action Traditionally believed to increase the synaptic concentration of norepinephrine (and to a lesser extent, serotonin) in the central nervous system by inhibition of its reuptake by the presynaptic neuronal membrane. However, additional receptor effects have been found including desensitization of adenyl cyclase, down regulation of beta-adrenergic receptors, and down regulation of serotonin receptors.

Pharmacodynamics/Kinetics

Onset of Action Depression: Initial effects may be observed within 1 to 2 weeks of treatment, with continued improvements through 4 to 6 weeks (Papakostas 2006; Posternak 2005; Szegedi 2009).

Half-life Elimination Adults: 15 to 24 hours (Weiner, 1981)

Time to Peak Plasma: ~6 hours (Weiner, 1981)

Pregnancy Considerations Animal reproduction studies are inconclusive. Tricyclic antidepressants may be associated with irritability, jitteriness, and convulsions (rare) in the neonate (Yonkers 2009).

The ACOG recommends that therapy for depression during pregnancy be individualized; treatment should incorporate the clinical expertise of the mental health clinician, obstetrician, primary health care provider, and pediatrician (ACOG 2008). According to the American Psychiatric Association (APA), the risks of medication treatment should be weighed against other treatment options and untreated depression. For women who discontinue antidepressant medications during pregnancy and who may be at high risk for postpartum depression, the medications can be restarted following delivery (APA 2010). Treatment algorithms have been developed by the ACOG and the APA for the management of depression in women prior to conception and during pregnancy (Yonkers 2009).

Pregnant women exposed to antidepressants during pregnancy are encouraged to enroll in the National Pregnancy Registry for Antidepressants (NPRAD). Women 18 to 45 years of age or their health care providers may contact the registry by calling 844-405-6185. Enrollment should be done as early in pregnancy as possible.

Dental Health Professional Considerations See Local Anesthetic/Vasoconstrictor Precautions

◆ **Desipramine HCl** *see* Desipramine *on page 458*

◆ **Desipramine Hydrochloride** *see* Desipramine *on page 458*

Desirudin (des i ROO din)

Related Information

Cardiovascular Diseases *on page 1654*

Brand Names: US Iprivask [DSC]

Pharmacologic Category Anticoagulant; Anticoagulant, Direct Thrombin Inhibitor

Use Deep vein thrombosis, prophylaxis: Prophylaxis of deep vein thrombosis (DVT) in patients undergoing hip-replacement surgery

Local Anesthetic/Vasoconstrictor Precautions No information available to require special precautions

Effects on Dental Treatment No significant effects or complications reported

Effects on Bleeding As with all anticoagulants, bleeding is a potential adverse effect of desirudin during dental surgery; risk is dependent on multiple variables, including the intensity of anticoagulation and patient susceptibility. Medical consult is suggested. It is unlikely that ambulatory patients presenting for dental treatment will be taking intravenous anticoagulant therapy such as desirudin.

Adverse Reactions As with all anticoagulants, bleeding is the major adverse effect. Hemorrhage may occur at any site.

2% to 10%:

Cardiovascular: Deep vein thrombophlebitis (2%)

Dermatologic: Wound secretion (4%)

Gastrointestinal: Nausea (2%)

Hematologic & oncologic: Hematoma (6%), anemia (3%), major hemorrhage (≤3%; may include hemophthalmos, intracranial hemorrhage, intraspinal hemorrhage, prosthetic joint hemorrhage, or retroperitoneal hemorrhage)

Local: Residual mass at injection site (4%)

<2%, postmarketing, and/or case reports: Anaphylactoid reaction, anaphylaxis, cerebrovascular disease, decreased hemoglobin, dizziness, epistaxis, fever, hematemesis, hematuria, hemorrhage (fatal), hypersensitivity reaction, hypotension, leg pain, lower extremity edema, thrombosis, vomiting, wound healing impairment

Mechanism of Action Desirudin is a direct, highly selective thrombin inhibitor. Reversibly binds to the active thrombin site of free and clot-associated thrombin. Inhibits fibrin formation, activation of coagulation factors V, VII, and XIII, and thrombin-induced platelet aggregation resulting in a dose-dependent prolongation of the activated partial thromboplastin time (aPTT).

Pharmacodynamics/Kinetics

Half-life Elimination ~2 hours; Prolonged with renal impairment (CrCl <31 mL/minute/1.73 m^2: Up to 12 hours)

Time to Peak Plasma: 1 to 3 hours

Pregnancy Risk Factor C

Pregnancy Considerations Adverse events have been observed in animal reproduction studies. Data are insufficient to evaluate the safety of thrombin inhibitors during pregnancy (Guyatt, 2012).

Product Availability Iprivask has been discontinued in the US for more than 1 year.

Desloratadine (des lor AT a deen)

Brand Names: US Clarinex

Pharmacologic Category Histamine H_1 Antagonist; Histamine H_1 Antagonist, Second Generation; Piperidine Derivative

Use

Allergic rhinitis: Relief of nasal and non-nasal symptoms of seasonal (SAR) and perennial (PAR) allergic rhinitis

Urticaria: Symptomatic relief of pruritus, reduction in number of hives, and reduction in size of hives associated with chronic idiopathic urticaria (CIU)

Local Anesthetic/Vasoconstrictor Precautions No information available to require special precautions

Effects on Dental Treatment Key adverse event(s) related to dental treatment: Xerostomia (normal salivary flow resumes upon discontinuation)

Effects on Bleeding No information available to require special precautions

Adverse Reactions

>10%:

Central nervous system: Headache (14%), irritability (infants: 12%)

Gastrointestinal: Diarrhea (infants: 15% to 20%)

Respiratory: Upper respiratory tract infection (infants: 11% to 21%), cough (infants: 11%)

Miscellaneous: Fever (infants: 12% to 17%)

1% to 10%:

Central nervous system: Drowsiness (infants: 9%), insomnia (infants: 5%), fatigue (2% to 5%), dizziness (4%), emotional lability (infants: 3%)

Dermatologic: Erythema of skin (infants: 3%), maculopapular rash (infants: 3%)

Gastrointestinal: Vomiting (infants: 6%), anorexia (infants: 5%), nausea (infants and children: 3% to 5%), dyspepsia (3%), increased appetite (infants: 3%), xerostomia (adults: 3%)

Genitourinary: Urinary tract infection (children: 4%)

Infection: Varicella zoster infection (4%), parasitic infection (infants: 3%)

Neuromuscular & skeletal: Myalgia (3%)

Otic: Otitis media (infants: 6%)

Respiratory: Bronchitis (infants: 6%), rhinorrhea (infants: 5%), pharyngitis (3% to 5%), epistaxis (infants: 3%)

Postmarketing and/or case reports: Dyspnea, hepatitis, hyperbilirubinemia, hypersensitivity reaction, increased liver enzymes, movement disorder, palpitations, pruritus, psychomotor agitation, seizure, skin rash, tachycardia

Mechanism of Action Desloratadine, a major active metabolite of loratadine, is a long-acting tricyclic antihistamine with selective peripheral histamine H_1 receptor antagonistic activity.

Pharmacodynamics/Kinetics

Onset of Action Within 1 hour

Duration of Action 24 hours

Half-life Elimination

Children 2 to 5 years: Mean: 16.4 hours (Gupta 2007).

Children 6 to 11 years: Mean: 19.4 hours (Gupta 2007).

Adults: 27 hours.

Time to Peak

Children 2 to 5 years: Mean: 3.17 hours (range: 1.5 to 8 hours) (Gupta 2007).

Children 6 to 11 years: Mean: 3.57 hours (range: 4 to 12 hours) (Gupta 2007).

Adults: 3 hours.

Pregnancy Considerations

Guidelines for the use of antihistamines in the treatment of allergic rhinitis or urticaria in pregnancy are generally the same as in nonpregnant females. Second generation antihistamines may be used for the treatment of allergic rhinitis and urticaria during pregnancy; however, information related to the use of desloratadine in pregnancy is limited and other medications may be preferred (BSACI [Powell 2015]; BSACI [Scadding 2017]; Zuberbier 2018).

◆ **Desmethylimipramine Hydrochloride** *see* Desipramine *on page 458*

Desmopressin (des moe PRES in)

Brand Names: US DDAVP; DDAVP Rhinal Tube; Nocdurna; Noctiva [DSC]; Stimate

Brand Names: Canada DDAVP; DDAVP Melt; DDAVP Rhinyle; Nocdurna; Octostim; PMS-Desmopressin; TEVA-Desmopressin [DSC]

Pharmacologic Category Antihemophilic Agent; Hemostatic Agent; Hormone, Posterior Pituitary; Vasopressin Analog, Synthetic

Use

Injection:

Diabetes insipidus: Antidiuretic replacement therapy in the management of central (cranial) diabetes insipidus; management of the temporary polyuria and polydipsia following head trauma or surgery in the pituitary region.

Limitations of use: Desmopressin is ineffective for the treatment of nephrogenic diabetes insipidus.

Hemophilia A: For use in patients with hemophilia A with factor VIII coagulant activity levels >5% to maintain hemostasis during surgical procedures and postoperatively when administered 30 minutes prior to the scheduled procedure and to also stop bleeding due to spontaneous or trauma-induced injuries, such as hemarthroses, intramuscular hematomas, or mucosal bleeding.

Limitations of use: Not indicated for the treatment of hemophilia A with factor VIII coagulant activity levels ≤5%, for the treatment of hemophilia B, or in patients who have factor VIII antibodies. In certain clinical situations, it may be justified to try desmopressin with careful monitoring in patients with factor VIII levels between 2% and 5%.

Von Willebrand disease (type 1): For use in patients with mild to moderate classic von Willebrand disease (type 1) with factor VIII coagulant activity levels >5% to maintain hemostasis during surgical procedures and postoperatively when administered 30 minutes prior to the scheduled procedure and to stop bleeding due to spontaneous or trauma-induced injuries, such as hemarthroses, intramuscular hematomas, or mucosal bleeding.

Limitations of use: Patients with von Willebrand disease who are least likely to respond are those with severe homozygous von Willebrand disease with factor VIII coagulant activity and factor VIII von Willebrand factor antigen levels <1%; other patients may respond (variable) depending on the type of molecular defect they have. Check bleeding time and factor VIII coagulant activity, ristocetin cofactor activity, and von Willebrand factor antigen during administration of desmopressin to ensure that adequate levels are being achieved. Not indicated for the treatment of severe classic von Willebrand disease (type I) or when there is evidence of an abnormal molecular form of factor VIII antigen.

Uremic bleeding (Octostim [Canadian product]): Prevention or treatment of bleeding in patients with uremia.

Intranasal:

Diabetes insipidus:

DDAVP Nasal Spray: Antidiuretic replacement therapy in the management of central diabetes insipidus in adults and children ≥4 years.

DDAVP Rhinal tube: Antidiuretic replacement therapy in the management of central diabetes insipidus; management of the temporary polyuria and polydipsia following head trauma or surgery in the pituitary region.

Limitation of use: Treatment of nephrogenic diabetes insipidus or primary nocturnal enuresis.

Hemophilia A (Stimate; Octostim [Canadian product]): For use in patients with hemophilia A with factor VIII coagulant activity levels >5% and to stop bleeding due to spontaneous or trauma-induced injuries, such as hemarthroses, intramuscular hematomas, or mucosal bleeding.

Limitations of use: Not indicated for the treatment of hemophilia A with factor VIII coagulant activity levels ≤5%, for the treatment of hemophilia B, or in patients who have factor VIII antibodies.

Nocturia (Noctiva): Treatment of nocturia due to nocturnal polyuria in adults who awaken at least 2 times per night to void.

Limitations of use: Has not been studied in patients <50 years of age.

von Willebrand disease (type 1) (Stimate; Octostim [Canadian product]): For use in patients with mild to moderate classic von Willebrand disease (type 1) with factor VIII coagulant activity levels >5% and to stop bleeding due to spontaneous or trauma-induced injuries, such as hemarthroses, intramuscular hematomas, mucosal bleeding, or menorrhagia.

Limitations of use: Not indicated for the treatment of severe classic von Willebrand disease (type 1) or when there is evidence of an abnormal molecular form of factor VIII antigen.

Oral:

Diabetes insipidus: Antidiuretic replacement therapy in the management of central diabetes insipidus; management of the temporary polyuria and polydipsia following head trauma or surgery in the pituitary region.

Limitation of use: Desmopressin is ineffective for the treatment of nephrogenic diabetes insipidus.

Nocturia (Nocdurna): Treatment of nocturia due to nocturnal polyuria in adults who awaken at least 2 times per night to void.

Primary nocturnal enuresis: Management of primary nocturnal enuresis, either alone or as an adjunct to behavioral conditioning or other nonpharmacologic intervention.

Local Anesthetic/Vasoconstrictor Precautions No information available to require special precautions

Effects on Dental Treatment Key adverse event(s) related to dental treatment: Frequent occurrence of xerostomia (normal salivary flow resumes upon discontinuance) with sublingual application has been reported.

Effects on Bleeding Rare reports of thrombotic events including thromboembolism have been associated with desmopressin, although no causality has been determined.

Adverse Reactions

>10%:

Endocrine & metabolic: Hyponatremia (<1%; intranasal: 2% to 12%; sublingual: 3% to 4%)

Gastrointestinal: Xerostomia (sublingual: ≤14%)

1% to 10%:
- Cardiovascular: Hypertension (intranasal: 2% to 3%)
- Central nervous system: Headache (2% to 5%), dizziness (intranasal, sublingual: 2% to 3%), chills (intranasal: 2%), nostril pain (intranasal: 2%)
- Gastrointestinal: Abdominal pain (intranasal: 2%), gastrointestinal disease (intranasal: 2%), nausea (intranasal: 2%)
- Neuromuscular & skeletal: Asthenia (intranasal: 2%), back pain (intranasal: 1% to 2%)
- Ophthalmic: Abnormal lacrimation (intranasal: 2%), conjunctivitis (intranasal: 2%), ocular edema (intranasal: 2%)
- Respiratory: Rhinitis (intranasal: 3% to 8%), nasal discomfort (intranasal: 6%), nasopharyngitis (intranasal: 4%), nasal congestion (intranasal: ≤3%), epistaxis (intranasal: 2% to 3%), sneezing (intranasal: 2% to 3%), bronchitis (intranasal: 2%)

Frequency not defined:
- Cardiovascular: Altered blood pressure, chest pain (intranasal), edema, facial flushing, flushing (intranasal), palpitations (intranasal), tachycardia (intranasal)
- Central nervous system: Abnormality in thinking, agitation (intranasal), drowsiness (intranasal), insomnia (intranasal), localized warm feeling (intranasal), pain (intranasal)
- Endocrine & metabolic: Weight gain
- Gastrointestinal: Abdominal cramps, diarrhea, dyspepsia (intranasal), sore throat (intranasal), vomiting (intranasal)
- Genitourinary: Balanitis (intranasal), vulvar pain
- Hepatic: Increased serum aspartate aminotransferase (oral; transient)
- Local: Burning sensation at injection site, erythema at injection site, swelling at injection site
- Ophthalmic: Eye pruritus (intranasal), photophobia (intranasal)
- Respiratory: Cough (intranasal), upper respiratory tract infection

<1%, postmarketing, and/or case reports: Anaphylaxis, atrial fibrillation, dysuria, serum hyposmolality, severe hypersensitivity, water intoxication

Mechanism of Action Synthetic analogue of the antidiuretic hormone arginine vasopressin. In a dose dependent manner, desmopressin increases cyclic adenosine monophosphate (cAMP) in renal tubular cells which increases water permeability resulting in decreased urine volume and increased urine osmolality; increases plasma levels of von Willebrand factor, factor VIII, and t-PA contributing to a shortened activated partial thromboplastin time (aPTT) and bleeding time.

Pharmacodynamics/Kinetics

Onset of Action

Intranasal: Antidiuretic: 15 to 30 minutes; Increased factor VIII and von Willebrand factor (vWF) activity (dose related): 30 minutes

Peak effect: Antidiuretic: 1 hour; Increased factor VIII and vWF activity: 1.5 hours; Nocturia: 0.25 to 0.75 hour

IV infusion: Increased factor VIII and vWF activity: 30 minutes (dose related)

Peak effect: 1.5 to 2 hours

Oral tablet: Antidiuretic: ~1 hour

Peak effect: 4 to 7 hours

Sublingual: Antidiuretic: ~30 minutes

Duration of Action Intranasal, Injection, Oral tablet, Sublingual: ~6 to 14 hours

Half-life Elimination 2 to 4 hours; Severe renal impairment: ~9 hours

Pregnancy Considerations

In vitro studies demonstrate poor placental transfer of desmopressin.

Desmopressin may be used throughout pregnancy for the treatment of diabetes insipidus (Aleksandrov 2010; Ananthakrishnan 2016; Brewster 2005; Schrier 2010). Information related to desmopressin for the treatment of von Willebrand disease in pregnancy is limited (NHLBI 2007); however, use is recommended for bleeding prophylaxis when otherwise indicated (Demers 2018; Pacheco 2010; Trigg 2012). Desmopressin is not recommended for nocturia caused by normal physiologic changes which occur during pregnancy.

◆ **Desmopressin Acetate** *see* Desmopressin *on page 460*

◆ **Desogen [DSC]** *see* Ethinyl Estradiol and Desogestrel *on page 609*

◆ **Desogestrel and Ethinyl Estradiol** *see* Ethinyl Estradiol and Desogestrel *on page 609*

◆ **Desonate** *see* Desonide *on page 461*

Desonide (DES oh nide)

Brand Names: US Desonate; DesOwen; LoKara [DSC]; Tridesilon; Verdeso

Brand Names: Canada PDP-Desonide; Tridesilon

Pharmacologic Category Corticosteroid, Topical

Use

Atopic dermatitis (foam and gel): Treatment of mild to moderate atopic dermatitis in patients 3 months and older

Corticosteroid-responsive dermatoses (cream, ointment, and lotion): Relief of inflammatory and pruritic manifestations of corticosteroid-responsive dermatoses.

Local Anesthetic/Vasoconstrictor Precautions No information available to require special precautions

Effects on Dental Treatment No significant effects or complications reported

Effects on Bleeding No information available to require special precautions

Adverse Reactions

1% to 10%:
- Cardiovascular: Increased blood pressure (2%)
- Central nervous system: Headache (2%), irritability (1%)
- Dermatologic: Stinging of the skin (≤3%), atopic dermatitis (<2%; exacerbation), contact dermatitis (<2%), exfoliation of skin (<2%), pruritus (<2%), skin irritation (<2%), xeroderma (<2%), skin rash (≤1%)
- Endocrine & metabolic: Hyperglycemia (2%), HPA-axis suppression (more common in pediatric patients)
- Hepatic: Abnormal liver function (1%)
- Infection: Viral infection (2%)
- Local: Application site reaction (1% to 6%), application site burning (≤3%), application site atrophy (1%)
- Respiratory: Upper respiratory tract infection (10%), cough (4%), asthma (1%), pharyngitis (1%)

<1%, postmarketing, and/or case reports: Application site erythema, application site induration, application site irritation, application-site pruritus, dermatological reaction, diaphoresis, erythema of skin, facial swelling, folliculitis, oily skin, pain, peripheral edema, pustular rash

Mechanism of Action Topical corticosteroids have anti-inflammatory, antipruritic, and vasoconstrictive properties. May depress the formation, release, and activity of endogenous chemical mediators of inflammation (kinins, histamine, liposomal enzymes, prostaglandins) through the induction of phospholipase A_2 inhibitory proteins (lipocortins) and sequential inhibition of the release of arachidonic acid. Desonide has low range potency.

- ◆ **DesOwen** *see* Desonide *on page 461*
- ◆ **Desoxyephedrine Hydrochloride** *see* Methamphetamine *on page 986*
- ◆ **Desoxyn** *see* Methamphetamine *on page 986*
- ◆ **Desoxyphenobarbital** *see* Primidone *on page 1276*
- ◆ **Desulfato-Hirudin** *see* Desirudin *on page 459*
- ◆ **Desulphatohirudin** *see* Desirudin *on page 459*

Desvenlafaxine (des ven la FAX een)

Related Information

Dentin Hypersensitivity, Acid Erosion, High Caries Index, Management of Alveolar Osteitis, and Xerostomia *on page 1762*

Vasoconstrictor Interactions With Antidepressants *on page 1821*

Brand Names: US Khedezla [DSC]; Pristiq

Brand Names: Canada APO-Desvenlafaxine; Pristiq

Pharmacologic Category Antidepressant, Serotonin/Norepinephrine Reuptake Inhibitor

Use Major depressive disorder: Treatment of major depressive disorder (MDD).

Local Anesthetic/Vasoconstrictor Precautions Part of the mechanism of desvenlafaxine is to block reuptake of norepinephrine along with dopamine. Because of the potential for norepinephrine elevation within CNS synapses, it is suggested that vasoconstrictor be administered with caution and to monitor vital signs in dental patients taking antidepressants that affect norepinephrine in this way. This is particularly important in patients taking desvenlafaxine, which has been noted to cause a sustained increase in blood pressure or heart rate. Dose-related increase in systolic and diastolic blood pressure have also been reported.

Effects on Dental Treatment Key adverse event(s) related to dental treatment: Significant xerostomia (normal salivary flow resumes upon discontinuation). See Effects on Bleeding.

Effects on Bleeding Platelet dysfunction (ie, impaired platelet aggregation) may occur during treatment with serotonin norepinephrine reuptake inhibitors (SNRIs), such as desvenlafaxine, due to platelet serotonin depletion, possibly increasing the risk of a bleeding complication. NSAIDs may increase this risk.

Adverse Reactions

>10%:

Central nervous system: Dizziness (10% to 13%), insomnia (9% to 12%)

Dermatologic: Hyperhidrosis (10% to 11%)

Gastrointestinal: Nausea (22% to 26%), xerostomia (11% to 17%)

1% to 10%:

Cardiovascular: Orthostatic hypotension (elderly 8%), syncope (<2%), tachycardia (<2%), hypertension (dose related; ≤1% of patients taking 50 to 100 mg daily had sustained diastolic BP ≥90 mm Hg)

Central nervous system: Drowsiness (≤9%), fatigue (7%), anxiety (3% to 5%), delayed ejaculation (1% to 5%), abnormal dreams (2% to 3%), anorgasmia (males ≤3%; females 1%), jitteriness (2%), vertigo (≤2%), depersonalization (<2%), dystonia (<2%), seizure (<2%), disturbance in attention (1%), yawning (1%), male sexual disorder (≤1%)

Dermatologic: Alopecia (<2%), skin photosensitivity (<2%), skin rash (<2%)

Endocrine & metabolic: Decreased libido (males 4% to 5%), increased serum cholesterol (increased by ≥50 mg/dL and ≥261 mg/dL: 3% to 4%), increased serum prolactin (<2%), weight gain (<2%), hot flash (1%), increased LDL cholesterol (increased by ≥50 mg/dL and ≥190 mg/dL: ≤1%)

Gastrointestinal: Constipation (9%), decreased appetite (5% to 8%), vomiting (≤4%), bruxism (<2%)

Genitourinary: Proteinuria (5% to 8%), erectile dysfunction (3% to 6%), urinary retention (<2%), ejaculation failure (≤1%), urinary hesitancy (≤1%)

Hepatic: Abnormal hepatic function tests (<2%)

Hypersensitivity: Angioedema (<2%)

Neuromuscular & skeletal: Tremor (≤3%), stiffness (<2%), weakness (<2%)

Ophthalmic: Blurred vision (3% to 4%), mydriasis (2%)

Otic: Tinnitus (≤2%)

Frequency not defined: Cardiovascular: Coronary occlusion, ischemic heart disease, myocardial infarction

<1%, postmarketing, and/or case reports: Acute pancreatitis, angle-closure glaucoma, cardiomyopathy (takotsubo), Stevens-Johnson syndrome

Mechanism of Action Desvenlafaxine is a potent and selective serotonin and norepinephrine reuptake inhibitor.

Pharmacodynamics/Kinetics

Onset of Action Depression: Initial effects may be observed within 1 to 2 weeks of treatment, with continued improvements through 4 to 6 weeks (Papakostas 2006; Posternak 2005; Szegedi 2009).

Half-life Elimination ~10 to 11 hours; prolonged in renal failure and hepatic failure

Pregnancy Considerations

Nonteratogenic effects in the newborn following SSRI/SNRI exposure late in the third trimester include respiratory distress, cyanosis, apnea, seizures, temperature instability, feeding difficulty, vomiting, hypoglycemia, hyper- or hypotonia, hyper-reflexia, jitteriness, irritability, constant crying, and tremor. Symptoms may be due to the toxicity of the SNRIs/SSRIs or a discontinuation syndrome and may be consistent with serotonin syndrome associated with treatment. The long-term effects of in utero SNRI/SSRI exposure on infant development and behavior are not known.

The ACOG recommends that therapy with SSRIs or SNRIs during pregnancy be individualized; treatment of depression during pregnancy should incorporate the clinical expertise of the mental health clinician, obstetrician, primary health care provider, and pediatrician. According to the American Psychiatric Association (APA), the risks of medication treatment should be weighed against other treatment options and untreated depression. For women who discontinue antidepressant medications during pregnancy and who may be at high risk for postpartum depression, the medications can be restarted following delivery. Treatment algorithms have been developed by the ACOG and the APA for the management of depression in women prior to conception and during pregnancy.

Desvenlafaxine is the major active metabolite of venlafaxine; also refer to the Venlafaxine monograph.

Pregnant women exposed to antidepressants during pregnancy are encouraged to enroll in the National Pregnancy Registry for Antidepressants (NPRAD). Women 18 to 45 years of age or their health care providers may contact the registry by calling 844-405-6185. Enrollment should be done as early in pregnancy as possible.

- ◆ **Desyrel** *see* TraZODone *on page 1481*
- ◆ **Detemir Insulin** *see* Insulin Detemir *on page 820*
- ◆ **Detrol** *see* Tolterodine *on page 1462*
- ◆ **Detrol LA** *see* Tolterodine *on page 1462*
- ◆ **Detryptoreline** *see* Triptorelin *on page 1500*
- ◆ **Dexabliss** *see* DexAMETHasone (Systemic) *on page 463*

DexAMETHasone (Systemic)

(deks a METH a sone)

Related Information

Respiratory Diseases *on page 1680*

Ulcerative, Erosive, and Painful Oral Mucosal Disorders *on page 1758*

Related Sample Prescriptions

Ulcerative and Erosive Disorders - Sample Prescriptions *on page 46*

Brand Names: US Active Injection D; Decadron; Dexabliss; Dexamethasone Intensol; DexPak 10 Day [DSC]; DexPak 13 Day [DSC]; DexPak 6 Day [DSC]; DoubleDex; Dxevo 11-Day; HiDex 6-Day; LoCort 11-Day [DSC]; LoCort 7-Day [DSC]; MAS Care-Pak; ReadySharp Dexamethasone; TaperDex 12-Day; TaperDex 6-Day; TaperDex 7-Day; TopiDex; Zodex 12-Day [DSC]; Zodex 6-Day [DSC]; ZonaCort 11 Day [DSC]; ZonaCort 7 Day [DSC]

Brand Names: Canada APO-Dexamethasone; Dexamethasone Omega Unidose; Dexamethasone-Omega; DOM-Dexamethasone; PMS-Dexamethasone; PMS-Dexamethasone Sod Phosphat; PRO-Dexamethasone-4 [DSC]; RATIO-Dexamethasone [DSC]

Generic Availability (US) May be product dependent

Pharmacologic Category Anti-inflammatory Agent; Antiemetic; Corticosteroid, Systemic

Dental Use Treatment of a variety of oral diseases of allergic, inflammatory or autoimmune origin; aphthous stomatitis (systemic dexamethasone used topically); lichen planus (erosive) and other oral vesiculoerosive diseases

Use

Oral, IV, or IM injection: Anti-inflammatory or immunosuppressant agent in the treatment of a variety of diseases, including those of allergic, hematologic (eg, immune thrombocytopenia), dermatologic, neoplastic, rheumatic, autoimmune, nervous system, renal, and respiratory origin; primary or secondary adrenocorticoid deficiency (not first line); management of shock, cerebral edema, and as a diagnostic agent.

Intra-articular or soft tissue injection: As adjunctive therapy for short-term administration in synovitis of osteoarthritis, rheumatoid arthritis, acute and subacute bursitis, acute gouty arthritis, epicondylitis, acute nonspecific tenosynovitis, and posttraumatic osteoarthritis.

Intralesional injection: Keloids; localized hypertrophic, infiltrated, inflammatory lesions of lichen planus, psoriatic plaques, granuloma annulare, and lichen simplex chronicus (neurodermatitis); discoid lupus erythematosus; necrobiosis lipoidica diabeticorum; alopecia areata; and cystic tumors of an aponeurosis or tendon (ganglia).

Local Anesthetic/Vasoconstrictor Precautions No information available to require special precautions

Effects on Dental Treatment No significant effects or complications reported

Effects on Bleeding No information available to require special precautions

Adverse Reactions Some reactions listed are based on reports for other agents in this same pharmacologic class and may not be specifically reported for dexamethasone.

Frequency not defined:

Cardiovascular: Bradycardia, cardiac arrhythmia, cardiac failure, cardiomegaly, circulatory shock, edema, embolism (fat), hypertension, hypertrophic cardiomyopathy (premature infants), myocardial rupture (post-MI), syncope, tachycardia, thromboembolism, thrombophlebitis, vasculitis

Central nervous system: Depression, emotional lability, euphoria, headache, increased intracranial pressure, insomnia, malaise, myasthenia, neuritis, neuropathy, paresthesia, personality changes, pseudotumor cerebri (usually following discontinuation), psychic disorder, seizure, vertigo

Dermatologic: Acne vulgaris, allergic dermatitis, alopecia, atrophic striae, diaphoresis, ecchymoses, erythema, facial erythema, fragile skin, hyperpigmentation, hypertrichosis, hypopigmentation, perianal skin irritation (itching, burning, tingling; following IV injection), petechiae, skin atrophy, skin rash, subcutaneous atrophy, suppression of skin test reaction, urticaria, xeroderma

Endocrine & metabolic: Adrenal suppression, carbohydrate intolerance, Cushing syndrome, decreased glucose tolerance, decreased serum potassium, diabetes mellitus, fluid retention, glycosuria, growth suppression (children), hirsutism, HPA-axis suppression, hyperglycemia, hypokalemic alkalosis, menstrual disease, moon face, negative nitrogen balance, protein catabolism, redistribution of body fat, sodium retention, weight gain

Gastrointestinal: Abdominal distention, gastrointestinal hemorrhage, gastrointestinal perforation, hiccups, increased appetite, nausea, pancreatitis, peptic ulcer, pruritus ani (following IV injection), ulcerative esophagitis

Genitourinary: Defective (increased or decreased) spermatogenesis

Hematologic & oncologic: Kaposi sarcoma, petechial, tumor lysis syndrome

Hepatic: Hepatomegaly, increased serum transaminases

Hypersensitivity: Anaphylactoid reaction, anaphylaxis, angioedema, hypersensitivity

Infection: Infection, sterile abscess

Local: Postinjection flare (intra-articular use)

Neuromuscular & skeletal: Amyotrophy, aseptic necrosis of bones (femoral and humoral heads), bone fractures, Charcot-like arthropathy, myasthenia, myopathy (particularly in conjunction with neuromuscular disease or neuromuscular-blocking agents), osteoporosis, rupture of tendon, steroid myopathy, vertebral compression fracture

Ophthalmic: Exophthalmos, glaucoma, increased intraocular pressure, subcapsular posterior cataract
Respiratory: Pulmonary edema
Miscellaneous: Wound healing impairment

Dental Usual Dosage

Erosive lichen planus and major aphthae: Oral: For 3 days, rinse with 15 mL dexamethasone (0.5 mg/5 mL) oral elixir 4 times/day and swallow; then for 3 days, rinse with 5 mL 4 times/day and swallow; then for 3 days, rinse with 5 mL 4 times/day and swallow every other time. Then for 3 days rinse with 5 mL 4 times/day and expectorate. Continue the rinse and expectorate mode for 2 minutes, but discontinue medication when mouth becomes completely comfortable.

Recurrent aphthous stomatitis: Rinse with 5 mL dexamethasone (0.5 mg/5 mL) oral elixir for 2 minutes 4 times/day and expectorate

Dosing

Adult

Note: Dosing: Evidence to support an optimal dose and duration is lacking for most indications; recommendations provided are general guidelines only and primarily based on expert opinion. In general, glucocorticoid dosing should be individualized and the minimum effective dose/duration should be used. For select indications with weight-based dosing, consider using ideal body weight in obese patients, especially with longer durations of therapy (Erstad 2004; Furst 2019a). **Hypothalamic-pituitary-adrenal (HPA) suppression:** Although some patients may become hypothalamic-pituitary-adrenal (HPA) suppressed with lower doses or briefer exposure, some experts consider HPA-axis suppression likely in any adult receiving >3 mg/day (daytime dosing) or ≥0.75 mg per 24 hours (evening or night dosing) for >3 weeks or with Cushingoid appearance (Furst 2019b; Joseph 2016); do not abruptly discontinue treatment in these patients; dose tapering may be necessary (Cooper 2003).

Usual dosage range: Oral, IV, IM: 4 to 20 mg/day given in a single daily dose or in 2 to 4 divided doses; *High dose:* 0.4 to 0.8 mg/**kg**/day (usually not to exceed 40 mg/day).

Indication-specific dosing:

Coronavirus disease 2019 (COVID-19), treatment (hospitalized patient) (off-label use):

Note: Dexamethasone is currently under investigation for use in the treatment of COVID-19 (see ClinicalTrials.gov). Based on a preliminary report, use of dexamethasone is recommended for treatment of COVID-19 in hospitalized patients who require mechanical ventilation or supplemental oxygen (IDSA [Bhimraj 2020]; NIH 2020; RECOVERY 2020).

IV, Oral: 6 mg once daily for up to 10 days (or until discharge if sooner); equivalent glucocorticoid dose may be substituted if dexamethasone is unavailable (Hornby 2020; IDSA [Bhimraj 2020]).

Acute mountain sickness/high-altitude cerebral edema (off-label use):

Prevention, moderate- to high-risk situations (alternative agent): **Note:** Use in addition to gradual ascent and start the day of ascent.

Oral: 2 mg every 6 hours **or** 4 mg every 12 hours; may be discontinued after staying at the same elevation for 2 to 4 days or if descent is initiated. Due to adverse effects, limit duration to ≤10 days (Luks 2014); some experts limit to ≤7 days (Gallagher 2019). In situations of rapid ascent to altitudes >3,500 meters (eg, rescue or military operations), 4 mg every 6 hours may be considered (Luks 2014).

Treatment:

Acute mountain sickness (moderate to severe): **Note**: Dexamethasone does not facilitate acclimatization; further ascent should be delayed until patient is asymptomatic off medication (Gallagher 2019; Luks 2014).

Oral, IM, IV: 4 mg every 6 hours, continue until 24 hours after symptoms resolve or descent completed (not longer than 7 days total) (Gallagher 2019; Luks 2014).

High-altitude cerebral edema: **Oral, IM, IV:** 8 mg as a single dose, followed by 4 mg every 6 hours until descent is complete and symptoms resolve (Luks 2014).

Acute respiratory distress syndrome, moderate to severe (off-label use): Note: May consider in most patients with persistent or refractory moderate to severe acute respiratory distress syndrome who are relatively early in the disease course (within 14 days) (Siegel 2020). Do not abruptly discontinue since this may cause deterioration due to inflammatory response (SCCM/ESICM [Annane 2017]).

IV: 20 mg once daily from days 1 to 5, then 10 mg once daily from days 6 to 10 (Villar 2020).

Adrenal insufficiency (adrenal crisis) (alternative agent): Note: Dexamethasone should only be used if hydrocortisone is unavailable. Corticosteroid therapy should be combined with adequate fluid resuscitation in patients with primary adrenal insufficiency (ES [Bornstein 2016]).

IV: 4 mg every 12 hours; transition to hydrocortisone as soon as possible (ES [Bornstein 2016]; Nieman 2019).

Antiemetic regimens: Chemotherapy-associated nausea and vomiting, prevention (off-label use): Note: When dexamethasone is given with rolapitant in a prechemotherapy regimen, the oral route for both is generally used.

Single-day IV chemotherapy regimens:

Highly emetogenic chemotherapy (>90% risk of emesis): Cisplatin and other highly emetogenic single agents:

Dexamethasone dose depends on specific neurokinin 1 (NK_1) receptor antagonist (ASCO [Hesketh 2017]; MASCC/ESMO [Roila 2016]):

Day of chemotherapy: Administer prior to chemotherapy **and** in combination with a NK_1 receptor antagonist, and a 5-HT_3 receptor antagonist, with or without olanzapine (ASCO [Hesketh 2017]; MASCC/ESMO [Roila 2016]).

In combination with aprepitant, fosaprepitant, netupitant/palonosetron (NEPA), or fosnetupitant/palonosetron: **Oral, IV:** 12 mg.

In combination with rolapitant: **Oral, IV:** 20 mg.

If NK_1 receptor antagonist not used: **Oral, IV:** 20 mg.

Postchemotherapy days:

If aprepitant given: **Oral, IV:** 8 mg once daily on days 2 to 4 (ASCO [Hesketh 2017]).

If fosaprepitant given: **Oral, IV:** 8 mg once on day 2, followed by 8 mg twice daily on days 3 and 4 (ASCO [Hesketh 2017]).

If NEPA or fosnetupitant/palonosetron given: Prophylaxis with dexamethasone on subsequent days is not needed unless regimen contained cisplatin: **Oral, IV:** 8 mg once daily on days 2 to 4 (Hesketh 2020).

If rolapitant given: **Oral, IV:** 8 mg twice daily on days 2 to 4 (ASCO [Hesketh 2017]).

If NK_1 receptor antagonist not used: **Oral, IV:** 8 mg twice daily on days 2 to 4 (ASCO [Hesketh 2017]).

Highly emetogenic chemotherapy (>90% risk of emesis): Breast cancer regimens that include an anthracycline combined with cyclophosphamide:

Dexamethasone dose depends on specific NK_1 receptor antagonist [ASCO [Hesketh 2017]; MASCC/ESMO [Roila 2016]):

Day of chemotherapy: Administer prior to chemotherapy **and** in combination with a NK_1 receptor antagonist, and a 5-HT_3 receptor antagonist, with or without olanzapine (ASCO [Hesketh 2017]; MASCC/ESMO [Roila 2016]).

In combination with aprepitant, fosaprepitant, NEPA, fosnetupitant/palonosetron: **Oral, IV:** 12 mg (ASCO [Hesketh 2017]; Hesketh 2020).

In combination with rolapitant: **Oral, IV:** 20 mg (ASCO [Hesketh 2017]).

If NK_1 receptor antagonist not used: **Oral, IV:** 20 mg (ASCO [Hesketh 2017]).

Postchemotherapy days: Dexamethasone use is not recommended (an alternative agent or agents is/are recommended) (ASCO [Hesketh 2017]; Hesketh 2020).

Moderately emetogenic chemotherapy (30% to 90% risk of emesis): Carboplatin-based regimens:

Dexamethasone dose depends on specific NK_1 receptor antagonist (ASCO [Hesketh 2017]; MASCC/ESMO [Roila 2016]):

Day of chemotherapy: Administer prior to chemotherapy **and** in combination with a NK_1 receptor antagonist and a 5-HT_3 receptor antagonist (ASCO [Hesketh 2017]; MASCC/ESMO [Roila 2016]).

In combination with aprepitant, fosaprepitant, NEPA, or fosnetupitant/palonosetron: **Oral, IV:** 12 mg (ASCO [Hesketh 2017]; Hesketh 2020).

In combination with rolapitant: **Oral, IV:** 20 mg (ASCO [Hesketh 2017]).

Postchemotherapy days: Prophylaxis is not necessary on subsequent days (ASCO [Hesketh 2017]; MASCC/ESMO [Roila 2016]).

Moderately emetogenic chemotherapy (30% to 90% risk of emesis): Non-carboplatin-based regimens:

Day of chemotherapy: Administer prior to chemotherapy **and** in combination with a 5-HT_3 receptor antagonist: **Oral, IV:** 8 mg (ASCO [Hesketh 2017]; MASCC/ESMO [Roila 2016]).

Postchemotherapy days: **Note:** Consider single-agent dexamethasone use for regimens containing agents with known potential to induce delayed emesis (eg, oxaliplatin, cyclophosphamide, doxorubicin) (ASCO [Hesketh 2017]; MASCC/ESMO [Roila 2016]); a single-day dexamethasone regimen may be employed when utilizing palonosetron (Komatsu 2015); however, if a first-generation 5-HT_3 antagonist was used on day 1 rather than palonosetron, some experts suggest the first-generation 5-HT_3 receptor antagonist be continued for postchemotherapy emetic prophylaxis on days 2 and 3 (Hesketh 2020).

Oral, IV: 8 mg on days 2 and 3 (ASCO [Hesketh 2017]; MASCC/ESMO [Roila 2016]).

Low emetogenic risk (10% to 30% risk of emesis): Oral, IV: 4 to 8 mg administered as a single agent in a single dose prior to chemotherapy; prophylaxis is not necessary on subsequent days (ASCO [Hesketh 2017]; Hesketh 2020; MASCC/ESMO [Roila 2016]).

Antiemetic regimens: Radiation therapy-associated nausea and vomiting, prevention (off-label use):

High emetogenic risk radiation therapy (total body irradiation):

Radiation day(s): **Oral, IV:** 4 mg once daily prior to each fraction of radiation; give in combination with a 5-HT_3 receptor antagonist (ASCO [Hesketh 2017]).

Postradiation days: **Oral, IV:** The appropriate duration of therapy following radiotherapy days is not well defined; ASCO guidelines recommend continuing dexamethasone 4 mg once on the day after each day of radiation if radiation is not planned for that day (ASCO [Hesketh 2017]).

Moderate emetogenic risk radiation therapy (upper abdomen, craniospinal irradiation):

Radiation day(s): **Oral, IV:** 4 mg once daily prior to each of the first 5 fractions of radiation; give in combination with a 5-HT_3 receptor antagonist (ASCO [Hesketh 2017]).

Asthma, acute exacerbation (alternative agent) (off-label use): Note: Alternative to a longer course of other corticosteroids in mild to moderate exacerbations or in patients who do not respond promptly and completely to short-acting beta-agonists; administer within 1 hour of presentation to emergency department (GINA 2020; NAEPP 2007).

Oral: 16 mg daily for 2 days only (Kravitz 2011); longer treatment at this dose may be associated with metabolic adverse effects (GINA 2020).

Cerebral (vasogenic) edema associated with brain tumor:

Moderate to severe symptoms (eg, lowered consciousness/brainstem dysfunction):

Initial: **IV:** 10 mg once followed by maintenance dosing (Vecht 1994).

Maintenance: **IV, Oral:** 4 mg every 6 hours (Chang 2019; Vecht 1994). **Note:** Consider taper after 7 days of therapy; taper slowly over several weeks (Ryken 2010; Vecht 1994).

Mild symptoms: **IV, Oral:** 4 to 8 mg/day in 1 to 4 divided doses (Chang 2019; Vecht 1994). **Note:** Consider taper after 7 days of therapy; taper slowly over several weeks (Ryken 2010; Vecht 1994).

Coronavirus disease 2019 (COVID-19), treatment (hospitalized patient) (off-label use): See above.

Cushing syndrome, diagnosis: Note: Interpretation requires evaluation of one or more of the following: serum cortisol concentration, serum dexamethasone concentration, urinary cortisol excretion, or 17-hydroxycorticosteroid excretion; consultation with a clinical endocrinologist is recommended (ES [Nieman 2008]).

Initial testing:

Overnight 1 mg dexamethasone suppression test: **Oral:** 1 mg given once between 11 PM and 12 AM (ES [Nieman 2008]).

Longer low-dose dexamethasone suppression test (2 mg/day for 48 hours): **Note:** May be preferred in patients with depression, anxiety, obsessive-compulsive disorder, morbid obesity, alcoholism, or diabetes mellitus (ES [Nieman 2008]).

Oral: 0.5 mg every 6 hours for 48 hours for a total of 8 doses; start time varies (eg, 9 AM **or** 12 PM) (ES [Nieman 2008]; Yanovski 1993).

Fetal lung maturation, acceleration of (maternal administration) (alternative to preferred agent [ie, betamethasone]) (off-label use): Note: Generally, for women between 24 and 34 weeks of gestation, including those with ruptured membranes or multiple gestations, who are at risk of delivering within 7 days. A single course may be appropriate in some women beginning at 23 weeks' gestation or late preterm (between 34 0/7 weeks' and 36 6/7 weeks' gestation) who are at risk of delivering within 7 days.

IM: 6 mg every 12 hours for a total of 4 doses. May repeat course in select patients (eg, women with pregnancies up to 34 weeks' gestation at risk for delivery within 7 days and >14 days have elapsed since initial course of antenatal corticosteroids) (ACOG 171 2016; ACOG 217 2020; ACOG 713 2017).

Immune thrombocytopenia (initial therapy): Note: Goal of therapy is to provide a safe platelet count to prevent clinically important bleeding rather than normalization of the platelet count (Arnold 2019).

Oral, IV: 40 mg once daily for 4 days and then stop (no taper); may repeat if inadequate response (ASH [Neunert 2011]; Mazzucconi 2007; Provan 2010; Wei 2016). For severe bleeding with thrombocytopenia, give in combination with other therapies (Arnold 2019).

Iodinated contrast media allergic-like reaction, prevention (alternative agent): Note: Generally for patients with a prior allergic-like or unknown-type iodinated contrast reaction who will be receiving another iodinated contrast agent. Nonurgent premedication with an oral corticosteroid (eg, prednisone) is generally preferred when contrast administration is scheduled to begin in ≥12 hours; however, consider an urgent (accelerated) regimen with an IV corticosteroid for those requiring contrast in <12 hours (ACR 2018).

Urgent (accelerated) regimen: IV: 7.5 mg every 4 hours until contrast medium administration in combination with IV diphenhydramine 50 mg (administered 1 hour prior to contrast) (ACR 2018).

Meningitis (bacterial), prevention of neurologic complications (off-label use): Note: Administer first dose of dexamethasone shortly before or at the same time as the first dose of antibacterials. If antibacterials have already been administered, do **not** administer dexamethasone. In patients with pneumococcal meningitis who receive dexamethasone, some experts recommend adding rifampin to the standard initial antibacterial regimen or adding rifampin if susceptibility tests, once available, show intermediate susceptibility (MIC ≥2 mcg/mL) to ceftriaxone and cefotaxime (IDSA [Tunkel 2004]; Sexton 2019).

Developed world (suspected or confirmed pneumococcal meningitis): **IV:** 0.15 mg/kg/dose **or** 10 mg every 6 hours for 4 days; discontinue if culture data reveal non-pneumococcal etiology (de Gans 2002; IDSA [Tunkel 2004]; SCCM/ESICM [Pastores 2018]; Sexton 2019).

Developing world (strongly suspected or confirmed bacterial meningitis): **IV:** 0.4 mg/kg/dose every 12 hours for 4 days; discontinue if culture data reveal non-pneumococcal etiology; not recommended in regions with high rates of HIV infection and/or malnutrition or in cases of delayed clinical presentation (Nguyen 2007; Sexton 2019).

Multiple myeloma (off-label use): Note: Multiple dexamethasone-containing regimens are available. Refer to literature/guidelines for additional details. For many regimens, dexamethasone is continued until disease progression or unacceptable toxicity. When administered weekly, dexamethasone is reduced to 20 mg once weekly for frail patients (eg, >75 years of age, BMI <18.5, poorly controlled diabetes, corticosteroid intolerance) (Dimopoulos 2016b; Palumbo 2016).

*Combination regimens that do **not** include a monoclonal antibody:*

Oral:

40 mg once weekly on days 1, 8, 15, and 22 every 28 days in combination with lenalidomide (Rajkumar 2010), pomalidomide (San Miguel 2013), ixazomib and lenalidomide (Moreau 2015), carfilzomib and lenalidomide (Stewart 2015), or bortezomib and lenalidomide (Rajkumar 2011) **or** 40 mg once weekly on days 1, 8, 15, and 22 every 28 days in cycles 1 to 9, and then 40 mg once weekly on days 1, 8, and 15 every 28 days beginning at cycle 10 (in combination with carfilzomib) (Moreau 2018).

or

20 mg on days 1, 2, 8, 9, 15, 16, 22, and 23 every 28 days (in combination with carfilzomib) (Dimopoulos 2016a).

or

20 mg on days 1 and 3 of each week (in combination with selinexor) (Chari 2019).

or

40 mg once daily on days 1 to 4, 9 to 12, and 17 to 20 in combination with bortezomib and doxorubicin for 3 cycles as induction (Sonneveld 2012). **Note:** Some experts reserve this dosing (for 1 cycle, followed by 40 mg once weekly thereafter) for patients with an aggressive disease presentation or acute renal failure from light chain cast nephropathy (Rajkumar 2019).

Combination regimens that include a monoclonal antibody:

Oral, IV:

40 mg weekly in combination with daratumumab and pomalidomide (Chari 2017) or daratumumab and lenalidomide (Dimopoulos 2016b; Facon 2019) **or** isatuximab and pomalidomide (Attal 2019) or 20 mg once daily on days 1, 2, 4, 5, 8, 9, 11, and 12 in combination with daratumumab and bortezomib (Palumbo 2016). **Note:** In some studies, the dexamethasone dose is split over 2 days (20 mg before daratumumab and 20 mg the day after daratumumab infusion).

or

40 mg weekly, except on days elotuzumab is administered (administer dexamethasone 28 mg orally [8 mg orally in patients >75 years of age] plus 8 mg IV prior to elotuzumab) in combination with elotuzumab and pomalidomide (Dimopoulos 2018) or elotuzumab and lenalidomide (Lonial 2015).

Neoplastic epidural spinal cord compression, symptomatic: Note: As an adjunct to definitive treatment (radiotherapy or surgery), particularly in patients with neurologic deficits (Loblaw 2012; NICE 2008).

IV (initial dose): 10 or 16 mg followed by oral dosing (Loblaw 2012; NICE 2008).

Oral (after IV dose): 16 mg/day (usually given in 2 to 4 divided doses). Once definitive treatment is underway, taper gradually over 1 to 2 weeks until discontinuation (George 2015; Kumar 2017; Loblaw 2012; NICE 2008).

Tuberculosis, central nervous system: Note: In general, steroids are indicated for patients with established or suspected tuberculous meningitis, regardless of HIV status (HHS [OI adult 2019]; WHO 2017).

IV: Initial dose: 0.3 to 0.4 mg/kg/day for 2 weeks, then 0.2 mg/kg/day for week 3, then 0.1 mg/kg/day for week 4, followed by **oral** therapy (Leonard 2019; Thwaites 2004).

Oral: Starting week 5 of treatment: 4 mg/day, then taper by 1 mg of the daily dose each week; total combined IV/oral therapy duration: ~8 weeks (Leonard 2019; Thwaites 2004).

Geriatric Refer to adult dosing. Use cautiously in the elderly at the lowest possible dose.

Renal Impairment: Adult There are no dosage adjustments provided in the manufacturer's labeling; use with caution.

Hemodialysis: Supplemental dose is not necessary (Aronoff 2007).

Peritoneal dialysis: Supplemental dose is not necessary (Aronoff 2007).

International Myeloma Working Group (IMWG) Recommendations: The International Myeloma Working Group (IMWG) recommendations suggest that dexamethasone may be administered without dosage adjustment in multiple myeloma patients with renal impairment, including those on dialysis. The IMWG recommends the use of the Chronic Kidney Disease Epidemiology Collaboration (CKD-EPI) equation (preferred) or the Modification of Diet in Renal Disease (MDRD) formula to evaluate renal function estimation in multiple myeloma patients with a stable serum creatinine (Dimopoulos 2016c).

Hepatic Impairment: Adult There are no dosage adjustments provided in the manufacturer's labeling.

Pediatric

Note: Dexamethasone is currently under investigation for use in the treatment of coronavirus disease 2019 (COVID-19) (see ClinicalTrials.gov). Based on a preliminary report, use of dexamethasone is recommended for treatment of COVID-19 in hospitalized adults who require mechanical ventilation or supplemental oxygen (IDSA [Bhimraj 2020]; NIH 2020; RECOVERY Collaborative Group 2020). Safety and efficacy in pediatric patients for this indication are unknown (NIH 2020); pediatric patients continue to be recruited in the pediatric component of the Recovery Trial (RECOVERY Collaborative Group 2020; Recovery Trial 2020). As data and experience in pediatric patients continue to rapidly evolve, dosing will be updated as appropriate.

Acute mountain sickness (AMS) (moderate)/high altitude cerebral edema (HACE); treatment: Limited data available: Infants, Children, and Adolescents: Oral, IM, IV: 0.15 mg/kg/dose every 6 hours; maximum dose: 4 mg/dose; consider using for high altitude pulmonary edema because of associated HACE with this condition (Luks 2010; Pollard 2001).

Airway edema or extubation: Limited data available: Infants, Children, and Adolescents: Oral, IM, IV: 0.5 mg/kg/dose (maximum dose: 10 mg/dose) administered 6 to 12 hours prior to extubation then every 6 hours for 6 doses (total dexamethasone dose: 3 mg/kg) (Anene 1996; Khemani 2009; Tellez 1991).

Anti-inflammatory: Infants, Children, and Adolescents: Oral, IM, IV: Initial dose range: 0.02 to 0.3 mg/kg/**day or** 0.6 to 9 mg/**m²/day** in divided doses every 6 to 12 hours; dose depends upon condition being treated and response of patient; dosage for infants and children should be based on disease severity and patient response; usual adult daily dose range: 0.75 to 9 mg/day.

Asthma exacerbation: Limited data available: Infants, Children, and Adolescents: Oral, IM, IV: 0.6 mg/kg once daily as a single dose or once daily for 2 days; maximum dose: 16 mg/dose (AAP [Hegenbarth 2008]; Keeney 2014; Qureshi 2001); single dose regimens as low as 0.3 mg/kg/dose and as high as 1.7 mg/kg/dose have also been reported (Keeney 2014; Qureshi 2001; Shefrin 2009). **Note:** Duration >2 days is not recommended due to increased risk of metabolic effects (GINA 2014).

Bacterial meningitis (*H. influenzae* type b): Limited data available: Infants >6 weeks and Children: IV: 0.15 mg/kg/dose every 6 hours for the first 2 to 4 days of antibiotic treatment; start dexamethasone 10 to 20 minutes before or with the first dose of antibiotic; if antibiotics have already been administered, dexamethasone use has not been shown to improve patient outcome and is not recommended (IDSA [Tunkel 2004]). **Note:** For pneumococcal meningitis, data has not shown clear benefit from dexamethasone administration; risk and benefits should be considered prior to use (*Red Book* [AAP 2012]).

Cerebral edema: Infants, Children, and Adolescents: Oral, IM, IV: Loading dose: 1 to 2 mg/kg/dose as a single dose; maintenance: 1 to 1.5 mg/kg/**day** in divided doses every 4 to 6 hours; maximum daily dose: 16 mg/**day** (Kliegman 2007).

Chemotherapy-induced nausea and vomiting, prevention: Refer to individual protocols and emetogenic potential: Infants, Children, and Adolescents:

POGO recommendations (Dupuis 2013): **Note:** Reduce dose by 50% if administered concomitantly with aprepitant:

Highly/severely emetogenic chemotherapy: Oral, IV: 6 mg/**m²**/dose every 6 hours.

Moderately emetogenic chemotherapy: Oral, IV:

BSA ≤0.6 m^2: 2 mg every 12 hours.

BSA >0.6 m^2: 4 mg every 12 hours.

Alternate dosing: *Highly/severely emetogenic chemotherapy:* IV: Usual: 10 mg/**m²**/dose once daily on days of chemotherapy; some patients may require every 12-hour dosing; usual range: 8 to 14 mg/**m²**/dose (Holdsworth 2006; Jordan 2010; Phillips 2010); others have used: Initial: 10 mg/**m²**/dose prior to chemotherapy (maximum dose: 20 mg) then 5 mg/**m²**/dose every 6 hours (Kliegman 2007).

Congenital adrenal hyperplasia: Adolescents (fully grown): Oral: 0.25 to 0.5 mg once daily; use of a liquid dosage form may be preferable to allow for better dose titration (AAP 2010; Speiser 2010). **Note:** For younger patients who are still growing, hydrocortisone or fludrocortisone are preferred.

Croup (laryngotracheobronchitis): Limited data available; dosing regimens variable: Infants and Children: Oral, IM, IV: 0.6 mg/kg once; reported maximum dose highly variable; usual maximum dose: 16 mg/dose (AAP [Hegenbarth 2008]); in trials, maximum doses of 10 to 20 mg/dose have been reported with similar efficacy findings for mild to moderate croup. The majority of reported experience in infants are those ≥3 months of age; data available in <3 months of age is very limited (AAP [Hegenbarth 2008]; Bjornson 2004; Cruz 1995; Petrocheilou 2014; Russell 2011). In one evaluation of 22 children >2 years of age, a maximum dose of 12 mg/dose (at 0.6 mg/kg/dose) did not decrease endogenous glucocorticoid levels (Gill 2017). A single oral dose of 0.15 mg/kg has also been shown effective in infants ≥3 months and children with mild to moderate croup (Russell 2004; Sparrow 2006).

Physiologic replacement: Infants, Children, and Adolescents: Oral, IM, IV: 0.03 to 0.15 mg/kg/**day** in divided doses every 6 to 12 hours (Kliegman 2007) **or** Initial: 0.2 to 0.25 mg/$\mathbf{m^2}$/**day** administered once daily; some patients may require 0.3 mg/$\mathbf{m^2}$/**day** (Gupta 2008).

Renal Impairment: Pediatric Infants, Children, and Adolescents: There are no dosage adjustments provided in the manufacturer's labeling; use with caution. Hemodialysis or peritoneal dialysis: Supplemental dose is not necessary.

Hepatic Impairment: Pediatric Infants, Children, and Adolescents: There are no dosage adjustments provided in the manufacturer's labeling.

Mechanism of Action Dexamethasone is a long acting corticosteroid with minimal sodium-retaining potential. It decreases inflammation by suppression of neutrophil migration, decreased production of inflammatory mediators, and reversal of increased capillary permeability; suppresses normal immune response. Dexamethasone's mechanism of antiemetic activity is unknown.

Contraindications

Hypersensitivity to dexamethasone or any component of the formulation; systemic fungal infections

Documentation of allergenic cross-reactivity for corticosteroids is limited. However, because of similarities in chemical structure and/or pharmacologic actions, the possibility of cross-sensitivity cannot be ruled out with certainty.

Warnings/Precautions Corticosteroids are not approved for epidural injection. Serious neurologic events (eg, spinal cord infarction, paraplegia, quadriplegia, cortical blindness, stroke), some resulting in death, have been reported with epidural injection of corticosteroids, with and without use of fluoroscopy. Intra-articular injection may produce systemic as well as local effects. Appropriate examination of any joint fluid present is necessary to exclude a septic process. Avoid injection into an infected site. Do not inject into unstable joints. Patients should not overuse joints in which symptomatic benefit has been obtained as long as the inflammatory process remains active. Frequent intra-articular injection may result in damage to joint tissues.

Use with caution in patients with thyroid disease, hepatic impairment, renal impairment, cardiovascular disease, diabetes, glaucoma, cataracts, myasthenia gravis, osteoporosis, seizures, or GI diseases (diverticulitis, fresh intestinal anastomoses, active or latent peptic ulcer, ulcerative colitis, abscess or other pyogenic infection) due to perforation risk. Use with caution in patients with systemic sclerosis; an increase in scleroderma renal crisis incidence has been observed with corticosteroid use. Monitor BP and renal function in patients with systemic sclerosis treated with corticosteroids (EULAR [Kowal-Bielecka 2017]). Use caution following acute myocardial infarction (corticosteroids have been associated with myocardial rupture). Use with caution in patients with a history of ocular herpes simplex; corneal perforation has occurred; do not use in active ocular herpes simplex. Not recommended for the treatment of optic neuritis; may increase frequency of new episodes. Use with caution in the elderly with the smallest possible effective dose for the shortest duration. May affect growth velocity; growth should be routinely monitored in pediatric patients. Withdraw therapy with gradual tapering of dose.

May cause hypercortisolism or suppression of hypothalamic-pituitary-adrenal (HPA) axis, particularly in younger children or in patients receiving high doses for prolonged periods. HPA axis suppression may lead to adrenal crisis. Withdrawal and discontinuation of a corticosteroid should be done slowly and carefully. Particular care is required when patients are transferred from systemic corticosteroids to inhaled products due to possible adrenal insufficiency or withdrawal from steroids, including an increase in allergic symptoms. Adult patients receiving >20 mg per day of prednisone (or equivalent) may be most susceptible. Fatalities have occurred due to adrenal insufficiency in asthmatic patients during and after transfer from systemic corticosteroids to aerosol steroids; aerosol steroids do not provide the systemic steroid needed to treat patients having trauma, surgery, or infections. Dexamethasone does not provide adequate mineralocorticoid activity in adrenal insufficiency (may be employed as a single dose while cortisol assays are performed). In the management/prevention of adrenal crisis in patients with known primary adrenal insufficiency, the Endocrine Society practice guidelines state dexamethasone (intravenous) is the least preferred alternative agent and should be used only if no other glucocorticoid is available. For the treatment of chronic primary adrenal insufficiency (ie, physiologic replacement), dexamethasone (oral) is not recommended due to the risk of Cushingoid side effects (ES [Bornstein 2016]). Rare cases of anaphylactoid reactions have been observed in patients receiving corticosteroids. Patients may require higher doses when subject to stress (ie, trauma, surgery, severe infection).

Acute myopathy has been reported with high-dose corticosteroids, usually in patients with neuromuscular transmission disorders; may involve ocular and/or respiratory muscles; monitor creatine kinase; recovery may be delayed. Perineal burning, tingling, pain and pruritus have been reported with IV administration. May occur more commonly in females, with higher doses, and with rapid administration. Symptom onset is sudden and usually resolves in <1 minute (Allan 1986; Neff 2002; Perron 2003; Singh 2011). Corticosteroid use may cause psychiatric disturbances, including depression, euphoria, insomnia, mood swings, severe depression to psychotic manifestations. Preexisting psychiatric conditions may be exacerbated by corticosteroid use. Prolonged use of corticosteroids may increase the incidence of secondary infection, cause activation of latent infections, mask acute infection (including fungal infections), prolong or exacerbate viral infections, or limit response to killed or inactivated vaccines. Exposure to chickenpox or measles should be avoided; corticosteroids should not be used to treat ocular herpes simplex. Corticosteroids should not be used for cerebral malaria, fungal infections, or viral hepatitis. Close observation is required in patients with latent tuberculosis and/or TB reactivity; restrict use in active TB (only fulminating or disseminated TB in conjunction with antituberculosis treatment). Amebiasis should be ruled out in any patient with recent travel to tropic climates or unexplained diarrhea prior to initiation of corticosteroids. Use with extreme caution in patients with Strongyloides infections; hyperinfection, dissemination and fatalities have occurred.

Prolonged treatment with corticosteroids has been associated with the development of Kaposi sarcoma (case reports); if noted, discontinuation of therapy should be considered (Goedert 2002). High-dose corticosteroids should not be used to manage acute head injury (BTF [Carney 2016]). Some products may contain sodium sulfite, a sulfite that may cause allergic-type reactions including anaphylaxis and life-threatening or less severe asthmatic episodes in susceptible patients. Potentially significant drug-drug interactions may exist, requiring dose or frequency adjustment, additional monitoring, and/or selection of alternative therapy. Some dosage forms may contain propylene glycol; large amounts are potentially toxic and have been associated hyperosmolality, lactic acidosis, seizures, and respiratory depression; use caution (AAP ["Inactive" 1997]; Zar 2007).

Benzyl alcohol and derivatives: Some dosage forms may contain sodium benzoate/benzoic acid; benzoic acid (benzoate) is a metabolite of benzyl alcohol; large amounts of benzyl alcohol (≥99 mg/kg/day) have been associated with a potentially fatal toxicity ("gasping syndrome") in neonates; the "gasping syndrome" consists of metabolic acidosis, respiratory distress, gasping respirations, CNS dysfunction (including convulsions, intracranial hemorrhage), hypotension, and cardiovascular collapse (AAP ["Inactive" 1997]; CDC 1982); some data suggest that benzoate displaces bilirubin from protein binding sites (Ahlfors 2001); avoid or use dosage forms containing benzyl alcohol derivative with caution in neonates. See manufacturer's labeling.

Warnings: Additional Pediatric Considerations May cause osteoporosis (at any age) or inhibition of bone growth in pediatric patients. Use with caution in patients with osteoporosis. In a population-based study of children, risk of fracture was shown to be increased with >4 courses of corticosteroids; underlying clinical condition may also impact bone health and osteoporotic effect of corticosteroids (Leonard, 2007). In premature neonates, the use of high-dose dexamethasone (approximately >0.5 mg/kg/day) for the prevention or treatment of BPD has been associated with adverse neurodevelopmental outcomes, including higher rates of cerebral palsy without additional clinical benefit over lower doses; current data does not support use of high doses, further studies are needed (Watterberg, 2010). Increased IOP may occur especially with prolonged use; in children, increased IOP has also been shown to be dose-dependent with a greater IOP observed in children <6 years than older children after ophthalmic dexamethasone application; monitor closely (Lam 2005).

Some dosage forms may contain propylene glycol; in neonates large amounts of propylene glycol delivered orally, intravenously (eg, >3,000 mg/day), or topically have been associated with potentially fatal toxicities which can include metabolic acidosis, seizures, renal failure, and CNS depression; toxicities have also been reported in children and adults including hyperosmolality, lactic acidosis, seizures and respiratory depression; use caution (AAP 1997; Shehab 2009).

Drug Interactions

Metabolism/Transport Effects **Substrate** of CYP3A4 (major), P-glycoprotein/ABCB1; **Note:** Assignment of Major/Minor substrate status based on clinically relevant drug interaction potential; **Induces** CYP3A4 (weak)

Avoid Concomitant Use

Avoid concomitant use of DexAMETHasone (Systemic) with any of the following: Abametapir; Aldesleukin; BCG (Intravesical); Cladribine; Conivaptan; Desmopressin; Disulfiram; Fexinidazole [INT]; Fusidic Acid (Systemic); Idelalisib; Indium 111 Capromab Pendetide; Lapatinib; Macimorelin; Methotrimeprazine; Mifamurtide; MiFEPRIStone; Natalizumab; Pimecrolimus; Rilpivirine; Simeprevir; Tacrolimus (Topical)

Increased Effect/Toxicity

DexAMETHasone (Systemic) may increase the levels/effects of: Acetylcholinesterase Inhibitors; Amphotericin B; Androgens; Baricitinib; CycloSPORINE (Systemic); Deferasirox; Desirudin; Desmopressin; Fexinidazole [INT]; Fingolimod; Fosphenytoin; Leflunomide; Lenalidomide; Loop Diuretics; Methotrimeprazine; Natalizumab; Nicorandil; Nonsteroidal Anti-Inflammatory Agents (COX-2 Selective); Nonsteroidal Anti-Inflammatory Agents (Nonselective); Ozanimod; Phenytoin; Quinolones; Ritodrine; Sargramostim; Siponimod; Thalidomide; Thiazide and Thiazide-Like Diuretics; Tofacitinib; Upadacitinib; Vaccines (Live); Vitamin K Antagonists

The levels/effects of DexAMETHasone (Systemic) may be increased by: Abametapir; Aprepitant; Asparaginase (E. coli); Asparaginase (Erwinia); Cladribine; Clofazimine; Conivaptan; CycloSPORINE (Systemic); CYP3A4 Inhibitors (Moderate); CYP3A4 Inhibitors (Strong); Denosumab; DiltIAZem; Disulfiram; Duvelisib; Erdafitinib; Estrogen Derivatives; Fosamprenavir; Fosaprepitant; Fosnetupitant; Fusidic Acid (Systemic); Idelalisib; Indacaterol; Inebilizumab; Larotrectinib; MiFEPRIStone; Netupitant; Neuromuscular-Blocking Agents (Nondepolarizing); Ocrelizumab; Palbociclib; Pimecrolimus; Roflumilast; Salicylates; Stiripentol; Tacrolimus (Topical); Trastuzumab

Decreased Effect

DexAMETHasone (Systemic) may decrease the levels/effects of: Aldesleukin; Antidiabetic Agents; Axicabtagene Ciloleucel; BCG (Intravesical); Calcitriol (Systemic); Caspofungin; CloZAPine; Cobicistat; Coccidioides immitis Skin Test; Corticorelin; Cosyntropin; CycloSPORINE (Systemic); Daclatasvir; Dasatinib; Elvitegravir; Fosamprenavir; Fosphenytoin; Hyaluronidase; Imatinib; Indium 111 Capromab Pendetide; Isoniazid; Ixabepilone; Lapatinib; Macimorelin; Mifamurtide; Nalmefene; NiMODipine; Nivolumab; Phenytoin; Pidotimod; Rilpivirine; Salicylates; Selpercatinib; Simeprevir; Sipuleucel-T; Somatropin; Tacrolimus (Systemic); Temsirolimus; Tertomotide; Tisagenlecleucel; Triazolam; Ubrogepant; Urea Cycle

Disorder Agents; Vaccines (Inactivated); Vaccines (Live); Voriconazole

The levels/effects of DexAMETHasone (Systemic) may be decreased by: Antacids; Bile Acid Sequestrants; CYP3A4 Inducers (Moderate); CYP3A4 Inducers (Strong); Dabrafenib; Deferasirox; Echinacea; Enzalutamide; EPHEDrine (Systemic); Erdafitinib; Fosphenytoin; Ivosidenib; MiFEPRIStone; Mitotane; Phenytoin; Sarilumab; Siltuximab; Tocilizumab

Dietary Considerations May be taken with meals to decrease GI upset. May need diet with increased potassium, pyridoxine, vitamin C, vitamin D, folate, calcium, and phosphorus.

Pharmacodynamics/Kinetics

Onset of Action

Acetate: IV: Rapid.

Immune thrombocytopenia: Oral: Initial response: 2 to 14 days; Peak response: 4 to 28 days (Neunert 2011).

Duration of Action IV: Short.

Half-life Elimination

Extremely low birth-weight infants with BPD: 9.26 ± 3.34 hours (range: 5.85 to 16.1 hours) (Charles 1993).

Children 4 months to 16 years: 4.34 ± 4.14 hours (range: 2.33 to 9.54 hours) (Richter 1983).

Adults: Oral: 4 ± 0.9 hours (Czock 2005); IV: ~1 to 5 hours (Hochhaus 2001; Miyabo 1981; Rohdewald 1987; Tóth 1999).

Time to Peak Serum: Oral: 1 to 2 hours (Czock 2005); IM: ~30 to 120 minutes (Egerman 1997; Hochhaus 2001); IV: 5 to 10 minutes (free dexamethasone) (Miyabo 1981; Rohdewald 1987).

Pregnancy Risk Factor C

Pregnancy Considerations

Dexamethasone crosses the placenta (Brownfoot 2013); and is partially metabolized by placental enzymes to an inactive metabolite (Murphy 2007).

Some studies have shown an association between first trimester systemic corticosteroid use and oral clefts or decreased birth weight; however, information is conflicting and may be influenced by maternal dose/indication for use (Lunghi 2010; Park-Wyllie 2000; Pradat 2003). Hypoadrenalism may occur in newborns following maternal use of corticosteroids during pregnancy; monitor.

Dexamethasone is classified as a fluorinated corticosteroid. When systemic corticosteroids are needed in pregnancy for rheumatic disorders, nonfluorinated corticosteroids (eg, prednisone) are preferred. Chronic high doses should be avoided (ACR [Sammaritano 2020]).

Antenatal corticosteroid administration promotes fetal lung maturity and is associated with the reduction of intraventricular hemorrhage, necrotizing enterocolitis, neonatal mortality, and respiratory distress syndrome. A single course of dexamethasone is recommended for women between 24 0/7 and 33 6/7 weeks' gestation who are at risk of delivering within 7 days. This recommendation includes those with ruptured membranes or multiple gestations. A single course of dexamethasone may be considered for women beginning at 23 0/7 weeks' gestation who are at risk of delivering within 7 days, in consultation with the family regarding resuscitation. In addition, a single course of dexamethasone may be given to women between 34 0/7 weeks and 36 6/7 weeks who are at risk of preterm delivery within 7 days and who have not previously received corticosteroids if induction or delivery will proceed ≥24 hours and ≤7 days; delivery should not be delayed for administration of antenatal corticosteroids. Use of concomitant tocolytics is not currently recommended and administration of late preterm corticosteroids has not been evaluated in women with intrauterine infection, multiple gestations, pregestational diabetes, or women who delivered previously by cesarean section at term. Multiple repeat courses are not recommended. However, in women with pregnancies less than 34 weeks' gestation at risk for delivery within 7 days and who had a course of antenatal corticosteroids >14 days prior, a single repeat course may be considered; use of a repeat course in women with preterm prelabor rupture of membranes is controversial (ACOG 171 2016; ACOG 217 2020; ACOG 713 2017). Modifications are not required in pregnant patients diagnosed with coronavirus disease 2019 (COVID-19) (ACOG FAQ 2020).

Dexamethasone is used off label to decrease mortality in hospitalized patients with COVID-19 who require supplemental oxygen or mechanical ventilation. Treatment should not be withheld in pregnant patients when otherwise indicated (ACOG FAQ 2020).

The American College of Obstetricians and Gynecologists (ACOG) and the Society for Maternal-Fetal Medicine (SMFM) have developed an algorithm to aid practitioners in assessing and managing pregnant women with suspected or confirmed COVID-19 (https://www.acog.org/topics/covid-19; https://www.-smfm.org/covid19). Interim guidance is also available from the CDC for pregnant women who are diagnosed with COVID-19 (https://www.cdc.gov/coronavirus/2019-ncov/hcp/inpatient-obstetric-healthcare-guidance.html).

Breastfeeding Considerations

Corticosteroids are present in breast milk; information specific to dexamethasone has not been located.

The manufacturer notes that when used systemically, maternal use of corticosteroids have the potential to cause adverse events in a breastfeeding infant (eg, growth suppression, interfere with endogenous corticosteroid production). Due to the potential for serious adverse reactions in the breastfeeding infant, the manufacturer recommends a decision be made whether to discontinue breastfeeding or to discontinue the drug, considering the importance of treatment to the mother.

Single doses of dexamethasone are considered compatible with breastfeeding; information related to prolonged use is not available (WHO 2002). If there is concern about exposure to the infant, some guidelines recommend waiting 4 hours after the maternal dose of an oral systemic corticosteroid before breastfeeding in order to decrease potential exposure to the breastfed infant (based on a study using prednisolone) (Bae 2012; Leachman 2006; Makol 2011; Ost 1985). Dexamethasone is classified as a fluorinated corticosteroid. When systemic corticosteroids are needed in a lactating woman for rheumatic disorders, low doses of nonfluorinated corticosteroids (eg, prednisone) are preferred (ACR [Sammaritano 2020]).

Product Availability Hemady 20 mg tablets: FDA approved October 2019; anticipated availability is currently unknown. Information pertaining to this product within the monograph is pending revision. Hemady is indicated in combination with other antimyeloma products for the treatment of adults with multiple myeloma. Consult the prescribing information for additional information.

Dosage Forms: US

Concentrate, Oral:
Dexamethasone Intensol: 1 mg/mL (30 mL)

Elixir, Oral:
Generic: 0.5 mg/5 mL (237 mL)

Kit, Injection:
ReadySharp Dexamethasone: 10 mg/mL
TopiDex: 10 mg/mL

Kit, Injection [preservative free]:
Active Injection D: 10 mg/mL
DoubleDex: 10 mg/mL
MAS Care-Pak: 10 mg/mL

Solution, Injection:
Generic: 4 mg/mL (1 mL); 20 mg/5 mL (5 mL); 120 mg/30 mL (30 mL); 10 mg/mL (1 mL); 100 mg/10 mL (10 mL)

Solution, Injection [preservative free]:
Generic: 4 mg/mL (1 mL); 10 mg/mL (1 mL)

Solution, Oral:
Generic: 0.5 mg/5 mL (240 mL, 500 mL)

Solution Prefilled Syringe, Injection [preservative free]:
Generic: 10 mg/mL (1 mL)

Tablet, Oral:
Decadron: 0.5 mg, 0.75 mg, 4 mg, 6 mg
Generic: 0.5 mg, 0.75 mg, 1 mg, 1.5 mg, 2 mg, 4 mg, 6 mg

Tablet Therapy Pack, Oral:
Dexabliss: 1.5 MG (39) (39 ea)
Dxevo 11-Day: 1.5 mg (39 ea)
HiDex 6-Day: 1.5 mg (21 ea)
TaperDex 12-Day: 1.5 mg (49 ea)
TaperDex 6-Day: 1.5 mg (21 ea)
TaperDex 7-Day: 1.5 mg (27 ea)
Generic: 1.5 mg (21 ea, 35 ea, 51 ea)

Dosage Forms: Canada

Elixir, Oral:
Generic: 0.5 mg/5 mL (100 ea)

Solution, Injection:
Generic: 4 mg/mL (5 mL); 10 mg/mL (1 mL, 10 mL)

Tablet, Oral:
Generic: 0.5 mg, 0.75 mg, 2 mg, 4 mg

◆ **Dexamethasone Intensol** *see* DexAMETHasone (Systemic) *on page 463*

◆ **Dexamethasone Sodium Phosphate** *see* DexAMETHasone (Systemic) *on page 463*

◆ **Dexamethasone Sod Phosphate** *see* DexAMETHasone (Systemic) *on page 463*

◆ **Dexbrompheniramine, Chlophedianol, and Pseudoephedrine** *see* Chlophedianol, Dexbrompheniramine, and Pseudoephedrine *on page 332*

◆ **Dexbrompheniramine, Pseudoephedrine, and Chlophedianol** *see* Chlophedianol, Dexbrompheniramine, and Pseudoephedrine *on page 332*

Dexchlorpheniramine (deks klor fen EER a meen)

Brand Names: US RyClora

Pharmacologic Category Alkylamine Derivative; Histamine H_1 Antagonist; Histamine H_1 Antagonist, First Generation

Use Hypersensitivity reactions: For the treatment of perennial and seasonal allergic rhinitis; vasomotor rhinitis; allergic conjunctivitis; mild, uncomplicated allergic skin manifestations of urticaria and angioedema; amelioration of allergic reactions to blood or plasma; dermatographism; adjunctive therapy for the management of anaphylactic reactions.

Local Anesthetic/Vasoconstrictor Precautions No information available to require special precautions

Effects on Dental Treatment Key adverse event(s) related to dental treatment: Significant xerostomia (normal salivary flow resumes upon discontinuation)

Effects on Bleeding No information available to require special precautions

Adverse Reactions Frequency not defined.

Cardiovascular: Chest tightness

Central nervous system: Ataxia, chills, confusion, convulsions, dizziness, drowsiness (slight to moderate), euphoria, excitement, fatigue, hysteria, insomnia, irritability, nervousness, neuritis, paresthesia, restlessness, sedation, vertigo

Dermatologic: Diaphoresis, skin photosensitivity, skin rash (due to drug), urticaria

Gastrointestinal: Anorexia, constipation, diarrhea, epigastric distress, nausea, vomiting, xerostomia

Genitourinary: Difficulty in micturition, early menses, urinary frequency, urinary retention

Hematologic & oncologic: Agranulocytosis, hemolytic anemia, thrombocytopenia

Hypersensitivity: Anaphylactic shock

Neuromuscular & skeletal: Tremor

Ophthalmic: Blurred vision, diplopia

Otic: Acute labyrinthitis, tinnitus

Respiratory: Dry nose, dry throat, nasal congestion, thickening of bronchial secretions, wheezing

Mechanism of Action Dexchlorpheniramine competes with histamine for H_1-receptor sites on effector cells in the gastrointestinal tract, blood vessels, and respiratory tract. Dexchlorpheniramine is the predominant active isomer of chlorpheniramine and is approximately twice as active as the racemic compound (Moreno 2010).

Pharmacodynamics/Kinetics

Half-life Elimination 20 to 30 hours (Moreno 2010)

Time to Peak ~3 hours (Moreno 2010)

Pregnancy Considerations

Maternal antihistamine use has generally not resulted in an increased risk of birth defects; however, information specific to dexchlorpheniramine is limited (Källén 2002).

Dexchlorpheniramine is not the preferred antihistamine for the treatment of rhinitis or urticaria in pregnant women (BSACI [Powell 2015]; BSACI [Scadding 2017]; Zuberbier 2018).

◆ **Dexchlorpheniramine Maleate** *see* Dexchlorpheniramine *on page 471*

◆ **Dexedrine** *see* Dextroamphetamine *on page 474*

◆ **Dexilant** *see* Dexlansoprazole *on page 471*

Dexlansoprazole (deks lan SOE pra zole)

Related Information

Gastrointestinal Disorders *on page 1678*

Brand Names: US Dexilant

Brand Names: Canada Dexilant

Pharmacologic Category Proton Pump Inhibitor; Substituted Benzimidazole

Use

Erosive esophagitis: Healing of all grades of erosive esophagitis in patients ≥12 years of age for up to 8 weeks; to maintain healing of erosive esophagitis and relief of heartburn for up to 6 months in adults and 16 weeks in patients 12 to 17 years of age.

Gastroesophageal reflux disease: Treatment of heartburn associated with symptomatic nonerosive gastroesophageal reflux disease (GERD) in patients ≥12 years of age for 4 weeks.

Local Anesthetic/Vasoconstrictor Precautions No information available to require special precautions

Effects on Dental Treatment Key adverse event(s) related to dental treatment: Xerostomia (normal salivary flow resumes upon discontinuation) and taste alteration has been reported in <2% of patients.

Effects on Bleeding No information available to require special precautions

Adverse Reactions Incidence reported for adults unless otherwise specified.

1% to 10%:

Cardiovascular: Angina pectoris (<2%), bradycardia (<2%), cardiac arrhythmia (<2%), chest pain (<2%), deep vein thrombosis (<2%), edema (<2%; including oral, facial, and pharyngeal), hypertension (<2%), palpitations (<2%), tachycardia (<2%)

Central nervous system: Headache (adolescents: ≥5%; adults: <2%), abnormal dreams (<2%), anxiety (<2%), chills (<2%), depression (<2%), dizziness (<2%), falling (<2%), feeling abnormal (<2%), insomnia (<2%), memory impairment (<2%), migraine (<2%), myocardial infarction (<2%), pain (<2%), painful defecation (<2%), procedural pain (<2%), psychomotor agitation (<2%), seizure (<2%), trigeminal neuralgia (<2%), vertigo (<2%)

Dermatologic: Acne vulgaris (<2%), dermatitis (<2%), erythema (<2%), pruritus (<2%), skin lesion (<2%), skin rash (<2%), sunburn (<2%), urticaria (<2%)

Endocrine & metabolic: Change in libido (<2%), goiter (<2%), heavy menstrual bleeding (<2%), hot flash (<2%), hypercalcemia (<2%), hypokalemia (<2%), increased gastrin (<2%), increased serum glucose (<2%), increased serum potassium (<2%), increased serum total protein (<2%), menstrual disease (<2%), weight gain (<2%)

Gastrointestinal: Abdominal pain (adolescents: ≥5%), diarrhea (adolescents and adults: ≥5%), flatulence (1% to 3%), abdominal distress (<2%), abdominal tenderness (<2%), abnormal bowel sounds (<2%), abnormal stools (<2%), anorectal pain (<2%), Barrett esophagus (<2%), bezoar formation (<2%), biliary colic (<2%), change in appetite (<2%), cholelithiasis (<2%), colitis (microscopic; <2%), colonic polyps (<2%), constipation (<2%), delayed gastric emptying (<2%), duodenitis (<2%), dysgeusia (<2%), dyspepsia (<2%), dysphagia (<2%), enteritis (<2%), eructation (<2%), esophagitis (<2%), gastric polyp (<2%), gastritis (<2%), gastroenteritis (<2%), gastroesophageal reflux disease (<2%), gastrointestinal disease (<2%), gastrointestinal hypermotility (<2%), gastrointestinal perforation (<2%), gastrointestinal ulcer (<2%), halitosis (<2%), hematemesis (<2%), hematochezia (<2%), hemorrhoids (<2%), hiccups (<2%), irritable bowel syndrome (<2%), mucosal inflammation (<2%), mucus stools (<2%), oral bullae (<2%), oral herpes simplex infection (<2%), oral paresthesia (<2%), proctitis (<2%), retching (<2%), sore throat (<2%), vomiting (2%), xerostomia (<2%)

Genitourinary: Dysmenorrhea (<2%), dyspareunia (<2%), dysuria (<2%), urinary urgency (<2%), vulvovaginal infection (<2%)

Hematologic & oncologic: Anemia (<2%), decreased platelet count (<2%), lymphadenopathy (<2%), rectal hemorrhage (<2%)

Hepatic: Abnormal hepatic function tests (<2%), decreased serum bilirubin (<2%), hepatomegaly (<2%), increased serum alkaline phosphatase (<2%), increased serum alanine aminotransferase (<2%), increased serum aspartate aminotransferase (<2%), increased serum bilirubin (<2%)

Hypersensitivity: Hypersensitivity reaction (<2%)

Infection: Candidiasis (<2%), influenza (<2%), viral infection (<2%)

Neuromuscular & skeletal: Arthralgia (<2%), arthritis (<2%), asthenia (<2%), bone fracture (<2%), joint sprain (<2%), muscle cramps (<2%), musculoskeletal pain (<2%), myalgia (<2%), tremor (<2%)

Ophthalmic: Eye irritation (<2%), swelling of eye (<2%)

Otic: Otalgia (<2%), tinnitus (<2%)

Renal: Increased serum creatinine (<2%)

Respiratory: Nasopharyngitis (adolescents: ≥5%; adults: <2%), oropharyngeal pain (adolescents: ≥5%), upper respiratory tract infection (2% to 3%), asthma (<2%), bronchitis (<2%), cough (<2%), dyspnea (<2%), hyperventilation (<2%), pharyngitis (<2%), pulmonary aspiration (<2%), respiratory congestion (<2%), sinusitis (<2%)

Miscellaneous: Fever (<2%), inflammation (<2%), nodule (<2%)

<1%, postmarketing, and/or case reports: Acute renal failure, anaphylactic shock, autoimmune hemolytic anemia, blurred vision, cerebrovascular accident, chronic renal failure (Lazarus 2016), *Clostridioides* (formerly *Clostridium*) *difficile*-associated diarrhea, constriction of the pharynx, deafness, exfoliative dermatitis, hepatitis, hepatotoxicity (idiosyncratic) (Chalasani 2014), hypersensitivity angiitis, hypomagnesemia, hyponatremia, immune thrombocytopenia, pancreatitis, polyp (fundic gland), Stevens-Johnson syndrome, toxic epidermal necrolysis, transient ischemic attacks

Mechanism of Action Proton pump inhibitor; decreases acid secretion in gastric parietal cells through inhibition of (H+, K+)-ATPase enzyme system, blocking the final step in gastric acid production

Pharmacodynamics/Kinetics

Half-life Elimination ~1 to 2 hours

Time to Peak Serum: Two distinct peaks secondary to dual release formulation: Initial peak between 1 and 2 hours and a second higher peak between 4 and 5 hours.

Pregnancy Considerations Adverse events have not been observed in animal reproduction studies.

Recommendations for the treatment of GERD in pregnancy are available. As in nonpregnant patients, lifestyle modifications followed by other medications are the initial treatments (Body 2016; Huerta-Iga 2016; Katz 2013; van der Woude 2014). Based on available data, PPIs may be used when clinically indicated (use of agents with more available data may be preferred) (Body 2016; Matok 2012; Pasternak 2010; van der Woude 2014).

DexMEDEtomidine (deks MED e toe mi deen)

Brand Names: US Precedex

Brand Names: Canada Precedex

Pharmacologic Category $Alpha_2$-Adrenergic Agonist; Sedative

Use

Intensive care unit sedation: Sedation of initially-intubated and mechanically-ventilated patients during treatment in an intensive care setting

Procedural sedation: Procedural sedation prior to and/or during awake fiberoptic intubation; sedation prior to and/or during surgical or other procedures of non-intubated patients

Local Anesthetic/Vasoconstrictor Precautions No information available to require special precautions

Effects on Dental Treatment Key adverse event(s) related to dental treatment: Xerostomia and changes in salivation (normal salivary flow resumes upon discontinuation)

Effects on Bleeding No information available to require special precautions

Adverse Reactions Frequency dependent upon dose, duration, and indication.

>10%:

Cardiovascular: Hypotension (24% to 56%), bradycardia (5% to 42%), systolic hypertension (28%), tachycardia (25%), hypertension (diastolic; 12%), hypertension (11%)

Central nervous system: Agitation (5% to 14%)

Gastrointestinal: Constipation (6% to 14%), nausea (3% to 11%)

Respiratory: Respiratory depression (37%; placebo 32%)

1% to 10%:

Cardiovascular: Atrial fibrillation (2% to 9%), peripheral edema (3% to 7%), hypovolemia (3%), edema (2%)

Central nervous system: Anxiety (5% to 9%)

Endocrine & metabolic: Hypokalemia (9%), hyperglycemia (7%), hypoglycemia (5%), increased thirst (2%), hypocalcemia (1%), hypomagnesemia (1%)

Gastrointestinal: Xerostomia (3% to 4%)

Genitourinary: Oliguria (2%)

Hematologic & oncologic: Anemia (3%)

Renal: Acute renal failure (2% to 3%), decreased urine output (1%)

Respiratory: Respiratory failure (2% to 10%), adult respiratory distress syndrome (1% to 9%), pleural effusion (2%), wheezing (≤1%)

Miscellaneous: Fever (5% to 7%), withdrawal syndrome (ICU sedation; 3% to 5%)

Postmarketing and/or case reports: Abdominal pain, acidosis, apnea, atrioventricular block, bronchospasm, cardiac arrhythmia, cardiac disease, chills, confusion, convulsions, decreased visual acuity, delirium, diaphoresis, diarrhea, dizziness, drug tolerance (use >24 hours), dyspnea, extrasystoles, hallucination, headache, heart block, hemorrhage, hepatic insufficiency, hyperbilirubinemia, hypercapnia, hyperkalemia, hypernatremia, hyperpyrexia, hypoventilation, hypoxia, illusion, increased blood urea nitrogen, increased gamma-glutamyl transferase, increased serum alkaline phosphatase, increased serum ALT, increased serum AST, inversion T-wave on ECG, myocardial infarction, neuralgia, neuritis, pain, photopsia, polyuria, prolonged QT interval on ECG, pulmonary congestion, respiratory acidosis, rigors, seizure, sinoatrial arrest, speech disturbance, supraventricular tachycardia, tachyphylaxis (use >24 hours), variable blood pressure, ventricular arrhythmia, ventricular tachycardia, visual disturbance, vomiting

Mechanism of Action Selective $alpha_2$-adrenoceptor agonist with anesthetic and sedative properties thought to be due to activation of G-proteins by $alpha_{2a}$-adrenoceptors in the brainstem resulting in inhibition of norepinephrine release; peripheral $alpha_{2b}$-adrenoceptors are activated at high doses or with rapid IV administration resulting in vasoconstriction.

Pharmacodynamics/Kinetics

Onset of Action

IV loading dose: 5 to 10 minutes

Intranasal: 45 to 60 minutes (Yuen 2007), may be faster in pediatric patients when administered via an atomizing device (Talon 2009)

Peak effect:

IV loading dose: 15 to 30 minutes

Intranasal: 90 to 105 minutes (Yuen 2007)

Duration of Action Dose dependent: 60 to 120 minutes

Half-life Elimination

Preterm Neonates (28 to <36 weeks GA): Terminal: 7.6 hours (range: 3 to 9.1 hours) (Chrysostomou 2014)

Term Neonates (36 to ≤44 weeks GA): Terminal: Median: 3.2 hours (range: 1 to 9.4 hours) (Chrysostomou 2014)

Infants and Children <2 years: Terminal: Median: 2.3 hours (range: 1.5 to 3.3 hours) (Vilo 2008)

Children 2 to 11 years: Terminal: Median: 1.6 hours (range: 1.2 to 2.3 hours) (Vilo 2008)

Adults: Distribution: ~6 minutes; Terminal: ~up to 3 hours (Venn 2002); significantly prolonged in patients with severe hepatic impairment (Cunningham 1999)

Time to Peak Serum: Intranasal: Median: 38 minutes (range: 15 to 60 minutes) (Iirola 2011)

Pregnancy Risk Factor C

Pregnancy Considerations

Dexmedetomidine is expected to cross the placenta. Information related to use during pregnancy is limited (El-Tahan 2012).

◆ **Dexmedetomidine HCl** *see* DexMEDEtomidine *on page 472*

◆ **Dexmedetomidine Hydrochloride** *see* DexMEDEtomidine *on page 472*

Dexmethylphenidate (dex meth il FEN i date)

Brand Names: US Focalin; Focalin XR

Pharmacologic Category Central Nervous System Stimulant

Use Attention-deficit/hyperactivity disorder: Treatment of attention-deficit/hyperactivity disorder.

Local Anesthetic/Vasoconstrictor Precautions No information available to require special precautions

Effects on Dental Treatment Key adverse event(s) related to dental treatment: Dexmethylphenidate causes tachycardia, increases in blood pressure, and palpitations. Consider monitoring blood pressure prior to using local anesthetic with a vasoconstrictor. Symptoms associated with bruxism have been observed in some patients.

Effects on Bleeding No information available to require special precautions

Adverse Reactions Actual frequency may be dependent upon dose and/or formulation. Also refer to Methylphenidate for adverse effects seen with other methylphenidate products.

>10%:

Central nervous system: Headache (adults: 26% to 39%; children and adolescents: 25%), insomnia (children and adolescents: 5% to 17%), jitteriness (adults: 12%), anxiety (5% to 11%)

Gastrointestinal: Decreased appetite (children and adolescents: 30%), xerostomia (adults: 7% to 20%), abdominal pain (children and adolescents: 15%)

1% to 10%:

Central nervous system: Dizziness (adults: 6%), irritability (children and adolescents: 2% to 5%), depression (children and adolescents: 3%), emotional lability (children and adolescents: 3%)

Dermatologic: Pruritus (children and adolescents: 3%)

Gastrointestinal: Nausea (children and adolescents: 9%), dyspepsia (5% to 9%), vomiting (children and adolescents: 2% to 9%), anorexia (children and adolescents: 5% to 7%)

Respiratory: Pharyngolaryngeal pain (adults: 4% to 7%), nasal congestion (children and adolescents: 5%)

Miscellaneous: Fever (children and adolescents: 5%)

Frequency not defined:

Central nervous system: Drug abuse, drug dependence

Endocrine & metabolic: Growth suppression, weight loss

<1%, postmarketing, and/or case reports: Anaphylaxis, angioedema, hypersensitivity reactions, peripheral vascular disease, Raynaud disease, rhabdomyolysis

Mechanism of Action Dexmethylphenidate is the more active, *d-threo*-enantiomer, of racemic methylphenidate. It is a CNS stimulant; blocks the reuptake of norepinephrine and dopamine, and increases their release into the extraneuronal space.

Pharmacodynamics/Kinetics

Onset of Action Rapid, within 1 to 2 hours of an effective dose

Duration of Action Immediate release: 3 to 5 hours; extended release: 9 to 12 hours (Dopheide 2009)

Half-life Elimination Immediate release: Children: 2 to 3 hours; Adults: 3 hours

Time to Peak Fasting:

Immediate release: 1 to 1.5 hours; after a high-fat meal: 2.9 hours

Extended release: First peak: 1.5 hours (range: 1 to 4 hours); Second peak: 6.5 hours (range: 4.5 to 7 hours)

Pregnancy Considerations Dexmethylphenidate is the more active *d-threo* enantiomer of racemic methylphenidate; refer to the methylphenidate monograph for additional information.

Controlled Substance C-II

- ◆ **Dexmethylphenidate HCl** *see* Dexmethylphenidate *on page 473*
- ◆ **Dexmethylphenidate Hydrochloride** *see* Dexmethylphenidate *on page 473*
- ◆ **DexPak 6 Day [DSC]** *see* DexAMETHasone (Systemic) *on page 463*
- ◆ **DexPak 10 Day [DSC]** *see* DexAMETHasone (Systemic) *on page 463*
- ◆ **DexPak 13 Day [DSC]** *see* DexAMETHasone (Systemic) *on page 463*
- ◆ **Dextroamphetam/Amphetam(Base)** *see* Dextroamphetamine and Amphetamine *on page 475*

Dextroamphetamine (deks troe am FET a meen)

Brand Names: US Dexedrine; ProCentra; Zenzedi

Brand Names: Canada ACT Dextroamphetamine SR; Dexedrine

Pharmacologic Category Central Nervous System Stimulant

Use

Attention-deficit/hyperactivity disorder: Treatment of attention-deficit/hyperactivity disorder as part of a total treatment program that typically includes other remedial measures (psychological, educational, social) for a stabilizing effect in pediatric patients 3 to 16 years (IR tablet, oral solution) or 6 to 16 years (ER capsule).

Narcolepsy: Treatment of narcolepsy.

Local Anesthetic/Vasoconstrictor Precautions Use vasoconstrictor with caution in patients taking dextroamphetamine. Amphetamines enhance the sympathomimetic response of epinephrine and norepinephrine leading to potential hypertension and cardiotoxicity.

Effects on Dental Treatment Key adverse event(s) related to dental treatment: Dextroamphetamine causes tachycardia, increases in blood pressure, and palpitations. Consider monitoring blood pressure prior to using local anesthetic with a vasoconstrictor. Symptoms associated with bruxism have been observed in some patients.

Effects on Bleeding No information available to require special precautions

Adverse Reactions Frequency not defined.

Cardiovascular: Cardiomyopathy, hypertension, palpitations, tachycardia

Central nervous system: Aggressive behavior, dizziness, dysphoria, euphoria, exacerbation of tics, Gilles de la Tourette syndrome, headache, insomnia, mania, overstimulation, psychosis, restlessness

Dermatologic: Alopecia, urticaria

Endocrine & metabolic: Change in libido, weight loss

Gastrointestinal: Anorexia, constipation, diarrhea, unpleasant taste, xerostomia

Genitourinary: Frequent erections, impotence, prolonged erection

Neuromuscular & skeletal: Dyskinesia, rhabdomyolysis, tremor

Ophthalmic: Accommodation disturbances, blurred vision

Mechanism of Action Amphetamines are noncatecholamine, sympathomimetic amines that promote release of catecholamines (primarily dopamine and norepinephrine) from their storage sites in the presynaptic nerve terminals. A less significant mechanism may include their ability to block the reuptake of catecholamines by competitive inhibition.

Pharmacodynamics/Kinetics

Duration of Action Immediate release: 4 to 6 hours; extended release: 8 hours (Dopheide 2009)

Half-life Elimination Adults: ~12 hours

Time to Peak Serum: Immediate release: ~3 hours; Sustained release: ~8 hours

Pregnancy Considerations

The majority of human data is based on illicit amphetamine/methamphetamine exposure and not from therapeutic maternal use (Golub 2005). Use of amphetamines during pregnancy may lead to an increased risk of premature birth and low birth weight; newborns may experience symptoms of withdrawal. Behavioral problems may also occur later in childhood (LaGasse 2012).

Controlled Substance C-II

- ◆ **Dextroamphetamine/Amphetamine** *see* Dextroamphetamine and Amphetamine *on page 475*

Dextroamphetamine and Amphetamine

(deks troe am FET a meen & am FET a meen)

Related Information

Dextroamphetamine *on page 474*

Brand Names: US Adderall; Adderall XR; Mydayis

Brand Names: Canada Adderall XR

Pharmacologic Category Central Nervous System Stimulant

Use

Attention-deficit/hyperactivity disorder: Treatment of attention-deficit/hyperactivity disorder (ADHD) as part of a total treatment program that typically includes other remedial measures (psychological, educational, social) for a stabilizing effect.

Narcolepsy, daytime sleepiness (immediate release only): Treatment of narcolepsy.

Local Anesthetic/Vasoconstrictor Precautions Use vasoconstrictor with caution in patients taking dextroamphetamine. Amphetamines enhance the sympathomimetic response of epinephrine and norepinephrine leading to potential hypertension and cardiotoxicity.

Effects on Dental Treatment Key adverse event(s) related to dental treatment: Frequent occurrence of xerostomia (normal salivary flow resumes upon discontinuance) has been reported. Infrequent occurrence of speech disturbances, tooth infections, and symptoms associated with clenching and bruxism have been observed in some patients. Rare occurrences of unpleasant taste and Stevens-Johnson syndrome have been reported.

Dextroamphetamine and amphetamine also cause tachycardia, increases in blood pressure, and palpitations. Consider monitoring blood pressure prior to using local anesthetic with a vasoconstrictor.

Effects on Bleeding No information available to require special precautions

Adverse Reactions Frequency not always defined.

Cardiovascular: Systolic hypertension (extended release; adolescents: 12% to 35%; dose related; transient), tachycardia (extended release; adults: ≤6%), palpitations (extended release: 2% to 4%), increased blood pressure, myocardial infarction, Raynaud's phenomenon

Central nervous system: Insomnia (extended release: 8% to 31%), headache (extended release; adults: ≤26%), emotional lability (extended release: 2% to 9%), anxiety (extended release; adults: 7% to 8%), agitation (extended release; adults: 2% to ≤8%), dizziness (extended release: 2% to 7%), irritability (6%), fatigue (extended release: 2% to 6%), drowsiness (extended release: 2% to 4%), speech disturbance (extended release: 2% to 4%), twitching (extended release: 2% to 4%), depression (3%), jitteriness (2%), aggressive behavior, dysphoria, euphoria, exacerbation of vocal tics, formication, outbursts of anger, overstimulation, paresthesia, psychosis, restlessness, talkativeness

Dermatologic: Diaphoresis (extended release: 2% to 4%), skin photosensitivity (extended release: 2% to 4%), alopecia, dermatillomania, skin rash, urticaria

Endocrine & metabolic: Weight loss (extended release: 4% to 10%), decreased libido (extended release: 2% to 4%), dysmenorrhea (extended release: 2% to 4%)

Gastrointestinal: Decreased appetite (extended release: 22% to 36%), xerostomia (extended release: 2% to 35%), abdominal pain (extended release: 11% to 14%), nausea (extended release: 2% to 8%), vomiting (extended release: 2% to 7%), diarrhea (extended release: 2% to 6%), constipation (extended release: 2% to 4%), dyspepsia (extended release: 2% to 4%), teeth clenching (extended release: ≤4%), tooth infection (extended release: ≤4%), anorexia (extended release: 2%), bruxism (2%), unpleasant taste

Genitourinary: Urinary tract infection (extended release: 5%), upper abdominal pain (adolescents: 4%), impotence (extended release: 2% to 4%), erectile dysfunction (2%), frequent erections, prolonged erections

Hypersensitivity: Anaphylaxis, angioedema, hypersensitivity reaction

Infection: Infection (extended release: 2% to 4%)

Neuromuscular & skeletal: Dyskinesia, rhabdomyolysis, tremor

Ophthalmic: Blurred vision, mydriasis

Respiratory: Dyspnea (extended release: 2% to 4%)

Miscellaneous: Fever (extended release: 5%), accidental injury (children and adolescents: 4%)

<1%, postmarketing, and/or case reports: Cardiomyopathy, cerebrovascular accident, exacerbation of Gilles de la Tourette's syndrome, exacerbation of vocal tics, peripheral vascular disease, seizure, Stevens-Johnson syndrome, toxic epidermal necrolysis

Mechanism of Action Amphetamines are noncatecholamine, sympathomimetic amines that promote release of catecholamines (primarily dopamine and norepinephrine) from their storage sites in the presynaptic nerve terminals. A less significant mechanism may include their ability to block the reuptake of catecholamines by competitive inhibition.

Pharmacodynamics/Kinetics

Duration of Action Immediate-release tablet: 4 to 6 hours (Dopheide 2009); Adderall XR: 8 to 12 hours (Jain 2017); Mydayis: ≤16 hours

Half-life Elimination

Children 6 to 12 years: d-amphetamine: 9 hours; l-amphetamine: 11 hours

Adolescents 13 to 17 years: d-amphetamine: 11 hours; l-amphetamine: 13 to 14 hours

Adults: d-amphetamine: 10 hours; l-amphetamine: 13 hours

Time to Peak Immediate release: 3 hours; Adderall XR: 7 hours; Mydayis: 7 to 10 hours (children and adolescents 6 to 17 years), 8 hours (adults)

Pregnancy Considerations

Outcome information related to the use of amphetamine/dextroamphetamine in pregnant women with attention-deficit/hyperactivity disorder is limited (Ornoy 2018).

Data collection to monitor pregnancy outcomes following exposure to amphetamine/dextroamphetamine is ongoing. Health care providers are encouraged to enroll females exposed to amphetamine/dextroamphetamine during pregnancy in the National Pregnancy Registry for Psychostimulants (1-866-961-2388 and/or https://womensmentalhealth.org/clinical-and-research-programs/pregnancyregistry/othermedications).

Refer to individual monographs for additional information.

Controlled Substance C-II

◆ **Dextroamphetamine Sulfate** *see* Dextroamphetamine *on page 474*

Dextromethorphan (deks troe meth OR fan)

Brand Names: US Buckleys Cough [OTC]; Cough DM [OTC]; Creomulsion Adult [OTC] [DSC]; Creomulsion for Children [OTC] [DSC]; Delsym Cough Childrens [OTC]; Delsym [OTC]; ElixSure Cough [OTC]; GoodSense Cough DM Childrens [OTC]; GoodSense Cough DM [OTC]; Hold [OTC]; Little Colds Cough Formula [OTC]; PediaCare Childrens Long-Act [OTC]; Robafen Cough [OTC]; Robitussin 12 Hour Cough Child [OTC]; Robitussin 12 Hour Cough [OTC]; Robitussin Childrens Cough LA [OTC]; Robitussin Lingering CoughGels [OTC]; Robitussin Lingering LA Cough [OTC] [DSC]; Scot-Tussin Diabetes CF [OTC] [DSC]; Silphen DM Cough [OTC]; Triaminic Long Acting Cough [OTC]; Trocal Cough Suppressant [OTC] [DSC]

Pharmacologic Category Antitussive; N-Methyl-D-Aspartate (NMDA) Receptor Antagonist

Use Cough (suppressant): Temporary control of cough due to minor throat and bronchial irritation associated with the common cold or inhaled irritants; temporary relief of cough impulse to improve sleep (extended release formulations)

Local Anesthetic/Vasoconstrictor Precautions No information available to require special precautions

Effects on Dental Treatment No significant effects or complications reported

Effects on Bleeding No information available to require special precautions

Adverse Reactions

Frequency not defined.

Central nervous system: Dizziness, drowsiness, nervousness, restlessness

Gastrointestinal: Gastrointestinal distress, nausea, stomach pain, vomiting

Mechanism of Action Decreases the sensitivity of cough receptors and interrupts cough impulse transmission by depressing the medullary cough center through sigma receptor stimulation; structurally related to codeine

Pharmacodynamics/Kinetics

Onset of Action Antitussive: 15 to 30 minutes.

Half-life Elimination

Dextromethorphan:

Pediatric patients: Excluding poor metabolizers (Guenin 2014).

Children 2 to 5 years: 4.09 ± 1.44 hours.

Children 6 to 11 years: 4.8 ± 1.59 hours.

Children ≥12 years and Adolescents: 6.41 ± 1.639 hours.

Adults: Extensive metabolizers: 2 to 4 hours; poor metabolizers: 24 hours.

Time to Peak

Children 2 to 5 years: 1.44 ± 0.563 hours (Guenin 2014).

Children 6 to 11 years: 2.12 ± 0.801 hours (Guenin 2014).

Children ≥12 years and Adolescents: 2.04 ± 0.865 hours (Guenin 2014).

Adults: Mean range: 2.1 to 2.6 hours (Silvasti 1987).

Peak concentration:

Pediatric patients: Excluding poor metabolizers (Guenin 2014).

Children 2 to 5 years (following doses of 7.5 to 11.25 mg): 1.47 ± 1.597 ng/mL.

Children 6 to 11 years (following doses of 15 to 24.75 mg): 1.26 ± 1.211 ng/mL.

Children ≥12 years and Adolescents (following doses of 30 mg): 4.9 ± 4.215 ng/mL.

Adults (following doses of 60 mg): Mean range: 5.2 to 5.8 ng/mL (Silvasti 1987).

Pregnancy Considerations Dextromethorphan is metabolized in the liver via CYP2D6 and CYP3A enzymes. The activity of both enzymes is increased in the mother during pregnancy (Tracy 2005; Wadelius 1997). In the fetus, CYP2D6 activity is low in the fetal liver and CYP3A4 activity is present by ~17 weeks' gestation (Jacqz-Aigrain 1992).

When an antitussive is needed during pregnancy, dextromethorphan at standard OTC doses is generally considered acceptable. Some sources recommend use be reserved for significant maternal need; products containing alcohol should be avoided (Chasnoff 1981; Conover 2003; Koren 1998; Ward 2005).

- **Dezocitidine** *see* Decitabine *on page* 447
- **DF** *see* Defibrotide *on page* 449
- **dFdC** *see* Gemcitabine *on page* 731
- **dFdCyd** *see* Gemcitabine *on page* 731
- **DHAD** *see* MitoXANTRONE *on page* 1042
- **DHAQ** *see* MitoXANTRONE *on page* 1042
- **DHE** *see* Dihydroergotamine *on page* 499
- **D.H.E. 45** *see* Dihydroergotamine *on page* 499
- **DHPG Sodium** *see* Ganciclovir (Systemic) *on page* 728
- **Diabeta** *see* GlyBURIDE *on page* 741
- **DiabetAid Pain and Tingling Relief [OTC]** *see* Capsaicin *on page* 284
- **Diacomit** *see* Stiripentol *on page* 1388
- **Dialyvite Omega-3 Concentrate [OTC]** *see* Omega-3 Fatty Acids *on page* 1137
- **Dialyvite Probiotic [OTC]** *see* *Lactobacillus* *on page* 869
- **Dialyvite Vitamin D 5000 [OTC]** *see* Cholecalciferol *on page* 344
- **Dialyvite Vitamin D3 Max [OTC]** *see* Cholecalciferol *on page* 344
- **Diaminocyclohexane Oxalatoplatinum** *see* Oxaliplatin *on page* 1151
- **Diaminodiphenylsulfone** *see* Dapsone (Systemic) *on page* 436
- **Diaminodiphenylsulfone** *see* Dapsone (Topical) *on page* 437
- **3,4-diaminopyridine** *see* Amifampridine *on page* 114
- **Diamode [OTC]** *see* Loperamide *on page* 928
- **Diamox Sequels [DSC]** *see* AcetaZOLAMIDE *on page* 73
- **Diaphenylsulfone** *see* Dapsone (Systemic) *on page* 436
- **Diaphenylsulfone** *see* Dapsone (Topical) *on page* 437
- **Diastat AcuDial** *see* DiazePAM *on page* 477
- **Diastat Pediatric** *see* DiazePAM *on page* 477
- **Diatx Zn** *see* Vitamins (Multiple/Oral) *on page* 1550

DiazePAM (dye AZ e pam)

Related Information

Dentin Hypersensitivity, Acid Erosion, High Caries Index, Management of Alveolar Osteitis, and Xerostomia *on page 1762*

Management of the Patient With Anxiety or Depression *on page 1778*

Temporomandibular Dysfunction (TMD), Chronic Pain, and Fibromyalgia *on page 1773*

Related Sample Prescriptions

Sedation (Prior to Dental Treatment) - Sample Prescriptions *on page 45*

Brand Names: US Diastat AcuDial; Diastat Pediatric; diazePAM Intensol; Valium; Valtoco 10 MG Dose; Valtoco 15 MG Dose; Valtoco 20 MG Dose; Valtoco 5 MG Dose

Brand Names: Canada BIO-Diazepam; Diastat; Diazepam 10 [DSC]; Diazepam 5 [DSC]; PMS-Diazepam; Valium

Generic Availability (US) May be product dependent

Pharmacologic Category Anticonvulsant, Benzodiazepine; Benzodiazepine

Dental Use Oral medication for preoperative dental anxiety; sedative component in IV conscious sedation in oral surgery patients; skeletal muscle relaxant

Use

Alcohol withdrawal syndrome (oral and injection): Symptomatic relief of acute agitation, tremor, impending or acute delirium, delirium tremens, and hallucinosis associated with alcohol withdrawal.

Anxiety, acute/severe (oral and injection): Short-term relief of severe anxiety symptoms.

Anxiety disorders (oral and injection): Management of anxiety disorders.

Muscle spasm, spasticity, and/or rigidity (oral and injection): As an adjunct for the relief of skeletal muscle spasm due to reflex spasm caused by local pathology (eg, inflammation of muscles or joints, secondary to trauma); spasticity caused by upper motor neuron disorders (eg, cerebral palsy, paraplegia); athetosis; stiff-man syndrome; and tetanus.

Procedural anxiety, premedication (injection): Relief of anxiety and tension in patients undergoing surgical procedures; prior to cardioversion for the relief of anxiety and tension and to diminish patient's recall (IV only); as an adjunct prior to endoscopic procedures for apprehension, anxiety, or acute stress reactions and to diminish patient's recall.

Note: Use of diazepam in patients undergoing cardioversion or endoscopic procedures has been superseded by agents with a more pharmacokinetically favorable profile (eg, midazolam) (Thomas 2014; Triantafillidis 2013).

Seizures, acute, active: Adjunct in convulsive disorders (oral); management of select, refractory epilepsy patients on stable regimens of antiepileptic drugs requiring intermittent use of diazepam to control episodes of increased seizure activity (rectal); treatment of intermittent, stereotypic episodes of frequent seizure activity (ie, seizure clusters, acute repetitive seizures) that are distinct from a patient's usual seizure pattern in patients with epilepsy (intranasal); adjunct in severe recurrent convulsive seizures (injection).

Status epilepticus (injection): Adjunct in status epilepticus.

Local Anesthetic/Vasoconstrictor Precautions No information available to require special precautions

Effects on Dental Treatment Key adverse event(s) related to dental treatment: Xerostomia and changes in salivation (normal salivary flow resumes upon discontinuation) (see Dental Health Professional Considerations)

Effects on Bleeding No information available to require special precautions

Adverse Reactions Adverse reactions may vary by route of administration.

>10%: Nervous system: Drowsiness (23%)

1% to 10%:

Cardiovascular: Hypotension (1% to 2%), vasodilation (1% to 2%)

Dermatologic: Skin rash (3%)

Gastrointestinal: Abdominal pain (≥1%), diarrhea (4%), dysgeusia (2%)

Nervous system: Abnormality in thinking (1% to 2%), agitation (≥1%), ataxia (3%), confusion (≥1%), dizziness (3%), emotional lability (≥1%), euphoria (3%), headache (5%), nervousness (≥1%), pain (≥1%), speech disturbance (≥1%)

Neuromuscular & skeletal: Asthenia (1% to 2%)

Respiratory: Asthma (2%), epistaxis (3%), nasal congestion (3%), nasal discomfort (6%), rhinitis (≥1%)

<1%:

Cardiovascular: Bradycardia, circulatory shock, syncope

Dermatologic: Diaphoresis, pruritus, urticaria

Gastrointestinal: Anorexia, vomiting

Genitourinary: Urinary tract infection

Hematologic & oncologic: Anemia, lymphadenopathy, neutropenia

Infection: Infection

Nervous system: Tonic clonic type of status epilepticus

Neuromuscular & skeletal: Hyperkinetic muscle activity

Ophthalmic: Mydriasis, nystagmus disorder

Respiratory: Cough

Frequency not defined:

Cardiovascular: ECG changes, localized phlebitis, venous thrombosis

Endocrine & metabolic: Change in libido

Gastrointestinal: Altered salivation, constipation, gastrointestinal distress, hiccups, nausea

Genitourinary: Urinary incontinence, urinary retention

Hematologic & oncologic: Neutropenia

Hepatic: Increased serum alkaline phosphatase, increased serum transaminases, jaundice

Nervous system: Anterograde amnesia, central nervous system depression, depression, drug dependence, drug withdrawal, dysarthria, fatigue, hypoactivity, myasthenia, paradoxical central nervous system stimulation, psychiatric signs and symptoms, slurred speech, vertigo

Neuromuscular & skeletal: Tremor

Ophthalmic: Blurred vision, diplopia

Dental Usual Dosage

Anxiety/sedation/skeletal muscle relaxant: Adults:

Oral: 2 to 10 mg 2 to 4 times daily

IM, IV: 2 to 10 mg, may repeat in 3 to 4 hours if needed

Anxiety: Elderly: Oral: Initial: 1 to 2 mg 1 to 2 times daily; increase gradually as needed, rarely need to use >10 mg daily (watch for hypotension and excessive sedation)

Skeletal muscle relaxant: Elderly: Oral: Initial: 2 to 5 mg 2 to 4 times daily

Dosing

Adult Note: Avoid use in patients with, or at risk for, substance abuse disorders, except for acute or emergency situations (eg, status epilepticus).

Anxiety:

Anxiety, acute/severe (monotherapy or adjunctive therapy):

IM, IV, Oral: 2 to 10 mg every 3 to 6 hours as needed up to 40 mg/day; adjust dose based on response and tolerability (Bystritsky 2019; WFSBP [Bandelow 2012]).

Anxiety disorders (monotherapy or adjunctive therapy) (alternative agent):

Note: Most commonly used short term for immediate symptom relief until concurrent therapy is effective (eg, ≤12 weeks). Long-term therapy may be considered for select patients only when other treatments are ineffective or poorly tolerated (Katzman 2014; WFSBP [Bandelow 2012]).

Oral: Initial: 2 to 5 mg once or twice daily; increase gradually based on response and tolerability up to 40 mg/day in 2 to 4 divided doses (Bystritsky 2019).

Procedural anxiety (premedication):

IV: 2 to 10 mg **or** 0.03 to 0.1 mg/kg once (maximum single dose: 10 mg) 5 to 15 minutes prior to procedure; if needed due to incomplete response and/or duration of procedure, may repeat the dose (usually 50% of the initial dose) after 5 to 30 minutes (Choy 2019; Ginsberg 1992; Zakko 1999). **Note:** In obese patients, non-weight-based dosing is preferred (Choy 2019).

Oral (off-label): 2 to 10 mg once 30 to 60 minutes prior to procedure; if needed due to incomplete response, may repeat the dose (usually 50% of the initial dose) after 30 to 60 minutes (Choy 2019).

Hydroxychloroquine/chloroquine toxicity (severe):

Note: Use is recommended in patients with severe toxicity (eg, hypotension, QTc prolongation, hypokalemia) in combination with other supportive measures (eg, mechanical ventilation, epinephrine, cardiovascular monitoring) (Barry 2019; Ling Ngan Wong 2008; Marquardt 2001; McBeth 2015; Riou 1988).

IV: 2 mg/kg once administered over 30 minutes, followed by 1 to 2 mg/kg/day for 2 to 4 days (Barry 2019; Marquardt 2001).

Intoxication (cocaine, methamphetamine, and other sympathomimetics) (off-label use): Based on limited data.

IV: 2 to 10 mg every 3 to 10 minutes as needed for agitation, sedation, seizures, hypertension, and tachycardia until desired symptom control achieved; doses up to 20 mg may be considered in severe agitation based on response and tolerability. Large, cumulative doses may be required for some patients; monitor for respiratory depression and hypotension. **Note :** If IV access is not possible, consider IM administration; however, IM diazepam time to peak drug levels is slower than IM midazolam (Arnold 2019; Boyer 2019b; Delgado 2020; Hall 1990; Wodarz 2017).

Muscle spasm, spasticity, and/or rigidity (alternative agent):

Oral: Initial: 2 mg twice daily **or** 5 mg at bedtime; increase gradually based on response and tolerability, up to 40 to 60 mg/day in 3 to 4 divided doses (Abrams 2019; Kita 2000; Olek 2020).

Neuroleptic malignant syndrome (adjunctive therapy) (off-label use): For management of muscle rigidity or anxiety in patients with severe symptoms at presentation (hyperthermia, evidence of rhabdomyolysis) and for those not responding to initial withdrawal of medication and supportive care.

IV: 10 mg every 8 hours until symptom resolution (Tsai 2010; Wijdicks 2019).

Seizures:

Note: If IV access is not available, IM diazepam is not recommended due to erratic absorption and slow time to peak drug levels (IM midazolam is recommended) (Leppik 2015; Wichliński 1985).

Acute active seizures (non-status epilepticus):

Intranasal: 0.2 mg/kg as a single dose; may repeat once based on response and tolerability after ≥4 hours. Maximum dose: Two doses per episode. Do not use for more than 1 episode every 5 days or more than 5 episodes per month.

The following table (derived from manufacturer labeling) provides acceptable weight ranges for each dose, such that patients will receive between 90% and 180% of the calculated recommended dose.

Recommended Intranasal Diazepam Dosage for Adults

Weight	Dose (rounded from 0.2 mg/kg)	Number of nasal spray devices	Number of sprays
28 to 50 kg	10 mg	One 10 mg device	One spray in one nostril
51 to 75 kg	15 mg	Two 7.5 mg devices	One spray in each nostril
76 kg and up	20 mg	Two 10 mg devices	One spray in each nostril

IV: 5 to 10 mg as a single dose given at a maximum infusion rate of 5 mg/minute; may repeat at 3- to 5-minute intervals up to a total dose of 30 mg (Drislane 2020; NCS [Brophy 2012]; manufacturer's labeling).

Rectal gel (generally for use in prehospital setting): 0.2 mg/kg (round dose up to the nearest 2.5 mg increment; maximum dose: 20 mg) **or** 10 to 20 mg as a single dose (Drappatz 2019; manufacturer's labeling).

Status epilepticus (alternative agent):

IV: 5 to 10 mg as a single dose given at a maximum infusion rate of 5 mg/minute; may repeat dose in 3 to 5 minutes if seizures continue; a nonbenzodiazepine antiseizure agent should follow to prevent seizure recurrence, even if seizures have ceased (AES [Glauser 2016]; Drislane 2020; NCS [Brophy 2012]).

Rectal gel (generally for use in prehospital setting) (off-label): 0.2 to 0.5 mg/kg (round dose up to the nearest 2.5 mg increment; maximum dose: 20 mg) as a single dose (AES [Glauser 2016]; Drislane 2020).

Serotonin syndrome (serotonin toxicity) (off-label use):

IV: 5 to 10 mg every 8 to 10 minutes until symptoms resolve (Boyer 2020).

Substance withdrawal:

Alcohol withdrawal syndrome:

Note: Symptom-triggered regimens preferred over fixed-dose regimens (WFSBP [Soyka 2017]). Dosage and frequency may vary based on institution-specific protocols. Some experts recommend avoiding IM administration due to variable absorption (Weintraub 2017).

Symptom-triggered regimen: **IV, Oral:** 5 to 20 mg as needed per institution-specific protocol until appropriate sedation achieved; dose and frequency determined by withdrawal symptom severity using a validated severity assessment scale, such as the Clinical Institute Withdrawal Assessment for Alcohol, revised scale (CIWA-Ar) (Hoffman 2019; Mayo-Smith 1997; WFSBP [Soyka 2017]).

Fixed-dose regimen: **IV, Oral:** 10 mg every 6 hours for 1 day, then 5 mg every 6 hours for 2 days; additional doses may be considered based on withdrawal symptoms and validated assessment scale scores (eg, CIWA-Ar) (Mayo-Smith 1997; WFSBP [Soyka 2017]).

Opioid withdrawal (autonomic instability and agitation) (alternative agent) (adjunctive therapy) (off-label use): Based on limited data.

IV: 10 to 20 mg every 5 to 10 minutes until hemodynamically stable and adequate sedation achieved (Stolbach 2019; Wightman 2018).

Vertigo, acute episodes, treatment (alternative agent) (off-label use):

IV, Oral: 1 to 5 mg every 12 hours as needed for 24 to 48 hours (Furman 2019; Hain 2003; Moskowitz 2020). If vomiting, may consider rectal administration (Robertson 2019).

Discontinuation of therapy: In patients receiving extended or higher-dose benzodiazepine therapy, unless safety concerns require a more rapid withdrawal, gradually withdraw to detect reemerging symptoms and minimize rebound and withdrawal symptoms. Taper total daily dose by 10% to 20% every 1 to 2 weeks based on response and tolerability. The optimal taper rate and duration will vary; durations up to 6 months may be necessary for some patients on higher doses (Bystritsky 2019; Lader 2011; VA/DoD 2015). For patients on high doses, taper more rapidly in the beginning and slow the reduction rate as the taper progresses because early stages of withdrawal are easier to tolerate. For example, reduce the dose weekly by 25% until half of the dose remains. Thereafter, continue to reduce by ~12% every 4 to 7 days (VA/DoD 2015).

Geriatric

Elderly and/or debilitated patients:

IM, IV: Initial: 2 to 5 mg; increase gradually based on response and tolerability.

Intranasal: Due to the increased half-life in elderly patients, consider reducing dose.

Oral: Initial: 2 to 2.5 mg 1 to 2 times daily; increase gradually based on response and tolerability.

Rectal gel: Due to the increased half-life in elderly and debilitated patients, consider reducing dose.

Renal Impairment: Adult There are no dosage adjustments provided in the manufacturer's labeling; use with caution.

Hemodialysis: Not dialyzable (0% to 5%); supplemental dose is not necessary.

Hepatic Impairment: Adult There are no dosage adjustments provided in the manufacturer's labeling; use with caution because distribution and half-life may increase, and clearance may decrease significantly. The oral tablets are contraindicated in severe hepatic impairment.

Pediatric

Seizures, acute:

Intranasal: Dosing varies with age; patients <12 years require a larger mg/kg/dose. May repeat dose in 4 hours; do not exceed 2 doses in 24 hours. Do not repeat dose if patient has difficulty breathing or excessive sedation. Do not exceed maximum treatment frequency of 1 episode **every 5 days** and 5 episodes per month.

Children 6 to 11 years:

Weight	Dose (mg)	Quantity and Type of Nasal Device	Number of Sprays
10 to <19 kg	5 mg	One 5 mg device	1 spray in 1 nostril
19 to <38 kg	10 mg	One 10 mg device	1 spray in 1 nostril
38 to <56 kg	15 mg	Two 7.5 mg devices	2 sprays delivered as 1 spray in each nostril
56 to 74 kg	20 mg	Two 10 mg devices	2 sprays delivered as 1 spray in each nostril

Children ≥12 years and Adolescents:

Weight	Dose (mg)	Quantity and Type of Nasal Device	Number of Sprays
14 to <28 kg	5 mg	One 5 mg device	1 spray in 1 nostril
28 to <51 kg	10 mg	One 10 mg device	1 spray in 1 nostril
51 to <76 kg	15 mg	Two 7.5 mg devices	2 sprays delivered as 1 spray in each nostril
≥76 kg	20 mg	Two 10 mg devices	2 sprays delivered as 1 spray in each nostril

Rectal gel formulation:

Infants and Children 6 months to 2 years: Rectal: Dose not established.

Children 2 to 5 years: Rectal: 0.5 mg/kg.

Children 6 to 11 years: Rectal: 0.3 mg/kg.

Children ≥12 years and Adolescents: Rectal: 0.2 mg/kg.

Note: Round dose up to the nearest 2.5 mg increment, not exceeding a 20 mg/dose; dose may be repeated in 4 to 12 hours if needed; do not use more than 5 times per month or more than once every 5 days.

Rectal: Undiluted 5 mg/mL parenteral formulation (filter if using ampul): Infants, Children, and Adolescents: 0.5 mg/kg/dose then 0.25 mg/kg/dose in 10 minutes if needed. Maximum dose: 20 mg/dose (Hegenbarth 2008; Kliegman 2007).

Status epilepticus:

IV (preferred route):

Weight-directed: Infants >30 days, Children, and Adolescents: IV: 0.15 to 0.2 mg/kg/dose slow IV; may repeat dose once in 5 minutes; maximum dose: 10 mg/dose (AES [Glauser 2016]; NCS [Brophy 2012]).

Fixed dosing: Manufacturer's labeling:

Infants >30 days and Children <5 years: IV: 0.2 to 0.5 mg slow IV every 2 to 5 minutes up to a maximum total dose of 5 mg; repeat in 2 to 4 hours if needed.

Children ≥5 years and Adolescents: IV: 1 mg slow IV every 2 to 5 minutes up to a maximum of 10 mg; repeat in 2 to 4 hours if needed.

Rectal (AES [Glauser 2016]; NCS [Brophy 2012]):

Note: For use when IV access unavailable.

Children 2 to 5 years: Rectal: 0.5 mg/kg; maximum dose: 20 mg/dose.

Children 6 to 11 years: Rectal: 0.3 mg/kg; maximum dose: 20 mg/dose.

Children ≥12 years and Adolescents: Rectal: 0.2 mg/kg; maximum dose: 20 mg/dose.

Febrile seizure, prophylaxis: Limited data available: Children: Oral: 1 mg/kg/day divided every 8 hours; initiate therapy at first sign of fever and continue for 24 hours after fever resolves (Rosman 1993; Steering Committee 2008).

Spasticity/muscle spasms:

General dosing: **Note:** Initiate therapy with lowest dose; dose should be individualized and titrated to effect and tolerability:

Manufacturer's labeling: Infants ≥6 months, Children, and Adolescents: Oral: Initial: 1 to 2.5 mg 3 to 4 times daily; increase gradually as needed and tolerated.

Alternate dosing (Kliegman 2016):

Oral:

Infants ≥6 months and Children <12 years: 0.12 to 0.8 mg/kg/day in divided doses every 6 to 8 hours; maximum dose: 10 mg/dose.

Children ≥12 years and Adolescents: 2 to 10 mg 2 to 4 times daily.

Cerebral palsy-associated spasticity: Limited data available. **Note:** Dose should be individualized and titrated to effect and tolerability:

Weight-based dosing: Children: Oral: 0.01 to 0.3 mg/kg/day divided 2 **or** 4 times daily (Kliegman 2016).

Low-dose fixed dosing (Mathew 2005): Children <12 years: Oral:

<8.5 kg: 0.5 to 1 mg at bedtime.

8.5 to 15 kg: 1 to 2 mg at bedtime.

Fixed dosing: Children ≥5 years and Adolescents: Oral: Initial: 1.25 mg 3 times daily; may titrate to 5 mg 4 times daily (Engle 1966).

Tetanus-associated spasm:

Manufacturer's labeling:

Infants >30 days and children <5 years: IV, IM: 1 to 2 mg every 3 to 4 hours as needed.

Children ≥5 years and Adolescents: IV, IM: 5 to 10 mg every 3 to 4 hours as needed.

Alternate dosing (WHO 2010):

Infants and Children: IV: Initial: 0.1 to 0.2 mg/kg/dose every 2 to 6 hours; titrate as needed.

Adolescents: IV: Initial: 5 mg every 2 to 6 hours, titrate as needed. Large doses may be required.

Muscle spasm/spasticity associated with chronic/terminal illness (eg, palliative care settings): Limited data available: Infants, Children, and Adolescents:

Oral: 0.12 to 0.8 mg/kg/day divided every 6 to 12 hours; maximum dose: 10 mg/dose (Wustoff 2007).

IM, IV: 0.05 to 0.2 mg/kg/dose every 6 to 12 hours; maximum total dose: 0.6 mg/kg cumulative in 8 hours (Wustoff 2007); **Note:** In palliative situations, the usual initial dose for children <5 years is 5 mg/dose and in children ≥5 years and adolescents is 10 mg/dose (Kliegman 2016).

Sedation, anxiolysis, and amnesia prior to procedure: Limited data available:

Oral:

Infants ≥6 months: 0.2 to 0.3 mg/kg 45 to 60 minutes prior to procedure. Maximum dose: 10 mg/dose (Zeltzer 1990).

Children: 0.2 to 0.5 mg/kg 45 to 60 minutes prior to procedure; maximum dose: 10 mg/dose (Everitt 2002; Fell 1985; Tyagi 2012; Zeltzer 1990).

Adolescents: 0.2 to 0.3 mg/kg 45 to 60 minutes prior to procedure. Maximum dose: 10 mg/dose (Zeltzer 1990).

IV:

Infants and Children: Initial: 0.05 to 0.1 mg/kg over 3 to 5 minutes, titrate slowly to effect (maximum total dose: 0.25 mg/kg) (Krauss 2006).

Adolescents: IV: 5 mg; may repeat with 2.5 mg if needed (Zeltzer 1990).

Renal Impairment: Pediatric There are no dosage adjustments provided in the manufacturer's labeling; use with caution.

Hemodialysis: Not dialyzable (0% to 5%); supplemental dose is not necessary.

Hepatic Impairment: Pediatric There are no dosage adjustments provided in the manufacturer's labeling; use with caution. The oral tablets are contraindicated in severe hepatic impairment.

Mechanism of Action Binds to stereospecific benzodiazepine receptors on the postsynaptic GABA neuron at several sites within the central nervous system, including the limbic system, reticular formation. Enhancement of the inhibitory effect of GABA on neuronal excitability results by increased neuronal membrane permeability to chloride ions. This shift in chloride ions results in hyperpolarization (a less excitable state) and stabilization. Benzodiazepine receptors and effects appear to be linked to the GABA-A receptors. Benzodiazepines do not bind to GABA-B receptors.

Contraindications

Hypersensitivity to diazepam or any component of the formulation; acute narrow-angle glaucoma.

Injection: Additional contraindications: Untreated open-angle glaucoma.

Oral: Additional contraindications: Untreated open-angle glaucoma; use in infants <6 months of age, myasthenia gravis, severe respiratory impairment, severe hepatic impairment, sleep apnea syndrome.

Documentation of allergenic cross-reactivity for benzodiazepines is limited. However, because of similarities in chemical structure and/or pharmacologic actions, the possibility of cross-sensitivity cannot be ruled out with certainty.

Warnings/Precautions When used as an adjunct in treating convulsive disorders, an increase in frequency/severity of tonic-clonic seizures may occur and require dose adjustment of anticonvulsant. Abrupt withdrawal may result in a temporary increase in the frequency and/or severity of seizures. Use with caution in debilitated patients, elderly patients, obese patients, patients with hepatic disease, or renal impairment. Active metabolites with extended half-lives may lead to delayed accumulation and adverse effects; limit dose to smallest effective amount and increase gradually and as tolerated to avoid adverse reactions. Elderly patients may be at an increased risk of death with use; risk has been found highest within the first 4 months of use in elderly dementia patients (Jennum 2015; Saarelainen 2018). Oral tablet is contraindicated in patients with severe hepatic impairment, severe respiratory impairment, or sleep apnea syndrome. Use with caution in patients with respiratory disease.

Use caution in patients with depression or anxiety associated with depression, particularly if suicidal risk may be present. Use with extreme caution in patients with a history of drug abuse or acute alcoholism; potential for drug dependency exists. Tolerance and psychological and physical dependence may occur with prolonged use (generally >10 days). Use with extreme caution in patients who are at risk of falls; benzodiazepines have been associated with falls and traumatic injury (Nelson 1999). Rebound or withdrawal symptoms may occur following abrupt discontinuation or large decreases in dose. Use caution when reducing dose or withdrawing therapy; decrease slowly and monitor for withdrawal symptoms. The benzodiazepine receptor antagonist flumazenil may cause withdrawal in patients receiving long-term benzodiazepine therapy. Diazepam is a long half-life benzodiazepine. Tolerance develops to the sedative, hypnotic, and anticonvulsant effects. It does not develop to the anxiolytic or skeletal muscle relaxing effects (Vinkers 2012). Chronic use of this agent may increase the perioperative benzodiazepine dose needed to achieve desired effect.

Benzodiazepines have been associated with anterograde amnesia (Nelson 1999). Paradoxical reactions, including hyperactive or aggressive behavior, have been reported with benzodiazepines; risk may be increased in adolescent/pediatric, geriatric patients, or patients with a history of alcohol use disorder or psychiatric/personality disorders (Mancuso 2004). Does not have analgesic, antidepressant, or antipsychotic properties. May be used in patients with open-angle glaucoma who are receiving appropriate therapy; contraindicated in acute narrow-angle glaucoma and untreated open-angle glaucoma. Potentially significant interactions may exist, requiring dose or frequency adjustment, additional monitoring, and/or selection of alternative therapy. **[US Boxed Warning]: Concomitant use of benzodiazepines and opioids may result in profound sedation, respiratory depression, coma, and death; reserve concomitant prescribing of these drugs for use in patients for whom alternative treatment options are inadequate, and limit dosages and durations to the minimum required. Follow patients for signs and symptoms of respiratory depression and sedation.**

May cause CNS depression, which may impair physical or mental abilities; patients must be cautioned about performing tasks that require mental alertness (eg, operating machinery, driving). Hazardous sleep-related activities such as sleep-driving, cooking and eating food, and making phone calls while asleep have been noted with benzodiazepines (Dolder 2008).

Intranasal: Pooled analysis of trials involving various antiepileptics (regardless of indication) showed an increased risk of suicidal thoughts/behavior (incidence rate: 0.43% of treated patients compared to 0.24% of patients receiving placebo); risk observed as early as 1 week after initiation and continued through duration of trials (most trials ≤24 weeks). Monitor all patients for notable changes in behavior that might indicate suicidal thoughts or depression; notify health care provider immediately if symptoms occur.

Parenteral: Vesicant; ensure proper needle or catheter placement prior to and during administration; avoid extravasation. Acute hypotension, muscle weakness, apnea, and/or cardiac arrest have occurred with parenteral administration. Acute effects may be more prevalent in patients receiving concurrent barbiturates, opioids, or ethanol. Appropriate resuscitative equipment and qualified personnel should be available during administration and monitoring. Avoid use of the injection in patients in shock, coma, or in acute ethanol intoxication with depression of vital signs. Intra-arterial injection should be avoided. Tonic status epilepticus has been precipitated in patients treated with diazepam IV for absence status or absence variant status.

Rectal gel: Administration of rectal gel should only be performed by individuals trained to recognize characteristic seizure activity and monitor response. Not recommended for chronic, daily use. Use with caution in patients with neurologic damage.

Some dosage forms may contain benzyl alcohol and/or sodium benzoate/benzoic acid; benzoic acid (benzoate) is a metabolite of benzyl alcohol; large amounts of benzyl alcohol (≥99 mg/kg/day) have been associated with a potentially fatal toxicity ("gasping syndrome") in neonates; the "gasping syndrome" consists of metabolic acidosis, respiratory distress, gasping respirations, CNS dysfunction (including convulsions, intracranial hemorrhage), hypotension, and cardiovascular collapse (AAP 1997; CDC 1982); some data suggest that benzoate displaces bilirubin from protein binding sites (Ahlfors 2001); avoid or use dosage forms containing benzyl alcohol and/or benzyl alcohol derivative with caution in neonates. See manufacturer's labeling.

Some dosage forms may contain propylene glycol; large amounts are potentially toxic and have been associated with hyperosmolality, lactic acidosis, seizures, and respiratory depression; use caution (AAP 1997; Wilson 2000; Wilson 2005; Zar 2007).

Warnings: Additional Pediatric Considerations Neonates and young infants have decreased metabolism of diazepam and desmethyldiazepam (active metabolite), both can accumulate with repeated use and cause increased toxicity.

Drug Interactions

Metabolism/Transport Effects Substrate of CYP1A2 (minor), CYP2B6 (minor), CYP2C19 (major), CYP2C9 (minor), CYP3A4 (major); **Note:** Assignment of Major/Minor substrate status based on clinically relevant drug interaction potential

Avoid Concomitant Use

Avoid concomitant use of DiazePAM with any of the following: Abametapir; Azelastine (Nasal); Bromperidol; Conivaptan; Fexinidazole [INT]; Fusidic Acid (Systemic); Idelalisib; Methotrimeprazine; MetroNIDAZOLE (Systemic); OLANZapine; Orphenadrine; Oxomemazine; Paraldehyde; Sodium Oxybate; Thalidomide

Increased Effect/Toxicity

DiazePAM may increase the levels/effects of: Ajmaline; Alcohol (Ethyl); Alfentanil; Azelastine (Nasal); Blonanserin; Brexanolone; Buprenorphine; CloZAPine; CNS Depressants; Flunitrazepam; Methadone; Methotrimeprazine; MetyroSINE; Opioid Agonists; Orphenadrine; OxyCODONE; Paraldehyde; Piribedil; Pramipexole; ROPINIRole; Rotigotine; Sodium Oxybate; Suvorexant; Thalidomide; Zolpidem

The levels/effects of DiazePAM may be increased by: Abametapir; Alizapride; Aprepitant; Brimonidine (Topical); Bromopride; Bromperidol; Cannabidiol; Cannabis; Chlormethiazole; Chlorphenesin Carbamate; Clofazimine; Conivaptan; Cosyntropin; CYP2C19 Inhibitors (Moderate); CYP2C19 Inhibitors (Strong); CYP3A4 Inhibitors (Moderate); CYP3A4 Inhibitors (Strong); Dimethindene (Topical); Disulfiram; Doxylamine; Dronabinol; Droperidol; Duvelisib; Erdafitinib; Esketamine; Fexinidazole [INT]; Fosamprenavir; Fosaprepitant; Fosnetupitant; Fusidic Acid (Systemic); HydrOXYzine; Idelalisib; Kava Kava; Larotrectinib; Lemborexant; Lisuride; Lofexidine; Magnesium Sulfate; Melatonin; MetroNIDAZOLE (Systemic); MiFEPRIStone; Minocycline (Systemic); Nabilone; Netupitant; OLANZapine; Oxomemazine; Palbociclib; Perampanel; Ritonavir; Rufinamide; Saquinavir;

Simeprevir; Stiripentol; Teduglutide; Tetrahydrocannabinol; Tetrahydrocannabinol and Cannabidiol; Trimeprazine

Decreased Effect

The levels/effects of DiazePAM may be decreased by: CYP2C19 Inducers (Moderate); CYP3A4 Inducers (Moderate); CYP3A4 Inducers (Strong); Dabrafenib; Deferasirox; Enzalutamide; Erdafitinib; Ivosidenib; Mitotane; Ombitasvir, Paritaprevir, and Ritonavir; Ombitasvir, Paritaprevir, Ritonavir, and Dasabuvir; Ritonavir; Sarilumab; Siltuximab; Theophylline Derivatives; Tocilizumab; Yohimbine

Pharmacodynamics/Kinetics

Onset of Action

Sedation: Pediatric patients: IV: 4 to 5 minutes (Krauss 2006)

Status epilepticus: IV: 1 to 3 minutes; Rectal: 2 to 10 minutes

Duration of Action

Sedation: Pediatric patients: 60 to 120 minutes (Krauss 2006)

Status epilepticus: 15 to 30 minutes

Half-life Elimination **Note:** Diazepam accumulates upon multiple dosing and the terminal elimination half-life is slightly prolonged.

IM:

Premature neonates (GA: 28 to 34 weeks): 54 hours.

Infants: ~30 hours (Morselli 1973).

Children 3 to 8 years: 18 hours (Morselli 1973).

Adults: Parent: ~60 to 72 hours; Desmethyldiazepam: ~152 to 174 hours (Lamson 2011).

Intranasal: ~49 hours.

IV: Parent: 33 to 45 hours; Desmethyldiazepam: 87 hours (Cloyd 1998; Greenblatt 1989a).

Oral: Parent: 44 to 48 hours; Desmethyldiazepam: 100 hours (Greenblatt 1989b).

Rectal: Parent: 45 to 46 hours; Desmethyldiazepam: 71 to 99 hours (Cloyd 1998).

Time to Peak

IM: Median: 1 hour (range: 0.25 to 2 hours) (Lamson 2011).

Intranasal: ~1.5 hours.

IV: ~1 minute (Cloyd 1998).

Oral: 15 minutes to 2.5 hours (1.25 hours when fasting; 2.5 hours with food) (Greenblatt 1989b).

Rectal: 1.5 hours.

Pregnancy Risk Factor D

Pregnancy Considerations

Diazepam and its metabolites (N-desmethyldiazepam, temazepam, and oxazepam) cross the placenta. Teratogenic effects have been observed with diazepam; however, additional studies are needed. The incidence of premature birth and low birth weights may be increased following maternal use of benzodiazepines; hypoglycemia and respiratory problems in the neonate may occur following exposure late in pregnancy. Neonatal withdrawal symptoms may occur within days to weeks after birth and "floppy infant syndrome" (which also includes withdrawal symptoms) has been reported with some benzodiazepines (including diazepam) (Bergman 1992; Iqbal 2002; Wikner 2007). A combination of factors influences the potential teratogenicity of anticonvulsant therapy. When treating women with epilepsy, monotherapy with the lowest effective dose and avoidance of medications known to have a high incidence of teratogenic effects is recommended (Harden 2009; Wlodarczyk 2012).

Patients exposed to diazepam during pregnancy are encouraged to enroll themselves into the North American Antiepileptic Drug (NAAED) Pregnancy Registry by calling 1-888-233-2334. Additional information is available at www.aedpregnancyregistry.org.

Breastfeeding Considerations Diazepam and its metabolites are present in breast milk.

Using data from one study, the relative infant dose (RID) of diazepam is 8.9% when compared to a weight-adjusted maternal dose of 10 mg/day.

In general, breastfeeding is considered acceptable when the RID of a medication is <10% (Anderson 2016; Ito 2000). However some sources note breastfeeding should only be considered if the RID is <5% for psychotropic agents (Larsen 2015).

The RID of diazepam was calculated using a milk concentration of 85 ng/mL, providing an estimated daily infant dose via breast milk of 0.01275 mg/kg/day. This was the highest milk concentration obtained in one study following maternal administration of diazepam 10 mg once daily at bedtime to four postpartum women (this sample was obtained after five maternal doses) (Brandt 1976). Higher milk concentrations have been reported; however, milk concentration related to maternal dose was not stated (Dusci 1990; Wesson 1985). The active metabolites of diazepam (desmethyldiazepam, oxazepam, and temazepam) have also been detected in breast milk and the urine of exposed infants (Brandt 1976; Cole 1975; Dusci 1990; Erkkola 1972; Wesson 1985). Relative infant doses of up to 11% have been reported (McElhatton 1994).

Sedation and weight loss have been observed in some infants exposed to diazepam via breast milk (Patrick 1972; Wesson 1985)

Diazepam has a long half-life and may accumulate in the breastfed infant, especially preterm infants or those exposed to chronic maternal doses (Davanzo 2013). Significant accumulation may occur even if the maternal dose is low (Wesson 1985). A single maternal dose may be compatible with breastfeeding (WHO 2002). If chronic use of a benzodiazepine is needed in breastfeeding women, use of shorter acting agents is preferred (Davanzo 2013; WHO 2002). Infants should be monitored for drowsiness, decreased feeding, and poor weight gain (Veiby 2015).

Controlled Substance C-IV

Dosage Forms: US

Concentrate, Oral:

diazePAM Intensol: 5 mg/mL (30 mL)

Generic: 5 mg/mL (30 mL)

Gel, Rectal:

Diastat AcuDial: 10 mg (1 ea); 20 mg (1 ea)

Diastat Pediatric: 2.5 mg (1 ea)

Generic: 2.5 mg (1 ea); 10 mg (1 ea); 20 mg (1 ea)

Liquid, Nasal:

Valtoco 10 MG Dose: 10 mg/0.1 mL (1 ea)

Valtoco 5 MG Dose: 5 mg/0.1 mL (1 ea)

Liquid Therapy Pack, Nasal:

Valtoco 15 MG Dose: 2 devices, 7.5 mg/0.1 mL each (1 ea)

Valtoco 20 MG Dose: 2 devices, 10 mg/0.1 mL each (1 ea)

Solution, Injection:

Generic: 5 mg/mL (2 mL, 10 mL)

Solution, Oral:

Generic: 5 mg/5 mL (500 mL)

Solution Auto-injector, Intramuscular:
Generic: 10 mg/2 mL (2 mL)
Tablet, Oral:
Valium: 2 mg, 5 mg, 10 mg
Generic: 2 mg, 5 mg, 10 mg
Dosage Forms: Canada
Gel, Rectal:
Diastat: 5 mg/mL (0.5 mL, 1 mL, 2 mL, 3 mL, 4 mL)
Solution, Injection:
Generic: 5 mg/mL (2 mL)
Solution, Oral:
Generic: 1 mg/mL (500 mL)
Tablet, Oral:
Valium: 5 mg
Generic: 2 mg, 5 mg, 10 mg
Dental Health Professional Considerations An adult companion should accompany the patient to and from dental office.

◆ **diazePAM Intensol** *see* DiazePAM *on page 477*

Dibucaine (DYE byoo kane)

Brand Names: US Nupercainal [OTC]
Generic Availability (US) Yes
Pharmacologic Category Antihemorrhoidal Agent; Local Anesthetic
Dental Use Amide derivative local anesthetic for minor skin conditions
Use
Dermal pain/itching: Temporary relief of pain and itching caused by sunburn, minor burns, minor cuts, scrapes, insect bites or minor skin irritation.
Hemorrhoids/anorectal disorders; rectal pain/itching: Temporary relief of pain and itching due to hemorrhoids and other anorectal disorders.
Local Anesthetic/Vasoconstrictor Precautions No information available to require special precautions
Effects on Dental Treatment No significant effects or complications reported
Effects on Bleeding No information available to require special precautions
Adverse Reactions Frequency not defined.
1% to 10%:
Central nervous system: Localized burning
Dermatologic: Contact dermatitis
Hypersensitivity: Angioedema
Dental Usual Dosage Local pain (local anesthetic): Children and Adults: Topical: Apply gently to the affected areas; no more than 30 g for adults or 7.5 g for children should be used in any 24-hour period
Dosing
Adult & Geriatric
Dermal pain/itching: Topical: Apply to affected area up to 3 or 4 times daily. Maximum daily dose: 30 g/**day**
Hemorrhoids/anorectal disorders; rectal pain/itching: Topical: Apply to affected external anal area up to 3 or 4 times daily.
Renal Impairment: Adult There are no dosage adjustments provided in the manufacturer's labeling.
Hepatic Impairment: Adult There are no dosage adjustments provided in the manufacturer's labeling.
Pediatric
Dermal pain/itching: Children ≥2 years weighing ≥16 kg and Adolescents: Topical: Apply to affected area up to 3 or 4 times daily. Maximum daily dose: 7.5 g/**day** for children and 30 g/**day** for adults
Hemorrhoids/anorectal disorders; rectal pain/itching: Children ≥12 years and Adolescents: Topical: Apply to affected external anal area up to 3 or 4 times daily
Renal Impairment: Pediatric There are no dosage adjustments provided in the manufacturer's labeling.
Hepatic Impairment: Pediatric There are no dosage adjustments provided in the manufacturer's labeling.
Mechanism of Action Blocks both the initiation and conduction of nerve impulses by decreasing the neuronal membrane's permeability to sodium ions, which results in inhibition of depolarization with resultant blockade of conduction.
Contraindications OTC labeling: When used for self-medication, do not use in or near the eyes or in children <2 years or weight <16 kg.
Documentation of allergenic cross-reactivity for amide local anesthetics limited. However, because of similarities in chemical structure and/or pharmacologic actions, the possibility of cross-sensitivity cannot be ruled out with certainty.
Warnings/Precautions When topical anesthetics are used prior to cosmetic or medical procedures, the lowest amount of anesthetic necessary for pain relief should be applied. High systemic levels and toxic effects (eg, methemoglobinemia, irregular heart beats, respiratory depression, seizures, death) have been reported in patients who (without supervision of a trained professional) have applied topical anesthetics in large amounts (or to large areas of the skin), left these products on for prolonged periods of time, or have used wraps/dressings to cover the skin following application.

Methemoglobinemia has been reported with local anesthetics; clinically significant methemoglobinemia requires immediate treatment along with discontinuation of the anesthetic and other oxidizing agents. Onset may be immediate or delayed (hours) after anesthetic exposure. Patients with glucose-6-phosphate dehydrogenase deficiency, congenital or idiopathic methemoglobinemia, cardiac or pulmonary compromise, exposure to oxidizing agents or their metabolites, or infants <6 months of age are more susceptible and should be closely monitored for signs and symptoms of methemoglobinemia (eg, cyanosis, headache, rapid pulse, shortness of breath, lightheadedness, fatigue).

Self-medication (OTC use): For external use only. When used for self-medication, notify health care provider and discontinue use if condition worsens, does not improve within 7 days, or if redness, irritation, swelling, bleeding, or other symptoms develop or increase. Do not put this product into the rectum using fingers or any mechanical device or applicator; do not exceed recommended dose unless directed by a health care provider. Do not use in large quantities, particularly over raw surfaces or blistered areas.
Drug Interactions
Metabolism/Transport Effects None known.
Avoid Concomitant Use There are no known interactions where it is recommended to avoid concomitant use.
Increased Effect/Toxicity
The levels/effects of Dibucaine may be increased by: Methemoglobinemia Associated Agents
Decreased Effect There are no known significant interactions involving a decrease in effect.
Pharmacodynamics/Kinetics
Onset of Action Within 15 minutes

Duration of Action 2 to 4 hours

Dosage Forms: US

Ointment, External:

Nupercainal [OTC]: 1% (28.4 g, 56.7 g, 60 g)

Generic: 1% (28 g, 28.35 g)

◆ **DIC** *see* Dacarbazine *on page 427*

Diclofenac (Systemic) (dye KLOE fen ak)

Related Information

Rheumatoid Arthritis, Osteoarthritis, and Osteoporosis *on page 1697*

Temporomandibular Dysfunction (TMD), Chronic Pain, and Fibromyalgia *on page 1773*

Brand Names: US Cambia; Dyloject [DSC]; Zipsor; Zorvolex

Brand Names: Canada APO-Diclo; APO-Diclo Rapide; APO-Diclo SR; Cambia; Diclofenac-50; DOM-Diclofenac; PMS-Diclofenac; PMS-Diclofenac K; PMS-Diclofenac-SR; PRO-Diclo Rapide-50 [DSC]; SANDOZ Diclofenac; SANDOZ Diclofenac Rapide; SANDOZ Diclofenac SR; TEVA-Diclofenac EC; TEVA-Diclofenac SR; TEVA-Diclofenac [DSC]; TEVA-Diclofenac-K; Voltaren; Voltaren Rapide; Voltaren SR

Generic Availability (US) May be product dependent

Pharmacologic Category Analgesic, Nonopioid; Nonsteroidal Anti-inflammatory Drug (NSAID); Nonsteroidal Anti-inflammatory Drug (NSAID), Oral

Dental Use Immediate-release tablets: Acute treatment of mild-to-moderate pain

Use

Ankylosing spondylitis (delayed-release tablets only): Acute or long-term use in the relief of signs and symptoms of ankylosing spondylitis.

Dysmenorrhea (immediate-release tablets only): Treatment of primary dysmenorrhea.

Migraine (powder for oral solution only): Acute treatment of migraine attacks with or without aura in adults.

Osteoarthritis (immediate-release, extended-release, and delayed-release tablets; capsules [Zorvolex]; and suppositories [Canadian product] only): Relief of signs and symptoms of osteoarthritis.

Pain

Capsules/immediate-release tablets only: Relief of mild to moderate acute pain.

Injection only: Management of mild to moderate pain and moderate to severe pain (alone or in combination with opioid analgesics) in adults.

Rheumatoid arthritis (immediate-release, extended-release, and delayed-release tablets; and suppositories [Canadian product] only): Relief of signs and symptoms of rheumatoid arthritis.

Local Anesthetic/Vasoconstrictor Precautions No information available to require special precautions

Effects on Dental Treatment The dentist should be aware of the potential of abnormal coagulation. Caution should also be exercised in the use of NSAIDs in patients already on anticoagulant therapy with drugs such as warfarin (Coumadin®). See Effects on Bleeding.

Effects on Bleeding Nonselective NSAIDs such as diclofenac (systemic) inhibit platelet aggregation and prolong bleeding time in some patients. Unlike aspirin, the NSAID effect on platelet function is quantitatively less, of shorter duration, and reversible. Normal platelet function should occur in ~5 elimination half-lives or in <10 hours after discontinuation of diclofenac (systemic). Concomitant use of other NSAIDs should be avoided.

Adverse Reactions

Injection: Frequency not always defined.

Cardiovascular: Edema (≤10%), cerebrovascular accident, hypertension, myocardial infarction, significant cardiovascular event

Central nervous system: Headache (≤10%), dizziness (8%)

Dermatologic: Pruritus (≤10%), skin rash (≤10%), exfoliative dermatitis, Stevens-Johnson syndrome, toxic epidermal necrolysis

Endocrine & metabolic: Fluid retention

Gastrointestinal: Constipation (13%), abdominal pain (≤10%), diarrhea (≤10%), dyspepsia (≤10%), esophageal perforation (≤10%), flatulence (≤10%), gastrointestinal ulcer (≤10%; including gastric/duodenal), heartburn (≤10%), intestinal perforation (≤10%), nausea (≤10%), vomiting (≤10%)

Hematologic & oncologic: Anemia (≤10%), hemorrhage (≤10%), prolonged bleeding time (≤10%)

Hepatic: Increased liver enzymes (≤10%), increased serum transaminases (15%), increased serum ALT (≤4%; >8X ULN: ≤1%), increased serum AST (2% to ≤4%; >8X ULN: ≤1%)

Hypersensitivity: Anaphylactoid reaction

Local: Infusion site reaction (10%), extravasation (3%)

Otic: Tinnitus (≤10%)

Renal: Renal insufficiency (≤10%)

Miscellaneous: Wound healing impairment (8%), gastrointestinal inflammation

<1%, postmarketing, and/or case reports: Abnormal Dreams, agranulocytosis, alopecia, anaphylaxis, angioedema, anxiety, aplastic anemia, asthma, auditory impairment, blurred vision, cardiac arrhythmia, cardiac failure, change in appetite, colitis, coma, confusion, conjunctivitis, convulsions, cystitis, depression, diaphoresis, drowsiness, dyspnea, dysuria, ecchymoses, eosinophilia, eructation, erythema multiforme, esophagitis, exfoliative dermatitis, fever, fulminant hepatitis, gastritis, gastrointestinal hemorrhage, glossitis, hallucination, hematemesis, hematuria, hemolytic anemia, hepatic failure, hepatic necrosis, hepatitis, hepatotoxicity, hyperglycemia, hypertension, hypotension, infection, insomnia, interstitial nephritis, jaundice, leukopenia, lymphadenopathy, malaise, melena, meningitis, nervousness, oliguria, palpitations, pancreatitis, pancytopenia, paresthesia, pneumonia, polyuria, proteinuria, purpura, rectal hemorrhage, renal failure, respiratory depression, sepsis, skin photosensitivity, stomatitis, syncope, tachycardia, thrombocytopenia, toxic epidermal necrolysis, tremor, urticaria, vasculitis, vertigo, weakness, weight changes

Oral: Frequency not always defined.

>10%:

Cardiovascular: Edema (33%)

Hepatic: Increased serum transaminases (≤3 x ULN; 15%)

1% to 10%:

Cardiovascular: Hypertension (2% to 3%)

Central nervous system: Headache (4% to 8%), procedural pain (3%), dizziness (2%), falling (2%)

Dermatologic: Pruritus (7%), skin rash

Gastrointestinal: Constipation (5% to 8%), nausea (6% to 7%), diarrhea (6%), GI adverse effects (gastric ulcer, hemorrhage, and perforation; ≤4%, risk increases with therapy duration), abdominal pain (2% to 3%), vomiting (3%), dyspepsia (2% to 3%), flatulence (2% to 3%), heartburn, abdominal discomfort (2%), duodenal ulcer

Genitourinary: Urinary tract infection (7%)

Hematologic & oncologic: Bruise (3%), anemia, prolonged bleeding time

Hepatic: Increased serum ALT (>3 x ULN: ≤4%; >8 x ULN: ≤1%), increased serum AST (>3 x ULN; ≤4%; >8 x ULN: ≤1%)

Infection: Influenza (3%)

Neuromuscular & skeletal: Osteoarthritis (5%), arthralgia (3%), back pain (3%), limb pain (3%)

Renal: Renal function abnormality

Otic: Tinnitus

Renal: Increased serum creatinine (2%), renal function abnormality

Respiratory: Upper respiratory tract infection (8%), nasopharyngitis (6%), sinusitis (3% to 5%), cough (4%), bronchitis (3%)

<1%, postmarketing, and/or case reports: Abnormal dreams, agranulocytosis, alopecia, anaphylactoid reaction, anaphylaxis, angioedema, anxiety, aplastic anemia, aseptic meningitis, asthma, auditory impairment, azotemia (Gurwitz, 1990), blurred vision, cardiac arrhythmia, cardiac failure, cerebrovascular accident, change in appetite, chest pain, colitis, coma, confusion, conjunctivitis, cystitis, decreased hemoglobin (Goldstein, 2011), depression, diaphoresis, diplopia, disorientation, drowsiness, dyspnea, dysuria, ecchymoses, eosinophilia, eructation, erythema multiforme, esophageal ulcer, esophagitis, exfoliative dermatitis, fever, fluid retention, fulminant hepatitis, gastritis, glossitis, hallucination, hearing loss, hematemesis, hematuria, hemolytic anemia, hepatic failure, hepatic necrosis, hepatitis, hepatotoxicity, hyperglycemia, hypotension, infection, insomnia, interstitial nephritis, intestinal perforation, jaundice, leukopenia, lymphadenopathy, malaise, melena, memory impairment, meningitis, myocardial infarction, nephrotic syndrome, nervousness, oliguria, palpitations, pancreatitis, pancytopenia, paresthesia, peptic ulcer, pneumonia, polyuria, proteinuria, psychotic reaction, purpura, rectal hemorrhage, renal failure, renal papillary necrosis, respiratory depression, seizure, sepsis, skin photosensitivity, Stevens-Johnson syndrome, stomatitis, syncope, tachycardia, taste disorder, thrombocytopenia, toxic epidermal necrolysis, tremor, urticaria, vasculitis, vertigo, weakness, weight changes, xerostomia

Rectal suppository [Canadian product]:

Also refer to adverse reactions associated with oral formulations.

<1%, postmarketing, and/or case reports: Hemorrhoids (exacerbation), local hemorrhage, proctitis, rectal irritation

Dental Usual Dosage Pain: Adults: Oral: Starting dose: 50 mg 3 times/day; maximum dose: 150 mg/day

Dosing

Adult Note: Use the lowest effective dose for the shortest duration of time, consistent with individual patient treatment goals. Due to an increased risk of cardiovascular events, use should generally be avoided in patients with established cardiovascular disease or risk factors for cardiovascular disease. Use should also be avoided in those with heart failure (Chan 2018; Schmidt 2016). Of note, Dyloject (diclofenac injection) has been discontinued in the United States for >1 year.

Note: For all indications, it has been recommended to not exceed 100 mg/day based on increased risk of vascular events (eg, stroke, nonfatal myocardial infarction) (Bhala 2013; Health Canada communication 2014).

Ankylosing spondylitis: Oral: Delayed-release tablet: 25 mg 4 times daily and 25 mg at bedtime as needed.

Gout, treatment (acute flares) (alternative agent) (off-label use): Oral: IR tablets or delayed-release tablets: 50 mg twice daily (Becker 2019); initiate within 24 to 48 hours of flare onset preferably; discontinue 2 to 3 days after resolution of clinical signs; usual duration: 5 to 7 days (ACR [Khanna 2012]; Becker 2019).

Migraine: Oral: Powder for oral solution: 50 mg (one packet) as a single dose; safety and efficacy of a second dose have not been established.

Osteoarthritis:

Oral:

Immediate-release tablet: 50 mg 2 to 3 times daily; Delayed-release tablet: 50 mg 2 to 3 times daily or 75 mg twice daily; Extended-release tablet: 100 mg once daily.

Immediate-release capsule: Zorvolex (diclofenac acid): 35 mg 3 times daily.

Rectal suppository [Canadian product]: Insert 50 mg or 100 mg rectally as single dose to substitute for final oral daily dose (maximum combined dose [rectal and oral]: 100 mg/day).

Pain:

Oral:

Immediate-release tablet: 50 mg 3 times daily; may administer 100 mg as an initial dose, followed by 50 mg 3 times daily.

Immediate-release capsule:

Zipsor (diclofenac potassium): 25 mg 4 times daily.

Zorvolex (diclofenac acid): 18 mg or 35 mg 3 times daily.

IV: 37.5 mg every 6 hours as needed; adjust frequency according to patient response (maximum: 150 mg/day).

Primary dysmenorrhea: Oral: Immediate-release tablet: 50 mg 3 times daily; may administer 100 mg as an initial dose, followed by 50 mg 3 times daily.

Rheumatoid arthritis:

Oral: Immediate-release tablet: 50 mg 3 to 4 times daily; Delayed-release tablet: 50 mg 3 to 4 times daily or 75 mg twice daily; Extended-release tablet: 100 mg once daily; may increase to 100 mg twice daily.

Rectal suppository [Canadian product]: Insert 50 mg or 100 mg rectally as single dose to substitute for final oral daily dose (maximum combined dose [rectal and oral]: 100 mg/day.

Geriatric Refer to adult dosing. Use with caution; initiate using lowest recommended dose and frequency.

Renal Impairment: Adult

Oral:

Mild or moderate impairment: No dosage adjustment necessary.

Significant impairment or advanced renal disease: Use is not recommended.

Injection:

Mild impairment: There are no dosage adjustments provided in the manufacturer's labeling.

Moderate to severe impairment: Use is not recommended; contraindicated in patients in the perioperative period and who are at risk for volume depletion.

KDIGO 2012 guidelines provide the following recommendations for NSAIDs:

eGFR 30 to <60 mL/minute/1.73 m^2: Temporarily discontinue in patients with intercurrent disease that increases risk of acute kidney injury.

eGFR <30 mL/minute/1.73 m^2: Avoid use.

Hepatic Impairment: Adult There are no dosage adjustments provided in the manufacturer's labeling; however, may require dosage adjustment due to extensive hepatic metabolism. Additional product-specific recommendations:

Cambia: Use the lowest effective dose for the shortest duration possible.

Zipsor/Zorvolex: Initial: Initiate treatment at the lowest dose; if efficacy is not achieved with the lowest dose, discontinue use.

Injection:

Mild impairment: No dosage adjustment necessary.

Moderate to severe impairment: Use is not recommended (has not been studied).

Pediatric Note: Different oral formulations are not bioequivalent; do not interchange products.

Juvenile idiopathic arthritis: Limited data available: Children and Adolescents: Oral: Immediate release tablet: 2 to 3 mg/kg/day in divided doses 2 to 4 times/day; maximum daily dose: 150 mg/**day** (Haapasaari 1983; Hashkes 2005; Leak 1996; Petty 2016)

Migraine: Adolescents ≥18 years: Oral: Oral solution: 50 mg (one packet) as a single dose at the time of migraine onset; safety and efficacy of a second dose have not been established

Renal Impairment: Pediatric

Children and Adolescents: There are no pediatric-specific dosage adjustments provided in the manufacturer's labeling; some experts have suggested the following:

KDIGO 2012 guidelines provide the following recommendations for NSAIDs (KDIGO 2013):

eGFR 30 to <60 mL/minute/1.73 m^2: Temporarily discontinue in patients with intercurrent disease that increases risk of acute kidney injury

eGFR <30 mL/minute/1.73 m^2: Avoid use.

Hepatic Impairment: Pediatric There are no dosage adjustments provided in the manufacturer's labeling; however, may require dosage adjustment due to extensive hepatic metabolism.

Mechanism of Action Reversibly inhibits cyclooxygenase-1 and 2 (COX-1 and 2) enzymes, which results in decreased formation of prostaglandin precursors; has antipyretic, analgesic, and anti-inflammatory properties

Other proposed mechanisms not fully elucidated (and possibly contributing to the anti-inflammatory effect to varying degrees), include inhibiting chemotaxis, altering lymphocyte activity, inhibiting neutrophil aggregation/activation, and decreasing proinflammatory cytokine levels.

Contraindications

Hypersensitivity to diclofenac (eg, anaphylactoid reactions, serious skin reactions) or bovine protein (Zipsor only) or any component of the formulation; history of asthma, urticaria, or other allergic-type reactions after taking aspirin or other NSAIDs; use in the setting of CABG surgery; patients with moderate to severe renal impairment in the perioperative period and who are at risk for volume depletion (injection only).

Canadian labeling: Additional contraindications (not in US labeling): Severe uncontrolled heart failure; active gastric/duodenal/peptic ulcer; active GI bleed or perforation, regional ulcer or enteritis, gastritis, ulcerative colitis, or recurrent ulceration; cerebrovascular bleeding or other bleeding disorders; inflammatory bowel disease; severe hepatic impairment; active hepatic disease; severe renal impairment (CrCl <30 mL/minute) or deteriorating renal disease; known hyperkalemia; patients <16 years of age (suppository, tablet) or <18 years of age (packet only); breastfeeding; pregnancy (third trimester); recent history of bleeding or inflammatory lesions of rectum/anus (suppository only)

Warnings/Precautions [US Boxed Warning]: Nonsteroidal anti-inflammatory drugs (NSAIDs) cause an increased risk of serious (and potentially fatal) adverse cardiovascular thrombotic events, including MI and stroke. Risk may occur early during treatment and may increase with duration of use. Relative risk appears to be similar in those with and without known cardiovascular disease or risk factors for cardiovascular disease; however, absolute incidence of serious cardiovascular thrombotic events (which may occur early during treatment) was higher in patients with known cardiovascular disease or risk factors and in those receiving higher doses. New onset hypertension or exacerbation of hypertension may occur (NSAIDs may also impair response to ACE inhibitors, thiazide diuretics, or loop diuretics); may contribute to cardiovascular events; monitor blood pressure; use with caution in patients with hypertension. May cause sodium and fluid retention; use with caution in patients with edema. Avoid use in heart failure (ACCF/AHA [Yancy 2013]). Avoid use in patients with recent MI unless benefits outweigh risk of cardiovascular thrombotic events. Use the lowest effective dose for the shortest duration of time, consistent with individual patient goals, to reduce risk of cardiovascular events; alternate therapies should be considered for patients at high risk. **[US Boxed Warning]: Use is contraindicated in the setting of coronary artery bypass graft (CABG) surgery.** Risk of MI and stroke may be increased with use following CABG surgery.

Clinical or population-based data regarding the risks of NSAIDs in the setting of coronavirus disease 2019 (COVID-19) are limited (FDA Safety Communication 2020; Kim 2020). Some experts recommend the use of acetaminophen as the preferred antipyretic agent, when possible, and if NSAIDs are needed, to use the lowest effective dose and shortest duration (EMA 2020; Kim 2020). In general, for patients already taking an NSAID for a comorbid condition, it is recommended to continue the NSAID as directed by their health care provider (EMA 2020; NIH 2020; WHO 2020).

NSAID use may compromise existing renal function; dose-dependent decreases in prostaglandin synthesis may result from NSAID use, reducing renal blood flow which may cause renal decompensation (usually reversible). Patients with impaired renal function, dehydration, hypovolemia, heart failure, hepatic impairment, those taking diuretics and ACE inhibitors, and the elderly are at greater risk of renal toxicity. Rehydrate patient before starting therapy; monitor function closely. Long-term NSAID use may result in renal papillary necrosis and other renal injury. NSAID use may increase the risk for hyperkalemia, particularly in elderly patients, diabetic patients, those with renal disease, and with concomitant use of other agents capable of inducing hyperkalemia (eg, ACE inhibitors). Monitor potassium closely. Avoid use in patients with advanced renal disease unless benefits are expected to outweigh risk of worsening renal function; monitor closely if therapy must be initiated. Injection is not recommended in patients with moderate to severe renal impairment and is contraindicated in patients with moderate to severe renal impairment in the perioperative period and who are at risk for volume depletion.

[US Boxed Warning]: NSAIDs cause an increased risk of serious GI inflammation, ulceration, bleeding, and perforation (may be fatal); elderly patients and patients with history of peptic ulcer disease and/or GI bleeding are at greater risk for serious GI events. These events may occur at any time during therapy and without warning. Avoid use in patients with active GI bleeding. In patients with a history of acute lower GI bleeding, avoid use of non-aspirin NSAIDs, especially if due to angioectasia or diverticulosis (Strate 2016). Use caution with a history of GI ulcers, concurrent therapy known to increase the risk of GI bleeding (eg, aspirin, anticoagulants and/or corticosteroids, selective serotonin reuptake inhibitors), advanced hepatic disease, coagulopathy, smoking, use of alcohol, or in elderly or debilitated patients. Use the lowest effective dose for the shortest duration of time, consistent with individual patient goals, to reduce risk of GI adverse events; alternate therapies should be considered for patients at high risk. When used concomitantly with aspirin, a substantial increase in the risk of gastrointestinal complications (eg, ulcer) occurs; concomitant gastroprotective therapy (eg, proton pump inhibitors) is recommended (Bhatt 2008). Avoid chronic use of oral nonselective NSAIDs in patients who have undergone bariatric surgery; development of anastomotic ulcerations/perforations may occur.

Use the lowest effective dose for the shortest duration of time, consistent with individual patient goals, to reduce risk of cardiovascular or GI adverse events. Alternate therapies should be considered for patients at high risk. Elderly patients are at greater risk for serious GI, cardiovascular, and/or renal adverse events.

NSAIDs may cause potentially fatal serious skin adverse events including exfoliative dermatitis, Stevens-Johnson syndrome (SJS), and toxic epidermal necrolysis (TEN); may occur without warning; discontinue use at first sign of skin rash (or any other hypersensitivity).

Anaphylactoid reactions may occur, even without prior exposure; patients with "aspirin triad" (bronchial asthma, aspirin intolerance, rhinitis) may be at increased risk. Use is contraindicated in patients who experience bronchospasm, asthma, rhinitis, or urticaria with NSAID or aspirin therapy. Use caution in other forms of asthma. Platelet adhesion and aggregation may be decreased; may prolong bleeding time; patients with coagulation disorders or who are receiving anticoagulants should be monitored closely. Anemia may occur; patients on long-term NSAID therapy should be monitored for anemia. Rarely, NSAID use may cause severe blood dyscrasias (eg, agranulocytosis, aplastic anemia, thrombocytopenia).

Use with caution in patients with hepatic impairment; reduced doses may be required due to extensive hepatic metabolism. Patients with advanced hepatic disease are at an increased risk of GI bleeding with NSAIDs. Transaminase elevations have been reported with use; closely monitor patients with any abnormal LFT. Rare, sometimes fatal, severe hepatic reactions (eg, fulminant hepatitis, hepatic necrosis, hepatic failure) have occurred with NSAID use; discontinue immediately if clinical signs or symptoms of liver disease develop or if systemic manifestations occur.

NSAIDS may cause drowsiness, dizziness, blurred vision, and other neurologic effects which may impair physical or mental abilities; patients must be cautioned about performing tasks which require mental alertness (eg, operating machinery or driving). Discontinue use with blurred or diminished vision and perform ophthalmologic exam. Monitor vision with long-term therapy. May increase the risk of aseptic meningitis, especially in patients with systemic lupus erythematosus (SLE) and mixed connective tissue disorders.

Withhold for at least 4 to 6 half-lives prior to surgical or dental procedures.

Different formulations of oral diclofenac are not bioequivalent, even if the milligram strength is the same; do not interchange products.

Zipsor (capsule) contains gelatin; use is contraindicated in patients with history of hypersensitivity to bovine protein.

Injection is not indicated for long-term use.

Oral solution: Indicated only for the acute treatment of migraine (not indicated for migraine prophylaxis or cluster headache). Acute migraine agents (eg, NSAIDs, triptans, opioids, ergotamine, or a combination of the agents) used for 10 or more days per month may lead to worsening of headaches (medication overuse headache); withdrawal treatment may be necessary in the setting of overuse. Product may contain phenylalanine.

Drug Interactions

Metabolism/Transport Effects Substrate of CYP1A2 (minor), CYP2B6 (minor), CYP2C19 (minor), CYP2C8 (minor), CYP2C9 (major), CYP2D6 (minor), CYP3A4 (minor); **Note:** Assignment of Major/Minor substrate status based on clinically relevant drug interaction potential; **Inhibits** UGT1A6

Avoid Concomitant Use

Avoid concomitant use of Diclofenac (Systemic) with any of the following: Acemetacin; Aminolevulinic Acid (Systemic); Deferiprone; Dexibuprofen; Dexketoprofen; Floctafenine; Ketorolac (Nasal); Ketorolac (Systemic); Macimorelin; Mifamurtide; Morniflumate; Nonsteroidal Anti-Inflammatory Agents (COX-2 Selective); Omacetaxine; Pelubiprofen; Phenylbutazone; Talniflumate; Tenoxicam; Urokinase; Zaltoprofen

Increased Effect/Toxicity

Diclofenac (Systemic) may increase the levels/effects of: 5-Aminosalicylic Acid Derivatives; Agents with Antiplatelet Properties; Aliskiren; Aminoglycosides; Aminolevulinic Acid (Systemic); Aminolevulinic Acid (Topical); Anticoagulants; Apixaban; Artesunate; Bemiparin; Bisphosphonate Derivatives; Cephalothin; Collagenase (Systemic); CycloSPORINE (Systemic); Dabigatran Etexilate; Deferasirox; Deferiprone; Deoxycholic Acid; Desmopressin; Dexibuprofen; Digoxin; Drospirenone; Edoxaban; Enoxaparin; Eplerenone; Haloperidol; Heparin; Ibritumomab Tiuxetan; Lithium; MetFORMIN; Methotrexate; Nalmefene; Nonsteroidal Anti-Inflammatory Agents; Nonsteroidal Anti-Inflammatory Agents (COX-2 Selective); Obinutuzumab; Omacetaxine; Porfimer; Potassium-Sparing Diuretics; PRALAtrexate; Quinolones; Rivaroxaban; Salicylates; Tacrolimus (Systemic); Tenofovir Products;

Thrombolytic Agents; Tolperisone; Urokinase; Vancomycin; Verteporfin; Vitamin K Antagonists

The levels/effects of Diclofenac (Systemic) may be increased by: Acalabrutinib; Acemetacin; Alcohol (Ethyl); Angiotensin II Receptor Blockers; Angiotensin-Converting Enzyme Inhibitors; Corticosteroids (Systemic); CycloSPORINE (Systemic); CYP2C9 Inhibitors (Moderate); Dasatinib; Dexketoprofen; Fat Emulsion (Fish Oil Based); Felbinac; Floctafenine; Glucosamine; Herbs (Anticoagulant/Antiplatelet Properties); Ibrutinib; Inotersen; Ketorolac (Nasal); Ketorolac (Systemic); Limaprost; Loop Diuretics; Lumacaftor and Ivacaftor; Morniflumate; Multivitamins/Fluoride (with ADE); Multivitamins/Minerals (with ADEK, Folate, Iron); Multivitamins/Minerals (with AE, No Iron); Naftazone; Omega-3 Fatty Acids; Pelubiprofen; Pentosan Polysulfate Sodium; Pentoxifylline; Phenylbutazone; Probenecid; Prostacyclin Analogues; Resveratrol; Selective Serotonin Reuptake Inhibitors; Selumetinib; Serotonin/Norepinephrine Reuptake Inhibitors; Sodium Phosphates; Talniflumate; Tenoxicam; Thiazide and Thiazide-Like Diuretics; Tipranavir; Tolperisone; Tricyclic Antidepressants (Tertiary Amine); Vitamin E (Systemic); Voriconazole; Zaltoprofen; Zanubrutinib

Decreased Effect

Diclofenac (Systemic) may decrease the levels/effects of: Aliskiren; Angiotensin II Receptor Blockers; Angiotensin-Converting Enzyme Inhibitors; Beta-Blockers; Eplerenone; HydrALAZINE; Loop Diuretics; Macimorelin; Mifamurtide; Potassium-Sparing Diuretics; Prostaglandins (Ophthalmic); Salicylates; Selective Serotonin Reuptake Inhibitors; Sincalide; Thiazide and Thiazide-Like Diuretics

The levels/effects of Diclofenac (Systemic) may be decreased by: Bile Acid Sequestrants; CYP2C9 Inducers (Moderate); Lumacaftor and Ivacaftor; Salicylates

Dietary Considerations Oral immediate-release formulations may be taken with food to decrease GI distress. However, food may reduce effectiveness of oral solution and diclofenac acid (capsule). Some products may contain phenylalanine.

Pharmacodynamics/Kinetics

Half-life Elimination Oral: ~2 hours, ~1 hour (liquid filled capsule [Zipsor]); Injection: ~1.4 hours

Time to Peak Serum: **Note:** Fasted values reported for oral products; may be delayed with food.

Cambia: ~0.25 hours

Cataflam, Zorvolex: ~1 hour

Zipsor: ~0.47 ± 0.17 hour

Injection: ~5 minutes

Tablet, delayed release (diclofenac sodium): 2.3 hours

Tablet, extended release (diclofenac sodium): 5.3 hours

Reproductive Considerations

The chronic use of NSAIDs, including diclofenac, in women of reproductive age may be associated with infertility that is reversible upon discontinuation of the medication. Consider discontinuing use in women having difficulty conceiving or those undergoing investigation of fertility.

Pregnancy Considerations

Diclofenac crosses the placenta. Birth defects have been observed following in utero NSAID exposure in some studies; however, data is conflicting (Bloor 2013). Nonteratogenic effects, including prenatal constriction of the ductus arteriosus, persistent pulmonary hypertension of the newborn, oligohydramnios, necrotizing enterocolitis, renal dysfunction or failure, and intracranial hemorrhage have been observed in the fetus/neonate following in utero NSAID exposure. In addition, nonclosure of the ductus arteriosus postnatally may occur and be resistant to medical management (Bermas 2014; Bloor 2013). Because they may cause premature closure of the ductus arteriosus, product labeling for diclofenac specifically states use should be avoided starting at 30 weeks' gestation.

Use of NSAIDs can be considered for the treatment of mild rheumatoid arthritis flares in pregnant women; however, use should be minimized or avoided early and late in pregnancy (Bermas 2014; Saavedra Salinas 2015). If treatment of migraine is needed in pregnant women, agents other than diclofenac are preferred (Amundsen 2015).

Breastfeeding Considerations Diclofenac may be present in breast milk.

The milk concentration of a woman treated with oral diclofenac 150 mg/day was reported to be 100 mcg/L (equivalent to an infant dose of ~0.03 mg/kg/day). Diclofenac was not detected in breast milk when 100 mg/day orally was administered to 12 women for 7 days or as a single dose of 50 mg IM immediately postpartum.

According to the manufacturer, the decision to breastfeed during therapy should consider the risk of infant exposure, the benefits of breastfeeding to the infant, and benefits of treatment to the mother. In general, NSAIDs may be used in postpartum women who wish to breastfeed; however, agents other than diclofenac may be preferred (ABM [Reece-Stremtan 2017]; Amundsen 2015) and use should be avoided in women breastfeeding infants with platelet dysfunction, thrombocytopenia (Bloor 2013; Sammaritano 2014), or ductal-dependent cardiac lesions (ABM [Reece-Stremtan 2017]).

Product Availability Dyloject (diclofenac injection) has been discontinued in the US for more than 1 year.

Dosage Forms: US

Capsule, Oral:

Zipsor: 25 mg

Zorvolex: 18 mg, 35 mg

Packet, Oral:

Cambia: 50 mg (1 ea, 9 ea)

Tablet, Oral:

Generic: 50 mg

Tablet Delayed Release, Oral:

Generic: 25 mg, 50 mg, 75 mg

Tablet Extended Release 24 Hour, Oral:

Generic: 100 mg

Dosage Forms: Canada

Packet, Oral:

Cambia: 50 mg (1 ea, 3 ea, 9 ea)

Suppository, Rectal:

Voltaren: 50 mg (30 ea); 100 mg (30 ea)

Generic: 50 mg (30 ea); 100 mg (30 ea)

Tablet, Oral:

Voltaren Rapide: 50 mg

Generic: 50 mg

Tablet Delayed Release, Oral:

Voltaren: 50 mg

Generic: 25 mg, 50 mg

Tablet Extended Release 24 Hour, Oral:

Voltaren SR: 75 mg, 100 mg

Generic: 75 mg, 100 mg

Diclofenac (Topical) (dye KLOE fen ak)

Brand Names: US Diclo Gel with Xrylix Sheets [DSC]; Diclo Gel [DSC]; Diclozor; DST Plus Pak [DSC]; EnovaRX-Diclofenac Sodium; Flector; Klofensaid II [DSC]; Lexixryl [DSC]; Pennsaid; Rexaphenac; Solaraze [DSC]; Voltaren; Voltaren [OTC]; Vopac MDS [DSC]; Xrylix

Brand Names: Canada JAMP Diclofenac; Pennsaid; PMS-Diclofenac; TARO-Diclofenac

Pharmacologic Category Nonsteroidal Anti-inflammatory Drug (NSAID); Nonsteroidal Anti-inflammatory Drug (NSAID), Topical

Use

Gel 1%:

Rx: Relief of osteoarthritis pain in joints amenable to topical therapy (eg, ankle, elbow, foot, hand, knee, wrist).

OTC: Temporary relief of arthritis pain in the hand, wrist, elbow, foot, ankle, or knee.

Gel 3%: Treatment of actinic keratosis in conjunction with sun avoidance.

Gel 1.16% (Voltaren Emulgel), 2.32% (Voltaren Emulgel Extra Strength) [Canadian products]: Relief of pain associated with acute, localized joint/muscle injuries (eg, sports injuries, strains) in patients ≥16 years of age (1.16% gel) or ≥18 years of age (2.32% gel).

Patch: Treatment of acute pain due to minor strains, sprains, and contusions in adults and children ≥6 years of age.

Solution: Treatment of osteoarthritis pain of the knee.

Local Anesthetic/Vasoconstrictor Precautions No information available to require special precautions

Effects on Dental Treatment No significant effects or complications reported

Effects on Bleeding No information available to require special precautions

Adverse Reactions

Topical gel:

>10%:

Dermatologic: Application-site scaling (6% to 24%), contact dermatitis (2%; application site: 33%), xeroderma (3%; application site: 27%)

Local: Application site pain (15% to 26%), application site pruritus (31% to 52%; nonapplication site: 4%), application site rash (35% to 46%; nonapplication site: 4%)

1% to 10%:

Cardiovascular: Chest pain (1% to 2%), hypertension (1% to 2%)

Dermatologic: Acne vulgaris (application site: 1%), alopecia (application site: 2%), dermal ulcer (1% to 2%), skin photosensitivity (application site: 3%), vesiculobullous dermatitis (4%)

Endocrine & metabolic: Hypercholesterolemia (1%), hyperglycemia (1%)

Gastrointestinal: Abdominal pain (1% to 2%), diarrhea (2%), dyspepsia (2%)

Genitourinary: Hematuria (2%)

Hepatic: Increased serum alanine aminotransferase (2%), increased serum aspartate aminotransferase (3%)

Hypersensitivity: Hypersensitivity reaction (1%)

Local: Application site edema (3% to 4%)

Nervous system: Headache (7%), hyperesthesia (application site: 3%), migraine (1%), paresthesia (≤8%; including application site)

Neuromuscular and skeletal: Arthralgia (2%), arthropathy (2%), asthenia (2%), back pain (4%), hypokinesia (2%), increased creatine phosphokinase in blood specimen (4%), myalgia (2% to 3%), neck pain (2%)

Ophthalmic: Eye pain (2%)

Respiratory: Asthma (2%), dyspnea (2%), sinusitis (2%)

<1%:

Dermatologic: Papule of skin (application site), seborrhea, skin hypertrophy, urticaria

Local: Application site irritation, application site reaction (skin carcinoma, hypertonia, skin hypertrophy lacrimation disorder, maculopapular rash, purpuric rash, vasodilation), application site vesicles

Topical solution:

>10%: Dermatologic: Xeroderma (application site: 22% to 32%; nonapplication site: 2%)

1% to 10%:

Cardiovascular: Edema (3%)

Dermatologic: Contact dermatitis (application site: 2% to 9%), desquamation (application site: 7%), ecchymosis (2%), pruritus (application site: 2% to 4%; nonapplication site: 2%), skin rash (2% to 3%; including application site)

Gastrointestinal: Abdominal pain (6%), constipation (3%), diarrhea (4%), dyspepsia (8%), flatulence (4%), halitosis (1%), nausea (2% to 4%)

Genitourinary: Urinary tract infection (3%)

Hematologic & oncologic: Bruise (2%)

Infection: Infection (3%)

Local: Application site erythema (4%), application site induration (2%), application site pain (2%), application site vesicles (2%)

Nervous system: Paresthesia (2%, including application site)

Respiratory: Paranasal sinus congestion (2%), sinusitis (1%)

Transdermal patch:

1% to 10%:

Dermatologic: Dermatitis (2%), hyperhidrosis (application site: ≤4%), localized erythema (application site: ≤4%), localized vesiculation (application site: ≤4%), skin discoloration (application site: ≤4%), xeroderma (application site: ≤4%)

Gastrointestinal: Constipation (≤3%), diarrhea (≤3%), dysgeusia (2%), gastritis (≤3%), nausea (3%), upper abdominal pain (≤3%), vomiting (≤3%), xerostomia (≤3%)

Local: Application site atrophy (≤4%), local irritation (application site: ≤4%)

Nervous system: Dizziness (≤1%), hypoesthesia (≤1%)

Neuromuscular & skeletal: Hyperkinetic muscle activity (≤1%)

Frequency not defined (any formulation):

Cardiovascular: Acute myocardial infarction, cerebrovascular accident, hypertension, thrombosis, vasodilation (application site)

Dermatologic: Acne vulgaris (application site), dermatological reaction, exfoliative dermatitis, Stevens-Johnson syndrome, toxic epidermal necrolysis, urticaria (application site)

Gastrointestinal: Esophageal perforation, gastrointestinal hemorrhage, gastrointestinal perforation, gastrointestinal ulcer

Hypersensitivity: Anaphylaxis

Postmarketing (any formulation):

Cardiovascular: Cardiac disorder, chest pain, facial edema, hypertension, increased blood pressure, lip edema, palpitations

Dermatologic: Burning sensation of skin, crusted skin, eczema, skin discoloration, urticaria

Gastrointestinal: Aphthous stomatitis, decreased appetite, dysgeusia, gastroenteritis, oral mucosa ulcer, xerostomia

Hematologic & oncologic: Rectal hemorrhage

Hepatic: Increased serum transaminases (Daniels 2018)

Hypersensitivity: Hypersensitivity reaction, tongue edema

Nervous system: Depression, dizziness, drowsiness, headache, lethargy

Neuromuscular & skeletal: Asthenia, back pain, lower limb cramp, myalgia, neck stiffness

Ophthalmic: Blurred vision, cataract, eye pain, visual disturbance

Otic: Otalgia

Renal: Increased serum creatinine

Respiratory: Asthma, dyspnea, laryngismus, laryngitis, pharyngeal edema, pharyngitis

Mechanism of Action

Reversibly inhibits cyclooxygenase-1 and 2 (COX-1 and 2) enzymes, which results in decreased formation of prostaglandin precursors; has antipyretic, analgesic, and anti-inflammatory properties

Other proposed mechanisms not fully elucidated (and possibly contributing to the anti-inflammatory effect to varying degrees), include inhibiting chemotaxis, altering lymphocyte activity, inhibiting neutrophil aggregation/activation, and decreasing proinflammatory cytokine levels.

Pharmacodynamics/Kinetics

Half-life Elimination Patch: ~12 hours; Solution 1.5%: 36.7 ± 20.8 hours (single application)

Time to Peak Serum: Patch: 10 to 20 hours; Solution 1.5%: 11 ± 6.4 hours (single application); Gel 3%: 4.5 ± 8 hours; Gel 1%: 10 to 14 hours.

Reproductive Considerations

The chronic use of NSAIDs in females of reproductive potential may be associated with infertility that is reversible upon discontinuation of the medication. Consider discontinuing use in females having difficulty conceiving or those undergoing investigation of fertility.

Pregnancy Considerations

Diclofenac crosses the placenta following systemic administration. The amount of diclofenac available systemically following topical application is less in comparison to oral doses. Reversible constriction of the ductus arteriosus in utero has been observed following topical application of diclofenac (Torloni 2006). Because NSAIDs may cause premature closure of the ductus arteriosus, product labeling for diclofenac specifically states use should be avoided starting at 30 weeks' gestation.

Product Availability

Solaraze gel has been discontinued in the United States for >1 year.

Diclofenac and Misoprostol

(dye KLOE fen ak & mye soe PROST ole)

Related Information

Diclofenac (Systemic) *on page 484*

MiSOPROStol *on page 1040*

Rheumatoid Arthritis, Osteoarthritis, and Osteoporosis *on page 1697*

Brand Names: US Arthrotec

Brand Names: Canada ACT Diclo-Miso [DSC]; Arthrotec; GD-Diclofenac/Misoprostol 50; GD-Diclofenac/Misoprostol 75; PMS-Diclofenac-Misoprostol

Pharmacologic Category Analgesic, Nonopioid; Nonsteroidal Anti-inflammatory Drug (NSAID), Oral; Prostaglandin

Use Osteoarthritis/rheumatoid arthritis: Treatment of the signs and symptoms of osteoarthritis or rheumatoid arthritis in patients at high risk for NSAID-induced gastric and duodenal ulcers and their complications.

Local Anesthetic/Vasoconstrictor Precautions No information available to require special precautions

Effects on Dental Treatment The dentist should be aware of the potential of abnormal coagulation. Caution should also be exercised in the use of NSAIDs in patients already on anticoagulant therapy with drugs such as warfarin (Coumadin). See Effects on Bleeding.

Effects on Bleeding Nonselective NSAIDs, such as diclofenac, inhibit platelet aggregation and prolong bleeding time in some patients. Unlike aspirin, the NSAID effect on platelet function is quantitatively less, of shorter duration, and reversible.

Adverse Reactions Percentages reported with combination product. Also see individual agents.

>10%: Gastrointestinal: Abdominal pain (21%), diarrhea (19%), dyspepsia (14%), nausea (11%)

1% to 10%:

Gastrointestinal: Flatulence (9%)

Hepatic: Increased serum ALT (2%)

Frequency not defined:

Central nervous system: Anxiety, depression, dizziness, drowsiness, fatigue, headache, insomnia, irritability, lack of concentration, malaise, paresthesia, vertigo

Dermatologic: Alopecia, diaphoresis, eczema, pemphigoid reaction, pruritus, skin photosensitivity

Endocrine & metabolic: Dehydration, hypermenorrhea, hyponatremia, menstrual disease

Gastrointestinal: Anorexia, benign gastrointestinal neoplasm, change in appetite, constipation, dysgeusia, dysphagia, eructation, esophageal ulcer, esophagitis, gastritis, gastroesophageal reflux disease, melena, peptic ulcer, tenesmus, vomiting, xerostomia

Genitourinary: Dysmenorrhea, dysuria, mastalgia, nocturia, proteinuria, urinary tract infection, vaginal hemorrhage

Hematologic & oncologic: Decreased hematocrit, leukopenia, purpura

Hepatic: Increased serum AST

Neuromuscular & skeletal: Arthralgia, increased serum alkaline phosphatase, myalgia, weakness

Ophthalmic: Diplopia

Otic: Tinnitus

Renal: Polyuria

Respiratory: Asthma, cough, epistaxis, hyperventilation

<1%, postmarketing, and/or case reports: Abnormal dreams, abnormal lacrimation, acne vulgaris, ageusia, agranulocytosis, amblyopia, anaphylactoid reaction, anaphylaxis, anemia, angioedema, aphthous stomatitis, aplastic anemia, aseptic meningitis, atrial fibrillation, auditory impairment, blurred vision, bruise, bullous rash, cardiac arrhythmia, cerebral hemorrhage, cerebrovascular accident, chills, coma, confusion, conjunctivitis, cystitis, decreased platelet aggregation, dermal ulcer, disorientation, dyspnea, ecchymosis, edema, enteritis, eosinophilia, erythema multiforme, exfoliative dermatitis, fever, fluid retention, fulminant hepatitis, gastrointestinal hemorrhage, gastrointestinal perforation, gastrointestinal ulcer, GI inflammation, glaucoma, glomerulonephritis, glomerulopathy (glomerulonephritis minimal lesion), glossitis, glycosuria, gout, hallucination, heartburn, hematemesis, hematuria, hemolytic anemia, hemorrhoids, hepatic failure, hepatic insufficiency, hepatic necrosis, hepatitis, hepatotoxicity (idiosyncratic) (Chalasani 2014), hyperbilirubinemia, hypercholesterolemia, hyperesthesia, hyperglycemia, hypersensitivity reaction, hypertension, hypertonia, hyperuricemia, hypoesthesia, hypoglycemia, hypotension, impotence, increased blood urea nitrogen, increased coagulation time, increased creatine phosphokinase, increased lactate dehydrogenase, infection, intermenstrual bleeding, interstitial nephritis, intestinal perforation, iritis, jaundice, laryngeal edema, leukocytosis, leukorrhea, lymphadenopathy, membranous glomerulonephritis, meningitis, migraine, mood changes, mucocutaneous eruptions, myocardial infarction, nephrotic syndrome, nervousness, neuralgia, nightmares, nocturnal amblyopia, oliguria, palpitations, pancreatitis, pancytopenia, paranoia, perineal pain, periorbital edema, pharyngeal edema, phlebitis, pneumonia, porphyria, pruritus ani, psychotic reaction, pulmonary embolism, rectal bleeding, reduced fertility (female), renal failure, renal insufficiency, renal papillary necrosis, respiratory depression, seizure, sepsis, skin rash, Stevens-Johnson syndrome, stomatitis, syncope, tachycardia, thrombocythemia, thrombocytopenia, toxic epidermal necrolysis, transient ischemic attacks, tremor, urinary frequency, urticaria, uterine cramps, uterine hemorrhage, vaginitis, vasculitis, ventricular premature contractions, visual disturbance, weight changes

Mechanism of Action

Diclofenac: Reversibly inhibits cyclooxygenase-1 and 2 (COX-1 and 2) enzymes, which results in decreased formation of prostaglandin precursors; has antipyretic, analgesic, and anti-inflammatory properties.

Misoprostol: Synthetic prostaglandin E1 analog that replaces the protective prostaglandins consumed with prostaglandin-inhibiting therapies (eg, NSAIDs).

Reproductive Considerations

[US Boxed Warning]: This product contains diclofenac and misoprostol. Do not use in women of childbearing potential unless the patient requires nonsteroidal anti-inflammatory drug (NSAID) therapy and is at high risk of developing gastric or duodenal ulceration or of developing complications from gastric or duodenal ulcers associated with the use of the NSAID. In such patients, this drug may be prescribed if the patient: Has had a negative serum pregnancy test within 2 weeks prior to beginning therapy; is capable of complying with effective contraceptive measures; has received both oral and written warnings of the hazards of misoprostol, risk of possible contraception failure, and danger to other women of childbearing potential if the drug is taken by mistake; and will begin using this product only on the second or third day of the next normal menstrual period. Patients must be advised of the abortifacient property and warned not to give the drug to others.

Refer to individual monographs for additional information.

Pregnancy Considerations

Use is contraindicated in pregnant women. **[US Boxed Warning]: This product contains diclofenac and misoprostol. Administration of misoprostol to women who are pregnant can cause abortion, premature birth, birth defects, or uterine rupture. Uterine rupture has been reported when misoprostol was administered to pregnant women to induce labor or to induce abortion. The risk of uterine rupture increases with advancing gestational ages and with prior uterine surgery, including cesarean delivery. Diclofenac/misoprostol should not be taken by pregnant women. Patients must be advised of the abortifacient property and warned not to give the drug to others.**

Refer to individual monographs for additional information.

- ◆ **Diclofenac Diethylamine [CAN]** *see* Diclofenac (Topical) *on page 489*
- ◆ **Diclofenac Epolamine** *see* Diclofenac (Topical) *on page 489*
- ◆ **Diclofenac Potassium** *see* Diclofenac (Systemic) *on page 484*
- ◆ **Diclofenac Sodium** *see* Diclofenac (Systemic) *on page 484*
- ◆ **Diclofenac Sodium** *see* Diclofenac (Topical) *on page 489*
- ◆ **Diclofenac Sodium/Misoprostol** *see* Diclofenac and Misoprostol *on page 490*
- ◆ **Diclo Gel [DSC]** *see* Diclofenac (Topical) *on page 489*
- ◆ **Diclo Gel with Xrylix Sheets [DSC]** *see* Diclofenac (Topical) *on page 489*

Dicloxacillin (dye kloks a SIL in)

Related Information

Bacterial Infections *on page 1739*

Pharmacologic Category Antibiotic, Penicillin

Use Staphylococcal infections: Treatment of infections caused by penicillinase-producing staphylococci.

Local Anesthetic/Vasoconstrictor Precautions No information available to require special precautions

Effects on Dental Treatment Key adverse event(s) related to dental treatment: Prolonged use of penicillins may lead to development of oral candidiasis.

Effects on Bleeding Thrombocytopenia has been reported.

Adverse Reactions Frequency not defined.

1% to 10%: Gastrointestinal: Abdominal pain diarrhea, nausea

<1%, postmarketing, and/or case reports: Agranulocytosis, anemia, eosinophilia, fever, hematuria, hemolytic anemia, hepatotoxicity, hypersensitivity reaction, increased blood urea nitrogen, increased liver enzymes (transient), increased serum creatinine, interstitial nephritis, leukopenia, neutropenia, prolonged prothrombin time, pseudomembranous colitis, seizure (with extremely high doses and/or renal

failure), serum sickness-like reaction, skin rash (maculopapular rash to exfoliative dermatitis), thrombocytopenia, vaginitis, vomiting

Mechanism of Action Inhibits bacterial cell wall synthesis by binding to one or more of the penicillin-binding proteins (PBPs) which in turn inhibits the final transpeptidation step of peptidoglycan synthesis in bacterial cell walls, thus inhibiting cell wall biosynthesis. Bacteria eventually lyse due to ongoing activity of cell wall autolytic enzymes (autolysins and murein hydrolases) while cell wall assembly is arrested.

Pharmacodynamics/Kinetics

Half-life Elimination ~0.7 hours; prolonged with renal impairment (Nauta 1976)

Time to Peak Serum: 1 to 1.5 hours

Pregnancy Risk Factor B

Pregnancy Considerations

Dicloxacillin crosses the placenta (Depp 1970). Maternal use of penicillins has generally not resulted in an increased risk of birth defects.

◆ **Dicloxacillin Sodium** *see* Dicloxacillin *on page 491*

◆ **Diclozor** *see* Diclofenac (Topical) *on page 489*

Dicyclomine (dye SYE kloe meen)

Related Information

Dentin Hypersensitivity, Acid Erosion, High Caries Index, Management of Alveolar Osteitis, and Xerostomia *on page 1762*

Brand Names: US Bentyl

Brand Names: Canada Bentylol [DSC]; JAMP-Dicyclomine HCl; Protylol; RIVA-Dicyclomine

Pharmacologic Category Anticholinergic Agent

Use Irritable bowel syndrome: Treatment of irritable bowel syndrome-associated abdominal pain.

Local Anesthetic/Vasoconstrictor Precautions No information available to require special precautions

Effects on Dental Treatment Key adverse event(s) related to dental treatment: Frequent occurrences of xerostomia and changes in salivation (normal salivary flow resumes upon discontinuation) have been reported. Rare occurrences of facial edema have also been observed.

Effects on Bleeding No information available to require special precautions

Adverse Reactions

>10%:

Central nervous system: Dizziness (40%)

Gastrointestinal: Xerostomia (33%), nausea (14%)

Ophthalmic: Blurred vision (27%)

1% to 10%:

Central nervous system: Drowsiness (9%), nervousness (6%)

Neuromuscular & skeletal: Weakness (7%)

Postmarketing and/or case reports: Abdominal distention, abdominal pain, anaphylactic shock, angioedema, confusion, constipation, cycloplegia, decreased lactation, delirium, dermatitis (allergic), dyspepsia, dyspnea, erythema, facial edema, fatigue, hallucination, headache, hypersensitivity, insomnia, malaise, mydriasis, nasal congestion, palpitations, skin rash, syncope, tachyarrhythmia, vomiting

Mechanism of Action Blocks the action of acetylcholine at parasympathetic sites in smooth muscle, secretory glands and the CNS

Pharmacodynamics/Kinetics

Onset of Action 1 to 2 hours

Duration of Action Up to 4 hours

Half-life Elimination Initial phase: ~1.8 hours; Terminal phase: Undetermined, but somewhat longer than the initial phase

Time to Peak Oral: 60 to 90 minutes

Pregnancy Considerations

In epidemiologic studies, birth defects were not observed following maternal doses up to 40 mg daily throughout the first trimester; information has not been located when used in pregnant women at recommended doses (80 to 160 mg daily). Antispasmodics are generally used to treat irritable bowel syndrome in pregnant patients only when symptoms are severe (Body 2016). Agents other than dicyclomine may be preferred for the treatment of irritable bowel syndrome in pregnant women (Enck 2016).

◆ **Dicyclomine Hydrochloride** *see* Dicyclomine *on page 492*

◆ **Dicycloverine Hydrochloride** *see* Dicyclomine *on page 492*

Didanosine (dye DAN oh seen)

Related Information

HIV Infection and AIDS *on page 1690*

Brand Names: US Videx EC [DSC]; Videx [DSC]

Brand Names: Canada Videx EC [DSC]

Pharmacologic Category Antiretroviral, Reverse Transcriptase Inhibitor, Nucleoside (Anti-HIV)

Use HIV-1 infection: Treatment of HIV-1 infection in combination with other antiretroviral agents. **Note:** Didanosine is no longer recommended for use in the treatment of HIV (HHS [adult] 2019).

Local Anesthetic/Vasoconstrictor Precautions No information available to require special precautions

Effects on Dental Treatment Key adverse event(s) related to dental treatment: Xerostomia (normal salivary flow resumes upon discontinuation).

Effects on Bleeding Thrombocytopenia has been reported in <1% of patients treated.

Adverse Reactions As reported in monotherapy studies; risk of toxicity may increase when combined with other agents.

>10%:

Central nervous system: Peripheral neuropathy (17% to 20%)

Endocrine & metabolic: Increased amylase (≥1.4 x ULN: 15% to 17%)

Gastrointestinal: Diarrhea (19% to 28%), abdominal pain (7% to 13%)

1% to 10%:

Dermatologic: Pruritus (≤9%), skin rash (≤9%)

Endocrine & metabolic: Increased uric acid (>12 mg/dL: 2% to 3%)

Gastrointestinal: Pancreatitis (6% to 7%)

Hepatic: Increased serum AST (>5 x ULN: 7% to 9%), increased serum ALT (>5 x ULN: 6% to 9%), increased serum alkaline phosphatase (>5 x ULN: 1% to 4%)

<1%, postmarketing, and/or case reports: Acute renal failure, alopecia, anaphylactoid reaction, anemia, anorexia, arthralgia, chills, diabetes mellitus, dyspepsia, fever, flatulence, hepatic failure, hepatitis, hyperglycemia, hypoglycemia, increased creatine phosphokinase, increased gamma-glutamyl transferase, lactic acidosis, leukopenia, lipoatrophy (buttocks, face, limbs), myalgia, myopathy, optic neuritis, pain, parotid gland enlargement, portal hypertension (noncirrhotic), retinal pigment changes (depigmentation),

rhabdomyolysis, severe hepatomegaly with steatosis, sialadenitis, symptomatic hyperlactatemia, thrombocytopenia, weakness, xerophthalmia, xerostomia

Mechanism of Action Didanosine, a purine nucleoside (adenosine) analog and the deamination product of dideoxyadenosine (ddA), inhibits HIV replication *in vitro* in both T cells and monocytes. Didanosine is converted within the cell to the mono-, di-, and triphosphates of ddA. These ddA triphosphates act as substrate and inhibitor of HIV reverse transcriptase substrate and inhibitor of HIV reverse transcriptase thereby blocking viral DNA synthesis and suppressing HIV replication.

Pharmacodynamics/Kinetics

Half-life Elimination

Plasma:

Newborns (1 day old): 2 ± 0.7 hours

Infants 2 weeks to 4 months: 1.2 ± 0.3 hours

Infants 8 months to Adolescents 19 years: 0.8 ± 0.3 hours

Adults with normal renal function: 1.5 ± 0.4 hours

Intracellular: Adults: 25 to 40 hours

Elimination: Increased as CrCl decreased

Children 20 kg to <25 kg: 0.75 ± 0.13 hours

Children 25 kg to <60 kg: 0.92 ± 0.09 hours

Children ≥60 kg: 1.26 ± 0.19 hours

Adults ≥60 kg: 1.19 ± 0.21 hours; 2 ± 0.3 hours (renal impairment [CrCl <30 mL/minute]); 4.1 ± 1.2 hours (dialysis)

Time to Peak Delayed release capsules: 2 hours; Powder for suspension: 0.25 to 1.5 hours

Reproductive Considerations

Based on the Health and Humans Services (HHS) perinatal HIV guidelines, didanosine is not one of the recommended antiretroviral agents for use in females living with HIV who are trying to conceive.

For males and females living with HIV and planning a pregnancy, maximum viral suppression below the limits of detection with antiretroviral therapy (ART), modification of therapy (if needed), optimization of the woman's health, and a discussion of the potential risks and benefits of ART therapy during pregnancy is recommended prior to conception (HHS [perinatal] 2019).

Pregnancy Considerations

[US Boxed Warning]: Fatal lactic acidosis has been reported in pregnant individuals using didanosine and stavudine in combination with other antiretroviral agents. The Health and Human Services (HHS) perinatal HIV guidelines do not recommend didanosine use in pregnant women due to toxicity, and women who are pregnant should be changed to a preferred or alternative therapy.

Didanosine crosses the human placenta.

Outcome information specific to didanosine use in pregnancy is no longer being reviewed and updated in the HHS perinatal guidelines. Maternal antiretroviral therapy (ART) may be associated with adverse pregnancy outcomes including preterm delivery, stillbirth, low birth weight, and small for gestational age infants. Actual risks may be influenced by maternal factors, such as disease severity, gestational age at initiation of therapy, and specific ART regimen, therefore close fetal monitoring is recommended. Because there is clear benefit to appropriate treatment, maternal ART should not be withheld due to concerns for adverse neonatal outcomes. Long-term follow-up is recommended for all infants exposed to antiretroviral medications; children without HIV but who were exposed to ART in utero and develop significant organ system abnormalities of unknown etiology (particularly of the CNS or heart) should be evaluated for potential mitochondrial dysfunction. Cases of lactic acidosis and hepatic steatosis have been reported in pregnant women with use of nucleoside reverse transcriptase inhibitors.

In general, ART is recommended for all pregnant females living with HIV to keep the viral load below the limit of detection and reduce the risk of perinatal transmission. Therapy should be individualized following a discussion of the potential risks and benefits of treatment during pregnancy. Monitoring of pregnant females is more frequent than in nonpregnant adults. ART should be continued postpartum for all females living with HIV and can be modified after delivery.

Health care providers are encouraged to enroll pregnant females exposed to antiretroviral medications as early in pregnancy as possible in the Antiretroviral Pregnancy Registry (1-800-258-4263 or http://www.APRegistry.com). Health care providers caring for pregnant females living with HIV and their infants may contact the National Perinatal HIV Hotline (888-448-8765) for clinical consultation (HHS [perinatal] 2019).

◆ **Dideoxyinosine** *see* Didanosine *on page 492*

◆ **Didronel** *see* Etidronate *on page 620*

Dienogest (dye EN oh jest)

Brand Names: Canada ASPEN-Dienogest; Visanne

Pharmacologic Category Antiandrogen

Use Note: Not approved in the US

Endometriosis: Management of pelvic pain associated with endometriosis

Local Anesthetic/Vasoconstrictor Precautions No information available to require special precautions

Effects on Dental Treatment No significant effects or complications reported

Effects on Bleeding No information available to require special precautions

Adverse Reactions

1% to 10%:

Central nervous system: Headache (7%), depression (3%), disturbed sleep (2%), irritability (1%), migraine (1%), nervousness (1%)

Dermatologic: Acne vulgaris (2%), alopecia (1%)

Endocrine & metabolic: Breast changes (discomfort: 5%), weight gain (4%), ovarian cyst (3%), decreased libido (2%)

Gastrointestinal: Nausea (4%), abdominal pain (2%)

Genitourinary: Vaginal hemorrhage (1%)

Neuromuscular & skeletal: Weakness (2%)

<1%, postmarketing, and/or case reports: Abdominal distress, anemia, anxiety, back pain, breast induration, constipation, decreased glucose tolerance, dermatitis, diarrhea, disturbance in attention, dysautonomia, edema, feeling of heaviness (extremities), fibrocystic breast disease, flatulence, genital discharge, GI inflammation, hot flash, increased appetite, limb pain, lump in breast, mood changes, muscle spasm, onychoclasis, ostealgia, palpitations, pelvic pain, pruritus, skin pigmentation, skin photosensitivity, tinnitus, urinary tract infection, vulvovaginal candidiasis, vomiting, vulvar dryness, xeroderma, xerophthalmia

Mechanism of Action Dienogest is a steroid with antiandrogen properties that lacks androgen, mineralocorticoid or glucocorticoid activity. Exhibits strong progestogenic effects although it binds uterine ▶

progesterone receptors with an affinity much lower (about one-tenth) than that of progesterone. Decreases estradiol production and thus suppresses estradiol's trophic effects on eutopic and ectopic endometrium. Inhibits cellular proliferation via direct antiproliferative, immunologic, and antiangiogenic effects.

Pharmacodynamics/Kinetics

Half-life Elimination ~9 to 10 hours

Time to Peak ~1.5 hours

Reproductive Considerations

Pregnancy status should be evaluated prior to use. Nonhormonal contraception should be used if contraception is needed; use of hormonal contraceptives is not recommended during dienogest therapy. Ovulation is often inhibited during therapy; however, this product is not intended for use as a contraceptive. Normal menstruation usually returns within 2 months of therapy discontinuation.

Pregnancy Considerations

Use is contraindicated during pregnancy. Based on limited data, inadvertent exposure in pregnancy has not shown adverse effects to the fetus.

Product Availability Not available in the US

◆ **Dienogest and Estradiol** *see* Estradiol and Dienogest *on page 597*

Diethylpropion (dye eth il PROE pee on)

Pharmacologic Category Anorexiant; Central Nervous System Stimulant; Sympathomimetic

Use

Obesity: Short-term (few weeks) adjunct in the management of exogenous obesity

Pharmacotherapy for weight loss is recommended only for obese patients with a body mass index ≥30 kg/m^2, or ≥27 kg/m^2 in the presence of other risk factors such as hypertension, diabetes, and/or dyslipidemia or a high waist circumference; therapy should be used in conjunction with a comprehensive weight management program.

Local Anesthetic/Vasoconstrictor Precautions

Use vasoconstrictor with caution in patients taking diethylpropion. Amphetamine-like drugs such as diethylpropion enhance the sympathomimetic response of epinephrine and norepinephrine leading to potential hypertension and cardiotoxicity.

Effects on Dental Treatment Key adverse event(s) related to dental treatment: Diethylpropion causes tachycardia, increases in blood pressure, and palpitations. Consider monitoring blood pressure prior to using local anesthetic with a vasoconstrictor. Symptoms associated with bruxism have been observed in some patients.

Effects on Bleeding No information available to require special precautions

Adverse Reactions Frequency not defined.

Cardiovascular: Cardiac arrhythmia, cerebrovascular accident, ECG changes, heart valve disease, hypertension, palpitations, tachycardia

Central nervous system: Anxiety, depression, dizziness, drowsiness, dysphoria, euphoria, headache, insomnia, jitteriness, malaise, nervousness, overstimulation, precordial pain, psychosis, restlessness, seizure

Dermatologic: Alopecia, diaphoresis, ecchymoses, erythema, skin rash, urticaria

Endocrine & metabolic: Changes in libido, gynecomastia, menstrual disease

Gastrointestinal: Abdominal distress, constipation, diarrhea, dysgeusia, nausea, vomiting, xerostomia

Genitourinary: Dysuria, impotence

Hematologic & oncologic: Agranulocytosis, bone marrow depression, leukopenia

Neuromuscular & skeletal: Dyskinesia, myalgia, tremor

Ophthalmic: Blurred vision, mydriasis

Renal: Polyuria

Respiratory: Dyspnea, pulmonary hypertension

Miscellaneous: Tachyphylaxis

Mechanism of Action Diethylpropion is a sympathomimetic amine with pharmacologic properties similar to the amphetamines. It is also structurally similar to bupropion. The mechanism of action in reducing appetite appears to be secondary to CNS effects, including stimulation of the hypothalamus to release norepinephrine

Pharmacodynamics/Kinetics

Half-life Elimination Aminoketone metabolites: ~4-6 hours

Pregnancy Risk Factor B

Pregnancy Considerations

Diethylpropion crosses the human placenta; spontaneous reports of congenital malformations have been reported, but an association with diethylpropion has not been established. Withdrawal symptoms may occur in the neonate following maternal use of diethylpropion.

Controlled Substance C-IV

◆ **Diethylpropion HCl** *see* Diethylpropion *on page 494*

◆ **Diethylpropion Hydrochloride** *see* Diethylpropion *on page 494*

◆ **Differin** *see* Adapalene *on page 85*

◆ **Dificid** *see* Fidaxomicin *on page 668*

◆ **Difimicin** *see* Fidaxomicin *on page 668*

Diflorasone (dye FLOR a sone)

Brand Names: US ApexiCon E; Psorcon

Pharmacologic Category Corticosteroid, Topical

Use Dermatoses: Treatment of inflammation and pruritic symptoms of corticosteroid-responsive dermatoses (high to very high potency topical corticosteroid)

Local Anesthetic/Vasoconstrictor Precautions

No information available to require special precautions

Effects on Dental Treatment No significant effects or complications reported

Effects on Bleeding No information available to require special precautions

Adverse Reactions Frequency not defined. Reactions listed are based on reports for other agents in this same pharmacologic class and may not be specifically reported for diflorasone. Diflorasone is classified as a potent topical steroid.

Central nervous system: Burning sensation

Dermatologic: Acneiform eruption, allergic contact dermatitis, atrophic striae, folliculitis, hypertrichosis, hypopigmentation, maceration of the skin, miliaria, perioral dermatitis, pruritus, skin atrophy, skin irritation, xeroderma

Endocrine & metabolic: HPA-axis suppression (children at greater risk)

Infection: Secondary infection

<1%, postmarketing and/or case reports: Acne rosacea (Hengge 2006), aggravation reaction (cutaneous candidiasis, herpes, dermodex) (Hengge 2006), cataract (Hengge 2006), dermal ulcer (Hengge 2006), glaucoma (Hengge 2006), hirsutism (Hengge 2006), hyperpigmentation (Hengge 2006), Kaposi's sarcoma (reactivation) (Hengge 2006), nonthrombocytopenic purpura (Hengge 2006), ocular hypertension (Hengge

2006), psoriasis flare (rebound) (Hengge 2006), purpura (Hengge 2006), skin photosensitivity (Hengge 2006), spontaneous star-shaped scar-like lesions (Hengge 2006), telangiectasia (Hengge 2006), tinea (tinea incognito) (Hengge 2006)

Mechanism of Action Topical corticosteroids have anti-inflammatory, antipruritic, and vasoconstrictive properties. May depress the formation, release, and activity of endogenous chemical mediators of inflammation (kinins, histamine, liposomal enzymes, prostaglandins) through the induction of phospholipase A_2 inhibitory proteins (lipocortins) and sequential inhibition of the release of arachidonic acid. Diflorasone has high range potency.

Pregnancy Considerations

Topical corticosteroids are not recommended for extensive use, in large quantities, or for long periods of time in pregnant women.

◆ **Diflorasone Diacetate** *see* Diflorasone *on page 494*

◆ **Diflucan** *see* Fluconazole *on page 674*

Diflunisal (dye FLOO ni sal)

Related Information

Oral Pain *on page 1734*

Rheumatoid Arthritis, Osteoarthritis, and Osteoporosis *on page 1697*

Temporomandibular Dysfunction (TMD), Chronic Pain, and Fibromyalgia *on page 1773*

Related Sample Prescriptions

Oral Pain - Sample Prescriptions *on page 30*

Brand Names: Canada NOVO-Diflunisal [DSC]

Generic Availability (US) Yes

Pharmacologic Category Analgesic, Nonopioid; Nonsteroidal Anti-inflammatory Drug (NSAID), Oral

Dental Use Treatment of postoperative pain

Use

Osteoarthritis/Rheumatoid arthritis (RA): Treatment of osteoarthritis and RA

Pain, mild to moderate: Treatment of mild to moderate pain

Local Anesthetic/Vasoconstrictor Precautions

No information available to require special precautions

Effects on Dental Treatment The dentist should be aware of the potential of abnormal coagulation. Caution should also be exercised in the use of NSAIDs in patients already on anticoagulant therapy with drugs such as warfarin (Coumadin®). See Effects on Bleeding.

Effects on Bleeding As an inhibitor of prostaglandin synthetase, diflunisal has a dose-related effect on platelet function and bleeding time. In healthy volunteers, 250 mg twice daily for 8 days had no effect on platelet function, and 500 mg twice daily (the usual recommended dose) had a slight effect. However, at 1000 mg twice daily (which exceeds the maximum recommended dosage), diflunisal inhibited platelet function. In contrast with aspirin, these effects of diflunisal were reversible because diflunisal is a salicylic acid derivative.

Adverse Reactions Frequency not always defined.

1% to 10%:

Central nervous system: Headache (3% to 9%), dizziness (1% to 3%), drowsiness (1% to 3%), fatigue (1% to 3%), insomnia (1% to 3%)

Dermatologic: Skin rash (3% to 9%)

Gastrointestinal: Diarrhea (3% to 9%), dyspepsia (3% to 9%), gastrointestinal pain (3% to 9%), nausea (3% to 9%), constipation (1% to 3%), flatulence (1% to 3%), vomiting (1% to 3%), gastrointestinal ulcer

Otic: Tinnitus (1% to 3%)

<1%, postmarketing, and/or case reports: Agranulocytosis, anaphylactic reaction (acute), angioedema, anorexia, auditory impairment, blurred vision, bronchospasm, chest pain, cholestasis, confusion, cystitis, depression, diaphoresis, disorientation, DRESS syndrome, dry mucous membranes, dyspnea, dysuria, edema, eructation, erythema multiforme, esophagitis, exfoliative dermatitis, flushing, gastritis, gastrointestinal hemorrhage, gastrointestinal perforation, hallucination, hearing loss, hematuria, hemolytic anemia, hepatitis, hepatotoxicity (idiosyncratic; Chalasani 2014), hypersensitivity angiitis, hypersensitivity reaction, interstitial nephritis, jaundice, muscle cramps, necrotizing fasciitis, nephrotic syndrome, nervousness, palpitations, paresthesia, peptic ulcer, peripheral neuropathy, proteinuria, pruritus, renal failure, renal insufficiency, seizure, skin photosensitivity, Stevens-Johnson syndrome, stomatitis, syncope, tachycardia, thrombocytopenia, toxic epidermal necrolysis, tremor, urticaria, vasculitis, vertigo, weakness, wheezing

Dental Usual Dosage Mild-to-moderate pain: Adults: Oral: Initial: 500-1000 mg followed by 250-500 mg every 8-12 hours; maximum daily dose: 1.5 g

Dosing

Adult

Osteoarthritis/Rheumatoid arthritis: Oral: 500 mg to 1,000 mg daily in 2 divided doses; maximum dose: 1,500 mg/day

Pain, mild to moderate: Oral: Initial: 1,000 mg, followed by 500 mg every 12 hours; maintenance doses of 500 mg every 8 hours may be necessary in some patients; maximum dose: 1,500 mg/day

Dosage adjustments: A lower dosage may be appropriate depending on pain severity, patient response, or weight; Initial: 500 mg, followed by 250 mg every 8 to 12 hours; maximum dose: 1,500 mg/day

Geriatric

Osteoarthritis/Rheumatoid arthritis: Refer to adult dosing.

Pain, mild to moderate: Oral: Initial: 500 mg, followed by 250 mg every 8 to 12 hours; maximum dose: 1,500 mg/day

Renal Impairment: Adult There are no dosage adjustments provided in the manufacturer's labeling; avoid use in patients with advanced renal disease.

The following adjustments have been used by some clinicians (Aronoff, 2007):

CrCl ≤50 mL/minute: Administer 50% of normal dose.

Hemodialysis: No supplement required.

CAPD: No supplement required.

KDIGO 2012 guidelines provide the following recommendations for NSAIDs:

eGFR 30 to <60 mL/minute/1.73 m^2: Temporarily discontinue in patients with intercurrent disease that increases risk of acute kidney injury.

eGFR <30 mL/minute/1.73 m^2: Avoid use.

Hepatic Impairment: Adult There are no dosage adjustments provided in the manufacturer's labeling; use with caution.

Pediatric

Osteoarthritis/Rheumatoid arthritis: Adolescents ≥12 years: Oral: Refer to adult dosing.

Pain, mild to moderate: Adolescents ≥12 years: Oral: Refer to adult dosing.

Renal Impairment: Pediatric

There are no dosage adjustments provided in the manufacturer's labeling; avoid use in advanced disease.

KDIGO 2012 guidelines provide the following recommendations for NSAIDs: Children ≥12 years and Adolescents:

eGFR 30 to <60 mL/minute/1.73 m^2: Avoid use in patients with intercurrent disease that increases risk of acute kidney injury

eGFR <30 mL/minute/1.73 m^2: Avoid use.

Hepatic Impairment: Pediatric There are no dosage adjustments provided in the manufacturer's labeling; use with caution.

Mechanism of Action Reversibly inhibits cyclooxygenase-1 and 2 (COX-1 and 2) enzymes, which results in decreased formation of prostaglandin precursors; has antipyretic, analgesic, and anti-inflammatory properties.

Other proposed mechanisms not fully elucidated (and possibly contributing to the anti-inflammatory effect to varying degrees) include inhibiting chemotaxis, altering lymphocyte activity, inhibiting neutrophil aggregation/activation, and decreasing proinflammatory cytokine levels.

Contraindications Known hypersensitivity to diflunisal or any component of the formulation; in the setting of coronary artery bypass graft (CABG) surgery; history of asthma, urticaria, or allergic-type reactions after taking aspirin or other NSAIDs.

Warnings/Precautions [US Boxed Warning]: Nonsteroidal anti-inflammatory drugs (NSAIDs) cause an increased risk of serious (and potentially fatal) adverse cardiovascular thrombotic events, including MI and stroke. Risk may occur early during treatment and may increase with duration of use. Relative risk appears to be similar in those with and without known cardiovascular disease or risk factors for cardiovascular disease; however, absolute incidence of serious cardiovascular thrombotic events (which may occur early during treatment) was higher in patients with known cardiovascular disease or risk factors and in those receiving higher doses. New onset hypertension or exacerbation of hypertension may occur (NSAIDs may also impair response to ACE inhibitors, thiazide diuretics, or loop diuretics); may contribute to cardiovascular events; monitor blood pressure; use with caution in patients with hypertension. May cause sodium and fluid retention; use with caution in patients with edema. Avoid use in heart failure (ACCF/AHA [Yancy 2013]). Avoid use in patients with recent MI unless benefits outweigh risk of cardiovascular thrombotic events. Use the lowest effective dose for the shortest duration of time, consistent with individual patient goals, to reduce risk of cardiovascular events; alternate therapies should be considered for patients at high risk.

[US Boxed Warning]: Use is contraindicated in the setting of coronary artery bypass graft (CABG) surgery. Risk of MI and stroke may be increased with use following CABG surgery.

Clinical or population-based data regarding the risks of NSAIDs in the setting of coronavirus disease 2019 (COVID 19) are limited (FDA Safety Communication 2020; Kim 2020). Some experts recommend the use of acetaminophen as the preferred antipyretic agent, when possible, and if NSAIDs are needed, to use the lowest effective dose and shortest duration (EMA 2020; Kim 2020). In general, for patients already taking an NSAID for a comorbid condition, it is recommended to continue the NSAID as directed by their health care provider (EMA 2020; NIH 2020; WHO 2020).

[US Boxed Warning]: NSAIDs cause an increased risk of serious GI inflammation, ulceration, bleeding, and perforation (may be fatal); elderly patients and patients with history of peptic ulcer disease and/or GI bleeding are at greater risk of serious GI events. These events may occur at any time during therapy and without warning. Avoid use in patients with active GI bleeding. In patients with a history of acute lower GI bleeding, avoid use of non-aspirin NSAIDs, especially if due to angioectasia or diverticulosis (Strate 2016). Use caution with a history of GI ulcers, concurrent therapy known to increase the risk of GI bleeding (eg, aspirin, anticoagulants and/or corticosteroids, selective serotonin reuptake inhibitors), advanced hepatic disease, coagulopathy, smoking, use of alcohol, or in elderly or debilitated patients. Use the lowest effective dose for the shortest duration of time, consistent with individual patient goals, to reduce risk of GI adverse events; alternate therapies should be considered for patients at high risk. When used concomitantly with aspirin, a substantial increase in the risk of GI complications (eg, ulcer) occurs; concomitant gastroprotective therapy (eg, proton pump inhibitors) is recommended (Bhatt 2008). Avoid chronic use of oral nonselective NSAIDs in patients who have undergone bariatric surgery; development of anastomotic ulcerations/perforations may occur.

Platelet adhesion and aggregation may be decreased; may prolong bleeding time; patients with coagulation disorders or who are receiving anticoagulants should be monitored closely. Anemia may occur; patients on long-term NSAID therapy should be monitored for anemia. Rarely, NSAID use has been associated with potentially severe blood dyscrasias (eg, agranulocytosis, thrombocytopenia, aplastic anemia).

NSAID use may compromise existing renal function; dose-dependent decreases in prostaglandin synthesis may result from NSAID use, reducing renal blood flow which may cause renal decompensation (usually reversible). Patients with impaired renal function, dehydration, hypovolemia, heart failure, hepatic impairment, those taking diuretics and ACE inhibitors, and elderly patients are at greater risk of renal toxicity. Rehydrate patient before starting therapy; monitor renal function closely. Long-term NSAID use may result in renal papillary necrosis and other renal injury. Avoid use in patients with advanced renal disease unless benefits are expected to outweigh risk of worsening renal function; monitor renal function closely if therapy must be initiated. NSAID use may increase the risk of hyperkalemia, particularly in the elderly, diabetics, renal disease, and with concomitant use of other agents capable of inducing hyperkalemia (eg, ACE-inhibitors). Monitor potassium closely.

Use with caution in patients with hepatic impairment; patients with advanced hepatic disease are at an increased risk of GI bleeding with NSAIDs. Transaminase elevations have been reported with use; closely monitor patients with any abnormal LFT. Rare, sometimes fatal severe hepatic reactions (eg, fulminant hepatitis, hepatic necrosis, hepatic failure) have occurred with NSAID use; discontinue immediately if clinical signs or symptoms of hepatic disease develop or if systemic manifestations occur.

Contraindicated in patients with aspirin-sensitive asthma; severe, potentially fatal bronchospasm may occur. Use caution in patients with other forms of asthma. May cause drowsiness, dizziness, blurred vision, and other neurologic effects which may impair physical or mental abilities; patients must be cautioned about performing tasks which require mental alertness (eg, operating machinery or driving). Blurred vision has been reported; refer for ophthalmologic evaluation if symptoms occur.

NSAIDs may cause potentially fatal, serious skin adverse events including exfoliative dermatitis, Stevens-Johnson syndrome (SJS), and toxic epidermal necrolysis (TEN); may occur without warning; discontinue use at first sign of skin rash (or any other hypersensitivity). A potentially life-threatening, hypersensitivity syndrome has been reported; monitor for constitutional symptoms and cutaneous findings; other organ dysfunction may be involved. Even in patients without prior exposure anaphylactoid reactions may occur; patients with "aspirin triad" (bronchial asthma, aspirin intolerance, rhinitis) may be at increased risk. Contraindicated in patients who experience bronchospasm, asthma, rhinitis, or urticaria with NSAID or aspirin therapy.

Diflunisal is a derivative of acetylsalicylic acid and therefore may be associated with Reye's syndrome. Elderly patients are at greater risk for serious GI, cardiovascular, and/or renal adverse events; use with caution. Withhold for at least 4 to 6 half-lives prior to surgical or dental procedures. Potentially significant interactions may exist, requiring dose or frequency adjustment, additional monitoring, and/or selection of alternative therapy.

Drug Interactions

Metabolism/Transport Effects None known.

Avoid Concomitant Use

Avoid concomitant use of Diflunisal with any of the following: Acemetacin; Aminolevulinic Acid (Systemic); Dexibuprofen; Dexketoprofen; Floctafenine; Ketorolac (Nasal); Ketorolac (Systemic); Macimorelin; Mifamurtide; Morniflumate; Nonsteroidal Anti-Inflammatory Agents (COX-2 Selective); Omacetaxine; Pelubiprofen; Phenylbutazone; Talniflumate; Tenoxicam; Urokinase; Zaltoprofen

Increased Effect/Toxicity

Diflunisal may increase the levels/effects of: 5-Aminosalicylic Acid Derivatives; Agents with Antiplatelet Properties; Aliskiren; Aminoglycosides; Aminolevulinic Acid (Systemic); Aminolevulinic Acid (Topical); Anticoagulants; Apixaban; Bemiparin; Bisphosphonate Derivatives; Cephalothin; Collagenase (Systemic); CycloSPORINE (Systemic); Dabigatran Etexilate; Deferasirox; Deoxycholic Acid; Desmopressin; Dexibuprofen; Digoxin; Drospirenone; Edoxaban; Enoxaparin; Eplerenone; Haloperidol; Heparin; Ibritumomab Tiuxetan; Lithium; MetFORMIN; Methotrexate; Nonsteroidal Anti-Inflammatory Agents (COX-2 Selective); Obinutuzumab; Omacetaxine; Porfimer; Potassium-Sparing Diuretics; PRALAtrexate; Quinolones; Rivaroxaban; Salicylates; Tacrolimus (Systemic); Tenofovir Products; Thrombolytic Agents; Tolperisone; Urokinase; Vancomycin; Verteporfin; Vitamin K Antagonists

The levels/effects of Diflunisal may be increased by: Acalabrutinib; Acemetacin; Alcohol (Ethyl); Angiotensin II Receptor Blockers; Angiotensin-Converting Enzyme Inhibitors; Corticosteroids (Systemic); CycloSPORINE (Systemic); Dasatinib; Dexketoprofen; Diclofenac (Systemic); Fat Emulsion (Fish Oil Based); Felbinac; Floctafenine; Glucosamine; Herbs (Anticoagulant/Antiplatelet Properties); Ibrutinib; Inotersen; Ketorolac (Nasal); Ketorolac (Systemic); Limaprost; Loop Diuretics; Morniflumate; Multivitamins/Fluoride (with ADE); Multivitamins/Minerals (with ADEK, Folate, Iron); Multivitamins/Minerals (with AE, No Iron); Naftazone; Omega-3 Fatty Acids; Pelubiprofen; Pentosan Polysulfate Sodium; Pentoxifylline; Phenylbutazone; Probenecid; Prostacyclin Analogues; Selective Serotonin Reuptake Inhibitors; Selumetinib; Serotonin/Norepinephrine Reuptake Inhibitors; Sodium Phosphates; Talniflumate; Tenoxicam; Thiazide and Thiazide-Like Diuretics; Tipranavir; Tolperisone; Tricyclic Antidepressants (Tertiary Amine); Vitamin E (Systemic); Zaltoprofen; Zanubrutinib

Decreased Effect

Diflunisal may decrease the levels/effects of: Aliskiren; Angiotensin II Receptor Blockers; Angiotensin-Converting Enzyme Inhibitors; Beta-Blockers; Eplerenone; HydrALAZINE; Loop Diuretics; Macimorelin; Mifamurtide; Potassium-Sparing Diuretics; Prostaglandins (Ophthalmic); Salicylates; Selective Serotonin Reuptake Inhibitors; Sincalide; Thiazide and Thiazide-Like Diuretics

The levels/effects of Diflunisal may be decreased by: Bile Acid Sequestrants; Salicylates

Dietary Considerations May administer with food or milk to decrease GI upset.

Pharmacodynamics/Kinetics

Onset of Action Analgesic: ~1 hour; maximal effect: 2 to 3 hours

Duration of Action 8 to 12 hours

Half-life Elimination 8 to 12 hours; prolonged with renal impairment (Brogden 1980)

Time to Peak Serum: 2 to 3 hours

Reproductive Considerations

The chronic use of NSAIDs in women of reproductive age may be associated with infertility that is reversible upon discontinuation of the medication (Micu 2011).

Pregnancy Risk Factor C

Pregnancy Considerations Birth defects have been observed following in utero NSAID exposure in some studies; however, data is conflicting (Bloor 2013). Nonteratogenic effects, including prenatal constriction of the ductus arteriosus, persistent pulmonary hypertension of the newborn, oligohydramnios, necrotizing enterocolitis, renal dysfunction or failure, and intracranial hemorrhage have been observed in the fetus/neonate following in utero NSAID exposure. In addition, nonclosure of the ductus arteriosus postnatally may occur and be resistant to medical management (Bermas 2014; Bloor 2013). Because they may cause premature closure of the ductus arteriosus, the use of NSAIDs late in pregnancy should be avoided. Use of NSAIDs can be considered for the treatment of mild rheumatoid arthritis flares in pregnant women; however, use should be minimized or avoided early and late in pregnancy (Bermas 2014; Saavedra Salinas 2015).

The use of NSAIDs close to conception may be associated with an increased risk of miscarriage (Bloor 2013; Bermas 2014).

Breastfeeding Considerations Diflunisal is present in breast milk at concentrations of 2% to 7% of those in maternal plasma. In general, NSAIDs may be used in postpartum women who wish to breastfeed; however, agents other than diflunisal are preferred (Montgomery 2012) and use should be avoided in women breastfeeding infants with platelet dysfunction or thrombocytopenia (Bloor 2013; Sammaritano 2014). According to the manufacturer, the decision to breastfeed during therapy should take into account the risk of exposure to the infant and the benefits of treatment to the mother.

Dosage Forms: US

Tablet, Oral:

Generic: 500 mg

Dosage Forms: Canada

Tablet, Oral:

Generic: 250 mg, 500 mg

Dental Health Professional Considerations The advantage of diflunisal as a pain reliever is its 12-hour duration of effect. In many cases, this long effect will ensure a full night sleep during the postoperative pain period.

◆ **Difluorodeoxycytidine Hydrochlorothiazide** *see* Gemcitabine *on page 731*

◆ **Digitalis** *see* Digoxin *on page 498*

◆ **Digitek** *see* Digoxin *on page 498*

◆ **Digox** *see* Digoxin *on page 498*

Digoxin (di JOKS in)

Related Information

Cardiovascular Diseases *on page 1654*

Brand Names: US Digitek; Digox; Lanoxin; Lanoxin Pediatric

Brand Names: Canada APO-Digoxin; Lanoxin; PMS-Digoxin [DSC]; Toloxin

Pharmacologic Category Antiarrhythmic Agent, Miscellaneous; Cardiac Glycoside

Use

Atrial fibrillation or atrial flutter, rate control: Control of ventricular response rate in adults with chronic atrial fibrillation.

Heart failure with reduced ejection fraction (HFrEF): Treatment of mild to moderate (or stage C as recommended by the ACCF/AHA) heart failure in adults; to increase myocardial contractility in pediatric patients with heart failure

Local Anesthetic/Vasoconstrictor Precautions Use vasoconstrictor with caution due to risk of cardiac arrhythmias with digoxin

Effects on Dental Treatment Sensitive gag reflex may cause difficulty in taking a dental impression.

Effects on Bleeding No information available to require special precautions

Adverse Reactions Incidence not always reported.

Cardiovascular: Accelerated junctional rhythm, asystole, atrial tachycardia with or without block, AV dissociation, first-, second- (Wenckebach), or third-degree heart block, facial edema, PR prolongation, PVCs (especially bigeminy or trigeminy), ST segment depression, ventricular tachycardia or ventricular fibrillation

Central nervous system: Dizziness (6%), mental disturbances (5%), headache (4%), apathy, anxiety, confusion, delirium, depression, fever, hallucinations

Dermatologic: Rash (erythematous, maculopapular [most common], papular, scarlatiniform, vesicular or bullous), pruritus, urticaria, angioneurotic edema

Gastrointestinal: Nausea (4%), vomiting (2%), diarrhea (4%), abdominal pain, anorexia

Neuromuscular & skeletal: Weakness

Ophthalmic: Visual disturbances (blurred or yellow vision)

Respiratory: Laryngeal edema

<1%, postmarketing, and/or case reports (limited to important or life-threatening): Asymmetric chorea, gynecomastia, thrombocytopenia, palpitation, intestinal ischemia, hemorrhagic necrosis of the intestines, vaginal cornification, eosinophilia, sexual dysfunction, diaphoresis

Mechanism of Action

Heart failure: Inhibition of the sodium/potassium ATPase pump in myocardial cells results in a transient increase of intracellular sodium, which in turn promotes calcium influx via the sodium-calcium exchange pump leading to increased contractility. May improve baroreflex sensitivity (Gheorghiade 1991).

Supraventricular arrhythmias: Direct suppression of the AV node conduction to increase effective refractory period and decrease conduction velocity - positive inotropic effect, enhanced vagal tone, and decreased ventricular rate to fast atrial arrhythmias. Atrial fibrillation may decrease sensitivity and increase tolerance to higher serum digoxin concentrations.

Pharmacodynamics/Kinetics

Onset of Action

Heart rate control: Oral: 1 to 2 hours; IV: 5 to 60 minutes

Peak effect: Heart rate control: Oral: 2 to 8 hours; IV: 1 to 6 hours; **Note:** In patients with atrial fibrillation, median time to ventricular rate control in one study was 6 hours (range: 3 to 15 hours) (Siu 2009)

Duration of Action Adults: 3 to 4 days

Half-life Elimination

Age, renal and cardiac function dependent:

Neonates: Premature: 61 to 170 hours; Full-term: 35 to 45 hours

Infants: 18 to 25 hours

Children: 18 to 36 hours

Adults: 36 to 48 hours

Adults, anephric: 3.5 to 5 days

Parent drug: 38 hours; Metabolites: Digoxigenin: 4 hours; Monodigitoxoside: 3 to 12 hours

Time to Peak Serum: Oral: 1 to 3 hours

Pregnancy Considerations Digoxin crosses the placenta.

Available guidelines note experience with digoxin in pregnancy is extensive (ESG [Regitz-Zagrosek 2018]). Based on available data, an increased risk of adverse pregnancy outcomes has not been observed. However, untreated maternal heart failure and atrial fibrillation may increase the risk of preterm birth and low birth weight, respectively. The manufacturer recommends monitoring neonates for signs and symptoms of digoxin toxicity following in utero exposure.

Due to pregnancy-induced physiologic changes, some pharmacokinetic properties of digoxin may be altered. Close monitoring of maternal serum digoxin is recommended (Hebert 2008; Luxford 1983; Martin-Suarez 2017); dose adjustments may be required during pregnancy and postpartum.

Heart failure and atrial fibrillation may worsen during pregnancy. Digoxin is recommended as a first-line agent for the chronic treatment of highly symptomatic supraventricular tachycardia (SVT) in pregnancy; the lowest effective dose is recommended (ACC/AHA/HRS [Page 2015]). Digoxin may be considered for long-term rate control of maternal atrial tachycardia or atrial fibrillation when preferred agents fail (ESG [Regitz-Zagrosek 2018]). Monitor for an increased risk of maternal arrhythmias during labor and delivery.

Digoxin may be considered for the in utero management of fetal SVT or atrial flutter with hydrops or ventricular dysfunction. Digoxin may also be considered for SVT without hydrops or ventricular dysfunction if heart rate is ≥200 bpm, atrial flutter, or other rare tachycardias with an average heart rate of ≥200 bpm (AHA [Donofrio 2014]).

- **Dihematoporphyrin Ether** *see* Porfimer *on page 1247*
- **Dihydroartemisinin Hemisuccinate Sodium** *see* Artesunate *on page 169*

Dihydroergotamine (dye hye droe er GOT a meen)

Brand Names: US D.H.E. 45; Migranal

Brand Names: Canada DHE; Migranal

Pharmacologic Category Antimigraine Agent; Ergot Derivative

Use

Cluster headaches (injection): Acute treatment of cluster headaches.

Migraines (intranasal; injection): Acute treatment of migraine headaches with or without aura; not intended for the prophylactic therapy of migraine or for the management of hemiplegic or basilar migraine.

Local Anesthetic/Vasoconstrictor Precautions Use vasoconstrictor with caution in patients taking dihydroergotamine; this ergot alkaloid derivative directly stimulates vascular smooth muscle resulting in vasoconstriction of peripheral vasculature

Effects on Dental Treatment Key adverse event(s) related to dental treatment: Rhinitis and abnormal taste.

Effects on Bleeding No information available to require special precautions

Adverse Reactions

>10%: Nasal spray: Respiratory: Rhinitis (26%)

1% to 10%: Nasal spray:

Central nervous system: Taste disorder (8%), dizziness (4%), drowsiness (3%)

Endocrine & metabolic: Hot flash (1%)

Gastrointestinal: Nausea (10%), vomiting (4%), diarrhea (2%)

Local: Application site reaction (6%)

Neuromuscular & skeletal: Stiffness (1%), weakness (1%)

Respiratory: Pharyngitis (3%)

<1%, postmarketing, and/or case reports (Limited to important or life-threatening): Injection and nasal spray: Abdominal pain, anxiety, cerebral hemorrhage, cerebrovascular accident, coronary artery vasospasm, diaphoresis, diarrhea, dizziness, dyspnea, edema, fibrothorax (prolonged use), flushing, headache, hyperkinesia, hypertension, ischemic heart disease, muscle cramps, myalgia, myasthenia, myocardial infarction, palpitations, paresthesia, peripheral cyanosis, peripheral ischemia, retroperitoneal fibrosis (prolonged use), skin rash, subarachnoid hemorrhage, tremor, valvular sclerosis (associated with ergot alkaloids), ventricular fibrillation, ventricular tachycardia (transient)

Mechanism of Action Efficacy in migraine is attributed to the activation of 5-HT_{1D} receptors located on intracranial blood vessels resulting in vasoconstriction and/or activation of 5-HT_{1D} receptors on sensory nerve endings of the trigeminal system resulting in the inhibition of pro-inflammatory neuropeptide release. Dihydroergotamine binds with high affinity to serotonin 5-$HT_{1D\alpha}$, 5-$HT_{1D\beta}$, 5-HT_{1A}, 5-HT_{2A}, and 5-HT_{2C} receptors, noradrenaline α_{2A}, α_{2B} and α_1 receptors, and dopamine D_{2L} and D_3 receptors. Dihydroergotamine also possesses oxytocic properties.

Pharmacodynamics/Kinetics

Half-life Elimination ~9 to 10 hours

Time to Peak Serum: IM: 24 minutes; IV: 1 to 2 minutes; Intranasal: 30 to 60 minutes (Saper 2006); SubQ 15 to 45 minutes (Schran 1985)

Pregnancy Risk Factor X

Pregnancy Considerations Dihydroergotamine is oxytocic and should not be used during pregnancy.

- **Dihydroergotamine Mesylate** *see* Dihydroergotamine *on page 499*
- **Dihydroergotoxine** *see* Ergoloid Mesylates *on page 582*
- **Dihydrogenated Ergot Alkaloids** *see* Ergoloid Mesylates *on page 582*
- **Dihydrohydroxycodeinone** *see* OxyCODONE *on page 1157*
- **Dihydromorphinone** *see* HYDROmorphone *on page 776*
- **Dihydroqinghaosu Hemisuccinate Sodium** *see* Artesunate *on page 169*
- **Dihydroxyanthracenedione** *see* MitoXANTRONE *on page 1042*
- **Dihydroxyanthracenedione Dihydrochloride** *see* MitoXANTRONE *on page 1042*
- **1,25 Dihydroxycholecalciferol** *see* Calcitriol (Systemic) *on page 279*
- **1,25 Dihydroxycholecalciferol** *see* Calcitriol (Topical) *on page 280*
- **Dihydroxydeoxynorvinkaleukoblastine** *see* Vinorelbine *on page 1547*
- **Dilantin** *see* Phenytoin *on page 1228*
- **Dilantin Infatabs** *see* Phenytoin *on page 1228*
- **Dilatrate-SR** *see* Isosorbide Dinitrate *on page 845*
- **Dilaudid** *see* HYDROmorphone *on page 776*
- **Dilaudid-HP [DSC]** *see* HYDROmorphone *on page 776*

DilTIAZem (dil TYE a zem)

Related Information

Calcium Channel Blockers and Gingival Hyperplasia *on page 1816*

Cardiovascular Diseases *on page 1654*

Brand Names: US Cardizem; Cardizem CD; Cardizem LA; Cartia XT; Dilt-XR; dilTIAZem CD [DSC]; Matzim LA; Taztia XT; Tiadylt ER; Tiazac

Brand Names: Canada AA-Diltiaz; ACT Diltiazem CD; ACT Diltiazem T; APO-Diltiaz CD; APO-Diltiaz SR [DSC]; APO-Diltiaz TZ; Cardizem CD; Diltiazem CD; Diltiazem TZ; Diltiazem-CD; MAR-Diltiazem CD; MAR-Diltiazem T; NU-Diltiaz-SR [DSC]; Pharma-Diltiaz; PMS-Diltiazem CD; SANDOZ Diltiazem CD; SANDOZ Diltiazem T; TEVA-Diltazem; TEVA-Diltiazem CD; TEVA-Diltiazem HCl ER; Tiazac; Tiazac XC

Pharmacologic Category Antianginal Agent; Antiarrhythmic Agent, Class IV; Antihypertensive; Calcium Channel Blocker; Calcium Channel Blocker, Nondihydropyridine

Use

Oral: Hypertension, chronic stable angina, vasospastic angina

Injection: Atrial fibrillation or atrial flutter for acute ventricular rate control, conversion of supraventricular tachycardia

Local Anesthetic/Vasoconstrictor Precautions No information available to require special precautions

Effects on Dental Treatment Key adverse event(s) related to dental treatment: Gingival hyperplasia (after consultation with physician, usually disappears with discontinuation), xerostomia (normal salivary flow resumes upon discontinuation), distortion of sense of taste (dysgeusia), and headache may occur.

Effects on Bleeding No information available to require special precautions

Adverse Reactions Incidences represent ranges for various dosage forms. Patients with impaired ventricular function and/or conduction abnormalities may have higher incidence of adverse reactions.

>10%: Cardiovascular: Peripheral edema (5% to 15%; dose-related)

1% to 10%:

Cardiovascular: Bradycardia (3% to 4%), bundle branch block (<2%), cardiac arrhythmia (1%), cardiac failure (<2%), complete atrioventricular block (<2%), ECG abnormality (<2%), edema (2% to 3%), extrasystoles (2%), first-degree atrioventricular block (3% to 4%), hypotension (3% to 4%), lower extremity edema (5% to 8%), palpitations (1% to 2%), second degree atrioventricular block (<2%), syncope (<2%), vasodilation (2% to 3%)

Dermatologic: Pruritus (<2%), skin photosensitivity (<2%) (Ramirez 2007), skin rash (1% to 2% [placebo: 0%]) (Tuchinda 2014)

Endocrine & metabolic: Albuminuria (<2%), gout (1% to 2%), gynecomastia (<2%), hyperglycemia (<2%), hyperuricemia (<2%), increased lactate dehydrogenase (<2%), increased thirst (<2%), weight gain (<2%)

Gastrointestinal: Abdominal swelling (2%), anorexia (<2%), constipation (<2%), diarrhea (1% to 2%), dysgeusia (<2%), dyspepsia (1% to 6%), nausea (2%), vomiting (<2%), xerostomia (<2%)

Genitourinary: Crystalluria (<2%), impotence (2%), nocturia (<2%), sexual difficulty (<2%)

Hematologic & oncologic: Petechia (<2%)

Hepatic: Increased serum alanine aminotransferase (<2%), increased serum alkaline phosphatase (<2%), increased serum aspartate transaminase (<2%)

Hypersensitivity: Hypersensitivity reaction (<2%)

Infection: Infection (1% to 6%)

Local: Burning sensation at injection site (≤4%), itching at injection site (≤4%)

Nervous system: Abnormal dreams (<2%), abnormal gait (<2%), amnesia (<2%), depression (<2%), dizziness (2% to 10%), drowsiness (<2%), fatigue (5%), hallucination (<2%), headache (2% to 8%), insomnia (<2%), nervousness (2%), pain (6%), paresthesia (<2%), personality changes (<2%)

Neuromuscular & skeletal: Asthenia (1% to 4%), increased creatine phosphokinase in blood specimen (<2%), muscle cramps (<2%), myalgia (2%), neck stiffness (<2%), osteoarthritis (<2%), tremor (<2%)

Ophthalmic: Amblyopia (<2%), conjunctivitis (2%), eye irritation (<2%)

Otic: Tinnitus (<2%)

Renal: Polyuria (<2%)

Respiratory: Bronchitis (1% to 4%), cough (1% to 2%), dyspnea (1% to 6%), epistaxis (<2%), flu-like symptoms (2%), paranasal sinus congestion (1% to 2%), pharyngitis (6%), rhinitis (<2%)

<1%:

Cardiovascular: Atrial flutter, sinus node dysfunction, ventricular fibrillation, ventricular tachycardia

Dermatologic: Urticaria

Frequency not defined: Hepatic: Hepatic injury (Deng 2013; Shallcross 1987), increased serum bilirubin

Postmarketing:

Cardiovascular: Asystole (Moser 1996; Subahi 2018), hypersensitivity angiitis, vasculitis (Sheehan-Dare 1988)

Dermatologic: Acute generalized exanthematous pustulosis (Gesierich 2006; Knowles 1998; Saenz de Santa Maria Garcia 2016; Vicente-Calleja 1997), alopecia, cutaneous lupus erythematosus (Crowson 1995; Srivastava 2003), erythema multiforme (Stern 1989; Wittal 1992), exfoliative dermatitis (Odeh 1997; Sousa-Basto 1993), Stevens-Johnson syndrome (Sanders 1993; Taylor 1990), toxic epidermal necrolysis

Gastrointestinal: Gingival hyperplasia (Bowman 1988; Steele 1994)

Hematologic & oncologic: Hemolytic anemia, leukopenia, prolonged bleeding time, purpuric disease (Inui 2001), thrombocytopenia (Michalets 1997)

Hypersensitivity: Angioedema

Nervous system: Extrapyramidal reaction

Neuromuscular & skeletal: Myopathy (Ahmad 1993)

Ophthalmic: Periorbital edema (Friedland 1993), retinopathy

Mechanism of Action Inhibits calcium ion from entering the "slow channels" or select voltage-sensitive areas of vascular smooth muscle and myocardium during depolarization; produces relaxation of coronary vascular smooth muscle and coronary vasodilation; increases myocardial oxygen delivery in patients with vasospastic angina.

Pharmacodynamics/Kinetics

Onset of Action Oral: Immediate release tablet: 30 to 60 minutes; IV: Bolus: 3 minutes

Duration of Action IV: Bolus: 1 to 3 hours; Continuous infusion (after discontinuation): 0.5 to 10 hours

Half-life Elimination Immediate release tablet: 3 to 4.5 hours; Extended release tablet: 6 to 9 hours; Extended release capsules: 4 to 9.5 hours; IV: single dose: ~3.4 hours; continuous infusion: 4 to 5 hours

Time to Peak Serum: Immediate release tablet: 2 to 4 hours; Extended release tablet: 11 to 18 hours; Extended release capsule: 10 to 14 hours

Pregnancy Risk Factor C

Pregnancy Considerations

Adverse events have been observed in animal reproduction studies.

Chronic maternal hypertension may increase the risk of birth defects, low birth weight, preterm delivery, stillbirth, and neonatal death. Actual fetal/neonatal risks may be related to duration and severity of maternal hypertension. Untreated hypertension may also increase the risks of adverse maternal outcomes, including gestational diabetes, myocardial infarction, preeclampsia, stroke, and delivery complications (ACOG 203 2019).

Calcium channel blockers may be used to treat hypertension in pregnant women; however, agents other than diltiazem are more commonly used (ACOG 203 2019; ESC [Regitz-Zagrosek 2018]). Females with preexisting hypertension may continue their medication during pregnancy unless contraindications exist (ESC [Regitz-Zagrosek 2018]).

◆ **dilTIAZem CD [DSC]** *see* DilTIAZem *on page 499*

◆ **Diltiazem Hcl/D5w** *see* DilTIAZem *on page 499*

◆ **Diltiazem HCl in 0.9% NaCl** *see* DilTIAZem *on page 499*

◆ **Diltiazem Hydrochloride** *see* DilTIAZem *on page 499*

◆ **Dilt-XR** *see* DilTIAZem *on page 499*

DimenhyDRINATE (dye men HYE dri nate)

Brand Names: US Dramamine [OTC]; Driminate [OTC]; GoodSense Motion Sickness [OTC]; Motion Sickness [OTC] [DSC]

Brand Names: Canada Gravol

Pharmacologic Category Ethanolamine Derivative; Histamine H_1 Antagonist; Histamine H_1 Antagonist, First Generation

Use

US labeling: **Motion sickness:** Treatment and prevention of nausea, vertigo, and vomiting associated with motion sickness.

Canadian labeling: **Nausea, vomiting and/or vertigo:** Treatment and prevention of nausea, vomiting and/or vertigo associated with motion sickness, radiation sickness, postoperative recovery, use of other drugs, Mènière disease and other labyrinthine disturbances.

Local Anesthetic/Vasoconstrictor Precautions No information available to require special precautions

Effects on Dental Treatment Key adverse event(s) related to dental treatment: Significant xerostomia (normal salivary flow resumes upon discontinuation).

Effects on Bleeding No information available to require special precautions

Adverse Reactions Frequency not defined.

Cardiovascular: Tachycardia

Central nervous system: Dizziness, drowsiness, excitement, headache, insomnia, lassitude, nervousness, restlessness

Dermatologic: Skin rash

Gastrointestinal: Anorexia, epigastric distress, nausea, xerostomia

Genitourinary: Dysuria

Ophthalmic: Blurred vision

Respiratory: Thickening of bronchial secretions

Mechanism of Action Competes with histamine for H_1-receptor sites on effector cells in the gastrointestinal tract, blood vessels, and respiratory tract; blocks chemoreceptor trigger zone, diminishes vestibular stimulation, and depresses labyrinthine function through its central anticholinergic activity

Pharmacodynamics/Kinetics

Onset of Action Antiemetic: IV: immediate; IM: 20 to 30 minutes; Oral: 15 to 30 minutes (Gravol Canadian labeling 2016)

Duration of Action 4 to 6 hours (Gravol Canadian labeling 2016)

Half-life Elimination 5 to 8 hours (Gravol Canadian labeling 2016)

Pregnancy Risk Factor B

Pregnancy Considerations

Dimenhydrinate crosses the placenta. The risk of fetal abnormalities was not increased following maternal use of dimenhydrinate during any trimester of pregnancy.

Dimenhydrinate may be used for the adjunctive treatment of nausea and vomiting of pregnancy (ACOG 189 2018; Campbell [SOGC] 2016). Dimenhydrinate may have an oxytocic effect if used during labor.

Dimethyl Fumarate (dye meth il FYOO ma rate)

Brand Names: US Tecfidera

Brand Names: Canada Tecfidera

Pharmacologic Category Fumaric Acid Derivative

Use Multiple sclerosis, relapsing: Treatment of patients with relapsing forms of multiple sclerosis, including clinically isolated syndrome, relapsing-remitting disease, and active secondary progressive disease.

Local Anesthetic/Vasoconstrictor Precautions No information available to require special precautions

Effects on Dental Treatment No significant effects or complications reported

Effects on Bleeding No information available to require special precautions

Adverse Reactions

>10%:

Cardiovascular: Flushing (40%)

Gastrointestinal: Abdominal pain (18%), diarrhea (14%), nausea (12%)

Infection: Infection (60%; similar to placebo)

1% to 10%:

Dermatologic: Pruritus (8%), skin rash (8%), erythema of skin (5%)

Endocrine & metabolic: Albuminuria (6%)

Gastrointestinal: Vomiting (9%), dyspepsia (5%)

Hematologic & oncologic: Lymphocytopenia (2% to 6%)

Hepatic: Increased serum aspartate aminotransferase (4%)

<1%, postmarketing, and/or case reports: Abnormal hepatic function tests, anaphylaxis, angioedema, aspergillosis, candidiasis, cytomegalovirus disease, eosinophilia (transient), hepatic injury, herpes meningoencephalitis, herpes simplex infection, herpes zoster infection, listeriosis, nocardiosis, opportunistic infection, progressive multifocal leukoencephalopathy, tuberculosis

Mechanism of Action DMF and its active metabolite, monomethyl fumarate (MMF), have been shown to activate the nuclear factor (erythroid-derived 2)-like 2 (Nrf2) pathway, which is involved in cellular response to oxidative stress. The mechanism by which dimethyl fumarate (DMF) exerts a therapeutic effect in MS is unknown, although it is believed to result from its anti-inflammatory and cytoprotective properties via activation of the Nrf2 pathway (Fox, 2012; Gold, 2012).

Pharmacodynamics/Kinetics

Half-life Elimination MMF: ~1 hour

Time to Peak 2 to 2.5 hours; delayed to 5.5 hours with food

Reproductive Considerations

In general, disease-modifying therapies for multiple sclerosis are stopped prior to a planned pregnancy except in females at high risk of multiple sclerosis activity (AAN [Rae-Grant 2018]). Consider use of agents other than dimethyl fumarate for females at high risk of disease reactivation who are planning a pregnancy. Delaying pregnancy is recommended for females with persistent high disease activity; when disease-modifying therapy is needed in these patients, other agents are preferred (ECTRIMS/EAN [Montalban 2018]).

Pregnancy Considerations

Information related to the use of dimethyl fumarate in pregnancy is limited (Gold 2015; MacDonald 2019; Nguyen 2019).

In general, disease-modifying therapies for multiple sclerosis are not initiated during pregnancy, except in females at high risk of multiple sclerosis activity (AAN [Rae-Grant 2018]). When disease-modifying therapy is needed in these patients, other agents are preferred (ECTRIMS/ EAN [Montalban 2018]).

Females exposed to dimethyl fumarate during pregnancy are encouraged to enroll in the Pregnancy Registry by calling 866-810-1462 or visiting www.tecfidera-pregnancyregistry.com.

- **Dimethylfumarate** *see* Dimethyl Fumarate *on page 501*
- **Dimethyl Triazeno Imidazole Carboxamide** *see* Dacarbazine *on page 427*
- **Diocto [OTC]** *see* Docusate *on page 509*
- **Dioctyl Calcium Sulfosuccinate** *see* Docusate *on page 509*
- **Dioctyl Sodium Sulfosuccinate** *see* Docusate *on page 509*
- **Diovan** *see* Valsartan *on page 1521*
- **Diphen** *see* DiphenhydrAMINE (Systemic) *on page 502*
- **Diphenhist [OTC]** *see* DiphenhydrAMINE (Systemic) *on page 502*

DiphenhydrAMINE (Systemic)

(dye fen HYE dra meen)

Related Information

Bacterial Infections *on page 1739*

Perioral Premalignant Lesions and Management of Patients Undergoing Cancer Therapy *on page 1781*

Ulcerative, Erosive, and Painful Oral Mucosal Disorders *on page 1758*

Viral Infections *on page 1754*

Brand Names: US Aler-Dryl [OTC]; Allergy Childrens [OTC]; Allergy Relief Childrens [OTC]; Allergy Relief [OTC]; Anti-Hist Allergy [OTC]; Aurodryl Allergy Childrens [OTC]; Banophen [OTC]; Benadryl Allergy Childrens [OTC]; Benadryl Allergy [OTC]; Complete Allergy Medication [OTC] [DSC]; Complete Allergy Relief [OTC]; Diphen; Diphen [OTC]; Diphenhist [OTC]; Genahist [OTC]; Geri-Dryl [OTC]; GoodSense Allergy Relief [OTC]; GoodSense Sleep Aid [OTC]; M-Dryl [OTC]; Naramin [OTC]; Nighttime Sleep Aid [OTC]; Nytol Maximum Strength [OTC]; Nytol [OTC]; Ormir [OTC]; PediaCare Childrens Allergy [OTC]; Pharbedryl [OTC]; Q-Dryl [OTC] [DSC]; Quenalin [OTC] [DSC]; Scot-Tussin Allergy Relief [OTC] [DSC]; Siladryl Allergy [OTC]; Silphen Cough [OTC] [DSC]; Simply Sleep [OTC]; Sleep Tabs [OTC]; Sominex [OTC] [DSC]; Tetra-Formula Nighttime Sleep [OTC]; Total Allergy Medicine [OTC]; Total Allergy [OTC]; Triaminic Cough/Runny Nose [OTC] [DSC]; ZzzQuil [OTC]

Brand Names: Canada Diphenist; PMS-DiphenhydrAMINE

Pharmacologic Category Ethanolamine Derivative; Histamine H_1 Antagonist; Histamine H_1 Antagonist, First Generation

Use

Symptomatic relief of allergic symptoms caused by histamine release, including nasal allergies and allergic dermatosis; adjunct to epinephrine in the treatment of anaphylaxis; insomnia, occasional; prevention or treatment of motion sickness; antitussive; management of parkinsonian syndrome including drug-induced extrapyramidal symptoms (dystonic reactions) alone or in combination with centrally acting anticholinergic agents

Guideline recommendations:

Anaphylaxis: Antihistamines are considered second-line treatment only after epinephrine administration in the adjunct management of anaphylaxis (AAAAI [Lieberman 2015]).

Insomnia: American Academy of Sleep Medicine guidelines for the treatment of chronic insomnia suggest diphenhydramine not be used for sleep-onset or sleep-maintenance insomnia in adults due to the absence of evidence for clinically significant improvement (AASM [Sateia 2017]).

Local Anesthetic/Vasoconstrictor Precautions

No information available to require special precautions

Effects on Dental Treatment Key adverse event(s) related to dental treatment: Xerostomia (normal salivary flow resumes upon discontinuation) and dry mucous membranes. Chronic use of antihistamines will inhibit salivary flow, particularly in elderly patients; may contribute to periodontal disease and oral discomfort. See Dental Health Professional Considerations.

Effects on Bleeding No information available to require special precautions

Adverse Reactions

Frequency not defined:

Cardiovascular: Chest tightness, extrasystoles, hypotension, palpitations, tachycardia

Central nervous system: Ataxia, chills, confusion, dizziness, drowsiness, euphoria, excitement, fatigue, headache, irritability, nervousness, neuritis, paradoxical excitation, paresthesia, restlessness, sedation, seizure, vertigo

Dermatologic: Diaphoresis, skin photosensitivity, skin rash, urticaria

Gastrointestinal: Anorexia, constipation, diarrhea, dry mucous membranes, epigastric distress, nausea, vomiting, xerostomia

Genitourinary: Difficulty in micturition, urinary frequency, urinary retention

Hematologic & oncologic: Agranulocytosis, hemolytic anemia, thrombocytopenia

Hypersensitivity: Anaphylactic shock

Neuromuscular & skeletal: Tremor

Ophthalmic: Blurred vision, diplopia

Respiratory: Nasal congestion, pharyngeal edema, thickening of bronchial secretions, wheezing

Mechanism of Action Competes with histamine for H_1-receptor sites on effector cells in the gastrointestinal tract, blood vessels, and respiratory tract; anticholinergic and sedative effects are also seen

Pharmacodynamics/Kinetics

Duration of Action

Histamine-induced wheal suppression: ≤10 hours (Simons 1990)

Histamine-induced flare suppression: ≤12 hours (Simons 1990)

Half-life Elimination Children: 5 hours (range: 4 to 7 hours); Adults: 9 hours (range: 7 to 12 hours); Elderly: 13.5 hours (range: 9 to 18 hours) (Blyden 1986; Simons 1990)

Time to Peak Serum: ~2 hours (Blyden 1986; Simons 1990)

Pregnancy Risk Factor B

Pregnancy Considerations

Diphenhydramine crosses the placenta (Miller 2000; Parkin 1974).

Diphenhydramine may be used for the treatment of allergic conditions in pregnant women when a first-generation antihistamine is indicated (Babalola 2013; Murase 2014). Diphenhydramine may be used as adjunctive therapy in the management of nausea and vomiting of pregnancy when the preferred agents do not provide initial symptom improvement (ACOG 189 2018).

Dental Health Professional Considerations 25 to 50 mg of diphenhydramine orally every 4 to 6 hours can be used to treat mild dermatologic manifestations of allergic reactions to penicillin and other antibiotics. Diphenhydramine is not recommended as local anesthetic for either infiltration route or nerve block since the vehicle has caused local necrosis upon injection. A 50:50 mixture of diphenhydramine liquid (12.5 mg/5 mL) in Kaopectate or Maalox is used as a local application for recurrent aphthous ulcers; swish 15 mL for 2 minutes 4 times/day.

DiphenhydrAMINE (Topical)

(dye fen HYE dra meen)

Brand Names: US Anti-Itch Maximum Strength [OTC] [DSC]; Anti-Itch [OTC]; Banophen [OTC]; Benadryl Itch Stopping [OTC]; Itch Relief [OTC]

Pharmacologic Category Ethanolamine Derivative; Histamine H_1 Antagonist; Histamine H_1 Antagonist, First Generation; Topical Skin Product

Use Relief of pain and itching: Temporary relief of pain and itching associated with insect bites; sunburn; scrapes; minor cuts, minor skin irritations, and minor burns; or rashes due to poison ivy, poison oak, and poison sumac

Local Anesthetic/Vasoconstrictor Precautions No information available to require special precautions

Effects on Dental Treatment No significant effects or complications reported

Effects on Bleeding No information available to require special precautions

Adverse Reactions Frequency not defined.

Dermatologic: Photosensitivity, rash, urticaria

Pregnancy Considerations When administered orally, diphenhydramine crosses the placenta. Diphenhydramine can also be measurable in the serum following topical administration to large areas of the body. Refer to the Diphenhydramine (Systemic) monograph.

- **Diphenhydramine Citrate** *see* DiphenhydrAMINE (Systemic) *on page 502*
- **Diphenhydramine HCl** *see* DiphenhydrAMINE (Systemic) *on page 502*
- **Diphenhydramine Hydrochloride** *see* DiphenhydrAMINE (Systemic) *on page 502*
- **Diphenhydramine Hydrochloride** *see* DiphenhydrAMINE (Topical) *on page 503*
- **Diphenhydramine Tannate** *see* DiphenhydrAMINE (Systemic) *on page 502*

Diphenoxylate and Atropine

(dye fen OKS i late & A troe peen)

Related Information

Dentin Hypersensitivity, Acid Erosion, High Caries Index, Management of Alveolar Osteitis, and Xerostomia *on page 1762*

Brand Names: US Lomotil

Brand Names: Canada Lomotil

Pharmacologic Category Antidiarrheal

Use Diarrhea, adjunct therapy: Adjunctive management of diarrhea in patients ≥13 years of age.

Local Anesthetic/Vasoconstrictor Precautions No information available to require special precautions

Effects on Dental Treatment Key adverse event(s) related to dental treatment: Significant xerostomia (normal salivary flow resumes upon discontinuation).

Effects on Bleeding No information available to require special precautions

Adverse Reactions Frequency not defined.

Cardiovascular: Flushing, tachycardia

Central nervous system: Confusion, depression, dizziness, drowsiness, euphoria, hallucination, headache, hyperthermia, lethargy, malaise, numbness, restlessness, sedation

Dermatologic: Pruritus, urticaria, xeroderma

Gastrointestinal: Abdominal distress, anorexia, gingival swelling, nausea, pancreatitis, paralytic ileus, toxic megacolon, vomiting, xerostomia

Genitourinary: Urinary retention

Hypersensitivity: Anaphylaxis, angioedema

Mechanism of Action Diphenoxylate inhibits excessive GI motility and GI propulsion; commercial preparations contain a subtherapeutic amount of atropine to discourage abuse

Pharmacodynamics/Kinetics

Onset of Action Within 45 to 60 minutes

Half-life Elimination Diphenoxylate: 2.5 hours; Diphenoxylic acid: 12 to 14 hours

Time to Peak Diphenoxylate: Serum: ~2 hours

Pregnancy Considerations Animal reproduction studies have not been conducted with this combination.

Controlled Substance C-V

- **Diphenylhydantoin** *see* Phenytoin *on page 1228*
- **Diprivan** *see* Propofol *on page 1286*
- **Diprolene** *see* Betamethasone (Topical) *on page 237*
- **Diprolene AF** *see* Betamethasone (Topical) *on page 237*
- **Dipropylacetic Acid** *see* Valproic Acid and Derivatives *on page 1518*

Dipyridamole (dye peer ID a mole)

Brand Names: Canada APO-Dipyridamole; APO-Dipyridamole SC; Persantine

Pharmacologic Category Antiplatelet Agent; Vasodilator

Use

Oral: Used with warfarin to decrease thrombosis in patients after artificial heart valve replacement

IV: Diagnostic agent in CAD

Local Anesthetic/Vasoconstrictor Precautions No information available to require special precautions

Effects on Dental Treatment No significant effects or complications reported

Effects on Bleeding Dipyridamole inhibits platelet aggregation and may increase the risk of bleeding.

Adverse Reactions

Oral: Frequency not always defined.

Cardiovascular: Angina pectoris, flushing

Central nervous system: Dizziness (14%), headache (2%)

Dermatologic: Skin rash (2%), pruritus

Gastrointestinal: Abdominal distress (6%), diarrhea, vomiting

Hepatic: Hepatic insufficiency

Postmarketing and/or case reports: Alopecia, arthritis, cholelithiasis, dyspepsia, fatigue, hepatitis, hypersensitivity reaction, hypotension, laryngeal edema, malaise, myalgia, nausea, palpitations, paresthesia, tachycardia, thrombocytopenia

IV:

>10%:

Cardiovascular: Exacerbation of angina pectoris (20%)

Central nervous system: Dizziness (12%), headache (12%)

1% to 10%:

Cardiovascular: ECG abnormality (5% to 8%; ST-T changes, extrasystoles), hypotension (5%), flushing (3%), tachycardia (3%), altered blood pressure (2%), hypertension (2%)

Central nervous system: Pain (3%), fatigue (1%), paresthesia (1%)

Gastrointestinal: Nausea (5%)

Respiratory: Dyspnea (3%)

<1%, postmarketing, and/or case reports (Limited to important or life-threatening): Abdominal pain, arthralgia, ataxia, back pain, bronchospasm, cardiac arrhythmia (ventricular tachycardia, bradycardia, AV block, SVT, atrial fibrillation, asystole), cardiomyopathy, cough, depersonalization, diaphoresis, dysgeusia, dyspepsia, dysphagia, ECG abnormality (unspecified), edema, eructation, flatulence, hypersensitivity reaction, hypertonia, hyperventilation, increased appetite, increased thirst, injection site reaction, leg cramps (intermittent claudication), malaise, mastalgia, muscle rigidity, myalgia, myocardial infarction, orthostatic hypotension, otalgia, palpitations, perineal pain, pharyngitis, pleuritic chest pain, pruritus, renal pain, rhinitis, skin rash, syncope, tenesmus, tinnitus, tremor, urticaria, vertigo, visual disturbance, vomiting, weakness, xerostomia

Mechanism of Action Inhibits the activity of adenosine deaminase and phosphodiesterase, which causes an accumulation of adenosine, adenine nucleotides, and cyclic AMP; these mediators then inhibit platelet aggregation and may cause vasodilation; may also stimulate release of prostacyclin or PGD_2; causes coronary vasodilation

Pharmacodynamics/Kinetics

Half-life Elimination Terminal: 10-12 hours

Time to Peak Serum: 2-2.5 hours

Pregnancy Considerations Adverse events have not been observed in animal reproduction studies.

◆ **Dipyridamole and Aspirin** *see* Aspirin and Dipyridamole *on page* 185

Diroximel Fumarate (dye ROX i mel FYOO ma rate)

Brand Names: US Vumerity

Pharmacologic Category Fumaric Acid Derivative

Use Multiple sclerosis, relapsing: Treatment of relapsing forms of multiple sclerosis, including clinically isolated syndrome, relapsing-remitting disease, and active secondary progressive disease, in adults.

Local Anesthetic/Vasoconstrictor Precautions No information available to require special precautions.

Effects on Dental Treatment No significant effects or complications reported.

Effects on Bleeding No information available to require special precautions.

Adverse Reactions All adverse reactions were reported with dimethyl fumarate delayed-release capsules, which have the same active metabolite as diroximel fumarate.

>10%:

Cardiovascular: Flushing (40%)

Gastrointestinal: Abdominal pain (18%), diarrhea (14%), nausea (12%)

Infection: Infection (60%; similar to placebo)

1% to 10%:

Dermatologic: Pruritus (8%), skin rash (8%), erythema of skin (5%)

Endocrine & metabolic: Albuminuria (6%)

Gastrointestinal: Vomiting (9%), dyspepsia (5%)

Hematologic & oncologic: Lymphocytopenia (2% to 6%)

Hepatic: Increased serum aspartate aminotransferase (4%)

Frequency not defined: Hematologic & oncologic: Eosinophilia (transient)

Postmarketing: Abnormal hepatic function tests, anaphylaxis, angioedema, progressive multifocal leukoencephalopathy

Mechanism of Action Diroximel fumarate and its active metabolite, monomethyl fumarate (MMF), have been shown to activate the nuclear factor (erythroid-derived 2)-like 2 (Nrf2) pathway, which is involved in cellular response to oxidative stress. The mechanism by which diroximel fumarate exerts a therapeutic effect in multiple sclerosis is unknown, although it is believed to result from its anti-inflammatory and cytoprotective properties via activation of the Nrf2 pathway (Fox 2012; Gold 2012). MMF has also been identified as a nicotinic acid receptor agonist in vitro.

Pharmacodynamics/Kinetics

Half-life Elimination Terminal: 1 hour.

Time to Peak 2.5 to 3 hours (fasting), 4.5 hours (with a 350 to 700 calorie and 10 to 30 g fat meal); 7 hours (with a >700 calorie and >30 g fat meal).

Reproductive Considerations

In general, disease-modifying therapies for multiple sclerosis are stopped prior to a planned pregnancy, except in females at high risk of multiple sclerosis activity (AAN [Rae-Grant 2018]). Consider use of agents other than diroximel fumarate for females at high risk of disease reactivation who are planning a pregnancy. Delaying pregnancy is recommended for females with persistent high disease activity; when disease-modifying therapy is needed in these patients, other agents are preferred (ECTRIMS/EAN [Montalban 2018]).

Pregnancy Considerations

Adverse events were observed in some animal reproduction studies.

In general, disease-modifying therapies for multiple sclerosis are not initiated during pregnancy, except in females at high risk of multiple sclerosis activity (AAN [Rae-Grant 2018]). When disease-modifying therapy is needed in these patients, other agents are preferred (ECTRIMS/ EAN [Montalban 2018]).

◆ **Disalcid [DSC]** *see* Salsalate *on page* 1356

- **Disalicylic Acid** *see* Salsalate *on page 1356*
- **Disodium Cromoglycate** *see* Cromolyn (Oral Inhalation) *on page 416*
- **Disodium Cromoglycate** *see* Cromolyn (Systemic) *on page 416*
- ***d*-Isoephedrine Hydrochloride** *see* Pseudoephedrine *on page 1291*

Disopyramide (dye soe PEER a mide)

Related Information

Clinical Risk Related to Drugs Prolonging QT Interval *on page 1675*

Brand Names: US Norpace; Norpace CR

Brand Names: Canada Rythmodan

Pharmacologic Category Antiarrhythmic Agent, Class Ia

Use Ventricular arrhythmias: Life-threatening ventricular arrhythmias (eg, sustained ventricular tachycardia).

Local Anesthetic/Vasoconstrictor Precautions Disopyramide is one of the drugs confirmed to prolong the QT interval and is accepted as having a risk of causing torsade de pointes. The risk of drug-induced torsade de pointes is extremely low when a single QT interval prolonging drug is prescribed. In terms of epinephrine, it is not known what effect vasoconstrictors in the local anesthetic regimen will have in patients with a known history of congenital prolonged QT interval or in patients taking any medication that prolongs the QT interval. Until more information is obtained, it is suggested that the clinician consult with the physician prior to the use of a vasoconstrictor in suspected patients, and that the vasoconstrictor (epinephrine, mepivacaine and levonordefrin [Carbocaine® 2% with Neo-Cobefrin®]) be used with caution.

Effects on Dental Treatment Key adverse event(s) related to dental treatment: Xerostomia (normal salivary flow resumes upon discontinuation).

Effects on Bleeding No information available to require special precautions

Adverse Reactions Frequency not always defined. The most common adverse effects are related to cholinergic blockade. The most serious adverse effects of disopyramide are hypotension and cardiac failure.

>10%:

Gastrointestinal: Xerostomia (32%), constipation (11%)

Genitourinary: Urinary hesitancy (14% to 23%)

1% to 10%:

Cardiovascular: Cardiac conduction disturbance, cardiac failure, chest pain, edema, hypotension, syncope

Central nervous system: Dizziness, fatigue, headache, malaise, myasthenia, nervousness

Dermatologic: Generalized dermatosis, pruritus, skin rash

Endocrine & metabolic: Hypokalemia, increased serum cholesterol, increased serum triglycerides, weight gain

Gastrointestinal: Abdominal distention, anorexia, bloating, diarrhea, flatulence, nausea, vomiting

Genitourinary: Impotence (1% to 3%), urinary frequency, urinary retention, urinary urgency

Neuromuscular & skeletal: Myalgia

Ophthalmic: Blurred vision, xerophthalmia

Respiratory: Dry throat, dyspnea

<1%, postmarketing, and/or case reports: Agranulocytosis, atrioventricular block, cardiac arrhythmia (new or worsened; proarrhythmic effect), cholestatic jaundice, decreased hematocrit, decreased hemoglobin, depression, dysuria, fever, gynecomastia, hepatotoxicity, hypoglycemia, increased blood urea nitrogen, increased serum creatinine, increased serum transaminases, insomnia, mydriasis, numbness, paresthesia, peripheral neuropathy, psychosis, psychotic reaction, respiratory distress, skin blister (toxic), systemic lupus erythematosus (rare; generally in patients previously receiving procainamide), thrombocytopenia, tingling sensation

Mechanism of Action Class Ia antiarrhythmic: Decreases myocardial excitability and conduction velocity; reduces disparity in refractory between normal and infarcted myocardium; possesses anticholinergic, peripheral vasoconstrictive, and negative inotropic effects

Pharmacodynamics/Kinetics

Onset of Action 0.5 to 3.5 hours

Duration of Action Immediate release: 1.5 to 8.5 hours

Half-life Elimination Children 5 to 12 years: 3.15 ± 0.64 hours (Chiba 1992); Adults: 4 to 10 hours; prolonged with heart failure and hepatic or renal impairment

Time to Peak Serum: Immediate release: Within 2 hours; Controlled release: 4 to 7 hours

Pregnancy Risk Factor C

Pregnancy Considerations

Disopyramide levels have been reported in human fetal blood. Disopyramide may stimulate contractions in pregnant women. In a case report, disopyramide use in the third trimester resulted in painful uterine contractions after the first dose and hemorrhage after the second dose (Abbi 1999).

Dental Health Professional Considerations See Local Anesthetic/Vasoconstrictor Precautions

- **Disopyramide Phosphate** *see* Disopyramide *on page 505*

Disulfiram (dye SUL fi ram)

Brand Names: US Antabuse

Pharmacologic Category Aldehyde Dehydrogenase Inhibitor

Use Alcohol use disorder: Management of chronic alcohol use disorder.

Note: Suggested for use in patients with alcohol use disorder (moderate to severe) who want to abstain from alcohol and either prefer disulfiram or are unable to tolerate or are unresponsive to naltrexone and acamprosate (APA [Reus 2018]).

Local Anesthetic/Vasoconstrictor Precautions No information available to require special precautions

Effects on Dental Treatment No significant effects or complications reported

Effects on Bleeding No information available to require special precautions

Adverse Reactions Frequency not defined.

Central nervous system: Bitter taste (garlic), drowsiness, fatigue, headache, metallic taste, peripheral neuritis, peripheral neuropathy, polyneuropathy, psychosis

Dermatologic: Acneiform eruption, allergic dermatitis, skin rash
Genitourinary: Impotence
Hepatic: Cholestatic hepatitis, fulminant hepatitis, hepatic failure (multiple case reports)
Ophthalmic: Optic neuritis

Mechanism of Action Disulfiram is a thiuram derivative which blocks the oxidation of alcohol at the acetaldehyde stage. When taken concomitantly with alcohol, there is an increase in serum acetaldehyde levels. High acetaldehyde causes uncomfortable symptoms including flushing, throbbing in head and neck, nausea, vomiting, diaphoresis, thirst, palpitations, chest pain, dyspnea, hyperventilation, tachycardia, syncope, weakness, blurred vision, confusion, vertigo, and hypotension. This reaction is the basis for disulfiram use in post-withdrawal long-term care of alcohol use disorder.

Pharmacodynamics/Kinetics

Onset of Action Full effect: 12 hours

Duration of Action ~1 to 2 weeks after last dose

Pregnancy Considerations

Safety in pregnancy has not been established; there is limited data on maternal use during pregnancy (Reitnauer 1997).

Pharmacological agents should not be used for the treatment of alcohol use disorder in pregnant women unless needed for the treatment of acute alcohol withdrawal or a coexisting disorder; agents other than disulfiram are recommended for acute alcohol withdrawal.

- ◆ **Ditropan** *see* Oxybutynin *on page 1156*
- ◆ **Ditropan XL** *see* Oxybutynin *on page 1156*
- ◆ **Diuril** *see* Chlorothiazide *on page 339*
- ◆ **Divalproex Sodium** *see* Valproic Acid and Derivatives *on page 1518*
- ◆ **Divigel** *see* Estradiol (Systemic) *on page 596*
- ◆ **5071-1DL(6)** *see* Megestrol *on page 956*
- ◆ ***dl*-Alpha Tocopherol** *see* Vitamin E (Systemic) *on page 1549*
- ◆ **DLV** *see* Delavirdine *on page 451*
- ◆ **DMF** *see* Dimethyl Fumarate *on page 501*
- ◆ **DMPA** *see* MedroxyPROGESTERone *on page 953*
- ◆ **DNA minor groove-binding agent PM01183** *see* Lurbinectedin *on page 944*

DOBUTamine (doe BYOO ta meen)

Brand Names: Canada DOBUTamine SDZ

Pharmacologic Category Adrenergic Agonist Agent; Inotrope

Use

Cardiac decompensation: Short-term management of patients with cardiac decompensation

Guideline recommendations:

Cardiogenic shock: The 2017 American Heart Association (AHA) scientific statement for the Contemporary Management of Cardiogenic Shock recommends dobutamine to maintain systemic perfusion and preserve end-organ performance in patients with cardiogenic shock. A vasopressor such as norepinephrine (preferred), vasopressin, or dopamine is typically the initial preferred therapy until hemodynamically stable. Once stable, consider adding or transitioning to an inotrope. However, an inotrope may be the preferred therapy for cardiogenic shock due to acute decompensated heart failure or in other cases when systolic blood pressure >90 mm Hg (ACCF/AHA [Yancy 2013]); AHA [van Diepen 2017]).

Inotropic support in advanced heart failure: Bridge therapy in stage D heart failure (HF) unresponsive to guideline-directed medical therapy and device therapy in patients awaiting heart transplant or mechanical circulatory support; short-term management of hospitalized patients with severe systolic dysfunction presenting with low blood pressure and significantly depressed cardiac output; long-term management (palliative therapy) in select patients with stage D HF unresponsive to guideline-directed medical therapy and device therapy who are not candidates for heart transplant or mechanical circulatory support (ACCF/AHA [Yancy 2013]).

Local Anesthetic/Vasoconstrictor Precautions
No information available to require special precautions

Effects on Dental Treatment No significant effects or complications reported

Effects on Bleeding No information available to require special precautions

Adverse Reactions

1% to 10%:

Cardiovascular: Increased heart rate (10%), increased systolic blood pressure (8%), ventricular premature contractions (5%), angina pectoris (1% to 3%), chest pain (1% to 3%), palpitations (1% to 3%)
Central nervous system: Headache (1% to 3%)
Gastrointestinal: Nausea (1% to 3%)
Respiratory: Dyspnea (1% to 3%)

Frequency not defined:

Cardiovascular: Hypotension, ventricular ectopy
Endocrine & metabolic: Decreased serum potassium

<1%, postmarketing, and/or case reports: Cardiomyopathy (stress), eosinophilia, hypersensitivity reaction, localized phlebitis

Mechanism of Action Dobutamine, a racemic mixture, stimulates myocardial $beta_1$-adrenergic receptors primarily by the (+) enantiomer and some $alpha_1$ receptor agonism by the (-) enantiomer, resulting in increased contractility and heart rate, and stimulates both $beta_2$- and $alpha_1$-receptors in the vasculature. Although $beta_2$ and $alpha_1$ adrenergic receptors are also activated, the effects of $beta_2$ receptor activation may equally offset or be slightly greater than the effects of $alpha_1$ stimulation, resulting in some vasodilation in addition to the inotropic and chronotropic actions (Leier 1988; Majerus 1989; Ruffolo 1987). Lowers central venous pressure and wedge pressure, but has little effect on pulmonary vascular resistance (Leier 1977; Leier 1978).

Pharmacodynamics/Kinetics

Onset of Action IV: 1 to 10 minutes; Peak effect: 10 to 20 minutes

Half-life Elimination 2 minutes

Pregnancy Considerations Dobutamine should not be used as a diagnostic agent for stress testing during pregnancy; use should be avoided when other options are available (ESC [Regitz-Zagrosek 2018]). Medications used for the treatment of cardiac arrest in pregnancy are the same as in the non-pregnant female. Appropriate medications should not be withheld due to concerns of fetal teratogenicity. Dobutamine use during the post-resuscitation phase may be considered; however, the effects of inotropic support on the fetus should also be considered. Doses and indications should follow current Advanced Cardiovascular Life Support (ACLS) guidelines (AHA [Jeejeebhoy 2015]).

- ◆ **Dobutamine HCl** *see* DOBUTamine *on page 506*
- ◆ **Dobutamine HCl/D5W** *see* DOBUTamine *on page 506*
- ◆ **Dobutamine Hydrochloride** *see* DOBUTamine *on page 506*
- ◆ **Docefrez [DSC]** *see* DOCEtaxel *on page 507*

DOCEtaxel (doe se TAKS el)

Brand Names: US Docefrez [DSC]; Taxotere

Brand Names: Canada Taxotere

Pharmacologic Category Antineoplastic Agent, Antimicrotubular; Antineoplastic Agent, Taxane Derivative

Use

Breast cancer: Treatment of breast cancer (locally advanced/metastatic) after prior chemotherapy failure; adjuvant treatment (in combination with doxorubicin and cyclophosphamide) of operable node-positive breast cancer

Gastric cancer: Treatment of advanced gastric adenocarcinoma, including gastroesophageal junction adenocarcinoma (in combination with cisplatin and fluorouracil) in patients who have not received prior chemotherapy for advanced disease

Head and neck cancer: Treatment (induction) of locally advanced squamous cell head and neck cancer (in combination with cisplatin and fluorouracil)

Non-small cell lung cancer: Treatment of locally advanced or metastatic non-small cell lung cancer (NSCLC) after failure of prior platinum-based chemotherapy; treatment of previously untreated unresectable locally advanced or metastatic NSCLC (in combination with cisplatin)

Prostate cancer: Treatment of metastatic castration-resistant prostate cancer (in combination with prednisone)

Local Anesthetic/Vasoconstrictor Precautions No information available to require special precautions

Effects on Dental Treatment Key adverse event(s) related to dental treatment: Mucositis, stomatitis, and taste perversion.

Effects on Bleeding Thrombocytopenia (8% to 14%) and bleeding episodes have been reported. A medical consult is recommended.

Adverse Reactions Percentages reported for docetaxel monotherapy; frequency may vary depending on diagnosis, dose, liver function, prior treatment, and premedication.

>10%:

Dermatologic: Alopecia (56% to 76%), dermatological reaction (20% to 48%), nail disease (11% to 41%)

Endocrine & metabolic: Fluid retention (26% to 60%)

Gastrointestinal: Stomatitis (26% to 53%; grades 3/4: 2%), diarrhea (23% to 43%), nausea (34% to 42%), vomiting (22% to 23%)

Hematologic & oncologic: Neutropenia (84% to 99%; grade 4: 75% to 86%; grades 3/4: 65%; nadir [median]: 7 days, duration [severe neutropenia]: 7 days), leukopenia (84% to 99%; grades 3/4: 49%; grade 4: 32% to 44%), anemia (87% to 97%; grades 3/4: 8% to 9%), thrombocytopenia (7% to 12%; grades 3/4: 3%; grade 4: 1%), febrile neutropenia (5% to 14%)

Hepatic: Increased serum transaminases (4% to 19%)

Hypersensitivity: Hypersensitivity reaction (6% to 21%)

Infection: Infection (22% to 34%; severe: 6%)

Neuromuscular & skeletal: Asthenia (53% to 66%), myalgia (6% to 23%), neuromuscular reaction (16%)

Respiratory: Pulmonary disorder (41%)

Miscellaneous: Fever (31% to 35%)

1% to 10%:

Cardiovascular: Hypotension (3%)

Gastrointestinal: Dysgeusia (6%)

Hepatic: Increased serum bilirubin (9%), increased serum alkaline phosphatase (7%)

Infection: Severe infection (2% to 6%)

Local: Infusion site reaction (4%)

Nervous system: Neurotoxicity (grades 3/4: 2% to 6%), peripheral motor neuropathy (4%; severe; mainly distal extremity weakness)

Neuromuscular and skeletal: Arthralgia (3% to 9%)

Frequency not defined:

Cardiovascular: Cardiac tamponade, decreased left ventricular ejection fraction, localized phlebitis, peripheral edema

Dermatologic: Exfoliation of skin, local dryness of skin, localized erythema of the extremities, nail depigmentation, nail hyperpigmentation, skin discoloration at injection site

Hepatic: Ascites

Local: Erythema at injection site, inflammation at injection site

Nervous system: Fatigue

Respiratory: Pleural effusion

<1%, postmarketing, and/or case reports: Abdominal pain, acute generalized exanthematous pustulosis, acute hepatic failure (Morgan 2011), acute myelocytic leukemia, acute myocardial infarction, acute respiratory distress, alcohol intoxication, alopecia (permanent), anaphylactic shock, anaphylaxis, anorexia, atrial fibrillation, atrial flutter, back pain, bleeding tendency disorder, bronchospasm, cardiac arrhythmia, cardiac failure, chest pain, chest tightness, chills, colitis, confusion, conjunctivitis, constipation, cutaneous lupus erythematosus, cystoid macular edema, deafness, deep vein thrombosis, dehydration, dermatological reaction (injection site recall at previous site of extravasation), disease of the lacrimal apparatus (duct obstruction), disseminated intravascular coagulation, drug fever, duodenal ulcer, dyspnea, ECG abnormality, electrolyte disorder, enterocolitis, epiphora (more common with weekly administration [Kintzel 2006]), erythema multiforme, esophagitis, flushing, gastrointestinal hemorrhage, gastrointestinal perforation, hearing loss, hepatitis, hypertension, hypocalcemia, hypokalemia, hypomagnesemia, hyponatremia, interstitial pulmonary disease, intestinal obstruction, ischemic colitis, lacrimation, loss of consciousness (transient), lymphedema (peripheral), multiorgan failure, myelodysplastic syndrome, neutropenic enterocolitis, non-Hodgkin's lymphoma, onycholysis, ototoxicity, pain, palmar-plantar erythrodysesthesia, pneumonia (interstitial), pneumonitis, pruritus, pulmonary edema, pulmonary embolism, pulmonary fibrosis, radiation pneumonitis, radiation recall phenomenon, renal failure syndrome, renal insufficiency, renal neoplasm, respiratory failure, seizure, sepsis, severe dermatological reaction, sinus tachycardia, skin changes (scleroderma-like), skin rash, Stevens-Johnson syndrome, syncope, tachycardia, thrombophlebitis, toxic epidermal necrolysis, unstable angina pectoris, ventricular arrhythmia, ventricular tachycardia, visual disturbance (transient)

Mechanism of Action Docetaxel promotes the assembly of microtubules from tubulin dimers, and inhibits the depolymerization of tubulin which stabilizes microtubules in the cell. This results in inhibition of DNA, RNA, and protein synthesis. Most activity occurs during the M phase of the cell cycle.

Pharmacodynamics/Kinetics

Half-life Elimination Terminal: ~11 hours

Reproductive Considerations

Evaluate pregnancy status prior to use in females of reproductive potential. Females of reproductive potential should use effective contraceptive measures before beginning treatment, during therapy, and for 6 months after the last docetaxel dose. Males with female partners of reproductive potential should use effective contraceptive measures during therapy and for 3 months after the last docetaxel dose.

Pregnancy Considerations

An ex vivo human placenta perfusion model illustrated that docetaxel crossed the placenta at term. Placental transfer was low and affected by the presence of albumin; higher albumin concentrations resulted in lower docetaxel placental transfer (Berveiller 2012).

Based on the mechanism of action and data from animal reproduction studies, in utero exposure to docetaxel may cause fetal harm. Formulations may contain alcohol, which is also associated with adverse fetal effects.

Some pharmacokinetic properties of docetaxel may be altered in pregnant women (van Hasselt 2014). Data related to the use of docetaxel for the treatment of breast cancer in pregnancy is limited. Use should be restricted for clinically urgent situations; use of other agents is preferred. The European Society for Medical Oncology has published guidelines for diagnosis, treatment, and follow-up of cancer during pregnancy; the guidelines recommend referral to a facility with expertise in cancer during pregnancy and encourage a multidisciplinary team (obstetrician, neonatologist, oncology team). In general, if chemotherapy is indicated, it should be avoided in the first trimester and there should be a 3-week time period between the last chemotherapy dose and anticipated delivery, and chemotherapy should not be administered beyond week 33 of gestation (Peccatori 2013).

A pregnancy registry is available for all cancers diagnosed during pregnancy at Cooper Health (877-635-4499).

Product Availability Docefrez has been discontinued in the US for more than 1 year.

◆ **Docetaxel** *see* DOCEtaxel *on page* 507

◆ **Docosahexaenoic Acid** *see* Omega-3 Fatty Acids *on page* 1137

Docosanol (doe KOE san ole)

Related Sample Prescriptions

Viral Infections - Sample Prescriptions *on page* 43

Brand Names: US Abreva [OTC]

Generic Availability (US) Yes

Pharmacologic Category Antiviral Agent, Topical

Dental Use Treatment of herpes simplex of the face or lips

Use Cold sore/fever blister: Treatment of cold sores/fever blisters on the face or lips.

Local Anesthetic/Vasoconstrictor Precautions No information available to require special precautions

Effects on Dental Treatment No significant effects or complications reported (see Dental Health Professional Considerations)

Effects on Bleeding No information available to require special precautions

Adverse Reactions Frequency not defined.

Hypersensitivity: Hypersensitivity reaction

Dental Usual Dosage Herpes simplex (face/lips): Children ≥12 years and Adults: Topical: Apply 5 times/day to affected area of face or lips. Start at first sign of cold sore or fever blister and continue until healed.

Dosing

Adult & Geriatric Cold sore/fever blister: Topical: Apply 5 times daily to affected area of face or lips. Start at first sign of cold sore or fever blister and continue until healed. If not healed within 10 days, discontinue use and contact health care provider.

Renal Impairment: Adult There are no dosage adjustments provided in the manufacturer's labeling.

Hepatic Impairment: Adult There are no dosage adjustments provided in the manufacturer's labeling.

Pediatric Cold sore/fever blister: Children ≥12 years and Adolescents: Refer to adult dosing.

Renal Impairment: Pediatric There are no dosage adjustments provided in the manufacturer's labeling.

Hepatic Impairment: Pediatric There are no dosage adjustments provided in the manufacturer's labeling.

Mechanism of Action Prevents viral entry and replication at the cellular level

Contraindications OTC labeling: When used for self-medication, do not use if you have hypersensitivity to docosanol or any component of the formulation

Warnings/Precautions For external use only; do not apply to inside of mouth or around eyes. Apply at the first sign of cold sore/fever blister (tingle); early treatment ensures best results. Do not share product with others. Discontinue use and contact a health care provider if the condition gets worse or is not healed within 10 days. Severe allergic reactions (eg, hives, facial swelling, wheezing/difficulty breathing, rash, shock) may occur with use; discontinue and seek medical attention immediately if an allergic reaction occurs.

Some dosage forms may contain benzyl alcohol; large amounts of benzyl alcohol (≥99 mg/kg/day) have been associated with a potentially fatal toxicity ("gasping syndrome") in neonates; the "gasping syndrome" consists of metabolic acidosis, respiratory distress, gasping respirations, CNS dysfunction (including convulsions, intracranial hemorrhage), hypotension and cardiovascular collapse (AAP ["Inactive" 1997]; CDC, 1982); some data suggests that benzoate displaces bilirubin from protein binding sites (Ahlfors, 2001); avoid or use dosage forms containing benzyl alcohol with caution in neonates. See manufacturer's labeling.

Drug Interactions

Metabolism/Transport Effects None known.

Avoid Concomitant Use There are no known interactions where it is recommended to avoid concomitant use.

Increased Effect/Toxicity There are no known significant interactions involving an increase in effect.

Decreased Effect

Docosanol may decrease the levels/effects of: Talimogene Laherparepvec

Dosage Forms: US

Cream, External:

Abreva [OTC]: 10% (2 g)

Generic: 10% (2 g)

Dental Health Professional Considerations Wash hands before and after applying cream. Begin treatment at first tingle of cold sore or fever blister. Rub into area gently, but completely. Do not apply directly to inside of mouth or around eyes. Contact healthcare provider if sore gets worse or does not heal within 10 days. Do not share this product with others, may spread infection. Notify healthcare professional if pregnant or breastfeeding.

- ◆ **DocQLace [OTC] [DSC]** *see* Docusate *on page 509*
- ◆ **Docu [OTC]** *see* Docusate *on page 509*
- ◆ **Docuprene [OTC] [DSC]** *see* Docusate *on page 509*

Docusate (DOK yoo sate)

Brand Names: US Colace Clear [OTC] [DSC]; Colace [OTC]; Diocto [OTC]; DocQLace [OTC] [DSC]; Docu Soft [OTC]; Docu [OTC]; Docuprene [OTC] [DSC]; Docusate Mini [OTC]; Docusil [OTC]; DocuSol Kids [OTC]; DocuSol Mini [OTC]; DOK [OTC]; Dulcolax Stool Softener [OTC]; Enemeez Mini [OTC]; GoodSense Stool Softener [OTC] [DSC]; Healthy Mama Move It Along [OTC]; Kao-Tin [OTC]; KS Stool Softener [OTC]; Laxa Basic [OTC]; Pedia-Lax [OTC]; Promolaxin [OTC]; Silace [OTC]; Sof-Lax [OTC] [DSC]; Stool Softener [OTC]

Pharmacologic Category Stool Softener

Use Stool softener: Prevention of straining during defecation and constipation associated with hard, dry stools; relief of occasional constipation

Local Anesthetic/Vasoconstrictor Precautions No information available to require special precautions

Effects on Dental Treatment Key adverse event(s) related to dental treatment: Throat irritation.

Effects on Bleeding No information available to require special precautions

Adverse Reactions 1% to 10%: Respiratory: Throat irritation (liquid)

Mechanism of Action Reduces surface tension of the oil-water interface of the stool resulting in enhanced incorporation of water and fat allowing for stool softening (Roering, 2010)

Pharmacodynamics/Kinetics

Onset of Action Oral: 12 to 72 hours; Rectal: 2 to 15 minutes

Pregnancy Considerations

Hypomagnesemia was reported in a newborn following chronic maternal overuse of docusate sodium throughout pregnancy (Schindler 1984).

Treatment of constipation in pregnant women is similar to that of nonpregnant patients and medications may be used when diet and lifestyle modifications are not effective. Agents other than docusate are recommended in pregnancy (Body 2016). Stool softeners may be used for the treatment of hemorrhoids (Shin 2015).

- ◆ **Docusate Calcium** *see* Docusate *on page 509*
- ◆ **Docusate Mini [OTC]** *see* Docusate *on page 509*
- ◆ **Docusate Potassium** *see* Docusate *on page 509*
- ◆ **Docusate Sodium** *see* Docusate *on page 509*
- ◆ **Docusil [OTC]** *see* Docusate *on page 509*
- ◆ **Docu Soft [OTC]** *see* Docusate *on page 509*
- ◆ **DocuSol Kids [OTC]** *see* Docusate *on page 509*
- ◆ **DocuSol Mini [OTC]** *see* Docusate *on page 509*

Dofetilide (doe FET il ide)

Related Information

Cardiovascular Diseases *on page 1654*

Clinical Risk Related to Drugs Prolonging QT Interval *on page 1675*

Brand Names: US Tikosyn

Pharmacologic Category Antiarrhythmic Agent, Class III

Use Atrial fibrillation/atrial flutter: Maintenance of normal sinus rhythm in patients with chronic atrial fibrillation/atrial flutter of longer than 1-week duration who have been converted to normal sinus rhythm; conversion of atrial fibrillation and atrial flutter to normal sinus rhythm.

Local Anesthetic/Vasoconstrictor Precautions Dofetilide is one of the drugs confirmed to prolong the QT interval and is accepted as having a risk of causing torsade de pointes. The risk of drug-induced torsade de pointes is extremely low when a single QT interval prolonging drug is prescribed. In terms of epinephrine, it is not known what effect vasoconstrictors in the local anesthetic regimen will have in patients with a known history of congenital prolonged QT interval or in patients taking any medication that prolongs the QT interval. Until more information is obtained, it is suggested that the clinician consult with the physician prior to the use of a vasoconstrictor in suspected patients, and that the vasoconstrictor (epinephrine, mepivacaine and levonordefrin [Carbocaine® 2% with Neo-Cobefrin®]) be used with caution.

Effects on Dental Treatment No significant effects or complications reported

Effects on Bleeding No information available to require special precautions

Adverse Reactions

>10%:

Cardiovascular: Torsades de pointes (patients receiving doses in excess of those recommended: ≤11%; cardiac failure patients: 3%; patients with recent myocardial infarction: <1%; occurs most frequently within the first 3 days of therapy)

Central nervous system: Headache (11%)

1% to 10%:

Cardiovascular: Chest pain (10%), ventricular fibrillation (≤5%), ventricular tachycardia (3% to 4%), bradycardia (≤2%), cardiac arrest (≤2%), cerebral ischemia (≤2%), cerebrovascular accident (≤2%), edema (≤2%), myocardial infarction (≤2%), syncope (≤2%), atrioventricular block (<2%), heart block (1%)

Central nervous system: Dizziness (8%), insomnia (4%), facial paralysis (≤2%), flaccid paralysis (≤2%), migraine (≤2%), paralysis (≤2%), paresthesia (≤2%)

Dermatologic: Skin rash (3%)

Gastrointestinal: Nausea (5%), abdominal pain (3%), diarrhea (3%)

Hepatic: Hepatotoxicity (≤2%), hepatic injury (<2%)

Hypersensitivity: Angioedema (≤2%)

Neuromuscular & skeletal: Back pain (3%)

Respiratory: Respiratory tract infection (7%), dyspnea (6%), flu-like symptoms (4%), increased cough (≤2%), cough (<2%)

Miscellaneous: Accidental injury (3%), surgery (3%)

<1%, postmarketing, and/or case reports: Bundle branch block

Mechanism of Action Vaughan Williams Class III antiarrhythmic activity. Blockade of the cardiac ion channel carrying the rapid component of the delayed rectifier potassium current. Dofetilide has no effect on sodium channels, adrenergic alpha-receptors, or adrenergic beta-receptors. It increases the monophasic action potential duration due to delayed repolarization. The increase in the QT interval is a function of prolongation of both effective and functional refractory periods in the His-Purkinje system and the ventricles. Changes in cardiac conduction velocity and sinus node function have not been observed in patients with or without structural heart disease. PR and QRS width remain the same in patients with preexisting heart block and or sick sinus syndrome.

Pharmacodynamics/Kinetics

Half-life Elimination ~10 hours; prolonged with renal impairment

Time to Peak Serum: Fasting: 2 to 3 hours

Pregnancy Considerations Adverse events have been observed in animal reproduction studies.

Dental Health Professional Considerations See Local Anesthetic/Vasoconstrictor Precautions

- **Dofus [OTC]** *see Lactobacillus on page 869*
- **Dojolvi** *see* Triheptanoin *on page 1498*
- **DOK [OTC]** *see* Docusate *on page 509*

Dolasetron (dol A se tron)

Related Information

Clinical Risk Related to Drugs Prolonging QT Interval *on page 1675*

Brand Names: US Anzemet

Pharmacologic Category Antiemetic; Selective 5-HT_3 Receptor Antagonist

Use

Chemotherapy-associated nausea and vomiting (oral): Prevention of nausea and vomiting associated with initial and repeat course of moderately emetogenic cancer chemotherapy in adults and children ≥2 years

Postoperative nausea and vomiting (injection): Prevention and treatment of postoperative nausea and vomiting (PONV) in adults and children ≥2 years

Limitations of use: Routine PONV prophylaxis is not recommended if there is little expectation that nausea and/or vomiting will occur postoperatively. In patients in whom nausea and/or vomiting must be avoided postoperatively, dolasetron (injection) is recommended even if the anticipated incidence of postoperative nausea and/or vomiting is low. If prophylaxis has failed, a repeat dose should not be utilized as rescue therapy.

Local Anesthetic/Vasoconstrictor Precautions Dolasetron is one of the drugs confirmed to prolong the QT interval and is accepted as having a risk of causing torsade de pointes. The risk of drug-induced torsade de pointes is extremely low when a single QT interval prolonging drug is prescribed. In terms of epinephrine, it is not known what effect vasoconstrictors in the local anesthetic regimen will have in patients with a known history of congenital prolonged QT interval or in patients taking any medication that prolongs the QT interval. Until more information is obtained, it is suggested that the clinician consult with the physician prior to the use of a vasoconstrictor in suspected patients, and that the vasoconstrictor (epinephrine, mepivacaine and levonordefrin [Carbocaine® 2% with Neo-Cobefrin®]) be used with caution.

Effects on Dental Treatment Key adverse event(s) related to dental treatment: Taste alterations.

Effects on Bleeding No information available to require special precautions

Adverse Reactions Adverse events may vary according to indication and route of administration.

>10%: Central nervous system: Headache (oral: 18% to 23%; IV: 9%)

1% to 10%:

Cardiovascular: Bradycardia (4% to 5%; may be severe after IV administration), tachycardia (≤3%), edema (<2%), facial edema (<2%), flushing (<2%), hypotension (<2%; may be severe after IV administration), orthostatic hypotension (<2%), peripheral edema (<2%), peripheral ischemia (<2%), phlebitis (<2%), sinus arrhythmia (<2%), thrombophlebitis (<2%)

Central nervous system: Fatigue (oral: 3% to 6%), dizziness (1% to 6%), pain (≤3%), abnormal dreams (<2%), agitation (<2%), anxiety (<2%), ataxia (<2%), chills (≤2%), confusion (<2%), depersonalization (<2%), paresthesia (<2%), shivering (≤2%), sleep disorder (<2%), twitching (<2%), vertigo (<2%)

Dermatologic: Diaphoresis (<2%), skin rash (<2%), urticaria (<2%)

Endocrine & metabolic: Increased gamma-glutamyl transferase (<2%)

Gastrointestinal: Diarrhea (oral: 2% to 5%), dyspepsia (≤3%), abdominal pain (<2%), anorexia (<2%), constipation (<2%), dysgeusia (<2%), pancreatitis (<2%)

Genitourinary: Dysuria (<2%), hematuria (<2%)

Hematologic and oncologic: Anemia (<2%), hematoma (<2%), prolonged prothrombin time (<2%), prolonged partial thromboplastin time (<2%), purpura (<2%), thrombocytopenia (<2%)

Hepatic: Hyperbilirubinemia (<2%), increased serum alkaline phosphatase (<2%)

Hypersensitivity: Anaphylaxis (<2%)

Local: Burning sensation at injection site (IV: <2%), pain at injection site (IV: <2%)

Neuromuscular & skeletal: Arthralgia (<2%), myalgia (<2%), tremor (<2%)

Ophthalmic: Photophobia (<2%), visual disturbance (<2%)

Otic: Tinnitus (<2%)

Renal: Acute renal failure (<2%), polyuria (<2%)

Respiratory: Bronchospasm (<2%), dyspnea (<2%), epistaxis (<2%)

<1%, postmarketing, and/or case reports: Abnormal T waves on ECG, appearance of U waves on ECG, atrial fibrillation, atrial flutter, atrioventricular block, bundle branch block (left and right), cardiac arrest, chest pain, extrasystoles (APCs or VPCs), increased serum ALT (transient), increased serum AST (transient), ischemic heart disease, nodal arrhythmia, palpitations, prolongation P-R interval on ECG (dose dependent), prolonged QT interval on ECG, serotonin syndrome, slow R wave progression, ST segment changes on ECG, syncope (may be severe after IV administration), torsades de pointes, ventricular arrhythmia, ventricular fibrillation cardiac arrest (IV), ventricular tachycardia (IV), wide complex tachycardia (IV), widened QRS complex on ECG (dose-dependent)

Mechanism of Action Dolasetron is a selective serotonin receptor (5-HT_3) antagonist which blocks serotonin both peripherally (primary site of action) and centrally at the chemoreceptor trigger zone

Pharmacodynamics/Kinetics

Half-life Elimination

Dolasetron: IV: ≤10 minutes

Hydrodolasetron:
Oral: Children: 5.5 hours; Adolescents: 6.4 hours; Adults: 8.1 hours
IV: Children: 4.8 hours; Adults: 7.3 hours
Severe renal impairment: 11 hours
Severe hepatic impairment: 11 hours

Time to Peak Hydrodolasetron: IV: 0.6 hours; Oral: ~1 hour

Pregnancy Considerations Adverse events have not been observed in animal reproduction studies.

Product Availability Anzemet injection has been discontinued in the US for more than 1 year.

Dental Health Professional Considerations See Local Anesthetic/Vasoconstrictor Precautions

◆ **Dolasetron Mesylate** *see* Dolasetron *on page 510*

◆ **Dolobid** *see* Diflunisal *on page 495*

◆ **Dolophine** *see* Methadone *on page 984*

◆ **Dolotranz [DSC]** *see* Lidocaine and Prilocaine *on page 911*

Dolutegravir (doe loo TEG ra vir)

Brand Names: US Tivicay; Tivicay PD

Brand Names: Canada Tivicay

Pharmacologic Category Antiretroviral, Integrase Inhibitor (Anti-HIV)

Use HIV-1 infection, treatment: Treatment of HIV-1 infection in combination with other antiretroviral agents in treatment-naïve or -experienced adult patients and treatment-naïve or -experienced pediatric patients (but integrase strand transfer inhibitor naïve) at least 4 weeks of age and weighing at least 3 kg, or in combination with rilpivirine in adults to replace the current antiretroviral regimen in those who are virologically suppressed (HIV-1 RNA <50 copies per mL) on a stable antiretroviral regimen for at least 6 months with no history of treatment failure or known substitutions associated with resistance to either antiretroviral agent.

Local Anesthetic/Vasoconstrictor Precautions No information available to require special precautions

Effects on Dental Treatment No significant effects or complications reported

Effects on Bleeding No information available to require special precautions

Adverse Reactions Adverse reactions reported with combination therapy.

>10%:
Endocrine & metabolic: Hyperglycemia (≤14%)
Hepatic: Increased serum alanine aminotransferase (≤18%; includes patients with hepatitis B and/or C infections)

1% to 10%:
Central nervous system: Insomnia (≤7%), fatigue (≤2%), headache (≤2%), suicidal ideation (<2%), suicidal tendencies (<2%), depression (≤1%)
Dermatologic: Pruritus (<2%)
Gastrointestinal: Increased serum lipase (2% to 10%), diarrhea (≤2%), abdominal distress (<2%), abdominal pain (<2%), flatulence (<2%), upper abdominal pain (<2%), vomiting (<2%), nausea (≤1%)
Hematologic & oncologic: Neutropenia (3% to 4%; grades 3/4: 2%), leukopenia (2% to 3%)
Hepatic: Increased serum aspartate aminotransferase (≤8%), hyperbilirubinemia (≤3%), hepatitis (<2%)
Hypersensitivity: Hypersensitivity reaction (≤1%)
Neuromuscular & skeletal: Increased creatine phosphokinase (1% to 7%), myositis (<2%)
Renal: Renal insufficiency (<2%)

<1%, postmarketing, and/or case reports: Abnormal dreams, acute hepatic failure, anxiety, arthralgia, dizziness, hepatotoxicity, immune reconstitution syndrome, increased serum creatinine, myalgia, skin rash, weight gain

Mechanism of Action Binds to the integrase active site and inhibits the strand transfer step of HIV-1 DNA integration necessary for the HIV replication cycle.

Pharmacodynamics/Kinetics

Half-life Elimination ~14 hours

Time to Peak 2 to 3 hours

Reproductive Considerations

Dolutegravir is recommended as an alternative agent for women living with HIV who are not yet pregnant but are trying to conceive. The potential risk of neural tube defects following in utero exposure should be discussed with the patient.

For males and females living with HIV and planning a pregnancy, maximum viral suppression below the limits of detection with antiretroviral therapy (ART), modification of therapy (if needed), optimization of the woman's health, and a discussion of the potential risks and benefits of ART therapy during pregnancy is recommended prior to conception (HHS [perinatal] 2019).

Pregnancy Considerations

Dolutegravir has a high level of transfer across the human placenta.

A small but significant increase in neural tube defects (NTDs) was observed following maternal use of dolutegravir in a study conducted in Botswana. The risk of NTDs was increased in women who became pregnant while taking dolutegravir, but not in women who started dolutegravir during pregnancy. Data from the study, completed in an area without routine folate fortification via food, may not predict the risk in the United States. It is not known if folic acid supplementation would decrease the risk of NTDs in women taking dolutegravir; however, daily folic acid is recommended for all women who are pregnant or who might conceive.

Maternal antiretroviral therapy (ART) may be associated with adverse pregnancy outcomes including preterm delivery, stillbirth, low birth weight, and small for gestational age infants. Actual risks may be influenced by maternal factors such as disease severity, gestational age at initiation of therapy, and specific ART regimen; therefore, close fetal monitoring is recommended. Because there is clear benefit to appropriate treatment, maternal ART should not be withheld due to concerns for adverse neonatal outcomes. Long-term follow-up is recommended for all infants exposed to antiretroviral medications; children without HIV but who were exposed to ART in utero and develop significant organ system abnormalities of unknown etiology (particularly of the CNS or heart) should be evaluated for potential mitochondrial dysfunction.

The Health and Human Services (HHS) Perinatal HIV Guidelines consider dolutegravir a preferred integrase strand transfer inhibitor (INSTI) for pregnant females living with HIV who are antiretroviral-naive, who have had ART therapy in the past but are restarting, and who require a new ART regimen (due to poor tolerance or poor virologic response of current regimen). In addition, females who become pregnant while taking dolutegravir may continue if viral suppression is effective and the regimen is well tolerated. Dolutegravir is also a preferred component of an initial regimen when acute HIV infection is detected during pregnancy. The HHS Perinatal HIV Guidelines consider dolutegravir in combination with abacavir and lamivudine to be a preferred INSTI regimen for initial therapy in antiretroviral-naive pregnant females. INSTIs can rapidly suppress viral load. A regimen with dolutegravir may be useful when drug interactions or the potential for preterm delivery with protease inhibitors are a concern. In addition, use of dolutegravir may be beneficial in women living with HIV who are not on ART and present for care late in pregnancy, as a fourth drug in women with high viral loads, or as part of a new regimen for a woman experiencing virologic failure on ART. The potential risk of NTDs following in utero exposure should be discussed with the patient. Pharmacokinetics of dolutegravir may be altered, but dosing adjustments are not needed during pregnancy.

In general, ART is recommended for all pregnant females living with HIV to keep the viral load below the limit of detection and reduce the risk of perinatal transmission. Therapy should be individualized following a discussion of the potential risks and benefits of treatment during pregnancy. Monitoring of pregnant females is more frequent than in nonpregnant adults. ART should be continued postpartum for all females living with HIV and can be modified after delivery.

Health care providers are encouraged to enroll pregnant females exposed to antiretroviral medications as early in pregnancy as possible in the Antiretroviral Pregnancy Registry (1-800-258-4263 or http://www.APRegistry.com). Health care providers caring for pregnant females living with HIV and their infants may contact the National Perinatal HIV Hotline (1-888-448-8765) for clinical consultation (HHS [perinatal] 2019).

Dolutegravir and Rilpivirine

(doe loo TEG ra vir & ril pi VIR een)

Brand Names: US Juluca

Brand Names: Canada Juluca

Pharmacologic Category Antiretroviral, Integrase Inhibitor (Anti-HIV); Antiretroviral, Reverse Transcriptase Inhibitor, Non-nucleoside (Anti-HIV)

Use HIV-1 infection, treatment: Treatment of HIV-1 infection in adults virologically suppressed on a stable antiretroviral regimen for ≥6 months with no history of treatment failure and no known resistance to the individual components

Local Anesthetic/Vasoconstrictor Precautions QTc prolongation: In healthy subjects, supratherapeutic doses of rilpivirine (ie, 75 mg daily, 300 mg daily) have been associated with QTc prolongation. The risk of drug-induced torsades de pointes is extremely low when a single QT interval prolonging drug is prescribed. In terms of epinephrine, it is not known what effect vasoconstrictors in the local anesthetic regimen will have in patients with a known history of congenital prolonged QT interval or in patients taking any medication that prolongs the QT interval. Until more information is obtained, it is suggested that the clinician consult with the physician prior to the use of a vasoconstrictor in suspected patients, and that the vasoconstrictor (epinephrine, mepivacaine, and levonordefrin [Carbocaine 2% with Neo-Cobefrin]) be used with caution.

Effects on Dental Treatment No significant effects or complications reported

Effects on Bleeding No information available to require special precautions

Adverse Reactions Also see individual agents.

1% to 10%:

Central nervous system: Headache (2%)

Endocrine & metabolic: Hyperglycemia (4%)

Gastrointestinal: Increased serum lipase (5%), diarrhea (2%)

Hepatic: Increased serum ALT (2%), increased serum bilirubin (2%)

Neuromuscular & skeletal: Decreased bone mineral density (2%), increased creatine phosphokinase (≤1%)

<1%, postmarketing, and/or case reports: Bone fracture, increased serum AST

Mechanism of Action Dolutegravir, an integrase inhibitor, inhibits HIV integrase by binding to the integrase active site and blocking the strand transfer step of retroviral DNA integration. Rilpivirine, a non-nucleoside reverse transcriptase inhibitor, binds to reverse transcriptase and blocks the RNA-dependent and DNA-dependent polymerase activities, including HIV-1 replication.

Reproductive Considerations

The Health and Human Services (HHS) Perinatal HIV Guidelines do not recommend use of this fixed-dose 2-drug combination in females living with HIV who are not yet pregnant but are trying to conceive (2-drug regimens are not recommended during pregnancy) (HHS [perinatal] 2019).

Refer to individual monographs for additional information.

Pregnancy Considerations

The Health and Human Services (HHS) Perinatal HIV Guidelines do not recommend use of this fixed-dose 2-drug combination in pregnant females living with HIV who are antiretroviral-naive, who have had antiretroviral therapy (ART) in the past but are restarting, or who require a new ART regimen (due to poor tolerance or poor virologic response of current regimen). For females who become pregnant while taking this combination as a complete regimen, the regimen should be changed or additional agents added (2-drug regimens are not recommended during pregnancy) (HHS [perinatal] 2019).

Refer to individual monographs for additional information.

◆ **Dolutegravir, Lamivudine, and Abacavir** *see* Abacavir, Dolutegravir, and Lamivudine *on page 51*

◆ **Dolutegravir Sodium** *see* Dolutegravir *on page 511*

◆ **Dolutegravir Sodium and Rilpivirine Hydrochloride** *see* Dolutegravir and Rilpivirine *on page 512*

Donepezil (doh NEP e zil)

Brand Names: US Aricept

Brand Names: Canada ACCEL-Donepezil [DSC]; ACT Donepezil ODT; ACT Donepezil [DSC]; APO-Donepezil; Aricept; Aricept RDT; Auro-Donepezil; BIO-Donepezil; JAMP-Donepezil; M-Donepezil; Mar-Donepezil; MINT-Donepezil; MYLAN-Donepezil [DSC]; NAT-Donepezil; PMS-Donepezil; RIVA-Donepezil [DSC]; SANDOZ Donepezil; SANDOZ Donepezil ODT; Septa-Donepezil; TARO-Donepezil; TEVA-Donepezil; VAN-Donepezil [DSC]

Pharmacologic Category Acetylcholinesterase Inhibitor (Central)

Use Alzheimer disease: Treatment of mild, moderate, or severe dementia of the Alzheimer type.

Local Anesthetic/Vasoconstrictor Precautions No information available to require special precautions

Effects on Dental Treatment No significant effects or complications reported.

Effects on Bleeding No information available to require special precautions

Adverse Reactions

>10%:

Gastrointestinal: Diarrhea (5% to 15%), nausea (3% to 19%)

Nervous system: Insomnia (2% to 14%)

Miscellaneous: Accidental injury (7% to 13%)

1% to 10%:

Cardiovascular: Chest pain (2%), hypertension (3%), syncope (2% [placebo: 1%])

Dermatologic: Ecchymosis (4% to 5%), eczema (3%)

Endocrine & metabolic: Hyperlipidemia (2%), weight loss (3% to 5% [placebo: 1%])

Gastrointestinal: Anorexia (2% to 8% [placebo: 2% to 4%]), gastrointestinal hemorrhage (1%), vomiting (3% to 9%)

Genitourinary: Urinary frequency (2%), urinary incontinence (1% to 3%)

Hematologic & oncologic: Bruise (2%), hemorrhage (2%)

Nervous system: Abnormal dreams (3%), confusion (2%), depression (2% to 3%), dizziness (2% to 8%), drowsiness (1% to 2%), emotional lability (2%), fatigue (1% to 8%), hallucination (3% [placebo: 1%]), headache (3% to 10%), hostility (3%), nervousness (3%), pain (3% to 9%), personality disorder (2%)

Neuromuscular & skeletal: Arthritis (2%), asthenia (1% to 2%), back pain (3%), increased creatine phosphokinase in blood specimen (3%), muscle cramps (3% to 8%)

Miscellaneous: Fever (2%)

<1%: Gastrointestinal: Peptic ulcer

Postmarketing:

Cardiovascular: Heart block, prolonged QT interval on ECG (Leitch 2007; Tanaka 2009), torsades de pointes (Tanaka 2009)

Dermatologic: Skin rash (Lim 2018)

Endocrine & metabolic: Hyponatremia (Shareef 2017)

Gastrointestinal: Abdominal pain, cholecystitis, pancreatitis (Niinomi 2019)

Hematologic & oncologic: Hemolytic anemia

Hepatic: Hepatitis (Dierckx 2008; Verrico 2000)

Nervous system: Aggressive behavior, agitation (Leung 2014), neuroleptic malignant syndrome (Matsumoto 2004; Warwick 2008), seizure (Babic 1999; Kumlien 2010)

Neuromuscular & skeletal: Rhabdomyolysis (Fleet 2019; Sahin 2014)

Mechanism of Action Alzheimer's disease is characterized by cholinergic deficiency in the cortex and basal forebrain, which contributes to cognitive deficits. Donepezil reversibly and noncompetitively inhibits centrally active acetylcholinesterase, the enzyme responsible for hydrolysis of acetylcholine. This appears to result in increased concentrations of acetylcholine available for synaptic transmission in the CNS.

Pharmacodynamics/Kinetics

Half-life Elimination 70 hours; time to steady-state: 15 days

Time to Peak Plasma: Tablet, 10 mg: 3 hours; Tablet, 23 mg: ~8 hours; **Note:** Peak plasma concentrations almost twofold higher for the 23 mg tablet compared to the 10 mg tablet

Pregnancy Considerations Adverse events have been observed in some animal reproduction studies.

◆ **Donepezil HCl** *see* Donepezil *on page 512*

◆ **Dopram** *see* Doxapram *on page 516*

◆ **Doral** *see* Quazepam *on page 1295*

Doravirine (DOR a VIR een)

Brand Names: US Pifeltro

Brand Names: Canada Pifeltro

Pharmacologic Category Antiretroviral, Reverse Transcriptase Inhibitor, Non-nucleoside (Anti-HIV)

Use HIV-1 infection, treatment: Treatment of HIV-1 infection in combination with other antiretroviral agents in adult patients with no prior antiretroviral treatment history or to replace the current antiretroviral regimen in those who are virologically suppressed (HIV-1 RNA <50 copies per mL) on a stable antiretroviral regimen with no history of treatment failure and no known substitutions associated with resistance to doravirine.

Local Anesthetic/Vasoconstrictor Precautions No information available to require special precautions

Effects on Dental Treatment No significant effects or complications reported

Effects on Bleeding No information available to require special precautions

Adverse Reactions Incidences reflect adverse reactions that occur with combination therapy.

1% to 10%:

Cardiovascular: Increased serum creatine kinase (3% to 5%)

Central nervous system: Fatigue (6%), headache (6%), dizziness (3%), abnormal dreams (1%), insomnia (1%)

Dermatologic: Skin rash (2%)

Endocrine & metabolic: Increased serum triglycerides (1%)

Gastrointestinal: Nausea (7%), increased serum lipase (3% to 7%), diarrhea (6%), abdominal pain (5%)

Hepatic: Increased serum bilirubin (≤6%), increased serum aspartate aminotransferase (2% to 5%), increased serum alanine aminotransferase (2% to 4%)

Renal: Increased serum creatinine (4%)

<1%, postmarketing, and/or case reports: Increased LDL cholesterol, increased serum alkaline phosphatase

Mechanism of Action Doravirine is a pyridinone non-nucleoside reverse transcriptase inhibitor that inhibits HIV-1 replication by noncompetitive inhibition of HIV-1 reverse transcriptase.

Pharmacodynamics/Kinetics

Half-life Elimination 15 hours

Time to Peak 2 hours

Reproductive Considerations

The Health and Human Services (HHS) perinatal HIV guidelines note data are insufficient to recommend doravirine for females living with HIV who are not yet pregnant but are trying to conceive.

For males and females living with HIV and planning a pregnancy, maximum viral suppression below the limits of detection with antiretroviral therapy (ART), modification of therapy (if needed), optimization of the woman's health, and a discussion of the potential risks and benefits of ART therapy during pregnancy is recommended prior to conception (HHS [perinatal] 2019).

Pregnancy Considerations

Data collected by the antiretroviral registry related to the use of doravirine in pregnancy are insufficient to evaluate teratogenicity.

Maternal antiretroviral therapy (ART) may be associated with adverse pregnancy outcomes including preterm delivery, stillbirth, low birth weight, and small for gestational age infants. Actual risks may be influenced by maternal factors, such as disease severity, gestational age at initiation of therapy, and specific ART regimen, therefore close fetal monitoring is recommended. Because there is clear benefit to appropriate treatment, maternal ART should not be withheld due to concerns for adverse neonatal outcomes. Long-term follow-up is recommended for all infants exposed to antiretroviral medications; children without HIV but who were exposed to ART in utero and develop significant organ system abnormalities of unknown etiology (particularly of the CNS or heart) should be evaluated for potential mitochondrial dysfunction. Hypersensitivity reactions (including hepatic toxicity and rash) are more common in women on NNRTI therapy; it is not known if pregnancy increases this risk.

The Health and Human Services (HHS) perinatal HIV guidelines note data are insufficient to recommend doravirine for pregnant females living with HIV who are antiretroviral naive, who have had ART therapy in the past but are restarting, who require a new ART regimen (due to poor tolerance or poor virologic response of current regimen), or who become pregnant during therapy. Pharmacokinetic studies of doravirine are not available to make dosing recommendations for pregnant females.

In general, ART is recommended for all pregnant females living with HIV to keep the viral load below the limit of detection and reduce the risk of perinatal transmission. Therapy should be individualized following a discussion of the potential risks and benefits of treatment during pregnancy. Monitoring of pregnant females is more frequent than in nonpregnant adults. ART should be continued postpartum for all females living with HIV and can be modified after delivery.

Health care providers are encouraged to enroll pregnant females exposed to antiretroviral medications as early in pregnancy as possible in the Antiretroviral Pregnancy Registry (1-800-258-4263 or http://www.APRegistry.com). Health care providers caring for pregnant females living with HIV and their infants may contact the National Perinatal HIV Hotline (1-888-448-8765) for clinical consultation (HHS [perinatal] 2019).

Doravirine, Lamivudine, and Tenofovir Disoproxil Fumarate

(DOR a VIR een, la MI vyoo deen & ten OF oh vir dye soe PROX il FUE ma rate)

Brand Names: US Delstrigo

Brand Names: Canada Delstrigo

Pharmacologic Category Antiretroviral, Reverse Transcriptase Inhibitor, Non-nucleoside (Anti-HIV); Antiretroviral, Reverse Transcriptase Inhibitor, Nucleoside (Anti-HIV); Antiretroviral, Reverse Transcriptase Inhibitor, Nucleotide (Anti-HIV)

Use HIV-1 infection, treatment: Treatment of HIV-1 infection in adult patients with no prior antiretroviral treatment history or to replace the current antiretroviral regimen in those who are virologically suppressed (HIV-1 RNA <50 copies per mL) on a stable antiretroviral regimen with no history of treatment failure and no known substitutions associated with resistance to doravirine, lamivudine, or tenofovir disoproxil fumarate.

Local Anesthetic/Vasoconstrictor Precautions No information available to require special precautions

Effects on Dental Treatment No significant effects or complications reported

Effects on Bleeding No information available to require special precautions

Adverse Reactions Also see individual agents.

>10%: Central nervous system: Sleep disorder (≤12%), sleep disturbance (≤12%)

1% to 10%:

- Cardiovascular: Increased serum creatine kinase (3% to 4%)
- Central nervous system: Dizziness (7% to 9%), abnormal dreams (5%), headache (4%), impaired consciousness (4%), insomnia (4%), depression (≤4%), suicidal tendencies (≤4%), drowsiness (3%)
- Dermatologic: Skin rash (2%)
- Endocrine & metabolic: Increased serum cholesterol (1%), increased serum triglycerides (1%)
- Gastrointestinal: Increased serum lipase (2% to 6%), nausea (5%), diarrhea (4%)
- Hepatic: Increased serum bilirubin (1% to 5%), increased serum alanine aminotransferase (1% to 4%), increased serum aspartate aminotransferase (1% to 3%)
- Renal: Increased serum creatinine (3%)

<1%: Increased LDL cholesterol, increased serum alkaline phosphatase

Mechanism of Action

Doravirine: Pyridinone non-nucleoside reverse transcriptase inhibitor that inhibits HIV-1 replication by non-competitive inhibition of HIV-1 reverse transcriptase.

Lamivudine: Cytosine analog that is phosphorylated intracellularly to its active 5'-triphosphate metabolite. The principal mode of action is inhibition of HIV reverse transcription via viral DNA chain termination; inhibits RNA- and DNA-dependent DNA polymerase activities of reverse transcriptase.

Tenofovir disoproxil fumarate: Nucleotide reverse transcriptase inhibitor; analog of adenosine 5' monophosphate that interferes with the HIV viral RNA dependent DNA polymerase resulting in inhibition of viral replication. TDF is first converted intracellularly by hydrolysis to tenofovir and subsequently phosphorylated to the active tenofovir diphosphate.

Reproductive Considerations

The Health and Human Services (HHS) perinatal HIV guidelines consider information related to this fixed-dose combination insufficient to make recommendations for use in females living with HIV who are not yet pregnant but are trying to conceive (HHS [perinatal] 2019).

Refer to individual monographs for additional information.

Pregnancy Considerations

The Health and Human Services (HHS) perinatal HIV guidelines consider information related to this fixed-dose combination insufficient to make recommendations for use in pregnant females living with HIV who are antiretroviral-naive, who have had antiretroviral therapy (ART) in the past but are restarting, who require a new ART regimen (due to poor tolerance or poor virologic response of current regimen), or who become pregnant while taking the regimen (HHS [perinatal] 2019).

Refer to individual monographs for additional information.

◆ **Doravirine, Tenofovir Disoproxil Fumarate, and Lamivudine** *see* Doravirine, Lamivudine, and Tenofovir Disoproxil Fumarate *on page 514*

◆ **Doribax [DSC]** *see* Doripenem *on page 515*

Doripenem (dore i PEN em)

Brand Names: US Doribax [DSC]

Pharmacologic Category Antibiotic, Carbapenem

Use

Intra-abdominal infections, complicated: Treatment of complicated intra-abdominal infections caused by *Bacteroides caccae, Bacteroides fragilis, Bacteroides thetaiotaomicron, Bacteroides uniformis, Bacteroides vulgatus, Escherichia coli, Klebsiella pneumoniae, Peptostreptococcus micros, Pseudomonas aeruginosa, Streptococcus intermedius,* and *Streptococcus constellatus.*

Urinary tract infections, complicated (including pyelonephritis): Treatment of complicated urinary tract infections (UTIs), including pyelonephritis, caused by *E. coli* (including cases with concurrent bacteremia), *Acinetobacter baumannii, K. pneumoniae, Proteus mirabilis,* and *P. aeruginosa.*

Local Anesthetic/Vasoconstrictor Precautions No information available to require special precautions

Effects on Dental Treatment Prolonged use of doripenem may lead to development of oral candidiasis.

Effects on Bleeding Thrombocytopenia has been reported through postmarketing surveillance

Adverse Reactions

>10%:

Central nervous system: Headache (3% to 16%)

Gastrointestinal: Diarrhea (6% to 12%), nausea (4% to 12%)

1% to 10%:

Cardiovascular: Phlebitis (2% to 8%)

Dermatologic: Skin rash (1% to 6%; includes allergic/bullous dermatitis, erythema, macular/papular eruptions, urticaria, and erythema multiforme), pruritus (1% to 3%)

Gastrointestinal: Oral candidiasis (1% to 3%), *Clostridioides* (formerly *Clostridium*) *difficile*-associated diarrhea (≤1%)

Genitourinary: Vaginal infection (1% to 2%)

Hematologic & oncologic: Anemia (2% to 10%)

Hepatic: Increased serum transaminases (2% to 7%)

<1%, postmarketing, and/or case reports: Anaphylaxis, interstitial pneumonitis, leukopenia, neutropenia, renal failure, renal insufficiency, seizure, Stevens-Johnson syndrome, thrombocytopenia, toxic epidermal necrolysis

Mechanism of Action Inhibits bacterial cell wall synthesis by binding to several of the penicillin-binding proteins (PBP-2, PBP-3, PBP-4), which in turn inhibits the final transpeptidation step of peptidoglycan synthesis in bacterial cell walls, thus inhibiting cell wall biosynthesis; bacteria eventually lyse due to ongoing activity of cell wall autolytic enzymes (autolysins and murein hydrolases) while cell wall assembly is arrested.

Pharmacodynamics/Kinetics

Half-life Elimination ~1 hour

Pregnancy Risk Factor B

Pregnancy Considerations Adverse events have not been observed in animal reproduction studies. Information related to use during pregnancy has not been located.

Dornase Alfa (DOOR nase AL fa)

Brand Names: US Pulmozyme

Brand Names: Canada Pulmozyme

Pharmacologic Category Enzyme; Mucolytic Agent

Use Cystic fibrosis: Management of cystic fibrosis patients, in conjunction with standard therapies, to improve pulmonary function; reduce the risk of respiratory tract infections requiring parenteral antibiotics in patients with a forced vital capacity (FVC) ≥40% of predicted.

Local Anesthetic/Vasoconstrictor Precautions No information available to require special precautions

Effects on Dental Treatment Key adverse event(s) related to dental treatment: Pharyngitis

Effects on Bleeding No information available to require special precautions

Adverse Reactions Adverse events were similar in children using the PARI BABY nebulizer (facemask as opposed to mouthpiece) with the addition of cough.

>10%:

Cardiovascular: Chest pain (18% to 25%)

Central nervous system: Voice disorder (12% to 18%)

Dermatologic: Skin rash (3% to 12%)

Respiratory: Cough (PARI-BABY nebulizer facemask: children 3 months to <5 years: 45%; children 5 to ≤10 years: 30%), pharyngitis (32% to 40%), rhinitis (30%; in patients with FVC: <40%), decrease in forced vital capacity (≥10% decrease of predicted: 22%; in patients with FVC: <40%), dyspnea (17%; in patients with FVC: <40%)

Miscellaneous: Fever (32% in patients with FVC <40%)

1% to 10%:

Gastrointestinal: Dyspepsia (≤3%)

Immunologic: Antibody development (to dornase alfa: 2% to 4%)

Ophthalmic: Conjunctivitis (1% to 5%)

Respiratory: Laryngitis (3% to 4%)

<1%, postmarketing and/or case reports: Headache, urticaria

Mechanism of Action The hallmark of cystic fibrosis lung disease is the presence of abundant, purulent airway secretions composed primarily of highly polymerized DNA. The principal source of this DNA is the nuclei of degenerating neutrophils, which is present in large concentrations in infected lung secretions. The presence of this DNA produces a viscous mucous that may contribute to the decreased mucociliary transport and persistent infections that are commonly seen in this population. Dornase alfa is a deoxyribonuclease (DNA) enzyme produced by recombinant gene technology. Dornase selectively cleaves DNA, thus reducing mucous viscosity and as a result, airflow in the lung is improved and the risk of bacterial infection may be decreased.

Pharmacodynamics/Kinetics

Onset of Action Nebulization: Enzyme levels are measured in sputum in ~15 minutes and decline rapidly thereafter

Duration of Action Sputum concentrations decline within 2 hours of inhalation

Pregnancy Considerations Adverse events have not been observed in animal reproduction studies.

- **Doryx** *see* Doxycycline *on page 522*
- **Doryx MPC** *see* Doxycycline *on page 522*

Dorzolamide and Timolol

(dor ZOLE a mide & TYE moe lole)

Brand Names: US Cosopt; Cosopt PF

Brand Names: Canada Apo-Dorzo-Timop; Cosopt; Cosopt Preservative Free; Sandoz-Dorzolamide/Timolol

Pharmacologic Category Beta-Adrenergic Blocker, Nonselective; Carbonic Anhydrase Inhibitor (Ophthalmic); Ophthalmic Agent, Antiglaucoma

Use Elevated intraocular pressure: Reduction of elevated intraocular pressure (IOP) in patients with open-angle glaucoma or ocular hypertension who are insufficiently responsive to beta-blockers

Local Anesthetic/Vasoconstrictor Precautions Epinephrine has interacted with nonselective beta-blockers, such as propranolol, to result in initial hypertensive episode followed by bradycardia. Timolol is also a nonselective beta-blocker. The significance of a potential systemic interaction with epinephrine is unknown. However, it is suggested that cautionary procedures be used, particularly if vasoconstrictor is used immediately following a dose of timolol taken by the patient.

Effects on Dental Treatment Key adverse event(s) related to dental treatment: Taste perversion.

Effects on Bleeding No information available to require special precautions

Adverse Reactions Frequency not always defined. Percentages as reported with combination product.

>5%:

Gastrointestinal: Dysgeusia (≤30%)

Ophthalmic: Burning sensation of eyes (≤30%), stinging of eyes (≤30%), blurred vision (5% to 15%), conjunctival hyperemia (5% to 15%), eye pruritus (5% to 15%), superficial punctate keratitis (5% to 15%)

1% to 5%:

Cardiovascular: Hypertension

Central nervous system: Dizziness, headache

Dermatologic: Erythema of eyelid

Gastrointestinal: Abdominal pain, dyspepsia, nausea

Genitourinary: Urinary tract infection

Infection: Influenza

Local: Local discoloration (lens nucleus)

Neuromuscular & skeletal: Back pain

Ophthalmic: Blepharitis, cataract (including post-subcapsular), cloudy vision, conjunctival discharge, conjunctival edema, conjunctivitis, corneal erosion, corneal staining, dry eye syndrome, eye discharge (including eyelid), eye disease (debris in eye), eye pain (includes eyelid), eyelid edema, follicular conjunctivitis, foreign body sensation of eye, lacrimation, ocular exudate (eyelid), optic disk cupping (glaucomatous), scaling of eyelid, visual field defect, vitreous detachment

Respiratory: Bronchitis, cough, pharyngitis, sinusitis, upper respiratory tract infection

<1%, postmarketing, and/or case reports: Bradycardia, cardiac failure, cerebrovascular accident, chest pain, choroidal detachment (following filtration procedures), depression, diarrhea, dyspnea, heart block, hypotension, iridocyclitis, myocardial infarction, nasal congestion, paresthesia, photophobia, respiratory failure, skin rash, Stevens-Johnson syndrome, toxic epidermal necrolysis, urolithiasis, vomiting, xerostomia

Mechanism of Action

Dorzolamide: Inhibits carbonic anhydrase in the ciliary processes of the eye resulting decreased bicarbonate ion formation which decreases sodium and fluid transport, thus decreasing aqueous humor secretion and reduces intraocular pressure.

Timolol: Blocks both $beta_1$- and $beta_2$-adrenergic receptors, reduces intraocular pressure by reducing aqueous humor production or possibly increases the outflow of aqueous humor

Pregnancy Risk Factor C

Pregnancy Considerations Reproductive studies have not been conducted with this combination.

- **Dorzolamide HCl/Timolol Maleate** *see* Dorzolamide and Timolol *on page 516*
- **DOSS** *see* Docusate *on page 509*
- **Dostinex** *see* Cabergoline *on page 276*
- **Dotti** *see* Estradiol (Systemic) *on page 596*
- **DoubleDex** *see* DexAMETHasone (Systemic) *on page 463*

Doxapram (DOKS a pram)

Brand Names: US Dopram

Pharmacologic Category Respiratory Stimulant

Use Respiratory stimulant for respiratory depression secondary to anesthesia, mild-to-moderate drug-induced respiratory and CNS depression; acute hypercapnia secondary to COPD

Note: In general, the use of doxapram as a respiratory stimulant in adults is limited; alternate therapies are preferred.

Local Anesthetic/Vasoconstrictor Precautions No information available to require special precautions

Effects on Dental Treatment No significant effects or complications reported

Effects on Bleeding No information available to require special precautions

Adverse Reactions Frequency not defined.

Cardiovascular: Cardiac arrhythmia, change in pulse, chest pain, chest tightness, flattened T wave on ECG, flushing, increased blood pressure, phlebitis, ventricular fibrillation, ventricular tachycardia

Central nervous system: Apprehension, clonus, disorientation, dizziness, hallucination, headache, hyperactivity, hyperreflexia, involuntary muscle movements, paresthesia, positive Babinski sign, seizure

Dermatologic: Burning sensation of skin, diaphoresis, pruritus

Endocrine & metabolic: Albuminuria

Gastrointestinal: Bowel urgency, diarrhea, hiccups, nausea, vomiting

Genitourinary: Urinary incontinence, urinary retention

Hematologic & oncologic: Decreased hematocrit, decreased hemoglobin, hemolysis, decreased red blood cells

Neuromuscular & skeletal: Fasciculations, laryngospasm, muscle spasm

Ophthalmic: Mydriasis

Renal: Increased blood urea nitrogen

Respiratory: Bronchospasm, cough, dyspnea, hyperventilation, hypoventilation (rebound), tachypnea

Miscellaneous: Fever

<1%, postmarketing, and/or case reports: Agitation (emergence), prolonged QT interval on ECG (premature neonates), second degree atrioventricular block (premature neonates)

Mechanism of Action Stimulates respiration through action on peripheral carotid chemoreceptors; respiratory center in medulla is also directly stimulated as dosage is increased

Pharmacodynamics/Kinetics

Onset of Action Respiratory stimulation: Single IV injection: 20 to 40 seconds; Peak effect: Single IV injection: 1 to 2 minutes

Duration of Action Single IV injection: 5 to 12 minutes

Half-life Elimination Serum: Neonates, premature: 6.6 to 12 hours; Adults: Mean: 3.4 hours (range: 2.4 to 4.1 hours)

Pregnancy Risk Factor B

Pregnancy Considerations Adverse events have not been observed in animal reproduction studies.

◆ **Doxapram Hydrochloride** *see* Doxapram *on page 516*

Doxazosin (doks AY zoe sin)

Related Information

Cardiovascular Diseases *on page 1654*

Brand Names: US Cardura; Cardura XL

Brand Names: Canada APO-Doxazosin; Cardura-1 [DSC]; Cardura-2 [DSC]; Cardura-4 [DSC]; DOM-Doxazosin; Doxazosin-1 [DSC]; Doxazosin-2 [DSC]; Doxazosin-4 [DSC]; JAMP-Doxazosin; MYLAN-Doxazosin [DSC]; PMS-Doxazosin; TEVA-Doxazosin

Pharmacologic Category Alpha$_1$ Blocker; Antihypertensive

Use

Benign prostatic hyperplasia: Treatment of signs and symptoms of benign prostatic hyperplasia (BPH).

Hypertension (immediate release only): Management of hypertension. **Note:** Alpha blockers are not recommended as first line therapy (ACC/AHA [Whelton 2017]).

Local Anesthetic/Vasoconstrictor Precautions No information available to require special precautions

Effects on Dental Treatment Key adverse event(s) related to dental treatment: Xerostomia (normal salivary flow resumes upon discontinuation); Patients may experience orthostatic hypotension as they stand up after treatment; especially if lying in dental chair for extended periods of time. Use caution with sudden changes in position during and after dental treatment.

Effects on Bleeding No information available to require special precautions

Adverse Reactions

>10%: Central nervous system: Dizziness (5% to 19%), malaise (≤12%), fatigue (8% to ≤12%), headache (6% to 10%)

1% to 10%:

Cardiovascular: Edema (3% to 4%), hypotension (1% to 2%), orthostatic hypotension (<1% to 2%), cardiac arrhythmia (1%), facial edema (1%), flushing (1%), palpitations (1%)

Central nervous system: Drowsiness (1% to 5%), vertigo (2% to 4%), pain (2%), anxiety (1%), ataxia (1%), hypertonia (1%), insomnia (1%), movement disorder (1%), myasthenia (1%)

Endocrine & metabolic: Sexual disorder (2%)

Gastrointestinal: Abdominal pain (2%), nausea (1% to 2%), dyspepsia (1%), xerostomia (1%)

Genitourinary: Urinary incontinence (1%), urinary tract infection (1%)

Neuromuscular & skeletal: Weakness (4% to 7%), muscle cramps (1%), myalgia (1%), arthralgia (≤1%), arthritis (≤1%)

Ophthalmic: Visual disturbance (2%)

Otic: Tinnitus (1%)

Renal: Polyuria (2%)

Respiratory: Respiratory tract infection (5%), rhinitis (3%), dyspnea (1% to 3%), epistaxis (1%)

<1%, postmarketing, and/or case reports: Abnormal hepatic function tests, abnormal lacrimation, abnormality in thinking, agitation, alopecia, altered sense of smell, amnesia, angina pectoris, anorexia, back pain, blurred vision, bradycardia, bronchospasm (aggravated), cerebrovascular accident, chest pain, cholestasis, cholestatic hepatitis, confusion, cough, decreased libido, depersonalization, diaphoresis, diarrhea, dysgeusia, dysuria, eczema, emotional lability, fecal incontinence, fever, flu-like symptoms, gastroenteritis, gastrointestinal obstruction, gout, gynecomastia, hematuria, hepatitis, hot flash, hypersensitivity reaction, hypoesthesia, hypokalemia, impotence, increased appetite, increased thirst, infection, intraoperative floppy iris syndrome (cataract surgery), jaundice, lack of concentration, leukopenia, lymphadenopathy, mastalgia, migraine, myocardial infarction, nephrolithiasis, nervousness, neutropenia, nocturia, orthostatic dizziness, otalgia, pallor, paranoia, paresis, paresthesia, peripheral ischemia, pharyngitis, photophobia, priapism, pruritus, purpura, rigors, sinusitis, skin rash, syncope, tachycardia, thrombocytopenia, tremor, twitching, urinary frequency, urination disorder, urticaria, vomiting, weight gain, weight loss, xeroderma

Mechanism of Action

Hypertension: Competitively inhibits postsynaptic alpha$_1$-adrenergic receptors which results in vasodilation of veins and arterioles and a decrease in total peripheral resistance and blood pressure; ~50% as potent on a weight by weight basis as prazosin.

BPH: Competitively inhibits postsynaptic alpha$_1$-adrenergic receptors in prostatic stromal and bladder neck tissues. This reduces the sympathetic tone-induced urethral stricture causing BPH symptoms.

Pharmacodynamics/Kinetics

Duration of Action >24 hours

Half-life Elimination Immediate release: ~22 hours; Extended release: 15 to 19 hours

Time to Peak Serum: Immediate release: 2 to 3 hours; Extended release: 8 ± 3.7 to 9 ± 4.7 hours

Pregnancy Considerations

Doxazosin crosses the placenta (Versmissen 2016).

Chronic maternal hypertension may increase the risk of birth defects, low birth weight, preterm delivery, stillbirth, and neonatal death. Actual fetal/neonatal risks may be related to duration and severity of maternal hypertension. Untreated hypertension may also increase the risks of adverse maternal outcomes, including gestational diabetes, myocardial infarction, preeclampsia, stroke, and delivery complications (ACOG 203 2019).

Agents other than doxazosin are more commonly used to treat hypertension in pregnancy (ACOG 203 2019; ESC [Regitz-Zagrosek 2018]). Females with preexisting hypertension may continue their medication during pregnancy unless contraindications exist (ESC

[Regitz-Zagrosek 2018]). Although rare, use of doxazosin for the treatment of hypertension due to a pheochromocytoma during pregnancy has been described; treatment was generally started after the first trimester (Lenders 2019; van der Weerd 2017).

◆ **Doxazosin Mesylate** *see* Doxazosin *on page 517*

Doxepin (Systemic) (DOKS e pin)

Related Information

Dentin Hypersensitivity, Acid Erosion, High Caries Index, Management of Alveolar Osteitis, and Xerostomia *on page 1762*

Management of the Patient With Anxiety or Depression *on page 1778*

Vasoconstrictor Interactions With Antidepressants *on page 1821*

Brand Names: US Silenor

Brand Names: Canada NOVO-Doxepin; Silenor; SINEquan

Pharmacologic Category Antidepressant, Tricyclic (Tertiary Amine)

Use

Insomnia, sleep maintenance (Silenor only): Treatment of insomnia characterized by difficulty with sleep maintenance.

Major depressive disorder (unipolar), treatment resistant (capsule and oral concentrate): Treatment of depression, including psychotic and bipolar depression.

Local Anesthetic/Vasoconstrictor Precautions Doxepin is one of the drugs confirmed to prolong the QT interval and is accepted as having a risk of causing torsade de pointes. In terms of epinephrine, it is not known what effect vasoconstrictors in the local anesthetic regimen will have in patients with a known history of congenital prolonged QT interval or in patients taking any medication that prolongs the QT interval. Until more information is obtained, it is suggested that the clinician consult with the physician prior to the use of a vasoconstrictor in suspected patients, and that the vasoconstrictor (epinephrine, mepivacaine, and levonordefrin [Carbocaine® 2% with Neo-Cobefrin®]) be used with caution.

Effects on Dental Treatment Key adverse event(s) related to dental treatment: Xerostomia and changes in salivation (normal salivary flow resumes upon discontinuation)

Oral: Aphthous stomatitis, unpleasant taste, trouble with gums

Long-term treatment with TCAs increases the risk of caries by reducing salivation and salivary buffer capacity.

Effects on Bleeding No information available to require special precautions

Adverse Reactions Actual frequency may be dependent on diagnosis.

Cardiovascular: Hypertension (chronic insomnia patients ≤3%), edema, flushing, hypotension, tachycardia

Central nervous system: Sedation (chronic insomnia patients 6% to 9%), dizziness (chronic insomnia patients ≥1%), ataxia, chills, confusion, disorientation, drowsiness, extrapyramidal reaction, fatigue, hallucination, headache, numbness, paresthesia, seizure, tardive dyskinesia

Dermatologic: Alopecia, diaphoresis (excessive), pruritus, skin photosensitivity, skin rash

Endocrine & metabolic: Altered serum glucose, change in libido, galactorrhea, gynecomastia, SIADH, weight gain

Gastrointestinal: Nausea (chronic insomnia patients 2%), gastroenteritis (chronic insomnia patients ≤2%), anorexia, aphthous stomatitis, constipation, diarrhea, dysgeusia, dyspepsia, vomiting, xerostomia

Genitourinary: Breast hypertrophy, testicular swelling, urinary retention

Hematologic & oncologic: Agranulocytosis, eosinophilia, leukopenia, purpura, thrombocytopenia

Hepatic: Jaundice

Neuromuscular & skeletal: Tremor, weakness

Ophthalmic: Blurred vision

Otic: Tinnitus

Respiratory: Upper respiratory tract infection (chronic insomnia patients 4%), exacerbation of asthma

<1%, postmarketing, and/or case reports: Abdominal pain, abnormal dreams, abnormal gait, acne rosacea, adenocarcinoma (lung, stage I), adjustment disorder, ageusia, altered blood pressure (inadequately controlled), anemia, angle-closure glaucoma, anxiety, arthralgia, atrioventricular block, back injury, back pain, blepharospasm, bone fracture, breast cyst, bronchitis, cerebrovascular accident, change in appetite, chest pain, confusion, cough, decreased heart rate, decreased lacrimation, decreased neutrophils, decreased performance on neuropsychometrics, decreased range of motion (joints), depression, dermatitis, diplopia, disturbance in attention, dysmenorrhea, dyspnea, dysuria, ECG abnormality (ST-T segment, QRS complex, QRS axis), erythema, eye infection, eye pain, eye redness, falling, feeling of heaviness, folliculitis, fungal infection, gastroesophageal reflux disease, gum line erosion, hematochezia, hematoma, hemoglobinuria, herpes zoster, hot flash, hyperbilirubinemia, hyperhidrosis, hyperkalemia, hypermagnesemia, hypersensitivity, hypoacusis, hypokalemia, increased serum ALT, increased serum transaminases, influenza, joint sprain, laceration, laryngitis, lethargy, limb pain, lip blister, lower respiratory tract infection, malignant melanoma, migraine, mood elevation, motion sickness, muscle cramps, myalgia, nasal congestion, nasopharyngeal disorder, neck pain, nightmares, nocturia, onychomycosis, otalgia, pallor, palpitations, perforated tympanic membrane, peripheral edema, pharyngitis, pharyngolaryngeal pain, pneumonia, rales, rhinorrhea, sinus congestion, sinusitis, skin irritation, sleep paralysis, somnambulism (complex sleep-related behavior [sleep-driving, cooking or eating food, making phone calls]), staphylococcal cellulitis, syncope, tenosynovitis, tooth infection, urinary incontinence, urinary tract infection, vasodepressor syncope, ventricular premature contractions, viral infection, wheezing

Mechanism of Action

Increases the synaptic concentration of serotonin and norepinephrine in the central nervous system by inhibition of their reuptake by the presynaptic neuronal membrane (Pinder 1977); antagonizes the histamine (H_1) receptor for sleep maintenance.

Efficacy of doxepin in the off-label use of chronic urticaria is believed to be related to its potent H_1 and H_2 receptor antagonist activity (Kozel 2004)

Pharmacodynamics/Kinetics

Onset of Action Depression: Initial effects may be observed within 1 to 2 weeks of treatment, with continued improvements through 4 to 6 weeks (Papakostas 2006; Posternak 2005; Szegedi 2009).

Half-life Elimination Adults: Doxepin: ~15 hours; N-desmethyldoxepin: 31 to 51 hours (Hiemke 2018)

Time to Peak Serum: Fasting: Silenor: 3.5 hours

Pregnancy Risk Factor C

Pregnancy Considerations

Tricyclic antidepressants may be associated with irritability, jitteriness, and convulsions (rare) in the neonate (Yonkers 2009).

The ACOG recommends that therapy for depression during pregnancy be individualized; treatment should incorporate the clinical expertise of the mental health clinician, obstetrician, primary health care provider, and pediatrician (ACOG 2008). According to the American Psychiatric Association (APA), the risks of medication treatment should be weighed against other treatment options and untreated depression. For women who discontinue antidepressant medications during pregnancy and who may be at high risk for postpartum depression, the medications can be restarted following delivery (APA 2010). Treatment algorithms have been developed by the ACOG and the APA for the management of depression in women prior to conception and during pregnancy (Yonkers 2009). Tricyclic antidepressants (TCAs) are not the preferred initial therapy for depression in pregnancy; if a TCA is needed, doxepin is not the recommended agent (Larsen 2015).

Pregnant women exposed to antidepressants during pregnancy are encouraged to enroll in the National Pregnancy Registry for Antidepressants (NPRAD). Women 18 to 45 years of age or their health care providers may contact the registry by calling 844-405-6185. Enrollment should be done as early in pregnancy as possible.

Dental Health Professional Considerations See Local Anesthetic/Vasoconstrictor Precautions

Doxepin (Topical) (DOKS e pin)

Brand Names: US Prudoxin; Zonalon

Pharmacologic Category Topical Skin Product

Use Pruritus: Short-term (≤8 days) management of moderate pruritus in adults with atopic dermatitis or lichen simplex chronicus.

Local Anesthetic/Vasoconstrictor Precautions No information available to require special precautions

Effects on Dental Treatment Key adverse event(s) related to dental treatment: Xerostomia and changes in salivation (normal salivary flow resumes upon discontinuation)

Topical: Taste alteration

Long-term treatment with TCAs increases the risk of caries by reducing salivation and salivary buffer capacity.

Effects on Bleeding No information available to require special precautions

Adverse Reactions

>10%:

Central nervous system: Drowsiness (22%)

Dermatologic: Burning sensation of skin (≤23%), stinging of the skin (≤23%)

1% to 10%:

Cardiovascular: Edema (1%)

Central nervous system: Dizziness (2%), emotional lability (2%)

Gastrointestinal: Xerostomia (10%), dysgeusia (2%)

<1%, postmarketing, and/or case reports: Anxiety, contact dermatitis, numbness of tongue

Mechanism of Action Doxepin has H_1 and H_2 histamine receptor blocking actions, the exact mechanism by which it exerts its antipruritic effect is unknown.

Pharmacodynamics/Kinetics

Half-life Elimination 28 to 52 hours (desmethyldoxepin)

Pregnancy Considerations

Following topical application, plasma levels may be similar to those achieved with oral administration. Also refer to the doxepin (systemic) monograph.

◆ **Doxepin HCl** *see* Doxepin (Systemic) *on page 518*

◆ **Doxepin HCl** *see* Doxepin (Topical) *on page 519*

◆ **Doxepin Hydrochloride** *see* Doxepin (Systemic) *on page 518*

◆ **Doxepin Hydrochloride** *see* Doxepin (Topical) *on page 519*

Doxercalciferol (doks er kal si fe FEER ole)

Brand Names: US Hectorol

Pharmacologic Category Vitamin D Analog

Use

Secondary hyperparathyroidism (patients on dialysis): Injection, oral: Treatment of secondary hyperparathyroidism in patients with chronic kidney disease (CKD) on dialysis

Secondary hyperparathyroidism (patients not on dialysis): Oral: Treatment of secondary hyperparathyroidism in patients with stage 3 or 4 CKD

Local Anesthetic/Vasoconstrictor Precautions No information available to require special precautions

Effects on Dental Treatment No significant effects or complications reported

Effects on Bleeding No information available to require special precautions

Adverse Reactions

>10%:

Cardiovascular: Edema (7% to 34%)

Central nervous system: Headache (28%), malaise (28%), insomnia (15%), paresthesia (15%), dizziness (12%), hypertonia (11%)

Gastrointestinal: Constipation (26%), nausea and vomiting (21%)

Hematologic & oncologic: Anemia (19%)

Infection: Infection (30%)

Neuromuscular & skeletal: Asthenia (15%)

Respiratory: Rhinitis (22%), cough (19%), dyspnea (12% to 19%)

1% to 10%:

Cardiovascular: Angina pectoris (8%), bradycardia (7%), chest pain (7%)

Central nervous system: Depression (7%), sleep disorder (3%)

Dermatologic: Pruritus (7% to 8%)

Endocrine & metabolic: Dehydration (7%), weight gain (5%)

Gastrointestinal: Dyspepsia (5% to 7%), anorexia (5%)

Genitourinary: Urinary tract infection (7%)

Hematologic & oncologic: Leukopenia (7%)

Infection: Abscess (3%)

Neuromuscular & skeletal: Arthralgia (5%)

Respiratory: Sinusitis (7%)

Frequency not defined:

Endocrine & metabolic: Hypercalcemia, hyperphosphatemia

<1%, postmarketing, and/or case reports: Anaphylaxis, angioedema, burning sensation of skin, chest discomfort, hypersensitivity reaction, hypotension, unresponsive to stimuli

Mechanism of Action Doxercalciferol is metabolized to the active form of vitamin D. The active form of vitamin D controls the intestinal absorption of dietary calcium, the tubular reabsorption of calcium by the kidneys, and in conjunction with PTH, the mobilization of calcium from the skeleton.

Pharmacodynamics/Kinetics

Half-life Elimination Major metabolite: ~32 to 37 hours (range: up to 96 hours)

Time to Peak Major metabolite: 8 hours (injection); 11 to 12 hours (oral).

Pregnancy Considerations Adverse events have not been observed in animal reproduction studies

◆ **Doxil** *see* DOXOrubicin (Liposomal) *on page 521*

DOXOrubicin (Conventional)

(doks oh ROO bi sin con VEN sha nal)

Related Information

DOXOrubicin (Liposomal) *on page 521*

Brand Names: US Adriamycin

Brand Names: Canada Adriamycin PFS; Myocet

Pharmacologic Category Antineoplastic Agent, Anthracycline; Antineoplastic Agent, Topoisomerase II Inhibitor

Use

Breast cancer, adjuvant therapy: Treatment component of adjuvant therapy (multi-agent) in women with evidence of axillary lymph node involvement following resection of primary breast cancer

Other cancers: Treatment of acute lymphoblastic leukemia, acute myeloid leukemia, bladder cancer (transitional cell, metastatic), bone sarcoma (metastatic), breast cancer (metastatic), bronchogenic carcinoma, (metastatic), gastric cancer (metastatic), Hodgkin lymphoma, non-Hodgkin lymphomas, neuroblastoma (metastatic), ovarian cancer (metastatic), soft tissue sarcoma (metastatic), thyroid carcinoma (metastatic), Wilms tumor (metastatic).

Local Anesthetic/Vasoconstrictor Precautions No information available to require special precautions

Effects on Dental Treatment Key adverse event(s) related to dental treatment: Stomatitis and mucositis.

Effects on Bleeding Severe myelosuppression with thrombocytopenia and anemia occur. Medical consult suggested.

Adverse Reactions Frequency not always defined.

Cardiovascular:

Acute cardiotoxicity: Atrioventricular block, bradycardia, bundle branch block, ECG abnormality, extrasystoles (atrial or ventricular), nonspecific ST or T wave changes on ECG, sinus tachycardia, supraventricular tachycardia, tachyarrhythmia, ventricular tachycardia

Delayed cardiotoxicity: Cardiac failure (manifestations include ascites, cardiomegaly, dyspnea, edema, gallop rhythm, hepatomegaly, oliguria, pleural effusion, pulmonary edema, tachycardia), decreased left ventricular ejection fraction, myocarditis, pericarditis

Central nervous system: Malaise

Dermatologic: Alopecia, discoloration of sweat, pruritus, skin photosensitivity, skin rash; urticaria

Endocrine & metabolic: Amenorrhea, dehydration, hyperuricemia

Gastrointestinal: Abdominal pain, anorexia, diarrhea, discoloration of saliva, gastrointestinal ulcer, mucositis, nausea, vomiting

Genitourinary: Urine discoloration, infertility (may be temporary)

Hematologic & oncologic: Leukopenia (≤75%; nadir: 10 to 14 days; recovery: by day 21), neutropenia (≤75%; nadir: 10 to 14 days; recovery: by day 21), anemia, thrombocytopenia

Local: Post-injection flare

Neuromuscular & skeletal: Weakness

Ophthalmic: Discoloration of tears

Miscellaneous: Necrosis (colon), radiation recall phenomenon

<1%, postmarketing, and/or case reports: Acute myelocytic leukemia (secondary), anaphylaxis, azoospermia, chills, coma (when in combination with cisplatin or vincristine), conjunctivitis, dysgeusia (Rehwaldt 2009), febrile neutropenia, fever, gonadal disease (gonadal impairment; children), growth suppression (prepubertal), hepatitis, hyperpigmentation (nail, oral mucosa, skin), hypersensitivity reaction (systemic; including angioedema, dysphagia, and dyspnea, pruritus, urticaria), increased serum bilirubin, increased serum transaminases, infection, keratitis, lacrimation, myelodysplastic syndrome, oligospermia, onycholysis, peripheral neurotoxicity (with intra-arterial doxorubicin), phlebosclerosis, pneumonitis (radiation recall; children), seizure (when in combination with cisplatin or vincristine), sepsis, shock, Stevens-Johnson syndrome, toxic epidermal necrolysis, typhlitis (neutropenic)

Mechanism of Action Doxorubicin inhibits DNA and RNA synthesis by intercalation between DNA base pairs by inhibition of topoisomerase II and by steric obstruction. Doxorubicin intercalates at points of local uncoiling of the double helix. Although the exact mechanism is unclear, it appears that direct binding to DNA (intercalation) and inhibition of DNA repair (topoisomerase II inhibition) result in blockade of DNA and RNA synthesis and fragmentation of DNA. Doxorubicin is also a powerful iron chelator; the iron-doxorubicin complex can bind DNA and cell membranes and produce free radicals that immediately cleave the DNA and cell membranes.

Pharmacodynamics/Kinetics

Half-life Elimination

Distribution: ~5 minutes

Terminal: 20 to 48 hours

Male: 54 hours; Female: 35 hours

Reproductive Considerations

Evaluate pregnancy status prior to use in females of reproductive potential.

Females of reproductive potential should use highly effective contraception during treatment and for 6 months after the last doxorubicin dose.

Males with female partners of reproductive potential should use effective contraception during treatment and for 3 to 6 months (depending on manufacturer) after the last doxorubicin dose. In addition, males with pregnant partners should use condoms during treatment and for at least 10 days after the last dose of doxorubicin.

Doxorubicin may impair fertility in males and females. In males, doxorubicin may damage spermatozoa and testicular tissue, resulting in possible genetic fetal abnormalities; may also result in oligospermia, azoospermia, and permanent loss of fertility (sperm counts have been reported to return to normal levels in some men, occurring several years after the end of therapy). In females of reproductive potential, doxorubicin may cause infertility and result in amenorrhea; premature menopause can occur.

Pregnancy Considerations

Doxorubicin crosses the placenta (Ryu 2014). First trimester exposure should be avoided (Azim 2010a; Azim 2010b). A neonatal echocardiogram and ECG are recommended following intrauterine anthracycline exposure (Amant 2019).

Some pharmacokinetic properties of doxorubicin may be altered in pregnant women (Ryu 2014; van Hasselt 2014). Use of doxorubicin in pregnant women has been described for indications such as acute myeloid leukemia, breast cancer, and aggressive Hodgkin and non-Hodgkin lymphomas (Ali 2015; Azim 2011; Lishner 2016; Ring 2005).

The European Society for Medical Oncology (ESMO) has published guidelines for diagnosis, treatment, and follow-up of cancer during pregnancy. The guidelines recommend referral to a facility with expertise in cancer during pregnancy and encourage a multidisciplinary team (obstetrician, neonatologist, oncology team). If chemotherapy is indicated, it should **not** be administered in the first trimester, but may begin in the second trimester. There should be a 3-week time period between the last chemotherapy dose and anticipated delivery, and chemotherapy should not be administered beyond week 33 of gestation (ESMO [Peccatori 2013]).

A pregnancy registry is available for all cancers diagnosed during pregnancy at Cooper Health (877-635-4499).

◆ **Doxorubicin HCl** *see* DOXOrubicin (Conventional) *on page 520*

◆ **DOXOrubicin HCl Peg-Liposomal** *see* DOXOrubicin (Liposomal) *on page 521*

◆ **Doxorubicin Hydrochloride** *see* DOXOrubicin (Conventional) *on page 520*

◆ **DOXOrubicin Hydrochloride (Liposomal)** *see* DOXOrubicin (Liposomal) *on page 521*

◆ **DOXOrubicin Hydrochloride Liposome** *see* DOXOrubicin (Liposomal) *on page 521*

DOXOrubicin (Liposomal)

(doks oh ROO bi sin lye po SO mal)

Related Information

DOXOrubicin (Conventional) *on page 520*

Brand Names: US Doxil; Lipodox 50 [DSC]

Brand Names: Canada Caelyx; TARO-Doxorubicin Liposomal

Pharmacologic Category Antineoplastic Agent, Anthracycline; Antineoplastic Agent, Topoisomerase II Inhibitor

Use

AIDS-related Kaposi sarcoma: Treatment of AIDS-related Kaposi sarcoma (after failure of or intolerance to prior systemic therapy)

Multiple myeloma: Treatment of multiple myeloma (in combination with bortezomib) in patients who are bortezomib-naïve and have received at least 1 prior therapy

Ovarian cancer, advanced: Treatment of progressive or recurrent ovarian cancer (after platinum-based treatment)

Local Anesthetic/Vasoconstrictor Precautions

No information available to require special precautions

Effects on Dental Treatment Key adverse event(s) related to dental treatment: Xerostomia (normal salivary flow resumes upon discontinuation), mucositis, gingivitis, glossitis, mouth ulceration, taste perversion, and stomatitis.

Effects on Bleeding Severe myelosuppression with thrombocytopenia and anemia occur. Medical consult suggested.

Adverse Reactions

>10%:

Cardiovascular: Cardiomyopathy (≤11%)

Central nervous system: Fatigue (>20%), headache (1% to 11%)

Dermatologic: Palmar-plantar erythrodysesthesia (ovarian cancer: 51%), skin rash (ovarian cancer: 29%, Kaposi sarcoma: 1% to 5%), alopecia (ovarian cancer: 19%; Kaposi sarcoma: 9%)

Gastrointestinal: Nausea (ovarian cancer: 46%; Kaposi sarcoma: 17%), stomatitis (ovarian cancer: 41%; ovarian cancer, grades 3/4: 8%: Kaposi sarcoma: 7%), vomiting (ovarian cancer: 33%; Kaposi sarcoma: 8%), diarrhea (ovarian cancer: 21%; Kaposi sarcoma: 8%), constipation (>20%), anorexia (20%; Kaposi sarcoma: 1% to 5%), mucous membrane disease (ovarian cancer: 14%), dyspepsia (ovarian cancer: 12%)

Hematologic & oncologic: Thrombocytopenia (Kaposi sarcoma: grade 3: 61%, grade 4: 4%; ovarian cancer: grade 3: 1%), anemia (Kaposi sarcoma: grade 3: 55%, grade 4: 18%; grade 3: 5%, grade 4: <1%), neutropenia (Kaposi sarcoma: grade 3: 49%, grade 4: 13%; ovarian cancer: grade 3: 8%, grade 4: 4%)

Infection: Infection (1% to 12%)

Neuromuscular & skeletal: Asthenia (ovarian cancer: 40%; Kaposi sarcoma: 10%), back pain (1% to 12%)

Respiratory: Pharyngitis (ovarian cancer: 16%; Kaposi sarcoma: <1%), dyspnea (ovarian cancer: 15%; Kaposi sarcoma: 1% to 5%)

Miscellaneous: Fever (ovarian cancer: 21%; Kaposi sarcoma: 9%), infusion related reaction (7% to 11%)

1% to 10%:

Cardiovascular: Deep vein thrombosis (ovarian cancer: 1% to 10%), hypotension (1% to 10%), tachycardia (1% to 10%), vasodilation (ovarian cancer: 1% to 10%), chest pain (1% to 5%), peripheral edema (ovarian cancer: 1% to 5%)

Central nervous system: Depression (ovarian cancer: 1% to 10%), dizziness (1% to 10%), drowsiness (1% to 10%), anxiety (ovarian cancer: 1% to 5%), chills (1% to 5%), emotional lability (Kaposi sarcoma: 1% to 5%), insomnia (ovarian cancer: 1% to 5%), malaise (ovarian cancer: 1% to 5%)

Dermatologic: Acne vulgaris (ovarian cancer: 1% to 10%), ecchymoses (ovarian cancer: 1% to 10%), exfoliative dermatitis (ovarian cancer: 1% to 10%), fungal dermatitis (ovarian cancer: 1% to 10%), furunculosis (ovarian cancer: 1% to 10%), herpes simplex dermatitis (1% to 10%), maculopapular rash (ovarian cancer: 1% to 10%; Kaposi sarcoma: <1%), pruritus (1% to 10%), skin discoloration (ovarian cancer: 1% to 10%), vesiculobullous dermatitis (ovarian cancer: 1% to 10%), xeroderma (ovarian cancer: 1% to 10%), diaphoresis (ovarian cancer: 1% to 5%)

Endocrine & metabolic: Dehydration (ovarian cancer: 1% to 10%; Kaposi sarcoma: <1%), hypercalcemia (ovarian cancer: 1% to 10%), hypokalemia (ovarian cancer: 1% to 10%), hyponatremia (ovarian cancer: 1% to 10%), weight loss (1% to 10%), albuminuria

(Kaposi sarcoma: 1% to 5%), hyperglycemia (Kaposi sarcoma: 1% to 5%), hypocalcemia (Kaposi sarcoma: 1% to 5%)

Gastrointestinal: Dysgeusia (ovarian cancer: 1% to 10%; Kaposi sarcoma: <1%), dysphagia (1% to 10%), esophagitis (ovarian cancer: 1% to 10%), intestinal obstruction (ovarian cancer: 1% to 10%), oral candidiasis (1% to 10%), oral mucosa ulcer (1% to 10%), abdominal pain (Kaposi sarcoma: 1% to 5%), aphthous stomatitis (Kaposi sarcoma: 1% to 5%), enlargement of abdomen (ovarian cancer 1% to 5%), glossitis (Kaposi sarcoma: 1% to 5%)

Genitourinary: Hematuria (ovarian cancer: 1% to 10%), urinary tract infection (ovarian cancer: 1% to 10%), vulvovaginal candidiasis (ovarian cancer: 1% to 10%)

Hematologic & oncologic: Rectal hemorrhage (ovarian cancer: 1% to 10%), hypochromic anemia (Kaposi sarcoma: ≥5%), hemolysis (Kaposi sarcoma: 1% to 5%), prolonged prothrombin time (Kaposi sarcoma: 1% to 5%)

Hepatic: Hyperbilirubinemia (1% to 10%), increased serum alkaline phosphatase (Kaposi sarcoma: 8%), increased serum alanine aminotransferase (Kaposi sarcoma: 1% to 5%)

Hypersensitivity: Hypersensitivity reaction (1% to 5%)

Infection: Herpes zoster infection (ovarian cancer: 1% to 10%; Kaposi sarcoma: <1%), paresthesia (5%), myalgia (ovarian cancer: 1% to 5%)

Ophthalmic: Conjunctivitis (ovarian cancer: 1% to 10%; Kaposi sarcoma: <1%), dry eye syndrome (ovarian cancer: 1% to 10%), retinitis (Kaposi sarcoma 1% to 5%)

Respiratory: Increased cough (ovarian cancer: 10%; Kaposi sarcoma: <1%), epistaxis (ovarian cancer: 1% to 10%), pneumonia (1% to 10%), rhinitis (ovarian cancer: 1% to 10%), sinusitis (ovarian cancer: 1% to 10%)

<1%: Bundle branch block, candidiasis, cardiac failure, cryptococcosis, hepatitis, palpitations, sepsis, thrombophlebitis, thrombosis, ventricular arrhythmia

Frequency not defined:

Hematologic & oncologic: Bone marrow depression, progression of cancer

Infection: Toxoplasmosis

Ophthalmic: Optic neuritis

Postmarketing: Erythema multiforme, lichenoid eruption (keratosis), muscle spasm, pulmonary embolism, secondary acute myelocytic leukemia, squamous cell carcinoma, Stevens-Johnson syndrome, toxic epidermal necrolysis

Mechanism of Action Doxorubicin inhibits DNA and RNA synthesis by intercalating between DNA base pairs causing steric obstruction and inhibits topoisomerase-II at the point of DNA cleavage. Doxorubicin is also a powerful iron chelator. The iron-doxorubicin complex can bind DNA and cell membranes, producing free hydroxyl (OH) radicals that cleave DNA and cell membranes. Active throughout entire cell cycle. Doxorubicin liposomal is a pegylated formulation which protects the liposomes, and thereby increases blood circulation time.

Pharmacodynamics/Kinetics

Half-life Elimination Terminal: Distribution: ~4.7 to 5.2 hours, Elimination: ~52 to 55 hours

Reproductive Considerations

Evaluate pregnancy status prior to use in females of reproductive potential. Women of reproductive potential and men with female partners of reproductive potential should use effective contraception during therapy and for 6 months after treatment. Doxorubicin liposomal may impair fertility in men and women. In men, doxorubicin may damage spermatozoa and testicular tissue, resulting in possible genetic fetal abnormalities; may also result in oligospermia, azoospermia, and permanent loss of fertility (sperm counts have been reported to return to normal levels in some men, occurring several years after the end of therapy). In females of reproductive potential, doxorubicin may cause infertility and result in amenorrhea; premature menopause can occur.

Pregnancy Considerations

Based on the mechanism of action and data from animal reproduction studies, doxorubicin (liposomal) may cause fetal harm if administered during pregnancy. Use during the first trimester should be avoided.

◆ **Doxy 100** *see* Doxycycline *on page 522*

Doxycycline (doks i SYE kleen)

Related Information

Periodontal Diseases *on page 1748*

Sexually-Transmitted Diseases *on page 1707*

Related Sample Prescriptions

Bacterial Infections and Periodontal Diseases - Sample Prescriptions *on page 35*

Brand Names: US Acticlate; Adoxa Pak 1/100 [DSC]; Adoxa Pak 1/150 [DSC]; Adoxa Pak 2/100 [DSC]; Adoxa [DSC]; Avidoxy; Doryx; Doryx MPC; Doxy 100; Mondoxyne NL; Monodox [DSC]; Morgidox; Okebo [DSC]; Oracea; Soloxide; TargaDOX; Vibramycin

Brand Names: Canada APO-Doxy; Apprilon; DOM-Doxycycline [DSC]; Doxycin; Doxytab; Periostat; PHL-Doxycycline [DSC]; PMS-Doxycycline [DSC]; TEVA-Doxycycline

Generic Availability (US) May be product dependent

Pharmacologic Category Antibiotic, Tetracycline Derivative

Dental Use Treatment of periodontitis associated with presence of *Actinobacillus actinomycetemcomitans* (AA); adjunct to scaling and root planing to promote attachment level gain and to reduce pocket depth in adult periodontitis (systemic levels are subinhibitory against bacteria)

Use

Acne: Adjunctive therapy in severe acne.

Actinomycosis: Treatment of actinomycosis caused by *Actinomyces israelii* when penicillin is contraindicated.

Acute intestinal amebiasis: Adjunct to amebicides in acute intestinal amebiasis.

Anthrax, including inhalational anthrax (postexposure): Treatment of anthrax caused by *Bacillus anthracis*, including inhalational (postexposure) prophylaxis; to reduce the incidence or progression of disease following exposure to aerosolized *B. anthracis*.

Cholera: Treatment of cholera infections caused by *Vibrio cholerae*.

Clostridium: Treatment of infections caused by *Clostridium* spp. when penicillin is contraindicated.

Gram-negative infections: Treatment of infections caused by *Escherichia coli*, *Enterobacter aerogenes*, *Shigella* spp., *Acinetobacter* spp., *Klebsiella* spp. (respiratory and urinary infections), and *Bacteroides* spp.; *Neisseria meningitidis* (when penicillin is contraindicated).

Gram-positive infections: Treatment of infections caused by *Streptococcus* spp., when susceptible.

Listeriosis: Treatment of listeriosis due to *Listeria monocytogenes* when penicillin is contraindicated.

Malaria, prophylaxis: Prophylaxis of malaria due to *Plasmodium falciparum* in short-term travelers (under 4 months) to areas with chloroquine and/or pyrimethamine-sulfadoxine-resistant strains.

Mycoplasma pneumoniae: Treatment of infections caused by *Mycoplasma pneumoniae*.

Ophthalmic infections: Treatment of inclusion conjunctivitis or trachoma caused by *Chlamydia trachomatis*.

Periodontitis (20 mg tablet and capsule [Periostat (Canadian product)] only): Adjunct to scaling and root planing to promote attachment level gain and to reduce pocket depth in patients with adult periodontitis.

Relapsing fever: Treatment of relapsing fever caused by *Borrelia recurrentis*.

Respiratory tract infections: Treatment of respiratory infections caused by *Haemophilus influenzae*, *Klebsiella* spp., or *Mycoplasma pneumoniae*; treatment of upper respiratory tract infections caused by *Streptococcus pneumoniae*; respiratory infections caused by *Staphylococcus aureus* (doxycycline is not the drug of choice in the treatment of any type of staphylococcal infection).

Rickettsial infections: Treatment of Rocky Mountain spotted fever, typhus fever and the typhus group, Q fever, rickettsialpox, and tick fevers caused by *Rickettsiae*.

Rosacea (Oracea, Apprilon [Canadian product] only): Treatment of only inflammatory lesions (papules and pustules) of rosacea in adults.

Sexually transmitted infections: Treatment of lymphogranuloma venereum and uncomplicated urethral, endocervical, or rectal infections caused by *Chlamydia trachomatis*; granuloma inguinale (donovanosis) caused by *Klebsiella granulomatis*; chancroid caused by *Haemophilus ducreyi*; nongonococcal urethritis caused by *Ureaplasma urealyticum*; when penicillin is contraindicated, uncomplicated gonorrhea caused by *Neisseria gonorrhea* and syphilis caused by *Treponema pallidum*.

Note: The CDC sexually transmitted disease guidelines recommend dual antimicrobial therapy be used for uncomplicated gonorrhea due to *N. gonorrhea* resistance concerns; ceftriaxone is the preferred cephalosporin and doxycycline is an alternative option for the second antimicrobial only in cases of azithromycin allergy (CDC [Workowski 2015]).

Skin and skin structure infections (Avidoxy only): Treatment of skin and skin structure infections caused by *Staphylococcus aureus* (doxycycline is not the drug of choice in the treatment of any type of staphylococcal infection).

Vincent infection: Treatment of Vincent infection caused by *Fusobacterium fusiforme* when penicillin is contraindicated.

Yaws: Treatment of yaws caused by *Treponema pallidum* subspecies *pertenue* when penicillin is contraindicated.

Zoonotic infections: Treatment of psittacosis (ornithosis) caused by *Chlamydophila psittaci*; plague due to *Yersinia pestis*; tularemia caused by *Francisella tularensis*; brucellosis caused by *Brucella* spp. (in conjunction with streptomycin); bartonellosis caused by *Bartonella bacilliformis*; infections caused by *Campylobacter fetus*.

Local Anesthetic/Vasoconstrictor Precautions No information available to require special precautions

Effects on Dental Treatment Key adverse event(s) related to dental treatment: Occurrence of xerostomia (normal salivation resumes upon discontinuation); occurrence of nasal congestion, sinusitis, and nasopharyngitis; rare occurrence of glossitis and tooth discoloration (children). Opportunistic "superinfection" with *Candida albicans*; tetracyclines are not recommended for use during pregnancy or in children ≤8 years of age since they have been reported to cause enamel hypoplasia and permanent teeth discoloration. The use of tetracyclines should only be used in these patients if other agents are contraindicated or alternative antimicrobials will not eradicate the organism.

Effects on Bleeding Hemolytic anemia and thrombocytopenia have been reported

Adverse Reactions

1% to 10%:

- Cardiovascular: Hypertension (3%)
- Central nervous system: Anxiety (2%), pain (2%)
- Endocrine & metabolic: Increased lactate dehydrogenase (2%), increased serum glucose (1%)
- Gastrointestinal: Diarrhea (5%), upper abdominal pain (2%), abdominal distention (1%), abdominal pain (1%), xerostomia (1%)
- Hepatic: Increased serum aspartate aminotransferase (2%)
- Infection: Fungal infection (2%), influenza (2%)
- Neuromuscular & skeletal: Back pain (1%)
- Respiratory: Nasopharyngitis (5%), sinusitis (3%), nasal congestion (2%), sinus headache (1%)

Frequency not defined:

- Dermatologic: Skin hyperpigmentation
- Gastrointestinal: Esophageal ulcer, esophagitis

<1%, postmarketing, and/or case reports: Anaphylactoid reaction, anaphylaxis, angioedema, anorexia, bulging fontanel, *Clostridioides difficile* associated diarrhea, *Clostridioides difficile* colitis, dental discoloration, DRESS syndrome, dysphagia, enamel hypoplasia, enterocolitis, eosinophilia, erythema multiforme, erythematous rash, exacerbation of systemic lupus erythematosus, exfoliative dermatitis, glossitis, headache, hemolytic anemia, hepatotoxicity, hypersensitivity reaction, increased blood urea nitrogen, increased serum alanine aminotransferase, inflammatory anogenital lesion, intracranial hypertension, Jarisch-Herxheimer reaction, maculopapular rash, nausea, neutropenia, pancreatitis, pericarditis, serum sickness, skin hyperpigmentation, skin photosensitivity, Stevens-Johnson syndrome, thrombocytopenia, thyroid disease (brown/black discoloration; no dysfunction reported), toxic epidermal necrolysis, urticaria, vomiting

Dental Usual Dosage Adults: Oral: Treatment of periodontitis (refractory): 100-200 mg once daily for 21 days (Jolkovsky 2006). **Note:** A specific formulation (Periostat [available in Canada]) containing a subantimicrobial dosage is also available for use as an adjunct to scaling and root planing. In addition, doxycycline gel (Atridox) is available for subgingival application (see Doxycycline Hyclate Periodontal Extended-Release Liquid monograph).

Dosing

Adult & Geriatric Note: Doxycycline is available as hyclate, monohydrate, and calcium salts. All doses are expressed as doxycycline base.

Usual dosage range:

Oral: IR and most ER formulations: 100 to 200 mg/day in 1 to 2 divided doses. **Note:** 120 mg of modified polymer coated tablet (Doryx MPC) is equivalent to 100 mg conventional delayed-release tablet.

IV: 100 mg every 12 hours. **Note:** IV form may cause phlebitis.

Acne vulgaris (moderate to severe, inflammatory) (off-label dose): Oral: Note: Use as an adjunct to topical acne therapy (AAD [Zaenglein 2016]).

Immediate release: 50 to 100 mg twice daily or 100 mg once daily (AAD [Zaenglein 2016]; Graber 2020).

Extended release: 100 mg twice daily on day 1, then 100 mg once daily (AAD [Zaenglein 2016]; Graber 2020).

Subantimicrobial dosing: 20 mg twice daily (immediate release) or 40 mg once daily (delayed release) (Moore 2015; Skidmore 2003).

Duration: Use the shortest possible duration to minimize risk of adverse effects and development of bacterial resistance; re-evaluate at 3 to 4 months (AAD [Zaenglein 2016]).

Actinomycosis (alternative agent): Oral, IV: 100 mg every 12 hours (Brook 2020; Cone 2003; Olson 2013). Duration of therapy is 2 to 6 months for mild infection and 6 to 12 months (including 4 to 6 weeks of parenteral therapy) for severe or extensive infection (Brook 2020).

Anaplasmosis and ehrlichiosis (off-label use): Oral, IV: 100 mg twice daily for 10 days (IDSA [Wormser 2006]) or at least 3 days after resolution of fever (CDC [Biggs 2016]).

Anthrax: Note: Consult public health officials for event-specific recommendations.

Inhalational exposure (postexposure prophylaxis [PEP]): **Oral:** 100 mg every 12 hours for 42 to 60 days (CDC [Hendricks 2014]).

Note: Anthrax vaccine should also be administered to exposed individuals (CDC [Bower 2019]; CDC [Hendricks 2014]). **Duration of therapy:** If the PEP anthrax vaccine series is administered on schedule (for all regimens), antibiotics may be discontinued in immunocompetent adults aged 18 to 65 years at 42 days after initiation of vaccine or 2 weeks after the last dose of the vaccine (whichever comes last and not to exceed 60 days); if the vaccination series cannot be completed, antibiotics should continue for 60 days (CDC [Bower 2019]). In addition, adults with immunocompromising conditions or receiving immunosuppressive therapy, patients >65 years of age, and patients who are pregnant or breastfeeding should receive antibiotics for 60 days (CDC [Bower 2019]).

Cutaneous (without systemic involvement), treatment: **Oral:** 100 mg every 12 hours for 7 to 10 days after naturally acquired infection; treat for 60 days for bioterrorism-related cases (CDC [Hendricks 2014]). **Note:** Patients with cutaneous lesions of the head or neck or extensive edema should be treated for systemic involvement.

Systemic (meningitis excluded; alternative agent), treatment: **IV:** Initial: 200 mg as a single dose, then 100 mg every 12 hours, in combination with a bactericidal agent; treat for 2 weeks or until clinically stable, whichever is longer. **Note:** Antitoxin should also be administered for systemic anthrax. Following a course of IV combination therapy, patients exposed to aerosolized spores require oral doxycycline monotherapy to complete an antimicrobial course of 60 days (CDC [Hendricks 2014]).

***Bartonella* spp. infection:**

HIV-infected: **Note:** Duration of therapy is at least 3 months; continuation of therapy depends on relapse occurrence and clinical condition (HHS [OI adult 2020]).

Bacillary angiomatosis, peliosis hepatis, bacteremia, and osteomyelitis: **Oral, IV:** 100 mg every 12 hours (HHS [OI adult 2020]). **Note:** Some experts recommend concomitant gentamicin for the first 2 weeks of therapy for patients with *Bartonella* bloodstream infection (Rolain 2004; Spach 2019a).

CNS infections: **Oral, IV:** 100 mg every 12 hours; may add rifampin therapy (HHS [OI adult 2020]).

Endocarditis: **Oral, IV:** 100 mg IV every 12 hours in combination with gentamicin for 2 weeks, then continue with doxycycline 100 mg IV or orally every 12 hours (HHS [OI adult 2020]).

Other severe infections: **Oral, IV:** 100 mg every 12 hours in combination with rifampin (HHS [OI adult 2020]).

HIV-uninfected:

Bacteremia without endocarditis: **Oral:** 200 mg once daily **or** 100 mg twice daily for 4 weeks with gentamicin once daily for first 2 weeks (Foucault 2003; Rolain 2004).

Cat-scratch disease, CNS infection, and neuroretinitis: **Oral, IV:** 100 mg twice daily in combination with rifampin (Rolain 2004).

Endocarditis: **Oral:** 100 mg every 12 hours for 6 to 12 weeks with gentamicin for first 2 weeks (Rolain 2004; Spach 2019b).

Bite wound infection, prophylaxis or treatment (animal or human bite) (alternative agent) (off-label use): Oral, IV: 100 mg twice daily. Duration is 3 to 5 days for prophylaxis (IDSA [Stevens 2014]); duration of treatment for established infection is typically 5 to 14 days (Baddour 2019a; Baddour 2019b). **Note:** Some experts use in combination with an appropriate agent for anaerobes (Baddour 2019a; Baddour 2019b; IDSA [Stevens 2014]).

Brucellosis:

Treatment:

Endocarditis or neurobrucellosis: Limited data available: **IV, Oral:** 100 mg twice daily for at least 12 weeks (may be needed for up to 6 months); use as part of an appropriate combination regimen (Bosilkovski 2019; Jia 2017; Zheng 2018).

Uncomplicated (nonfocal): **Oral:** 100 mg twice daily for 6 weeks as part of an appropriate combination regimen (Ariza 2007; Hasanjani Roushan 2006; Skalsky 2008).

Spondylitis: **Oral:** 100 mg twice daily for at least 12 weeks as part of an appropriate combination regimen (Bosilkovski 2019; Colmenero 1994).

Postexposure prophylaxis (high-risk laboratory exposure): **Oral:** 100 mg twice daily with rifampin for 3 weeks (CDC 2012); for exposure to *B. abortus* RB51 strains, some experts give doxycycline plus trimethoprim-sulfamethoxazole (Bosilkovski 2019).

Cellulitis, mild to moderate (outpatient treatment; empiric coverage of MRSA) (off-label use): Oral: 100 mg twice daily for 5 to 14 days (IDSA [Liu 2011]; IDSA [Stevens 2014]). **Note:** For empiric therapy of nonpurulent cellulitis, an additional agent (eg, amoxicillin, cephalexin) for coverage of beta-hemolytic streptococci is needed.

Cholera (*Vibrio cholerae*), treatment (adjunctive therapy for severely ill patients): Oral: 300 mg as a single dose. **Note**: Due to resistance concerns, antimicrobial therapy during an outbreak or epidemic should be guided by isolate susceptibility (CDC 2015; WHO 2010).

Chronic obstructive pulmonary disease, acute exacerbation: Oral: 200 mg once daily for 5 to 7 days (Daniels 2010; GOLD 2020). **Note:** Some experts reserve for patients with uncomplicated COPD (eg, age <65 years without major comorbidities, FEV_1 >50% predicted, infrequent exacerbations) (Anzueto 2007; Sethi 2008).

Hidradenitis suppurativa (off-label use): Oral: 100 mg once or twice daily (Ingram 2020; Vural 2019).

Lyme disease (*Borrelia* spp. infection) (off-label use):

Prophylaxis: **Oral:** 200 mg as a single dose. **Note:** Prophylaxis is used only in patients who meet **all** of the following criteria: Deer tick attached for ≥36 hours, prophylaxis can be given within 72 hours of tick removal, local rate of deer tick infection with *Borrelia burgdorferi* is ≥20%, and there are no contraindications to doxycycline (Hu 2017; IDSA [Wormser 2006]).

Treatment, early localized disease (single erythema migrans lesion): **Oral:** 100 mg twice daily for 10 to 21 days (IDSA [Wormser 2006]); some experts prefer a 10-day duration (Sanchez 2016; Wormser 2003).

Treatment, early disseminated disease (multiple erythema migrans lesions): **Oral:**100 mg twice daily for 14 to 21 days (Hu 2019).

Treatment, early disseminated neurologic disease (isolated facial nerve palsy, meningitis, or radiculoneuropathy): **Oral:** 100 mg twice daily for 14 days (range: 14 to 28 days) (Hu 2019; IDSA [Wormser 2006]).

Treatment, early disseminated carditis (initial therapy for mild disease [first-degree atrioventricular block with PR interval <300 msec] or step-down therapy after initial parenteral treatment for more severe disease once PR interval <300 msec): **Oral:** 100 mg twice daily for 14 to 21 days (IDSA [Wormser 2006], although some experts extend the duration up to 28 days in those with serious disease (Hu 2019).

Treatment, arthritis without neurologic involvement: **Oral:** 100 mg twice daily for 28 days (IDSA [Wormser 2006]).

Malaria:

Prophylaxis: **Oral** (immediate release and delayed release): 100 mg daily; initiate 1 to 2 days prior to travel to endemic area; continue daily during travel and for 4 weeks after leaving endemic area.

Treatment (alternative agent) (off-label use): **Oral:** 100 mg twice daily for 7 days in combination with quinine sulfate (quinine sulfate duration is region specific). **Note:** If used for *P. vivax* or *P. ovale*, use in combination with primaquine. If used for severe malaria (after completion of IV therapy), use full 7-day schedule of doxycycline (CDC 2020).

Otitis media, acute (alternative agent if unable to tolerate penicillins and cephalosporins) (off-label use): Oral: 100 mg every 12 hours; duration of therapy is 5 to 7 days (mild to moderate infection) **or** 10 days (severe infection) (Limb 2019).

Periodontitis, chronic: *Subantimicrobial dosing:* **Oral:** 20 mg twice daily (immediate release) for 3 to 9 months as an adjunct to periodontal debridement (Smiley 2015).

Plague (*Yersinia pestis*) (alternative agent): Oral, IV: 200 mg initially then 100 mg twice daily **or** 200 mg once daily for 10 to 14 days and at least until 2 days after patient has defervesced (CDC 2015; IDSA [Stevens 2014]; Inglesby 2000; Sexton 2019a).

Pleurodesis, chemical (sclerosing agent for pleural effusion) (off-label use): Intrapleural: 500 mg as a single dose in 30 to 100 mL NS (Porcel 2006; Robinson 1993); may require a repeat dose (Kvale 2007); some experts combine with or administer following instillation of a local anesthetic (eg, lidocaine, 10 mL [100 mg] of 1% solution [Robinson 1993] or mepivacaine 20 mL [400 mg] of 2% solution [Porcel 2006]).

Pneumonia, community-acquired, empiric therapy:

Outpatients with no risk factors for antibiotic resistant pathogens: **Oral:** 100 mg twice daily; must be used as part of an appropriate combination regimen in outpatients with comorbidities (ATS/IDSA [Metlay 2019]). Some experts prefer to use as part of an appropriate combination regimen in all outpatients, regardless of comorbidities (File 2019).

Inpatients (alternative agent): **Oral, IV:** 100 mg twice daily as part of an appropriate combination regimen (ATS/IDSA [Metlay 2019]).

Duration: Minimum of 5 days; patients should be clinically stable with normal vital signs before discontinuing therapy (ATS/IDSA [Metlay 2019]).

Prosthetic joint infection (off-label use):

Treatment: Oral continuation therapy for S. aureus (following pathogen-specific IV therapy in patients undergoing 1-stage exchange or debridement with retention of prosthesis) (alternative agent): **Oral:** 100 mg twice daily in combination with rifampin; duration is a minimum of 3 months, depending on patient-specific factors (Berbari 2019; IDSA [Osmon 2013]).

Chronic suppression for staphylococci (methicillin resistant) and Cutibacterium acnes (alternative agent for C. acnes): **Oral:** 100 mg twice daily (IDSA [Osmon 2013]).

Q fever: Oral:

Acute: 100 mg every 12 hours for 14 days (CDC [Anderson 2013]). **Note:** In patients with valvulopathy/cardiomyopathy, some experts recommend extending treatment to 12 months in combination with hydroxychloroquine to prevent progression to persistent infection (Million 2013; Raoult 2020).

Persistent localized infection (endocarditis, vascular infection): **Oral:** 100 mg every 12 hours in combination with hydroxychloroquine for ≥18 months depending on site of infection and serologic response (CDC [Anderson 2013]).

Rhinosinusitis, acute bacterial (alternative agent for beta-lactam intolerance): Oral: 200 mg/day in 1 to 2 divided doses for 5 to 7 days (IDSA [Chow 2012]). **Note:** In uncomplicated acute bacterial rhinosinusitis, initial observation and symptom management without antibiotic therapy is appropriate in most patients (ACP/CDC [Harris 2016]).

Rocky Mountain spotted fever: Oral, IV: 100 mg twice daily for 5 to 7 days or for at least 3 days after fever subsides, whichever is longer; initiate treatment as soon as possible. Severe or complicated disease may require longer treatment (CDC [Biggs 2016]). **Note:** A loading dose of 200 mg IV is recommended for critically ill patients (Sexton 2019b).

Rosacea, moderate to severe or unresponsive to topical therapy: Oral:

Traditional dosing (off-label dose): Initial: 50 to 100 mg twice daily for 4 to 12 weeks; may follow with a topical agent and/or subantimicrobial doxycycline dosing for long-term management. Alternatively, may initiate therapy with subantimicrobial dosing (Akhyani 2008; Maier 2019).

Subantimicrobial dosing: 40 mg once daily (delayed release; Oracea) or 20 mg twice daily (immediate release) (Sanchez 2005).

Sexually transmitted infections:

Cervicitis or urethritis:

Chlamydia trachomatis: **Oral:** 100 mg twice daily for 7 days (CDC [Workowski 2015]) **or** 200 mg delayed release once daily for 7 days (Geisler 2012); consider concurrent treatment for gonorrhea with a single dose of ceftriaxone based on individual risk factors, if local prevalence is elevated (>5%), or if intracellular gram-negative diplococci on Gram stain (CDC [Workowski 2015]; Marrazzo 2017). **Note:** Directly observed single-dose azithromycin is preferred for the treatment of uncomplicated genital chlamydial infections by some experts (Marrazzo 2017).

Neisseria gonorrhea (alternative agent [due to resistance]; reserve for patients with azithromycin intolerance): **Oral:** 100 mg twice daily for 7 days in combination with a single dose of ceftriaxone (CDC [Workowski 2015]).

Epididymitis, acute (off-label use): Empiric or pathogen-directed therapy for chlamydia and/or gonorrhea: **Oral:** 100 mg twice daily for 10 days with single dose of ceftriaxone (CDC [Workowski 2015]). **Note:** An alternative regimen is recommended in patients who practice insertive anal sex (Eyre 2019; Marrazzo 2017).

Granuloma inguinale (donovanosis) (alternative agent): **Oral:** 100 mg twice daily for at least 3 weeks and until all lesions have healed. **Note:** If symptoms do not improve within the first few days of therapy, another agent (eg, aminoglycoside) can be added (CDC [Workowski 2015]).

Lymphogranuloma venereum: **Oral:** 100 mg twice daily for 21 days (CDC [Workowski 2015]).

Pelvic inflammatory disease (off-label use):

Inpatient (severe PID): **IV, Oral:** 100 mg every 12 hours in combination with cefoxitin or cefotetan; transition to oral therapy after >24 hours improvement to complete a 14-day total course. If pelvic abscess, anaerobic coverage is warranted (CDC [Workowski 2015]).

Outpatient (mild to moderate PID): **Oral:** 100 mg every 12 hours for 14 days in combination with a single dose of ceftriaxone (preferred) (Wiesenfeld 2019) **or** single dose of cefoxitin plus oral probenecid or other third generation cephalosporin; if *Trichomonas vaginalis* or recent uterine instrumentation, add metronidazole (CDC [Workowski 2015]).

Proctitis, acute or proctocolitis (off-label use): Empiric or pathogen-directed therapy for chlamydia and/or gonorrhea: **Oral:** 100 mg twice daily for 7 days plus a single dose of ceftriaxone. **Note:** Provide 21 days of doxycycline if polymerase chain reaction (PCR) for lymphogranuloma venereum (LGV) confirmed or as presumptive therapy for LGV if patient has severe rectal symptoms (eg, bloody discharge, perianal ulcers, or mucosal ulcers), and either a positive rectal chlamydia NAAT or HIV infection. Additional coverage for herpes simplex virus is warranted in patients with perianal or mucosal ulcers (CDC [Workowski 2015]).

Syphilis, penicillin-allergic patients: **Note:** Limited data support use of alternatives to penicillin and close serologic and clinical follow up is warranted (CDC [Workowski 2015]; Hicks 2019).

Early syphilis (primary, secondary, and early latent): **Oral:** 100 mg twice daily for 14 days (CDC [Workowski 2015]).

Late syphilis (late latent): **Oral:** 100 mg twice daily for 28 days (CDC [Workowski 2015]).

Surgical prophylaxis, uterine evacuation (induced abortion or pregnancy loss) (off-label use): Oral: 200 mg as a single dose 1 hour prior to uterine aspiration (ACOG 195 2018); may be administered up to 12 hours before the procedure (Achilles 2011). **Note:** The optimal dosing regimen has not been established; various protocols are in use (Achilles 2011; RCOG 2015; White 2018; White 2019).

Tularemia (*Francisella tularensis*):

Treatment (mild infection) (alternative agent): **Oral:** 100 mg twice daily for 14 to 21 days (IDSA [Stevens 2014]; Penn 2019).

Postexposure prophylaxis (nonbioterrorism event, high-risk exposure): **Oral:** 100 mg twice daily for 14 days (Penn 2019).

Bioterrorism event: **Note:** Consult public health officials for event-specific recommendations.

Mass casualty management or postexposure prophylaxis (when used as a biological weapon): **Oral:** 100 mg twice daily for 14 days (Dennis 2001).

Contained casualty management (when used as a biological weapon): **IV** (may transition to oral if clinically appropriate): 100 mg every 12 hours for 14 to 21 days (Dennis 2001).

Renal Impairment: Adult

The renal dosing recommendations are based upon the best available evidence and clinical expertise. Senior Editorial Team: Bruce Mueller, PharmD, FCCP, FASN, FNKF; Jason Roberts, PhD, BPharm (Hons), B App Sc, FSHP, FISAC; Michael Heung, MD, MS.

IV, Oral:

Mild to severe impairment: No dosage adjustment necessary (Alestig 1973; Lee 1972).

Hemodialysis, intermittent (thrice weekly): Poorly dialyzed (0% to 5%); no supplemental dose or dosage adjustment necessary (Houin 1983; Lee 1972; Letteri 1973).

Peritoneal dialysis: Poorly dialyzed; no dosage adjustment necessary (Letteri 1973).

CRRT: No dosage adjustment necessary (Heintz 2009).

PIRRT (eg, sustained, low-efficiency diafiltration): No dosage adjustment necessary (expert opinion).

Hepatic Impairment: Adult There are no dosage adjustments provided in the manufacturer's labeling.

Pediatric Note: Doxycycline is available as hyclate, monohydrate, and calcium salts. All doses are expressed as doxycycline base.

General dosing:

Children and Adolescents: Oral, IV: 2.2 mg/kg/dose every 12 hours, maximum dose: 100 mg/dose. **Note:** Use of doxycycline in children <8 years should be reserved for severe, potentially life-threatening infections, or when better alternatives are unavailable (*Red Book* [AAP 2018]; manufacturer's labeling).

Acne vulgaris, moderate to severe, treatment: Limited data available: Children ≥8 years and Adolescents: Oral: 50 to 100 mg once or twice daily or 150 mg once daily (Eichenfeld 2013).

Anthrax (AAP [Bradley 2014]): **Note:** Consult public health officials for event-specific recommendations.

Prophylaxis; postexposure (inhalation or cutaneous); prior to susceptibility testing or penicillin-resistant strains: **Note:** Doxycycline is a preferred option or ciprofloxacin: Infants, Children, and Adolescents: Treatment duration: 60 days.

Patient weight <45 kg: Oral: 2.2 mg/kg/dose every 12 hours.

Patient weight ≥45 kg: Oral: 100 mg every 12 hours.

Treatment; susceptible strains:

Cutaneous infection without systemic involvement: **Note:** Doxycycline is an option if first-line therapy (ie, ciprofloxacin) is unavailable or patient unable to tolerate; for naturally-occurring infection, usual treatment duration is 7 to 10 days; in the event of biological weapon exposure, additional therapy (as prophylaxis for inhaled spores) is necessary for a total course of 60 days from onset of illness.

Infants, Children, and Adolescents:

Patient weight <45 kg: Oral: 2.2 mg/kg/dose every 12 hours.

Patient weight ≥45 kg: Oral: 100 mg every 12 hours.

Systemic anthrax, excluding meningitis: **Note:** Not recommended for meningitis or disseminated infection when meningitis cannot be ruled out. Doxycycline is an alternative to clindamycin as protein synthesis inhibitor and should be used in combination with a bactericidal antimicrobial (eg, fluoroquinolone, carbapenem, vancomycin). Duration of therapy at least 14 days or longer until patient clinically stable; additional therapy (as prophylaxis for inhaled spores) is necessary for a total course of 60 days from onset of illness.

Infants, Children, and Adolescents:

Patient weight <45 kg:

Initial: IV: Loading dose: 4.4 mg/kg once, then 2.2 mg/kg/dose every 12 hours; may transition to oral therapy for patients without signs of active infection who are able to tolerate oral therapy and patient/caregiver adherent to therapy.

Step-down: Oral: 2.2 mg/kg/dose every 12 hours.

Patient weight ≥45 kg:

Initial: IV: Loading dose: 200 mg once, then 100 mg every 12 hours; may transition to oral therapy for patients without signs of active infection who are able to tolerate oral therapy and patient/caregiver adherent to therapy.

Step-down: Oral: 100 mg every 12 hours.

Brucellosis: Limited data available: Children ≥8 years and Adolescents: Oral: 2.2 mg/kg/dose twice daily for at least 6 weeks; maximum dose: 100 mg/dose; use in combination with rifampin; for serious infections, an aminoglycoside should be added for initial 1 to 2 weeks and therapy may be extended for up to 4 to 6 months (AAP [Bradley 2019]; *Red Book* [AAP 2018]).

Chlamydial infections, uncomplicated (sexually transmitted *C. trachomatis*):

Children ≥8 years: Oral: 2.2 mg/kg/dose twice daily for 7 days. Maximum dose: 100 mg/dose (AAP [Bradley 2019]).

Adolescents: Oral: 100 mg twice daily for 7 days (CDC [Workowski 2015]).

Lyme disease: Limited data available:

Prophylaxis, postexposure: Children and Adolescents: Oral: 4.4 mg/kg/dose once as a single dose; maximum dose: 200 mg/dose; initiate within 72 hours of tick removal (CDC 2019).

Treatment:

Early Lyme disease: **Note:** The American Academy of Pediatrics (AAP) recommends the use of doxycycline in ages <8 years for treatment courses ≤21 days; this recommendation is based upon data in younger children treated for Rocky Mountain spotted fever that suggest short courses of doxycycline are unlikely to cause visible teeth staining or enamel hyperplasia (*Red Book* [AAP 2018]).

Erythema migrans: Children ≥8 years and Adolescents: Oral: 2 mg/kg/dose twice daily for 10 to 21 days (usual duration: 14 days); maximum dose: 100 mg/dose (IDSA [Wormser 2006]).

Meningitis, neurologic Lyme disease: Children ≥8 years and Adolescents: Oral: 2 to 4 mg/kg/dose twice daily for 10 to 28 days; maximum dose: 200 mg/dose (IDSA [Wormser 2006]).

Borrelial lymphocytoma: Children ≥8 years and Adolescents: Oral: 2 mg/kg/dose twice daily for 10 to 21 days (usual duration: 14 days); maximum dose: 100 mg/dose (IDSA [Wormser 2006]).

Late Lyme disease: Lyme arthritis (no neurologic involvement): Children ≥8 years and Adolescents: Oral: 2 mg/kg/dose twice daily for 28 days; maximum dose: 100 mg/dose (IDSA [Wormser 2006]).

Malaria:

Prophylaxis: Children ≥8 years and Adolescents: Oral: 2.2 mg/kg/dose once daily starting 1 to 2 days before travel to the area with endemic infection, continuing daily during travel and for 4 weeks after leaving endemic area; maximum daily dose: 100 mg/**day** (CDC [Tan 2019]).

Treatment: Children and Adolescents: Oral, IV: 2.2 mg/kg/dose twice daily for 7 days; maximum dose: 100 mg/dose; use in combination with quinine sulfate (plus primaquine for *Plasmodium vivax*) (CDC 2019). **Note:** Use of doxycycline in children <8 years should be reserved for when alternatives are not available or are not tolerated; benefits should outweigh risks.

Pneumonia, community-acquired; presumed or proven atypical infection (*Mycoplasma pneumoniae, Chlamydophila pneumoniae*): Children ≥8 years and Adolescents: Oral: 1 to 2 mg/kg/dose twice daily for 10 days (IDSA [Bradley 2011]).

Q fever *(Coxiella burnetii)* (preferred therapy): Children and Adolescents: Oral: 2.2 mg/kg/dose twice daily for 14 days; maximum dose: 100 mg/dose; in children <8 years with mild or uncomplicated disease, may consider treatment duration of 5 days, and if longer treatment required, may consider alternate therapy (trimethoprim/sulfamethoxazole) (CDC [Anderson 2013]).

Skin/soft tissue infections; MRSA or community-acquired cellulitis (purulent) (IDSA [Liu 2011]): Children ≥8 years and Adolescents:

≤45 kg: Oral: 2 mg/kg/dose every 12 hours for 5 to 10 days.

>45 kg: Oral: 100 mg twice daily for 5 to 10 days.

Tickborne rickettsial disease (Rocky Mountain spotted fever), ehrlichiosis, or anaplasmosis: Children and Adolescents: Oral, IV: 2.2 mg/kg/dose every 12 hours; maximum dose: 100 mg/dose; treat for minimum of 5 to 7 days; continue for at least 3 days after defervescence and clinical improvement observed. Severe or complicated disease may require longer treatment; anaplasmosis should be treated for 10 days (CDC [Biggs 2016]).

Renal Impairment: Pediatric

Children and Adolescents: IV, Oral: Limited data available:

Mild to severe kidney impairment: Based on adult information, no dosage adjustment is necessary (Alestig 1973; Lee 1972).

Hemodialysis, intermittent (thrice weekly): Poorly dialyzed (0% to 5%); based on adult information, no supplemental dose or dosage adjustment necessary (Houin 1983; Lee 1972; Letteri 1973).

Peritoneal dialysis: Poorly dialyzed; based on adult information, no dosage adjustment necessary (Letteri 1973).

Continuous renal replacement therapy (CRRT): Based on adult information, no dosage adjustment necessary (Heintz 2009).

Hepatic Impairment: Pediatric There are no dosage adjustments provided in the manufacturer's labeling.

Mechanism of Action

Inhibits protein synthesis by binding with the 30S and possibly the 50S ribosomal subunit(s) of susceptible bacteria; may also cause alterations in the cytoplasmic membrane

20 mg tablets and capsules (Periostat [Canadian product]): Proposed mechanism: Has been shown to inhibit collagenase activity in vitro. Also has been noted to reduce elevated collagenase activity in the gingival crevicular fluid of patients with periodontal disease. Systemic levels do not reach inhibitory concentrations against bacteria.

Contraindications

Hypersensitivity to doxycycline, other tetracyclines, or any component of the formulation

Periostat, Apprilon [Canadian products]: Additional contraindications: Use in infants and children <8 years of age or during second or third trimester of pregnancy; breastfeeding

Warnings/Precautions Photosensitivity reaction may occur with this drug; discontinue at first sign of skin erythema. Use skin protection and avoid prolonged exposure to sunlight and ultraviolet light. May be associated with increases in BUN secondary to antianabolic effects; this does not occur with use of doxycycline in patients with renal impairment. Severe skin reactions (eg, exfoliative dermatitis, erythema multiforme, Stevens-Johnson syndrome, toxic epidermal necrolysis, drug reaction with eosinophilia and systemic symptoms [DRESS]) have been reported; discontinue use for serious hypersensitivity reactions. Hepatotoxicity rarely occurs; if symptomatic, assess LFTs and discontinue drug. Intracranial hypertension (pseudotumor cerebri) has been associated with use; headache, blurred vision, diplopia, vision loss, and/or papilledema may occur. Women of childbearing age who are overweight or have a history of intracranial hypertension are at greater risk. Intracranial hypertension typically resolves after discontinuation of treatment; however, permanent visual loss is possible. If visual symptoms develop during treatment, prompt ophthalmologic evaluation is warranted. Intracranial pressure can remain elevated for weeks after drug discontinuation; monitor patient until stable. Esophagitis and ulcerations (sometimes severe) may occur; patients with dysphagia and/or retrosternal pain may require assessment for esophageal lesions.

Prolonged use may result in fungal or bacterial superinfection, including *C. difficile*-associated diarrhea (CDAD) and pseudomembranous colitis; CDAD has been observed >2 months postantibiotic treatment. May induce hyperpigmentation in many organs, including nails, bone, skin (diffuse pigmentation as well as over sites of scars and injury), eyes, thyroid, visceral tissue, oral cavity (adult teeth, mucosa, alveolar bone), sclerae, and heart valves independently of time or amount of drug administration. Safety and effectiveness have not been established for treatment of periodontitis in patients with coexistent oral candidiasis; use with caution in patients with a history or predisposition to oral candidiasis. May cause tissue hyperpigmentation, tooth enamel hypoplasia, or permanent tooth discoloration (more common with long-term use, but observed with repeated, short courses) when used during tooth development (last half of pregnancy, infancy, and childhood ≤8 years of age); manufacturer states to use in children ≤8 years of age only when the potential benefits outweigh the risks in severe or life threatening conditions (eg, anthrax, Rocky Mountain spotted fever), particularly when there are no alternative therapies. Limited use between 6 to 7 years of age has minimal effect on the color of permanent incisors (CDC [Biggs 2016]). Recommended in prevention and treatment of anthrax (AAP [Bradley 2014]), treatment of tickborne rickettsial diseases (CDC [Biggs 2016]), and Q fever (CDC 2013). When used for malaria prophylaxis, does not completely suppress asexual blood stages of *Plasmodium* strains. Doxycycline does not suppress *P. falciparum's* sexual blood stage gametocytes. Patients completing a regimen may still transmit the infection to mosquitoes outside endemic areas. Potentially significant drug-drug interactions may exist, requiring dose or frequency adjustment, additional monitoring, and/or selection of alternative therapy.

Acne: The American Academy of Dermatology acne guidelines recommend doxycycline as adjunctive treatment for moderate and severe acne and forms of inflammatory acne that are resistant to topical treatments. Concomitant topical therapy with benzoyl peroxide or a retinoid should be administered with systemic antibiotic therapy (eg, doxycycline) and continued for maintenance after the antibiotic course is completed (AAD [Zaenglein 2016]).

Oracea or Apprilon (Canadian product): Do not be use for the treatment or prophylaxis of bacterial infections (dose may be subefficacious and promote resistance).

Syrup contains sodium metabisulfite, which may cause allergic reactions in certain individuals (eg, asthmatic patients).

Warnings: Additional Pediatric Considerations Tooth staining or enamel hypoplasia of developing teeth is a known concern with the use of tetracycline-class of antibiotics in children <8 years of age based on experience with older tetracyclines which bind to calcium more readily than doxycycline. A cohort analysis of 58 children who were exposed to doxycycline for treatment of Rocky Mountain Spotted Fever when <8 years of age reported no visible tetracycline-like tooth staining of permanent teeth at recommended dose and duration compared to a control group of 213 children not exposed to doxycycline; the cohort received a total of 107 courses of doxycycline (multiple courses), mean duration: 7.3 days (range: 1 to 10 days), and mean dose: 2.3 mg/kg/day (Todd 2015). An analysis of 31 asthmatic children who received doxycycline also reported no evidence of tooth staining. A meta-analysis of the combined data reported a 0% prevalence rate for tooth staining (CDC [Biggs 2016]; Todd 2015). Retrospective data suggests that at standard doses, children <8 years could receive up to 5 courses of doxycycline without detectable evidence of tooth staining (AAP [Bradley 2014]). The American Academy of Pediatrics recommends the use of doxycycline in children <8 years of age for short durations (≤21 days) when appropriate (*Red Book* [AAP 2018]).

Administration of tetracycline 25 mg/kg/day was associated with decreased fibular growth rate in premature infants (reversible with discontinuation of drug); bulging fontanels have been reported in infants.

Some dosage forms may contain propylene glycol; in neonates large amounts of propylene glycol delivered orally, intravenously (eg, >3,000 mg/day), or topically have been associated with potentially fatal toxicities which can include metabolic acidosis, seizures, renal failure, and CNS depression; toxicities have also been reported in children and adults including hyperosmolality, lactic acidosis, seizures, and respiratory depression; use caution (AAP 1997; Shehab 2009).

Drug Interactions

Metabolism/Transport Effects None known.

Avoid Concomitant Use

Avoid concomitant use of Doxycycline with any of the following: Aminolevulinic Acid (Systemic); BCG (Intravesical); Cholera Vaccine; Mecamylamine; Methoxyflurane; Retinoic Acid Derivatives; Strontium Ranelate

Increased Effect/Toxicity

Doxycycline may increase the levels/effects of: Aminolevulinic Acid (Systemic); Aminolevulinic Acid (Topical); Lithium; Mecamylamine; Methoxyflurane; Mipomersen; Neuromuscular-Blocking Agents; Porfimer; Retinoic Acid Derivatives; Verteporfin; Vitamin K Antagonists

Decreased Effect

Doxycycline may decrease the levels/effects of: BCG (Intravesical); BCG Vaccine (Immunization); Cholera Vaccine; Iron Preparations; Lactobacillus and Estriol; Penicillins; Sodium Picosulfate; Typhoid Vaccine

The levels/effects of Doxycycline may be decreased by: Antacids; Barbiturates; Bile Acid Sequestrants; Bismuth Subcitrate; Bismuth Subsalicylate; Calcium Salts; CarBAMazepine; Fosphenytoin; Iron Preparations; Lanthanum; Magnesium Salts; Multivitamins/Minerals (with ADEK, Folate, Iron); Multivitamins/Minerals (with AE, No Iron); Phenytoin; Proton Pump Inhibitors; Quinapril; RifAMPin; Strontium Ranelate; Sucralfate; Sucroferric Oxyhydroxide

Food Interactions

Ethanol: Chronic ethanol ingestion may reduce the serum concentration of doxycycline.

Food: Doxycycline serum levels may be slightly decreased if taken with high-fat meal or milk. Administration with iron or calcium may decrease doxycycline absorption. May decrease absorption of calcium, iron, magnesium, zinc, and amino acids. Management: Administer Doryx and Doryx MPC without regard to meals. Administer Oracea and doxycycline 20 mg tablet on an empty stomach 1 hour before or 2 hours after meals.

Dietary Considerations

Tetracyclines (in general): Take with food if gastric irritation occurs. While administration with food may decrease GI absorption of doxycycline by up to 20%, administration on an empty stomach is generally not recommended due to GI intolerance. Of currently available tetracyclines, doxycycline has the least affinity for calcium.

Doxycycline 20 mg tablet, Oracea, Apprilon [Canadian product]: Manufacturer states to take on an empty stomach 1 hour before or 2 hours after meals. Take with food if gastric irritation occurs.

Periostat [Canadian product]: Manufacturer states to take at least 1 hour before morning and evening meals. Take with food if gastric irritation occurs.

Some products may contain sodium.

Pharmacodynamics/Kinetics

Half-life Elimination 18 to 22 hours; End-stage renal disease: 18 to 25 hours

Time to Peak Serum: Oral: Immediate release: 1.5 to 4 hours; delayed-release tablets: 2.8 to 3 hours

Reproductive Considerations Doxycycline can be detected in semen (Zakhem 2019). The manufacturer does not recommend use of doxycycline for the treatment of rosacea in males with female partners who plan to become pregnant.

Pregnancy Considerations Tetracyclines cross the placenta (Mylonas 2011).

Therapeutic doses of doxycycline during pregnancy are unlikely to produce substantial teratogenic risk, but data are insufficient to say that there is no risk. In general, reports of exposure have been limited to short durations of therapy in the first trimester. Tetracyclines accumulate in developing teeth and long tubular bones (Mylonas 2011). Permanent discoloration of teeth (yellow, gray, brown) can occur following in utero exposure and is more likely to occur following long-term or repeated exposure.

Doxycycline is the recommended agent for the treatment of Rocky Mountain spotted fever (RMSF) in pregnant women (CDC [Biggs 2016]). For other indications, many guidelines consider use of doxycycline to be contraindicated during pregnancy, or to be a relative contraindication in pregnant women if other agents are available and appropriate for use (CDC [Anderson 2013]; CDC 2020; CDC [Workowski 2015]; HHS [OI adult 2019]; IDSA [Stevens 2014]). Doxycycline should not be used for the treatment of acne or rosacea in pregnant women (AAD [Zaenglein 2016]). When systemic antibiotics are needed for dermatologic conditions, other agents are preferred (Kong 2013; Murase 2014). As a class, tetracyclines are generally considered second-line antibiotics in pregnant women and their use should be avoided (Mylonas 2011).

Breastfeeding Considerations Doxycycline is present in breast milk.

The relative infant dose (RID) of doxycycline is 6.14% when calculated using the highest average breast milk concentration located and compared to an infant therapeutic dose of 4.4 mg/kg/day.

In general, breastfeeding is considered acceptable when the RID is <10%; when an RID is >25% breastfeeding should generally be avoided (Anderson 2016; Ito 2000).

Using the highest average milk concentration (1.8 mcg/mL), the estimated daily infant dose via breast milk is 0.27 mg/kg/day. This milk concentration was obtained following maternal administration of a single oral dose of doxycycline 200 mg (Tokuda 1969). Concentrations of doxycycline in breast milk may increase with duration of therapy (Anderson 1991).

Oral absorption of doxycycline is not markedly influenced by simultaneous ingestion of milk; therefore, oral absorption of doxycycline by the breastfeeding infant would not be expected to be diminished by the calcium in the maternal milk.

The therapeutic use of doxycycline should be avoided during tooth development (children <8 years) unless there are no alternative therapies due to the potential for tissue hyperpigmentation, tooth enamel hypoplasia, or permanent tooth discoloration. Theoretically, this risk is also present in breastfeeding infants exposed to doxycycline via breast milk. Although breastfeeding is not specifically contraindicated, the effects of long-term exposure via breast milk are not known. According to the manufacturer, the decision to continue or discontinue breastfeeding during therapy should take into account the risk of infant exposure, the benefits of breastfeeding to the infant, and benefits of treatment to the mother. The World Health Organization (WHO) states that maternal use of doxycycline should be avoided if possible but that a single dose or the short-term use of doxycycline is probably safe; there exists a possibility of dental staining and inhibition of bone growth in the infant, especially with prolonged use (WHO 2002). In general, antibiotics that are present in breast milk may cause nondose-related modification of bowel flora. Monitor infants for GI disturbances, such as thrush and diarrhea (WHO 2002).

Current guidelines note that the short-term use of doxycycline for the treatment of RMSF is considered compatible with breastfeeding (CDC [Biggs 2016]). If used for the treatment or prophylaxis of malaria, breastfeeding during doxycycline therapy is considered compatible; however, the theoretical risk of dental staining and inhibition of long bone growth in the breastfeeding infant should be considered (WHO 2002). Breastfeeding is not recommended when doxycycline is being used for maternal treatment of acne (AAD [Zaenglein 2016]).

Product Availability LymePak (doxycycline tablets): FDA approved June 2018; anticipated availability is currently unknown. Information pertaining to this product within the monograph is pending revision. LymePak is indicated for the treatment of early Lyme disease due to *Borrelia burgdorferi* in adults and pediatric patients ≥8 years of age weighing ≥45 kg. Consult the prescribing information for additional information.

Dosage Forms Considerations

Morgidox kits contain doxycycline capsules 100 mg, plus AcuWash moisturizing Daily Cleanser

NizAzel Doxy kits contain doxycycline tablets 100 mg, plus NicAzel FORTE dietary supplement tablets

Dosage Forms: US

Capsule, Oral:
- Mondoxyne NL: 50 mg, 75 mg, 100 mg
- Morgidox: 50 mg, 100 mg
- Vibramycin: 100 mg
- Generic: 50 mg, 75 mg, 100 mg, 150 mg

Capsule Delayed Release, Oral:
- Oracea: 40 mg
- Generic: 40 mg

Kit, Combination:
- Morgidox: 1 x 50 mg, 1 x 100 mg, 2 x 100 mg

Solution Reconstituted, Intravenous [preservative free]:
- Doxy 100: 100 mg (1 ea)
- Generic: 100 mg (1 ea)

Suspension Reconstituted, Oral:
- Vibramycin: 25 mg/5 mL (60 mL)
- Generic: 25 mg/5 mL (60 mL)

Syrup, Oral:
- Vibramycin: 50 mg/5 mL (473 mL)

Tablet, Oral:
- Acticlate: 75 mg, 150 mg
- Avidoxy: 100 mg
- TargaDOX: 50 mg
- Generic: 20 mg, 50 mg, 75 mg, 100 mg, 150 mg

Tablet Delayed Release, Oral:
- Doryx: 50 mg, 200 mg
- Doryx MPC: 120 mg
- Soloxide: 150 mg
- Generic: 50 mg, 75 mg, 100 mg, 150 mg, 200 mg

Dosage Forms: Canada

Capsule, Oral:
- Periostat: 20 mg
- Generic: 100 mg

Capsule Delayed Release, Oral:
- Apprilon: 40 mg

Tablet, Oral:
- Generic: 100 mg

◆ **Doxycycline Calcium** *see* Doxycycline *on page 522*

◆ **Doxycycline Hyclate** *see* Doxycycline *on page 522*

Doxycycline Hyclate Periodontal Extended-Release Liquid

(doks i SYE kleen HI klayt per ee oh DON tal ik STEN did ri LES LIK wid)

Related Information

Doxycycline *on page 522*

Periodontal Diseases *on page 1748*

Brand Names: Canada Atridox

Generic Availability (US) May be product dependent

Pharmacologic Category Antibiotic, Tetracycline Derivative

Dental Use Treatment of chronic adult periodontitis for gain in clinical attachment, reduction in probing depth, and reduction in bleeding upon probing

Use Periodontitis: Treatment of chronic adult periodontitis for a gain in clinical attachment, reduction in probing depth, and reduction in bleeding on probing (John 2017).

Local Anesthetic/Vasoconstrictor Precautions No information available to require special precautions

Effects on Dental Treatment Key adverse event(s) related to dental treatment: Discoloration of teeth (in children), gum discomfort, toothache, periodontal abscess, tooth sensitivity, broken tooth, tooth mobility, endodontic abscess, and jaw pain

Mechanical oral hygiene procedures (ie, tooth brushing, flossing) should be avoided in any treated area for 7 days.

Effects reported in clinical trials were similar in incidence between doxycycline-containing product and vehicle alone; comparable to standard therapies including scaling and root planing or oral hygiene. Although there is no known relationship between doxycycline and hypertension, unspecified primary hypertension was noted in 1.6% of the doxycycline gel group, as compared to 0.2% in the vehicle group (allergic reactions to the vehicle were also reported in two patients).

Effects on Bleeding No information available to require special precautions

Adverse Reactions

>10%:

Central nervous system: Headache (27%)

Gastrointestinal: Minor gum irritation (18%), toothache (14%; pressure sensitivity)

1% to 10%:

Cardiovascular: Hypertension (<1% to 2%)

Central nervous system: Local discomfort (sensitive teeth: 8%), sore mouth (4%; soft tissue erythema, unspecified pain), insomnia (3%), tension headache (2%)

Dermatologic: Dermatitis (1%), skin infection (1%)

Endocrine & metabolic: Premenstrual syndrome (4%)

Gastrointestinal: Periodontal abscess (10%), sore throat (6%), injury of tooth (5%), dyspepsia (4%), gingivitis (4%), diarrhea (3%), nausea (2%), periodontal abscess (2%; lesion), vomiting (2%), dental bleeding (1%)

Infection: Common cold (26%), influenza (3% to 6%), tooth abscess (2%; pulpitis)

Neuromuscular & skeletal: Myalgia (6%), back pain (4%), arm pain (2%), leg pain (2%), lower back pain (2%), muscle tenderness (2%), jaw pain (1%), neck pain (1%), shoulder pain (1%)

Respiratory: Sinus congestion (6%), sinus infection (5%), cough (4%), bronchitis (2%), ENT infection (2%), allergic rhinitis (1%)

Miscellaneous: Fever (1%)

<1%, postmarketing, and/or case reports: Aphthous stomatitis, enamel hypoplasia, fistula, hypersensitivity reaction, permanent dental discoloration, skin photosensitivity, tooth loss

Dental Usual Dosage Oral, subgingival: Dose depends on size, shape and number of pockets treated. Application may be repeated four months after initial treatment. The delivery system consists of 2 separate syringes in a single pouch. Syringe A contains 450 mg of a bioabsorbable polymer gel; syringe B contains doxycycline hyclate 50 mg. To prepare for instillation, couple syringe A to syringe B. Inject contents of syringe A (purple stripe) into syringe B, then push contents back into syringe A. Repeat this mixing cycle at a rate of one cycle per second for 100 cycles. If syringes are stored prior to use (a maximum of 3 days), repeat mixing cycle 10 times before use. After appropriate mixing, contents should be in syringe A. Holding syringes vertically, with syringe A at the bottom, pull back on the syringe A plunger, allowing contents to flow down barrel for several seconds. Uncouple syringes and attach enclosed blunt cannula to syringe A. Local anesthesia is not required for placement. Cannula tip may be bent to resemble periodontal probe and used to explore pocket. Express product from syringe until pocket is filled. To separate tip from formulation, turn tip towards the tooth and press against tooth surface to achieve separation. An appropriate dental instrument may be used to pack gel into the pocket. Pockets may be covered with either Coe-pak or Octyldentdental adhesive.

Dosing

Adult & Geriatric

Periodontitis: Subgingival application: Dose depends on size, shape and number of pockets treated. Contains 50 mg doxycycline hyclate per 500 mg of formulation in each final blended syringe product.

Atridox subgingival controlled-release product: Local anesthesia is not required for placement. Cannula tip may be bent to resemble periodontal probe and used to explore pocket. Express product from syringe until pocket is filled. To separate tip from formulation, turn tip towards the tooth and press against tooth surface to achieve separation. An appropriate dental instrument may be used to pack gel into the pocket. Pockets may be covered with either Coe-Pak or Octyldent dental adhesive. Application may be repeated 4 months after initial treatment.

Mechanism of Action Inhibits protein synthesis by binding with the 30S and possibly the 50S ribosomal subunit(s) of susceptible bacteria; may also cause alterations in the cytoplasmic membrane

Doxycycline inhibits collagenase *in vitro* and has been shown to inhibit collagenase in the gingival crevicular fluid in adults with periodontitis

Contraindications

Hypersensitivity to doxycycline, tetracycline or any component of the formulation; children <8 years of age.

Canadian labeling: Additional contraindications (not in US labeling): Children <12 years of age; pregnancy; breastfeeding.

Warnings/Precautions Photosensitivity reaction may occur with this drug; avoid prolonged exposure to sunlight or tanning equipment. Prolonged use may result in fungal or bacterial superinfection, including *C. difficile*-associated diarrhea (CDAD) and pseudomembranous colitis; CDAD has been observed >2 months postantibiotic treatment. May cause tissue hyperpigmentation, enamel hypoplasia, or permanent tooth discoloration; use of tetracyclines should be avoided during tooth development (children <8 years of age) unless other drugs are not likely to be effective or are contraindicated.

Additional specific warnings for doxycycline gel (Atridox) for subgingival application: This product has not been evaluated or tested in immunocompromised patients, in patients with oral candidiasis, or in conditions characterized by severe periodontal defects with little remaining periodontium. May result in overgrowth of nonsusceptible organisms, including fungi. Effects of treatment >9 months have not been evaluated. Has not been evaluated for use in regeneration of alveolar bone

Drug Interactions

Metabolism/Transport Effects None known.

Avoid Concomitant Use There are no known interactions where it is recommended to avoid concomitant use.

Increased Effect/Toxicity There are no known significant interactions involving an increase in effect.

Decreased Effect There are no known significant interactions involving a decrease in effect.

Pregnancy Risk Factor D

Pregnancy Considerations
Tetracyclines cross the placenta (Mylonas 2011). Tetracyclines accumulate in developing teeth and long tubular bones. Permanent discoloration of teeth (yellow, gray, brown) can occur following in utero exposure and is more likely to occur following long-term or repeated exposure. Serum concentrations following subgingival use are significantly less than with oral tablets. Use of this product should be avoided in pregnant patients unless other options are not likely to be effective or are contraindicated.

Refer to the Doxycycline monograph for additional information.

Breastfeeding Considerations
It is not known if doxycycline is present in breast milk following subgingival application.
Doxycycline is present in breast milk following systemic use. Due to the potential for serious adverse reactions in the breastfed infant, the manufacturer recommends a decision be made to discontinue breastfeeding or to discontinue the drug, considering the importance of treatment to the mother.
Refer to the Doxycycline monograph for additional information.

Dosage Forms: Canada
Gel, Mouth/Throat:
Atridox: 44 mg/0.5 mL (0.5 mL)

◆ **Doxycycline Monohydrate** *see* Doxycycline *on page 522*

Doxylamine (dox IL a meen)

Brand Names: US Sleep Aid [OTC]
Pharmacologic Category Ethanolamine Derivative; Histamine H_1 Antagonist; Histamine H_1 Antagonist, First Generation
Use Insomnia: Reduce difficulty falling asleep
Local Anesthetic/Vasoconstrictor Precautions No information available to require special precautions
Effects on Dental Treatment Key adverse event(s) related to dental treatment: Dry mucous membranes and significant xerostomia (normal salivary flow resumes upon discontinuation)
Effects on Bleeding No information available to require special precautions
Adverse Reactions Frequency not defined.
Cardiovascular: Palpitations, tachycardia
Central nervous system: Disorientation, dizziness, drowsiness, headache, paradoxical central nervous system stimulation, vertigo
Gastrointestinal: Anorexia, constipation, diarrhea, dry mucous membranes, epigastric pain, xerostomia
Genitourinary: Dysuria, urinary retention
Ophthalmic: Blurred vision, diplopia
Mechanism of Action Doxylamine competes with histamine for H_1-receptor sites on effector cells; blocks chemoreceptor trigger zone, diminishes vestibular stimulation, and depresses labyrinthine function through its central anticholinergic activity.
Pharmacodynamics/Kinetics
Half-life Elimination 10-12 hours (Paton, 1985; Friedman, 1985); may be increased in the elderly (Friedman, 1989)
Time to Peak 2-4 hours (Paton, 1985; Friedman, 1985; Friedman, 1989)

Pregnancy Considerations
Maternal use of doxylamine in combination with pyridoxine during pregnancy has not been shown to increase the baseline risk of major malformations. Doxylamine may be used for the treatment of nausea and vomiting of pregnancy (ACOG 189 2018).

◆ **Doxylamine Succinate** *see* Doxylamine *on page 532*
◆ **DPA** *see* Valproic Acid and Derivatives *on page 1518*
◆ **DPH** *see* Phenytoin *on page 1228*
◆ **Dramamine [OTC]** *see* DimenhyDRINATE *on page 501*
◆ **Dramamine Less Drowsy [OTC]** *see* Meclizine *on page 952*
◆ **Dr Gs Clear Nail [OTC]** *see* Tolnaftate *on page 1462*
◆ **Driminate [OTC]** *see* DimenhyDRINATE *on page 501*
◆ **Drinkables Fruits and Vegetables [OTC]** *see* Vitamins (Multiple/Oral) *on page 1550*
◆ **Drinkables MultiVitamins [OTC]** *see* Vitamins (Multiple/Oral) *on page 1550*
◆ **Drisdol** *see* Ergocalciferol *on page 582*
◆ **Dristan Spray [OTC]** *see* Oxymetazoline (Nasal) *on page 1173*
◆ **Drizalma Sprinkle** *see* DULoxetine *on page 536*
◆ **Dr Manzanilla Antihistamine [OTC] [DSC]** *see* Triprolidine *on page 1500*

Dronabinol (droe NAB i nol)

Brand Names: US Marinol; Syndros
Pharmacologic Category Antiemetic; Appetite Stimulant; Cannabinoid
Use
Anorexia in patients with AIDS: Treatment of anorexia associated with weight loss in patients with AIDS.
Chemotherapy-induced nausea and vomiting: Treatment of nausea and vomiting associated with cancer chemotherapy in patients who have failed to respond adequately to conventional antiemetic treatments.
Local Anesthetic/Vasoconstrictor Precautions No information available to require special precautions
Effects on Dental Treatment Key adverse event(s) related to dental treatment: Xerostomia (normal salivary flow resumes upon discontinuation); Patients may experience orthostatic hypotension as they stand up after treatment; especially if lying in dental chair for extended periods of time. Use caution with sudden changes in position during and after dental treatment.
Effects on Bleeding No information available to require special precautions
Adverse Reactions Frequency not always defined.
>10%: Central nervous system: Euphoria (antiemetic: 24%; appetite stimulant: 8%)
1% to 10%:
Cardiovascular: Facial flushing (>1%), palpitations (>1%), tachycardia (>1%), vasodilation (>1%), flushing (≤1%), hypotension (≤1%)
Central nervous system: Abnormality in thinking (3% to 10%), dizziness (3% to 10%), drowsiness (3% to 10%), paranoia (3% to 10%), amnesia (>1%), anxiety (>1%), ataxia (>1%), confusion (>1%), depersonalization (>1%), hallucination (>1%), nervousness (>1%), chills (≤1%), depression (≤1%), headache (≤1%), malaise (≤1%), nightmares (≤1%), speech disturbance (≤1%)
Dermatologic: Diaphoresis (≤1%)

Gastrointestinal: Abdominal pain (3% to 10%), nausea (3% to 10%), vomiting (3% to 10%), anorexia (≤1%), diarrhea (≤1%), fecal incontinence (≤1%)
Hepatic: Increased liver enzymes (≤1%)
Neuromuscular & skeletal: Weakness (>1%), myalgia (≤1%)
Ophthalmic: Conjunctival injection (≤1%), conjunctivitis (≤1%), visual disturbance (≤1%)
Otic: Tinnitus (≤1%)
Respiratory: Cough (≤1%), rhinitis (≤1%), sinusitis (≤1%)

<1%, postmarketing, and/or case reports: Burning sensation of skin, delirium, disorientation, exacerbation of depression, falling, fatigue, insomnia, loss of consciousness, mental status changes (exacerbation of mania or schizophrenia), movement disorder, oral lesion, panic attack, pharyngeal edema, seizure, skin rash, swelling of lips, syncope, urticaria, visual disturbance

Mechanism of Action Dronabinol (synthetic delta-9-tetrahydrocannabinol [delta-9-THC]), an active cannabinoid and natural occurring component of *Cannabis sativa L.* (marijuana), activates cannabinoid receptors CB_1 and CB_2. Activation of the CB_1 receptor produces marijuana-like effects on psyche and circulation, whereas activation of the CB_2 receptor does not. Dronabinol has approximately equal affinity for the CB_1 and CB_2 receptors; however, efficacy is less at CB_2 receptors. Activation of the cannabinoid system with dronabinol causes psychological effects that can be divided into 4 groups: affective (euphoria and easy laughter); sensory (increased perception of external stimuli and of the person's own body); somatic (feeling of the body floating or sinking in the bed); and cognitive (distortion of time perception, memory lapses, difficulty in concentration). Most effects (eg, analgesia, appetite enhancement, muscle relaxation, hormonal actions) are mediated by central cannabinoid receptors (CB_1), their distribution reflecting many of the medicinal benefits and adverse effects (Grotenhermen 2003).

Pharmacodynamics/Kinetics

Onset of Action ~0.5 to 1 hour; Peak effect: 2 to 4 hours

Duration of Action 4 to 6 hours (psychoactive effects); ≥24 hours (appetite stimulation)

Half-life Elimination Biphasic: Alpha: 4 to 5 hours; Terminal: 25 to 36 hours

Time to Peak Serum: 0.5 to 4 hours

Pregnancy Considerations Although information related to the use of synthetic cannabinoids during pregnancy is limited, cannabinoids cross the placenta. Maternal use may increase the risk of adverse fetal/neonatal outcomes including growth restriction, low birth weight, preterm birth, and stillbirth. Some dosage forms also contain a significant amount of alcohol.

Controlled Substance Marinol: C-III; Syndros: C-II

Dronedarone (droe NE da rone)

Related Information

Cardiovascular Diseases *on page 1654*
Clinical Risk Related to Drugs Prolonging QT Interval *on page 1675*

Brand Names: US Multaq

Brand Names: Canada Multaq

Pharmacologic Category Antiarrhythmic Agent, Class III

Use Paroxysmal or persistent atrial fibrillation: To reduce the risk of hospitalization for atrial fibrillation (AF) in patients in sinus rhythm with a history of paroxysmal or persistent AF

Local Anesthetic/Vasoconstrictor Precautions Dronedarone is one of the drugs confirmed to prolong the QT interval and is accepted as having a risk of causing torsade de pointes. The risk of drug-induced torsade de pointes is extremely low when a single QT interval prolonging drug is prescribed. In terms of epinephrine, it is not known what effect vasoconstrictors in the local anesthetic regimen will have in patients with a known history of congenital prolonged QT interval or in patients taking any medication that prolongs the QT interval. Until more information is obtained, it is suggested that the clinician consult with the physician prior to the use of a vasoconstrictor in suspected patients, and that the vasoconstrictor (epinephrine, mepivacaine and levonordefrin [Carbocaine® 2% with Neo-Cobefrin®]) be used with caution.

Effects on Dental Treatment No significant effects or complications reported

Effects on Bleeding No information available to require special precautions

Adverse Reactions

>10%:
Cardiovascular: Prolonged QT interval on ECG (Bazett; 28% [placebo: 19%]; defined as >450 msec in males or >470 msec in female)
Renal: Increased serum creatinine (51%; increased >10%; occurred 5 days after initiation)

1% to 10%:
Cardiovascular: Bradycardia (3%)
Dermatologic: Allergic dermatitis (≤5%), dermatitis (≤5%), eczema (≤5%), pruritus (≤5%), skin rash (≤5%; described as generalized, macular, maculopapular, erythematous)
Gastrointestinal: Diarrhea (9%), nausea (5%), abdominal pain (4%), dyspepsia (2%), vomiting (2%)
Neuromuscular & skeletal: Weakness (7%)

<1%, postmarketing, and/or case reports: Acute hepatic failure (requiring transplant), anaphylaxis, angioedema, atrial flutter (with 1:1 atrioventricular conduction), cardiac failure (new or worsened), dysgeusia, hepatic injury, hyperbilirubinemia, hypersensitivity angiitis, increased blood urea nitrogen, increased liver enzymes, interstitial pulmonary disease, pneumonitis, pulmonary fibrosis, skin photosensitivity, vasculitis

Mechanism of Action A noniodinated antiarrhythmic agent structurally related to amiodarone exhibiting properties of all 4 antiarrhythmic classes. Dronedarone inhibits sodium (I_{Na}) and potassium (I_{kr}, I_{kS}, I_{k1}, and $I_{k\text{-}ACh}$) channels resulting in prolongation of the action potential and refractory period in myocardial tissue without reverse-use dependent effects; decreases AV conduction and sinus node function through inhibition of calcium ($I_{Ca\text{-}L}$) channels and $beta_1$-receptor blocking activity. Similar to amiodarone, dronedarone also inhibits $alpha_1$-receptor mediated increases in blood pressure.

Pharmacodynamics/Kinetics

Half-life Elimination 13 to 19 hours

Time to Peak Plasma: 3 to 6 hours

Reproductive Considerations

Use is contraindicated in women who may become pregnant. Women of reproductive potential should use effective contraception during treatment.

Pregnancy Risk Factor X

Pregnancy Considerations
Studies in animals have shown evidence of fetal abnormalities and use is contraindicated in women who are pregnant.

Dental Health Professional Considerations See Local Anesthetic/Vasoconstrictor Precautions

◆ **Dronedarone Hydrochloride** *see* Dronedarone *on page 533*

Droperidol (droe PER i dole)

Related Information
Clinical Risk Related to Drugs Prolonging QT Interval *on page 1675*

Pharmacologic Category Antiemetic; First Generation (Typical) Antipsychotic

Use Postoperative nausea/vomiting (PONV): Prevention and/or treatment of nausea and vomiting from surgical and diagnostic procedures

Local Anesthetic/Vasoconstrictor Precautions
Droperidol is one of the drugs confirmed to prolong the QT interval and is accepted as having a risk of causing torsade de pointes. The risk of drug-induced torsade de pointes is extremely low when a single QT interval prolonging drug is prescribed. In terms of epinephrine, it is not known what effect vasoconstrictors in the local anesthetic regimen will have in patients with a known history of congenital prolonged QT interval or in patients taking any medication that prolongs the QT interval. Until more information is obtained, it is suggested that the clinician consult with the physician prior to the use of a vasoconstrictor in suspected patients, and that the vasoconstrictor (epinephrine, mepivacaine and levonordefrin [Carbocaine® 2% with Neo-Cobefrin®]) be used with caution.

Effects on Dental Treatment Key adverse event(s) related to dental treatment: Patients may experience orthostatic hypotension as they stand up after treatment; especially if lying in dental chair for extended periods of time. Use caution with sudden changes in position during and after dental treatment.

Effects on Bleeding No information available to require special precautions

Adverse Reactions Frequency not defined.
Cardiovascular: Cardiac arrest, hypertension, hypotension (especially orthostatic), QT_c prolongation (dose dependent), tachycardia, torsade de pointes, ventricular tachycardia
Central nervous system: Anxiety, chills, depression (postoperative, transient), dizziness, drowsiness (postoperative) increased, dysphoria, extrapyramidal symptoms (akathisia, dystonia, oculogyric crisis), hallucinations (postoperative), hyperactivity, neuroleptic malignant syndrome (NMS) (rare), restlessness
Respiratory: Bronchospasm, laryngospasm
Miscellaneous: Anaphylaxis, shivering

Mechanism of Action Droperidol is a butyrophenone antipsychotic; antiemetic effect is a result of blockade of dopamine stimulation of the chemoreceptor trigger zone. Other effects include alpha-adrenergic blockade, peripheral vascular dilation, and reduction of the pressor effect of epinephrine resulting in hypotension and decreased peripheral vascular resistance; may also reduce pulmonary artery pressure

Pharmacodynamics/Kinetics
Onset of Action 3 to 10 minutes; Peak effect: Within 30 minutes
Duration of Action 2 to 4 hours, may extend to 12 hours
Half-life Elimination Children ~1.7 hours; Adults: ~2 hours (McKeage 2006)

Pregnancy Risk Factor C

Pregnancy Considerations
Droperidol has been evaluated for the adjunctive management of hyperemesis gravidarum (Ferreira 2003; Nageotte 1996); however, use for the treatment of persistent symptoms of nausea and vomiting in pregnancy is not recommended (ACOG 189 2018).

Dental Health Professional Considerations See Local Anesthetic/Vasoconstrictor Precautions

Drospirenone (droe SPYE re none)

Brand Names: US Slynd

Pharmacologic Category Contraceptive; Progestin

Use Contraception: Prevention of pregnancy in females of reproductive potential

Local Anesthetic/Vasoconstrictor Precautions
No information available to require special precautions

Effects on Dental Treatment No significant effects or complications reported

Effects on Bleeding No information available to require special precautions

Adverse Reactions
1% to 10%:
Central nervous system: Headache (3%)
Dermatologic: Acne vulgaris (4%)
Endocrine & metabolic: Weight gain (2%), decreased libido (1%), menstrual disease (1%)
Gastrointestinal: Nausea (2%)
Genitourinary: Breakthrough bleeding (64%), abnormal uterine bleeding (3%), dysmenorrhea (2%), mastalgia (2%), vaginal hemorrhage (2%), breast tenderness (1%)
Frequency not defined: Endocrine & metabolic: Decreased plasma estradiol concentration
<1%, postmarketing, and/or case reports: Hyperkalemia

Mechanism of Action Drospirenone is a spironolactone analogue with antimineralocorticoid and antiandrogenic activity that provides contraception primarily by suppressing ovulation.

Pharmacodynamics/Kinetics
Half-life Elimination Terminal: ~30 hours
Time to Peak 2 to 6 hours

Pregnancy Considerations Use is contraindicated in pregnancy. Drospirenone is used to prevent pregnancy; treatment should be discontinued if pregnancy occurs. In general, the use of progestin contraceptives, when inadvertently used early in pregnancy, have not been associated adverse fetal effects.

Drospirenone and Estradiol
(droh SPYE re none & es tra DYE ole)

Related Information
Estradiol (Systemic) *on page 596*

Brand Names: US Angeliq

Brand Names: Canada Angeliq

Pharmacologic Category Estrogen and Progestin Combination

Use
Vasomotor symptoms associated with menopause: Treatment of moderate to severe vasomotor symptoms associated with menopause in women with a uterus.

Vulvar and vaginal atrophy associated with menopause: Treatment of moderate to severe vulvar and vaginal atrophy due to menopause in women with a uterus.

Limitations of use: When used solely for the treatment of vulvar and vaginal atrophy, topical vaginal products should be considered.

Note: The International Society for the Study of Women's Sexual Health and The North American Menopause Society have endorsed the term genitourinary syndrome of menopause (GSM) as new terminology for vulvovaginal atrophy. The term GSM encompasses all genital and urinary signs and symptoms associated with a loss of estrogen due to menopause Portman 2014.

Local Anesthetic/Vasoconstrictor Precautions No information available to require special precautions

Effects on Bleeding No information available to require special precautions related to hemostasis in dental procedures.

Adverse Reactions

>10%:

Genitourinary: Mastalgia (6% to 18%), genital bleeding (3% to 14%)

1% to 10%:

Central nervous system: Emotional lability (1%), migraine (≤1%)

Gastrointestinal: Abdominal pain (≤4% to 7%), gastrointestinal pain (≤4% to 7%)

Genitourinary: Cervical polyp (≤1%)

<1%, postmarketing, and/or case reports: Cerebral infarction, cerebrovascular accident, embolism, hypersensitivity reaction, malignant neoplasm of breast, myocardial infarction, pulmonary vascular occlusion, pruritus, skin rash, thromboembolism, urticaria, venous obstruction (peripheral deep vein)

Mechanism of Action

Drospirenone is a synthetic progestin and spironolactone analog with antimineralocorticoid and antiandrogenic activity. Counteracts estrogen effects causing endometrial thinning.

Estrogens are responsible for the development and maintenance of the female reproductive system and secondary sexual characteristics. Estradiol is the principal intracellular human estrogen and is more potent than estrone and estriol at the receptor level; it is the primary estrogen secreted prior to menopause. Following menopause, estrone and estrone sulfate are more highly produced. Estrogens modulate the pituitary secretion of gonadotropins, luteinizing hormone, and follicle-stimulating hormone through a negative feedback system; estrogen replacement reduces elevated levels of these hormones in postmenopausal women.

Pharmacodynamics/Kinetics

Half-life Elimination Drospirenone: ~36-42 hours

Time to Peak Plasma: Drospirenone: 1 hour; Estradiol: ~2 hours (range 0.3-10 hours)

Pregnancy Considerations Use is contraindicated in pregnant women.

- **Drospirenone and Ethinyl Estradiol** *see* Ethinyl Estradiol and Drospirenone *on page* *610*
- **Drospirenone/Estradiol** *see* Drospirenone and Estradiol *on page* *534*
- **Drospirenone, Ethinyl Estradiol, and Levomefolate Calcium** *see* Ethinyl Estradiol, Drospirenone, and Levomefolate *on page* *618*

Droxidopa (drox i DOE pa)

Brand Names: US Northera

Pharmacologic Category Alpha/Beta Agonist

Use Neurogenic orthostatic hypotension: Treatment of orthostatic dizziness, light-headedness, or the "feeling that you are about to black out" in adults with symptomatic neurogenic orthostatic hypotension (NOH) caused by primary autonomic failure (Parkinson disease [PD], multiple system atrophy [MSA], and pure autonomic failure [PAF]), dopamine beta-hydroxylase deficiency, and nondiabetic autonomic neuropathy.

Local Anesthetic/Vasoconstrictor Precautions Droxidopa is converted to norepinephrine in tissues to result in possible hypertension; use vasoconstrictor with caution since epinephrine or levonordefrin may increase the hypertensive effects of Droxidopa.

Effects on Dental Treatment Key adverse event(s) related to dental treatment: Dizziness, syncope, falling have all been observed; special precautions should be taken when patient suddenly arises from the dental chair

Effects on Bleeding No information available to require special precautions

Adverse Reactions

>10%: Central nervous system: Headache (6% to 13%)

1% to 10%:

Cardiovascular: Hypertension (2% to 7%)

Central nervous system: Dizziness (4% to 10%)

Gastrointestinal: Nausea (9%)

Postmarketing and/or case reports: Abdominal pain, agitation, blurred vision, cerebrovascular accident, chest pain, confusion, delirium, diarrhea, fatigue, hallucination, hyperpyrexia, hypersensitivity reaction (including anaphylaxis, angioedema, bronchospasm, skin rash, urticaria), memory impairment, pancreatitis, psychosis, vomiting

Mechanism of Action A synthetic amino acid analog that is directly metabolized to norepinephrine by dopadecarboxylase. Droxidopa is believed to exert its pharmacological effects through norepinephrine. Norepinephrine increases blood pressure by inducing peripheral arterial and venous vasoconstriction.

Pharmacodynamics/Kinetics

Half-life Elimination ~2.5 hours

Time to Peak

Plasma: 1 to 4 hours

Pregnancy Considerations Adverse events have been observed in some animal reproduction studies.

- **DRV** *see* Darunavir *on page* *441*
- **DS-8201** *see* Fam-Trastuzumab Deruxtecan *on page* *636*
- **DS-8201a** *see* Fam-Trastuzumab Deruxtecan *on page* *636*
- **DS8201-A-J101** *see* Fam-Trastuzumab Deruxtecan *on page* *636*
- **DSCG** *see* Cromolyn (Oral Inhalation) *on page* *416*
- **DSCG** *see* Cromolyn (Systemic) *on page* *416*
- **DSS** *see* Docusate *on page* *509*
- **DST Plus Pak [DSC]** *see* Diclofenac (Topical) *on page* *489*
- **Dsuvia** *see* SUFentanil *on page* *1390*
- **DTC 101** *see* Cytarabine (Liposomal) *on page* *425*
- **DTIC** *see* Dacarbazine *on page* *427*
- **DTIC-Dome** *see* Dacarbazine *on page* *427*

- ◆ **D-Trp(6)-LHRH** *see* Triptorelin *on page 1500*
- ◆ **Duac [DSC]** *see* Clindamycin and Benzoyl Peroxide *on page 375*
- ◆ **Duavee** *see* Estrogens (Conjugated/Equine) and Bazedoxifene *on page 603*
- ◆ **Duetact** *see* Pioglitazone and Glimepiride *on page 1235*
- ◆ **Dulcolax Stool Softener [OTC]** *see* Docusate *on page 509*
- ◆ **Dulera** *see* Mometasone and Formoterol *on page 1047*

DULoxetine (doo LOX e teen)

Related Information

Dentin Hypersensitivity, Acid Erosion, High Caries Index, Management of Alveolar Osteitis, and Xerostomia *on page 1762*

Vasoconstrictor Interactions With Antidepressants *on page 1821*

Brand Names: US Cymbalta; Drizalma Sprinkle

Brand Names: Canada AG-Duloxetine; APO-Duloxetine; Auro-Duloxetine; Cymbalta; JAMP-Duloxetine; M-Duloxetine; Mar-Duloxetine; MINT-Duloxetine; MYLAN-Duloxetine [DSC]; NRA-Duloxetine; PMS-Duloxetine; PRIVA-Duloxetine; RAN-Duloxetine; RIVA-Duloxetine; SANDOZ Duloxetine; TEVA-Duloxetine

Pharmacologic Category Antidepressant, Serotonin/Norepinephrine Reuptake Inhibitor

Use

Fibromyalgia (delayed-release particles capsule only): Management of fibromyalgia in adult and pediatric patients ≥13 years of age.

Generalized anxiety disorder: Treatment of generalized anxiety disorder in adult and pediatric patients ≥7 years of age.

Major depressive disorder (unipolar): Treatment of unipolar major depressive disorder in adults.

Musculoskeletal pain, chronic: Management of chronic musculoskeletal pain including osteoarthritis of the knee and low back pain in adults.

Neuropathic pain associated with diabetes mellitus: Management of pain associated with diabetic peripheral neuropathy in adults.

Local Anesthetic/Vasoconstrictor Precautions Although duloxetine is not a tricyclic antidepressant, it does block norepinephrine reuptake within the CNS synapses as part of its mechanism. It has been suggested that vasoconstrictors be administered with caution and to monitor vital signs in dental patients taking antidepressants that affect norepinephrine in this way.

Effects on Dental Treatment Key adverse event(s) related to dental treatment: Xerostomia and changes in salivation (normal salivary flow resumes upon discontinuation). See Effects on Bleeding.

Effects on Bleeding Platelet dysfunction (ie, impaired platelet aggregation) may occur during treatment with serotonin norepinephrine reuptake inhibitors (SNRIs) such as duloxetine due to platelet serotonin depletion, possibly increasing the risk of a bleeding complication. Concurrent NSAID use may increase this risk.

Adverse Reactions

>10%:

Endocrine & metabolic: Weight loss (children and adolescents: 14% to 15%; adults: ≥1%)

Gastrointestinal: Abdominal pain (children and adolescents: 13%; adults: 5%), decreased appetite (6% to 15%; dose related), nausea (18% to 25%; dose related), vomiting (children and adolescents: 9% to 15%; adults: 3% to 4%), xerostomia (adults: 11% to 14%, dose related; children and adolescents: 2%)

Nervous system: Drowsiness (9% to 11%; dose related), fatigue (5% to 11%; dose related), headache (13% to 18%)

1% to 10%:

Cardiovascular: Flushing (3%), increased blood pressure (2%), palpitations (2%)

Dermatologic: Diaphoresis (6%), pruritus (≥1%)

Endocrine & metabolic: Decreased libido (3% [placebo: 1%]), hot flash (≥1%), orgasm abnormal (2% [placebo: <1%]), weight gain (≥1%)

Gastrointestinal: Constipation (9% to 10%; dose related), diarrhea (6% to 9%), dysgeusia (≥1%), dyspepsia (2%), flatulence (≥1%), viral gastroenteritis (adolescents: 5%)

Genitourinary: Ejaculatory disorder (2%), erectile dysfunction (4% [placebo: 1%]), urinary frequency (≥1%)

Hepatic: Increased serum alanine aminotransferase (>3 x ULN: 1%)

Nervous system: Abnormal dreams (≥1%), agitation (3% to 4%), anorgasmia (≥1%), anxiety (3%), chills (≥1%), delayed ejaculation (2% [placebo: 1%]; dose related), dizziness (8% to 9%), hypoesthesia (≥1%), insomnia (7% to 10%), lethargy (≥1%), paresthesia (≥1%), rigors (≥1%), sleep disorder (≥1%), vertigo (≥1%), yawning (2%)

Neuromuscular & skeletal: Musculoskeletal pain (≥1%), tremor (2% to 3%)

Ophthalmic: Blurred vision (3%)

Respiratory: Cough (children and adolescents: 3%), nasopharyngitis (adolescents: 9%), oropharyngeal pain (children and adolescents: 4%; adults: ≥1%), upper respiratory tract infection (adolescents: 7%)

<1%:

Cardiovascular: Acute myocardial infarction, cardiomyopathy (Takotsubo), cold extremity, orthostatic hypotension, tachycardia

Dermatologic: Contact dermatitis, ecchymoses, erythema of skin, night sweats, skin photosensitivity

Endocrine & metabolic: Dehydration, dyslipidemia, hyperlipidemia, hypothyroidism, increased serum cholesterol, increased thirst, menstrual disease

Gastrointestinal: Bruxism, dysphagia, eructation, gastric ulcer, gastritis, gastroenteritis, gastrointestinal hemorrhage, halitosis, stomatitis

Genitourinary: Dysuria, malodorous urine, menopausal symptoms, nocturia, sexual disorder, urinary urgency

Hematologic & oncologic: Nonthrombocytopenic purpura

Nervous system: Abnormal gait, apathy, confusion, disorientation, disturbance in attention, dysarthria, falling, feeling abnormal, irritability, malaise, myoclonus, sensation of cold, suicidal tendencies

Neuromuscular & skeletal: Asthenia, dyskinesia, muscle spasm, muscle twitching

Ophthalmic: Diplopia, dry eye syndrome, visual impairment

Otic: Otalgia, tinnitus

Renal: Polyuria

Respiratory: Laryngitis, pharyngeal edema

Frequency not defined:

Endocrine & metabolic: Decreased serum potassium, increased serum bicarbonate, increased serum potassium

Hepatic: Increased serum alkaline phosphatase, increased serum aspartate aminotransferase
Nervous system: Suicidal ideation (Parikh 2008)
Neuromuscular & skeletal: Bone fracture, increased creatinine phosphokinase in blood specimen
Postmarketing:
Cardiovascular: Cerebrovascular accident (Leong 2017), hypersensitivity angiitis, hypertensive crisis, supraventricular cardiac arrhythmia, syncope
Dermatologic: Erythema multiforme, skin rash, Stevens-Johnson syndrome (Strawn 2011), urticaria
Endocrine & metabolic: Galactorrhea not associated with childbirth, hyperglycemia, hyperprolactinemia, hyponatremia (Hu 2018), SIADH (Mori 2014)
Gastrointestinal: Acute pancreatitis, colitis, gingival hemorrhage (Balhara 2007; Gicquel 2017)
Genitourinary: Gynecological bleeding, postpartum hemorrhage (Huybrechts 2020), priapism (Wilkening 2016), urinary retention
Hepatic: Acute hepatic failure (Hanje 2006), cholestatic hepatitis (Vuppalanchi 2010), cholestatic jaundice (Park 2010), hepatic necrosis (LiverTox NIH 2018), hepatitis (LiverTox NIH 2018), hepatocellular hepatitis (Vuppalanchi 2010), hepatotoxicity (Park 2013), increased serum transaminases (Kang 2011)
Hypersensitivity: Anaphylaxis, angioedema, hypersensitivity reaction
Nervous system: Aggressive behavior (particularly early in treatment or after treatment discontinuation), extrapyramidal reaction, hypomania (Peritogiannis 2008), mania (Dunner 2005), outbursts of anger (particularly early in treatment or after treatment discontinuation), restless leg syndrome, seizure (with treatment discontinuation), serotonin syndrome (Gelener 2011), sleep disorder (rapid eye movement) (Tan 2017), trismus, withdrawal syndrome (Perahia 2005)
Ophthalmic: Acute angle-closure glaucoma (Mahmut 2017), cataract (Erie 2014)
Renal: Renal colic (Wilkening 2017)

Mechanism of Action Duloxetine is a potent inhibitor of neuronal serotonin and norepinephrine reuptake and a weak inhibitor of dopamine reuptake. Duloxetine has no significant activity for muscarinic cholinergic, H_1-histaminergic, or alpha$_2$-adrenergic receptors. Duloxetine does not possess MAO-inhibitory activity.

Pharmacodynamics/Kinetics

Onset of Action

Onset of action: Anxiety disorders (generalized anxiety disorder): Initial effects may be observed within 2 weeks of treatment, with continued improvements through 4 to 6 weeks (WFSBP [Bandelow 2012]); some experts suggest up to 12 weeks of treatment may be necessary for response (BAP [Baldwin 2014]; Katzman 2014; WFSBP [Bandelow 2012]).
Depression: Initial effects may be observed within 1 to 2 weeks of treatment, with continued improvements through 4 to 6 weeks (Papakostas 2006; Posternak 2005; Szegedi 2009).

Half-life Elimination

Children ≥7 years and Adolescents: 10.4 hours (Lobo 2014).
Adults: ~12 hours (range: 8 to 22 hours); ~4 hours longer in elderly women.

Time to Peak 5 to 6 hours; food delays by 1.7 to 4 hours.

Reproductive Considerations

If treatment for major depressive disorder is initiated for the first time in females planning a pregnancy, agents other than duloxetine are preferred (Larsen 2015).

Pregnancy Considerations

Duloxetine crosses the placenta (Boyce 2011; Briggs 2009; Collin-Lévesque 2018).

Nonteratogenic adverse events have been observed with venlafaxine or other SNRIs/SSRIs when used during pregnancy. Cyanosis, apnea, respiratory distress, seizures, temperature instability, feeding difficulty, vomiting, hypoglycemia, hypo- or hypertonia, hyperreflexia, jitteriness, irritability, constant crying, and tremor have been reported in the neonate immediately following delivery after exposure to venlafaxine, SSRIs, or other SNRIs late in the third trimester. Prolonged hospitalization, respiratory support, or tube feedings may be required. Some symptoms may be due to the toxicity of the SNRIs/SSRIs or a discontinuation syndrome and may be consistent with serotonin syndrome associated with treatment.

Duloxetine may impair platelet aggregation, resulting in an increased risk of bleeding; the risk of postpartum hemorrhage may be increased when used within the month prior to delivery.

Untreated or inadequately treated mental illness may lead to poor compliance with prenatal care. The ACOG recommends that therapy with SSRIs or SNRIs during pregnancy be individualized. Use of a single agent is preferred. According to their recommendations, treatment of depression during pregnancy should incorporate the clinical expertise of the mental health clinician, obstetrician, primary care provider, and pediatrician (ACOG 2008). If treatment for major depressive disorder is initiated for the first time during pregnancy, agents other than duloxetine are preferred (Larsen 2015; MacQueen 2016).

Untreated fibromyalgia may be associated with adverse pregnancy outcomes, including placental abruption, venous thrombosis, premature rupture of membranes, preterm birth, and intrauterine growth restriction/small for gestational age. It is not known if these outcomes are due specifically to fibromyalgia or comorbid conditions. Due to limited data, use of duloxetine for the treatment of fibromyalgia syndrome (FMS) in pregnancy should be reserved for women with severe forms of FMS complicated by depressive symptoms which worsen during pregnancy. Close monitoring is recommended (Gentile 2019).

Health care providers are encouraged to enroll women exposed to duloxetine during pregnancy in the Cymbalta Pregnancy Registry (866-814-6975 or http://cymbaltapregnancyregistry.com).

Pregnant women exposed to antidepressants during pregnancy are encouraged to enroll in the National Pregnancy Registry for Antidepressants (NPRAD). Women 18 to 45 years of age or their health care providers may contact the registry by calling 844-405-6185. Enrollment should be done as early in pregnancy as possible.

- **Duloxetine HCl** *see* DULoxetine *on page 536*
- **Duloxetine Hydrochloride** *see* DULoxetine *on page 536*
- **Duoneb** *see* Ipratropium and Albuterol *on page 839*
- **Duopa** *see* Carbidopa and Levodopa *on page 290*
- **DuP 753** *see* Losartan *on page 938*

Dupilumab (doo PIL ue mab)

Brand Names: US Dupixent

Brand Names: Canada Dupixent

Pharmacologic Category Interleukin-4 Receptor Antagonist; Monoclonal Antibody; Monoclonal Antibody, Anti-Asthmatic

Use

Asthma: Add-on maintenance treatment of moderate to severe asthma in adults and pediatric patients ≥12 years of age with an eosinophilic phenotype or with corticosteroid dependent asthma.

Limitations of use: Not indicated for the relief of acute bronchospasm or status asthmaticus.

Atopic dermatitis: Treatment of moderate to severe atopic dermatitis in adults and pediatric patients ≥6 years of age whose disease is not adequately controlled with topical prescription therapies or when those therapies are not advisable.

Rhinosinusitis (chronic) with nasal polyposis: Add-on maintenance treatment in adults with inadequately controlled chronic rhinosinusitis with nasal polyposis.

Local Anesthetic/Vasoconstrictor Precautions No information available to require special precautions

Effects on Dental Treatment No significant effects or complications reported

Effects on Bleeding No information available to require special precautions

Adverse Reactions

>10%:

Immunologic: Antibody development (5% to 16%; neutralizing: 2% to 5%)

Local: Injection site reaction (6% to 18%)

1% to 10%:

Central nervous system: Insomnia (1%)

Gastrointestinal: Oral herpes simplex infection (4%), gastritis (2%), toothache (1%)

Hematologic & oncologic: Eosinophilia (≤2%)

Infection: Herpes simplex infection (2%)

Neuromuscular & skeletal: Arthralgia (3%)

Ophthalmic: Conjunctivitis (2% to 10%), eye pruritus (1%)

Respiratory: Oropharyngeal pain (2%)

<1%, postmarketing, and/or case reports: Anaphylaxis, dry eye syndrome, eosinophilic granulomatosis with polyangiitis, eosinophilic pneumonitis, erythema nodosum, hypersensitivity reaction, keratitis, serum sickness, serum sickness-like reaction, significant cardiovascular event, vasculitis

Mechanism of Action Dupilumab is a human monoclonal IgG4 antibody that inhibits interleukin-4 (IL-4) and interleukin-13 (IL-13) signaling by binding to the IL-4Rα subunit. Blocking IL-4Rα with dupilumab inhibits IL-4 and IL-13 cytokine-induced inflammatory responses, including the release of proinflammatory cytokines, chemokines, nitric oxide and IgE; however, the mechanism of dupilumab action in asthma has not been definitively established.

Pharmacodynamics/Kinetics

Time to Peak ~1 week

Pregnancy Considerations

Dupilumab is a humanized monoclonal antibody (IgG_4). Placental transfer of human IgG is dependent upon the IgG subclass, maternal serum concentrations, newborn birth weight, and gestational age, generally increasing as pregnancy progresses. The lowest exposure would be expected during the period of organogenesis (Palmeira 2012; Pentsuk 2009).

Uncontrolled asthma is associated with adverse events on pregnancy (increased risk of perinatal mortality, preeclampsia, preterm birth, low birth weight infants, cesarean delivery, and the development of gestational diabetes). Poorly controlled asthma or asthma exacerbations may have a greater fetal/maternal risk than what is associated with appropriately used asthma medications. Maternal treatment improves pregnancy outcomes by reducing the risk of some adverse events (eg, preterm birth, gestational diabetes). Maternal asthma symptoms should be monitored monthly during pregnancy (ERS/TSANZ [Middleton 2020]; GINA 2020).

Use of monoclonal antibodies for the treatment of asthma in pregnancy may be considered when conventional therapies are insufficient; use of an agent other than dupilumab may be preferred (ERS/TSANZ [Middleton 2020]).

Data collection to monitor pregnancy and infant outcomes following exposure to dupilumab is ongoing. Health care providers are encouraged to enroll exposed pregnant females in the MotherToBaby Pregnancy Studies conducted by the Organization of Teratology Information Specialists (877-311-8972 or https://mothertobaby.org). Patients may also enroll themselves.

- ◆ **Dupixent** *see* Dupilumab *on page 538*
- ◆ **Duraclon** *see* CloNIDine *on page 389*
- ◆ **Duragesic** *see* FentaNYL *on page 642*
- ◆ **Duramorph** *see* Morphine (Systemic) *on page 1050*
- ◆ **Duricef** *see* Cefadroxil *on page 299*
- ◆ **Durlaza** *see* Aspirin *on page 177*
- ◆ **Durolane** *see* Hyaluronate and Derivatives *on page 761*

Durvalumab (dur VAL ue mab)

Brand Names: US Imfinzi

Brand Names: Canada Imfinzi

Pharmacologic Category Antineoplastic Agent, Anti-PD-L1 Monoclonal Antibody; Antineoplastic Agent, Monoclonal Antibody

Use

Non-small cell lung cancer, unresectable: Treatment of unresectable stage III non-small cell lung cancer in adults whose disease has not progressed following concurrent platinum-based chemotherapy and radiation therapy.

Small cell lung cancer, extensive stage: First-line treatment of extensive-stage small cell lung cancer in combination with etoposide and either carboplatin or cisplatin in adults.

Urothelial carcinoma, locally advanced or metastatic: Treatment of locally advanced or metastatic urothelial carcinoma in adults who have disease progression during or following platinum-containing chemotherapy, or disease progression within 12 months of neoadjuvant or adjuvant treatment with platinum-containing chemotherapy.

Local Anesthetic/Vasoconstrictor Precautions No information available to require special precautions

Effects on Dental Treatment No significant effects or complications reported

Effects on Bleeding No information available to require special precautions

Adverse Reactions

>10%:

Cardiovascular: Peripheral edema (≤15%)

Dermatologic: Dermatitis (≤26%), pruritus (12%), skin rash (≤26%; including immune mediated rashes)

Endocrine & metabolic: Hyperglycemia (52%), hyperkalemia (32%), hypocalcemia (46%), hyponatremia (33%), hypothyroidism (11% to 12%, including immune mediated), increased gamma-glutamyl transferase (24%)

Gastrointestinal: Abdominal pain (10% to 14%; severe abdominal pain: 3%), colitis (≤18%, including immune mediated), constipation (21%), decreased appetite (19%), diarrhea (≤18%, including immune mediated), nausea (16%)

Genitourinary: Urinary tract infection (15%)

Hematologic & oncologic: Lymphocytopenia (43%; grades 3/4: 11% to 17%)

Hepatic: Hepatitis (12%, including immune mediated), increased serum alanine aminotransferase (39%), increased serum aspartate aminotransferase (36%)

Infection: Infection (38% to 56%)

Nervous system: Fatigue (34% to 39%)

Neuromuscular & skeletal: Musculoskeletal pain (24%)

Respiratory: Cough (≤40%), dyspnea (≤25%), dyspnea on exertion (≤25%), pneumonia (17%), pneumonitis (≤34%, including immune mediated), productive cough (≤40%), radiation pneumonitis (≤34%), upper respiratory tract infection (26%)

Miscellaneous: Fever (≤15%; including tumor-associated fever)

1% to 10%:

Dermatologic: Night sweats (<10%)

Endocrine & metabolic: Dehydration (grades 3/4: ≤3%), hypercalcemia (grades 3/4: 3%), hypermagnesemia (grades 3/4: 4%), hyperthyroidism (7%, including immune mediated), hypoalbuminemia (grades 3/4: 1%), hypokalemia (grades 3/4: 1%)

Genitourinary: Dysuria (<10%)

Hematologic & oncologic: Anemia (grades 3/4: 8%), neutropenia (grades 3/4: 1%)

Hepatic: Hyperbilirubinemia (grades 3/4: 1%), increased serum alkaline phosphatase (grades 3/4: 4%), severe hepatic insufficiency (3%)

Immunologic: Antibody development (3%; neutralizing: <1%)

Infection: Increased susceptibility to infection (<10%), sepsis (>2%)

Nervous system: Voice disorder (<10%)

Renal: Acute renal failure (5%), increased serum creatinine (grades 3/4: 1%), nephritis (6%; immune mediated)

Miscellaneous: Infusion related reaction (2%)

<1%:

Cardiovascular: Myocarditis (immune mediated)

Endocrine & metabolic: Adrenocortical insufficiency (immune mediated), pituitary insufficiency (immune mediated), thyroiditis (immune mediated), type 1 diabetes mellitus (immune mediated)

Hematologic & oncologic: Hemolytic anemia (immune mediated), immune thrombocytopenia

Nervous system: Aseptic meningitis (immune mediated), myasthenia gravis (immune mediated)

Neuromuscular & skeletal: Myositis (immune mediated)

Ophthalmic: Ophthalmic inflammation (immune mediated; including uveitis and keratitis)

Frequency not defined:

Endocrine & metabolic: Hypophysitis (immune mediated)

Hepatic: Hepatic injury

Mechanism of Action Durvalumab is a human immunoglobulin G1 kappa monoclonal antibody which blocks programmed cell death ligand 1 (PD-L1) binding to PD-1 and CD80 (B7.1); PD-L1 blockade leads to increased T-cell activation, allowing T-cells to kill tumor cells (Massard 2016). PD-L1 is an immune check point protein expressed on tumor cells and tumor infiltrating cells and down regulates anti-tumor t-cell function by binding to PD-1 and B7.1; blocking PD-1 and B7.1 interactions restores antitumor t-cell function (Fehrenbacher 2016; Rosenberg 2016).

Pharmacodynamics/Kinetics

Half-life Elimination Terminal half-life: ~18 days

Reproductive Considerations

Females of reproductive potential should use effective contraception during therapy and for at least 3 months after the last durvalumab dose.

Pregnancy Considerations

Based on the mechanism of action, and data from animal reproduction studies, in utero exposure to durvalumab may cause fetal harm. Durvalumab is a humanized monoclonal antibody (IgG_1). Potential placental transfer of human IgG is dependent upon the IgG subclass and gestational age, generally increasing as pregnancy progresses. The lowest exposure would be expected during the period of organogenesis (Palmeira 2012; Pentsuk 2009).

Dutasteride (doo TAS teer ide)

Brand Names: US Avodart

Brand Names: Canada ACT Dutasteride; APO-Dutasteride; AURO-Dutasteride; Avodart; JAMP Dutasteride; MED-Dutasteride; MINT-Dutasteride; PMS-Dutasteride; PRIVA-Dutasteride; RIVA-Dutasteride; SANDOZ Dutasteride; TEVA-Dutasteride

Pharmacologic Category 5 Alpha-Reductase Inhibitor

Use

Benign prostatic hyperplasia: Treatment of symptomatic benign prostatic hyperplasia (BPH) as monotherapy (to improve symptoms, reduce the risk of acute urinary retention, and to reduce the risk of need for BPH-related surgery) or combination therapy with tamsulosin

Limitations of use: Not approved for the prevention of prostate cancer.

Local Anesthetic/Vasoconstrictor Precautions No information available to require special precautions

Effects on Dental Treatment No significant effects or complications reported

Effects on Bleeding No information available to require special precautions

Adverse Reactions Frequency of most adverse events (except prostate cancer high grade) tends to decrease with continued use (>6 months). Frequency not always defined.

1% to 10%:

Endocrine & metabolic: Decreased libido (≤3%; incidence highest during first 6 months of therapy), gynecomastia (including breast tenderness, breast enlargement; ≤1%), increased luteinizing hormone, increased testosterone level, increased thyroid stimulating hormone level

Genitourinary: Impotence (≤5%; incidence highest during first 6 months of therapy), ejaculatory disorder (≤2%)

Hematologic & oncologic: Prostate cancer high grade (≤1%)

<1%, postmarketing, and/or case reports: Angioedema, cardiac failure, depressed mood, dermatological reaction (serious), dizziness, hypersensitivity, localized edema, malignant neoplasm of breast (males), pruritus, skin rash, testicular pain, testicular swelling, urticaria

Mechanism of Action Dutasteride is a 4-azo analog of testosterone and is a competitive, selective inhibitor of both reproductive tissues (type 2) and skin and hepatic (type 1) 5α-reductase. This results in inhibition of the conversion of testosterone to dihydrotestosterone and markedly suppresses serum dihydrotestosterone levels.

Pharmacodynamics/Kinetics

Half-life Elimination Terminal: ~5 weeks

Time to Peak 2-3 hours

Reproductive Considerations

Dutasteride can be detected in semen; sperm count, semen volume, and sperm movement may be decreased, but the effect on male fertility is unknown.

Pregnancy Considerations

Based on the mechanism of action and data from animal reproduction studies, in utero exposure to dutasteride may cause fetal harm. Use is contraindicated in pregnant women.

Capsules should not be handled by pregnant women or women who may be pregnant; if contact with a leaking capsule occurs, wash area immediately with soap and water.

Dutasteride and Tamsulosin

(doo TAS teer ide & tam SOO loe sin)

Related Information

Dutasteride *on page 539*

Tamsulosin *on page 1405*

Brand Names: US Jalyn

Brand Names: Canada Jalyn

Pharmacologic Category 5 Alpha-Reductase Inhibitor; Alpha$_1$ Blocker

Use

Benign prostatic hyperplasia: Treatment of symptomatic benign prostatic hyperplasia (BPH) in men with an enlarged prostate.

Limitations of use: Dutasteride-containing products are not approved for the prevention of prostate cancer.

Local Anesthetic/Vasoconstrictor Precautions No information available to require special precautions

Effects on Dental Treatment Key adverse event(s) related to dental treatment: Tamsulosin: Patients may experience orthostatic hypotension as they stand up after treatment; especially if lying in dental chair for extended periods of time. Use caution with sudden changes in position during and after dental treatment.

Effects on Bleeding No information available to require special precautions

Adverse Reactions Frequencies reported for when products used in combination. Also see individual agents.

1% to 10%:

Central nervous system: Dizziness (2%)

Endocrine & metabolic: Decreased libido (5% to 6%), breast changes (3% to 5%, including breast hypertrophy, breast swelling, breast tenderness, gynecomastia, mastalgia, nipple pain, nipple swelling)

Genitourinary: Ejaculatory disorder (10% to 11%), impotence (8% to 10%)

<1%, postmarketing, and/or case reports: Malignant neoplasm of prostate (high-grade)

Mechanism of Action

Dutasteride is a 4-azo analog of testosterone and is a competitive, selective inhibitor of both reproductive tissues (type 2) and skin and hepatic (type 1) 5α-reductase. This results in inhibition of the conversion of testosterone to dihydrotestosterone and markedly suppresses serum dihydrotestosterone levels.

Tamsulosin is an antagonist of alpha$_{1A}$-adrenoreceptors in the prostate. Smooth muscle tone in the prostate is mediated by alpha$_{1A}$-adrenoreceptors; blocking them leads to relaxation of smooth muscle in the bladder neck and prostate, causing an improvement of urine flow and decreased symptoms of BPH. Approximately 75% of the alpha$_1$-receptors in the prostate are of the alpha$_{1A}$ subtype.

Reproductive Considerations

Women trying to conceive should not handle the product; if contact with a leaking capsule occurs, wash area immediately with soap and water. Use is contraindicated in females of reproductive potential.

Dutasteride can be detected in semen; the effect on male fertility is unknown. Refer to the dutasteride monograph for additional information.

Pregnancy Risk Factor X

Pregnancy Considerations Pregnant women should not handle the product; if contact with a leaking capsule occurs, wash area immediately with soap and water; dutasteride may negatively impact fetal development. Use is contraindicated during pregnancy. Refer to individual monographs for additional information.

- **Dutasteride/Tamsulosin HCl** *see* Dutasteride and Tamsulosin *on page 540*

Duvelisib

(DOO ve LIS ib)

Brand Names: US Copiktra

Pharmacologic Category Antineoplastic Agent, Phosphatidylinositol 3-Kinase Inhibitor

Use

Chronic lymphocytic leukemia/small lymphocytic lymphoma, relapsed or refractory: Treatment of relapsed or refractory chronic lymphocytic leukemia (CLL) or small lymphocytic lymphoma (SLL) in adult patients after at least 2 prior therapies.

Follicular lymphoma, relapsed or refractory: Treatment of relapsed or refractory follicular lymphoma (FL) in adult patients after at least 2 prior systemic therapies.

Local Anesthetic/Vasoconstrictor Precautions No information available to require special precautions

Effects on Dental Treatment Key adverse event(s) related to dental treatment: Frequent occurrence of mucositis

Effects on Bleeding Chemotherapy may result in significant myelosuppression; leukopenia, neutropenia, and thrombocytopenia are significant (see adverse reactions); in patients under active treatment with duvelisib, medical consult is suggested.

Adverse Reactions

>10%:

Cardiovascular: Edema (11% to 14%)

Central nervous system: Fatigue (25% to 29%), headache (12%)

Dermatologic: Skin rash (27% to 31%)

Endocrine & metabolic: Hypophosphatemia (31%), hyponatremia (27% to 31%), hyperkalemia (26% to 31%), hypoalbuminemia (25% to 31%), hypocalcemia (23% to 25%), hypokalemia (10% to 20%), weight loss (11%)

Gastrointestinal: Colitis (≤57%), diarrhea (≤57%), increased serum lipase (36% to 37%), increased serum amylase (28% to 31%), nausea (23% to 24%), abdominal pain (16% to 18%), constipation (13% to 17%), vomiting (15% to 16%), mucositis (14%), decreased appetite (13% to 14%)

Hematologic & oncologic: Neutropenia (34% to 67%; grade ≥3: 30% to 49%; grade 4: 18% to 32%), anemia (20% to 55%; grade ≥3: 11% to 20%), thrombocytopenia (17% to 43%; grade ≥3: 10% to 16%; grade 4: 6% to 7%), lymphocytosis (30%; grade ≥3: 21% to 22%), leukopenia (29%; grade ≥3: 8%; grade 4: 2%), lymphocytopenia (21%; grade ≥3: 9%; grade 4: 3%)

Hepatic: Increased serum alanine aminotransferase (40% to 42%), increased serum aspartate aminotransferase (36% to 37%), decreased serum alkaline phosphatase (34%), increased serum alkaline phosphatase (27% to 29%), increased serum transaminases (11% to 15%)

Infection: Sepsis (≤58%), serious infection (31%)

Neuromuscular & skeletal: Musculoskeletal pain (17% to 20%)

Renal: Renal insufficiency (≤58%), increased serum creatinine (24% to 29%)

Respiratory: Upper respiratory tract infection (21% to 28%), pneumonia (21% to 27%), cough (23% to 25%), lower respiratory tract infection (10% to 18%), dyspnea (12%)

Miscellaneous: Fever (26% to 29%)

1% to 10%:

Dermatologic: Dermatological reaction (5%)

Infection: Cytomegalovirus disease (1%)

Neuromuscular & skeletal: Arthralgia (10%)

Respiratory: Pneumonitis (5%), pneumonia due to *Pneumocystis jiroveci* (1%)

Mechanism of Action Duvelisib is an oral PI3K inhibitor with dual inhibitory activity primarily against PI3K-δ and PI3K-γ which are expressed in hematologic malignancies. Inhibition of PI3K-δ reduced tumor cell proliferation while allowing survival of normal cells. Inhibition of PI3K-γ reduces differentiation and migration of tumor microenvironment support cells (Flinn 2018). Duvelisib resulted in reduced viability of cell lines derived from malignant B-cells and CLL cells. Additionally, duvelisib inhibits B-cell receptor signaling pathways and CXCR12-mediated chemotaxis of malignant B-cells as well as CXCL12-induced T cell migration and M-CSF and IL-4 driven M2 macrophage polarization.

Pharmacodynamics/Kinetics

Half-life Elimination 4.7 hours

Time to Peak 1 to 2 hours

Reproductive Considerations

Pregnancy status should be evaluated prior to treatment. Females of reproductive potential, and males with female partners of reproductive potential, should use effective contraception during therapy and for at least 1 month after the last duvelisib dose.

Pregnancy Considerations

Based on the mechanism of action and adverse events observed in animal reproduction studies, fetal harm may occur if administered to a pregnant female.

- **Duzallo [DSC]** *see* Lesinurad and Allopurinol *on page 887*
- **D-Vi-Sol [OTC]** *see* Cholecalciferol *on page 344*
- **D-Vita [OTC] [DSC]** *see* Cholecalciferol *on page 344*
- **D-Vite Pediatric [OTC]** *see* Cholecalciferol *on page 344*
- **DW286** *see* Gemifloxacin *on page 733*
- **Dxevo 11-Day** *see* DexAMETHasone (Systemic) *on page 463*
- **Dyanavel XR** *see* Amphetamine *on page 135*
- **Dyazide** *see* Hydrochlorothiazide and Triamterene *on page 763*
- **Dyloject [DSC]** *see* Diclofenac (Systemic) *on page 484*
- **Dynacin** *see* Minocycline (Systemic) *on page 1032*
- **Dyna-Hex 2 [OTC]** *see* Chlorhexidine Gluconate (Topical) *on page 335*
- **Dyna-Hex 4 [OTC]** *see* Chlorhexidine Gluconate (Topical) *on page 335*
- **Dyrenium** *see* Triamterene *on page 1493*
- **Dyspel [OTC]** *see* Ibuprofen *on page 786*
- **Dysport** *see* AbobotulinumtoxinA *on page 55*
- **E2** *see* Estradiol (Systemic) *on page 596*
- **E2 and DRSP** *see* Drospirenone and Estradiol *on page 534*
- **E-400 [OTC] [DSC]** *see* Vitamin E (Systemic) *on page 1549*
- **E-400-Clear [OTC]** *see* Vitamin E (Systemic) *on page 1549*
- **E-400-Mixed [OTC]** *see* Vitamin E (Systemic) *on page 1549*
- **E2020** *see* Donepezil *on page 512*
- **E 2080** *see* Rufinamide *on page 1350*
- **E7080** *see* Lenvatinib *on page 885*
- **E7389** *see* EriBULin *on page 584*
- **E7438** *see* Tazemetostat *on page 1408*
- **EACA** *see* Aminocaproic Acid *on page 116*
- **Ear Drops [OTC]** *see* Carbamide Peroxide *on page 289*
- **Ear Drops Earwax Aid [OTC]** *see* Carbamide Peroxide *on page 289*
- **Earwax Treatment Drops [OTC] [DSC]** *see* Carbamide Peroxide *on page 289*
- **ECMS** *see* Mycophenolate *on page 1067*
- **EC-Naprosyn** *see* Naproxen *on page 1080*
- **EC-Naproxen** *see* Naproxen *on page 1080*
- ***E. coli* Asparaginase** *see* Asparaginase (*E. coli*) *on page 175*

Econazole (e KONE a zole)

Brand Names: US Ecoza; Zolpak

Pharmacologic Category Antifungal Agent, Imidazole Derivative; Antifungal Agent, Topical

Use Fungal infection:

Cream: Treatment of tinea pedis, tinea cruris, and tinea corporis caused by *Trichophyton rubrum*, *Trichophyton mentagrophytes*, *Trichophyton tonsurans*, *Microsporum canis*, *Microsporum audouini*, *Microsporum gypseum*, and *Epidermophyton floccosum* in the treatment of cutaneous candidiasis, and in the treatment of tinea versicolor.

Foam: Treatment of interdigital tinea pedis caused by *Trichophyton rubrum*, *Trichophyton mentagrophytes*, and *Epidermophyton floccosum* in patients 12 years and older

Local Anesthetic/Vasoconstrictor Precautions No information available to require special precautions

Effects on Dental Treatment No significant effects or complications reported

Effects on Bleeding No information available to require special precautions

Adverse Reactions

1% to 10%: Dermatologic: Burning sensation of skin (3%), erythema (3%), pruritus (3%), stinging of the skin (3%)

<1%, postmarketing, and/or case reports: Application site reaction, pruritic rash

Mechanism of Action Alters fungal cell wall membrane permeability; may interfere with RNA and protein synthesis, and lipid metabolism

Pharmacodynamics/Kinetics

Time to Peak Foam: 6.8 ± 5.1 hours

Pregnancy Considerations Information related to econazole use in pregnancy is primarily from use for other indications and route of administration. Until more data are available, it is suggested to avoid use in the first trimester and apply sparingly during the second and third trimesters if needed for topical fungal infections (Patel 2017).

- ◆ **Econazole Nitrate** *see* Econazole *on page 542*
- ◆ **Ecotrin [OTC]** *see* Aspirin *on page 177*
- ◆ **Ecotrin Arthritis Strength [OTC]** *see* Aspirin *on page 177*
- ◆ **Ecotrin Low Strength [OTC]** *see* Aspirin *on page 177*
- ◆ **Ecoza** *see* Econazole *on page 542*

Edaravone (e DAR a vone)

Brand Names: US Radicava

Brand Names: Canada Radicava

Pharmacologic Category Free Radical Scavenger

Use Amyotrophic lateral sclerosis: Treatment of amyotrophic lateral sclerosis (ALS)

Local Anesthetic/Vasoconstrictor Precautions No information available to require special precautions

Effects on Dental Treatment No significant effects or complications reported

Effects on Bleeding No information available to require special precautions

Adverse Reactions

>10%:

Central nervous system: Abnormal gait (13%)

Hematologic & oncologic: Bruise (15%)

1% to 10%:

Central nervous system: Headache (10%)

Dermatologic: Dermatitis (8%), eczema (7%), tinea (4%)

Endocrine & metabolic: Glycosuria (4%)

Respiratory: Dyspnea (≤6%), hypoxia (≤6%), respiratory failure (≤6%)

<1%, postmarketing, and/or case reports: Anaphylaxis, hypersensitivity reaction

Mechanism of Action The mechanism by which edaravone slows the decline of physical function in patients with ALS is unknown. Edaravone is a free radical and peroxynitrite scavenger that prevents oxidative damage to cell membranes and may contribute to inhibiting the progression of ALS (Nagase 2016).

Pharmacodynamics/Kinetics

Half-life Elimination 4.5 to 6 hours

Time to Peak 1 hour

Pregnancy Considerations Adverse events were observed in some animal reproduction studies.

- ◆ **Edarbi** *see* Azilsartan *on page 202*
- ◆ **Ed ChlorPed [OTC] [DSC]** *see* Chlorpheniramine *on page 340*
- ◆ **Ed Chlorped Jr [OTC]** *see* Chlorpheniramine *on page 340*
- ◆ **Ed-Chlortan [OTC] [DSC]** *see* Chlorpheniramine *on page 340*
- ◆ **Edecrin** *see* Ethacrynic Acid *on page 608*
- ◆ **Edex** *see* Alprostadil *on page 110*
- ◆ **Edluar** *see* Zolpidem *on page 1582*

Edoxaban (e DOX a ban)

Related Information

Antiplatelet and Anticoagulation Considerations in Dentistry *on page 1666*

Brand Names: US Savaysa

Brand Names: Canada Lixiana

Pharmacologic Category Anticoagulant; Anticoagulant, Factor Xa Inhibitor; Direct Oral Anticoagulant (DOAC)

Use

Nonvalvular atrial fibrillation: To reduce the risk of stroke and systemic embolism in patients with nonvalvular atrial fibrillation (AF).

Limitations of use: Do not use in nonvalvular AF patients with CrCl >95 mL/minute because of an increased risk of ischemic stroke compared to warfarin.

Venous thromboembolism (deep vein thrombosis and pulmonary embolism): Treatment of deep vein thrombosis and pulmonary embolism following 5 to 10 days of initial therapy with a parenteral anticoagulant.

Local Anesthetic/Vasoconstrictor Precautions No information available to require special precautions

Effects on Dental Treatment Key adverse event(s) related to dental treatment: Surgical site bleeding may occur. See effects on bleeding.

Effects on Bleeding Edoxaban inhibits platelet activation and fibrin clot formation via direct, selective, and reversible inhibition of factor Xa. As with all anticoagulants, bleeding is the major adverse effect of edoxaban. Hemorrhage may occur at virtually any site; risk is dependent on multiple variables including the intensity of anticoagulation and patient susceptibility. Medical consult is suggested.

Adverse Reactions

>10%: Hematologic and oncologic: Hemorrhage (22% to 26%), major hemorrhage (1% to 13%), minor hemorrhage (7% to 13%)

1% to 10%:

Dermatologic: Dermal hemorrhage (6%), skin rash (4%)

Gastrointestinal: Gastrointestinal hemorrhage (≤4%)

Genitourinary: Gross hematuria (≤2%), urethral bleeding (≤2%), vaginal hemorrhage (9%)

Hematologic and oncologic: Anemia (2%), oral hemorrhage (≤3%), puncture site bleeding (1%)

Hepatic: Abnormal hepatic function tests (5% to 8%)

Respiratory: Epistaxis (5%), pharyngeal bleeding (≤3%)

<1%:

Nervous system: Intracranial hemorrhage

Respiratory: Interstitial pulmonary disease

Frequency not defined:

Cardiovascular: Ischemia (with premature discontinuation)

Hematologic & oncologic: Spinal hematoma (in patients receiving neuraxial anesthesia or undergoing spinal puncture)

Nervous system: Epidural intracranial hemorrhage (in patients receiving neuraxial anesthesia or undergoing spinal puncture)

Postmarketing:

Dermatologic: Urticaria

Gastrointestinal: Abdominal pain

Hematologic & oncologic: Thrombocytopenia

Hypersensitivity: Angioedema, hypersensitivity reaction

Nervous system: Dizziness, headache

Mechanism of Action Edoxaban, a selective factor Xa inhibitor, inhibits free factor Xa and prothrombinase activity and inhibits thrombin-induced platelet aggregation. Inhibition of factor Xa in the coagulation cascade reduces thrombin generation and thrombus formation.

Pharmacodynamics/Kinetics

Half-life Elimination 10 to 14 hours

Time to Peak 1 to 2 hours

Reproductive Considerations

Information related to the use of direct acting oral anticoagulants in pregnancy is limited; until safety data are available, adequate contraception is recommended during therapy for females of childbearing potential. Females planning a pregnancy should be switched to alternative anticoagulants prior to conception (Cohen 2016).

Pregnancy Considerations

Information related to the use of edoxaban in pregnancy is limited (Beyer-Westendorf 2016; Lameijer 2018; Sakai 2019). Use of direct acting oral anticoagulants increases the risk of bleeding in all patients. When used in pregnancy, there is also the potential for fetal bleeding or subclinical placental bleeding which may increase the risk of miscarriage, preterm delivery, fetal compromise, or stillbirth (Cohen 2016).

Data are insufficient to evaluate the safety of direct acting oral anticoagulants during pregnancy (Bates 2012) and use in pregnant females is not recommended (Regitz-Zagrosek [ESC 2018]). Agents other than edoxaban are preferred for the treatment of AF or VTE in pregnant patients (Kearon 2016; Lip 2018; Regitz-Zagrosek [ESC 2018]). Patients should be switched to an alternative anticoagulant if pregnancy occurs during therapy. Fetal monitoring that includes evaluations for fetal bleeding and assessments for risk of preterm delivery are recommended if the direct acting oral anticoagulant is continued (Cohen 2016).

Dental Health Professional Considerations Routine coagulation testing (INR) is not required, or necessary, for Direct-Acting Oral Anticoagulants (DOAC).

- ◆ **Edoxaban Tosylate** *see* Edoxaban *on page 542*
- ◆ **Edurant** *see* Rilpivirine *on page 1327*
- ◆ **EEMT** *see* Estrogens (Esterified) and Methyltestosterone *on page 605*
- ◆ **EEMT HS** *see* Estrogens (Esterified) and Methyltestosterone *on page 605*
- ◆ **E.E.S. 400** *see* Erythromycin (Systemic) *on page 588*
- ◆ **E.E.S. Granules** *see* Erythromycin (Systemic) *on page 588*

Efavirenz (e FAV e renz)

Related Information

HIV Infection and AIDS *on page 1690*

Brand Names: US Sustiva

Brand Names: Canada Auro-Efavirenz; JAMP-Efavirenz; MYLAN-Efavirenz; Sustiva; TEVA-Efavirenz

Pharmacologic Category Antiretroviral, Reverse Transcriptase Inhibitor, Non-nucleoside (Anti-HIV)

Use HIV-1 infection: Treatment of HIV-1 infection in combination with other antiretroviral agents in adults and pediatric patients at least 3 months old and weighing at least 3.5 kg

Local Anesthetic/Vasoconstrictor Precautions No information available to require special precautions

Effects on Dental Treatment Key adverse event(s) related to dental treatment: Abnormal taste

Effects on Bleeding No information available to require special precautions related to hemostasis.

Adverse Reactions Frequency of adverse events is as reported for patients receiving combination antiretroviral therapy.

>10%:

Dermatologic: Skin rash (5% to 32%)

Endocrine & metabolic: Increased serum cholesterol (20% to 40%), increased HDL cholesterol (25% to 35%), increased serum triglycerides (≥751 mg/dL: 6% to 11%)

Gastrointestinal: Diarrhea (3% to 14%)

Nervous system: Central nervous system toxicity (53%), dizziness (2% to 28%), depression (3% to 19%), insomnia (7% to 16%), anxiety (2% to 13%), pain (1% to 13%)

1% to 10%:

Dermatologic: Pruritus (≤9%), erythema multiforme (≤2%)

Endocrine & metabolic: Increased gamma-glutamyl transferase (grades 3/4: 5% to 8%), increased amylase (grades 3/4: grades 3/4: 4% to 6%), hyperglycemia (>250 mg/dL: 2% to 5%)

Gastrointestinal: Nausea (2% to 10%), vomiting (3% to 6%), dyspepsia (4%), abdominal pain (2% to 3%), anorexia (≤2%)

Hematologic & oncologic: Neutropenia (grades 3/4: 2% to 10%)

Hepatic: Increased serum aspartate aminotransferase (grades 3/4: 5% to 8%; incidence higher with hepatitis B and/or C coinfection), increased serum alanine aminotransferase (grades 3/4: 2% to 8%; incidence higher with hepatitis B and/or C coinfection)

Nervous system: Lack of concentration (3% to 8%), fatigue (2% to 8%), headache (2% to 8%), drowsiness (2% to 7%), nervousness (2% to 7%), abnormal dreams (1% to 6%), severe depression (2%), hallucination (1%)

Frequency not defined: Cardiovascular: Prolonged QT interval on ECG

<1%, postmarketing, and/or case reports: Aggressive behavior, agitation, arthralgia, asthenia, ataxia, catatonia, cerebellar ataxia, constipation, delusion, dyspnea, emotional lability, encephalopathy, flushing, fulminant hepatitis, gynecomastia, hepatic failure, hepatitis, hypersensitivity reaction, hypoesthesia, immune reconstitution syndrome, lipotrophy, loss of balance, malabsorption, mania, myalgia, myopathy, neuropathy, palpitations, pancreatitis, paranoid ideation, paresthesia, photodermatitis, psychoneurosis, psychosis, redistribution of body fat, seizure, Stevens-Johnson syndrome, suicidal ideation, suicidal tendencies, tinnitus, tremor, vertigo, visual disturbance

Mechanism of Action As a non-nucleoside reverse transcriptase inhibitor, efavirenz has activity against HIV-1 by binding to reverse transcriptase. It consequently blocks the RNA-dependent and DNA-dependent DNA polymerase activities including HIV-1 replication. It does not require intracellular phosphorylation for antiviral activity.

Pharmacodynamics/Kinetics

Half-life Elimination Single dose: 52 to 76 hours; Multiple doses: 40 to 55 hours

Time to Peak 3 to 5 hours

Reproductive Considerations

The Health and Human Services (HHS) perinatal HIV guidelines consider efavirenz an alternative antiretroviral therapy for females living with HIV who are not yet pregnant but are trying to conceive.

Females living with HIV not planning a pregnancy may use any available type of contraception, considering possible drug interactions and contraindications of the specific method. Consult drug interactions database for more detailed information specific to use of efavirenz and specific contraceptives (HHS [perinatal] 2019). The manufacturer recommends women of reproductive potential undergo pregnancy testing prior to initiation of efavirenz. Barrier contraception should be used in combination with other (hormonal) methods of contraception during therapy and for 12 weeks after efavirenz is discontinued. However, current HHS perinatal HIV guidelines do not restrict use in females planning a pregnancy.

For males and females living with HIV and planning a pregnancy, maximum viral suppression below the limits of detection with antiretroviral therapy (ART), modification of therapy (if needed), optimization of the woman's health, and a discussion of the potential risks and benefits of ART therapy during pregnancy is recommended prior to conception (HHS [perinatal] 2019).

Pregnancy Considerations

Efavirenz has a moderate level of transfer across the human placenta.

Based on data from the Antiretroviral Pregnancy Registry, an increased risk of overall birth defects has not been observed following first trimester exposure to efavirenz. Neural tube and other CNS defects have been reported; however, a meta-analysis has shown that the risk for neural tube defects after efavirenz exposure in the first trimester are not greater than those in the general population. Maternal antiretroviral therapy (ART) may be associated with adverse pregnancy outcomes including preterm delivery, stillbirth, low birth weight, and small for gestational age infants. Actual risks may be influenced by maternal factors, such as disease severity, gestational age at initiation of therapy, and specific ART regimen, therefore close fetal monitoring is recommended. Because there is clear benefit to appropriate treatment, maternal ART should not be withheld due to concerns for adverse neonatal outcomes. Long-term follow-up is recommended for all infants exposed to antiretroviral medications; children without HIV but who were exposed to ART in utero and develop significant organ system abnormalities of unknown etiology (particularly of the CNS or heart) should be evaluated for potential mitochondrial dysfunction. Hypersensitivity reactions (including hepatic toxicity and rash) are more common in women on non-nucleoside reverse transcriptase inhibitor therapy; it is not known if pregnancy increases this risk.

The Health and Human Services (HHS) perinatal HIV guidelines consider efavirenz an alternative ART for pregnant females living with HIV who are antiretroviral-naive, who have had ART therapy in the past but are restarting, or who require a new ART regimen (due to poor tolerance or poor virologic response of current regimen). Females who become pregnant while taking efavirenz may continue if viral suppression is effective and the regimen is well tolerated. Pharmacokinetic data from available studies do not suggest dose alterations are needed during pregnancy.

Use may be considered for females having drug interactions with other medications or who require the convenience of once daily dosing (and are not eligible for dolutegravir or rilpivirine); screening for antenatal and postpartum depression is recommended. Although not recommended by the manufacturer, HHS guidelines do not restrict the use of efavirenz in the first trimester.

In general, ART is recommended for all pregnant females living with HIV to keep the viral load below the limit of detection and reduce the risk of perinatal transmission. Therapy should be individualized following a discussion of the potential risks and benefits of treatment during pregnancy. Monitoring of pregnant females is more frequent than in nonpregnant adults. ART should be continued postpartum for all females living with HIV and can be modified after delivery.

Health care providers are encouraged to enroll pregnant females exposed to antiretroviral medications as early in pregnancy as possible in the Antiretroviral Pregnancy Registry (1-800-258-4263 or http://www.APRegistry.com). Health care providers caring for pregnant females living with HIV and their infants may contact the National Perinatal HIV Hotline (1-888-448-8765) for clinical consultation (HHS [perinatal] 2019).

Prescribing and Access Restrictions Efavirenz oral solution is available only through an expanded access (compassionate use) program. Enrollment information may be obtained by calling 877-372-7097.

Efavirenz, Emtricitabine, and Tenofovir Disoproxil Fumarate

(e FAV e renz, em trye SYE ta been, & ten OF oh vir dye soe PROX il FUE ma rate)

Related Information

Efavirenz *on page 543*
Emtricitabine *on page 556*
HIV Infection and AIDS *on page 1690*
Tenofovir Disoproxil Fumarate *on page 1419*

Brand Names: US Atripla

Brand Names: Canada Atripla

Pharmacologic Category Antiretroviral, Reverse Transcriptase Inhibitor, Non-nucleoside (Anti-HIV); Antiretroviral, Reverse Transcriptase Inhibitor, Nucleoside (Anti-HIV); Antiretroviral, Reverse Transcriptase Inhibitor, Nucleotide (Anti-HIV)

Use HIV-1 infection, treatment: Treatment of HIV-1 infection in adult and pediatric patients weighing ≥40 kg (may be used alone or in combination with other antiretroviral agents).

Local Anesthetic/Vasoconstrictor Precautions No information available to require special precautions

Effects on Dental Treatment Key adverse event(s) related to dental treatment: Efavirenz alone has caused xerostomia (normal salivary flow resumes upon discontinuation) and abnormal taste (see individual monograph). No significant effects or complications reported with combination drug.

Effects on Bleeding No information available to require special precautions related to hemostasis.

Adverse Reactions The complete adverse reaction profile of combination therapy has not been established. Also see individual agents. The following adverse effects were noted in clinical trials with combination therapy.

>10%:

- Central nervous system: Abnormal dreams
- Endocrine & metabolic: Hypercholesterolemia (22%)

1% to 10%:

- Cardiovascular: Increased serum creatine kinase (9%)
- Central nervous system: Depression (9%), fatigue (9%), dizziness (8%), headache (6%), anxiety (5%), insomnia (5%)
- Dermatologic: Skin rash (7%)
- Endocrine & metabolic: Increased serum triglycerides (4%), hyperglycemia (2%)
- Gastrointestinal: Diarrhea (9%), nausea (9%), increased serum amylase (8%), vomiting (2%)
- Genitourinary: Hematuria (3%)
- Hematologic & oncologic: Decreased neutrophils (3%)
- Hepatic: Increased serum aspartate aminotransferase (3%), increased serum alanine aminotransferase (2%), increased serum alkaline phosphatase (1%)
- Respiratory: Sinusitis (8%), upper respiratory tract infection (8%), nasopharyngitis (5%)

<1%: Glycosuria

Mechanism of Action

Efavirenz: Non-nucleoside reverse transcriptase inhibitor of HIV-1. It consequently blocks the RNA-dependent and DNA-dependent DNA polymerase activities including HIV-1 replication.

Emtricitabine: Nucleoside reverse transcriptase inhibitor; cytosine analogue that is phosphorylated intracellularly to emtricitabine 5'-triphosphate which interferes with HIV viral RNA dependent DNA polymerase resulting in inhibition of viral replication.

Tenofovir disoproxil fumarate: Nucleotide reverse transcriptase inhibitor; analog of adenosine 5'-monophosphate that interferes with the HIV viral RNA dependent DNA polymerase resulting in inhibition of viral replication. TDF is first converted intracellularly by hydrolysis to tenofovir and subsequently phosphorylated to the active tenofovir diphosphate. Tenofovir inhibits replication of HBV by inhibiting HBV polymerase.

Reproductive Considerations

The Health and Human Services (HHS) perinatal HIV guidelines consider this fixed-dose combination an alternative regimen for females living with HIV who are not yet pregnant but are trying to conceive (HHS [perinatal] 2019).

Females living with HIV not planning a pregnancy may use any available type of contraception, considering possible drug interactions and contraindications of the specific method. Consult drug interactions database for more detailed information specific to use of this combination and specific contraceptives (HHS [perinatal] 2019). The manufacturer's labeling recommends pregnancy testing prior to therapy, and effective contraception in females of reproductive potential during treatment and for 12 weeks after therapy is discontinued.

Refer to individual monographs for additional information.

Pregnancy Considerations

The Health and Human Services (HHS) perinatal HIV guidelines consider this fixed-dose combination an alternative regimen for pregnant females living with HIV who are antiretroviral-naive, who have had antiretroviral therapy (ART) in the past but are restarting, or who require a new ART regimen (due to poor tolerance or poor virologic response of current regimen). In addition, females who become pregnant while taking this fixed-dose combination may continue if viral suppression is effective and the regimen is well tolerated. This fixed dose combination may be considered for women when significant drug interactions would occur with preferred agents or in women who need the convenience of a co-formulated single dose tablet in a once daily regimen but are not eligible for preferred agents (HHS [perinatal] 2019).

Refer to individual monographs for additional information.

◆ **Efavirenz/Emtricitab/Tenofovir** *see* Efavirenz, Emtricitabine, and Tenofovir Disoproxil Fumarate *on page 545*

Efavirenz, Lamivudine, and Tenofovir Disoproxil Fumarate

(e FAV e renz la MI vyoo deen & ten OF oh vir dye soe PROX il FUE ma rate)

Brand Names: US Symfi; Symfi Lo

Pharmacologic Category Antiretroviral, Reverse Transcriptase Inhibitor, Non-nucleoside (Anti-HIV); Antiretroviral, Reverse Transcriptase Inhibitor, Nucleoside (Anti-HIV); Antiretroviral, Reverse Transcriptase Inhibitor, Nucleotide (Anti-HIV)

Use HIV-1 infection, treatment: Treatment of HIV-1 infection in adult and pediatric patients weighing ≥40 kg (Symfi) or ≥35 kg (Symfi Lo).

Local Anesthetic/Vasoconstrictor Precautions No information available to require special precautions

Effects on Dental Treatment No significant effects or complications reported

Effects on Bleeding No information available to require special precautions

Adverse Reactions Also see individual agents.

>10%:

Cardiovascular: Increased serum creatine kinase (grades 3/4: 12%)

Dermatologic: Skin rash (18%)

Endocrine & metabolic: Increased serum cholesterol (grades 3/4: 19%)

Gastrointestinal: Diarrhea (11%)

Nervous system: Headache (14%), pain (13%), depression (11%)

Neuromuscular & skeletal: Decreased bone mineral density (28%)

1% to 10%:

Endocrine & metabolic: Increased amylase (grades 3/4: 9%), increased serum triglycerides (grades 3/4: 1%), lipodystrophy (1%)

Gastrointestinal: Nausea (8%), abdominal pain (7%), vomiting (5%), dyspepsia (4%)

Genitourinary: Hematuria (grades 3/4: 7%)

Hematologic & oncologic: Decreased neutrophils (grades 3/4: 3%)

Hepatic: Increased serum aspartate aminotransferase (grades 3/4: 5%), increased serum alanine aminotransferase (grades 3/4: 4%)

Nervous system: Anxiety (6%), insomnia (5%), dizziness (3%), peripheral neuropathy (1%)

Neuromuscular & skeletal: Back pain (9%), asthenia (6%), arthralgia (5%), myalgia (3%)

Respiratory: Pneumonia (5%)

Miscellaneous: Fever (8%)

Frequency not defined: Hepatic: Exacerbation of hepatitis B

Mechanism of Action

Efavirenz: Non-nucleoside reverse transcriptase inhibitor of HIV-1. It consequently blocks the RNA-dependent and DNA-dependent DNA polymerase activities including HIV-1 replication.

Lamivudine: Cytosine analog that is phosphorylated intracellularly to its active 5"-triphosphate metabolite. The principle mode of action is inhibition of HIV reverse transcription via viral DNA chain termination; inhibits RNA- and DNA-dependent DNA polymerase activities of reverse transcriptase.

Tenofovir disoproxil fumarate: Nucleotide reverse transcriptase inhibitor; analog of adenosine 5' monophosphate that interferes with the HIV viral RNA dependent DNA polymerase resulting in inhibition of viral replication. TDF is first converted intracellularly by hydrolysis to tenofovir and subsequently phosphorylated to the active tenofovir diphosphate. Tenofovir inhibits replication of HBV by inhibiting HBV polymerase.

Reproductive Considerations

The Health and Human Services perinatal HIV guidelines consider this fixed-dose combination an alternative regimen for females living with HIV who are not yet pregnant but are trying to conceive (HHS [perinatal] 2019).

Females living with HIV not planning a pregnancy may use any available type of contraception, considering possible drug interactions and contraindications of the specific method. Consult drug interactions database for more detailed information specific to use of this combination and specific contraceptives (HHS [perinatal] 2019). The manufacturer's labeling recommends pregnancy testing prior to therapy and effective contraception (including a barrier method) in females of reproductive potential during treatment and for 12 weeks after therapy is discontinued.

Refer to individual monographs for additional information.

Pregnancy Considerations

The Health and Human Services perinatal HIV guidelines consider this fixed-dose combination an alternative regimen for pregnant females living with HIV who are antiretroviral-naive, who have had antiretroviral therapy (ART) in the past but are restarting, or who require a new ART regimen (due to poor tolerance or poor virologic response of current regimen). In addition, females who become pregnant while taking this fixed-dose combination may continue if viral suppression is effective and the regimen is well tolerated. This fixed dose combination may be considered for women when significant drug interactions would occur with preferred agents or in women who need the convenience of a co-formulated single dose tablet in a once daily regimen but are not eligible for preferred agents (HHS [perinatal] 2019).

Refer to individual monographs for additional information.

◆ **Effexor XR** *see* Venlafaxine *on page 1539*

◆ **Effient** *see* Prasugrel *on page 1252*

Efinaconazole (ef in a KON a zole)

Brand Names: US Jublia

Brand Names: Canada Jublia

Pharmacologic Category Antifungal Agent, Topical

Use Onychomycosis: Topical treatment of onychomycosis of the toenail(s) due to *Trichophyton rubrum* and *Trichophyton mentagrophytes*

Local Anesthetic/Vasoconstrictor Precautions No information available to require special precautions

Effects on Dental Treatment No significant effects or complications reported

Effects on Bleeding No information available to require special precautions

Adverse Reactions 1% to 10%:

Dermatologic: Ingrown nail (2%)

Local: Application site dermatitis (2%), application site vesicles (2%), application site pain (1%)

Mechanism of Action An azole antifungal; inhibits fungal lanosterol 14alpha-demethylase involved in the biosynthesis of ergosterol, a constituent of fungal cell membranes, resulting in fungal cell death.

Pharmacodynamics/Kinetics

Half-life Elimination 29.9 hours.

Pregnancy Considerations Small amounts of efinaconazole are absorbed systemically following topical administration. If antifungal treatment cannot be delayed until after pregnancy, topical therapy, when appropriate, is preferred over systemic treatment (Kaul 2017). Information specific to efinaconazole in pregnancy has not been located (Lipner 2015).

◆ **Efmoroctocog Alfa** *see* Antihemophilic Factor (Recombinant [Fc Fusion Protein]) *on page 154*

◆ **Eformoterol** *see* Formoterol *on page 711*

◆ **Eformoterol and Budesonide** *see* Budesonide and Formoterol *on page 255*

◆ **Eformoterol and Mometasone** *see* Mometasone and Formoterol *on page 1047*

◆ **Eha** *see* Lidocaine (Topical) *on page 902*

- ◆ **EHDP** *see* Etidronate *on page 620*
- ◆ **Eicosapentaenoic Acid** *see* Omega-3 Fatty Acids *on page 1137*
- ◆ **EL-970** *see* Dalfampridine *on page 431*

Elagolix (EL a GOE lix)

Brand Names: US Orilissa

Brand Names: Canada Orilissa

Pharmacologic Category Gonadotropin Releasing Hormone Antagonist

Use Endometriosis: Management of moderate to severe pain associated with endometriosis.

Local Anesthetic/Vasoconstrictor Precautions No information available to require special precautions

Effects on Dental Treatment No significant effects or complications reported

Effects on Bleeding No information available to require special precautions

Adverse Reactions

>10%:

Central nervous system: Headache (17% to 20%)

Dermatologic: Night sweats (≤46%)

Endocrine & metabolic: Amenorrhea (4% to 57%), hot flash (≤46%)

Gastrointestinal: Nausea (16%)

Neuromuscular & skeletal: Decreased bone mineral density (≤21%)

1% to 10%:

Central nervous system: Insomnia (6% to 9%), depressed mood (≤6%), depression (≤6%), emotional lability (≤6%), lacrimation (≤6%; including tearfulness), mood changes (≤6%), anxiety (5%), dizziness (≥3% to <5%), irritability (≥3% to <5%)

Endocrine & metabolic: Decreased libido (≥3% to <5%), weight gain (≥3% to <5%)

Gastrointestinal: Abdominal pain (≥3% to <5%), constipation (≥3% to <5%), diarrhea (≥3% to <5%)

Hepatic: Increased serum alanine aminotransferase (≥3 x ULN: 1%)

Neuromuscular & skeletal: Arthralgia (5%)

Frequency not defined:

Endocrine & metabolic: Increased HDL cholesterol, increased LDL cholesterol, increased serum cholesterol, increased triglycerides

Genitourinary: Menstrual flow (reduction in the amount, intensity, or duration of menstrual bleeding)

<1%, postmarketing, and/or case reports: Appendicitis, back pain, suicidal ideation

Mechanism of Action Elagolix is a short-acting, nonpeptide, gonadotropin-releasing hormone antagonist that suppresses pituitary and ovarian hormone function in a dose-dependent manner. Concentrations of LH, FSH, and estradiol are decreased during therapy and rapidly return to previous levels once treatment is discontinued. In patients with endometriosis, these actions reduce dysmenorrhea and nonmenstrual pelvic pain (Ng 2017; Struthers 2009; Taylor 2017).

Pharmacodynamics/Kinetics

Onset of Action FSH, LH, and estradiol suppression: Within hours of day 1 (initial) administration (Ng 2017)

Duration of Action FSH, LH, and estradiol concentrations return to baseline or higher within 24 to 48 hours after discontinuation (Ng 2017)

Half-life Elimination 4 to 6 hours

Time to Peak 1 hour

Reproductive Considerations

Evaluate pregnancy status prior to use. Exclude pregnancy prior to treatment or start elagolix within 7 days from the onset of menses. Treatment with elagolix may reduce the amount, intensity, or duration of menstrual bleeding, which may make it more difficult to recognize pregnancy. Perform pregnancy testing if pregnancy is suspected during elagolix therapy.

Ovulation is not fully suppressed during elagolix therapy (Taylor 2017). Nonhormonal contraceptives should be used during therapy and for 1 week after elagolix treatment is discontinued.

Pregnancy Considerations

Use is contraindicated during pregnancy.

Information related to inadvertent exposure in pregnancy is limited. Elagolix may increase the risk of early pregnancy loss.

Data collection to monitor pregnancy and infant outcomes following exposure to elagolix is ongoing. Health care providers are encouraged to enroll females exposed to elagolix during pregnancy in the pregnancy registry (833-782-7241).

Elagolix, Estradiol, and Norethindrone

(EL a GOE lix, ES tra DYE ol, & nor ETH in drone)

Brand Names: US Oriahnn

Pharmacologic Category Estrogen and Progestin Combination; Estrogen Derivative; Gonadotropin Releasing Hormone Receptor Antagonist; Progestin

Use

Heavy menstrual bleeding: Management of heavy menstrual bleeding associated with uterine leiomyomas (fibroids) in premenopausal women.

Limitation of use: Use should be limited to 24 months due to the risk of continued bone loss, which may not be reversible.

Local Anesthetic/Vasoconstrictor Precautions No information available to require special precautions.

Effects on Dental Treatment No significant effects or complications reported.

Effects on Bleeding No information available to require special precautions.

Adverse Reactions Also see individual drugs.

>10%: Endocrine & metabolic: Hot flash (22%)

1% to 10%:

Cardiovascular: Hypertension (≥3% to <5%; severe hypertension: <1%), hypertensive crisis (4%)

Dermatologic: Alopecia (≥3% to <5%), loss of scalp hair (4%), thinning hair (4%)

Endocrine & metabolic: Decreased libido (≥3% to <5%), heavy menstrual bleeding (≥3% to <5%), weight gain (≥3% to <5%)

Gastrointestinal: Abdominal distention (≥3% to <5%), vomiting (≥3% to <5%)

Genitourinary: Uterine hemorrhage (5%)

Hepatic: Increased serum alanine aminotransferase (1%), increased serum aspartate aminotransferase (1%)

Infection: Influenza (≥3% to <5%)

Nervous system: Depressed mood (3%), depression (3%), emotional lability (≥3% to <5%), fatigue (6%), headache (9%)

Neuromuscular & skeletal: Arthralgia (≥3% to <5%), bone fracture (2%)

Respiratory: Upper respiratory tract infection (≥3% to <5%)

Miscellaneous: Crying (3%)

Frequency not defined:

Cardiovascular: Acute myocardial infarction, angina pectoris, cerebrovascular accident, deep vein thrombosis, pulmonary embolism, thromboembolic disease, thrombosis

Endocrine & metabolic: Increased apolipoprotein B, increased LDL cholesterol, increased serum cholesterol, increased serum triglycerides

Gastrointestinal: Nausea

Hematologic & oncologic: Malignant neoplasm of the breast

Nervous system: Homicidal ideation, irritability

Neuromuscular & skeletal: Decreased bone mineral density

Mechanism of Action Combination of elagolix, estradiol, and norethindrone. Elagolix is a short-acting, nonpeptide, gonadotropin-releasing hormone antagonist that suppresses pituitary and ovarian hormone function in a dose-dependent manner. Concentrations of luteinizing hormone, follicle stimulating hormone, estradiol, and progesterone are decreased during therapy, reducing bleeding associated with uterine fibroids. Estradiol may reduce the bone loss associated with elagolix. Norethindrone may protect the uterus from adverse endometrial effects of unopposed estrogen. A significant decrease in menstrual blood loss and an increase in hemoglobin was observed after 3 months of therapy (Schlaff 2020).

Reproductive Considerations

Exclude pregnancy prior to use or initiate therapy within 7 days of the onset of menses.

Use of this combination may alter menstrual bleeding patterns, delaying the ability to detect a pregnancy; if pregnancy is suspected during treatment, pregnancy testing is recommended.

Nonhormonal contraception is recommended during treatment and for 1 week after therapy is discontinued.

Pregnancy Considerations

Based on the mechanism of action and limited human data, exposure during early pregnancy may increase the risk of early pregnancy loss. Use is contraindicated during pregnancy. Discontinue use if pregnancy occurs during therapy.

Also refer to the Elagolix and Norethindrone monographs for additional information.

Data collection to monitor pregnancy and infant outcomes following inadvertent exposure to Oriahnn is ongoing. Health care providers are encouraged to enroll females exposed to Oriahnn during pregnancy in the Pregnancy Registry (833-782-7241).

◆ **Elagolix Sodium** *see* Elagolix *on page 547*

◆ **Elagolix sodium, estradiol, and norethindrone** *see* Elagolix, Estradiol, and Norethindrone *on page 547*

◆ **Elavil** *see* Amitriptyline *on page 120*

◆ **Elavil [DSC]** *see* Amitriptyline *on page 120*

Elbasvir and Grazoprevir

(ELB as vir & graz OH pre vir)

Brand Names: US Zepatier

Brand Names: Canada Zepatier

Pharmacologic Category Antihepaciviral, NS3/4A Protease Inhibitor (Anti-HCV); Antihepaciviral, NS5A Inhibitor; NS3/4A Inhibitor; NS5A Inhibitor

Use Chronic hepatitis C: Treatment of chronic hepatitis C virus (HCV) genotype 1 or 4 infection in adults; used with ribavirin in certain patient populations.

Local Anesthetic/Vasoconstrictor Precautions No information available to require special precautions

Effects on Dental Treatment Key adverse event(s) related to dental treatment: Xerostomia; normal salivary flow resumes upon discontinuation

Effects on Bleeding No information available to require special precautions

Adverse Reactions

>10%: Nervous system: Fatigue (11%)

1% to 10%:

Hepatic: Increased serum alanine aminotransferase (1%)

Nervous system: Headache (10%)

<1%, postmarketing, and/or case reports: Acute hepatic failure (FDA Safety Alert, August 28, 2019), angioedema, decreased hemoglobin, increased serum bilirubin, reactivation of HBV, severe hepatic disease (FDA Safety Alert, August 28, 2019)

Mechanism of Action

Elbasvir is an inhibitor of HCV NS5A, which is essential for viral replication and virion assembly.

Grazoprevir is an inhibitor of HCV NS3/4A protease, necessary for the proteolytic cleavage of the HCV-encoded polyprotein (into mature forms of the NS3, NS4A, NS4B, NS5A, and NS5B proteins) and is essential for viral replication.

Pharmacodynamics/Kinetics

Half-life Elimination Elbasvir: ~24 hours; Grazoprevir: ~31 hours

Time to Peak Elbasvir: Median: 3 hours (range: 3 to 6 hours); Grazoprevir: Median: 2 hours (range: 30 minutes to 3 hours)

Reproductive Considerations

HCV-infected females of childbearing potential should consider postponing pregnancy until therapy is complete to reduce the risk of HCV transmission (AASLD/IDSA 2018).

If used in combination with ribavirin, all warnings related to the use of ribavirin and contraception should be followed. Refer to the ribavirin monograph for additional information.

Pregnancy Considerations

Use in combination with ribavirin is contraindicated in pregnant women and males whose female partners are pregnant.

Treatment of hepatitis C is not currently recommended to treat maternal infection or to decrease the risk of mother-to-child transmission during pregnancy (Tran 2016). When HCV infection is detected during pregnancy, treatment should be deferred until after delivery. Direct-acting antiviral medications should not be used in pregnant females outside of clinical trials until safety and efficacy information is available (SMFM [Hughes 2017]).

If used in combination with ribavirin, all warnings related to the use of ribavirin and pregnancy should be followed. Refer to the ribavirin monograph for additional information.

◆ **Eldepryl [DSC]** *see* Selegiline *on page 1363*

◆ **Elepsia XR** *see* LevETIRAcetam *on page 894*

◆ **Elestat [DSC]** *see* Epinastine *on page 569*

◆ **Elestrin** *see* Estradiol (Systemic) *on page 596*

Eletriptan (el e TRIP tan)

Related Information

Temporomandibular Dysfunction (TMD), Chronic Pain, and Fibromyalgia *on page 1773*

Brand Names: US Relpax

Brand Names: Canada APO-Eletriptan; AURO-Eletriptan; GD-Eletriptan; PMS-Eletriptan; Relpax; TEVA-Eletriptan

Pharmacologic Category Antimigraine Agent; Serotonin 5-$HT_{1B, 1D}$ Receptor Agonist

Use Migraines: Acute treatment of migraine, with or without aura in adults

Local Anesthetic/Vasoconstrictor Precautions No information available to require special precautions

Effects on Dental Treatment Key adverse event(s) related to dental treatment: Xerostomia (normal salivary flow resumes upon discontinuation)

Effects on Bleeding No information available to require special precautions

Adverse Reactions

1% to 10%:

Cardiovascular: Chest pain (2% to 4%; chest tightness, pain, and pressure), palpitations

Central nervous system: Dizziness (6% to 7%), drowsiness (6% to 7%), headache (4%), paresthesia (3% to 4%), chills, hypertonia, hypoesthesia, pain, vertigo

Dermatologic: Diaphoresis

Gastrointestinal: Nausea (8%), xerostomia (3% to 4%), abdominal pain (2%; pain, discomfort, stomach pain, cramps, and pressure), dyspepsia (2%), dysphagia (1% to 2%)

Neuromuscular & skeletal: Weakness (4% to 10%), back pain

Respiratory: Pharyngitis

<1%, postmarketing, and/or case reports (limited to important or life-threatening): Abnormal dreams, abnormal hepatic function tests, agitation, alopecia, amnesia, anaphylactoid reaction, anaphylaxis, anemia, angina pectoris, angioedema, aphasia, ataxia, cardiac arrhythmia, confusion, constipation, depersonalization, depression, diarrhea, diplopia, dysgeusia, dyspnea, dystonia, edema, emotional lability, esophagitis, euphoria, gingivitis, hallucination, hyperesthesia, hyperglycemia, hyperkinesia, hypersensitivity reaction, hypertension, impotence, increased creatine phosphokinase, insomnia, ischemic colitis, lacrimation, manic behavior, myalgia, myasthenia, myocardial infarction, nervousness, paralysis, peripheral edema, peripheral vascular disorder, photophobia, polyuria, Prinzmetal angina, pruritus, purpura, seizure, sensation of pressure (chest/neck/throat/jaw), shock, sialorrhea, skin discoloration, skin rash, speech disturbance, stupor, syncope, tachycardia, thrombophlebitis, tinnitus, tongue edema, tremor, twitching, urinary frequency, urticaria, vasospasm, ventricular fibrillation, visual disturbance, vomiting

Mechanism of Action Selective agonist for serotonin (5-HT_{1B}, 5-HT_{1D}, and 5-HT_{1F} receptors) in cranial arteries; causes vasoconstriction and reduces sterile inflammation associated with antidromic neuronal transmission correlating with relief of migraine

Pharmacodynamics/Kinetics

Half-life Elimination ~4 hours (Elderly: 4.4 to 5.7 hours); Metabolite: ~13 hours

Time to Peak Plasma: 1.5 to 2 hours

Pregnancy Considerations

In comparison to other medications in this class, information related to eletriptan use in pregnancy is limited (Källén 2011; Nezvalová-Henriksen, 2010; Nezvalová-Henriksen 2012; Spielmann 2018).

Until additional information is available, other agents are preferred for the acute management of migraine in pregnancy (CHS [Worthington 2013]; MacGregor 2014).

- ◆ **Eletriptan Hydrobromide** *see* Eletriptan *on page 549*
- ◆ **Elfolate** *see* Methylfolate *on page 996*
- ◆ **Elidel** *see* Pimecrolimus *on page 1232*
- ◆ **Eligard** *see* Leuprolide *on page 890*

Eliglustat (el i GLOO stat)

Brand Names: US Cerdelga

Brand Names: Canada Cerdelga

Pharmacologic Category Enzyme Inhibitor; Glucosylceramide Synthase Inhibitor

Use

Gaucher disease: Treatment of adult patients with Gaucher disease type 1 (GD1) who are CYP2D6 extensive metabolizers (EMs), intermediate metabolizers (IMs), or poor metabolizers (PMs).

Limitations of use: Patients who are CYP2D6 ultra-rapid metabolizers (URMs) may not achieve adequate concentrations of eliglustat to achieve a therapeutic effect. A specific dosage cannot be recommended for those patients whose CYP2D6 genotype cannot be determined (indeterminate metabolizers).

Local Anesthetic/Vasoconstrictor Precautions No information available to require special precautions

Effects on Dental Treatment Key adverse event(s) related to dental treatment: Oropharyngeal pain has been reported in up to 10% of patients receiving the drug

Effects on Bleeding No information available to require special precautions

Adverse Reactions

>10%:

Central nervous system: Headache (13% to 40%), fatigue (14%)

Gastrointestinal: Diarrhea (12%), nausea (10% to 12%)

Neuromuscular & skeletal: Arthralgia (45%), back pain (12%), limb pain (11%)

1% to 10%:

Cardiovascular: Palpitations (5%)

Central nervous system: Migraine (10%), dizziness (8%)

Dermatologic: Skin rash (5%)

Gastrointestinal: Flatulence (10%), upper abdominal pain (10%), dyspepsia (7%), gastroesophageal reflux disease (7%), constipation (5%)

Neuromuscular & skeletal: Weakness (8%)

Respiratory: Oropharyngeal pain (10%), cough (7%)

Mechanism of Action Eliglustat inhibits the enzyme needed to produce glycosphingolipids and decreases the rate of glycosphingolipid glucosylceramide formation. Glucosylceramide accumulates in type 1 Gaucher disease, causing complications specific to this disease.

Pharmacodynamics/Kinetics

Half-life Elimination EMs: 6.5 hours; PMs: 8.9 hours.

Time to Peak EMs: 1.5 to 2 hours; PMs: 3 hours

Pregnancy Considerations
Adverse events were observed in some animal reproduction studies.

Uncontrolled type 1 Gaucher disease is associated with an increased risk of spontaneous abortion; maternal hepatosplenomegaly and thrombocytopenia may also occur and lead to adverse pregnancy outcomes.

- **Eliglustat Tartrate** *see* Eliglustat *on page 549*
- **Elinest** *see* Ethinyl Estradiol and Norgestrel *on page 617*
- **Eliquis** *see* Apixaban *on page 159*
- **Eliquis DVT/PE Starter Pack** *see* Apixaban *on page 159*
- **Elitek** *see* Rasburicase *on page 1312*
- **Elixophyllin** *see* Theophylline *on page 1437*
- **ElixSure Cough [OTC]** *see* Dextromethorphan *on page 476*
- **Ella** *see* Ulipristal *on page 1506*
- **Ellence** *see* EpiRUBicin *on page 576*
- **Elmiron** *see* Pentosan Polysulfate Sodium *on page 1214*
- **Eloctate** *see* Antihemophilic Factor (Recombinant [Fc Fusion Protein]) *on page 154*

Elosulfase Alfa (el oh SUL fase AL fa)

Brand Names: US Vimizim
Brand Names: Canada Vimizim
Pharmacologic Category Enzyme
Use Mucopolysaccharidosis type IVA: Treatment of mucopolysaccharidosis type IVA (MPS IVA; Morquio A syndrome)
Local Anesthetic/Vasoconstrictor Precautions No information available to require special precautions
Effects on Dental Treatment No significant effects or complications reported
Effects on Bleeding No information available to require special precautions
Adverse Reactions
>10%:
Gastrointestinal: Vomiting (31%), nausea (24%), abdominal pain (21%)
Hypersensitivity: Hypersensitivity reaction (19%)
Immunologic: Antibody development (100%; neutralizing: 100%)
Nervous system: Headache (26%)
Miscellaneous: Fever (33%)
1% to 10%:
Hypersensitivity: Anaphylaxis (8%)
Nervous system: Chills (10%), fatigue (10%)

Mechanism of Action Elosulfase alfa is a recombinant form of N-acetylgalactosamine-6-sulfatase, produced in Chinese hamster cells. A deficiency of this enzyme leads to accumulation of the glycosaminoglycan (GAG) substrates (keratan sulfate and chondroitin-6-sulfate) in tissues, causing cellular, tissue and organ dysfunction. Elosulfase alfa provides the exogenous enzyme (N-acetylgalactosamine-6-sulfatase) that is taken into lysosomes and thereby increases the catabolism of the GAG substrates (eg, keratan sulfate and chondroitin-6-sulfate).

Pharmacodynamics/Kinetics
Half-life Elimination Week 0: ~8 minutes; Week 22: ~36 minutes
Time to Peak Week 0: 172 minutes; Week 22: 202 minutes

Pregnancy Risk Factor C
Pregnancy Considerations
Adverse events were observed in some animal reproduction studies. Mucopolysaccharidosis type IVA (MPS IVA) has the potential to cause adverse events in both the mother and fetus.

A pregnancy registry is available for women who may be exposed to elosulfase alfa for the treatment of MPS IVA during pregnancy (MARS@bmrn.com or 1-800-983-4587).

- **Elosulfase alfa** *see* Elosulfase Alfa *on page 550*

Elotuzumab (el oh TOOZ ue mab)

Brand Names: US Empliciti
Pharmacologic Category Antineoplastic Agent, Anti-SLAMF7; Antineoplastic Agent, Monoclonal Antibody
Use Multiple myeloma, relapsed/refractory: Treatment of multiple myeloma (in combination with lenalidomide and dexamethasone) in patients who have received 1 to 3 prior therapies; treatment of multiple myeloma (in combination with pomalidomide and dexamethasone) in patients who have received at least 2 prior therapies, including lenalidomide and a proteasome inhibitor
Local Anesthetic/Vasoconstrictor Precautions No information available to require special precautions
Effects on Dental Treatment No significant effects or complications reported
Effects on Bleeding Cytopenias including thrombocytopenia (grades 3/4, 19%) has been reported. Medical consult is recommended.
Adverse Reactions All incidences reported with combination therapy.
>10%:
Cardiovascular: Decreased heart rate (43% to 66%; <60 bpm), increased heart rate (23% to 48%; ≥100 bpm), altered blood pressure (systolic ≥160 mmHg: 18% to 33%; systolic <90 mmHg: 7% to 29%; diastolic ≥100 mmHg: 8% to 17%), peripheral edema (13%)
Central nervous system: Fatigue (62%), peripheral neuropathy (27%; grades 3/4: 4%), headache (15%)
Endocrine & metabolic: Hyperglycemia (20% to 89%), hypocalcemia (58% to 78%), hypoalbuminemia (65% to 73%), decreased serum bicarbonate (63%), hyponatremia (40%), hyperkalemia (32%), hypokalemia (23%), weight loss (14%)
Gastrointestinal: Diarrhea (18% to 47%), constipation (22% to 36%), decreased appetite (21%), vomiting (14%)
Hematologic & oncologic: Lymphocytopenia (10% to 99%; grades 3/4: 8% to 77%), leukopenia (80% to 91%; grades 3/4: 32% to 52%), thrombocytopenia (78% to 84%; grades 3/4: 17% to 19%)
Hepatic: Increased serum alkaline phosphatase (39%)
Immunologic: Antibody development (19% to 36%; neutralizing: 4% to 6%)
Infection: Infection (65% to 81%), opportunistic infection (10% to 22%), herpes zoster infection (5% to 14%), fungal infection (10%)
Neuromuscular & skeletal: Limb pain (16%), ostealgia (15%), muscle spasm (13%)
Ophthalmic: Cataract (12%)
Respiratory: Cough (34%), nasopharyngitis (25%), upper respiratory tract infection (23%), pneumonia (13% to 20%), respiratory tract infection (3% to 17%), dyspnea (15%), oropharyngeal pain (10%)

Miscellaneous: Fever (7% to 37%), infusion related reaction (3% to 10%)

1% to 10%:

Cardiovascular: Chest pain (≥5%), pulmonary embolism (3%)

Central nervous system: Hypoesthesia (≥5%), mood changes (≥5%)

Dermatologic: Night sweats (≥5%)

Hematologic & oncologic: Second primary malignant neoplasm (9%), malignant neoplasm of skin (4%), malignant solid tumor (4%), anemia (3%), malignant neoplasm (hematologic: 2%)

Hepatic: Hepatotoxicity (3%)

Hypersensitivity: Hypersensitivity reaction (≥5%)

Renal: Acute renal failure (3%)

Mechanism of Action Elotuzumab is a humanized IgG1 immunostimulatory monoclonal antibody directed against signaling lymphocytic activation molecule family member 7 (SLAMF7, also called CS1 [cell surface glycoprotein CD2 subset 1). SLAMF7 is expressed on most myeloma and natural killer cells, but not on normal tissues; more than 95% of bone marrow myeloma cells express SLAMF7 (Lonial 2015). Elotuzumab directly activates natural killer cells through both the SLAMF7 pathway and Fc receptors. It also targets SLAMF7 on myeloma cells and mediates antibody-dependent cellular cytotoxicity (ADCC) through the CD16 pathway (Lonial 2015). This immunostimulatory activity, through the increased activation of natural killer cells, increases anti-tumor activity.

Pharmacodynamics/Kinetics

Half-life Elimination ~97% of the maximum steady-state concentration is expected to be eliminated with a geometric mean (CV%) of 78 to 82.4 days.

Reproductive Considerations

Elotuzumab is indicated for use in combination with lenalidomide or pomalidomide. Due to its potential to cause fetal harm, lenalidomide and pomalidomide are only available through a REMS program. Males and females of reproductive potential using these combinations must be able to comply with pregnancy testing and contraception requirements for lenalidomide or pomalidomide. Refer to the lenalidomide or pomalidomide monograph for additional information.

Pregnancy Considerations

Animal reproduction studies have not been conducted. Elotuzumab is indicated for use in combination with lenalidomide or pomalidomide. Due to its potential to cause fetal harm, lenalidomide and pomalidomide are only available through a REMS program. Refer to the lenalidomide or pomalidomide monograph for additional information.

◆ **Eloxatin** *see* Oxaliplatin *on page 1151*

◆ **Elspar** *see* Asparaginase (*E. coli*) *on page 175*

Eltrombopag (el TROM boe pag)

Brand Names: US Promacta

Brand Names: Canada Revolade

Pharmacologic Category Colony Stimulating Factor; Hematopoietic Agent; Thrombopoietic Agent; Thrombopoietin Receptor Agonist

Use

Aplastic anemia, severe: First-line treatment (in combination with standard immunosuppressive therapy) of severe aplastic anemia in patients ≥2 years of age; treatment of severe (refractory) aplastic anemia in patients who have had an insufficient response to immunosuppressive therapy

Chronic hepatitis C infection-associated thrombocytopenia: Treatment of thrombocytopenia in patients with chronic hepatitis C (CHC) to allow the initiation and maintenance of interferon-based therapy.

Chronic immune thrombocytopenia: Treatment of thrombocytopenia in adult and pediatric patients ≥1 year of age with chronic immune thrombocytopenia (ITP) who have had insufficient response to corticosteroids, immunoglobulins, or splenectomy.

Limitations of use: For ITP, eltrombopag should only be used if the degree of thrombocytopenia and clinical condition increase the risk for bleeding. For CHC, eltrombopag should only be used if the degree of thrombocytopenia prevents initiation of or limits the ability to maintain interferon-based therapy. Safety and efficacy have not been established when used in combination with direct-acting antiviral agents without interferon for treatment of CHC infection. Eltrombopag is not indicated for the treatment of myelodysplastic syndromes (MDS).

Local Anesthetic/Vasoconstrictor Precautions No information available to require special precautions

Effects on Dental Treatment Key adverse event(s) related to dental treatment: Risk of bleeding in soft tissues upon discontinuation of therapy due to rebound thrombocytopenia; monitor for at least 4 weeks after discontinuation of treatment.

Effects on Bleeding Eltrombopag is used in the management of severe thrombocytopenia. Medical consultation is warranted.

Adverse Reactions

>10%:

Hepatic: Abnormal hepatic function tests (adults: 11%)

Respiratory: Upper respiratory tract infection (children and adolescents: 17%; adults: 7%), nasopharyngitis (children and adolescents: 12%)

1% to 10%:

Cardiovascular: Thromboembolic disease (adults: 6%), thrombosis (adults: 3%), portal vein thrombosis (adults: 2%)

Dermatologic: Skin rash (3% to 5%), alopecia (adults: 2%)

Gastrointestinal: Diarrhea (9%), nausea (adults: 9%), abdominal pain (children and adolescents: 8%), toothache (children and adolescents: 6%), vomiting (adults: 6%), xerostomia (adults: 2%)

Genitourinary: Urinary tract infection (adults: 5%)

Hepatic: Increased serum alanine aminotransferase (5% to 6%), increased serum aspartate aminotransferase (4%), increased serum alkaline phosphatase (adults: 2%), hepatotoxicity (≤1%)

Infection: Influenza (adults: 3%)

Neuromuscular & skeletal: Myalgia (adults: 5%), back pain (adults: 3%), paresthesia (adults: 3%), musculoskeletal pain (adults: 2%)

Ophthalmic: Cataract (children and adolescents: 1%)

Respiratory: Cough (children and adolescents: 9%), oropharyngeal pain (4% to 8%), pharyngitis (adults: 4%), rhinorrhea (children and adolescents: 4%)

Miscellaneous: Fever (children and adolescents: 9%)

Frequency not defined: Hematologic & oncologic: Hemorrhage

<1%, postmarketing, and/or case reports: Skin discoloration (including hyperpigmentation and skin yellowing), thrombotic microangiopathy (with acute renal failure)

Mechanism of Action Eltrombopag is a thrombopoietin (TPO) nonpeptide agonist which increases platelet counts by binding to and activating the human TPO receptor. Activates intracellular signal transduction pathways to increase proliferation and differentiation of marrow progenitor cells.

Pharmacodynamics/Kinetics

Onset of Action Platelet count increase: Within 1 to 2 weeks

Duration of Action Platelets return to baseline: 1 to 2 weeks after last dose

Half-life Elimination ~21 to 32 hours in healthy individuals; ~26 to 35 hours in patients with ITP

Time to Peak 2 to 6 hours

Reproductive Considerations

Females of reproductive potential should use effective contraception (methods that result in <1% pregnancy rates) during eltrombopag therapy and for at least 7 days after the last eltrombopag dose.

If used in combination with ribavirin, all warnings related to the use of ribavirin contraception should be followed. Refer to the ribavirin monograph for additional information.

Pregnancy Considerations

Information related to the use of eltrombopag for the treatment of thrombocytopenia in pregnancy is limited (Favier 2018; Purushothaman 2016; Suzuki 2018).

If used in combination with ribavirin, all warnings related to the use of ribavirin and pregnancy should be followed. Refer to the ribavirin monograph for additional information.

- ◆ **Eltrombopag Olamine** *see* Eltrombopag *on page 551*
- ◆ **EluRyng** *see* Ethinyl Estradiol and Etonogestrel *on page 612*
- ◆ **Elviteg/Cobi/Emtric/Tenofo Ala** *see* Elvitegravir, Cobicistat, Emtricitabine, and Tenofovir Alafenamide *on page 553*

Elvitegravir (el vi TEG ra vir)

Brand Names: US Vitekta [DSC]

Brand Names: Canada Vitekta [DSC]

Pharmacologic Category Antiretroviral, Integrase Inhibitor (Anti-HIV)

Use HIV-1 infection: In combination with an HIV protease inhibitor coadministered with ritonavir and with other antiretroviral drug(s) for the treatment of HIV-1 infection in antiretroviral treatment-experienced adults

Local Anesthetic/Vasoconstrictor Precautions No information available to require special precautions

Effects on Dental Treatment No significant effects or complications reported

Effects on Bleeding No information available to require special precautions

Adverse Reactions Percentages are reported for antiretroviral treatment experienced adults.

1% to 10%:

Central nervous system: Headache (3%), depression (<2%), fatigue (<2%), insomnia (<2%), suicidal ideation (<2%)

Dermatologic: Skin rash (<2%)

Gastrointestinal: Diarrhea (7%), nausea (4%), abdominal pain (<2%), dyspepsia (<2%), vomiting (<2%)

Immunologic: Immune reconstitution syndrome

Mechanism of Action Integrase is an HIV-1 encoded enzyme that is required for viral replication. Inhibition of integrase prevents the integration of HIV-1 DNA into host genomic DNA, blocking the formation of the HIV-1 provirus and propagation of the viral infection. Elvitegravir does not inhibit human topoisomerases I or II.

Pharmacodynamics/Kinetics

Half-life Elimination Terminal: ~9 hours

Time to Peak Plasma: ~4 hours

Reproductive Considerations

The Health and Human Services perinatal HIV guidelines do not recommend an elvitegravir-containing regimen for females living with HIV who are not yet pregnant but are trying to conceive (HHS [perinatal] 2019).

For males and females living with HIV and planning a pregnancy, maximum viral suppression below the limits of detection with antiretroviral therapy (ART), modification of therapy (if needed), optimization of the woman's health, and a discussion of the potential risks and benefits of ART therapy during pregnancy is recommended prior to conception (HHS [perinatal] 2019).

Pregnancy Risk Factor B

Pregnancy Considerations

Elvitegravir has a high level of transfer across the placenta.

Data collected by the antiretroviral pregnancy registry are insufficient to evaluate teratogenic risk. Maternal antiretroviral therapy (ART) may be associated with adverse pregnancy outcomes including preterm delivery, stillbirth, low birth -weight, and small-for-gestational-age infants. Actual risks may be influenced by maternal factors such as disease severity, gestational age at initiation of therapy, and specific ART regimen, therefore close fetal monitoring is recommended. Because there is clear benefit to appropriate treatment, maternal ART should not be withheld due to concerns for adverse neonatal outcomes. Long-term follow-up is recommended for all infants exposed to antiretroviral medications; children without HIV but who were exposed to ART in utero and develop significant organ system abnormalities of unknown etiology (particularly of the CNS or heart) should be evaluated for potential mitochondrial dysfunction.

The Health and Human Services perinatal HIV guidelines do not recommend an elvitegravir-containing regimen in pregnant females living with HIV due to inadequate serum concentrations observed during pregnancy. Pharmacokinetic data are insufficient to make dosing recommendations during pregnancy. If pregnancy occurs during therapy, consideration should be given to changing to a more effective regimen. If continued, close monitoring, including more frequent therapeutic drug monitoring if available, is recommended. Do not administer within 2 hours of iron or calcium containing preparations, including prenatal vitamins.

In general, ART is recommended for all pregnant females living with HIV to keep the viral load below the limit of detection and reduce the risk of perinatal transmission. Therapy should be individualized following a discussion of the potential risks and benefits of treatment during pregnancy. Monitoring of pregnant females is more frequent than in nonpregnant adults. ART should be continued postpartum for all females living with HIV and can be modified after delivery.

Health care providers are encouraged to enroll pregnant females exposed to antiretroviral medications as early in pregnancy as possible in the Antiretroviral Pregnancy Registry (1-800-258-4263 or http://www.-APRegistry.com). Health care providers caring for pregnant females living with HIV and their infants may contact the National Perinatal HIV Hotline (888-448-8765) for clinical consultation (HHS [perinatal] 2019).

Product Availability Vitekta has been discontinued in the US for more than 1 year.

Elvitegravir, Cobicistat, Emtricitabine, and Tenofovir Alafenamide

(el vi TEG ra vir, koe BIK i stat, em trye SYE ta been, & ten OF oh vir al a FEN a mide)

Brand Names: US Genvoya

Brand Names: Canada Genvoya

Pharmacologic Category Antiretroviral, Integrase Inhibitor (Anti-HIV); Antiretroviral, Reverse Transcriptase Inhibitor, Nucleoside (Anti-HIV); Antiretroviral, Reverse Transcriptase Inhibitor, Nucleotide (Anti-HIV); Cytochrome P-450 Inhibitor

Use HIV-1 infection, treatment: Treatment of HIV-1 infection in adult and pediatric patients weighing ≥25 kg who have no antiretroviral treatment history or to replace the current antiretroviral regimen in those who are virologically-suppressed (HIV-1 RNA <50 copies per mL) on a stable antiretroviral regimen for ≥6 months with no history of treatment failure and no known substitutions associated with resistance to elvitegravir, cobicistat, emtricitabine, or tenofovir alafenamide.

Local Anesthetic/Vasoconstrictor Precautions No information available to require special precautions

Effects on Dental Treatment No significant effects or complications reported

Effects on Bleeding No information available to require special precautions

Adverse Reactions Includes data from both treatment-naive and treatment-experienced patients. Also see individual agents.

>10%:

Endocrine & metabolic: Increased LDL cholesterol (grades 3/4: 11%)

Gastrointestinal: Nausea (11%)

Neuromuscular & skeletal: Decreased bone mineral density (≥5% decrease at lumbar spine: 12%; ≥7% decrease at femoral neck: 11%), increased serum creatine kinase (grades 3/4: 11%)

1% to 10%:

Central nervous system: Headache (6%), fatigue (5%)

Endocrine & metabolic: Increased serum cholesterol (grades 3/4: 4%)

Gastrointestinal: Diarrhea (7%)

Genitourinary: Hematuria (grades 3/4: 3%)

Hepatic: Increased serum alanine aminotransferase (grades 3/4: 3%), increased serum amylase (grades 3/4: 3%), increased serum aspartate aminotransferase (grades 3/4: 3%)

Frequency not defined:

Endocrine & metabolic: Increased HDL cholesterol, increased serum triglycerides

Hepatic: Exacerbation of hepatitis B

Renal: Increased serum creatinine (mean increase 0.1 mg/dL)

<1%, postmarketing, and/or case reports: Angioedema, skin rash, urticaria

Mechanism of Action Integrase strand transfer inhibitor, CYP3A enzyme inhibitor plus nucleoside and nucleotide reverse transcriptase inhibitor combination; the viral cDNA strand produced by reverse transcriptase is processed and inserted into the human genome by the enzyme HIV-1 integrase. Elvitegravir inhibits the catalytic activity of integrase, thus preventing integration of the proviral gene into human DNA. Cobicistat inhibits enzymes of the CYP3A subfamily and enhances systemic exposure to elvitegravir. Emtricitabine is a cytosine analogue and tenofovir alafenamide is converted to tenofovir in vivo; tenofovir is an analog of adenosine 5'-monophosphate. Emtricitabine and tenofovir interfere with HIV viral RNA dependent DNA polymerase activities resulting in inhibition of viral replication.

Pharmacodynamics/Kinetics

Half-life Elimination Elvitegravir: 12.9 hours; Cobicistat: 3.5 hours; Emtricitabine: 10 hours; Tenofovir alafenamide: 0.51 hours

Time to Peak Elvitegravir: 4 hours; Cobicistat: 3 hours; Emtricitabine: 3 hours; Tenofovir alafenamide: 1 hour

Reproductive Considerations

The Health and Human Services perinatal HIV guidelines do not recommend this fixed dose combination for females living with HIV who are not yet pregnant but are trying to conceive (HHS [perinatal] 2019).

Refer to individual monographs for additional information.

Pregnancy Considerations

The Health and Human Services Perinatal HIV Guidelines do not recommend this fixed dose combination for pregnant females living with HIV who are antiretroviral-naïve, who have had antiretroviral therapy (ART) in the past but are restarting, or who require a new ART regimen (due to poor tolerance or poor virologic response of current regimen) due to inadequate serum concentrations of elvitegravir and cobicistat observed during pregnancy. For females who become pregnant while taking this combination, consider altering the regimen, or continue with more frequent monitoring if viral suppression is effective and the regimen is well tolerated. Do not administer within 2 hours of iron or calcium containing preparations, including prenatal vitamins (HHS [perinatal] 2019).

Refer to individual monographs for additional information.

Elvitegravir, Cobicistat, Emtricitabine, and Tenofovir Disoproxil Fumarate

(el vi TEG ra vir, koe BIK i stat, em trye SYE ta been, & ten OF oh vir dye soe PROX il FUE ma rate)

Related Information

HIV Infection and AIDS *on page 1690*

Brand Names: US Stribild

Brand Names: Canada Stribild

Pharmacologic Category Antiretroviral, Integrase Inhibitor (Anti-HIV); Antiretroviral, Reverse Transcriptase Inhibitor, Nucleoside (Anti-HIV); Antiretroviral, Reverse Transcriptase Inhibitor, Nucleotide (Anti-HIV); Cytochrome P-450 Inhibitor

Use HIV-1 infection, treatment: Treatment of HIV-1 infection in adults and pediatric patients ≥12 years weighing ≥35 kg who are antiretroviral treatment-naïve; as a replacement for the current antiretroviral regimen in patients who are virologically-suppressed (HIV-1 RNA <50 copies/mL) on a stable antiretroviral regimen for ≥6 months with no history of treatment failure and no known substitutions associated with resistance to elvitegravir, cobicistat, emtricitabine, or tenofovir disoproxil fumarate.

Local Anesthetic/Vasoconstrictor Precautions No information available to require special precautions

Effects on Dental Treatment No significant effects or complications reported

Effects on Bleeding No information available to require special precautions

Adverse Reactions

>10%:

Gastrointestinal: Nausea (4% to 16%), diarrhea (12%)

Genitourinary: Proteinuria (52%)

Renal: Increased serum creatinine (12%)

1% to 10%:

Central nervous system: Abnormal dreams (9%), headache (2% to 7%), fatigue (4%), dizziness (3%), insomnia (3%), drowsiness (1%)

Dermatologic: Skin rash (4%)

Endocrine & metabolic: Increased amylase (3%)

Gastrointestinal: Flatulence (2%)

Genitourinary: Hematuria (4%)

Hepatic: Increased serum AST (3%), increased serum ALT (2%)

Neuromuscular & skeletal: Increased creatine phosphokinase (8%), bone fracture (4%)

Frequency not defined:

Endocrine & metabolic: Increased serum cholesterol, increased serum triglycerides

Gastrointestinal: Increased serum lipase

<1%, postmarketing, and/or case reports: Acute renal failure, Fanconi syndrome, immune reconstitution syndrome, renal failure, renal tubular disease (proximal), scleral icterus, suicidal ideation

Mechanism of Action Integrase strand transfer inhibitor, CYP3A enzyme inhibitor plus nucleoside and nucleotide reverse transcriptase inhibitor combination; the viral cDNA strand produced by reverse transcriptase is processed and inserted into the human genome by the enzyme HIV-1 integrase. Elvitegravir inhibits the catalytic activity of integrase, thus preventing integration of the proviral gene into human DNA. Cobicistat inhibits enzymes of the CYP3A subfamily and enhances systemic exposure to elvitegravir. Emtricitabine is a cytosine analogue and tenofovir disoproxil fumarate (TDF) is an analog of adenosine 5'-monophosphate. Emtricitabine and tenofovir interfere with HIV viral RNA dependent DNA polymerase activities resulting in inhibition of viral replication.

Pharmacodynamics/Kinetics

Half-life Elimination Elvitegravir: 12.9 hours; Cobicistat: 3.5 hours; Emtricitabine: 10 hours; Tenofovir: 12 to 18 hours

Time to Peak Plasma: Elvitegravir: 4 hours; Cobicistat: 3 hours; Emtricitabine: 3 hours; Tenofovir: 2 hours

Reproductive Considerations

The Health and Human Services perinatal HIV guidelines do not recommend this fixed-dose combination for females living with HIV who are not yet pregnant but are trying to conceive (HHS [perinatal] 2019).

Refer to individual monographs for additional information.

Pregnancy Considerations

The Health and Human Services perinatal HIV guidelines do not recommend this fixed-dose combination for pregnant females living with HIV who are antiretroviral-naive, who have had antiretroviral therapy (ART) in the past but are restarting, or who require a new ART regimen (due to poor tolerance or poor virologic response of current regimen) due to inadequate serum concentrations of elvitegravir and cobicistat observed during pregnancy. For females who become pregnant while taking this combination, consider altering the regimen, or continue with more frequent monitoring if viral suppression is effective and the regimen is well tolerated. Do not administer within 2 hours of iron or calcium containing preparations, including prenatal vitamins (HHS [perinatal] 2019).

Refer to individual monographs for additional information.

◆ **Elvitegravir, Cobicistat, Tenofovir Alafenamide, and Emtricitabine** *see* Elvitegravir, Cobicistat, Emtricitabine, and Tenofovir Alafenamide *on page 553*

◆ **Elyxyb** *see* Celecoxib *on page 318*

Emapalumab (EM a PAL ue mab)

Brand Names: US Gamifant

Pharmacologic Category Monoclonal Antibody

Use Primary hemophagocytic lymphohistiocytosis: Treatment of primary hemophagocytic lymphohistiocytosis (HLH) in adult and pediatric (newborn and older) patients with refractory, recurrent or progressive disease or intolerance to conventional HLH therapy.

Local Anesthetic/Vasoconstrictor Precautions No information available to require special precautions

Effects on Dental Treatment No significant effects or complications reported

Effects on Bleeding No information available to require special precautions

Adverse Reactions

>10%:

Cardiovascular: Hypertension (41%), tachycardia (12%)

Central nervous system: Irritability (12%)

Dermatologic: Skin rash (12%)

Endocrine & metabolic: Hypokalemia (15%)

Gastrointestinal: Appendicitis (≤32%), constipation (15%), abdominal pain (12%), diarrhea (12%)

Hematologic & oncologic: Lymphocytosis (12%)

Infection: Infection (56%), viral infection (32% to 41%), bacterial infection (35%), bacteremia (≤32%), histoplasmosis (≤32%), necrotizing fasciitis (≤32%), sepsis (≤32%), cytomegalovirus disease (12%)

Respiratory: Pneumonia (≤32%), cough (12%), tachypnea (12%)

Miscellaneous: Infusion related reaction (27%), fever (24%)

1% to 10%:

Cardiovascular: Bradycardia (<10%), peripheral edema (<10%)

Gastrointestinal: Gastrointestinal hemorrhage (<10%), vomiting (<10%)
Immunologic: Antibody development (3% to 5%)
Infection: Fungal infection (9%)
Neuromuscular & skeletal: Asthenia (<10%)
Renal: Acute renal failure (<10%)
Respiratory: Dyspnea (<10%), epistaxis (<10%)
Miscellaneous: Multi-organ failure (≥3%)

Mechanism of Action Emapalumab is an interferon gamma (IFNγ) blocking monoclonal antibody. IFNγ is hypersecreted in hemophagocytic lymphohistiocytosis (HLH); emapalumab binds to IFNγ and neutralizes it.

Pharmacodynamics/Kinetics

Half-life Elimination Healthy subjects: ~22 days; Patients with hemophagocytic lymphohistiocytosis (HLH): 2.5 to 18.9 days

Pregnancy Considerations Adverse events were not observed in animal reproduction studies.

- **Emapalumab-lzsg** *see* Emapalumab *on page 554*
- **E-Max-1000 [OTC]** *see* Vitamin E (Systemic) *on page 1549*
- **Emcyt** *see* Estramustine *on page 600*
- **EMD 68843** *see* Vilazodone *on page 1544*
- **Emend** *see* Aprepitant *on page 162*
- **Emend** *see* Fosaprepitant *on page 713*
- **Emend Tri-Pack** *see* Aprepitant *on page 162*
- **Emerphed** *see* EPHEDrine (Systemic) *on page 568*
- **Emflaza** *see* Deflazacort *on page 449*
- **Emgality** *see* Galcanezumab *on page 728*
- **Emgality (300 MG Dose)** *see* Galcanezumab *on page 728*
- **Emoquette** *see* Ethinyl Estradiol and Desogestrel *on page 609*

Empagliflozin (em pa gli FLOE zin)

Brand Names: US Jardiance

Brand Names: Canada Jardiance

Pharmacologic Category Antidiabetic Agent, Sodium-Glucose Cotransporter 2 (SGLT2) Inhibitor; Sodium-Glucose Cotransporter 2 (SGLT2) Inhibitor

Use

Diabetes mellitus, type 2, treatment: As an adjunct to diet and exercise to improve glycemic control in adults with type 2 diabetes mellitus; risk reduction of cardiovascular mortality in adults with type 2 diabetes mellitus and established cardiovascular disease.

Local Anesthetic/Vasoconstrictor Precautions No information available to require special precautions

Effects on Dental Treatment Key adverse event(s) related to dental treatment: Dizziness and syncope have been reported; patients may experience orthostatic hypotension as they stand up after treatment; especially if lying in dental chair for extended periods of time. Use caution with sudden changes in position during and after dental treatment.

Empagliflozin-dependent patients with diabetes (noninsulin dependent, type 2) should be questioned by the dental professional at each dental visit to assess their risk for stress-induced hypoglycemia. The dental professional should inquire about the patient's routine (ie, work, sleep schedule, eating patterns), history of hypoglycemia, time of last medication dose, last meal, and most recent blood sugar assessment. Keep a supply of glucose tablets and other carbohydrates in the office to prepare for a hypoglycemic event. Seek medical attention when necessary (American Diabetes Association 2016).

Effects on Bleeding No information available to require special precautions

Adverse Reactions

>10%: Genitourinary: Urinary tract infection (9%; females: 18%; males: 4%)

1% to 10%:

Endocrine & metabolic: Dyslipidemia (4%), increased thirst (2%)
Gastrointestinal: Nausea (2%)
Genitourinary: Increased urine output (3%)
Hematologic & oncologic: Increased hematocrit (3% to 4%)
Infection: Genitourinary fungal infection (2% to 6%)

Frequency not defined: Endocrine & metabolic: Increased LDL cholesterol

<1%, postmarketing, and/or case reports: Acute renal failure, angioedema, decreased estimated GFR (eGFR), hypersensitivity reaction, hypovolemia, increased serum creatinine, ketoacidosis, necrotizing fasciitis (perineum), phimosis, pyelonephritis, skin rash, urinary tract infection with sepsis, urticaria

Mechanism of Action By inhibiting sodium-glucose cotransporter 2 (SGLT2) in the proximal renal tubules, empagliflozin reduces reabsorption of filtered glucose from the tubular lumen and lowers the renal threshold for glucose (RT_G). SGLT2 is the main site of filtered glucose reabsorption; reduction of filtered glucose reabsorption and lowering of RT_G result in increased urinary excretion of glucose, thereby reducing plasma glucose concentrations.

Pharmacodynamics/Kinetics

Duration of Action Following discontinuation, urinary glucose excretion returns to baseline within ~3 days for the 10 mg and 25 mg doses.

Half-life Elimination 12.4 hours.

Time to Peak 1.5 hours.

Pregnancy Considerations

Information related to the use of empagliflozin in pregnancy is limited (Formoso 2018). Due to adverse effects on renal development observed in animal studies, the manufacturer does not recommend use of empagliflozin during the second and third trimesters of pregnancy.

Poorly controlled diabetes during pregnancy can be associated with an increased risk of adverse maternal and fetal outcomes, including diabetic ketoacidosis, preeclampsia, spontaneous abortion, preterm delivery, delivery complications, major birth defects, stillbirth, and macrosomia. To prevent adverse outcomes, prior to conception and throughout pregnancy, maternal blood glucose and HbA_{1c} should be kept as close to target goals as possible but without causing significant hypoglycemia (ADA 2020; Blumer 2013).

Agents other than empagliflozin are currently recommended to treat diabetes mellitus in pregnancy (ADA 2020).

Empagliflozin, Linagliptin, and Metformin

(EM pa gli FLOE zin, LIN a GLIP tin, & met FOR min)

Brand Names: US Trijardy XR

Pharmacologic Category Antidiabetic Agent, Biguanide; Antidiabetic Agent, Dipeptidyl Peptidase 4 (DPP-4) Inhibitor; Antidiabetic Agent, Sodium-Glucose

Cotransporter 2 (SGLT2) Inhibitor; Sodium-Glucose Cotransporter 2 (SGLT2) Inhibitor

Use Diabetes mellitus, type 2, treatment: Adjunct to diet and exercise to improve glycemic control in adults with type 2 diabetes mellitus. **Note:** Empagliflozin is also indicated to reduce the risk of cardiovascular death in adults with type 2 diabetes mellitus and established cardiovascular disease.

Local Anesthetic/Vasoconstrictor Precautions No information available to require special precautions.

Effects on Dental Treatment Key adverse event(s) related to dental treatment: Empagliflozin, as sole agent, has caused dizziness, orthostatic hypotension, and syncope (see individual monograph); empagliflozin, linagliptin, metformin-dependent patients with diabetes (noninsulin dependent type 2) should be appointed for dental treatment in the morning in order to minimize chance of stress-induced hypoglycemia.

Effects on Bleeding No information available to require special precautions.

Adverse Reactions Also see individual agents.

1% to 10%:

Gastrointestinal: Diarrhea (2% to 7%), constipation (5% to 6%), gastroenteritis (3% to 6%)

Genitourinary: Urinary tract infection (10%)

Nervous system: Headache (5%)

Respiratory: Upper respiratory tract infection (8% to 10%), nasopharyngitis (6% to 8%)

<1%: Hypoglycemia

Postmarketing: Lactic acidosis

Mechanism of Action See individual agents.

Reproductive Considerations

Ovulation rates may increase in some anovulatory females following use of metformin.

Refer to individual monographs for additional information.

Pregnancy Considerations

Due to adverse effects on renal development observed in animal studies following use of empagliflozin, the manufacturer does not recommend use of this combination product during the second and third trimesters of pregnancy.

Refer to individual monographs for additional information.

◆ **Empagliflozin, metformin hydrochloride, and linagliptin** *see* Empagliflozin, Linagliptin, and Metformin *on page* 555

◆ **Empliciti** *see* Elotuzumab *on page* 550

◆ **Emsam** *see* Selegiline *on page* 1363

◆ **Emtec** *see* Acetaminophen and Codeine *on page* 65

Emtricitabine (em trye SYE ta been)

Related Information

HIV Infection and AIDS *on page* 1690

Brand Names: US Emtriva

Brand Names: Canada Emtriva

Pharmacologic Category Antiretroviral, Reverse Transcriptase Inhibitor, Nucleoside (Anti-HIV)

Use HIV-1 infection, treatment: Treatment of HIV-1 infection in combination with other antiretroviral agents.

Local Anesthetic/Vasoconstrictor Precautions No information available to require special precautions

Effects on Dental Treatment No significant effects or complications reported

Effects on Bleeding No information available to require special precautions related to hemostasis.

Adverse Reactions Clinical trials were conducted in patients receiving other antiretroviral agents, and it is not possible to correlate frequency of adverse events with emtricitabine alone. The range of frequencies of adverse events is generally comparable to comparator groups, with the exception of hyperpigmentation, which occurred more frequently in patients receiving emtricitabine. Unless otherwise noted, percentages are as reported in adults.

>10%:

Central nervous system: Dizziness (4% to 25%), headache (6% to 22%), insomnia (5% to 16%), abnormal dreams (2% to 11%)

Dermatologic: Hyperpigmentation (children: 32%; adults: 2% to 4%; primarily of palms and/or soles but may include tongue, arms, lip and nails; generally mild and nonprogressive without associated local reactions such as pruritus or rash), skin rash (17% to 30%; includes hypersensitivity reaction, maculopapular rash, pruritus, pustular rash, vesiculobullous rash)

Gastrointestinal: Diarrhea (children: 20%; adults: 9% to 23%), vomiting (children: 23%; adults: 9%), nausea (13% to 18%), abdominal pain (8% to 14%), gastroenteritis (children: 11%)

Infection: Infection (children: 44%)

Neuromuscular & skeletal: Weakness (12% to 16%), increased creatine phosphokinase (grades 3/4: 11% to 12%)

Otic: Otitis media (children: 23%)

Respiratory: Cough (children: 28%; adults; 14%), rhinitis (children: 20%; adults: 12% to 18%), pneumonia (children: 15%)

Miscellaneous: Fever (children: 18%)

1% to 10%:

Central nervous system: Depression (6% to 9%), paresthesia (5% to 6%), neuritis (≤4%), neuropathy (≤4%)

Endocrine & metabolic: Increased serum triglycerides (grades 3/4: 4% to 10%), increased amylase (grades 3/4: children: 9%; adults: 2% to 5%), hyperglycemia (grades 3/4: 2% to 3%)

Gastrointestinal: Dyspepsia (4% to 8%), increased serum lipase (grades 3/4: ≤1%)

Genitourinary: Hematuria (grades 3/4: 3%)

Hematologic & oncologic: Anemia (children: 7%), neutropenia (grades 3/4: children: 2%; adults: 5%)

Hepatic: Increased serum transaminases (grades 3/4: 2% to 6%), increased serum alkaline phosphatase (>550 units/L: 1%), increased serum bilirubin (grades 3/4: 1%)

Neuromuscular & skeletal: Myalgia (4% to 6%), arthralgia (3% to 5%)

Respiratory: Sinusitis (8%), upper respiratory tract infection (8%), pharyngitis (5%)

<1%, postmarketing, and/or case reports: Immune reconstitution syndrome

Mechanism of Action Nucleoside reverse transcriptase inhibitor; emtricitabine is a cytosine analogue which is phosphorylated intracellularly to emtricitabine 5'-triphosphate which interferes with HIV viral RNA dependent DNA polymerase resulting in inhibition of viral replication.

Pharmacodynamics/Kinetics

Half-life Elimination Normal renal function:

Infants, Children, and Adolescents: Elimination half-life (emtricitabine):

- Single dose: 11 hours
- Multiple dose: 7.9 to 9.5 hours
- Infants 0 to 3 months (n=20; median age: 26 days): 12.1 ± 3.1 hours
- Infants 3 to 24 months (n=14): 8.9 ± 3.2 hours
- Children 25 months to 6 years (n=19): 11.3 ± 6.4 hours
- Children 7 to 12 years (n=17): 8.2 ± 3.2 hours
- Adolescents 13 to 17 years (n=27): 8.9 ± 3.3 hours

Adults: Emtricitabine: 10 hours; Intracellular half-life (emtricitabine 5'-triphosphate): 39 hours

Time to Peak Plasma: 1 to 2 hours

Reproductive Considerations

The Health and Human Services (HHS) perinatal HIV guidelines consider emtricitabine a preferred nucleoside reverse transcriptase inhibitor for females living with HIV who are not yet pregnant but are trying to conceive.

Emtricitabine is one of the agents recommended for preexposure prophylaxis in couples with discordant HIV status who are planning a pregnancy. The partner without HIV should begin therapy 1 month prior to attempting conception and continue therapy for 1 month after attempting conception.

For males and females living with HIV and planning a pregnancy, maximum viral suppression below the limits of detection with antiretroviral therapy (ART), modification of therapy (if needed), optimization of the woman's health, and a discussion of the potential risks and benefits of ART therapy during pregnancy is recommended prior to conception (HHS [perinatal] 2019).

Pregnancy Considerations

Emtricitabine has a high level of transfer across the human placenta.

No increased risk of overall birth defects has been observed according to data collected by the antiretroviral pregnancy registry. Maternal antiretroviral therapy (ART) may be associated with adverse pregnancy outcomes including preterm delivery, stillbirth, low birth weight, and small for gestational age infants. Actual risks may be influenced by maternal factors, such as disease severity, gestational age at initiation of therapy, and specific ART regimen, therefore close fetal monitoring is recommended. Because there is clear benefit to appropriate treatment, maternal ART should not be withheld due to concerns for adverse neonatal outcomes. Long-term follow-up is recommended for all infants exposed to antiretroviral medications; children without HIV but who were exposed to ART in utero and develop significant organ system abnormalities of unknown etiology (particularly of the CNS or heart) should be evaluated for potential mitochondrial dysfunction. Cases of lactic acidosis and hepatic steatosis have been reported in pregnant women with use of nucleoside reverse transcriptase inhibitors (NRTIs).

The Health and Human Services (HHS) perinatal HIV guidelines consider emtricitabine a preferred NRTI for pregnant females living with HIV who are antiretroviral-naive, who have had ART therapy in the past but are restarting, or who require a new ART regimen (due to poor tolerance or poor virologic response of current regimen). In addition, females who become pregnant while taking emtricitabine may continue if viral suppression is effective and the regimen is well tolerated. The pharmacokinetics of emtricitabine are not significantly altered during pregnancy and dosing adjustments are not needed.

The HHS perinatal HIV guidelines consider emtricitabine with tenofovir disoproxil fumarate to be a preferred NRTI backbone for initial therapy in antiretroviral-naive pregnant females. The guidelines also consider emtricitabine plus tenofovir disoproxil fumarate a recommended dual NRTI backbone in regimens for HIV/hepatitis B virus-coinfected pregnant females. Use caution with hepatitis B coinfection; hepatitis B flare may occur if emtricitabine is discontinued. Emtricitabine is also a preferred component of an initial regimen when acute HIV infection is detected during pregnancy.

In general, ART is recommended for all pregnant females living with HIV to keep the viral load below the limit of detection and reduce the risk of perinatal transmission. Therapy should be individualized following a discussion of the potential risks and benefits of treatment during pregnancy. Monitoring of pregnant females is more frequent than in nonpregnant adults. ART should be continued postpartum for all females living with HIV and can be modified after delivery.

Health care providers are encouraged to enroll pregnant females exposed to antiretroviral medications as early in pregnancy as possible in the Antiretroviral Pregnancy Registry (1-800-258-4263 or http://www.APRegistry.com). Health care providers caring for pregnant females living with HIV and their infants may contact the National Perinatal HIV Hotline (888-448-8765) for clinical consultation (HHS [perinatal] 2019).

Emtricitabine and Tenofovir Alafenamide

(em trye SYE ta been & ten OF oh vir al a FEN a mide)

Brand Names: US Descovy

Brand Names: Canada Descovy

Pharmacologic Category Antiretroviral, Reverse Transcriptase Inhibitor, Nucleoside (Anti-HIV); Antiretroviral, Reverse Transcriptase Inhibitor, Nucleotide (Anti-HIV)

Use

HIV-1 infection, treatment: Treatment of HIV-1 infection in combination with other antiretroviral agents in adults and pediatric patients weighing ≥35 kg; in combination with other antiretroviral agents (other than protease inhibitors that require a CYP3A inhibitor) in pediatric patients weighing ≥25 kg and <35 kg.

HIV-1 infection, preexposure prophylaxis: Preexposure prophylaxis to reduce the risk of sexually acquired HIV-1 infection in at-risk adults and adolescents weighing ≥35 kg.

Limitations of use: Not indicated for individuals at risk from receptive vaginal sex.

Local Anesthetic/Vasoconstrictor Precautions No information available to require special precautions

Effects on Dental Treatment Key adverse event(s) related to dental treatment: Nausea reported in 10% of patients

Effects on Bleeding No information available to require special precautions

Adverse Reactions Also see individual agents.

1% to 10%:

- Central nervous system: Headache (2%)
- Gastrointestinal: Diarrhea (5%), nausea (4%), abdominal pain (2%), fatigue (2%)

Neuromuscular & skeletal: Decreased bone mineral density (≥5% decrease at lumbar spine: 4%; ≥7% decrease at femoral neck: 1%)

Frequency not defined:

Endocrine & metabolic: Increased serum triglycerides

Hepatic: Exacerbation of hepatitis B

Postmarketing: Angioedema, skin rash, urticaria

Mechanism of Action Nucleoside and nucleotide reverse transcriptase inhibitor combination; emtricitabine is a cytosine analogue while tenofovir alafenamide fumarate (TAF) is an analog of adenosine 5'-monophosphate. Each drug interferes with HIV viral RNA dependent DNA polymerase activities resulting in inhibition of viral replication.

Pharmacodynamics/Kinetics

Half-life Elimination Emtricitabine: 10 hours; TAF: 0.51 hours

Reproductive Considerations

The Health and Human Services perinatal HIV guidelines note there are insufficient data to recommend tenofovir alafenamide in females living with HIV who are not yet pregnant but are trying to conceive (HHS [perinatal] 2019).

Refer to individual monographs for additional information.

Pregnancy Considerations

The Health and Human Services perinatal HIV guidelines note there are insufficient data to recommend use of this fixed dose combination product as an initial regimen in antiretroviral-naive pregnant females.

In general, females who become pregnant on a stable antiretroviral therapy (ART) regimen may continue that regimen if viral suppression is effective, appropriate drug exposure can be achieved, contraindications for use in pregnancy are not present, and the regimen is well tolerated (HHS [perinatal] 2019).

Refer to individual monographs for additional information.

Emtricitabine and Tenofovir Disoproxil Fumarate

(em trye SYE ta been & ten OF oh vir dye soe PROX il FUE ma rate)

Related Information

Emtricitabine *on page 556*

HIV Infection and AIDS *on page 1690*

Tenofovir Disoproxil Fumarate *on page 1419*

Brand Names: US Truvada

Brand Names: Canada Truvada

Pharmacologic Category Antiretroviral, Reverse Transcriptase Inhibitor, Nucleoside (Anti-HIV); Antiretroviral, Reverse Transcriptase Inhibitor, Nucleotide (Anti-HIV)

Use

HIV-1 infection, treatment: Treatment of HIV-1 infection in combination with other antiretroviral agents in adults and pediatric patients weighing ≥17 kg

HIV-1 infection, preexposure prophylaxis: Preexposure prophylaxis (PrEP) to reduce the risk of sexually acquired HIV-1 infection in at-risk adults and adolescents weighing ≥35 kg (must have negative HIV-1 test immediately prior to initiation of emtricitabine/tenofovir disoproxil fumarate for HIV-1 PrEP).

Local Anesthetic/Vasoconstrictor Precautions No information available to require special precautions

Effects on Dental Treatment No significant effects or complications reported

Effects on Bleeding No information available to require special precautions related to hemostasis.

Adverse Reactions Also see individual agents.

>10%: Neuromuscular & skeletal: Decreased bone mineral density (13%)

1% to 10%:

Central nervous system: Headache (7%)

Endocrine & metabolic: Weight loss (3%)

Gastrointestinal: Abdominal pain (4%)

Hematologic & oncologic: Abnormal phosphorus levels (<2.0 mg/dL: 10%), decreased neutrophils (5%)

Neuromuscular & skeletal: Bone fracture (2%)

<1%, postmarketing, and/or case reports: Glycosuria, immune reconstitution syndrome, proteinuria

Mechanism of Action Nucleoside and nucleotide reverse transcriptase inhibitor combination; emtricitabine is a cytosine analogue while tenofovir is an analog of adenosine 5'-monophosphate. Each drug interferes with HIV viral RNA dependent DNA polymerase resulting in inhibition of viral replication.

Reproductive Considerations

The Health and Human Services (HHS) perinatal HIV guidelines consider this a preferred combination for females living with HIV who are not yet pregnant but are trying to conceive.

This combination is recommended for pre-exposure prophylaxis in couples with discordant HIV status who are planning a pregnancy. The partner without HIV should begin therapy 1 month prior to and continue for 1 month after conception is attempted (HHS [perinatal] 2019).

Refer to individual monographs for additional information.

Pregnancy Considerations

The Health and Human Services (HHS) perinatal HIV guidelines consider emtricitabine with tenofovir disoproxil fumarate to be a preferred nucleoside reverse transcriptase inhibitor backbone for initial therapy in antiretroviral-naive pregnant females. Emtricitabine with tenofovir disoproxil fumarate may also be recommended as part of a regimen when acute HIV infection is detected during pregnancy. In addition, this combination is preferred for use in pregnant females living with HIV who have had antiretroviral therapy (ART) in the past but are restarting, or who require a new ART regimen (due to poor tolerance or poor virologic response of current regimen). Females who become pregnant while taking this combination may continue if viral suppression is effective and the regimen is well tolerated.

The HHS perinatal guidelines also recommend emtricitabine plus tenofovir disoproxil fumarate as a component of regimens for HIV/hepatitis B virus-coinfected pregnant females.

Refer to individual monographs for additional information.

- ◆ **Emtricitabine, Efavirenz, and Tenofovir Disoproxil Fumarate** *see* Efavirenz, Emtricitabine, and Tenofovir Disoproxil Fumarate *on page 545*
- ◆ **Emtricitabine, Elvitegravir, Cobicistat, and Tenofovir Alafenamide** *see* Elvitegravir, Cobicistat, Emtricitabine, and Tenofovir Alafenamide *on page 553*

Emtricitabine, Rilpivirine, and Tenofovir Alafenamide

(em trye SYE ta been, ril pi VIR een, & ten OF oh vir al a FEN a mide)

Brand Names: US Odefsey

Brand Names: Canada Odefsey

Pharmacologic Category Antiretroviral, Reverse Transcriptase Inhibitor, Non-nucleoside (Anti-HIV); Antiretroviral, Reverse Transcriptase Inhibitor, Nucleoside (Anti-HIV); Antiretroviral, Reverse Transcriptase Inhibitor, Nucleotide (Anti-HIV)

Use

HIV-1 infection, treatment: Treatment of HIV-1 infection (as a complete regimen) in patients ≥12 years of age as initial therapy in those with no antiretroviral treatment history with HIV-1 RNA ≤100,000 copies/mL; or to replace a stable antiretroviral regimen in those who are virologically suppressed (HIV-1 RNA <50 copies/mL) for ≥6 months with no history of treatment failure and no known substitutions associated with resistance to the individual components.

Limitations of use: More rilpivirine-treated patients with no history of antiretroviral treatment with HIV-1 RNA >100,000 copies/mL at therapy initiation experienced virologic failure (HIV-1 RNA ≥50 copies/mL) compared to rilpivirine-treated patients with HIV-1 RNA ≤100,000 copies/mL.

Local Anesthetic/Vasoconstrictor Precautions No information available to require special precautions

Effects on Dental Treatment No significant effects or complications reported

Effects on Bleeding No information available to require special precautions

Adverse Reactions Also see individual agents.

1% to 10%:

Central nervous system: Headache (2%), sleep disorder (2%), abnormal dreams (1%)

Gastrointestinal: Diarrhea (1%), nausea (1%), flatulence (≤1%)

Neuromuscular & skeletal: Decreased bone mineral density (1% to 2%)

Frequency not defined: Endocrine: Decreased HDL cholesterol, decreased LDL cholesterol, decreased serum cholesterol, decreased serum triglycerides, increased HDL cholesterol, increased LDL cholesterol, increased serum cholesterol, increased serum triglycerides

Mechanism of Action Non-nucleoside, nucleoside, and nucleotide reverse transcriptase inhibitor combination; rilpivirine binds to reverse transcriptase and does not require intracellular phosphorylation for antiviral activity; emtricitabine is a cytosine analogue while tenofovir alafenamide fumarate (TAF) is an analog of adenosine 5'-monophosphate. Each drug interferes with HIV viral RNA dependent DNA polymerase activities resulting in inhibition of viral replication.

Reproductive Considerations

The Health and Human Services (HHS) perinatal HIV guidelines do not recommend this fixed-dose combination for females living with HIV who are not yet pregnant but are trying to conceive (HHS [perinatal] 2019).

Refer to individual monographs for additional information.

Pregnancy Considerations

The Health and Human Services (HHS) perinatal HIV guidelines note data are insufficient to recommend this fixed-dose combination for initiation in pregnant females living with HIV who are antiretroviral naive, who have had antiretroviral therapy (ART) in the past but are restarting, or who require a new ART regimen (due to poor tolerance or poor virologic response of current regimen). Females who become pregnant while taking this combination may continue if viral suppression is effective and the regimen is well tolerated; however, more frequent monitoring is recommended. Alternately, consider changing tenofovir alafenamide to tenofovir disoproxil fumarate (HHS [perinatal] 2019).

Refer to individual monographs for additional information.

Emtricitabine, Rilpivirine, and Tenofovir Disoproxil Fumarate

(em trye SYE ta been, ril pi VIR een, & ten OF oh vir dye soe PROX il FUE ma rate)

Related Information

HIV Infection and AIDS *on page 1690*

Brand Names: US Complera

Brand Names: Canada Complera

Pharmacologic Category Antiretroviral, Reverse Transcriptase Inhibitor, Non-nucleoside (Anti-HIV); Antiretroviral, Reverse Transcriptase Inhibitor, Nucleoside (Anti-HIV); Antiretroviral, Reverse Transcriptase Inhibitor, Nucleotide (Anti-HIV)

Use HIV-1 infection, treatment: Treatment of HIV-1 infection (as a complete regimen) in adult and pediatric patients >35 kg as initial therapy in antiretroviral treatment-naive patients with HIV-1 RNA ≤100,000 copies/mL at the start of therapy, and in certain virologically suppressed (HIV-1 RNA <50 copies/mL) patients on a stable antiretroviral regimen for ≥6 months with no treatment failure or substitutions due to resistance to emtricitabine, rilpivirine, or tenofovir disoproxil fumarate in order to replace their current antiretroviral treatment regimen.

Local Anesthetic/Vasoconstrictor Precautions No information available to require special precautions

Effects on Dental Treatment No significant effects or complications reported

Effects on Bleeding No information available to require special precautions

Adverse Reactions Observed in patients receiving the same doses of emtricitabine, rilpivirine, and tenofovir as the combination product; also see individual agents.

>10%:

Endocrine & metabolic: Increased serum cholesterol (≤14%), increased LDL cholesterol (1% to 13%)

Hepatic: Increased serum alanine aminotransferase (1% to 19%), increased serum aspartate aminotransferase (1% to 16%)

1% to 10%:

Central nervous system: Depression (2% to 9%), headache (2%), insomnia (2%), abnormal dreams (1%), dizziness (1%)

Dermatologic: Skin rash (1%)

Endocrine & metabolic: Adrenocortical insufficiency (7%), increased serum triglycerides (1%)

Gastrointestinal: Nausea (1%)

Hepatic: Increased serum bilirubin (1% to 6%)

Renal: Increased serum creatinine (≤6%)

Frequency not defined:

Central nervous system: Anxiety, drowsiness, fatigue, sleep disorder

Gastrointestinal: Abdominal distress, abdominal pain, cholecystitis, cholelithiasis, decreased appetite, diarrhea, vomiting

Renal: Glomerulonephritis (membranous and mesangioproliferative), nephrolithiasis

<1%, postmarketing, and/or case reports: DRESS syndrome, hypersensitivity reaction, immune reconstitution syndrome, severe dermatological reaction, suicidal ideation, suicidal tendencies, weight gain

Mechanism of Action Non-nucleoside, nucleoside, and nucleotide reverse transcriptase inhibitor combination; rilpivirine binds to reverse transcriptase and does not require intracellular phosphorylation for antiviral activity; emtricitabine is a cytosine analogue while tenofovir disoproxil fumarate (TDF) is an analog of adenosine 5'-monophosphate. Each drug interferes with HIV viral RNA dependent DNA polymerase activities resulting in inhibition of viral replication.

Reproductive Considerations

The Health and Human Services (HHS) perinatal HIV guidelines consider this fixed-dose combination an alternative regimen for females living with HIV who are not yet pregnant but are trying to conceive (HHS [perinatal] 2019).

Refer to individual monographs for additional information.

Pregnancy Considerations

The Health and Human Services (HHS) perinatal HIV guidelines recommend this fixed-dose combination an alternative regimen for initial use in pregnant females living with HIV who are antiretroviral naive, who have had antiretroviral therapy (ART) in the past but are restarting, or who require a new ART regimen (due to poor tolerance or poor virologic response of current regimen). Females who become pregnant while taking this combination may continue if viral suppression is effective and the regimen is well tolerated. More frequent monitoring is recommended during pregnancy. This combination should not be used in pregnant females with a pretreatment HIV RNA ≤100,000 copies/mL or CD4 cell count ≥200 cells/mm^3 (HHS [perinatal] 2019).

Refer to individual monographs for additional information.

◆ **Emtricitabine/Tenofov Alafenam** *see* Emtricitabine and Tenofovir Alafenamide *on page 557*

◆ **Emtricitabine, Tenofovir Alafenamide, Darunavir, and Cobicistat** *see* Darunavir, Cobicistat, Emtricitabine, and Tenofovir Alafenamide *on page 442*

◆ **Emtricitabine, Tenofovir Disoproxil Fumarate, Elvitegravir, and Cobicistat** *see* Elvitegravir, Cobicistat, Emtricitabine, and Tenofovir Disoproxil Fumarate *on page 553*

◆ **Emtricitab/Rilpiviri/Tenof Ala** *see* Emtricitabine, Rilpivirine, and Tenofovir Alafenamide *on page 559*

◆ **Emtriva** *see* Emtricitabine *on page 556*

◆ **ENA 713** *see* Rivastigmine *on page 1341*

◆ **Enablex** *see* Darifenacin *on page 441*

Enalapril (e NAL a pril)

Related Information

Cardiovascular Diseases *on page 1654*

Brand Names: US Epaned; Vasotec

Brand Names: Canada ACT Enalapril; APO-Enalapril; JAMP Enalapril; MAR-Enalapril; MYLAN-Enalapril [DSC]; NOVO-Enalapril; PMS-Enalapril [DSC]; PRO-Enalapril-10; PRO-Enalapril-2.5; PRO-Enalapril-20; PRO-Enalapril-5; RAN-Enalapril; RIVA-Enalapril; SANDOZ Enalapril; TARO-Enalapril; TEVA-Enalapril [DSC]; Vasotec

Pharmacologic Category Angiotensin-Converting Enzyme (ACE) Inhibitor; Antihypertensive

Use

Heart failure: Treatment of symptomatic heart failure with reduced ejection fraction (HFrEF) to improve symptoms, increase survival, and decrease hospitalizations. In patients with stable asymptomatic HFrEF, enalapril decreases the risk of developing overt heart failure and the incidence of heart failure hospitalizations.

Hypertension: Management of hypertension, alone or in combination with other antihypertensive agents

Local Anesthetic/Vasoconstrictor Precautions

No information available to require special precautions

Effects on Dental Treatment Key adverse event(s) related to dental treatment: Abnormal taste; Patients may experience orthostatic hypotension as they stand up after treatment; especially if lying in dental chair for extended periods of time. Use caution with sudden changes in position during and after dental treatment.

An angiotensin-converting enzyme (ACE) Inhibitor cough is a dry, hacking, nonproductive cough that can potentially interfere with longer dental procedures if patient has this side effect.

Effects on Bleeding No information available to require special precautions

Adverse Reactions Note: Frequency ranges include data from hypertension and heart failure trials. Higher rates of adverse reactions have generally been noted in patients with CHF. However, the frequency of adverse effects associated with placebo is also increased in this population.

>10%: Renal: Increased serum creatinine (≤20%)

1% to 10%:

Cardiovascular: Hypotension (1% to 7%), chest pain (2%), orthostatic effect (1% to 2%), orthostatic hypotension (2%), syncope (≤2%)

Central nervous system: Dizziness (4% to 8%), headache (2% to 5%), fatigue (2% to 3%)

Dermatologic: Skin rash (1% to 2%)

Gastrointestinal: Abdominal pain, anorexia, constipation, diarrhea, dysgeusia, nausea, vomiting

Neuromuscular & skeletal: Weakness

Renal: Renal insufficiency (in patients with bilateral renal artery stenosis or hypovolemia)

Respiratory: Bronchitis (1% to 2%), cough (1% to 2%), dyspnea (1% to 2%)

<1%, postmarketing, and/or case reports: Abnormal dreams, acute generalized exanthematous pustulosis, agranulocytosis, alopecia, anaphylactoid reaction, angina pectoris, angioedema, anosmia, arthralgia, arthritis, asthma, ataxia, atrial fibrillation, atrial tachycardia, blurred vision, bone marrow depression, bradycardia, bronchospasm, cardiac arrest, cardiac arrhythmia, cerebrovascular accident, cholestatic jaundice, confusion, conjunctivitis, depression, diaphoresis, drowsiness, dry eye syndrome, dyspepsia, eosinophilia, eosinophilic pneumonitis, erythema multiforme, exfoliative dermatitis, fever, flank pain, flushing, giant-cell arteritis, glossitis, gynecomastia, hallucination, hemolysis (with G6PD), hepatitis, herpes zoster, hoarseness, IgA vasculitis, increased erythrocyte sedimentation rate, intestinal obstruction, impotence, insomnia, interstitial nephritis, jaundice, lacrimation, leukocytosis, lichenoid eruption, melena, muscle cramps, myocardial infarction, myalgia, myositis, nervousness, neutropenia, ototoxicity,

palpitations, pancreatitis, paresthesia, pemphigus, pemphigus foliaceus, peripheral neuropathy, positive ANA titer, pruritus, psychosis, pulmonary edema, pulmonary embolism, pulmonary infarct, pulmonary infiltrates, Raynaud's phenomenon, rhinorrhea, serositis, Sjogren's syndrome, skin photosensitivity, sore throat, Stevens-Johnson syndrome, stomatitis, systemic lupus erythematosus, thrombocytopenia, tinnitus, toxic epidermal necrolysis, upper respiratory tract infection, urticaria, vasculitis, vertigo, visual hallucination (Doane, 2013), xerostomia

Mechanism of Action Competitive inhibitor of angiotensin-converting enzyme (ACE); prevents conversion of angiotensin I to angiotensin II, a potent vasoconstrictor; results in lower levels of angiotensin II which causes an increase in plasma renin activity and a reduction in aldosterone secretion

Pharmacodynamics/Kinetics

Onset of Action ~1 hour; Peak effect: 4 to 6 hours

Duration of Action 12 to 24 hours

Half-life Elimination

Enalapril: CHF: Neonates (n=3, PNA: 10 to 19 days): 10.3 hours (range: 4.2 to 13.4 hours) (Nakamura 1994); CHF: Infants and Children ≤6.5 years of age (n=11): 2.7 hours (range: 1.3 to 6.3 hours) (Nakamura 1994); Adults: Healthy: 2 hours; CHF: 3.4 to 5.8 hours

Enalaprilat: CHF: Neonates (n=3, PNA: 10 to 19 days): 11.9 hours (range: 5.9 to 15.6 hours) (Nakamura 1994); CHF: Infants and Children ≤6.5 years of age (n=11): 11.1 hours (range: 5.1 to 20.8 hours) (Nakamura 1994); Infants 6 weeks to 8 months of age: 6 to 10 hours (Lloyd 1989); Adults: ~35 hours (Till 1984; Ulm 1982)

Time to Peak Serum: Oral: Enalapril: 0.5 to 1.5 hours; Enalaprilat (active metabolite): 3 to 4.5 hours

Reproductive Considerations

Angiotensin-converting enzyme (ACE) inhibitors should be avoided in sexually active females of reproductive potential not using effective contraception (ADA 2020).

ACE inhibitors should generally be avoided for the treatment of hypertension in women planning a pregnancy; use should only be considered for cases of hypertension refractory to other medications (ACOG 203 2019).

Pregnancy Considerations

Enalapril crosses the placenta; the active metabolite enalaprilat can be detected in the newborn (Schubiger 1988).

Exposure to an angiotensin-converting enzyme (ACE) inhibitor during the first trimester of pregnancy may be associated with an increased risk of fetal malformations (ACOG 203 2019; ESC [Regitz-Zagrosek 2018]); however, outcomes observed may also be influenced by maternal disease (ACC/AHA [Whelton 2017]).

[US Boxed Warning]: Drugs that act on the renin-angiotensin system can cause injury and death to the developing fetus. Discontinue as soon as possible once pregnancy is detected.

Drugs that act on the renin-angiotensin system are associated with oligohydramnios. Oligohydramnios, due to decreased fetal renal function, may lead to fetal lung hypoplasia and skeletal malformations. The use of these drugs in pregnancy is also associated with anuria, hypotension, renal failure, skull hypoplasia, and death in the fetus/neonate. Infants exposed to an ACE inhibitor in utero should be monitored for hyperkalemia, hypotension, and oliguria. Oligohydramnios may not appear until after irreversible fetal injury has occurred. Exchange transfusions or dialysis may be required to reverse hypotension or improve renal function, although data related to the effectiveness in neonates is limited.

Chronic maternal hypertension is also associated with adverse events in the fetus/infant. Chronic maternal hypertension may increase the risk of birth defects, low birth weight, premature delivery, stillbirth, and neonatal death. Actual fetal/neonatal risks may be related to duration and severity of maternal hypertension. Untreated chronic hypertension may also increase the risks of adverse maternal outcomes, including gestational diabetes, preeclampsia, delivery complications, stroke, and myocardial infarction (ACOG 203 2019).

When treatment of hypertension in pregnancy is indicated, ACE inhibitors should generally be avoided due to their adverse fetal events; use in pregnant women should only be considered for cases of hypertension refractory to other medications (ACOG 203 2019). ACE inhibitors are not recommended for the treatment of heart failure in pregnancy (Regitz-Zagrosek [ESC 2018]).

When treatment is needed in females of reproductive potential with diabetic nephropathy, the ACE inhibitor should be discontinued at the first positive pregnancy test (Cabiddu 2016; Spotti 2018).

Enalaprilat (en AL a pril at)

Brand Names: Canada Vasotec IV

Pharmacologic Category Angiotensin-Converting Enzyme (ACE) Inhibitor; Antihypertensive

Use Hypertension: Management of hypertension when oral therapy is not practical

Local Anesthetic/Vasoconstrictor Precautions No information available to require special precautions

Effects on Dental Treatment Key adverse event(s) related to dental treatment: Abnormal taste; Patients may experience orthostatic hypotension as they stand up after treatment; especially if lying in dental chair for extended periods of time. Use caution with sudden changes in position during and after dental treatment.

An angiotensin-converting enzyme (ACE) Inhibitor cough is a dry, hacking, nonproductive cough that can potentially interfere with longer dental procedures if patient has this side effect.

Effects on Bleeding No information available to require special precautions

Adverse Reactions Since enalapril is converted to enalaprilat, adverse reactions associated with enalapril may also occur with enalaprilat (also refer to Enalapril monograph). Frequency ranges include data from hypertension and cardiac failure trials. Higher rates of adverse reactions have generally been noted in patients with cardiac failure. However, the frequency of adverse effects associated with placebo is also increased in this population.

1% to 10%:

Cardiovascular: Hypotension (2% to 5%)

Central nervous system: Headache (3%)

Gastrointestinal: Nausea (1%)

<1%, postmarketing, and/or case reports: Angioedema, constipation, cough, dizziness, fatigue, fever, myocardial infarction, skin rash

Mechanism of Action Competitive inhibitor of angiotensin-converting enzyme (ACE); prevents conversion of angiotensin I to angiotensin II, a potent vasoconstrictor; results in lower levels of angiotensin II which causes an increase in plasma renin activity and a reduction in aldosterone secretion

Pharmacodynamics/Kinetics

Onset of Action IV: ≤15 minutes; Peak effect: IV: 1-4 hours

Duration of Action IV: ~6 hours (dose-dependent)

Half-life Elimination CHF: Neonates (n=3; PNA: 10-19 days): 11.9 hours (range: 5.9-15.6 hours) (Nakamura, 1994); CHF: Infants and Children ≤6.5 years of age (n=11): 11.1 hours (range: 5.1-20.8 hours) (Nakamura, 1994); Infants 6 weeks to 8 months of age: 6-10 hours (Lloyd, 1989); Adults: ~35 hours (Till, 1984; Ulm, 1982)

Reproductive Considerations

Angiotensin-converting enzyme (ACE) inhibitors should be avoided in sexually active females of reproductive potential not using effective contraception (ADA 2020).

ACE inhibitors should generally be avoided for the treatment of hypertension in women planning a pregnancy; use should only be considered for cases of hypertension refractory to other medications (ACOG 203 2019).

Pregnancy Considerations

Enalapril crosses the placenta; the active metabolite enalaprilat can be detected in the newborn (Schubiger 1988).

Exposure to an angiotensin-converting enzyme (ACE) inhibitor during the first trimester of pregnancy may be associated with an increased risk of fetal malformations (ACOG 203 2019; ESC [Regitz-Zagrosek 2018]); however, outcomes observed may also be influenced by maternal disease (ACC/AHA [Whelton 2017]).

[US Boxed Warning]: Drugs that act on the renin-angiotensin system can cause injury and death to the developing fetus. Discontinue as soon as possible once pregnancy is detected. Drugs that act on the renin-angiotensin system are associated with oligohydramnios. Oligohydramnios, due to decreased fetal renal function, may lead to fetal lung hypoplasia and skeletal malformations. The use of these drugs in pregnancy is also associated with anuria, hypotension, renal failure, skull hypoplasia, and death in the fetus/neonate. Infants exposed to an ACE inhibitor in utero should be monitored for hyperkalemia, hypotension, and oliguria. Oligohydramnios may not appear until after irreversible fetal injury has occurred. Exchange transfusions or dialysis may be required to reverse hypotension or improve renal function, although data related to the effectiveness in neonates is limited.

Chronic maternal hypertension is also associated with adverse events in the fetus/infant. Chronic maternal hypertension may increase the risk of birth defects, low birth weight, premature delivery, stillbirth, and neonatal death. Actual fetal/neonatal risks may be related to duration and severity of maternal hypertension. Untreated chronic hypertension may also increase the risks of adverse maternal outcomes, including gestational diabetes, pre-eclampsia, delivery complications, stroke and myocardial infarction (ACOG 203 2019).

When treatment of hypertension in pregnancy is indicated, ACE inhibitors should generally be avoided due to their adverse fetal events; use in pregnant women should only be considered for cases of hypertension refractory to other medications (ACOG 203 2019).

◆ **Enalapril Maleate** *see* Enalapril *on page 560*

Enasidenib (en a SID a nib)

Brand Names: US IDHIFA

Brand Names: Canada IDHIFA

Pharmacologic Category Antineoplastic Agent, IDH2 Inhibitor

Use Acute myeloid leukemia (relapsed/refractory): Treatment of relapsed or refractory acute myeloid leukemia (AML) in patients with an isocitrate dehydrogenase-2 (IDH2) mutation as detected by an approved test

Local Anesthetic/Vasoconstrictor Precautions No information available to require special precautions

Effects on Dental Treatment No significant effects or complications reported

Effects on Bleeding No information available to require special precautions

Adverse Reactions

>10%:

Endocrine & metabolic: Decreased serum calcium (74%), decreased serum potassium (41%)

Gastrointestinal: Nausea (50%), diarrhea (43%), decreased appetite (34%), vomiting (34%), dysgeusia (12%)

Hematologic & oncologic: Abnormal phosphorus levels (27%; ≥3 grade: 8%; decreased), differentiation syndrome (14%), leukocytosis (12%; ≥3 grade: 6%; noninfectious)

Hepatic: Increased serum bilirubin (81%)

1% to 10%:

Hematologic & oncologic: Tumor lysis syndrome (6%)

Respiratory: Acute respiratory distress (≤10%), pulmonary edema (≤10%)

Mechanism of Action Enasidenib is a small molecule inhibitor of the enzyme isocitrate dehydrogenase 2 (IDH2); it targets the mutant IDH2 variants R140Q, R172S, and R172K at ~40-fold lower concentrations than the wild-type enzyme. Mutant IDH2 inhibition results in decreased 2-hydroxyglutarate (2-HG) levels, reduced abnormal histone hypermethylation, and restored myeloid differentiation (Stein 2017). Additionally, enasidenib reduces blast counts and increases percentages of mature myeloid cells.

Pharmacodynamics/Kinetics

Half-life Elimination Terminal: 7.9 days.

Time to Peak 4 hours

Reproductive Considerations

Women of reproductive potential should have a pregnancy test prior to treatment initiation; effective contraception should be used during therapy and for at least 2 months after the last dose. Male patients with female partners of reproductive potential should also use effective contraception during therapy and for at least 2 months after the last dose.

Pregnancy Considerations

Based on the mechanism of action and data from animal reproduction studies, the use of enasidenib in pregnancy may cause fetal harm.

Prescribing and Access Restrictions Enasidenib is available through select specialty pharmacies and authorized distributors. Refer to http://www.idhifa.com for further information.

◆ **Enasidenib Mesylate** *see* Enasidenib *on page 562*
◆ **Enbrel** *see* Etanercept *on page 607*
◆ **Enbrel Mini** *see* Etanercept *on page 607*
◆ **Enbrel SureClick** *see* Etanercept *on page 607*
◆ **Encora** *see* Vitamins (Multiple/Oral) *on page 1550*

Encorafenib (en koe RAF e nib)

Brand Names: US Braftovi

Pharmacologic Category Antineoplastic Agent, BRAF Kinase Inhibitor

Use

Colorectal cancer, metastatic: Treatment of metastatic colorectal cancer in adults with a BRAF V600E mutation (in combination with cetuximab) as detected by an approved test, after prior therapy.

Melanoma, unresectable or metastatic: Treatment of unresectable or metastatic melanoma with a BRAF V600E or V600K mutation (in combination with binimetinib) as detected by an approved test.

Limitations of use: Encorafenib is not indicated for treatment of wild-type BRAF melanoma or wild-type BRAF colorectal cancer.

Local Anesthetic/Vasoconstrictor Precautions BRAF kinase inhibitors, including encorafinib, are associated with prolonging the QT interval. Encorafenib is one of the drugs confirmed to prolong the QT interval and is accepted as having a risk of causing torsade de pointes. The risk of drug-induced torsade de pointes is extremely low when a single QT interval-prolonging drug is prescribed. In terms of epinephrine, it is not known what effect vasoconstrictors in the local anesthetic regimen will have in patients with a known history of congenital prolonged QT interval or in patients taking any medication that prolongs the QT interval. Until more information is obtained, it is suggested that the clinician consult with the physician prior to the use of a vasoconstrictor in suspected patients, and that the vasoconstrictor (epinephrine, mepivacaine, and levonordefrin [Carbocaine 2% with Neo-Cobefrin]) be used with caution.

Effects on Dental Treatment Key adverse event(s) related to dental treatment: Facial paresis has been reported

Effects on Bleeding Hemorrhage has been reported; none involving the oral cavity

Adverse Reactions Incidence of adverse reactions for encorafenib are in combination therapy with either binimetinib or cetixumab, unless otherwise noted. Encorafenib as a single agent is associated with an increased risk of certain adverse reactions.

>10%:

Dermatologic: Acneiform eruption (combination therapy: 3% to 32%; single agent: 8%), alopecia (single agent: 56%; combination therapy: 14%), dermatological reaction (grades 3/4: single agent: 21%; combination therapy: 2%), erythema of skin (single agent: 16%; combination therapy: 7%), hyperkeratosis (single agent: 57%; combination therapy: 23%), melanocytic nevus (14%), palmar-plantar erythrodysesthesia (single agent: 51%; combination therapy: 7%), pruritus (single agent: 31%; combination therapy: 13% to 14%), skin rash (single agent: 41%; combination therapy: 22% to 26%), xeroderma (single agent: 38%; combination therapy: 13% to 16%)

Endocrine & metabolic: Hyperglycemia (28%), hypokalemia (12%), hypomagnesemia (19%), hyponatremia (11% to 18%), increased gamma-glutamyl transferase (45%)

Gastrointestinal: Abdominal pain (28% to 30%), constipation (15% to 22%), decreased appetite (27%), diarrhea (33%), dysgeusia (single agent: 13%, combination therapy: 6%), nausea (34% to 41%), vomiting (21% to 30%)

Hematologic & oncologic: Anemia (34% to 36%; grades 3/4: 4%), hemorrhage (19%; grades 3/4: 2% to 3%), leukopenia (13%), lymphocytopenia (13% to 24%; grades 3/4: 2% to 7%), neutropenia (13%; grades 3/4: 3%), prolonged partial thromboplastin time (13%; grades 3/4: 1%)

Hepatic: Increased serum alanine aminotransferase (17% to 29%), increased serum alkaline phosphatase (18% to 21%), increased serum aspartate aminotransferase (15% to 27%)

Nervous system: Dizziness (15%), fatigue (43% to 51%), headache (20% to 22%), insomnia (13%), peripheral neuropathy (12%; grades 3/4: 1%)

Neuromuscular & skeletal: Arthralgia (single agent: 44%; combination therapy: 26% to 27%), back pain (single agent: 15%; combination therapy: 9%), limb pain (10% to 11%), myopathy (single agent: 33%; combination therapy: 15% to 23%)

Renal: Increased serum creatinine (93%)

Miscellaneous: Fever (17% to 18%)

1% to 10%:

Endocrine & metabolic: Hypermagnesemia (10%)

Gastrointestinal: Hematochezia (2% to 3%), hemorrhoidal bleeding (1% to 2%), pancreatitis (<10%)

Hematologic & oncologic: Basal cell carcinoma of skin (combination therapy: 2%; single agent: 1%), keratoacanthoma (single agent: ≤8%; combination therapy: ≤3%), malignant melanoma (single agent: 5%; combination therapy: 1%), rectal hemorrhage (4%), squamous cell carcinoma of skin (single agent: ≤8%; combination therapy: ≤3%)

Hypersensitivity: Hypersensitivity reaction (<10%)

Nervous system: Facial paresis (<10%)

Neuromuscular & skeletal: Panniculitis (<10%)

Ophthalmic: Uveitis (4%, including iritis and iridocyclitis)

Respiratory: Epistaxis (7%)

<1%: Cardiovascular: Prolonged QT interval on ECG

Frequency not defined:

Gastrointestinal: Gastrointestinal hemorrhage

Nervous system: Intracranial hemorrhage

Mechanism of Action Encorafenib is an ATP-competitive inhibitor of protein kinase B-raf (BRAF) which suppresses the MAPK pathway (Dummer 2018). Encorafenib targets BRAF V600E, V600 D, and V600 K, and has a longer dissociation half-life than other BRAF inhibitors, allowing for sustained inhibition (Dummer 2018). BRAF V600 mutations result in constitutive activation of the BRAF pathway (which may stimulate tumor growth); BRAF inhibition inhibits tumor cell growth. The combination of encorafenib and binimetinib allows for greater antitumor activity in BRAF V600 mutant cell lines; in animal studies, the combination also delayed the emergence of resistance in BRAF V600E mutant cells compared to either drug alone. In BRAF-mutant colorectal cancer, EGFR-mediated MAPK pathway activation is a resistance mechanism to BRAF inhibitors; the combination of a BRAF inhibitor and anti-EGFR agents has been shown to overcome this resistance mechanism (in nonclinical models). The combination of encorafenib and cetuximab had an antitumor effect greater than either agent alone (in an animal model).

Pharmacodynamics/Kinetics

Half-life Elimination 3.5 hours

Time to Peak 2 hours

Reproductive Considerations

Verify pregnancy status in females of reproductive potential prior to initiating encorafenib therapy. Females of reproductive potential should use a highly effective nonhormonal contraceptive during therapy and for at least 2 weeks after the last encorafenib dose; hormonal contraceptives may not be effective.

Pregnancy Considerations

Based on its mechanism of action and on findings in animal reproduction studies, encorafenib may cause fetal harm if administered during pregnancy.

Prescribing and Access Restrictions Encorafenib is available through a network of select specialty pharmacies. Refer to https://www.braftovimektovi.com/hcp/ for more information.

- ◆ **Endo Avitene** *see* Collagen Hemostat *on page 410*
- ◆ **Endocet** *see* Oxycodone and Acetaminophen *on page 1164*
- ◆ **Endometrin** *see* Progesterone *on page 1280*
- ◆ **Enemeez Mini [OTC]** *see* Docusate *on page 509*

Enfortumab Vedotin (en FORT ue mab ve DOE tin)

Brand Names: US Padcev

Pharmacologic Category Antineoplastic Agent, Anti-Nectin-4; Antineoplastic Agent, Antibody Drug Conjugate; Antineoplastic Agent, Monoclonal Antibody

Use Urothelial cancer, locally advanced or metastatic: Treatment of locally advanced or metastatic urothelial cancer in adults who have previously received a programmed death receptor-1 or programmed death-ligand 1 inhibitor, and a platinum-containing chemotherapy in the neoadjuvant/adjuvant, locally advanced or metastatic setting.

Local Anesthetic/Vasoconstrictor Precautions

No information available to require special precautions.

Effects on Dental Treatment Key adverse event(s) related to dental treatment: Distorted sense of taste (dysgeusia).

Effects on Bleeding Therapy with enfortumab vedotin can result in significant hematologic toxicities including anemia, lymphocytopenia, neutropenia, and leukopenia. In patients under active treatment with enfortumab vedotin, medical consult is suggested.

Adverse Reactions

>10%:

Central nervous system: Fatigue (56%), peripheral neuropathy (49% to 56%; grade 3/4: 4%)

Dermatologic: Skin rash (52% to 54%; including symmetrical drug-related intertriginous and flexural exanthema), alopecia (50%), pruritus (26% to 30%), maculopapular rash (26%), xeroderma (26%)

Endocrine & metabolic: Decreased serum phosphate (34%), decreased serum potassium (19%)

Gastrointestinal: Decreased appetite (52%), nausea (45%), diarrhea (42%), dysgeusia (42%), vomiting (18%), increased serum lipase (14%)

Hematologic & oncologic: Decreased hemoglobin (34%; grade 3/4: 10%), lymphocytopenia (32%; grade 3/4: 10%), decreased neutrophils (14%; grade 3/4: 5%), leukopenia (14%; grade 3/4: 4%)

Ophthalmic: Ocular toxicity (46%), dry eye syndrome (36% to 40%), blurred vision (14%)

Renal: Increased serum creatinine (20%)

1% to 10%:

Dermatologic: Cellulitis (5%)

Endocrine & metabolic: Decreased serum sodium (8%), hyperglycemia (grade 3/4: 8%), increased uric acid (7%)

Gastrointestinal: Severe diarrhea (4%)

Genitourinary: Urinary tract infection (6%)

Hematologic & oncologic: Febrile neutropenia (4%)

Immunologic: Antibody development (≤1%)

Infection: Herpes zoster infection (3%), sepsis (3%)

Renal: Acute renal failure (3%)

Respiratory: Dyspnea (3%)

Frequency not defined:

Central nervous system: Abnormal gait, hypoesthesia, peripheral motor neuropathy, peripheral sensory neuropathy

Dermatologic: Acneiform eruption, bullous dermatitis, contact dermatitis, erythema multiforme, erythematous rash, exfoliation of skin, exfoliative dermatitis, palmar-plantar erythrodysesthesia, pustular rash, skin photosensitivity, stasis dermatitis, urticaria, vesicular eruption

Endocrine & metabolic: Diabetic ketoacidosis

Neuromuscular & skeletal: Asthenia

Ophthalmic: Blepharitis, conjunctivitis, eye irritation, increased lacrimation, keratitis, punctate keratitis

Mechanism of Action Enfortumab vedotin is an antibody drug conjugate (ADC) directed at Nectin-4 (an adhesion protein located on cell surfaces). Nectin-4 is highly expressed in urothelial carcinoma as well as breast, gastric, and lung cancers (Rosenberg 2019). It contains an IgG1 anti-Nectin-4 antibody conjugated to a microtubule-disrupting agent, monomethyl auristatin E (MMAE). MMAE is attached to the antibody via a protease cleavable linker. The ADC binds to Nectin-4 expressing cells to form a complex which is internalized within the cell. Released MMAE binds to the tubules and disrupts the cellular microtubule network, inducing cell cycle arrest and apoptosis of Nectin-4 expressing cells (Rosenberg 2019).

Pharmacodynamics/Kinetics

Half-life Elimination Antibody drug conjugate: 3.4 days; monomethyl auristatin E: 2.4 days.

Time to Peak Antibody drug conjugate: At the end of the infusion; monomethyl auristatin E: at ~2 days after a dose.

Reproductive Considerations

Evaluate pregnancy status prior to use in females of reproductive potential. Females of reproductive potential should use effective contraception during therapy and for 2 months after the last enfortumab vedotin dose. Males with female partners of reproductive potential should use effective contraception during therapy and for 4 months after the last dose of enfortumab vedotin.

Pregnancy Considerations

Based on the mechanism of action and data from animal reproduction studies, in utero exposure to enfortumab vedotin may cause fetal harm.

- ◆ **Enfortumab vedotin-ejfv** *see* Enfortumab Vedotin *on page 564*

Enfuvirtide (en FYOO vir tide)

Related Information

HIV Infection and AIDS *on page 1690*

Brand Names: US Fuzeon

Brand Names: Canada Fuzeon

Pharmacologic Category Antiretroviral, Fusion Protein Inhibitor (Anti-HIV)

Use HIV-1 infection, treatment: Treatment of HIV-1 infection in combination with other antiretroviral agents in treatment-experienced patients with evidence of HIV-1 replication despite ongoing antiretroviral therapy.

Local Anesthetic/Vasoconstrictor Precautions No information available to require special precautions

Effects on Dental Treatment Key adverse event(s) related to dental treatment: Xerostomia (normal salivary flow resumes upon discontinuation) and taste disturbance

Effects on Bleeding No information available to require special precautions related to hemostasis.

Adverse Reactions

>10%:

Central nervous system: Fatigue (20%), insomnia (11%)

Gastrointestinal: Diarrhea (32%), nausea (23%)

Local: Injection site reaction (98%; may include cyst at injection site, erythema at injection site, induration at injection site, injection site ecchymosis, injection site nodule, injection site pruritus, pain at injection site), injection site infection (children: 11%, adults: 2%)

1% to 10%:

Dermatologic: Folliculitis (2%)

Endocrine & metabolic: Weight loss (7%)

Gastrointestinal: Abdominal pain (4%), decreased appetite (3%), pancreatitis (3%), anorexia (2%), xerostomia (2%)

Hematologic & oncologic: Eosinophilia (2% to 9%)

Hepatic: Increased serum transaminases (4%, grade 4: 1%)

Infection: Infection (4% to 6%), herpes simplex infection (4%)

Neuromuscular & skeletal: Increased creatine phosphokinase (3% to 7%), limb pain (3%), myalgia (3%)

Ophthalmic: Conjunctivitis (2%)

Respiratory: Sinusitis (6%), cough (4%), bacterial pneumonia (3%), flu-like symptoms (2%)

<1%, postmarketing, and/or case reports: Amyloidosis (cutaneous; at the injection site), angina pectoris, anxiety, constipation, depression, dysgeusia, glomerulonephritis, Guillain-Barré syndrome, hyperglycemia; hypersensitivity exacerbation (to abacavir), hypersensitivity reaction (symptoms may include fever, hypotension, increased serum transaminases, nausea, skin rash, vomiting); increased amylase, increased gamma-glutamyl transferase, insomnia, increased serum lipase, increased serum triglycerides, liver steatosis, lymphadenopathy, neutropenia, peripheral neuropathy, pulmonary disease, renal failure, renal insufficiency, renal tubular necrosis, respiratory distress, sepsis, sixth nerve palsy, suicidal tendencies, thrombocytopenia, toxic hepatitis, weakness

Mechanism of Action Binds to the first heptad-repeat (HR1) in the gp41 subunit of the viral envelope glycoprotein. Inhibits the fusion of HIV-1 virus with CD4 cells by blocking the conformational change in gp41 required for membrane fusion and entry into CD4 cells

Pharmacodynamics/Kinetics

Half-life Elimination 3.8 ± 0.6 hours

Time to Peak SubQ: Single dose: Median: 8 hours (range: 3 to 12 hours); Multiple dosing: Median: 4 hours (range: 4 to 8 hours)

Reproductive Considerations

The Health and Human Services (HHS) perinatal HIV guidelines do not recommend enfuvirtide (except in special circumstances) for females living with HIV who are not yet pregnant but are trying to conceive.

For males and females living with HIV and planning a pregnancy, maximum viral suppression below the limits of detection with antiretroviral therapy (ART), modification of therapy (if needed), optimization of the woman's health, and a discussion of the potential risks and benefits of ART therapy during pregnancy is recommended prior to conception (HHS [perinatal] 2019).

Pregnancy Considerations

Enfuvirtide has minimal to low transfer across the human placenta.

Data collected by the antiretroviral pregnancy registry are insufficient to evaluate human teratogenic risk. Maternal antiretroviral therapy (ART) may be associated with adverse pregnancy outcomes, including preterm delivery, stillbirth, low birth weight, and small for gestational age infants. Actual risks may be influenced by maternal factors, such as disease severity, gestational age at initiation of therapy, and specific ART regimen; therefore, close fetal monitoring is recommended. Because there is clear benefit to appropriate treatment, maternal ART should not be withheld due to concerns for adverse neonatal outcomes. Long-term follow-up is recommended for all infants exposed to antiretroviral medications; children without HIV but who were exposed to ART in utero and develop significant organ system abnormalities of unknown etiology (particularly of the CNS or heart) should be evaluated for potential mitochondrial dysfunction.

The Health and Human Services (HHS) perinatal HIV guidelines do not recommend enfuvirtide as initial therapy for patients living with HIV (including pregnant females); enfuvirtide is not recommended (except in special circumstances) in pregnant females who have had ART therapy in the past but are restarting, or who require a new ART regimen (due to poor tolerance or poor virologic response of current regimen). Females who become pregnant while taking enfuvirtide may continue if viral suppression is effective and the regimen is well tolerated. Pharmacokinetic data are insufficient to make dosing recommendations during pregnancy.

In general, ART is recommended for all pregnant females living with HIV to keep the viral load below the limit of detection and reduce the risk of perinatal transmission. Therapy should be individualized following a discussion of the potential risks and benefits of treatment during pregnancy. Monitoring of pregnant females is more frequent than in nonpregnant adults. ART should be continued postpartum for all females living with HIV and can be modified after delivery.

Health care providers are encouraged to enroll pregnant females exposed to antiretroviral medications as early in pregnancy as possible in the Antiretroviral Pregnancy Registry (1-800-258-4263 or http://www.-APRegistry.com). Health care providers caring for pregnant females living with HIV and their infants may contact the National Perinatal HIV Hotline (888-448-8765) for clinical consultation (HHS [perinatal] 2019).

- **ENG** *see* Etonogestrel *on page 625*
- **Engerix-B** *see* Hepatitis B Vaccine (Recombinant) *on page 757*
- **Engerix-B and Havrix** *see* Hepatitis A and Hepatitis B Recombinant Vaccine *on page 754*
- **Enhanced-Potency Inactivated Poliovirus Vaccine** *see* Poliovirus Vaccine (Inactivated) *on page 1243*

◆ **Enhertu** *see* Fam-Trastuzumab Deruxtecan *on page 636*

◆ **EnovaRX-Diclofenac Sodium** *see* Diclofenac (Topical) *on page 489*

Enoxaparin (ee noks a PA rin)

Related Information

Cardiovascular Diseases *on page 1654*

Brand Names: US Lovenox

Brand Names: Canada Lovenox; Lovenox HP

Pharmacologic Category Anticoagulant; Anticoagulant, Low Molecular Weight Heparin

Use

Acute coronary syndromes: Unstable angina, non-ST-elevation myocardial infarction, and ST-elevation myocardial infarction.

Deep vein thrombosis treatment (acute): Inpatient treatment (patients with or without pulmonary embolism [PE]) and outpatient treatment (patients without PE).

Venous thromboembolism prophylaxis: Following hip or knee replacement surgery, abdominal surgery, or in medical patients with severely restricted mobility during acute illness who are at risk for thromboembolic complications.

Local Anesthetic/Vasoconstrictor Precautions No information available to require special precautions

Effects on Dental Treatment Key adverse event(s) related to dental treatment: Bleeding is the major adverse effect of enoxaparin. See Effects on Bleeding.

Effects on Bleeding As with all anticoagulants, bleeding is the major adverse effect of enoxaparin. Hemorrhage may occur at virtually any site. Routine coagulation tests, such as prothrombin time (PT) and aPTT, are relatively insensitive measures of enoxaparin injection activity and, therefore, unsuitable for monitoring. Moderate thrombocytopenia occurred at a rate of ~1%. Medical consult is suggested.

Adverse Reactions As with all anticoagulants, bleeding is the major adverse effect of enoxaparin. Hemorrhage may occur at virtually any site. Risk is dependent on multiple variables. At the recommended doses, single injections of enoxaparin do not significantly influence platelet aggregation or affect global clotting time (ie, PT or aPTT).

>10%: Hematologic & oncologic: Anemia (≤16%), hemorrhage (4% to 13%)

1% to 10%:

Cardiovascular: Peripheral edema (6%)

Central nervous system: Confusion (2%)

Gastrointestinal: Nausea (3%)

Hematologic & oncologic: Major hemorrhage (<1% to 4%; includes cases of intracranial [up to 0.8%], retroperitoneal, or intraocular hemorrhage; incidence varies with indication/population), ecchymoses (3%), thrombocytopenia (1% to 2%)

Hepatic: Increased serum ALT (>3 x ULN: 6%), increased serum AST (>3 x ULN: 6%)

Local: Hematoma at injection site (9%), bleeding at injection site (3% to 5%), pain at injection site (2%)

Renal: Hematuria (≤2%)

Miscellaneous: Fever (≤8%)

<1%, postmarketing, and/or case reports: Acute posthemorrhagic anemia, alopecia, anaphylactoid reaction, anaphylaxis, atrial fibrillation, bruising at injection site, eosinophilia, epidural hematoma (spinal; after neuroaxial anesthesia or spinal puncture; risk may be increased with indwelling epidural catheter or concomitant use of other drugs affecting hemostasis), erythema at injection site, headache, hepatic injury (hepatocellular and cholestatic), hyperkalemia, hyperlipidemia (very rare), hypersensitivity angiitis, hypersensitivity reaction, hypertriglyceridemia, injection site reactions (including nodules, inflammation, oozing), irritation at injection site, osteoporosis (following long-term therapy), pneumonia, pruritus, pulmonary edema, purpura, shock, skin necrosis, thrombocythemia, thrombosis in heparin-induced thrombocytopenia, thrombosis (prosthetic value [in pregnant females] or associated with enoxaparin-induced thrombocytopenia; can cause limb ischemia or organ infarction), urticaria, vesicobullous rash

Mechanism of Action Standard heparin consists of components with molecular weights ranging from 4000 to 30,000 daltons with a mean of 16,000 daltons. Heparin acts as an anticoagulant by enhancing the inhibition rate of clotting proteases by antithrombin III impairing normal hemostasis and inhibition of factor Xa. Low molecular weight heparins have a small effect on the activated partial thromboplastin time and strongly inhibit factor Xa. Enoxaparin is derived from porcine heparin that undergoes benzylation followed by alkaline depolymerization. The average molecular weight of enoxaparin is 4500 daltons which is distributed as (≤20%) 2000 daltons (≥68%) 2000 to 8000 daltons, and (≤18%) >8000 daltons. Enoxaparin has a higher ratio of anti-factor Xa to anti-factor IIa activity than unfractionated heparin.

Pharmacodynamics/Kinetics

Onset of Action Peak effect: SubQ: Anti-factor Xa and antithrombin (anti-factor IIa): 3 to 5 hours

Duration of Action 40 mg dose: Anti-factor Xa activity: ~12 hours

Half-life Elimination Plasma: 2 to 4 times longer than standard heparin, independent of dose; based on anti-factor Xa activity: 4.5 to 7 hours

Reproductive Considerations

Venous thromboembolism (VTE) prophylaxis is not routinely recommended for women undergoing assisted reproduction therapy; however, LMWH therapy is recommended for women who develop severe ovarian hyperstimulation syndrome (Bates 2012).

Pregnancy Considerations

Low molecular weight heparin (LMWH) does not cross the placenta; increased risks of fetal bleeding or teratogenic effects have not been reported (Bates 2012).

LMWH is recommended over unfractionated heparin for the treatment of acute VTE in pregnant women. LMWH is also recommended over unfractionated heparin for VTE prophylaxis in pregnant women with certain risk factors (eg, homozygous factor V Leiden, antiphospholipid antibody syndrome with ≥3 previous pregnancy losses). For women undergoing cesarean section and who have additional risk factors for developing VTE, the prophylactic use of LMWH may be considered (Bates 2012). Consult current recommendations for appropriate use in pregnant women.

LMWH may also be used in women with mechanical heart valves (consult current guidelines for details) (Bates 2012; Nishimura 2014). Women who require long-term anticoagulation with warfarin and who are considering pregnancy, LMWH substitution should be done prior to conception when possible. When choosing therapy, fetal outcomes (ie, pregnancy loss, malformations), maternal outcomes (ie, VTE, hemorrhage), burden of therapy, and maternal preference should be considered (Bates 2012). Monitoring anti-factor Xa levels is recommended (Bates 2012; Nishimura 2014).

Multiple-dose vials contain benzyl alcohol (avoid in pregnant women due to association with gasping syndrome in premature infants); use of preservative-free formulations is recommended.

◆ **Enoxaparin Sodium** *see* Enoxaparin *on page 566*

◆ **Enpresse-28** *see* Ethinyl Estradiol and Levonorgestrel *on page 612*

◆ **Enskyce** *see* Ethinyl Estradiol and Desogestrel *on page 609*

Entacapone (en TA ka pone)

Brand Names: US Comtan

Brand Names: Canada Comtan; MYLAN-Entacapone [DSC]; SANDOZ Entacapone; TEVA-Entacapone

Pharmacologic Category Anti-Parkinson Agent, COMT Inhibitor

Use Parkinson disease: Adjunct to levodopa/carbidopa therapy in patients with idiopathic Parkinson disease who experience "wearing-off" symptoms at the end of a dosing interval

Local Anesthetic/Vasoconstrictor Precautions No information available to require special precautions

Effects on Dental Treatment Key adverse event(s) related to dental treatment: Abnormal taste; Dopaminergic therapy in Parkinson's disease (ie, treatment with levodopa) is associated with orthostatic hypotension. Entacapone enhances levodopa bioavailability and may increase the occurrence of hypotension/syncope in the dental patient. Patients may experience orthostatic hypotension as they stand up after treatment; especially if lying in dental chair for extended periods of time. Use caution with sudden changes in position during and after dental treatment.

Effects on Bleeding No information available to require special precautions

Adverse Reactions

>10%:

Gastrointestinal: Nausea (14%)

Neuromuscular & skeletal: Dyskinesia (25%)

1% to 10%:

Cardiovascular: Syncope (1%)

Central nervous system: Dizziness (8%), fatigue (6%), anxiety (2%), drowsiness (2%), agitation (1%), hallucination (≤1%)

Dermatologic: Diaphoresis (increased; 2%)

Gastrointestinal: Diarrhea (10%), abdominal pain (8%), constipation (6%), vomiting (4%), xerostomia (3%), dyspepsia (2%), flatulence (2%), dysgeusia (1%), gastritis (1%), gastrointestinal disease (1%)

Genitourinary: Urine discoloration (brown-orange; 10%)

Hematologic & oncologic: Purpura (2%)

Infection: Bacterial infection (1%)

Neuromuscular & skeletal: Hyperkinesia (10%), hypokinesia (9%), back pain (2% to 4%), weakness (2%)

Respiratory: Dyspnea (3%)

<1%, postmarketing, and/or case reports: Behavioral changes (including psychotic-like behavior), hepatitis (mainly cholestatic features), impulse control disorder (eg, pathological gambling, hypersexuality, spending money), mental status changes, neurological signs and symptoms (hyperpyrexia and confusion [resembling neuroleptic malignant syndrome]), orthostatic hypotension, pulmonary fibrosis, retroperitoneal fibrosis, rhabdomyolysis, sudden onset of sleep

Mechanism of Action Entacapone is a reversible and selective inhibitor of catechol-O-methyltransferase (COMT). When entacapone is taken with levodopa, the pharmacokinetics are altered, resulting in more sustained levodopa serum levels compared to levodopa taken alone. The resulting levels of levodopa provide for increased concentrations available for absorption across the blood-brain barrier, thereby providing for increased CNS levels of dopamine, the active metabolite of levodopa.

Pharmacodynamics/Kinetics

Onset of Action Rapid

Half-life Elimination Beta phase: 0.4 to 0.7 hours; gamma phase: 2.4 hours

Time to Peak Serum: 1 hour

Pregnancy Considerations The incidence of Parkinson disease in pregnancy is relatively rare and information related to the use of entacapone in pregnant women is very limited (Kranick 2010; Tüfekçioğlu 2018).

◆ **Entacapone, Carbidopa, and Levodopa** *see* Levodopa, Carbidopa, and Entacapone *on page 897*

Entecavir (en TE ka veer)

Related Information

HIV Infection and AIDS *on page 1690*

Systemic Viral Diseases *on page 1709*

Brand Names: US Baraclude

Brand Names: Canada ACCEL-Entecavir; APO-Entecavir; Auro-Entecavir; Baraclude; JAMP-Entecavir; MINT-Entecavir; PMS-Entecavir

Pharmacologic Category Antihepadnaviral, Reverse Transcriptase Inhibitor, Nucleoside (Anti-HBV)

Use

Chronic hepatitis B: Treatment of chronic hepatitis B virus (HBV) infection in adults and pediatric patients ≥2 years of age with evidence of active viral replication and either evidence of persistent transaminase elevations or histologically-active disease.

Note: In adults, indication is based on data in patients with compensated and decompensated liver disease; in children, indication is based on data in patients with compensated, HBeAg-positive liver disease.

Local Anesthetic/Vasoconstrictor Precautions No information available to require special precautions

Effects on Dental Treatment No significant effects or complications reported

Effects on Bleeding No information available to require special precautions related to hemostasis.

Adverse Reactions As reported with adult patients, unless otherwise noted.

>10%: Hepatic: Increased serum alanine aminotransferase (>5 x ULN: 11% to 12%; >10 x ULN and >2 x baseline: 2%)

1% to 10%:

Central nervous system: Headache (2% to 4%), fatigue (1% to 3%)

Dermatologic: Skin rash (>1%)

Endocrine & metabolic: Glycosuria (4%), hyperglycemia (2% to 3%)

Gastrointestinal: Increased serum lipase (7%), abdominal pain (children and adolescents: >1%), diarrhea (children and adolescents: >1%; adults: ≤1%), nausea (children and adolescents: >1%; adults: <1%), unpleasant taste (children and adolescents: >1%), vomiting (children and adolescents: >1%; adults: <1%), dyspepsia (≤1%)

Genitourinary: Hematuria (9%)
Hepatic: Increased serum bilirubin (2% to 3%)
Renal: Increased serum creatinine (1% to 2%)

<1%, postmarketing, and/or case reports: Alopecia, anaphylactoid shock, dizziness, drowsiness, hepatomegaly, hepatomegaly with steatosis, hypoalbuminemia, increased serum transaminases, insomnia, lactic acidosis, macular edema (Muqit 2011), thrombocytopenia

Mechanism of Action Entecavir is intracellularly phosphorylated to guanosine triphosphate which competes with natural substrates to effectively inhibit hepatitis B viral polymerase; enzyme inhibition blocks reverse transcriptase activity thereby reducing viral DNA synthesis.

Pharmacodynamics/Kinetics

Half-life Elimination Terminal: ~5 to 6 days; accumulation: ~24 hours

Time to Peak 0.5 to 1.5 hours

Pregnancy Considerations

Teratogenic effects have been observed in animal studies. Information related to use in pregnancy is limited. Other agents may be preferred for the treatment of chronic hepatitis B in pregnancy (AASLD [Terrault 2016]).

Pregnant women taking entecavir should enroll in the pregnancy registry by calling 1-800-258-4263.

- ◆ **Entereg** *see* Alvimopan *on page 112*
- ◆ **Entertainer's Secret [OTC]** *see* Saliva Substitute *on page 1354*
- ◆ **Entocort EC** *see* Budesonide (Systemic) *on page 252*
- ◆ **Entresto** *see* Sacubitril and Valsartan *on page 1353*
- ◆ **Entyvio** *see* Vedolizumab *on page 1536*
- ◆ **Envarsus XR** *see* Tacrolimus (Systemic) *on page 1398*

Enzalutamide (en za LOO ta mide)

Brand Names: US Xtandi

Brand Names: Canada Xtandi

Pharmacologic Category Antineoplastic Agent, Antiandrogen

Use Prostate cancer: Treatment of castration-resistant prostate cancer; treatment of metastatic castration-sensitive prostate cancer.

Local Anesthetic/Vasoconstrictor Precautions No information available to require special precautions

Effects on Dental Treatment No significant effects or complications reported

Effects on Bleeding Although significant myelosuppression with associated altered hemostasis has been reported for many chemotherapeutic agents, myelosuppression is not common with enzalutamide and no specific precautions appear to necessary.

Adverse Reactions

>10%:

Cardiovascular: Peripheral edema (12% to 15%), hypertension (6% to 14%)
Central nervous system: Fatigue (≤51%), falling (5% to 13%), dizziness (10% to 12%), headache (9% to 12%)
Endocrine & metabolic: Hyperglycemia (83%), hot flash (13% to 27%), hypermagnesemia (16%), hyponatremia (13%), weight loss (6% to 12%)
Gastrointestinal: Constipation (9% to 23%), diarrhea (12% to 22%), decreased appetite (5% to 19%), nausea (11% to 14%)
Hematologic & oncologic: Decreased neutrophils (20%; grades 3/4: <1%), decreased white blood cell count (17%; grades 3/4: <1%)
Neuromuscular & skeletal: Asthenia (≤51%), back pain (19% to 29%), arthralgia (21%), musculoskeletal pain (6% to 16%)
Respiratory: Upper respiratory tract infection (11% to 16%), dyspnea (11%)

1% to 10%:

Cardiovascular: Ischemic heart disease (3%)
Central nervous system: Myasthenia (10%), insomnia (8% to 9%), paresthesia (7%), cauda equina syndrome (≤7%), spinal cord compression (≤7%), anxiety (3% to 7%), altered mental status (4% to 6%), cognitive dysfunction (5%), hypoesthesia (4%), restless leg syndrome (2%)
Dermatologic: Pruritus (4%), xeroderma (4%)
Endocrine & metabolic: Hypercalcemia (7%), gynecomastia (3%)
Gastrointestinal: Dysgeusia (8%)
Genitourinary: Hematuria (7% to 9%), pollakiuria (5%)
Neuromuscular & skeletal: Bone fracture (4% to 10%), muscle rigidity (3%)
Respiratory: Lower respiratory tract infection (8% to 9%), epistaxis (3%)

<1%, postmarketing, and/or case reports: Angioedema, hypersensitivity reaction, reversible posterior leukoencephalopathy syndrome, seizure, skin rash, vomiting

Mechanism of Action Enzalutamide is a pure androgen receptor signaling inhibitor; unlike other antiandrogen therapies, it has no known agonistic properties. It inhibits androgen receptor nuclear translocation, DNA binding, and coactivator mobilization, leading to cellular apoptosis and decreased prostate tumor volume.

Pharmacodynamics/Kinetics

Half-life Elimination Parent drug: 5.8 days (range: 2.8 to 10.2 days); N-desmethyl enzalutamide: 7.8 to 8.6 days

Time to Peak 1 hour (range: 0.5 to 3 hours)

Reproductive Considerations

Male patients with female partners of reproductive potential should use effective contraception during treatment and for 3 months after the last enzalutamide dose.

Pregnancy Considerations

Based on the mechanism of action and data from animal reproduction studies, in utero exposure to enzalutamide may cause fetal harm and loss of pregnancy.

- ◆ **Epaned** *see* Enalapril *on page 560*
- ◆ **Epclusa** *see* Sofosbuvir and Velpatasvir *on page 1379*
- ◆ **EPEG** *see* Etoposide *on page 626*

EPHEDrine (Systemic) (e FED rin)

Brand Names: US Akovaz; Emerphed

Pharmacologic Category Alpha/Beta Agonist

Use Hypotension, anesthesia-induced: Treatment of anesthesia-induced hypotension.

Local Anesthetic/Vasoconstrictor Precautions Use vasoconstrictor with caution since ephedrine may enhance cardiostimulation and vasopressor effects of sympathomimetics such as epinephrine

Effects on Dental Treatment Key adverse event(s) related to dental treatment: Xerostomia (normal salivary flow resumes upon discontinuation)

Effects on Bleeding No information available to require special precautions

Adverse Reactions Frequency not defined.

Cardiovascular: Angina pectoris, bradycardia, cardiac arrhythmia, hypertension, palpitations, pulse irregularity, tachycardia, ventricular ectopy, visceral vasoconstriction (renal)

Central nervous system: Anxiety, confusion, delirium, dizziness, hallucination, headache, insomnia, intracranial hemorrhage, nervousness, precordial pain, restlessness, tension, vertigo

Dermatologic: Diaphoresis, pallor

Gastrointestinal: Anorexia, nausea, vomiting

Genitourinary: Dysuria, oliguria, urinary retention (males with prostatism)

Neuromuscular & skeletal: Tremor, vesicle sphincter spasm, weakness

Respiratory: Dyspnea

Miscellaneous: Tachyphylaxis

Mechanism of Action Releases tissue stores of norepinephrine and thereby produces an alpha- and beta-adrenergic stimulation; longer-acting and less potent than epinephrine

Pharmacodynamics/Kinetics

Onset of Action IM: Within 10 to 20 minutes.

Duration of Action Pressor/cardiac effects: SubQ: 1 hour.

Half-life Elimination Dependent upon urinary pH; Urine pH 5: ~3 hours; Urine pH 6.3: ~6 hours.

Pregnancy Considerations

Metabolic acidosis has been reported in neonates following maternal use of ephedrine; monitor.

Untreated maternal hypotension during cesarean delivery is associated with adverse events, including maternal nausea and vomiting, and bradycardia and acidosis in the fetus. Ephedrine injection is used at delivery for the prevention and/or treatment of maternal hypotension associated with spinal anesthesia in women undergoing cesarean delivery (ASA 2016). Serious postpartum hypertension and possibly stroke may occur if administered with oxytocic medications.

- **Ephedrine Sulfate** *see* EPHEDrine (Systemic) *on page 568*
- **E-Pherol [OTC] [DSC]** *see* Vitamin E (Systemic) *on page 1549*
- **Epidiolex** *see* Cannabidiol *on page 283*
- **Epidoxorubicin** *see* EpiRUBicin *on page 576*

Epinastine (ep i NAS teen)

Brand Names: US Elestat [DSC]

Pharmacologic Category Histamine H_1 Antagonist; Histamine H_1 Antagonist, Second Generation

Use Treatment of allergic conjunctivitis

Local Anesthetic/Vasoconstrictor Precautions No information available to require special precautions

Effects on Dental Treatment No significant effects or complications reported

Effects on Bleeding No information available to require special precautions

Adverse Reactions Frequency not always defined.

1% to 10%:

Central nervous system: Headache (1% to 3%)

Infection: Infection (10%; defined as cold symptoms and upper respiratory tract infection)

Ophthalmic: Burning sensation of eyes, eye pruritus, follicular conjunctivitis, ocular hyperemia

Respiratory: Cough (1% to 3%), pharyngitis (1% to 3%), rhinitis (1% to 3%), sinusitis (1% to 3%)

<1%, postmarketing, and/or case reports: Increased lacrimation

Mechanism of Action Selective H_1-receptor antagonist; inhibits release of histamine from the mast cell; also has affinity for the H_2, alpha$_1$, alpha$_2$, and the 5-HT_2 receptors

Pharmacodynamics/Kinetics

Onset of Action 3-5 minutes

Duration of Action 8 hours

Half-life Elimination 12 hours

Pregnancy Risk Factor C

Pregnancy Considerations Adverse events were observed in some animal reproduction studies.

- **Epinastine Hydrochloride** *see* Epinastine *on page 569*
- **Epinastrine HCl** *see* Epinastine *on page 569*

EPINEPHrine (Systemic) (ep i NEF rin)

Brand Names: US Adrenaclick [DSC]; Adrenalin; Adyphren; Adyphren Amp; Adyphren Amp II; Adyphren II; Auvi-Q; Epinephrine Professional; EpinephrineSnap-EMS; Epinephrinesnap-v; EpiPen 2-Pak; EpiPen Jr 2-Pak; EPIsnap; EPY II [DSC]; EPY [DSC]; Symjepi

Brand Names: Canada Adrenalin Chloride; Allerject; Anapen; Anapen Junior; EpiPen; EpiPen Jr; TARO-Epinephrine

Generic Availability (US) Yes

Pharmacologic Category Alpha/Beta Agonist

Dental Use Emergency drug for treatment of anaphylactic reactions; used as vasoconstrictor to prolong local anesthesia

Use

Hypersensitivity reaction: Treatment of type I allergic reactions, including anaphylactic reactions.

Mydriasis during intraocular surgery (product specific): Induction and maintenance of mydriasis during intraocular surgery. **Note:** Not all formulations of epinephrine injection are suitable for intraocular use; consult the prescribing information.

Shock/Hypotension: Treatment of hypotension associated with septic shock in adults (increase mean arterial BP).

Local Anesthetic/Vasoconstrictor Precautions No information available to require special precautions

Effects on Dental Treatment Key adverse event(s) related to dental treatment: Xerostomia (normal salivary flow resumes upon discontinuation) and dry throat.

Effects on Bleeding No information available to require special precautions

Adverse Reactions Frequency not defined:

Cardiovascular: Angina pectoris, cardiac arrhythmia, cardiomyopathy (stress), cerebrovascular accident, chest pain, hypertension, increased cardiac work, ischemic heart disease, limb ischemia, localized blanching, myocardial infarction, palpitations, peripheral vasoconstriction, supraventricular tachycardia, tachyarrhythmia, tachycardia, vasoconstriction, ventricular arrhythmia, ventricular ectopy, ventricular fibrillation

Central nervous system: Anxiety, apprehension, cerebral hemorrhage, disorientation, dizziness, drowsiness, exacerbation of Parkinson disease, headache, memory impairment, panic, paresthesia, psychomotor agitation, restlessness, tingling sensation

Dermatologic: Diaphoresis, gangrene of skin or other tissue (at injection site), pallor, piloerection

Endocrine & metabolic: Hyperglycemia, hypoglycemia, hypokalemia, insulin resistance, lactic acidosis
Gastrointestinal: Nausea, vomiting
Local: Tissue necrosis at injection site
Neuromuscular & skeletal: Asthenia, tremor
Renal: Renal insufficiency
Respiratory: Dyspnea, pulmonary edema, rales

Dental Usual Dosage Hypersensitivity reaction: Self-administration following severe allergic reactions (eg, insect stings, food): **Note:** World Health Organization (WHO) and Anaphylaxis Canada recommend the availability of 1 dose for every 10 to 20 minutes of travel time to a medical emergency facility. More than 2 sequential doses should only be administered under direct medical supervision.

Children:

Adrenaclick: IM, SubQ:

Children 15 to 29 kg: 0.15 mg

Children ≥30 kg: 0.3 mg

Auvi-Q: IM, SubQ:

Children 15 to 29 kg: 0.15 mg; if anaphylactic symptoms persist, dose may be repeated

Children ≥30 kg: 0.3 mg; if anaphylactic symptoms persist, dose may be repeated

EpiPen Jr: IM, SubQ: Children 15 to 29 kg: 0.15 mg; if anaphylactic symptoms persist, dose may be repeated in 5 to 15 minutes using an additional EpiPen Jr

EpiPen: IM, SubQ: Children ≥30 kg: 0.3 mg; if anaphylactic symptoms persist, dose may be repeated in 5 to 15 minutes using an additional EpiPen

Twinject: IM SubQ:

Children 15 to 29 kg: 0.15 mg; if anaphylactic symptoms persist, dose may be repeated in 5 to 15 minutes using the same device after partial disassembly

Children ≥30 kg: 0.3 mg; if anaphylactic symptoms persist, dose may be repeated in 5 to 15 minutes using the same device after partial disassembly

Adults:

Adrenaclick: IM, SubQ: 0.3 mg

Auvi-Q: IM, SubQ: 0.3 mg; if anaphylactic symptoms persist, dose may be repeated

EpiPen: IM, SubQ: 0.3 mg; if anaphylactic symptoms persist, dose may be repeated in 5 to 15 minutes using an additional EpiPen

Twinject: IM, SubQ: 0.3 mg; if anaphylactic symptoms persist, dose may be repeated in 5 to 15 minutes using the same device after partial disassembly

Dosing

Adult & Geriatric Note: Adrenaclick has been discontinued in the US for more than 1 year.

Note: As of May 1, 2016, ratio expressions of epinephrine concentrations are prohibited on drug labels. Ampules, vials, and syringes of epinephrine with ratio expressions may, however, remain in inventory until replaced by products with revised labeling. Therefore, the ratio expression of 1:1,000 is equivalent to 1 mg/mL and 1:10,000 is equivalent to 0.1 mg/mL (ISMP 2015).

Asthma, acute severe, unresponsive to inhaled beta-agonist (off-label use): IM, SubQ: 0.01 mg/kg divided into 3 doses of approximately 0.3 to 0.5 mg every 20 minutes; the **1 mg/mL** concentration is recommended (AHA [Vanden Hoek 2010]; Cydulka 2016; Shah 2012).

Asystole/pulseless cardiac arrest, ventricular fibrillation, or pulseless ventricular tachycardia (off-label use):

IV, Intraosseous: 1 mg (using the **0.1 mg/mL** solution) every 3 to 5 minutes until return of spontaneous circulation (AHA [Panchal 2019]).

Endotracheal (alternative route): 2 to 2.5 mg every 3 to 5 minutes until IV/intraosseous access established or return of spontaneous circulation; dilute in 5 to 10 mL NS or sterile water. **Note:** Absorption may be greater with sterile water (Naganobu 2000). May cause false-negative reading with exhaled CO_2 detectors; use second method to confirm tube placement if CO_2 is not detected (AHA [Neumar 2010]).

Bradycardia, symptomatic, unresponsive to atropine or pacing (off-label use): IV: Continuous infusion: 0.1 to 0.5 mcg/kg/minute (7 to 35 mcg/minute in a 70 kg patient); titrate to desired effect (ACC/AHA/HRS [Kusumoto 2019]).

Hypersensitivity reaction (eg, anaphylaxis): Note: IM administration in the anterolateral aspect of the middle third of the thigh is preferred in the setting of anaphylaxis (AHA [Vanden Hoek 2010]; WAO [Simons 2011]).

Endotracheal (alternative route): 2 to 2.5 mg every 3 to 5 minutes until IV/intraosseous access established; dilute in 5 to 10 mL NS or sterile water (AAAAI [Lieberman 2015]; AHA [Neumar 2010]; Campbell 2014). **Note:** Absorption may be greater with sterile water (Naganobu 2000).

IM: 0.2 to 0.5 mg **or** 0.01 mg/kg (maximum dose: 0.5 mg) using the **1 mg/mL** solution; repeat every 5 to 15 minutes in the absence of clinical improvement (AAAAI [Lieberman 2015]; AHA [Vanden Hoek 2010]; WAO [Simons 2011]). **Note:** May administer epinephrine as a continuous IV infusion in patients not responding to IM injections (AAAAI [Lieberman 2015]; Campbell 2014).

IV: **Note:** In general, IV administration should only be done in patients who are unresponsive or profoundly hypotensive after failure to respond to IV fluid replacement and several epinephrine IM injections (WAO [Simons 2011]).

Slow IV bolus (off-label dose): 0.05 to 0.1 mg using the **0.1 mg/mL** solution (further diluted in 10 mL of NS) administered over 5 to 10 minutes (AHA [Vanden Hoek 2010]; Barach 1984). If the patient is in cardiopulmonary arrest, use of higher IV/intraosseous bolus doses (ie, 1 mg every 3 to 5 minutes) should be employed (AAAAI [Lieberman 2015]; AHA [Neumar 2010]; Campbell 2014). **Note:** Rapid IV bolus administration is associated with cardiac arrhythmias, only use in this way if absolutely necessary (Campbell 2014).

Continuous infusion (off-label dose): May initiate with an infusion at 1 to 15 mcg/minute (with fluid resuscitation) (AAAAI [Lieberman 2015]; AHA [Vanden Hoek 2010]; Brown 2004; Campbell 2014).

Self-administration following severe allergic reactions (eg, insect stings, food): **Note:** The World Health Organization (WHO) and Anaphylaxis Canada recommend the availability of one dose for every 10 to 20 minutes of travel time to a medical emergency facility. If anaphylactic symptoms persist after first dose, may repeat dose in 5 to 15 minutes (AHA [Vanden Hoek 2010]; WAO [Simons 2011]); more than 2 sequential doses should only be administered under direct medical supervision.

Adrenaclick: IM, SubQ: 0.3 mg; if anaphylactic symptoms persist, dose may be repeated using an additional Adrenaclick injector.

Allerject [Canadian product]: IM: 0.3 mg; if anaphylactic symptoms persist, dose may be repeated using an additional Allerject injector.

Auvi-Q: IM, SubQ: Weight ≥30 kg: 0.3 mg; if anaphylactic symptoms persist, dose may be repeated.

EpiPen: IM, SubQ: 0.3 mg; if anaphylactic symptoms persist, dose may be repeated using an additional EpiPen.

Symjepi: IM, SubQ: Weight ≥30 kg: 0.3 mg; if anaphylactic symptoms persist, dose may be repeated.

Twinject [Canadian product]: IM, SubQ: 0.3 mg; if anaphylactic symptoms persist, dose may be repeated in 5 to 15 minutes using the same device after partial disassembly.

Inotropic support (off-label use): IV: Continuous infusion: Initial: 0.01 to 0.5 mcg/kg/minute; titrate to desired response (AHA [Peberdy 2010]; Gillies 2005; Hollenberg 2004). **Note:** Inotropic actions predominate at lower doses with vasoconstrictive actions at higher doses (Hollenberg 2004; Manaker 2019).

Mydriasis during intraocular surgery, induction and maintenance (product specific): Intraocular: Must dilute 1 mL of a 1 mg/mL single-use solution to a concentration of 1 to 10 **mcg**/mL prior to intraocular use: May use as an irrigation solution as needed during the procedure or may administer intracamerally (ie, directly into the anterior chamber of the eye) with a bolus dose of 0.1 mL of a 2.5 to 10 **mcg**/mL dilution. **Note:** Not all formulations of epinephrine injection are suitable for intraocular use; consult the prescribing information (ISMP 2017).

Shock/Hypotension: Note: Vasopressors should be used if patient is hypotensive during or after fluid resuscitation to maintain goal mean arterial pressure (MAP) ≥65 mm Hg (AHA [Peberdy 2010]; Levy 2018). Titrate to lowest effective dose. Institutional protocols may vary with weight-based or nonweight dose regimens.

Cardiogenic shock or post-cardiac arrest (off-label dose): IV: Continuous infusion: 0.01 to 0.5 mcg/kg/minute (AHA [Peberdy 2010]; AHA [van Diepen 2017]). **Note:** Consider for initial use in patients with bradycardia or evidence of end organ hypoperfusion and shock (AHA [Peberdy 2010]; AHA [van Diepen 2017]).

Septic shock (adjunctive agent) (off-label dose): IV: Continuous infusion: 0.01 to 0.7 mcg/kg/minute (Annane 2007; Dellinger 2017). **Note:** Consider for use in addition to norepinephrine (preferred vasopressor for septic shock) to achieve target MAP (SCCM [Rhodes 2017]).

Manufacturer's labeling: Dosing in the prescribing information may not reflect current clinical practice. IV: Continuous infusion: Initial: 0.05 to 2 mcg/kg/minute (3.5 to 140 mcg/minute in a 70 kg patient); titrate to desired MAP. May adjust dose every 10 to 15 minutes by 0.05 to 0.2 mcg/kg/minute to achieve desired BP goal.

Renal Impairment: Adult There are no dosage adjustments provided in the manufacturer's labeling.

Hepatic Impairment: Adult There are no dosage adjustments provided in the manufacturer's labeling.

Pediatric Note: As of May 1, 2016, ratio expressions of epinephrine concentrations are prohibited on drug labels. Ampules, vials, and syringes of epinephrine with ratio expressions may, however, remain in inventory until replaced by products with revised labeling. Therefore, the ratio expression of 1:1,000 is equivalent to 1 mg/mL and 1:10,000 is equivalent to 0.1 mg/mL (ISMP 2015). Adrenaclick has been discontinued in the US for more than 1 year.

Asystole or pulseless arrest (PALS [Duff 2018]; PALS [Kleinman 2010]): Infants, Children, and Adolescents:

IV, Intraosseous: 0.01 mg/kg (0.1 mL/kg of **0.1 mg/mL** solution) (maximum single dose: 1 mg); every 3 to 5 minutes until return of spontaneous circulation.

Endotracheal: 0.1 mg/kg (0.1 mL/kg of **1 mg/mL** solution) (maximum single dose: 2.5 mg) every 3 to 5 minutes until return of spontaneous circulation or IV/intraosseous access established. **Note:** Recent clinical studies suggest that lower epinephrine concentrations delivered by endotracheal administration may produce transient beta 2-adrenergic effects which may be detrimental (eg, hypotension, lower coronary artery perfusion pressure). IV or intraosseous are the preferred methods of administration.

Bradycardia (PALS [Kleinman 2010]): Infants, Children, and Adolescents:

IV, Intraosseous: 0.01 mg/kg (0.1 mL/kg of **0.1 mg/mL** solution) (maximum dose: 1 mg or 10 mL); may repeat every 3 to 5 minutes as needed.

Endotracheal: 0.1 mg/kg (0.1 mL/kg of **1 mg/mL** solution) (maximum single dose: 2.5 mg); doses as high as 0.2 mg/kg may be effective; may repeat every 3 to 5 minutes as needed until IV/intraosseous access established. **Note:** Recent clinical studies suggest that lower epinephrine concentrations delivered by endotracheal administration may produce transient beta 2-adrenergic effects which may be detrimental (eg, hypotension, lower coronary artery perfusion pressure). IV or intraosseous are the preferred methods of administration.

Cardiac output increase or maintenance/post-resuscitation stabilization: Infants, Children, and Adolescents: Continuous IV or intraosseous infusion: 0.05 to 1 **mcg**/kg/**minute**; doses <0.3 **mcg**/kg/**minute** generally produce beta-adrenergic effects and higher doses (>0.3 **mcg**/kg/**minute**) generally produce alpha-adrenergic vasoconstriction; titrate dosage to desired effect (ACCM [Davis 2017]; PALS [Kleinman 2010]).

Hypersensitivity reaction/Anaphylaxis: Infants, Children, and Adolescents: **Note:** The preferred route of administration is IM administration in the anterolateral aspect of the middle third of the thigh; SubQ administration results in slower absorption and is less reliable (Campbell 2014; AAAAI [Lieberman 2015]; WAO [Simons 2011]).

General dosing or health care settings: IM, SubQ: 0.01 mg/kg (0.01 mL/kg/dose of **1 mg/mL** solution) not to exceed: Prepubertal child: 0.3 mg/dose; adolescent: 0.5 mg/dose; administered every 5 to 15 minutes (Hegenbarth 2008; AAP [Sicherer 2017]; WAO [Simons 2011]).

Self/caregiver-administration following severe allergic reactions (eg, insect stings, food): Autoinjector dose: **Note:** If anaphylactic symptoms persist after first dose, may repeat dose in 5 to 15 minutes (WAO [Simons 2011]).

Manufacturer's labeling (eg, Adrenaclick, Auvi-Q, EpiPen Jr, EpiPen): IM, SubQ:

7.5 to <15 kg: 0.1 mg; if anaphylactic symptoms persist, dose may be repeated based on severity and response to initial dose; more than 2 sequential doses should only be administered under direct medical supervision.

15 to <30 kg: 0.15 mg; if anaphylactic symptoms persist, dose may be repeated based on severity and response to initial dose; more than 2 sequential doses should only be administered under direct medical supervision.

≥30 kg: 0.3 mg; if anaphylactic symptoms persist, dose may be repeated based on severity and response to initial dose; more than 2 sequential doses should only be administered under direct medical supervision.

Alternate dosing: AAP Recommendations (Sicherer 2017): Limited data available:

7.5 to <25 kg: 0.15 mg.

≥25 kg: 0.3 mg.

Refractory cases (unresponsive to IM doses): Continuous IV infusion: Prepared 1 **mcg**/mL solution: Initial: 0.1 **mcg**/kg/**minute**; titrate dose to response. Usual range: 0.1 to 1 **mcg**/kg/**minute**; maximum dose: 10 **mcg/minute** (Campbell 2014; Cheng 2011; AAAAI [Lieberman 2015]). **Note:** Suggested concentration of initial solution is more dilute than those typically utilized in other clinical conditions; evaluate infusion concentration with continued therapy and patient fluid status.

Hypotension/shock, fluid-resistant: Infants, Children, and Adolescents:

Continuous IV infusion: 0.1 to 1 **mcg**/kg/**minute**; rates >0.3 **mcg**/kg/**minute** associated with vasopressor activity; doses up to 5 mcg/kg/minute may rarely be necessary; for fluid-resistant shock, may be combined with inotropic support (ACCM [Davis 2017]; Hegenbarth 2008).

SubQ: 0.01 mg/kg (0.01 mL/kg of **1 mg/mL** solution) (maximum single dose: 0.5 mg) every 20 minutes for 3 doses (Hegenbarth 2008).

Mydriasis during intraocular surgery, induction, and maintenance (product specific): Note: Not all formulations of epinephrine injection are suitable for intraocular use; consult product labeling prior to use. Infants, Children, and Adolescents: Intraocular: Must dilute 1 mL of a 1 mg/mL preservative-/sulfite-free, single-use solution to a concentration of 1 **mcg**/mL to 10 **mcg**/mL prior to intraocular use: May use as an irrigation solution as needed during the procedure or may administer intracamerally (ie, directly into the anterior chamber of the eye) with a bolus dose of 0.1 mL of a 2.5 **mcg**/mL to 10 **mcg**/mL dilution.

Renal Impairment: Pediatric There are no dosage adjustments provided in the manufacturer's labeling.

Hepatic Impairment: Pediatric There are no dosage adjustments provided in the manufacturer's labeling.

Mechanism of Action Stimulates alpha-, beta$_1$-, and beta$_2$-adrenergic receptors resulting in relaxation of smooth muscle of the bronchial tree, cardiac stimulation (increasing myocardial oxygen consumption), and dilation of skeletal muscle vasculature; small doses can cause vasodilation via beta$_2$-vascular receptors; large doses may produce constriction of skeletal and vascular smooth muscle

Contraindications

There are no absolute contraindications to the use of injectable epinephrine (including Adrenaclick, Auvi-Q, EpiPen, EpiPen Jr, Symjepi, Allerject [Canadian product], and Twinject [Canadian product]) in a life-threatening situation. Some products include the following contraindications: Hypersensitivity to sympathomimetic amines; general anesthesia with halogenated hydrocarbons (eg, halothane) or cyclopropane; narrow angle glaucoma; nonanaphylactic shock; in combination with local anesthesia of certain areas such as fingers, toes, and ears; use in situations where vasopressors may be contraindicated (eg, thyrotoxicosis, diabetes, in obstetrics when maternal blood pressure is in excess of 130/80 mm Hg and in hypertension and other cardiovascular disorders).

Injectable solution (Adrenalin, Epinephrine injection, USP): There are no contraindications listed in the manufacturer's labeling.

Warnings/Precautions Use with caution in elderly patients, patients with diabetes mellitus, cardiovascular diseases (eg, coronary artery disease, arrhythmias, cerebrovascular disease, heart disease hypertension), thyroid disease, pheochromocytoma, or Parkinson disease. May precipitate or aggravate angina pectoris or induce cardiac arrhythmias; use with caution especially in patients with cardiac disease or those receiving drugs that sensitize the myocardium. Due to peripheral constriction and cardiac stimulation, pulmonary edema may occur. Due to renal blood vessel constriction, decreased urine output may occur. In hypovolemic patients, correct blood volume depletion before administering any vasopressor. Some products contain sulfites as preservatives; the presence of sulfites in some products should not deter administration during a serious allergic or other emergency situation even if the patient is sulfite-sensitive. Potentially significant drug-drug interactions may exist, requiring dose or frequency adjustment, additional monitoring, and/or selection of alternative therapy.

Hypersensitivity reactions: Do not inject into the buttock; may not effectively treat anaphylaxis and has been associated with Clostridial infections (gas gangrene). Serious skin and soft tissue infections, including necrotizing fasciitis and myonecrosis caused by Clostridia (gas gangrene), have been reported rarely at the injection site. Cleansing skin with alcohol may reduce bacteria at the injection site, but alcohol cleansing does not kill *Clostridium* spores. Preferred injection site is anterolateral aspect of the thigh. Do not administer repeated injections at the same site (tissue necrosis may occur). Monitor for signs/symptoms of injection-site infection. Lacerations, bent needles, and embedded needles have been reported in young children who are uncooperative during injection for hypersensitivity reaction. To minimize risk, hold the child's leg firmly in place and limit movement prior to and during injection. Although the manufacturers of auto-injectors recommend varying lengths of time for holding the device in the thigh (range: 2 to 10 seconds), longer times have occasionally resulted in injury. For all devices, the needle should remain in the thigh for the least amount of time as possible (~3 seconds) (Brown 2016).

IV administration: Rapid IV administration may cause death from cerebrovascular hemorrhage or cardiac arrhythmias. However, rapid IV administration during pulseless arrest is necessary. Vesicant; ensure proper needle or catheter placement prior to and during infusion; avoid extravasation. Accidental injection into digits, hands, or feet may result in local reactions, including injection-site pallor, coldness, and hypoesthesia or injury, resulting in bruising, bleeding, discoloration, erythema, or skeletal injury; patient should seek immediate medical attention if this occurs.

Intraocular administration: Not all formulations of epinephrine injection are suitable for intraocular use; consult the prescribing information prior to selecting a product. Appropriate products should have an indication for induction and maintenance of mydriasis during intraocular surgery, and should not contain any sulfites or preservatives (ISMP 2017). Prior to intraocular use of an appropriate product, must dilute single-use 1 mg/mL (1 mL) solution to a concentration of 1 mcg/mL to 10 mcg/mL. Corneal endothelial damage has occurred when products containing sodium bisulfite have been used undiluted; therefore, dilution is advised prior to any intraocular use. In addition, products containing chlorobutanol must also not be used intraocularly (may be harmful to corneal endothelium).

Drug Interactions

Metabolism/Transport Effects **Substrate** of COMT

Avoid Concomitant Use

Avoid concomitant use of EPINEPHrine (Systemic) with any of the following: Blonanserin; Bromperidol; Ergot Derivatives; Lurasidone

Increased Effect/Toxicity

EPINEPHrine (Systemic) may increase the levels/effects of: Doxofylline; Lurasidone; Solriamfetol; Sympathomimetics

The levels/effects of EPINEPHrine (Systemic) may be increased by: AtoMOXetine; Beta-Blockers (Nonselective); Bretylium; Cannabinoid-Containing Products; Chloroprocaine; Cocaine (Topical); COMT Inhibitors; Ergot Derivatives; Guanethidine; Hyaluronidase; Inhalational Anesthetics; Linezolid; Monoamine Oxidase Inhibitors; Ozanimod; Procarbazine; Serotonin/Norepinephrine Reuptake Inhibitors; Tedizolid; Tricyclic Antidepressants

Decreased Effect

EPINEPHrine (Systemic) may decrease the levels/effects of: Antidiabetic Agents; Benzylpenicilloyl Polylysine

The levels/effects of EPINEPHrine (Systemic) may be decreased by: Alpha1-Blockers; Benperidol; Beta-Blockers (Beta1 Selective); Beta-Blockers (with Alpha-Blocking Properties); Blonanserin; Bromperidol; CloZAPine; Haloperidol; Promethazine; Spironolactone

Pharmacodynamics/Kinetics

Onset of Action Bronchodilation: SubQ: ~5 to 10 minutes

Half-life Elimination IV: <5 minutes

Pregnancy Considerations

Epinephrine crosses the placenta (Sandler 1964).

Epinephrine is recommended for the treatment of anaphylaxis in pregnant women. Specific dosing is not available; use with caution and monitor hemodynamic response (Hepner 2013). Medications used for the treatment of cardiac arrest in pregnancy are the same as in the non-pregnant woman. Doses and indications should follow current Advanced Cardiovascular Life Support guidelines. Appropriate medications should not be withheld due to concerns of fetal teratogenicity (Jeejeebhoy [AHA] 2015).

Breastfeeding Considerations It is not known if epinephrine is present in breast milk.

Epinephrine is generally considered compatible in breastfeeding and is recommended for the treatment of anaphylaxis in breastfeeding women (WHO 2002).

Product Availability Adrenaclick: Adrenaclick has been discontinued in the US for more than 1 year.

Dosage Forms: US

Kit, Injection:

Adyphren Amp: 1 mg/mL
Adyphren Amp II: 1 mg/mL
Adyphren II: 1 mg/mL
Epinephrine Professional: 1 mg/mL
EpinephrineSnap-EMS: 1 mg/mL
Epinephrinesnap-v: 1 mg/mL
EPIsnap: 1 mg/mL

Kit, Injection [preservative free]:

Adyphren: 1 mg/mL
Epinephrinesnap-v: 1 mg/mL

Solution, Injection:

Adrenalin: 30 mg/30 mL (30 mL)
Generic: 30 mg/30 mL (30 mL)

Solution, Injection [preservative free]:

Adrenalin: 1 mg/mL (1 mL)
Generic: 1 mg/mL (1 mL)

Solution Auto-injector, Injection:

Auvi-Q: 0.1 mg/0.1 mL (2 ea); 0.15 mg/0.15 mL (2 ea); 0.3 mg/0.3 mL (2 ea)
EpiPen 2-Pak: 0.3 mg/0.3 mL (2 ea)
EpiPen Jr 2-Pak: 0.15 mg/0.3 mL (2 ea)
Generic: 0.15 mg/0.3 mL (1 ea, 2 ea); 0.15 mg/0.15 mL (2 ea); 0.3 mg/0.3 mL (1 ea, 2 ea)

Solution Auto-injector, Injection [preservative free]:

Generic: 0.15 mg/0.3 mL (1 ea, 2 ea)

Solution Prefilled Syringe, Injection [preservative free]:

Symjepi: 0.15 mg/0.3 mL (1 ea); 0.3 mg/0.3 mL (2 ea)
Generic: 1 mg/10 mL (10 mL)

Dosage Forms: Canada

Solution, Injection:

Adrenalin Chloride: 1 mg/mL (1 mL, 30 mL)
Generic: 1 mg/10 mL (10 mL); 1 mg/mL (1 mL, 10 mL)

Solution Auto-injector, Intramuscular:

Allerject: 0.15 mg/0.15 mL (1 ea); 0.3 mg/0.3 mL (1 ea)
Anapen: 0.3 mg/0.3 mL (0.3 mL)
Anapen Junior: 0.15 mg/0.3 mL (0.3 mL)
EpiPen: 0.3 mg/0.3 mL (2 mL)
EpiPen Jr: 0.15 mg/0.3 mL (2 mL)
Generic: 0.15 mg/0.3 mL (0.3 mL); 0.3 mg/0.3 mL (0.3 mL)

EPINEPHrine (Oral Inhalation) (ep i NEF rin)

Brand Names: US Asthmanefrin Refill [OTC]; S2 (Racepinephrine) [OTC]

Brand Names: Canada S2 (Racepinephrine) [DSC]

Generic Availability (US) No

Pharmacologic Category Alpha/Beta Agonist

Dental Use Emergency drug for treatment of anaphylactic reactions; used as vasoconstrictor to prolong local anesthesia

Use **Bronchospasm, relief of mild asthma symptoms:** Temporary relief of mild symptoms of intermittent asthma (ie, shortness of breath, tightness of chest, wheezing). **Note:** Primary utility is in acute anaphylaxis with edema; not recommended for routine management and treatment of asthma (GINA 2020; NAEPP 2007).

Local Anesthetic/Vasoconstrictor Precautions No information available to require special precautions

Effects on Dental Treatment Key adverse event(s) related to dental treatment: Xerostomia (normal salivary flow resumes upon discontinuation) and dry throat.

Effects on Bleeding No information available to require special precautions

Adverse Reactions There are no adverse reactions listed in the manufacturer's labeling.

Dosing

Adult & Geriatric

Bronchospasm, relief of mild asthma symptoms: **Note:** Primary utility is in acute anaphylaxis with edema; not recommended for routine management and treatment of asthma (GINA 2020; NAEPP 2007).

Metered-dose inhaler: Oral inhalation: 1 inhalation (0.125 mg) once; if symptoms not relieved after 1 minute, may repeat; wait ≥4 hours between additional doses (maximum dose: 8 inhalations/24 hours).

Nebulization solution: Hand-bulb nebulizer: 1 to 3 inhalations of 2.25% (1 vial); may repeat dose after ≥3 hours as needed (maximum dose: 12 inhalations/24 hours).

Renal Impairment: Adult There are no dosage adjustment provided in the manufacturer's labeling.

Hepatic Impairment: Adult There are no dosage adjustment provided in the manufacturer's labeling.

Pediatric

Bronchospasm, relief of mild asthma symptoms: **Note:** Not recommended for routine management and treatment of asthma (GINA 2018; NAEPP 2007).

Nebulization solution: Children ≥4 years and Adolescents: Handheld bulb nebulizer: Add 0.5 mL (1 vial) of 2.25% solution to nebulizer; 1 to 3 inhalations; may repeat dose after at least 3 hours if needed. Maximum daily dose: 12 inhalations/24 hours.

Metered-dose inhaler: Children ≥12 years and Adolescents: Oral inhalation: 1 inhalation once; if symptoms not relieved after 1 minute, may repeat 1 inhalation; wait ≥4 hours between additional doses; maximum daily dose: 8 inhalations/24 hours

Croup (laryngotracheobronchitis), airway edema; moderate to severe: Limited data available: Infants, Children, and Adolescents: **Note:** Typically relief of symptoms occurs within 10 to 30 minutes and lasts 2 to 3 hours; patients should be observed for rapid symptom recurrence and possible repeat treatment.

Racemic epinephrine (2.25% solution): Nebulization: 0.05 to 0.1 mL/kg (maximum dose: 0.5 mL) diluted in 2 to 3 mL NS, may repeat dose every 20 minutes; others have reported use of 0.5 mL as a fixed dose for all patients; use lower end of dosing range for younger infants (Hegenbarth 2008; Kliegman 2016; Rosekrans 1998; Rotta 2003; Wright 2002)

L-epinephrine (using parenteral 1 mg/mL solution): Nebulization: 0.5 mL/kg of **1:1,000** solution (maximum dose: 5 mL) diluted in NS, may repeat dose every 20 minutes; **Note:** Racemic epinephrine 10 mg = 5 mg L-epinephrine (Hegenbarth 2008)

Renal Impairment: Pediatric There are no dosage adjustments provided in the manufacturer's labeling.

Hepatic Impairment: Pediatric There are no dosage adjustments provided in the manufacturer's labeling.

Mechanism of Action Stimulates alpha-, $beta_1$-, and $beta_2$-adrenergic receptors resulting in relaxation of smooth muscle of the bronchial tree, cardiac stimulation (increasing myocardial oxygen consumption), and dilation of skeletal muscle vasculature; small doses can cause vasodilation via $beta_2$-vascular receptors; large doses may produce constriction of skeletal and vascular smooth muscle

Contraindications

OTC labeling: When used for self-medication, do not use with or within 2 weeks of discontinuing an MAOI or in patients without a diagnosis of asthma.

Documentation of allergenic cross-reactivity for sympathomimetics is limited. However, because of similarities in chemical structure and/or pharmacologic actions, the possibility of cross-sensitivity cannot be ruled out with certainty.

Warnings/Precautions Use with caution in patients with diabetes mellitus, heart disease and/or hypertension, increased intraocular pressure or glaucoma, thyroid disease, cerebrovascular disease, prostatic hyperplasia and/or urinary retention, psychiatric or emotional conditions, or in patients with seizure disorders. Do not use if product is brown in color or cloudy.

Self-medication (OTC use): When used for self-medication (OTC), notify health care provider if symptoms are not relieved in 20 minutes or become worse; if >8 inhalations of Primatene Mist, >12 inhalations of Asthmanefrin, S2 are needed in 24 hours; if >9 inhalations in 24 hours for ≥3 days a week of Asthmanefrin, S2 are needed, or if >2 asthma attacks have occurred within a week. Discontinue use and notify health care provider if your asthma is getting worse, or if difficulty sleeping, rapid heartbeat, tremors, nervousness, or seizure occur. The product should not be used more frequently or at higher doses than recommended.

Drug Interactions

Metabolism/Transport Effects **Substrate** of COMT

Avoid Concomitant Use

Avoid concomitant use of EPINEPHrine (Oral Inhalation) with any of the following: Ergot Derivatives; Monoamine Oxidase Inhibitors

Increased Effect/Toxicity

EPINEPHrine (Oral Inhalation) may increase the levels/effects of: Doxofylline; Solriamfetol; Sympathomimetics

The levels/effects of EPINEPHrine (Oral Inhalation) may be increased by: AtoMOXetine; Beta-Blockers (Nonselective); Cannabinoid-Containing Products; Chloroprocaine; Cocaine (Topical); COMT Inhibitors; Ergot Derivatives; Guanethidine; Inhalational Anesthetics; Monoamine Oxidase Inhibitors; Ozanimod; Procarbazine; Serotonin/Norepinephrine Reuptake Inhibitors; Tedizolid; Tricyclic Antidepressants

Decreased Effect

The levels/effects of EPINEPHrine (Oral Inhalation) may be decreased by: Alpha1-Blockers; Beta-Blockers (Beta1 Selective); Beta-Blockers (with Alpha-Blocking Properties); Promethazine; Spironolactone

Food Interactions Avoid food or beverages that contain caffeine.

Dietary Considerations Avoid food or beverages that contain caffeine.

Pharmacodynamics/Kinetics

Onset of Action Bronchodilation: Inhalation: ~1 minute

Pregnancy Considerations Epinephrine crosses the placenta following injection (Sandler 1964).

Uncontrolled asthma is associated with adverse events on pregnancy (increased risk of perinatal mortality, preeclampsia, preterm birth, low birth weight infants, cesarean delivery, and the development of gestational diabetes). Poorly controlled asthma or asthma exacerbations may have a greater fetal/maternal risk than what is associated with appropriately used asthma medications. Maternal treatment improves pregnancy outcomes by reducing the risk of some adverse events (eg, preterm birth, gestational diabetes). Maternal asthma symptoms should be monitored monthly during pregnancy. However, epinephrine inhalation is not recommended for routine management and treatment of asthma (ERS/TSANZ [Middleton 2020]; GINA 2020).

Breastfeeding Considerations Breastfeeding females with asthma should be encouraged to breastfeed (GINA 2020). Use of epinephrine is generally considered acceptable in breastfeeding females (WHO 2002).

Dosage Forms: US

Nebulization Solution, Inhalation:

Asthmanefrin Refill [OTC]: 2.25% (1 ea)

Nebulization Solution, Inhalation [preservative free]:

S2 (Racepinephrine) [OTC]: 2.25% (1 ea)

◆ **Epinephrine and Lidocaine** *see* Lidocaine and Epinephrine *on page 908*

◆ **Epinephrine and Lignocaine** *see* Lidocaine and Epinephrine *on page 908*

◆ **Epinephrine Bitartrate** *see* EPINEPHrine (Systemic) *on page 569*

◆ **Epinephrine Bitartrate and Articaine Hydrochloride** *see* Articaine and Epinephrine *on page 170*

◆ **Epinephrine Bitartrate and Bupivacaine Hydrochloride** *see* Bupivacaine and Epinephrine *on page 257*

◆ **Epinephrine HCl/D5W** *see* EPINEPHrine (Systemic) *on page 569*

◆ **Epinephrine Hydrochloride** *see* EPINEPHrine (Systemic) *on page 569*

◆ **Epinephrine Professional** *see* EPINEPHrine (Systemic) *on page 569*

Epinephrine (Racemic) and Aluminum Potassium Sulfate

(ep i NEF rin, ra SEE mik and a LOO mi num poe TASS ee um SUL fate)

Related Information

EPINEPHrine (Systemic) *on page 569*

Brand Names: US GingiBRAID+

Generic Availability (US) No

Pharmacologic Category Adrenergic Agonist Agent; Alpha/Beta Agonist; Astringent; Vasoconstrictor

Dental Use Gingival retraction

Use Dental aid: Aids in temporary gingival retraction and hemostasis procedures

Local Anesthetic/Vasoconstrictor Precautions No information available to require special precautions

Effects on Dental Treatment Key adverse event(s) related to dental treatment: Tissue retraction around base of the tooth (therapeutic effect).

Effects on Bleeding No information available to require special precautions

Adverse Reactions No data reported.

Dental Usual Dosage Gingival retraction: Adults: Pass the impregnated cord around the neck of the tooth and place into gingival sulcus; normal tissue moisture, water, or gingival retraction solutions activate impregnated cord. Limit use to one quadrant of the mouth at a time; recommended use is for 3-8 minutes in the mouth.

Dosing

Adult & Geriatric Dental aid: Pass the impregnated cord around the neck of the tooth and place into gingival sulcus; leave cord in sulcus for up to 5 minutes; normal tissue moisture, water, or gingival retraction solutions activate impregnated cord. Limit use to one quadrant of the mouth at a time.

Mechanism of Action Epinephrine stimulates alpha$_1$ adrenergic receptors to cause vasoconstriction in blood vessels in gingiva; aluminum potassium sulfate, precipitates tissue and blood proteins

Contraindications Hypersensitivity to epinephrine, sulfites, aluminum-containing products, or any component of the formulation; cardiovascular disease, hypertension, hyperthyroidism, diabetes, or congestive glaucoma; concurrent antidepressant use; do not apply to areas of heavy or deep bleeding or overexposed bone

Warnings/Precautions Caution should be exercised whenever using gingival retraction cords with epinephrine since it delivers vasoconstrictor doses of racemic epinephrine to patients; the general medical history should be thoroughly evaluated before using in any patient

Drug Interactions

Metabolism/Transport Effects None known.

Avoid Concomitant Use There are no known interactions where it is recommended to avoid concomitant use.

Increased Effect/Toxicity

The levels/effects of Epinephrine (Racemic) and Aluminum Potassium Sulfate may be increased by: Beta-Blockers (Nonselective); Monoamine Oxidase Inhibitors

Decreased Effect

The levels/effects of Epinephrine (Racemic) and Aluminum Potassium Sulfate may be decreased by: Beta-Blockers (Beta1 Selective); Beta-Blockers (with Alpha-Blocking Properties); Promethazine

Dosage Forms: US

Retraction cord, for gingival sulcus placement:

GingiBRAID+:

0e fine: Epinephrine 0.10 – 0.30 mg and aluminum potassium sulfate 0.05 – 0.25 mg per inch

1e small: Epinephrine 0.20 – 0.60 mg and aluminum potassium sulfate 0.15 – 0.35 mg per inch

2e medium: Epinephrine 0.40 – 0.80 mg and aluminum potassium sulfate 0.20 – 0.50 mg per inch

3e large: Epinephrine 0.60 – 1.20 mg and aluminum potassium sulfate 0.30 – 0.80 mg per inch

◆ **EpinephrineSnap-EMS** *see* EPINEPHrine (Systemic) *on page 569*

◆ **Epinephrinesnap-v** *see* EPINEPHrine (Systemic) *on page 569*

◆ **EpiPen 2-Pak** *see* EPINEPHrine (Systemic) *on page 569*

◆ **EpiPen Jr 2-Pak** *see* EPINEPHrine (Systemic) *on page 569*

◆ **Epipodophyllotoxin** *see* Etoposide *on page 626*

◆ **Epipodophyllotoxin** *see* Etoposide Phosphate *on page 626*

EpiRUBicin (ep i ROO bi sin)

Brand Names: US Ellence

Brand Names: Canada Pharmorubicin PFS; PMS-EpiRUBicin

Pharmacologic Category Antineoplastic Agent, Anthracycline; Antineoplastic Agent, Topoisomerase II Inhibitor

Use Breast cancer, adjuvant treatment: Adjuvant therapy component for primary breast cancer in patients with evidence of axillary node tumor involvement

Local Anesthetic/Vasoconstrictor Precautions No information available to require special precautions

Effects on Dental Treatment Key adverse event(s) related to dental treatment: Mucositis

Effects on Bleeding Causes severe myelosuppression, including severe thrombocytopenia (grades 3/4: <5%) and anemia. In patients who are under active treatment with this agent, medical consult is suggested.

Adverse Reactions Frequency not always defined. Percentages reported as part of combination chemotherapy regimens.

Cardiovascular: Decreased left ventricular ejection fraction (asymptomatic; delayed: 1% to 2%), cardiac failure (≤2%), atrioventricular block, bradycardia, bundle branch block, cardiac arrhythmia, cardiomyopathy, ECG abnormality, myocarditis, non-specific T wave on ECG, sinus tachycardia, ST segment changes on ECG, tachyarrhythmia, thromboembolism, ventricular premature contractions, ventricular tachycardia

Central nervous system: Lethargy (1% to 46%)

Dermatologic: Alopecia (70% to 96%), skin rash (1% to 9%), skin changes (1% to 5%)

Endocrine & metabolic: Amenorrhea (69% to 72%), hot flash (5% to 39%)

Gastrointestinal: Nausea and vomiting (83% to 92%; grades 3/4: 22% to 25%), mucositis (9% to 59%; grades 3/4: ≤9%), diarrhea (7% to 25%), anorexia (2% to 3%), abdominal pain, esophagitis, neutropenic enterocolitis, stomatitis, toxic megacolon

Genitourinary: Menopause (premature or early)

Hematologic & oncologic: Neutropenia (54% to 80%; grades 3/4: 11% to 67%; nadir: 10 to 14 days; recovery: by day 21), leukopenia (50% to 80%; grades 3/4: 2% to 59%), anemia (13% to 72%; grades 3/4: ≤6%), thrombocytopenia (5% to 49%; grades 3/4: ≤5%), febrile neutropenia (grades 3/4: ≤6%), acute lymphocytic leukemia, acute myelocytic leukemia, myelodysplastic syndrome

Hepatic: Ascites, hepatomegaly, increased serum transaminases

Hypersensitivity: Hypersensitivity reaction

Infection: Infection (15% to 22%; grades 3/4: ≤2%)

Local: Injection site reaction (3% to 20%; grades 3/4: <1%)

Ophthalmic: Conjunctivitis (1% to 15%)

Respiratory: Dyspnea, pulmonary edema

Miscellaneous: Fever (1% to 5%)

<1%, postmarketing, case reports: Anaphylaxis, arterial embolism, burning sensation of gastrointestinal tract, chills, dehydration, erythema, flushing, gastrointestinal erosion, gastrointestinal hemorrhage, gastrointestinal pain, gastrointestinal ulcer, hyperuricemia, nail hyperpigmentation, oral mucosa hyperpigmentation, phlebitis, pneumonia, pulmonary embolism, radiation recall phenomenon, red urine discoloration, sepsis, shock, skin hyperpigmentation, skin photosensitivity, thrombophlebitis, urticaria

Mechanism of Action Epirubicin is an anthracycline antineoplastic agent; known to inhibit DNA and RNA synthesis by steric obstruction after intercalating between DNA base pairs; active throughout entire cell cycle. Intercalation triggers DNA cleavage by topoisomerase II, resulting in cytocidal activity. Also inhibits DNA helicase, and generates cytotoxic free radicals.

Pharmacodynamics/Kinetics

Half-life Elimination Triphasic; Mean terminal: 33 hours

Reproductive Considerations

Women of reproductive potential should be advised to use effective contraception and avoid becoming pregnant during treatment. Men with female partners of reproductive potential should use effective contraception during and after treatment. Epirubicin may cause irreversible amenorrhea in premenopausal women.

Pregnancy Considerations

Adverse events were observed in animal reproduction studies. Pregnant women should avoid handling epirubicin.

Limited information is available from a retrospective study of women who received epirubicin (in combination with cyclophosphamide or weekly as a single-agent) during the second or third (prior to week 35) trimester for the treatment of pregnancy-associated breast cancer (Ring 2005) and from a study of women who received epirubicin (weekly as a single-agent) at gestational weeks 16 through 30 for the treatment of pregnancy-associated breast cancer (Peccatori 2009). Some pharmacokinetic properties of epirubicin may be altered in pregnant women (van Hasselt 2014). The European Society for Medical Oncology (ESMO) has published guidelines for diagnosis, treatment, and follow-up of cancer during pregnancy (Peccatori 2013); the guidelines recommend referral to a facility with expertise in cancer during pregnancy and encourage a multidisciplinary team (obstetrician, neonatologist, oncology team). If chemotherapy is indicated, it should not be administered in the first trimester, but may begin in the second trimester. There should be a 3-week time period between the last chemotherapy dose and anticipated delivery, and chemotherapy should not be administered beyond week 33 of gestation.

A pregnancy registry is available for all cancers diagnosed during pregnancy at Cooper Health (877-635-4499).

- ◆ **Epirubicin HCl** *see* EpiRUBicin *on page* *576*
- ◆ **Epirubicin Hydrochloride** *see* EpiRUBicin *on page* *576*
- ◆ **Episil** *see* Mucosal Coating Agent *on page* *1066*
- ◆ **EPIsnap** *see* EPINEPHrine (Systemic) *on page* *569*
- ◆ **Epitol** *see* CarBAMazepine *on page* *288*
- ◆ **Epivir** *see* LamiVUDine *on page* *872*
- ◆ **Epivir HBV** *see* LamiVUDine *on page* *872*

Eplerenone (e PLER en one)

Related Information

Cardiovascular Diseases *on page* *1654*

Brand Names: US Inspra

Brand Names: Canada Inspra; MINT-Eplerenone

Pharmacologic Category Antihypertensive; Diuretic, Potassium-Sparing; Mineralocorticoid (Aldosterone) Receptor Antagonists

Use

Hypertension: Management of hypertension. **Note: Not** recommended for the initial treatment of hypertension (ACC/AHA [Whelton 2018]).

Post myocardial infarction, complicated by heart failure with reduced ejection fraction: To improve survival of stable patients with symptomatic heart failure (left ventricular ejection fraction ≤40%) following acute myocardial infarction.

Local Anesthetic/Vasoconstrictor Precautions No information available to require special precautions

Effects on Dental Treatment No significant effects or complications reported

Effects on Bleeding No information available to require special precautions

Adverse Reactions

>10%: Endocrine & metabolic: Hyperkalemia ([cardiac failure, post-myocardial infarction: >5.5 mEq/L: 16%; ≥6 mEq/L: 6%], [hypertension, >5.5 mEq/L: at dose of 400 mg: 9%; dose ≤200 mg: ≤1%]), hypertriglyceridemia (1% to 15%; dose-related)

1% to 10%:

Central nervous system: Dizziness (3%), fatigue (2%)

Endocrine & metabolic: Hyponatremia (2%; dose-related), albuminuria (1%), gynecomastia (≤1%), hypercholesterolemia (≤1%)

Gastrointestinal: Diarrhea (2%), abdominal pain (1%)

Genitourinary: Abnormal vaginal hemorrhage (≤2%), mastalgia (males: ≤1%)

Renal: Increased serum creatinine (cardiac failure, post-myocardial infarction: 6%)

Respiratory: Cough (2%), flu-like symptoms (2%)

<1%, postmarketing, and/or case reports: Angioedema, increased blood urea nitrogen, increased liver enzymes, increased uric acid, skin rash

Mechanism of Action Aldosterone, a mineralocorticoid, increases blood pressure primarily by inducing sodium and water retention. Overexpression of aldosterone is thought to contribute to myocardial fibrosis (especially following myocardial infarction) and vascular fibrosis. Mineralocorticoid receptors are located in the kidney, heart, blood vessels, and brain. Eplerenone selectively blocks mineralocorticoid receptors reducing blood pressure in a dose-dependent manner and appears to prevent myocardial and vascular fibrosis.

Pharmacodynamics/Kinetics

Half-life Elimination ~3 to 6 hours

Time to Peak Plasma: ~1.5 to 2 hours; may take up to 4 weeks for full antihypertensive effect

Pregnancy Considerations

Information related to eplerenone use in pregnancy is limited to case reports (Cabassi 2012; Gunganah 2015; Hutter 2006; Morton 2011; Morton 2017).

Chronic maternal hypertension is associated with adverse events in the fetus/infant. The risk of birth defects, low birth weight, premature delivery, stillbirth, and neonatal death may be increased with chronic hypertension in pregnancy. Actual risks may be related to duration and severity of maternal hypertension. The use of mineralocorticoid receptor antagonists for the treatment of hypertension in pregnancy is generally not recommended (ACOG 203 2019).

The treatment of edema associated with chronic heart failure during pregnancy is similar to that of nonpregnant patients. However, the use of mineralocorticoid receptor antagonists is not recommended. Patients diagnosed after delivery can be treated according to heart failure guidelines (ESC [Bauersachs 2016]; ESC [Regitz-Zagrosek 2018]).

Information related to the use of mineralocorticoid receptor antagonists for the treatment of primary hyperaldosteronism in pregnancy is limited. Use of eplerenone may be considered in some cases (Riester 2015).

◆ **EPO** *see* Epoetin Alfa *on page* 577

Epoetin Alfa (e POE e tin AL fa)

Brand Names: US Epogen; Procrit; Retacrit

Brand Names: Canada Eprex

Pharmacologic Category Colony Stimulating Factor; Erythropoiesis-Stimulating Agent (ESA); Hematopoietic Agent

Use

Anemia due to chemotherapy in patients with cancer: Treatment of anemia in patients with nonmyeloid malignancies in which anemia is due to the effect of concomitant myelosuppressive chemotherapy, and upon initiation, there is a minimum of 2 additional months of planned chemotherapy.

Anemia due to chronic kidney disease: Treatment of anemia due to chronic kidney disease, including patients on dialysis and not on dialysis, to decrease the need for RBC transfusion.

Anemia due to zidovudine in HIV-infected patients: Treatment of anemia due to zidovudine administered at ≤4.2 g/week in HIV-infected patients with endogenous serum erythropoietin levels of ≤500 milliunits/mL.

Reduction of allogeneic RBC transfusion in patients undergoing elective, noncardiac, nonvascular surgery: To reduce the need for allogeneic RBC transfusions among patients with perioperative hemoglobin >10 to ≤13 g/dL who are at high risk of perioperative blood loss from elective, noncardiac, nonvascular surgery. Epoetin alfa is not indicated for patients who are willing to donate autologous blood preoperatively.

Limitations of use: Epoetin alfa has not been shown to improve quality of life, fatigue, or patient well-being. Epoetin alfa is **not** indicated for use under the following conditions:

- Cancer patients receiving hormonal therapy, therapeutic biologic products, or radiation therapy unless also receiving concurrent myelosuppressive chemotherapy
- Cancer patients receiving myelosuppressive chemotherapy when the expected outcome is curative
- Cancer patients receiving myelosuppressive chemotherapy when anemia can be managed by transfusion
- Surgery patients who are willing to donate autologous blood
- Surgery patients undergoing cardiac or vascular surgery
- As a substitute for RBC transfusion in patients requiring immediate correction of anemia

Note: Retacrit (epoetin alfa-epbx) is approved as a biosimilar to Epogen (epoetin alfa) and Procrit (epoetin alfa).

Local Anesthetic/Vasoconstrictor Precautions No information available to require special precautions

Effects on Dental Treatment No significant effects or complications reported

Effects on Bleeding Although ESAs have been associated with thromboembolic events, there is no information available to require special precautions for dental procedures.

Adverse Reactions

>10%:

Cardiovascular: Hypertension (6% to 28%)

Central nervous system: Headache (5% to 18%)

Dermatologic: Pruritus (16% to 21%), skin rash (2% to 19%)

Gastrointestinal: Nausea (35% to 56%), vomiting (19% to 28%)

Local: Injection site pain (9% to 13%)

Neuromuscular & skeletal: Arthralgia (10% to 16%)

Respiratory: Cough (4% to 26%)

Miscellaneous: Fever (10% to 42%)

1% to 10%:

Cardiovascular: Thrombosis of hemodialysis vascular access (8%), thrombosis (≤6%), deep vein thrombosis (5% to 6%), edema (3%)

Central nervous system: Dizziness (10%), chills (4% to 7%), insomnia (6%), depression (5%)

Dermatologic: Urticaria (3%)

Endocrine & metabolic: Weight loss (9%), hyperglycemia (6%), hypokalemia (5%)

Gastrointestinal: Stomatitis (10%), dysphagia (5%)

Hematologic & oncologic: Leukopenia (8%)

Local: Irritation at injection site (7%)

Neuromuscular & skeletal: Myalgia (10%), muscle spasm (7%), ostealgia (7%)

Respiratory: Upper respiratory tract infection (7%)

<1%, postmarketing, and/or case reports: Antibody development (neutralizing), cardiac failure, cerebrovascular accident, erythema, erythema multiforme, exfoliation of skin, hypertensive encephalopathy, myocardial infarction, porphyria, pure red cell aplasia, seizure, severe anemia, skin blister, Stevens-Johnson syndrome, toxic epidermal necrolysis

Mechanism of Action Epoetin alfa induces erythropoiesis by stimulating the division and differentiation of committed erythroid progenitor cells; induces the release of reticulocytes from the bone marrow into the bloodstream, where they mature to erythrocytes. There is a dose response relationship with this effect. This results in an increase in reticulocyte counts followed by a rise in hematocrit and hemoglobin levels.

Pharmacodynamics/Kinetics

Onset of Action Reticulocyte count increase: Within 10 days; Peak effect: Hemoglobin level: 2 to 6 weeks

Half-life Elimination

Neonates: With high doses, nonlinear kinetics have been observed (Wu 2012)

Anemia of prematurity:

Post menstrual age (PMA) <32 week (weight: 800 ± 206 grams): IV: 8.1 ± 2.7 hours; SubQ: 7.1 ± 4.1 hours (Brown 1993)

PMA ≥32 weeks (weight range: 1,330 to 1,740 g): SubQ: Median: 7.9 hours (range: 5.6 to 19.4 hours) (Krishnan 1996)

Neuroprotective/hypoxic ischemia encephalopathy (HIE) (Wu 2012): ≥36 weeks GA; IV:

250 units/kg: 7.6 ± 6.9 hours

500 units/kg: 7.2 ± 1.9 hours

1,000 units/kg: 15 ± 4.5 hours

2,500 units/kg: 18.7 ± 4.7 hours

Infants, Children, and Adolescents: Chronic kidney disease: IV; 4 to 13 hours

Adults: Cancer: SubQ: 16 to 67 hours; Chronic kidney disease: IV: 4 to 13 hours

Time to Peak Serum: Pediatric patients >1 month and Adults: Chronic kidney disease: SubQ: 5 to 24 hours

Pregnancy Considerations

In vitro studies suggest that recombinant erythropoietin does not cross the human placenta (Reisenberger 1997). Polyhydramnios and intrauterine growth retardation have been reported with use in females with chronic kidney disease (CKD) (adverse effects also associated with maternal disease).

Recombinant erythropoietin alfa has been evaluated as adjunctive treatment for severe pregnancy associated iron deficiency anemia (Breymann 2001; Krafft 2009) and has been used in pregnant females with iron-deficiency anemia associated with CKD (Furaz-Czerpak 2012; Josephson 2007).

Multidose formulations containing benzyl alcohol are contraindicated for use in pregnant females; if treatment during pregnancy is needed, single-dose preparations should be used.

◆ **Epoetin Alfa-epbx** *see* Epoetin Alfa *on page* 577

◆ **Epoetin Alfa, Recombinant** *see* Epoetin Alfa *on page* 577

◆ **Epogen** *see* Epoetin Alfa *on page* 577

Epoprostenol (e poe PROST en ole)

Brand Names: US Flolan; Veletri

Brand Names: Canada Caripul; Flolan

Pharmacologic Category Prostacyclin; Prostaglandin; Vasodilator

Use Pulmonary arterial hypertension: Treatment of pulmonary arterial hypertension (PAH) (WHO Group I) in patients with NYHA Class III or IV symptoms to improve exercise capacity.

Local Anesthetic/Vasoconstrictor Precautions No information available to require special precautions

Effects on Dental Treatment No significant effects or complications reported. Epoprostenol is an inhibitor of platelet aggregation and may enhance the risk of bleeding with other antiplatelet agents (such as aspirin and/or NSAIDs).

Effects on Bleeding Epoprostenol is a potent inhibitor of platelet aggregation and increases the risk of hemorrhagic complications. A medical consult is suggested.

Adverse Reactions

>10%:

Cardiovascular: Flushing (23% to 58%), tachycardia (1% to 43%), hypotension (13% to 27%), chest pain (11%)

Central nervous system: Headache (46% to 83%), dizziness (8% to 83%), chills (≤25%), anxiety (≤21%), nervousness (≤21%), hyperesthesia (≤12%), hypoesthesia (≤12%), paresthesia (≤12%), agitation (11%)

Dermatologic: Dermal ulcer (39%), eczema (≤10% to ≤25%), skin rash (≤10% to ≤25%), urticaria (≤10% to ≤25%)

Gastrointestinal: Nausea and vomiting (32% to 67%), anorexia (25% to 66%), diarrhea (37% to 50%)

Infection: Sepsis (≤25%)

Neuromuscular & skeletal: Musculoskeletal pain (3% to 84%), arthralgia (≤84%), neck pain (≤84%), jaw pain (54% to 75%), myalgia (44%), hyperkinesia (≤21%), tremor (≤21%)

Respiratory: Flu-like symptoms (≤25%)

Miscellaneous: Fever (≤25%)

1% to 10%:

Cardiovascular: Bradycardia (5%)

Dermatologic: Diaphoresis (1%)

Gastrointestinal: Abdominal pain (5%), dyspepsia (1%)

Neuromuscular & skeletal: Back pain (2%)

Respiratory: Dyspnea (2%)

<1%, postmarketing, and/or case reports: Anemia, cardiac failure, fatigue, hemorrhage, hepatic failure, hypersplenism, hyperthyroidism, increased pulmonary artery pressure, pallor, pancytopenia, pulmonary edema, pulmonary embolism, splenomegaly, thrombocytopenia

Mechanism of Action Epoprostenol is also known as prostacyclin and PGI_2. It is a strong vasodilator of all vascular beds. In addition, it is a potent endogenous inhibitor of platelet aggregation. The reduction in platelet aggregation results from epoprostenol's activation of intracellular adenylate cyclase and the resultant increase in cyclic adenosine monophosphate concentrations within the platelets. Additionally, it is capable of decreasing thrombogenesis and platelet clumping in the lungs by inhibiting platelet aggregation.

Pharmacodynamics/Kinetics

Half-life Elimination ~6 minutes

Pregnancy Considerations

Information related to the use of epoprostenol in pregnancy is limited (Geohas 2003; Kawabe 2018; Martinez 2013; Smith 2012; Timofeev 2013); however, the manufacturer notes adverse maternal or fetal outcomes have not been associated with its use based on the available data.

Untreated pulmonary arterial hypertension (PAH) is associated with adverse pregnancy outcomes, including heart failure, stroke, preterm delivery, and maternal and fetal death.

Prescribing and Access Restrictions Orders for epoprostenol are distributed by two sources in the United States. Information on orders or reimbursement assistance may be obtained from either Accredo Health, Inc (1-866-344-4874) or CVS Caremark (1-877-242-2738).

- **Epoprostenol Sodium** *see* Epoprostenol *on page 578*
- **Epoprostenol Sodium (Arginine)** *see* Epoprostenol *on page 578*
- **Epothilone B Lactam** *see* Ixabepilone *on page 852*

Eprosartan (ep roe SAR tan)

Related Information

Cardiovascular Diseases *on page 1654*

Brand Names: Canada Teveten

Pharmacologic Category Angiotensin II Receptor Blocker; Antihypertensive

Use Hypertension: Management of hypertension

Local Anesthetic/Vasoconstrictor Precautions

No information available to require special precautions

Effects on Dental Treatment Key adverse event(s) related to dental treatment: Patients may experience orthostatic hypotension as they stand up after treatment; especially if lying in dental chair for extended periods of time. Use caution with sudden changes in position during and after dental treatment.

Effects on Bleeding No information available to require special precautions

Adverse Reactions

1% to 10%:

Cardiovascular: Chest pain (≥1%)

Central nervous system: Fatigue (2%), dizziness (≥1%), headache (≥1%), depression (1%)

Endocrine & metabolic: Dependent edema (≥1%), hypertriglyceridemia (1%)

Gastrointestinal: Abdominal pain (2%), diarrhea (≥1%), dyspepsia (≥1%)

Genitourinary: Urinary tract infection (1%)

Infection: Viral infection (2%)

Neuromuscular & skeletal: Arthralgia (2%), myalgia (≥1%)

Renal: Increased blood urea nitrogen (1%)

Respiratory: Upper respiratory tract infection (8%), pharyngitis (4%), rhinitis (4%), cough (ARBs: 3%; Matchar 2008), bronchitis (≥1%), sinusitis (≥1%)

Miscellaneous: Accidental injury (2%)

<1%, postmarketing, and/or case reports: Albuminuria, alcohol intolerance, anemia, angina pectoris, anorexia, anxiety, arthritis, asthenia, asthma, ataxia, atrial fibrillation, back pain, bradycardia, conjunctivitis, constipation, cystitis, decreased hemoglobin (>20% decrease), diabetes mellitus, diaphoresis, drowsiness, ECG abnormality, eczema, epistaxis, esophagitis, exacerbation of arthritis, extrasystoles, facial edema, fever, flatulence, flu-like symptoms, flushing sensation, furunculosis, gastritis, gastroenteritis, gingivitis, glycosuria, gout, hematuria, herpes simplex infection, hypercholesterolemia, hyperglycemia, hyperkalemia, hypokalemia, hyponatremia, hypotension, increased creatine phosphokinase, increased serum alanine aminotransferase, increased serum aspartate aminotransferase, insomnia, lower limb cramp, maculopapular rash, malaise, migraine, nausea, nephrolithiasis, nervousness, neuritis, nonthrombocytopenic purpura, orthostatic hypotension, osteoarthritis, otitis externa, otitis media, pain, palpitations, paresthesia, periodontitis, peripheral edema, peripheral ischemia, polyuria, pruritus, rigors, skeletal pain, skin rash, substernal pain, tachycardia, tendonitis, thrombocytopenia, tinnitus, toothache, tremor, urinary frequency, urinary incontinence, vertigo, visual disturbance, vomiting, xerophthalmia, xerostomia

Mechanism of Action Angiotensin II is formed from angiotensin I in a reaction catalyzed by angiotensin-converting enzyme (ACE, kininase II). Angiotensin II is the principal pressor agent of the renin-angiotensin system, with effects that include vasoconstriction, stimulation of synthesis and release of aldosterone, cardiac stimulation, and renal reabsorption of sodium. Eprosartan blocks the vasoconstrictor and aldosterone-secreting effects of angiotensin II by selectively blocking the binding of angiotensin II to the AT1 receptor in many tissues, such as vascular smooth muscle and the adrenal gland. Its action is therefore independent of the pathways for angiotensin II synthesis. Blockade of the renin-angiotensin system with ACE inhibitors, which inhibit the biosynthesis of angiotensin II from angiotensin I, is widely used in the treatment of hypertension. ACE inhibitors also inhibit the degradation of bradykinin, a reaction also catalyzed by ACE. Because eprosartan does not inhibit ACE (kininase II), it does not affect the response to bradykinin. Whether this difference has clinical relevance is not yet known. Eprosartan does not bind to or block other hormone receptors or ion channels known to be important in cardiovascular regulation.

Pharmacodynamics/Kinetics

Half-life Elimination Terminal: 5 to 9 hours (Bottorff, 1999)

Time to Peak Serum: Fasting: 1 to 2 hours

Reproductive Considerations
The use of angiotensin II receptor blockers should generally be avoided in women planning a pregnancy (ACOG 203 2019).

Pregnancy Risk Factor D

Pregnancy Considerations

[US Boxed Warning]: Drugs that act on the renin-angiotensin system can cause injury and death to the developing fetus. When pregnancy is detected, discontinue as soon as possible. The use of drugs which act on the renin-angiotensin system are associated with oligohydramnios. Oligohydramnios, due to decreased fetal renal function, may lead to fetal lung hypoplasia and skeletal malformations. Oligohydramnios may not appear until after irreversible fetal injury has occurred. Use in pregnancy is also associated with anuria, hypotension, renal failure, skull hypoplasia, and death in the fetus/neonate. The exposed fetus should be monitored for fetal growth, amniotic fluid volume, and organ formation. Infants exposed in utero should be monitored for hyperkalemia, hypotension, and oliguria (exchange transfusions or dialysis may be needed). These adverse events are generally associated with maternal use in the second and third trimesters.

Chronic maternal hypertension itself is also associated with adverse events in the fetus/infant. The risk of birth defects, low birth weight, premature delivery, stillbirth, and neonatal death may be increased with chronic hypertension in pregnancy. Actual risks may be related to duration and severity of maternal hypertension (ACOG 203 2019).

The use of angiotensin II receptor blockers is generally not recommended to treat chronic hypertension in pregnant women (ACOG 203 2019).

◆ **Epsilon Aminocaproic Acid** *see* Aminocaproic Acid *on page 116*

◆ **EPT** *see* Teniposide *on page 1417*

Eptifibatide (ep TIF i ba tide)

Related Information
Cardiovascular Diseases *on page 1654*

Brand Names: US Integrilin

Brand Names: Canada Integrilin

Pharmacologic Category Antiplatelet Agent, Glycoprotein IIb/IIIa Inhibitor

Use

Non-ST elevation acute coronary syndromes: Treatment of patients with unstable angina or non-ST-segment elevation myocardial infarction (UA/NSTEMI), including patients who are to be managed medically and those undergoing percutaneous coronary intervention (PCI).

Percutaneous coronary intervention with or without coronary stenting: Treatment of patients undergoing PCI, including those undergoing coronary stenting.

Local Anesthetic/Vasoconstrictor Precautions
No information available to require special precautions

Effects on Dental Treatment Key adverse event(s) related to dental treatment: Bleeding; patients weighing <70 kg may have an increased risk of major bleeding. See Effects on Bleeding.

Effects on Bleeding Bleeding is the most common complication. Eptifibatide inhibits platelet aggregation. Vascular and other trauma should be avoided. It is unlikely that dental work would be performed in patients undergoing treatment for acute coronary syndrome.

Adverse Reactions Frequency not always defined. Bleeding is the major drug-related adverse effect. Access site is often primary source of bleeding complications. Incidence of bleeding is also related to heparin intensity. Patients weighing <70 kg may have an increased risk of major bleeding.

>10%: Hematologic: & oncologic: Hemorrhage (major: 1% to 11%; minor: 3% to 14%; transfusion required: 2% to 13%)

1% to 10%:

Cardiovascular: Hypotension (≤7%)

Hematologic & oncologic: Thrombocytopenia (1% to 3%; includes acute profound thrombocytopenia, immune-mediated thrombocytopenia)

Local: Injection site reaction

<1%, postmarketing and/or case reports: Anaphylaxis, cerebrovascular accident, gastrointestinal hemorrhage, intracranial hemorrhage, pulmonary hemorrhage

Mechanism of Action Eptifibatide is a cyclic heptapeptide which blocks the platelet glycoprotein IIb/IIIa receptor, the binding site for fibrinogen, von Willebrand factor, and other ligands. Inhibition of binding at this final common receptor reversibly blocks platelet aggregation and prevents thrombosis.

Pharmacodynamics/Kinetics

Onset of Action Immediate after initial bolus (>80% inhibition of ADP-induced aggregation achieved 5 minutes after bolus dose); maximal effect achieved within 1 hour (Gilchrist, 2001; Tardiff, 2001)

Duration of Action Platelet function restored ~4 to 8 hours following discontinuation (Tardiff, 2001)

Half-life Elimination ~2.5 hours

Pregnancy Risk Factor B

Pregnancy Considerations Adverse events have not been observed in animal reproduction studies.

Eptinezumab (EP ti NEZ ue mab)

Brand Names: US Vyepti

Pharmacologic Category Antimigraine Agent; Calcitonin Gene-Related Peptide (CGRP) Receptor Antagonist; Monoclonal Antibody, CGRP Antagonist

Use Migraine prophylaxis: Preventive treatment of migraine in adults.

Local Anesthetic/Vasoconstrictor Precautions
No information available to require special precautions.

Effects on Dental Treatment Key adverse event(s) related to dental treatment: Occurrence of nasopharyngitis.

Effects on Bleeding No information available to require special precautions.

Adverse Reactions

>10%: Immunologic: Antibody development (18% to 21%; neutralizing: 35% to 41%)

1% to 10%:

Gastrointestinal: Nausea (2% [Lipton 2020])

Hypersensitivity: Hypersensitivity reaction (1% to 2% [placebo: 0%])

Nervous system: Fatigue (2% [Lipton 2020])

Respiratory: Nasopharyngitis (8%)

Frequency not defined: Hypersensitivity: Angioedema

Mechanism of Action Eptinezumab is a humanized monoclonal antibody that binds to calcitonin gene-related peptide ligand and blocks its binding to the receptor.

Pharmacodynamics/Kinetics

Onset of Action ~1 day (Ashina 2020).

Half-life Elimination ~27 days.

Time to Peak Immediately following infusion (Baker 2020).

Pregnancy Considerations

Eptinezumab is a humanized monoclonal antibody (IgG_1). Placental transfer of human IgG is dependent upon the IgG subclass, maternal serum concentrations, birth weight, and gestational age, generally increasing as pregnancy progresses. The lowest exposure would be expected during the period of organogenesis (Palmeira 2012; Pentsuk 2009).

Agents other than eptinezumab are currently recommended for the prophylaxis of migraine in pregnant women (Burch 2019; Negro 2017).

- **Eptinezumab-jjmr** *see* Eptinezumab *on page 580*
- **EPY [DSC]** *see* EPINEPHrine (Systemic) *on page 569*
- **EPY II [DSC]** *see* EPINEPHrine (Systemic) *on page 569*
- **EPZ-6438** *see* Tazemetostat *on page 1408*
- **Epzicom** *see* Abacavir and Lamivudine *on page 51*
- **Equetro** *see* CarBAMazepine *on page 288*
- **ER-086526** *see* EriBULin *on page 584*

Eravacycline (ER a va SYE kleen)

Brand Names: US Xerava

Pharmacologic Category Antibiotic, Tetracycline Derivative

Use

Intra-abdominal infections, complicated: Treatment of complicated intra-abdominal infections caused by susceptible microorganisms: *Escherichia coli, Klebsiella pneumoniae, Citrobacter freundii, Enterobacter cloacae, Klebsiella oxytoca, Enterococcus faecalis, Enterococcus faecium, Staphylococcus aureus, Streptococcus anginosus* group, *Clostridium perfringens, Bacteroides* species, and *Parabacteroides distasonis* in patients ≥18 years.

Limitations of use: Not indicated for the treatment of complicated urinary tract infections.

Local Anesthetic/Vasoconstrictor Precautions No information available to require special precautions

Effects on Dental Treatment Key adverse event(s) related to dental treatment: Although ervacycline is a member of the tetracycline family, there is no dental indication for its use. Therefore, the concerns of tetracyclines in dental patients relative to enamel incorporation in pediatrics are not applicable for ervacycline. Use may result in fungal or bacterial superinfection.

Effects on Bleeding No information available to require special precautions

Adverse Reactions

1% to 10%:

Cardiovascular: Hypotension (1%)

Gastrointestinal: Nausea (7%), vomiting (4%), diarrhea (2%)

Local: Infusion site reaction (8%)

Miscellaneous: Wound dehiscence (1%)

<1%, postmarketing, and/or case reports: Acute pancreatitis, anaphylaxis, anxiety, chest pain, decreased creatinine clearance, decreased white blood cell count, depression, dizziness, dysgeusia, dyspnea, hyperhidrosis, hypersensitivity reaction, hypocalcemia, increased amylase, increased gamma-glutamyl transferase, increased serum alanine aminotransferase, increased serum lipase, insomnia, neutropenia, palpitations, pancreatic necrosis, pleural effusion, prolonged partial thromboplastin time, skin rash

Mechanism of Action Eravacycline is a fluorocycline antibiotic within the tetracycline class that binds to the 30S ribosomal subunit and prevents the incorporation of amino acid residues into elongating peptide chains, thereby, inhibiting bacterial protein synthesis.

Pharmacodynamics/Kinetics

Half-life Elimination 20 hours

Pregnancy Considerations Tetracyclines cross the placenta.

As a class, tetracyclines accumulate in developing teeth and long tubular bones (Mylonas 2011). Exposure during the second and third trimesters of pregnancy may cause reversible inhibition of bone growth. Permanent discoloration of teeth (yellow, gray, brown) can occur following in utero exposure and is more likely to occur following long-term or repeated exposure.

- **Eraxis** *see* Anidulafungin *on page 152*
- **Erbitux** *see* Cetuximab *on page 329*
- **Erelzi** *see* Etanercept *on page 607*

Erenumab (e REN ue mab)

Brand Names: US Aimovig; Aimovig (140 MG Dose) [DSC]

Brand Names: Canada Aimovig

Pharmacologic Category Antimigraine Agent; Calcitonin Gene-Related Peptide (CGRP) Receptor Antagonist; Monoclonal Antibody, CGRP Antagonist

Use Migraine prophylaxis: Preventive treatment of migraine in adults

Local Anesthetic/Vasoconstrictor Precautions No information available to require special precautions

Effects on Dental Treatment No significant effects or complications reported

Effects on Bleeding No information available to require special precautions

Adverse Reactions

1% to 10%:

Gastrointestinal: Constipation (3%; with serious complications)

Immunologic: Antibody development (3% to 6%; neutralizing: <1%)

Local: Injection site reaction (5% to 6%)

Neuromuscular & skeletal: Muscle cramps (≤2%), muscle spasm (≤2%)

Frequency not defined:

Dermatologic: Injection site pruritus

Local: Erythema at injection site, pain at injection site

Postmarketing:

Cardiovascular: Exacerbation of hypertension, hypertension

Dermatologic: Skin rash

Hypersensitivity: Anaphylaxis, angioedema, hypersensitivity reaction

Mechanism of Action Erenumab is a human monoclonal antibody that antagonizes calcitonin gene-related peptide (CGRP) receptor function.

Pharmacodynamics/Kinetics

Half-life Elimination 28 days

Time to Peak ~6 days

Pregnancy Considerations Adverse events were not observed in animal reproduction studies.

- **Erenumab-aooe** *see* Erenumab *on page 581*
- **Ergocal** *see* Ergocalciferol *on page 582*

Ergocalciferol (er goe kal SIF e role)

Brand Names: US Calcidol [OTC]; Calciferol [OTC]; Drisdol; Ergocal

Brand Names: Canada D-Forte; Osto-D2 [DSC]; SANDOZ D-Forte

Pharmacologic Category Vitamin D Analog

Use

Dietary supplement: For use as a vitamin D supplement.

Hypoparathyroidism: Treatment of hypoparathyroidism. **Note:** Since parathyroid hormone (PTH) is required for the conversion of vitamin D (ergocalciferol or cholecalciferol) to the active metabolite of vitamin D (1,25-dihydroxyvitamin D), alternative vitamin D preparations not dependent on this conversion (eg, alfacalcidol, calcitriol) are recommended for routine use (Endocrine Society [Brandi 2016]).

Local Anesthetic/Vasoconstrictor Precautions No information available to require special precautions

Effects on Dental Treatment Key adverse event(s) related to dental treatment: Metallic taste and xerostomia (normal salivary flow resumes upon discontinuation).

Effects on Bleeding No information available to require special precautions

Adverse Reactions Frequency not defined: Endocrine & metabolic: Hypervitaminosis D

Mechanism of Action Ergocalciferol (vitamin D_2) is a provitamin. The active metabolite, 1,25-dihydroxyvitamin D (calcitriol), stimulates calcium and phosphate absorption from the small intestine, promotes secretion of calcium from bone to blood; promotes renal tubule phosphate resorption.

Pharmacodynamics/Kinetics

Onset of Action 10 to 24 hours; Maximum effect: ~1 month following daily doses

Half-life Elimination Circulating: 25(OH)D: 2 to 3 weeks; 1,25-dihydroxyvitamin D ~4 hours

Pregnancy Considerations

The ergocalciferol (vitamin D_2) metabolite, 25(OH)D, crosses the placenta; maternal serum concentrations correlate with fetal concentrations at birth (Misra 2008; Wagner 2008).

Vitamin D deficiency in a pregnant woman may lead to a vitamin D deficiency in the neonate (Misra 2008; Wagner 2008). Serum 25(OH)D concentrations should be measured in pregnant women considered to be at increased risk of deficiency (ACOG 2011). The amount of vitamin D contained in prenatal vitamins may not be adequate to treat a deficiency during pregnancy; although larger doses may be needed, current guidelines recommend a total of 1000 to 2000 units/day until more safety data is available (ACOG 2011). In women not at risk for deficiency, doses larger than the RDA should be avoided during pregnancy (ACOG 2011).

Maternal vitamin D requirements are the same for breastfeeding and nonbreastfeeding females (IOM 2011). The maternal dose of vitamin D needed to provide the infant with an adequate amount of vitamin D is still under study (Wagner 2008)

Ergoloid Mesylates (ER goe loid MES i lates)

Brand Names: Canada Hydergine

Pharmacologic Category Ergot Derivative

Use

Mental capacity decline: Treatment of signs and symptoms of an idiopathic decline in mental capacity. **Note:** Individuals who do respond come from groups of patients who would be considered clinically to suffer from some ill-defined process related to aging or to have some underlying dementing condition (ie, primary progressive dementia, Alzheimer dementia, senile onset, multi-infarct dementia).

Local Anesthetic/Vasoconstrictor Precautions Although ergoloid mesylates are derivatives of the natural ergot alkaloids, they lack any vasoconstricting effects; there is no information available to require special precautions with vasoconstrictor

Effects on Dental Treatment Key adverse event(s) related to dental treatment: Patients may experience orthostatic hypotension as they stand up after treatment; especially if lying in dental chair for extended periods of time. Use caution with sudden changes in position during and after dental treatment.

Effects on Bleeding No information available to require special precautions

Adverse Reactions Frequency not defined. Adverse effects are minimal.

Cardiovascular: Bradycardia, flushing, orthostatic hypotension

Dermatologic: Skin rash

Gastrointestinal: Gastrointestinal distress (sublingual administration), nausea (sublingual administration; transient)

Local: Local irritation (sublingual administration)

Ophthalmic: Blurred vision

Respiratory: Nasal congestion

Mechanism of Action Ergoloid mesylates do not have the vasoconstrictor effects of the natural ergot alkaloids; exact mechanism in dementia is unknown; originally classed as peripheral and cerebral vasodilator, now considered a "metabolic enhancer"; there is no specific evidence that clearly establishes the mechanism by which ergoloid mesylate preparations produce mental effects, nor is there conclusive evidence that the drug particularly affects cerebral arteriosclerosis or cerebrovascular insufficiency.

Pharmacodynamics/Kinetics

Half-life Elimination Serum: ~2.6 to 5.1 hours

Time to Peak Serum: 1.5 to 3 hours

◆ **Ergomar** *see* Ergotamine *on page 583*

◆ **Ergometrine Maleate** *see* Ergonovine *on page 582*

Ergonovine (er goe NOE veen)

Pharmacologic Category Ergot Derivative; Oxytocic Agent

Use Note: Not approved in the US

Postpartum or postabortion hemorrhage: Prevention and treatment of postpartum and postabortion hemorrhage caused by uterine atony

Local Anesthetic/Vasoconstrictor Precautions Use vasoconstrictor with caution in patients taking ergonovine; this ergot alkaloid derivative causes constriction of peripheral blood vessels

Effects on Dental Treatment No significant effects or complications reported

Effects on Bleeding Rare but significant events related to hemorrhage (cerebral hemorrhage, subarachnoid hemorrhage, and stroke) have occurred following injection of some agents in this class. However, there is no information related to special precautions associated with bleeding related to dental procedures.

Adverse Reactions Frequency not defined.

Cardiovascular: Angina pectoris (transient), bradycardia, hypertension, myocardial infarction, palpitations, shock, thrombophlebitis

Central nervous system: Dizziness, hallucination, headache, vertigo

Dermatologic: Diaphoresis

Endocrine & metabolic: Water intoxication

Gastrointestinal: Abdominal pain, diarrhea, nausea, vomiting

Genitourinary: Hematuria

Hypersensitivity: Hypersensitivity reaction

Respiratory: Dyspnea

Miscellaneous: Ergot alkaloids toxicity

Mechanism of Action Similar smooth muscle actions as seen with ergotamine; however, it affects primarily uterine smooth muscles producing sustained contractions and thereby shortens the third stage of labor. Has slight alpha-adrenergic blocking activity and produces less vasoconstriction than ergotamine.

Pharmacodynamics/Kinetics

Onset of Action IM: 2 to 5 minutes; IV: Immediate

Duration of Action IM: Uterine effect: ≥3 hours; IV: ~45 minute

Pregnancy Considerations Ergonovine is used in the third stage of labor for the prevention or treatment of postpartum hemorrhage and should not be used prior to delivery of the placenta. Prior to administration, the placenta should be delivered and the possibility of twin pregnancy ruled out. Administration causes hyperstimulation of the uterus and may cause uterine tetany, decreased uteroplacental blood flow, uterine rupture, cervical and perineal lacerations, amniotic fluid embolism, and possible trauma to the infant.

Product Availability Not available in the US

◆ **Ergonovine Maleate** *see* Ergonovine *on page 582*

Ergotamine (er GOT a meen)

Related Information

Dentin Hypersensitivity, Acid Erosion, High Caries Index, Management of Alveolar Osteitis, and Xerostomia *on page 1762*

Brand Names: US Ergomar

Pharmacologic Category Antimigraine Agent; Ergot Derivative

Use Vascular headache: Abort or prevent vascular headaches, such as migraine, migraine variants, or so-called "histaminic cephalalgia"

Local Anesthetic/Vasoconstrictor Precautions Use vasoconstrictor with caution in patients taking ergotamine; this ergot alkaloid derivative causes constriction of peripheral blood vessels

Effects on Dental Treatment No significant effects or complications reported

Effects on Bleeding No information available to require special precautions

Adverse Reactions Frequency not defined.

Cardiovascular: Bradycardia, cold extremities, ECG changes, edema, hypertension, ischemia, tachycardia, valvular sclerosis, vasospasm

Central nervous system: Numbness, paresthesia, precordial pain, vertigo

Dermatologic: Gangrene of skin or other tissue, pruritus

Gastrointestinal: Nausea, vomiting

Genitourinary: Retroperitoneal fibrosis

Neuromuscular & skeletal: Myalgia, weakness

Respiratory: Cyanosis, pleuropulmonary fibrosis

Mechanism of Action Has partial agonist and/or antagonist activity against tryptaminergic, dopaminergic and alpha-adrenergic receptors depending upon their site; is a highly active uterine stimulant; it causes constriction of peripheral and cranial blood vessels and produces depression of central vasomotor centers

Pharmacodynamics/Kinetics

Half-life Elimination 2-2.5 hours (Perrin 1985)

Time to Peak Serum: Oral: 2 hours (Perrin 1985)

Pregnancy Risk Factor X

Pregnancy Considerations

Ergotamine crosses the placenta. Use is contraindicated in pregnancy. Ergotamine may cause prolonged constriction of the uterine vessels and/or increased myometrial tone leading to reduced placental blood flow. This has contributed to fetal growth retardation in animals.

Ergotamine and Caffeine

(er GOT a meen & KAF een)

Related Information

Caffeine *on page 277*

Ergotamine *on page 583*

Brand Names: US Cafergot; Migergot

Brand Names: Canada Cafergor

Pharmacologic Category Antimigraine Agent; Central Nervous System Stimulant; Ergot Derivative

Use Vascular headache: Prevention or treatment of vascular headaches, such as migraine, migraine variants, or so-called "histaminic cephalalgia"

Local Anesthetic/Vasoconstrictor Precautions Use vasoconstrictor with caution in patients taking ergotamine; this ergot alkaloid derivative causes constriction of peripheral blood vessels

Effects on Dental Treatment Key adverse event(s) related to dental treatment: Ergotamine and caffeine cause tachycardia, increases in blood pressure, and palpitations. Consider monitoring blood pressure prior to using local anesthetic with a vasoconstrictor. Symptoms associated with bruxism have been observed in some patients.

Effects on Bleeding No information available to require special precautions

Adverse Reactions Frequency not defined.

Cardiovascular: Bradycardia, cold extremities, ECG changes, edema, hypertension, ischemia, tachycardia, valvular sclerosis, vasospasm

Central nervous system: Numbness, paresthesia, precordial pain, vertigo

Dermatologic: Gangrene of skin or other tissue, pruritus

Gastrointestinal: Anal fissure (with overuse of suppository), nausea, rectal ulcer (with overuse of suppository), vomiting

Genitourinary: Retroperitoneal fibrosis

Neuromuscular & skeletal: Myalgia, weakness

Respiratory: Cyanosis, pleuropulmonary fibrosis

Mechanism of Action Has partial agonist and/or antagonist activity against tryptaminergic, dopaminergic and alpha-adrenergic receptors depending upon their site; is a highly active uterine stimulant; it causes constriction of peripheral and cranial blood vessels and produces depression of central vasomotor centers

Pharmacodynamics/Kinetics

Half-life Elimination 2 to 2.5 hours (Perrin, 1985)

Time to Peak Serum: Ergotamine: 2 hours (Perrin, 1985)

Pregnancy Considerations

Ergotamine and caffeine both cross the placenta. Use is contraindicated in pregnant women. Refer to individual monographs for additional information.

- ◆ **Ergotamine Tartrate** *see* Ergotamine *on page* *583*
- ◆ **Ergotamine Tartrate and Caffeine** *see* Ergotamine and Caffeine *on page* *583*
- ◆ **Ergotamine Tartrate/Caffeine** *see* Ergotamine and Caffeine *on page* *583*

EriBULin (er i BUE lin)

Brand Names: US Halaven

Brand Names: Canada Halaven

Pharmacologic Category Antineoplastic Agent, Antimicrotubular

Use

Breast cancer, metastatic: Treatment of metastatic breast cancer in patients who have received at least 2 prior chemotherapy regimens for the treatment of metastatic disease (prior treatment should have included an anthracycline and a taxane in either the adjuvant or metastatic setting)

Liposarcoma, unresectable or metastatic: Treatment of unresectable or metastatic liposarcoma in patients who have received a prior anthracycline-containing regimen

Local Anesthetic/Vasoconstrictor Precautions

No information available to require special precautions

Effects on Dental Treatment Key adverse event(s) related to dental treatment: Xerostomia (normal salivary flow resumes upon discontinuation), stomatitis, mucosal inflammation, or taste alteration.

Effects on Bleeding Anemia is a primary adverse effect. A medical consult is suggested.

Adverse Reactions

>10%:

Cardiovascular: Peripheral edema (≥5% to 12%)

Central nervous system: Fatigue (≤62%), peripheral neuropathy (29% to 35%; grades 3/4: 3% to 8%), headache (18% to 19%)

Dermatologic: Alopecia (35% to 45%)

Endocrine & metabolic: Hypokalemia (≥5% to 30%), hypocalcemia (28%), weight loss (21%), hypophosphatemia (20%)

Gastrointestinal: Nausea (35% to 41%), constipation (25% to 32%), abdominal pain (≥5% to 29%), anorexia (20%), decreased appetite (19%), vomiting (18% to 19%), diarrhea (17% to 18%), stomatitis (≥5% to 14%)

Genitourinary: Urinary tract infection (10% to 11%)

Hematologic & oncologic: Neutropenia (63% to 82%; grade 4: 29% grades 3/4: 12% to 57%; nadir: 13 days; recovery: 8 days), anemia (58% to 70%; grades 3/4: 2% to 4%)

Hepatic: Increased serum ALT (18% to 43%), increased serum AST (36%)

Neuromuscular & skeletal: Weakness (≤62%), arthralgia (≤22%), myalgia (≤22%), back pain (16%), ostealgia (12%), limb pain (11%)

Respiratory: Cough (14% to 18%), dyspnea (16%)

Miscellaneous: Fever (21% to 28%)

1% to 10%:

Cardiovascular: Hypotension (≥5% to <10%)

Central nervous system: Anxiety (≥5% to <10%), depression (≥5% to <10%), dizziness (≥5% to <10%), insomnia (≥5% to <10%), myasthenia (≥5% to <10%)

Dermatologic: Skin rash (≥5% to <10%)

Endocrine & metabolic: Hyperglycemia (≥5% to <10%)

Gastrointestinal: Dysgeusia (≥5% to <10%), dyspepsia (≥5% to <10%), xerostomia (≥5% to <10%), mucosal inflammation (9%)

Hematologic & oncologic: Thrombocytopenia (≥5% to <10%; grades ≥3: 1%), febrile neutropenia (≤5%)

Neuromuscular & skeletal: Muscle spasm (≥5% to <10%), musculoskeletal pain (≥5% to <10%),

Ophthalmic: Increased lacrimation (≥5% to <10%)

Respiratory: Oropharyngeal pain (≥5% to <10%), upper respiratory tract infection (≥5% to <10%)

<1%, postmarketing, and/or case reports: Dehydration, drug-induced hypersensitivity, hepatotoxicity, hypomagnesemia, interstitial pulmonary disease, lymphocytopenia, neutropenic sepsis, pancreatitis, pneumonia, prolonged QT interval on ECG, pruritus, sepsis, Stevens-Johnson syndrome, toxic epidermal necrolysis

Mechanism of Action Eribulin is a non-taxane microtubule inhibitor which is a halichondrin B analog. It inhibits the growth phase of the microtubule by inhibiting formation of mitotic spindles causing mitotic blockage and arresting the cell cycle at the G_2/M phase; suppresses microtubule polymerization yet does not affect depolymerization.

Pharmacodynamics/Kinetics

Half-life Elimination ~40 hours

Reproductive Considerations

Women of reproductive potential should use effective contraception to avoid pregnancy during eribulin treatment and for at least 2 weeks following the last eribulin dose; males with female partners of reproductive potential should use effective contraception during eribulin treatment and for 3.5 months following the last dose.

Pregnancy Considerations

Based on the mechanism of action, and data from animal reproduction studies, in utero exposure to eribulin may cause fetal harm.

- ◆ **Eribulin Mesylate** *see* EriBULin *on page* *584*
- ◆ **Erismodegib** *see* Sonidegib *on page* *1382*
- ◆ **Erivedge** *see* Vismodegib *on page* *1548*
- ◆ **Erleada** *see* Apalutamide *on page* *158*

Erlotinib (er LOE tye nib)

Brand Names: US Tarceva

Brand Names: Canada APO-Erlotinib; NAT-Erlotinib; PMS-Erlotinib; Tarceva; TEVA-Erlotinib

Pharmacologic Category Antineoplastic Agent, Epidermal Growth Factor Receptor (EGFR) Inhibitor; Antineoplastic Agent, Tyrosine Kinase Inhibitor

Use

Non-small cell lung cancer, metastatic: Treatment of metastatic non-small cell lung cancer (NSCLC) in tumors with epidermal growth factor receptor (EGFR) exon 19 deletions or exon 21 (L858R) substitution mutations as detected by an approved test either as first-line, maintenance, or as second or greater line treatment after progression following at least 1 prior chemotherapy regimen.

Limitations of use: Use in combination with platinum-based chemotherapy is not recommended. Safety and efficacy of treatment for metastatic NSCLC with EGFR mutations other than exon 19 deletion or exon 21 (L858R) substitution have not been established.

Pancreatic cancer, locally advanced, unresectable or metastatic: First-line treatment of locally advanced, unresectable, or metastatic pancreatic cancer (in combination with gemcitabine).

Guideline recommendations:

According to American Society of Clinical Oncology (ASCO) guidelines for locally advanced, unresectable pancreatic cancer, if disease progression occurs following induction with an initial systemic combination therapy regimen, treatment according to guidelines for metastatic pancreatic cancer should be offered (in appropriate patients) (ASCO [Balaban 2016]).

The updated ASCO guidelines for metastatic pancreatic cancer recommend gemcitabine monotherapy as first-line therapy (when there is a preference for cancer-directed treatment) in patients with an ECOG performance status of 2 or a comorbidity profile that prohibits more aggressive therapy; erlotinib may be added to gemcitabine in this setting (ASCO [Sohal 2018]).

Local Anesthetic/Vasoconstrictor Precautions

No information available to require special precautions

Effects on Dental Treatment Key adverse event(s) related to dental treatment: Xerostomia (normal salivary flow resumes upon discontinuation), mucositis, abnormal taste, and stomatitis.

Effects on Bleeding In treatment of pancreatic carcinoma, has been noted to cause microangiopathic hemolytic anemia with thrombocytopenia

Adverse Reactions

Adverse reactions reported with monotherapy:

>10%:

Cardiovascular: Chest pain (≤18%)

Central nervous system: Fatigue (9% to 52%)

Dermatologic: Skin rash (49% to 85%; grade 3: 5% to 13%; grade 4: <1%; median onset: 8 days), xeroderma (4% to 21%), pruritus (7% to 16%), paronychia (4% to 16%), alopecia (14% to 15%), acne vulgaris (6% to 12%)

Gastrointestinal: Diarrhea (20% to 62%; grade 3: 2% to 6%; grade 4: <1%; median onset: 12 days), anorexia (9% to 52%), nausea (23% to 33%), decreased appetite (≤28%), vomiting (13% to 23%), mucositis (≤18%), stomatitis (11% to 17%), abdominal pain (3% to 11%), constipation (≤8%)

Genitourinary: Urinary tract infection (≤4%)

Hematologic & oncologic: Anemia (≤11%; grade 4: 1%)

Infection: Increased susceptibility to infection (4% to 24%)

Neuromuscular & skeletal: Weakness (≤53%), back pain (19%), arthralgia (≤13%), musculoskeletal pain (11%)

Ophthalmic: Conjunctivitis (12% to 18%), keratoconjunctivitis sicca (12%)

Respiratory: Cough (33% to 48%), dyspnea (41% to 45%; grades 3/4: 8% to 28%)

Miscellaneous: Fever (≤11%)

1% to 10%:

Cardiovascular: Peripheral edema (≤5%)

Central nervous system: Pain (≤9%), headache (≤7%), anxiety (≤5%), dizziness (≤4%), insomnia (≤4%), neurotoxicity (≤4%), paresthesia (≤4%), voice disorder (≤4%)

Dermatologic: Folliculitis (≤8%), nail disease (≤7%), exfoliative dermatitis (5%), hypertrichosis (5%), skin fissure (5%), acneiform eruption (4% to 5%), erythema (≤5%), dermatitis (4%), erythematous rash (≤4%), palmar-plantar erythrodysesthesia (≤4%), bullous dermatitis

Endocrine & metabolic: Weight loss (4% to 5%)

Gastrointestinal: Dyspepsia (≤5%), xerostomia (≤3%), taste disorder (≤1%)

Hematologic & oncologic: Lymphocytopenia (≤4%; grade 3: 1%), leukopenia (≤3%), thrombocytopenia (≤1%)

Hepatic: Hyperbilirubinemia (7%; grade 3: ≤1%), increased serum ALT (grade 2: 2% to 4%; grade 3: 1% to 3%), increased gamma-glutamyl transferase (≤4%), hepatic failure (≤1%)

Neuromuscular & skeletal: Muscle spasm (≤4%), musculoskeletal chest pain (≤4%), ostealgia (≤4%)

Otic: Tinnitus (≤1%)

Renal: Increased serum creatinine (≤1%), renal failure (≤1%),

Respiratory: Nasopharyngitis (≤7%), epistaxis (≤4%), pulmonary embolism (≤4%), respiratory tract infection (≤4%), pneumonitis (3%), pulmonary fibrosis (3%)

<1%: Interstitial pulmonary disease

Adverse reactions reported with combination (erlotinib plus gemcitabine) therapy:

>10%:

Cardiovascular: Edema (37%), thrombosis (grades 3/4: 11%)

Central nervous system: Fatigue (73% to 79%), depression (19%), dizziness (15%), headache (15%), anxiety (13%)

Dermatologic: Skin rash (70%), alopecia (14%)

Gastrointestinal: Nausea (60%), anorexia (52%), diarrhea (48%), abdominal pain (46%), vomiting (42%), weight loss (39%), stomatitis (22%), dyspepsia (17%), flatulence (13%)

Hepatic: Increased serum ALT (grade 2: 31%, grade 3: 13%, grade 4: <1%), increased serum AST (grade 2: 24%, grade 3: 10%, grade 4 <1%), hyperbilirubinemia (grade 2: 17%, grade 3: 10%, grade 4: <1%)

Infection: Increased susceptibility to infection (39%)

Neuromuscular & skeletal: Ostealgia (25%), myalgia (21%), neuropathy (13%), rigors (12%)

Respiratory: Dyspnea (24%), cough (16%)

Miscellaneous: Fever (36%)

1% to 10%:

Cardiovascular: Cardiac arrhythmia (<5%), syncope (<5%), deep vein thrombosis (4%), cerebrovascular accident (3%; including cerebral hemorrhage), myocardial infarction (2%)

Gastrointestinal: Intestinal obstruction (<5%), pancreatitis (<5%)

Hematologic & oncologic: Hemolytic anemia (<5%), microangiopathic hemolytic anemia with thrombocytopenia (1%)

Renal: Renal insufficiency (<5%), renal failure (1%)

Respiratory: Interstitial pulmonary disease (<3%)

<1%: Bullous dermatitis, exfoliative dermatitis, hepatic failure

Mono- or combination therapy: <1%, postmarketing, and/or case reports: Acute peptic ulcer with hemorrhage, bronchiolitis, corneal perforation, corneal ulcer, decreased lacrimation, episcleritis, gastritis, gastrointestinal hemorrhage, gastrointestinal perforation, hearing loss, hematemesis, hematochezia, hepatorenal syndrome, hepatotoxicity, hirsutism, hyperpigmentation, hypokalemia, increased eyelash thickness, increased growth in number of eyelashes, keratitis, melena, misdirected growth of eyelashes, myopathy (in combination with statin therapy), ocular inflammation, peptic ulcer, rhabdomyolysis (in combination with statin therapy), skin photosensitivity, skin rash (acneiform; sparing prior radiation field), Stevens-Johnson syndrome, toxic epidermal necrolysis, tympanic membrane perforation, uveitis

Mechanism of Action Erlotinib reversibly inhibits overall epidermal growth factor receptor (HER1/EGFR) - tyrosine kinase activity. Intracellular phosphorylation is inhibited which prevents further downstream signaling, resulting in cell death. Erlotinib has higher binding affinity for EGFR exon 19 deletion or exon 21 (L858R) mutations than for the wild type receptor.

Pharmacodynamics/Kinetics

Half-life Elimination 36.2 hours

Time to Peak Plasma: 4 hours

Reproductive Considerations

Females of reproductive potential should use effective contraception during treatment and for at least 1 month after the last erlotinib dose.

Pregnancy Considerations

Erlotinib crosses the placenta (Ji 2015; Jovelet 2015). Information related to the use of erlotinib in pregnancy is limited (Ji 2015; Rivas 2012; Zambelli 2008). Based on the mechanism of action and data from animal reproduction studies, erlotinib may cause fetal harm if administered in pregnancy.

◆ **Erlotinib Hydrochloride** *see* Erlotinib *on page 584*

◆ **E-R-O Ear Drops [OTC] [DSC]** *see* Carbamide Peroxide *on page 289*

◆ **E-R-O Ear Wax Removal System [OTC] [DSC]** *see* Carbamide Peroxide *on page 289*

◆ **Errin** *see* Norethindrone *on page 1117*

◆ **Ertaczo** *see* Sertaconazole *on page 1367*

Ertapenem (er ta PEN em)

Brand Names: US INVanz

Brand Names: Canada INVanz

Pharmacologic Category Antibiotic, Carbapenem

Use

Intra-abdominal infection, complicated: For the treatment of complicated intra-abdominal infections caused by *Clostridium clostridioforme*, *Escherichia coli, Eubacterium lentum*, *Peptostreptococcus* spp, *Bacteroides distasonis*, *Bacteroides fragilis*, *Bacteroides ovatus*, *Bacteroides thetaiotaomicron*, or *Bacteroides uniformis*.

Pelvic infection: For the treatment of acute pelvic infections, including postpartum endomyometritis, septic abortion, and postsurgical gynecologic infections caused by *Streptococcus agalactiae*, *E. coli*, *B. fragilis*, *Porphyromonas asaccharolytica*, *Peptostreptococcus* spp, or *Prevotella bivia*.

Pneumonia, community acquired: For the treatment of community-acquired pneumonia (CAP) caused by *Streptococcus pneumoniae* (penicillin-susceptible isolates only), including cases with concurrent bacteremia; *Haemophilus influenzae* (beta-lactamase-negative isolates only); or *Moraxella catarrhalis*.

Skin and skin structure infection, complicated: For the treatment of complicated skin and skin structure infections, including diabetic foot infections without osteomyelitis caused by *Staphylococcus aureus* (methicillin-susceptible isolates only), *S. agalactiae*, *Streptococcus pyogenes*, *E. coli*, *Klebsiella pneumoniae*, *Proteus mirabilis*, *B. fragilis*, *Peptostreptococcus* spp, *P. asaccharolytica*, or *P. bivia*. Ertapenem has not been studied in diabetic foot infections with concomitant osteomyelitis.

Surgical prophylaxis: For the prophylaxis of surgical site infection in adults following elective colorectal surgery.

Urinary tract infection, complicated: For the treatment of complicated urinary tract infections (UTIs), including pyelonephritis caused by *E. coli*, including cases with concurrent bacteremia or *K. pneumoniae*.

Note: Methicillin-resistant *Staphylococcus aureus*, *Enterococcus* spp, *Acinetobacter*, *Pseudomonas aeruginosa*, and penicillin-resistant strains of *Streptococcus pneumoniae* are **resistant** to ertapenem while most extended-spectrum beta-lactamase (ESBL)-producing bacteria remain sensitive to ertapenem.

Local Anesthetic/Vasoconstrictor Precautions

No information available to require special precautions

Effects on Dental Treatment Key adverse event(s) related to dental treatment: Oral candidiasis

Effects on Bleeding No information available to require special precautions

Adverse Reactions

>10%: Gastrointestinal: Diarrhea (6% to 12%)

1% to 10%:

Cardiovascular: Edema (≤3%), chest pain (<2%), phlebitis (<2%), thrombophlebitis (<2%), hypotension (1% to 2%)

Dermatologic: Diaper rash (infants and children: 5%), skin rash (2% to 3%), pruritus (1% to 2%), genital rash (infants, children, and adolescents: <2%), skin lesion (infants, children, and adolescents: <2%)

Endocrine & metabolic: Decreased serum potassium (<2%), increased serum glucose (<2%), increased serum potassium (<2%)

Gastrointestinal: Vomiting (4% to 10%), nausea (6% to 9%), abdominal pain (4% to 5%), constipation (2% to 4%), decreased appetite (infants, children, and adolescents: <2%)

Genitourinary: Vaginitis (1% to 3%), proteinuria (infants, children, and adolescents: <2%)

Hematologic & oncologic: Thrombocythemia (4% to 7%), decreased neutrophils (6%), decreased hemoglobin (5%), decreased hematocrit (3%), leukocyturia (2% to 3%), decreased platelet count (<2%), decreased white blood cell count (<2%), prolonged partial thromboplastin time (<2%), prolonged prothrombin time (<2%), eosinophilia (1% to 2%)

Hepatic: Increased serum alanine aminotransferase (1% to 9%), increased serum aspartate transaminase (4% to 8%), increased serum alkaline phosphatase (4% to 7%)

Infection: Candidiasis (<2%), herpes simplex infection (infants, children, and adolescents: <2%)

Local: Infused vein complication (7%), infusion-site pain (infants, children, and adolescents: 7%), erythema at injection site (infants, children, and adolescents: 4%)
Nervous system: Headache (4% to 7%), altered mental status (3% to 5%), insomnia (3%), dizziness (2%), hypothermia (infants, children, and adolescents: <2%)
Neuromuscular & skeletal: Arthralgia (infants, children, and adolescents: <2%)
Otic: Otic infection (infants, children, and adolescents: <2%)
Respiratory: Cough (≤4%), dyspnea (1% to 3%), nasopharyngitis (infants, children, and adolescents: <2%), rhinitis (infants, children, and adolescents: <2%), rhinorrhea (infants, children, and adolescents: <2%), upper respiratory tract infection (infants, children, and adolescents: 2%), wheezing (infants, children, and adolescents: <2%)
Miscellaneous: Fever (2% to 5%), swelling (≤3%)

Frequency not defined: Central nervous system: Agitation, confusion, decreased mental acuity, disorientation, drowsiness, stupor

<1%, postmarketing, and/or case reports: Abdominal distention, acid regurgitation, acute generalized exanthematous pustulosis, aggressive behavior, anaphylaxis, anorexia, anuria, anxiety, asthenia, asthma, asystole, ataxia, atrial fibrillation, bladder dysfunction, bradycardia, bronchoconstriction, cardiac arrhythmia, cardiac failure, chills, cholelithiasis, *Clostridioides difficile* associated diarrhea, decreased serum albumin, dehydration, delirium, dental discoloration, depression, dermatitis, desquamation, diaphoresis, drug reaction with eosinophilia and systemic symptoms, duodenitis, dysgeusia, dyskinesia, dyspepsia, dysphagia, epistaxis, erythema of skin, esophagitis, facial edema, fatigue, flank pain, flatulence, flushing, gastritis, gastrointestinal hemorrhage, gout, hallucination, heart murmur, hematoma, hematuria, hemoptysis, hemorrhoids, hiccups, hypertension, hypoesthesia, hypoglycemia (Kennedy 2019), hypoxemia, impaired consciousness, increased blood urea nitrogen, increased serum bilirubin, increased serum creatinine, increased serum sodium, induration at injection site, intestinal obstruction, jaundice, lower extremity pain, malaise, muscle spasm, myoclonus, nervousness, nonimmune anaphylaxis, oliguria, oral candidiasis, oral mucosa ulcer, pain, pain at injection site, pancreatitis, paresthesia, pharyngitis, pleural effusion, pleuritic chest pain, pyloric stenosis, rales, renal insufficiency, respiratory distress, rhonchi, seizure, septicemia, septic shock, sore throat, stomatitis, subdural hematoma, syncope, tachycardia, tissue necrosis, tremor, unsteady gait, urinary retention, urticaria, ventricular tachycardia, vertigo, voice disorder, vulvovaginal candidiasis, vulvovaginal pruritus, vulvovaginitis, weight loss

Mechanism of Action Inhibits bacterial cell wall synthesis by binding to one or more of the penicillin-binding proteins; which in turn inhibits the final transpeptidation step of peptidoglycan synthesis in bacterial cell walls, thus inhibiting cell wall biosynthesis. Bacteria eventually lyse due to ongoing activity of cell wall autolytic enzymes (autolysins and murein hydrolases) while cell wall assembly is arrested.

Pharmacodynamics/Kinetics

Half-life Elimination

Infants ≥3 months and Children: ~2.5 hours
Adolescents and Adults: ~4 hours

Time to Peak IM: ~2.3 hours

Pregnancy Considerations Ertapenem is approved for the treatment of postpartum endomyometritis, septic abortion, and postsurgical infections. Ertapenem may be considered for use as an alternative antibiotic in the treatment of intraamniotic infection (ACOG 712 2017).

◆ **Ertapenem Sodium** *see* Ertapenem *on page 586*

Ertugliflozin (er too gli FLOE zin)

Brand Names: US Steglatro
Brand Names: Canada Steglatro

Pharmacologic Category Antidiabetic Agent, Sodium-Glucose Cotransporter 2 (SGLT2) Inhibitor; Sodium-Glucose Cotransporter 2 (SGLT2) Inhibitor

Use Diabetes mellitus, type 2, treatment: As an adjunct to diet and exercise to improve glycemic control in adults with type 2 diabetes mellitus.

Local Anesthetic/Vasoconstrictor Precautions No information available to require special precautions

Effects on Dental Treatment Key adverse event(s) related to dental treatment: Schedule type 1 and type 2 diabetic patients for dental treatment in the morning in order to minimize chance of stress-induced hypoglycemia.

Effects on Bleeding No information available to require special precautions

Adverse Reactions Incidences may include ertugliflozin used as add on therapy.

>10%: Genitourinary: Genitourinary fungal infection (females: 9% to 12%; males: 4%)

1% to 10%:
Central nervous system: Headache (3% to 4%)
Endocrine & metabolic: Hypovolemia (2% to 4%), hypoglycemia (3%), increased thirst (1% to 3%), weight loss (2%), severe hypoglycemia (1%)
Genitourinary: Increased urine output (2% to 3%), vulvovaginal pruritus (2% to 3%)
Neuromuscular & skeletal: Back pain (3%)
Renal: Renal insufficiency (1% to 3%)
Respiratory: Nasopharyngitis (3%)

Frequency not defined:
Endocrine & metabolic: Increased LDL cholesterol, increased serum phosphate
Genitourinary: Decreased estimated GFR (eGFR)
Renal: Increased serum creatinine

<1%, postmarketing, and/or case reports: Acute renal failure, increased hemoglobin, ketoacidosis, pyelonephritis, urinary tract infection, urinary tract infection with sepsis

Mechanism of Action By inhibiting sodium-glucose cotransporter 2 (SGLT2) in the proximal renal tubules, ertugliflozin reduces reabsorption of filtered glucose from the tubular lumen and lowers the renal threshold for glucose (RT_G). SGLT2 is the main site of filtered glucose reabsorption; reduction of filtered glucose reabsorption and lowering of RT_G result in increased urinary excretion of glucose, thereby reducing plasma glucose concentrations.

Pharmacodynamics/Kinetics

Half-life Elimination 16.6 hours

Time to Peak Plasma: 1 hour (fasting); 2 hours (administered with high-fat, high-calorie meal)

Pregnancy Considerations

Due to adverse effects on renal development observed in animal studies, the manufacturer does not recommend use of ertugliflozin during the second and third trimesters of pregnancy

Poorly controlled diabetes during pregnancy can be associated with an increased risk of adverse maternal and fetal outcomes, including diabetic ketoacidosis, preeclampsia, spontaneous abortion, preterm delivery, delivery complications, major birth defects, stillbirth, and macrosomia. To prevent adverse outcomes, prior to conception and throughout pregnancy, maternal blood glucose and HbA_{1c} should be kept as close to target goals as possible but without causing significant hypoglycemia (ADA 2020; Blumer 2013).

Agents other than ertugliflozin are currently recommended to treat diabetes mellitus in pregnancy (ADA 2020).

Ertugliflozin and Metformin

(er too gli FLOE zin & met FOR min)

Brand Names: US Segluromet

Brand Names: Canada Segluromet

Pharmacologic Category Antidiabetic Agent, Biguanide; Antidiabetic Agent, Sodium-Glucose Cotransporter 2 (SGLT2) Inhibitor; Sodium-Glucose Cotransporter 2 (SGLT2) Inhibitor

Use Diabetes mellitus, type 2, treatment: As an adjunct to diet and exercise to improve glycemic control in adults with type 2 diabetes mellitus who are not adequately controlled on a regimen containing ertugliflozin or metformin or who are already treated with both ertugliflozin and metformin

Local Anesthetic/Vasoconstrictor Precautions No information available to require special precautions

Effects on Dental Treatment Key adverse event(s) related to dental treatment: Schedule type 1 and type 2 diabetic patients for dental treatment in the morning in order to minimize chance of stress-induced hypoglycemia.

Effects on Bleeding No information available to require special precautions

Adverse Reactions See individual agents.

Mechanism of Action

Ertugliflozin: By inhibiting sodium-glucose cotransporter 2 (SGLT2) in the proximal renal tubules, ertugliflozin reduces reabsorption of filtered glucose from the tubular lumen and lowers the renal threshold for glucose (RT_G). SGLT2 is the main site of filtered glucose reabsorption; reduction of filtered glucose reabsorption and lowering of RT_G result in increased urinary excretion of glucose, thereby reducing plasma glucose concentrations.

Metformin: Decreases hepatic glucose production, decreasing intestinal absorption of glucose and improves insulin sensitivity (increases peripheral glucose uptake and utilization).

Pregnancy Considerations

Metformin crosses the placenta (ADA 2020). Refer to individual monographs for additional information.

Ertugliflozin and Sitagliptin

(er too gli FLOE zin & sit a GLIP tin)

Brand Names: US Steglujan

Brand Names: Canada Steglujan

Pharmacologic Category Antidiabetic Agent, Dipeptidyl Peptidase 4 (DPP-4) Inhibitor; Antidiabetic Agent, Sodium-Glucose Cotransporter 2 (SGLT2) Inhibitor; Sodium-Glucose Cotransporter 2 (SGLT2) Inhibitor

Use Diabetes mellitus, type 2, treatment: As an adjunct to diet and exercise to improve glycemic control in adults with type 2 diabetes mellitus when treatment with both ertugliflozin and sitagliptin is appropriate.

Local Anesthetic/Vasoconstrictor Precautions No information available to require special precautions

Effects on Dental Treatment Key adverse event(s) related to dental treatment: Schedule type 1 and type 2 diabetic patients for dental treatment in the morning in order to minimize chance of stress-induced hypoglycemia.

Effects on Bleeding No information available to require special precautions

Adverse Reactions See individual agents.

Mechanism of Action

Ertugliflozin: By inhibiting sodium-glucose cotransporter 2 (SGLT2) in the proximal renal tubules, ertugliflozin reduces reabsorption of filtered glucose from the tubular lumen and lowers the renal threshold for glucose (RTG). SGLT2 is the main site of filtered glucose reabsorption; reduction of filtered glucose reabsorption and lowering of RTG result in increased urinary excretion of glucose, thereby reducing plasma glucose concentrations.

Sitagliptin: Inhibits dipeptidyl peptidase 4 (DPP-4) enzyme resulting in prolonged active incretin levels. Incretin hormones (eg, glucagon-like peptide-1 [GLP-1] and glucose-dependent insulinotropic polypeptide [GIP]) regulate glucose homeostasis by increasing insulin synthesis and release from pancreatic beta cells and decreasing glucagon secretion from pancreatic alpha cells. Decreased glucagon secretion results in decreased hepatic glucose production. Under normal physiologic circumstances, incretin hormones are released by the intestine throughout the day and levels are increased in response to a meal; incretin hormones are rapidly inactivated by the DPP-4 enzyme.

Pregnancy Considerations

Animal reproduction studies have not been conducted with this combination. Refer to individual monographs.

Health care providers are encouraged to report any prenatal exposure to sitagliptin to the pregnancy registry (1-800-986-8999).

- ◆ **Erwinaze** *see* Asparaginase (*Erwinia*) *on page 176*
- ◆ ***Erwinia chrysanthemi*** *see* Asparaginase (*Erwinia*) *on page 176*
- ◆ **Eryc** *see* Erythromycin (Systemic) *on page 588*
- ◆ **EryPed 200** *see* Erythromycin (Systemic) *on page 588*
- ◆ **EryPed 400** *see* Erythromycin (Systemic) *on page 588*
- ◆ **Ery-Tab** *see* Erythromycin (Systemic) *on page 588*
- ◆ **Erythrocin Lactobionate** *see* Erythromycin (Systemic) *on page 588*
- ◆ **Erythrocin Stearate** *see* Erythromycin (Systemic) *on page 588*

Erythromycin (Systemic) (er ith roe MYE sin)

Related Information

Bacterial Infections *on page 1739*

Clinical Risk Related to Drugs Prolonging QT Interval *on page 1675*

Brand Names: US E.E.S. 400; E.E.S. Granules; Ery-Tab; EryPed 200; EryPed 400; Erythrocin Lactobionate; Erythrocin Stearate; PCE [DSC]

Brand Names: Canada EES 200 [DSC]; EES 400 [DSC]; EES 600 [DSC]; Erybid [DSC]; Eryc; Erythro-Base; Erythro-ES [DSC]; Erythro-S; Erythrocin; NOVO-Rythro Estolate [DSC]; PCE [DSC]

Pharmacologic Category Antibiotic, Macrolide

Use

Bacterial infections: Treatment of susceptible bacterial infections, including *S. pyogenes*, some *S. pneumoniae,* some *S. aureus*, *M. pneumoniae*, *Legionella pneumophila*, diphtheria, pertussis, *Chlamydia*, erythrasma, *N. gonorrhoeae*, *E. histolytica*, syphilis and nongonococcal urethritis, and *Campylobacter* gastroenteritis; used in conjunction with neomycin for decontaminating the bowel

Surgical (preoperative) prophylaxis (colorectal): Colorectal decontamination, in conjunction with other agents, prior to surgical intervention

Local Anesthetic/Vasoconstrictor Precautions Erythromycin is one of the drugs confirmed to prolong the QT interval and is accepted as having a risk of causing torsade de pointes. In terms of epinephrine, it is not known what effect vasoconstrictors in the local anesthetic regimen will have in patients with a known history of congenital prolonged QT interval or in patients taking any medication that prolongs the QT interval. Until more information is obtained, it is suggested that the clinician consult with the physician prior to the use of a vasoconstrictor in suspected patients, and that the vasoconstrictor (epinephrine, mepivacaine and levonordefrin [Carbocaine® 2% with Neo-Cobefrin®]) be used with caution. See Dental Health Professional Considerations.

Effects on Dental Treatment Key adverse event(s) related to dental treatment: Oral candidiasis.

Effects on Bleeding No information available to require special precautions

Adverse Reactions Frequency not defined. Incidence may vary with formulation.

Cardiovascular: QT_c prolongation, torsade de pointes, ventricular arrhythmia, ventricular tachycardia

Central nervous system: Seizure

Dermatologic: Erythema multiforme, pruritus, skin rash, Stevens-Johnson syndrome, toxic epidermal necrolysis, urticaria

Gastrointestinal: Abdominal pain, anorexia, diarrhea, nausea, oral candidiasis, pancreatitis, pseudomembranous colitis, pyloric stenosis (infantile hypertrophic), vomiting

Hepatic: Abnormal hepatic function tests, cholestatic jaundice (most common with estolate), hepatitis

Hypersensitivity: Anaphylaxis, hypersensitivity reaction

Local: Injection site phlebitis

Neuromuscular & skeletal: Weakness

Otic: Hearing loss

Renal: Interstitial nephritis

Postmarketing and/or case reports: Hepatotoxicity (idiosyncratic) (Chalasani 2014)

Mechanism of Action Inhibits RNA-dependent protein synthesis at the chain elongation step; binds to the 50S ribosomal subunit resulting in blockage of transpeptidation

Pharmacodynamics/Kinetics

Half-life Elimination Neonates (≤15 days of age): 2.1 hours; Adults: Peak: 1.5-2 hours; End-stage renal disease: 5-6 hours

Time to Peak Serum: Base: 4 hours; Ethylsuccinate: 0.5 to 2.5 hours; Stearate: 3 hours (Steigbigel 2000); delayed with food due to differences in absorption

Pregnancy Considerations Erythromycin crosses the placenta.

Cardiovascular anomalies following exposure in early pregnancy have been reported in some observational studies.

Serum concentrations of erythromycin may be variable in pregnant women (Kiefer 1955; Philipson 1976).

Erythromycin is the antibiotic of choice for preterm prelabor rupture of membranes <34 0/7 weeks' gestation) (ACOG 188 2018), the treatment of lymphogranuloma venereum in pregnancy, and the treatment of or long-term suppression of *Bartonella* infection in HIV-infected pregnant patients. Erythromycin is one of the antibiotics that may be used for the treatment of chancroid or granuloma inguinale during pregnancy, and may be appropriate as an alternative agent for the treatment of chlamydial infections in pregnant women (consult current guidelines) (CDC [Workowski 2015]; HHS [OI adult 2020]). Agents other than systemic erythromycin are preferred for the treatment of acne during pregnancy (AAD [Zaenglein 2016]).

Product Availability PCE tablets have been discontinued in the US for more than 1 year.

Dental Health Professional Considerations Many patients cannot tolerate erythromycin because of abdominal pain and nausea; the mechanism of this adverse effect appears to be the motilin agonistic properties of erythromycin in the GI tract. For these patients, clindamycin is indicated as the alternative antibiotic for treatment of orofacial infections.

HMG-CoA reductase inhibitors, also known as the statins, effectively decrease the hepatic cholesterol biosynthesis resulting in the reduction of blood LDL-cholesterol concentrations. The AUC of atorvastatin (Lipitor®) was increased 33% by erythromycin administration. Combination of erythromycin and lovastatin (Mevacor®) has been associated with rhabdomyolysis (Ayanian, et al). The mechanism of erythromycin is inhibiting the CYP3A4 metabolism of atorvastatin, lovastatin, and cerivastatin. Simvastatin (Zocor®) would likely be affected in a similar manner by the coadministration of erythromycin. Clarithromycin (Biaxin®) may exert a similar effect as erythromycin on atorvastatin, lovastatin, cerivastatin, and simvastatin.

Also see Local Anesthetic/Vasoconstrictor Precautions

◆ **Erythromycin Base** *see* Erythromycin (Systemic) *on page 588*

◆ **Erythromycin Ethylsuccinate** *see* Erythromycin (Systemic) *on page 588*

◆ **Erythromycin Lactobionate** *see* Erythromycin (Systemic) *on page 588*

◆ **Erythromycin Stearate** *see* Erythromycin (Systemic) *on page 588*

◆ **Erythropoiesis-Stimulating Agent (ESA)** *see* Darbepoetin Alfa *on page 440*

◆ **Erythropoiesis-Stimulating Agent (ESA)** *see* Epoetin Alfa *on page 577*

◆ **Erythropoiesis-Stimulating Agent (ESA)** *see* Methoxy Polyethylene Glycol-Epoetin Beta *on page 993*

◆ **Erythropoiesis-Stimulating Protein** *see* Darbepoetin Alfa *on page 440*

◆ **Erythropoietin** *see* Epoetin Alfa *on page 577*

Escitalopram (es sye TAL oh pram)

Related Information

Citalopram *on page 353*

Clinical Risk Related to Drugs Prolonging QT Interval *on page 1675*

Vasoconstrictor Interactions With Antidepressants *on page 1821*

Brand Names: US Lexapro

Brand Names: Canada ACH-Escitalopram; ACT Escitalopram ODT; ACT Escitalopram [DSC]; AG-Escitalopram; APO-Escitalopram; Auro-Escitalopram; BIO-Escitalopram; Cipralex; Cipralex Meltz [DSC]; JAMP-Escitalopram; M-Escitalopram; Mar-Escitalopram; MINT-Escitalopram; MYLAN-Escitalopram; NAT-Escitalopram; NRA-Escitalopram; PMS-Escitalopram; Priva-Escitalopram; RAN-Escitalopram; RIVA-Escitalopram; SANDOZ Escitalopram; TEVA-Escitalopram

Pharmacologic Category Antidepressant, Selective Serotonin Reuptake Inhibitor

Use

Major depressive disorder (unipolar): Acute and maintenance treatment of unipolar major depressive disorder (MDD)

Generalized anxiety disorder: Acute treatment of generalized anxiety disorder (GAD)

Local Anesthetic/Vasoconstrictor Precautions Although caution should be used in patients taking tricyclic antidepressants, no interactions have been reported with vasoconstrictors and escitalopram, a non-tricyclic antidepressant which acts to increase serotonin; no precautions appear to be needed

Escitalopram is one of the drugs confirmed to prolong the QT interval and is accepted as having a risk of causing torsade de pointes. The risk of drug-induced torsade de pointes is extremely low when a single QT interval prolonging drug is prescribed. In terms of epinephrine, it is not known what effect vasoconstrictors in the local anesthetic regimen will have in patients with a known history of congenital prolonged QT interval or in patients taking any medication that prolongs the QT interval. Until more information is obtained, it is suggested that the clinician consult with the physician prior to the use of a vasoconstrictor in suspected patients, and that the vasoconstrictor (epinephrine, mepivacaine, and levonordefrin [Carbocaine® 2% with Neo-Cobefrin®]) be used with caution.

Effects on Dental Treatment Key adverse event(s) related to dental treatment: Xerostomia (normal salivary flow resumes upon discontinuation) and toothache (see Effects on Bleeding and Dental Health Professional Considerations)

Effects on Bleeding Selective serotonin reuptake inhibitors such as escitalopram may impair platelet aggregation due to platelet serotonin depletion, possibly increasing the risk of a bleeding complication. The risk of a bleeding complication can be increased by coadministration of other antiplatelet agents such as NSAIDs and aspirin.

Adverse Reactions

>10%:

Gastrointestinal: Diarrhea (6% to 14%), nausea (15% to 18%)

Genitourinary: Ejaculatory disorder (9% to 14% [placebo: <1% to 2%])

Nervous system: Drowsiness (4% to 13%; literature suggests incidence is lower in children and adolescents compared to adults [Safer 2006]), headache (24%), insomnia (7% to 14%)

1% to 10%:

Dermatologic: Diaphoresis (3% to 8%)

Endocrine & metabolic: Decreased libido (3% to 7% [placebo: 1% to 2%]), menstrual disease (2%)

Gastrointestinal: Abdominal pain (2%), constipation (3% to 6%), decreased appetite (3%), dyspepsia (2% to 6%), flatulence (2%), toothache (2%), vomiting (3%; literature suggests incidence is higher in adolescents compared to adults, and is two- to threefold higher in children compared to adolescents [Safer 2006]), xerostomia (4% to 9%)

Genitourinary: Impotence (2% to 3% [placebo: <1%]), urinary tract infection (children ≥2%)

Nervous system: Abnormal dreams (3%), anorgasmia (2% to 6% [placebo: <1%]), dizziness (4% to 7%), fatigue (2% to 8%), lethargy (3%), paresthesia (2%), yawning (2%)

Neuromuscular & skeletal: Back pain (children ≥2%), neck pain (≤3%), shoulder pain (≤3%)

Respiratory: Flu-like symptoms (5%), nasal congestion (children ≥2%), rhinitis (5%), sinusitis (3%)

<1%:

Cardiovascular: Chest pain, hypertension, palpitations

Dermatologic: Skin rash

Endocrine & metabolic: Hot flash, weight gain

Gastrointestinal: Abdominal cramps, gastroenteritis, heartburn, increased appetite

Genitourinary: Dysmenorrhea, urinary frequency

Hypersensitivity: Hypersensitivity reaction

Nervous system: Irritability, lack of concentration, migraine

Neuromuscular & skeletal: Arthralgia, jaw tightness, limb pain, myalgia

Ophthalmic: Blurred vision

Otic: Tinnitus

Respiratory: Bronchitis, cough, paranasal sinus congestion, sinus headache

Miscellaneous: Fever

Postmarketing:

Cardiovascular: Acute myocardial infarction, atrial fibrillation, bradycardia, cardiac failure, cerebrovascular accident, deep vein thrombosis, edema, flushing, hypertensive crisis, hypotension, orthostatic hypotension, phlebitis, prolonged QT interval on ECG (Funk 2013), pulmonary embolism, syncope, tachycardia, thrombosis, torsades de pointes, ventricular arrhythmia, ventricular tachycardia

Dermatologic: Alopecia, dermatitis, ecchymoses, erythema multiforme, skin photosensitivity, Stevens-Johnson syndrome, toxic epidermal necrolysis, urticaria

Endocrine & metabolic: Diabetes mellitus, heavy menstrual bleeding, hypercholesterolemia, hyperglycemia, hyperprolactinemia, hypoglycemia, hypokalemia, hyponatremia (Rawal 2017), SIADH (Raj 2018)

Gastrointestinal: Dysphagia, gastroesophageal reflux disease, gastrointestinal hemorrhage (Kumar 2009), pancreatitis

Genitourinary: Dysuria, erectile dysfunction, orgasm disturbance, priapism (Budak 2019), sexual disorder (Roy 2019), spontaneous abortion, urinary retention
Hematologic & oncologic: Agranulocytosis, anemia, aplastic anemia, hemolytic anemia, hypoprothrombinemia, immune thrombocytopenia, increased INR, leukopenia, rectal hemorrhage, thrombocytopenia
Hepatic: Hepatic failure, hepatic necrosis, hepatitis, increased liver enzymes, increased serum bilirubin
Hypersensitivity: Anaphylaxis, angioedema
Nervous system: Abnormal gait, aggressive behavior, agitated depression, agitation, akathisia, amnesia, anxiety, apathy, ataxia, choreoathetosis, delirium, delusion, depersonalization, dystonia, extrapyramidal reaction, hallucination, hypoesthesia, hypomania (Sharma 2009b), mania (Prapotnik 2004), myasthenia, myoclonus, neuroleptic malignant syndrome (Stevens 2008), nightmares, panic, paranoid ideation, parkinsonism, psychosis, restless leg syndrome, seizure, serotonin syndrome (Huska 2007; Sanyal 2010), suicidal ideation (Madsen 2019), suicidal tendencies, tardive dyskinesia, vertigo, withdrawal syndrome (De Berardis 2014)
Neuromuscular & skeletal: Bone fracture (fragility) (Khanassov 2018), dyskinesia, rhabdomyolysis, tremor
Ophthalmic: Acute angle-closure glaucoma (AlQuorain 2016; Zelefsky 2006), diplopia, mydriasis, nystagmus disorder, subconjunctival hemorrhage (Sharma 2009a), visual disturbance
Renal: Acute renal failure
Respiratory: Dyspnea, epistaxis (Lake 2000)

Mechanism of Action Escitalopram is the S-enantiomer of the racemic derivative citalopram, which selectively inhibits the reuptake of serotonin with little to no effect on norepinephrine or dopamine reuptake. It has no or very low affinity for 5-HT_{1-7}, alpha- and beta-adrenergic, D_{1-5}, H_{1-3}, M_{1-5}, and benzodiazepine receptors. Escitalopram does not bind to or has low affinity for Na^+, K^+, Cl^-, and Ca^{++} ion channels.

Pharmacodynamics/Kinetics

Onset of Action

Anxiety disorders (generalized anxiety, obsessive-compulsive, panic, and posttraumatic stress disorder): Initial effects may be observed within 2 weeks of treatment, with continued improvements through 4 to 6 weeks (Issari 2016; Varigonda 2016; WFSBP [Bandelow 2012]); some experts suggest up to 12 weeks of treatment may be necessary for response, particularly in patients with obsessive-compulsive disorder and posttraumatic stress disorder (BAP [Baldwin 2014]; Katzman 2014; WFSBP [Bandelow 2012]).

Body dysmorphic disorder: Initial effects may be observed within 2 weeks; some experts suggest up to 12 to 16 weeks of treatment may be necessary for response in some patients (Phillips 2008).

Depression: Initial effects may be observed within 1 to 2 weeks of treatment, with continued improvements through 4 to 6 weeks (Papakostas 2006; Posternak 2005; Szegedi 2009; Taylor 2006).

Premenstrual dysphoric disorder: Initial effects may be observed within the first few days of treatment, with response at the first menstrual cycle of treatment (ISPMD [Nevatte 2013]).

Half-life Elimination Mean: Adolescents: 19 hours; Adults: ~27 to 32 hours (increased ~50% in the elderly and doubled in patients with hepatic impairment)

Time to Peak Escitalopram: Adolescents: 2.9 hours; Adults: ~5 hours

Pregnancy Considerations

Escitalopram crosses the placenta and is distributed into the amniotic fluid. An increased risk of teratogenic effects, including cardiovascular defects, may be associated with maternal use of escitalopram or other SSRIs; however, available information is conflicting. Nonteratogenic effects in the newborn following SSRI/SNRI exposure late in the third trimester include respiratory distress, cyanosis, apnea, seizures, temperature instability, feeding difficulty, vomiting, hypoglycemia, hypo- or hypertonia, hyper-reflexia, jitteriness, irritability, constant crying, and tremor. Symptoms may be due to the toxicity of the SSRIs/SNRIs or a discontinuation syndrome and may be consistent with serotonin syndrome associated with SSRI treatment. Persistent pulmonary hypertension of the newborn (PPHN) has also been reported with SSRI exposure. The long-term effects of in utero SSRI exposure on infant development and behavior are not known. Escitalopram is the S-enantiomer of the racemic derivative citalopram; also refer to the Citalopram monograph.

Due to pregnancy-induced physiologic changes, some pharmacokinetic parameters of escitalopram may be altered. The ACOG recommends that therapy with SSRIs or SNRIs during pregnancy be individualized; treatment of depression during pregnancy should incorporate the clinical expertise of the mental health clinician, obstetrician, primary health care provider, and pediatrician. According to the American Psychiatric Association (APA), the risks of medication treatment should be weighed against other treatment options and untreated depression. For women who discontinue antidepressant medications during pregnancy and who may be at high risk for postpartum depression, the medications can be restarted following delivery. Treatment algorithms have been developed by the ACOG and the APA for the management of depression in women prior to conception and during pregnancy.

Pregnant women exposed to antidepressants during pregnancy are encouraged to enroll in the National Pregnancy Registry for Antidepressants (NPRAD). Women 18 to 45 years of age or their health care providers may contact the registry by calling 844-405-6185. Enrollment should be done as early in pregnancy as possible.

Dental Health Professional Considerations Problems with SSRI-induced bruxism have been reported and may preclude their use; clinicians attempting to evaluate any patient with bruxism or involuntary muscle movement, who is simultaneously being treated with an SSRI drug, should be aware of the potential association (see Local Anesthetic/Vasoconstrictor Precautions)

◆ **Escitalopram Oxalate** *see* Escitalopram *on page* 590
◆ **Eserine Salicylate** *see* Physostigmine *on page* 1229
◆ **Eskalith** *see* Lithium *on page* 923
◆ **Eskata** *see* Hydrogen Peroxide *on page* 776

Esketamine (es KET a meen)

Brand Names: US Spravato (56 MG Dose); Spravato (84 MG Dose)

Brand Names: Canada Spravato

Pharmacologic Category N-Methyl-D-Aspartate (NMDA) Receptor Antagonist

Use

Depression, treatment-resistant: Treatment of treatment-resistant depression in adults, in conjunction with an oral antidepressant.

Major depressive disorder (unipolar) with suicidality: Treatment of depressive symptoms in adults with major depressive disorder with suicidal ideation or behavior.

Limitations of use: Not approved as an anesthetic agent. The safety and effectiveness of esketamine as an anesthetic agent have not been established. Additionally, esketamine treats depressive symptoms; effectiveness of esketamine in preventing suicide or decreasing suicidal ideation has not been shown.

Local Anesthetic/Vasoconstrictor Precautions Increases in systolic and/or diastolic blood pressure have been observed at all recommended doses of esketamine. Monitor blood pressure when using local anesthetic with vasoconstrictor; medical consult is suggested.

Effects on Dental Treatment Key adverse event(s) related to dental treatment: Frequent occurrence of dysgeusia (altered sense of taste); occurrence of xerostomia (normal salivary flow resumes upon discontinuation); occurrence of oropharyngeal pain, and throat irritation.

Effects on Bleeding No information available to require special precautions

Adverse Reactions

>10%:

Cardiovascular: Increased systolic blood pressure (3% to 17%), increased diastolic blood pressure (4% to 14%)

Central nervous system: Depersonalization (≤75%), derealization (≤75%), dissociative reaction (41% to 75%), sedated state (23% to 61%), dizziness (29%), vertigo (23%), headache (20%), hypoesthesia (18%), anxiety (13%), lethargy (11%)

Gastrointestinal: Nausea (27% to 32%), dysgeusia (19%), vomiting (6% to 12%)

1% to 10%:

Cardiovascular: Increased blood pressure (10%), tachycardia (2%)

Central nervous system: Insomnia (8%), intoxicated feeling (5%), dysarthria (4%), euphoria (4%), feeling abnormal (3%), mental deficiency (3%)

Dermatologic: Hyperhidrosis (4%)

Gastrointestinal: Diarrhea (7%), xerostomia (5%), constipation (3%), severe nausea (3%), severe vomiting (3%)

Genitourinary: Pollakiuria (3%)

Neuromuscular & skeletal: Tremor (3%)

Respiratory: Nasal discomfort (7%), throat irritation (7%), oropharyngeal pain (3%)

Frequency not defined:

Central nervous system: Cognitive dysfunction, drug abuse

Genitourinary: Cystitis, dysuria, nocturia, urinary urgency

<1%, postmarketing, and/or case reports: Loss of consciousness

Mechanism of Action Esketamine (S-enantiomer of racemic ketamine) is a nonselective, noncompetitive N-methyl-D-aspartate (NMDA) receptor antagonist. The mechanism by which it exerts its antidepressant effect is unknown. The major circulating metabolite noresketamine demonstrated activity at the same receptor with less affinity.

Pharmacodynamics/Kinetics

Half-life Elimination Esketamine: 7 to 12 hours; Noresketamine (active metabolite): ~8 hours

Time to Peak Plasma: 20 to 40 minutes

Reproductive Considerations

Based on adverse events observed in animal reproduction studies, the manufacturer recommends females of reproductive potential consider pregnancy planning and prevention during esketamine therapy.

Pregnancy Considerations

Based on animal data, use of medications that block N-methyl-D-aspartate (NMDA) receptors and/or potentiate gamma-aminobutyric acid (GABA) activity, may affect brain development.

The ACOG recommends treatment of depression during pregnancy should be individualized and incorporate the clinical expertise of the mental health clinician, obstetrician, primary health care provider, and pediatrician. According to the American Psychiatric Association (APA), the risks of medication treatment should be weighed against other treatment options and untreated depression. For women who discontinue antidepressant medications during pregnancy and who may be at high risk for postpartum depression, the medications can be restarted following delivery. Treatment algorithms have been developed by the ACOG and the APA for the management of depression in women prior to conception and during pregnancy (ACOG 2008; APA 2010; Yonkers 2009)

Pregnant females exposed to antidepressants during pregnancy are encouraged to enroll in the National Pregnancy Registry for Antidepressants (NPRAD). Females 18 to 45 years of age or their health care providers may contact the registry by calling 1-844-405-6185 or online at https://womensmentalhealth.org/clinical-and-researchprograms/pregnancyregistry/antidepressants/. Enrollment should be done as early in pregnancy as possible.

Controlled Substance C-III

Prescribing and Access Restrictions In Canada, Spravato is only available through the JANSSEN JOURNEY Program. Patients, pharmacists, and physicians must all be enrolled in the program prior to prescribing and dispensing. More information can be obtained by contacting the JANSSEN JOURNEY Program at 1-833-257-7191 or https://www.JanssenJourneyHCP.ca.

◆ **Esketamine Hydrochloride** *see* Esketamine *on page 591*

Eslicarbazepine (es li kar BAZ e peen)

Brand Names: US Aptiom

Brand Names: Canada Aptiom

Pharmacologic Category Anticonvulsant, Miscellaneous

Use Partial-onset seizures (epilepsy): Monotherapy or adjunctive therapy in the treatment of partial-onset seizures in adults and pediatric patients ≥4 years of age

Local Anesthetic/Vasoconstrictor Precautions No information available to require special precautions

Effects on Dental Treatment No significant effects or complications reported

Effects on Bleeding No information available to require special precautions

Adverse Reactions

>10%:

Central nervous system: Dizziness (20% to 28%), drowsiness (11% to 28%), headache (13% to 15%)

Gastrointestinal: Nausea (10% to 16%)

Ophthalmic: Diplopia (9% to 11%)

1% to 10%:

Cardiovascular: Hypertension (2%), peripheral edema (2%)

Central nervous system: Fatigue (7%), cognitive dysfunction (4% to 7%), ataxia (4% to 6%), vertigo (2% to 6%), depression (3%), equilibrium disturbance (3%), falling (3%), abnormal gait (2%), insomnia (2%), dysarthria (1% to 2%), memory impairment (1% to 2%)

Dermatologic: Skin rash (3%)

Endocrine & metabolic: Hyponatremia (serum sodium <125 mEq/L: 1% to 2%)

Gastrointestinal: Vomiting (6% to 10%), diarrhea (4%), abdominal pain (2%), constipation (2%), gastritis (2%)

Genitourinary: Urinary tract infection (2%)

Neuromuscular & skeletal: Tremor (2% to 4%), weakness (3%)

Ophthalmic: Blurred vision (5% to 6%), decreased visual acuity (2%), nystagmus (1% to 2%)

Respiratory: Cough (2%)

Frequency not defined:

Endocrine & metabolic: Hypercholesterolemia, hypochloremia (concurrent with hyponatremia), increased LDL cholesterol, increased serum triglycerides

Hematologic & oncologic: Decreased hematocrit, decreased hemoglobin

Neuromuscular & skeletal: Increased creatine phosphokinase

<1%, postmarketing, and/or case reports: Agranulocytosis, anaphylaxis, angioedema, decreased T3 level, decreased T4 (free and total), DRESS syndrome, increased serum bilirubin (>2 x ULN), increased serum transaminases (>3 x ULN), leukopenia, megaloblastic anemia, pancytopenia, prolongation P-R interval on ECG (mild [Vas-Da-Silva 2012]), severe dermatological reaction, SIADH, Stevens-Johnson syndrome, thrombocytopenia, toxic epidermal necrolysis

Mechanism of Action Eslicarbazepine acetate is extensively converted to eslicarbazepine, which is considered responsible for therapeutic effects. A precise mechanism has not been defined, but is thought to involve inhibition of voltage-gated sodium channels.

Pharmacodynamics/Kinetics

Half-life Elimination Pediatric patients 4 to 17 years: 10 to 16 hours; Adults: 13 to 20 hours

Time to Peak Eslicarbazepine: Pediatric patients 4 to 17 years: 1 to 3 hours; Adults: 1 to 4 hours

Reproductive Considerations

Eslicarbazepine may decrease plasma concentrations of hormonal contraceptives; additional or alternative nonhormonal contraceptives are recommended in women of reproductive potential.

Pregnancy Considerations

Adverse events have been observed in animal reproduction studies.

Patients exposed to eslicarbazepine during pregnancy are encouraged to enroll themselves into the North American Antiepileptic Drug (NAAED) Pregnancy Registry by calling 1-888-233-2334. Additional information is available at http://www.aedpregnancyregistry.org.

◆ **Eslicarbazepine Acetate** *see* Eslicarbazepine *on page 592*

Esmolol (ES moe lol)

Brand Names: US Brevibloc; Brevibloc in NaCl; Brevibloc Premixed; Brevibloc Premixed DS

Brand Names: Canada Brevibloc

Pharmacologic Category Antiarrhythmic Agent, Class II; Antihypertensive; Beta-Blocker, Beta-1 Selective

Use

Intraoperative and postoperative tachycardia and/or hypertension: Treatment of intraoperative and postoperative tachycardia and/or hypertension

Sinus tachycardia: Treatment of noncompensatory sinus tachycardia

Supraventricular tachycardia and atrial fibrillation/flutter: Control of ventricular rate in patients with supraventricular tachycardia or atrial fibrillation/flutter

Local Anesthetic/Vasoconstrictor Precautions No information available to require special precautions

Effects on Dental Treatment Esmolol is a cardioselective beta-blocker. Local anesthetic with vasoconstrictor can be safely used in patients medicated with esmolol. Nonselective beta-blockers (ie, propranolol, nadolol) enhance the pressor response to epinephrine, resulting in hypertension and bradycardia; this has not been reported for esmolol. Many nonsteroidal anti-inflammatory drugs, such as ibuprofen and indomethacin, can reduce the hypotensive effect of beta-blockers after 3 or more weeks of therapy with the NSAID. Short-term NSAID use (ie, 3 days) requires no special precautions in patients taking beta-blockers.

Effects on Bleeding No information available to require special precautions

Adverse Reactions

>10%: Cardiovascular: Asymptomatic hypotension (25%), symptomatic hypotension (12%)

1% to 10%:

Cardiovascular: Peripheral ischemia (1%)

Central nervous system: Dizziness (≤3%), drowsiness (3%), headache (2%), agitation (≤2%), confusion (≤2%)

Gastrointestinal: Nausea (7%), vomiting (1%)

Local: Infusion site reaction (8%; including inflammation and induration)

<1%, postmarketing, and/or case reports: Abdominal distress, abnormality in thinking, angioedema, anxiety, bradycardia, constipation, coronary artery vasospasm, depression, dyspepsia, flushing, heart block, hyperkalemia, increased heart rate (moderate increase above pretreatment levels 30 minutes after discontinuation), infusion site irritation, local thrombophlebitis (at infusion site), local tissue necrosis (at infusion site), pallor, paresthesia, psoriasis, renal tubular acidosis (hyperkalemic), seizure, severe bradycardia, sinus pause, skin blister (at infusion site), syncope, urinary retention, urticaria, voice disorder, xerostomia

Mechanism of Action Class II antiarrhythmic: Competitively blocks response to $beta_1$-adrenergic stimulation with little or no effect of $beta_2$-receptors except at high doses, no intrinsic sympathomimetic activity, no membrane stabilizing activity

Pharmacodynamics/Kinetics

Onset of Action Beta-blockade: IV: 2-10 minutes (quickest when loading doses are administered)

Duration of Action Hemodynamic effects: 10-30 minutes; prolonged following higher cumulative doses, extended duration of use

Half-life Elimination

Children ≥18 months and Adolescents ≤16 years: Variable; mean range: 2.7 to 4.8 minutes (reported full range: 0.2 to 9.9 minutes) (Cuneo 1994; Tabbutt 2008; Wiest 1991; Wiest 1998)

Adults: Esmolol: 9 minutes; Acid metabolite: 3.7 hours; elimination of metabolite decreases with end-stage renal disease

Pregnancy Considerations

Exposure to esmolol may cause fetal bradycardia which may continue after esmolol is discontinued. If maternal use of a beta-blocker is needed, fetal growth should be monitored during pregnancy and the newborn should be monitored for 48 hours after delivery for bradycardia, hypoglycemia, and respiratory depression (ESC [Regitz-Zagrosek 2018]).

Esmolol is a short-acting beta-blocker and not indicated for the chronic treatment of hypertension; however, use may be considered as an alternative agent for hypertensive emergencies in pregnancy (ACOG 767 2019). Agents other than esmolol may be preferred for the treatment of supraventricular tachycardia, atrial fibrillation, atrial flutter, and ventricular tachycardia in pregnancy. Consult current guidelines for indication specific recommendations (ACC/AHA/HRS [Page 2016]; ESC [Regitz-Zagrosek 2018]).

◆ **Esmolol HCl** *see* Esmolol *on page 593*

◆ **Esmolol Hydrochloride** *see* Esmolol *on page 593*

◆ **Esomep-EZS** *see* Esomeprazole *on page 594*

Esomeprazole (es oh ME pray zol)

Related Information

Gastrointestinal Disorders *on page 1678*

Omeprazole *on page 1139*

Brand Names: US Esomep-EZS; GoodSense Esomeprazole [OTC]; NexIUM; NexIUM 24HR Clear Minis [OTC]; NexIUM 24HR [OTC]; NexIUM I.V.

Brand Names: Canada APO-Esomeprazole; MYL-Esomeprazole; MYLAN-Esomeprazole [DSC]; NexIUM; PMS-Esomeprazole DR; RAN-Esomeprazole; SANDOZ Esomeprazole; TEVA-Esomeprazole

Pharmacologic Category Proton Pump Inhibitor; Substituted Benzimidazole

Use

Oral, IV:

Peptic ulcer disease, treatment of bleeding ulcers: Decrease the risk of rebleeding after successful endoscopy for acute bleeding gastric or duodenal ulcers in adults.

Oral:

Esomeprazole magnesium and esomeprazole strontium:

Gastroesophageal reflux disease (Rx only):

Healing of erosive esophagitis: Short-term (4 to 8 weeks) treatment of erosive esophagitis

Maintenance of healing of erosive esophagitis: Maintaining symptom resolution and healing of erosive esophagitis

Symptomatic gastroesophageal reflux disease: Short-term (4 to 8 weeks) treatment of symptomatic gastroesophageal reflux disease (GERD)

***Helicobacter pylori* eradication (Rx only):** As part of a multidrug regimen for *Helicobacter pylori* eradication in patients with duodenal ulcer disease (active or history of within the past 5 years)

Risk reduction of nonsteroidal anti-inflammatory drug-associated gastric ulcer (Rx only): Prevention of gastric ulcers associated with continuous NSAID therapy in patients at risk (age ≥60 years and/or history of gastric ulcer)

Pathological hypersecretory conditions, including Zollinger-Ellison syndrome (Rx only): Treatment (long-term) of pathological hypersecretory conditions including Zollinger-Ellison syndrome

Esomeprazole magnesium:

Heartburn (OTC labeling): Treatment of frequent heartburn (≥2 days per week).

IV: Esomeprazole sodium:

Gastroesophageal reflux disease (Rx only): Short-term (≤10 days) treatment of gastroesophageal reflux disease (GERD) with erosive esophagitis in pediatric patients 1 month to 17 years of age and adults when oral therapy is not possible or appropriate.

Local Anesthetic/Vasoconstrictor Precautions

No information available to require special precautions

Effects on Dental Treatment Key adverse event(s) related to dental treatment: Xerostomia (normal salivary flow resumes upon discontinuation)

Effects on Bleeding No information available to require special precautions

Adverse Reactions Unless otherwise specified, percentages represent adverse reactions identified in clinical trials evaluating the oral formulation.

>10%: Central nervous system: Headache (2% to 11%)

1% to 10%:

Central nervous system: Irritability (infants: ≥5%), dizziness (intravenous: ≤3%; oral: <1%), vertigo (intravenous: ≤3%), drowsiness (children: 2%; adults: <1%)

Dermatologic: Pruritus (intravenous: 1%; oral: <1%)

Endocrine & metabolic: Altered thyroid hormone levels (increased thyroxine: ≤1%), decreased serum potassium (≤1%), decreased serum sodium (≤1%), decreased thyroid hormones (thyroxine: ≤1%), increased gastrin (≤1%), increased serum potassium (≤1%), increased serum sodium (≤1%), increased thyroid stimulating hormone level (≤1%), increased uric acid (≤1%)

Gastrointestinal: Flatulence (intravenous: 10%; oral: ≥1%), diarrhea (2% to 4%), abdominal pain (1% to 6%), nausea (intravenous: 6%; oral: ≥1% to 2%), vomiting (infants: 1% to ≥5%; adults: <1%), xerostomia (intravenous: 4%; oral: ≥1%), constipation (intravenous: 3%; oral: ≥1%)

Hematologic & oncologic: Quantitative disorders of platelets (≤1%)

Hepatic: Increased serum alkaline phosphatase (≤1%), increased serum alanine aminotransferase (≤1%), increased serum aspartate aminotransferase (≤1%)

Local: Injection site reaction (intravenous: 2% to 4%)

Renal: Increased serum creatinine (≤1%)

Respiratory: Cough (intravenous: 1%; oral: <1%), tachypnea (infants, oral: 1%)

Miscellaneous: Fever (intravenous: 4%; oral: <1%)

Frequency not defined:

Cardiovascular: Esophageal varices

Gastrointestinal: Barrett esophagus, duodenitis, esophageal stenosis, esophageal ulcer, esophagitis, gastritis, mucosal discoloration

Hematologic & oncologic: Benign polyp
Miscellaneous: Benign nodule
<1%, postmarketing, and/or case reports: Acne vulgaris, acute interstitial nephritis, aggressive behavior, ageusia, agitation, agranulocytosis, albuminuria, alopecia, altered sense of smell, anaphylactic shock, anaphylaxis, anemia, angioedema, anorexia, apathy, aphthous stomatitis, arthralgia, arthropathy, asthenia, back pain, blurred vision, bone fracture, bronchospasm, candidiasis (urogenital), cervical lymphadenopathy, change in bowel habits, chest pain, *Clostridioides* (formerly *Clostridium*) *difficile*-associated diarrhea, colitis (microscopic), confusion, conjunctivitis, cutaneous lupus erythematosus (including exacerbations), cyanocobalamin deficiency, cystitis, depression, dermatitis, diaphoresis, dysgeusia, dysmenorrhea, dyspepsia, dysphagia, dyspnea, dysuria, edema, enlargement of abdomen, epigastric pain, epistaxis, eructation, erythema multiforme, erythematous rash, exacerbation of arthritis, exacerbation of asthma, facial edema, fatigue, fibromyalgia syndrome, flu-like symptoms, flushing, frequent bowel movements, fungal infection, gastroenteritis, gastrointestinal candidiasis, gastrointestinal dysplasia, gastrointestinal hemorrhage, genital candidiasis, glycosuria, goiter, gynecomastia, hallucination, hematuria, hepatic encephalopathy, hepatic failure, hepatitis, hepatotoxicity (idiosyncratic) (Chalasani 2014), hernia of abdominal cavity, hiccups, hot flash, hyperbilirubinemia, hyperhidrosis, hypersensitivity reaction, hypertension, hypertonia, hyperuricemia, hypochromic anemia, hypoesthesia, hypomagnesemia (with or without hypocalcemia and/or hypokalemia), hyponatremia, impotence, increased appetite, increased thirst, insomnia, interstitial nephritis, jaundice, laryngeal edema, leukocytosis, leukopenia, maculopapular rash, malaise, melena, menstrual disease, migraine, mouth disease, muscle cramps, myalgia, myasthenia, nervousness, otalgia, otitis media, pain, pancreatitis, pancytopenia, paresthesia, pathological fracture due to osteoporosis, peripheral edema, pharyngeal disease, pharyngitis, polymyalgia rheumatica, polyp (fundic gland), polyuria, pruritus ani, rectal disease, renal disease (chronic; [Lazarus 2016]), rhinitis, rigors, sinusitis, skin photosensitivity, skin rash, sleep disorder, Stevens-Johnson syndrome, stomatitis, systemic lupus erythematosus (including exacerbations), tachycardia, thrombocytopenia, tinnitus, tongue disease, tongue edema, toxic epidermal necrolysis, tremor, urinary frequency, urine abnormality, urticaria, vaginitis, vertigo, visual disturbance, visual field defect, weight gain, weight loss

Mechanism of Action Proton pump inhibitor suppresses gastric acid secretion by inhibition of the H^+/K^+-ATPase in the gastric parietal cell. Esomeprazole is the S-isomer of omeprazole.

Pharmacodynamics/Kinetics

Half-life Elimination

Infants: 0.93 hours
Children 1 to 5 years: 0.42 to 0.74 hours (Zhao 2006)
Children 6 to 11 years: 0.73 to 0.88 hours (Zhao 2006)
Children ≥12 years and Adolescents ≤17 years: 0.82 to 1.22 hours (Li 2006)
Adults: ~1 to 1.5 hours

Time to Peak Oral:

Infants: Median: 3 hours
Children 1 to 5 years: 1.33 to 1.44 hours (Zhao 2006)
Children 6 to 11 years: 1.75 to 1.79 hours (Zhao 2006)
Children ≥12 years and Adolescents ≤17 years: 1.96 to 2.04 hours (Li 2006)
Adults: 1.5 to 2 hours

Pregnancy Considerations Esomeprazole crosses the placenta (Saito 2020).

Following a maternal dose of esomeprazole 10 mg/day throughout pregnancy, cord blood concentrations at delivery were ~40% of those in the maternal serum (~12 hours after the last maternal dose). Twelve hours after delivery (~23 hours after the last maternal dose), esomeprazole was no longer detected in the infant serum (Saito 2020).

Recommendations for the treatment of GERD in pregnancy are available. As in nonpregnant patients, lifestyle modifications followed by other medications are the initial recommended treatments (Body 2016; Huerta-Iga 2016; Katz 2013; van der Woude 2014). Based on available data, PPIs may be used when clinically indicated (use of an agent with more data in pregnancy may be preferred) (Body 2016; Matok 2012; Pasternak 2010; van der Woude 2014).

◆ **Esomeprazole and Naproxen** *see* Naproxen and Esomeprazole *on page 1084*

◆ **Esomeprazole Magnesium** *see* Esomeprazole *on page 594*

◆ **Esomeprazole Sodium** *see* Esomeprazole *on page 594*

◆ **Esomeprazole Strontium** *see* Esomeprazole *on page 594*

◆ **Estarylla** *see* Ethinyl Estradiol and Norgestimate *on page 616*

Estazolam (es TA zoe lam)

Related Information

Dentin Hypersensitivity, Acid Erosion, High Caries Index, Management of Alveolar Osteitis, and Xerostomia *on page 1762*

Pharmacologic Category Benzodiazepine

Use Insomnia: Short-term management of insomnia characterized by difficulty in falling asleep, frequent nocturnal awakenings, and/or early morning awakenings.

Local Anesthetic/Vasoconstrictor Precautions No information available to require special precautions

Effects on Dental Treatment Key adverse event(s) related to dental treatment: Significant xerostomia (normal salivary flow resumes upon discontinuation)

Effects on Bleeding No information available to require special precautions

Adverse Reactions

>10%: Central nervous system: Drowsiness (42%)
1% to 10%:
Central nervous system: Dizziness (7%), ataxia (4%), hangover effect (3%), abnormality in thinking (2%), confusion (2%), anxiety (≥1%)
Dermatologic: Pruritus (1%)
Gastrointestinal: Constipation (≥1%), xerostomia (≥1%)
Neuromuscular & skeletal: Hypokinesia (8%), leg pain (3%), stiffness (1%)

<1%, postmarketing, and/or case reports: Acne vulgaris, adenopathy, agitation, agranulocytosis, amnesia, apathy, arm pain, arthralgia, arthritis, asthma, auditory impairment, breast swelling, cardiac arrhythmia, chills, cough, decreased appetite, decreased libido, diaphoresis, diplopia, dysgeusia, dyspnea, edema, emotional lability, enterocolitis, epistaxis, euphoria, eye irritation, eye pain, fever, flatulence, flushing, gastritis, genital discharge, hallucination, hematuria, hostility, hypersensitivity reaction, hyperventilation, hyporeflexia, increased appetite, increased serum AST, increased thirst, jaw pain, laryngitis, leukopenia, melena, muscle spasm, myalgia, neck pain, neuritis, nocturia, nystagmus, oliguria, oral mucosa ulcer, oral paresthesia, otalgia, palpitations, paresthesia, pelvic cramps (menstrual cramps), photophobia, polyuria, purpura, rhinitis, scotoma, seizure, sinusitis, skin photosensitivity, skin rash, sleep disorder, Stevens-Johnson syndrome, stupor, swelling of eye, syncope, thyroid nodule, tinnitus, tremor, twitching, urinary hesitancy, urinary incontinence, urinary urgency, urticaria, visual disturbance, vomiting, vulvovaginal pruritus, weight gain, weight loss, xeroderma

Mechanism of Action Binds to stereospecific benzodiazepine receptors on the postsynaptic GABA neuron at several sites within the central nervous system, including the limbic system, reticular formation. Enhancement of the inhibitory effect of GABA on neuronal excitability results by increased neuronal membrane permeability to chloride ions. This shift in chloride ions results in hyperpolarization (a less excitable state) and stabilization. Benzodiazepine receptors and effects appear to be linked to the GABA-A receptors. Benzodiazepines do not bind to GABA-B receptors (Vinkers 2012).

Pharmacodynamics/Kinetics

Duration of Action Variable

Half-life Elimination 10 to 24 hours

Time to Peak Serum: ~2 hours (range: 0.5 to 6 hours)

Pregnancy Risk Factor X

Pregnancy Considerations Although information specific to estazolam has not been located, all benzodiazepines are assumed to cross the placenta. Teratogenic effects have been observed with some benzodiazepines; however, additional studies are needed. The incidence of premature birth and low birth weights may be increased following maternal use of benzodiazepines; hypoglycemia and respiratory problems in the neonate may occur following exposure late in pregnancy. Neonatal withdrawal symptoms may occur within days to weeks after birth and "floppy infant syndrome" (which also includes withdrawal symptoms) has been reported with some benzodiazepines (Bergman 1992; Iqbal 2002; Wikner 2007). The use of estazolam is contraindicated in pregnant women.

Controlled Substance C-IV

- **Esterified Estrogen and Methyltestosterone** *see* Estrogens (Esterified) and Methyltestosterone *on page 605*
- **Esterified Estrogens** *see* Estrogens (Esterified) *on page 604*
- **Estiripentol** *see* Stiripentol *on page 1388*
- **Estrace** *see* Estradiol (Systemic) *on page 596*
- **Estradiol** *see* Estradiol (Systemic) *on page 596*

Estradiol (Systemic) (es tra DYE ole)

Related Information

Endocrine Disorders and Pregnancy *on page 1684*

Rheumatoid Arthritis, Osteoarthritis, and Osteoporosis *on page 1697*

Brand Names: US Alora; Climara; Delestrogen; Depo-Estradiol; Divigel; Dotti; Elestrin; Estrace; Estrogel; Evamist; Femring; Menostar; Minivelle; Vivelle-Dot

Brand Names: Canada Climara 100 [DSC]; Climara 25; Climara 50; Climara 75; Divigel; Estrace; Estradot 100; Estradot 25; Estradot 37.5; Estradot 50; Estradot 75; Estrogel; Lupin-Estradiol; Oesclim; PMS-Estradiol Valerate [DSC]; SANDOZ Estradiol Derm 100; SANDOZ Estradiol Derm 50; SANDOZ Estradiol Derm 75

Pharmacologic Category Estrogen Derivative

Use

Breast cancer, metastatic: Treatment of metastatic breast cancer (palliation) in appropriately selected men and postmenopausal women.

Hypoestrogenism (female): Treatment of hypoestrogenism due to hypogonadism, castration, or primary ovarian failure.

Osteoporosis prevention (female): Prevention of postmenopausal osteoporosis.

Limitations of use: For use only in women at significant risk of postmenopausal osteoporosis; consider use of nonestrogen medications.

Prostate cancer, advanced: Treatment of androgen-dependent advanced prostatic cancer (palliation).

Vasomotor symptoms associated with menopause: Treatment of moderate to severe vasomotor symptoms associated with menopause.

Vulvar and vaginal atrophy associated with menopause: Treatment of moderate to severe vulvar and vaginal atrophy associated with menopause.

Limitations of use: When used solely for the treatment of vulvar and vaginal atrophy, consider topical vaginal products.

Note: The International Society for the Study of Women's Sexual Health and The North American Menopause Society have endorsed the term genitourinary syndrome of menopause (GSM) as new terminology for vulvovaginal atrophy. The term GSM encompasses all genital and urinary signs and symptoms associated with a loss of estrogen due to menopause Portman 2014.

Local Anesthetic/Vasoconstrictor Precautions No information available to require special precautions

Effects on Dental Treatment No significant effects or complications reported

Effects on Bleeding No information available to require special precautions

Adverse Reactions Frequency not always defined. Some adverse reactions observed with estrogen and/or progestin combination therapy.

Cardiovascular: Edema (10% to 13%), hypertension (3% to 7%), cerebrovascular accident, deep vein thrombosis, local thrombophlebitis, myocardial infarction, pulmonary thromboembolism, retinal thrombosis, thrombophlebitis, venous thromboembolism

Central nervous system: Headache (9% to 50%), pain (6% to 13%), depression (1% to 11%), anxiety (4% to 10%), dizziness (≤8%), migraine (7%), nipple pain (1% to 7%), hypoesthesia (3%), chorea, dementia, exacerbation of epilepsy, irritability, mood disorder, nervousness

Dermatologic: Skin rash (7% to 9%), pruritus (4% to 7%), chloasma, erythema multiforme, erythema nodosum, localized erythema (transdermal patch), loss of scalp hair, skin discoloration (melasma), urticaria
Endocrine & metabolic: Weight gain (4% to 9%), hot flash (6%), hirsutism (≤5%), change in libido, change in menstrual flow (alterations in frequency and flow of bleeding patterns), exacerbation of diabetes mellitus, exacerbation of porphyria, fibrocystic breast changes, fluid retention, galactorrhea, hypocalcemia, increased serum triglycerides, weight loss
Gastrointestinal: Abdominal pain (6% to 16%), dyspepsia (3% to 9%), constipation (4% to 7%), flatulence (3% to 7%), nausea (3% to 7%), gastroenteritis (3% to 4%), diarrhea (3%), abdominal cramps, bloating, carbohydrate intolerance, gallbladder disease, pancreatitis, vomiting
Genitourinary: Mastalgia (5% to 35%), vaginal hemorrhage (33%), breast tenderness (3% to 17%), endometrium disease (15%), breakthrough bleeding (6% to 11%), leukorrhea (2% to 11%), abnormal uterine bleeding (4% to 10%), breast hypertrophy (7%), dysmenorrhea (7%), cervical polyp (6%), vulvovaginal candidiasis (6%), urinary tract infection (4% to 6%), change in cervical ectropion, change in cervical secretions, endometrial hyperplasia, nipple discharge, spotting, uterine fibroids (size increased), uterine pain, vaginal discomfort (vaginal ring; burning, irritation, itching), vaginitis
Hematologic & oncologic: Hemorrhagic eruption, hypercoagulability state, malignant neoplasm of breast, ovarian cancer
Hepatic: Cholestatic jaundice, exacerbation of hepatic hemangioma
Hypersensitivity: Hypersensitivity reaction (4% to 5%), anaphylactoid reaction, anaphylaxis, angioedema
Infection: Infection (3% to 12%), fungal infection (3% to 10%)
Local: Application site reaction (gel, spray, transdermal patch ≤1%)
Neuromuscular & skeletal: Arthralgia (4% to 12%), back pain (3% to 11%), weakness (8%), limb pain (7% to 8%), myalgia (5% to 6%), neck pain (3% to 6%), arthropathy (4% to 5%), exacerbation of systemic lupus erythematosus, leg cramps
Ophthalmic: Conjunctivitis (3%), change in corneal curvature (steepening), contact lens intolerance
Otic: Otitis media (3%)
Respiratory: Nasopharyngitis (4% to 20%), upper respiratory tract infection (6% to 17%), flu-like symptoms (8% to 13%), sinusitis (4% to 13%), sinus headache (9% to 11%), bronchitis (6% to 8%), sinus congestion (7%), pharyngitis (2% to 7%), rhinitis (2% to 6%), cough (3% to 4%), asthma (3%), exacerbation of asthma
Miscellaneous: Accidental injury (7% to 14%), cyst (7%)
Postmarketing and/or case reports: Abnormal gait, abnormal hepatic function tests, aphasia, blindness, bowel obstruction (vaginal ring), chest pain, cholecystitis, cholelithiasis, cognitive dysfunction, dyspnea, emotional lability, fatigue, genitourinary complaint (inadvertent ring insertion into the bladder should be considered with unexplained urinary complaints), hemorrhage, hepatitis, hyperhidrosis, hypermenorrhea, ischemic heart disease, lip swelling, local irritation (transdermal patch), localized erythema (transdermal patch), malaise, mechanical complication of genitourinary device (ring adherence to vaginal or bladder wall), meningioma, muscle spasm, myoclonus, night sweats, oral paresthesia, ovarian cyst, palpitations, paresthesia, peripheral edema, pharyngeal edema, phlebitis, portal vein thrombosis, purpura, retinal vein occlusion, soft tissue sarcoma (malignant mesenchymoma), swollen tongue, tachyphylaxis, toxic shock syndrome (vaginal ring), transient ischemic attacks, unstable angina pectoris, uterine enlargement, uterine neoplasm, vaginal discharge

Mechanism of Action Estrogens are responsible for the development and maintenance of the female reproductive system and secondary sexual characteristics. Estradiol is the principle intracellular human estrogen and is more potent than estrone and estriol at the receptor level; it is the primary estrogen secreted prior to menopause. Following menopause, estrone and estrone sulfate are more highly produced. Estrogens modulate the pituitary secretion of gonadotropins, luteinizing hormone, and follicle-stimulating hormone through a negative feedback system; estrogen replacement reduces elevated levels of these hormones in postmenopausal women.

Pregnancy Considerations

Products approved for use only in postmenopausal women are not appropriate for use in pregnancy; use of some products is specifically contraindicated in the manufacturer's labeling.

In general, the use of estrogen and progestin as in combination hormonal contraceptives has not been associated with teratogenic effects when inadvertently taken early in pregnancy.

◆ **Estradiol Acetate** *see* Estradiol (Systemic) *on page 596*

Estradiol and Dienogest

(es tra DYE ole & dye EN oh jest)

Related Information

Dienogest *on page 493*
Endocrine Disorders and Pregnancy *on page 1684*
Estradiol (Systemic) *on page 596*

Brand Names: US Natazia

Pharmacologic Category Contraceptive; Estrogen and Progestin Combination

Use

Contraception: Prevention of pregnancy.

Limitations of use: Efficacy has not been evaluated in women with a BMI >30 kg/m^2.

Heavy menstrual bleeding: Treatment of heavy menstrual bleeding in women without organic pathology who choose to use an oral contraceptive as their method for contraception.

Local Anesthetic/Vasoconstrictor Precautions No information available to require special precautions

Effects on Dental Treatment No significant effects or complications reported

Effects on Bleeding No information available to require special precautions

Adverse Reactions

>10%: Central nervous system: Headache (13%, including migraine)

1% to 10%:

Central nervous system: Mood changes (3%, including depression)
Dermatologic: Acne vulgaris (4%)
Endocrine & metabolic: Menstrual disease (≤7% to 8%), breast changes (discomfort: ≤7%), weight gain (3%)
Gastrointestinal: Nausea (≤7%), vomiting (≤7%)

Genitourinary: Uterine hemorrhage (≤7% to 8%), breast tenderness (≤7%), mastalgia (≤7%)

Mechanism of Action Combination hormonal contraceptives inhibit ovulation and may also cause changes in the cervical mucus, rendering it unfavorable for sperm penetration even if ovulation occurs. The four-phasic formulation provides the estrogen in decreasing concentrations and the progestin in increasing concentrations over the 28-day cycle.

Pharmacodynamics/Kinetics

Half-life Elimination Estradiol: ~14 hours; Dienogest: ~11 hours

Time to Peak Estradiol: ~6 hours; Dienogest: ~1 hour

Reproductive Considerations

The manufacturer does not recommend use until ≥4 weeks after delivery in women who choose not to breastfeed or ≥4 weeks after a second trimester abortion.

Due to the increased risk of venous thromboembolism (VTE) postpartum, combination hormonal contraceptives should not be started in any woman <21 days following delivery. The risk decreases to baseline by postpartum day 42. Use of combination hormonal contraceptives in women between 21 and 42 days after delivery should take into consideration the individual woman's risk factors for VTE (eg, age ≥35 years, previous VTE, thrombophilia, immobility, preeclampsia, transfusion at delivery, cesarean delivery, peripartum cardiomyopathy, BMI ≥30 kg/m^2, postpartum hemorrhage, smoking) (Curtis 2016b).

Pregnancy Considerations

Use is contraindicated in pregnant women. Combination hormonal contraceptives are used to prevent pregnancy; treatment should be discontinued if pregnancy occurs. In general, the use of combination hormonal contraceptives when inadvertently taken early in pregnancy has not been associated with adverse fetal or maternal effects (Curtis 2016b).

◆ **Estradiol and Drospirenone** *see* Drospirenone and Estradiol *on page 534*

Estradiol and Levonorgestrel

(es tra DYE ole & LEE voe nor jes trel)

Related Information

Endocrine Disorders and Pregnancy *on page 1684*

Estradiol (Systemic) *on page 596*

Brand Names: US Climara Pro

Brand Names: Canada Climara Pro

Pharmacologic Category Estrogen and Progestin Combination

Use

Moderate to severe vasomotor symptoms: Treatment of moderate to severe vasomotor symptoms associated with menopause in women with an intact uterus

Osteoporosis prevention: Prevention of postmenopausal osteoporosis in women with an intact uterus

Limitations of use: Osteoporosis: For use only in women at significant risk of osteoporosis and for whom other nonestrogen medications are not considered appropriate

Local Anesthetic/Vasoconstrictor Precautions No information available to require special precautions

Effects on Dental Treatment No significant effects or complications reported

Effects on Bleeding No information available to require special precautions related to hemostasis in dental procedures.

Adverse Reactions Percentages reported as greater in ClimaraPro when compared to estradiol alone.

>10%:

Central nervous system: Depression (12%)

Genitourinary: Vaginal hemorrhage (78%), mastalgia (40%)

Local: Application site reaction (86%)

Neuromuscular & skeletal: Back pain (13%)

Respiratory: Upper respiratory tract infection (28%)

1% to 10%: Cardiovascular: Edema (8%)

Mechanism of Action Estrogens are responsible for the development and maintenance of the female reproductive system and secondary sexual characteristics. Estradiol is the principle intracellular human estrogen and is more potent than estrone and estriol at the receptor level; it is the primary estrogen secreted prior to menopause. Following menopause, estrone and estrone sulfate are more highly produced. Estrogens modulate the pituitary secretion of gonadotropins, luteinizing hormone, and follicle-stimulating hormone through a negative feedback system; estrogen replacement reduces elevated levels of these hormones in postmenopausal women.

Levonorgestrel inhibits gonadotropin production; when used in this combination, it counteracts the proliferative effects of estradiol on the endometrium.

Pharmacodynamics/Kinetics

Half-life Elimination Estradiol: 3 ± 0.67 hours; Levonorgestrel: 28 ± 6.4 hours

Time to Peak Serum: Topical: Estradiol (mean): 2-2.5 days; Levonorgestrel: 2.5 days

Pregnancy Considerations

Use during pregnancy is contraindicated.

Refer to individual monographs.

◆ **Estradiol and NGM** *see* Estradiol and Norgestimate *on page 599*

Estradiol and Norethindrone

(es tra DYE ole & nor eth IN drone)

Related Information

Endocrine Disorders and Pregnancy *on page 1684*

Estradiol (Systemic) *on page 596*

Norethindrone *on page 1117*

Brand Names: US Activella; Amabelz; CombiPatch; Lopreeza; Mimvey; Mimvey Lo [DSC]

Brand Names: Canada Activelle; Activelle LD; Estalis

Pharmacologic Category Estrogen and Progestin Combination

Use

Hypoestrogenism (female) (patch): Treatment of hypoestrogenism due to hypogonadism, castration, or primary ovarian failure

Osteoporosis prevention (females): (tablet): Prevention of postmenopausal osteoporosis

Limitations of use: For use only in women at significant risk of postmenopausal osteoporosis; consider use of nonestrogen medications.

Vasomotor symptoms associated with menopause (patch, tablet): Treatment of moderate to severe vasomotor symptoms associated with menopause

Vulvar and vaginal atrophy associated with menopause (patch, tablet): Treatment of moderate to severe vulvar and vaginal atrophy associated with menopause

Limitations of use: When used solely for the treatment of vulvar and vaginal atrophy, topical vaginal products should be considered.

Note: The International Society for the Study of Women's Sexual Health and The North American Menopause Society have endorsed the term genitourinary syndrome of menopause (GSM) as new terminology for vulvovaginal atrophy. The term GSM encompasses all genital and urinary signs and symptoms associated with a loss of estrogen due to menopause Portman 2014.

Local Anesthetic/Vasoconstrictor Precautions No information available to require special precautions

Effects on Dental Treatment No significant effects or complications reported

Effects on Bleeding No information available to require special precautions related to hemostasis in dental procedures.

Adverse Reactions Frequency not always defined.

Cardiovascular: Peripheral edema (transdermal: 6%)

Central nervous system: Headache (11% to 25%), pain (transdermal: 15% to 19%), depression (transdermal: 8% to 9%), insomnia (6% to 8%), dizziness (transdermal: 6% to 7%), nervousness (transdermal: 3% to 6%), emotional lability (oral: 1% to 6%)

Dermatologic: Skin rash (transdermal: 5% to 6%), acne vulgaris (transdermal: 4% to 5%)

Endocrine & metabolic: Menstrual disease (transdermal: 6% to 19%), weight gain (oral: ≤9%), ovarian cyst (oral: 3% to 7%), breast hypertrophy (transdermal: 2% to 7%), hypermenorrhea (transdermal: 2% to 5%)

Gastrointestinal: Diarrhea (transdermal: 9% to 14%), abdominal pain (transdermal: 6% to 14%), nausea (3% to 12%), dyspepsia (transdermal: 6% to 8%), flatulence (transdermal: 5% to 7%), gastroenteritis (oral: 2% to 6%), constipation (transdermal: 2% to 5%)

Genitourinary: Mastalgia (transdermal: 25% to 48%; oral: 17% to 24%), dysmenorrhea (transdermal: 20% to 31%), vaginal hemorrhage (oral: 26%; transdermal: 3% to 6%), vaginitis (transdermal: 6% to 13%), postmenopausal bleeding (oral: 5% to 11%), leukorrhea (transdermal: 5% to 10%), endometrial hyperplasia (oral: ≤1% to 10%), abnormal pap smear (transdermal: 8%), vulvovaginal candidiasis (oral: 4% to 6%)

Hematologic & oncologic: Uterine fibroids (oral: 5%)

Infection: Infection (transdermal: 3% to 5%), viral infection (oral: 4%)

Local: Application site reaction (transdermal: 6% to 23%)

Neuromuscular & skeletal: Back pain (6% to 15%), weakness (transdermal: 8% to 13%), arthralgia (transdermal: 6%), limb pain (oral: 5%)

Respiratory: Rhinitis (transdermal: 13% to 22%), nasopharyngitis (oral: 21%), upper respiratory tract infection (oral: 10% to 18%), sinusitis (7% to 15%), flu-like symptoms (transdermal: 9% to 14%), respiratory tract disease (transdermal: 9% to 13%), pharyngitis (transdermal: 4% to 10%), bronchitis (transdermal: 3% to 5%)

Miscellaneous: Accidental injury (3% to 17%)

<1%, postmarketing, and/or case reports: Alopecia, altered blood pressure, anaphylactoid reaction, anaphylaxis, angioedema, bloating, breast tenderness, carbohydrate intolerance, cerebrovascular accident, cervical polyp, change in appetite, change in cervical secretions, change in corneal curvature, change in libido, chloasma, cholelithiasis, cholestatic jaundice, chorea, contact lens intolerance, cystitis-like syndrome, dementia, edema, endometrial carcinoma, erythema multiforme, erythema nodosum, exacerbation of asthma, exacerbation of endometriosis, exacerbation of porphyria, fallopian tube disease (cyst), fatigue, fibrocystic breast changes, galactorrhea, gallbladder disease, hemorrhagic eruption, hirsutism, hypersensitivity, hypertension, increased serum transaminases, increased serum triglycerides, irregular menses, irritability, leg cramps, loss of scalp hair, malignant neoplasm of breast, migraine, mood changes, myalgia, myocardial infarction, nipple discharge, ovarian carcinoma, pancreatitis, paresthesia, premenstrual-like syndrome, pruritus, pulmonary thromboembolism, retinal thrombosis, seborrhea, significant cardiovascular event, skin discoloration, stomach cramps, thrombophlebitis, uterine fibroids (size increased), uterine spasm, varicose veins, venous thromboembolism, vertigo, vomiting, weight loss

Pharmacodynamics/Kinetics

Half-life Elimination Oral tablet: Estradiol: 12 to 14 hours; Norethindrone: 8 to 11 hours

Time to Peak Oral tablet: Estradiol: 5 to 8 hours; Norethindrone: 0.5 to 1.5 hours

Pregnancy Considerations Use during pregnancy is contraindicated.

Not for use prior to menopause. Refer to individual monographs.

Estradiol and Norgestimate

(es tra DYE ole & nor JES ti mate)

Related Information

Endocrine Disorders and Pregnancy *on page 1684*

Estradiol (Systemic) *on page 596*

Rheumatoid Arthritis, Osteoarthritis, and Osteoporosis *on page 1697*

Brand Names: US Prefest

Pharmacologic Category Estrogen and Progestin Combination

Use

Osteoporosis prevention: Prevention of osteoporosis

Limitations of use: For use only in women at significant risk of postmenopausal osteoporosis; consider use of nonestrogen medications.

Vasomotor symptoms associated with menopause: Treatment of moderate to severe vasomotor symptoms

Vulvar and vaginal atrophy associated with menopause: Treatment of moderate to severe symptoms of vulvar and vaginal atrophy

Limitations of use: When used solely for the treatment of vulvar and vaginal atrophy, topical vaginal products should be considered.

Note: The International Society for the Study of Women's Sexual Health and The North American Menopause Society have endorsed the term genitourinary syndrome of menopause (GSM) as new terminology for vulvovaginal atrophy. The term GSM encompasses all genital and urinary signs and symptoms associated with a loss of estrogen due to menopause Portman 2014.

Local Anesthetic/Vasoconstrictor Precautions No information available to require special precautions

Effects on Dental Treatment No significant effects or complications reported

Effects on Bleeding No information available to require special precautions related to hemostasis in dental procedures.

Adverse Reactions

>10%:

Central nervous system: Headache (23%)

Gastrointestinal: Abdominal pain (12%)

Genitourinary: Mastalgia (16%)

Neuromuscular & skeletal: Back pain (12%)

Respiratory: Upper respiratory tract infection (21%), flu-like symptoms (11%)

1% to 10%:

Central nervous system: Fatigue (6%), pain (6%), depression (5%), dizziness (5%)

Gastrointestinal: Nausea (6%), flatulence (5%)

Genitourinary: Vaginal hemorrhage (9%), dysmenorrhea (8%), vaginitis (7%)

Infection: Viral infection (6%)

Neuromuscular & skeletal: Arthralgia (9%), myalgia (5%)

Respiratory: Sinusitis (8%), pharyngitis (7%), cough (5%)

Mechanism of Action Estrogens are responsible for the development and maintenance of the female reproductive system and secondary sexual characteristics. Estradiol is the principle intracellular human estrogen and is more potent than estrone and estriol at the receptor level; it is the primary estrogen secreted prior to menopause. Following menopause, estrone and estrone sulfate are more highly produced. Estrogens modulate the pituitary secretion of gonadotropins, luteinizing hormone, and follicle-stimulating hormone through a negative feedback system; estrogen replacement reduces elevated levels of these hormones in postmenopausal women.

Progestins inhibit gonadotropin production which then prevents follicular maturation and ovulation. In women with adequate estrogen, progestins transform a proliferative endometrium into a secretory endometrium; when administered with estradiol, reduces the incidence of endometrial hyperplasia and risk of adenocarcinoma.

Pharmacodynamics/Kinetics

Half-life Elimination Norgestimate: 17-deacetylnorgestimate: 37 hours

Time to Peak Norgestimate: ~2 hours

Pregnancy Considerations Use is contraindicated in pregnant women.

In general, the use of estrogen and progestin as in combination hormonal contraceptives has not been associated with teratogenic effects when inadvertently taken early in pregnancy.

◆ **Estradiol, elagolix, and norethindrone** *see* Elagolix, Estradiol, and Norethindrone *on page* *547*

◆ **Estradiol/Levonorgestrel** *see* Estradiol and Levonorgestrel *on page* *598*

◆ **Estradiol/Norethindrone Acet** *see* Estradiol and Norethindrone *on page* *598*

◆ **Estradiol, norethindrone, and elagolix** *see* Elagolix, Estradiol, and Norethindrone *on page* *547*

◆ **Estradiol Transdermal** *see* Estradiol (Systemic) *on page* *596*

◆ **Estradiol Valerate** *see* Estradiol (Systemic) *on page* *596*

◆ **Estradiol Valerate and Dienogest** *see* Estradiol and Dienogest *on page* *597*

◆ **Estradiol Valerate/Dienogest** *see* Estradiol and Dienogest *on page* *597*

Estramustine (es tra MUS teen)

Brand Names: US Emcyt

Brand Names: Canada Emcyt [DSC]

Pharmacologic Category Antineoplastic Agent, Alkylating Agent; Antineoplastic Agent, Antimicrotubular; Antineoplastic Agent, Hormone (Estrogen/Nitrogen Mustard)

Local Anesthetic/Vasoconstrictor Precautions No information available to require special precautions

Effects on Dental Treatment No significant effects or complications reported

Effects on Bleeding Thrombocytopenia has been reported in a small number of patients

Adverse Reactions Frequency not always defined.

>10%:

Cardiovascular: Edema (20%)

Endocrine & metabolic: Gynecomastia (75%), increased lactate dehydrogenase (2% to 33%), decreased libido

Gastrointestinal: Nausea (16%), diarrhea (13%), gastrointestinal irritation (12%)

Genitourinary: Breast tenderness (71%)

Hepatic: Increased serum AST (2% to 33%)

Respiratory: Dyspnea (12%)

1% to 10%:

Cardiovascular: Cardiac failure (3%), local thrombophlebitis (3%), myocardial infarction (3%), cerebrovascular accident (2%), pulmonary embolism (2%), chest pain (1%), flushing (1%)

Central nervous system: Lethargy (4%), insomnia (3%), emotional lability (2%), anxiety (1%), headache (1%)

Dermatologic: Pruritus (2%), xeroderma (2%), exfoliation of skin (1%), skin rash (1%), thinning hair (1%)

Endocrine & metabolic: Increased thirst (1%)

Gastrointestinal: Anorexia (4%), flatulence (2%), gastrointestinal hemorrhage (1%), sore throat (1%), vomiting (1%)

Hematologic & oncologic: Leukopenia (4%), bruise (3%), thrombocytopenia (1%)

Hepatic: Increased serum bilirubin (1% to 2%)

Neuromuscular & skeletal: Leg cramps (9%)

Ophthalmic: Lacrimation (1%)

Respiratory: Hoarseness (1%), rhinorrhea (1%)

<1%, postmarketing, and/or case reports: Anemia, angina pectoris, angioedema, cerebral ischemia, confusion, depression, decreased glucose tolerance, hypercalcemia, hypocalcemia, hypersensitivity reaction, hypertension, impotence, ischemic heart disease, myasthenia, venous thrombosis

Mechanism of Action Estramustine is an estradiol and nornitrogen mustard carbamate-linked combination which has antiandrogen effects (due to estradiol) and antimicrotubule effects (due to nornitrogen mustard); it causes a marked decrease in plasma testosterone and an increase in estrogen levels.

Pharmacodynamics/Kinetics

Half-life Elimination Estromustine: 13.6 hours (range: 9 to 23 hours); Estrone: 16.5 hours (Bergenheim 1998)

Time to Peak 2 to 3 hours (Bergenheim 1998)

Reproductive Considerations
Some men who were impotent on estrogen therapy have regained potency while taking estramustine; effective contraception should be used for male patients with partners of childbearing potential.
Pregnancy Considerations Estramustine is not indicated for use in women.

- ◆ **Estramustine Phosphate** *see* Estramustine *on page 600*
- ◆ **Estramustine Phosphate Sodium** *see* Estramustine *on page 600*
- ◆ **Estratest** *see* Estrogens (Esterified) and Methyltestosterone *on page 605*
- ◆ **Estrogel** *see* Estradiol (Systemic) *on page 596*
- ◆ **Estrogenic Substances, Conjugated** *see* Estrogens (Conjugated/Equine, Systemic) *on page 601*
- ◆ **Estrogenic Substances, Conjugated** *see* Estrogens (Conjugated/Equine, Topical) *on page 602*

Estrogens (Conjugated B/Synthetic)
(ES troe jenz, KON joo gate ed, bee, sin THET ik)

Related Information
Endocrine Disorders and Pregnancy *on page 1684*
Pharmacologic Category Estrogen Derivative
Use
Vasomotor symptoms associated with menopause: Treatment of moderate to severe vasomotor symptoms associated with menopause
Vulvar and vaginal atrophy associated with menopause: Treatment of moderate to severe vaginal dryness and pain with intercourse, symptoms of vulvar and vaginal atrophy, associated with menopause
Limitations of use: When used solely for the treatment of vulvar and vaginal atrophy, topical vaginal products should be considered.
Note: The International Society for the Study of Women's Sexual Health and The North American Menopause Society have endorsed the term genitourinary syndrome of menopause (GSM) as new terminology for vulvovaginal atrophy. The term GSM encompasses all genital and urinary signs and symptoms associated with a loss of estrogen due to menopause (Portman 2014).
Local Anesthetic/Vasoconstrictor Precautions No information available to require special precautions
Effects on Dental Treatment No significant effects or complications reported
Effects on Bleeding No information available to require special precautions related to hemostasis in dental procedures.
Adverse Reactions
>10%:
Central nervous system: Headache (25%), pain (10% to 19%)
Gastrointestinal: Abdominal pain (4% to 15%), nausea (10% to 12%)
Genitourinary: Mastalgia (13% to 15%)
1% to 10%:
Cardiovascular: Peripheral edema (4%), chest pain (3% to 4%)
Central nervous system: Dizziness (7%), paresthesia (1% to 6%), chills (4%), depression (3% to 4%), emotional lability (3% to 4%)
Dermatologic: Pruritus (6%), fungal dermatitis (2% to 4%), acne vulgaris (1% to 4%)
Gastrointestinal: Flatulence (4% to 7%), constipation (4%)
Genitourinary: Dysmenorrhea (8%), vaginitis (7%), breast tenderness (4%)
Neuromuscular & skeletal: Back pain (4%), weakness (3% to 4%)
Respiratory: Bronchitis (7%), rhinitis (7%), flu-like symptoms (6% to 7%), sinusitis (4% to 7%), increased cough (4%), upper respiratory tract infection (4%), pharyngitis (3% to 4%)
Miscellaneous: Accidental injury (9%)
<1%, postmarketing, and/or case reports: Abdominal distention, abdominal distress, alopecia, anaphylaxis, deep vein thrombosis, dementia, exacerbation of endometriosis (including malignant transformation), gallbladder disease, hypercalcemia, hypersensitivity reaction, insomnia, muscle spasm, retinal thrombosis, skin rash, thrombosis, urticaria
Mechanism of Action Conjugated B/synthetic estrogens contain a mixture of 10 synthetic estrogen substances, including sodium estrone sulfate, sodium equilin sulfate, sodium 17-alpha-dihydroequilin, sodium 17-alpha-estradiol, and sodium 17-beta-dihydroequilin. Estrogens are responsible for the development and maintenance of the female reproductive system and secondary sexual characteristics. Estradiol is the principle intracellular human estrogen and is more potent than estrone and estriol at the receptor level; it is the primary estrogen secreted prior to menopause. Following menopause, estrone and estrone sulfate are more highly produced. Estrogens modulate the pituitary secretion of gonadotropins, luteinizing hormone, and follicle-stimulating hormone through a negative feedback system; estrogen replacement reduces elevated levels of these hormones in postmenopausal women.
Pharmacodynamics/Kinetics
Half-life Elimination Conjugated estrone: 8-20 hours; conjugated equilin: 5-17 hours
Pregnancy Considerations Use is contraindicated in pregnant women.

In general, the use of estrogen and progestin as in combination hormonal contraceptives have not been associated with teratogenic effects when inadvertently taken early in pregnancy.
Product Availability Enjuvia has been discontinued in the US for more than 1 year.

Estrogens (Conjugated/Equine, Systemic)
(ES troe jenz KON joo gate ed, EE kwine)

Related Information
Endocrine Disorders and Pregnancy *on page 1684*
Brand Names: US Premarin
Brand Names: Canada C.E.S.; Congest; PMS-Conjugated Estrogens [DSC]; Premarin
Pharmacologic Category Estrogen Derivative
Use
Abnormal uterine bleeding (injection only): Treatment of abnormal uterine bleeding due to hormonal imbalance in the absence of organic pathology.
Limitations of use: For short term use only to provide a rapid and temporary increase in estrogen levels.
Breast cancer, metastatic: Treatment of breast cancer (palliation) in appropriately selected men and postmenopausal women.
Hypoestrogenism (female): Treatment of hypoestrogenism due to hypogonadism, castration, or primary ovarian failure.
Osteoporosis prevention (female): Prevention of postmenopausal osteoporosis.

Limitations of use: For use only in women at significant risk of osteoporosis; consider use of nonestrogen medications.

Prostate cancer, advanced: Treatment of androgen-dependent prostatic cancer (palliation).

Vasomotor symptoms associated with menopause: Treatment of moderate to severe vasomotor symptoms associated with menopause.

Vulvar and vaginal atrophy associated with menopause: Treatment of moderate to severe vulvar and vaginal atrophy due to menopause.

Limitations of use: When used solely for the treatment of vulvar and vaginal atrophy, topical vaginal products should be considered.

Note: The International Society for the Study of Women's Sexual Health and The North American Menopause Society have endorsed the term genitourinary syndrome of menopause (GSM) as new terminology for vulvovaginal atrophy. The term GSM encompasses all genital and urinary signs and symptoms associated with a loss of estrogen due to menopause (Portman 2014).

Local Anesthetic/Vasoconstrictor Precautions No information available to require special precautions

Effects on Dental Treatment No significant effects or complications reported

Effects on Bleeding No information available to require special precautions

Adverse Reactions Percentages reported in postmenopausal women following oral use.

>10%:

Central nervous system: Headache (26% to 32%), pain (17% to 20%)

Gastrointestinal: Abdominal pain (15% to 17%)

Genitourinary: Vaginal hemorrhage (2% to 14%), mastalgia (7% to 12%)

Neuromuscular & skeletal: Back pain (13% to 14%), arthralgia (7% to 14%)

Respiratory: Pharyngitis (10% to 12%), sinusitis (6% to 11%)

1% to 10%:

Central nervous system: Depression (5% to 8%), dizziness (4% to 6%), nervousness (2% to 5%)

Dermatologic: Pruritus (4% to 5%)

Gastrointestinal: Diarrhea (6% to 7%), flatulence (6% to 7%)

Genitourinary: Vaginitis (5% to 7%), leukorrhea (4% to 7%), vulvovaginal candidiasis (5% to 6%)

Neuromuscular & skeletal: Weakness (7% to 8%), leg cramps (3% to 7%)

Respiratory: Increased cough (4% to 7%)

Frequency not defined (injection): Local: Injection site phlebitis, pain at injection site, swelling at injection site

<1%, postmarketing, and/or case reports: Abnormal uterine bleeding, alopecia, anaphylaxis, angioedema, bloating, breast hypertrophy, breast tenderness, cerebrovascular accident, change in cervical secretions, change in libido, chloasma, cholestatic jaundice, contact lens intolerance, decreased glucose tolerance, deep vein thrombosis, dementia, dysmenorrhea, edema, endometrial carcinoma, endometrial hyperplasia, erythema multiforme, erythema nodosum, exacerbation of asthma, exacerbation of epilepsy, exacerbation of hepatic hemangioma, exacerbation of porphyria, fibrocystic breast changes, galactorrhea, gallbladder disease, growth potentiation of benign meningioma, gynecomastia, hirsutism, hypersensitivity reaction, hypertension, increased serum triglycerides, irritability, ischemic colitis, malignant neoplasm of breast, migraine, mood changes, myocardial infarction, nausea, nipple discharge, ovarian carcinoma, pancreatitis, pelvic pain, pulmonary embolism, retinal thrombosis, skin rash, superficial venous thrombosis, thrombophlebitis, urticaria, uterine fibroids (increased size), vomiting, vulvovaginal candidiasis, weight changes

Mechanism of Action Conjugated estrogens contain a mixture of estrone sulfate, equilin sulfate, 17 alpha-dihydroequilin, 17 alpha-estradiol and 17 beta-dihydroequilin. Estrogens are responsible for the development and maintenance of the female reproductive system and secondary sexual characteristics. Estradiol is the principle intracellular human estrogen and is more potent than estrone and estriol at the receptor level; it is the primary estrogen secreted prior to menopause. Following menopause, estrone and estrone sulfate are more highly produced. Estrogens modulate the pituitary secretion of gonadotropins, luteinizing hormone, and follicle-stimulating hormone through a negative feedback system; estrogen replacement reduces elevated levels of these hormones in postmenopausal women.

Pharmacodynamics/Kinetics

Half-life Elimination Total estrone: 27 hours

Time to Peak Total estrone: 7 hours

Pregnancy Considerations Use is contraindicated during pregnancy.

Estrogens are not indicated for use during pregnancy or immediately postpartum. In general, the use of estrogen and progestin as in combination hormonal contraceptives have not been associated with teratogenic effects when inadvertently taken early in pregnancy.

Estrogens (Conjugated/Equine, Topical) (ES troe jenz KON joo gate ed, EE kwine)

Brand Names: US Premarin

Brand Names: Canada Premarin

Pharmacologic Category Estrogen Derivative

Use

Vulvar and vaginal atrophy associated with menopause: Treatment of atrophic vaginitis and kraurosis vulvae and moderate-to-severe dyspareunia (pain during intercourse) due to vaginal/vulvar atrophy of menopause

Note: The International Society for the Study of Women's Sexual Health and The North American Menopause Society have endorsed the term genitourinary syndrome of menopause (GSM) as new terminology for vulvovaginal atrophy. The term GSM encompasses all genital and urinary signs and symptoms associated with a loss of estrogen due to menopause (Portman 2014).

Local Anesthetic/Vasoconstrictor Precautions No information available to require special precautions

Effects on Dental Treatment No significant effects or complications reported

Effects on Bleeding No information available to require special precautions

Adverse Reactions Due to systemic absorption, other adverse effects associated with systemic therapy may also occur. Frequency of adverse events reported with daily use.

1% to 10%:

Cardiovascular: Vasodilation (4%)

Central nervous system: Pain (7%)

Gastrointestinal: Abdominal pain (8%)

Genitourinary: Mastalgia (6%), vaginitis (6%)

Neuromuscular & skeletal: Weakness (6%), back pain (5%)

<1%, postmarketing, and/or case reports: Abdominal cramps, abnormal uterine bleeding, acne vulgaris, alopecia, anaphylaxis, application site reaction (application site burning, application site irritation, genital pruritus), arthralgia, bloating, breast hypertrophy, breast tenderness, cerebrovascular accident, change in cervical secretions, change in libido, chloasma, contact lens intolerance, cystitis-like syndrome, decreased glucose tolerance, deep vein thrombosis, dementia, depression, dizziness, dysmenorrhea, dysuria, edema, endometrial carcinoma, endometrial hyperplasia, exacerbation of asthma, fibrocystic breast changes, gallbladder disease, gynecomastia, headache, hirsutism, hypersensitivity reaction, hypertension, increased serum triglycerides, irritability, leg cramps, leukorrhea, malignant neoplasm of breast, migraine, mood disorder, muscle cramps, myocardial infarction, nausea, nervousness, nipple discharge, pelvic pain, polyuria, precocious puberty, pulmonary embolism, retinal thrombosis, skin rash, spotting, urinary tract infection, urinary urgency, urticaria, uterine fibroids (increase in size), vomiting, vulvovaginal disease, weight changes

Mechanism of Action Conjugated estrogens contain a mixture of estrone sulfate, equilin sulfate, 17 alpha-dihydroequilin, 17 alpha-estradiol and 17 beta-dihydroequilin. Estrogens are responsible for the development and maintenance of the female reproductive system and secondary sexual characteristics. Estradiol is the principle intracellular human estrogen and is more potent than estrone and estriol at the receptor level; it is the primary estrogen secreted prior to menopause. Following menopause, estrone and estrone sulfate are more highly produced. Estrogens modulate the pituitary secretion of gonadotropins, luteinizing hormone, and follicle-stimulating hormone through a negative feedback system; estrogen replacement reduces elevated levels of these hormones in postmenopausal women.

Pharmacodynamics/Kinetics

Time to Peak Total estrone: 6 hours

Reproductive Considerations

Use of the vaginal cream may weaken latex found in condoms, diaphragms, or cervical caps.

Pregnancy Considerations Use is contraindicated during pregnancy.

In general, the use of estrogen and progestin as in combination hormonal contraceptives have not been associated with teratogenic effects when inadvertently taken early in pregnancy.

Estrogens (Conjugated/Equine) and Bazedoxifene

(ES troe jenz, KON joo gate ed/EE kwine & ba ze DOX i feen)

Brand Names: US Duavee

Brand Names: Canada Duavive

Pharmacologic Category Estrogen Derivative; Selective Estrogen Receptor Modulator (SERM); Tissue-Selective Estrogen Complex (TSEC)

Use

Osteoporosis, prevention: Prevention of postmenopausal osteoporosis in females with a uterus.

Limitations of use: For use only in women at significant risk of postmenopausal osteoporosis; consider use of nonestrogen medications.

Vasomotor symptoms: Treatment of moderate-to-severe vasomotor symptoms associated with menopause in females with a uterus.

Local Anesthetic/Vasoconstrictor Precautions No information available to require special precautions

Effects on Dental Treatment No significant effects or complications reported

Effects on Bleeding No information available to require special precautions

Adverse Reactions Percentages as reported with combination product.

1% to 10%:

Central nervous system: Dizziness (5%)

Gastrointestinal: Diarrhea (8%), nausea (8%), dyspepsia (7%), upper abdominal pain (7%)

Neuromuscular & skeletal: Muscle spasm (9%), neck pain (5%)

Respiratory: Oropharyngeal pain (7%)

Mechanism of Action Conjugated estrogens contain a mixture of estrone sulfate, equilin sulfate, 17 alpha-dihydroequilin, 17 alpha-estradiol and 17 beta-dihydroequilin. Bazedoxifene is a selective estrogen receptor modulator (SERM). Conjugated estrogens act as an estrogen agonist and bazedoxifene acts as an estrogen agonist/antagonist depending on the specific tissue. The combination of a SERM and estrogen [referred to as a tissue-selective estrogen complex (TSEC)] provides relief of vasomotor symptoms and maintenance of bone mineral density in postmenopausal females with a uterus, while reducing the risk of endometrial hyperplasia observed with estrogen use alone (Pickar 2009).

Pharmacodynamics/Kinetics

Onset of Action

Relief of vasomotor symptoms: A significant reduction in the number and severity of moderate/severe hot flashes was observed after 4 weeks of therapy (Pinkerton, 2009).

Osteoporosis: A significant increase in BMD measured at the lumbar spine and hip was observed at 12 months of therapy (Lindsay, 2009).

Half-life Elimination

Bazedoxifene: ~30 hours

Total estrone: ~17 hours

Time to Peak

Bazedoxifene: ~2.5 hours

Total estrone: ~6.5 hours

Pregnancy Considerations

This combination product is approved for use in postmenopausal women only. Use is contraindicated during pregnancy.

◆ **Estrogens (Conjugated/Equine) and Bazedoxifene Acetate** *see* Estrogens (Conjugated/Equine) and Bazedoxifene *on page 603*

Estrogens (Conjugated/Equine) and Medroxyprogesterone

(ES troe jenz KON joo gate ed/EE kwine & me DROKS ee proe JES te rone)

Related Information

Endocrine Disorders and Pregnancy *on page 1684*

Estrogens (Conjugated/Equine, Systemic) *on page 601*

MedroxyPROGESTERone *on page 953*

Brand Names: US Premphase; Prempro

Brand Names: Canada Premplus [DSC]

Pharmacologic Category Estrogen and Progestin Combination

Use

Osteoporosis prevention (female): Prevention of postmenopausal osteoporosis

Limitations of use: For use only in women at significant risk of postmenopausal osteoporosis; consider use of nonestrogen medications.

Vasomotor symptoms associated with menopause: Treatment of moderate to severe vasomotor symptoms associated with menopause.

Vulvar and vaginal atrophy associated with menopause: Treatment of moderate to severe vulvar and vaginal atrophy associated with menopause.

Limitations of use: When used solely for the treatment of vulvar and vaginal atrophy, topical vaginal products should be considered.

Note: The International Society for the Study of Women's Sexual Health and The North American Menopause Society have endorsed the term genitourinary syndrome of menopause (GSM) as new terminology for vulvovaginal atrophy. The term GSM encompasses all genital and urinary signs and symptoms associated with a loss of estrogen due to menopause (Portman 2014).

Guideline recommendations: Due to safety considerations, when a progesterone is needed, use of micronized progesterone is preferred over medroxyprogesterone acetate (AACE [Goodman 2011]; AACE/ACE [Cobin 2017]).

Local Anesthetic/Vasoconstrictor Precautions No information available to require special precautions

Effects on Dental Treatment No significant effects or complications reported

Effects on Bleeding No information available to require special precautions related to hemostasis in dental procedures.

Adverse Reactions Also see individual agents.

>10%:

Central nervous system: Headache (15% to 19%)

Gastrointestinal: Abdominal pain (7% to 17%)

Genitourinary: Mastalgia (13% to 36%), dysmenorrhea (3% to 13%)

1% to 10%:

Cardiovascular: Edema (≤4%), peripheral edema (2% to 3%), hypertension (2%), vasodilation (≤2%), chest pain (1%), palpitations (≤1%)

Central nervous system: Depression (7% to 8%), pain (5%), emotional lability (3%), dizziness (2% to 3%), migraine (2% to 3%), nervousness (1% to 3%), anxiety (2%), hypertonia (1% to 2%), insomnia (1% to 2%)

Dermatologic: Pruritus (2% to 6%), skin rash (2%), acne vulgaris (≤2%), alopecia (≤2%), skin discoloration (1% to 2%), diaphoresis (≤1%), xeroderma (≤1%)

Endocrine & metabolic: Weight gain (3%), decreased glucose tolerance (≤1%), hypermenorrhea (≤1%)

Gastrointestinal: Nausea (6% to 8%), flatulence (4% to 8%), diarrhea (≤6%), constipation (2%), increased appetite (≤2%), eructation (≤1%)

Genitourinary: Leukorrhea (3% to 8%), breast hypertrophy (2% to 5%), pelvic pain (2% to 5%), vaginal hemorrhage (≤5%), vaginitis (2% to 4%), breakthrough bleeding (1% to 4%), uterine spasm (1% to 4%), vulvovaginal candidiasis (1% to 4%), cervical changes (1% to 3%), abnormal Pap smear (≤2%), breast engorgement (≤1%), urinary incontinence (≤1%)

Hematologic & oncologic: Malignant neoplasm of breast (≤1%)

Infection: Candidiasis (≤2%), infection (≤1%)

Neuromuscular & skeletal: Weakness (3% to 6%), back pain (2% to 7%), leg cramps (2% to 4%)

Respiratory: Pharyngitis (>5%), sinusitis (>5%), flu-like symptoms (≤1%)

<1%, postmarketing, and/or case reports: Abnormal uterine bleeding, amenorrhea, anaphylactoid reaction, anaphylaxis, angioedema, bloating, breast tenderness, cerebrovascular accident, change in appetite, change in cervical secretions, change in libido, chloasma, cholestatic jaundice, contact lens intolerance, cough, deep vein thrombosis, dementia, endometrial carcinoma, endometrial hyperplasia, erythema multiforme, erythema nodosum, exacerbation of asthma, exacerbation of epilepsy, exacerbation of tics, fibrocystic breast changes, galactorrhea, gallbladder disease, hirsutism, hypersensitivity reaction, increased serum triglycerides, irritability, ischemic colitis, malignant neoplasm of ovary, meningioma (benign; possible growth), myalgia, myocardial infarction, nipple discharge, pancreatitis, pulmonary embolism, retinal thrombosis, rhinitis, superficial venous thrombosis, thrombophlebitis, upper respiratory tract infection, urticaria, uterine fibroids (increase in size), vomiting, vulvovaginal candidiasis, weight loss

Mechanism of Action See individual agents.

Pregnancy Considerations Use is contraindicated in pregnant women.

In general, the use of estrogen and progestin as in combination hormonal contraceptives have not been associated with teratogenic effects when inadvertently taken early in pregnancy.

Estrogens (Esterified) (ES troe jenz, es TER i fied)

Related Information

Endocrine Disorders and Pregnancy *on page 1684*

Brand Names: US Menest

Brand Names: Canada Estragyn

Pharmacologic Category Estrogen Derivative

Use

Breast cancer, metastatic: Treatment of metastatic breast cancer (palliation) in appropriately selected men and postmenopausal women

Hypoestrogenism (female): Treatment of hypoestrogenism due to hypogonadism, castration, or primary ovarian failure

Prostate cancer: Palliative therapy of advanced prostatic carcinoma

Vasomotor symptoms associated with menopause: Treatment of moderate to severe vasomotor symptoms associated with menopause

Vulvar and vaginal atrophy associated with menopause: Treatment of moderate to severe symptoms of vulvar and vaginal atrophy associated with menopause

Limitations of use: When used solely for the treatment of vulvar and vaginal atrophy, topical vaginal products should be considered

Note: The International Society for the Study of Women's Sexual Health and The North American Menopause Society have endorsed the term genitourinary syndrome of menopause (GSM) as new terminology for vulvovaginal atrophy. The term GSM encompasses all genital and urinary signs and symptoms associated with a loss of estrogen due to menopause (Portman 2014).

Local Anesthetic/Vasoconstrictor Precautions No information available to require special precautions

Effects on Dental Treatment No significant effects or complications reported

Effects on Bleeding No information available to require special precautions related to hemostasis in dental procedures.

Adverse Reactions Frequency not defined.

Cardiovascular: Cerebrovascular accident, edema, hypertension, local thrombophlebitis, myocardial infarction, pulmonary embolism, retinal thrombosis, venous thromboembolism

Central nervous system: Chorea, dementia (exacerbation), depression, dizziness, exacerbation of epilepsy, headache, irritability, migraine, mood disorder, nervousness

Dermatologic: Chloasma, erythema multiforme, erythema nodosum, pruritus, loss of scalp hair, skin rash, urticaria

Endocrine & metabolic: Change in libido, exacerbation of porphyria, fibrocystic breast changes, galactorrhea, hirsutism, hypocalcemia, menstrual disease (alterations in frequency and flow of menstrual patterns), premenstrual-like syndrome, weight gain, weight loss

Gastrointestinal: Abdominal cramps, bloating, carbohydrate intolerance, gallbladder disease, nausea, pancreatitis, vomiting

Genitourinary: Breakthrough bleeding, breast hypertrophy, breast tenderness, change in cervical ectropion, change in cervical secretions, cystitis-like syndrome, dysmenorrhea, endometrial hyperplasia, nipple discharge, vulvovaginal candidiasis, vaginitis

Hematologic & oncologic: Endometrial carcinoma, hemorrhagic eruption, malignant neoplasm of breast, malignant neoplasm of ovary, uterine fibroids (increased size)

Hepatic: Cholestatic jaundice, exacerbation of hepatic hemangioma (enlargement)

Hypersensitivity: Anaphylactoid reaction, anaphylaxis, angioedema

Neuromuscular & skeletal: Arthralgia, leg cramps

Ophthalmic: Contact lens intolerance, change in corneal curvature (steepening)

Respiratory: Exacerbation of asthma

Mechanism of Action Esterified estrogens contain a mixture of estrogenic substances; the principle component is estrone. Preparations contain 75% to 85% sodium estrone sulfate and 6% to 15% sodium equilin sulfate such that the total is not <90%. Estrogens are responsible for the development and maintenance of the female reproductive system and secondary sexual characteristics. Estradiol is the principle intracellular human estrogen and is more potent than estrone and estriol at the receptor level; it is the primary estrogen secreted prior to menopause. In males and following menopause in females, estrone and estrone sulfate are more highly produced. Estrogens modulate the pituitary secretion of gonadotropins, luteinizing hormone, and follicle-stimulating hormone through a negative feedback system; estrogen replacement reduces elevated levels of these hormones.

Pregnancy Considerations

Estrogens esterified are contraindicated for use during pregnancy.

In general, the use of estrogen and progestin as in combination hormonal contraceptives have not been associated with teratogenic effects when inadvertently taken early in pregnancy.

Estrogens (Esterified) and Methyltestosterone

(ES troe jenz es TER i fied & meth il tes TOS te rone)

Related Information

Endocrine Disorders and Pregnancy *on page 1684*
Estrogens (Esterified) *on page 604*
MethylTESTOSTERone *on page 1006*

Brand Names: US Covaryx; Covaryx H.S.; EEMT; EEMT HS

Pharmacologic Category Estrogen and Androgen Combination

Use Vasomotor symptoms associated with menopause: Treatment of moderate to severe vasomotor symptoms associated with menopause not improved by estrogens alone

Local Anesthetic/Vasoconstrictor Precautions No information available to require special precautions

Effects on Dental Treatment No significant effects or complications reported

Effects on Bleeding No information available to require special precautions related to hemostasis in dental procedures.

Adverse Reactions Refer to the Estrogens (Esterified) and the Testosterone monographs.

Mechanism of Action

Conjugated estrogens: Activate estrogen receptors (DNA protein complex) located in estrogen-responsive tissues. Once activated, regulate transcription of certain genes leading to observed effects.

Testosterone: Increases synthesis of DNA, RNA, and various proteins in target tissues

Pregnancy Risk Factor X

Pregnancy Considerations [US Boxed Warning]: Estrogens should not be used during pregnancy. This product is specifically contraindicated during pregnancy.

Refer to the Estrogens (Esterified) monograph and the Testosterone monograph for additional information.

Controlled Substance C-III or nonscheduled (DEA exemption status dependent)

Estropipate (ES troe pih pate)

Related Information

Endocrine Disorders and Pregnancy *on page 1684*

Pharmacologic Category Estrogen Derivative

Use

Hypoestrogenism, female: Treatment of hypoestrogenism due to hypogonadism, castration, or primary ovarian failure.

Osteoporosis prevention: Prevention of postmenopausal osteoporosis.

Limitations of use: For use only in women at significant risk of postmenopausal osteoporosis; consider use of nonestrogen medications.

Vasomotor symptoms due to menopause: Treatment of moderate to severe vasomotor symptoms due to menopause.

Vulvar and vaginal atrophy due to menopause: Treatment of moderate to severe symptoms of vulvar and vaginal atrophy due to menopause.

Limitations of use: When used solely for the treatment of vulvar and vaginal atrophy, topical vaginal products should be considered.

Note: The International Society for the Study of Womens Sexual Health and The North American Menopause Society have endorsed the term genitourinary syndrome of menopause (GSM) as new terminology for vulvovaginal atrophy. The term GSM encompasses all genital and urinary signs and symptoms associated with a loss of estrogen due to menopause (Portman 2014).

Local Anesthetic/Vasoconstrictor Precautions No information available to require special precautions

Effects on Dental Treatment No significant effects or complications reported

Effects on Bleeding No information available to require special precautions related to hemostasis in dental procedures.

Adverse Reactions Frequency not defined.

Cardiovascular: Edema, hypertension, pulmonary thromboembolism, venous thromboembolism

Central nervous system: Chorea, depression, dizziness, headache, migraine

Dermatologic: Chloasma, erythema multiforme, erythema nodosum, loss of scalp hair

Endocrine & metabolic: Change in libido, exacerbation of porphyria, hirsutism, hypercalcemia, impaired glucose tolerance, increased HDL cholesterol, decreased LDL cholesterol, increased serum triglycerides, increased T4, increased thyroxine binding globulin, menstrual disease (alterations in frequency and flow of menses), phospholipidemia, weight gain, weight loss

Gastrointestinal: Abdominal cramps, bloating, carbohydrate intolerance, cholecystitis, cholelithiasis, gallbladder disease, nausea, pancreatitis, vomiting

Genitourinary: Breast hypertrophy, breast tenderness, vulvovaginal candidiasis

Hematologic & oncologic: Change in platelet count (increase), decreased antifactor Xa, decreased antithrombin III plasma level, endometrial carcinoma, hemorrhagic eruption, increased clotting factor VII, increased clotting factor VIII, increased clotting factor IX, increased clotting factor X, increased platelet aggregation, increased serum fibrinogen, prolonged prothrombin time, uterine fibroids (increased size)

Hepatic: Cholestatic jaundice

Ophthalmic: Change in corneal curvature (steepening), contact lens intolerance

Mechanism of Action Estropipate is prepared from naturally occurring estrone. Estrogens are responsible for the development and maintenance of the female reproductive system and secondary sexual characteristics. Estradiol is the principle intracellular human estrogen and is more potent than estrone and estriol at the receptor level; it is the primary estrogen secreted prior to menopause. In males and following menopause in females, estrone and estrone sulfate are more highly produced. Estrogens modulate the pituitary secretion of gonadotropins, luteinizing hormone, and follicle-stimulating hormone through a negative feedback system; estrogen replacement reduces elevated levels of these hormones. Estropipate is prepared from purified crystalline estrone that has been solubilized as the sulfate and stabilized with piperazine.

Pregnancy Considerations Use is contraindicated in pregnant women.

In general, the use of estrogen and progestin as in combination hormonal contraceptives has not been associated with teratogenic effects when inadvertently taken early in pregnancy.

- ◆ **Estrostep 21** *see* Ethinyl Estradiol and Norethindrone *on page 614*
- ◆ **Estrostep Fe** *see* Ethinyl Estradiol and Norethindrone *on page 614*

Eszopiclone (es zoe PIK lone)

Brand Names: US Lunesta

Pharmacologic Category Hypnotic, Miscellaneous

Use Insomnia: Treatment of insomnia

Local Anesthetic/Vasoconstrictor Precautions No information available to require special precautions

Effects on Dental Treatment Key adverse event(s) related to dental treatment: Unpleasant taste and xerostomia (normal salivary flow resumes upon discontinuation).

Effects on Bleeding No information available to require special precautions

Adverse Reactions

>10%:

Central nervous system: Headache (15% to 21%)

Gastrointestinal: Dysgeusia (8% to 34%)

1% to 10%:

Cardiovascular: Chest pain (≥1%), peripheral edema (≥1%)

Central nervous system: Drowsiness (8% to 10%), dizziness (5% to 7%), pain (4% to 5%), nervousness (≤5%), depression (1% to 4%), confusion (≤3%), neuralgia (≤3%), abnormal dreams (1% to 3%), anxiety (1% to 3%), hallucination (1% to 3%), migraine

Dermatologic: Skin rash (3% to 4%), pruritus (1% to 4%)

Endocrine & metabolic: Decreased libido (≤3%), gynecomastia (≤3%)

Gastrointestinal: Xerostomia (3% to 7%), dyspepsia (2% to 6%), nausea (4% to 5%), diarrhea (2% to 4%), vomiting (≤3%)

Genitourinary: Dysmenorrhea (≤3%), urinary tract infection (≤3%)

Infection: Infection (5% to 10%), viral infection (3%)

Miscellaneous: Accidental injury (≤3%)

<1%, postmarketing, and/or case reports: Abnormal gait, abnormality in thinking, agitation, alopecia, altered sense of smell, amenorrhea, anaphylaxis, anemia, angioedema, anorexia, apathy, aphthous stomatitis, arthritis, asthma, ataxia, blepharoptosis, breast hypertrophy, breast neoplasm, bronchitis, bursitis, cholelithiasis, colitis, complex sleep-related disorder, conjunctivitis, contact dermatitis, cystitis, dehydration, diaphoresis, dry eye syndrome, dysphagia, dyspnea, dysuria, eczema, emotional lability, epistaxis, erythema multiforme, euphoria, facial edema, fever, gastric ulcer, gastritis, gout, halitosis, heatstroke, heavy menstrual bleeding, hematuria, hepatic disease, hepatitis, hepatomegaly, herpes zoster infection, hirsutism, hostility, hypercholesterolemia, hypersensitivity reaction, hypertension, hypokalemia, hyporeflexia, increased appetite, increased thirst, insomnia, laryngitis, lymphadenopathy, maculopapular rash, malaise, mastalgia, mastitis, melena, memory impairment, myasthenia, mydriasis, myopathy, neck stiffness, nephrolithiasis, neuritis, neuropathy, neurosis, nystagmus disorder, oliguria, paresthesia, photophobia, pyelonephritis, rectal hemorrhage, renal pain, skin discoloration, skin photosensitivity, swelling, thrombophlebitis, tinnitus, tongue edema, tremor, twitching, urethritis, urinary frequency, urinary incontinence, urticaria, uterine hemorrhage, vaginal

hemorrhage, vaginitis, vertigo, vesiculobullous dermatitis, vestibular disturbance

Mechanism of Action May interact with GABA-receptor complexes at binding domains located close to or allosterically coupled to benzodiazepine receptors.

Pharmacodynamics/Kinetics

Half-life Elimination ~6 hours; Elderly (≥65 years): ~9 hours

Time to Peak ~1 hour

Pregnancy Considerations

Eszopiclone is the S-isomer of the racemic derivative zopiclone. Available data related to zopiclone (not available in the United States) and similar medications note the potential for preterm birth, low birth weight, and/or small for gestational age infants following maternal use.

Long-term use of medications in this class is not recommended during pregnancy and a planned discontinuation should be done to prevent rebound insomnia (Okun 2015).

Controlled Substance C-IV

Etanercept (et a NER sept)

Related Information

Rheumatoid Arthritis, Osteoarthritis, and Osteoporosis *on page 1697*

Brand Names: US Enbrel; Enbrel Mini; Enbrel SureClick

Brand Names: Canada Brenzys; Enbrel; Erelzi

Pharmacologic Category Antirheumatic, Disease Modifying; Tumor Necrosis Factor (TNF) Blocking Agent

Use

Ankylosing spondylitis: Reducing signs and symptoms in patients with active ankylosing spondylitis.

Plaque psoriasis (Enbrel): Treatment of patients ≥4 years of age with chronic moderate to severe plaque psoriasis who are candidates for systemic therapy or phototherapy.

Polyarticular juvenile idiopathic arthritis: Reducing signs and symptoms of moderately to severely active polyarticular juvenile idiopathic arthritis in patients ≥2 years of age.

Psoriatic arthritis (Enbrel): Reducing signs and symptoms, inhibiting the progression of structural damage of active arthritis, and improving physical function in patients with psoriatic arthritis. Etanercept can be used with or without methotrexate.

Rheumatoid arthritis: Reducing signs and symptoms, inducing major clinical response, inhibiting the progression of structural damage, and improving physical function in patients with moderately to severely active rheumatoid arthritis (RA). Etanercept can be initiated in combination with methotrexate or used alone.

Local Anesthetic/Vasoconstrictor Precautions

No information available to require special precautions

Effects on Dental Treatment Key adverse event(s) related to dental treatment: Etanercept belongs to the class of disease-modifying antirheumatic drugs and, as such, has immunosuppressive properties. Consider a medical consult prior to any invasive treatment for patients under active treatment with etanercept. Delayed wound healing due to the immunosuppressive effects and increased potential for postsurgical infection may be of concern.

Effects on Bleeding No information available to require special precautions

Adverse Reactions

>10%:

Dermatologic: Skin rash (3% to 13%)

Gastrointestinal: Diarrhea (3% to 16%)

Infection: Infection (50% to 81%)

Local: Injection site reaction (adults: 15% to 43%; children: 7%; bleeding, bruising, erythema, itching, pain, or swelling; mild to moderate and usually decreases with subsequent injections)

Respiratory: Upper respiratory tract infection (38% to 65%), respiratory tract infection (21% to 54%)

Miscellaneous: Antibody development (non-neutralizing; 4% to 16%), positive ANA titer (11%)

1% to 10%:

Dermatologic: Pruritus (2% to 5%), urticaria (2%)

Hypersensitivity: Hypersensitivity reaction (1%)

Miscellaneous: Fever (2% to 3%)

Frequency not defined:

Dermatologic: Cellulitis

Gastrointestinal: Gastroenteritis

Infection: Abscess, influenza, sepsis

Neuromuscular & skeletal: Osteomyelitis, septic arthritis

Renal: Pyelonephritis

Respiratory: Bronchitis, pneumonia, sinusitis

<1%, postmarketing, and/or case reports: Anemia, angioedema, aplastic anemia, aseptic meningitis, aspergillosis, autoimmune hepatitis, cardiac failure, chest pain, cutaneous lupus erythematous, demyelinating disease of the central nervous system, erythema multiforme, fungal infection (including histoplasmosis), Guillain-Barré syndrome, hepatotoxicity (idiosyncratic) (Chalasani 2014), herpes zoster, increased serum transaminases, inflammatory bowel disease, interstitial pulmonary disease, leukemia, leukopenia, lupus-like syndrome, lymphadenopathy, malignant lymphoma, malignant melanoma, malignant neoplasm, Merkel cell carcinoma, multiple sclerosis, neutropenia, optic neuritis, pancytopenia, paresthesia, pneumonia due to *Pneumocystis carinii*, psoriasis (including new onset, palmoplantar, pustular, or exacerbation), reactivation of HBV, sarcoidosis, scleritis, seizure, skin carcinoma, Stevens-Johnson syndrome, subcutaneous nodule, thrombocytopenia, toxic epidermal necrolysis, transverse myelitis, tuberculosis (including pulmonary and extrapulmonary), uveitis, varicella zoster infection, vasculitis (cutaneous and systemic)

Mechanism of Action Etanercept is a recombinant DNA-derived protein composed of tumor necrosis factor receptor (TNFR) linked to the Fc portion of human IgG1. Etanercept binds tumor necrosis factor (TNF) and blocks its interaction with cell surface receptors. TNF plays an important role in the inflammatory processes and the resulting joint pathology of rheumatoid arthritis (RA), polyarticular-course juvenile idiopathic arthritis (JIA), ankylosing spondylitis (AS), and plaque psoriasis.

Pharmacodynamics/Kinetics

Onset of Action ~2 to 3 weeks; RA: 1 to 2 weeks; Maximum effect: RA: Full effect is usually seen within 3 months

Half-life Elimination Half-life elimination: SubQ: Children ≥4 years and Adolescents (JIA): Mean range: 70 to 94.8 hours (range: 31.2 to 104.8 hours) (Yim 2005); Adults (RA): 102 ± 30 hours

Time to Peak RA: SubQ: 69 ± 34 hours

Reproductive Considerations

The American Academy of Dermatology considers tumor necrosis factor alpha (TNFα) blocking agents for the treatment of psoriasis to be compatible for use in male patients planning to father a child (AAD-NPF [Menter 2019]).

Women with well-controlled psoriasis planning a pregnancy who wish to avoid fetal exposure can consider discontinuing etanercept 15 days prior to attempting pregnancy (Rademaker 2018).

Pregnancy Considerations Etanercept crosses the placenta.

Following in utero exposure, etanercept concentrations in the newborn at delivery are 3% to 32% of the maternal serum concentration. A case report describes maternal use of subcutaneous etanercept 25 mg twice weekly throughout pregnancy. Maternal concentrations remained stable throughout each trimester. Maternal and cord blood concentrations at delivery were 2,239 ng/mL and 81 ng/mL, respectively. Etanercept concentrations in the neonate were 21 ng/mL, 1 week after delivery and not detectable 12 weeks later even though the child was breastfed and etanercept was present in breast milk (3.5 ng/mL) (Murashima 2009).

Outcome information following maternal use of etanercept in pregnancy is available. Information related to this class of medications is emerging, but based on available data, tumor necrosis factor alpha (TNFα) blocking agents are considered to have low to moderate risk when used in pregnancy (ACOG 776 2019).

The risk of immunosuppression may be increased following third trimester maternal use of TNFα blocking agents; the fetus, neonate/infant should be considered immunosuppressed for 1 to 3 months following in utero exposure (AAD-NPF [Menter 2019]).

Use of immune modulating therapies in pregnancy should be individualized to optimize maternal disease and pregnancy outcomes (ACOG 776 2019). The American Academy of Dermatology considers TNFα blocking agents for the treatment of psoriasis to be compatible with pregnancy (AAD-NPF [Menter 2019]).

Product Availability

Erelzi (etanercept-szzs): FDA approved August 2016; anticipated availability is currently unknown. Erelzi is approved as biosimilar to Enbrel, but not as an interchangeable product.

Eticovo (etanercept-ykro): FDA approved April 2019; anticipated availability is currently unknown. Eticovo is approved as biosimilar to Enbrel, but not as an interchangeable product.

◆ **Etanercept-szzs** *see* Etanercept *on page 607*

◆ **Etanercept-ykro** *see* Etanercept *on page 607*

◆ **Ethacrynate Sodium** *see* Ethacrynic Acid *on page 608*

Ethacrynic Acid (eth a KRIN ik AS id)

Brand Names: US Edecrin; Sodium Edecrin

Brand Names: Canada Edecrin; Sodium Edecrin; VPI-Ethacrynate Sodium

Pharmacologic Category Diuretic, Loop

Use

Oral: Management of edema associated with congestive heart failure; hepatic cirrhosis or renal disease; short-term management of ascites due to malignancy, idiopathic edema, and lymphedema; short-term management of hospitalized pediatric patients, other than infants, with congenital heart disease or the nephrotic syndrome

IV: Indicated when a rapid onset of diuresis is desired (eg, in acute pulmonary edema, or when gastrointestinal absorption is impaired or oral medication is not feasible)

Local Anesthetic/Vasoconstrictor Precautions No information available to require special precautions

Effects on Dental Treatment No significant effects or complications reported

Effects on Bleeding No information available to require special precautions

Adverse Reactions Frequency not defined.

Cardiovascular: Thrombophlebitis (with intravenous use)

Central nervous system: Apprehension, brain disease (patients with preexisting liver disease), chills, confusion, fatigue, headache, vertigo

Dermatologic: IgA vasculitis (in patient with rheumatic heart disease), skin rash

Endocrine & metabolic: Abnormal phosphorus levels (variations), abnormal serum calcium (variations), gout, hyperglycemia, hyperuricemia (reversible), hypoglycemia (occurred in two uremic patients who received doses above those recommended), hyponatremia, variations in bicarbonate, variations in CO_2 content

Gastrointestinal: Abdominal distress, abdominal pain, anorexia, diarrhea, dysphagia, gastrointestinal hemorrhage, malaise, nausea, vomiting, acute pancreatitis (rare)

Genitourinary: Hematuria

Hematologic & oncologic: Agranulocytosis, severe neutropenia, thrombocytopenia

Hepatic: Abnormal hepatic function tests, jaundice

Local: Local irritation, local pain

Ophthalmic: Blurred vision

Otic: Deafness (temporary or permanent), tinnitus

Renal: Increased serum creatinine

Miscellaneous: Fever

Mechanism of Action Inhibits reabsorption of sodium and chloride in the ascending loop of Henle and distal renal tubule, interfering with the chloride-binding cotransport system, thus causing increased excretion of water, sodium, chloride, magnesium, and calcium

Pharmacodynamics/Kinetics

Onset of Action Diuresis: Oral: ~30 minutes; IV: 5 minutes; Peak effect: Oral: 2 hours; IV: 30 minutes

Duration of Action Oral: 12 hours; IV: 2 hours

Half-life Elimination Normal renal function: 2-4 hours

Pregnancy Risk Factor B

Pregnancy Considerations Adverse events have not been observed in animal reproduction studies.

Ethambutol (e THAM byoo tole)

Brand Names: US Myambutol

Brand Names: Canada Etibi

Pharmacologic Category Antitubercular Agent

Use Treatment of pulmonary tuberculosis in conjunction with other antituberculosis agents

Local Anesthetic/Vasoconstrictor Precautions No information available to require special precautions

Effects on Dental Treatment No significant effects or complications reported

Effects on Bleeding No information available to require special precautions

Adverse Reactions Frequency not defined.

Cardiovascular: Myocarditis, pericarditis

Central nervous system: Confusion, disorientation, dizziness, hallucination, headache, malaise, peripheral neuritis
Dermatologic: Dermatitis, erythema multiforme, exfoliative dermatitis, pruritus, skin rash
Endocrine & metabolic: Acute gout attack, hyperuricemia
Gastrointestinal: Abdominal pain, anorexia, gastric distress, nausea, vomiting
Hematologic & oncologic: Eosinophilia, leukopenia, lymphadenopathy, neutropenia, thrombocytopenia
Hepatic: Abnormal hepatic function tests, hepatitis, hepatotoxicity (possibly related to concurrent therapy)
Hypersensitivity: Anaphylaxis, anaphylactoid reaction, hypersensitivity reaction (syndrome includes cutaneous reactions, eosinophilia, and organ-specific inflammation)
Neuromuscular & skeletal: Arthralgia
Ophthalmic: Color blindness, decreased visual acuity, optic neuritis, scotoma, visual disturbance (usually reversible with discontinuation; irreversible blindness has been described)
Renal: Nephritis
Respiratory: Pneumonitis, pulmonary infiltrates (with or without eosinophilia)
Miscellaneous: Fever

Mechanism of Action Inhibits arabinosyl transferase resulting in impaired mycobacterial cell wall synthesis

Pharmacodynamics/Kinetics

Half-life Elimination 2.5-3.6 hours; End-stage renal disease: 7-15 hours

Time to Peak Serum: 2-4 hours

Pregnancy Risk Factor C

Pregnancy Considerations Adverse events were observed in animal reproduction studies. Ophthalmic abnormalities have been reported in infants born to women receiving ethambutol as a component of antituberculous therapy. Due to the risk of untreated tuberculosis to the mother and fetus, treatment is recommended when the probability of maternal disease is moderate to high. Ethambutol is one of the recommended agents to treat tuberculosis in pregnant women (Nahid 2016).

◆ **Ethambutol HCl** *see* Ethambutol *on page 608*

◆ **Ethambutol Hydrochloride** *see* Ethambutol *on page 608*

◆ **Ethamolin** *see* Ethanolamine Oleate *on page 609*

Ethanolamine Oleate

(ETH a nol a meen OH lee ate)

Brand Names: US Ethamolin

Pharmacologic Category Sclerosing Agent

Use Esophageal varices: Treatment of esophageal varices that have recently bled, to prevent rebleeding.

Local Anesthetic/Vasoconstrictor Precautions No information available to require special precautions

Effects on Dental Treatment No significant effects or complications reported

Effects on Bleeding No information available to require special precautions

Adverse Reactions

1% to 10%:
Cardiovascular: Substernal pain (2%)
Gastrointestinal: Esophageal ulcer (2%), esophageal stenosis (1%)
Respiratory: Pleural effusion (2%), pneumonia (1%)
Miscellaneous: Fever (2%)

<1%, postmarketing, and/or case reports: Acute renal failure, anaphylaxis, esophageal perforation, esophagitis, tissue necrosis at injection site

Mechanism of Action Ethanolamine oleate produces a sterile dose-related inflammatory response resulting in fibrosis and possible occlusion of the vein; a dose-related extravascular inflammatory reaction occurs when the drug diffuses through the venous wall.

Pregnancy Risk Factor C

Pregnancy Considerations Animal reproduction studies have not been conducted.

◆ **Eth Estradiol/Norethindr/Iron** *see* Ethinyl Estradiol and Norethindrone *on page 614*

Ethinyl Estradiol and Desogestrel

(ETH in il es tra DYE ole & des oh JES trel)

Brand Names: US Apri; Azurette; Bekyree; Caziant; Cyclessa [DSC]; Cyred; Cyred EQ; Desogen [DSC]; Emoquette; Enskyce; Isibloom; Juleber; Kalliga; Kariva; Kimidess [DSC]; Mircette; Pimtrea; Reclipsen; Simliya; Velivet; Viorele; Volnea

Brand Names: Canada Apri 21; Apri 28; Freya 21; Freya 28; Linessa 21; Linessa 28; Marvelon; Mirvala 21; Mirvala 28; Reclipsen 21 [DSC]; Reclipsen 28 [DSC]

Pharmacologic Category Contraceptive; Estrogen and Progestin Combination

Use Contraception: Prevention of pregnancy.

Local Anesthetic/Vasoconstrictor Precautions No information available to require special precautions

Effects on Dental Treatment When prescribing antibiotics, patient must be warned to use additional methods of birth control if on oral contraceptives.

Effects on Bleeding No information available to require special precautions

Adverse Reactions Frequency not defined. Reactions listed are based on reports in clinical trials or observational studies with ethinyl estradiol/desogestrel or other oral contraceptives.

Central nervous system: Depression, headache, migraine, mood changes
Dermatologic: Erythema multiforme, erythema nodosum, skin rash, urticaria
Endocrine & metabolic: Decreased libido, fluid retention, increased libido, weight gain, weight loss
Gastrointestinal: Abdominal pain, diarrhea, nausea, vomiting
Genitourinary: Breast hypertrophy, breast tenderness, mastalgia, vaginal discharge
Hypersensitivity: Hypersensitivity reaction
Ophthalmic: Contact lens intolerance

Mechanism of Action Combination hormonal contraceptives inhibit ovulation via a negative feedback mechanism on the hypothalamus, which alters the normal pattern of gonadotropin secretion of a follicle-stimulating hormone (FSH) and luteinizing hormone by the anterior pituitary. The follicular phase FSH and midcycle surge of gonadotropins are inhibited. In addition, combination hormonal contraceptives produce alterations in the genital tract, including changes in the cervical mucus, rendering it unfavorable for sperm penetration even if ovulation occurs. Changes in the endometrium may also occur, producing an unfavorable environment for nidation. Combination hormonal contraceptive drugs may alter the tubal transport of the ova through the fallopian tubes. Progestational agents may also alter sperm fertility.

Pharmacodynamics/Kinetics

Half-life Elimination Monophasic preparations: Etonogestrel: 38 ± 20 hours; Ethinyl estradiol: 26 ± 6.8 hours

Time to Peak Monophasic preparations: Etonogestrel: 1.4 ± 0.8 hours; Ethinyl estradiol: 1.5 ± 0.8 hours; Time to peak of etonogestrel and ethinyl estradiol varies by day in cycle for biphasic and triphasic preparations

Reproductive Considerations

Due to the increased risk of venous thromboembolism (VTE) postpartum, combination hormonal contraceptives should not be started in any woman <21 days following delivery. The risk decreases to baseline by postpartum day 42. Use of combination hormonal contraceptives in women between 21 and 42 days after delivery should take into consideration the individual woman's risk factors for VTE (eg, age ≥35 years, previous VTE, thrombophilia, immobility, preeclampsia, transfusion at delivery, cesarean delivery, peripartum cardiomyopathy, BMI ≥30 kg/m^2, postpartum hemorrhage, or smoking) (Curtis 2016b).

Pregnancy Considerations

Use is contraindicated in pregnant women. Combination hormonal contraceptives are used to prevent pregnancy; treatment should be discontinued if pregnancy occurs. In general, the use of combination hormonal contraceptives, when inadvertently used early in pregnancy, have not been associated adverse fetal or maternal effects (Curtis 2016b).

Ethinyl Estradiol and Drospirenone

(ETH in il es tra DYE ole & droh SPYE re none)

Related Information

Endocrine Disorders and Pregnancy *on page 1684*

Brand Names: US Gianvi; Jasmiel; Lo-Zumandimine; Loryna; Nikki; Ocella; Syeda; Vestura [DSC]; Yasmin 28; YAZ; Zarah; Zumandimine

Brand Names: Canada MYA; Yasmin 21; Yasmin 28; YAZ; Zamine 21; Zamine 28; Zarah 21 [DSC]; Zarah 28 [DSC]

Pharmacologic Category Contraceptive; Estrogen and Progestin Combination

Use

Acne vulgaris (Gianvi, Loryna, Nikki, Vestura, Yaz): Treatment of moderate acne vulgaris in women 14 years and older only if the patient desires an oral contraceptive for birth control

Contraception: Prevention of pregnancy

Premenstrual dysphoric disorder (Gianvi, Yaz): Treatment of premenstrual dysphoric disorder (PMDD) for women who choose to use an oral contraceptive for contraception

Local Anesthetic/Vasoconstrictor Precautions

No information available to require special precautions

Effects on Dental Treatment When prescribing antibiotics, patient must be warned to use additional methods of birth control if on oral contraceptives.

Effects on Bleeding No information available to require special precautions

Adverse Reactions Frequency not defined. Reactions listed are based on reports for other agents in this same pharmacologic class (oral contraceptives) and may not be specifically reported for drospirenone/ethinyl estradiol.

Increased risk or evidence of association with use:

Cardiovascular: Arterial thromboembolism, cerebral thrombosis, hypertension, local thrombophlebitis, mesenteric thrombosis, myocardial infarction, pulmonary embolism, retinal thrombosis

Central nervous system: Cerebral hemorrhage

Gastrointestinal: Gallbladder disease

Hepatic: Hepatic adenoma, hepatic neoplasm (benign)

Adverse reactions considered drug related:

Cardiovascular: Edema, worsening of varicose veins

Central nervous system: Depression, exacerbation of tics, migraine

Dermatologic: Allergic skin rash, chloasma

Endocrine & metabolic: Amenorrhea, breast changes (breast hypertrophy, breast secretion, breast tenderness, mastalgia), decreased serum folate level, exacerbation of porphyria, menstrual disease (menstrual flow changes), weight changes

Gastrointestinal: Abdominal cramps, bloating, carbohydrate intolerance, nausea, vomiting

Genitourinary: Breakthrough bleeding, cervical ectropion, cervical erosion, change in cervical secretions, decreased lactation (with use immediately postpartum), infertility (temporary), spotting, vulvovaginal candidiasis

Hepatic: Cholestatic jaundice

Hypersensitivity: Anaphylaxis/anaphylactoid reaction (including angioedema, circulatory shock, respiratory collapse, urticaria)

Neuromuscular & skeletal: Exacerbation of systemic lupus erythematosus

Ophthalmic: Change in corneal curvature (steepening), contact lens intolerance

Adverse reactions in which association is not confirmed or denied:

Cardiovascular: Budd-Chiari syndrome

Central nervous system: Dizziness, headache, nervousness

Dermatologic: Acne vulgaris, erythema multiforme, erythema nodosum, loss of scalp hair

Endocrine & metabolic: Change in libido, hirsutism, porphyria, premenstrual syndrome

Gastrointestinal: Change in appetite, colitis, pancreatitis

Genitourinary: Cystitis-like syndrome, dysmenorrhea, vaginitis

Hematologic & oncologic: Hemolytic-uremic syndrome, hemorrhagic eruption

Ophthalmic: Cataract, optic neuritis (with or without partial or complete loss of vision)

Renal: Renal insufficiency

Mechanism of Action Combination oral contraceptives inhibit ovulation via a negative feedback mechanism on the hypothalamus, which alters the normal pattern of gonadotropin secretion of a follicle-stimulating hormone (FSH) and luteinizing hormone by the anterior pituitary. The follicular phase FSH and midcycle surge of gonadotropins are inhibited. In addition, oral contraceptives produce alterations in the genital tract, including changes in the cervical mucus, rendering it unfavorable for sperm penetration even if ovulation occurs. Changes in the endometrium may also occur, producing an unfavorable environment for nidation. Oral contraceptive drugs may alter the tubal transport of the ova through the fallopian tubes. Progestational agents may also alter sperm fertility. Drospirenone is a spironolactone analogue with antimineralocorticoid and antiandrogenic activity.

Pharmacodynamics/Kinetics

Half-life Elimination Terminal: Drospirenone: ~30 hours; Ethinyl estradiol: ~24 hours

Time to Peak 1 to 2 hours

Reproductive Considerations

The manufacturer states that combination hormonal contraceptives should not be started until ≥4 weeks after delivery in women who choose not to breastfeed, or ≥4 weeks after a second trimester abortion or miscarriage.

Due to the increased risk of venous thromboembolism (VTE) postpartum, combination hormonal contraceptives should not be started in any woman <21 days following delivery. The risk decreases to baseline by postpartum day 42. Use of combination hormonal contraceptives in women between 21 and 42 days after delivery should take into consideration the individual woman's risk factors for VTE (eg, age ≥35 years, previous VTE, thrombophilia, immobility, preeclampsia, transfusion at delivery, cesarean delivery, peripartum cardiomyopathy, BMI ≥30 kg/m^2, postpartum hemorrhage, or smoking) (Curtis 2016b).

Pregnancy Considerations

Use is contraindicated in pregnant women. Combination hormonal contraceptives are used to prevent pregnancy; treatment should be discontinued if pregnancy occurs. In general, the use of combination hormonal contraceptives, when inadvertently used early in pregnancy, have not been associated adverse fetal or maternal effects (Curtis 2016b).

Ethinyl Estradiol and Ethynodiol Diacetate

(ETH in il es tra DYE ole & e thye noe DYE ole dye AS e tate)

Related Information

Endocrine Disorders and Pregnancy *on page 1684*

Brand Names: US Kelnor 1/35; Kelnor 1/50; Zovia 1/35E (28); Zovia 1/50E (28) [DSC]

Brand Names: Canada Demulen 30 [DSC]

Pharmacologic Category Contraceptive; Estrogen and Progestin Combination

Use Contraception: For the prevention of pregnancy

Limitation of use: Products containing the equivalent of estrogen 50 mcg should not be used unless medically indicated.

Local Anesthetic/Vasoconstrictor Precautions No information available to require special precautions

Effects on Dental Treatment When prescribing antibiotics, patient must be warned to use additional methods of birth control if on oral contraceptives.

Effects on Bleeding No information available to require special precautions

Adverse Reactions Frequency not defined.

Cardiovascular: Arterial thromboembolism, Budd-Chiari syndrome, cerebral thrombosis, cerebrovascular accident, edema, hypertension, local thrombophlebitis, mesenteric thrombosis, myocardial infarction, pulmonary thromboembolism, retinal thrombosis

Central nervous system: Cerebral hemorrhage, depression, dizziness, headache, migraine, nervousness

Dermatologic: Acne vulgaris, allergic skin rash, chloasma (may persist), erythema multiforme, erythema nodosum, loss of scalp hair

Endocrine & metabolic: Amenorrhea, change in libido, change in menstrual flow, decreased glucose tolerance, decreased serum folate level, hirsutism, increased serum triglycerides, increased sex hormone binding globulins, increased thyroxine binding globulin, porphyria, premenstrual syndrome, weight gain, weight loss

Gastrointestinal: Abdominal cramps, bloating, carbohydrate intolerance, change in appetite, cholestasis, colitis, gallbladder disease, nausea, vomiting

Genitourinary: Breakthrough bleeding, breast hypertrophy, breast secretion, breast tenderness, change in cervical erosion, change in cervical secretions, cystitis-like syndrome, decreased lactation (postpartum), spotting, transient infertility (following discontinuation), vaginitis, vulvovaginal candidiasis

Hematologic & oncologic: Decreased antithrombin III plasma level, hemolytic-uremic syndrome, hemorrhagic eruption, increased clotting factor VII, increased clotting factor VIII, increased clotting factor IX, increased clotting factor X, increased norepinephrine-induced platelet aggregation, prolonged prothrombin time

Hepatic: Cholestatic jaundice, hepatic adenoma, hepatic neoplasm (benign), jaundice

Ophthalmic: Cataract, change in corneal curvature (steepening), contact lens intolerance, optic neuritis

Renal: Renal insufficiency

Mechanism of Action Combination hormonal contraceptives inhibit ovulation via a negative feedback mechanism on the hypothalamus, which alters the normal pattern of gonadotropin secretion of a follicle-stimulating hormone (FSH) and luteinizing hormone by the anterior pituitary. The follicular phase FSH and midcycle surge of gonadotropins are inhibited. In addition, combination hormonal contraceptives produce alterations in the genital tract, including changes in the cervical mucus, rendering it unfavorable for sperm penetration even if ovulation occurs. Changes in the endometrium may also occur, producing an unfavorable environment for nidation. Combination hormonal contraceptive drugs may alter the tubal transport of the ova through the fallopian tubes. Progestational agents may also alter sperm fertility.

Reproductive Considerations

The manufacturer states that combination hormonal contraceptives should not be started until ≥4 to 6 weeks after delivery in women who choose not to breastfeed.

Due to the increased risk of venous thromboembolism (VTE) postpartum, combination hormonal contraceptives should not be started in any woman <21 days following delivery. The risk decreases to baseline by postpartum day 42. Use of combination hormonal contraceptives in women between 21 and 42 days after delivery should take into consideration the individual woman's risk factors for VTE (eg, age ≥35 years, previous VTE, thrombophilia, immobility, preeclampsia, transfusion at delivery, cesarean delivery, peripartum cardiomyopathy, BMI ≥30 kg/m^2, postpartum hemorrhage, or smoking) (Curtis 2016b).

Pregnancy Risk Factor X

Pregnancy Considerations

Use is contraindicated in pregnant women. Combination hormonal contraceptives are used to prevent pregnancy; treatment should be discontinued if pregnancy occurs. In general, the use of combination hormonal contraceptives, when inadvertently used early in pregnancy, have not been associated adverse fetal or maternal effects (Curtis 2016b).

Ethinyl Estradiol and Etonogestrel

(ETH in il es tra DYE ole & et oh noe JES trel)

Related Information

Endocrine Disorders and Pregnancy *on page 1684*

Etonogestrel *on page 625*

Brand Names: US EluRyng; NuvaRing

Brand Names: Canada NuvaRing

Pharmacologic Category Contraceptive; Estrogen and Progestin Combination

Use Contraception: Prevention of pregnancy.

Local Anesthetic/Vasoconstrictor Precautions No information available to require special precautions

Effects on Dental Treatment When prescribing antibiotics, patient must be warned to use additional methods of birth control if on oral contraceptives.

Effects on Bleeding No information available to require special precautions

Adverse Reactions

>10%:

Central nervous system: Headache (11%)

Endocrine & metabolic: Intermenstrual bleeding (7% to 12%)

Genitourinary: Vaginitis (14%)

1% to 10%:

Central nervous system: Mood changes (6%)

Dermatologic: Acne vulgaris (2%)

Endocrine & metabolic: Weight gain (5%), amenorrhea (≤4%), decreased libido (2%)

Gastrointestinal: Nausea (≤6%), vomiting (≤6%), abdominal pain (3%)

Genitourinary: Vaginal discharge (6%), dysmenorrhea (4%), vaginal discomfort (4%), breast tenderness (≤4%), mastalgia (≤4%)

Frequency not defined:

Cardiovascular: Deep vein thrombosis

Central nervous system: Anxiety

Gastrointestinal: Cholelithiasis

<1%, postmarketing, and/or case reports: Acute myocardial infarction, anaphylaxis, angioedema, arterial thromboembolism, cerebrovascular accident, chloasma, galactorrhea not associated with childbirth, hypersensitivity reaction, toxic shock syndrome, urticaria, venous thromboembolism, worsening of varicose veins

Mechanism of Action Combination hormonal contraceptives inhibit ovulation via a negative feedback mechanism on the hypothalamus, which alters the normal pattern of gonadotropin secretion of a follicle-stimulating hormone (FSH) and luteinizing hormone by the anterior pituitary. The follicular phase FSH and midcycle surge of gonadotropins are inhibited. In addition, combination hormonal contraceptives produce alterations in the genital tract, including changes in the cervical mucus, rendering it unfavorable for sperm penetration even if ovulation occurs. Changes in the endometrium may also occur, producing an unfavorable environment for nidation. Combination hormonal contraceptive drugs may alter the tubal transport of the ova through the fallopian tubes. Progestational agents may also alter sperm fertility (Rivera 1999).

Pharmacodynamics/Kinetics

Duration of Action Serum levels (contraceptive effectiveness) decrease after 3 weeks of continuous use

Half-life Elimination Ethinyl estradiol: 45 hours; Etonogestrel: 29 hours

Time to Peak Vaginal: Ethinyl estradiol: 59 hours; Etonogestrel: 200 hours

Reproductive Considerations

The manufacturer states that combination hormonal contraceptives should not be started until ≥4 weeks after delivery in women who choose not to breastfeed, or ≥4 weeks after a second trimester abortion or miscarriage.

Due to the increased risk of venous thromboembolism (VTE) postpartum, combination hormonal contraceptives should not be started in any woman <21 days following delivery. The risk decreases to baseline by postpartum day 42. Use of combination hormonal contraceptives in women between 21 and 42 days after delivery should take into consideration the individual woman's risk factors for VTE (eg, age ≥35 years, previous VTE, thrombophilia, immobility, preeclampsia, transfusion at delivery, cesarean delivery, peripartum cardiomyopathy, BMI ≥30 kg/m^2, postpartum hemorrhage, smoking) (Curtis 2016b).

Pregnancy Considerations

Use is contraindicated in pregnant women. Combination hormonal contraceptives are used to prevent pregnancy; treatment should be discontinued if pregnancy occurs. In general, the use of combination hormonal contraceptives, when inadvertently used early in pregnancy, have not been associated adverse fetal or maternal effects (Curtis 2016b).

Ethinyl Estradiol and Levonorgestrel

(ETH in il es tra DYE ole & LEE voe nor jes trel)

Related Information

Endocrine Disorders and Pregnancy *on page 1684*

Brand Names: US Afirmelle; Altavera; Amethia; Amethia Lo; Amethyst; Ashlyna; Aubra; Aubra EQ; Aviane; Ayuna; Balcoltra; Camrese; Camrese Lo; Chateal; Chateal EQ; Daysee; Delyla; Enpresse-28; FaLessa; Falmina; Fayosim; Introvale; Jaimiess; Jolessa; Kurvelo; Larissia; Lessina; Levonest; Levora 0.15/30 (28); Lillow; LoJaimiess; LoSeasonique; Lutera; Marlissa; Myzilra [DSC]; Orsythia; Portia-28; Quartette; Quasense [DSC]; Rivelsa; Seasonique; Setlakin; Simpesse; Sronyx; Trivora (28); Twirla; Vienva

Brand Names: Canada Alesse 21; Alesse 28; Alysena 21; Alysena 28; Aviane; ESME 21 [DSC]; ESME 28 [DSC]; Indayo; Lutera 21 [DSC]; Lutera 28 [DSC]; Min Ovral 21; Min Ovral 28; Ovima 21; Ovima 28; Portia 21; Portia 28; Seasonale; Seasonique; Triquilar 21; Triquilar 28

Pharmacologic Category Contraceptive; Estrogen and Progestin Combination

Use

Contraception: Prevention of pregnancy.

Emergency contraception: Postcoital emergency contraception.

Limitations of use: Ethinyl estradiol in combination with levonorgestrel is effective and recommended as an alternative method for the management of emergency contraception when other methods are not available. The use of other methods is preferred due to increased side effects and decreased efficacy observed with this combination (AAP 2012; ACOG 2015)

Local Anesthetic/Vasoconstrictor Precautions No information available to require special precautions

Effects on Dental Treatment When prescribing antibiotics, patient must be warned to use additional methods of birth control if on oral contraceptives.

Effects on Bleeding No information available to require special precautions

Adverse Reactions Frequency not defined. Reactions listed are based on reports for other agents in this same pharmacologic class (oral contraceptives) and may not be specifically reported for ethinyl estradiol/levonorgestrel.

Increased risk or evidence of association with use:

Cardiovascular: Arterial thromboembolism, cerebral thrombosis, hypertension, local thrombophlebitis, mesenteric thrombosis, myocardial infarction, pulmonary embolism, retinal thrombosis, venous thrombosis (with or without embolism)

Central nervous system: Cerebral hemorrhage

Gastrointestinal: Gallbladder disease

Hepatic: Hepatic adenoma, hepatic neoplasm (benign)

Adverse reactions considered drug related:

Cardiovascular: Edema, worsening of varicose veins

Central nervous system: Depression, exacerbation of tics, migraine, mood changes

Dermatologic: Allergic skin rash, chloasma

Endocrine & metabolic: Amenorrhea, breast changes (breast hypertrophy, breast secretion, breast tenderness, mastalgia), carbohydrate intolerance, decreased lactation (with use immediately postpartum), decreased serum folate level, exacerbation of porphyria, fluid retention, menstrual disease (menstrual flow changes), weight changes

Gastrointestinal: Abdominal cramps, abdominal pain, bloating, change in appetite, nausea, vomiting

Genitourinary: Breakthrough bleeding, cervical ectropion, cervical erosion, change in cervical secretions, endocervical hyperplasia, infertility (temporary), spotting, vulvovaginal candidiasis, vaginitis

Hematologic & oncologic: Uterine fibroid enlargement

Hepatic: Cholestatic jaundice, hepatic focal nodular hyperplasia

Hypersensitivity: Anaphylaxis/Anaphylactoid reaction (including angioedema, circulatory shock, respiratory collapse, urticaria)

Neuromuscular & skeletal: Exacerbation of systemic lupus erythematosus

Ophthalmic: Change in corneal curvature (steepening), contact lens intolerance

Respiratory: Rhinitis

Adverse reactions in which association is not confirmed or denied:

Cardiovascular: Budd-Chiari syndrome

Central nervous system: Dizziness, headache, nervousness

Dermatologic: Acne vulgaris, erythema multiforme, erythema nodosum, loss of scalp hair

Endocrine & metabolic: Change in libido, hirsutism, premenstrual syndrome

Gastrointestinal: Colitis, pancreatitis

Genitourinary: Abnormal Pap smear, cystitis-like syndrome, dysmenorrhea

Hematologic & oncologic: Hemolytic-uremic syndrome, hemorrhagic eruption

Ophthalmic: Cataract, optic neuritis (with or without partial or complete loss of vision)

Otic: Auditory disturbance

Renal: Renal insufficiency

Mechanism of Action Combination hormonal contraceptives inhibit ovulation via a negative feedback mechanism on the hypothalamus, which alters the normal pattern of gonadotropin secretion of a follicle-stimulating hormone (FSH) and luteinizing hormone by the anterior pituitary. The follicular phase FSH and midcycle surge of gonadotropins are inhibited. In addition, combination hormonal contraceptives produce alterations in the genital tract, including changes in the cervical mucus, rendering it unfavorable for sperm penetration even if ovulation occurs. Changes in the endometrium may also occur, producing an unfavorable environment for nidation. Combination hormonal contraceptive drugs may alter the tubal transport of the ova through the fallopian tubes. Progestational agents may also alter sperm fertility.

Pharmacodynamics/Kinetics

Half-life Elimination Ethinyl estradiol: 12-23 hours; Levonorgestrel: 22-49 hours

Reproductive Considerations

Some manufacturers recommend waiting at least 4 to 6 weeks' postpartum before starting this combination.

Due to the increased risk of venous thromboembolism (VTE) postpartum, combination hormonal contraceptives should not be started in any woman <21 days following delivery. The risk decreases to baseline by postpartum day 42. Use of combination hormonal contraceptives in women between 21 and 42 days after delivery should take into consideration the individual woman's risk factors for VTE (eg, age ≥35 years, previous VTE, thrombophilia, immobility, preeclampsia, transfusion at delivery, cesarean delivery, peripartum cardiomyopathy, BMI ≥30 kg/m^2, postpartum hemorrhage, smoking) (Curtis 2016b).

When used for emergency contraception, a barrier contraceptive is recommended immediately following use. Any regular (nonemergency) contraceptive method can be started immediately after combined estrogen/progestin emergency contraception; however, a barrier method (or abstinence from sexual intercourse) is also needed for 7 days (ACOG 2015; Curtis 2016a).

Pregnancy Considerations

Use is contraindicated in pregnant women. Combination hormonal contraceptives are used to prevent pregnancy; treatment should be discontinued if pregnancy occurs. In general, the use of combination hormonal contraceptives, when inadvertently used early in pregnancy, have not been associated adverse fetal or maternal effects (Curtis 2016b).

Product Availability Twirla transdermal system: FDA approved February 2020; availability anticipated in the 4th quarter of 2020. Twirla is indicated as a method of contraception for use in women of reproductive potential with a BMI <30 kg/m^2 for whom a combined hormonal contraceptive is appropriate. Information pertaining to this product within the monograph is pending revision. Consult the prescribing information for additional information.

◆ **Ethinyl Estradiol and NGM** *see* Ethinyl Estradiol and Norgestimate *on page 616*

Ethinyl Estradiol and Norelgestromin

(ETH in il es tra DYE ole & nor el JES troe min)

Brand Names: US Xulane

Brand Names: Canada Evra

Pharmacologic Category Contraceptive; Estrogen and Progestin Combination

Use

Contraception: For the prevention of pregnancy in women with a BMI <30 kg/m^2.

Limitations of use: The patch is contraindicated for use in women with BMI ≥30 kg/m^2. In addition, the patch may be less effective in patients weighing ≥90 kg.

Local Anesthetic/Vasoconstrictor Precautions

No information available to require special precautions

Effects on Dental Treatment When prescribing antibiotics, patient must be warned to use additional methods of birth control if on oral contraceptives.

Effects on Bleeding No information available to require special precautions

Adverse Reactions The following reactions have been reported with the contraceptive patch. Adverse reactions associated with oral combination hormonal contraceptive agents are also likely to appear with the topical contraceptive patch (frequency difficult to anticipate). See individual oral contraceptive monographs for additional information.

>10%:

- Central nervous system: Headache (21%)
- Endocrine & metabolic: Breast changes (22%; including breast engorgement, discomfort, mastalgia)
- Gastrointestinal: Nausea (17%)
- Local: Application site reaction (17%)

1% to 10%:

- Cardiovascular: Increased blood pressure (<3%), pulmonary embolism (<3%)
- Central nervous system: Anxiety (≤6%), mood disorder (≤6%), dizziness (3%), fatigue (3%), migraine (3%), insomnia (<3%), malaise (<3%)
- Dermatologic: Acne vulgaris (3%), pruritus (3%), chloasma (<3%), contact dermatitis (<3%), erythema (<3%), skin irritation (<3%)
- Endocrine & metabolic: Menstrual disease (6%), weight gain (3%), change in libido (<3%), dyslipidemia (<3%), fluid retention (<3%), galactorrhea (<3%), premenstrual syndrome (<3%)
- Gastrointestinal: Abdominal pain (8%), vomiting (5%), diarrhea (4%), abdominal distention (<3%), cholecystitis (<3%)
- Genitourinary: Dysmenorrhea (8%), vaginal hemorrhage (6%), vulvovaginal candidiasis (4%), genital discharge (<3%), uterine spasm (<3%), vaginal dryness (<3%), vulvar dryness (<3%)
- Neuromuscular & skeletal: Muscle spasm (<3%)

<1%, postmarketing, and/or case reports: Alopecia, altered serum glucose, arterial thrombosis, benign mammary fibroadenoma, blood cholesterol abnormal, cerebrovascular accident, cervical dysplasia, cholelithiasis, cholestasis, cholestatic jaundice, colitis, contact lens intolerance (or complication), decreased lactation, deep vein thrombosis, dermatological reaction, dysgeusia, eczema, edema, emotional disturbance, erythema multiforme, erythema nodosum, hepatic adenoma, hepatic neoplasm, hyperglycemia, hyperirritability, hypersensitivity reaction, hypertension, hypertensive crisis, increased appetite, increased LDL cholesterol, insulin resistance, intracranial hemorrhage, irritability, lesion (hepatic), malignant neoplasm of breast, malignant neoplasm of cervix, mass (breast), migraine (with aura), myocardial infarction, outbursts of anger, seborrheic dermatitis, skin photosensitivity, skin rash, thrombosis, urticaria, uterine fibroids

Mechanism of Action Combination hormonal contraceptives inhibit ovulation via a negative feedback mechanism on the hypothalamus, which alters the normal pattern of gonadotropin secretion of a follicle-stimulating hormone (FSH) and luteinizing hormone by the anterior pituitary. The follicular phase FSH and midcycle surge of gonadotropins are inhibited. In addition, combination hormonal contraceptives produce alterations in the genital tract, including changes in the cervical mucus, rendering it unfavorable for sperm penetration even if ovulation occurs. Changes in the endometrium may also occur, producing an unfavorable environment for nidation. Combination hormonal contraceptive drugs may alter the tubal transport of the ova through the fallopian tubes. Progestational agents may also alter sperm fertility.

Pharmacodynamics/Kinetics

Half-life Elimination Topical: Ethinyl estradiol: ~17 hours; Norelgestromin: ~28 hours

Reproductive Considerations

The manufacturer states that combination hormonal contraceptives should not be started until ≥4 weeks after delivery in women who choose not to breastfeed, or ≥4 weeks after a second trimester abortion or miscarriage.

Due to the increased risk of venous thromboembolism (VTE) postpartum, combination hormonal contraceptives should not be started in any woman <21 days following delivery. The risk decreases to baseline by postpartum day 42. Use of combination hormonal contraceptives in women between 21 and 42 days after delivery should take into consideration the individual woman's risk factors for VTE (eg, age ≥35 years, previous VTE, thrombophilia, immobility, preeclampsia, transfusion at delivery, cesarean delivery, peripartum cardiomyopathy, BMI ≥30 kg/m², postpartum hemorrhage, smoking) (Curtis 2016b).

[US Boxed Warning]: Norelgestromin/ethinyl estradiol is contraindicated in women with a BMI ≥30 kg/m². The risk of VTE may be greater with norelgestromin/ethinyl estradiol in women with a BMI ≥30 kg/m² compared to women with a lower BMI. In addition, the patch may be less effective in patients weighing ≥90 kg (198 lb). **Combination oral contraceptives, including norelgestromin/ethinyl estradiol, are contraindicated in women who are over 35 years of age and smoke.**

Pregnancy Considerations

Use is contraindicated in pregnant women. Combination hormonal contraceptives are used to prevent pregnancy; treatment should be discontinued if pregnancy occurs. In general, the use of combination hormonal contraceptives, when inadvertently used early in pregnancy, have not been associated with adverse fetal or maternal effects (Curtis 2016b).

Ethinyl Estradiol and Norethindrone

(ETH in il es tra DYE ole & nor eth IN drone)

Related Information

Endocrine Disorders and Pregnancy *on page 1684*
Norethindrone *on page 1117*
Rheumatoid Arthritis, Osteoarthritis, and Osteoporosis *on page 1697*

Brand Names: US Alyacen 1/35; Alyacen 7/7/7; Aranelle; Aurovela 1.5/30; Aurovela 1/20; Aurovela 24 FE; Aurovela Fe 1.5/30; Aurovela FE 1/20; Balziva; Blisovi 24 Fe; Blisovi Fe 1.5/30; Blisovi FE 1/20; Brevicon (28) [DSC]; Briellyn; Charlotte 24 Fe; Cyclafem 1/35; Cyclafem 7/7/7; Dasetta 1/35; Dasetta 7/7/7; Estrostep Fe; Femcon Fe [DSC]; Femhrt Low Dose; Fyavolv; Generess FE; Gildagia [DSC]; Gildess 1.5/30 [DSC]; Gildess 1/20 [DSC]; Gildess 24 FE [DSC]; Gildess FE 1.5/30 [DSC]; Gildess FE 1/20 [DSC]; Hailey 1.5/30; Hailey 24 Fe; Hailey FE 1.5/30; Hailey FE 1/20; Jevantique Lo [DSC]; Jinteli; Junel 1.5/30; Junel 1/20; Junel FE 1.5/30; Junel FE 1/20; Junel Fe 24; Kaitlib Fe; Larin 1.5/30; Larin 1/20; Larin 24 FE; Larin Fe 1.5/30; Larin Fe 1/20; Layolis FE; Leena; Lo Loestrin Fe; Loestrin 1.5/30 (21); Loestrin 1/20 (21); Loestrin Fe 1.5/30;

Loestrin Fe 1/20; Lomedia 24 FE [DSC]; Melodetta 24 Fe; Mibelas 24 Fe; Microgestin 1.5/30; Microgestin 1/20; Microgestin 24 Fe [DSC]; Microgestin FE 1.5/30; Microgestin FE 1/20; Minastrin 24 Fe; Modicon (28) [DSC]; Necon 0.5/35 (28); Necon 1/35 (28) [DSC]; Necon 10/11 (28) [DSC]; Necon 7/7/7 [DSC]; Norinyl 1 +35 (28) [DSC]; Nortrel 0.5/35 (28); Nortrel 1/35 (21); Nortrel 1/35 (28); Nortrel 7/7/7; Ortho-Novum 1/35 (28) [DSC]; Ortho-Novum 7/7/7 (28) [DSC]; Ovcon-35 (28) [DSC]; Philith; Pirmella 1/35; Pirmella 7/7/7; Tarina 24 Fe; Tarina FE 1/20; Tarina FE 1/20 EQ; Taytulla; Tilia Fe; Tri-Legest Fe; Tri-Norinyl (28) [DSC]; Vyfemla; Wera; Wymzya Fe; Zenchent FE [DSC]; Zenchent [DSC]

Brand Names: Canada Brevicon 0.5/35; Brevicon 1/35; Loestrin 1.5/30; Lolo; Minestrin 1/20; Ortho 0.5/35 [DSC]; Ortho 1/35 [DSC]; Ortho 7/7/7 [DSC]; Select 1/35; Synphasic

Pharmacologic Category Contraceptive; Estrogen and Progestin Combination

Use

Acne vulgaris (Estrostep Fe, Tilia Fe, Tri-Legest Fe): Treatment of moderate acne vulgaris in females at least 15 years.

Limitations of use: When used for acne, use only in females ≥15 years who have achieved menarche, who also desire combination hormonal contraceptive therapy, are unresponsive to topical treatments, have no contraindications to combination hormonal contraceptive use, and plan to stay on therapy for ≥6 months.

Contraception: Prevention of pregnancy.

Limitations of use: The efficacy of some products has not been established in women with a BMI >35 kg/m^2.

Osteoporosis prevention (female) (femhrt, Jevantique Lo, Jinteli): Prevention of postmenopausal osteoporosis.

Limitations of use: For use only in women at significant risk of postmenopausal osteoporosis; consider use of nonestrogen medications.

Vasomotor symptoms associated with menopause (femhrt, Jevantique Lo, Jinteli): Treatment of moderate to severe vasomotor symptoms associated with menopause.

Local Anesthetic/Vasoconstrictor Precautions No information available to require special precautions

Effects on Dental Treatment When prescribing antibiotics, patient must be warned to use additional methods of birth control if on oral contraceptives.

Effects on Bleeding No information available to require special precautions

Adverse Reactions

Menopausal vasomotor symptoms and osteoporosis prevention:

>10%: Endocrine & metabolic: Increased sex hormone binding globulin (22%)

1% to 10%:

Cardiovascular: Edema (5%)

Central nervous system: Headache (6%)

Gastrointestinal: Abdominal pain (5% to 7%)

Genitourinary: Mastalgia (8% to 9%), endometrial hyperplasia (≤1%)

Contraception and Acne:

>10%:

Endocrine & metabolic: Change in menstrual flow (including absence of withdrawal bleeding: 31% to 41%), amenorrhea (8% to 36%)

Genitourinary: Breakthrough bleeding (≤86%), spotting (≤86%)

1% to 10%:

Central nervous system: Headache (≤8%), migraine (≤8%), depression (≤4%), mood changes (≤4%), mood disorder (≤3%), anxiety (≤2%)

Dermatologic: Acne vulgaris (3%)

Endocrine & metabolic: Heavy menstrual bleeding (≤5%), weight changes (4%), weight gain (2%)

Gastrointestinal: Nausea (≤9%), vomiting (≤9%), abdominal pain (3%)

Genitourinary: Vulvovaginal candidiasis (6%), abnormal uterine bleeding (≤5%), irregular menses (≤5%), vaginal hemorrhage (≤5%), dysmenorrhea (4%), uterine cramps (4%), abnormal cervical or vaginal Papanicolaou smear (3%), bacterial vaginosis (3%), breast tenderness (≤3%), mastalgia (≤2%)

Frequency not defined:

Cardiovascular: Hypertension

Endocrine & metabolic: Decreased libido

<1%, postmarketing, and/or case reports: Abdominal cramps, abnormal sensory symptoms, allergic skin rash, alopecia, altered serum glucose, anaphylaxis, anemia, angina pectoris, angioedema, arthralgia, back pain, benign breast nodule, bipolar mood disorder, bloating, blurred vision, breast changes, breast disease, breast hypertrophy, breast secretion, burning sensation of skin, cerebral embolism, cerebral thrombosis, cerebrovascular accident, change in appetite, change in cervical ectropion, change in cervical secretions, change in corneal curvature (steepening), change in libido, chest pain, chloasma, cholecystitis, cholelithiasis, cholestatic jaundice, chorea, constipation, contact lens intolerance, corneal thinning, coronary thrombosis, cystitis-like syndrome, deep vein thrombosis, dementia, diabetes mellitus, dissociative reaction, dizziness, drowsiness, dyspnea, dysuria, embolism, endometrial carcinoma, erythema, erythema multiforme, erythema nodosum, exacerbation of asthma, exacerbation of epilepsy, exacerbation of hepatic hemangioma, exacerbation of porphyria, facial swelling, fatigue, fibrocystic breast changes, fungal infection, galactorrhea not associated with childbirth, gallbladder disease, hemangioma (hepatic), hemiparesis, hemorrhagic eruption, hepatic adenoma, hirsutism, homicidal ideation, hot flash, hyperesthesia, hypersensitivity reaction, hyperthyroidism, hypocalcemia, hypoesthesia, hypoglycemia, hypothyroidism, impaired glucose tolerance/prediabetes, increased blood pressure, increased serum triglycerides, insomnia, irregular pulse, irritability, ischemic stroke, localized edema (pelvic), loss of consciousness, loss of scalp hair, lower limb cramp, malaise, malignant neoplasm of breast, malignant neoplasm of ovary, malignant neoplasm of uterus, myalgia, myocardial infarction, nervousness, night sweats, nipple discharge, nipple pain, nonimmune anaphylaxis, ovarian cyst, palpitations, pancreatitis, panic attack, paresthesia, pelvic pain, peripheral edema, pollakiuria, premenstrual syndrome, pruritus, pulmonary embolism, retinal thrombosis, rupture of ovarian cyst, skin discoloration, skin rash, suicidal ideation, superficial venous thrombosis, swelling of lips, tachycardia, thrombophlebitis, thrombosis (including ovarian), transient blindness, transient ischemic attacks, urticaria, uterine fibroid enlargement, uterine hypertrophy, vaginal infection, vaginitis, visual impairment, weight loss

Mechanism of Action Combination oral contraceptives inhibit ovulation via a negative feedback mechanism on the hypothalamus, which alters the normal pattern of gonadotropin secretion of a follicle-stimulating hormone (FSH) and luteinizing hormone by the anterior pituitary. The follicular phase FSH and midcycle surge of gonadotropins are inhibited. In addition, combination hormonal contraceptives produce alterations in the genital tract, including changes in the cervical mucus, rendering it unfavorable for sperm penetration even if ovulation occurs. Changes in the endometrium may also occur, producing an unfavorable environment for nidation. Combination hormonal contraceptive drugs may alter the tubal transport of the ova through the fallopian tubes. Progestational agents may also alter sperm fertility.

In postmenopausal women, exogenous estrogen is used to replace decreased endogenous production. The addition of progestin reduces the incidence of endometrial hyperplasia and risk of endometrial cancer in women with an intact uterus.

Pharmacodynamics/Kinetics

Half-life Elimination Ethinyl estradiol: 19 to 24 hours

Reproductive Considerations

The manufacturer states that combination hormonal contraceptives should not be started until ≥4 weeks after delivery in women who choose not to breastfeed.

Due to the increased risk of venous thromboembolism (VTE) postpartum, combination hormonal contraceptives should not be started in any woman <21 days following delivery. The risk decreases to baseline by postpartum day 42. Use of combination hormonal contraceptives in women between 21 and 42 days after delivery should take into consideration the individual woman's risk factors for VTE (eg, age ≥35 years, previous VTE, thrombophilia, immobility, preeclampsia, transfusion at delivery, cesarean delivery, peripartum cardiomyopathy, BMI ≥30 kg/m^2, postpartum hemorrhage, smoking) (Curtis 2016b).

Pregnancy Risk Factor X

Pregnancy Considerations

Use is contraindicated in pregnant women. Combination hormonal contraceptives are used to prevent pregnancy; treatment should be discontinued if pregnancy occurs. In general, the use of combination hormonal contraceptives, when inadvertently used early in pregnancy, have not been associated adverse fetal or maternal effects (Curtis 2016b).

Dental Health Professional Considerations Current hormone contraceptives should not be considered a risk factor for gingival or periodontal disease (Preshaw 2013).

Ethinyl Estradiol and Norgestimate

(ETH in il es tra DYE ole & nor JES ti mate)

Related Information

Endocrine Disorders and Pregnancy *on page 1684*

Brand Names: US Estarylla; Femynor; Mili; Mono-Linyah; MonoNessa [DSC]; Ortho Tri-Cyclen (28) [DSC]; Ortho Tri-Cyclen Lo [DSC]; Ortho-Cyclen (28) [DSC]; Previfem; Sprintec 28; Tri Femynor; Tri-Estarylla; Tri-Linyah; Tri-Lo-Estarylla; Tri-Lo-Marzia; Tri-Lo-Mili; Tri-Lo-Sprintec; Tri-Mili; Tri-Previfem; Tri-Sprintec; Tri-VyLibra; Tri-VyLibra Lo; TriNessa (28) [DSC]; Tri-Nessa Lo [DSC]; VyLibra

Brand Names: Canada Cyclen; Tri-Cyclen Lo; Tri-Cyclen [DSC]; TRI-Jordyna 21; TRI-Jordyna 28; Tricira Lo 21; Tricira Lo 28

Pharmacologic Category Contraceptive; Estrogen and Progestin Combination

Use

Acne vulgaris: Treatment of moderate acne vulgaris in females at least 15 years of age

Limitations of use: When used for acne, use only in females ≥15 years of age who achieved menarche, who also desire combination hormonal contraceptive therapy, and have no contraindications to combination hormonal contraceptive use

Contraception: Prevention of pregnancy.

Local Anesthetic/Vasoconstrictor Precautions No information available to require special precautions

Effects on Dental Treatment When prescribing antibiotics, patient must be warned to use additional methods of birth control if on oral contraceptives.

Effects on Bleeding No information available to require special precautions

Adverse Reactions

>10%:

Central nervous system: Headache (≤34%), migraine (≤34%)

Gastrointestinal: Nausea (≤16%), vomiting (≤16%)

Genitourinary: Breakthrough bleeding (7% to 38%)

1% to 10%:

Central nervous system: Nipple pain (≤10%), depression (≤8%), emotional lability (≤8%), mood changes (≤8%), mood disorder (≤8%), nervousness (3%), fatigue (2%)

Dermatologic: Acne vulgaris (5%), skin rash (3%)

Endocrine & metabolic: Menstrual disease (≤9%), weight changes (≤3%), weight gain (≤3%), weight loss (≤3%)

Gastrointestinal: Abdominal pain (≤9%), gastrointestinal pain (≤8%), abdominal distention (3%), flatulence (3%)

Genitourinary: Breast cyst (≤10%), breast hypertrophy (≤10%), breast swelling (≤10%), breast tenderness (≤10%), mastalgia (≤10%), nipple discharge (≤10%), dysmenorrhea (≤9%), vaginal infection (7% to 8%), genital discharge (3% to 7%), vulvovaginal infection (4%)

Frequency not defined:

Cardiovascular: Hypertension, venous thromboembolism

Central nervous system: Irritability

Endocrine & metabolic: Amenorrhea, premenstrual syndrome

Genitourinary: Abnormal uterine bleeding, cervical carcinoma (in situ), cervical dysplasia

<1%, postmarketing, and/or case reports: Angioedema, anxiety, arterial thromboembolism, asthenia, back pain, breast neoplasm (benign), cerebrovascular accident, chest pain, constipation, contact lens intolerance, deep vein thrombosis, diarrhea, dizziness, dyslipidemia, dyspnea, erythema nodosum, hepatic adenoma, hepatic focal nodular hyperplasia, hepatitis, hirsutism, hot flash, hyperhidrosis, hypersensitivity reaction, insomnia, lactation insufficiency, limb pain, malignant neoplasm of breast, muscle spasm, myalgia, myocardial infarction, night sweats, ovarian cyst, palpitations, pancreatitis, paresthesia, pruritus, pulmonary embolism, retinal thrombosis, seizure, skin photosensitivity, syncope, tachycardia, urinary tract infection, urticaria, vaginal dryness, vertigo, visual impairment, vulvar dryness, xerophthalmia

Mechanism of Action Combination hormonal contraceptives inhibit ovulation via a negative feedback mechanism on the hypothalamus, which alters the normal pattern of gonadotropin secretion of a follicle-stimulating hormone (FSH) and luteinizing hormone by the anterior pituitary. The follicular phase FSH and midcycle surge of gonadotropins are inhibited. In addition, combination hormonal contraceptives produce alterations in the genital tract, including changes in the cervical mucus, rendering it unfavorable for sperm penetration even if ovulation occurs. Changes in the endometrium may also occur, producing an unfavorable environment for nidation. Combination hormonal contraceptive drugs may alter the tubal transport of the ova through the fallopian tubes. Progestational agents may also alter sperm fertility.

Pharmacodynamics/Kinetics

Half-life Elimination EE: 10-16 hours; NGMN: 18-25 hours; NG: 38-45 hours

Time to Peak EE and NGM: ~2 hours

Reproductive Considerations

The manufacturer states that combination hormonal contraceptives should not be started until ≥4 weeks after delivery in women who choose not to breastfeed. Due to the increased risk of venous thromboembolism (VTE) postpartum, combination hormonal contraceptives should not be started in any woman <21 days following delivery. The risk decreases to baseline by postpartum day 42. Use of combination hormonal contraceptives in women between 21 and 42 days after delivery should take into consideration the individual woman's risk factors for VTE (eg, age ≥35 years, previous VTE, thrombophilia, immobility, preeclampsia, transfusion at delivery, cesarean delivery, peripartum cardiomyopathy, BMI ≥30 kg/m^2, postpartum hemorrhage, smoking) (Curtis 2016b).

Pregnancy Considerations

Use is contraindicated in pregnant women. Combination hormonal contraceptives are used to prevent pregnancy; treatment should be discontinued if pregnancy occurs. In general, the use of combination hormonal contraceptives, when inadvertently used early in pregnancy, have not been associated adverse fetal or maternal effects (Curtis 2016b).

Dental Health Professional Considerations Current hormone contraceptives should not be considered a risk factor for gingival or periodontal disease (Preshaw, 2013).

Ethinyl Estradiol and Norgestrel

(ETH in il es tra DYE ole & nor JES trel)

Related Information

Endocrine Disorders and Pregnancy *on page 1684*

Brand Names: US Cryselle-28; Elinest; Low-Ogestrel; Ogestrel [DSC]

Pharmacologic Category Contraceptive; Estrogen and Progestin Combination

Use Contraception: Prevention of pregnancy

Local Anesthetic/Vasoconstrictor Precautions

No information available to require special precautions

Effects on Dental Treatment When prescribing antibiotics, patient must be warned to use additional methods of birth control if on oral contraceptives.

Effects on Bleeding No information available to require special precautions

Adverse Reactions Frequency not defined.

Cardiovascular: Arterial thromboembolism, Budd-Chiari syndrome, cerebral thrombosis, cerebrovascular accident, edema, hypertension, local thrombophlebitis, mesenteric thrombosis, myocardial infarction, pulmonary thromboembolism, retinal thrombosis

Central nervous system: Cerebral hemorrhage, depression, dizziness, headache, migraine, nervousness

Dermatologic: Acne vulgaris, allergic skin rash, chloasma (may persist), erythema multiforme, erythema nodosum, loss of scalp hair

Endocrine & metabolic: Amenorrhea, change in libido, decreased glucose tolerance, decreased serum folate level, hirsutism, increased serum triglycerides, increased sex hormone binding globulin, increased thyroxine binding globulin, menstrual disease (flow changes), porphyria, premenstrual syndrome, weight gain, weight loss

Gastrointestinal: Abdominal cramps, bloating, carbohydrate intolerance, change in appetite, cholestasis, colitis, gallbladder disease, nausea, vomiting

Genitourinary: Breakthrough bleeding, breast hypertrophy, breast secretion, breast tenderness, change in cervical erosion, change in cervical secretions, cystitis-like syndrome, decreased lactation (postpartum), spotting, transient infertility (following discontinuation), vaginitis, vulvovaginal candidiasis

Hematologic & oncologic: Decreased antithrombin III plasma level, hemolytic-uremic syndrome, hemorrhagic eruption, increased clotting factor VII, increased clotting factor VIII, increased clotting factor IX, increased clotting factor X, increased norepinephrine-induced platelet aggregation, prolonged prothrombin time

Hepatic: Cholestatic jaundice, hepatic adenoma, hepatic neoplasm (benign), jaundice

Ophthalmic: Cataract, change in corneal curvature (steepening), contact lens intolerance, optic neuritis

Renal: Renal insufficiency

Mechanism of Action Combination hormonal contraceptives inhibit ovulation via a negative feedback mechanism on the hypothalamus, which alters the normal pattern of gonadotropin secretion of a follicle-stimulating hormone (FSH) and luteinizing hormone by the anterior pituitary. The follicular phase FSH and midcycle surge of gonadotropins are inhibited. In addition, combination hormonal contraceptives produce alterations in the genital tract, including changes in the cervical mucus, rendering it unfavorable for sperm penetration even if ovulation occurs. Changes in the endometrium may also occur, producing an unfavorable environment for nidation. Combination hormonal contraceptive drugs may alter the tubal transport of the ova through the fallopian tubes. Progestational agents may also alter sperm fertility.

Reproductive Considerations

The manufacturer states that combination hormonal contraceptives should not be started until ≥4 to 6 weeks after delivery in women who choose not to breastfeed. Due to the increased risk of venous thromboembolism (VTE) postpartum, combination hormonal contraceptives should not be started in any woman <21 days following delivery. The risk decreases to baseline by postpartum day 42. Use of combination hormonal contraceptives in women between 21 and 42 days after delivery should take into consideration the individual woman's risk factors for VTE (eg, age ≥35 years, previous VTE, thrombophilia, immobility, preeclampsia, transfusion at delivery, cesarean delivery, peripartum cardiomyopathy, BMI ≥30 kg/m^2, postpartum hemorrhage, smoking) (Curtis 2016b).

Pregnancy Risk Factor X

Pregnancy Considerations

Use is contraindicated in pregnant women. Combination hormonal contraceptives are used to prevent pregnancy; treatment should be discontinued if pregnancy occurs. In general, the use of combination hormonal contraceptives, when inadvertently used early in pregnancy, have not been associated adverse fetal or maternal effects (Curtis 2016b).

Dental Health Professional Considerations Current hormone contraceptives should not be considered a risk factor for gingival or periodontal disease (Preshaw, 2013).

◆ **Ethinyl Estradiol and Segesterone Acetate** *see* Segesterone Acetate and Ethinyl Estradiol *on page 1362*

◆ **Ethinyl Estradiol/Desogestrel** *see* Ethinyl Estradiol and Desogestrel *on page 609*

◆ **Ethinyl Estradiol/Drospirenone** *see* Ethinyl Estradiol and Drospirenone *on page 610*

Ethinyl Estradiol, Drospirenone, and Levomefolate

(ETH in il es tra DYE ole, droh SPYE re none, & lee voe me FOE late)

Related Information

Endocrine Disorders and Pregnancy *on page 1684*

Brand Names: US Beyaz; Rajani [DSC]; Safyral; Tydemy

Brand Names: Canada YAZ Plus

Pharmacologic Category Contraceptive; Estrogen and Progestin Combination

Use

Acne vulgaris (Beyaz, Rajani): Treatment of moderate acne vulgaris in women 14 years and older who have achieved menarche and who desire an oral contraceptive for birth control.

Contraception: Prevention of pregnancy.

Folate supplementation: To increase folate concentrations in women choosing an oral contraceptive for birth control, in order to reduce the risk of neural tube defects in pregnancies conceived during therapy or soon after treatment is discontinued.

Premenstrual dysphoric disorder (Beyaz, Rajani): Treatment of symptoms of premenstrual dysphoric disorder (PMDD) in women who choose to use an oral contraceptive for contraception.

Limitations of use: The effectiveness of use for more than 3 menstrual cycles has not been evaluated. Has not been evaluated for the treatment of premenstrual syndrome (PMS).

Local Anesthetic/Vasoconstrictor Precautions No information available to require special precautions

Effects on Dental Treatment When prescribing antibiotics, patient must be warned to use additional methods of birth control if on oral contraceptives.

Effects on Bleeding No information available to require special precautions

Adverse Reactions Frequency not always defined. Percentages reported with Beyaz. For additional adverse events and postmarketing reports, refer to the Ethinyl Estradiol and Drospirenone (Yasmin, Yaz) monograph.

Central nervous system: Headache (≤6% to 13%), migraine (≤6% to 13%), fatigue (4%), irritability (3%), emotional lability (2%)

Endocrine & metabolic: Menstrual disease (4% to 25%, including menorrhagia, spotting, uterine hemorrhage, vaginal hemorrhage), decreased libido (3%), weight gain (3%)

Gastrointestinal: Nausea (≤4% to 16%), vomiting (≤4% to 16%)

Genitourinary: Breast tenderness (≤3% to 11%), mastalgia (≤3% to 11%), cervical carcinoma (stage 0), cervical dysplasia

Mechanism of Action Combination oral contraceptives inhibit ovulation via a negative feedback mechanism on the hypothalamus, which alters the normal pattern of gonadotropin secretion of a follicle-stimulating hormone (FSH) and luteinizing hormone by the anterior pituitary. The follicular phase FSH and midcycle surge of gonadotropins are inhibited. In addition, oral contraceptives produce alterations in the genital tract, including changes in the cervical mucus, rendering it unfavorable for sperm penetration even if ovulation occurs. Changes in the endometrium may also occur, producing an unfavorable environment for nidation. Oral contraceptive drugs may alter the tubal transport of the ova through the fallopian tubes. Progestational agents may also alter sperm fertility. Drospirenone is a spironolactone analogue with antimineralocorticoid and antiandrogenic activity.

Pharmacodynamics/Kinetics

Half-life Elimination Terminal: Drospirenone: ~31 hours; Ethinyl estradiol: ~24 hours; levomefolate calcium: ~4-5 hours

Time to Peak Drospirenone, ethinyl estradiol: 1-2 hours; Levomefolate calcium: 0.5-1.5 hours

Reproductive Considerations

The manufacturer states that combination hormonal contraceptives should not be started until ≥4 weeks after delivery in women who choose not to breastfeed, or ≥4 weeks after a second trimester abortion or miscarriage.

Due to the increased risk of venous thromboembolism (VTE) postpartum, combination hormonal contraceptives should not be started in any woman <21 days following delivery. The risk decreases to baseline by postpartum day 42. Use of combination hormonal contraceptives in women between 21 and 42 days after delivery should take into consideration the individual woman's risk factors for VTE (eg, age ≥35 years, previous VTE, thrombophilia, immobility, preeclampsia, transfusion at delivery, cesarean delivery, peripartum cardiomyopathy, BMI ≥30 kg/m^2, postpartum hemorrhage, smoking) (Curtis 2016b).

Pregnancy Considerations

Use is contraindicated in pregnant women. Combination hormonal contraceptives are used to prevent pregnancy; treatment should be discontinued if pregnancy occurs. In general, the use of combination hormonal contraceptives, when inadvertently used early in pregnancy, have not been associated adverse fetal or maternal effects (Curtis 2016b). The addition of levomefolate in this product is intended to decrease the risk of neural tube defects if pregnancy inadvertently occurs during therapy or shortly after discontinuation.

◆ **Ethinyl Estradiol, Drospirenone, and Levomefolate Calcium** *see* Ethinyl Estradiol, Drospirenone, and Levomefolate *on page 618*

◆ **Ethinyl Estradiol/Norethindr** *see* Ethinyl Estradiol and Norethindrone *on page 614*

Ethosuximide (eth oh SUKS i mide)

Brand Names: US Zarontin
Brand Names: Canada Zarontin
Pharmacologic Category Anticonvulsant, Succinimide
Use Absence (petit mal) seizures: Management of absence (petit mal) seizures
Local Anesthetic/Vasoconstrictor Precautions No information available to require special precautions
Effects on Dental Treatment No significant effects or complications reported
Effects on Bleeding No information available to require special precautions
Adverse Reactions Frequency not defined.

Central nervous system: Aggressive behavior, ataxia, delusional paranoid disorder, depression (with cases of overt suicidal intentions), disturbed sleep dizziness, drowsiness, euphoria, fatigue, headache, hyperactivity, irritability, lack of concentration, lethargy, night terrors
Dermatologic: Pruritus, skin rash, Stevens-Johnson syndrome, urticaria
Endocrine & metabolic: Hirsutism, increased libido, weight loss
Gastrointestinal: Abdominal pain, anorexia, abdominal cramps, diarrhea, epigastric pain, gastric distress, gingival hyperplasia, hiccups, nausea, swollen tongue, vomiting
Genitourinary: Occult blood in urine, vaginal hemorrhage
Hematologic & oncologic: Agranulocytosis, eosinophilia, leukopenia, pancytopenia
Hypersensitivity: Hypersensitivity reaction
Immunologic: DRESS syndrome (drug rash with eosinophilia and systemic symptoms)
Neuromuscular & skeletal: Systemic lupus erythematosus
Ophthalmic: Myopia

Mechanism of Action Increases the seizure threshold and suppresses paroxysmal spike-and-wave pattern in absence seizures; depresses nerve transmission in the motor cortex
Pharmacodynamics/Kinetics
Half-life Elimination Serum: Children: 30 hours; Adults: 50 to 60 hours
Time to Peak Serum: 1 to 7 hours
Reproductive Considerations
Women with epilepsy who are planning a pregnancy in advance should have baseline serum concentrations measured once or twice prior to pregnancy during a period when seizure control is optimal (Patsalos 2008; Patsalos 2018).
Pregnancy Considerations
Ethosuximide crosses the placenta. Birth defects have been reported in infants. Epilepsy itself, the number of medications, genetic factors, or a combination of these may influence the teratogenicity of anticonvulsant therapy. In general, polytherapy may increase the risk of congenital malformations; monotherapy with the lowest effective dose is recommended (Harden 2009). Monitoring of serum concentrations should begin prior to pregnancy and continue up to once a month during pregnancy in women with stable seizure control (Patsalos 2008; Patsalos 2018).

Patients exposed to ethosuximide during pregnancy are encouraged to enroll themselves into the NAAED Pregnancy Registry by calling 1-888-233-2334. Additional information is available at www.aedpregnancyregistry.org.

Ethotoin (ETH oh toyn)

Brand Names: US Peganone
Pharmacologic Category Anticonvulsant, Hydantoin
Use Seizures: Control of generalized tonic-clonic (grand mal) and complex-partial (psychomotor) seizures
Local Anesthetic/Vasoconstrictor Precautions No information available to require special precautions
Effects on Dental Treatment No significant effects or complications reported
Effects on Bleeding No information available to require special precautions
Adverse Reactions Frequency not defined.

Cardiovascular: Chest pain
Central nervous system: Ataxia, dizziness, fatigue, headache, insomnia, numbness
Dermatologic: Skin rash, Stevens-Johnson syndrome
Gastrointestinal: Diarrhea, gingival hyperplasia, nausea, vomiting
Hematologic & oncologic: Hematologic disease, lymphadenopathy
Neuromuscular & skeletal: Lupus-like syndrome
Ophthalmic: Diplopia, nystagmus
Miscellaneous: Fever

Mechanism of Action Stabilizes the seizure threshold and prevents the spread of seizure activity
Pharmacodynamics/Kinetics
Half-life Elimination 3 to 9 hours
Pregnancy Considerations Adverse fetal effects may occur following maternal use of ethotoin. Cleft lip and cleft palate observed with other hydantoins has also been reported following in utero exposure to ethotoin (Zablen 1977). Maternal ingestion of antiepileptic agents has been associated with neonatal coagulation defects/bleeding usually within 24 hours of birth..

Patients exposed to ethotoin during pregnancy are encouraged to enroll themselves into the AED Pregnancy Registry by calling 1-888-233-2334. Additional information is available at www.aedpregnancy- registry.org.

- **Ethyl Aminobenzoate** *see* Benzocaine *on page 228*
- **Ethyl Eicosapentaenoate** *see* Omega-3 Fatty Acids *on page 1137*
- **Ethyl-Eicosapentaenoic Acid** *see* Omega-3 Fatty Acids *on page 1137*
- **Ethyl-EPA** *see* Omega-3 Fatty Acids *on page 1137*
- **Ethyl Esters of Omega-3 Fatty Acids** *see* Omega-3 Fatty Acids *on page 1137*
- **Ethyl Icosapentate** *see* Omega-3 Fatty Acids *on page 1137*
- **Ethynodiol Diacetate and Ethinyl Estradiol** *see* Ethinyl Estradiol and Ethynodiol Diacetate *on page 611*
- **Eticovo** *see* Etanercept *on page 607*

Etidronate (e ti DROE nate)

Related Information

Osteonecrosis of the Jaw *on page 1699*

Brand Names: Canada ACT Etidronate; APO-Etidronate [DSC]; CO Etidronate; MYLAN-Etidronate [DSC]

Pharmacologic Category Bisphosphonate Derivative

Use

Heterotopic ossification: Prevention and treatment of heterotopic ossification due to spinal cord injury or after total hip replacement

Paget disease: Symptomatic treatment of Paget disease of bone

Note: Not generally a recommended treatment option; guidelines recommend the use of more potent bisphosphonate therapy (eg, zoledronic acid) (Endocrine Society [Singer 2014]; Ralston 2019).

Local Anesthetic/Vasoconstrictor Precautions No information available to require special precautions

Effects on Dental Treatment Key adverse event(s) related to dental treatment: Abnormal taste.

Osteonecrosis of the jaw (ONJ), generally associated with local infection and/or tooth extraction and often with delayed healing, has been reported in patients taking bisphosphonates. Symptoms included nonhealing extraction socket or an exposed jawbone. Most reported cases of bisphosphonate-associated osteonecrosis have been in cancer patients treated with intravenous bisphosphonates. However, some have occurred in patients with postmenopausal osteoporosis taking oral bisphosphonates. Dental surgery, particularly tooth extraction, may increase the risk for ONJ. Patients who develop ONJ while on bisphosphonate therapy should receive care by an oral surgeon. See Dental Health Professional Considerations.

Effects on Bleeding No information available to require special precautions

Adverse Reactions

Gastrointestinal: Diarrhea (≤30%; dose dependent), nausea (≤30%; dose dependent)

Neuromuscular & skeletal: Ostealgia (10% to 20%; dose dependent)

Postmarketing and/or case reports: Agranulocytosis, alopecia, amnesia, angioedema, arthralgia, arthritis, bone fracture, confusion, depression, erythema multiforme, esophagitis, exacerbation of asthma, exacerbation of peptic ulcer, folliculitis, gastritis, glossitis, glossopyrosis, hallucination, headache, hypersensitivity reaction, leg cramps, leukemia, leukopenia, maculopapular rash, osteomalacia, osteonecrosis of the jaw, pancytopenia, paresthesia, pruritus, skin rash (macular), Stevens-Johnson syndrome, toxic epidermal necrolysis, urticaria

Mechanism of Action Decreases bone resorption by inhibiting osteocytic osteolysis; decreases mineral release and matrix or collagen breakdown in bone

Pharmacodynamics/Kinetics

Onset of Action 1 to 3 months

Duration of Action Can persist for 12 months without continuous therapy

Half-life Elimination 1 to 6 hours

Reproductive Considerations

Bisphosphonates are incorporated into the bone matrix and gradually released over time. Because exposure prior to pregnancy may theoretically increase the risk of fetal harm, use in premenopausal females should be reserved for special circumstances when rapid bone loss is occurring (Bhalla 2010; Pereira 2012; Stathopoulos 2011).

Pregnancy Considerations

It is not known if bisphosphonates cross the placenta, but based on their lower molecular weight, fetal exposure is expected (Djokanovic 2008; Stathopoulos 2011).

Information related to the use of etidronate in pregnancy is available from case reports and small retrospective studies (Agarwal 2020; Levy 2009; Sokal 2019; Vujasinovic-Stupar 2012).

Bisphosphonates are incorporated into the bone matrix and gradually released over time. The amount available in the systemic circulation varies by drug, dose, and duration of therapy. Theoretically, there may be a risk of fetal harm when pregnancy follows the completion of therapy (hypocalcemia, low birth weight, and decreased gestation have been observed in some case reports); however, available data have not shown that exposure to bisphosphonates during pregnancy significantly increases the risk of adverse fetal events (Djokanovic 2008; Green 2014; Levy 2009; Machairiotis 2019; Sokal 2019; Stathopoulos 2011). Exposed infants should be monitored for hypocalcemia after birth (Djokanovic 2008; Stathopoulos 2011).

Dental Health Professional Considerations A review of 2,408 published cases of bisphosphonate-associated osteonecrosis of the jaw bone (BP-associated ONJ) was done by Filleul 2010. BP therapy was associated with 89% of the cases to treat malignancies and 11% of the cases to treat nonmalignant conditions. Information on the specific bisphosphonate used was available for 1,694 of the patients. Intravenous therapy (primarily zoledronic acid) was received by 88% of the patients and 12% received oral treatment (primarily alendronate). Of all the cases of BP-associated ONJ, 67% were preceded by tooth extraction and for 26% of patients, there was no predisposing factor identified.

A 2010 retrospective case review reported the prevalence of BP-associated ONJ in patients using alendronate-type drugs was one out of 952 patients or ~0.1% (Lo 2010). Of the 8,572 respondents, nine cases of ONJ were identified; five had developed ONJ spontaneously and four developed ONJ after tooth extraction. When extrapolated to patient-years of bisphosphonate exposure, this prevalence rate of 0.1% equates to a frequency of 28 cases per 100,000 person-years of oral bisphosphonate treatment. An Australian group (Mavrokokki 2007), identified the frequency of BP-associated ONJ in osteoporotic patients, mainly taking weekly oral alendronate, was 1 in 8,470 to 1 in 2,260 (0.01% to 0.04%) patients. If extractions were carried out, the calculated frequency was 1 in 1,130 to 1 in 296 (0.09% to 0.34%) patients. The median time to onset of ONJ in alendronate patients was 24 months.

According to the 2011 report by the American Dental Association (ADA), the incidence of BP-associated ONJ remains low and the benefits of using oral bisphosphonates significantly outweighs the risk of developing BP-associated ONJ for treatment and prevention of osteoporosis and cancer treatment (Hellstein 2011). The full 47-page report can be accessed at http://www.ada.org/~/media/ADA/Member%20Center/FIles/topics_ARONJ_report.ashx.

The ADA review of 2011 stated the incidence of oral BP-associated ONJ was one case for every 1,000 individuals exposed to oral bisphosphonates (0.1%) (Hellstein 2011).

The most comprehensive review to date on osteonecrosis of the jaw bone (ONJ) has been published in the *Journal of Bone and Mineral Research* (Khan 2015), and written by an International Task Force of authors, totaling 34, from academe; industry; clinical medical and dental practice; oral and maxillofacial surgery; bone and mineral research; epidemiology; medical and dental oncology; orthopedic surgery; osteoporosis research; muscle and bone research; endocrinology and diagnostic sciences. The work provides a systematic review of the literature and international consensus on the classification, incidence, pathophysiology, diagnosis, and management of ONJ in both oncology and osteoporosis patient populations. This review of the literature from January 2003 to April 2014, with 299 references, offers recommendations for management of ONJ based on multidisciplinary international consensus.

Prevalence and incidence of ONJ in osteoporosis patients from the Task Force report:

Prevalence – the percent of osteoporotic population affected with ONJ

After reviewing all literature reports on this subject, the Task Force concluded that the prevalence of ONJ in patients prescribed oral BPs for the treatment of osteoporosis ranges from 0% to 0.04% with the majority being below 0.001%. However, the Task Force does cite the study of (Lo et al) that evaluated the Kaiser Permanente database and found the prevalence of ONJ in those receiving BPs for more than 2 years to range from 0.05% to 0.21% and appeared to be related to duration of exposure. As mentioned above, the American Dental Association has previously reported that the prevalence of ONJ in osteoporosis patients using oral BPs to be 1 out of 1,000 or 0.1% (Hellstein 2011).

Incidence - the rate at which ONJ occurs or the number of times it happens

From currently available data, the incidence of ONJ in the osteoporosis patient population appears to be low ranging from 0.15% to less than 0.001% person-years drug exposure. In terms of the osteoporosis patient population taking oral BPs, the incidence ranges from 1.04 to 69 per 100,000 patient years of drug exposure.

Etidronate and Calcium Carbonate

(e ti DROE nate & KAL see um KAR bun ate)

Related Information

Etidronate *on page 620*

Brand Names: Canada ACT Etidrocal; MYLAN-Eti-Cal Carepac [DSC]; NOVO-Etidronatecal [DSC]

Pharmacologic Category Bisphosphonate Derivative; Calcium Salt

Use Note: Not approved in the US

Corticosteroid-induced osteoporosis: Prevention of corticosteroid-induced osteoporosis

Postmenopausal osteoporosis: Treatment and prevention of established postmenopausal osteoporosis

Local Anesthetic/Vasoconstrictor Precautions No information available to require special precautions

Effects on Dental Treatment Osteonecrosis of the jaw (ONJ), generally associated with local infection and/or tooth extraction and often with delayed healing, has been reported in patients taking bisphosphonates. Symptoms included nonhealing extraction socket or an exposed jawbone. Most reported cases of bisphosphonate-associated osteonecrosis have been in cancer patients treated with intravenous bisphosphonates. However, some have occurred in patients with postmenopausal osteoporosis taking oral bisphosphonates. Dental surgery, particularly tooth extraction, may increase the risk for ONJ. Patients who develop ONJ while on bisphosphonate therapy should receive care by an oral surgeon. See Dental Health Professional Considerations.

Effects on Bleeding No information available to require special precautions

Adverse Reactions

>10%:

Central nervous system: Dizziness (16%), headache (13%)

Gastrointestinal: Diarrhea (37%), nausea (18%), flatulence (17%), constipation (13%), dyspepsia (12%), vomiting (11%)

<1%, postmarketing, and/or case reports: Agranulocytosis, alopecia, amnesia, angioedema, arthropathy, bone fracture, confusion, depression, erythema multiforme, esophagitis, exacerbation of asthma, exacerbation of peptic ulcer, folliculitis, glossitis, glossopyrosis, hallucination, leukemia (1 in 100,000 patients), leukopenia, maculopapular rash, malignant neoplasm of esophagus, musculoskeletal pain, pancytopenia, paresthesia, Stevens-Johnson syndrome, urticaria

Mechanism of Action See individual agents.

Reproductive Considerations

Bisphosphonates are incorporated into the bone matrix and gradually released over time. Because exposure prior to pregnancy may theoretically increase the risk of fetal harm, most sources recommend discontinuing bisphosphonate therapy in females of reproductive potential as early as possible prior to a planned pregnancy. Use in premenopausal females should be reserved for special circumstances when rapid bone loss is occurring; a bisphosphonate with the shortest half-life should then be used (Bhalla 2010; Pereira 2012; Stathopoulos 2011).

Oral bisphosphonates can be considered for the prevention of glucocorticoid-induced osteoporosis in premenopausal females with moderate to high risk of fracture who do not plan to become pregnant during the treatment period and who are using effective birth control (or are not sexually active); intravenous therapy should be reserved for high risk patients only (Buckley [ACR 2017]).

Pregnancy Considerations

It is not known if bisphosphonates cross the placenta, but based on their lower molecular weight, fetal exposure is expected (Djokanovic 2008; Stathopoulos 2011).

Information related to the use of etidronate in pregnancy is available from case reports and small retrospective studies (Levy 2009; Sokol 2019; Vjuasinovic-Stupar 2012).

Bisphosphonates are incorporated into the bone matrix and gradually released over time. The amount available in the systemic circulation varies by drug, dose, and duration of therapy. Theoretically, there may be a risk of fetal harm when pregnancy follows the completion of therapy (hypocalcemia, low birth weight, and decreased gestation have been observed in some case reports); however, available data have not shown that exposure to bisphosphonates during pregnancy significantly increases the risk of adverse fetal events (Djokanovic 2008; Green 2014; Levy 2009; Sokal 2019;

Stathopoulos 2011). Exposed infants should be monitored for hypocalcemia after birth (Djokanovic 2008; Stathopoulos 2011).

This product is not intended for use in pregnant women.

Product Availability Not available in the US

Dental Health Professional Considerations See Etidronate monograph.

◆ **Etidronate Disodium** *see* Etidronate *on page 620*

◆ **Etidronate Disodium and Calcium** *see* Etidronate and Calcium Carbonate *on page 621*

Etodolac (ee toe DOE lak)

Related Information

Oral Pain *on page 1734*

Rheumatoid Arthritis, Osteoarthritis, and Osteoporosis *on page 1697*

Temporomandibular Dysfunction (TMD), Chronic Pain, and Fibromyalgia *on page 1773*

Brand Names: US Lodine

Brand Names: Canada NU-Etodolac [DSC]; TARO-Etodolac

Generic Availability (US) Yes

Pharmacologic Category Analgesic, Nonopioid; Nonsteroidal Anti-inflammatory Drug (NSAID), Oral

Dental Use Management of postoperative pain

Use

Acute pain: Management of acute pain (immediate release only).

Arthritis: Relief of the signs and symptoms of osteoarthritis, rheumatoid arthritis, and juvenile arthritis (ER only).

Local Anesthetic/Vasoconstrictor Precautions No information available to require special precautions

Effects on Dental Treatment The dentist should be aware of the potential of abnormal coagulation. Caution should also be exercised in the use of NSAIDs in patients already on anticoagulant therapy with drugs such as warfarin (Coumadin®). See Effects on Bleeding.

Effects on Bleeding Nonselective NSAIDs such as etodolac inhibit platelet aggregation and prolong bleeding time in some patients. Unlike aspirin, the NSAID effect on platelet function is quantitatively less, of shorter duration, and reversible.

Adverse Reactions

1% to 10%:

Central nervous system: Dizziness (3% to 9%), chills (≤3%), depression (1% to 3%), nervousness (1% to 3%)

Dermatologic: Skin rash (1% to 3%), pruritus (1% to 3%)

Gastrointestinal: Dyspepsia (10%), abdominal cramps (3% to 9%), diarrhea (3% to 9%), flatulence (3% to 9%), nausea (3% to 9%), vomiting (1% to 3%), constipation (1% to 3%), melena (1% to 3%), gastritis (1% to 3%)

Genitourinary: Dysuria (1% to 3%)

Neuromuscular & skeletal: Weakness (3% to 9%)

Ophthalmic: Blurred vision (1% to 3%)

Otic: Tinnitus (1% to 3%)

Renal: Polyuria (1% to 3%)

Miscellaneous: Fever (≤3%)

<1%: Abnormal uterine bleeding, agranulocytosis, alopecia, anaphylactoid reaction, anaphylaxis, anemia, angioedema, anorexia, aphthous stomatitis, aseptic meningitis, asthma, cardiac arrhythmia, cardiac failure, cerebrovascular accident, confusion, conjunctivitis, cystitis, duodenitis, dyspnea, ecchymosis, edema, erythema multiforme, esophagitis (+/- stricture or cardiospasm), exfoliative dermatitis, gastrointestinal ulceration, hallucination, headache, hearing loss, hematemesis, hematuria, hepatic failure, hepatitis, hepatotoxicity (idiosyncratic) (Chalasani, 2014), hyperglycemia (in controlled patients with diabetes), hyperpigmentation, hypersensitivity angiitis, hypersensitivity reaction, hypertension, increased liver function tests, infection, insomnia, interstitial nephritis, jaundice, leukopenia, myocardial infarction, necrotizing angiitis, nephrolithiasis, palpitations, pancreatitis, pancytopenia, paresthesia, peptic ulcer (+/- bleeding/perforation), peripheral neuropathy, photophobia, prolonged bleeding time, pulmonary infiltrates (eosinophilia), rectal bleeding, renal failure, renal insufficiency, shock, skin photosensitivity, Stevens-Johnson syndrome, syncope, thrombocytopenia, toxic epidermal necrolysis, urticaria, vesiculobullous dermatitis, renal papillary necrosis, visual disturbance

Dental Usual Dosage Acute pain: Adults: Oral: Immediate release formulation: 200 to 400 mg every 6 to 8 hours, as needed, not to exceed total daily doses of 1000 mg

Dosing

Adult Note: For chronic conditions, response is usually observed within 1 to 2 weeks.

Acute pain: Oral: Immediate release: 200 to 400 mg every 6 to 8 hours; maximum: 1,000 mg daily.

Osteoarthritis, rheumatoid arthritis: Oral:

Immediate release: 400 mg 2 times daily **or** 300 mg 2 to 3 times daily **or** 500 mg 2 times daily.

Extended release: Initial: 400 to 1,000 mg once daily.

Geriatric Refer to adult dosing, use with caution. Elderly patients are more sensitive to antiprostaglandin effects and may need dosage adjustments.

Renal Impairment: Adult

CrCl >88 mL/minute: No dosage adjustment necessary.

CrCl 37 to 88 mL/minute: No dosage adjustment necessary; however, use with caution.

CrCl <37 mL/minute: There are no specific dosage adjustments provided in the manufacturer's labeling; if use must be initiated, use with caution. Avoid use in patients with advanced renal disease unless benefits are expected to outweigh risk of worsening renal function.

Hemodialysis: Not significantly removed.

KDIGO 2012 guidelines provide the following recommendations for NSAIDs:

eGFR 30 to <60 mL/minute/1.73 m^2: Temporarily discontinue in patients with intercurrent disease that increases risk of acute kidney injury.

eGFR <30 mL/minute/1.73 m^2: Avoid use.

Hepatic Impairment: Adult No dosage adjustment necessary. However, reduced doses may be required due to extensive hepatic metabolism.

Pediatric Note: Dosage should be titrated to the lowest effective dose for the shortest duration possible. For chronic conditions, therapeutic response may take 1 to 2 weeks of treatment.

Analgesia, acute pain:

Children and Adolescents <18 years: Limited data available (American Pain Society 2016): Oral: Immediate release:

Patient weight <50 kg: 7.5 to 10 mg/kg/dose every 12 hours; maximum daily dose: 1,000 mg/**day**

Patient weight ≥50 kg: 300 to 400 mg every 8 to 12 hours; maximum daily dose: 1,000 mg/**day**

Adolescents ≥18 years: Oral: Immediate release: 200 to 400 mg every 6 to 8 hours, as needed; maximum daily dose: 1,000 mg/**day**

Juvenile idiopathic arthritis: Children ≥6 years weighing at least 20 kg and Adolescents: Oral: Extended-release tablets:

20 to 30 kg: 400 mg once daily

31 to 45 kg: 600 mg once daily

46 to 60 kg: 800 mg once daily

>60 kg: 1,000 mg once daily

Rheumatoid arthritis, osteoarthritis: Adolescents ≥18 years: Oral:

Immediate release: 300 to 500 mg twice daily or 300 mg 3 times daily; maximum daily dose: 1,000 mg/**day**

Extended-release tablets: 400 to 1,000 mg once daily

Renal Impairment: Pediatric

KDIGO 2012 guidelines provide the following recommendations for NSAIDs (KDIGO 2013): Children and Adolescents:

eGFR 30 to <60 mL/minute/1.73 m^2: Temporarily discontinue in patients with intercurrent disease that increases risk of acute kidney injury

eGFR <30 mL/minute/1.73 m^2: Avoid use

Manufacturer's labeling:

Adolescents ≥18 years: Immediate release:

CrCl >88 mL/minute: No adjustment required

CrCl 37 to 88 mL/minute: No dosage adjustment necessary; however, use with caution.

CrCl <37 mL/minute: There are no specific dosage adjustments provided in the manufacturer's labeling; if use must be initiated, use with caution. Avoid use in patients with advanced renal disease unless benefits are expected to outweigh risk of worsening renal function.

Hemodialysis: Not significantly removed

Extended release: There are no dosing adjustments provided in the manufacturer's labeling; has not been studied

Hepatic Impairment: Pediatric No adjustment required; in adult patients, reduced doses may be required due to extensive hepatic metabolism.

Mechanism of Action Reversibly inhibits cyclooxygenase-1 and 2 (COX-1 and 2) enzymes, which results in decreased formation of prostaglandin precursors; has antipyretic, analgesic, and anti-inflammatory properties

Other proposed mechanisms not fully elucidated (and possibly contributing to the anti-inflammatory effect to varying degrees), include inhibiting chemotaxis, altering lymphocyte activity, inhibiting neutrophil aggregation/activation, and decreasing proinflammatory cytokine levels.

Contraindications

Hypersensitivity to etodolac, or any component of the formulation; history of asthma, urticaria, or allergic-type reactions after taking aspirin or other NSAID agents; use in the setting of coronary artery bypass graft (CABG) surgery.

Canadian labeling: Additional contraindications (not in US labeling): Active peptic ulcer; inflammatory diseases of the GI tract

Warnings/Precautions [US Boxed Warning]: Nonsteroidal anti-inflammatory drugs (NSAIDs) cause an increased risk of serious (and potentially fatal) adverse cardiovascular thrombotic events, including MI and stroke. Risk may occur early during treatment and may increase with duration of use. Relative risk appears to be similar in those with and without known cardiovascular disease or risk factors for cardiovascular disease; however, absolute incidence of serious cardiovascular thrombotic events (which may occur early during treatment) was higher in patients with known cardiovascular disease or risk factors and in those receiving higher doses. New onset hypertension or exacerbation of hypertension may occur (NSAIDs may also impair response to ACE inhibitors, thiazide diuretics, or loop diuretics); may contribute to cardiovascular events; monitor blood pressure; use with caution in patients with hypertension. May cause sodium and fluid retention; use with caution in patients with edema. Avoid use in heart failure (ACCF/AHA [Yancy, 2013]). Avoid use in patients with recent MI unless benefits outweigh risk of cardiovascular thrombotic events. Use the lowest effective dose for the shortest duration of time, consistent with individual patient goals, to reduce risk of cardiovascular events; alternate therapies should be considered for patients at high risk. **[US Boxed Warning]: Use is contraindicated in the setting of coronary artery bypass graft (CABG) surgery.** Risk of MI and stroke may be increased with use following CABG surgery.

Clinical or population-based data regarding the risks of NSAIDs in the setting of coronavirus disease 2019 (COVID-19) are limited (FDA Safety Communication 2020; Kim 2020). Some experts recommend the use of acetaminophen as the preferred antipyretic agent, when possible, and if NSAIDs are needed, to use the lowest effective dose and shortest duration (EMA 2020; Kim 2020). In general, for patients already taking an NSAID for a comorbid condition, it is recommended to continue the NSAID as directed by their health care provider (EMA 2020; NIH 2020; WHO 2020).

[US Boxed Warning]: NSAIDs cause increased risk of serious GI inflammation, ulceration, bleeding, and perforation (may be fatal); elderly patients and patients with history of peptic ulcer disease and/or GI bleeding are at greater risk for serious GI events. These events may occur at any time during therapy and without warning. Avoid use in patients with active GI bleeding. In patients with a history of acute lower GI bleeding, avoid use of non-aspirin NSAIDs, especially if due to angioectasia or diverticulosis (Strate 2016). Use caution with a history of GI ulcers, concurrent therapy known to increase the risk of GI bleeding (eg, aspirin, anticoagulants and/or corticosteroids, selective serotonin reuptake inhibitors), advanced hepatic disease, coagulopathy, smoking, use of alcohol, or in elderly or debilitated patients. Use the lowest effective dose for the shortest duration of time, consistent with individual patient goals, to reduce risk of GI adverse events; alternate therapies should be considered for patients at high risk. When used concomitantly with aspirin, a substantial increase in the risk of GI complications (eg, ulcer) occurs; concomitant gastroprotective therapy (eg, proton pump inhibitors) is recommended (Bhatt, 2008). Avoid chronic use of oral nonselective NSAIDs in patients who have undergone bariatric surgery; development of anastomotic ulcerations/perforations may occur.

Platelet adhesion and aggregation may be decreased; may prolong bleeding time; patients with coagulation disorders or who are receiving anticoagulants should be monitored closely. Anemia may occur; patients on long-term NSAID therapy should be monitored for anemia. Rarely, NSAID use may cause severe blood dyscrasias (eg, agranulocytosis, aplastic anemia, thrombocytopenia). May increase the risk of aseptic meningitis, especially in patients with systemic lupus erythematosus (SLE) and mixed connective tissue disorders.

NSAID use may compromise existing renal function; dose-dependent decreases in prostaglandin synthesis may result from NSAID use, reducing renal blood flow which may cause renal decompensation (usually reversible). Patients with impaired renal function, dehydration, hypovolemia, heart failure, hepatic impairment, those taking diuretics, and ACE inhibitors, and the elderly are at greater risk of renal toxicity. Rehydrate patient before starting therapy; monitor renal function closely. Long-term NSAID use may result in renal papillary necrosis and other renal injury. Avoid use in patients with advanced renal disease unless benefits are expected to outweigh risk of worsening renal function; monitor closely if therapy must be initiated.

Elderly patients are at greater risk for serious GI, cardiovascular, and/or renal events; use with caution.

NSAIDs may cause potentially fatal serious skin adverse events including exfoliative dermatitis, Stevens-Johnson syndrome (SJS), and toxic epidermal necrolysis (TEN); may occur without warning; discontinue use at first sign of skin rash (or any other hypersensitivity). Even in patients without prior exposure anaphylactoid reactions may occur; patients with "aspirin triad" (bronchial asthma, aspirin intolerance, rhinitis) may be at increased risk. Contraindicated in patients who experience bronchospasm, asthma, rhinitis, or urticaria with NSAID or aspirin therapy. Contraindicated in patients with aspirin-sensitive asthma; severe and potentially fatal bronchospasm may occur. Use caution in patients with other forms of asthma.

Transaminase elevations have been reported with use; closely monitor patients with any abnormal LFT. Rare (sometimes fatal) severe hepatic reactions (eg, fulminant hepatitis, hepatic necrosis, hepatic failure) have occurred with NSAID use; discontinue immediately if clinical signs or symptoms of liver disease develop or if systemic manifestations occur. Use with caution in patients with hepatic impairment; reduced doses may be required due to extensive hepatic metabolism. Patients with advanced hepatic disease are at an increased risk of GI bleeding with NSAIDs. NSAIDS may cause drowsiness, dizziness, blurred vision and other neurologic effects which may impair physical or mental abilities; patients must be cautioned about performing tasks which require mental alertness (eg, operating machinery or driving).

Withhold for at least 4 to 6 half-lives prior to surgical or dental procedures. Potentially significant interactions may exist, requiring dose or frequency adjustment, additional monitoring, and/or selection of alternative therapy.

Use of extended release product consisting of a nondeformable matrix should be avoided in patients with stricture/narrowing of the GI tract; symptoms of obstruction have been associated with nondeformable products.

Drug Interactions

Metabolism/Transport Effects None known.

Avoid Concomitant Use

Avoid concomitant use of Etodolac with any of the following: Acemetacin; Aminolevulinic Acid (Systemic); Dexibuprofen; Dexketoprofen; Floctafenine; Ketorolac (Nasal); Ketorolac (Systemic); Macimorelin; Mifamurtide; Morniflumate; Nonsteroidal Anti-Inflammatory Agents (COX-2 Selective); Omacetaxine; Pelubiprofen; Phenylbutazone; Talniflumate; Tenoxicam; Urokinase; Zaltoprofen

Increased Effect/Toxicity

Etodolac may increase the levels/effects of: 5-Aminosalicylic Acid Derivatives; Agents with Antiplatelet Properties; Aliskiren; Aminoglycosides; Aminolevulinic Acid (Systemic); Aminolevulinic Acid (Topical); Anticoagulants; Apixaban; Bemiparin; Bisphosphonate Derivatives; Cephalothin; Collagenase (Systemic); CycloSPORINE (Systemic); Dabigatran Etexilate; Deferasirox; Deoxycholic Acid; Desmopressin; Dexibuprofen; Digoxin; Drospirenone; Edoxaban; Enoxaparin; Eplerenone; Haloperidol; Heparin; Ibritumomab Tiuxetan; Lithium; MetFORMIN; Methotrexate; Nonsteroidal Anti-Inflammatory Agents (COX-2 Selective); Obinutuzumab; Omacetaxine; Porfimer; Potassium-Sparing Diuretics; PRALAtrexate; Quinolones; Rivaroxaban; Salicylates; Tacrolimus (Systemic); Tenofovir Products; Thrombolytic Agents; Tolperisone; Urokinase; Vancomycin; Verteporfin; Vitamin K Antagonists

The levels/effects of Etodolac may be increased by: Acalabrutinib; Acemetacin; Alcohol (Ethyl); Angiotensin II Receptor Blockers; Angiotensin-Converting Enzyme Inhibitors; Corticosteroids (Systemic); CycloSPORINE (Systemic); Dasatinib; Dexketoprofen; Diclofenac (Systemic); Fat Emulsion (Fish Oil Based); Felbinac; Floctafenine; Glucosamine; Herbs (Anticoagulant/Antiplatelet Properties); Ibrutinib; Inotersen; Ketorolac (Nasal); Ketorolac (Systemic); Limaprost; Loop Diuretics; Morniflumate; Multivitamins/Fluoride (with ADE); Multivitamins/Minerals (with ADEK, Folate, Iron); Multivitamins/Minerals (with AE, No Iron); Naftazone; Omega-3 Fatty Acids; Pelubiprofen; Pentosan Polysulfate Sodium; Pentoxifylline; Phenylbutazone; Probenecid; Prostacyclin Analogues; Selective Serotonin Reuptake Inhibitors; Selumetinib; Serotonin/Norepinephrine Reuptake Inhibitors; Sodium Phosphates; Talniflumate; Tenoxicam; Thiazide and Thiazide-Like Diuretics; Tipranavir; Tolperisone; Tricyclic Antidepressants (Tertiary Amine); Vitamin E (Systemic); Zaltoprofen; Zanubrutinib

Decreased Effect

Etodolac may decrease the levels/effects of: Aliskiren; Angiotensin II Receptor Blockers; Angiotensin-Converting Enzyme Inhibitors; Beta-Blockers; Eplerenone; HydrALAZINE; Loop Diuretics; Macimorelin; Mifamurtide; Potassium-Sparing Diuretics; Prostaglandins (Ophthalmic); Salicylates; Selective Serotonin Reuptake Inhibitors; Sincalide; Thiazide and Thiazide-Like Diuretics

The levels/effects of Etodolac may be decreased by: Bile Acid Sequestrants; Salicylates

Food Interactions Etodolac peak serum levels may be decreased if taken with food. Management: Administer with food to decrease GI upset.

Pharmacodynamics/Kinetics

Onset of Action Analgesia: Immediate release: ~0.5 hour; Arthritis (chronic management): Typically within 2 weeks; Maximum effect: Analgesia: 1 to 2 hours

Duration of Action Mean range: 4 to 6 hours

Half-life Elimination Terminal:

Immediate release: Children (6 to 16 years, n=11): 6.5 hours (Boni 1999); Adults: 6.4 hours

Extended release: Children (6 to 16 years, n=72): 12 hours; Adults: 8.4 hours

Time to Peak Serum:

Immediate release: Children (6 to 16 years, n=11): 1.4 hours (Boni 1999); Adults: ~1 to 2 hours, increased 1.4 to 3.8 hours with food

Extended release: ~5 to 7 hours

Reproductive Considerations

The chronic use of NSAIDs in women of reproductive age may be associated with infertility that is reversible upon discontinuation of the medication (Micu 2011).

Pregnancy Risk Factor C

Pregnancy Considerations

Birth defects have been observed following in utero NSAID exposure in some studies; however, data is conflicting (Bloor 2013). Nonteratogenic effects, including prenatal constriction of the ductus arteriosus, persistent pulmonary hypertension of the newborn, oligohydramnios, necrotizing enterocolitis, renal dysfunction or failure, and intracranial hemorrhage have been observed in the fetus/neonate following in utero NSAID exposure. In addition, nonclosure of the ductus arteriosus postnatally may occur and be resistant to medical management (Bermas 2014; Bloor 2013). Because they may cause premature closure of the ductus arteriosus, the use of NSAIDs late in pregnancy (the third trimester) should be avoided. Use of NSAIDs can be considered for the treatment of mild rheumatoid arthritis flares in pregnant women; however, use should be minimized or avoided early and late in pregnancy (Bermas 2014; Saavedra Salinas 2015).

The use of NSAIDs close to conception may be associated with an increased risk of miscarriage (Bloor 2013; Bermas 2014).

Breastfeeding Considerations It is not known if etodolac is present in breast milk. In general, NSAIDs may be used in postpartum women who wish to breastfeed; however, agents other than etodolac are preferred (Montgomery 2012) and use should be avoided in women breastfeeding infants with platelet dysfunction or thrombocytopenia (Bloor 2013; Sammaritano 2014). Due to the potential for serious adverse reactions in the breastfeeding infant, the manufacturer recommends a decision be made whether to discontinue breastfeeding or to discontinue the drug, taking into account the importance of treatment to the mother.

Dosage Forms: US

Capsule, Oral:

Generic: 200 mg, 300 mg

Tablet, Oral:

Lodine: 400 mg

Generic: 400 mg, 500 mg

Tablet Extended Release 24 Hour, Oral:

Generic: 400 mg, 500 mg, 600 mg

Dosage Forms: Canada

Capsule, Oral:

Generic: 200 mg, 300 mg

◆ **Etodolic Acid** *see* Etodolac *on page* 622

Etonogestrel (e toe noe JES trel)

Brand Names: US Nexplanon

Pharmacologic Category Contraceptive; Progestin

Use Contraception: Prevention of pregnancy

Local Anesthetic/Vasoconstrictor Precautions No information available to require special precautions

Effects on Dental Treatment Key adverse event(s) related to dental treatment: Until more is known about the mechanism of interaction, use caution in prescribing antibiotics to female patients taking progestin-only contraceptives.

Effects on Bleeding No information available to require special precautions

Adverse Reactions

>10%:

Dermatologic: Acne vulgaris (14%)

Endocrine & metabolic: Menstrual disease (<3 episodes/90 days: 34%; prolonged menstrual bleeding lasting >14 days: 18%; >5 episodes/90 days: 7%), amenorrhea (no bleeding in 90 days: 22%), weight gain (14%)

Gastrointestinal: Abdominal pain (11%)

Genitourinary: Vaginitis (15%), mastalgia (13%)

Nervous system: Headache (25%)

Respiratory: Pharyngitis (11%)

1% to 10%:

Dermatologic: Localized erythema (implant site: ≤3%)

Endocrine & metabolic: Dysmenorrhea (7%)

Gastrointestinal: Nausea (6%)

Genitourinary: Leukorrhea (10%)

Hypersensitivity: Hypersensitivity reaction (5%)

Local: Application site reaction (implant site: 4% to 9%), local pain (implant site: 1% to 5%), hematoma at injection site (implant site: ≤3%), bruising at injection site (implant site: 2%)

Nervous system: Dizziness (7%), emotional lability (7%), depression (6%), nervousness (6%), pain (6%)

Neuromuscular & skeletal: Back pain (7%)

Respiratory: Flu-like symptoms (8%)

<1%, postmarketing, and/or case reports: Abscess, acute myocardial infarction, alopecia, anaphylaxis, angioedema (including exacerbation of hereditary angioedema), anxiety, arthralgia, breast hypertrophy, cerebrovascular accident, chloasma, cicatrix of skin, constipation, decreased libido, deep vein thrombosis, diarrhea, drowsiness, dysuria, edema, fatigue, fever, fibrosis (implant site), flatulence, genital pruritus, hot flash, hypertension, hypertrichosis, increased appetite, insomnia, intracranial hypertension (Tan 2019), migraine, musculoskeletal pain, myalgia, nipple discharge, ovarian cyst, paresthesia, pruritus, pulmonary embolism, rhinitis, seborrhea, seizure, skin rash, swelling (implant site), urinary tract infection, urticaria, vaginal discomfort, vomiting, weight loss

Mechanism of Action Etonogestrel is the active metabolite of desogestrel. It prevents pregnancy by suppressing ovulation, increasing the viscosity of cervical mucous, and inhibiting endometrial proliferation.

Pharmacodynamics/Kinetics

Duration of Action Each implant maintains etonogestrel levels sufficient to inhibit ovulation for 3 years

Half-life Elimination ~25 hours

Reproductive Considerations Evaluate pregnancy status prior to use.

Due to the risk of thromboembolism associated with pregnancy and the immediate postpartum period, the manufacturer does not recommend insertion <21 days' postpartum. However, available guidelines state that progestin-only implants may be inserted at any time if it is reasonably certain the woman is not pregnant, including immediately postpartum or post abortion (Curtis 2016a). Administration immediately postpartum (prior to hospital discharge) may be offered regardless of breastfeeding status and may help prevent rapid repeat and unintended pregnancies (ACOG 186 2017).

Etonogestrel serum concentrations decrease by 1 week after removal of the implant; pregnancies have been reported as early as 7 to 14 days after removal. Restart contraception immediately after removal if continued contraception is desired.

Pregnancy Considerations Use is contraindicated in pregnant women.

Etonogestrel is used to prevent pregnancy; the implant should be removed if pregnancy occurs. In general, the use of combination hormonal contraceptives, when inadvertently used early in pregnancy, have not been associated with teratogenic effects. There is no evidence that the risk is different with etonogestrel.

◆ **Etonogestrel and Ethinyl Estradiol** *see* Ethinyl Estradiol and Etonogestrel *on page 612*

◆ **ETOP** *see* Etoposide Phosphate *on page 626*

◆ **Etopophos** *see* Etoposide Phosphate *on page 626*

Etoposide (e toe POE side)

Brand Names: US Toposar

Brand Names: Canada GEN-Etoposide; VePesid

Pharmacologic Category Antineoplastic Agent, Podophyllotoxin Derivative; Antineoplastic Agent, Topoisomerase II Inhibitor

Use

Small cell lung cancer (oral and IV): Treatment (first-line) of small cell lung cancer (in combination with other chemotherapeutic agents).

Testicular cancer (IV): Treatment of refractory testicular tumors (injectable formulation) (in combination with other chemotherapeutic agents).

Local Anesthetic/Vasoconstrictor Precautions No information available to require special precautions

Effects on Dental Treatment Key adverse event(s) related to dental treatment: Mucositis (especially at high doses) and stomatitis.

Effects on Bleeding Myelosuppression is dose related. When thrombocytopenia occurs, platelet nadirs develop 9-16 days after drug administration. Bone marrow recovery is usually complete by day 20, and no cumulative toxicity has been reported.

Adverse Reactions The following may occur with higher doses used in stem cell transplantation: Alopecia, ethanol intoxication, hepatitis, hypotension (infusion-related), metabolic acidosis, mucositis, nausea and vomiting (severe), secondary malignancy, skin lesions (resembling Stevens-Johnson syndrome).

>10%:

Dermatologic: Alopecia (8% to 66%)

Gastrointestinal: Nausea and vomiting (31% to 43%), anorexia (10% to 13%), diarrhea (1% to 13%)

Hematologic & oncologic: Leukopenia (60% to 91%; grade 4: 3% to 17%; nadir: 7 to 14 days; recovery: by day 20), thrombocytopenia (22% to 41%; grades 3/4: 1% to 20%; nadir: 9 to 16 days; recovery: by day 20), anemia (≤33%)

1% to 10%:

Cardiovascular: Hypotension (1% to 2%; due to rapid infusion)

Central nervous system: Peripheral neuropathy (1% to 2%)

Gastrointestinal: Stomatitis (1% to 6%), abdominal pain (≤2%)

Hepatic: Hepatotoxicity (≤3%)

Hypersensitivity: Anaphylactoid reaction (intravenous: 1% to 2%; oral capsules: <1%; including bronchospasm, chills, dyspnea, fever, tachycardia)

<1%, postmarketing, and/or case reports: Amenorrhea, apnea (hypersensitivity-associated), back pain, constipation, cortical blindness (transient), cough, cyanosis, diaphoresis, drowsiness, dysphagia, erythema, esophagitis, extravasation (induration/necrosis), facial swelling, fatigue, fever, hyperpigmentation, hypersensitivity reaction, interstitial pneumonitis, ischemic heart disease, laryngospasm, maculopapular rash, malaise, metabolic acidosis, mucositis, myocardial infarction, optic neuritis, ovarian failure, pruritic erythematous rash, pruritus, pulmonary fibrosis, radiation-recall phenomenon (dermatitis), reversible posterior leukoencephalopathy syndrome (RPLS), seizure, skin rash, Stevens-Johnson syndrome, tongue edema, toxic epidermal necrolysis, toxic megacolon, urticaria, vasospasm, weakness

Mechanism of Action Etoposide has been shown to delay transit of cells through the S phase and arrest cells in late S or early G_2 phase. The drug may inhibit mitochondrial transport at the NADH dehydrogenase level or inhibit uptake of nucleosides into HeLa cells. It is a topoisomerase II inhibitor and appears to cause DNA strand breaks. Etoposide does not inhibit microtubular assembly.

Pharmacodynamics/Kinetics

Half-life Elimination Terminal: IV: Normal renal/hepatic function: Children: 6 to 8 hours: Adults: 4 to 11 hours

Reproductive Considerations

In females of reproductive potential, product labeling for etoposide phosphate notes that it may cause amenorrhea, infertility, or premature menopause; effective contraception should be used during therapy and for at least 6 months after the last dose. In males, azoospermia, oligospermia, or permanent loss of fertility may occur. In addition, spermatozoa and testicular tissue may be damaged. Males with female partners of reproductive potential should use condoms during therapy and for at least 4 months after the last dose.

Pregnancy Risk Factor D

Pregnancy Considerations

Adverse events were observed in animal reproduction studies. Fetal growth restriction and newborn myelosuppression have been observed following maternal use of regimens containing etoposide during pregnancy (NTP 2013; Peccatori 2013).

The European Society for Medical Oncology has published guidelines for diagnosis, treatment, and follow-up of cancer during pregnancy. The guidelines recommend referral to a facility with expertise in cancer during pregnancy and encourage a multidisciplinary team (obstetrician, neonatologist, oncology team). In general, if chemotherapy is indicated, it should be avoided during in the first trimester, there should be a 3-week time period between the last chemotherapy dose and anticipated delivery, and chemotherapy should not be administered beyond week 33 of gestation (Peccatori 2013).

Etoposide Phosphate (e toe POE side FOS fate)

Related Information

Etoposide *on page 626*

Brand Names: US Etopophos

Pharmacologic Category Antineoplastic Agent, Podophyllotoxin Derivative; Antineoplastic Agent, Topoisomerase II Inhibitor

Use

Small cell lung cancer: First-line treatment of small cell lung cancer (in combination with cisplatin)

Testicular cancer, refractory: Treatment of refractory testicular tumors (in combination with other chemotherapy agents)

Local Anesthetic/Vasoconstrictor Precautions No information available to require special precautions

Effects on Dental Treatment Key adverse event(s) related to dental treatment: Mucositis (especially at high doses), stomatitis, and taste perversion.

Effects on Bleeding Myelosuppression is dose related. When thrombocytopenia occurs, platelet nadirs develop 10-15 days after drug administration. Bone marrow recovery is usually complete by day 21, and no cumulative toxicity has been reported.

Adverse Reactions Also see adverse reactions for etoposide; etoposide phosphate is converted to etoposide, adverse reactions experienced with etoposide would also be expected with etoposide phosphate.

Frequency not defined:

- Central nervous system: Seizure, unusual taste
- Dermatologic: Skin abnormalities related to radiation recall, skin pigmentation, Stevens-Johnson syndrome, toxic epidermal necrolysis
- Gastrointestinal: Abdominal pain, constipation, dysphagia, nausea, vomiting
- Hematologic & oncologic: Bone marrow depression, major hemorrhage (life-threatening), neutropenia, secondary acute myelocytic leukemia, thrombocytopenia
- Hepatic: Hepatotoxicity
- Hypersensitivity: Anaphylaxis, hypersensitivity reaction
- Infection: Infection
- Ophthalmic: Cortical blindness (transient), optic neuritis
- Respiratory: Interstitial pneumonitis, pulmonary fibrosis
- Miscellaneous: Fever

<1%, postmarketing, and/or case reports: Extravasation injury

Mechanism of Action Etoposide phosphate is converted *in vivo* to the active moiety, etoposide, by dephosphorylation. Etoposide inhibits mitotic activity; inhibits cells from entering prophase; inhibits DNA synthesis. Initially thought to be mitotic inhibitors similar to podophyllotoxin, but actually have no effect on microtubule assembly. However, later shown to induce DNA strand breakage and inhibition of topoisomerase II (an enzyme which breaks and repairs DNA); etoposide acts in late S or early G2 phases.

Pharmacodynamics/Kinetics

Half-life Elimination Terminal: 4 to 11 hours; Children: Normal renal/hepatic function: 6 to 8 hours

Reproductive Considerations

Females of reproductive potential should avoid pregnancy during treatment. Etoposide phosphate may cause amenorrhea, infertility, or premature menopause; effective contraception should be used during therapy and for at least 6 months after the last dose.

In males, azoospermia, oligospermia, or permanent loss of fertility may occur. In addition, spermatozoa and testicular tissue may be damaged. Males with female partners of reproductive potential should use condoms during therapy and for 4 months after the last dose.

Pregnancy Considerations

Based on animal reproduction studies and the mechanism of action, etoposide phosphate may cause fetal harm if administered during pregnancy. Fetal growth restriction and newborn myelosuppression have been observed following maternal use of regimens containing etoposide during pregnancy (NTP 2013; Peccatori 2013).

The European Society for Medical Oncology has published guidelines for diagnosis, treatment, and follow-up of cancer during pregnancy. The guidelines recommend referral to a facility with expertise in cancer during pregnancy and encourage a multidisciplinary team (obstetrician, neonatologist, oncology team). In general, if chemotherapy is indicated, it should be avoided during in the first trimester, there should be a 3-week time period between the last chemotherapy dose and anticipated delivery, and chemotherapy should not be administered beyond week 33 of gestation. Guidelines for the treatment of SCLC are not provided (Peccatori 2013).

A pregnancy registry is available for all cancers diagnosed during pregnancy at Cooper Health (877-635-4499).

◆ **ETR** *see* Etravirine *on page 627*

Etravirine (et ra VIR een)

Related Information

HIV Infection and AIDS *on page 1690*

Brand Names: US Intelence

Brand Names: Canada Intelence

Pharmacologic Category Antiretroviral, Reverse Transcriptase Inhibitor, Non-nucleoside (Anti-HIV)

Use HIV-1 infection, treatment: Treatment of HIV-1 infection in combination with other antiretroviral agents in treatment-experienced patients ≥2 years of age.

Local Anesthetic/Vasoconstrictor Precautions No information available to require special precautions

Effects on Dental Treatment Key adverse event(s) related to dental treatment: Stomatitis has been reported.

Effects on Bleeding No information available to require special precautions related to hemostasis.

Adverse Reactions

>10%:

- Dermatologic: Skin rash (10% to 15%)
- Endocrine & metabolic: Increased serum cholesterol (grades 2/3: 8% to 20%), increased serum glucose (grades 2/3: 4% to 15%), increased LDL cholesterol (13%)

1% to 10%:

- Cardiovascular: Angina pectoris (<2%), atrial fibrillation (<2%), facial edema (<2%), myocardial infarction (<2%), syncope (<2%)
- Central nervous system: Peripheral neuropathy (4%), abnormal dreams (<2%), amnesia (<2%), anxiety (<2%), confusion (<2%), disorientation (<2%), disturbance in attention (<2%), drowsiness (<2%), hypersomnia (<2%), hypoesthesia (<2%), lethargy (<2%), nervousness (<2%), nightmares (<2%), paresthesia (<2%), seizure (<2%), sleep disturbance (<2%), vertigo (<2%)
- Dermatologic: Hyperhidrosis (<2%), night sweats (<2%), prurigo (<2%), xeroderma (<2%)

Endocrine & metabolic: Increased serum triglycerides (grades 2 to 4: 4% to 9%), increased amylase (grade 4: 2%), diabetes mellitus (<2%), dyslipidemia (<2%), gynecomastia (<2%), lipohypertrophy (<2%)

Gastrointestinal: Diarrhea (children and adolescents: ≥2%), abdominal distention (<2%), anorexia (<2%), constipation (<2%), flatulence (<2%), gastritis (<2%), gastroesophageal reflux disease (<2%), hematemesis (<2%), pancreatitis (<2%), retching (<2%), stomatitis (<2%), xerostomia (<2%), increased serum lipase (grade 4: 1%)

Hematologic & oncologic: Hemolytic anemia (<2%), decreased white blood cell count (grade 4: 1%)

Hepatic: Increased serum alanine aminotransferase (grades 2 to 4: 1% to 6%), increased serum aspartate aminotransferase (grade 3: 3%), hepatic failure (<2%), hepatitis (<2%), hepatomegaly (<2%), liver steatosis (<2%)

Hypersensitivity: Hypersensitivity reaction (<2%)

Immunologic: Immune reconstitution syndrome (<2%)

Neuromuscular & skeletal: Tremor (<2%)

Ophthalmic: Blurred vision (<2%)

Renal: Increased serum creatinine (grades 2/3: 2% to 6%), acute renal failure (<2%)

Respiratory: Bronchospasm (<2%), dyspnea on exertion (<2%)

<1%, postmarketing, and/or case reports: Angioedema, DRESS syndrome, erythema multiforme, hemorrhagic stroke, lipodystrophy, rhabdomyolysis, Stevens-Johnson syndrome, toxic epidermal necrolysis

Mechanism of Action As a non-nucleoside reverse transcriptase inhibitor, etravirine has activity against HIV-1 by binding to reverse transcriptase. It consequently blocks the RNA-dependent and DNA-dependent DNA polymerase activities, including HIV-1 replication. It does not require intracellular phosphorylation for antiviral activity.

Pharmacodynamics/Kinetics

Half-life Elimination 41 hours (± 20 hours)

Time to Peak 2.5 to 4 hours

Reproductive Considerations

The Health and Human Services (HHS) perinatal HIV guidelines do not recommend use of etravirine (except in special circumstances) for females living with HIV who are not yet pregnant but are trying to conceive.

For males and females living with HIV and planning a pregnancy, maximum viral suppression below the limits of detection with antiretroviral therapy (ART), modification of therapy (if needed), optimization of the woman's health, and a discussion of the potential risks and benefits of ART therapy during pregnancy is recommended prior to conception (HHS [perinatal] 2019).

Pregnancy Considerations

Etravirine has a variable (moderate to high) level of transfer across the human placenta.

Only limited data have been reported to the antiretroviral pregnancy registry and information is insufficient to evaluate teratogenic effects in humans. Maternal antiretroviral therapy (ART) may be associated with adverse pregnancy outcomes, including preterm delivery, stillbirth, low birth weight, and small for gestational age infants. Actual risks may be influenced by maternal factors, such as disease severity, gestational age at initiation of therapy, and specific ART regimen; therefore, close fetal monitoring is recommended. Because there is clear benefit to appropriate treatment, maternal ART should not be withheld due to concerns for adverse neonatal outcomes. Long-term follow-up is recommended for all infants exposed to antiretroviral medications; children without HIV but who were exposed to ART in utero and develop significant organ system abnormalities of unknown etiology (particularly of the CNS or heart) should be evaluated for potential mitochondrial dysfunction. Hypersensitivity reactions (including hepatic toxicity and rash) are more common in women on nonnucleoside reverse transcriptase inhibitor therapy; it is not known if pregnancy increases this risk.

The Health and Human Services (HHS) perinatal HIV guidelines do not recommend use in antiretroviral-naive pregnant females; use is not recommended (except in special circumstances) in pregnant females who have had ART therapy in the past but are restarting, or who require a new ART regimen (due to poor tolerance or poor virologic response of current regimen). In addition, females who become pregnant while taking etravirine may continue if viral suppression is effective and the regimen is well tolerated. The pharmacokinetics of etravirine are not significantly altered in pregnancy and dosing adjustment is not needed (limited data).

In general, ART is recommended for all pregnant females living with HIV to keep the viral load below the limit of detection and reduce the risk of perinatal transmission. Therapy should be individualized following a discussion of the potential risks and benefits of treatment during pregnancy. Monitoring of pregnant females is more frequent than in nonpregnant adults. ART should be continued postpartum for all females living with HIV and can be modified after delivery.

Health care providers are encouraged to enroll pregnant females exposed to antiretroviral medications as early in pregnancy as possible in the Antiretroviral Pregnancy Registry (1-800-258-4263 or http://www.APRegistry.com). Health care providers caring for pregnant females living with HIV and their infants may contact the National Perinatal HIV Hotline (888-448-8765) for clinical consultation (HHS [perinatal] 2019).

- ◆ **Euflexxa** *see* Hyaluronate and Derivatives *on page 761*
- ◆ **Eulexin** *see* Flutamide *on page 702*
- ◆ **Eutectic Mixture of Lidocaine and Tetracaine** *see* Lidocaine and Tetracaine *on page 914*
- ◆ **Euthyrox** *see* Levothyroxine *on page 900*
- ◆ **Evamist** *see* Estradiol (Systemic) *on page 596*
- ◆ **Evarrest** *see* Fibrin Sealant *on page 667*
- ◆ **Evekeo** *see* Amphetamine *on page 135*
- ◆ **Evekeo ODT** *see* Amphetamine *on page 135*
- ◆ **Evenity** *see* Romosozumab *on page 1344*

Everolimus (e ver OH li mus)

Related Information

Dentin Hypersensitivity, Acid Erosion, High Caries Index, Management of Alveolar Osteitis, and Xerostomia *on page 1762*

Osteonecrosis of the Jaw *on page 1699*

Brand Names: US Afinitor; Afinitor Disperz; Zortress

Brand Names: Canada Afinitor; Afinitor Disperz; TEVA-Everolimus

Pharmacologic Category Antineoplastic Agent, mTOR Kinase Inhibitor; Immunosuppressant Agent; mTOR Kinase Inhibitor

Use

Breast cancer, advanced (Afinitor only): Treatment of advanced hormone receptor-positive, HER2-negative breast cancer in postmenopausal women (in combination with exemestane and after letrozole or anastrozole failure)

Liver transplantation (Zortress only): Prophylaxis of allograft rejection in liver transplantation (in combination with corticosteroids and reduced doses of tacrolimus, everolimus should not be administered earlier than 30 days post-transplant)

Neuroendocrine tumors (Afinitor only): Treatment of locally advanced, metastatic or unresectable progressive pancreatic neuroendocrine tumors (PNET); treatment of progressive, well-differentiated, nonfunctional GI or lung neuroendocrine tumors in patients with unresectable, locally advanced or metastatic disease

Limitations of use: Not indicated for the treatment of functional carcinoid tumors.

Renal cell carcinoma, advanced (Afinitor only): Treatment of advanced renal cell cancer (RCC) after sunitinib or sorafenib failure

Renal transplantation (Zortress only): Prophylaxis of organ rejection in renal transplant patients at low to moderate immunologic risk (in combination with basiliximab induction and concurrent with corticosteroids and reduced doses of cyclosporine)

Tuberous sclerosis complex-associated partial-onset seizures (Afinitor Disperz only): Adjunctive treatment of partial-onset seizures associated with tuberous sclerosis complex (TSC) in adult and pediatric patients ≥2 years of age

Tuberous sclerosis complex-associated renal angiomyolipoma (Afinitor only): Treatment of renal angiomyolipoma with TSC not requiring immediate surgery

Tuberous sclerosis complex-associated subependymal giant cell astrocytoma (Afinitor or Afinitor Disperz only): Treatment of subependymal giant cell astrocytoma (SEGA) associated with TSC in adults and pediatric patients ≥1 year of age which requires therapeutic intervention, but cannot be curatively resected

Local Anesthetic/Vasoconstrictor Precautions

No information available to require special precautions

Effects on Dental Treatment Key adverse event(s) related to dental treatment: High incidence of mouth ulcers, mucositis, and stomatitis; xerostomia and taste alterations have been observed (normal salivary flow resumes upon discontinuation) (see Dental Health Professional Considerations)

Effects on Bleeding No information available to require special precautions

Adverse Reactions

Transplantation:

Reactions occur in kidney and liver transplantation unless otherwise specified. Reported as a part of combination therapy.

>10%:

Cardiovascular: Hypertension (17% to 30%), peripheral edema (kidney transplant: 45%; liver transplant: 18% to 20%)

Endocrine & metabolic: Diabetes mellitus (new onset: liver transplant: 32%, kidney transplant: 9%), hypercholesterolemia (9% to 17%), hyperglycemia (kidney transplant: 12%), hyperkalemia (renal transplant: 18%), hypokalemia (kidney transplant: 12%), hypomagnesemia (kidney transplant: 14%), hypophosphatemia (kidney transplant: 13%)

Gastrointestinal: Abdominal pain (13% to 15%), constipation (kidney transplant: 38%), diarrhea (19% to 24%), nausea (kidney transplant: 29%; liver transplant: 14% to 15%), vomiting (kidney transplant: 15%)

Genitourinary: Dysuria (kidney transplant: 11%), hematuria (kidney transplant: 12%), urinary tract infection (kidney transplant: 22%)

Hematologic & oncologic: Anemia (kidney transplant: 26%), leukopenia (3% to 13%)

Infection: Bacterial infection (liver transplant: 16%), hepatitis C (liver transplant: 11% to 14%), infection (kidney transplant: 62% to 64%; liver transplant: 50%), viral infection (liver transplant: 17%; kidney transplant: 10%)

Nervous system: Fatigue (9% to 11%), headache (18% to 22%), insomnia (kidney transplant: 17%; liver transplant: 6% to 7%)

Neuromuscular & skeletal: Back pain (kidney transplant: 11%), limb pain (kidney transplant: 12%)

Renal: Increased serum creatinine (kidney transplant: 18%)

Respiratory: Upper respiratory tract infection (kidney transplant: 16%)

Miscellaneous: Fever (13% to 19%), wound healing impairment (kidney transplant: 35%; liver transplant: 11%; includes dehiscence, incisional hernia, lymphocele, seroma)

1% to 10%:

Cardiovascular: Angina pectoris, atrial fibrillation, cardiac failure, chest discomfort, chest pain, deep vein thrombosis, edema, hypertensive crisis, hypotension, palpitations, phlebitis, pulmonary embolism, renal artery thrombosis, syncope, tachycardia, venous thromboembolism

Dermatologic: Acne vulgaris, acneiform eruption, alopecia, cellulitis, diaphoresis, ecchymoses, folliculitis, hypertrichosis, night sweats, onychomycosis, pruritus, skin rash, tinea pedis

Endocrine & metabolic: Acidosis, amenorrhea, cushingoid appearance, cyanocobalamin deficiency, dehydration, fluid retention, gout, hirsutism, hypercalcemia, hyperparathyroidism, hypertriglyceridemia, hyperuricemia, hypocalcemia, hypoglycemia, hyponatremia, hypothyroidism, iron deficiency, ovarian cyst

Gastrointestinal: Abdominal distention, anorexia, biliary obstruction, cholangitis, cholestasis, decreased appetite, dyspepsia (kidney transplant: 4%), dysphagia, epigastric distress, flatulence, gastritis, gastroenteritis, gastroesophageal reflux disease, gingival hyperplasia, hematemesis, hemorrhoids, hernia of abdominal cavity, inguinal hernia, intestinal obstruction, oral candidiasis, oral herpes simplex infection, oral mucosa ulcer, peritoneal effusion, peritonitis, stomatitis (kidney transplant: 8%), upper abdominal pain (kidney transplant: 3%)

Genitourinary: Benign prostatic hypertrophy, bladder spasm, erectile dysfunction (kidney transplant: 5%), nocturia, perinephric abscess, perinephric hematoma, pollakiuria, proteinuria, pyuria, scrotal edema, urethritis, urinary retention, urinary urgency

Hematologic & oncologic: Benign neoplasm (≤4%), leukocytosis, lymphadenopathy, lymphorrhea, malignant neoplasm (≤4%), neutropenia, pancytopenia, thrombocythemia, thrombocytopenia

Hepatic: Abnormal hepatic function tests (liver transplant: 7% to 8%), ascites (liver transplant: 4%), hepatitis (noninfectious), increased liver enzymes, increased serum alkaline phosphatase, increased serum bilirubin

Infection: Bacteremia, BK virus (kidney transplant: 1%), candidiasis, cytomegalovirus disease (1%), fungal infection (liver transplant: 2%), herpes virus infection, influenza, sepsis, wound infection

Nervous system: Agitation, anxiety, chills, depression, dizziness, drowsiness, hallucination, hemiparesis, hypoesthesia, lethargy, malaise, migraine, myasthenia, neuralgia, pain, paresthesia

Neuromuscular & skeletal: Arthralgia, asthenia, joint swelling, muscle spasm, musculoskeletal pain, myalgia, osteoarthritis, osteomyelitis, osteonecrosis, osteoporosis, spondylitis, tremor (8% to 10%)

Ophthalmic: Blurred vision, cataract, conjunctivitis

Renal: Hydronephrosis, increased blood urea nitrogen, interstitial nephritis, polyuria, pyelonephritis, renal failure syndrome (5% to 10%; may be acute), renal insufficiency, renal tubular necrosis

Respiratory: Atelectasis, bronchitis, cough (kidney transplant: 7%), dyspnea, epistaxis, lower respiratory tract infection, nasal congestion, nasopharyngitis, oropharyngeal pain, paranasal sinus congestion, pleural effusion (liver transplant: 5%), pneumonia, pulmonary edema, rhinorrhea, sinusitis, wheezing

<1%:

Cardiovascular: Pericardial effusion

Gastrointestinal: Pancreatitis

Hematologic & oncologic: Hemolytic-uremic syndrome, hepatocellular neoplasm, lymphoproliferative disorder, thrombotic microangiopathy, thrombotic thrombocytopenic purpura

Hypersensitivity: Angioedema

Respiratory: Interstitial pulmonary disease

Frequency not defined:

Cardiovascular: Venous thrombosis

Endocrine & metabolic: Decreased plasma testosterone, increased follicle-stimulating hormone

Hematologic & oncologic: Malignant lymphoma, malignant neoplasm of skin

Infection: Polyomavirus infection

Antineoplastic:

Antineoplastic indications include advanced hormone receptor-positive, advanced nonfunctional NET of gastrointestinal or lung origin, pancreatic neuroendocrine tumors, renal cell carcinoma, and tuberous sclerosis complex associated renal angiomyolipoma, subependymal giant cell astrocytoma, or seizures.

>10%:

Cardiovascular: Edema (≤39%), hypertension (4% to 13%), peripheral edema (13% to 39%)

Dermatologic: Acne vulgaris (10% to 22%), nail disease (5% to 22%), pruritus (12% to 21%), skin rash (21% to 59%), xeroderma (13%)

Endocrine & metabolic: Amenorrhea (15% to 17%), decreased serum bicarbonate (56%), decreased serum fibrinogen (8% to 38%), hypercholesterolemia (66% to 85%), hyperglycemia (13% to 75%), hypertriglyceridemia (27% to 73%), hypoalbuminemia (13% to 18%), hypocalcemia (37%), hypokalemia (23% to 27%), hypophosphatemia (9% to 49%)

Gastrointestinal: Abdominal pain (5% to 36%), anorexia (25%), constipation (10% to 14%), decreased appetite (6% to 30%), diarrhea (14% to 50%), dysgeusia (5% to 19%), gastroenteritis (10% to 12%), nausea (8% to 26%), stomatitis (44% to 78%; grades 3/4: 4% to 9%), vomiting (15% to 29%), weight loss (5% to 28%), xerostomia (8%)

Genitourinary: Irregular menses (10% to 11%), proteinuria (2% to 18%), urinary tract infection (9% to 31%)

Hematologic & oncologic: Anemia (41% to 92%; grades 3/4: ≤15%), leukopenia (37% to 49%; grades 3/4: 2%), lymphocytopenia (20% to 66%, grades 3/4: 1% to 18%), neutropenia (14% to 46%, grades 3/4: ≤9%), prolonged partial thromboplastin time (63% to 72%; grades 3/4: 3%), prolonged prothrombin time (40%), thrombocytopenia (19% to 45%; grades 3/4: ≤3%)

Hepatic: Increased serum alanine aminotransaminase (18% to 48%), increased serum alkaline phosphatase (32% to 74%), increased serum aspartate aminotransferase (23% to 57%)

Infection: Infection (37% to 58%)

Nervous system: Aggressive behavior (≤21%), anxiety (≤21%), behavioral problems (≤21%; includes abnormal behavior, agitation, obsessive compulsive symptoms, panic attack), dizziness (7% to 12%), fatigue (14% to 45%), headache (≤30%), insomnia (6% to 14%), malaise (≤45%), migraine (≤30%)

Neuromuscular & skeletal: Arthralgia (13% to 15%), asthenia (23% to 33%), back pain (15%), limb pain (8% to 14%), myalgia (11%)

Renal: Increased serum creatinine (5% to 50%)

Respiratory: Cough (20% to 30%; includes productive cough), dyspnea (20% to 24%; includes dyspnea on exertion), epistaxis (5% to 22%), nasopharyngitis (≤25%), oropharyngeal pain (11%), pneumonia (6% to 19%), pneumonitis (1% to 17%; may include interstitial pulmonary disease, pulmonary alveolar hemorrhage, pulmonary alveolitis, pulmonary fibrosis, pulmonary infiltrates, pulmonary toxicity, restrictive pulmonary disease), respiratory tract infection (31%), rhinitis (≤25%), upper respiratory tract infection (≤25%)

Miscellaneous: Fever (20% to 31%)

1% to 10%:

Cardiovascular: Cardiac failure (1%), chest pain (5%), tachycardia (3%)

Dermatologic: Acneiform eruption (3%), cellulitis (6%), erythema of skin (4%), onychoclasis (4%), palmar-plantar erythrodysesthesia (5%), skin lesion (4%)

Endocrine & metabolic: Diabetes mellitus (10%; new onset: <1%), exacerbation of diabetes mellitus (2%), heavy menstrual bleeding (6% to 10%), increased follicle-stimulating hormone (3%), increased luteinizing hormone (1% to 4%), menstrual disease (6% to 10%), ovarian cyst (3%)

Gastrointestinal: Dysphagia (4%), hemorrhoids (5%)

Genitourinary: Abnormal uterine bleeding (6%), azoospermia, dysmenorrhea (6%), vaginal hemorrhage (8%)

Hematologic & oncologic: Hemorrhage (3%)

Hepatic: Increased serum bilirubin (3%)

Hypersensitivity: Anaphylaxis, angioedema (≤1%), hypersensitivity reaction (≤3%)

Nervous system: Chills (4%), depression (5%), paresthesia (5%)

Neuromuscular & skeletal: Jaw pain (3%), muscle spasm (10%)

Ophthalmic: Conjunctivitis (2%), eyelid edema (4%)

Otic: Otitis media (6%)

Renal: Renal failure syndrome (3%)
Respiratory: Pharyngolaryngeal pain (4%), pleural effusion (7%), rhinorrhea (3%), streptococcal pharyngitis (10%)
<1%:
Cardiovascular: Deep vein thrombosis
Infection: Candidiasis, hepatitis C, sepsis
Respiratory: Respiratory distress
Miscellaneous: Wound healing impairment
Postmarketing (any indication):
Cardiovascular: Arterial thrombosis, hypersensitivity angiitis, septic shock, thrombosis of vascular graft (kidney)
Gastrointestinal: Acute pancreatitis, cholecystitis, cholelithiasis
Genitourinary: Male infertility, nephrotoxicity, oligospermia
Hematologic & oncologic: Thrombotic microangiopathy
Infection: Aspergillosis, polyomavirus infection, reactivation of HBV
Nervous system: Complex regional pain syndrome, progressive multifocal leukoencephalopathy

Mechanism of Action Everolimus is a macrolide immunosuppressant and a mechanistic target of rapamycin (mTOR) inhibitor which has antiproliferative and antiangiogenic properties, and also reduces lipoma volume in patients with angiomyolipoma. Reduces protein synthesis and cell proliferation by binding to the FK binding protein-12 (FKBP-12), an intracellular protein, to form a complex that inhibits activation of mTOR (mechanistic target of rapamycin) serine-threonine kinase activity. Also reduces angiogenesis by inhibiting vascular endothelial growth factor (VEGF) and hypoxia-inducible factor (HIF-1) expression. Angiomyolipomas may occur due to unregulated mTOR activity in TSC-associated renal angiomyolipoma (Budde 2012); everolimus reduces lipoma volume (Bissler 2013).

Pharmacodynamics/Kinetics

Half-life Elimination ~30 hours (Afinitor and Zortress); in pediatric renal transplant patients (3 to 16 years), half-life similar to adult data (Van Damme-Lombaerts 2002)

Time to Peak 1 to 2 hours (Afinitor and Zortress)

Reproductive Considerations

Verify pregnancy status in females of reproductive potential prior to initiating therapy. Females of reproductive potential should be advised to avoid pregnancy and use highly effective birth control during treatment and for 8 weeks after the last everolimus dose. Male patients with female partners of reproductive potential should use effective contraception during treatment and for 4 weeks after the last everolimus dose.

Everolimus may cause infertility. In females, menstrual irregularities, secondary amenorrhea, and increases in luteinizing hormone and follicle-stimulating hormone have occurred. Azoospermia and oligospermia have been observed in males.

Pregnancy Considerations

Based on the mechanism of action and data from animal reproduction studies, everolimus may cause fetal harm if administered during pregnancy. Information related to the use of everolimus in pregnancy is limited (Yamamura 2017).

The Transplant Pregnancy Registry International (TPR) is a registry that follows pregnancies that occur in maternal transplant recipients or those fathered by male transplant recipients. The TPR encourages reporting of pregnancies following solid organ transplant by contacting them at 1-877-955-6877 or https://www.transplantpregnancyregistry.org.

Dental Health Professional Considerations Consider a medical consultation prior to any invasive dental procedure in patients who have received an organ transplant; delayed wound healing due to the immunosuppressive effects and an increased potential for postoperative infection may be of concern.

◆ **EVG/COBI/FTC/TDF** *see* Elvitegravir, Cobicistat, Emtricitabine, and Tenofovir Disoproxil Fumarate *on page 553*
◆ **Evicel** *see* Fibrin Sealant *on page 667*
◆ **Evista** *see* Raloxifene *on page 1304*
◆ **Evithrom [DSC]** *see* Thrombin (Topical) *on page 1440*
◆ **Evoclin** *see* Clindamycin (Topical) *on page 375*

Evolocumab (e voe LOK ue mab)

Brand Names: US Repatha; Repatha Pushtronex System; Repatha SureClick

Brand Names: Canada Repatha

Pharmacologic Category Antilipemic Agent, PCSK9 Inhibitor; Monoclonal Antibody

Use

Homozygous familial hypercholesterolemia: Adjunct to diet and other LDL-lowering therapies (eg, statins, ezetimibe, LDL apheresis) for the treatment of patients with homozygous familial hypercholesterolemia who require additional lowering of LDL-C

Hyperlipidemia, primary: Adjunct to diet, alone or in combination with other lipid-lowering therapies (eg, maximum tolerated dose of statins), for the treatment of adults with primary hyperlipidemia, including heterozygous familial hyperlipidemia, to reduce LDL-C (Sabatine 2015)

Prevention of cardiovascular events in patients with established cardiovascular disease: To reduce the risk of MI, stroke, and coronary revascularization in adults with established cardiovascular disease. **Note:** Use in combination with an optimized regimen of lipid-lowering therapy (eg, high-intensity statin) (Sabatine 2017).

Local Anesthetic/Vasoconstrictor Precautions No information available to require special precautions

Effects on Dental Treatment Key adverse event(s) related to dental treatment: Nasopharyngitis has been reported

Effects on Bleeding No information available to require special precautions

Adverse Reactions

>10%: Respiratory: Nasopharyngitis (6% to 11%)
1% to 10%:
Cardiovascular: Hypertension (3%)
Central nervous system: Dizziness (4%), fatigue (2%)
Dermatologic: Skin rash (1%)
Endocrine & metabolic: Diabetes mellitus (9%)
Gastrointestinal: Gastroenteritis (3% to 6%), nausea (2%)
Genitourinary: Urinary tract infection (5%)
Hematologic & oncologic: Bruise (1%)
Infection: Influenza (8% to 9%)
Local: Injection site reaction (6%)
Neuromuscular & skeletal: Myalgia (4%)

Respiratory: Upper respiratory tract infection (9%), cough (1% to 5%), sinusitis (4%)

<1%, postmarketing, and/or case reports: Angioedema, antibody development, flu-like symptoms, hypersensitivity reaction

Mechanism of Action Evolocumab is a human monoclonal antibody (IgG2 isotype) that binds to proprotein convertase subtilisin kexin type 9 (PCSK9). PCSK9 binds to the low-density lipoprotein receptors (LDLR) on hepatocyte surfaces to promote LDLR degradation within the liver. LDLR is the primary receptor that clears circulating LDL; therefore, the decrease in LDLR levels by PCSK9 results in higher blood levels of LDL-cholesterol (LDL-C). By inhibiting the binding of PCSK9 to LDLR, evolocumab increases the number of LDLRs available to clear LDL from the blood, thereby lowering LDL-C levels.

Pharmacodynamics/Kinetics

Onset of Action Peak effect: Proprotein convertase subtilisin kexin type 9 (PCSK9) suppression: 4 hours

Half-life Elimination 11 to 17 days

Time to Peak SubQ: 3 to 4 days

Pregnancy Considerations

Evolocumab is a humanized monoclonal antibody (IgG_2). Potential placental transfer of human IgG is dependent upon the IgG subclass and gestational age, generally increasing as pregnancy progresses. The lowest exposure would be expected during the period of organogenesis (Palmeira 2012; Pentsuk 2009).

Data collection to monitor pregnancy and infant outcomes following exposure to evolocumab is ongoing. Health care providers are encouraged to enroll females exposed to evolocumab during pregnancy in the Pregnancy Registry (1-877-311-8972 or https://mothertobaby.org/ongoing-study/repatha).

- **Evomela** *see* Melphalan *on page 961*
- **Evotaz** *see* Atazanavir and Cobicistat *on page 188*
- **Evoxac** *see* Cevimeline *on page 330*
- **Evzio** *see* Naloxone *on page 1074*
- **Exalgo [DSC]** *see* HYDROmorphone *on page 776*
- **ExCel AP [OTC] [DSC]** *see* Povidone-Iodine (Topical) *on page 1249*
- **Exelderm** *see* Sulconazole *on page 1391*
- **Exelon** *see* Rivastigmine *on page 1341*

Exemestane (ex e MES tane)

Brand Names: US Aromasin

Brand Names: Canada ACT Exemestane; APO-Exemestane; Aromasin; MED-Exemestane; TEVA-Exemestane

Pharmacologic Category Antineoplastic Agent, Aromatase Inhibitor

Use Breast cancer: Treatment of advanced breast cancer in postmenopausal women whose disease has progressed following tamoxifen therapy; adjuvant treatment of postmenopausal women with estrogen receptor-positive early breast cancer following 2 to 3 years of tamoxifen (for a total of 5 consecutive years of adjuvant therapy)

Local Anesthetic/Vasoconstrictor Precautions No information available to require special precautions

Effects on Dental Treatment No significant effects or complications reported

Effects on Bleeding No information available to require special precautions

Adverse Reactions

Frequency not always defined. *Incidence not specifically defined, but reported in the range of 1% to 10%.

Cardiovascular: Hypertension (5% to 15%), edema (6% to 7%), ischemic heart disease (2%; angina pectoris, myocardial infarction), chest pain*

Central nervous system: Fatigue (8% to 22%), insomnia (11% to 14%), pain (13%), headache (7% to 13%), depression (6% to 13%), dizziness (8% to 10%), anxiety (4% to 10%), paresthesia (3%), carpal tunnel syndrome (2%), confusion,* hypoesthesia*

Dermatological: Hyperhidrosis (4% to 18%), alopecia (15%), dermatitis (8%), pruritus,* skin rash*

Endocrine & metabolic: Hot flash (13% to 33%), weight gain (8%), increased follicle-stimulating hormone, increased luteinizing hormone, increased sex hormone binding globulin (with daily doses of ≥2.5 mg; dose-dependent)

Gastrointestinal: Nausea (9% to 18%), abdominal pain (6% to 11%), diarrhea (4% to 10%), vomiting (7%), anorexia (6%), constipation (5%), increased appetite (3%), dyspepsia*

Genitourinary: Urinary tract infection (2% to 5%)

Hematologic & oncologic: Lymphedema*

Hepatic: Increased serum alkaline phosphatase (14% to 15%), increased serum bilirubin (5% to 7%)

Infection: Infection*

Neuromuscular & skeletal: Arthralgia (15% to 29%), back pain (9%), limb pain (9%), myalgia (6%), osteoarthritis (6%), weakness (6%), osteoporosis (5%), pathological fracture (4%), muscle cramps (2%)

Ophthalmic: Visual disturbance (5%)

Renal: Increased serum creatinine (6%)

Respiratory: Dyspnea (10%), cough (6%), flu-like symptoms (6%), bronchitis,* pharyngitis,* rhinitis,* sinusitis,* upper respiratory tract infection*

Miscellaneous: Fever (5%)

<1%, postmarketing, and/or case reports: Abnormal bone growth (osteochondrosis), acute generalized exanthematous pustulosis, cardiac failure, cholestatic hepatitis, endometrial hyperplasia, endometrial polyps, gastric ulcer, hepatitis, hypersensitivity reaction, increased gamma-glutamyl transferase, increased serum transaminases, neuropathy, tenosynovitis (fingers), thromboembolism, urticaria

Mechanism of Action Exemestane is an irreversible, steroidal aromatase inactivator. It is structurally related to androstenedione, and is converted to an intermediate that irreversibly blocks the active site of the aromatase enzyme, leading to inactivation ("suicide inhibition") and thus preventing conversion of androgens to estrogens in peripheral tissues. Significantly lowers circulating estrogens in postmenopausal breast cancers where growth is estrogen-dependent.

Pharmacodynamics/Kinetics

Half-life Elimination ~24 hours

Time to Peak Women with breast cancer: 1.2 hours

Reproductive Considerations

Evaluate pregnancy status prior to use. Pregnancy testing is recommended for females of reproductive potential within 7 days prior to therapy initiation. Women of reproductive potential should use effective contraception during treatment and for 1 month after the final dose.

Pregnancy Considerations

Exemestane is not indicated for use in premenopausal women. Based on the mechanism of action and on animal data, exemestane is expected to cause fetal harm if administered to a pregnant woman.

Exenatide (ex EN a tide)

Related Information

Endocrine Disorders and Pregnancy *on page 1684*

Brand Names: US Bydureon; Bydureon BCise; Byetta 10 MCG Pen; Byetta 5 MCG Pen

Brand Names: Canada Bydureon; Byetta 10 MCG Pen; Byetta 5 MCG Pen

Pharmacologic Category Antidiabetic Agent, Glucagon-Like Peptide-1 (GLP-1) Receptor Agonist

Use Diabetes mellitus, type 2, treatment: As an adjunct to diet and exercise to improve glycemic control in adults with type 2 diabetes mellitus.

Local Anesthetic/Vasoconstrictor Precautions No information available to require special precautions

Effects on Dental Treatment No significant effects or complications reported

Effects on Bleeding No information available to require special precautions

Adverse Reactions Incidence rates are for the extended release formulation unless otherwise noted.

>10%:

Gastrointestinal: Nausea (extended release: 8% to 11%; immediate release: 8%), diarrhea (extended release: 4% to 11%; immediate release: ≥1% to 2%)

Immunologic: Immunogenicity (20%, injection site reaction)

Local: Injection site reaction (17%), injection site nodule (11%)

1% to 10%:

Central nervous system: Headache (4% to 8%), dizziness (extended release: 3%; immediate release: ≥1% to 2%)

Dermatologic: Injection site pruritus (3%)

Endocrine & metabolic: Hypoglycemia (4% to 5%), severe hypoglycemia (≤2%)

Gastrointestinal: Constipation (2% to 9%), dyspepsia (extended release: 7%; immediate release: 3%), vomiting (immediate release: 4%, extended release: 3%), decreased appetite (immediate release: ≥1% to <2%)

Immunologic: Antibody development (extended release: 6%; immediate release: 1%; associated with glycemic response)

Local: Erythema at injection site (2% to 5%)

Frequency not defined: Cardiovascular: Increased heart rate (Robinson 2013)

<1%, postmarketing, and/or case reports (all formulations): Abdominal distention, abdominal pain, abscess at injection site, acute pancreatitis, acute renal failure, alopecia, anaphylaxis, angioedema, cellulitis at injection site, drowsiness, dysgeusia, eructation, exacerbation of renal failure, flatulence, hemorrhagic pancreatitis, hypersensitivity reaction, increased serum creatinine, kidney transplant dysfunction, macular eruption, necrotizing pancreatitis, papular rash, prolongation P-R Interval on ECG (Linnebjerg 2011), pruritus, renal function abnormality, renal insufficiency, tissue necrosis at injection site, urticaria

Mechanism of Action Exenatide is an analog of the hormone incretin (glucagon-like peptide 1 or GLP-1) which increases glucose-dependent insulin secretion, decreases inappropriate glucagon secretion, increases B-cell growth/replication, slows gastric emptying, and decreases food intake. Exenatide administration results in decreases in hemoglobin A_{1c} by approximately 0.5% to 1% (immediate release) or 1.5% to 1.9% (extended release).

Pharmacodynamics/Kinetics

Half-life Elimination

Immediate release (daily) formulation: 2.4 hours

Extended release (weekly) formulation: ~2 weeks

Time to Peak SubQ:

Immediate release (daily) formulation: 2.1 hours

Extended release (weekly) formulation: Single dose: Initial period of release of surface-bound exenatide is followed by a gradual release from microspheres with peaks at week 2 and week 6 to 7 respectively; with once-weekly dosing steady state is achieved at 6 to 7 weeks (Bydureon) and 10 weeks (Bydureon BCise).

Pregnancy Considerations

Based on in vitro data, exenatide has a low potential to cross the placenta (Hiles 2003).

Poorly controlled diabetes during pregnancy can be associated with an increased risk of adverse maternal and fetal outcomes, including diabetic ketoacidosis, preeclampsia, spontaneous abortion, preterm delivery, delivery complications, major birth defects, stillbirth, and macrosomia. To prevent adverse outcomes, prior to conception and throughout pregnancy, maternal blood glucose and HbA_{1c} should be kept as close to target goals as possible but without causing significant hypoglycemia (ADA 2020; Blumer 2013).

Agents other than exenatide are currently recommended to treat diabetes mellitus in pregnancy (ADA 2020).

- ◆ **Exendin-4** *see* Exenatide *on page 633*
- ◆ **Exparel** *see* Bupivacaine (Liposomal) *on page 259*
- ◆ **Exservan** *see* Riluzole *on page 1328*
- ◆ **Extavia** *see* Interferon Beta-1b *on page 835*
- ◆ **Extina** *see* Ketoconazole (Topical) *on page 859*
- ◆ **EYE001** *see* Pegaptanib *on page 1198*
- ◆ **Ezallor** *see* Rosuvastatin *on page 1348*
- ◆ **Ezallor Sprinkle** *see* Rosuvastatin *on page 1348*

Ezetimibe (ez ET i mibe)

Related Information

Cardiovascular Diseases *on page 1654*

Brand Names: US Zetia

Brand Names: Canada ACH-Ezetimibe; ACT Ezetimibe [DSC]; AG-Ezetimibe; APO-Ezetimibe; AURO-Ezetimibe; BIO-Ezetimibe; Ezetrol; GLN-Ezetimibe; JAMP-Ezetimibe; M-Ezetimibe [DSC]; Mar-Ezetimibe; MINT-Ezetimibe; MYLAN-Ezetimibe [DSC]; NRA-Ezetimibe; PMS-Ezetimibe; Priva-Ezetimibe; RAN-Ezetimibe; RIVA-Ezetimibe [DSC]; SANDOZ Ezetimibe; TEVA-Ezetimibe

Pharmacologic Category Antilipemic Agent, 2-Azetidinone

Use

Homozygous familial hypercholesterolemia: In combination with a high-intensity statin (eg, atorvastatin) for the reduction of elevated total cholesterol (total-C) and low-density lipoprotein cholesterol (LDL-C) levels in patients with homozygous familial hypercholesterolemia as an adjunct to other lipid-lowering treatments (eg, LDL apheresis) or if such treatments are unavailable.

Homozygous sitosterolemia: As adjunctive therapy to diet for the reduction of elevated sitosterol and campesterol levels in patients with homozygous familial sitosterolemia.

Primary hyperlipidemia: As adjunctive therapy to diet and an HMG-CoA reductase inhibitor or as monotherapy if an HMG-CoA reductase inhibitor is not tolerated for the reduction of total-C, LDL-C, apolipoprotein B, and nonhigh-density lipoprotein cholesterol in patients with primary (heterozygous familial and nonfamilial) hyperlipidemia or mixed hyperlipidemia.

Local Anesthetic/Vasoconstrictor Precautions No information available to require special precautions

Effects on Dental Treatment No significant effects or complications reported

Effects on Bleeding No information available to require special precautions

Adverse Reactions

1% to 10%:

- Central nervous system: Fatigue (2%)
- Gastrointestinal: Diarrhea (4%)
- Hepatic: Increased serum transaminases (with HMG-CoA reductase inhibitors; ≥3 x ULN: 1%)
- Infection: Influenza (2%)
- Neuromuscular & skeletal: Arthralgia (3%), limb pain (3%)
- Respiratory: Upper respiratory tract infection (4%), sinusitis (3%)

<1%, postmarketing, and/or case reports: Abdominal pain, anaphylaxis, angioedema, autoimmune hepatitis (Stolk 2006), cholecystitis, cholelithiasis, cholestatic hepatitis (Stolk 2006), depression, dizziness, erythema multiforme, headache, hepatitis, hypersensitivity reaction, increased creatine phosphokinase, myalgia, myopathy, nausea, pancreatitis, paresthesia, rhabdomyolysis, skin rash, thrombocytopenia, urticaria

Mechanism of Action Inhibits absorption of cholesterol at the brush border of the small intestine via the sterol transporter, Niemann-Pick C1-Like1 (NPC1L1). This leads to a decreased delivery of cholesterol to the liver, reduction of hepatic cholesterol stores and an increased clearance of cholesterol from the blood; decreases total C, LDL-cholesterol (LDL-C), ApoB, and triglycerides (TG) while increasing HDL-cholesterol (HDL-C).

Pharmacodynamics/Kinetics

Onset of Action Within 1 week; Maximum effect: 2-4 weeks

Half-life Elimination 22 hours (ezetimibe and metabolite)

Time to Peak Plasma: 4-12 hours (ezetimibe); 1-2 hours (active metabolite); Effects: ~2 weeks

Pregnancy Risk Factor C

Pregnancy Considerations

Adverse events were observed in some animal reproduction studies. Use is contraindicated in pregnant women who require combination therapy with an HMG-CoA reductase inhibitor. If treatment for familial hypercholesterolemia is needed during pregnancy, other agents are preferred (Wiegman 2015).

◆ **Ezetimibe and Bempedoic Acid** *see* Bempedoic Acid and Ezetimibe *on page 224*

Ezetimibe and Simvastatin

(ez ET i mibe & SIM va stat in)

Related Information

Ezetimibe *on page 633*

Simvastatin *on page 1372*

Brand Names: US Vytorin

Pharmacologic Category Antilipemic Agent, 2-Azetidinone; Antilipemic Agent, HMG-CoA Reductase Inhibitor

Use

Homozygous familial hypercholesterolemia: As an adjunct to diet for the reduction of elevated total cholesterol (total-C) and low-density lipoprotein cholesterol (LDL-C) in patients with homozygous familial hypercholesterolemia, as an adjunct to other lipid-lowering treatments (eg, LDL apheresis), or if such treatments are unavailable.

Primary hyperlipidemia: As an adjunct to diet for the reduction of elevated total-C, LDL-C, apolipoprotein B (apo B), triglycerides, and non-high-density lipoprotein cholesterol (HDL-C), and to increase HDL-C in patients with primary (heterozygous familial and nonfamilial) hyperlipidemia or mixed hyperlipidemia.

Limitations of use: No incremental benefit of ezetimibe/simvastatin on cardiovascular morbidity and mortality over and above that demonstrated for simvastatin has been established. Ezetimibe/simvastatin has not been studied in Fredrickson type I, III, IV, and V dyslipidemias.

Local Anesthetic/Vasoconstrictor Precautions No information available to require special precautions

Effects on Dental Treatment Key adverse event(s) related to dental treatment: Assess unusual presentations of muscle weakness or myopathy resulting from lipid therapy such as patient having a difficult time brushing teeth or weakness with chewing. Refer patient back to their physician for evaluation and adjustment of lipid therapy.

Effects on Bleeding No information available to require special precautions

Adverse Reactions Incidences refer to combination, Vytorin. Also see individual agents.

1% to 10%:

- Central nervous system: Headache (6%)
- Gastrointestinal: Diarrhea (3%)
- Hepatic: Increased serum ALT (4%)
- Infection: Influenza (2%)
- Neuromuscular & skeletal: Myalgia (4%), limb pain (2%), myopathy
- Respiratory: Upper respiratory infection (4%)

Mechanism of Action

Ezetimibe: Inhibits absorption of cholesterol at the brush border of the small intestine, leading to a decreased delivery of cholesterol to the liver. Ezetimibe inhibits the enzyme Niemann-Pick C1-Like1 (NPC1L1), a sterol transporter.

Simvastatin: A methylated derivative of lovastatin that acts by competitively inhibiting 3-hydroxy-3-methylglutaryl-coenzyme A (HMG-CoA) reductase, the enzyme that catalyzes the rate-limiting step in cholesterol biosynthesis. In addition to the ability of HMG-CoA reductase inhibitors to decrease levels of high-sensitivity C-reactive protein (hsCRP), they also possess pleiotropic properties including improved endothelial function, reduced inflammation at the site of the coronary plaque, inhibition of platelet aggregation, and anticoagulant effects (de Denus 2002; Ray 2005).

Reproductive Considerations

Use is contraindicated in women who may become pregnant.

Pregnancy Risk Factor X

Pregnancy Considerations

Use is contraindicated in pregnant women. See individual monographs for additional information.

- **EZN-2285** *see* Calaspargase Pegol *on page 278*
- **F_3T** *see* Trifluridine *on page 1497*
- **FA-8 [OTC]** *see* Folic Acid *on page 709*
- **Fabior** *see* Tazarotene *on page 1408*
- **Factive [DSC]** *see* Gemifloxacin *on page 733*
- **Factor VIII Concentrate** *see* Antihemophilic Factor/von Willebrand Factor Complex (Human) *on page 154*
- **Factor VIII (Human)** *see* Antihemophilic Factor (Human) *on page 152*
- **Factor VIII (Human)/von Willebrand Factor** *see* Antihemophilic Factor/von Willebrand Factor Complex (Human) *on page 154*
- **Factor VIII Inhibitor Bypassing Activity** *see* Anti-inhibitor Coagulant Complex (Human) *on page 156*
- **Factor VIII (Recombinant [Fc Fusion Protein])** *see* Antihemophilic Factor (Recombinant [Fc Fusion Protein]) *on page 154*
- **Factor VIII (Recombinant)** *see* Antihemophilic Factor (Recombinant) *on page 153*
- **Factor Eight Inhibitor Bypassing Activity** *see* Anti-inhibitor Coagulant Complex (Human) *on page 156*
- **FAG-201** *see* Dimethyl Fumarate *on page 501*
- **FaLessa** *see* Ethinyl Estradiol and Levonorgestrel *on page 612*
- **Falmina** *see* Ethinyl Estradiol and Levonorgestrel *on page 612*

Famciclovir (fam SYE kloe veer)

Related Information

Systemic Viral Diseases *on page 1709*

Viral Infections *on page 1754*

Brand Names: US Famvir [DSC]

Brand Names: Canada ACT Famciclovir; APO-Famciclovir; Famvir; PMS-Famciclovir; SANDOZ Famciclovir

Pharmacologic Category Antiviral Agent

Use Treatment of acute herpes zoster (shingles) in immunocompetent patients; treatment and suppression of recurrent episodes of genital herpes in immunocompetent patients; treatment of herpes labialis (cold sores) in immunocompetent patients; treatment of recurrent orolabial/genital (mucocutaneous) herpes simplex in adult patients with HIV.

Local Anesthetic/Vasoconstrictor Precautions

No information available to require special precautions

Effects on Dental Treatment No significant effects or complications reported

Effects on Bleeding No information available to require special precautions

Adverse Reactions Frequencies vary with dose and duration.

>10%:

Central nervous system: Headache (9% to 23%)

Gastrointestinal: Nausea (11% to 13%)

1% to 10%:

Central nervous system: Fatigue (≤5%), migraine (≤3%), paresthesia (≤3%)

Dermatologic: Pruritus (2% to 4%), skin rash (3%)

Gastrointestinal: Diarrhea (2% to 8%), flatulence (≤5%), vomiting (≤5%)

Genitourinary: Dysmenorrhea (≤8%)

Hematologic & oncologic: Neutropenia (3%), leukopenia (1%)

Hepatic: Increased serum ALT (3%), increased serum AST (2%), increased serum bilirubin (2%)

<1%, postmarketing, and/or case reports: Abnormal hepatic function tests, anaphylactic shock, anaphylaxis, anemia, angioedema (eyelid edema, facial edema, periorbital edema, pharyngeal edema), cholestatic jaundice, confusion, delirium, disorientation, dizziness, drowsiness, erythema multiforme, hallucination, hypersensitivity angiitis, palpitations, seizure, Stevens-Johnson syndrome, thrombocytopenia, toxic epidermal necrolysis, urticaria

Mechanism of Action Famciclovir undergoes rapid biotransformation to the active compound, penciclovir (prodrug), which is phosphorylated by viral thymidine kinase in HSV-1, HSV-2, and VZV-infected cells to a monophosphate form; this is then converted to penciclovir triphosphate and competes with deoxyguanosine triphosphate to inhibit HSV-2 polymerase, therefore, herpes viral DNA synthesis/replication is selectively inhibited.

Pharmacodynamics/Kinetics

Half-life Elimination

Penciclovir: 2 to 4 hours; Prolonged in renal impairment:

CrCl 40 to 59 mL/minute: ~3.4 hours

CrCl 20 to 39 mL/minute: ~6.2 hours

CrCl <20 mL/minute: ~13.4 hours

Intracellular penciclovir triphosphate: HSV 1: 10 hours; HSV 2: 20 hours; VZV: 7 hours

Time to Peak Penciclovir: ~1 hour

Pregnancy Considerations

Based on available data, use during pregnancy appears to be well tolerated; however, other agents are preferred when treatment is needed (CDC [Workowski 2015]; Werner 2017).

Health care providers are encouraged to enroll women exposed to famciclovir during pregnancy in the Famvir Pregnancy reporting system (888-669-6682).

Famotidine (fa MOE ti deen)

Related Information

Gastrointestinal Disorders *on page 1678*

Brand Names: US Acid Controller Max St [OTC]; Acid Controller Original Str [OTC]; Acid Reducer Maximum Strength [OTC]; Acid Reducer [OTC]; Heartburn Relief Max St [OTC]; Heartburn Relief [OTC]; Pepcid; Pepcid AC Maximum Strength [OTC]

Brand Names: Canada ALTI-Famotidine; APO-Famotidine; BCI-Famotidine [DSC]; CO Famotidine; Famotidine Omega W-O Preserv; Famotidine Omega W-Preserv; GMD-Famotidine; MYLAN-Famotidine [DSC]; TEVA-Famotidine

Pharmacologic Category Histamine H_2 Antagonist

Use

Oral:

Gastroesophageal reflux disease: Treatment of gastroesophageal reflux disease (GERD) and esophagitis due to GERD.

Heartburn (OTC only): Relief of heartburn, acid indigestion, and sour stomach.

Peptic ulcer disease: Treatment of active duodenal or gastric ulcers. **Note:** Although a labeled indication, proton pump inhibitors (PPIs) are considered the standard of care for treatment of peptic ulcer disease (PUD) rather than H_2-receptor antagonists (eg, famotidine) (Lanas 2017; Vakil 2019).

Injection:

Patients not able to take oral medication: As an alternative to the oral dosage form for short-term use in patients who are unable to take oral medication.

Local Anesthetic/Vasoconstrictor Precautions No information available to require special precautions

Effects on Dental Treatment Key adverse event(s) related to dental treatment: Rare occurrence of Stevens-Johnson syndrome, taste disorder, and xerostomia (normal salivary flow resumes upon discontinuation) have been reported.

Effects on Bleeding No information available to require special precautions

Adverse Reactions All reported ADRs are for the oral formulations unless otherwise noted.

>10%: Central nervous system: Agitation (infants: ≤14%; adults: <1%)

1% to 10%:

Central nervous system: Headache (5%), dizziness (1%)

Gastrointestinal: Diarrhea (2%), constipation (1%), necrotizing enterocolitis (very low birth weight neonates; Guillet 2006)

Frequency not defined: Local: Irritation at injection site (IV)

<1%, postmarketing, and/or case reports: Abdominal distress, acne vulgaris, agranulocytosis, alopecia, anaphylaxis, angioedema, anorexia, anxiety, arthralgia, asthenia, atrioventricular block, bronchospasm, cardiac arrhythmia, cholestatic jaundice, confusion, conjunctival injection, decreased libido, depression, drowsiness, facial edema, fatigue, fever, flushing, hallucination, hepatitis, hypersensitivity reaction, impotence, increased liver enzymes, insomnia, interstitial pneumonitis, leukopenia, muscle cramps, musculoskeletal pain, nausea, palpitations, pancytopenia, paresthesia, periorbital edema, prolonged QT interval on ECG, pruritus, psychiatric disturbance, rhabdomyolysis, seizure, skin rash, Stevens-Johnson syndrome, taste disorder, thrombocytopenia, tinnitus, toxic epidermal necrolysis, urticaria, vomiting, xeroderma, xerostomia

Mechanism of Action Competitive inhibition of histamine at H_2 receptors of the gastric parietal cells, which inhibits gastric acid secretion

Pharmacodynamics/Kinetics

Onset of Action Antisecretory effect: Oral: Within 1 hour; Peak effect: Antisecretory effect: Oral: Within 1 to 3 hours (dose-dependent); IV: Within 30 minutes

Duration of Action Antisecretory effect: IV, Oral: 10 to 12 hours

Half-life Elimination IV:

Infants: ≤3 months: 8.1 ± 3.5 hours to 10.5 ± 5.4 hours; >3 to 12 months: 4.5 ± 1.1 hours

Children <11 years: 3.38 ± 2.6 hours

Children ≥11 years and Adolescents ≤15 years: 2.3 ± 0.4 hours

Adults: 2.5 to 3.5 hours; prolonged with renal impairment; Oliguria: >20 hours; Anuria: 24 hours

Time to Peak Serum: Oral: ~1 to 3 hours

Pregnancy Considerations Famotidine crosses the placenta (Wang 2013).

Due to pregnancy-induced physiologic changes, renal clearance of famotidine may be increased (Wang 2011).

Histamine H_2 antagonists have been evaluated for the treatment of gastroesophageal reflux disease (GERD) during pregnancy. Agents other than famotidine may be preferred for initial therapy (Richter 2005; van der Woude 2014). Histamine H_2 antagonists may be used for aspiration prophylaxis prior to cesarean delivery (ASA 2016).

◆ **Fampridine** *see* Dalfampridine *on page 431*

◆ **Fampridine-SR** *see* Dalfampridine *on page 431*

Fam-Trastuzumab Deruxtecan

(fam tras TU zoo mab de RUX teh can)

Brand Names: US Enhertu

Pharmacologic Category Antineoplastic Agent, Anti-HER2; Antineoplastic Agent, Antibody Drug Conjugate; Antineoplastic Agent, Monoclonal Antibody; Antineoplastic Agent, Topoisomerase I Inhibitor

Use

Breast cancer, unresectable or metastatic: Treatment of unresectable or metastatic human epidermal growth factor receptor 2 (HER2)-positive breast cancer in adults who previously received 2 or more prior anti-HER2-based regimens in the metastatic setting.

Local Anesthetic/Vasoconstrictor Precautions No information available to require special precautions.

Effects on Dental Treatment Key adverse event(s) related to dental treatment: Frequent occurrence of stomatitis.

Effects on Bleeding Thrombocytopenia (20%) has been associated with use; severe thrombocytopenia (rare) may be associated with delayed coagulation. Consultation to ensure adequate platelet counts may be considered.

Adverse Reactions

>10%:

Central nervous system: Fatigue (59%), headache (19%)

Dermatologic: Alopecia (46%)

Endocrine & metabolic: Hypokalemia (12% to 26%)

Gastrointestinal: Nausea (79%), vomiting (47%), constipation (35%), decreased appetite (32%), diarrhea (29%), abdominal pain (19%), stomatitis (14%; grades 3/4: <1%), dyspepsia (12%)

Hematologic & oncologic: Anemia (31%; grades 3/4: 7%), neutropenia (30%; grades 3/4: 16%), leukopenia (22%; grades 3/4: 6%), thrombocytopenia (20%; grades 3/4: 3%)

Hepatic: Increased serum aspartate aminotransferase (14% to 41%), increased serum alanine aminotransferase (10% to 38%)

Ophthalmic: Dry eye syndrome (11%)

Respiratory: Cough (20%), upper respiratory tract infection (15%), dyspnea (13%), epistaxis (13%)

1% to 10%:

Central nervous system: Dizziness (10%)

Dermatologic: Skin rash (10%), cellulitis (>1%)

Gastrointestinal: Intestinal obstruction (>1%)

Hematologic & oncologic: Febrile neutropenia (2%)

Respiratory: Interstitial pulmonary disease (9%), pneumonia (>1%)

Miscellaneous: Infusion related reaction (3%)

<1%: Antibody development, decreased left ventricular ejection fraction

Frequency not defined: Respiratory: Pneumonitis

Mechanism of Action Fam-trastuzumab deruxtecan is a human epidermal growth factor receptor 2 (HER2)-directed antibody-drug conjugate composed of a humanized IgG1 monoclonal antibody, which has the same amino acid sequence as trastuzumab (and targets HER2), a cleavable tetrapeptide-based linker, and the cytotoxic component, a topoisomerase I inhibitor (Modi 2020). The deruxtecan component is a cleavable linker and the topoisomerase inhibitor, DXd (an exatecan derivative). Upon binding to HER2 on tumor cells, fam-trastuzumab deruxtecan undergoes internalization and intracellular linker cleavage by lysosomal enzymes, releasing DXd and resulting in DNA damage and cell death.

Pharmacodynamics/Kinetics

Half-life Elimination Fam-trastuzumab deruxtecan: ~5.7 days; DXd: 5.8 days.

Reproductive Considerations

[US Boxed Warning]: Exposure to fam-trastuzumab deruxtecan during pregnancy can result in embryo-fetal harm. Advise patients of these risks and the need for effective contraception.

Evaluate pregnancy status prior to use in females of reproductive potential. Females of reproductive potential should use effective contraception during therapy and for at least 7 months after the last fam-trastuzumab deruxtecan dose. Males with female partners of reproductive potential should use effective contraception during therapy and for at least 4 months after the last dose of fam-trastuzumab deruxtecan.

Pregnancy Considerations

[US Boxed Warning]: Exposure to fam-trastuzumab deruxtecan during pregnancy can result in embryo-fetal harm. Advise patients of these risks and the need for effective contraception.

Oligohydramnios and oligohydramnios sequence (manifested as pulmonary hypoplasia, skeletal malformations, and neonatal death) were observed following trastuzumab exposure during pregnancy (trastuzumab is the antibody component of fam-trastuzumab deruxtecan). Monitor for oligohydramnios if trastuzumab exposure occurs during pregnancy or within 7 months prior to conception; conduct appropriate fetal testing if oligohydramnios occurs.

- ◆ **Fam-Trastuzumab Deruxtecan-nxki** *see* Fam-Trastuzumab Deruxtecan *on page* 636
- ◆ **Famvir [DSC]** *see* Famciclovir *on page* 635
- ◆ **Fanapt** *see* Iloperidone *on page* 796
- ◆ **Fanapt Titration Pack** *see* Iloperidone *on page* 796
- ◆ **2F-ara-AMP** *see* Fludarabine *on page* 682
- ◆ **Fareston** *see* Toremifene *on page* 1466
- ◆ **Faridak** *see* Panobinostat *on page* 1188
- ◆ **Farxiga** *see* Dapagliflozin *on page* 435
- ◆ **Farydak** *see* Panobinostat *on page* 1188
- ◆ **Fasenra** *see* Benralizumab *on page* 227
- ◆ **Fasenra Pen** *see* Benralizumab *on page* 227
- ◆ **Faslodex** *see* Fulvestrant *on page* 721
- ◆ **Fast-Acting Insulin Aspart** *see* Insulin Aspart *on page* 817
- ◆ **Faster Aspart** *see* Insulin Aspart *on page* 817
- ◆ **Fayosim** *see* Ethinyl Estradiol and Levonorgestrel *on page* 612
- ◆ **FazaClo [DSC]** *see* CloZAPine *on page* 399
- ◆ **5-FC** *see* Flucytosine *on page* 682
- ◆ **FC1157a** *see* Toremifene *on page* 1466
- ◆ **FC1271a** *see* Ospemifene *on page* 1150
- ◆ **FdUrD** *see* Floxuridine *on page* 673
- ◆ **FE200486** *see* Degarelix *on page* 450

Febuxostat (feb UX oh stat)

Brand Names: US Uloric

Brand Names: Canada JAMP Febuxostat; MAR-Febuxostat; TEVA-Febuxostat; Uloric

Pharmacologic Category Antigout Agent; Xanthine Oxidase Inhibitor

Use

Hyperuricemia: Chronic management of hyperuricemia in patients with gout who have an inadequate response to a maximally titrated dose of allopurinol, who are intolerant to allopurinol, or for whom treatment with allopurinol is not advisable

Limitations of use: Not recommended for treatment of asymptomatic hyperuricemia.

Local Anesthetic/Vasoconstrictor Precautions No information available to require special precautions

Effects on Dental Treatment Key adverse event(s) related to dental treatment: Xerostomia (normal salivary flow resumes upon discontinuation) and taste alteration has been reported in <1% of patients.

Effects on Bleeding No information available to require special precautions

Adverse Reactions

1% to 10%:

Dermatologic: Skin rash (2%)

Gastrointestinal: Nausea (1%)

Hepatic: Hepatic insufficiency (5% to 7%), increased serum alanine aminotransferase (3%), increased serum aspartate aminotransferase (2%)

Neuromuscular & skeletal: Arthralgia (≤1%)

Frequency not defined: Endocrine & metabolic: Acute gout attack

<1%, postmarketing, and/or case reports: Abdominal distention, abdominal pain, abnormal electroencephalogram, abnormal gait, abnormal hepatic function tests, abnormal skin odor, aggressive behavior, agitation, agranulocytosis, alopecia, altered sense of smell, anaphylaxis, anemia, angina pectoris, angioedema, anorexia, anxiety, arthritis, asthenia, atrial fibrillation, atrial flutter, blood coagulation test abnormality, blurred vision, bronchitis, bruise, casts in urine, cerebral infarction (lacunar), cerebrovascular accident, chest discomfort, chest pain, cholecystitis, cholelithiasis, constipation, cough, deafness, decreased appetite, decreased libido, decreased mental acuity, decreased serum bicarbonate, decreased urine output, dehydration, depression, dermatitis, diabetes mellitus, drowsiness, drug reaction with eosinophilia and systemic symptoms, dry nose, dysgeusia, dyspepsia, dyspnea, ecchymoses, ECG abnormality, eczema, edema, eosinophilia, epistaxis, equilibrium disturbance, erectile dysfunction, erythema multiforme, exfoliation of skin, fatigue, feeling abnormal, flatulence, flu-like symptoms, flushing, frequent bowel movements, gastric hyperacidity, gastritis, gastroesophageal reflux disease, gastrointestinal distress, gingival pain, Guillain-Barré syndrome, gynecomastia, hair discoloration, headache, heart murmur, hematemesis, hematochezia, hematuria, hemiparesis, hepatic disease, hepatic failure, hepatitis, hepatomegaly, herpes

zoster, hirsutism, hot flash, hypercholesterolemia, hyperglycemia, hyperhidrosis, hyperlipidemia, hypersensitivity reaction, hypertension, hypertonia, hypertriglyceridemia, hypoesthesia, hypokalemia, hypotension, immune thrombocytopenia, increased amylase, increased appetite, increased blood urea nitrogen, increased creatine phosphokinase in blood specimen, increased lactate dehydrogenase, increased LDL cholesterol, increased MCV, increased serum alkaline phosphatase, increased serum creatinine, increased serum glucose, increased serum potassium, increased serum sodium, increased thirst, increased thyroid stimulating hormone level, increased urine output, insomnia, interstitial nephritis, irritability, jaundice, joint stiffness, joint swelling, lethargy, leukocytosis, leukocyturia, leukopenia, liver steatosis, lymphocytopenia, mass, mastalgia, migraine, muscle rigidity, muscle spasm, muscle twitching, musculoskeletal pain, myalgia, myasthenia, nephrolithiasis, nervousness, neutropenia, oral mucosa ulcer, pain, palpitations, pancreatitis, pancytopenia, panic attack, paranasal sinus hypersecretion, paresthesia, peptic ulcer, personality changes, petechia, pharyngeal edema, pollakiuria, prolonged partial thromboplastin time, prolonged prothrombin time, prostate specific antigen increase, proteinuria, pruritus, psychotic symptoms, purpuric disease, renal failure syndrome, renal insufficiency, respiratory congestion, rhabdomyolysis, sinus bradycardia, skin discoloration, skin lesion, skin photosensitivity, sneezing, splenomegaly, Stevens-Johnson syndrome, tachycardia, throat irritation, thrombocytopenia, tinnitus, toxic epidermal necrolysis, transient ischemic attacks, tremor, upper respiratory tract infection, urinary incontinence, urinary urgency, urticaria (including dermographism), vertigo, vomiting, weight gain, weight loss, xerostomia

Mechanism of Action Selectively inhibits xanthine oxidase, the enzyme responsible for the conversion of hypoxanthine to xanthine to uric acid thereby decreasing uric acid. At therapeutic concentration does not inhibit other enzymes involved in purine and pyrimidine synthesis.

Pharmacodynamics/Kinetics

Half-life Elimination ~5 to 8 hours

Time to Peak Plasma: 1 to 1.5 hours

Pregnancy Considerations Adverse events were observed in some animal reproduction studies.

- **FEIBA** *see* Anti-inhibitor Coagulant Complex (Human) *on page 156*
- **FEIBA NF** *see* Anti-inhibitor Coagulant Complex (Human) *on page 156*
- **FEIBA VH** *see* Anti-inhibitor Coagulant Complex (Human) *on page 156*

Felbamate (FEL ba mate)

Brand Names: US Felbatol

Pharmacologic Category Anticonvulsant, Miscellaneous

Use

Partial seizures (monotherapy or adjunctive): Monotherapy or adjunctive therapy in the treatment of partial seizures (with and without generalization) in adults and adolescents 14 years and older

Lennox-Gastaut syndrome: Adjunctive therapy in the treatment of partial and generalized seizures associated with Lennox-Gastaut syndrome in children

Limitations of use: Not indicated for use as first-line treatment

Local Anesthetic/Vasoconstrictor Precautions No information available to require special precautions

Effects on Dental Treatment Key adverse event(s) related to dental treatment: Xerostomia (normal salivary flow resumes upon discontinuation) and abnormal taste.

Effects on Bleeding Associated with marked increase in aplastic anemia and may present with signs of infection, bleeding, or anemia; therefore, incidents of abnormal bleeding should be reported to prescribing physician. Incidence of thrombocytopenia is ≤1%.

Adverse Reactions

>10%:

Central nervous system: Drowsiness (children: 48%; adults: 19%), headache (adults: 7% to 37%; children: 7%), dizziness (18%), insomnia (9% to 18%), fatigue (7% to 17%), nervousness (children: 16%; adults: 7%)

Gastrointestinal: Anorexia (children: 55%; adults: 19%), vomiting (children: 39%; adults: 9% to 17%), nausea (adults: 34%; children: 7%), dyspepsia (9% to 12%), constipation (7% to 11%)

Hematologic & oncologic: Purpura (children: 13%)

Respiratory: Upper respiratory infection (children: 45%; adults: 5% to 9%)

Miscellaneous: Fever (children: 23%; adults: 3%)

1% to 10%:

Cardiovascular: Chest pain (3%), facial edema (3%), palpitations (≥1%), tachycardia (≥1%)

Central nervous system: Abnormal gait (children: 10%; adults: 5%), abnormality in thinking (children: 7%), ataxia (children: 7%; adults: 4%), emotional lability (children: 7%), pain (children: 7%), anxiety (5%), depression (5%), paresthesia (4%), stupor (3%), aggressive behavior (≥1%), agitation (≥1%), malaise (≥1%), psychological disorder (≥1%), attempted suicide (≤1%), dystonia (≤1%), euphoria (≤1%), hallucination (≤1%), migraine (≤1%)

Dermatologic: Skin rash (children: 10%; adults: 3% to 4%), acne vulgaris (3%), pruritus (≥1%), bullous rash (≤1%), urticaria (≤1%)

Endocrine and metabolic: Menstrual disease (3%), hypophosphatemia (≤3%), hypokalemia (≤1%), hyponatremia (≤1%), increased lactate dehydrogenase (≤1%)

Gastrointestinal: Hiccups (children: 10%), weight loss (children: 7%; adults: 3%), dysgeusia (6%), abdominal pain (5%), diarrhea (5%), xerostomia (3%), weight gain (≥1%), esophagitis (≤1%), increased appetite (≤1%)

Genitourinary: Urinary tract infection (3%)

Hematologic & oncologic: Leukopenia (children: 7%; adults: ≤1%), granulocytopenia (≤1%), leukocytosis (≤1%), lymphadenopathy (≤1%), thrombocytopenia (≤1%)

Hepatic: Increased liver enzymes (1% to 5%), increased serum alkaline phosphatase (≤1%)

Neuromuscular & skeletal: Tremor (6%), myalgia (3%), weakness (≥1%)

Ophthalmic: Miosis (children: 7%), diplopia (3% to 6%), visual disturbance (5%)

Otic: Otitis media (children: 10%; adults: 3%)

Respiratory: Pharyngitis (children: 10%; adults: 3%), cough (children: 7%), rhinitis (7%), sinusitis (4%), flu-like symptoms (≥1%)

<1%, postmarketing, and/or case reports: Acute renal failure, agranulocytosis, alopecia, anaphylactoid reaction, anemia, apathy, aphthous stomatitis, aplastic

anemia, atrial arrhythmia, atrial fibrillation, blood coagulation disorder, blood platelet disorder, body odor, bradycardia, brain disease, buccal mucous membrane swelling, cardiac failure, cerebral edema, cerebrovascular disease, choreoathetosis, coma, confusion, delusions, diaphoresis, disseminated intravascular coagulation (DIC), dysarthria, dyskinesia, dysphagia, dyspnea, dysuria, embolism, enteritis, eosinophilia, epistaxis, exacerbation of asthma, extrapyramidal reaction, flatulence, flushing, gastric ulcer, gastritis, gastroesophageal reflux disease, gastrointestinal hemorrhage, gingival hemorrhage, glossitis, hematemesis, hematuria, hemianopia, hemolytic anemia, hepatic failure, hepatitis, hepatorenal syndrome, hyperammonemia, hyperglycemia, hypernatremia, hypersensitivity reaction, hypertension, hypocalcemia, hypoglycemia, hypomagnesemia, hypotension, hypoxia, IgA vasculitis, increased creatine phosphokinase, intestinal obstruction, jaundice, lack of concentration, leukemia, lichen planus, livedo reticularis, manic reaction, nephrosis, neuritis (mononeuritis), nystagmus, pancreatitis, pancytopenia, paralysis, paranoia, peripheral ischemia (potentially leading to necrosis), pleural effusion, pneumonitis, psychosis, pulmonary hemorrhage, rectal hemorrhage, renal insufficiency, respiratory depression, rhabdomyolysis, SIADH (syndrome of inappropriate antidiuretic hormone secretion), skin photosensitivity, status epilepticus, Stevens-Johnson syndrome, suicidal ideation, suicidal tendencies, supraventricular tachycardia, thrombophlebitis, torsades de pointes, toxic epidermal necrolysis, urinary retention, urticaria, vaginal hemorrhage

Mechanism of Action Mechanism of action is unknown but has properties in common with other marketed anticonvulsants; has weak inhibitory effects on GABA-receptor binding, benzodiazepine receptor binding, and is devoid of activity at the MK-801 receptor binding site of the NMDA receptor-ionophore complex.

Pharmacodynamics/Kinetics

Half-life Elimination 20 to 23 hours (average); prolonged by 9 to 15 hours in patients with renal impairment

Time to Peak Serum: 2 to 6 hours (Patsalos 2018).

Pregnancy Risk Factor C

Pregnancy Considerations

Postmarketing case reports in humans include fetal death, genital malformation, anencephaly, encephalocele, and placental disorder.

Patients exposed to felbamate during pregnancy are encouraged to enroll themselves into the North American Antiepileptic Drug (AED) Pregnancy Registry by calling 1-888-233-2334. Additional information is available at www.aedpregnancyregistry.org.

Prescribing and Access Restrictions A patient "informed consent" form should be completed and signed by the patient and physician. Copies are available from MEDA Pharmaceuticals by calling 800-526-3840.

◆ **Felbatol** *see* Felbamate *on page 638*

◆ **Feldene** *see* Piroxicam (Systemic) *on page 1237*

Felodipine (fe LOE di peen)

Related Information

Calcium Channel Blockers and Gingival Hyperplasia *on page 1816*

Cardiovascular Diseases *on page 1654*

Brand Names: Canada APO-Felodipine; Plendil; SANDOZ Felodipine

Pharmacologic Category Antihypertensive; Calcium Channel Blocker; Calcium Channel Blocker, Dihydropyridine

Use Hypertension: Management of hypertension

Local Anesthetic/Vasoconstrictor Precautions No information available to require special precautions

Effects on Dental Treatment Key adverse event(s) related to dental treatment: Gingival hyperplasia (fewer reports than other CCBs, resolves upon discontinuation, consultation with physician is suggested).

Effects on Bleeding No information available to require special precautions

Adverse Reactions

>10%:

Cardiovascular: Peripheral edema (2% to 17%)

Central nervous system: Headache (11% to 15%)

1% to 10%: Cardiovascular: Flushing (4% to 7%), tachycardia (≤3%)

<1%, postmarketing, and/or case reports: Abdominal pain, acid regurgitation, anemia, angina pectoris, angioedema, anxiety disorder, arm pain, arthralgia, back pain, bronchitis, bruise, cardiac arrhythmia, cardiac failure, cerebrovascular accident, chest pain, constipation, decreased libido, depression, diarrhea, dizziness, drowsiness, dyspnea, dysuria, epistaxis, erythema, extrasystoles, facial edema, flatulence, flu-like symptoms, flushing, foot pain, gingival hyperplasia, gynecomastia, hip pain, hypersensitivity angiitis, hypotension, impotence, influenza, insomnia, irritability, knee pain, leg pain, muscle cramps, myalgia, myocardial infarction, nausea, nervousness, palpitations, paresthesia, pharyngitis, polyuria, respiratory tract infection, sinusitis, syncope, urinary frequency, urinary urgency, urticaria, visual disturbance, vomiting, xerostomia

Mechanism of Action Inhibits calcium ions from entering the "slow channels" or select voltage-sensitive areas of vascular smooth muscle and myocardium during depolarization, producing a relaxation of coronary vascular smooth muscle and coronary vasodilation; increases myocardial oxygen delivery in patients with vasospastic angina

Pharmacodynamics/Kinetics

Onset of Action Antihypertensive: 2 to 5 hours

Duration of Action Antihypertensive effect: 24 hours

Half-life Elimination Immediate release: 11 to 16 hours

Time to Peak 2.5 to 5 hours

Pregnancy Risk Factor C

Pregnancy Considerations

Adverse events were observed in animal reproduction studies.

Chronic maternal hypertension may increase the risk of birth defects, low birth weight, preterm delivery, stillbirth, and neonatal death. Actual fetal/neonatal risks may be related to duration and severity of maternal hypertension. Untreated hypertension may also increase the risks of adverse maternal outcomes, including gestational diabetes, myocardial infarction, preeclampsia, stroke, and delivery complications (ACOG 203 2019).

Calcium channel blockers may be used to treat hypertension in pregnant women; however, agents other than felodipine are more commonly used (ACOG 203 2019; ESC [Regitz-Zagrosek 2018]). Females with preexisting hypertension may continue their medication during pregnancy unless contraindications exist (ESC [Regitz-Zagrosek 2018]).

◆ **Femara** *see* Letrozole *on page 888*

◆ **Femcon Fe [DSC]** *see* Ethinyl Estradiol and Norethindrone *on page 614*

◆ **Femhrt Low Dose** *see* Ethinyl Estradiol and Norethindrone *on page 614*

◆ **Femring** *see* Estradiol (Systemic) *on page 596*

◆ **Femynor** *see* Ethinyl Estradiol and Norgestimate *on page 616*

Fenfluramine (fen FLUR a meen)

Brand Names: US Fintepla

Pharmacologic Category Anticonvulsant, Miscellaneous; Serotonin 5HT-2 Receptor Agonist

Use Dravet syndrome–associated seizures: Treatment of seizures associated with Dravet syndrome in patients ≥2 years of age.

Local Anesthetic/Vasoconstrictor Precautions Fenfluramine causes tachycardia and increases in blood pressure; consider monitoring blood pressure prior to using local anesthetic with vasoconstrictor.

Effects on Dental Treatment Key adverse event(s) related to dental treatment: Increased salivary flow/drooling.

Effects on Bleeding No information available to require special precautions.

Adverse Reactions

>10%:

Cardiovascular: Aortic insufficiency (≤23%), increased blood pressure (8% to 13%), mitral valve insufficiency (≤23%)

Endocrine & metabolic: Weight loss (5% to 13%, dose-related)

Gastrointestinal: Decreased appetite (23% to 38%), diarrhea (15% to 31%), sialorrhea (≤13%)

Nervous system: Drooling (≤13%), drowsiness (≤26%), fatigue (≤15%), lethargy (≤26%), malaise (≤15%), sedated state (≤26%)

Neuromuscular & skeletal: Asthenia (≤15%)

Respiratory: Upper respiratory tract infection (5% to 21%)

Miscellaneous: Fever (5% to 15%)

1% to 10%:

Cardiovascular: Increased heart rate (3% to 5%)

Dermatologic: Skin rash (8%)

Endocrine & metabolic: Dehydration (5%), increased serum prolactin (5%)

Gastrointestinal: Constipation (3% to 10%), gastroenteritis (3% to 8%), vomiting (5% to 10%)

Genitourinary: Urinary incontinence (3% to 5%), urinary tract infection (5%)

Hematologic & oncologic: Bruise (5%)

Nervous system: Abnormal behavior (8%; stereotypy: 5%), abnormal gait (≤10%), ataxia (≤10%), balance impairment (≤10%), chills (5%), falling (10%), headache (8%), hypoactivity (5%), hypotonia (8%), insomnia (5%), irritability (3%), mood changes (negativism: 5%), status epilepticus (3%)

Neuromuscular & skeletal: Tremor (3%)

Otic: Otic infection (3% to 8%)

Respiratory: Bronchitis (3%), croup (3% to 5%), rhinitis (3% to 8%)

Frequency not defined:

Cardiovascular: Heart valve disease, hypertensive crisis

Nervous system: Serotonin syndrome, suicidal ideation, suicidal tendencies

Ophthalmic: Angle-closure glaucoma, mydriasis

Respiratory: Pulmonary hypertension (arterial)

Mechanism of Action The mechanisms by which fenfluramine exerts its therapeutic effects in the treatment of seizures associated with Dravet syndrome are unknown. Fenfluramine and the metabolite, norfenfluramine, increase extracellular levels of serotonin through interaction with serotonin transporter proteins, and exhibit agonist activity at serotonin 5HT-2 receptors.

Pharmacodynamics/Kinetics

Half-life Elimination 20 hours.

Time to Peak 4 to 5 hours.

Pregnancy Considerations

Information related to inadvertent maternal use of fenfluramine in pregnancy is available from previous reports when used to treat obesity (Jones 2002; Vial 1992). Fenfluramine is associated with an increased risk of pulmonary arterial hypertension, which has also been reported following exposure in pregnancy (Bonnin 2005).

Data collection to monitor pregnancy and infant outcomes following exposure to antiepileptic drugs is ongoing. Patients exposed to fenfluramine during pregnancy are encouraged to enroll in the North American Antiepileptic Drug (NAAED) Pregnancy Registry (888-233-2334 or http://www.aedpregnancyregistry.org).

◆ **Fenfluramine hydrochloride** *see* Fenfluramine *on page 640*

Fenofibrate and Derivatives
(fen oh FYE brate & dah RIV ah tives)

Related Information

Cardiovascular Diseases *on page 1654*

Brand Names: US Antara; Fenoglide; Fibricor; Lipofen; Lofibra [DSC]; Tricor; Triglide; Trilipix

Brand Names: Canada AA-Feno-Micro; APO-Feno-Super; APO-Fenofibrate; DOM-Fenofibrate Micro [DSC]; Feno-Micro-200 [DSC]; Fenofibrate Micro; Fenomax; Lipidil EZ; Lipidil Micro [DSC]; Lipidil Supra; MINT-Fenofibrate E [DSC]; MYLAN-Fenofibrate Micro [DSC]; NU-Feno-Micro [DSC]; PHL-Fenofibrate Micro [DSC]; PMS-Fenofibrate; PMS-Fenofibrate Micro; PRO-Feno-Super-100 [DSC]; PRO-Feno-Super-160 [DSC]; RATIO-Fenofibrate MC [DSC]; SANDOZ Fenofibrate E; SANDOZ Fenofibrate S; TEVA-Fenofibrate-S [DSC]

Pharmacologic Category Antilipemic Agent, Fibric Acid

Use

Hypercholesterolemia or mixed dyslipidemia: Adjunctive therapy to diet for the reduction of low-density lipoprotein cholesterol (LDL-C), total cholesterol (total-C), triglycerides, and apolipoprotein B (apo B), and to increase high-density lipoprotein cholesterol (HDL-C) in adults with primary hypercholesterolemia or mixed dyslipidemia (Fredrickson types IIa and IIb). Use lipid-altering agents in addition to a diet restricted in saturated fat and cholesterol when response to diet and nonpharmacological interventions alone has been inadequate.

Note: While FDA-approved for hypercholesterolemia, fenofibrate is not a first- or second-line choice; other agents may be more suitable (ACC/AHA [Stone 2013]). In addition, use is not recommended to lower LDL-C or raise HDL-C in the absence of hypertriglyceridemia.

Hypertriglyceridemia: Adjunctive therapy to diet for treatment of adult patients with severe hypertriglyceridemia (Fredrickson types IV and V hyperlipidemia).

Local Anesthetic/Vasoconstrictor Precautions No information available to require special precautions

Effects on Dental Treatment Key adverse event(s) related to dental treatment: Dry mouth

Effects on Bleeding Thrombocytopenia has been reported through postmarketing surveillance.

Adverse Reactions

>10%: Hepatic: Increased serum transaminases (≥3 x ULN: 5% to 13%)

1% to 10%:

Cardiovascular: Pulmonary embolism (≤5%), thrombophlebitis (≤5%)

Central nervous system: Dizziness (≥3%), pain (≥3%)

Dermatologic: Skin rash (1%), urticaria (1%)

Gastrointestinal: Abdominal pain (5%), diarrhea (≥3%), dyspepsia (≥3%), constipation (2%)

Hepatic: Abnormal hepatic function tests (8%), increased serum alanine aminotransferase (3%), increased serum aspartate aminotransferase (3%)

Neuromuscular & skeletal: Arthralgia (≥3%), limb pain (≥3%), myalgia (≥3%), increased creatine phosphokinase in blood specimen (3%)

Respiratory: Nasopharyngitis (≥3%), sinusitis (≥3%), upper respiratory tract infection (≥3%), rhinitis (2%)

<1%, postmarketing, and/or case reports: Acute renal failure, agranulocytosis, anaphylaxis, anemia, angioedema, asthenia, cholestatic hepatitis, chronic active hepatitis, decreased HDL cholesterol (severe), decreased hematocrit, decreased hemoglobin, decreased white blood cell count, drug reaction with eosinophilia and systemic symptoms, headache, hepatic cirrhosis, hepatitis, hepatocellular hepatitis, hypersensitivity reaction, increased serum creatinine, interstitial pulmonary disease, muscle spasm, myopathy, pancreatitis, renal failure syndrome, rhabdomyolysis, severe dermatological reaction (severe cutaneous adverse reactions [SCAR]), skin photosensitivity, Stevens-Johnson syndrome, thrombocytopenia, toxic epidermal necrolysis

Mechanism of Action Fenofibric acid, an agonist for the nuclear transcription factor peroxisome proliferator-activated receptor-alpha (PPAR-alpha), downregulates apoprotein C-III (an inhibitor of lipoprotein lipase) and upregulates the synthesis of apolipoprotein A-I, fatty acid transport protein, and lipoprotein lipase resulting in an increase in VLDL catabolism, fatty acid oxidation, and elimination of triglyceride-rich particles; as a result of a decrease in VLDL levels, total plasma triglycerides are reduced by 30% to 60%; modest increase in HDL occurs in some hypertriglyceridemic patients.

Pharmacodynamics/Kinetics

Half-life Elimination Half-life elimination: Fenofibric acid: Mean: 20 hours (range: 10 to 35 hours); half-life prolonged in patients with renal impairment

Time to Peak 2 to 8 hours

Pregnancy Considerations Triglyceride and lipid concentrations increase during pregnancy as required for normal fetal development. When increases are greater than expected, supervised dietary intervention should be initiated. In women who develop very severe hypertriglyceridemia and are at risk for pancreatitis, use of fenofibrate beginning in the second trimester is one intervention that may be considered. Agents other than fenofibrate should be used for hypercholesterolemia (Avis 2009; Berglund 2012; Jacobson 2015; Wong 2015).

- **Fenofibric Acid** *see* Fenofibrate and Derivatives *on page 640*
- **Fenoglide** *see* Fenofibrate and Derivatives *on page 640*

Fenoldopam (fe NOL doe pam)

Brand Names: US Corlopam

Pharmacologic Category Antihypertensive; Dopamine Agonist

Use Severe hypertension: Short-term treatment of severe hypertension (up to 48 hours in adults while in hospital), including patients with malignant hypertension with deteriorating end-organ function; short-term (up to 4 hours while in hospital) blood pressure reduction in pediatric patients while in hospital

Local Anesthetic/Vasoconstrictor Precautions No information available to require special precautions

Effects on Dental Treatment Key adverse event(s) related to dental treatment: Xerostomia and changes in salivation (normal salivary flow resumes upon discontinuation).

Effects on Bleeding No information available to require special precautions

Adverse Reactions Frequency not defined.

≥5%:

Cardiovascular: Flushing, hypotension

Central nervous system: Headache

Gastrointestinal: Nausea

<5%:

Cardiovascular: Angina pectoris, bradycardia, cardiac failure, chest pain, ECG abnormality (ST-T abnormalities), extrasystoles, inversion T wave on ECG, myocardial infarction, orthostatic hypotension, palpitations, tachycardia

Central nervous system: Anxiety, dizziness, insomnia

Dermatologic: Diaphoresis

Endocrine & metabolic: Hyperglycemia, hypokalemia, increased lactate dehydrogenase

Gastrointestinal: Abdominal distention, abdominal pain, constipation, diarrhea, vomiting

Genitourinary: Oliguria, urinary tract infection

Hematologic & oncologic: Hemorrhage, leukocytosis

Hepatic: Increased serum transaminases

Local: Injection site reaction

Neuromuscular & skeletal: Back pain, muscle cramps (limbs)

Ophthalmic: Increased intraocular pressure

Renal: Increased blood urea nitrogen, increased serum creatinine

Respiratory: Dyspnea, nasal congestion

Miscellaneous: Fever

Mechanism of Action A selective postsynaptic dopamine agonist (D_1-receptors) which exerts hypotensive effects by decreasing peripheral vasculature resistance with increased renal blood flow, diuresis, and natriuresis; 6 times as potent as dopamine in producing renal vasodilatation; has minimal adrenergic effects

Pharmacodynamics/Kinetics

Onset of Action IV: Children: 5 minutes; Adults: 10 minutes; **Note:** Majority of effect of a given infusion rate is attained within 15 minutes.

Duration of Action IV: 1 hour

Half-life Elimination IV: Children: 3 to 5 minutes; Adults: ~5 minutes

Pregnancy Risk Factor B

Pregnancy Considerations

Adverse events were not observed in animal reproduction studies.

◆ **Fenoldopam Mesylate** *see* Fenoldopam *on page 641*

Fenoprofen (fen oh PROE fen)

Related Information

Rheumatoid Arthritis, Osteoarthritis, and Osteoporosis *on page 1697*

Temporomandibular Dysfunction (TMD), Chronic Pain, and Fibromyalgia *on page 1773*

Brand Names: US Fenortho; Nalfon; ProFeno [DSC]

Pharmacologic Category Analgesic, Nonopioid; Nonsteroidal Anti-inflammatory Drug (NSAID), Oral

Use

Osteoarthritis: Relief of the signs and symptoms of osteoarthritis.

Pain: Relief of mild to moderate pain in adults.

Rheumatoid arthritis (RA): Relief of the signs and symptoms of RA.

Local Anesthetic/Vasoconstrictor Precautions No information available to require special precautions

Effects on Dental Treatment The dentist should be aware of the potential of abnormal coagulation. Caution should also be exercised in the use of NSAIDs in patients already on anticoagulant therapy with drugs such as warfarin (Coumadin®). See Effects on Bleeding.

Effects on Bleeding Nonselective NSAIDs such as fenoprofen inhibit platelet aggregation and prolong bleeding time in some patients. Unlike aspirin, the NSAID effect on platelet function is quantitatively less, of shorter duration, and reversible.

Adverse Reactions

1% to 10%:

Cardiovascular: Peripheral edema (5%), palpitations (3%)

Central nervous system: Drowsiness (9%), headache (9%), dizziness (7%), nervousness (6%), fatigue (2%), confusion (1%)

Dermatologic: Diaphoresis (5%), pruritus (4%), skin rash (4%)

Gastrointestinal: Dyspepsia (10%), nausea (8%), constipation (7%), vomiting (3%), abdominal pain (2%)

Neuromuscular & skeletal: Weakness (5%), tremor (2%)

Ophthalmic: Blurred vision (2%)

Otic: Tinnitus (5%), auditory impairment (2%)

Respiratory: Dyspnea (3%), nasopharyngitis (1%)

<1%, postmarketing, and/or case reports: Agranulocytosis, alopecia, anaphylaxis, anemia, angioedema (angioneurotic edema), anorexia, anuria, aphthous stomatitis, aplastic anemia, atrial fibrillation, azotemia, bloody stools, bruise, cholestatic hepatitis, cystitis, depression, diplopia, disorientation, dysgeusia, dysuria, ECG changes, exfoliative dermatitis, fever, flatulence, gastritis, gastrointestinal hemorrhage, gastrointestinal perforation, gastrointestinal ulcer, glossopyrosis, hematuria, hemolytic anemia, hemorrhage, hepatotoxicity (idiosyncratic; Chalasani, 2014), hypertension, increased lactate dehydrogenase, increased serum alkaline phosphatase, increased serum AST, insomnia, interstitial nephritis, jaundice, lymphadenopathy, malaise, mastalgia, nephrosis, oliguria, optic neuritis, pancreatitis, pancytopenia, peptic ulcer, pulmonary edema, purpura, renal failure, renal papillary necrosis, seizure, Stevens-Johnson syndrome, supraventricular tachycardia, tachycardia, thrombocytopenia, toxic epidermal necrolysis, trigeminal neuralgia, urticaria, xerostomia

Mechanism of Action Reversibly inhibits cyclooxygenase-1 and 2 (COX-1 and 2) enzymes, which results in decreased formation of prostaglandin precursors; has antipyretic, analgesic, and anti-inflammatory properties

Other proposed mechanisms not fully elucidated (and possibly contributing to the anti-inflammatory effect to varying degrees), include inhibiting chemotaxis, altering lymphocyte activity, inhibiting neutrophil aggregation/activation, and decreasing proinflammatory cytokine levels.

Pharmacodynamics/Kinetics

Onset of Action A few days; full benefit: up to 2 to 3 weeks

Half-life Elimination ~3 hours

Time to Peak Serum: ~2 hours

Reproductive Considerations

The chronic use of NSAIDs in women of reproductive age may be associated with infertility that is reversible upon discontinuation of the medication. Consider discontinuing use in women having difficulty conceiving or those undergoing investigation of fertility.

Pregnancy Considerations

Birth defects have been observed following in utero NSAID exposure in some studies; however, data is conflicting (Bloor 2013). Nonteratogenic effects, including prenatal constriction of the ductus arteriosus, persistent pulmonary hypertension of the newborn, oligohydramnios, necrotizing enterocolitis, renal dysfunction or failure, and intracranial hemorrhage have been observed in the fetus/neonate following in utero NSAID exposure. In addition, nonclosure of the ductus arteriosus postnatally may occur and be resistant to medical management (Bermas 2014; Bloor 2013). Because NSAIDs may cause premature closure of the ductus arteriosus, product labeling for fenoprofen specifically states use should be avoided starting at 30-weeks gestation. Use of NSAIDs can be considered for the treatment of mild rheumatoid arthritis flares in pregnant women; however, use should be minimized or avoided early and late in pregnancy (Bermas 2014; Saavedra Salinas 2015).

The use of NSAIDs close to conception may be associated with an increased risk of miscarriage (Bermas 2014; Bloor 2013).

◆ **Fenoprofen Calcium** *see* Fenoprofen *on page 642*

◆ **Fenortho** *see* Fenoprofen *on page 642*

◆ **Fenoterol and Ipratropium** *see* Ipratropium and Fenoterol *on page 839*

◆ **Fenoterol Hydrobromide and Ipratropium Bromide** *see* Ipratropium and Fenoterol *on page 839*

◆ **Fensolvi (6 Month)** *see* Leuprolide *on page 890*

FentaNYL (FEN ta nil)

Related Information

Management of the Chemically Dependent Patient *on page 1724*

Brand Names: US Abstral; Actiq; Duragesic; Fentora; Ionsys [DSC]; Lazanda; Sublimaze; Subsys

Brand Names: Canada Abstral; Duragesic; Fentora

Generic Availability (US) Yes: Injection, lozenge, patch

Pharmacologic Category Analgesic, Opioid; Anilidopiperidine Opioid; General Anesthetic

Dental Use Adjunct in preoperative intravenous conscious sedation in patients undergoing dental surgery

Use

Pain management, acute and chronic pain:

***Injection:* Surgery:** Adjunct to general or regional anesthesia; preoperative medication; analgesic during anesthesia and in the immediate postoperative period.

***Transdermal device (eg, Ionsys):* Postoperative pain, acute:** Short-term management of acute postoperative pain severe enough to require an opioid analgesic in the hospital and for which alternative treatments are inadequate.

Limitations of use: Reserve for use in patients for whom alternative treatment options (eg, nonopioid analgesics) are ineffective, not tolerated, or would be otherwise inadequate to provide sufficient management of pain. Only for use in patients who are alert enough and have adequate cognitive ability to understand the directions for use. Not for home use. Transdermal device is for use only in patients in the hospital. Discontinue treatment with the device before patients leave the hospital. The device is for use after patients have been titrated to an acceptable level of analgesia using alternate opioid analgesics.

***Transdermal patch (eg, Duragesic):* Chronic pain:** Management of pain in opioid-tolerant patients, severe enough to require daily, around-the-clock, long-term opioid treatment and for which alternative treatment options are inadequate.

Limitations of use: Reserve for use in patients for whom alternative treatment options (eg, nonopioid analgesics, immediate-release opioids) are ineffective, not tolerated, or would be otherwise inadequate to provide sufficient management of pain. Not indicated as an as-needed analgesic.

***Transmucosal lozenge (eg, Actiq), buccal tablet (Fentora), intranasal (Lazanda), sublingual tablet (Abstral), sublingual spray (Subsys):* Cancer pain, breakthrough:** Management of breakthrough cancer pain in opioid-tolerant patients ≥18 years (Abstral, Fentora, Lazanda, Subsys) and ≥16 years (Actiq) of age who are already receiving and who are tolerant to around-the-clock opioid therapy for their underlying persistent cancer pain.

Limitations of use: Not for use in opioid non-tolerant patients. Not for use in the management of acute or postoperative pain, including headache/migraine, dental pain, or in the emergency department. As a part of the TIRF REMS Access program, these products may be dispensed only to outpatients enrolled in the program. For inpatient administration (eg, hospitals, hospices, and long-term care facilities that prescribe for inpatient use), patient and prescriber enrollment is not required.

Note: "Opioid-tolerant" patients are defined as patients who are taking at least:
Oral morphine 60 mg/day, **or**
Transdermal fentanyl 25 mcg/hour, **or**
Oral oxycodone 30 mg/day, **or**
Oral hydromorphone 8 mg/day, **or**
Oral oxymorphone 25 mg/day, **or**
Oral hydrocodone 60 mg/day, **or**
Equianalgesic dose of another opioid for at least 1 week

Local Anesthetic/Vasoconstrictor Precautions No information available to require special precautions

Effects on Dental Treatment Key adverse event(s) related to dental treatment: Occurrence of xerostomia, changes in salivation (normal salivary flow resumes upon discontinuation), and orthostatic hypotension as patient stands up after treatment, especially if lying in dental chair for extended periods of time, have been reported. Use caution with sudden changes in position during and after dental treatment. Occurrence of taste alteration; oral ulcers of the gingiva; lip, mouth, and gingival pain; gingivitis; glossitis; periodontal abscess; stomatitis; tongue disease; and sinusitis have all been reported, usually with transmucosal use, nasal, buccal tablet, sublingual film, sublingual spray, sublingual tablet, or lozenge. Rare occurrence of dental caries, gingival hemorrhage, gingival recession, Stevens-Johnson syndrome, swollen tongue, tooth loss, and voice disorders have been reported.

Actiq may contribute to dental caries due to sugar and acid content of oral lozenge; advise patients to maintain good oral hygiene and have regular dental examinations. See Dental Health Professional Considerations.

Effects on Bleeding No information available to require special precautions

Adverse Reactions

>10%:

Central nervous system: Confusion, dizziness, drowsiness, fatigue, headache, sedated state
Endocrine & metabolic: Dehydration
Gastrointestinal: Constipation, nausea, vomiting
Local: Application site erythema (transdermal device)
Neuromuscular & skeletal: Asthenia
Respiratory: Dyspnea

1% to 10%:

Cardiovascular: Atrial fibrillation, bigeminy, cardiac arrhythmia, chest pain, deep vein thrombosis, edema, hypertension, hypotension, myocardial infarction, orthostatic hypotension, palpitations, peripheral edema, pulmonary embolism (nasal spray), sinus tachycardia, syncope, tachycardia, vasodilation

Central nervous system: Abnormal dreams, abnormal gait, abnormality in thinking, agitation, altered sense of smell, amnesia, anxiety, ataxia, chills, depression, disorientation, dysphoria, euphoria, hallucination, hypertonia, hypoesthesia, hypothermia, insomnia, irritability, lack of concentration, lethargy, malaise, mental status changes, migraine, nervousness, neuropathy, paranoia, paresthesia, restlessness, speech disturbance, stupor, vertigo, withdrawal syndrome

Dermatologic: Alopecia, cellulitis, decubitus ulcer, diaphoresis, erythema, exfoliation of skin (application site, transdermal device), hyperhidrosis, night sweats, pallor, papule (application site, transdermal device), pruritus, pustules (application site, transdermal device), skin rash, vesicobullous rash (application site, transdermal device)

Endocrine & metabolic: Hot flash, hypercalcemia, hyperglycemia, hypoalbuminemia, hypocalcemia, hypokalemia, hypomagnesemia, hyponatremia, weight loss

Gastrointestinal: Abdominal distention, abdominal pain, anorexia, decreased appetite, diarrhea, dysgeusia, dyspepsia, dysphagia (buccal tablet/film/sublingual spray), flatulence, gastritis, gastroenteritis, gastroesophageal reflux disease, gastrointestinal hemorrhage, gastrointestinal ulcer (gingival, lip, mouth; transmucosal use/nasal spray), gingival pain (buccal tablet), gingivitis (lozenge), glossitis (lozenge), hematemesis, intestinal obstruction, periodontal abscess (lozenge/buccal tablet), rectal pain, stomatitis (lozenge/buccal tablet/sublingual tablet/sublingual spray), tongue disease (sublingual tablet), xerostomia

Genitourinary: Urinary retention (3%), difficulty in micturition, dysuria, erectile dysfunction, mastalgia, urinary incontinence, urinary tract infection, urinary urgency, vaginal hemorrhage, vaginitis

Hematologic & oncologic: Anemia (3%), bruise, leukopenia, lymphadenopathy, neutropenia, thrombocytopenia

Hepatic: Ascites, increased serum alkaline phosphatase, increased serum AST, jaundice

Hypersensitivity: Hypersensitivity reaction

Infection: Abscess

Local: Application site burning (transdermal device), application site discharge (transdermal device), application site edema (transdermal device), application site irritation, application site itching (transdermal device), application site pain, application site rash (transdermal device), application site vesicles (transdermal device)

Neuromuscular & skeletal: Arthralgia, back pain, lower limb cramp, limb pain, myalgia, tremor

Ophthalmic: Blepharoptosis, blurred vision, diplopia, dry eye syndrome, strabismus, swelling of eye, visual disturbance

Renal: Renal failure syndrome

Respiratory: Apnea, asthma, atelectasis, bronchitis, cough, dyspnea on exertion, epistaxis, flu-like symptoms, hemoptysis, hyperventilation, hypoventilation, hypoxia, laryngitis, nasal congestion (nasal spray), nasal discomfort (nasal spray), nasopharyngitis, pharyngitis, pharyngolaryngeal pain, pneumonia, post nasal drip (nasal spray), rhinitis, rhinorrhea (nasal spray), sinusitis, upper respiratory tract infection, wheezing

Miscellaneous: Fever

<1%, postmarketing, and/or case reports: Allergic dermatitis, anaphylactoid shock, anaphylaxis, angina pectoris, bradycardia, bronchoconstriction, candidiasis, chest wall rigidity, clonus, contact dermatitis, crusted skin, cyanosis, decreased libido, dental caries, dermatitis, drug dependence (physical and psychological; with prolonged use), eczema, emotional lability, eructation, esophageal stenosis, exfoliative dermatitis, falling, fecal impaction, flank pain, flushing, genitourinary tract spasm, gingival hemorrhage, gingival recession, hematuria, hiccups, hostility, hyperesthesia, hypoglycemia, hypogonadism (Brennan 2013; Debono 2011), impaired consciousness, increased bronchial secretions, joint swelling, local hemorrhage, local hypersensitivity reaction, localized infection, local skin hyperpigmentation (lasted 2 to 3 weeks), local tissue necrosis, loss of consciousness, miosis, muscle rigidity (transient; observed in infants whose mothers were treated with IV fentanyl), muscle spasm, muscle twitching, myasthenia, nocturia, oliguria, pancytopenia, pleural effusion, polyuria, respiratory depression, respiratory distress, seizure, sexual disorder, skin erosion, Stevens-Johnson syndrome, swelling, swollen tongue, tonic-clonic epilepsy, tooth loss, upper abdominal pain, urticaria, voice disorder

Dental Usual Dosage Surgery: Adults:

Premedication: IM, slow IV: 25 to 100 mcg/dose 30 to 60 minutes prior to surgery

Adjunct to regional anesthesia: Slow IV: 25 to 100 mcg/dose over 1 to 2 minutes. **Note:** An IV should be in place with regional anesthesia so the IM route is rarely used but still maintained as an option in the package labeling.

Dosing

Adult

<u>Analgesia and sedation:</u>

Critically ill patients in the ICU (analgesia and sedation) (off-label use): Note: Multimodal approaches (eg, a combination of analgesics and techniques) should typically be employed for pain control in this setting. Pain should be monitored using validated scales (eg, behavioral pain scale, critical-care pain observation tool) in ICU patients who are unable to self-report (SCCM [Devlin 2018]). In patients who are obese, standard non–weight-based initial dosing is preferred (Pandharipande 2019).

Intermittent dosing:

Loading dose: IV: 25 to 100 mcg **or** 1 to 2 mcg/**kg**; may repeat dose if severe pain persists and adverse effects are minimal at the time of expected peak effect (eg, ~5 minutes after administration) (Pandharipande 2019). Follow with intermittent maintenance dose or a continuous infusion.

Maintenance dose: IV: 25 to 50 mcg **or** 0.35 to 0.5 mcg/**kg** every 30 to 60 minutes as needed (Pandharipande 2019; SCCM [Barr 2013]).

Continuous infusion:

IV: After initial loading dose (see **Intermittent dosing:** *Loading dose*), begin continuous infusion at an initial rate of 25 to 50 mcg/hour; titrate every 30 to 60 minutes to clinical effect (ie, pain control and/or sedation). Usual dosing range: 50 to 200 mcg/hour (some patients may require doses as high as 300 mcg/hour); weight-based dosing range: 0.7 to 10 mcg/**kg**/hour (Pandharipande 2019; SCCM [Barr 2013]). **Note:** Fentanyl can accumulate in lipid stores when used for extended periods of time and may result in prolonged sedation and reduced ability to liberate from mechanical ventilator (Pandharipande 2019). May administer an additional small bolus dose (eg, 25 mcg) prior to increasing the infusion rate (Peng 1999; Salomäki 1991).

Procedural sedation and analgesia:

Outside the operating room (alternative agent) (off-label use): IV: 0.5 to 1 mcg/**kg** every 2 minutes until desired level of sedation and analgesia achieved (Bahn 2005; Frank 2019); generally, the maximum total dose is 250 mcg. If administered with other sedatives (eg, etomidate, propofol, midazolam), do not exceed single doses of 0.5 mcg/**kg** (Frank 2019).

Analgesia during monitored anesthesia care or regional anesthesia: IV: Usual initial dose range: 0.5 to 2 mcg/**kg**, administered in incremental boluses of 25 to 50 mcg, titrated to effect. When used in combination with a sedative (eg, midazolam), consider dosage reduction (Rosero 2019). **Note:** Since an IV should be in place with anesthesia, the IM route is rarely used but still maintained as an option in the manufacturer's labeling. If IM route is used, the dose is equivalent to the recommended IV dose.

General anesthesia:

Preinduction: IV: 25 mcg; may repeat in increments of 25 mcg (typical total dose is ≤100 mcg) to provide pain relief or if patient requires a regional anesthesia procedure prior to surgery (Casserly 2019; Roberts 2019).

Induction: IV: 25 to 100 mcg (or 0.5 to 1 mcg/**kg**) (Casserly 2019; King 2019). Some use a high-dose opioid induction technique (eg, 10 to 25 mcg/**kg**) for select patients (eg, those with poor myocardial function) who will remain intubated for several hours postoperatively (Casserly 2019).

Maintenance:

Intermittent: IV: 25 to 50 mcg bolus as needed; may be used to provide supplemental analgesia during maintenance of general anesthesia with inhaled agents. For opioid-naive patients, do not exceed 1 mcg/**kg**/hour based on ideal body weight (Casserly 2019).

Continuous infusion: IV: 1 to 2 mcg/**kg**/hour as supplement to total IV anesthesia (TIVA) when controlled postoperative ventilation is planned (Casserly 2019).

Rapid sequence intubation (pretreatment) (off-label use): IV: Usual dose: 50 to 200 mcg (or 1 to 3 mcg/**kg**) over 30 to 60 seconds administered ~3 minutes prior to induction. In patients with tenuous hemodynamic status, use lower doses (eg, 1 mcg/**kg** [or 50 mcg]) or avoid use; in patients with elevated intracranial pressure, use higher doses (eg, 3 mcg/**kg** [or 200 mcg]) (Caro 2019; Groth 2018; Roberts 2019; Stollings 2014).

Pain management, severe pain: Note: Opioids may be part of a comprehensive, multimodal, patient-specific treatment plan for pain. Maximize nonopioid analgesia, if appropriate, prior to initiation of opioid analgesia (CDC [Dowell 2016]; Hill 2018). Dosing provided is based on typical doses and some patients may require higher or lower doses. Individualize dosing and dosing intervals based on patient-specific factors (eg, comorbidities, severity of pain, concomitant medications, general condition, degree of opioid experience/tolerance) and titrate to patient-specific treatment goals (eg, improvement in function and quality of life, decrease in pain using a validated pain rating scale). Use the lowest effective dose for the shortest period of time. For acute non–cancer-related pain severe enough to require an opioid, do not prescribe fentanyl for use on an outpatient basis; consider the use of other oral opioids. Before starting opioid therapy for chronic pain, establish realistic treatment goals for pain and function, and consider how therapy will be discontinued if benefits do not outweigh risks (CDC [Dowell 2016]).

Acute pain (including ICU, postoperative, and other closely monitored settings):

Patient-controlled analgesia (alternative agent): Note: Generally, the preferred opioid for patients with severe kidney or hepatic dysfunction and/or for patients who are unable to tolerate morphine or hydromorphone (Mariano 2019).

IV:

Example IV Patient-Controlled Analgesia Initial Dose Ranges for Opioid-Naive Patients[a]	
Usual concentration	10 mcg/mL
Demand dose	Usual range: 5 to 20 mcg
Basal dose	In general, a continuous (basal) infusion is **not** recommended in an opioid-naive patient (ISMP 2009)[b]
Lockout interval	4 to 10 minutes
Maximum cumulative dose	75 mcg within 1 hour (or 300 mcg within a 4-hour period)

[a]For use to maintain pain control after initial pain control achieved. May adjust dosing and provide rescue bolus doses (eg, 5 to 20 mcg) if analgesia is inadequate (Mariano 2019).

[b]The use of a continuous background infusion for patient-controlled analgesia is generally **not** recommended for most patients because of the risk of respiratory depression, and use should be limited to carefully selected patients who are opioid tolerant and/or receiving care in a critical care unit, or if required to maintain baseline opioid dosing during intervals when oral or transdermal opioid administration is not possible (Arnold 2019; Mariano 2019).

Postoperative pain:

Postoperative recovery/Postanesthesia care unit (ie, immediate postoperative period):

IV: 25 to 50 mcg every 5 minutes (moderate pain) or 50 to 100 mcg every 2 to 5 minutes (severe pain) until pain is relieved or unwanted side effects appear; after initial pain control, readdress postoperative analgesic regimen to optimize comfort (Casserly 2019).

IM: 50 to 100 mcg every 1 to 2 hours as needed. **Note:** IM route should only be used if IV administration is not available (eg, loss of IV access).

Transdermal device (Ionsys): Note: For hospital use only by patients under medical supervision for whom alternative treatments are inadequate and only after patients have been titrated to an acceptable level of analgesia using another opioid analgesic.

Apply 1 device to chest or upper outer arm only. Only the patient may activate the device (40 mcg dose of fentanyl per activation, delivered over 10 minutes; maximum: 6 doses per hour). Only 1 device may be applied at a time and operates for up to 24 hours or 80 doses, whichever comes first. Reapply every 24 hours, as necessary, with each subsequent device applied to a different skin site; maximum duration: 72 hours. If inadequate analgesia is achieved with 1 device, either provide additional supplemental analgesia or replace with an alternative analgesic. Refer to manufacturer's labeling for activation instructions and application sites.

Severe pain (nonoperative):

Intermittent dosing: IV, IM: 25 to 50 mcg **or** 0.35 to 0.5 mcg/**kg** every 30 to 60 minutes as needed (Pandharipande 2019; SCCM [Barr 2013]). **Note:** More frequent administration may be necessary when used by the IV route due to short duration of activity. IM route should only be used if IV administration is not available (eg, loss of IV access).

Chronic pain, including chronic cancer pain:

Note: Opioids, including fentanyl, are **not** the preferred therapy for chronic noncancer pain due to insufficient evidence of benefit and risk of serious harm; nonpharmacologic treatment and nonopioid analgesics are preferred, with the exception of chronic pain from sickle cell disease and end-of-life care. Opioids, including fentanyl, should **only** be considered in patients with chronic, noncancer pain who are expected to experience clinically meaningful improvement in pain and function that outweighs patient safety risks (CDC [Dowell 2016]; Dowell [CDC letter] 2019).

SubQ continuous infusion: Note: For progressive illnesses (eg, cancer), a continuous SubQ infusion, with or without a patient-controlled analgesia option, can be used as pain requirements increase. In general, SubQ continuous infusion dose is equivalent to IV continuous infusion dose (Anderson 2004). Individualize dose based on previous opioid intake and appropriate opioid analgesic equivalents; titrate further, if needed, based on level of pain. Reported dosing varies greatly and is based on practice and patient needs; refer to institutional protocols (Miller 1995; Oosten 2016; Paix 1995; Portenoy 2019b).

Transdermal patch: Discontinue or taper all other around-the-clock or extended-release opioids when initiating therapy with fentanyl transdermal patch.

Initial: To convert patients from oral or parenteral opioids to fentanyl transdermal patch, a 24-hour analgesic requirement should be calculated (based on prior opioid use). Using the table below, the appropriate initial dose can be determined. The initial fentanyl dosage may be approximated from the 24-hour morphine dosage equivalent and titrated to minimize adverse effects and provide analgesia. While there are useful tables of opioid equivalents available, substantial interpatient variability exists in relative potency of different opioids and products. Therefore, it is safer to underestimate the daily fentanyl requirement and provide breakthrough pain relief with rescue medication (eg, immediate-release opioid) than to overestimate requirements, which could result in adverse reactions. With the initial application, the absorption of transdermal fentanyl requires several hours to reach plateau; therefore, transdermal fentanyl is inappropriate for management of acute pain. Change patch every 72 hours. The majority of patients may be controlled on every-72-hour administration; however, some patients may require every-48-hour administration because of more breakthrough pain in the last 24 hours of each cycle.

Conversion from continuous IV infusion of fentanyl: In patients who have adequate pain relief with IV fentanyl infusion, may convert to transdermal dosing at a rate equivalent to the IV rate using a 2-step taper of the infusion to be completed over 12 hours after the patch is applied. Six hours after the application of the first patch, decrease the infusion to 50% of the original rate; discontinue infusion 12 hours after patch application (Kornick 2001).

Titration: Do not titrate more frequently than every 3 days after the initial application or every 6 days thereafter. Short-acting opioids may be required until analgesic efficacy is established and/or as supplements for breakthrough pain. The number and quantity of supplemental doses should be closely monitored. When increasing the dose, base the new dose on the daily requirement of supplemental opioids required by the patient during the second or third day of initial application. For example, if 24-hour oral morphine requirement for breakthrough pain is 50 mg, then may increase transdermal fentanyl dose by 25 mcg/hour (McPherson 2016).

Dose conversion guidelines for transdermal fentanyl (see table below):

Note: Using the manufacturer's recommended dose conversion guidelines, based upon the daily oral morphine dose, may underestimate the transdermal fentanyl strength required and result in the need for supplemental immediate-release opioid therapy for breakthrough pain or in the patient experiencing withdrawal syndrome (Skaer 2004). The manufacturers recommend a ratio of approximately 45 mg/24 hours of oral morphine to a 12 mcg/hour fentanyl dosage (US labeling) or the ratio of 45 to 59 mg/24 hours of oral morphine to a 12 mcg/hour fentanyl dosage (Canadian labeling). Below is a less conservative dosing conversion strategy based on a 2:1 ratio of oral morphine to transdermal fentanyl (McPherson 2016; Portenoy 2019a). For the more conservative dose conversion strategy, see the manufacturer's labeling. The table is only to be used for the conversion from current opioid therapy to transdermal fentanyl. **Do not use this table to convert from transdermal fentanyl to another opioid (doing so may lead to fatal overdose due to overestimation of the new opioid).** This is **not** a table of equianalgesic doses.

Step 1: Determine the patient's 24-hour oral morphine requirement. If patient was not receiving oral morphine, must convert the 24-hour requirement to the oral morphine equivalent using a conversion chart or tool.

Step 2: Once the 24-hour oral morphine requirement is determined, use the Dose Conversion Guidelines to determine the appropriate fentanyl transdermal dose (mcg/hour).

Dose Conversion Guidelines: Recommended Initial Fentanyl Transdermal Dose Based Upon Daily Oral Morphine Dose[a,b,c]

Oral 24-Hour Morphine Dose (mg/day)	Fentanyl Transdermal Dose (mcg/hour)
25	12
50	25
100	50
150	75
200	100
250	125
300	150
350	175
400	200
450	225
500	250
550	275
600	300

[a]Portenoy 2019a.
[b]The table should **not** be used to convert from transdermal fentanyl to other opioid analgesics. Rather, following removal of the patch, titrate the dose of the new opioid until adequate analgesia is achieved.
[c]Suggested doses for conversion to transdermal fentanyl from other opioids are less conservative than recommendations in the US product labeling. The recommendations in this table are based on guidance available at experienced centers.

Cancer pain, breakthrough:

Transmucosal:

Note: For patients who are tolerant to and currently receiving opioid therapy for persistent cancer pain; dosing should be individually titrated to provide adequate analgesia with minimal side effects. Dose titration should be done if patient requires more than 1 dose per breakthrough pain episode for several consecutive episodes. Patients experiencing >4 breakthrough pain episodes per day should have the dose of their long-term opioid reevaluated. **Patients must remain on around-the-clock opioids during use** (Portenoy 2019b).

Lozenge (Actiq): Note: Do **not** convert patients from any other fentanyl product to Actiq on a mcg-per-mcg basis. Patients previously using another fentanyl product should be initiated at a dose of 200 mcg; individually titrate to provide adequate analgesia while minimizing adverse effects.

Initial dose: 200 mcg (consumed over 15 minutes) for all patients; if after 30 minutes from the start of the lozenge (ie, 15 minutes following the completion of the lozenge) pain is unrelieved, a second 200 mcg dose may be given over 15 minutes. A maximum of 1 additional dose can be given per pain episode; **must wait at least 4 hours before treating another episode**. To limit the number of units in the home during titration, only prescribe an initial titration supply of six 200 mcg lozenges.

Dose titration: From the initial dose, closely monitor patients and modify the dose until patient reaches a dose providing adequate analgesia using a single dosage unit per breakthrough cancer pain episode. If signs/symptoms of excessive opioid effects (eg, respiratory depression) occur, immediately remove the dosage unit from the patient's mouth, dispose of properly, and reduce subsequent doses. If adequate relief is not achieved 15 minutes after completion of the first dose (ie, 30 minutes after the start of the lozenge), only 1 additional lozenge of the same strength may be given for that episode; **must wait at least 4 hours before treating another episode.**

Maintenance dose: Once titrated to an effective dose, patients should generally use a single dosage unit per breakthrough pain episode. During any pain episode, if adequate relief is not achieved 15 minutes after completion of the first dose (ie, 30 minutes after the start of the lozenge), only 1 additional lozenge of the same strength may be given over 15 minutes for that episode; **must wait at least 4 hours before treating another episode**. Consumption should be limited to ≤4 units per day (once an effective breakthrough dose is found). If adequate analgesia is **not** provided after treating several episodes of breakthrough pain using the same dose, increase dose to next highest lozenge strength (initially dispense no more than 6 units of the new strength). Reevaluate the around-the-clock opioid therapy in patients experiencing >4 breakthrough pain episodes per day. If signs/symptoms of excessive opioid effects (eg, respiratory depression) occur, immediately remove the dosage unit from the patient's mouth, dispose of properly, and reduce subsequent doses.

Buccal tablet (Fentora): Note: Do **not** convert patients from any other fentanyl product to Fentora on a mcg-per-mcg basis. Patients previously using another fentanyl product should be initiated at a dose of 100 mcg (except Actiq); individually titrate to provide adequate analgesia while minimizing adverse effects. For patients previously using the transmucosal lozenge (Actiq), the initial dose should be selected using the conversions listed; see *Conversion from lozenge (Actiq) to buccal tablet (Fentora).*

Initial dose: 100 mcg for all patients unless patient is already using Actiq; see *Conversion from lozenge (Actiq) to buccal tablet (Fentora).* If after 30 minutes pain is unrelieved, a second 100 mcg dose may be administered (US labeling) or an alternative analgesic rescue medication (other than Fentora) may be given (Canadian labeling). A maximum of 2 doses (or 1 dose [Canadian labeling]) can be given per breakthrough pain episode. **Must wait at least 4 hours before treating another episode with buccal tablet.**

Dose titration: If titration required, the 100 mcg dose may be increased to 200 mcg using two 100 mcg tablets (one on each side of mouth) with the next breakthrough pain episode. If 200 mcg dose is not successful, patient can use four 100 mcg tablets (two on each side of mouth) with the next breakthrough pain episode. If titration requires >400 mcg per dose, titrate using 200 mcg tablets; do not use more than 4 tablets simultaneously (maximum single dose: 800 mcg). During any breakthrough pain episode, if adequate relief is not achieved 30 minutes after buccal tablet application, a second dose of same strength for that breakthrough pain episode may be used (US labeling) or an alternative analgesic rescue medication (other than Fentora) may be given (Canadian labeling). **Must wait at least 4 hours before treating another episode with buccal tablet.**

Maintenance dose: Following titration, the effective maintenance dose using 1 tablet of the appropriate strength should be administered once per episode; if after 30 minutes pain is unrelieved, may administer a second dose of the same strength (US labeling) or an alternative analgesic rescue medication (other than Fentora) may be given (Canadian labeling). **Must wait at least 4 hours before treating another episode with buccal tablet.** Limit to 4 applications per day. Reevaluate the around-the-clock opioid therapy in patients experiencing >4 breakthrough pain episodes per day. Once an effective maintenance dose has been established, the buccal tablet may be administered sublingually (alternative route). To prevent confusion, patient should only have one strength available at a time. Once maintenance dose is determined, all other unused tablets should be disposed of and that strength (using a single tablet) should be used. Using more than 4 buccal tablets at a time has not been studied.

Conversion from lozenge (Actiq) to buccal tablet (Fentora):

Lozenge dose 200 or 400 mcg: Initial buccal tablet dose is 100 mcg; may titrate using multiples of 100 mcg.

Lozenge dose 600 or 800 mcg: Initial buccal tablet dose is 200 mcg; may titrate using multiples of 200 mcg.

Lozenge dose 1,200 or 1,600 mcg: Initial buccal tablet dose is 400 mcg (using two 200 mcg tablets); may titrate using multiples of 200 mcg.

Intranasal (Lazanda): Note: Do **not** convert patients from any other fentanyl product to Lazanda on a mcg-per-mcg basis. Patients previously using another fentanyl product should be initiated at a dose of 100 mcg (except Actiq); individually titrate to provide adequate analgesia while minimizing adverse effects.

Initial dose: 100 mcg (one 100 mcg spray in one nostril) for all patients; if after 30 minutes pain is unrelieved, an alternative rescue medication may be used. **Must wait at least 2 hours before treating another episode with fentanyl intranasal.** However, for the next pain episode, increase to a higher dose using the recommended dose titration steps.

Dose titration: If titration required, increase to a higher dose for the next pain episode using the following titration steps **(Note: Must wait at least 2 hours before treating another episode with fentanyl intranasal)**: If no relief with 100 mcg dose, increase to 200 mcg dose per episode (one 100 mcg spray in each nostril); if no relief with 200 mcg dose, increase to 300 mcg dose per episode (alternating one 100 mcg spray in right nostril, one 100 mcg spray in left nostril, and one 100 mcg spray in the right nostril); if no relief with 300 mcg dose, increase to 400 mcg dose per episode (one 400 mcg spray in one nostril or alternating two 100 mcg sprays in each nostril); if no relief with 400 mcg dose, increase to 600 mcg dose per episode (one 300 mcg spray in each nostril); if no relief with 600 mcg dose, increase to 800 mcg dose per episode (one 400 mcg spray in each nostril). **Note:** Single doses >800 mcg have not been evaluated. Avoid use of a combination of dose strengths to treat an episode, as this may cause confusion and dosing errors.

Maintenance dose: Once maintenance dose for breakthrough pain episode has been determined, use that dose for subsequent episodes. For pain that is not relieved 30 minutes after Lazanda administration or if a separate breakthrough pain episode occurs within the 2-hour window before the next Lazanda dose is permitted, a rescue medication may be used. Limit Lazanda use to ≤4 doses per day. If patient is experiencing >4 breakthrough pain episodes per day, consider increasing the around-the-clock, long-acting opioid therapy; if long-acting opioid therapy dose is altered, reevaluate and retitrate Lazanda dose as needed. If response to maintenance dose changes (increase in adverse reactions or alterations in pain relief), dose readjustment may be necessary.

Sublingual:

Sublingual spray (Subsys): Note: Do **not** convert patients from any other fentanyl product to Subsys on a mcg-per-mcg basis. Patients previously using another fentanyl product should be initiated at a dose of 100 mcg (except Actiq); individually titrate to provide adequate analgesia while minimizing adverse effects. For patients previously using the transmucosal lozenge (Actiq), the initial dose should be selected using the conversions listed; see *Conversion from lozenge (Actiq) to sublingual spray (Subsys).*

Initial dose: 100 mcg for all patients unless patient is already using Actiq; see *Conversion from lozenge (Actiq) to sublingual spray (Subsys).* If after 30 minutes pain is unrelieved, 1 additional 100 mcg dose may be given. A maximum of 2 doses can be given per breakthrough pain episode. **Must wait at least 4 hours before treating another episode with sublingual spray.**

Dose titration: If titration required, titrate to a dose that provides adequate analgesia (with tolerable side effects) using the following titration steps: If no relief with 100 mcg dose, increase to 200 mcg dose (using one 200 mcg unit); if no relief with 200 mcg dose, increase to 400 mcg dose (using one 400 mcg unit); if no relief with 400 mcg dose, increase to 600 mcg dose (using one 600 mcg unit); if no relief with 600 mcg dose, increase to 800 mcg dose (using one 800 mcg unit); if no relief with 800 mcg dose, increase to 1,200 mcg dose (using two 600 mcg units); if no relief with 1,200 mcg dose, increase to 1,600 mcg dose (using two 800 mcg units). During dose titration, if breakthrough pain is unrelieved 30 minutes after Subsys administration, 1 additional dose using the same strength may be administered (maximum: 2 doses per breakthrough pain episode); **patient must wait 4 hours before treating another breakthrough pain episode with sublingual spray.**

Maintenance dose: Once maintenance dose for breakthrough pain episode has been determined, use that dose for subsequent episodes. If occasional episodes of unrelieved breakthrough pain occur 30 minutes after Subsys administration, 1 additional dose using the same strength may be administered (maximum: 2 doses per breakthrough pain episode); **patient must wait 4 hours before treating another breakthrough pain episode with sublingual spray.** Once maintenance dose is determined, limit Subsys use to ≤4 doses per day. If response to maintenance dose changes (increase in adverse reactions or alterations in pain relief), dose readjustment may be necessary. If patient is experiencing >4 breakthrough pain episodes per day, reevaluate the around-the-clock, long-acting opioid therapy.

Conversion from lozenge (Actiq) to sublingual spray (Subsys):

Lozenge dose 200 or 400 mcg: Initial sublingual spray dose is 100 mcg; may titrate using multiples of 100 mcg.

Lozenge dose 600 or 800 mcg: Initial sublingual spray dose is 200 mcg; may titrate using multiples of 200 mcg.

Lozenge dose 1,200 or 1,600 mcg: Initial sublingual spray dose is 400 mcg; may titrate using multiples of 400 mcg.

Sublingual tablet (Abstral): Note: Do **not** convert patients from any other fentanyl product to Abstral on a mcg-per-mcg basis. Patients previously using another fentanyl product should be initiated at a dose of 100 mcg (except Actiq); individually titrate to provide adequate analgesia while minimizing adverse effects. For patients previously using the transmucosal lozenge (Actiq), the initial dose should be selected using the conversions listed; see *Conversion from lozenge (Actiq) to sublingual tablet (Abstral).*

Initial dose: 100 mcg for all patients unless patient is already using Actiq; see *Conversion from lozenge (Actiq) to sublingual tablet (Abstral).* If after 30 minutes pain is unrelieved, a second 100 mcg dose may be given (US labeling) or an alternative rescue medication (other than Abstral) may be given (Canadian labeling). A maximum of 2 doses (or 1 dose [Canadian labeling]) can be given per breakthrough pain episode. **Must wait at least 2 hours before treating another episode with sublingual tablet.**

Dose titration: If titration required, increase in 100 mcg increments (up to 400 mcg) over consecutive breakthrough episodes. If titration requires >400 mcg per dose, increase in increments of 200 mcg, starting with a 600 mcg dose and titrating up to 800 mcg. During titration, patients may use multiples of 100 mcg and/or 200 mcg tablets for any single dose; do not exceed 4 tablets at one time; safety and efficacy of doses >800 mcg have not been evaluated. During dose titration, if breakthrough pain is unrelieved 30 minutes after sublingual tablet administration, 1 additional dose using the same strength may be administered (US labeling) or an alternative rescue medication (other than Abstral) may be given (Canadian labeling). A maximum of 2 doses (or 1 dose [Canadian labeling]) can be given per breakthrough pain episode. **Must wait 2 hours before treating another breakthrough pain episode with sublingual tablet.**

Maintenance dose: Once maintenance dose for breakthrough pain episode has been determined, use only 1 tablet of the appropriate strength per episode; if pain is unrelieved with maintenance dose, a second dose may be given after 30 minutes (US labeling) or an alternative rescue medication (other than Abstral) may be given (Canadian labeling). A maximum of 2 doses (or 1 dose [Canadian labeling]) can be given per breakthrough pain episode. Separate treatment of subsequent episodes by ≥2 hours; limit Abstral use to ≤4 doses per day. Consider reevaluating the around-the-clock, long-acting opioid therapy in patients experiencing >4 breakthrough pain episodes per day; if long-acting opioid therapy dose altered, reevaluate and retitrate Abstral dose as needed.

Conversion from lozenge (Actiq) to sublingual tablet (Abstral):

Lozenge dose of 200 mcg: Initial sublingual tablet dose is 100 mcg; may titrate using multiples of 100 mcg.

Lozenge dose of 400, 600, 800, or 1,200 mcg: Initial sublingual tablet dose is 200 mcg; may titrate using multiples of 200 mcg.

Lozenge dose of 1,600 mcg: Initial sublingual tablet dose is 400 mcg; may titrate using multiples of 400 mcg.

Discontinuation of pain management therapy:

When reducing the dose or discontinuing chronic opioid therapy, the dose should be gradually tapered down. An optimal tapering schedule has not been established (CDC [Dowell 2016]). Proposed schedules range from slow (eg, 10% reduction per week) to rapid (eg, 25% to 50% reduction every few days) (CDC 2019). When discontinuing transdermal fentanyl and not converting to another opioid, particularly in patients who are physically opioid dependent, use a gradual downward titration (eg, decrease the dose by 25% every 2 to 4 weeks) (manufacturer's labeling). Upon system removal of transdermal fentanyl, ≥17 hours are required for a 50% decrease in fentanyl levels. Individualize discontinuation to minimize withdrawal, while considering patient-specific goals and concerns, as well as the opioid's pharmacokinetics. Slower tapers may be appropriate after long-term use (eg, years), particularly in the final stage of tapering, whereas more rapid tapers may be appropriate in patients experiencing severe adverse events (CDC [Dowell 2016]). Monitor carefully for signs/symptoms of withdrawal. If the patient displays withdrawal symptoms, consider slowing the taper schedule; alterations may include increasing the interval between dose reductions, decreasing amount of daily dose reduction, pausing the taper and restarting when the patient is ready, and/or coadministration of an alpha-2 agonist (eg, clonidine) to blunt withdrawal symptoms (Berna 2015; CDC [Dowell 2016]). Continue to offer nonopioid analgesics as needed for pain management during the taper; consider nonopioid adjunctive treatments for withdrawal symptoms (eg, GI complaints, muscle spasm) as needed (Berna 2015; Sevarino 2019). In patients who continue to take chronic opioid therapy but no longer require fentanyl for breakthrough pain, fentanyl can usually be discontinued without a taper.

Neuraxial analgesia:

Epidural: **Note:** Reserve use for patients with severe acute pain (eg, after major abdominal surgery, cancer pain, during labor and delivery). Must be administered by health care providers skilled in the care of patients receiving intraspinal opioids (APS [Chou 2016]). Use a **preservative-free** formulation intended for neuraxial use (Mariano 2019).

Single dose: 25 to 100 mcg; may provide adequate relief for up to 8 hours. May repeat with additional 100 mcg boluses on demand (US labeling) or alternatively may administer by a continuous infusion (APS 2008; Canadian labeling).

Continuous infusion: 25 to 100 mcg/hour (fentanyl alone). When combined with a local anesthetic (eg, bupivacaine), fentanyl requirement is less (APS 2008; Manion 2011).

Intrathecal: **Note:** Reserve use for patients with severe acute pain (eg, after major abdominal surgery, cancer pain, during labor and delivery). Must be administered by health care providers skilled in the care of patients receiving intraspinal opioids (APS [Chou 2016]). Use a **preservative-free** formulation intended for neuraxial use (Mariano 2019).

Single dose: 15 to 25 mcg; may provide adequate relief for up to 6 hours. When combined with a local anesthetic (eg, bupivacaine), fentanyl dose requirement is less (eg, 10 to 15 mcg instead of 15 to 25 mcg) (APS 2008; d'Arby Toledano 2019).

Geriatric Elderly patients have been found to be twice as sensitive as younger patients to the effects of fentanyl. A wide range of doses may be used. When choosing a dose, take into consideration the following patient factors: age, weight, physical status, underlying disease states, other drugs used, type of anesthesia used, and the surgical procedure to be performed.

Transmucosal lozenge (eg, Actiq): In clinical trials, patients who were >65 years of age were titrated to a mean dose that was 200 mcg less than that of younger patients.

Renal Impairment: Adult Note: Although limited pharmacokinetic data exists in patients with renal insufficiency, <7% to 10% of fentanyl is excreted as unchanged drug and its metabolites are inactive. Fentanyl may be used in patients with renal impairment with careful monitoring for accumulation and adverse effects. In critically ill patients with renal impairment, fentanyl or hydromorphone are preferred (Dean 2004; Jacobi 2002; Koncicki 2017; Van Nimmen 2010).

Injection: CrCl <50 mL/minute: May need to decrease dose to avoid accumulation, especially with continuous infusions; titrate to clinical effect with careful monitoring for adverse effects (Jacobi 2002).

Transdermal (patch):

CrCl 10 to 50 mL/minute: Initial: 75% of normal dose (Koncicki 2017)

CrCl <10 mL/minute: Initial: 50% of normal dose (Koncicki 2017)

Intermittent hemodialysis: Initial: 50% of normal dose (Koncicki 2017)

Manufacturer's labeling:

Injection: There are no dosage adjustments provided in the manufacturer's labeling; use with caution.

Transdermal (device): There are no dosage adjustments provided in the manufacturer's labeling (has not been studied); fentanyl pharmacokinetics may be altered in renal disease.

Transdermal (patch): Degree of impairment (ie, CrCl) not defined in manufacturer's labeling.

Mild to moderate impairment: Initial: Reduce dose by 50%.

Severe impairment: Use not recommended.

Transmucosal (buccal tablet, sublingual spray/tablet, lozenge) and intranasal: There are no dosage adjustments provided in the manufacturer's labeling; use with caution. Although fentanyl pharmacokinetics may be altered in renal disease, fentanyl can be used successfully in the management of breakthrough cancer pain. Doses should be titrated to reach clinical effect with careful monitoring of patients with severe renal disease.

Hepatic Impairment: Adult

Injection: There are no dosage adjustments provided in the manufacturer's labeling; use with caution.

Transdermal (device): There are no dosage adjustments provided in the manufacturer's labeling (has not been studied); fentanyl pharmacokinetics may be altered in hepatic disease.

Transdermal (patch):

Mild to moderate impairment: Initial: Reduce dose by 50%.

Severe impairment: Use not recommended.

Transmucosal (buccal tablet, sublingual spray/tablet, lozenge) and intranasal: There are no dosage adjustments provided in the manufacturer's labeling; use with caution. Although fentanyl pharmacokinetics may be altered in hepatic disease, fentanyl can be used successfully in the management of breakthrough cancer pain. Doses should be titrated to reach clinical effect with careful monitoring of patients with severe hepatic disease.

Pediatric Note: Doses should be titrated to appropriate effects; wide range of doses exist, dependent upon desired degree of analgesia/anesthesia, clinical environment, patient's status, and presence of opioid tolerance.

Infants, Children, and Adolescents <18 years of age:

Acute, short-term uses:

Acute pain: Opioid-naïve:

Infants: Limited data available: IV: Initial: 1 to 2 mcg/kg/dose; may repeat at 2 to 4 hour intervals; in opioid-tolerant or younger infants, titration to higher doses may be required (up to 4 mcg/kg/dose) (Hegenbarth 2008; Nelson 1996; WHO 2012).

Children: Limited data available in <2 years of age: IV: Initial: 1 to 2 mcg/kg/dose; may repeat at 30- to 60-minute intervals; in opioid-tolerant children, titration to higher doses may be required. **Note:** Usual adolescent starting dose is 25 to 50 mcg (Hegenbarth 2008; Nelson 1996; WHO 2012).

Adolescents <18 years: **Note:** After the first dose, if severe pain persists and adverse effects are minimal at the time of expected peak effect, may repeat dose (APS 2008).

<50 kg: Initial: IV: 0.5 to 1 mcg/kg/dose may repeat every 1 to 2 hours although some patients may require more frequent dosing (eg, 30-minute intervals) (APS 2008; Berde 2002).

≥50 kg: Initial: IV: 25 to 50 mcg every 1 to 2 hours although some patients may require more frequent dosing (eg, 30-minute intervals) (APS 2008; Berde 2002).

Analgesia for minor procedures/sedation:

Parenteral:

Infants and Children: Limited data available in <2 years of age: IM, IV: 1 to 2 mcg/kg/dose; administer 3 minutes before the procedure; maximum dose: 50 mcg/dose; may repeat 1/2 original dose every 3 to 5 minutes if necessary; titrate to effect (Cramton 2012; Krauss 2006; Zeltzer 1990).

Adolescents <18 years: IV: 0.5 to 1 mcg/kg/dose; may repeat after 30 to 60 minutes; or 25 to 50 mcg, repeat full dose in 5 minutes if needed, may repeat 4 to 5 times with 25 mcg at 5-minute intervals if needed. **Note:** Higher doses are used for major procedures.

Intranasal (using parenteral preparation): Limited data available: Infants and Children weighing ≥10 kg: Intranasal: 1.5 mcg/kg once (maximum: 100 mcg/dose); reported range: 1 to 2 mcg/kg; some studies that used an initial dose of 1.5 mcg/kg allowed for additional incremental doses of 0.3 to 0.5 mcg/kg to be administered every 5 minutes, not to exceed a total dose of 3 mcg/kg depending on pain type and severity (Borland 2002; Borland 2005; Borland 2007; Chung 2010; Cole 2009; Crellin 2010; Herd 2009; Manjushree 2002; Saunders 2010).

Anesthesia, general; adjunct:

Children 2 to 12 years: IM, IV: 2 to 3 mcg/kg/dose; **Note:** An IV should be in place with general anesthesia so the IM route is rarely used but still maintained as an option in the manufacturer's labeling.

Adolescents <18 years: IV:

Low dose: 0.5 to 2 mcg/kg/dose depending on the indication.

Moderate dose: Initial: 2 to 20 mcg/kg/dose; Maintenance (bolus or infusion): 1 to 2 mcg/kg/**hour**. Discontinuing fentanyl infusion 30 to 60 minutes prior to the end of surgery will usually allow adequate ventilation upon emergence from anesthesia. For "fast-tracking" and early extubation following major surgery, total fentanyl doses are limited to 10 to 15 mcg/kg.

High dose: 20 to 50 mcg/kg/dose; **Note:** High-dose fentanyl as an adjunct to general anesthesia is rarely used, but is still described in the manufacturer's label.

Anesthesia, general without additional anesthetic agents: Adolescents <18 years: IV: 50 to 100 mcg/kg/dose with O_2 and skeletal muscle relaxant.

Anesthesia, regional; adjunct: Adolescents <18 years: IM, IV: 50 to 100 mcg; **Note:** An IV should be in place with regional anesthesia so the IM route is rarely used but still maintained as an option in the manufacturer's labeling.

Continuous analgesia/sedation:

Infants and Children: Limited data available in <2 years of age: Initial IV bolus: 1 to 2 mcg/kg followed by continuous IV infusion at initial rate: 1 mcg/kg/**hour**; titrate to effect; usual range: 1 to 3 mcg/kg/**hour**; some patients may require higher rates (5 mcg/kg/**hour**) (WHO 2012).

Adolescents <18 years:

≤50 kg: Initial IV bolus: 0.5 to 2 mcg/kg followed by continuous IV infusion at initial rate: 0.5 to 2 mcg/kg/**hour** based on expert recommendations for children and pediatric patients ≤50 kg (APS 2008; Berde 2002; WHO 2012).

>50 kg: Initial IV bolus: 25 to 100 mcg/dose followed by continuous IV infusion at initial rate: 25 to 200 mcg/**hour** based on expert recommendations for pediatric patients and experience in adult patients (APS 2008; Berde 2002; Liu 2003; Peng 1999).

Endotracheal intubation, emergent: Limited data available: Infants and Children: IV: 1 to 5 mcg/kg/dose (Hegenbarth 2008).

Preoperative sedation: Adolescents <18 years: IM, IV: 50 to 100 mcg administered 30 to 60 minutes prior to surgery or slow IV: 25 to 50 mcg given shortly before induction (Barash 2009).

Patient-controlled analgesia (PCA): Limited data available: Children ≥5 years and Adolescents <18 years; opioid-naïve: **Note:** PCA has been used in children as young as 5 years; however, clinicians need to assess children 5 to 8 years of age to determine if they are able to use the PCA device correctly. All patients should receive an initial loading dose of an analgesic (to attain adequate control of pain) before starting PCA for maintenance. Adjust doses, lockouts, and limits based on required loading dose, age, state of health, and presence of opioid tolerance. Use lower end of dosing range for opioid-naïve. Assess patient and pain control at regular intervals and adjust settings if needed (APS 2008): IV:

Patient weight ≤50 kg:

Usual concentration: Determined by weight; some centers use the following:

Children <12 kg: 10 mcg/mL.

Children 12 to 30 kg: 25 mcg/mL.

Children >30 kg: 50 mcg/mL.

Demand dose: Usual initial: 0.5 to 1 mcg/kg/dose; usual range: 0.5 to 1 mcg/kg/dose.

Lockout: Usual initial: 5 doses/hour.

Lockout interval: Range: 6 to 8 minutes.

Usual basal rate: 0 to 0.5 mcg/kg/**hour.**

Patient weight >50 kg:

Usual concentration: 50 mcg/mL.

Demand dose: Usual initial: 20 mcg; usual range: 10 to 50 mcg.

Lockout interval: Usual initial: 6 minutes; usual range: 5 to 8 minutes.

Usual basal rate: ≤50 mcg/**hour.**

Chronic uses or opioid-tolerant patients (eg, cancer pain):

Chronic pain, moderate to severe (opioid-tolerant): Transdermal patch: Duragesic: Children ≥2 years and Adolescents <18 years who are opioid-tolerant receiving at least 60 mg oral morphine equivalents per day: **Note:** Discontinue or taper all other around-the-clock or extended release opioids when initiating therapy with fentanyl transdermal patch:

Initial: 25 mcg/**hour** system or higher based on previous opioid dosing. To convert patients from oral or parenteral opioids to transdermal patch, a 24-hour analgesic requirement should be calculated (based on prior opioid use). Using the following tables, the appropriate initial dose can be determined. The initial fentanyl dosage may be approximated from the 24-hour morphine dosage equivalent and titrated to minimize adverse effects and provide analgesia. Substantial interpatient variability exists in relative potency. Therefore, it is safer to underestimate a patient's daily fentanyl requirement and provide breakthrough pain relief with rescue medication (eg, immediate release opioid) than to overestimate requirements. With the initial application, the absorption of transdermal fentanyl requires several hours to reach plateau; therefore, transdermal fentanyl is inappropriate for management of acute pain. Change patch every 72 hours.

Conversion from continuous infusion of fentanyl: In patients who have adequate pain relief with a fentanyl infusion, fentanyl may be converted to transdermal dosing at a rate equivalent to the intravenous rate. Based on experience in adults, a two-step taper of the infusion to be completed over 12 hours may be considered (Kornick 2001) after the patch is applied. The infusion is decreased to 50% of the original rate 6 hours after the application of the first patch, and subsequently discontinued twelve hours after application.

Titration: Short-acting agents may be required until analgesic efficacy is established and/or as supplements for "breakthrough" pain. The amount of supplemental doses should be closely monitored. Appropriate dosage increases may be based on daily supplemental dosage using the ratio of 45 mg/24 hours of oral morphine to a 12.5 mcg/hour increase in fentanyl dosage.

Frequency of adjustment: The dosage should not be titrated more frequently than every 3 days after the initial dose or every 6 days thereafter. Titrate dose based on the daily dose of supplemental opioids required by the patient on the second or third day of the initial application. **Note:** Upon discontinuation, ~17 hours are required for a 50% decrease in fentanyl levels.

Frequency of application: The majority of patients may be controlled on every 72-hour administration; however, a small number of adult patients have required every 48-hour administration.

Discontinuation: When discontinuing transdermal fentanyl and not converting to another opioid, use a gradual downward titration, such as decreasing the dose by 50% every 6 days, to reduce the possibility of withdrawal symptoms.

Dose conversion guidelines for transdermal fentanyl from other opioids (see tables).

Note: The conversion factors in these tables are only to be used for the conversion from current opioid therapy to Duragesic patch. Conversion factors in this table cannot be used to convert from Duragesic to another opioid (doing so may lead to fatal overdose due to overestimation of the new opioid). US and Canadian dose conversion guidelines differ; consult table for US recommendations. The Canadian product is not approved in pediatric patients. **These are not tables of equianalgesic doses**.

US Labeling: Dose Conversion Guidelines: Recommended Initial Duragesic Dose Based Upon Daily Oral Morphine Dose[a]

Oral 24-Hour Morphine (mg/day)	Duragesic Dose[b,c] (mcg/hour)
60 to 134	25
135 to 224	50
225 to 314	75
315 to 404	100
405 to 494	125
495 to 584	150
585 to 674	175
675 to 764	200
765 to 854	225
855 to 944	250
945 to 1,034	275
1,035 to 1,124	300

[a]The table should NOT be used to convert from transdermal fentanyl (Duragesic) to other opioid analgesics. Rather, following removal of the patch, titrate the dose of the new opioid until adequate analgesia is achieved.

[b]Pediatric patients initiating therapy on a 25 mcg/hour Duragesic system should be opioid-tolerant and receiving at least 60 mg oral morphine equivalents per day.

[c]A fentanyl 37.5 mcg/hour transdermal system is also available and may be considered during conversion from prior opioids or dose titration.

US Labeling: Dose Conversion Guidelines[a]

Current Analgesic	Daily Dosage (mg/day)			
Morphine (IM/IV)	10 to 22	23 to 37	38 to 52	53 to 67
Oxycodone (oral)	30 to 67	67.5 to 112	112.5 to 157	157.5 to 202
Codeine (oral)	150 to 447	-	-	-
Hydromorphone (oral)	8 to 17	17.1 to 28	28.1 to 39	39.1 to 51
Hydromorphone (IV)	1.5 to 3.4	3.5 to 5.6	5.7 to 7.9	8 to 10
Meperidine (IM)	75 to 165	166 to 278	279 to 390	391 to 503
Methadone (oral)	20 to 44	45 to 74	75 to 104	105 to 134
Duragesic (fentanyl transdermal) recommended dose (mcg/hour)	**25 mcg/hour**	**50 mcg/hour**	**75 mcg/hour**	**100 mcg/hour**

[a]The table should NOT be used to convert from transdermal fentanyl (Duragesic) to other opioid analgesics. Rather, following removal of the patch, titrate the dose of the new opioid until adequate analgesia is achieved.

Cancer pain; breakthrough: Transmucosal lozenge: Actiq: Adolescents ≥16 years: **Note:** For patients who are tolerant to and currently receiving opioid therapy for persistent cancer pain; dosing should be individually titrated to provide adequate analgesia with minimal side effects. **Patients must remain on around-the-clock opioids during use.** Initial dose: 200 mcg (consumed over 15 minutes) for all patients; if after 30 minutes from the start of the lozenge (ie, 15 minutes following the completion of the lozenge), the pain is unrelieved, a second 200 mcg dose may be given over 15 minutes. A maximum of 1 additional dose can be given per pain episode; **must wait at least 4 hours before treating another episode.** To limit the number of units in the home during titration, only prescribe an initial titration supply of six 200 mcg lozenges. **Note:** Do not convert patients from any other fentanyl product to Actiq on a mcg-per-mcg basis. Patients previously using another fentanyl product should be initiated at a dose of 200 mcg; individually titrate to provide adequate analgesia while minimizing adverse effects.

Dose titration: Dose titration should be done if patient requires more than 1 dose/breakthrough pain episode for several consecutive episodes. From the initial dose, closely follow patients and modify the dose until patient reaches a dose providing adequate analgesia using a single dosage unit per breakthrough cancer pain episode. If signs/symptoms of excessive opioid effects (eg, respiratory depression) occur, immediately remove the dosage unit from the patient's mouth, dispose of properly, and reduce subsequent doses. If adequate relief is not achieved 15 minutes after completion of the first dose (ie, 30 minutes after the start of the lozenge), only 1 additional lozenge of the same strength may be given for that episode; **must wait at least 4 hours before treating another episode.**

Maintenance dose: Once titrated to an effective dose, patients should generally use a single dosage unit per breakthrough pain episode. During any pain episode, if adequate relief is not achieved 15 minutes after completion of the first dose (ie, 30 minutes after the start of the lozenge), only 1 additional lozenge of the same strength may be given over 15 minutes for that episode; **must wait at least 4 hours before treating another episode**. Consumption should be limited to ≤4 units per day (once an effective breakthrough dose is found). If adequate analgesia is **not** provided after treating several episodes of breakthrough pain using the same dose, increase dose to next highest lozenge strength (initially dispense no more than 6 units of the new strength). Consider increasing the around-the-clock opioid therapy in patients experiencing >4 breakthrough pain episodes per day and have their long-term opioid re-evaluated. If signs/symptoms of excessive opioid effects (eg, respiratory depression) occur, immediately remove the dosage unit from the patient's mouth, dispose of properly, and reduce subsequent doses.

Adolescents ≥18 years:

Note: Ranges listed may not represent the maximum doses that may be required in some patients. Doses and dosage intervals should be titrated to pain relief/prevention. Monitor vital signs routinely. Single IM doses have duration of 1 to 2 hours; single IV doses last 0.5 to 1 hour.

Surgery:

Premedication: IM, slow IV: 50 to 100 mcg administered 30 to 60 minutes prior to surgery **or** slow IV: 25 to 50 mcg given shortly before induction (Barash 2009).

Adjunct to general anesthesia: Slow IV:

Low dose: 1 to 2 mcg/**kg** depending on the indication (Miller 2010); additional maintenance doses are generally not needed.

Moderate dose (fentanyl plus a sedative/hypnotic): Initial: 2 to 4 mcg/**kg**; Maintenance (bolus or infusion): 25 to 50 mcg every 15 to 30 minutes or 0.5 to 2 mcg/kg/**hour**. Discontinuing fentanyl infusion 30 to 60 minutes prior to the end of surgery will usually allow adequate ventilation upon emergence from anesthesia.

High dose (opioid anesthesia): 4 to 20 mcg/**kg** bolus then 2 to 10 mcg/kg/**hour** (Miller 2010); **Note:** High-dose fentanyl (ie, 20 to 50 mcg/kg) is rarely used, but is still described in the manufacturer's label. The concept of fast-tracking and early extubation following cardiac surgery has essentially replaced high-dose fentanyl anesthesia.

Adjunct to regional anesthesia: 50 to 100 mcg IM or slow IV over 1 to 2 minutes. **Note:** An IV should be in place with regional anesthesia so the IM route is rarely used but still maintained as an option in the manufacturer's labeling.

Postoperative recovery: IM, slow IV: 50 to 100 mcg every 1 to 2 hours as needed.

Pain management:

Postoperative pain, acute: Transdermal device (Ionsys): Apply one device to chest or upper outer arm only. Only the patient may activate the device (40 mcg dose of fentanyl per activation; maximum: 6 doses per hour). Only one device may be applied at a time for up to 24 hours or 80 doses, whichever comes first. May be used for a maximum of 72 hours, with each subsequent device applied to a different skin site. If inadequate analgesia is achieved with one device, either provide additional supplemental analgesic medication or replace with an alternate analgesic medication. Refer to manufacturer's labeling for activation instructions.

Note: For hospital use only by patients under medical supervision and direction and only after patients have been titrated to an acceptable level of analgesia using another opioid analgesic.

Severe pain:

Intermittent dosing: IM, IV: Slow IV: 25 to 35 mcg (based on ~70 kg patient) **or** 0.35 to 0.5 mcg/kg every 30 to 60 minutes as needed (SCCM [Barr 2013]). **Note:** After the first dose, if severe pain persists and adverse effects are minimal at the time of expected peak effect (eg, ~5 minutes after IV administration), may repeat dose (APS 2008). In addition, since the duration of activity with IV administration is 30 to 60 minutes, more frequent administration may be necessary when administered by this route.

Patient-controlled analgesia (PCA) (APS 2008; Miller 2010): Opioid-naive: IV:

Usual concentration: 10 mcg/mL.

Demand dose: Usual: 10 to 20 mcg.

Lockout interval: 4 to 10 minutes.

Usual basal rate: ≤50 mcg/hour. **Note:** Continuous basal infusions are not recommended for initial programming and should rarely be used; consider limiting infusion rate to 10 mcg/hour if used (Grass 2005).

Cancer pain; breakthrough: Transmucosal: Opioid-tolerant patients: For patients who are tolerant to and currently receiving opioid therapy for persistent cancer pain; dosing should be individually titrated to provide adequate analgesia with minimal side effects. Dose titration should be done if patient requires more than 1 dose/breakthrough pain episode for several consecutive episodes. Patients experiencing >4 breakthrough pain episodes/day should have the dose of their long-term opioid re-evaluated. **Patients must remain on around-the-clock opioids during use.**

Lozenge (eg, Actiq): **Note:** Do **not** convert patients from any other fentanyl product to Actiq on a mcg-per-mcg basis. Patients previously using another fentanyl product should be initiated at a dose of 200 mcg; individually titrate to provide adequate analgesia while minimizing adverse effects.

Initial dose: 200 mcg (consumed over 15 minutes) for all patients; if after 30 minutes from the start of the lozenge (ie, 15 minutes following the completion of the lozenge), the pain is unrelieved, a second 200 mcg dose may be given over 15 minutes. A maximum of 1 additional dose can be given per pain episode; **must wait at least 4 hours before treating another episode**. To limit the number of units in the home during titration, only prescribe an initial titration supply of six 200 mcg lozenges.

Dose titration: From the initial dose, closely follow patients and modify the dose until patient reaches a dose providing adequate analgesia using a single dosage unit per breakthrough cancer pain episode. If signs/symptoms of excessive opioid effects (eg, respiratory depression) occur, immediately remove the dosage unit from the patient's mouth, dispose of properly, and reduce subsequent doses. If adequate relief is not achieved 15 minutes after completion of the first dose (ie, 30 minutes after the start of the lozenge), only 1 additional lozenge of the same strength may be given for that episode; **must wait at least 4 hours before treating another episode.**

Maintenance dose: Once titrated to an effective dose, patients should generally use a single dosage unit per breakthrough pain episode. During any pain episode, if adequate relief is not achieved 15 minutes after completion of the first dose (ie, 30 minutes after the start of the lozenge), only 1 additional lozenge of the same strength may be given over 15 minutes for that episode; **must wait at least 4 hours before treating another episode.** Consumption should be limited to ≤4 units per day (once an effective breakthrough dose is found). If adequate analgesia is **not** provided after treating several episodes of breakthrough pain using the same dose, increase dose to next highest lozenge strength (initially dispense no more than 6 units of the new strength). Consider increasing the around-the-clock opioid therapy in patients experiencing >4 breakthrough pain episodes per day. If signs/symptoms of excessive opioid effects (eg, respiratory depression) occur, immediately remove the dosage unit from the patient's mouth, dispose of properly, and reduce subsequent doses.

Buccal tablets (Fentora): **Note:** Do **not** convert patients from any other fentanyl product to Fentora on a mcg-per-mcg basis. Patients previously using another fentanyl product should be initiated at a dose of 100 mcg; individually titrate to provide adequate analgesia while minimizing adverse effects. For patients previously using the transmucosal lozenge (Actiq), the initial dose should be selected using the conversions listed; see *Conversion from lozenge (Actiq) to buccal tablet (Fentora)*.

Initial dose: 100 mcg for all patients unless patient already using Actiq; see *Conversion from lozenge (Actiq) to buccal tablet (Fentora)*; if after 30 minutes pain is unrelieved, a second 100 mcg dose may be administered (maximum of 2 doses per breakthrough pain episode). **Must wait at least 4 hours before treating another episode with Fentora buccal tablet.**

Dose titration: If titration required, 100 mcg dose may be increased to 200 mcg using two 100 mcg tablets (one on each side of mouth) with the next breakthrough pain episode. If 200 mcg dose is not successful, patient can use four 100 mcg tablets (two on each side of mouth) with the next breakthrough pain episode. If titration requires >400 mcg per dose, titrate using 200 mcg tablets; do not use more than 4 tablets simultaneously (maximum single dose: 800 mcg). During any pain episode, if adequate relief is not achieved after 30 minutes following buccal tablet application, a second dose of same strength per breakthrough pain episode may be used. **Must wait at least 4 hours before treating another episode with Fentora buccal tablet.**

Maintenance dose: Following titration, the effective maintenance dose using 1 tablet of the appropriate strength should be administered once per episode; if after 30 minutes pain is unrelieved, may administer a second dose of the same strength. **Must wait ≥4 hours before treating another episode with Fentora buccal tablet.** Limit to 4 applications per day. Consider increasing the around-the-clock opioid therapy in patients experiencing >4 breakthrough pain episodes per day. Once an effective maintenance dose has been established, the buccal tablet may be administered sublingually (alternate route). To prevent confusion, patient should only have one strength available at a time. Once maintenance dose is determined, all other unused tablets should be disposed of and that strength (using a single tablet) should be used. Using more than four buccal tablets at a time has not been studied.

Conversion from lozenge (Actiq) to buccal tablet (Fentora):

Lozenge dose 200 to 400 mcg: Initial buccal tablet dose is 100 mcg; may titrate using multiples of 100 mcg.

Lozenge dose 600 to 800 mcg: Initial buccal tablet dose is 200 mcg; may titrate using multiples of 200 mcg.

Lozenge dose 1,200 to 1,600 mcg: Initial buccal tablet dose is 400 mcg (using two 200 mcg tablets); may titrate using multiples of 200 mcg.

Nasal spray (Lazanda): **Note:** Do **not** convert patients from any other fentanyl product to Lazanda on a mcg-per-mcg basis. Patients previously using another fentanyl product should be initiated at a dose of 100 mcg; individually titrate to provide adequate analgesia while minimizing adverse effects.

Initial dose: 100 mcg (one 100 mcg spray in one nostril) for all patients; if after 30 minutes pain is unrelieved, an alternative rescue medication may be used as directed by their health care provider. **Must wait at least 2 hours before treating another episode with Lazanda nasal spray.** However, for the next pain episode, increase to a higher dose using the recommended dose titration steps.

Dose titration: If titration required, increase to a higher dose using the recommended titration steps. **(Note: Must wait at least 2 hours before treating another episode with nasal spray.)** Dose titration steps: If no relief with 100 mcg dose, increase to 200 mcg dose per episode (one 100 mcg spray in each nostril); if no relief with 200 mcg dose, increase to 300 mcg dose per episode (alternating one 100 mcg spray in right nostril, one 100 mcg spray in left nostril, and one 100 mcg spray in the right nostril); if no relief with 300 mcg dose, increase to 400 mcg per episode (one 400 mcg spray in one nostril **or** two 100 mcg sprays in each nostril); if no relief with 400 mcg dose, increase to 600 mcg dose per episode (one 300 mcg spray in each nostril); if no relief with 600 mcg dose, increase to 800 mcg dose per episode (one 400 mcg spray in each nostril). **Note:** Single doses >800 mcg have not been evaluated. There are no data supporting the use of a combination of dose strengths. Avoid use of a combination of dose strengths to treat an episode.

Maintenance dose: Once maintenance dose for breakthrough pain episode has been determined, use that dose for subsequent episodes. For pain that is not relieved after 30 minutes of Lazanda administration or if a separate breakthrough pain episode occurs within the 2 hour window before the next Lazanda dose is permitted, a rescue medication may be used. Limit Lazanda use to ≤4 episodes of breakthrough pain per day. If patient is experiencing >4 breakthrough pain episodes/day, consider increasing the around-the-clock, long-acting opioid therapy; if long-acting opioid therapy dose is altered, re-evaluate and retitrate Lazanda dose as needed. If response to maintenance dose changes (increase in adverse reactions or alterations in pain relief), dose readjustment may be necessary.

Sublingual spray (Subsys): **Note:** Do **not** convert patients from any other fentanyl product to Subsys on a mcg-per-mcg basis. Patients previously using another fentanyl product should be initiated at a dose of 100 mcg; individually titrate to provide adequate analgesia while minimizing adverse effects. For patients previously using the transmucosal lozenge (Actiq), the initial dose should be selected using the conversions listed; see *Conversion from lozenge (Actiq) to sublingual spray (Subsys)*.

Initial dose: 100 mcg for all patients unless patient already using Actiq; see *Conversion from lozenge (Actiq) to sublingual spray (Subsys)* If pain is unrelieved, one additional 100 mcg dose may be given 30 minutes after administration of the first dose. A maximum of two doses can be given per breakthrough pain episode. **Must wait at least 4 hours before treating another episode with sublingual spray**.

Dose titration: If titration required, titrate to a dose that provides adequate analgesia (with tolerable side effects) using the following titration steps: If no relief with 100 mcg dose, increase to 200 mcg dose per episode (one 200 mcg unit); if no relief with 200 mcg dose, increase to 400 mcg per episode (one 400 mcg unit); if no relief with 400 mcg dose, increase to 600 mcg dose per episode (one 600 mcg unit); if no relief with 600 mcg dose, increase to 800 mcg dose per episode (one 800 mcg unit); if no relief with 800 mcg dose, increase to 1,200 mcg dose per episode (two 600 mcg units); if no relief with 1,200 mcg dose, increase to 1,600 mcg per episode (two 800 mcg units). During dose titration, if breakthrough pain unrelieved 30 minutes after Subsys administration, 1 additional dose using the same strength may be administered (maximum: 2 doses per breakthrough pain episode); **patient must wait 4 hours before treating another breakthrough pain episode with sublingual spray.**

Maintenance dose: Once maintenance dose for breakthrough pain episode has been determined, use that dose for subsequent episodes. If occasional episodes of unrelieved breakthrough pain occur following 30 minutes of Subsys administration, one additional dose using the same strength may be administered (maximum: Two doses per breakthrough pain episode); patient must wait 4 hours before treating another breakthrough pain episode with Subsys. Once maintenance dose is determined, limit Subsys use to ≤4 episodes of breakthrough pain per day. If response to maintenance dose changes (increase in adverse reactions or alterations in pain relief), dose readjustment may be necessary. If patient is experiencing >4 breakthrough pain episodes/day, consider increasing the around-the-clock, long-acting opioid therapy.

Conversion from lozenge (Actiq) to sublingual spray (Subsys):

Lozenge dose 200 to 400 mcg: Initial sublingual spray dose is 100 mcg; may titrate using multiples of 100 mcg.

Lozenge dose 600 to 800 mcg: Initial sublingual spray dose is 200 mcg; may titrate using multiples of 200 mcg.

Lozenge dose 1,200 to 1,600 mcg: Initial sublingual spray dose is 400 mcg; may titrate using multiples of 400 mcg.

Sublingual tablet (Abstral): **Note:** Do **not** convert patients from any other fentanyl product to Abstral on a mcg-per-mcg basis. Patients previously using another fentanyl product should be initiated at a dose of 100 mcg (except Actiq); individually titrate to provide adequate analgesia while minimizing adverse effects.

Initial dose: 100 mcg for all patients unless patient already using Actiq; see *Conversion from lozenge (Actiq) to sublingual tablet (Abstral)*; if pain is unrelieved, a second dose may be given 30 minutes after administration of the first dose. A maximum of two doses can be given per breakthrough pain episode. **Must wait at least 2 hours before treating another episode.**

Dose titration: If titration required, increase in 100 mcg increments (up to 400 mcg) over consecutive breakthrough episodes. If titration requires >400 mcg/dose, increase in increments of 200 mcg, starting with 600 mcg dose and titrating up to 800 mcg. During titration, patients may use multiples of 100 mcg and/or 200 mcg tablets for any single dose; do not exceed 4 tablets at one time; safety and efficacy of doses >800 mcg have not been evaluated. During dose titration, if breakthrough pain unrelieved 30 minutes after sublingual tablet administration, one additional dose using the same strength may be administered (maximum: 2 doses per breakthrough pain episode). **Patient must wait 2 hours before treating another breakthrough pain episode with sublingual tablet.**

Maintenance dose: Once maintenance dose for breakthrough pain episode has been determined, use only one tablet in the appropriate strength per episode. If pain is unrelieved with maintenance dose, a second dose may be given after 30 minutes; maximum of 2 doses/episode of breakthrough pain; separate treatment of subsequent episodes by ≥2 hours; limit treatment to ≤4 breakthrough episodes/day. Consider increasing the around-the-clock, long-acting opioid therapy in patients experiencing >4 breakthrough pain episodes/day; if long-acting opioid therapy dose altered, re-evaluate and retitrate Abstral dose as needed.

Conversion from lozenge (Actiq) to sublingual tablet (Abstral):

Lozenge dose 200 mcg: Initial sublingual tablet dose is 100 mcg; may titrate using multiples of 100 mcg.

Lozenge dose 400 to 1,200 mcg: Initial sublingual tablet dose is 200 mcg; may titrate using multiples of 200 mcg.

Lozenge dose 1,600 mcg: Initial sublingual tablet dose is 400 mcg; may titrate using multiples of 400 mcg.

Chronic pain management (opioid-tolerant patients only): Transdermal patch: Discontinue or taper all other around-the-clock or extended release opioids when initiating therapy with fentanyl transdermal patch.

Initial: To convert patients from oral or parenteral opioids to transdermal patch, a 24-hour analgesic requirement should be calculated (based on prior opioid use). Using the following tables, the appropriate initial dose can be determined. The initial fentanyl dosage may be approximated from the 24-hour morphine dosage equivalent and titrated to minimize adverse effects and provide analgesia. Substantial interpatient variability exists in relative potency. Therefore, it is safer to underestimate a patient's daily fentanyl requirement and provide breakthrough pain relief with rescue medication (eg, immediate release opioid) than to overestimate requirements. With the initial application, the absorption of transdermal fentanyl requires several hours to reach plateau; therefore, transdermal fentanyl is inappropriate for management of acute pain. Change patch every 72 hours.

Conversion from continuous infusion of fentanyl: In patients who have adequate pain relief with a fentanyl infusion, fentanyl may be converted to transdermal dosing at a rate equivalent to the intravenous rate. A two-step taper of the infusion to be completed over 12 hours has been recommended (Kornick 2001) after the patch is applied. The infusion is decreased to 50% of the original rate six hours after the application of the first patch, and subsequently discontinued 12 hours after application.

Titration: Short-acting agents may be required until analgesic efficacy is established and/or as supplements for "breakthrough" pain. The amount of supplemental doses should be closely monitored. Appropriate dosage increases may be based on daily supplemental dosage using the ratio of 45 mg/24 hours of oral morphine to a 12.5 mcg/hour increase in fentanyl dosage.

Frequency of adjustment: The dosage should not be titrated more frequently than every 3 days after the initial dose or every 6 days thereafter. Titrate dose based on the daily dose of supplemental opioids required by the patient on the second or third day of the initial application. **Note:** Upon discontinuation, ~17 hours are required for a 50% decrease in fentanyl levels.

Frequency of application: The majority of patients may be controlled on every 72-hour administration; however, a small number of adult patients require every 48-hour administration.

Discontinuation: When discontinuing transdermal fentanyl and not converting to another opioid, use a gradual downward titration, such as decreasing the dose by 50% every 6 days, to reduce the possibility of withdrawal symptoms.

Dose conversion guidelines for transdermal fentanyl (see tables). **Note:** The conversion factors in these tables are only to be used for the conversion from current opioid therapy to Duragesic (US labeling). Conversion factors in this table cannot be used to convert from Duragesic to another opioid (doing so may lead to fatal overdose due to overestimation of the new opioid). These are not tables of equianalgesic doses.

US Labeling: Dose Conversion Guidelines: Recommended Initial Duragesic Dose Based Upon Daily Oral Morphine Dose[a]

Oral 24-Hour Morphine (mg/day)	Duragesic Dose[b] (mcg/hour)
60 to 134	25
135 to 224	50
225 to 314	75
315 to 404	100
405 to 494	125
495 to 584	150
585 to 674	175
675 to 764	200
765 to 854	225
855 to 944	250
945 to 1,034	275
1,035 to 1,124	300

[a]The table should NOT be used to convert from transdermal fentanyl (Duragesic) to other opioid analgesics. Rather, following removal of the patch, titrate the dose of the new opioid until adequate analgesia is achieved.

[b]A fentanyl 37.5 mcg/hour transdermal system is also available and may be considered during conversion from prior opioids or dose titration.

US Labeling: Dose Conversion Guidelines[a]

Current Analgesic	Daily Dosage (mg/day)			
Morphine (IM/IV)	10 to 22	23 to 37	38 to 52	53 to 67
Oxycodone (oral)	30 to 67	67.5 to 112	112.5 to 157	157.5 to 202
Codeine (oral)	150 to 447	-	-	-
Hydromorphone (oral)	8 to 17	17.1 to 28	28.1 to 39	39.1 to 51
Hydromorphone (IV)	1.5 to 3.4	3.5 to 5.6	5.7 to 7.9	8 to 10
Meperidine (IM)	75 to 165	166 to 278	279 to 390	391 to 503
Methadone (oral)	20 to 44	45 to 74	75 to 104	105 to 134
Duragesic (fentanyl transdermal) recommended dose (mcg/hour)	**25 mcg/hour**	**50 mcg/hour**	**75 mcg/hour**	**100 mcg/hour**

[a]The table should NOT be used to convert from transdermal fentanyl (Duragesic) to other opioid analgesics. Rather, following removal of the patch, titrate the dose of the new opioid until adequate analgesia is achieved.

Renal Impairment: Pediatric

Injection: There are no dosage adjustments provided in the manufacturer's labeling; however, the following guidelines have been used by some clinicians (Aronoff 2007):

Infants, Children, and Adolescents: The following assumes dosages of 0.5 to 2 mcg/kg/dose or 1 to 5 mcg/kg/**hour** in normal renal function: IV:

GFR >50 mL/minute/1.73 m^2: No adjustment required

GFR 10 to 50 mL/minute/1.73 m^2: Administer 75% of usual dose

GFR <10 mL/minute/1.73 m^2: Administer 50% of usual dose

Intermittent hemodialysis: Administer 50% of usual dose

Peritoneal dialysis (PD): Administer 50% of usual dose

Continuous renal replacement therapy (CRRT): Administer 75% of usual dose

Transdermal (device): Adolescents ≥18 years: There are no dosage adjustments provided in the manufacturer's labeling (has not been studied); fentanyl pharmacokinetics may be altered in renal disease.

Transdermal (patch): Pediatric patients ≥2 years: Degree of impairment (ie, CrCl) not defined in manufacturer's labeling.

Mild to moderate impairment: Initial: Reduce dose by 50%

Severe impairment: Use not recommended

Transmucosal (buccal tablet, sublingual spray/tablet, lozenge) and nasal spray: Adolescents ≥18 years: Although fentanyl pharmacokinetics may be altered in renal disease, fentanyl can be used successfully in the management of breakthrough cancer pain. Use with caution; reduce initial dose and titrate to reach clinical effect with careful monitoring of patients, especially those with severe renal disease.

Hepatic Impairment: Pediatric

Injection: There are no dosage adjustments provided in the manufacturer's labeling.

Transdermal (device): Adolescents ≥18 years: There are no dosage adjustments provided in the manufacturer's labeling (has not been studied); fentanyl pharmacokinetics may be altered in hepatic disease.

Transdermal (patch): Pediatric patients ≥2 years:

Mild to moderate impairment: Initial: Reduce dose by 50%.

Severe impairment: Use not recommended.

Transmucosal (buccal tablet, sublingual spray/tablet, lozenge) and nasal spray: Adolescents ≥18 years: Although fentanyl pharmacokinetics may be altered in hepatic disease, fentanyl can be used successfully in the management of breakthrough cancer pain. Use with caution; reduce initial dose and titrate to reach clinical effect with careful monitoring of patients, especially those with severe hepatic disease.

Mechanism of Action Binds with stereospecific receptors at many sites within the CNS, increases pain threshold, alters pain reception, inhibits ascending pain pathways

Contraindications

Hypersensitivity (eg, anaphylaxis, hypersensitivity) to fentanyl or any component of the formulation.

Additional contraindications for transdermal device (Ionsys): Significant respiratory depression; acute or severe bronchial asthma in an unmonitored setting or in the absence of resuscitative equipment; gastrointestinal obstruction, including paralytic ileus (known or suspected); hypersensitivity to cetylpyridinium chloride (eg, Cepacol).

Additional contraindications for transdermal patch (Duragesic): Significant respiratory depression; acute or severe bronchial asthma in an unmonitored setting or in the absence of resuscitative equipment; gastrointestinal obstruction, including paralytic ileus (known or suspected); patients requiring short-term therapy, management of acute or intermittent pain, postoperative or mild pain; patients who are **not** opioid tolerant.

Additional contraindications for transmucosal buccal tablets (Fentora), lozenges (Actiq), sublingual tablets (Abstral), sublingual spray (Subsys), intranasal (Lazanda): Significant respiratory depression (Actiq, Fentora only); acute or severe bronchial asthma in an unmonitored setting or in the absence of resuscitative equipment; gastrointestinal obstruction, including paralytic ileus (known or suspected); acute or postoperative pain (including headache, migraine, or dental pain); patients who are **not** opioid tolerant; acute pain management in the emergency room.

Canadian labeling: Additional contraindication (not in US labeling):

Injection: Septicemia; severe hemorrhage or shock; local infection at proposed injection site; disturbances in blood morphology and/or anticoagulant therapy or other concomitant drug therapy or medical conditions which could contraindicate the technique of epidural administration

Sublingual tablets (Abstral): Severe bronchial asthma, chronic obstructive airway, or status asthmaticus; acute respiratory depression; hypercapnia; cor pulmonale; known or suspected mechanical GI obstruction (eg, bowel obstruction or strictures) or any diseases/conditions that affect bowel transit (eg, ileus of any type); suspected surgical abdomen (eg, acute appendicitis or pancreatitis); mild pain that can be managed with other pain medications; acute pain management other than breakthrough or postoperative pain (including headache or migraine, dental pain or emergency room use); acute alcoholism, delirium tremens, and convulsive disorders; severe CNS depression, increased cerebrospinal or intracranial pressure and head injury; concurrent use or use within 14 days of a monoamine oxidase (MAO) inhibitor; breastfeeding women; during labor and delivery; opioid-nontolerant patients (including patients on intermittent or as needed opioid dosing).

Transdermal patch: Hypersensitivity to other opioids; suspected surgical abdomen (eg, acute appendicitis, pancreatitis); known or suspected mechanical GI obstruction (eg, bowel obstruction, strictures) or any diseases/conditions that affect bowel transit (eg, ileus of any type); acute alcoholism, delirium tremens, and convulsive disorders; severe CNS depression, increased cerebrospinal or intracranial pressure and head injury; concurrent use of MAO inhibitors or within 14 days of therapy; perioperative pain; women who are nursing, pregnant, or during labor and delivery

Transmucosal buccal tablets (Fentora): Hypersensitivity to other opioids; acute pain management in the emergency room; known or suspected mechanical GI obstruction (eg, bowel obstruction or strictures) or any diseases/conditions that affect bowel transit (eg, ileus of any type); suspected surgical abdomen (eg, acute appendicitis or pancreatitis); acute or severe bronchial asthma, chronic obstructive airway, status asthmaticus; acute respiratory depression; hypercapnia; cor pulmonale; acute alcoholism, delirium tremens, and convulsive disorders; severe CNS depression, increased cerebrospinal or intracranial pressure and head injury; concurrent use or use within 14 days of an MAO inhibitor

Documentation of allergenic cross-reactivity for opioids is limited. However, because of similarities in chemical structure and/or pharmacologic actions, the possibility of cross-sensitivity cannot be ruled out with certainty.

Warnings/Precautions An opioid-containing analgesic regimen should be tailored to each patient's needs and based upon the type of pain being treated (acute versus chronic), the route of administration, degree of tolerance for opioids (naive versus chronic user), age, weight, and medical condition. The optimal analgesic dose varies widely among patients. Doses should be titrated to pain relief/prevention. May cause CNS depression, which may impair physical or mental abilities; patients must be cautioned about performing tasks which require mental alertness (eg, operating machinery or driving). **[US Boxed Warning]: Concomitant use of opioids with benzodiazepines or other CNS depressants, including alcohol, may result in profound sedation, respiratory depression, coma, and death. Reserve concomitant prescribing of oxycodone/acetaminophen and benzodiazepines or other CNS depressants for use in patients for whom alternative treatment options are inadequate. Limit dosage and durations to the minimum required and follow patients for signs and symptoms of respiratory depression and sedation. [US Boxed Warning]: The concomitant use of fentanyl with all cytochrome P450 3A4 inhibitors may result in an increase in fentanyl plasma concentrations, which could increase or prolong adverse reactions and may cause potentially fatal respiratory depression. In addition, discontinuation of a concomitantly used cytochrome P450 3A4 inducer may result in an increase in fentanyl plasma concentration. Monitor patients receiving fentanyl and any CYP3A4 inhibitor or inducer.** Potentially significant drug/drug interactions may exist, requiring dose or frequency adjustment, additional monitoring, and/or selection of alternative therapy. Rapid IV infusion may result in skeletal muscle and chest wall rigidity leading to respiratory distress and/or apnea, bronchoconstriction, laryngospasm; inject slowly over 1 to 2 minutes. **[US Boxed Warning]: Use exposes patients and other users to the risks of opioid addiction, abuse, and misuse, which can lead to overdose and death. Assess each patient's risk prior to prescribing fentanyl and monitor all patients regularly for the development of these behaviors and conditions.** Use with caution in patients with a history of drug abuse or acute alcoholism; potential for drug dependency exists. Consider offering naloxone prescriptions in patients with factors associated with an increased risk for overdose, such as history of overdose or substance use disorder, higher opioid dosages (≥50 morphine milligram equivalents/day orally), and concomitant benzodiazepine use (Dowell [CDC 2016]). **[US Boxed Warning]: Accidental ingestion of even one dose, especially by children, can result in a fatal overdose of fentanyl. Fentanyl must be kept out of reach of children.** Use opioids with caution in chronic pain in patients with mental health conditions (eg, depression, anxiety disorders, post-traumatic stress disorder) due to increased risk for opioid use disorder and overdose; more frequent monitoring is recommended (Dowell [CDC 2016]). Use with caution in the elderly; may be more sensitive to adverse effects. Decrease initial dose. Use opioids for chronic pain with caution in this age group; monitor closely due to an increased potential for risks, including certain risks such as falls/fracture, cognitive impairment, and constipation. Clearance may also be reduced in older adults (with or without renal impairment) resulting in a narrow therapeutic window and increasing the risk for respiratory depression or overdose (Dowell [CDC 2016]). Consider the use of alternative nonopioid analgesics in these patients.

Use caution with adrenal insufficiency (including Addison disease), biliary tract impairment (including acute pancreatitis), bradycardia or bradyarrhythmias, head injuries, intracranial lesions, elevated intracranial pressure, history of seizure disorders, morbid obesity, thyroid dysfunction, delirium tremens, toxic psychosis, prostatic hyperplasia and/or urinary stricture. Use with caution in patients with renal or hepatic impairment; avoid transdermal (patch) in patients with severe hepatic impairment. Abrupt discontinuation in patients who are physically dependent on opioids has been associated with serious withdrawal symptoms, uncontrolled pain, attempts to find other opioids (including illicit), and suicide. Use a collaborative, patient-specific taper schedule that minimizes the risk of withdrawal, considering factors such as current opioid dose, duration of use, type of pain, and physical and psychological factors. Monitor pain control, withdrawal symptoms, mood changes, suicidal ideation, and for use of other substances and provide care as needed. Concurrent use of mixed agonist/antagonist analgesics (eg, pentazocine, nalbuphine, butorphanol) or partial agonist (eg, buprenorphine) analgesics may also precipitate withdrawal symptoms and/or reduced analgesic efficacy in patients following prolonged therapy with mu opioid agonists. Opioid use increases the risk for sleep-related disorders (eg, central sleep apnea [CSA], hypoxemia) in a dose-dependent fashion. Use with caution for chronic pain and titrate dosage cautiously in patients with risk factors for sleep-disordered breathing (eg, heart failure, obesity). Consider dose reduction in patients presenting with CSA. Avoid opioids in patients with moderate to severe sleep-disordered breathing (Dowell [CDC 2016]). May cause severe hypotension (including orthostatic hypotension and syncope); use with caution in patients with hypovolemia, cardiovascular disease (including acute MI), or drugs which may exaggerate hypotensive effects (including phenothiazines or general anesthetics). Monitor for symptoms of hypotension following initiation or dose titration. Avoid use in patients with circulatory shock. Opioids decrease bowel motility; monitor for decreased bowel motility in postop patients receiving opioids. Use with caution in the perioperative setting; individualize treatment when transitioning from parenteral to oral analgesics. Opioids may obscure diagnosis or clinical course of patients with acute abdominal conditions.

Chronic pain (outside of end-of-life or palliative care, active cancer treatment, sickle cell disease, or medication-assisted treatment for opioid use disorder) in outpatient setting in adults: Opioids should not be used as first-line therapy for chronic pain management (pain >3-month duration or beyond time of normal tissue healing) due to limited short-term benefits, undetermined long-term benefits, and association with serious risks (eg, overdose, MI, auto accidents, risk of developing opioid use disorder). Preferred management includes nonpharmacologic therapy and nonopioid therapy (eg, NSAIDs, acetaminophen, certain anticonvulsants and antidepressants). If opioid therapy is initiated, it should be combined with nonpharmacologic and nonopioid therapy, as appropriate. Prior to initiation, known risks of opioid therapy should be discussed and realistic treatment goals for pain/function should be established, including consideration for discontinuation if benefits do not outweigh risks. Therapy should be continued only if clinically meaningful improvement in pain/function outweighs risks. Therapy should be initiated at the lowest effective dosage using immediate-release opioids (instead of extended-release/long-acting opioids). Risk associated with use increases with higher opioid dosages. Risks and benefits should be re-evaluated when increasing dosage to ≥50 morphine milligram equivalents (MME)/day orally; dosages ≥90 MME/day orally should be avoided unless carefully justified (Dowell [CDC 2016]).

[US Boxed Warning]: Buccal tablet, intranasal, sublingual tablet, sublingual spray, and lozenge preparations contain an amount of medication that can be fatal to children. Keep all used and unused products out of the reach of children at all times and discard products properly. Patients and caregivers should be counseled on the dangers to children including the risk of exposure to partially-consumed products. **[US Boxed Warning]: Prolonged use of opioids during pregnancy can cause neonatal withdrawal syndrome in the newborn which may be life-threatening if not recognized and treated according to protocols developed by neonatology experts. If opioid use is required for a prolonged period in a pregnant woman, advise the patient of the risk of neonatal opioid withdrawal syndrome and ensure that appropriate treatment will be available.** Signs and symptoms include irritability, hyperactivity and abnormal sleep pattern, high pitched cry, tremor, vomiting, diarrhea and failure to gain weight. Onset, duration and severity depend on the drug used, duration of use, maternal dose, and rate of drug elimination by the newborn. Use with caution in cachectic or debilitated patients; there is a greater potential for critical respiratory depression, even at therapeutic dosages. Consider the use of alternative nonopioid analgesics in these patients. Avoid use in patients with impaired consciousness or coma as these patients are susceptible to intracranial effects of CO_2 retention.

[US Boxed Warning]: Serious, life-threatening, or fatal respiratory depression may occur, including following use in opioid non-tolerant patients and improper dosing. Monitor closely for respiratory depression, especially during initiation or dose escalation. Abstral, Actiq, Duragesic, Fentora, Lazanda, or Subsys should only be prescribed for opioid-tolerant patients. Risk of respiratory depression usually occurs after administration of initial dose in nontolerant patients or when given with other drugs that depress respiratory function. Carbon dioxide retention from opioid-induced respiratory depression can exacerbate the sedating effects of opioids. Use with caution and monitor for respiratory depression in patients with significant chronic obstructive pulmonary disease or cor pulmonale, and those with a substantially decreased respiratory reserve, hypoxia, hypercapnia, or preexisting respiratory depression, particularly when initiating and titrating therapy; critical respiratory depression may occur, even at therapeutic dosages. Consider the use of alternative nonopioid analgesics in these patients.

Transmucosal (buccal tablet, sublingual spray/tablet, lozenge) and intranasal: **[US Boxed Warning]: Transmucosal and nasal fentanyl formulations are contraindicated in the management of acute or postoperative pain and in opioid nontolerant patients.** Should be used only for the care of opioid-tolerant cancer patients with breakthrough pain and is intended for use by specialists who are knowledgeable in treating cancer pain. **[US Boxed Warning]: Substantial differences exist in the pharmacokinetic profile of fentanyl products that result in clinically important differences in the extent of absorption of fentanyl. When prescribing or dispensing fentanyl, do not convert patients on a mcg-per-mcg basis from one fentanyl product to another fentanyl product; the substitution of one fentanyl product for another fentanyl product may result in a fatal overdose. Death has been reported in children who have accidentally ingested transmucosal immediate-release fentanyl products. Strict adherence to the recommended handling and disposal instructions is of the utmost importance to prevent accidental exposure. [US Boxed Warning]: Available only through the TIRF REMS ACCESS program, a restricted distribution program with outpatients, prescribers who prescribe to outpatients, pharmacies (inpatient and outpatient), and distributor-required enrollment.** Titration of intranasal fentanyl is not recommended during use of nasal decongestants (eg, oxymetazoline). Avoid use of sublingual spray in cancer patients with grade 2 or higher mucositis (fentanyl exposure increased); use with caution in patients with grade 1 mucositis, and closely monitor for respiratory and CNS depression. Application site reactions, ranging from paresthesia to ulcerations and bleeding, occurred with buccal tablet (Fentora).

Transdermal iontophoretic system (Ionsys): **[US Boxed Warning]: Available only through a restricted program under a Risk Evaluation and Mitigation Strategy (REMS) called the Ionsys REMS Program. Healthcare facilities that dispense Ionsys must be certified in this program and comply with the REMS requirements. [US Boxed Warning]: For use only in patients in the hospital. Discontinue treatment before patients leave the hospital. Only the patient should activate Ionsys dosing. Accidental exposure to an intact Ionsys device or to the hydrogel component, especially by children, through contact with skin or contact with mucous membranes, can result in a fatal overdose of fentanyl.** Following accidental contact with the device or its components, immediately rinse the affected area thoroughly with water. Do not use soap, alcohol, or other solvent because they may enhance the drug's ability to penetrate the skin; monitor for signs of respiratory or CNS depression. If the device is not handled correctly using gloves, healthcare professionals are at risk of accidental exposure to a fatal overdose of fentanyl. Ionsys device is considered magnetic resonance unsafe. The device contains metal parts and must be removed and properly disposed of before an MRI procedure to avoid injury to the patient and damage to device. It is unknown if exposure to an MRI procedure increases release of fentanyl from the device. Monitor any patients wearing the device with inadvertent exposure to an MRI for signs of CNS and respiratory depression. Use of Ionsys device during cardioversion, defibrillation, X-ray, CT, or diathermy can damage the device from the strong electromagnetic fields set up by these procedures. The device contains radio-opaque components and may interfere with an X-ray image or CT scan. Remove and properly dispose of the device prior to cardioversion, defibrillation, X-ray, CT, or diathermy. Avoid contact with synthetic materials (such as carpeted flooring) to reduce the possibility of electrostatic discharge and damage to the device. Avoid exposing the device to electronic security systems to reduce the possibility of damage. Use near communications equipment (eg, base stations for radio telephones and land mobile radios, amateur radio, AM and FM radio broadcast and TV broadcast Radio) and Radio Frequency Identification (RFID) transmitters can damage the device. Depending on the rated maximum output power and frequency of the transmitter, the recommended separation distance between the device and communications equipment or the RFID transmitter ranges between 0.12 and 23 meters. The low-level electrical current provided by the device does not result in electromagnetic interference with other electromechanical devices like pacemakers or electrical monitoring equipment. If exposure to the procedures listed above, electronic security systems, electrostatic discharge, communications equipment, or RFID transmitters occurs, and if the device does not appear to function normally, remove and replace with a new device. Topical skin reactions (erythema, sweating, vesicles, papules/pustules) may occur with use and are typically limited to the application site area. If a severe skin reaction is observed, remove device and discontinue further use.

Transdermal patch (Duragesic): **[US Boxed Warning]: Transdermal patch is contraindicated for use as an as-needed analgesic, in acute or postoperative pain, or in patients who are opioid nontolerant. Monitor closely for respiratory depression during use, particularly during initiation of therapy or after dose increases.** Should only be prescribed by health care professionals who are knowledgeable in the use of potent opioids in the management of chronic pain. **[US Boxed Warning]: Exposure of application site and surrounding area to direct external heat sources (eg, heating pads, electric blankets, heat or tanning lamps, sunbathing, hot baths, hot tubs, heated water beds, saunas) may increase fentanyl absorption and has resulted in fatalities. Warn patients to avoid exposing the application site and surrounding area to direct external heat sources.** Serum fentanyl concentrations may increase by approximately one-third for patients with a body temperature of 40°C (104°F) secondary to a temperature-dependent increase in fentanyl release from the patch and increased skin permeability. **[US Boxed Warning]: Deaths due to a fatal overdose of fentanyl have occurred when children and adults were accidentally exposed to fentanyl transdermal patch. Strict adherence to recommended handling and disposal instructions is necessary to prevent accidental exposures.** Avoid unclothed/unwashed application site exposure, inadvertent person-to-person patch transfer (eg, while hugging), incidental exposure (eg, sharing same bed, sitting on patch), intentional exposure (eg, chewing), or accidental exposure by caregivers when applying/removing patch. **[US Boxed Warning]: To ensure that the benefits of opioid analgesics outweigh the risks of addiction, abuse, and misuse, the FDA has required a Risk Evaluation and Mitigation Strategy (REMS) for these products. Under the requirements of the REMS, drug companies with**

approved opioid analgesic products must make REMS-compliant education programs available to health care providers. Health care providers are strongly encouraged to complete a REMS-compliant education program; counsel patients and/or their caregivers, with every prescription, on safe use, serious risks, storage, and disposal of these products; emphasize to patients and their caregivers the importance of reading the Medication Guide every time it is provided by their pharmacist; and consider other tools to improve patient, household, and community safety. Should be applied only to intact skin. Use of a patch that has been cut, damaged, or altered in any way may result in overdosage. Patients who experience adverse reactions should be monitored for at least 24 hours after removal of the patch. Drug continues to be absorbed from the skin for 24 hours or more following removal of the patch. May contain conducting metal (eg, aluminum); remove patch prior to MRI.

Warnings: Additional Pediatric Considerations Opioid withdrawal may occur after conversion of one dosage form to another or after dosage adjustment; with prolonged use, taper dose to prevent withdrawal symptoms. Neonates who receive a total fentanyl dose >1.6 mg/kg or continuous infusion duration >5 days are more likely to develop opioid withdrawal symptoms; for infants and children 1 week to 22 months of age, those who receive a total dose of 1.5 mg/kg or duration >5 days have a 50% chance of developing opioid withdrawal and those receiving a total dose >2.5 mg/kg or duration of infusion >9 days have a 100% chance of developing withdrawal.

Dosage form specific:

Use transdermal patch in pediatric patients only if they are opioid-tolerant, receiving at least 60 mg oral morphine equivalents per day, and ≥2 years of age.

Use of Actiq was evaluated in a clinical trial of 15 opioid-tolerant pediatric patients (age: 5 to 15 years) with breakthrough pain; 12 of the 15 patients received doses of 200 mcg to 600 mcg; no conclusions about safety and efficacy could be drawn due to the small sample size.

Some dosage forms may contain propylene glycol; in neonates large amounts of propylene glycol delivered orally, intravenously (eg, >3,000 mg/day), or topically have been associated with potentially fatal toxicities which can include metabolic acidosis, seizures, renal failure, and CNS depression; toxicities have also been reported in children and adults including hyperosmolality, lactic acidosis, seizures, and respiratory depression; use caution (AAP 1997; Shehab 2009).

Drug Interactions

Metabolism/Transport Effects **Substrate** of CYP3A4 (major); **Note:** Assignment of Major/Minor substrate status based on clinically relevant drug interaction potential

Avoid Concomitant Use

Avoid concomitant use of FentaNYL with any of the following: Abametapir; Azelastine (Nasal); Bromperidol; Conivaptan; Dapoxetine; Eluxadoline; Enzalutamide; Fexinidazole [INT]; Fusidic Acid (Systemic); Idelalisib; MiFEPRIStone; Monoamine Oxidase Inhibitors (Antidepressant); Monoamine Oxidase Inhibitors (Type B); Opioids (Mixed Agonist / Antagonist); Orphenadrine; Oxomemazine; Paraldehyde; Thalidomide

Increased Effect/Toxicity

FentaNYL may increase the levels/effects of: Alvimopan; Azelastine (Nasal); Blonanserin; Bradycardia-Causing Agents; Ceritinib; Desmopressin; Diuretics; Eluxadoline; Fexinidazole [INT]; Flunitrazepam; Ivabradine; Lacosamide; Methotrimeprazine; MetyroSINE; Monoamine Oxidase Inhibitors (Antidepressant); Monoamine Oxidase Inhibitors (Type B); Nefazodone; Opioid Agonists; Orphenadrine; Oxitriptan; OxyCODONE; Paraldehyde; Piribedil; Pramipexole; Ramosetron; ROPINIRole; Rotigotine; Selective Serotonin Reuptake Inhibitors; Serotonergic Agents (High Risk, Miscellaneous); Serotonin/Norepinephrine Reuptake Inhibitors; Siponimod; Suvorexant; Thalidomide; TraMADol; Tricyclic Antidepressants; Zolpidem

The levels/effects of FentaNYL may be increased by: Abametapir; Alizapride; Almotriptan; Alosetron; Amphetamines; Anticholinergic Agents; Antiemetics (5HT3 Antagonists); Brimonidine (Topical); Bromopride; Bromperidol; BusPIRone; Cannabidiol; Cannabis; Chlormethiazole; Chlorphenesin Carbamate; Clofazimine; CNS Depressants; Conivaptan; CYP3A4 Inhibitors (Moderate); CYP3A4 Inhibitors (Strong); Dapoxetine; Dexmethylphenidate-Methylphenidate; Dextromethorphan; Dimethindene (Topical); Dronabinol; Droperidol; Eletriptan; Erdafitinib; Ergot Derivatives; Fosaprepitant; Fusidic Acid (Systemic); Idelalisib; Kava Kava; Larotrectinib; Lemborexant; Linezolid; Lisuride; Lofexidine; Lorcaserin (Withdrawn From US Market); Magnesium Sulfate; Meperidine; Methotrimeprazine; Methylene Blue; Metoclopramide; Midodrine; MiFEPRIStone; Minocycline (Systemic); Nabilone; Nefazodone; Ondansetron; Oxomemazine; Ozanimod; Palbociclib; Perampanel; PHENobarbital; Primidone; Propofol; Ramosetron; Rufinamide; Ruxolitinib; Serotonergic Non-Opioid CNS Depressants; Serotonin 5-HT1D Receptor Agonists (Triptans); Simeprevir; Sodium Oxybate; St John's Wort; Stiripentol; Succinylcholine; Syrian Rue; Terlipressin; Tetrahydrocannabinol; Tetrahydrocannabinol and Cannabidiol; Tofacitinib; Tricyclic Antidepressants

Decreased Effect

FentaNYL may decrease the levels/effects of: Antiplatelet Agents (P2Y12 Inhibitors); Diuretics; Gastrointestinal Agents (Prokinetic); Ioflupane I 123; Pegvisomant; Sincalide

The levels/effects of FentaNYL may be decreased by: Alpha-/Beta-Agonists (Indirect-Acting); Alpha1-Agonists; CYP3A4 Inducers (Moderate); CYP3A4 Inducers (Strong); Enzalutamide; Nalmefene; Naltrexone; Opioids (Mixed Agonist / Antagonist); PHENobarbital; Primidone; St John's Wort

Dietary Considerations Transmucosal lozenge contains 2 g sugar per unit.

Pharmacodynamics/Kinetics

Onset of Action

Children 3 to 12 years: Intranasal: 5 to 10 minutes (Borland 2002)

Adults: Analgesic: IM: 7 to 8 minutes; IV: Almost immediate (maximal analgesic and respiratory depressant effects may not be seen for several minutes); Transdermal patch (initial placement): 6 hours; Transmucosal: 5 to 15 minutes

Duration of Action IM: 1 to 2 hours; IV: 0.5 to 1 hour; Transdermal (removal of patch/no replacement): Related to blood level; some effects may last 72 to 96 hours due to extended half-life and absorption from the skin, fentanyl concentrations decrease by ~50% in 20 to 27 hours; Transmucosal: Related to blood level;

respiratory depressant effect may last longer than analgesic effect

Half-life Elimination

IV:

Pediatric patients 5 months to 4.5 years: 2.4 hours

Pediatric patients 6 months to 14 years (after long-term continuous infusion): ~21 hours (range: 11 to 36 hours)

Adults: 2 to 4 hours; when administered as a continuous infusion, the half-life prolongs with infusion duration due to the large volume of distribution (Sessler 2008)

SubQ bolus injection: 10 hours (Capper 2010)

Transdermal device: Terminal: ~16 hours

Transdermal patch: 20 to 27 hours (apparent half-life is influenced by continued fentanyl absorption from skin)

Transmucosal products: 3 to 14 hours (dose dependent)

Intranasal: 15 to 25 hours (based on a multiple-dose pharmacokinetic study when doses are administered in the same nostril and separated by a 1-, 2-, or 4-hour time lapse)

Buccal tablet: 100 to 200 mcg: 3 to 4 hours; 400 to 800 mcg: 11 to 12 hours

Time to Peak

Buccal tablet: 20 to 240 minutes (median: 47 minutes)

Lozenge: 20 to 480 minutes (median: 20 to 40 minutes)

Intranasal: Median: 15 to 21 minutes

Sublingual spray: 10 to 120 minutes (median: 90 minutes)

Sublingual tablet: 15 to 240 minutes (median: 30 to 60 minutes)

SubQ bolus injection: 10 to 30 minutes (median: 15 minutes) (Capper 2010)

Transdermal patch: 20 to 72 hours; steady state serum concentrations are reached after two sequential 72-hour applications

Reproductive Considerations

Long-term opioid use may cause secondary hypogonadism, which may lead to sexual dysfunction or infertility (Brennan 2013).

Pregnancy Considerations

Fentanyl crosses the placenta (Leuschen 1990). Fentanyl can be detected in neonatal urine 24 hours after maternal epidural administration (Moore 2016).

According to some studies, maternal use of opioids may be associated with birth defects (including neural tube defects, congenital heart defects, and gastroschisis), poor fetal growth, stillbirth, and preterm delivery (CDC [Dowell 2016]). Opioids used as part of obstetric analgesia/anesthesia during labor and delivery may temporarily affect the fetal heart rate (ACOG 209 2019). Transient muscular rigidity has been observed in the neonate following maternal administration of IV fentanyl; symptoms of respiratory or neurological depression were not different than those observed in infants of untreated mothers following IV or epidural use during labor.

[US Boxed Warning]: Prolonged use of fentanyl during pregnancy can result in neonatal opioid withdrawal syndrome, which may be life-threatening if not recognized and treated, and requires management according to protocols developed by neonatology experts. If opioid use is required for a prolonged period in a pregnant woman, advise the patient of the risk of neonatal opioid withdrawal syndrome and ensure that appropriate treatment will be available. If chronic opioid exposure occurs in pregnancy, adverse events in the newborn (including withdrawal) may occur (Chou 2009). Symptoms of neonatal abstinence syndrome (NAS) following opioid exposure may be autonomic (eg, fever, temperature instability), gastrointestinal (eg, diarrhea, vomiting, poor feeding/weight gain), or neurologic (eg, high-pitched crying, hyperactivity, increased muscle tone, increased wakefulness/abnormal sleep pattern, irritability, sneezing, seizure, tremor, yawning) (Dow 2012; Hudak 2012). Mothers who are physically dependent on opioids may give birth to infants who are also physically dependent. Opioids may cause respiratory depression and psychophysiologic effects in the neonate; newborns of mothers receiving opioids during labor should be monitored.

Fentanyl IM and IV injection are commonly used to treat maternal pain during labor and immediately postpartum; the intranasal route has also been studied (ACOG 209 2019; Jabalameli 2016). Not all formulations are recommended.

The ACOG recommends that pregnant women should not be denied medically necessary surgery, regardless of trimester. If the procedure is elective, it should be delayed until after delivery (ACOG 775 2019).

Breastfeeding Considerations

Fentanyl and norfentanyl are present in breast milk (Cohen 2009).

The actual amount received by a breastfeeding infant varies. Reports are available following IV or epidural use during labor (Goma 2008; Leuschen 1990; Nitsun 2006; Steer 1992) or chronic maternal use of the transdermal patch (Cohen 2009). Not all studies evaluated concentrations of the active metabolite.

Nonopioid analgesics are preferred for breastfeeding females who require pain control peripartum or for surgery outside of the postpartum period (ABM [Martin 2018]; ABM [Reece-Stremtan 2017]). Fentanyl may be used when an opioid is needed (ABM [Martin 2018]; ABM [Reece-Stremtan 2017]).

When opioids are needed in breastfeeding women, the lowest effective dose for the shortest duration of time should be used to limit adverse events in the mother and breastfeeding infant. In general, a single occasional dose of an opioid analgesic may be compatible with breastfeeding (WHO 2002). Breastfeeding women using opioids for postpartum pain or for the treatment of chronic maternal pain should monitor their infants for drowsiness, sedation, feeding difficulties, or limpness (ACOG 209 2019). Withdrawal symptoms may occur when maternal use is discontinued, or breastfeeding is stopped.

The Academy of Breast Feeding Medicine recommends postponing elective surgery until milk supply and breastfeeding are established. Milk should be expressed ahead of surgery when possible. In general, when the child is healthy and full term, breastfeeding may resume, or milk may be expressed once the mother is awake and in recovery. For children who are at risk for apnea, hypotension, or hypotonia, milk may be saved for later use when the child is at lower risk (ABM [Reece-Stremtan 2017]).

Controlled Substance C-II

Prescribing and Access Restrictions

As a requirement of the REMS program, access is restricted.

Transmucosal immediate-release fentanyl products (eg, sublingual tablets and spray, oral lozenges, buccal tablets, intranasal) are only available through the Transmucosal Immediate-Release Fentanyl (TIRF)

REMS ACCESS program. Enrollment in the program is required for outpatients, prescribers for outpatient use, pharmacies (inpatient and outpatient), and distributors. Enrollment is not required for inpatient administration (eg, hospitals, hospices, long-term care facilities), inpatients, and prescribers who prescribe to inpatients. Further information is available at 1-866-822-1483 or at www.TIRFREMSaccess.com

Note: Effective December, 2011, individual REMs programs for TIRF products were combined into a single access program (TIRF REMS Access). Prescribers and pharmacies that were enrolled in at least one individual REMS program for these products will automatically be transitioned to the single access program.

Dosage Forms: US

Injection, solution [preservative free]:

Sublimaze: 100 mcg/2 mL (2 mL); 250 mcg/5 mL (5 mL)

Generic: 100 mcg/2 mL (2 mL); 250 mcg/5 mL (5 mL); 500 mcg/10 mL (10 mL); 500 mcg/50 mL (50 mL); 1000 mcg/ 20 mL (20 mL); 1250 mcg/250 mL (250 mL); 2500 mcg/50 mL (50 mL)

Liquid, sublingual, [spray]:

Subsys: 100 mcg (30s); 200 mcg (30s); 400 mcg (30s); 600 mcg (30s); 800 mcg (30s)

Lozenge, oral:

Actiq: 200 mcg (30s); 400 mcg (30s); 600 mcg (30s); 800 mcg (30s); 1200 mcg (30s); 1600 mcg (30s)

Generic: 200 mcg (30s); 400 mcg (30s); 600 mcg (30s); 800 mcg (30s); 1200 mcg (30s); 1600 mcg (30s)

Patch, transdermal:

Duragesic: 12 [delivers 12.5 mcg/hr] (5s); 25 [delivers 25 mcg/hr] (5s); 50 [delivers 50 mcg/hr] (5s); 75 [delivers 75 mcg/hr] (5s); 100 [delivers 100 mcg/hr] (5s)

Generic: 12 [delivers 12.5 mcg/hr] (5s); 25 [delivers 25 mcg/hr] (5s); 37.5 [delivers 37.5 mcg/hr]; 50 [delivers 50 mcg/hr] (5s); 62.5 [delivers 62.5 mcg/hr]; 75 [delivers 75 mcg/hr] (5s); 87.5 [delivers 87.5 mcg/hr] (5s); 100 [delivers 100 mcg/hr] (5s)

Powder, for prescription compounding: USP: 100% (1 g)

Solution, intranasal, as citrate [spray]:

Lazanda: 100 mcg/spray (5 mL); 300 mcg/spray (5 mL); 400 mcg/spray (5 mL) [delivers 8 metered sprays]

Tablet, for buccal application:

Fentora: 100 mcg (28s); 200 mcg (28s); 400 mcg (28s); 600 mcg (28s); 800 mcg (28s)

Tablet, sublingual:

Abstral: 100 mcg (12s, 32s); 200 mcg (12s, 32s); 300 mcg (12s, 32s); 400 mcg (12s, 32s); 600 mcg (32s); 800 mcg (32s)

Dosage Forms: Canada Patch, transdermal, as base: 37 mcg/hr (5s)

Dental Health Professional Considerations Transdermal fentanyl should not be used as a pain reliever in dentistry due to danger of hypoventilation

Actiq is a solid formulation of fentanyl with a high sugar content of 2 g hydrated dextrates per unit. Frequent use of Actiq could result in significant dental problems including risk of dental decay. Dry mouth caused by fentanyl could add to the risk of caries. Oral adverse reactions reported in clinical trials have included tooth caries, gum hemorrhage, mouth ulcerations, oral moniliasis, dry mouth, and cheilitis.

Sedation: There is a subsequent slow release from muscle and fat which results in a terminal half-life that is beyond that of morphine. Fentanyl does not induce the release of histamine; therefore, fentanyl is preferable in patients with a predisposition to bronchospasm. Fentanyl is a good choice for use in cardiac patients because it lacks direct myocardial depression. The incidence of nausea is less than that reported with morphine or meperidine. The clinician should wait 2 to 3 minutes between doses to allow time for observation of the clinical effects of each administered dose.

- ◆ **Fentanyl Citrate** *see* FentaNYL *on page 642*
- ◆ **Fentanyl HCl** *see* FentaNYL *on page 642*
- ◆ **Fentanyl Hydrochloride** *see* FentaNYL *on page 642*
- ◆ **Fentanyl Patch** *see* FentaNYL *on page 642*
- ◆ **Fentora** *see* FentaNYL *on page 642*
- ◆ **Feosol Original** *see* Ferrous Sulfate *on page 664*
- ◆ **Feraheme** *see* Ferumoxytol *on page 665*
- ◆ **Fer-In-Sol [OTC]** *see* Ferrous Sulfate *on page 664*
- ◆ **Fer-Iron [OTC] [DSC]** *see* Ferrous Sulfate *on page 664*
- ◆ **FeRiva** *see* Vitamins (Multiple/Oral) *on page 1550*
- ◆ **FeRiva 21/7** *see* Vitamins (Multiple/Oral) *on page 1550*
- ◆ **FeRivaFA** *see* Vitamins (Multiple/Oral) *on page 1550*
- ◆ **FeroSul [OTC]** *see* Ferrous Sulfate *on page 664*
- ◆ **Ferralet 90** *see* Vitamins (Multiple/Oral) *on page 1550*

Ferric Maltol (FER ik MAWL tol)

Pharmacologic Category Iron Preparations

Use Iron deficiency: Treatment of iron deficiency in adults.

Local Anesthetic/Vasoconstrictor Precautions No information available to require special precautions

Effects on Dental Treatment No significant effects or complications reported

Effects on Bleeding No information available to require special precautions

Adverse Reactions

1% to 10%:

Gastrointestinal: Flatulence (5%), constipation (4%), diarrhea (4%), fecal discoloration (4%), abdominal pain (3%), nausea (2%), vomiting (2%), abdominal distention (1%), abdominal distress (1%)

Mechanism of Action Ferric maltol delivers iron for uptake across the intestinal wall and transfer to transferrin and ferritin. Replaces iron, found in hemoglobin, myoglobin, and other enzymes; allows the transportation of oxygen via hemoglobin.

Pharmacodynamics/Kinetics

Time to Peak Iron: 1.5 to 3 hours.

Pregnancy Considerations

Iron and maltol are absorbed separately following maternal ingestion; the fetus is not expected to be exposed to the ferric maltol complex.

Maternal iron requirements increase during pregnancy. Adequate iron concentrations to the fetus can be maintained regardless of maternal iron status, except in severe cases of anemia (IOM 2001). Untreated iron deficiency and iron deficiency anemia (IDA) in a pregnant female may be associated with adverse events, including low birth weight, preterm birth, or increased perinatal mortality (ACOG 95 2008; BSH [Pavord 2019]; IOM 2001).

In general, treatment of iron deficiency or IDA in pregnancy is the same as in nonpregnant females (USPSTF [Siu 2015]). Ferrous salts are preferred over ferric salts for the oral management of IDA in pregnancy due to better absorption and bioavailability (BSH [Pavord 2019]). Iron supplementation is recommended for 3 months once hemoglobin is within the normal range, and for at least 6 months postpartum to replenish maternal iron stores (BSH [Pavord 2019]; FIGO 2019). The majority of studies note iron therapy improves maternal hematologic parameters; however, information related to clinical outcomes in the mother and neonate is limited (FIGO 2019; Peña-Rosas 2015; Reveiz 2011; USPSTF [Siu 2015]). Oral preparations are generally sufficient; however, parenteral iron therapy may be used in females who cannot tolerate or will not take oral iron, in cases of severe iron deficiency, or when malabsorption is present (ACOG 95 2008; BSH [Pavord 2019]).

Product Availability Accrufer: FDA approved July 2019; anticipated availability is currently unknown.

◆ **Ferric Pyrophosphate** *see* Ferric Pyrophosphate Citrate *on page 664*

Ferric Pyrophosphate Citrate
(FER ik pye roe FOS fate SIT rate)

Brand Names: US Triferic

Pharmacologic Category Iron Preparations

Use

Iron replacement therapy in hemodialysis-dependent patients: Replacement of iron to maintain hemoglobin in adult patients with hemodialysis-dependent chronic kidney disease (HDD-CKD)

Limitations of use: Not intended for use in patients receiving peritoneal dialysis; has not been studied in patients receiving home hemodialysis

Local Anesthetic/Vasoconstrictor Precautions No information available to require special precautions

Effects on Dental Treatment No significant effects or complications reported

Effects on Bleeding No information available to require special precautions

Adverse Reactions Note: Frequency not always defined.

>10%: Cardiovascular: Procedural hypotension (22%)

1% to 10%:

Cardiovascular: Peripheral edema (7%), clotted AV fistula (3%), dialysis access hemorrhage (3%)

Central nervous system: Headache (9%), fatigue (4%), dizziness

Dermatologic: Pruritus

Gastrointestinal: Constipation, nausea

Genitourinary: Urinary tract infection (5%)

Neuromuscular & skeletal: Muscle spasm (10%), limb pain (7%), back pain (5%), weakness (4%)

Respiratory: Dyspnea (6%)

Miscellaneous: Fever (5%)

<1%, postmarketing, and/or case reports: Anaphylaxis, hypersensitivity

Mechanism of Action Iron in the form of ferric pyrophosphate citrate and added to hemodialysate solution is administered to patients by transfer across the dialyzer membrane. Iron delivered into the circulation binds to transferrin for transport to erythroid precursor cells to be incorporated into hemoglobin.

Pharmacodynamics/Kinetics

Half-life Elimination ~1.48 hours

Reproductive Considerations

The manufacturer recommends effective contraception during therapy and for at least 2 weeks after treatment is complete in females of reproductive potential.

Pregnancy Considerations

Adverse events were observed in some animal reproduction studies.

Maternal iron requirements increase during pregnancy. Adequate iron concentrations to the fetus can be maintained regardless of maternal iron status, except in severe cases of anemia (IOM 2001).

Product Availability

Triferic AVNU: FDA approved March 2020; anticipated availability is currently unknown. Triferic AVNU is a ferric pyrophosphate citrate formulation approved for IV administration. Information pertaining to this product within the monograph is pending revision. Consult the prescribing information for additional information.

◆ **Ferric Sulfate** *see* Ferrous Sulfate *on page 664*

◆ **Ferro-Bob [OTC] [DSC]** *see* Ferrous Sulfate *on page 664*

Ferrous Sulfate (FER us SUL fate)

Brand Names: US BProtected Pedia Iron [OTC]; Fer-In-Sol [OTC]; Fer-Iron [OTC] [DSC]; FeroSul [OTC]; Ferro-Bob [OTC] [DSC]; FerrouSul [OTC]; Iron Supplement Childrens [OTC]; Iron Supplement [OTC]; Slow Fe [OTC]; Slow Iron [OTC]

Brand Names: Canada PMS-Ferrous Sulfate

Pharmacologic Category Iron Preparations

Use Iron-deficiency anemia: Prevention and treatment of iron-deficiency anemias

Local Anesthetic/Vasoconstrictor Precautions No information available to require special precautions

Effects on Dental Treatment Do not prescribe tetracyclines simultaneously with iron since GI tract absorption of both tetracycline and iron may be inhibited. Liquid preparations may temporarily stain the teeth.

Effects on Bleeding No information available to require special precautions

Adverse Reactions

>10%: Gastrointestinal: Darkening of stools (≤80%; Tolkien 2015), abdominal pain (≤70%; Tolkien 2015), heartburn (1% to 68%; Tolkien 2015), nausea (≤63%; Tolkien 2015), constipation (≤39%; Tolkien 2015), flatulence (≤36%; Tolkien 2015), vomiting (≤34%; Tolkien 2015), diarrhea (≤23%; Tolkien 2015)

<1%, postmarketing, and/or case reports: Abdominal discomfort (Tolkien 2015)

Mechanism of Action Replaces iron, found in hemoglobin, myoglobin, and other enzymes; allows the transportation of oxygen via hemoglobin

Pharmacodynamics/Kinetics

Onset of Action Hematologic response: Oral: ~3 to 10 days

Peak effect: Reticulocytosis: 5 to 10 days; hemoglobin increases within 2 to 4 weeks

Pregnancy Considerations

Maternal iron requirements increase during pregnancy. Adequate iron concentrations to the fetus can be maintained regardless of maternal iron status, except in severe cases of anemia (IOM 2001). Untreated iron deficiency and iron deficiency anemia (IDA) in a pregnant female may be associated with adverse events, including low birth weight, preterm birth, or increased perinatal mortality (ACOG 95 2008; BSH [Pavord 2019]; IOM 2001).

In general, treatment of iron deficiency or IDA in pregnancy is the same as in non-pregnant females (USPSTF [Siu 2015]). Ferrous salts are preferred for oral management of IDA in pregnancy (BSH [Pavord 2019]). Continued supplementation is recommended for 3 months once hemoglobin is within the normal range, and for at least 6 months postpartum to replenish maternal iron stores (BSH [Pavord 2019]; FIGO 2019). The majority of studies note iron therapy improves maternal hematologic parameters; however, information related to clinical outcomes in the mother and neonate is limited (FIGO 2019; Peña-Rosas 2015; Reveiz 2011; USPSTF [Siu 2015]). Oral preparations are generally sufficient; however, parenteral iron therapy may be used in females who cannot tolerate or will not take oral iron, in cases of severe iron deficiency, or when malabsorption is present (ACOG 95 2008; BSH [Pavord 2019]). Ferrous sulfate has been evaluated in multiple studies as an iron supplement or for the treatment of IDA in pregnancy (Peña-Rosas 2015; Reveiz 2011). Enteric-coated and slow/sustained-release preparations may be less effective and use should be avoided (ACOG 95 2008; BSH [Pavord 2019]).

◆ **Ferrous Sulphate** *see* Ferrous Sulfate *on page 664*

◆ **FerrouSul [OTC]** *see* Ferrous Sulfate *on page 664*

Ferumoxytol (fer ue MOX i tol)

Brand Names: US Feraheme
Brand Names: Canada Feraheme [DSC]
Pharmacologic Category Iron Preparations
Use Iron-deficiency anemia: Treatment of iron-deficiency anemia in adults with an intolerance or unsatisfactory response to oral iron or who have chronic kidney disease
Local Anesthetic/Vasoconstrictor Precautions No information available to require special precautions
Effects on Dental Treatment No significant effects or complications reported
Effects on Bleeding No information available to require special precautions
Adverse Reactions
1% to 10%:
Cardiovascular: Hypotension (≤3%), edema (2%), peripheral edema (2%), chest pain (1%), hypertension (1%)
Central nervous system: Dizziness (2% to 3%), headache (2% to 3%), fatigue (2%)
Dermatologic: Pruritus (1%), skin rash (1%)
Gastrointestinal: Diarrhea (1% to 4%), nausea (2% to 3%), constipation (2%), vomiting (2%), abdominal pain (1%)
Hypersensitivity: Hypersensitivity reaction (≤4%; serious hypersensitivity: <1%)
Neuromuscular & skeletal: Back pain (1%), muscle spasm (1%)
Respiratory: Cough (1%), dyspnea (1%)
Miscellaneous: Fever (1%)
<1%, postmarketing, and/or case reports: Anaphylaxis, angioedema, cardiac arrhythmia, cardiac failure, cyanosis, ischemic heart disease, loss of consciousness, syncope, tachycardia, unresponsive to stimuli, urticaria, wheezing
Mechanism of Action Superparamagnetic iron oxide coated with a low molecular weight semisynthetic carbohydrate; iron-carbohydrate complex enters the reticuloendothelial system macrophages of the liver, spleen, and bone marrow where the iron is released from the complex. The released iron is either transported into storage pools or is transported via plasma transferrin for incorporation into hemoglobin.
Pharmacodynamics/Kinetics
Half-life Elimination ~15 hours; ferumoxytol is not removed by hemodialysis
Pregnancy Considerations
Maternal iron requirements increase during pregnancy. Adequate iron concentrations to the fetus can be maintained regardless of maternal iron status, except in severe cases of anemia (IOM 2001). Untreated iron deficiency and iron deficiency anemia (IDA) in a pregnant female may be associated with adverse events, including low birth weight, preterm birth, or increased perinatal mortality (ACOG 95 2008; BSH [Pavord 2020]; IOM 2001).

In general, treatment of iron deficiency or IDA in pregnancy is the same as in nonpregnant females (USPSTF [Siu 2015]). The majority of studies note iron therapy improves maternal hematologic parameters; however, information related to clinical outcomes in the mother and neonate is limited (FIGO 2019; USPSTF [Siu 2015]). Oral preparations are generally sufficient; however, parenteral iron therapy may be used in females who cannot tolerate or will not take oral iron, in cases of severe iron deficiency, or when malabsorption is present (ACOG 95 2008; BSH [Pavord 2020]). Due to limited safety data in early pregnancy, use of IV iron products is generally not started until the second or third trimester (BSH [Pavord 2020]; FIGO 2019).

◆ **FESO** *see* Fesoterodine *on page 665*

◆ **$FeSO_4$** *see* Ferrous Sulfate *on page 664*

Fesoterodine (fes oh TER oh deen)

Brand Names: US Toviaz
Brand Names: Canada Toviaz
Pharmacologic Category Anticholinergic Agent
Use Overactive bladder: Treatment of patients with an overactive bladder with symptoms of urinary frequency, urgency, or urge incontinence.
Local Anesthetic/Vasoconstrictor Precautions No information available to require special precautions
Effects on Dental Treatment Key adverse event(s) related to dental treatment: Prolonged use will cause significant xerostomia (normal salivary flow resumes upon discontinuation).
Effects on Bleeding No information available to require special precautions
Adverse Reactions
>10%: Gastrointestinal: Xerostomia (19% to 35%; dose-related)
1% to 10%:
Cardiovascular: Peripheral edema (1%)
Central nervous system: Insomnia (1%)
Dermatological: Skin rash (1%)
Endocrine & metabolic: Increased gamma-glutamyl transferase (1%)
Gastrointestinal: Constipation (4% to 6%), dyspepsia (2%), nausea (1% to 2%), abdominal pain (1%)
Genitourinary: Urinary tract infection (3% to 4%), dysuria (1% to 2%), urinary retention (1%)
Hepatic: Increased serum ALT (1%)
Neuromuscular & skeletal: Back pain (1% to 2%)
Ophthalmic: Dry eye syndrome (1% to 4%)
Respiratory: Upper respiratory tract infection (2% to 3%), cough (1% to 2%), dry throat (1% to 2%)

<1%, postmarketing, and/or case reports: Angina pectoris, angioedema, blurred vision, chest pain, diverticulitis, dizziness, drowsiness, facial edema, gastroenteritis, headache, heat exhaustion, hypersensitivity reaction, increased heart rate (dose-related), irritable bowel syndrome, palpitations, prolonged QT interval on ECG, pruritus, urticaria

Mechanism of Action Fesoterodine acts as a prodrug and is converted to an active metabolite, 5-hydroxymethyl tolterodine (5-HMT); 5-HMT is responsible for fesoterodine's antimuscarinic activity and acts as a competitive antagonist of muscarinic receptors.

Urinary bladder contractions are mediated by muscarinic receptors; fesoterodine inhibits the receptors in the bladder preventing symptoms of urgency and frequency.

Pharmacodynamics/Kinetics

Half-life Elimination ~7 hours

Time to Peak Plasma: 5-HMT: ~5 hours; C_{max} higher in poor CYP2D6 metabolizers

Pregnancy Considerations Adverse effects have been observed in some animal reproduction studies.

- ◆ **Fesoterodine Fumarate** *see* Fesoterodine *on page 665*
- ◆ **Fetroja** *see* Cefiderocol *on page 308*
- ◆ **Fetzima** *see* Levomilnacipran *on page 899*
- ◆ **Fetzima Titration** *see* Levomilnacipran *on page 899*
- ◆ **FeverAll Adult [OTC]** *see* Acetaminophen *on page 59*
- ◆ **FeverAll Children's [OTC]** *see* Acetaminophen *on page 59*
- ◆ **FeverAll Infants' [OTC]** *see* Acetaminophen *on page 59*
- ◆ **FeverAll Junior Strength [OTC]** *see* Acetaminophen *on page 59*
- ◆ **Fexmid** *see* Cyclobenzaprine *on page 418*

Fexofenadine (feks oh FEN a deen)

Brand Names: US Allegra Allergy Childrens [OTC]; Allegra Allergy [OTC]; Allergy 24-HR [OTC]; Allergy Relief [OTC]; Allergy Relief/Indoor/Outdoor [OTC]; Fexofenadine HCl Childrens [OTC] [DSC]; Mucinex Allergy [OTC] [DSC]

Pharmacologic Category Histamine H_1 Antagonist; Histamine H_1 Antagonist, Second Generation; Piperidine Derivative

Use Upper respiratory allergies: Temporary relief of runny nose, sneezing, itching of the nose or throat, and/or itchy, watery eyes due to hay fever or other upper respiratory allergies.

Local Anesthetic/Vasoconstrictor Precautions No information available to require special precautions

Effects on Dental Treatment No significant effects or complications reported

Effects on Bleeding No information available to require special precautions

Adverse Reactions

>10%:

Central nervous system: Headache (5% to 11%)

Gastrointestinal: Vomiting (children 6 months to 5 years: 4% to 12%)

1% to 10%:

Central nervous system: Drowsiness (1% to 3%), fatigue (1% to 3%), dizziness (2%), pain (2%)

Gastrointestinal: Diarrhea (3% to 4%), nausea (2%), dyspepsia (1% to 2%)

Genitourinary: Dysmenorrhea (2%)

Infection: Viral infection (3%)

Neuromuscular & skeletal: Myalgia (3%), back pain (2% to 3%), limb pain (2%)

Otic: Otitis media (2% to 4%)

Respiratory: Upper respiratory tract infection (3% to 4%), cough (2% to 4%), rhinorrhea (1% to 2%)

Miscellaneous: Fever (2%)

<1%, postmarketing, and/or case reports: Hypersensitivity reaction (including anaphylaxis, angioedema, chest tightness, dyspnea, flushing, pruritus, skin rash, urticaria), insomnia, nervousness, nightmares, sleep disorder

Mechanism of Action Fexofenadine is an active metabolite of terfenadine and like terfenadine it competes with histamine for H_1-receptor sites on effector cells in the gastrointestinal tract, blood vessels and respiratory tract; it appears that fexofenadine does not cross the blood-brain barrier to any appreciable degree, resulting in a reduced potential for sedation

Pharmacodynamics/Kinetics

Onset of Action 2 hours (Simons 2004)

Duration of Action 24 hours (Simons 2004)

Half-life Elimination 14.4 hours (59% longer in patients with mild to moderate renal impairment [CrCl 41 to 80 mL/minute]; 72% longer in patients with severe renal impairment [CrCl 11 to 40 mL/minute]) (Markham 1998; Simons 2004)

Time to Peak Serum: ODT: 2 hours (4 hours with high-fat meal); Tablet: ~2.6 hours (Simons 2004); Suspension: ~1 hour

Pregnancy Considerations Limited information is available related to the use of fexofenadine in pregnancy. When a second generation antihistamine is needed, other agents with more information available regarding their use in pregnancy are currently preferred (Murase 2014; Powell 2015; Scadding 2008; Wallace 2008; Zuberbier 2014).

- ◆ **Fexofenadine HCl Childrens [OTC] [DSC]** *see* Fexofenadine *on page 666*
- ◆ **Fexofenadine Hydrochloride** *see* Fexofenadine *on page 666*
- ◆ **FGFR inhibitor INCB054828** *see* Pemigatinib *on page 1207*
- ◆ **Fiasp** *see* Insulin Aspart *on page 817*
- ◆ **Fiasp FlexTouch** *see* Insulin Aspart *on page 817*
- ◆ **Fiasp PenFill** *see* Insulin Aspart *on page 817*
- ◆ **Fibricor** *see* Fenofibrate and Derivatives *on page 640*

Fibrinogen Concentrate (Human)

(fi BRIN o gin KON suhn trate HYU man)

Brand Names: US Fibryga; RiaSTAP

Brand Names: Canada Fibryga; RiaSTAP

Pharmacologic Category Blood Product Derivative

Use Congenital fibrinogen deficiency: Treatment of acute bleeding episodes in patients with congenital fibrinogen deficiency, including afibrinogenemia and hypofibrinogenemia.

Local Anesthetic/Vasoconstrictor Precautions No information available to require special precautions

Effects on Dental Treatment No significant effects or complications reported

Effects on Bleeding Serious thromboembolism and thrombosis have been reported.

Adverse Reactions

1% to 10%:

Central nervous system: Headache (>1%)

Dermatologic: Erythema (≤8%), pruritus (≤8%)

Gastrointestinal: Vomiting (>5%)

Neuromuscular & skeletal: Weakness (>5%)

Miscellaneous: Fever (>5%)

<1%, postmarketing, and/or case reports: Anaphylaxis, arterial thrombosis, chills, deep vein thrombosis, dyspnea, hypersensitivity reaction, myocardial infarction, nausea, pulmonary embolism, skin rash, thromboembolism

Mechanism of Action Fibrinogen (coagulation factor I), a protein found in normal plasma, is required to clot blood. Fibrinogen concentrate made from pooled human plasma replaces this protein which is missing or reduced in patients with a congenital fibrinogen deficiency.

Pharmacodynamics/Kinetics

Half-life Elimination Similar to biological fibrinogen

Biological fibrinogen: 100 hours (Kamath 2003)

Fibryga: Patients 12 to 53 years: 75.9 ± 23.8 (40 to 157 hours)

RiaSTAP:

Patients <16 years: 69.9 ± 8.5 hours

Patients ≥16 years: 82.5 ± 20 hours

Reproductive Considerations

Patients with congenital fibrinogen deficiency may have an increased risk of bleeding, thrombosis, and pregnancy loss; replacement therapy may be initiated prior to conception (RCOG [Pavord 2017]).

Pregnancy Considerations

Pregnant patients with congenital fibrinogen deficiency may have an increased risk of bleeding, thrombosis, and pregnancy loss; therefore, close surveillance is recommended. Maternal fibrinogen concentrations increase during pregnancy but do not protect against potential complications. Prophylaxis throughout pregnancy may be needed and higher doses may be required as pregnancy progresses. Plasma derived fibrinogen concentrate may be used for treatment or prevention of bleeding in patients with severe deficiency (RCOG [Pavord 2017]).

Fibrin Sealant (FI brin SEEL ent)

Related Information

Antiplatelet and Anticoagulation Considerations in Dentistry *on page 1666*

Brand Names: US Artiss; Evarrest; Evicel; Raplixa [DSC]; TachoSil; Tisseel

Brand Names: Canada Artiss; Evicel; Tisseel

Pharmacologic Category Blood Product Derivative; Hemostatic Agent

Use

Colonic anastomosis sealing (Tisseel only): As an adjunct to standard surgical techniques (such as suture and ligature) to prevent leakage from colonic anastomoses following the reversal of temporary colostomies

Facial rhytidectomy (Artiss only): To adhere tissue flaps during facial rhytidectomy surgery (face lift)

Hemostasis, adjunct:

Artiss: Not indicated as an adjunct to hemostasis

Evarrest, Evicel: As an adjunct to hemostasis for use in patients undergoing surgery when control of bleeding by conventional surgical techniques (such as suture, ligature, and cautery) is ineffective or impractical

Raplixa: As an adjunct to hemostasis for mild to moderate bleeding in adults undergoing surgery when control of bleeding by standard surgical techniques (such as suture, ligature, and cautery) is ineffective or impractical

TachoSil: As an adjunct to hemostasis for use with manual compression in adults and pediatric patients ≥1 month in cardiovascular and hepatic surgery when control of bleeding by standard surgical techniques (such as suture, ligature, or cautery) is ineffective or impractical

Tisseel: As an adjunct to hemostasis in adult and pediatric patients (≥1 month) undergoing surgery when control of bleeding by conventional surgical techniques, including suture, ligature, and cautery, is ineffective or impractical. Tisseel is effective in heparinized patients.

Skin graft adhesion (Artiss only): To adhere autologous skin grafts to surgically prepared wound beds resulting from burns in adults and pediatric patients ≥1 year

Local Anesthetic/Vasoconstrictor Precautions No information available to require special precautions

Effects on Dental Treatment No significant effects or complications reported

Effects on Bleeding No information available to require special precautions

Adverse Reactions Frequency may vary by product and patient age.

>10%:

Cardiovascular: Atrial fibrillation (29%), hypertension (children: 17%)

Gastrointestinal: Nausea (30%), diarrhea (children: 17%)

Hematologic & oncologic: Anemia (23%)

Hepatic: Increased serum transaminases (children: 11%)

Immunologic: Antibody development (equine collagen: 26% human thrombin: 2%, human fibrinogen: 1%)

Respiratory: Pleural effusion (23%)

1% to 10%:

Cardiovascular: Bradycardia (≥5%), peripheral edema (≥5%), thromboembolism (≤3%), deep vein thrombosis (≤1%)

Dermatologic: Pruritus (1%)

Immunologic: Graft complications (skin graft failure in burn patients: 3%)

Infection: Localized infection (grafts: ≥5%)

Miscellaneous: Postoperative complication (bile leakage after hepatic surgery; 7%), fever (6% to 7%), procedural complications (seroma; ≤4%)

Frequency not defined:

Hematologic & oncologic: Decreased hemoglobin, hematoma

Infection: Abscess (abdomen), staphylococcal infection

Local: Incision site hemorrhage

<1%, postmarketing, and/or case reports: Abdominal distension, anaphylactic shock, anaphylactoid reaction, anaphylaxis, angioedema, ascites, bile leakage (postprocedural), bronchospasm, catheter complication, cerebral embolism, cerebral infarction, chest discomfort, chills, dyspnea, edema, eosinophilia, erythema, flushing, gastrointestinal hemorrhage, granuloma, hemorrhage (internal, postprocedural), hemothorax, hepatitis C, hypersensitivity reaction, hypotension, inflammation, ischemic bowel disease, laryngeal edema, local hemorrhage (spleen), multiorgan failure, mydriasis, nerve compression, paralysis, parathyroid disease, paresthesia, procedural

complications (thoracic cavity drainage), pulmonary embolism, renal artery thrombosis, renal failure, respiratory distress, tachycardia, thrombosis, urticaria, wheezing

Mechanism of Action Formation of a biodegradable adhesive is done by duplicating the last step of the coagulation cascade, the formation of fibrin from fibrinogen. Fibrinogen is the main component of the sealant solution. The solution also contains thrombin, which transforms fibrinogen from the sealer protein solution into fibrin, and fibrinolysis inhibitor (aprotinin), which prevents the premature degradation of fibrin. When mixed as directed, a viscous solution forms that sets into an elastic coagulum. Patches contain fibrinogen and thrombin that, in contact with bleeding surfaces, hydrate, form active fibrin, then produce a fibrin clot.

Pharmacodynamics/Kinetics

Onset of Action Artiss: Full adherence achieved: ~2 hours

Time to hemostasis: Evarrest: 4 minutes; Evicel: 4 to 10 minutes; Raplixa: 5 minutes; TachoSil: 3 to 6 minutes; Tisseel: 5 minutes

Pregnancy Risk Factor C (manufacturer dependent)

Pregnancy Considerations Animal reproduction studies have not been conducted.

◆ **Fibrin Sealant (Human)** *see* Fibrin Sealant *on page 667*

◆ **Fibryga** *see* Fibrinogen Concentrate (Human) *on page 666*

Fidaxomicin (fye DAX oh mye sin)

Brand Names: US Dificid

Brand Names: Canada Dificid

Pharmacologic Category Antibiotic, Macrolide

Use

Clostridioides (formerly Clostridium) difficile infection: Treatment of *Clostridioides* (formerly *Clostridium*) *difficile* infection (CDI) in adult and pediatric patients ≥6 months of age.

Note: The 2017 Infectious Diseases Society of America (IDSA) and Society for Healthcare Epidemiology of America (SHEA) guidelines for CDI in adults and children recommend fidaxomicin as a treatment option for the initial episode of CDI (nonsevere and severe), first recurrence (if vancomycin given for the initial episode), and second or subsequent recurrence (IDSA/SHEA [McDonald 2018]).

Local Anesthetic/Vasoconstrictor Precautions No information available to require special precautions

Effects on Dental Treatment No significant effects or complications reported

Effects on Bleeding No information available to require special precautions

Adverse Reactions

>10%:

Gastrointestinal: Nausea (adults 11%)

Miscellaneous: Fever (infants, children, and adolescents: 13%)

1% to 10%:

Dermatologic: Pruritus (<5%), skin rash (adults: <2%), urticaria (infants, children, and adolescents: <5%)

Endocrine & metabolic: Decreased serum bicarbonate (adults: <2%), hyperglycemia (adults: <2%), metabolic acidosis (adults: <2%)

Gastrointestinal: Abdominal distention (adults: <2%), abdominal pain (6% to 8%), abdominal tenderness (adults: <2%), constipation (infants, children, and adolescents: 5%), diarrhea (infants, children, and adolescents: 7%), dyspepsia (adults: <2%), dysphagia (adults: <2%), flatulence (adults: <2%), gastrointestinal hemorrhage (adults: 4%), intestinal obstruction (adults: <2%), non-Hirschsprung megacolon (adults: <2%), vomiting (7%)

Hematologic & oncologic: Anemia (adults: 2%), decreased platelet count (adults: <2%), neutropenia (adults: 2%)

Hepatic: Increased liver enzymes (adults: ≤5%), increased serum alkaline phosphatase (adults: <2%), increased serum transaminases (infants, children, and adolescents: 5%)

Hypersensitivity: Fixed drug eruption (adults: <2%)

Postmarketing:

Hepatic: Hepatotoxicity (idiosyncratic) (Chalasani 2014)

Hypersensitivity: Angioedema, hypersensitivity reaction

Mechanism of Action Inhibits RNA polymerase sigma subunit resulting in inhibition of protein synthesis and cell death in susceptible organisms including *C. difficile*; bactericidal

Pregnancy Considerations The limited systemic absorption of fidaxomicin may limit potential fetal exposure.

Product Availability Dificid 200 mg/5 mL oral suspension: FDA approved January 2020; availability anticipated in October 2020. Dificid oral suspension is indicated for the treatment of *Clostridioides* (formerly *Clostridium*) *difficile* infection (CDI) in adults and pediatric patients ≥6 months. Consult the prescribing information for additional information.

Filgrastim (fil GRA stim)

Brand Names: US Granix; Neupogen; Nivestym; Zarxio

Brand Names: Canada Grastofil; Neupogen; Nivestym

Pharmacologic Category Colony Stimulating Factor; Hematopoietic Agent

Use

Chemotherapy-induced myelosuppression in nonmyeloid malignancies:

Neupogen and filgrastim biosimilars: To decrease the incidence of infection (neutropenic fever) in patients with nonmyeloid malignancies receiving myelosuppressive chemotherapy associated with a significant incidence of severe neutropenia with fever

Tbo-filgrastim: To decrease the duration of severe neutropenia in adult and pediatric patients ≥1 month of age with nonmyeloid malignancies receiving myelosuppressive chemotherapy associated with a clinically significant incidence of neutropenic fever

Acute myeloid leukemia (AML) following induction or consolidation chemotherapy (Neupogen and filgrastim biosimilars): To reduce the time to neutrophil recovery and the duration of fever following induction or consolidation chemotherapy in adults with AML

Bone marrow transplantation (Neupogen and filgrastim biosimilars): To reduce the duration of neutropenia and neutropenia-related events (eg, neutropenic fever) in patients with nonmyeloid malignancies receiving myeloablative chemotherapy followed by marrow transplantation

Hematopoietic radiation injury syndrome, acute (Neupogen only): To increase survival in patients acutely exposed to myelosuppressive doses of radiation

Peripheral blood progenitor cell collection and therapy (Neupogen and filgrastim biosimilars): Mobilization of autologous hematopoietic progenitor cells into the peripheral blood for apheresis collection

Severe chronic neutropenia (Neupogen and filgrastim biosimilars): Long-term administration to reduce the incidence and duration of neutropenic complications (eg, fever, infections, oropharyngeal ulcers) in symptomatic patients with congenital, cyclic, or idiopathic neutropenia

Note: Nivestym (filgrastim-aafi) and Zarxio (filgrastim-sndz) are approved as biosimilars to Neupogen (filgrastim). In Canada, Grastofil is a biosimilar to Neupogen (filgrastim).

Local Anesthetic/Vasoconstrictor Precautions No information available to require special precautions

Effects on Dental Treatment No significant effects or complications reported

Effects on Bleeding No information available to require special precautions. Medical consultation may be considered to confirm adequate platelet counts.

Adverse Reactions

>10%:

Cardiovascular: Chest pain (5% to 13%)

Central nervous system: Fatigue (20%), dizziness (14%), pain (12%)

Dermatologic: Skin rash (2% to 14%)

Gastrointestinal: Nausea (43%)

Hematologic & oncologic: Thrombocytopenia (5% to 38%), splenomegaly (≥5%; severe chronic neutropenia: 30%)

Hepatic: Increased serum alkaline phosphatase (6% to 11%)

Neuromuscular & skeletal: Ostealgia (11% to 30%), back pain (2% to 15%)

Respiratory: Epistaxis (≥5%), cough (14%), dyspnea (13%)

Miscellaneous: Fever (8% to 48%)

1% to 10%:

Cardiovascular: Peripheral edema (≥5%), hypertension (≥5%)

Central nervous system: Headache (6% to 10%), hypoesthesia (≥5%), insomnia (≥5%), malaise (≥5%), mouth pain (≥5%)

Dermatologic: Alopecia (≥5%), erythema (≥2%), maculopapular rash (≥2%)

Endocrine & metabolic: Increased lactate dehydrogenase (6%)

Gastrointestinal: Vomiting (≥5%), decreased appetite (≥5%), constipation (≥2%), diarrhea (≥2%)

Genitourinary: Urinary tract infection (≥5%)

Hematologic & oncologic: Anemia (≥5%), decreased hemoglobin (≥5%), leukocytosis (≤2%)

Hypersensitivity: Transfusion reaction (≥2%), hypersensitivity reaction (≥5%)

Immunologic: Antibody development (2% to 3%; no evidence of neutralizing response)

Infection: Sepsis (≥5%)

Neuromuscular & skeletal: Arthralgia (5% to 9%), limb pain (2% to 7%), muscle spasm (≥5%), musculoskeletal pain (≥5%) asthenia (≥5%)

Respiratory: Bronchitis (≥5%), oropharyngeal pain (≥5%), upper respiratory tract infection (≥5%)

<1%, postmarketing, and/or case reports: Acute respiratory distress syndrome, anaphylaxis, capillary leak syndrome, decreased bone mineral density, glomerulonephritis, hemoptysis, hypersensitivity angiitis, myalgia, osteoporosis, pulmonary alveolar hemorrhage, pulmonary infiltrates, sickle cell crisis, splenic rupture, Sweet syndrome, vasculitis (aortitis)

Mechanism of Action Filgrastim is a granulocyte colony-stimulating factor (G-CSF) produced by recombinant DNA technology. G-CSFs stimulate the production, maturation, and activation of neutrophils to increase both their migration and cytotoxicity.

Pharmacodynamics/Kinetics

Onset of Action

Filgrastim: 1 to 2 days

Tbo-filgrastim: Time to maximum ANC: 3 to 5 days

Duration of Action

Filgrastim: Neutrophil counts generally return to baseline within 4 days

Tbo-filgrastim: ANC returned to baseline by 21 days after completion of chemotherapy

Half-life Elimination

Neonates: 4.4 ± 0.4 hours (Gillan 1994)

Adults: Filgrastim: ~3.5 hours; Tbo-filgrastim: 3 to 3.5 hours

Time to Peak Serum: Filgrastim: SubQ: 2 to 8 hours; Tbo-filgrastim: 4 to 6 hours

Pregnancy Considerations Filgrastim crosses the placenta.

Available data do not suggest an association between the use of filgrastim during pregnancy and an increased risk of miscarriage, preterm labor, or adverse fetal outcomes (birth weight or infection) following maternal use for severe chronic neutropenia. Information related to the use of granulocyte-colony stimulating factor (G-CSF) in pregnant patients with congenital, cyclic, or idiopathic neutropenia (Boxer 2015; Zeidler 2014) and G-CSF-induced allogeneic peripheral blood stem cells donation is limited (Leitner 2001; Shibata 2003).

Data collected from the Severe Chronic Neutropenia International Registry (SCNIR) note dosing for chronic conditions may need adjusted in pregnant women; the lowest effective dose to maintain the absolute neutrophil count is recommended (Zeidler 2014). An international consensus panel has published guidelines for hematologic malignancies during pregnancy that suggest that although data are limited, administration of granulocyte growth factors during pregnancy may be acceptable (Lishner 2016). One review suggests when utilizing for hematopoietic stem cell mobilization (in healthy donors; not a labeled use) avoiding use during the first trimester until additional outcome information is available (Pessach 2013).

- **Filgrastim-aafi** *see* Filgrastim *on page 668*
- **Filgrastim-sndz** *see* Filgrastim *on page 668*

Finasteride (fi NAS teer ide)

Brand Names: US Propecia; Proscar

Brand Names: Canada ACH-Finasteride; ACT Finasteride [DSC]; AG-Finasteride; APO-Finasteride; Auro-Finasteride; DOM-Finasteride; JAMP-Finasteride; MINT-Finasteride; MYLAN-Finasteride HG [DSC]; MYLAN-Finasteride [DSC]; PMS-Finasteride; Propecia; Proscar; RAN-Finasteride; RATIO-Finasteride [DSC]; RIVA-Finasteride; SANDOZ Finasteride; SANDOZ Finasteride A; TEVA-Finasteride; VAN-Finasteride [DSC]

Pharmacologic Category 5 Alpha-Reductase Inhibitor

Use

Androgenetic alopecia (male pattern hair loss): Treatment of male pattern hair loss in men.

Limitations of use: Efficacy in bitemporal recession has not been established.

Benign prostatic hyperplasia: Treatment (monotherapy) of symptomatic benign prostatic hyperplasia (BPH) to improve symptoms, reduce the risk of acute urinary retention, and reduce the risk of need for BPH-related surgery; used in combination with an alpha-blocker (doxazosin) to reduce the risk of symptomatic progression.

Limitations of use: Not approved for the prevention of prostate cancer.

Local Anesthetic/Vasoconstrictor Precautions No information available to require special precautions

Effects on Dental Treatment No significant effects or complications reported

Effects on Bleeding No information available to require special precautions

Adverse Reactions

>10%: Genitourinary: Impotence (monotherapy: 5% to 19%)

1% to 10%:

Cardiovascular: Orthostatic hypotension (monotherapy: 9%), peripheral edema (monotherapy: 1%), hypotension (monotherapy: 1%)

Endocrine & metabolic: Decreased libido (monotherapy: 2% to 10%), gynecomastia (monotherapy: 1% to 2%)

Genitourinary: Ejaculatory disorder (monotherapy: <1% to 7%), decreased ejaculate volume (monotherapy: 2% to 4%), sexual disorder (3%), breast tenderness (monotherapy: ≤1%)

Hematologic & oncologic: Prostate cancer (high grade: 2%)

Respiratory: Rhinitis (monotherapy: 1%)

<1%, postmarketing, and/or case reports: Altered mental status, breast hypertrophy, change in libido, depression, hypersensitivity reaction, male infertility (temporary), malignant neoplasm of the breast (men), suicidal ideation (Welk 2017), suicidal tendencies (Welk 2017), testicular pain

Mechanism of Action Finasteride competitively inhibits type II 5-alpha reductase, resulting in inhibition of the conversion of testosterone to dihydrotestosterone and markedly suppresses serum dihydrotestosterone levels

Pharmacodynamics/Kinetics

Duration of Action Dihydrotestosterone levels return to normal within 14 days of discontinuation of treatment; BPH: Prostate volume returns to baseline within ~3 months after discontinuation; Male pattern baldness: Reversal of increased hair count within 12 months

Half-life Elimination 5 to 6 hours (range: 3 to 16 hours); Elderly (≥70 years): 8 hours (range: 6 to 15 hours)

Time to Peak Serum: 1 to 2 hours

Reproductive Considerations

Use is contraindicated in females of childbearing potential. Adequate contraception is recommended if used off label in the management hirsutism in females associated with polycystic ovary syndrome (ACOG 194 2018). Females of childbearing potential should not touch or handle crushed or broken tablets.

Finasteride is present in semen. Male infertility and poor seminal quality have been reported and may be reversible upon discontinuation of finasteride. Adverse events may be dose related and, less likely, associated with doses used for male pattern hair loss (Zakhem 2019).

Pregnancy Risk Factor X

Pregnancy Considerations

Based on the mechanism of action and data from animal reproduction studies, in utero exposure to finasteride may lead to abnormal development of the male genital tract. Use is contraindicated during pregnancy. Pregnant females are advised to avoid contact with crushed or broken tablets.

Fingolimod (fin GOL i mod)

Brand Names: US Gilenya

Brand Names: Canada ACH-Fingolimod; APO-Fingolimod; Gilenya; JAMP Fingolimod; MAR-Fingolimod; MYLAN-Fingolimod; PMS-Fingolimod; SANDOZ Fingolimod; TARO-Fingolimod; TEVA-Fingolimod

Pharmacologic Category Sphingosine 1-Phosphate (S1P) Receptor Modulator

Use Multiple sclerosis, relapsing: Treatment of relapsing forms of multiple sclerosis (MS), including clinically isolated syndrome, relapsing-remitting disease, and active secondary progressive disease, in patients ≥10 years.

Local Anesthetic/Vasoconstrictor Precautions No information available to require special precautions

Effects on Dental Treatment Key adverse event(s) related to dental treatment: Increased blood pressure may occur with fingolimod; assess and plan treatment according to patient's blood pressure. Fingolimod causes immune suppression; medical consult needed prior to dental surgery.

Effects on Bleeding No information available to require special precautions

Adverse Reactions As reported in adults, unless otherwise noted.

>10%:

Endocrine & metabolic: Increased gamma-glutamyl transfer (≤15%)

Gastrointestinal: Diarrhea (13%), nausea (13%), abdominal pain (11%)

Hepatic: Increased serum alanine aminotransferase (≤15%), increased serum aspartate transaminase (≤15%)

Infection: Influenza (11%)

Nervous system: Headache (25%)

Respiratory: Cough (12%), sinusitis (11%)

1% to 10%:

Cardiovascular: Hypertension (8%), first degree atrioventricular block (5%), second degree atrioventricular block (4%), bradycardia (3%)

Dermatologic: Alopecia (3%), actinic keratosis (2%), pityriasis versicolor (2%)

Endocrine & metabolic: Increased serum triglycerides (3%)

Hematologic & oncologic: Lymphocytopenia (7%), cutaneous papilloma (3%), leukopenia (2%), basal cell carcinoma of skin (2%)

Infection: Herpes virus infection (9%), herpes zoster infection (2%)

Nervous system: Seizure (children and adolescents: 6%), migraine (6%)

Neuromuscular & skeletal: Back pain (10%), limb pain (10%), asthenia (2%)

Ophthalmic: Blurred vision (4%)

Respiratory: Dyspnea (9%), bronchitis (8%), decreased lung function (3%; diffusion lung capacity for carbon monoxide), reduced forced expiratory volume (3%)

<1%, postmarketing, and/or case reports: Acute exacerbations of multiple sclerosis (tumefactive), angioedema, arthralgia, asystole, bacterial infection, cerebrovascular accident, complete atrioventricular block, cryptococcosis, fungal infection, hemolytic anemia, hepatic injury, herpes simplex encephalitis, human papilloma virus infection (including related cancer), hypersensitivity reaction, increased serum bilirubin, JC virus infection, Kaposi sarcoma, macular edema, malignant lymphoma (including B-cell), malignant melanoma, Merkel cell carcinoma, multiorgan failure, myalgia, neoplasm, non-Hodgkin lymphoma, peripheral arterial disease, pneumonia, progressive multifocal leukoencephalopathy, prolonged QT interval on ECG, reversible posterior leukoencephalopathy syndrome, skin rash, squamous cell carcinoma, status epilepticus, syncope, T-cell lymphoma (including cutaneous T-cell lymphoma and mycosis fungoides), thrombocytopenia, urticaria

Mechanism of Action Fingolimod-phosphate, active metabolite of fingolimod, binds to sphingosine 1-phosphate receptors 1, 3, 4, and 5. Fingolimod-phosphate blocks the lymphocytes' ability to emerge from lymph nodes; therefore, the amount of lymphocytes available to the central nervous system is decreased, which reduces central inflammation.

Pharmacodynamics/Kinetics

Half-life Elimination 6 to 9 days; prolonged by approximately 50% in patients with moderate or severe hepatic impairment

Time to Peak Plasma: 12 to 16 hours

Reproductive Considerations

Evaluate pregnancy status prior to use in females of reproductive potential. Elimination of fingolimod takes approximately 2 months; to avoid potential fetal harm, females of childbearing potential should use effective contraception to avoid pregnancy during therapy and for 2 months after discontinuing treatment.

In general, disease-modifying therapies for multiple sclerosis (MS) are stopped prior to a planned pregnancy except in females at high risk of MS activity (AAN [Rae-Grant 2018]). Consider use of agents other than fingolimod in females at high risk of disease reactivation who are planning a pregnancy. Delaying pregnancy is recommended for females with persistent high disease activity; when disease-modifying therapy is needed in these patients, other agents are preferred (ECTRIMS/EAN [Montalban 2018]). Females who are considering stopping fingolimod when planning pregnancy should be counseled on the possibility of severe worsening of disability. Patients should seek immediate medical attention if they experience new or worsened symptoms of MS after fingolimod is stopped.

Pregnancy Considerations

Outcome information related to the use of fingolimod in pregnancy is limited (Geissbühler 2018; Karlsson 2014; Navardi 2018; Nguyen 2019). Based on data from animal reproduction studies, in utero exposure to fingolimod may cause fetal harm.

In general, disease-modifying therapies for multiple sclerosis (MS) are not initiated during pregnancy, except in females at high risk of MS activity (AAN [Rae-Grant 2018]). When disease-modifying therapy is needed in these patients, other agents are preferred (ECTRIMS/EAN [Montalban 2018]). Clinical rebound (new neurologic symptoms and increased lesions) has been reported when fingolimod treatment was discontinued during pregnancy (Meinl 2018; Novi 2017; Sempere 2013). Females who are considering stopping fingolimod because of pregnancy should be counseled on the possibility of severe worsening of disability. Patients should seek immediate medical attention if they experience new or worsened symptoms of MS after fingolimod is stopped.

Data collection to monitor pregnancy and infant outcomes following exposure to fingolimod is ongoing. Health care providers are encouraged to enroll females exposed during pregnancy in the Gilenya Pregnancy Registry (1-877-598-7237 or https://www.gilenyapregnancyregistry.com). Pregnant females may also enroll themselves.

- **Fingolimod HCl** *see* Fingolimod *on page 670*
- **Fintepla** *see* Fenfluramine *on page 640*
- **Fioricet/Codeine** *see* Butalbital, Acetaminophen, Caffeine, and Codeine *on page 274*
- **Firazyr** *see* Icatibant *on page 795*
- **Firdapse** *see* Amifampridine *on page 114*
- **Firmagon** *see* Degarelix *on page 450*
- **Firmagon (240 MG Dose)** *see* Degarelix *on page 450*
- **First Care Pain Relief [OTC]** *see* Lidocaine (Topical) *on page 902*
- **Firvanq** *see* Vancomycin *on page 1522*
- **Fisalamine** *see* Mesalamine *on page 980*
- **Fish Oil** *see* Omega-3 Fatty Acids *on page 1137*
- **Fish Oil Concentrate [OTC]** *see* Omega-3 Fatty Acids *on page 1137*
- **FK228** *see* RomiDEPsin *on page 1343*
- **FK506** *see* Tacrolimus (Systemic) *on page 1398*
- **Flagyl** *see* MetroNIDAZOLE (Systemic) *on page 1011*
- **Flanax Pain Relief** *see* Naproxen *on page 1080*
- **Flarex** *see* Fluorometholone *on page 695*
- **Flebogamma DIF** *see* Immune Globulin *on page 803*

Flecainide (fle KAY nide)

Related Information

Clinical Risk Related to Drugs Prolonging QT Interval *on page 1675*

Brand Names: Canada APO-Flecainide; Auro-Flecainide; Tambocor

Pharmacologic Category Antiarrhythmic Agent, Class Ic

Use

Paroxysmal atrial fibrillation/flutter and paroxysmal supraventricular tachycardias (prevention): Prevention of paroxysmal atrial fibrillation/flutter associated with disabling symptoms and paroxysmal supraventricular tachycardias (PSVT), including atrioventricular nodal reentrant tachycardia, atrioventricular reentrant tachycardia, and other supraventricular tachycardias of unspecified mechanism associated with disabling symptoms in patients without structural heart disease.

Guideline recommendations: Due to safety risks, flecainide should be reserved for symptomatic supraventricular tachycardias (SVTs) in patients without structural or ischemic heart disease who are not candidates for, or prefer not to undergo, catheter ablation and in whom other therapies have failed or are contraindicated (ACC/AHA/HRS [Page 2015]).

Ventricular arrhythmias (prevention): Prevention of documented life-threatening ventricular tachyarrhythmias (eg, sustained ventricular tachycardia) in patients without structural heart disease.

Guideline recommendations: Flecainide is an appropriate adjunctive therapy in patients with type 3 long QT syndrome or catecholaminergic polymorphic ventricular tachycardia who are already taking a maximally tolerated beta-blocker but still experiencing symptoms (AHA/ACC/HRS [Al-Khatib 2017]; Ben-horin 2000; Chorin 2018; Van der Werf 2011; Watanabe 2013)

Limitations of use: Use of flecainide is not recommended in patients with less severe ventricular arrhythmias, even if symptomatic. Because of the proarrhythmic effects of flecainide, its use should be reserved for patients in whom the benefits of treatment outweigh the risks. Flecainide should not be used in patients with permanent atrial fibrillation (not adequately studied) or recent myocardial infarction. No evidence from controlled trials have demonstrated favorable effects of flecainide on survival or the incidence of sudden death.

Local Anesthetic/Vasoconstrictor Precautions Flecainide is one of the drugs confirmed to prolong the QT interval and is accepted as having a risk of causing torsade de pointes. The risk of drug-induced torsade de pointes is extremely low when a single QT interval prolonging drug is prescribed. In terms of epinephrine, it is not known what effect vasoconstrictors in the local anesthetic regimen will have in patients with a known history of congenital prolonged QT interval or in patients taking any medication that prolongs the QT interval. Until more information is obtained, it is suggested that the clinician consult with the physician prior to the use of a vasoconstrictor in suspected patients, and that the vasoconstrictor (epinephrine, mepivacaine and levonordefrin [Carbocaine® 2% with Neo-Cobefrin®]) be used with caution.

Effects on Dental Treatment No significant effects or complications reported

Effects on Bleeding No information available to require special precautions

Adverse Reactions

>10%:

Central nervous system: Dizziness (19% to 30%)

Ocular: Visual disturbances (16%)

Respiratory: Dyspnea (~10%)

1% to 10%:

Cardiovascular: Palpitation (6%), chest pain (5%), edema (3.5%), tachycardia (1% to 3%), proarrhythmic (4% to 12%), sinus node dysfunction (1.2%), syncope

Central nervous system: Headache (4% to 10%), fatigue (8%), nervousness (5%) additional symptoms occurring at a frequency between 1% and 3%: fever, malaise, hypoesthesia, paresis, ataxia, vertigo, somnolence, tinnitus, anxiety, insomnia, depression

Dermatologic: Rash (1% to 3%)

Gastrointestinal: Nausea (9%), constipation (1%), abdominal pain (3%), anorexia (1% to 3%), diarrhea (0.7% to 3%)

Neuromuscular & skeletal: Tremor (5%), weakness (5%), paresthesia (1%)

Ophthalmic: Diplopia (1% to 3%), blurred vision

<1% (Limited to important or life-threatening): Bradycardia, paradoxical increase in ventricular rate in atrial fibrillation/flutter, heart block, increased P-R, QRS duration, ventricular arrhythmia, CHF, flushing, AV block, angina, hyper-/hypotension, amnesia, confusion, decreased libido, depersonalization, euphoria, apathy, nervousness, twitching, neuropathy, weakness, taste disturbance, urticaria, exfoliative dermatitis, pruritus, alopecia, flatulence, xerostomia, blood dyscrasias, possible hepatic dysfunction, paresthesia, eye pain, photophobia, bronchospasm, pneumonitis, swollen lips/tongue/mouth, arthralgia, myalgia, polyuria, urinary retention, leukopenia, granulocytopenia, thrombocytopenia, metallic taste, alters pacing threshold

Postmarketing and/or case reports: Tardive dyskinesia, corneal deposits

Mechanism of Action Class Ic antiarrhythmic; slows conduction in cardiac tissue by altering transport of ions across cell membranes; causes slight prolongation of refractory periods; decreases the rate of rise of the action potential without affecting its duration; increases electrical stimulation threshold of ventricle, His-Purkinje system; possesses local anesthetic and moderate negative inotropic effects

Pharmacodynamics/Kinetics

Half-life Elimination

Newborns: Up to ≤29 hours; 3 months: 11 to 12 hours; 12 months: 6 hours

Children: ~8 hours

Adolescents 12 to 15 years: ~11 to 12 hours

Adults: ~20 hours (range: 12 to 27 hours); increased in patients with heart failure (NYHA Class III) or renal dysfunction

Time to Peak Serum: ~3 hours (range: 1 to 6 hours)

Pregnancy Considerations

Flecainide crosses the placenta (Palmer 1990). Placental transfer is not decreased when fetal hydrops is present. Neonatal conduction abnormalities have been reported (AHA [Donofrio 2014]).

Untreated maternal arrhythmias may cause adverse events in the mother and fetus. Flecainide may be used for the ongoing management of pregnant women with highly symptomatic supraventricular tachycardia (SVT). The lowest effective dose is recommended; avoid use during the first trimester if possible (ACC/AHA/HRS [Page 2015]). Use is also recommended for the prevention of SVT in patients with Wolff-Parkinson-White (WPW) syndrome. Until more information is available, when prevention of SVT in patients without WPW syndrome, atrial tachycardia, or atrial fibrillation is needed in pregnancy, flecainide is generally reserved for use when other agents are not effective (ESC [Regitz-Zagrosek 2018]).

Flecainide (administered maternally) may be considered for the in utero management of fetal SVT or atrial flutter with hydrops or ventricular dysfunction. Flecainide may also be considered for SVT without hydrops or ventricular dysfunction if heart rate is ≥200 bpm, or other rare tachycardias with an average heart rate of ≥200 bpm. In addition, flecainide may be considered for fetal ventricular tachycardia (VT) with normal QTc with or without hydrops but is contraindicated for the treatment of fetal VT when long QT syndrome is suspected or confirmed (AHA [Donofrio 2014]).

Dental Health Professional Considerations See Local Anesthetic/Vasoconstrictor Precautions

◆ **Flecainide Acetate** *see* Flecainide *on page 671*

◆ **Flector** *see* Diclofenac (Topical) *on page 489*

◆ **Flexeril** *see* Cyclobenzaprine *on page 418*

- **Flexin** *see* Capsaicin *on page 284*
- **Floctafenina** *see* Floctafenine *on page 673*

Floctafenine (flok ta FEN een)

Related Information

Rheumatoid Arthritis, Osteoarthritis, and Osteoporosis *on page 1697*

Pharmacologic Category Analgesic, Nonopioid; Nonsteroidal Anti-inflammatory Drug (NSAID), Oral

Use Note: Not approved in the US

Pain: Short-term management of acute, mild-to-moderate pain

Local Anesthetic/Vasoconstrictor Precautions No information available to require special precautions

Effects on Dental Treatment Key adverse event(s) related to dental treatment: Xerostomia and changes in salivation (normal salivary flow resumes upon discontinuation), bitter taste. See Effects on Bleeding.

Effects on Bleeding Nonselective NSAIDs are known to reversibly decrease platelet aggregation via mechanisms different than observed with aspirin. Platelet function is restored as the drug is eliminated from the body. Dental professionals should be aware that recommendations differ between dental and general medical surgery. NSAIDs should be avoided (if possible) in general medical surgery patients for 3 to 5 half-lives of the drug (usually 1 to 3 days) prior to surgery to reduce the risk of excessive bleeding. However, there is no scientific evidence to warrant discontinuance of NSAIDs prior to dental surgery. In medically complicated patients or extensive oral surgery, the decision to interrupt therapy must be based on the risk to benefit in an individual patient and a medical consult is suggested. Routine interruption of NSAID therapy for most dental procedures is not warranted. If therapy is continued without interruption, the clinician should anticipate the potential for slower clotting times.

Adverse Reactions Frequency not defined.

Cardiovascular: Edema, flushing, tachycardia

Central nervous system: Bitter taste, depression, dizziness, drowsiness, fatigue, headache, insomnia, irritability, malaise, nervousness, vertigo

Dermatologic: Diaphoresis, pruritus, skin rash, urticaria

Endocrine & metabolic: Fluid retention, hyperkalemia, increased thirst

Gastrointestinal: Abdominal pain, constipation, diarrhea, dyspepsia, flatulence, gastrointestinal hemorrhage, gastrointestinal perforation (with gross bleeding), gastrointestinal ulcer, heartburn, nausea, vomiting, xerostomia

Genitourinary: Burning sensation on urination, cystitis, dysuria, hematuria

Hematologic & oncologic: Agranulocytosis, aplastic anemia, hemorrhage, leukopenia, neutropenia, thrombocytopenia

Hepatic: Hepatotoxicity, increased liver enzymes

Hypersensitivity: Anaphylaxis, angioedema

Ophthalmic: Blurred vision, vision loss

Otic: Tinnitus

Renal: Interstitial nephritis, polyuria, renal insufficiency (acute, reversible; with or without oliguria or anuria), urethritis, urine abnormality (strong smell)

Respiratory: Dyspnea (asthmatic-type)

Mechanism of Action Reversibly inhibits cyclooxygenase-1 and 2 (COX-1 and 2) enzymes, which results in decreased formation of prostaglandin precursors; has antipyretic, analgesic, and anti-inflammatory properties

Other proposed mechanisms not fully elucidated (and possibly contributing to the anti-inflammatory effect to varying degrees), include inhibiting chemotaxis, altering lymphocyte activity, inhibiting neutrophil aggregation/activation, and decreasing proinflammatory cytokine levels.

Pharmacodynamics/Kinetics

Duration of Action 6 to 8 hours

Half-life Elimination Initial phase (distribution): 1 hour; second phase (elimination): 8 hours

Time to Peak Plasma: Floctafenic acid: 1 to 2 hours

Pregnancy Considerations Floctafenic acid, the active metabolite of floctafenine crosses the placenta. In late pregnancy, NSAIDs may cause premature closure of the ductus arteriosus.

Product Availability Not available in the US

- **Floctafeninum** *see* Floctafenine *on page 673*
- **Flolan** *see* Epoprostenol *on page 578*
- **FloLipid** *see* Simvastatin *on page 1372*
- **Flomax** *see* Tamsulosin *on page 1405*
- **Flonase Allergy Relief [OTC]** *see* Fluticasone (Nasal) *on page 703*
- **Flonase Sensimist** *see* Fluticasone (Nasal) *on page 703*
- **Flonase Sensimist [OTC]** *see* Fluticasone (Nasal) *on page 703*
- **Floranex [OTC]** *see Lactobacillus on page 869*
- **Flovent** *see* Fluticasone (Oral Inhalation) *on page 703*
- **Flovent Diskus** *see* Fluticasone (Oral Inhalation) *on page 703*
- **Flovent HFA** *see* Fluticasone (Oral Inhalation) *on page 703*
- **Floxuridin** *see* Floxuridine *on page 673*

Floxuridine (floks YOOR i deen)

Pharmacologic Category Antineoplastic Agent, Antimetabolite; Antineoplastic Agent, Antimetabolite (Pyrimidine Analog)

Use

Colorectal cancer, hepatic metastases: Palliative management of hepatic metastases of colorectal cancer (administered by continuous regional hepatic intra-arterial infusion) in select patients considered incurable by surgical resection or other means.

Limitation of use: Patients with known disease extending beyond an area capable of a single artery infusion should (in most cases) be considered for systemic chemotherapy with other agents.

Local Anesthetic/Vasoconstrictor Precautions No information available to require special precautions

Effects on Dental Treatment Key adverse event(s) related to dental treatment: Stomatitis.

Effects on Bleeding Thrombocytopenia and anemia can occur.

Adverse Reactions

>10%:

Gastrointestinal: Diarrhea (may be dose limiting), stomatitis

Hematologic & oncologic: Anemia, bone marrow depression (nadir: 7-10 days; may be dose limiting), leukopenia, thrombocytopenia

1% to 10%:

Dermatologic: Alopecia, dermatitis, localized erythema, skin hyperpigmentation, skin photosensitivity

Gastrointestinal: Anorexia, biliary sclerosis, cholecystitis
Hepatic: Jaundice

<1%, postmarketing, and/or case reports: Abdominal cramps, abdominal pain, BSP abnormality, change in prothrombin time, decreased erythrocyte sedimentation rate, decreased serum total protein, duodenal ulcer, duodenitis, enteritis, fever, gastritis, gastroenteritis, gastrointestinal hemorrhage, gastrointestinal ulcer, glossitis, hemorrhage, hepatic abscess, increased erythrocyte sedimentation rate, increased lactate dehydrogenase, increased serum alkaline phosphatase, increased serum bilirubin, increased serum total protein, increased serum transaminases, infusion related reaction (arterial aneurysm; arterial ischemia; arterial thrombosis; embolism; fibromyositis; thrombophlebitis; hepatic necrosis; abscesses; infection at catheter site; bleeding at catheter site; catheter blocked, displaced, or leaking), ischemic heart disease, lethargy, malaise, nausea, pharyngitis, skin rash, vomiting, weakness

Mechanism of Action Floxuridine is catabolized to fluorouracil after intra-arterial administration, resulting in activity similar to fluorouracil; inhibits thymidylate synthetase and disrupts DNA and RNA synthesis.

Reproductive Considerations
Females of reproductive potential should avoid pregnancy during floxuridine treatment.

Pregnancy Risk Factor D

Pregnancy Considerations
Adverse effects have been observed in animal reproduction studies. Floxuridine may cause fetal harm if administered during pregnancy. Medications that inhibit DNA synthesis are known to be teratogenic in humans.

- **Fluad** *see* Influenza Virus Vaccine (Inactivated) *on page 812*
- **Fluarix Quadrivalent** *see* Influenza Virus Vaccine (Inactivated) *on page 812*
- **Flubenisolone** *see* Betamethasone (Systemic) *on page 233*
- **Flublok [DSC]** *see* Influenza Virus Vaccine (Recombinant) *on page 815*
- **Flublok Quadrivalent** *see* Influenza Virus Vaccine (Recombinant) *on page 815*
- **Flucelvax [DSC]** *see* Influenza Virus Vaccine (Inactivated) *on page 812*
- **Flucelvax Quadrivalent** *see* Influenza Virus Vaccine (Inactivated) *on page 812*
- **Flucinom** *see* Flutamide *on page 702*

Fluconazole (floo KOE na zole)

Related Information
Clinical Risk Related to Drugs Prolonging QT Interval *on page 1675*
Fungal Infections *on page 1752*

Related Sample Prescriptions
Fungal Infections - Sample Prescriptions *on page 38*

Brand Names: US Diflucan

Brand Names: Canada ACT Fluconazole; APO-Fluconazole; Diflucan; DOM-Fluconazole; Fluconazole Omega; Fluconazole SDZ; MYLAN-Fluconazole; PHL-Fluconazole [DSC]; PMS-Fluconazole; PRO-Fluconazole; TARO-Fluconazole; TEVA-Fluconazole

Generic Availability (US) Yes

Pharmacologic Category Antifungal Agent, Oral; Antifungal Agent, Parenteral

Dental Use Treatment of susceptible fungal infections in the oral cavity including candidiasis, oral thrush, and chronic mucocutaneous candidiasis treatment of esophageal and oropharyngeal candidiasis caused by *Candida* species; treatment of severe, chronic mucocutaneous candidiasis caused by *Candida* species

Use Treatment of candidiasis (esophageal, oropharyngeal, peritoneal, urinary tract, vaginal); systemic candida infections (eg, candidemia, disseminated candidiasis, pneumonia); and cryptococcal meningitis; and antifungal prophylaxis in allogeneic hematopoietic cell transplant recipients

Local Anesthetic/Vasoconstrictor Precautions
Fluconazole is one of the drugs confirmed to prolong the QT interval and is accepted as having a risk of causing torsade de pointes. The risk of drug-induced torsade de pointes is extremely low when a single QT interval prolonging drug is prescribed. In terms of epinephrine, it is not known what effect vasoconstrictors in the local anesthetic regimen will have in patients with a known history of congenital prolonged QT interval or in patients taking any medication that prolongs the QT interval. Until more information is obtained, it is suggested that the clinician consult with the physician prior to the use of a vasoconstrictor in suspected patients, and that the vasoconstrictor (epinephrine, mepivacaine and levonordefrin [Carbocaine® 2% with Neo-Cobefrin®]) be used with caution.

Effects on Dental Treatment Key adverse event(s) related to dental treatment: Abnormal taste.

Effects on Bleeding No information available to require special precautions

Adverse Reactions
>10%: Central nervous system: Headache (adults: 2% to 13%)
1% to 10%:
Central nervous system: Dizziness (adults: 1%)
Dermatologic: Skin rash (adults: 2%)
Gastrointestinal: Nausea (adults: 4% to 7%; children and adolescents: 2%), abdominal pain (2% to 6%), vomiting (2% to 5%), diarrhea (2% to 3%), dysgeusia (adults: 1%), dyspepsia (adults: 1%)

Frequency not defined: Hepatic: Fulminant hepatitis, hepatitis, increased serum alkaline phosphatase, increased serum aspartate aminotransferase, increased serum transaminases, jaundice

<1%, postmarketing, and/or case reports: Acute generalized exanthematous pustulosis, agranulocytosis, alopecia, anaphylaxis, angioedema, asthenia, cholestasis, diaphoresis, DRESS syndrome, drowsiness, exfoliative dermatitis, fatigue, fever, fixed drug eruption, hepatic failure, hepatotoxicity, hypercholesterolemia, hypertriglyceridemia, hypokalemia, insomnia, leukopenia, malaise, myalgia, neutropenia, paresthesia, prolonged QT interval on ECG, seizure, Stevens-Johnson syndrome, thrombocytopenia, torsades de pointes, toxic epidermal necrolysis, tremor, vertigo, xerostomia

Dental Usual Dosage Candidiasis: Adults:
Usual dosage range: 200 to 400 mg/day; duration and dosage depends on severity of infection
Oropharyngeal (long-term suppression): 200 mg/day; chronic therapy is recommended in immunocompromised patients with history of oropharyngeal candidiasis (OPC)

Dosing

Adult & Geriatric

Blastomycosis (off-label use):

CNS disease (alternative agent): Step-down therapy: Oral: 800 mg once daily for ≥12 months and until resolution of cerebrospinal (CSF) abnormalities (Bradsher 2020; IDSA [Chapman 2008]).

Pulmonary disease (alternative agent if unable to tolerate itraconazole): Oral: 400 to 800 mg once daily for 6 to 12 months (IDSA [Chapman 2008]; Pappas 1997).

Candidiasis, treatment: Note: Consider weight-based dosing for patients <50 kg or >90 kg (Rex 1994; Rex 2003). A maximum dose has not been established, but based on a small number of patients, doses up to 1.6 g/day appear to be well tolerated (Anaissie 1995).

Candidemia (neutropenic and non-neutropenic patients):

Initial therapy (alternative to echinocandin if no previous azole exposure, noncritically ill, and not at high risk of fluconazole-resistant isolate): IV, Oral: Loading dose of 800 mg (12 mg/kg) on day 1, then 400 mg (6 mg/kg) once daily; if fluconazole-susceptible *Candida glabrata* isolated, transition to 800 mg (12 mg/kg) once daily (IDSA [Pappas 2016]).

Step-down therapy:

Isolates other than *C. glabrata*: Oral: 400 mg (6 mg/kg) once daily (IDSA [Pappas 2016]).

Isolates of *C. glabrata* (if fluconazole-susceptible or susceptible dose-dependent): Oral: 800 mg (12 mg/kg) once daily (IDSA [Pappas 2016]; Kauffman 2020a).

Duration: Continue for ≥14 days after first negative blood culture and resolution of signs/symptoms (longer duration required in patients with metastatic complications); step-down therapy to oral fluconazole (eg, after initial therapy with an echinocandin) is recommended after 5 to 7 days in stable patients with negative repeat cultures and fluconazole-susceptible isolates (IDSA [Pappas 2016]; Kauffman 2020a).

Candidiasis, invasive (empiric therapy) and/or critically ill non-neutropenic patients in the ICU at risk of invasive candidiasis with fever and unidentified etiology (alternative to echinocandin if not critically ill and unlikely to be colonized with a fluconazole-resistant isolate): IV, Oral: Loading dose of 800 mg (12 mg/kg) on day 1, then 400 mg (6 mg/kg) once daily; continue for ≥14 days in patients with clinical improvement. Consider discontinuing after 4 to 5 days in patients with no clinical response and no evidence of invasive candidiasis (IDSA [Pappas 2016]; Kauffman 2020a).

Cardiac device infection (eg, implantable cardiac defibrillator, pacemaker, ventricular assist device [VAD]): Step-down therapy: IV, Oral: 400 to 800 mg (6 to 12 mg/kg) once daily for 4 to 6 weeks after device removal (4 weeks for infections limited to generator pockets and ≥6 weeks for infections involving wires). **Note:** If VAD cannot be removed, chronic suppressive therapy with fluconazole 400 to 800 mg (6 to 12 mg/kg) once daily should be used (IDSA [Pappas 2016]).

Chronic, disseminated (hepatosplenic): Step-down therapy: Oral: 400 mg (6 mg/kg) once daily; continue until lesion resolution (usually several months) and through periods of immunosuppression (IDSA [Pappas 2016]).

CNS: Step-down therapy (fluconazole-susceptible isolates): IV, Oral: 400 to 800 mg (6 to 12 mg/kg) once daily; continue until signs/symptoms and CSF/radiologic abnormalities have resolved (IDSA [Pappas 2016]; IDSA [Tunkel 2017]).

Endocarditis, native or prosthetic valve: Step-down therapy (fluconazole-susceptible isolates): IV, Oral: 400 to 800 mg (6 to 12 mg/kg) once daily for ≥6 weeks after valve replacement surgery (longer durations recommended in patients with perivalvular abscesses or other complications). **Note:** In patients who cannot undergo valve replacement surgery or with prosthetic valve endocarditis, chronic suppressive therapy with fluconazole 400 to 800 mg (6 to 12 mg/kg) once daily should be used (IDSA [Pappas 2016]).

Endophthalmitis, endogenous (with or without vitritis) (fluconazole-susceptible isolates): IV, Oral: Loading dose of 800 mg (12 mg/kg) on day 1, then 400 to 800 mg (6 to 12 mg/kg) once daily for ≥4 to 6 weeks and until examination indicates resolution (longer duration may be needed for patients with vitritis); for patients with vitritis or macular involvement, intravitreal antifungal therapy is also recommended (IDSA [Pappas 2016]; Kauffman 2020b).

Esophageal: IV, Oral: Loading dose of 400 mg (6 mg/kg) on day 1, then 200 to 400 mg (3 to 6 mg/kg) once daily for 14 to 21 days; for patients with HIV with recurrent infections who have not attained immune reconstitution on antiretroviral therapy, chronic suppressive therapy of 100 to 200 mg 3 times weekly may be used (Goldman 2005; IDSA [Pappas 2016]; Kauffman 2018).

Intertrigo, refractory to topical therapy (off-label use): Oral: 150 mg once weekly for 4 weeks (Brodell 2018; Nozickova 1998; Stengel 1994).

Intra-abdominal infections (alternative to echinocandin if no previous azole exposure, noncritically ill, and not at high risk of fluconazole-resistant isolate): IV, Oral: Loading dose of 800 mg (12 mg/kg) on day 1, then 400 mg (6 mg/kg) once daily; duration is for ≥2 weeks **and** until all signs of infection have resolved. Step-down therapy (after patient has responded to initial therapy [eg, echinocandin]) with fluconazole is recommended in stable patients with a fluconazole-susceptible isolate (IDSA [Pappas 2016]; Kauffman 2020c).

Oropharyngeal: IV, Oral: Loading dose of 200 mg on day 1, then 100 to 200 mg once daily for 7 to 14 days; recommended for patients unresponsive to topical therapy or those with moderate to severe infection, recurrent infection, or risk for esophageal candidiasis (eg, patients with HIV with CD4 counts <100 cells/mm^3). In patients with recurrent infection, chronic suppressive therapy (100 mg 3 times weekly) may be considered, but is usually unnecessary (IDSA [Pappas 2016]; Kauffman 2018).

Osteoarticular (osteomyelitis or septic arthritis) (fluconazole-susceptible isolates): Initial or step-down therapy: IV, Oral: 400 mg (6 mg/kg) once daily. Duration for osteomyelitis is 6 to 12 months and for septic arthritis is 6 weeks. Course may include 2 weeks of initial treatment with a lipid formulation of amphotericin B or an echinocandin. For prosthetic joints that cannot be removed, chronic suppressive therapy with fluconazole 400 mg (6 mg/kg) once daily is recommended (IDSA [Pappas 2016]).

Peritonitis, associated with peritoneal dialysis: **Note:** Use for empiric treatment if no prior azole exposure or for directed therapy against fluconazole-susceptible isolates (Glickman 2019):

IV, Oral: 200 mg on day 1, then 100 to 200 mg once daily for 2 to 4 weeks (Chen 2004; Glickman 2019; ISPD [Li 2016]; Wang 2000).

Thrombophlebitis, suppurative: Initial or step-down therapy: IV, Oral: 400 to 800 mg (6 to 12 mg/kg) once daily for ≥2 weeks after candidemia (if present) has cleared (IDSA [Pappas 2016]).

Urinary tract infection:

Candiduria (asymptomatic):

Patients with neutropenia: Treat as if patient has candidemia (Georgiadou 2013; IDSA [Pappas 2016]).

Patients undergoing a urologic procedure: Oral: 400 mg (6 mg/kg) once daily several days before and after the procedure (IDSA [Pappas 2016]).

Cystitis (symptomatic): Oral: 200 mg (3 mg/kg) once daily for 2 weeks (IDSA [Pappas 2016]).

Pyelonephritis: Oral: 200 to 400 mg (3 to 6 mg/kg) once daily for 2 weeks (IDSA [Pappas 2016]).

Urinary tract infection associated with fungus balls: Oral: 200 to 400 mg (3 to 6 mg/kg) once daily; concomitant amphotericin B deoxycholate irrigation via nephrostomy tubes, if present, is also recommended, along with surgical management (IDSA [Pappas 2016]).

Vaginal/Vulvovaginal:

Uncomplicated: Oral: 150 mg as a single dose (IDSA [Pappas 2016]; manufacturer's labeling).

Complicated or severe: Oral: 150 mg every 72 hours for 2 or 3 doses (CDC [Workowski 2015]; IDSA [Pappas 2016]).

Recurrent: Oral: 150 mg every 72 hours for 10 to 14 days, followed by 150 mg once weekly for 6 months (IDSA [Pappas 2016]; Sobel 2004) **or** 100 mg, 150 mg, or 200 mg every 72 hours for 3 doses, then 100 mg, 150 mg, or 200 mg once weekly for 6 months (CDC [Workowski 2015]).

Candidiasis, prophylaxis:

Hematologic malignancy patients (off-label use) or hematopoietic cell transplant (HCT) recipients who do **not** warrant mold-active prophylaxis (off-label use): Oral: 400 mg once daily. Duration is at least until resolution of neutropenia and/or through day 75 in allogeneic HCT recipients (ASBMT [Tomblyn 2009]; ASCO/IDSA [Taplitz 2018]; Glasmacher 2006; Wingard 2019).

ICU patients (high risk) in units with a high rate (>5%) of invasive candidiasis (off-label use): Oral, IV: Loading dose of 800 mg (12 mg/kg) once on day 1, then 400 mg (6 mg/kg) once daily (IDSA [Pappas 2016]). **Note:** Some experts do not routinely use prophylaxis in this setting (Kauffman 2020a).

Peritoneal dialysis-associated infection (concurrently treated with antibacterials), prevention of secondary fungal infection: Oral: 200 mg every other day or 100 mg once daily (Burkart 2018; Glickman 2019; Restrepo 2010).

Solid organ transplant recipients (selected patients at high-risk for *Candida* infection) (off-label use): Oral, IV: 400 mg (6 mg/kg) given perioperatively and continued once daily postoperatively; indications and duration vary among transplant centers (ASHP/IDSA/SIS/SHEA [Bratzler 2013]; Fishman 2020; Winston 2002).

Coccidioidomycosis, treatment (off-label use):

Bone and/or joint infection: Initial or step-down therapy: Oral: 800 mg once daily for ≥3 years; in some cases, lifelong treatment is needed; duration depends on severity and host immunocompetence (IDSA [Galgiani 2016]).

Meningitis: Oral: 400 mg to 1.2 g once daily, depending on severity (IDSA [Galgiani 2016]); some experts favor a starting dose of ≥800 mg once daily (AST-IDCOP [Miller 2019]; Blair 2020). Continue lifelong as there is a high relapse rate when the dose is decreased or treatment is discontinued (HHS [OI adult 2020]; IDSA [Galgiani 2016]).

Pneumonia, primary infection: **Note:** Only for patients with significantly debilitating illness, extensive pulmonary involvement, concurrent diabetes, frailty due to age or comorbidities, or HIV (HHS [OI adult 2020]; IDSA [Galgiani 2016]):

Oral: Usual dose: 400 mg once daily; IDSA guidelines state that some experts recommend 800 mg once daily. Duration of therapy is 3 to 6 months for immunocompetent patients; immunocompromised patients require a longer duration of therapy (sometimes lifelong) (HHS [adult OI 2020]; IDSA [Galgiani 2016]).

Pneumonia, symptomatic chronic cavitary and/or cavitary disease in immunocompromised patients: Oral: 400 mg once daily for ≥12 months. In patients with ruptured cavities, the duration may be shorter, but depends upon the postoperative course (IDSA [Galgiani 2016]; Jaroszewski 2020).

Soft tissue infection (not associated with bone infection): Oral: 400 mg once daily; some experts give up to 800 mg once daily; duration is for ≥6 to 12 months (IDSA [Galgiani 2016]).

Coccidioidomycosis, prophylaxis (off-label use):

Patients with HIV: **Note:** Primary prophylaxis is not recommended; yearly or twice-yearly serologic testing should be performed in patients living in endemic areas.

Patients with a CD4 count <250 cells/mm^3 who have a new positive serology: Oral: 400 mg once daily until antiretroviral therapy has fully suppressed HIV replication and the CD4 count is ≥250 cells/mm^3 (HHS [OI adult 2020]).

Solid organ transplant recipients:

Seronegative patients in endemic areas (regardless of clinical history of coccidioidomycosis): Oral: 200 mg once daily for 6 to 12 months following transplantation (AST-IDCOP [Miller 2019]; IDSA [Galgiani 2016]); some experts favor 400 mg once daily (Ampel 2020).

Seropositive patients in endemic areas: Oral: 400 mg once daily for 6 to 12 months following transplantation (AST-IDCOP [Miller 2019]; IDSA [Galgiani 2016]); some experts favor 400 mg once daily for 12 months posttransplantation followed by 200 mg once daily for the duration of immunosuppressive therapy (Ampel 2020).

Cryptococcal meningitis: Note: Treatment involves induction, consolidation, and maintenance phases of therapy.

Patients with HIV:

Induction: Oral:

Resource-rich settings, alternative regimens:

If flucytosine is unavailable or not tolerated: 800 mg once daily in combination with amphotericin B (lipid formulation preferred) for ≥2 weeks (HHS [OI adult 2020]); **or**

If amphotericin B is unavailable or not tolerated: 800 mg to 1.2 g once daily in combination with flucytosine for ≥2 weeks (IDSA [Perfect 2010]; Molloy 2018; Nussbaum 2010); **or**

If flucytosine and amphotericin B are unavailable or not tolerated: 1.2 g once daily as monotherapy for ≥2 weeks (HHS [OI adult 2020]).

Resource-limited settings:

Amphotericin B deoxycholate in combination with flucytosine for 1 week followed by fluconazole 1.2 g once daily for 1 week (preferred regimen) (WHO 2018); **or**

If IV therapy is difficult to administer: 1.2 g once daily as a 2-week induction regimen in combination with flucytosine for 2 weeks (WHO 2018); **or**

If flucytosine is unavailable: 1.2 g once daily in combination with amphotericin B deoxycholate for 2 weeks (WHO 2018).

Note: Induction therapy should be continued beyond the durations listed above if clinical improvement is not observed and/or if CSF cultures remain positive (Cox 2018).

Consolidation: Oral: 400 mg once daily for ≥8 weeks following induction with the preferred regimen of amphotericin B and flucytosine (HHS [OI adult 2020]; IDSA [Perfect 2010]); patients receiving any other induction regimen should receive 800 mg once daily for ≥8 weeks (Cox 2018; IDSA [Perfect 2010]; WHO 2018).

Maintenance (suppression): Oral: 200 mg once daily for ≥12 months; may discontinue if completed induction, consolidation, and ≥12 months of maintenance therapy, patient remains asymptomatic, and CD4 count has been ≥100 cells/mm^3 for ≥3 months and HIV RNA is suppressed in response to effective antiretroviral therapy (HHS [OI adult 2020]).

HIV-uninfected patients:

Induction (alternative regimens): Oral:

If flucytosine is unavailable or not tolerated: 800 mg once daily in combination with amphotericin B for 2 weeks (Cox 2020a); **or**

If amphotericin B is unavailable or not tolerated: 800 mg to 1.2 g once daily in combination with flucytosine for 2 to 10 weeks, depending on severity and response to therapy (Cox 2020a); **or**

If amphotericin B and flucytosine are unavailable or not tolerated: 1.2 g once daily as monotherapy for ≥10 weeks (Cox 2020a).

Consolidation: Oral: 400 to 800 mg once daily for 8 weeks (800 mg once daily preferred for patients who receive a 2-week induction course) (AST-IDCOP [Baddley 2019]; Cox 2020a; IDSA [Perfect 2010]).

Maintenance (suppression): Oral: 200 to 400 mg once daily for 6 to 12 months (AST-IDCOP [Baddley 2019]; IDSA [Perfect 2010]). A longer duration may be warranted for patients receiving very high doses of immunosuppression (eg, high-dose steroids or biologic agents [eg, alemtuzumab]) or with radiographic evidence of cryptococcoma (AST-IDCOP [Baddley 2019]; Cox 2020a).

Cryptococcosis, pulmonary infection (off-label use):

Mild to moderate symptoms (if severe pneumonia, treat like CNS infection): Immunocompetent or immunocompromised patients without diffuse pulmonary infiltrates or disseminated infection: Oral: 400 mg once daily for 6 to 12 months (AST-IDCOP [Baddley 2019]; Cox 2020b; IDSA [Perfect 2010]); for patients with HIV, some experts recommend a duration of 12 months (HHS [OI adult 2020]). Chronic suppressive therapy may be warranted for patients with ongoing immunosuppression (AST-IDCOP [Baddley 2019]; Cox 2020b; HHS [OI adult 2020]).

Tinea:

Tinea corporis or cruris: Oral: 150 to 200 mg once weekly for 2 to 4 weeks (Goldstein 2020; Kotogyan 1996; Montero-Gei 1992; Stary 1998).

Tinea pedis: Oral: 150 mg once weekly for 2 to 6 weeks (Gupta 2008; Kotogyan 1996; Montero-Gei 1992).

Tinea versicolor: Oral: 300 mg once weekly for 2 weeks (Karakas 2005).

Renal Impairment: Adult

The renal dosing recommendations are based upon the best available evidence and clinical expertise. Senior Editorial Team: Bruce Mueller, PharmD, FCCP, FASN, FNKF; Jason Roberts, PhD, BPharm (Hons), B App Sc, FSHP, FISAC; Michael Heung, MD, MS.

Note: Renal function estimated using the Cockcroft-Gault formula.

No adjustment for vaginal candidiasis single-dose therapy.

For multiple dosing, administer 100% of the indication-specific loading/initial dose recommended in the adult dosing section, then adjust daily doses as follows: IV, Oral (Berl 1995; manufacturer's labeling):

CrCl >50 mL/minute: No dosage adjustment necessary.

CrCl ≤50 mL/minute: Reduce dose by 50%.

Hemodialysis, intermittent (thrice weekly): IV, Oral: Dialyzable (33% to 38% with low-flux dialyzers [Oono 1992; Toon 1990]): No dosage adjustment necessary for indication-specific loading/initial or maintenance dose recommended in the adult dosing section; however, only administer maintenance doses 3 times/week (on dialysis days) after the hemodialysis session (Berl 1995).

Peritoneal dialysis:

IV, Oral: Initial: Administer 100% of the indication-specific loading/initial dose recommended in the adult dosing section; reduce maintenance doses by 50% (Cousin 2003; expert opinion).

CRRT: Note: Drug clearance is dependent on the effluent flow rate, filter type, and method of renal replacement. Recommendations are based on high-flux dialyzers and effluent flow rates of 20 to 25 mL/kg/hour (or ~1,500 to 3,000 mL/hour), unless otherwise noted. Appropriate dosing requires consideration of adequate drug concentrations (eg, site of infection) and consideration of initial loading doses. Close monitoring of response and adverse reactions due to drug accumulation is important.

CVVH/CVVHD/CVVHDF: IV, Oral:

If the usual recommended dose is 200 mg once daily, administer 400 mg once daily (expert opinion; see note regarding increased clearance in patients receiving renal replacement therapy below).

If the usual recommended dose is 400 mg once daily, administer an 800 mg loading dose, followed by maintenance doses of 800 mg/day in 1 to 2 divided doses (Bergner 2006; Kishino 2001; Muhl 2000; Patel 2011).

If the usual recommended dose is 800 mg once daily, administer a 1.2 g loading dose, followed by maintenance doses of 1.2 g/day in 1 to 2 divided doses (expert opinion; see note regarding increased clearance in patients receiving renal replacement therapy below).

Note: Fluconazole undergoes substantial tubular reabsorption in patients with normal kidney function. Because this reabsorption is absent in anuric patients receiving renal replacement therapy, total fluconazole clearance during CRRT with rates of 1,500 to 3,000 mL/hour is **1.5 to 2.3** times that reported in healthy volunteers (Bergner 2006; Kishino 2001; Muhl 2000; Patel 2011; Valtonen 1997).

PIRRT (eg, sustained, low-efficiency diafiltration): Note: Drug clearance is dependent on the effluent flow rate, filter type, and method of renal replacement. Appropriate dosing requires consideration of adequate drug concentrations (eg, site of infection) and consideration of initial loading doses. Close monitoring of response and adverse reactions due to drug accumulation is important.

PIRRT (effluent flow rate 4 to 5 L/hour, 8- to 10-hour session given every day):

IV, Oral:

Loading dose:

Administer 100% of the recommended indication-specific loading dose recommended in the adult dosing section.

Maintenance dose: **Note:** Optimal dose not well established. Select dose based on pathogen, minimum inhibitory concentration, immunocompromised state, and disease severity.

400 mg once (Sinnollareddy 2015; expert opinion) or twice daily (Gharibian 2016).

Hepatic Impairment: Adult There are no dosage adjustments provided in the manufacturer's labeling; use with caution.

Pediatric

General dosing, susceptible infection: Infants, Children, and Adolescents: IV, Oral: Initial: 6 to 12 mg/kg/dose, followed by 3 to 12 mg/kg/dose once daily; duration and dosage depends on severity of infection; the manufacturer suggests limiting dose to 600 mg/dose.

Candida infections, prophylaxis:

Oncology patients at high risk of invasive candidiasis (eg, AML, recurrent ALL, myelodysplastic syndrome [MDS], HSCT recipients): Limited data available: Infants, Children, and Adolescents: IV, Oral: 6 to 12 mg/kg/dose once daily; maximum dose: 400 mg/dose; duration dependent upon type of transplant and/or chemotherapy, consult institution-specific protocols (ESCMID [Hope 2012]; Science 2014).

Surgical prophylaxis , high-risk patients undergoing liver, pancreas, kidney, or pancreas-kidney transplantation: Infants, Children, and Adolescents: IV: 6 mg/kg as a single dose 60 minutes before procedure; maximum dose: 400 mg/dose; time of initiation and duration varies with transplant type, consult institution-specific protocols (ASHP/IDSA [Bratzler 2013]).

Candidiasis, systemic (including Candidemia and invasive candidiasis), treatment: Infants, Children, and Adolescents: IV, Oral: 12 mg/kg/dose once daily; maximum dose: 800 mg/dose; continue treatment for 14 days after documented clearance and resolution of symptoms (ESCMID [Hope 2012]; IDSA [Pappas 2016]; *Red Book* [AAP 2018]).

Candidiasis, chronic, disseminated (hepatosplenic), step-down therapy: Infants, Children, and Adolescents: Oral: 6 mg/kg/dose once daily following several weeks of initial therapy with an amphotericin B lipid formulation or an echinocandin; treatment should continue until lesion resolution (usually several months); maximum dose: 400 mg/dose (IDSA [Pappas 2016]).

Candidiasis, CNS candidiasis, step-down therapy: Infants, Children, and Adolescents: Oral, IV: 12 mg/kg/dose once daily following initial therapy with liposomal amphotericin B (with or without flucytosine); maximum dose: 800 mg/dose; treatment should continue until all signs, symptoms, and CSF and radiological abnormalities have resolved (IDSA [Pappas 2016]; IDSA [Tunkel 2017]; *Red Book* [AAP 2018]).

Candidiasis, endophthalmitis, treatment: Oral, IV: Infants, Children, and Adolescents: 12 mg/kg/dose on day 1 followed by 6 to 12 mg/kg/dose once daily for at least 4 to 6 weeks until examination indicates resolution; maximum dose 800 mg/dose. **Note:** Use in combination with intravitreal injection of voriconazole or amphotericin B deoxycholate when vitritis or macular involvement is present (IDSA [Pappas 2016]).

Candidiasis, esophageal, treatment:

Non-HIV-exposed/-positive: Infants, Children, and Adolescents: IV, Oral: 6 mg/kg/dose once daily for 14 to 21 days. **Note:** Usual adult dose is 200 to 400 mg/day (IDSA [Pappas 2016]; *Red Book* [AAP 2018]).

HIV-exposed/-positive:

Infants and Children: IV, Oral: 6 to 12 mg/kg/dose once daily for 14 days following symptom resolution (minimum duration: 21 days); maximum dose: 600 mg/dose (HHS [OI pediatric 2018]).

Adolescents: IV, Oral: 100 to 400 mg once daily for 14 to 21 days; may follow with chronic suppressive therapy of 100 to 200 mg once daily for patients with frequent or severe recurrences (HHS [OI adult 2018]).

Candidiasis, oropharyngeal:

Non-HIV-exposed/-positive: Infants, Children, and Adolescents: IV, Oral: 6 mg/kg/dose on day 1 followed by 3 to 6 mg/kg/dose once daily for 7 to 14 days (IDSA [Pappas 2016]; *Red Book* [AAP 2018]). **Note:** Usual adult dose is 100 to 200 mg/day.

HIV-exposed/-positive:

Treatment:

Infants and Children: IV, Oral: 6 to 12 mg/kg/dose once daily for 7 to 14 days; maximum dose: 400 mg/dose (HHS [OI pediatric 2018]).

Adolescents: Oral: 100 mg once daily for 7 to 14 days; may follow with chronic suppressive therapy of 100 mg once daily **or** 3 times weekly for patients with frequent or severe recurrences (HHS [OI adult 2018]).

Secondary prophylaxis, recurrent severe: Infants and Children: Oral: 3 to 6 mg/kg/dose once daily; maximum dose: 200 mg/dose (HHS [OI pediatric 2018]).

Candidiasis, peritoneal dialysis-related infections (ISPD [Warady 2012]):

Peritonitis:

Treatment: Intraperitoneal, IV, Oral: 6 to 12 mg/kg/dose every 24 to 48 hours; maximum dose: 400 mg/dose.

Prophylaxis for high-risk situations (eg, during antibiotic therapy or PEG placement): IV, Oral: 3 to 6 mg/kg/dose every 24 to 48 hours; maximum dose: 200 mg/dose.

Exit-site or tunnel infection, treatment: Oral: 6 mg/kg/dose every 24 to 48 hours; maximum dose: 400 mg/dose.

Candidiasis, vulvovaginal infection:

Uncomplicated infections, treatment (independent of HIV status): Adolescents: Oral: 150 mg as a single dose (CDC [Workowski 2015]; HHS [OI adult 2018]).

Severe infections, treatment:

Non-HIV-exposed/-positive: Adolescents: Oral: 150 mg every 72 hours for 2 to 3 doses (CDC [Workowski 2015]; IDSA [Pappas 2016]).

HIV-exposed/-positive: Adolescents: Oral: 100 to 200 mg once daily for ≥7 days; may follow with chronic suppressive therapy of 150 mg once weekly (HHS [OI adult 2018]).

Recurrent infection, treatment:

Non HIV-exposed/-positive: Adolescents: Oral: Initial: 100 to 200 mg every 72 hours for 3 doses; followed by maintenance of 100 to 200 mg once weekly for 6 months (CDC [Workowski 2015]; IDSA [Pappas 2016]).

HIV-exposed/-positive: Adolescents: Oral: 100 to 200 mg once daily for ≥7 days; may follow with chronic suppressive therapy of 150 mg once weekly (HHS [OI adult 2018]).

Coccidioidomycosis (HIV-exposed/-positive) (HHS [OI adult 2018]; HHS [OI pediatric 2018]):

Mild to moderate non-meningeal infection (eg, focal pneumonia):

Infants and Children: IV, Oral: 6 to 12 mg/kg/dose once daily; maximum dose: 400 mg/dose.

Adolescents: Oral: 400 mg once daily for ≥6 months.

Severe illness (diffuse pulmonary or disseminated non-meningitic disease) initial therapy if unable to use amphotericin or as step-down therapy: Infants and Children: IV, Oral: 12 mg/kg/dose once daily; maximum dose: 800 mg/dose for a total of 1 year of treatment followed by secondary prophylaxis.

Meningeal infection:

Infants and Children: IV, Oral: 12 mg/kg/dose once daily; maximum dose: 800 mg/dose, followed by lifelong secondary prophylaxis.

Adolescents: IV, Oral: 400 to 800 mg once daily, followed by lifelong suppressive therapy.

Secondary prophylaxis/chromic suppressive therapy: Infants, Children, and Adolescents: Oral: 6 mg/kg/dose once daily; maximum dose: 400 mg/dose.

Cryptococcal infection:

Mild to moderate localized infection including pneumonia (not CNS), treatment:

Non HIV-exposed/-positive: Infants, Children, and Adolescents: Oral: 6 to 12 mg/kg/dose once daily for 6 to 12 months. Usual adult dose is 400 mg/dose (IDSA [Perfect 2010]).

HIV-exposed/-positive:

Infants and Children: IV, Oral: 12 mg/kg on day 1, then 6 to 12 mg/kg/dose once daily; maximum dose: 600 mg/dose; duration depends on severity and clinical response (HHS [OI pediatric 2018].

Adolescents: Oral: 400 mg daily for 12 months (HHS [OI adult 2018]).

CNS, severe pulmonary or disseminate infection, treatment:

Induction therapy: HIV-exposed/-positive (not first-line therapy):

Infants and Children: IV: 12 mg/kg on day 1, then 10 to 12 mg/kg/dose once daily in combination with amphotericin B or flucytosine for ≥14 days; maximum dose: 800 mg/dose (HHS [OI pediatric 2018]).

Adolescents: IV, Oral: 400 to 800 mg once daily in combination with flucytosine for ≥14 days **or** 800 mg once daily in combination with amphotericin for ≥14 days **or** 1,200 mg once daily as monotherapy for at least 2 weeks (HHS [OI adult 2018]).

Consolidation:

Non-HIV-exposed/-positive: Infants, Children, and Adolescents: IV, Oral: 10 to 12 mg/kg/**day** once daily or in divided doses twice daily for 8 weeks; maximum dose: 800 mg/dose (IDSA [Perfect 2010]; *Red Book* [AAP 2018]).

HIV-exposed/-positive:

Infants and Children: IV, Oral: 12 mg/kg on day 1, then 10 to 12 mg/kg/day once daily for ≥8 weeks; maximum daily dose: 800 mg/dose (HHS [OI pediatric 2018]).

Adolescents: IV, Oral: 400 mg once daily for ≥8 weeks (HHS [OI adult 2018]).

Secondary prophylaxis/chronic suppressive maintenance therapy:

Non-HIV-exposed/-positive: Infants, Children, and Adolescents: Oral: 6 mg/kg/dose once daily for 6 to 12 months; maximum dose: 200 mg/dose (IDSA [Perfect 2010]).

HIV-exposed/-positive: Infants, Children, and Adolescents: Oral: 6 mg/kg/dose once daily for ≥12 months; maximum dose: 200 mg/dose (HHS [OI adult 2018]; HHS [OI pediatric 2018]).

Histoplasmosis: HIV-exposed/-positive patients, alternative therapy (HHS [OI adult 2018]; HHS [OI pediatric 2018]):

Pulmonary, acute primary disease: Infants and Children: Oral: 3 to 6 mg/kg/dose once daily; maximum dose: 200 mg/dose.

Disseminated disease, mild to moderate:

Infants and Children: IV, Oral: 5 to 6 mg/kg/dose twice daily for 12 months; maximum dose: 300 mg/dose.

Adolescents: Oral: 800 mg once daily.

Secondary prophylaxis/chronic suppressive therapy:

Infants and Children: Oral: 3 to 6 mg/kg/dose once daily for ≥12 months; maximum dose: 200 mg/dose.

Adolescents: Oral: 400 mg once daily for ≥12 months.

Renal Impairment: Pediatric

Altered kidney function: Note: Kidney function estimated using the Schwartz equation.

Single-dose therapy: Adolescents: Oral: No adjustment required for vaginal candidiasis single-dose therapy.

Multiple-dose therapy: Infants, Children, and Adolescents: IV, Oral: Administer 100% of the indication-specific loading/initial dose recommended in the dosing section, then adjust daily doses as follows:

CrCl >50 mL/minute/1.73 m^2: No adjustment necessary.

CrCl ≤50 mL/minute/1.73 m^2: Reduce dose by 50%.

Hemodialysis, intermittent: Note: Based on adult information, fluconazole is dialyzable (33% to 38% with low-flux dialyzers [Oono 1992; Toon 1990]) or approximately 50% after a 3-hour session (manufacturer labeling).

Infants, Children, and Adolescents: IV, Oral: Dialysis days: No dosage adjustment necessary for indication-specific loading/initial or maintenance dose recommended in the dosing section; administer dose after hemodialysis.

Peritoneal dialysis: Infants, Children, and Adolescents: IV, Oral: Administer 50% of recommended dose every 48 hours (Aronoff 2007).

Continuous renal replacement therapy (CRRT) (Veltri 2004): Limited data available: Children and Adolescents: IV, Oral:

<1,500 mL/m^2/**hour** (<25 mL/m^2/minute):

Loading dose: Usual dose: 6 to 10 mg/kg/dose once.

Maintenance dose: 3 to 12 mg/kg/dose once daily depending on indication.

≥1,500 mL/m^2/**hour** (≥25 mL/m^2/minute):

Loading dose: Usual dose: 6 to 10 mg/kg/dose once.

Maintenance dose: 6 to 12 mg/kg/dose once daily depending on indication.

Prolonged intermittent renal replacement therapy (PIRRT) (eg, sustained, low-efficiency diafiltration): There are no pediatric-specific recommendations for dosing in patients receiving PIRRT; based on adult experience, dose adjustment may be necessary.

Hepatic Impairment: Pediatric There are no dosage adjustments provided in manufacturer's labeling; use with caution.

Mechanism of Action Interferes with fungal cytochrome P450 activity (lanosterol 14-α-demethylase), decreasing ergosterol synthesis (principal sterol in fungal cell membrane) and inhibiting cell membrane formation

Contraindications Hypersensitivity to fluconazole or any component of the formulation (cross-reaction with other azole antifungal agents may occur, but has not been established; use caution); coadministration of terfenadine in adult patients receiving multiple doses of 400 mg or higher or with CYP3A4 substrates which may lead to QTc prolongation (eg, astemizole, cisapride, erythromycin, pimozide, or quinidine)

Warnings/Precautions Serious (and sometimes fatal) hepatic toxicity (eg, hepatitis, cholestasis, fulminant hepatic failure) has been observed. Use with caution in patients with renal and hepatic dysfunction or previous hepatotoxicity from other azole derivatives. Patients who develop abnormal liver function tests during fluconazole therapy should be monitored closely and discontinued if symptoms consistent with liver disease develop. Rare exfoliative skin disorders have been observed; fatal outcomes have been reported in patients with serious concomitant diseases. Monitor patients with deep seated fungal infections closely for rash development and discontinue if lesions progress. In patients with superficial fungal infections who develop a rash attributable to fluconazole, treatment should also be discontinued. Cases of QTc prolongation and torsade de pointes associated with fluconazole use have been reported (usually high dose or in combination with agents known to prolong the QT interval); use caution in patients with concomitant medications or conditions which are arrhythmogenic. Anaphylaxis has been reported rarely; use with caution in patients with hypersensitivity to other azoles. Potentially significant drug-drug interactions may exist, requiring dose or frequency adjustment, additional monitoring, and/or selection of alternative therapy. May occasionally cause dizziness or seizures; use caution driving or operating machines.

Powder for oral suspension contains sucrose; use caution with fructose intolerance, sucrose-isomaltase deficiency, or glucose-galactose malabsorption.

Benzyl alcohol and derivatives: Some dosage forms may contain sodium benzoate/benzoic acid; benzoic acid (benzoate) is a metabolite of benzyl alcohol; large amounts of benzyl alcohol (≥99 mg/kg/day) have been associated with a potentially fatal toxicity ("gasping syndrome") in neonates; the "gasping syndrome" consists of metabolic acidosis, respiratory distress, gasping respirations, CNS dysfunction (including convulsions, intracranial hemorrhage), hypotension, and cardiovascular collapse (AAP 1997; CDC 1982); some data suggests that benzoate displaces bilirubin from protein binding sites (Ahlfors 2001); avoid or use dosage forms containing benzyl alcohol derivative with caution in neonates. See manufacturer's labeling.

Drug Interactions

Metabolism/Transport Effects Inhibits CYP2C19 (strong), CYP2C9 (moderate), CYP3A4 (moderate)

Avoid Concomitant Use

Avoid concomitant use of Fluconazole with any of the following: Aprepitant; Astemizole; Asunaprevir; Bosentan; Bosutinib; Budesonide (Systemic); Cisapride; Domperidone; Entrectinib; Erythromycin (Systemic); Fedratinib; Fexinidazole [INT]; Flibanserin; Fosaprepitant; Ivabradine; Lemborexant; Lomitapide; Lumateperone; Mizolastine; Ospemifene; Pimozide; QuiNIDine; Saccharomyces boulardii; Simeprevir; Siponimod; Ulipristal; Voriconazole

Increased Effect/Toxicity

Fluconazole may increase the levels/effects of: Abemaciclib; Acalabrutinib; Alfentanil; Alitretinoin (Systemic); Amiodarone; Amitriptyline; AmLODIPine; Apixaban; Aprepitant; ARIPiprazole; Astemizole; Asunaprevir; AtorvaSTATin; Avanafil; Avapritinib; Avatrombopag; Axitinib; Benzhydrocodone; Blonanserin; Bosentan; Bosutinib; Brexpiprazole; Brigatinib; Brivaracetam; Bromocriptine; Budesonide (Systemic); Budesonide (Topical); Busulfan; Calcium Channel Blockers; Cannabidiol; Cannabis; CarBAMazepine; Carisoprodol; Carvedilol; Celecoxib; Ceritinib; Cilostazol; Cisapride; Citalopram; CloBAZam; Cobimetinib; Codeine; Colchicine; Copanlisib; Crizotinib; CycloSPORINE (Systemic); CYP3A4 Substrates (High risk with Inhibitors); Dabigatran Etexilate; Dapoxetine; Darifenacin; Deflazacort; Dexlansoprazole; DiazePAM; Dichlorphenamide; Diclofenac (Systemic); Domperidone; DOXOrubicin (Conventional); Dronabinol; Dronedarone; Eletriptan; Elexacaftor, Tezacaftor, and Ivacaftor; Eliglustat; Encorafenib; Entrectinib; Eplerenone; Erdafitinib; Erythromycin (Systemic); Estrogen

Derivatives; Etizolam; Etravirine; Everolimus; Fedratinib; FentaNYL; Flibanserin; Flurbiprofen (Systemic); Fluvastatin; Fosaprepitant; Fosphenytoin-Phenytoin; GuanFACINE; Haloperidol; HYDROcodone; Ibrutinib; Ibuprofen; Imatinib; Ivabradine; Ivacaftor; Ivosidenib; Lansoprazole; Lapatinib; Larotrectinib; Lefamulin; Lemborexant; Lercanidipine; Lesinurad; Levamlodipine; Levomethadone; Lomitapide; Lorlatinib; Lornoxicam; Losartan; Lovastatin; Lumateperone; Lurasidone; Lurbinectedin; Macitentan; Manidipine; Meloxicam; Meperidine; Methadone; Mirodenafil; Mizolastine; Moclobemide; Naldemedine; Nalfurafine; Nalmefene; Naloxegol; Nateglinide; Nelfinavir; Neratinib; Nevirapine; NiMODipine; Olaparib; Omeprazole; Ospemifene; OxyCODONE; Parecoxib; PAZOPanib; Pemigatinib; Pexidartinib; Pimecrolimus; Pimozide; PredniSONE; Proguanil; QT-prolonging Antipsychotics (Moderate Risk); QT-prolonging Class IA Antiarrhythmics (Highest Risk); QT-prolonging Class III Antiarrhythmics (Highest Risk); QT-prolonging Kinase Inhibitors (Highest Risk); QT-prolonging Kinase Inhibitors (Moderate Risk); QT-prolonging Miscellaneous Agents (Highest Risk); QT-prolonging Miscellaneous Agents (Moderate Risk); QT-prolonging Moderate CYP3A4 Inhibitors (Moderate Risk); QT-prolonging Strong CYP3A4 Inhibitors (Moderate Risk); QUEtiapine; QuiNIDine; Ramelteon; Ranolazine; Red Yeast Rice; Rifamycin Derivatives; Rimegepant; Rupatadine; Ruxolitinib; Salmeterol; SAXagliptin; Selpercatinib; Selumetinib; Sildenafil; Silodosin; Simeprevir; Simvastatin; Siponimod; Sirolimus; Sonidegib; Sulfonylureas; Suvorexant; Tacrolimus (Systemic); Tadalafil; Tamsulosin; Tazemetostat; Telithromycin; Temsirolimus; Terfenadine; Tetrahydrocannabinol; Tetrahydrocannabinol and Cannabidiol; Tezacaftor and Ivacaftor; Theophylline Derivatives; Ticagrelor; Tipranavir; Tofacitinib; Tolvaptan; Torsemide; Trabectedin; Triazolam; Ubrogepant; Udenafil; Ulipristal; Vardenafil; Venetoclax; Vilazodone; VinCRIStine; Vindesine; Vitamin K Antagonists; Voriconazole; Voxelotor; Zanubrutinib; Zidovudine; Zopiclone

The levels/effects of Fluconazole may be increased by: Amisulpride (Oral); Amitriptyline; Ceritinib; Domperidone; Encorafenib; Entrectinib; Fexinidazole [INT]; Ivosidenib; Methadone; Ondansetron; Pentamidine (Systemic); Pimozide; QT-prolonging Antidepressants (Moderate Risk); QT-prolonging Class IC Antiarrhythmics (Moderate Risk); QT-prolonging Class III Antiarrhythmics (Highest Risk); QT-prolonging Kinase Inhibitors (Highest Risk); QT-prolonging Miscellaneous Agents (Highest Risk); QT-prolonging Quinolone Antibiotics (Moderate Risk)

Decreased Effect

Fluconazole may decrease the levels/effects of: Amphotericin B; Carisoprodol; Clopidogrel; Ifosfamide; Losartan; Proguanil; Saccharomyces boulardii

The levels/effects of Fluconazole may be decreased by: Rifamycin Derivatives

Pharmacodynamics/Kinetics

Half-life Elimination Normal renal function: ~30 hours (range: 20 to 50 hours); Elderly: 46.2 hours; Neonates (gestational age 26 to 29 weeks): 73.6 to 46.6 hours (decreases with increasing postnatal age); Pediatric patients 9 months to 15 years: 19.5 to 25 hours

Time to Peak Oral: 1 to 2 hours

Reproductive Considerations

The manufacturer recommends females of childbearing potential taking higher doses (≥400 mg/day) use effective contraception during therapy and for ~1 week after the final fluconazole dose.

Pregnancy Considerations

Following exposure during the first trimester, malformations have been noted in humans when maternal fluconazole was used in higher doses (≥400 mg/day). Abnormalities reported include brachycephaly, abnormal facies, abnormal calvarial development, cleft palate, femoral bowing, thin ribs and long bones, arthrogryposis, and congenital heart disease. Fetal outcomes following exposure to lower doses is less clear and additional study is needed to confirm an association between maternal use of low dose fluconazole and an increased risk of birth defects. However, epidemiological studies of fluconazole ≤150 mg as a single dose or repeated doses in the first trimester suggest a potential risk of spontaneous abortion and malformations (Liu 2020; Zhang 2019; Zhu 2020).

Oral fluconazole for the treatment of vaginal candidiasis is not recommended during pregnancy. Topical therapy for oral or vaginal candidiasis is recommended in pregnant women whenever possible (HHS [OI adult 2020]; Workowski [CDC 2015]). Fluconazole is not the treatment of choice for invasive candidiasis in pregnant women (IDSA [Pappas 2016]). Fluconazole may be used for the treatment of cryptococcosis or coccidioidomycosis after the first trimester if otherwise appropriate (IDSA [Galgiani 2016]; IDSA [Perfect 2010]; Pastick 2020). Systemic fluconazole is not preferred for the treatment of blastomycosis in pregnant women (IDSA Chapman 2008]).

Breastfeeding Considerations Fluconazole is present in breast milk.

The relative infant dose (RID) of fluconazole is 5% to 21% when calculated using the highest breast milk concentration located and compared to an infant therapeutic dose of 3 to 12 mg/kg/day.

In general, breastfeeding is considered acceptable when the RID is <10%; when an RID is >25% breastfeeding should generally be avoided (Anderson 2016; Ito 2000).

The RID of fluconazole was calculated using a milk concentration of 4.1 mcg/mL, providing an estimated daily infant dose via breast milk of 0.62 mg/kg/day. This milk concentration was obtained following maternal administration of oral fluconazole 200 mg daily for 18 days; the apparent elimination half-life of fluconazole in breast milk was 26.9 hours (Schilling 1993). In another study, peak breast milk concentrations following a single oral dose of fluconazole 150 mg to 10 lactating women, 5 days' to 19 months' postpartum, were reported as 1.57 to 3.65 mcg/mL

Serious adverse events in breastfeeding infants have not been reported following maternal use of fluconazole for nipple or breast candidiasis (Bodley 1997; Chetwynd 2002; Moorhead 2011); flushed cheeks, GI upset, loose stools, mucous feces, and somnolence have been reported in breastfed infants (Moorhead 2011).

Although the manufacturer recommends that caution be exercised when administering fluconazole to breastfeeding women, existing recommendations state that fluconazole is considered compatible with breastfeeding when used in usual recommended doses (WHO 2002). Treatment of breastfeeding women with nipple or breast candidiasis with oral fluconazole is common, especially in persistent or recurring infections (Brent

2001). Untreated candida nipple or breast infections may be painful for the mother and can contribute to premature weaning (Brent 2001). The amount of fluconazole contained in the breast milk is not sufficient to treat mucocutaneous candidiasis in the infant (Force 1995; Schilling 1993); concurrent treatment of both the breastfeeding infant and mother may be required (Chetwynd 2002).

Dosage Forms: US

Solution, Intravenous:
Generic: 200 mg (100 mL); 200 mg/100 mL in NaCl 0.9% (100 mL); 400 mg (200 mL)

Solution, Intravenous [preservative free]:
Generic: 200 mg (100 mL); 200 mg/100 mL in NaCl 0.9% (100 mL); 400 mg (200 mL); 400 mg/200 mL in NaCl 0.9% (200 mL)

Suspension Reconstituted, Oral:
Diflucan: 10 mg/mL (35 mL); 40 mg/mL (35 mL)
Generic: 10 mg/mL (35 mL); 40 mg/mL (35 mL)

Tablet, Oral:
Diflucan: 50 mg, 100 mg, 150 mg, 200 mg
Generic: 50 mg, 100 mg, 150 mg, 200 mg

Dosage Forms: Canada

Solution, Intravenous:
Diflucan: 2 mg/mL (100 mL)
Generic: 2 mg/mL (50 mL, 100 mL, 200 mL)

Suspension Reconstituted, Oral:
Diflucan: 10 mg/mL (35 mL)

Tablet, Oral:
Diflucan: 50 mg, 100 mg
Generic: 50 mg, 100 mg, 200 mg

Dental Health Professional Considerations See Local Anesthetic/Vasoconstrictor Precautions

Flucytosine (floo SYE toe seen)

Brand Names: US Ancobon

Pharmacologic Category Antifungal Agent, Oral

Use Candida/Cryptococcus infections: Adjunctive treatment of systemic fungal infections (eg, septicemia, endocarditis, UTI, meningitis, or pulmonary) caused by susceptible strains of *Candida* or *Cryptococcus*

Local Anesthetic/Vasoconstrictor Precautions No information available to require special precautions

Effects on Dental Treatment No significant effects or complications reported

Effects on Bleeding No information available to require special precautions

Adverse Reactions Frequency not defined.

Cardiovascular: Cardiotoxicity, chest pain, ventricular dysfunction
Central nervous system: Ataxia, confusion, fatigue, hallucination, headache, paresthesia, parkinsonian-like syndrome, peripheral neuropathy, psychosis, sedation, seizure, vertigo
Dermatologic: Pruritus, skin photosensitivity, skin rash, toxic epidermal necrolysis, urticaria
Endocrine & metabolic: Hypoglycemia, hypokalemia
Gastrointestinal: Abdominal pain, anorexia, diarrhea, duodenal ulcer, enterocolitis, gastrointestinal hemorrhage, nausea, ulcerative colitis, vomiting, xerostomia
Genitourinary: Azotemia, crystalluria
Hematologic & oncologic: Agranulocytosis, anemia, aplastic anemia, bone marrow aplasia, eosinophilia, leukopenia, pancytopenia, thrombocytopenia
Hepatic: Hepatic injury (acute), hepatic insufficiency, hepatic necrosis, increased liver enzymes, increased serum bilirubin, jaundice
Hypersensitivity: Hypersensitivity reaction
Neuromuscular & skeletal: Weakness
Otic: Hearing loss
Renal: Increased blood urea nitrogen, increased serum creatinine, renal failure
Respiratory: Dyspnea
Miscellaneous: Fever

Mechanism of Action Penetrates fungal cells and is converted to fluorouracil which competes with uracil interfering with fungal RNA and protein synthesis

Pharmacodynamics/Kinetics

Half-life Elimination Neonates: 4 to 34 hours (Baley, 1990); Infants: 7.4 hours; Adults: 2 to 5 hours; Anuria: 85 hours (range: 30 to 250); End-stage renal disease (ESRD): 75 to 200 hours

Time to Peak Serum: Neonates: 2.5 ± 1.3 hours; Adults: ~1 to 2 hours

Pregnancy Considerations Adverse events have been observed in some animal reproduction studies. Flucytosine is metabolized to fluorouracil which may cause adverse events if administered during pregnancy; refer to the Fluorouracil (Systemic) monograph for additional information.

◆ **Fludara** *see* Fludarabine *on page* 682

Fludarabine (floo DARE a been)

Brand Names: Canada Fludara

Pharmacologic Category Antineoplastic Agent, Antimetabolite; Antineoplastic Agent, Antimetabolite (Purine Analog)

Use Chronic lymphocytic leukemia (refractory or progressive): Treatment of B-cell chronic lymphocytic leukemia (CLL) in adults who have not responded to or have progressed during treatment with at least one standard regimen containing an alkylating agent.

Local Anesthetic/Vasoconstrictor Precautions No information available to require special precautions

Effects on Dental Treatment Key adverse event(s) related to dental treatment: Stomatitis.

Effects on Bleeding Thrombocytopenia (nadir: 16 days) and anemia reported in the majority of patients.

Adverse Reactions Frequency not always defined.

>10%:

Cardiovascular: Edema (8% to 19%)
Central nervous system: Fatigue (10% to 38%), neurological signs and symptoms (doses >96 mg/m^2/day for 5 to 7 days: 36%; doses <125 mg/m^2/cycle: <1%; characterized by cortical blindness, coma, and paralysis; symptom onset may be delayed for 3 to 4 weeks), pain (20% to 22%), chills (11% to 19%), paresthesia (4% to 12%)
Dermatologic: Skin rash (15%), diaphoresis (1% to 13%)
Gastrointestinal: Nausea and vomiting (31% to 36%), anorexia (7% to 34%), diarrhea (13% to 15%), gastrointestinal hemorrhage (3% to 13%)
Genitourinary: Urinary tract infection (2% to 15%)
Hematologic & oncologic: Anemia (60%), neutropenia (grade 4: 59%; nadir: ~13 days), thrombocytopenia (55%; nadir: ~16 days), bone marrow depression (nadir: 10 to 14 days; recovery: 5 to 7 weeks; dose-limiting toxicity)
Infection: Infection (33% to 44%)
Neuromuscular & skeletal: Asthenia (9% to 65%), myalgia (4% to 16%)
Ophthalmic: Visual disturbance (3% to 15%)
Respiratory: Cough (10% to 44%), pneumonia (16% to 22%), dyspnea (9% to 22%), upper respiratory tract infection (2% to 16%)

Miscellaneous: Fever (60% to 69%)

1% to 10%:

Cardiovascular: Angina pectoris (≤6%), cardiac arrhythmia (≤3%), cardiac failure (≤3%), cerebrovascular accident (≤3%), myocardial infarction (≤3%), supraventricular tachycardia (≤3%), deep vein thrombosis (1% to 3%), phlebitis (1% to 3%), aneurysm (≤1%), transient ischemic attacks (≤1%)

Central nervous system: Malaise (6% to 8%), headache (≤3%), sleep disorder (1% to 3%), cerebellar syndrome (≤1%), depression (≤1%), difficulty thinking (≤1%)

Dermatologic: Alopecia (≤3%), pruritus (1% to 3%), seborrhea (≤1%)

Endocrine & metabolic: Hyperglycemia (1% to 6%), dehydration (≤1%)

Gastrointestinal: Stomatitis (≤9%), cholelithiasis (≤3%), esophagitis (≤3%), constipation (1% to 3%), mucositis (≤2%), dysphagia (≤1%)

Genitourinary: Dysuria (3% to 4%), urinary hesitancy (≤3%), hematuria (2% to 3%), proteinuria (≤1%)

Hematologic & oncologic: Hemorrhage (≤1%), tumor lysis syndrome (≤1%)

Hepatic: Abnormal hepatic function tests (1% to 3%), hepatic failure (≤1%)

Hypersensitivity: Anaphylaxis (≤1%)

Neuromuscular & skeletal: Osteoporosis (≤2%), arthralgia (≤1%)

Otic: Hearing loss (2% to 6%)

Renal: Renal failure (≤1%), renal function test abnormality (≤1%)

Respiratory: Pharyngitis (≤9%), hypersensitivity pneumonitis (≤6%), hemoptysis (1% to 6%), sinusitis (≤5%), bronchitis (≤1%), epistaxis (≤1%), hypoxia (≤1%)

<1%, postmarketing, and/or case reports: Acquired blood coagulation disorder, acute myelocytic leukemia (usually associated with prior or concurrent treatment with other anticancer agents), adult respiratory distress syndrome, agitation, autoimmune hemolytic anemia, autoimmune thrombocytopenia, blindness, bone marrow aplasia (trilineage), bone marrow depression (trilineage), cerebral hemorrhage, coma, confusion, Epstein-Barr-associated lymphoproliferative disorder, erythema multiforme, Evans syndrome, flank pain, hemorrhagic cystitis, herpes zoster infection (reactivation), hyperkalemia, hyperphosphatemia, hyperuricemia, hypocalcemia, immune thrombocytopenia (autoimmune), increased liver enzymes, interstitial pneumonitis, lactic acidosis (Smith 2019), malignant neoplasm of skin (new-onset or exacerbation), metabolic acidosis, myelodysplastic syndrome (usually associated with prior or concurrent treatment with other anticancer agents), myelofibrosis, opportunistic infection, optic neuritis, optic neuropathy, pancreatic disease (pancreatic enzymes abnormal), pancytopenia, pemphigus, pericardial effusion, peripheral neuropathy, pneumonitis, progressive multifocal leukoencephalopathy (PML), pulmonary fibrosis, pulmonary hemorrhage, reactivation of latent Epstein-Barr virus, respiratory distress, respiratory failure, seizure, Stevens-Johnson syndrome, toxic epidermal necrolysis, urate crystalluria, wrist-drop

Mechanism of Action Fludarabine inhibits DNA synthesis by inhibition of DNA polymerase and ribonucleotide reductase; also inhibits DNA primase and DNA ligase I

Pharmacodynamics/Kinetics

Half-life Elimination 2-fluoro-ara-A: Adults: ~20 hours

Time to Peak Oral: 1 to 2 hours

Reproductive Considerations

Females of reproductive potential should use effective contraception during therapy and for at least 6 months after the last fludarabine dose.

Fludarabine may damage testicular tissue and spermatozoa. Males with female partners of reproductive potential should use contraception during therapy and for at least 6 months after the last fludarabine dose (duration of effect is uncertain).

Pregnancy Considerations

Based on the mechanism of action, fludarabine may cause fetal harm if administered during pregnancy.

◆ **Fludarabine Monophosphate** *see* Fludarabine *on page 682*

◆ **Fludarabine Phosphate** *see* Fludarabine *on page 682*

Fludrocortisone (floo droe KOR ti sone)

Brand Names: Canada Florinef

Generic Availability (US) Yes

Pharmacologic Category Corticosteroid, Systemic

Use

Adrenal insufficiency, primary (Addison disease): Partial replacement therapy for primary adrenocortical insufficiency

Congenital adrenal hyperplasia, classic (salt-losing adrenogenital syndrome): Treatment of classic congenital adrenal hyperplasia (salt-losing adrenogenital syndrome)

Local Anesthetic/Vasoconstrictor Precautions

No information available to require special precautions

Effects on Dental Treatment No significant effects or complications reported

Effects on Bleeding No information available to require special precautions

Adverse Reactions Frequency not defined.

Cardiovascular: Cardiac failure, cardiomegaly, edema, hypertension

Central nervous system: Delirium, depression, emotional lability, euphoria, hallucination, headache, increased intracranial pressure, insomnia, malaise, nervousness, personality changes, pseudotumor cerebri, psychiatric disturbance, psychosis, seizure, vertigo

Dermatologic: Acne vulgaris, atrophic striae, diaphoresis, erythema, hyperpigmentation, maculopapular rash, skin atrophy, skin rash, suppression of skin test reaction, urticaria

Endocrine & metabolic: Cushing's syndrome, diabetes mellitus, glycosuria, growth suppression, hirsutism, HPA-axis suppression, hyperglycemia, hypokalemia, hypokalemic alkalosis, impaired glucose tolerance, menstrual disease, negative nitrogen balance

Gastrointestinal: Abdominal distention, esophageal ulcer, pancreatitis, peptic ulcer

Hematologic & oncologic: Bruise, petechia, purpura

Hypersensitivity: Anaphylaxis (generalized)

Local: Lipoatrophy at injection site

Neuromuscular & skeletal: Amyotrophy, bone fracture, myasthenia, myopathy, osteonecrosis (femoral and humeral heads), osteoporosis, vertebral compression fracture

Ophthalmic: Cataract, exophthalmos, glaucoma, increased intraocular pressure

Miscellaneous: Wound healing impairment

Dosing

Adult & Geriatric

Adrenal insufficiency, primary (Addison disease): Oral: Initial: 0.05 to 0.1 mg once daily in the morning (in combination with hydrocortisone or cortisone). Usual maintenance dose: 0.05 to 0.2 mg once daily. If hypertension develops, dose reduction is suggested; an antihypertensive may be necessary if hypertension remains uncontrolled (Endocrine Society [Bornstein 2016]).

Manufacturer's labeling: Dosing in the prescribing information may not reflect current clinical practice. 0.1 mg daily; if transient hypertension develops, reduce dose to 0.05 mg daily; maintenance dosage range: 0.1 mg 3 times weekly to 0.2 mg daily.

Congenital adrenal hyperplasia, classic (salt-losing adrenogenital syndrome): Oral: 0.05 to 0.2 mg/day in 1 or 2 divided doses (in combination with glucocorticoid therapy) (Endocrine Society [Speiser 2018])

Orthostatic hypotension (off-label use; Kearney 2009; Lahrmann 2006; Lanier 2011): Oral: Initial: 0.1 mg daily in conjunction with a high-salt diet and adequate fluid intake; may be increased in increments of 0.1 mg per week; maximum dose: 1 mg daily. **Note:** Doses exceeding 0.3 mg daily may not be beneficial and predispose patient to unwanted side effects (eg, hypertension, hypokalemia).

Septic shock (off-label use): Note: Corticosteroids should only be used for septic shock that is not responsive to volume resuscitation and vasopressors (Rhodes 2017; SCCM/ESICM [Annane 2017]). Oral: 0.05 mg once daily (via nasogastric tube) for 7 days (in combination with IV hydrocortisone) (Annane 2002; Annane 2018).

Renal Impairment: Adult There are no dosage adjustments provided in the manufacturer's labeling; use with caution.

Hepatic Impairment: Adult There are no dosage adjustments provided in the manufacturer's labeling; use with caution.

Pediatric Note: Dosing should be individualized to lowest effective dose.

Adrenal insufficiency, autoimmune (primary adrenal insufficiency, aldosterone deficiency component Addison disease); replacement therapy: Limited data available: Infants, Children, and Adolescents: Oral: 0.05 to 0.2 mg daily (Betterle 2002; Endocrine Society [Bornstein 2016]; Kliegman 2020).

Congenital adrenal hyperplasia (salt losers) (eg, 21-hydroxylase deficiency): Limited data available: **Note:** Use in combination with glucocorticoid therapy (eg, hydrocortisone); concurrent sodium replacement therapy may be required, particularly in young infants.

Maintenance therapy:

Infants, Children, and Adolescents (actively growing): Oral: Usual range: 0.05 to 0.2 mg daily in 1 or 2 divided doses; doses as high as 0.3 mg/day may be necessary (AAP 2000; Endocrine Society [Speiser 2018]).

Adolescents (fully grown): Oral: 0.05 to 0.2 mg once daily (Endocrine Society [Speiser 2018]).

Renal Impairment: Pediatric There are no dosage adjustments provided in the manufacturer's labeling; use with caution.

Hepatic Impairment: Pediatric There are no dosage adjustments provided in the manufacturer's labeling.

Mechanism of Action Very potent mineralocorticoid with high glucocorticoid activity; used primarily for its mineralocorticoid effects. Promotes increased reabsorption of sodium and loss of potassium from renal distal tubules.

Contraindications

Hypersensitivity to fludrocortisone or any component of the formulation; systemic fungal infections

Documentation of allergenic cross-reactivity for corticosteroids is limited. However, because of similarities in chemical structure and/or pharmacologic actions, the possibility of cross-sensitivity cannot be ruled out with certainty.

Warnings/Precautions May cause hypercortisolism or suppression of hypothalamic-pituitary-adrenal (HPA) axis, particularly in younger children or in patients receiving high doses for prolonged periods. HPA axis suppression may lead to adrenal crisis. Withdrawal and discontinuation of a corticosteroid should be done slowly and carefully. Rare cases of anaphylactoid reactions have been observed in patients receiving corticosteroids.

Prolonged use may increase risk of infection, mask acute infection (including fungal infections), prolong or exacerbate viral infections, or limit response to killed or inactivated vaccines. Exposure to chickenpox or measles should be avoided. Corticosteroids should not be used for cerebral malaria or viral hepatitis. Close observation is required in patients with latent tuberculosis (TB) and/or TB reactivity. Restrict use in active TB (only fulminating or disseminated TB in conjunction with antituberculosis treatment). Amebiasis should be ruled out in any patient with recent travel to tropic climates or unexplained diarrhea prior to initiation of corticosteroids. Use with extreme caution in patients with Strongyloides infections; hyperinfection, dissemination and fatalities have occurred.

Prolonged treatment with corticosteroids has been associated with the development of Kaposi sarcoma (case reports); if noted, discontinuation of therapy should be considered (Goedert 2002). Acute myopathy has been reported with high-dose corticosteroids, usually in patients with neuromuscular transmission disorders; may involve ocular and/or respiratory muscles; monitor creatine kinase; recovery may be delayed. Corticosteroid use may cause psychiatric disturbances, including euphoria, insomnia, mood swings, personality changes, severe depression to psychotic manifestation. Preexisting psychiatric conditions may be exacerbated by corticosteroid use.

Use with caution in patients with GI diseases (diverticulitis, fresh intestinal anastomoses, active or latent peptic ulcer, ulcerative colitis, abscess or other pyogenic infection) due to perforation risk. Use with caution in patients with a history of ocular herpes simplex; corneal perforation has occurred; do not use in active ocular herpes simplex. Use with caution in patients with renal impairment; hepatic impairment; history of seizure disorder; myasthenia gravis; osteoporosis; diabetes mellitus; thyroid disease; HF and/or hypertension; in patients with cataracts and/or glaucoma; and the elderly. Use with caution following acute MI; corticosteroids have been associated with myocardial rupture. Potentially significant interactions may exist, requiring dose or frequency adjustment, additional monitoring, and/or selection of alternative therapy. When discontinuing therapy, withdraw therapy with gradual tapering of dose. Patients may require higher doses when subject to stress (ie, trauma, surgery, severe illness). Use with caution in patients with systemic sclerosis; an increase in scleroderma renal crisis incidence has been observed with corticosteroid use. Monitor BP and renal function in patients with systemic sclerosis treated with corticosteroids (EULAR [Kowal-Bielecka 2017]).

Warnings: Additional Pediatric Considerations May cause osteoporosis (at any age) or inhibition of bone growth in pediatric patients. Use with caution in patients with osteoporosis. In a population-based study of children, risk of fracture was shown to be increased with >4 courses of corticosteroids; underlying clinical condition may also impact bone health and osteoporotic effect of corticosteroids (Leonard 2007). Hypertrophic cardiomyopathy has been reported in premature neonates.

Drug Interactions

Metabolism/Transport Effects None known.

Avoid Concomitant Use

Avoid concomitant use of Fludrocortisone with any of the following: Aldesleukin; BCG (Intravesical); Cladribine; Desmopressin; Fexinidazole [INT]; Indium 111 Capromab Pendetide; Macimorelin; Mifamurtide; MiFEPRIStone; Natalizumab; Pimecrolimus; Tacrolimus (Topical)

Increased Effect/Toxicity

Fludrocortisone may increase the levels/effects of: Acetylcholinesterase Inhibitors; Amphotericin B; Androgens; Baricitinib; Deferasirox; Desirudin; Desmopressin; Fexinidazole [INT]; Fingolimod; Leflunomide; Loop Diuretics; Natalizumab; Nicorandil; Nonsteroidal Anti-Inflammatory Agents (COX-2 Selective); Nonsteroidal Anti-Inflammatory Agents (Nonselective); Ozanimod; Quinolones; Ritodrine; Sargramostim; Siponimod; Thiazide and Thiazide-Like Diuretics; Tofacitinib; Upadacitinib; Vaccines (Live); Vitamin K Antagonists

The levels/effects of Fludrocortisone may be increased by: Aprepitant; Cladribine; CYP3A4 Inhibitors (Strong); Denosumab; DilTIAZem; Estrogen Derivatives; Fosaprepitant; Indacaterol; Inebilizumab; MiFEPRIStone; Neuromuscular-Blocking Agents (Nondepolarizing); Ocrelizumab; Pimecrolimus; Roflumilast; Salicylates; Tacrolimus (Topical); Trastuzumab

Decreased Effect

Fludrocortisone may decrease the levels/effects of: Aldesleukin; Antidiabetic Agents; Axicabtagene Ciloleucel; BCG (Intravesical); Calcitriol (Systemic); Coccidioides immitis Skin Test; Corticorelin; Cosyntropin; Hyaluronidase; Indium 111 Capromab Pendetide; Isoniazid; Macimorelin; Mifamurtide; Nivolumab; Pidotimod; Salicylates; Sipuleucel-T; Somatropin; Tacrolimus (Systemic); Tertomotide; Tisagenlecleucel; Urea Cycle Disorder Agents; Vaccines (Inactivated); Vaccines (Live)

The levels/effects of Fludrocortisone may be decreased by: Antacids; Bile Acid Sequestrants; CYP3A4 Inducers (Strong); Echinacea; MiFEPRIStone; Mitotane

Dietary Considerations Systemic use of mineralocorticoids/corticosteroids may require a diet with increased potassium, vitamins A, B_6, C, D, folate, calcium, zinc, and phosphorus, and decreased sodium. With fludrocortisone, a decrease in dietary sodium is often not required as the increased retention of sodium is usually the desired therapeutic effect.

Pharmacodynamics/Kinetics

Half-life Elimination Plasma: ≥3.5 hours; Biological: 18 to 36 hours

Pregnancy Risk Factor C

Pregnancy Considerations

Animal reproduction studies have not been conducted with fludrocortisone; adverse events have been observed with corticosteroids in animal reproduction studies. Some studies have shown an association between first trimester systemic corticosteroid use and oral clefts (Park-Wyllie 2000; Pradat 2003). Systemic corticosteroids may also influence fetal growth (decreased birth weight); however, information is conflicting (Lunghi 2010). Hypoadrenalism may occur in newborns following maternal use of corticosteroids in pregnancy; monitor.

When systemic corticosteroids are needed in pregnancy, it is generally recommended to use the lowest effective dose for the shortest duration of time, avoiding high doses during the first trimester (Leachman 2006; Lunghi 2010). Fludrocortisone may be used to treat women during pregnancy who require therapy for congenital adrenal hyperplasia or primary adrenal insufficiency (Endocrine Society [Bornstein 2016; Speiser 2018]).

Breastfeeding Considerations It is not known if fludrocortisone is excreted in breast milk; corticosteroids are excreted in breast milk. The manufacturer recommends that caution be exercised when administering fludrocortisone to nursing women.

Dosage Forms: US

Tablet, Oral:

Generic: 0.1 mg

Dosage Forms: Canada

Tablet, Oral:

Florinef: 0.1 mg

◆ **Fludrocortisone Acetate** *see* Fludrocortisone *on page 683*

◆ **Flugerel** *see* Flutamide *on page 702*

◆ **FluLaval Quadrivalent** *see* Influenza Virus Vaccine (Inactivated) *on page 812*

◆ **Flumadine [DSC]** *see* RiMANTAdine *on page 1329*

Flumazenil (FLOO may ze nil)

Generic Availability (US) Yes

Pharmacologic Category Antidote

Use

Benzodiazepine reversal when used in conscious sedation or general anesthesia: Complete or partial reversal of the sedative effects of benzodiazepines used in conscious sedation and general anesthesia.

Management of benzodiazepine overdose: Treatment of benzodiazepine overdose.

Local Anesthetic/Vasoconstrictor Precautions No information available to require special precautions

Effects on Dental Treatment Key adverse event(s) related to dental treatment: Xerostomia (normal salivary flow resumes upon discontinuation).

Effects on Bleeding No information available to require special precautions

Adverse Reactions

>10%: Gastrointestinal: Vomiting (11%)

1% to 10%:

Cardiovascular: Palpitation (3% to 9%), flushing (1% to 3%), thrombophlebitis (1% to 3%), vasodilation (1% to 3%)

Central nervous system: Ataxia (10%), dizziness (10%), vertigo (10%), agitation (3% to 9%), anxiety (3% to 9%), insomnia (3% to 9%), nervousness (3% to 9%), depersonalization (1% to 3%), depression (1% to 3%), dysphoria (1% to 3%), emotional lability (1% to 3%; including crying), euphoria (1% to 3%), fatigue (1% to 3%), headache (1% to 3%), hypoesthesia (1% to 3%), malaise (1% to 3%), paranoia (1% to 3%), paresthesia (1% to 3%)

Dermatologic: Dermatological disease (skin abnormality: 1% to 3%), diaphoresis (1% to 3%), skin rash (1% to 3%)

Endocrine & metabolic: Hot flash (1% to 3%)

Gastrointestinal: Xerostomia (3% to 9%), nausea (1% to 3%)

Local: Pain at injection site (3% to 9%), injection site reaction (1% to 3%)

Neuromuscular & skeletal: Weakness (1% to 3%), tremor

Ophthalmic: Blurred vision (3% to 9%), lacrimation (1% to 3%), visual disturbance (1% to 3%)

Respiratory: Dyspnea (3% to 9%), hyperventilation (3% to 9%)

<1%, postmarketing, and/or case reports: Atrial tachycardia (paroxysmal), auditory disturbance, bradycardia, cardiac arrhythmia, chest pain, confusion, decreased blood pressure, delirium, drowsiness, fear, hiccups, hyperacusis, hypertension, increased blood pressure, lack of concentration, panic attack, reversible hearing loss, rigors, seizure (including generalized), sensation of cold, shivering, stupor, tachycardia, tinnitus, tongue edema, ventricular tachycardia, voice disorder, withdrawal syndrome

Dosing

Adult

Benzodiazepine reversal when used in conscious sedation or general anesthesia: IV:

Initial dose: 0.2 mg over 15 seconds

Repeat doses (maximum: 4 doses): If the desired level of consciousness is not obtained, 0.2 mg may be repeated at 1-minute intervals.

Maximum total cumulative dose: 1 mg (usual total dose: 0.6 to 1 mg). In the event of resedation: Repeat doses may be given at 20-minute intervals as needed at 0.2 mg per minute to a maximum of 1 mg total dose and 3 mg in 1 hour.

Management of benzodiazepine overdose: IV:

Initial dose: 0.2 mg over 30 seconds; if the desired level of consciousness is not obtained 30 seconds after the dose, 0.3 mg can be given over 30 seconds

Repeat doses: 0.5 mg over 30 seconds repeated at 1-minute intervals

Maximum total cumulative dose: 3 mg (usual total dose: 1 to 3 mg).

Patients with a partial response at 3 mg may require (rare) additional titration up to a total dose of 5 mg (although doses >3 mg do not reliably produce additional effects). If a patient has not responded 5 minutes after a cumulative dose of 5 mg, the major cause of sedation is not likely due to benzodiazepines or may be due to exposure to additional CNS depressants (eg, opioids). In the event of resedation, repeat doses may be given at 20-minute intervals if needed, at 0.5 mg per minute to a maximum of 1 mg total dose and 3 mg in 1 hour.

Geriatric Refer to adult dosing. No differences in safety or efficacy have been reported; however, increased sensitivity may occur in some elderly patients.

Renal Impairment: Adult No dosage adjustment provided in manufacturer's labeling; however, pharmacokinetics are not significantly affected by renal failure (CrCl <10 mL/minute) or hemodialysis.

Hepatic Impairment: Adult Initial reversal: No dosage adjustment necessary. Repeat doses: Reduce dose or frequency.

Pediatric

Benzodiazepine reversal when used in conscious sedation or general anesthesia: Infants, Children, and Adolescents: IV: Initial dose: 0.01 mg/kg (maximum dose: 0.2 mg) given over 15 seconds; may repeat 0.01 mg/kg (maximum dose: 0.2 mg) after 45 seconds, and then every minute to a maximum total cumulative dose of 0.05 mg/kg or 1 mg, whichever is lower; usual total dose: 0.08 to 1 mg (mean: 0.65 mg)

Suspected benzodiazepine overdose: Limited data available: Infants, Children, and Adolescents: Initial dose: 0.01 mg/kg (maximum dose: 0.2 mg) with repeat doses of 0.01 mg/kg (maximum dose: 0.2 mg) given every minute to a maximum total cumulative dose of 1 mg; as an alternative to repeat bolus doses, follow up continuous infusions of 0.005-0.01 mg/kg/**hour** have been used (Clark 1995; Richard 1991; Roald 1989; Sugarman 1994)

Renal Impairment: Pediatric There are no dosage adjustments provided in the manufacturer's labeling; adult pharmacokinetic data suggests drug not significantly affected by renal failure (CrCl <10 mL/minute) or hemodialysis.

Hepatic Impairment: Pediatric Initial reversal dose: Use normal dose; repeat doses should be decreased in size or frequency

Mechanism of Action Competitively inhibits the activity at the benzodiazepine receptor site on the GABA/benzodiazepine receptor complex. Flumazenil does not antagonize the CNS effect of drugs affecting GABA-ergic neurons by means other than the benzodiazepine receptor (ethanol, barbiturates, general anesthetics) and does not reverse the effects of opioids

Contraindications Hypersensitivity to flumazenil, benzodiazepines, or any component of the formulation; patients given benzodiazepines for control of potentially life-threatening conditions (eg, control of intracranial pressure or status epilepticus); patients who may have ingested or are showing signs of cyclic-antidepressant overdosage.

Warnings/Precautions [US Boxed Warning]: Benzodiazepine reversal may result in seizures; seizures may occur more frequently in patients on benzodiazepines for long-term sedation or following tricyclic antidepressant overdose. Dose should be individualized and practitioners should be prepared to manage seizures. Seizures may also develop in patients with concurrent major sedative-hypnotic drug withdrawal, recent therapy with repeated doses of parenteral benzodiazepines, myoclonic jerking or seizure activity prior to flumazenil administration. Use with caution in patients relying on a benzodiazepine for seizure control. May cause CNS depression, which may impair physical or mental abilities; patients must be cautioned about performing tasks which require mental alertness (eg, operating machinery or driving) for 24 hours after discharge.

Flumazenil may not reliably reverse respiratory depression/hypoventilation. Flumazenil is not a substitute for evaluation of oxygenation; establishing an airway and assisting ventilation, as necessary, is always the initial step in overdose management. Resedation occurs more frequently in patients where a large single dose or cumulative dose of a benzodiazepine is administered along with a neuromuscular-blocking agent and multiple anesthetic agents. Flumazenil should be used with caution in the intensive care unit because of increased risk of unrecognized benzodiazepine dependence in such settings. Should not be used to diagnose benzodiazepine-induced sedation. Reverse neuromuscular blockade before considering use. Flumazenil does not antagonize the CNS effects of other GABA agonists (such as ethanol, barbiturates, or general anesthetics); nor does it reverse opioids. Flumazenil does not consistently reverse amnesia; patient may not recall verbal instructions after procedure.

Use with caution in patients with a history of panic disorder; may provoke panic attacks. Use caution in drug and ethanol-dependent patients; these patients may also be dependent on benzodiazepines. Not recommended for treatment of benzodiazepine dependence. Use with caution in patients with a head injury; may alter cerebral blood flow or precipitate convulsions in patients receiving benzodiazepines. Use caution in patients with mixed drug overdoses; toxic effects of other drugs taken may emerge once benzodiazepine effects are reversed. Use caution in hepatic dysfunction; repeated doses of the drug should be reduced in frequency or amount.

Warnings: Additional Pediatric Considerations Pediatric patients (especially 1 to 5 years of age) may experience resedation; these patients may require repeat bolus doses or continuous infusion.

Drug Interactions

Metabolism/Transport Effects None known.

Avoid Concomitant Use There are no known interactions where it is recommended to avoid concomitant use.

Increased Effect/Toxicity There are no known significant interactions involving an increase in effect.

Decreased Effect There are no known significant interactions involving a decrease in effect.

Dietary Considerations Avoid alcohol for the first 24 hours after administration or as long as the effects of benzodiazepines exist.

Pharmacodynamics/Kinetics

Onset of Action 1-2 minutes; 80% response within 3 minutes; Peak effect: 6-10 minutes

Duration of Action Resedation occurs after ~1 hour (range: 19-50 minutes); duration related to dose given and benzodiazepine plasma concentrations; reversal effects of flumazenil may wear off before effects of benzodiazepine

Half-life Elimination

Children: Terminal: 20-75 minutes (mean: 40 minutes)

Adults: Alpha: 4-11 minutes; Terminal: 40-80 minutes

Moderate hepatic dysfunction: 1.3 hours

Severe hepatic impairment: 2.4 hours

Pregnancy Risk Factor C

Pregnancy Considerations Teratogenic effects were not seen in animal reproduction studies. Embryocidal effects were seen at large doses. Use during labor and delivery is not recommended. In general, medications used as antidotes should take into consideration the health and prognosis of the mother; antidotes should be administered to pregnant women if there is a clear indication for use and should not be withheld because of fears of teratogenicity (Bailey 2003).

Breastfeeding Considerations It is not known if flumazenil is excreted in breast milk. The manufacturer recommends that caution be used if administering to breastfeeding women.

Dosage Forms: US

Solution, Intravenous:

Generic: 0.5 mg/5 mL (5 mL); 1 mg/10 mL (10 mL)

Dosage Forms: Canada

Solution, Intravenous:

Generic: 0.1 mg/mL (5 mL)

Dental Health Professional Considerations **Sedation:** Patients should be monitored for at least 1 hour following administration of flumazenil to ensure full recovery. Flumazenil should only be used in an emergency situation and not as a means of hastening recovery from conscious sedation. When used to hasten recovery, emergence can be sudden and unpleasant. Flumazenil should be used with caution in patients routinely taking benzodiazepines for other therapeutic uses, withdrawal symptoms will be induced.

◆ **FluMist Quadrivalent** *see* Influenza Virus Vaccine (Live/Attenuated) *on page 813*

Flunarizine (floo NAR i zeen)

Pharmacologic Category Calcium Channel Blocker

Use Note: Not approved in the US

Migraine: Prophylaxis of migraine (with and without aura) in patients with frequent and severe attacks, who have not responded satisfactorily to other treatments, and/or do not tolerate other therapy (due to unacceptable adverse effects).

Limitation of use: Not indicated for treatment of acute attacks.

Local Anesthetic/Vasoconstrictor Precautions No information available to require special precautions

Effects on Dental Treatment Key adverse event(s) related to dental treatment: Xerostomia and changes in salivation (normal salivary flow resumes upon discontinuation).

Effects on Bleeding No information available to require special precautions

Adverse Reactions Frequency not always defined.

Central nervous system: Drowsiness (20%), anxiety, depression, dizziness, extrapyramidal reaction, fatigue, insomnia, motor dysfunction, sedation, sleep disorder, vertigo

Dermatologic: Skin rash

Endocrine & metabolic: Weight gain (15%), galactorrhea, increased serum prolactin, menstrual disease

Gastrointestinal: Heartburn, increased appetite, nausea, stomach pain, vomiting, xerostomia

Neuromuscular & skeletal: Myalgia, weakness

Mechanism of Action Flunarizine is a selective calcium channel blocker that prevents cellular calcium overload by reducing excessive transmembrane calcium influx; also has antihistamine properties. Has greater effect on decreasing the frequency of migraine attacks than on decreasing the severity or duration of attacks.

Pharmacodynamics/Kinetics

Half-life Elimination Variable; Alpha: ~2.4 to 5.5 hours (single dose); Beta: ~4 days (single dose), ~19 days (multidose)

Time to Peak 2 to 4 hours

Pregnancy Considerations Adverse events have been observed in animal reproduction studies.

Product Availability Not available in the US

◆ **Flunarizine Hydrochloride** *see* Flunarizine *on page 687*

Flunisolide (Nasal) (floo NISS oh lide)

Brand Names: Canada APO-Flunisolide [DSC]

Pharmacologic Category Corticosteroid, Nasal

Use Rhinitis: Management of the nasal symptoms associated with seasonal or perennial rhinitis

Local Anesthetic/Vasoconstrictor Precautions No information available to require special precautions

Effects on Dental Treatment Key adverse event(s) related to dental treatment: *Candida* infections of the nose, atrophic rhinitis, sneezing, nasal congestion, nasal dryness and burning, increased susceptibility to infections, dry throat, epistaxis

Effects on Bleeding No information available to require special precautions

Adverse Reactions Frequency not always defined.

>10%:

Dermatologic: Burning sensation of the nose (≤13%)

Respiratory: Nasal congestion (15%), stinging sensation of the nose (≤13%)

1% to 10%:

Central nervous system: Anosmia

Respiratory: Dry nose, nasal mucosa irritation, rhinitis, sneezing

<1%, postmarketing, and/or case reports: Nasal mucosa ulcer

Mechanism of Action Decreases inflammation by suppression of migration of polymorphonuclear leukocytes and reversal of increased capillary permeability; does not depress hypothalamus

Pregnancy Considerations An agent with less systemic absorption is preferred for the treatment of allergic rhinitis during pregnancy (BSACI [Scadding 2017]).

Flunisolide (Oral Inhalation) (floo NISS oh lide)

Related Information

Respiratory Diseases *on page 1680*

Brand Names: US Aerospan [DSC]

Pharmacologic Category Corticosteroid, Inhalant (Oral)

Use

Asthma: Maintenance treatment of asthma as prophylactic therapy in patients ≥6 years.

Limitations of use: Not indicated for relief of acute bronchospasm.

Local Anesthetic/Vasoconstrictor Precautions No information available to require special precautions

Effects on Dental Treatment Key adverse event(s) related to dental treatment: *Candida* infections of the pharynx, sore throat, bitter taste, palpitations, dizziness, headache, nervousness, GI irritation, sneezing, coughing, upper respiratory tract infection, bronchitis, increased susceptibility to infections, xerostomia (normal salivary flow resumes upon discontinuation), dry throat, loss of taste, and diaphoresis.

Effects on Bleeding No information available to require special precautions

Adverse Reactions Frequency not always defined.

>10%:

Central nervous system: Headache (9% to 14%)

Respiratory: Pharyngitis (17% to 18%), rhinitis (4% to 16%)

1% to 10%:

Cardiovascular: Chest pain (1% to 3%), edema (1% to 3%), capillary fragility (≥1%), chest tightness (≥1%), hypertension (≥1%), palpitations (≥1%), peripheral edema (≥1%), tachycardia (≥1%)

Central nervous system: Pain (2% to 5%), dizziness (1% to 3%), insomnia (1% to 3%), migraine (1% to 3%), voice disorder (1% to 3%), anosmia (≥1%), anxiety (≥1%), depression (≥1%), fatigue (≥1%), hyperactivity (≥1%), hypoactivity (≥1%), irritability (≥1%), malaise (≥1%), mood changes (≥1%), numbness (≥1%), shakiness (≥1%), vertigo (≥1%)

Dermatologic: Skin rash (2% to 4%), erythema multiforme (1% to 3%), acne vulgaris (≥1%), diaphoresis (≥1%), eczema (≥1%), pruritus (≥1%), urticaria (≥1%)

Endocrine & metabolic: Weight gain (≥1%), adrenal suppression, adrenocortical insufficiency, growth suppression (children and adolescents), hypercorticoidism

Gastrointestinal: Vomiting (≤5%), dyspepsia (2% to 4%), abdominal pain (1% to 3%), diarrhea (1% to 3%), dysgeusia (1% to 3%), gastroenteritis (1% to 3%), nausea (1% to 3%), oral candidiasis (1% to 3%), ageusia (≥1%), constipation (≥1%), decreased appetite (≥1%), epigastric fullness (≥1%), flatulence (≥1%), glossitis (≥1%), heartburn (≥1%), mouth irritation (≥1%), sore throat (≥1%), stomach discomfort (≥1%), oropharyngeal candidiasis

Genitourinary: Urinary tract infection (1% to 4%), dysmenorrhea (1% to 3%), vaginitis (1% to 3%)

Hematologic & oncologic: Lymphadenopathy (≥1%)

Hypersensitivity: Hypersensitivity reaction (4% to 5%)

Infection: Bacterial infection (4%), infection (1% to 3%), cold symptoms (≥1%), influenza (≥1%)

Neuromuscular & skeletal: Back pain (1% to 3%), myalgia (1% to 3%), neck pain (1% to 3%), weakness (≥1%), decreased bone mineral density

Ophthalmic: Conjunctivitis (1% to 3%), blurred vision (≥1%), eye discomfort (≥1%), eye infection (≥1%), cataract, glaucoma, increased intraocular pressure

Otic: Otalgia (1% to 3%), otitis (≥1%)

Respiratory: Cough (9%), sinusitis (7% to 9%), epistaxis (3%), bronchitis (1% to 3%), laryngitis (1% to 3%), bronchospasm (≥1%), chest congestion (≥1%), dry throat (≥1%), dyspnea (≥1%), hoarseness (≥1%), increased bronchial secretions (≥1%), nasal congestion (≥1%), nasal mucosa irritation (≥1%), pleurisy (≥1%), pneumonia (≥1%), rhinorrhea (≥1%), sinus congestion (≥1%), sinus discomfort (≥1%), sinus drainage (≥1%), sinus infection (≥1%), sneezing (≥1%), throat irritation (≥1%), upper respiratory tract infection (≥1%), wheezing (≥1%), exacerbation of asthma

Miscellaneous: Fever (1% to 7%)

Mechanism of Action Decreases airway inflammation by suppression of endogenous inflammatory mediators (kinins, histamine, liposomal enzymes, prostaglandins). Inhibits inflammatory cell migration and reverses increased capillary permeability to decrease access of inflammatory cells to the site of inflammation; does not depress hypothalamus.

Pharmacodynamics/Kinetics

Half-life Elimination 1.3-1.7 hours

Time to Peak Within 5-10 minutes

Pregnancy Considerations

Maternal use of inhaled corticosteroids (ICS) in usual doses is not associated with an increased risk of fetal malformations; a small risk of malformations was observed in one study following high maternal doses of an alternative ICS. Uncontrolled asthma is associated with adverse events in pregnancy (increased risk of perinatal mortality, preeclampsia, preterm birth, low birth weight infants, cesarean delivery, and the development of gestational diabetes). Poorly controlled asthma or asthma exacerbations may have a greater fetal/maternal risk than what is associated with appropriately used asthma medications. Maternal treatment improves pregnancy outcomes by reducing the risk of some adverse events (eg, preterm birth, gestational diabetes) (ERS/TSANZ [Middleton 2020]; GINA 2020).

ICS are recommended for the treatment of asthma during pregnancy (GINA 2020). Pregnant females adequately controlled on flunisolide for asthma may continue therapy; if initiating treatment during pregnancy, use of an agent with more data in pregnant females may be preferred. The lowest dose that maintains asthma control should be used. Maternal asthma symptoms should be monitored monthly during pregnancy (ERS/TSANZ [Middleton 2020]).

Data collection to monitor pregnancy and infant outcomes associated with asthma and the medications used to treat asthma in pregnancy is ongoing. Health care providers are encouraged to enroll exposed pregnant females in the MotherToBaby Pregnancy Studies conducted by the Organization of Teratology Information Specialists (OTIS) (877-311-8972 or https://mothertobaby.org). Patients may also enroll themselves.

Product Availability Aerospan has been discontinued in the US for more than 1 year.

◆ **Flunisolide Hemihydrate** *see* Flunisolide (Oral Inhalation) *on page 688*

Fluocinolone (Topical) (floo oh SIN oh lone)

Brand Names: US Capex; Derma-Smoothe/FS Body; Derma-Smoothe/FS Scalp; Synalar; Synalar (Cream); Synalar (Ointment); Synalar TS; Xilapak [DSC]

Brand Names: Canada Derma-Smoothe/FS; Fluoderm; Synalar; Synalar Mild

Generic Availability (US) May be product dependent

Pharmacologic Category Corticosteroid, Topical

Dental Use Relief of inflammatory and pruritic manifestations (low, medium, high potency topical corticosteroid)

Use

Body oil: Treatment of moderate to severe atopic dermatitis in pediatric patients ≥3 months; treatment of atopic dermatitis in adults

Cream, ointment, topical solution: Relief of inflammatory and pruritic manifestations of corticosteroid-responsive dermatoses

Scalp oil: Treatment of psoriasis of the scalp in adults

Shampoo: Treatment of seborrheic dermatitis of the scalp

Local Anesthetic/Vasoconstrictor Precautions No information available to require special precautions

Effects on Dental Treatment No significant effects or complications reported

Effects on Bleeding No information available to require special precautions

Adverse Reactions Frequency not defined.

Cardiovascular: Intracranial hypertension (rare)

Central nervous system: Telangiectasia

Dermatologic: Acneiform eruptions, allergic contact dermatitis, atopic dermatitis (secondary), burning, dryness, erythema, folliculitis, irritation, itching, hypertrichosis, hypopigmentation, keratosis pilaris, miliaria, papules, perioral dermatitis, pustules, shiny skin, skin atrophy, striae

Endocrine & metabolic: Cushing's syndrome, HPA axis suppression

Otic: Ear infection

Miscellaneous: Herpes simplex, secondary infection

Dental Usual Dosage Inflammatory and pruritic manifestations: Adults: Topical: Apply to oral lesion 4 times/day, after meals and at bedtime

Dosing

Adult & Geriatric Note: Dosage should be based on severity of disease and patient response; use smallest amount for shortest period of time. Therapy should be discontinued when control is achieved.

Atopic dermatitis: Topical: Body oil: Apply thin film to affected area 3 times daily

Corticosteroid-responsive dermatoses: Topical: Cream, ointment, solution: Apply a thin layer to affected area 2 to 4 times daily; may use occlusive dressings to manage psoriasis or recalcitrant conditions

Scalp psoriasis: Topical: Scalp oil: Massage thoroughly into wet or dampened hair/scalp; cover with shower cap. Leave on overnight (or for at least 4 hours). Remove by washing hair with shampoo and rinsing thoroughly.

Seborrheic dermatitis of the scalp: Topical: Shampoo: Apply no more than 1 ounce to scalp once daily; work into lather and allow to remain on scalp for ~5 minutes. Remove from hair and scalp by rinsing thoroughly with water.

Renal Impairment: Adult There are no dosage adjustments provided in the manufacturer's labeling.

Hepatic Impairment: Adult There are no dosage adjustments provided in the manufacturer's labeling.

Pediatric Note: Dosage should be based on severity of disease and patient response; use smallest amount for shortest period of time to avoid HPA axis suppression. Therapy should be discontinued when control is achieved.

Atopic dermatitis, moderate to severe:

Derma-Smoothe/FS body oil (0.01%): Infants ≥3 months, Children, and Adolescents: Topical: Moisten skin; apply a thin film to affected area twice daily; do not use for longer than 4 weeks

Derma-Smoothe/FS scalp oil (0.01%): Limited data available: Children ≥2 years and Adolescents: Topical: Apply a thin film to affected area twice daily; do not use longer than 4 weeks

Corticosteroid-responsive dermatoses: Synalar cream (0.025%), ointment (0.025%), topical solution (0.01%): Children and Adolescents: Topical: Apply thin layer 2 to 4 times daily to affected area; may use occlusive dressings to manage psoriasis or recalcitrant conditions

Renal Impairment: Pediatric There are no dosage adjustments provided in the manufacturer's labeling.

Hepatic Impairment: Pediatric There are no dosage adjustments provided in the manufacturer's labeling.

Mechanism of Action Topical corticosteroids have anti-inflammatory, antipruritic, and vasoconstrictive properties. May depress the formation, release, and activity of endogenous chemical mediators of inflammation (kinins, histamine, liposomal enzymes, prostaglandins) through the induction of phospholipase A_2 inhibitory proteins (lipocortins) and sequential inhibition of the release of arachidonic acid. Fluocinolone has low to intermediate range potency (dosage-form dependent).

Contraindications

Hypersensitivity to fluocinolone or any component of the formulation

Documentation of allergenic cross-reactivity for corticosteroids is limited. However, because of similarities in chemical structure and/or pharmacologic actions, the possibility of cross-sensitivity cannot be ruled out with certainty.

Canadian labeling: Additional contraindications (not in US labeling): Viral (eg, herpes, varicella) lesions of the skin; bacterial or fungal skin infections; parasitic infections; skin manifestations relating to tuberculosis or syphilis; eruptions following vaccinations; application to the eye

Warnings/Precautions Topical corticosteroids may be absorbed percutaneously. Absorption of topical corticosteroids may cause manifestations of Cushing syndrome, hyperglycemia, or glycosuria. Absorption is increased by the use of occlusive dressings, application to denuded skin, or application to large surface areas. May cause hypercortisolism or suppression of hypothalamic-pituitary-adrenal (HPA) axis, particularly in younger children or in patients receiving high doses for prolonged periods. HPA axis suppression may lead to adrenal crisis. HPA axis suppression, intracranial hypertension, and Cushing syndrome have been reported in children receiving topical corticosteroids. Prolonged use may affect growth velocity; growth should be routinely monitored in pediatric patients. Allergic contact dermatitis can occur, it is usually diagnosed by failure to heal rather than clinical exacerbation. Prolonged treatment with corticosteroids has been associated with the development of Kaposi sarcoma (case reports); if noted, discontinuation of therapy should be considered (Goedert 2002). Local adverse reactions may occur (eg, skin atrophy, striae, telangiectasias, burning, itching, irritation, dryness, folliculitis, acneiform eruptions, hypopigmentation, perioral dermatitis, allergic contact dermatitis, secondary infection miliaria); may be irreversible. Local adverse reactions are more likely to occur with occlusive and/or prolonged use. If irritation develops, discontinued use and institute appropriate therapy. Concomitant skin infections may be present or develop during therapy; discontinue if dermatological infection persists despite appropriate antimicrobial therapy. Not for oral, ophthalmic, or intravaginal use; do not apply to the face, axillae, groin, or diaper area unless directed by health care provider. Use the least amount needed to cover the affected area; discontinue when control is achieved. If improvement is not seen within 2 weeks, reassess.

Derma-Smoothe/FS products may contain peanut oil; use caution in peanut-sensitive individuals.

Shampoo: Has not been proven to be effective in corticosteroid responsive dermatoses other than seborrheic dermatitis of the scalp.

Warnings: Additional Pediatric Considerations Topical corticosteroids may be absorbed percutaneously. The extent of absorption is dependent on several factors, including epidermal integrity (intact vs abraded skin), formulation, age of the patient, prolonged duration of use, and the use of occlusive dressings. Percutaneous absorption of topical steroids is increased in neonates (especially preterm neonates), infants, and young children. Hypothalamic-pituitary-adrenal (HPA) suppression may occur, particularly in younger children or in patients receiving high doses for prolonged periods; acute adrenal insufficiency (adrenal crisis) may occur with abrupt withdrawal after long-term therapy or with stress. Infants and small children may be more susceptible to HPA axis suppression or other systemic toxicities due to larger skin surface area to body mass ratio; use with caution in pediatric patients.

Some dosage forms may contain propylene glycol; in neonates large amounts of propylene glycol delivered orally, intravenously (eg, >3,000 mg/day), or topically have been associated with potentially fatal toxicities which can include metabolic acidosis, seizures, renal failure, and CNS depression; toxicities have also been reported in children and adults including hyperosmolality, lactic acidosis, seizures, and respiratory depression; use caution (AAP, 1997; Shehab, 2009).

Drug Interactions

Metabolism/Transport Effects None known.

Avoid Concomitant Use

Avoid concomitant use of Fluocinolone (Topical) with any of the following: Aldesleukin

Increased Effect/Toxicity

Fluocinolone (Topical) may increase the levels/effects of: Deferasirox; Ritodrine

Decreased Effect

Fluocinolone (Topical) may decrease the levels/effects of: Aldesleukin; Corticorelin; Hyaluronidase

Pregnancy Risk Factor C

Pregnancy Considerations Adverse events have been observed with corticosteroids in animal reproduction studies. In general, the use of topical corticosteroids during pregnancy is not considered to have significant risk; however, intrauterine growth retardation in the infant has been reported (rare). The use of large amounts or for prolonged periods of time should be avoided (Reed 1997).

Breastfeeding Considerations Systemic corticosteroids are excreted in human milk. It is not known if sufficient quantities of fluocinolone are absorbed following topical administration to produce detectable amounts in breast milk. Hypertension in the breastfeeding infant has been reported following corticosteroid ointment applied to the nipples (Reed 1997). The manufacturer recommends that caution be exercised when administering fluocinolone to breastfeeding women.

Dosage Forms: US

Cream, External:

Synalar: 0.025% (120 g)

Generic: 0.01% (15 g, 60 g); 0.025% (15 g, 60 g)

Kit, External:

Synalar (Cream): 0.025%

Synalar (Ointment): 0.025%

Synalar TS: 0.01%

Oil, External:

Derma-Smoothe/FS Body: 0.01% (118.28 mL)

Derma-Smoothe/FS Scalp: 0.01% (118.28 mL)

Generic: 0.01% (118.28 mL)

Ointment, External:

Synalar: 0.025% (120 g)

Generic: 0.025% (15 g, 60 g)

Shampoo, External:
Capex: 0.01% (120 mL)
Solution, External:
Synalar: 0.01% (60 mL, 90 mL)
Generic: 0.01% (60 mL)

Dosage Forms: Canada

Cream, External:
Fluoderm: 0.01% (15 g, 500 g); 0.025% (15 g, 500 g)
Oil, External:
Derma-Smoothe/FS: 0.01% (118 mL, 120 mL, 355 mL)
Ointment, External:
Fluoderm: 0.025% (15 g, 454 g)
Synalar: 0.025% (60 g)
Synalar Mild: 0.01% (60 g)
Solution, External:
Synalar: 0.01% (20 mL, 60 mL)

◆ **Fluocinolone Acetonide** *see* Fluocinolone (Topical) *on page 689*

◆ **Fluocinolone and Ciprofloxacin** *see* Ciprofloxacin and Fluocinolone *on page 351*

Fluocinonide (floo oh SIN oh nide)

Related Information
Ulcerative, Erosive, and Painful Oral Mucosal Disorders *on page 1758*

Related Sample Prescriptions
Ulcerative and Erosive Disorders - Sample Prescriptions *on page 46*

Brand Names: US Vanos

Brand Names: Canada Lidemol; Lidex; Lyderm; Tiamol; Topactin Emollient; Topactin [DSC]

Generic Availability (US) Yes

Pharmacologic Category Corticosteroid, Topical

Dental Use Relief of inflammatory and pruritic manifestations (high potency topical corticosteroid)

Use Inflammatory and pruritic dermatologic conditions: Relief of the inflammatory and pruritic manifestations of corticosteroid-responsive dermatoses.

Local Anesthetic/Vasoconstrictor Precautions No information available to require special precautions

Effects on Dental Treatment No significant effects or complications reported

Effects on Bleeding No information available to require special precautions

Adverse Reactions Frequency not defined.

Central nervous system: Intracranial hypertension, localized burning
Dermatologic: Acne vulgaris, allergic dermatitis, atrophic striae, contact dermatitis, folliculitis, hypertrichosis, hypopigmentation, maceration of the skin, miliaria, perioral dermatitis, pruritus, skin atrophy, telangiectasia, xeroderma
Endocrine & metabolic: Cushing's syndrome, glycosuria, growth suppression, HPA-axis suppression, hyperglycemia
Infection: Secondary infection
Local: Local irritation

Dental Usual Dosage Pruritus and inflammation: Children and Adults: Topical (0.05% cream): Apply thin layer to affected area 2-4 times/day depending on the severity of the condition. Therapy should be discontinued when control is achieved; if no improvement is seen, reassessment of diagnosis may be necessary.

Dosing

Adult & Geriatric

Atopic dermatitis: Topical:
Cream, gel, ointment, solution (0.05%): Apply thin layer to affected area 2 to 4 times daily.
Cream (0.1%): Apply thin layer to affected areas once daily. Not recommended for use >2 consecutive weeks or >60 g/week total exposure. Therapy should be discontinued when control is achieved; if no improvement is seen within 2 weeks, reassessment of diagnosis may be necessary.

Psoriasis: Topical:
Cream, gel, ointment, solution (0.05%): Apply thin layer to affected area 2 to 4 times daily.
Cream (0.1%): Apply a thin layer once or twice daily to affected areas. Not recommended for use >2 consecutive weeks or >60 g/week total exposure. Therapy should be discontinued when control is achieved; if no improvement is seen within 2 weeks, reassess diagnosis.

Other inflammatory and pruritic dermatologic conditions besides atopic dermatitis or psoriasis: Topical:
Cream, gel, ointment, solution (0.05%): Apply thin layer to affected area 2 to 4 times daily.
Cream (0.1%): Apply thin layer to affected area once or twice daily. Not recommended for use >2 consecutive weeks or >60 g/week total exposure. Therapy should be discontinued when control is achieved; if no improvement is seen within 2 weeks, reassess diagnosis.

Renal Impairment: Adult There are no dosage adjustments provided in the manufacturer's labeling.

Hepatic Impairment: Adult There are no dosage adjustments provided in the manufacturer's labeling.

Pediatric

Atopic dermatitis:
Cream, gel, ointment, topical solution (0.05%): Children and Adolescents: Topical: Apply thin layer to affected area 2 to 4 times daily depending on the severity of the condition. **Note:** In children <12 years, NICE guidelines recommend applying only once or twice daily (NICE 2007).
Cream (0.1%): Children ≥12 years and Adolescents: Topical: Apply a thin layer once daily to affected areas. Not recommended for use >2 consecutive weeks or >60 g/week total exposure. Therapy should be discontinued when control is achieved; if no improvement is seen within 2 weeks, reassessment of diagnosis may be necessary.

Corticosteroid-responsive dermatoses (including psoriasis):
Cream, gel, ointment, topical solution (0.05%): Children and Adolescents: Topical: Apply thin layer to affected area 2 to 4 times daily depending on the severity of the condition; may use occlusive dressings to manage psoriasis or recalcitrant conditions
Cream (0.1%): Children ≥12 years and Adolescents: Topical: Apply a thin layer once or twice daily to affected areas. Not recommended for use >2 consecutive weeks or >60 g/week total exposure. Therapy should be discontinued when control is achieved; if no improvement is seen within 2 weeks, reassess diagnosis.

Renal Impairment: Pediatric There are no dosage adjustments provided in the manufacturer's labeling.

Hepatic Impairment: Pediatric There are no dosage adjustments provided in the manufacturer's labeling.

Mechanism of Action Topical corticosteroids have anti-inflammatory, antipruritic, and vasoconstrictive properties. May depress the formation, release, and activity of endogenous chemical mediators of inflammation (kinins, histamine, liposomal enzymes, prostaglandins) through the induction of phospholipase A_2 inhibitory proteins (lipocortins) and sequential inhibition of the release of arachidonic acid. Fluocinonide is fluorinated corticosteroid considered to be of high potency.

Contraindications Hypersensitivity to fluocinonide or any component of the formulation

Warnings/Precautions May cause hypercortisolism or suppression of hypothalamic-pituitary-adrenal (HPA) axis, particularly in younger children or in patients receiving high doses for prolonged periods. HPA axis suppression may lead to adrenal crisis. Absorption of topical corticosteroids may cause manifestations of Cushing syndrome, hyperglycemia, or glycosuria. Absorption is increased by the use of occlusive dressings, application to denuded skin, or application to large surface areas.

Allergic contact dermatitis can occur, it is usually diagnosed by failure to heal rather than clinical exacerbation. Local adverse reactions may occur (eg, skin atrophy, striae, telangiectasias, burning, itching, irritation, dryness, folliculitis, acneiform eruptions, hypopigmentation, perioral dermatitis, allergic contact dermatitis, secondary infection miliaria); may be irreversible. Local adverse reactions are more likely to occur with occlusive and/or prolonged use. If irritation develops, discontinued use and institute appropriate therapy. Concomitant skin infections may be present or develop during therapy; discontinue if dermatological infection persists despite appropriate antimicrobial therapy. Prolonged treatment with corticosteroids has been associated with the development of Kaposi sarcoma (case reports); if noted, discontinuation of therapy should be considered. Lower-strength formulations (0.05%) may be used cautiously on face or opposing skin surfaces that may rub or touch (eg, skin folds of the groin, axilla, and breasts); higher-strength (0.1%) should not be used on the face, groin, or axillae. Children may absorb proportionally larger amounts after topical application and may be more prone to systemic effects. HPA axis suppression, intracranial hypertension, and Cushing syndrome have been reported in children receiving topical corticosteroids. Prolonged use may affect growth velocity; growth should be routinely monitored in pediatric patients. Treatment beyond 2 consecutive weeks with the 0.1% cream is not recommended and the total dosage should not exceed 60 g per week; therapy should be discontinued when control of the disease is achieved; if no improvement is seen within 2 weeks, reassess diagnosis; do not use more than half of the 120 g tube per week; should not be used in the treatment of rosacea or perioral dermatitis.

Warnings: Additional Pediatric Considerations Topical corticosteroids may be absorbed percutaneously. The extent of absorption is dependent on several factors, including epidermal integrity (intact vs abraded skin), formulation, age of the patient, prolonged duration of use, and the use of occlusive dressings. Percutaneous absorption of topical steroids is increased in neonates (especially preterm neonates), infants, and young children. Hypothalamic-pituitary-adrenal (HPA) suppression may occur, particularly in younger children or in patients receiving high doses for prolonged periods; acute adrenal insufficiency (adrenal crisis) may occur with abrupt withdrawal after long-term therapy or with stress. Infants and small children may be more susceptible to HPA axis suppression or other systemic toxicities due to larger skin surface area to body mass ratio; use with caution in pediatric patients.

Some dosage forms may contain propylene glycol; in neonates large amounts of propylene glycol delivered orally, intravenously (eg, >3,000 mg/day), or topically have been associated with potentially fatal toxicities which can include metabolic acidosis, seizures, renal failure, and CNS depression; toxicities have also been reported in children and adults including hyperosmolality, lactic acidosis, seizures and respiratory depression; use caution (AAP 1997; Shehab 2009).

Drug Interactions

Metabolism/Transport Effects None known.

Avoid Concomitant Use

Avoid concomitant use of Fluocinonide with any of the following: Aldesleukin

Increased Effect/Toxicity

Fluocinonide may increase the levels/effects of: Deferasirox; Ritodrine

Decreased Effect

Fluocinonide may decrease the levels/effects of: Aldesleukin; Corticorelin; Hyaluronidase

Pregnancy Risk Factor C

Pregnancy Considerations Adverse events have been observed with corticosteroids in animal reproduction studies. Topical corticosteroids are preferred over systemic for treating conditions, such as psoriasis or atopic dermatitis in pregnant women; high-potency corticosteroids are not recommended during the first trimester. Topical products are not recommended for extensive use, in large quantities, or for long periods of time in pregnant women (Bae 2011; Koutroulis 2011; Leachman 2006). Information specific to the use of fluocinonide during pregnancy is limited (Valkova 2006).

Breastfeeding Considerations Systemic corticosteroids are excreted in human milk. It is not known if sufficient quantities of fluocinonide are absorbed following topical administration to produce detectable amounts in breast milk. Do not apply topical corticosteroids to nipples; hypertension was noted in a breastfeeding infant exposed to a topical corticosteroid while breastfeeding (Leachman 2006).

The manufacturer recommends that caution be exercised when administering fluocinonide 0.05% to nursing women. Because maternal use of systemic corticosteroids have the potential to cause adverse events in a breastfeeding infant (eg, growth suppression, interfere with endogenous corticosteroid production), the manufacturer recommends that a decision be made whether to discontinue breastfeeding or to discontinue the drug, taking into account the importance of treatment to the mother when using the fluocinonide 0.1%.

Dosage Forms: US

Cream, External:

Vanos: 0.1% (30 g, 60 g, 120 g)

Generic: 0.05% (15 g, 30 g, 60 g, 120 g); 0.1% (30 g, 60 g, 120 g)

Gel, External:

Generic: 0.05% (15 g, 30 g, 60 g)

Ointment, External:

Generic: 0.05% (15 g, 30 g, 60 g)

Solution, External:

Generic: 0.05% (20 mL, 60 mL)

Dosage Forms: Canada

Cream, External:

Lidemol: 0.05% (15 g, 30 g, 60 g, 100 g)

Lidex: 0.05% (60 g, 400 g)

Lyderm: 0.05% (15 g, 60 g, 400 g)

Tiamol: 0.05% (25 g, 100 g)

Topactin Emollient: 0.05% (60 g, 225 g)

Gel, External:

Lidex: 0.05% (60 g)

Lyderm: 0.05% (15 g, 60 g)

Ointment, External:

Lidex: 0.05% (60 g)

Lyderm: 0.05% (60 g)

◆ **Fluohydrisone Acetate** *see* Fludrocortisone *on page 683*

◆ **Fluohydrocortisone Acetate** *see* Fludrocortisone *on page 683*

◆ **Fluorabon** *see* Fluoride *on page 693*

◆ **Fluor-A-Day [DSC]** *see* Fluoride *on page 693*

Fluoride (FLOR ide)

Related Information

Dentifrices Without Sodium Lauryl Sulfate (SLS)[a] *on page 1819*

Dentin Hypersensitivity, Acid Erosion, High Caries Index, Management of Alveolar Osteitis, and Xerostomia *on page 1762*

Brand Names: US Act Kids [OTC]; Act Restoring [OTC]; Act Total Care Dry Mouth [OTC]; Act Total Care Sensitive [OTC]; Act Total Care [OTC]; Act [OTC]; CaviRinse [DSC]; Clinpro 5000; Denta 5000 Plus; DentaGel; Fluor-A-Day [DSC]; Fluorabon; Fluoridex; Fluoridex Daily Renewal; Fluoridex Enhanced Whitening; Fluorinse; Fluoritab; Flura-Drops; Gel-Kam Rinse; Gel-Kam [OTC]; Just For Kids [OTC]; Lozi-Flur [DSC]; NeutraCare; NeutraGard Advanced [DSC]; Omni Gel [OTC]; OrthoWash; parodontax [OTC]; PerioMed; Phos-Flur Rinse [OTC]; Phos-Flur [DSC]; PreviDent; PreviDent 5000 Booster Plus; PreviDent 5000 Booster [DSC]; PreviDent 5000 Dry Mouth; PreviDent 5000 Plus; Sensodyne Repair & Protect [OTC]; StanGard Perio

Brand Names: Canada Fluor-A-Day

Generic Availability (US) Yes: Excludes lozenge

Pharmacologic Category Nutritional Supplement

Dental Use Prevention of dental caries

Use Prevention of dental caries

Local Anesthetic/Vasoconstrictor Precautions No information available to require special precautions

Effects on Dental Treatment Key adverse event(s) related to dental treatment: Products containing stannous fluoride may stain teeth. See Dental Health Professional Considerations.

Effects on Bleeding No information available to require special precautions

Adverse Reactions Frequency not defined.

Dermatologic: Skin rash

Gastrointestinal: Dental discoloration (with products containing stannous fluoride; temporary), nausea

Hypersensitivity: Hypersensitivity reaction

Dosing

Adult & Geriatric

Cream or paste:

Clinpro 5000 paste, Control Rx 1.1%, Denta 5000 Plus: Once daily, in place of conventional toothpaste, brush teeth with a thin ribbon or pea-sized amount of paste for at least 2 minutes. Brush teeth with cream or paste once daily regardless of fluoride content of drinking water

Prevident 5000 Sensitive: Twice daily, brush teeth with a 1 inch strip of toothpaste for at least 1 minute. After brushing, expectorate and rinse mouth thoroughly. Brush teeth twice daily regardless of fluoride content of drinking water

Dental rinse or gel:

ACT Restoring 0.02% rinse, ACT Total Care 0.02% rinse: Twice daily after brushing, rinse 10 mL around and between teeth for 1 minute, then spit. Do not eat, drink, or rinse mouth for at least 30 minutes after treatment; do not swallow

ACT 0.05% rinse, Phos-Flur Rinse: Once daily after brushing, rinse 10 mL around and between teeth for 1 minute, then spit. Do not eat, drink, or rinse mouth for at least 30 minutes after treatment; do not swallow

Cavirinse, PreviDent rinse: Once weekly, rinse 10 mL vigorously around and between teeth for 1 minute, then spit; this should be done preferably at bedtime, after thoroughly brushing teeth; do not swallow. For maximum benefit with PreviDent rinse, do not eat, drink, or rinse mouth for at least 30 minutes after treatment.

Gel-Kam rinse: After diluting solution as directed, rinse with 15 mL for 1 minute at least daily, then spit. Repeat with remaining solution.

Lozenge: Lozi-Flur: One lozenge daily regardless of fluoride content of drinking water

Pediatric Note: Dosages below may be presented as fluoride ion, sodium fluoride, or stannous fluoride; use caution to ensure the correct product is ordered or administered.

Dental caries, prevention:

Systemic therapy:

Drops/tablets: Oral: The recommended oral daily dose of fluoride ion is adjusted in proportion to the fluoride content of available drinking water (ppm of fluoride in drinking water):

Birth to 6 months: No supplement required regardless of fluoride content of drinking water.

6 months to 3 years:

<0.3 ppm: 0.25 mg fluoride ion once daily.

≥0.3 ppm: No supplement required.

3 to 6 years:

<0.3 ppm: 0.5 mg fluoride ion once daily.

0.3 to 0.6 ppm: 0.25 mg fluoride ion once daily.

>0.6 ppm: No supplement required.

6 to 16 years:

<0.3 ppm: 1 mg fluoride ion once daily.

0.3 to 0.6 ppm: 0.5 mg fluoride ion once daily.

>0.6 ppm: No supplement required.

Lozenges (Lozi-Flur): Children ≥6 years and Adolescents: Oral: 1 lozenge daily; allow lozenge to dissolve slowly in the mouth and swallow with saliva. **Note:** For use in areas where the fluoride content of drinking water is <0.3 ppm.

Topical therapy:

Dental rinse: **Note:** Do not eat, drink, or rinse mouth for at least 30 minutes after treatment; do not swallow.

Sodium fluoride: Topical:

0.02% Sodium fluoride: Children ≥6 years and Adolescents: 10 mL swish and spit twice daily after brushing.

0.04% Sodium fluoride: Children ≥6 years and Adolescents: 10 mL once daily after brushing; swish between teeth for 1 minute, then spit.

0.05% Sodium fluoride: Children ≥6 years and Adolescents: 10 mL swish and spit once daily after brushing.

0.2% Neutral sodium fluoride: Children ≥6 years and Adolescents: 10 mL swish and spit once **weekly**, preferably at bedtime after brushing.

Stannous fluoride 0.63%: Children ≥6 years and Adolescents: Topical: After diluting solution as directed, rinse with 15 mL (1/2 of the prepared solution) for 1 minute, then spit out; repeat with remaining solution. Use once daily.

Gel:

Stannous fluoride 0.4%: Children ≥6 years and Adolescents: Topical: Once daily after brushing, apply a pea-sized amount of gel to teeth and brush thoroughly. Allow gel to remain on teeth for 1 minute prior to spitting out.

Sodium fluoride 1.1%: Children ≥6 years and Adolescents: Topical: Once daily after brushing, apply a thin ribbon of gel to teeth with a toothbrush or mouth tray. Allow gel to remain on teeth for 1 minute then expectorate; children ≥6 years and adolescents <16 years should also rinse mouth thoroughly with water.

Paste or cream:

Sodium fluoride:

1.1% Neutral sodium fluoride: Children ≥6 years and Adolescents: Topical: Once daily, preferably at bedtime, in place of conventional toothpaste; brush teeth with a thin ribbon or pea-sized amount of toothpaste for at least 2 minutes then expectorate; some products recommend children ≥6 years and adolescents <16 years should also rinse mouth thoroughly with water after use.

Sodium fluoride and potassium nitrate:

0.25% Sodium fluoride/5% Potassium nitrate: Children ≥12 years and Adolescents: Topical: Brush teeth with a 1-inch strip of toothpaste for at least 1 minute 2 to 3 times daily then expectorate.

1.1% Sodium fluoride /5% Potassium nitrate: Children ≥12 years and Adolescents: Topical: Twice daily, brush teeth with a 1-inch strip of toothpaste for at least 1 minute. After brushing, expectorate and rinse mouth thoroughly.

Stannous fluoride 0.454%: Children ≥2 years and Adolescents: Topical: Brush teeth with a pea-sized amount of toothpaste 2 to 3 times daily, preferably after meals. Expectorate after brushing.

Dental varnish: 5% Sodium fluoride (2.26% Fluoride ion): Infants (after primary tooth eruption), Children, and Adolescents: Topical: Apply a thin layer of varnish to surfaces of teeth at least every 3 to 6 months (ADA [Weyant 2013]). **Note:** Must be professionally applied; USPSTF recommends dental varnish may be applied by primary care practitioners to the primary teeth of all infants and children starting at the age of primary tooth eruption through 5 years of age (USPSTF 2014).

Mechanism of Action Promotes remineralization of decalcified enamel; inhibits the cariogenic microbial process in dental plaque; increases tooth resistance to acid dissolution

Contraindications

Fluor-A-Day: When fluoride content of drinking water exceeds 0.6 ppm; patients with arthralgia, GI ulceration, chronic renal insufficiency and failure, or osteomalacia

Fluorabon: When fluoride content of drinking water exceeds 0.6 ppm

Fluoritab: Patients with dental fluorosis

Flura-Drops, Loziflur: When fluoride content of drinking water is ≥0.3 ppm

Warnings/Precautions Prolonged ingestion with excessive doses may result in dental fluorosis and osseous changes; do **not** exceed recommended dosage. Dietary fluoride supplements are recommended for children at high risk of developing dental caries. They are not recommended for use in children <6 months of age, or any child at low risk. All sources of fluoride should be considered prior to preventive intervention (Rozier 2010). Some dosage forms may contain propylene glycol; large amounts are potentially toxic and have been associated with hyperosmolality, lactic acidosis, seizures, and respiratory depression; use caution (AAP 1997; Zar 2007). Some products contain tartrazine.

Benzyl alcohol and derivatives: Some dosage forms may contain sodium benzoate/benzoic acid; benzoic acid (benzoate) is a metabolite of benzyl alcohol; large amounts of benzyl alcohol (≥99 mg/kg/day) have been associated with a potentially fatal toxicity ("gasping syndrome") in neonates; the "gasping syndrome" consists of metabolic acidosis, respiratory distress, gasping respirations, CNS dysfunction (including convulsions, intracranial hemorrhage), hypotension, and cardiovascular collapse (AAP ["Inactive" 1997]; CDC, 1982); some data suggests that benzoate displaces bilirubin from protein binding sites (Ahlfors, 2001); avoid or use dosage forms containing benzyl alcohol derivative with caution in neonates. See manufacturer's labeling.

Polysorbate 80: Some dosage forms may contain polysorbate 80 (also known as Tweens). Hypersensitivity reactions, usually a delayed reaction, have been reported following exposure to pharmaceutical products containing polysorbate 80 in certain individuals (Isaksson, 2002; Lucente 2000; Shelley, 1995). Thrombocytopenia, ascites, pulmonary deterioration, and renal and hepatic failure have been reported in premature neonates after receiving parenteral products containing polysorbate 80 (Alade, 1986; CDC, 1984). See manufacturer's labeling.

OTC products: Swallowing should be minimized with topical products (eg, creams, gels, rinses). OTC products are generally not recommended for use in children <6 years of age unless as directed by a health care provider.

Warnings: Additional Pediatric Considerations Supervise children <12 years of age using topical fluoride products, especially children <6 years old, to prevent repeated swallowing; swallowing should be minimized with topical products (eg, creams, gels, rinses).

Some dosage forms may contain propylene glycol; in neonates, large amounts of propylene glycol delivered orally, intravenously (eg, >3,000 mg/day), or topically have been associated with potentially fatal toxicities which can include metabolic acidosis, seizures, renal failure, and CNS depression; toxicities have also been reported in children and adults including hyperosmolality, lactic acidosis, seizures, and respiratory depression; use caution (AAP 1997; Shehab 2009).

Drug Interactions

Metabolism/Transport Effects None known.

Avoid Concomitant Use There are no known interactions where it is recommended to avoid concomitant use.

Increased Effect/Toxicity There are no known significant interactions involving an increase in effect.

Decreased Effect There are no known significant interactions involving a decrease in effect.

Dietary Considerations Do not administer with dairy products.

Dietary adequate intake (AI) (IOM 1997):

1 to 6 months: 0.01 mg/day; additional supplementation is not recommended in infants <6 months of age.

7 to 12 months: 0.5 mg/day.

1 to 3 years: 0.7 mg/day.

4 to 8 years: 1 mg/day.

9 to 13 years: 2 mg/day.

14 to 18 years: 3 mg/day.

Pregnancy Risk Factor B

Pregnancy Considerations Fluoride crosses the placenta and can be found in the fetal circulation (IOM, 1997). Adverse events have not been observed in animal reproduction studies; epidemiological studies in areas with high levels of fluorinated water have not shown an increase in adverse effects. Heavy exposure *in utero* may be linked to skeletal fluorosis seen later in childhood.

Breastfeeding Considerations Low concentrations of fluoride can be found in breast milk and the amount is not significantly affected by supplementation or concentrations in drinking water (IOM, 1997). The manufacturer recommends that caution be exercised when administering fluoride to nursing women.

Dosage Forms: US

Cream, oral:

Denta 5000 Plus: 1.1% (51 g)

PreviDent 5000 Plus: 1.1% (51 g)

Gel, oral:

PreviDent 5000 Booster Plus: 1.1% (100 mL)

PreviDent 5000 Dry Mouth: 1.1% (100 mL)

Generic: 1.1% (56 g)

Gel, topical:

DentaGel: 1.1% (56 g)

Gel-Kam [OTC]: 0.4% (122 g)

Just For Kids [OTC]: 0.4% (122 g)

NeutraCare: 1.1% (60 g)

Omni Gel [OTC]: 0.4% (122 g); 0.4% (122 g)

PreviDent: 1.1% (56 g)

Paste, oral:

Clinpro 5000: 1.1% (113 g)

Fluoridex: 1.1% (112 g)

Fluoridex Enhanced Whitening: 1.1% (112 g)

parodontax [OTC]: 0.454% (96.4 g)

Sensodyne Repair & Protect [OTC]: 0.454% (96.4 g)

Solution, oral:

Act [OTC]: 0.05% (532 mL)

Act Kids [OTC]: 0.05% (500 mL, 532 mL)

Act Restoring [OTC]: 0.02% (1000 mL); 0.05% (532 mL)

Act Total Care [OTC]: 0.05% (90 mL, 532 mL, 1000 mL)

Fluorabon: 0.55 mg/0.6 mL (60 mL)

Fluoridex Daily Renewal: 0.63% (248 mL)

Fluorinse: 0.2% (480 mL)

Fluoritab: 0.275 mg/drop

Flura-Drops: 0.55 mg/drop (24 mL)

Gel-Kam Rinse: 0.63% (300 mL)

OrthoWash: 0.044% (480 mL)

PerioMed: 0.63% (284 mL)

Phos-Flur Rinse [OTC]: 0.044% (473 mL, 500 mL)

PreviDent: 0.2% (473 mL)

StanGard Perio: 0.63% (284 mL)

Tablet, chewable, oral:

Fluoritab: 1.1 mg, 2.2 mg

Generic: 0.55 mg, 1.1 mg, 2.2 mg

Dental Health Professional Considerations Neutral pH fluoride preparations are preferred in patients with oral mucositis to reduce tissue irritation; long-term use of acidulated fluorides has been associated with enamel demineralization and damage to porcelain crowns

◆ **Fluoridex** *see* Fluoride *on page 693*

◆ **Fluoridex Daily Renewal** *see* Fluoride *on page 693*

◆ **Fluoridex Enhanced Whitening** *see* Fluoride *on page 693*

◆ **Fluorinse** *see* Fluoride *on page 693*

◆ **Fluoritab** *see* Fluoride *on page 693*

◆ **5-Fluorocytosine** *see* Flucytosine *on page 682*

◆ **Fluorodeoxyuridine** *see* Floxuridine *on page 673*

◆ **9α-Fluorohydrocortisone Acetate** *see* Fludrocortisone *on page 683*

Fluorometholone (flure oh METH oh lone)

Brand Names: US Flarex; FML; FML Forte; FML Liquifilm

Brand Names: Canada Flarex; FML; PMS-Fluorometholone [DSC]; SANDOZ Fluorometholone

Pharmacologic Category Corticosteroid, Ophthalmic

Use Ocular inflammation: Treatment of steroid-responsive inflammation of the palpebral and bulbar conjunctiva, cornea, and anterior segment of the eye

Local Anesthetic/Vasoconstrictor Precautions No information available to require special precautions

Effects on Dental Treatment No significant effects or complications reported

Effects on Bleeding No information available to require special precautions

Adverse Reactions Frequency not defined.

Dermatologic: Skin rash

Endocrine & metabolic: Hypercorticoidism (rare)

Gastrointestinal: Dysgeusia

Hypersensitivity: Hypersensitivity reaction

Ophthalmic: Bacterial eye infection (secondary), blurred vision, burning sensation of eyes, cataract, decreased visual acuity, erythema of eyelid, eye discharge, eye irritation, eyelid edema, eye pain, eye pruritus, foreign body sensation of eye, fungal eye infection (secondary), glaucoma, increased intraocular pressure, increased lacrimation, optic nerve damage, stinging of eyes, swelling of eye, viral eye infection (secondary), visual field defect, wound healing impairment

Mechanism of Action Corticosteroids inhibit the inflammatory response including edema, capillary dilation, leukocyte migration, and scar formation. Fluorometholone penetrates cells readily to induce the production of lipocortins. These proteins modulate the activity of prostaglandins and leukotrienes.

Pregnancy Considerations

Adverse events were observed in animal reproduction studies following use of ophthalmic fluorometholone. The extent of systemic absorption following topical application of the ophthalmic drops is not known. If ophthalmic agents are needed during pregnancy, the minimum effective dose should be used in combination with punctal occlusion to decrease potential exposure to the fetus (Samples 1988).

◆ **Fluoro Uracil** *see* Fluorouracil (Systemic) *on page 696*

◆ **5-Fluorouracil** *see* Fluorouracil (Systemic) *on page 696*

Fluorouracil (Systemic) (flure oh YOOR a sil)

Brand Names: US Adrucil [DSC]

Pharmacologic Category Antineoplastic Agent, Antimetabolite; Antineoplastic Agent, Antimetabolite (Pyrimidine Analog)

Use

Breast cancer: Management of breast cancer

Colon and rectal cancer: Management of colon and rectal cancer

Gastric cancer: Management of stomach (gastric) cancer

Pancreatic cancer: Management of pancreatic cancer

Guideline recommendations: American Society of Clinical Oncology:

Potentially curable pancreatic cancer: American Society of Clinical Oncology (ASCO) guidelines (ASCO [Khorana 2019]) recommend fluorouracil as part of the modified FOLFIRINOX regimen (fluorouracil, leucovorin, oxaliplatin, and irinotecan), as the preferred adjuvant therapy in patients without concerns for toxicity or tolerance, and in the absence of medical or surgical contraindications. Alternatively, if there are concerns of toxicity or tolerance, fluorouracil (plus leucovorin calcium) is an option that may be offered.

Locally advanced, unresectable pancreatic cancer: According to the ASCO guidelines for locally advanced, unresectable pancreatic cancer (ASCO [Balaban 2016]), induction with ≥6 months of initial systemic therapy (with a combination regimen) is recommended in patients with an Eastern Cancer Cooperative Group (ECOG) performance status of 0 or 1, a favorable comorbidity profile, a preference for aggressive therapy, and a suitable support system; there is no clear evidence to encourage one regimen over another. If disease progression occurs, treatment according to guidelines for metastatic pancreatic cancer should be offered.

Metastatic pancreatic cancer: ASCO guidelines (ASCO [Sohal 2018]) recommend the FOLFIRINOX regimen (fluorouracil, leucovorin, oxaliplatin, and irinotecan) as first-line therapy in patients with an ECOG performance status of 0 or 1, a favorable comorbidity profile, a preference for aggressive therapy, a suitable support system, and access to a chemotherapy port/infusion pump management service. For patients who received an alternative first-line therapy and meet the above criteria, preferred second-line therapy includes fluorouracil in combination with irinotecan (liposomal) or conventional irinotecan (if liposomal irinotecan is unavailable), or fluorouracil in combination with oxaliplatin may also be considered. For patients with a performance status of 2 or with comorbidities, fluorouracil (with leucovorin) may be considered as an option for second-line therapy.

Local Anesthetic/Vasoconstrictor Precautions No information available to require special precautions

Effects on Dental Treatment Key adverse event(s) related to dental treatment: Stomatitis.

Effects on Bleeding Thrombocytopenia and anemia can occur during systemic therapy.

Adverse Reactions Frequency not defined. Toxicity depends on duration of treatment and/or rate of administration.

Cardiovascular: Angina pectoris, cardiac arrhythmia, cardiac failure, cerebrovascular accident, ischemic heart disease, local thrombophlebitis, myocardial infarction, vasospasm, ventricular ectopy

Central nervous system: Cerebellar syndrome (acute), confusion, disorientation, euphoria, headache

Dermatologic: Alopecia, changes in nails (including nail loss), dermatitis, hyperpigmentation (supravenous), maculopapular rash (pruritic), palmar-plantar erythrodysesthesia, skin fissure, skin photosensitivity, Stevens-Johnson syndrome, toxic epidermal necrolysis, xeroderma

Gastrointestinal: Anorexia, diarrhea, esophagopharyngitis, gastrointestinal hemorrhage, gastrointestinal ulcer, mesenteric ischemia (acute), nausea, stomatitis, tissue sloughing (gastrointestinal), vomiting

Hematologic & oncologic: Agranulocytosis, anemia, leukopenia (nadir: days 9 to 14; recovery by day 30), pancytopenia, thrombocytopenia

Hypersensitivity: Anaphylaxis, hypersensitivity reaction (generalized)

Ophthalmic: Lacrimal stenosis, lacrimation, nystagmus, photophobia, visual disturbance

Respiratory: Epistaxis

<1%, postmarketing, and/or case reports: Dysgeusia (Syed 2016)

Mechanism of Action Fluorouracil is a pyrimidine analog antimetabolite that interferes with DNA and RNA synthesis; after activation, F-UMP (an active metabolite) is incorporated into RNA to replace uracil and inhibit cell growth; the active metabolite F-dUMP, inhibits thymidylate synthetase, depleting thymidine triphosphate (a necessary component of DNA synthesis).

Pharmacodynamics/Kinetics

Half-life Elimination Following bolus infusion: 8 to 20 minutes

Reproductive Considerations

Females of reproductive potential and males with female partners of reproductive potential should use effective contraception during treatment and for 3 months following cessation of fluorouracil therapy.

Pregnancy Risk Factor D

Pregnancy Considerations

Based on the mechanism of action, fluorouracil may cause fetal harm if administered during pregnancy.

Chemotherapy, if indicated, may be administered to pregnant women with breast cancer as part of a combination chemotherapy regimen (common regimens administered during pregnancy include doxorubicin [or epirubicin], cyclophosphamide, and fluorouracil); chemotherapy should not be administered during the first trimester, after 35 weeks' gestation, or within 3 weeks of planned delivery (Amant 2010; Loibl 2006). The European Society for Medical Oncology has published guidelines for diagnosis, treatment, and follow-up of cancer during pregnancy. The guidelines recommend referral to a facility with expertise in cancer during pregnancy and encourage a multidisciplinary team (obstetrician, neonatologist, oncology team). In general, if chemotherapy is indicated, it should be avoided during in the first trimester, there should be a 3-week time period between the last chemotherapy dose and anticipated delivery, and chemotherapy should not be administered beyond week 33 of gestation (Peccatori 2013).

- ◆ **Fluorouridine deoxyribose** *see* Floxuridine *on page 673*
- ◆ **Fluouracil** *see* Fluorouracil (Systemic) *on page 696*

FLUoxetine (floo OKS e teen)

Related Information

Clinical Risk Related to Drugs Prolonging QT Interval *on page 1675*

Management of the Patient With Anxiety or Depression *on page 1778*

Vasoconstrictor Interactions With Antidepressants *on page 1821*

Brand Names: US PROzac; PROzac Weekly [DSC]; Sarafem

Brand Names: Canada ACCEL-FLUoxetine [DSC]; ACH-FLUoxetine; ACT FLUoxetine; AG-Fluoxetine; APO-FLUoxetine; Auro-FLUoxetine; BCI FLUoxetine [DSC]; BIO-FLUoxetine; DOM-FLUoxetine; JAMP-FLUoxetine; Mar-FLUoxetine [DSC]; MINT-FLUoxetine; MYLAN-FLUoxetine [DSC]; Odan-FLUoxetine; PHL-FLUoxetine [DSC]; PMS-FLUoxetine; PRIVA-FLUoxetine; PRO-FLUoxetine; PROzac; RAN-FLUoxetine; RIVA-FLUoxetine; SANDOZ FLUoxetine; TEVA-FLUoxetine; VAN-FLUoxetine [DSC]

Pharmacologic Category Antidepressant, Selective Serotonin Reuptake Inhibitor

Use

Bipolar major depression (excluding Sarafem): Acute treatment of major depressive episodes (in combination with olanzapine [preferred], other antipsychotics, or antimanic agents) (WFSBP [Grunze 2010]) associated with bipolar I disorder

Bulimia nervosa (excluding Sarafem): Acute and maintenance treatment of binge eating and vomiting behaviors in patients with moderate to severe bulimia nervosa

Major depressive disorder (unipolar) (excluding Sarafem): Acute and maintenance treatment of unipolar major depressive disorder (MDD)

Obsessive-compulsive disorder (excluding Sarafem): Acute and maintenance treatment of obsessions and compulsions in patients with obsessive-compulsive disorder

Panic disorder (excluding Sarafem): Acute treatment of panic disorder with or without agoraphobia

Premenstrual dysphoric disorder (Sarafem only): Treatment of premenstrual dysphoric disorder

Treatment-resistant depression (excluding Sarafem): Acute treatment of treatment-resistant depression (patients with MDD who do not respond to 2 separate trials of different antidepressants of adequate dose and duration in the current episode) in combination with olanzapine or other antipsychotics (APA 2010)

Local Anesthetic/Vasoconstrictor Precautions Although caution should be used in patients taking tricyclic antidepressants, no interactions have been reported with vasoconstrictors and fluoxetine, a nontricyclic antidepressant which acts to increase serotonin; no precautions appear to be needed. Fluoxetine is one of the drugs confirmed to prolong the QT interval and is accepted as having a risk of causing torsade de pointes. The risk of drug-induced torsade de pointes is extremely low when a single QT interval prolonging drug is prescribed. In terms of epinephrine, it is not known what effect vasoconstrictors in the local anesthetic regimen will have in patients with a known history of congenital prolonged QT interval or in patients taking any medication that prolongs the QT interval. Until more information is obtained, it is suggested that the clinician consult with the physician prior to the use of a vasoconstrictor in suspected patients, and that the vasoconstrictor (epinephrine, mepivacaine and levonordefrin [Carbocaine 2% with Neo-Cobefrin]) be used with caution.

Effects on Dental Treatment Key adverse event(s) related to dental treatment: Xerostomia (normal salivary flow resumes upon discontinuation) and taste perversion. Problems with SSRI-induced bruxism have been reported and may preclude their use. Clinicians attempting to evaluate any patient with bruxism or involuntary muscle movement, who is simultaneously being treated with an SSRI drug, should be aware of this potential association (see Effects on Bleeding and Dental Health Professional Considerations)

Effects on Bleeding Selective serotonin reuptake inhibitors such as fluoxetine may impair platelet aggregation due to platelet serotonin depletion, possibly increasing the risk of a bleeding complication. The risk of a bleeding complication can be increased by coadministration of other antiplatelet agents such as NSAIDs and aspirin.

Adverse Reactions As reported in adults, unless otherwise noted.

>10%:

Central nervous system: Insomnia (10% to 33%), headache (21%), drowsiness (5% to 17%), anxiety (6% to 15%), nervousness (8% to 14%), yawning (≤11%)

Endocrine & metabolic: Decreased libido (4% to 11%)

Gastrointestinal: Nausea (12% to 29%), diarrhea (8% to 18%), anorexia (4% to 17%), xerostomia (9% to 12%)

Neuromuscular & skeletal: Weakness (9% to 21%), tremor (3% to 13%)

Respiratory: Pharyngitis (10% to 11%)

1% to 10%:

Cardiovascular: Vasodilation (1% to 5%), palpitations (≥1%), prolonged QT interval on ECG (≥1%; QTcF ≥450 msec[3]), chest pain, hypertension

Central nervous system: Dizziness (9%), abnormal dreams (5%), agitation (children and adolescents: ≥2%), personality disorder (children and adolescents: ≥2%), abnormality in thinking (2%), chills (≥1%), emotional lability (≥1%), amnesia, confusion, sleep disorder

Dermatologic: Diaphoresis (7% to 8%), skin rash (4% to 6%), pruritus (3%)

Endocrine & metabolic: Hypermenorrhea (children and adolescents: ≥2%), increased thirst (children and adolescents: ≥2%), weight loss (2%), weight gain

Gastrointestinal: Dyspepsia (6% to 10%), constipation (5%), flatulence (3%), vomiting (3%), dysgeusia (≥1%), increased appetite

Genitourinary: Ejaculatory disorder (≤7%), impotence (≤7%), urinary frequency (children and adolescents: ≥2%), urination disorder (≥1%)

Neuromuscular & skeletal: Hyperkinesia (children and adolescents: ≥2%)

Ophthalmic: Visual disturbance (2%)
Otic: Otalgia, tinnitus
Respiratory: Flu-like symptoms (8% to 10%), sinusitis (5% to 6%), epistaxis (children and adolescents: ≥2%)

<1%, postmarketing, and/or case reports: Abnormal hepatic function tests, acne vulgaris, acute abdominal condition, akathisia, albuminuria, alopecia, amenorrhea, anaphylactoid reaction, anemia, angina pectoris, angle-closure glaucoma, aphthous stomatitis, aplastic anemia, arthritis, asthma, ataxia, atrial fibrillation, bruise, bruxism, bursitis, cardiac arrhythmia, cardiac failure, cataract, cerebrovascular accident, cholelithiasis, cholestatic jaundice, colitis, dehydration, delusions, depersonalization, dyskinesia, dysphagia, dysuria, ecchymoses, edema, eosinophilic pneumonitis, equilibrium disturbance, erythema multiforme, erythema nodosum, esophagitis, euphoria, exfoliative dermatitis, extrapyramidal reaction (rare), gastritis, gastroenteritis, gastrointestinal ulcer, glossitis, gout, gynecological bleeding, gynecomastia, hallucination, hemolytic anemia (immune-related), hepatic failure, hepatic necrosis, hepatitis, hiccups, hostility, hypercholesteremia, hyperprolactinemia, hypersensitivity reaction, hypertonia, hyperventilation, hypoglycemia, hypokalemia, hyponatremia (possibly in association with SIADH), hypotension, hypothyroidism, immune thrombocytopenia, laryngeal edema, laryngospasm, leg cramps, lupus-like syndrome, malaise, melena, memory impairment, migraine, mydriasis, myocardial infarction, myoclonus, neuroleptic malignant syndrome (Stevens 2008), optic neuritis, orthostatic hypotension, ostealgia, pancreatitis, pancytopenia, paranoia, petechia, priapism, pulmonary embolism, pulmonary fibrosis, pulmonary hypertension, purpuric rash, renal failure, serotonin syndrome, sexual disorder (may persist after discontinuation), skin photosensitivity, Stevens-Johnson syndrome, suicidal ideation, syncope, tachycardia, thrombocytopenia, toxic epidermal necrolysis, vasculitis, ventricular tachycardia (including torsades de pointes), violent behavior

Mechanism of Action Inhibits CNS neuron serotonin reuptake; minimal or no effect on reuptake of norepinephrine or dopamine; does not significantly bind to alpha-adrenergic, histamine, or cholinergic receptors

Pharmacodynamics/Kinetics

Onset of Action

Anxiety disorders (generalized anxiety, panic, obsessive-compulsive disorder, posttraumatic stress disorder): Initial effects may be observed within 2 weeks of treatment, with continued improvements through 4 to 6 weeks (Issari 2016; Varigonda 2016; WFSBP [Bandelow 2012]); some experts suggest up to 12 weeks of treatment may be necessary for response, particularly in patients with obsessive-compulsive disorder and posttraumatic stress disorder (BAP [Baldwin 2014]; Katzman 2014; WFSBP [Bandelow 2012]).

Body dysmorphic disorder: Initial effects may be observed within 2 weeks; some experts suggest up to 12 to 16 weeks of treatment may be necessary for response in some patients (Phillips 2008).

Depression: Initial effects may be observed within 1 to 2 weeks of treatment, with continued improvements through 4 to 6 weeks (Papakostas 2006; Posternak 2005; Szegedi 2009; Taylor 2006).

Premenstrual dysphoric disorder: Initial effects may be observed within the first few days of treatment, with response at the first menstrual cycle of treatment (ISPMD [Nevatte 2013]).

Half-life Elimination Adults: Parent drug: 1 to 3 days (acute), 4 to 6 days (chronic), 7.6 days (cirrhosis); Metabolite (norfluoxetine): 9.3 days (range: 4 to 16 days), 12 days (cirrhosis)

Time to Peak Serum: 6 to 8 hours

Reproductive Considerations

If treatment for major depressive disorder is initiated for the first time in females planning a pregnancy, agents other than fluoxetine are preferred (use of fluoxetine is not preferred in pregnant women) (Larsen 2015).

Selective serotonin reuptake inhibitors may be associated with male and female sexual dysfunction (WFSBP [Bauer 2013]). This may also be a manifestation of the psychiatric disorder. The actual risk associated with fluoxetine is not known. Fluoxetine is used off label for the treatment of premature ejaculation (Althof 2014; Siroosbakht 2019).

Pregnancy Considerations Fluoxetine and its metabolite cross the placenta.

Available studies evaluating teratogenic effects following maternal use of fluoxetine in the first trimester have shown inconsistent results. An increased risk of cardiovascular events was observed in one study; however, no specific pattern was observed and a causal relationship has not been established. Nonteratogenic effects in the newborn following selective serotonin reuptake inhibitor (SSRI)/serotonin–norepinephrine reuptake inhibitor (SNRI) exposure late in the third trimester include respiratory distress, cyanosis, apnea, seizures, temperature instability, feeding difficulty, vomiting, hypoglycemia, hypo- or hypertonia, hyper-reflexia, jitteriness, irritability, constant crying, and tremor. Prolonged hospitalization, respiratory support, or tube feedings may be required. Symptoms may be due to the toxicity of the SSRIs/SNRIs or a discontinuation syndrome and may be consistent with serotonin syndrome associated with SSRI treatment. Persistent pulmonary hypertension of the newborn has also been reported with SSRI exposure. The long-term effects of in utero SSRI exposure on infant development and behavior are not known (CANMAT [MacQueen 2016]).

Due to pregnancy-induced physiologic changes, some pharmacokinetic parameters of fluoxetine may be altered (Heikkinen 2003; Hostetter 2000; Kim 2006; Sit 2010). However, dose adjustments may only be needed if symptoms recur or worsen during pregnancy. If dosing is increased during pregnancy, a gradual taper to the prepregnancy range should be done postpartum (Betcher 2020; Schoretsanitis 2020; Sit 2010).

Untreated or inadequately treated psychiatric illness may lead to poor compliance with prenatal care. Therapy with antidepressants during pregnancy should be individualized (ACOG 92 2008; CANMAT [MacQueen 2016]). Psychotherapy or other nonmedication therapies may be considered for some women; however, antidepressant medication should be considered for pregnant women with moderate to severe major depressive disorder (APA 2010). If treatment for major depressive disorder is initiated for the first time during pregnancy, fluoxetine is not recommended (CANMAT [MacQueen 2016]; Larsen 2015; WFSBP [Bauer 2013]); fluoxetine is considered a third-line agent for the treatment of mild to moderate depression during pregnancy (CANMAT [MacQueen 2016]). If pregnancy occurs during fluoxetine therapy, a change in treatment is only recommended if it can be safely done in relation to maternal disease (Larsen 2015).

Data collection to monitor pregnancy and infant outcomes following exposure to antidepressants is ongoing. Pregnant women exposed to antidepressants during pregnancy are encouraged to enroll in the National Pregnancy Registry for Antidepressants (NPRAD). Women 18 to 45 years of age or their health care providers may contact the registry by calling 1-844-405-6185. Enrollment should be done as early in pregnancy as possible.

Dental Health Professional Considerations Problems with SSRI-induced bruxism have been reported and may preclude their use; clinicians attempting to evaluate any patient with bruxism or involuntary muscle movement, who is simultaneously being treated with an SSRI drug, should be aware of the potential association (see Local Anesthetic/Vasoconstrictor Precautions)

◆ **Fluoxetine Hydrochloride** *see* FLUoxetine *on page 697*

Fluoxymesterone (floo oks i MES te rone)

Brand Names: US Androxy [DSC]

Pharmacologic Category Androgen

Use

Breast cancer, metastatic (females): Salvage treatment of inoperable metastatic breast cancer in postmenopausal females.

Delayed puberty (males): Replacement therapy in the treatment of delayed male puberty.

Local Anesthetic/Vasoconstrictor Precautions No information available to require special precautions

Effects on Dental Treatment No significant effects or complications reported

Effects on Bleeding No information available to require special precautions

Adverse Reactions Frequency not defined.

Cardiovascular: Edema

Central nervous system: Anxiety, depression, headache, paresthesia

Dermatologic: Acne vulgaris, androgenetic alopecia

Endocrine & metabolic: Change in libido (decreased libido or increased libido), electrolyte disturbance (calcium, chloride, inorganic phosphate, potassium, and sodium retention), fluid retention, gynecomastia (males), hirsutism, hypercholesterolemia, menstrual disease (females; including amenorrhea)

Gastrointestinal: Gastrointestinal irritation, nausea, vomiting

Genitourinary: Benign prostatic hypertrophy (males), oligospermia (males; at higher doses), priapism (males), testicular atrophy (males), virilization (females; including clitoromegaly, deepening of the voice in females)

Hematologic & oncologic: Clotting factors suppression, polycythemia, prostate carcinoma (males)

Hepatic: Abnormal hepatic function tests, cholestatic jaundice, hepatic insufficiency

Hypersensitivity: Anaphylactoid reaction (non-immunologic anaphylaxis), hypersensitivity reaction

<1%, postmarketing, and/or case reports: Hepatic coma, hepatocellular neoplasm, hepatotoxicity (idiosyncratic; Chalasani 2014), peliosis hepatitis

Mechanism of Action Synthetic derivative of testosterone; responsible for the normal growth and development of male sex hormones, male sex organs, and maintenance of secondary sex characteristics; large doses suppress endogenous testosterone release

Pharmacodynamics/Kinetics

Half-life Elimination 10 hours (range: 10-100 minutes)

Reproductive Considerations

Use is contraindicated in women who may become pregnant.

Pregnancy Risk Factor X

Pregnancy Considerations

Use is contraindicated in women who are pregnant. May cause androgenic effects to the female fetus; clitoral hypertrophy, labial fusion, urogenital sinus defect, vaginal atresia, and ambiguous genitalia have been reported.

Product Availability Androxy has been discontinued in the US for more than 1 year.

Controlled Substance C-III

FluPHENAZine (floo FEN a zeen)

Brand Names: Canada APO-Fluphenazine [DSC]; FluPHENAZine Omega; Modecate Concentrate [DSC]; PMS-Fluphenazine; PMS-Fluphenazine Decanoate

Pharmacologic Category First Generation (Typical) Antipsychotic; Phenothiazine Derivative

Use

Psychotic disorders: For the management of manifestations of psychotic disorders; decanoate injection is intended for use in the management of patients requiring prolonged therapy.

Limitations of use: Fluphenazine has not been shown to be effective in the management of behavioral complications in patients with mental retardation.

Local Anesthetic/Vasoconstrictor Precautions No information available to require special precautions

Effects on Dental Treatment Key adverse event(s) related to dental treatment: Xerostomia and increased salivation (normal salivary flow resumes upon discontinuation); nasal congestion is possible; since the drug is a dopamine antagonist, extrapyramidal symptoms of the TMJ are a possibility. Patients may experience orthostatic hypotension as they stand up after treatment; especially if lying in dental chair for extended periods of time. Use caution with sudden changes in position during and after dental treatment.

Effects on Bleeding No information available to require special precautions

Adverse Reactions Frequency not defined.

Cardiovascular: Cardiac arrhythmia, edema, hypertension, hypotension, tachycardia, variable blood pressure

Central nervous system: Akathisia, bizarre dream, cerebral edema, depression, disruption of body temperature regulation, dizziness, drowsiness, dystonia, EEG pattern changes, excitement, headache, hyperreflexia, lethargy, neuroleptic malignant syndrome, Parkinsonian-like syndrome, restlessness, seizure, tardive dyskinesia

Dermatologic: Dermatitis, eczema, erythema, pruritus, seborrhea, skin photosensitivity, skin pigmentation, skin rash, urticaria

Endocrine & metabolic: Amenorrhea, change in libido, galactorrhea, gynecomastia, increased serum prolactin, menstrual disease, SIADH (syndrome of inappropriate antidiuretic hormone secretion), weight gain

Gastrointestinal: Anorexia, constipation, paralytic ileus, salivation, xerostomia

Genitourinary: Bladder paralysis, ejaculatory disorder, impotence, mastalgia, urinary incontinence
Hematologic & oncologic: Agranulocytosis, eosinophilia, leukopenia, nonthrombocytopenic purpura, pancytopenia, thrombocytopenia
Hepatic: Cholestatic jaundice, hepatotoxicity
Neuromuscular & skeletal: Muscle spasm (neck), systemic lupus erythematosus, tremor (fingers)
Ophthalmic: Blurred vision, corneal changes, glaucoma, lens disease, retinitis pigmentosa
Renal: Polyuria
Respiratory: Asthma, laryngeal edema, nasal congestion

Mechanism of Action Fluphenazine is a piperazine phenothiazine antipsychotic which blocks nonselectively postsynaptic mesolimbic dopaminergic D_2 receptors in the brain (Risch 1996); fluphenazine has limited activity on histaminergic, muscarinic and alpha receptors (Richelson 1999)

Pharmacodynamics/Kinetics

Onset of Action Decanoate: 24 to 72 hours; Peak effect: Decanoate: 48 to 96 hours

Duration of Action Decanoate: ~4 to 6 weeks

Half-life Elimination Derivative dependent: Hydrochloride: Oral: 14.4 to 16.4 hours (Dysken 1981; Koytchev 1996); Decanoate: ~14 days (Altamura 2003)

Time to Peak Serum: Hydrochloride: Oral: 2.8 hours (Koytchev 1996); Decanoate: 8 to 10 hours (Altamura 2003)

Pregnancy Considerations Antipsychotic use during the third trimester of pregnancy has a risk for abnormal muscle movements (extrapyramidal symptoms [EPS]) and withdrawal symptoms in newborns following delivery. Symptoms in the newborn may include agitation, feeding disorder, hypertonia, hypotonia, respiratory distress, somnolence, and tremor; these effects may be self-limiting or require hospitalization. The ACOG recommends that therapy during pregnancy be individualized; treatment with psychiatric medications during pregnancy should incorporate the clinical expertise of the mental health clinician, obstetrician, primary healthcare provider, and pediatrician (ACOG 2008).

◆ **Fluphenazine Decanoate** *see* FluPHENAZine *on page 699*

◆ **Fluphenazine HCl** *see* FluPHENAZine *on page 699*

◆ **Fluphenazine Hydrochloride** *see* FluPHENAZine *on page 699*

◆ **5-Fluracil** *see* Fluorouracil (Systemic) *on page 696*

◆ **Flura-Drops** *see* Fluoride *on page 693*

Flurandrenolide (flure an DREN oh lide)

Brand Names: US Cordran; Nolix

Pharmacologic Category Corticosteroid, Topical

Use Corticosteroid-responsive dermatoses: Relief of inflammatory and pruritic manifestations of corticosteroid-responsive dermatoses

Local Anesthetic/Vasoconstrictor Precautions No information available to require special precautions

Effects on Dental Treatment No significant effects or complications reported

Effects on Bleeding No information available to require special precautions

Adverse Reactions Frequency not defined.
Central nervous system: Burning sensation
Dermatologic: Acne vulgaris, acneiform eruptions, allergic contact dermatitis, atrophic striae, folliculitis, hypopigmentation, hypertrichosis, maceration of the skin, miliaria, perioral dermatitis, pruritus, skin atrophy, xeroderma
Infection: Secondary infection
Local: Local irritation
Postmarketing and/or case reports: Hypersensitivity, skin discoloration

Mechanism of Action Topical corticosteroids have anti-inflammatory, antipruritic, and vasoconstrictive properties. May depress the formation, release, and activity of endogenous chemical mediators of inflammation (kinins, histamine, liposomal enzymes, prostaglandins) through the induction of phospholipase A_2 inhibitory proteins (lipocortins) and sequential inhibition of the release of arachidonic acid. Flurandrenolide has intermediate range potency.

Pregnancy Risk Factor C

Pregnancy Considerations Adverse events have been observed with corticosteroids in animal reproduction studies. When topical corticosteroids are needed during pregnancy, low- to mid-potency preparations are preferred; higher-potency preparations should be used for the shortest time possible and fetal growth should be monitored (Chi 2011; Chi 2013). Topical products are not recommended for extensive use, in large quantities, or for long periods of time in pregnant women (Leachman 2006).

◆ **Flurandrenolone** *see* Flurandrenolide *on page 700*

Flurazepam (flure AZ e pam)

Related Information
Dentin Hypersensitivity, Acid Erosion, High Caries Index, Management of Alveolar Osteitis, and Xerostomia *on page 1762*

Brand Names: Canada BIO-Flurazepam; PMS-Flurazepam; Som-Pam

Pharmacologic Category Hypnotic, Benzodiazepine

Use Insomnia: For the treatment of insomnia characterized by difficulty in falling asleep, frequent nocturnal awakenings, and/or early-morning awakenings.

Local Anesthetic/Vasoconstrictor Precautions No information available to require special precautions

Effects on Dental Treatment Key adverse event(s) related to dental treatment: Xerostomia and changes in salivation (normal salivary flow resumes upon discontinuation), and bitter taste.

Effects on Bleeding No information available to require special precautions

Adverse Reactions Frequency not defined.
Cardiovascular: Chest pain, flushing, hypotension, palpitations, syncope
Central nervous system: Abnormal reflexes (slowing), apprehension, ataxia, bitter taste, body pain, confusion, depression, dizziness, drowsiness, drug dependence, dysarthria, euphoria, falling, hallucination, hangover effect, headache, irritability, memory impairment, nervousness, paradoxical reaction, restlessness, slurred speech, staggering, talkativeness
Dermatologic: Diaphoresis, pruritus, skin rash
Endocrine & metabolic: Weight gain, weight loss
Gastrointestinal: Constipation, decreased appetite, diarrhea, gastric distress, gastrointestinal pain, heartburn, increased appetite, nausea, sialorrhea, vomiting, xerostomia

Hematologic & oncologic: Granulocytopenia, leukopenia
Hepatic: Abnormal bilirubin levels (total bilirubin increased), cholestatic jaundice, increased serum alkaline phosphatase, increased serum ALT, increased serum AST
Neuromuscular & skeletal: Arthralgia, weakness
Ophthalmic: Accommodation disturbance, blurred vision, burning sensation of eyes
Respiratory: Apnea, dyspnea
<1%, postmarketing, and/or case reports: Anaphylaxis, angioedema, parasomnias (cooking while sleeping, making phone calls while sleeping, sleep driving, sleep eating)

Mechanism of Action Binds to stereospecific benzodiazepine receptors on the postsynaptic GABA neuron at several sites within the central nervous system, including the limbic system, reticular formation. Enhancement of the inhibitory effect of GABA on neuronal excitability results by increased neuronal membrane permeability to chloride ions. This shift in chloride ions results in hyperpolarization (a less excitable state) and stabilization. Benzodiazepine receptors and effects appear to be linked to the GABA-A receptors. Benzodiazepines do not bind to GABA-B receptors (Vinkers, 2012).

Pharmacodynamics/Kinetics

Half-life Elimination
Flurazepam: 2.3 hours
N-desalkylflurazepam:
Adults: Single dose: 74 to 90 hours; Multiple doses: 111 to 113 hours
Elderly (61 to 85 years): Single dose: 120 to 160 hours; Multiple doses: 126 to 158 hours

Time to Peak Flurazepam: 30 to 60 minutes; N-desalkylflurazepam: 10.6 hours (range: 7.6 to 13.6 hours); N-hydroxyethylflurazepam: ~1 hour (Greenblatt, 1989)

Pregnancy Risk Factor C

Pregnancy Considerations
All benzodiazepines are assumed to cross the placenta. Teratogenic effects have been observed with some benzodiazepines; however, additional studies are needed. The incidence of premature birth and low birth weights may be increased following maternal use of benzodiazepines; hypoglycemia and respiratory problems in the neonate may occur following exposure late in pregnancy. Neonatal withdrawal symptoms may occur within days to weeks after birth and "floppy infant syndrome" (which also includes withdrawal symptoms) has been reported with some benzodiazepines (Bergman 1992; Iqbal 2002; Wikner 2007). Neonatal depression has been observed, specifically following exposure to flurazepam when used maternally for 10 consecutive days prior to delivery. Serum levels of N-desalkylflurazepam were measurable in the infant during the first 4 days of life. Use of flurazepam during pregnancy is contraindicated.

Patients exposed to flurazepam during pregnancy are encouraged to enroll themselves into the North American Antiepileptic Drug (NAAED) Pregnancy Registry by calling 1-888-233-2334. Additional information is available at http://www.aedpregnancyregistry.org.

Controlled Substance C-IV

◆ **Flurazepam Hydrochloride** *see* Flurazepam *on page 700*

Flurbiprofen (Systemic) (flure BI proe fen)

Related Information
Rheumatoid Arthritis, Osteoarthritis, and Osteoporosis *on page 1697*
Temporomandibular Dysfunction (TMD), Chronic Pain, and Fibromyalgia *on page 1773*

Brand Names: Canada TEVA-Flurbiprofen

Pharmacologic Category Analgesic, Nonopioid; Nonsteroidal Anti-inflammatory Drug (NSAID), Oral

Use
Rheumatoid arthritis, osteoarthritis: Relief of the signs and symptoms of rheumatoid arthritis (RA) and osteoarthritis (OA)
Canadian labeling: Additional use (not in US labeling): Relief of signs and symptoms of ankylosing spondylitis; relief of pain associated with dysmenorrhea; relief of mild to moderate pain accompanied by inflammation (eg, bursitis, tendinitis, soft tissue trauma)

Local Anesthetic/Vasoconstrictor Precautions
No information available to require special precautions

Effects on Dental Treatment The dentist should be aware of the potential of abnormal coagulation. Caution should also be exercised in the use of NSAIDs in patients already on anticoagulant therapy with drugs such as warfarin (Coumadin®). See Effects on Bleeding.

Effects on Bleeding Nonselective NSAIDs such as flurbiprofen inhibit platelet aggregation and prolong bleeding time in some patients. Unlike aspirin, the NSAID effect on platelet function is quantitatively less, of shorter duration, and reversible.

Adverse Reactions Frequency not defined.
>1%:
Cardiovascular: Edema
Central nervous system: Amnesia, anxiety, depression, dizziness, drowsiness, headache, hyperreflexia, insomnia, malaise, nervousness, vertigo
Dermatologic: Skin rash
Endocrine & metabolic: Weight changes
Gastrointestinal: Abdominal pain, constipation, diarrhea, dyspepsia, flatulence, gastrointestinal bleeding, nausea, vomiting
Hepatic: Increased liver enzymes
Neuromuscular & skeletal: Tremor, weakness
Ophthalmic: Visual disturbance
Otic: Tinnitus
Respiratory: Rhinitis
<1%, postmarketing, and/or case reports: Altered sense of smell, anaphylaxis, anemia, angioedema, asthma, bruise, cardiac failure, cerebral ischemia, confusion, decreased hematocrit, decreased hemoglobin, eczema, eosinophilia, epistaxis, exfoliative dermatitis, fever, gastric ulcer, hematuria, hepatitis, hepatotoxicity (idiosyncratic; Chalasani 2014), hypertension, hyperuricemia, interstitial nephritis, jaundice, leukopenia, paresthesia, peptic ulcer, pruritus, purpura, renal failure, skin photosensitivity, stomatitis, thrombocytopenia, toxic epidermal necrolysis, urticaria, vasodilation

Mechanism of Action Reversibly inhibits cyclooxygenase-1 and 2 (COX-1 and 2) enzymes, which results in decreased formation of prostaglandin precursors; has antipyretic, analgesic, and anti-inflammatory properties

Other proposed mechanisms not fully elucidated (and possibly contributing to the anti-inflammatory effect to varying degrees), include inhibiting chemotaxis, altering lymphocyte activity, inhibiting neutrophil aggregation/activation, and decreasing proinflammatory cytokine levels.

Pharmacodynamics/Kinetics

Half-life Elimination 4.7 to 5.7 hours

Time to Peak ~2 hours

Reproductive Considerations

The chronic use of NSAIDs in women of reproductive age may be associated with infertility that is reversible upon discontinuation of the medication. Consider discontinuing use in women having difficulty conceiving or those undergoing investigation of fertility

Pregnancy Considerations Birth defects have been observed following in utero NSAID exposure in some studies; however, data is conflicting (Bloor 2013). Nonteratogenic effects, including prenatal constriction of the ductus arteriosus, persistent pulmonary hypertension of the newborn (PPHN), oligohydramnios, necrotizing enterocolitis, renal dysfunction or failure, and intracranial hemorrhage, have been observed in the fetus/neonate following in utero NSAID exposure. In addition, nonclosure of the ductus arteriosus postnatally may occur and be resistant to medical management (Bermas 2014; Bloor 2013). Because NSAIDs may cause premature closure of the ductus arteriosus, product labeling for flurbiprofen specifically states use should be avoided starting at 30 weeks' gestation.

Use of NSAIDs can be considered for the treatment of mild rheumatoid arthritis flares in pregnant women; however, use should be minimized or avoided early and late in pregnancy (Bermas 2014; Saavedra Salinas 2015).

The use of NSAIDs close to conception may be associated with an increased risk of miscarriage (Bermas 2014; Bloor 2013).

◆ **Flurbiprofen Sodium** *see* Flurbiprofen (Systemic) *on page 701*

◆ **5-Flurocytosine** *see* Flucytosine *on page 682*

Flutamide (FLOO ta mide)

Brand Names: Canada DOM-Flutamide; NU-Flutamide [DSC]; PMS-Flutamide; TEVA-Flutamide [DSC]

Pharmacologic Category Antineoplastic Agent, Antiandrogen

Use

Prostate cancer (metastatic): Management of locally confined Stage B_2 to C and Stage D_2 metastatic prostate cancer (in combination with a luteinizing hormone-releasing hormone [LHRH] agonist). For Stage B_2 to C prostate cancer, flutamide treatment (and goserelin) should start 8 weeks prior to initiating radiation therapy and continue during radiation therapy. To achieve treatment benefit in Stage D_2 metastatic prostate cancer, initiate flutamide with the LHRH agonist and continue until disease progression.

Guideline recommendations: The American Society of Clinical Oncology and Cancer Care Ontario clinical practice guideline for systemic therapy in men with metastatic castration-resistant prostate cancer suggests that data regarding the clinical benefit of older antiandrogens (including flutamide) are limited, and that older antiandrogen agents may be less efficacious compared to contemporary antiandrogen agents. However, older antiandrogen agents may be offered in patients with low prostate cancer disease burden or limited therapy options (ASCO [Basch 2014]).

Local Anesthetic/Vasoconstrictor Precautions

No information available to require special precautions

Effects on Dental Treatment No significant effects or complications reported

Effects on Bleeding Hemolytic anemia has been reported.

Adverse Reactions

>10%:

Endocrine & metabolic: Hot flash (46% to 61%), galactorrhea (9% to 42%), decreased libido (36%), increased lactate dehydrogenase (transient; mild)

Gastrointestinal: Diarrhea (12% to 40%), vomiting (11% to 12%)

Genitourinary: Impotence (33%), cystitis (16%), breast tenderness

Hematologic & oncologic: Rectal hemorrhage (14%), tumor flare

Hepatic: Increased serum AST (transient; mild)

1% to 10%:

Cardiovascular: Edema (4%), hypertension (1%)

Central nervous system: Anxiety, confusion, depression, dizziness, drowsiness, headache, insomnia, nervousness

Dermatologic: Skin rash (3% to 8%), ecchymoses, pruritus

Endocrine & metabolic: Gynecomastia (9%)

Gastrointestinal: Nausea (9%), proctitis (8%), gastric distress (4% to 6%), anorexia (4%), constipation, dyspepsia, increased appetite

Genitourinary: Hematuria (7%)

Hematologic & oncologic: Anemia (6%), leukopenia (3%), thrombocytopenia (1%)

Infection: Herpes zoster

Neuromuscular & skeletal: Weakness (1%)

<1%, postmarketing, and case reports: Cholestatic jaundice, hemolytic anemia, hepatic encephalopathy, hepatic failure, hepatic necrosis, hepatitis, hypersensitivity pneumonitis, increased blood urea nitrogen, increased gamma-glutamyl transferase, increased serum ALT, increased serum bilirubin, increased serum creatinine, jaundice, macrocytic anemia, malignant neoplasm of breast (male), methemoglobinemia, myocardial infarction, oligospermia, pulmonary embolism, skin photosensitivity, sulfhemoglobinemia, thrombophlebitis, urine discoloration (amber, yellow-green)

Mechanism of Action Flutamide is a nonsteroidal antiandrogen that inhibits androgen uptake and/or inhibits binding of androgen in target tissues.

Pharmacodynamics/Kinetics

Half-life Elimination ~6 hours (2-hydroxyflutamide [active metabolite])

Time to Peak ~2 hours (2-hydroxyflutamide [active metabolite])

Reproductive Considerations

Although flutamide is not indicated for use in females, it has been used off label for acne, hirsutism, polycystic ovary syndrome (PCOS), and female pattern hair loss in women. Due to the potential for serious toxicity and the availability of other treatment options, off-label use for these conditions is not recommended (Azarchi 2019; ES [Goodman 2015]); ES [Martin 2018]). Effective contraception is recommended if used in females for these conditions (Azarchi 2019).

Women treated with flutamide for PCOS may have a return of regular menses and ovulatory cycles (Paradisi 2013).

Pregnancy Risk Factor D

Pregnancy Considerations

Based on the mechanism of action and data from animal reproduction studies, in utero exposure to flutamide may cause fetal harm.

Fluticasone (Nasal) (floo TIK a sone)

Brand Names: US Flonase Allergy Relief [OTC]; Flonase Sensimist [OTC]; GoodSense Nasoflow [OTC] [DSC]; Ticaspray [DSC]; Veramyst [DSC]; Xhance

Brand Names: Canada APO-Fluticasone; Avamys; Flonase [DSC]; RATIO-Fluticasone; TEVA-Fluticasone

Pharmacologic Category Corticosteroid, Nasal

Use

Rx products:

Allergic rhinitis (Veramyst, Avamys [Canadian product], Flonase [Canadian product]): Management of seasonal and perennial allergic rhinitis in adults and children ≥2 years of age (Veramyst, Avamys) and in patients 4 to 17 years of age (Flonase)

Nasal polyps (Xhance): Treatment of nasal polyps in patients ≥18 years of age

Nonallergic rhinitis (Flonase): Management of the nasal symptoms of perennial nonallergic rhinitis in adults and pediatric patients ≥4 years of age

OTC products:

Upper respiratory allergies: Relief of hay fever or other upper respiratory allergies (eg, itchy and watery eyes, nasal congestion, runny nose, sneezing, itchy nose) in adults and children ≥4 years of age (Clarispray, Flonase Allergy Relief, Good Sense Nasoflow) or children ≥2 years of age (Flonase Sensimist)

Local Anesthetic/Vasoconstrictor Precautions
No information available to require special precautions

Effects on Dental Treatment No significant effects or complications reported

Effects on Bleeding No information available to require special precautions

Adverse Reactions

>10%: Central nervous system: Headache (4% to 16%)

1% to 10%:

Central nervous system: Body pain (1% to 3%), dizziness (1% to 3%), generalized ache (1% to 3%)

Endocrine & metabolic: Weight gain (1% to <3%)

Gastrointestinal: Nausea and vomiting (3% to 5%), abdominal pain (1% to 3%), diarrhea (1% to 3%), abdominal distress (1% to <3%), toothache (1% to <3%)

Local: Local irritation (nose: 4% to 6%)

Ophthalmic: Increased intraocular pressure (1% to <3%)

Respiratory: Epistaxis (6% to 12%), nasal mucosa ulcer (3% to 8%; includes nasal septal ulceration), pharyngitis (3% to 8%), nasopharyngitis (8%), acute asthma (7%), nasal congestion (6%), acute sinusitis (5%), cough (4%), blood in nasal mucosa (1% to 3%), bronchitis (1% to 3%), flu-like symptoms (1% to 3%), rhinorrhea (1% to 3%), dry nose (1% to <3%), oropharyngeal pain (1% to <3%), sinusitis (1% to <3%)

Miscellaneous: Fever (1% to 3%)

<1%, postmarketing, and/or case reports: Altered sense of smell, anaphylactoid reaction, anaphylaxis, angioedema, blurred vision, bronchospasm, cataract, conjunctivitis, contact dermatitis, dry eye syndrome, dry throat, dysgeusia, dyspnea, esophageal candidiasis, eye irritation, facial edema, glaucoma, growth suppression, hoarseness, hypersensitivity reaction, intestinal candidiasis, nasal candidiasis, nasal septum perforation, pharyngeal candidiasis, pruritus, skin rash, sore throat, throat irritation, tongue edema, urticaria, voice disorder, wheezing

Mechanism of Action Fluticasone belongs to a group of corticosteroids which utilizes a fluorocarbothioate ester linkage at the 17 carbon position; extremely potent vasoconstrictive and anti-inflammatory activity

Pharmacodynamics/Kinetics

Onset of Action Maximal benefit may take several days or several months (Xhance)

Half-life Elimination IV: Fluticasone propionate: ~8 hours (~7.8 hours [Xhance]); Fluticasone furoate: ~15 hours

Pregnancy Considerations

Fluticasone can be detected in cord blood following maternal use via oral inhalation during pregnancy; one woman in the study was also using intranasal fluticasone (Battista 2016).

Maternal use of intranasal corticosteroids in usual doses are not associated with an increased risk of fetal malformations or preterm birth (ERS/TSANZ [Middleton 2020]). Systemic absorption of fluticasone nasal is limited. Use of intranasal fluticasone is likely acceptable for the treatment of allergic rhinitis during pregnancy (Alhussien 2018; BSACI [Scadding 2017]; ERS/TSANZ [Middleton 2020]).

Fluticasone (Oral Inhalation) (floo TIK a sone)

Related Information

Respiratory Diseases *on page 1680*

Brand Names: US ArmonAir RespiClick 113 [DSC]; ArmonAir RespiClick 232 [DSC]; ArmonAir RespiClick 55 [DSC]; Arnuity Ellipta; Flovent Diskus; Flovent HFA

Brand Names: Canada Arnuity Ellipta; Flovent Diskus; Flovent HFA

Pharmacologic Category Corticosteroid, Inhalant (Oral)

Use

Asthma:

ArmonAir Digihaler, ArmonAir RespiClick, and Arnuity Ellipta: Maintenance treatment of asthma as prophylactic therapy in patients ≥5 years of age (Arnuity Ellipta) or ≥12 years of age (ArmonAir Digihaler and ArmonAir RespiClick).

Flovent Diskus and Flovent HFA: Maintenance treatment of asthma as prophylactic therapy in patients ≥4 years of age.

Limitations of use: Not indicated for relief of acute bronchospasm.

Local Anesthetic/Vasoconstrictor Precautions
No information available to require special precautions

Effects on Dental Treatment Key adverse event(s) related to dental treatment: Localized infections with *Candida albicans* or *Aspergillus niger* have occurred frequently in the mouth and pharynx with repetitive use of oral inhaler of corticosteroids. These infections may require treatment with appropriate antifungal therapy or discontinuance of treatment with corticosteroid inhaler.

Effects on Bleeding No information available to require special precautions

Adverse Reactions

>10%:

Central nervous system: Fatigue (≤16%), malaise (≤16%), headache (5% to 14%)

Gastrointestinal: Oral candidiasis (2% to 31%)

Neuromuscular & skeletal: Arthralgia (17%), musculoskeletal pain (3% to 12%)

Respiratory: Sinus infection (≤33%), sinusitis (≤33%), upper respiratory tract infection (6% to 31%), throat irritation (≤22%), nasal congestion (16%), rhinitis (3% to 13%)

1% to 10%:

Cardiovascular: Hypertension (<3%), subarachnoid hemorrhage (≤1%)

Central nervous system: Pain (10%), voice disorder (≤9%), dizziness (<3%)

Dermatologic: Skin rash (8%), pruritus (6%)

Gastrointestinal: Nausea and vomiting (8% to 9%), viral gastrointestinal infection (3% to 5%), gastrointestinal distress (≤4%), gastrointestinal pain (≤4%), oropharyngeal candidiasis (3%), toothache (3%), viral gastroenteritis (3%)

Hematologic & oncologic: Malignant neoplasm of breast (≤1%)

Infection: Viral infection (5%), influenza (<3%), abscess (≤1%)

Neuromuscular & skeletal: Muscle injury (2% to 5%), limb pain (<3%), muscle spasm (<3%), sprain (<3%)

Respiratory: Hoarseness (≤9%), cough (5% to 9%), viral respiratory tract infection (5% to 9%), nasopharyngitis (5% to 8%), bronchitis (2% to 8%), pharyngitis (4%), upper respiratory tract inflammation (2% to 5%), oropharyngeal pain (3%), epistaxis (<3%), respiratory tract infection (<3%)

Miscellaneous: Fever (≤7%), accidental injury (2% to 5%)

Frequency not defined:

Cardiovascular: Edema, palpitations

Central nervous system: Migraine, mood disorder, mouth pain

Dermatologic: Acne vulgaris, dermatitis, dermatologic disorders, eczema, folliculitis, photodermatitis, viral skin infection

Endocrine & metabolic: Cushingoid appearance, fluid volume disorder, weight gain

Gastrointestinal: Change in appetite, diarrhea, dyspepsia, gastrointestinal signs and symptoms, oral mucosal erythema, oral mucosa ulcer, oral rash, tongue disease

Genitourinary: Urinary tract infection

Hematologic & oncologic: Polyp (ENT)

Infection: Bacterial infection, bacterial reproductive infection, fungal infection

Ophthalmic: Blepharoconjunctivitis, conjunctivitis, keratitis

Respiratory: Allergic rhinitis, constriction of the pharynx, ENT signs and symptoms, laryngitis, rhinorrhea

Miscellaneous: Soft tissue injury, swelling

<1%, postmarketing, and/or case reports: Aggressive behavior, agitation, allergic skin reaction, anaphylaxis, angioedema, anxiety, aphonia, behavioral changes, blurred vision, bronchospasm, bruise, cataract, chest symptoms, chest tightness, decreased linear skeletal growth rate, dental caries, dental discomfort, depression, dyspnea, ecchymoses, esophageal candidiasis, exacerbation of asthma, facial edema, gastrointestinal disease, glaucoma, hyperactive behavior, hyperglycemia, hypersensitivity reaction, increased intraocular pressure, irritability, mouth disease, oropharyngeal edema, osteoporosis, paradoxical bronchospasm, pneumonia, restlessness, retinopathy (central serous), sore throat, staining of tooth, type IV hypersensitivity reaction, wheezing

Mechanism of Action Fluticasone belongs to a group of corticosteroids which utilizes a fluorocarbothioate ester linkage at the 17 carbon position; extremely potent vasoconstrictive and anti-inflammatory activity. The effectiveness of inhaled fluticasone is due to its direct local effect.

Pharmacodynamics/Kinetics

Onset of Action Maximal benefit may take 1 to 2 weeks or longer

Half-life Elimination IV: ~8 hours; Oral inhalation: Fluticasone furoate: 24 hours (plasma elimination phase following repeat dosing); Fluticasone propionate: ~11.2 hours (terminal half-life).

Time to Peak 0.5 to 1 hour

Pregnancy Considerations

Fluticasone can be detected in cord blood following maternal use via oral inhalation during pregnancy (Battista 2016).

Maternal use of inhaled corticosteroids (ICS) in usual doses is not associated with an increased risk of fetal malformations; a small risk of malformations was observed in one study following high maternal doses of an alternative ICS. Uncontrolled asthma is associated with adverse events in pregnancy (increased risk of perinatal mortality, preeclampsia, preterm birth, low birth weight infants, cesarean delivery, and the development of gestational diabetes). Poorly controlled asthma or asthma exacerbations may have a greater fetal/maternal risk than what is associated with appropriately used asthma medications. Maternal treatment improves pregnancy outcomes by reducing the risk of some adverse events (eg, preterm birth, gestational diabetes) (ERS/TSANZ [Middleton 2020]; GINA 2020).

ICS are recommended for the treatment of asthma during pregnancy (GINA 2020). Fluticasone oral inhalation is considered compatible for use during pregnancy. Pregnant females adequately controlled on fluticasone for asthma may continue therapy; if initiating treatment during pregnancy, use of an agent with more data in pregnant females may be preferred. The lowest dose that maintains asthma control should be used. Maternal asthma symptoms should be monitored monthly during pregnancy (ERS/TSANZ [Middleton 2020]).

Data collection to monitor pregnancy and infant outcomes associated with asthma and the medications used to treat asthma in pregnancy is ongoing. Health care providers are encouraged to enroll exposed pregnant females in the MotherToBaby Pregnancy Studies conducted by the Organization of Teratology Information Specialists (877-311-8972 or https://mothertobaby.org). Patients may also enroll themselves.

Product Availability

ArmonAir Digihaler: FDA approved February 2020; anticipated availability currently unknown. Consult the prescribing information for additional information.

ArmonAir RespiClick has been discontinued in the United States for >1 year.

Fluticasone and Salmeterol

(floo TIK a sone & sal ME te role)

Related Information

Fluticasone (Oral Inhalation) *on page 703*

Salmeterol *on page 1355*

Brand Names: US Advair Diskus; Advair HFA; AirDuo RespiClick; Wixela Inhub

Brand Names: Canada Advair; Advair Diskus

Pharmacologic Category $Beta_2$ Agonist; $Beta_2$-Adrenergic Agonist, Long-Acting; Corticosteroid, Inhalant (Oral)

Use

Asthma: Treatment of asthma in patients ≥4 years of age (Advair Diskus, Wixela Inhub) and in patients ≥12 years of age (Advair HFA, AirDuo Digihaler, AirDuo RespiClick).

Chronic obstructive pulmonary disease (Advair Diskus and Wixela Inhub only): Maintenance treatment of airflow obstruction in patients with chronic obstructive pulmonary disease (COPD), including chronic bronchitis and/or emphysema. Fluticasone 250 mcg/salmeterol 50 mcg is also indicated to reduce exacerbations of COPD in patients with a history of exacerbations.

Fluticasone 250 mcg/salmeterol 50 mcg (Advair Diskus, Wixela Inhub) twice daily is the only approved dosage for the treatment of COPD because an efficacy advantage of the higher strength fluticasone 500 mcg/salmeterol 50 mcg over fluticasone 250 mcg/salmeterol 50 mcg has not been demonstrated.

Limitations of use: Fluticasone/salmeterol is not indicated for the relief of acute bronchospasm.

Local Anesthetic/Vasoconstrictor Precautions No information available to require special precautions

Effects on Dental Treatment Key adverse event(s) related to dental treatment: Localized infections with *Candida albicans* or *Aspergillus niger* have occurred frequently in the mouth and pharynx with repetitive use of oral inhaler of corticosteroids. These infections may require treatment with appropriate antifungal therapy or discontinuance of treatment with corticosteroid inhaler.

Effects on Bleeding No information available to require special precautions

Adverse Reactions Adverse reactions occur in adults and adolescents unless otherwise specified.

>10%:

Central nervous system: Headache (5% to 21%)

Respiratory: Upper respiratory tract infection (16% to 27%), pneumonia (4% to 18%; higher incidence is associated with older adults), pharyngitis (≤13%)

1% to 10%:

Cardiovascular: Cardiac arrhythmia (1% to 3%), myocardial infarction (1% to 3%), tachycardia (1% to 3%), palpitations (<3%)

Central nervous system: Voice disorder (≤5%), dizziness (≤4%), migraine (1% to 3%), sleep disorder (1% to 3%)

Dermatologic: Dermatitis (1% to 3%), dermatologic disease (1% to 3%; includes dermatosis and disorder of sweat and sebum), eczema (1% to 3%), contact dermatitis (<3%), pruritus (1%)

Endocrine & metabolic: Weight gain (1% to 3%)

Gastrointestinal: Oral candidiasis (1% to 10%; including mouth and throat infections), nausea and vomiting (4% to 6%), nausea (>5%), gastrointestinal distress (≤4%), viral gastrointestinal infection (3% to 4%), diarrhea (2% to 4%), abdominal distress (1% to 3%), abdominal pain (1% to 3%), dental discomfort (1% to 3%), dental disease (disorder of hard tissue of teeth: 1% to 3%), gastrointestinal infection (1% to 3%), infection of mouth (unspecified oropharyngeal plaque: 1% to 3%), toothache (1% to 3%), xerostomia (1% to 3%), dyspepsia (<3%), upper abdominal pain (<3%)

Genitourinary: Genitourinary infection (1% to 3%), urinary tract infection (1% to 3%)

Hypersensitivity: Hypersensitivity reaction (1% to 3%; can be immediate or delayed), local ocular hypersensitivity (1% to 3%)

Infection: Candidiasis (3%), bacterial infection (1% to 3%), viral infection (1% to 3%), influenza (<3%)

Neuromuscular & skeletal: Musculoskeletal pain (4% to 7%), myalgia (≤4%), back pain (3%), arthralgia (1% to 3%), arthritis (1% to 3%), muscle injury (1% to 3%), muscle spasm (1% to 3%), ostealgia (1% to 3%), skeletal muscle disease (inflammation: 1% to 3%), skeletal pain (1% to 3%), limb pain (<3%), muscle cramps (≤3%)

Ophthalmic: Ocular edema (1% to 3%)

Otic: Ear sign or symptom (1% to 3%)

Respiratory: Throat irritation (8% to 9%; children: ≥3%), nasopharyngitis (5% to 9%), bronchitis (8%), upper respiratory tract inflammation (4% to 7%; includes upper respiratory tract irritation), cough (4% to 6%), viral respiratory tract infection (4% to 6%), hoarseness (≤5%), sinusitis (≤5%), ENT infection (children: ≥3%), dry nose (1% to 3%), epistaxis (1% to 3%), laryngitis (1% to 3%), lower respiratory signs and symptoms (1% to 3%), lower respiratory tract infection (1% to 3%), postnasal drip (1% to 3%), respiratory tract hemorrhage (lower respiratory tract: 1% to 3%), nasal congestion (≤3%), allergic rhinitis (<3%), oropharyngeal pain (<3%), respiratory tract infection (<3%), rhinitis (<3%), rhinorrhea (1% to 3%)

Miscellaneous: Fever (4%), inflammation (1% to 3%), laceration (1% to 3%), postoperative complication (1% to 3%), soft tissue injury (1% to 3%), wound (1% to 3%)

Frequency not defined:

Cardiovascular: Edema

Central nervous system: Hypertonia, mouth pain, pain

Dermatologic: Acquired ichthyosis, exfoliation of skin, viral skin infection

Endocrine & metabolic: Fluid retention, hyperglycemia, hypothyroidism

Gastrointestinal: Dysgeusia, oral discomfort, oral lesion, oral mucosa ulcer

Hematologic & oncologic: Hematoma, lymphadenopathy

Hepatic: Increased liver enzymes (incidence may be higher in children but were transient)

Neuromuscular & skeletal: Bone fracture, connective tissue disease (cartilage disorder), muscle rigidity

Ophthalmic: Conjunctivitis, eye infection, keratitis, xerophthalmia

Respiratory: Nasal signs and symptoms, paranasal sinus disease

<1%, postmarketing, and/or case reports: Abnormal hepatic function tests, aggressive behavior, agitation, anaphylaxis, angioedema, anxiety, aphonia, asthma, atrial fibrillation, behavioral changes, blurred vision, bronchospasm (may be immediate), bruise, cataract, chest congestion, chest tightness, choking sensation, cushingoid appearance, Cushing syndrome, decreased linear skeletal growth rate, depression, dysmenorrhea, dyspnea, ecchymoses, esophageal candidiasis, exacerbation of asthma (can be serious), extrasystoles, facial edema, glaucoma, hyperactivity,

hypercorticoidism, hypertension, irregular menses, irritability, laryngeal edema, laryngospasm, myositis, oropharyngeal edema, osteoporosis, otalgia, pallor, paradoxical bronchospasm, paresthesia, pelvic inflammatory disease, photodermatitis, restlessness, retinopathy (central serous), sinus pain, skin rash, sore throat, stridor, supraventricular tachycardia, syncope, tonsillitis, tracheitis, upper airway swelling, vaginitis, ventricular tachycardia, vulvovaginal candidiasis, vulvovaginitis, wheezing

Mechanism of Action Combination of fluticasone (corticosteroid) and salmeterol (long-acting beta$_2$-agonist) designed to improve pulmonary function and control over what is produced by either agent when used alone. Because fluticasone and salmeterol act locally in the lung, plasma levels do not predict therapeutic effect.

Fluticasone: The mechanism of action for all topical corticosteroids is believed to be a combination of three important properties: Anti-inflammatory activity, immunosuppressive properties, and antiproliferative actions. Fluticasone has extremely potent vasoconstrictive and anti-inflammatory activity.

Salmeterol: Relaxes bronchial smooth muscle by selective action on beta$_2$-receptors with little effect on heart rate

Pregnancy Considerations

Adverse events were observed in animal reproduction studies using this combination. Refer to individual agents.

Product Availability AirDuo Digihaler: FDA approved July 2019; availability anticipated in 2020. Consult the prescribing information for additional information.

Fluticasone and Vilanterol

(floo TIK a sone & VYE lan ter ol)

Brand Names: US Breo Ellipta

Brand Names: Canada Breo Ellipta

Pharmacologic Category Beta$_2$ Agonist; Beta$_2$-Adrenergic Agonist, Long-Acting; Corticosteroid, Inhalant (Oral)

Use

Asthma: Treatment of asthma in patients ≥18 years.

Chronic obstructive pulmonary disease: Maintenance treatment of airflow obstruction in patients with chronic obstructive pulmonary disease (COPD), including chronic bronchitis and/or emphysema; to reduce exacerbations of COPD in patients with a history of exacerbations

Fluticasone 100 mcg/vilanterol 25 mcg is the only strength indicated for the treatment of COPD.

Limitations of use: Not indicated for the relief of acute bronchospasm.

Local Anesthetic/Vasoconstrictor Precautions

No information available to require special precautions.

Effects on Dental Treatment Key adverse event(s) related to dental treatment: Infections with *Candida albicans* in the mouth and throat (thrush).

Effects on Bleeding No information available to require special precautions.

Adverse Reactions Also see fluticasone (oral inhalation) monograph.

1% to 10%:

Cardiovascular: Hypertension (≥3%), extrasystoles (≥2%), supraventricular extrasystole (≥2%), ventricular premature contractions (≥2%)

Central nervous system: Headache (5% to 8%), voice disorder (2%)

Gastrointestinal: Oropharyngeal candidiasis (2% to 5%), upper abdominal pain (≥2%)

Infection: Influenza (≥3%)

Neuromuscular & skeletal: Arthralgia (≥2%), back pain (≥2%), bone fracture (2%)

Respiratory: Nasopharyngitis (6% to 10%), pneumonia (2% to 7%), upper respiratory tract infection (2% to 7%), acute sinusitis (≥2%), allergic rhinitis (≥2%), oropharyngeal pain (≥2%), pharyngitis (≥2%), rhinitis (≥2%), viral respiratory tract infection (≥2%), cough (≥1%), sinusitis (≥1%), bronchitis

Miscellaneous: Fever (≥2%)

<1%, postmarketing, and/or case reports: Anaphylaxis, angioedema, hyperglycemia, hypersensitivity reaction, muscle spasm, nervousness, palpitations, paradoxical bronchospasm, skin rash, tachycardia, tremor, urticaria

Mechanism of Action

Fluticasone: A corticosteroid with anti-inflammatory activity, immunosuppressive properties, and antiproliferative actions.

Vilanterol: A long-acting beta$_2$-agonist, relaxes bronchial smooth muscle by selective action on beta$_2$-receptors with little effect on heart rate.

Pregnancy Considerations Adverse events have not been observed in animal reproduction studies. Hypoadrenalism may occur in infants born to mothers receiving corticosteroids during pregnancy (refer to the fluticasone, oral inhalation monograph for additional details). Beta-agonists have the potential to affect uterine contractility if administered during labor. Uncontrolled asthma is associated with adverse events in pregnancy (increased risk of perinatal mortality, preeclampsia, preterm birth, low birth weight infants).

◆ **Fluticasone Furoate** *see* Fluticasone (Nasal) *on page 703*

◆ **Fluticasone Furoate** *see* Fluticasone (Oral Inhalation) *on page 703*

◆ **Fluticasone Furoate and Vilanterol** *see* Fluticasone and Vilanterol *on page 706*

◆ **Fluticasone Propionate** *see* Fluticasone (Nasal) *on page 703*

◆ **Fluticasone Propionate** *see* Fluticasone (Oral Inhalation) *on page 703*

◆ **Fluticasone Propionate and Salmeterol Xinafoate** *see* Fluticasone and Salmeterol *on page 705*

◆ **Fluticasone/Salmeterol** *see* Fluticasone and Salmeterol *on page 705*

◆ **Fluticasone/Vilanterol** *see* Fluticasone and Vilanterol *on page 706*

◆ **Flu Vaccine** *see* Influenza Virus Vaccine (Inactivated) *on page 812*

◆ **Flu Vaccine** *see* Influenza Virus Vaccine (Live/Attenuated) *on page 813*

◆ **Flu Vaccine** *see* Influenza Virus Vaccine (Recombinant) *on page 815*

Fluvastatin (FLOO va sta tin)

Related Information

Cardiovascular Diseases *on page 1654*

Brand Names: US Lescol XL

Brand Names: Canada Lescol XL; Lescol [DSC]; SANDOZ Fluvastatin [DSC]; TEVA-Fluvastatin

Pharmacologic Category Antilipemic Agent, HMG-CoA Reductase Inhibitor

Use

Dyslipidemias:

Heterozygous familial and nonfamilial hypercholesterolemia and mixed dyslipidemia: Adjunct to diet to reduce elevated total cholesterol (total-C), low-density lipoprotein-cholesterol (LDL-C), triglyceride, and apolipoprotein B (apo-B) levels and to increase HDL-C in adults with primary hypercholesterolemia and mixed dyslipidemia (Fredrickson types IIa and IIb)

Heterozygous familial hypercholesterolemia: As an adjunct to diet to reduce total-C, LDL-C, and apo B levels in children ≥10 years and adolescents ≤16 years of age (female patients must be at least 1 year postmenarche) with heterozygous familial hypercholesterolemia and an LDL-C that remains ≥190 mg/dL or ≥160 mg/dL (with ≥2 cardiovascular risk factors or a positive family history of premature cardiovascular disease).

Prevention of cardiovascular disease (CVD):

Secondary prevention of CVD: To slow the progression of coronary atherosclerosis in patients with coronary heart disease; reduce risk of coronary revascularization procedures in patients with coronary heart disease

Limitations of use: Has not been studied in conditions where the major abnormality is elevation of chylomicrons, very low-density lipoprotein (VLDL), or intermediate density lipoprotein (IDL) (ie, hyperlipoproteinemia types I, III, IV, or V).

Local Anesthetic/Vasoconstrictor Precautions No information available to require special precautions

Effects on Dental Treatment Key adverse event(s) related to dental treatment: Assess unusual presentations of muscle weakness or myopathy resulting from lipid therapy such as patient having a difficult time brushing teeth or weakness with chewing. Refer patient back to their physician for evaluation and adjustment of lipid therapy.

Effects on Bleeding No information available to require special precautions

Adverse Reactions Frequency not always defined. The following adverse events were reported with fluvastatin capsules; in general, adverse reactions reported with fluvastatin extended release tablet were similar, but incidences were lower. <1%/Postmarketing adverse reactions include additional class-related events that were not necessarily reported with fluvastatin therapy.

1% to 10%:

Central nervous system: Headache (9%), fatigue (3%), insomnia (3%)

Gastrointestinal: Dyspepsia (8%), abdominal pain (5%), diarrhea (5%), nausea (3%)

Genitourinary: Urinary tract infection (2%)

Neuromuscular & skeletal: Myalgia (5%)

Respiratory: Sinusitis (3%), bronchitis (2%)

<1%, postmarketing, and/or case reports: Alopecia, amnesia (reversible), anaphylaxis, angioedema, anorexia, anxiety, arthralgia, arthritis, blurred vision, cataract, changes in nails, chills, cholestatic jaundice, cognitive dysfunction (reversible), cystitis (interstitial; Huang 2015), decreased libido, depression, dermatomyositis, dizziness, dry mucous membranes, dysgeusia, dyspnea, elevated glycosylated hemoglobin (HbA_{1c}), eosinophilia, erectile dysfunction, erythema multiforme, facial paresis, fever, flushing, fulminant hepatic necrosis, gynecomastia, hemolytic anemia, hepatic cirrhosis, hepatic neoplasm, hepatitis, hyperbilirubinemia, hypersensitivity reaction, immune-mediated necrotizing myopathy (IMNM), impairment of extraocular movement, impotence, increased creatine phosphokinase (>10x normal), increased erythrocyte sedimentation rate, increased gamma-glutamyl transferase, increased serum alkaline phosphatase, increased serum glucose, increased serum transaminases, interstitial pulmonary disease, leukopenia, liver steatosis, lupus-like syndrome, malaise, memory impairment (reversible), muscle cramps, myopathy, nodule, ophthalmoplegia, pancreatitis, paresthesia, peripheral nerve palsy, peripheral neuropathy, polymyalgia rheumatica, positive ANA titer, pruritus, psychic disorder, purpura, reversible confusional state, rhabdomyolysis, skin discoloration, skin photosensitivity, skin rash, Stevens-Johnson syndrome, thrombocytopenia, thyroid dysfunction, toxic epidermal necrolysis, tremor, urticaria, vasculitis, vertigo, vomiting, xeroderma

Mechanism of Action Acts by competitively inhibiting 3-hydroxyl-3-methylglutaryl-coenzyme A (HMG-CoA) reductase, the enzyme that catalyzes the reduction of HMG-CoA to mevalonate; this is an early rate-limiting step in cholesterol biosynthesis. HDL is increased while total, LDL, and VLDL cholesterols; apolipoprotein B; and plasma triglycerides are decreased. In addition to the ability of HMG-CoA reductase inhibitors to decrease levels of high-sensitivity C-reactive protein (hsCRP), they also possess pleiotropic properties including improved endothelial function, reduced inflammation at the site of the coronary plaque, inhibition of platelet aggregation, and anticoagulant effects (de Denus 2002; Ray 2005).

Pharmacodynamics/Kinetics

Onset of Action Peak effect: Maximal LDL-C reductions achieved within 4 weeks

Half-life Elimination Immediate-release: ~3 hours; Extended-release: 7.3 to 10.5 hours (due to prolonged absorption time) (Barilla 2004)

Time to Peak

Immediate-release: <1 hour (delayed more than 2-fold when administered with food as compared to administering 4 hours after the evening meal)

Extended-release: ~3 hours (minimally affected by low-fat meals; however, with a high-fat meal, delayed by 2-fold)

Reproductive Considerations

Fluvastatin is contraindicated in females who may become pregnant.

Adequate contraception is recommended if an HMG-CoA reductase inhibitor is required in females of reproductive potential. Females planning a pregnancy should discontinue the HMG-CoA reductase inhibitor 1 to 2 months prior to attempting to conceive (AHA/ACC [Grundy 2018]).

Pregnancy Risk Factor X

Pregnancy Considerations Fluvastatin is contraindicated in pregnant females.

Studies in pregnant women have shown evidence of fetal abnormalities and use is contraindicated in women who are or may become pregnant. There are reports of congenital anomalies following maternal use of HMG-CoA reductase inhibitors in pregnancy; however, maternal disease, differences in specific agents used, and the low rates of exposure limit the interpretation of the available data (Godfrey 2012; Lecarpentier 2012). Cholesterol biosynthesis may be important in fetal development; serum cholesterol and triglycerides increase normally during pregnancy. The discontinuation of lipid lowering medications temporarily during pregnancy is not expected to have significant impact on the long term outcomes of primary hypercholesterolemia treatment.

Fluvastatin should be discontinued immediately if an unplanned pregnancy occurs during treatment.

- ◆ **Fluvastatin Sodium** *see* Fluvastatin *on page 706*
- ◆ **Fluvirin [DSC]** *see* Influenza Virus Vaccine (Inactivated) *on page 812*

FluvoxaMINE (floo VOKS a meen)

Related Information

Management of the Patient With Anxiety or Depression *on page 1778*

Vasoconstrictor Interactions With Antidepressants *on page 1821*

Brand Names: Canada ACT Fluvoxamine; APO-Fluvoxamine; DOM-Fluvoxamine [DSC]; Luvox; NOVO-Fluvoxamine [DSC]; PHL-Fluvoxamine [DSC]; PMS-Fluvoxamine [DSC]; RATIO-Fluvoxamine [DSC]; RIVA-Fluvox; SANDOZ Fluvoxamine [DSC]

Pharmacologic Category Antidepressant, Selective Serotonin Reuptake Inhibitor

Use Obsessive-compulsive disorder: Treatment of obsessive-compulsive disorder (OCD) in pediatric patients 8 to 17 years of age and adults.

Local Anesthetic/Vasoconstrictor Precautions Although caution should be used in patients taking tricyclic antidepressants, no interactions have been reported with vasoconstrictors and fluvoxamine, a non-tricyclic antidepressant which acts to increase serotonin; no precautions appear to be needed

Effects on Dental Treatment Key adverse event(s) related to dental treatment: Xerostomia (normal salivary flow resumes upon discontinuation) and abnormal taste. Problems with SSRI-induced bruxism have been reported and may preclude their use; clinicians attempting to evaluate any patient with bruxism or involuntary muscle movement, who is simultaneously being treated with an SSRI drug, should be aware of the potential association. See Effects on Bleeding and Dental Health Professional Considerations.

Effects on Bleeding Selective serotonin reuptake inhibitors such as fluvoxamine may impair platelet aggregation due to platelet serotonin depletion, possibly increasing the risk of a bleeding complication. The risk of a bleeding complication can be increased by coadministration of other antiplatelet agents such as NSAIDs and aspirin.

Adverse Reactions Frequency varies by dosage form and indication. Adverse reactions reported as a composite of all indications.

>10%:

Central nervous system: Headache (22% to 35%), insomnia (21% to 35%), drowsiness (22% to 27%), dizziness (11% to 15%), nervousness (10% to 12%)

Gastrointestinal: Nausea (34% to 40%), diarrhea (11% to 18%), xerostomia (10% to 14%), anorexia (6% to 14%)

Genitourinary: Ejaculatory disorder (8% to 11%)

Neuromuscular & skeletal: Weakness (14% to 26%)

1% to 10%:

Cardiovascular: Chest pain (3%), palpitations (3%), vasodilation (2% to 3%), hypertension (1% to 2%), edema (≥1%), hypotension (≥1%), syncope (≥1%)

Central nervous system: Pain (10%), anxiety (5% to 8%), anorgasmia (2% to 5%), yawning (2% to 5%), abnormal dreams (3%), abnormality in thinking (3%), paresthesia (3%), agitation (2% to 3%), apathy (≥1% to 3%), central nervous system stimulation (2%), chills (2%), depression (2%), hypertonia (2%), psychoneurosis (2%), twitching (2%), amnesia (≥1%), manic reaction (≥1%), myoclonus (≥1%), psychotic reaction (≥1%), malaise (≤1%)

Dermatologic: Diaphoresis (6% to 7%), ecchymoses (4%), acne vulgaris (2%)

Endocrine & metabolic: Decreased libido (2% to 10%; incidence higher in males), hypermenorrhea (3%), weight loss (≥1% to 2%), weight gain (≥1%)

Gastrointestinal: Dyspepsia (8% to 10%), constipation (4% to 10%), vomiting (5% to 6%), abdominal pain (5%), flatulence (4%), dental caries (≤3%), tooth loss (≤3%), toothache (≤3%), dysgeusia (2% to 3%), dysphagia (2%), gingivitis (2%)

Genitourinary: Urinary frequency (3%), sexual disorder (2% to 3%), impotence (2%), urinary tract infection (2%), urinary retention (1%)

Hepatic: Abnormal hepatic function tests (2%)

Infection: Tooth abscess (≤3%), viral infection (2%)

Neuromuscular & skeletal: Tremor (5% to 8%), myalgia (5%), hyperkinesia (≥1%), hypokinesia (≥1%)

Ophthalmic: Amblyopia (2% to 3%)

Renal: Polyuria (2%)

Respiratory: Upper respiratory tract infection (9%), pharyngitis (6%), flu-like symptoms (3%), laryngitis (3%), bronchitis (2%), dyspnea (2%), epistaxis (2%), increased cough (≥1%), sinusitis (≥1%)

<1%, postmarketing, and/or case reports: Abnormal gait, activation syndrome, acute renal failure, aggressive behavior, agranulocytosis, akinesia, amenorrhea, anaphylaxis, anemia, angina pectoris, angioedema, angle-closure glaucoma, anuria, aplastic anemia, apnea, asthma, ataxia, blurred vision, bradycardia, bruxism, bullous skin disease, cardiac conduction delay, cardiomyopathy, cardiorespiratory arrest, cerebrovascular accident, cholecystitis, cholelithiasis, colitis, crying, decreased white blood cell count, delirium, diplopia, drowsiness (neonatal), dysarthria, dyskinesia, dystonia, extrapyramidal reaction, fatigue, fever, first degree atrioventricular block, gastroesophageal reflux disease, gastrointestinal hemorrhage, glossalgia, goiter, hallucination, hematemesis, hematuria, hemoptysis, hepatitis, homicidal ideation, hypercholesterolemia, hyperglycemia, hypersensitivity reaction, hypoglycemia, hypokalemia, hyponatremia, hypothyroidism, IgA vasculitis, impulsivity, interstitial pulmonary disease, intestinal obstruction, intoxicated feeling, irritability, jaundice, jitteriness, laryngismus, lethargy, leukocytosis, leukopenia, loss of consciousness, lymphadenopathy, melena, myasthenia, myocardial infarction, myopathy, neuroleptic malignant syndrome (Stevens 2008), outbursts of anger, pancreatitis, paralysis, Parkinsonian-like syndrome, pericarditis, porphyria, priapism, prolonged QT interval on ECG, purpura, Raynaud's phenomenon (Khouri 2016; Peiró 2007), renal insufficiency, rhabdomyolysis, seizure, serotonin syndrome, shock, SIADH, ST segment changes on ECG, Stevens-Johnson syndrome, suicidal tendencies, supraventricular extrasystole, tachycardia, tardive dyskinesia, thrombocytopenia, thromboembolism, toxic epidermal necrolysis, vasculitis, ventricular arrhythmia, ventricular tachycardia (including torsades de pointes)

Mechanism of Action Inhibits CNS neuron serotonin uptake; minimal or no effect on reuptake of norepinephrine or dopamine; does not significantly bind to alpha-adrenergic, histamine or cholinergic receptors

Pharmacodynamics/Kinetics

Onset of Action

Anxiety disorders (obsessive-compulsive, panic, and posttraumatic stress disorder): Initial effects may be observed within 2 weeks of treatment, with continued improvements through 4 to 6 weeks (Issari 2016; Varigonda 2016; WFSBP [Bandelow 2012]); some experts suggest up to 12 weeks of treatment may be necessary for response, particularly in patients with obsessive-compulsive disorder and posttraumatic stress disorder (BAP [Baldwin 2014]; Katzman 2014; WFSBP [Bandelow 2012]).

Depression: Initial effects may be observed within 1 to 2 weeks of treatment, with continued improvements through 4 to 6 weeks (Papakostas 2006; Posternak 2005; Szegedi 2009; Taylor 2006).

Half-life Elimination ~14 to 16 hours; ~17 to 26 hours in the elderly

Time to Peak Plasma: 3 to 8 hours

Reproductive Considerations

If treatment for major depressive disorder is initiated for the first time in females planning a pregnancy, agents other than fluvoxamine are preferred (Larsen 2015).

Pregnancy Considerations

Fluvoxamine crosses the human placenta (Newport 2003).

Nonteratogenic effects in the newborn following selective serotonin reuptake inhibitor (SSRI)/serotonin and norepinephrine reuptake inhibitor (SNRI) exposure late in the third trimester include respiratory distress, cyanosis, apnea, seizures, temperature instability, feeding difficulty, vomiting, hypoglycemia, hypo- or hypertonia, hyper-reflexia, jitteriness, irritability, constant crying, and tremor. Symptoms may be due to the toxicity of the SSRIs/SNRIs or a discontinuation syndrome and may be consistent with serotonin syndrome associated with SSRI treatment. Persistent pulmonary hypertension of the newborn (PPHN) has also been reported with SSRI exposure.

Untreated or inadequately treated mental illness may lead to poor compliance with prenatal care. The American College of Obstetricians and Gynecologists recommends that therapy with SSRIs or SNRIs during pregnancy be individualized. Use of a single agent is preferred. According to their recommendations, treatment of depression during pregnancy should incorporate the clinical expertise of the mental health clinician, obstetrician, primary care provider, and pediatrician (ACOG 2008). If treatment for major depressive disorder is initiated for the first time during pregnancy, agents other than fluvoxamine are preferred (Larsen 2015; MacQueen 2016).

Pregnant women exposed to antidepressants during pregnancy are encouraged to enroll in the National Pregnancy Registry for Antidepressants (NPRAD). Women 18 to 45 years of age or their health care providers may contact the registry by calling 844-405-6185. Enrollment should be done as early in pregnancy as possible.

Dental Health Professional Considerations Problems with SSRI-induced bruxism have been reported and may preclude their use. Clinicians attempting to evaluate any patient with bruxism or involuntary muscle movement, who is simultaneously being treated with an SSRI drug, should be aware of the potential association.

- **Fluvoxamine Maleate** *see* FluvoxaMINE *on page 708*
- **Fluzone [DSC]** *see* Influenza Virus Vaccine (Inactivated) *on page 812*
- **Fluzone High-Dose** *see* Influenza Virus Vaccine (Inactivated) *on page 812*
- **Fluzone Intradermal Quadrivalent [DSC]** *see* Influenza Virus Vaccine (Inactivated) *on page 812*
- **Fluzone Quadrivalent** *see* Influenza Virus Vaccine (Inactivated) *on page 812*
- **FML** *see* Fluorometholone *on page 695*
- **FML Forte** *see* Fluorometholone *on page 695*
- **FML Liquifilm** *see* Fluorometholone *on page 695*
- **Focalin** *see* Dexmethylphenidate *on page 473*
- **Focalin XR** *see* Dexmethylphenidate *on page 473*
- **Foille [OTC] [DSC]** *see* Benzocaine *on page 228*
- **Folacin** *see* Folic Acid *on page 709*
- **Folate** *see* Folic Acid *on page 709*

Folic Acid (FOE lik AS id)

Brand Names: US FA-8 [OTC]

Brand Names: Canada JAMP-Folic Acid; SANDOZ Folic Acid

Pharmacologic Category Vitamin, Water Soluble

Use Megaloblastic and macrocytic anemias due to folate deficiency: Treatment of megaloblastic and macrocytic anemias due to folate deficiency

Local Anesthetic/Vasoconstrictor Precautions

No information available to require special precautions

Effects on Dental Treatment No significant effects or complications reported

Effects on Bleeding No information available to require special precautions

Adverse Reactions Frequency not defined.

Cardiovascular: Flushing (slight)

Central nervous system: Malaise (general)

Dermatologic: Erythema, pruritus, skin rash

Hypersensitivity: Hypersensitivity reaction

Respiratory: Bronchospasm

Mechanism of Action

Folic acid is necessary for formation of a number of coenzymes in many metabolic systems, particularly for purine and pyrimidine synthesis; required for nucleoprotein synthesis and maintenance in erythropoiesis; stimulates WBC and platelet production in folate deficiency anemia.

In the treatment of methanol intoxication, folic acid enhances the metabolism of formic acid, the toxic metabolite of methanol, to nontoxic metabolites (Barceloux 2002).

Pharmacodynamics/Kinetics

Time to Peak Oral: 1 hour

Reproductive Considerations

Folate supplementation during the periconceptual period decreases the risk of neural tube defects. All females planning a pregnancy or who may potentially become pregnant should begin folic acid supplementation prior to conception. Higher doses are required in females at high risk of neural tube defects (ACOG 187 2017; USPSTF 2017).

Pregnancy Considerations

Water soluble vitamins cross the placenta (IOM 1998).

Folate requirements increase during pregnancy (IOM 1998). Folate supplementation during the periconceptual period decreases the risk of neural tube defects. Higher doses are required in females at high risk of neural tube defects (ACOG 187 2017; USPSTF 2017). Folic acid is also indicated for the treatment of anemias due to folate deficiency in pregnant women.

- ◆ **Folinate Calcium** *see* Leucovorin Calcium *on page 889*
- ◆ **Folinic Acid (error prone synonym)** *see* Leucovorin Calcium *on page 889*
- ◆ **Follicle-Stimulating Hormone, Human** *see* Urofollitropin *on page 1509*
- ◆ **Folotyn** *see* PRALAtrexate *on page 1250*
- ◆ **Foltrin** *see* Vitamins (Multiple/Oral) *on page 1550*

Fomepizole (foe ME pi zole)

Brand Names: US Antizol

Brand Names: Canada Antizol

Pharmacologic Category Antidote

Use

Ethylene glycol or methanol poisoning: Treatment of methanol or ethylene glycol poisoning alone or in combination with hemodialysis

Note: Fomepizole is the preferred antidote for known or suspected ethylene glycol poisoning or methanol poisoning. If fomepizole is unavailable or if the patient is intolerant to fomepizole, ethanol therapy may be considered. Ethanol as an antidote is effective in the management of methanol and ethylene glycol poisoning (Thanacoody 2016; Zakharov 2015); however, ethanol is associated with a higher incidence of adverse events and medication errors (Bestic 2009; Lepik 2009; Lepik 2011).

Local Anesthetic/Vasoconstrictor Precautions

No information available to require special precautions

Effects on Dental Treatment Key adverse event(s) related to dental treatment: Bad/metallic taste.

Effects on Bleeding No information available to require special precautions

Adverse Reactions

>10%:

Central nervous system: Headache (14%)

Gastrointestinal: Nausea (11%)

1% to 10% (≤3% unless otherwise noted):

Cardiovascular: Bradycardia, facial flushing, hypotension, phlebitis, shock, tachycardia

Central nervous system: Dizziness (6%), drowsiness (6%), metallic taste (≤6%), agitation, altered sense of smell, anxiety, seizure, speech disturbance, vertigo

Dermatologic: Skin rash

Gastrointestinal: Unpleasant taste (≤6%), abdominal pain, decreased appetite, diarrhea, heartburn, hiccups, vomiting

Genitourinary: Anuria

Hematologic & oncologic: Anemia, disseminated intravascular coagulation (DIC), eosinophilia, lymphangitis

Hepatic: Increased liver enzymes

Local: Application site reaction, inflammation at injection site, pain at injection site

Neuromuscular & skeletal: Back pain

Ophthalmic: Nystagmus, transient blurred vision, visual disturbance

Respiratory: Pharyngitis

Miscellaneous: Fever, multi-organ failure

<1%, postmarketing and/or case reports: Hypersensitivity reaction (mild; mild rash, eosinophilia)

Mechanism of Action Fomepizole competitively inhibits alcohol dehydrogenase, an enzyme which catalyzes the metabolism of ethanol, ethylene glycol, and methanol to their toxic metabolites. Ethylene glycol is metabolized to glycoaldehyde, then oxidized to glycolate, glyoxylate, and oxalate. Glycolate and oxalate are responsible for metabolic acidosis and renal damage. Methanol is metabolized to formaldehyde, then oxidized to formic acid. Formic acid is responsible for metabolic acidosis and visual disturbances.

Pharmacodynamics/Kinetics

Onset of Action Peak effect: Maximum: 1.5-2 hours

Half-life Elimination Has not been calculated; varies with dose

Pregnancy Risk Factor C

Pregnancy Considerations Animal reproduction studies have not been conducted. In general, medications used as antidotes should take into consideration the health and prognosis of the mother; antidotes should be administered to pregnant women if there is a clear indication for use and should not be withheld because of fears of teratogenicity (Bailey, 2003).

Fondaparinux (fon da PARE i nuks)

Brand Names: US Arixtra

Brand Names: Canada Arixtra

Pharmacologic Category Anticoagulant; Anticoagulant, Factor Xa Inhibitor; Pentasaccharide, Synthetic

Use

Deep vein thrombosis: Treatment of acute deep vein thrombosis in conjunction with warfarin.

Pulmonary embolism: Treatment of acute pulmonary embolism in conjunction with warfarin.

Venous thromboembolism prophylaxis in surgical patients: Prophylaxis of venous thromboembolism in patients undergoing surgery for hip replacement, knee replacement, hip fracture (including extended prophylaxis following hip fracture surgery), or abdominal surgery (in patients at risk for thromboembolic complications).

Local Anesthetic/Vasoconstrictor Precautions

No information available to require special precautions

Effects on Dental Treatment Key adverse event(s) related to dental treatment: Hemorrhage may occur at any site. See Effects on Bleeding.

Effects on Bleeding Dose related bleeding is the most common adverse event. Bleeding from the gums is reported (3%). Moderate thrombocytopenia occurs in 3% of patients and severe thrombocytopenia in 0.2%. Medical consult recommended.

Adverse Reactions As with all anticoagulants, bleeding is the major adverse effect. Hemorrhage may occur at any site. Risk appears increased by a number of factors including renal dysfunction, age (>75 years), and weight (<50 kg).

>10%: Hematologic & oncologic: Anemia (2% to 20%)

1% to 10%:

Cardiovascular: Hypotension (≤4%)

Central nervous system: Insomnia (≤5%), dizziness (≤4%), confusion (1% to 3%)

Dermatologic: Increased wound secretion (≤5%), skin blister (≤3%)

Endocrine & metabolic: Hypokalemia (≤4%)
Hematologic & oncologic: Purpura (≤4%), thrombocytopenia (50,000 to 100,000/mm^3: 3%), hematoma (2% to 3%), minor hemorrhage (2% to 3%), major hemorrhage (1% to 3%; risk of major hemorrhage increased as high as 5% in patients receiving initial dose <6 hours following surgery), postoperative hemorrhage (≤2%)
Hepatic: Increased serum ALT (>3 × ULN: 1% to 3%), increased serum AST (>3 × ULN: <1% to ≤2%)
Infection: postoperative wound infection (abdominal surgery: 5%)
Respiratory: Epistaxis (VTE: 1%)

<1%, postmarketing, and/or case reports: Anaphylactoid reaction, anaphylaxis, angioedema, catheter site thrombosis (during PCI; without heparin), elevated aPTT associated with bleeding, epidural hematoma, hemorrhagic death, injection site reaction (bleeding at injection site, skin rash, pruritus), intracranial hemorrhage, reoperation due to bleeding, severe thrombocytopenia (<50,000/mm^3), spinal hematoma, thrombocytopenia (with thrombosis)

Mechanism of Action Fondaparinux is a synthetic pentasaccharide that causes an antithrombin III-mediated selective inhibition of factor Xa. Neutralization of factor Xa interrupts the blood coagulation cascade and inhibits thrombin formation and thrombus development.

Pharmacodynamics/Kinetics

Half-life Elimination 17 to 21 hours; prolonged with renal impairment and in the elderly

Time to Peak SubQ: ~2 to 3 hours

Pregnancy Considerations Based on case reports, small amounts of fondaparinux have been detected in the umbilical cord following multiple doses during pregnancy (Dempfle 2004). Use of fondaparinux in pregnancy should be limited to those women who have severe allergic reactions to heparin, including heparin-induced thrombocytopenia, and who cannot receive danaparoid (Guyatt 2012).

◆ **Fondaparinux Sodium** *see* Fondaparinux *on page 710*

◆ **Forfivo XL** *see* BuPROPion *on page 271*

Formoterol (for MOH te rol)

Related Information

Respiratory Diseases *on page 1680*

Brand Names: US Perforomist

Brand Names: Canada Foradil; Oxeze Turbuhaler

Pharmacologic Category Beta$_2$ Agonist; Beta$_2$-Adrenergic Agonist, Long-Acting

Use

US labeling:

Asthma: Treatment of asthma (only as concomitant therapy with an inhaled corticosteroid) in patients with reversible obstructive airway disease, including patients with symptoms of nocturnal asthma (Foradil Aerolizer).

Chronic obstructive pulmonary disease (COPD): Maintenance treatment of bronchoconstriction in patients with COPD (Foradil Aerolizer, Perforomist).

Exercise-induced bronchospasm: Prevention of exercise-induced bronchospasm when administered on an as-needed basis (monotherapy may be indicated in patients without persistent asthma) (Foradil Aerolizer).

Canadian labeling:

Asthma: Treatment of asthma (only as concomitant therapy with an inhaled corticosteroid) in patients with reversible obstructive airway disease, including patients with symptoms of nocturnal asthma (Foradil, Oxeze Turbuhaler).

COPD: Maintenance treatment of COPD (Foradil).

Exercise-induced bronchospasm: Prevention of exercise-induced bronchospasm when administered on an as-needed basis (monotherapy may be indicated in patients without persistent asthma) (Oxeze Turbuhaler).

Local Anesthetic/Vasoconstrictor Precautions No information available to require special precautions

Effects on Dental Treatment Key adverse event(s) related to dental treatment: Xerostomia (normal salivary flow resumes upon discontinuation).

Effects on Bleeding No information available to require special precautions

Adverse Reactions

1% to 10%:

Cardiovascular: Chest pain (2% to 3%)
Central nervous system: Anxiety (2%), dizziness (2%), insomnia (2%), voice disorder (1%), headache
Dermatologic: Pruritus (2%), skin rash (1%)
Gastrointestinal: Diarrhea (5%), nausea (5%), xerostomia (1% to 3%), vomiting (2%), abdominal pain, dyspepsia, gastroenteritis
Neuromuscular & skeletal: Muscle cramps (2%), tremor
Respiratory: Respiratory tract infection (3% to 7%), exacerbation of asthma (ages 5 to 12 years: 5% to 6%; age >12 years: <4%; acute deterioration: <1%), bronchitis (5%), pharyngitis (3% to 4%), sinusitis (3%), dyspnea (2%), tonsillitis (1%)
Miscellaneous: Fever (2%)

<1%, postmarketing, and/or case reports: Agitation, anaphylaxis (including severe hypotension/angioedema), angina pectoris, atrial fibrillation, behavioral changes, cardiac arrhythmia, cough, decreased glucose tolerance, dermatitis, disturbed sleep, dysgeusia, fatigue, hyperglycemia, hypertension, hypokalemia, malaise, metabolic acidosis, muscle spasm, nervousness, palpitations, paradoxical bronchospasm, prolonged QT interval on ECG, restlessness, tachycardia, urticaria, variable blood pressure, ventricular premature contractions

Mechanism of Action Relaxes bronchial smooth muscle by selective action on beta$_2$ receptors with little effect on heart rate. Formoterol has a long-acting effect.

Pharmacodynamics/Kinetics

Onset of Action Dry powder inhaler: Within 3 minutes.

Peak effect: Dry powder inhaler: 80% of peak effect within 15 minutes; Nebulization solution: 2 hours.

Duration of Action Improvement in FEV$_1$ observed for 12 hours in most patients

Half-life Elimination Dry powder inhaler: ~10 to 14 hours; Nebulization solution: ~7 hours.

Time to Peak Maximum improvement in FEV$_1$ in 1-3 hours

Pregnancy Considerations

Maternal use of beta-2 agonists is not associated with an increased risk of fetal malformations (GINA 2020). Uncontrolled asthma is associated with adverse events in pregnancy (increased risk of perinatal mortality, pre-eclampsia, preterm birth, low birth weight infants, cesarean delivery, and the development of gestational diabetes). Poorly controlled asthma or asthma exacerbations may have a greater fetal/maternal risk than what is associated with appropriately used asthma medications. Maternal treatment improves pregnancy outcomes by reducing the risk of some adverse events (eg, preterm birth, gestational diabetes) (ERS/TSANZ [Middleton 2020]; GINA 2020).

Short-acting beta-2 agonists are preferred over long-acting agents when treatment for asthma is needed during pregnancy. Pregnant females adequately controlled on formoterol for asthma may continue therapy; if initiating treatment during pregnancy, use of an agent with more data in pregnant females may be preferred. Maternal asthma symptoms should be monitored monthly during pregnancy (ERS/TSANZ [Middleton 2020]).

Beta agonists may interfere with uterine contractility if administered during labor.

Data collection to monitor pregnancy and infant outcomes associated with asthma and the medications used to treat asthma in pregnancy is ongoing. Health care providers are encouraged to enroll exposed pregnant females in the MotherToBaby Pregnancy Studies conducted by the Organization of Teratology Information Specialists (877-311-8972 or https://mothertobaby.org). Patients may also enroll themselves.

Product Availability Foradil Aerolizer is no longer available in the US.

- ◆ **Formoterol and Budesonide** *see* Budesonide and Formoterol *on page 255*
- ◆ **Formoterol and Glycopyrrolate** *see* Glycopyrrolate and Formoterol *on page 743*
- ◆ **Formoterol and Mometasone** *see* Mometasone and Formoterol *on page 1047*
- ◆ **Formoterol and Mometasone Furoate** *see* Mometasone and Formoterol *on page 1047*
- ◆ **Formoterol Fumarate** *see* Formoterol *on page 711*
- ◆ **Formoterol Fumarate and Glycopyrronium Bromide** *see* Glycopyrrolate and Formoterol *on page 743*
- ◆ **Formoterol Fumarate Dihydrate** *see* Formoterol *on page 711*
- ◆ **Formoterol Fumarate Dihydrate and Budesonide** *see* Budesonide and Formoterol *on page 255*
- ◆ **Formoterol Fumarate Dihydrate and Mometasone** *see* Mometasone and Formoterol *on page 1047*
- ◆ **Formula E 400 [OTC]** *see* Vitamin E (Systemic) *on page 1549*
- ◆ **5-Formyl Tetrahydrofolate** *see* Leucovorin Calcium *on page 889*
- ◆ **Fortamet** *see* MetFORMIN *on page 983*
- ◆ **Fortaz** *see* CefTAZidime *on page 313*
- ◆ **Fortaz in D5W [DSC]** *see* CefTAZidime *on page 313*
- ◆ **Forteo** *see* Teriparatide *on page 1424*
- ◆ **Fortesta** *see* Testosterone *on page 1425*
- ◆ **Fortovase** *see* Saquinavir *on page 1357*
- ◆ **Fosamax** *see* Alendronate *on page 95*
- ◆ **Fosamax Plus D** *see* Alendronate and Cholecalciferol *on page 100*

Fosamprenavir (FOS am pren a veer)

Related Information

HIV Infection and AIDS *on page 1690*

Brand Names: US Lexiva

Brand Names: Canada Telzir

Pharmacologic Category Antiretroviral, Protease Inhibitor (Anti-HIV)

Use HIV-1 infection, treatment: Treatment of HIV-1 infection, in combination with other antiretroviral agents. **Note:** Fosamprenavir is not recommended as a component of initial therapy for the treatment of HIV (HHS [adults] 2019).

Local Anesthetic/Vasoconstrictor Precautions No information available to require special precautions

Effects on Dental Treatment No significant effects or complications reported

Effects on Bleeding No information available to require special precautions

Adverse Reactions

>10%:

Dermatologic: Skin rash (≤19%; onset: ~11 days; duration: ~13 days)

Endocrine & metabolic: Hypertriglyceridemia (>750 mg/dL: ≤11%)

Gastrointestinal: Diarrhea (5% to 13%; moderate-to-severe)

1% to 10%:

Central nervous system: Fatigue (2% to 4%; moderate-to-severe), headache (2% to 4%; moderate-to-severe)

Dermatologic: Pruritus (7% to 8%)

Endocrine & metabolic: Hyperglycemia (>251 mg/dL: ≤2%)

Gastrointestinal: Increased serum lipase (>2x ULN: 5% to 8%), nausea (3% to 7%; moderate-to-severe), vomiting (2% to 6%; moderate-to-severe), abdominal pain (≤2%; moderate-to-severe)

Hematologic & oncologic: Neutropenia (<750 cells/mm^3: 3%)

Hepatic: Increased serum transaminases (>5x ULN: 4% to 8%)

<1%, postmarketing, and/or case reports: Angioedema, cerebrovascular accident, hypercholesterolemia, myocardial infarction, nephrolithiasis, oral paresthesia, Stevens-Johnson syndrome

Mechanism of Action Fosamprenavir is rapidly and almost completely converted to amprenavir by cellular phosphatases *in vivo*. Amprenavir binds to the site of HIV-1 protease activity and inhibits cleavage of viral Gag-Pol polyprotein precursors into individual functional proteins required for infectious HIV. This results in the formation of immature, noninfectious viral particles.

Pharmacodynamics/Kinetics

Half-life Elimination ~7.7 hours (amprenavir)

Time to Peak 1.5 to 4 hours (median: 2.5 hours)

Reproductive Considerations

Based on the Health and Humans Services (HHS) perinatal HIV guidelines, fosamprenavir (boosted or unboosted) is not one of the recommended antiretroviral agents for use in females living with HIV who are trying to conceive.

Females living with HIV not planning a pregnancy may use any available type of contraception, considering possible drug interactions and contraindications of the specific method. Consult drug interactions database for more detailed information specific to use of fosamprenavir and specific contraceptive methods (HHS [perinatal] 2019).

Pregnancy Considerations Fosamprenavir crosses the human placenta.

Outcome information specific to fosamprenavir use in pregnancy is no longer being reviewed and updated in the Health and Human Services (HHS) perinatal guidelines. Maternal antiretroviral therapy (ART) may be associated with adverse pregnancy outcomes, including preterm delivery, stillbirth, low birth weight, and small for gestational age infants. Actual risks may be influenced by maternal factors such as disease severity, gestational age at initiation of therapy, and specific ART regimen; therefore, close fetal monitoring is recommended. Because there is clear benefit to appropriate treatment, maternal ART should not be withheld due to concerns for adverse neonatal outcomes. Long-term follow-up is recommended for all infants exposed to antiretroviral medications; children without HIV but who were exposed to ART in utero and develop significant organ system abnormalities of unknown etiology (particularly of the CNS or heart) should be evaluated for potential mitochondrial dysfunction. Hyperglycemia, new onset of diabetes mellitus, or diabetic ketoacidosis have been reported with protease inhibitors; it is not clear if pregnancy increases this risk. Consider performing the standard glucose screening test earlier in pregnancy in women who initiated protease inhibitor therapy prior to conception.

Based on the HHS perinatal HIV guidelines, fosamprenavir (boosted or unboosted), is not one of the recommended antiretroviral agents for use during pregnancy.

In general, ART is recommended for all pregnant females living with HIV to keep the viral load below the limit of detection and reduce the risk of perinatal transmission. Therapy should be individualized following a discussion of the potential risks and benefits of treatment during pregnancy. Monitoring of pregnant females is more frequent than in nonpregnant adults. ART should be continued postpartum for all females living with HIV and can be modified after delivery.

Health care providers are encouraged to enroll pregnant females exposed to antiretroviral medications as early in pregnancy as possible in the Antiretroviral Pregnancy Registry (1-800-258-4263 or http://www.APRegistry.com). Health care providers caring for pregnant females living with HIV and their infants may contact the National Perinatal HIV Hotline (1-888-448-8765) for clinical consultation (HHS [perinatal] 2019).

◆ **Fosamprenavir Calcium** *see* Fosamprenavir *on page 712*

Fosaprepitant (fos a PRE pi tant)

Brand Names: US Emend

Brand Names: Canada Emend

Pharmacologic Category Antiemetic; Substance P/Neurokinin 1 Receptor Antagonist

Use

Prevention of chemotherapy-induced nausea and vomiting:

Prevention of acute and delayed nausea and vomiting associated with highly emetogenic chemotherapy, including high-dose cisplatin (initial and repeat courses; in combination with other antiemetics) in patients ≥6 months of age

Prevention of delayed nausea and vomiting associated with moderately emetogenic chemotherapy (initial and repeat courses; in combination with other antiemetics) in patients ≥6 months of age

Limitations of use: Fosaprepitant has not been studied for the management of existing nausea and vomiting.

Local Anesthetic/Vasoconstrictor Precautions No information available to require special precautions

Effects on Dental Treatment Key adverse event(s) related to dental treatment: Stomatitis, taste disturbances, xerostomia (normal salivary flow resumes upon discontinuation).

Effects on Bleeding No information available to require special precautions

Adverse Reactions Adverse reactions reported with fosaprepitant (as part of a combination chemotherapy regimen) occurring at a higher frequency than standard antiemetic therapy. Also see aprepitant monograph for additional adverse reactions.

>10%:

Central nervous system: Fatigue (15%)

Gastrointestinal: Diarrhea (13%)

1% to 10%:

Central nervous system: Peripheral neuropathy (3%)

Gastrointestinal: Dyspepsia (2%)

Genitourinary: Urinary tract infection (2%)

Hematologic & oncologic: Neutropenia (8%), anemia (3%), leukopenia (2%)

Local: Infusion-site reaction (2% to 3%; includes induration at injection site, infusion-site pain, local pruritus, localized erythema)

Neuromuscular & skeletal: Weakness (4%), limb pain (2%)

<1%, postmarketing, and/or case reports: Anaphylactic shock, anaphylaxis, dyspnea, erythema, flushing, hypersensitivity reaction, hypotension, pruritus, skin rash, Stevens-Johnson syndrome, syncope, toxic epidermal necrolysis, urticaria

Mechanism of Action Fosaprepitant is a prodrug of aprepitant, a substance P/neurokinin 1 (NK1) receptor antagonist. Fosaprepitant is rapidly converted to aprepitant, which prevents acute and delayed vomiting by inhibiting the substance P/neurokinin 1 (NK1) receptor; also augments the antiemetic activity of the 5-HT_3 receptor antagonist and corticosteroid activity and inhibits chemotherapy-induced emesis.

Pharmacodynamics/Kinetics

Half-life Elimination Aprepitant: ~9 to 13 hours

Time to Peak Fosaprepitant is converted to aprepitant within 30 minutes after the end of infusion

Reproductive Considerations

Efficacy of hormonal contraceptive may be reduced; alternative or additional methods of contraception should be used during treatment with fosaprepitant and for at least 1 month following the last fosaprepitant dose.

Pregnancy Considerations

Adverse events were not observed in animal reproduction studies.

◆ **Fosaprepitant Dimeglumine** *see* Fosaprepitant *on page 713*

Foscarnet (fos KAR net)

Related Information

Systemic Viral Diseases *on page 1709*

Brand Names: US Foscavir

Pharmacologic Category Antiviral Agent

Use

Cytomegalovirus treatment, ophthalmic disease (retinitis): Treatment of cytomegalovirus (CMV) retinitis in persons with AIDS

Herpes simplex virus: Treatment of acyclovir-resistant mucocutaneous herpes simplex virus (HSV) infection in immunocompromised persons (eg, with advanced AIDS)

Local Anesthetic/Vasoconstrictor Precautions Foscarnet is one of the drugs confirmed to prolong the QT interval and is accepted as having a risk of causing torsade de pointes. In terms of epinephrine, it is not known what effect vasoconstrictors in the local anesthetic regimen will have in patients with a known history of congenital prolonged QT interval or in patients taking any medication that prolongs the QT interval. Until more information is obtained, it is suggested that the clinician consult with the physician prior to the use of a vasoconstrictor in suspected patients, and that the vasoconstrictor (epinephrine, mepivacaine and levonordefrin [Carbocaine® 2% with Neo-Cobefrin®]) be used with caution.

Effects on Dental Treatment Key adverse event(s) related to dental treatment: Xerostomia (normal salivary flow resumes upon discontinuation), taste perversion, and ulcerative stomatitis.

Effects on Bleeding No information available to require special precautions

Adverse Reactions

>10%:

Central nervous system: Headache (26%)

Endocrine & metabolic: Hypokalemia (16% to 48%), hypocalcemia (15% to 30%), hypomagnesemia (15% to 30%), hypophosphatemia (8% to 26%)

Gastrointestinal: Nausea (47%), diarrhea (30%), vomiting (26%)

Hematologic & oncologic: Anemia (33%), granulocytopenia (17%)

Renal: Renal insufficiency (27%)

Miscellaneous: Fever (65%)

1% to 10%:

Cardiovascular: Chest pain (1% to 5%; including transient chest pain as part of infusion reactions), edema (1% to 5%), facial edema (1% to 5%), first degree atrioventricular block (1% to 5%), flushing (1% to 5%), hypertension (1% to 5%), hypotension (1% to 5%), palpitations (1% to 5%), sinus tachycardia (1% to 5%), ST segment changes on ECG (1% to 5%), thrombosis (1% to 5%)

Central nervous system: Seizure (10%), anxiety (≥5%), confusion (≥5%), depression (≥5%), dizziness (≥5%), fatigue (≥5%), hypoesthesia (≥5%), malaise (≥5%), neuropathy (≥5%), pain (≥5%), paresthesia (≥5%), rigors (≥5%), abnormal electroencephalogram (1% to 5%), aggressive behavior (1% to 5%), agitation (1% to 5%), amnesia (1% to 5%), aphasia (1% to 5%), ataxia (1% to 5%), cerebrovascular disease (1% to 5%), dementia (1% to 5%), hallucination (1% to 5%), insomnia (1% to 5%), meningitis (1% to 5%), nervousness (1% to 5%), sensory disturbance (1% to 5%), somnolence (1% to 5%), stupor (1% to 5%)

Dermatologic: Diaphoresis (≥5%), skin rash (≥5%), dermal ulcer (1% to 5%), erythematous rash (1% to 5%), maculopapular rash (1% to 5%), pruritus (1% to 5%), seborrhea (1% to 5%), skin discoloration (1% to 5%)

Endocrine & metabolic: Hyperphosphatemia (6%), electrolyte disturbance (≥5%), abnormal albumin-Globulin ratio (1% to 5%), acidosis (1% to 5%), albuminuria (1% to 5%), cachexia (1% to 5%), hyponatremia (1% to 5%), increased lactate dehydrogenase (1% to 5%), increased thirst (1% to 5%), weight loss (1% to 5%)

Gastrointestinal: Abdominal pain (≥5%), anorexia (≥5%), aphthous stomatitis (1% to 5%), cachexia (1% to 5%), constipation (1% to 5%), dysgeusia (1% to 5%), dyspepsia (1% to 5%), dysphagia (1% to 5%), flatulence (1% to 5%), melena (1% to 5%), pancreatitis (1% to 5%), xerostomia (1% to 5%)

Genitourinary: Nephrotoxicity (8%), dysuria (1% to 5%), nocturia (1% to 5%), urinary retention (1% to 5%), urinary tract infection (1% to 5%)

Hematologic & oncologic: Bone marrow suppression (10%), leukopenia (≥5%), mineral abnormalities (≥5%), neutropenia (≥5%), abnormal white cell differential (1% to 5%), altered platelet function (1% to 5%), lymphadenopathy (1% to 5%), pseudolymphoma (1% to 5%), rectal hemorrhage (1% to 5%), sarcoma (1% to 5%), thrombocytopenia (1% to 5%)

Hepatic: Abnormal hepatic function tests (1% to 5%), increased lactate dehydrogenase (1% to 5%), increased serum alkaline phosphatase (1% to 5%), increased serum ALT (1% to 5%), increased serum AST (1% to 5%)

Infection: Infection (≥5%), sepsis (≥5%), abscess, bacterial infection (1% to 5%), fungal infection (1% to 5%)

Local: Inflammation at injection site (1% to 5%), pain at injection site (1% to 5%)

Neuromuscular & skeletal: Muscle spasm (≥5%), neuropathy (peripheral; ≥5%), weakness (≥5%), arthralgia (1% to 5%), back pain (1% to 5%), leg cramps (1% to 5%), myalgia (1% to 5%), tremor (1% to 5%)

Ophthalmic: Visual disturbance (≥5%), conjunctivitis (1% to 5%), eye pain (1% to 5%)

Renal: Decreased creatinine clearance (≥5%), increased serum creatinine (≥5%), acute renal failure (1% to 5%), increased blood urea nitrogen (1% to 5%), polyuria (1% to 5%)

Respiratory: Cough (≥5%), dyspnea (≥5%), bronchospasm (1% to 5%), flu-like symptoms (1% to 5%), hemoptysis (1% to 5%), pharyngitis (1% to 5%), pneumonia (1% to 5%), pneumothorax (1% to 5%), pulmonary infiltrates (1% to 5%), respiratory failure (1% to 5%), respiratory insufficiency (1% to 5%), rhinitis (1% to 5%), sinusitis (1% to 5%), stridor (1% to 5%)

<1%, postmarketing, and/or case reports: Coma, dehydration, diabetes insipidus (usually nephrogenic), erythema multiforme, esophageal ulcer, extravasation, Fanconi syndrome, gastrointestinal hemorrhage, glomerulonephritis, hematuria, hypercalcemia, hypersensitivity reaction (including anaphylactic shock, angioedema, urticaria), hypoproteinemia, increased amylase, increased creatine phosphokinase, increased gamma-glutamyl transferase, increased serum lipase, local irritation (genitals), localized edema, myasthenia, myopathy, myositis, nephrolithiasis, nephrotic syndrome, pancytopenia, penile ulceration, prolonged QT interval on ECG, proteinuria, renal disease (crystal-induced), renal tubular acidosis, renal tubular necrosis, rhabdomyolysis, SIADH, status epilepticus, Stevens-Johnson syndrome, torsades de pointes, toxic epidermal necrolysis, vaginal ulcer, ventricular arrhythmia

Mechanism of Action Pyrophosphate analogue which acts as a noncompetitive inhibitor of many viral RNA and DNA polymerases as well as HIV reverse transcriptase. Similar to ganciclovir, foscarnet is a virostatic agent. Foscarnet does not require activation by thymidine kinase.

Pharmacodynamics/Kinetics

Half-life Elimination Elimination: ~3 to 4 hours; terminal: ~88 hours (due to bone deposition)

Pregnancy Considerations

Information related to use of foscarnet in pregnancy is limited (Alvarez-McLeod 1999).

Foscarnet is not the preferred treatment of cytomegalovirus infection in pregnant women. Monitoring of amniotic fluid volumes by ultrasound is recommended weekly after 20 weeks of gestation to detect oligohydramnios if foscarnet is used. In general, intravitreous injections for local therapy are preferred for retinal disease to limit systemic exposure (HHS [OI adult 2019]).

Dental Health Professional Considerations See Local Anesthetic/Vasoconstrictor Precautions

◆ **Foscavir** *see* Foscarnet *on page 713*

Fosfomycin (fos foe MYE sin)

Brand Names: US Monurol

Brand Names: Canada Ivozfo; JAMP-Fosfomycin; Monurol

Pharmacologic Category Antibiotic, Miscellaneous

Use

Oral packet:

Cystitis, acute uncomplicated: Treatment of uncomplicated urinary tract infections (acute cystitis) in women due to susceptible strains of *Escherichia coli* and *Enterococcus faecalis*.

Limitations of use: Not indicated for the treatment of pyelonephritis or perinephric abscess. If persistence or reappearance of bacteriuria occurs after treatment with fosfomycin, other therapeutic agents should be selected.

IV [Canadian product]: Note: Reserve for use when it is considered inappropriate to use commonly recommended antibacterial agents, or when these alternative antibacterial agents have failed to demonstrate efficacy. Fosfomycin should usually be used as part of a combination antibacterial regimen.

Meningitis, bacterial: Treatment of bacterial meningitis and associated bacteremia.

Osteomyelitis: Treatment of osteomyelitis and associated bacteremia.

Pneumonia, hospital-acquired: Treatment of lower respiratory tract infection and associated bacteremia.

Urinary tract infection, complicated: Treatment of complicated urinary tract infection and associated bacteremia.

Local Anesthetic/Vasoconstrictor Precautions

No information available to require special precautions

Effects on Dental Treatment No significant effects or complications reported

Effects on Bleeding No information available to require special precautions

Adverse Reactions

1% to 10%:

Central nervous system: Headache (4% to 10%), pain (2%), dizziness (1% to 2%)

Dermatologic: Skin rash (1%)

Gastrointestinal: Diarrhea (9% to 10%), nausea (4% to 5%), abdominal pain (2%), dyspepsia (1% to 2%)

Genitourinary: Vaginitis (6% to 8%), dysmenorrhea (3%)

Neuromuscular & skeletal: Back pain (3%), weakness (1% to 2%)

Respiratory: Rhinitis (5%), pharyngitis (3%)

<1%, postmarketing, and/or case reports: Abnormal stools, anaphylaxis, angioedema, anorexia, aplastic anemia, cholestatic jaundice, constipation, dermatological disease, drowsiness, dysuria, ear disease, exacerbation of asthma, fatigue, fever, flatulence, flu-like symptoms, hearing loss, hematuria, hepatic necrosis, increased serum ALT, insomnia, lymphadenopathy, menstrual disease, migraine, myalgia, nervousness, optic neuritis, paresthesia, pruritus, toxic megacolon, vomiting, xerostomia

Mechanism of Action As a phosphonic acid derivative, fosfomycin inhibits bacterial wall synthesis (bactericidal) by inactivating the enzyme, pyruvyl transferase, which is critical in the synthesis of cell walls by bacteria.

Pharmacodynamics/Kinetics

Half-life Elimination

Oral: 3 to 8 hours; CrCl <54 mL/minute: 50 hours; Hemodialysis patients: 40 hours

IV [Canadian product]: 2 hours; Elderly and/or critically ill patients: 3.6 to 3.8 hours; CVVHF: 12 hours

Time to Peak Serum: Oral: 2 hours; Within 4 hours with high-fat meal.

Pregnancy Considerations Fosfomycin crosses the placenta.

Single dose fosfomycin has been shown to clear bacteria in the urine of pregnant females treated for asymptomatic bacteriuria. However, clinical outcomes (such as pyelonephritis and preterm labor) following single dose therapy are not well studied in pregnancy. When treatment is needed, a 4- to 7-day regimen with an appropriate antibiotic is currently recommended (Nicolle [IDSA 2019]).

◆ **Fosfomycin Sodium** *see* Fosfomycin *on page 715*

◆ **Fosfomycin Tromethamine** *see* Fosfomycin *on page 715*

Fosinopril (foe SIN oh pril)

Related Information

Cardiovascular Diseases *on page 1654*

Brand Names: Canada APO-Fosinopril; CO Fosinopril; Fosinopril-10; Fosinopril-20; JAMP-Fosinopril; MYLAN-Fosinopril [DSC]; PMS-Fosinopril; RAN-Fosinopril; TEVA-Fosinopril

Pharmacologic Category Angiotensin-Converting Enzyme (ACE) Inhibitor; Antihypertensive

Use

Heart failure: Adjunctive treatment of heart failure (HF)

Guideline recommendations: The American College of Cardiology/American Heart Association (ACC/AHA) 2013 Heart Failure Guidelines recommend the use of ACE inhibitors, along with other guideline-directed medical therapies, to prevent progression of HF and reduced ejection fraction in asymptomatic patients with or without a history of myocardial infarction (Stage B HF), or to treat those with symptomatic heart failure and reduced ejection fraction to reduce morbidity and mortality (Stage C HFrEF).

Hypertension: Management of hypertension

Guideline recommendations: The 2017 Guideline for the Prevention, Detection, Evaluation, and Management of High Blood Pressure in Adults recommends if monotherapy is warranted, in the absence of comorbidities (eg, cerebrovascular disease, chronic kidney disease, diabetes, heart failure, ischemic heart disease, etc.), that thiazide-like diuretics or dihydropyridine calcium channel blockers may be preferred options due to improved cardiovascular endpoints (eg, prevention of heart failure and stroke). ACE inhibitors and ARBs are also acceptable for monotherapy. Combination therapy may be required to achieve blood pressure goals and is initially preferred in patients at high risk (stage 2 hypertension or atherosclerotic cardiovascular disease [ASCVD] risk ≥10%) (ACC/AHA [Whelton 2017]).

Local Anesthetic/Vasoconstrictor Precautions No information available to require special precautions

Effects on Dental Treatment Key adverse event(s) related to dental treatment: Patients may experience orthostatic hypotension as they stand up after treatment; especially if lying in dental chair for extended periods of time. Use caution with sudden changes in position during and after dental treatment.

An angiotensin-converting enzyme (ACE) Inhibitor cough is a dry, hacking, nonproductive cough that can potentially interfere with longer dental procedures if patient has this side effect.

Effects on Bleeding No information available to require special precautions

Adverse Reactions Frequency not always defined. Frequency ranges include data from hypertension and heart failure trials. Higher rates of adverse reactions have generally been noted in patients with CHF. However, the frequency of adverse effects associated with placebo is also increased in this population.

>10%: Central nervous system: Dizziness (1% to 2%; cardiac failure patients: ≤12%)

1% to 10%:

- Cardiovascular: Orthostatic hypotension (1% to 2%), palpitations (1%)
- Central nervous system: Headache (3%), noncardiac chest pain (≤2%), fatigue (1% to 2%)
- Endocrine & metabolic: Hyperkalemia (3%)
- Gastrointestinal: Diarrhea (2%), nausea and vomiting (1% to 2%)
- Hepatic: Increased serum transaminases
- Neuromuscular & skeletal: Musculoskeletal pain (≤3%), weakness (1%)
- Renal: Increased serum creatinine, renal function decompensation (patients with bilateral renal artery stenosis or hypovolemia)
- Respiratory: Cough (2% to 10%), upper respiratory infection (2%)

<1%, postmarketing, and/or case reports: Abdominal distention, anaphylactoid reaction, angina pectoris, angioedema, arthralgia, behavioral changes, bradycardia, bronchospasm, cerebral infarction, cerebrovascular accident, claudication, confusion, constipation, decreased libido, drowsiness, dysgeusia, dysphagia, edema, eosinophilia, epistaxis, eye irritation, flatulence, flushing, gout, heartburn, hepatitis, hepatomegaly, hyperhidrosis, hypertension, hypertensive crisis, hypotension, insomnia, laryngitis, lower extremity edema, lymphadenopathy, memory impairment, mood changes, myalgia, myocardial infarction, numbness, pancreatitis, paranasal sinus disease (abnormality), paresthesia, pharyngitis, pleuritic chest pain, pruritus, renal insufficiency, shock, skin photosensitivity, skin rash, sleep disorder, syncope, tachycardia, tinnitus, tracheobronchitis, transient ischemic attacks, tremor, urinary frequency, urticaria, vertigo, visual disturbance, weight gain, xerostomia

Mechanism of Action Competitive inhibitor of angiotensin-converting enzyme (ACE); prevents conversion of angiotensin I to angiotensin II, a potent vasoconstrictor; results in lower levels of angiotensin II which causes an increase in plasma renin activity and a reduction in aldosterone secretion; a CNS mechanism may also be involved in hypotensive effect as angiotensin II increases adrenergic outflow from CNS; vasoactive kallikreins may be decreased in conversion to active hormones by ACE inhibitors, thus reducing blood pressure

Pharmacodynamics/Kinetics

Onset of Action 1 hour

Duration of Action 24 hours

Half-life Elimination Serum (fosinoprilat):

Children and Adolescents 6-16 years: 11-13 hours
Adults: 12 hours
Adults with CHF: 14 hours

Time to Peak Serum: ~3 hours

Reproductive Considerations

Angiotensin-converting enzyme (ACE) inhibitors should be avoided in sexually active females of reproductive potential not using effective contraception (ADA 2020).

ACE inhibitors should generally be avoided for the treatment of hypertension in women planning a pregnancy; use should only be considered for cases of hypertension refractory to other medications (ACOG 203 2019).

Pregnancy Risk Factor D

Pregnancy Considerations Fosinopril crosses the placenta.

Exposure to an angiotensin-converting enzyme (ACE) inhibitor during the first trimester of pregnancy may be associated with an increased risk of fetal malformations (ACOG 203 2019; ESC [Regitz-Zagrosek 2018]); however, outcomes observed may also be influenced by maternal disease (ACC/AHA [Whelton 2018]).

[US Boxed Warning]: Drugs that act on the renin-angiotensin system can cause injury and death to the developing fetus. Discontinue as soon as possible once pregnancy is detected. Drugs that act on the renin-angiotensin system are associated with oligohydramnios. Oligohydramnios, due to decreased fetal renal function, may lead to fetal lung hypoplasia and skeletal malformations. The use of these drugs in pregnancy is also associated with anuria, hypotension, renal failure, skull hypoplasia, and death in the fetus/neonate. Infants exposed to an ACE inhibitor in utero should be monitored for hyperkalemia, hypotension, and oliguria. Oligohydramnios may not appear until after irreversible fetal injury has occurred. Exchange transfusions or dialysis may be required to reverse hypotension or improve renal function, although data related to the effectiveness in neonates is limited.

Chronic maternal hypertension is also associated with adverse events in the fetus/infant. Chronic maternal hypertension may increase the risk of birth defects, low birth weight, premature delivery, stillbirth, and neonatal death. Actual fetal/neonatal risks may be related to duration and severity of maternal hypertension. Untreated chronic hypertension may also increase the risks of adverse maternal outcomes, including gestational diabetes, preeclampsia, delivery complications, stroke, and myocardial infarction (ACOG 203 2019).

When treatment of hypertension in pregnancy is indicated, ACE inhibitors should generally be avoided due to their adverse fetal events; use in pregnant women should only be considered for cases of hypertension refractory to other medications (ACOG 203 2019). ACE inhibitors are not recommended for the treatment of heart failure in pregnancy (Regitz-Zagrosek [ESC 2018]).

◆ **Fosinopril Sodium** *see* Fosinopril *on page 715*

Fosnetupitant and Palonosetron

(fos net UE pi tant & pal oh NOE se tron)

Brand Names: US Akynzeo

Pharmacologic Category Antiemetic; Selective 5-HT_3 Receptor Antagonist; Substance P/Neurokinin 1 Receptor Antagonist

Use

Chemotherapy-induced nausea and vomiting: Prevention of acute and delayed nausea and vomiting associated with initial and repeat courses of highly emetogenic chemotherapy (in combination with dexamethasone).

Limitations of use: Has not been studied for the prevention of nausea and vomiting associated with anthracycline plus cyclophosphamide (AC) chemotherapy.

Local Anesthetic/Vasoconstrictor Precautions No information available to require special precautions

Effects on Dental Treatment No significant effects or complications reported

Effects on Bleeding No information available to require special precautions

Adverse Reactions See Palonosetron monograph.

Mechanism of Action Fosnetupitant is a prodrug of netupitant, a selective substance P/neurokinin (NK_1) receptor antagonist, which augments the antiemetic activity of 5-HT_3 receptor antagonists and corticosteroids to inhibit acute and delayed chemotherapy-induced emesis. Palonosetron is a selective 5-HT_3 receptor antagonist, which blocks serotonin, both on vagal nerve terminals in the periphery and centrally in the chemoreceptor trigger zone. Palonosetron inhibits the cross-talk between the 5-HT_3 and NK_1 receptors. The combination of palonosetron and netupitant works synergistically to inhibit substance P response to a greater extent than either agent alone (Aapro 2014).

Pharmacodynamics/Kinetics

Half-life Elimination Fosnetupitant: 0.75 ± 0.4 hours; Netupitant: 144 ± 73 hours; Palonosetron: 58 ± 27 hours

Time to Peak At end of the 30-minute infusion

Pregnancy Considerations Adverse events were observed in some animal reproduction studies using the components of this combination product.

◆ **Fosnetupitant/Palonosetron** *see* Fosnetupitant and Palonosetron *on page 717*

Fosphenytoin (FOS fen i toyn)

Related Information

Phenytoin *on page 1228*

Brand Names: US Cerebyx

Brand Names: Canada Cerebyx

Pharmacologic Category Anticonvulsant, Hydantoin

Use Seizures: Control of generalized tonic-clonic status epilepticus and the prevention and treatment of seizures occurring during neurosurgery (eg, prophylaxis during craniotomy); may be used for short-term parenteral administration (eg, focal [partial] onset seizures or generalized onset seizures) when oral phenytoin is not possible.

Local Anesthetic/Vasoconstrictor Precautions No information available to require special precautions

Effects on Dental Treatment Key adverse event(s) related to dental treatment: Tongue disorder and dry mouth.

Effects on Bleeding No information available to require special precautions

Adverse Reactions Also refer to the phenytoin monograph for additional adverse reactions.

>10%:

Central nervous system: Burning sensation (≤44%), paresthesia (≤44%), dizziness (IV: 31%; IM: 5%), drowsiness (IV: 20%; IM: 7%), ataxia (IV: 4% to 11%; IM: 8%)

Dermatologic: Pruritus (IV: 49%; IM: 3%; generally transient; often reported in groin area)

Ophthalmic: Nystagmus disorder (IV: 44%; IM: 15%)

1% to 10%:

Cardiovascular: Hypotension (IV: 8%), vasodilation (IV: 6%), tachycardia (IV: 2%), facial edema (>1%), hypertension (>1%), atrial flutter (≤1%), bundle branch block (≤1%), cardiac failure (≤1%), cardiomegaly (≤1%), cerebral infarction (≤1%), edema (≤1%), orthostatic hypotension (≤1%), palpitations (≤1%), prolonged QT interval on ECG (≤1%), pulmonary embolism (≤1%), shock (≤1%), sinus bradycardia (≤1%), subdural hematoma (≤1%), syncope (≤1%), thrombophlebitis (≤1%), ventricular premature contractions (≤1%)

Central nervous system: Headache (IM: 9%; IV: 2%), stupor (IV: 8%), paresthesia (4%; generally transient; often reported in groin area; may be more common with IV), extrapyramidal reaction (≤4%; more common with IV), absent reflexes (IM: 3%), agitation (IV: 3%), vertigo (IV: 2%), cerebral edema (≤2%; more common with IV), dysarthria (≤2%), hypoesthesia (≤2%; more common with IV), abnormality in thinking (>1%), chills (>1%), hyperreflexia (>1%), intracranial hypertension (>1%), myasthenia (>1%), nervousness (>1%), speech disturbance (>1%), akathisia (≤1%), altered sense of smell (≤1%), amnesia (≤1%), aphasia (≤1%), brain disease (≤1%), central nervous system depression (≤1%), cerebral hemorrhage (≤1%), coma (≤1%), confusion (≤1%), delirium (≤1%), depersonalization (≤1%), depression (≤1%), emotional lability (≤1%), encephalitis (≤1%), hemiplegia (≤1%), hostility (≤1%), hyperacusis (≤1%), hyperesthesia (≤1%), hypotonia (≤1%), insomnia (≤1%), malaise (≤1%), meningitis (≤1%), migraine (≤1%), myoclonus (≤1%), paralysis (≤1%), personality disorder (≤1%), positive Babinski sign (≤1%), psychoneurosis (≤1%), psychosis (≤1%), seizure (≤1%), twitching (≤1%)

Dermatologic: Ecchymoses (IM: 7%), skin rash (>1%), contact dermatitis (≤1%), cutaneous nodule (≤1%), diaphoresis (≤1%), maculopapular rash (≤1%), pustular rash (≤1%), skin discoloration (≤1%), skin photosensitivity (≤1%), urticaria (≤1%)

Endocrine & metabolic: Hypokalemia (>1%), acidosis (≤1%), albuminuria (≤1%), alkalosis (≤1%), cachexia (≤1%), dehydration (≤1%), diabetes insipidus (≤1%), hyperglycemia (≤1%), hyperkalemia (≤1%), hypophosphatemia (≤1%), ketosis (≤1%)

Gastrointestinal: Nausea (IV: 9%; IM: 5%), tongue disease (IV: 4%), xerostomia (IV: 4%), dysgeusia (3%), vomiting (IM: 3%; IV: 2%), constipation (>1%), ageusia (≤1%), anorexia (≤1%), diarrhea (≤1%), dyspepsia (≤1%), dysphagia (≤1%), flatulence (≤1%), gastritis (≤1%), gastrointestinal hemorrhage (≤1%), intestinal obstruction (≤1%), oral paresthesia (≤1%), sialorrhea (≤1%), tenesmus (≤1%)

Genitourinary: Pelvic pain (IV: 4%), dysuria (≤1%), genital edema (≤1%), oliguria (≤1%), urethral pain (≤1%), urinary incontinence (≤1%), urinary retention (≤1%), vaginitis (≤1%), vulvovaginal candidiasis (≤1%)

Hematologic & oncologic: Anemia (≤1%), hypochromic anemia (≤1%), leukocytosis (≤1%), leukopenia (≤1%), lymphadenopathy (≤1%), petechia (≤1%), thrombocytopenia (≤1%)

Hepatic: Abnormal hepatic function tests (≤1%)

Hypersensitivity: Tongue edema (≤1%)

Infection: Infection (>1%), cryptococcosis (≤1%), sepsis (≤1%)

Local: Injection site reaction (>1%), pain at injection site (>1%), bleeding at injection site (≤1%), inflammation at injection site (≤1%), swelling at injection site (≤1%)

Neuromuscular & skeletal: Tremor (IM: 10%; IV: 3%), asthenia (IM: 9%; IV: 2%), back pain (IV: 2%), arthralgia (≤1%), hyperkinetic muscle activity (≤1%), hypokinesia (≤1%), lower limb cramp (≤1%), myalgia (≤1%), myopathy (≤1%)

Ophthalmic: Diplopia (IV: 3%), amblyopia (IV: 2%), conjunctivitis (≤1%), eye pain (≤1%), mydriasis (≤1%), photophobia (≤1%), visual field defect (≤1%)

Otic: Tinnitus (IV: 9%), deafness (≤2%; more common with IV), otalgia (≤1%)

Renal: Polyuria (≤1%), renal failure syndrome (≤1%)

Respiratory: Pneumonia (>1%), apnea (≤1%), aspiration pneumonia (≤1%), asthma (≤1%), atelectasis (≤1%), bronchitis (≤1%), cyanosis (≤1%), dyspnea (≤1%), epistaxis (≤1%), flu-like symptoms (≤1%), hemoptysis (≤1%), hyperventilation (≤1%), hypoxia (≤1%), increased bronchial secretions (≤1%), increased cough (≤1%), pharyngitis (≤1%), pneumothorax (≤1%), rhinitis (≤1%), sinusitis (≤1%)

Miscellaneous: Fever (>1%)

Frequency not defined: Cardiovascular: Cardiac arrhythmia, severe hypotension

<1%, postmarketing, and/or case reports: Acute generalized exanthematous pustulosis, anaphylaxis, angioedema, drug reaction with eosinophilia and systemic symptoms, dyskinesia, severe dermatological reaction, signs and symptoms of injection site (purple glove syndrome), Stevens-Johnson syndrome, toxic epidermal necrolysis

Mechanism of Action Diphosphate ester salt of phenytoin that acts as a water-soluble prodrug of phenytoin; after administration, plasma esterases convert fosphenytoin to phosphate, formaldehyde (not expected to be clinically consequential [Fierro 1996]), and phenytoin as the active moiety. Phenytoin works by stabilizing neuronal membranes and decreasing seizure activity by increasing efflux or decreasing influx of sodium ions across cell membranes in the motor cortex during generation of nerve impulses

Pharmacodynamics/Kinetics

Half-life Elimination

Pediatric patients (ages: 1 day to 16.7 years): 8.3 minutes (range: 2.5 to 18.5 minutes) (Fischer 2003).

Adults:

Fosphenytoin: IV: ~15 minutes; IM: ~30 minutes.

Phenytoin: Variable (mean: 12 to 29 hours); pharmacokinetics of phenytoin are saturable.

Time to Peak Conversion to phenytoin:

IV: Adults: Following IV administration (maximum rate of administration): ~15 minutes.

IM:

Neonates and infants ≤6 months of age: 1 to 2.4 hours was reported in a case series (n=3; postnatal age: 15 to 47 days) (Hatzopoulos 1998).

Pediatric patients >7 months of age: Therapeutic concentrations within 30 minutes; time to maximum serum concentration not reported (Fischer 2003).

Adults: ~3 hours; Therapeutic phenytoin concentrations may be achieved as early as 5 to 20 minutes following IM (gluteal) administration (Pryor 2001).

Reproductive Considerations

Females of reproductive potential who are not planning a pregnancy should use effective contraception; hormonal contraceptives may be less effective.

Pregnancy Considerations

Fosphenytoin is the prodrug of phenytoin. An increased risk of congenital malformations and adverse outcomes may occur following in utero phenytoin exposure. Reported malformations include orofacial clefts, cardiac defects, dysmorphic facial features, nail/digit hypoplasia, growth abnormalities including microcephaly, and mental deficiency. Isolated cases of malignancies (including neuroblastoma) and coagulation defects in the neonate (may be life threatening) following delivery have also been reported. Potentially life-threatening bleeding disorders in the newborn may also occur due to decreased concentrations of vitamin K-dependent clotting factors following phenytoin exposure in utero; vitamin K administration to the mother prior to delivery and the newborn after birth is recommended.

Due to pregnancy-induced physiologic changes, the pharmacokinetics may be changed; additional monitoring is needed.

Also refer to the Phenytoin monograph for additional information.

Patients exposed to fosphenytoin during pregnancy are encouraged to enroll themselves into the North American Antiepileptic Drug (NAAED) Pregnancy Registry by calling 1-888-233-2334. Additional information is available at http://www.aedpregnancyregistry.org/.

◆ **Fosphenytoin Sodium** *see* Fosphenytoin *on page 717*

Fostamatinib (fos ta ma ti nib)

Brand Names: US Tavalisse

Pharmacologic Category Spleen Tyrosine Kinase (Syk) Inhibitor; Tyrosine Kinase Inhibitor

Use Immune thrombocytopenia (ITP) (chronic, refractory): Treatment of thrombocytopenia in adults with chronic immune thrombocytopenia (ITP) who have had an insufficient response to a previous treatment.

Local Anesthetic/Vasoconstrictor Precautions
No information available to require special precautions

Effects on Dental Treatment Key adverse event(s) related to dental treatment: Tooth ache has been reported

Effects on Bleeding No information available to require special precautions

Adverse Reactions

>10%:

Cardiovascular: Hypertension (28%)

Central nervous system: Dizziness (11%)

Gastrointestinal: Diarrhea (31%), nausea (19%)

Hepatic: Increased serum ALT (11%)

Respiratory: Respiratory tract infection (11%)

1% to 10%:

Cardiovascular: Chest pain (6%), hypertensive crisis (1%), syncope (1%, serious)

Central nervous system: Fatigue (6%)

Dermatologic: Skin rash (9%)

Gastrointestinal: Abdominal pain (6%), toothache (1%, serious)

Hematologic & oncologic: Neutropenia (6%), febrile neutropenia (1%)

Hepatic: Increased serum AST (9%)

Neuromuscular & skeletal: Arthralgia (1%, serious), limb pain (1%, serious)

Renal: Nephrolithiasis (1%, serious)

Respiratory: Dyspnea (2%, serious), hypoxia (1%, serious)

Mechanism of Action Fostamatinib is a small molecule spleen tyrosine kinase (Syk) inhibitor. Syk affects cellular proliferation, differentiation, survival and immune regulation via IgG Fc-receptor signaling and is also linked to B-cell receptor signaling and autoantibody production (Bussel 2018). The major active metabolite of fostamatinib, R406, inhibits signal transduction of Fc-activating receptors and B-cell receptor and reduces antibody-mediated destruction of platelets.

Pharmacodynamics/Kinetics

Onset of Action Median time to response (platelets ≥50,000/mm^3): 15 days (Bussel 2018)

Half-life Elimination R406: 15 (± 4.3) hours

Time to Peak R406: ~1.5 hours (range: 1 to 4 hours)

Reproductive Considerations

Evaluate pregnancy status in females of reproductive potential prior to therapy; effective contraception should be used during treatment and for at least 1 month after the last fostamatinib dose.

Pregnancy Considerations

Based on the mechanism of action and information from animal reproduction studies, fostamatinib may cause fetal harm if exposure occurs during pregnancy.

◆ **Fostamatinib Disodium Hexahydrate** *see* Fostamatinib *on page 718*

Fostemsavir (fos TEM sa vir)

Brand Names: US Rukobia

Pharmacologic Category Antiretroviral Agent, gp120 Attachment Inhibitor

Use HIV-1 infection, treatment: Treatment of HIV-1 infection, in combination with other antiretrovirals, in heavily treatment-experienced adults with multidrug-resistant HIV-1 infection failing their current antiretroviral regimen.

Local Anesthetic/Vasoconstrictor Precautions No information available to require special precautions.

Effects on Dental Treatment No significant effects or complications reported.

Effects on Bleeding No information available to require special precautions.

Adverse Reactions Frequency of adverse events is as reported in adults receiving combination antiretroviral therapy.

>10%:

Hepatic: Increased serum alanine aminotransferase (grades 3/4: ≤14%), increased serum aspartate aminotransferase (grades 3/4: ≤14%)

Renal: Increased serum creatinine (grades 3/4: 19%)

1% to 10%:

Cardiovascular: Increased serum creatine kinase (grades 3/4: 2%), prolonged QT interval on ECG (<2%)

Dermatologic: Pruritus (<2%), skin rash (3%)

Endocrine & metabolic: Hypercholesterolemia (grade 3: 5%), hyperglycemia (grades 3/4: 4%), increased LDL cholesterol (grades 3/4: 4%), increased serum triglycerides (grades 3/4: 5%), increased uric acid (grades 3/4: 3%)

Gastrointestinal: Abdominal pain (3%), diarrhea (4%), dysgeusia (<2%), dyspepsia (3%), increased serum lipase (grades 3/4: 5%), nausea (10%), vomiting (2%)

Hematologic & oncologic: Decreased hemoglobin (grades 3/4: 6%), decreased neutrophils (grades 3/4: 4%), leukocyte disorder (grades 3/4: 1%)

Hepatic: Increased direct serum bilirubin (grade 3: 7%), increased serum bilirubin (grades 3/4: 3%)

Immunologic: Immune reconstitution syndrome (2%)

Nervous system: Dizziness (<2%), drowsiness (2%), fatigue (3%), headache (4%), peripheral neuropathy (<2%), peripheral sensory neuropathy (<2%), sleep disturbance (3%)

Neuromuscular & skeletal: Myalgia (<2%)

Frequency not defined:

Infection: Infection, reactivation of HBV

Mechanism of Action Fostemsavir is hydrolyzed to the active moiety, temsavir, which is a gp120 attachment inhibitor. Temsavir binds to the HIV-1 envelope protein gp120 subunit and selectively inhibits the interaction between the virus and cellular CD4 receptors, preventing host cell attachment. In addition, temsavir can inhibit gp120-dependent postattachment steps required for viral entry into host cells.

Pharmacodynamics/Kinetics

Half-life Elimination 11 hours.

Time to Peak 2 hours.

Reproductive Considerations

Information specific to fostemsavir use in females or males planning a pregnancy is not yet available from the antiretroviral pregnancy registry.

Based on the Health and Human Services perinatal HIV guidelines, fostemsavir is not one of the recommended antiretroviral agents for use in females or males planning a pregnancy.

For males and females living with HIV and planning a pregnancy, maximum viral suppression below the limits of detection with antiretroviral therapy (ART), modification of therapy (if needed), optimization of the woman's health, and a discussion of the potential risks and benefits of ART therapy during pregnancy is recommended prior to conception (HHS [perinatal] 2020).

Pregnancy Considerations

Outcome information specific to fostemsavir in pregnancy is not yet available from the antiretroviral pregnancy registry.

In general, maternal antiretroviral therapy (ART) may be associated with adverse pregnancy outcomes including preterm delivery, stillbirth, low birthweight, and small-for-gestational-age infants. Actual risks may be influenced by maternal factors such as disease severity, gestational age at initiation of therapy, and specific

ART regimen, therefore, close fetal monitoring is recommended. Because there is clear benefit to appropriate treatment, maternal ART should not be withheld due to concerns for adverse neonatal outcomes. Long-term follow-up is recommended for all infants exposed to antiretroviral medications; children without HIV but who were exposed to ART in utero and develop significant organ system abnormalities of unknown etiology (particularly of the CNS or heart) should be evaluated for potential mitochondrial dysfunction.

Based on the Health and Human Services perinatal HIV guidelines, fostemsavir is not one of the recommended antiretroviral agents for use during pregnancy.

In general, ART is recommended for all pregnant females living with HIV to keep the viral load below the limit of detection and reduce the risk of perinatal transmission. Therapy should be individualized following a discussion of the potential risks and benefits of treatment during pregnancy. Monitoring of pregnant females is more frequent than in nonpregnant adults. ART should be continued postpartum for all females living with HIV and can be modified after delivery.

Health care providers are encouraged to enroll pregnant females exposed to antiretroviral medications as early in pregnancy as possible in the Antiretroviral Pregnancy Registry (1-800-258-4263 or http://www.APRegistry.com). Health care providers caring for pregnant females living with HIV and their infants may contact the National Perinatal HIV Hotline (888-448-8765) for clinical consultation (HHS [perinatal] 2020).

- ◆ **Fostemsavir Tromethamine** *see* Fostemsavir *on page 719*
- ◆ **FR901228** *see* RomiDEPsin *on page 1343*
- ◆ **Fragmin** *see* Dalteparin *on page 431*
- ◆ **Freedavite [OTC]** *see* Vitamins (Multiple/Oral) *on page 1550*
- ◆ **Fresenius Propoven** *see* Propofol *on page 1286*
- ◆ **Frova** *see* Frovatriptan *on page 720*

Frovatriptan (froe va TRIP tan)

Related Information

Temporomandibular Dysfunction (TMD), Chronic Pain, and Fibromyalgia *on page 1773*

Brand Names: US Frova

Brand Names: Canada APO-Frovatriptan; Frova; TEVA-Frovatriptan

Pharmacologic Category Antimigraine Agent; Serotonin 5-$HT_{1B, 1D}$ Receptor Agonist

Use

Migraines: Acute treatment of migraine with or without aura in adults

Limitations of use: For use only in patients with a clear diagnosis of migraine. Not indicated for prevention of migraine attacks or the treatment of cluster headache.

Local Anesthetic/Vasoconstrictor Precautions No information available to require special precautions

Effects on Dental Treatment No significant effects or complications reported

Effects on Bleeding No information available to require special precautions

Adverse Reactions

1% to 10%:

Cardiovascular: Flushing (4%), hot or cold flashes (3%), chest pain (2%), palpitations (1%)

Central nervous system: Dizziness (8%), fatigue (5%), headache (4%), paresthesia (4%), drowsiness (≥2%), anxiety (1%), dysesthesia (1%), hypoesthesia (1%), insomnia (1%), pain (1%)

Dermatologic: Diaphoresis (1%)

Gastrointestinal: Xerostomia (3%), nausea (≥2%), dyspepsia (2%), abdominal pain (1%), diarrhea (1%), vomiting (1%)

Neuromuscular & skeletal: Musculoskeletal pain (3%)

Ophthalmic: Visual disturbance (1%)

Otic: Tinnitus (1%)

Respiratory: Rhinitis (1%), sinusitis (1%)

<1%, postmarketing, and/or case reports: Abnormal dreams, abnormal gait, abnormal lacrimation, abnormal reflexes, agitation, amnesia, anaphylactoid reaction, anaphylaxis, anorexia, arthralgia, ataxia, back pain, bradycardia, bullous rash, change in bowel habits, cheilitis, chest tightness, confusion, conjunctivitis, constipation, dehydration, depersonalization, depression, dysgeusia, dysphagia, dyspnea, ECG changes, emotional lability, epistaxis, eructation, esophageal spasm, euphoria, eye pain, fever, flatulence, gastroesophageal reflux disease, hiccups, hyperacusis, hyperesthesia, hypersensitivity reaction (including angioedema), hypertonia, hyperventilation, hypocalcemia, hypoglycemia, hypotonia, increased thirst, involuntary muscle movements, jaw tightness, lack of concentration, laryngitis, leg pain, malaise, mouth edema, myalgia, myasthenia, myocardial infarction, nervousness, nocturia, osteoarthritis, otalgia, peptic ulcer, personality disorder, pharyngitis, polyuria, pruritus, purpura, renal pain, rigors, salivary gland pain, seizure, sialorrhea, significant cardiovascular event, speech disturbance, stomatitis, syncope, tachycardia, tightness in chest and throat, tongue paralysis, toothache, tremor, urinary frequency, urine abnormality, vertigo, weakness

Mechanism of Action Selective agonist for serotonin (5-HT_{1B} and 5-HT_{1D} receptors) in cranial arteries; causes vasoconstriction and reduces sterile inflammation associated with antidromic neuronal transmission correlating with relief of migraine.

Pharmacodynamics/Kinetics

Half-life Elimination ~26 hours

Time to Peak 2-4 hours

Pregnancy Considerations Adverse events were observed in animal reproduction studies. Information related to the use of frovatriptan in pregnancy has not been located. Until additional information is available, other agents are preferred for the initial treatment of migraine in pregnancy (Da Silva 2012; MacGregor 2012; Williams 2012).

- ◆ **Frovatriptan Succinate** *see* Frovatriptan *on page 720*
- ◆ **Frusemide** *see* Furosemide *on page 721*
- ◆ **FS** *see* Fibrin Sealant *on page 667*
- ◆ **FSH** *see* Urofollitropin *on page 1509*
- ◆ **FS VH S/D** *see* Fibrin Sealant *on page 667*
- ◆ **FTC** *see* Emtricitabine *on page 556*
- ◆ **FTC/RPV/TDF** *see* Emtricitabine, Rilpivirine, and Tenofovir Disoproxil Fumarate *on page 559*
- ◆ **FTC, TDF, and EFV** *see* Efavirenz, Emtricitabine, and Tenofovir Disoproxil Fumarate *on page 545*
- ◆ **FTY720** *see* Fingolimod *on page 670*
- ◆ **FU** *see* Fluorouracil (Systemic) *on page 696*
- ◆ **5-FU** *see* Fluorouracil (Systemic) *on page 696*
- ◆ **FUDF** *see* Floxuridine *on page 673*

◆ **FUDR** *see* Floxuridine *on page 673*

◆ **5-FUDR** *see* Floxuridine *on page 673*

◆ **Fulphila** *see* Pegfilgrastim *on page 1200*

Fulvestrant (fool VES trant)

Brand Names: US Faslodex

Brand Names: Canada Faslodex; TEVA-Fulvestrant

Pharmacologic Category Antineoplastic Agent, Estrogen Receptor Antagonist

Use

Breast cancer (monotherapy):

Treatment of hormone-receptor (HR)-positive advanced breast cancer in postmenopausal women with disease progression following endocrine therapy

Treatment of HR-positive, human epidermal growth factor receptor 2 (HER2)-negative advanced breast cancer in postmenopausal women not previously treated with endocrine therapy

Breast cancer (combination therapy):

Treatment of HR-positive, HER2-negative advanced or metastatic breast cancer (in combination with ribociclib) in postmenopausal women as initial endocrine-based therapy or following disease progression on endocrine therapy

Treatment of HR-positive, HER2-negative advanced or metastatic breast cancer (in combination with palbociclib or abemaciclib) in women with disease progression following endocrine therapy

Local Anesthetic/Vasoconstrictor Precautions No information available to require special precautions

Effects on Dental Treatment No significant effects or complications reported

Effects on Bleeding No information available to require special precautions

Adverse Reactions

>10%:

Central nervous system: Fatigue (8% to 32%), headache (8% to 15%)

Endocrine & metabolic: Increased gamma-glutamyl transferase (49%), decreased serum glucose (18%), hot flash (7% to 11%)

Gastrointestinal: Nausea (10% to 28%), diarrhea (6% to 25%), abdominal pain (13% to 16%), vomiting (6% to 15%), stomatitis (10% to 13%), decreased appetite (8% to 13%), constipation (5% to 12%)

Hematologic & oncologic: Anemia (4% to 40%; grade 3: ≤2%), lymphocytopenia (35%; grade 3: 2%)

Hepatic: Increased serum aspartate aminotransferase (5% to 48%), increased serum alanine aminotransferase (5% to 37%), increased liver enzymes (>15%)

Infection: Infection (25% to 31%)

Local: Pain at injection site (12%)

Neuromuscular & skeletal: Arthralgia (8% to 17%)

Renal: Increased serum creatinine (≤74%)

Respiratory: Cough (5% to 15%), dyspnea (4% to 12%)

1% to 10%:

Cardiovascular: Peripheral edema (7%)

Central nervous system: Dizziness (6% to 8%)

Dermatologic: Pruritus (6% to 7%), skin rash (4% to 7%), alopecia (2% to 6%)

Endocrine & metabolic: Decreased serum albumin (8%), decreased serum phosphate (8%), weight loss (2%)

Gastrointestinal: Anorexia (6%), dysgeusia (3%)

Hematologic & oncologic: Leukopenia (≤5%; grade 3: 1%; grade 4: 1%), thrombocytopenia (3%; grade 4: <1%), neutropenia (2%; grade 3: 1%; grade 4: <1%)

Neuromuscular & skeletal: Ostealgia (9%), back pain (8% to 9%), myalgia (7%), limb pain (6% to 7%), musculoskeletal pain (6%), asthenia (5% to 6%)

Miscellaneous: Fever (5% to 7%)

Frequency not defined: Central nervous system: Neuralgia, peripheral neuropathy, sciatica

<1%, postmarketing, and/or case reports: Hepatic failure, hepatitis, increased serum bilirubin, vaginal hemorrhage, venous thromboembolism

Mechanism of Action Fulvestrant is an estrogen receptor antagonist; competitively binds to estrogen receptors on tumors and other tissue targets, producing a nuclear complex that causes a dose-related down-regulation of estrogen receptors and inhibits tumor growth.

Pharmacodynamics/Kinetics

Duration of Action IM: Steady state concentrations reached within first month, when administered with additional dose given 2 weeks following the initial dose; plasma levels maintained for at least 1 month

Half-life Elimination

Children 1.7 to 8.5 years: 70.4 ± 8.1 days (Sims 2012)

Adults: 250 mg: ~40 days

Reproductive Considerations

For females of reproductive potential, pregnancy testing is recommended within 7 days prior to initiation of fulvestrant and effective contraception should be used during treatment and for 1 year after the last fulvestrant dose.

Pregnancy Considerations

Based on findings from animal reproduction studies and the mechanism of action, fulvestrant may cause fetal harm if administered during pregnancy.

◆ **Fungi-Guard [OTC]** *see* Tolnaftate *on page 1462*

◆ **Fungoid-D [OTC] [DSC]** *see* Tolnaftate *on page 1462*

◆ **Fungoid Tincture [OTC]** *see* Miconazole (Topical) *on page 1019*

◆ **Furadantin [DSC]** *see* Nitrofurantoin *on page 1111*

◆ **Furazosin** *see* Prazosin *on page 1254*

Furosemide (fyoor OH se mide)

Related Information

Cardiovascular Diseases *on page 1654*

Brand Names: US Lasix

Brand Names: Canada APO-Furosemide; BIO-Furosemide; Furosemide Special; Lasix Oral; Lasix Special; MINT-Furosemide; PMS-Furosemide; TEVA-Furosemide

Pharmacologic Category Antihypertensive; Diuretic, Loop

Use

Edema: Management of edema associated with heart failure, cirrhosis of the liver (ie, ascites), or renal disease (including nephrotic syndrome); acute pulmonary edema.

Local Anesthetic/Vasoconstrictor Precautions No information available to require special precautions

Effects on Dental Treatment No significant effects or complications reported

Effects on Bleeding No information available to require special precautions

Adverse Reactions

Frequency not defined:

Cardiovascular: Necrotizing angiitis, orthostatic hypotension, thrombophlebitis, vasculitis

Central nervous system: Dizziness, headache, paresthesia, restlessness, vertigo
Dermatologic: Acute generalized exanthematous pustulosis, bullous pemphigoid, erythema multiforme, exfoliative dermatitis, pruritus, skin photosensitivity, skin rash, Stevens-Johnson syndrome, toxic epidermal necrolysis, urticaria
Endocrine & metabolic: Glycosuria, hyperglycemia, hyperuricemia, increased serum cholesterol, increased serum triglycerides
Gastrointestinal: Abdominal cramps, anorexia, constipation, diarrhea, gastric irritation, mouth irritation, nausea, pancreatitis, vomiting
Genitourinary: Bladder spasm
Hematologic & oncologic: Agranulocytosis, anemia, aplastic anemia, eosinophilia, hemolytic anemia, leukopenia, purpura, thrombocytopenia
Hepatic: Hepatic encephalopathy, intrahepatic cholestatic jaundice, liver enzymes increased
Hypersensitivity: Anaphylaxis, anaphylactoid reaction, anaphylactic shock
Immunologic: DRESS syndrome
Neuromuscular & skeletal: Muscle spasm, weakness
Ophthalmic: Blurred vision, xanthopsia
Otic: Deafness, tinnitus
Renal: Interstitial nephritis (allergic), renal disease
Miscellaneous: Fever

Mechanism of Action Primarily inhibits reabsorption of sodium and chloride in the ascending loop of Henle and proximal and distal renal tubules, interfering with the chloride-binding cotransport system, thus causing its natriuretic effect (Rose 1991).

Pharmacodynamics/Kinetics

Onset of Action Diuresis: Oral, sublingual: 30 to 60 minutes.

Symptomatic improvement with acute pulmonary edema: Within 15 to 20 minutes; occurs prior to diuretic effect.

Peak effect: Oral, SL: 1 to 2 hours; IV: 0.5 hours.

Duration of Action Oral, sublingual: 6 to 8 hours; IV: 2 hours

Half-life Elimination Normal renal function: 0.5 to 2 hours; End-stage renal disease (ESRD): 9 hours

Pregnancy Considerations

Furosemide crosses the placenta (Beerman 1978; Riva 1978).

Monitor fetal growth if used during pregnancy (ESC [Regitz-Zagrosek 2018]).

Chronic maternal hypertension is associated with adverse events in the fetus/infant. The risk of birth defects, low birth weight, premature delivery, stillbirth, and neonatal death may be increased with chronic hypertension in pregnancy. Actual risks may be related to duration and severity of maternal hypertension. If a diuretic is needed for the treatment of hypertension in pregnancy, other agents are preferred (ACOG 203 2019). Low dose furosemide may be considered in patients with preeclampsia and oliguria (ESC [Regitz-Zagrosek 2018]).

The treatment of edema associated with chronic heart failure during pregnancy is similar to that of nonpregnant patients. Use of diuretics may be considered but use with caution due to the potential reduction in placental blood flow. Patients diagnosed after delivery can be treated according to heart failure guidelines (ESC [Bauersachs 2016]; ESC [Regitz-Zagrosek 2018]).

◆ **Fusilev [DSC]** *see* LEVOleucovorin *on page 899*

◆ **Fusion [OTC]** *see* Vitamins (Multiple/Oral) *on page 1550*

◆ **Fusion Plus** *see* Vitamins (Multiple/Oral) *on page 1550*

◆ **Fuzeon** *see* Enfuvirtide *on page 564*

◆ **FVIII/vWF** *see* Antihemophilic Factor/von Willebrand Factor Complex (Human) *on page 154*

◆ **Fyavolv** *see* Ethinyl Estradiol and Norethindrone *on page 614*

◆ **Fycompa** *see* Perampanel *on page 1216*

◆ **GA101** *see* Obinutuzumab *on page 1124*

Gabapentin (GA ba pen tin)

Related Information

Temporomandibular Dysfunction (TMD), Chronic Pain, and Fibromyalgia *on page 1773*

Brand Names: US Gralise; Gralise Starter; Neurontin

Brand Names: Canada ACT Gabapentin [DSC]; AG-Gabapentin; APO-Gabapentin; Auro-Gabapentin; BCI Gabapentin [DSC]; BIO-Gabapentin; DOM-Gabapentin; GD-Gabapentin; GLN-Gabapentin; JAMP-Gabapentin; Mar-Gabapentin; MYLAN-Gabapentin [DSC]; Neurontin; PMS-Gabapentin; Priva-Gabapentin; PRO-Gabapentin; RAN-Gabapentin; RIVA-Gabapentin; TARO-Gabapentin; TEVA-Gabapentin; VAN-Gabapentin [DSC]

Generic Availability (US) May be product dependent

Pharmacologic Category Anticonvulsant, Miscellaneous; GABA Analog

Dental Use Neuropathic pain (consult with physician)

Use

Postherpetic neuralgia: Management of postherpetic neuralgia (PHN) in adults.

Seizures, focal (partial) onset (immediate release only): As adjunctive therapy in the treatment of focal (partial) seizures with and without secondary generalization in adults and pediatric patients 3 years of age and older with epilepsy.

Local Anesthetic/Vasoconstrictor Precautions

No information available to require special precautions

Effects on Dental Treatment Key adverse event(s) related to dental treatment: Xerostomia (normal salivary flow resumes upon discontinuation), dry throat, and dental abnormalities.

Effects on Bleeding No information available to require special precautions

Adverse Reactions

>10%:

Infection: Viral infection (IR, children: 11%)
Nervous system: Ataxia (IR, adolescents and adults: 1% to 13%), dizziness (IR, adolescents and adults: 17% to 28% [placebo: 7% to 8%]; ER, adults: 11% [placebo: 2%]; IR, children: 3% [placebo: 2%]), drowsiness (IR, adolescents and adults: 19% to 21% [placebo: 5% to 9%]; IR, children: 8% [placebo: 5%]; ER, adults: 5% [placebo: 3%]), fatigue (IR, adolescents and adults: 11%; IR, children: 3%)

1% to 10%:

Cardiovascular: Hypertension (ER, adults: >1%), increased blood pressure (ER, adults: >1%), peripheral edema (adolescents and adults: 2% to 8%), vasodilation (IR, adolescents and adults: 1%)
Dermatologic: Excoriation of skin (IR, adolescents and adults: 1%), skin rash (ER, adults: >1%)
Endocrine & metabolic: Hyperglycemia (IR, adults: 1%), weight gain (2% to 3%)

Gastrointestinal: Constipation (adolescents and adults: 1% to 4%), dental disease (IR, adolescents and adults: 2%), diarrhea (IR, adults: 6%), dyspepsia (adolescents and adults: 1% to 2%), nausea (IR: ≤8%; ER, adults: >1%), viral gastroenteritis (ER, adults: >1%), vomiting (IR: ≤8%), xerostomia (adolescents and adults: ≤5%)

Genitourinary: Impotence (IR, adolescents and adults: 2%), urinary tract infection (ER, adults: 2%)

Infection: Herpes zoster infection (ER, adults: >1%), infection (IR, adults: 5%)

Nervous system: Abnormal gait (IR, adults: 2%), abnormality in thinking (IR: 2% to 3% [placebo: ≤1%]), amnesia (IR, adolescents and adults: 2%), confusion (ER, adults: >1%), depression (IR, adolescents and adults: 2%), dysarthria (IR, adolescents and adults: 2%), emotional lability (IR: 4% to 6% [placebo: 1% to 2%]), hostility (IR: 5% to 8% [placebo: 1% to 2%]), lethargy (ER, adults: 1%), memory impairment (ER, adults: >1%), pain (ER, adults: 1%), status epilepticus (IR, adolescents and adults: 2%), vertigo (ER, adults: 1%)

Neuromuscular & skeletal: Asthenia (IR, adults: 6%), back pain (adolescents and adults: 2%), hyperkinetic muscle activity (IR: 3% to 5% [placebo: 1% to 3%]), joint swelling (ER, adults: >1%), limb pain (ER, adults: 2%), tremor (IR, adolescents and adults: 7%)

Ophthalmic: Amblyopia (IR: 3% to 4%), conjunctivitis (IR, adults: 1%), diplopia (IR, adolescents and adults: 1% to 6%), nystagmus disorder (IR, adolescents and adults: 8%)

Otic: Otitis media (IR, adults: 1%)

Respiratory: Bronchitis (IR, children: 3%), cough (IR, adolescents and adults: 2%), dry throat (IR, adolescents and adults: ≤2%), nasopharyngitis (ER, adults: 3%), pharyngitis (IR, adolescents and adults: 1% to 3%), pneumonia (ER, adults: >1%), respiratory tract infection (IR, children: 3%), upper respiratory tract infection (ER, adults: >1%)

Miscellaneous: Accidental injury (IR, adults: 3% [placebo: 1%]), fever (IR, children: 10%; ER, adults: >1%)

<1%:

Hypersensitivity: Anaphylaxis, angioedema

Immunologic: Drug reaction with eosinophilia and systemic symptoms (Ragucci 2001; Scaparotta 2011)

Nervous system: Suicidal ideation (Molero 2019), suicidal tendencies (Molero 2019)

Postmarketing:

Cardiovascular: Cardiomyopathy (Tellor 2019), hypersensitivity angiitis (Sahin 2008)

Dermatologic: Bullous pemphigoid (Flamm 2017), dermatitis (interstitial granulomatous [Georgesen 2014]), erythema multiforme, Stevens-Johnson syndrome (Gonzales-Sicilia 1998)

Endocrine & metabolic: Altered serum glucose, amenorrhea (Berger 2004), change in libido, hypoglycemia (Penumalee 2003; Scholl 2015), hyponatremia (Falhammar 2018; Lu 2017; Wilton 2002), thyroiditis (Fyre 1999)

Genitourinary: Breast hypertrophy (Zylicz 2000), ejaculation failure (Labbate 1999), ejaculatory disorder, urinary incontinence (Rissardo 2019)

Hematologic & oncologic: Thrombocytopenia (Ataki 2015)

Hepatic: Hepatotoxicity (Jackson 2018), increased liver enzymes (Jackson 2018; Lasso-de-la-Vega 2001)

Infection: Parasitic infection (Lopez 2010)

Nervous system: Agitation (Childers 1997), anorgasmia (Labbate 1999), coma (Abdennour 2017; Butler 2003; Dogukan 2006), encephalopathy (Beauvais 2015), movement disorder (Allford 2007; Attupurath 2009; Palomeras 2000; Pina 2005; Raju 2007; Rohman 2014; Souzdalnitski 2014; Twardowschy 2008; Zesiewicz 2008), myoclonus (facial) (Hampton 2019; Hui 2019; Yeddi 2019), polyneuropathy (Gould 1998), stuttering (Nissani 1997), visual hallucination (Parsons 2016)

Neuromuscular & skeletal: Increased creatine phosphokinase in blood specimen, rhabdomyolysis (Bilgir 2009; Choi 2017; Coupal 2017; Lipson 2005; Tuccori 2007)

Respiratory: Respiratory depression (FDA Safety Alert, December 19, 2019)

Dental Usual Dosage

Pain (off-label use): Children >12 years and Adults: Oral: 300-1800 mg/day given in 3 divided doses has been the most common dosage range

Postherpetic neuralgia or neuropathic pain: Adults: Oral: Day 1: 300 mg, Day 2: 300 mg twice daily, Day 3: 300 mg 3 times/day; dose may be titrated as needed for pain relief (range: 1800-3600 mg/day, daily doses >1800 mg do not generally show greater benefit)

Dosing

Adult Note: For patients with respiratory disease, initiate therapy at the lowest dose (FDA 2019).

Alcohol use disorder, moderate to severe (alternative agent) (off-label use): Immediate release: **Oral:** Initial: 300 mg once daily; increase dose based on response and tolerability in increments of 300 mg every 1 to 2 days up to a target dose of 600 mg 3 times daily (Brower 2008; Mason 2014; VA/DoD 2015). **Note:** Gabapentin is suggested by some experts as an alternative when first-line agents cannot be used (Johnson 2019; VA/DoD 2015). Gabapentin may be misused by some patients with substance use disorders; evaluate for risk and signs of addiction and dependence (Mersfelder 2016).

Alcohol withdrawal, mild (alternative agent) (off-label use):

Note: Withdrawal will progress at different rates in some patients; flexibility in dosing and duration is warranted (Holt 2018; VA/DoD 2015). The following is one suggested regimen based on a single randomized, double-blind trial:

Immediate release: **Oral:** Initial: 300 to 400 mg 3 times daily on days 1 through 3, then 300 to 400 mg twice daily on day 4, then discontinue. For breakthrough symptoms during days 1 through 4, consider providing single doses of 100 mg, which may be administered up to 3 times daily, and a 300 mg dose reserved for the evening (Myrick 2009).

Cough, chronic refractory (alternative agent) (off-label use): Immediate release: **Oral:** Initial: 300 mg once daily; increase dose gradually based on response and tolerability in increments of 300 mg to a maximum dose of 900 mg twice daily (ACCP [Gibson 2016]; Ryan 2012). Re-evaluate therapeutic need after 6 months (ACCP [Gibson 2016]).

Fibromyalgia (alternative agent) (off-label use):
Note: For patients who do not respond to or tolerate preferred agents (Goldenberg 2020):
Immediate release: **Oral:** Initial: 100 to 300 mg once daily at bedtime; increase dose gradually based on response and tolerability every 1 to 2 weeks to a target dose of 1.2 to 2.4 g/day in divided doses (Arnold 2007; Goldenberg 2020).
Hiccups (singultus) (off-label use): Immediate release: **Oral:** Usual dose range: 300 mg to 1.2 g/day in 3 to 4 divided doses (Hernández 2004; Jatzko 2007; Moretti 2004; Porzio 2010; Schuchmann 2007). Can be discontinued the day after hiccups subside; long-term therapy may be warranted for persistent or relapsing hiccups (eg, palliative care) (Lembo 2018). **Note:** In patients with refractory hiccups, may use in combination with a proton pump inhibitor, baclofen, or metoclopramide (Kohse 2017).
Neuropathic pain:
General dosing recommendations (for other than postherpetic neuralgia) (off-label use):
Note: For chronic use, an adequate trial with gabapentin may require 2 months or more (Bone 2002; Tauben 2020). For critically ill patients with neuropathic pain, gabapentin may be a useful component of multimodal pain control (SCCM [Devlin 2018]).
Immediate release: **Oral:** Initial: 100 to 300 mg 1 to 3 times daily (ADA [Pop-Busui 2017]; Dolgun 2014; Mishra 2012); increase dose based on response and tolerability to a target dose range of 300 mg to 1.2 g 3 times daily (AAN [Bril 2011]; ADA [Pop-Busui 2017]; EFNS [Attal 2010]; IASP [Finnerup 2015]).
Extended release: **Oral:** Initial: 300 mg at bedtime; increase dose based on response and tolerability to a target dose of 900 mg to 3.6 g once daily (IASP [Finnerup 2015]; Sandercock 2012).
Postherpetic neuralgia:
Immediate release: **Oral:** 300 mg once on day 1, 300 mg twice daily on day 2, and 300 mg 3 times daily on day 3, then increase as needed up to 1.8 to 3.6 g/day in divided doses. Additional benefit of doses >1.8 g/day has not been established.
Extended release: **Oral:** Initial: 300 mg once daily; increase by 300 mg each day up to 900 mg once daily. Further increase as needed up to 1.8 g once daily. Additional benefit of doses >1.8 g/day has not been established.
Postoperative pain (off-label use): Immediate release: **Oral:** 300 mg to 1.2 g as a single dose, given 1 to 2 hours prior to surgery or immediately following surgery as part of a multimodal analgesia regimen (Chou 2016; Doleman 2015; Peng 2007; Yu 2013). **Note:** Some experts avoid use in patients with sleep-disordered breathing (eg, obstructive sleep apnea) (Joshi 2020; Mariano 2018).
Pruritus, chronic (alternative agent) (off-label use):
Note: For patients with pruritus resistant to preferred therapies (Matsuda 2016; Weisshaar 2012):
Neuropathic (eg, brachioradial pruritus, notalgia paresthetica) or malignancy-related pruritus: Immediate release: **Oral:** Initial: 300 mg/day in 1 to 3 divided doses; increase dose based on response and tolerability up to 1.8 g/day in divided doses (Kanitakis 2006; Winhoven 2004; Yilmaz 2010). Higher doses up to 3.6 g/day have been used in oncology populations (Demierre 2006; Lee 2010).
Uremic pruritus: Immediate release: **Oral:** Initial: 100 mg after dialysis on hemodialysis days; may increase dose based on response and tolerability up to 300 mg after dialysis on hemodialysis days (Gunal 2004; Kobrin 2018; Nofal 2016; Razeghi 2009).
Restless legs syndrome (off-label use): Immediate release: **Oral:** Initial: 100 to 300 mg once daily 2 hours before bedtime; may increase dose every 1 to 2 weeks until symptom relief is achieved (range: 300 mg to 2.4 g/day). Suggested maintenance dosing schedule for doses ≥600 mg/day: One-third of total daily dose given midday, remaining two-thirds of the total daily dose given in the evening (Garcia-Borreguero 2002; Happe 2003; IRLSSG/EURLSSG/RLS-F [Garcia-Borreguero 2016]; Saletu 2010; Silber 2018; Vignatelli 2006).
Seizures, focal (partial) onset: Immediate release: **Oral:** Initial: 300 mg 3 times daily; increase dose based on response and tolerability. Usual dosage: 300 to 600 mg 3 times daily; doses up to 2.4 g/day and 3.6 g/day have been tolerated in long-term and short-term clinical studies, respectively. Some experts recommend a lower starting dose (eg, 100 mg 3 times daily) with titration as tolerated (Schachter 2018).
Social anxiety disorder (alternative agent) (off-label use):
Note: Monotherapy or adjunctive therapy for patients who do not tolerate or respond to preferred agents (Stein 2020):
Immediate release: **Oral:** Initial: 300 mg twice daily; increase dose based on response and tolerability in increments of no more than 300 mg/day up to a maximum of 3.6 g/day in 3 divided doses (Pande 1999). Some experts recommend initiating with 100 mg 3 times daily in patients with respiratory disease (Stein 2020).
Vasomotor symptoms associated with menopause (off-label use):
Immediate release: **Oral:** Initial: 300 to 400 mg once daily at bedtime; some experts use an initial dose of 100 mg once daily to avoid adverse effects (Santen 2018); increase gradually (eg, over 3 to 12 days) based on response and tolerability up to 600 mg to 2.4 g/day in 2 to 3 divided doses (ACOG 2014; NAMS 2015; Reddy 2006; Toulis 2009). Some experts suggest gabapentin for women whose symptoms occur primarily at night and favor a maximum dose of 900 mg to 1.2 g, given as one dose at bedtime (ES [Stuenkel 2015]; Santen 2018).
Extended release: **Oral:** Initial: 600 mg once daily at bedtime; increase gradually (eg, 600 mg every 3 days) to target dose of 600 mg in the morning and 1.2 g at bedtime (Pinkerton 2014).

Discontinuation of therapy: In patients receiving gabapentin chronically, unless safety concerns require a more rapid withdrawal, gabapentin should be withdrawn gradually over ≥1 week to minimize the potential of increased seizure frequency (in patients with epilepsy) or other withdrawal symptoms (eg, confusion, irritability, tachycardia, diaphoresis) (Norton 2001; Tran 2005).

Geriatric
Restless legs syndrome (off-label use): Immediate release: Oral: Initial: 100 mg once daily (IRLSSG/EURLSSG/RLS-F [Garcia-Borreguero 2016]).

Other indications: Initiate therapy at the lowest dose (FDA 2019). Refer to adult dosing. For postoperative pain (off-label use), some experts avoid use in patients >65 years of age (Joshi 2020).

Discontinuation of therapy: Refer to adult dosing.

Renal Impairment: Adult

The renal dosing recommendations are based upon the best available evidence and clinical expertise. Senior Editorial Team: Bruce Mueller, PharmD, FCCP, FASN, FNKF; Jason Roberts, PhD, BPharm (Hons), B App Sc, FSHP, FISAC; Michael Heung, MD, MS.

Oral: Immediate release:

Note: Initial doses of gabapentin should be conservative and titrated based on effectiveness and tolerability.

Gabapentin Dose Adjustments for Kidney Impairment[a,b]

CrCl (mL/minute)[c]	Approximate Maintenance Dose Adjustment	Maximum Maintenance Dose
>79	No dose adjustment necessary	3,600 mg/day in 3 divided doses
50 to 79	No dose adjustment necessary	1,800 mg/day in 3 divided doses
30 to 49	~50% reduction	900 mg/day in 2 to 3 divided doses
15 to 29	~75% reduction	600 mg/day in 1 to 2 divided doses
<15	~90% reduction	300 mg/**day** in 1 dose

[a]Choose normal dose based on indication (see Adult dosing), then choose the adjusted dose from the column corresponding to the patient's CrCl.

[b]Expert opinion derived from Blum 1994, Davison 2014, Davison 2019, manufacturer's labeling.

[c]Estimation of renal function for dosing adjustments should be done using the Cockcroft Gault formula.

Hemodialysis, intermittent (thrice weekly): Dialyzable (50% over 4 hours [Wong 1995]):

Initial: 100 mg 3 times per week after hemodialysis. Titrate to effect up to 300 mg 3 times per week given after hemodialysis on dialysis days (Atalay 2013; Gunal 2004; Kobrin 2018; Koncicki 2015; Nofal 2016; Razeghi 2009; Spaia 2009).

Note: Some experts recommend cautious titration to a maximum of 300 mg/day in select patients requiring additional pain control (Koncicki 2017; Kurella 2003; Davison 2019).

Peritoneal dialysis:

Initial: 100 mg every other day. Titrate to effect up to 300 mg every other day (Koncicki 2015; expert opinion).

Note: Some experts recommend cautious titration to a maximum of 300 mg/day in select patients requiring additional pain control (Koncicki 2017; Kurella 2003; Davison 2019).

CRRT:

Note: Drug clearance is dependent on the effluent flow rate, filter type, and method of renal replacement. Recommendations are based on high-flux dialyzers and effluent flow rates of 20 to 25 mL/kg/hour (or approximately 1,500 to 3,000 mL/hour) unless otherwise noted.

CVVH/CVVHD/CVVHDF:

Note: Dosing based on expert opinion; no evidence available. Pharmacokinetic characteristics and one case report suggest gabapentin is cleared by CRRT (Guddati 2012).

Initial: 100 mg twice daily and titrate to effect. Suggested maximum dose: 300 mg twice daily.

Oral: Extended release:

Note: Follow initial dose titration schedule if treatment naive. Estimation of renal function for dosing adjustments should be done using the Cockcroft-Gault formula. Renally adjusted dose recommendations are based on doses up to 1.8 g/day.

CrCl ≥60 mL/minute: Oral: No dosage adjustment necessary.

CrCl >30 to 59 mL/minute: Oral: 600 mg to 1.8 g once daily; dependent on tolerability and clinical response.

CrCl <30 mL/minute: Use is not recommended.

End-stage renal disease requiring hemodialysis: Use is not recommended.

Peritoneal dialysis: Use is not recommended.

Hepatic Impairment: Adult There are no dosage adjustments provided in the manufacturer's labeling; however, gabapentin is not hepatically metabolized.

Pediatric Note: Do not exceed 12 hours between doses with 3 times daily dosing. Pediatric doses presented as mg/kg/day and mg/kg/dose; use precaution.

Seizures, partial onset; adjunctive therapy: Oral: Immediate release: **Note:** If gabapentin is discontinued or if another anticonvulsant is added to therapy, it should be done slowly over a minimum of 1 week.

Children 3 to <12 years:

Initial: 10 to 15 mg/kg/**day** divided into 3 doses daily; titrate dose upward over ~3 days

Maintenance usual dose:

Children 3 to 4 years: 40 mg/kg/**day** divided into 3 doses daily; maximum daily dose: In one long-term study, doses up to 50 mg/kg/**day** were well-tolerated

Children 5 to <12 years: 25 to 35 mg/kg/**day** divided into 3 doses daily; maximum daily dose: In one long-term study, doses up to 50 mg/kg/**day** were well-tolerated

Children ≥12 years and Adolescents: Initial: 300 mg 3 times daily; titrate dose upward if needed; usual maintenance dose: 900 to 1,800 mg/day divided into 3 doses daily; doses up to 2,400 mg/day divided into 3 doses daily are well tolerated long-term; maximum daily dose: Doses up to 3,600 mg/**day** have been tolerated in short-term studies.

Neuropathic pain: Limited data available: Oral: Immediate release: Children and Adolescents: Initial: 5 mg/kg/dose up to 300 mg at bedtime; day 2: Increase to 5 mg/kg/dose twice daily (up to 300 mg twice daily); day 3: Increase to 5 mg/kg/dose 3 times daily (up to 300 mg 3 times daily); further titrate with dosage increases (not frequency) to effect; American Pain Society (APS) recommends a lower initial dose of 2 mg/kg/**day** which may be considered if concurrent analgesics are also sedating; usual dosage range: 8 to 35 mg/kg/**day** divided into 3 doses daily (APS, 2008; Galloway, 2000); maximum daily dose: 3,600 mg/**day**

Renal Impairment: Pediatric

Immediate release:

Children <12 years: There are no dosing adjustments provided in the manufacturer's labeling (has not been studied).

Children ≥12 years and Adolescents: See table.

Gabapentin Dosing Adjustments in Renal Impairment

Creatinine Clearance (mL/minute)	Total Daily Dose Range (mg/day)	Dosage Regimens (Maintenance Doses) (mg)				
≥60	900 to 3,600	300 3 times/day	400 3 times/day	600 3 times/day	800 3 times/day	1,200 3 times/day
>30 to 59	400 to 1,400	200 twice daily	300 twice daily	400 twice daily	500 twice daily	700 twice daily
>15 to 29	200 to 700	200 daily	300 daily	400 daily	500 daily	700 daily
15[A]	100 to 300	100 daily	125 daily	150 daily	200 daily	300 daily
Hemodialysis[B]		Posthemodialysis Supplemental Dose				
		125 mg	150 mg	200 mg	250 mg	350 mg

[A]CrCl <15 mL/minute: Reduce daily dose in proportion to creatinine clearance.

[B]Supplemental dose should be administered after each 4 hours of hemodialysis (patients on hemodialysis should also receive maintenance doses based on renal function as listed in the upper portion of the table).

Hepatic Impairment: Pediatric There are no dosage adjustments provided in the manufacturer's labeling; however, adjustment not necessary since gabapentin is not hepatically metabolized.

Mechanism of Action Gabapentin is structurally related to GABA. However, it does not bind to $GABA_A$ or $GABA_B$ receptors, and it does not appear to influence degradation or uptake of GABA. High affinity gabapentin binding sites have been located throughout the brain; these sites correspond to the presence of voltage-gated calcium channels specifically possessing the alpha-2-delta-1 subunit. This channel appears to be located presynaptically, and may modulate the release of excitatory neurotransmitters which participate in epileptogenesis and nociception. These effects on restless leg syndrome are unknown.

Contraindications Hypersensitivity to gabapentin or any component of the formulation

Warnings/Precautions Serious, life-threatening, and fatal respiratory depression may occur in patients using gabapentin; risk may be increased with conditions such as chronic obstructive pulmonary disease, in the elderly, and with the concomitant use of opioids and other CNS depressants. Initiate gabapentin at the lowest dose and monitor patients for symptoms of respiratory depression and sedation in patients with underlying respiratory disease (FDA 2019). Antiepileptics are associated with an increased risk of suicidal behavior/thoughts with use (regardless of indication); patients should be monitored for signs/symptoms of depression, suicidal tendencies, and other unusual behavior changes during therapy and instructed to inform their healthcare provider immediately if symptoms occur. Avoid abrupt withdrawal; may precipitate seizures or other withdrawal symptoms; decrease dose slowly over ≥1 week (Norton 2001; Tran 2005). Use cautiously in patients with renal dysfunction; male rat studies demonstrated an association with pancreatic adenocarcinoma (clinical implication unknown). May cause CNS depression, including somnolence and dizziness, that may impair physical or mental abilities. Patients must be cautioned about performing tasks which require mental alertness (eg, operating machinery or driving). Pediatric patients have shown increased incidence of CNS-related adverse effects, including emotional lability, hostility, changes in behavior and thinking, and hyperkinesia. IR and ER products are not interchangeable with each other **or** with gabapentin enacarbil. Use with caution in patients with myasthenia gravis; may exacerbate condition (Mehrizi 2012). The safety and efficacy of the ER formulation has not been studied in patients with epilepsy. Potentially serious, sometimes fatal multiorgan hypersensitivity (also known as drug reaction with eosinophilia and systemic symptoms) has been reported with some antiepileptic drugs, including gabapentin; may affect lymphatic, hepatic, renal, cardiac, and/or hematologic systems; fever, rash, and eosinophilia may also be present. Discontinue immediately if suspected. Anaphylaxis and/or angioedema may occur after the first dose or at any time during treatment; discontinue therapy and seek immediate medical care if signs or symptoms of anaphylaxis or angioedema occur. Use with caution in patients with a history of substance abuse, including alcohol, benzodiazepines, cannabis, cocaine, and opioids; potential for drug dependency exists. Gabapentin may cause respiratory depression; use caution and initiate with the lowest recommended dose in elderly patients and those with respiratory disease (FDA 2019). Tolerance, psychological and physical dependence may occur (Evoy 2017; Mersfelder 2016). Potentially significant drug-drug interactions may exist, requiring dose or frequency adjustment, additional monitoring, and/or selection of alternative therapy.

Warnings: Additional Pediatric Considerations Neuropsychiatric adverse events, such as emotional lability (eg, behavioral problems), hostility, aggressive behaviors, thought disorders (eg, problems with concentration and school performance), and hyperkinesia (eg, hyperactivity and restlessness), have been reported in clinical trials of pediatric patients ages 3 to 12 years. Most of these pediatric neuropsychiatric adverse events are mild to moderate in terms of intensity but discontinuation of gabapentin may be required; children with mental retardation and attention-deficit disorders may be at increased risk for behavioral side effects (Lee 1996).

Drug Interactions

Metabolism/Transport Effects None known.

Avoid Concomitant Use

Avoid concomitant use of Gabapentin with any of the following: Azelastine (Nasal); Bromperidol; Orphenadrine; Oxomemazine; Paraldehyde; Thalidomide

Increased Effect/Toxicity

Gabapentin may increase the levels/effects of: Alcohol (Ethyl); Azelastine (Nasal); Blonanserin; Brexanolone; Buprenorphine; CNS Depressants; Flunitrazepam; Methotrimeprazine; MetyroSINE; Morphine (Systemic); Opioid Agonists; Orphenadrine; OxyCODONE; Paraldehyde; Piribedil; Pramipexole; ROPINIRole; Rotigotine; Suvorexant; Thalidomide; Zolpidem

The levels/effects of Gabapentin may be increased by: Alizapride; Brimonidine (Topical); Bromopride; Bromperidol; Cannabidiol; Cannabis; Chlormethiazole; Chlorphenesin Carbamate; Dimethindene (Topical); Doxylamine; Dronabinol; Droperidol; Esketamine; HydrOXYzine; Kava Kava; Lemborexant; Lisuride; Lofexidine; Magnesium Salts; Methotrimeprazine; Metoclopramide; Minocycline (Systemic); Morphine (Systemic); Nabilone; Oxomemazine; Perampanel; Rufinamide; Sodium Oxybate; Tetrahydrocannabinol; Tetrahydrocannabinol and Cannabidiol; Trimeprazine

Decreased Effect

The levels/effects of Gabapentin may be decreased by: Aluminum Hydroxide; Magnesium Salts; Mefloquine; Mianserin; Orlistat

Food Interactions Tablet, solution (immediate release): No significant effect on rate or extent of absorption; extended release tablet: Increases rate and extent of absorption. Management: Administer immediate release products without regard to food. Administer extended release with food.

Dietary Considerations Extended release tablet should be taken with food.

Pharmacodynamics/Kinetics

Half-life Elimination

Infants 1 month to Children 12 years: 4.7 hours

Adults, normal: 5 to 7 hours; increased half-life with decreased renal function; anuric adult patients: 132 hours; adults during hemodialysis: 3.8 hours

Time to Peak Immediate release: Infants 1 month to Children 12 years: 2 to 3 hours; Adults: 2 to 4 hours; Extended release: 8 hours

Reproductive Considerations

Folic acid supplementation is recommended prior to pregnancy in women using gabapentin (Borgelt 2016; Picchietti 2015).

Pregnancy Risk Factor C

Pregnancy Considerations

Gabapentin crosses the placenta. In a small study (n=6), the umbilical/maternal plasma concentration ratio was ~1.74. Neonatal concentrations declined quickly after delivery and at 24 hours of life were ~27% of the cord blood concentrations at birth (gabapentin neonatal half-life ~14 hours) (Ohman 2005). Pregnancy registry outcome data following maternal use of gabapentin during pregnancy is limited (Holmes 2012). Folic acid supplementation is recommended during pregnancy in women using gabapentin (Borgelt 2016; Picchietti 2015).

Gabapentin is used off-label for the treatment of restless leg syndrome; however, current guidelines note there is insufficient evidence to recommend its use in pregnant women for this indication (Picchietti 2015). Pharmacological agents should not be used for the treatment of alcohol use disorder in pregnant women unless needed for the treatment of acute alcohol withdrawal or a coexisting disorder.

Patients exposed to gabapentin during pregnancy are encouraged to enroll in the North American Antiepileptic Drug (NAAED) Pregnancy Registry by calling 1-888-233-2334. Additional information is available at www.aedpregnancyregistry.org.

Breastfeeding Considerations Gabapentin is present in breast milk.

The relative infant dose (RID) of gabapentin is 8.7% to 13% when calculated using the highest breast milk concentration located and compared to an infant therapeutic dose of 10 to 15 mg/kg/day. In general, breastfeeding is considered acceptable when the RID is <10%; when an RID is >25% breastfeeding should generally be avoided (Anderson 2016; Ito 2000).

The RID of gabapentin was calculated using a milk concentration of 8.7 mcg/mL, providing an estimated daily infant dose via breast milk of 1.3 mg/kg/day. This milk concentration was obtained following maternal administration of oral gabapentin 2,100 mg/day. Gabapentin was detected in the serum of two breastfeeding infants 2 to 3 weeks after delivery and in one infant after 3 months of breastfeeding. Adverse events were not reported in the breastfed infants (Ohman 2005).

Manufacturer recommendations may vary; the decision to breastfeed during therapy should consider the risk of infant exposure, the benefits of breastfeeding to the infant, and benefits of treatment to the mother. Based on limited information, gabapentin is considered relatively compatible with breastfeeding; infants should be monitored for drowsiness, adequate weight gain, and developmental milestones (Davanzo 2013; Veiby 2015). Available guidelines state gabapentin may be considered for the treatment of refractory restless leg syndrome in breastfeeding women (Picchietti 2015). Pharmacological agents should not be used for the treatment of alcohol use disorder in breastfeeding women unless needed for the treatment of acute alcohol withdrawal or a coexisting disorder (APA [Reus 2018]).

Dosage Forms Considerations

Gralise is the extended release formulation.

Fanatrex FusePaq is a compounding kit for the preparation of an oral suspension. Refer to manufacturer's labeling for compounding instructions.

Neuraptine cream is compounded from a kit. Refer to manufacturer's labeling for compounding instructions.

Dosage Forms: US

Capsule, Oral:

Neurontin: 100 mg, 300 mg, 400 mg

Generic: 100 mg, 300 mg, 400 mg

Miscellaneous, Oral:

Gralise Starter: 300 & 600 mg (78 ea)

Solution, Oral:

Neurontin: 250 mg/5 mL (470 mL); 250 mg/5 mL (470 mL)

Generic: 250 mg/5 mL (473 mL); 300 mg/6 mL (6 mL); 250 mg/5 mL (5 mL, 6 mL, 470 mL)

Tablet, Oral:

Gralise: 300 mg, 600 mg

Neurontin: 600 mg, 800 mg

Generic: 600 mg, 800 mg

Dosage Forms: Canada

Capsule, Oral:

Neurontin: 100 mg, 300 mg, 400 mg

Generic: 100 mg, 300 mg, 400 mg

Tablet, Oral:

Neurontin: 600 mg, 800 mg

Generic: 600 mg, 800 mg

Gabapentin Enacarbil (gab a PEN tin en a KAR bil)

Brand Names: US Horizant

Pharmacologic Category Anticonvulsant, Miscellaneous

Use

Postherpetic neuralgia: Management of postherpetic neuralgia.

Restless legs syndrome: Treatment of moderate to severe restless leg syndrome.

Local Anesthetic/Vasoconstrictor Precautions No information available to require special precautions

Effects on Dental Treatment Key adverse event(s) related to dental treatment: Infrequent occurrence of xerostomia (normal salivary flow resumes upon discontinuation) has been reported.

Effects on Bleeding No information available to require special precautions

Adverse Reactions Percentages reported are for restless leg syndrome (RLS) 600 mg daily and postherpetic neuralgia (PHN) 1200 mg daily.

>10%: Central nervous system: Drowsiness (RLS: ≤20%; PHN: ≤10%), sedated state (RLS: ≤20%; PHN: ≤10%), dizziness (13% to 17%), headache (10% to 12%)

1% to 10%:

Cardiovascular: Peripheral edema (PHN: 6%; RLS: <1%)

Central nervous system: Fatigue (6%), irritability (≤4%), insomnia (PHN: 3%), equilibrium disturbance (<2%), depression (<2%), disorientation (<2%), intoxicated feeling (<2%), lethargy (<2%), vertigo (<2%)

Endocrine & metabolic: Weight gain (2% to 3%)

Gastrointestinal: Nausea (6% to 8%), flatulence (≤3%), xerostomia (≤3%), increased appetite (≤2%)

Ophthalmic: Blurred vision (≤2%)

<1%, postmarketing, and/or case reports: Breast hypertrophy (gabapentin), decreased libido, feeling abnormal, gynecomastia (gabapentin), increased creatine phosphokinase in blood specimen (gabapentin), respiratory depression (FDA Safety Alert, Dec 19, 2019)

Mechanism of Action Gabapentin enacarbil is a prodrug of gabapentin. Gabapentin is structurally related to GABA. However, it does not bind to $GABA_A$ or $GABA_B$ receptors, and it does not appear to influence degradation or uptake of GABA. High affinity gabapentin binding sites have been located throughout the brain; these sites correspond to the presence of voltage-gated calcium channels specifically possessing the alpha-2-delta-1 subunit. This channel appears to be located presynaptically, and may modulate the release of excitatory neurotransmitters. These effects on restless leg syndrome are unknown.

Pharmacodynamics/Kinetics

Half-life Elimination 5-6 hours

Time to Peak Plasma: With food: 7.3 hours; Fasting: 5 hours

Pregnancy Considerations Gabapentin enacarbil is the prodrug of gabapentin; bioavailability following gabapentin enacarbil is increased in comparison to gabapentin (Backonja 2011). Current guidelines note there is insufficient evidence to recommend gabapentin enacarbil in pregnant women for the treatment of restless legs syndrome (Picchietti 2015); use should be avoided (Garcia-Borreguero 2016).

Refer to Gabapentin monograph for information related to gabapentin exposure during pregnancy.

- ◆ **Gabitril** *see* TiaGABine *on page 1443*
- ◆ **Gablofen** *see* Baclofen *on page 213*
- ◆ **Galafold** *see* Migalastat *on page 1030*

Galcanezumab (GAL ka NEZ ue mab)

Brand Names: US Emgality; Emgality (300 MG Dose)

Brand Names: Canada Emgality

Pharmacologic Category Antimigraine Agent; Calcitonin Gene-Related Peptide (CGRP) Receptor Antagonist; Monoclonal Antibody, CGRP Antagonist

Use

Cluster headache (prevention): Preventative treatment of cluster headache during cluster episodes in adults.

Migraine prophylaxis: Preventive treatment of migraine in adults.

Local Anesthetic/Vasoconstrictor Precautions No information available to require special precautions

Effects on Dental Treatment No significant effects or complications reported

Effects on Bleeding No information available to require special precautions

Adverse Reactions

>10%:

Immunologic: Antibody development (5% to 13%; neutralizing: ≥50%)

Local: Injection site reaction (18%)

Frequency not defined: Hypersensitivity: Hypersensitivity reaction

Postmarketing: Anaphylaxis, angioedema, skin rash

Mechanism of Action Galcanezumab is a humanized monoclonal antibody that binds to calcitonin gene-related peptide (CGRP) ligand and blocks its binding to the receptor.

Pharmacodynamics/Kinetics

Half-life Elimination 27 days

Time to Peak 5 days

Reproductive Considerations

Consider the long half-life prior to use in females who may become pregnant until information related to pregnancy is available (Tepper 2018).

Pregnancy Considerations

Adverse events were not observed in animal reproduction studies.

Galcanezumab is a humanized monoclonal antibody (IgG_4). Potential placental transfer of human IgG is dependent upon the IgG subclass and gestational age, generally increasing as pregnancy progresses. The lowest exposure would be expected during the period of organogenesis (Palmeira 2012; Pentsuk 2009).

Consider the long half-life prior to use in females who are pregnant until information related to pregnancy is available (Tepper 2018).

- ◆ **Galcanezumab-gnlm** *see* Galcanezumab *on page 728*
- ◆ **GamaSTAN** *see* Immune Globulin *on page 803*
- ◆ **Gamifant** *see* Emapalumab *on page 554*
- ◆ **Gammagard** *see* Immune Globulin *on page 803*
- ◆ **Gammagard S/D Less IgA** *see* Immune Globulin *on page 803*
- ◆ **Gamma Globulin** *see* Immune Globulin *on page 803*
- ◆ **Gamma Hydroxybutyric Acid** *see* Sodium Oxybate *on page 1377*
- ◆ **Gammaked** *see* Immune Globulin *on page 803*
- ◆ **Gammaplex** *see* Immune Globulin *on page 803*
- ◆ **Gamunex-C** *see* Immune Globulin *on page 803*

Ganciclovir (Systemic) (gan SYE kloe veer)

Related Information

Systemic Viral Diseases *on page 1709*

ValGANciclovir *on page 1517*

Brand Names: US Cytovene

Brand Names: Canada Cytovene

Pharmacologic Category Antiviral Agent

Use

Cytomegalovirus disease, prophylaxis (transplant patients): Prevention of cytomegalovirus (CMV) disease in adult transplant recipients at risk for CMV disease.

Cytomegalovirus retinitis (immunocompromised patients): Treatment of CMV retinitis in immunocompromised adult patients, including patients with AIDS.

Local Anesthetic/Vasoconstrictor Precautions No information available to require special precautions

Effects on Dental Treatment No significant effects or complications reported

Effects on Bleeding Anemia (15% to 25%), thrombocytopenia (57% in bone marrow transplant patients; less common in other populations [8%]), and unusual bleeding are frequently reported.

Adverse Reactions

>10%:

Dermatologic: Hyperhidrosis (12%)

Gastrointestinal: Diarrhea (44%), anorexia (14%), vomiting (13%)

Hematologic & oncologic: Thrombocytopenia (6%; ≤50,000/mcL: 8% to 57%; <25,000/mcL: 3% to 32%), leukopenia (41%), neutropenia (ANC <500/mcL: 4% to 25%; 500 to 1,000/mcL: 14% to 29%), anemia (25%; hemoglobin <6.5 g/dL: 5%)

Infection: Sepsis (15%), infection (13%)

Ophthalmic: Retinal detachment (11%; relationship to ganciclovir not established)

Renal: Increased serum creatinine (2% to 50%; ≥2.5 mg/dL: 2% to 20%)

Miscellaneous: Fever (48%)

1% to 10%:

Central nervous system: Chills (10%), peripheral neuropathy (9%)

Dermatologic: Pruritus (5%)

Infection: Catheter sepsis (8%)

Local: Catheter infection (9%), catheter-site reaction (5%)

Frequency not defined:

Cardiovascular: Cardiac arrhythmia, chest pain, edema, hypertension, hypotension, phlebitis, vasodilation

Central nervous system: Abnormal dreams, abnormality in thinking, agitation, anxiety, confusion, depression, dizziness, drowsiness, fatigue, headache, hypoesthesia, insomnia, malaise, myasthenia, pain, paresthesia, psychosis, seizure

Dermatologic: Alopecia, cellulitis, dermatitis, skin rash, urticaria, xeroderma

Endocrine & metabolic: Weight loss

Gastrointestinal: Abdominal distention, abdominal pain, aphthous stomatitis, constipation, dysgeusia, dyspepsia, dysphagia, eructation, flatulence, gastrointestinal perforation, nausea, oral candidiasis, oral mucosa ulcer, pancreatitis, xerostomia

Genitourinary: Hematuria, urinary frequency, urinary tract infection

Hematologic & oncologic: Bone marrow failure

Hepatic: Abnormal hepatic function tests, increased serum alanine aminotransferase, increased serum aspartate aminotransferase, increased serum alkaline phosphatase

Infection: Candidiasis, influenza

Local: Inflammation at injection site

Neuromuscular & skeletal: Arthralgia, asthenia, back pain, lower limb cramp, muscle spasm, myalgia, tremor

Ophthalmic: Conjunctivitis, eye disease (vitreous disorder), eye pain, macular edema, visual impairment

Otic: Deafness, otalgia, tinnitus

Renal: Decreased creatinine clearance, renal failure syndrome, renal function abnormality

Respiratory: Cough, dyspnea, upper respiratory tract infection

Miscellaneous: Multiorgan failure

<1%, postmarketing, and/or case reports: Acidosis, agranulocytosis, amnesia, anaphylaxis, anosmia, aphasia, arthritis, bronchospasm, cardiac conduction disturbance, cataract, cerebrovascular accident, cholelithiasis, cholestasis, cranial nerve palsy (third), dysesthesia, dysphasia, encephalopathy, exfoliative dermatitis, extrapyramidal reaction, facial nerve paralysis, granulocytopenia, hallucination, hemolytic anemia, hemolytic-uremic syndrome, hepatic failure, hepatitis, hypercalcemia, hypersensitivity reaction, hyponatremia, increased serum triglycerides, infertility, intracranial hypertension, irritability, myelopathy, oculomotor nerve paralysis, pancytopenia, peripheral ischemia, pulmonary fibrosis, renal tubular disease, rhabdomyolysis, SIADH, Stevens-Johnson syndrome, testicular hypotrophy, torsades de pointes, ulcerative bowel lesion, vasculitis, ventricular tachycardia, xerophthalmia

Mechanism of Action Ganciclovir is phosphorylated to a substrate which competitively inhibits the binding of deoxyguanosine triphosphate to DNA polymerase resulting in inhibition of viral DNA synthesis

Pharmacodynamics/Kinetics

Half-life Elimination

Neonates 2 to 49 days of age: 2.4 hours

Children 9 months to 12 years: 2.4 ± 0.7 hours

Adults: Mean: IV: 3.5 ± 0.9 hours; Oral: 4.8 ± 0.9 hours; CrCl <25 mL/minute: 10.7 ± 5.7 hours

Reproductive Considerations

[US Boxed Warning]: Based on animal data and limited human data, ganciclovir may cause temporary or permanent inhibition of spermatogenesis in males and suppression of fertility in females.

Female patients should undergo pregnancy testing prior to initiation and use effective contraception during and for at least 30 days after therapy. Male patients should use a barrier contraceptive during and for at least 90 days after therapy.

Pregnancy Considerations

Ganciclovir crosses the placenta. **[US Boxed Warning]: Based on animal data, ganciclovir has the potential to cause birth defects in humans.**

Adverse events following congenital cytomegalovirus (CMV) infection may also occur. Hearing loss, mental retardation, microcephaly, seizures, and other medical problems have been observed in infants with congenital CMV infection.

The indications for treating maternal CMV retinitis during pregnancy are the same as in nonpregnant HIV infected women. In general, intravitreous injections for local therapy are preferred for retinal disease to limit systemic exposure during the first trimester when possible. Ganciclovir is not the preferred systemic therapy in pregnant women. Close fetal monitoring is recommended (HHS [OI adult 2019]).

◆ **Ganciclovir Sodium** *see* Ganciclovir (Systemic) *on page 728*

◆ **GAR-936** *see* Tigecycline *on page 1447*

◆ **Gastrocrom** *see* Cromolyn (Systemic) *on page 416*

Gatifloxacin (gat i FLOKS a sin)

Related Information

Bacterial Infections *on page 1739*

Brand Names: US Zymaxid

Brand Names: Canada APO-Gatifloxacin; Zymar

Pharmacologic Category Antibiotic, Fluoroquinolone; Antibiotic, Ophthalmic

Use Conjunctivitis: Treatment of bacterial conjunctivitis caused by *Staphylococcus aureus*, *Staphylococcus epidermidis*, *Streptococcus mitis* group, *Streptococcus oralis*, *Streptococcus pneumoniae*, and *Haemophilus influenzae*.

Local Anesthetic/Vasoconstrictor Precautions No information available to require special precautions

Effects on Dental Treatment Key adverse event(s) related to dental treatment: Taste disturbance.

Effects on Bleeding No information available to require special precautions

Adverse Reactions

1% to 10%:

Central nervous system: Headache

Endocrine & metabolic: Chemosis

Gastrointestinal: Dysgeusia

Ophthalmic: Conjunctival hemorrhage, conjunctival irritation, conjunctivitis (worsening), decreased visual acuity, dry eye syndrome, eye discharge, eye irritation, eye pain, eye redness, eyelid edema, increased lacrimation, keratitis, papillary conjunctivitis

<1%, postmarketing, and/or case reports: Anaphylaxis, angioedema (including facial edema, oral edema, pharyngeal edema), blepharitis, blurred vision, dyspnea, eye pruritus, hypersensitivity reaction (including allergic dermatitis, eye allergy), nausea, pruritus (including skin rash), Stevens-Johnson syndrome, swelling of eye (including corneal edema, conjunctival edema), urticaria

Mechanism of Action Gatifloxacin is a DNA gyrase inhibitor, and also inhibits topoisomerase IV. DNA gyrase (topoisomerase II) is an essential bacterial enzyme that maintains the superhelical structure of DNA. DNA gyrase is required for DNA replication and transcription, DNA repair, recombination, and transposition; inhibition is bactericidal.

Pregnancy Considerations

Systemic concentrations of gatifloxacin following ophthalmic administration are below the limit of quantification. If ophthalmic agents are needed during pregnancy, the minimum effective dose should be used in combination with punctal occlusion for 3 to 5 minutes after application to decrease potential exposure to the fetus (Samples 1988).

- **Gattex** *see* Teduglutide *on page* *1410*
- **Gazyva** *see* Obinutuzumab *on page* *1124*
- **GBT 440** *see* Voxelotor *on page* *1556*
- **GCR-8015** *see* Moxetumomab Pasudotox *on page* *1063*
- **G-CSF** *see* Filgrastim *on page* *668*
- **G-CSF (PEG Conjugate)** *see* Pegfilgrastim *on page* *1200*
- **GCV Sodium** *see* Ganciclovir (Systemic) *on page* *728*
- **GDC-0199** *see* Venetoclax *on page* *1538*
- **GDC-0449** *see* Vismodegib *on page* *1548*
- **GDC-0973** *see* Cobimetinib *on page* *402*

Gefitinib (ge FI tye nib)

Brand Names: US Iressa

Brand Names: Canada APO-Gefitinib; Iressa; NAT-Gefitinib; SANDOZ Gefitinib

Pharmacologic Category Antineoplastic Agent, Epidermal Growth Factor Receptor (EGFR) Inhibitor; Antineoplastic Agent, Tyrosine Kinase Inhibitor

Use

Non-small cell lung cancer: First-line treatment of metastatic non-small cell lung cancer (NSCLC) in tumors with epidermal growth factor receptor (EGFR) exon 19 deletions or exon 21 (L858R) substitution mutations as detected in tumor or plasma specimen by an approved test.

Limitation of use: Safety and efficacy have not been established in patients with metastatic NSCLC whose tumors have EGFR mutations other than exon 19 deletions or exon 21 (L858R) substitution mutations

Local Anesthetic/Vasoconstrictor Precautions No information available to require special precautions

Effects on Dental Treatment Key adverse event(s) related to dental treatment: Mouth ulceration.

Effects on Bleeding Bleeding has been reported in <1% of patients, but can be serious.

Adverse Reactions

>10%:

Central nervous system: Insomnia (15%), fatigue (14%)

Dermatologic: Dermatological reaction (47% to 58%), skin rash (52%), xeroderma (24%), pruritus (18%), paronychia (14%), acne vulgaris (11%), alopecia (5% to 11%)

Gastrointestinal: Diarrhea (29% to 47%; grades 3/4: 3%), anorexia (19% to 20%), nausea (17% to 18%), decreased appetite (17%), vomiting (13% to 14%), stomatitis (7% to 13%), constipation (12%)

Genitourinary: Proteinuria (8% to 35%)

Hepatic: Increased serum AST (8% to 40%; grades 3/4: 2% to 3%), increased serum ALT (11% to 38%; grades 3/4: 2% to 5%)

Neuromuscular & skeletal: Weakness (18%)

1% to 10%:

Central nervous system: Hypoesthesia (4%), peripheral sensory neuropathy (4%), peripheral neuropathy (2%)

Dermatologic: Nail disease (5% to 8%), acneiform eruption (6%)

Endocrine & metabolic: Dehydration (2%; secondary to diarrhea, nausea, vomiting, or anorexia)

Gastrointestinal: Xerostomia (2%)

Genitourinary: Cystitis (1%)

Hematologic & oncologic: Anemia (7%), pulmonary hemorrhage (4% to 5%), hemorrhage (4%; including epistaxis, hematuria), neutropenia (3%), leukopenia (2%), thrombocytopenia (1%)

Hepatic: Increased serum bilirubin (3%; grades 3/4: <1%)

Neuromuscular & skeletal: Myalgia (8%), arthralgia (6%)

Ophthalmic: Eye disease (6% to 7%; grades 3/4: <1%; including conjunctivitis, blepharitis, and dry eye)

Renal: Increased serum creatinine (2%)

Respiratory: Cough (9%), interstitial pulmonary disease (1%; grades 3/4: 3%)

Miscellaneous: Fever (9%)

<1%, postmarketing, and/or case reports: Angioedema, bullous skin disease, corneal erosion (reversible; may be associated with aberrant eyelash growth), decreased white blood cell count, erythema multiforme, fulminant hepatitis, gastrointestinal perforation, hemorrhagic cystitis, hepatic failure, hepatitis, hypersensitivity angiitis, hypersensitivity reaction, keratitis, keratoconjunctivitis sicca, pancreatitis, renal failure, skin fissure, Stevens-Johnson syndrome, toxic epidermal necrolysis, urticaria

Mechanism of Action Gefitinib is a tyrosine kinase inhibitor (TKI) which reversibly inhibits kinase activity of wild-type and select activation mutations of epidermal growth factor receptor (EGFR). EGFR is expressed on cell surfaces of normal and cancer cells and has a role in cell growth and proliferation. Gefitinib prevents autophosphorylation of tyrosine residues associated with the EGFR receptor, which blocks downstream signaling and EGFR-dependent proliferation. Gefitinib has a higher binding affinity for EGFR exon 19 deletion and exon 21 (L858R) substitution mutation than for wild-type EGFR.

Pharmacodynamics/Kinetics

Half-life Elimination Oral: 48 hours

Time to Peak Plasma: Oral: 3 to 7 hours

Reproductive Considerations

Females of reproductive potential should use effective contraception during and for at least 2 weeks following gefitinib treatment.

Pregnancy Considerations

Adverse events have been observed in animal reproduction studies. Gefitinib may cause fetal harm when administered to a pregnant female.

◆ **Gelatin** *see* Gelatin (Absorbable) *on page 731*

Gelatin (Absorbable) (JEL a tin, ab SORB a ble)

Related Information

Antiplatelet and Anticoagulation Considerations in Dentistry *on page 1666*

Brand Names: US Gel-Flow NT; Gelfilm; Gelfoam; Gelfoam Dental; Surgifoam; Surgifoam Hermorrhoidectomy

Pharmacologic Category Hemostatic Agent

Use

Hemostasis (adjunct): Adjunct to provide hemostasis in surgical procedures (except ophthalmic) when control of bleeding by pressure, ligature and other conventional techniques are ineffective; adjunct in neuro, thoracic, or ocular surgeries to promote tissue repair and/or prevent adhesions (Gelfilm).

Note: May be moistened with sterile saline or sterile topical thrombin.

Local Anesthetic/Vasoconstrictor Precautions

No information available to require special precautions

Effects on Dental Treatment Key adverse event(s) related to dental treatment: Local infection and abscess formation.

Effects on Bleeding Used as adjunct to enhance hemostasis.

Adverse Reactions Cardiopulmonary bypass surgery (Gelfoam):

>10%: Cardiovascular: Atrial fibrillation (13%)

1% to 10%:

Cardiovascular: Cardiac failure (4%), atrial flutter (2%), peripheral vascular disease (2%), ventricular tachycardia (2%), heart block (1%)

Infection: Wound infection (6%)

Respiratory: Pneumothorax (2%), respiratory failure (2%)

Miscellaneous: Fever (1%)

Frequency not defined (Gelfoam was used in cited surgical procedures):

Central nervous system: Arachnoiditis (laminectomy operations), cauda equina syndrome (laminectomy operations), headache (laminectomy operations), meningitis (laminectomy operations), pain (laminectomy operations), paresthesia (laminectomy operations), spinal cord compression (brain implant surgery)

Gastrointestinal: Gastrointestinal disease (laminectomy operations)

Genitourinary: Bladder dysfunction (laminectomy operations), impotence (laminectomy operations)

Hematologic & oncologic: Hematoma

Infection: Abscess, localized infection, toxic shock syndrome (nasal surgery)

Local: Injection site granuloma (brain; brain implant surgery), localized edema (includes encapsulation of fluid and fluid accumulation in the brain and spinal cord; brain implant surgery and laminectomy operations)

Neuromuscular & skeletal: Tendon disease (prolonged fixation of tendon post severed tendon repair)

Otic: Hearing loss (tympanoplasty)

Miscellaneous: Fever, fibrosis (tendon repair), foreign body reaction

Mechanism of Action Arrests bleeding by forming artificial clot and producing mechanical matrix which facilitates clotting

Pregnancy Considerations When administered topically, gelatin is completely absorbed; however, the amount of gelatin available systemically following topical application is unknown.

◆ **Gelclair** *see* Mucosal Coating Agent *on page 1066*

◆ **Gelfilm** *see* Gelatin (Absorbable) *on page 731*

◆ **Gel-Flow NT** *see* Gelatin (Absorbable) *on page 731*

◆ **Gelfoam** *see* Gelatin (Absorbable) *on page 731*

◆ **Gelfoam Dental** *see* Gelatin (Absorbable) *on page 731*

◆ **Gel-Kam [OTC]** *see* Fluoride *on page 693*

◆ **Gel-Kam Rinse** *see* Fluoride *on page 693*

◆ **Gelnique** *see* Oxybutynin *on page 1156*

◆ **Gelnique Pump [DSC]** *see* Oxybutynin *on page 1156*

◆ **Gel-One** *see* Hyaluronate and Derivatives *on page 761*

◆ **Gelsyn-3** *see* Hyaluronate and Derivatives *on page 761*

Gemcitabine (jem SITE a been)

Brand Names: US Gemzar [DSC]; Infugem

Brand Names: Canada ACT Gemcitabine [DSC]; Gemcitabine SUN

Pharmacologic Category Antineoplastic Agent, Antimetabolite; Antineoplastic Agent, Antimetabolite (Pyrimidine Analog)

Use

Breast cancer (metastatic): First-line treatment of metastatic breast cancer (in combination with paclitaxel) after failure of adjuvant chemotherapy that contained an anthracycline (unless anthracyclines are contraindicated).

Non-small cell lung cancer (inoperable, locally advanced, or metastatic): First-line treatment (in combination with cisplatin) of inoperable, locally advanced (stage IIIA or IIIB) or metastatic (stage IV) non-small cell lung cancer (NSCLC).

Ovarian cancer (advanced): Treatment of advanced ovarian cancer (in combination with carboplatin) that has relapsed at least 6 months following completion of platinum-based chemotherapy.

Pancreatic cancer (locally advanced or metastatic): First-line treatment of locally advanced (nonresectable stage II or III) or metastatic (stage IV) pancreatic adenocarcinoma. Gemcitabine is indicated for patients previously treated with fluorouracil.

Guideline recommendations:

Metastatic pancreatic cancer: American Society of Clinical Oncology (ASCO) guidelines for metastatic pancreatic cancer (ASCO [Sohal 2018]) recommend gemcitabine (in combination with paclitaxel [protein bound]) as first-line therapy in patients with Eastern Cooperative Oncology Group (ECOG) performance status of 0 or 1, a relatively favorable comorbidity profile, a preference for relatively aggressive therapy, and a suitable support system. First-line therapy with single-agent gemcitabine is recommended in patients with ECOG performance status of 2 or a comorbidity profile prohibiting more aggressive therapy when there is a preference for cancer-directed therapy; capecitabine or erlotinib (added to gemcitabine) may also be offered in this situation. Gemcitabine (in combination with paclitaxel [protein bound]) may be utilized as second-line therapy in patients who received first-line FOLFIRINOX therapy, have an ECOG performance status of 0 or 1, have a relatively favorable comorbidity profile, a preference for aggressive therapy, and a suitable support system. Second-line therapy with gemcitabine (alone) may also be considered as an option in patients with ECOG performance status of 2 or a comorbidity profile prohibiting more aggressive regimens when there is a preference to pursue cancer-directed therapy.

Locally advanced, unresectable pancreatic cancer: According to the ASCO guidelines for locally advanced, unresectable pancreatic cancer (ASCO [Balaban 2016]), induction with 6 months of initial systemic therapy (with a combination regimen) is generally recommended, although there is not enough evidence to encourage one regimen over another, and gemcitabine-based therapies recommended in the metastatic setting have not been evaluated in randomized controlled studies for locally advanced unresectable pancreatic cancer. If disease progression occurs, treatment according to guidelines for metastatic pancreatic cancer should be offered.

Local Anesthetic/Vasoconstrictor Precautions No information available to require special precautions

Effects on Dental Treatment Key adverse event(s) related to dental treatment: Stomatitis.

Effects on Bleeding Bleeding occurs in 2% to 17% of patients. Anemia (68% to 73%) and thrombocytopenia (24% to 36%) frequently occur. Medical consult is recommended.

Adverse Reactions Frequency of adverse reactions reported for single-agent use of gemcitabine only.

>10%:

Cardiovascular: Peripheral edema (20%), edema (≤13%)

Central nervous system: Drowsiness (11%)

Dermatologic: Skin rash (30%), alopecia (15%)

Gastrointestinal: Nausea and vomiting (69%), diarrhea (19%), stomatitis (11%; grade 3: <1%)

Genitourinary: Proteinuria (45%), hematuria (35%)

Hematologic & oncologic: Anemia (68%; grade 3: 7%; grade 4: 1%), neutropenia (63%; grade 3: 19%; grade 4: 6%), thrombocytopenia (24%; grade 3: 4%; grade 4: 1%), hemorrhage (17%; grade 3: <1%; grade 4: <1%)

Hepatic: Increased serum alanine aminotransferase (68%), increased serum aspartate aminotransferase (67%), increased serum alkaline phosphatase (55%), hyperbilirubinemia (13%)

Infection: Infection (16%)

Renal: Increased blood urea nitrogen (16%)

Respiratory: Dyspnea (23%), flu-like symptoms (19%)

Miscellaneous: Fever (41%)

1% to 10%:

Central nervous system: Paresthesia (10%)

Local: Injection site reaction (4%)

Renal: Increased serum creatinine (8%)

Respiratory: Bronchospasm (<2%)

Frequency not defined:

Hypersensitivity: Nonimmune anaphylaxis

<1%, postmarketing, and/or case reports (reported with single-agent use or with combination therapy): Acute myocardial infarction, acute respiratory distress syndrome, bullous skin disease, capillary leak syndrome, cardiac arrhythmia, cardiac failure, cellulitis (including pseudocellulitis), cerebrovascular accident (Kuenen 2002), desquamation, eosinophilic pneumonitis, gangrene of skin and/or subcutaneous tissues, hemolytic-uremic syndrome, hepatic failure, hepatic sinusoidal obstruction syndrome, hepatotoxicity, interstitial pneumonitis, petechia (Nishijima 2013; Zupancic 2007), pruritus (Curtis 2016), pulmonary edema, pulmonary fibrosis, radiation recall phenomenon, renal failure syndrome, respiratory failure, reversible posterior leukoencephalopathy syndrome, sepsis, severe dermatological reaction, supraventricular cardiac arrhythmia, thrombotic microangiopathy, thrombotic thrombocytopenic purpura (Nishijima 2013; Zupancic 2007), vasculitis (peripheral)

Mechanism of Action Gemcitabine is a pyrimidine antimetabolite that inhibits DNA synthesis by inhibition of DNA polymerase and ribonucleotide reductase, cell cycle-specific for the S-phase of the cycle (also blocks cellular progression at G1/S-phase). Gemcitabine is phosphorylated intracellularly by deoxycytidine kinase to gemcitabine monophosphate, which is further phosphorylated to active metabolites gemcitabine diphosphate and gemcitabine triphosphate. Gemcitabine diphosphate inhibits DNA synthesis by inhibiting ribonucleotide reductase; gemcitabine triphosphate incorporates into DNA and inhibits DNA polymerase.

Pharmacodynamics/Kinetics

Half-life Elimination

Gemcitabine: Infusion time ≤70 minutes: 42 to 94 minutes; infusion time 3 to 4 hours: 4 to 10.5 hours (affected by age and gender)

Metabolite (gemcitabine triphosphate), terminal phase: 1.7 to 19.4 hours

Time to Peak 30 minutes after completion of infusion

Reproductive Considerations

Verify pregnancy status (with pregnancy test) prior to treatment initiation in females of reproductive potential. Females of reproductive potential should use effective contraception during treatment and for 6 months after the final gemcitabine dose. Males with female partners of reproductive potential should use effective contraception during treatment and for 3 months after the final gemcitabine dose.

Pregnancy Considerations

Based on the mechanism of action and on findings from animal reproduction studies, gemcitabine may cause fetal harm if administered during pregnancy.

Information related to the use of gemcitabine in pregnancy is limited (Lubner 2011; Wiesweg 2014).

A pregnancy registry is available for all cancers diagnosed during pregnancy at Cooper Health (877-635-4499).

- ◆ **Gemcitabine HCl** *see* Gemcitabine *on page 731*
- ◆ **Gemcitabine Hydrochloride** *see* Gemcitabine *on page 731*

Gemfibrozil (jem FI broe zil)

Related Information

Cardiovascular Diseases *on page 1654*

Brand Names: US Lopid

Brand Names: Canada APO-Gemfibrozil; DOM-Gemfibrozil; MYLAN-Gemfibrozil [DSC]; PHL-Gemfibrozil [DSC]; PMS-Gemfibrozil; TEVA-Gemfibrozil

Pharmacologic Category Antilipemic Agent, Fibric Acid

Use Treatment of hypertriglyceridemia in Fredrickson types IV and V hyperlipidemia for patients who are at greater risk for pancreatitis and who have not responded to dietary intervention; to reduce the risk of CHD development in Fredrickson type IIb patients without a history or symptoms of existing CHD who have not responded to dietary and other interventions (including pharmacologic treatment) and who have decreased HDL, increased LDL, and increased triglycerides

Local Anesthetic/Vasoconstrictor Precautions No information available to require special precautions

Effects on Dental Treatment No significant effects or complications reported

Effects on Bleeding Anemia has been reported in <1% of patients.

Adverse Reactions

>10%: Gastrointestinal: Dyspepsia (20%)

1% to 10%:

Cardiovascular: Atrial fibrillation (1%)

Central nervous system: Fatigue (4%), vertigo (2%)

Dermatologic: Eczema (2%), skin rash (2%)

Gastrointestinal: Abdominal pain (10%), nausea and vomiting (3%)

<1%, postmarketing and/or case reports (probable causation): Anemia, angioedema, arthralgia, blurred vision, bone marrow depression, cholecystitis, cholelithiasis, cholestatic jaundice, decreased libido, depression, dermatitis, dermatomyositis, dizziness, drowsiness, dysgeusia, eosinophilia, exfoliative dermatitis, headache, hypoesthesia, hypokalemia, impotence, increased creatine phosphokinase, increased serum alkaline phosphatase, increased serum bilirubin, increased serum transaminases, laryngeal edema, leukopenia, limb pain, myalgia, myasthenia, myopathy, nephrotoxicity, paresthesia, peripheral neuritis, polymyositis, pruritus, Raynaud phenomenon, rhabdomyolysis, synovitis, urticaria

Reports where causal relationship has not been established: Alopecia, anaphylaxis, cataract, colitis, confusion, extrasystoles, hepatic neoplasm, intracranial hemorrhage, lupus-like syndrome, pancreatitis, peripheral vascular disease, positive ANA titer, reduced fertility (male), renal insufficiency, retinal edema, seizure, skin photosensitivity, syncope, thrombocytopenia, vasculitis, weight loss

Mechanism of Action The exact mechanism of action of gemfibrozil is unknown, however, several theories exist regarding the VLDL effect; it can inhibit lipolysis and decrease subsequent hepatic fatty acid uptake as well as inhibit hepatic secretion of VLDL; together these actions decrease serum VLDL levels; increases HDL-cholesterol; the mechanism behind HDL elevation is currently unknown

Pharmacodynamics/Kinetics

Onset of Action May require several days

Half-life Elimination 1.5 hours

Time to Peak Serum: 1 to 2 hours

Pregnancy Considerations

Gemfibrozil crosses the placenta (Tsai 2004).

Triglyceride concentrations increase during pregnancy as required for normal fetal development. When increases are greater than expected, supervised dietary intervention should be initiated. In women who develop very severe hypertriglyceridemia and are at risk for pancreatitis, use of gemfibrozil beginning in the second trimester is one intervention that may be considered (Avis 2009; Berglund 2012; Jacobson 2015; Wong 2015).

Gemifloxacin (je mi FLOKS a sin)

Related Information

Bacterial Infections *on page 1739*

Clinical Risk Related to Drugs Prolonging QT Interval *on page 1675*

Brand Names: US Factive [DSC]

Pharmacologic Category Antibiotic, Fluoroquinolone; Antibiotic, Respiratory Fluoroquinolone

Use

Treatment of acute exacerbation of chronic bronchitis; treatment of community-acquired pneumonia (CAP), including pneumonia caused by multidrug-resistant strains of *S. pneumoniae* (MDRSP)

Limitations of use: Because fluoroquinolones have been associated with disabling and potentially irreversible serious adverse reactions (eg, tendinitis and tendon rupture, peripheral neuropathy, CNS effects), reserve gemifloxacin for use in patients who have no alternative treatment options for acute bacterial exacerbation of chronic bronchitis.

Local Anesthetic/Vasoconstrictor Precautions Gemifloxacin is one of the drugs confirmed to prolong the QT interval and is accepted as having a risk of causing torsade de pointes. The risk of drug-induced torsade de pointes is extremely low when a single QT interval prolonging drug is prescribed. In terms of epinephrine, it is not known what effect vasoconstrictors in the local anesthetic regimen will have in patients with a known history of congenital prolonged QT interval or in patients taking any medication that prolongs the QT interval. Until more information is obtained, it is suggested that the clinician consult with the physician prior to the use of a vasoconstrictor in suspected patients, and that the vasoconstrictor (epinephrine, mepivacaine and levonordefrin [Carbocaine® 2% with Neo-Cobefrin®]) be used with caution.

Effects on Dental Treatment No significant effects or complications reported

Effects on Bleeding No information available to require special precautions

Adverse Reactions

1% to 10%:

Central nervous system: Headache (4%), dizziness (≤2%)

Dermatologic: Skin rash (≤4%)

Gastrointestinal: Diarrhea (5%), nausea (4%), abdominal pain (≤2%), vomiting (≤2%)

Hematologic & oncologic: Thrombocythemia (1%)
Hepatic: Increased serum alanine aminotransferase (≤4%), increased serum aspartate aminotransferase (≤1%)

Frequency not defined: Central nervous system: Agitation, anxiety, confusion, delirium, depression, disorientation, disturbance in attention, hallucination, idiopathic intracranial hypertension, memory impairment, paranoid ideation, restlessness, seizure, suicidal ideation, suicidal tendencies, toxic psychosis

<1%, postmarketing, and/or case reports: Acute renal failure, agranulocytosis, anaphylaxis, anemia, angioedema, anorexia, antibiotic-associated colitis, aplastic anemia, arthralgia, asthenia, axonal peripheral polyneuropathy, back pain, candidiasis, *Clostridioides difficile* associated diarrhea, *Clostridioides difficile* colitis, constipation, decreased hematocrit, decreased hemoglobin, decreased neutrophils, decreased serum albumin, decreased serum calcium, decreased serum potassium, decreased serum sodium, decreased serum total protein, dermatitis, drowsiness, dysesthesia, dysgeusia, dyspepsia, dyspnea, eczema, eosinophilia, eosinophilic pneumonitis, erythema multiforme, exacerbation of myasthenia gravis, exfoliation of skin, facial edema, fatigue, fever, flatulence, flushing, fungal infection, gastritis, gastroenteritis, genital candidiasis, genital pruritus, granulocytopenia, hemolytic anemia, hemorrhage, hepatic necrosis, hepatitis, hepatotoxicity, hot flash, hyperbilirubinemia, hyperglycemia, hypersensitivity reaction, hypoesthesia, increased blood urea nitrogen, increased creatine phosphokinase in blood specimen, increased gamma-glutamyl transferase, increased hematocrit, increased hemoglobin, increased INR, increased intracranial pressure, increased lactate dehydrogenase, increased neutrophils, increased nonprotein nitrogen, increased serum alkaline phosphatase, increased serum bilirubin, increased serum calcium, increased serum creatinine, increased serum potassium, increased serum sodium, insomnia, interstitial nephritis, jaundice, leukopenia, lower limb cramp, myalgia, nervousness, pain, pancytopenia, paresthesia, peripheral edema, peripheral neuropathy, pharyngitis, pneumonia, prolonged QT interval on ECG, pruritus, renal failure syndrome, retinal hemorrhage, rupture of tendon, serum sickness, severe dermatological reaction, skin photosensitivity, Stevens-Johnson syndrome, supraventricular tachycardia, syncope, tendonitis, thrombocythemia, thrombocytopenia, thrombotic thrombocytopenic purpura, toxic epidermal necrolysis, transient ischemic attacks, tremor, urine abnormality, urticaria, vaginitis, vertigo, visual disturbance, xerostomia

Mechanism of Action Gemifloxacin is a DNA gyrase inhibitor and also inhibits topoisomerase IV. DNA gyrase (topoisomerase IV) is an essential bacterial enzyme that maintains the superhelical structure of DNA. DNA gyrase is required for DNA replication and transcription, DNA repair, recombination, and transposition; bactericidal

Pharmacodynamics/Kinetics

Half-life Elimination 7 hours (range 4-12 hours)

Time to Peak Plasma: 0.5-2 hours

Pregnancy Considerations Adverse events have been observed in some animal reproduction studies.

Product Availability Factive is no longer available in the United States.

Dental Health Professional Considerations See Local Anesthetic/Vasoconstrictor Precautions

◆ **Gemifloxacin Mesylate** *see* Gemifloxacin *on page 733*

Gemtuzumab Ozogamicin

(gem TOO zoo mab oh zog a MY sin)

Brand Names: US Mylotarg

Brand Names: Canada Mylotarg

Pharmacologic Category Antineoplastic Agent, Anti-CD33; Antineoplastic Agent, Antibody Drug Conjugate; Antineoplastic Agent, Monoclonal Antibody

Use

Acute myeloid leukemia, CD33-positive (newly diagnosed de novo): Treatment of newly diagnosed CD33-positive acute myeloid leukemia (AML) in adults and pediatric patients ≥1 month of age.

Acute myeloid leukemia, CD33-positive (relapsed/refractory): Treatment of relapsed or refractory CD33-positive AML in adults and pediatric patients ≥2 years of age.

Local Anesthetic/Vasoconstrictor Precautions No information available to require special precautions

Effects on Dental Treatment Key adverse event(s) related to dental treatment: Mucositis and stomatitis have been reported

Effects on Bleeding Bleeding reported in 13% of patients with gum hemorrhage reported in 9%. Bone marrow suppression with anemia and thrombocytopenia are common. Recovery of platelets may be delayed. Medical consult recommended.

Adverse Reactions

>10%:

Cardiovascular: Cardiotoxicity (28%)
Central nervous system: Fatigue (44%), headache (19%)
Dermatologic: Skin rash (16%)
Gastrointestinal: Constipation (21%), mucositis (21%), nausea and vomiting (21%)
Hematologic & oncologic: Hemorrhage (23% to 25%; ≥ grade 3: 7% to 13%), febrile neutropenia (18%; ≥ grade 3: 18%)
Hepatic: Hepatotoxicity (51%), increased serum AST (40%), increased serum ALT (16%)
Infection: Infection (42% to 44%)
Miscellaneous: Fever (79%)

1% to 10%:

Genitourinary: Nephrotoxicity (6%)
Hepatic: Hyperbilirubinemia

<1%, postmarketing and/or case reports: Bacterial infection, hemorrhagic cystitis, hepatic veno-occlusive disease, interstitial pneumonitis, neutropenic enterocolitis, pulmonary infection, pneumonia due to *Pneumocystis carinii*

Mechanism of Action Gemtuzumab ozogamicin is a humanized CD-33 directed monoclonal antibody-drug conjugate, which is composed of the IgG4 kappa antibody gemtuzumab linked to a cytotoxic calicheamicin derivative. CD33 is expressed on leukemic cells in over 80% of patients with AML (Castaigne 2012). Gemtuzumab ozogamicin binds to the CD33 antigen, resulting in internalization of the antibody-antigen complex. Following internalization, the calicheamicin derivative is released inside the myeloid cell. The calicheamlcin derivative binds to DNA resulting in double strand breaks, inducing cell cycle arrest and apoptosis.

Pharmacodynamics/Kinetics

Half-life Elimination Based on a 9 mg/m^2 dose: Antibody portion: 62 hours (after first dose); 90 hours (after second dose)

Reproductive Considerations
Evaluate pregnancy status prior to use in females of reproductive potential. Females of reproductive potential should use effective contraception during treatment and for at least 6 months after the last gemtuzumab ozogamicin dose. Males with female partners of reproductive potential should use effective contraception during therapy and for at least 3 months after the last gemtuzumab ozogamicin dose.

Pregnancy Considerations
Based on the mechanism of action and data animal reproduction studies, in utero exposure to gemtuzumab ozogamicin may cause fetal harm.

Prescribing and Access Restrictions In Canada, gemtuzumab is available through a special access program (access information is available from Health Canada).

- **Gemzar** *see* Gemcitabine *on page 731*
- **Gemzar [DSC]** *see* Gemcitabine *on page 731*
- **Gen7T** *see* Lidocaine (Topical) *on page 902*
- **Genahist [OTC]** *see* DiphenhydrAMINE (Systemic) *on page 502*
- **Genaphed [OTC]** *see* Pseudoephedrine *on page 1291*
- **Generess FE** *see* Ethinyl Estradiol and Norethindrone *on page 614*
- **Gengraf** *see* CycloSPORINE (Systemic) *on page 421*
- **Genicin Vita-Q** *see* Vitamins (Multiple/Oral) *on page 1550*
- **Genotropin** *see* Somatropin *on page 1381*
- **Genotropin MiniQuick** *see* Somatropin *on page 1381*
- **Genpril [OTC]** *see* Ibuprofen *on page 786*

Gentamicin (Systemic) (jen ta MYE sin)

Pharmacologic Category Antibiotic, Aminoglycoside

Use Serious infections: Treatment of serious infections (eg, sepsis, meningitis, urinary tract infections, respiratory tract infections, peritonitis, bone infections, skin and soft tissue infections) caused by susceptible strains of the following microorganisms: *Pseudomonas aeruginosa*, *Proteus* species (indole-positive and indole-negative), *Escherichia coli*, *Klebsiella* species, *Enterobacter* species, *Serratia* species, *Citrobacter* species, and *Staphylococcus* species (coagulase-positive and coagulase-negative); treatment of infective endocarditis caused by enterococci, in combination with other antibiotics.

Local Anesthetic/Vasoconstrictor Precautions
No information available to require special precautions

Effects on Dental Treatment No significant effects or complications reported

Effects on Bleeding No information available to require special precautions

Adverse Reactions Frequency not defined.

Cardiovascular: Edema, hypertension, hypotension, phlebitis, thrombophlebitis

Central nervous system: Abnormal gait, ataxia, brain disease, confusion, depression, dizziness, drowsiness, headache, lethargy, myasthenia, numbness, paresthesia, peripheral neuropathy, pseudomotor cerebri, seizure, vertigo

Dermatologic: Alopecia, erythema, pruritus, skin rash, urticaria

Endocrine & metabolic: Hypocalcemia, hypokalemia, hypomagnesemia, hyponatremia, weight loss

Gastrointestinal: Anorexia, *Clostridioides* (formerly *Clostridium*) *difficile*-associated diarrhea, decreased appetite, enterocolitis, nausea, sialorrhea, stomatitis, vomiting

Genitourinary: Casts in urine (hyaline, granular), Fanconi-like syndrome (infants and adults; high dose, prolonged course), oliguria, proteinuria

Hematologic & oncologic: Agranulocytosis, anemia, eosinophilia, granulocytopenia, leukopenia, purpura, reticulocytopenia, reticulocytosis, splenomegaly, thrombocytopenia

Hepatic: Hepatomegaly, increased liver enzymes

Hypersensitivity: Anaphylaxis, anaphylactoid reaction, hypersensitivity reaction

Local: Injection site reaction, pain at injection site

Neuromuscular & skeletal: Arthralgia, muscle cramps, muscle fatigue (myasthenia gravis-like syndrome), muscle twitching, tremor, weakness

Ophthalmic: Visual disturbance

Otic: Auditory impairment, hearing loss (associated with persistently increased serum concentrations; early toxicity usually affects high-pitched sound), tinnitus

Renal: Decreased creatinine clearance, decreased urine specific gravity, increased blood urea nitrogen, increased serum creatinine, polyuria, renal failure (high trough serum concentrations), renal tubular necrosis

Respiratory: Dyspnea, laryngeal edema, pulmonary fibrosis, respiratory depression

Miscellaneous: Fever

Mechanism of Action Interferes with bacterial protein synthesis by binding to 30S ribosomal subunit resulting in a defective bacterial cell membrane

Pharmacodynamics/Kinetics

Half-life Elimination

Neonates: <1 week: 3 to 11.5 hours; 1 week to 1 month: 3 to 6 hours

Infants: 4 ± 1 hour

Children: 2 ± 1 hour

Adolescents: 1.5 ± 1 hour

Adults: ~2 hours (Regamey 1973); Renal failure: mean: 41 ± 24 hours; Range: 6 to 127 hours (Dager 2006)

Time to Peak Serum: IM: 30 to 90 minutes; IV: 30 minutes after 30-minute infusion (MacDougall 2011); **Note:** Distribution is prolonged after larger doses (≥90 minutes after 30- to 60-minute infusion of 7 mg/kg) (Demczar 1997; McNamara 2001; Wallace 2002).

Pregnancy Risk Factor D

Pregnancy Considerations Gentamicin crosses the placenta.

[US Boxed Warning]: Aminoglycosides may cause fetal harm if administered to a pregnant woman. There are several reports of total irreversible bilateral congenital deafness in children whose mothers received another aminoglycoside (streptomycin) during pregnancy. Although serious side effects to the fetus/infant have not been reported following maternal use of all aminoglycosides, a potential for harm exists.

Due to pregnancy-induced physiologic changes, some pharmacokinetic parameters of gentamicin may be altered (Popović 2007). Gentamicin use has been evaluated for various infections in pregnant women including the treatment of acute pyelonephritis (Jolley 2010) and as an alternative antibiotic for prophylactic use prior to cesarean delivery (Bratzler 2013).

- **Gentamicin Sulfate** *see* Gentamicin (Systemic) *on page 735*

- ◆ **GenVisc 850** *see* Hyaluronate and Derivatives *on page 761*
- ◆ **Genvoya** *see* Elvitegravir, Cobicistat, Emtricitabine, and Tenofovir Alafenamide *on page 553*
- ◆ **Genz-112638** *see* Eliglustat *on page 549*
- ◆ **Geodon** *see* Ziprasidone *on page 1572*
- ◆ **Geriation [OTC]** *see* Vitamins (Multiple/Oral) *on page 1550*
- ◆ **Geri-Dryl [OTC]** *see* DiphenhydrAMINE (Systemic) *on page 502*
- ◆ **Geri-Freeda [OTC]** *see* Vitamins (Multiple/Oral) *on page 1550*
- ◆ **Geritol Complete [OTC]** *see* Vitamins (Multiple/Oral) *on page 1550*
- ◆ **Geritol Extend [OTC]** *see* Vitamins (Multiple/Oral) *on page 1550*
- ◆ **Geritol Tonic [OTC]** *see* Vitamins (Multiple/Oral) *on page 1550*
- ◆ **GF196960** *see* Tadalafil *on page 1401*
- ◆ **GHB** *see* Sodium Oxybate *on page 1377*
- ◆ **GI87084B** *see* Remifentanil *on page 1315*
- ◆ **Gianvi** *see* Ethinyl Estradiol and Drospirenone *on page 610*
- ◆ **Giazo [DSC]** *see* Balsalazide *on page 214*
- ◆ **Gildagia [DSC]** *see* Ethinyl Estradiol and Norethindrone *on page 614*
- ◆ **Gildess 1.5/30 [DSC]** *see* Ethinyl Estradiol and Norethindrone *on page 614*
- ◆ **Gildess 1/20 [DSC]** *see* Ethinyl Estradiol and Norethindrone *on page 614*
- ◆ **Gildess 24 FE [DSC]** *see* Ethinyl Estradiol and Norethindrone *on page 614*
- ◆ **Gildess FE 1.5/30 [DSC]** *see* Ethinyl Estradiol and Norethindrone *on page 614*
- ◆ **Gildess FE 1/20 [DSC]** *see* Ethinyl Estradiol and Norethindrone *on page 614*
- ◆ **Gilenya** *see* Fingolimod *on page 670*

Gilteritinib (GIL te RI ti nib)

Brand Names: US Xospata

Brand Names: Canada Xospata

Pharmacologic Category Antineoplastic Agent, FLT3 Inhibitor; Antineoplastic Agent, Tyrosine Kinase Inhibitor

Use Acute myeloid leukemia, relapsed or refractory: Treatment of relapsed or refractory acute myeloid leukemia (AML) in adult patients with an FMS-like tyrosine kinase 3 (FLT3) mutation as detected by an approved test.

Local Anesthetic/Vasoconstrictor Precautions Gilteritinib is one of the drugs confirmed to prolong the QT interval and is accepted as having a risk of causing torsades de pointes. The risk of drug-induced torsades de pointes is extremely low when a single QT interval prolonging drug is prescribed. In terms of epinephrine, it is not known what effect vasoconstrictors in the local anesthetic regimen will have in patients with a known history of congenital prolonged QT interval or in patients taking any medication that prolongs the QT interval. Until more information is obtained, it is suggested that the clinician consult with the physician prior to the use of a vasoconstrictor in suspected patients, and that the vasoconstrictor (epinephrine, mepivacaine, and levonordefrin [Carbocaine 2% with Neo-Cobefrin]) be used with caution.

Effects on Dental Treatment Key adverse event(s) related to dental treatment: Frequent occurrence of stomatitis

Effects on Bleeding Chemotherapy with other antineoplastic FLT3 inhibitor midostaurin has resulted in significant myelosuppression, potentially including significant reduction in platelet counts and altered hemostasis. So far there are no reports of the FLT3 inhibitor gilteritinib causing any effects on bleeding.

Adverse Reactions

>10%:

Cardiovascular: Edema (40%), hypotension (22%)

Central nervous system: Fatigue (≤44%), malaise (≤44%), headache (24%), dizziness (22%), neuropathy (18%), insomnia (15%)

Dermatologic: Skin rash (36%)

Endocrine & metabolic: Decreased serum phosphate (grades 3/4: 14%), decreased serum sodium (grades 3/4: 12%)

Gastrointestinal: Stomatitis (41%; grades ≥3: 7%), diarrhea (35%), nausea (30%), constipation (28%), vomiting (21%), abdominal pain (18%), decreased appetite (15%), dysgeusia (11%)

Hematologic & oncologic: Febrile neutropenia (17% to 27%; grade ≥3: 17% to 26%)

Hepatic: Increased serum transaminases (51%), increased serum alanine aminotransferase (grade 3/4: 13%)

Neuromuscular & skeletal: Arthralgia (≤50%), myalgia (≤50%)

Ophthalmic: Eye disease (25%)

Renal: Renal insufficiency (21%)

Respiratory: Dyspnea (35%), cough (28%)

Miscellaneous: Fever (41%)

1% to 10%:

Cardiovascular: Prolonged QT interval on ECG (1% to 10%), increased serum creatine kinase (grades 3/4: 6%), cardiac failure (4%), pericardial effusion (4%), myocarditis (≤2%), pericarditis (≤2%)

Central nervous system: Reversible posterior leukoencephalopathy syndrome (1%)

Dermatologic: Dermatologic disorder (acute febrile neutrophilic dermatosis: 3%)

Endocrine & metabolic: Decreased serum calcium (grades 3/4: 6%), increased serum triglycerides (grades 3/4: 6%)

Gastrointestinal: Pancreatitis (4%), gastrointestinal perforation (1%)

Hematologic & oncologic: Differentiation syndrome (3%)

Hepatic: Increased serum aspartate aminotransferase (grades 3/4: 10%), increased serum alkaline phosphatase (grades 3/4: 2%)

Hypersensitivity: Hypersensitivity condition (8%)

Renal: Increased serum creatinine (grades 3/4: 3%)

Frequency not defined:

Hypersensitivity: Anaphylaxis, angioedema, drug-induced hypersensitivity reaction

Mechanism of Action Gilteritinib is a tyrosine kinase inhibitor which inhibits multiple tyrosine kinases, such as FMS-like tyrosine kinase 3 (FLT3). Gilteritinib inhibits FLT3 receptor signaling and proliferation in cells expressing FLT3 (including FLT3-ITD), tyrosine kinase domain mutations (TKD) FLT3-D835Y and FLT3-ITD-D835Y; it induces apoptosis in FLT3-ITD-expressing leukemia cells.

Pharmacodynamics/Kinetics

Onset of Action Inhibition of FLT3 phosphorylation: Rapid (within 24 hours after the initial dose)

Half-life Elimination 113 hours

Time to Peak ~4 to 6 hours

Reproductive Considerations Pregnancy status should be evaluated within 7 days prior to starting therapy in females of reproductive potential. Females of reproductive potential should use effective contraception during treatment and for at least 6 months after the last gilteritinib dose. Males with female partners of reproductive potential should use effective contraception during treatment and for at least 4 months after the last gilteritinib dose.

Pregnancy Considerations

Based on the mechanism of action and information from animal reproductions studies, gilteritinib may cause fetal harm following maternal use during pregnancy.

- **Gilteritinib Fumarate** *see* Gilteritinib *on page 736*
- **GingiBRAID** [+] *see* Epinephrine (Racemic) and Aluminum Potassium Sulfate *on page 575*
- **Givlaari** *see* Givosiran *on page 737*

Givosiran (GIV o si ran)

Brand Names: US Givlaari

Pharmacologic Category Aminolevulinate Synthase 1-Directed Small Interfering Ribonucleic Acid (siRNA)

Use Acute hepatic porphyria: Treatment of adults with acute hepatic porphyria.

Local Anesthetic/Vasoconstrictor Precautions
No information available to require special precautions.

Effects on Dental Treatment No significant effects or complications reported.

Effects on Bleeding No information available to require special precautions.

Adverse Reactions

>10%:

Dermatologic: Skin rash (17%)

Gastrointestinal: Nausea (27%)

Hepatic: Increased serum alanine aminotransferase (≥3 x ULN: 15%), increased serum transaminases (13%)

Local: Injection site reaction (25%)

Renal: Renal function abnormality (15%), decreased estimated GFR (eGFR) (≤15%), increased serum creatinine (≤15%)

1% to 10%: Central nervous system: Fatigue (10%)

<1%: Anaphylaxis, antibody development, hypersensitivity reaction

Mechanism of Action Givosiran causes degradation of aminolevulinate synthase 1 (ALAS1) messenger RNA (mRNA) in hepatocytes through RNA interference, reducing the elevated levels of liver ALAS1 mRNA. This leads to reduced circulating levels of neurotoxic intermediates aminolevulinic acid and porphobilinogen, factors associated with attacks and other disease manifestations of acute hepatic porphyria.

Pharmacodynamics/Kinetics

Half-life Elimination 6 hours.

Time to Peak Givosiran: 3 hours (range: 0.5 to 8 hours); AS(N-1)3' givosiran: 7 hours (range: 1.5 to 12 hours).

Pregnancy Considerations

Adverse events were observed in animal reproduction studies.

Outcome information following exposure to givosiran in pregnancy is limited (Sardh 2019).

- **Glargine Insulin** *see* Insulin Glargine *on page 822*
- **Glargine Insulin and Lixisenatide** *see* Insulin Glargine and Lixisenatide *on page 823*

Glasdegib (glas DEG ib)

Brand Names: US Daurismo

Pharmacologic Category Antineoplastic Agent, Hedgehog Pathway Inhibitor

Use

Acute myeloid leukemia: Treatment of newly diagnosed acute myeloid leukemia (in combination with low-dose cytarabine) in adult patients who are ≥75 years of age or who have comorbidities that preclude use of intensive induction chemotherapy.

Local Anesthetic/Vasoconstrictor Precautions
Glasdegib is one of the drugs confirmed to prolong the QT interval and is accepted as having a risk of causing torsades de pointes. The risk of drug-induced torsades de pointes is extremely low when a single QT interval prolonging drug is prescribed. In terms of epinephrine, it is not known what effect vasoconstrictors in the local anesthetic regimen will have in patients with a known history of congenital prolonged QT interval or in patients taking any medication that prolongs the QT interval. Until more information is obtained, it is suggested that the clinician consult with the physician prior to the use of a vasoconstrictor in suspected patients, and that the vasoconstrictor (epinephrine, mepivacaine, and levonordefrin [Carbocaine 2% with Neo-Cobefrin]) be used with caution.

Effects on Dental Treatment Key adverse event(s) related to dental treatment: Frequent occurrence of mucositis

Effects on Bleeding Bone marrow depression (eg, anemia, neutropenia, thrombocytopenia, and hemorrhage) has been reported. In patients under active treatment with glasdegib, medical consult is suggested.

Adverse Reactions

>10%:

Cardiovascular: Edema (30%), atrial arrhythmia (13%), chest pain (12%)

Central nervous system: Fatigue (36%), dizziness (18%), headache (12%)

Dermatologic: Skin rash (20%)

Endocrine & metabolic: Hyponatremia (11% to 54%), hypomagnesemia (33%), hyperkalemia (16%), hypokalemia (15%), weight loss (13%)

Gastrointestinal: Nausea (29%), decreased appetite (21%), dysgeusia (21%), mucositis (21%; grade ≥3: 1%), constipation (20%), abdominal pain (19%), diarrhea (18%), vomiting (18%)

Hematologic & oncologic: Anemia (43%; grade ≥3: 41%), hemorrhage (36%; grade ≥3: 6%), febrile neutropenia (31%; grade ≥3: 31%), thrombocytopenia (30%; grade ≥3: 30%), decreased white blood cell count (11%; grade ≥3: 11%)

Hepatic: Increased serum aspartate aminotransferase (28%), increased serum bilirubin (25%), increased serum alanine aminotransferase (24%), increased serum alkaline phosphatase (23%)

Neuromuscular & skeletal: Musculoskeletal pain (30%), increased creatine phosphokinase in blood specimen (16%), muscle spasm (15%)

Renal: Increased serum creatinine (96%), renal insufficiency (19%)

Respiratory: Dyspnea (23%), pneumonia (19%), cough (18%)

Miscellaneous: Fever (18%)

1% to 10%:

Cardiovascular: Prolonged QT interval on ECG (4% to 5%)

Infection: Sepsis (7%)

Frequency not defined: Endocrine & metabolic: Hypophosphatemia

Mechanism of Action Glasdegib is a small molecule inhibitor of the Hedgehog pathway. Glasdegib binds to and inhibits Smoothened (SMO), which is a transmembrane protein involved in hedgehog signal transduction. Glasdegib blocks the translocation of SMO into cilia and prevents SMO-mediated activation of downstream Hedgehog targets (Cortes 2018). In an animal AML model, glasdegib (in combination with low-dose cytarabine) reduced the percentage of CD45+/CD33+ blasts in the bone marrow and inhibited increases in tumor size to a greater extent than either agent alone.

Pharmacodynamics/Kinetics

Half-life Elimination 17.4 hours ± 3.7 hours

Time to Peak 1.3 to 1.8 hours

Reproductive Considerations

[US Boxed Warning]: Conduct pregnancy testing in females of reproductive potential prior to initiation of glasdegib treatment. Pregnancy testing should be conducted within 7 days prior to starting glasdegib treatment. **Advise females of reproductive potential to use effective contraception during treatment and for at least 30 days after the last glasdegib dose.**

[US Boxed Warning]: Advise males of the potential risk of glasdegib exposure through semen and to use condoms with a pregnant partner or a female partner of reproductive potential during glasdegib treatment and for at least 30 days after the last glasdegib dose to avoid potential drug exposure. Effective contraception, including a condom, should be used by males even after vasectomy. Semen should not be donated during treatment and for at least 30 days after the last dose of glasdegib. Based on animal data, males should consider effective fertility preservation prior to therapy.

Pregnancy Considerations

Glasdegib use is not recommended in pregnant females. **[US Boxed Warning]: Glasdegib can cause embryo-fetal death or severe birth defects when administered to a pregnant woman. Glasdegib is embryotoxic, fetotoxic, and teratogenic in animals.** Glasdegib inhibits the Hedgehog pathway, which is critical to fetal development (Walterhouse 1999).

Data collection to monitor pregnancy and infant outcomes following exposure to glasdegib is ongoing. Health care providers are encouraged to enroll females inadvertently exposed to glasdegib during pregnancy to the Pfizer pregnancy registry (800-438-1985).

◆ **Glasdegib Maleate** *see* Glasdegib *on page 737*

Glecaprevir and Pibrentasvir

(glek A pre vir & pi BRENT as vir)

Brand Names: US Mavyret

Brand Names: Canada Maviret

Pharmacologic Category Antihepaciviral, NS3/4A Protease Inhibitor (Anti-HCV); Antihepaciviral, NS5A Inhibitor; NS3/4A Inhibitor; NS5A Inhibitor

Use Chronic hepatitis C: Treatment of chronic hepatitis C virus (HCV) genotype 1, 2, 3, 4, 5, or 6 infection in adults and pediatric patients ≥12 years of age or weighing ≥45 kg, without cirrhosis or with compensated cirrhosis (Child-Pugh class A); HCV genotype 1 infection in adults and pediatric patients ≥12 years of age or weighing ≥45 kg, previously treated with a regimen containing an HCV NS5A inhibitor or an NS3/4A protease inhibitor, but not both.

Local Anesthetic/Vasoconstrictor Precautions No information available to require special precautions

Effects on Dental Treatment No significant effects or complications reported

Effects on Bleeding No information available to require special precautions

Adverse Reactions As reported in adults, unless otherwise noted.

>10%:

Gastrointestinal: Nausea (6% to 12%)

Nervous system: Fatigue (adults: 8% to 15%; adolescents: 6%), headache (6% to 17%)

1% to 10%:

Dermatologic: Pruritus (6% to 7%)

Gastrointestinal: Diarrhea (3% to 7%)

Hepatic: Increased serum bilirubin (≥2 x ULN: 4%)

Frequency not defined: Infection: Reactivation of HBV

Postmarketing:

Hepatic: Acute hepatic failure (FDA Safety Alert, August 28, 2019), decompensated liver disease, severe hepatic disease (FDA Safety Alert, August 28, 2019)

Hypersensitivity: Angioedema

Mechanism of Action

Glecaprevir is an inhibitor of hepatitis C virus (HCV) NS3/4A protease, necessary for the proteolytic cleavage of the HCV-encoded polyprotein (into mature forms of the NS3, NS4A, NS4B, NS5A, and NS5B proteins) and is essential for viral replication.

Pibrentasvir is an inhibitor of HCV NS5A, essential for viral RNA replication and virion assembly.

Pharmacodynamics/Kinetics

Half-life Elimination Glecaprevir: 6 hours; Pibrentasvir: 13 hours

Time to Peak 5 hours

Reproductive Considerations

HCV-infected females of childbearing potential should consider postponing pregnancy until therapy is complete to reduce the risk of HCV transmission (AASLD/IDSA 2018).

Pregnancy Considerations

Adverse events were not observed in animal reproduction studies with glecaprevir or pibrentasvir as individual agents.

Treatment of hepatitis C is not currently recommended to treat maternal infection or to decrease the risk of mother-to-child transmission during pregnancy (Tran 2016). When HCV infection is detected during pregnancy, treatment should be deferred until after delivery. Direct-acting antiviral medications should not be used in pregnant females outside of clinical trials until safety and efficacy information is available (SMFM [Hughes 2017]).

◆ **Gleevec** *see* Imatinib *on page 797*

◆ **Gleostine** *see* Lomustine *on page 927*

◆ **G-levOCARNitine S/F [OTC]** *see* LevOCARNitine *on page 896*

◆ **Glibenclamide** *see* GlyBURIDE *on page 741*

Gliclazide (GLYE kla zide)

Brand Names: Canada APO-Gliclazide; APO-Gliclazide MR; Diamicron; Diamicron MR; Gliclazide-80; GPC-Gliclazide MR; MINT-Gliclazide MR; MYLAN-Gliclazide MR; MYLAN-Gliclazide [DSC]; PMS-Gliclazide; SANDOZ Gliclazide MR; TARO-Gliclazide MR; TEVA-Gliclazide

Pharmacologic Category Antidiabetic Agent, Sulfonylurea

Use Note: Not approved in the United States.

Diabetes mellitus, type 2, treatment: Adjunct to diet and exercise to improve glycemic control in adults with type 2 diabetes mellitus.

Local Anesthetic/Vasoconstrictor Precautions No information available to require special precautions

Effects on Dental Treatment Key adverse event(s) related to dental treatment: Patients with diabetes should be questioned by the dental professional at each dental visit to assess their risk for stress-induced hypoglycemia. The dental professional should inquire about the patient's routine (ie, work, sleep schedule, eating patterns), history of hypoglycemia, time of last medication dose, last meal, and most recent blood sugar assessment. Keep a supply of glucose tablets and other carbohydrates in the office to prepare for a hypoglycemic event. Seek medical attention when necessary (American Diabetes Association 2018).

Effects on Bleeding No information available to require special precautions

Adverse Reactions

>10%: Endocrine & metabolic: Hypoglycemia (11% to 12%)

1% to 10%:

Cardiovascular: Hypertension (3% to 4%), angina pectoris (2%), peripheral edema (1%)

Central nervous system: Headache (4% to 5%), dizziness (2%), depression (1% to 2%), insomnia (1% to 2%), neuralgia (≤1%)

Dermatologic: Dermatological disorders (2%), dermatitis (1% to 2%), skin rash (1%; includes maculopapular rash, morbilliform rash), pruritus (≤1%)

Endocrine & metabolic: Hyperglycemia (2%), hyperlipidemia (≤1%), lipid metabolism disorder (≤1%)

Gastrointestinal: Diarrhea (2% to 3%), constipation (1% to 2%), gastroenteritis (1% to 2%), abdominal pain (1%), gastritis (1%), nausea (≤1%)

Genitourinary: Urinary tract infection (3%)

Infection: Viral infection (6% to 8%)

Neuromuscular & skeletal: Back pain (4% to 5%), arthralgia (3% to 4%), asthenia (2% to 3%), arthropathy (2%), myalgia (2%), arthritis (1% to 2%), tendonitis (1%)

Ophthalmic: Conjunctivitis (1%)

Otic: Otitis media (≤1%)

Respiratory: Bronchitis (4% to 5%), rhinitis (4% to 5%), pharyngitis (4%), upper respiratory tract infection (3% to 4%), cough (2%), pneumonia (1% to 2%), sinusitis (1% to 2%)

Frequency not defined:

Endocrine & metabolic: Increased lactate dehydrogenase

Renal: Increased serum creatinine

<1%, postmarketing, and/or case reports: Abnormal lacrimation, acute myocardial infarction, acute pancreatitis, agranulocytosis, albuminuria, anal fissure, anemia, angioedema, anxiety, arteritis, asthma, auditory disturbance, balanitis, bone disease (spine malformation), breast neoplasm (female; benign), bullous rash, bursitis, cardiac failure, carpal tunnel syndrome, cataract, cerebrovascular disease, chest pain, cholestatic jaundice, colitis, confusion, conjunctival hemorrhage, coronary artery disease, cystitis, dermal ulcer, diplopia, disulfiram-like reaction, drug reaction with eosinophilia and systemic symptoms, duodenal ulcer, dyspepsia, dyspnea, eczema, epigastric fullness, epistaxis, erythema of skin, erythrocytopenia, esophagitis, fecal incontinence, fever, flatulence, fungal dermatitis, fungal infection, gastroesophageal reflux disease, gastrointestinal neoplasm (benign), glaucoma, glycosuria, gout, hemolytic anemia, hemorrhoids, hepatitis, hepatomegaly, hypercholesterolemia, hyperkeratosis, hypersensitivity angiitis, hypersensitivity reaction, hypertriglyceridemia, hypoglycemic coma, hyponatremia, hypotension, hypothyroidism, impotence, increased appetite, increased serum alanine aminotransferase, increased serum alkaline phosphatase, increased serum aspartate aminotransferase, increased serum transaminases, increased thirst, infection, leukopenia, lower extremity pain, malaise, mastitis, melena, menstrual disease, nail disease, nephrolithiasis, nervousness, neuropathy, nocturia, onychomycosis, pain, palpitations, pancytopenia, polyuria, prostatic disease, renal cyst, retinopathy, sialorrhea, skeletal pain, Stevens-Johnson syndrome, tachycardia, thrombocytopenia, thrombophlebitis, tinnitus, toothache, toxic epidermal necrolysis, tracheitis, urticaria, vaginitis, vascular disease (vein disorder), visual disturbance, vitreous disorder, vomiting, weight gain, xeroderma, xerophthalmia, xerostomia

Mechanism of Action Stimulates insulin release from the pancreatic beta cells; reduces glucose output from the liver; insulin sensitivity is increased at peripheral target sites.

Pharmacodynamics/Kinetics

Duration of Action Modified-release tablet: 24 hours

Half-life Elimination Immediate-release tablet: 10.4 hours; Modified-release tablet: 16 hours (range: 12 to 20 hours)

Time to Peak Immediate-release tablet: 4 to 6 hours; Modified-release tablet: ~6 hours

Pregnancy Considerations

Gliclazide is contraindicated for use during pregnancy.

Poorly controlled diabetes during pregnancy can be associated with an increased risk of adverse maternal and fetal outcomes, including diabetic ketoacidosis, preeclampsia, spontaneous abortion, preterm delivery, delivery complications, major birth defects, stillbirth, and macrosomia (ACOG 201 2018). To prevent adverse outcomes, prior to conception and throughout pregnancy, maternal blood glucose and HbA_{1c} should be kept as close to target goals as possible but without causing significant hypoglycemia (ADA 2020; Blumer 2013).

Agents other than gliclazide are currently recommended to treat diabetes mellitus in pregnancy (ADA 2020).

Product Availability Not available in the US

Glimepiride (GLYE me pye ride)

Related Information

Endocrine Disorders and Pregnancy *on page 1684*

Brand Names: US Amaryl

Brand Names: Canada Amaryl [DSC]; APO-Glimepiride; GEN-Glimepiride; PMS-Glimepiride [DSC]; RATIO-Glimepiride [DSC]; SANDOZ Glimepiride

Pharmacologic Category Antidiabetic Agent, Sulfonylurea

Use Diabetes mellitus, type 2, treatment: As an adjunct to diet and exercise to improve glycemic control in adults with type 2 diabetes mellitus.

Local Anesthetic/Vasoconstrictor Precautions
No information available to require special precautions

Effects on Dental Treatment Key adverse event(s) related to dental treatment: Patients with diabetes should be questioned by the dental professional at each dental visit to assess their risk for stress-induced hypoglycemia. The dental professional should inquire about the patient's routine (ie, work, sleep schedule, eating patterns), history of hypoglycemia, time of last medication dose, last meal, and most recent blood sugar assessment. Keep a supply of glucose tablets and other carbohydrates in the office to prepare for a hypoglycemic event. Seek medical attention when necessary (American Diabetes Association, 2018).

Effects on Bleeding No information available to require special precautions

Adverse Reactions

>10%: Endocrine & metabolic: Hypoglycemia (4% to 20%)

1% to 10%:

Central nervous system: Dizziness (2%), headache
Gastrointestinal: Nausea (5%)
Hepatic: Increased serum ALT (2%)
Respiratory: Flu-like symptoms (5%)
Miscellaneous: Accidental injury (6%)

<1%, postmarketing, and/or case reports: Abnormal hepatic function tests, accommodation disturbance (early treatment), agranulocytosis, alopecia, anaphylaxis, angioedema, aplastic anemia, cholestatic jaundice, diarrhea, disulfiram-like reaction, dysgeusia, dyspnea, erythema, gastrointestinal pain, hemolytic anemia, hepatic failure, hepatic insufficiency, hepatic porphyria, hepatitis, hypersensitivity, hypersensitivity angiitis, hyponatremia, hypotension, immune thrombocytopenia, leukopenia, maculopapular rash, morbilliform rash, pancytopenia, porphyria cutanea tarda, pruritus, shock, SIADH, skin photosensitivity, Stevens-Johnson syndrome, thrombocytopenia, urticaria, vomiting, weight gain

Mechanism of Action Stimulates insulin release from the pancreatic beta cells; reduces glucose output from the liver; insulin sensitivity is increased at peripheral target sites

Pharmacodynamics/Kinetics

Onset of Action Peak effect: Blood glucose reductions: 2 to 3 hours

Duration of Action 24 hours

Half-life Elimination 5 to 9 hours

Time to Peak 2 to 3 hours

Pregnancy Considerations

Information related to the use of glimepiride during pregnancy is limited (Balaguer Santamaría 2000; Kalyoncu 2005). Severe hypoglycemia lasting 4 to 10 days has been noted in infants born to mothers taking a sulfonylurea at the time of delivery. If exposure during pregnancy occurs, discontinue at least 2 weeks prior to delivery.

Poorly controlled diabetes during pregnancy can be associated with an increased risk of adverse maternal and fetal outcomes, including diabetic ketoacidosis, preeclampsia, spontaneous abortion, preterm delivery, delivery complications, major birth defects, stillbirth, and macrosomia. To prevent adverse outcomes, prior to conception and throughout pregnancy, maternal blood glucose and HbA_{1c} should be kept as close to target goals as possible but without causing significant hypoglycemia (ADA 2020; Blumer 2013).

Agents other than glimepiride are currently recommended to treat diabetes mellitus in pregnancy (ADA 2020).

◆ **Glimepiride and Pioglitazone** *see* Pioglitazone and Glimepiride *on page 1235*

◆ **Glimepiride and Pioglitazone Hydrochloride** *see* Pioglitazone and Glimepiride *on page 1235*

GlipiZIDE (GLIP i zide)

Related Information

Endocrine Disorders and Pregnancy *on page 1684*

Brand Names: US glipiZIDE XL; Glucotrol; Glucotrol XL

Brand Names: Canada Glucotrol XL

Pharmacologic Category Antidiabetic Agent, Sulfonylurea

Use Diabetes mellitus, type 2, treatment: Adjunct to diet and exercise to improve glycemic control in adults with type 2 diabetes mellitus

Local Anesthetic/Vasoconstrictor Precautions
No information available to require special precautions

Effects on Dental Treatment Key adverse event(s) related to dental treatment: Patients with diabetes should be questioned by the dental professional at each dental visit to assess their risk for stress-induced hypoglycemia. The dental professional should inquire about the patient's routine (ie, work, sleep schedule, eating patterns), history of hypoglycemia, time of last medication dose, last meal, and most recent blood sugar assessment. Keep a supply of glucose tablets and other carbohydrates in the office to prepare for a hypoglycemic event. Seek medical attention when necessary (American Diabetes Association, 2018).

Effects on Bleeding No information available to require special precautions

Adverse Reactions Frequency not always defined.

Cardiovascular: Syncope (<3%)

Central nervous system: Dizziness (2% to 7%), nervousness (4%), anxiety (<3%), depression (<3%), hypoesthesia (<3%), insomnia (<3%), pain (<3%), paresthesia (<3%), drowsiness (2%), headache (2%)

Dermatologic: Diaphoresis (<3%), pruritus (1% to <3%), eczema (1%), erythema (1%), maculopapular rash (1%), morbilliform rash (1%), skin rash (1%), urticaria (1%)

Endocrine & metabolic: Hypoglycemia (<3%), increased lactate dehydrogenase

Gastrointestinal: Diarrhea (1% to 5%), flatulence (3%), dyspepsia (<3%), vomiting (<3%), constipation (1% to <3%), nausea (1% to <3%), abdominal pain (1%)

Hepatic: Increased serum alkaline phosphatase, increased serum AST

Neuromuscular & skeletal: Tremor (4%), arthralgia (<3%), leg cramps (<3%), myalgia (<3%)

Ophthalmic: Blurred vision (<3%)

Renal: Increased blood urea nitrogen, increased serum creatinine

Respiratory: Rhinitis (<3%)

1%, postmarketing, and/or case reports: Agranulocytosis, anorexia, aplastic anemia, bloody stools, cardiac arrhythmia, chills, cholestatic jaundice, confusion, conjunctivitis, decreased libido, disulfiram-like reaction, dyspnea, dysuria, edema, eye pain, flushing, hemolytic anemia, hepatic injury, hypertension, hypertonia, hyponatremia, jaundice, leukopenia, migraine, pancytopenia, pharyngitis, porphyria, retinal hemorrhage, SIADH (syndrome of inappropriate antidiuretic hormone secretion), skin photosensitivity, thrombocytopenia, unsteady gait, vertigo

Mechanism of Action Stimulates insulin release from the pancreatic beta cells; reduces glucose output from the liver; insulin sensitivity is increased at peripheral target sites

Pharmacodynamics/Kinetics

Duration of Action 12 to 24 hours

Half-life Elimination 2 to 5 hours

Time to Peak 1 to 3 hours; extended release tablets: 6 to 12 hours

Pregnancy Considerations

Glipizide was found to cross the placenta in vitro (Elliott 1994).

Severe hypoglycemia lasting 4 to 10 days has been noted in infants born to mothers taking a sulfonylurea at the time of delivery. The manufacturer recommends if glipizide is used during pregnancy, it should be discontinued at least 2 weeks before the expected delivery date.

Poorly controlled diabetes during pregnancy can be associated with an increased risk of adverse maternal and fetal outcomes, including diabetic ketoacidosis, preeclampsia, spontaneous abortion, preterm delivery, delivery complications, major birth defects, stillbirth, and macrosomia. To prevent adverse outcomes, prior to conception and throughout pregnancy, maternal blood glucose and HbA_{1c} should be kept as close to target goals as possible but without causing significant hypoglycemia (ADA 2020; Blumer 2013).

Agents other than glipizide are currently recommended to treat diabetes mellitus in pregnancy (ADA 2020).

- **glipiZIDE XL** *see* GlipiZIDE *on page 740*
- **Glivec** *see* Imatinib *on page 797*
- **Gloperba** *see* Colchicine *on page 405*
- **Gloperba** *see* Levamlodipine *on page 893*
- **Glucophage** *see* MetFORMIN *on page 983*
- **Glucophage XR** *see* MetFORMIN *on page 983*
- **Glucotrol** *see* GlipiZIDE *on page 740*
- **Glucotrol XL** *see* GlipiZIDE *on page 740*
- **Glucovance [DSC]** *see* Glyburide and Metformin *on page 742*
- **Glulisine Insulin** *see* Insulin Glulisine *on page 823*
- **Glumetza** *see* MetFORMIN *on page 983*
- **Glutofac-MX** *see* Vitamins (Multiple/Oral) *on page 1550*
- **Glybenclamide** *see* GlyBURIDE *on page 741*
- **Glybenzcyclamide** *see* GlyBURIDE *on page 741*

GlyBURIDE (GLYE byoor ide)

Related Information

Endocrine Disorders and Pregnancy *on page 1684*

Brand Names: US Glynase

Brand Names: Canada APO-GlyBURIDE; Diabeta [DSC]; DOM-GlyBURIDE; Euglucon; MYLAN-Glybe [DSC]; PMS-GlyBURIDE; PRO-Glyburide [DSC]; RIVA-GlyBURIDE [DSC]; SANDOZ GlyBURIDE [DSC]; TEVA-GlyBURIDE; TRIA-GlyBURIDE

Pharmacologic Category Antidiabetic Agent, Sulfonylurea

Use Diabetes mellitus, type 2: Adjunct to diet and exercise to improve glycemic control in adults with type 2 diabetes mellitus

Local Anesthetic/Vasoconstrictor Precautions No information available to require special precautions

Effects on Dental Treatment Key adverse event(s) related to dental treatment: Patients with diabetes should be questioned by the dental professional at each dental visit to assess their risk for stress-induced hypoglycemia. The dental professional should inquire about the patient's routine (ie, work, sleep schedule, eating patterns), history of hypoglycemia, time of last medication dose, last meal, and most recent blood sugar assessment. Keep a supply of glucose tablets and other carbohydrates in the office to prepare for a hypoglycemic event. Seek medical attention when necessary (American Diabetes Association, 2018).

Effects on Bleeding No information available to require special precautions

Adverse Reactions

1% to 10%:

Gastrointestinal: Epigastric fullness (≤2%), heartburn (≤2%), nausea (≤2%)

Hypersensitivity: Hypersensitivity reaction (2%; including erythema, maculopapular rash, morbilliform rash, pruritus, urticaria)

Frequency not defined:

Central nervous system: Disulfiram-like reaction

Endocrine & metabolic: Hypoglycemia, hyponatremia, weight gain

Genitourinary: Diuresis (minor)

Hematologic & oncologic: Hemolytic anemia

Hepatic: Cholestatic jaundice, hepatic failure, hepatitis

<1%, postmarketing, and/or case reports: Accommodation disturbance, angioedema, arthralgia, blurred vision, bullous rash, erythema multiforme, exfoliative dermatitis, increased serum transaminases, myalgia, vasculitis

Mechanism of Action Stimulates insulin release from the pancreatic beta cells; reduces glucose output from the liver; insulin sensitivity is increased at peripheral target sites

Pharmacodynamics/Kinetics

Onset of Action Serum insulin levels begin to increase 15-60 minutes after a single dose

Duration of Action ≤24 hours

Half-life Elimination Diaβeta: 10 hours; Glynase PresTab: ~4 hours; may be prolonged with renal or hepatic impairment

Time to Peak Serum: Adults: 2-4 hours

Pregnancy Considerations Glyburide crosses the placenta.

Severe hypoglycemia lasting 4 to 10 days has been noted in infants born to mothers taking a sulfonylurea at the time of delivery. Additional adverse maternal and fetal events have been noted in some studies and may be influenced by maternal glycemic control and/or differences in study design (Bertini 2005; Ekpebegh 2007; Joy 2012; Langer 2000; Langer 2005). According to the manufacturer, if glyburide is used during pregnancy, it should be discontinued at least 2 weeks before the expected delivery date. Due to pregnancy-induced physiologic changes, some pharmacokinetic properties of glyburide may be altered (Hebert 2009).

Poorly controlled diabetes during pregnancy can be associated with an increased risk of adverse maternal and fetal outcomes, including diabetic ketoacidosis, preeclampsia, spontaneous abortion, preterm delivery, delivery complications, major birth defects, stillbirth, and macrosomia (ACOG 201 2018). To prevent adverse outcomes, prior to conception and throughout pregnancy, maternal blood glucose and HbA_{1c} should be kept as close to target goals as possible but without causing significant hypoglycemia (ADA 2020; Blumer 2013).

Glyburide has been evaluated for the treatment of gestational diabetes mellitus. However, because glyburide crosses the placenta, long-term safety data are not available, and adverse events have been observed, glyburide should not be recommended as an initial alternative therapy (ACOG 190 2018; ADA 2020).

Agents other than glyburide are currently recommended to treat diabetes mellitus in pregnancy (ADA 2020).

Glyburide and Metformin

(GLYE byoor ide & met FOR min)

Related Information

GlyBURIDE *on page 741*

MetFORMIN *on page 983*

Brand Names: US Glucovance [DSC]

Pharmacologic Category Antidiabetic Agent, Biguanide; Antidiabetic Agent, Sulfonylurea

Use Diabetes mellitus, type 2: As an adjunct to diet and exercise, to improve glycemic control in adults with type 2 diabetes

Local Anesthetic/Vasoconstrictor Precautions No information available to require special precautions

Effects on Dental Treatment Key adverse event(s) related to dental treatment: Patients with diabetes should be questioned by the dental professional at each dental visit to assess their risk for stress-induced hypoglycemia. The dental professional should inquire about the patient's routine (ie, work, sleep schedule, eating patterns), history of hypoglycemia, time of last medication dose, last meal, and most recent blood sugar assessment. Keep a supply of glucose tablets and other carbohydrates in the office to prepare for a hypoglycemic event. Seek medical attention when necessary (American Diabetes Association, 2018).

Effects on Bleeding No information available to require special precautions

Adverse Reactions Also see individual agents.

>10%:

Endocrine & metabolic: Hypoglycemia (11% to 38%, effects higher when increased doses were used as initial therapy)

Gastrointestinal: Gastrointestinal symptoms (38%; combined GI effects increased to 38% in patients taking high doses as initial therapy), diarrhea (17%)

Respiratory: Upper respiratory infection (17%)

1% to 10%:

Central nervous system: Headache (9%), dizziness (6%)

Gastrointestinal: Nausea (8%), vomiting (8%), abdominal pain (7%)

<1%, postmarketing, and/or case reports: Cholestatic jaundice, hepatitis

Mechanism of Action The combination of glyburide and metformin is used to improve glycemic control in patients with type 2 diabetes mellitus by using two different, but complementary, mechanisms of action:

Glyburide: Stimulates insulin release from the pancreatic beta cells; reduces glucose output from the liver; insulin sensitivity is increased at peripheral target sites

Metformin: Decreases hepatic glucose production, decreasing intestinal absorption of glucose and improves insulin sensitivity (increases peripheral glucose uptake and utilization)

Pharmacodynamics/Kinetics

Time to Peak Glucovance: 2.75 hours when taken with food

Reproductive Considerations

Based on the metformin component, ovulation rates may increase in some anovulatory females; contraception should be discussed for women who do not wish to conceive (ACOG 194 2018).

Pregnancy Considerations

If exposure during pregnancy occurs, discontinue at least 2 weeks prior to expected delivery. Refer to individual monographs for additional information.

◆ **Glyburide and Metformin Hydrochloride** *see* Glyburide and Metformin *on page 742*

◆ **Glyburide/Metformin** *see* Glyburide and Metformin *on page 742*

◆ **Glycate** *see* Glycopyrrolate (Systemic) *on page 742*

◆ **Glyceryl Trinitrate** *see* Nitroglycerin *on page 1112*

◆ **Glycopyrrolate** *see* Glycopyrrolate (Oral Inhalation) *on page 743*

Glycopyrrolate (Systemic)

(glye koe PYE roe late)

Brand Names: US Cuvposa; Glycate; Glyrx-PF; Robinul [DSC]; Robinul-Forte [DSC]

Brand Names: Canada Cuvposa

Pharmacologic Category Anticholinergic Agent

Use

Chronic drooling (Cuvposa only): To reduce chronic, severe drooling in pediatric patients 3 to 16 years with neurologic conditions (eg, cerebral palsy) associated with problem drooling

Reduction of secretions (injection only): To reduce salivary, tracheobronchial, and pharyngeal secretions and to reduce the volume and acidity of gastric secretions during induction of anesthesia and intubation

Reversal of bradycardia, vagal reflexes (injection only): To block cardiac vagal inhibitory reflexes during induction of anesthesia and intubation; intraoperatively to counteract surgically or drug-induced or vagal reflexes associated arrhythmias

Reversal of muscarinic effects of cholinergic agents (injection only): Protects against the peripheral muscarinic effects (eg, bradycardia, excessive secretions) of cholinergic agents (eg, neostigmine, pyridostigmine) given to reverse the neuromuscular blockade due to non-depolarizing muscle relaxants

Local Anesthetic/Vasoconstrictor Precautions No information available to require special precautions

Effects on Dental Treatment Key adverse event(s) related to dental treatment: Significant xerostomia (normal salivary flow resumes upon discontinuation).

Effects on Bleeding No information available to require special precautions

Adverse Reactions Frequency not always defined.

Cardiovascular: Flushing (30%), pallor (≤2%), cardiac arrhythmias, heart block, hypertension, hypotension, palpitation, tachycardia

Central nervous system: Headache (15%), aggressiveness (≤2%), agitation (≤2%), crying (abnormal; ≤2%), irritability (≤2%), mood changes (≤2%), pain (≤2%), restlessness (≤2%), confusion, dizziness, drowsiness, excitement (higher incidence in older adults), insomnia, nervousness

Dermatologic: Dry skin (≤2%), pruritus (≤2%), rash (≤2%), hypohidrosis, urticaria

Endocrine & metabolic: Dehydration (≤2%)

Gastrointestinal: Vomiting (40%), xerostomia (40%), constipation (35%), abdominal distention (≤2%), abdominal pain (≤2%), flatulence (≤2%), retching (≤2%), intestinal obstruction, loss of taste, nausea, pseudo-obstruction

Genitourinary: Urinary retention (15%), urinary tract infection (≤2%), decreased lactation, impotence, urinary hesitancy

Neuromuscular & skeletal: Weakness

Ophthalmic: Nystagmus (≤2%), blurred vision, cycloplegia, increased intraocular pressure, mydriasis

Respiratory: Nasal congestion (30%), sinusitis (15%), upper respiratory tract infection (15%), bronchial secretion (thickening; ≤2%), nasal dryness (≤2%), pneumonia (≤2%)

<1%, postmarketing, and/or case reports: Arrhythmias, hypertension, hypotension, malignant hyperthermia, seizure

Mechanism of Action Blocks the action of acetylcholine at parasympathetic sites in smooth muscle, secretory glands, and the CNS; indirectly reduces the rate of salivation by preventing the stimulation of acetylcholine receptors

Pharmacodynamics/Kinetics

Onset of Action IM: 15 to 30 minutes; IV: Within 1 minute; Peak effect: IM: Within ~30 to 45 minutes

Duration of Action Vagal effect: 2 to 3 hours; Inhibition of salivation: Up to 7 hours; Parenteral: 7 hours

Half-life Elimination IV: Infants: 21.6 to 130 minutes; Children: 19.2 to 99.2 minutes; IM: Adults: 0.55 to 1.25 hours; IV: 0.83 ± 0.27 hour; Oral solution: Adults: 3 hours

Time to Peak 3.1 hours

Pregnancy Risk Factor B (injection)

Pregnancy Considerations Glycopyrrolate does not appear to penetrate through the placental barrier in significant amounts. Glycopyrrolate in doses of 0.004 mg/kg has not been found to affect fetal heart rate or fetal heart rate variability to a significant degree.

Product Availability Glyrx-PF (glycopyrrolate 0.2 mg/mL injection): FDA approved July 2018; availability anticipated in the third quarter 2018.

Glycopyrrolate (Oral Inhalation)

(glye koe PYE roe late)

Brand Names: US Lonhala Magnair Refill Kit; Lonhala Magnair Starter Kit; Seebri Neohaler

Brand Names: Canada Seebri Breezhaler

Pharmacologic Category Anticholinergic Agent; Anticholinergic Agent, Long-Acting

Use Chronic obstructive pulmonary disease: Maintenance treatment of airflow obstruction in patients with chronic obstructive pulmonary disease (COPD), including chronic bronchitis and/or emphysema.

Local Anesthetic/Vasoconstrictor Precautions No information available to require special precautions

Effects on Dental Treatment Key adverse event(s) related to dental treatment: Significant xerostomia (normal salivary flow resumes upon discontinuation).

Effects on Bleeding No information available to require special precautions

Adverse Reactions

1% to 10%:

Cardiovascular: Peripheral edema (<2%)

Central nervous system: Fatigue (≥2%)

Gastrointestinal: Diarrhea (≥2%), nausea (≥2%), upper abdominal pain (≥2%)

Genitourinary: Urinary tract infection (2%)

Neuromuscular & skeletal: Arthralgia (≥2%), back pain (≥2%)

Respiratory: Dyspnea (≤5%), upper respiratory tract infection (2% to 3%), bronchitis (≥2%), nasopharyngitis (≥2%), pneumonia (≥2%), rhinitis (≥2%), wheezing (≥2%), oropharyngeal pain (2%), sinusitis (1%)

<1% postmarketing, and/or case reports: Angioedema, atrial fibrillation, cough, diabetes mellitus, dysuria, gastroenteritis, hypersensitivity reaction, insomnia, limb pain, paradoxical bronchospasm, productive cough, pruritus, skin rash, voice disorder, vomiting

Mechanism of Action Competitively and reversibly inhibits the action of acetylcholine at muscarinic receptor subtypes 1 to 3 (greater affinity for subtypes 1 and 3) in bronchial smooth muscle thereby causing bronchodilation

Pharmacodynamics/Kinetics

Half-life Elimination 33 to 53 hours

Time to Peak Plasma: Dry powder inhaler (capsule): 5 minutes; Nebulization solution: <20 minutes

Pregnancy Risk Factor C

Pregnancy Considerations Adverse events have been observed in some animal reproduction studies. Small amounts of glycopyrrolate cross the human placenta following IM injection.

Glycopyrrolate and Formoterol

(glye koe PYE roe late & for MOH te rol)

Brand Names: US Bevespi Aerosphere

Pharmacologic Category Anticholinergic Agent; Anticholinergic Agent, Long-Acting; Beta2 Agonist; $Beta_2$-Adrenergic Agonist, Long-Acting

Use Chronic obstructive pulmonary disease: Maintenance treatment of airflow obstruction in patients with chronic obstructive pulmonary disease (COPD), including chronic bronchitis and/or emphysema

Local Anesthetic/Vasoconstrictor Precautions No information available to require special precautions

Effects on Dental Treatment No significant effects or complications reported

Effects on Bleeding No information available to require special precautions

Adverse Reactions See individual agents.

1% to 10%:

Cardiovascular: Chest pain (1% to <2%)

Central nervous system: Anxiety (1% to <2%), dizziness (1% to <2%), falling (1% to <2%), fatigue (1% to <2%), headache (1% to <2%)

Gastrointestinal: Vomiting (1% to <2%), xerostomia (1% to <2%)

Genitourinary: Urinary tract infection (3%)
Hematologic & oncologic: Bruise (1% to <2%)
Infection: Influenza (1% to <2%), tooth abscess (1% to <2%)
Neuromuscular & skeletal: Arthralgia (1% to <2%), limb pain (1% to <2%), muscle spasm (1% to <2%)
Respiratory: Cough (4%), acute sinusitis (1% to <2%), oropharyngeal pain (1% to <2%)

Frequency not defined: Respiratory: Paradoxical bronchospasm

<1%, postmarketing, and/or case reports: Hypersensitivity reaction, urinary retention

Mechanism of Action

Glycopyrrolate: In COPD, competitively and reversibly inhibits the action of acetylcholine at muscarinic receptor subtypes 1-3 (greater affinity for subtypes 1 and 3) in bronchial smooth muscle thereby causing bronchodilation.

Formoterol: Relaxes bronchial smooth muscle by selective action on $beta_2$ receptors with little effect on heart rate. Formoterol has a long-acting effect.

Pregnancy Risk Factor C

Pregnancy Considerations

Animal reproduction studies have not been conducted with this combination. Beta-agonists have the potential to affect uterine contractility if administered during labor. Refer to individual monographs for additional information.

- **Glycopyrrolate and Formoterol Fumarate** *see* Glycopyrrolate and Formoterol *on page* 743
- **Glycopyrronium and Formoterol** *see* Glycopyrrolate and Formoterol *on page* 743
- **Glycopyrronium Bromide** *see* Glycopyrrolate (Oral Inhalation) *on page* 743
- **Glycopyrronium Bromide** *see* Glycopyrrolate (Systemic) *on page* 742
- **Glycopyrronium Bromide and Formoterol Fumarate** *see* Glycopyrrolate and Formoterol *on page* 743
- **Glydiazinamide** *see* GlipiZIDE *on page* 740
- **Glydo** *see* Lidocaine (Topical) *on page* 902
- **Glynase** *see* GlyBURIDE *on page* 741
- **Gly-Oxide [OTC]** *see* Carbamide Peroxide *on page* 289
- **Glyrx-PF** *see* Glycopyrrolate (Systemic) *on page* 742
- **Glyset** *see* Miglitol *on page* 1030
- **GM-CSF** *see* Sargramostim *on page* 1358
- **GM-CSF-Encoding Oncolytic Herpes Simplex Virus** *see* Talimogene Laherparepvec *on page* 1403
- **GnRH** *see* Gonadorelin *on page* 746
- **GnRH Agonist** *see* Histrelin *on page* 759
- **Gocovri** *see* Amantadine *on page* 112

Golimumab (goe LIM ue mab)

Related Information

Rheumatoid Arthritis, Osteoarthritis, and Osteoporosis *on page* 1697

Brand Names: US Simponi; Simponi Aria

Brand Names: Canada Simponi; Simponi I.V.

Pharmacologic Category Antipsoriatic Agent; Antirheumatic, Disease Modifying; Monoclonal Antibody; Tumor Necrosis Factor (TNF) Blocking Agent

Use

Ankylosing spondylitis (Simponi, Simponi Aria): Treatment of adults with active ankylosing spondylitis (alone or in combination with methotrexate).

Psoriatic arthritis (Simponi, Simponi Aria): Treatment of adults with active psoriatic arthritis (alone or in combination with methotrexate).

Rheumatoid arthritis (Simponi, Simponi Aria): Treatment of adults with moderately-to-severely active rheumatoid arthritis (in combination with methotrexate).

Ulcerative colitis (Simponi): Treatment of moderately to severely active ulcerative colitis in adults with corticosteroid dependence or who have had an inadequate response to conventional therapy (to induce and maintain clinical response, improve mucosal appearance during induction, induce clinical remission, and achieve and sustain remission in induction responders).

Local Anesthetic/Vasoconstrictor Precautions

No information available to require special precautions

Effects on Dental Treatment Key adverse event(s) related to dental treatment: Golimumab belongs to the class of disease-modifying antirheumatic drugs and, as such, has immunosuppressive properties. Consider a medical consult prior to any invasive treatment for patients under active treatment with golimumab. Delayed wound healing due to the immunosuppressive effects and increased potential for postsurgical infection may be of concern.

Effects on Bleeding No information available to require special precautions

Adverse Reactions As reported with combination therapy.

>10%:

Hematologic & oncologic: Positive ANA titer (IV: 17%, anti-dsDNA: <1%; subcutaneous: 4%, anti-dsDNA: <1%)
Immunologic: Antibody development (subcutaneous: Drug-tolerant EIA: 16% to 38%; IV: Drug-tolerant EIA: 19% to 21%; approximately 1/3 were neutralizing)
Infection: Infection (27% to 28%)
Respiratory: Upper respiratory tract infection (13% to 16%)

1% to 10%:

Cardiovascular: Hypertension (3%)
Central nervous system: Dizziness (≤2%), paresthesia (≤2%)
Dermatologic: Skin rash (3%)
Gastrointestinal: Constipation (≤1%)
Hematologic & oncologic: Decreased neutrophils (≤5%), leukopenia (1%)
Hepatic: Increased serum alanine aminotransferase (≤8%), increased serum aspartate aminotransferase (≤5%)
Infection: Viral infection (4% to 5%; includes herpes and influenza), fungal infection (≤2%; may be invasive or superficial), bacterial infection (1%)
Local: Injection site reaction (subcutaneous: 3% to 6%)
Respiratory: Nasopharyngitis (≤6%), bronchitis (2% to 3%), sinusitis (≤2%)
Miscellaneous: Fever (2%), infusion-related reaction (intravenous: 1%)

Frequency not defined:

Dermatologic: Cellulitis
Infection: Opportunistic infections, sepsis, serious infection

Respiratory: Activated tuberculosis, reactivated tuberculosis

<1%, postmarketing, and/or case reports: Abscess, agranulocytosis, anaphylaxis, aplastic anemia, atypical serious infection, bullous skin disease, cardiac failure, demyelinating disease of the central nervous system, dyspnea, exfoliation of skin, Guillain-Barre syndrome, hepatitis B, hepatotoxicity (idiosyncratic), hypersensitivity angiitis, hypersensitivity reaction, infective bursitis, interstitial pulmonary disease, leukemia, lichenoid eruption, lupus-like syndrome, malignant lymphoma, malignant melanoma, malignant neoplasm, Merkel cell carcinoma, multiple sclerosis, mycobacterial infection, nausea, neutropenia, non-Hodgkin's lymphoma, optic neuritis, pancytopenia, peripheral demyelinating polyneuropathy, pneumonia, pruritus, psoriasis (including new onset, palmoplantar, pustular, or exacerbation), pyelonephritis, sarcoidosis, septic arthritis, septic shock, thrombocytopenia, urticaria, vasculitis

Mechanism of Action Human monoclonal antibody that binds to human tumor necrosis factor alpha (TNFα), thereby interfering with endogenous TNFα activity. Biological activities of TNFα include the induction of proinflammatory cytokines (interleukin [IL]-6, IL-8, Granulocyte-colony stimulating factor, granulocyte-macrophage colony stimulating factor), expression of adhesion molecules (E-selectin, vascular cell adhesion molecule [VCAM]-1, intercellular adhesion molecule [ICAM]-1) necessary for leukocyte infiltration, activation of neutrophils and eosinophils.

Pharmacodynamics/Kinetics

Half-life Elimination ~2 weeks

Time to Peak SubQ: 2-6 days

Reproductive Considerations

Treatment algorithms are available for use of biologics in female patients with Crohn disease who are planning a pregnancy (Weizman 2019). Serum levels should be optimized prior to conception (Mahadevan 2019).

Pregnancy Considerations Golimumab crosses the placenta (Benoit 2019).

Golimumab is a humanized monoclonal antibody (IgG_1). Placental transfer of human IgG is dependent upon the IgG subclass, maternal serum concentrations, birth weight, and gestational age, generally increasing as pregnancy progresses. The lowest exposure would be expected during the period of organogenesis (Palmeira 2012; Pentsuk 2009).

Following administration of golimumab 100 mg every 2 weeks throughout pregnancy to a patient with ulcerative colitis, cord blood concentrations of golimumab were 121% of the maternal serum concentration at delivery. Delivery occurred 3 days after the last maternal dose (Benoit 2019).

Information related to this class of medications is emerging, but based on available data, tumor necrosis factor alpha (TNFα) blocking agents are considered to have low to moderate risk when used in pregnancy (ACOG 776 2019).

Vaccination with live vaccines (eg, rotavirus vaccine) should be avoided for the first 6 months of life if exposure to a biologic agent occurs during the third trimester of pregnancy (eg, >27 weeks' gestation) (Mahadevan 2019).

Inflammatory bowel disease is associated with adverse pregnancy outcomes including an increased risk of miscarriage, premature delivery, delivery of a low birth weight infant, and poor maternal weight gain. Management of maternal disease should be optimized prior to pregnancy. Treatment decreases disease flares, disease activity, and the incidence of adverse pregnancy outcomes (Mahadevan 2019).

Use of immune modulating therapies in pregnancy should be individualized to optimize maternal disease and pregnancy outcomes (ACOG 776 2019). When treatment for inflammatory bowel disease is needed in pregnant women, appropriate biologic therapy can be continued without interruption. Serum levels should be evaluated prior to conception and optimized to avoid subtherapeutic concentrations or high levels which may increase placental transfer. Dosing can be adjusted so delivery occurs at the lowest serum concentration. For golimumab, the final injection can be given 4 to 6 weeks prior to the estimated date of delivery, then continued 48 hours' postpartum (Mahadevan 2019).

Golodirsen (GOE loe DIR sen)

Brand Names: US Vyondys 53

Pharmacologic Category Antisense Oligonucleotide

Use Duchenne muscular dystrophy: Treatment of Duchenne muscular dystrophy (DMD) in patients who have a confirmed mutation of the DMD gene that is amenable to exon 53 skipping.

Local Anesthetic/Vasoconstrictor Precautions No information available to require special precautions.

Effects on Dental Treatment Key adverse event(s) related to dental treatment: Frequent occurrence of nasopharyngitis; infrequent occurrence of oropharyngeal pain.

Effects on Bleeding No information available to require special precautions.

Adverse Reactions

>10%:

Central nervous system: Headache (41%), falling (29%)

Gastrointestinal: Abdominal pain (27%), vomiting (27%), nausea (20%)

Respiratory: Cough (27%), nasopharyngitis (27%)

Miscellaneous: Fever (41%)

1% to 10%:

Cardiovascular: Tachycardia (>5%)

Central nervous system: Dizziness (>5%), pain (>5%)

Dermatologic: Excoriation of skin (>5%)

Gastrointestinal: Constipation (>5%), diarrhea (>5%)

Hematologic & oncologic: Bruise (>5%)

Hypersensitivity: Seasonal allergy (>5%)

Infection: Influenza (>5%)

Local: Catheter-site reaction (>5%), infusion-site pain (>5%)

Neuromuscular & skeletal: Back pain (>5%), bone fracture (>5%), sprain (>5%)

Otic: Otic infection (>5%)

Respiratory: Oropharyngeal pain (>5%), rhinitis (>5%)

Frequency not defined:

Dermatologic: Dermatitis, exfoliation of skin, pruritus, skin rash, urticaria

Hypersensitivity: Hypersensitivity reaction

Mechanism of Action Binds to exon 53 of dystrophin pre-messenger RNA (mRNA), resulting in exclusion of this exon during mRNA processing. Exon 53 skipping allows for production of an internally truncated dystrophin protein in patients with genetic mutations that are amenable to exon 53 skipping.

Pharmacodynamics/Kinetics

Half-life Elimination 3.4 hours.

Pregnancy Considerations
Animal reproduction studies or studies in females have not been conducted.

Gonadorelin (goe nad oh RELL in)

Brand Names: Canada Lutrepulse; Relisorm [DSC]
Pharmacologic Category Gonadotropin
Use Note: Not approved in the US
Induction of ovulation in females with hypothalamic amenorrhea
Local Anesthetic/Vasoconstrictor Precautions No information available to require special precautions
Effects on Dental Treatment No significant effects or complications reported
Effects on Bleeding No information available to require special precautions
Adverse Reactions Frequency not defined.
Cardiovascular: Superficial thrombophlebitis
Local: Injection site irritation
<1%, postmarketing, and/or case reports: Abdominal pain, anaphylactic shock, anaphylaxis, antibody development (with long-term therapy, resulting in therapy failure), erythema at injection site, fever, headache, hypermenorrhea, inflammation at injection site (mild and severe), nausea, ovarian hyperstimulation syndrome (moderate)
Mechanism of Action Stimulates the release of luteinizing hormone (LH) from the anterior pituitary gland
Pharmacodynamics/Kinetics
Onset of Action Response to therapy usually observed within 2-3 weeks
Half-life Elimination Terminal: ~10-40 minutes; increased in patients with renal impairment
Pregnancy Considerations
The risk of fetal harm appears remote if gonadorelin is used during pregnancy. Clinical studies of pregnant women have not demonstrated an increased risk of fetal abnormalities during the first trimester. Follow-up reports of infants born to exposed mothers revealed no adverse effects or complications attributed to gonadorelin therapy. Based on its indicated use, gonadorelin treatment is continued for 2 weeks following ovulation to maintain the corpus luteum; initiation of treatment is not appropriate if pregnancy has been established.
Product Availability Not available in the US

- ◆ **Gonadorelin Acetate** *see* Gonadorelin *on page* 746
- ◆ **Gonadotropin Releasing Hormone** *see* Gonadorelin *on page* 746
- ◆ **GoNitro** *see* Nitroglycerin *on page* 1112
- ◆ **GoodSense All Day Allergy [OTC]** *see* Cetirizine (Systemic) *on page* 328
- ◆ **GoodSense Allergy Relief [OTC]** *see* DiphenhydrAMINE (Systemic) *on page* 502
- ◆ **GoodSense Allergy Relief [OTC]** *see* Loratadine *on page* 930
- ◆ **GoodSense Clear Anti-Itch [OTC]** *see* Pramoxine *on page* 1252
- ◆ **GoodSense Cough DM [OTC]** *see* Dextromethorphan *on page* 476
- ◆ **GoodSense Cough DM Childrens [OTC]** *see* Dextromethorphan *on page* 476
- ◆ **GoodSense Ear Wax Kit [OTC]** *see* Carbamide Peroxide *on page* 289
- ◆ **GoodSense Ear Wax Removal [OTC]** *see* Carbamide Peroxide *on page* 289
- ◆ **GoodSense Esomeprazole [OTC]** *see* Esomeprazole *on page* 594
- ◆ **GoodSense Hemorrhoidal [OTC]** *see* Phenylephrine (Topical) *on page* 1227
- ◆ **GoodSense Hydrogen Peroxide [OTC]** *see* Hydrogen Peroxide *on page* 776
- ◆ **GoodSense Ibuprofen [OTC]** *see* Ibuprofen *on page* 786
- ◆ **GoodSense Ibuprofen Childrens [OTC]** *see* Ibuprofen *on page* 786
- ◆ **GoodSense Lansoprazole [OTC]** *see* Lansoprazole *on page* 876
- ◆ **GoodSense Low Dose [OTC]** *see* Aspirin *on page* 177
- ◆ **GoodSense Miconazole 1 [OTC]** *see* Miconazole (Topical) *on page* 1019
- ◆ **GoodSense Motion Sickness [OTC]** *see* DimenhyDRINATE *on page* 501
- ◆ **GoodSense Naproxen Sodium [OTC]** *see* Naproxen *on page* 1080
- ◆ **GoodSense Nasal Allergy Spray [OTC]** *see* Triamcinolone (Nasal) *on page* 1489
- ◆ **GoodSense Nasoflow [OTC] [DSC]** *see* Fluticasone (Nasal) *on page* 703
- ◆ **GoodSense Nicotine [OTC]** *see* Nicotine *on page* 1101
- ◆ **GoodSense Oral Pain Relief [OTC]** *see* Benzocaine *on page* 228
- ◆ **GoodSense Oral Rinse [OTC]** *see* Cetylpyridinium *on page* 330
- ◆ **GoodSense Pain Relief** *see* Acetaminophen *on page* 59
- ◆ **GoodSense Pain Relief Extra Strength [OTC]** *see* Acetaminophen *on page* 59
- ◆ **GoodSense Sleep Aid [OTC]** *see* DiphenhydrAMINE (Systemic) *on page* 502
- ◆ **GoodSense Stool Softener [OTC] [DSC]** *see* Docusate *on page* 509
- ◆ **Goprelto** *see* Cocaine (Topical) *on page* 403
- ◆ **Gordons-Vite A [OTC]** *see* Vitamin A *on page* 1549

Goserelin (GOE se rel in)

Brand Names: US Zoladex
Brand Names: Canada Zoladex; Zoladex LA
Pharmacologic Category Antineoplastic Agent, Gonadotropin-Releasing Hormone Agonist; Gonadotropin Releasing Hormone Agonist
Use
Breast cancer, advanced (3.6 mg only): Palliative treatment of advanced breast cancer in pre- and perimenopausal women (estrogen and progesterone receptor values may help to predict if goserelin is likely to be beneficial).
Endometrial thinning (3.6 mg only): Endometrial-thinning agent prior to endometrial ablation for dysfunctional uterine bleeding.
Endometriosis (3.6 mg only): Management of endometriosis, including pain relief and reduction of endometriotic lesions for the duration of therapy (goserelin experience for endometriosis has been limited to women 18 years and older treated for 6 months).

Prostate cancer, advanced (3.6 mg or 10.8 mg): Palliative treatment of advanced carcinoma of the prostate.

Prostate cancer, stage B2 to C (3.6 mg or 10.8 mg): Management of locally confined stage T2b to T4 (stage B2 to C) prostate cancer (in combination with an antiandrogen [eg, flutamide]); begin goserelin and antiandrogen therapy 8 weeks prior to initiating radiation therapy and continue during radiation therapy.

Local Anesthetic/Vasoconstrictor Precautions

No information available to require special precautions

Effects on Dental Treatment Key adverse event(s) related to dental treatment: Xerostomia (normal salivary flow resumes upon discontinuation) and taste disturbances.

Effects on Bleeding No information available to require special precautions

Adverse Reactions Some frequencies not defined. Percentages reported with the 1-month implant:

>10%:

- Cardiovascular: Vasodilation (females 57%), peripheral edema (females 21%)
- Central nervous system: Headache (females 32% to 75%; males 1% to 5%), emotional lability (females 60%), depression (females 54%; males 1% to 5%), pain (8% to 17%), dyspareunia (females 14%), insomnia (5% to 11%)
- Dermatologic: Diaphoresis (females 16% to 45%; males 6%), acne vulgaris (females 42%; usually within 1 month after starting treatment), seborrhea (females 26%)
- Endocrine & metabolic: Hot flash (females 57% to 96%; males 64%), decreased libido (females 48% to 61%), increased libido (females 12%)
- Gastrointestinal: Abdominal pain (females 7% to 11%), nausea (5% to 11%)
- Genitourinary: Vaginitis (75%), breast atrophy (females 33%), sexual disorder (males 21%), breast hypertrophy (females 18%), decrease in erectile frequency (18%), pelvic symptoms (females 18%), genitourinary signs and symptoms (lower; males 13%)
- Hematologic & oncologic: Tumor flare (females 23%; males: Incidence not reported)
- Infection: Infection (females 13%; males: Incidence not reported)
- Neuromuscular & skeletal: Decreased bone mineral density (females 23%; ~4% decrease from baseline in 6 months; male: Incidence not reported), weakness (females 11%)

1% to 10%:

- Cardiovascular: Edema (females 5%; male 7%), hypertension (1% to 6%), cardiac failure (males 5%), cardiac arrhythmia (males >1% to <5%), cerebrovascular accident (males >1% to <5%), peripheral vascular disease (males >1% to <5%), varicose veins (males >1% to <5%), chest pain (1% to <5%), myocardial infarction (males <1% to <5%), palpitations, tachycardia (females)
- Central nervous system: Lethargy (females ≤8%), migraine (females 1% to 7%), dizziness (females 6%; male 5%), malaise (females ≤5%), chills (males >1% to <5%), anxiety (1% to <5%), nervousness (females 3% to 5%), voice disorder (females 3%), abnormality in thinking, drowsiness, paresthesia
- Dermatologic: Skin rash (males 6% to 8%; female frequency not reported), hair disease (females 4%), pruritus (females 2%), alopecia, skin discoloration, xeroderma
- Endocrine & metabolic: Gynecomastia (males 8%), hirsutism (7%), gout (males >1% to <5%), hyperglycemia (males >1% to <5%), weight gain (>1% to <5%)
- Gastrointestinal: Anorexia (1% to 5%), gastric ulcer (males >1% to <5%), constipation (1% to <5%), diarrhea (1% to <5%), vomiting (1% to <5%), increased appetite (females 2%), dyspepsia, flatulence, xerostomia
- Genitourinary: Pelvic pain (females 9%; males 6%), mastalgia (>1% to 7%), uterine hemorrhage (6%), vulvovaginitis (5%), breast swelling (males >1% to <5%), urinary tract obstruction (males: >1% to <5%), urinary tract infection (1% to <5%), urinary frequency, vaginal hemorrhage
- Hematologic & oncologic: Anemia (males >1% to <5%), bruise, hemorrhage
- Hypersensitivity: Hypersensitivity reaction
- Infection: Sepsis (males >1% to <5%)
- Local: Application site reaction (females 6%)
- Neuromuscular & skeletal: Myalgia (females 3%, males frequency not reported), leg cramps (females 2%, males frequency not reported), hypertonia (females 1%; male frequency not reported), arthralgia, arthropathy
- Ophthalmic: Amblyopia, dry eye syndrome
- Renal: Renal insufficiency (<1% to >5%)
- Respiratory: Upper respiratory tract infection (males 7%), chronic obstructive pulmonary disease (males 5%), flu-like symptoms (females 5%, male frequency not reported), pharyngitis (females 5%), sinusitis (females ≥1%; male frequency not reported), bronchitis, cough, epistaxis, rhinitis
- Miscellaneous: Fever

<1%, postmarketing, and/or case reports (with monthly or 3-month implant): Anaphylaxis, bone fracture, convulsions, decreased glucose tolerance, decreased HDL cholesterol, deep vein thrombosis, diabetes mellitus, hypercalcemia, hypercholesterolemia, hyperlipidemia, hypotension, increased HDL cholesterol, increased LDL cholesterol, increased serum ALT, increased serum AST, increased serum triglycerides, injection site reaction (including vascular injury, pain, hematoma, hemorrhage, hemorrhagic shock), osteoporosis, ovarian cyst, ovarian hyperstimulation syndrome, pituitary apoplexy, pituitary neoplasm (including adenoma), pulmonary embolism, psychotic reaction, transient ischemic attacks

Mechanism of Action Goserelin (a gonadotropin-releasing hormone [GnRH] analog) causes an initial increase in luteinizing hormone (LH) and follicle stimulating hormone (FSH), chronic administration of goserelin results in a sustained suppression of pituitary gonadotropins. Serum testosterone falls to levels comparable to surgical castration. The exact mechanism of this effect is unknown, but may be related to changes in the control of LH or down-regulation of LH receptors.

Pharmacodynamics/Kinetics

Onset of Action

Females: Estradiol suppression reaches postmenopausal levels within 3 weeks and FSH and LH are suppressed to follicular phase levels within 4 weeks of initiation.

Males: Testosterone suppression reaches castrate levels within 2 to 4 weeks after initiation.

Duration of Action

Females: Estradiol, LH and FSH generally return to baseline levels within 12 weeks following the last monthly implant.

Males: Testosterone levels maintained at castrate levels throughout the duration of therapy.

Time to Peak SubQ: Male: 12 to 15 days, Female: 8 to 22 days

Reproductive Considerations

When used for endometriosis or endometrial thinning, females of reproductive potential should not receive goserelin until pregnancy has been excluded. Nonhormonal contraception is recommended for premenopausal women during therapy and for 12 weeks after therapy is discontinued. Although ovulation is usually inhibited and menstruation may stop, pregnancy prevention is not ensured during goserelin therapy. Changes in reproductive function may occur following chronic administration.

Goserelin may prevent premature ovarian failure when added to chemotherapy in women with early stage hormone receptor negative breast cancer. In one study, women followed for 5 years were less likely to experience ovarian failure and more likely to become pregnant than women who did not receive goserelin in addition to their chemotherapy. The desire to become pregnant and the incidence of prior pregnancies was not considered in the analysis, and pregnancies occurred in some women who were not attempting to conceive (Moore 2015; Moore 2019). Use of gonadotropin-releasing hormone (GnRH) agonists such as goserelin for preserving ovarian function and potentially maintaining future fertility may be considered for some premenopausal women undergoing chemotherapy (ACOG 747 2018).

Pregnancy Considerations

Goserelin induces hormonal changes, which increase the risk for fetal loss.

Use is contraindicated during pregnancy for the treatment of endometriosis or endometrial thinning. If used for the palliative treatment of breast cancer during pregnancy, the potential for increased fetal loss should be discussed with the patient. Outcome information following inadvertent goserelin exposure during pregnancy is limited (Ishizuka 2016).

◆ **Goserelin Acetate** *see* Goserelin *on page 746*
◆ **GP 47680** *see* OXcarbazepine *on page 1154*
◆ **GR38032R** *see* Ondansetron *on page 1143*
◆ **Gralise** *see* Gabapentin *on page 722*
◆ **Gralise Starter** *see* Gabapentin *on page 722*

Granisetron (gra NI se tron)

Related Information

Clinical Risk Related to Drugs Prolonging QT Interval *on page 1675*

Brand Names: US Sancuso; Sustol

Brand Names: Canada APO-Granisetron; NAT-Granisetron

Pharmacologic Category Antiemetic; Selective 5-HT_3 Receptor Antagonist

Use

Chemotherapy-associated nausea and vomiting: Prevention of nausea and vomiting associated with initial and repeat courses of emetogenic chemotherapy, including high-dose cisplatin (injection and tablets); prevention of nausea and vomiting associated with anthracycline/cyclophosphamide chemotherapy regimens; prevention of nausea and vomiting associated with moderately and/or highly emetogenic chemotherapy regimens of up to 5 consecutive days of duration (transdermal).

Radiation-associated nausea and vomiting: Prevention of nausea and vomiting associated with radiation therapy, including total body radiation and fractionated abdominal radiation (tablets).

Local Anesthetic/Vasoconstrictor Precautions Granisetron is one of the drugs confirmed to prolong the QT interval and is accepted as having a risk of causing torsade de pointes. The risk of drug-induced torsade de pointes is extremely low when a single QT interval prolonging drug is prescribed. In terms of epinephrine, it is not known what effect vasoconstrictors in the local anesthetic regimen will have in patients with a known history of congenital prolonged QT interval or in patients taking any medication that prolongs the QT interval. Until more information is obtained, it is suggested that the clinician consult with the physician prior to the use of a vasoconstrictor in suspected patients, and that the vasoconstrictor (epinephrine, mepivacaine and levonordefrin [Carbocaine® 2% with Neo-Cobefrin®]) be used with caution.

Effects on Dental Treatment No significant effects or complications reported

Effects on Bleeding No information available to require special precautions

Adverse Reactions

>10%:

Central nervous system: Headache (oral and IV: 3% to 21%; transdermal: <1%)

Gastrointestinal: Nausea (20%), constipation (oral and IV: 3% to 18%; transdermal: 5%), vomiting (12%)

Neuromuscular & skeletal: Weakness (oral: 14% to 18%; IV: 5%)

1% to 10%:

Cardiovascular: Prolonged QT interval on ECG (1% to 3%; >450 milliseconds, not associated with any arrhythmias), hypertension (oral and IV: 1% to 2%)

Central nervous system: Dizziness (5%), insomnia (oral and IV: ≤5%), drowsiness (1% to 4%), anxiety (oral and IV: ≤2%), agitation (IV: <2%), central nervous system stimulation (IV: <2%)

Dermatologic: Alopecia (3%), skin rash (IV: 1%)

Gastrointestinal: Diarrhea (oral and IV: 4% to 9%), decreased appetite (6%), dyspepsia (oral: 6%), abdominal pain (4% to 6%), dysgeusia (IV: 2%)

Hematologic & oncologic: Leukopenia (9%), anemia (4%), thrombocytopenia (2%)

Hepatic: Increased serum ALT (>2 x ULN: 3% to 6%), increased serum AST (>2 x ULN: 3% to 5%)

Miscellaneous: Fever (3% to 9%)

<1%, postmarketing, and/or case reports (all routes): Angina pectoris, application site reaction (including allergic rash, burn, discoloration, erythema, erythematous rash, irritation, macular rash, pain, papular rash, pruritus, urticaria, vesicles), atrial fibrillation, atrioventricular block, bradycardia, cardiac arrhythmia, chest pain, ECG abnormality, extrapyramidal reaction, hypersensitivity reaction (includes anaphylaxis, dyspnea, hypotension, urticaria), hypotension, palpitations, serotonin syndrome, sick sinus syndrome, sinus bradycardia, syncope, ventricular ectopy (includes nonsustained tachycardia)

Mechanism of Action Selective 5-HT_3-receptor antagonist, blocking serotonin, both peripherally on vagal nerve terminals and centrally in the chemoreceptor trigger zone

Pharmacodynamics/Kinetics

Onset of Action IV: 1 to 3 minutes

Duration of Action Oral, IV: Generally up to 24 hours; SubQ (extended-release): Remains detectable in the plasma for 7 days

Half-life Elimination Oral: 6 hours; IV: Mean range: 5 to 9 hours; SubQ (extended-release): ~24 hours

Time to Peak Transdermal patch: Maximum systemic concentrations: ~48 hours after application (range: 24 to 168 hours); SubQ (extended-release): ~24 hours

Pregnancy Risk Factor B

Pregnancy Considerations Adverse events have not been observed in animal reproduction studies. In an ex vivo placental perfusion study, granisetron was shown to cross the placenta in a concentration (dose) dependent manner (Julius 2014). Initial studies note the pharmacokinetics of the transdermal system may be different in pregnant women. A relationship between granisetron plasma concentrations and relief of symptoms of nausea and vomiting of pregnancy was also observed (Caritis 2016). Some dosage forms (injection) may contain benzyl alcohol.

Product Availability Granisol oral solution has been discontinued in the US for more than 1 year.

Dental Health Professional Considerations See Local Anesthetic/Vasoconstrictor Precautions

- **Granisetron HCl** *see* Granisetron *on page* 748
- **Granisetron Hydrochloride** *see* Granisetron *on page* 748
- **Granisol** *see* Granisetron *on page* 748
- **Granix** *see* Filgrastim *on page* 668
- **Granulocyte Colony Stimulating Factor** *see* Filgrastim *on page* 668
- **Granulocyte Colony Stimulating Factor (PEG Conjugate)** *see* Pegfilgrastim *on page* 1200
- **Granulocyte-Macrophage Colony Stimulating Factor** *see* Sargramostim *on page* 1358
- **Grazoprevir and Elbasvir** *see* Elbasvir and Grazoprevir *on page* 548
- **Grifulvin V** *see* Griseofulvin *on page* 749

Griseofulvin (gri see oh FUL vin)

Brand Names: US Gris-PEG [DSC]

Pharmacologic Category Antifungal Agent, Oral

Use

Dermatophyte infections: Treatment of the following dermatophyte infections of the skin, hair, and nails not adequately treated by topical therapy: Tinea corporis, tinea pedis, tinea cruris, tinea barbae, tinea capitis, tinea unguium (onychomycosis) when caused by one or more of the following species of fungi: *Trichophyton rubrum, Trichophyton tonsurans, Trichophyton mentagrophytes, Trichophyton interdigitalis, Trichophyton verrucosum, Trichophyton megnini, Trichophyton gallinae, Trichophyton crateriform, Trichophyton sulphureum, Trichophyton schoenleini, Microsporum audouini, Microsporum canis, Microsporum gypseum,* and *Epidermophyton floccosum.*

Limitations of use: Use for the prophylaxis of fungal infections has not been established; not effective for the treatment of tinea versicolor.

Local Anesthetic/Vasoconstrictor Precautions No information available to require special precautions

Effects on Dental Treatment Key adverse event(s) related to dental treatment: May cause soreness or irritation of mouth or tongue. May cause oral thrush.

Effects on Bleeding No information available to require special precautions

Adverse Reactions Frequency not defined.

Central nervous system: Confusion, dizziness, fatigue, headache, insomnia

Dermatologic: Dermatological reaction (erythema multiforme-like drug reaction), skin photosensitivity, skin rash (most common), urticaria (most common)

Gastrointestinal: Diarrhea, epigastric distress, gastrointestinal hemorrhage, nausea, oral candidiasis, vomiting

Genitourinary: Nephrosis

Hematologic & oncologic: Granulocytopenia

Hepatic: Hepatotoxicity

<1%, postmarketing, and/or case reports: Angioedema, increased serum bilirubin, increased serum transaminases, leukopenia, lupus-like syndrome, paresthesia, proteinuria, Stevens-Johnson syndrome, toxic epidermal necrolysis

Mechanism of Action Inhibits fungal cell mitosis at metaphase; binds to human keratin making it resistant to fungal invasion

Pharmacodynamics/Kinetics

Half-life Elimination 9 to 24 hours

Time to Peak Serum: 4 hours

Reproductive Considerations

Females of reproductive potential should use affective contraception during therapy (estrogen containing contraceptives may be less effective). Men should avoid fathering a child for at least 6 months after therapy.

Pregnancy Risk Factor X

Pregnancy Considerations

Griseofulvin crosses the placenta (Pacifici 2006). Adverse events have been observed in humans (two cases of conjoined twins); therefore, use during pregnancy is contraindicated.

- **Griseofulvin Microsize** *see* Griseofulvin *on page* 749
- **Griseofulvin Ultramicrosize** *see* Griseofulvin *on page* 749
- **Gris-PEG [DSC]** *see* Griseofulvin *on page* 749
- **Growth Hormone, Human** *see* Somatropin *on page* 1381
- **GRX Hemorrhoidal [OTC]** *see* Phenylephrine (Topical) *on page* 1227
- **GS-1101** *see* Idelalisib *on page* 795
- **GS-7340** *see* Tenofovir Alafenamide *on page* 1418
- **GSK-580299** *see* Papillomavirus (Types 16, 18) Vaccine (Human, Recombinant) *on page* 1191
- **GSK1120212** *see* Trametinib *on page* 1475
- **GSK 1838262** *see* Gabapentin Enacarbil *on page* 727
- **GTN** *see* Nitroglycerin *on page* 1112
- **GTx 011** *see* Voxelotor *on page* 1556

GuanFACINE (GWAHN fa seen)

Related Information

Cardiovascular Diseases *on page* 1654

Dentin Hypersensitivity, Acid Erosion, High Caries Index, Management of Alveolar Osteitis, and Xerostomia *on page* 1762

Brand Names: US Intuniv; Tenex [DSC]

Brand Names: Canada Intuniv XR

Pharmacologic Category $Alpha_2$-Adrenergic Agonist; Antihypertensive

Use

Attention-deficit/hyperactivity disorder (extended release only): Treatment of attention-deficit/hyperactivity disorder (ADHD) as monotherapy and as adjunctive therapy to stimulant medications.

Hypertension (immediate release only): Management of hypertension. **Note: Not** recommended for the initial treatment of hypertension (ACC/AHA [Whelton 2017]).

Local Anesthetic/Vasoconstrictor Precautions No information available to require special precautions

Effects on Dental Treatment Key adverse event(s) related to dental treatment: Xerostomia and changes in salivation (normal salivary flow resumes upon discontinuation).

Effects on Bleeding No information available to require special precautions

Adverse Reactions Adverse events occurred with children and adolescents 6 to 17 years of age unless otherwise specified.

>10%:

Central nervous system: Drowsiness (28% to 57%), headache (16% to 28%), fatigue (10% to 22%), dizziness (4% to 16%), insomnia (2% to 13%)

Gastrointestinal: Abdominal pain (8% to 19%), decreased appetite (5% to 15%)

1% to 10%:

Cardiovascular: Hypotension (4% to 9%), bradycardia (2% to 5%), orthostatic hypotension (1% to 5%), first-degree atrioventricular block (≥2%), sinus arrhythmia (≥2%), tachycardia (≥2%), syncope (1% to ≥2%)

Central nervous system: Irritability (5% to 8%), lethargy (3% to 8%), anxiety (2% to 5%), nightmares (3% to 4%), emotional lability (2% to 3%), agitation (≥2%), depression (≥2%), increased blood pressure (≥2%), loss of consciousness (children: ≥2%)

Dermatologic: Skin rash (2% to 3%), pruritus (2%)

Endocrine & metabolic: Weight gain (2% to 3%)

Gastrointestinal: Xerostomia (3% to 8%), nausea (5% to 7%), vomiting (2% to 7%), diarrhea (2% to 6%), constipation (2% to 4%), abdominal distress (≥2%), dyspepsia (≥2%), stomach discomfort (≥2%)

Genitourinary: Urinary incontinence (2% to 5%)

Respiratory: Asthma (≥2%)

Miscellaneous: Fever (8%; Biederman 2008)

Frequency not defined:

Cardiovascular: Atrioventricular block, chest pain, hypertension

Central nervous system: Seizure

Dermatologic: Pallor

Genitourinary: Urinary frequency

Hepatic: Increased serum ALT

Hypersensitivity: Hypersensitivity reaction

Neuromuscular & skeletal: Weakness

<1%, postmarketing, and/or case reports: Alopecia, arthralgia, blurred vision, confusion, dermatitis, dysgeusia, dyspnea, edema, erectile dysfunction, exfoliative dermatitis, hallucination, hypertensive encephalopathy (with abrupt discontinuation), leg cramps, leg pain, malaise, myalgia, palpitations, paresthesia, rebound hypertension (with abrupt discontinuation), sedation, tremor, vertigo

Mechanism of Action Guanfacine is a selective alpha$_{2A}$-adrenoreceptor agonist that reduces sympathetic nerve impulses, resulting in reduced sympathetic outflow and a subsequent decrease in vasomotor tone and heart rate. In addition, guanfacine preferentially binds postsynaptic alpha$_{2A}$-adrenoreceptors in the prefrontal cortex and has been theorized to improve delay-related firing of prefrontal cortex neurons. As a result, underlying working memory and behavioral inhibition are affected; thereby improving symptoms associated with ADHD. Guanfacine is not a CNS stimulant.

Pharmacodynamics/Kinetics

Duration of Action Antihypertensive effect: 24 hours following single dose

Half-life Elimination

Immediate release: ~17 hours (range: 10 to 30 hours)

Extended release: Children ≥6 years: 14.4 hours; Adolescents: 18 hours (Boellner 2007); Adults: 18 ± 4 hours

Time to Peak Serum:

Immediate release: 2.6 hours (range: 1 to 4 hours)

Extended release: Children ≥6 years and Adolescents: 5 hours (Boellner 2007); Adults: 4 to 8 hours

Pregnancy Considerations

Information related to guanfacine use during pregnancy is limited (Karesoja 1981; Philipp 1980). In one study of 30 women treated with guanfacine for hypertension during pregnancy, the majority (n=25) experience sedation; dry mouth and dizziness were also reported (Philipp 1980).

Chronic maternal hypertension may increase the risk of birth defects, low birth weight, preterm delivery, stillbirth, and neonatal death. Actual fetal/neonatal risks may be related to duration and severity of maternal hypertension. Untreated hypertension may also increase the risks of adverse maternal outcomes, including gestational diabetes, myocardial infarction, preeclampsia, stroke, and delivery complications (ACOG 203 2019).

Agents other than guanfacine are more commonly used to treat hypertension in pregnancy (ACOG 203 2019; ESC [Regitz-Zagrosek 2018]). Females with preexisting hypertension may continue their medication during pregnancy unless contraindications exist (ESC [Regitz-Zagrosek 2018]).

If treatment for attention-deficit/hyperactivity disorder (ADHD) during pregnancy is needed, other agents are preferred (Ornoy 2018).

◆ **Guanfacine HCl** *see* GuanFACINE *on page 749*

◆ **Guanfacine Hydrochloride** *see* GuanFACINE *on page 749*

Guselkumab (gue sel KOO mab)

Brand Names: US Tremfya

Brand Names: Canada Tremfya

Pharmacologic Category Antipsoriatic Agent; Interleukin-23 Inhibitor; Monoclonal Antibody

Use

Plaque psoriasis: Treatment of moderate to severe plaque psoriasis in adults who are candidates for systemic therapy or phototherapy.

Psoriatic arthritis: Treatment of active psoriatic arthritis in adults.

Local Anesthetic/Vasoconstrictor Precautions No information available to require special precautions

Effects on Dental Treatment No significant effects or complications reported

Effects on Bleeding No information available to require special precautions

Adverse Reactions

>10%:

Infection: Infection (23%)

Respiratory: Upper respiratory tract infection (14%)

1% to 10%:

Dermatologic: Tinea (1%)

Gastrointestinal: Diarrhea (2%), gastroenteritis (1%)
Hepatic: Increased liver enzymes (3%)
Immunologic: Antibody development (6% to 9%; neutralizing antibodies: 6% to 7%; efficacy of guselkumab may be affected)
Infection: Herpes simplex infection (1%)
Local: Injection site reaction (5%)
Nervous system: Headache (5%)
Neuromuscular & skeletal: Arthralgia (3%)

<1%:
Dermatologic: Urticaria
Infection: Candidiasis
Nervous system: Migraine

<1%, postmarketing, and/or case reports: Anaphylaxis, hypersensitivity reaction, severe hypersensitivity reaction, skin rash

Mechanism of Action Human IgG1 monoclonal antibody selectively binds with IL-23, thereby reducing serum levels of IL-17A, IL-17F, and IL-22. Guselkumab inhibits the release of proinflammatory cytokines and chemokines.

Pharmacodynamics/Kinetics
Half-life Elimination 15 to 18 days
Time to Peak 5.5 days

Pregnancy Considerations
Guselkumab is a humanized monoclonal antibody (IgG_1). Placental transfer of human IgG is dependent upon the IgG subclass, maternal serum concentrations, birth weight, and gestational age, generally increasing as pregnancy progresses. The lowest exposure would be expected during the period of organogenesis (Palmeira 2012; Pentsuk 2009).

Agents other than guselkumab are currently recommended for the treatment of psoriasis in pregnancy (Menter 2019; Yeung 2020).

Data collection to monitor pregnancy and infant outcomes following exposure to guselkumab is ongoing. Patients exposed to guselkumab during pregnancy are encouraged to enroll themselves in the pregnancy registry (1-877-311-8972).

- ◆ **GW506U78** *see* Nelarabine *on page 1091*
- ◆ **GW-1000** *see* Tetrahydrocannabinol and Cannabidiol *on page 1434*
- ◆ **GW433908G** *see* Fosamprenavir *on page 712*
- ◆ **GW572016** *see* Lapatinib *on page 877*
- ◆ **GW786034** *see* PAZOPanib *on page 1196*
- ◆ **Gynazole-1** *see* Butoconazole *on page 275*
- ◆ **Gyne-Lotrimin [OTC]** *see* Clotrimazole (Topical) *on page 397*
- ◆ **Gyne-Lotrimin 3 [OTC]** *see* Clotrimazole (Topical) *on page 397*
- ◆ **Gynodiol** *see* Estradiol (Systemic) *on page 596*
- ◆ **Gynovite Plus [OTC]** *see* Vitamins (Multiple/Oral) *on page 1550*
- ◆ **H1N1 Influenza Vaccine** *see* Influenza Virus Vaccine (Inactivated) *on page 812*
- ◆ **H1N1 Influenza Vaccine** *see* Influenza Virus Vaccine (Live/Attenuated) *on page 813*
- ◆ **H_2O_2** *see* Hydrogen Peroxide *on page 776*
- ◆ **H5N1 Influenza Vaccine** *see* Influenza A Virus Vaccine (H5N1) *on page 811*
- ◆ **HA22** *see* Moxetumomab Pasudotox *on page 1063*
- ◆ **Habitrol** *see* Nicotine *on page 1101*
- ◆ **Haemophilus influenzae Type b** *see* Meningococcal Polysaccharide (Groups C and Y) and *Haemophilus* b Tetanus Toxoid Conjugate Vaccine *on page 965*
- ◆ **Hailey 1.5/30** *see* Ethinyl Estradiol and Norethindrone *on page 614*
- ◆ **Hailey 24 Fe** *see* Ethinyl Estradiol and Norethindrone *on page 614*
- ◆ **Hailey FE 1.5/30** *see* Ethinyl Estradiol and Norethindrone *on page 614*
- ◆ **Hailey FE 1/20** *see* Ethinyl Estradiol and Norethindrone *on page 614*
- ◆ **Halaven** *see* EriBULin *on page 584*
- ◆ **Halcion** *see* Triazolam *on page 1493*
- ◆ **Haldol** *see* Haloperidol *on page 751*
- ◆ **Haldol Decanoate** *see* Haloperidol *on page 751*
- ◆ **Halfprin [OTC] [DSC]** *see* Aspirin *on page 177*
- ◆ **Halichondrin B Analog** *see* EriBULin *on page 584*

Haloperidol (ha loe PER i dole)

Related Information
Clinical Risk Related to Drugs Prolonging QT Interval *on page 1675*

Brand Names: US Haldol; Haldol Decanoate

Brand Names: Canada APO-Haloperidol; Haloperidol-LA Omega; PMS-Haloperidol; PMS-Haloperidol LA; TEVA-Haloperidol

Pharmacologic Category First Generation (Typical) Antipsychotic

Use
Behavioral disorders, nonpsychotic (tablet, concentrate): Treatment of severe behavioral problems in children with combative, explosive hyperexcitability that cannot be accounted for by immediate provocation. Reserve for use in these children only after failure to respond to psychotherapy or medications other than antipsychotics.

Hyperactivity (tablet, concentrate): Short-term treatment of hyperactive children who show excessive motor activity with accompanying conduct disorders consisting of some or all of the following symptoms: impulsivity, difficulty sustaining attention, aggression, mood lability, or poor frustration tolerance. Reserve for use in these children only after failure to respond to psychotherapy or medications other than antipsychotics.

Schizophrenia:
IM lactate: Treatment of schizophrenia.
IM decanoate: Treatment of patients with schizophrenia who require prolonged parenteral antipsychotic therapy.
Tablet, concentrate: Treatment of manifestations of psychotic disorders such as schizophrenia.

Tourette syndrome, management of tics (tablet, concentrate, IM lactate): Control of tics and vocal utterances in Tourette syndrome in adults and children.

Local Anesthetic/Vasoconstrictor Precautions
Manufacturer's information states that haloperidol may block vasopressor activity of epinephrine. This has not been observed during use of epinephrine as a vasoconstrictor in local anesthesia. Haloperidol is one of the drugs confirmed to prolong the QT interval and is accepted as having a risk of causing torsade de pointes. The risk of drug-induced torsade de pointes is extremely low when a single QT interval prolonging drug is prescribed. In terms of epinephrine, it is not

known what effect vasoconstrictors in the local anesthetic regimen will have in patients with a known history of congenital prolonged QT interval or in patients taking any medication that prolongs the QT interval. Until more information is obtained, it is suggested that the clinician consult with the physician prior to the use of a vasoconstrictor in suspected patients, and that the vasoconstrictor (epinephrine, mepivacaine and levonordefrin [Carbocaine® 2% with Neo-Cobefrin®]) be used with caution.

Effects on Dental Treatment Key adverse event(s) related to dental treatment: Infrequent occurrence of xerostomia (normal salivary flow resumes upon discontinuation) has been reported. Rare occurrence of orthostatic hypotension (use caution with sudden changes in position during and after dental treatment), tardive dyskinesia, trismus, and nasal congestion have also been reported.

Note: Since the drug is a dopamine antagonist, extrapyramidal symptoms of the TMJ are a possibility.

Effects on Bleeding No information available to require special precautions

Adverse Reactions

>10%: Central nervous system: Extrapyramidal reaction (lactate: 51%; oral: <1%), parkinsonism (decanoate: 31%; lactate and oral: <1%)

1% to 10%:

Central nervous system: Dystonia (lactate: 7%; decanoate and oral: <1%), hypertonia (lactate: 7%; decanoate and oral: <1%), drowsiness (lactate: 5%; decanoate and oral: <1%), akathisia (decanoate: 3%; lactate and oral: <1%), headache (decanoate: 3%; lactate and oral: <1%)

Gastrointestinal: Constipation (lactate: 4%; decanoate and oral: <1%), abdominal pain (decanoate: 3%), xerostomia (≤2%), sialorrhea (≤1%)

Neuromuscular & skeletal: Hyperkinetic muscle activity (lactate: 10%), tremor (3% to 8%), bradykinesia (lactate: 4%), akinesia (decanoate: 3%)

Ophthalmic: Oculogyric crisis (decanoate: 6%; lactate: <1%)

Frequency not defined:

Central nervous system: Anxiety, euphoria, lethargy, psychotic symptoms (exacerbation), vertigo

Dermatologic: Diaphoresis

Endocrine & metabolic: Hyperglycemia, hyponatremia, increased libido, menstrual disease

Gastrointestinal: Anorexia, diarrhea, dyspepsia

Genitourinary: Breast engorgement, impotence, lactation

Ophthalmic: Cataract, retinopathy, visual disturbance

Respiratory: Increased depth of respiration

<1%, postmarketing, and/or case reports: Abnormal hepatic function tests, abscess at injection site, acneiform eruption, acute hepatic failure, agitation, agranulocytosis, akathisia, alopecia, amenorrhea, anaphylaxis, anemia, angioedema, blurred vision, bronchopneumonia, bronchospasm, cardiac arrhythmia, cholestasis, cogwheel rigidity, confusion, decreased libido, depression, dizziness, dyskinesia, dysmenorrhea, dyspnea, edema, erectile dysfunction, exfoliative dermatitis, extrasystoles, facial edema, galactorrhea not associated with childbirth, gynecomastia, heatstroke, heavy menstrual bleeding, hepatic insufficiency, hepatitis, hyperammonemia, hyperhidrosis, hyperprolactinemia, hyperpyrexia, hypersensitivity angiitis, hypersensitivity reaction, hypertension, hyperthermia, hypoglycemia, hypokinesia, hypotension, hypothermia, injection site reaction, insomnia, jaundice, laryngeal edema, laryngospasm, leukocytosis, leukopenia, lymphocytosis with monocytosis, maculopapular rash, mask-like face, mastalgia, motor dysfunction, muscle rigidity, muscle twitching, nausea, neonatal withdrawal, neuroleptic malignant syndrome, neutropenia, nystagmus, opisthotonus, orthostatic hypotension, pancytopenia, priapism, prolonged QT interval on ECG, pruritus, restlessness, rhabdomyolysis, sedated state, seizure, SIADH, skin photosensitivity, skin rash, tachycardia, tardive dyskinesia, tardive dystonia, thrombocytopenia, torsades de pointes, torticollis, trismus, urinary retention, urticaria, ventricular arrhythmia, ventricular fibrillation, ventricular tachycardia, vomiting, weight gain, weight loss

Mechanism of Action Haloperidol is a butyrophenone antipsychotic that nonselectively blocks postsynaptic dopaminergic D_2 receptors in the brain (Richelson 1999; Risch 1996).

Pharmacodynamics/Kinetics

Onset of Action

Lactate:

IM: Sedation: Mean: 28.3 minutes (Nobay 2004).

IV: Sedation: 3 to 20 minutes (Jacobi 2002).

Peak effect: Lactate: IV: Sedation: ~30 minutes (Forsman 1976; Jacobi 2002; Magliozzi 1985).

Duration of Action

Lactate (dose dependent):

IM: Sedation: Mean: 126.5 minutes (Nobay 2004).

IV: Sedation: 3 to 24 hours (Magliozzi 1985).

Half-life Elimination

Decanoate: 21 days.

Lactate:

IM: 20 hours (Kudo 1999).

IV: 14 to 26 hours (Kudo 1999).

Oral: 14 to 37 hours (Kudo 1999).

Time to Peak

Decanoate: 6 days.

Lactate:

IM: 20 minutes (Kudo 1999).

Oral: 2 to 6 hours (Kudo 1999).

Pregnancy Considerations

Haloperidol crosses the placenta in humans (Newport 2007). Although haloperidol has not been found to be a major human teratogen, an association with limb malformations following first trimester exposure in humans cannot be ruled out (ACOG 2008; Diav-Citrin 2005). Antipsychotic use during the third trimester of pregnancy has a risk for abnormal muscle movements (extrapyramidal symptoms) and withdrawal symptoms in newborns following delivery. Symptoms in the newborn may include agitation, feeding disorder, hypertonia, hypotonia, respiratory distress, somnolence, and tremor; these effects may be self-limiting or require hospitalization. If needed, the minimum effective maternal dose should be used in order to decrease the risk of EPS (ACOG 2008).

Dental Health Professional Considerations See Local Anesthetic/Vasoconstrictor Precautions

◆ **Haloperidol Decanoate** *see* Haloperidol *on page* 751

◆ **Haloperidol Lactate** *see* Haloperidol *on page* 751

◆ **Halotestin** *see* Fluoxymesterone *on page* 699

◆ **Harkoseride** *see* Lacosamide *on page* 868

◆ **Havrix** *see* Hepatitis A Vaccine *on page* 755

◆ **Havrix and Engerix-B** *see* Hepatitis A and Hepatitis B Recombinant Vaccine *on page* 754

◆ **HBIG** *see* Hepatitis B Immune Globulin (Human) *on page* 756

◆ **hBNP** *see* Nesiritide *on page* 1094

- ◆ **25-HCC** *see* Calcifediol *on page 279*
- ◆ **HCTZ (error-prone abbreviation)** *see* HydroCHLOROthiazide *on page 762*
- ◆ **HDCV** *see* Rabies Vaccine *on page 1303*
- ◆ **Healon** *see* Hyaluronate and Derivatives *on page 761*
- ◆ **Healon5** *see* Hyaluronate and Derivatives *on page 761*
- ◆ **Healon EndoCoat** *see* Hyaluronate and Derivatives *on page 761*
- ◆ **Healon GV** *see* Hyaluronate and Derivatives *on page 761*
- ◆ **Healthy Mama Move It Along [OTC]** *see* Docusate *on page 509*
- ◆ **Heartburn Relief [OTC]** *see* Famotidine *on page 635*
- ◆ **Heartburn Relief Max St [OTC]** *see* Famotidine *on page 635*
- ◆ **Heartburn Treatment 24 Hour [OTC]** *see* Lansoprazole *on page 876*
- ◆ **Heather** *see* Norethindrone *on page 1117*
- ◆ **Hectorol** *see* Doxercalciferol *on page 519*
- ◆ **Hedgehog Antagonist GDC-0449** *see* Vismodegib *on page 1548*
- ◆ **HeliCote** *see* Collagen (Absorbable) *on page 408*
- ◆ **Helidac** *see* Tetracycline, Bismuth Subsalicylate, and Metronidazole *on page 1433*
- ◆ **Helidac Therapy** *see* Tetracycline, Bismuth Subsalicylate, and Metronidazole *on page 1433*
- ◆ **HeliPlug** *see* Collagen (Absorbable) *on page 408*
- ◆ **HeliTape** *see* Collagen (Absorbable) *on page 408*
- ◆ **Helixate FS [DSC]** *see* Antihemophilic Factor (Recombinant) *on page 153*
- ◆ **Hemady** *see* DexAMETHasone (Systemic) *on page 463*
- ◆ **Hemangeol** *see* Propranolol *on page 1287*
- ◆ **Hemmorex-HC** *see* Hydrocortisone (Topical) *on page 775*
- ◆ **Hemocyte Plus** *see* Vitamins (Multiple/Oral) *on page 1550*
- ◆ **Hemofil M** *see* Antihemophilic Factor (Human) *on page 152*
- ◆ **Hemorrhoidal [OTC]** *see* Phenylephrine (Topical) *on page 1227*
- ◆ **Hemorrhoidal Cooling [OTC]** *see* Phenylephrine (Topical) *on page 1227*
- ◆ **Hemorrhoidal HC** *see* Hydrocortisone (Topical) *on page 775*
- ◆ **HepA** *see* Hepatitis A and Hepatitis B Recombinant Vaccine *on page 754*
- ◆ **HepA** *see* Hepatitis A Vaccine *on page 755*
- ◆ **HepaGam B** *see* Hepatitis B Immune Globulin (Human) *on page 756*
- ◆ **HepA-HepB** *see* Hepatitis A and Hepatitis B Recombinant Vaccine *on page 754*

Heparin (HEP a rin)

Related Information

Cardiovascular Diseases *on page 1654*

Brand Names: Canada Heparin Leo

Pharmacologic Category Anticoagulant

Use

Anticoagulation: Prophylaxis and treatment of thromboembolic disorders (eg, venous thromboembolism, pulmonary embolism) and thromboembolic complications associated with atrial fibrillation; prevention of clotting in arterial and cardiac surgery; as an anticoagulant for blood transfusions, extracorporeal circulation, and dialysis procedures.

Note: Heparin lock flush solution is intended only to maintain patency of IV devices and is **not** to be used for systemic anticoagulant therapy.

Local Anesthetic/Vasoconstrictor Precautions
No information available to require special precautions

Effects on Dental Treatment Key adverse event(s) related to dental treatment: Bleeding. See Effects on Bleeding.

Effects on Bleeding The most serious adverse effect is bleeding, including bleeding from the gums. Medical consult is recommended.

Adverse Reactions Thrombocytopenia has been reported to occur at an incidence between 0% and 30%. It is often of no clinical significance; however, immunologically mediated heparin-induced thrombocytopenia (HIT) has been estimated to occur in 1% to 2% of patients and is marked by a progressive fall in platelet counts and, in some cases, thromboembolic complications (skin necrosis, pulmonary embolism, gangrene of the extremities, cerebrovascular accident, or myocardial infarction).

>10%: Hematologic & oncologic: Thrombocytopenia (≤30%)

1% to 10%: Hematologic & oncologic: Heparin-induced thrombocytopenia (1% to 2%)

Frequency not defined: Miscellaneous: Drug tolerance

Postmarketing: Adrenal hemorrhage, anaphylactic shock, burning sensation of feet, cyanotic extremities, dermal ulcer, hematoma, hemorrhage, hypersensitivity reaction, increased serum alanine aminotransferase, increased serum aspartate aminotransferase, limb pain, local irritation, localized erythema, local pain, nonimmune anaphylaxis, osteoporosis, ovarian hemorrhage, peripheral ischemia, priapism, pruritus (feet), retroperitoneal hemorrhage, skin necrosis, suppression of aldosterone synthesis, thrombosis in heparin-induced thrombocytopenia, transient alopecia

Mechanism of Action Potentiates the action of antithrombin III and thereby inactivates thrombin (as well as other coagulation factors IXa, Xa, XIa, XIIa, and plasmin) and prevents the conversion of fibrinogen to fibrin; heparin also stimulates release of lipoprotein lipase (lipoprotein lipase hydrolyzes triglycerides to glycerol and free fatty acids)

Pharmacodynamics/Kinetics

Onset of Action Anticoagulation: IV: Immediate; SubQ: ~20 to 30 minutes

Half-life Elimination

Age-related: Shorter half-life reported in premature neonates compared to adult patients.

Premature neonates gestational age 25 to 36 weeks (data based on single dose of 100 units/kg within 4 hours of birth): Mean range: 35.5 to 41.6 minutes (McDonald 1981).

Dose-dependent: IV bolus: 25 units/kg: 30 minutes (Bjornsson 1982); 100 units/kg: 60 minutes (de Swart 1982); 400 units/kg: 150 minutes (Olsson 1963).

Mean: 1.5 hours; Range: 1 to 2 hours; affected by obesity, renal function, malignancy, presence of pulmonary embolism, and infections.

Note: At therapeutic doses, elimination occurs rapidly via nonrenal mechanisms. With very high doses, renal elimination may play more of a role; however, dosage adjustment remains unnecessary for patients with renal impairment (Kandrotas 1992).

Pregnancy Considerations

Heparin does not cross the placenta (ESC [Regitz-Zagrosek 2018]).

Heparin may be used for anticoagulation in pregnancy (ACOG 196 2018). Due to a better safety profile and ease of administration, the use of low molecular weight heparin (LMWH) is generally preferred over heparin (unfractionated heparin [UFH]) in pregnancy (ACOG 196 2018; Bates 2018; ESC [Regitz-Zagrosek 2018]). Anticoagulant therapy for the prevention and treatment of thromboembolism in pregnant females can be discontinued prior to induction of labor or a planned cesarean delivery (Bates 2018) or LMWH can be converted to UFH in higher risk women (ESC [Regitz-Zagrosek 2018]). UFH or LMWH may be used in pregnant patients with mechanical heart valves (ESC [Regitz-Zagrosek 2018]; Nishimura 2014).

Some products contain benzyl alcohol as a preservative; their use in pregnant females is contraindicated by some manufacturers; use of a preservative-free formulation is recommended.

- ◆ **Heparin Calcium** *see* Heparin *on page* 753
- ◆ **Heparinized Saline** *see* Heparin *on page* 753
- ◆ **Heparin Lock Flush** *see* Heparin *on page* 753
- ◆ **Heparin Sodium** *see* Heparin *on page* 753
- ◆ **Hepatitis A** *see* Hepatitis A and Hepatitis B Recombinant Vaccine *on page* 754

Hepatitis A and Hepatitis B Recombinant Vaccine

(hep a TYE tis aye & hep a TYE tis bee ree KOM be nant vak SEEN)

Related Information

Systemic Viral Diseases *on page* 1709

Brand Names: US Twinrix

Brand Names: Canada Twinrix; Twinrix Junior

Pharmacologic Category Vaccine; Vaccine, Inactivated (Viral)

Use

Hepatitis A and B diseases prevention:

Twinrix: Active immunization of persons 18 years and older (US labeling) or 19 years and older (Canadian labeling) against disease caused by hepatitis A virus and hepatitis B virus (all known subtypes)

Canadian labeling: Additional uses (not in US labeling): Approved for active immunization of children and adolescents ages 1 to 15 years.

Twinrix Junior [Canadian product]: Active immunization of children and adolescents ages 1 to 18 years against disease caused by hepatitis A virus and hepatitis B virus (all known subtypes).

Limitations of use: Hepatitis A/hepatitis B vaccine cannot be used for postexposure prophylaxis.

Local Anesthetic/Vasoconstrictor Precautions No information available to require special precautions

Effects on Dental Treatment Key adverse event(s) related to dental treatment: Flu-like syndrome and upper respiratory tract infection.

Effects on Bleeding No information available to require special precautions

Adverse Reactions Incidence of adverse effects of the combination product were similar to those occurring after administration of hepatitis A vaccine and hepatitis B vaccine alone. (Incidence reported is not versus placebo.) Also see individual agents.

>10%:

Central nervous system: Headache (13% to 22%), fatigue (11% to 14%)

Local: Local soreness/soreness at injection site (35% to 41%), erythema at injection site (8% to 11%)

1% to 10%:

Dermatologic: Skin sclerosis (at injection site)

Gastrointestinal: Diarrhea (4% to 6%), nausea (2% to 4%), vomiting (≤1%)

Local: Local swelling (at injection site: 4% to 6%)

Respiratory: Upper respiratory tract infection

Miscellaneous: Fever (2% to 4%)

<1%, postmarketing, and/or case reports: Abdominal pain, abnormal hepatic function tests, agitation, alopecia, anaphylactoid reaction, anaphylaxis, angioedema, anorexia, arthralgia, arthritis, back pain, Bell's palsy, brain disease, bronchospasm, bruise, bruising at injection site, chills, conjunctivitis, diaphoresis, dizziness, drowsiness, dyspepsia, dyspnea (including asthma-like symptoms), eczema, encephalitis, erythema, erythema multiforme, erythema nodosum, flu-like symptoms, flushing, Guillain-Barre syndrome, hepatitis, herpes zoster, hyperhidrosis, hypersensitivity reaction, hypoesthesia, immune thrombocytopenia, injection site pruritus, injection site reaction (burning sensation at injection site, pain at injection site), insomnia, irritability, jaundice, lichen planus, malaise, meningitis, migraine, multiple sclerosis, myalgia, myasthenia, myelitis, neuropathy, neuritis, optic neuritis, otalgia, palpitations, paralysis, paresis, paresthesia, petechiae, respiratory tract disease, seizure, serum sickness-like reaction (days to weeks after vaccination), skin rash, syncope, tachycardia, thrombocytopenia, tinnitus, transverse myelitis, urticaria, vasculitis, vertigo, visual disturbance, weakness

Mechanism of Action

Hepatitis A vaccine, an inactivated virus vaccine, offers active immunization against hepatitis A virus infection at an effective immune response rate in up to 99% of subjects.

Recombinant hepatitis B vaccine is a noninfectious subunit viral vaccine. The vaccine is derived from hepatitis B surface antigen (HBsAg) produced through recombinant DNA techniques from yeast cells. The portion of the hepatitis B gene which codes for HBsAg is cloned into yeast which is then cultured to produce hepatitis B vaccine.

In immunocompetent people, Twinrix provides active immunization against hepatitis A virus infection (at an effective immune response rate >99% of subjects) and against hepatitis B virus infection (at an effective immune response rate of 93% to 97%) 30 days after completion of the 3-dose series. This is comparable to using hepatitis A vaccine and hepatitis B vaccine concomitantly.

Pharmacodynamics/Kinetics

Onset of Action Seroconversion for antibodies against HAV and HBV were detected 1 month after completion of the 3-dose series.

Duration of Action HAV and HBV seropositivity have been observed for 15 years in adults and for 10 years in children (Diaz-Mitoma 2008, Van Herck 2007).

Pregnancy Considerations

Based on data collected from a pregnancy registry between 2001 and 2015, an increased risk of major birth defects or miscarriage was not observed following maternal use of hepatitis A and hepatitis B vaccine.

Inactivated vaccines have not been shown to cause increased risks to the fetus (ACIP [Ezeanolue 2020]). Refer to current immunization schedule for vaccinating pregnant females.

◆ **Hepatitis A and Typhoid Vaccine** *see* Typhoid and Hepatitis A Vaccine *on page 1505*

Hepatitis A Vaccine (hep a TYE tis aye vak SEEN)

Related Information

Systemic Viral Diseases *on page 1709*

Brand Names: US Havrix; VAQTA

Brand Names: Canada Avaxim; Avaxim-Pediatric; HAVRIX; VAQTA

Pharmacologic Category Vaccine; Vaccine, Inactivated (Viral)

Use Hepatitis A virus disease prevention:

For active immunization of persons 12 months and older against disease caused by hepatitis A virus (HAV).

The Advisory Committee on Immunization Practices (ACIP) recommends vaccination for:

- All children 12 to 23 months of age (CDC/ACIP [Fiore 2006], ACIP [Robinson 2020]).
- All unvaccinated children and adolescents 2 through 18 years of age (ACIP [Robinson 2020]).
- All unvaccinated adults requesting protection from HAV infection (CDC/ACIP [Fiore 2006]).
- Unvaccinated adults with any of the following: Men who have sex with men; injection and non-injection drug users; persons who work with HAV-infected primates or with HAV in a research laboratory setting; persons with HIV; persons with chronic liver disease (eg, persons with hepatitis B or C infection, cirrhosis, fatty liver disease, alcoholic liver disease, autoimmune hepatitis, ALT or AST > twice the upper limit of normal); patients experiencing homelessness; pregnant patients at risk for infection or severe outcome from infection during pregnancy; workers in health care settings targeting services to injection or non-injection drug users or group homes and nonresidential day care facilities for developmentally disabled persons (ACIP [Freedman 2020]; ACIP [Robinson 2020]; CDC/ACIP [Doshani 2019]; CDC/ACIP [Fiore 2006]).
- Unvaccinated persons ≥6 months traveling to or working in countries with high or intermediate levels of endemic HAV infection (CDC/ACIP [Nelson 2018]).
- Unvaccinated persons who anticipate close personal contact with international adoptee from a country of intermediate to high endemicity of HAV, during their first 60 days of arrival into the United States (eg, household contacts, babysitters) (CDC/ACIP 58 [36] 2009).
- A component of hepatitis A outbreak response, or as postexposure prophylaxis to patients ≥12 months of age within 14 days of exposure, as determined by local public health authorities (CDC/ACIP [Fiore 2006]; CDC/ACIP [Nelson 2018]).

The Canadian National Advisory Committee on Immunization (NACI) also recommends vaccination for the following (NACI 2016):

- Persons ≥6 months at risk for hepatitis A infection (eg, traveling to or from endemic countries) or severe hepatitis A (eg, underlying hepatic disease of idiopathic, metabolic, infectious or cholestatic etiology).
- Infants ≥6 months living with an individual at risk for hepatitis A infection or severe hepatitis A.
- Postexposure prophylaxis:
  - Healthy patients ≥6 months (vaccine is preferred over immune globulin [Ig]).
  - Within 14 days of exposure of susceptible adults ≥60 years of age who are household or close contacts of a case (Ig may also be given).
  - Susceptible individuals with chronic liver disease (Ig should also be administered within 14 days of exposure).
- May be considered in patients who receive repeat administration of plasma-derived clotting factors.

Local Anesthetic/Vasoconstrictor Precautions

No information available to require special precautions

Effects on Dental Treatment No significant effects or complications reported

Effects on Bleeding No information available to require special precautions

Adverse Reactions All serious adverse reactions must be reported to the US Department of Health and Human Services (DHHS) Vaccine Adverse Event Reporting System (VAERS) at 1-800-822-7967 or online at https://vaers.hhs.gov/esub/index. In Canada, adverse reactions may be reported to local provincial/territorial health agencies or to the Vaccine Safety Section at Public Health Agency of Canada (1-866-844-0018).

Frequency dependent upon age, product used, and concomitant vaccine administration. In general, headache and injection site reactions were less common in younger children.

>10%:

Central nervous system: Drowsiness, headache, irritability

Gastrointestinal: Decreased appetite

Local: Erythema at injection site, injection site reaction (soreness, warmth), pain at injection site, swelling at injection site, tenderness at injection site

Neuromuscular & skeletal: Weakness

Miscellaneous: Fever (≥100.4°F [1-5 days postvaccination], >98.6°F [1-14 days postvaccination])

1% to 10%:

Central nervous system: Chills, fatigue, insomnia, malaise

Dermatologic: Skin rash

Endocrine & metabolic: Menstrual disease

Gastrointestinal: Abdominal pain, anorexia, constipation, diarrhea, gastroenteritis, nausea, vomiting

Local: Bruising at injection site, induration at injection site

Neuromuscular & skeletal: Arm pain, back pain, myalgia, stiffness

Ophthalmic: Conjunctivitis

Otic: Otitis media

Respiratory: Asthma, cough, nasal congestion, nasopharyngitis, pharyngitis, rhinitis, rhinorrhea, upper respiratory tract infection

Miscellaneous: Excessive crying, fever ≥102°F (1-5 days postvaccination)

<1%, postmarketing, and/or case reports: Anaphylaxis, angioedema, arthralgia, ataxia (cerebellar), bronchiolitis, bronchoconstriction, croup, dehydration,

dermatitis, dizziness, dysgeusia, dyspnea, encephalitis, erythema multiforme, eye irritation, flu-like symptoms, Guillain-Barre syndrome, hematoma at injection site, hepatitis, hyperhidrosis, hypersensitivity reaction, hypertonia, hypoesthesia, increased creatine kinase, increased serum transaminases (transient), injection site reaction (nodule), insomnia, jaundice, lymphadenopathy, multiple sclerosis, myelitis, neuropathy, otitis, paresthesia, photophobia, pneumonia, pruritus, rash at injection site, respiratory congestion, seizure, serum sickness-like reaction, syncope, thrombocytopenia, urticaria, vasculitis, vertigo, viral exanthem, wheezing

Mechanism of Action As an inactivated virus vaccine, hepatitis A vaccine induces active immunity against hepatitis A virus infection

Pharmacodynamics/Kinetics

Onset of Action Protective antibodies develop in 95% of adults after the first dose and in 100% of adults after the second dose of the vaccine; ≥97% of children and adolescents will be seropositive within 1 month of the first dose and 100% will develop protective antibodies after receiving two doses. The efficacy of preventing hepatitis A disease in children living in highly infected areas is 94% to 100% (CDC 2015).

Duration of Action Protective antibodies induced by the vaccine have been observed to persist for ≥20 years (Plumb 2017; Theeten 2015).

Pregnancy Considerations

In general, maternal use of inactivated vaccines are not associated with increased risks to the fetus (ACIP [Ezeanolue 2020]). In addition, an increased risk of most adverse maternal or fetal events, including miscarriage or major birth defects, has not been observed following maternal use of the hepatitis A vaccine (Groom 2019; Nasser 2019).

The Centers for Disease Control and Prevention recommends immunization for pregnant patients at risk for hepatitis A infection or patients who are at risk for severe outcomes from infection during pregnancy (ACIP [Freedman 2020]). Refer to current immunization schedule for vaccinating pregnant females.

◆ **Hepatitis B** *see* Hepatitis A and Hepatitis B Recombinant Vaccine *on page 754*

◆ **Hepatitis B and Hepatitis A Vaccine** *see* Hepatitis A and Hepatitis B Recombinant Vaccine *on page 754*

Hepatitis B Immune Globulin (Human)

(hep a TYE tis bee i MYUN GLOB yoo lin YU man)

Related Information

Systemic Viral Diseases *on page 1709*

Brand Names: US HepaGam B; HyperHEP B S/D; Nabi-HB

Brand Names: Canada HyperHep B S/D

Pharmacologic Category Blood Product Derivative; Immune Globulin

Use

Postexposure prophylaxis following acute exposure to hepatitis B surface antigen (HBsAg) blood, plasma, or serum (eg, parenteral exposure, direct mucus membrane contact, oral ingestion); perinatal exposure of infants born to HBsAg-positive mothers; sexual exposure to HBsAg-positive persons; and household exposure to persons with acute HBV infection

In addition, the Advisory Committee on Immunization Practices (ACIP) also recommends administration to neonates born to mothers in which HBsAg test results are not available and other evidence suggests possible maternal HBV infection; postexposure prophylaxis to a health care provider (HCP) in which the source has an unknown HBsAg status; in a nonoccupational setting, postexposure prophylaxis to a person who has not been completely vaccinated (CDC/ACIP [Schillie 2018]).

Prevention of hepatitis B virus recurrence after liver transplantation in HBsAg-positive transplant patients (HepaGam B only)

Note: Hepatitis B immune globulin is not indicated for treatment of active hepatitis B infection and is ineffective in the treatment of chronic active hepatitis B infection.

Local Anesthetic/Vasoconstrictor Precautions No information available to require special precautions

Effects on Dental Treatment No significant effects or complications reported

Effects on Bleeding No information available to require special precautions

Adverse Reactions Reported with postexposure prophylaxis. Adverse events reported in liver transplant patients included tremor and hypotension, were associated with a single infusion during the first week of treatment, and did not recur with additional infusions.

>10%:

Central nervous system: Headache (14%)
Dermatologic: Erythema (12%)

1% to 10%:

Cardiovascular: Hypotension (2%)
Central nervous system: Malaise (6%)
Dermatologic: Ecchymoses (2%)
Gastrointestinal: Nausea (2% to 4%), vomiting (2%)
Hematologic & oncologic: Change in WBC count (2%)
Hepatic: Increased serum alkaline phosphatase (4%), increased liver enzymes (2%)
Local: Pain at injection site (4%)
Neuromuscular & skeletal: Myalgia (10%), joint stiffness (2%)
Renal: Increased serum creatinine (2%)

<1%, postmarketing, and/or case reports: Abdominal pain, anaphylactic reaction (rare), angioedema, back pain, chills, diaphoresis, dizziness, dyspnea, fever, flu-like symptoms, hypersensitivity, increased serum lipase, increased serum transaminases, sinus tachycardia, tenderness at injection site, urticaria

Mechanism of Action Hepatitis B immune globulin (HBIG) is a nonpyrogenic sterile solution containing immunoglobulin G (IgG) specific to hepatitis B surface antigen (HBsAg). HBIG differs from immune globulin in the amount of anti-HBs. Immune globulin is prepared from plasma that is not preselected for anti-HBs content. HBIG is prepared from plasma preselected for high titer anti-HBs. In the US, HBIG has an anti-HBs high titer >1:100,000 by IRA.

Pharmacodynamics/Kinetics

Duration of Action Postexposure prophylaxis: 3 to 6 months

Half-life Elimination 17 to 25 days

Time to Peak Serum: IM: 2 to 10 days

Pregnancy Risk Factor C

Pregnancy Considerations

Use of HBIG is not contraindicated in pregnant females and may be used for postexposure prophylaxis when indicated (CDC 2001). In addition, use of HBIG has been evaluated to reduce maternal to fetal transmission of hepatis B virus during pregnancy (ACOG 2007)

◆ **Hepatitis B Inactivated Virus Vaccine (recombinant DNA)** *see* Hepatitis B Vaccine (Recombinant) *on page 757*

Hepatitis B Vaccine (Recombinant)

(hep a TYE tis bee vak SEEN ree KOM be nant)

Related Information

Systemic Viral Diseases *on page 1709*

Brand Names: US Engerix-B; Recombivax HB

Brand Names: Canada Engerix-B; Recombivax HB

Pharmacologic Category Vaccine; Vaccine, Inactivated (Viral); Vaccine, Recombinant

Use Hepatitis B disease prevention: Active immunization against infection caused by all known subtypes of hepatitis B virus (HBV).

The Advisory Committee on Immunization Practices (ACIP) recommends routine vaccination for the following (CDC/ACIP [Schillie 2018]):

- All neonates (regardless of weight) born to either hepatitis B surface antigen (HBsAg) positive mother or mother with unknown status (administer first dose within 12 hours of birth).
- All neonates weighing ≥2 kg (eg, term) born to HBsAg negative mother (administer first dose within 24 hours of birth).
- All neonates weighing <2 kg (eg, preterm) born to HBsAg negative mother (administer first dose at 1 month of age or prior to hospital discharge).
- All unvaccinated infants, children, and adolescents <19 years of age.
- All unvaccinated adults requesting protection from HBV infection.
- All unvaccinated adults at risk for HBV infection such as those with:

  Behavioral risks: Sexually-active persons with >1 partner in a 6-month period; persons seeking evaluation or treatment for a sexually transmitted disease; men who have sex with men; injection drug users.

  Occupational risks: Health care personnel and public safety workers with reasonably anticipated risk for exposure to blood or blood contaminated body fluids.

  Medical risks: Persons with end-stage renal disease (including predialysis, hemodialysis, peritoneal dialysis, and home dialysis); persons with HIV infection; persons with chronic liver disease (eg, hepatitis C virus infection, cirrhosis, fatty liver disease, alcoholic liver disease, autoimmune hepatitis, ALT or AST level >2 times the upper limit of normal). Adults (19 through 59 years of age) with diabetes mellitus type 1 or type 2 should be vaccinated as soon as possible following diagnosis. Adults ≥60 years of age with diabetes mellitus may also be vaccinated at the discretion of their treating clinician based on the likelihood of acquiring HBV infection.

  Other risks: Household contacts or sex partners of persons who are HBsAg-positive; residents and staff of facilities for developmentally disabled persons; international travelers to regions with high or intermediate levels of endemic HBV infection; incarcerated persons.

  Pregnant patients at risk for infection or severe outcome from infection during pregnancy (ACIP [Freedman 2020]).

In addition, the ACIP recommends vaccination for any persons who are wounded in bombings or similar mass casualty events who have penetrating injuries or nonintact skin exposure, or who have contact with mucous membranes (exception - superficial contact with intact skin), and who cannot confirm receipt of a hepatitis B vaccination (CDC [Chapman 2008]).

Local Anesthetic/Vasoconstrictor Precautions No information available to require special precautions

Effects on Dental Treatment No significant effects or complications reported

Effects on Bleeding No information available to require special precautions

Adverse Reactions All serious adverse reactions must be reported to the US Department of Health and Human Services (DHHS) Vaccine Adverse Event Reporting System (VAERS) at 1-800-822-7967 or online at https://vaers.hhs.gov/esub/index.

Frequency not defined. The most common adverse effects reported with both products included injection site reactions (>10%).

Cardiovascular: Flushing, hypotension

Central nervous system: Body pain, chills, dizziness, drowsiness, fatigue, headache, insomnia, irritability, malaise, paresthesia, tingling sensation, vertigo

Dermatologic: Diaphoresis, pruritus, skin rash, urticaria

Gastrointestinal: Abdominal pain, anorexia, decreased appetite, diarrhea, dyspepsia, nausea, stomach cramps, vomiting

Genitourinary: Dysuria

Hematologic & oncologic: Lymphadenopathy

Hypersensitivity: Angioedema

Infection: Influenza

Local: Bruising at injection site, erythema at injection site, induration at injection site, injection site nodule, itching at injection site, local soreness/soreness at injection site, pain at injection site, swelling at injection site, tenderness at injection site, warm sensation at injection site

Neuromuscular & skeletal: Arthralgia, back pain, myalgia, neck pain, neck stiffness, shoulder pain, weakness

Otic: Otalgia

Respiratory: Cough, pharyngitis, rhinitis, upper respiratory tract infection

Miscellaneous: Fever (≥37.5°C/100°F)

Postmarketing and/or case reports: Abnormal hepatic function tests, acute exacerbations of multiple sclerosis, agitation, alopecia, anaphylactoid reaction, anaphylaxis, apnea, arthritis, Bell's palsy, brain disease, bronchospasm, conjunctivitis, constipation, convulsions, eczema, encephalitis, erythema nodosum, erythema multiforme, febrile seizures, Guillain-Barre syndrome, herpes zoster, hypersensitivity reaction, hypoesthesia, increased erythrocyte sedimentation rate, increased liver enzymes, keratitis, lichen planus, limb pain, lupus-like syndrome, meningitis, migraine, multiple sclerosis, myasthenia, myelitis, neuritis, neuropathy, optic neuritis, palpitations, paralysis, paresis, periarteritis nodosa, peripheral neuropathy, petechiae, purpura, radiculopathy, seizure, serum sickness-like reaction (may be delayed days to weeks), Stevens-Johnson syndrome, syncope, systemic lupus erythematosus, tachycardia, thrombocytopenia, tinnitus, transverse myelitis, uveitis, vasculitis, visual disturbance

Mechanism of Action Recombinant hepatitis B vaccine is a noninfectious subunit viral vaccine, which confers active immunity via formation of antihepatitis B antibodies. The vaccine is derived from hepatitis B surface antigen (HBsAg) produced through recombinant DNA techniques from yeast cells. The portion of the hepatitis B gene which codes for HBsAg is cloned into yeast, which is then cultured to produce hepatitis B vaccine.

Pharmacodynamics/Kinetics

Duration of Action Duration of protection against hepatitis B has been shown to be ≥30 years for immunocompetent persons who originally responded to the full three dose hepatitis B vaccine series (CDC/ACIP [Schillie 2018]).

Pregnancy Considerations

An increased risk of adverse maternal or fetal events, including miscarriage or major birth defects, has not been observed following maternal use of the hepatitis B vaccine (Groom 2018).

The Advisory Committee on Immunization Practices recommends hepatitis B surface antigen (HBsAg) testing for all pregnant females. Pregnancy itself is not a contraindication to vaccination (CDC/ACIP [Schillie 2018]). The Centers for Disease Control and Prevention recommends immunization for pregnant patients at risk for hepatitis B infection or severe outcome from infection during pregnancy (ACIP [Freedman 2020]). Refer to current immunization schedule for vaccinating pregnant females.

Dental Health Professional Considerations Immunization is recommended for dentists, oral surgeons, dental hygienists, dental nurses, and dental students

Hepatitis B Vaccine (Recombinant [Adjuvanted])

(hep a TYE tis bee vak SEEN ree KOM be nant ad ju VANT ed)

Brand Names: US Heplisav-B

Pharmacologic Category Vaccine; Vaccine, Inactivated (Viral); Vaccine, Recombinant

Use Hepatitis B virus disease prevention : Prevention of infection caused by all known subtypes of hepatitis B virus in adults

The Advisory Committee on Immunization Practices (ACIP) recommends routine vaccination for the following (CDC/ACIP [Schillie 2018b]):

- All unvaccinated adults requesting protection from HBV infection
- All unvaccinated adults at risk for HBV infection such as those with:
  - Behavioral risks: Sexually active persons not in a long-term, mutually monogamous relationship; persons seeking evaluation or treatment for a sexually transmitted disease; men who have sex with men; injection drug users
  - Occupational risks: Health care personnel (HCP) and public safety workers with reasonably anticipated risk for exposure to blood or blood contaminated body fluids
  - Medical risks: Persons with ESRD (including predialysis, hemodialysis, peritoneal dialysis, and home dialysis); persons with HIV infection; persons with chronic liver disease (eg, hepatitis C virus infection, cirrhosis, fatty liver disease, alcoholic liver disease, autoimmune hepatitis, ALT or AST level >2 times the upper limit of normal); adults (<60 years of age) with diabetes mellitus; adults ≥60 years of age with diabetes mellitus may also be vaccinated at the discretion of their treating clinician
  - Other risks: Household contacts or sex partners of persons who are HBsAg-positive; residents and staff of facilities for developmentally disabled persons; international travelers to regions with high or intermediate levels of endemic HBV infection; incarcerated persons

Local Anesthetic/Vasoconstrictor Precautions No information available to require special precautions

Effects on Dental Treatment No significant effects or complications reported

Effects on Bleeding No information available to require special precautions

Adverse Reactions

>10%

- Central nervous system: Fatigue (11% to 17%), headache (8% to 17%)
- Local: Pain at injection site (23% to 39%)

1% to 10%:

- Central nervous system: Malaise (7% to 9%)
- Local: Erythema at injection site (≤4%), swelling at injection site (≤2%)
- Neuromuscular & skeletal: Myalgia (6% to 9%)
- Miscellaneous: Fever (≤2%)

<1%, postmarketing, and/or case reports: Graves disease, Guillain-Barre syndrome, herpes zoster, lichen planus, myocardial infarction, Wegener granulomatosis

Mechanism of Action Recombinant (adjuvanted) hepatitis B vaccine is a noninfectious viral vaccine, which confers active immunity via formation of antihepatitis B antibodies.

Pregnancy Considerations

The ACIP recommends HBsAg testing for all pregnant women (CDC/ACIP [Schillie 2018a]). When vaccination is clinically indicated, the ACIP recommends use of a different hepatitis B vaccine until additional information related to this formulation in pregnancy is available (CDC/ACIP [Schillie 2018b]).

Females exposed to this vaccine during pregnancy are encouraged to enroll in the HEPLISAV-B Pregnancy Registry 1-844-443-7734.

- ◆ **HepB** *see* Hepatitis A and Hepatitis B Recombinant Vaccine *on page* 754
- ◆ **HepB** *see* Hepatitis B Vaccine (Recombinant [Adjuvanted]) *on page* 758
- ◆ **HepB** *see* Hepatitis B Vaccine (Recombinant) *on page* 757
- ◆ **HepB-CpG** *see* Hepatitis B Vaccine (Recombinant [Adjuvanted]) *on page* 758
- ◆ **Heplisav-B** *see* Hepatitis B Vaccine (Recombinant [Adjuvanted]) *on page* 758
- ◆ **Hepsera** *see* Adefovir *on page* 86
- ◆ **Herceptin** *see* Trastuzumab *on page* 1479
- ◆ **Herpes Zoster Vaccine** *see* Zoster Vaccine (Live/Attenuated) *on page* 1585
- ◆ **Herpes Zoster Vaccine** *see* Zoster Vaccine (Recombinant) *on page* 1586
- ◆ **Herzuma** *see* Trastuzumab *on page* 1479
- ◆ **Hetlioz** *see* Tasimelteon *on page* 1407
- ◆ **Hexamethylenetetramine** *see* Methenamine *on page* 987
- ◆ **hFSH** *see* Urofollitropin *on page* 1509
- ◆ **hGH** *see* Somatropin *on page* 1381
- ◆ **HHT** *see* Omacetaxine *on page* 1133
- ◆ **Hib** *see* Meningococcal Polysaccharide (Groups C and Y) and *Haemophilus* b Tetanus Toxoid Conjugate Vaccine *on page* 965
- ◆ **Hibiclens [OTC]** *see* Chlorhexidine Gluconate (Topical) *on page* 335

- ◆ **Hib-MenCY** *see* Meningococcal Polysaccharide (Groups C and Y) and *Haemophilus* b Tetanus Toxoid Conjugate Vaccine *on page 965*
- ◆ **Hib-MenCY-TT** *see* Meningococcal Polysaccharide (Groups C and Y) and *Haemophilus* b Tetanus Toxoid Conjugate Vaccine *on page 965*
- ◆ **HiDex 6-Day** *see* DexAMETHasone (Systemic) *on page 463*
- ◆ **Highly Pathogenic Avian Influenza (HPAI) A (H5N1) Virus Vaccine** *see* Influenza A Virus Vaccine (H5N1) *on page 811*
- ◆ **Hi-Kovite [OTC]** *see* Vitamins (Multiple/Oral) *on page 1550*
- ◆ **Hiprex** *see* Methenamine *on page 987*
- ◆ **Hirulog** *see* Bivalirudin *on page 246*
- ◆ **Histex [OTC]** *see* Triprolidine *on page 1500*
- ◆ **Histex PD [OTC]** *see* Triprolidine *on page 1500*
- ◆ **Histex PDX [OTC] [DSC]** *see* Triprolidine *on page 1500*
- ◆ **Histone methyl transferase EZH2 inhibitor E7438** *see* Tazemetostat *on page 1408*

Histrelin (his TREL in)

Brand Names: US Supprelin LA; Vantas

Brand Names: Canada Vantas [DSC]

Pharmacologic Category Antineoplastic Agent, Gonadotropin-Releasing Hormone Agonist; Gonadotropin Releasing Hormone Agonist

Use

Central precocious puberty (Supprelin LA): Treatment of children with central precocious puberty

Prostate cancer, advanced (Vantas): Palliative treatment of advanced prostate cancer

Local Anesthetic/Vasoconstrictor Precautions No information available to require special precautions

Effects on Dental Treatment No significant effects or complications reported

Effects on Bleeding Anemia reported in <2% of patients

Adverse Reactions

CPP:

>10%: Dermatologic: Dermatological reaction (51%; insertion site reaction includes bruise, discomfort, erythema, pain, protrusion of implant area, pruritus, soreness, swelling, tingling)

1% to 10%:

Central nervous system: Emotional lability (≤2%), headache (≤2%), migraine (≤2%), sensation of cold (≤2%)

Dermatologic: Cicatrix of skin (6%), pruritus (≤2%)

Endocrine & metabolic: Gynecomastia (≤2%), heavy menstrual bleeding (≤2%), weight gain (≤2%)

Genitourinary: Uterine hemorrhage (4%), breast tenderness (≤2%), dysmenorrhea (≤2%), precocious puberty (≤2%; progression of central precocious puberty)

Hematologic & oncologic: Pituitary neoplasm (≤2%)

Infection: Localized infection (≤2%; implant site)

Local: Application site pain (4%)

Neuromuscular & skeletal: Keloid-like scar (6%)

Respiratory: Epistaxis (≤2%), flu-like symptoms (≤2%)

Miscellaneous: Procedural complications (6%; suture-related), postoperative pain (4%)

Frequency not defined: Endocrine & metabolic: Altered hormone levels

<1%, postmarketing, and/or case reports: Aggressive behavior, amblyopia, crying, hostility, irritability, seizure, suicidal ideation

Prostate cancer:

>10%:

Dermatologic: Dermatological reaction (3% to 14%)

Endocrine & metabolic: Hot flash (66%)

1% to 10%:

Cardiovascular: Flushing (<2%), palpitations (<2%), peripheral edema (<2%), ventricular premature contractions (<2%)

Central nervous system: Fatigue (10%), headache (3%), insomnia (3%), depression (<2%), dizziness (<2%), irritability (<2%), lethargy (<2%), malaise (<2%), pain (<2%), sensation of cold (<2%)

Dermatologic: Diaphoresis (<2%), genital pruritus (<2%), hypotrichosis (<2%), night sweats (<2%), pruritus (<2%)

Endocrine & metabolic: Gynecomastia (4%), decreased libido (2%), weight gain (2%), fluid retention (<2%), hypercalcemia (<2%), hypercholesterolemia (<2%), increased lactate dehydrogenase (<2%), increased prostatic acid phosphatase (<2%), increased serum glucose (<2%), weight loss (<2%)

Gastrointestinal: Constipation (4%), abdominal distress (<2%), food cravings (<2%), increased appetite (<2%), nausea (<2%)

Genitourinary: Testicular atrophy (5%; expected pharmacological consequence of testosterone suppression), erectile dysfunction (4%), breast tenderness (<2%), dysuria (<2%), exacerbation of gynecomastia (<2%), exacerbation of hematuria (<2%), exacerbation of urinary frequency (<2%), hematuria (<2%), mastalgia (<2%), urinary frequency (<2%), urinary retention (<2%)

Hematologic & oncologic: Anemia (<2%), bruise (<2%), hematoma (<2%)

Hepatic: Hepatic disease (<2%), increased serum AST (<2%)

Local: Bruising at injection site (7%), pain at injection site (≤4%), tenderness at injection site (≤4%), erythema at injection site (3%), inflammation at injection site (1%), injection site infection (1%)

Neuromuscular & skeletal: Arthralgia (<2%), asthenia (<2%), back pain (<2%), exacerbation of back pain (<2%), limb pain (<2%), muscle twitching (<2%), myalgia (<2%), neck pain (<2%), ostealgia (<2%), tremor (<2%)

Renal: Renal insufficiency (5%), decreased creatinine clearance (<2%), exacerbation of renal failure (<2%), nephrolithiasis (<2%)

Respiratory: Dyspnea on exertion (<2%)

Miscellaneous: Stent occlusion (<2%)

<1%, postmarketing, and/or case reports: Decreased bone mineral density, hepatic injury (severe), increased testosterone level, swelling at injection site

Mechanism of Action Potent inhibitor of gonadotropin secretion; continuous administration results in, after an initiation phase, the suppression of luteinizing hormone (LH), follicle-stimulating hormone (FSH), and a subsequent decrease in testosterone and dihydrotestosterone (males) and estrone and estradiol (premenopausal females). Testosterone levels are reduced to castrate levels in males (treated for prostate cancer) within 2 to 4 weeks. Additionally, in patients with CPP, linear growth velocity is slowed (improves chance of attaining predicted adult height).

Pharmacodynamics/Kinetics

Onset of Action Prostate cancer: Chemical castration: Within 2 to 4 weeks; CPP: Progression of sexual development stops and growth is decreased within 1 month

Duration of Action 12 months (plus a few additional weeks of histrelin release)

Half-life Elimination Adults: Terminal: ~4 hours

Time to Peak Adults: 12 hours

Reproductive Considerations

Histrelin is contraindicated for use in women who may become pregnant.

Pregnancy Risk Factor X

Pregnancy Considerations

Histrelin is contraindicated for use during pregnancy. May cause fetal harm or spontaneous abortion if administered during pregnancy.

- ◆ **Histrelin Acetate** *see* Histrelin *on page 759*
- ◆ **Hizentra** *see* Immune Globulin *on page 803*
- ◆ **HKI-272** *see* Neratinib *on page 1094*
- ◆ **hMG** *see* Menotropins *on page 965*
- ◆ **HMR1726** *see* Teriflunomide *on page 1423*
- ◆ **HMR 3647** *see* Telithromycin *on page 1412*
- ◆ **HOE 140** *see* Icatibant *on page 795*
- ◆ **Hold [OTC]** *see* Dextromethorphan *on page 476*
- ◆ **Homoharringtonine** *see* Omacetaxine *on page 1133*
- ◆ **Horizant** *see* Gabapentin Enacarbil *on page 727*
- ◆ **Horse Antihuman Thymocyte Gamma Globulin** *see* Antithymocyte Globulin (Equine) *on page 157*
- ◆ **12 Hour Decongestant [OTC]** *see* Oxymetazoline (Nasal) *on page 1173*
- ◆ **12 Hour Nasal Decongestant [OTC]** *see* Oxymetazoline (Nasal) *on page 1173*
- ◆ **12 Hour Nasal Relief Spray [OTC]** *see* Oxymetazoline (Nasal) *on page 1173*
- ◆ **12 Hour Nasal Spray [OTC]** *see* Oxymetazoline (Nasal) *on page 1173*
- ◆ **hpAT** *see* Antithrombin *on page 156*
- ◆ **HPV2** *see* Papillomavirus (Types 16, 18) Vaccine (Human, Recombinant) *on page 1191*
- ◆ **HPV4** *see* Papillomavirus (Types 6, 11, 16, 18) Vaccine (Human, Recombinant) *on page 1190*
- ◆ **HPV 16/18 L1 VLP/AS04 VAC** *see* Papillomavirus (Types 16, 18) Vaccine (Human, Recombinant) *on page 1191*
- ◆ **HPV Vaccine (Bivalent)** *see* Papillomavirus (Types 16, 18) Vaccine (Human, Recombinant) *on page 1191*
- ◆ **HPV Vaccine (Quadrivalent)** *see* Papillomavirus (Types 6, 11, 16, 18) Vaccine (Human, Recombinant) *on page 1190*
- ◆ **HRIG** *see* Rabies Immune Globulin (Human) *on page 1302*
- ◆ **hRS7-SN38 Antibody-drug Conjugate** *see* Sacituzumab Govitecan *on page 1352*
- ◆ **HTF919** *see* Tegaserod *on page 1411*
- ◆ **HuLuc63** *see* Elotuzumab *on page 550*
- ◆ **HumaLOG** *see* Insulin Lispro *on page 824*
- ◆ **HumaLOG Junior KwikPen** *see* Insulin Lispro *on page 824*
- ◆ **HumaLOG KwikPen** *see* Insulin Lispro *on page 824*
- ◆ **Humalog Mix** *see* Insulin Lispro Protamine and Insulin Lispro *on page 826*
- ◆ **HumaLOG Mix** *see* Insulin Lispro Protamine and Insulin Lispro *on page 826*
- ◆ **HumaLOG Mix 50/50** *see* Insulin Lispro Protamine and Insulin Lispro *on page 826*
- ◆ **HumaLOG Mix 50/50 KwikPen** *see* Insulin Lispro Protamine and Insulin Lispro *on page 826*
- ◆ **Humalog Mix 75/25** *see* Insulin Lispro Protamine and Insulin Lispro *on page 826*
- ◆ **HumaLOG Mix 75/25** *see* Insulin Lispro Protamine and Insulin Lispro *on page 826*
- ◆ **HumaLOG Mix 75/25 KwikPen** *see* Insulin Lispro Protamine and Insulin Lispro *on page 826*
- ◆ **Human Antitumor Necrosis Factor Alpha** *see* Adalimumab *on page 83*
- ◆ **Human Corticotrophin-Releasing Hormone, Analogue** *see* Corticorelin *on page 411*
- ◆ **Human Diploid Cell Cultures Rabies Vaccine** *see* Rabies Vaccine *on page 1303*
- ◆ **Human Growth Hormone** *see* Somatropin *on page 1381*
- ◆ **Humanized IgG1 Anti-CD52 Monoclonal Antibody** *see* Alemtuzumab *on page 93*
- ◆ **Human Menopausal Gonadotropin** *see* Menotropins *on page 965*
- ◆ **Human Normal Immunoglobulin** *see* Immune Globulin *on page 803*
- ◆ **Human Papillomavirus Vaccine (Bivalent)** *see* Papillomavirus (Types 16, 18) Vaccine (Human, Recombinant) *on page 1191*
- ◆ **Human Papillomavirus Vaccine (Quadrivalent)** *see* Papillomavirus (Types 6, 11, 16, 18) Vaccine (Human, Recombinant) *on page 1190*
- ◆ **Human Rotavirus Vaccine, Attenuated (HRV)** *see* Rotavirus Vaccine *on page 1349*
- ◆ **Human Thyroid Stimulating Hormone** *see* Thyrotropin Alpha *on page 1442*
- ◆ **Humate-P** *see* Antihemophilic Factor/von Willebrand Factor Complex (Human) *on page 154*
- ◆ **Humatrope** *see* Somatropin *on page 1381*
- ◆ **HuMax-CD20** *see* Ofatumumab *on page 1126*
- ◆ **HuMax-CD38-rHuPH20** *see* Daratumumab and Hyaluronidase *on page 439*
- ◆ **Hum Insulin Nph/Reg Insulin Hm** *see* Insulin NPH and Insulin Regular *on page 828*
- ◆ **Humira** *see* Adalimumab *on page 83*
- ◆ **Humira Pediatric Crohns Start** *see* Adalimumab *on page 83*
- ◆ **Humira Pen** *see* Adalimumab *on page 83*
- ◆ **Humira Pen-CD/UC/HS Starter** *see* Adalimumab *on page 83*
- ◆ **Humira Pen-Ps/UV/Adol HS Start** *see* Adalimumab *on page 83*
- ◆ **HumuLIN 70/30** *see* Insulin NPH and Insulin Regular *on page 828*
- ◆ **HumuLIN 70/30 KwikPen** *see* Insulin NPH and Insulin Regular *on page 828*
- ◆ **HumuLIN N [OTC]** *see* Insulin NPH *on page 827*
- ◆ **HumuLIN N KwikPen [OTC]** *see* Insulin NPH *on page 827*
- ◆ **HumuLIN R [OTC]** *see* Insulin Regular *on page 829*
- ◆ **HumuLIN R U-500 (CONCENTRATED)** *see* Insulin Regular *on page 829*

- ◆ **HumuLIN R U-500 KwikPen** *see* Insulin Regular *on page 829*
- ◆ **Hurricaine [OTC]** *see* Benzocaine *on page 228*
- ◆ **HurriCaine One [OTC]** *see* Benzocaine *on page 228*
- ◆ **HurriPak Starter Kit [OTC]** *see* Benzocaine *on page 228*
- ◆ **Hyalgan** *see* Hyaluronate and Derivatives *on page 761*
- ◆ **Hyaluronan** *see* Hyaluronate and Derivatives *on page 761*

Hyaluronate and Derivatives

(hye al yoor ON ate & dah RIV ah tives)

Brand Names: US Amvisc; Amvisc Plus; Bionect; Durolane; Euflexxa; Gel-One; Gelsyn-3; GenVisc 850; Healon; Healon EndoCoat; Healon GV; Healon5; Hyalgan; HyGel [DSC]; Hylinate; Hymovis; Juvederm Ultra; Juvederm Ultra Plus; Juvederm Ultra Plus XC; Juvederm Ultra XC; Juvederm Voluma XC; Monovisc; Orthovisc; Perlane [DSC]; Perlane-L [DSC]; Provisc; Restylane Lyft; Restylane Silk; Restylane [DSC]; Restylane-L [DSC]; Supartz FX; Supartz [DSC]; Synvisc; Synvisc-One; Therapevo [DSC]; Triluron

Brand Names: Canada Cystistat; Durolane; Ortho-Visc; Suplasyn

Pharmacologic Category Antirheumatic Miscellaneous; Cosmetic Agent, Implant; Ophthalmic Agent, Viscoelastic; Skin and Mucous Membrane Agent, Miscellaneous

Use

Intra-articular injection: Treatment of pain in osteoarthritis of the knee in patients who have failed nonpharmacologic treatment or simple analgesics (Durolane, Euflexxa, Gel-One, Gelsyn-3, GenVisc 850, Hyalgan, Hymovis, Monovisc, OrthoVisc, Supartz, Supartz FX, Synvisc, Synvisc-One, Triluron, TriVisc, Visco-3) or nonsteroidal anti-inflammatory drugs (Gel-One).

Intradermal:

Juvederm (all formulations except Volbella XC and Voluma XC), Perlane, Restylane, Restylane Defyne, Restylane Lyft, Restylane-L, Restylane Refyne: Correction of moderate to severe facial wrinkles or folds.

Juvederm Volbella XC, Restylane Kysse, and Restylane Silk: Correction of perioral rhytids in adults >21 years.

Subcutaneous: Restylane Lyft: Correction of volume deficit of the dorsal hand in adults >21 years.

Subcutaneous/supraperiosteal: Juvederm Voluma XC, Restylane Lyft: Correction of age-related volume deficit (deep [subcutaneous and/or supraperiosteal] injection) for cheek augmentation in the mid-face in adults >21 years.

Ophthalmic: Surgical aid in cataract extraction (Amvisc, Amvisc Plus, Biolon, Provisc); intraocular lens implantation (Amvisc, Amvisc Plus, Biolon, Provisc); corneal transplant (Amvisc, Amvisc Plus); glaucoma filtration (Amvisc, Amvisc Plus); and retinal attachment surgery (Amvisc, Amvisc Plus); anterior segment surgery (Biolon, Healon [all formulations]).

Submucosal: Lip augmentation in adults >21 years (Restylane, Restylane-L, Restylane Kysse, Restylane Silk, Juvederm Ultra XC, Juvederm Volbella XC).

Topical cream, gel: Management of skin ulcers and wounds (Bionect, Therapevo); management and relief of symptoms associated with dermatoses (eg, atopic dermatitis, allergic contact dermatitis, radiodermatitis), including burning, itching, and pain (Therapevo).

Topical lotion: Treatment of symptoms associated with xerosis.

Local Anesthetic/Vasoconstrictor Precautions No information available to require special precautions

Effects on Dental Treatment No significant effects or complications reported

Effects on Bleeding No information available to require special precautions

Adverse Reactions Type of local reactions may vary by formulation and site of application/injection. Some reports include concomitant lidocaine.

>10%:

Central nervous system: Headache (≤18%)

Dermatologic: Skin discoloration at injection site (4% to 78%), ecchymoses (≤14%), skin rash (≤14%)

Hematologic & oncologic: Bruise (≤28%; more common in older patients)

Local: Swelling at injection site (3% to 98%), tenderness at injection site (17% to 95%), bruising at injection site (3% to 93%), erythema at injection site (≤93%), induration at injection site (6% to 92%), pain at injection site (≤92%), residual mass at injection site (3% to 90%), itching at injection site (7% to 47%), muscle rigidity at injection site (25%), hematoma at injection site (8% to 18%)

Neuromuscular & skeletal: Arthralgia (1% to 25%), joint swelling (knee; ≤14%), joint effusion (≤11%)

Miscellaneous: Swelling (18% to 28%)

1% to 10%:

Cardiovascular: Presyncope (≤5%), hypertension (4%), increased blood pressure (4%), edema (1%)

Central nervous system: Dizziness (≤5%), hyperesthesia (injection site; ≤5%), hypoesthesia (≤5%), malaise (≤5%), tingling in the lips (≤5%), falling (≤4%), fatigue (1%), paresthesia (1%), sciatica (1%)

Dermatologic: Hyperpigmentation (≤9%; postinflammatory; in patients of African-American heritage and Fitzpatrick Skin Types IV, V, and VI), exfoliation of skin (2% to 8%), cheilosis (≤5%), fine wrinkling (≤5%), local acneiform eruptions (≤5%), local dryness of skin (≤5%), papule of skin (injection site; ≤5%), rash at injection site (≤5%), skin tightness (≤5%), xanthoderma (≤5%)

Gastrointestinal: Oral herpes simplex infection (≤5%), toothache (4%), abdominal pain (≤4%), diarrhea (≤4%), dyspepsia (≤4%), nausea (≤4%)

Genitourinary: Urinary tract infection (4%)

Infection: Infection (1% to 4%), influenza (2%), herpes zoster infection (1%)

Local: Bleeding at injection site (5% to 7%), injection site reaction (1% to 6%), injection site nodule (≤5%), injection site numbness (≤5%), local skin exfoliation (≤5%), injection site infection (1%)

Neuromuscular & skeletal: Back pain (≤10%), limb pain (≤8%), puffiness of cheeks (≤5%), arthropathy (≤4%; including joint crepitation), connective tissue disease (≤4%), lower extremity pain (≤4%), musculoskeletal disease (≤4%; including pain and discomfort), musculoskeletal pain (2%), osteoarthritis (2%), tendonitis (2%), localized osteoarthritis (≤2%), muscle strain (1%), joint stiffness (≤1%)

Ophthalmic: Increased intraocular pressure (requiring treatment: 7%), punctate keratitis (≤4%; conjunctival), superficial keratitis (≤4%), cystoid macular edema (3%), opacity of ocular lens capsule (3%), conjunctivitis (1%), corneal edema (1%), corneal erosion (1%), corneal injury (1%; including Seidel Phenomenon and corneo-scleral leak), injury to eye region (1%; ocular sphincter), uveitis (1%)

Respiratory: Nasopharyngitis (2% to 10%), upper respiratory tract infection (1% to 6%), flu-like symptoms (1% to ≤4%), bronchitis (≤4%), rhinitis (≤4%), sinusitis (≤4%), cough (2%), oropharyngeal pain (2%), respiratory tract infection (2%)
Miscellaneous: Laceration (injection site; ≤5%), soft tissue injury (lips; ≤5%), wound (≤5%), accidental injury (≤4%), fever (3%)
Frequency not defined:
Central nervous system: Tingling sensation
Ophthalmic: Ophthalmic inflammation (postoperative; iritis, hypopyon)
<1%, postmarketing, and/or case reports: Abnormal gait, abnormal sensory symptoms, abscess, acne vulgaris, anaphylactic shock, anaphylaxis, angioedema, anterior chamber fibrin deposition, anxiety, application site reaction (implant migration), atrophy at injection site, bacterial infection, blindness, blurred vision, burning sensation, bursitis, capillary fragility, central nervous system disease, cerebrovascular accident, cerebrovascular occlusion, cutaneous nodule, cystitis, depression, dermatitis, dislocation (joint), dyspnea, edema, erythema of skin, eyelid edema, eye pain, facial swelling, feeling of heaviness, fistula, gouty arthritis, granuloma, hemarthrosis, hematoma, herpetic lesion, hypersensitivity reaction, hypotension, increased serum alanine aminotransferase, increased serum glucose, inflammation, injection site infection (abscess/necrosis), injection site ischemia, injection site scarring, keloids, leukocytosis, metallic taste, mouth edema, muscle spasm (knee), myalgia, myasthenia, neck pain, nervousness, neuralgia, nonimmune anaphylaxis, peripheral edema, popliteal cyst, pruritic rash, pruritus, red face, rhinorrhea, sensation of cold (knee), skin blister, skin or other tissue necrosis, sore throat, subconjunctival hemorrhage (including hyphema and hematic Tyndall), subcutaneous nodule, swelling of extremities, swelling of eye, syncope, synechiae of iris, synovitis (knee), telangiectasia, thrombocytopenia (rare), tissue necrosis, urticaria, vasodepressor syncope, vertebral disk disease (protrusion), viral infection, visual disturbance, vitreous disorder (anterior chamber), vomiting, wound secretion, xeroderma

Mechanism of Action Sodium hyaluronate is a biological polysaccharide which is distributed widely in the extracellular matrix of connective tissue in man (vitreous and aqueous humor of the eye, synovial fluid, skin, and umbilical cord). Sodium hyaluronate and its derivatives form a viscoelastic solution in water (at physiological pH and ionic strength) which makes it suitable for aqueous and vitreous humor in ophthalmic surgery, and functions as a tissue and/or joint lubricant which plays an important role in modulating the interactions between adjacent tissues. Intradermal injection may decrease the depth of facial wrinkles. Transcutaneous injection for lip augmentation may correct perioral rhytids. Subcutaneous and/or supraperiosteal injection for cheek augmentation may correct age-related volume deficit. In the topical management of wounds and ulcers, sodium hyaluronate protects the skin against friction and abrasion.

Pregnancy Considerations
Adverse events were not observed in animal reproduction studies.

- **Hyaluronate Sodium** *see* Hyaluronate and Derivatives *on page 761*
- **Hyaluronic Acid** *see* Hyaluronate and Derivatives *on page 761*
- **Hyaluronidase and daratumumab** *see* Daratumumab and Hyaluronidase *on page 439*
- **Hyaluronidase and Rituximab** *see* Rituximab and Hyaluronidase *on page 1338*
- **Hyaluronidase, pertuzumab, and trastuzumab** *see* Pertuzumab, Trastuzumab, and Hyaluronidase *on page 1221*
- **Hyaluronidase, trastuzumab, and pertuzumab** *see* Pertuzumab, Trastuzumab, and Hyaluronidase *on page 1221*
- **Hycamptamine** *see* Topotecan *on page 1465*
- **Hycamtin** *see* Topotecan *on page 1465*
- **Hydergine [DSC]** *see* Ergoloid Mesylates *on page 582*

HydroCHLOROthiazide

(hye droe klor oh THYE a zide)

Related Information
Cardiovascular Diseases *on page 1654*

Brand Names: US Microzide [DSC]

Brand Names: Canada APO-Hydro; BIO-Hydrochlorothiazide; MINT-Hydrochlorothiazide; PMS-Hydrochlorothiazide; TEVA-Hydrochlorothiazide; Urozide

Pharmacologic Category Antihypertensive; Diuretic, Thiazide

Use
Edema: Treatment of edema due to heart failure, various forms of renal dysfunction (eg, nephrotic syndrome, acute glomerulosclerosis, chronic renal failure), or corticosteroid or estrogen therapy. **Note:** Loop diuretics are typically favored, but hydrochlorothiazide may be used as an adjunctive agent for refractory edema (Brater 2011).
Hypertension: Management of mild to moderate hypertension.

Local Anesthetic/Vasoconstrictor Precautions No information available to require special precautions

Effects on Dental Treatment Key adverse event(s) related to dental treatment: Hypotension; Patients may experience orthostatic hypotension as they stand up after treatment; especially if lying in dental chair for extended periods of time. Use caution with sudden changes in position during and after dental treatment.

Effects on Bleeding No information available to require special precautions

Adverse Reactions Frequency not defined; the occurrence of adverse events are dose related, with the majority occurring with doses ≥25 mg.
Cardiovascular: Hypotension, necrotizing angiitis, orthostatic hypotension
Central nervous system: Dizziness, headache, paresthesia, restlessness, vertigo
Dermatologic: Alopecia, erythema multiforme, exfoliative dermatitis, skin photosensitivity, skin rash, Stevens-Johnson syndrome, toxic epidermal necrolysis, urticaria
Endocrine & metabolic: Glycosuria, hypercalcemia, hyperglycemia, hyperuricemia, hypochloremic alkalosis, hypokalemia, hypomagnesemia, hyponatremia
Gastrointestinal: Abdominal cramps, anorexia, constipation, diarrhea, gastric irritation, nausea, pancreatitis, sialadenitis, vomiting
Genitourinary: Impotence
Hematologic & oncologic: Agranulocytosis, aplastic anemia, hemolytic anemia, leukopenia, purpura, thrombocytopenia
Hepatic: Jaundice

Hypersensitivity: Anaphylaxis
Neuromuscular & skeletal: Muscle spasm, weakness
Ophthalmic: Transient blurred vision, xanthopsia
Renal: Interstitial nephritis, renal failure, renal insufficiency
Respiratory: Respiratory distress, pneumonitis, pulmonary edema
Miscellaneous: Fever
<1%, postmarketing, and/or case reports: Allergic myocarditis, eosinophilic pneumonitis, hepatic insufficiency, malignant neoplasm of lip (Friedman 2012), skin carcinoma (Pedersen 2018), systemic lupus erythematosus

Mechanism of Action Inhibits sodium reabsorption in the distal tubules causing increased excretion of sodium and water as well as potassium and hydrogen ions

Pharmacodynamics/Kinetics

Onset of Action Diuresis: Infants: 2 to 6 hours (Chemtob 1989); Adults: ~2 hours; Peak effect: 4 to 6 hours.

Duration of Action Infants: 8 hours (Chemtob 1989); Adults: 6 to 12 hours.

Half-life Elimination ~6 to 15 hours.

Time to Peak ~1 to 5 hours.

Pregnancy Considerations

Hydrochlorothiazide crosses the placenta (Beerman 1980).

Maternal use may cause fetal or neonatal jaundice, thrombocytopenia, or other adverse events observed in adults.

Use of thiazide diuretics to treat edema during normal pregnancies is not appropriate; use may be considered when edema is due to pathologic causes (as in the nonpregnant patient); monitor.

Chronic maternal hypertension is associated with adverse events in the fetus/infant. The risk of birth defects, low birth weight, premature delivery, stillbirth, and neonatal death may be increased with chronic hypertension in pregnancy. Actual risks may be related to duration and severity of maternal hypertension. Diuretics are considered second-line therapy for treating chronic hypertension in pregnancy (ACOG 203 2019).

The treatment of edema associated with chronic heart failure during pregnancy is similar to that of nonpregnant patients. Use of thiazide diuretics may be considered but use with caution due to the potential reduction in placental blood flow. Patients diagnosed after delivery can be treated according to heart failure guidelines (ESC [Bauersachs 2016]; ESC [Regitz-Zagrosek 2018]).

◆ **Hydrochlorothiazide and Losartan** *see* Losartan and Hydrochlorothiazide *on page* 939

Hydrochlorothiazide and Triamterene

(hye droe klor oh THYE a zide & trye AM ter een)

Related Information

HydroCHLOROthiazide *on page* 762
Triamterene *on page* 1493

Brand Names: US Dyazide; Maxzide; Maxzide-25

Pharmacologic Category Antihypertensive; Diuretic, Potassium-Sparing; Diuretic, Thiazide

Use Hypertension, edema: Treatment of hypertension or edema (not recommended for initial treatment) when hypokalemia has developed on hydrochlorothiazide alone or when the development of hypokalemia must be avoided.

Local Anesthetic/Vasoconstrictor Precautions No information available to require special precautions

Effects on Dental Treatment No significant effects or complications reported

Effects on Bleeding No information available to require special precautions

Adverse Reactions Also see individual agents. Frequency not defined.

Cardiovascular: Angina pectoris, cardiac arrhythmia, necrotizing angiitis, orthostatic hypotension, tachycardia
Central nervous system: Anxiety, depression, dizziness, fatigue, glossopyrosis, headache, insomnia, paresthesia, restlessness, vertigo
Dermatologic: Skin photosensitivity, skin rash, urticaria
Endocrine & metabolic: Acidosis, diabetes mellitus, glycosuria, hypercalcemia, hyperglycemia, hyperkalemia, hyperuricemia, hypochloremia, hypokalemia, hypomagnesemia, hyponatremia
Gastrointestinal: Abdominal pain, anorexia, constipation, diarrhea, dysgeusia, gastric distress, nausea, pancreatitis, sialadenitis, stomach cramps, tongue discoloration (bright orange), vomiting, xerostomia
Genitourinary: Impotence, urine discoloration, urine sedimentation abnormality
Hematologic & oncologic: Agranulocytosis, aplastic anemia, hemolytic anemia, leukopenia, megaloblastic anemia, purpura, thrombocytopenia
Hepatic: Abnormal liver function tests, jaundice
Hypersensitivity: Anaphylaxis
Neuromuscular & skeletal: Exacerbation of systemic lupus erythematosus, lupus-like syndrome (subacute, cutaneous), muscle cramps, weakness
Ophthalmic: Transient blurred vision, xanthopsia
Renal: Acute renal failure, increased blood urea nitrogen, increased serum creatinine, interstitial nephritis, nephrolithiasis
Respiratory: Dyspnea, hypersensitivity pneumonitis, pulmonary edema, respiratory distress
Miscellaneous: Fever
<1%, postmarketing, and/or case reports: Malignant neoplasm of lip (Friedman 2012)

Mechanism of Action

Hydrochlorothiazide: Inhibits sodium reabsorption in the distal tubules causing increased excretion of sodium and water as well as potassium and hydrogen ions.

Triamterene: Blocks epithelial sodium channels in the late distal convoluted tubule (DCT) and collecting duct which inhibits sodium reabsorption from the lumen. This effectively reduces intracellular sodium, decreasing the function of Na+/K+ ATPase, leading to potassium retention and decreased calcium, magnesium, and hydrogen excretion. As sodium uptake capacity in the DCT/collecting duct is limited, the natriuretic, diuretic, and antihypertensive effects are generally considered weak.

Pregnancy Risk Factor C

Pregnancy Considerations Animal reproduction studies have not been conducted with this combination product. See individual monographs.

Hydrocodone and Acetaminophen

(hye droe KOE done & a seet a MIN oh fen)

Related Information

Acetaminophen *on page 59*

Oral Pain *on page 1734*

Related Sample Prescriptions

Oral Pain - Sample Prescriptions *on page 30*

Brand Names: US Lorcet; Lorcet HD; Lorcet Plus; Lortab; Norco; Verdrocet; Vicodin; Vicodin ES; Vicodin HP; Xodol 10/300; Xodol 5/300; Xodol 7.5/300; Zamicet [DSC]

Generic Availability (US) Yes: Oral solution, tablet

Pharmacologic Category Analgesic Combination (Opioid); Analgesic, Opioid

Dental Use Treatment of postoperative pain

Use

Pain management: Management of pain severe enough to require an opioid analgesic and for which alternative treatments are inadequate.

Limitations of use: Generally, 3 days or less of treatment with the lowest effective dose is recommended for acute pain, and rarely should use exceed 7 days. For chronic pain, nonpharmacologic and nonopioid pharmacologic treatment are first-line therapy and opioid prescriptions should be accompanied by established goals for pain and function and a discussion of risks and benefits (Dowell 2016).

Local Anesthetic/Vasoconstrictor Precautions No information available to require special precautions

Effects on Dental Treatment No significant effects or complications reported (see Dental Health Professional Considerations)

Effects on Bleeding As a single agent, acetaminophen does not appear to affect bleeding or platelet aggregation. Acetaminophen may prolong the INR and increase bleeding in patients taking warfarin (Coumadin). For patients taking warfarin, single acetaminophen doses or acetaminophen therapy of short duration should be safe, but if large (>1.3 g/day) doses are administered for longer than 10-14 days, then the INR should be monitored (see Dental Health Professional Considerations).

Adverse Reactions Frequency not defined.

Cardiovascular: Bradycardia, cardiac arrest, circulatory shock, hypotension

Central nervous system: Anxiety, clouding of consciousness, coma, dizziness, drowsiness, drug dependence, dysphoria, euphoria, fear, lethargy, malaise, mental deficiency, mood changes, sedation, stupor

Dermatologic: Cold and clammy skin, diaphoresis, pruritus, skin rash

Endocrine & metabolic: Hypoglycemic coma

Gastrointestinal: Abdominal pain, constipation, gastric distress, heartburn, nausea, occult blood in stools, peptic ulcer, vomiting

Genitourinary: Nephrotoxicity, ureteral spasm, urinary retention

Hematologic & oncologic: Agranulocytosis, hemolytic anemia, iron deficiency anemia, prolonged bleeding time, thrombocytopenia

Hepatic: Hepatic necrosis, hepatitis

Hypersensitivity: Hypersensitivity reaction

Neuromuscular & skeletal: Vesicle sphincter spasm

Otic: Hearing loss (chronic overdose)

Renal: Renal tubular necrosis

Respiratory: Airway obstruction, apnea, dyspnea, respiratory depression (dose related)

Postmarketing and/or case reports: Hypogonadism (Brennan, 2013; Debono, 2011)

Dental Usual Dosage Postoperative pain: Oral:

Children and Adults ≥50 kg: Average starting dose in opioid naive patients: Hydrocodone 5-10 mg 4 times/day; the dosage of acetaminophen should be limited to ≤4 g/day (and possibly less in patients with hepatic impairment or ethanol use).

Dosage ranges (based on specific product labeling): Hydrocodone 2.5-10 mg every 4-6 hours; maximum: 60 mg hydrocodone/day (maximum dose of hydrocodone may be limited by the acetaminophen content of specific product)

Elderly: Doses should be titrated to appropriate analgesic effect; 2.5-5 mg of the hydrocodone component every 4-6 hours. Do not exceed 4 g/day of acetaminophen.

Dosing

Adult

Pain management: Oral: **Note:** Pain relief and adverse events should be assessed frequently. Individually titrate to a dose that provides adequate analgesia and minimizes adverse reactions. Use of higher starting doses in patients who are not opioid tolerant may cause fatal respiratory depression.

Dosage ranges (based on specific product labeling): Hydrocodone 2.5 to 10 mg every 4 to 6 hours as needed (maximum dose of hydrocodone may be limited by the acetaminophen content of specific product; refer to manufacturer's labeling); the dosage of acetaminophen should be limited to ≤4 g/day. Use the lowest effective dose. Start at the lower end of dosing range for opioid-naive patients; for acute pain, use a low dose for ≤3 to 7 days (CDC [Dowell 2016]).

Discontinuation of therapy: When discontinuing chronic opioid therapy, the dose should be gradually tapered down. An optimal universal tapering schedule for all patients has not been established (CDC [Dowell 2016]). Proposed schedules range from slow (eg, 10% reductions per week) to rapid (eg, 25% to 50% reduction every few days) (CDC 2015). Tapering schedules should be individualized to minimize opioid withdrawal while considering patient-specific goals and concerns as well as the pharmacokinetics of the opioid being tapered. An even slower taper may be appropriate in patients who have been receiving opioids for a long duration (eg, years), particularly in the final stage of tapering, whereas more rapid tapers may be appropriate in patients experiencing severe adverse events (CDC [Dowell 2016]). Monitor carefully for signs/symptoms of withdrawal. If the patient displays withdrawal symptoms, consider slowing the taper schedule; alterations may include increasing the interval between dose reductions, decreasing amount of daily dose reduction, pausing the taper and restarting when the patient is ready, and/or coadministration of an alpha-2 agonist (eg, clonidine) to blunt withdrawal symptoms (Berna 2015; CDC [Dowell 2016]). Continue to offer nonopioid analgesics as needed for pain management during the taper; consider nonopioid adjunctive treatments for withdrawal symptoms (eg, GI complaints, muscle spasm) as needed (Berna 2015; Sevarino 2018).

Geriatric Refer to adult dosing. Initiate dosing at the lower end of the dosage range. Monitor closely.

Renal Impairment: Adult There are no specific dosage adjustments provided in the manufacturer's labeling; use with caution. Initiate therapy with a low dose and monitor closely. Also refer to individual agents.

Hepatic Impairment: Adult There are no specific dosage adjustments provided in the manufacturer's labeling; use with caution. Initiate therapy with a low dose and monitor closely. Also refer to individual agents.

Pediatric Note: Doses based on hydrocodone; titrate to appropriate analgesic effect. All sources of acetaminophen (eg, prescription, OTC, combination products) should be considered when evaluating a patient's maximum daily dose. To lower the risk for hepatotoxicity, limit daily dose to ≤75 mg/kg/**day** (maximum of 5 daily doses), not to exceed 4,000 mg/**day**; while recommended doses are generally considered safe, hepatotoxicity has been reported (rarely) even with doses below recommendations (AAP [Sullivan 2011]; Heard 2014; Lavonas 2010).

Analgesic; opioid-naive patients (Coté 2018; Kliegman 2020; Thigpen 2019): Infants, Children, and Adolescents: Limited data available in infants and children <2 years:

Patient weight:

<50 kg: Oral: Usual initial dose: Hydrocodone 0.1 to 0.2 mg/kg/dose every 4 to 6 hours; in infants, reduced doses and close monitoring should be considered due to possible increased sensitivity to respiratory depressant effects; use with caution in infants.

≥50 kg: Oral: Usual initial dose: Hydrocodone 5 to 10 mg every 4 to 6 hours.

Discontinuation of therapy: Do not abruptly discontinue therapy in patients who are physically dependent; dose should be gradually tapered to avoid withdrawal. An optimal tapering schedule has not been established. The taper should be individualized to minimize withdrawal and should be based on total daily opioid dose, length of opioid exposure, and patient response. Monitor patients for signs and symptoms of opioid withdrawal (D'Souza 2018).

Renal Impairment: Pediatric There are no specific dosage adjustments provided in the manufacturer's labeling; use with caution as plasma hydrocodone concentrations may be higher than in patients with normal renal function. Initiate therapy with a low dose and monitor closely; may also consider extending dosing intervals.

Hepatic Impairment: Pediatric There are no specific dosage adjustments provided in the manufacturer's labeling; use with caution as plasma hydrocodone concentrations may be higher than in patients with normal hepatic function. Initiate therapy with a low dose and monitor closely. For acetaminophen, limited, low-dose therapy is usually well-tolerated in hepatic disease/cirrhosis; however, cases of hepatotoxicity at daily acetaminophen dosages <4,000 mg/day have been reported. Avoid chronic use in hepatic impairment. See individual monograph.

Mechanism of Action

Hydrocodone: Binds to opiate receptors in the CNS, altering the perception of and response to pain; suppresses cough in medullary center; produces generalized CNS depression.

Acetaminophen: Although not fully elucidated, the analgesic effects are believed to be due to activation of descending serotonergic inhibitory pathways in the CNS. Interactions with other nociceptive systems may be involved as well (Smith 2009). Antipyresis is produced from inhibition of the hypothalamic heat-regulating center.

Contraindications

Hypersensitivity (eg, anaphylaxis) to hydrocodone, acetaminophen, or any component of the formulation; significant respiratory depression; acute or severe bronchial asthma in an unmonitored setting or in the absence of resuscitative equipment; GI obstruction, including paralytic ileus (known or suspected)

Documentation of allergenic cross-reactivity for opioids is limited. However, because of similarities in chemical structure and/or pharmacologic actions, the possibility of cross-sensitivity cannot be ruled out with certainty. Consider an opioid from an alternative structural class (eg, phenylpiperidine, diphenylheptane) (DeDea 2012).

Warnings/Precautions [US Boxed Warning]: Serious, life-threatening, or fatal respiratory depression may occur. Monitor closely for respiratory depression, especially during initiation or following a dose increase. Carbon dioxide retention from opioid-induced respiratory depression can exacerbate the sedating effects of opioids. Use opioids with caution and monitor for respiratory depression in patients with significant chronic obstructive pulmonary disease or cor pulmonale, and those having a substantially decreased respiratory reserve, hypoxia, hypercapnia, or preexisting respiratory depression, particularly when initiating therapy and titrating therapy; critical respiratory depression may occur, even at therapeutic dosages. Consider the use of alternative nonopioid analgesics in these patients. Use is contraindicated in patients with acute or severe bronchial asthma in an unmonitored setting or without resuscitative equipment. Avoid use in patients with impaired consciousness or coma as these patients are susceptible to intracranial effects of CO_2 retention. May cause severe hypotension (including orthostatic hypotension and syncope); use with caution in patients with hypovolemia, cardiovascular disease (including acute myocardial infarction [MI]), or drugs which may exaggerate hypotensive effects (including phenothiazines or general anesthetics). Monitor for symptoms of hypotension following initiation or dose titration. Avoid use in patients with circulatory shock. May cause CNS depression, which may impair physical or mental abilities; patients must be cautioned about performing tasks which require mental alertness (eg, operating machinery or driving).

[US Boxed Warning]: Prolonged use of opioids during pregnancy can cause neonatal withdrawal syndrome, which may be life-threatening if not recognized and treated according to protocols developed by neonatology experts. If opioid use is required for a prolonged period in a pregnant woman, advise the patient of the risk of neonatal opioid withdrawal syndrome and ensure that appropriate treatment will be available. Signs and symptoms include irritability, hyperactivity and abnormal sleep pattern, high-pitched cry, tremor, vomiting, diarrhea, and failure to gain weight. Onset, duration, and severity depend on the drug used, duration of use, maternal dose, and rate of drug elimination by the newborn.

Use with caution in patients with hypersensitivity reactions to other phenanthrene derivative opioid agonists (morphine, hydromorphone, levorphanol, oxycodone, oxymorphone). Abrupt discontinuation in patients who are physically dependent on opioids has been associated with serious withdrawal symptoms, uncontrolled pain, attempts to find other opioids (including illicit), and suicide. Use a collaborative, patient-specific taper schedule that minimizes the risk of withdrawal, considering factors such as current opioid dose, duration of use, type of pain, and physical and psychological factors. Monitor pain control, withdrawal symptoms, mood changes, suicidal ideation, and for use of other substances and provide care as needed. Concurrent use of mixed agonist/antagonist analgesics (eg, pentazocine, nalbuphine, butorphanol) or partial agonist analgesics (eg, buprenorphine) may also precipitate withdrawal symptoms and/or reduced analgesic efficacy in patients following prolonged therapy with mu opioid agonists. **[US Boxed Warning]: Use exposes patients and other users to the risks of addiction, abuse, and misuse, potentially leading to overdose and death. Assess each patient's risk prior to prescribing; monitor all patients regularly for development of these behaviors or conditions. Use with caution in patients with a personal or family history of substance abuse (drugs or alcohol); potential for drug dependency exists. Other factors associated with increased risk include younger age, concomitant mental illness such as depression (major), and psychotropic medication use. Consider offering naloxone prescriptions in patients with factors associated with an increased risk for overdose, such as history of overdose or substance use disorder, higher opioid dosages (≥50 morphine milligram equivalents/day orally), and concomitant benzodiazepine use (Dowell [CDC 2016]).**

Opioid use increases the risk for sleep-related disorders (eg, central sleep apnea [CSA], hypoxemia) in a dose-dependent fashion. Use with caution for chronic pain and titrate dosage cautiously in patients with risk factors for sleep-disordered breathing (eg, heart failure, obesity). Consider dose reduction in patients presenting with CSA. Avoid opioids in patients with moderate to severe sleep-disordered breathing (Dowell [CDC 2016]). Use caution in patients with adrenal insufficiency (including Addison disease), biliary tract impairment, acute pancreatitis, delirium tremens, history of seizure disorders, alcoholic liver disease, toxic psychosis, thyroid dysfunction, prostatic hyperplasia and/or urinary stricture, hepatic and/or renal disease, and in cachectic or debilitated patients. Hydrocodone may cause constipation which may be problematic in patients with unstable angina and patients post-myocardial infarction. Use with extreme caution in patients with head injury, intracranial lesions, or elevated intracranial pressure; exaggerated elevation of ICP may occur. Use with caution in patients who are morbidly obese. May obscure diagnosis or clinical course of patients with acute abdominal conditions. Use with caution in patients with underlying intestinal motility disorders; may result in constipation or obstructive bowel disease. Use is contraindicated with known or suspected GI obstruction, including paralytic ileus. Use with caution in elderly patients; may be more sensitive to adverse effects; use opioids for chronic pain with caution in this age group; monitor closely due to an increased potential for risks, including certain risks such as falls/fracture, cognitive impairment, and constipation. Clearance may also be reduced in older adults (with or without renal impairment) resulting in a narrow therapeutic window and increasing the risk for respiratory depression or overdose (Dowell [CDC 2016]).

[US Boxed Warning]: Concomitant use of opioids with benzodiazepines or other CNS depressants, including alcohol, may result in profound sedation, respiratory depression, coma, and death. Reserve concomitant prescribing of hydrocodone/acetaminophen and benzodiazepines or other CNS depressants for use in patients for whom alternative treatment options are inadequate. Limit dosage and durations to the minimum required and follow patients for signs and symptoms of respiratory depression and sedation. [US Boxed Warning]: Use with all CYP3A4 inhibitors may result in an increase in hydrocodone plasma concentrations, which could increase or prolong adverse drug effects and may cause potentially fatal respiratory depression. In addition, discontinuation of a concomitantly used CYP3A4 inducer may result in increased hydrocodone plasma concentrations. Monitor patients receiving hydrocodone/acetaminophen and any CYP3A4 inhibitor or inducer for signs of respiratory depression or sedation. Potentially significant interactions may exist, requiring dose or frequency adjustment, additional monitoring, and/or selection of alternative therapy.

Rarely, acetaminophen may cause serious and potentially fatal skin reactions such as acute generalized exanthematous pustulosis, Stevens-Johnson syndrome, and toxic epidermal necrolysis. Discontinue treatment if severe skin reactions develop.

Due to the role of CYP2D6 in the metabolism of hydrocodone to hydromorphone (an active metabolite with higher binding affinity to mu-opioid receptors compared to hydrocodone), patients with genetic variations of CYP2D6, including "poor metabolizers" or "extensive metabolizers," may have decreased or increased hydromorphone formation, respectively. Variable effects in positive and negative opioid effects have been reported in these patients; however, limited data exists to determine if clinically significant differences of analgesia and toxicity can be predicted based on CYP2D6 phenotype (Hutchinson 2004; Otton 1993; Zhou 2009).

[US Boxed Warning]: Acetaminophen has been associated with cases of acute liver failure, at times resulting in liver transplant and death. Most of the cases of liver injury are associated with the use of acetaminophen at doses that exceed >4 g/day, and often involve more than one acetaminophen-containing product. Risk is increased with alcohol use and preexisting liver disease. Chronic daily dosing in adults has also resulted in liver damage in some patients. Hypersensitivity and anaphylactic reactions have been reported with acetaminophen use; discontinue immediately if symptoms of allergic or hypersensitivity reactions occur. Use acetaminophen caution in patients with known G6PD deficiency. Limit acetaminophen dose from all sources (prescription and OTC) to <4 g/day in adults.

[US Boxed Warning]: To ensure that the benefits of opioid analgesics outweigh the risks of addiction, abuse, and misuse, a REMS is required. Drug companies with approved opioid analgesic products must make REMS-compliant education programs available to health care providers. Health care providers are encouraged to complete a REMS-compliant education program; counsel patients and/or their caregivers, with every prescription, on safe use, serious risks, storage, and disposal of these products; emphasize to patients and their

caregivers the importance of reading the Medication Guide every time it is provided by their pharmacist; and consider other tools to improve patient, household, and community safety.

An opioid-containing analgesic regimen should be tailored to each patient's needs and based upon the type of pain being treated (acute versus chronic), the route of administration, degree of tolerance for opioids (naive versus chronic user), age, weight, and medical condition. The optimal analgesic dose varies widely among patients; doses should be titrated to pain relief/prevention. Opioids decrease bowel motility; monitor for decreased bowel motility in postop patients receiving opioids. Use with caution in the perioperative setting; individualize treatment when transitioning from parenteral to oral analgesics. Some dosage forms may contain propylene glycol; large amounts are potentially toxic and have been associated hyperosmolality, lactic acidosis, seizures and respiratory depression; use caution (AAP 1997; Zar 2007).

Chronic pain: Opioids should not be used as first-line therapy for chronic pain management (pain >3-month duration or beyond time of normal tissue healing) due to limited short-term benefits, undetermined long-term benefits, and association with serious risks (eg, overdose, MI, auto accidents, risk of developing opioid use disorder). Preferred management includes nonpharmacologic therapy and nonopioid therapy (eg, nonsteroidal anti-inflammatory drugs, acetaminophen, certain anticonvulsants and antidepressants). If opioid therapy is initiated, it should be combined with nonpharmacologic and nonopioid therapy, as appropriate. Prior to initiation, known risks of opioid therapy should be discussed and realistic treatment goals for pain/function should be established, including consideration for discontinuation if benefits do not outweigh risks. Therapy should be continued only if clinically meaningful improvement in pain/function outweighs risks. Therapy should be initiated at the lowest effective dosage using immediate-release opioids (instead of extended-release/long-acting opioids). Risk associated with use increases with higher opioid dosages. Risks and benefits should be re-evaluated when increasing dosage to ≥50 morphine milligram equivalents/day; dosages ≥90 morphine milligram equivalents/day should be avoided unless carefully justified (Dowell [CDC 2016]).

Warnings: Additional Pediatric Considerations

Hepatoxicity has been reported in patients using acetaminophen. In pediatric patients, this is most commonly associated with supratherapeutic dosing, more frequent administration than recommended, and use of multiple acetaminophen-containing products; however, hepatotoxicity has been rarely reported with recommended dosages (AAP [Sullivan 2011]; Heard 2014). All sources of acetaminophen (eg, prescription, OTC, combination) should be considered when evaluating a patient's maximum daily dose. To lower the risk for hepatotoxicity, the maximum daily acetaminophen dose should be limited to ≤75 mg/kg/day (maximum of 5 daily doses), not to exceed 4,000 mg/day (AAP [Sullivan 2011]; Heard 2014; Krenzelok 2012; Lavonas 2010). Acetaminophen avoidance or a lower total daily dose (2,000 to 3,000 mg/day) has been suggested for adults with increased risk for acetaminophen hepatotoxicity (eg, malnutrition, certain liver diseases, use of drugs that interact with acetaminophen metabolism); similar data are unavailable in pediatric patients (Hayward 2016; Larson 2007; Worriax 2007).

Infants born to women physically dependent on opioids will also be physically dependent and may experience respiratory difficulties or opioid withdrawal symptoms (neonatal abstinence syndrome [NAS]). Onset, duration, and severity of NAS depend upon the drug used (maternal), duration of use, maternal dose, and rate of drug elimination by the newborn. Symptoms of opioid withdrawal may include excessive crying, diarrhea, fever, hyper-reflexia, irritability, tremors, or vomiting or failure to gain weight. Opioid withdrawal syndrome in the neonate may be life-threatening and should be promptly treated.

Some dosage forms may contain propylene glycol; in neonates large amounts of propylene glycol delivered orally, intravenously (eg, >3,000 mg/day), or topically have been associated with potentially fatal toxicities which can include metabolic acidosis, seizures, renal failure, and CNS depression; toxicities have also been reported in children and adults including hyperosmolality, lactic acidosis, seizures and respiratory depression; use caution (AAP 1997; Shehab 2009).

Drug Interactions

Metabolism/Transport Effects Refer to individual components.

Avoid Concomitant Use

Avoid concomitant use of Hydrocodone and Acetaminophen with any of the following: Abametapir; Alcohol (Ethyl); Azelastine (Nasal); Bromperidol; Conivaptan; Eluxadoline; Fusidic Acid (Systemic); Idelalisib; Opioids (Mixed Agonist / Antagonist); Orphenadrine; Oxomemazine; Paraldehyde; Thalidomide

Increased Effect/Toxicity

Hydrocodone and Acetaminophen may increase the levels/effects of: Alvimopan; Azelastine (Nasal); Blonanserin; Busulfan; Dasatinib; Desmopressin; Diuretics; Eluxadoline; Flunitrazepam; Imatinib; Local Anesthetics; Methotrimeprazine; MetyroSINE; Mipomersen; Opioid Agonists; Orphenadrine; OxyCODONE; Paraldehyde; Phenylephrine (Systemic); Piribedil; Pramipexole; Prilocaine; Ramosetron; ROPINIRole; Rotigotine; Serotonergic Agents (High Risk); Sodium Nitrite; SORAfenib; Suvorexant; Thalidomide; Vitamin K Antagonists; Zolpidem

The levels/effects of Hydrocodone and Acetaminophen may be increased by: Abametapir; Alcohol (Ethyl); Alizapride; Amphetamines; Anticholinergic Agents; Aprepitant; Brimonidine (Topical); Bromopride; Bromperidol; Cannabidiol; Cannabis; Chlormethiazole; Chlorphenesin Carbamate; Clofazimine; CNS Depressants; Conivaptan; CYP3A4 Inhibitors (Moderate); CYP3A4 Inhibitors (Strong); Dapsone (Topical); Dasatinib; Dimethindene (Topical); Dronabinol; Droperidol; Duvelisib; Erdafitinib; Flucloxacillin; Fosaprepitant; Fosnetupitant; Fusidic Acid (Systemic); Idelalisib; Isoniazid; Kava Kava; Larotrectinib; Lemborexant; Lisuride; Lofexidine; Magnesium Sulfate; Methotrimeprazine; Metoclopramide; MetyraPONE; MiFEPRIStone; Minocycline (Systemic); Monoamine Oxidase Inhibitors; Nabilone; Netupitant; Nitric Oxide; Ombitasvir, Paritaprevir, and Ritonavir; Ombitasvir, Paritaprevir, Ritonavir, and Dasabuvir; Oxomemazine; Palbociclib; Perampanel; PHENobarbital; Primidone; Probenecid; Rufinamide; Simeprevir; Sodium Oxybate; SORAfenib; Stiripentol; Succinylcholine; Tetrahydrocannabinol; Tetrahydrocannabinol and Cannabidiol

Decreased Effect

Hydrocodone and Acetaminophen may decrease the levels/effects of: Diuretics; Gastrointestinal Agents (Prokinetic); Pegvisomant; Sincalide

The levels/effects of Hydrocodone and Acetaminophen may be decreased by: CarBAMazepine; CYP2D6 Inhibitors (Strong); CYP3A4 Inducers (Moderate); CYP3A4 Inducers (Strong); Dabrafenib; Deferasirox; Enzalutamide; Erdafitinib; Fosphenytoin-Phenytoin; Isoniazid; Ivosidenib; Lorlatinib; Mitotane; Nalmefene; Naltrexone; Opioids (Mixed Agonist / Antagonist); PHENobarbital; Primidone; Sarilumab; Siltuximab; Tocilizumab

Pharmacodynamics/Kinetics

Half-life Elimination Hydrocodone: ~4 hours

Time to Peak

Hydrocodone: Serum: ~1 hour

Reproductive Considerations

Long-term opioid use may cause secondary hypogonadism, which may lead to sexual dysfunction or infertility in men and women (Brennan 2013).

Pregnancy Considerations

[US Boxed Warning]: Prolonged use of opioids during pregnancy can cause neonatal withdrawal syndrome, which may be life-threatening if not recognized and treated according to protocols developed by neonatology experts. If opioid use is required for a prolonged period in a pregnant woman, advise the patient of the risk of neonatal opioid withdrawal syndrome and ensure that appropriate treatment will be available.

Refer to individual monographs for additional information.

Breastfeeding Considerations

Acetaminophen and hydrocodone are present in breast milk. According to the manufacturer, the decision to continue or discontinue breastfeeding during therapy should take into account the risk of infant exposure, the benefits of breastfeeding to the infant, and benefits of treatment to the mother. See individual agents.

Controlled Substance C-II

Dosage Forms: US

Elixir, oral:

Lortab: Hydrocodone bitartrate 10 mg and acetaminophen 300 mg per 15 mL (473 mL) [contains ethanol 7%, propylene glycol; tropical fruit punch flavor]

Solution, oral:

Generic: Hydrocodone 7.5 mg and acetaminophen 325 mg per 15 mL; 10 mg and acetaminophen 325 mg per 15 mL

Tablet, oral:

Brands:

Lorcet: Hydrocodone 5 mg and acetaminophen 325 mg

Lorcet HD: Hydrocodone 10 mg and acetaminophen 325 mg

Lorcet Plus: Hydrocodone 7.5 mg and acetaminophen 325 mg

Norco: Hydrocodone 5 mg and acetaminophen 325 mg; hydrocodone 7.5 mg and acetaminophen 325 mg; hydrocodone 10 mg and acetaminophen 325 mg

Verdrocet: Hydrocodone 2.5 mg and acetaminophen 325 mg

Vicodin: Hydrocodone 5 mg and acetaminophen 300 mg

Vicodin ES: Hydrocodone 7.5 mg and acetaminophen 300 mg

Vicodin HP: Hydrocodone 10 mg and acetaminophen 300 mg

Xodol: 7.5/300: Hydrocodone 7.5 mg and acetaminophen 300 mg; 10/300: Hydrocodone 10 mg and acetaminophen 300 mg

Generics:

Hydrocodone 2.5 mg and acetaminophen 325 mg
Hydrocodone 5 mg and acetaminophen 300 mg
Hydrocodone 5 mg and acetaminophen 325 mg
Hydrocodone 7.5 mg and acetaminophen 300 mg
Hydrocodone 7.5 mg and acetaminophen 325 mg
Hydrocodone 10 mg and acetaminophen 300 mg
Hydrocodone 10 mg and acetaminophen 325 mg

Dental Health Professional Considerations

Although the ***OTC product labeling*** for acetaminophen products state to limit the maximum dose to 3,000 mg daily (for extra strength) or 3,250 mg (for regular strength) (see this site for details: http://www.-tylenolprofessional.com/products-and-dosages.html), it is still appropriate for patients to take up to 4,000 mg daily "under the direction of a health care provider" (http://www.tylenolprofessional.com/dosage.html).

Neither hydrocodone nor acetaminophen elicit anti-inflammatory effects. Because of addiction liability of opioid analgesics, the use of hydrocodone should be limited to 2-3 days postoperatively for treatment of dental pain. Nausea is the most common adverse effect seen after use in dental patients; sedation and constipation are second. Nausea elicited by opioid analgesics is centrally mediated and the presence or absence of food will not affect the degree nor incidence of nausea.

The acetaminophen component requires use with caution in patients who use alcohol, with preexisting liver disease, and those receiving more than one source of acetaminophen-containing medication.

Hepatotoxicity caused by acetaminophen is potentiated by chronic alcohol consumption. People who are taking acetaminophen, even at therapeutic doses, and consume alcohol are at risk of developing hepatotoxicity.

Acetaminophen may increase the levels and enhance the anticoagulant effects of vitamin K antagonists acenocoumarol and warfarin (Coumadin®). Studies have reported that acetaminophen has increased the INR in warfarin treated patients with daily acetaminophen doses as low as 2 g, particularly when taking acetaminophen for >1 week (Antlitz, 1968; Boeijinga, 1982; Gebauer, 2003; Hylek, 1998; Rubin, 1984). In addition, case reports of bleeding as a result of increased INR have been published (Bagheri, 1999; Bartle, 1991). There is no known mechanism of the interaction; furthermore, some studies have failed to demonstrate this interaction (Gadisseur, 2003; Kwan, 1995; van den Bemt, 2002). In terms of risk, the data suggest that acetaminophen and warfarin could interact in some clinically significant manner but that the benefits of concomitant use of acetaminophen for pain control in dental patients taking warfarin usually outweigh the risks. An appropriate monitoring plan should be in place to identify potential negative effects and dosage adjustments may be necessary in a minority of patients. The interaction may be more likely to occur with daily acetaminophen doses of >1.3 g for >1 week.

There are no reports of acetaminophen interacting with antiplatelet drugs such as aspirin, clopidogrel (Plavix®), or prasugrel (Effient™). Also, there are no reports of acetaminophen in combination with hydrocodone, codeine, or oxycodone interacting with warfarin (Coumadin®).

Hydrocodone and Ibuprofen

(hye droe KOE done & eye byoo PROE fen)

Related Information

Ibuprofen *on page 786*

Oral Pain *on page 1734*

Related Sample Prescriptions

Oral Pain - Sample Prescriptions *on page 30*

Brand Names: US Ibudone [DSC]; Reprexain [DSC]; Xylon [DSC]

Brand Names: Canada Vicoprofen

Generic Availability (US) Yes

Pharmacologic Category Analgesic Combination (Opioid); Nonsteroidal Anti-inflammatory Drug (NSAID), Oral

Dental Use Short-term management (generally <10 days) of moderate-to-severe acute postoperative dental pain where an anti-inflammatory effect is desired

Use

Pain management: Short-term (generally <10 days) management of acute pain severe enough to require an opioid analgesic and for which alternative treatments are inadequate.

Limitations of use: Do not use hydrocodone/ibuprofen for the treatment of conditions such as osteoarthritis or rheumatoid arthritis. Reserve hydrocodone/ibuprofen for use in patients for whom alternative treatment options (eg, nonopioid analgesics) are ineffective, not tolerated, or would be otherwise inadequate to provide sufficient management of pain.

Local Anesthetic/Vasoconstrictor Precautions No information available to require special precautions

Effects on Dental Treatment Key adverse event(s) related to dental treatment: Xerostomia (normal salivary flow resumes upon discontinuation). See Effects on Bleeding.

Effects on Bleeding Nonselective NSAIDs such as ibuprofen inhibit platelet aggregation and prolong bleeding time in some patients. Unlike aspirin, the NSAID effect on platelet function is quantitatively less, of shorter duration, and reversible.

Adverse Reactions

>10%:

Central nervous system: Headache (27%), drowsiness (22%), dizziness (14%)

Gastrointestinal: Constipation (22%), nausea (21%), dyspepsia (12%)

1% to 10%:

Cardiovascular: Edema (3% to 9%), palpitations (<3%), vasodilation (<3%)

Central nervous system: Anxiety (3% to 9%), insomnia (3% to 9%), nervousness (3% to 9%), abnormality in thinking (<3%), confusion (<3%), hypertonia (<3%), pain (<3%), paresthesia (<3%)

Dermatologic: Diaphoresis (3% to 9%), pruritus (3% to 9%)

Endocrine & metabolic: Increased thirst (<3%)

Gastrointestinal: Abdominal pain (3% to 9%), diarrhea (3% to 9%), flatulence (3% to 9%), hiccups (3% to 9%), vomiting (3% to 9%), xerostomia (3% to 9%), anorexia (<3%), gastritis (<3%), melena (<3%), oral mucosa ulcer (<3%)

Infection: Infection (3% to 9%)

Neuromuscular & skeletal: Weakness (3% to 9%)

Otic: Tinnitus (<3%)

Renal: Polyuria (<3%)

Respiratory: Flu-like symptoms (3% to 9%), dyspnea (<3%), pharyngitis (<3%), rhinitis (<3%)

Miscellaneous: Fever (<3%)

<1%, postmarketing, and/or case reports: Abnormal dreams, agitation, arthralgia, asthma, bronchitis, cardiac arrhythmia, chalky stools, cough, cystitis, decreased libido, depression, drug dependence (with prolonged use), dry eye syndrome, dysphagia, esophageal spasm, esophagitis, euphoria, exfoliative dermatitis, gastroenteritis, gastrointestinal hemorrhage, gastrointestinal perforation, GI inflammation, glossitis, glycosuria, hepatotoxicity (idiosyncratic) (Chalasani, 2014), hoarseness, hypersensitivity reaction, hypertension, hypogonadism (Brennan, 2013; Debono, 2011), hypotension, impotence, increased liver enzymes, mood changes, myalgia, neuralgia, pneumonia, pulmonary congestion, respiratory depression, sinusitis, skin rash, slurred speech, Stevens-Johnson syndrome, tachycardia, teeth clenching, toxic epidermal necrolysis, tremor, ulcer, unpleasant taste, urinary incontinence, urinary retention, urticaria, vertigo, visual disturbance, weight loss

Dental Usual Dosage Moderate-to-severe acute postoperative dental pain: Adults: Oral: 1-2 tablets every 4-6 hours as needed for pain; maximum: 5 tablets/day

Dosing

Adult

Pain management: Oral: One tablet (hydrocodone 5 mg to 10 mg/ibuprofen 200 mg) every 4 to 6 hours as needed; (maximum: 5 tablets [hydrocodone 25 to 50 mg/ibuprofen 1,000 mg] per 24 hours). **Note:** Short-term use is recommended (<10 days total therapy).

Discontinuation of therapy: When discontinuing chronic opioid therapy, the dose should be gradually tapered down. An optimal universal tapering schedule for all patients has not been established (CDC [Dowell 2016]). Proposed schedules range from slow (eg, 10% reductions per week) to rapid (eg, 25% to 50% reduction every few days) (CDC 2015). Tapering schedules should be individualized to minimize opioid withdrawal while considering patient-specific goals and concerns as well as the pharmacokinetics of the opioid being tapered. An even slower taper may be appropriate in patients who have been receiving opioids for a long duration (eg, years), particularly in the final stage of tapering, whereas more rapid tapers may be appropriate in patients experiencing severe adverse events (CDC [Dowell 2016]). Monitor carefully for signs/symptoms of withdrawal. If the patient displays withdrawal symptoms, consider slowing the taper schedule; alterations may include increasing the interval between dose reductions, decreasing amount of daily dose reduction, pausing the taper and restarting when the patient is ready, and/or coadministration of an alpha-2 agonist (eg, clonidine) to blunt withdrawal symptoms (Berna 2015; CDC [Dowell 2016]). Continue to offer nonopioid analgesics as needed for pain management during the taper; consider nonopioid adjunctive treatments for withdrawal symptoms (eg, GI complaints, muscle spasm) as needed (Berna 2015; Sevarino 2018).

Geriatric Refer to adult dosing. Initiate dosing at the lower end of the dosage range. Monitor closely.

Renal Impairment: Adult There are no dosage adjustments provided in the manufacturer's labeling. Initiate therapy with a low dose and monitor closely. Avoid use in advanced renal disease.

Hepatic Impairment: Adult There are no dosage adjustments provided in the manufacturer's labeling; use with caution; initiate therapy with a low dose and monitor closely in severe impairment.

Pediatric Pain management: Oral: Adolescents ≥16 years: Refer to adult dosing.

Renal Impairment: Pediatric There are no dosage adjustments provided in the manufacturer's labeling. Initiate therapy with a low dose and monitor closely. Avoid use in advanced renal disease.

Hepatic Impairment: Pediatric There are no dosage adjustments provided in the manufacturer's labeling; use with caution; initiate therapy with a low dose and monitor closely in severe impairment.

Mechanism of Action

Hydrocodone: Binds to opiate receptors in the CNS, altering the perception of and response to pain; suppresses cough in medullary center; produces generalized CNS depression

Ibuprofen: Reversibly inhibits cyclooxygenase-1 and 2 (COX-1 and 2) enzymes, which result in decreased formation of prostaglandin precursors; has antipyretic, analgesic, and anti-inflammatory properties

Contraindications

Hypersensitivity (eg, anaphylactic reactions, serious skin reactions) to hydrocodone, ibuprofen, or any component of the formulation; significant respiratory depression; acute or severe bronchial asthma in an unmonitored setting or in the absence of resuscitative equipment; GI obstruction, including paralytic ileus (known or suspected); history of asthma, urticaria, or allergic-type reactions to aspirin or other NSAIDs; in the setting of coronary artery bypass graft (CABG) surgery.

Documentation of allergenic cross-reactivity for opioids is limited. However, because of similarities in chemical structure and/or pharmacologic actions, the possibility of cross-sensitivity cannot be ruled out with certainty.

Warnings/Precautions **[US Boxed Warning]: Serious, life-threatening, or fatal respiratory depression may occur. Monitor closely for respiratory depression, especially during initiation or dose escalation.** Carbon dioxide retention from opioid-induced respiratory depression can exacerbate the sedating effects of opioids. Use with caution and monitor for respiratory depression in patients with significant chronic obstructive pulmonary disease or cor pulmonale, and those having a substantially decreased respiratory reserve, hypoxia, hypercarbia, or preexisting respiratory depression, particularly when initiating therapy and titrating therapy; critical respiratory depression may occur, even at therapeutic dosages. Consider the use of alternative nonopioid analgesics in these patients. Avoid use in patients with impaired consciousness or coma as these patients are susceptible to intracranial effects of carbon dioxide retention. **[US Boxed Warning]: Concomitant use of opioids with benzodiazepines or other CNS depressants, including alcohol, may result in profound sedation, respiratory depression, coma, and death. Reserve concomitant prescribing of hydrocodone/ibuprofen and benzodiazepines or other CNS depressants for use in patients for whom alternative treatment options are inadequate. Limit dosage and durations to the minimum required and follow patients for signs and symptoms of respiratory depression and sedation. [US Boxed Warning]: Use with all CYP3A4 inhibitors may result in an increase in hydrocodone plasma concentrations, which could increase or prolong adverse drug effects and may cause potentially fatal respiratory depression. In addition, discontinuation of a concomitant CYP3A4 inducer may result in increased hydrocodone concentrations. Monitor patients receiving hydrocodone/ibuprofen and any CYP3A4 inhibitor or inducer.** Potentially significant interactions may exist, requiring dose or frequency adjustment, additional monitoring, and/or selection of alternative therapy. **[US Boxed Warning]: Use exposes patients and other users to the risks of addiction, abuse, and misuse, potentially leading to overdose and death. Assess each patient's risk prior to prescribing; monitor all patients regularly for development of these behaviors or conditions.** Use with caution in patients with a history of drug abuse or acute alcoholism; potential for drug dependency exists. Other factors associated with increased risk include younger age, concomitant depression (major), and psychotropic medication use. **[US Boxed Warning]: Accidental ingestion of even one dose, especially in children, can result in a fatal overdose of hydrocodone.**

Even in patients without prior exposure anaphylactoid reactions may occur; patients with "aspirin triad" (bronchial asthma, aspirin intolerance, rhinitis) may be at increased risk. Contraindicated in patients who experience bronchospasm, asthma, rhinitis, or urticaria with NSAID or aspirin therapy. Avoid chronic use of oral nonselective NSAIDs in patients who have undergone bariatric surgery; development of anastomotic ulcerations/perforations may occur. **[US Boxed Warning]: NSAIDs cause an increased risk of serious (and potentially fatal) adverse cardiovascular thrombotic events, including fatal MI and stroke. Risk may occur early during treatment and may increase with duration of use.** Relative risk appears to be similar in those with and without known cardiovascular disease or risk factors for cardiovascular disease; however, absolute incidence of cardiovascular events (which may occur early during treatment) was higher in patients with known cardiovascular disease or risk factors. New-onset hypertension or exacerbation of hypertension may occur (NSAIDS may also impair response to ACE inhibitors, thiazide diuretics, or loop diuretics); may contribute to cardiovascular events; monitor blood pressure; use with caution in patients with hypertension. May cause sodium and fluid retention; use with caution in patients with edema. Avoid use in heart failure (ACCF/AHA [Yancy 2013]). Avoid use in patients with a recent MI unless benefits outweigh risk of cardiovascular thrombotic events. Use the lowest effective dose for the shortest duration of time, consistent with individual patient goals, to reduce risk of cardiovascular events; alternate therapies should be considered for patients at high risk. **[US Boxed Warning]: NSAIDs cause an increased risk of serious GI inflammation, ulceration, bleeding, and perforation (may be fatal); elderly patients and patients with history of peptic ulcer disease and/or GI bleeding are at greater risk for serious GI events. These events may occur at any time during therapy and without warning.** Avoid use in patients with active GI bleeding. In patients with a history of acute lower GI bleeding, avoid use of non-aspirin NSAIDs, especially if due to angioectasia or diverticulosis (Strate 2016). Use caution with a history of GI ulcers, concurrent therapy known to increase the risk of GI bleeding (eg, aspirin, anticoagulants and/or corticosteroids, selective serotonin reuptake inhibitors), advanced hepatic disease, coagulopathy, smoking, use of alcohol, or in elderly or debilitated patients. Use the lowest effective dose for the shortest duration of time, consistent with individual patient goals, to reduce risk of GI adverse events; alternate therapies should be considered for patients at high risk. When used concomitantly with aspirin, a substantial increase in the risk of GI complications (eg, ulcer) occurs; concomitant gastroprotective therapy (eg, proton pump inhibitors) is recommended (Bhatt 2008). Platelet adhesion and aggregation may be decreased; may prolong bleeding time; patients with coagulation disorders or who are receiving anticoagulants should be monitored closely. Anemia may occur; patients on long-term NSAID therapy should be monitored for anemia. Rarely, NSAID use has been associated with potentially severe blood dyscrasias (eg, agranulocytosis, thrombocytopenia, aplastic anemia). Transaminase elevations have been reported with use; closely monitor patients with any abnormal LFT. Rare (sometimes fatal) severe hepatic reactions (eg, fulminant hepatitis, liver necrosis, hepatic failure) have occurred with NSAID use; discontinue immediately if signs or symptoms of hepatic disease develop or if systemic manifestations occur. NSAID use may increase the risk of hyperkalemia, particularly in the elderly, diabetics, renal disease, and with concomitant use of other agents capable of inducing hyperkalemia (eg, ACE-inhibitors). Monitor potassium closely. Blurred/diminished vision, scotomata, and changes in color vision have been reported with ibuprofen. Discontinue therapy and refer for ophthalmologic evaluation if symptoms occur. NSAID use may compromise existing renal function; dose-dependent decreases in prostaglandin synthesis may result from NSAID use, reducing renal blood flow which may cause renal decompensation (usually reversible). Patients with impaired renal function, dehydration, hypovolemia, heart failure, hepatic impairment, those taking diuretics and ACE inhibitors, and the elderly are at greater risk of renal toxicity. Rehydrate patient before starting therapy; monitor renal function closely. Long-term NSAID use may result in renal papillary necrosis and other renal injury. **[US Boxed Warning]: Use is contraindicated in the setting of coronary artery bypass graft (CABG) surgery.** Risk of MI and stroke may be increased with use following CABG surgery. Clinical or population-based data regarding the risks of NSAIDs in the setting of coronavirus disease 2019 (COVID-19) are limited (FDA Safety Communication 2020; Kim 2020). Some experts recommend the use of acetaminophen as the preferred antipyretic agent, when possible, and if NSAIDs are needed, to use the lowest effective dose and shortest duration (EMA 2020; Kim 2020). In general, for patients already taking an NSAID for a comorbid condition, it is recommended to continue the NSAID as directed by their health care provider (EMA 2020; NIH 2020; WHO 2020). NSAIDs may cause serious skin adverse events including exfoliative dermatitis, Stevens-Johnson syndrome (SJS), and toxic epidermal necrolysis (TEN), which can be fatal and may occur without warning; discontinue use at first sign of skin rash (or any other hypersensitivity). NSAIDs may increase the risk of aseptic meningitis, especially in patients with systemic lupus erythematosus (SLE) and mixed connective tissue disorders. NSAID use may compromise existing renal function. Avoid use in patients with advanced renal disease.

May cause CNS depression, which may impair physical or mental abilities; patients must be cautioned about performing tasks which require mental alertness (eg, operating machinery or driving). May cause severe hypotension (including orthostatic hypotension and syncope); use with caution in patients with hypovolemia, cardiovascular disease (including acute MI), or drugs which may exaggerate hypotensive effects (including phenothiazines or general anesthetics). Monitor for symptoms of hypotension following initiation or dose titration. Avoid use in patients with circulatory shock. Use with caution in patients with hypersensitivity reactions to other phenanthrene derivative opioid agonists (codeine, hydromorphone, levorphanol, oxycodone, oxymorphone). May obscure diagnosis or clinical course of patients with acute abdominal conditions. Use with caution in patients who are morbidly obese (APS 2008). Use with caution in patients with adrenocortical insufficiency (including Addison disease), asthma, biliary tract dysfunction or including acute pancreatitis, delirium tremens, head injury, intracranial lesions, or elevated intracranial pressure (ICP); hepatic impairment; prostatic hyperplasia and/or urinary stricture; toxic psychosis; history of seizure disorder; and/or thyroid dysfunction. Use with caution in cachectic or debilitated patients and in the elderly; consider the use of alternative nonopioid analgesics in these patients. Opioid clearance may be reduced in older adults (with or without renal impairment) resulting in a narrow therapeutic window and increasing the risk for respiratory depression or overdose (CDC [Dowell 2016]). Opioid use increases the risk for sleep-related disorders (eg, central sleep apnea [CSA], hypoxemia) in a dose-dependent fashion. Use with caution for chronic pain and titrate dosage cautiously in patients with risk factors for sleep-disordered breathing (eg, heart failure, obesity). Consider dose reduction in patients presenting with CSA. Avoid opioids in patients with moderate to severe sleep-disordered breathing (CDC [Dowell 2016]).

Due to the role of CYP2D6 in the metabolism of hydrocodone to hydromorphone (an active metabolite with higher binding affinity to mu-opioid receptors compared to hydrocodone), patients with genetic variations of CYP2D6, including "poor metabolizers" or "extensive metabolizers," may have decreased or increased hydromorphone formation, respectively. Variable effects in positive and negative opioid effects have been reported in these patients; however, limited data exists to determine if clinically significant differences of analgesia and toxicity can be predicted based on CYP2D6 phenotype (Hutchinson 2004; Otton 1993; Zhou 2009).

[US Boxed Warning]: Prolonged use of opioids during pregnancy can cause neonatal withdrawal syndrome, which may be life-threatening if not recognized and treated according to protocols developed by neonatology experts. If opioid use is required for a prolonged period in a pregnant woman, advise the patient of the risk of neonatal opioid withdrawal syndrome and ensure that appropriate treatment will be available. Signs and symptoms include irritability, hyperactivity and abnormal sleep pattern, high-pitched cry, tremor, vomiting, diarrhea, and failure to gain weight. Onset, duration, and severity depend on the drug used, duration of use, maternal dose, and rate of drug elimination by the newborn.

An opioid-containing analgesic regimen should be tailored to each patient's needs and based upon the type of pain being treated (acute versus chronic), the route of administration, degree of tolerance for opioids (naive versus chronic user), age, weight, and medical condition. The optimal analgesic dose varies widely among patients; doses should be titrated to pain relief/prevention. **To ensure that the benefits of opioid analgesics outweigh the risks of addiction, abuse, and misuse, a REMS is required. Drug companies with approved opioid analgesic products must make REMS-compliant education programs available to health care providers. Health care providers are encouraged to complete a REMS-compliant education program; counsel patients and/or their caregivers, with every prescription, on safe use, serious risks, storage, and disposal of these products; emphasize to patients and their caregivers the importance of reading the Medication Guide every time it is provided by their pharmacist; and consider other tools to improve patient, household, and community safety.** Withhold for at least 4 to 6 half-lives prior to surgical or dental procedures (Douketis 2008). Opioids decrease bowel motility; monitor for decrease bowel motility in postop patients receiving opioids. Use with caution in the perioperative setting; individualize treatment when transitioning from parenteral to oral analgesics. Abrupt discontinuation in patients who are physically dependent on opioids has been associated with serious withdrawal symptoms, uncontrolled pain, attempts to find other opioids (including illicit), and suicide. Use a collaborative, patient-specific taper schedule that minimizes the risk of withdrawal, considering factors such as current opioid dose, duration of use, type of pain, and physical and psychological factors. Monitor pain control, withdrawal symptoms, mood changes, suicidal ideation, and for use of other substances; provide care as needed. Concurrent use of mixed agonist/antagonist analgesics (eg, pentazocine, nalbuphine, butorphanol) or partial agonist (eg, buprenorphine) analgesics may also precipitate withdrawal symptoms and/or reduced analgesic efficacy in patients following prolonged therapy with mu opioid agonists.

Drug Interactions

Metabolism/Transport Effects Refer to individual components.

Avoid Concomitant Use

Avoid concomitant use of Hydrocodone and Ibuprofen with any of the following: Abametapir; Acemetacin; Alcohol (Ethyl); Aminolevulinic Acid (Systemic); Azelastine (Nasal); Bromperidol; Conivaptan; Dexibuprofen; Dexketoprofen; Eluxadoline; Floctafenine; Fusidic Acid (Systemic); Idelalisib; Ketorolac (Nasal); Ketorolac (Systemic); Macimorelin; Mifamurtide; Morniflumate; Nonsteroidal Anti-Inflammatory Agents (COX-2 Selective); Omacetaxine; Opioids (Mixed Agonist / Antagonist); Orphenadrine; Oxomemazine; Paraldehyde; Pelubiprofen; Phenylbutazone; Talniflumate; Tenoxicam; Thalidomide; Urokinase; Zaltoprofen

Increased Effect/Toxicity

Hydrocodone and Ibuprofen may increase the levels/effects of: 5-Aminosalicylic Acid Derivatives; Agents with Antiplatelet Properties; Aliskiren; Alvimopan; Aminoglycosides; Aminolevulinic Acid (Systemic); Aminolevulinic Acid (Topical); Anticoagulants; Apixaban; Azelastine (Nasal); Bemiparin; Bisphosphonate Derivatives; Blonanserin; Cephalothin; Collagenase (Systemic); CycloSPORINE (Systemic); Dabigatran Etexilate; Deferasirox; Deoxycholic Acid; Desmopressin; Dexibuprofen; Dichlorphenamide; Digoxin; Diuretics; Drospirenone; Edoxaban; Eluxadoline; Enoxaparin; Eplerenone; Flunitrazepam; Heparin; Ibritumomab Tiuxetan; Lithium; MetFORMIN; Methotrexate; Methotrimeprazine; MetyroSINE; Nonsteroidal Anti-Inflammatory Agents (COX-2 Selective); Obinutuzumab; Omacetaxine; Opioid Agonists; Orphenadrine; OxyCODONE; Paraldehyde; PEMEtrexed; Piribedil; Porfimer; Potassium-Sparing Diuretics; PRALAtrexate; Pramipexole; Quinolones; Ramosetron; Rivaroxaban; ROPINIRole; Rotigotine; Salicylates; Serotonergic Agents (High Risk); Suvorexant; Tacrolimus (Systemic); Tenofovir Products; Thalidomide; Thrombolytic Agents; Tolperisone; Urokinase; Vancomycin; Verteporfin; Vitamin K Antagonists; Zolpidem

The levels/effects of Hydrocodone and Ibuprofen may be increased by: Abametapir; Acalabrutinib; Acemetacin; Alcohol (Ethyl); Alizapride; Amphetamines; Angiotensin II Receptor Blockers; Angiotensin-Converting Enzyme Inhibitors; Anticholinergic Agents; Aprepitant; Brimonidine (Topical); Bromopride; Bromperidol; Cannabidiol; Cannabis; Chlormethiazole; Chlorphenesin Carbamate; Clofazimine; CNS Depressants; Conivaptan; Corticosteroids (Systemic); CycloSPORINE (Systemic); CYP3A4 Inhibitors (Moderate); CYP3A4 Inhibitors (Strong); Dasatinib; Dexketoprofen; Diclofenac (Systemic); Dimethindene (Topical); Dronabinol; Droperidol; Duvelisib; Erdafitinib; Fat Emulsion (Fish Oil Based); Felbinac; Floctafenine; Fluconazole; Fosaprepitant; Fosnetupitant; Fusidic Acid (Systemic); Glucosamine; Herbs (Anticoagulant/Antiplatelet Properties); Ibrutinib; Idelalisib; Inotersen; Kava Kava; Ketorolac (Nasal); Ketorolac (Systemic); Larotrectinib; Lemborexant; Limaprost; Lisuride; Lofexidine; Loop Diuretics; Magnesium Sulfate; Methotrimeprazine; Metoclopramide; MiFEPRIStone; Minocycline (Systemic); Monoamine Oxidase Inhibitors; Morniflumate; Multivitamins/Fluoride (with ADE); Multivitamins/Minerals (with ADEK, Folate, Iron); Multivitamins/Minerals (with AE, No Iron); Nabilone; Naftazone; Netupitant; Ombitasvir, Paritaprevir, and Ritonavir; Ombitasvir, Paritaprevir, Ritonavir, and Dasabuvir; Omega-3 Fatty Acids; Oxomemazine; Palbociclib; Pelubiprofen; Pentosan Polysulfate Sodium; Pentoxifylline; Perampanel; PHENobarbital; Phenylbutazone; Primidone; Probenecid; Prostacyclin Analogues; Rufinamide; Selective Serotonin Reuptake Inhibitors; Selumetinib; Serotonin/Norepinephrine Reuptake Inhibitors; Simeprevir; Sodium Oxybate; Sodium Phosphates; Stiripentol; Succinylcholine; Talniflumate; Tenoxicam; Tetrahydrocannabinol; Tetrahydrocannabinol and Cannabidiol; Thiazide and Thiazide-Like Diuretics; Tipranavir; Tolperisone; Vitamin E (Systemic); Voriconazole; Zaltoprofen; Zanubrutinib

Decreased Effect

Hydrocodone and Ibuprofen may decrease the levels/effects of: Aliskiren; Angiotensin II Receptor Blockers; Angiotensin-Converting Enzyme Inhibitors; Beta-Blockers; Diuretics; Eplerenone; Gastrointestinal Agents (Prokinetic); HydrALAZINE; Imatinib; Loop Diuretics; Macimorelin; Mifamurtide; Pegvisomant; Potassium-Sparing Diuretics; Prostaglandins (Ophthalmic); Salicylates; Selective Serotonin Reuptake Inhibitors; Sincalide; Thiazide and Thiazide-Like Diuretics

The levels/effects of Hydrocodone and Ibuprofen may be decreased by: Bile Acid Sequestrants; CYP2D6 Inhibitors (Strong); CYP3A4 Inducers (Moderate); CYP3A4 Inducers (Strong); Dabrafenib; Deferasirox; Enzalutamide; Erdafitinib; Ivosidenib; Lumacaftor and Ivacaftor; Mitotane; Nalmefene; Naltrexone; Opioids (Mixed Agonist / Antagonist); PHENobarbital; Primidone; Salicylates; Sarilumab; Siltuximab; Tocilizumab

Food Interactions See individual agents.

Pharmacodynamics/Kinetics

Onset of Action Hydrocodone: Opioid analgesic: 10 to 20 minutes

Duration of Action Hydrocodone: 4 to 8 hours

Half-life Elimination Hydrocodone: 4.5 hours

Time to Peak Hydrocodone: 1.7 hours

Reproductive Considerations

Long-term opioid use may cause secondary hypogonadism, which may lead to sexual dysfunction and infertility (Brennan 2013).

Pregnancy Considerations

[US Boxed Warning]: Prolonged use of opioids during pregnancy can cause neonatal withdrawal syndrome, which may be life-threatening if not recognized and treated according to protocols developed by neonatology experts. If opioid use is required for a prolonged period in a pregnant woman, advise the patient of the risk of neonatal opioid withdrawal syndrome and ensure treatment that appropriate treatment will be available.

Refer to individual monographs for additional information.

Breastfeeding Considerations

Hydrocodone and ibuprofen are excreted in breast milk. According to the manufacturer, the decision to continue or discontinue breastfeeding during therapy should take into account the risk of infant exposure, the benefits of breastfeeding to the infant, and benefits of treatment to the mother. See individual agents.

Controlled Substance C-II

Dosage Forms: US

Tablet, oral:

Xylon: 10/200: Hydrocodone 10 mg and ibuprofen 200 mg

Generic: Hydrocodone 5 mg and ibuprofen 200 mg; Hydrocodone 7.5 mg and ibuprofen 200 mg; Hydrocodone 10 mg and ibuprofen 200 mg

Hydrocodone and Phenyltoloxamine

(hye droe KOE done & fen il to LOKS a meen)

Brand Names: Canada Tussionex [DSC]

Pharmacologic Category Alkylamine Derivative; Analgesic, Opioid; Antitussive; Histamine H_1 Antagonist; Histamine H_1 Antagonist, First Generation

Use Note: Not approved in the US

Cough: Symptomatic relief of exhausting or nonproductive cough associated with cold or upper respiratory allergies that does not respond to nonopioid antitussives

Local Anesthetic/Vasoconstrictor Precautions

No information available to require special precautions

Effects on Dental Treatment No significant effects or complications reported

Effects on Bleeding No information available to require special precautions

Adverse Reactions Frequency not defined.

Cardiovascular: Tachycardia

Central nervous system: Drowsiness, drug dependence, hallucination, seizure

Dermatologic: Facial pruritus

Gastrointestinal: Constipation, nausea

Hypersensitivity: Hypersensitivity reaction

Respiratory: Dyspnea, respiratory depression

Postmarketing and/or case reports: Hypogonadism (Brennan 2013; Debono 2011)

Mechanism of Action

Hydrocodone binds to opiate receptors in the CNS, altering the perception of and response to pain; suppresses cough in medullary center; produces generalized CNS depression.

Phenyltoloxamine competes with histamine for H_1-receptor sites on effector cells. May potentiate the antitussive effects of hydrocodone; sedative effects are also seen.

Pharmacodynamics/Kinetics

Duration of Action Antitussive effects: ≥8 hours

Half-life Elimination Hydrocodone: ~4 hours (Tussionex Pennkinetic US prescribing information 2008).

Reproductive Considerations

Long-term opioid use may cause secondary hypogonadism, which may lead to sexual dysfunction and infertility (Brennan 2013).

Pregnancy Considerations

[Canadian Boxed Warning]: Prolonged use of opioids during pregnancy can cause neonatal withdrawal syndrome, which may be life-threatening if not recognized and treated according to protocols developed by neonatology experts. If opioid use is required for a prolonged period in a pregnant woman, advise the patient of the risk of neonatal opioid withdrawal syndrome and ensure that appropriate treatment will be available.

Product Availability Tussionex represents a different product in Canada than it does in the US. In Canada, Tussionex contains hydrocodone and phenyltoloxamine while in the US Tussionex (Pennkinetic) contains hydrocodone and chlorpheniramine.

Controlled Substance CDSA I

- **Hydrocodone Bit/Acetaminophen** *see* Hydrocodone and Acetaminophen *on page* *764*
- **Hydrocodone Bitartrate and Ibuprofen** *see* Hydrocodone and Ibuprofen *on page* *769*
- **Hydrocodone Bitartrate and Phenyltoloxamine Citrate** *see* Hydrocodone and Phenyltoloxamine *on page* *773*
- **Hydrocodone Bit/Ibuprofen** *see* Hydrocodone and Ibuprofen *on page* *769*
- **Hydrocodone/Ibuprofen** *see* Hydrocodone and Ibuprofen *on page* *769*
- **Hydrocodone Resin Complex and Phenyltoloxamine Resin Complex** *see* Hydrocodone and Phenyltoloxamine *on page* *773*

Hydrocortisone (Systemic)

(hye droe KOR ti sone)

Brand Names: US Cortef; Solu-CORTEF

Brand Names: Canada Cortef; Solu-CORTEF

Pharmacologic Category Corticosteroid, Systemic

Use

Allergic states: Control of severe or incapacitating allergic conditions intractable to adequate trials of conventional treatment in drug hypersensitivity reactions, perennial or seasonal allergic rhinitis, serum sickness, transfusion reactions, or acute noninfectious laryngeal edema (epinephrine is the drug of first choice).

Dermatologic diseases: Atopic dermatitis; bullous dermatitis herpetiformis; contact dermatitis; exfoliative dermatitis; exfoliative erythroderma; pemphigus; severe erythema multiforme (Stevens-Johnson syndrome); severe psoriasis; severe seborrheic dermatitis; mycosis fungoides.

Edematous states: To induce diuresis or remission of proteinuria in the nephrotic syndrome, without uremia, of the idiopathic type or that due to lupus erythematosus.

Endocrine disorders: Acute adrenocortical insufficiency; congenital adrenal hyperplasia; hypercalcemia associated with cancer; nonsuppurative thyroiditis; primary or secondary adrenocortical insufficiency; preoperatively and in the event of serious trauma or illness, in patients with known adrenal insufficiency or when adrenocortical reserve is doubtful; shock unresponsive to conventional therapy if adrenocortical insufficiency exists or is suspected.

GI diseases: To tide the patient over a critical period of the disease in ulcerative colitis and regional enteritis.

Hematologic disorders: Acquired (autoimmune) hemolytic anemia; congenital (erythroid) hypoplastic anemia (Diamond Blackfan anemia); erythroblastopenia (RBC anemia); immune thrombocytopenia (formerly known as idiopathic thrombocytopenic purpura) in adults; pure red cell aplasia; select cases of secondary thrombocytopenia.

Neoplastic diseases: Palliative management of leukemias and lymphomas (adults); acute leukemia of childhood.

Nervous system: Cerebral edema associated with primary or metastatic brain tumor, or craniotomy.

Ophthalmic diseases: Severe acute and chronic allergic and inflammatory processes involving the eye, such as allergic conjunctivitis; allergic corneal marginal ulcers; anterior segment inflammation; chorioretinitis; diffuse posterior uveitis and choroiditis; herpes zoster ophthalmicus; iritis and iridocyclitis; keratitis; optic neuritis; sympathetic ophthalmia; other ocular inflammatory conditions unresponsive to topical corticosteroids.

Respiratory diseases: Aspiration pneumonitis; bronchial asthma; berylliosis; fulminating or disseminated pulmonary tuberculosis when used concurrently with appropriate antituberculous chemotherapy; idiopathic eosinophilic pneumonias; Loeffler syndrome (not manageable by other means); symptomatic sarcoidosis.

Rheumatic disorders: As adjunctive therapy for short-term administration in acute and subacute bursitis, acute gouty arthritis, acute nonspecific tenosynovitis, ankylosing spondylitis, epicondylitis, posttraumatic osteoarthritis, psoriatic arthritis, rheumatoid arthritis, including juvenile rheumatoid arthritis, synovitis of osteoarthritis; during an exacerbation or as maintenance therapy in acute rheumatic carditis, dermatomyositis (polymyositis), temporal arteritis, and systemic lupus erythematosus.

Miscellaneous: Trichinosis with neurologic or myocardial involvement; tuberculous meningitis with subarachnoid block or impending block when used concurrently with appropriate antituberculous chemotherapy.

Local Anesthetic/Vasoconstrictor Precautions No information available to require special precautions

Effects on Dental Treatment No significant effects or complications reported

Effects on Bleeding No information available to require special precautions

Adverse Reactions Frequency not defined.

Cardiovascular: Atheromatous embolism, bradycardia, cardiac arrhythmia, cardiac failure (especially in susceptible patients), cardiomegaly, circulatory shock, hypertension, hypertrophic cardiomyopathy (premature infants), myocardial rupture (post-myocardial infarction), syncope, tachycardia, thromboembolism, thrombophlebitis, vasculitis

Central nervous system: Arachnoiditis (intrathecal administration), depression, emotional lability, euphoria, headache, increased intracranial pressure (with pseudotumor cerebri; usually following discontinuation), insomnia, malaise, meningitis (intrathecal administration), myasthenia, neuritis, neuropathy, paraplegia (intrathecal administration), paresthesia, personality changes, psychic disorder, seizure, sensory disturbance (intrathecal administration), tingling of skin (especially in the perineal area after IV injection), vertigo

Dermatologic: Acne vulgaris, allergic dermatitis, alopecia, atrophic striae, burning sensation of skin (especially in the perineal area after IV injection), diaphoresis, ecchymosis, erythema (including facial), exfoliation of skin, hyperpigmentation, hypertrichosis, hypopigmentation, skin atrophy, skin rash, suppression of skin test reaction, urticaria, xeroderma

Endocrine & metabolic: Adrenal suppression, Cushing syndrome, diabetes mellitus (latent), fluid retention, glycosuria, growth suppression, hirsutism, HPA-axis suppression, hypercalcemia (associated with cancers), hyperglycemia (including increased requirements for insulin or oral hypoglycemic agents in diabetes mellitus), hypokalemia, hypokalemic alkalosis, impaired glucose tolerance, lipodystrophy, lipomatosis (epidural), menstrual disease (menstrual irregularities), moon face, negative nitrogen balance, protein catabolism, sodium retention, weight gain

Gastrointestinal: Abdominal distention, carbohydrate intolerance, dyspepsia, gastrointestinal disease (intrathecal administration), gastrointestinal perforation (small and large intestine, particularly in patients with inflammatory bowel disease), hiccups, increased appetite, nausea, pancreatitis, peptic ulcer (with possible perforation and hemorrhage), ulcerative esophagitis, vomiting

Genitourinary: Asthenospermia, bladder dysfunction (intrathecal administration)

Hematologic & oncologic: Leukocytosis, petechia

Hepatic: Hepatomegaly, increased serum transaminases (usually mild elevations and reversible on discontinuation)

Hypersensitivity: Anaphylaxis, angioedema, hypersensitivity reaction

Infection: Increased susceptibility to infection, infection, sterile abscess

Local: Atrophy at injection site (cutaneous and subcutaneous), postinjection flare (intra-articular use), skin edema

Neuromuscular & skeletal: Amyotrophy, Charcot-like arthropathy, lower extremity weakness (intrathecal administration), osteonecrosis (aseptic necrosis of femoral and humoral heads), osteoporosis, pathological fracture (long bones), rupture of tendon (particularly Achilles tendon), steroid myopathy, vertebral compression fracture

Ophthalmic: Cataract (posterior subcapsular), exophthalmos, glaucoma, increased intraocular pressure, retinopathy (central serous chorioretinopathy)

Respiratory: Pulmonary edema

Miscellaneous: Wound healing impairment

<1%, postmarketing, and/or case reports: Anaphylactoid reaction, blindness (periocular injection)

Mechanism of Action Short-acting corticosteroid with minimal sodium-retaining potential; decreases inflammation by suppression of migration of polymorphonuclear leukocytes and reversal of increased capillary permeability

Pharmacodynamics/Kinetics

Onset of Action IV: 1 hour

Half-life Elimination IV: 2 ± 0.3 hours; Oral: 1.8 ± 0.5 hours (Czock 2005)

Time to Peak Plasma: Oral: 1.2 ± 0.4 hours (Czock 2005)

Pregnancy Considerations

Some studies have shown an association between first trimester systemic corticosteroid use and oral clefts or decreased birth weight; however, information is conflicting and may be influenced by maternal dose/indication for use (Lunghi 2010; Park-Wyllie 2000; Pradat 2003). Hypoadrenalism may occur in newborns following maternal use of corticosteroids in pregnancy; monitor.

When treating women with adrenal insufficiency (primary or central or congenital adrenal hyperplasia) during pregnancy, hydrocortisone is the preferred corticosteroid. Doses may need to be adjusted as pregnancy progresses, and stress doses may be required during active labor. Pregnant women with adrenal insufficiency should be monitored at least once each trimester (ES [Bornstein 2016]; ES [Fleseriu 2016]; ES [Speiser 2018]).

Uncontrolled asthma is associated with adverse events on pregnancy (increased risk of perinatal mortality, preeclampsia, preterm birth, low birth weight infants, cesarean delivery, and the development of gestational diabetes). Poorly controlled asthma or asthma exacerbations may have a greater fetal/maternal risk than what is associated with appropriately used asthma medications. Maternal treatment improves pregnancy outcomes by reducing the risk of some adverse events (eg, preterm birth and gestational diabetes). Maternal asthma symptoms should be monitored monthly during pregnancy. Inhaled corticosteroids are recommended for the treatment of asthma during pregnancy; however, systemic corticosteroids should be used to control acute exacerbations or treat severe persistent asthma. Hydrocortisone may be used when parenteral administration is required (ERS/TSANZ [Middleton 2019]; GINA 2020). Women who require systemic corticosteroids for management of their asthma should be given intravenous corticosteroids, such as hydrocortisone, during labor and for 24 hours after delivery to prevent adrenal crisis (ACOG 2008; ERS/TSANZ [Middleton 2019]).

When systemic corticosteroids are needed in pregnancy for rheumatic disorders, it is generally recommended to use the lowest effective dose for the shortest duration of time, avoiding high doses during the first trimester (Götestam Skorpen 2016; Makol 2011; Østensen 2009).

For dermatologic disorders in pregnant women, systemic corticosteroids are generally not preferred for initial therapy; should be avoided during the first trimester; and used during the second or third trimester at the lowest effective dose (Bae 2012; Leachman 2006).

Hydrocortisone (Topical) (hye droe KOR ti sone)

Brand Names: US Advanced Allergy Collection; Ala Scalp; Ala-Cort; Anti-Itch Maximum Strength [OTC]; Anucort-HC; Anusol-HC; Aquanil HC [OTC]; Beta HC [OTC]; Colocort [DSC]; Cortaid Maximum Strength [OTC]; Cortenema; Corticool [OTC] [DSC]; Cortifoam; Curad Hydrocortisone [OTC]; Dermasorb HC [DSC]; Hemmorex-HC; Hydrocortisone Anti-Itch [OTC]; Hydrocortisone in Absorbase [DSC]; Hydrocortisone Max St [OTC]; Hydrocortisone Max St/12 Moist [OTC]; HydroSKIN [OTC]; Instacort 5 [OTC]; Locoid; Locoid Lipocream; Med-Derm Hydrocortisone [OTC] [DSC]; Medi-First Hydrocortisone [OTC] [DSC]; MiCort-HC; NuCort; Pandel; Preparation H [OTC]; Procto-Med HC; Procto-Pak; Proctocort; Proctosol HC; Proctozone-HC; Recort Plus [OTC]; Rederm [OTC] [DSC]; Sarnol-HC [OTC]; Scalacort DK; Scalacort [DSC]; Scalpicin Maximum Strength [OTC]; Texacort; Westcort [DSC]

Brand Names: Canada Barriere-HC; Cortenema; Cortifoam [DSC]; Cortoderm; Emo Cort; Hyderm; Hydroval; NOVO-Hydrocort; Prevex HC; SANDOZ Hydrocortisone; Sarna HC; Topiderm [DSC]

Pharmacologic Category Antihemorrhoidal Agent; Corticosteroid, Rectal; Corticosteroid, Topical

Use

Anal and genital pruritus, external: Topical: Use in external genital and anal itching.

Corticosteroid-responsive dermatoses (eg, atopic dermatitis, contact dermatitis, vulvar dermatitis, psoriasis, seborrheic dermatitis): Topical: Relief of inflammatory and pruritic manifestations of corticosteroid-responsive dermatoses.

Hemorrhoids: Rectal: Use in inflamed hemorrhoids.

Ulcerative colitis: Rectal: Treatment of ulcerative colitis, especially distal forms, including ulcerative proctitis, ulcerative proctosigmoiditis, and left-sided ulcerative colitis.

Local Anesthetic/Vasoconstrictor Precautions No information available to require special precautions

Effects on Dental Treatment No significant effects or complications reported

Effects on Bleeding No information available to require special precautions

Adverse Reactions Frequency not defined. Local adverse events presented. Adverse events similar to those observed with systemic absorption are also observed, especially following rectal use. Refer to the Hydrocortisone (Systemic) monograph for details.

Cream, ointment: Dermatologic: Acneiform eruption, atrophic striae, burning sensation of skin, folliculitis, hypertrichosis, hypopigmentation, maceration of the skin, miliaria, perioral dermatitis, pruritus, secondary skin infection, skin atrophy, skin irritation, xeroderma

Enema:

Central nervous system: Localized burning

Hematologic & oncologic: Rectal hemorrhage

Local: Local pain

Suppositories:

Central nervous system: Localized burning

Dermatologic: Allergic contact dermatitis, folliculitis, hypopigmentation, pruritus, xeroderma

Infection: Secondary infection

Mechanism of Action Topical corticosteroids have anti-inflammatory, antipruritic, and vasoconstrictive properties. May depress the formation, release, and activity of endogenous chemical mediators of inflammation (kinins, histamine, liposomal enzymes,

Pregnancy Considerations
Based on the radioactivity, Y-90 ibritumomab may cause fetal harm if administered during pregnancy. In addition, ibritumomab tiuxetan is a humanized monoclonal antibody (IgG_1). Potential placental transfer of human IgG is dependent upon the IgG subclass and gestational age, generally increasing as pregnancy progresses. The lowest exposure would be expected during the period of organogenesis (Palmeira 2012; Pentsuk 2009).

Ibrutinib (eye BROO ti nib)

Brand Names: US Imbruvica
Brand Names: Canada Imbruvica
Pharmacologic Category Antineoplastic Agent; Antineoplastic Agent, Bruton Tyrosine Kinase Inhibitor; Antineoplastic Agent, Tyrosine Kinase Inhibitor
Use
Chronic graft-versus-host disease (refractory): Treatment of chronic graft-versus-host disease in adults after failure of ≥1 lines of systemic therapy.
Chronic lymphocytic leukemia/small lymphocytic lymphoma: Treatment of chronic lymphocytic leukemia/small lymphocytic lymphoma (CLL/SLL) in adults; treatment of CLL/SLL in adults with 17p deletion.
Mantle cell lymphoma, previously treated: Treatment of mantle cell lymphoma in adults who have received at least 1 prior therapy.
Marginal zone lymphoma, relapsed/refractory: Treatment of marginal zone lymphoma in adults who require systemic therapy and have received at least 1 prior anti-CD20-based therapy.
Waldenström macroglobulinemia: Treatment of Waldenström macroglobulinemia in adults.
Local Anesthetic/Vasoconstrictor Precautions
No information available to require special precautions
Effects on Dental Treatment Key adverse event(s) related to dental treatment: Stomatitis has been reported
Effects on Bleeding Bleeding has been reported in up to 48% of patients, including gastrointestinal bleeding; decreased platelet count (57%; grades 3/4: 17%), decreased hemoglobin (41%; grades 3/4: 9%), bruise (30%), neutropenia (47%; grades 3/4: 29%), petechia (11%). Medical consult is recommended.
Adverse Reactions
>10%:
Cardiovascular: Peripheral edema (12% to 35%), hypertension (12% to 16%)
Dermatologic: Skin rash (12% to 29%), skin infection (14% to 18%), pruritus (11% to 14%)
Endocrine & metabolic: Hyperuricemia (15% to 16%), hypoalbuminemia (14%), hypokalemia (12% to 13%), dehydration (12%)
Gastrointestinal: Diarrhea (36% to 59%), nausea (20% to 31%), stomatitis (14% to 29%; grades ≥3: 1% to 2%), constipation (12% to 25%), abdominal pain (13% to 24%), vomiting (11% to 23%), decreased appetite (16% to 21%), dyspepsia (11% to 19%), gastroesophageal reflux disease (12%), upper abdominal pain (13%)
Genitourinary: Urinary tract infection (10% to 14%)
Hematologic & oncologic: Thrombocytopenia (33% to 69%; grades 3/4: 5% to 17%; grade 4: 3% to 8%), neutropenia (22% to 53%; grades 3/4: 13% to 29%; grade 4: 2% to 13%), bruise (12% to 51%; grades 3/4: ≤2%), hemorrhage (≤44%; grades ≥3: ≤6%), decreased hemoglobin (13% to 43%; grades 3/4: ≤13%), petechia (11% to 16%), second primary malignant neoplasm (10% to 12%; grades ≥3: 2%)
Infection: Infection (grade ≥3: 24%)
Nervous system: Fatigue (18% to 57%), dizziness (11% to 20%), headache (12% to 18%), anxiety (16%), chills (12%)
Neuromuscular & skeletal: Musculoskeletal pain (14% to 40%), muscle spasm (11% to 29%), arthralgia (11% to 24%), asthenia (14%), arthropathy (13%)
Ophthalmic: Dry eye syndrome (17%), increased lacrimation (13%), blurred vision (10% to 13%), decreased visual acuity (11%)
Respiratory: Upper respiratory tract infection (16% to 47%), dyspnea (10% to 27%), cough (13% to 22%), sinusitis (11% to 22%), pneumonia (11% to 21%), epistaxis (11% to 19%), oropharyngeal pain (14%), bronchitis (11%)
Miscellaneous: Fever (12% to 25%), falling (17%)
1% to 10%:
Cardiovascular: Atrial fibrillation (≤9%), atrial flutter (≤9%), subdural hematoma (grades ≥3: ≤3%), ventricular tachycardia (1%)
Endocrine & metabolic: Weight loss (10%)
Gastrointestinal: Gastrointestinal hemorrhage (grades ≥3: ≤3%)
Genitourinary: Hematuria (grades ≥3: ≤3%)
Hematologic & oncologic: Skin carcinoma (non-melanoma; 6%), anemia (grades 3/4: 3%), postprocedural hemorrhage (grades ≥3: ≤3%)
Infection: Sepsis (10%)
Nervous system: Intracranial hemorrhage (grades ≥3: ≤3%)
Renal: Increased serum creatinine (1.5 to 3 x ULN: 9%)
<1%, postmarketing, and/or case reports: Abnormal platelet aggregation (Kamel 2015), acute anaphylactic shock, angioedema, hepatic cirrhosis, hepatic failure, hyponatremia (Burger 2015), interstitial pulmonary disease, onychoclasis, panniculitis, peripheral neuropathy, pneumonia due to Pneumocystis jirovecii, pneumonitis (Mato 2016), progressive multifocal leukoencephalopathy, reactivation of HBV, renal failure syndrome, Stevens-Johnson syndrome, tumor lysis syndrome, urticaria
Mechanism of Action Ibrutinib is a potent and irreversible inhibitor of Bruton's tyrosine kinase (BTK), an integral component of the B-cell receptor (BCR) and cytokine receptor pathways. Constitutive activation of B-cell receptor signaling is important for survival of malignant B-cells; BTK inhibition results in decreased malignant B-cell proliferation and survival.
Pharmacodynamics/Kinetics
Half-life Elimination 4 to 6 hours
Time to Peak 1 to 2 hours (4 hours under fed conditions [de Jong 2015])
Reproductive Considerations Verify pregnancy status in females of reproductive potential prior to treatment initiation. Females of reproductive potential should use effective contraception during treatment and for 1 month after the last ibrutinib dose; males with female partners of reproductive potential should use effective contraception during treatment and for 1 month after the last ibrutinib dose.

Pregnancy Considerations
Based on the mechanism of action and data from animal reproduction studies, ibrutinib may cause fetal harm if administered during pregnancy.

- ◆ **Ibsrela** *see* Tenapanor *on page 1417*
- ◆ **IBU** *see* Ibuprofen *on page 786*
- ◆ **IBU-200 [OTC]** *see* Ibuprofen *on page 786*
- ◆ **IBU 600-EZS** *see* Ibuprofen *on page 786*
- ◆ **Ibudone [DSC]** *see* Hydrocodone and Ibuprofen *on page 769*

Ibuprofen (eye byoo PROE fen)

Related Information

Antiplatelet and Anticoagulation Considerations in Dentistry *on page 1666*
Oral Pain *on page 1734*
Rheumatoid Arthritis, Osteoarthritis, and Osteoporosis *on page 1697*
Temporomandibular Dysfunction (TMD), Chronic Pain, and Fibromyalgia *on page 1773*

Related Sample Prescriptions

Oral Pain - Sample Prescriptions *on page 30*

Brand Names: US Addaprin [OTC]; Advil Junior Strength [OTC]; Advil Liqui-Gels minis [OTC]; Advil Migraine [OTC]; Advil [OTC]; Caldolor; Childrens Advil [OTC]; Childrens Motrin [OTC]; Dyspel [OTC]; Genpril [OTC]; GoodSense Ibuprofen Childrens [OTC]; GoodSense Ibuprofen [OTC]; I-Prin [OTC] [DSC]; IBU; IBU 600-EZS; IBU-200 [OTC]; Ibuprofen Childrens [OTC]; Ibuprofen Comfort Pac [DSC]; Infants Advil [OTC]; KS Ibuprofen [OTC]; Motrin Childrens [OTC]; Motrin IB [OTC]; Motrin Infants Drops [OTC]; NeoProfen; Provil [OTC]

Brand Names: Canada APO-Ibuprofen FC; Caldolor; PMS-Ibuprofen; TEVA-Profen

Generic Availability (US) May be product dependent

Pharmacologic Category Analgesic, Nonopioid; Nonsteroidal Anti-inflammatory Drug (NSAID), Oral; Nonsteroidal Anti-inflammatory Drug (NSAID), Parenteral

Dental Use Management of pain and swelling

Use
Oral: Inflammatory diseases and rheumatoid disorders, mild to moderate pain, fever, dysmenorrhea, osteoarthritis

Ibuprofen injection (Caldolor): Management of mild to moderate pain and management of moderate to severe pain as an adjunct to opioid analgesics in adults and children 6 months and older; reduction of fever in adults and children 6 months and older.

Ibuprofen lysine injection (NeoProfen): Patent ductus arteriosus (PDA): To close a clinically significant PDA in premature infants weighing between 500-1500 g who are no more than 32 weeks of gestational age when usual medical management (eg, diuretics, fluid restriction, respiratory support) is ineffective.

OTC labeling: Reduction of fever; management of pain due to headache, migraine, sore throat, arthritis, physical or athletic overexertion (eg, sprains/strains), menstrual pain, dental pain, minor muscle/bone/joint pain, backache, pain due to the common cold and flu

Local Anesthetic/Vasoconstrictor Precautions No information available to require special precautions

Effects on Dental Treatment Key adverse event(s) related to dental treatment: Glossitis reported (frequency not defined). NSAIDs such as ibuprofen are known to reversibly decrease platelet aggregation via mechanisms different than observed with aspirin. The dentist should be aware of the potential of abnormal coagulation.

The FDA notified consumers and healthcare professionals that the administration of ibuprofen for pain relief to patients taking aspirin for cardioprotection may interfere with aspirin's cardiovascular benefits. The FDA states that ibuprofen can interfere with the antiplatelet effect of low-dose aspirin (81 mg/day). This could result in diminished effectiveness of aspirin as used for cardioprotection and stroke prevention. The FDA adds that although ibuprofen and aspirin can be taken together, it is recommended that consumers talk with their healthcare providers for additional information. For more information, including how to advise aspirin patients requiring ibuprofen for pain relief, see Effects on Bleeding and Dental Health Professional Considerations. (http://www.fda.gov/Drugs/DrugSafety/PostmarketDrugSafetyInformationforPatientsandProviders/ucm110510.htm)

Effects on Bleeding Nonselective NSAIDs such as ibuprofen inhibit platelet aggregation and prolong bleeding time in some patients. Unlike aspirin, the NSAID effect on platelet function is quantitatively less, of shorter duration, and reversible.

Adverse Reactions
Oral:
>10%:
Hematologic & oncologic: Decreased hemoglobin (7% to 23%)
Hepatic: Increased serum alanine aminotransferase (≤15%), increased serum aspartate aminotransferase (≤15%)
1% to 10%:
Cardiovascular: Edema
Central nervous system: Dizziness (3% to 9%), headache, nervousness
Dermatologic: Skin rash (3% to 9%), maculopapular rash, pruritus
Endocrine & metabolic: Fluid retention
Gastrointestinal: Epigastric pain (3% to 9%), heartburn (3% to 9%), nausea (3% to 9%), abdominal cramps, abdominal distress, abdominal pain, bloating, constipation, decreased appetite, diarrhea, dyspepsia, flatulence, nausea and vomiting, vomiting
Hematologic & oncologic: Anemia, prolonged bleeding time
Hepatic: Increased liver enzymes
Otic: Tinnitus (<3%)
Renal: Renal function abnormality
Frequency not defined:
Cardiovascular: Hypertension, syncope, tachycardia
Central nervous system: Anxiety, malaise, vertigo
Dermatologic: Diaphoresis, ecchymoses
Endocrine & metabolic: Weight changes
Gastrointestinal: Duodenitis, esophagitis, glossitis, hematemesis, rectal hemorrhage, stomatitis
Genitourinary: Dysuria, oliguria, proteinuria
Hematologic & oncologic: Leukopenia
Infection: Infection, sepsis
Neuromuscular & skeletal: Asthenia, tremor
Renal: Interstitial nephritis
Respiratory: Asthma, dyspnea
<1%, postmarketing, and/or case reports: Abnormal dreams, abnormal hepatic function tests, acidosis, acute renal failure, agranulocytosis, alopecia, amblyopia, anaphylactoid shock, anaphylaxis, anemia, angioedema, aplastic anemia, apnea, aseptic meningitis, auditory impairment, azotemia, blurred

vision, bronchospasm, cardiac arrhythmia, cardiac failure, cataract, cerebrovascular accident, change in appetite, chills, coma, confusion, conjunctivitis, cystitis, decreased creatinine clearance, decreased hematocrit, depression, diplopia, DRESS syndrome (Koca 2016; Roales-Gómez 2014), drowsiness, duodenal ulcer, emotional lability, eosinophilia, epistaxis, eructation, erythema multiforme, exfoliative dermatitis, fever, gastric ulcer, gastritis, gastrointestinal hemorrhage, gastrointestinal perforation, gastrointestinal ulcer, gingival ulceration, glomerulonephritis, gynecomastia, hallucination, hearing loss, heavy menstrual bleeding, hematuria, hemolytic anemia, hemorrhage, Henoch-Schonlein purpura, hepatic failure, hepatic necrosis, hepatitis, hepatorenal syndrome, hepatotoxicity (idiosyncratic) (Chalasani 2014), hyperglycemia, hypoglycemia, hypotension, increased serum creatinine, insomnia, jaundice, lymphadenopathy, melena, myocardial infarction, neutropenia, nonthrombocytopenic purpura, occult blood in stools, optic neuritis, palpitations, pancreatitis, pancytopenia, paresthesia, pneumonia, polyuria, pseudotumor cerebri, renal papillary necrosis, renal tubular necrosis, respiratory depression, rhinitis, scotoma, seizure, serum sickness, sinus bradycardia, sinus tachycardia, skin photosensitivity, Stevens-Johnson syndrome, systemic lupus erythematosus, thrombocytopenia, thrombosis, toxic epidermal necrolysis, urticaria, vasculitis, vesiculobullous dermatitis, vision color changes, vision loss, xerophthalmia, xerostomia

Injection: Ibuprofen (Caldolor):

>10%:

Central nervous system: Headache (12%; children: ≥2%)

Endocrine & metabolic: Hypokalemia (4% to 19%)

Gastrointestinal: Vomiting (22%; children: ≥2%), flatulence (16%)

Hematologic & oncologic: Anemia (4% to 36%; children: ≥2%), eosinophilia (26%), neutropenia (13%), hypoproteinemia (10% to 13%)

Hepatic: Increased serum alanine aminotransferase (≤15%), increased serum aspartate aminotransferase (≤15%)

Infection: Bacteremia (13%)

1% to 10%:

Cardiovascular: Hypertension (10%), hypotension (7% to 10%), peripheral edema (3%)

Central nervous system: Dizziness (4% to 6%), infusion-site pain (children: ≥2%)

Endocrine & metabolic: Hypoalbuminemia (10%), hypernatremia (7% to 10%), increased lactate dehydrogenase (7% to 10%)

Gastrointestinal: Diarrhea (10%), dyspepsia (1% to 4%), abdominal distress (≤3%), nausea (children: ≥2%)

Genitourinary: Urinary retention (5%)

Hematologic & oncologic: Hemorrhage (10%), thrombocythemia (3% to 10%), wound hemorrhage (3%), decreased hemoglobin (2% to 3%)

Renal: Increased blood urea nitrogen (10%)

Respiratory: Bacterial pneumonia (3% to 10%), cough (3%)

Frequency not defined:

Dermatologic: Exfoliative dermatitis, skin rash, Stevens-Johnson syndrome, toxic epidermal necrolysis

Hypersensitivity: Hypersensitivity reaction

<1%, postmarketing, and/or case reports: Abdominal pain, anaphylaxis, cerebrovascular accident, esophageal perforation, gastrointestinal hemorrhage, gastrointestinal inflammation, gastrointestinal tract perforation, gastrointestinal ulcer, hepatotoxicity (idiosyncratic) (Chalasani 2014), myocardial infarction, nasal congestion, thrombosis

Injection: Ibuprofen lysine (NeoProfen):

>10%:

Central nervous system: Intraventricular hemorrhage (29%)

Dermatologic: Skin irritation (≤16%), skin lesion (≤16%)

Endocrine & metabolic: Hypocalcemia (12%), hypoglycemia (12%)

Gastrointestinal: Enterocolitis (22%)

Hematologic & oncologic: Anemia (32%)

Infection: Sepsis (43%)

Respiratory: Apnea (28%), respiratory tract infection (19%)

1% to 10%:

Cardiovascular: Edema (4%)

Endocrine & metabolic: Adrenocortical insufficiency (7%), hypernatremia (7%)

Genitourinary: Urinary tract infection (9%), decreased urine output (3%)

Renal: Increased blood urea nitrogen (7%), renal insufficiency (6%), increased serum creatinine (3%)

Respiratory: Respiratory failure (10%), atelectasis (4%)

Frequency not defined:

Cardiovascular: Cardiac failure, hypotension, tachycardia

Central nervous system: Seizure

Endocrine & metabolic: Hyperglycemia

Gastrointestinal: Abdominal distention, cholestasis, gastritis, gastroesophageal reflux disease, inguinal hernia, intestinal obstruction

Genitourinary: Oliguria

Hematologic & oncologic: Neutropenia, prolonged bleeding time, thrombocytopenia

Hepatic: Jaundice

Infection: Infection

Local: Injection site reaction

Renal: Renal failure syndrome

Miscellaneous: Reduced intake of food/fluids

<1%, postmarketing, and/or case reports: Gastrointestinal perforation, hepatotoxicity (idiosyncratic) (Chalasani 2014), necrotizing enterocolitis, pulmonary hypertension

Dental Usual Dosage

Analgesic/pain/fever/dysmenorrhea: Oral:

Children: 4-10 mg/kg/dose every 6-8 hours

Adults: 200-400 mg/dose every 4-6 hours (maximum daily dose: 1.2 g, unless directed by physician; under physician supervision daily doses ≤3.2 g may be used)

OTC labeling (analgesic, antipyretic): **Note:** Treatment for >10 days is not recommended unless directed by healthcare provider. Oral:

Children 6 months to 11 years: See table; use of weight to select dose is preferred; doses may be repeated every 6-8 hours (maximum: 4 doses/day)

Children ≥12 years and Adults: 200 mg every 4-6 hours as needed (maximum: 1200 mg/24 hours)

Ibuprofen Dosing (Infants and Children 6 months to 11 years)

Weight (Preferred)[a]		Age	Dosage (mg)
kg	lb		
5.4 to 8.1	12 to 17	6 to 11 mo	50
8.2 to 10.8	18 to 23	12 to 23 mo	75
10.9 to 16.3	24 to 35	2 to 3 y	100
16.4 to 21.7	36 to 47	4 to 5 y	150
21.8 to 27.2	48 to 59	6 to 8 y	200
27.3 to 32.6	60 to 71	9 to 10 y	250
32.7 to 43.2	72 to 95	11 y	300

[a]Manufacturer's recommendations are based on weight in pounds (OTC labeling); weight in kg listed here is derived from pounds and rounded; kg weight listed also is adjusted to allow for continuous weight ranges in kg.

Dosing

Adult

Analgesia (mild to moderate pain):

Oral:

200 to 800 mg 3 to 4 times daily; usual dose: 400 mg; usual daily dose: 1,200 to 2,400 mg/day (Becker 2010; Blondell 2013; Derry 2009; Roelofs 2008); maximum: 3,200 mg/day (Blondell 2013; Derry 2009)

American Pain Society: 200 to 400 mg every 4 to 6 hours; maximum: 3,200 mg/day (APS 2016)

IV (Caldolor): 400 to 800 mg every 6 hours as needed (maximum: 3,200 mg/day). **Note:** Patients should be well hydrated prior to administration.

Antipyretic: IV (Caldolor): **Note**: Patients should be well hydrated prior to administration. Initial: 400 mg, then every 4 to 6 hours or 100 to 200 mg every 4 hours as needed (maximum: 3,200 mg/day)

Dysmenorrhea: Oral:

200 to 800 mg three to four times daily; usual daily dose: 1,200 to 2,400 mg/day; most sources did not exceed a daily dose of 2,400 mg/day and a maximum duration of 3 to 5 days (Majoribanks 2010).

Manufacturer's labeling: Dosing in the prescribing information may not reflect current clinical practice. 400 mg every 4 hours as needed; maximum: 3,200 mg/day

Gout, acute flares (alternative agent) (off-label use): Oral: 800 mg three times daily; initiate within 24 to 48 hours of flare onset preferably; discontinue 2 to 3 days after resolution of clinical signs; usual duration: 5 to 7 days (ACR [Khanna 2012]; Becker 2018)

Osteoarthritis: Oral: 400 to 800 mg 3 to 4 times daily (maximum: 3,200 mg/day)

Rheumatoid arthritis: Oral: 400 to 800 mg 3 to 4 times daily (maximum: 3,200 mg/day)

OTC labeling:

Analgesic, antipyretic: Oral: 200 mg every 4 to 6 hours as needed; if no relief may increase to 400 mg every 4 to 6 hours as needed (maximum: 1,200 mg/day); Duration: treatment for >10 days as an analgesic or >3 days as an antipyretic is not recommended unless directed by health care provider.

Migraine: Oral: 400 mg at onset of symptoms (maximum: 400 mg/24 hours unless directed by health care provider)

Pericarditis (off-label use): Oral: **Note:** Administer in combination with colchicine therapy. Concurrent gastroduodenal prophylaxis with a proton pump inhibitor has been used and is recommended (ESC [Adler 2015]; Imazio 2013; Imazio 2005). With pericarditis postmyocardial infarction, the ACCF/AHA prefers the use of aspirin (ACCF/AHA [O'Gara 2013]).

Acute pericarditis: 600 mg every 8 hours for 7 to 14 days followed by a gradual tapering of the dose by 200 to 400 mg every 1 to 2 weeks (ESC [Adler 2015])

Recurrent pericarditis: 600 mg every 8 hours (range: 1,200 to 2,400 mg) for weeks to months until complete symptom resolution followed by a gradual tapering of the dose by 200 to 400 mg every 1 to 2 weeks (ESC [Adler 2015])

Geriatric Refer to adult dosing. Use with caution; consider reduced initial dosage.

Renal Impairment: Adult There are no dosage adjustments provided in the manufacturer's labeling; use with caution; avoid use in advanced renal disease. KDIGO 2012 guidelines provide the following recommendations for NSAIDs:

eGFR 30 to <60 mL/minute/1.73 m^2: Avoid use in patients with intercurrent disease that increases risk of acute kidney injury.

eGFR <30 mL/minute/1.73 m^2: Avoid use.

Hemodialysis: Not dialyzable (NCS/SCCM [Frontera 2016])

Hepatic Impairment: Adult There are no dosage adjustments provided in the manufacturer's labeling; use caution and discontinue if hepatic function worsens.

Pediatric Note: To reduce the risk of adverse cardiovascular and GI effects, use the lowest effective dose for the shortest period of time to achieve treatment goals. Oral liquid products are available in two concentrations (ie, concentrated infant drops: 50 mg/1.25 mL and suspension: 100 mg/5 mL); precautions should be taken to verify and avoid confusion between the different concentrations; dose should be clearly presented as "mg".

Analgesic:

IV: Ibuprofen injection (Caldolor): **Note:** Patients should be well hydrated prior to administration.

Infants 6 months to Children <12 years: 10 mg/kg/dose (maximum dose: 400 mg/dose) every 4 to 6 hours as needed; maximum daily dose: 40 mg/kg/**day** or 2,400 mg/**day**, whichever is less.

Children and Adolescents 12 to 17 years: 400 mg every 4 to 6 hours as needed; maximum daily dose: 2,400 mg/**day**.

Oral:

Weight-directed dosing: Infants and Children <50 kg: Limited data available in infants <6 months: 4 to 10 mg/kg/dose every 6 to 8 hours; maximum single dose: 400 mg; maximum daily dose: 40 mg/kg/**day** (APS 2008; Berde 1990; Berde 2002; Kliegman 2011).

Fixed dosing:

Infants and Children 6 months to 11 years: See table based upon manufacturer's labeling; use of weight to select dose is preferred; if weight is not available, then use age; doses may be repeated every 6 to 8 hours; maximum: 4 doses/day; treatment of sore throat for >2 days or use in infants and children <3 years of age with sore throat is not recommended, unless directed by health care provider.

Ibuprofen Dosing

Weight (preferred)[A]		Age	Dosage (mg)
kg	lbs		
5.4 to 8.1	12 to 17	6 to 11 months	50
8.2 to 10.8	18 to 23	12 to 23 months	75 to 80
10.9 to 16.3	24 to 35	2 to 3 years	100
16.4 to 21.7	36 to 47	4 to 5 years	150
21.8 to 27.2	48 to 59	6 to 8 years	200
27.3 to 32.6	60 to 71	9 to 10 years	200 to 250
32.7 to 43.2	72 to 95	11 years	300

[A]Manufacturer's recommendations are based on weight in pounds (OTC labeling); weight in kg listed here is derived from pounds and rounded; kg weight listed also is adjusted to allow for continuous weight ranges in kg.

Children ≥12 years and Adolescents: Oral: 200 mg every 4 to 6 hours as needed; if pain does not respond may increase to 400 mg; maximum daily dose: 1,200 mg/**day**; treatment of pain for >10 days is not recommended, unless directed by health care provider.

Antipyretic:

IV: Ibuprofen injection (Caldolor): **Note:** Patients should be well hydrated prior to administration.

Infants 6 months to Children <12 years: 10 mg/kg/dose (maximum dose: 400 mg/dose) every 4 to 6 hours as needed; maximum daily dose: 40 mg/kg/**day** or 2,400 mg/**day**, whichever is less.

Children and Adolescents 12 to 17 years: 400 mg every 4 to 6 hours as needed; maximum daily dose: 2,400 mg/**day**.

Oral:

Weight-directed dosing: Infants ≥6 months, Children, and Adolescents: 5 to 10 mg/kg/dose every 6 to 8 hours; maximum single dose: 400 mg; maximum daily dose: 40 mg/kg/**day** up to 1,200 mg, unless directed by physician; under physician supervision daily doses ≤2,400 mg may be used (Kliegman 2011; Litalien 2001; Sullivan 2011).

Fixed dosing:

Infants and Children 6 months to 11 years: Oral: See table based upon manufacturer's labeling; use of weight to select dose is preferred; if weight is not available, then use age; doses may be repeated every 6 to 8 hours; maximum: 4 doses/day; treatment for >3 days is not recommended unless directed by health care provider.

Weight (preferred)[A]		Age	Dosage (mg)
kg	lbs		
5.4 to 8.1	12 to 17	6 to 11 months	50
8.2 to 10.8	18 to 23	12 to 23 months	75 to 80
10.9 to 16.3	24 to 35	2 to 3 years	100
16.4 to 21.7	36 to 47	4 to 5 years	150
21.8 to 27.2	48 to 59	6 to 8 years	200
27.3 to 32.6	60 to 71	9 to 10 years	200 to 250
32.7 to 43.2	72 to 95	11 years	300

[A]Manufacturer's recommendations are based on weight in pounds (OTC labeling); weight in kg listed here is derived from pounds and rounded; kg weight listed also is adjusted to allow for continuous weight ranges in kg.

Children ≥12 years and Adolescents: Oral: 200 mg every 4 to 6 hours as needed; if fever does not respond may increase to 400 mg; maximum daily dose: 1,200 mg/day; treatment of fever >3 days is not recommended, unless directed by health care provider.

Cystic fibrosis, mild disease (to slow lung disease progression): Limited data available: Children and Adolescents 6 to 17 years with FEV_1 >60% predicted (Mogayzel 2013): Oral: Initial: 20 to 30 mg/kg/dose twice daily; titrate to achieve peak plasma concentrations of 50 to 100 mcg/mL; should not eat or take pancreatic enzymes for 2 hours after the ibuprofen dose. Dosing based on a study of 41 patients (ages: 5 to 39 years); mean required dose: ~25 mg/kg/dose twice daily, reported range: 16.2 to 31.6 mg/kg/dose every 12 hours required to achieve target concentration; results showed that chronic ibuprofen use (over 4 years) slowed the rate of decline in FEV_1; patients 5 to 13 years old with mild lung disease were observed to have greatest benefit; (Konstan 1995). A follow up observational study (n=1,365; ages: 6 to 17 years) under noncontrolled conditions (real world) showed significant improvement in the rate of decline of lung disease progression with chronic ibuprofen therapy (Konstan 2007). **Note:** Timing of blood sampling postdose is based on dosage form: Oral suspension: Obtain blood samples at 30, 45, and 60 minutes postdose; tablets: Obtain blood samples at 1, 2, and 3 hours postdose (Litalien 2001; Scott 1999).

Juvenile idiopathic arthritis (JIA): Children and Adolescents: Usual range: 30 to 40 mg/kg/**day** in 3 to 4 divided doses; start at lower end of dosing range and titrate; patients with milder disease may be treated with 20 mg/kg/**day**; patients with more severe disease may require up to 50 mg/kg/**day**; maximum single dose: 800 mg; maximum daily dose: 2,400 mg/**day** (Giannini 1990; Kliegman 2011; Litalien 2001).

Renal Impairment: Pediatric

Infants, Children, and Adolescents: Oral, IV (Caldolor): There are no dosage adjustments provided in the manufacturer's labeling; avoid use in advanced disease.

KDIGO 2012 guidelines provide the following recommendations for NSAIDs (KDIGO 2013):

eGFR 30 to <60 mL/minute/1.73 m^2: Avoid use in patients with intercurrent disease that increases risk of acute kidney injury

eGFR <30 mL/minute/1.73 m^2: Avoid use

Hepatic Impairment: Pediatric There are no dosage adjustments provided in the manufacturer's labeling; use caution and discontinue if hepatic function worsens.

Mechanism of Action Reversibly inhibits cyclooxygenase-1 and 2 (COX-1 and 2) enzymes, which results in decreased formation of prostaglandin precursors; has antipyretic, analgesic, and anti-inflammatory properties

Other proposed mechanisms not fully elucidated (and possibly contributing to the anti-inflammatory effect to varying degrees), include inhibiting chemotaxis, altering lymphocyte activity, inhibiting neutrophil aggregation/activation, and decreasing proinflammatory cytokine levels.

Contraindications

Hypersensitivity to ibuprofen (eg, anaphylactic reactions, serious skin reactions) or any component of the formulation; history of asthma, urticaria, or allergic-type reaction to aspirin or other NSAIDs; aspirin triad (eg, bronchial asthma, aspirin intolerance, rhinitis); use in the setting of coronary artery bypass graft (CABG) surgery

Ibuprofen lysine (NeoProfen): Preterm neonates: With proven or suspected infection that is untreated; congenital heart disease in whom patency of the PDA is necessary for satisfactory pulmonary or systemic blood flow (eg, pulmonary atresia, severe coarctation of the aorta, severe tetralogy of Fallot); bleeding (especially those with active intracranial hemorrhage or GI bleeding); thrombocytopenia; coagulation defects; proven or suspected necrotizing enterocolitis; or significant renal function impairment.

Canadian labeling: Additional contraindications (not in US labeling): Cerebrovascular bleeding or other bleeding disorders; active gastric/duodenal/peptic ulcer, active GI bleeding; inflammatory bowel disease; uncontrolled heart failure; moderate [IV formulation only] to severe renal impairment (creatinine clearance [CrCl] <30 mL/minute); deteriorating renal disease; moderate [IV formulation only] to severe hepatic impairment; active hepatic disease; hyperkalemia; third trimester of pregnancy; breastfeeding; patients <18 years of age [IV formulation only]; patients <12 years of age [oral formulation only]; systemic lupus erythematosus [oral formulation only]; children suffering from dehydration as a result of acute diarrhea, vomiting, or lack of fluid intake

OTC labeling: When used for self-medication, do not use if previous allergic reaction to any other pain reliever/fever reducer; prior to or following cardiac surgery.

Warnings/Precautions **[US Boxed Warning]: Use is contraindicated in the setting of coronary artery bypass graft (CABG) surgery.** Risk of MI and stroke may be increased with use following CABG surgery. **[US Boxed Warning]: NSAIDs cause an increased risk of serious (and potentially fatal) adverse cardiovascular thrombotic events, including fatal MI and stroke. Risk may occur early during treatment and may increase with duration of use.** Relative risk appears to be similar in those with and without known cardiovascular disease or risk factors for cardiovascular disease; however, absolute incidence of cardiovascular events (which may occur early during treatment) was higher in patients with known cardiovascular disease or risk factors. New-onset hypertension or exacerbation of hypertension may occur (NSAIDS may also impair response to ACE inhibitors, thiazide diuretics, or loop diuretics); may contribute to cardiovascular events; monitor blood pressure; use with caution in patients with hypertension. May cause sodium and fluid retention; use with caution in patients with edema. Avoid use in heart failure (ACCF/AHA [Yancy 2013]). Avoid use in patients with a recent MI unless benefits outweigh risk of cardiovascular thrombotic events. Use the lowest effective dose for the shortest duration of time, consistent with individual patient goals, to reduce risk of cardiovascular events; alternate therapies should be considered for patients at high risk. Avoid chronic use of oral nonselective NSAIDs in patients who have undergone bariatric surgery; development of anastomotic ulcerations/perforations may occur.

Clinical or population-based data regarding the risks of NSAIDs in the setting of coronavirus disease 2019 (COVID-19) are limited (FDA Safety Communication 2020; Kim 2020). Some experts recommend the use of acetaminophen as the preferred antipyretic agent, when possible, and if NSAIDs are needed, to use the lowest effective dose and shortest duration (EMA 2020; Kim 2020). In general, for patients already taking an NSAID for a comorbid condition, it is recommended to continue the NSAID as directed by their health care provider (EMA 2020; NIH 2020; WHO 2020).

May increase the risk of aseptic meningitis, especially in patients with systemic lupus erythematosus (SLE) and mixed connective tissue disorders. Platelet adhesion and aggregation may be decreased; may prolong bleeding time; patients with coagulation disorders or who are receiving anticoagulants should be monitored closely. Anemia may occur; patients on long-term NSAID therapy should be monitored for anemia. Rarely, NSAID use may cause severe blood dyscrasias (eg, agranulocytosis, aplastic anemia, thrombocytopenia).

NSAID use may compromise existing renal function; dose-dependent decreases in prostaglandin synthesis may result from NSAID use, reducing renal blood flow, which may cause renal decompensation (usually reversible). NSAID use may increase the risk for hyperkalemia. Patients with impaired renal function, dehydration, hypovolemia, heart failure, hepatic impairment, those taking diuretics and ACE inhibitors, and the elderly are at greater risk of renal toxicity and hyperkalemia. Rehydrate patient before starting therapy; monitor renal function closely. Avoid use in patients with advanced renal disease; discontinue use with persistent or worsening abnormal renal function tests. Use of ibuprofen lysine (NeoProfen) is contraindicated in preterm infants with significant renal impairment. Long-term NSAID use may result in renal papillary necrosis and other renal injury.

[US Boxed Warning]: NSAIDs cause an increased risk of serious gastrointestinal inflammation, ulceration, bleeding, and perforation (may be fatal); elderly patients and patients with history of peptic ulcer disease and/or GI bleeding are at greater risk for serious GI events. These events may occur at any time during therapy and without warning. Avoid use in patients with active GI bleeding. In patients with a history of acute lower GI bleeding, avoid use of non-aspirin NSAIDs, especially if due to angioectasia or diverticulosis (Strate 2016). Use caution with a history of GI ulcers, concurrent therapy known to increase the risk of GI bleeding (eg, aspirin, anticoagulants and/or corticosteroids, selective serotonin reuptake inhibitors), advanced hepatic disease, coagulopathy, smoking, use of alcohol, or in elderly or debilitated patients. Use the lowest effective dose for the shortest duration of time, consistent with individual patient goals, to reduce risk of GI adverse events; alternate therapies should be considered for patients at high risk. When used concomitantly with aspirin, a substantial increase in the risk of gastrointestinal complications (eg, ulcer) occurs; concomitant gastroprotective therapy (eg, proton pump inhibitors) is recommended (Bhatt 2008).

NSAIDs may cause potentially fatal serious skin adverse events including exfoliative dermatitis, Stevens-Johnson Syndrome (SJS) and toxic epidermal necrolysis (TEN); discontinue use at first sign of skin rash (or other hypersensitivity). Anaphylactoid reactions may occur, even without prior exposure; patients with "aspirin triad" (bronchial asthma, aspirin intolerance, rhinitis) may be at increased risk. Contraindicated in patients who experience bronchospasm, asthma, rhinitis, or urticaria with NSAID or aspirin therapy. Use caution in other forms of asthma.

May cause drowsiness, dizziness, blurred vision and other neurologic effects which may impair physical or mental abilities; patients must be cautioned about performing tasks which require mental alertness (eg, operating machinery or driving). Monitor vision with long-term therapy. Blurred/diminished vision, scotomata, and changes in color vision have been reported. Discontinue use with altered vision and perform ophthalmologic exam.

Use with caution in patients with hepatic impairment. Transaminase elevations have been reported with use; closely monitor patients with any abnormal LFT. Rare (sometimes fatal) severe hepatic reactions (eg, fulminant hepatitis, liver necrosis, hepatic failure) have occurred with NSAID use; discontinue immediately if signs or symptoms of hepatic disease develop or if systemic manifestations occur.

Some products may contain phenylalanine. Potentially significant drug interactions may exist, requiring dose or frequency adjustment, additional monitoring, and/or selection of alternative therapy. Withhold for at least 4 to 6 half-lives prior to surgical or dental procedures.

Ibuprofen injection (Caldolor) must be diluted prior to administration; hemolysis can occur if not diluted.

Ibuprofen lysine injection (NeoProfen): Hold second or third doses if urinary output is <0.6 mL/kg/hour. May alter signs of infection. May inhibit platelet aggregation; monitor for signs of bleeding. May displace bilirubin; use caution when total bilirubin is elevated. Long-term evaluations of neurodevelopment, growth, or diseases associated with prematurity following treatment have not been conducted. A second course of treatment, alternative pharmacologic therapy or surgery may be needed if the ductus arteriosus fails to close or reopens following the initial course of therapy.

Some dosage forms may contain sodium benzoate/benzoic acid; benzoic acid (benzoate) is a metabolite of benzyl alcohol; large amounts of benzyl alcohol (≥99 mg/kg/day) have been associated with a potentially fatal toxicity ("gasping syndrome") in neonates; the "gasping syndrome" consists of metabolic acidosis, respiratory distress, gasping respirations, CNS dysfunction (including convulsions, intracranial hemorrhage), hypotension, and cardiovascular collapse (AAP ["Inactive" 1997]; CDC 1982); some data suggests that benzoate displaces bilirubin from protein binding sites (Ahlfors 2001); avoid or use dosage forms containing benzyl alcohol derivative with caution in neonates. See manufacturer's labeling.

Some dosage forms may contain propylene glycol; large amounts are potentially toxic and have been associated hyperosmolality, lactic acidosis, seizures and respiratory depression; use caution (AAP ["Inactive" 1997]; Zar 2007).

Some dosage forms may contain polysorbate 80 (also known as Tweens). Hypersensitivity reactions, usually a delayed reaction, have been reported following exposure to pharmaceutical products containing polysorbate 80 in certain individuals (Isaksson 2002; Lucente 2000; Shelley 1995). Thrombocytopenia, ascites, pulmonary deterioration, and renal and hepatic failure have been reported in premature neonates after receiving parenteral products containing polysorbate 80 (Alade 1986; CDC 1984). See manufacturer's labeling.

Self-medication (OTC use): Prior to self-medication, patients should contact health care provider if they have had recurring stomach pain or upset, ulcers, bleeding problems, high blood pressure, heart or kidney disease, other serious medical problems, are currently taking a diuretic, aspirin, anticoagulant, or are ≥60 years of age. If patients are using for migraines, they should also contact health care provider if they have not had a migraine diagnosis by health care provider, a headache that is different from usual migraine, worst headache of life, fever and neck stiffness, headache from head injury or coughing, first headache at ≥50 years of age, daily headache, or migraine requiring bed rest. Recommended dosages should not be exceeded, due to an increased risk of GI bleeding. Stop use and consult a health care provider if symptoms do not improve within first 24 hours of use (children), get worse, newly appear, fever lasts for >3 days or pain lasts >3 days (children) and >10 days (adults). Do not give for >10 days unless instructed by health care provider. Consuming ≥3 alcoholic beverages/day or taking longer than recommended may increase the risk of GI bleeding.

Warnings: Additional Pediatric Considerations Oral liquid products are available in two concentrations (ie, concentrated infant drops: 50 mg/1.25 mL and suspension: 100 mg/5 mL); precautions should be taken to verify and avoid confusion between the different concentrations; dose should be clearly presented as "mg".

A single-center, 10-year, retrospective review of pediatric patients diagnosed with acute kidney injury (AKI) (n=1,015; ages: ≤18 years) reported NSAIDS as a potential cause of AKI in 2.7% of patients (n=27); a higher incidence (6.6%) was reported when additional exclusion factors were included in the data analysis. Dosing information was available for 74% of the NSAID-associated AKI cases (n=20); dosing was within the recommended range in 75% (n=15) of these cases. The median age of children with NSAID-associated AKI was 14.7 years (range: 0.5 to 17.7 years) and 15% of patients were <5 years and more likely to require dialysis than the older patients. Some experts suggest the incidence of NSAID-associated AKI found in this study is conservative due to aggressive exclusion criteria (eg, concurrent aminoglycoside or other nephrotoxic therapy) and the actual incidence may be higher (Brophy 2013; Misurac 2013). IV ibuprofen is as effective as IV indomethacin for the treatment of PDA in preterm neonates, but is less likely to cause adverse effects on renal function (eg, oliguria, increased serum creatinine) (Aranda 2006; Lago 2002; Ohlsson 2013;

Van Overmeire 2000). Ibuprofen (compared to indomethacin) also has been shown to decrease the risk of developing NEC (Ohlsson 2013).

In neonates, pulmonary hypertension has occurred following use for treatment of PDA; ten cases have been reported; three following early (prophylactic) administration of tromethamine ibuprofen (not available in US) and seven cases following L-lysine ibuprofen therapy (Bellini 2006; Gournay 2002; Ohlsson 2013). Avoid extravasation of ibuprofen lysine injection (NeoProfen); IV solution may be irritating to tissues. Use with caution in neonates with controlled infection or those at risk for infection; ibuprofen may alter the usual signs of infection. Use with caution in neonates when total bilirubin is elevated; ibuprofen may displace bilirubin from albumin-binding sites. Intraventricular hemorrhage has been reported; overall incidence: 29%; grade 3/4: 15%. Long-term evaluations of neurodevelopmental outcome, growth, or diseases associated with prematurity (eg, chronic lung disease, retinopathy of prematurity) following treatment have not been conducted.

Some dosage forms may contain propylene glycol; in neonates large amounts of propylene glycol delivered orally, intravenously (eg, >3,000 mg/day), or topically have been associated with potentially fatal toxicities which can include metabolic acidosis, seizures, renal failure, and CNS depression; toxicities have also been reported in children and adults including hyperosmolality, lactic acidosis, seizures and respiratory depression; use caution (AAP 1997; Shehab 2009).

Drug Interactions

Metabolism/Transport Effects **Substrate** of CYP2C19 (minor), CYP2C9 (minor); **Note:** Assignment of Major/Minor substrate status based on clinically relevant drug interaction potential; **Inhibits** OAT1/3

Avoid Concomitant Use

Avoid concomitant use of Ibuprofen with any of the following: Acemetacin; Aminolevulinic Acid (Systemic); Dexibuprofen; Dexketoprofen; Floctafenine; Ketorolac (Nasal); Ketorolac (Systemic); Macimorelin; Mifamurtide; Morniflumate; Nonsteroidal Anti-Inflammatory Agents (COX-2 Selective); Omacetaxine; Pelubiprofen; Phenylbutazone; Talniflumate; Tenoxicam; Urokinase; Zaltoprofen

Increased Effect/Toxicity

Ibuprofen may increase the levels/effects of: 5-Aminosalicylic Acid Derivatives; Agents with Antiplatelet Properties; Aliskiren; Aminoglycosides; Aminolevulinic Acid (Systemic); Aminolevulinic Acid (Topical); Anticoagulants; Apixaban; Bemiparin; Bisphosphonate Derivatives; Cephalothin; Collagenase (Systemic); CycloSPORINE (Systemic); Dabigatran Etexilate; Deferasirox; Deoxycholic Acid; Desmopressin; Dexibuprofen; Dichlorphenamide; Digoxin; Drospirenone; Edoxaban; Enoxaparin; Eplerenone; Haloperidol; Heparin; Ibritumomab Tiuxetan; Lithium; MetFORMIN; Methotrexate; Nonsteroidal Anti-Inflammatory Agents (COX-2 Selective); Obinutuzumab; Omacetaxine; PEMEtrexed; Porfimer; Potassium-Sparing Diuretics; PRALAtrexate; Quinolones; Rivaroxaban; Salicylates; Tacrolimus (Systemic); Tenofovir Products; Thrombolytic Agents; Tolperisone; Urokinase; Vancomycin; Verteporfin; Vitamin K Antagonists

The levels/effects of Ibuprofen may be increased by: Acalabrutinib; Acemetacin; Alcohol (Ethyl); Angiotensin II Receptor Blockers; Angiotensin-Converting Enzyme Inhibitors; Corticosteroids (Systemic); CycloSPORINE (Systemic); Dasatinib; Dexketoprofen; Diclofenac (Systemic); Fat Emulsion (Fish Oil Based); Felbinac; Floctafenine; Fluconazole; Glucosamine; Herbs (Anticoagulant/Antiplatelet Properties); Ibrutinib; Inotersen; Ketorolac (Nasal); Ketorolac (Systemic); Limaprost; Loop Diuretics; Morniflumate; Multivitamins/Fluoride (with ADE); Multivitamins/Minerals (with ADEK, Folate, Iron); Multivitamins/Minerals (with AE, No Iron); Naftazone; Omega-3 Fatty Acids; Pelubiprofen; Pentosan Polysulfate Sodium; Pentoxifylline; Phenylbutazone; Probenecid; Prostacyclin Analogues; Selective Serotonin Reuptake Inhibitors; Selumetinib; Serotonin/Norepinephrine Reuptake Inhibitors; Sodium Phosphates; Talniflumate; Tenoxicam; Thiazide and Thiazide-Like Diuretics; Tipranavir; Tolperisone; Tricyclic Antidepressants (Tertiary Amine); Vitamin E (Systemic); Voriconazole; Zaltoprofen; Zanubrutinib

Decreased Effect

Ibuprofen may decrease the levels/effects of: Aliskiren; Angiotensin II Receptor Blockers; Angiotensin-Converting Enzyme Inhibitors; Beta-Blockers; Eplerenone; HydrALAZINE; Imatinib; Loop Diuretics; Macimorelin; Mifamurtide; Potassium-Sparing Diuretics; Prostaglandins (Ophthalmic); Salicylates; Selective Serotonin Reuptake Inhibitors; Sincalide; Thiazide and Thiazide-Like Diuretics

The levels/effects of Ibuprofen may be decreased by: Bile Acid Sequestrants; Lumacaftor and Ivacaftor; Salicylates

Food Interactions Ibuprofen peak serum levels may be decreased if taken with food. Management: Administer with food.

Dietary Considerations Some products may contain phenylalanine and/or potassium.

Pharmacodynamics/Kinetics

Onset of Action

Onset of Action: Oral: Analgesic: Within 30 to 60 minutes (Davies 1998; Mehlisch 2013); Antipyretic: Single oral dose 8 mg/kg (Kauffman 1992): Infants ≤1 year: 69 ± 22 minutes; Children ≥6 years: Single oral dose 8 mg/kg (Kauffman 1992): 109 ± 64 minutes; Adults: <1 hour (Sullivan 2011)

Maximum effect: Antipyretic: 2-4 hours

Duration of Action Oral: Antipyretic: 6 to 8 hours (Sullivan 2011)

Half-life Elimination

IV:

Ibuprofen (Caldor):

- Pediatric patients: 6 months to <2 years: 1.8 hours; 2 to 16 years: ~1.5 hours
- Adults: 2.22 to 2.44 hours

Ibuprofen lysine (Neoprofen):

- Premature neonates, GA <32 weeks: Reported data highly variable
- R-enantiomer: 10 hours; S-enantiomer: 25.5 hours (Gregoire 2004)
  - Age-based observations:
    - PNA <1 day: 30.5 ± 4.2 hours (Aranda 1997)
    - PNA 3 days: 43.1 ± 26.1 hours (Van Overmeire 2001)
    - PNA 5 days: 26.8 ± 23.6 hours (Van Overmeire 2001)

Oral:

- Children 3 months to 10 years: Oral suspension: 1.6 ± 0.7 hours (Kauffman 1992)
- Adults: ~2 hours; End-stage renal disease: Unchanged (Aronoff 2007)

Time to Peak

Tablets: 1 to 2 hours; suspension: 1 hour

Children with cystic fibrosis (Scott 1999):

Suspension (n=22): 0.74 ± 0.43 hours (median: 30 minutes)

Chewable tablet (n=4): 1.5 ± 0.58 hours (median: 1.5 hours)

Tablet (n=12): 1.33 ± 0.95 hours (median: 1 hour)

Reproductive Considerations

The chronic use of NSAIDs in women of reproductive age may be associated with infertility that is reversible upon discontinuation of the medication. Consider discontinuing use in women having difficulty conceiving or those undergoing investigation of fertility.

Pregnancy Considerations Birth defects have been observed following in utero NSAID exposure in some studies; however, data is conflicting (Bloor 2013). Nonteratogenic effects, including prenatal constriction of the ductus arteriosus, persistent pulmonary hypertension of the newborn, oligohydramnios, necrotizing enterocolitis, renal dysfunction or failure, and intracranial hemorrhage have been observed in the fetus/neonate following in utero NSAID exposure. In addition, nonclosure of the ductus arteriosus postnatally may occur and be resistant to medical management (Bermas 2014; Bloor 2013). Because NSAIDs cause premature closure of the ductus arteriosus, prescribing information for ibuprofen specifically states use should be avoided starting at 30-weeks gestation.

Use of NSAIDs can be considered for the treatment of mild rheumatoid arthritis flares in pregnant women; however, use should be minimized or avoided early and late in pregnancy (Bermas 2014; Saavedra Salinas 2015). If treatment of migraine is needed in pregnant women, ibuprofen is preferred when an NSAID is required; however, other agents are recommended as initial therapy (Amundsen 2015).

The use of NSAIDs close to conception may be associated with an increased risk of miscarriage (Bloor 2013; Bermas 2014).

Breastfeeding Considerations Ibuprofen is present in breast milk.

The relative infant dose (RID) of ibuprofen is 0.6% to 0.9% when calculated using the highest breast milk concentration located and compared to an infant therapeutic dose of 10 to 15 mg/kg/day. In general, breastfeeding is considered acceptable when the RID is <10%; when an RID is >25%, breastfeeding should generally be avoided (Anderson 2016; Ito 2000). Using the highest milk concentration (0.59 mcg/mL), the estimated daily infant dose via breast milk is 0.089 mg/kg/day. This milk concentration was obtained following maternal administration of oral ibuprofen ≥600 mg/day (Rigourd 2014).

Based on the available data, adverse events have not been reported in breastfeeding infants and milk production is not affected.

In general, NSAIDs may be used in postpartum women who wish to breastfeed and if needed for postpartum pain, ibuprofen is the preferred agent (Montgomery 2012). Ibuprofen is considered compatible with breastfeeding when used in usual recommended doses (WHO 2002). Use should be avoided in women breastfeeding infants with platelet dysfunction or thrombocytopenia (Bloor 2013; Sammaritano 2014). The manufacturer recommends that the decision to breastfeed during therapy consider the risk of infant exposure, the benefits of breastfeeding to the infant, and benefits of treatment to the mother.

Dosage Forms Considerations EnovaRX-Ibuprofen cream is compounded from a kit. Refer to manufacturer's labeling for compounding instructions.

Dosage Forms: US

Capsule, Oral:

Advil [OTC]: 200 mg

Advil Liqui-Gels minis [OTC]: 200 mg

Advil Migraine [OTC]: 200 mg

GoodSense Ibuprofen [OTC]: 200 mg

KS Ibuprofen [OTC]: 200 mg

Motrin IB [OTC]: 200 mg

Generic: 200 mg

Kit, Oral:

IBU 600-EZS: 600 mg

Solution, Intravenous [preservative free]:

Caldolor: 800 mg/200 mL (200 mL); 800 mg/8 mL (8 mL)

NeoProfen: 10 mg/mL (2 mL)

Generic: 10 mg/mL (2 mL)

Suspension, Oral:

Childrens Advil [OTC]: 100 mg/5 mL (30 mL, 120 mL)

Childrens Motrin [OTC]: 100 mg/5 mL (30 mL, 120 mL)

GoodSense Ibuprofen Childrens [OTC]: 100 mg/5 mL (120 mL)

Ibuprofen Childrens [OTC]: 100 mg/5 mL (5 mL, 10 mL, 118 mL, 120 mL, 237 mL, 240 mL)

Infants Advil [OTC]: 50 mg/1.25 mL (15 mL, 30 mL)

Motrin Infants Drops [OTC]: 50 mg/1.25 mL (15 mL, 30 mL)

Generic: 100 mg/5 mL (5 mL, 118 mL, 120 mL, 473 mL)

Tablet, Oral:

Addaprin [OTC]: 200 mg

Advil [OTC]: 200 mg

Advil Junior Strength [OTC]: 100 mg

Dyspel [OTC]: 200 mg

Genpril [OTC]: 200 mg

GoodSense Ibuprofen [OTC]: 200 mg

IBU-200 [OTC]: 200 mg

IBU: 400 mg, 600 mg, 800 mg

Motrin IB [OTC]: 200 mg

Provil [OTC]: 200 mg

Generic: 200 mg, 400 mg, 600 mg, 800 mg

Tablet Chewable, Oral:

Advil Junior Strength [OTC]: 100 mg

Motrin Childrens [OTC]: 100 mg

Dosage Forms: Canada

Solution, Intravenous:

Caldolor: 100 mg/mL (4 mL, 8 mL)

Tablet, Oral:

Generic: 600 mg

Dental Health Professional Considerations Preoperative use of ibuprofen at a dose of 400-600 mg every 6 hours 24 hours before the appointment decreases postoperative edema and hastens healing time.

New information from the FDA states that ibuprofen can interfere with the antiplatelet effect of low-dose aspirin (81 mg/day), potentially rendering aspirin less effective when used for cardioprotection and stroke protection. In situations where these drugs could be used concomitantly, the FDA has provided the following information.

Patients who use immediate release aspirin (not enteric-coated aspirin) and take a single dose or chronic doses of ibuprofen 400 mg, should dose the ibuprofen at least **30 minutes or longer after aspirin ingestion or more than 8 hours before aspirin ingestion** to avoid attenuation of aspirin's effect.

At this time, recommendations about the timing of ibuprofen 400 mg in patients taking enteric-coated low-dose aspirin cannot be made based on available data. One study however, showed that the antiplatelet effect of enteric-coated low-dose aspirin was attenuated when ibuprofen 400 mg was dosed 2, 7, and 12 hours after aspirin (Catella-Lawson 2001).

With occasional use of ibuprofen, there is likely to be minimal risk from any attenuation of the antiplatelet effect of low-dose aspirin, because of a long-lasting effect of aspirin on platelets.

Other over-the-counter (OTC) NSAIDs (ie, naproxen sodium and ketoprofen) should be viewed as having the potential to interfere with the antiplatelet effect of low-dose aspirin until proven otherwise. However, the FDA is unaware of any studies that have looked at the same type of interference by ketoprofen with low-dose aspirin. One study of naproxen and low-dose aspirin has suggested that naproxen may interfere with aspirin's antiplatelet activity when they are coadministered (Steinhubl 2005). However, naproxen 500 mg administered 2 hours before or after aspirin 100 mg, did not interfere with aspirin's antiplatelet effect. The FDA stated that there is no data looking at doses of naproxen <500 mg. Naproxen OTC strength is 220 mg tablets.

Ibuprofen, prescription dose of 800 mg 3 times daily, significantly diminishes the antiplatelet effects of low-dose aspirin (baby) in healthy volunteers. Diclofenac (Systemic), 50 mg 3 times daily, did not interfere with the antiplatelet effects of low-dose aspirin (baby) in healthy volunteers. Ibuprofen, and possibly other non-selective NSAIDs, may reduce the cardioprotective effects of aspirin. It seems prudent to avoid regular, frequent use of ibuprofen in patients receiving aspirin for its cardioprotective effects. Alternative analgesics (eg, acetaminophen) or prescription diclofenac in place of prescription ibuprofen may be a safer choice.

◆ **Ibuprofen and Hydrocodone** *see* Hydrocodone and Ibuprofen *on page 769*

◆ **Ibuprofen and Pseudoephedrine** *see* Pseudoephedrine and Ibuprofen *on page 1292*

◆ **Ibuprofen Childrens [OTC]** *see* Ibuprofen *on page 786*

◆ **Ibuprofen Comfort Pac [DSC]** *see* Ibuprofen *on page 786*

◆ **Ibuprofen Lysine** *see* Ibuprofen *on page 786*

Ibutilide (i BYOO ti lide)

Related Information

Clinical Risk Related to Drugs Prolonging QT Interval *on page 1675*

Brand Names: US Corvert

Brand Names: Canada Corvert

Pharmacologic Category Antiarrhythmic Agent, Class III

Use

Atrial fibrillation/flutter: Rapid conversion of atrial fibrillation or atrial flutter of recent onset to sinus rhythm (effectiveness has not been determined in patients with arrhythmias >90 days in duration).

Note: According to the American Heart Association/American College of Cardiology/Heart Rhythm Society guidelines for the management of atrial fibrillation, in patients with pre-excited atrial fibrillation and rapid ventricular response who are not hemodynamically compromised, the use of ibutilide to restore sinus rhythm or slow the ventricular rate is recommended (AHA/ACC/HRS [January 2014]).

Local Anesthetic/Vasoconstrictor Precautions

Ibutilide is one of the drugs confirmed to prolong the QT interval and is accepted as having a risk of causing torsade de pointes. The risk of drug-induced torsade de pointes is extremely low when a single QT interval prolonging drug is prescribed. In terms of epinephrine, it is not known what effect vasoconstrictors in the local anesthetic regimen will have in patients with a known history of congenital prolonged QT interval or in patients taking any medication that prolongs the QT interval. Until more information is obtained, it is suggested that the clinician consult with the physician prior to the use of a vasoconstrictor in suspected patients, and that the vasoconstrictor (epinephrine, mepivacaine and levonordefrin [Carbocaine® 2% with Neo-Cobefrin®]) be used with caution.

Effects on Dental Treatment No significant effects or complications reported

Effects on Bleeding No information available to require special precautions

Adverse Reactions

1% to 10%:

Cardiovascular: Nonsustained monomorphic ventricular tachycardia (5%), ventricular premature contractions (5), unsustained polymorphic ventricular tachycardia (3%), supraventricular tachycardia (≤3%), tachycardia (≤3%), atrioventricular block (2%), bundle branch block (2%), hypotension (2%), sustained polymorphic ventricular tachycardia (2%; eg, torsade de pointes; often requiring cardioversion), bradycardia (1%), hypertension (1%), palpitations (1%), prolonged QT interval on ECG (1%)

Central nervous system: Headache (4%)

Gastrointestinal: Nausea (>1%)

<1%, postmarketing, and/or case reports: Bullous rash (erythematous), cardiac failure, idioventricular rhythm, nodal arrhythmia, renal failure, supraventricular extrasystole, sustained monomorphic ventricular tachycardia

Mechanism of Action Vaughan Williams class III antiarrhythmic agent that prolongs myocardial action potential duration (APD) and increases atrial and ventricular refractoriness primarily by activation of a slow inward sodium current (INa-s), in contrast to other agents in this class. Ibutilide also delays repolarization by inhibiting the rapid component of the delayed rectifier potassium current (IKr), though the relative contribution of this mechanism to the antiarrhythmic activity of ibutilide is not known (Cimini 1992; Foster 1997; Lee 1992; Yang 1995).

Pharmacodynamics/Kinetics

Onset of Action Conversion to sinus rhythm: ≤90 minutes after start of infusion

Half-life Elimination ~6 hours (range: 2 to 12 hours)

Pregnancy Considerations

Use in pregnancy may be considered (Regitz-Zagrosek [ESC 2018]); however, information related to the use of ibutilide in pregnancy is limited (Burkart 2007; Kockova 2007).

Dental Health Professional Considerations See Local Anesthetic/Vasoconstrictor Precautions

◆ **Ibutilide Fumarate** *see* Ibutilide *on page 794*

Icatibant (eye KAT i bant)

Brand Names: US Firazyr
Brand Names: Canada Firazyr
Pharmacologic Category Selective Bradykinin B2 Receptor Antagonist
Use Hereditary angioedema: Treatment of acute attacks of hereditary angioedema (HAE)
Local Anesthetic/Vasoconstrictor Precautions No information available to require special precautions
Effects on Dental Treatment No significant effects or complications reported
Effects on Bleeding No information available to require special precautions
Adverse Reactions
>10%: Local: Injection site reaction (97%)
1% to 10%:
Hepatic: Increased serum transaminase (4%)
Immunologic: Antibody development (4%; anti-icatibant, no association with efficacy observed)
Nervous system: Dizziness (3%)
Miscellaneous: Fever (4%)
Frequency not defined:
Dermatologic: Skin rash
Gastrointestinal: Nausea
Nervous system: Headache
Postmarketing: Dermatologic: Urticaria
Mechanism of Action Icatibant is a selective competitive antagonist for the bradykinin B_2 receptor. Patients with HAE have an absence or dysfunction of C1-esterase-inhibitor which leads to the production of bradykinin. The presence of bradykinin may cause symptoms of localized swelling, inflammation, and pain. Icatibant inhibits bradykinin from binding at the B_2 receptor, thereby treating the symptoms associated with acute attack.
Pharmacodynamics/Kinetics
Onset of Action Median time to 50% decrease of symptoms: ~2 hours
Duration of Action Inhibits symptoms caused by bradykinin for ~6 hours
Half-life Elimination
Children ≥2 years: 0.8 ± 0.04 hours (Farkas 2017)
Adolescents: 1.34 ± 0.96 hours (Farkas 2017)
Adults: 1.4 ± 0.4 hours
Time to Peak
Children ≥2 years: 0.42 ± 0.13 hours (Farkas 2017)
Adolescents: 0.55 ± 0.19 hours (Farkas 2017)
Adults: ~0.75 hours
Pregnancy Considerations
Information related to the use of icatibant in pregnancy is limited (Boufleur 2014; Farkas 2016; Hakl 2018; Kaminsky 2017; Tran 2013; Zanichelli 2015).

When treatment for hereditary angioedema in pregnancy is needed, other agents are recommended (Betschel 2019; WAO/EEACI [Maurer 2018]).

◆ **Icatibant Acetate** *see* Icatibant *on page 795*
◆ **ICI-182,780** *see* Fulvestrant *on page 721*
◆ **ICI-204,219** *see* Zafirlukast *on page 1565*
◆ **ICI-46474** *see* Tamoxifen *on page 1404*
◆ **ICI-118630** *see* Goserelin *on page 746*
◆ **ICI-D1033** *see* Anastrozole *on page 150*
◆ **Iclusig** *see* PONATinib *on page 1246*
◆ **Icosapent Ethyl** *see* Omega-3 Fatty Acids *on page 1137*

IdaruCIZUmab (eye da roo SIZ uh mab)

Brand Names: US Praxbind
Brand Names: Canada Praxbind
Pharmacologic Category Antidote; Monoclonal Antibody
Use Reversal of dabigatran: Reversal of the anticoagulant effects of dabigatran for emergency surgery/urgent procedures or in life-threatening or uncontrolled bleeding.
Local Anesthetic/Vasoconstrictor Precautions No information available to require special precautions
Effects on Dental Treatment No significant effects or complications reported
Effects on Bleeding No information available to require special precautions
Adverse Reactions
1% to 10%:
Central nervous system: Headache (5%)
Gastrointestinal: Constipation (7%), nausea (5%)
Frequency not defined:
Hypersensitivity: Hypersensitivity reaction (including bronchospasm, fever, hyperventilation, pruritus, skin rash)
<1%, postmarketing, and/or case reports (Pollack 2015): Acute ischemic stroke, circulatory shock, deep vein thrombosis, intracardiac thrombus (left atrium), multiorgan failure, myocardial infarction (NSTEMI), pulmonary edema, pulmonary embolism, right heart failure, thromboembolic complications (Pollack 2017)
Mechanism of Action Idarucizumab, a specific reversal agent for dabigatran, is a humanized monoclonal antibody fragment (Fab) that binds specifically to dabigatran and its acylglucuronide metabolites with an affinity for dabigatran that is ~350 times greater than that of thrombin, and neutralizes the anticoagulant effect within minutes (Das 2015; Schiele 2013).
Pharmacodynamics/Kinetics
Onset of Action Uncontrolled bleeding: Effects observed within minutes and hemostasis is restored at a median of 11.4 hours (Pollack 2015)
Duration of Action Usually at least 24 hours
Half-life Elimination 47 minutes (initial); 10.3 hours (terminal)
Pregnancy Considerations Animal reproduction studies have not been conducted.

◆ **IDEC-C2B8** *see* RiTUXimab *on page 1336*
◆ **IDEC-Y2B8** *see* Ibritumomab Tiuxetan *on page 784*

Idelalisib (eye del a LIS ib)

Brand Names: US Zydelig
Brand Names: Canada Zydelig
Pharmacologic Category Antineoplastic Agent, Phosphatidylinositol 3-Kinase Inhibitor
Use
Chronic lymphocytic leukemia: Treatment of relapsed chronic lymphocytic leukemia (CLL) (in combination with rituximab) when rituximab alone is appropriate therapy due to other comorbidities
Follicular B-cell non-Hodgkin lymphoma: Treatment of relapsed follicular B-cell non-Hodgkin lymphoma (NHL) after at least 2 prior systemic therapies

Small lymphocytic lymphoma: Treatment of relapsed small lymphocytic lymphoma (SLL) after at least 2 prior systemic therapies

Limitations of use: Idelalisib is not indicated or recommended for first-line treatment of CLL, follicular B-cell NHL, or SLL. Idelalisib is not indicated and is not recommended in combination with bendamustine and/or rituximab for the treatment of follicular NHL.

Local Anesthetic/Vasoconstrictor Precautions No information available to require special precautions

Effects on Dental Treatment No significant effects or complications reported

Effects on Bleeding Chemotherapy may result in significant myelosuppression, potentially including significant reduction in platelet counts and altered hemostasis. In patients who are under active treatment with these agents, medical consult is suggested.

Adverse Reactions As reported with monotherapy.

>10%:

Central nervous system: Fatigue (30%), insomnia (12%), headache (11%)

Dermatologic: Skin rash (21%), night sweats (12%)

Gastrointestinal: Diarrhea (47%), nausea (29%), abdominal pain (26%), decreased appetite (16%), vomiting (15%)

Hematologic & oncologic: Decreased hemoglobin (28%; grade 3: 2%), decreased platelet count (26%; grade 3: 3%; grade 4: 3%), neutropenia (25%; grades 3/4)

Hepatic: Increased serum ALT (50%), increased serum AST (41%), severe hepatotoxicity (18%)

Infection: Severe infection (21%; including sepsis, febrile neutropenia)

Neuromuscular & skeletal: Weakness (12%)

Respiratory: Cough (29%), pneumonia (15% to 25%), dyspnea (17%), upper respiratory tract infection (12%)

Miscellaneous: Fever (28%)

1% to 10%:

Cardiovascular: Peripheral edema (10%)

Respiratory: Pneumonitis (4%)

<1%, postmarketing, and/or case reports: Anaphylaxis, cytomegalovirus disease, erythematous rash, exfoliative dermatitis, hypersensitivity reaction, intestinal perforation, macular eruption, maculopapular rash, papular rash, pneumonia due to pneumocystic carinii, progressive multifocal leukoencephalopathy (Raisch 2016), pruritic rash, Stevens-Johnson syndrome, toxic epidermal necrolysis

Mechanism of Action Idelalisib is a potent small molecule inhibitor of the delta isoform of phosphatidylinositol 3-kinase (PI3Kδ), which is highly expressed in malignant lymphoid B-cells. PI3Kδ inhibition results in apoptosis of malignant tumor cells. In addition, idelalisib inhibits several signaling pathways, including B-cell receptor, CXCR4 and CXCR5 signaling which may play important roles in CLL pathophysiology (Furman 2014).

Pharmacodynamics/Kinetics

Half-life Elimination 8.2 hours

Time to Peak Median: 1.5 hours

Reproductive Considerations

Verify pregnancy status in females of reproductive potential prior to initiating treatment with idelalisib. Females of reproductive potential should use effective contraception during therapy and for at least 1 month after the final idelalisib dose. Males with female partners of reproductive potential should use effective contraception during therapy and for 3 months after the final idelalisib dose.

Pregnancy Considerations

Based on findings in animal reproduction studies and the mechanism of action, idelalisib may cause fetal harm if administered during pregnancy.

Prescribing and Access Restrictions Available through specialty pharmacies. Further information may be obtained at http://www.zydeligaccessconnect.com/.

- ◆ **IDH1 Inhibitor AG-120** *see* Ivosidenib *on page 851*
- ◆ **IDH2 inhibitor** *see* Enasidenib *on page 562*
- ◆ **Idhifa** *see* Enasidenib *on page 562*
- ◆ **IDHIFA** *see* Enasidenib *on page 562*
- ◆ **IDV** *see* Indinavir *on page 807*
- ◆ **IG** *see* Immune Globulin *on page 803*
- ◆ **IgG4-Kappa Monoclonal Antibody** *see* Natalizumab *on page 1086*
- ◆ **IGIM** *see* Immune Globulin *on page 803*
- ◆ **IGIV** *see* Immune Globulin *on page 803*
- ◆ **IGSC** *see* Immune Globulin *on page 803*
- ◆ **IIV** *see* Influenza Virus Vaccine (Inactivated) *on page 812*
- ◆ **IIV3** *see* Influenza Virus Vaccine (Inactivated) *on page 812*
- ◆ **IIV4** *see* Influenza Virus Vaccine (Inactivated) *on page 812*
- ◆ **IL-1Ra** *see* Anakinra *on page 149*
- ◆ **IL-2** *see* Aldesleukin *on page 91*
- ◆ **Ilevro** *see* Nepafenac *on page 1093*

Iloperidone (eye loe PER i done)

Related Information

Clinical Risk Related to Drugs Prolonging QT Interval *on page 1675*

Brand Names: US Fanapt; Fanapt Titration Pack

Pharmacologic Category Second Generation (Atypical) Antipsychotic

Use Schizophrenia: Treatment of adults with schizophrenia

Local Anesthetic/Vasoconstrictor Precautions Iloperidone is one of the drugs confirmed to prolong the QT interval and is accepted as having a risk of causing torsade de pointes. The risk of drug-induced torsade de pointes is extremely low when a single QT interval prolonging drug is prescribed. In terms of epinephrine, it is not known what effect vasoconstrictors in the local anesthetic regimen will have in patients with a known history of congenital prolonged QT interval or in patients taking any medication that prolongs the QT interval. Until more information is obtained, it is suggested that the clinician consult with the physician prior to the use of a vasoconstrictor in suspected patients, and that the vasoconstrictor (epinephrine, mepivacaine and levonordefrin [Carbocaine 2% with Neo-Cobefrin]) be used with caution.

Effects on Dental Treatment Key adverse event(s) related to dental treatment: Xerostomia and changes in salivation (normal salivary flow resumes upon discontinuation); Patients may experience orthostatic hypotension as they stand up after treatment; especially if lying in dental chair for extended periods of time. Use caution with sudden changes in position during and after dental treatment.

Effects on Bleeding No information available to require special precautions

Adverse Reactions

>10%:

Cardiovascular: Tachycardia (3% to 12%; dose-related)

Central nervous system: Dizziness (10% to 20%; dose-related), drowsiness (9% to 15%)

Endocrine & metabolic: Increased serum prolactin (26%), weight gain (9% to 18%; dose-related)

1% to 10%:

Cardiovascular: Orthostatic hypotension (3% to 5%), hypotension (3%; dose-related), palpitations (≥1%)

Central nervous system: Fatigue (4% to 6%), extrapyramidal reaction (4% to 5%), lethargy (3%), aggressive behavior (≥1%), delusions (≥1%), restlessness (≥1%), dystonia (≤1%)

Dermatologic: Skin rash (3%)

Endocrine & metabolic: Increased serum triglycerides (10%), increased serum cholesterol (4%), weight loss (≥1%)

Gastrointestinal: Nausea (10%), xerostomia (8% to 10%), diarrhea (5% to 7%), abdominal distress (3%; dose-related)

Genitourinary: Ejaculation failure (2%), erectile dysfunction (≥1%), urinary incontinence (≥1%)

Hematologic & oncologic: Decreased hematocrit (≤1%)

Neuromuscular & skeletal: Arthralgia (3%), muscle rigidity (3%; dose-related), tremor (3%), muscle spasm (≥1%), myalgia (≥1%)

Ophthalmic: Blurred vision (3%), conjunctivitis (≥1%; including allergic)

Respiratory: Nasal congestion (5% to 8%), nasopharyngitis (≤4%), upper respiratory tract infection (2% to 3%), dyspnea (2%)

Frequency not defined: Genitourinary: Priapism

<1%, postmarketing, and/or case reports: Abnormal gait, acute renal failure, amenorrhea, amnesia, anemia, anorgasmia, aphthous stomatitis, asthma, blepharitis, bradykinesia, bulimia nervosa, cardiac arrhythmia, cataract, catatonia, cholelithiasis, confusion, decreased hemoglobin, decreased libido, dehydration, delirium, dry nose, duodenal ulcer, dyspnea on exertion, dysuria, edema, emotional lability, epistaxis, eyelid edema, fecal incontinence, first degree atrioventricular block, fluid retention, gastritis, gastroesophageal reflux disease, gynecomastia, hiatal hernia, hostility, hyperacidity, hyperemia (including conjunctival), hyperglycemia, hypermenorrhea, hypersensitivity reaction (including anaphylaxis; angioedema; throat tightness; oropharyngeal swelling; swelling of the face, lips, mouth, and tongue; urticaria; pruritus), hyperthermia, hypokalemia, hypothyroidism, impulse control disorder, increased appetite, increased neutrophils, increased thirst, iron deficiency anemia, leukopenia, major depressive disorder, mania, mastalgia, menstrual disease, nephrolithiasis, neuroleptic malignant syndrome, nystagmus, obsessive compulsive disorder, oral mucosa ulcer, panic attack, paranoia, paresthesia, Parkinson's disease, pollakiuria, polydipsia (psychogenic), postmenopausal bleeding, prolonged QT interval on ECG, prostatitis, psychomotor agitation, restless leg syndrome, retrograde ejaculation, rhinorrhea, salivation, sinus congestion, sleep apnea, stomatitis, swelling of eye, syncope, testicular pain, tinnitus, torticollis, urinary retention, uterine hemorrhage, vertigo, xerophthalmia

Mechanism of Action Iloperidone is a piperidinyl-benzisoxazole atypical antipsychotic with mixed D_2/5-HT_2 antagonist activity. It exhibits high affinity for 5-HT_{2A}, $NE_{\alpha1}$, D_2, and D_3 receptors, low to moderate affinity for D_1, D_4, H_1, 5-HT_{1A}, 5-HT_6, and 5-HT_7 receptors, and no affinity for muscarinic receptors. The addition of serotonin antagonism to dopamine antagonism (classic neuroleptic mechanism) is thought to improve negative symptoms of psychoses and reduce the incidence of extrapyramidal side effects (Huttunen 1995). Iloperidone's low affinity for histamine H_1 receptors may decrease the risk for weight gain and somnolence while its affinity for $NE_{\alpha1/\alpha2C}$ may improve cognitive function but increase the risk for orthostasis (Arif 2011, Huttunen 1995, Nasrallah 2008).

Pharmacodynamics/Kinetics

Half-life Elimination

Extensive metabolizers: Iloperidone: 18 hours; P88: 26 hours; P95: 23 hours

Poor metabolizers: Iloperidone: 33 hours; P88: 37 hours; P95: 31 hours

Time to Peak Plasma: 2 to 4 hours

Reproductive Considerations

Iloperidone may cause hyperprolactinemia, which may decrease reproductive function in both males and females.

Pregnancy Considerations

Antipsychotic use during the third trimester of pregnancy has a risk for abnormal muscle movements (extrapyramidal symptoms [EPS]) and/or withdrawal symptoms in newborns following delivery. Symptoms in the newborn may include agitation, feeding disorder, hypertonia, hypotonia, respiratory distress, somnolence, and tremor; these effects may be self-limiting or require hospitalization.

The ACOG recommends that therapy during pregnancy be individualized; treatment with psychiatric medications during pregnancy should incorporate the clinical expertise of the mental health clinician, obstetrician, primary healthcare provider, and pediatrician. Safety data related to atypical antipsychotics during pregnancy is limited and routine use is not recommended. However, if a woman is inadvertently exposed to an atypical antipsychotic while pregnant, continuing therapy may be preferable to switching to a typical antipsychotic that the fetus has not yet been exposed to; consider risk: benefit (ACOG 2008).

Health care providers are encouraged to enroll women 18 to 45 years of age exposed to iloperidone during pregnancy in the Atypical Antipsychotics Pregnancy Registry (1-866-961-2388 or http://www.womensmentalhealth.org/pregnancyregistry).

Dental Health Professional Considerations See Local Anesthetic/Vasoconstrictor Precautions

◆ **Ilumya** *see* Tildrakizumab *on page 1448*

Imatinib (eye MAT eh nib)

Brand Names: US Gleevec

Brand Names: Canada APO-Imatinib; Gleevec; MINT-Imatinib; NAT-Imatinib; PMS-Imatinib; TEVA-Imatinib

Pharmacologic Category Antineoplastic Agent, BCR-ABL Tyrosine Kinase Inhibitor; Antineoplastic Agent, Tyrosine Kinase Inhibitor

Use

Acute lymphoblastic leukemia: Treatment of relapsed or refractory Philadelphia chromosome-positive (Ph+) acute lymphoblastic leukemia (ALL) in adults

Treatment of newly diagnosed Ph+ ALL in children (in combination with chemotherapy)

Aggressive systemic mastocytosis: Treatment of aggressive systemic mastocytosis in adults without D816V c-Kit mutation (as determined by an approved test) or with c-Kit mutational status unknown.

Chronic myeloid leukemia:

Treatment of Ph+ chronic myeloid leukemia (CML) in chronic phase (newly diagnosed) in adults and children

Treatment of Ph+ CML in blast crisis, accelerated phase, or chronic phase after failure of interferon-alfa therapy

Dermatofibrosarcoma protuberans: Treatment of unresectable, recurrent, and/or metastatic dermatofibrosarcoma protuberans (DFSP) in adults

Gastrointestinal stromal tumors: Treatment of Kit (CD117)-positive unresectable and/or metastatic malignant gastrointestinal stromal tumors (GIST)

Adjuvant treatment of Kit (CD117)-positive GIST following complete gross resection

Hypereosinophilic syndrome and/or chronic eosinophilic leukemia: Treatment of hypereosinophilic syndrome (HES) and/or chronic eosinophilic leukemia (CEL) in adult patients who have the FIP1L1–platelet-derived growth factor (PDGF) receptor alpha fusion kinase (mutational analysis or fluorescent in situ hybridization [FISH] demonstration of CHIC2 allele deletion) and for patients with HES and/or CEL who are FIP1L1-PDGF receptor alpha fusion kinase negative or unknown

Myelodysplastic/Myeloproliferative diseases: Treatment of myelodysplastic syndrome/myeloproliferative diseases (MDS/MPD) associated with PDGF receptor gene rearrangements as determined by an approved test in adults

Local Anesthetic/Vasoconstrictor Precautions No information available to require special precautions

Effects on Dental Treatment Key adverse event(s) related to dental treatment: Mouth ulceration and taste disturbance.

Effects on Bleeding Bleeding was reported in 12% to 53% of patients. Cytopenias including thrombocytopenia (grade 4 severe: <33%) and anemia (25% to 80%; grade 4: <11%) have been reported. Medical consult is recommended.

Adverse Reactions

>10%:

Cardiovascular: Edema (11% to 86%), peripheral edema (20% to 41%), facial edema (≤17%), chest pain (7% to 11%)

Central nervous system: Fatigue (20% to 75%), pain (≤47%), headache (8% to 37%), dizziness (5% to 19%), insomnia (9% to 15%), depression (3% to 15%), taste disorder (≤13%), rigors (10% to 12%), anxiety (8% to 12%), paresthesia (≤12%), chills (≤11%)

Dermatologic: Skin rash (9% to 50%), dermatitis (≤39%), pruritus (7% to 26%), night sweats (13% to 17%), alopecia (7% to 15%), diaphoresis (≤13%)

Endocrine & metabolic: Fluid retention (2% to 76%), increased lactate dehydrogenase (≤60%), weight gain (5% to 32%), decreased serum albumin (≤21%), hypokalemia (6% to 13%)

Gastrointestinal: Nausea (41% to 73%), diarrhea (25% to 59%), vomiting (11% to 58%), abdominal pain (3% to 57%), anorexia (≤36%), dyspepsia (11% to 27%), flatulence (≤25%), abdominal distension (≤19%), constipation (8% to 16%), upper abdominal pain (14%), stomatitis (≤10%)

Hematologic & oncologic: Hemorrhage (3% to 53%; grades 3/4: ≤19%), neutropenia (≤16%; grades 3/4: 3% to 48%), leukopenia (GIST: 5% to 47%; grades 3/4: 2%), anemia (32% to 35%; grades 3/4: 1% to 42%), thrombocytopenia (grades 3/4: ≤33%), hypoproteinemia (≤32%)

Hepatic: Increased serum aspartate aminotransferase (≤38%), increased serum alanine aminotransferase (≤34%), increased alkaline phosphatase (≤17%), increased serum bilirubin (≤13%)

Infection: Infection (14% to 28%), influenza (≤14%)

Neuromuscular & skeletal: Muscle cramps (16% to 62%), musculoskeletal pain (adults: 38% to 49%; children: 21%), muscle spasm (16% to 49%), arthralgia (11% to 40%), myalgia (9% to 32%), asthenia (≤21%), back pain (≤17%), limb pain (≤16%), ostealgia (≤11%)

Ophthalmic: Periorbital edema (15% to 74%), increased lacrimation (≤25%), eyelid edema (19%), blurred vision (≤11%)

Renal: Increased serum creatinine (≤44%)

Respiratory: Nasopharyngitis (1% to 31%), cough (11% to 27%), upper respiratory tract infection (3% to 21%), dyspnea (≤21%), pharyngolaryngeal pain (≤18%), rhinitis (17%), pharyngitis (10% to 15%), flu-like symptoms (1% to 14%), pneumonia (4% to 13%), sinusitis (4% to 11%)

Miscellaneous: Fever (6% to 41%)

1% to 10%:

Cardiovascular: Palpitations (≤5%), hypertension (≤4%), cardiac failure (1%), hypotension (≤1%), flushing

Central nervous system: Cerebral hemorrhage (≤9%), hypoesthesia, peripheral neuropathy

Dermatologic: Skin photosensitivity (4% to 7%), xeroderma (≤7%), erythema, nail disease

Endocrine & metabolic: Hypophosphatemia (10%), hyperglycemia (≤10%), weight loss (≤10%), hypocalcemia (≤6%), hyperkalemia (1%)

Gastrointestinal: Decreased appetite (10%), gastroenteritis (≤10%), gastrointestinal hemorrhage (1% to 8%), increased serum lipase (grades 3/4: 4%), gastritis, gastroesophageal reflux disease, xerostomia

Hematologic & oncologic: Lymphocytopenia (≤10%; grades 3/4: 1% to 2%), eosinophilia, febrile neutropenia, pancytopenia, purpuric rash

Neuromuscular & skeletal: Joint swelling

Ophthalmic: Conjunctivitis (5% to 8%), conjunctival hemorrhage, dry eyes

Respiratory: Oropharyngeal pain (≤6%), interstitial pneumonitis (≤1%), pleural effusion (≤1%), epistaxis

<1%, postmarketing, and/or case reports: Actinic keratosis, acute generalized exanthematous pustulosis, anaphylactic shock, angina pectoris, angioedema, aplastic anemia, arthritis, ascites, atrial fibrillation, avascular necrosis of bones, blepharitis, bullous rash, cardiac arrhythmia, cardiac tamponade, cardiogenic shock, cataract, cellulitis, cerebral edema, cheilitis, cold extremities, colitis, confusion, decreased libido, decreased linear skeletal growth rate (children), dehydration, diverticulitis of the gastrointestinal tract, DRESS syndrome, drowsiness, dyschromia, dysphagia, embolism, eructation, erythema multiforme, esophagitis, exfoliative dermatitis, folliculitis, fungal infection, gastric ulcer, gastrointestinal obstruction, gastrointestinal perforation, glaucoma, gout, gynecomastia, hearing loss, heavy menstrual bleeding, hematemesis, hematoma, hematuria, hemolytic anemia, Henoch-Schonlein purpura, hepatic failure, hepatic

necrosis, hepatitis, hepatotoxicity, herpes simplex infection, herpes zoster infection, hypercalcemia, hypersensitivity angiitis, hyperuricemia, hypomagnesemia, hyponatremia, hypothyroidism, increased creatine phosphokinase, increased intracranial pressure, inflammatory bowel disease, interstitial pulmonary disease, intestinal obstruction, jaundice, left ventricular dysfunction, lichen planus, lower respiratory tract infection, lymphadenopathy, macular edema, melena, memory impairment, menstrual disease, migraine, myocardial infarction, myopathy, onychoclasis, optic neuritis, oral mucosa ulcer, osteonecrosis (hip), ovarian cyst (hemorrhagic), palmar-plantar erythrodysesthesia, pancreatitis, papilledema, pericarditis, petechia, pleuritic chest pain, polyuria, pseudoporphyria, psoriasis, pulmonary fibrosis, pulmonary hemorrhage, pulmonary hypertension, Raynaud disease, reactivation of HBV, renal failure syndrome, respiratory failure, restless leg syndrome, retinal hemorrhage, rhabdomyolysis, ruptured corpus luteal cyst, sciatica, scrotal edema, seizure, sepsis, sexual disorder, Stevens-Johnson syndrome, subconjunctival hemorrhage, subdural hematoma, Sweet syndrome, syncope, tachycardia, telangiectasia (gastric antral), thrombocythemia, thrombosis, thrombotic microangiopathy, tinnitus, toxic epidermal necrolysis, tremor, tumor hemorrhage (GIST), tumor lysis syndrome, urinary tract infection, urticaria, vertigo, vesicular eruption, vitreous hemorrhage

Mechanism of Action Imatinib inhibits Bcr-Abl tyrosine kinase, the constitutive abnormal gene product of the Philadelphia chromosome in chronic myeloid leukemia (CML). Inhibition of this enzyme blocks proliferation and induces apoptosis in Bcr-Abl positive cell lines as well as in fresh leukemic cells in Philadelphia chromosome positive CML. Also inhibits tyrosine kinase for platelet-derived growth factor (PDGF), stem cell factor (SCF), c-Kit, and cellular events mediated by PDGF and SCF.

Pharmacodynamics/Kinetics

Half-life Elimination Adults: Parent drug: ~18 hours; N-desmethyl metabolite: ~40 hours; Children: Parent drug: ~15 hours

Time to Peak 2 to 4 hours

Reproductive Considerations

Pregnancy should be avoided during imatinib treatment. Pregnancy testing should be conducted in females of reproductive potential prior to treatment; women of reproductive potential should use highly effective contraception during imatinib treatment (methods with <1% pregnancy rates) and for 2 weeks after the last imatinib dose.

Pregnancy Considerations

Imatinib crosses the placenta (Burwick 2017). Spontaneous abortion and congenital anomalies (including skeletal, renal, and GI malformations [Lishner 2016]) have been reported (case reports) following imatinib exposure during pregnancy.

The European Society for Medical Oncology (ESMO) has published guidelines for diagnosis, treatment, and follow-up of cancer during pregnancy. The guidelines suggest that imatinib should only be used for the treatment of chronic myeloid leukemia (CML) in the second and third trimester and recommend referral to a facility with expertise in cancer during pregnancy; a multidisciplinary team (obstetrician, neonatologist, oncology team) is encouraged (Peccatori 2013). An international consensus panel suggests delaying treatment until WBC and platelet counts have risen to a level associated with CML symptom onset and then utilizing approaches other than tyrosine kinase inhibitors (Lishner 2016).

◆ **Imatinib Mesylate** *see* Imatinib *on page 797*
◆ **Imbruvica** *see* Ibrutinib *on page 785*
◆ **IMC-3G3** *see* Olaratumab *on page 1131*
◆ **IMC-11F8** *see* Necitumumab *on page 1089*
◆ **IMC-1121B** *see* Ramucirumab *on page 1308*
◆ **IMC-C225** *see* Cetuximab *on page 329*
◆ **Imdur** *see* Isosorbide Mononitrate *on page 845*
◆ **Imfinzi** *see* Durvalumab *on page 538*
◆ **IMI-28** *see* EpiRUBicin *on page 576*
◆ **IMid-1** *see* Lenalidomide *on page 883*
◆ **Imidazole Carboxamide** *see* Dacarbazine *on page 427*
◆ **Imidazole Carboxamide Dimethyltriazene** *see* Dacarbazine *on page 427*
◆ **IMIG** *see* Immune Globulin *on page 803*
◆ **Imipemide** *see* Imipenem and Cilastatin *on page 799*

Imipenem and Cilastatin

(i mi PEN em & sye la STAT in)

Brand Names: US Primaxin I.V.

Brand Names: Canada Imipenem and Cilastatin for Injection; Imipenem and Cilastatin for Injection, USP; Primaxin; RAN-Imipenem-Cilastatin

Pharmacologic Category Antibiotic, Carbapenem

Use

Bacterial septicemia: Treatment of septicemia caused by *Enterococcus faecalis, Staphylococcus aureus* (penicillinase-producing), *Escherichia coli, Klebsiella* species, *Pseudomonas aeruginosa, Serratia* species, *Enterobacter* species, *Bacteroides* species (including *Bacteroides fragilis*).

Bone and joint infections: Treatment of bone and joint infections caused by *E. faecalis, S. aureus* (penicillinase-producing), *Staphylococcus epidermidis, Enterobacter* species, *P. aeruginosa.*

Endocarditis: Treatment of endocarditis caused by *S. aureus* (penicillinase-producing).

Gynecologic infections: Treatment of gynecologic infections caused by *E. faecalis; S. aureus* (penicillinase-producing), *S. epidermidis, Streptococcus agalactiae* (group B streptococci), *E. coli, Klebsiella* species, *Proteus* species, *Enterobacter* species, *Bifidobacterium* species, *Bacteroides* species (including *B. fragilis), Gardnerella vaginalis*; *Peptococcus* species, *Peptostreptococcus* species, *Cutibacterium* species.

Intra-abdominal infections: Treatment of intra-abdominal infections caused by *E. faecalis, S. aureus* (penicillinase-producing), *S. epidermidis, E. coli, Klebsiella* species, *Enterobacter* species, *Proteus* species, *Morganella morganii, P. aeruginosa, Citrobacter* species, *Clostridium* species, *Bacteroides* species (including *B. fragilis*), *Fusobacterium* species, *Peptococcus* species, *Peptostreptococcus* species, *Eubacterium* species, *Cutibacterium* species, *Bifidobacterium* species.

Lower respiratory tract infections: Treatment of lower respiratory tract infections caused by *S. aureus* (penicillinase-producing), *E. coli, Klebsiella* species, *Enterobacter* species, *Haemophilus influenzae, Haemophilus parainfluenzae, Acinetobacter* species, *Serratia marcescens.*

Skin and skin structure infections: Treatment of skin and skin structure infections caused by *E. faecalis, S. aureus* (penicillinase-producing), S. *epidermidis, E. coli, Klebsiella* species, *Enterobacter species, Proteus vulgaris, Providencia rettgeri, M. morganii, P. aeruginosa, Serratia* species, *Citrobacter* species, *Acinetobacter* species, *Bacteroides* species (including *B. fragilis*), *Fusobacterium* species, *Peptococcus* species, *Peptostreptococcus* species.

Urinary tract infections (complicated and uncomplicated): Treatment of uncomplicated and complicated urinary tract infections caused by *E. faecalis, S. aureus* (penicillinase-producing), *E. coli, Klebsiella* species, *Enterobacter* species, *P. vulgaris, Providencia rettgeri, M. morganii, P. aeruginosa.*

Limitations of use: Not indicated in patients with meningitis because safety and efficacy have not been established; not recommend in pediatric patients with CNS infections because of the risk of seizures.

Local Anesthetic/Vasoconstrictor Precautions No information available to require special precautions

Effects on Dental Treatment No significant effects or complications reported

Effects on Bleeding No information available to require special precautions

Adverse Reactions

>10%

Hematologic & oncologic: Decreased hematocrit (infants and children 3 months to 12 years: 18%; neonates and infants <3 months: 2%), decreased hemoglobin (infants and children 3 months to 12 years: 15%), eosinophilia (neonates, infants, and children to 12 years: 9% to 13%), thrombocythemia (infants and children 3 months to 12 years: 13%; neonates and infants <3 months: 4%)

Hepatic: Increased serum AST (infants and children 3 months to 12 years: 18%; neonates and infants <3 months: 6%), increased serum ALT (infants and children 3 months to 12 years: 11%; neonates and infants <3 months: 3%)

1% to 10%:

Cardiovascular: Phlebitis (2% to 3%), tachycardia (neonates and infants ≤3 months: 2%; adults <1%)

Central nervous system: Seizure (neonates and infants ≤3 months: 6%; adults <1%)

Dermatologic: Skin rash (≤2%)

Gastrointestinal: Diarrhea (neonates, infants, and children to 12 years: 3% to 4%; adults 2%), nausea (2%), oral candidiasis (neonates and infants ≤3 months: 2%), vomiting (≤1% to 2%), gastroenteritis (≤1%)

Genitourinary: Proteinuria (infants and children 3 months to 12 years: 8%), urine discoloration (≤1%), oliguria (neonates and infants ≤3 months: 2%; adults <1%)

Hematologic & oncologic: Neutropenia (infants and children 3 months to 12 years: 3%; adults <1%), decreased platelet count (neonates and infants <3 months: 2%), increased hematocrit (neonates and infants <3 months: 1%)

Hepatic: Increased serum alkaline phosphatase (neonates and infants <3 months: 3%), increased serum bilirubin (neonates and infants <3 months: 3%), decreased serum bilirubin (neonates and infants <3 months: 1%)

Local: Irritation at injection site (infants, children, and adolescents 3 months to 16 years: 1%)

Renal: Increased serum creatinine (neonates and infants <3 months: 5%)

<1%, postmarketing and/or case reports: Abdominal pain, acute renal failure, agitation, agranulocytosis, anaphylaxis, angioedema, back pain (thoracic spinal), basophilia, bilirubinuria, bone marrow depression, brain disease, candidiasis, casts in urine, change in prothrombin time, chest discomfort, *Clostridioides* (formerly *Clostridium*) *difficile*-associated diarrhea, confusion, cyanosis, decreased serum sodium, dental discoloration, dizziness, drowsiness, drug fever, dysgeusia, dyskinesia, dyspnea, erythema at injection site, erythema multiforme, fever, flushing, glossitis, hallucination, headache, hearing loss, heartburn, hematuria, hemolytic anemia, hemorrhagic colitis, hepatic failure, hepatitis (including fulminant onset), hyperchloremia, hyperhidrosis, hypersensitivity, hyperventilation, hypotension, increased blood urea nitrogen, increased lactate dehydrogenase, increased monocytes, increased serum potassium, increased urinary urobilinogen, induration at injection site, injection site infection, jaundice, leukocytosis, leukocyturia, leukopenia, lymphocytosis, myoclonus, neutropenia, pain at injection site, palpitations, pancytopenia, paresthesia, polyarthralgia, polyuria, positive direct Coombs' test, pruritus, pruritus vulvae, pseudomembranous colitis, pseudomonas infection (resistant P. aeruginosa), psychiatric disturbances, sialorrhea, skin changes (texture), sore throat, Stevens-Johnson syndrome, thrombocytopenia, tinnitus, tongue changes (papillar hypertrophy), tongue discoloration, toxic epidermal necrolysis, tremor, urticaria, vertigo, weakness

Mechanism of Action Inhibits bacterial cell wall synthesis by binding to one or more of the penicillin-binding proteins (PBPs); which in turn inhibits the final transpeptidation step of peptidoglycan synthesis in bacterial cell walls, thus inhibiting cell wall biosynthesis. Bacteria eventually lyse due to ongoing activity of cell wall autolytic enzymes (autolysins and murein hydrolases) while cell wall assembly is arrested. Cilastatin prevents renal metabolism of imipenem by competitive inhibition of dehydropeptidase along the brush border of the renal tubules.

Pharmacodynamics/Kinetics

Half-life Elimination IV: Both drugs: Prolonged with renal impairment:

Neonates: Imipenem: 1.7 to 2.4 hours; Cilastatin: 3.9 to 6.3 hours (Freij 1985)

Infants and Children: Imipenem: 1.2 hours (Blumer 1996)

Adults: ~60 minutes

Pregnancy Considerations

Imipenem and cilastatin cross the placenta (Cho 1988; Heikkilä 1992)

Due to pregnancy-induced physiologic changes, some pharmacokinetic parameters of imipenem/cilastatin may be altered (Heikkilä 1992).

Imipenem is not one of the preferred antibiotics for the management of cystic fibrosis in pregnant females; however, it may be used when a safer alternative is not available (Panchaud 2016).

◆ **Imipenem/Cilastatin** *see* Imipenem and Cilastatin *on page 799*

Imipenem, Cilastatin, and Relebactam

(IM i PEN em, SYE la STAT in, & REL e BAK tam)

Brand Names: US Recarbrio

Pharmacologic Category Antibiotic, Carbapenem; Beta-Lactamase Inhibitor

Use

Intra-abdominal infection, complicated: Treatment of complicated intra-abdominal infections in patients ≥18 years of age with limited or no alternative options caused by the following susceptible gram-negative microorganisms: *Bacteroides caccae, Bacteroides fragilis, Bacteroides ovatus, Bacteroides thetaiotaomicron, Bacteroides uniformis, Bacteroides vulgatus, Bifidobacterium stercoris, Citrobacter freundii, Enterobacter cloacae, Escherichia coli, Fusobacterium nucleatum, Klebsiella aerogenes, Klebsiella oxytoca, Klebsiella pneumoniae, Parabacteroides distasonis,* and *Pseudomonas aeruginosa.*

Pneumonia, hospital acquired or ventilator associated: Treatment of hospital-acquired pneumonia (HAP) and ventilator-associated pneumonia (VAP) in patients ≥18 years of age caused by the following susceptible gram-negative microorganisms: *Acinetobacter calcoaceticus-baumannii* complex, *E. cloacae, E. coli, Haemophilus influenzae, K. aerogenes, K. oxytoca, K. pneumoniae, P. aeruginosa,* and *Serratia marcescens.*

Urinary tract infection, complicated (including pyelonephritis): Treatment of complicated urinary tract infections, including pyelonephritis, in patients ≥18 years of age with limited or no alternative options caused by the following susceptible gram-negative microorganisms: *E. cloacae, E. coli, K. aerogenes, K. pneumoniae,* and *P. aeruginosa.*

Local Anesthetic/Vasoconstrictor Precautions

No information available to require special precautions

Effects on Dental Treatment No significant effects or complications reported

Effects on Bleeding No information available to require special precautions

Adverse Reactions

1% to 10%:

- Cardiovascular: Phlebitis (≤2%)
- Central nervous system: Headache (4%)
- Gastrointestinal: Diarrhea (6%), vomiting (3%)
- Hepatic: Increased serum alanine aminotransferase (3%), increased serum aspartate aminotransferase (3%)
- Local: Erythema at injection site (≤2%), infusion site pain (≤2%)
- Miscellaneous: Fever (2%)

Frequency not defined:

- Gastrointestinal: *Clostridioides difficile* associated diarrhea

Mechanism of Action

Imipenem: Binds to PBP 2 and PBP 1B in Enterobacteriaceae and *P. aeruginosa* and subsequently inhibits penicillin-binding proteins, leading to the disruption of bacterial cell wall synthesis.

Cilastatin: Renal dehydropeptidase inhibitor that limits renal metabolism of imipenem.

Relebactam: Beta-lactamase inhibitor that protects imipenem from degradation by certain serine beta-lactamases (eg, Sulhydryl Variable, Temoneira, Cefotaximase-Munich, *E. cloacae* P99, Pseudomonas-derived cephalosporinase, and Klebsiella-pneumoniae carbapenemase).

Pharmacodynamics/Kinetics

Half-life Elimination Imipenem: 1 hour; relebactam: 1.2 hours.

Pregnancy Considerations

Imipenem and cilastatin cross the placenta (Cho 1988; Heikkilä 1992). Information specific to relebactam has not been located.

Also refer to the imipenem/cilastatin monograph for additional information.

- ◆ **Imipenem Monohydrate, Cilastatin Sodium, and Relebactam Monohydrate** *see* Imipenem, Cilastatin, and Relebactam *on page 800*
- ◆ **Imipenem, Relebactam, and Cilastatin** *see* Imipenem, Cilastatin, and Relebactam *on page 800*

Imipramine (im IP ra meen)

Related Information

Vasoconstrictor Interactions With Antidepressants *on page 1821*

Brand Names: US Tofranil [DSC]

Brand Names: Canada NOVO-Pramine [DSC]; PMS-Imipramine [DSC]

Pharmacologic Category Antidepressant, Tricyclic (Tertiary Amine)

Use

Childhood enuresis (imipramine hydrochloride only): As temporary adjunctive therapy in reducing enuresis in children ≥6 years of age, after possible organic causes have been excluded by appropriate tests

Major depressive disorder (unipolar): Treatment of unipolar major depressive disorder (MDD)

Local Anesthetic/Vasoconstrictor Precautions

Use with caution; epinephrine and levonordefrin have been shown to have an increased pressor response in combination with TCAs. Imipramine is one of the drugs confirmed to prolong the QT interval and is accepted as having a risk of causing torsade de pointes. The risk of drug-induced torsade de pointes is extremely low when a single QT interval prolonging drug is prescribed. In terms of epinephrine, it is not known what effect vasoconstrictors in the local anesthetic regimen will have in patients with a known history of congenital prolonged QT interval or in patients taking any medication that prolongs the QT interval. Until more information is obtained, it is suggested that the clinician consult with the physician prior to the use of a vasoconstrictor in suspected patients, and that the vasoconstrictor (epinephrine, mepivacaine and levonordefrin [Carbocaine® 2% with Neo-Cobefrin®]) be used with caution.

Effects on Dental Treatment Key adverse event(s) related to dental treatment: Xerostomia and changes in salivation (normal salivary flow resumes upon discontinuation). Long-term treatment with TCAs, such as imipramine, increases the risk of caries by reducing salivation and salivary buffer capacity. In a study by Rundergren, et al, pathological alterations were observed in the oral mucosa of 72% of 58 patients; 55% had new carious lesions after taking TCAs for a median of 5 1/2 years. Current research is investigating the use of the salivary stimulant pilocarpine to overcome the xerostomia from imipramine.

Effects on Bleeding No information available to require special precautions

Adverse Reactions Reported for tricyclic antidepressants in general. Frequency not defined.

- Cardiovascular: Cardiac arrhythmia, cardiac failure, cerebrovascular accident, ECG changes, heart block, hypertension, myocardial infarction, orthostatic hypotension, palpitations, tachycardia

Central nervous system: Agitation, anxiety, ataxia, confusion, delusions, disorientation, dizziness, drowsiness, EEG pattern changes, extrapyramidal reaction, falling, fatigue, hallucination, headache, hypomania, insomnia, nightmares, numbness, paresthesia, peripheral neuropathy, psychosis, restlessness, seizure, taste disorder, tingling sensation

Dermatologic: Alopecia, diaphoresis, pruritus, skin photosensitivity, skin rash, urticaria

Endocrine & metabolic: Decreased libido, decreased serum glucose, galactorrhea, gynecomastia, increased libido, increased serum glucose, SIADH, weight gain, weight loss

Gastrointestinal: Abdominal cramps, anorexia, constipation, diarrhea, epigastric distress, intestinal obstruction, melanoglossia, nausea, stomatitis, sublingual adenitis, vomiting, xerostomia

Genitourinary: Breast hypertrophy, impotence, testicular swelling, urinary hesitancy, urinary retention, urinary tract dilation

Hematologic & oncologic: Agranulocytosis, eosinophilia, petechia, purpura, thrombocytopenia

Hepatic: Cholestatic jaundice, increased serum transaminases

Hypersensitivity: Hypersensitivity (eg, drug fever, edema)

Neuromuscular & skeletal: Tremor, weakness

Ophthalmic: Accommodation disturbance, angle-closure glaucoma, blurred vision, mydriasis

Otic: Tinnitus

Mechanism of Action Traditionally believed to increase the synaptic concentration of serotonin and/or norepinephrine in the central nervous system by inhibition of their reuptake by the presynaptic neuronal membrane. However, additional receptor effects have been found including desensitization of adenyl cyclase, down regulation of beta-adrenergic receptors, and down regulation of serotonin receptors.

Pharmacodynamics/Kinetics

Onset of Action

Anxiety disorders (panic disorder): Initial effects may be observed within 2 weeks of treatment, with continued improvements through 4 to 6 weeks (WFSBP [Bandelow 2012]); some experts suggest up to 12 weeks of treatment may be necessary for response (BAP [Baldwin 2014]; Katzman 2014; WFSBP [Bandelow 2012]).

Depression: Initial effects may be observed within 1 to 2 weeks of treatment, with continued improvements through 4 to 6 weeks (Papakostas 2006; Posternak 2005; Szegedi 2009).

Half-life Elimination 8 to 21 hours (Salle 1990); Mean: Children: 11 hours; Adults: 16 to 17 hours; Desipramine (active metabolite): 22 to 28 hours

Time to Peak Serum: 2 to 6 hours (Sallee 1990)

Pregnancy Considerations

Congenital abnormalities have been reported in humans; however, a causal relationship has not been established. Tricyclic antidepressants may be associated with irritability, jitteriness, and convulsions (rare) in the neonate (Yonkers 2009). Due to pregnancy-induced physiologic changes, women who are pregnant may require dose adjustments late in pregnancy to achieve euthymia (Altshuler 1996).

The ACOG recommends that therapy for depression during pregnancy be individualized; treatment should incorporate the clinical expertise of the mental health clinician, obstetrician, primary health care provider, and pediatrician (ACOG 2008). According to the American Psychiatric Association (APA), the risks of medication treatment should be weighed against other treatment options and untreated depression. For women who discontinue antidepressant medications during pregnancy and who may be at high risk for postpartum depression, the medications can be restarted following delivery (APA 2010). Treatment algorithms have been developed by the ACOG and the APA for the management of depression in women prior to conception and during pregnancy (Yonkers 2009).

Pregnant women exposed to antidepressants during pregnancy are encouraged to enroll in the National Pregnancy Registry for Antidepressants (NPRAD). Women 18 to 45 years of age or their health care providers may contact the registry by calling 844-405-6185. Enrollment should be done as early in pregnancy as possible.

Dental Health Professional Considerations See Local Anesthetic/Vasoconstrictor Precautions

- **Imipramine HCl** *see* Imipramine *on page 801*
- **Imipramine Hydrochloride** *see* Imipramine *on page 801*
- **Imipramine Pamoate** *see* Imipramine *on page 801*

Imiquimod (i mi KWI mod)

Related Information

Systemic Viral Diseases *on page 1709*

Viral Infections *on page 1754*

Brand Names: US Aldara; Zyclara; Zyclara Pump

Brand Names: Canada Aldara P; APO-Imiquimod; TARO-Imiquimod Pump; Vyloma; Zyclara

Pharmacologic Category Skin and Mucous Membrane Agent; Topical Skin Product

Use

Actinic keratosis (2.5%, 3.75%, and 5% cream): Topical treatment of clinically typical, nonhyperkeratotic, nonhypertrophic, visible or palpable actinic keratoses on the full face or scalp in immunocompetent adults.

Genital and perianal warts (3.75% and 5% cream): Treatment of external genital and perianal warts (condyloma acuminata) in patients 12 years and older.

Superficial basal cell carcinoma (Aldara 5% cream): Topical treatment of biopsy-confirmed, primary superficial basal cell carcinoma in immunocompetent adults with a maximum tumor diameter of 2 cm located on the trunk (excluding anogenital skin), neck, or extremities (excluding hands and feet), only when surgical methods are medically less appropriate and patient follow-up can be reasonably assured.

Limitations of use: Safety and efficacy has not been established in immunosuppressed patients and in patients with basal cell nevus syndrome or xeroderma pigmentosum, or for prevention or transmission of HPV. Imiquimod should be used with caution in patients with preexisting autoimmune conditions. Imiquimod has been evaluated in pediatrics ages 2 to 12 with molluscum, contagiosum, however, studies failed to demonstrate efficacy.

Local Anesthetic/Vasoconstrictor Precautions No information available to require special precautions

Effects on Dental Treatment No significant effects or complications reported

Effects on Bleeding No information available to require special precautions

Adverse Reactions Note: Frequency of reactions vary and are related to the degree of inflammation associated with the treated disease, number of weekly applications, product formulation, and individual sensitivity.

>10%:

- Dermatologic: Localized erythema (58% to 100%; remote: 2%), xeroderma (local; including flaking, scaling; 18% to 93%; remote: 1%), crusted skin (local; 4% to 93%), skin sclerosis (local; 5% to 84%), dermal ulcer (local; 4% to 62%; remote: 2%), localized vesiculation (2% to 31%), excoriation (local; remote: 1%)
- Infection: Fungal infection (2% to 11%)
- Local: Localized edema (12% to 78%; remote: 1%), application site discharge (22% to 51%), local pruritus (3% to 32%), localized burning (9% to 26%)
- Respiratory: Upper respiratory tract infection (15% to 33%)

1% to 10%:

- Cardiovascular: Chest pain, localized blanching
- Central nervous system: Headache (2% to 6%), fatigue (1% to 4%), dizziness (<1% to 3%), local discomfort (soreness; ≤3%), rigors (1%), anxiety, pain, tingling of skin (local)
- Dermatologic: Skin pain (local; 1% to 8%), skin hypertrophy (local; 3%), skin infection (local; 1% to 3%), eczema (2%), cheilitis (≤2%), alopecia (1%), dermal hemorrhage (local), localized rash, papule (local), seborrhoeic keratosis, skin tenderness (local), stinging of the skin (local), tinea (cruris)
- Endocrine & metabolic: Increased serum glucose
- Gastrointestinal: Nausea (1% to 4%), diarrhea (1% to 3%), anorexia (≤3%), vomiting (1%), dyspepsia
- Genitourinary: Bacterial vaginosis (3%), urinary tract infection (1%)
- Hematologic & oncologic: Squamous cell carcinoma (4%), lymphadenopathy (2% to 3%)
- Infection: Herpes simplex (≤3%)
- Local: Local irritation (3% to 6%)
- Neuromuscular & skeletal: Arthralgia (1% to 3%), myalgia (≥1%), back pain
- Respiratory: Sinusitis (7%), flu-like symptoms (<1% to 4%), cough, pharyngitis, rhinitis
- Miscellaneous: Fever (≤3%)

Postmarketing and/or case reports: Abdominal pain, acute exacerbations of multiple sclerosis, agitation, anemia, angioedema, atrial fibrillation, capillary leak syndrome, cardiac failure, cardiomyopathy, cellulitis (local), cerebrovascular accident, chills, depression, dermatitis, dyspnea, dysuria, erythema multiforme, erythema (scrotal), exacerbation of psoriasis, exacerbation of ulcerative colitis, exfoliative dermatitis, febrile seizures, Henoch-Schönlein purpura (IgA vasculitis), hepatic insufficiency, herpes zoster, hyperpigmentation, immune thrombocytopenia (ITP), insomnia, ischemia, lethargy, leukopenia, malignant lymphoma, myocardial infarction, pain (scrotal), palpitations, pancytopenia, paresis, proteinuria, psoriasis, pulmonary edema, scrotal edema, seizure, squamous cell carcinoma, supraventricular tachycardia, syncope, tachycardia, thrombocytopenia, thyroiditis, ulcerative colitis, ulcer (scrotal), urinary retention, urticaria, vertebral disk disease (spondylitis onset or exacerbated)

Mechanism of Action Imiquimod, an immune response modifier, is a Toll-like receptor 7 agonist that activates immune cells. Topical application to the skin is associated with increases in markers for cytokines and immune cells.

Pharmacodynamics/Kinetics

Time to Peak 9 to 12 hours

Reproductive Considerations

Imiquimod may weaken condoms and vaginal diaphragms.

Pregnancy Risk Factor C

Pregnancy Considerations

Adverse events were observed in some animal reproduction studies following oral administration. Imiquimod appears to pose a low risk, but use in pregnant women should be avoided until additional data are available (CDC [Workowski 2015]).

Dental Health Professional Considerations Imiquimod cream 5% has been used for actinic cheilitis or keratosis. Imiquimod 2.5% and 3.75% cream is FDA approved to treat actinic keratosis. Adverse events of erosion/ulcerations have been reported with topical use. Imiquimod use in the treatment of oral papilloma virus remains inadequately studied.

◆ **Imitrex** *see* SUMAtriptan *on page 1394*

◆ **Imitrex STATdose Refill** *see* SUMAtriptan *on page 1394*

◆ **Imitrex STATdose System** *see* SUMAtriptan *on page 1394*

◆ **Imlygic** *see* Talimogene Laherparepvec *on page 1403*

◆ **IMMU-132** *see* Sacituzumab Govitecan *on page 1352*

Immune Globulin (i MYUN GLOB yoo lin)

Related Information

Systemic Viral Diseases *on page 1709*

Brand Names: US Asceniv; Bivigam; Carimune NF; Cutaquig; Cuvitru; Flebogamma DIF; GamaSTAN; Gammagard; Gammagard S/D Less IgA; Gammaked; Gammaplex; Gamunex-C; Hizentra; Hyqvia; Octagam; Panzyga; Privigen; Xembify

Brand Names: Canada Cutaquig; Cuvitru; Gamastan S/D; Gammagard; Gammagard S/D; Gamunex; Hizentra; IGIVnex; Iveegam Immuno; Octagam; Panzyga; Privigen

Pharmacologic Category Blood Product Derivative; Immune Globulin

Use

Chronic inflammatory demyelinating polyneuropathy: Gammaked, Gamunex-C, Hizentra, Privigen: Treatment of chronic inflammatory demyelinating polyneuropathy.

Chronic lymphocytic leukemia: Gammagard S/D: Prevention of bacterial infection in patients with hypogammaglobulinemia and/or recurrent bacterial infections with B-cell chronic lymphocytic leukemia.

Immune thrombocytopenia:

- Carimune NF, Gammaked, Gamunex-C: Treatment of acute immune thrombocytopenia (ITP).
- Carimune NF, Flebogamma DIF 10%, Gammagard S/D, Gammaked, Gammaplex, Gamunex-C, Octagam 10%, Panzyga, Privigen: Treatment of chronic ITP.

Immunodeficiency syndromes: Asceniv, Bivigam, Carimune NF, Cutaquig, Cuvitru, Flebogamma DIF, HyQvia, Gammagard Liquid, Gammagard S/D, Gammaked, Gammaplex, Gamunex-C, Hizentra, Octagam 5%, Panzyga, Privigen, Xembify: Treatment of primary humoral immunodeficiency syndromes (congenital agammaglobulinemia, severe combined immunodeficiency syndromes, common variable immunodeficiency, X-linked agammaglobulinemia, Wiskott-Aldrich syndrome).

Kawasaki syndrome: Gammagard S/D: Prevention of coronary artery aneurysms associated with Kawasaki syndrome (in combination with aspirin).

Multifocal motor neuropathy: Gammagard Liquid: Treatment of multifocal motor neuropathy.

Passive immunity: GamaSTAN, GamaSTAN S/D: Provision of passive immunity in the following susceptible individuals:

Hepatitis A: Preexposure prophylaxis; postexposure: within 14 days and/or prior to manifestation of disease.

Measles: For use within 6 days of exposure in an unvaccinated person who has not previously had measles.

ACIP recommendations: The Advisory Committee on Immunization Practices (ACIP) recommends postexposure prophylaxis with immune globulin (IG) to any nonimmune person exposed to measles. The following patient groups are at risk for severe measles complications and should receive IG therapy: Infants <12 months of age, pregnant women without evidence of immunity; severely compromised persons (eg, persons with severe primary immunodeficiency; some bone marrow transplant patients; some ALL patients; and some patients with AIDS or HIV infection [refer to guidelines for additional details]). Although prophylaxis may be given to any nonimmune person, priority should be given to those at greatest risk for measles complications and also to persons exposed in settings with intense, prolonged, close contact (eg, households, daycare centers, classrooms). IG therapy is not indicated for any person who already received one dose of a measles-containing vaccine at ≥12 months of age unless they are severely immunocompromised (CDC 2013).

Rubella: Postexposure prophylaxis to reduce the risk of infection and fetal damage in exposed pregnant women who will not consider therapeutic abortion.

Varicella: For immunosuppressed patients when varicella zoster immune globulin is not available.

Local Anesthetic/Vasoconstrictor Precautions No information available to require special precautions

Effects on Dental Treatment No significant effects or complications reported

Effects on Bleeding No information available to require special precautions

Adverse Reactions Adverse effects are reported as class effects rather than for specific products. Some clinical trials were extremely small and skewed the incidence upward ("≤" indicates this trend).

>10%:

Cardiovascular: Hypotension (children and adolescents: 25%; adults: ≤14%), tachycardia (children and adolescents: 25%; adults: 5%), decreased diastolic blood pressure (children and adolescents: 21%; adults: 5%), decreased heart rate (16%), hypertension (≤14%), increased systolic blood pressure (≤14%)

Central nervous system: Headache (≤75%), fatigue (≤29%), chills (5% to 19%), pain (5% to 15%), rigors (7% to 13%), dizziness (≤13%)

Dermatologic: Injection site pruritus (2% to 15%)

Gastrointestinal: Sore throat (11% to 35%), abdominal pain (≤33%), diarrhea (adults: ≤28%; children and adolescents: 8%), vomiting (adults: ≤26%; children and adolescents: 8%), viral gastroenteritis (22%), nausea (adults: ≤22%; children and adolescents: 8%), upper abdominal pain (≤20%)

Hematologic & oncologic: Positive direct Coombs test (≤47%), hemorrhage (29%), anemia (6% to 11%)

Hepatic: Increased serum alanine aminotransferase (adults: ≤18%; children and adolescents: ≤7%), hemolysis (7% to 14%), increased serum alkaline phosphatase (≤13%), hyperbilirubinemia (5%)

Immunologic: Antibody development (18%)

Local: Infusion site reaction (≤100%; higher incidences seen with subcutaneous administration and children and adolescents), erythema at injection site (3% to 39%), pain at injection site (≤21%), infusion-site pain (18%), bruising at injection site (16%), injection site nodule (16%), local swelling (at injection/infusion site: ≤16%)

Neuromuscular and skeletal: Arthralgia (≤20%), limb pain (2% to 15%), asthenia (≤14%), muscle cramps (≤14%), back pain (≤11%)

Otic: Otalgia (6% to 18%)

Renal: Nephrolithiasis (≤16%)

Respiratory: Cough (5% to 54%), nasal congestion (≤52%), sinusitis (≤50%), pharyngitis (2% to 41%), asthma (2% to 29%), upper respiratory tract infection (≤25%), rhinitis (4% to 24%), epistaxis (5% to 23%), bronchitis (≤22%), nasopharyngitis (3% to 22%), rhinorrhea (7% to 17%), paranasal sinus congestion (15%), nasal mucosa swelling (≤13%), wheezing (≤11%)

Miscellaneous: Fever (1% to 33%), accidental injury (13%)

1% to 10%:

Cardiovascular: Chest pain (≤9%), peripheral edema (8%), heart murmur (7%), chest discomfort (≤7%), flushing (6%), thrombosis (≤2%)

Central nervous system: Insomnia (9%), myasthenia (7%), migraine (≤7%), depression (≤6%), lethargy (≤6%), fibromyalgia syndrome (5%), falling (2% to 5%), malaise (≤5%), vertigo (≤5%)

Dermatologic: Skin rash (≤10%), xeroderma (≤9%), dermatitis (8%), cellulitis (≤8%), urticaria (≤8%), excoriation of skin (7%), hyperhidrosis (6%), allergic dermatitis (subcutaneous: ≤6%), erythema of skin (≤6%), pruritus (5%), eczema (≤5%)

Endocrine & metabolic: Thyroiditis (children and adolescents: ≤9%), ketonuria (≤8%), dehydration (≤6%), increased lactate dehydrogenase (5%)

Gastrointestinal: Dyspepsia (6% to 9%), *Clostridioides difficile* colitis (≤8%), gastroenteritis (≤8%), gastritis (6%), stomach discomfort (6%), abdominal distress (≤4%)

Genitourinary: Vulvovaginal candidiasis (9%), urinary tract infection (≤9%), cystitis (≤5%), dysuria (≤5%)

Hematologic & oncologic: Bruise (≤4%), hematoma (≤4%)

Hepatic: Increased serum aspartate aminotransferase (≤9%), leukopenia (7%), decreased serum alkaline phosphatase (≤3%)

Hypersensitivity: Hypersensitivity reaction (≤9%)

Infection: Fungal infection (7% to 9%), influenza (children and adolescents: ≤9%), infection (≤8%), viral infection (≤6%)

Local: Induration at injection site (8%), local inflammation (7%), localized edema (infusion site: 6%)

Neuromuscular & skeletal: Myalgia (≤8%), muscle spasm (7%), joint effusion (≤6%), joint swelling (≤6%)

Ophthalmic: Conjunctivitis (9%), eye discharge (7%), eye irritation (7%)

Otic: Otitis media (7% to 8%)

Renal: Increased serum creatinine (9%)

Respiratory: Exacerbation of asthma (7% to 9%), viral upper respiratory tract infection (children and adolescents: ≤9%), tonsil disease (children: 8%), dyspnea (7% to 8%), pharyngolaryngeal pain (5% to 8%), pneumonia (≤8%), oropharyngeal pain (≤9%), post nasal drip (7%), throat irritation (7%), flu-like symptoms (6% to 7%)

Frequency not defined:

Cardiovascular: Facial flushing

Central nervous system: Drowsiness

Dermatologic: Papule of skin

Hematologic & oncologic: Hyperproteinemia, increased serum immunoglobulins (hyperviscosity)

Local: Localized tenderness, local pain

Neuromuscular & skeletal: Lower limb cramp

Ophthalmic: Blurred vision

Renal: Increased blood urea nitrogen, renal insufficiency

<1%, postmarketing, and/or case reports: Abdominal distension, acute myocardial infarction, acute renal failure, acute respiratory distress syndrome, agitation, alopecia, altered blood pressure, anaphylactic shock, anaphylaxis, angina pectoris, angioedema, anorexia, anxiety, apnea, aseptic meningitis, bradycardia, bronchospasm, bullous dermatitis, burning sensation, cerebrovascular accident, chronic inflammatory demyelinating polyneuropathy (exacerbation), circulatory shock, coma, confusion, cyanosis, decreased haptoglobins, decreased neutrophils, deep vein thrombosis, delirium, disseminated intravascular coagulation (intravenous, subcutaneous, intramuscular), edema, epidermolysis, erythema multiforme, erythematous rash, exacerbation of autoimmune pure red cell aplasia, exfoliation of skin, facial edema, hematuria, hemoglobinuria, hemolytic anemia, hepatic insufficiency, hot and cold flashes, hypervolemia, hypoesthesia, hyponatremia (Daphnis 2007; Nguyen 2006; Steinberger 2003), hypoxemia, hypoxia, increased hemoglobin, increased liver enzymes, infusion related reaction, injection site extravasation, laryngospasm, loss of consciousness, mass (skin), muscle rigidity, musculoskeletal pain, neck pain, nervousness, nonimmune anaphylaxis, oral paresthesia, osmotic nephrosis, oxygen saturation decreased, pallor, palpitations, pancytopenia, paresthesia, peripheral vascular insufficiency, pharyngeal edema, phlebitis, photophobia, proximal tubular nephropathy, pseudohyponatremia (Daphnis 2007; Nguyen 2006; Steinberger 2003), pulmonary edema, pulmonary embolism, rash at injection site, renal failure syndrome, renal pain, renal tubular necrosis, respiratory distress, respiratory failure, seizure, skin discoloration, skin ulceration at injection site, Stevens-Johnson syndrome, thromboembolism, tissue necrosis at injection site, transfusion-related acute lung injury, transient ischemic attacks, translocational hyponatremia (Daphnis 2007; Nguyen 2006; Steinberger 2003), tremor, urine discoloration, voice disorder

Mechanism of Action Replacement therapy for primary and secondary immunodeficiencies, and IgG antibodies against bacteria, viral, parasitic and mycoplasma antigens; interference with F_c receptors on the cells of the reticuloendothelial system for autoimmune cytopenias and ITP; provides passive immunity by increasing the antibody titer and antigen-antibody reaction potential

Pharmacodynamics/Kinetics

Onset of Action IV: Provides immediate antibody levels

Immune thrombocytopenia: Initial response: 1 to 3 days; Peak response: 2 to 7 days (Neunert 2011)

Duration of Action IM, IV: Immune effects: 3 to 4 weeks (variable)

Half-life Elimination IM: ~23 days; SubQ: ~59 days (HyQvia): IV: IgG (variable among patients): Healthy subjects: 14 to 24 days; Patients with congenital humoral immunodeficiencies: 26 to 40 days; hypermetabolism associated with fever and infection have coincided with a shortened half-life

Time to Peak

Plasma: SubQ: Cutaquig: ~2 days; Cuvitru: ~4.4 days; Gammagard Liquid: 2.9 days; Hizentra: 2.9 days; HyQvia: ~5 days; Xembify: ~3 days.

Serum: IM: ~48 hours.

Pregnancy Considerations

Placental transfer of human IgG is dependent upon the IgG subclass and gestational age, generally increasing as pregnancy progresses. The lowest exposure would be expected during the period of organogenesis (Palmeira 2012; Pentsuk 2009). In a study of two women treated with IV immune globulin (IVIG) for common variable immunodeficiency, exogenous immune globulin was shown to cross the placenta similar to endogenous immune globulin (Palmeira 2012).

IV immune globulin has been recommended for use in fetal-neonatal alloimmune thrombocytopenia and pregnancy-associated immune thrombocytopenia (ITP) (ACOG 207 2019; Anderson 2007; Neunert 2011); use is appropriate for ITP in cases refractory to corticosteroids, when side effects to corticosteroids are significant, or when a rapid increase in platelets is needed (ACOG 207 2019). Intravenous immune globulin is recommended to prevent measles in nonimmune women exposed during pregnancy (CDC 2013). May also be used in postexposure prophylaxis for rubella to reduce the risk of infection and fetal damage in exposed pregnant females who will not consider therapeutic abortion (per GamaSTAN, GamaSTAN S/D product labeling; use for postexposure rubella prophylaxis is not currently recommended [CDC 2013]). IV immune globulin may be used when a prompt response for the treatment of myasthenia gravis is needed during pregnancy (Sanders 2016).

HyQvia: Data collection to monitor pregnancy and infant outcomes following exposure to HyQvia is ongoing. Patients may enroll themselves in the HyQvia pregnancy registry by calling (866) 424-6724.

◆ **Immune Globulin IV** *see* Immune Globulin *on page 803*

◆ **Immune Globulin (Human)-klhw** *see* Immune Globulin *on page 803*

◆ **Immune Globulin (Human)-slra** *see* Immune Globulin *on page 803*

◆ **Immune Globulin Subcutaneous (Human)** *see* Immune Globulin *on page 803*

◆ **Immune Serum Globulin** *see* Immune Globulin *on page 803*

◆ **Immunotoxin CAT-8015** *see* Moxetumomab Pasudotox *on page 1063*

◆ **Imodium A-D [OTC]** *see* Loperamide *on page 928*

◆ **Imogam Rabies-HT** *see* Rabies Immune Globulin (Human) *on page 1302*

◆ **Imovax Rabies** *see* Rabies Vaccine *on page 1303*

◆ **Implanon** *see* Etonogestrel *on page 625*

◆ **Impoyz** *see* Clobetasol *on page 377*

- ◆ **Imuran** *see* AzaTHIOprine *on page 199*
- ◆ **Inactivated Influenza Vaccine** *see* Influenza Virus Vaccine (Inactivated) *on page 812*
- ◆ **Inapsine** *see* Droperidol *on page 534*
- ◆ **INC280** *see* Capmatinib *on page 283*
- ◆ **Incassia** *see* Norethindrone *on page 1117*
- ◆ **INCB424** *see* Ruxolitinib *on page 1351*
- ◆ **INCB 18424** *see* Ruxolitinib *on page 1351*
- ◆ **INCB028060** *see* Capmatinib *on page 283*
- ◆ **INCB054828** *see* Pemigatinib *on page 1207*

IncobotulinumtoxinA

(in kuh BOT yoo lin num TOKS in aye)

Related Information

Dentin Hypersensitivity, Acid Erosion, High Caries Index, Management of Alveolar Osteitis, and Xerostomia *on page 1762*

Brand Names: US Xeomin

Brand Names: Canada Xeomin; Xeomin Cosmetic

Pharmacologic Category Neuromuscular Blocker Agent, Toxin; Ophthalmic Agent, Toxin

Use

US labeling:

Blepharospasm: Treatment of adults with blepharospasm.

Cervical dystonia: Treatment of adults with cervical dystonia.

Glabellar lines: Temporary improvement in the appearance of moderate to severe glabellar lines associated with corrugator and/or procerus muscle activity in adult patients.

Sialorrhea: Treatment of chronic sialorrhea in adults.

Upper limb spasticity: Treatment of upper limb spasticity in adult patients.

Canadian labeling:

Xeomin:

Cervical dystonia: Treatment of cervical dystonia (spasmodic torticollis) in adults.

Hypertonicity disorders: Treatment of hypertonicity disorders of the seventh nerve (eg, blepharospasm, hemifacial spasm) in adults.

Upper limb spasticity: Treatment of poststroke spasticity of upper limb(s) in adults.

Xeomin Cosmetic: **Glabellar lines:** Temporary improvement in the appearance of moderate to severe glabellar lines in adults.

Local Anesthetic/Vasoconstrictor Precautions No information available to require special precautions

Effects on Dental Treatment Key adverse event(s) related to dental treatment: Xerostomia (normal salivary flow resumes upon discontinuation).

Effects on Bleeding No information available to require special precautions

Adverse Reactions

Upper limb spasticity and cervical dystonia:

>10%:

Central nervous system: Myasthenia (cervical dystonia: 7% to 11%)

Gastrointestinal: Dysphagia (cervical dystonia: 13% to 18%)

Infection: Infection (cervical dystonia: 13% to 14%)

Neuromuscular & skeletal: Neck pain (cervical dystonia: 7% to 15%)

Respiratory: Respiratory system disorder (cervical dystonia: 10% to 13%)

1% to 10%:

Central nervous system: Seizure (upper limb spasticity: 3%)

Gastrointestinal: Xerostomia (upper limb spasticity: 2%)

Immunologic: Antibody development (neutralizing; cervical dystonia, upper limb spasticity: ≤2%)

Local: Pain at injection site (cervical dystonia: 9%)

Neuromuscular & skeletal: Musculoskeletal pain (cervical dystonia: 4% to 7%)

Respiratory: Nasopharyngitis (upper limb spasticity: 2%), upper respiratory tract infection (upper limb spasticity: 2%)

Blepharospasm, chronic sialorrhea, and glabellar lines:

>10%:

Gastrointestinal: Xerostomia (blepharospasm: 16%; chronic sialorrhea: 4%)

Ophthalmic: Blepharoptosis (blepharospasm: 19%; reduction of glabellar lines: <1%), dry eye syndrome (blepharospasm: 16%; chronic sialorrhea: 3%), visual disturbance (blepharospasm: 12%)

1% to 10%:

Cardiovascular: Hypertension (chronic sialorrhea: 4%)

Central nervous system: Headache (blepharospasm: 7%; reduction of glabellar lines: 5%), falling (chronic sialorrhea: 3%), voice disorder (chronic sialorrhea: 3%)

Gastrointestinal: Diarrhea (blepharospasm, chronic sialorrhea: 4% to 8%), tooth loss (chronic sialorrhea: 5%)

Neuromuscular & skeletal: Back pain (chronic sialorrhea: 3%)

Respiratory: Dyspnea (blepharospasm: 5%), nasopharyngitis (blepharospasm: 5%), respiratory tract infection (blepharospasm: 5%), bronchitis (chronic sialorrhea: 3%)

<1%, postmarketing and/or case reports: Any indication. Allergic dermatitis, anaphylaxis, antibody development (neutralizing; blepharospasm, chronic sialorrhea), asthenia, blepharospasm, blurred vision, corneal perforation, diplopia, dysarthria, dysphagia, dyspnea, ecchymoses, edema, erythema of skin, eye disease, eyelid edema, facial pain, facial paresis, flu-like symptoms, hematoma at injection site, herpes zoster infection, hypersensitivity reaction, inflammation at injection site, injection site reaction, local hypersensitivity reaction, muscle spasm, myalgia, nausea, pain at injection site, pruritus, reduced blinking (leading to corneal ulceration), respiratory failure, serum sickness, skin rash, swelling of eye, urinary incontinence, urticaria

Mechanism of Action IncobotulinumtoxinA is a neurotoxin produced from *Clostridium botulinum* that inhibits acetylcholine release from peripheral cholinergic nerve endings. Inhibition occurs sequentially via binding and internalization of the neurotoxin into presynaptic cholinergic nerve terminals, translocation to the nerve terminal cytosol, and enzymatic cleavage of SNAP25, a protein necessary for acetylcholine release. Inhibition of acetylcholine release at the neuromuscular junction produces a state of denervation. Muscle inactivation persists until new fibrils grow from the nerve and form junction plates on new areas of the muscle-cell walls.

Pharmacodynamics/Kinetics

Onset of Action Improvement: ~4 to 7 days

Duration of Action ~3 to 4 months

Pregnancy Considerations
Adverse events were observed in some animal reproduction studies.

◆ **Increlex** *see* Mecasermin *on page 951*

◆ **Incruse Ellipta** *see* Umeclidinium *on page 1507*

Indacaterol (in da KA ter ol)

Related Information
Respiratory Diseases *on page 1680*
Brand Names: US Arcapta Neohaler
Brand Names: Canada Onbrez Breezhaler
Pharmacologic Category $Beta_2$ Agonist; $Beta_2$-Adrenergic Agonist, Long-Acting
Use Chronic obstructive pulmonary disease (maintenance): Long-term maintenance treatment of airflow obstruction in chronic obstructive pulmonary disease (COPD), including chronic bronchitis and/or emphysema
Local Anesthetic/Vasoconstrictor Precautions
No information available to require special precautions
Effects on Dental Treatment Key adverse event(s) related to dental treatment: oropharyngeal pain has been reported
Effects on Bleeding No information available to require special precautions
Adverse Reactions
>10%: Respiratory: Cough (post-inhalation 7% to 24%)
1% to 10%:
Central nervous system: Headache (5%)
Gastrointestinal: Nausea (2%)
Respiratory: Nasopharyngitis (5%), oropharyngeal pain (2%)
<1%, postmarketing, and/or case reports: Dizziness, hypersensitivity reaction, palpitations, paradoxical bronchospasm, pruritus, skin rash, tachycardia
Mechanism of Action Relaxes bronchial smooth muscle by selective action on $beta_2$-receptors with little effect on heart rate; acts locally in the lung.
Pharmacodynamics/Kinetics
Onset of Action 5 minutes; Peak effect: 1-4 hours
Duration of Action 24 hours
Half-life Elimination 40-56 hours
Time to Peak Serum: ~15 minutes
Pregnancy Risk Factor C
Pregnancy Considerations Adverse events were not observed in animal reproduction studies. Beta-agonists may interfere with uterine contractility if administered during labor.

◆ **Indacaterol Maleate** *see* Indacaterol *on page 807*

◆ **Inderal** *see* Propranolol *on page 1287*

◆ **Inderal XL** *see* Propranolol *on page 1287*

◆ **Inderal LA** *see* Propranolol *on page 1287*

Indinavir (in DIN a veer)

Related Information
HIV Infection and AIDS *on page 1690*
Brand Names: US Crixivan
Brand Names: Canada Crixivan [DSC]
Pharmacologic Category Antiretroviral, Protease Inhibitor (Anti-HIV)
Use
HIV-1 infection: Treatment of HIV infection in combination with other antiretroviral agents.
Note: Indinavir is no longer recommended for use in the treatment of HIV (HHS [adult] 2019a).
Local Anesthetic/Vasoconstrictor Precautions
No information available to require special precautions
Effects on Dental Treatment Key adverse event(s) related to dental treatment: Abnormal taste.
Effects on Bleeding Spontaneous bleeding has been reported in patients with hemophilia and concurrent HIV infection. Medical consult recommended.
Adverse Reactions
>10%:
Gastrointestinal: Abdominal pain (17%), nausea (12%)
Hepatic: Hyperbilirubinemia (12% to 14%; dose dependent)
Renal: Nephrolithiasis (including flank pain with/without hematuria; ≤29% pediatric patients; ≤12% adult patients; dose dependent), urolithiasis (including flank pain with/without hematuria; ≤29% pediatric patients; ≤12% adult patients; dose dependent)
1% to 10%:
Central nervous system: Headache (5%), dizziness (3%), drowsiness (2%), malaise (2%), fatigue (≤2%)
Dermatologic: Pruritus (4%), skin rash (1%)
Gastrointestinal: Vomiting (8%), anorexia (3%), diarrhea (3%), dysgeusia (3%), gastroesophageal reflux disease (3%), dyspepsia (2%), increased appetite (2%), increased serum amylase (2%)
Genitourinary: Dysuria (2%)
Hematologic & oncologic: Neutropenia (2%), anemia (1%)
Hepatic: Increased serum transaminases (4% to 5%), jaundice (2%)
Neuromuscular & skeletal: Back pain (8%), weakness (≤2%)
Renal: Hydronephrosis (3%)
Respiratory: Cough (2%)
Miscellaneous: Fever (2%)
<1%, postmarketing, and/or case reports: Abdominal distention, acute renal failure, alopecia, anaphylactoid reaction, angina pectoris, arthralgia, cerebrovascular disease, crystalluria, decreased hemoglobin, depression, diabetes mellitus, erythema multiforme, hemolytic anemia, hemorrhage (spontaneous in patients with hemophilia A or B), hepatic failure, hepatitis, hyperglycemia, hyperpigmentation, immune reconstitution syndrome, increased serum cholesterol, increased serum triglycerides, interstitial nephritis (with medullary calcification and cortical atrophy), leukocyturia (severe and asymptomatic), myocardial infarction, oral paresthesia, pancreatitis, paronychia, periarthritis, pharyngitis, prolonged QT interval on ECG, pyelonephritis, redistribution of body fat, renal failure, renal insufficiency, Stevens-Johnson syndrome, thrombocytopenia, torsades de pointes, upper respiratory tract infection, urticaria, vasculitis, xeroderma
Mechanism of Action Binds to the site of HIV-1 protease activity and inhibits cleavage of viral Gag-Pol polyprotein precursors into individual functional proteins required for infectious HIV. This results in the formation of immature, noninfectious viral particles.
Pharmacodynamics/Kinetics
Half-life Elimination Children 4 to 17 years (n=18): 1.1 hours; Adults: 1.8 ± 0.4 hours; Adults with hepatic insufficiency: 2.8 ± 0.5 hours
Time to Peak 0.8 ± 0.3 hours

Reproductive Considerations

Based on the Health and Humans Services (HHS) perinatal HIV guidelines, indinavir is not one of the recommended antiretroviral agents for use in females living with HIV who are trying to conceive.

For males and females living with HIV and planning a pregnancy, maximum viral suppression below the limits of detection with antiretroviral therapy (ART), modification of therapy (if needed), optimization of the woman's health, and a discussion of the potential risks and benefits of ART therapy during pregnancy is recommended prior to conception (HHS [perinatal] 2019).

Pregnancy Considerations Placental transfer in humans is minimal.

Outcome information specific to use in pregnancy is no longer being reviewed and updated in the Health and Humans Services (HHS) perinatal guidelines. Maternal antiretroviral therapy (ART) may be associated with adverse pregnancy outcomes, including preterm delivery, stillbirth, low birth weight, and small for gestational age infants. Actual risks may be influenced by maternal factors such as disease severity, gestational age at initiation of therapy, and specific ART regimen; therefore, close fetal monitoring is recommended. Because there is clear benefit to appropriate treatment, maternal ART should not be withheld due to concerns for adverse neonatal outcomes. Long-term follow-up is recommended for all infants exposed to antiretroviral medications; children without HIV but who were exposed to ART in utero and develop significant organ system abnormalities of unknown etiology (particularly of the CNS or heart) should be evaluated for potential mitochondrial dysfunction. Hyperbilirubinemia has been reported following therapy; it is not known if this will occur in neonates following in utero exposure to indinavir. Hyperglycemia, new onset of diabetes mellitus, or diabetic ketoacidosis have been reported with protease inhibitors (PIs); it is not clear if pregnancy increases this risk. Consider performing the standard glucose screening test earlier in pregnancy in women who initiated PI therapy prior to conception.

Based on the HHS perinatal HIV guidelines, indinavir is not one of the recommended antiretroviral agents for use during pregnancy.

In general, ART is recommended for all pregnant females living with HIV to keep the viral load below the limit of detection and reduce the risk of perinatal transmission. Therapy should be individualized following a discussion of the potential risks and benefits of treatment during pregnancy. Monitoring of pregnant females is more frequent than in nonpregnant adults. ART should be continued postpartum for all females living with HIV and can be modified after delivery.

Health care providers are encouraged to enroll pregnant females exposed to antiretroviral medications as early in pregnancy as possible in the Antiretroviral Pregnancy Registry (1-800-258-4263 or http://www.APRegistry.com). Health care providers caring for pregnant females living with HIV and their infants may contact the National Perinatal HIV Hotline (1-888-448-8765) for clinical consultation (HHS [perinatal] 2019).

◆ **Indinavir Sulfate** *see* Indinavir *on page 807*

Inebilizumab (in EB i LIZ ue mab)

Brand Names: US Uplizna

Pharmacologic Category Anti-CD19 Monoclonal Antibody; Monoclonal Antibody

Use Neuromyelitis optica spectrum disorder: Treatment of neuromyelitis optica spectrum disorder (NMOSD) in adults who are anti-aquaporin-4 (AQP4) antibody positive.

Local Anesthetic/Vasoconstrictor Precautions No information available to require special precautions.

Effects on Dental Treatment No significant effects or complications reported.

Effects on Bleeding Chemotherapy may result in myelosuppression. In patients under active treatment a medical consult is suggested.

Adverse Reactions

>10%:

- Genitourinary: Urinary tract infection (11%)
- Hematologic & oncologic: Decreased neutrophils (2% to 12%)

1% to 10%:

- Hematologic & oncologic: Lymphocytopenia (5%)
- Immunologic: Antibody development (6%)
- Local: Infusion site reaction (9%)
- Neuromuscular & skeletal: Arthralgia (10%), back pain (7%)

Frequency not defined:

- Hematologic & oncologic: Decreased serum immunoglobulins
- Infection: Influenza
- Respiratory: Nasopharyngitis, upper respiratory tract infection

Mechanism of Action Inebilizumab is an anti-CD19 monoclonal antibody directed against pre-B and mature B-cell lymphocytes, which express the cell surface antigen CD19. Following binding to CD19, inebilizumab causes antibody-dependent cellular cytolysis.

Pharmacodynamics/Kinetics

Half-life Elimination Terminal: 18 days.

Reproductive Considerations Females of reproductive potential should use effective contraception during therapy and for at least 6 months after the last inebilizumab dose.

Pregnancy Considerations

Inebilizumab is a humanized monoclonal antibody (IgG_1). Placental transfer of human IgG is dependent upon the IgG subclass, maternal serum concentrations, newborn birth weight, and gestational age, generally increasing as pregnancy progresses. The lowest exposure would be expected during the period of organogenesis (Palmeira 2012; Pentsuk 2009).

Based on data from animal reproduction studies, in utero exposure to inebilizumab may cause fetal harm. Transient B-cell depletion and lymphocytopenia may occur in infants following in utero exposure to inebilizumab.

Maternal neuromyelitis optica spectrum disorder (NMOSD) may be associated with adverse pregnancy outcomes. Information related to the treatment of NMOSD in pregnancy is limited; agents other than inebilizumab may be preferred (Borisow 2018; Chang 2020; Zhu 2020).

◆ **Inebilizumab-cdon** *see* Inebilizumab *on page 808*
◆ **INF-alpha 2** *see* Interferon Alfa-2b *on page 831*
◆ **Infants Advil [OTC]** *see* Ibuprofen *on page 786*
◆ **Inflectra** *see* InFLIXimab *on page 809*

InFLIXimab (in FLIKS e mab)

Related Information

Rheumatoid Arthritis, Osteoarthritis, and Osteoporosis *on page 1697*

Brand Names: US Avsola; Inflectra; Remicade; Renflexis

Brand Names: Canada Avsola; Inflectra; Remicade; Renflexis

Pharmacologic Category Antirheumatic, Disease Modifying; Gastrointestinal Agent, Miscellaneous; Immunosuppressant Agent; Monoclonal Antibody; Tumor Necrosis Factor (TNF) Blocking Agent

Use

Ankylosing spondylitis: Treatment of adults with active ankylosing spondylitis (to reduce signs/symptoms).

Crohn disease: Treatment of adults and pediatric patients ≥6 years of age with moderately to severely active Crohn disease who have had inadequate responses to conventional therapy (to reduce signs/symptoms and induce and maintain clinical remission) or to reduce the number of draining enterocutaneous and rectovaginal fistulas and maintain fistula closure in adults.

Plaque psoriasis: Treatment of adults with chronic, severe (extensive and/or disabling) plaque psoriasis as an alternative to other systemic therapy.

Psoriatic arthritis: Treatment of adults with psoriatic arthritis (to reduce signs/symptoms of active arthritis and inhibit progression of structural damage and improve physical function).

Rheumatoid arthritis: Treatment of adults with moderately to severely active rheumatoid arthritis (with methotrexate) (to reduce signs/symptoms of active arthritis and inhibit progression of structural damage and improve physical function).

Ulcerative colitis: Treatment of adults and pediatric patients ≥6 years of age with moderately to severely active ulcerative colitis with inadequate response to conventional therapy (to reduce signs/symptoms and induce and maintain clinical remission) or to induce/maintain mucosal healing and eliminate corticosteroid use in adults.

Note: Avsola (infliximab-axxq), Inflectra (infliximab-dyyb), and Renflexis (infliximab-abda) are approved as biosimilars to Remicade (infliximab). In Canada, Avsola, Inflectra, and Renflexis are also approved as biosimilars to Remicade (infliximab).

Local Anesthetic/Vasoconstrictor Precautions No information available to require special precautions

Effects on Dental Treatment Key adverse event(s) related to dental treatment: Infliximab belongs to the class of disease-modifying antirheumatic drugs and, as such, has immunosuppressive properties. Consider a medical consult prior to any invasive treatment for patients under active treatment with infliximab. Delayed wound healing due to the immunosuppressive effects and increased potential for postsurgical infection may be of concern.

Effects on Bleeding Has been associated with thrombocytopenia, anemia, and hemolytic anemia, but incidence may vary with indication.

Adverse Reactions As reported in adults with rheumatoid arthritis, unless otherwise noted.

>10%:

Central nervous system: Headache (18%)

Gastrointestinal: Abdominal pain (Crohn disease: 26%; rheumatoid arthritis: 12%), nausea (21%)

Hematologic & oncologic: Anemia (children and adolescents with Crohn disease: 11%; adults: <1%)

Hepatic: Increased serum alanine aminotransferase (<3 x ULN: 17% to 51%; ≥3 x ULN: 2% to 10%; ≥5x ULN: 1% to 4%)

Immunologic: Antibody development (10% to 52%), increased ANA titer (~50%), antibody development (double-stranded DNA, ~20%)

Infection: Infection (children and adolescents: 38% to 74%; other indications: 27% to 59%; adults with Crohn disease: 50%), serious infection (children and adolescents: 12% to 60%; adults: 5%), abscess (Crohn disease patients with fistulizing disease: 15%)

Respiratory: Upper respiratory tract infection (rheumatoid arthritis: 32%; children and adolescents with ulcerative colitis: 12%), sinusitis (14%), cough (12%), pharyngitis (8% to 12%)

Miscellaneous: Infusion related reaction (≤18%; severe: <1%)

1% to 10%:

Cardiovascular: Flushing (children and adolescents with Crohn disease: 9%), hypertension (7%)

Central nervous system: Fatigue (9%), pain (8%)

Dermatologic: Skin rash (10%), pruritus (7%)

Gastrointestinal: Dyspepsia (10%)

Genitourinary: Urinary tract infection (8%)

Hematologic & oncologic: Leukopenia (children and adolescents with Crohn disease: 9%; other indications: <1%), neutropenia (children and adolescents with Crohn disease: 7%)

Hypersensitivity: Hypersensitivity reaction (children and adolescents with Crohn disease: 6%; other indications: <1%), type IV hypersensitivity reaction (plaque psoriasis: 1%), serum sickness (≤1%)

Infection: Viral infection (children and adolescents with Crohn disease: 8%), bacterial infection (children and adolescents with Crohn disease: 6%), candidiasis (5%)

Neuromuscular & skeletal: Arthralgia (8%), bone fracture (children and adolescents with Crohn disease: 7%)

Respiratory: Bronchitis (10%), pneumonia (≤2%)

Miscellaneous: Fever (7%)

<1%, postmarketing, and/or case reports: Acute hepatic failure, acute myocardial infarction, agranulocytosis, anaphylactic shock, anaphylaxis, aspergillosis, autoimmune hepatitis, bacterial pneumonia (legionnaires' disease), blastomycosis, bradycardia, bronchospasm, bullous dermatitis (linear IgA) (Bryant 2016), cardiac arrhythmia, cellulitis, cerebrovascular accident, cholestasis, chronic inflammatory demyelinating polyneuropathy, coccidioidomycosis, constipation, cryptococcosis, cytomegalovirus disease, dehydration, demyelinating disease of the central nervous system, demyelinating disease (peripheral), dermal ulcer, diaphoresis, dizziness, edema, erythema multiforme, erythematous rash, exacerbation of psoriasis, fungal infection, gastrointestinal infection (salmonellosis), Guillain-Barre syndrome, hemolytic anemia, hepatic failure, hepatic injury, hepatitis, hepatotoxicity (idiosyncratic), hepatosplenic T-cell lymphomas (mainly young adult or adolescent males), herpes zoster infection, histoplasmosis, Hodgkin lymphoma,

hypotension, immune thrombocytopenia, increased serum aspartate aminotransferase, interstitial pulmonary disease, intestinal obstruction, ischemic heart disease, jaundice, laryngeal edema, leukemia, listeriosis, liver enzyme disorder (transient), lower respiratory tract infection, lupus-like syndrome, lymphadenopathy, malignant lymphoma, malignant melanoma, malignant neoplasm, malignant neoplasm of breast, malignant neoplasm of cervix, malignant neoplasm of colon or rectum, Merkel cell carcinoma, multiple sclerosis, neuropathy (includes multifocal motor), nocardiosis, non-Hodgkin lymphoma, opportunistic infection, optic neuritis, pancytopenia, pericardial effusion, pharyngeal edema, pleurisy, pneumonia due to *Pneumocystis jirovecii*, psoriasis (including new onset, palmoplantar, pustular), pulmonary edema, pulmonary fibrosis, reactivated tuberculosis, reactivation of HBV, sarcoidosis, seizure, sepsis, Stevens-Johnson syndrome, temporary vision loss, thrombocytopenia, thrombophlebitis, thrombotic thrombocytopenic purpura, toxic epidermal necrolysis, transverse myelitis, tuberculosis, urticaria, vasculitis (systemic and cutaneous)

Mechanism of Action Infliximab is a chimeric monoclonal antibody that binds to human tumor necrosis factor alpha (TNFα), thereby interfering with endogenous TNFα activity. Elevated TNFα levels have been found in involved tissues/fluids of patients with rheumatoid arthritis, ankylosing spondylitis, psoriatic arthritis, plaque psoriasis, Crohn disease and ulcerative colitis. Biological activities of TNFα include the induction of proinflammatory cytokines (interleukins), enhancement of leukocyte migration, activation of neutrophils and eosinophils, and the induction of acute phase reactants and tissue degrading enzymes. Animal models have shown TNFα expression causes polyarthritis, and infliximab can prevent disease as well as allow diseased joints to heal.

Pharmacodynamics/Kinetics

Onset of Action Crohn disease: 1 to 2 weeks; Rheumatoid arthritis: 3 to 7 days

Duration of Action Crohn disease: 8 to 48 weeks; Rheumatoid arthritis: 6 to 12 weeks

Half-life Elimination 7 to 12 days (Klotz 2007)

Reproductive Considerations

Infliximab may be used in females with rheumatic and musculoskeletal diseases who are planning a pregnancy. Conception should be planned during a period of quiescent/low disease activity (ACR [Sammaritano 2020]).

Women with psoriasis planning a pregnancy may continue treatment with infliximab. Women with well-controlled psoriasis who wish to avoid fetal exposure can consider discontinuing infliximab 50 days prior to attempting pregnancy (Rademaker 2018).

Treatment algorithms are available for use of biologics in female patients with Crohn disease who are planning a pregnancy (Weizman 2019). Serum levels should be optimized prior to conception (Mahadevan 2019).

Infliximab is recommended for use in males with rheumatic and musculoskeletal diseases who are planning to father a child (ACR [Sammaritano 2020]).

The American Academy of Dermatology considers tumor necrosis factor alpha (TNFα)-blocking agents for the treatment of psoriasis to be compatible for use in male patients planning to father a child (AAD-NPF [Menter 2019]).

Pregnancy Considerations Infliximab crosses the placenta.

Infliximab is a humanized monoclonal antibody (IgG_1). Placental transfer of human IgG is dependent upon the IgG subclass, maternal serum concentrations, birth weight, and gestational age, generally increasing as pregnancy progresses. The lowest exposure would be expected during the period of organogenesis (Palmeira 2012; Pentsuk 2009).

Following administration to pregnant patients with inflammatory bowel disease, cord blood and newborn concentrations of infliximab are greater than maternal serum at delivery (Julsgaard 2016; Mahadevan 2013). The mean time to infliximab clearance was 7.3 months (range: 6.2 to 8.3 months) in a study in 44 infants exposed in utero. Infliximab serum concentrations remained detectable in one infant until 12 months of age (Julsgaard 2016).

A paper describes agranulocytosis requiring treatment with granulocyte colony stimulating factor in four infants (three of which were triplets) exposed to infliximab in utero. In the singleton pregnancy, infliximab was present in the newborn serum 13 weeks after the last maternal pregnancy dose, but concentrations were not measurable in the mother. Infliximab serum concentrations were not evaluated in the triplets (Guiddir 2014). Information related to this class of medications is emerging, but based on available data, tumor necrosis factor alpha (TNFα)-blocking agents are considered to have low to moderate risk when used in pregnancy (ACOG 776 2019).

A fatal outcome has been reported in an infant who received a live vaccine (BCG) after in utero exposure to infliximab. The mother was treated with infliximab 10 mg/kg once weekly as monotherapy for steroid refractory Crohn disease. The infant was well at delivery and was not breastfed. BCG vaccination occurred at 3 months of age; the infant died at 4.5 months of age due to disseminated BCG (Cheent 2010). The risk of immunosuppression may be increased following third trimester maternal use of TNFα blocking agents; the fetus, neonate/infant should be considered immunosuppressed for 1 to 3 months following in utero exposure (AAD-NPF [Menter 2019]). Vaccination with live vaccines (eg, rotavirus vaccine) should be avoided for the first 6 months of life if exposure to a biologic agent occurs during the third trimester of pregnancy (eg, >27 weeks' gestation) (Mahadevan 2019).

Inflammatory bowel disease is associated with adverse pregnancy outcomes including an increased risk of miscarriage, premature delivery, delivery of a low birth weight infant, and poor maternal weight gain. Management of maternal disease should be optimized prior to pregnancy. Treatment decreases disease flares, disease activity, and the incidence of adverse pregnancy outcomes (Mahadevan 2019).

Use of immune-modulating therapies in pregnancy should be individualized to optimize maternal disease and pregnancy outcomes (ACOG 776 2019). The American Academy of Dermatology (AAD) considers TNFα-blocking agents for the treatment of psoriasis to be compatible with pregnancy (AAD-NPF [Menter 2019]).

When treatment for inflammatory bowel disease is needed in pregnant women, appropriate biologic therapy can be continued without interruption. Weight based dosing can be done using prepregnancy body weight and adjusted as needed based on disease activity and serum concentrations. Serum levels should be evaluated prior to conception and optimized to avoid subtherapeutic concentrations or high levels which may increase placental transfer. Dosing can be adjusted so delivery occurs at the lowest serum concentration. For infliximab, the final injection can be given 6 to 10 weeks prior to the estimated date of delivery, then continued 48 hours' postpartum (Mahadevan 2019).

Infliximab may be continued during the first and second trimesters of pregnancy in females with rheumatic and musculoskeletal diseases. Use should be discontinued during the third trimester in women with well-controlled disease. Newborn exposure should be considered if treatment cannot be discontinued due to active disease (ACR [Sammaritano 2020]).

Data collection to monitor pregnancy and infant outcomes following exposure to infliximab is ongoing. Health care providers are also encouraged to enroll females exposed to infliximab during pregnancy in the MotherToBaby Autoimmune Diseases Study by contacting the Organization of Teratology Information Specialists (OTIS) (877-311-8972).

Product Availability

Ixifi (infliximab-qbtx): FDA approved December 2017; anticipated availability is currently undetermined.

- ◆ **Infliximab-abda** *see* InFLIXimab *on page 809*
- ◆ **Infliximab-axxq** *see* InFLIXimab *on page 809*
- ◆ **Infliximab-dyyb** *see* InFLIXimab *on page 809*
- ◆ **Infliximab-qbtx** *see* InFLIXimab *on page 809*
- ◆ **Infliximab, Recombinant** *see* InFLIXimab *on page 809*

Influenza A Virus Vaccine (H5N1)

(in floo EN za aye VYE rus vak SEEN H5N1)

Pharmacologic Category Vaccine; Vaccine, Inactivated (Viral)

Use Influenza A (H5N1) prevention:

Seqirus (Audenz) and GlaxoSmithKline products (adjuvanted): Active immunization of persons ≥6 months of age at increased risk of exposure to the influenza A (H5N1) virus subtype contained in the vaccine.

Note: Audenz: Use in persons 6 months through 17 years of age received accelerated approval based on the immune response elicited by Audenz. Effectiveness of the seasonal vaccine made by the same process has not been confirmed for this age group. Continued approval for use in this age group may be contingent upon verification and description of clinical benefit in confirmatory trials.

Sanofi Pasteur product: Active immunization of persons 18 to 64 years of age at increased risk of exposure to the influenza A (H5N1) virus subtype contained in the vaccine.

Local Anesthetic/Vasoconstrictor Precautions No information available to require special precautions

Effects on Dental Treatment No significant effects or complications reported

Effects on Bleeding No information available to require special precautions

Adverse Reactions Actual percentages may vary by product and age group.

>10%:

Dermatologic: Diaphoresis (6% to 11%)

Gastrointestinal: Abdominal pain (children and adolescents: ≤17%), anorexia (children and adolescents: 14% to 29%), change in appetite (infants and children: 18%), diarrhea (≤17%), nausea (≤17%), vomiting (children and adolescents: ≤17%)

Local: Erythema at injection site (≤34%), induration at injection site (≤15%), pain at injection site (36% to 83%), swelling at injection site (adults: ≤15%; infants, children, and adolescents: 28% to 29%), tenderness at injection site (adults: 70%; infants and children: 56%)

Nervous system: Drowsiness (infants and children: 25% to 38%), fatigue (20% to 34%), headache (3% to 35%), irritability (infants and children: ≤51%), malaise (16% to 25%), shivering (adults: 17%; children and adolescents: 4% to 10%)

Neuromuscular & skeletal: Arthralgia (10% to 25%), myalgia (9% to 45%)

Miscellaneous: Fever (3% to 22%), fussiness in an infant or toddler (≤51%)

1% to 10%:

Gastrointestinal: Gastroenteritis (children and adolescents: 1%)

Local: Itching at injection site (adults: 2%), warm sensation at injection site (adults: 1%)

Nervous system: Chills (older adults: 4%), dizziness (adults: 1%)

<1%:

Dermatologic: Skin rash (adults)

Local: Bruising at injection site (adults)

Mechanism of Action Promotes active immunity to influenza A H5N1 (avian).

Pharmacodynamics/Kinetics

Onset of Action

Audenz: 4-fold increase in antibody titers (measured by hemagglutination inhibition [HI]) occurred in up to 96% of patients 6 months to 17 years of age, 95% of patients 18 to 64 years of age, and 86% of patients ≥65 years of age 21 days after the second dose.

GlaxoSmithKline product (adjuvanted): 4-fold increase in antibody titers (measured by HI) occurred in up to 90% of patients 18 to 64 years of age and 74% of patients ≥65 years of age 21 days after the second dose.

Sanofi Pasteur product: 4-fold increase in antibody titers (measured by HI) occurred in up to 58% of patients 28 days after the second dose (Treanor 2006).

Pregnancy Risk Factor C (Sanofi Pasteur product)

Pregnancy Considerations Adverse events were not observed in animal reproduction studies using the H5N1 vaccine GlaxoSmithKline adjuvanted product; animal reproduction studies have not been conducted with the Sanofi Pasteur product. Inactivated viral vaccines have not been shown to cause increased risks to the fetus (ACIP [Ezeanolue 2020]).

Product Availability Products will not be commercially available; distribution will be limited as part of the US Strategic National Stockpile.

Prescribing and Access Restrictions Commercial distribution is not planned. The vaccine will be included as part of the US Strategic National Stockpile. It will be distributed by public health officials if needed.

- ◆ **Influenza Vaccine** *see* Influenza Virus Vaccine (Inactivated) *on page 812*
- ◆ **Influenza Vaccine** *see* Influenza Virus Vaccine (Live/Attenuated) *on page 813*
- ◆ **Influenza Vaccine** *see* Influenza Virus Vaccine (Recombinant) *on page 815*

◆ **Influenza Virus Vaccine (H5N1)** *see* Influenza A Virus Vaccine (H5N1) *on page 811*

Influenza Virus Vaccine (Inactivated)

(in floo EN za VYE rus vak SEEN, in ak ti VAY ted)

Brand Names: US Afluria Quadrivalent; Afluria [DSC]; Fluad; Fluarix Quadrivalent; Flucelvax Quadrivalent; Flucelvax [DSC]; FluLaval Quadrivalent; Fluvirin [DSC]; Fluzone High-Dose; Fluzone Intradermal Quadrivalent [DSC]; Fluzone Quadrivalent; Fluzone [DSC]

Brand Names: Canada Afluria Tetra; Agriflu; Fluad; Fluad Pediatric; Flulaval Tetra; Fluviral; Fluzone High-Dose; Fluzone Quadrivalent; Influvac

Pharmacologic Category Vaccine; Vaccine, Inactivated (Viral)

Use Influenza disease prevention: Active immunization against influenza disease caused by influenza virus subtypes A and type B contained in the vaccine in the following persons:

US labeling:

- ≥6 months of age (Afluria Quadrivalent, Fluarix Quadrivalent, FluLaval Quadrivalent, Fluzone Quadrivalent)
- ≥4 years of age (Flucelvax Quadrivalent)
- ≥65 years of age (Fluad, Fluad Quadrivalent, Fluzone High-Dose Quadrivalent)

Canadian labeling:

- 6 months to <2 years of age (Fluad Pediatric)
- ≥6 months of age (Agriflu, FluLaval Tetra, Fluviral, Fluzone Quadrivalent)
- ≥3 years of age (Influvac Tetra)
- ≥5 years of age (Afluria Tetra)
- ≥65 years of age (Fluad, Fluzone High-Dose Quadrivalent)

The Advisory Committee on Immunization Practices (ACIP) recommends routine annual vaccination with the seasonal influenza vaccine for all persons ≥6 months of age who do not otherwise have contraindications to the vaccine. The ACIP and American Academy of Pediatrics (AAP) recommend use of any age and risk factor appropriate product and do not have a preferential recommendation for an influenza vaccine product; in addition to inactivated influenza vaccines (IIV3, IIV4), the live attenuated vaccine (LAIV4) may be used for persons ≥2 years of age and recombinant influenza vaccine (RIV) can be used in persons ≥18 years of age (AAP 2019; CDC/ACIP [Grohskopf 2019]).

The Canadian National Advisory Committee on Immunization (NACI) recommends the following (NACI 2019): Annual vaccination with seasonal influenza vaccine for all persons ≥6 months who do not otherwise have contraindications to the vaccine. Healthy, nonpregnant persons aged 2 to 59 years may receive vaccination with the seasonal live, attenuated influenza vaccine (LAIV) (nasal spray). The following influenza vaccine preferences should be considered:

- Persons 6 to 23 months of age: Quadrivalent inactivated influenza vaccine (IIV4) is preferred or trivalent inactivated influenza vaccine (IIV3) if IIV4 is not available.
- Persons 2 to 17 years of age: Either IIV4 or LAIV is preferred (IIV3 may be considered if neither IIV4 nor LAIV are available).
- Persons ≥65 years of age: IIV3-HD (high dose) is preferred over IIV3-SD (standard dose); however, any available IIV3 or IIV4 vaccine may be used for public health program-level decision making.
- Health care workers: Either IIV4 or IIV3 are recommended; LAIV should not be used.

When vaccine supply is limited, target groups for vaccination (those at higher risk of complications from influenza infection and their close contacts) include the following (CDC/ACIP [Grohskopf 2019]):

- All infants and children 6 to 59 months of age
- Persons ≥50 years of age
- Infants, children, and adolescents (6 months to 18 years of age) who are receiving long-term aspirin or salicylate therapy, and therefore, may be at risk for developing Reye syndrome after influenza
- Women who are or will be pregnant during the influenza season
- Patients with chronic pulmonary disorders (including asthma) or cardiovascular systems disorders (except isolated hypertension), renal, hepatic, neurologic, hematologic, or metabolic disorders (including diabetes mellitus)
- Persons who have immunosuppression due to any cause (including immunosuppression caused by medications or HIV)
- Residents of nursing homes and other long-term care facilities
- American Indians/Alaska Natives
- Extremely obese (BMI ≥40)
- Health care personnel, including students in these professions, who will have contact with patients and other persons not directly involved in patient care but may be exposed to infectious agents (eg, clerical, housekeeping, volunteers)
- Household contacts (including children) and caregivers of neonates, infants, and children <5 years of age (particularly neonates and infants <6 months of age) and adults ≥50 years of age
- Household contacts (including children) and caregivers of persons with medical conditions which put them at higher risk of severe complications from influenza infection

In addition, the NACI also recommends vaccination of patients with neurologic or neurodevelopment conditions including neuromuscular/neurovascular/neurodegenerative conditions, seizure disorders (including febrile seizures in pediatric patients and isolated developmental delay) but excluding migraines and psychiatric conditions without neurological conditions (NACI 2018).

Local Anesthetic/Vasoconstrictor Precautions No information available to require special precautions

Effects on Dental Treatment No significant effects or complications reported

Effects on Bleeding No information available to require special precautions

Adverse Reactions Incidence of adverse events for the second dose of vaccine (when warranted) was typically milder than first dose.

>10%:

Gastrointestinal: Anorexia (infants, children, and adolescents: 9% to 32%; adults and older adults: 4% to 8%), diarrhea (4% to 13%), nausea (≤12%), vomiting (infants, children, and adolescents: ≤15%; adults and older adults: ≤3%)

Local: Erythema at injection site (1% to 37%), induration at injection site (≤17%), pain at injection site (17% to 67%), swelling at injection site (≤25%), tenderness at injection site (21% to 69%)

Nervous system: Drowsiness (infants and children: 8% to 38%), fatigue (≤22%), headache (1% to 27%), irritability (infants and children: 2% to 54%), malaise (≤38%), uncontrolled crying (infants and children: 33% to 41%)
Neuromuscular & skeletal: Arthralgia (4% to 15%), myalgia (8% to 40%)
Respiratory: Cough (infants, children, and adolescents: 1% to 15%), rhinorrhea (infants and children: 1% to 11%), wheezing
Miscellaneous: Fever (infants, children, and adolescents: 1% to 16%; adults and older adults: ≤4%)

1% to 10%:
Dermatologic: Skin rash (infants and children: 1%)
Gastrointestinal: Change in appetite (children: 10%)
Local: Bruising at injection site (≤9%)
Nervous system: Chills (≤7%), shivering (≤9%)
Respiratory: Flu-like symptoms (infants and children: 1%), nasal congestion (infants, children, and adolescents: 2% to 6%), nasopharyngitis (infants and children: 2%), oropharyngeal pain (adolescents and adults: 2% to 7%)

Frequency not defined: Local: Hematoma at injection site, itching at injection site

Postmarketing:
Cardiovascular: Chest pain, facial edema, flushing, presyncope, swelling of injected limb (lasting >1 week), syncope (shortly after vaccination), tachycardia, vasculitis (including transient renal involvement), vasodilation
Dermatologic: Diaphoresis, ecchymoses, erythema multiforme, erythema of skin, pallor, pruritus, rash at injection site, Stevens-Johnson syndrome, urticaria
Endocrine & metabolic: Hot flash
Gastrointestinal: Abdominal distress, abdominal pain, dysphagia, gastroenteritis, swollen tongue
Hematologic & oncologic: Henoch-Schönlein purpura, lymphadenopathy (local), thrombocytopenia
Hypersensitivity: Anaphylactic shock, anaphylaxis, angioedema, hypersensitivity reaction (including oculorespiratory syndrome, an acute, self-limited reaction with ocular and respiratory symptoms) (CDC/ACIP [Grohskopf 2013]), nonimmune anaphylaxis, serum sickness
Local: Abscess at injection site, cellulitis at injection site, inflammation at injection site, warm sensation at injection site
Nervous system: Bell's palsy, body pain, cranial nerve palsy, dizziness, encephalopathy, facial nerve paralysis, feeling hot, Guillain-Barre syndrome, hypoesthesia, insomnia, myasthenia, neuralgia, neuritis, neuropathy (including brachial plexus), paralysis (including limb), paresthesia, seizure, transverse myelitis, vertigo, voice disorder
Neuromuscular & skeletal: Asthenia, hypokinesia, limb pain, myelitis (including encephalomyelitis), tremor
Ophthalmic: Eyelid edema, eye pain, ocular hyperemia, optic neuritis, optic neuropathy, photophobia, swelling of eye
Respiratory: Bronchospasm, dyspnea, pharyngeal edema, pharyngitis, rhinitis, tonsillitis
Miscellaneous: Febrile seizure

Mechanism of Action Promotes immunity to seasonal influenza virus by inducing specific antibody production. Preparations from previous seasons must not be used.

Pharmacodynamics/Kinetics

Onset of Action Most adults have antibody protection within 2 weeks of vaccination (CDC/ACIP [Grohskopf 2019]).

Duration of Action Vaccine effectiveness declines at a variable rate, depending on virus subtypes, patient age, and other confounding factors (CDC/ACIP [Grohskopf 2019]).

Reproductive Considerations

Influenza vaccination with any licensed, recommended, age-appropriate vaccine is recommended for all females who may become pregnant during the influenza season and who do not otherwise have contraindications to the vaccine (CDC/ACIP [Grohskopf 2019]).

Pregnancy Considerations

Inactivated influenza vaccine (IIV) has not been shown to cause fetal harm when given to pregnant women, although information related to use in the first trimester is relatively limited (CDC/ACIP [Grohskopf 2019]).

Following maternal immunization with IIV, vaccine-specific antibodies are observed in the newborn (CDC 2018). Most studies evaluating the use of inactivated influenza vaccines during pregnancy have not shown an increased risk of adverse pregnancy events (CDC/ACIP [Grohskopf 2019]).

The risk for severe illness and complications from influenza infection is increased during pregnancy, particularly during the second and third trimesters (CDC/ACIP [Grohskopf 2019]). Influenza vaccination decreases the risk of laboratory-confirmed influenza in pregnant women (Thompson 2014) and infants <6 months of age whose mothers have been vaccinated (CDC 2018).

Influenza vaccination with any licensed, recommended, age-appropriate vaccine is recommended for all females who are pregnant during the influenza season and who do not otherwise have contraindications to the vaccine (CDC/ACIP [Grohskopf 2019]). Use of an inactivated vaccine is recommended; vaccination may be done during any trimester of pregnancy (ACOG 732 2018).

Pregnant females should observe the same precautions as nonpregnant patients to reduce the risk of exposure to influenza and other respiratory infections (CDC/HHS 2019). When vaccine supply is limited, focus on delivering the vaccine should be given to females who are pregnant or will be pregnant during the flu season, as well as mothers of newborns and contacts or caregivers of children <5 years of age (CDC/ACIP [Grohskopf 2019]).

Women exposed to FluLaval Quadrivalent or Fluarix Quadrivalent vaccine during pregnancy or their health care provider may contact the GlaxoSmithKline registry at 888-452-9622.

Women exposed to Afluria Quadrivalent or Flucelvax Quadrivalent vaccine during pregnancy may contact the Seqirus registry at 855-358-8966 or via email at us.-medicalinformation@seqirus.com.

Health care providers may enroll women exposed to Fluzone Quadrivalent during pregnancy in the Sanofi Pasteur vaccination registry at 800-822-2463.

Influenza Virus Vaccine (Live/Attenuated)

(in floo EN za VYE rus vak SEEN live ah TEN yoo aye ted)

Brand Names: US FluMist Quadrivalent

Pharmacologic Category Vaccine; Vaccine, Live (Viral)

Use Influenza disease prevention:

US labeling: Active immunization of individuals 2 to 49 years of age against influenza disease caused by influenza virus subtypes A and type B contained in the vaccine.

The Advisory Committee on Immunization Practices (ACIP) recommends routine annual vaccination with seasonal influenza vaccine for all persons ≥6 months of age who do not otherwise have contraindications to vaccination. Live attenuated influenza vaccine (LAIV4) is an option for the 2019-2020 influenza season in healthy persons aged 2 to 49 years (CDC/ACIP [Grohskopf 2019]). ACIP and American Academy of Pediatrics (AAP) do not express any preference for an influenza vaccine product when age and risk factors are accounted for (AAP 2019; CDC/ACIP [Grohskopf 2019]).

Canadian labeling: Active immunization of individuals 2 to 59 years of age against influenza disease caused by influenza virus subtypes A and type B contained in the vaccine.

The Canadian National Advisory Committee on Immunization (NACI) recommends the following (NACI 2019): Annual vaccination with seasonal influenza vaccine for all persons ≥6 months of age who do not otherwise have contraindications to the vaccine. Healthy, nonpregnant persons aged 2 to 59 years may receive vaccination with the seasonal live, attenuated influenza vaccine (LAIV) (nasal spray). The following influenza vaccine preferences should be considered:

- Persons 6 months to 23 months of age: Quadrivalent inactivated influenza vaccine (IIV4) is preferred or trivalent inactivated influenza vaccine (IIV3) if IIV4 is not available.
- Persons 2 to 17 years of age: Either IIV4 or LAIV is preferred (IIV3 may be considered if neither IIV4 nor LAIV are available).
- Persons ≥65 years of age: IIV3-HD (high dose) is preferred over IIV3-SD (standard dose); however, any available IIV3 or IIV4 vaccine may be used for public health program-level decision making.
- Health care workers: Either IIV4 or IIV3 are recommended; LAIV should not be used.

When vaccine supply is limited, target groups for vaccination (those at higher risk of complications from influenza infection and their close contacts) include the following (CDC/ACIP [Grohskopf 2019]): **Note:** Only use LAIV if appropriate:

- All infants and children 6 to 59 months of age
- Persons ≥50 years of age
- Infants, children, and adolescents (6 months to 18 years of age) who are receiving long-term aspirin therapy, and therefore, may be at risk for developing Reye syndrome after influenza
- Women who are or will be pregnant during the influenza season
- Patients with chronic pulmonary disorders (including asthma) or cardiovascular systems disorders (except isolated hypertension), renal, hepatic, neurologic, or metabolic disorders (including diabetes mellitus)
- Persons who have immunosuppression due to any cause (including immunosuppression caused by medications or HIV)
- Residents of nursing homes and other long-term care facilities
- American Indians/Alaska Natives
- Extremely obese (BMI ≥40)
- Health care personnel including students in these professions who will have contact with patients and other persons not directly involved in patient care but may be exposed to infectious agents (eg, clerical, housekeeping, volunteers)
- Household contacts (including children) and caregivers of neonates, infants, and children <5 years (particularly neonates and infants <6 months) and adults ≥50 years
- Household contacts (including children) and caregivers of persons with medical conditions which put them at high risk of complications from influenza infection

In addition, the NACI also recommends vaccination of patients with neurologic or neurodevelopment conditions including neuromuscular/neurovascular/neurodegenerative conditions, seizure disorders (including febrile seizures in pediatric patients and isolated developmental delay), but excluding migraines and psychiatric conditions without neurological conditions (NACI 2019).

Local Anesthetic/Vasoconstrictor Precautions No information available to require special precautions

Effects on Dental Treatment No significant effects or complications reported

Effects on Bleeding No information available to require special precautions

Adverse Reactions Frequency of events reported within 10 days.

>10%:

Central nervous system: Headache (adults: 40%; children: 3% to 9%), irritability (children: 12% to 21%), lethargy (children: 7% to 14%)

Gastrointestinal: Sore throat (adults: 28%; children: 5% to 11%), decreased appetite (children: 13% to 21%), abdominal pain (children: 2% to 12%)

Neuromuscular & skeletal: Fatigue (adults: ≤26%), weakness (adults: ≤26%), myalgia (adults: 17%; children: 2% to 6%)

Respiratory: Nasal congestion (children: ≤58%; adults: ≤44%), rhinorrhea (children: ≤58%; adults: ≤44%), cough (adults: 14%)

1% to 10%:

Central nervous system: Chills (adults: 9%; children: 2% to 4%)

Otic: Otitis media (children: 3%)

Respiratory: Wheezing (children: 6 to 23 months: 6%; 24 to 59 months: 2%), sinusitis (adults: 4%), sneezing (children: 2%)

Miscellaneous: Fever (children: 100°F to 101°F: 6% to 9%; >101°F: 1% to 4%)

<1%, postmarketing, and/or case reports: Anaphylaxis, Bell's palsy, diarrhea, encephalitis (vaccine-associated), epistaxis, exacerbation of asthma, facial edema, Guillain-Barre syndrome, hypersensitivity reaction, meningitis (including eosinophilic meningitis), nausea, pericarditis, skin rash, subacute necrotizing encephalomyelopathy (Leigh syndrome exacerbation), urticaria, vomiting

Mechanism of Action The vaccine contains live attenuated viruses which infect and replicate within the cells lining the nasopharynx. Promotes immunity to seasonal influenza virus by inducing specific antibody production. Preparations from previous seasons must not be used.

Pharmacodynamics/Kinetics

Onset of Action Most adults have antibody protection within 2 weeks of vaccination (CDC/ACIP [Grohskopf 2019])

Duration of Action Vaccine effectiveness declines at a variable rate, depending on virus subtypes, patient age, and other confounding factors (CDC/ACIP [Grohskopf 2019]).

Pregnancy Considerations

The Advisory Committee on Immunization Practices contraindicates use of live attenuated influenza vaccine during pregnancy (CDC/ACIP [Grohskopf 2019]).

This vaccine is not systemically absorbed following maternal nasal administration and is not expected to result in exposure to the fetus.

◆ **Influenza Virus Vaccine (Monovalent)** *see* Influenza A Virus Vaccine (H5N1) *on page 811*

◆ **Influenza Virus Vaccine (Purified Surface Antigen)** *see* Influenza Virus Vaccine (Inactivated) *on page 812*

Influenza Virus Vaccine (Recombinant)

(in floo EN za VYE rus vak SEEN ree KOM be nant)

Brand Names: US Flublok Quadrivalent; Flublok [DSC]

Pharmacologic Category Vaccine; Vaccine, Recombinant

Use Influenza disease prevention: Active immunization against influenza disease caused by influenza virus subtypes A and type B contained in the vaccine in persons ≥18 years of age

The Advisory Committee on Immunization Practices (ACIP) recommends routine annual vaccination with seasonal influenza vaccine for all persons ≥6 months who do not otherwise have contraindications to the vaccine. ACIP recommends use of any age and risk factor appropriate product and does not express any preference for an influenza vaccine product. Persons ≥18 years may receive vaccination with the recombinant influenza vaccine (RIV). In addition to RIV, other products are available for certain patient populations: Persons ≥6 months of age may receive the trivalent inactivated influenza vaccine or the quadrivalent inactivated influenza vaccine. Live attenuated influenza vaccine is also an option for the 2019 to 2020 influenza season in persons 2 to 49 years of age (CDC/ACIP [Grohskopf 2019]).

When vaccine supply is limited, target groups for vaccination (those at higher risk of complications from influenza infection and their close contacts) include the following (CDC/ACIP [Grohskopf 2019]): **Note:** Only use RIV if appropriate.

- All infants and children 6 to 59 months of age
- Persons ≥50 years of age
- Infants, children, and adolescents (6 months to 18 years of age) who are receiving long-term aspirin or salicylate therapy, and therefore, may be at risk for developing Reye syndrome after influenza
- Residents of nursing homes and other long-term care facilities
- Patients with chronic pulmonary disorders (including asthma) or cardiovascular systems disorders (except isolated hypertension), renal, hepatic, neurologic, hematologic, or metabolic disorders (including diabetes mellitus)
- Persons who have immunosuppression due to any cause (including immunosuppression caused by medications or HIV)
- Infants, children, and adolescents (6 months to 18 years of age) who are receiving long-term aspirin or salicylate therapy, and therefore, may be at risk for developing Reye syndrome after influenza
- Women who are or will be pregnant during the influenza season
- Health care personnel, including students in these professions who will have contact with patients and other persons not directly involved in patient care but may be exposed to infectious agents (eg, clerical, housekeeping, volunteers)
- Household contacts (including children) and caregivers of neonates, infants, and children <5 years (particularly neonates and infants <6 months) and adults ≥50 years
- Household contacts (including children) and caregivers of persons with medical conditions that put them at higher risk of severe complications from influenza infection
- American Indians/Alaska Natives
- Extremely obese (BMI ≥40)

Local Anesthetic/Vasoconstrictor Precautions No information available to require special precautions

Effects on Dental Treatment No significant effects or complications reported

Effects on Bleeding No information available to require special precautions

Adverse Reactions All serious adverse reactions must be reported to the US Department of Health and Human Services (DHHS) Vaccine Adverse Event Reporting System (VAERS) 1-800-822-7967 or online at https://vaers.hhs.gov/esub/index. In Canada, adverse reactions may be reported to local provincial/territorial health agencies or to the Vaccine Safety Section at Public Health Agency of Canada (1-866-844-0018).

Note: Older adults refers to adults ≥50 years of age

>10%:

Central nervous system: Headache (older adults 10% to 17%), fatigue (13% to 15%)

Local: Pain at injection site (37%, older adults 19% to 32%)

Neuromuscular & skeletal: Myalgia (8% to 11%)

1% to 10%:

Central nervous system: Chills (older adults 5%)

Gastrointestinal: Nausea (4% to 6%)

Local: Injection site reactions (3% to 7%; includes redness, swelling and firmness)

Neuromuscular & skeletal: Arthralgia (older adults 6% to 8%)

Respiratory: Cough (1% to 2%), nasal congestion (1% to 2%), nasopharyngitis (1% to 2%), pharyngolaryngeal pain (1% to 2%), rhinorrhea (1% to 2%), upper respiratory tract infection (1% to 2%)

<1%, postmarketing and/or case reports: Anaphylactoid reaction, anaphylaxis, hypersensitivity, hypersensitivity reaction, pleuropericarditis

Mechanism of Action Promotes immunity to seasonal influenza virus by inducing specific antibody production. Preparations from previous seasons must not be used.

Pharmacodynamics/Kinetics

Onset of Action Most adults have antibody protection within 2 weeks of vaccination (CDC/ACIP [Grohskopf 2019]).

Duration of Action Vaccine effectiveness declines at a variable rate, depending on virus subtypes, patient age, and other confounding factors (CDC/ACIP [Grohskopf 2019]).

Reproductive Considerations
Influenza vaccination with any licensed, recommended, age-appropriate vaccine is recommended for all females who may become pregnant during the influenza season and who do not otherwise have contraindications to the vaccine (CDC/ACIP [Grohskopf 2019]).

Pregnancy Considerations Information specific to the use of recombinant influenza vaccine in pregnancy is limited (CDC/ACIP [Grohskopf 2019]).

The risk for severe illness and complications from influenza infection is increased during pregnancy, particularly during the second and third trimesters (CDC/ACIP [Grohskopf 2019]). Influenza vaccination decreases the risk of laboratory-confirmed influenza in pregnant women (Thompson 2014) and infants <6 months of age whose mothers have been vaccinated (CDC 2018).

Influenza vaccination with any licensed, recommended, age-appropriate vaccine is recommended for all females who are pregnant during the influenza season and who do not otherwise have contraindications to the vaccine (CDC/ACIP [Grohskopf 2019]). Use of an inactivated vaccine is recommended; vaccination may be done during any trimester of pregnancy (ACOG 2018).

Pregnant females should observe the same precautions as nonpregnant patients to reduce the risk of exposure to influenza and other respiratory infections (CDC/HHS 2019). When vaccine supply is limited, focus on delivering the vaccine should be given to females who are pregnant or will be pregnant during the flu season, as well as mothers of newborns and contacts or caregivers of children <5 years of age (CDC/ACIP [Grohskopf 2019]).

Women exposed to this vaccine during pregnancy may contact the Flublok pregnancy registry at 1-800-822-2463.

- ◆ **Influenza Virus Vaccine (Split-Virus)** *see* Influenza Virus Vaccine (Inactivated) *on page 812*
- ◆ **Infugem** *see* Gemcitabine *on page 731*
- ◆ **Infumorph 200** *see* Morphine (Systemic) *on page 1050*
- ◆ **Infumorph 500** *see* Morphine (Systemic) *on page 1050*
- ◆ **Ingrezza** *see* Valbenazine *on page 1516*
- ◆ **INH** *see* Isoniazid *on page 844*
- ◆ **Inhaled Insulin** *see* Insulin (Oral Inhalation) *on page 828*
- ◆ **INK-1197** *see* Duvelisib *on page 540*
- ◆ **Inlyta** *see* Axitinib *on page 197*
- ◆ **InnoPran XL** *see* Propranolol *on page 1287*

Inotersen (in oh TER sen)

Brand Names: US Tegsedi

Brand Names: Canada Tegsedi

Pharmacologic Category Antisense Oligonucleotide

Use Polyneuropathy of hereditary transthyretin mediated amyloidosis: Treatment of the polyneuropathy of hereditary transthyretin mediated amyloidosis in adults

Local Anesthetic/Vasoconstrictor Precautions
No information available to require special precautions

Effects on Dental Treatment Key adverse event(s) related to dental treatment: Inotersen has antiplatelet properties and NSAIDs used as dental pain relievers have the potential to enhance the antiplatelet effect; NSAIDs are not contraindicated, but caution is suggested (ie, use lowest effective pain relieving dose at the shortest period of time); xerostomia has been reported and normal salivary flow resumes with drug discontinuation; patients may experience orthostatic hypotension as they stand up after treatment especially if lying in dental chair for extended periods of time. Use caution with sudden changes in position during and after dental treatment.

Effects on Bleeding Exposure to antisense oligonucleotides may result in significant myelosuppression including reduction in platelet counts (thrombocytopenia) and altered hemostasis. In patients under active treatment with this agent, medical consult is suggested.

Adverse Reactions
>10%:
Cardiovascular: Peripheral edema (19%), cardiac arrhythmia (13%), presyncope (≤13%), syncope (≤13%)
Central nervous system: Headache (26%), fatigue (25%), chills (18%), paresthesia (10%)
Gastrointestinal: Nausea (31%), vomiting (15%).
Hematologic & oncologic: Thrombocytopenia (24%; severe thrombocytopenia: 3%), anemia (17%)
Immunologic: Antibody development (30%)
Local: Injection site reaction (49%)
Neuromuscular & skeletal: Myalgia (15%), arthralgia (13%)
Renal: Renal insufficiency (14%)
Miscellaneous: Fever (20%)
1% to 10%:
Cardiovascular: Orthostatic hypotension (8%)
Gastrointestinal: Decreased appetite (10%), xerostomia (5%)
Hematologic & oncologic: Bruise (7%), eosinophilia (5%)
Hepatic: Increased liver enzymes (9%)
Infection: Increased serum alanine aminotransferase (≥3 x ULN: 8%; ≥8 x ULN: 3%), bacterial infection (7%)
Renal: Glomerulonephritis (3%)
Respiratory: Dyspnea (9%), flu-like symptoms (8%)
Frequency not defined: Endocrine & metabolic: Vitamin A deficiency
<1%, postmarketing, and/or case reports: Autoimmune hepatitis, cerebrovascular accident, coronary artery dissection, hepatobiliary disease, hypersensitivity reaction, immune thrombocytopenia, lower back pain, paraplegia, speech disturbance, vasculitis (antineutrophil cytoplasmic autoantibody - positive systemic vasculitis), weight loss

Mechanism of Action Inotersen is an antisense oligonucleotide that causes degradation of mutant and wild type TTR mRNA through binding to the TTR mRNA, which results in a reduction of serum TTR protein and TTR protein deposits in tissues.

Pharmacodynamics/Kinetics

Half-life Elimination 32.3 days (range: 29.4 to 35.5 days)

Time to Peak 2 to 4 hours (median)

Reproductive Considerations
Females of reproductive potential and males with female partners of reproductive potential were required to use effective contraception during clinical trials of inotersen (Benson 2018).

Pregnancy Considerations
Adverse events were observed in some animal reproduction studies.

Inotersen decreases serum vitamin A levels; appropriate concentrations of vitamin A are required for fetal development.

Data collection to monitor pregnancy and infant outcomes following exposure to inotersen is ongoing. Health care providers are encouraged to enroll females exposed to inotersen during pregnancy in the pregnancy registry (1-877-465-7510, tegsedi-pregnancy@ubc.com, or www.tegsedipregnancystudy.com); patients may also enroll themselves.

◆ **Inotersen Sodium** *see* Inotersen *on page 816*
◆ **Inqovi** *see* Decitabine and Cedazuridine *on page 448*
◆ **Inspra** *see* Eplerenone *on page 576*
◆ **Instacort 5 [OTC]** *see* Hydrocortisone (Topical) *on page 775*

Insulin Aspart (IN soo lin AS part)

Related Information
Endocrine Disorders and Pregnancy *on page 1684*
Insulin Regular *on page 829*

Brand Names: US Fiasp; Fiasp FlexTouch; Fiasp PenFill; NovoLOG; NovoLOG FlexPen; NovoLOG PenFill

Brand Names: Canada Fiasp; NovoRapid

Pharmacologic Category Insulin, Rapid-Acting

Use Diabetes mellitus, types 1 and 2, treatment: Treatment of type 1 diabetes mellitus and type 2 diabetes mellitus to improve glycemic control.

Local Anesthetic/Vasoconstrictor Precautions No information available to require special precautions

Effects on Dental Treatment Key adverse event(s) related to dental treatment: In general, morning appointments are advisable in patients with diabetes since endogenous cortisol levels are typically higher at this time; because cortisol increases blood sugar levels, the risk of hypoglycemia is less. It is important to confirm that the patient has eaten normally prior to the appointment and has taken all scheduled medications. If a procedure is planned with the expectation that the patient will alter normal eating habits ahead of time (eg, conscious sedation), diabetes medication dose may need to be modified in consultation with the patient's physician. Patients with well-controlled diabetes can usually be managed conventionally for most surgical procedures. Although patients with diabetes usually recognize signs and symptoms of hypoglycemia and self-intervene before changes in or loss of consciousness occurs, they may not. Staff should be trained to recognize the signs (eg, unusual behavior or profuse sweating in patients who have diabetes) and treat patients who have hypoglycemia; a glucometer should be used to test patient blood glucose levels. Every dental office should have a protocol for managing hypoglycemia in conscious and unconscious patients. Having snack foods or oral glucose tablets or gels available, especially in practices where a large number of surgical procedures are performed, is also prudent (American Diabetes Association 2017).

Effects on Bleeding No information available to require special precautions

Adverse Reactions Rates of adverse reactions were defined during combination therapy with other insulins (NPH, detemir, or glargine). Adverse reactions are reported for adults, unless otherwise noted.

>10%:
- Endocrine & metabolic: Severe hypoglycemia (adults, children, and adolescents: Type 1: 1% to 17%, Type 2: 3% to 10%)
- Immunologic: Antibody development (adults: 3% to 28%; children and adolescents: 3%)
- Nervous system: Headache (adults: 5% to 12%; children and adolescents: 6% to 10%), hyporeflexia (11%)
- Respiratory: Nasopharyngitis (20% to 24%), viral respiratory tract infection (children and adolescents: 21% to 23%)
- Miscellaneous: Accidental injury (11%)

1% to 10%:
- Cardiovascular: Chest pain (5%)
- Dermatologic: Onychomycosis (10%), dermatological disorder (5%), allergic skin rash (2%)
- Gastrointestinal: Vomiting (children and adolescents: 3% to 8%), nausea (5% to 7%), abdominal pain (5%), diarrhea (3% to 5%)
- Genitourinary: Urinary tract infection (6% to 8%)
- Hypersensitivity: Hypersensitivity reaction (4%)
- Infection: Influenza (children and adolescents: 6% to 8%)
- Local: Infusion site reaction (10%), injection site reaction (children and adolescents: 4%; adults: 2%), lipoatrophy at injection site (children and adolescents: 2%; adults: <1%)
- Nervous system: Abnormal sensory symptoms (9%)
- Neuromuscular & skeletal: Back pain (4% to 5%)
- Respiratory: Upper respiratory tract infection (children and adolescents: 8% to 12%; adults: 7% to 9%), rhinitis (children and adolescents: 4% to 6%), sinusitis (5%)
- Miscellaneous: Fever (children and adolescents: 6% to 8%)

<1%: Facial edema, peripheral edema

Frequency not defined:
- Endocrine & metabolic: Diabetic retinopathy, weight gain
- Local: Erythema at injection site, injection site pruritus, swelling at injection site
- Nervous system: Peripheral neuropathy
- Ophthalmic: Error of refraction

Postmarketing: Amyloidosis (localized cutaneous at injection site), anaphylaxis

Mechanism of Action Insulin acts via specific membrane-bound receptors on target tissues to regulate metabolism of carbohydrate, protein, and fats. Target organs for insulin include the liver, skeletal muscle, and adipose tissue.

Within the liver, insulin stimulates hepatic glycogen synthesis. Insulin promotes hepatic synthesis of fatty acids, which are released into the circulation as lipoproteins. Skeletal muscle effects of insulin include increased protein synthesis and increased glycogen synthesis. Within adipose tissue, insulin stimulates the processing of circulating lipoproteins to provide free fatty acids, facilitating triglyceride synthesis and storage by adipocytes; it also directly inhibits the hydrolysis of triglycerides. In addition, insulin stimulates the cellular uptake of amino acids and increases cellular permeability to several ions, including potassium, magnesium, and phosphate. By activating sodium-potassium ATPases, insulin promotes the intracellular movement of potassium.

Normally secreted by the pancreas, insulin products are manufactured for pharmacologic use through recombinant DNA technology using either *E. coli* or *Saccharomyces cerevisiae*. Insulin aspart differs from human insulin by containing aspartic acid at position B28 in comparison to the proline found in human insulin. Insulins are categorized based on the onset, peak, and duration of effect (eg, rapid-, short-, intermediate-, and long-acting insulin). Insulin aspart is a rapid-acting insulin analog.

Pharmacodynamics/Kinetics

Onset of Action

SubQ: ~0.2 to 0.3 hours; onset of glucose-lowering effect occurred ~5 minutes earlier with Fiasp compared to conventional insulin aspart (Heise 2017).

Peak effect: SubQ: Fiasp: ~1.5 to 2.2 hours; the peak glucose-lowering effect occurred ~10 minutes earlier with Fiasp compared to conventional insulin aspart (Heise 2017); NovoLOG: 1 to 3 hours.

Duration of Action SubQ: Fiasp: ~5 to 7 hours; NovoLOG: 3 to 5 hours.

Half-life Elimination SubQ: Fiasp: 1.1 hours; NovoLOG: 81 minutes.

Time to Peak

Plasma: SubQ:

Fiasp: ~63 minutes; peak plasma concentration occurred 7.3 minutes earlier with Fiasp compared to conventional insulin aspart (Heise 2017).

NovoLOG: 40 to 50 minutes.

Reproductive Considerations

Females with diabetes mellitus who wish to conceive should use adequate contraception until glycemic control is achieved (ADA 2020). Rapid acting insulin aspart is one of the preferred insulins for use in females with diabetes mellitus planning a pregnancy (Blumer 2013).

Pregnancy Considerations

Rapid-acting insulin aspart (NovoLOG) can be detected in cord blood (Pettitt 2007).

Poorly controlled diabetes during pregnancy can be associated with an increased risk of adverse maternal and fetal outcomes, including diabetic ketoacidosis, preeclampsia, spontaneous abortion, preterm delivery, delivery complications, major birth defects, stillbirth, and macrosomia. To prevent adverse outcomes, prior to conception and throughout pregnancy, maternal blood glucose and HbA_{1c} should be kept as close to target goals as possible but without causing significant hypoglycemia (ADA 2020; Blumer 2013).

Due to pregnancy-induced physiologic changes, insulin requirements tend to increase as pregnancy progresses, requiring frequent monitoring and dosage adjustments. Following delivery, insulin requirements decrease rapidly (ACOG 201 2018; ADA 2020).

Insulin is the preferred treatment of type 1 and type 2 diabetes mellitus in pregnancy, as well as gestational diabetes mellitus when pharmacologic therapy is needed (ACOG 190 2018; ACOG 201 2018; ADA 2020). Rapid-acting insulin aspart is one of the preferred insulins for use in pregnancy (ACOG 190 2018; ACOG 201 2018; Blumer 2013).

Maternal use of faster-acting insulin aspart (Fiasp) compared to rapid-acting insulin aspart (NovoLog) in pregnancy is under study (NCT03770767).

◆ **Insulin Aspart and Insulin Aspart Protamine** *see* Insulin Aspart Protamine and Insulin Aspart *on page 818*

Insulin Aspart Protamine and Insulin Aspart (IN soo lin AS part PROE ta meen & IN soo lin AS part)

Related Information

Insulin Regular *on page 829*

Brand Names: US NovoLOG Mix 70/30; NovoLOG Mix 70/30 FlexPen

Brand Names: Canada NovoMix 30

Pharmacologic Category Insulin, Combination

Use Diabetes mellitus, types 1 and 2: Treatment of type 1 diabetes mellitus and type 2 diabetes mellitus to improve glycemic control

Local Anesthetic/Vasoconstrictor Precautions No information available to require special precautions

Effects on Dental Treatment Key adverse event(s) related to dental treatment: In general, morning appointments are advisable in patients with diabetes since endogenous cortisol levels are typically higher at this time; because cortisol increases blood sugar levels, the risk of hypoglycemia is less. It is important to confirm that the patient has eaten normally prior to the appointment and has taken all scheduled medications. If a procedure is planned with the expectation that the patient will alter normal eating habits ahead of time (eg, conscious sedation), diabetes medication dose may need to be modified in consultation with the patient's physician. Patients with well-controlled diabetes can usually be managed conventionally for most surgical procedures. Although patients with diabetes usually recognize signs and symptoms of hypoglycemia and self-intervene before changes in or loss of consciousness occurs, they may not. Staff should be trained to recognize the signs (eg, unusual behavior or profuse sweating in patients who have diabetes) and treat patients who have hypoglycemia; a glucometer should be used to test patient blood glucose levels. Every dental office should have a protocol for managing hypoglycemia in conscious and unconscious patients. Having snack foods or oral glucose tablets or gels available, especially in practices where a large number of surgical procedures are performed, is also prudent (American Diabetes Association 2017).

Effects on Bleeding No information available to require special precautions

Adverse Reactions

>10%: Endocrine & metabolic: Hypoglycemia (47% to 75%), severe hypoglycemia (4% to 16%)

Frequency not defined:

Cardiovascular: Peripheral edema

Endocrine & metabolic: Hypokalemia, weight gain

Hypersensitivity: Anaphylaxis, hypersensitivity reaction

Immunologic: Antibody development

Local: Hypersensitivity at injection site (including edema, erythema, or pruritus), lipoatrophy at injection site, lipotrophy at injection site

Mechanism of Action Insulin acts via specific membrane-bound receptors on target tissues to regulate metabolism of carbohydrate, protein, and fats. Target organs for insulin include the liver, skeletal muscle, and adipose tissue.

Within the liver, insulin stimulates hepatic glycogen synthesis. Insulin promotes hepatic synthesis of fatty acids, which are released into the circulation as lipoproteins. Skeletal muscle effects of insulin include increased protein synthesis and increased glycogen synthesis. Within adipose tissue, insulin stimulates the processing of circulating lipoproteins to provide free fatty acids, facilitating triglyceride synthesis and storage by adipocytes; also directly inhibits the hydrolysis of triglycerides. In addition, insulin stimulates the cellular uptake of amino acids and increases cellular permeability to several ions, including potassium, magnesium, and phosphate. By activating sodium-potassium ATPases, insulin promotes the intracellular movement of potassium.

Normally secreted by the pancreas, insulin products are manufactured for pharmacologic use through recombinant DNA technology using either *E. coli* or *Saccharomyces cerevisiae*. Insulin aspart differs from human insulin by containing aspartic acid at position B28 in comparison to the proline found in human insulin. Insulins are categorized based on the onset, peak, and duration of effect (eg, rapid-, short-, intermediate-, and long-acting insulin). Insulin aspart protamine and insulin aspart is an intermediate-acting combination product with a more rapid onset and similar duration of action as compared to that of insulin NPH and insulin regular combination products.

Pharmacodynamics/Kinetics

Onset of Action 10 to 20 minutes; Peak effect: 1 to 4 hours

Duration of Action NovoLog Mix 70/30: 18 to 24 hours.

Half-life Elimination NovoLog Mix 70/30: ~8 to 9 hours.

Time to Peak 1 to 1.5 hours

Pregnancy Considerations

Biphasic insulin aspart (insulin aspart protamine suspension 70% [intermediate acting] and insulin aspart solution 30% [rapid acting]) was found to be comparable to biphasic human insulin (Insulin NPH suspension 70% [intermediate acting] and insulin regular solution 30% [short acting]) in initial studies of women with gestational diabetes mellitus (Balaji 2010; Balaji 2012).

Poorly controlled diabetes during pregnancy can be associated with an increased risk of adverse maternal and fetal outcomes, including diabetic ketoacidosis, preeclampsia, spontaneous abortion, preterm delivery, delivery complications, major birth defects, stillbirth, and macrosomia. To prevent adverse outcomes, prior to conception and throughout pregnancy, maternal blood glucose and HbA_{1c} should be kept as close to target goals as possible but without causing significant hypoglycemia (ADA 2020; Blumer 2013).

Due to pregnancy-induced physiologic changes, insulin requirements tend to increase as pregnancy progresses, requiring frequent monitoring and dosage adjustments. Following delivery, insulin requirements decrease rapidly (ACOG 201 2018; ADA 2020).

Insulin is the preferred treatment of type 1 and type 2 diabetes mellitus in pregnancy, as well as gestational diabetes mellitus when pharmacologic therapy is needed (ACOG 190 2018; ACOG 201 2018; ADA 2020).

Insulin Degludec (IN su lin de GLOO dek)

Brand Names: US Tresiba; Tresiba FlexTouch

Brand Names: Canada Tresiba

Pharmacologic Category Insulin, Long-Acting

Use Diabetes mellitus, types 1 and 2, treatment: To improve glycemic control in patients ≥1 year of age with type 1 or type 2 diabetes mellitus.

Local Anesthetic/Vasoconstrictor Precautions No information available to require special precautions

Effects on Dental Treatment Key adverse event(s) related to dental treatment: In general, morning appointments are advisable in patients with diabetes since endogenous cortisol levels are typically higher at this time; because cortisol increases blood sugar levels, the risk of hypoglycemia is less. It is important to confirm that the patient has eaten normally prior to the appointment and has taken all scheduled medications. If a procedure is planned with the expectation that the patient will alter normal eating habits ahead of time (eg, conscious sedation), diabetes medication dose may need to be modified in consultation with the patient's physician. Patients with well-controlled diabetes can usually be managed conventionally for most surgical procedures. Although patients with diabetes usually recognize signs and symptoms of hypoglycemia and self-intervene before changes in or loss of consciousness occurs, they may not. Staff should be trained to recognize the signs (eg, unusual behavior or profuse sweating in patients who have diabetes) and treat patients who have hypoglycemia; a glucometer should be used to test patient blood glucose levels. Every dental office should have a protocol for managing hypoglycemia in conscious and unconscious patients. Having snack foods or oral glucose tablets or gels available, especially in practices where a large number of surgical procedures are performed, is also prudent (American Diabetes Association 2017).

Effects on Bleeding No information available to require special precautions

Adverse Reactions

10%:

Central nervous system: Headache (9% to 12%)

Endocrine & metabolic: Severe hypoglycemia (type 1 diabetics on combination insulin therapy: 10% to 18%; type 2 diabetics on combination therapy: ≤5%)

Immunologic: Antibody development

Respiratory: Nasopharyngitis (13% to 24%), upper respiratory tract infection (8% to 12%)

1% to 10%:

Cardiovascular: Peripheral edema (type 2 diabetes: 3%; type 1 diabetes: <1%)

Gastrointestinal: Diarrhea (type 2 diabetes: 6%), gastroenteritis (type 1 diabetes: 5%)

Local: Injection site reaction (4%; including discoloration, erythema, hematoma, hemorrhage, mass, nodules, pain, pruritus)

Respiratory: Sinusitis (type 1 diabetes: 5%)

Frequency not defined: Endocrine & metabolic: Hypokalemia, weight gain

<1%, postmarketing and/or case reports: Hypersensitivity reaction, hypertrophy at injection site (lipohypertrophy), lipoatrophy at injection site, urticaria

Mechanism of Action Insulin acts via specific membrane-bound receptors on target tissues to regulate metabolism of carbohydrate, protein, and fats. Target organs for insulin include the liver, skeletal muscle, and adipose tissue.

Within the liver, insulin stimulates hepatic glycogen synthesis. Insulin promotes hepatic synthesis of fatty acids, which are released into the circulation as lipoproteins. Skeletal muscle effects of insulin include increased protein synthesis and increased glycogen synthesis. Within adipose tissue, insulin stimulates the processing of circulating lipoproteins to provide free fatty acids, facilitating triglyceride synthesis and storage by adipocytes; also directly inhibits the hydrolysis of triglycerides. In addition, insulin stimulates the cellular uptake of amino acids and increases cellular permeability to several ions, including potassium, magnesium, and phosphate. By activating sodium-potassium ATPases, insulin promotes the intracellular movement of potassium.

Normally secreted by the pancreas, insulin products are manufactured for pharmacologic use through recombinant DNA technology using either *E. coli* or *Saccharomyces cerevisiae*. Insulin degludec differs from human insulin by the omission of the amino acid threonine in position B-30 of the B-chain, and the subsequent addition of a side chain composed of glutamic acid and a C16 fatty acid. Insulins are categorized based on the onset, peak, and duration of effect (eg, rapid-, short-, intermediate-, and long-acting insulin). Insulin degludec is a long-acting, human insulin analog.

Pharmacodynamics/Kinetics

Onset of Action ~1 hour

Half-life Elimination ~25 hours (independent of dose)

Time to Peak 9 hours

Pregnancy Considerations

Information specific to the use of insulin degludec in pregnancy is limited (Bonora 2018; Formoso 2018; Hiranput 2018; Milluzzo 2017).

Poorly controlled diabetes during pregnancy can be associated with an increased risk of adverse maternal and fetal outcomes, including diabetic ketoacidosis, preeclampsia, spontaneous abortion, preterm delivery, delivery complications, major birth defects, stillbirth, and macrosomia. To prevent adverse outcomes, prior to conception and throughout pregnancy, maternal blood glucose and HbA_{1c} should be kept as close to target goals as possible but without causing significant hypoglycemia (ADA 2020; Blumer 2013).

Due to pregnancy-induced physiologic changes, insulin requirements tend to increase as pregnancy progresses, requiring frequent monitoring and dosage adjustments. Following delivery, insulin requirements decrease rapidly (ACOG 201 2018; ADA 2020).

Insulin is the preferred treatment of type 1 and type 2 diabetes mellitus in pregnancy, as well as gestational diabetes mellitus when pharmacologic therapy is needed. Agents other than insulin degludec are currently recommended to treat diabetes mellitus in pregnancy (ACOG 190 2018; ACOG 201 2018; ADA 2020).

Insulin Degludec and Liraglutide

(IN su lin de GLOO dek & lir a GLOO tide)

Brand Names: US Xultophy

Brand Names: Canada Xultophy

Pharmacologic Category Antidiabetic Agent, Glucagon-Like Peptide-1 (GLP-1) Receptor Agonist; Insulin, Long-Acting

Use Diabetes mellitus, type 2: As an adjunct to diet and exercise to improve glycemic control in adults with type 2 diabetes mellitus.

Local Anesthetic/Vasoconstrictor Precautions No information available to require special precautions

Effects on Dental Treatment Key adverse event(s) related to dental treatment: In general, morning appointments are advisable in patients with diabetes since endogenous cortisol levels are typically higher at this time; because cortisol increases blood sugar levels, the risk of hypoglycemia is less. It is important to confirm that the patient has eaten normally prior to the appointment and has taken all scheduled medications. If a procedure is planned with the expectation that the patient will alter normal eating habits ahead of time (eg, conscious sedation), diabetes medication dose may need to be modified in consultation with the patient's physician. Patients with well-controlled diabetes can usually be managed conventionally for most surgical procedures. Although patients with diabetes usually recognize signs and symptoms of hypoglycemia and self-intervene before changes in or loss of consciousness occurs, they may not. Staff should be trained to recognize the signs (eg, unusual behavior or profuse sweating in patients who have diabetes) and treat patients who have hypoglycemia; a glucometer should be used to test patient blood glucose levels. Every dental office should have a protocol for managing hypoglycemia in conscious and unconscious patients. Having snack foods or oral glucose tablets or gels available, especially in practices where a large number of surgical procedures are performed, is also prudent (American Diabetes Association 2017).

Effects on Bleeding No information available to require special precautions

Adverse Reactions Also see individual agents.

>10%:

Endocrine & metabolic: Hypoglycemia (22% to 37%)

Immunologic: Antibody development (2% to 11%; antibody formation has not been associated with reduced efficacy)

1% to 10%:

Central nervous system: Headache (9%)

Gastrointestinal: Diarrhea (8%), nausea (8%), increased serum lipase (7%)

Local: Injection site reaction (3%; mild and transitory)

Respiratory: Nasopharyngitis (10%), upper respiratory tract infection (6%)

Frequency not defined:

Cardiovascular: Increased heart rate

Local: Hypertrophy at injection site, lipoatrophy at injection site

<1%, postmarketing, and/or case reports: Abdominal distension, abdominal pain, allergic skin reaction, anaphylaxis, angioedema, constipation, decreased appetite, dyspepsia, eructation, flatulence, gastritis, gastroesophageal reflux disease, hypersensitivity reaction, severe hypoglycemia, urticaria, vomiting

Mechanism of Action Refer to individual agents.

Pregnancy Considerations Adverse events were observed in some animal reproduction studies. Refer to individual agents.

Insulin Detemir (IN soo lin DE te mir)

Related Information

Endocrine Disorders and Pregnancy *on page 1684*
Insulin Regular *on page 829*

Brand Names: US Levemir; Levemir FlexTouch

Brand Names: Canada Levemir FlexTouch; Levemir Penfill

Pharmacologic Category Insulin, Long-Acting

Use Diabetes mellitus, types 1 and 2: Treatment of type 1 diabetes mellitus and type 2 diabetes mellitus to improve glycemic control

Local Anesthetic/Vasoconstrictor Precautions No information available to require special precautions

Effects on Dental Treatment Key adverse event(s) related to dental treatment: In general, morning appointments are advisable in patients with diabetes since endogenous cortisol levels are typically higher at this time; because cortisol increases blood sugar levels, the risk of hypoglycemia is less. It is important to confirm that the patient has eaten normally prior to the appointment and has taken all scheduled medications. If a procedure is planned with the expectation that the patient will alter normal eating habits ahead of time (eg, conscious sedation), diabetes medication dose may need to be modified in consultation with the patient's physician. Patients with well-controlled diabetes can usually be managed conventionally for most surgical procedures. Although patients with diabetes usually recognize signs and symptoms of hypoglycemia and self-intervene before changes in or loss of consciousness occurs, they may not. Staff should be trained to recognize the signs (eg, unusual behavior or profuse sweating in patients who have diabetes) and treat patients who have hypoglycemia; a glucometer should be used to test patient blood glucose levels. Every dental office should have a protocol for managing hypoglycemia in conscious and unconscious patients. Having snack foods or oral glucose tablets or gels available, especially in practices where a large number of surgical procedures are performed, is also prudent (American Diabetes Association 2017).

Effects on Bleeding No information available to require special precautions

Adverse Reactions

>10%:

Central nervous system: Headache (adults: 7% to 23%, children: 31%)

Endocrine & metabolic: Hypoglycemia (Type 1 combination regimens: children & adolescents: 93% to 95%, adults: 82% to 88%; Type 2 combination regimens: adults: 9% to 41%), severe hypoglycemia (Type 1 combination regimens: children & adolescents: 2% to 16%; adults 5% to 9%; Type 2 combination regimens: adults: ≤2%)

Gastrointestinal: Gastroenteritis (children & adolescents: 17%), abdominal pain (6%; children & adolescents: 13%)

Respiratory: Upper respiratory tract infection (13% to 26%; children & adolescents: 36%), pharyngitis (10%; children & adolescents: 17%), flu-like symptoms (8%; children & adolescents: 14%)

1% to 10%:

Gastrointestinal: Nausea (children & adolescents: 7%), vomiting (children & adolescents: 7%)

Infection: Viral infection (children & adolescents: 7%)

Respiratory: Cough (children & adolescents: 8%), rhinitis (children & adolescents: 7%)

Miscellaneous: Fever (children & adolescents: 10%)

<1%: Pain at injection site

Frequency not defined: Immunologic: Antibody development

Postmarketing: Amyloidosis (localized cutaneous at injection site)

Mechanism of Action Insulin acts via specific membrane-bound receptors on target tissues to regulate metabolism of carbohydrate, protein, and fats. Target organs for insulin include the liver, skeletal muscle, and adipose tissue.

Within the liver, insulin stimulates hepatic glycogen synthesis. Insulin promotes hepatic synthesis of fatty acids, which are released into the circulation as lipoproteins. Skeletal muscle effects of insulin include increased protein synthesis and increased glycogen synthesis. Within adipose tissue, insulin stimulates the processing of circulating lipoproteins to provide free fatty acids, facilitating triglyceride synthesis and storage by adipocytes; also directly inhibits the hydrolysis of triglycerides. In addition, insulin stimulates the cellular uptake of amino acids and increases cellular permeability to several ions, including potassium, magnesium, and phosphate. By activating sodium-potassium ATPases, insulin promotes the intracellular movement of potassium.

Normally secreted by the pancreas, insulin products are manufactured for pharmacologic use through recombinant DNA technology using either *E. coli* or *Saccharomyces cerevisiae*. Insulin detemir differs from human insulin by the omission of threonine in position B30 and the addition of a C14 fatty acid chain to the amino acid located at position B29. Insulins are categorized based on the onset, peak, and duration of effect (eg, rapid-, short-, intermediate-, and long-acting insulin).

Pharmacodynamics/Kinetics

Onset of Action 3 to 4 hours; Peak effect: 3 to 9 hours (Plank 2005)

Duration of Action Dose dependent: 6 to 23 hours; **Note:** At lower dosages (0.1 to 0.2 units/kg), mean duration is variable (5.7 to 12.1 hours). At 0.4 units/kg, the mean duration was 19.9 hours. At high dosages (≥0.8 units/kg) the duration is longer and less variable (mean of 22 to 23 hours) (Plank 2005).

Half-life Elimination 5 to 7 hours (dose-dependent)

Time to Peak Plasma: 6 to 8 hours

Reproductive Considerations

Females with diabetes who wish to conceive should use adequate contraception until glycemic control is achieved (ADA 2020). Females successfully using long acting insulin detemir prior to conception may continue use (Blumer 2013).

Pregnancy Considerations Insulin detemir can be detected in cord blood.

An increased risk of fetal abnormalities has not been observed following the use of insulin detemir in pregnant females with type 1 diabetes mellitus.

Poorly controlled diabetes during pregnancy can be associated with an increased risk of adverse maternal and fetal outcomes, including diabetic ketoacidosis, preeclampsia, spontaneous abortion, preterm delivery, delivery complications, major birth defects, stillbirth, and macrosomia (ACOG 201 2018). To prevent adverse outcomes, prior to conception and throughout pregnancy, maternal blood glucose and HbA_{1c} should be kept as close to target goals as possible but without causing significant hypoglycemia (ADA 2020; Blumer 2013).

Due to pregnancy-induced physiologic changes, insulin requirements tend to increase as pregnancy progresses, requiring frequent monitoring and dosage adjustments. Following delivery, insulin requirements decrease rapidly (ACOG 201 2018; ADA 2020).

Insulin is the preferred treatment of type 1 and type 2 diabetes mellitus in pregnancy, as well as gestational diabetes mellitus when pharmacologic therapy is needed (ACOG 190 2018; ACOG 201 2018; ADA 2020). Pregnancy outcomes are similar following maternal use of insulin detemir and NPH insulin in pregnant females with type 1 diabetes mellitus. Outcomes are likely to be similar in pregnant females with type 2 diabetes and insulin detemir may be used when clinically appropriate (ACOG 201 2018). Females may be switched to insulin detemir during pregnancy when NPH insulin is not adequate (Blumer 2013).

Females successfully using long acting insulin detemir prior to conception may continue use during pregnancy (Blumer 2013).

Insulin Glargine (IN soo lin GLAR jeen)

Related Information

Endocrine Disorders and Pregnancy *on page 1684*

Insulin Regular *on page 829*

Brand Names: US Basaglar KwikPen; Lantus; Lantus SoloStar; Toujeo Max SoloStar; Toujeo SoloStar

Brand Names: Canada Basaglar; Basaglar KwikPen; Lantus; Lantus SoloStar; Toujeo Doublestar; Toujeo SoloStar

Pharmacologic Category Insulin, Long-Acting

Use Diabetes mellitus, types 1 and 2: To improve glycemic control in pediatric patients ≥6 years of age and adults with type 1 diabetes mellitus; to improve glycemic control in pediatric patients ≥6 years of age (Toujeo only) and adults with type 2 diabetes mellitus.

Local Anesthetic/Vasoconstrictor Precautions No information available to require special precautions

Effects on Dental Treatment Key adverse event(s) related to dental treatment: In general, morning appointments are advisable in patients with diabetes since endogenous cortisol levels are typically higher at this time; because cortisol increases blood sugar levels, the risk of hypoglycemia is less. It is important to confirm that the patient has eaten normally prior to the appointment and has taken all scheduled medications. If a procedure is planned with the expectation that the patient will alter normal eating habits ahead of time (eg, conscious sedation), diabetes medication dose may need to be modified in consultation with the patient's physician. Patients with well-controlled diabetes can usually be managed conventionally for most surgical procedures. Although patients with diabetes usually recognize signs and symptoms of hypoglycemia and self-intervene before changes in or loss of consciousness occurs, they may not. Staff should be trained to recognize the signs (eg, unusual behavior or profuse sweating in patients who have diabetes) and treat patients who have hypoglycemia; a glucometer should be used to test patient blood glucose levels. Every dental office should have a protocol for managing hypoglycemia in conscious and unconscious patients. Having snack foods or oral glucose tablets or gels available, especially in practices where a large number of surgical procedures are performed, is also prudent (American Diabetes Association 2017).

Effects on Bleeding No information available to require special precautions

Adverse Reactions Incidence rates are from glargine administered with concomitant antidiabetic agents (insulin or oral products).

>10%

Cardiovascular: Hypertension (20%), peripheral edema (20%)

Central nervous system: Depression (11%)

Endocrine & metabolic: Severe hypoglycemia (Type I on combination regimens: 4% to 69%; Type II on combination regimens: ≤37%; monotherapy in adults ≥50 years old: 6% [ORIGIN trial])

Gastrointestinal: Diarrhea (11%)

Genitourinary: Urinary tract infection (11%)

Immunologic: Antibody development (12% to 44%)

Infection: Infection (9% to 24%), influenza (19%)

Neuromuscular & skeletal: Arthralgia (14%), back pain (13%), limb pain (13%)

Ophthalmic: Cataract (18%)

Respiratory: Upper respiratory tract infection (5% to 29%), sinusitis (19%), nasopharyngitis (6% to 16%), bronchitis (15%), cough (12%)

1% to 10%:

Cardiovascular: Retinal vascular disease (6%)

Central nervous system: Headache (6% to 10%)

Local: Pain at injection site (3%)

Respiratory: Pharyngitis (children and adolescents: 8%), rhinitis (children and adolescents: 5%)

Miscellaneous: Accidental injury (6%)

Frequency not defined:

Dermatologic: Urticaria at injection site

Endocrine & metabolic: Sodium retention, weight gain

Hypersensitivity: Anaphylaxis, angioedema, hypersensitivity reaction

Local: Erythema at injection site, hypertrophy at injection site, inflammation at injection site, itching at injection site, lipoatrophy at injection site, localized edema, swelling at injection site

Postmarketing: Amyloidosis (localized cutaneous at injection site)

Mechanism of Action Insulin acts via specific membrane-bound receptors on target tissues to regulate metabolism of carbohydrate, protein, and fats. Target organs for insulin include the liver, skeletal muscle, and adipose tissue.

Within the liver, insulin stimulates hepatic glycogen synthesis. Insulin promotes hepatic synthesis of fatty acids, which are released into the circulation as lipoproteins. Skeletal muscle effects of insulin include increased protein synthesis and increased glycogen synthesis. Within adipose tissue, insulin stimulates the processing of circulating lipoproteins to provide free fatty acids, facilitating triglyceride synthesis and storage by adipocytes; also directly inhibits the hydrolysis of triglycerides. In addition, insulin stimulates the cellular uptake of amino acids and increases cellular permeability to several ions, including potassium, magnesium, and phosphate. By activating sodium-potassium ATPases, insulin promotes the intracellular movement of potassium.

Normally secreted by the pancreas, insulin products are manufactured for pharmacologic use through recombinant DNA technology using either *E. coli* or *Saccharomyces cerevisiae*. Insulin glargine differs from human insulin by adding two arginines to the C-terminus of the B-chain in addition to containing glycine at position A21 in comparison to the asparagine found in human insulin. Insulins are categorized based on the onset, peak, and duration of effect (eg, rapid-, short-, intermediate-, and long-acting insulin). Insulin glargine is a long-acting insulin analog.

Pharmacodynamics/Kinetics

Onset of Action

Basaglar, Lantus, Semglee: Peak effect: No pronounced peak.

Lantus: 3 to 4 hours; Peak effect: No pronounced peak.

Toujeo: 6 hours; Peak effect: Maximum glucose lowering effect may take up to 5 days with repeat dosing; at steady state, the 24-hour glucose lowering effect is ~27% lower than that of Lantus at equivalent doses.

Duration of Action Basaglar, Lantus, Semglee: Generally 24 hours or longer; reported range (Lantus): 10.8 to >24 hours (up to ~30 hours documented in some studies) (Heinemann 2000); Toujeo: >24 hours.

Time to Peak Plasma: Lantus: No pronounced peak; Basaglar, Semglee: Median: ~12 hours; Toujeo: Median of 12 to 16 hours (dose dependent).

Reproductive Considerations

Females with diabetes mellitus who wish to conceive should use adequate contraception until glycemic control is achieved (ADA 2020). Because insulin glargine has an increased affinity to the insulin-like growth factor (IGF-I) receptor, there are theoretical concerns that it may contribute to adverse events when used during pregnancy (Blumer 2013). Females who are stable on insulin glargine prior to conception may continue it during pregnancy. Theoretical concerns of adverse events associated with insulin glargine during pregnancy should be discussed prior to conception (Blumer 2013).

Pregnancy Considerations

Because insulin glargine has an increased affinity to the insulin-like growth factor (IGF-I) receptor, there are theoretical concerns that it may contribute to adverse events when used during pregnancy (Blumer 2013).

Poorly controlled diabetes during pregnancy can be associated with an increased risk of adverse maternal and fetal outcomes, including diabetic ketoacidosis, preeclampsia, spontaneous abortion, preterm delivery, delivery complications, major birth defects, stillbirth, and macrosomia. To prevent adverse outcomes, prior to conception and throughout pregnancy, maternal blood glucose and HbA_{1c} should be kept as close to target goals as possible but without causing significant hypoglycemia (ADA 2020; Blumer 2013).

Due to pregnancy-induced physiologic changes, insulin requirements tend to increase as pregnancy progresses, requiring frequent monitoring and dosage adjustments. Following delivery, insulin requirements decrease rapidly (ACOG 201 2018; ADA 2020).

Insulin is the preferred treatment of type 1 and type 2 diabetes mellitus in pregnancy, as well as gestational diabetes mellitus when pharmacologic therapy is needed (ACOG 190 2018; ACOG 201 2018; ADA 2020). Pregnancy outcomes are similar following maternal use of insulin glargine and NPH insulin in pregnant females with type 1 diabetes mellitus. Outcomes are likely to be similar in pregnant females with type 2 diabetes and insulin glargine may be used when clinically indicated (ACOG 201 2018).

Product Availability

Basaglar Tempo Pen: FDA approved November 2019; anticipated availability is currently unknown. The Tempo Pen contains a component that allows for data connectivity when used with a compatible transmitter. Consult the prescribing information for additional information.

Semglee: FDA approved June 2020; anticipated availability currently unknown.

Insulin Glargine and Lixisenatide

(IN soo lin GLAR jeen & lix i SEN a tide)

Brand Names: US Soliqua

Brand Names: Canada Soliqua

Pharmacologic Category Antidiabetic Agent, Glucagon-Like Peptide-1 (GLP-1) Receptor Agonist; Insulin, Long-Acting

Use Diabetes mellitus, type 2: As an adjunct to diet and exercise to improve glycemic control in adults with type 2 diabetes mellitus

Local Anesthetic/Vasoconstrictor Precautions No information available to require special precautions

Effects on Dental Treatment Key adverse event(s) related to dental treatment: In general, morning appointments are advisable in patients with diabetes since endogenous cortisol levels are typically higher at this time; because cortisol increases blood sugar levels, the risk of hypoglycemia is less. It is important to confirm that the patient has eaten normally prior to the appointment and has taken all scheduled medications. If a procedure is planned with the expectation that the patient will alter normal eating habits ahead of time (eg, conscious sedation), diabetes medication dose may need to be modified in consultation with the patient's physician. Patients with well-controlled diabetes can usually be managed conventionally for most surgical procedures. Although patients with diabetes usually recognize signs and symptoms of hypoglycemia and self-intervene before changes in or loss of consciousness occurs, they may not. Staff should be trained to recognize the signs (eg, unusual behavior or profuse sweating in patients who have diabetes) and treat patients who have hypoglycemia; a glucometer should be used to test patient blood glucose levels. Every dental office should have a protocol for managing hypoglycemia in conscious and unconscious patients. Having snack foods or oral glucose tablets or gels available, especially in practices where a large number of surgical procedures are performed, is also prudent (American Diabetes Association 2017).

Effects on Bleeding No information available to require special precautions

Adverse Reactions Also see individual agents.

>10%:

- Endocrine & metabolic: Hypoglycemia (8% to 40%)
- Immunologic: Antibody development (21% to 26%)

1% to 10%:

- Central nervous system: Headache (5%)
- Endocrine & metabolic: Severe hypoglycemia (≤1%)
- Gastrointestinal: Nausea (10%), diarrhea (7%), vomiting (3%)
- Local: Injection site reaction (2%)
- Respiratory: Nasopharyngitis (7%), upper respiratory tract infection (6%)

Frequency not defined: Local: Hypertrophy at injection site, lipoatrophy at injection site

<1%, postmarketing, and/or case reports: Abdominal distention, abdominal pain, constipation, decreased appetite, dyspepsia, flatulence, gastritis, gastroesophageal reflux disease

Mechanism of Action Refer to individual agents.

Pregnancy Considerations Adverse events were observed in some animal reproduction studies. Refer to individual monographs.

Insulin Glulisine (IN soo lin gloo LIS een)

Related Information

Endocrine Disorders and Pregnancy *on page 1684*

Insulin Regular *on page 829*

Brand Names: US Apidra; Apidra SoloStar

Brand Names: Canada Apidra; Apidra Optiset [DSC]; Apidra SoloStar

Pharmacologic Category Insulin, Rapid-Acting

Use Diabetes mellitus, types 1 and 2, treatment: Treatment of type 1 diabetes mellitus and type 2 diabetes mellitus to improve glycemic control

Local Anesthetic/Vasoconstrictor Precautions No information available to require special precautions

Effects on Dental Treatment Key adverse event(s) related to dental treatment: In general, morning appointments are advisable in patients with diabetes since endogenous cortisol levels are typically higher at this time; because cortisol increases blood sugar levels, the risk of hypoglycemia is less. It is important to confirm that the patient has eaten normally prior to the appointment and has taken all scheduled medications. If a procedure is planned with the expectation that the patient will alter normal eating habits ahead of time (eg, conscious sedation), diabetes medication dose may need to be modified in consultation with the patient's physician. Patients with well-controlled diabetes can usually be managed conventionally for most surgical procedures. Although patients with diabetes usually recognize signs and symptoms of hypoglycemia and self-intervene before changes in or loss of consciousness occurs, they may not. Staff should be trained to recognize the signs (eg, unusual behavior or profuse sweating in patients who have diabetes) and treat patients who have hypoglycemia; a glucometer should be used to test patient blood glucose levels. Every dental office should have a protocol for managing hypoglycemia in conscious and unconscious patients. Having snack foods or oral glucose tablets or gels available, especially in practices where a large number of surgical procedures are performed, is also prudent (American Diabetes Association 2017).

Effects on Bleeding No information available to require special precautions

Adverse Reactions

>10%:

- Endocrine & metabolic: Severe hypoglycemia (7% to 16%; type 1 diabetes)
- Respiratory: Nasopharyngitis (8% to 11%), upper respiratory tract infection (7% to 11%)

1% to 10%:

- Cardiovascular: Peripheral edema (8%; adults, type 2 diabetes), hypertension (4%; adults, type 2 diabetes)
- Hypersensitivity: Hypersensitivity reaction (4%)
- Infection: Influenza (4% to 6%)
- Local: Infusion site reaction (10%)
- Nervous system: Headache (7%; children and adolescents, type 1 diabetes), hypoglycemic seizure (6%; children and adolescents, type 1 diabetes)
- Neuromuscular & skeletal: Arthralgia (6%; adults, type 2 diabetes)

Frequency not defined:

- Endocrine & metabolic: Weight gain
- Hypersensitivity: Anaphylaxis
- Immunologic: Antibody development (no effect on drug efficacy)
- Local: Erythema at injection site, hypertrophy at injection site, itching at injection site, lipoatrophy at injection site, swelling at injection site

<1%, postmarketing, and/or case reports: Amyloidosis (cutaneous at injection site), catheter complication

Mechanism of Action Insulin acts via specific membrane-bound receptors on target tissues to regulate metabolism of carbohydrate, protein, and fats. Target organs for insulin include the liver, skeletal muscle, and adipose tissue.

Within the liver, insulin stimulates hepatic glycogen synthesis. Insulin promotes hepatic synthesis of fatty acids, which are released into the circulation as lipoproteins. Skeletal muscle effects of insulin include increased protein synthesis and increased glycogen synthesis. Within adipose tissue, insulin stimulates the processing of circulating lipoproteins to provide free fatty acids, facilitating triglyceride synthesis and storage by adipocytes; also directly inhibits the hydrolysis of triglycerides. In addition, insulin stimulates the cellular uptake of amino acids and increases cellular permeability to several ions, including potassium, magnesium, and phosphate. By activating sodium-potassium ATPases, insulin promotes the intracellular movement of potassium.

Normally secreted by the pancreas, insulin products are manufactured for pharmacologic use through recombinant DNA technology using either *E. coli* or *Saccharomyces cerevisiae*. Insulin glulisine differs from human insulin by containing a lysine and glutamic acid at positions B3 and B29, respectively, in comparison to the asparagine and lysine found at B3 and B29 in human insulin. Insulins are categorized based on the onset, peak, and duration of effect (eg, rapid-, short-, intermediate-, and long-acting insulin). Insulin glulisine is a rapid-acting insulin analog.

Pharmacodynamics/Kinetics

Onset of Action 0.2-0.5 hours; Peak effect: 1.6-2.8 hours

Duration of Action 3-4 hours

Half-life Elimination

IV: 13 minutes

SubQ: 42 minutes

Time to Peak Plasma: 60 minutes (range: 40-120 minutes)

Pregnancy Considerations

Based on available information, maternal use of insulin glulisine is not associated with an increased risk of adverse pregnancy outcomes (Doder 2015).

Poorly controlled diabetes during pregnancy can be associated with an increased risk of adverse maternal and fetal outcomes, including diabetic ketoacidosis, preeclampsia, spontaneous abortion, preterm delivery, delivery complications, major birth defects, stillbirth, and macrosomia. To prevent adverse outcomes, prior to conception and throughout pregnancy, maternal blood glucose and HbA_{1c} should be kept as close to target goals as possible but without causing significant hypoglycemia (ADA 2020; Blumer 2013).

Due to pregnancy-induced physiologic changes, insulin requirements tend to increase as pregnancy progresses, requiring frequent monitoring and dosage adjustments. Following delivery, insulin requirements decrease rapidly (ACOG 201 2018; ADA 2020).

Insulin is the preferred treatment of type 1 and type 2 diabetes mellitus in pregnancy, as well as gestational diabetes mellitus when pharmacologic therapy is needed (ACOG 190 2018; ACOG 201 2018; ADA 2020). Agents other than insulin glulisine are currently recommended to treat diabetes mellitus in pregnancy (ACOG 190 2018; ACOG 201 2018; Blumer 2013).

◆ **Insulin Human (Regular)** *see* Insulin Regular *on page 829*

Insulin Lispro (IN soo lin LYE sproe)

Related Information

Endocrine Disorders and Pregnancy *on page 1684*
Insulin Regular *on page 829*

Brand Names: US Admelog; Admelog SoloStar; HumaLOG; HumaLOG Junior KwikPen; HumaLOG KwikPen; Lyumjev; Lyumjev KwikPen

Brand Names: Canada Admelog; Admelog SoloStar; HumaLOG; HumaLOG KwikPen

Pharmacologic Category Insulin, Rapid-Acting

Use Diabetes mellitus, types 1 and 2, treatment: To improve glycemic control in pediatric patients ≥3 years of age (Admelog and Humalog only) and adults with type 1 diabetes mellitus; to improve glycemic control in adults with type 2 diabetes mellitus.

Local Anesthetic/Vasoconstrictor Precautions No information available to require special precautions

Effects on Dental Treatment Key adverse event(s) related to dental treatment: In general, morning appointments are advisable in patients with diabetes since endogenous cortisol levels are typically higher at this time; because cortisol increases blood sugar levels, the risk of hypoglycemia is less. It is important to confirm that the patient has eaten normally prior to the appointment and has taken all scheduled medications. If a procedure is planned with the expectation that the patient will alter normal eating habits ahead of time (eg, conscious sedation), diabetes medication dose may need to be modified in consultation with the patient's physician. Patients with well-controlled diabetes can usually be managed conventionally for most surgical procedures. Although patients with diabetes usually recognize signs and symptoms of hypoglycemia and self-intervene before changes in or loss of consciousness occurs, they may not. Staff should be trained to recognize the signs (eg, unusual behavior or profuse sweating in patients who have diabetes) and treat patients who have hypoglycemia; a glucometer should be used to test patient blood glucose levels. Every dental office should have a protocol for managing hypoglycemia in conscious and unconscious patients. Having snack foods or oral glucose tablets or gels available, especially in practices where a large number of surgical procedures are performed, is also prudent (American Diabetes Association 2017).

Effects on Bleeding No information available to require special precautions

Adverse Reactions

>10%:

- Endocrine & metabolic: Severe hypoglycemia (2% to 14%)
- Immunologic: Antibody development (19% to 23%)
- Local: Infusion site reaction (21% to 24%; includes erythema at injection site and occlusion)
- Nervous system: Headache
- Respiratory: Nasopharyngitis

1% to 10%:

- Gastrointestinal: Abdominal pain, nausea
- Genitourinary: Dysmenorrhea
- Neuromuscular & skeletal: Asthenia, myalgia (may be secondary to excipient metacresol)

Frequency not defined:

- Cardiovascular: Peripheral edema
- Endocrine & metabolic: Hypokalemia, weight gain
- Hypersensitivity: Hypersensitivity reaction
- Local: Hypertrophy at injection site, injection site reaction (including local reactions secondary to excipient metacresol), lipoatrophy at injection site

Postmarketing: Endocrine & metabolic: Amyloidosis (localized cutaneous)

Mechanism of Action Insulin acts via specific membrane-bound receptors on target tissues to regulate metabolism of carbohydrate, protein, and fats. Target organs for insulin include the liver, skeletal muscle, and adipose tissue.

Within the liver, insulin stimulates hepatic glycogen synthesis. Insulin promotes hepatic synthesis of fatty acids, which are released into the circulation as lipoproteins. Skeletal muscle effects of insulin include increased protein synthesis and increased glycogen synthesis. Within adipose tissue, insulin stimulates the processing of circulating lipoproteins to provide free fatty acids, facilitating triglyceride synthesis and storage by adipocytes; also directly inhibits the hydrolysis of triglycerides. In addition, insulin stimulates the cellular uptake of amino acids and increases cellular permeability to several ions, including potassium, magnesium, and phosphate. By activating sodium-potassium ATPases, insulin promotes the intracellular movement of potassium.

Normally secreted by the pancreas, insulin products are manufactured for pharmacologic use through recombinant DNA technology using either *E. coli* or *Saccharomyces cerevisiae*. Insulin lispro differs from human insulin by containing a lysine and proline at positions B28 and B29, respectively, in comparison to the proline and lysine found at B28 and B29 in human insulin. Insulins are categorized based on the onset, peak, and duration of effect (eg, rapid-, short-, intermediate-, and long-acting insulin). Insulin lispro is a rapid-acting insulin analog.

Pharmacodynamics/Kinetics

Onset of Action

SubQ:

- Admelog: Similar onset to Humalog (Kapitza 2017).
- Humalog: 31 minutes (patients with type 1 diabetes) (Linnebjerg 2020); 45 minutes (patients with type 2 diabetes) (Leohr 2020).
- Lyumjev: ~15 to 17 minutes (manufacturer's labeling); 20.1 minutes (patients with type 1 diabetes) (Linnebjerg 2020); 32 minutes (patients with type 2 diabetes) (Leohr 2020).

Peak effect:

- Admelog: ~2.1 hours.
- Humalog: 2.4 to 2.8 hours.
- Lyumjev: ~2 to 2.9 hours.

Duration of Action

SubQ:

- Admelog: ~6.9 hours (patients with type 1 diabetes) (Kapitza 2017).
- Humalog: ~5.7 to 6.6 hours (patients with type 1 diabetes) (Kapitza 2017; Linnebjerg 2020); ~6.7 hours (patients with type 2 diabetes) (Leohr 2020).
- Lyumjev: ~4.6 to 7.3 hours (manufacturer's labeling); ~5 hours (patients with type 1 diabetes) (Linnebjerg 2020); ~6.4 hours (patients with type 2 diabetes) (Leohr 2020).

Half-life Elimination Admelog, Humalog: 51 to 60 minutes; Lyumjev: 44 minutes.

Time to Peak

Plasma: SubQ:

- Admelog, Humalog: Median: ~50 minutes (Kapitza 2017; manufacturer's labeling [Admelog]); range: 30 to 90 minutes (manufacturer's labeling [Humalog]).
- Lyumjev: 57 minutes; time to reach 50% of peak plasma concentration was 14 minutes shorter compared to Humalog in patients with type 1 diabetes (14.8 vs 29 minutes, respectively) (Linnebjerg 2020) and 11 minutes shorter compared to Humalog in patients with type 2 diabetes (18.6 vs 29.6 minutes respectively) (Leohr 2020).

Reproductive Considerations

Females with diabetes mellitus who wish to conceive should use adequate contraception until glycemic control is achieved (ADA 2019).

Insulin lispro is one of the preferred insulins for use in females with diabetes mellitus planning a pregnancy (Blumer 2013).

Pregnancy Considerations

Insulin lispro has not been shown to cross the placenta at standard clinical doses (Boskovic 2003; Holcberg 2004; Jovanovic 1999).

Poorly controlled diabetes during pregnancy can be associated with an increased risk of adverse maternal and fetal outcomes, including diabetic ketoacidosis, preeclampsia, spontaneous abortion, preterm delivery, delivery complications, major birth defects, stillbirth, and macrosomia (ACOG 201 2018). To prevent adverse outcomes prior to conception and throughout pregnancy, maternal blood glucose and HbA_{1c} should be kept as close to target goals as possible but without causing significant hypoglycemia (ADA 2020; Blumer 2013).

Due to pregnancy-induced physiologic changes, insulin requirements tend to increase as pregnancy progresses, requiring frequent monitoring and dosage adjustments. Following delivery, insulin requirements decrease rapidly (ACOG 201 2018; ADA 2020).

Insulin is the preferred treatment of type 1 and type 2 diabetes mellitus in pregnancy, as well as gestational diabetes mellitus when pharmacologic therapy is needed (ACOG 190 2018; ACOG 201 2018; ADA 2020). Insulin lispro is one of the preferred insulins for use in pregnancy (ACOG 190 2018; ACOG 201 2018; Blumer 2013).

Product Availability

Humalog Tempo Pen: FDA approved November 2019; anticipated availability is currently unknown. Information pertaining to this product within the monograph is pending revision. The Tempo Pen contains a component that allows for data connectivity when used with a compatible transmitter. Consult the prescribing information for additional information.

Lyumjev: FDA approved June 2020; availability anticipated in July 2020. Information pertaining to this product within the monograph is pending revision. Consult the prescribing information for additional information.

- **Insulin Lispro-aabc** *see* Insulin Lispro *on page 824*
- **Insulin Lispro and Insulin Lispro Protamine** *see* Insulin Lispro Protamine and Insulin Lispro *on page 826*

Insulin Lispro Protamine and Insulin Lispro

(IN soo lin LYE sproe PROE ta meen & IN soo lin LYE sproe)

Related Information

Insulin Regular *on page 829*

Brand Names: US HumaLOG Mix; HumaLOG Mix 50/50; HumaLOG Mix 50/50 KwikPen; HumaLOG Mix 75/25; HumaLOG Mix 75/25 KwikPen

Brand Names: Canada Humalog Mix 25; Humalog Mix 50

Pharmacologic Category Insulin, Combination

Use Diabetes mellitus, types 1 and 2: Treatment of type 1 diabetes mellitus and type 2 diabetes mellitus to improve glycemic control

Local Anesthetic/Vasoconstrictor Precautions

No information available to require special precautions

Effects on Dental Treatment Key adverse event(s) related to dental treatment: In general, morning appointments are advisable in patients with diabetes since endogenous cortisol levels are typically higher at this time; because cortisol increases blood sugar levels, the risk of hypoglycemia is less. It is important to confirm that the patient has eaten normally prior to the appointment and has taken all scheduled medications. If a procedure is planned with the expectation that the patient will alter normal eating habits ahead of time (eg, conscious sedation), diabetes medication dose may need to be modified in consultation with the patient's physician. Patients with well-controlled diabetes can usually be managed conventionally for most surgical procedures. Although patients with diabetes usually recognize signs and symptoms of hypoglycemia and self-intervene before changes in or loss of consciousness occurs, they may not. Staff should be trained to recognize the signs (eg, unusual behavior or profuse sweating in patients who have diabetes) and treat patients who have hypoglycemia; a glucometer should be used to test patient blood glucose levels. Every dental office should have a protocol for managing hypoglycemia in conscious and unconscious patients. Having snack foods or oral glucose tablets or gels available, especially in practices where a large number of surgical procedures are performed, is also prudent (American Diabetes Association 2017).

Effects on Bleeding No information available to require special precautions

Adverse Reactions Also see insulin lispro for additional reactions.

Postmarketing: Amyloidosis (cutaneous at injection site), anaphylaxis, erythema at injection site, hypersensitivity reaction, injection site pruritus, injection site reaction, lipohypertrophy, lipotrophy at injection site, skin rash, swelling at injection site, weight gain

Mechanism of Action Insulin acts via specific membrane-bound receptors on target tissues to regulate metabolism of carbohydrate, protein, and fats. Target organs for insulin include the liver, skeletal muscle, and adipose tissue.

Within the liver, insulin stimulates hepatic glycogen synthesis. Insulin promotes hepatic synthesis of fatty acids, which are released into the circulation as lipoproteins. Skeletal muscle effects of insulin include increased protein synthesis and increased glycogen synthesis. Within adipose tissue, insulin stimulates the processing of circulating lipoproteins to provide free fatty acids, facilitating triglyceride synthesis and storage by adipocytes; also directly inhibits the hydrolysis of triglycerides. In addition, insulin stimulates the cellular uptake of amino acids and increases cellular permeability to several ions, including potassium, magnesium, and phosphate. By activating sodium-potassium ATPases, insulin promotes the intracellular movement of potassium.

Normally secreted by the pancreas, insulin products are manufactured for pharmacologic use through recombinant DNA technology using either *E. coli* or *Saccharomyces cerevisiae*. Insulin lispro differs from human insulin by containing a lysine and proline at positions B28 and B29, respectively, in comparison to the proline and lysine found at B28 and B29 in human insulin. Insulins are categorized based on the onset, peak, and duration of effect (eg, rapid-, short-, intermediate-, and long-acting insulin). Insulin lispro protamine and insulin lispro is an intermediate-acting combination product with a more rapid onset and similar duration of action as compared to that of insulin NPH and insulin regular combination products.

Pharmacodynamics/Kinetics

Onset of Action 0.25 to 0.5 hours; Peak effect: Humalog Mix 50/50: 0.8 to 4.8 hours; Humalog Mix 75/25: 1 to 6.5 hours

Duration of Action 14 to 24 hours

Time to Peak Plasma: Humalog Mix 50/50: 0.75 to 13.5 hours; Humalog Mix 75/25: 0.5 to 4 hours

Pregnancy Considerations

Insulin lispro has not been shown to cross the placenta at standard clinical doses (Boskovic 2003; Holcberg 2004; Jovanovic 1999).

Refer to Insulin Lispro monograph for additional information.

Insulin NPH (IN soo lin N P H)

Related Information

Endocrine Disorders and Pregnancy *on page 1684*

Insulin Regular *on page 829*

Brand Names: US HumuLIN N KwikPen [OTC]; HumuLIN N [OTC]; NovoLIN N FlexPen ReliOn [OTC]; NovoLIN N FlexPen [OTC]; NovoLIN N ReliOn [OTC]; NovoLIN N [OTC]

Pharmacologic Category Insulin, Intermediate-Acting

Use Diabetes mellitus, types 1 and 2: Treatment of types 1 and 2 diabetes mellitus to improve glycemic control in adults and pediatric patients

Local Anesthetic/Vasoconstrictor Precautions

No information available to require special precautions

Effects on Dental Treatment Key adverse event(s) related to dental treatment: In general, morning appointments are advisable in patients with diabetes since endogenous cortisol levels are typically higher at this time; because cortisol increases blood sugar levels, the risk of hypoglycemia is less. It is important to confirm that the patient has eaten normally prior to the appointment and has taken all scheduled medications. If a procedure is planned with the expectation that the patient will alter normal eating habits ahead of time (eg, conscious sedation), diabetes medication dose may need to be modified in consultation with the patient's physician. Patients with well-controlled diabetes can usually be managed conventionally for most surgical procedures. Although patients with diabetes usually recognize signs and symptoms of hypoglycemia and self-intervene before changes in or loss of consciousness occurs, they may not. Staff should be trained to recognize the signs (eg, unusual behavior or profuse sweating in patients who have diabetes) and treat patients who have hypoglycemia; a glucometer should be used to test patient blood glucose levels. Every dental office should have a protocol for managing hypoglycemia in conscious and unconscious patients. Having snack foods or oral glucose tablets or gels available, especially in practices where a large number of surgical procedures are performed, is also prudent (American Diabetes Association 2017).

Effects on Bleeding No information available to require special precautions

Adverse Reactions

Frequency not defined:

Cardiovascular: Peripheral edema

Dermatologic: Injection site pruritus

Endocrine & metabolic: Amyloidosis (cutaneous at injection site), hypoglycemia, hypokalemia, lipodystrophy, lipohypertrophy, weight gain

Hypersensitivity: Anaphylaxis, hypersensitivity reaction

Immunologic: Immunogenicity

Local: Atrophy at injection site, erythema at injection site, hypertrophy at injection site, injection site reaction, swelling at injection site

Neuromuscular & skeletal: Swelling of extremities

Ophthalmic: Visual disturbance

Mechanism of Action Insulin acts via specific membrane-bound receptors on target tissues to regulate metabolism of carbohydrate, protein, and fats. Target organs for insulin include the liver, skeletal muscle, and adipose tissue.

Within the liver, insulin stimulates hepatic glycogen synthesis. Insulin promotes hepatic synthesis of fatty acids, which are released into the circulation as lipoproteins. Skeletal muscle effects of insulin include increased protein synthesis and increased glycogen synthesis. Within adipose tissue, insulin stimulates the processing of circulating lipoproteins to provide free fatty acids, facilitating triglyceride synthesis and storage by adipocytes; also directly inhibits the hydrolysis of triglycerides. In addition, insulin stimulates the cellular uptake of amino acids and increases cellular permeability to several ions, including potassium, magnesium, and phosphate. By activating sodium-potassium ATPases, insulin promotes the intracellular movement of potassium.

Normally secreted by the pancreas, insulin products are manufactured for pharmacologic use through recombinant DNA technology using either *E. coli* or *Saccharomyces cerevisiae*. Insulins are categorized based on the onset, peak, and duration of effect (eg, rapid-, short-, intermediate-, and long-acting insulin). Insulin NPH, an isophane suspension of human insulin, is an intermediate-acting insulin.

Pharmacodynamics/Kinetics

Onset of Action 1 to 2 hours; Peak effect: 4 to 12 hours

Duration of Action 14 to 24 hours

Time to Peak Plasma: 6 to 10 hours

Pregnancy Considerations

Poorly controlled diabetes during pregnancy can be associated with an increased risk of adverse maternal and fetal outcomes, including diabetic ketoacidosis, preeclampsia, spontaneous abortion, preterm delivery, delivery complications, major birth defects, stillbirth, and macrosomia (ACOG 201 2018). To prevent adverse outcomes, prior to conception and throughout pregnancy, maternal blood glucose and HbA_{1c} should be kept as close to target goals as possible but without causing significant hypoglycemia (ADA 2020; Blumer 2013).

Due to pregnancy-induced physiologic changes, insulin requirements tend to increase as pregnancy progresses, requiring frequent monitoring and dosage adjustments. Following delivery, insulin requirements decrease rapidly (ACOG 201 2018; ADA 2020).

Insulin is the preferred treatment of type 1 and type 2 diabetes mellitus in pregnancy, as well as gestational diabetes mellitus, when pharmacologic therapy is needed (ACOG 190 2018; ACOG 201 2018; ADA 2020). NPH insulin may be used to treat diabetes mellitus in pregnancy (ACOG 190 2018; ACOG 201 2018; Blumer 2013)

Insulin NPH and Insulin Regular

(IN soo lin N P H & IN soo lin REG yoo ler)

Related Information

Insulin Regular *on page 829*

Brand Names: US HumuLIN 70/30; HumuLIN 70/30 KwikPen; NovoLIN 70/30; NovoLIN 70/30 FlexPen; NovoLIN 70/30 FlexPen Relion

Brand Names: Canada Humulin 70/30; Novolin ge 30/70; Novolin ge 40/60; Novolin ge 50/50

Pharmacologic Category Insulin, Combination

Use Diabetes mellitus, types 1 and 2: Treatment of types 1 and 2 diabetes mellitus to improve glycemic control

Local Anesthetic/Vasoconstrictor Precautions

No information available to require special precautions

Effects on Dental Treatment Key adverse event(s) related to dental treatment: In general, morning appointments are advisable in patients with diabetes since endogenous cortisol levels are typically higher at this time; because cortisol increases blood sugar levels, the risk of hypoglycemia is less. It is important to confirm that the patient has eaten normally prior to the appointment and has taken all scheduled medications. If a procedure is planned with the expectation that the patient will alter normal eating habits ahead of time (eg, conscious sedation), diabetes medication dose may need to be modified in consultation with the patient's physician. Patients with well-controlled diabetes can usually be managed conventionally for most surgical procedures. Although patients with diabetes usually recognize signs and symptoms of hypoglycemia and self-intervene before changes in or loss of consciousness occurs, they may not. Staff should be trained to recognize the signs (eg, unusual behavior or profuse sweating in patients who have diabetes) and treat patients who have hypoglycemia; a glucometer should be used to test patient blood glucose levels. Every dental office should have a protocol for managing hypoglycemia in conscious and unconscious patients. Having snack foods or oral glucose tablets or gels available, especially in practices where a large number of surgical procedures are performed, is also prudent (American Diabetes Association 2017).

Effects on Bleeding No information available to require special precautions

Adverse Reactions See individual agents.

Frequency not defined:

Cardiovascular: Peripheral edema

Dermatologic: Injection site pruritus

Endocrine & metabolic: Amyloidosis (cutaneous at injection site), hypoglycemia, hypokalemia, weight gain

Hypersensitivity: Anaphylaxis, hypersensitivity reaction

Immunologic: Immunogenicity

Local: Erythema at injection site, hypertrophy at injection site, lipoatrophy at injection site, swelling at injection site

Mechanism of Action Insulin acts via specific membrane-bound receptors on target tissues to regulate metabolism of carbohydrate, protein, and fats. Target organs for insulin include the liver, skeletal muscle, and adipose tissue.

Within the liver, insulin stimulates hepatic glycogen synthesis. Insulin promotes hepatic synthesis of fatty acids, which are released into the circulation as lipoproteins. Skeletal muscle effects of insulin include increased protein synthesis and increased glycogen synthesis. Within adipose tissue, insulin stimulates the processing of circulating lipoproteins to provide free fatty acids, facilitating triglyceride synthesis and storage by adipocytes; also directly inhibits the hydrolysis of triglycerides. In addition, insulin stimulates the cellular uptake of amino acids and increases cellular permeability to several ions, including potassium, magnesium, and phosphate. By activating sodium-potassium ATPases, insulin promotes the intracellular movement of potassium.

Normally secreted by the pancreas, insulin products are manufactured for pharmacologic use through recombinant DNA technology using either *E. coli* or *Saccharomyces cerevisiae*. Insulins are categorized based on the onset, peak, and duration of effect (eg, rapid-, short-, intermediate-, and long-acting insulin). Insulin NPH (an isophane suspension of human insulin) and insulin regular is an intermediate-acting combination insulin product with a more rapid onset than that of insulin NPH alone.

Pharmacodynamics/Kinetics

Onset of Action 0.5 hours; Peak effect: 2 to 12 hours

Duration of Action 18 to 24 hours

Time to Peak Based on individual components:

Insulin regular: 0.8 to 2 hours

Insulin NPH: 6 to 10 hours

Pregnancy Considerations

Poorly controlled diabetes during pregnancy can be associated with an increased risk of adverse maternal and fetal outcomes, including diabetic ketoacidosis, preeclampsia, spontaneous abortion, preterm delivery, delivery complications, major birth defects, stillbirth, and macrosomia (ACOG 201 2018). To prevent adverse outcomes, prior to conception and throughout pregnancy, maternal blood glucose and HbA_{1c} should be kept as close to target goals as possible but without causing significant hypoglycemia (ADA 2020; Blumer 2013).

Due to pregnancy-induced physiologic changes, insulin requirements tend to increase as pregnancy progresses, requiring frequent monitoring and dosage adjustments. Following delivery, insulin requirements decrease rapidly (ACOG 201 2018; ADA 2020).

Insulin is the preferred treatment of type 1 and type 2 diabetes mellitus in pregnancy, as well as gestational diabetes mellitus when pharmacologic therapy is needed (ACOG 190 2018; ACOG 201 2018; ADA 2020). Also refer to individual monographs for additional information.

Insulin (Oral Inhalation)

(IN soo lin)

Brand Names: US Afrezza

Pharmacologic Category Insulin, Rapid-Acting

Use Diabetes mellitus, type 1 or type 2, treatment: Treatment of type 1 diabetes mellitus and type 2 diabetes mellitus to improve glycemic control.

Local Anesthetic/Vasoconstrictor Precautions

No information available to require special precautions

Effects on Dental Treatment Key adverse event(s) related to dental treatment: In general, morning appointments are advisable in patients with diabetes since endogenous cortisol levels are typically higher at this time; because cortisol increases blood sugar levels, the risk of hypoglycemia is less. It is important to confirm that the patient has eaten normally prior to the appointment and has taken all scheduled medications. If a procedure is planned with the expectation that the patient will alter normal eating habits ahead of time (eg, conscious sedation), diabetes medication dose may need to be modified in consultation with the patient's physician. Patients with well-controlled diabetes can usually be managed conventionally for most surgical procedures. Although patients with diabetes usually recognize signs and symptoms of hypoglycemia and self-intervene before changes in or loss of consciousness occurs, they may not. Staff should be trained to recognize the signs (eg, unusual behavior or profuse sweating in patients who have diabetes) and treat patients who have hypoglycemia; a glucometer should be used to test patient blood glucose levels. Every dental office should have a protocol for managing hypoglycemia in conscious and unconscious patients. Having snack foods or oral glucose tablets or gels available, especially in practices where a large number of surgical procedures are performed, is also prudent (American Diabetes Association 2017).

Effects on Bleeding No information available to require special precautions

Adverse Reactions

>10%:

Endocrine & metabolic: Hypoglycemia (67%)

Respiratory: Acute bronchospasm (patients with asthma: 29%), cough (26% to 29%)

1% to 10%:

Central nervous system: Headache (5%), fatigue (2%)

Endocrine & metabolic: Severe hypoglycemia (5%)

Gastrointestinal: Sore throat (≤6%), diarrhea (3%), nausea (2%)

Genitourinary: Urinary tract infection (2%)

Respiratory: Reduced forced expiratory volume (6%; ≥15% decline), throat irritation (≤6%), bronchitis (3%), decreased lung function (3%), productive cough (2%)

<1%, postmarketing, and/or case reports: Antibody development (drug efficacy not affected), diabetic ketoacidosis (diabetes mellitus, type 1), hypersensitivity reaction, hypokalemia

Mechanism of Action

Insulin acts via specific membrane-bound receptors on target tissues to regulate metabolism of carbohydrate, protein, and fats. Target organs for insulin include the liver, skeletal muscle, and adipose tissue.

Within the liver, insulin stimulates hepatic glycogen synthesis. Insulin promotes hepatic synthesis of fatty acids, which are released into the circulation as lipoproteins. Skeletal muscle effects of insulin include increased protein synthesis and increased glycogen synthesis. Within adipose tissue, insulin stimulates the processing of circulating lipoproteins to provide free fatty acids, facilitating triglyceride synthesis and storage by adipocytes; also directly inhibits the hydrolysis of triglycerides. In addition, insulin stimulates the cellular uptake of amino acids and increases cellular permeability to several ions, including potassium, magnesium, and phosphate. By activating sodium-potassium ATPases, insulin promotes the intracellular movement of potassium.

Normally secreted by the pancreas, insulin products are manufactured for pharmacologic use through recombinant DNA technology using either *E. coli* or *Saccharomyces cerevisiae*. Inhaled human insulin has an identical structure to that of native human insulin and is adsorbed onto carrier particles which dissolve within the lungs after inhalation leading to rapid absorption of insulin in the systemic circulation. Insulins are categorized based on the onset, peak, and duration of effect (eg, rapid-, short-, intermediate-, and long-acting insulin). Inhaled insulin is an ultra-rapid acting insulin.

Pharmacodynamics/Kinetics

Onset of Action ~12 minutes; Peak effect: ~35 to 55 minutes

Duration of Action ~90 to 270 minutes (proportional to dose)

Half-life Elimination 120 to 206 minutes (apparent terminal half-life)

Time to Peak 10 to 20 minutes

Pregnancy Considerations

Information specific to the use of inhaled insulin during pregnancy is limited (Makam 2009).

Poorly controlled diabetes during pregnancy can be associated with an increased risk of adverse maternal and fetal outcomes, including diabetic ketoacidosis, preeclampsia, spontaneous abortion, preterm delivery, delivery complications, major birth defects, stillbirth, and macrosomia (ACOG 201 2018). To prevent adverse outcomes, prior to conception and throughout pregnancy, maternal blood glucose and HbA_{1c} should be kept as close to target goals as possible but without causing significant hypoglycemia (ADA 2020; Blumer 2013).

Due to pregnancy-induced physiologic changes, insulin requirements tend to increase as pregnancy progresses, requiring frequent monitoring and dosage adjustments. Following delivery, insulin requirements decrease rapidly (ACOG 201 2018; ADA 2020).

Insulin is the preferred treatment of type 1 and type 2 diabetes mellitus in pregnancy, as well as gestational diabetes mellitus when pharmacologic therapy is needed. Agents other than inhaled insulin are currently preferred (ACOG 190 2018; ACOG 201 2018; ADA 2020).

Refer to the Insulin Regular monograph for additional information related to the use of insulin in pregnancy.

Insulin Regular (IN soo lin REG yoo ler)

Related Information

Endocrine Disorders and Pregnancy *on page 1684*
Insulin Aspart *on page 817*
Insulin Aspart Protamine and Insulin Aspart *on page 818*
Insulin Detemir *on page 820*
Insulin Glargine *on page 822*
Insulin Glulisine *on page 823*
Insulin Lispro *on page 824*
Insulin Lispro Protamine and Insulin Lispro *on page 826*
Insulin NPH *on page 827*
Insulin NPH and Insulin Regular *on page 828*

Brand Names: US HumuLIN R U-500 (CONCENTRATED); HumuLIN R U-500 KwikPen; HumuLIN R [OTC]; Myxredlin; NovoLIN R FlexPen ReliOn [OTC]; NovoLIN R FlexPen [OTC]; NovoLIN R ReliOn [OTC]; NovoLIN R [OTC]

Brand Names: Canada Entuzity Kwikpen

Pharmacologic Category Insulin, Short-Acting

Use

Diabetes mellitus, types 1 and 2, treatment: Treatment of type 1 diabetes mellitus and type 2 diabetes mellitus to improve glycemic control.

Note: Concentrated U-500 regular insulin is indicated only in patients requiring more than 200 units of insulin per day.

Local Anesthetic/Vasoconstrictor Precautions No information available to require special precautions

Effects on Dental Treatment Key adverse event(s) related to dental treatment: In general, morning appointments are advisable in patients with diabetes since endogenous cortisol levels are typically higher at this time; because cortisol increases blood sugar levels, the risk of hypoglycemia is less. It is important to confirm that the patient has eaten normally prior to the appointment and has taken all scheduled medications. If a procedure is planned with the expectation that the patient will alter normal eating habits ahead of time (eg, conscious sedation), diabetes medication dose may need to be modified in consultation with the patient's physician. Patients with well-controlled diabetes can usually be managed conventionally for most surgical procedures. Although patients with diabetes usually recognize signs and symptoms of hypoglycemia and self-intervene before changes in or loss of consciousness occurs, they may not. Staff should be trained to recognize the signs (eg, unusual behavior or profuse sweating in patients who have diabetes) and treat patients who have hypoglycemia; a glucometer should be used to test patient blood glucose levels. Every dental office should have a protocol for managing hypoglycemia in conscious and unconscious patients. Having snack foods or oral glucose tablets or gels available, especially in practices where a large number of surgical procedures are performed, is also prudent (American Diabetes Association 2017).

Effects on Bleeding No information available to require special precautions

Adverse Reactions

Frequency not defined:

Cardiovascular: Peripheral edema

Dermatologic: Injection site pruritus

Endocrine & metabolic: Amyloidosis (localized at injection site), hypoglycemia, hypokalemia, weight gain

Hypersensitivity: Anaphylaxis, hypersensitivity reaction

Immunologic: Immunogenicity

Local: Erythema at injection site, hypertrophy at injection site, lipoatrophy at injection site, swelling at injection site

Mechanism of Action Insulin acts via specific membrane-bound receptors on target tissues to regulate metabolism of carbohydrate, protein, and fats. Target organs for insulin include the liver, skeletal muscle, and adipose tissue.

Within the liver, insulin stimulates hepatic glycogen synthesis. Insulin promotes hepatic synthesis of fatty acids, which are released into the circulation as lipoproteins. Skeletal muscle effects of insulin include increased protein synthesis and increased glycogen synthesis. Within adipose tissue, insulin stimulates the processing of circulating lipoproteins to provide free fatty acids, facilitating triglyceride synthesis and storage by adipocytes; also directly inhibits the hydrolysis of triglycerides. In addition, insulin stimulates the cellular uptake of amino acids and increases cellular permeability to several ions, including potassium, magnesium, and phosphate. By activating sodium-potassium ATPases, insulin promotes the intracellular movement of potassium.

Normally secreted by the pancreas, insulin products are manufactured for pharmacologic use through recombinant DNA technology using either *E. coli* or *Saccharomyces cerevisiae*. Regular insulin has an identical structure to that of native human insulin. Insulins are categorized based on the onset, peak, and duration of effect (eg, rapid-, short-, intermediate-, and long-acting insulin). Insulin regular is a short-acting insulin analog.

Pharmacodynamics/Kinetics

Onset of Action SubQ: 0.25 to 0.5 hours; Peak effect: SubQ: U-100: 2.5 to 5 hours; U-500: 4 to 8 hours

Duration of Action

IV: U-100: 2 to 6 hours

SubQ: U-100: 4 to 12 hours (may increase with dose); U-500: 13 to 24 hours

Half-life Elimination IV: ~0.5 to 1 hour (dose-dependent); SubQ: 1.5 hours

Time to Peak Plasma: SubQ: 0.8 to 2 hours

Reproductive Considerations

Females diagnosed with diabetes who wish to conceive should use adequate contraception until glycemic control is achieved (ADA 2020). Rapid acting insulin analogs are preferred over short acting regular insulin in females planning a pregnancy (Blumer 2013).

Pregnancy Considerations

Exogenous insulin bound to anti-insulin antibodies can be detected in cord blood (Menon 1990).

Poorly controlled diabetes during pregnancy can be associated with an increased risk of adverse maternal and fetal outcomes, including diabetic ketoacidosis, preeclampsia, spontaneous abortion, preterm delivery, delivery complications, major birth defects, stillbirth, and macrosomia. To prevent adverse outcomes, prior to conception and throughout pregnancy, maternal blood glucose and HbA_{1c} should be kept as close to target goals as possible but without causing significant hypoglycemia (ADA 2020; Blumer 2013).

Due to pregnancy-induced physiologic changes, insulin requirements tend to increase as pregnancy progresses, requiring frequent monitoring and dosage adjustments. Following delivery, insulin requirements decrease rapidly (ACOG 201 2018; ADA 2020).

Insulin is the preferred treatment of type 1 and type 2 diabetes mellitus in pregnancy, as well as gestational diabetes mellitus when pharmacologic therapy is needed (ACOG 190 2018; ACOG 201 2018; ADA 2020). Rapid acting insulin analogs are preferred over short acting regular insulin when treatment is needed during pregnancy due to improved outcomes and increased compliance (ACOG 198 2018; ACOG 201 2018; Blumer 2013). Regular insulin is used intravenously for glycemic control during labor.

◆ **Insulin Regular and Insulin NPH** *see* Insulin NPH and Insulin Regular *on page* 828

◆ **Intal** *see* Cromolyn (Oral Inhalation) *on page* 416

◆ **Integrilin** *see* Eptifibatide *on page* 580

◆ **Intelence** *see* Etravirine *on page* 627

◆ **Interceed** *see* Cellulose (Oxidized/Regenerated) *on page* 320

◆ **Interferon Alfa-2a (PEG Conjugate)** *see* Peginterferon Alfa-2a *on page* 1201

◆ **Interferon Alfa-2b (PEG Conjugate)** *see* Peginterferon Alfa-2b *on page* 1202

Interferon Alfa-2b (in ter FEER on AL fa too bee)

Related Information

Dentin Hypersensitivity, Acid Erosion, High Caries Index, Management of Alveolar Osteitis, and Xerostomia *on page 1762*

Systemic Viral Diseases *on page 1709*

Brand Names: US Intron A

Brand Names: Canada Intron A; Intron A (Hsa-Free); Intron A Pen [DSC]

Pharmacologic Category Antineoplastic Agent, Biological Response Modulator; Biological Response Modulator; Interferon

Use

AIDS-related Kaposi sarcoma: Treatment of AIDS-related Kaposi sarcoma in select patients ≥18 years of age.

Chronic hepatitis B: Treatment of chronic hepatitis B in patients ≥1 year of age with compensated liver disease.

Condylomata acuminata: Treatment of condylomata acuminata involving external surfaces of the genital and perianal areas in patients ≥18 years of age.

Follicular lymphoma: Initial treatment of clinically aggressive follicular non-Hodgkin lymphoma in conjunction with anthracycline-containing combination chemotherapy in patients ≥18 years of age. **Note:** Indications in the manufacturer's labeling may not reflect current clinical practices.

Hairy cell leukemia: Treatment of hairy cell leukemia in patients ≥18 years of age.

Melanoma (malignant): Adjuvant to surgical treatment of malignant melanoma in patients ≥18 years of age who are free of disease but at high risk for systemic recurrence within 56 days of surgery. **Note:** Indications in the manufacturer's labeling may not reflect current clinical practices.

Local Anesthetic/Vasoconstrictor Precautions No information available to require special precautions

Effects on Dental Treatment Key adverse event(s) related to dental treatment: Xerostomia (normal salivary flow resumes upon discontinuation), metallic taste, taste alteration, and gingivitis.

Effects on Bleeding Hematologic toxicity associated with dose and disease being treated. Thrombocytopenia may be as high as 15%. Medical consult recommended.

Adverse Reactions

>10%:

Central nervous system: Fatigue (8% to 96%), headache (21% to 62%), chills (45% to 54%), rigors (2% to 42%), depression (3% to 40%), drowsiness (1% to 33%), dizziness (≤23%), vertigo (≤23%), irritability (≤22%), pain (3% to 18%), right upper quadrant pain (≤15%), malaise (3% to 14%), paresthesia (≤13%), confusion (≤12%), insomnia (≤12%)

Dermatologic: Alopecia (8% to 38%), skin rash (1% to 25%), diaphoresis (1% to 13%), pruritus (1% to 11%)

Endocrine & metabolic: Weight loss (≤13%), amenorrhea (≤12%)

Gastrointestinal: Anorexia (1% to 69%), nausea and vomiting (66%; children: 40%), nausea (17% to 66%), gastrointestinal disease (≤7%; children: 46%), diarrhea (2% to 35%), vomiting (2% to 40%), dysgeusia (≤24%), xerostomia (1% to 22%), abdominal pain (≤20%), constipation (≤14%)

Hematologic & oncologic: Neutropenia (≤92%; grades 3/4: 26%; children: 13% to 14%), granulocytopenia (31% to 92%), decreased white blood cell count (9% to 68%), leukopenia (<5%; malignant melanoma, grades 3/4: ≤26%), anemia (≤22%), decreased platelet count (1% to 15%), thrombocytopenia (≤10%; children: 3%)

Hepatic: Increased serum aspartate aminotransferase (4% to 63%), increased serum alkaline phosphatase (4% to 13%), increased serum alanine aminotransferase (2% to 13%)

Local: Injection site reaction (≤20%; children: 5%)

Neuromuscular & skeletal: Myalgia (16% to 75%), asthenia (≤63%), musculoskeletal pain (1% to 21%), arthralgia (3% to 19%), back pain (1% to 19%)

Renal: Increased blood urea nitrogen (2% to 12%)

Respiratory: Flu-like symptoms (≤45%; children: 100%), dyspnea (≤15%), cough (≤13%)

Miscellaneous: Fever (34% to 94%)

1% to 10%:

Cardiovascular: Hypertension (≤9%), chest pain (≤8%; includes substernal), peripheral edema (≤6%), edema (≤5%), peripheral vascular insufficiency (≤5%), angina pectoris (<5%), arteritis (<5%), atrial fibrillation (<5%), bradycardia (<5%), cardiac arrhythmia (<5%), cardiac failure (<5%), cardiomegaly (<5%), cardiomyopathy (<5%), cerebrovascular accident (<5%), coronary artery disease (<5%), extrasystoles (<5%), flushing (<5%), heart valve disease (<5%), hypotension (<5%), orthostatic hypotension (<5%), palpitations (<5%), polyarteritis nodosa (<5%), peripheral ischemia (<5%), phlebitis (<5%), pulmonary embolism (<5%), Raynaud disease (<5%), syncope (<5%), tachycardia (<5%), thrombosis (<5%), varicose veins (<5%), facial edema (≤3%)

Central nervous system: Anxiety (≤9%), lack of concentration (≤8), agitation (≤7%), hypothermia (≤5%), abnormal dreams (<5%), abnormal gait (<5%), abnormality in thinking (<5%), aggressive behavior (<5%), altered sense of smell (<5%), amnesia (<5%), apathy (<5%), aphasia (<5%), ataxia (<5%), Bell palsy (<5%), carpal tunnel syndrome (<5%), central nervous system dysfunction (<5%), coma (<5%), delirium (<5%), dysphasia (<5%), emotional lability (<5%), exacerbation of depression (<5%), extrapyramidal reaction (<5%), hyperesthesia (<5%), hyperthermia (<5%), hypertonia (<5%), hypoesthesia (<5%), hyporeflexia (<5%), intoxicated feeling (<5%), loss of consciousness (<5%), manic depressive reaction (<5%), manic reaction (<5%), migraine (<5%), myasthenia (<5%), neuralgia (<5%), neuritis (<5%), neuropathy (<5%), nightmares (<5%), paresis (<5%), personality disorder (<5%), polyneuropathy (<5%), psychoneurosis (<5%), psychosis (<5%), seizure (<5%), speech disturbance (<5%), twitching (<5%), voice disorder (<5%), nervousness (1% to 3%), attempted suicide (≤2%), suicidal ideation (≤2%),

Dermatologic: Xeroderma (≤9%), dermatitis (1% to 8%), injection site pruritus (≤5%), abnormal hair texture (<5%), acne vulgaris (<5%), cellulitis (<5%), cold and clammy skin (<5%), eczema (<5%), epidermal cyst of skin (<5%), erythema (<5%), erythema nodosum (<5%), erythematous rash (<5%), exacerbation of psoriasis (<5%), folliculitis (<5%), furunculosis (<5%), genital pruritus (<5%), lichenoid dermatitis (<5%), maculopapular rash (<5%), nail disease (<5%), pallor (<5%), psoriasis (<5%), skin depigmentation (<5%), skin discoloration (<5%), skin photosensitivity (<5%), toxic epidermal necrolysis (<5%), urticaria (<5%), vitiligo (<5%)

Endocrine & metabolic: Cachexia (≤5%), decreased libido (≤5%), dehydration (≤5%), hypercalcemia (≤5%), hyperglycemia (≤5%), increased thirst (≤5%), weight gain (≤5%), albuminuria (<5%), cutaneous nodule (<5%), exacerbation of diabetes mellitus (<5%), goiter (<5%), gynecomastia (<5%), heavy menstrual bleeding (<5%), hypertrichosis (<5%), hot flash (<5%), hyperthyroidism (<5%), hypertriglyceridemia (<5%), hypothyroidism (<5%), menstrual disease (<5%), increased lactate dehydrogenase (≤1%)

Gastrointestinal: Dyspepsia (2% to 8%), gingivitis (1% to 7%), hernia of abdominal cavity (≤5%), abdominal distention (<5%), ageusia (<5%), aphthous stomatitis (<5%; including non-herpetic cold sore), biliary colic (<5%), cholelithiasis (<5%), colitis (<5%), dental disease (<5%), dysphagia (<5%), eructation (<5%), esophagitis (<5%), flatulence (<5%), gastric ulcer (<5%), gastritis (<5%), gastroenteritis (<5%), gastrointestinal hemorrhage (<5%), gingival hemorrhage (<5%), gingival hyperplasia (<5%), halitosis (<5%), hemorrhoids (<5%), increased appetite (<5%), melanosis (<5%), melena (<5%), mucositis (<5%), oral leukoplakia (<5%), oral mucosa ulcer (<5%), sialorrhea (<5%), stomatitis (<5%), tongue disease (<5%), loose stools (≤2%)

Genitourinary: Mastitis (≤5%), penile swelling (≤5%), scrotal edema (≤5%), urinary tract infection (≤5%), herpes genitalis (1% to 5%), cystitis (<5%), dysmenorrhea (<5%), dysuria (<5%), hematuria (<5%), impotence (<5%), leukorrhea (<5%), nocturia (<5%), pelvic pain (<5%), penile disease (<5%), proteinuria (<5%), sexual disorder (<5%), urinary frequency (<5%), urinary incontinence (<5%), urination disorder (<5%), uterine hemorrhage (<5%), vaginal dryness (<5%), virilization (<5%), genital candidiasis (≤1%)

Hematologic & oncologic: Lymphadenitis (≤5%), lymphadenopathy (≤5%), purpuric rash (≤5%), hematoma (<5%), hemolytic anemia (<5%), hypochromic anemia (<5%), lipoma (<5%), lymphocytosis (<5%), oral hemorrhage (<5%), rectal hemorrhage (<5%), thrombotic thrombocytopenic purpura (<5%)

Hepatic: Abnormal hepatic function tests (<5%), ascites (<5%), hepatic encephalopathy (<5%), hepatic failure (<5%), hepatitis (<5%), hyperbilirubinemia (<5%), jaundice (<5%)

Hypersensitivity: Hypersensitivity reaction (≤5%; includes acute reaction)

Infection: Infection (≤7%; including hemophilus), viral infection (7%), abscess (<5%), bacterial infection (<5%), fungal infection (<5%), herpes zoster infection (<5%), parasitic infection (including trichomonas), sepsis (<5%)

Local: Bleeding at injection site (≤5%), burning sensation at injection site (≤5%), local pain (pleural: ≤5%), pain at injection site (≤5%), inflammation at injection site (1% to 5%), local discoloration (gastrointestinal mucosa: <5%)

Neuromuscular & skeletal: Amyotrophy (<5%), arthritis (<5%), bone disease (<5%), exacerbation of arthritis (<5%), hyperkinesia (<5%), hypokinesia (<5%), lower limb cramp (<5%), ostealgia (<5%), osteoarthritis (<5%), rheumatoid arthritis (<5%), spondylitis (<5%), tendonitis (<5%), tremor (<5%)

Ophthalmic: Periorbital edema (≤5%), blurred vision (<5%), conjunctivitis (<5%), diplopia (<5%), eye pain (<5%), hordeolum (<5%), lacrimation (<5%), nystagmus (<5%), photophobia (<5%), visual disturbance (<5%), xerophthalmia (<5%)

Otic: Otalgia (≤5%), auditory impairment (<5%), labyrinth disease (<5%), otitis media (<5%), tinnitus (<5%)

Renal: Polyuria (≤10%), increased serum creatinine (2% to 6%), renal insufficiency (<5%)

Respiratory: Bronchitis (≤10%), pharyngitis (≤8%), epistaxis (≤7%), nasal congestion (≤7%), asthma (≤5%), bronchospasm (≤5%), cyanosis (≤5%), hemoptysis (≤5%), hypoventilation (≤5%), laryngitis (≤5%), orthopnea (≤5%), pleural effusion (≤5%), pneumonia (≤5%), pneumonitis (≤5%), pneumothorax (≤5%), pulmonary fibrosis (≤5%), rales (≤5%), respiratory insufficiency (≤5%), respiratory tract disease (≤5%), sneezing (≤5%), tonsillitis (≤5%), tracheitis (≤5%), wheezing (≤5%), rhinitis (<5%), rhinorrhea (<5%), upper respiratory tract infection (<5%), sinusitis (1% to 4%)

Miscellaneous: Inflammation (≤5%), alcohol intolerance (<5%)

<1%, postmarketing, and/or case reports: Anaphylaxis, angioedema, aplastic anemia, autoimmune disease, bronchoconstriction, encephalopathy, erythema multiforme, exacerbation of sarcoidosis, hallucination, hepatotoxicity, homicidal ideation, immune thrombocytopenia, ischemic changes (cerebrovascular events), leukemia (intralesional administration), macular edema, myocardial infarction, myositis, nephrotic syndrome, optic neuritis, pancreatitis, pancytopenia, pericarditis, peripheral neuropathy, pituitary insufficiency, pulmonary hypertension, pulmonary infiltrates, pure red cell aplasia, reactivation of HBV, reduced ejection fraction, renal failure syndrome, retinal detachment (serous), rhabdomyolysis, sarcoidosis, Stevens-Johnson syndrome, suicidal tendencies, supraventricular cardiac arrhythmia, systemic lupus erythematosus, tissue necrosis at injection site, tongue discoloration, vasculitis, Vogt-Koyanagi-Harada syndrome

Mechanism of Action Interferon alfas bind to a specific receptor on the cell membrane to initiate intracellular activity; multiple effects can be detected including induction of gene transcription. It inhibits cellular growth, alters the state of cellular differentiation, interferes with oncogene expression, alters cell surface antigen expression, increases phagocytic activity of macrophages, and augments cytotoxicity of lymphocytes for target cells

Pharmacodynamics/Kinetics

Half-life Elimination IV: ~2 hours; IM, SubQ: ~2 to 3 hours

Time to Peak Serum: IM, SubQ: ~3 to 12 hours; IV: By the end of a 30-minute infusion

Reproductive Considerations

Verify pregnancy status prior to administration in females of reproductive potential. Disruption of the normal menstrual cycle may occur. Female patients of reproductive potential should use effective contraception during treatment.

If used in combination with ribavirin, all warnings related to the use of ribavirin and contraception should be followed. Refer to the Ribavirin monograph for additional information.

Pregnancy Considerations

Alfa interferon is endogenous to normal amniotic fluid (Lebon 1982); however, placenta perfusion studies note exogenous interferon alfa does not cross the placenta (Waysbort 1993).

Essential thrombocythemia is associated with an increased risk of thrombosis, bleeding and, when untreated, may increase the risk of pregnancy loss. Maternal use of interferon alfas may improve pregnancy outcomes; use of interferon alfa-2b may be considered in pregnant women when other agents are not appropriate (Lapoirie 2020; Maze 2019; Sakai 2018; Tefferi 2019; Yazdani Brojeni 2012; Yoshida 2017).

The European Society for Medical Oncology (ESMO) has published guidelines for diagnosis, treatment, and follow-up of cancer during pregnancy. The guidelines suggest that interferon-alfa may be used for the treatment of chronic myeloid leukemia (CML) during pregnancy and recommend referral to a facility with expertise in cancer during pregnancy; a multidisciplinary team (obstetrician, neonatologist, oncology team) is encouraged (ESMO [Peccatori 2013]). An international consensus panel suggests use of interferon-alfa in pregnant patients once WBC and platelet counts have risen to a level associated with CML symptom onset (Lishner 2016).

Interferon alfa-2b in combination with ribavirin is contraindicated in pregnant females and males whose female partners are pregnant. Combination therapy with ribavirin may cause birth defects and death in an unborn child. If used in combination with ribavirin, all warnings related to the use of ribavirin and pregnancy should be followed. Refer to the Ribavirin monograph for additional information.

◆ **Interferon Alfa n3** *see* Interferon Alfa-n3 *on page 833*

Interferon Alfa-n3 (in ter FEER on AL fa en three)

Related Information

Dentin Hypersensitivity, Acid Erosion, High Caries Index, Management of Alveolar Osteitis, and Xerostomia *on page 1762*

Systemic Viral Diseases *on page 1709*

Brand Names: US Alferon N

Pharmacologic Category Interferon

Use Condylomata acuminata: Intralesional treatment of refractory or recurring external condylomata acuminata (venereal or genital warts) in patients 18 years of age or older.

Local Anesthetic/Vasoconstrictor Precautions No information available to require special precautions

Effects on Dental Treatment Key adverse event(s) related to dental treatment: Xerostomia (normal salivary flow resumes upon discontinuation), metallic taste, tongue hyperesthesia, abnormal taste, thirst, rhinitis, pharyngitis, nosebleed, increased diaphoresis, taste disturbance, and gingivitis.

Effects on Bleeding No information available to require special precautions

Adverse Reactions Adverse reaction incidence noted below is specific to intralesional administration in patients with condylomata acuminata.

>10%:

- Central nervous system: Headache (31%), chills (14%), fatigue (14%)
- Hematologic & oncologic: Decreased white blood cell count (11%)
- Neuromuscular & skeletal: Myalgia (45%)
- Respiratory: Flu-like symptoms (30%; includes headache, fever, and/or myalgia; abated with repeated dosing)
- Miscellaneous: Fever (40%)

1% to 10%:

- Central nervous system: Malaise (9%), dizziness (9%), depression (2%), insomnia (2%), vasodepressor syncope (2%), hyperesthesia (tongue: 1%), paresthesia (1%)
- Dermatologic: Diaphoresis (2%), pruritus (2%)
- Endocrine & metabolic: Increased thirst (1%)
- Gastrointestinal: Nausea (4%), vomiting (3%), dyspepsia (3%), diarrhea (2%), dysgeusia (1%)
- Hematologic & oncologic: Adenopathy (groin: 1%)
- Neuromuscular & skeletal: Arthralgia (5%), back pain (4%), muscle cramps (1%)
- Ophthalmic: Visual disturbance (1%)
- Respiratory: Rhinitis (2%), epistaxis (1%), pharyngitis (1%)

<1%, postmarketing, and/or case reports: Dysuria, hepatotoxicity (idiosyncratic; Chalasani 2014), hot flash, lack of concentration, nervousness, skin photosensitivity

Mechanism of Action Interferons interact with cells through high affinity cell surface receptors. Following activation, multiple effects can be detected including induction of gene transcription. Inhibits cellular growth, alters the state of cellular differentiation, interferes with oncogene expression, alters cell surface antigen expression, increases phagocytic activity of macrophages, and augments cytotoxicity of lymphocytes for target cells

Reproductive Considerations

Menstrual irregularities have been reported; effective contraception is recommended during treatment.

Pregnancy Risk Factor C

Pregnancy Considerations

Animal reproduction studies have not been conducted.

◆ **Interferon Alpha 2b** *see* Interferon Alfa-2b *on page 831*

◆ **Interferon beta 1a** *see* Interferon Beta-1a *on page 833*

◆ **Interferon Beta 1b** *see* Interferon Beta-1b *on page 835*

Interferon Beta-1a (in ter FEER on BAY ta won aye)

Brand Names: US Avonex; Avonex Pen; Rebif; Rebif Rebidose; Rebif Rebidose Titration Pack; Rebif Titration Pack

Brand Names: Canada Avonex; Rebif

Pharmacologic Category Interferon

Use

US labeling:

Multiple sclerosis, relapsing: Treatment of relapsing forms of multiple sclerosis (MS), including clinically isolated syndrome, relapsing-remitting disease, and active secondary progressive disease

Canadian labeling:

Treatment of relapsing forms of MS to decrease the frequency of clinical exacerbations, delay the accumulation of physical disability, reduce the requirement for steroids, reduce the number of hospitalizations, and reduce disease burden

To decrease the number and volume of active brain lesions, decrease overall disease burden, and delay onset of clinically definite MS in patients who have experienced a single demyelinating event

Local Anesthetic/Vasoconstrictor Precautions

No information available to require special precautions

Effects on Dental Treatment Key adverse event(s) related to dental treatment: Xerostomia and changes in salivation (normal salivary flow resumes upon discontinuation), and toothache.

Effects on Bleeding Thrombocytopenia has been reported in 2% to 8% of patients. Medical consult recommended.

Adverse Reactions Adverse reactions reported as a composite of both commercially-available products. Spectrum and incidence of reactions is generally similar between products, but consult individual product labels for specific incidence.

>10%:

Central nervous system: Headache (58% to 70%), fatigue (33% to 41%), depression (18% to 25%), pain (23%), chills (19%), dizziness (14%)

Gastrointestinal: Nausea (23%), abdominal pain (8% to 22%)

Genitourinary: Urinary tract infection (17%)

Hematologic & oncologic: Leukopenia (28% to 36%), lymphadenopathy (11% to 12%)

Hepatic: Increased serum ALT (20% to 27%), increased serum AST (10% to 17%)

Immunologic: Antibody development (neutralizing; significance not known; Rebif: 24% to 31%; Avonex: 5%)

Local: Injection site reaction (3% to 92%)

Neuromuscular & skeletal: Myalgia (25% to 29%), back pain (23% to 25%), weakness (24%), skeletal pain (10% to 15%), rigors (6% to 13%)

Ophthalmic: Visual disturbance (7% to 13%)

Respiratory: Flu-like symptoms (49% to 59%), sinusitis (14%), upper respiratory tract infection (14%)

Miscellaneous: Fever (20% to 28%)

1% to 10%:

Cardiovascular: Chest pain (5% to 8%), vasodilation (2%)

Central nervous system: Hypertonia (6% to 7%), migraine (5%), ataxia (4% to 5%), drowsiness (4% to 5%), malaise (4% to 5%), seizure (1% to 5%), suicidal tendencies (4%)

Dermatologic: Erythematous rash (5% to 7%), maculopapular rash (4% to 5%), alopecia (4%), hyperhidrosis (4%), urticaria

Endocrine & metabolic: Thyroid disease (4% to 6%)

Gastrointestinal: Xerostomia (1% to 5%), toothache (3%)

Genitourinary: Urinary frequency (2% to 7%), urinary incontinence (2% to 4%), urine abnormality (3%)

Hematologic & oncologic: Thrombocytopenia (2% to 8%), anemia (3% to 5%)

Hepatic: Hyperbilirubinemia (2% to 3%)

Infection: Infection (7%)

Local: Pain at injection site (8%), bruising at injection site (6%), inflammation at injection site (6%), tissue necrosis at injection site (1% to 3%)

Neuromuscular & skeletal: Arthralgia (9%)

Ophthalmic: Eye disease (4%), xerophthalmia (1% to 3%)

Respiratory: Bronchitis (8%)

<1%, postmarketing, and/or case reports: Abnormal gait, abnormal healing, abnormal hepatic function tests, abscess, abscess at injection site, amnesia, anaphylaxis, angioedema, anxiety, arteritis, arthritis, ascites, autoimmune hepatitis, basal cell carcinoma, Bell's palsy, bloody stools, breast fibroadenosis, cardiac arrhythmia, cardiac failure, cardiomyopathy, cellulitis, cellulitis at injection site, clumsiness, cold and clammy skin, colitis, confusion, conjunctivitis, constipation, contact dermatitis, dehydration, depersonalization, dermal ulcer, diaphoresis, diverticulitis, drug dependence, dyspnea, dysuria, ecchymoses, emotional lability, emphysema, epididymitis, erythema, erythema multiforme, eye pain, facial edema, facial paralysis, fibrocystic breast changes, fibrosis at injection site, furunculosis, gallbladder disease, gastritis, gastrointestinal hemorrhage, genital pruritus, gingival hemorrhage, gingivitis, gynecomastia, hematuria, hemolytic-uremic syndrome, hemoptysis, hemorrhage, hepatic failure, hepatic injury, hepatic neoplasm, hepatitis, hepatomegaly, hepatotoxicity (idiosyncratic) (Chalasani 2014), hernia, hiccups, hyperesthesia, hypermenorrhea, hypersensitivity reaction at injection site, hyperthyroidism, hyperventilation, hypoglycemia, hypokalemia, hypomagnesemia, hypotension, hypothyroidism, immune thrombocytopenia, increased appetite, increased coagulation time, increased libido, increased thirst, intestinal obstruction, intestinal perforation, labyrinthitis, laryngitis, leukorrhea, lipoma, lump in breast, lupus erythematosus, menopause, myasthenia, neoplasm, nephrolithiasis, neurological signs and symptoms (transient; may mimic multiple sclerosis exacerbations), nevus, nocturia, orolingual edema, orthostatic hypotension, osteonecrosis, otalgia, palpitations, pancytopenia, paresthesia, pelvic inflammatory disease, penile disease, pericarditis, periodontal abscess, periodontitis, peripheral ischemia, peripheral vascular disease, petechia, Peyronie disease, pharyngeal edema, pneumonia, polyuria, postmenopausal bleeding, proctitis, prostatic disease, pruritus, psychiatric disturbance (new or worsening; including suicidal ideation), psychoneurosis, pulmonary embolism, pulmonary hypertension (Govern 2015; Health Canada Nov. 2, 2016), pyelonephritis, renal pain, retinal vascular disease, seborrhea, sepsis, severe weakness (transient), skin blister, skin discoloration, skin photosensitivity, skin rash, spider telangiectasia, Stevens-Johnson syndrome, synovitis, tachycardia, telangiectasia, testicular disease, thromboembolism, thrombotic thrombocytopenic purpura, tongue disease, urethral pain, urinary retention, urinary urgency, uterine fibroids, uterine hemorrhage, vaginal hemorrhage, vascular disease, vesicular eruption, vitreous opacity, vomiting

Mechanism of Action Interferon beta differs from naturally occurring human protein by a single amino acid substitution and the lack of carbohydrate side chains; alters the expression and response to surface antigens and can enhance immune cell activities. Properties of interferon beta that modify biologic responses are mediated by cell surface receptor interactions; mechanism in the treatment of MS is unknown.

Pharmacodynamics/Kinetics

Onset of Action Avonex: 12 hours (based on biological response markers)

Duration of Action Avonex: 4 days (based on biological response markers)

Half-life Elimination Avonex: ~19 hours (range: 8-54 hours); Rebif: 69 hours

Time to Peak Serum: Avonex (IM): ~15 hours (range: 6-36 hours); Rebif (SubQ): 16 hours

Reproductive Considerations

In general, disease-modifying therapies for multiple sclerosis (MS) are stopped prior to a planned pregnancy except in females at high risk of MS activity (AAN [Rae-Grant 2018]). When disease-modifying therapy is needed in females planning a pregnancy (eg, high risk of disease reactivation), interferon beta-1a may be considered until pregnancy is confirmed, and in select cases (eg, female with active disease), use may be continued during pregnancy. Delaying pregnancy is recommended for females with persistent high disease activity (ECTRIMS/EAN [Montalban 2018]).

Pregnancy Considerations

Based on available data, an increased risk of adverse fetal events has not been observed when exposure occurs during pregnancy (Burkill 2019; Foulds 2010; Nguyen 2019; Richman 2012; Sandberg-Wollheim 2011; Tomczyk 2013).

In general, disease-modifying therapies for multiple sclerosis (MS) are not initiated during pregnancy, except in females at high risk of MS activity (AAN [Rae-Grant 2018]). When disease-modifying therapy is needed in females planning a pregnancy (eg, high risk of disease reactivation), interferon beta-1a may be considered until pregnancy is confirmed, and in select cases (eg, female with active disease), use may be continued during pregnancy (ECTRIMS/EAN [Montalban 2018]).

Interferon Beta-1b (in ter FEER on BAY ta won bee)

Brand Names: US Betaseron; Extavia

Brand Names: Canada Betaseron; Extavia

Pharmacologic Category Interferon

Use

Multiple sclerosis, relapsing: Treatment of relapsing forms of multiple sclerosis, including clinically isolated syndrome, relapsing-remitting disease, and active secondary progressive disease in adults.

Local Anesthetic/Vasoconstrictor Precautions

No information available to require special precautions

Effects on Dental Treatment No significant effects or complications reported

Effects on Bleeding Thrombocytopenia has been reported. Medical consult recommended.

Adverse Reactions

>10%:

Cardiovascular: Peripheral edema (12%)

Dermatologic: Skin rash (21%)

Gastrointestinal: Abdominal pain (16%)

Genitourinary: Urinary urgency (11%)

Hematologic & oncologic: Leukopenia (13%), lymphocytopenia (86%), neutropenia (13%)

Hepatic: Increased serum alanine aminotransferase (>5x baseline: 12%)

Immunologic: Antibody development (17% to 45%, neutralizing)

Local: Inflammation at injection site (42%), injection site reaction (78%), pain at injection site (16%)

Nervous system: Ataxia (17%), chills (21%), headache (50%), hypertonia (40%), insomnia (21%), pain (42%)

Neuromuscular & skeletal: Asthenia (53%), myalgia (23%)

Respiratory: Flu-like symptoms (57%)

Miscellaneous: Fever (31%)

1% to 10%:

Cardiovascular: Chest pain (9%), hypertension (6%)

Dermatologic: Alopecia (2%), dermatologic disorder (10%)

Genitourinary: Impotence (8%), uterine hemorrhage (9%)

Hematologic & oncologic: Lymphadenopathy (6%)

Hepatic: Increased serum aspartate aminotransferase (>5x baseline: 4%)

Local: Hypersensitivity reaction at injection site (4%), residual mass at injection site (2%), swelling at injection site (2%), tissue necrosis at injection site (4%)

Nervous system: Malaise (6%)

Respiratory: Dyspnea (6%)

<1%: Nervous system: Suicidal ideation

Frequency not defined:

Cardiovascular: Palpitations, peripheral vascular disease, tachycardia, vasodilation

Dermatologic: Urticaria

Endocrine & metabolic: Heavy menstrual bleeding, weight gain

Gastrointestinal: Constipation, diarrhea, dyspepsia, nausea

Genitourinary: Dysmenorrhea, prostatic disease, urinary frequency

Hypersensitivity: Tongue edema

Nervous system: Anxiety, dizziness, myasthenia, nervousness

Neuromuscular & skeletal: Arthralgia, lower limb cramp

Respiratory: Bronchospasm

Postmarketing (any indication): Anaphylaxis, anemia, anorexia, autoimmune hepatitis, capillary leak syndrome, cardiac failure, cardiomyopathy, confusion, depression, emotional lability, hemolytic-uremic syndrome, hepatic failure, hepatic injury, hepatitis, hepatotoxicity, hyperthyroidism, hypothyroidism, increased gamma-glutamyl transferase, increased serum triglycerides, lupus erythematosus, pancreatitis, pruritus, psychotic symptoms, seizure, skin discoloration, thrombocytopenia, thrombotic microangiopathy, thrombotic thrombocytopenic purpura, thyroid dysfunction, vomiting, weight loss

Mechanism of Action Interferon beta-1b differs from naturally occurring human protein by a single amino acid substitution and the lack of carbohydrate side chains; mechanism in the treatment of MS is unknown; however, immunomodulatory effects attributed to interferon beta-1b include enhancement of suppressor T cell activity, reduction of proinflammatory cytokines, down-regulation of antigen presentation, and reduced trafficking of lymphocytes into the central nervous system. Improves MRI lesions, decreases relapse rate, and disease severity in patients with secondary progressive MS.

Pharmacodynamics/Kinetics

Half-life Elimination 8 minutes to 4.3 hours

Time to Peak 1-8 hours

Reproductive Considerations

In general, disease-modifying therapies for multiple sclerosis (MS) are stopped prior to a planned pregnancy, except in females at high risk of MS activity (AAN [Rae-Grant 2018]). When disease-modifying therapy is needed in females planning a pregnancy (eg, high risk of disease reactivation), interferon beta-1b may be considered until pregnancy is confirmed, and in select cases (eg, women with active disease), use may be continued during pregnancy. Delaying pregnancy is recommended for females with persistent high disease activity (ECTRIMS/EAN [Montalban 2018]).

Pregnancy Considerations

Data from available pregnancy registries have not observed an increased risk or pattern of major birth defects, preterm birth, or decreased birth weight following maternal use of interferon beta-1b (Coyle 2014; Romero 2015; Thiel 2016). In most cases, therapy was stopped during the first trimester after pregnancy was detected (Thiel 2016).

In general, disease-modifying therapies for multiple sclerosis (MS) are not initiated during pregnancy, except in females at high risk of MS activity (AAN [Rae-Grant 2018]). When disease-modifying therapy is needed in females planning a pregnancy (eg, high risk of disease reactivation), interferon beta-1b may be considered until pregnancy is confirmed, and in select cases (eg, women with active disease), use may be continued during pregnancy (ECTRIMS/EAN [Montalban 2018]).

- **Interferon Gamma 1b** *see* Interferon Gamma-1b *on page 836*

Interferon Gamma-1b

(in ter FEER on GAM ah won bee)

Brand Names: US Actimmune

Pharmacologic Category Interferon

Use

Chronic granulomatous disease: Reduction in the frequency and severity of serious infections associated with chronic granulomatous disease

Malignant osteopetrosis (severe): To delay time to disease progression in patients with severe, malignant osteopetrosis

Local Anesthetic/Vasoconstrictor Precautions No information available to require special precautions

Effects on Dental Treatment No significant effects or complications reported

Effects on Bleeding Dose related (>100 mcg/m^2 administered 3 times weekly) thrombocytopenia has been reported. Medical consult recommended.

Adverse Reactions Based on 50 mcg/m^2 dose administered 3 times weekly for chronic granulomatous disease

>10%:

Central nervous system: Fever (52%), headache (33%), chills (14%), fatigue (14%)

Dermatologic: Rash (17%)

Gastrointestinal: Diarrhea (14%), vomiting (13%)

Local: Injection site erythema or tenderness (14%)

1% to 10%:

Central nervous system: Depression (3%)

Gastrointestinal: Nausea (10%), abdominal pain (8%)

Neuromuscular & skeletal: Myalgia (6%), arthralgia (2%), back pain (2%)

<1%, postmarketing, and/or case reports: Alkaline phosphatase elevated, atopic dermatitis, granulomatous colitis, hepatomegaly, hypersensitivity reactions, hypokalemia, neutropenia, Stevens-Johnson syndrome

Additional adverse reactions noted at doses >100 mcg/m^2 administered 3 times weekly: ALT increased, AST increased, autoantibodies increased, bronchospasm, chest discomfort, confusion, dermatomyositis exacerbation, disorientation, DVT, gait disturbance, GI bleeding, hallucinations, heart block, heart failure, hepatic insufficiency, hyperglycemia, hypertriglyceridemia, hyponatremia, hypotension, interstitial pneumonitis, lupus-like syndrome, MI, neutropenia, pancreatitis (may be fatal), Parkinsonian symptoms, PE, proteinuria, renal insufficiency (reversible), seizure, syncope, tachyarrhythmia, tachypnea, thrombocytopenia, TIA

Mechanism of Action Interferon gamma participates in immunoregulation by enhancing the oxidative metabolism of macrophages; it also enhances antibody dependent cellular cytotoxicity, activates natural killer cells and has a role in the expression of Fc receptors and major histocompatibility antigens.

Pharmacodynamics/Kinetics

Half-life Elimination IM: ~3 hours, SubQ: ~6 hours

Time to Peak Plasma: IM: ~4 hours (1.5 ng/mL); SubQ: ~7 hours (0.6 ng/mL)

Pregnancy Considerations Adverse events have been observed in animal reproduction studies.

- **Interleukin-1 Receptor Antagonist** *see* Anakinra *on page 149*
- **Interleukin 2** *see* Aldesleukin *on page 91*
- **Intermezzo** *see* Zolpidem *on page 1582*
- **Intrauterine Copper Device** *see* Copper IUD *on page 410*
- **Intrifiban** *see* Eptifibatide *on page 580*
- **Intron A** *see* Interferon Alfa-2b *on page 831*
- **Introvale** *see* Ethinyl Estradiol and Levonorgestrel *on page 612*
- **Intuniv** *see* GuanFACINE *on page 749*
- **INVanz** *see* Ertapenem *on page 586*
- **Invega** *see* Paliperidone *on page 1182*
- **Invega Sustenna** *see* Paliperidone *on page 1182*
- **Invega Trinza** *see* Paliperidone *on page 1182*
- **Invirase** *see* Saquinavir *on page 1357*
- **Invokana** *see* Canagliflozin *on page 281*

Iodoquinol and Hydrocortisone

(eye oh doe KWIN ole & hye droe KOR ti sone)

Related Information

Hydrocortisone (Topical) *on page 775*

Brand Names: US Alcortin A; Dermazene; Vytone

Pharmacologic Category Antifungal Agent, Topical; Corticosteroid, Topical

Use Dermatoses: Treatment of eczema (including impetiginized, nuchal, and nummular); acne urticata; anogenital pruritus (vulvae, scroti, ani); atopic or contact dermatitis; endogenous chronic infectious dermatitis; chronic eczematoid otitis externa; folliculitis; intertrigo; lichen simplex chronicus; moniliasis; dermatoses (mycotic or bacterial); neurodermatitis (localized or systemic); pyoderma, stasis dermatitis.

Local Anesthetic/Vasoconstrictor Precautions No information available to require special precautions

Effects on Dental Treatment No significant effects or complications reported

Effects on Bleeding No information available to require special precautions

Adverse Reactions See individual agents.

Mechanism of Action

Iodoquinol: Amebicide that has antifungal and antibacterial properties.

Hydrocortisone: Decreases inflammation by suppression of migration of polymorphonuclear leukocytes and reversal of increased capillary permeability.

Pregnancy Risk Factor C

Pregnancy Considerations Animal reproduction studies have not been conducted with this combination. Refer to individual monographs.

- **Ionsys [DSC]** *see* FentaNYL *on page 642*
- **Iopidine** *see* Apraclonidine *on page 161*
- **IPI-145** *see* Duvelisib *on page 540*

Ipilimumab (ip i LIM u mab)

Brand Names: US Yervoy

Brand Names: Canada Yervoy

Pharmacologic Category Antineoplastic Agent, Monoclonal Antibody

Use

Colorectal cancer, metastatic (microsatellite instability-high or mismatch repair deficient): Treatment (in combination with nivolumab) of microsatellite instability-high (MSI-H) or mismatch repair deficient (dMMR) metastatic colorectal cancer (CRC) that has progressed following treatment with a fluoropyrimidine, oxaliplatin, and irinotecan in adults and pediatric patients ≥12 years of age.

Hepatocellular carcinoma: Treatment of hepatocellular carcinoma (in combination with nivolumab) in patients who have been previously treated with sorafenib.

Melanoma, adjuvant treatment: Adjuvant treatment of cutaneous melanoma in patients with pathologic involvement of regional lymph nodes of >1 mm who have undergone complete resection, including total lymphadenectomy.

Melanoma, unresectable or metastatic: Treatment of unresectable or metastatic melanoma in adult and pediatric patients ≥12 years of age.

Non-small cell lung cancer, metastatic: First-line treatment of metastatic non-small cell lung cancer (in combination with nivolumab) in adults whose tumors express PD-L1 (≥1%) as determined by an approved test, and with no epidermal growth factor receptor (EGFR) or anaplastic lymphoma kinase (ALK) genomic tumor aberrations.

Non-small cell lung cancer, metastatic or recurrent: First-line treatment of metastatic or recurrent non-small cell lung cancer (in combination with nivolumab and 2 cycles of platinum doublet chemotherapy) in adults with no EGFR or ALK genomic tumor aberrations.

Renal cell carcinoma, advanced: Treatment of intermediate or poor risk, previously untreated advanced renal cell carcinoma (in combination with nivolumab).

Local Anesthetic/Vasoconstrictor Precautions No information available to require special precautions

Effects on Dental Treatment No significant effects or complications reported

Effects on Bleeding No information available to require special precautions

Adverse Reactions

>10%:

Dermatologic: Dermatitis (3% to 21%), pruritus (24% to 45%) (Hodi 2010), skin rash (19% to 50%) (Hodi 2010)

Endocrine & metabolic: Weight loss (32%)

Gastrointestinal: Abdominal pain (15%) (Hodi 2010), colitis (8% to 16%), constipation (21%) (Hodi 2010), decreased appetite (14% to 27%) (Hodi 2010), diarrhea (32% to 49%), enterocolitis (5% to 16%), increased serum amylase (17%), increased serum lipase (26%), nausea (25% to 35%) (Hodi 2010), vomiting (13% to 24%) (Hodi 2010)

Hematologic & oncologic: Anemia (12%) (Hodi 2010)

Hepatic: Hepatitis (5% to 11%), increased serum alanine aminotransferase (≤46%) (Hodi 2010), increased serum alkaline phosphatase (17%), increased serum aspartate aminotransferase (≤38%) (Hodi 2010), increased serum bilirubin (11%)

Nervous system: Fatigue (41% to 46%), headache (15% to 33%) (Hodi 2010)

Respiratory: Cough (16%) (Hodi 2010), dyspnea (15%) (Hodi 2010)

Miscellaneous: Fever (12% to 18%) (Hodi 2010)

1% to 10%:

Dermatologic: Urticaria (2%), vitiligo (2%) (Hodi 2010)

Endocrine & metabolic: Adrenocortical insufficiency (≤2%) (Hodi 2010), endocrine disease (2% to 8%), hypophysitis (2%) (Hodi 2010), hypothyroidism (≤2%) (Hodi 2010), pituitary insufficiency (4% to 7%)

Gastrointestinal: Intestinal perforation (1% to 2%), pancreatitis (1%)

Genitourinary: Hypogonadism (≤2%)

Hematologic & oncologic: Eosinophilia (1% to 2%)

Hepatic: Hepatotoxicity (1% to 3%)

Immunologic: Antibody development (1%)

Nervous system: Insomnia (10%), neuropathy (≤2%)

Renal: Increased serum creatinine (10%)

<1%:

Cardiovascular: Myocarditis, pericarditis

Endocrine & metabolic: Cushing's syndrome, hyperthyroidism, thyroiditis (autoimmune)

Gastrointestinal: Esophagitis, ulcerative bowel lesion

Hematologic & oncologic: Cytopenia, sarcoidosis

Hepatic: Hepatic failure

Nervous system: Encephalitis, meningitis, myasthenia gravis, peripheral motor neuropathy

Ophthalmic: Graves' ophthalmopathy, iritis, uveitis

Renal: Nephritis, renal failure syndrome

Respiratory: Acute respiratory distress syndrome, pneumonitis

Miscellaneous: Infusion related reaction

Frequency not defined:

Cardiovascular: Capillary leak syndrome (Hodi 2010)

Dermatologic: Stevens-Johnson syndrome, toxic epidermal necrolysis

Nervous system: Guillain-Barré syndrome

Postmarketing:

Dermatologic: Drug reaction with eosinophilia and systemic symptoms

Hematologic & oncologic: Immunological signs and symptoms (hemophagocytic lymphohistiocytosis) (Hantel 2018)

Immunologic: Graft versus host disease

Respiratory: Bronchiolitis obliterans organizing pneumonia (Barjaktarevic 2013)

Mechanism of Action Ipilimumab is a recombinant human IgG1 immunoglobulin monoclonal antibody that binds to the cytotoxic T-lymphocyte associated antigen 4 (CTLA-4). CTLA-4 is a down-regulator of T-cell activation pathways. Blocking CTLA-4 allows for enhanced T-cell activation and proliferation. In melanoma, ipilimumab may indirectly mediate T-cell immune responses against tumors. Combining ipilimumab (anti-CTLA-4) with nivolumab (anti-PD-1) results in enhanced T-cell function that is greater than that of either antibody alone, resulting in improved antitumor responses in metastatic melanoma and advanced renal cell carcinoma.

Pharmacodynamics/Kinetics

Half-life Elimination Terminal: 15.4 days

Reproductive Considerations

Verify pregnancy status in females of reproductive potential prior to ipilimumab treatment initiation. Females of reproductive potential should use effective contraception during treatment and for 3 months following the last ipilimumab dose.

Pituitary dysfunction, secondary to autoimmune hypophysitis, may occur with ipilimumab therapy; male and female fertility may be impaired (Grunewald 2015).

Pregnancy Considerations

Based on the mechanism of action and findings from animal reproduction studies, in utero exposure to ipilimumab may cause fetal harm. Ipilimumab is a humanized monoclonal antibody (IgG_1). Potential placental transfer of human IgG is dependent upon the IgG subclass and gestational age, generally increasing as pregnancy progresses. The lowest exposure would be expected during the period of organogenesis (Palmeira 2012; Pentsuk 2009).

Information related to ipilimumab in pregnancy is limited to case reports describing use in patients with metastatic melanoma (Burotto 2018; Mehta 2018; Menzer 2018).

Guidelines are available for the diagnosis, treatment, and follow-up of cancer during pregnancy; the guidelines recommend referral to a facility with expertise in cancer during pregnancy and encourage a multidisciplinary team (obstetrician, neonatologist, oncology team) (ESMO [Peccatori 2013]; Swetter 2019). Until additional information is available, use of ipilimumab for the treatment of melanoma during pregnancy is not recommended (ESMO [Peccatori 2013]).

A pregnancy registry has been established to collect information about women exposed to ipilimumab during pregnancy. Ipilimumab exposures during pregnancy should be reported to the manufacturer by calling 1-844-593-7869.

◆ **Ipilimumab, inj** *see* Ipilimumab *on page 836*

◆ **IPOL** *see* Poliovirus Vaccine (Inactivated) *on page 1243*

Ipratropium (Nasal) (i pra TROE pee um)

Brand Names: Canada Atrovent Nasal [DSC]; DOM-Ipratropium; Ipravent; PMS-Ipratropium

Pharmacologic Category Anticholinergic Agent

Use

Allergic/nonallergic perennial rhinitis (0.03% solution): Symptomatic relief of rhinorrhea associated with allergic and nonallergic perennial rhinitis in adults and children ≥6 years.

Colds (0.06% solution): Symptomatic relief of rhinorrhea associated with the common cold in adults and children ≥5 years.

Seasonal allergic rhinitis (0.06% solution): Symptomatic relief of rhinorrhea associated with seasonal allergic rhinitis in adults and children ≥5 years.

Local Anesthetic/Vasoconstrictor Precautions No information available to require special precautions

Effects on Dental Treatment No significant effects or complications reported

Effects on Bleeding No information available to require special precautions

Adverse Reactions

1% to 10%:

Central nervous system: Headache (4% to 10%)

Gastrointestinal: Dysgeusia (≤4%), xerostomia (1% to 4%), diarrhea (2%), nausea (2%)

Respiratory: Upper respiratory tract infection (5% to 10%), epistaxis (6% to 9%), pharyngitis (≤8%), dry nose (≤5%), nasal mucosa irritation (2%), nasal congestion (1%)

<2%, postmarketing, and/or case reports: Anaphylaxis, angioedema, blurred vision, burning sensation of the nose, conjunctivitis, cough, dizziness, eye irritation, hoarseness, increased thirst, laryngospasm, palpitations, skin rash, tachycardia, tinnitus, urticaria

Mechanism of Action Local application to nasal mucosa inhibits serous and seromucous gland secretions.

Pharmacodynamics/Kinetics

Onset of Action 15 minutes

Pregnancy Risk Factor B

Pregnancy Considerations Adverse events have not been observed in animal reproduction studies.

Ipratropium (Oral Inhalation)
(i pra TROE pee um)

Related Information

Dentin Hypersensitivity, Acid Erosion, High Caries Index, Management of Alveolar Osteitis, and Xerostomia *on page 1762*

Respiratory Diseases *on page 1680*

Brand Names: US Atrovent HFA

Brand Names: Canada APO-Ipravent; APO-Ipravent Sterules; Atrovent HFA; PHL-Ipratropium [DSC]; PMS-Ipratropium; RATIO-Ipratropium UDV [DSC]; RATIO-Ipratropium [DSC]; TEVA-Ipratropium Bromide

Pharmacologic Category Anticholinergic Agent

Use Chronic obstructive pulmonary disease: Maintenance treatment of bronchospasm associated with chronic obstructive pulmonary disease (COPD), including chronic bronchitis and emphysema

Local Anesthetic/Vasoconstrictor Precautions No information available to require special precautions

Effects on Dental Treatment Key adverse event(s) related to dental treatment: Xerostomia and changes in salivation (normal salivary flow resumes upon discontinuation), and dry mucous membranes.

Effects on Bleeding No information available to require special precautions

Adverse Reactions

>10%: Respiratory: Bronchitis (10% to 23%), exacerbation of chronic obstructive pulmonary disease (8% to 23%), sinusitis (1% to 11%)

1% to 10%:

Central nervous system: Headache (6% to 7%), dizziness (3%)

Gastrointestinal: Dyspepsia (1% to 5%), nausea (4%), xerostomia (2% to 4%), dysgeusia (1%)

Genitourinary: Urinary tract infection (2% to 10%)

Neuromuscular & skeletal: Back pain (2% to 7%)

Respiratory: Dyspnea (7% to 8%), flu-like symptoms (4% to 8%), cough (>3%), rhinitis (>3%), upper respiratory tract infection (>3%)

<1%, postmarketing, and/or case reports: Accommodation disturbance, acute eye pain, anaphylaxis, angioedema, blurred vision, bronchospasm, conjunctival hyperemia, constipation, corneal edema, decreased gastrointestinal motility, diarrhea, dry throat, glaucoma, hypersensitivity reaction, hypotension, increased intraocular pressure, laryngospasm, mouth edema, mydriasis, nausea, palpitations, pharyngeal edema, pruritus, skin rash, stomatitis, tachycardia, throat irritation, urinary retention, urticaria, visual halos around lights, vomiting

Mechanism of Action Blocks the action of acetylcholine at parasympathetic sites in bronchial smooth muscle causing bronchodilation; local application to nasal mucosa inhibits serous and seromucous gland secretions.

Pharmacodynamics/Kinetics

Onset of Action Bronchodilation: Within 15 minutes; Peak effect: 1 to 2 hours

Duration of Action Metered-dose inhaler: 2 to 4 hours; Nebulization solution: 4 to 5 hours, up to 7 to 8 hours in some patients

Half-life Elimination 2 hours

Pregnancy Considerations Systemic exposure following inhalation is negligible; maternal use is not expected to result in fetal exposure. Based on available information, an increased risk of adverse maternal or fetal outcomes has not been observed following use during pregnancy.

◆ **Ipratropium/Albuterol Sulfate** *see* Ipratropium and Albuterol *on page 839*

Ipratropium and Albuterol

(i pra TROE pee um & al BYOO ter ole)

Related Information

Albuterol *on page 90*

Ipratropium (Oral Inhalation) *on page 838*

Brand Names: US Combivent Respimat

Brand Names: Canada Apo-Salvent-Ipravent Sterules; Combivent Respimat; Combivent UDV; ratio-Ipra Sal UDV; Teva-Combo Sterinebs

Pharmacologic Category Anticholinergic Agent; Beta$_2$-Adrenergic Agonist

Use Chronic obstructive pulmonary disease: Treatment of chronic obstructive pulmonary disease (COPD) in those patients who are currently on a regular bronchodilator who continue to have bronchospasms and require a second bronchodilator

Local Anesthetic/Vasoconstrictor Precautions No information available to require special precautions

Effects on Dental Treatment Key adverse event(s) related to dental treatment: Xerostomia (normal salivary flow resumes upon discontinuation), dry mucous membrane, and unusual taste.

Effects on Bleeding No information available to require special precautions

Adverse Reactions Also see individual agents.

1% to 10%:

Cardiovascular: Angina pectoris (<2%), cardiac arrhythmia (<2%), chest discomfort (<2%), edema (<2%), hypertension (<2%), palpitations (<2%), tachycardia (<2%)

Central nervous system: Headache (3%), pain (≥2%), dizziness (<2%), fatigue (<2%), insomnia (<2%), nervousness (<2%), voice disorder (<2%)

Dermatologic: Pruritus (<2%), skin rash (<2%)

Endocrine & metabolic: Hypokalemia (<2%)

Gastrointestinal: Constipation (<2%), diarrhea (<2%), dysgeusia (<2%), dyspepsia (<2%), vomiting (<2%), xerostomia (<2%)

Genitourinary: Dysuria (<2%), urinary tract infection (<2%)

Neuromuscular & skeletal: Arthralgia (<2%), asthenia (<2%), muscle spasm (<2%), myalgia (<2%), tremor (<2%)

Ophthalmic: Eye pain (<2%)

Respiratory: Cough (3% to 7%), nasopharyngitis (4%), bronchitis (3%), upper respiratory tract infection (3%), pharyngitis (≥2%), respiratory insufficiency (≥2%), sinusitis (≥2%), dyspnea (2%), bronchospasm (<2%), dry throat (<2%), flu-like symptoms (<2%), increased bronchial secretions (<2%), pharyngolaryngeal pain (<2%), wheezing (<2%)

Frequency not defined: Gastrointestinal: Nausea

<1%, postmarketing, and/or case reports: Accommodation disturbance, anaphylaxis, angioedema, blurred vision, central nervous system stimulation, conjunctival hyperemia, corneal edema, decreased diastolic blood pressure, dry secretions, eye irritation, gastrointestinal motility disorder, glaucoma, hyperhidrosis, hypersensitivity reaction, increased systolic blood pressure, ischemic heart disease, mouth edema, myasthenia, mydriasis, nasal congestion, paradoxical bronchospasm, pharyngeal edema, psychiatric disturbance, stomatitis, throat irritation, urinary retention, visual halos around lights

Mechanism of Action See individual agents.

Pregnancy Risk Factor C

Pregnancy Considerations Animal reproduction studies have not been conducted with this combination. See individual agents.

Ipratropium and Fenoterol

(i pra TROE pee um & fen oh TER ole)

Related Information

Ipratropium (Oral Inhalation) *on page 838*

Brand Names: Canada Duovent UDV [DSC]

Pharmacologic Category Anticholinergic Agent; Beta$_2$-Adrenergic Agonist

Use Note: Not approved in the US

Bronchospasm: Treatment of bronchospasm associated with acute severe exacerbation of COPD or bronchial asthma in patients ≥12 years of age

Local Anesthetic/Vasoconstrictor Precautions No information available to require special precautions

Effects on Dental Treatment Key adverse event(s) related to dental treatment: Xerostomia (normal salivary flow resumes upon discontinuation).

Effects on Bleeding No information available to require special precautions

Adverse Reactions Frequency not defined.

Cardiovascular: Atrial fibrillation, cardiac arrhythmia, hypertension, hypotension, ischemic heart disease, palpitations, prolonged QT interval on ECG, supraventricular tachycardia, tachycardia

Central nervous system: Dizziness, headache, nervousness, psychological disorder

Dermatologic: Diaphoresis

Endocrine & metabolic: Hyperglycemia, hypokalemia

Gastrointestinal: Constipation, diarrhea, nausea, vomiting, xerostomia

Genitourinary: Urinary retention

Hypersensitivity: Hypersensitivity reaction (anaphylaxis, angioedema, bronchospasm, laryngospasm, oropharyngeal edema, skin rash, urticaria)

Neuromuscular & skeletal: Muscle cramps, myalgia, tremor, weakness

Ophthalmic: Accommodation disturbance, acute angle-closure glaucoma, eye pain, increased intraocular pressure, mydriasis

Respiratory: Bronchospasm (inhalation-induced), cough, pharyngitis, throat irritation

Mechanism of Action

Ipratropium: Blocks the action of acetylcholine at parasympathetic sites in bronchial smooth muscle causing bronchodilation

Fenoterol: Relaxes bronchial smooth muscle by action on beta$_2$-receptors

Pharmacodynamics/Kinetics

Onset of Action

Ipratropium: Bronchodilation: Within 15 minutes; Peak effect: 1 to 2 hours

Fenoterol: Bronchodilation: 5 minutes; Peak effect: 30 to 60 minutes

Duration of Action

Ipratropium: 4 to 8 hours

Fenoterol: 6 to 8 hours

Half-life Elimination
Ipratropium: 1.6 hours
Fenoterol: ~3 hours

Pregnancy Considerations Adverse events were not observed in animal reproduction studies using this combination via inhalation. Adverse events were observed in animal reproduction studies using oral formulations of each component.

Product Availability Not available in the US

- **Ipratropium Bromide** *see* Ipratropium (Nasal) *on page 838*
- **Ipratropium Bromide** *see* Ipratropium (Oral Inhalation) *on page 838*
- **Ipratropium Bromide and Fenoterol Hydrobromide** *see* Ipratropium and Fenoterol *on page 839*
- **I-Prin [OTC] [DSC]** *see* Ibuprofen *on page 786*
- **Iprivask [DSC]** *see* Desirudin *on page 459*
- **Iproveratril Hydrochloride** *see* Verapamil *on page 1540*
- **IPV** *see* Poliovirus Vaccine (Inactivated) *on page 1243*

Irbesartan (ir be SAR tan)

Related Information
Cardiovascular Diseases *on page 1654*

Brand Names: US Avapro

Brand Names: Canada ACT Irbesartan [DSC]; AG-Irbesartan; APO-Irbesartan; Auro-Irbesartan; Avapro; BIO-Irbesartan; DOM-Irbesartan [DSC]; JAMP-Irbesartan; MINT-Irbesartan; MYLAN-Irbesartan [DSC]; PMS-Irbesartan; Priva-Irbesartan; RIVA-Irbesartan [DSC]; SANDOZ Irbesartan; TARO-Irbesartan; TEVA-Irbesartan; VAN-Irbesartan [DSC]

Pharmacologic Category Angiotensin II Receptor Blocker; Antihypertensive

Use

Diabetic nephropathy: Treatment of diabetic nephropathy with an elevated serum creatinine and proteinuria (>300 mg/day) in patients with type 2 diabetes and hypertension

Hypertension: Management of hypertension

Guideline recommendations: The 2017 Guideline for the Prevention, Detection, Evaluation, and Management of High Blood Pressure in Adults recommends if monotherapy is warranted, in the absence of comorbidities (eg, cerebrovascular disease, chronic kidney disease, diabetes, heart failure, ischemic heart disease, etc.), that thiazide-like diuretics or dihydropyridine calcium channel blockers may be preferred options due to improved cardiovascular endpoints (eg, prevention of heart failure and stroke). ACE inhibitors and ARBs are also acceptable for monotherapy. Combination therapy may be required to achieve blood pressure goals and is initially preferred in patients at high risk (stage 2 hypertension or atherosclerotic cardiovascular disease [ASCVD] risk ≥10%) (ACC/AHA [Whelton 2017]).

Local Anesthetic/Vasoconstrictor Precautions
No information available to require special precautions

Effects on Dental Treatment Key adverse event(s) related to dental treatment: Patients may experience orthostatic hypotension as they stand up after treatment; especially if lying in dental chair for extended periods of time. Use caution with sudden changes in position during and after dental treatment.

Effects on Bleeding No information available to require special precautions

Adverse Reactions Unless otherwise indicated, incidences are reported for patients with hypertension.

>10%: Endocrine & metabolic: Hyperkalemia (diabetic nephropathy: 19%)

1% to 10%:

Cardiovascular: Orthostatic dizziness (diabetic nephropathy: 5%), orthostatic hypotension (diabetic nephropathy: 5%)

Central nervous system: Dizziness (diabetic nephropathy: 10%), fatigue (4%)

Gastrointestinal: Diarrhea (3%), dyspepsia (≤2%), heartburn (≤2%)

<1%, postmarketing, and/or case reports: Anaphylactic shock, anaphylaxis, anemia (case report; Simonetti 2007), angioedema, facial edema, hepatitis, increased creatine phosphokinase, increased liver enzymes, jaundice, lip edema, pharyngeal edema, thrombocytopenia, tinnitus, tongue edema, urticaria

Mechanism of Action Irbesartan is an angiotensin receptor antagonist. Angiotensin II acts as a vasoconstrictor. In addition to causing direct vasoconstriction, angiotensin II also stimulates the release of aldosterone. Once aldosterone is released, sodium as well as water are reabsorbed. The end result is an elevation in blood pressure. Irbesartan binds to the AT1 angiotensin II receptor. This binding prevents angiotensin II from binding to the receptor thereby blocking the vasoconstriction and the aldosterone secreting effects of angiotensin II.

Pharmacodynamics/Kinetics

Onset of Action
Peak levels in 1 to 2 hours
Maximum effect: 3-6 hours postdose; with chronic dosing maximum effect: ~2 weeks

Duration of Action >24 hours

Half-life Elimination Terminal: 11 to 15 hours

Time to Peak Serum: 1.5 to 2 hours

Reproductive Considerations
The use of angiotensin II receptor blockers should generally be avoided in women planning a pregnancy (ACOG 203 2019).

Pregnancy Risk Factor D

Pregnancy Considerations
[US Boxed Warning]: Drugs that act on the renin-angiotensin system can cause injury and death to the developing fetus. When pregnancy is detected, discontinue as soon as possible. The use of drugs which act on the renin-angiotensin system are associated with oligohydramnios. Oligohydramnios, due to decreased fetal renal function, may lead to fetal lung hypoplasia and skeletal malformations. Oligohydramnios may not appear until after irreversible fetal injury has occurred. Use in pregnancy is also associated with anuria, hypotension, renal failure, skull hypoplasia, and death in the fetus/neonate. The exposed fetus should be monitored for fetal growth, amniotic fluid volume, and organ formation. Infants exposed in utero should be monitored for hyperkalemia, hypotension, and oliguria (exchange transfusions or dialysis may be needed). These adverse events are generally associated with maternal use in the second and third trimesters.

Chronic maternal hypertension itself is also associated with adverse events in the fetus/infant. The risk of birth defects, low birth weight, premature delivery, stillbirth, and neonatal death may be increased with chronic hypertension in pregnancy. Actual risks may be related to duration and severity of maternal hypertension (ACOG 203 2019).

The use of angiotensin II receptor blockers is generally not recommended to treat chronic hypertension in pregnant women (ACOG 203 2019).

- **Irbinitinib** *see* Tucatinib *on page 1503*
- **Iressa** *see* Gefitinib *on page 730*

Irinotecan (Conventional)

(eye rye no TEE kan con VEN sha nal)

Brand Names: US Camptosar

Brand Names: Canada Camptosar

Pharmacologic Category Antineoplastic Agent, Camptothecin; Antineoplastic Agent, Topoisomerase I Inhibitor

Use Colorectal cancer, metastatic: Treatment of metastatic carcinoma of the colon or rectum, either as first-line therapy (in combination with fluorouracil and leucovorin), or for recurrent disease following initial fluorouracil-based treatment.

Local Anesthetic/Vasoconstrictor Precautions No information available to require special precautions

Effects on Dental Treatment Key adverse event(s) related to dental treatment: Increased salivation, mucositis, and stomatitis.

Effects on Bleeding Hematologic adverse effects include anemia (60% to 97%) and thrombocytopenia (96%; grades 3/4: 1% to 4%). Bleeding and hemorrhage have been noted in 1% to 5% of patients. Medical consult recommended.

Adverse Reactions Frequency of adverse reactions reported for single-agent use of irinotecan only. In limited pediatric experience, dehydration (often associated with severe hypokalemia and hyponatremia) was among the most significant grade 3/4 adverse events, with a frequency up to 29%. In addition, grade 3/4 infection was reported in 24%.

>10%:

Cardiovascular: Vasodilation (9% to 11%)

Central nervous system: Cholinergic syndrome (47%; includes diaphoresis, flushing, increased peristalsis, lacrimation, miosis, rhinitis, sialorrhea), pain (23% to 24%), dizziness (15% to 21%), insomnia (19%), headache (17%), chills (14%)

Dermatologic: Alopecia (46% to 72%), diaphoresis (16%), skin rash (13% to 14%)

Endocrine & metabolic: Weight loss (30%), dehydration (15%)

Gastrointestinal: Diarrhea (late: 83% to 88%, grades 3/4: 14% to 31%; early: 43% to 51%, grades 3/4: 7% to 22%), nausea (70% to 86%), abdominal pain (57% to 68%), vomiting (62% to 67%), abdominal cramps (57%), anorexia (44% to 55%), constipation (30% to 32%), mucositis (30%), flatulence (12%), stomatitis (12%)

Hematologic & oncologic: Anemia (60% to 97%; grades 3/4: 5% to 7%), leukopenia (63% to 96%, grades 3/4: 14% to 28%), thrombocytopenia (96%, grades 3/4: 1% to 4%), neutropenia (30% to 96%; grades 3/4: 14% to 31%)

Hepatic: Increased serum bilirubin (84%), increased serum alkaline phosphatase (13%)

Infection: Infection (14%)

Neuromuscular & skeletal: Weakness (69% to 76%), back pain (14%)

Respiratory: Dyspnea (22%), cough (17% to 20%), rhinitis (16%)

Miscellaneous: Fever (44% to 45%)

1% to 10%:

Cardiovascular: Edema (10%), hypotension (6%), thromboembolism (5%)

Central nervous system: Drowsiness (9%), confusion (3%)

Gastrointestinal: Abdominal distention (10%), dyspepsia (10%)

Hematologic & oncologic: Febrile neutropenia (grades 3/4: 2% to 6%), hemorrhage (grades 3/4: 1% to 5%), neutropenic infection (grades 3/4: 1% to 2%)

Hepatic: Increased serum AST (10%), ascites (grades 3/4: ≤9%), jaundice (grades 3/4: ≤9%)

Respiratory: Pneumonia (4%)

<1%, postmarketing, and/or case reports: Acute renal failure, anaphylactoid reaction, anaphylaxis, angina pectoris, arterial thrombosis, bradycardia, cardiac arrhythmia, cerebral infarction, cerebrovascular accident, circulatory shock, colitis, deep vein thrombophlebitis, dysarthria, embolism, gastrointestinal hemorrhage, gastrointestinal obstruction, hepatomegaly, hiccups, hyperglycemia, hypersensitivity reaction, hyponatremia, immune thrombocytopenia, increased amylase, increased serum ALT, increased serum lipase, interstitial pulmonary disease, intestinal obstruction, intestinal perforation, ischemic colitis, ischemic heart disease, lymphocytopenia, megacolon, muscle cramps, myocardial infarction, pancreatitis, paresthesia, peripheral vascular disease, pulmonary embolism; pulmonary toxicity (includes dyspnea, fever, reticulonodular infiltrates on chest x-ray), renal insufficiency, syncope, thrombophlebitis, thrombosis, typhlitis (including neutropenic typhlitis), ulcer, ulcerative colitis, vertigo

Mechanism of Action Irinotecan and its active metabolite (SN-38) bind reversibly to topoisomerase I-DNA complex preventing religation of the cleaved DNA strand. This results in the accumulation of cleavable complexes and double-strand DNA breaks. As mammalian cells cannot efficiently repair these breaks, cell death consistent with S-phase cell cycle specificity occurs, leading to termination of cellular replication.

Pharmacodynamics/Kinetics

Half-life Elimination

Children and Adolescents (Ma 2000): Irinotecan: 2.66 hours (range: 1.82 to 4.47 hours); SN-38 (active metabolite): 1.58 hours (range: 0.29 to 8.28 hours)

Adults: Irinotecan: 6 to 12 hours; SN-38: ~10 to 20 hours

Time to Peak

Irinotecan: Oral: Children and Adolescents: 3 hours (Wagner 2010a)

SN-38: Following 90-minute infusion: ~1 hour

Reproductive Considerations

Evaluate pregnancy status prior to use in females of reproductive potential. Females of reproductive potential should use highly effective contraception during therapy and for 6 months after the last irinotecan dose. Males with female partners of reproductive potential should use condoms during therapy and for 3 months after the last dose of irinotecan.

Menstrual cycle changes and impairment of female fertility may occur with irinotecan therapy.

Pregnancy Considerations

Based on the mechanism of action and data from animal reproduction studies, in utero exposure to irinotecan may cause fetal harm.

Information related to the use of irinotecan (conventional) during pregnancy is limited (Cirillo 2012; Taylor 2009).

Evaluate pregnancy status prior to use in females of reproductive potential. Females of reproductive potential should use highly effective contraception during therapy and for 6 months after the last irinotecan dose. Males with female partners of reproductive potential should use condoms during therapy and for 3 months after the last dose of irinotecan.

Menstrual cycle changes and impairment of female fertility may occur with irinotecan therapy.

Irinotecan (Liposomal)

(eye rye no TEE kan lye po SO mal)

Brand Names: US Onivyde

Brand Names: Canada Onivyde

Pharmacologic Category Antineoplastic Agent, Camptothecin; Antineoplastic Agent, Topoisomerase I Inhibitor

Use

Pancreatic adenocarcinoma, metastatic: Treatment of metastatic adenocarcinoma of the pancreas (in combination with fluorouracil and leucovorin) after disease progression following gemcitabine-based therapy.

Limitations of use: Irinotecan (liposomal) is not indicated as a single agent for the treatment of metastatic adenocarcinoma of the pancreas.

Guideline recommendations:

The American Society of Clinical Oncology (ASCO) guidelines for metastatic pancreatic cancer recommend fluorouracil in combination with irinotecan (liposomal) as preferred second-line therapy in patients with Eastern Cancer Cooperative Group (ECOG) performance status of 2 or a comorbidity profile prohibiting more aggressive therapy who received an alternative (gemcitabine-based) first-line therapy (ASCO [Sohal 2018]).

According to ASCO guidelines for locally advanced, unresectable pancreatic cancer, if disease progression occurs following induction with an initial systemic combination therapy regimen, treatment according to guidelines for metastatic pancreatic cancer should be offered (in appropriate patients) (ASCO [Balaban 2016]).

Local Anesthetic/Vasoconstrictor Precautions No information available to require special precautions

Effects on Dental Treatment Key adverse event(s) related to dental treatment: Stomatitis has been reported

Effects on Bleeding Hematologic adverse effects include anemia (97%), neutropenia (52%) and thrombocytopenia (41%)

Adverse Reactions Frequency not always defined. Percentages reported as part of combination chemotherapy regimens.

Cardiovascular: Septic shock (≥2%)

Central nervous system: Fatigue (≤56%)

Dermatologic: Alopecia (14%)

Endocrine & metabolic: Hypoalbuminemia (43%), hypomagnesemia (35%), hypocalcemia (32%), hypokalemia (32%), hypophosphatemia (29%), hyponatremia (27%), weight loss (17%), dehydration (8%)

Gastrointestinal: Diarrhea (59%, grade 3/4: 13%; early onset 30%, grade 3/4: 3%; late onset 43%, grade 3/4: 9%), vomiting (52%), nausea (51%), decreased appetite (44%), stomatitis (32%), gastroenteritis (3%)

Hematologic & oncologic: Anemia (97%, grades 3/4: 6%), lymphocytopenia (81%, grades 3/4: 27%), neutropenia (52%, grades 3/4: 20%; incidence of neutropenia was higher among Asian patients), thrombocytopenia (41%, grades 3/4: 2%), febrile neutropenia (≤3%, grades 3/4: ≤3%)

Hepatic: Increased serum ALT (51%)

Hypersensitivity: Severe hypersensitivity

Infection: Sepsis (4%, grades 3/4: 3%), neutropenic sepsis (≤3%, grades 3/4: ≤3%)

Local: Catheter infection (3%)

Neuromuscular & skeletal: Weakness (≤56%)

Renal: Increased creatinine clearance (18%), acute renal failure (≥2%)

Respiratory: Pneumonia (≥2%), interstitial pulmonary disease

Miscellaneous: Fever (23%)

Mechanism of Action Irinotecan (liposomal) is a topoisomerase 1 inhibitor encapsulated in a lipid bilayer (liposome). Irinotecan and its active metabolite (SN-38) bind reversibly to topoisomerase I-DNA complex preventing re-ligation of the cleaved DNA strand. This results in the accumulation of cleavable complexes and double-strand DNA breaks. As mammalian cells cannot efficiently repair these breaks, cell death consistent with S-phase cell cycle specificity occurs, leading to termination of cellular replication.

Pharmacodynamics/Kinetics

Half-life Elimination Total irinotecan: ~26 hours; SN-38: ~68 hours

Reproductive Considerations

Women of childbearing potential should use effective contraception while receiving treatment and avoid pregnancy for 1 month following the last dose. Males with female partners of reproductive potential should use condoms during therapy and for 4 months following the last dose.

Pregnancy Considerations

Based on the mechanism of action as well as animal data using irinotecan (conventional), irinotecan (liposomal) may cause fetal harm if administered during pregnancy.

- **Irinotecan HCl** *see* Irinotecan (Conventional) *on page 841*
- **Irinotecan Hydrochloride** *see* Irinotecan (Conventional) *on page 841*
- **Irinotecan Liposome** *see* Irinotecan (Liposomal) *on page 842*
- **Iron Sulfate** *see* Ferrous Sulfate *on page 664*
- **Iron Supplement [OTC]** *see* Ferrous Sulfate *on page 664*
- **Iron Supplement Childrens [OTC]** *see* Ferrous Sulfate *on page 664*

Isatuximab (EYE sa TUX i mab)

Brand Names: US Sarclisa

Brand Names: Canada Sarclisa

Pharmacologic Category Antineoplastic Agent, Anti-CD38; Antineoplastic Agent, Monoclonal Antibody

Use Multiple myeloma (relapsed or refractory): Treatment of multiple myeloma (in combination with pomalidomide and dexamethasone) in adults who have received ≥2 prior therapies including lenalidomide and a proteasome inhibitor.

Local Anesthetic/Vasoconstrictor Precautions No information available to require special precautions.

Effects on Dental Treatment No significant effects or complications reported.

Effects on Bleeding Chemotherapy may result in significant myelosuppression, including thrombocytopenia. In patients under active treatment a medical consult is suggested.

Adverse Reactions As reported in combination with pomalidomide plus dexamethasone. Comparator: Pomalidomide plus dexamethasone.

>10%:

Gastrointestinal: Diarrhea (26%), nausea (15%), vomiting (12%)

Hematologic & oncologic: Anemia (99%; grade 3: 32%), febrile neutropenia (12% [comparator: 2%]), lymphocytopenia (92%; grade 3: 42%; grade 4: 13%), neutropenia (96% [comparator: 92%]; grade 3: 24% [comparator: 38%]; grade 4: 61% [comparator: 31%]), thrombocytopenia (84%; grade 3: 14%; grade 4: 16%)

Infection: Infection (grades 3/4: 43%)

Respiratory: Dyspnea (17% [comparator: 12%]), pneumonia (31% [comparator: 23%]), upper respiratory tract infection (57% [comparator: 42%])

Miscellaneous: Infusion related reaction (38% to 40%)

1% to 10%:

Hematologic & oncologic: Squamous cell carcinoma (3% [comparator: 0.7%])

Immunologic: Antibody development (2%)

<1%:

Hematologic & oncologic: Malignant neoplasm of breast (angiosarcoma), myelodysplastic syndrome

Mechanism of Action Isatuximab is an IgG1-derived monoclonal antibody directed against CD38. CD38 is expressed on the surface of hematopoietic and tumor cells, including multiple myeloma cells. Isatuximab has antitumor activity via antibody-dependent, cell-mediated cytotoxicity; complement-dependent cytotoxicity; and antibody-dependent cellular phagocytosis and directly inhibits activity of CD38 ectoenzymes (Attal 2019). Isatuximab can activate natural killer cells in the absence of CD38-positive target tumor cells and suppresses CD38-positive T-regulatory cells. The combination of isatuximab plus pomalidomide enhanced antibody-dependent, cell-mediated cytotoxicity activity and direct tumor cell killing compared to isatuximab alone (in vitro) and enhanced antitumor activity compared to isatuximab or pomalidomide activities alone in animal models.

Reproductive Considerations

Evaluate pregnancy status prior to use in females of reproductive potential. Females of reproductive potential should use effective contraception during therapy and for ≥5 months after the last isatuximab dose.

Isatuximab is used in combination with pomalidomide; also refer to the pomalidomide monograph for additional information related to use in females of reproductive potential and males with female partners of reproductive potential.

Pregnancy Considerations

Isatuximab is a monoclonal antibody (IgG_1). Placental transfer of human IgG is dependent upon the IgG subclass, maternal serum concentrations, birth weight, and gestational age, generally increasing as pregnancy progresses. The lowest exposure would be expected during the period of organogenesis (Palmeira 2012; Pentsuk 2009).

Based on the mechanism of action, in utero exposure to isatuximab may cause fetal harm, including depletion of fetal CD38-positive immune cells and decreased bone density.

Isatuximab is used in combination with pomalidomide; pomalidomide is contraindicated for use during pregnancy. Refer to the pomalidomide monograph for additional information.

Prescribing and Access Restrictions

Available through authorized specialty distributors and specialty pharmacies. Information regarding distribution is available from the manufacturer at SanofiCareAssist.com/hcp/Sarclisa or at 1-833-930-2273.

◆ **Isatuximab-irfc** *see* Isatuximab *on page 842*

◆ **Isavuconazole** *see* Isavuconazonium Sulfate *on page 843*

Isavuconazonium Sulfate

(eye sa vue koe na ZOE nee um sul FATE)

Brand Names: US Cresemba

Brand Names: Canada Cresemba

Pharmacologic Category Antifungal Agent, Azole Derivative; Antifungal Agent, Oral; Antifungal Agent, Parenteral

Use

Aspergillosis: Treatment of invasive aspergillosis in adults

Mucormycosis: Treatment of invasive mucormycosis in adults

Local Anesthetic/Vasoconstrictor Precautions

No information available to require special precautions

Effects on Dental Treatment No significant effects or complications reported

Effects on Bleeding No information available to require special precautions

Adverse Reactions Frequency not always defined.

>10%:

Cardiovascular: Peripheral edema (11% to 15%)

Central nervous system: Headache (17%), fatigue (11%), insomnia (11%)

Endocrine & metabolic: Hypokalemia (14% to 19%)

Gastrointestinal: Nausea (26% to 28%), vomiting (25%), diarrhea (22% to 24%), abdominal pain (17%), constipation (13% to 14%)

Hepatic: Increased liver enzymes (16% to 17%)

Respiratory: Dyspnea (12% to 17%), cough (12%)

1% to 10%:

Cardiovascular: Chest pain (9%), hypotension (8%), atrial fibrillation (<5%), atrial flutter (<5%), bradycardia (<5%), cardiac arrest (<5%), catheter site thrombosis (<5%), extrasystoles (<5%), palpitations (<5%), shortened QT interval (<5%), supraventricular extrasystole (<5%), supraventricular tachycardia (<5%), syncope (<5%), thrombophlebitis (<5%), ventricular premature contractions (<5%)

Central nervous system: Delirium (9%), anxiety (8%), brain disease (<5%), chills (<5%), confusion (<5%), convulsions (<5%), depression (<5%), drowsiness (<5%), falling (<5%), hallucination (<5%), hypoesthesia (<5%), malaise (<5%), migraine (<5%), peripheral neuropathy (<5%), stupor (<5%), vertigo (<5%), dizziness, hypoesthesia, paresthesia

Dermatologic: Skin rash (9%), pruritus (8%), alopecia (<5%), dermatitis (<5%), erythema (<5%), exfoliative dermatitis (<5%), urticaria (<5%)

Endocrine & metabolic: Hypomagnesemia (5%), hypoalbuminemia (<5%), hypoglycemia (<5%), hyponatremia (<5%)

Gastrointestinal: Decreased appetite (9%), dyspepsia (6%), abdominal distention (<5%), cholecystitis (<5%), cholelithiasis (<5%), cholestasis (<5%), dysgeusia (<5%), gastritis (<5%), gingivitis (<5%), stomatitis (<5%)

Genitourinary: Hematuria (<5%), proteinuria (<5%)

Hematologic & oncologic: Agranulocytosis (<5%), leukopenia (<5%), pancytopenia (<5%), petechia (<5%)

Hepatic: Hepatitis (<5%), hepatomegaly (<5%), increased serum ALT (>3x ULN ≤4%; >10x ULN ≤1%), increased serum AST (>3x ULN ≤4%; >10x ULN ≤1%), hepatic failure, increased serum transaminases

Hypersensitivity: Hypersensitivity (<5%)

Local: Injection site reaction (6%)

Neuromuscular & Skeletal: Back pain (10%), myositis (<5%), neck pain (<5%), ostealgia (<5%), tremor (<5%)

Ophthalmic: Optic neuropathy (<5%)

Otic: Tinnitus (<5%)

Respiratory: Acute respiratory tract failure (7%), bronchospasm (<5%), tachypnea (<5%)

Mechanism of Action Isavuconazonium sulfate is a prodrug that is rapidly hydrolyzed in the blood to active isavuconazole. Isavuconazole inhibits the synthesis of ergosterol, a key component of the fungal cell membrane, through the inhibition of cytochrome P-450 dependent enzyme lanosterol 14-alpha-demethylase. This enzyme is responsible for the conversion of lanosterol to ergosterol. An accumulation of methylated sterol precursors and a depletion of ergosterol within the fungal cell membrane weakens the membrane structure and function.

Pharmacodynamics/Kinetics

Half-life Elimination IV: 130 hours

Time to Peak Oral: 2 to 3 hours

Reproductive Considerations

Evaluate pregnancy status prior to use in females of reproductive potential. Females of reproductive potential should use effective contraception during therapy and for 28 days after the last isavuconazonium sulfate dose.

Pregnancy Considerations

Based on data from animal reproduction studies, in utero exposure to isavuconazonium sulfate may cause fetal harm.

Use of alternative antifungals is recommended in pregnant women (HHS [OI 2019]).

- **ISD** *see* Isosorbide Dinitrate *on page* 845
- **ISDN** *see* Isosorbide Dinitrate *on page* 845
- **Isentress** *see* Raltegravir *on page* 1306
- **Isentress HD** *see* Raltegravir *on page* 1306
- **ISG** *see* Immune Globulin *on page* 803
- **Isibloom** *see* Ethinyl Estradiol and Desogestrel *on page* 609
- **ISIS 301012** *see* Mipomersen *on page* 1037
- **ISMN** *see* Isosorbide Mononitrate *on page* 845
- **Isoamyl Nitrite** *see* Amyl Nitrite *on page* 148
- **Isobamate** *see* Carisoprodol *on page* 293

Isoniazid (eye soe NYE a zid)

Brand Names: Canada DOM-Isoniazid; Isotamine; PDP-Isoniazid

Pharmacologic Category Antitubercular Agent

Use

Active tuberculosis infections: Treatment of susceptible active tuberculosis (eg, *Mycobacterium tuberculosis*) infections.

Latent tuberculosis infection: Treatment of latent tuberculosis infection (LTBI) caused by *Mycobacterium tuberculosis* (also referred to as prophylaxis or preventive therapy). **Note:** To identify candidates for LTBI treatment, refer to CDC guidelines (https://www.cdc.gov/tb/publications/ltbi/default.htm) for current recommendations.

Local Anesthetic/Vasoconstrictor Precautions No information available to require special precautions

Effects on Dental Treatment Key adverse event(s) related to dental treatment: Xerostomia (normal salivary flow resumes upon discontinuation).

Effects on Bleeding Anemia and thrombocytopenia have been reported.

Adverse Reactions

>10%: Hepatic: Increased serum transaminases (mild and transient 10% to 20%)

Frequency not defined.

Cardiovascular: Vasculitis

Central nervous system: Brain disease, memory impairment, paresthesia, peripheral neuropathy, psychosis, seizure

Dermatologic: Skin rash (morbilliform, maculopapular, pruritic, or exfoliative), toxic epidermal necrolysis

Endocrine & metabolic: Gynecomastia, hyperglycemia, metabolic acidosis, pellagra, pyridoxine deficiency

Gastrointestinal: Epigastric distress, nausea, pancreatitis, vomiting

Genitourinary: Bilirubinuria

Hematologic & oncologic: Agranulocytosis, anemia (sideroblastic, hemolytic, or aplastic), eosinophilia, lymphadenopathy, thrombocytopenia

Hepatic: Hepatitis (risk increases with age; 2% in patients ≥50 years), hyperbilirubinemia, jaundice

Immunologic: DRESS syndrome

Neuromuscular & skeletal: Lupus-like syndrome, rheumatic disease

Ophthalmic: Optic atrophy, optic neuritis

Miscellaneous: Fever

Postmarketing and/or case reports: Hepatotoxicity (idiosyncratic) (Chalasani 2014)

Mechanism of Action Isoniazid inhibits the synthesis of mycoloic acids, an essential component of the bacterial cell wall. At therapeutic levels isoniazid is bactericidal against actively growing intracellular and extracellular *Mycobacterium tuberculosis* organisms.

Pharmacodynamics/Kinetics

Half-life Elimination May be prolonged in patients with impaired hepatic function or severe renal impairment

Fast acetylators: 30 to 100 minutes; Slow acetylators: 2 to 5 hours

Time to Peak Serum: 1 to 2 hours

Pregnancy Considerations Isoniazid crosses the human placenta.

Due to the risk of tuberculosis to the fetus, treatment is recommended when the probability of maternal disease is moderate to high. Drug-susceptible TB guidelines recommend isoniazid as part of the initial treatment regimen; close monitoring is recommended during pregnancy and postpartum (due to increased risk of hepatitis). Isoniazid is also recommended for the treatment of TB in pregnant women with HIV-coinfection. Pyridoxine supplementation is recommended to decrease the risk of peripheral neurotoxicity (ATC/CDC/IDSA 2003; Nahid 2016). Due to biologic changes during pregnancy and early postpartum, pregnant women may have increased susceptibility to tuberculosis infection or reactivation of latent disease (Mathad 2012).

- ◆ **Isoniazid and Rifampin** *see* Rifampin and Isoniazid *on page 1325*
- ◆ **Isonicotinic Acid Hydrazide** *see* Isoniazid *on page 844*
- ◆ **Isonipecaine Hydrochloride** *see* Meperidine *on page 966*
- ◆ **Isophane Insulin** *see* Insulin NPH *on page 827*
- ◆ **Isophane Insulin and Regular Insulin** *see* Insulin NPH and Insulin Regular *on page 828*
- ◆ **Isordil Titradose** *see* Isosorbide Dinitrate *on page 845*

Isosorbide Dinitrate

(eye soe SOR bide dye NYE trate)

Related Information

Cardiovascular Diseases *on page 1654*

Isosorbide Mononitrate *on page 845*

Brand Names: US Dilatrate-SR; Isordil Titradose

Brand Names: Canada ISDN; PMS-Isosorbide

Pharmacologic Category Antianginal Agent; Vasodilator

Use

Angina pectoris, prevention: Prevention of angina pectoris due to coronary artery disease.

Note: Due to slower onset of action, isosorbide dinitrate is not the drug of choice to abort an acute anginal episode.

Local Anesthetic/Vasoconstrictor Precautions No information available to require special precautions

Effects on Dental Treatment Key adverse event(s) related to dental treatment: Xerostomia and changes in salivation (normal salivary flow resumes upon discontinuation).

Effects on Bleeding No information available to require special precautions

Adverse Reactions

Frequency not defined.

Cardiovascular: Hypotension, rebound hypertension, syncope, unstable angina pectoris

Central nervous system: Headache

Mechanism of Action Isosorbide dinitrate and other nitrates form free radical nitric oxide. In smooth muscle, nitric oxide activates guanylate cyclase which increases guanosine 3'5' monophosphate (cGMP) leading to dephosphorylation of myosin light chains and smooth muscle relaxation. Produces a vasodilator effect on the peripheral veins and arteries with more prominent effects on the veins. Primarily reduces cardiac oxygen demand by decreasing preload (left ventricular end-diastolic pressure); may modestly reduce afterload. Additionally, coronary artery dilation improves collateral flow to ischemic regions.

Pharmacodynamics/Kinetics

Onset of Action Sublingual tablet: ~2 to 5 minutes; Oral tablet and capsule (includes extended-release formulations): ~1 hour

Duration of Action Sublingual tablet: 1 to 2 hours; Oral tablet and capsule (includes extended-release formulations): Up to 8 hours

Half-life Elimination Parent drug: ~1 hour; Metabolites (5-mononitrate: 5 hours; 2-mononitrate: 2 hours)

Pregnancy Considerations Adverse events have been observed in some animal reproduction studies. Nitric oxide donors, such as isosorbide, have been evaluated for pre-eclampsia and cervical ripening; isosorbide dinitrate use in these conditions is not currently recommended (Kalidindi 2012; Ramirez 2011).

Isosorbide Mononitrate

(eye soe SOR bide mon oh NYE trate)

Related Information

Cardiovascular Diseases *on page 1654*

Isosorbide Dinitrate *on page 845*

Brand Names: Canada APO-ISMN; Imdur; ISMN [DSC]; PMS-ISMN; PRO-ISMN-60

Pharmacologic Category Antianginal Agent; Vasodilator

Use Angina pectoris: Treatment (immediate-release only) and prevention of angina pectoris caused by coronary artery disease. **Note:** The onset of action of oral isosorbide mononitrate is not sufficiently rapid for this product to be useful in aborting an acute anginal episode.

Local Anesthetic/Vasoconstrictor Precautions No information available to require special precautions

Effects on Dental Treatment No significant effects or complications reported

Effects on Bleeding No information available to require special precautions

Adverse Reactions

>10%: Central nervous system: Headache (≤57%), dizziness (≤11%)

1% to 10%:

Cardiovascular: Abnormal heart sounds (≤5%), atrial arrhythmia (≤5%), atrial fibrillation (≤5%), bradycardia (≤5%), bundle branch block (≤5%), cardiac arrhythmia (≤5%), cardiac failure (≤5%), chest pain (≤5%), ECG abnormality (Q wave: ≤5%), edema (≤5%), exacerbation of angina pectoris (≤5%), extrasystoles (≤5%), flushing (≤5%), heart murmur (≤5%), hypertension (≤5%), hypotension (≤5%), intermittent claudication (≤5%), myocardial infarction (≤5%), palpitations (≤5%), tachycardia (≤5%), varicose veins (≤5%), ventricular tachycardia (≤5%), cardiovascular toxicity (2%)

Central nervous system: Anxiety (≤5%), confusion (≤5%), depression (≤5%), drowsiness (≤5%), fatigue (≤5%), hypoesthesia (≤5%), insomnia (≤5%), lack of concentration (≤5%), malaise (≤5%), migraine (≤5%), myasthenia (≤5%), nervousness (≤5%), neuritis (≤5%), nightmares (≤5%), paresis (≤5%), paresthesia (≤5%), rigors (≤5%), vertigo (≤5%), pain (4%), emotional lability (2%)

Dermatologic: Abnormal hair texture (≤5%), acne vulgaris (≤5%), diaphoresis (≤5%), leg ulcer (≤5%), pruritus (≤5%), skin rash (≤5%)

Endocrine & metabolic: Decreased libido (≤5%), hot flash (≤5%), hyperuricemia (≤5%), hypokalemia (≤5%)

Gastrointestinal: Abdominal pain (≤5%), constipation (≤5%), diarrhea (≤5%), dyspepsia (≤5%), flatulence (≤5%), gastric ulcer (≤5%), gastric ulcer with hemorrhage (≤5%), gastritis (≤5%), glossitis (≤5%), hemorrhoids (≤5%), loose stools (≤5%), melena (≤5%), nausea (≤5%), vomiting (≤5%), xerostomia (≤5%)

Genitourinary: Atrophic vaginitis (≤5%), impotence (≤5%), mastalgia (≤5%), urinary tract infection (≤5%)

Hematologic & oncologic: Hypochromic anemia (≤5%), nonthrombocytopenic purpura (≤5%), thrombocytopenia (≤5%)
Hepatic: Increased serum alanine aminotransferase (≤5%), increased serum aspartate aminotransferase (≤5%)
Hypersensitivity: Hypersensitivity reaction (2%)
Infection: Bacterial infection (≤5%), candidiasis (≤5%), viral infection (≤5%)
Neuromuscular & skeletal: Arthralgia (≤5%), asthenia (≤5%), back pain (≤5%), musculoskeletal pain (≤5%), myalgia (≤5%), myositis (≤5%), shoulder stiffness (frozen shoulder: ≤5%), tendon disease (≤5%), torticollis (≤5%), tremor (≤5%)
Ophthalmic: Blepharoptosis (≤5%), conjunctivitis (≤5%), photophobia (≤5%), visual disturbance (≤5%)
Otic: Otalgia (≤5%), perforated tympanic membrane (≤5%), tinnitus (≤5%)
Renal: Nephrolithiasis (≤5%), polyuria (≤5%)
Respiratory: Bronchitis (≤5%), bronchospasm (≤5%), cough (≤5%), dyspnea (≤5%), flu-like symptoms (≤5%), increased bronchial secretions (≤5%), nasal congestion (≤5%), pharyngitis (≤5%), pneumonia (≤5%), pulmonary infiltrates (≤5%), rales (≤5%), rhinitis (≤5%), sinusitis (≤5%), upper respiratory infection (1% to 4%), increased cough (2%)
Miscellaneous: Fever (≤5%), nodule (≤5%)

<1%, postmarketing, and/or case reports: Acute myocardial infarction, amblyopia, anorexia, asthma, bitter taste, cerebrovascular accident, increased thirst, muscle cramps, neck pain, pallor, prostatic disease, restlessness, syncope, weight loss

Mechanism of Action Nitroglycerin and other nitrates form free radical nitric oxide. In smooth muscle, nitric oxide activates guanylate cyclase which increases guanosine 3'5' monophosphate (cGMP) leading to dephosphorylation of myosin light chains and smooth muscle relaxation. Produces a vasodilator effect on the peripheral veins and arteries with more prominent effects on the veins. Primarily reduces cardiac oxygen demand by decreasing preload (left ventricular end-diastolic pressure); may modestly reduce afterload; dilates coronary arteries and improves collateral flow to ischemic regions.

Pharmacodynamics/Kinetics

Onset of Action 30 to 45 minutes (Thadani 1987)

Duration of Action Immediate release: ≥6 hours (Thadani 1987); Extended release: ≥12 to 24 hours (Anderson 2007)

Half-life Elimination ~5 to 6 hours (Thadani 1987)

Time to Peak Plasma: 30 to 60 minutes

Pregnancy Risk Factor B

Pregnancy Considerations Adverse events have been observed in some animal reproduction studies. Nitric oxide donors, such as isosorbide, have been evaluated for pre-eclampsia and cervical ripening; isosorbide mononitrate use in these conditions is not currently recommended (Kalidindi 2012; Ramirez 2011).

ISOtretinoin (Systemic) (eye soe TRET i noyn)

Related Information

Dentin Hypersensitivity, Acid Erosion, High Caries Index, Management of Alveolar Osteitis, and Xerostomia *on page 1762*

Brand Names: US Absorica; Absorica LD; Amnesteem; Claravis; Myorisan; Zenatane

Brand Names: Canada Accutane Roche; ALTI-Isotretinoin; Clarus; Epuris

Pharmacologic Category Acne Products; Antineoplastic Agent, Retinoic Acid Derivative; Retinoic Acid Derivative

Use Acne, severe recalcitrant nodular: Treatment of severe recalcitrant nodular acne unresponsive to conventional therapy (including systemic antibiotics)

Local Anesthetic/Vasoconstrictor Precautions No information available to require special precautions

Effects on Dental Treatment Key adverse event(s) related to dental treatment: Xerostomia and changes in salivation (normal salivary flow resumes upon discontinuation).

Effects on Bleeding No information available to require special precautions

Adverse Reactions

>10%:
Endocrine & metabolic: Increased serum triglycerides (25% including cases reported >800 mg/dL), increased creatine phosphokinase in blood specimen (adults: 24%; adolescents: 12%), decreased HDL cholesterol (15%)
Hepatic: Increased liver enzymes (15%)
Neuromuscular & skeletal: Back pain (children: 29%), arthralgia (≤22%), musculoskeletal disease (16%)

1% to 10%:
Endocrine & metabolic: Increased serum cholesterol (7%)
Neuromuscular & skeletal: Decreased bone mineral density (adolescents: 9%), severe arthralgia (children: 8%)

Frequency not defined:
Cardiovascular: Cerebrovascular accident, chest pain, edema, flushing, palpitations, syncope, tachycardia, thrombosis, vasculitis
Dermatologic: Acne fulminans, alopecia, cheilitis, cheilosis, contact dermatitis, dermatitis, diaphoresis, eczema, erythema of skin, facial erythema, fragile skin, hair disease, nail disease, paronychia, pruritus, pyogenic granuloma, scaling of skin of feet, seborrhea, skin photosensitivity, skin rash, sunburn, superficial peeling of palms, urticaria, xeroderma
Endocrine & metabolic: Altered serum glucose, decreased libido, eruptive xanthoma, hirsutism, increased gamma-glutamyl transferase, increased lactate dehydrogenase, increased LDL cholesterol, increased serum glucose, hyperuricemia, menstrual disease, weight loss
Gastrointestinal: Abdominal pain, colitis, constipation, decreased appetite, diarrhea, esophagitis, esophageal ulcer, gingival hemorrhage, gingivitis, ileitis, inflammatory bowel disease, nausea, pancreatitis, vomiting, xerostomia
Genitourinary: Erectile dysfunction, gross hematuria, microscopic hematuria, proteinuria, pyuria, sexual disorder
Hematologic & oncologic: Anemia, bruise, decreased white blood cell count, increased erythrocyte sedimentation rate, lymphadenopathy, purpuric disease, severe neutropenia, thrombocythemia, thrombocytopenia
Hepatic: Increased serum alanine aminotransferase, increased serum alkaline phosphatase, increased serum aspartate aminotransferase, increased serum bilirubin
Infection: Herpes simplex infection (disseminated), infection

Nervous system: Aggressive behavior, anxiety, auditory hallucinations, depression, dizziness, drowsiness, emotional lability, euphoria, fatigue, headache, idiopathic intracranial hypertension, insomnia, irritability, lethargy, malaise, nervousness, outbursts of anger, pain, panic attack, paresthesia, psychosis, seizure, suicidal ideation, suicidal tendencies, violent behavior, voice disorder

Neuromuscular & skeletal: Asthenia, arthritis, bone fracture, calcification of ligament, calcification of tendon, granulomatosis with polyangiitis, limb pain, musculoskeletal pain, myalgia, neck pain, osteopenia, osteoporosis, premature epiphyseal closure, skeletal hyperostosis, stiffness, tendonitis

Ophthalmic: Asthenopia, blepharitis, blurred vision, cataract, conjunctivitis, corneal opacity, decreased visual acuity, eye irritation, eye pruritus, hordeolum, increased lacrimation, keratitis, ocular hyperemia, optic neuritis, photophobia, vision color changes, visual disturbance

Otic: Tinnitus

Renal: Glomerulonephritis

Respiratory: Bronchospasm, dry nose, epistaxis, nasopharyngitis, respiratory tract infection, upper respiratory tract infection

Miscellaneous: Wound healing impairment

Postmarketing: Acute pancreatitis, agranulocytosis, allergic skin reaction, anaphylaxis, auditory impairment, dry eye syndrome, erythema multiforme, eyelid disease (meibomian gland dysfunction/atrophy; Neudorfer 2012), hepatitis, hypersensitivity angiitis, hypersensitivity reaction, intracranial hypertension (Tan 2019), night blindness, rhabdomyolysis, Stevens-Johnson syndrome, toxic epidermal necrolysis

Mechanism of Action Reduces sebaceous gland size and reduces sebum production in acne treatment; in neuroblastoma, decreases cell proliferation and induces differentiation

Pharmacodynamics/Kinetics

Half-life Elimination Terminal: Parent drug: 21 hours; Metabolite: 21 to 24 hours

Time to Peak Serum: 3 to 5 hours

Reproductive Considerations

[US Boxed Warning]: Isotretinoin must not be used by patients who may become pregnant.

Patients of childbearing potential must be able to comply with the guidelines of the iPLEDGE™ pregnancy prevention program. Females of childbearing potential must have 2 negative pregnancy tests with a sensitivity of ≥25 milliunits/mL prior to beginning therapy, and testing should continue monthly during therapy. Patients of childbearing potential should not become pregnant during therapy or for 1 month following discontinuation of isotretinoin. Upon discontinuation of treatment, patients of childbearing potential should have a pregnancy test after their last dose and again 1 month after their last dose.

All patients (male and female), must be registered in the iPLEDGE™ risk management program. Patients of childbearing potential must receive oral and written information reviewing the hazards of therapy and the effects that isotretinoin can have on a fetus. Therapy should not begin without 2 negative pregnancy tests ≥19 days apart. Two forms of contraception (a primary and secondary form as described in the iPLEDGE™ program materials) must be used simultaneously beginning 1 month prior to treatment, during treatment, and for 1 month after therapy is discontinued; limitations to their use must be explained. Micro-dosed progesterone products that do not contain an estrogen ("mini-pills") are not an acceptable form of contraception during isotretinoin treatment. Prescriptions should be written for no more than a 30-day supply, and pregnancy testing and counseling should be repeated monthly. During therapy, pregnancy tests must be conducted by a CLIA-certified laboratory. Prescriptions must be filled and picked up from the pharmacy within 7 days of specimen collection for pregnancy test for patients of childbearing potential. Prescriptions for patients of nonchildbearing potential (male and female) must be filled and picked up within 30 days of prescribing.

Any cases of accidental pregnancy should be reported to the iPLEDGE™ program or FDA MedWatch. All patients (male and female) must read and sign the informed consent material provided in the pregnancy prevention program.

Pregnancy Risk Factor X

Pregnancy Considerations

Isotretinoin and its metabolites can be detected in fetal tissue following maternal use during pregnancy (Benifla 1995; Kraft 1989).

Use is contraindicated in pregnant women. **[US Boxed Warning]: Isotretinoin must not be used by patients who are pregnant. There is an extremely high risk that severe birth defects can result if pregnancy occurs while taking isotretinoin in any amount, even for short periods of time. Potentially, any fetus exposed during pregnancy can be affected. There are no accurate means of determining whether an exposed fetus has been affected. Birth defects that have been documented following isotretinoin exposure include abnormalities of the face, eyes, ears, skull, CNS, cardiovascular system, and thymus and parathyroid glands. Cases of intelligence quotient (IQ) scores less than 85 with or without other abnormalities have been reported. There is an increased risk of spontaneous abortion, and premature births have been reported. Documented external abnormalities include skull abnormality; ear abnormalities (including anotia, micropinna, small or absent external auditory canals); eye abnormalities (including microphthalmia); facial dysmorphia; cleft palate. Documented internal abnormalities include CNS abnormalities (including cerebral abnormalities, cerebellar malformation, hydrocephalus, microcephaly, cranial nerve deficit); cardiovascular abnormalities; thymus gland abnormality; parathyroid hormone deficiency. In some cases, death has occurred with some of the abnormalities previously noted.**

If pregnancy does occur during treatment of a patient who is taking isotretinoin, isotretinoin must be discontinued immediately and the patient should be referred to an obstetrician-gynecologist experienced in reproductive toxicity for further evaluation and counseling.

Any pregnancies should be reported to the iPLEDGE™ program (www.ipledgeprogram.com or 866-495-0654) and the FDA through MedWatch (800-FDA-1088).

◆ **Isotretinoinum** *see* ISOtretinoin (Systemic) *on page 846*

Isoxsuprine (eye SOKS syoo preen)

Pharmacologic Category Vasodilator

Use

Cerebrovascular insufficiency: Relief of symptoms associated with cerebrovascular insufficiency.

Peripheral vascular diseases: Treatment of peripheral vascular diseases, such as arteriosclerosis obliterans, thromboangiitis obliterans (Buerger disease), and Raynaud disease.

Note: More appropriate therapies (medical or surgical) should be considered; efficacy of isoxsuprine in the treatment of these conditions has not been well established.

Local Anesthetic/Vasoconstrictor Precautions No information available to require special precautions

Effects on Dental Treatment May enhance effects of other vasodilators.

Effects on Bleeding No information available to require special precautions

Adverse Reactions Frequency not defined.

Cardiovascular: Chest pain, hypotension, tachycardia

Central nervous system: Dizziness

Dermatologic: Skin rash

Gastrointestinal: Abdominal distress, nausea, vomiting

Mechanism of Action Isoxsuprine increases muscle blood flow, but skin blood flow is usually unaffected. Rather than increasing muscle blood flow by beta-receptor stimulation, isoxsuprine probably has a direct action on vascular smooth muscle. The generally accepted mechanism of action of isoxsuprine on the uterus is beta-adrenergic stimulation (Kaindl 1959; Samuels 1959).

Pharmacodynamics/Kinetics

Time to Peak Time to peak, serum: ~1 hour; serum concentrations maintained for at least 3 hours (Kaindl 1959)

Pregnancy Considerations Isoxsuprine crosses the placenta. Adverse effects (eg, hypocalcemia, hypoglycemia, hypotension, and ileus) requiring treatment have been observed in infants born to mothers who received isoxsuprine during pregnancy. Maternal and fetal tachycardia have occurred with use and pulmonary edema has been reported with maternal use of beta stimulants (Brazy 1979; Brazy 1981). Although isoxsuprine has been evaluated for the treatment of preterm labor, use for this indication is not currently recommended (ACOG 171 2016).

◆ **Isoxsuprine HCl** *see* Isoxsuprine *on page 847*

◆ **Isoxsuprine Hydrochloride** *see* Isoxsuprine *on page 847*

Isradipine (iz RA di peen)

Related Information

Calcium Channel Blockers and Gingival Hyperplasia *on page 1816*

Cardiovascular Diseases *on page 1654*

Pharmacologic Category Antihypertensive; Calcium Channel Blocker; Calcium Channel Blocker, Dihydropyridine

Use Hypertension: Management of hypertension.

Guideline recommendations: The 2017 Guideline for the Prevention, Detection, Evaluation, and Management of High Blood Pressure in Adults recommends if monotherapy is warranted, in the absence of comorbidities (eg, cerebrovascular disease, chronic kidney disease, diabetes, heart failure, ischemic heart disease), that thiazide-like diuretics or dihydropyridine calcium channel blockers may be preferred options due to improved cardiovascular end points (eg, prevention of heart failure and stroke). ACE inhibitors and ARBs are also acceptable for monotherapy. Combination therapy may be required to achieve blood pressure goals and is initially preferred in patients at high risk (stage 2 hypertension or atherosclerotic cardiovascular disease [ASCVD] risk ≥10%) (ACC/AHA [Whelton 2017]).

Local Anesthetic/Vasoconstrictor Precautions Isradipine is one of the drugs confirmed to prolong the QT interval and is accepted as having a risk of causing torsade de pointes. The risk of drug-induced torsade de pointes is extremely low when a single QT interval prolonging drug is prescribed. In terms of epinephrine, it is not known what effect vasoconstrictors in the local anesthetic regimen will have in patients with a known history of congenital prolonged QT interval or in patients taking any medication that prolongs the QT interval. Until more information is obtained, it is suggested that the clinician consult with the physician prior to the use of a vasoconstrictor in suspected patients, and that the vasoconstrictor (epinephrine, mepivacaine and levonordefrin [Carbocaine® 2% with Neo-Cobefrin®]) be used with caution.

Effects on Dental Treatment Unlike other calcium channel blockers, information is sparse as to whether isradipine causes gingival hyperplasia. Consultation with physician is suggested if hyperplasia is observed in patients taking isradipine.

Effects on Bleeding No information available to require special precautions

Adverse Reactions

>10%: Central nervous system: Headache (dose related 2% to 22%)

1% to 10%:

Cardiovascular: Edema (dose related 1% to 9%), flushing (dose related 1% to 5%), palpitations (dose related 1% to 5%), chest pain (3%), tachycardia (1% to 3%)

Central nervous system: Fatigue (dose related ≤9%), dizziness (2% to 8%)

Dermatologic: Skin rash (2%)

Gastrointestinal: Nausea (3% to 5%), abdominal distress (≤3%), diarrhea (≤3%), vomiting (≤1%)

Neuromuscular & skeletal: Weakness (≤1%)

Renal: Urinary frequency (1% to 3%)

Respiratory: Dyspnea (3%)

<1%, postmarketing, and/or case reports: Atrial fibrillation, cardiac failure, cerebrovascular accident, constipation, cough, decreased libido, depression, drowsiness, foot cramps, hyperhidrosis, hypotension, impotence, increased liver enzymes, insomnia, leg cramps, lethargy, leukopenia, myocardial infarction, nervousness, nocturia, numbness, paresthesia, pruritus, sore throat, syncope, transient ischemic attacks, urticaria, ventricular fibrillation, visual disturbance, xerostomia

Mechanism of Action Inhibits calcium ion from entering the "slow channels" or select voltage-sensitive areas of vascular smooth muscle and myocardium during depolarization, producing relaxation of vascular smooth muscle, resulting in coronary vasodilation and reduced blood pressure; increases myocardial oxygen delivery in patients with vasospastic angina

Pharmacodynamics/Kinetics

Onset of Action 2 to 3 hours; **Note:** Full hypotensive effect may not occur for 2 to 4 weeks

Duration of Action >12 hours

Half-life Elimination Alpha half-life: 1.5 to 2 hours; Terminal half-life: 8 hours

Time to Peak Serum: 1 to 1.5 hours

Pregnancy Risk Factor C

Pregnancy Considerations

Isradipine crosses the human placenta. In a study of 16 women, umbilical cord concentrations were less than maternal serum (Lunell 1993).

Chronic maternal hypertension may increase the risk of birth defects, low birth weight, preterm delivery, stillbirth, and neonatal death. Actual fetal/neonatal risks may be related to duration and severity of maternal hypertension. Untreated hypertension may also increase the risks of adverse maternal outcomes, including gestational diabetes, myocardial infarction, preeclampsia, stroke, and delivery complications (ACOG 203 2019).

Calcium channel blockers may be used to treat hypertension in pregnant women; however, agents other than isradipine are more commonly used (ACOG 203 2019; ESC [Regitz-Zagrosek 2018]). Females with preexisting hypertension may continue their medication during pregnancy unless contraindications exist (ESC [Regitz-Zagrosek 2018]).

Dental Health Professional Considerations See Local Anesthetic/Vasoconstrictor Precautions

◆ **Istodax [DSC]** *see* RomiDEPsin *on page 1343*

◆ **Istodax (Overfill)** *see* RomiDEPsin *on page 1343*

Istradefylline (IS tra DEF i lin)

Brand Names: US Nourianz

Pharmacologic Category Anti-Parkinson Agent, Adenosine Receptor Antagonist

Use Parkinson disease, "off" episode: Treatment of Parkinson disease, in combination with levodopa/carbidopa, in adult patients experiencing "off" episodes.

Local Anesthetic/Vasoconstrictor Precautions No information available to require special precautions

Effects on Dental Treatment Key adverse event(s) related to dental treatment: Occurrence of oropharyngeal pain

Effects on Bleeding No information available to require special precautions

Adverse Reactions Frequencies noted refer to experience with combination therapy.

>10%: Neuromuscular & skeletal: Dyskinesia (15% to 17%)

1% to 10%:

Central nervous system: Insomnia (6%), dizziness (3% to 6%), auditory hallucination (≤6%), hallucination (≤6%), visual hallucination (≤6%), abnormal behavior (≤2%), abnormality in thinking (≤2%), aggressive behavior (≤2%), agitation (≤2%), confusion (≤2%), delirium (≤2%), delusion (≤2%), disorientation (≤2%), mania (≤2%), paranoid ideation (≤2%)

Dermatologic: Skin rash (2%)

Endocrine & metabolic: Increased serum glucose (1% to 2%)

Gastrointestinal: Nausea (6%), constipation (5% to 6%), decreased appetite (3%), diarrhea (2%)

Hepatic: Increased serum alkaline phosphatase (2%)

Renal: Increased blood urea nitrogen (1% to 2%)

Respiratory: Upper respiratory tract inflammation (1% to 2%)

<1%: Impulse control disorder

Postmarketing: Increased libido

Mechanism of Action The mechanism of action of istradefylline is unknown. In *in vitro* studies and in *in vivo* animal studies, istradefylline was demonstrated to be an adenosine A_{2A} receptor antagonist.

Pharmacodynamics/Kinetics

Half-life Elimination ~83 hours

Time to Peak Median: 3 to 4 hours

Reproductive Considerations

Females of reproductive potential should use effective contraception during therapy.

Pregnancy Considerations

Based on data from animal reproduction studies, in utero exposure to istradefylline may cause fetal harm.

◆ **Isturisa** *see* Osilodrostat *on page 1148*

◆ **Itch-X [OTC]** *see* Pramoxine *on page 1252*

◆ **Itch Relief [OTC]** *see* DiphenhydrAMINE (Topical) *on page 503*

Itraconazole (i tra KOE na zole)

Brand Names: US Onmel [DSC]; Sporanox; Sporanox Pulsepak; Tolsura

Brand Names: Canada JAMP Itraconazole; MINT-Itraconazole; ODAN Itraconazole; Sporanox

Pharmacologic Category Antifungal Agent, Azole Derivative; Antifungal Agent, Oral

Use

Aspergillosis (capsules): Treatment of pulmonary and extrapulmonary aspergillosis in immunocompromised and nonimmunocompromised patients who are intolerant of or refractory to amphotericin B therapy. **Note:** IDSA Aspergillosis guidelines recommend amphotericin B formulations for invasive aspergillosis (initial or salvage) only when voriconazole is contraindicated or not tolerated (IDSA [Patterson 2016]).

Blastomycosis (capsules): Treatment of pulmonary and extrapulmonary blastomycosis in immunocompromised and nonimmunocompromised patients.

Histoplasmosis (capsules): Treatment of histoplasmosis, including chronic cavitary pulmonary disease and disseminated, nonmeningeal histoplasmosis in immunocompromised and nonimmunocompromised patients.

Onychomycosis:

Capsules (100 mg [Sporanox]): Treatment of onychomycosis of the toenail, with or without fingernail involvement, and onychomycosis of the fingernail caused by dermatophytes (tinea unguium) in nonimmunocompromised patients

Tablets: Treatment of onychomycosis of the toenail caused by *Trichophyton rubrum* or *Trichophyton mentagrophytes* in nonimmunocompromised patients

Oropharyngeal/Esophageal candidiasis (oral solution): Treatment of oropharyngeal and esophageal candidiasis

Canadian labeling: **Oral capsules: Additional indications (not in US labeling):**

Candidiasis, oral and/or esophageal: Treatment of oral and/or esophageal candidiasis in immunocompromised and immunocompetent patients

Chromomycosis: Treatment of chromomycosis in immunocompromised and immunocompetent patients

Dermatomycoses: Treatment of dermatomycoses due to tinea pedis, tinea cruris, tinea corporis, and of pityriasis versicolor in patients for whom oral therapy is appropriate

Onychomycosis: Treatment of onychomycosis in immunocompromised and immunocompetent patients

Paracoccidioidomycosis: Treatment of paracoccidioidomycosis in immunocompromised and immunocompetent patients

Sporotrichosis: Treatment of cutaneous and lymphatic sporotrichosis in immunocompromised and immunocompetent patients

Local Anesthetic/Vasoconstrictor Precautions No information available to require special precautions

Effects on Dental Treatment No significant effects or complications reported

Effects on Bleeding No information available to require special precautions

Adverse Reactions

>10%: Gastrointestinal: Diarrhea (3% to 11%), nausea (3% to 11%)

1% to 10%:

Cardiovascular: Edema (4%), chest pain (3%), hypertension (2% to 3%),

Central nervous system: Headache (1% to 10%), dizziness (2% to 4%), anxiety (3%), depression (2% to 3%), fatigue (2% to 3%), pain (2% to 3%), malaise (1% to 3%), abnormal dreams (2%)

Dermatologic: Skin rash (3% to 9%), pruritus (≤5%), diaphoresis (3%)

Endocrine & metabolic: Hypertriglyceridemia (≤3%), hypokalemia (2%)

Gastrointestinal: Vomiting (5% to 7%), abdominal pain (2% to 6%), dyspepsia (≤4%), flatulence (≤4%), gastrointestinal disease (≤4%), gingivitis (3%), aphthous stomatitis (≤3%), constipation (2% to 3%), gastritis (2%), gastroenteritis (2%), increased appetite (2%)

Genitourinary: Cystitis (2%), urinary tract infection (2%)

Hepatic: Abnormal hepatic function tests (3%), increased liver enzymes (4%)

Infection: Herpes zoster (2%)

Neuromuscular & skeletal: Bursitis (3%), myalgia (≤3%), tremor (2%)

Respiratory: Rhinitis (5% to 9%), upper respiratory tract infection (8%), sinusitis (2% to 7%), cough (4%), dyspnea (2%), pneumonia (2%), pharyngitis (≤2%)

Miscellaneous: Fever (2% to 7%)

<2%, postmarketing, and/or case reports: Abnormal urinalysis, acute generalized exanthematous pustulosis, adrenocortical insufficiency, albuminuria, alopecia, anaphylactoid reaction, anaphylaxis, angioedema, anorexia, arthralgia, blurred vision, cardiac arrhythmia, cardiac failure, chills, confusion, decreased libido, dehydration, diplopia, drowsiness, dysgeusia, dysphagia, erectile dysfunction, erythema multiforme, erythematous rash, exfoliative dermatitis, facial edema, gynecomastia, hearing loss, hematuria, hepatic failure, hepatitis, hepatotoxicity, hot flash, hyperbilirubinemia, hyperglycemia, hyperhidrosis, hyperkalemia, hypersensitivity angiitis, hypersensitivity reaction, hypoesthesia, hypomagnesemia, hypotension, impotence, increased blood urea nitrogen, increased creatine phosphokinase, increased gamma-glutamyl transferase, increased lactate dehydrogenase, increased serum alkaline phosphatase, increased serum ALT, increased serum AST, insomnia, jaundice, left heart failure, leukopenia, menstrual disease, mucosal inflammation, neutropenia, orthostatic hypotension, pancreatitis, paresthesia, peripheral edema, peripheral neuropathy, pharyngolaryngeal pain, pollakiuria, pulmonary edema, renal insufficiency, rigors, serum sickness, sinus bradycardia, skin photosensitivity, Stevens-Johnson syndrome, tachycardia, thrombocytopenia, tinnitus, toxic epidermal necrolysis, urinary incontinence, urticaria, vasculitis, vertigo, voice disorder

Mechanism of Action Interferes with cytochrome P450 activity, decreasing ergosterol synthesis (principal sterol in fungal cell membrane) and inhibiting cell membrane formation

Pharmacodynamics/Kinetics

Half-life Elimination

Children (6 months to 12 years): Oral solution: ~36 hours; Metabolite hydroxy-itraconazole: ~18 hours

Adults: Oral: Single dose: 16 to 28 hours, Multiple doses: 34 to 42 hours; Cirrhosis (single dose): 37 hours (range: 20 to 54 hours)

Time to Peak Plasma: Capsules/tablets: 2 to 5 hours; Oral solution: 2.5 hours

Reproductive Considerations

Use is contraindicated in females planning a pregnancy. Due to the potential risk of congenital malformations, the manufacturer recommends that when used for the treatment of onychomycosis in females of reproductive potential, effective contraception should be used during treatment and for 2 months following treatment. Therapy should begin on the second or third day following menses.

Pregnancy Considerations

Congenital abnormalities (eg, skeletal, genitourinary tract, cardiovascular and ophthalmic malformations, chromosomal abnormalities, and multiple malformations) have been reported during postmarketing surveillance; however, a causal relationship has not been established.

Itraconazole is contraindicated for the treatment of onychomycosis during pregnancy. Although itraconazole is approved for the treatment of various fungal infections, when treatment of a systemic fungal infection is needed in pregnant females, itraconazole should be avoided, especially during the first trimester (Chapman 2008; Galgiani 2016; HHS [OI adult 2017]; Pappas 2016; Perfect 2010; Wheat 2007).

Product Availability Onmel has been discontinued in the US for more than 1 year.

◆ **IUD, Copper** *see* Copper IUD *on page 410*

Ivabradine (eye VAB ra deen)

Brand Names: US Corlanor

Brand Names: Canada Lancora

Pharmacologic Category Cardiovascular Agent, Miscellaneous

Use Heart failure: To reduce the risk of hospitalization for worsening heart failure in adult patients with stable, symptomatic (NYHA class II to III according to the ACC/AHA/HFSA heart failure guidelines [Yancy 2016]) chronic heart failure with left ventricular ejection fraction ≤35%, who are in sinus rhythm with resting heart rate ≥70 beats per minute (bpm) and either are on maximally tolerated doses of beta blockers or have a contraindication to beta-blocker use.

Local Anesthetic/Vasoconstrictor Precautions No information available to require special precautions

Effects on Dental Treatment No significant effects or complications reported

Effects on Bleeding No information available to require special precautions

Adverse Reactions

1% to 10%:

Cardiovascular: Bradycardia (4% to 10%), hypertension (9%), atrial fibrillation (8%)

Central nervous system: Phosphene (3%)

Frequency not defined: Cardiovascular: Heart block, sinoatrial arrest

<1%, postmarketing, and/or case reports: Angioedema, diplopia, erythema, hypotension, pruritus, skin rash, syncope, torsades de pointes, urticaria, ventricular fibrillation, ventricular tachycardia, vertigo, visual impairment

Mechanism of Action Selective and specific inhibition of the hyperpolarization-activated cyclic nucleotide-gated (HCN) channels (f-channels) within the sinoatrial (SA) node of cardiac tissue resulting in disruption of I_f ion current flow prolonging diastolic depolarization, slowing firing in the SA node, and ultimately reducing heart rate. Has not demonstrated effects on myocardial contractility or relaxation, ventricular repolarization, or conduction apart from the sinus node effects. Partial inhibition of the retinal I_h current (similar to the cardiac I_f current) may explain visual disturbances (eg, phosphenes) (Nawarskas 2015).

Pharmacodynamics/Kinetics

Half-life Elimination Distribution half-life: 2 hours; Effective half-life: ~6 hours

Time to Peak Plasma: ~1 hour (fasting); ~2 hours (with food)

Reproductive Considerations

Effective contraception is recommended in women of reproductive potential.

Pregnancy Considerations

Adverse events have been observed in animal reproduction studies, and fetal harm may occur if ivabradine is administered to pregnant women. If treatment is needed during pregnancy, closely monitor for destabilization of heart failure that could potentially result from heart rate slowing caused by ivabradine, especially during the first trimester. Pregnant women with chronic heart failure should also be monitored for preterm birth.

Prescribing and Access Restrictions Corlanor oral solution (for outpatient use) is exclusively distributed through Avella Specialty Pharmacy. Call 1-844-6CORLANOR or visit https://www.corlanorhcp.com/pediatric-indication for additional information.

- **Ivabradine HCl** *see* Ivabradine *on page 850*
- **Ivabradine Hydrochloride** *see* Ivabradine *on page 850*
- **IVIG** *see* Immune Globulin *on page 803*
- **IV Immune Globulin** *see* Immune Globulin *on page 803*
- **IV NEPA** *see* Fosnetupitant and Palonosetron *on page 717*

Ivosidenib (EYE voe SID e nib)

Brand Names: US Tibsovo

Pharmacologic Category Antineoplastic Agent, IDH1 Inhibitor

Use

Acute myeloid leukemia (newly diagnosed): Treatment of newly diagnosed acute myeloid leukemia (AML) in adults ≥75 years of age (or with comorbidities that preclude use of intensive induction chemotherapy) with a susceptible isocitrate dehydrogenase-1 (IDH1) mutation as detected by an approved test.

AML (relapsed/refractory): Treatment of relapsed or refractory AML in adults with a susceptible IDH1 mutation as detected by an approved test.

Local Anesthetic/Vasoconstrictor Precautions

Frequent occurrence of prolonged QT interval has been reported for Ivosidenib. The risk of drug-induced torsades de pointes (arrhythmias) is low when a single QT interval prolonging drug is prescribed. In terms of epinephrine, it is not known what effect vasoconstrictors in the local anesthetic regimen will have in patients with a known history of congenital prolonged QT interval or in patients taking any medication that prolongs the QT interval. Until more information is obtained, it is suggested that the clinician consult with the physician prior to the use of a vasoconstrictor in suspected patients, and that the vasoconstrictor (epinephrine, levonordefrin [Neo-Cobefrin]) be used with caution.

Effects on Dental Treatment Key adverse event(s) related to dental treatment: Orthostatic hypotension has been reported, patients may experience hypotension as they arise from the dental chair; monitor patient for signs of dizziness.

Frequent occurrence of mucositis in patients medicated with Ivosidenib. Mucositis and stomatitis (also known as mucosal barrier injury) are general terms for the erythema, edema, desquamation, and ulceration of the gastrointestinal tract caused by many antineoplastic drugs and external beam radiation therapy (radiotherapy). Stomatitis refers to the finding of mucositis in the mouth or oropharynx. Gastrointestinal complications of mucositis include pain, xerostomia, bloating, diarrhea, malabsorption, and dysmotility. Ivosidenib is a target-specific antineoplastic drug. Oral care for patients taking target-specific agents should align with basic oral care for mucositis due to standard chemotherapy. For management see Ulcerative, Erosive, and Painful Oral Mucosal Disorders on page 1758 and Perioral Premalignant Lesions and Management of Patients Undergoing Cancer Therapy on page 1781.

Effects on Bleeding Target-specific antineoplastics such as Ivosidenib can cause significant myelosuppression including decreased hemoglobin, leukocytosis, and differentiation syndrome.

Adverse Reactions

>10%:

Cardiovascular: Edema (32% to 43%), prolonged QT interval on ECG (21% to 26%), chest pain (16%), hypotension (12%)

Central nervous system: Fatigue (39% to 50%), dizziness (21%), headache (11% to 16%), neuropathy (12% to 14%)

Dermatologic: Skin rash (14% to 26%), pruritis (14%)

Endocrine & metabolic: Decreased serum potassium (31% to 43%), decreased serum sodium (39%), decreased serum magnesium (25% to 38%), increased uric acid (29% to 32%), decreased serum calcium (25%), decreased serum phosphate (21% to 25%), weight loss (11%)

Gastrointestinal: Diarrhea (34% to 61%), decreased appetite (18% to 39%), nausea (31% to 36%), abdominal pain (16% to 29%), stomatitis (21% to 28%; grades ≥3: 3%), constipation (20% to 21%), vomiting (18% to 21%), dyspepsia (11%)

Hematologic & oncologic: Decreased hemoglobin (54% to 60%; ≥3 grade: 43% to 46%), leukocytosis (36% to 38%; ≥3 grade: 7% to 8%), differentiation syndrome (19% to 25%; ≥3 grade: 11% to 13%)

Hepatic: Increased serum alkaline phosphatase (27% to 46%), increased serum aspartate aminotransferase (27% to 29%), increased serum bilirubin (16%), increased serum alanine aminotransferase (14% to 15%)
Neuromuscular & skeletal: Arthralgia (32% to 36%), myalgia (18% to 25%)
Renal: Increased serum creatinine (23% to 29%)
Respiratory: Dyspnea (29% to 33%), cough (14% to 22%), pleural effusion (13%)
Miscellaneous: Fever (23%)

1% to 10%: Hematologic & oncologic: Tumor lysis syndrome (8%; ≥3 grade: 6%)

Frequency not defined:
Cardiovascular: Facial edema, orthostatic hypotension, peripheral edema
Central nervous system: Ataxia, reversible posterior leukoencephalopathy syndrome
Dermatologic: Acneiform eruption, dermal ulcer, exfoliation of skin, urticaria
Endocrine & metabolic: Hypovolemia
Gastrointestinal: Esophageal pain, rectal pain
Neuromuscular & skeletal: Asthenia
Respiratory: Oropharyngeal pain

<1%, postmarketing, and/or case reports: Guillain-Barré syndrome, progressive multifocal leukoencephalopathy, ventricular arrhythmia, ventricular fibrillation

Mechanism of Action Ivosidenib is an oral small-molecule inhibitor of the mutant isocitrate dehydrogenase 1 (IDH1) enzyme. Susceptible IDH1 mutations can lead to increased levels of 2-hydroxyglutarate (2-HG) in leukemia cells. 2-HG inhibits alpha-ketoglutarate-dependent enzymes, resulting in impaired hematopoietic differentiation (DiNardo 2018). In IDH1 mutated AML blood samples, ivosidenib decreased intracellular levels of 2-HG, reduced blast counts, and induced differentiation (resulting in increased percentages of mature myeloid cells). IDH1 mutations occur in ~6% to10% of patients with acute myeloid leukemia (DiNardo 2018).

Pharmacodynamics/Kinetics

Onset of Action
Maximal inhibition of 2-hydroxyglutarate: By day 14 (DiNardo 2018)
Median time to response: 1.9 months; range: 0.8 to 4.7 months (DiNardo 2018)
Median time to complete remission: 2.8 months; range: 0.9 to 8.3 months (DiNardo 2018)

Duration of Action
Median duration of response: 6.5 months (DiNardo 2018)
Median duration of complete remission: 9.3 months (DiNardo 2018)

Half-life Elimination 93 hours

Time to Peak ~3 hours

Pregnancy Considerations Adverse events were observed in animal reproduction studies. The use of ivosidenib during pregnancy may cause fetal harm.

Product Availability Tibsovo: FDA approved July 2018; anticipated availability is currently unknown.

Prescribing and Access Restrictions Ivosidenib is available through a network of select specialty pharmacies. Please refer to http://www.myagios.com or call 844-409-1411 for more information.

Dental Health Professional Considerations Target-specific antineoplastics are differentiated from general chemotherapeutic agents in their specificity for molecular targets and genetic mutations in neoplastic cells. Ivosidenib targets the mutant isocitrate dehydrogenase 1 (IDH1) enzyme.The overall result is effectiveness in treatment of relapsed or refractory acute myeloid leukemia (AML) in adult patients with a susceptible isocitrate dehydrogenase-1 (IDH1) mutation as detected by an approved test. Like chemotherapeutic agents, the target-specific agents can induce mucositis.

Airway compromise can result from mucositis due to severe tissue damage and inflammation. Mucositis is defined as severe (grade 3 to 4) when the pain and anatomic damage prevent adequate oral hydration and oral nutrition, or airway compromise is evident. Severe mucositis increases the risk of infectious complications. Moreover, some opportunistic infections, such as herpes virus, cause and exacerbate mucositis. In addition, severe and prolonged mucositis contributes to anticancer treatment dosage reductions and delays, and increases the cost of therapy.

◆ **IV-VIG** *see* Vaccinia Immune Globulin (Intravenous) *on page 1511*

◆ **Ivy-Rid [OTC]** *see* Benzocaine *on page 228*

◆ **Ivy Wash Poison Ivy Cleanser [OTC]** *see* Pramoxine *on page 1252*

Ixabepilone (ix ab EP i lone)

Brand Names: US Ixempra Kit

Pharmacologic Category Antineoplastic Agent, Antimicrotubular; Antineoplastic Agent, Epothilone B Analog

Use Breast cancer (metastatic or locally advanced): Treatment (in combination with capecitabine) of metastatic or locally advanced breast cancer that is resistant to an anthracycline and a taxane, or that is taxane-resistant and when further anthracycline therapy is contraindicated; treatment (as a single agent) of metastatic or locally advanced breast cancer that is resistant or refractory to anthracyclines, taxanes, and capecitabine.

Anthracycline resistance is defined as progression while on treatment or within 3 months in the metastatic setting or within 6 months in the adjuvant setting. Taxane resistance is defined as progression while on treatment or within 4 months in the metastatic setting or within 12 months in the adjuvant setting.

Local Anesthetic/Vasoconstrictor Precautions No information available to require special precautions

Effects on Dental Treatment Key adverse event(s) related to dental treatment: Stomatitis, mucositis, and taste perversion.

Effects on Bleeding Anemia and thrombocytopenia (grades 3/4: 2% to 5%) are dose-limiting toxicities. Medical consult recommended.

Adverse Reactions

Percentages reported with monotherapy.

>10%:
Central nervous system: Peripheral neuropathy (63%; grades 3/4: 14%; grade 3/4 median onset: Cycle 4), peripheral sensory neuropathy (62%; grades 3/4: 14%), headache (11%)
Dermatologic: Alopecia (48%)
Gastrointestinal: Nausea (42%), vomiting (29%), mucositis (≤29%), stomatitis (≤29%), diarrhea (22%), anorexia (19%), constipation (16%), abdominal pain (13%)

Hematologic & oncologic: Leukopenia (grade 3: 36%; grade 4: 13%), neutropenia (grade 3: 31%; grade 4: 23%)
Neuromuscular & skeletal: Weakness (56%), arthralgia (≤49%), myalgia (≤49%), musculoskeletal pain (20%)
1% to 10%:
Cardiovascular: Edema (9%), chest pain (5%)
Central nervous system: Peripheral motor neuropathy (10%; grade 3: 1%), pain (8%), dizziness (7%), insomnia (5%)
Dermatologic: Nail disease (9%), skin rash (9%), palmar-plantar erythrodysesthesia (8%), pruritus (6%), desquamation (2%), hyperpigmentation (2%)
Endocrine & metabolic: Hot flash (6%), weight loss (6%), dehydration (2%)
Gastrointestinal: Dysgeusia (6%), gastroesophageal reflux (6%)
Hematologic & oncologic: Anemia (grade 3: 6%; grade 4: 2%), febrile neutropenia (3%; grade 3: 3%), thrombocytopenia (grade 3: 5%; grade 4: 2%)
Hypersensitivity: Hypersensitivity (5%; grade 3: 1%)
Infection: Infection (5%)
Ophthalmic: Increased lacrimation (4%)
Respiratory: Dyspnea (9%), upper respiratory tract infection (6%), cough (2%)
Miscellaneous: Fever (8%)

Mono- and combination therapy: <1%, postmarketing, and/or case reports: Acute hepatic failure, acute pulmonary edema, angina pectoris, atrial flutter, autonomic neuropathy, blood coagulation disorder, cardiomyopathy, cerebral hemorrhage, colitis, delayed gastric emptying, dysphagia, embolism, enterocolitis, erythema multiforme, gastrointestinal hemorrhage, hemorrhage, hypokalemia, hyponatremia, hypotension, hypovolemia, hypovolemic shock, hypoxia, increased gamma-glutamyl transferase, increased serum alkaline phosphatase, increased serum transaminases, interstitial pneumonitis, intestinal obstruction, jaundice, left ventricular dysfunction, metabolic acidosis, myocardial infarction, nephrolithiasis, neutropenic infection, orthostatic hypotension, pneumonia, pneumonitis, radiation recall phenomenon, renal failure, respiratory failure, sepsis, septic shock, supraventricular cardiac arrhythmia, syncope, thrombosis, trismus, urinary tract infection, vasculitis, voice disorder

Mechanism of Action Ixabepilone is an epothilone B analog, which binds to the beta-tubulin subunit of the microtubule, stabilizing microtubular promoting tubulin polymerization and stabilizing microtubular function, thus arresting the cell cycle (at the G2/M phase) and inducing apoptosis. Activity in taxane-resistant cells has been demonstrated.

Pharmacodynamics/Kinetics

Half-life Elimination ~52 hours

Time to Peak At the end of the 3-hour infusion

Reproductive Considerations

Females of reproductive potential should be advised to use effective contraception during treatment.

Pregnancy Risk Factor D

Pregnancy Considerations

Adverse events were observed in animal reproduction studies. May cause fetal harm if administered during pregnancy.

Ixazomib (ix AZ oh mib)

Brand Names: US Ninlaro
Brand Names: Canada Ninlaro

Pharmacologic Category Antineoplastic Agent, Proteasome Inhibitor

Use Multiple myeloma: Treatment of multiple myeloma (in combination with lenalidomide and dexamethasone) in patients who have received at least one prior therapy

Local Anesthetic/Vasoconstrictor Precautions No information available to require special precautions

Effects on Dental Treatment No significant effects or complications reported

Effects on Bleeding Cytopenias including thrombocytopenia (grades 3/4, 26%) has been reported. Medical consult is recommended.

Adverse Reactions Adverse reaction percentages reported as part of a combination regimen with lenalidomide and dexamethasone.

>10%:
Cardiovascular: Peripheral edema (25%)
Dermatologic: Skin rash (19%)
Gastrointestinal: Constipation (34%), diarrhea (42%), nausea (26%), vomiting (22%)
Hematologic & oncologic: Neutropenia (67%; grades 3/4: 26%), thrombocytopenia (78%; grades 3/4: 26%)
Nervous system: Peripheral neuropathy (28%; grade 3: 2%), peripheral sensory neuropathy (19%)
Neuromuscular & skeletal: Back pain (21%)
Ophthalmic: Eye disease (26%)
Respiratory: Upper respiratory tract infection (19%)
1% to 10%:
Hepatic: Hepatic insufficiency (6%)
Infection: Herpes zoster infection (4%; <1% with antiviral prophylaxis)
Ophthalmic: Blurred vision (6%), conjunctivitis (6%), xerophthalmia (5%)
<1%:
Hepatic: Cholestatic hepatitis, hepatocellular hepatitis, hepatotoxicity, liver steatosis
Nervous system: Peripheral motor neuropathy
Postmarketing:
Dermatologic: Stevens-Johnson syndrome, Sweet's syndrome
Hematologic & oncologic: Hemolytic-uremic syndrome, thrombotic microangiopathy, thrombotic thrombocytopenic purpura, tumor lysis syndrome
Nervous system: Reversible posterior leukoencephalopathy syndrome, transverse myelitis

Mechanism of Action Ixazomib reversibly inhibits proteasomes, enzyme complexes which regulate protein homeostasis within the cell. Specifically, it reversibly inhibits chymotrypsin-like activity of the beta 5 subunit of the 20S proteasome, leading to activation of signaling cascades, cell-cycle arrest, and apoptosis.

Pharmacodynamics/Kinetics

Half-life Elimination Terminal: 9.5 days

Time to Peak Median: 1 hour

Reproductive Considerations

Males and females of reproductive potential should use effective contraception during therapy and for 90 days after the last dose. Women using hormonal contraception should also use a barrier method.

Pregnancy Considerations

Based on the mechanism of action and data from animal reproduction studies, in utero exposure to ixazomib may cause fetal harm.

When used for the treatment of multiple myeloma, ixazomib is indicated to be used with lenalidomide and dexamethasone. Lenalidomide is contraindicated for use during pregnancy (refer to Lenalidomide monograph for details).

Prescribing and Access Restrictions Available through specialty pharmacies and distributors. Further information may be obtained from the manufacturer, Takeda Oncology, at 1-800-390-5663 or at http://www.-ninlarohcp.com.

◆ **Ixazomib Citrate** *see* Ixazomib *on page 853*

Ixekizumab (ix ee KIZ ue mab)

Brand Names: US Taltz

Brand Names: Canada Taltz

Pharmacologic Category Anti-interleukin 17A Monoclonal Antibody; Antipsoriatic Agent; Monoclonal Antibody

Use

Ankylosing spondylitis: Treatment of active ankylosing spondylitis in adult patients.

Nonradiographic axial spondyloarthritis: Treatment of active nonradiographic axial spondyloarthritis with objective signs of inflammation in adult patients.

Plaque psoriasis: Treatment of moderate to severe plaque psoriasis in adult and pediatric patients ≥6 years of age who are candidates for systemic therapy or phototherapy.

Psoriatic arthritis: Treatment of active psoriatic arthritis in adult patients.

Local Anesthetic/Vasoconstrictor Precautions

No information available to require special precautions

Effects on Dental Treatment No significant effects or complications reported

Effects on Bleeding No information available to require special precautions

Adverse Reactions

>10%:

Hematologic & oncologic: Neutropenia (11%; grades ≥3: <1%)

Immunologic: Antibody development (5% to 22%; neutralizing antibodies associated with decreased drug concentration and loss of efficacy: 2%)

Infection: Infection (27% to 38%; maintenance period: 57%; serious infection: <1%)

Local: Injection site reaction (17%; includes erythema at injection site, pain at injection site)

Respiratory: Upper respiratory tract infection (14%)

1% to 10%:

Dermatologic: Tinea (2%)

Gastrointestinal: Crohn's disease (≤1%), nausea (2%)

Hematologic & oncologic: Thrombocytopenia (3%)

Infection: Influenza (≤1%)

Ophthalmic: Conjunctivitis (adults: ≤1%; children and adolescents: 3%)

<1%:

Dermatologic: Urticaria

Gastrointestinal: Inflammatory bowel disease, oral candidiasis, ulcerative colitis

Hypersensitivity: Angioedema, severe hypersensitivity reaction

Respiratory: Rhinitis

Postmarketing: Hypersensitivity: Anaphylaxis

Mechanism of Action Ixekizumab is a humanized IgG4 monoclonal antibody that selectively binds with the interleukin 17A (IL-17A) cytokine and inhibits its interaction with the IL-17 receptor. IL-17A is a naturally occurring cytokine that is involved in normal inflammatory and immune responses. Ixekizumab inhibits the release of proinflammatory cytokines and chemokines.

Pharmacodynamics/Kinetics

Half-life Elimination 13 days

Time to Peak ~4 days

Reproductive Considerations

The American Academy of Dermatology considers ixekizumab for the treatment of psoriasis to be likely compatible for use in male patients planning to father a child (AAD-NPF [Menter 2019]).

Women and men with well-controlled psoriasis who are planning a pregnancy and wish to avoid fetal exposure can consider discontinuing ixekizumab 9 weeks prior to attempting pregnancy (Rademaker 2018).

Pregnancy Considerations

Ixekizumab is a humanized monoclonal antibody (IgG_4). Placental transfer of human IgG is dependent upon the IgG subclass, maternal serum concentrations, birth weight, and gestational age, generally increasing as pregnancy progresses. The lowest exposure would be expected during the period of organogenesis (Palmeira 2012; Pentsuk 2009).

◆ **Ixempra Kit** *see* Ixabepilone *on page 852*

◆ **Ixifi** *see* InFLIXimab *on page 809*

◆ **Jaimiess** *see* Ethinyl Estradiol and Levonorgestrel *on page 612*

◆ **Jakafi** *see* Ruxolitinib *on page 1351*

◆ **Jalyn** *see* Dutasteride and Tamsulosin *on page 540*

◆ **Jantoven** *see* Warfarin *on page 1557*

◆ **Janumet** *see* Sitagliptin and Metformin *on page 1376*

◆ **Janumet XR** *see* Sitagliptin and Metformin *on page 1376*

◆ **Januvia** *see* SITagliptin *on page 1376*

◆ **Jardiance** *see* Empagliflozin *on page 555*

◆ **Jasmiel** *see* Ethinyl Estradiol and Drospirenone *on page 610*

◆ **Jatenzo** *see* Testosterone *on page 1425*

◆ **Jelmyto** *see* MitoMYcin (Systemic) *on page 1041*

◆ **Jencycla** *see* Norethindrone *on page 1117*

◆ **Jentadueto** *see* Linagliptin and Metformin *on page 917*

◆ **Jentadueto XR** *see* Linagliptin and Metformin *on page 917*

◆ **Jevantique Lo [DSC]** *see* Ethinyl Estradiol and Norethindrone *on page 614*

◆ **Jinteli** *see* Ethinyl Estradiol and Norethindrone *on page 614*

◆ **JNJ-54767414** *see* Daratumumab *on page 438*

◆ **JNJ-56021927** *see* Apalutamide *on page 158*

◆ **Jock Itch Spray [OTC]** *see* Tolnaftate *on page 1462*

◆ **Jolessa** *see* Ethinyl Estradiol and Levonorgestrel *on page 612*

◆ **Jolivette [DSC]** *see* Norethindrone *on page 1117*

◆ **Jornay PM** *see* Methylphenidate *on page 997*

◆ **Jublia** *see* Efinaconazole *on page 546*

◆ **Juleber** *see* Ethinyl Estradiol and Desogestrel *on page 609*

◆ **Juluca** *see* Dolutegravir and Rilpivirine *on page 512*

◆ **Junel 1.5/30** *see* Ethinyl Estradiol and Norethindrone *on page 614*

◆ **Junel 1/20** *see* Ethinyl Estradiol and Norethindrone *on page 614*

◆ **Junel FE 1.5/30** *see* Ethinyl Estradiol and Norethindrone *on page 614*

◆ **Junel FE 1/20** *see* Ethinyl Estradiol and Norethindrone *on page 614*

- ◆ **Junel Fe 24** *see* Ethinyl Estradiol and Norethindrone *on page 614*
- ◆ **Just For Kids [OTC]** *see* Fluoride *on page 693*
- ◆ **Juvederm Ultra** *see* Hyaluronate and Derivatives *on page 761*
- ◆ **Juvederm Ultra XC** *see* Hyaluronate and Derivatives *on page 761*
- ◆ **Juvederm Ultra Plus** *see* Hyaluronate and Derivatives *on page 761*
- ◆ **Juvederm Ultra Plus XC** *see* Hyaluronate and Derivatives *on page 761*
- ◆ **Juvederm Voluma XC** *see* Hyaluronate and Derivatives *on page 761*
- ◆ **Juxtapid** *see* Lomitapide *on page 927*
- ◆ **Jynarque** *see* Tolvaptan *on page 1463*
- ◆ **Kadcyla** *see* Ado-Trastuzumab Emtansine *on page 86*
- ◆ **Kadian** *see* Morphine (Systemic) *on page 1050*
- ◆ **Kaitlib Fe** *see* Ethinyl Estradiol and Norethindrone *on page 614*
- ◆ **Kala [OTC]** *see Lactobacillus on page 869*
- ◆ **Kaletra** *see* Lopinavir and Ritonavir *on page 929*
- ◆ **Kalliga** *see* Ethinyl Estradiol and Desogestrel *on page 609*
- ◆ **Kanjinti** *see* Trastuzumab *on page 1479*
- ◆ **Kank-A Mouth Pain [OTC] [DSC]** *see* Benzocaine *on page 228*
- ◆ **Kao-Tin [OTC]** *see* Docusate *on page 509*
- ◆ **Kapidex** *see* Dexlansoprazole *on page 471*
- ◆ **Kapspargo Sprinkle** *see* Metoprolol *on page 1009*
- ◆ **Kapvay** *see* CloNIDine *on page 389*
- ◆ **Karbinal ER** *see* Carbinoxamine *on page 292*
- ◆ **Kariva** *see* Ethinyl Estradiol and Desogestrel *on page 609*
- ◆ **Katerzia** *see* AmLODIPine *on page 121*
- ◆ **KCl** *see* Potassium Chloride *on page 1249*
- ◆ **Kdur** *see* Potassium Chloride *on page 1249*
- ◆ **Kedrab** *see* Rabies Immune Globulin (Human) *on page 1302*
- ◆ **Keep Alert [OTC]** *see* Caffeine *on page 277*
- ◆ **Keflex** *see* Cephalexin *on page 322*
- ◆ **Kefzol** *see* CeFAZolin *on page 301*
- ◆ **Kelnor 1/35** *see* Ethinyl Estradiol and Ethynodiol Diacetate *on page 611*
- ◆ **Kelnor 1/50** *see* Ethinyl Estradiol and Ethynodiol Diacetate *on page 611*
- ◆ **Kenalog** *see* Triamcinolone (Systemic) *on page 1485*
- ◆ **Kenalog** *see* Triamcinolone (Topical) *on page 1490*
- ◆ **Kenalog-80** *see* Triamcinolone (Systemic) *on page 1485*
- ◆ **Kengreal** *see* Cangrelor *on page 282*
- ◆ **Keoxifene Hydrochloride** *see* Raloxifene *on page 1304*
- ◆ **Kepivance** *see* Palifermin *on page 1181*
- ◆ **Keppra** *see* LevETIRAcetam *on page 894*
- ◆ **Keppra XR** *see* LevETIRAcetam *on page 894*
- ◆ **Keratinocyte Growth Factor, Recombinant Human** *see* Palifermin *on page 1181*
- ◆ **Kerlone** *see* Betaxolol (Systemic) *on page 240*
- ◆ **Ketalar** *see* Ketamine *on page 855*

Ketamine (KEET a meen)

Brand Names: US Ketalar

Brand Names: Canada Ketalar

Pharmacologic Category General Anesthetic

Use Anesthesia: Induction and maintenance of general anesthesia.

Local Anesthetic/Vasoconstrictor Precautions No information available to require special precautions

Effects on Dental Treatment Key adverse event(s) related to dental treatment: Increased salivation.

Effects on Bleeding No information available to require special precautions

Adverse Reactions

>10%: Central nervous system: Prolonged emergence from anesthesia (12%; includes confusion, delirium, dreamlike state, excitement, hallucinations, irrational behavior, vivid imagery)

Frequency not defined:

Cardiovascular: Bradycardia, cardiac arrhythmia, hypotension, increased blood pressure, increased pulse

Central nervous system: Drug dependence, hypertonia (tonic-clonic movements sometimes resembling seizures), increased cerebrospinal fluid pressure

Dermatologic: Erythema, morbilliform rash, rash at injection site

Endocrine & metabolic: Central diabetes insipidus (Hatab 2014)

Gastrointestinal: Anorexia, nausea, sialorrhea (Hatab 2014), vomiting

Genitourinary: Bladder dysfunction (reduced capacity), cystitis (including cystitis noninfective, cystitis interstitial, cystitis ulcerative, cystitis erosive, cystitis hemorrhagic), dysuria, hematuria, urinary frequency, urinary incontinence, urinary urgency

Hypersensitivity: Anaphylaxis

Local: Pain at injection site

Neuromuscular & skeletal: Laryngospasm

Ophthalmic: Diplopia, increased intraocular pressure, nystagmus

Renal: Hydronephrosis

Respiratory: Airway obstruction, apnea, respiratory depression

Mechanism of Action Produces a cataleptic-like state in which the patient is dissociated from the surrounding environment by direct action on the cortex and limbic system. Ketamine is a noncompetitive NMDA receptor antagonist that blocks glutamate. Low (subanesthetic) doses produce analgesia, and modulate central sensitization, hyperalgesia and opioid tolerance. Reduces polysynaptic spinal reflexes.

Pharmacodynamics/Kinetics

Onset of Action

IV: Anesthetic effect: Within 30 seconds

IM: Anesthetic effect: 3 to 4 minutes; Analgesia: Within 10 to 15 minutes

Intranasal: Analgesic effect: Within 10 minutes (Carr 2004); Sedation: Children 2 to 6 years: 5 to 8 minutes (Bahetwar 2011)

Oral: Analgesia: Within 30 minutes; Sedation: Children 2 to 8 years (Turhanoglu 2003):

4 mg/kg/dose: 12.9 ± 1.9 minutes

6 mg/kg/dose: 10.4 ± 2.9 minutes

8 mg/kg/dose: 9.5 ± 1.9 minutes

Duration of Action

IV: Anesthetic effect: 5 to 10 minutes; Recovery: 1 to 2 hours

IM: Anesthetic effect: 12 to 25 minutes; Analgesia: 15 to 30 minutes; Recovery: 3 to 4 hours

Intranasal: Analgesic effect: Up to 60 minutes (Carr 2004); Recovery: Children 2 to 6 years: 34 to 46 minutes (Bahetwar 2011)

Half-life Elimination Alpha: 10 to 15 minutes; Beta: 2.5 hours

Time to Peak

Plasma:

IM: 5 to 30 minutes (Clements 1982)

Intranasal: 10 to 14 minutes (Huge 2010); Children 2 to 9 years: ~20 minutes (Malinovsky 1996)

Oral: ~30 minutes (Soto 2012)

Rectal: Children 2 to 9 years: ~45 minutes (Malinovsky 1996)

Pregnancy Considerations

Ketamine crosses the placenta (Ellingson 1977; Little 1972).

Ketamine produces dose dependent increases in uterine contractions; effects may vary by trimester. The plasma clearance of ketamine is reduced during pregnancy. Dose related neonatal depression and decreased Apgar scores have been reported with large doses administered at delivery (Little 1972; Neuman 2013; White 1982).

Based on animal data, repeated or prolonged use of general anesthetic and sedation medications that block N-methyl-D-aspartate (NMDA) receptors and/or potentiate gamma-aminobutyric acid (GABA) activity may affect brain development. Evaluate benefits and potential risks of fetal exposure to ketamine when duration of surgery is expected to be >3 hours (Olutoye 2018).

Although obstetric use is not recommended by the manufacturer, ketamine has been evaluated for use during cesarean and vaginal delivery (ACOG 209 2019; Akamatsu 1974; Galbert 1973). Ketamine may be considered as an alternative induction agent in females requiring general anesthesia for cesarean delivery who are hemodynamically unstable (Devroe 2015). Use of ketamine as an adjunctive analgesic in cesarean section has also been evaluated; however, use for this purpose may require additional studies (Carvalho 2017; Heesen 2015). When sedation and analgesia is needed for other procedures during pregnancy, low doses of ketamine may be used, but other agents are preferred (Neuman 2013; Schwenk 2018). Use of ketamine infusion for the treatment of refractory status epilepticus in a pregnant patient has been noted in a case report (Talahma 2018).

The ACOG recommends that pregnant women should not be denied medically necessary surgery, regardless of trimester. If the procedure is elective, it should be delayed until after delivery (ACOG 775 2019).

Controlled Substance C-III

◆ **Ketamine HCl** *see* Ketamine *on page* 855

◆ **Ketamine Hydrochloride** *see* Ketamine *on page* 855

◆ **Ketek [DSC]** *see* Telithromycin *on page* 1412

Ketoconazole (Systemic) (kee toe KOE na zole)

Related Information

Fungal Infections *on page* 1752

Related Sample Prescriptions

Fungal Infections - Sample Prescriptions *on page* 38

Brand Names: Canada APO-Ketoconazole; Ketoconazole-200; TEVA-Ketoconazole

Generic Availability (US) Yes

Pharmacologic Category Antifungal Agent, Imidazole Derivative; Antifungal Agent, Oral

Dental Use Treatment of susceptible fungal infections in the oral cavity including candidiasis, oral thrush, and chronic mucocutaneous candidiasis

Use Fungal infections (systemic):

US labeling: Treatment of susceptible systemic fungal infections, including blastomycosis, histoplasmosis, paracoccidioidomycosis, coccidioidomycosis, and chromomycosis in patients who have failed or who are intolerant to other antifungal therapies

Limitations of use: Ketoconazole should only be used when other effective antifungal therapy is not available or tolerated **and** the potential benefits outweigh the potential risks. Ketoconazole tablets are not indicated for the treatment of onychomycosis, cutaneous dermatophyte infections, or Candida infections.

Canadian labeling: Treatment of serious or life-threatening systemic fungal infections (eg, systemic candidiasis, chronic mucocutaneous candidiasis, coccidioidomycosis, paracoccidioidomycosis, histoplasmosis, and chromomycosis) where alternate therapy is inappropriate or ineffective; may be considered for severe dermatophytoses unresponsive to other therapy

Local Anesthetic/Vasoconstrictor Precautions No information available to require special precautions

Effects on Dental Treatment No significant effects or complications reported

Effects on Bleeding No information available to require special precautions

Adverse Reactions Frequency not always defined.

Cardiovascular: Orthostatic hypotension, peripheral edema

Central nervous system: Fatigue, insomnia, malaise, nervousness, paresthesia

Dermatologic: Pruritus (2%), alopecia, dermatitis, erythema, erythema multiforme, skin rash, urticaria, xeroderma

Endocrine & metabolic: Hot flash, hyperlipidemia, menstrual disease

Gastrointestinal: Nausea (3%), vomiting (3%), abdominal pain (1%), anorexia, constipation, dysgeusia, dyspepsia, flatulence, increased appetite, tongue discoloration, upper abdominal pain, xerostomia

Hematologic & oncologic: Decreased platelet count

Hepatic: Jaundice

Hypersensitivity: Anaphylactoid reaction

Neuromuscular & skeletal: Myalgia, weakness

Respiratory: Epistaxis

Miscellaneous: Alcohol intolerance

<1%, postmarketing, and/or case reports: Acute generalized exanthematous pustulosis, adrenocortical insufficiency (≥400 mg/day), anaphylactic shock, anaphylaxis, angioedema, arthralgia, azoospermia, bulging fontanel (infants), chills, cholestatic hepatitis, cirrhosis, decreased plasma testosterone (impaired at 800 mg/day), depression, diarrhea, dizziness, drowsiness, erectile dysfunction (doses >200-400 mg/day),

fever, gynecomastia, headache, hemolytic anemia, hepatic failure, hepatic necrosis, hepatitis, hepatotoxicity, hypertriglyceridemia, hypersensitivity reaction, impotence, increased intracranial pressure (reversible), leukopenia, myopathy, papilledema, photophobia, prolonged QT interval on ECG, skin photosensitivity, suicidal tendencies, thrombocytopenia

Dental Usual Dosage Oral fungal infections: Oral:

Children ≥2 years: 3.3-6.6 mg/kg/day as a single dose for 1-2 weeks for candidiasis, for at least 4 weeks in recalcitrant dermatophyte infections, and for up to 6 months for other systemic mycoses

Adults: 200-400 mg/day as a single daily dose for durations as stated above

Dosing

Adult & Geriatric

Fungal infections (systemic): Oral: 200 mg once daily; may increase to 400 mg once daily if response is insufficient. Continue until active fungal infection is resolved; some infections may require a treatment duration of up to 6 months.

Prostate cancer, advanced (off-label use): Oral: 400 mg 3 times daily (in combination with oral hydrocortisone) until disease progression (Ryan 2007; Small 2004)

Cushing syndrome (off-label use): Oral: Initial: 400 to 600 mg daily in 2 or 3 divided doses; may increase dose by 200 mg daily every 7 to 28 days up to a maximum of 1,200 mg daily in 2 or 3 divided doses; dosage range: 200 to 1,200 mg daily; mean effective dose in most studies: 600 to 800 mg daily in 2 divided doses (Castinetti 2014; ES [Nieman 2015]; Miller 1993)

Renal Impairment: Adult

The renal dosing recommendations are based upon the best available evidence and clinical expertise. Senior Editorial Team: Bruce Mueller, PharmD, FCCP, FASN, FNKF; Jason Roberts, PhD, BPharm (Hons), B App Sc, FSHP, FISAC; Michael Heung, MD, MS.

Mild to severe impairment: No dosage adjustment necessary because ketoconazole pharmacokinetics are not significantly altered in patients with kidney impairment (Daneshmend 1988).

Hemodialysis: Minimally dialyzable: No dosage adjustment necessary because ketoconazole pharmacokinetics are not significantly altered in patients on hemodialysis (Brass 1982).

Hepatic Impairment: Adult

Use is contraindicated in acute or chronic liver disease.

Hepatotoxicity during treatment:

US labeling: If ALT >ULN or 30% above baseline (or if patient is symptomatic), interrupt therapy and obtain full hepatic function panel. Upon normalization of liver function, may consider resuming therapy if benefit outweighs risk (hepatotoxicity has been reported on rechallenge).

Canadian labeling: Discontinue therapy for liver function tests >3 times ULN or if abnormalities persist, worsen, or are associated with hepatotoxicity symptoms.

Pediatric

Fungal infections (systemic): Children ≥2 years and Adolescents: Oral: 3.3 to 6.6 mg/kg/day once daily; maximum daily dose: 400 mg/**day**; duration of therapy variable based on pathogen, patient, and disease-specific factors. **Note:** Usual adult dose: 200 mg/**day**; systemic ketoconazole should only be used when other effective antifungal therapy is not available or tolerated due to potential for serious adverse reactions.

Peripheral precocious puberty (gonadotropin-independent): Very limited data available, optimal dose not defined: Children ≥2 years and Adolescents: Oral: 10 to 20 mg/kg/day in 3 divided doses (Schoelwer 2016; Kliegman 2020). Reported doses in patients with familial male-limited precocious puberty or McCune-Albright syndrome vary widely; however, all describe response with decreased testosterone levels and cessation of puberty; some authors report flat doses of 400 to 600 mg/**day** divided 2 to 3 times daily (Holland 1987; Messina 2008; Syed 1999); others describe weight-based doses as high as 30 mg/kg/day in 3 divided doses (Almeida 2008; Soriano-Guillén 2005).

Cushing syndrome, second-line therapy: Very limited data available: Children ≥12 years and Adolescents: Oral: Initial: 400 to 600 mg/**day** in 2 or 3 divided doses; doses can be increased by 200 mg/**day** every 7 to 28 days based on patient response (urinary or plasma cortisol) and tolerability to 800 to 1,200 mg/**day** in 2 or 3 divided doses (Young 2018; European Medicines Agency 2020). In one compassionate use trial of adult and pediatric patients with Cushing syndrome (n=108; mean age: 51.3 years; range: 11 to 86 years), median final dose of ketoconazole was 600 mg/**day** (range: 200 to 1,200 mg/**day**) in divided doses (Young 2018).

Renal Impairment: Pediatric

Altered kidney function: Children ≥2 years and Adolescents: Oral:

Mild to severe impairment: No dosage adjustment necessary.

Hemodialysis: Minimally dialyzable: There are no dosage adjustments provided in the manufacturer's labeling; ketoconazole pharmacokinetics are not significantly altered in patients on hemodialysis, and, as a result, no dosage adjustments are necessary (Brass 1982).

Hepatic Impairment: Pediatric

Children ≥2 years and Adolescents:

Baseline hepatic impairment: There are no dosage adjustments provided in manufacturer's labeling; use with extreme caution due to risks of hepatotoxicity; use is contraindicated with acute or chronic liver disease.

Hepatotoxicity during treatment: If ALT > ULN or 30% above baseline (or if patient is symptomatic), interrupt therapy and obtain full hepatic function panel. Upon normalization of liver function, may consider resuming therapy if benefit outweighs risk (hepatotoxicity has been reported on rechallenge).

Mechanism of Action Alters the permeability of the cell wall by blocking fungal cytochrome P450; inhibits biosynthesis of triglycerides and phospholipids by fungi; inhibits several fungal enzymes that results in a build-up of toxic concentrations of hydrogen peroxide; for management of prostate cancer, ketoconazole inhibits androgen synthesis

Contraindications

Hypersensitivity to ketoconazole or any component of the formulation; acute or chronic liver disease; coadministration with alprazolam, cisapride, colchicine, disopyramide, dofetilide, dronedarone, eplerenone, ergot alkaloids (eg, dihydroergotamine, ergometrine, ergotamine, methylergometrine), felodipine, HMG-CoA reductase inhibitors (eg, lovastatin, simvastatin), irinotecan, lurasidone, methadone, oral midazolam, nisoldipine, pimozide, quinidine, ranolazine, tolvaptan, triazolam

Canadian labeling: Additional contraindications (not in US labeling): Women of childbearing potential unless effective forms of contraception are used; coadministration with astemizole or terfenadine

Warnings/Precautions [US Boxed Warning]: Ketoconazole tablets are not indicated for the treatment of onychomycosis, cutaneous dermatophyte infections, or Candida infections. Use only when other effective antifungal therapy is unavailable or not tolerated and the benefits of ketoconazole treatment are considered to outweigh the risks. Ketoconazole oral tablets are only approved to treat systemic fungal infections and should not be prescribed to treat skin and nail fungal infections; the risks of serious liver damage, adrenal gland problems and drug-drug interactions outweigh any potential benefit. Ketoconazole has poor penetration into cerebral-spinal fluid and should not be used to treat fungal meningitis.

[US Boxed Warning]: Ketoconazole has been associated with hepatotoxicity, including fatal cases and cases requiring liver transplantation; some patients had no apparent risk factors for hepatic disease. Patients should be advised of the hepatotoxicity risks and monitored closely. Toxicity was observed after a median duration of therapy of ~4 weeks but has also been noted after as little as 3 days; may occur when patients receive high doses for short durations or low doses for long durations. Cases have been reported in patients treated with ketoconazole for onychomycosis, cutaneous dermatophyte infections, or Candida infections. Use with caution in patients with preexisting hepatic impairment, those on prolonged therapy and/or taking other hepatotoxic drugs concurrently. Hepatic dysfunction is typically (but not always) reversible upon discontinuation. Obtain liver function tests at baseline and frequently throughout therapy; serum ALT should be monitored weekly throughout therapy. Discontinue therapy for elevated hepatic enzymes that persist or worsen or if accompanied by signs/symptoms (eg, jaundice, nausea/vomiting, dark urine) of hepatic injury.

High doses of ketoconazole may depress adrenocortical function; returns to baseline upon discontinuation of therapy. Recommended maximum dosing should not be exceeded. Monitor adrenal function as clinically necessary, particularly in patients with adrenal insufficiency and in patients under prolonged stress (eg, intensive care, major surgery). In European clinical trials of men with metastatic prostate cancer, fatalities were reported in a small number of study participants within 14 days of initiating high-dose ketoconazole (1,200 mg daily); a causal effect has not been established. In animal studies, increased long bone fragility with cases of fracture has been observed with high-dose ketoconazole. Careful dose selection may be advisable for patients susceptible to bone fragility (eg, postmenopausal women, elderly). Cases of hypersensitivity reactions (including rare cases of anaphylaxis) have been reported; some reactions occurred after the initial dose.

[US Boxed Warning]: Concomitant use with cisapride, disopyramide, dofetilide, dronedarone, methadone, pimozide, quinidine, and ranolazine is contraindicated due to the possible occurrence of life-threatening ventricular arrhythmias such as torsade de pointes. Concomitant use with HMG-CoA reductase inhibitors (eg, lovastatin, simvastatin) or with oral midazolam, triazolam, and alprazolam is contraindicated. Absorption is reduced in patients with achlorhydria; administer with acidic liquids (eg, soda pop). Avoid concomitant use of drugs that decrease gastric acidity (eg, proton pump inhibitors, antacids, H_2-blockers). Other potentially significant interactions may exist, requiring dose or frequency adjustment, additional monitoring, and/or selection of alternative therapy.

Drug Interactions

Metabolism/Transport Effects Substrate of CYP3A4 (major); **Note:** Assignment of Major/Minor substrate status based on clinically relevant drug interaction potential; **Inhibits** CYP2C19 (weak), CYP2C8 (weak), CYP3A4 (strong), P-glycoprotein/ABCB1

Avoid Concomitant Use

Avoid concomitant use of Ketoconazole (Systemic) with any of the following: Abemaciclib; Acalabrutinib; Ado-Trastuzumab Emtansine; Alfuzosin; ALPRAZolam; Aprepitant; Astemizole; Asunaprevir; Avanafil; Avapritinib; Barnidipine; Bilastine; Blonanserin; Bosutinib; Bromocriptine; Budesonide (Systemic); Cisapride; Cobimetinib; Conivaptan; Dabrafenib; Dapoxetine; Dihydroergotamine; Disopyramide; Dofetilide; Domperidone; DOXOrubicin (Conventional); Dronedarone; Efavirenz; Elagolix, Estradiol, and Norethindrone; Elbasvir; Eletriptan; Eplerenone; Ergoloid Mesylates; Ergonovine; Ergotamine; Estazolam; Everolimus; Felodipine; Flibanserin; Fluticasone (Nasal); Fosaprepitant; Grazoprevir; Halofantrine; Ibrutinib; Indium 111 Capromab Pendetide; Irinotecan Products; Isavuconazonium Sulfate; Ivabradine; Ivosidenib; Lefamulin; Lemborexant; Lercanidipine; Lomitapide; Lovastatin; Lumateperone; Lurasidone; Lurbinectedin; Macitentan; Methadone; Methylergonovine; Midazolam; Mizolastine; Naloxegol; Neratinib; Nevirapine; NiMODipine; Nisoldipine; PAZOPanib; Pimozide; QuiNIDine; Radotinib; Ranolazine; Red Yeast Rice; Regorafenib; Rimegepant; Rivaroxaban; Rupatadine; Saccharomyces boulardii; Salmeterol; Silodosin; Simeprevir; Simvastatin; Sonidegib; Suvorexant; Tamsulosin; Tazemetostat; Telithromycin; Terfenadine; Ticagrelor; Tolvaptan; Topotecan; Trabectedin; Triazolam; Ubrogepant; Udenafil; Ulipristal; VinCRIStine (Liposomal); Vinflunine; Vorapaxar

Increased Effect/Toxicity

Ketoconazole (Systemic) may increase the levels/effects of: Abemaciclib; Acalabrutinib; Ado-Trastuzumab Emtansine; Afatinib; Alcohol (Ethyl); Alfuzosin; Aliskiren; Alitretinoin (Systemic); Almotriptan; Alosetron; ALPRAZolam; Antihepaciviral Combination Products; Apixaban; Aprepitant; ARIPiprazole; ARIPiprazole Lauroxil; Astemizole; Asunaprevir; AtorvaSTATin; Avanafil; Avapritinib; Axitinib; Barnidipine; Bedaquiline; Benperidol; Benzhydrocodone; Betamethasone (Ophthalmic); Betrixaban; Bictegravir; Bilastine; Blonanserin; Bortezomib; Bosentan; Bosutinib; Brentuximab Vedotin; Brexpiprazole; Brigatinib; Brinzolamide; Bromocriptine; Budesonide (Nasal); Budesonide (Oral Inhalation); Budesonide (Systemic); Budesonide (Topical); Buprenorphine; BusPIRone; Busulfan; Cabazitaxel; Cabozantinib; Calcifediol; Calcium Channel Blockers; Cannabidiol; Cannabis; Capmatinib; Carbocisteine; Cariprazine; Celiprolol; Ceritinib; Cilostazol; Cinacalcet; Cisapride; CloBAZam; CloZAPine; Cobicistat; Cobimetinib; Codeine; Colchicine; Conivaptan; Copanlisib; Corticosteroids (Orally Inhaled); Corticosteroids (Systemic); Crizotinib; CycloSPORINE (Systemic); CYP3A4 Substrates (High risk with Inhibitors); Dabigatran Etexilate; Dabrafenib; Daclatasvir; Dapoxetine; Darifenacin;

Darolutamide; Darunavir; Dasatinib; Deflazacort; Delamanid; DexAMETHasone (Ophthalmic); Dichlorphenamide; Dienogest; Dihydroergotamine; Disopyramide; DOCEtaxel; Dofetilide; Domperidone; DOXOrubicin (Conventional); Dronabinol; Dronedarone; Drospirenone; Dutasteride; Duvelisib; Edoxaban; Elagolix; Elagolix, Estradiol, and Norethindrone; Elbasvir; Eletriptan; Elexacaftor, Tezacaftor, and Ivacaftor; Eliglustat; Elvitegravir; Emedastine (Systemic); Encorafenib; Enfortumab Vedotin; Entrectinib; Eplerenone; Erdafitinib; Ergoloid Mesylates; Ergonovine; Ergotamine; Erlotinib; Estazolam; Estrogen Derivatives; Eszopiclone; Etizolam; Etoposide; Etoposide Phosphate; Etravirine; Everolimus; Evogliptin; Fedratinib; Felodipine; FentaNYL; Fesoterodine; Fexofenadine; Fimasartan; Fingolimod; Flibanserin; Fluticasone (Nasal); Fluticasone (Oral Inhalation); Fosamprenavir; Fosaprepitant; Fostamatinib; Galantamine; Gefitinib; Gilteritinib; Glasdegib; Glecaprevir and Pibrentasvir; Grazoprevir; GuanFACINE; Halofantrine; HYDROcodone; Ibrutinib; Idelalisib; Iloperidone; Imatinib; Imidafenacin; Indinavir; Irinotecan Products; Isavuconazonium Sulfate; Istradefylline; Ivabradine; Ivacaftor; Ivosidenib; Ixabepilone; Lapatinib; Larotrectinib; Lefamulin; Lemborexant; Lercanidipine; Levobupivacaine; Levomilnacipran; Lomitapide; Lopinavir; Loratadine; Lorlatinib; Lovastatin; Lumateperone; Lumefantrine; Lurasidone; Lurbinectedin; Macitentan; Manidipine; Maraviroc; MedroxyPROGESTERone; Meperidine; Methadone; Methylergonovine; MethylPREDNISolone; Midazolam; Midostaurin; MiFEPRIStone; Mirabegron; Mirodenafil; Mirtazapine; Mizolastine; Morphine (Systemic); Nadolol; Naldemedine; Nalfurafine; Naloxegol; Neratinib; Nilotinib; NiMODipine; Nintedanib; Nisoldipine; Olaparib; Osilodrostat; Ospemifene; Oxybutynin; Palbociclib; Panobinostat; Parecoxib; Paricalcitol; PAZOPanib; Pemigatinib; Pexidartinib; P-glycoprotein/ABCB1 Substrates; Pimavanserin; Pimecrolimus; Pimozide; Piperaquine; Polatuzumab Vedotin; PONATinib; Pranlukast; Praziquantel; PrednisoLONE (Systemic); PredniSONE; Propafenone; Proton Pump Inhibitors; QUEtiapine; QuiNIDine; Radotinib; Ramelteon; Ranolazine; Red Yeast Rice; Regorafenib; Repaglinide; Retapamulin; Ribociclib; Rifamycin Derivatives; RifAXIMin; Rilpivirine; Rimegepant; Riociguat; Ripretinib; RisperiDONE; Rivaroxaban; RomiDEPsin; Rupatadine; Ruxolitinib; Salmeterol; Saquinavir; SAXagliptin; Selpercatinib; Selumetinib; Sibutramine; Sildenafil; Silodosin; Simeprevir; Simvastatin; Sirolimus; Solifenacin; Sonidegib; SORAfenib; SUFentanil; SUNItinib; Suvorexant; Tacrolimus (Systemic); Tacrolimus (Topical); Tadalafil; Talazoparib; Tamsulosin; Tasimelteon; Tazemetostat; Tegaserod; Telithromycin; Temsirolimus; Teneligliptin; Terfenadine; Tetrahydrocannabinol; Tetrahydrocannabinol and Cannabidiol; Tezacaftor and Ivacaftor; Thiotepa; Ticagrelor; Tofacitinib; Tolterodine; Tolvaptan; Topotecan; Toremifene; Trabectedin; TraMADol; TraZODone; Triazolam; Ubrogepant; Udenafil; Ulipristal; Upadacitinib; Valbenazine; Vardenafil; Vemurafenib; Venetoclax; Vilazodone; VinCRIStine (Liposomal); Vindesine; Vinflunine; Vinorelbine; Vitamin K Antagonists; Vorapaxar; Voxelotor; Zanubrutinib; Zolpidem; Zopiclone

The levels/effects of Ketoconazole (Systemic) may be increased by: Antihepaciviral Combination Products; AtorvaSTATin; Cobicistat; Darunavir; Fosamprenavir; Indinavir; Lopinavir; Ritonavir; Saquinavir; Telithromycin; Tipranavir; Vilanterol

Decreased Effect

Ketoconazole (Systemic) may decrease the levels/effects of: Amphotericin B; Choline C 11; Doxercalciferol; Ifosfamide; Indium 111 Capromab Pendetide; Saccharomyces boulardii; Thiotepa; Ticagrelor

The levels/effects of Ketoconazole (Systemic) may be decreased by: Antacids; CYP3A4 Inducers (Moderate); CYP3A4 Inducers (Strong); Deferasirox; Didanosine; Efavirenz; Enzalutamide; Etravirine; Histamine H2 Receptor Antagonists; Hyoscyamine; Isoniazid; Ivosidenib; Lumacaftor and Ivacaftor; Mitotane; Nevirapine; Proton Pump Inhibitors; Rifamycin Derivatives; Rilpivirine; Sarilumab; Siltuximab; Sucralfate; Tocilizumab

Pharmacodynamics/Kinetics

Half-life Elimination Biphasic: Initial: 2 hours; Terminal: 8 hours

Time to Peak Serum: 1-2 hours

Reproductive Considerations

Women with Cushing syndrome often experience oligomenorrhea or amenorrhea due to the pathological cortisol excess associated with this disease. Patients treated with ketoconazole may experience a decrease in ovulatory disturbances and should be informed of the potential return of fertility (Berwaerts 1999; Boronat 2011; Costenaro 2015).

The use of ketoconazole in male patients has been associated with decreased testosterone concentrations. Adverse effects have included reversible gynecomastia, oligospermia, impotence, and decreased libido.

Pregnancy Considerations

Due to the teratogenicity reported in animal reproduction studies and its antiandrogenic effects, ketoconazole is not recommended for the treatment of systemic fungal infections in pregnant women. Other agents are more frequently used to treat Cushing syndrome in pregnancy (Bronstein 2015; Brue 2018; Galgiani 2016; HHS [OI adult]; Pilmis 2015).

Breastfeeding Considerations Ketoconazole is present in breast milk.

Milk concentrations following an oral ketoconazole dose of 200 mg daily for 10 days were ≤0.22 mcg/mL in a case report. Using the reported peak milk concentration of 0.22 mcg/mL in this patient, authors of the study calculated the estimated exposure to the breastfeeding infant to be 0.033 mg/kg/day (relative infant dose: 1.4% based on the weight-adjusted maternal dose of 200 mg/day) (Moretti 1995).

Breastfeeding is not recommended by the manufacturer.

Dosage Forms: US

Tablet, Oral:

Generic: 200 mg

Dosage Forms: Canada

Tablet, Oral:

Generic: 200 mg

Ketoconazole (Topical) (kee toe KOE na zole)

Related Information

Fungal Infections *on page 1752*

Brand Names: US Extina; Ketodan; Nizoral A-D [OTC]; Nizoral [DSC]; Xolegel

Brand Names: Canada Ketoderm

Pharmacologic Category Antifungal Agent, Imidazole Derivative; Antifungal Agent, Topical

Use

Cream: Treatment of tinea corporis (ringworm), tinea cruris (jock itch), and tinea pedis (athlete's foot) caused by *Trichophyton rubrum*, *Trichophyton mentagrophytes*, and *Epidermophyton floccosum*; treatment of tinea (pityriasis) versicolor caused by *Pityrosporum orbiculare* (also known as *Malassezia furfur*); treatment of cutaneous candidiasis caused by *Candida* sp; treatment of seborrheic dermatitis

Foam, gel: Treatment of seborrheic dermatitis in immunocompetent adults and children 12 years and older

Limitations of use: Safety and efficacy for the treatment of fungal infections have not been established.

Shampoo:

US labeling: Treatment of tinea versicolor caused by or presumed to be caused by *P. orbiculare* (*M. furfur* or *Malassezia orbiculare*)

Canadian labeling: Treatment and prophylaxis of conditions caused by *Pityrosporum* (eg, pityriasis capitis [dandruff]); treatment of seborrheic dermatitis

OTC labeling: Controls flaking, scaling, and itching associated with dandruff

Local Anesthetic/Vasoconstrictor Precautions No information available to require special precautions

Effects on Dental Treatment No significant effects or complications reported

Effects on Bleeding No information available to require special precautions

Adverse Reactions

1% to 10%:

Dermatologic: Application-site pruritus (cream: ≤5%; shampoo: 1% to 3%; foam, gel: <1%), stinging of the skin (cream: ≤5%), xeroderma (shampoo: 1% to 3%; foam, gel: <1%)

Local: Application site reaction (foam: 6%; shampoo: 1% to 3%), local irritation (cream: ≤5%; foam, shampoo <1%), application site burning (gel: 4%; foam, shampoo: <1%)

Frequency not defined: Dermatologic: Dry hair, dry scalp, oily hair

<1%, postmarketing, and/or case reports: Abnormal hair texture, acne vulgaris, alopecia, anaphylaxis, angioedema, application-site dermatitis, application site discharge, application site erythema, application site pain, cheilitis, contact dermatitis, dizziness, eye irritation, facial swelling, hair discoloration, headache, hypersensitivity reaction, impetigo, keratoconjunctivitis sicca, localized warm feeling, nail discoloration, paresthesia, pustules, pyogenic granuloma, skin irritation, skin rash, swelling of eye, urticaria

Mechanism of Action Alters the permeability of the cell wall by blocking fungal cytochrome P450; inhibits biosynthesis of triglycerides and phospholipids by fungi; inhibits several fungal enzymes that results in a build-up of toxic concentrations of hydrogen peroxide; also inhibits androgen synthesis

Pregnancy Considerations

Ketoconazole is not detectable in the plasma following chronic use of the shampoo.

Topical ketoconazole may be used for the treatment of infectious atopic dermatitis complications in pregnant women (Vestergaard 2019).

◆ **Ketodan** *see* Ketoconazole (Topical) *on page 859*

◆ **3-Keto-desogestrel** *see* Etonogestrel *on page 625*

Ketoprofen (kee toe PROE fen)

Related Information

Oral Pain *on page 1734*

Rheumatoid Arthritis, Osteoarthritis, and Osteoporosis *on page 1697*

Temporomandibular Dysfunction (TMD), Chronic Pain, and Fibromyalgia *on page 1773*

Brand Names: Canada Anafen; Ketoprofen-E; NU-Ketoprofen-SR [DSC]; PMS-Ketoprofen; PMS-Ketoprofen-E

Pharmacologic Category Analgesic, Nonopioid; Nonsteroidal Anti-inflammatory Drug (NSAID), Oral

Use

Osteoarthritis: Management of the signs and symptoms of osteoarthritis

Pain (immediate release only): Management of pain

Primary dysmenorrhea (immediate release only): Treatment of primary dysmenorrhea

Rheumatoid arthritis: Management of the signs and symptoms of rheumatoid arthritis

Local Anesthetic/Vasoconstrictor Precautions No information available to require special precautions

Effects on Dental Treatment Key adverse event(s) related to dental treatment: Stomatitis.

According to the FDA, the over-the-counter NSAID ketoprofen should be viewed as having the potential to interfere with the antiplatelet effect of low-dose aspirin until proven otherwise. This statement was provided in the same warning from the FDA that ibuprofen can interfere with the antiplatelet effect of low-dose aspirin (81 mg/day), potentially rendering aspirin less effective when used for cardioprotection and stroke protection. In situations where these drugs could be used concomitantly, the FDA has provided the following information: Patients who use immediate release aspirin (not enteric-coated aspirin) and take single doses of ibuprofen 400 mg, should dose the ibuprofen at least 30 minutes or longer after aspirin ingestion or more than 8 hours before aspirin ingestion to avoid attenuation of aspirin's effect. Similar recommendations may hold for concomitant ketoprofen and aspirin use. See Effects on Bleeding.

At this time, recommendations about the timing of ibuprofen 400 mg or other NSAIDs (such as ketoprofen) in patients taking enteric-coated low-dose aspirin cannot be made based on available data.

Effects on Bleeding Nonselective NSAIDs such as ketoprofen inhibit platelet aggregation and prolong bleeding time in some patients. Unlike aspirin, the NSAID effect on platelet function is quantitatively less, of shorter duration, and reversible.

Adverse Reactions

>10%:

Gastrointestinal: Dyspepsia (11%)

Hepatic: Abnormal hepatic function tests (≤15%)

1% to 10%:

Cardiovascular: Peripheral edema (2%)

Central nervous system: Headache (3% to 9%), dizziness (>1%), abnormal dreams, depression, drowsiness, insomnia, malaise, nervousness

Dermatologic: Skin rash (>1%)

Gastrointestinal: Abdominal pain (3% to 9%), constipation (3% to 9%), diarrhea (3% to 9%), flatulence (3% to 9%), nausea (3% to 9%), gastrointestinal hemorrhage (>2%), peptic ulcer (>2%), anorexia (>1%), stomatitis (>1%), vomiting (>1%)

Genitourinary: Urinary tract irritation (>1%)

Ophthalmic: Visual disturbance (>1%)

Otic: Tinnitus (>1%)

Renal: Renal insufficiency (3% to 9%)

<1%, postmarketing, and/or case reports: Acute renal tubular disease, agranulocytosis, allergic rhinitis, alopecia, anaphylaxis, anemia, angioedema, aseptic meningitis, auditory impairment, blurred vision, bone marrow depression, bronchospasm, buccal necrosis, bullous rash, cardiac arrhythmia, cardiac failure, change in libido, chills, cholestatic hepatitis, confusion, conjunctivitis, cystitis, dysphoria, dyspnea, eczema, edema, epistaxis, erythema multiforme, exacerbation of diabetes mellitus, exfoliative dermatitis, facial edema, fluid retention, gastritis, gastrointestinal perforation, gastrointestinal ulcer, gynecomastia, hallucination, hematemesis, hematuria, hemolytic anemia, hemoptysis, hepatic insufficiency, hepatitis, hepatotoxicity (idiosyncratic; Chalasani 2014), hot flash, hypersensitivity reaction, hypertension, hyponatremia, impotence, infection, interstitial nephritis, jaundice, laryngeal edema, leukopenia, melena, microvesicular steatosis, migraine, myocardial infarction, nephrotic syndrome, occult blood in stools, onycholysis, palpitations, pancreatitis, peripheral neuropathy, peripheral vascular disease, polydipsia, polyuria, pruritus, purpura, purpuric rash, renal failure, renal papillary necrosis, retinal hemorrhage, septicemia, shock, skin photosensitivity, Stevens-Johnson syndrome, tachycardia, thrombocytopenia, toxic amblyopia, toxic epidermal necrolysis, ulcerative bowel lesion, ulcerative colitis, urticaria, vasodilation, xerostomia

Mechanism of Action Reversibly inhibits cyclooxygenase-1 and 2 (COX-1 and 2) enzymes, which results in decreased formation of prostaglandin precursors; has antipyretic, analgesic, and anti-inflammatory properties

Other proposed mechanisms not fully elucidated (and possibly contributing to the anti-inflammatory effect to varying degrees), include inhibiting chemotaxis, altering lymphocyte activity, inhibiting neutrophil aggregation/activation, and decreasing proinflammatory cytokine levels.

Pharmacodynamics/Kinetics

Onset of Action Regular release: <30 minutes

Duration of Action Regular release: Up to 6 hours

Half-life Elimination

Regular release: 2 to 4 hours; Renal impairment: Mild: 3 hours; moderate to severe: 5 to 9 hours

Enteric coated tablet [Canadian product]: 2 hours

Extended release: ~3 to 7.5 hours

Rectal suppository [Canadian product]: ~2 to 2.5 hours

Time to Peak Regular release: 0.5 to 2 hours; Extended release capsule: 6 to 7 hours; Extended release tablet [Canadian product]: 5 to 6 hours; Enteric coated tablet [Canadian product]: 1 to 2 hours; Rectal suppository [Canadian product]: ~1 hour

Reproductive Considerations

The chronic use of NSAIDs in women of reproductive age may be associated with infertility that is reversible upon discontinuation of the medication (Micu 2011).

Pregnancy Risk Factor C

Pregnancy Considerations

Ketoprofen crosses the placenta (Bannwarth 1999). Birth defects have been observed following in utero NSAID exposure in some studies; however, data is conflicting (Bloor 2013). Nonteratogenic effects, including prenatal constriction of the ductus arteriosus, persistent pulmonary hypertension of the newborn, oligohydramnios, necrotizing enterocolitis, renal dysfunction or failure, and intracranial hemorrhage have been observed in the fetus/neonate following in utero NSAID exposure. In addition, nonclosure of the ductus arteriosus postnatally may occur and be resistant to medical management (Bermas 2014; Bloor 2013). Because they may cause premature closure of the ductus arteriosus, the use of NSAIDs late in pregnancy should be avoided. Use of NSAIDs can be considered for the treatment of mild rheumatoid arthritis flares in pregnant women; however, use should be minimized or avoided early and late in pregnancy (Bermas 2014; Saavedra Salinas 2015).

The use of NSAIDs close to conception may be associated with an increased risk of miscarriage (Bloor 2013; Bermas 2014).

Ketorolac (Systemic) (KEE toe role ak)

Related Information

Oral Pain *on page 1734*

Rheumatoid Arthritis, Osteoarthritis, and Osteoporosis *on page 1697*

Temporomandibular Dysfunction (TMD), Chronic Pain, and Fibromyalgia *on page 1773*

Brand Names: US ReadySharp Ketorolac

Brand Names: Canada ALTI-Ketorolac; APO-Ketorolac; Mar-Ketorolac; MINT-Ketorolac; Toradol

Generic Availability (US) May be product dependent

Pharmacologic Category Analgesic, Nonopioid; Nonsteroidal Anti-inflammatory Drug (NSAID), Oral; Nonsteroidal Anti-inflammatory Drug (NSAID), Parenteral

Dental Use Short-term (≤5 days) management of moderate to severe acute pain

Use Pain management (acute; moderately severe): Short-term (≤5 days) management of moderate to severe acute pain

Local Anesthetic/Vasoconstrictor Precautions No information available to require special precautions

Effects on Dental Treatment Key adverse event(s) related to dental treatment: Xerostomia (normal salivary flow resumes upon discontinuation) and stomatitis. Rare occurrence of glossitis, ulcerative stomatitis, tongue edema.

NSAID formulations are known to reversibly decrease platelet aggregation via mechanisms different than observed with aspirin. The dentist should be aware of the potential of abnormal coagulation. Caution should also be exercised in the use of NSAIDs in patients already on anticoagulant therapy with drugs such as warfarin (Coumadin®). See Dental Health Professional Considerations.

Effects on Bleeding Nonselective NSAIDs such as ketorolac inhibit platelet aggregation and prolong bleeding time in some patients. Unlike aspirin, the NSAID effect on platelet function is quantitatively less, of shorter duration, and reversible due to shorter duration of treatment with ketorolac.

Adverse Reactions Frequencies noted for parenteral administration:

>10%:

Central nervous system: Headache (17%)

Gastrointestinal: Gastrointestinal pain (13%), dyspepsia (12%), nausea (12%)

>1% to 10%:

Cardiovascular: Edema (4%), hypertension

Central nervous system: Dizziness (7%), drowsiness (6%)

Dermatologic: Diaphoresis, pruritus, skin rash

Gastrointestinal: Diarrhea (7%), constipation, flatulence, gastrointestinal fullness, gastrointestinal hemorrhage, gastrointestinal perforation, gastrointestinal ulcer, heartburn, stomatitis, vomiting
Hematologic & oncologic: Anemia, prolonged bleeding time, purpura
Hepatic: Increased liver enzymes
Local: Pain at injection site (2%)
Otic: Tinnitus
Renal: Renal function abnormality
<1%, postmarketing, and/or case reports: Abnormality in thinking, acute pancreatitis, acute renal failure, agranulocytosis, alopecia, anaphylactoid reaction, anaphylaxis, angioedema, anxiety, aplastic anemia, aseptic meningitis, asthma, azotemia, blurred vision, bradycardia, bronchospasm, bruise, cardiac arrhythmia, cardiac failure, chest pain, cholestatic jaundice, coma, confusion, conjunctivitis, cough, cystitis, depression, dyspnea, dysuria, eosinophilia, epistaxis, eructation, erythema multiforme, esophagitis, euphoria, exacerbation of urinary frequency, exfoliative dermatitis, extrapyramidal reaction, fever, flank pain, flushing, gastritis, glossitis, hallucination, hearing loss, hematemesis, hematuria, hemolytic anemia, hemolytic-uremic syndrome, hepatic failure, hepatitis, hepatotoxicity (idiosyncratic) (Chalasani, 2014), hyperglycemia, hyperkalemia, hyperkinesis, hypersensitivity reaction, hyponatremia, hypotension, increased susceptibility to infection, increased thirst, infertility, inflammatory bowel disease, insomnia, interstitial nephritis, jaundice, lack of concentration, laryngeal edema, leukopenia, lymphadenopathy, maculopapular rash, melena, myocardial infarction, nephritis, nervousness, oliguria, pallor, palpitations, pancytopenia, paresthesia, pneumonia, polyuria, proteinuria, psychosis, pulmonary edema, rectal hemorrhage, renal failure, respiratory depression, rhinitis, seizure, sepsis, skin photosensitivity, Stevens-Johnson syndrome, stomatitis (ulcerative), stupor, syncope, tachycardia, thrombocytopenia, tongue edema, toxic epidermal necrolysis, tremor, urinary retention, urticaria, vasculitis, vertigo, weakness, weight gain, wound hemorrhage (postoperative), xerostomia

Dental Usual Dosage

Short-term (≤5 days) management of moderate to severe acute pain (**Note:** The maximum combined duration of treatment (for parenteral and oral) is 5 days; do not increase dose or frequency; supplement with low-dose opioids if needed for breakthrough pain). For patients <50 kg and/or ≥65 years, see Geriatric dosing.

Adults:

IM: 60 mg as a single dose or 30 mg every 6 hours (maximum daily dose: 120 mg)

IV: 30 mg as a single dose or 30 mg every 6 hours (maximum daily dose: 120 mg)

Oral: 20 mg, followed by 10 mg every 4-6 hours; do not exceed 40 mg/day; oral dosing is intended to be a continuation of IM or IV therapy only

Dosage adjustments in elderly (≥65 years), renal insufficiency, or low body weight (<50 kg): Note: These groups have an increased incidence of GI bleeding, ulceration, and perforation. The maximum combined duration of treatment (for parenteral and oral) is 5 days.

IM: 30 mg as a single dose or 15 mg every 6 hours (maximum daily dose: 60 mg)

IV: 15 mg as a single dose or 15 mg every 6 hours (maximum daily dose: 60 mg)

Oral: 10 mg, followed by 10 mg every 4-6 hours; do not exceed 40 mg/day; oral dosing is intended to be a continuation of IM or IV therapy only

Dosing

Adult

Pain management (acute; moderately severe) in patients ≥50 kg: Note: The maximum combined duration of treatment (for parenteral and oral) is 5 days; do not increase dose or frequency; supplement with low-dose opioids if needed for breakthrough pain. Oral formulation should not be given as an initial dose.

IM: 60 mg as a single dose or 30 mg every 6 hours; alternatively, an initial dose of 10 to 30 mg (as single dose) and then every 4 to 6 hours as needed has been recommended (Toradol IM Canadian product labeling 2015). Maximum: 120 mg/day

IV: 30 mg as a single dose or 30 mg every 6 hours (maximum: 120 mg/day)

Note: A randomized, double-blind trial (n=240) demonstrated that a lower dose of ketorolac 10 mg IV produced similar analgesic effects as 15 mg and 30 mg IV doses in patients with acute pain in the ED (Motov 2017); consideration for lower doses may be appropriate.

Oral: 20 mg, followed by 10 mg every 4 to 6 hours as needed; maximum: 40 mg/day; oral dosing is intended to be a continuation of IM or IV therapy only

Patient population-specific dosing:

Critically ill patients (off-label dose): IM, IV: 30 mg once, followed by 15 to 30 mg every 6 hours for up to 5 days (maximum: 120 mg/day) (SCCM [Barr 2013]; Tietze 2019).

Perioperative patients (off-label dose): IV: **Note:** Multimodal perioperative pain management strategies should be employed. Maximum daily dose should not exceed 120 mg/day. Perioperative dosing strategies described in the literature have included bolus dose of 10 to 30 mg, followed by a continuous infusion of 2 to 5 mg/hour for 24 hours (Etches 1995; Howard 2018; Ready 1994). One study administered 3.6 mg/hour for 48 hours (Schwinghammer 2017).

Dosage adjustment for low body weight (<50 kg): Note: May have an increased incidence of GI bleeding, ulceration, and perforation. The maximum combined duration of treatment (for parenteral and oral) is 5 days. Oral formulation should not be given as an initial dose.

IM: 30 mg as a single dose or 15 mg every 6 hours (maximum: 60 mg/day)

IV: 15 mg as a single dose or 15 mg every 6 hours (maximum: 60 mg/day)

Oral: 10 mg, followed by 10 mg every 4 to 6 hours as needed (maximum: 40 mg/day). Oral dosing is intended to be a continuation of IM or IV therapy only.

Geriatric Avoid use (Beers Criteria [AGS 2019]).

Renal Impairment: Adult

Dosage adjustment recommendations:

Manufacturer's labeling:

Renally impaired patients: **Note:** The specific degree of renal impairment where use is permitted is not defined in the product labeling; however, use is contraindicated in patients with advanced renal impairment or those at risk for renal failure due to volume depletion.

IM: 30 mg as a single dose or 15 mg every 6 hours (maximum: 60 mg/day)

IV: 15 mg as a single dose or 15 mg every 6 hours (maximum: 60 mg/day)
Oral: 10 mg, followed by 10 mg every 4 to 6 hours as needed; maximum: 40 mg/day; oral dosing is intended to be a continuation of IM or IV therapy only
Advanced impairment or patients at risk for renal failure due to volume depletion: Use is contraindicated.

Alternative recommendations:
GFR >50 mL/minute/1.73 m^2: 15 to 30 mg IM or IV every 6 hours (Golightly 2013)
GFR 10 to 50 mL/minute/1.73 m^2: Preferably avoid **or** administer 7.5 to 15 mg IM or IV every 6 hours (Golightly 2013)
GFR <10 mL/minute/1.73 m^2: Preferably avoid (Golightly 2013)
Hemodialysis: Preferably avoid (Golightly 2013)
CAPD: Preferably avoid (Golightly 2013)
CRRT: 7.5 to 15 mg IM or IV every 6 hours (Golightly 2013)

Hepatic Impairment: Adult There are no dosage adjustments provided in the manufacturer's labeling. Use with caution, may cause elevation of liver enzymes; discontinue if clinical signs and symptoms of liver disease develop.

Pediatric Note: To reduce the risk of adverse cardiovascular and GI effects, use the lowest effective dose for the shortest period of time.

Pain management (acute; moderately severe):
Infants and Children <2 years: Limited data available: Multiple-dose treatment: IV: 0.5 mg/kg/dose every 6 to 8 hours, not to exceed 48 to 72 hours of treatment; has been used postoperatively primarily following cardiac and abdominal surgery (Burd 2002; Dawkins 2009; Gupta 2004; Moffett 2006)
Children ≥2 years and Adolescents ≤16 years: Limited data available:
IM, IV: 0.5 mg/kg/dose every 6 hours; maximum dose: 30 mg/dose, usual reported duration: 48 to 72 hours; not to exceed 5 days of treatment (APS 2016; Buck 1994; Dsida 2002; Gupta 2004; Gupta 2005)
Oral: 1 mg/kg as a single dose; maximum dose: 10 mg/dose has been reported in children preoperatively (eg, bilateral myringotomy) (Forrest 1997; Watcha 1992)
Adolescents ≥17 years: **Note:** The maximum combined duration of treatment (for parenteral and oral) is 5 days; do not increase dose or frequency; supplement with low-dose opioids if needed for breakthrough pain.
<50 kg:
IM: 30 mg as a single dose or 15 mg every 6 hours; maximum daily dose: 60 mg/**day**
IV: 15 mg as a single dose or 15 mg every 6 hours; maximum daily dose: 60 mg/**day**
Oral: Initial: 10 mg, then 10 mg every 4 to 6 hours; maximum daily dose: 40 mg/**day**
≥50 kg:
IM: 60 mg as a single dose or 30 mg every 6 hours; maximum daily dose: 120 mg/**day**
IV: 30 mg as a single dose or 30 mg every 6 hours; maximum daily dose: 120 mg/**day**
Oral: Initial: 20 mg, then 10 mg every 4 to 6 hours; maximum daily dose: 40 mg/**day**

Renal Impairment: Pediatric There are no pediatric-specific dosage adjustments provided in the manufacturer's labeling; however, dosage adjustments are recommended for adult patients. The specific degree of renal impairment where use is permitted is not defined in the product labeling; however, use is contraindicated in patients with advanced renal impairment or those at risk for renal failure due to volume depletion; some experts have suggested the following:
Infants, Children, and Adolescents:
Aronoff 2007 recommendations: **Note:** Renally adjusted dose recommendations are based on doses of IV, IM: 0.25 to 1 mg/kg/dose every 6 hours (Aronoff 2007).
GFR ≥30 mL/minute/1.73 m^2: No dosage adjustment necessary
GFR 10 to 29 mL/minute/1.73 m^2: Administer 50% of dose
GFR <10 mL/minute/1.73 m^2: Administer 25% to 50% of dose
Intermittent hemodialysis: Avoid use
Peritoneal dialysis: Avoid use
KDIGO 2012 guidelines provide the following recommendations for NSAIDs (KDIGO 2013):
eGFR 30 to <60 mL/minute/1.73 m^2: Temporarily discontinue in patients with intercurrent disease that increases risk of acute kidney injury
eGFR <30 mL/minute/1.73 m^2: Avoid use

Hepatic Impairment: Pediatric There are no dosage adjustments provided in the manufacturer's labeling. Use with caution, may cause elevation of liver enzymes; discontinue if clinical signs and symptoms of liver disease develop.

Mechanism of Action Reversibly inhibits cyclooxygenase-1 and 2 (COX-1 and 2) enzymes, which results in decreased formation of prostaglandin precursors; has antipyretic, analgesic, and anti-inflammatory properties

Other proposed mechanisms not fully elucidated (and possibly contributing to the anti-inflammatory effect to varying degrees), include inhibiting chemotaxis, altering lymphocyte activity, inhibiting neutrophil aggregation/activation, and decreasing proinflammatory cytokine levels.

Contraindications
Hypersensitivity to ketorolac, aspirin, other NSAIDs, or any component of the formulation; active or history of peptic ulcer disease; recent or history of GI bleeding or perforation; history of asthma, urticaria, or allergic-type reactions after taking aspirin or other NSAIDs; advanced renal disease or patients at risk for renal failure due to volume depletion; prophylactic analgesic before any major surgery; suspected or confirmed cerebrovascular bleeding, hemorrhagic diathesis, incomplete hemostasis, or high risk of bleeding; concurrent use with aspirin, other NSAIDs, probenecid, or pentoxifylline; epidural or intrathecal administration (injection only); use in the setting of coronary artery bypass graft (CABG) surgery; labor and delivery.

Canadian labeling: Additional contraindications (not in US labeling): Intraoperative use; coagulation disorders; active GI bleeding; postoperative patients with high-bleeding risk; severe uncontrolled heart failure; inflammatory bowel disease; severe hepatic impairment or active hepatic disease; moderate to severe renal impairment (serum creatinine >442 micromol/L and/or creatinine clearance <30 mL/minute) or deteriorating renal disease; known hyperkalemia; third trimester of pregnancy; breastfeeding; use in children and adolescents <18 years of age

Warnings/Precautions [US Boxed Warning]: Inhibits platelet function; contraindicated in patients with cerebrovascular bleeding (suspected or confirmed), hemorrhagic diathesis, incomplete hemostasis and patients at high risk for bleeding. Platelet adhesion and aggregation may be decreased; may prolong bleeding time; patients with coagulation disorders or who are receiving anticoagulants should be monitored closely. Anemia may occur; patients on long-term nonsteroidal anti-inflammatory drug (NSAID) therapy should be monitored for anemia. Rarely, NSAID use has been associated with potentially severe blood dyscrasias (eg, agranulocytosis, thrombocytopenia, aplastic anemia). **[US Boxed Warning]: NSAIDs cause an increased risk of serious (and potentially fatal) adverse cardiovascular thrombotic events, including MI and stroke. Risk may occur early during treatment and may increase with duration of use.** Relative risk appears to be similar in those with and without known cardiovascular disease or risk factors for cardiovascular disease; however, absolute incidence of serious cardiovascular thrombotic events (which may occur early during treatment) was higher in patients with known cardiovascular disease or risk factors and in those receiving higher doses. New onset hypertension or exacerbation of hypertension may occur (NSAIDs may also impair response to ACE inhibitors, thiazide diuretics, or loop diuretics); may contribute to cardiovascular events; monitor blood pressure; use with caution in patients with hypertension. May cause sodium and fluid retention, use with caution in patients with edema. Avoid use in heart failure (ACCF/AHA [Yancy 2013]). Avoid use in patients with a recent MI unless benefits outweigh risk of cardiovascular thrombotic events. Use the lowest effective dose for the shortest duration of time, consistent with individual patient goals, to reduce risk of cardiovascular events; alternate therapies should be considered for patients at high risk. **[US Boxed Warning]: Use is contraindicated as prophylactic analgesic before any major surgery and is contraindicated in the setting of coronary artery bypass graft (CABG) surgery.** Risk of MI and stroke may be increased with use following CABG surgery. Wound bleeding and postoperative hematomas have been associated with ketorolac use in the perioperative setting.

[US Boxed Warning]: Ketorolac is contraindicated in patients with advanced renal impairment and in patients at risk for renal failure due to volume depletion. NSAID use may compromise existing renal function; dose-dependent decreases in prostaglandin synthesis may result from NSAID use, reducing renal blood flow, which may cause renal decompensation (usually reversible). Patients with impaired renal function, dehydration, hypovolemia, heart failure, hepatic impairment, those taking diuretics and ACE inhibitors, and the elderly are at greater risk of renal toxicity. Rehydrate patient before starting therapy; monitor renal function closely. Acute renal failure, interstitial nephritis, and nephrotic syndrome have been reported with ketorolac use; papillary necrosis and renal injury have been reported with long-term use of NSAIDs. Use with caution in patients with renal impairment or history of kidney disease. Dosage adjustment is required in patients with moderate elevation in serum creatinine.

[US Boxed Warning]: Ketorolac can cause peptic ulcers, GI bleeding, and/or perforation of the stomach or intestines, which can be fatal. These events can occur at any time during use and without warning symptoms. Therefore, ketorolac is contraindicated in patients with active peptic ulcer disease, recent GI bleeding or perforation, and a history of peptic ulcer disease or GI bleeding. Elderly patients and patients with a prior history of peptic ulcer disease and/or GI bleeding are at greater risk for serious GI events. Avoid use in patients with active GI bleeding. In patients with a history of acute lower GI bleeding, avoid use of nonaspirin NSAIDs, especially if due to angioectasia or diverticulosis (Strate 2016). Use caution with a history of GI ulcers, inflammatory bowel disease, concurrent therapy known to increase the risk of GI bleeding (eg, aspirin, anticoagulants and/or corticosteroids, selective serotonin reuptake inhibitors), advanced hepatic disease, coagulopathy, smoking, use of alcohol, or in the elderly or debilitated patients. Use the lowest effective dose for the shortest duration of time, consistent with individual patient goals, to reduce risk of GI adverse events; alternate therapies should be considered for patients at high risk. When used concomitantly with aspirin, a substantial increase in the risk of gastrointestinal complications (eg, ulcer) occurs; concomitant gastroprotective therapy (eg, proton pump inhibitors) is recommended (Bhatt 2008). **[US Boxed Warning]: Ketorolac injection is contraindicated in patients with prior hypersensitivity reaction to aspirin or NSAIDs.** NSAIDs may cause potentially fatal serious skin adverse events including exfoliative dermatitis, Stevens-Johnson syndrome (SJS), and toxic epidermal necrolysis (TEN); may occur without warning; discontinue use at first sign of skin rash (or any other hypersensitivity). Hypersensitivity or anaphylactoid reactions may occur, even without prior exposure; patients with "aspirin triad" (bronchial asthma, aspirin intolerance, rhinitis) may be at increased risk. Contraindicated in patients who experience bronchospasm, asthma, rhinitis, or urticaria with NSAID or aspirin therapy. Use caution in other forms of asthma.

Use with caution in patients with hepatic impairment or a history of hepatic disease; patients with advanced hepatic disease are at an increased risk of GI bleeding with NSAIDs. Transaminase elevations have been reported with use; closely monitor patients with any abnormal LFT. Rare (sometimes fatal) severe hepatic reactions (eg, jaundice, fulminant hepatitis, hepatic necrosis, hepatic failure) have occurred with NSAID use; discontinue immediately if signs or symptoms of hepatic disease develop or if systemic manifestations occur. NSAID use may increase the risk of hyperkalemia, particularly in the elderly, diabetics, renal disease, and with concomitant use of other agents capable of inducing hyperkalemia (eg, ACE-inhibitors). Monitor potassium closely.

[US Boxed Warning]: Dosage adjustment is required for patients ≥65 years of age. Elderly patients are at greater risk for serious GI, cardiovascular, and/or renal adverse events; use with caution. **[US Boxed Warning]: Dosage adjustment is required for patients weighing <50 kg (<110 pounds). [US Boxed Warning]: The use of ketorolac in labor and delivery is contraindicated because it may adversely affect fetal circulation and inhibit uterine contractions. [US Boxed Warning]: Concurrent use of ketorolac with aspirin or other NSAIDs is contraindicated due to the increased risk of adverse reactions.**

[US Boxed Warning]: Contraindicated for epidural or intrathecal administration (formulation contains alcohol). [US Boxed Warning]: Systemic ketorolac

is indicated for short-term (≤5 days) use in adults for treatment of moderately severe acute pain requiring opioid-level analgesia. The combined therapy duration (oral and parenteral) should not exceed 5 days due to the increased risk of serious adverse events. The recommended total daily dose of ketorolac tablets (maximum 40 mg) is significantly lower than for ketorolac injection (maximum 120 mg). [US Boxed Warning]: Oral therapy is only indicated for use as continuation treatment, following parenteral ketorolac and is not indicated for minor or chronic painful conditions. [US Boxed Warning]: Ketorolac is not indicated for use in pediatric patients.

Potentially significant drug-drug interactions may exist, requiring dose or frequency adjustment, additional monitoring, and/or selection of alternative therapy.

NSAIDs may increase the risk of aseptic meningitis, especially in patients with systemic lupus erythematosus (SLE) and mixed connective tissue disorders. May cause drowsiness, dizziness, blurred vision and other neurologic effects which may impair physical or mental abilities; patients must be cautioned about performing tasks which require mental alertness (eg, operating machinery or driving). Withhold for at least 4 to 6 half-lives prior to surgical or dental procedures. Avoid chronic use of oral nonselective NSAIDs in patients who have undergone bariatric surgery; development of anastomotic ulcerations/perforations may occur. Short-term use of celecoxib or IV ketorolac are recommended as part of a multimodal pain management strategy for postoperative pain.

Clinical or population-based data regarding the risks of NSAIDs in the setting of coronavirus disease 2019 (COVID-19) are limited (FDA Safety Communication 2020; Kim 2020). Some experts recommend the use of acetaminophen as the preferred antipyretic agent, when possible, and if NSAIDs are needed, to use the lowest effective dose and shortest duration (EMA 2020; Kim 2020). In general, for patients already taking an NSAID for a comorbid condition, it is recommended to continue the NSAID as directed by their health care provider (EMA 2020; NIH 2020; WHO 2020).

Warnings: Additional Pediatric Considerations In neonates, bleeding events have been reported; in a retrospective analysis of 57 postsurgical neonates and infants (age range: 0 to 3 months), 17.2% of patients experienced a bleeding event, most were PNA <21 days and those with PNA <14 days had a significantly higher risk than older neonates (Aldrink 2011). Acute kidney injury (AKI) has been observed in pediatric patients; with ketorolac use following cardiothoracic surgery, an increased risk of AKI was observed in neonates and infants who underwent a bidirectional Glenn procedure and were receiving concomitant aspirin therapy (Moffett 2013).

Drug Interactions

Metabolism/Transport Effects None known.

Avoid Concomitant Use

Avoid concomitant use of Ketorolac (Systemic) with any of the following: Acemetacin; Aminolevulinic Acid (Systemic); Aspirin; Dexibuprofen; Dexketoprofen; Floctafenine; Ketorolac (Nasal); Macimorelin; Mifamurtide; Morniflumate; Nonsteroidal Anti-Inflammatory Agents; Omacetaxine; Pelubiprofen; Pentoxifylline; Phenylbutazone; Probenecid; Talniflumate; Tenoxicam; Urokinase; Zaltoprofen

Increased Effect/Toxicity

Ketorolac (Systemic) may increase the levels/effects of: 5-Aminosalicylic Acid Derivatives; Agents with Antiplatelet Properties; Aliskiren; Aminoglycosides; Aminolevulinic Acid (Systemic); Aminolevulinic Acid (Topical); Anticoagulants; Apixaban; Aspirin; Bemiparin; Bisphosphonate Derivatives; Cephalothin; Collagenase (Systemic); CycloSPORINE (Systemic); Dabigatran Etexilate; Deferasirox; Deoxycholic Acid; Desmopressin; Dexibuprofen; Digoxin; Drospirenone; Edoxaban; Enoxaparin; Eplerenone; Haloperidol; Heparin; Ibritumomab Tiuxetan; Lithium; MetFORMIN; Methotrexate; Neuromuscular-Blocking Agents (Nondepolarizing); Nonsteroidal Anti-Inflammatory Agents; Obinutuzumab; Omacetaxine; Pentoxifylline; Porfimer; Potassium-Sparing Diuretics; PRALAtrexate; Quinolones; Rivaroxaban; Salicylates; Tacrolimus (Systemic); Tenofovir Products; Thrombolytic Agents; Tolperisone; Urokinase; Vancomycin; Verteporfin; Vitamin K Antagonists

The levels/effects of Ketorolac (Systemic) may be increased by: Acalabrutinib; Acemetacin; Alcohol (Ethyl); Angiotensin II Receptor Blockers; Angiotensin-Converting Enzyme Inhibitors; Corticosteroids (Systemic); CycloSPORINE (Systemic); Dasatinib; Dexketoprofen; Fat Emulsion (Fish Oil Based); Felbinac; Floctafenine; Glucosamine; Herbs (Anticoagulant/Antiplatelet Properties); Ibrutinib; Inotersen; Ketorolac (Nasal); Limaprost; Loop Diuretics; Morniflumate; Multivitamins/Fluoride (with ADE); Multivitamins/Minerals (with ADEK, Folate, Iron); Multivitamins/Minerals (with AE, No Iron); Naftazone; Omega-3 Fatty Acids; Pelubiprofen; Pentosan Polysulfate Sodium; Phenylbutazone; Probenecid; Prostacyclin Analogues; Selective Serotonin Reuptake Inhibitors; Selumetinib; Serotonin/Norepinephrine Reuptake Inhibitors; Sodium Phosphates; Talniflumate; Tenoxicam; Thiazide and Thiazide-Like Diuretics; Tipranavir; Tolperisone; Tricyclic Antidepressants (Tertiary Amine); Vitamin E (Systemic); Zaltoprofen; Zanubrutinib

Decreased Effect

Ketorolac (Systemic) may decrease the levels/effects of: Aliskiren; Angiotensin II Receptor Blockers; Angiotensin-Converting Enzyme Inhibitors; Aspirin; Beta-Blockers; Eplerenone; HydrALAZINE; Loop Diuretics; Macimorelin; Mifamurtide; Potassium-Sparing Diuretics; Prostaglandins (Ophthalmic); Salicylates; Selective Serotonin Reuptake Inhibitors; Sincalide; Thiazide and Thiazide-Like Diuretics

The levels/effects of Ketorolac (Systemic) may be decreased by: Bile Acid Sequestrants; Salicylates

Food Interactions High-fat meals may delay time to peak (by ~1 hour) and decrease peak concentrations. Management: Administer tablet with food or milk to decrease gastrointestinal distress.

Dietary Considerations Administer tablet with food or milk to decrease gastrointestinal distress.

Pharmacodynamics/Kinetics

Onset of Action Analgesic: Oral: 30 to 60 minutes; IM, IV: ~30 minutes; Peak effect: Analgesic: Oral: 2 to 3 hours; IM, IV: ≤2 to 3 hours

Duration of Action Analgesic: 4 to 6 hours

Half-life Elimination

Infants 6 to 18 months of age (n=25): S-enantiomer: 0.83 ± 0.7 hours; R-enantiomer: 4 ± 0.8 hours (Lynn 2007)

Children:

1 to 16 years (n=36): Mean: 3 ± 1.1 hours (Dsida 2002)

3 to 18 years (n=24): Mean: 3.8 ± 2.6 hours

4 to 8 years (n=10): Mean: ~6 hours; Range: 3.5 to 10 hours

Adults:

Mean: ~5 hours; Range: 2 to 9 hours [S-enantiomer ~2.5 hours (biologically active); R-enantiomer ~5 hours]

With renal impairment: S_{cr} 1.9 to 5 mg/dL: Mean: ~11 hours; Range: 4 to 19 hours

Renal dialysis patients: Mean: ~14 hours; Range: 8 to 40 hours

Time to Peak Serum: Oral: ~45 minutes; IM: 30 to 60 minutes; IV: 1 to 3 minutes

Reproductive Considerations

The chronic use of NSAIDs in women of reproductive age may be associated with infertility that is reversible upon discontinuation of the medication. Consider discontinuing use in women having difficulty conceiving or those undergoing investigation of fertility.

Pregnancy Considerations

[US Boxed Warning]: The use of ketorolac in labor and delivery is contraindicated because it may adversely affect fetal circulation and inhibit uterine contractions.

Ketorolac crosses the placenta (Walker 1988).

The use of nonsteroidal anti-inflammatory drugs (NSAIDs) close to conception may be associated with an increased risk of miscarriage (Bermas 2014; Bloor 2013).

Birth defects have been observed following in utero NSAID exposure in some studies; however, data is conflicting (Bloor 2013). Nonteratogenic effects, including prenatal constriction of the ductus arteriosus, persistent pulmonary hypertension of the newborn, oligohydramnios, necrotizing enterocolitis, renal dysfunction or failure, and intracranial hemorrhage have been observed in the fetus/neonate following in utero NSAID exposure. In addition, nonclosure of the ductus arteriosus postnatally may occur and be resistant to medical management (Bermas 2014; Bloor 2013). Because they may cause premature closure of the ductus arteriosus, the use of NSAIDs late in pregnancy should be avoided.

Due to pregnancy-induced physiologic changes, some pharmacokinetic properties of ketorolac may be altered (Välitalo 2017).

NSAIDs may be used as part of multimodal pain management following cesarean delivery. Use of a specific agent should consider potential breastfeeding status (ACOG 209 2019; Carvalho 2017; Sutton 2017).

Breastfeeding Considerations

Ketorolac is present in breast milk (Wischnik 1989).

The relative infant dose (RID) of ketorolac is 0.21% when calculated using the highest breast milk concentration located and compared to a weight-adjusted maternal dose of 40 mg/day.

In general, breastfeeding is considered acceptable when the RID is <10% (Anderson 2016; Ito 2000).

Using the highest milk concentration (7.9 ng/mL), the estimated daily infant dose via breast milk is 1.185 mcg/kg/day. This milk concentration was obtained following maternal administration of oral ketorolac 10 mg four times a day for 2 days in women 2 to 6 days postpartum (Wischnik 1989).

In general, nonsteroidal anti-inflammatory drugs may be used in postpartum women who wish to breastfeed; however, agents other than ketorolac are preferred in women at risk of hemorrhage (ABM [Reece-Stremtan 2017]), and use should be avoided in women breastfeeding infants with platelet dysfunction or thrombocytopenia (Bloor 2013; Sammaritano 2014). The manufacturer recommends that caution be used if administered to breastfeeding women.

Dosage Forms: US

Kit, Injection:

ReadySharp Ketorolac: 15 mg/mL

Solution, Injection:

Generic: 15 mg/mL (1 mL); 30 mg/mL (1 mL)

Solution, Injection [preservative free]:

Generic: 15 mg/mL (1 mL); 30 mg/mL (1 mL)

Solution, Intramuscular:

Generic: 60 mg/2 mL (2 mL)

Solution, Intramuscular [preservative free]:

Generic: 60 mg/2 mL (2 mL)

Tablet, Oral:

Generic: 10 mg

Dosage Forms: Canada

Solution, Injection:

Generic: 30 mg/mL (1 mL)

Solution, Intramuscular:

Toradol: 10 mg/mL (1 mL)

Generic: 30 mg/mL (1 mL, 10 mL)

Tablet, Oral:

Toradol: 10 mg

Generic: 10 mg

Dental Health Professional Considerations

According to the manufacturer, ketorolac has been used inappropriately by physicians in the past. According to the manufacturer, ketorolac has been prescribed to NSAID-sensitive patients, patients with GI bleeding, and for long-term use, which is not recommended. A warning has been issued regarding increased incidence and severity of GI complications with increasing doses and duration of use. Labeling now includes the statement that ketorolac inhibits platelet function and is indicated for up to 5 days use only.

◆ **Ketorolac Tromethamine** *see* Ketorolac (Systemic) *on page 861*

Ketotifen (Systemic) (kee toe TYE fen)

Related Information

Respiratory Diseases *on page 1680*

Brand Names: Canada APO-Ketotifen [DSC]; Zaditen

Pharmacologic Category Histamine H_1 Antagonist; Histamine H_1 Antagonist, Second Generation; Mast Cell Stabilizer; Piperidine Derivative

Use Note: Not approved in the US

Atopic asthma: Adjunctive therapy in the chronic treatment of mild, atopic asthma in children

Limitations of use: Not indicated for acute prevention or treatment of acute asthma attacks.

Local Anesthetic/Vasoconstrictor Precautions

No information available to require special precautions

Effects on Dental Treatment No significant effects or complications reported

Effects on Bleeding No information available to require special precautions

Adverse Reactions

1% to 10%:

Central nervous system: Disturbed sleep (1%), headache (1%)

Dermatologic: Skin rash (4%), urticaria (1%)

Endocrine & metabolic: Weight gain (5%)
Gastrointestinal: Abdominal pain (1%), increased appetite (1%)
Infection: Influenza (3%)
Ophthalmic: Eyelid edema (1%)
Respiratory: Respiratory tract infection (4%), epistaxis (1%)

<1%, postmarketing, and/or case reports: Cystitis, dizziness, erythema multiforme, excitement, hepatitis, increased serum transaminases, insomnia, irritability, nervousness, Stevens-Johnson syndrome, thrombocytopenia, xerostomia

Mechanism of Action Exhibits noncompetitive H_1-receptor antagonist and mast cell stabilizer properties. Efficacy in asthma likely results from a combination of anti-inflammatory and antihistaminergic actions including interference with chemokine-induced migration of eosinophils into inflamed airways, inhibition of airway hyper-reactivity due to platelet activating factor (PAF), antagonism of leukotriene-induced bronchoconstriction.

Pharmacodynamics/Kinetics

Half-life Elimination Biphasic: Distribution: 3 to 5 hours; Elimination: 21 hours

Time to Peak Plasma: 2 to 4 hours

Pregnancy Considerations Adverse events have been observed in some animal studies.

Product Availability Not available in the US

- **Ketotifen Fumarate** *see* Ketotifen (Systemic) *on page 866*
- **Kevzara** *see* Sarilumab *on page 1359*
- **Keytruda** *see* Pembrolizumab *on page 1204*
- **Khapzory** *see* LEVOleucovorin *on page 899*
- **Khedezla [DSC]** *see* Desvenlafaxine *on page 462*
- **Khloditan** *see* Mitotane *on page 1041*
- **Kimidess [DSC]** *see* Ethinyl Estradiol and Desogestrel *on page 609*
- **Kineret** *see* Anakinra *on page 149*
- **Kisqali (200 MG Dose)** *see* Ribociclib *on page 1322*
- **Kisqali (400 MG Dose)** *see* Ribociclib *on page 1322*
- **Kisqali (600 MG Dose)** *see* Ribociclib *on page 1322*
- **Kitabis Pak** *see* Tobramycin (Oral Inhalation) *on page 1456*
- **KIT/PDGFR Inhibitor DCC-2618** *see* Ripretinib *on page 1330*
- **Klofensaid II [DSC]** *see* Diclofenac (Topical) *on page 489*
- **KlonoPIN** *see* ClonazePAM *on page 385*
- **Klor-Con** *see* Potassium Chloride *on page 1249*
- **Klor-Con 10** *see* Potassium Chloride *on page 1249*
- **Klor-Con M10** *see* Potassium Chloride *on page 1249*
- **Klor-Con M15** *see* Potassium Chloride *on page 1249*
- **Klor-Con M20** *see* Potassium Chloride *on page 1249*
- **Klor-Con Sprinkle** *see* Potassium Chloride *on page 1249*
- **KMD 3213** *see* Silodosin *on page 1370*
- **Koate** *see* Antihemophilic Factor (Human) *on page 152*
- **Koate DVI** *see* Antihemophilic Factor (Human) *on page 152*
- **Koate-DVI** *see* Antihemophilic Factor (Human) *on page 152*
- **Kogenate FS** *see* Antihemophilic Factor (Recombinant) *on page 153*
- **Kogenate FS Bio-Set [DSC]** *see* Antihemophilic Factor (Recombinant) *on page 153*
- **Kombiglyze XR** *see* Saxagliptin and Metformin *on page 1360*
- **Korlym** *see* MiFEPRIStone *on page 1028*
- **Koselugo** *see* Selumetinib *on page 1365*
- **Kovaltry** *see* Antihemophilic Factor (Recombinant) *on page 153*
- **Kovanaze** *see* Tetracaine and Oxymetazoline *on page 1429*
- **Krintafel** *see* Tafenoquine *on page 1402*
- **Krystexxa** *see* Pegloticase *on page 1203*
- **KS Ibuprofen [OTC]** *see* Ibuprofen *on page 786*
- **KS Stool Softener [OTC]** *see* Docusate *on page 509*
- **K-Tab** *see* Potassium Chloride *on page 1249*
- **K-Tan Plus** *see* Vitamins (Multiple/Oral) *on page 1550*
- **KTE-C19** *see* Axicabtagene Ciloleucel *on page 196*
- **KTE-C19 CAR** *see* Axicabtagene Ciloleucel *on page 196*
- **KU-0059436** *see* Olaparib *on page 1130*
- **Kurvelo** *see* Ethinyl Estradiol and Levonorgestrel *on page 612*
- **Kymriah** *see* Tisagenlecleucel *on page 1454*
- **Kynamro** *see* Mipomersen *on page 1037*
- **Kynmobi** *see* Apomorphine *on page 160*
- **Kynmobi Titration Kit** *see* Apomorphine *on page 160*
- **Kytril** *see* Granisetron *on page 748*
- **L-749,345** *see* Ertapenem *on page 586*
- **L-758,298** *see* Fosaprepitant *on page 713*
- **L 754030** *see* Aprepitant *on page 162*
- **LA 20304a** *see* Gemifloxacin *on page 733*

Labetalol (la BET a lole)

Related Information

Cardiovascular Diseases *on page 1654*

Brand Names: Canada APO-Labetalol; RIVA-Labetalol; Trandate

Pharmacologic Category Antihypertensive; Beta-Blocker With Alpha-Blocking Activity

Use Hypertension: Management of hypertension (IV indicated for severe hypertension only [eg, hypertensive emergencies]). **Note:** Beta-blockers are **not** recommended as first-line therapy (ACC/AHA [Whelton 2018]).

Local Anesthetic/Vasoconstrictor Precautions Use with caution; epinephrine has interacted with nonselective beta-blockers to result in initial hypertensive episode followed by bradycardia

Effects on Dental Treatment Key adverse event(s) related to dental treatment: Taste disorder.

Many nonsteroidal anti-inflammatory drugs, such as ibuprofen and indomethacin, can reduce the hypotensive effect of beta-blockers after 3 or more weeks of therapy with the NSAID. Short-term NSAID use (ie, 3 days) requires no special precautions in patients taking beta-blockers.

Effects on Bleeding No information available to require special precautions

Adverse Reactions

>10%:

Cardiovascular: Orthostatic hypotension (intravenous: 58%; tablet: 1%)

Central nervous system: Dizziness (1% to 20%), fatigue (1% to 11%)
Gastrointestinal: Nausea (≤19%)

1% to 10%:

Cardiovascular: Edema (1% to 2%), flushing (1%), hypotension (1%), ventricular arrhythmia (intravenous: 1%)
Central nervous system: Paresthesia (≤7%), drowsiness (≤3%), yawning (≤3%), headache (2%), vertigo (1% to 2%), hypoesthesia (1%)
Dermatologic: Diaphoresis (≤4%), pruritus (1%), skin rash (1%)
Gastrointestinal: Dyspepsia (≤4%), vomiting (≤4%), dysgeusia (1%)
Genitourinary: Ejaculatory failure (1% to 5%), impotence (1% to 4%)
Hepatic: Increased serum transaminases (4%)
Neuromuscular & skeletal: Asthenia (1%)
Ophthalmic: Visual disturbance (1%)
Renal: Increased blood urea nitrogen (≤8%), increased serum creatinine (≤8%)
Respiratory: Nasal congestion (1% to 6%), dyspnea (2%), wheezing (1%)

<1%, postmarketing, and/or case reports: Anaphylactoid reaction, angioedema, antibody development (antimitochondrial), bradycardia, bronchospasm, cardiac failure, cholestatic jaundice, diabetes mellitus, diarrhea, difficulty in micturition, facial erythema, fever, heart block, hepatic injury, hepatic necrosis, hepatitis, hypersensitivity reaction, increased liver enzymes, jaundice, lichenoid eruption, lichen planus, maculopapular rash, muscle cramps, myopathy, Peyronie disease, positive ANA titer, psoriasiform eruption, syncope, systemic lupus erythematosus, transient alopecia, urinary retention, urticaria, xerophthalmia

Mechanism of Action Blocks alpha$_1$-, beta$_1$-, and beta$_2$-adrenergic receptor sites; elevated renins are reduced. The ratios of alpha- to beta-blockade differ depending on the route of administration estimated to be 1:3 (oral) and 1:7 (IV) (Goa 1989).

Pharmacodynamics/Kinetics

Onset of Action Oral: 20 minutes to 2 hours (McNeil 1984); IV: Within 5 minutes (Goa 1989); Peak effect: Oral: 2 to 4 hours; IV: 5 to 15 minutes (Goa 1989)

Duration of Action Blood pressure response:
Oral: 8 to 12 hours (dose dependent)
IV: Average: 16 to 18 hours (dose dependent)

Half-life Elimination Oral: 6 to 8 hours; IV: ~5.5 hours

Time to Peak Plasma: Oral: 1 to 2 hours

Pregnancy Risk Factor C

Pregnancy Considerations Labetalol crosses the placenta.

Exposure to labetalol during pregnancy may increase the risk for adverse events in the neonate. If maternal use of a beta-blocker is needed, fetal growth should be monitored during pregnancy and the newborn should be monitored for 48 hours after delivery for bradycardia, hypoglycemia, and respiratory depression (ESC [Regitz-Zagrosek 2018]).

Chronic maternal hypertension is also associated with adverse events in the fetus/infant. Chronic maternal hypertension may increase the risk of birth defects, low birth weight, premature delivery, stillbirth, and neonatal death. Actual fetal/neonatal risks may be related to duration and severity of maternal hypertension. Untreated chronic hypertension may also increase the risks of adverse maternal outcomes, including gestational diabetes, preeclampsia, delivery complications, stroke, and myocardial infarction (ACOG 203 2019).

Most pharmacokinetic properties of labetalol are not significantly changed by pregnancy (Fischer 2014; Rogers 1990; Rubin 1983; Saotome 1993).

Oral labetalol is considered appropriate for the treatment of chronic hypertension in pregnancy (ACOG 203 2019; Magee 2014). Intravenous labetalol is recommended for use in the management of acute onset, severe hypertension (systolic BP ≥160 mm Hg or diastolic BP ≥110 mm Hg) in pregnant and postpartum women. In general, avoid use of labetalol in women with asthma or heart failure (ACOG 202 2019; ACOG 767 2019; Magee 2014).

◆ **Labetalol HCl** *see* Labetalol *on page 867*

◆ **Labetalol Hydrochloride** *see* Labetalol *on page 867*

Lacosamide (la KOE sa mide)

Brand Names: US Vimpat

Brand Names: Canada APO-Lacosamide; Auro-Lacosamide; JAMP-Lacosamide; MAR-Lacosamide; MINT-Lacosamide; Pharma-Lacosamide; SANDOZ Lacosamide; TEVA-Lacosamide; Vimpat

Pharmacologic Category Anticonvulsant, Miscellaneous

Use Focal (partial) onset seizures: Monotherapy or adjunctive therapy in the treatment of focal (partial) onset seizures in children 4 years or older and adults.

Local Anesthetic/Vasoconstrictor Precautions Lacosamide may prolong PR interval resulting in cardiac conduction problems; it is not known what effect vasoconstrictors will have in patients taking medications that could prolong PR interval. It is suggested that the clinician consult with the physician prior to use of vasoconstrictor in suspected patients; use vasoconstrictor with caution.

Effects on Dental Treatment No significant effects or complications reported

Effects on Bleeding No information available to require special precautions

Adverse Reactions

>10%:

Central nervous system: Dizziness (16% to 30%), headache (11% to 14%)
Gastrointestinal: Nausea (7% to 11%)

1% to 10%:

Central nervous system: Drowsiness (8%), fatigue (7%), ataxia (4% to 7%), vertigo (3% to 5%), equilibrium disturbance (1% to 5%), abnormal gait (2%), depression (2%)
Dermatologic: Pruritus (2% to 3%)
Gastrointestinal: Vomiting (6% to 9%), diarrhea (5%)
Hematologic & oncologic: Bruise (4%)
Local: Pain at injection site (IV: 3%), local irritation (IV: 1%)
Neuromuscular & skeletal: Tremor (6%), asthenia (2%)
Ophthalmic: Diplopia (6% to 10%), blurred vision (9%), nystagmus (5%)
Miscellaneous: Laceration (3%)

Frequency not defined:
Cardiovascular: Palpitations, syncope
Central nervous system: Cerebellar syndrome, cognitive dysfunction, confusion, disturbance in attention, dysarthria, falling, hypoesthesia, intoxicated feeling, irritability, mood changes, paresthesia, suicidal ideation, suicidal tendencies
Gastrointestinal: Constipation, dyspepsia, oral hypoesthesia, xerostomia
Hematologic & oncologic: Anemia, neutropenia
Neuromuscular & skeletal: Muscle spasm
Otic: Tinnitus
Miscellaneous: Fever
<1%, postmarketing, and/or case reports: Abnormal hepatic function tests, acute psychosis, aggressive behavior, agitation, agranulocytosis, angioedema, atrial fibrillation, atrial flutter, atrioventricular block, bradycardia, cardiac arrhythmia, DRESS syndrome, erythema at injection site, euphoria, first degree atrioventricular block, hallucination, hepatitis, increased serum alanine aminotransferase, insomnia, nephritis, prolongation P-R interval on ECG, seizure, skin rash, Stevens-Johnson syndrome, toxic epidermal necrolysis, urticaria, ventricular tachyarrhythmia

Mechanism of Action *In vitro* studies have shown that lacosamide stabilizes hyperexcitable neuronal membranes and inhibits repetitive neuronal firing by enhancing the slow inactivation of sodium channels (with no effects on fast inactivation of sodium channels).

Pharmacodynamics/Kinetics

Half-life Elimination

Children ≥4 years and Adolescents:
Mean weight 11 kg: 7.4 hours
Mean weight 28.9 kg: 10.6 hours
Mean weight 70 kg: 14.8 hours
Adults: ~13 hours

Time to Peak Oral: 1 to 4 hours

Pregnancy Considerations

Lacosamide crosses the placenta (Ylikotila 2015; Zárubová 2016).

Due to pregnancy-induced physiologic changes, some pharmacokinetic properties of lacosamide may be altered (Zárubová 2016). Information related to pregnancy outcomes following maternal use of lacosamide is limited (Hoeltzenbein 2011; Lattanzi 2017; Zárubová 2016). In general, maternal polytherapy with antiepileptic drugs may increase the risk of congenital malformations; monotherapy with the lowest effective dose is recommended. Newborns of women taking antiepileptic medications may be at an increased risk of adverse events (Harden 2009).

Patients exposed to lacosamide during pregnancy are encouraged to enroll themselves into the North American Antiepileptic Drug (NAAED) Pregnancy Registry by calling 1-888-233-2334. Additional information is available at http://www.aedpregnancyregistry.org.

Controlled Substance C-V

◆ **Lactinex [OTC]** *see Lactobacillus on page 869*

Lactitol (LAK ti tol)

Pharmacologic Category Ammonium Detoxicant; Laxative, Osmotic

Use Chronic idiopathic constipation: Treatment of chronic idiopathic constipation (CIC) in adult patients.

Local Anesthetic/Vasoconstrictor Precautions No information available to require special precautions.

Effects on Dental Treatment No significant effects or complications reported.

Effects on Bleeding No information available to require special precautions.

Adverse Reactions

1% to 10%:
Cardiovascular: Increased blood pressure (3%)
Gastrointestinal: Flatulence (8%), diarrhea (4%), abdominal distention (3%), abdominal pain (3%), severe diarrhea (1%)
Genitourinary: Urinary tract infection (5%)
Neuromuscular & skeletal: Increased creatine phosphokinase in blood specimen (4%)
Respiratory: Upper respiratory tract infection (9%)
Postmarketing: Hypersensitivity reaction, pruritus, skin rash

Mechanism of Action Simple monosaccharide sugar; produces laxative effect in colon by causing water influx into small intestine.

Pharmacodynamics/Kinetics

Half-life Elimination 2.4 hours.

Pregnancy Considerations

Lactitol has minimal systemic absorption.

Treatment of constipation in pregnant women is similar to that of nonpregnant patients, and medications may be used when diet and lifestyle modifications are not effective. In general, osmotic laxatives are not initial therapy and should be used with caution and only for short durations in pregnancy due to the risk of electrolyte abnormalities (Body 2016).

Product Availability Pizensy: FDA approved February 2020; anticipated availability is currently unknown.

◆ **Lactitol Monohydrate** *see* Lactitol *on page 869*

Lactobacillus (lak toe ba SIL us)

Related Information

Ulcerative, Erosive, and Painful Oral Mucosal Disorders *on page 1758*

Brand Names: US Advanced Probiotic [OTC]; Culturelle Baby [OTC]; Culturelle [OTC]; Dialyvite Probiotic [OTC]; Dofus [OTC]; Floranex [OTC]; Kala [OTC]; Lactinex [OTC]; Lacto-Bifidus [OTC]; Lacto-Key [OTC]; Lacto-Pectin [OTC]; Lacto-TriBlend [OTC]; Megadophilus [OTC]; MoreDophilus [OTC]; Pedia-Lax Probiotic Yums [OTC]; Prodigen; Promella in Prebiotic; ReZyst IM [DSC]; Risa-Bid [OTC]; RisaQuad [OTC]; RisaQuad-2 [OTC]; Superdophilus [OTC]; Visbiome [OTC]; VSL #3 [OTC]; VSL #3-DS

Brand Names: Canada Bacid; Bio-K+; Fermalac

Generic Availability (US) Yes

Pharmacologic Category Dietary Supplement; Probiotic

Dental Use Treatment of uncomplicated diarrhea, particularly that caused by antibiotic therapy; re-establish normal physiologic and bacterial flora of the intestinal tract

Use

Dietary supplement: Probiotic to promote normal bacterial flora of the intestinal tract; probiotic supplement for breastfed or partially breastfed infants experiencing excessive crying, colic, and fussiness (Gerber Soothe Colic only).

Medical food:

Visbiome: Dietary management of pouchitis, ulcerative colitis, and irritable bowel syndrome.
VSL#3: Dietary management of an ileal pouch or ulcerative colitis.

Local Anesthetic/Vasoconstrictor Precautions No information available to require special precautions

Effects on Dental Treatment No significant effects or complications reported

Effects on Bleeding No information available to require special precautions

Adverse Reactions Frequency not defined.

Gastrointestinal: Bloating (intestinal), flatulence

Dental Usual Dosage Dietary supplement: Oral: Dosing varies by manufacturer; consult product labeling

Children (Culturelle): 1 capsule daily

Adults:

Bacid: 2 caplets/day

Culturelle: 1 capsule daily; may increase to twice daily

Flora-Q: 1 capsule/day

Lacto-Key 100 or 600: 1-2 capsules/day

Lactinex: 1 packet or 4 tablets 3-4 times/day

VSL #3: 1-8 sachets or 2-32 capsules/day

VSL #3-DS: 1-4 packets/day

Dosing

Adult & Geriatric

Dietary supplement/medical food: Oral: Dosing varies by manufacturer; consult product labeling.

Acidophilus products: 2 capsules 2 to 4 times daily or 1 to 2 wafers 2 to 4 times daily

Culturelle Digestive Health capsule and chewable tablet: 1 capsule or chewable tablet once daily; may increase chewable tablet to twice daily to alleviate digestive distress or during travel

Floranex: 4 tablets 3 to 4 times daily

Lactinex: 1 packet or 4 tablets 3 to 4 times daily

Visbiome:

Irritable bowel syndrome: 2 to 4 capsules or 1/2 to 1 packet per day

Pouchitis: 2 to 4 packets/day

Ulcerative colitis (active): 4 to 8 packets/day

Ulcerative colitis (maintenance): 4 to 8 capsules or 1 to 2 packets per day

VSL #3: 1 to 8 packets or 2 to 8 capsules/day

VSL #3-DS: 1 to 4 packets/day

Renal Impairment: Adult There are no dosage adjustments provided in the manufacturer's labeling.

Hepatic Impairment: Adult There are no dosage adjustments provided in the manufacturer's labeling.

Pediatric

Dietary supplement: Note: Product formulations and labeling for use in pediatric patients may vary among available formulations; consult product labeling.

Culturelle:

Baby Grow and Thrive Drops: *Lactobacillus rhamnosus* GG 400 million CFU, *Bifidobacterium animalis* 100 million CFU, and cholecalciferol 2 mcg/drop: Infants: Oral: 5 drops once daily.

Baby Grow and Thrive Packets: *Lactobacillus rhamnosus* GG 3 billion CFU, *Bifidobacterium animalis* 500 million CFU, and cholecalciferol 10 mcg/packet: Children ≤2 years: Oral: 1 packet once daily.

Kids Daily Probiotic Packets: *Lactobacillus rhamnosus* GG 5 billion CFU/packet: Children <3 years: Oral: 1 packet once or twice daily.

Kids Daily Probiotic Chewables: *Lactobacillus rhamnosus* GG 5 billion CFU/tablet: Children ≥3 years and Adolescents: Oral: 1 tablet once or twice daily.

Digestive Health Daily Probiotic Chewable: *Lactobacillus rhamnosus* GG 10 billion CFU, inulin 200 mg, and vitamin C 6 mg/tablet: Children ≥12 years and Adolescents: Oral: 1 tablet once or twice daily.

Digestive Health Daily Probiotic Capsule: *Lactobacillus rhamnosus* GG 10 billion CFU and inulin 200 mg/capsule: Children ≥12 years and Adolescents: Oral: 1 capsule once or twice daily.

Digestive Health Extra Strength: *Lactobacillus rhamnosus* GG 20 billion CFU and inulin 200 mg/capsule: Children ≥12 years and Adolescents: Oral: 1 capsule once daily.

Gerber:

Soothe Probiotic Colic Drops: *Lactobacillus reuteri* 20 million CFU/drop: Infants: Oral: 5 drops once daily.

Soothe Vitamin D and Probiotic Drops: *Lactobacillus reuteri* 20 million CFU and cholecalciferol 2 mcg/drop: Infants: Oral: 5 drops once daily.

Good Start Toddler Digestive and Immune Support Probiotic Packet: *Lactobacillus reuteri* 100 million CFU/packet: Children: Oral: 1 packet once daily.

Good Start Kids Digestive and Immune Support Probiotic Tablet: *Lactobacillus reuteri* 100 million CFU/tablet: Children ≥3 years: Oral: 1 tablet once daily.

Renal Impairment: Pediatric There are no dosage adjustments provided in the manufacturer's labeling.

Hepatic Impairment: Pediatric There are no dosage adjustments provided in the manufacturer's labeling.

Mechanism of Action Helps re-establish normal intestinal flora; suppresses the growth of potentially pathogenic microorganisms by producing lactic acid which favors the establishment of an aciduric flora.

Contraindications OTC labeling: When used for self-medication, do not use if sensitive to milk protein (product specific).

Warnings/Precautions Probiotics are classified as dietary supplements; therefore, there are no safety reviews or approved therapeutic indications by the FDA. Use dietary supplements containing live bacteria or yeast with caution in immunocompromised patients. A fatal case of GI mucormycosis caused by the mold *Rhizopus oryzae* has been previously reported in a premature infant administered a dietary supplement containing 3 species of live bacteria (FDA Safety Information 2014). There is no conclusive evidence to support widespread use in the treatment of diarrhea. Significant differences may exist from one preparation compared to another with respect to biologic activity and composition. Some products may contain lactose; use with caution in patients with lactose intolerance.

Warnings: Additional Pediatric Considerations Dietary supplements containing live bacteria or yeast may be associated with a risk of invasive fungal disease in the immunocompromised. A premature neonate developed a fatal case of GI mucormycosis caused by *Rhizopus oryzae*; this mold was found in an unopened bottle of ABC Dophilus powder that was used to treat the infant (FDA Safety Information 2014). Case reports of *Lactobacillus* sepsis have also been reported in at least 5 pediatric patients (ages 18 days to 17 years) treated with *Lactobacillus Rhamnosus* GG (Dani 2016; Land 2005; Vahabnezhad 2013). The AAP recommends avoiding use of probiotics in pediatric patients who are seriously or chronically ill, including ill preterm neonates and patients with indwelling medical devices or IV catheters (AAP [Thomas 2010]).

Other trials evaluating the addition of probiotic formulations (various live bacteria/yeast have been reported) to infant formula have reported no adverse effects when used in healthy infants. Use with caution; *Lactobacillus*-containing products are considered a dietary supplement and therefore less regulated by the FDA in terms of production, safety and efficacy, and definitive data reporting in these areas are lacking.

Drug Interactions

Metabolism/Transport Effects None known.

Avoid Concomitant Use There are no known interactions where it is recommended to avoid concomitant use.

Increased Effect/Toxicity There are no known significant interactions involving an increase in effect.

Decreased Effect There are no known significant interactions involving a decrease in effect.

Dietary Considerations Some products may contain lactose, potassium, and/or sodium.

Dosage Forms: US

Capsule:

Advanced Probiotic [OTC]: *L. acidophilus, L. casei, L. delbrueckii,* and *L. rhamnosus* GG 10 billion live cultures

Culturelle [OTC]: *L. rhamnosus* GG 10 billion colony-forming units

Dofus [OTC]: *L. acidophilus* and *L. bifidus* 10:1 ratio

Lacto-Key [OTC]:

100: *L. acidophilus* 1 billion colony-forming units

600: *L. acidophilus* 6 billion colony-forming units

Lacto-Bifidus [OTC]:

100: *L. bifidus* 1 billion colony-forming units

600: *L. bifidus* 6 billion colony-forming units

Lacto-Pectin [OTC]: *L. acidophilus, L. casei, L. plantarum, L. rhamnosus, Bifidobacterium breve, and B. longum* 20 billion colony-forming units

Lacto-TriBlend [OTC]:

100: *L. acidophilus, L. bifidus,* and *L. bulgaricus* 1 billion colony-forming units

600: *L. acidophilus, L. bifidus,* and *L. bulgaricus* 6 billion colony-forming units

Megadophilus [OTC], Superdophilus [OTC]: *L. acidophilus* 2 billion units

Prodigen: *L. acidophilus* 42 billion colony-forming units and *Bifidobacterium lactis* 39 billion colony-forming units

Promella in Prebiotic: *L. acidophilus* and *Bifidobacterium animalis lactis* 64 billion colony-forming units

RisaQuad [OTC]: *L. acidophilus* and *L. paracasei* 8 billion colony-forming units

RisaQuad-2 [OTC]: *L. acidophilus* and *L. paracasei* 16 billion colony-forming units

Visbiome [OTC]: *L. acidophilus, L. plantarum, L. paracasei, L. bulgaricus, Bifidobacterium breve, B. longum, B. infantis, and Streptococcus thermophilus* 112 billion live cells

VSL #3 [OTC]: *L. acidophilus, L. plantarum, L. paracasei, L. bulgaricus, Bifidobacterium breve, B. longum, B. infantis, and Streptococcus thermophilus* 112 billion live cells

Caplet:

Risa-Bid [OTC]: *L. acidophilus* and *L. bulgaricus* [also contains *Bifidobacterium bifidum* and *Streptococcus thermophilus*]

Granules:

Culturelle Baby Grow + Thrive [OTC]: *L. rhamnosus* and *Bifidobacterium animalis* 3.5 billion colony-forming untis with cholecalciferol 400 IU per packet (30s)

Floranex [OTC], Lactinex [OTC]: *L. acidophilus* and *L. bulgaricus* 100 million live cells per 1 g packet (12s)

Liquid:

Culturelle Baby Grow + Thrive: *L. rhamnosus* and *Bifidobacterium animalis* 2.5 billion colony-forming units with cholecalciferol 400 IU per 5 drops (9 mL)

Powder:

Lacto-TriBlend [OTC]: *L. acidophilus, L. bifidus,* and *L. bulgaricus* 10 billion colony-forming units per 1/4 teaspoon

Megadophilus [OTC], Superdophilus [OTC]: *L. acidophilus* 2 billion units per half-teaspoon

MoreDophilus [OTC]: *L. acidophilus* 12.4 billion units per teaspoon

VSL #3 [OTC]: *L. acidophilus, L. plantarum, L. paracasei, L. bulgaricus* 450 billion live cells

VSL #3-DS: *L. acidophilus, L. plantarum, L. paracasei, L. bulgaricus* 900 billion live cells

Tablet:

Floranex [OTC]: *L. acidophilus* and *L. bulgaricus* 1 million colony-forming units

Kala [OTC]: *L. acidophilus* 200 million units

Tablet, chewable:

Dialyvite Probiotic: *L. acidophilus* and *Bifidobacterium lactis* 10 billion cells

Lactinex [OTC]: *L. acidophilus* and *L. bulgaricus* 1 million live cells

Pedia-Lax Probiotic Yums [OTC]: *L. reuteri* 100 million organisms

Wafer: *L. acidophilus* 90 mg and *L. bifidus* 25 mg (100s)

- ***Lactobacillus acidophilus*** *see Lactobacillus on page 869*
- ***Lactobacillus bifidus*** *see Lactobacillus on page 869*
- ***Lactobacillus bulgaricus*** *see Lactobacillus on page 869*
- ***Lactobacillus casei*** *see Lactobacillus on page 869*
- ***Lactobacillus paracasei*** *see Lactobacillus on page 869*
- ***Lactobacillus plantarum*** *see Lactobacillus on page 869*
- ***Lactobacillus reuteri*** *see Lactobacillus on page 869*
- ***Lactobacillus rhamnosus* GG** *see Lactobacillus on page 869*
- **Lacto-Bifidus [OTC]** *see Lactobacillus on page 869*
- **Lactoflavin** *see* Riboflavin *on page 1323*
- **Lacto-Key [OTC]** *see Lactobacillus on page 869*
- **Lacto-Pectin [OTC]** *see Lactobacillus on page 869*
- **Lacto-TriBlend [OTC]** *see Lactobacillus on page 869*
- **Ladakamycin** *see* AzaCITIDine *on page 198*
- **LAIV** *see* Influenza Virus Vaccine (Live/Attenuated) *on page 813*
- **LAIV4** *see* Influenza Virus Vaccine (Live/Attenuated) *on page 813*
- **L-AmB** *see* Amphotericin B (Liposomal) *on page 138*
- **Lambrolizumab** *see* Pembrolizumab *on page 1204*
- **LaMICtal** *see* LamoTRIgine *on page 874*
- **LaMICtal ODT** *see* LamoTRIgine *on page 874*
- **LaMICtal Starter** *see* LamoTRIgine *on page 874*
- **LaMICtal XR** *see* LamoTRIgine *on page 874*
- **LamISIL [DSC]** *see* Terbinafine (Systemic) *on page 1421*
- **LamISIL AF Defense [OTC] [DSC]** *see* Tolnaftate *on page 1462*

LamiVUDine (la MI vyoo deen)

Related Information

HIV Infection and AIDS *on page 1690*

Systemic Viral Diseases *on page 1709*

Brand Names: US Epivir; Epivir HBV

Brand Names: Canada 3TC; APO-LamiVUDine; APO-LamiVUDine HBV; Heptovir

Pharmacologic Category Antihepadnaviral, Reverse Transcriptase Inhibitor, Nucleoside (Anti-HBV); Antiretroviral, Reverse Transcriptase Inhibitor, Nucleoside (Anti-HIV)

Use

Chronic hepatitis B (Epivir HBV): Treatment of chronic hepatitis B associated with evidence of hepatitis B viral replication and active liver inflammation

Limitations of use: Use only when an alternative antiviral agent with a higher genetic barrier to resistance is not available or appropriate. Lamivudine-HBV has not been evaluated in patients coinfected with HIV, hepatitis C virus, or hepatitis delta virus; with decompensated liver disease; or in liver transplant recipients.

HIV-1 infection, treatment (Epivir): Treatment of HIV-1 in combination with other antiretroviral agents

Local Anesthetic/Vasoconstrictor Precautions No information available to require special precautions

Effects on Dental Treatment No significant effects or complications reported

Effects on Bleeding No information available to require special precautions relative to hemostasis.

Adverse Reactions Incidence data include patients on combination therapy with other antiretroviral agents.

>10%:

Central nervous system: Headache (35%), fatigue (≤27%), malaise (≤27%), paresthesia (≤15%), peripheral neuropathy (≤15%), neuropathy (12%), insomnia (≤11%), sleep disorder (≤11%)

Dermatologic: Skin rash (9% to 12%)

Gastrointestinal: Nausea (≤33%), diarrhea (adults: 14% to 18%, children: 8%), pancreatitis (≤18%; higher percentage in pediatric patients), sore throat (13%), vomiting (≤13%)

Hematologic & oncologic: Neutropenia (7% to 15%)

Hepatic: Increased serum alanine aminotransferase (adults: 4% to 27%, children: 1%), hepatomegaly (children: 11%, adults: <1%)

Infection: infection (25%; includes ear, nose, and throat)

Neuromuscular & skeletal: Musculoskeletal pain (12%)

Respiratory: Nasal signs and symptoms (8% to 20%), cough (15% to 18%)

Miscellaneous: Fever (children: 25%, adults: ≤10%)

1% to 10%:

Central nervous system: Dizziness (10%), chills (≤10%), depression (9%)

Endocrine & metabolic: Increased amylase (2% to 4%)

Gastrointestinal: Increased serum lipase (adults: 10%, children: 3%), anorexia (≤10%), decreased appetite (≤10%), abdominal pain (9%), abdominal cramps (6%), stomatitis (children: 6%, adults: <1%), dyspepsia (5%)

Hematologic & oncologic: Lymphadenopathy (children: 9%), splenomegaly (children 5%, adults <1%), thrombocytopenia (adults: 4%, children: 1%), decreased hemoglobin (2% to 4%)

Hepatic: Increased serum aspartate aminotransferase (2% to 4%)

Neuromuscular & skeletal: Increased creatine phosphokinase (9%), myalgia (8%), arthralgia (5%)

Otic: Ear disease (children: 7%)

Respiratory: Abnormal breath sounds (children: ≤7%; adults: <1%), wheezing (children: ≤7%, adults: <1%)

<1%, postmarketing, and/or case reports: Alopecia, anaphylaxis, anemia, asthenia, cramps, exacerbation of hepatitis B, hyperbilirubinemia, hyperglycemia, immune reconstitution syndrome, lactic acidosis, liver steatosis, muscle cramps, myasthenia, pruritus, pure red cell aplasia, redistribution of body fat, rhabdomyolysis, urticaria

Mechanism of Action Lamivudine is a cytosine analog. In vitro, lamivudine is triphosphorylated, the principle mode of action is inhibition of HIV reverse transcription via viral DNA chain termination; inhibits RNA- and DNA-dependent DNA polymerase activities of reverse transcriptase. In hepatitis B, the monophosphate form of lamivudine is incorporated into the viral DNA by hepatitis B virus polymerase, resulting in DNA chain termination.

Pharmacodynamics/Kinetics

Half-life Elimination

Intracellular: 10 to 15 hours

Elimination:

Children 4 months to 14 years: 2 ± 0.6 hours

Adults: 5 to 7 hours; increased with renal impairment

Time to Peak

Pediatric patients 0.5 to 17 years: Median: 1.5 hours (range: 0.5 to 4 hours) (Lewis 1996)

Adolescents 13 to 17 years: 0.5 to 1 hour

Adults: Fed: 3.2 hours; Fasted: 0.9 hours

Reproductive Considerations

The Health and Human Services perinatal HIV guidelines consider lamivudine a preferred nucleoside reverse transcriptase inhibitor for females living with HIV who are not yet pregnant but are trying to conceive.

For males and females living with HIV and planning a pregnancy, maximum viral suppression below the limits of detection with antiretroviral therapy (ART), modification of therapy (if needed), optimization of the woman's health, and a discussion of the potential risks and benefits of ART therapy during pregnancy is recommended prior to conception (HHS [perinatal] 2019).

Pregnancy Considerations

Lamivudine has a high level of transfer across the human placenta.

No increased risk of overall birth defects has been observed following first trimester exposure according to data collected by the antiretroviral pregnancy registry. Maternal antiretroviral therapy (ART) may be associated with adverse pregnancy outcomes, including preterm delivery, stillbirth, low birth weight, and small for gestational age infants. Actual risks may be influenced by maternal factors such as disease severity, gestational age at initiation of therapy, and specific ART regimen; therefore, close fetal monitoring is recommended. Based on data collected by the antiretroviral pregnancy registry, the risk of spontaneous abortions, induced abortions, and preterm birth is less in lamivudine-containing regimens compared with regimens without lamivudine. Because there is clear benefit to appropriate treatment, maternal ART should not be withheld due to concerns for adverse neonatal outcomes. Long-term follow-up is recommended for all infants exposed to antiretroviral medications; children without HIV but who were exposed to ART in utero and develop significant organ system abnormalities of unknown etiology (particularly of the CNS or heart) should be evaluated for potential mitochondrial dysfunction. Cases of lactic acidosis and hepatic steatosis have been reported in pregnant women with use of nucleoside reverse transcriptase inhibitors (NRTIs).

The Health and Human Services (HHS) perinatal HIV guidelines consider lamivudine a preferred NRTI for pregnant females living with HIV who are antiretroviral-naive, who have had ART therapy in the past but are restarting, or who require a new ART regimen (due to poor tolerance or poor virologic response of current regimen). In addition, females who become pregnant while taking lamivudine may continue if viral suppression is effective and the regimen is well tolerated. The pharmacokinetics of lamivudine during pregnancy are not significantly altered, and dosage adjustment is not required.

The HHS perinatal HIV guidelines consider lamivudine in combination with either abacavir or tenofovir disoproxil fumarate to be a preferred NRTI backbone for initial therapy in antiretroviral-naive pregnant females. The lamivudine/abacavir backbone is not recommended with atazanavir/ritonavir or efavirenz if pretreatment HIV RNA is >100,000 copies/mL. In addition, the HHS perinatal HIV guidelines consider lamivudine in combination with abacavir and dolutegravir to be a preferred INSTI regimen for initial therapy in antiretroviral-naive pregnant females. The guidelines consider lamivudine with zidovudine to be an alternative NRTI backbone for initial therapy in antiretroviral-naive pregnant females. The guidelines also consider lamivudine plus tenofovir disoproxil fumarate a recommended dual NRTI backbone in regimens for HIV/hepatitis B virus (HBV)-coinfected pregnant females. Use caution with hepatitis B coinfection; hepatitis B flare may occur if lamivudine is discontinued.

In general, ART is recommended for all pregnant females living with HIV to keep the viral load below the limit of detection and reduce the risk of perinatal transmission. Therapy should be individualized following a discussion of the potential risks and benefits of treatment during pregnancy. Monitoring of pregnant females is more frequent than in nonpregnant adults. ART should be continued postpartum for all females living with HIV and can be modified after delivery.

In hepatitis B-infected women (not coinfected with HIV), the American Association for the Study of Liver Diseases (AASLD) chronic hepatitis B treatment guidelines suggest antiviral therapy to reduce the risk of perinatal transmission of hepatitis B in HBsAg-positive pregnant women with an HBV DNA >200,000 units/mL. There are limited data on the level of HBV DNA for when antiviral therapy is routinely recommended (>200,000 units/mL is a conservative recommendation); however, the AASLD recommends against antiviral therapy to reduce the risk of perinatal transmission in HBsAg-positive pregnant women with an HBV DNA ≤200,000 units/mL. Lamivudine is one of the antivirals that has been studied in pregnant women, with most studies initiating antiviral therapy at 28 to 32 weeks gestation and discontinuing antiviral therapy between birth to 3 months postpartum (monitor for ALT flares every 3 months for 6 months following discontinuation). There are insufficient long-term safety data in infants born to mothers who took antiviral agents during pregnancy (AASLD [Terrault 2016]).

Health care providers are encouraged to enroll pregnant females exposed to antiretroviral medications as early in pregnancy as possible in the Antiretroviral Pregnancy Registry (1-800-258-4263 or http://www.APRegistry.com). Health care providers caring for pregnant females living with HIV and their infants may contact the National Perinatal HIV Hotline (888-448-8765) for clinical consultation (HHS [perinatal] 2019).

- **Lamivudine, Abacavir, and Dolutegravir** *see* Abacavir, Dolutegravir, and Lamivudine *on page 51*
- **Lamivudine, Abacavir, and Zidovudine** *see* Abacavir, Lamivudine, and Zidovudine *on page 52*
- **Lamivudine and Abacavir** *see* Abacavir and Lamivudine *on page 51*

Lamivudine and Tenofovir Disoproxil Fumarate

(la MI vyoo deen & ten OF oh vir dye soe PROX il FUE ma rate)

Brand Names: US Cimduo; Temixys

Pharmacologic Category Antiretroviral, Reverse Transcriptase Inhibitor, Nucleoside (Anti-HIV); Antiretroviral, Reverse Transcriptase Inhibitor, Nucleotide (Anti-HIV)

Use HIV-1 infection, treatment: Treatment of HIV-1 infection in combination with other antiretroviral agents in adult and pediatric patients weighing ≥35 kg.

Local Anesthetic/Vasoconstrictor Precautions No information available to require special precautions

Effects on Dental Treatment No significant effects or complications reported

Effects on Bleeding No information available to require special precautions

Adverse Reactions See individual agents.

Mechanism of Action

Lamivudine: Cytosine analog that is phosphorylated intracellularly to its active 5'-triphosphate metabolite. The principal mode of action is inhibition of HIV reverse transcription via viral DNA chain termination; inhibits RNA- and DNA-dependent DNA polymerase activities of reverse transcriptase.

Tenofovir disoproxil fumarate: Nucleotide reverse transcriptase inhibitor; analog of adenosine 5' monophosphate that interferes with the HIV viral RNA dependent DNA polymerase resulting in inhibition of viral replication. TDF is first converted intracellularly by hydrolysis to tenofovir and subsequently phosphorylated to the active tenofovir diphosphate.

Reproductive Considerations

The Health and Human Services (HHS) Perinatal HIV Guidelines consider lamivudine in combination with tenofovir disoproxil fumarate a preferred combination for females living with HIV who are not yet pregnant but are trying to conceive (HHS [perinatal] 2019).

Refer to individual monographs for additional information.

Pregnancy Considerations

The Health and Human Services (HHS) Perinatal HIV Guidelines consider lamivudine in combination with tenofovir disoproxil fumarate to be one of the preferred NRTI backbone for initial therapy in antiretroviral-naive pregnant females. This combination is also preferred for pregnant females who have had antiretroviral therapy (ART) in the past but are restarting, or who require a new ART regimen (due to poor tolerance or poor virologic response of current regimen). Females who become pregnant while taking this combination may continue if viral suppression is effective and the regimen is well tolerated. The guidelines also consider lamivudine plus tenofovir disoproxil fumarate to be a recommended dual NRTI backbone in regimens for HIV/HBV-coinfected pregnant females (HHS [perinatal] 2019).

Refer to individual monographs for additional information.

Lamivudine and Zidovudine

(la MI vyoo deen & zye DOE vyoo deen)

Related Information

HIV Infection and AIDS *on page 1690*
LamiVUDine *on page 872*
Zidovudine *on page 1569*

Brand Names: US Combivir

Brand Names: Canada APO-Lamivudine-Zidovudine; Auro-Lamivudine/Zidovudine; Combivir; TEVA-Lamivudine/Zidovudine

Pharmacologic Category Antiretroviral, Reverse Transcriptase Inhibitor, Nucleoside (Anti-HIV)

Use HIV-1 infection, treatment: Treatment of HIV-1 infection in combination with other antiretrovirals.

Local Anesthetic/Vasoconstrictor Precautions No information available to require special precautions

Effects on Dental Treatment No significant effects or complications reported

Effects on Bleeding No information available to require special precautions relative to hemostasis.

Adverse Reactions See individual agents.

Mechanism of Action The combination of zidovudine and lamivudine is believed to act synergistically to inhibit reverse transcriptase via DNA chain termination after incorporation of the nucleoside analogue as well as to delay the emergence of mutations conferring resistance

Reproductive Considerations

The Health and Human Services (HHS) Perinatal HIV Guidelines consider this combination an alternative regimen for females living with HIV who are not yet pregnant but are trying to conceive (HHS [perinatal] 2019).

Refer to individual monographs for additional information.

Pregnancy Considerations

The Health and Human Services (HHS) Perinatal HIV Guidelines consider lamivudine in combination with zidovudine an alternative NRTI backbone for pregnant females who are antiretroviral-naive, females who have had antiretroviral therapy (ART) in the past but are restarting, ot who require a new ART regimen (due to poor tolerance or poor virologic response of current regimen). Females who become pregnant while taking this combination may continue if viral suppression is effective and the regimen is well tolerated. Although use of this combination has the most experience for use in pregnancy, it has an increased potential for hematologic toxicity and requires twice-daily dosing (HHS [perinatal] 2019).

Refer to individual monographs for additional information.

◆ **Lamivudine, Doravirine, and Tenofovir Disoproxil Fumarate** *see* Doravirine, Lamivudine, and Tenofovir Disoproxil Fumarate *on page 514*

◆ **Lamivudine, Efavirenz, and Tenofovir Disoproxil Fumarate** *see* Efavirenz, Lamivudine, and Tenofovir Disoproxil Fumarate *on page 545*

◆ **Lamivudine, Tenofovir Disoproxil Fumarate, and Doravirine** *see* Doravirine, Lamivudine, and Tenofovir Disoproxil Fumarate *on page 514*

◆ **Lamivudine/Zidovudine** *see* Lamivudine and Zidovudine *on page 874*

LamoTRIgine (la MOE tri jeen)

Brand Names: US LaMICtal; LaMICtal ODT; LaMICtal Starter; LaMICtal XR; Subvenite; Subvenite Starter Kit-Blue; Subvenite Starter Kit-Green; Subvenite Starter Kit-Orange

Brand Names: Canada APO-LamoTRIgine; Auro-LamoTRIgine; LaMICtal; LamoTRIgine-100; LamoTRIgine-150; LamoTRIgine-25; MYLAN-LamoTRIgine; PMS-LamoTRIgine; RATIO-LamoTRIgine [DSC]; TEVA-LamoTRIgine

Pharmacologic Category Anticonvulsant, Miscellaneous

Use

Bipolar disorder: Maintenance treatment of bipolar disorder to delay the time to occurrence of mood episodes (depression, mania, hypomania, mixed episodes), as monotherapy or adjunctive therapy.

Focal (partial) onset seizures and generalized onset seizures: Treatment of Lennox-Gastaut syndrome (adjunctive therapy only), primary generalized tonic-clonic seizures (adjunctive therapy only), and focal onset seizures (monotherapy or adjunctive therapy). May be used off-label for other seizure types.

Local Anesthetic/Vasoconstrictor Precautions No information available to require special precautions

Effects on Dental Treatment Key adverse event(s) related to dental treatment: Xerostomia (normal salivary flow resumes upon discontinuation). Occurence of nasophayngitis; rare occurrence of taste alteration, gingival hemorrhage, gingival hyperplasia, gingivitis, glossitis, oral mucosa ulcer, orthostatic hypotension, stomatitis, tongue edema.

Effects on Bleeding Rare reports of thrombocytopenia and anemia.

Adverse Reactions Percentages reported in adults on monotherapy for epilepsy or bipolar disorder.

>10%: Gastrointestinal: Nausea (7% to 14%)

1% to 10%:

Cardiovascular: Chest pain (2% to 5%), peripheral edema (2% to 5%), edema (1% to 5%)

Central nervous system: Insomnia (5% to 10%), drowsiness (9%), fatigue (8%), dizziness (7%), ataxia (2% to 7%), anxiety (5%), pain (5%), irritability (2% to 5%), suicidal ideation (2% to 5%), abnormal dreams (1% to 5%), abnormality in thinking (1% to 5%), agitation (1% to 5%), amnesia (1% to 5%), depression (1% to 5%), emotional lability (1% to 5%), hypoesthesia (1% to 5%), migraine (1% to 5%), neurologic abnormality (dyspraxia) (1% to 5%), hyperreflexia (>2% to <5%), hyporeflexia (>2% to <5%), confusion (≥1%), paresthesia (≥1%)

Dermatologic: Skin rash (nonserious: 7%; requiring hospitalization: ≤1%), contact dermatitis (2% to 5%), diaphoresis (2% to 5%), xeroderma (2% to 5%)

Endocrine & metabolic: Increased libido (2% to 5%), weight loss (2% to 5%), weight gain (1% to 5%)

Gastrointestinal: Vomiting (5% to 9%), dyspepsia (7%), abdominal pain (6%), xerostomia (2% to 6%), constipation (5%), anorexia (2% to 5%), peptic ulcer (2% to 5%), flatulence (1% to 5%)
Genitourinary: Dysmenorrhea (2% to 5%), urinary frequency (1% to 5%)
Hematologic & oncologic: Rectal hemorrhage (2% to 5%)
Infection: Infection (5%)
Neuromuscular & skeletal: Back pain (8%), asthenia (2% to 5%), arthralgia (1% to 5%), myalgia (1% to 5%), neck pain (1% to 5%)
Ophthalmic: Nystagmus disorder (2% to 5%), visual disturbance (2% to 5%), amblyopia (≥1%)
Respiratory: Rhinitis (7%), cough (5%), pharyngitis (5%), bronchitis (2% to 5%), dyspnea (2% to 5%), epistaxis (2% to 5%), sinusitis (1% to 5%), nasopharyngitis (≥3%), upper respiratory tract infection (≥3%)
Miscellaneous: Fever (1% to 5%)

Frequency not defined:
Dermatologic: Severe dermatological reaction
Hematologic & oncologic: Natural killer cell count increased (hemophagocytic lymphohistiocytosis)

<1%, postmarketing and/or case reports (any indication): Abnormal hepatic function tests, abnormal lacrimation, accommodation disturbance, acne vulgaris, acute renal failure, ageusia, aggressive behavior, agranulocytosis, akathisia, alcohol intolerance, alopecia, altered sense of smell, amyotrophy, anemia, angioedema, anorgasmia, apathy, aphasia, aplastic anemia, apnea, arthritis, aseptic meningitis, blepharoptosis, breast abscess, breast neoplasm, bursitis, central nervous system depression, chills, choreoathetosis, conjunctivitis, cystitis, deafness, decreased fibrin, decreased libido, decreased serum fibrinogen, delirium, delusion, depersonalization, dermatitis (exfoliative, fungal), drug reaction with eosinophilia and systemic symptoms syndrome, dry eye syndrome, dysarthria, dysgeusia, dyskinesia, dysphagia, dysphoria, dystonia, dysuria, ecchymosis, ejaculatory disorder, eosinophilia, epididymitis, eructation, erythema multiforme, erythema of skin, esophagitis, euphoria, exacerbation of Parkinson disease, extrapyramidal reaction, flushing, gastric ulcer, gastritis, gastrointestinal hemorrhage, gingival hemorrhage, gingival hyperplasia, gingivitis, glossitis, goiter, hallucination, heavy menstrual bleeding, hematemesis, hematuria, hemiplegia, hemolytic anemia, hemorrhagic colitis, hepatitis, hepatotoxicity (idiosyncratic) (Chalasani 2014), herpes zoster infection, hiccups, hirsutism, hostility, hot flash, hyperalgesia, hyperbilirubinemia, hyperesthesia, hyperglycemia, hyperkinetic muscle activity, hypersensitivity reaction, hypertension, hypertonia, hyperventilation, hypogammaglobulinemia, hypokinesia, hypothyroidism, hypotonia, immunosuppression (progressive), impotence, increased appetite, increased gamma-glutamyl transferase, increased serum alkaline phosphatase, increased serum alanine aminotransferase, increased serum aspartate aminotransferase, increased serum creatinine, iron deficiency anemia, lactation, leukocytosis, leukoderma, leukopenia, lower limb cramp, lupus-like syndrome, lymphadenopathy, lymphocytosis, macrocytic anemia, maculopapular rash, malaise, manic depressive reaction, melena, memory impairment, movement disorder, multiorgan failure, muscle spasm, myasthenia, myoclonus, neuralgia, neutropenia, nocturia, oral mucosa ulcer, orthostatic hypotension, oscillopsia, otalgia, palpitations, pancreatitis, pancytopenia, panic attack, paralysis, paranoid ideation, pathological fracture, peripheral neuritis, personality disorder, petechia, petechial rash, photophobia, polyuria, pruritus, psychoneurosis, psychosis, pure red cell aplasia, pustular rash, racing mind, renal pain, rhabdomyolysis, sialorrhea, skin discoloration, sleep disorder, status epilepticus, Stevens-Johnson syndrome, stomatitis, strabismus, stupor, suicidal tendencies, syncope, tachycardia, tendinous contracture, thrombocytopenia, tic disorder, tinnitus, tongue edema, tonic clonic epilepsy (exacerbation), toxic epidermal necrolysis, twitching, urinary incontinence, urinary retention, urinary urgency, urticaria, uveitis, vasculitis, vasodilation, vesiculobullous dermatitis, visual field defect, withdrawal syndrome (seizures with abrupt withdrawal), yawning

Mechanism of Action A triazine derivative which inhibits release of glutamate (an excitatory amino acid) and inhibits voltage-sensitive sodium channels, which stabilizes neuronal membranes. Lamotrigine has weak inhibitory effect on the 5-HT_3 receptor; *in vitro* inhibits dihydrofolate reductase.

Pharmacodynamics/Kinetics

Half-life Elimination

Pediatric patients:
No concomitant enzyme-inducing AED (ie, phenytoin, phenobarbital, carbamazepine, primidone):
Infants and Children 10 months to 5 years: 19 hours (range: 13 to 27 hours)
Concomitant valproate derivative therapy:
Infants and Children 10 months to 5 years: 45 hours (range: 30 to 52 hours)
Children 5 to 11 years: 66 hours (50 to 74 hours)
Concomitant enzyme-inducing AEDs (ie, phenytoin, phenobarbital, carbamazepine, primidone):
Infants and Children 10 months to 5 years: 7.7 hours (range: 6 to 11 hours)
Children 5 to 11 years: 7 hours (range: 4 to 10 hours)
Concomitant enzyme-inducing AEDs plus valproate derivative therapy: Children 5 to 11 years: 19 hours (range: 7 to 31 hours)

Adults:
Immediate release: 25 to 33 hours, Elderly: 25 to 43 hours; Extended release: Similar to immediate release
Concomitant valproic acid therapy: 48 to 70 hours
Concomitant phenytoin, phenobarbital, primidone, or carbamazepine therapy: 13 to 14 hours
Concomitant phenytoin, phenobarbital, primidone, or carbamazepine plus valproate therapy: 27 hours
Chronic renal failure: 43 hours
Hemodialysis: 13 hours during dialysis; 57 hours between dialysis (~20% of a dose is eliminated in a 4-hour dialysis session)
Hepatic impairment:
Mild: 46 ± 20 hours
Moderate: 72 ± 44 hours
Severe without ascites: 67 ± 11 hours
Severe with ascites: 100 ± 48 hours

Time to Peak Plasma: Immediate release: 1 to 5 hours (dependent on adjunct therapy); Extended release: 4 to 11 hours (dependent on adjunct therapy)

Reproductive Considerations

For women with epilepsy who are planning a pregnancy in advance, baseline serum concentrations should be measured once or twice prior to pregnancy during a period when seizure control is optimal (Patsalos 2008; Patsalos 2018).

Potentially significant interactions may exist with hormone-containing contraceptives.

Pregnancy Considerations

Lamotrigine crosses the human placenta and can be measured in the plasma of exposed newborns (Harden and Pennell 2009; Ohman 2000). An overall increase in the risk for major congenital malformations has not been observed in available studies; however, an increased risk for cleft lip or cleft palate has not been ruled out (Cunnington 2011; Hernández-Díaz 2012; Holmes 2012). An increased risk of malformations following maternal lamotrigine use may be associated with larger doses (Cunnington 2007; Tomson 2011). Polytherapy may increase the risk of congenital malformations; monotherapy with the lowest effective dose is recommended (Harden and Meader 2009).

Due to pregnancy-induced physiologic changes, women who are pregnant may require dose adjustments of lamotrigine in order to maintain clinical response; monitoring during pregnancy should be considered (Harden and Pennell 2009). Baseline serum concentrations should be measured once or twice prior to pregnancy during a period when seizure control is optimal. Monitoring can then be continued up to once a month during pregnancy and every second day during the first week postpartum (Patsalos 2008; Patsalos 2018).

Pregnancy registries are available for women who have been exposed to lamotrigine. Patients may enroll themselves in the North American Antiepileptic Drug (NAAED) Pregnancy Registry by calling (888) 233-2334. Additional information is available at www.aedpregnancyregistry.org.

- **Lanoxicaps** *see* Digoxin *on page 498*
- **Lanoxin** *see* Digoxin *on page 498*
- **Lanoxin Pediatric** *see* Digoxin *on page 498*

Lansoprazole (lan SOE pra zole)

Related Information

Gastrointestinal Disorders *on page 1678*

Brand Names: US GoodSense Lansoprazole [OTC]; Heartburn Treatment 24 Hour [OTC]; Prevacid; Prevacid 24HR [OTC]; Prevacid SoluTab

Brand Names: Canada APO-Lansoprazole; DOM-Lansoprazole; M-Lansoprazole; MYLAN-Lansoprazole; PMS-Lansoprazole; Prevacid; Prevacid FasTab; RIVA-Lansoprazole; SANDOZ Lansoprazole; TARO-Lansoprazole; TEVA-Lansoprazole

Pharmacologic Category Proton Pump Inhibitor; Substituted Benzimidazole

Use

Gastroesophageal reflux disease (GERD): Short-term (up to 8 weeks) treatment of symptomatic GERD in children ≥1 year of age and adults; short-term (up to 8 weeks in children ≥12 years and adults; up to 12 weeks in children 1 to 11 years) treatment for all grades of erosive esophagitis; to maintain healing of erosive esophagitis in adults

Hypersecretory conditions: Long-term treatment of pathological hypersecretory conditions, including Zollinger-Ellison syndrome in adults

Peptic ulcer disease: Short-term (4 weeks) treatment of active duodenal ulcers in adults; maintenance treatment of healed duodenal ulcers in adults; as part of a multidrug regimen for *Helicobacter pylori* eradication to reduce the risk of duodenal ulcer recurrence in adults; short-term (up to 8 weeks) treatment of active benign gastric ulcer in adults; treatment of NSAID-associated gastric ulcer; to reduce the risk of NSAID-associated gastric ulcer in adults with a history of gastric ulcer who require an NSAID

OTC labeling: Relief of frequent heartburn (≥2 days/week)

Local Anesthetic/Vasoconstrictor Precautions No information available to require special precautions

Effects on Dental Treatment No significant effects or complications reported

Effects on Bleeding No information available to require special precautions

Adverse Reactions

1% to 10%:

Central nervous system: Headache (3% to 7%), dizziness (adolescents: 3%; adults: <1%)

Gastrointestinal: Diarrhea (≤7%), abdominal pain (2% to 5%), constipation (children: 5%; adults 1%), nausea (adolescents: 3%; adults <1%)

Frequency not defined:

Endocrine & metabolic: Abnormal albumin-globulin ratio, albuminuria, decreased serum cholesterol, hyperlipidemia, increased gamma-glutamyl transferase, increased gastrin, increased lactate dehydrogenase, increased serum glucocorticoids, increased serum potassium

Gastrointestinal: Occult blood in stools

Genitourinary: Crystalluria, hematuria

Hematologic & oncologic: Abnormal erythrocytes, blood platelet disorder (abnormal platelets), leukocyte disorder, leukocytosis

Hepatic: Abnormal hepatic function tests, hyperbilirubinemia, increased serum alkaline phosphatase, increased serum ALT, increased serum AST

Immunologic: Increased serum globulins

Renal: Acute interstitial nephritis, increased blood urea nitrogen, increased serum creatinine

<1%, postmarketing, and/or case reports: Abdominal distention, abnormal dreams, abnormal stools, abnormality in thinking, acne vulgaris, ageusia, agitation, agranulocytosis, alopecia, altered sense of smell, amblyopia, amnesia, anaphylactoid reaction, anaphylaxis, anemia, angina pectoris, anorexia, anxiety, apathy, aphthous stomatitis, aplastic anemia, arthralgia, arthritis, arthropathy, asthma, back pain, bezoar formation, blepharitis, blepharoptosis, blurred vision, bone disease, bone fracture, bradycardia, breast hypertrophy, breast tenderness, bronchitis, candidiasis, carcinoma, cardiac arrhythmia, cataract, cerebral infarction, cerebrovascular accident, change in platelet count (decreased/increased), chest pain, chills, cholelithiasis, circulatory shock, *Clostridioides* (formerly *Clostridium*) *difficile*-associated diarrhea, colitis, confusion, conjunctivitis, contact dermatitis, cough, cutaneous lupus erythematosus, deafness, decreased libido, dehydration, dementia, depersonalization, depression, dermatological disease, diabetes mellitus, diaphoresis, difficulty in micturition, diplopia, dizziness, drowsiness, dry eye syndrome, dysgeusia, dysmenorrhea, dyspepsia, dysphagia, dyspnea, dysuria, ear disease, edema, electrolyte disturbance (decreased/increased), emotional lability, enteritis, eosinophilia, epistaxis, eructation, erythema

multiforme, esophageal achalasia, esophageal stenosis, esophageal ulcer, esophagitis, eye pain, fecal discoloration, fever, fixed drug eruption, flatulence, flu-like symptoms, gastritis, gastroenteritis, gastrointestinal hemorrhage, GI moniliasis, gingival hemorrhage, glaucoma, glossitis, glycosuria, goiter, gout, gynecomastia, hair disease, halitosis, hallucination, hematemesis, hemiplegia, hemolysis, hemolytic anemia, hemoptysis, hepatotoxicity, hiccups, hostility, hyperkinesia, hypermenorrhea, hypersensitivity reaction, hypertension, hypertonia, hypoesthesia, hypoglycemia, hypomagnesemia, hypotension, hypothyroidism, impotence, increased appetite, increased libido, increased thirst, infection, insomnia, interstitial nephritis, leg cramps, leukopenia, leukorrhea, lymphadenopathy, maculopapular rash, malaise, malignant neoplasm of larynx, mastalgia, melena, menstrual disease (includes abnormal menses), migraine, musculoskeletal pain, myalgia, myasthenia, myocardial infarction, myositis, nail disease, neck pain, neck stiffness, nephrolithiasis, nervousness, neutropenia, oral mucosa ulcer, otitis media, pain, palpitations, pancreatitis, pancytopenia, paresthesia, pelvic pain, penile disease, peripheral edema, pharyngitis, photophobia, pleural disease, pneumonia, polyp (gastric nodules and fundic gland polyp), polyuria, pruritus, psychoneurosis, pulmonary fibrosis, rectal disease, rectal hemorrhage, renal disease (chronic; Lazarus 2016), renal pain, respiratory tract disease, retinal degeneration, retinopathy, rhinitis, seizure, sialorrhea, sinusitis, skin carcinoma, skin rash, sleep disorder, speech disturbance, Stevens-Johnson syndrome, stomatitis, stridor, syncope, synovitis, systemic lupus erythematosus, tachycardia, tenesmus, testicular disease, thrombocytopenia, thrombotic thrombocytopenic purpura, tinnitus, tremor, tongue disease, toxic epidermal necrolysis, ulcerative colitis, upper respiratory tract inflammation, upper respiratory tract infection, urethral pain, urinary frequency, urinary retention, urinary tract infection, urinary urgency, urticaria, vaginitis, vasodilation, vertigo, visual disturbance, visual field defect, vitamin deficiency, vomiting, weakness, weight gain, weight loss, xeroderma, xerostomia

Mechanism of Action Decreases acid secretion in gastric parietal cells through inhibition of (H+, K+)-ATPase enzyme system, blocking the final step in gastric acid production.

Pharmacodynamics/Kinetics

Onset of Action Gastric acid suppression: Oral: 1 to 3 hours

Duration of Action Gastric acid suppression: Oral: >1 day

Half-life Elimination Children: 1.2 to 1.5 hours; Adults: 1.5 ± 1 hour; Elderly: 1.9 to 2.9 hours; Hepatic impairment: 4 to 7.2 hours

Time to Peak Plasma: 1.7 hours

Pregnancy Considerations

Available data have not shown an increased risk of major birth defects following maternal use of lansoprazole during pregnancy.

Recommendations for the treatment of GERD in pregnancy are available. As in nonpregnant patients, lifestyle modifications followed by other medications are the initial treatments (ACG [Katz 2013]; Body 2016; Huerta-Iga 2016; van der Woude 2014). Based on available data, proton pump inhibitors may be used when clinically indicated (Body 2016; Matok 2012; Pasternak 2010; van der Woude 2014).

Lansoprazole, Amoxicillin, and Clarithromycin

(lan SOE pra zole, a moks i SIL in, & kla RITH roe mye sin)

Related Information

Amoxicillin *on page 124*
Clarithromycin *on page 361*
Gastrointestinal Disorders *on page 1678*
Lansoprazole *on page 876*

Brand Names: US Prevpac

Brand Names: Canada Hp-PAC

Pharmacologic Category Antibiotic, Macrolide Combination; Antibiotic, Penicillin; Gastrointestinal Agent, Miscellaneous; Proton Pump Inhibitor; Substituted Benzimidazole

Use ***Helicobacter pylori* eradication:** Eradication of *H. pylori* infection to reduce the risk of recurrent duodenal ulcer in patients with active or 1-year history of duodenal ulcer

Local Anesthetic/Vasoconstrictor Precautions No information available to require special precautions

Effects on Dental Treatment Key adverse event(s) related to dental treatment: Taste perversion.

Effects on Bleeding No information available to require special precautions

Adverse Reactions Also see individual agents.

3% to 10%:

Central nervous system: Headache (6%), confusion (<3%), dizziness (<3%)
Dermatologic: Dermatological reaction (<3%)
Endocrine & metabolic: Increased thirst (<3%)
Gastrointestinal: Diarrhea (7%), dysgeusia (5%), abdominal pain (<3%), anorectal pruritus (<3%), darkening of stools (<3%), glossitis (<3%), nausea (<3%), oral candidiasis (<3%), stomatitis (<3%), tongue discoloration (<3%), tongue disease (<3%), vomiting (<3%), xerostomia (<3%)
Genitourinary: Vaginitis (<3%), vulvovaginal candidiasis (<3%)
Neuromuscular & skeletal: Myalgia (<3%)

<3%, postmarketing, and/or case reports: Hepatotoxicity (idiosyncratic) (Chalasani 2014)

Mechanism of Action

Lansoprazole: Suppresses gastric acid secretion by blocking the acid (proton) pump within gastric parietal cells.

Amoxicillin: Inhibits bacterial cell wall mucopeptide synthesis.

Clarithromycin: Inhibits microbial protein synthesis.

Pregnancy Risk Factor C

Pregnancy Considerations

Adverse events have been observed in some animal reproduction studies. Refer to individual monographs.

◆ **Lansoprazole/Amoxiciln/Clarith** *see* Lansoprazole, Amoxicillin, and Clarithromycin *on page 877*

◆ **Lantus** *see* Insulin Glargine *on page 822*

◆ **Lantus SoloStar** *see* Insulin Glargine *on page 822*

Lapatinib (la PA ti nib)

Related Information

Clinical Risk Related to Drugs Prolonging QT Interval *on page 1675*

Brand Names: US Tykerb

Brand Names: Canada Tykerb

Pharmacologic Category Antineoplastic Agent, Anti-HER2; Antineoplastic Agent, Epidermal Growth Factor

Receptor (EGFR) Inhibitor; Antineoplastic Agent, Tyrosine Kinase Inhibitor

Use

Breast cancer: Treatment of human epidermal growth receptor type 2 (HER2) overexpressing advanced or metastatic breast cancer (in combination with capecitabine) in patients who have received prior therapy (with an anthracycline, a taxane, and trastuzumab); HER2 overexpressing hormone receptor-positive metastatic breast cancer in postmenopausal women where hormone therapy is indicated (in combination with letrozole)

Limitations of use: Patients should have disease progression on trastuzumab prior to initiation of treatment with lapatinib in combination with capecitabine.

Local Anesthetic/Vasoconstrictor Precautions Lapatinib is one of the drugs confirmed to prolong the QT interval and is accepted as having a risk of causing torsade de pointes. The risk of drug-induced torsade de pointes is extremely low when a single QT interval prolonging drug is prescribed. In terms of epinephrine, it is not known what effect vasoconstrictors in the local anesthetic regimen will have in patients with a known history of congenital prolonged QT interval or in patients taking any medication that prolongs the QT interval. Until more information is obtained, it is suggested that the clinician consult with the physician prior to the use of a vasoconstrictor in suspected patients, and that the vasoconstrictor (epinephrine, mepivacaine and levonordefrin [Carbocaine® 2% with Neo-Cobefrin®]) be used with caution.

Effects on Dental Treatment Key adverse event(s) related to dental treatment: Stomatitis.

Effects on Bleeding Anemia and thrombocytopenia have been reported. Medical consult recommended.

Adverse Reactions Percentages reported for combination therapy.

>10%:

Central nervous system: Fatigue (≤20%), headache (14%)

Dermatologic: Palmar-plantar erythrodysesthesia (with capecitabine: 53%), skin rash (28% to 44%), alopecia (13%), xeroderma (10% to 13%), pruritus (12%), nail disease (11%)

Gastrointestinal: Diarrhea (64% to 65%), nausea (31% to 44%), vomiting (17% to 26%), mucositis (15%), stomatitis (14%), anorexia (11%), dyspepsia (11%)

Hematologic & oncologic: Decreased hemoglobin (with capecitabine: 56%; grade 3: <1%), decreased neutrophils (with capecitabine: 22%; grade 3: 3%; grade 4: <1%), decreased platelet count (with capecitabine: 18%; grade 3: <1%)

Hepatic: Increased serum aspartate aminotransferase (49% to 53%), increased serum alanine aminotransferase (37% to 46%), increased serum bilirubin (22% to 45%)

Neuromuscular & skeletal: Asthenia (12%), limb pain (12%), back pain (11%)

Respiratory: Dyspnea (12%), epistaxis (11%)

1% to 10%:

Cardiovascular: Decreased left ventricular ejection fraction (with letrozole: 5%; with capecitabine: grade 2: 2%; grade 3: <1%)

Central nervous system: Insomnia (10%)

<1%, postmarketing, and/or case reports: Anaphylaxis, hepatotoxicity, hypersensitivity reaction, interstitial pulmonary disease, paronychia, pneumonitis, prolonged QT interval on ECG, severe dermatological reaction, Stevens-Johnson syndrome, torsades de pointes, toxic epidermal necrolysis, ventricular arrhythmia

Mechanism of Action Tyrosine kinase (dual kinase) inhibitor; inhibits EGFR (ErbB1) and HER2 (ErbB2) by reversibly binding to tyrosine kinase, blocking phosphorylation and activation of downstream second messengers (Erk1/2 and Akt), regulating cellular proliferation and survival in ErbB- and ErbB2-expressing tumors. Combination therapy with lapatinib and endocrine therapy may overcome endocrine resistance occurring in HER2+ and hormone receptor positive disease.

Pharmacodynamics/Kinetics

Half-life Elimination ~24 hours

Time to Peak ~4 hours (Burris 2009)

Reproductive Considerations

Pregnancy status should be determined prior to initiation of lapatinib. Females of reproductive potential and male patients with female partners of reproductive potential should be advised to use effective contraception during treatment and for 1 week after the last lapatinib dose. Females of reproductive potential should be advised of the potential risk to the fetus should pregnancy occur.

Pregnancy Considerations

Based on the mechanism of action and data from animal reproduction studies, in utero exposure to lapatinib may cause fetal harm. Pregnant females should be advised of the potential risk to the fetus.

European Society for Medical Oncology (ESMO) guidelines for cancer during pregnancy recommend delaying treatment with HER-2 targeted agents until after delivery in pregnant patients with HER-2 positive disease (Peccatori 2013).

Dental Health Professional Considerations See Local Anesthetic/Vasoconstrictor Precautions

- **Lapatinib Ditosylate** *see* Lapatinib *on page 877*
- **Lariam** *see* Mefloquine *on page 955*
- **Larin 1.5/30** *see* Ethinyl Estradiol and Norethindrone *on page 614*
- **Larin 1/20** *see* Ethinyl Estradiol and Norethindrone *on page 614*
- **Larin 24 FE** *see* Ethinyl Estradiol and Norethindrone *on page 614*
- **Larin Fe 1.5/30** *see* Ethinyl Estradiol and Norethindrone *on page 614*
- **Larin Fe 1/20** *see* Ethinyl Estradiol and Norethindrone *on page 614*
- **Larissia** *see* Ethinyl Estradiol and Levonorgestrel *on page 612*

Laronidase (lair OH ni days)

Brand Names: US Aldurazyme

Brand Names: Canada Aldurazyme

Pharmacologic Category Enzyme

Use **Mucopolysaccharidosis I (Hurler syndrome, Hurler-Scheie, and Scheie forms):** Treatment of Hurler and Hurler-Scheie forms of mucopolysaccharidosis I (MPS I); treatment of Scheie form of MPS I in patients with moderate to severe symptoms

Local Anesthetic/Vasoconstrictor Precautions No information available to require special precautions

Effects on Dental Treatment No significant effects or complications reported

Effects on Bleeding Thrombocytopenia has been reported.

Adverse Reactions Unless otherwise noted, adverse reactions were reported in patients ≥6 years of age.

>10%:

Cardiovascular: Flushing (11% to 23%), venous irritation (poor venous access: 14%)

Central nervous system: Chills (infants and children 6 months to 5 years: 20%), hyperreflexia (14%), paresthesia (14%)

Dermatologic: Skin rash (13% to 36%; infants and children 6 months to 5 years: ≥5%)

Immunologic: Antibody development (93% to 97%; infants and children 6 months to 5 years: 100%)

Local: Injection site reaction (18%)

Otic: Otitis media (infants and children 6 months to 5 years: 20%)

Respiratory: Upper respiratory tract infection (32%)

Miscellaneous: Infusion-related reaction (32% to 49%; may be severe; infants and children 6 months to 5 years: 35%), fever (11%; infants and children 6 months to 5 years: 30%)

1% to 10%:

Cardiovascular: Hypertension (infants and children 6 months to 5 years: 10%), oxygen saturation decreased (infants and children 6 months to 5 years: 10%), tachycardia (infants and children 6 months to 5 years: 10%), chest pain (9%), edema (9%), facial edema (9%), hypotension (9%), hot and cold flashes (7%)

Central nervous system: Headache (9%)

Dermatologic: Pallor (infants and children 6 months to 5 years: ≥5%), pruritus (4%), urticaria (4%), hyperhidrosis

Gastrointestinal: Abdominal pain (≤9%), abdominal distress (≤9%), diarrhea (7%), vomiting (4%)

Hematologic & oncologic: Thrombocytopenia (9%)

Hepatic: Hyperbilirubinemia (9%)

Hypersensitivity: Severe hypersensitivity (1%)

Local: Abscess at injection site (9%), pain at injection site (9%)

Neuromuscular & skeletal: Tremor (infants and children 6 months to 5 years: ≥5%), arthralgia (4%), back pain, musculoskeletal pain

Ophthalmic: Corneal opacity (9%)

Respiratory: Rales (infants and children 6 months to 5 years: ≥5%), respiratory distress (infants and children 6 months to 5 years: ≥5%), wheezing (infants and children 6 months to 5 years: ≥5%), bronchospasm, cough, dyspnea

<1%, postmarketing, and/or case reports: Anaphylaxis, angioedema, cardiac failure, cyanosis, erythema, fatigue, laryngeal edema, peripheral edema, pneumonia, respiratory failure

Mechanism of Action Laronidase is a recombinant (replacement) form of alpha-L-iduronidase derived from Chinese hamster cells. Alpha-L-iduronidase is an enzyme needed to break down endogenous glycosaminoglycans (GAGs) within lysosomes. A deficiency of alpha-L-iduronidase leads to an accumulation of GAGs, causing cellular, tissue, and organ dysfunction as seen in MPS I. Improved pulmonary function and walking capacity have been demonstrated with the administration of laronidase to patients with Hurler, Hurler-Scheie, or Scheie (with moderate-to-severe symptoms) forms of MPS.

Pharmacodynamics/Kinetics

Half-life Elimination

Infants and Children 6 months to 5 years: 0.3-1.9 hours

Children ≥6 years and Adults: 1.5-3.6 hours

Pregnancy Considerations

Information related to the use of laronidase in pregnancy is limited (Anbu 2006; Castorina 2015).

Pregnant patients are encouraged to enroll in the mucopolysaccharidosis I registry (1-800-745-4447, extension 15500 or www.registrynxt.com).

Larotrectinib (LAR oh TREK ti nib)

Brand Names: US Vitrakvi

Brand Names: Canada Vitrakvi

Pharmacologic Category Antineoplastic Agent, Tropomyosin Receptor Kinase (TRK) Inhibitor; Antineoplastic Agent, Tyrosine Kinase Inhibitor

Use Solid tumors: Treatment of solid tumors (in adult and pediatric patients) that have a neurotrophic receptor tyrosine kinase (NTRK) gene fusion without a known acquired resistance mutation; are metastatic or where surgical resection is likely to result in severe morbidity; and have no satisfactory alternative treatments or that have progressed following treatment.

Local Anesthetic/Vasoconstrictor Precautions No information available to require special precautions

Effects on Dental Treatment Key adverse event(s) related to dental treatment: Nasal congestion has been reported.

Effects on Bleeding Bone marrow depression (eg, anemia, neutropenia) has been reported. In patients under active treatment with larotrectinib, medical consult is suggested.

Adverse Reactions

>10%:

Cardiovascular: Peripheral edema (15%), hypertension (11%)

Central nervous system: Neurotoxicity (53%), fatigue (37%), dizziness (28%), headache (14%), myasthenia (13%)

Endocrine & metabolic: Hypoalbuminemia (35%), weight gain (15%)

Gastrointestinal: Nausea (29%), vomiting (26%), constipation (23%), diarrhea (22%), abdominal pain (13%), decreased appetite (13%)

Hematologic & oncologic: Anemia (42%; grades 3/4: 10%), neutropenia (23%; grades 3/4: 7%)

Hepatic: Increased serum alanine aminotransferase (45%), increased serum aspartate aminotransferase (45%), increased serum alkaline phosphatase (30%)

Neuromuscular & skeletal: Arthralgia (14%), myalgia (14%), back pain (12%), limb pain (12%)

Respiratory: Cough (26%), dyspnea (18%)

Miscellaneous: Fever (18%)

1% to 10%:

Central nervous system: Falling (10%), delirium (grade 3: 2%), abnormal gait (grade 3: 1%), dysarthria (grade 3: 1%), paresthesia (grade 3: 1%)

Respiratory: Nasal congestion (10%)

Frequency not defined:

Cardiovascular: Pericardial effusion, syncope

Central nervous system: Cerebral edema, memory impairment

Dermatologic: Cellulitis, enterocutaneous fistula

Endocrine & metabolic: Dehydration, hyponatremia, increased amylase, increased serum lipase

Gastrointestinal: Intestinal obstruction (small intestine), intestinal perforation

Hematologic & oncologic: Acute myelocytic leukemia

Hepatic: Jaundice

Infection: Sepsis

Neuromuscular & skeletal: Asthenia, tremor

Respiratory: Pleural effusion

<1%, postmarketing, and/or case reports: Encephalopathy

Mechanism of Action Larotrectinib is a potent and highly selective small-molecule inhibitor of the 3 tropomyosin receptor kinase (TRK) proteins, TRKA, TRKB, and TRKC (Drilon 2018). TRKA, TRKB, and TRKC are encoded by neurotrophic receptor tyrosine kinase (NTRK) genes, NTRK1, NTRK2, and NTRK3. Chromosomal rearrangements involving fusions of NTRK genes may result in constitutively-activated chimeric TRK fusion proteins, acting as an oncogenic driver to promote cell proliferation and survival in tumor cell lines. Larotrectinib has anti-tumor activity in cells with constitutive activation of TRK proteins resulting from gene fusions, deletion of a protein regulatory domain, or in cells with TRK protein overexpression.

Pharmacodynamics/Kinetics

Half-life Elimination 2.9 hours

Time to Peak ~1 hour

Reproductive Considerations

Pregnancy status should be evaluated prior to therapy; females of reproductive potential should use effective contraception during therapy and for at least 1 week after the final larotrectinib dose. Males with female partners of reproductive potential should also use effective contraception during therapy and for 1 week after the final larotrectinib dose.

Pregnancy Considerations

Based the mechanism of action and available human and animal data, larotrectinib may cause fetal harm if administered to a pregnant female.

Larotrectinib interferes with TRK signaling; obesity, developmental delays, cognitive impairment, insensitivity to pain, and anhidrosis have been observed in persons with congenital mutations in TRK pathway proteins.

◆ **Larotrectinib Sulfate** *see* Larotrectinib *on page 879*

◆ **Lartruvo** *see* Olaratumab *on page 1131*

◆ **Larynex [OTC]** *see* Cetylpyridinium *on page 330*

◆ **LAS-34273** *see* Aclidinium *on page 74*

◆ **LAS-34273 Micronized** *see* Aclidinium *on page 74*

◆ **Lasix** *see* Furosemide *on page 721*

Lasmiditan (las MID i tan)

Brand Names: US Reyvow

Pharmacologic Category Antimigraine Agent; Serotonin 5-HT1F Receptor Agonist

Use

Migraine, treatment: Acute treatment of migraine with or without aura in adults.

Limitations of use: Lasmiditan is not indicated for preventive treatment of migraine.

Local Anesthetic/Vasoconstrictor Precautions
Infrequent occurrence of palpitations, increase in blood pressure (frequency not defined) – monitor blood pressure and use caution if necessary when injecting local anesthetic with vasoconstrictor.

Effects on Dental Treatment No significant effects or complications reported.

Effects on Bleeding No information available to require special precautions.

Adverse Reactions

>10%: Central nervous system: Dizziness (9% to 17%)

1% to 10%:

Cardiovascular: Chest discomfort (<2%), palpitations (<2%)

Central nervous system: Paresthesia (3% to 9%), drowsiness (6% to 7%), fatigue (4% to 6%), abnormal dreams (<2%), anxiety (<2%), ataxia (<2%), cognitive dysfunction (<2%), confusion (<2%), euphoria (<2%), feeling abnormal (<2%), hallucination (<2%), lethargy (<2%), local discomfort (limb: <2%), restlessness (<2%), sleep disturbance (<2%), speech disturbance (<2%), vertigo (<2%), myasthenia (1% to 2%)

Gastrointestinal: Nausea (≤4%), vomiting (≤4%)

Neuromuscular & skeletal: Muscle spasm (<2%), tremor (<2%)

Ophthalmic: Visual impairment (<2%)

Respiratory: Dyspnea (<2%)

<1%: Angioedema, hypersensitivity reaction, skin photosensitivity, skin rash

Frequency not defined:

Cardiovascular: Decreased heart rate, increased blood pressure

Central nervous system: Central nervous system depression

Mechanism of Action Lasmiditan is a high-affinity, highly selective 5-HT_{1F} receptor agonist. Selective targeting of the 5-HT_{1F} receptor is hypothesized to decrease stimulation of the trigeminal system and treat migraine pain without causing vasoconstriction (Nelson 2010).

Pharmacodynamics/Kinetics

Onset of Action 30 to 60 minutes (100 and 200 mg doses) (Ashina 2019).

Half-life Elimination ~5.7 hours.

Time to Peak 1.8 hours.

Pregnancy Considerations Adverse events were observed in animal reproduction studies.

Product Availability

Reyvow: FDA approved October 2019; anticipated availability is currently unknown.

Controlled Substance C-V

◆ **Lasmiditan hemisuccinate** *see* Lasmiditan *on page 880*

◆ **L-ASP** *see* Asparaginase (*E. coli*) *on page 175*

◆ **L-asparaginase (*E. coli*)** *see* Asparaginase (*E. coli*) *on page 175*

◆ **L-asparaginase (*Erwinia*)** *see* Asparaginase (*Erwinia*) *on page 176*

◆ **L-asparaginase with Polyethylene Glycol** *see* Pegaspargase *on page 1199*

◆ **LAS-W-330** *see* Aclidinium *on page 74*

Latanoprost (la TA noe prost)

Brand Names: US Xalatan; Xelpros

Brand Names: Canada APO-Latanoprost; GD-Latanoprost; JAMP Latanoprost; MED-Latanoprost; Monoprost; PMS-Latanoprost; RIVA-Latanoprost; SANDOZ Latanoprost; TEVA-Latanoprost; Xalatan

Pharmacologic Category Ophthalmic Agent, Antiglaucoma; Prostaglandin, Ophthalmic

Use Elevated intraocular pressure: Reduction of elevated intraocular pressure (IOP) in patients with open-angle glaucoma and ocular hypertension.

Local Anesthetic/Vasoconstrictor Precautions
No information available to require special precautions

Effects on Dental Treatment No significant effects or complications reported

Effects on Bleeding No information available to require special precautions

Adverse Reactions

>10%:

Central nervous system: Foreign body sensation of eye (2% to 13%)

Ophthalmic: Eye pain (≤55%), stinging of eyes (≤55%), ocular hyperemia (41%), conjunctival hyperemia (8% to 15%), eye discharge (12%), increased eyelash length (11%)

1% to 10%:

Dermatologic: Erythema of eyelid (3%), hyperpigmentation of eyelashes (1%), allergic skin reaction (≤1%, including eyelid), skin rash (≤1%)

Infection: Influenza (≤3%)

Neuromuscular & skeletal: Arthralgia (≤1%), back pain (≤1%), myalgia (≤1%)

Ophthalmic: Punctate keratitis (1% to 10%), blurred vision (8%), increased eyelash thickness (8%), eye pruritus (5% to 8%), burning sensation of eyes (7%), iris hyperpigmentation (7%), decreased visual acuity (4%), eyelid pain (4%), lacrimation (4%), crusting of eyelid (3%), dry eye syndrome (3%), photophobia (2%), eyelid edema (1% to 2%), conjunctival edema (1%)

Respiratory: Nasopharyngitis (≤3%), upper respiratory tract infection (≤3%)

<1%, postmarketing, and/or case reports: Angina pectoris, asthma, bacterial keratitis, chest pain, conjunctivitis (including pseudopemphigoid of the ocular conjunctiva), corneal edema, corneal erosion, dizziness, dyspnea, exacerbation of asthma, eye disease (periorbital and lid changes resulting in deepening of the eyelid sulcus), headache, herpes simplex keratitis, hyperpigmentation of eyelids, increased growth in number of eyelashes, iris cyst, iritis, keratitis, macular edema (including cystoid macular edema), misdirected growth of eyelashes (including trichiasis), palpitations, pruritus, toxic epidermal necrolysis, unstable angina pectoris, uveitis

Mechanism of Action Latanoprost is a prostaglandin F_2-alpha analog believed to reduce intraocular pressure by increasing the outflow of the aqueous humor

Pharmacodynamics/Kinetics

Onset of Action 3 to 4 hours; Peak effect: Maximum: 8 to 12 hours

Half-life Elimination 17 minutes

Pregnancy Considerations

Information related to use in pregnancy is limited (DeSantis 2004).

In general, if ophthalmic agents are needed in pregnancy, the minimum effective dose should be used in combination with punctal occlusion to decrease exposure to the fetus (Samples 1988).

Latanoprostene Bunod

(la tan oh PROS teen BU nod)

Brand Names: US Vyzulta

Brand Names: Canada Vyzulta

Pharmacologic Category Ophthalmic Agent, Antiglaucoma; Prostaglandin, Ophthalmic

Use Elevated intraocular pressure: Reduction of elevated intraocular pressure (IOP) in patients with open-angle glaucoma and ocular hypertension.

Local Anesthetic/Vasoconstrictor Precautions No information available to require special precautions

Effects on Dental Treatment No significant effects or complications reported

Effects on Bleeding No information available to require special precautions

Adverse Reactions

1% to 10%:

Local: Application site pain (2%)

Ophthalmic: Conjunctival hyperemia (6%), eye irritation (4%), eye pain (3%)

Mechanism of Action Latanoprostene bunod is rapidly metabolized in the eye to latanoprost acid, an F_2 alpha prostaglandin analog and to butanediol mononitrate; latanoprost acid is thought to lower intraocular pressure by increasing outflow of aqueous humor through both the trabecular meshwork and uveoscleral routes.

Pharmacodynamics/Kinetics

Onset of Action Onset of action: 1 to 3 hours; peak effect: 11 to 13 hours

Time to Peak Latanoprost acid: 5 minutes

Pregnancy Considerations Adverse events were observed in animal reproduction studies. Agents other than latanoprostene bunod may be preferred in pregnant women (Prum 2016; Sethi 2016).

- **Latuda** *see* Lurasidone *on page 943*
- **Laxa Basic [OTC]** *see* Docusate *on page 509*
- **Layolis FE** *see* Ethinyl Estradiol and Norethindrone *on page 614*
- **Lazanda** *see* FentaNYL *on page 642*
- **LBH589** *see* Panobinostat *on page 1188*
- **LC-4 Lidocaine [OTC] [DSC]** *see* Lidocaine (Topical) *on page 902*
- **LC-5 Lidocaine [OTC]** *see* Lidocaine (Topical) *on page 902*
- **L-Carnitine** *see* LevOCARNitine *on page 896*
- **LCM** *see* Lacosamide *on page 868*
- **LCZ696** *see* Sacubitril and Valsartan *on page 1353*
- **LDE225** *see* Sonidegib *on page 1382*
- **L-Deoxythymidine** *see* Telbivudine *on page 1412*
- **L-Deprenyl** *see* Selegiline *on page 1363*
- **L-Dihydroxyphenylserine** *see* Droxidopa *on page 535*
- **LDK378** *see* Ceritinib *on page 326*
- **LDO Plus** *see* Lidocaine (Topical) *on page 902*
- **L-DOPS** *see* Droxidopa *on page 535*
- **LDP-341** *see* Bortezomib *on page 248*
- **LdT** *see* Telbivudine *on page 1412*
- **LEA29Y** *see* Belatacept *on page 221*
- **LEE-011** *see* Ribociclib *on page 1322*
- **Leena** *see* Ethinyl Estradiol and Norethindrone *on page 614*

Lefamulin (le FAM ue lin)

Brand Names: US Xenleta

Pharmacologic Category Antibiotic, Pleuromutilin

Use Pneumonia, community-acquired: Treatment of adults with community-acquired bacterial pneumonia caused by the following susceptible microorganisms: *Streptococcus pneumoniae*, *Staphylococcus aureus* (methicillin-susceptible isolates), *Haemophilus influenzae*, *Legionella pneumophila*, *Mycoplasma pneumoniae*, and *Chlamydophila pneumoniae*.

Local Anesthetic/Vasoconstrictor Precautions Lefamulin is one of the drugs confirmed to prolong the QT interval and is accepted as having a risk of causing torsade de pointes. The risk of drug-induced torsade de pointes is extremely low when a single QT interval prolonging drug is prescribed. In terms of epinephrine, it is not known what effect vasoconstrictors in the local anesthetic regimen will have in patients with a known history of congenital prolonged QT interval or in patients taking any medication that prolongs the QT interval. Until more information is obtained, it is suggested that the clinician consult with the physician prior to the use of a vasoconstrictor in suspected patients, and that the vasoconstrictor (epinephrine, mepivacaine and levonordefrin [Carbocaine 2% with Neo-Cobefrin]) be used with caution.

Effects on Dental Treatment Key adverse event(s) related to dental treatment: Occurrence of oropharyngeal candidiasis.

Effects on Bleeding Occurrence of anemia and thrombocytopenia. Medical consult suggested.

Adverse Reactions

>10%:

Gastrointestinal: Diarrhea (12%)

1% to 10%:

Cardiovascular: Atrial fibrillation (<2%), palpitations (<2%), prolonged QT interval on ECG (<2%)

Central nervous system: Insomnia (3%), headache (2%), anxiety (<2%), drowsiness (<2%)

Endocrine & metabolic: Hypokalemia (3%), increased gamma-glutamyl transferase (<2%)

Gastrointestinal: Nausea (3% to 5%), vomiting (3%), abdominal pain (<2%), *Clostridioides difficile* associated diarrhea (<2%), constipation (<2%), dyspepsia (<2%), epigastric discomfort (<2%), gastritis (<2%), oropharyngeal candidiasis (<2%)

Genitourinary: Urinary retention (<2%), vulvovaginal candidiasis (<2%)

Hematologic & oncologic: Anemia (<2%), thrombocytopenia (<2%)

Hepatic: Increased liver enzymes (≤3), increased serum alanine aminotransferase (≤3), increased serum aspartate aminotransferase (≤3), increased serum alkaline phosphatase (<2%)

Local: Infusion-site pain (≤7%), injection site phlebitis (≤7%), injection site reaction (≤7%)

Neuromuscular & skeletal: Increased creatine phosphokinase in blood specimen (<2%)

Mechanism of Action Lefamulin is a pleuromutilin that inhibits bacterial protein synthesis through interactions (hydrogen bonds, hydrophobic interactions, and Van der Waals forces) with the A- and P- sites of the peptidyl transferase center in domain V of the 23s ribosomal RNA of the 50S subunit. The binding pocket of the bacterial ribosome closes around the mutilin core for an induced fit that prevents correct positioning of transfer RNA.

Pharmacodynamics/Kinetics

Half-life Elimination ~8 hours (range: 3 to 20 hours); 17.5 hours in patients with severe hepatic impairment after IV administration.

Time to Peak Oral: 0.88 to 2 hours.

Reproductive Considerations

Evaluate pregnancy status prior to use in females of reproductive potential. Females of reproductive potential should use effective contraception during therapy and for 2 days after the last dose.

Pregnancy Considerations

Based on data from animal reproduction studies, in utero exposure to lefamulin may cause fetal harm.

Data collection to monitor pregnancy and infant outcomes following exposure to lefamulin is ongoing. Health care providers are encouraged to enroll females exposed to lefamulin during pregnancy in the pregnancy pharmacovigilance program (1-855-5NABRIVA).

◆ **Lefamulin acetate** *see* Lefamulin *on page 881*

Leflunomide (le FLOO noh mide)

Related Information

Rheumatoid Arthritis, Osteoarthritis, and Osteoporosis *on page 1697*

Brand Names: US Arava

Brand Names: Canada ACCEL-Leflunomide; APO-Leflunomide; Arava; MYLAN-Leflunomide [DSC]; PMS-Leflunomide; SANDOZ Leflunomide; TEVA-Leflunomide

Pharmacologic Category Antirheumatic, Disease Modifying

Use Rheumatoid arthritis: Treatment of adults with active rheumatoid arthritis (RA).

Local Anesthetic/Vasoconstrictor Precautions No information available to require special precautions

Effects on Dental Treatment Key adverse event(s) related to dental treatment: Xerostomia (normal salivary flow resumes upon discontinuation), stomatitis, oral candidiasis, abnormal taste, enlarged salivary gland, esophagitis, and gingivitis.

Effects on Bleeding There have been rare reports of thrombocytopenia.

Adverse Reactions

>10%:

Central nervous system: Headache (7% to 13%)

Dermatologic: Alopecia (9% to 17%), skin rash (10% to 12%)

Gastrointestinal: Diarrhea (17% to 27%), nausea (9% to 13%)

1% to 10%:

Cardiovascular: Hypertension (9% to 10%)

Central nervous system: Dizziness (4% to 7%)

Dermatologic: Pruritus (4% to 6%)

Gastrointestinal: Gastrointestinal pain (5% to 8%), abdominal pain (5% to 6%), oral mucosa ulcer (3% to 5%), vomiting (3% to 5%)

Hepatic: Abnormal hepatic function tests (5% to 10%), increased serum ALT (>3 x ULN: 2% to 4%; reversible)

Hypersensitivity: Hypersensitivity reaction (1% to 5%)

Neuromuscular & skeletal: Back pain (5% to 8%), weakness (3% to 6%), tenosynovitis (2% to 5%)

Respiratory: Bronchitis (5% to 8%), rhinitis (2% to 5%)

Frequency not defined:

Cardiovascular: Chest pain, increased blood pressure, leg thrombophlebitis, palpitations, varicose veins

Central nervous system: Drowsiness, malaise

Endocrine & metabolic: Increased gamma-glutamyl transferase

Gastrointestinal: Anorexia, enlargement of salivary glands, flatulence, sore throat, xerostomia

Genitourinary: Vulvovaginal candidiasis

Hematologic & oncologic: Leukocytosis, thrombocytopenia

Hepatic: Hyperbilirubinemia, increased serum alkaline phosphatase, increased serum AST

Hypersensitivity: Anaphylaxis

Infection: Abscess

Ophthalmic: Blurred vision, eye disease, papilledema, retinal hemorrhage, retinopathy

Respiratory: Dyspnea, flu-like symptoms

<1%, postmarketing and/or case reports: Agranulocytosis, angioedema, cholestasis, colitis (including microscopic colitis), cutaneous lupus erythematosus, DRESS syndrome, erythema multiforme, exacerbation of psoriasis, hepatitis, hepatotoxicity (rare, including hepatic necrosis and hepatic failure), interstitial pneumonitis, interstitial pulmonary disease, jaundice, leukopenia, necrotizing angiitis (cutaneous), neutropenia, opportunistic infection, pancreatitis, pancytopenia, peripheral neuropathy, pulmonary fibrosis, pulmonary hypertension, pustular psoriasis, sepsis (including *Pneumocystis jirovecii* pneumonia and aspergillosis), severe infection, Stevens-Johnson syndrome, toxic epidermal necrolysis, vasculitis

Mechanism of Action Leflunomide is an immunomodulatory agent that inhibits pyrimidine synthesis, resulting in antiproliferative and anti-inflammatory effects. Leflunomide is a prodrug; the active metabolite is responsible for activity. For CMV, may interfere with virion assembly.

Pharmacodynamics/Kinetics

Half-life Elimination Teriflunomide: Mean: 18 to 19 days; enterohepatic recycling appears to contribute to the long half-life of this agent, since activated charcoal and cholestyramine substantially reduce plasma half-life

Time to Peak Teriflunomide: 6 to 12 hours

Reproductive Considerations

[US Boxed Warning]: Exclude pregnancy before the start of treatment in females of reproductive potential. Advise females of reproductive potential to use effective contraception during treatment and during an accelerated elimination procedure after treatment is discontinued. Females of reproductive potential should not receive therapy until pregnancy has been excluded, they have been counseled concerning fetal risk, and reliable contraceptive measures have been confirmed. Following treatment, pregnancy should be avoided until undetectable serum concentrations (<0.02 mg/L) are verified. This may be accomplished by the use of an enhanced drug elimination procedure using cholestyramine. Serum concentrations <0.02 mg/L should be verified by 2 separate tests performed at least 14 days apart. If serum concentrations are >0.02 mg/L, additional cholestyramine treatment should be considered. Use of the accelerated elimination procedure is recommended in all females of reproductive potential upon discontinuation of leflunomide.

Pregnancy Considerations

[US Boxed Warning]: Leflunomide is contraindicated in pregnant females because of the potential for fetal harm. Adverse events were observed in animal reproduction studies with doses lower than the expected human exposure. Discontinue leflunomide and use an accelerated elimination procedure if pregnancy occurs during treatment. The accelerated elimination procedure may decrease potential risks to the fetus by decreasing the plasma concentration teriflunomide, of the active metabolite of leflunomide. Following treatment, pregnancy should be avoided until undetectable serum concentrations (<0.02 mg/L) are verified. Limited outcome information following in utero fetal exposure to leflunomide is available (Bérard 2018; Chambers 2010; Weber-Schoendorfer 2017).

Health care providers are encouraged to enroll women exposed to leflunomide during pregnancy in the Pregnancy Registry (877-311-8972 or http://www.-pregnancystudies.org/participate-ina-study/).

Lemborexant (lem boe REX ant)

Brand Names: US DayVigo

Pharmacologic Category Hypnotic, Miscellaneous; Orexin Receptor Antagonist

Use Insomnia: Treatment of insomnia characterized by difficulties with sleep onset and/or sleep maintenance in adults.

Local Anesthetic/Vasoconstrictor Precautions No information available to require special precautions.

Effects on Dental Treatment No significant effects or complications reported.

Effects on Bleeding No information available to require special precautions.

Adverse Reactions

1% to 10%: Central nervous system: Drowsiness (≤10%), fatigue (≤10%), headache (5% to 6%), abnormal dreams (≤2%), nightmares (≤2%), sleep paralysis (1% to 2%)

<1%: Hypnogenic hallucinations

Frequency not defined:

Cardiovascular: Palpitations

Central nervous system: Cataplexy, central nervous system depression

Postmarketing: Complex sleep-related disorder

Mechanism of Action Lemborexant blocks the binding of wake-promoting neuropeptides orexin A and orexin B to receptors OX1R and OX2R, which is thought to suppress wake drive.

Pharmacodynamics/Kinetics

Onset of Action ~15 to 20 minutes.

Half-life Elimination 17 to 19 hours.

Time to Peak ~1 to 3 hours.

Pregnancy Considerations

Adverse events were observed in some animal reproduction studies.

Data collection to monitor pregnancy and infant outcomes following exposure to lemborexant is ongoing. Health care providers are encouraged to enroll females exposed to lemborexant during pregnancy in the Dayvigo Pregnancy Registry (888-274-2378).

Controlled Substance C-IV

◆ **Lemtrada** *see* Alemtuzumab *on page* 93

Lenalidomide (le na LID oh mide)

Brand Names: US Revlimid

Brand Names: Canada Revlimid

Pharmacologic Category Angiogenesis Inhibitor; Antineoplastic Agent

Use

Follicular lymphoma (previously treated): Treatment of previously treated follicular lymphoma (in combination with a rituximab product) in adults.

Mantle cell lymphoma (relapsed or progressive): Treatment of mantle cell lymphoma in adults that has relapsed or progressed after 2 prior therapies (one of which included bortezomib).

Marginal zone lymphoma (previously treated): Treatment of previously treated marginal zone lymphoma (in combination with a rituximab product) in adults.

Multiple myeloma: Treatment of multiple myeloma (in combination with dexamethasone) in adults; maintenance therapy following autologous hematopoietic stem cell transplantation in adults.

Myelodysplastic syndromes: Treatment of adults with transfusion-dependent anemia due to low- or intermediate-1-risk myelodysplastic syndromes (MDS) associated with a deletion 5q (del 5q) cytogenetic abnormality with or without additional cytogenetic abnormalities.

Limitations of use: Lenalidomide is not indicated and is not recommended for the treatment of chronic lymphocytic leukemia (CLL) outside of controlled clinical trials.

Local Anesthetic/Vasoconstrictor Precautions No information available to require special precautions

Effects on Dental Treatment Key adverse event(s) related to dental treatment: Xerostomia (normal salivary flow resumes upon discontinuation), taste perversion.

Effects on Bleeding Associated with significant thrombocytopenia and anemia. Medical consult recommended.

Adverse Reactions May vary based on indication.

>10%:

Cardiovascular: Peripheral edema (16% to 20%)

Central nervous system: Fatigue (11% to 34%), dizziness (20%), headache (9% to 20%), paresthesia (13%)

Dermatologic: Pruritus (MDS: 42%; MCL: 17%), skin rash (8% to 36%), xeroderma (≤11%)

Endocrine & metabolic: Weight loss (13%), hypokalemia (7% to 13%)

Gastrointestinal: Diarrhea (MM maintenance, MDS: 39% to 49%; MCL: 31%), nausea (11% to 30%), constipation (13% to 24%), gastroenteritis (23%), decreased appetite (14%), abdominal pain (10% to 12%), vomiting (6% to 12%)

Genitourinary: Urinary tract infection (4% to 11%)

Hematologic & oncologic: Thrombocytopenia (24% to 62%; grades 3/4: 13% to 50%), neutropenia (49% to 61%; grades 3/4: 43% to 54%), leukopenia (8% to 32%; grades 3/4: 5% to 24%), anemia (MCL: 31%, grades 3/4: 11%, MDS, MM maintenance: 9% to 12%, grades 3/4: 4% to 6%)

Infection: Influenza (13%)

Neuromuscular & skeletal: Muscle spasm (MM maintenance: 33%; MCL: 13%), asthenia (14% to 30%), arthralgia (MDS: 22%; MCL: 8%), back pain (13% to 21%), muscle cramps (18%), limb pain (11%)

Respiratory: Bronchitis (MM: 44%; MDS: 6%), nasopharyngitis (≤35%), cough (20% to 28%), pneumonia (12% to 17%), dyspnea (6% to 17%; includes exacerbation), pharyngitis (16%), epistaxis (15%), upper respiratory tract infection (11% to 15%), rhinitis (7% to 15%), sinusitis (≤14%)

Miscellaneous: Fever (21% to 23%; may be intermittent)

1% to 10%:

Cardiovascular: Edema (10%), hypotension (7%), hypertension (6%), chest pain (5%), palpitations (5%), deep vein thrombosis (2% to 4%), pulmonary embolism (1% to 2%), cardiac failure

Central nervous system: Insomnia (10%), peripheral neuropathy (5% to 10%), hypoesthesia (7%), pain (7%), myasthenia (6%), rigors (6%), chills, lethargy, vertigo

Dermatologic: Night sweats (8%), diaphoresis (7%), ecchymoses (5%), erythema of skin (5%), cellulitis (2% to 5%)

Endocrine & metabolic: Dehydration (7%), hypothyroidism (7%), hypomagnesemia (6%), hypocalcemia (3%), hyponatremia (2%)

Gastrointestinal: Anorexia (10%), upper abdominal pain (7% to 8%), xerostomia (7%), dysgeusia (6%), loose stools (6%), oral herpes simplex infection

Genitourinary: Dysuria (7%), urolithiasis (ureter)

Hematologic & oncologic: Tumor flare (10%), bruise (8%), lymphocytopenia (4% to 7%; grades 3/4: 4%), febrile neutropenia (2% to 6%; grades 3/4: 2% to 6%), pancytopenia (4%; grades 3/4: 2%), squamous cell carcinoma of skin (3%), granulocytopenia (grades 3/4: 2%), myelodysplastic syndrome (≤1%)

Hepatic: Increased serum alanine aminotransferase (8%), hyperbilirubinemia (1%)

Hypersensitivity: Hypersensitivity reaction

Infection: Herpes zoster infection (10%), infection (6%), sepsis (1% to 2%; including *enterobacter, klebsiella, staphylococcus*), bacteremia (1%)

Neuromuscular & skeletal: Myalgia (7% to 9%), swelling of extremities (8%), musculoskeletal pain (7%)

Renal: Renal failure syndrome (4%)

Respiratory: Oropharyngeal pain (10%), dyspnea on exertion (7%), pleural effusion (7%), rhinorrhea (5%), pulmonary infection (3%), hypoxia (2%), respiratory distress (1%), respiratory tract infection

Miscellaneous: Physical health deterioration (2%), troponin increased in blood specimen (troponin I)

Frequency not defined:

Cardiovascular: Acute myocardial infarction, angina pectoris, arterial thromboembolism, atrial fibrillation (including exacerbation), bradycardia, cardiac disorder (aortic disorder), cardiogenic shock, cardiomyopathy, cerebral infarction, cerebrovascular accident, ischemia, ischemic heart disease, septic shock, subarachnoid hemorrhage, superficial thrombophlebitis, supraventricular cardiac arrhythmia, supraventricular tachycardia, tachyarrhythmia, thrombosis, transient ischemic attacks, venous thromboembolism, ventricular dysfunction

Central nervous system: Abnormal gait, aphasia, cerebellar infarction, confusion, depression, dysarthria, falling, impaired consciousness, migraine, spinal cord compression

Dermatologic: Erythema multiforme, erythematous rash, exfoliative dermatitis, follicular rash, macular eruption, maculopapular rash, papular rash, pruritic rash, pustular rash, Sweet's syndrome

Endocrine & metabolic: Gout, gouty arthritis, Graves' disease, hypernatremia, hypoglycemia

Gastrointestinal: Biliary obstruction, cholecystitis (may be acute), *Clostridioides difficile* associated diarrhea, *Clostridioides difficile* colitis, colonic polyps, diverticulitis of the gastrointestinal tract, dysphagia, gastritis, gastrointestinal hemorrhage, gastrointestinal pain, gastrointestinal reflux disease, infection of mouth, inguinal hernia (obstructive), intestinal obstruction (small intestine), intestinal perforation, irritable bowel syndrome, ischemic colitis, lower abdominal pain, melena, pancreatitis

Genitourinary: Abscess of rectum and/or peri-rectal area, azotemia, hematuria, pelvic pain, urinary tract infection with sepsis

Hematologic & oncologic: Acquired blood coagulation disorder, acute leukemia, basal cell carcinoma of skin, bone marrow depression, bronchogenic carcinoma, decreased hemoglobin, hemolysis, hemolytic anemia, malignant lymphoma, malignant neoplasm of lung, myeloid leukemia (acute), postprocedural hemorrhage, progression of cancer, prostate carcinoma, rectal hemorrhage, splenic infarction, warm antibody immunohemolytic anemia

Hepatic: Abnormal hepatic function tests (may be transient), hepatic failure
Hypersensitivity: Transfusion reaction
Infection: Fungal infection, herpes virus infection, kidney infection, localized infection, pseudomonas infection, staphylococcal infection
Local: Catheter infection
Neuromuscular & skeletal: Arthritis (including exacerbation), bone fracture (femur, femoral neck, pelvis, hip, rib, spinal compression), calcium pyrophosphate deposition disease, neck pain
Otic: Otic infection
Renal: Acute renal failure, increased serum creatinine
Respiratory: Acute sinusitis, chronic obstructive pulmonary disease (includes exacerbation), interstitial pulmonary disease, lobar pneumonia, pulmonary edema, pulmonary infiltrates, respiratory failure, wheezing
Miscellaneous: Accidental injury (traffic accident), mass (renal), nodule

<1%, postmarketing, and/or case reports: Anaphylaxis, angioedema, cholestatic hepatitis, drug reaction with eosinophilia and systemic symptoms, graft versus host disease, hematologic disease (impaired stem cell mobilization), hepatic cytolysis, hyperthyroidism, organ transplant rejection, pneumonitis, progressive multifocal leukoencephalopathy, reactivation of HPV, Stevens-Johnson syndrome, toxic epidermal necrolysis, toxic hepatitis, tumor lysis syndrome

Mechanism of Action Lenalidomide has immunomodulatory, antiangiogenic, and antineoplastic characteristics via multiple mechanisms. It selectively inhibits secretion of proinflammatory cytokines (potent inhibitor of tumor necrosis factor-alpha secretion); enhances cell-mediated immunity by stimulating proliferation of anti-CD3 stimulated T cells (resulting in increased IL-2 and interferon gamma secretion); inhibits trophic signals to angiogenic factors in cells. Inhibits the growth of myeloma, myelodysplastic, and lymphoma tumor cells by inducing cell cycle arrest and cell death. The addition of lenalidomide to rituximab increases antibody dependent cell-mediated cytotoxicity in follicular lymphoma and marginal zone lymphoma and increases tumor cell apoptosis in follicular lymphoma (compared to rituximab alone).

Pharmacodynamics/Kinetics

Half-life Elimination 3 to 5 hours

Time to Peak MDS or myeloma patients: 0.5 to 6 hours

Reproductive Considerations

[US Boxed Warning]: In females of reproductive potential, obtain 2 negative pregnancy tests before starting lenalidomide treatment. Females of reproductive potential must use 2 forms of contraception or continuously abstain from heterosexual sex during and for 4 weeks after lenalidomide treatment. To avoid embryo-fetal exposure to lenalidomide, it is only available under a restricted distribution program called Revlimid REMS program.

Females of reproductive potential should be treated only if they are able to comply with the conditions of the Revlimid REMS program. Females of reproductive potential must avoid pregnancy beginning 4 weeks prior to therapy, during therapy, during therapy interruptions, and for at least 4 weeks after therapy is discontinued. Two forms of effective/reliable contraception (eg, tubal ligation, IUD, hormonal birth control methods, male latex or synthetic condom, diaphragm, or cervical cap) or total abstinence from heterosexual intercourse must be used by females who are not infertile or who have not had a hysterectomy. A negative pregnancy test (sensitivity of at least 50 milliunits/mL) 10 to 14 days prior to therapy, within 24 hours prior to beginning therapy, weekly during the first 4 weeks, and every 4 weeks (every 2 weeks for females with irregular menstrual cycles) thereafter is required for females of reproductive potential. Lenalidomide must be immediately discontinued for a missed period, abnormal pregnancy test or abnormal menstrual bleeding; refer patient to a reproductive toxicity specialist if pregnancy occurs during treatment. False-positive pregnancy tests have been reported during lenalidomide therapy (Castaneda 2018).

Lenalidomide is also present in the semen of males. Males (including those vasectomized) should use a latex or synthetic condom during any sexual contact with females of reproductive age during treatment, during treatment interruptions, and for 4 weeks after discontinuation. Male patients should not donate sperm during, for 4 weeks after treatment, and during therapy interruptions.

Pregnancy Considerations

Use is contraindicated in pregnancy. **[US Boxed Warning]: Do not use lenalidomide during pregnancy. Lenalidomide, a thalidomide analogue, caused limb abnormalities in a developmental monkey study. Thalidomide is a known human teratogen that causes severe, life-threatening human birth defects. If lenalidomide is used during pregnancy, it may cause birth defects or embryo-fetal death. To avoid embryo-fetal exposure to lenalidomide, it is only available under a restricted distribution program called Revlimid REMS program.**

A pregnancy exposure registry has been created to monitor outcomes in females exposed to lenalidomide during pregnancy and female partners of male patients and to understand the root cause for the pregnancy. The pregnancy exposure registry may be contacted at 1-888-423-5436. The parent or legal guardian for patients between 12 and 18 years of age must agree to ensure compliance with the required guidelines. Any suspected fetal exposure should be reported to the FDA via the MedWatch program (1-800-FDA-1088) and to Celgene Corporation (1-888-423-5436).

Prescribing and Access Restrictions In Canada, distribution is restricted through RevAid (www.RevAid.ca or 1-888-738-2431).

Lenvatinib (len VA ti nib)

Brand Names: US Lenvima (10 MG Daily Dose); Lenvima (12 MG Daily Dose); Lenvima (14 MG Daily Dose); Lenvima (18 MG Daily Dose); Lenvima (20 MG Daily Dose); Lenvima (24 MG Daily Dose); Lenvima (4 MG Daily Dose); Lenvima (8 MG Daily Dose)

Brand Names: Canada Lenvima (10 MG Daily Dose); Lenvima (12 MG Daily Dose); Lenvima (14 MG Daily Dose); Lenvima (18 MG Daily Dose); Lenvima (20 MG Daily Dose); Lenvima (24 MG Daily Dose); Lenvima (4 MG Daily Dose); Lenvima (8 MG Daily Dose)

Pharmacologic Category Antineoplastic Agent, Tyrosine Kinase Inhibitor; Antineoplastic Agent, Vascular Endothelial Growth Factor (VEGF) Inhibitor

Use

Endometrial carcinoma, advanced: Treatment of advanced endometrial carcinoma (in combination with pembrolizumab) that is not microsatellite instability-high or mismatch repair deficient, in patients who have disease progression following prior systemic therapy and are not candidates for curative surgery or radiation.

Hepatocellular carcinoma, unresectable: First-line treatment of unresectable hepatocellular carcinoma.

Renal cell carcinoma, advanced: Treatment of advanced renal cell carcinoma (in combination with everolimus) following one prior anti-angiogenic therapy.

Thyroid cancer, differentiated: Treatment of locally recurrent or metastatic, progressive, radioactive iodine-refractory differentiated thyroid cancer.

Local Anesthetic/Vasoconstrictor Precautions Hypertension can occur in significant numbers of patients; monitor for hypertension prior to using local anesthetic with vasoconstrictor; medical consult if necessary.

Lenvatinib is one of the drugs confirmed to prolong the QT interval and is accepted as having a risk of causing torsade de pointes. The risk of drug-induced torsade de pointes is extremely low when a single QT interval prolonging drug is prescribed. In terms of epinephrine, it is not known what effect vasoconstrictors in the local anesthetic regimen will have in patients with a known history of congenital prolonged QT interval or in patients taking any medication that prolongs the QT interval. Until more information is obtained, it is suggested that the clinician consult with the physician prior to the use of a vasoconstrictor in suspected patients, and that the vasoconstrictor (epinephrine, mepivacaine, and levonordefrin [Carbocaine 2% with Neo-Cobefrin]) be used with caution.

Effects on Dental Treatment Key adverse event(s) related to dental treatment: Xerostomia (normal salivary flow resumes after discontinuation). Mouth pain, stomatitis, infection of the mouth have been reported.

Effects on Bleeding Chemotherapy may result in significant myelosuppression, potentially including reduction in platelet counts (grades 3/4: 2%); Bleeding has been reported in 35% of patients. In patients who are under active treatment with these agents, medical consult is suggested.

Adverse Reactions

>10%:

Cardiovascular: Hypertension (45% to 73%), peripheral edema (14% to 21%)

Central nervous system: Fatigue (44% to 67%), headache (10% to 38%), voice disorder (24% to 31%), mouth pain (25%), dizziness (15%), insomnia (12%)

Dermatologic: Palmar-plantar erythrodysesthesia (27% to 32%), skin rash (14% to 21%), alopecia (12%)

Endocrine & metabolic: Increased thyroid stimulating hormone level (57% to 70%), weight loss (31% to 51%), hypothyroidism (21%), increased gamma-glutamyl transferase (grades 3/4: 17%), hyponatremia (grades 3/4: 15%)

Gastrointestinal: Diarrhea (39% to 67%), decreased appetite (34% to 54%), nausea (20% to 47%), stomatitis (11% to 41%; grades 3/4: <1%), vomiting (16% to 36%), abdominal pain (30% to 31%), constipation (16% to 29%), dysgeusia (18%), xerostomia (17%), dyspepsia (13%)

Genitourinary: Proteinuria (26% to 34%), urinary tract infection (11%)

Hematologic & oncologic: Hemorrhage (23% to 35%, including carotid artery hemorrhage; grades ≥3: 2%)

Hepatic: Increased serum aspartate aminotransferase (grades ≥3: 5% to 12%)

Neuromuscular & skeletal: Arthralgia (≤62%), myalgia (≤62%)

Renal: Renal insufficiency (7% to 14%)

Respiratory: Cough (24%), epistaxis (12%)

Miscellaneous: Fever (15%)

1% to 10%:

Cardiovascular: Hypotension (9%), prolonged QT interval on ECG (8% to 9%; >500 msec: 2%), cardiac failure (≤7%), ventricular dysfunction (≤7%), arterial thromboembolism (2% to 5%), cardiac abnormality (≤ grade 3: 3%), pulmonary embolism (3%), reduced ejection fraction (ejection fraction reduced by >20%: 2%)

Dermatologic: Hyperkeratosis (7%)

Endocrine & metabolic: Dehydration (9%), hypocalcemia (grades 3/4: 9%), hypokalemia (grades 3/4: 3% to 6%), hypercalcemia (>5%), hypercholesterolemia (>5%), hyperkalemia (>5%), hypoalbuminemia (3% to >5%), hypoglycemia (>5%), hypomagnesemia (>5%)

Gastrointestinal: Infection of mouth (≤10%), increased serum lipase (grades 3/4: 4% to 6%), increased serum amylase (>5%), gastrointestinal fistula (≤2%), gastrointestinal perforation (≤2%)

Hematologic & oncologic: Thrombocytopenia (grades 3/4: 2% to 10%), lymphocytopenia (grades 3/4: 8%), neutropenia (grades 3/4: 7%), anemia (grades 3/4: 4%)

Hepatic: Hepatic encephalopathy (8%), hyperbilirubinemia (>5%), increased serum alanine aminotransferase (grades ≥3: 4% to 8%), increased serum alkaline phosphatase (>5%), hepatic failure (3%)

Renal: Increased serum creatinine (grades 3/4: 2% to 3%)

Respiratory: Pulmonary edema (≤7%), pneumonia (4%)

<1%, postmarketing, and/or case reports: Aortic dissection, cholecystitis, fistula, hepatitis, nephrotic syndrome, pancreatitis, pneumothorax, reversible posterior leukoencephalopathy syndrome, tumor hemorrhage, wound healing impairment

Mechanism of Action Lenvatinib is a multitargeted tyrosine kinase inhibitor of vascular endothelial growth factor (VEGF) receptors VEGFR1 (FLT1), VEGFR2 (KDR), VEGFR3 (FLT4), fibroblast growth factor (FGF) receptors FGFR1, 2, 3, and 4, platelet derived growth factor receptor alpha (PDGFRα), KIT, and RET. Inhibition of these receptor tyrosine kinases leads to decreased tumor growth and slowing of cancer progression. In hepatocellular carcinoma cell lines dependent on activated FGFR signaling (with a concurrent inhibition of FGF-receptor substrate 2α phosphorylation), lenvatinib exhibited antiproliferative activity. Combining lenvatinib with everolimus has demonstrated increased antiangiogenic and antitumor activity by decreasing human endothelial cell proliferation, tube formation, and VEGF signaling (in vitro) compared to either drug alone.

Pharmacodynamics/Kinetics

Half-life Elimination ~28 hours

Time to Peak 1 to 4 hours

Reproductive Considerations
Verify pregnancy status prior to initiating lenvatinib in females of reproductive potential. Females of reproductive potential should use effective contraception during lenvatinib treatment and for at least 30 days after completion of therapy.

Pregnancy Considerations
Based on the mechanism of action and findings from animal reproduction studies, lenvatinib may cause fetal harm if administered in pregnancy.

Prescribing and Access Restrictions Lenvatinib is available only through specialty pharmacies. For further information on patient assistance, product availability, and prescribing instructions, please refer to the following website: http://www.eisaireimbursement.com/patient/lenvima

- **Lenvatinib Mesylate** *see* Lenvatinib *on page 885*
- **Lenvima (4 MG Daily Dose)** *see* Lenvatinib *on page 885*
- **Lenvima (8 MG Daily Dose)** *see* Lenvatinib *on page 885*
- **Lenvima (10 MG Daily Dose)** *see* Lenvatinib *on page 885*
- **Lenvima (12 MG Daily Dose)** *see* Lenvatinib *on page 885*
- **Lenvima (14 MG Daily Dose)** *see* Lenvatinib *on page 885*
- **Lenvima (18 MG Daily Dose)** *see* Lenvatinib *on page 885*
- **Lenvima (20 MG Daily Dose)** *see* Lenvatinib *on page 885*
- **Lenvima (24 MG Daily Dose)** *see* Lenvatinib *on page 885*
- **Lescol XL** *see* Fluvastatin *on page 706*

Lesinurad (le SIN ure ad)

Brand Names: US Zurampic

Pharmacologic Category Antigout Agent; Uric Acid Transporter 1 (URAT1) Inhibitor

Use

Hyperuricemia associated with gout: Treatment of hyperuricemia associated with gout (in combination with a xanthine oxidase inhibitor) in patients who have not achieved target serum uric acid levels with a xanthine oxidase inhibitor alone.

Limitations of use: Lesinurad is not recommended for the treatment of asymptomatic hyperuricemia. Lesinurad should not be used as monotherapy.

Local Anesthetic/Vasoconstrictor Precautions
No information available to require special precautions

Effects on Dental Treatment No significant effects or complications reported

Effects on Bleeding No information available to require special precautions

Adverse Reactions Incidence reported in combination with a xanthine oxidase inhibitor.

1% to 10%:
- Central nervous system: Headache (5%)
- Gastrointestinal: Gastroesophageal reflux disease (3%)
- Infection: Influenza (5%)
- Renal: Increased serum creatinine (≤6%; 1.5 x to <2.0 x baseline: 4%; ≥2.0 x baseline: 2%; most elevations were transient and resolved without therapy interruption), renal failure (2%)

Frequency not defined:
- Cardiovascular: Cerebrovascular accident, myocardial infarction
- Renal: Acute renal failure

<1%, postmarketing, and/or case reports: Nephrolithiasis

Mechanism of Action Lesinurad inhibits the function of transporter proteins involved in renal uric acid reabsorption (uric acid transporter 1 [URAT1] and organic anion transporter 4 [OAT4]), and lowers serum uric acid levels and increases renal clearance and fractional excretion of uric acid in patients with gout.

Pharmacodynamics/Kinetics

Half-life Elimination ~5 hours

Time to Peak Within 1 to 4 hours

Reproductive Considerations
All forms of hormonal contraceptives (eg, oral, injectable, topical) may be less effective during therapy with lesinurad. Additional methods of contraception are recommended during therapy.

Pregnancy Considerations
Adverse events were not observed in animal reproduction studies.

Lesinurad and Allopurinol
(le SIN ure ad & al oh PURE i nole)

Brand Names: US Duzallo [DSC]

Pharmacologic Category Antigout Agent; Uric Acid Transporter 1 (URAT1) Inhibitor; Xanthine Oxidase Inhibitor

Use

Hyperuricemia associated with gout: Treatment of hyperuricemia associated with gout in patients who have not achieved target serum uric acid levels with a medically appropriate daily dose of allopurinol alone.

Limitations of use: Not recommended for the treatment of asymptomatic hyperuricemia.

Local Anesthetic/Vasoconstrictor Precautions
No information available to require special precautions

Effects on Dental Treatment No significant effects or complications reported

Effects on Bleeding No information available to require special precautions

Adverse Reactions See individual agents.

Mechanism of Action

Lesinurad/allopurinol: Lowers serum uric acid levels by increasing excretion and inhibiting production of uric acid.

Allopurinol: Allopurinol inhibits xanthine oxidase, the enzyme responsible for the conversion of hypoxanthine to xanthine to uric acid. Allopurinol is metabolized to oxypurinol which is also an inhibitor of xanthine oxidase; allopurinol acts on purine catabolism, reducing the production of uric acid without disrupting the biosynthesis of vital purines.

Lesinurad: Lesinurad inhibits the function of transporter proteins involved in renal uric acid reabsorption (uric acid transporter 1 [URAT1] and organic anion transporter 4 [OAT4]), and lowers serum uric acid levels and increases renal clearance and fractional excretion of uric acid in patients with gout.

Pharmacodynamics/Kinetics

Half-life Elimination Allopurinol: ~1 to 2 hours; Oxypurinol: ~26 hours; lesinurad: ~5 hours

Time to Peak Allopurinol: 1.5 hours; Oxypurinol: 4.5 hours

Reproductive Considerations
All forms of hormonal contraceptives (eg, oral, injectable, topical) may be less effective during therapy with lesinurad. Additional methods of contraception are recommended during therapy.

Pregnancy Considerations
Animal reproduction studies have not been conducted with this combination. See individual monographs for additional information.

Product Availability Duzallo has been discontinued in the United States for >1 year.

- **Lessina** *see* Ethinyl Estradiol and Levonorgestrel *on page 612*
- **Letairis** *see* Ambrisentan *on page 113*

Letermovir (le term oh vir)

Brand Names: US Prevymis

Brand Names: Canada Prevymis

Pharmacologic Category Antiviral Agent

Use Cytomegalovirus (prophylaxis): Prophylaxis of cytomegalovirus (CMV) infection and disease in adult CMV-seropositive recipients [R+] of an allogeneic hematopoietic stem cell transplant (HSCT)

Local Anesthetic/Vasoconstrictor Precautions
No information available to require special precautions

Effects on Dental Treatment No significant effects or complications reported

Effects on Bleeding Decreased hemoglobin (grade 4: 2%), decreased platelet count (grade 4: 27%)

Adverse Reactions

>10%:

Cardiovascular: Peripheral edema (14%)

Central nervous system: Headache (14%), fatigue (13%)

Gastrointestinal: Nausea (27%), diarrhea (26%), vomiting (19%), abdominal pain (12%)

Hematologic & oncologic: Decreased platelet count (grade 4: 27%)

Respiratory: Cough (14%)

1% to 10%:

Cardiovascular: Tachycardia (4%), atrial fibrillation (3%)

Hematologic & oncologic: Decreased hemoglobin (grade 4: 2%)

<1%, postmarketing, and/or case reports: Hypersensitivity reaction

Mechanism of Action Letermovir inhibits cytomegalovirus (CMV) replication by targeting the CMV DNA terminase complex (pUL51, pUL56, pUL89), which is required for viral DNA processing and packaging. Letermovir affects production of genome unit lengths and alters virion maturation.

Pharmacodynamics/Kinetics

Half-life Elimination 12 hours

Time to Peak 1.5 to 3 hours

Pregnancy Considerations Adverse events were observed in some animal reproduction studies.

Letrozole (LET roe zole)

Brand Names: US Femara

Brand Names: Canada ACH-Letrozole; APO-Letrozole; BIO-Letrozole; CCP-Letrozole; Femara; JAMP-Letrozole; Mar-Letrozole; MED-Letrozole; NAT-Letrozole; PMS-Letrozole; RAN-Letrozole; RIVA-Letrozole; SANDOZ Letrozole; TEVA-Letrozole; VAN-Letrozole [DSC]; Zinda-Letrozole

Pharmacologic Category Antineoplastic Agent, Aromatase Inhibitor

Use Breast cancer in postmenopausal women: Adjuvant treatment of hormone receptor-positive early breast cancer, extended adjuvant treatment of early breast cancer after 5 years of tamoxifen; treatment of advanced breast cancer with disease progression following antiestrogen therapy; first-line treatment of hormone receptor-positive or hormone receptor-unknown, locally-advanced, or metastatic breast cancer

Local Anesthetic/Vasoconstrictor Precautions
No information available to require special precautions

Effects on Dental Treatment No significant effects or complications reported

Effects on Bleeding Thrombocytopenia has been reported but relationship to letrozole is unclear.

Adverse Reactions

>10%:

Cardiovascular: Flushing (50%), edema (7% to 18%)

Central nervous system: Headache (4% to 20%), dizziness (3% to 14%), fatigue (10% to 13%)

Dermatologic: Diaphoresis (24%), night sweats (15%)

Endocrine & metabolic: Hypercholesterolemia (3% to 52%), hot flash (6% to 34%), weight gain (2% to 13%)

Gastrointestinal: Nausea (9% to 17%), constipation (2% to 11%)

Neuromuscular & skeletal: Weakness (4% to 34%), arthralgia (8% to 25%), arthritis (7% to 25%), ostealgia (5% to 22%), musculoskeletal pain (21%), back pain (5% to 18%), bone fracture (10% to 15%), osteoporosis (5% to 15%)

Respiratory: Dyspnea (6% to 18%), cough (6% to 13%)

1% to 10%:

Cardiovascular: Chest pain (6% to 8%), hypertension (5% to 8%), chest wall pain (6%), peripheral edema (5%), cerebrovascular accident (2% to 3%), thromboembolism (≤3%; including portal vein thrombosis, pulmonary embolism, thrombophlebitis, venous thrombosis), transient ischemic attacks (≤3%), angina pectoris (≤2%), hemorrhagic stroke (≤2%), ischemic heart disease (≤2%), thrombotic stroke (≤2%), cardiac failure (1% to 2%), myocardial infarction (1% to 2%)

Central nervous system: Insomnia (6% to 7%), pain (5%), anxiety (<5%), depression (<5%), vertigo (<5%), drowsiness (3%), hemiparesis (≤2%)

Dermatologic: Skin rash (5%), alopecia (<5%), pruritus (1%)

Endocrine & metabolic: Weight loss (6% to 7%), hypercalcemia (<5%)

Gastrointestinal: Diarrhea (5% to 8%), vomiting (3% to 7%), abdominal pain (6%), anorexia (1% to 5%), dyspepsia (3%)

Genitourinary: Mastalgia (2% to 7%), urinary tract infection (6%), vaginal dryness (5%), vaginal hemorrhage (5%), vaginal irritation (5%)

Hematologic & oncologic: Lymphedema (7%; post-mastectomy), second primary malignant neoplasm (2% to 5%)

Infection: Infection (7%), influenza (6%), viral infection (6%)

Neuromuscular & skeletal: Limb pain (4% to 10%), myalgia (7% to 9%), osteopenia (4%)

Ophthalmic: Cataract (2%)

Renal: Renal disease (5%)

Respiratory: Pleural effusion (<5%)

<1%, postmarketing, and/or case reports: Anaphylaxis, angioedema, arterial thrombosis, blurred vision, carpal tunnel syndrome, dysesthesia, dysgeusia, endometrial carcinoma, endometrium disease, endometrial hyperplasia, erythema multiforme, eye irritation, fever, hepatitis, hypersensitivity reaction, increased appetite, increased liver enzymes, increased thirst, irritability, leukopenia, memory impairment, nervousness, ovarian cyst, palpitations, paresthesia, spontaneous abortion, stomatitis, tachycardia, tenosynovitis (trigger finger), thrombocytopenia, toxic epidermal necrolysis, urinary frequency, urticaria, vaginal discharge, xeroderma, xerostomia

Mechanism of Action Letrozole is a nonsteroidal competitive inhibitor of the aromatase enzyme system which binds to the heme group of aromatase, a cytochrome P450 enzyme which catalyzes conversion of androgens to estrogens (specifically, androstenedione to estrone and testosterone to estradiol). This leads to inhibition of the enzyme and a significant reduction in plasma estrogen (estrone, estradiol and estrone sulfate) levels. Letrozole does not appear to affect synthesis of adrenal or thyroid hormones, aldosterone, or androgens.

Pharmacodynamics/Kinetics

Half-life Elimination Terminal: ~2 days

Time to Peak Steady state, plasma: 2 to 6 weeks; steady state serum concentrations are 1.5 to 2 times higher than single-dose values. In girls 3 to 9 years, steady state concentrations were 25% to 67% that of the mean adult values (Feuillan 2007)

Reproductive Considerations

A pregnancy test is recommended prior to starting letrozole therapy in all females of reproductive potential.

When used for breast cancer, effective contraception should be used during letrozole therapy and for at least 3 weeks following the last letrozole dose.

Letrozole is used off-label for ovulation induction in females with polycystic ovarian syndrome (PCOS) and anovulatory infertility when no other causes of infertility are present (ACOG 194 2018; Teede 2018). Baseline pregnancy testing is done prior to letrozole therapy to rule out unexpected ovulation, which prevents exposure in early pregnancy (Legro 2016). Because information related to newborn outcomes following maternal use is limited, guidelines recommend counseling females of the off-label status prior to use (ACOG 194 2018).

Pregnancy Considerations

Use is contraindicated in women with an established pregnancy.

Letrozole is approved for the treatment of breast cancer in postmenopausal women. Based on the mechanism of action and data from animal reproduction studies, letrozole may cause fetal harm if used during pregnancy.

◆ **Leucovorin** *see* Leucovorin Calcium *on page 889*

Leucovorin Calcium (loo koe VOR in KAL see um)

Brand Names: Canada Lederle Leucovorin; RIVA Leucovorin

Pharmacologic Category Antidote; Chemotherapy Modulating Agent; Rescue Agent (Chemotherapy); Vitamin, Water Soluble

Use

Colorectal cancer, advanced: Injection: Palliative treatment of advanced colorectal cancer to prolong survival (in combination with fluorouracil).

Megaloblastic anemia: Injection: Treatment of megaloblastic anemias due to folic acid deficiency (when oral therapy is not feasible).

Methotrexate toxicity:

Injection: Rescue agent after high-dose methotrexate treatment in osteosarcoma and to diminish the toxicity and counteract the effects of impaired methotrexate elimination and of inadvertent overdosage of folic acid antagonists.

Oral: Rescue agent to diminish toxicity and counteract effects of impaired methotrexate elimination and inadvertent overdoses of folic acid antagonists.

Local Anesthetic/Vasoconstrictor Precautions No information available to require special precautions

Effects on Dental Treatment No significant effects or complications reported

Effects on Bleeding No information available to require special precautions

Adverse Reactions As reported in combination with 5-fluorouracil.

>10%:

Central nervous system: Fatigue (≤13%), lethargy (≤13%), malaise (≤13%)

Dermatologic: Alopecia (42% to 43%), dermatitis (21% to 25%)

Gastrointestinal: Stomatitis (75% to 84%; grades ≥3: 27% to 29%), nausea (74% to 80%), diarrhea (66% to 67%), vomiting (44% to 46%), anorexia (14% to 22%)

Miscellaneous: Drug toxicity

1% to 10%:

Gastrointestinal: Constipation (3% to 4%)

Infection: Infection (3% to 8%)

Frequency not defined: Gastrointestinal: Gastrointestinal toxicity

Postmarketing: Anaphylactic shock, anaphylaxis, hypersensitivity reaction, nonimmune anaphylaxis, seizure, syncope, urticaria

Mechanism of Action Leucovorin calcium is a reduced form of folic acid, leucovorin supplies the necessary cofactor blocked by methotrexate. Leucovorin actively competes with methotrexate for transport sites, displaces methotrexate from intracellular binding sites, and restores active folate stores required for DNA/RNA synthesis. Leucovorin stabilizes the binding of 5-dUMP and thymidylate synthetase, enhancing the activity of fluorouracil. When administered with pyrimethamine for the treatment of opportunistic infections, leucovorin reduces the risk for hematologic toxicity (HHS [OI adult 2020]).

Methanol toxicity treatment: Formic acid (methanol's toxic metabolite) is normally metabolized to carbon dioxide and water by 10-formyltetrahydrofolate dehydrogenase after being bound to tetrahydrofolate. Administering a source of tetrahydrofolate may aid the body in eliminating formic acid (AACT [Barceloux] 2002).

Pharmacodynamics/Kinetics

Half-life Elimination ~4 to 8 hours

Time to Peak Oral: ~2 hours; IV: Total folates: 10 minutes; 5MTHF: ~1 hour; IM: Total folates: 52 minutes; 5MTHF: 2.8 hours

Pregnancy Risk Factor C

Pregnancy Considerations Animal reproduction studies have not been conducted. Leucovorin is a biologically active form of folic acid. Adequate amounts of folic acid are recommended during pregnancy. Refer to Folic Acid monograph.

♦ **Leukeran** *see* Chlorambucil *on page 332*

♦ **Leukine** *see* Sargramostim *on page 1358*

Leuprolide (loo PROE lide)

Brand Names: US Eligard; Fensolvi (6 Month); Lupron Depot (1-Month); Lupron Depot (3-Month); Lupron Depot (4-Month); Lupron Depot (6-Month); Lupron Depot-Ped (1-Month); Lupron Depot-Ped (3-Month)

Brand Names: Canada Eligard; Lupron; Lupron Depot; Lupron Depot (1-Month); Lupron Depot (3-Month); Lupron Depot 3 Month Kit; Zeulide Depot

Pharmacologic Category Antineoplastic Agent, Gonadotropin-Releasing Hormone Agonist; Gonadotropin Releasing Hormone Agonist

Use

Central precocious puberty: Treatment of pediatric patients ≥2 years of age with central precocious puberty (CPP). CPP is defined as early onset of secondary sexual characteristics (usually <8 years of age in girls and <9 years of age in boys) associated with pubertal pituitary gonadotropin activation; may have a significantly advanced bone age resulting in diminished adult height.

Limitations of use: Prior to treatment initiation, confirm clinical diagnosis of CPP with blood concentrations of luteinizing hormone (basal or stimulated with a gonadotropin-releasing hormone), sex steroids, and bone age assessment (versus chronological age). Baseline evaluations should include height and weight measurements, diagnostic brain imaging (to rule out intracranial tumor), pelvic/testicular/adrenal ultrasound (to rule out steroid-secreting tumors), human chorionic gonadotropin levels (to rule out a chorionic gonadotropin-secreting tumor), and adrenal steroid measurements (to exclude congenital adrenal hyperplasia).

Endometriosis: Management of endometriosis, including pain relief and reduction of endometriotic lesions. Initial management of endometriosis and symptom recurrence (in combination with norethindrone acetate as add-back therapy).

Limitations of use: Initial treatment (maximum 6 months) may be as monotherapy or combination therapy with norethindrone acetate (used as add-back therapy to reduce the loss of bone mineral density). A single retreatment course (maximum 6 months) of leuprolide in combination with norethindrone acetate may be considered if symptoms recur. Monotherapy is not recommended for retreatment. Total duration of therapy should not exceed 12 months.

Prostate cancer, advanced: Palliative treatment of advanced prostate cancer.

Uterine leiomyomata (fibroids): Treatment (preoperative) of anemia caused by uterine leiomyomata (fibroids).

Limitations of use: For use in combination with supplemental iron in females with inadequate response to iron alone.

Local Anesthetic/Vasoconstrictor Precautions No information available to require special precautions

Effects on Dental Treatment Key adverse event(s) related to dental treatment: Gum hemorrhage, gingivitis, dry mucous membranes, and dysphagia.

Effects on Bleeding Decreased and increased platelet count has been reported.

Adverse Reactions

Children (percentages based on 1-month and 3-month pediatric formulations combined):

>10%: Local: Pain at injection site (19% to 20%)

1% to 10%:

Cardiovascular: Vasodilation (2%), bradycardia (<2%), hypertension (<2%), peripheral edema (<2%), peripheral vascular disease (<2%), syncope (<2%)

Central nervous system: Headache (2% to 7%), emotional lability (5%), mood changes (5%), pain (3%), depression (<2%), drowsiness (<2%), nervousness (<2%)

Dermatologic: Skin rash (3%), acne vulgaris (≤3%), erythema multiforme (≤3%), seborrhea (≤3%), alopecia (<2%), body odor (<2%), hair disease (<2%), leukoderma (<2%), nail disease (<2%), nonthrombocytopenic purpura (<2%), skin hypertrophy (<2%)

Endocrine & metabolic: Weight gain (≤7%), feminization (<2%), goiter (<2%), growth suppression (<2%), gynecomastia (<2%), hirsutism (<2%), menstrual disease (females: <2%)

Gastrointestinal: Constipation (<2%), dyspepsia (<2%), dysphagia (<2%), gingivitis (<2%), increased appetite (<2%), nausea (<2%), vomiting (<2%)

Genitourinary: Vaginal discharge (females: ≤3%), vaginal hemorrhage (females: ≤3%), vaginitis (females: ≤3%), breast disease (<2%), cervical neoplasm (females: <2%), cervix disease (females: <2%), dysmenorrhea (females: <2%), urinary incontinence (<2%)

Hematologic & oncologic: Increased erythrocyte sedimentation rate (<2%), tumor flare (<2%)

Hypersensitivity: Hypersensitivity reaction (<2%)

Immunologic: Increased ANA titer (<2%)

Infection: Infection (<2%)

Local: Abscess at injection site (≤9%), injection site reaction (≤9%), swelling at injection site (2%)

Neuromuscular & skeletal: Arthralgia (<2%), arthropathy (<2%), hyperkinesia (<2%), myalgia (<2%), myopathy (<2%)

Ophthalmic: Visual disturbance (<2%)

Respiratory: Asthma (<2%), epistaxis (<2%), flu-like symptoms (<2%), pharyngitis (<2%), rhinitis (<2%), sinusitis (<2%)

Miscellaneous: Fever (<2%)

Frequency not defined:

Cardiovascular: Flushing

Central nervous system: Abnormal gait

Dermatologic: Diaphoresis

Endocrine & metabolic: Diabetes mellitus, hot flash

Adults:

>10%:

Cardiovascular: Flushing (≤58%), ECG changes (≤19%), ischemia (≤19%), edema (≤14%), peripheral edema (≤12%)

Central nervous system: Headache (≤65%), migraine (≤65%), pain (8% to 33%), depression (≤31%), emotional lability (≤31%), insomnia (≤31%), sleep disorder (≤31%), fatigue (≤18%), malaise (≤18%), dizziness (≤16%), vertigo (≤16%), lethargy (≤12%), local discomfort (injection site: ≤11%)

Dermatologic: Diaphoresis (≤98%), allergic skin reaction (≤12%)
Endocrine & metabolic: Hot flash (≤98%), increased serum cholesterol (7% to 59%), increased serum triglycerides (5% to 32%), weight loss (13%), weight gain (≤13%), decreased libido (≤11%)
Gastrointestinal: Nausea (≤25%), vomiting (≤25%), gastrointestinal disease (≤16%), constipation (≤14%), diarrhea (≤14%)
Genitourinary: Vaginitis (females: 11% to 28%), testicular atrophy (males: ≤20%), genitourinary complaint (10% to 15%)
Hematologic & oncologic: Decreased hemoglobin (≤44%; grades 3/4: 1%)
Local: Pain at injection site (≤18%), injection site reaction (≤14%), erythema at injection site (2% to 13%), bruising at injection site (3% to 12%)
Neuromuscular & skeletal: Asthenia (≤18%), arthropathy (8% to 16%)
Respiratory: Flu-like symptoms (≤12%), respiratory tract disease (6% to 11%)

1% to 10%:
Cardiovascular: Hypertension (≤8%), angina pectoris (<5%), atrial fibrillation (<5%), bradycardia (<5%), cardiac arrhythmia (<5%), cardiac failure (<5%), deep vein thrombophlebitis (<5%), hypotension (<5%), myocardial infarction (<5%), palpitations (<5%), pulmonary embolism (<5%), syncope (<5%), tachycardia (<5%), varicose veins (<5%), heart murmur (3%), phlebitis (≤2%), thrombosis (≤2%)
Central nervous system: Anxiety (≤8%), nervousness (≤8%), paresthesia (≤8%), memory impairment (≤6%), ostealgia (<2% to 5%), abnormality in thinking (<5%), agitation (<5%), amnesia (<5%), chills (<5%), confusion (<5%), delusions (<5%), dementia (<5%), hypoesthesia (<5%), loss of consciousness (<5%), neuropathy (<5%), numbness (<5%), paralysis (<5%), peripheral neuropathy (<5%), personality disorder (<5%), seizure (<5%), voice disorder (<5%), altered sense of smell (<2%), rigors (<2%)
Dermatologic: Acne vulgaris (≤10%), dermatological reaction (≤10%), injection site pruritus (≤9%), dermatitis (5%), body odor (<5%), cellulitis (<5%), ecchymoses (<5%), hair disease (<5%), hyperpigmentation (<5%), nail disease (<5%), skin lesion (<5%), xeroderma (<5%), alopecia (≤4%), cold and clammy skin (≤4%), night sweats (≤3%), pruritus (≤3%), skin rash (2%)
Endocrine & metabolic: Decreased HDL cholesterol (2% to 10%), increased LDL cholesterol (8%), dehydration (≤8%), gynecomastia (males: ≤7%), breast changes (≤6%), decreased serum albumin (≥5%), decreased serum bicarbonate (≥5%), decreased serum total protein (≥5%), hypercholesterolemia (≥5%), hyperglycemia (≥5%), hyperlipidemia (≥5%), hyperphosphatemia (≥5%), hyperuricemia (≥5%), increased gamma-glutamyl transferase (≥5%), increased lactate dehydrogenase (≥5%), increased prostatic acid phosphatase (males: ≥5%), diabetes mellitus (≤5%), goiter (<5%), hypercalcemia (<5%), hypoglycemia (<5%), increased thirst (<5%), androgen-like effect (females: ≤4%), menstrual disease (females: ≤2%), loss of libido (<2%), pitting edema (≤1%)
Gastrointestinal: Anorexia (≤6%), abdominal distention (<5%), duodenal ulcer (<5%), dysgeusia (<5%), dysphagia (<5%), eructation (<5%), gastrointestinal hemorrhage (<5%), gingival hemorrhage (<5%), gingivitis (<5%), hernia of abdominal cavity (<5%), hiccups (<5%), increased appetite (<5%), intestinal obstruction (<5%), melanosis (<5%), peptic ulcer (<5%), periodontal abscess (<5%), rectal polyp (<5%), xerostomia (<5%), change in appetite (4%), flatulence (≤4%), mucous membrane abnormality (≤4%), dyspepsia (<4%), colitis (≤3%), gastroenteritis (≤3%)
Genitourinary: Decreased testicular size (males: 7%), mastalgia (≤7%), breast tenderness (≤6%), hematuria (≤6%), urinary frequency (≤6%), urinary urgency (≤6%), impotence (males: ≤5%), balanitis (males: <5%), bladder spasm (<5%), breast hypertrophy (<5%), dysuria (<5%), epididymitis (males: <5%), lactation (females: <5%), penile disease (males: <5%), prostatic disease (males: <5%), testicular disease (males: <5%), urinary incontinence (<5%), urinary tract obstruction (<5%), urinary tract infection (3%), nocturia (≤2%), testicular pain (males: ≤2%), difficulty in micturition (<2%), erectile dysfunction (males: <2%), oliguria (<2%), reduction in penile size (males: <2%), urinary retention (<2%)
Hematologic & oncologic: Decreased prostatic acid phosphatase (males: ≥5%), eosinophilia (≥5%), leukopenia (≥5%), prolonged partial thromboplastin time (≥5%), prolonged prothrombin time (≥5%), thrombocythemia (≥5%), anemia (≤5%), bladder carcinoma (<5%), carcinoma (<5%), lymphadenopathy (<5%), lymphedema (<5%), neoplasm (<5%), skin carcinoma (<5%)
Hepatic: Abnormal hepatic function tests (≥5%), increased liver enzymes (≥5%), increased serum alanine aminotransferase (≥5%), increased serum aspartate aminotransferase (≥5%), hepatomegaly (<5%), increased serum transaminases (3%)
Hypersensitivity: Hypersensitivity reaction (<5%)
Infection: Infection (≤5%), abscess (<5%), herpes zoster infection (<5%)
Local: Induration at injection site (3%)
Neuromuscular & skeletal: Neuromuscular disease (≤10%), myalgia (≤8%), ostealgia (5%), lower limb cramp (≤5%), bone disease (temporal bone swelling: <5%), neck pain (<5%), pathological fracture (<5%), arthralgia (1% to 3%), limb pain (≤3%), musculoskeletal pain (≤2%), amyotrophy (<2%), back pain (<2%), tremor (<2%)
Ophthalmic: Amblyopia (<5%), blepharoptosis (<5%), blurred vision (<5%), conjunctivitis (<5%), ophthalmic signs and symptoms (<5%), visual disturbance (<5%), xerophthalmia (<5%)
Otic: Tinnitus (<5%)
Renal: Decreased urine specific gravity (≥5%), increased urine specific gravity (≥5%)
Respiratory: Paranasal sinus congestion (5%), sinusitis (≤5%), asthma (<5%), bronchitis (<5%), emphysema (<5%), epistaxis (<5%), hemoptysis (<5%), hypoxia (<5%), increased bronchial secretions (<5%), pharyngitis (<5%), pleural effusion (<5%), pleural rub (<5%), pneumonia (<5%), pulmonary disease (<5%), pulmonary edema (<5%), pulmonary fibrosis (<5%), rhinitis (<5%), dyspnea (≤2%), sinus headache (≤2%), cough (1%), dyspnea on exertion (≤1%)
Miscellaneous: Abnormal healing (<5%), accidental injury (<5%), cyst (<5%), fever (<5%), inflammation (<5%)

Frequency not defined:

Cardiovascular: Aortic aneurysm (ruptured), auditory hallucination, carotid stenosis, chest tightness, extrasystoles, facial edema

Central nervous system: Anosmia, burning sensation of feet, euphoria, hyperreflexia, hyporeflexia, motor dysfunction

Dermatologic: Dyschromia, facial swelling, hyperkeratosis, pallor, spider telangiectasia

Endocrine & metabolic: Decreased serum potassium, galactorrhea not associated with childbirth (females), hyperkalemia, increased libido, increased serum albumin, increased serum total protein, thyroid nodule

Gastrointestinal: Glossitis, inguinal hernia, occult blood in stools, rectal fistula, rectal irritation

Genitourinary: Blisters on penis (males), increased post-void residual urine volume, penile swelling (males), prostate pain (males), pyuria, uricosuria

Hematologic & oncologic: Bruise, decreased hematocrit, decreased red blood cells, hypoproteinemia, leukocytosis, second primary malignant neoplasm, thrombocytopenia

Hepatic: Hepatitis, increased serum alkaline phosphatase, increased serum bilirubin

Infection: Influenza

Neuromuscular & skeletal: Ankylosing spondylitis, arthritis, bone fracture, knee effusion, muscle cramps, muscle rigidity, muscle spasm, muscle tenderness

Ophthalmic: Eyelid edema, papilledema, retinal vascular disease (perivascular cuffing)

Renal: Increased blood urea nitrogen, increased serum creatinine, nephrolithiasis, pyelonephritis

Respiratory: Abnormal breath sounds (decreased), chronic obstructive pulmonary disease, dry throat, pleuritic chest pain, pulmonary infiltrates, rales, rhonchi, streptococcal pharyngitis, wheezing

Miscellaneous: Fibrosis (pelvic), mass

<1%, postmarketing, and/or case reports: Abdominal pain, abnormal gait, adenoma (pituitary), aggressive behavior, anaphylactoid shock, anaphylaxis, attempted suicide, auditory disturbance, cerebrovascular accident, chest pain, coronary artery disease, decreased appetite, decreased bone mineral density, decreased white blood cell count, deep vein thrombosis, exacerbation of hematuria, fibromyalgia syndrome, gastrointestinal distress, hematoma at injection site, hepatic injury, hepatic insufficiency, hirsutism, hostility, hyperhidrosis, hypertrichosis, increased testosterone level, induration at injection site, interstitial pulmonary disease, intracranial hypertension (Tan 2019), irritability, lower extremity weakness, nodule (throat), obesity, pituitary apoplexy, severe hepatotoxicity, skin photosensitivity, skin ulceration at injection site, sterile abscess at injection site, suicidal ideation, tenosynovitis (symptoms), thromboembolism, tingling of extremities, transient ischemic attacks, urticaria, venous thrombosis, vertebral column fracture, warm sensation at injection site

Mechanism of Action Leuprolide, is an agonist of gonadotropin releasing hormone (GnRH) receptors. Acting as a potent inhibitor of gonadotropin secretion, leuprolide produces an initial increase in luteinizing hormone (LH) and follicle stimulating hormone (FSH), which leads to a transient increase (5 to 12 days [Cook 2000]) in testosterone and dihydrotestosterone (in males) and estrone and estradione (in premenopausal females). Continuous leuprolide administration then results in suppression of ovarian and testicular steroidogenesis due to decreased levels of LH and FSH with subsequent decrease in testosterone (male) and estrogen (female) levels. In males, testosterone levels are reduced to below castrate levels. Leuprolide may also have a direct inhibitory effect on the testes, and act by a different mechanism not directly related to reduction in serum testosterone.

Pharmacodynamics/Kinetics

Onset of Action

Onset of action: Following transient increase, testosterone suppression occurs in ~2 to 4 weeks of continued therapy

Onset of therapeutic suppression for precocious puberty: Leuprolide: 2 to 4 weeks; Leuprolide depot: 1 month

Half-life Elimination ~3 hours

Reproductive Considerations

Evaluate pregnancy status prior to use and throughout treatment in females of reproductive potential; pregnancy should be excluded prior to use. Although leuprolide usually inhibits ovulation and stops menstruation, contraception is not ensured and a nonhormonal contraceptive should be used during therapy.

Based on the mechanism of action, fertility may be impaired; suppression of fertility is reversible following discontinuation of leuprolide.

Pregnancy Risk Factor X

Pregnancy Considerations

Use is contraindicated during pregnancy.

Based on the mechanism of action and data from animal reproduction studies, adverse fetal events may occur following maternal use during pregnancy.

◆ **Leuprolide Acetate** *see* Leuprolide *on page 890*

◆ **Leuprorelin Acetate** *see* Leuprolide *on page 890*

◆ **Leurocristine Sulfate** *see* VinCRIStine *on page 1546*

◆ **Leustatin** *see* Cladribine *on page 359*

Levalbuterol (leve al BYOO ter ole)

Related Information

Respiratory Diseases *on page 1680*

Brand Names: US Xopenex; Xopenex Concentrate; Xopenex HFA

Pharmacologic Category $Beta_2$ Agonist

Use Bronchospasm: Treatment or prevention of bronchospasm in patients with reversible obstructive airway disease (eg, asthma).

Local Anesthetic/Vasoconstrictor Precautions

No information available to require special precautions

Effects on Dental Treatment No significant effects or complications reported

Effects on Bleeding No information available to require special precautions

Adverse Reactions

>10%:

Central nervous system: Headache (children: 12%)

Gastrointestinal: Vomiting (children: 11%)

Infection: Viral infection (≤12%)

Respiratory: Rhinitis (6% to 11%)

>2% to 10%:

Cardiovascular: Tachycardia (adolescents and adults: 3%)

Central nervous system: Nervousness (adolescents and adults: 3% to 10%), dizziness (adolescents and adults: 3%), migraine (adolescents and adults: 3%), anxiety (adolescents and adults: ≤3%), pain (adolescents and adults: ≤3%)
Dermatologic: Skin rash (children: 8%), urticaria (children: 3%)
Gastrointestinal: Diarrhea (children: 2% to 6%; adolescents and adults: <2%), dyspepsia (adolescents and adults: ≤3%)
Hematologic & oncologic: Lymphadenopathy (≤3%)
Neuromuscular & skeletal: Tremor (adolescents and adults: ≤7%), leg cramps (adolescents and adults: ≤3%), weakness (children: 3%), myalgia (≤2%)
Respiratory: Pharyngitis (7% to 10%), asthma (9%), cough (adolescents and adults: 4%), sinusitis (adolescents and adults: 4%), flu-like symptoms (adolescents and adults: ≤4%), bronchitis (children: 3%), nasal mucosa swelling (1% to 3%)
Miscellaneous: Fever (children: 9%), accidental injury (children 5% to 9%; adolescents and adults: 3%)

Frequency not defined:
Endocrine & metabolic: Decreased serum potassium, increased heart rate, increased serum glucose, paradoxical bronchospasm
Hypersensitivity: Hypersensitivity reaction (including bronchospasm, oropharyngeal edema)

<2%, postmarketing, and/or case reports: Acne vulgaris, anaphylaxis, angina pectoris, angioedema, atrial fibrillation, cardiac arrhythmia, chest pain, chills, constipation, conjunctivitis, dry throat, dysmenorrhea, dyspnea, ECG abnormality, epistaxis, extrasystoles, eye pruritus, gastroenteritis, gastroesophageal reflux disease, hematuria, hyperesthesia (hand), hypertension, hypokalemia, hypotension, insomnia, metabolic acidosis, nausea, otalgia, paresthesia, pulmonary disease, supraventricular cardiac arrhythmia, syncope, vertigo, voice disorder, vulvovaginal candidiasis, xerostomia

Mechanism of Action Relaxes bronchial smooth muscle by action on $beta_2$-receptors with little effect on heart rate

Pharmacodynamics/Kinetics

Onset of Action Measured as a 15% increase in FEV_1:
Metered-dose inhaler: 5.5 to 10.2 minutes; Peak effect: 76 to 78 minutes
Nebulization solution: 10 to 17 minutes; Peak effect: 1.5 hours

Duration of Action Measured as a 15% increase in FEV_1:
Metered-dose inhaler: 3 to 4 hours (up to 6 hours in some patients)
Nebulization solution: 5 to 6 hours (up to 8 hours in some patients)

Half-life Elimination 3.3 to 4 hours

Time to Peak Nebulization solution: Children: 0.3 to 0.6 hours, Adults: 0.2 hours

Pregnancy Considerations

Maternal use of $beta_2$ agonists are not associated with an increased risk of fetal malformations (GINA 2020).

Uncontrolled asthma is associated with adverse events on pregnancy (increased risk of perinatal mortality, preeclampsia, preterm birth, low birth weight infants, cesarean delivery, and the development of gestational diabetes). Poorly controlled asthma or asthma exacerbations may have a greater fetal/maternal risk than what is associated with appropriately used asthma medications. Maternal treatment improves pregnancy outcomes by reducing the risk of some adverse events (eg, preterm birth and gestational diabetes) (ERS/TSANZ [Middleton 2019]; GINA 2020).

Short-acting beta-2 agonists (SABA) should be used to treat acute asthma exacerbations in pregnant women (GINA 2020). SABA are preferred over long-acting agents when treatment for asthma is needed during pregnancy; maternal asthma symptoms should be monitored monthly during pregnancy (ERS/TSANZ [Middleton 2019]). If high doses of SABA are needed during the last 48 hours of labor and delivery, monitor blood glucose in the newborn for 24 hours after birth (GINA 2020). Levalbuterol is not approved for the management of preterm labor.

Data collection to monitor pregnancy and infant outcomes associated with asthma and the medications used to treat asthma in pregnancy is ongoing. Health care providers are encouraged to enroll exposed pregnant females in the MotherToBaby Pregnancy Studies conducted by the Organization of Teratology Information Specialists (OTIS) (877-311-8972 or http://mothertobaby.org). Patients may also enroll themselves.

◆ **Levalbuterol HCl** *see* Levalbuterol *on page 892*
◆ **Levalbuterol Hydrochloride** *see* Levalbuterol *on page 892*
◆ **Levalbuterol Tartrate** *see* Levalbuterol *on page 892*

Levamlodipine (lev am LOE di peen)

Pharmacologic Category Antihypertensive; Calcium Channel Blocker; Calcium Channel Blocker, Dihydropyridine

Use Hypertension: Treatment of hypertension, alone or in combination with other antihypertensive agents, in adults and pediatric patients ≥6 years of age.

Local Anesthetic/Vasoconstrictor Precautions No information available to require special precautions.

Effects on Dental Treatment Key adverse event(s) related to dental treatment: Levamlodipine is the pharmacologically active isomer of amlodipine. Information for amlodipine indicates that there are fewer reports of gingival hyperplasia with amlodipine than with other calcium channel blockers (usually resolves upon discontinuation). Consultation with physician is suggested if gingival hypoplasia is observed.

Effects on Bleeding No information available to require special precautions.

Adverse Reactions All adverse reactions were reported with amlodipine, as levamlodipine is the pharmacologically active isomer of amlodipine.

>10%: Cardiovascular: Edema (2% to 11%)

1% to 10%:
Cardiovascular: Palpitations (1% to 5%), flushing (≤3%)
Central nervous system: Fatigue (5%), dizziness (3%), drowsiness (1%)
Gastrointestinal: Nausea (3%), abdominal pain (2%)

<1%: Abnormal dreams, angioedema, anorexia, anxiety, arthralgia, arthropathy, asthenia, atrial fibrillation, back pain, bradycardia, cardiac arrhythmia, chest pain, conjunctivitis, constipation, depersonalization, depression, diaphoresis, diarrhea, diplopia, dysphagia, dyspnea, epistaxis, erythema multiforme, erythematous rash, eye pain, female sexual disorder, flatulence, gingival hyperplasia, hot flash, hyperglycemia, hypersensitivity reaction, hypoesthesia,

increased thirst, insomnia, leukopenia, maculopapular rash, malaise, male sexual disorder, muscle cramps, myalgia, nervousness, nocturia, pain, pancreatitis, paresthesia, peripheral ischemia, peripheral neuropathy, pruritus, purpuric disease, rigors, skin rash, syncope, tachycardia, thrombocytopenia, tinnitus, tremor, urinary frequency, urination disorder, vasculitis, ventricular tachycardia, vertigo, visual disturbance, vomiting, weight gain, weight loss, xerostomia

Frequency not defined: Cardiovascular: Peripheral edema

Postmarketing: Extrapyramidal reaction, gynecomastia, increased liver enzymes, jaundice

Mechanism of Action Amlodipine is a 1:1 racemic mixture of levamlodipine and dextro amlodipine; it has been demonstrated that levamlodipine is the pharmacologically active, antihypertensive isomer. Amlodipine is a dihydropyridine calcium channel blocker that exerts its effect by blocking the transmembrane influx of calcium ions primarily into vascular smooth muscle cells and to a lesser extent into cardiac muscle cells. It reduces peripheral vascular resistance and lowers BP by acting directly on vascular smooth muscle.

Pharmacodynamics/Kinetics

Onset of Action Gradual.

Duration of Action ≥24 hours.

Half-life Elimination Terminal (biphasic): ~30 to 50 hours; increased with hepatic dysfunction.

Time to Peak 6 to 12 hours.

Pregnancy Considerations

Amlodipine is a racemic mixture of levamlodipine and dextro amlodipine; levamlodipine is the pharmacologically active isomer. Amlodipine crosses the placenta (Morgan 2017; Morgan 2018).

Refer to the amlodipine monograph for additional information,

Product Availability Conjupri: FDA approved December 2019; anticipated availability is currently undetermined.

◆ **Levamlodipine Maleate** *see* Levamlodipine *on page 893*

◆ **Levaquin [DSC]** *see* LevoFLOXacin (Systemic) *on page 898*

◆ **Levarterenol Bitartrate** *see* Norepinephrine *on page 1116*

◆ **Leva Set [DSC]** *see* Lidocaine and Prilocaine *on page 911*

◆ **Levatio** *see* Capsaicin *on page 284*

◆ **Levemir** *see* Insulin Detemir *on page 820*

◆ **Levemir FlexTouch** *see* Insulin Detemir *on page 820*

LevETIRAcetam (lee va tye RA se tam)

Brand Names: US Keppra; Keppra XR; Roweepra; Roweepra XR; Spritam

Brand Names: Canada ACT Levetiracetam; APO-Levetiracetam; Auro-Levetiracetam; BIO-Levetiracetam; DOM-Levetiracetam; JAMP-Levetiracetam; Keppra; NAT-Levetiracetam; PDP-Levetiracetam; PMS-Levetiracetam; Priva-Levetiracetam; PRO-Levetiracetam-250; PRO-Levetiracetam-500; PRO-Levetiracetam-750; RAN-Levetiracetam; RIVA-Levetiracetam; SANDOZ Levetiracetam; VAN-Levetiracetam [DSC]

Pharmacologic Category Anticonvulsant, Miscellaneous

Use

Focal (partial) onset:

IR tablets/oral solution: Treatment of focal (partial) onset seizures in adults, adolescents, children, and infants ≥1 month of age with epilepsy.

Tablets for oral suspension: Adjunctive therapy in the treatment of focal (partial) onset seizures in adults and children ≥4 years of age and >20 kg with epilepsy.

ER tablets: Treatment of focal (partial) onset seizures in adults and adolescents ≥12 years of age with epilepsy.

IV: Treatment of focal (partial) onset seizures in adults and children ≥1 month of age with epilepsy.

Limitation of use: IV use is only as an alternative when oral administration is temporarily not feasible.

Generalized onset:

Juvenile myoclonic epilepsy:

Immediate-release tablets/oral solution/tablets for oral suspension: Adjunctive therapy in the treatment of myoclonic seizures in adults and adolescents 12 years and older with juvenile myoclonic epilepsy.

IV: Adjunctive therapy in the treatment of myoclonic seizures in adults and adolescents 12 years and older with juvenile myoclonic epilepsy.

Primary generalized tonic-clonic seizures:

Immediate-release tablets/oral solution/tablets for oral suspension: Adjunctive therapy in the treatment of primary generalized tonic-clonic seizures in adults and children 6 years and older with idiopathic generalized epilepsy.

IV: Adjunctive therapy in the treatment of primary generalized tonic-clonic seizures in adults and children 6 years and older with idiopathic generalized epilepsy.

Local Anesthetic/Vasoconstrictor Precautions

No information available to require special precautions

Effects on Dental Treatment No significant effects or complications reported

Effects on Bleeding No information available to require special precautions

Adverse Reactions Incidences are for all indications and populations (adults and children) unless otherwise specified.

>10%:

Cardiovascular: Increased blood pressure (diastolic; infants and children: 17%)

Central nervous system: Behavioral problems (includes aggression, agitation, anger, anxiety, apathy, depersonalization, emotional lability, irritability, neurosis; children and adolescents: 7% to 38%; adults: 7% to 13%), headache (14% to 19%), psychotic symptoms (infants and children: 17%; adults: 1%), drowsiness (8% to 15%; immediate release 4 g/day, no titration: 45%; serious [patients hospitalized]: <1%), irritability (infants, children, and adolescents: 6% to 12%), fatigue (10% to 11%)

Gastrointestinal: Vomiting (children and adolescents: 15%)

Infection: Infection (13%)

Neuromuscular & skeletal: Weakness (15%)

Respiratory: Nasopharyngitis (7% to 15%)

1% to 10%:

Central nervous system: Aggressive behavior (children and adolescents: 10%; adults: 1%), dizziness (5% to 9%), pain (7%), lethargy (children and adolescents: 6%), insomnia (children and adolescents: 5%), depression (3% to 5%), vertigo (3% to 5%), emotional lability (2% to 5%), agitation (children and adolescents: 4%), nervousness (4%), ataxia (partial-onset seizures: 3%; includes abnormal gait, incoordination), falling (children and adolescents: 3%), mood changes (children and adolescents: 3%), confusion (2% to 3%), amnesia (2%), anxiety (2%), hostility (2%), paranoia (children and adolescents: 2%), paresthesia (2%), sedation (children and adolescents: 2%)

Gastrointestinal: Upper abdominal pain (children and adolescents: 9%), decreased appetite (children and adolescents: 8%), diarrhea (6% to 8%), nausea (5%), anorexia (3% to 4%), constipation (children and adolescents: 3%), gastroenteritis (children and adolescents: 2%)

Hematologic & oncologic: Eosinophilia (children and adolescents: 9%), bruise (children and adolescents: 3%), decreased white blood cell count (3%), decreased neutrophils (2%)

Infection: Influenza (3% to 8%)

Neuromuscular & skeletal: Neck pain (2% to 8%), arthralgia (children and adolescents: 2%), joint sprain (children and adolescents: 2%)

Ophthalmic: Conjunctivitis (children and adolescents: 2%), diplopia (2%)

Otic: Otalgia (children and adolescents: 2%)

Respiratory: Nasal congestion (children and adolescents: 9%), cough (2% to 9%), pharyngolaryngeal pain (children and adolescents: 7%), pharyngitis (6% to 7%), rhinitis (2% to 4%), sinusitis (2%)

Miscellaneous: Head trauma (children and adolescents: 4%)

<1%, postmarketing and/or case reports: Abnormal hepatic function tests, acute renal failure, agranulocytosis, alopecia, anaphylaxis, angioedema, blurred vision, choreoathetosis, decreased hematocrit, decreased hemoglobin, decreased red blood cells, disturbance in attention, DRESS syndrome, dyskinesia, eczema, equilibrium disturbance, erythema multiforme, granulomatous interstitial nephritis (Chau 2012), hepatic failure, hepatitis, hyperkinesia, hyponatremia, leukopenia, memory impairment, myalgia, myasthenia, neutropenia, pancreatitis, pancytopenia (with bone marrow suppression in some cases), panic attack, personality disorder, pruritus, psychosis, skin rash, Stevens-Johnson syndrome, suicidal ideation, suicidal tendencies, thrombocytopenia, toxic epidermal necrolysis, weight loss

Mechanism of Action The precise mechanism by which levetiracetam exerts its antiepileptic effect is unknown. However, several studies have suggested the mechanism may involve one or more of the following central pharmacologic effects: inhibition of voltage-dependent N-type calcium channels; facilitation of GABA-ergic inhibitory transmission through displacement of negative modulators; reduction of delayed rectifier potassium current; and/or binding to synaptic proteins which modulate neurotransmitter release.

Pharmacodynamics/Kinetics

Onset of Action Peak effect: Oral: 1 hour

Half-life Elimination Increased in patients with renal impairment

Infants and Children <4 years: 5.3 ± 1.3 hours (Glauser 2007)

Children 4 to 12 years: 6 ± 1.1 hours (Pellock 2001)

Adults: ~6 to 8 hours; extended release tablet: ~7 hours

Time to Peak

IV: 5 to 30 minutes (Ramael 2006).

Oral solution: Fasting infants and children <4 years of age: 1.4 ± 0.9 hours.

Oral: Immediate release: Fasting adults and children: ~1 hour.

Oral: Extended release: ~4 hours; median time to peak is 2 hours longer in the fed state.

Pregnancy Considerations

Levetiracetam crosses the placenta and can be detected in the newborn following delivery (Johannessen 2005; López-Fraile 2009; Tomson 2007). An increase in the overall rate of major congenital malformations has not been observed following maternal use of levetiracetam. Available studies have not been large enough to determine if there is an increased risk of specific birth defects (Hernández-Díaz 2012; Mawhinney 2013; Mølgaard-Nielsen 2011; Vajda 2012). In general, maternal polytherapy with antiepileptic drugs may increase the risk of congenital malformations; monotherapy with the lowest effective dose is recommended. Newborns of women taking antiepileptic medications may be at an increased risk of SGA and a 1 minute APGAR score <7 (Harden 2009).

Due to pregnancy-induced physiologic changes, plasma concentrations of levetiracetam gradually decrease during pregnancy, especially during the third trimester; patients should be closely monitored during pregnancy and postpartum.

A registry is available for women exposed to levetiracetam during pregnancy: Pregnant women may enroll themselves into the North American Antiepileptic Drug (AED) Pregnancy Registry (888-233-2334 or http://www.aedpregnancyregistry.org/).

Product Availability Elepsia XR: FDA approved December 2018; anticipated availability is currently unknown. Information pertaining to this product within the monograph is pending revision. Consult the prescribing information for additional information.

◆ **LevigoSP [OTC]** *see* Lidocaine (Topical) *on page 902*

◆ **Levitra** *see* Vardenafil *on page 1532*

◆ **Levlen** *see* Ethinyl Estradiol and Levonorgestrel *on page 612*

◆ **Levocabastine Hydrochloride** *see* Levocabastine (Nasal) *on page 895*

Levocabastine (Nasal) (LEE voe kab as teen)

Brand Names: Canada Livostin

Pharmacologic Category Histamine H_1 Antagonist; Histamine H_1 Antagonist, Second Generation; Piperidine Derivative

Use Note: Not approved in the US

Allergic rhinitis: Symptomatic treatment of allergic rhinitis in patients 12 years and older.

Local Anesthetic/Vasoconstrictor Precautions

No information available to require special precautions

Effects on Dental Treatment Key adverse event(s) related to dental treatment: Xerostomia (normal salivary flow resumes upon discontinuation)

Effects on Bleeding No information available to require special precautions

Adverse Reactions Most adverse reactions are transient. Frequency not always defined.

1% to 10%:

Central nervous system: Fatigue (1%)

Local: Application site burning, application site irritation, application site pain, application site reaction (dryness, discomfort)

Ophthalmic: Eye irritation (3%; mostly with concomitant levocabastine eye drop administration)

Respiratory: Epistaxis (1%), pharyngolaryngeal pain, sinusitis

<1%, postmarketing, and/or case reports: Abdominal pain, anaphylaxis, application site reactions (nasal edema), bronchospasm, cough, dry nose, dysgeusia, dyspnea, eyelid edema, facial edema, hearing loss, hypersensitivity, increased appetite, malaise, nasal congestion, nasal obstruction (aggravated), nausea, palpitations, pruritus of ear (external), pruritus of nose, respiratory tract disease, rhinorrhea, skin rash, tachycardia, throat irritation, weight gain

Mechanism of Action Potent, selective histamine H_1-receptor antagonist

Pharmacodynamics/Kinetics

Onset of Action 10 minutes

Half-life Elimination 35 to 40 hours

Time to Peak 3 hours

Pregnancy Considerations Adverse events were observed in some animal reproduction studies when using oral doses much larger than the equivalent maximum human nasal dose.

Product Availability Not available in the US

LevOCARNitine (lee voe KAR ni teen)

Brand Names: US Carnitor; Carnitor SF; G-levOCARNitine S/F [OTC]; McCarnitine [OTC] [DSC]

Brand Names: Canada Carnitor; ODAN Levocarnitine

Pharmacologic Category Dietary Supplement

Use

Carnitine deficiency in patients with end-stage renal disease requiring hemodialysis (injection only): Prevention and treatment of carnitine deficiency in patients with end-stage renal disease (ESRD) who are undergoing dialysis.

Dietary supplement (OTC only): As a levocarnitine dietary supplement.

Primary systemic carnitine deficiency (oral [Rx] only): Treatment of primary systemic carnitine deficiency.

Secondary carnitine deficiency (oral [Rx] and injection): Acute and chronic treatment of patients with an inborn error of metabolism which results in a secondary carnitine deficiency.

Local Anesthetic/Vasoconstrictor Precautions No information available to require special precautions

Effects on Dental Treatment Key adverse event(s) related to dental treatment: Taste perversion.

Effects on Bleeding No information available to require special precautions

Adverse Reactions Frequencies noted with hemodialysis patients.

>10%:

Cardiovascular: Hypertension (intravenous: 18% to 21%), chest pain (intravenous: 15%)

Central nervous system: Headache (intravenous: 37%), dizziness (intravenous: 15% to 18%), paresthesia (intravenous: 12%)

Endocrine & metabolic: Hypercalcemia (intravenous: 6% to 15%)

Gastrointestinal: Diarrhea (intravenous: 35%), abdominal pain (intravenous: 21%), vomiting (intravenous: 21%), nausea (intravenous: 12%)

Hematologic & oncologic: Anemia (intravenous: 5% to 12%)

Infection: Infection (intravenous: 24%)

Neuromuscular & skeletal: Weakness (intravenous: 9% to 12%)

Respiratory: Cough (intravenous: 18%), rhinitis (intravenous: 11%)

Miscellaneous: Accidental injury (intravenous: 12%), fever (intravenous: 6% to 12%)

1% to 10%:

Cardiovascular: Tachycardia (intravenous: 6% to 9%), palpitations (intravenous: 3% to 8%), vascular disease (intravenous: 6%), peripheral edema (intravenous: 5% to 6%), ECG abnormality (intravenous: 3% to 6%), atrial fibrillation (intravenous: 2% to 6%)

Central nervous system: Drug dependence (intravenous: 6%), vertigo (intravenous: 6%), depression (intravenous: 5% to 6%)

Dermatologic: Skin rash (intravenous: 5%)

Endocrine & metabolic: Weight loss (intravenous: 8%), parathyroid disorder (intravenous: 6%), weight gain (intravenous: 3% to 6%)

Gastrointestinal: Dysgeusia (intravenous: 2% to 9%), melena (intravenous: 6%), anorexia (intravenous: 5% to 6%), gastrointestinal disorder (intravenous: 3% to 6%)

Hematologic & oncologic: Hemorrhage (intravenous: 9%)

Hypersensitivity: Hypersensitivity reaction (intravenous: 6%)

Ophthalmic: Amblyopia (intravenous: 6%), eye disease (intravenous: 3% to 6%)

Renal: Renal failure (intravenous: 6%)

Respiratory: Bronchitis (intravenous: 3% to 5%)

Frequency not defined:

Gastrointestinal: Gastritis (intravenous)

Miscellaneous: Body odor

<1%, postmarketing, and/or case reports: Abdominal cramps, anaphylaxis, bronchospasm, facial edema, laryngeal edema, myasthenia (uremic patients), seizure, urticaria

Mechanism of Action Carnitine is a naturally occurring metabolic compound which functions as a carrier molecule for long-chain fatty acids within the mitochondria, facilitating energy production. Carnitine deficiency is associated with accumulation of excess acyl CoA esters and disruption of intermediary metabolism.

Pharmacodynamics/Kinetics

Half-life Elimination 17.4 hours

Time to Peak Oral: 3.3 hours

Pregnancy Considerations Teratogenic effects were not observed in animal studies. Carnitine is a naturally occurring substance in mammalian metabolism.

◆ **Levocarnitine Tartrate** *see* LevOCARNitine *on page 896*

Levocetirizine (LEE vo se TI ra zeen)

Brand Names: US Xyzal Allergy 24HR Childrens [OTC]; Xyzal Allergy 24HR [OTC]; Xyzal [DSC]

Pharmacologic Category Histamine H_1 Antagonist; Histamine H_1 Antagonist, Second Generation; Piperazine Derivative

Use

Chronic idiopathic urticaria: Treatment of uncomplicated skin manifestations of chronic idiopathic urticaria in adults and pediatric patients 6 months and older

Perennial allergic rhinitis: Relief of symptoms associated with perennial allergic rhinitis in adults and pediatric patients 6 months to 2 years

Allergic rhinitis (OTC only): Temporary relief of symptoms due to hay fever or other respiratory allergies (including rhinitis, sneezing, itchy/watery eyes, or itching of the throat/nose) in adults and pediatric patients 2 years and older

Local Anesthetic/Vasoconstrictor Precautions No information available to require special precautions

Effects on Dental Treatment Key adverse event(s) related to dental treatment: Xerostomia and changes in salivation (normal salivary flow resumes upon discontinuation).

Effects on Bleeding No information available to require special precautions

Adverse Reactions

>10%: Gastrointestinal: Diarrhea (infants: 13%; children: 4%)

1% to 10%:

- Central nervous system: Drowsiness (3% to 6%), fatigue (adolescents and adults: 4%)
- Gastrointestinal: Constipation (infants: 7%), vomiting (4%), xerostomia (adolescents and adults: 2% to 3%)
- Otic: Otitis media (children: 3%)
- Respiratory: Nasopharyngitis (adolescents and adults: 4% to 6%), cough (children: 3%), epistaxis (children: 2%), pharyngitis (adolescents and adults: 2%)
- Miscellaneous: Fever (children: 4%)

Frequency not defined: Neuromuscular & skeletal: Weakness

<1%, postmarketing, and/or case reports: Aggressive behavior, agitation, anaphylaxis, angioedema, arthralgia, blurred vision, depression, dizziness, dysgeusia, dyspnea, dysuria, edema, febrile seizures, fixed drug eruption, hallucination, hepatitis, hypersensitivity reaction, increased appetite, increased serum bilirubin, increased serum transaminases, insomnia, movement disorder (including dystonia and oculogyric crisis), myalgia, nausea, nightmares, palpitations, paresthesia, pruritus, seizure, skin rash, suicidal ideation, syncope, tachycardia, tremor, urinary retention, urticaria, vertigo, visual disturbances, weight gain

Mechanism of Action Levocetirizine is an antihistamine which selectively competes with histamine for H_1-receptor sites on effector cells in the gastrointestinal tract, blood vessels, and respiratory tract. Levocetirizine, the active enantiomer of cetirizine, has twice the binding affinity at the H_1-receptor compared to cetirizine.

Pharmacodynamics/Kinetics

Onset of Action 1 hour (Devillier 2008)

Duration of Action 24 hours (Devillier 2008)

Half-life Elimination Children 1 to 2 years: Oral solution: 4.09 ± 0.67 hours (Cranswick 2005); Children 6 to 11 years: Oral tablet: 5.7 ± 0.2 hours (Simons 2005); Adults: ~8 to 9 hours

Time to Peak Children 1 to 2 years: Oral solution: Median: 1 hour (range: 1 to 6 hours) (Cranswick 2005); Children 6 to 11 years: Oral tablet: 1.2 ± 0.2 hours (Simons 2005); Adults: Oral solution: 0.5 hours; Tablet: 0.9 hours

Pregnancy Considerations

Guidelines for the use of antihistamines in the treatment of allergic rhinitis or urticaria in pregnancy are generally the same as in nonpregnant females. Second generation antihistamines may be used for the treatment of allergic rhinitis and urticaria during pregnancy; however, information related to the use of levocetirizine in pregnancy is limited and other medications may be preferred (Wallace 2008; Zuberbier 2018).

Levocetirizine is the active enantiomer of cetirizine.

◆ **Levocetirizine Dihydrochloride** *see* Levocetirizine *on page 896*

◆ **Levodopa and Carbidopa** *see* Carbidopa and Levodopa *on page 290*

Levodopa, Carbidopa, and Entacapone

(lee voe DOE pa, kar bi DOE pa, & en TA ka pone)

Related Information

Carbidopa *on page 289*

Entacapone *on page 567*

Brand Names: US Stalevo

Brand Names: Canada Stalevo

Pharmacologic Category Anti-Parkinson Agent, COMT Inhibitor; Anti-Parkinson Agent, Decarboxylase Inhibitor; Anti-Parkinson Agent, Dopamine Precursor

Use Parkinson disease: Treatment of Parkinson disease.

Local Anesthetic/Vasoconstrictor Precautions No information available to require special precautions

Effects on Dental Treatment No significant effects or complications reported

Effects on Bleeding No information available to require special precautions

Adverse Reactions See individual agents.

Mechanism of Action

Levodopa: The metabolic precursor of dopamine, a chemical depleted in Parkinson's disease. Levodopa is able to circulate in the plasma and cross the blood-brain-barrier (BBB), where it is converted by striatal enzymes to dopamine.

Carbidopa: Inhibits the peripheral plasma breakdown of levodopa by inhibiting its decarboxylation; increases available levodopa at the BBB

Entacapone: A reversible and selective inhibitor of catechol-O-methyltransferase (COMT). Alters the pharmacokinetics of levodopa, resulting in more sustained levodopa serum levels and increased concentrations available for absorption across the BBB.

Pharmacodynamics/Kinetics

Half-life Elimination Levodopa: 1.7 hours (range: 1.1 to 3.2 hours); Carbidopa: 1.6 to 2 hours (range ~1 to 4 hours); Entacapone: ~1 hour (range: 0.3 to 4.5 hours)

Time to Peak Levodopa: ~1 to 2 hours; Carbidopa: 2.5 to 3.4 hours; Entacapone: ~1 hour

Pregnancy Considerations

The incidence of Parkinson disease in pregnancy is relatively rare and information related to the use of carbidopa/levodopa/entacapone in pregnant women is limited (Seier 2017; Tüfekçioglu 2018).

Refer to the entacapone and the carbidopa/levodopa monographs for additional information.

LevoFLOXacin (Systemic)

(lee voe FLOKS a sin)

Related Information

Clinical Risk Related to Drugs Prolonging QT Interval *on page 1675*

Gastrointestinal Disorders *on page 1678*

Brand Names: US Levaquin [DSC]

Brand Names: Canada ACT Levofloxacin; APO-Levofloxacin; Auro-Levofloxacin; MYLAN-Levofloxacin [DSC]; PMS-Levofloxacin; RIVA-Levofloxacin; SANDOZ Levofloxacin; TEVA-Levofloxacin [DSC]

Pharmacologic Category Antibiotic, Fluoroquinolone; Antibiotic, Respiratory Fluoroquinolone

Use

Treatment of community-acquired pneumonia, including multidrug-resistant strains of *Streptococcus pneumoniae* (MDRSP); nosocomial pneumonia; chronic obstructive pulmonary disease, acute exacerbation; rhinosinusitis, acute bacterial (ABRS); prostatitis (chronic bacterial); urinary tract infection (uncomplicated or complicated); acute pyelonephritis; skin or skin structure infections (uncomplicated or complicated); inhalational anthrax (postexposure) to reduce incidence or disease progression; prophylaxis and treatment of plague (pneumonic and septicemic) due to *Yersinia pestis*

Limitations of use: Because fluoroquinolones have been associated with disabling and potentially irreversible serious adverse reactions (eg, tendinitis and tendon rupture, peripheral neuropathy, CNS effects), reserve levofloxacin for use in patients who have no alternative treatment options for acute exacerbation of chronic bronchitis, acute bacterial sinusitis, and uncomplicated urinary tract infections.

Local Anesthetic/Vasoconstrictor Precautions Levofloxacin is one of the drugs confirmed to prolong the QT interval and is accepted as having a risk of causing torsade de pointes. The risk of drug-induced torsade de pointes is extremely low when a single QT interval prolonging drug is prescribed. In terms of epinephrine, it is not known what effect vasoconstrictors in the local anesthetic regimen will have in patients with a known history of congenital prolonged QT interval or in patients taking any medication that prolongs the QT interval. Until more information is obtained, it is suggested that the clinician consult with the physician prior to the use of a vasoconstrictor in suspected patients, and that the vasoconstrictor (epinephrine, mepivacaine and levonordefrin [Carbocaine® 2% with Neo-Cobefrin®]) be used with caution.

Effects on Dental Treatment No significant effects or complications reported

Effects on Bleeding No information available to require special precautions

Adverse Reactions

1% to 10%:

Cardiovascular: Chest pain (1%), edema (1%)

Dermatologic: Pruritus (1%), skin rash (2%)

Gastrointestinal: Abdominal pain (2%), constipation (3%), diarrhea (5%), dyspepsia (2%), nausea (7%), vomiting (2%)

Genitourinary: Vaginitis (1%)

Infection: Candidiasis (1%)

Local: Injection site reaction (1%)

Nervous system: Dizziness (3%), headache (6%), insomnia (4%)

Respiratory: Dyspnea (1%)

<1%:

Cardiovascular: Palpitations, phlebitis, syncope, ventricular arrhythmia, ventricular tachycardia

Dermatologic: Urticaria

Endocrine & metabolic: Hyperglycemia, hyperkalemia, hypoglycemia

Gastrointestinal: Anorexia, *Clostridioides difficile* colitis, esophagitis, gastritis, gastroenteritis, glossitis, pancreatitis, stomatitis

Genitourinary: Genital candidiasis

Hematologic & oncologic: Anemia, granulocytopenia, thrombocytopenia (Sim 2018)

Hepatic: Hepatic insufficiency, increased liver enzymes, increased serum alkaline phosphatase

Hypersensitivity: Hypersensitivity reaction

Nervous system: Abnormal dreams, abnormal gait, agitation, anxiety, confusion, depression, drowsiness, hallucination, hypertonia, nightmares, paresthesia, seizure, sleep disorder, vertigo

Neuromuscular & skeletal: Arthralgia, hyperkinetic muscle activity, myalgia, skeletal pain, tendonitis, tremor

Renal: Acute renal failure, renal function abnormality

Respiratory: Epistaxis

Postmarketing:

Cardiovascular: Cardiac arrhythmia, hypersensitivity angiitis, hypotension, prolonged QT interval on ECG, tachycardia, torsades de pointes, vasodilation

Dermatologic: Acute generalized exanthematous pustulosis, dermatologic disorder, erythema multiforme, phototoxicity, skin photosensitivity, Stevens-Johnson syndrome, toxic epidermal necrolysis

Gastrointestinal: Ageusia, *Clostridioides difficile* associated diarrhea, dysgeusia

Genitourinary: Casts in urine, crystalluria

Hematologic & oncologic: Agranulocytosis, aplastic anemia, eosinophilia, hemolytic anemia, increased INR, leukopenia, pancytopenia, prolonged prothrombin time, thrombotic thrombocytopenic purpura

Hepatic: Hepatic failure, hepatitis, hepatotoxicity (idiosyncratic) (Chalasani 2014; Gulen 2015; Schloss 2018)

Hypersensitivity: Anaphylactic shock, anaphylaxis, angioedema, fixed drug eruption, jaundice, nonimmune anaphylaxis, serum sickness

Immunologic: Drug reaction with eosinophilia and systemic symptoms (Charfi 2015)

Nervous system: Abnormal electroencephalogram, altered sense of smell, anosmia, delirium, disorientation, disturbance in attention, encephalopathy (rare), exacerbation of myasthenia gravis, idiopathic intracranial hypertension, increased intracranial pressure, memory impairment, nervousness, paranoid ideation, peripheral neuropathy (may be irreversible), psychosis, restlessness, suicidal ideation, suicidal tendencies, toxic psychosis, voice disorder

Neuromuscular & skeletal: Elevation in serum levels of skeletal-muscle enzymes, muscle injury, muscular paralysis (musculospiral) (Pan 2017), rhabdomyolysis, rupture of tendon

Ophthalmic: Blurred vision, decreased visual acuity, diplopia, scotoma, uveitis, visual disturbance

Otic: Hypoacusis, tinnitus

Renal: Interstitial nephritis

Respiratory: Bronchospasm, hypersensitivity pneumonitis

Miscellaneous: Fever, multi-organ failure

Mechanism of Action As the S(-) enantiomer of the fluoroquinolone, ofloxacin, levofloxacin, inhibits DNA-gyrase in susceptible organisms thereby inhibits relaxation of supercoiled DNA and promotes breakage of DNA strands. DNA gyrase (topoisomerase II), is an essential bacterial enzyme that maintains the superhelical structure of DNA and is required for DNA replication and transcription, DNA repair, recombination, and transposition.

Pharmacodynamics/Kinetics

Half-life Elimination

Infants ≥6 months and Children ≤5 years: ~4 hours (Chien 2005)

Children 5 to 10 years: 4.8 hours (Chien 2005)

Children 10 to 12 years: 5.4 hours (Chien 2005)

Children 12 to 16 years: 6 hours (Chien 2005)

Adults: ~6 to 8 hours

Adults, renal impairment: 27 ± 10 hours (CrCl 20 to 49 mL/minute); 35 ± 5 hours (CrCl <20 mL/minute)

Time to Peak 1 to 2 hours

Pregnancy Considerations Levofloxacin crosses the placenta and can be detected in the amniotic fluid and cord blood (Ozyüncü 2010a; Ozyüncü 2010b). Information specific to levofloxacin use during pregnancy is limited (Padberg 2014).

Dental Health Professional Considerations See Local Anesthetic/Vasoconstrictor Precautions

- **Levo-folinic Acid** *see* LEVOleucovorin *on page 899*

LEVOleucovorin (lee voe loo koe VOR in)

Brand Names: US Fusilev [DSC]; Khapzory

Pharmacologic Category Antidote; Chemotherapy Modulating Agent; Rescue Agent (Chemotherapy)

Use

Colorectal cancer, metastatic: Treatment of adults with advanced, metastatic colorectal cancer (in combination with fluorouracil).

Folic acid antagonist overdose: Antidote to diminish toxicity associated with overdosage of folic acid antagonists in adult and pediatric patients.

High-dose methotrexate rescue: Rescue agent after high-dose methotrexate therapy in adult and pediatric patients with osteosarcoma.

Impaired methotrexate elimination: Antidote to diminish toxicity associated with impaired methotrexate elimination in adult and pediatric patients.

Limitations of use: Levoleucovorin is not indicated for pernicious anemia or megaloblastic anemias secondary to the lack of vitamin B_{12} (due to the risk of progressive neurologic manifestations despite hematologic remission).

Local Anesthetic/Vasoconstrictor Precautions No information available to require special precautions

Effects on Dental Treatment Key adverse event(s) related to dental treatment: Stomatitis and taste perversion.

Effects on Bleeding No information available to require special precautions

Adverse Reactions Adverse reactions reported with levoleucovorin either as a part of combination chemotherapy or following chemotherapy.

>10%:

Dermatologic: Dermatitis (6% to 29%), alopecia (26%)

Gastrointestinal: Stomatitis (38% to 72%; grades ≥3: 6% to 12%), diarrhea (6% to 70%), nausea (19% to 62%), vomiting (38% to 40%), anorexia (≤24%), decreased appetite (≤24%), abdominal pain (14%)

Nervous system: Fatigue (≤29%), malaise (≤29%)

Neuromuscular & skeletal: Asthenia (≤29%)

1% to 10%:

Gastrointestinal: Dysgeusia (6%), dyspepsia (6%), neutropenic typhlitis (6%)

Nervous system: Confusion (6%), neuropathy (6%)

Renal: Renal insufficiency (6%)

Respiratory: Dyspnea (6%)

<1%, postmarketing, and/or case reports: Disruption of body temperature regulation, hypersensitivity reaction, pruritus, rigors, skin rash

Mechanism of Action Levoleucovorin counteracts the toxic (and therapeutic) effects of folic acid antagonists (eg, methotrexate) which act by inhibiting dihydrofolate reductase. Levoleucovorin is the levo isomeric and pharmacologic active form of leucovorin (levoleucovorin does not require reduction by dihydrofolate reductase). A reduced derivative of folic acid, leucovorin supplies the necessary cofactor blocked by methotrexate.

Leucovorin enhances the activity (and toxicity) of fluorouracil by stabilizing the binding of 5-fluoro-2'-deoxyuridine-5'-monophosphate (FdUMP; a fluorouracil metabolite) to thymidylate synthetase resulting in inhibition of this enzyme.

Pharmacodynamics/Kinetics

Half-life Elimination Total-tetrahydrofolate: 5.1 hours; (6)-5-methyl-5,6,7,8-tetrahydrofolate: 6.8 hours

Time to Peak Serum: IV (healthy volunteers; 15 mg dose): 0.9 hours

Pregnancy Considerations

Information related to levoleucovorin use in pregnancy is limited. Levoleucovorin is administered in combination with either methotrexate or fluorouracil; also refer to the Methotrexate or Fluorouracil monographs for additional information.

- **Levo-leucovorin** *see* LEVOleucovorin *on page 899*
- **Levoleucovorin Calcium Pentahydrate** *see* LEVOleucovorin *on page 899*
- **Levomefolate Calcium, Drospirenone, and Ethinyl Estradiol** *see* Ethinyl Estradiol, Drospirenone, and Levomefolate *on page 618*
- **Levomefolate, Drospirenone, and Ethinyl Estradiol** *see* Ethinyl Estradiol, Drospirenone, and Levomefolate *on page 618*
- **Levomepromazine** *see* Methotrimeprazine *on page 992*

Levomilnacipran (lee voe mil NA si pran)

Brand Names: US Fetzima; Fetzima Titration

Brand Names: Canada Fetzima

Pharmacologic Category Antidepressant, Serotonin/ Norepinephrine Reuptake Inhibitor

Use Major depressive disorder: Treatment of major depressive disorder (MDD)

Local Anesthetic/Vasoconstrictor Precautions

Although levomilnacipran is not a tricyclic antidepressant, it blocks norepinephrine reuptake within the CNS synapses as part of the mechanism of action. It has been suggested that vasoconstrictors be administered with caution and vital signs monitored in dental patients taking antidepressants that affect norepinephrine in this way.

Effects on Dental Treatment Key adverse events(s) related to dental treatment: Bruxism (<2%) has been reported; Patients may experience orthostatic hypotension (6% to 12%) as they stand up after treatment; especially if lying in dental chair for extended periods of time. Use caution with sudden changes in position during and after dental treatment.

Effects on Bleeding Serotonin/norepinephrine reuptake inhibitors (SNRIs) may impair platelet aggregation resulting in increased risk of bleeding events, particularly if used concomitantly with aspirin or NSAIDs.

Adverse Reactions

>10%:

Cardiovascular: Orthostatic hypotension (6% to 12%; dose related)

Gastrointestinal: Nausea (17%)

1% to 10%:

Cardiovascular: Increased heart rate (6%), tachycardia (6%), palpitations (5%), hypertension (3%), hypotension (3%), increased blood pressure (3%), angina pectoris (<2%), chest pain (<2%), supraventricular extrasystole (<2%), syncope (<2%), ventricular premature contractions (<2%)

Central nervous system: Aggressive behavior (<2%), agitation (<2%), extrapyramidal reaction (<2%), migraine (<2%), outbursts of anger (<2%), panic attack (<2%), paresthesia (<2%), tension (<2%), yawning (<2%)

Dermatologic: Hyperhidrosis (9%), skin rash (2%), pruritus (<2%), urticaria (<2%), xeroderma (<2%)

Endocrine & metabolic: Hot flash (3%), hypercholesterolemia (<2%), increased thirst (<2%)

Gastrointestinal: Constipation (9%), vomiting (5%), decreased appetite (3%), abdominal pain (<2%), bruxism (<2%), flatulence (<2%)

Genitourinary: Erectile dysfunction (6% to 10%; dose related), urinary hesitancy (4% to 6%; dose related), ejaculatory disorder (5%), testicular pain (4%), hematuria (<2%), pollakiuria (<2%), proteinuria (<2%)

Hepatic: Abnormal hepatic function tests (<2%)

Ophthalmic: Blurred vision (<2%), conjunctival hemorrhage (<2%), dry eye syndrome (<2%)

<1%, postmarketing, and/or case reports: Angle-closure glaucoma, cardiomyopathy (takotsubo), hemorrhagic diathesis, mydriasis, seizure

Mechanism of Action Levomilnacipran, the more active enantiomer of milnacipran, is a potent inhibitor of norepinephrine and serotonin reuptake (Montgomery, 2013).

Pharmacodynamics/Kinetics

Onset of Action Depression: Initial effects may be observed within 1 to 2 weeks of treatment, with continued improvements through 4 to 6 weeks (Papakostas 2006; Posternak 2005; Szegedi 2009).

Half-life Elimination 12 hours

Time to Peak 6 to 8 hours

Pregnancy Risk Factor C

Pregnancy Considerations

Nonteratogenic effects in the newborn following SSRI/SNRI exposure late in the third trimester include respiratory distress, cyanosis, apnea, seizures, temperature instability, feeding difficulty, vomiting, hypoglycemia, hypo- or hypertonia, hyper-reflexia, jitteriness, irritability, constant crying, and tremor. Symptoms may be due to the toxicity of the SSRIs/SNRIs or a discontinuation syndrome and may be consistent with serotonin syndrome associated with SSRI treatment.

Women treated for major depression and who are euthymic prior to pregnancy are more likely to experience a relapse when medication is discontinued as compared to pregnant women who continue taking antidepressant medications (Cohen 2006). The ACOG recommends that therapy with SSRIs or SNRIs during pregnancy be individualized; treatment of depression during pregnancy should incorporate the clinical expertise of the mental health clinician, obstetrician, primary health care provider, and pediatrician. According to the American Psychiatric Association (APA), the risks of medication treatment should be weighed against other treatment options and untreated depression. For women who discontinue antidepressant medications during pregnancy and who may be at high risk for postpartum depression, the medications can be restarted following delivery. Treatment algorithms have been developed by the ACOG and the APA for the management of depression in women prior to conception and during pregnancy (ACOG 2008; APA 2010; Yonkers 2009).

Pregnant women exposed to antidepressants during pregnancy are encouraged to enroll in the National Pregnancy Registry for Antidepressants (NPRAD). Women 18 to 45 years of age or their health care providers may contact the registry by calling 844-405-6185. Enrollment should be done as early in pregnancy as possible.

- ◆ **Levonest** *see* Ethinyl Estradiol and Levonorgestrel *on page 612*
- ◆ **Levonordefrin and Mepivacaine Hydrochloride** *see* Mepivacaine and Levonordefrin *on page 975*
- ◆ **Levonorgestrel and Estradiol** *see* Estradiol and Levonorgestrel *on page 598*
- ◆ **Levonorgestrel and Ethinyl Estradiol** *see* Ethinyl Estradiol and Levonorgestrel *on page 612*
- ◆ **Levophed** *see* Norepinephrine *on page 1116*
- ◆ **Levora 0.15/30 (28)** *see* Ethinyl Estradiol and Levonorgestrel *on page 612*
- ◆ **Levosalbutamol** *see* Levalbuterol *on page 892*
- ◆ **Levothroid** *see* Levothyroxine *on page 900*

Levothyroxine (lee voe thye ROKS een)

Related Information

Endocrine Disorders and Pregnancy *on page 1684*

Brand Names: US Euthyrox; Levoxyl; Synthroid; Tirosint; Tirosint-SOL; Unithroid; Unithroid Direct [DSC]

Brand Names: Canada Eltroxin; Euthyrox; Soloxine [DSC]; Synthroid

Pharmacologic Category Thyroid Product

Use

Oral:

Hypothyroidism: Replacement or supplemental therapy in congenital or acquired hypothyroidism of any etiology. Specific indications include primary (thyroidal), secondary (pituitary), and tertiary (hypothalamic) hypothyroidism. **Note:** Levothyroxine monotherapy is recommended as the preferred thyroid preparation for the treatment of hypothyroidism (ATA [Jonklaas 2014]; ES [Fleseriu 2016]).

Pituitary thyrotropin-stimulating hormone suppression: An adjunct to surgery and radioiodine therapy in the management of thyrotropin-dependent well-differentiated thyroid cancer.

Injectable: Treatment of myxedema coma

Local Anesthetic/Vasoconstrictor Precautions No precautions with vasoconstrictor are necessary if patient is well controlled with levothyroxine

Effects on Dental Treatment No significant effects or complications reported

Effects on Bleeding No information available to require special precautions

Adverse Reactions

Adverse reactions are primarily those of hyperthyroidism due to therapeutic overdosage.

Frequency not defined:

Cardiovascular: Angina pectoris, cardiac arrhythmia, cardiac failure, flushing, increased blood pressure, increased pulse, myocardial infarction, palpitations, tachycardia

Central nervous system: Anxiety, emotional lability, fatigue, headache, heat intolerance, hyperactivity, insomnia, irritability, myasthenia, nervousness, pseudotumor cerebri (children)

Dermatologic: Alopecia, diaphoresis, skin rash

Endocrine & metabolic: Goiter (exophthalmic; IV), menstrual disease, weight loss

Gastrointestinal: Abdominal cramps, diarrhea, increased appetite, vomiting

Genitourinary: Reduced fertility

Hepatic: Increased liver enzymes

Neuromuscular & skeletal: Decreased bone mineral density, muscle spasm, slipped capital femoral epiphysis (children), tremor

Respiratory: Dyspnea

Miscellaneous: Fever

<1%, postmarketing, and/or case reports: Dysgeusia (Syed 2016), seizure

Mechanism of Action Levothyroxine (T_4) is a synthetic form of thyroxine, an endogenous hormone secreted by the thyroid gland. T_4 is converted to its active metabolite, L-triiodothyronine (T_3). Thyroid hormones (T_4 and T_3) then bind to thyroid receptor proteins in the cell nucleus and exert metabolic effects through control of DNA transcription and protein synthesis; involved in normal metabolism, growth, and development; promotes gluconeogenesis, increases utilization and mobilization of glycogen stores, and stimulates protein synthesis, increases basal metabolic rate

Pharmacodynamics/Kinetics

Onset of Action Oral: 3 to 5 days; peak therapeutic effect may require 4 to 6 weeks; IV: Within 6 to 8 hours

Half-life Elimination Euthyroid: 6 to 7 days; Hypothyroid: 9 to 10 days; Hyperthyroid: 3 to 4 days

Time to Peak Serum: 2 to 4 hours

Reproductive Considerations Overt hypothyroidism increases the risk of irregular menses and infertility; treatment with levothyroxine is recommended to normalize thyroid function in infertile females with overt hypothyroidism who desire pregnancy. Levothyroxine may also be used in infertile females with subclinical hypothyroidism using assisted reproductive techniques (ATA [Alexander 2017]).

Pregnancy Considerations

Levothyroxine has not been shown to increase the risk of congenital abnormalities or miscarriage. Maternal hypothyroidism, however, can be associated with adverse effects in the mother and fetus, including spontaneous abortion, stillbirth, premature birth, low birth weight, impaired neurocognitive development in the offspring, abruptio placentae, gestational hypertension, and preeclampsia (ACOG 148 2015; ATA [Alexander 2017]).

Thyroid replacement therapy minimizes the risk of adverse pregnancy outcomes in females with overt hypothyroidism and treatment is recommended during pregnancy (ACOG 148 2015; ATA [Alexander 2017]). Levothyroxine is the preferred treatment of maternal hypothyroidism; other agents should not be used in pregnant females (ACOG 148 2015; ATA [Alexander 2017]; ES [De Groot 2012]). Levothyroxine is also recommended in some cases of subclinical hypothyroidism during pregnancy, and overt hypothyroidism in females with postpartum thyroiditis (ACOG 148 2015; ATA [Alexander 2017]; ES [De Groot 2012]).

Due to alterations of endogenous maternal thyroid hormones, hypothyroid patients treated with levothyroxine prior to pregnancy require a dose increase as soon as pregnancy is confirmed (ATA [Alexander 2017]; ES [De Groot 2012]). Close monitoring of pregnant patients is recommended (ATA [Alexander 2017]).

- **Levothyroxine and Liothyronine** *see* Liotrix *on page 919*
- **Levothyroxine and Liothyronine** *see* Thyroid, Desiccated *on page 1442*
- **Levothyroxine Sodium** *see* Levothyroxine *on page 900*
- **Levoxyl** *see* Levothyroxine *on page 900*
- **Levulan Kerastick** *see* Aminolevulinic Acid (Topical) *on page 117*
- **Lexapro** *see* Escitalopram *on page 590*
- **Lexiva** *see* Fosamprenavir *on page 712*
- **Lexixryl [DSC]** *see* Diclofenac (Topical) *on page 489*
- **LGX 818** *see* Encorafenib *on page 563*
- **LHRH** *see* Gonadorelin *on page 746*
- **LH-RH Agonist** *see* Histrelin *on page 759*
- **Lialda** *see* Mesalamine *on page 980*
- **Librium** *see* ChlordiazePOXIDE *on page 333*
- **Libtayo** *see* Cemiplimab *on page 320*
- **LiceMD Complete [OTC]** *see* Pyrethrins and Piperonyl Butoxide *on page 1293*
- **LiceMD Treatment [OTC]** *see* Pyrethrins and Piperonyl Butoxide *on page 1293*
- **Licide [OTC]** *see* Pyrethrins and Piperonyl Butoxide *on page 1293*
- **Lidex** *see* Fluocinonide *on page 691*
- **Lido BDK** *see* Lidocaine and Prilocaine *on page 911*

Lidocaine (Systemic) (LYE doe kane)

Related Information

Oral Pain *on page 1734*

Brand Names: US P-Care X; ReadySharp Lidocaine; Xylocaine; Xylocaine (Cardiac) [DSC]; Xylocaine-MPF

Brand Names: Canada Xylocaine; Xylocaine Plain; Xylocard

Pharmacologic Category Antiarrhythmic Agent, Class Ib; Local Anesthetic

Use

Local and regional anesthesia by infiltration, nerve block, epidural, or spinal techniques; acute treatment of ventricular arrhythmias (eg, due to acute myocardial infarction [MI] or during cardiac manipulation [eg, cardiac surgery]).

Note: The routine prophylactic use of lidocaine to prevent arrhythmia associated during ST-elevation MI or to suppress isolated ventricular premature beats, couplets, runs of accelerated idioventricular rhythm, and nonsustained ventricular tachycardia is not recommended (ACCF/AHA [O'Gara, 2013]).

Local Anesthetic/Vasoconstrictor Precautions No information available to require special precautions

Effects on Dental Treatment Key adverse event(s) related to dental treatment: Metallic taste.

Effects on Bleeding No information available to require special precautions

Adverse Reactions Effects vary with route of administration. Many effects are dose-related.

1% to 10%:

Central nervous system: Headache (positional headache following spinal anesthesia: 3%), shivering (following spinal anesthesia: 2%), radiculopathy (≤2%; transient pain; subarachnoid administration)

Frequency not defined:

Cardiovascular: Bradycardia, cardiac arrhythmia, circulatory shock, coronary artery vasospasm, edema, flushing, heart block, hypotension (including following spinal anesthesia), local thrombophlebitis, vascular insufficiency (periarticular injections)

Central nervous system: Agitation, anxiety, apprehension, cauda equina syndrome (following spinal anesthesia), coma, confusion, disorientation, dizziness, drowsiness, euphoria, hallucination, hyperesthesia, hypoesthesia, intolerance to temperature, lethargy, loss of consciousness, metallic taste, nervousness, paresthesia, peripheral neuropathy (following spinal anesthesia), psychosis, seizure, slurred speech, twitching

Gastrointestinal: Nausea (including following spinal anesthesia), vomiting

Hypersensitivity: Anaphylactoid reaction, anaphylaxis, hypersensitivity reaction

Neuromuscular & skeletal: Tremor, weakness

Otic: Tinnitus

Respiratory: Bronchospasm, dyspnea, respiratory depression, respiratory insufficiency (following spinal anesthesia)

<1%, postmarketing, and/or case reports: Asystole, dermatological reaction, diplopia (following spinal anesthesia), methemoglobinemia

Mechanism of Action Class Ib antiarrhythmic; suppresses automaticity of conduction tissue, by increasing electrical stimulation threshold of ventricle, His-Purkinje system, and spontaneous depolarization of the ventricles during diastole by a direct action on the tissues; blocks both the initiation and conduction of nerve impulses by decreasing the neuronal membrane's permeability to sodium ions, which results in inhibition of depolarization with resultant blockade of conduction

Pharmacodynamics/Kinetics

Onset of Action Single bolus dose: 45 to 90 seconds

Duration of Action 10 to 20 minutes

Half-life Elimination Biphasic: Prolonged with congestive heart failure, liver disease, shock, severe renal disease; Initial: 7 to 30 minutes; Terminal: Infants, premature: 3.2 hours, Adults: 1.5 to 2 hours

Pregnancy Considerations

Lidocaine and its metabolites cross the placenta and can be detected in the fetal circulation following maternal injection for anesthesia prior to delivery (Cavalli 2004; Mitani 1987).

Adverse reactions in the fetus/neonate may affect the CNS, heart, or peripheral vascular tone. Fetal heart monitoring is recommended by the manufacturer.

Lidocaine injection is approved for obstetric analgesia (eg, prior to epidural or spinal anesthesia). Lidocaine administered by local infiltration is used to provide analgesia prior to episiotomy and during repair of obstetric lacerations (ACOG 209 2019). Administration by the perineal route may result in greater absorption than administration by the epidural route (Cavalli 2004). Cumulative exposure from all routes of administration should be considered. The ACOG recommends that pregnant women should not be denied medically necessary surgery regardless of trimester. If the procedure is elective, it should be delayed until after delivery (ACOG 775 2019).

Medications used for the treatment of cardiac arrest in pregnancy are the same as in the nonpregnant woman. Doses and indications should follow current Advanced Cardiovascular Life Support guidelines. Appropriate medications should not be withheld due to concerns of fetal teratogenicity (AHA [Jeejeebhoy 2015]).

Lidocaine (Topical) (LYE doe kane)

Related Information

Perioral Premalignant Lesions and Management of Patients Undergoing Cancer Therapy *on page 1781*

Viral Infections *on page 1754*

Brand Names: US 7T Lido; Alocane Emergency Burn Max Str [OTC]; Anastia [DSC]; AneCream [OTC]; AneCream5 [OTC]; Asperflex Max St [OTC]; Astero; Blue Tube/ Aloe [OTC]; CidalEaze [DSC]; Eha; First Care Pain Relief [OTC]; Gen7T; Glydo; LC-4 Lidocaine [OTC] [DSC]; LC-5 Lidocaine [OTC]; LDO Plus; LevigoSP [OTC]; Lido King [OTC]; Lido-K [DSC]; Lido-Sorb; Lidocaine Max St 24 Hours [OTC]; Lidocaine Pain Relief [OTC]; Lidocaine PAK [DSC]; Lidocaine Plus [OTC]; Lidoderm; LidoDose Pediatric Bulk Pack [OTC]; LidoDose [OTC]; Lidopac; Lidopin; LidoPure Patch; LidoRx; Lidotral; Lidotrans 5 Pak [DSC]; Lidotrex; Lidovex [DSC]; Lidovin [DSC]; Lidozion [DSC]; Lidozol [DSC]; Lipocaine 5 [OTC]; LMX 4 Plus [OTC]; LMX 4 [OTC]; LMX 5 [OTC]; Lubricaine [OTC]; Lydexa; NeuroMed7 [OTC]; Numbonex [DSC]; Pain Relief Maximum Strength [OTC]; Pain Relieving [OTC]; Predator [OTC]; Premium Lidocaine; Re-Lieved Maximum Strength [OTC]; RectaSmoothe [OTC]; RectiCare [OTC]; Salonpas Pain Relieving [OTC]; TheraCare Pain Relief [OTC]; Topicaine 5 [OTC]; Topicaine [OTC]; Tranzarel [DSC]; Venipuncture Px1 Phlebotomy; Xolido XP [OTC]; Xolido [OTC]; Xryliderm [DSC]; Zeyocaine [DSC]; Zingo; Zionodil; Zionodil 100; ZTlido

Brand Names: Canada Cathejell; Jelido; Lidodan; Xylocaine

Generic Availability (US) Yes

Pharmacologic Category Analgesic, Topical; Local Anesthetic

Dental Use Topical local anesthetic

Patch: Production of mild topical anesthesia of accessible mucous membranes of the mouth prior to superficial dental procedures

Oral topical solution (viscous): Reduce gagging during dental impressions and x-rays

Use

Intradermal injection (Zingo): Topical local analgesia prior to venipuncture or peripheral IV cannulation in children ≥3 years of age; topical local analgesia prior to venipuncture in adults.

Jelly: Prevention and control of pain in procedures involving the male and female urethra; for topical treatment of painful urethritis; lubricant for endotracheal intubation (oral, nasal) (Glydo only).

Oral topical solution (2% viscous): Topical anesthesia of irritated or inflamed oral mucous membranes and pharyngeal tissue, reducing gagging during the taking of x-ray. **Note:** Not approved for relief of teething pain and discomfort in infants and children; serious adverse (toxic) effects have been reported (AAP 2011; AAPD 2012; ISMP 2014).

Oral topical solution (4%): Topical anesthesia of accessible mucous membranes of the oral and nasal cavities and proximal portions of the digestive tract. **Note:** Not approved for relief of teething pain and discomfort in infants and children; serious adverse (toxic) effects have been reported (AAP 2011; AAPD 2012; ISMP 2014).

Oral topical solution (metered-dose spray) [Canadian product]: Topical anesthesia of accessible mucous membranes of the oral and nasal cavities and proximal portions of the digestive tract.

Patch (Lidoderm, ZTlido): Relief of pain associated with postherpetic neuralgia.

Patch (OTC 4%): Temporary relief of minor localized pain.

Rectal: Temporary relief of pain and itching due to anorectal disorders.

Topical: Local anesthetic for mucous membrane of the oropharynx; lubricant for intubation; use in laser/cosmetic surgeries; pruritus, pruritic eczemas, insect bites, pain, soreness, minor burns (including sunburns), cuts, and abrasions of the skin; discomfort due to pruritus ani, pruritus vulvae, hemorrhoids, anal fissures, and similar conditions of the skin and mucous membranes; local management of skin wounds, including pressure ulcers, venous stasis ulcers, first- and second-degree burns, and superficial wounds and scrapes. Indications may vary by product; also refer to manufacturer's labeling.

Local Anesthetic/Vasoconstrictor Precautions
No information available to require special precautions

Effects on Dental Treatment Key adverse event(s) related to dental treatment: Metallic taste.

Effects on Bleeding No information available to require special precautions

Adverse Reactions Adverse effects vary with formulation and extent of systemic absorption; children may be at increased risk.

>10%:

Dermatologic: Erythema (intradermal powder: adults - 67%; children & adolescents - 53%)

Hematologic & oncologic: Petechia (intradermal powder: 44% to 46%)

1% to 10%:

Cardiovascular: Edema (intradermal powder: 4% to 8%)

Dermatologic: Pruritus (intradermal powder: 9%; also occurs with topical patch)

Gastrointestinal: Nausea (intradermal powder: 2%; also occurs with topical patch), vomiting

Frequency not defined:

Cardiovascular: Bradycardia, circulatory shock, flushing (topical patch), hypotension, shock

Central nervous system: Apprehension, central nervous system depression, confusion, disorientation (topical patch), dizziness, drowsiness, euphoria, excitement, headache (topical patch), hyperesthesia (topical patch), hypoesthesia (topical patch), localized warm feeling, loss of consciousness, metallic taste (topical patch), nervousness, numbness, pain (exacerbation; topical patch), paresthesia, seizure, sensation disorder (topical patch), sensation of cold, twitching

Dermatologic: Dermatitis, exfoliation of skin (topical patch), papule (topical patch), skin blister (topical patch), skin depigmentation (topical patch), skin edema (topical patch), skin erosion (topical patch), urticaria

Gastrointestinal: Dysgeusia (topical patch)

Hematologic & oncologic: Bruise (topical patch), methemoglobinemia

Hypersensitivity: Anaphylactoid shock, angioedema, hypersensitivity reaction

Local: Application site burning (topical patch), application site erythema (topical patch), application site vesicles (topical patch), local discoloration (topical patch), local irritation (topical patch)

Neuromuscular & skeletal: Asthenia, laryngospasm, tremor

Ophthalmic: Blurred vision, diplopia

Otic: Tinnitus

Respiratory: Bronchospasm, dyspnea, respiratory depression

Dental Usual Dosage

Anesthesia, topical:

Oral topical solution (viscous): **Note:** Not approved for relief of teething pain and discomfort in infants and children; serious adverse (toxic) effects have been reported; AAP, AAPD, and ISMP strongly discourage use (AAP 2011; AAPD 2012; ISMP 2014).

Infants and Children <3 years: ≤1.2 mL applied to area with a cotton-tipped applicator no more frequently than every 3 hours (maximum: 4 doses per 12-hour period); use only if the underlying condition requires treatment with product volume of ≤1.2 mL)

Children ≥3 years and Adolescents: Should not exceed 4.5mg/kg/dose (or 300mg/dose); swished in the mouth and spit out no more frequently than every 3 hours (maximum: 4 doses per 12-hour period)

Adults: Anesthesia of the mouth: 15 mL swished in the mouth and spit out no more frequently than every 3 hours (maximum: 8 doses per 24-hour period)

Postherpetic neuralgia: Adults: Patch: Apply patch to most painful area. Up to 3 patches may be applied in a single application. Patch may remain in place for up to 12 hours in any 24-hour period.

Dosing

Adult Anesthesia, topical: Note: Not all available products may be represented in dosing; also refer to manufacturer's labeling.

Cream:

Aspercreme: Pain: Apply a thin layer to affected area every 6 to 8 hours, not to exceed 3 applications in a 24-hour period.

Blue Tube, LMX 4: Skin irritation: Apply up to 3 to 4 times daily to intact skin.

Lidocaine 4.12%, Lidovex: Skin irritation: Apply a thin film to affected area 2 to 3 times daily as needed.

Lipocaine 5, LMX 5: Relief of anorectal pain and itching: Apply to affected area up to 6 times daily.

Gel: Usual dosage: Apply to affected area ≤4 times daily as needed (maximum dose: 4.5 mg/kg, not to exceed 300 mg).

Product-specific dosing:

Astero 4%; Apply 1 to 4 pumps to affected area; each pump provides 0.25 mL (lidocaine 10 mg) and covers a 2 × 2 inch area. Maximum single application: 4 pumps (lidocaine 40 mg); maximum daily application: 12 pumps/day (lidocaine 120 mg/day).

LidoRx 3%: Apply 1 to 4 pumps to affected area 3 to 4 times daily; each pump provides 0.25 mL (lidocaine 7.5 mg) and covers a 2 × 2 inch area. Maximum single application: 4 pumps (lidocaine 30 mg); maximum daily application: 16 pumps/day (lidocaine 120 mg/day).

Topicaine 5%: Apply to affected area up to 6 times daily.

Intradermal injection: Apply one intradermal lidocaine (0.5 mg) device to the site planned for venipuncture, 1 to 3 minutes prior to needle insertion.

Jelly: Maximum dose: 30 mL (600 mg) in any 12-hour period:

Anesthesia of male urethra: 5 to 30 mL (100 to 600 mg).

Anesthesia of female urethra: 3 to 5 mL (60 to 100 mg).

Lubricant, endotracheal intubation (Glydo): Apply moderate amount to external surface of the endotracheal tube prior to insertion.

Lotion: Apply a thin film to affected area 2 to 4 times daily; product-specific application frequency may vary; also refer to manufacturer's labeling.

Ointment: Apply as a single application not exceeding 5 g of ointment (equivalent to lidocaine base 250 mg); maximum: 20 g of ointment/day (equivalent to lidocaine base 1,000 mg/day).

Oral topical solution (2% viscous):

Anesthesia of the mouth: 15 mL swished in the mouth and spit out no more frequently than every 3 hours (maximum: 4.5 mg/kg [or 300 mg per dose]; 8 doses per 24-hour period).

Anesthesia of the pharynx: 15 mL gargled no more frequently than every 3 hours (maximum: 4.5 mg/kg [or 300 mg per dose]; 8 doses per 24-hour period); may be swallowed.

Oral topical solution (4%): **Note:** For use in mucous membranes of oral and nasal cavities and proximal GI tract. Apply 1 to 5 mL (40 to 200 mg) to affected area (maximum dose: 4.5 mg/kg, not to exceed 300 mg per dose).

Oral topical endotracheal solution, metered-dose spray (10 mg/actuation) [Canadian product]:

Nasal: 20 to 60 mg (maximum dose: 500 mg for procedure <1 minute or 600 mg for procedure >5 minutes).

Oropharyngeal: 20 to 200 mg (maximum dose: 500 mg for procedure <1 minute or 600 mg for procedure >5 minutes).

Respiratory tract: 50 to 400 mg (maximum dose: 400 mg for procedure <1 minute or 600 mg for procedure >5 minutes).

Trachea, larynx, bronchi: 50 to 200 mg (maximum dose: 200 mg for procedure <1 minute or 400 mg for procedure >5 minutes).

Patch: **Note:** One ZTlido 1.8% patch provides equivalent lidocaine exposure to one Lidoderm 5% patch.

Gel-patch (OTC 4%): Pain (localized): Apply 1 patch to painful area up to 4 times daily. Each patch may remain in place for up to 8 hours. No more than 1 patch should be used at a time.

Lidoderm, ZTlido: Postherpetic neuralgia: Apply patch to most painful area. Up to 3 patches may be applied in a single application. Patch(es) may remain in place for up to 12 hours in any 24-hour period.

OTC 4%, Rx 3.5% (Gen7T): Pain (localized): Apply patch to painful area. Patch may remain in place for up to 12 hours in any 24-hour period. No more than 1 patch should be used in a 24-hour period.

Topical solution (OTC 4% [products labeled for external use only]): Apply thin layer to affected area every 6 to 8 hours; maximum of 3 applications in 24 hours.

Geriatric Refer to adult dosing. Administer reduced doses commensurate with age and physical status.

Renal Impairment: Adult There are no dosage adjustments provided in the manufacturer's labeling.

Hepatic Impairment: Adult There are no dosage adjustments provided in the manufacturer's labeling; use caution in patients with severe hepatic disease.

Pediatric

Note: Smaller areas of treatment are recommended in younger or smaller patients (<12 months or <10 kg) or those with impaired elimination (Fein 2012); use lowest effective dose

Anesthetic: Topical: Dose varies with age, weight, and physical condition.

Cream:

Lidovex (lidocaine 3.75%), Lidocaine 4.12%: Infants, Children, and Adolescents: Apply a thin film to affected area 2 to 3 times daily as needed; maximum dose: 4.5 mg/kg/dose; not to exceed 300 mg/dose

LMX 4 (lidocaine 4%, liposomal): Children >2 years and Adolescents: Apply a thin film to affected area up to 3 to 4 times daily as needed; maximum dose: 4.5 mg/kg/dose; not to exceed 300 mg/dose

Gel: Children ≥2 years and Adolescents: Apply to affected area up to 3 to 4 times daily as needed; maximum dose: 4.5 mg/kg/dose; not to exceed 300 mg/dose

Jelly: Children and Adolescents: Dose varies with age and weight; maximum dose: 4.5 mg/kg/dose; not to exceed 600 mg in a 12-hour period

Lotion: Children and Adolescents: Apply to affected area up to 2 to 3 times daily as needed; maximum dose: 4.5 mg/kg/dose; not to exceed 300 mg/dose

Ointment: Children and Adolescents: Apply to affected area; maximum dose: 4.5 mg/kg/dose; not to exceed 300 mg/dose

Patch: OTC 4%: Children ≥12 years and Adolescents: Apply patch to painful area. Patch may remain in place for up to 12 hours. No more than 1 patch should be used in a 24-hour period.

Minor dermal procedures (eg, peripheral IV cannulation, venipuncture, lumbar puncture, abscess drainage, joint aspiration); anesthetic: Limited data available:

Intradermal injection: Zingo: Venipuncture or peripheral IV catheter insertion: Children ≥3 years and Adolescents: Apply one intradermal lidocaine (0.5 mg) device to the site planned for venipuncture, administer 1 to 3 minutes prior to the IV needle insertion; perform procedure within 10 minutes of application

Topical: Cream LMX 4 (lidocaine 4%):

Infants and Children <4 years: Apply 1 **g** of cream to site 30 minutes prior to procedure (Fein 2012; Taddio 2005)

Children ≥4 years and Adolescents ≤17 years: Apply 1 to 2.5 **g** of cream to site 30 minutes prior to procedure (Eichenfield 2002; Fein 2012; Koh 2004; Luhmann 2004; Taddio 2005)

Note: For peripheral IV cannulation, some have recommended application to 6.25 cm^2 of skin (Sobanko 2012).

Oral inflammation or irritation: Topical: **Note:** Not approved for relief of teething pain and discomfort in infants and children; serious adverse (toxic) effects, including fatalities, have been reported; AAP, AAPD, and ISMP strongly discourage use (AAP 2011; AAPD 2012; ISMP 2014).

Oral solution (2% viscous): Dose should be adjusted according to patient's age, weight, and physical condition:

Infants and Children <3 years: 24 mg/dose (1.2 mL) applied to area with a cotton-tipped applicator no more frequently than every 3 hours; maximum dose: 4 doses per 12-hour period; should not be swallowed

Children ≥3 years and Adolescents: Do not exceed 4.5 mg/kg/dose; maximum dose: 300 mg/dose; swished in the mouth and spit out no more frequently than every 3 hours; maximum dose: 4 doses per 12-hour period

Topical solution (4%): **Note:** For use on mucous membranes of the oral and nasal cavities and proximal portions of the digestive tract; use lowest effective dose. Children and Adolescents: Do not exceed 4.5 mg/kg/dose; maximum dose: 300 mg/dose; applied with cotton applicator, cotton pack, or via spray; should not be swallowed

Topical endotracheal solution, metered-dose spray (10 mg/actuation) [Canadian product]: Children 2 to <12 years: Topical: Dose varies with age, weight, and application site.

Maximum dose:

Laryngotracheal: 3 mg/kg/dose

Nasal/oropharyngeal: 4 to 5 mg/kg/dose

Rectal pain, itching: Topical:

Cream: LMX 5 (lidocaine 5%): Children ≥12 years and Adolescents: Apply to affected area up to 6 times daily

Gel: Topicaine (lidocaine 5%): Children ≥12 years and Adolescents: Apply to affected area up to 6 times daily

Skin irritation: Topical: Cream: LMX 4 (lidocaine 4%): Children ≥2 years and Adolescents: Apply up to 3 to 4 times daily to intact skin

Renal Impairment: Pediatric There are no dosage adjustments provided in the manufacturer's labeling. Use caution in patients with severe renal impairment; accumulation of active metabolites may occur with long-term treatment.

Hepatic Impairment: Pediatric There are no dosage adjustments provided in the manufacturer's labeling; use caution in patients with severe hepatic disease.

Mechanism of Action Blocks both the initiation and conduction of nerve impulses by decreasing the neuronal membrane's permeability to sodium ions, which results in inhibition of depolarization with resultant blockade of conduction

Contraindications Hypersensitivity to lidocaine or any component of the formulation; hypersensitivity to another local anesthetic of the amide type; traumatized mucosa, bacterial infection at the site of application (lotion, LidoRx and Lidovex only); tuberculous or fungal lesions of skin vaccinia, varicella and acute herpes simplex (4.12% cream only).

Warnings/Precautions Use with caution in patients with known drug sensitivities. Allergic reactions (cutaneous lesions, urticaria, edema, or anaphylactoid reactions) may be a result of sensitivity to lidocaine (rare) or preservatives used in formulations. Patients allergic to para-aminobenzoic acid (PABA) derivatives (eg, procaine, tetracaine, benzocaine) have not shown cross sensitivity to lidocaine. Potentially life-threatening side effects (eg, irregular heartbeat, seizures, coma, respiratory depression, death) have occurred when used prior to cosmetic procedures. Excessive dosing for any indication (eg, application to large areas, use above recommended dose, application to denuded or inflamed skin, or wearing of device for longer than recommended), smaller patients, and/or impaired elimination may lead to increased absorption and systemic toxicity; patient should adhere strictly to recommended dosage and administration guidelines; serious adverse effects may require the use of supportive care and resuscitative equipment. Use caution in patients with severe hepatic disease and/or pseudocholinesterase deficiency due to diminished ability to metabolize systemically-absorbed lidocaine. Use with caution in patients with severe shock or heart block. Use with extreme caution in the presence of sepsis/or severely traumatized mucosa due to an increased risk of rapid systemic absorption at application site. Elderly, debilitated patients, children, and acutely ill patients should be given reduced doses commensurate with their age and physical status. Use intradermal injection with caution in patients with bleeding tendencies/platelet disorders; may have a higher risk of superficial dermal bleeding. May potentially trigger malignant hyperthermia; follow standard protocol for identification and treatment.

Methemoglobinemia has been reported with local anesthetics; clinically significant methemoglobinemia requires immediate treatment along with discontinuation of the anesthetic and other oxidizing agents. Onset may be immediate or delayed (hours) after anesthetic exposure. Patients with glucose-6-phosphate dehydrogenase deficiency, congenital or idiopathic methemoglobinemia, cardiac or pulmonary compromise, exposure to oxidizing agents or their metabolites, or infants <6 months are more susceptible and should be closely monitored for signs and symptoms of methemoglobinemia (eg, cyanosis, headache, rapid pulse, shortness of breath, lightheadedness, fatigue).

When topical anesthetics are used prior to cosmetic or medical procedures, the lowest amount of anesthetic necessary for pain relief should be applied. High systemic levels and toxic effects (eg, methemoglobinemia, irregular heartbeats, respiratory depression, seizures, death) have been reported in patients who (without supervision of a trained professional) have applied topical anesthetics in large amounts (or to large areas of the skin), left these products on for prolonged periods of time, or have used wraps/dressings to cover the skin following application. Irritation, sensitivity and/or infection may occur at the site of application; discontinue use and institute appropriate therapy if local effects occur. Mild and transient application site reactions may occur during or immediately after treatment with patch; spontaneously resolves within a few minutes to hours; may include blisters, bruising, burning sensation, depigmentation, dermatitis, discoloration, edema, erythema, exfoliation, irritation, papules, petechial, pruritus, vesicles, or the area may be the locus of abnormal sensation. Potentially significant interactions may exist, requiring dose or frequency adjustment, additional monitoring, and/or selection of alternative therapy.

Topical cream, liquid, lotion, gel, and ointment: Do not leave on large body areas for >2 hours. Not for ophthalmic use. Some products are not recommended for use on mucous membranes; consult specific product labeling.

Intradermal injection: Only use on skin locations where an adequate seal can be maintained. Do not use on body orifices, mucous membranes, around the eyes, or on areas with a compromised skin barrier.

Topical oral solution/viscous: **[US Boxed Warning]: Life-threatening and fatal events in infants and young children:** Postmarketing cases of seizures, cardiopulmonary arrest, and death in patients <3 years of age have been reported with use of lidocaine 2% viscous solution when it was not administered in strict adherence to the dosing and administration recommendations. Lidocaine 2% viscous solution should generally not be used for teething pain. For other conditions, the use of lidocaine 2% viscous solution in patients <3 years of age should be limited to those situations where safer alternatives are not available or have been tried but failed. To decrease the risk of serious adverse events, instruct caregivers to strictly adhere to the prescribed dose and frequency of administration, and store the prescription bottle safely out of reach of children. Multiple cases of seizures (including fatalities) have occurred in pediatric patients using viscous lidocaine for oral discomfort, including teething pain and stomatitis (Curtis 2009; Giard 1983; Gonzalez del Ray 1994; Hess 1988; Mofenson 1983; Puczynski 1985; Rothstein 1982; Smith 1992). The FDA recommends against using topical OTC medications for teething pain as some products may cause harm. The American Academy of Pediatrics (AAP) recommends managing teething pain with a chilled (not frozen) teething ring or gently rubbing/massaging with the caregiver's finger.

When used in mouth or throat, topical anesthesia may impair swallowing and increase aspiration risk. Avoid food for ≥60 minutes following oral or throat application. This is especially important in the pediatric population. Numbness may increase the danger of tongue/buccal biting trauma; ingesting food or chewing gum should be avoided while mouth or throat is anesthetized. Excessive doses or frequent application may result in high plasma levels and serious adverse effects; strictly adhere to dosing instructions. Use measuring devices to measure the correct volume, if applicable, to ensure accuracy of dose.

Use of topical anesthetics for teething is discouraged by the AAP, the American Academy of Pediatric Dentistry, and the ISMP (AAP 2012; AAPD 2012; ISMP 2014).

Topical patch: Apply only on intact skin. Do not use around or in the eyes. To avoid accidental ingestion by children, store and dispose of products out of the reach of children. Avoid exposing application site to external heat sources (eg, heating pad, electric blanket, heat lamp, hot tub).

Benzyl alcohol and derivatives: Some dosage forms may contain benzyl alcohol; large amounts of benzyl alcohol (≥99 mg/kg/day) have been associated with a potentially fatal toxicity ("gasping syndrome") in neonates; the "gasping syndrome" consists of metabolic acidosis, respiratory distress, gasping respirations, CNS dysfunction (including convulsions, intracranial hemorrhage), hypotension, and cardiovascular collapse (AAP ["Inactive" 1997]; CDC 1982); some data suggests that benzoate displaces bilirubin from protein binding sites (Ahlfors 2001); avoid or use dosage forms containing benzyl alcohol with caution in neonates.

Some dosage forms may contain polysorbate 80 (also known as Tweens). Hypersensitivity reactions, usually a delayed reaction, have been reported following exposure to pharmaceutical products containing polysorbate 80 in certain individuals (Isaksson 2002; Lucente 2000; Shelley 1995). Thrombocytopenia, ascites, pulmonary deterioration, and renal and hepatic failure have been reported in premature neonates after receiving parenteral products containing polysorbate 80 (Alade 1986; CDC 1984). See manufacturer's labeling.

Warnings: Additional Pediatric Considerations In infants and children, seizures (some fatal) have been reported following topical lidocaine ingestion at serum concentrations within the therapeutic range of 1 to 5 mcg/mL (Curtis 2009); others have reported toxic effects with excessive doses or frequent application of topical oral lidocaine solution that resulted in high plasma concentrations. Multiple cases of seizures, including fatalities, have occurred in pediatric patients using viscous lidocaine for oral discomfort (eg, teething pain, herpetic gingivostomatitis) (Curtis 2009; Giard 1983; Gonzalez del Rey 1994; Hess 1988; Mofenson 1983; Puczynski 1985; Rothstein 1982; Smith 1992). Lidocaine oral solution is not approved for treatment of teething pain or discomfort; off-label use is strongly discouraged and should be avoided. When used for oral irritation, the solution should not be swallowed, but should be applied topically with a cotton swab to individual lesions or the excess should be expectorated (swish and spit). Toxicology data suggests that in infants and children<6 years, ingestion of as little as 5 mL of lidocaine may result in serious toxicity and emergency care should be sought (Curtis 2009). Additionally, the FDA recommends against using topical OTC medications for teething pain as some products may cause harm; the use of OTC topical anesthetics (eg, benzocaine) for teething pain is also discouraged by AAP, and The American Academy of Pediatric Dentistry (AAP 2011; AAPD 2012). The AAP recommends managing teething pain with a chilled (not frozen) teething ring or gently rubbing/massaging with the caregiver's finger.

Topical patches (both used and unused) may cause toxicities in children; used patches still contain large amounts of lidocaine; store and dispose patches out of the reach of children; efficacy of patches in pediatric patients has not been evaluated due to safety concerns.

Some dosage forms may contain propylene glycol; in neonates large amounts of propylene glycol delivered orally, intravenously (eg, >3,000 mg/day), or topically have been associated with potentially fatal toxicities which can include metabolic acidosis, seizures, renal failure, and CNS depression; toxicities have also been reported in children and adults including hyperosmolality, lactic acidosis, seizures, and respiratory depression; use caution (AAP 1997; Shehab 2009).

Drug Interactions

Metabolism/Transport Effects **Substrate** of CYP1A2 (minor), CYP2A6 (minor), CYP2B6 (minor), CYP2C9 (minor), CYP3A4 (major); **Note:** Assignment of Major/Minor substrate status based on clinically relevant drug interaction potential

Avoid Concomitant Use

Avoid concomitant use of Lidocaine (Topical) with any of the following: Abametapir; Conivaptan; Fusidic Acid (Systemic); Idelalisib

Increased Effect/Toxicity

Lidocaine (Topical) may increase the levels/effects of: Antiarrhythmic Agents (Class III); Local Anesthetics; Prilocaine; Sodium Nitrite

The levels/effects of Lidocaine (Topical) may be increased by: Abametapir; Antiarrhythmic Agents (Class III); Aprepitant; Beta-Blockers; Clofazimine; Conivaptan; CYP3A4 Inhibitors (Moderate); CYP3A4 Inhibitors (Strong); Dapsone (Topical); Disopyramide; Duvelisib; Erdafitinib; Fosaprepitant; Fosnetupitant;

Fusidic Acid (Systemic); Idelalisib; Larotrectinib; Methemoglobinemia Associated Agents; MiFEPRIStone; Netupitant; Nitric Oxide; Palbociclib; Simeprevir; Stiripentol

Decreased Effect There are no known significant interactions involving a decrease in effect.

Pharmacodynamics/Kinetics

Onset of Action Intradermal injection: 1 to 3 minutes; Topical: 3 to 5 minutes; Transdermal: ~4 hours (Davies 2004)

Duration of Action Intradermal injection: 10 minutes

Half-life Elimination IV: 1.5 to 2 hours; prolonged 2-fold or more in hepatic impairment

Time to Peak Transdermal (5%): 11 hours (following application of 3 patches); Transdermal (1.8%): ~14 hours (following application of 3 patches)

Pregnancy Risk Factor B

Pregnancy Considerations

Lidocaine and its metabolites cross the placenta and can be detected in the fetal circulation following injection (Cavalli 2004; Mitani 1987). The amount of lidocaine absorbed topically (and therefore available systemically to potentially reach the fetus) varies by dose administered, duration of exposure, and site of application. Cumulative exposure from all routes of administration should be considered.

Breastfeeding Considerations

Information regarding the presence of lidocaine in breast milk following topical administration has not been located. Lidocaine is present in breast milk following systemic administration (Dryden 2000; Giuliani 2001; Lebedevs 1993; Ortega 1999; Zeisler 1986). However, the oral bioavailability is low and rapid biotransformation occurs via the liver. The amount of lidocaine to reach the bloodstream of a breastfed infant is expected to be low and would be unlikely to cause adverse effects (Dryden 2000; Giuliani 2001; Lebedevs 1993; Ortega 1999).

Lidocaine is considered compatible with breastfeeding (WHO 2002). The manufacturer recommends caution be used when administering topical lidocaine to breastfeeding women. Cumulative exposure from all routes of administration should be considered.

Dosage Forms Considerations EnovaRX-Lidocaine, and Lidtopic Max creams are compounded from kits. Refer to manufacturer's package insert for compounding instructions.

Dosage Forms: US

Cream, External:

AneCream [OTC]: 4% (5 g, 15 g, 30 g)
AneCream5 [OTC]: 5% (15 g)
Blue Tube/ Aloe [OTC]: 4% (30 g)
LC-5 Lidocaine [OTC]: 5% (45 g)
Lidocaine Plus [OTC]: 4% (120 g)
Lidopin: 3% (28 g, 85 g); 3.25% (28 g, 85 g)
Lidotral: 3.88% (85 g)
Lipocaine 5 [OTC]: 5% (30 g, 113 g)
LMX 4 [OTC]: 4% (5 g, 15 g, 30 g)
LMX 5 [OTC]: 5% (15 g, 30 g)
Lydexa: 4.12% (28.3 g)
NeuroMed7 [OTC]: 4% (63 g)
Pain Relieving [OTC]: 4% (15 g)
Predator [OTC]: 4% (63 g)
RectaSmoothe [OTC]: 5% (30 g)
RectiCare [OTC]: 5% (15 g, 30 g)
Xolido [OTC]: 2% (118 mL)
Xolido XP [OTC]: 4% (118 mL)
Generic: 3% (28.3 g, 28.35 g, 85 g); 4% (5 g, 15 g, 30 g, 120 g); 4.12% (28.3 g, 85 g); 5% (15 g, 28.35 g, 30 g)

Gel, External:

Alocane Emergency Burn Max Str [OTC]: 4% (75 mL)
Astero: 4% (90 mL)
LDO Plus: 4% (30 mL)
LidoDose [OTC]: 3% (1 mL)
LidoDose Pediatric Bulk Pack [OTC]: 3% (1 mL)
LidoRx: 3% (10 mL, 30 mL, 90 mL)
Lidotrex: 2% (28.33 g)
Lubricaine [OTC]: 4% (113 g); 5% (113 g)
7T Lido: 2% (85 g)
Topicaine [OTC]: 4% (10 g, 30 g, 113 g)
Topicaine 5 [OTC]: 5% (10 g, 30 g, 113 g)
Generic: 2% (5 mL, 30 mL)

Jet-injector, Intradermal [preservative free]:

Zingo: 0.5 mg (1 ea)
Generic: 0.5 mg (1 ea)

Kit, External:

AneCream [OTC]: 4%
Lidopac: 5%
LidoPure Patch: 5%
LMX 4 Plus [OTC]: 4%
Venipuncture Px1 Phlebotomy: 2%
Generic: 4%

Liquid, External:

LevigoSP [OTC]: 2.5% (150 mL)

Lotion, External:

Eha: 4% (88 mL)
Gen7T: 3.5% (120 g)
Lido-Sorb: 3% (177 mL)
Zionodil: 3% (177 mL)
Zionodil 100: 3% (177 mL)
Generic: 3% (118 mL, 177 mL)

Ointment, External:

Premium Lidocaine: 5% (50 g)
Generic: 5% (30 g, 35.44 g, 50 g, 150 g, 250 g, 2500 g)

Patch, External:

Asperflex Max St [OTC]: 4% (6 ea)
First Care Pain Relief [OTC]: 4% (5 ea)
Gen7T: 3.5% (15 ea)
Lido King [OTC]: 4% (5 ea)
Lidocaine Max St 24 Hours [OTC]: 4% (15 ea)
Lidocaine Pain Relief [OTC]: 4% (5 ea)
Lidoderm: 5% (1 ea, 30 ea)
Pain Relief Maximum Strength [OTC]: 4% (5 ea)
Re-Lieved Maximum Strength [OTC]: 4% (6 ea)
Salonpas Pain Relieving [OTC]: 4% (6 ea)
TheraCare Pain Relief [OTC]: 4% (5 ea)
ZTlido: 1.8% (1 ea, 30 ea)
Generic: 4% (10 ea); 5% (1 ea, 15 ea, 30 ea)

Prefilled Syringe, External:

Generic: 2% (20 mL)

Prefilled Syringe, External [preservative free]:

Glydo: 2% (6 mL, 11 mL)
Generic: 2% (5 mL, 10 mL)

Solution, External:

Generic: 4% (50 mL)

Solution, Mouth/Throat:

Generic: 2% (15 mL, 100 mL)

Solution, Mouth/Throat [preservative free]:

Generic: 4% (4 mL)

Dosage Forms: Canada

Gel, External:
Lidodan: 2% (10 mL)
Xylocaine: 2% (30 mL)

Ointment, External:
Lidodan: 5% (15 g, 30 g, 35 g)
Xylocaine: 5% (35 g)

Prefilled Syringe, External:
Jelido: 2% (6 mL, 11 mL)
Xylocaine: 2% (10 mL)
Generic: 2% (12.5 g, 12.5 mL)

Lidocaine and Epinephrine

(LYE doe kane & ep i NEF rin)

Related Information

EPINEPHrine (Systemic) *on page 569*
Lidocaine (Systemic) *on page 901*
Oral Pain *on page 1734*

Brand Names: US D-Care 100X; Lignospan Forte; Lignospan Standard; Xylocaine MPF With Epinephrine; Xylocaine With Epinephrine

Brand Names: Canada Xylocaine With Epinephrine

Generic Availability (US) Yes

Pharmacologic Category Local Anesthetic

Dental Use Amide-type anesthetic used for local infiltration anesthesia injection near nerve trunks to produce nerve block

Use Anesthesia, local: Production of local anesthesia by nerve block or infiltration for dental procedures.

Local Anesthetic/Vasoconstrictor Precautions No information available to require special precautions

Effects on Dental Treatment It is common to misinterpret psychogenic responses to local anesthetic injection as an allergic reaction. Intraoral injections are perceived by many patients as a stressful procedure in dentistry. Common symptoms to this stress are diaphoresis, palpitations, hyperventilation. Patients may exhibit hypersensitivity to bisulfites contained in local anesthetic solution to prevent oxidation of epinephrine. In general, patients reacting to bisulfites have a history of asthma and their airways are hyper-reactive to asthmatic syndrome.

Degree of adverse effects in the CNS and cardiovascular system is directly related to the blood levels of lidocaine: Bradycardia, hypersensitivity reactions (rare; may be manifest as dermatologic reactions and edema at injection site), asthmatic syndromes

High blood levels: Anxiety, restlessness, disorientation, confusion, dizziness, tremors, seizures, CNS depression (resulting in somnolence, unconsciousness and possible respiratory arrest), nausea, and vomiting.

Effects on Bleeding No information available to require special precautions

Adverse Reactions Also see individual agents.

<1%, postmarketing, and/or case reports: Methemoglobinemia

Dental Usual Dosage Dosage varies with the anesthetic procedure, degree of anesthesia needed, vascularity of tissue, duration of anesthesia required, and physical condition of patient.

Dental anesthesia, infiltration, or conduction block:

Children <12 years: 20-30 mg (1-1.5 mL) of lidocaine hydrochloride as a 2% solution with epinephrine 1:100,000; maximum: 4.5 mg of lidocaine hydrochloride/kg of body weight or 100-150 mg as a single dose

Children ≥12 years and Adults: Do not exceed 7 mg/kg body weight or 300 mg of lidocaine hydrochloride and 3 mcg (0.003 mg) of epinephrine/kg of body weight or 0.2 mg epinephrine per dental appointment. The effective anesthetic dose varies with procedure, intensity of anesthesia needed, duration of anesthesia required, and physical condition of the patient. Always use the lowest effective dose along with careful aspiration.

The following numbers of dental carpules (1.7 mL or 1.8 mL) provide the indicated amounts of lidocaine hydrochloride 2% and epinephrine 1:100,000 (see table):

# of Cartridges (1.7 mL or 1.8 mL)	Lidocaine HCl (2%) (mg)		Epinephrine 1:100,000 (mg)	
	(1.7 mL cartridge)	(1.8 mL cartridge)	(1.7 mL cartridge)	(1.8 mL cartridge)
1	34	36	0.017	0.018
2	68	72	0.034	0.036
3	102	108	0.051	0.054
4	136	144	0.068	0.072
5	170	180	0.085	0.090
6	204	216	0.102	0.108
7	238	252	0.119	0.126
8	272	288	0.136	0.144
9	306	324	0.153	0.162
10	340	360	0.170	0.180

For most routine dental procedures, lidocaine hydrochloride 2% with epinephrine 1:100,000 is preferred. When a more pronounced hemostasis is required, a 1:50,000 epinephrine concentration should be used. The following numbers of dental cartridges (1.7 mL or 1.8 mL) provide the indicated amounts of lidocaine hydrochloride 2% and epinephrine 1:50,000.

# of Cartridges (1.7 mL or 1.8 mL)	Lidocaine HCl (2%) (mg)		Epinephrine 1:50,000 (mg)	
	(1.7 mL cartridge)	(1.8 mL cartridge)	(1.7 mL cartridge)	(1.8 mL cartridge)
1	34	36	0.034	0.036
2	68	72	0.068	0.072
3	102	108	0.102	0.108
4	136	144	0.136	0.144
5	170	180	0.170	0.180
6	204	216	0.204	0.216

Dosing

Adult

Anesthesia:

Dental: Oral infiltration/mandibular block: Initial: 1 to 5 mL (lidocaine 20 mg to 100 mg). **Note:** For most routine dental procedures, lidocaine 2% with epinephrine 1:100,000 is preferred. When a more pronounced hemostasis is required, use a 1:50,000 epinephrine concentration. Do not exceed 7 mg/kg body weight, up to a maximum range of 300 mg (usual dental practice) to 500 mg (approved product labeling) of lidocaine and 3 mcg (0.003 mg) of epinephrine/kg of body weight or 0.2 mg epinephrine per dental appointment.

Epidural: Administer a test dose (eg, 2 to 3 mL of lidocaine 1.5%) at least 5 minutes prior to injecting the total volume required for a lumbar or caudal block. Dosage varies with the number of dermatomes to be anesthetized (generally 2 to 3 mL of lidocaine 1%, 1.5%, or 2% with epinephrine [1:200,000] per dermatome). For continuous epidural or caudal anesthesia, the maximum dose should not be administered at intervals of <90 minutes. Maximum total dose for paracervical block: 200 mg/90 minutes (50% of the total dose to each side, with 5 minutes between sides).

Local: Infiltration: Dosage varies with procedure, degree of anesthesia needed, vascularity of tissue, duration of anesthesia required, and physical condition of patient. Maximum dose of lidocaine: 7 mg/kg (up to 500 mg). Use lidocaine 1%, 1.5%, or 2% with epinephrine (1:200,000) as single dose units.

Geriatric Refer to adult dosing; use with caution and at reduced dosages.

Renal Impairment: Adult

There are no dosage adjustments provided in the manufacturer's labeling. However, accumulation of metabolites may be increased in renal impairment.

Dialysis: Not dialyzable (0% to 5%) by hemo- or peritoneal dialysis; supplemental dose is not necessary (Aronoff 2007).

Hepatic Impairment: Adult There are no dosage adjustments provided in the manufacturer's labeling; use with caution (hepatically metabolized); patients with severe hepatic impairment are at greater risk of lidocaine toxicity.

Pediatric Note: Dose varies with procedure, depth of anesthesia, vascularity of tissues, duration of anesthesia, and condition of patient should only be administered under the supervision of a qualified physician experienced in the use of anesthetics. Dosing units variable (mL/kg, **mg/kg**); use extra precaution to ensure accuracy.

Note: Dosing should be based on lean body mass (Cote 2013). Due to shorter duration of action and potential toxicity with repeat dosing, lidocaine is not typically used for central (spinal) or regional (epidural/caudal) anesthesia (Cote 2013; Miller 2015).

Local anesthesia; dermal/cutaneous infiltration: Infants, Children, and Adolescents: Usual concentration ≤2% (eg, 1% or 2%) solution: Infiltrate area locally; maximum dose is 7 mg/kg, not to exceed adult maximum dose of 500 mg (Cote 2013; Kliegman 2016). **Note:** Aspiration should be performed prior to each injection; however, absence of blood in the syringe does not guarantee that intravascular injection has been avoided (Mulroy 2010).

Peripheral nerve block; excluding digital or penile: Infants ≥6 months, Children, and Adolescents: Usual concentrations ≤1%: Dosage (concentration [0.25, 0.5 or 1%]) and volume varies with procedure, degree of anesthesia needed, vascularity of tissue, duration of anesthesia required, and physical condition of patient. Maximum dose of lidocaine: 7 mg/kg, not to exceed adult maximum of 500 mg (Cote 2013; Kliegman 2016). For infants <6 months, maximum doses should be reduced by 30% (Cote 2013; Miller 2015).

Dental anesthesia; oral infiltration/mandibular block: Note: For most routine dental procedures, lidocaine 2% with epinephrine 1:100,000 is preferred. When a more pronounced hemostasis is required, a 1:50,000 epinephrine concentration should be used.

Children <10 years: Lidocaine 2% with epinephrine solution: ≤0.9 to 1 mL (lidocaine 18 mg to 20 mg) per procedure; maximum dose: 4.4 mg/kg not to exceed 300 mg (AAPD 2009); dosing is for procedures involving a single tooth, maxillary infiltration for 2 to 3 teeth, or mandibular block of an entire quadrant; it is rare that a patient would require a higher dose (ie, >1 mL)

Children ≥10 years and Adolescents: Lidocaine 2% with epinephrine solution: Initial: 1 to 5 mL (lidocaine 20 mg to 100 mg). Do not exceed usual dental guideline recommended maximum dose of 4.4 mg/kg up to a maximum total dose of 300 mg (AAPD 2009); some suggest a higher maximum of 7 mg/kg up to total maximum of 500 mg (approved product labeling) of lidocaine and 3 mcg (0.003 mg) of epinephrine/kg of body weight or 0.2 mg epinephrine per dental appointment.

Renal Impairment: Pediatric There are no dosage adjustments provided in the manufacturer's labeling; however, accumulation of metabolites may be increased in renal impairment. Not dialyzable (0% to 5%) by hemo- or peritoneal dialysis; supplemental dose is not necessary (Aronoff 2007).

Hepatic Impairment: Pediatric Use with caution; reduce dose; use with caution (hepatically metabolized); patients with severe hepatic impairment are at greater risk of lidocaine toxicity.

Mechanism of Action

Lidocaine: Blocks both the initiation and conduction of nerve impulses by decreasing the neuronal membrane's permeability to sodium ions, which results in inhibition of depolarization with resultant blockade of conduction.

Epinephrine: Increases the duration of action of lidocaine by causing vasoconstriction (via alpha effects) which slows the vascular absorption of lidocaine.

Contraindications

Hypersensitivity to lidocaine, other local anesthetics of the amide type, epinephrine, or any component of the formulation.

Canadian labeling: Additional contraindications (not in US labeling): Hypersensitivity to para amino benzoic acid (PABA).

Warnings/Precautions Lidocaine can cause cardiac depression (eg, bradycardia, hypotension); patients with hypovolemia may be at increased risk. Careful and constant monitoring of the patient's state of consciousness should be done following each local anesthetic injection; at such times, restlessness, anxiety, tinnitus, dizziness, blurred vision, tremors, depression, drowsiness, may be early warning signs of CNS toxicity. Treatment is primarily symptomatic and supportive. Use with caution in patients with bradycardia, severe shock, heart block, or impaired cardiovascular function; use with caution in areas of the body supplied by end arteries or having otherwise compromised blood supply. Patients with peripheral vascular disease or hypertensive vascular disease may exhibit exaggerated vasoconstrictor response. Ischemic injury (eg, exfoliating, ulcerating lesions) or necrosis may result.

Anaphylactic reactions may occur following administration. Continuous intra-articular infusion of local anesthetics after arthroscopic or other surgical procedures is not an approved use; chondrolysis (primarily in the shoulder joint) has occurred following infusion, with some cases requiring arthroplasty or shoulder replacement. Methemoglobinemia has been reported with local anesthetics; clinically significant methemoglobinemia requires immediate treatment along with discontinuation of the anesthetic and other oxidizing agents. Onset may be immediate or delayed (hours) after anesthetic exposure. Patients with G6PD deficiency, congenital or idiopathic methemoglobinemia, cardiac or pulmonary compromise, exposure to oxidizing agents or their metabolites, or infants <6 months of age are more susceptible and should be closely monitored for signs and symptoms of methemoglobinemia (eg, cyanosis, headache, rapid pulse, shortness of breath, lightheadedness, fatigue). Local anesthetics have been associated with occurrences of respiratory arrest. Use with caution in patients with severe renal impairment, hepatic impairment, diabetes and in patients with poorly controlled hyperthyroidism. Use with caution in children, the elderly and in acutely ill or debilitated patients; reduce dose consistent with age and physical status. Potentially significant interactions may exist, requiring dose or frequency adjustment, additional monitoring, and/or selection of alternative therapy.

Avoid intravascular injections. Aspirate the syringe prior to administration; the needle must be repositioned until no return of blood can be elicited by aspiration; however, absence of blood in the syringe does not guarantee that intravascular injection has been avoided. Use with caution when there is inflammation and/or sepsis in the region of the proposed injection. Do not use injections containing preservatives (eg, methylparaben) for epidural or spinal anesthesia, or for any route of administration that would introduce solution into the cerebrospinal fluid. Use lumbar and caudal epidural anesthesia with extreme caution in patients with existing neurological disease, spinal deformities, septicemia, and impaired cardiovascular function (eg, severe hypertension). Repeat doses of lidocaine may cause significant increases in blood levels with each repeated dose due to slow accumulation of the drug or its metabolites. Tolerance to elevated blood levels varies with the status of the patient. Dental practitioners and/or clinicians using local anesthetic agents should be well trained in diagnosis and management of emergencies that may arise from the use of these agents. Resuscitative equipment, oxygen, and other resuscitative drugs should be available for immediate use.

Some dosage forms may contain benzyl alcohol; large amounts of benzyl alcohol (≥99 mg/kg/day) have been associated with a potentially fatal toxicity ("gasping syndrome") in neonates; the "gasping syndrome" consists of metabolic acidosis, respiratory distress, gasping respirations, CNS dysfunction (including convulsions, intracranial hemorrhage), hypotension and cardiovascular collapse (AAP 1997; CDC 1982); some data suggests that benzoate displaces bilirubin from protein binding sites (Ahlfors 2001); avoid or use dosage forms containing benzyl alcohol with caution in neonates See manufacturer's labeling. May contain sodium metabisulfite; use caution in patients with a sulfite allergy.

Drug Interactions

Metabolism/Transport Effects Refer to individual components.

Avoid Concomitant Use

Avoid concomitant use of Lidocaine and Epinephrine with any of the following: Blonanserin; Bromperidol; Ergot Derivatives; Lurasidone

Increased Effect/Toxicity

Lidocaine and Epinephrine may increase the levels/effects of: Doxofylline; Lurasidone; Solriamfetol; Sympathomimetics

The levels/effects of Lidocaine and Epinephrine may be increased by: AtoMOXetine; Beta-Blockers (Nonselective); Bretylium; Cannabinoid-Containing Products; Chloroprocaine; Cocaine (Topical); COMT Inhibitors; Ergot Derivatives; Guanethidine; Hyaluronidase; Inhalational Anesthetics; Linezolid; Monoamine Oxidase Inhibitors; Ozanimod; Procarbazine; Serotonin/Norepinephrine Reuptake Inhibitors; Tedizolid; Tricyclic Antidepressants

Decreased Effect

Lidocaine and Epinephrine may decrease the levels/effects of: Antidiabetic Agents; Benzylpenicilloyl Polylysine

The levels/effects of Lidocaine and Epinephrine may be decreased by: Alpha1-Blockers; Benperidol; Beta-Blockers (Beta1 Selective); Beta-Blockers (with Alpha-Blocking Properties); Blonanserin; Bromperidol; CloZAPine; Haloperidol; Promethazine; Spironolactone

Pharmacodynamics/Kinetics

Onset of Action Dental: ≤2 to 4 minutes

Duration of Action Dental: ~2.5 hours (infiltration); 3 to 3.5 hours (nerve block); dose and anesthetic procedure dependent

Pregnancy Risk Factor B

Pregnancy Considerations Adverse events have not been observed in animal reproduction studies. See individual agents.

Breastfeeding Considerations It is not known if lidocaine/epinephrine is excreted in breast milk. The manufacturer recommends that caution be exercised when administering lidocaine/epinephrine to nursing women. See individual agents.

Dosage Forms: US

Injection, solution:

Xylocaine with Epinephrine:

0.5% / 1:200,000: Lidocaine hydrochloride 0.5% [5 mg/mL] and epinephrine 1:200,000 (50 mL)

1% / 1:100,000: Lidocaine hydrochloride 1% [10 mg/mL] and epinephrine 1:100,000 (10 mL, 20 mL, 50 mL)

2% / 1:100,000: Lidocaine hydrochloride 2% [20 mg/mL] and epinephrine 1:100,000 (10 mL, 20 mL, 50 mL)

Generic:

0.5% / 1:200,000: Lidocaine hydrochloride 0.5% [5 mg/mL] and epinephrine 1:200,000 (50 mL)

1% / 1:100,000: Lidocaine hydrochloride 1% [10 mg/mL] and epinephrine 1:100,000 (20 mL, 30 mL, 50 mL)

1.5% / 1:200,000: Lidocaine hydrochloride 1.5% [15 mg/mL] and epinephrine 1:200,000 (5 mL) [contains sodium metabisulfite]

2% / 1:100,000: Lidocaine hydrochloride 2% [20 mg/mL] and epinephrine 1:100,000 (30 mL, 50 mL)

Injection, solution [preservative free]:

Xylocaine-MPF with Epinephrine:

1% / 1:200,000: Lidocaine hydrochloride 1% [10 mg/mL] and epinephrine 1:200,000 (5 mL, 10 mL, 30 mL)

1.5% / 1:200,000: Lidocaine hydrochloride 1.5% [15 mg/mL] and epinephrine 1:200,000 (5 mL, 10 mL, 30 mL)

2% / 1:200,000: Lidocaine hydrochloride 2% [20 mg/mL] and epinephrine 1:200,000 (5 mL, 10 mL, 20 mL)

Generic:

1.5% / 1:200,000: Lidocaine hydrochloride 1.5% [15 mg/mL] and epinephrine 1:200,000 (5 mL, 30 mL)

2% / 1:200,000: Lidocaine hydrochloride 2% [20 mg/mL] and epinephrine 1:200,000 (20 mL)

Injection, solution [for dental use]:

Lignospan Forte: 2% / 1:50,000: Lidocaine hydrochloride 2% [20 mg/mL] and epinephrine 1:50,000 (1.7 mL)

Lignospan Standard: 2% / 1:100,000: Lidocaine hydrochloride 2% [20 mg/mL] and epinephrine 1:100,000 (1.7 mL)

Xylocaine Dental with Epinephrine:

2% / 1:50,000: Lidocaine hydrochloride 2% [20 mg/mL] and epinephrine 1:50,000 (1.7 mL)

2% / 1:100,000: Lidocaine hydrochloride 2% [20 mg/mL] and epinephrine 1:100,000 (1.7 mL)

Generic:

2% / 1:50,000: Lidocaine hydrochloride 2% [20 mg/mL] and epinephrine 1:50,000 (1.7 mL, 1.8 mL)

2% / 1:100,000: Lidocaine hydrochloride 2% [20 mg/mL] and epinephrine 1:100,000 (1.7 mL, 1.8 mL)

Kit, Injection:

D-Care 100X: 1% / 1:200,000: Lidocaine hydrochloride 1% [10 mg/mL] and epinephrine 1:200,000

Dental Health Professional Considerations Oral paresthesia: The occurrence of oral paresthesia associated with 4% solutions of prilocaine or articaine, although rare, continue to be slightly more frequent than other local anesthetics. From 1999-2008, there were 182 cases of nonsurgical paresthesia (Gaffen, 2009). Of the cases, 172 involved mandibular block injection only. Another eight cases involved mandibular block combined with at least one other type of anesthetic injection. A single case involved infiltration around tooth number 35 (European numbering system; tooth number 20 for Universal numbering system) and the final case involved infiltration and intraligamentary injection in the maxillary anterior region.

A 2010 report, reviewed adverse events submitted voluntarily over a 10-year period involving the dental local anesthetics articaine, bupivacaine, lidocaine, mepivacaine, and prilocaine in the United States. Lidocaine reported incidence: One case per 181,076,673 cartridges sold. The reported incidence of paresthesia was one case for 13,800,970 cartridges of all local anesthetics sold in the U.S. (Garisto, 2010).

Lidocaine and Prilocaine

(LYE doe kane & PRIL oh kane)

Related Information

Lidocaine (Topical) *on page 902*

Prilocaine *on page 1274*

Brand Names: US AgonEaze; Anodyne LPT; DermacinRx Empricaine; DermacinRx Prizopak; Dolotranz [DSC]; Leva Set [DSC]; Lido BDK; Lidopril; Lidopril XR; LiProZonePak; Livixil Pak; LP Lite Pak [DSC]; Medolor Pak; Oraqix; Prikaan; Prikaan Lite; Prilolid; Prilovix; Priloxx LP [DSC]; Prizotral II; Relador Pak; Venipuncture CPI [DSC]

Brand Names: Canada EMLA; Oraqix

Generic Availability (US) Yes: Cream

Pharmacologic Category Local Anesthetic

Dental Use

Periodontal gel (Oraqix®): Use in adults who require localized anesthesia in periodontal pockets during scaling and/or root planing.

Topical: Amide-type topical anesthetic for use on normal intact skin to provide local analgesia for minor procedures such as IV cannulation or venipuncture

Use

US labeling:

Cream: Topical anesthetic for use on normal intact skin to provide local analgesia; for use on genital mucous membranes for superficial minor surgery; and as pretreatment for infiltration anesthesia.

Periodontal gel: Topical anesthetic for use in periodontal pockets during scaling and/or root planing procedures

Canadian labeling:

Cream: Topical anesthetic for use on intact skin in connection with: IV cannulation or venipuncture; superficial surgical procedures (eg, split skin grafting, electrolysis, removal of molluscum contagiosum); laser treatment for superficial skin surgery (eg, telangiectasia, port wine stains, warts, moles, skin nodules, scar tissue); surgical procedures of genital mucosa (≤10 minutes) on small superficial localized lesions (eg, removal of condylomata by laser or cautery, biopsies); local infiltration anesthesia in genital mucous membranes; mechanical cleansing/debridement of leg ulcers; vaccination with measles-mumps-rubella (MMR), diphtheria-pertussis-tetanus-poliovirus (DPTP), *Haemophilus influenzae* b, and hepatitis B.

Patch: Topical anesthetic for use on intact skin in connection with IV cannulation or venipuncture; vaccination with measles-mumps-rubella (MMR), diphtheria-pertussis-tetanus-poliovirus (DPTP), *Haemophilus influenzae* b, and hepatitis B.

Periodontal gel: Topical anesthetic for use in periodontal pockets during scaling and/or root planing procedures

Local Anesthetic/Vasoconstrictor Precautions

No information available to require special precautions

Effects on Dental Treatment Key adverse event(s) related to dental treatment: Application site reactions in the oral cavity in 52/391 patients (13%) included pain, soreness, irritation, numbness, ulcerations, vesicles, edema, abscess and/or redness in the treated area. The 13% represented adverse effects occurring in more than one patient. Each patient was counted only once per adverse event. Taste perversion also reported (2%) including complaints of bad or bitter taste for up to 4 hours after administration.

Effects on Bleeding No information available to require special precautions

Adverse Reactions

Cream/patch:

>10%:

Dermatologic: Pallor (local: 37%)

Local: Application site erythema (21% to 30%), application site burning (17%)

1% to 10%:

Central nervous system: Local alterations in temperature sensations (7%)

Local: Application site edema (6% to 10%), application site pruritus (2%)

Frequency not defined:

Dermatologic: Hyperpigmentation, stinging of the skin (local), urticaria

Hematologic & oncologic: Local purpuric or petechial reaction

<1%, postmarketing, and/or case reports: Anaphylactic shock, angioedema, application site rash, blistering of foreskin, bronchospasm, central nervous system depression, central nervous system stimulation, central nervous system toxicity (high dose), circulatory shock (high dose), hypotension, local hypersensitivity reaction, methemoglobinemia (high dose)

Periodontal gel:

>10%: Local: Application site reaction (13%, includes abscess, edema, irritation, numbness, pain, ulceration, vesicles)

1% to 10%:

Central nervous system: Bitter taste (2%), fatigue (1%)

Gastrointestinal: Nausea (1%)

Hypersensitivity: Local hypersensitivity reaction

Respiratory: Flu-like symptoms (1%), respiratory tract infection (1%)

Dental Usual Dosage Oraqix: Gel: Apply on gingival margin around selected teeth using the blunt-tipped applicator included in package. Wait 30 seconds, then fill the periodontal pockets using the blunt-tipped applicator until gel becomes visible at the gingival margin. Wait another 30 seconds before starting treatment. Maximum recommended dose: One treatment session: 5 cartridges (8.5 g)

Dosing

Adult Anesthetic: Topical:

Cream (intact skin): **Note:** Apply a thick layer to intact skin and cover with an occlusive dressing. Dermal analgesia can be expected to increase for up to 3 hours under occlusive dressing and persist for 1 to 2 hours after removal of the cream.

US labeling:

Minor dermal procedures (eg, IV cannulation or venipuncture): Apply 2.5 g (1/2 of the 5 g tube) over 20 to 25 cm^2 of skin surface area) for at least 1 hour

Major dermal procedures (eg, more painful dermatological procedures involving a larger skin area such as split thickness skin graft harvesting): Apply 2 g per 10 cm^2 of skin and allow to remain in contact with the skin for at least 2 hours.

Adult male genital skin (eg, pretreatment prior to local anesthetic infiltration): Apply 1 g per 10 cm^2 to the skin surface for 15 minutes. Local anesthetic infiltration should be performed immediately after removal of cream.

Adult female genital mucous membranes: Minor procedures (eg, removal of condylomata acuminata, pretreatment for local anesthetic infiltration): Apply 5 to 10 g for 5 to 10 minutes. The local anesthetic infiltration or procedure should be performed immediately after removal of cream.

Canadian labeling:

Minor dermal procedures (eg, IV cannulation, venipuncture, surgical or laser treatment): Apply 2 g (~1/2 of the 5 g tube) over ~13.5 cm^2 for at least 1 hour but no longer than 5 hours

Major dermal procedures (eg, split-skin grafting): 1.5 to 2 g per 10 cm^2 (maximum: 60 g per 400 cm^2) for at least 2 hours but no longer than 5 hours

Genital mucosa (eg, surgical procedures ≤10 minutes such as localized wart removal, and prior to local anesthetic infiltration): Apply 2 g (~1/2 of 5 g tube) per lesion (maximum: 10 g) for 5 to 10 minutes. Initiate procedure immediately after removing cream.

Leg ulcers (eg, mechanical cleansing/surgical debridement): Apply ~1 to 2 g per 10 cm^2 (maximum: 10 g) for at least 30 minutes and up to 60 minutes for necrotic tissue that is more difficult to penetrate. Initiate procedure immediately after removing cream.

Periodontal gel (Oraqix): Apply on gingival margin around selected teeth using the blunt-tipped applicator included in package. Wait 30 seconds, then fill the periodontal pockets using the blunt-tipped applicator until gel becomes visible at the gingival margin. Wait another 30 seconds before starting treatment. May reapply; maximum recommended dose: One treatment session: 5 cartridges (8.5 g)

Transdermal patch [Canadian product]: Minor procedures (eg, needle insertion): Apply 1 or more patches to intact skin surface area <10 cm^2 for at least 1 hour (maximum application time: 5 hours)

Geriatric Smaller areas of treatment may be necessary depending on status of patient (eg, debilitated, impaired hepatic function). Refer to adult dosing.

Renal Impairment: Adult There are no dosage adjustments provided in the manufacturer labeling. Lidocaine and prilocaine primarily undergo hepatic metabolism and their pharmacokinetics are not expected to be changed significantly in renal impairment.

Hepatic Impairment: Adult Smaller areas of treatment are recommended for patients with severe hepatic impairment.

Pediatric Note: Smaller areas of treatment recommended in smaller or debilitated patients or patients with impaired elimination; decreasing the duration of application may decrease analgesic effect, however maximum application duration times should not be exceeded.

US labeling:

Minor dermal procedures (eg, IV access, venipuncture, IM injection); anesthetic: Note: General dosing information provided, dose should be individualized based on procedure and area to be anesthetized.

Infants and Children: Topical:

<5 kg: Apply ≤1 g per 10 cm^2 area; cover with an occlusive dressing for usual duration of application of 60 minutes prior to procedure. Maximum dosing information for a 24-hour period: Maximum total dose (for all sites combined): 1 g; maximum application area: 10 cm^2; maximum application time: 1 hour.

5 kg to 10 kg: Apply 1 to 2 g per 10 cm^2 area; cover with occlusive dressing for at least 60 minutes. Maximum dosing information for a 24-hour period: Maximum total dose (for all sites combined): 2 g; maximum application area: 20 cm^2; maximum application time: 4 hours.

>10 kg to 20 kg: Apply 1 to 2 g per 10 cm^2 area; cover with occlusive dressing for at least 60 minutes. Maximum dosing information for a 24-hour period: Maximum total dose (for all sites combined): 10 g; maximum application area: 100 cm^2; maximum application time: 4 hours.

>20 kg: Apply 1 to 2 g per 10 cm^2 area; cover with occlusive dressing for at least 60 minutes. Maximum dosing information for a 24-hour period: Maximum total dose (for all sites combined): 20 g; maximum application area: 200 cm^2; maximum application time: 4 hours.

Adolescents: Apply 2.5 g of cream (1/2 of the 5 g tube) over 20 to 25 cm^2 of skin surface area for at least 1 hour.

Major dermal procedures (eg, more painful dermatological procedures involving a larger skin area such as split thickness skin graft harvesting); anesthetic: Adolescents: Topical: Apply 2 g of cream per 10 cm^2 of skin and allow to remain in contact with the skin for at least 2 hours.

Male genital skin (eg, pretreatment prior to local anesthetic infiltration): Adolescents: Topical: Apply 1 g per 10 cm^2 to the skin surface for 15 minutes. Local anesthetic infiltration should be performed immediately after removal of cream.

Female genital mucous membranes: Minor procedures (eg, removal of condylomata acuminata, pretreatment for local anesthetic infiltration): Adolescents: Topical: Apply 5 to 10 g of cream for 5 to 10 minutes.

Canadian labeling: **Local anesthetic:** General dosing information provided, dose should be individualized based on procedure and area to be anesthetized.

Transdermal patch [Canadian product]: **Note:** Dosing is based on child's age and weight; if a patient is ≥3 months and is smaller than weight requirement, defer to maximum dose for the patient's weight.

Apply patch(es) to skin area(s) <10 cm^2:

Infants <3 months or <5 kg: Topical: Apply 1 patch and leave on for ~1 hour; maximum dose: 1 patch; maximum application time: 1 hour. Do not apply more than 1 patch at same time.

Infants ≥3 months and >5 kg: Topical: Apply 1 to 2 patches for ~1 hour; maximum dose: 2 patches; maximum application time: 4 hours.

Children ≤6 years and >10 kg: Topical: Apply 1 or more patches for minimum of 1 hour; maximum dose: 10 patches; maximum application time: 5 hours.

Children ≥7 years and >20 kg and Adolescents: Topical: Apply 1 or more patches for a minimum of 1 hour; maximum dose: 20 patches; maximum application time: 5 hours.

Renal Impairment: Pediatric There are no dosage adjustments provided in the manufacturer labeling. Lidocaine and prilocaine primarily undergo hepatic metabolism and their pharmacokinetics are not expected to be changed significantly in renal impairment.

Hepatic Impairment: Pediatric Smaller areas of treatment are recommended for patients with severe hepatic impairment.

Mechanism of Action Local anesthetic action occurs by stabilization of neuronal membranes and inhibiting the ionic fluxes required for the initiation and conduction of impulses

Contraindications

Hypersensitivity to local anesthetics of the amide type or any component of the formulation

Canadian labeling: Additional contraindications (not in US labeling): Congenital or idiopathic methemoglobinemia.

Cream and patch only: Infants ≤12 months of age who require treatment with methemoglobin-inducing agents; preterm infants (gestational age <37 weeks); procedures requiring large amounts over a large body area that are not conducted in a facility with health care professionals trained in the diagnosis and management of dose-related toxicity and other acute emergencies, and with appropriate resuscitative treatments and equipment.

Warnings/Precautions Methemoglobinemia has been reported with local anesthetics; clinically significant methemoglobinemia requires immediate treatment along with discontinuation of the anesthetic and other oxidizing agents. Onset may be immediate or delayed (hours) after anesthetic exposure. Patients with glucose-6-phosphate dehydrogenase deficiency, congenital or idiopathic methemoglobinemia, cardiac or pulmonary compromise, exposure to oxidizing agents or their metabolites, or infants <6 months of age are more susceptible and should be closely monitored for signs and symptoms of methemoglobinemia (eg, cyanosis, headache, rapid pulse, shortness of breath, lightheadedness, fatigue). Patients with glucose-6-phosphate dehydrogenase (G6PD) deficiency may be more susceptible to drug-induced methemoglobinemia. Allergic and anaphylactic reactions may occur. Patients allergic to paraaminobenzoic acid derivatives (eg, procaine, tetracaine, benzocaine) have not shown cross sensitivity to lidocaine and/or prilocaine; use with caution in patients with a history of drug sensitivities.

Although the incidence of systemic adverse reactions with use of the cream is very low, caution should be exercised, particularly when applying over large areas and leaving on for longer than 2 hours. When used prior to cosmetic or medical procedures, the smallest amount of cream necessary for pain relief should be applied. High systemic levels and toxic effects (eg, methemoglobinemia, irregular heartbeats, respiratory depression, seizures, death) have been reported in patients who (without supervision of a trained professional) have applied topical anesthetics in large amounts (or to large areas of the skin), left these products on for a prolonged time, or have used wraps/dressings to cover the skin following application. Do not apply to broken or inflamed skin, open wounds or near the eyes. Avoid use in situations where penetration or migration past the tympanic membrane into the middle ear is possible; ototoxicity has been observed in animal studies. Avoid inadvertent trauma to the treated area (eg, scratching, rubbing, exposure to extreme hot or cold temperatures) until complete sensation has returned.

Use with caution in patients with severe hepatic impairment; smaller treatment area may be required due to risk of increased systemic exposure. Use with caution in patients with severe impairment of impulse initiation and conduction in the heart (eg, grade II and III AV block, pronounced bradycardia). Use with caution in patients with atopic dermatitis; rapid and greater absorption through the skin is observed in these patients; a shorter application time should be used. Use with caution in the debilitated or acutely ill patients and elderly patients; smaller treatment area may be required. Potentially significant drug-drug interactions may exist, requiring dose or frequency adjustment, additional monitoring, and/or selection of alternative therapy.

Do not use periodontal gel with standard dental syringes; only use with the supplied blunt-tipped applicator.

Warnings: Additional Pediatric Considerations Adjust dose in patients with increased risk for methemoglobinemia; use smaller areas for application in small children (especially infants <3 months of age). In small infants and children, an occlusive bandage may prevent the child from placing the cream in his/her mouth or smearing the cream on the eyes.

Drug Interactions

Metabolism/Transport Effects Refer to individual components.

Avoid Concomitant Use

Avoid concomitant use of Lidocaine and Prilocaine with any of the following: Abametapir; Bupivacaine (Liposomal); Conivaptan; Fusidic Acid (Systemic); Idelalisib

Increased Effect/Toxicity

Lidocaine and Prilocaine may increase the levels/effects of: Antiarrhythmic Agents (Class III); Bupivacaine (Liposomal); Local Anesthetics; Neuromuscular-Blocking Agents; Prilocaine; Sodium Nitrite

The levels/effects of Lidocaine and Prilocaine may be increased by: Abametapir; Antiarrhythmic Agents (Class III); Aprepitant; Beta-Blockers; Clofazimine; Conivaptan; CYP3A4 Inhibitors (Moderate); CYP3A4 Inhibitors (Strong); Dapsone (Topical); Disopyramide; Duvelisib; Erdafitinib; Fosaprepitant; Fosnetupitant; Fusidic Acid (Systemic); Hyaluronidase; Idelalisib; Larotrectinib; Methemoglobinemia Associated Agents; MiFEPRIStone; Netupitant; Nitric Oxide; Palbociclib; Simeprevir; Stiripentol

Decreased Effect

Lidocaine and Prilocaine may decrease the levels/effects of: Technetium Tc 99m Tilmanocept

Pharmacodynamics/Kinetics

Onset of Action

EMLA: 1 hour (more rapid in genital mucosa: 5 to 10 minutes); Peak effect: 2 to 3 hours

Oraqix: ≤30 seconds

Duration of Action

EMLA: 1 to 2 hours after removal; Genital mucosa: 15 to 20 minutes after application (range: 5 to 45 minutes)

Oraqix: ~20 minutes

Pregnancy Risk Factor B

Pregnancy Considerations Animal reproduction studies have not been conducted with this combination. Lidocaine and prilocaine cross the placenta. Their use is not contraindicated during labor and delivery. Refer to individual agents.

Breastfeeding Considerations Lidocaine is excreted in breast milk; excretion of prilocaine in breast milk unknown; however, systemic absorption following topical application is expected to be low. The manufacturer recommends that caution be exercised when administering to nursing women. Refer to individual agents.

Dosage Forms: US

Cream, topical:

AgonEaze: Lidocaine 2.5% and prilocaine 2.5% (2 x 30 g)

Anodyne LPT: Lidocaine 2.5% and prilocaine 2.5% (3 x 30 g)

DermacinRx Empricaine: Lidocaine 2.5% and prilocaine 2.5% (1 x 30 g)

DermacinRx Prizopak: Lidocaine 2.5% and prilocaine 2.5% (3 x 30 g)

Lido BDK: Lidocaine 2.5% and prilocaine 2.5% (5 g)

Lidopril: Lidocaine 2.5% and prilocaine 2.5% (3 x 30 g)

Lidopril XR: Lidocaine 2.5% and prilocaine 2.5% (2 x 30 g)

LiProZonePak: Lidocaine 2.5% and prilocaine 2.5% (3 x 30 g)

Livixil Pak: Lidocaine 2.5% and prilocaine 2.5% (3 x 30 g)

Medolor Pak: Lidocaine 2.5% and prilocaine 2.5% (3 x 30 g)

Prilolid: Lidocaine 2.5% and prilocaine 2.5% (1 x 30 g)

Prilovix Versipac: Lidocaine 2.5% and prilocaine 2.5% (3 x 30 g) [packaged with occlusive dressing]

Prizotral II: Lidocaine 2.5% and prilocaine 2.5% (3 x 30 g) with lidocaine HCl 3.88% (85 g)

Relador Pak: Lidocaine 2.5% and prilocaine 2.5% (3 x 30 g)

Generic: Lidocaine 2.5% and prilocaine 2.5% (5 g, 30 g, 5800 g, 18,000 g)

Gel, periodontal:

Oraqix: Lidocaine 2.5% and prilocaine 2.5% (1.7 g)

Dosage Forms: Canada

Patch, transdermal:

EMLA Patch: Lidocaine 2.5% and prilocaine 2.5% per patch (2s, 20s)

Lidocaine and Tetracaine

(LYE doe kane & TET ra kane)

Related Information

Lidocaine (Topical) *on page 902*

Tetracaine (Topical) *on page 1428*

Brand Names: US Pliaglis; Synera

Brand Names: Canada Pliaglis

Generic Availability (US) Yes: cream

Pharmacologic Category Analgesic, Topical; Local Anesthetic

Use Anesthesia, topical:

Cream: For use on intact skin in adults to provide topical local analgesia for superficial dermatological procedures, including dermal filler injection, pulsed dye laser therapy, facial laser resurfacing, and laser-assisted tattoo removal.

Patch: For use on intact skin in patients ≥3 years to provide local analgesia for superficial venous access and superficial dermatological procedures, including excision, electrodesiccation, and shave biopsy of skin lesions.

Local Anesthetic/Vasoconstrictor Precautions No information available to require special precautions

Effects on Dental Treatment No significant effects or complications reported

Effects on Bleeding No information available to require special precautions

Adverse Reactions Also see individual agents.

>10%:

Cardiovascular: Localized blanching (12% to 16%)
Dermatologic: Erythema (47% to 71%)
Local: Skin edema (12% to 14%)

1% to 10%:

Central nervous system: Dizziness (≤1%), drowsiness (≤1%), headache (≤1%), paresthesia (≤1%)
Dermatologic: Acne vulgaris (≤1%), contact dermatitis (≤1%), ecchymosis (≤1%), maculopapular rash (≤1%), skin blister (≤1%), urticaria (≤1%), vesicobullous dermatitis (≤1%), xeroderma (≤1%)
Gastrointestinal: Nausea (≤1%), vomiting (≤1%)
Hematologic & oncologic: Petechial rash (≤1%)
Hypersensitivity: Hypersensitivity reaction (≤1%)
Infection: Infection (≤1%)
Local: Application-site dermatitis (<4%), application site rash (<4%), local discoloration (<4%), application site pain (≤1%), application-site pruritus (≤1%)

<1%, postmarketing, and/or case reports: Anaphylactoid shock, angioedema, blepharitis, bronchospasm, burning sensation of skin, confusion, dehydration, diaphoresis, fever, hyperventilation, hypotension, nervousness, pallor, pharyngitis, stupor, syncope, tremor

Dosing

Adult & Geriatric Anesthesia, topical:

Cream: Superficial dermatological procedures: Prior to procedure, apply to intact skin for 20 to 60 minutes. Amount of cream varies depending on size of the surface area to be treated; see manufacturer's labeling for detailed information.

Patch:

Venipuncture or intravenous cannulation: Prior to procedure, apply to intact skin for 20 to 30 minutes; **Note:** May use another patch at a new location to facilitate venous access after a failed attempt; remove previous patch.

Superficial dermatological procedures: Prior to procedure, apply to intact skin for 30 minutes

Renal Impairment: Adult There are no dosage adjustments provided in the manufacturer's labeling. Lidocaine primarily undergoes hepatic metabolism and its pharmacokinetics are not expected to be changed significantly following topical administration of recommended doses in renal impairment.

Hepatic Impairment: Adult There are no dosage adjustments provided in the manufacturer's labeling (has not been studied). Use caution in patients with severe hepatic dysfunction.

Pediatric

Anesthesia, topical: Children ≥3 years and Adolescents: Patch:

Venipuncture or IV cannulation: Prior to procedure, apply to intact skin for 20 to 30 minutes. **Note:** May use another patch at a new location to facilitate venous access after a failed attempt; remove previous patch. Otherwise, simultaneous or sequential application of multiple patches is not recommended.

Superficial dermatologic procedures: Prior to procedure, apply to intact skin for 30 minutes.

Renal Impairment: Pediatric There are no dosage adjustments provided in the manufacturer's labeling. Lidocaine primarily undergoes hepatic metabolism and its pharmacokinetics are not expected to be changed significantly following topical administration of recommended doses in renal impairment.

Hepatic Impairment: Pediatric There are no dosage adjustments provided in the manufacturer's labeling (has not been studied). Use caution in patients with severe hepatic dysfunction.

Mechanism of Action Local anesthetic action occurs by stabilization of neuronal membranes and inhibiting the sodium ion fluxes required for the initiation and conduction of impulses.

Contraindications

Hypersensitivity to lidocaine, tetracaine, amide or ester-type anesthetic agents, para-aminobenzoic acid (PABA), or any other component of the formulation

Canadian labeling: Additional contraindications (not in US labeling): Cream: Congenital or idiopathic methemoglobinemia; procedures requiring large amounts over large areas of the body (>400 cm^2).

Warnings/Precautions Hypersensitivity or anaphylactic reactions may occur. Use with caution in patients who may be sensitive to systemic effects (eg, acutely ill, debilitated, elderly). If being used with other products containing local anesthetic, consider potential for additive effects. Avoid contact with eye and lip; loss of protective reflexes may predispose to corneal irritation and/or abrasion. Application to broken or inflamed skin or mucous membranes may lead to increased systemic absorption. Use caution in patients with severe hepatic disease or pseudocholinesterase deficiency. Not for use at home. Methemoglobinemia has been reported with local anesthetics; clinically significant methemoglobinemia requires immediate treatment along with discontinuation of the anesthetic and other oxidizing agents. Onset may be immediate or delayed (hours) after anesthetic exposure. Patients with glucose-6-phosphate dehydrogenase deficiency, congenital or idiopathic methemoglobinemia, cardiac or pulmonary compromise, exposure to oxidizing agents or their metabolites, or infants <6 months are more susceptible and should be closely monitored for signs and symptoms of methemoglobinemia (eg, cyanosis, headache, rapid pulse, shortness of breath, lightheadedness, fatigue).

Application of patch for longer duration than recommended, or simultaneous or sequential application of multiple patches is not recommended because of the risk for increased drug absorption and possible adverse reactions. May contain conducting metal (eg, iron); remove patch prior to MRI. Proper storage and disposal of used patches are essential to prevent accidental exposures, especially in children; accidental exposure may result in serious adverse effects.

Application of cream for longer duration than recommended, or application over larger surface areas is not recommended because of the risk for increased drug absorption and possible adverse reactions.

Warnings: Additional Pediatric Considerations In a clinical trial, lidocaine/tetracaine cream (Pliaglis) applied for 30 minutes was not shown to be effective at providing venipuncture analgesia in pediatric patients 5 to 17 years. Topical patches and cream (both used and unused) may cause toxicities in children; used patches and cream still contain large amounts of lidocaine and tetracaine; store and dispose out of the reach of children.

Drug Interactions

Metabolism/Transport Effects Refer to individual components.

Avoid Concomitant Use

Avoid concomitant use of Lidocaine and Tetracaine with any of the following: Abametapir; Conivaptan; Fusidic Acid (Systemic); Idelalisib

Increased Effect/Toxicity

Lidocaine and Tetracaine may increase the levels/effects of: Antiarrhythmic Agents (Class III); Local Anesthetics; Prilocaine; Sodium Nitrite

The levels/effects of Lidocaine and Tetracaine may be increased by: Abametapir; Antiarrhythmic Agents (Class III); Aprepitant; Beta-Blockers; Clofazimine; Conivaptan; CYP3A4 Inhibitors (Moderate); CYP3A4 Inhibitors (Strong); Dapsone (Topical); Disopyramide; Duvelisib; Erdafitinib; Fosaprepitant; Fosnetupitant; Fusidic Acid (Systemic); Idelalisib; Larotrectinib; Methemoglobinemia Associated Agents; MiFEPRIStone; Netupitant; Nitric Oxide; Palbociclib; Simeprevir; Stiripentol

Decreased Effect There are no known significant interactions involving a decrease in effect.

Pharmacodynamics/Kinetics

Onset of Action Within 20 to 30 minutes

Duration of Action Cream: 11 hours

Half-life Elimination Lidocaine: Adults: 1.8 hours

Pregnancy Considerations

Systemic absorption following topical application is expected to be low compared to parenteral administration, and is related to duration of exposure and surface area of application site. Systemic absorption would be required in order for lidocaine and tetracaine to cross the placenta and reach the fetus.

Refer to Lidocaine (Systemic), Lidocaine (Topical), and Tetracaine (Systemic) monographs.

Breastfeeding Considerations

Lidocaine is present in breast milk; it is not known if tetracaine is present in breast milk.

The amount of lidocaine in breast milk following topical application is not known. Systemic absorption following topical application is expected to be low compared to parenteral administration, and is related to duration of exposure and surface area of application site. Do not apply to the nipple or surrounding breast area to avoid direct exposure to the breastfeeding infant. According to the manufacturer, the decision to breastfeed during therapy should consider the risk of infant exposure, the benefits of breastfeeding to the infant, and benefits of treatment to the mother.

Refer to Lidocaine (Systemic), Lidocaine (Topical), and Tetracaine (Systemic) monographs.

Dosage Forms: US

Cream, external:

Pliaglis: Lidocaine 7% and tetracaine 7% (30 g)

Generic: Lidocaine 7% and tetracaine 7% (30 g)

Patch, transdermal:

Synera: Lidocaine 70 mg and tetracaine 70 mg (10s)

◆ **Lidocaine/Epinephrine** *see* Lidocaine and Epinephrine *on page 908*

◆ **Lidocaine HCl** *see* Lidocaine (Systemic) *on page 901*

◆ **Lidocaine HCl** *see* Lidocaine (Topical) *on page 902*

◆ **Lidocaine HCl/Epinephrine Bit** *see* Lidocaine and Epinephrine *on page 908*

◆ **Lidocaine Hydrochloride** *see* Lidocaine (Systemic) *on page 901*

◆ **Lidocaine Hydrochloride** *see* Lidocaine (Topical) *on page 902*

◆ **Lidocaine Hydrochloride and Epinephrine Bitartrate** *see* Lidocaine and Epinephrine *on page 908*

◆ **Lidocaine Max St 24 Hours [OTC]** *see* Lidocaine (Topical) *on page 902*

◆ **Lidocaine Pain Relief [OTC]** *see* Lidocaine (Topical) *on page 902*

◆ **Lidocaine PAK [DSC]** *see* Lidocaine (Topical) *on page 902*

◆ **Lidocaine Patch** *see* Lidocaine (Topical) *on page 902*

◆ **Lidocaine Plus [OTC]** *see* Lidocaine (Topical) *on page 902*

◆ **Lidocaine/Prilocaine** *see* Lidocaine and Prilocaine *on page 911*

◆ **Lidocaine/Tetracaine** *see* Lidocaine and Tetracaine *on page 914*

◆ **Lidoderm** *see* Lidocaine (Topical) *on page 902*

◆ **LidoDose [OTC]** *see* Lidocaine (Topical) *on page 902*

◆ **LidoDose Pediatric Bulk Pack [OTC]** *see* Lidocaine (Topical) *on page 902*

◆ **Lido-K [DSC]** *see* Lidocaine (Topical) *on page 902*

◆ **Lido King [OTC]** *see* Lidocaine (Topical) *on page 902*

◆ **Lidopac** *see* Lidocaine (Topical) *on page 902*

◆ **Lidopin** *see* Lidocaine (Topical) *on page 902*

◆ **Lidopril** *see* Lidocaine and Prilocaine *on page 911*

◆ **Lidopril XR** *see* Lidocaine and Prilocaine *on page 911*

◆ **LidoPure Patch** *see* Lidocaine (Topical) *on page 902*

◆ **LidoRx** *see* Lidocaine (Topical) *on page 902*

◆ **Lido-Sorb** *see* Lidocaine (Topical) *on page 902*

◆ **Lidotral** *see* Lidocaine (Topical) *on page 902*

◆ **Lidotrans 5 Pak [DSC]** *see* Lidocaine (Topical) *on page 902*

◆ **Lidotrex** *see* Lidocaine (Topical) *on page 902*

◆ **Lidovex [DSC]** *see* Lidocaine (Topical) *on page 902*

◆ **Lidovin [DSC]** *see* Lidocaine (Topical) *on page 902*

◆ **Lidozion [DSC]** *see* Lidocaine (Topical) *on page 902*

◆ **Lidozol [DSC]** *see* Lidocaine (Topical) *on page 902*

◆ **Lignocaine and Epinephrine** *see* Lidocaine and Epinephrine *on page 908*

◆ **Lignocaine and Prilocaine** *see* Lidocaine and Prilocaine *on page 911*

◆ **Lignocaine and Tetracaine** *see* Lidocaine and Tetracaine *on page 914*

◆ **Lignocaine Hydrochloride** *see* Lidocaine (Systemic) *on page 901*

◆ **Lignocaine Hydrochloride** *see* Lidocaine (Topical) *on page 902*

◆ **Lignospan Forte** *see* Lidocaine and Epinephrine *on page 908*

◆ **Lignospan Standard** *see* Lidocaine and Epinephrine *on page 908*

◆ **Lillow** *see* Ethinyl Estradiol and Levonorgestrel *on page 612*

LinaCLOtide (lin AK loe tide)

Brand Names: US Linzess

Brand Names: Canada Constella

Pharmacologic Category Gastrointestinal Agent, Miscellaneous; Guanylate Cyclase-C (GC-C) Agonist

Use

Chronic idiopathic constipation: Treatment of chronic idiopathic constipation (CIC) in adults

Irritable bowel syndrome with constipation: Treatment of irritable bowel syndrome with constipation (IBS-C) in adults

Local Anesthetic/Vasoconstrictor Precautions No information available to require special precautions

Effects on Dental Treatment Key adverse event(s) related to dental treatment: Upper respiratory tract infection and sinusitis

Effects on Bleeding No information available to require special precautions

Adverse Reactions Adverse reactions reported with use in IBS-C and CIC.

>10%: Gastrointestinal: Diarrhea (16% to 22%)

1% to 10%:

Central nervous system: Headache (4%), fatigue (<2%)

Endocrine & metabolic: Dehydration (≤1%)

Gastrointestinal: Abdominal pain (7%), flatulence (4% to 6%), abdominal distension (2% to 3%), viral gastroenteritis (≤3%), severe diarrhea (2%), dyspepsia (<2%), fecal incontinence (<2%), gastroesophageal reflux disease (<2%), vomiting (<2%)

Respiratory: Upper respiratory tract infection (5%), sinusitis (3%)

<1%, postmarketing, and/or case reports: Hematochezia, hypersensitivity reaction, melena, nausea, rectal hemorrhage, urticaria

Mechanism of Action Linaclotide and its active metabolite bind and agonize guanylate cyclase-C on the luminal surface of intestinal epithelium. Intracellular and extracellular cyclic guanosine monophosphate (cGMP) concentrations are subsequently increased resulting in chloride and bicarbonate secretion into the intestinal lumen. Intestinal fluid increases and GI transit is accelerated. Increased extracellular cGMP may decrease visceral pain by reducing pain-sensing nerve activity.

Pregnancy Considerations Linaclotide and its metabolite are not measurable in plasma when used at recommended doses. Maternal use is not expected to result in fetal exposure.

◆ **Linaclotide Acetate** *see* LinaCLOtide *on page 916*

LinaGLIPtin (lin a GLIP tin)

Related Information

Endocrine Disorders and Pregnancy *on page 1684*

Brand Names: US Tradjenta

Brand Names: Canada Trajenta

Pharmacologic Category Antidiabetic Agent, Dipeptidyl Peptidase 4 (DPP-4) Inhibitor

Use Diabetes mellitus, type 2, treatment: As an adjunct to diet and exercise to improve glycemic control in adults with type 2 diabetes as monotherapy or in combination with other antidiabetic agents.

Local Anesthetic/Vasoconstrictor Precautions No information available to require special precautions

Effects on Dental Treatment Linagliptin-dependent patients with diabetes should be appointed for dental treatment in the morning in order to minimize chance of stress-induced hypoglycemia.

Effects on Bleeding No information available to require special precautions

Adverse Reactions Incidences may include use in combination therapy regimens.

1% to 10%:

Endocrine & metabolic: Hypoglycemia (7%), increased uric acid (3%)

Gastrointestinal: Increased serum lipase (8%; >3x upper limit of normal)

Respiratory: Nasopharyngitis (7%), cough (2%)

Frequency not defined:

Dermatologic: Urticaria

Neuromuscular & skeletal: Myalgia

Respiratory: Bronchoconstriction

Postmarketing: Acute pancreatitis, anaphylaxis, angioedema, bullous pemphigoid, exfoliation of skin, oral mucosa ulcer, rhabdomyolysis, severe arthralgia, severe hypersensitivity, skin rash, stomatitis

Mechanism of Action Linagliptin inhibits dipeptidyl peptidase 4 (DPP-4) enzyme resulting in prolonged active incretin levels. Incretin hormones (eg, glucagon-like peptide-1 [GLP-1] and glucose-dependent insulinotropic polypeptide [GIP]) regulate glucose homeostasis by increasing insulin synthesis and release from pancreatic beta cells and decreasing glucagon secretion from pancreatic alpha cells. Decreased glucagon secretion results in decreased hepatic glucose production. Under normal physiologic circumstances, incretin hormones are released by the intestine throughout the day and levels are increased in response to a meal; incretin hormones are rapidly inactivated by the DPP-4 enzyme.

Pharmacodynamics/Kinetics

Half-life Elimination ~11 hours; Terminal (DPP-4 saturable binding): ~200 hours.

Time to Peak 1.5 hours

Pregnancy Considerations

Poorly controlled diabetes during pregnancy can be associated with an increased risk of adverse maternal and fetal outcomes, including diabetic ketoacidosis, preeclampsia, spontaneous abortion, preterm delivery, delivery complications, major birth defects, stillbirth, and macrosomia (ACOG 201 2018). To prevent adverse outcomes, prior to conception and throughout pregnancy, maternal blood glucose and HbA_{1c} should be kept as close to target goals as possible but without causing significant hypoglycemia (ADA 2020; Blumer 2013).

Agents other than linagliptin are currently recommended to treat diabetes mellitus in pregnancy (ADA 2020).

Linagliptin and Metformin
(lin a GLIP tin & met FOR min)

Related Information

LinaGLIPtin *on page 917*

MetFORMIN *on page 983*

Brand Names: US Jentadueto; Jentadueto XR

Brand Names: Canada Jentadueto

Pharmacologic Category Antidiabetic Agent, Biguanide; Antidiabetic Agent, Dipeptidyl Peptidase 4 (DPP-4) Inhibitor

Use Diabetes mellitus type 2, treatment: As an adjunct to diet and exercise to improve glycemic control in adults with type 2 diabetes mellitus.

Local Anesthetic/Vasoconstrictor Precautions No information available to require special precautions

Effects on Dental Treatment

Linagliptin-dependent patients with diabetes should be appointed for dental treatment in the morning in order to minimize chance of stress-induced hypoglycemia.

Metformin-dependent patients with diabetes (noninsulin dependent, Type 2) should be appointed for dental treatment in the morning in order to minimize chance of stress-induced hypoglycemia.

Effects on Bleeding No information available to require special precautions

Adverse Reactions Reactions/percentages reported with combination product; also see individual agents. Frequency not always defined.

Dermatologic: Pruritus

Gastrointestinal: Diarrhea (6%), decreased appetite, nausea, pancreatitis, vomiting

Hypersensitivity: Hypersensitivity reaction

Respiratory: Nasopharyngitis (6%), cough

<1%, postmarketing, and/or case reports: Severe arthralgia (FDA Safety Alert, Aug 28, 2015)

Mechanism of Action

Linagliptin inhibits dipeptidyl peptidase 4 (DPP-4) enzymes resulting in prolonged active incretin levels. Incretin hormones [eg, glucagon-like peptide-1 (GLP-1) and glucose-dependent insulinotropic polypeptide (GIP) regulate glucose homeostasis by increasing insulin synthesis and release from pancreatic beta cells and decreasing glucagon secretion from pancreatic alpha cells. Decreased glucagon secretion results in decreased hepatic glucose production. Under normal physiologic circumstances, incretin hormones are released by the intestine throughout the day and levels are increased in response to a meal; incretin hormones are rapidly inactivated by DPP-4 enzymes.

Metformin decreases hepatic glucose production, decreasing intestinal absorption of glucose, and improves insulin sensitivity (increases peripheral glucose uptake and utilization).

Pregnancy Considerations

Metformin crosses the placenta (ADA 2020). Refer to individual monographs for additional information.

- **Linagliptin and Metformin Hydrochloride** *see* Linagliptin and Metformin *on page 917*
- **Linagliptin, empagliflozin, and metformin hydrochloride** *see* Empagliflozin, Linagliptin, and Metformin *on page 555*
- **Linagliptin/Metformin HCl** *see* Linagliptin and Metformin *on page 917*
- **Linagliptin, metformin hydrochloride, and empagliflozin** *see* Empagliflozin, Linagliptin, and Metformin *on page 555*

Linezolid (li NE zoh lid)

Brand Names: US Zyvox

Brand Names: Canada APO-Linezolid; SANDOZ Linezolid; Zyvoxam

Pharmacologic Category Antibiotic, Oxazolidinone

Use

Enterococcal infections (vancomycin-resistant): Treatment of vancomycin-resistant *Enterococcus faecium* infections, including cases with concurrent bacteremia. **Note:** Not a preferred agent in resistant *Enterococcus faecalis* infections, which are usually susceptible to beta-lactams (O'Driscoll 2015).

Pneumonia:

Treatment of community-acquired pneumonia caused by *Streptococcus pneumoniae*, including cases with concurrent bacteremia, or *Staphylococcus aureus* (methicillin-susceptible isolates only).

Treatment of hospital-acquired or health care-associated pneumonia caused by *S. aureus* (methicillin-susceptible and methicillin-resistant isolates) or *S. pneumoniae*.

Skin and skin structure infections:

Complicated: Treatment of complicated skin and skin structure infections, including diabetic foot infections, without concomitant osteomyelitis, caused by *S. aureus* (methicillin-susceptible and methicillin-resistant isolates), *Streptococcus pyogenes*, or *Streptococcus agalactiae*.

Uncomplicated: Treatment of uncomplicated skin and skin structure infections caused by *S. aureus* (methicillin-susceptible isolates) or *S. pyogenes*.

Limitations of use: Linezolid has not been studied in the treatment of decubitus ulcers. Linezolid is not indicated for treatment of gram-negative infections; if a concomitant gram-negative pathogen is documented or suspected, initiate specific therapy immediately.

Local Anesthetic/Vasoconstrictor Precautions Linezolid has mild monoamine oxidase inhibitor properties. The clinician is reminded that vasoconstrictors have the potential to interact with MAO-Is to result in elevation of blood pressure. Caution is suggested.

Effects on Dental Treatment Key adverse event(s) related to dental treatment: Infrequent occurrence of oral *Candida* infection, taste alteration, and tongue discoloration; rare occurrence of tooth discoloration.

Effects on Bleeding Mylosuppression has been reported and usually dependant on duration of therapy; thrombocytopenia is the most frequently observed blood dyscrasia.

Adverse Reactions

>10%:

Gastrointestinal: Diarrhea (8% to 11%)

Hematologic & oncologic: Decreased white blood cells (neonates, infants, and children: 12%; children, adolescents, and adults: ≤2%), decreased platelet count (adults: ≤10%)

1% to 10%:

Central nervous system: Headache (children, adolescents, and adults: 6% to 9%; neonates, infants, and children: <1%), dizziness (adults: 2% to 3%), vertigo (children and adolescents: 1%)

Dermatologic: Skin rash (adults: 1% to 2%), pruritus (neonates, infants, children, and adolescents: ≤1%; nonapplication site)

Endocrine & metabolic: Increased amylase (≤2%), increased lactate dehydrogenase (adults: ≤2%)

Gastrointestinal: Vomiting (3% to 9%), nausea (2% to 7%), increased serum lipase (adults: 3% to 4%; children and adolescents: <1%), loose stools (neonates, infants, children, and adolescents: 2%), abdominal pain (≤2%), oral candidiasis (adults: ≤2%), dysgeusia (adults: 1% to 2%), tongue discoloration (≤1%)

Genitourinary: Vulvovaginal candidiasis (adults: 1% to 2%)

Hematologic & oncologic: Anemia (neonates, infants, and children: 6%; adults ≤2%), decreased neutrophils (neonates, infants, and children: 6%; children, adolescents, and adults: ≤1%), thrombocytopenia (neonates, infants, and children: 5%), eosinophilia (neonates, infants, children, and adolescents: ≤2%)

Hepatic: Increased serum ALT (2% to 10%), increased serum bilirubin (neonates, infants, and children: 6%; adults: <1%), increased serum AST (adults: 2% to 5%), increased serum alkaline phosphatase (adults: ≤4%), abnormal hepatic function tests (adults: ≤2%)

Infection: Fungal infection (adults: ≤2%)

Renal: Increased blood urea nitrogen (adults: ≤2%), increased serum creatinine (≤2%)

<1%, postmarketing, and/or case reports: Anaphylaxis, angioedema, blurred vision, bone marrow depression, bullous skin disease, *Clostridioides* (formerly *Clostridium*) *difficile*-associated diarrhea, dental discoloration, hypoglycemia, lactic acidosis, optic neuropathy, pancytopenia, peripheral neuropathy, seizure, serotonin syndrome (with concurrent use of other serotonergic agents), severe dermatological reaction, sideroblastic anemia, Stevens-Johnson syndrome, toxic epidermal necrolysis, vision loss

Mechanism of Action Inhibits bacterial protein synthesis by binding to bacterial 23S ribosomal RNA of the 50S subunit. This prevents the formation of a functional 70S initiation complex that is essential for the bacterial translation process. Linezolid is bacteriostatic against enterococci and staphylococci and bactericidal against most strains of streptococci.

Pharmacodynamics/Kinetics

Half-life Elimination

Preterm neonates <1 week: 5.6 hours

Full-term neonates <1 week: 3 hours

Full-term neonates ≥1 week to ≤28 days: 1.5 hours

Infants >28 days to <3 months: 1.8 hours

Infants and Children 3 months to 11 years: 2.9 hours

Adolescents: 4.1 hours

Adults: 4.9 hours

Time to Peak Adults: Oral: 1 to 2 hours

Pregnancy Considerations

Information related to linezolid use during pregnancy is limited (Jaspard 2017; Mercieri 2010). Due to pregnancy-induced physiologic changes, some pharmacokinetic properties of linezolid may be altered (van Kampenhout 2017).

◆ **Linzess** *see* LinaCLOtide *on page 916*

◆ **Lioresal** *see* Baclofen *on page 213*

Liothyronine (lye oh THYE roe neen)

Related Information

Endocrine Disorders and Pregnancy *on page 1684*

Brand Names: US Cytomel; Triostat

Brand Names: Canada Cytomel

Pharmacologic Category Thyroid Product

Use

Thyroid disorders: Oral: Replacement therapy in primary (thyroidal), secondary (pituitary), and tertiary (hypothalamic) congenital or acquired hypothyroidism; adjunct to surgery and radioiodine therapy in the management of well-differentiated thyroid cancer; a diagnostic agent in suppression tests to differentiate suspected mild hyperthyroidism or thyroid gland autonomy.

Limitations of use: Not indicated for suppression of benign thyroid nodules and nontoxic diffuse goiter in iodine-sufficient patients; not indicated for treatment of hypothyroidism during the recovery phase of subacute thyroiditis.

Myxedema coma: IV: Treatment of myxedema coma.

Note: May be used in patients allergic to desiccated thyroid or thyroid extract derived from pork or beef.

Local Anesthetic/Vasoconstrictor Precautions No precautions with vasoconstrictor are necessary if patient is well controlled with liothyronine

Effects on Dental Treatment No significant effects or complications reported

Effects on Bleeding No information available to require special precautions

Adverse Reactions

1% to 10%: Cardiovascular: Cardiac arrhythmia (6%), tachycardia (3%), hypotension (≤2%), myocardial infarction (≤2%)

<1%, postmarketing, and/or case reports: Allergic skin reaction, angina pectoris, cardiac failure, fever, hypertension, phlebitis, twitching

Mechanism of Action Exact mechanism of action is unknown; however, it is believed the thyroid hormone exerts its many metabolic effects through control of DNA transcription and protein synthesis; involved in normal metabolism, growth, and development; promotes gluconeogenesis, increases utilization and mobilization of glycogen stores, and stimulates protein synthesis, increases basal metabolic rate

Pharmacodynamics/Kinetics

Onset of Action

Oral: Within a few hours

Peak response: Oral: 2 to 3 days

Half-life Elimination 0.75 days (Brent 2011)

Pregnancy Considerations

Liothyronine has not been found to increase the risk of teratogenic or adverse effects following maternal use during pregnancy.

Uncontrolled maternal hypothyroidism may result in adverse neonatal and maternal outcomes. To prevent adverse events, normal maternal thyroid function should be maintained prior to conception and throughout pregnancy. Levothyroxine is considered the treatment of choice for the control of hypothyroidism during pregnancy (Stagnaro-Green 2011).

◆ **Liothyronine and Levothyroxine** *see* Liotrix *on page 919*

◆ **Liothyronine Sodium** *see* Liothyronine *on page 919*

Liotrix (LYE oh triks)

Related Information

Endocrine Disorders and Pregnancy *on page 1684*

Brand Names: US Thyrolar

Pharmacologic Category Thyroid Product

Use

Hypothyroidism: Replacement or supplemental therapy in hypothyroidism

Note: Clinical practice guidelines currently do not recommend routine use of levothyroxine/liothyronine combinations over levothyroxine monotherapy in the management of hypothyroidism (ATA [Jonklaas 2014]).

Local Anesthetic/Vasoconstrictor Precautions No precautions with vasoconstrictor are necessary if patient is well controlled with liotrix

Effects on Dental Treatment No significant effects or complications reported

Effects on Bleeding No information available to require special precautions

Adverse Reactions Frequency not defined.

Cardiovascular: Cardiac arrhythmia, chest pain, increased blood pressure, palpitations, tachycardia

Central nervous system: Anxiety, ataxia, headache, insomnia, nervousness
Dermatologic: Alopecia, diaphoresis, pruritus, urticaria
Endocrine & metabolic: Menstrual disease, weight loss
Gastrointestinal: Abdominal cramps, constipation, diarrhea, increased appetite, nausea, vomiting
Neuromuscular & skeletal: Myalgia, tremor, tremor of hands
Respiratory: Dyspnea
Miscellaneous: Fever
<1%, postmarketing, and/or case reports: Allergic skin reaction

Mechanism of Action The primary active compound is T_3 (triiodothyronine), which may be converted from T_4 (thyroxine) and then circulates throughout the body to influence growth and maturation of various tissues. Liotrix is uniform mixture of synthetic T_4 and T_3 in 4:1 ratio; exact mechanism of action is unknown; however, it is believed the thyroid hormone exerts its many metabolic effects through control of DNA transcription and protein synthesis; involved in normal metabolism, growth, and development; promotes gluconeogenesis, increases utilization and mobilization of glycogen stores and stimulates protein synthesis, increases basal metabolic rate

Pharmacodynamics/Kinetics

Onset of Action Liothyronine (T_3): ~3 hours

Half-life Elimination

T_4: Euthyroid: 6-7 days; Hyperthyroid: 3-4 days; Hypothyroid: 9-10 days
T_3: 2.5 days

Time to Peak Serum: T_4: 2-4 hours; T_3: 2-3 days

Pregnancy Considerations

Endogenous thyroid hormones minimally cross the placenta; the fetal thyroid becomes active around the end of the first trimester. Liotrix has not been found to increase the risk of adverse effects following maternal use during pregnancy.

Uncontrolled maternal hypothyroidism may result in adverse neonatal and maternal outcomes. To prevent adverse events, normal maternal thyroid function should be maintained prior to conception and throughout pregnancy. Levothyroxine is considered the treatment of choice for the control of hypothyroidism during pregnancy.

- ◆ **Lipiarrmycin** *see* Fidaxomicin *on page 668*
- ◆ **Lipitor** *see* AtorvaSTATin *on page 191*
- ◆ **Lipocaine 5 [OTC]** *see* Lidocaine (Topical) *on page 902*
- ◆ **Lipodox** *see* DOXOrubicin (Liposomal) *on page 521*
- ◆ **Lipodox 50 [DSC]** *see* DOXOrubicin (Liposomal) *on page 521*
- ◆ **Lipofen** *see* Fenofibrate and Derivatives *on page 640*
- ◆ **Liposomal Amphotericin** *see* Amphotericin B (Liposomal) *on page 138*
- ◆ **Liposomal Amphotericin B** *see* Amphotericin B (Liposomal) *on page 138*
- ◆ **Liposomal Bupivacaine** *see* Bupivacaine (Liposomal) *on page 259*
- ◆ **Liposomal Cytarabine** *see* Cytarabine (Liposomal) *on page 425*
- ◆ **Liposomal Cytarabine and Daunorubicin** *see* Daunorubicin and Cytarabine (Liposomal) *on page 445*
- ◆ **Liposomal Cytarabine-Daunorubicin** *see* Daunorubicin and Cytarabine (Liposomal) *on page 445*
- ◆ **Liposomal DAUNOrubicin** *see* DAUNOrubicin (Liposomal) *on page 446*
- ◆ **Liposomal Daunorubicin and Cytarabine** *see* Daunorubicin and Cytarabine (Liposomal) *on page 445*
- ◆ **Liposomal DOXOrubicin** *see* DOXOrubicin (Liposomal) *on page 521*
- ◆ **Liposomal Irinotecan** *see* Irinotecan (Liposomal) *on page 842*
- ◆ **Liposomal Vincristine** *see* VinCRIStine (Liposomal) *on page 1546*
- ◆ **Liposome-Encapsulated Daunorubicin-Cytarabine** *see* Daunorubicin and Cytarabine (Liposomal) *on page 445*
- ◆ **Liposome-Encapsulated Irinotecan Hydrochloride PEP02** *see* Irinotecan (Liposomal) *on page 842*
- ◆ **Liposome Vincristine** *see* VinCRIStine (Liposomal) *on page 1546*
- ◆ **LiProZonePak** *see* Lidocaine and Prilocaine *on page 911*
- ◆ **Liquigen [OTC]** *see* Medium Chain Triglycerides *on page 953*

Liraglutide (lir a GLOO tide)

Related Information

Endocrine Disorders and Pregnancy *on page 1684*

Brand Names: US Saxenda; Victoza

Brand Names: Canada Saxenda; Victoza

Pharmacologic Category Antidiabetic Agent, Glucagon-Like Peptide-1 (GLP-1) Receptor Agonist

Use

Chronic weight management (Saxenda): As an adjunct to a reduced-calorie diet and increased physical activity for chronic weight management in adult patients with an initial body mass index of ≥30 kg/m^2 (obesity) or ≥27 kg/m^2 (overweight) in the presence of at least 1 weight-related comorbid condition (eg, hypertension, type 2 diabetes mellitus, dyslipidemia).

Diabetes mellitus, type 2, treatment (Victoza): As an adjunct to diet and exercise to improve glycemic control in children ≥10 years of age, adolescents, and adults with type 2 diabetes mellitus; risk reduction of major cardiovascular events (cardiovascular death, nonfatal myocardial infarction, nonfatal stroke) in adults with type 2 diabetes mellitus and established cardiovascular disease.

Local Anesthetic/Vasoconstrictor Precautions No information available to require special precautions

Effects on Dental Treatment Key adverse event(s) related to dental treatment: Schedule type 1 and type 2 diabetic patients for dental treatment in the morning in order to minimize chance of stress-induced hypoglycemia. Occurrence of xerostomia during treatment for obesity (normal salivary flow resumes upon discontinuance). Type 2 diabetes, occurrence of nasopharyngitis; rare occurrence of distortion of the sense of taste (dysgeusia), facial edema, oropharyngeal edema.

Effects on Bleeding No information available to require special precautions

Adverse Reactions

Obesity:

>10%:

Cardiovascular: Increased heart rate (>10 bpm from baseline: 34%; >20 bpm from baseline: 5%)
Central nervous system: Headache (14%)

Endocrine & metabolic: Hypoglycemia (obesity patients with type 2 diabetics: combination therapy with sulfonylurea: 44%; monotherapy: 16%; nondiabetic patients: 2% to 3%)
Gastrointestinal: Nausea (39%), diarrhea (21%), constipation (19%), vomiting (16%)
Local: Injection site reaction (3% to 14%)
1% to 10%:
Cardiovascular: Tachycardia (6%; one resting heart rate >100 bpm)
Central nervous system: Fatigue (8%), dizziness (7%)
Dermatologic: Injection site pruritus (1% to 3%), rash at injection site (1% to 3%)
Endocrine & metabolic: Altered hormone level (1%; increased serum calcitonin)
Gastrointestinal: Decreased appetite (10%), dyspepsia (10%), abdominal distension (5%), abdominal pain (5%), eructation (5%), gastroenteritis (5%), gastroesophageal reflux disease (5%), upper abdominal pain (5%), increased serum lipase (2% to 5%), flatulence (4%), viral gastroenteritis (3%), cholelithiasis (2%), xerostomia (2%)
Genitourinary: Urinary tract infection (4%)
Immunologic: Antibody development (3%; neutralizing: 1%)
Local: Erythema at injection site (1% to 3%)
Neuromuscular & skeletal: Asthenia (2%)

Type 2 diabetes mellitus: Incidence reported with adult patients in monotherapy trials unless otherwise specified.
>10%:
Central nervous system: Headache (10% to 11%)
Endocrine & metabolic: Hypoglycemia (children and adolescents: 21%)
Gastrointestinal: Gastrointestinal disease (43%), nausea (18% to 20%), diarrhea (10% to 12%)
Infection: Infection (patients with antibodies: 40%)
Respiratory: Upper respiratory tract infection (7%; patients with antibodies: 11%)
1% to 10%:
Dermatologic: Rash at injection site
Gastrointestinal: Decreased appetite (9% to 10%), dyspepsia (combination trials: 9%, monotherapy: 4% to 7%), vomiting (6% to 9%), increased serum lipase (8%), constipation (5%), cholelithiasis (2%), cholecystitis (1%), increased amylase (1%)
Hepatic: Hyperbilirubinemia (monotherapy and combination trials: 4%)
Immunologic: Antibody development (≤9%; neutralizing antibodies: 2%)
Local: Injection site reaction (monotherapy and combination trials: 2%), erythema at injection site
Neuromuscular & skeletal: Back pain (4% to 5%)
Respiratory: Nasopharyngitis (9% to 10%)

<1%, postmarketing, and/or case reports (any indication): Acute pancreatitis, acute renal failure, anaphylaxis, angioedema, asthma, benign gastrointestinal neoplasm (colorectal), bronchospasm, cholecystitis, cholestasis, dehydration, dysgeusia, exacerbation of renal failure, facial edema, first degree atrioventricular block, hemorrhagic pancreatitis, hepatitis, hypersensitivity reaction, increased liver enzymes, increased serum creatinine, increased susceptibility to infection, left bundle branch block, malaise, malignant neoplasm, malignant neoplasm of breast, malignant neoplasm of colon or rectum, medullary thyroid carcinoma, necrotizing pancreatitis, oropharyngeal edema, pancreatitis, papillary thyroid carcinoma, pharyngeal edema, pruritus, right bundle branch block, skin rash, suicidal ideation, systolic hypotension, thyroid disease (C-cell hyperplasia), urticaria

Mechanism of Action Liraglutide is a long acting analog of human glucagon-like peptide-1 (GLP-1) (an incretin hormone) which increases glucose-dependent insulin secretion, decreases inappropriate glucagon secretion, increases B-cell growth/replication, slows gastric emptying, and decreases food intake. Liraglutide administration results in decreases in hemoglobin A_{1c} by approximately 1%.

Pharmacodynamics/Kinetics

Half-life Elimination ~13 hours

Time to Peak Plasma: SubQ: 8 to 12 hours

Pregnancy Considerations

Use of liraglutide for chronic weight management is contraindicated in pregnant women (lack of potential benefit and possible fetal harm). An increased risk of adverse maternal and fetal outcomes is associated with obesity; however, medications for weight loss therapy are not recommended at conception or during pregnancy (ACOG 156 2015).

Poorly controlled diabetes during pregnancy can be associated with an increased risk of adverse maternal and fetal outcomes, including diabetic ketoacidosis, preeclampsia, spontaneous abortion, preterm delivery, delivery complications, major birth defects, stillbirth, and macrosomia (ACOG 201 2018). To prevent adverse outcomes, prior to conception and throughout pregnancy, maternal blood glucose and HbA_{1c} should be kept as close to target goals as possible but without causing significant hypoglycemia (ADA 2020; Blumer 2013).

Agents other than liraglutide are currently recommended to treat diabetes in pregnant women (ADA 2020).

◆ **Liraglutide and Insulin Degludec** *see* Insulin Degludec and Liraglutide *on page 820*

Lisdexamfetamine (lis dex am FET a meen)

Brand Names: US Vyvanse

Brand Names: Canada Vyvanse

Pharmacologic Category Central Nervous System Stimulant

Use

Attention-deficit/hyperactivity disorder: Treatment of attention-deficit/hyperactivity disorder (ADHD).

Binge eating disorder: Treatment of moderate to severe binge eating disorder in adults.

Local Anesthetic/Vasoconstrictor Precautions Use vasoconstrictor with caution in patients taking lisdexamfetamine. Amphetamines enhance the sympathomimetic response of epinephrine or mepivacaine and levonordefrin (Carbocaine® 2% with Neo-Cobefrin®) leading to potential hypertension and cardiotoxicity.

Effects on Dental Treatment Key adverse event(s) related to dental treatment: Lisdexamfetamine causes tachycardia, increases in blood pressure, and palpitations. Consider monitoring blood pressure prior to using local anesthetic with a vasoconstrictor. Symptoms associated with bruxism have been observed in some patients.

Effects on Bleeding No information available to require special precautions

Adverse Reactions

>10%:
Central nervous system: Insomnia (13% to 27%)

Gastrointestinal: Decreased appetite (children and adolescents 34% to 39%; adults 8% to 27%), xerostomia (adults: 26% to 36%; children and adolescents: 4% to 5%), upper abdominal pain (children: 12%; adults: 2%)

1% to 10%:

Cardiovascular: Increased heart rate (adults: 2% to 7%), increased blood pressure (adults: 3%), palpitations (2%)

Central nervous system: Irritability (children: 10%), anxiety (adults: 5% to 6%), jitteriness (adults: 4% to 6%), dizziness (children: 5%), agitation (adults: 3%), emotional lability (children: 3%), restlessness (adults: 2% to 3%), drowsiness (children: 2%), increased energy (adults: 2%), nightmares (adults: 2%), paresthesia (adults: 2%), tic disorder (children: 2%)

Dermatologic: Hyperhidrosis (adults: 3% to 4%), skin rash (children: 3%), pruritus (adults: 2%)

Endocrine & metabolic: Weight loss (children and adolescents: 9%; adults: 3% to 4%), decreased libido (adults: 2%)

Gastrointestinal: Vomiting (children: 9%; adults: 2%), diarrhea (adults: 4% to 7%), nausea (6% to 7%), constipation (adults: 6%), anorexia (2% to 5%), gastroenteritis (adults: 2%)

Genitourinary: Erectile dysfunction (adults: 3%), urinary tract infection (adults: 2%)

Neuromuscular & skeletal: Tremor (2%)

Respiratory: Dyspnea (adults: 2%), oropharyngeal pain (2%)

Miscellaneous: Fever (children: 2%)

Frequency not defined:

Central nervous system: Drug abuse, drug dependence, talkativeness

<1%, postmarketing, and/or case reports: Accommodation disturbance, aggressive behavior, alopecia, anaphylaxis, angioedema, blurred vision, bruxism, cardiomyopathy, chest pain, decreased linear skeletal growth rate, depression, dermatillomania, diplopia, dysgeusia, dyskinesia, frequent erections, hepatitis (eosinophilic), hypersensitivity condition, mydriasis, peripheral vascular insufficiency, prolonged erection, rhabdomyolysis, Raynaud's disease, seizure, Stevens-Johnson syndrome, urticaria

Mechanism of Action The exact mechanism of lisdexamfetamine in ADHD and binge eating disorder is not known. Lisdexamfetamine dimesylate is a prodrug that is converted to the active component dextroamphetamine (a noncatecholamine, sympathomimetic amine). Amphetamines are noncatecholamine, sympathomimetic amines that cause release of catecholamines (primarily dopamine and norepinephrine) from their storage sites in the presynaptic nerve terminals. A less significant mechanism may include their ability to block the reuptake of catecholamines by competitive inhibition.

Pharmacodynamics/Kinetics

Duration of Action 8 to 14 hours (Jain 2017)

Half-life Elimination Lisdexamfetamine: <1 hour; Dextroamphetamine: 10 to 13 hours

Time to Peak

Capsule: T_{max}: Lisdexamfetamine: Children 6 to 12 years: 1 hour (fasting); Adults: ~1 hour; Dextroamphetamine: Children 6 to 12 years: 3.5 hours (fasting); Adults: 3.8 hours (fasting), 4.7 hours (after a high-fat meal)

Chewable tablet: T_{max}: Lisdexamfetamine: 1 hour (fasting); Dextroamphetamine: 3.9 to 4.4 hours (fasting); 4.9 hours (after a high-fat meal)

Pregnancy Considerations Lisdexamfetamine is converted to dextroamphetamine. The majority of human data is based on illicit amphetamine/methamphetamine exposure and not from therapeutic maternal use (Golub 2005). Use of amphetamines during pregnancy may lead to an increased risk of premature birth and low birth weight; newborns may experience symptoms of withdrawal. Behavioral problems may also occur later in childhood (LaGasse 2012).

Controlled Substance C-II

◆ **Lisdexamfetamine Dimesylate** *see* Lisdexamfetamine *on page 921*

◆ **Lisdexamphetamine** *see* Lisdexamfetamine *on page 921*

Lisinopril (lyse IN oh pril)

Related Information

Cardiovascular Diseases *on page 1654*

Brand Names: US Prinivil; Qbrelis; Zestril

Brand Names: Canada ACT Lisinopril [DSC]; APO-Lisinopril; Auro-Lisinopril; DOM-Lisinopril; JAMP-Lisinopril; MYLAN-Lisinopril [DSC]; PMS-Lisinopril; Prinivil; PRO-Lisinopril-10; PRO-Lisinopril-20; PRO-Lisinopril-5; RAN-Lisinopril; RIVA-Lisinopril [DSC]; SANDOZ Lisinopril; TEVA-Lisinopril (Type P); TEVA-Lisinopril (Type Z); Zestril

Pharmacologic Category Angiotensin-Converting Enzyme (ACE) Inhibitor; Antihypertensive

Use

Heart failure with reduced ejection fraction: Adjunctive therapy to reduce signs and symptoms of systolic heart failure.

Hypertension: Management of hypertension in adult and pediatric patients ≥6 years of age.

ST-elevation myocardial infarction: Treatment of acute MI within 24 hours in hemodynamically stable patients to improve survival.

Local Anesthetic/Vasoconstrictor Precautions

No information available to require special precautions

Effects on Dental Treatment Key adverse event(s) related to dental treatment: Infrequent occurrences of xerostomia, cough, Stevens-Johnson syndrome, and dysgeusia. Orthostatic hypotension may occur; use caution with sudden changes in position during and after dental treatment.

An angiotensin-converting enzyme (ACE) Inhibitor cough is a dry, hacking, nonproductive cough that can potentially interfere with longer dental procedures if patient has this side effect.

Effects on Bleeding No information available to require special precautions

Adverse Reactions

>10%:

Cardiovascular: Hypotension (4% to 11%)

Central nervous system: Dizziness (4% to 19%)

Renal: Increased serum creatinine (≤10%; transient), increased blood urea nitrogen (≤2%; transient)

1% to 10%:

Cardiovascular: Syncope (5% to 7%), chest pain (2% to 3%), flushing (≥1%), orthostatic effect (≥1%), vasculitis (≥1%)

Central nervous system: Headache (4% to 6%), altered sense of smell (≥1%), fatigue (≥1%), paresthesia (≥1%), vertigo (≥1%)

Dermatologic: Skin rash (≥1% to 2%), alopecia (≥1%), diaphoresis (≥1%), erythema (≥1%), pruritus (≥1%), skin photosensitivity (≥1%), Stevens-Johnson syndrome (≥1%), toxic epidermal necrolysis (≥1%), urticaria (≥1%)
Endocrine & metabolic: Hyperkalemia (2% to 6%), diabetes mellitus (≥1%), gout (≥1%), SIADH (≥1%)
Gastrointestinal: Diarrhea (≥1% to 4%), constipation (≥1%), dysgeusia (≥1%), flatulence (≥1%), pancreatitis (≥1%), xerostomia (≥1%)
Genitourinary: Impotence (≥1%)
Hematologic & oncologic: Bone marrow depression (≥1%), eosinophilia (≥1%), hemolytic anemia (≥1%), increased erythrocyte sedimentation rate (≥1%), leukocytosis (≥1%), leukopenia (≥1%), neutropenia (≥1%), positive ANA titer (≥1%), thrombocytopenia (≥1%; mean decrease of 0.4 mg/dL)
Neuromuscular & skeletal: Arthralgia (≥1%), arthritis (≥1%), myalgia (≥1%), weakness (≥1%)
Ophthalmic: Blurred vision (≥1%), diplopia (≥1%), photophobia (≥1%), vision loss (≥1%)
Otic: Tinnitus (≥1%)
Renal: Renal insufficiency (in patients with acute myocardial infarction: 1% to 2%)
Respiratory: Cough (3% to 4%)

Frequency not defined:
Hematologic & oncologic: Decreased hematocrit, decreased hemoglobin (mean decrease of 1.3%)
Hepatic: Increased liver enzymes, increased serum bilirubin

<1%, postmarketing, and/or case reports: Acute renal failure, angioedema, confusion, cutaneous pseudolymphoma, dehydration, fever, hallucination, hypoglycemia (diabetic patients on oral antidiabetic agents or insulin), hyponatremia, mood changes (including depressive symptoms), psoriasis, visual hallucination

Mechanism of Action Competitive inhibitor of angiotensin-converting enzyme (ACE); prevents conversion of angiotensin I to angiotensin II, a potent vasoconstrictor; results in lower levels of angiotensin II which causes an increase in plasma renin activity and a reduction in aldosterone secretion; a CNS mechanism may also be involved in hypotensive effect as angiotensin II increases adrenergic outflow from CNS; vasoactive kallikreins may be decreased in conversion to active hormones by ACE inhibitors, thus reducing blood pressure

Pharmacodynamics/Kinetics

Onset of Action 1 hour; Peak effect: Hypotensive: Oral: ~6 hours

Duration of Action 24 hours

Half-life Elimination 12 hours

Time to Peak

Pediatric patients 6 months to 15 years: Median (range): 5 to 6 hours (Hogg 2007)
Adults: ~7 hours

Reproductive Considerations

Angiotensin-converting enzyme (ACE) inhibitors should be avoided in sexually active females of reproductive potential not using effective contraception (ADA 2020).

ACE inhibitors should generally be avoided for the treatment of hypertension in women planning a pregnancy; use should only be considered for cases of hypertension refractory to other medications (ACOG 203 2019).

Pregnancy Considerations

Lisinopril crosses the placenta (Bhatt-Mehta 1993; Filler 2003).

Exposure to an angiotensin-converting enzyme (ACE) inhibitor during the first trimester of pregnancy may be associated with an increased risk of fetal malformations (ACOG 203 2019; ESC [Regitz-Zagrosek 2018]); however, outcomes observed may also be influenced by maternal disease (ACC/AHA [Whelton 2017]).

[US Boxed Warning]: Drugs that act on the renin-angiotensin system can cause injury and death to the developing fetus. Discontinue as soon as possible once pregnancy is detected.

Drugs that act on the renin-angiotensin system are associated with oligohydramnios. Oligohydramnios, due to decreased fetal renal function, may lead to fetal lung hypoplasia and skeletal malformations. The use of these drugs in pregnancy is also associated with anuria, hypotension, renal failure, skull hypoplasia, and death in the fetus/neonate. Infants exposed to an ACE inhibitor in utero should be monitored for hyperkalemia, hypotension, and oliguria. Oligohydramnios may not appear until after irreversible fetal injury has occurred. Exchange transfusions or dialysis may be required to reverse hypotension or improve renal function, although data related to the effectiveness in neonates is limited.

Chronic maternal hypertension is also associated with adverse events in the fetus/infant. Chronic maternal hypertension may increase the risk of birth defects, low birth weight, premature delivery, stillbirth, and neonatal death. Actual fetal/neonatal risks may be related to duration and severity of maternal hypertension. Untreated chronic hypertension may also increase the risks of adverse maternal outcomes, including gestational diabetes, pre-eclampsia, delivery complications, stroke and myocardial infarction (ACOG 203 2019).

When treatment of hypertension in pregnancy is indicated, ACE inhibitors should generally be avoided due to their adverse fetal events; use in pregnant women should only be considered for cases of hypertension refractory to other medications (ACOG 203 2019). ACE inhibitors are not recommended for the treatment of heart failure in pregnancy (Regitz-Zagrosek [ESC 2018]).

- ◆ **Lispro Insulin** *see* Insulin Lispro *on page 824*
- ◆ **Lispro Insulin and Insulin Lispro Protamine** *see* Insulin Lispro Protamine and Insulin Lispro *on page 826*
- ◆ **Listerine Antiseptic [OTC]** *see* Mouthwash (Antiseptic) *on page 1062*
- ◆ **Listerine Naturals Antiseptic [OTC]** *see* Mouthwash (Antiseptic) *on page 1062*
- ◆ **Listerine Ultraclean Antiseptic [OTC]** *see* Mouthwash (Antiseptic) *on page 1062*

Lithium (LITH ee um)

Brand Names: US Lithobid

Brand Names: Canada APO-Lithium Carbonate; Carbolith; DOM-Lithium Carbonate; Lithane; Lithmax; PMS-Lithium Carbonate; PMS-Lithium Citrate

Pharmacologic Category Antimanic Agent

Use

Bipolar disorder:

Immediate release: Treatment of manic and mixed episodes and maintenance treatment in patients ≥7 years of age with a diagnosis of bipolar disorder.

Extended release: Treatment of manic episodes and maintenance treatment in patients ≥12 years of age with a diagnosis of bipolar disorder.

Local Anesthetic/Vasoconstrictor Precautions No information available to require special precautions

Effects on Dental Treatment Key adverse event(s) related to dental treatment: Xerostomia and changes in salivation (normal salivary flow resumes upon discontinuation), salivary gland swelling, and metallic taste. Avoid NSAIDs if analgesics are required since lithium toxicity has been reported with concomitant administration; acetaminophen products (ie, singly or with opioids) are recommended.

Effects on Bleeding No information available to require special precautions

Adverse Reactions

>10%: Endocrine & metabolic: Hypothyroidism (females: 14%; males: 5% [Johnston 1999]; children and adolescents: <1% [Findling 2015])

Frequency not defined:

Cardiovascular: Abnormal T waves on ECG, bradycardia, cardiac arrhythmia (including unmasking of Brugada Syndrome), chest tightness, circulatory shock, cold extremities, edema, hypotension, myxedema, sinus node dysfunction, syncope

Dermatologic: Alopecia, dermal ulcer, dry and/or thinning hair, exacerbation of psoriasis, folliculitis, pruritus, psoriasis, skin rash, xeroderma

Endocrine & metabolic: Albuminuria, dehydration, diabetes insipidus, euthyroid goiter, glycosuria, hypercalcemia (including secondary to hyperparathyroidism [McKnight 2012]), hyperglycemia, hyperparathyroidism, hyperthyroidism, increased thirst, nephrogenic diabetes insipidus, polydipsia, weight gain, weight loss

Gastrointestinal: Abdominal pain, anorexia, dental caries, diarrhea, dysgeusia, dyspepsia, fecal incontinence, flatulence, gastritis, nausea, salivary gland disease (swelling), sialorrhea, swelling of lips, tongue changes (movement), vomiting, xerostomia

Genitourinary: Glomerulopathy (fibrosis), impotence, incontinence, nephron atrophy, nephrotic syndrome, oliguria, sexual disorder

Hematologic & oncologic: Leukocytosis

Hypersensitivity: Angioedema

Immunologic: Drug reaction with eosinophilia and systemic symptoms

Local: Localized edema (ankles and wrists), local pain (fingers and toes), local skin discoloration (fingers and toes)

Nervous system: Abnormal electroencephalogram (diffuse slowing, potentiation, disorganization of background rhythm), ataxia, blackout spells, cogwheel rigidity, coma, confusion, decreased mental acuity (worsening of organic brain syndromes), dizziness, drowsiness, dystonic reaction, extrapyramidal reaction, fatigue, hallucination, headache, hyperactive behavior (startled response), hyperactive deep tendon reflex, hypertonia, idiopathic intracranial hypertension, involuntary choreoathetoid movements, lethargy, local anesthesia (skin), memory impairment, metallic taste, psychomotor impairment, reduced intellectual ability, restlessness, salty taste, sedated state, seizure, slowed intellectual functioning, slurred speech, stupor, tics, vertigo

Neuromuscular & skeletal: Joint swelling, muscle hyperirritability, polyarthralgia, tremor

Ophthalmic: Blurred vision, exophthalmos, nystagmus, transient scotoma

Otic: Tinnitus

Renal: Decreased creatinine clearance, polyuria, renal concentrating defect

Miscellaneous: Fever, interstitial fibrosis, iodism (elevated iodine uptake)

Postmarketing: Intracranial hypertension (Tan 2019), lupus-like syndrome (Shukla 1982)

Mechanism of Action The precise mechanism of action in mood disorders is unknown. Traditionally thought to alter cation transport across cell membranes in nerve and muscle cells, influence the reuptake of serotonin and/or norepinephrine, and inhibit second messenger systems involving the phosphatidylinositol cycle (Ward 1994). May also provide neuroprotective effects by increasing glutamate clearance, inhibiting apoptotic glycogen synthase kinase activity, increasing the levels of antiapoptotic protein Bcl-2 and, enhancing the expression of neurotropic factors, including brain-derived neurotrophic factor (Sanacora 2008).

Pharmacodynamics/Kinetics

Half-life Elimination

Pediatric patients 7 to 17 years: $t_{1/2\ (beta)}$: 27 hours (Findling 2010)

Adults: 18 to 36 hours; prolonged in elderly patients (28.5 hours) (Ward 1994)

Time to Peak Serum: Nonsustained release: ~0.5 to 3 hours; Extended release: 2 to 6 hours; Solution: 15 to 60 minutes (Ward 1994)

Pregnancy Considerations Lithium crosses the placenta in concentrations similar to those in the maternal plasma (Newport 2005).

Cardiac malformations in the infant, including Ebstein anomaly, are associated with use of lithium during the first trimester of pregnancy. Other adverse events including polyhydramnios, fetal/neonatal cardiac arrhythmias, hypoglycemia, diabetes insipidus, changes in thyroid function, premature delivery, floppy infant syndrome, or neonatal lithium toxicity are associated with lithium exposure when used later in pregnancy (ACOG 2008). The incidence of adverse events may be associated with higher maternal doses (Newport 2005). Fetal echocardiography should be considered if first trimester exposure occurs (ACOG 2008).

Due to pregnancy-induced physiologic changes, women who are pregnant may require dose adjustments of lithium to achieve euthymia and avoid toxicity (ACOG 2008; Grandjean 2009; Yonkers 2011).

For planned pregnancies, use of lithium during the first trimester should be avoided if possible (Grandjean 2009). However, the absolute risk of Ebstein anomaly is small and treatment for bipolar disorder should not be withheld when clinically indicated (Larsen 2015). If lithium is needed during pregnancy, the minimum effective dose should be used, maternal serum concentrations should be monitored, and consideration should be given to start therapy after the period of organogenesis; lithium should be suspended 24 to 48 hours prior to delivery or at the onset of labor when delivery is spontaneous, then restarted when the patient is medically stable after delivery (ACOG 2008; Grandjean 2009; Newport 2005).

- **Lithium Carbonate** *see* Lithium *on page 923*
- **Lithium Citrate** *see* Lithium *on page 923*
- **Lithobid** *see* Lithium *on page 923*
- **Little Colds Cough Formula [OTC]** *see* Dextromethorphan *on page 476*
- **Little Colds Decongestant [OTC]** *see* Phenylephrine (Systemic) *on page 1227*

- **Little Fevers [OTC]** *see* Acetaminophen *on page 59*
- **Livalo** *see* Pitavastatin *on page 1238*
- **Live Attenuated Influenza Vaccine** *see* Influenza Virus Vaccine (Live/Attenuated) *on page 813*
- **Live Attenuated Influenza Vaccine (Quadrivalent)** *see* Influenza Virus Vaccine (Live/Attenuated) *on page 813*
- **Livixil Pak** *see* Lidocaine and Prilocaine *on page 911*

Lixisenatide (lix i SEN a tide)

Brand Names: US Adlyxin; Adlyxin Starter Pack

Brand Names: Canada Adlyxin; Adlyxin Starter Pack [DSC]

Pharmacologic Category Antidiabetic Agent, Glucagon-Like Peptide-1 (GLP-1) Receptor Agonist

Use Diabetes mellitus, type 2, treatment: As an adjunct to diet and exercise to improve glycemic control in adults with type 2 diabetes mellitus.

Local Anesthetic/Vasoconstrictor Precautions No information available to require special precautions

Effects on Dental Treatment No significant effects or complications reported

Effects on Bleeding No information available to require special precautions

Adverse Reactions

>10%:

Gastrointestinal: Gastrointestinal symptoms (40%; most were mild to moderate and within the first 3 weeks of starting treatment), nausea (25%)

Immunologic: Antibody development (70%: 2% had high antibody concentrations [>100 nmol/L] and experienced an attenuated glycemic response)

1% to 10%:

Central nervous system: Headache (9%), dizziness (7%)

Gastrointestinal: Vomiting (10%), diarrhea (8%), constipation (3%), dyspepsia (3%), abdominal distension (2%), upper abdominal pain (2%)

Local: Injection site reaction (4%; including pain, pruritus, and erythema)

<1%, postmarketing, and/or case reports: Acute renal injury, hypersensitivity reaction, pancreatitis (acute, chronic, and edematous), renal insufficiency

Mechanism of Action Lixisenatide is a selective glucagon-like peptide-1 (GLP-1) receptor agonist. Acting on the same receptor as the endogenous hormone incretin, lixisenatide increases glucose-dependent insulin secretion, decreases inappropriate glucagon secretion, and slows gastric emptying.

Pharmacodynamics/Kinetics

Half-life Elimination ~3 hours

Time to Peak 1 to 3.5 hours

Pregnancy Considerations

Poorly controlled diabetes during pregnancy can be associated with an increased risk of adverse maternal and fetal outcomes, including diabetic ketoacidosis, preeclampsia, spontaneous abortion, preterm delivery, delivery complications, major birth defects, stillbirth, and macrosomia (ACOG 201 2018). To prevent adverse outcomes, prior to conception and throughout pregnancy, maternal blood glucose and HbA_{1c} should be kept as close to target goals as possible but without causing significant hypoglycemia (ADA 2020; Blumer 2013).

Agents other than lixisenatide are currently recommended to treat diabetes mellitus in pregnancy (ADA 2020).

- **Lixisenatide and Insulin Glargine** *see* Insulin Glargine and Lixisenatide *on page 823*
- **L-leucovorin** *see* LEVOleucovorin *on page 899*

L-Lysine (el LYE seen)

Related Information

Viral Infections *on page 1754*

Brand Names: US Lysine4000 [OTC]

Generic Availability (US) Yes

Pharmacologic Category Nutritional Supplement

Dental Use Prevention of recurrent herpes simplex infection

Use Dietary supplement: Essential amino acid that regulates immune response helping to manage stress in body.

Local Anesthetic/Vasoconstrictor Precautions No information available to require special precautions

Effects on Dental Treatment No significant effects or complications reported

Effects on Bleeding No information available to require special precautions

Dental Usual Dosage Recurrent herpes simplex infection: Adults: Oral: 500-3000 mg/day; begin treatment during early stage of recurrence.

Dosing

Adult & Geriatric

Dietary supplement: Oral: **Note:** Dosage varies; also consult specific product information.

Capsule: One capsule 1 to 3 times daily

Powder: 1/4 level teaspoonful once daily

Tablet: 1 to 2 tablets daily

Renal Impairment: Adult There are no dosage adjustments provided in the manufacturer's labeling.

Hepatic Impairment: Adult There are no dosage adjustments provided in the manufacturer's labeling.

Pregnancy Considerations L-lysine crosses the placenta in humans (Ronzoni, 1999; Schneider, 1979). Lysine is an essential amino acid. The RDA for lysine is increased in pregnant women (IOM, 2005).

Breastfeeding Considerations Lysine is an essential amino acid and is found in breast milk. The RDA for lysine is increased in breastfeeding women (IOM, 2005).

Dosage Forms: US

Capsule, Oral:

Generic: 500 mg

Packet, Oral:

Lysine4000 [OTC]: 4000 mg (30 ea)

Tablet, Oral:

Generic: 500 mg, 1000 mg

- **L-Lysine Hydrochloride** *see* L-Lysine *on page 925*
- **LM3100** *see* Plerixafor *on page 1241*
- **L-methylfolate** *see* Methylfolate *on page 996*
- **L-Methylfolate Formula 7.5 [DSC]** *see* Methylfolate *on page 996*
- **L-Methylfolate Formula 15 [DSC]** *see* Methylfolate *on page 996*
- **L-Methylfolate Forte** *see* Methylfolate *on page 996*
- **LMX 4 [OTC]** *see* Lidocaine (Topical) *on page 902*
- **LMX 4 Plus [OTC]** *see* Lidocaine (Topical) *on page 902*
- **LMX 5 [OTC]** *see* Lidocaine (Topical) *on page 902*
- **Locoid** *see* Hydrocortisone (Topical) *on page 775*

◆ **Locoid Lipocream** *see* Hydrocortisone (Topical) *on page 775*

◆ **LoCort 7-Day [DSC]** *see* DexAMETHasone (Systemic) *on page 463*

◆ **LoCort 11-Day [DSC]** *see* DexAMETHasone (Systemic) *on page 463*

◆ **Lodine** *see* Etodolac *on page 622*

◆ **Lodosyn** *see* Carbidopa *on page 289*

Lodoxamide (loe DOKS a mide)

Brand Names: US Alomide
Brand Names: Canada Alomide
Pharmacologic Category Mast Cell Stabilizer
Use Ocular disorders: Treatment of the ocular disorders referred to by the terms vernal keratoconjunctivitis, vernal conjunctivitis, and vernal keratitis

Local Anesthetic/Vasoconstrictor Precautions No information available to require special precautions

Effects on Dental Treatment No significant effects or complications reported

Effects on Bleeding No information available to require special precautions

Adverse Reactions

>10%: Ophthalmic: Burning sensation of eyes (transient), eye discomfort (transient), stinging of eyes (transient)

1% to 10%:

Central nervous system: Foreign body sensation of eye, headache

Ophthalmic: Blurred vision, crystalline eye deposits, eye pruritus, lacrimation, ocular hyperemia, ocular edema, xerophthalmia

1%, postmarketing, and/or case reports: Asthenopia, blepharitis, chemosis, corneal abrasion, corneal erosion, corneal ulcer, dizziness, drowsiness, dry nose, epitheliopathy, eye pain, keratitis, nausea, ocular warming sensation, skin rash, sneezing, stomach discomfort, swelling of eye

Mechanism of Action Mast cell stabilizer that inhibits the *in vivo* type I immediate hypersensitivity reaction to increase cutaneous vascular permeability associated with IgE and antigen-mediated reactions

Pharmacodynamics/Kinetics

Half-life Elimination 8.5 hours

Pregnancy Considerations Adverse events have not been observed in animal reproduction studies following oral administration. The amount of lodoxamide available systemically following ophthalmic administration is below the level of detection.

◆ **Lodoxamide Tromethamine** *see* Lodoxamide *on page 926*

◆ **Loestrin 1.5/30 (21)** *see* Ethinyl Estradiol and Norethindrone *on page 614*

◆ **Loestrin 1/20 (21)** *see* Ethinyl Estradiol and Norethindrone *on page 614*

◆ **Loestrin Fe 1.5/30** *see* Ethinyl Estradiol and Norethindrone *on page 614*

◆ **Loestrin Fe 1/20** *see* Ethinyl Estradiol and Norethindrone *on page 614*

Lofexidine (loe FEX i deen)

Brand Names: US Lucemyra
Pharmacologic Category $Alpha_2$-Adrenergic Agonist
Use Opioid withdrawal: Mitigation of opioid withdrawal symptoms to facilitate abrupt opioid discontinuation in adults.

Local Anesthetic/Vasoconstrictor Precautions Rare occurrence of prolonged QT interval has been reported for lofexidine. The risk of drug-induced torsades de pointes (arrhythmias) is extremely low when a single QT interval prolonging drug is prescribed. In terms of epinephrine, it is not known what effect vasoconstrictors in the local anesthetic regimen will have in patients with a known history of congenital prolonged QT interval or in patients taking any medication that prolongs the QT interval. Until more information is obtained, it is suggested that the clinician consult with the physician prior to the use of a vasoconstrictor in suspected patients, and that the vasoconstrictor (epinephrine, levonordefrin [Neo-Cobefrin]) be used with caution.

Effects on Dental Treatment Key adverse event(s) related to dental treatment: Frequent occurrence of xerostomia; normal salivation resumes with discontinuation; orthostatic hypotension has been reported, patients may experience hypotension as they arise from the dental chair; monitor patient for signs of dizziness.

Effects on Bleeding No information available to require special precautions

Adverse Reactions

>10%:

Cardiovascular: Orthostatic hypotension (29% to 42%), bradycardia (24% to 32%), hypotension (30%)

Central nervous system: Insomnia (51% to 55%), dizziness (19% to 23%), sedation (12% to 13%), drowsiness (11% to 13%)

Gastrointestinal: Xerostomia (10% to 11%)

1% to 10%:

Cardiovascular: Syncope (≤1%)

Otic: Tinnitus (≤3%)

<1%, postmarketing, and/or case reports: Prolonged QT interval on ECG, torsades de pointes

Mechanism of Action Lofexidine is a central alpha-2 adrenergic agonist that reduces the release of norepinephrine and decreases sympathetic tone. It binds to alpha-2A (k_i=7.2 nM) and alpha-2C (k_i=12 nM) adrenoreceptors. Due to its high selectivity for the alpha-2A receptor, lofexidine is thought to be associated with less anti-hypertensive activity than clonidine (Gish 2010).

Pharmacodynamics/Kinetics

Half-life Elimination 11 to 13 hours (first dose); 17 to 22 hours (steady state)

Time to Peak 3 to 5 hours

Pregnancy Considerations Information related to the use of lofexidine in pregnancy is limited (Akhurst 2000). Abrupt discontinuation of opioid therapy in dependent females is generally not recommended during pregnancy (Kampman 2015).

Dental Health Professional Considerations Lofexidine is a nonopioid agent approved for opioid detoxification. It is an $alpha_2$-agonist structurally related to clonidine. This family of drugs was originally approved as antihypertensive agents, but it was observed that lofexidine was not an effective antihypertensive drug. The effects of lofexidine is to decrease the CNS sympathetic outflow responsible for many opioid withdrawal symptoms. According to a Cochrane review of controlled trials, lofexidine was more effective than placebo for the management of withdrawal from heroin or methadone. There was no significant difference in the efficacy between treatment regimens based on clonidine or lofexidine and those based on reducing doses of methadone over a period of around 10 days. Lofexidine had a better safety profile than clonidine.

◆ **Lofexidine Hydrochloride** *see* Lofexidine *on page 926*

◆ **Lofibra [DSC]** *see* Fenofibrate and Derivatives *on page 640*

◆ **LoHist-D [OTC]** *see* Chlorpheniramine and Pseudoephedrine *on page 341*

◆ **L-OHP** *see* Oxaliplatin *on page 1151*

◆ **LoJaimiess** *see* Ethinyl Estradiol and Levonorgestrel *on page 612*

◆ **LoKara [DSC]** *see* Desonide *on page 461*

◆ **Lo Loestrin Fe** *see* Ethinyl Estradiol and Norethindrone *on page 614*

◆ **Lomaira** *see* Phentermine *on page 1224*

◆ **Lomedia 24 FE [DSC]** *see* Ethinyl Estradiol and Norethindrone *on page 614*

Lomitapide (loe MI ta pide)

Related Information

Cardiovascular Diseases *on page 1654*

Brand Names: US Juxtapid

Brand Names: Canada Juxtapid

Pharmacologic Category Antilipemic Agent, Microsomal Triglyceride Transfer Protein (MTP) Inhibitor

Use

Homozygous familial hypercholesterolemia: Adjunct to a low-fat diet and other lipid-lowering treatments, including low-density lipoprotein (LDL) apheresis where available, to reduce low-density lipoprotein cholesterol (LDL-C), total cholesterol, apolipoprotein B (apo B), and non-high-density lipoprotein cholesterol (non-HDL-C) in patients with homozygous familial hypercholesterolemia (HoFH).

Guideline recommendations: Lomitapide may be useful in patients with HoFH not responsive to PCSK9 inhibitor therapy (AACE [Jellinger 2017]). In addition, lomitapide may be considered in patients with ASCVD and baseline LDL-C ≥190 mg/dL who have an inadequate response to statins (with or without ezetimibe and PCSK9 inhibitors) (ACC [Lloyd-Jones 2016]).

Local Anesthetic/Vasoconstrictor Precautions

No information available to require special precautions

Effects on Dental Treatment Key adverse event(s) related to dental treatment: Nasal congestion, nasopharyngitis, and pharyngolaryngeal pain

Effects on Bleeding No information available to require special precautions

Adverse Reactions

>10%:

Cardiovascular: Chest pain (24%)

Central nervous system: Fatigue (17%)

Gastrointestinal: Diarrhea (79%; severe: 14%), nausea (65%), dyspepsia (38%), vomiting (34%; severe: 10%), abdominal pain (34%; severe: 7%), weight loss (24%), abdominal discomfort (21%; severe: 7%), abdominal distension (21%; severe: 7%), constipation (21%), flatulence (21%), gastroenteritis (14%)

Hepatic: Liver steatosis (increase in hepatic fat >5%: 78%; >20% fat increase: 13%), increased serum transaminases (≥3 times upper limit of normal: 34%; ≥5 times upper limit of normal: 14%)

Infection: Influenza (21%)

Neuromuscular & skeletal: Back pain (14%)

Respiratory: Nasopharyngitis (17%), pharyngolaryngeal pain (14%)

1% to 10%:

Cardiovascular: Angina pectoris (10%), palpitations (10%)

Central nervous system: Dizziness (10%), headache (10%)

Gastrointestinal: Bowel urgency (10%), gastroesophageal reflux disease (10%), rectal tenesmus (10%)

Hepatic: Hepatotoxicity (severe: 10%)

Respiratory: Nasal congestion (10%)

Miscellaneous: Fever (10%)

<1%, postmarketing, and/or case reports: Alopecia, myalgia

Mechanism of Action Lomitapide directly binds to and inhibits microsomal triglyceride transfer protein (MTP) which is located in the lumen of the endoplasmic reticulum. MTP inhibition prevents the assembly of apo-B containing lipoproteins in enterocytes and hepatocytes resulting in reduced production of chylomicrons and VLDL and subsequently reduces plasma LDL-C concentrations.

Pharmacodynamics/Kinetics

Half-life Elimination 39.7 hours

Time to Peak ~6 hours

Reproductive Considerations

Evaluate pregnancy status prior to use in females of reproductive potential. Women of reproductive potential should have a negative pregnancy test prior to therapy and effective contraception must be used during treatment and for 2 weeks after the final lomitapide dose. Dose adjustment may be required for women using oral contraceptives. In addition, females using oral contraceptives should also use an effective, alternate form of contraception for 7 days after the resolution of symptoms if nausea or diarrhea occur during lomitapide treatment.

Pregnancy Considerations

Based on data from animal reproduction studies, in utero exposure to lomitapide may cause fetal harm. Use is contraindicated in pregnant women. Discontinue if pregnancy occurs during treatment.

Data collection to monitor pregnancy and infant outcomes following exposure to lomitapide is ongoing. Health care providers are encouraged to enroll women exposed to lomitapide during pregnancy in the Global Lomitapide Pregnancy Exposure Registry by calling 1-877-902-4099.

◆ **Lomitapide Mesylate** *see* Lomitapide *on page 927*

◆ **Lomotil** *see* Diphenoxylate and Atropine *on page 503*

Lomustine (loe MUS teen)

Brand Names: US Gleostine

Brand Names: Canada CeeNU

Pharmacologic Category Antineoplastic Agent, Alkylating Agent; Antineoplastic Agent, Alkylating Agent (Nitrosourea)

Use

Brain tumors: Treatment of primary and metastatic brain tumors (after appropriate surgical and/or radiotherapeutic procedures).

Hodgkin lymphoma: Treatment (in combination with other chemotherapy agents) of Hodgkin lymphoma which has progressed following initial chemotherapy; however, the use of lomustine in the management of Hodgkin lymphoma is limited due to efficacy of other chemotherapy agents/regimens.

Local Anesthetic/Vasoconstrictor Precautions
No information available to require special precautions

Effects on Dental Treatment No significant effects or complications reported

Effects on Bleeding Delayed and cumulative myelosuppression is the major adverse effect and includes thrombocytopenia and anemia. Medical consult recommended.

Adverse Reactions

>10%:

Gastrointestinal: Nausea and vomiting, (onset: 3 to 6 hours after oral administration; duration: <24 hours)

Hematologic & oncologic: Leukopenia (65%; nadir: 5 to 6 weeks; recovery 6 to 8 weeks), bone marrow depression (dose-limiting, delayed, cumulative), thrombocytopenia (nadir: 4 weeks; recovery 5 to 6 weeks)

Frequency not defined:

Central nervous system: Ataxia, disorientation, dysarthria, lethargy

Dermatologic: Alopecia

Gastrointestinal: Stomatitis

Genitourinary: Azotemia (progressive), nephron atrophy, nephrotoxicity

Hematologic & oncologic: Acute leukemia, anemia, bone marrow dysplasia

Hepatic: Hepatotoxicity, increased serum alkaline phosphatase, increased serum bilirubin, increased serum transaminases

Ophthalmic: Blindness, optic atrophy, visual disturbance

Renal: Renal failure

Respiratory: Pulmonary fibrosis, pulmonary infiltrates

Mechanism of Action Inhibits DNA, RNA, and protein synthesis via alkylation and carbamylation of DNA and RNA; lomustine is cell cycle non-specific (Perry 2012)

Pharmacodynamics/Kinetics

Half-life Elimination Metabolites: 16 to 48 hours

Time to Peak Serum: ~3 hours (Perry 2012)

Reproductive Considerations
Women of reproductive potential should use effective contraception during treatment and for 2 weeks after the final lomustine dose. Males with female partners of reproductive potential should use effective contraception during treatment and for 3.5 months after the final lomustine dose.

Pregnancy Considerations
Based on the mechanism of action and data from animal reproduction studies, in utero exposure to lomustine may cause fetal harm.

◆ **Lomustinum** *see* Lomustine *on page 927*

◆ **Long Lasting Nasal Spray [OTC]** *see* Oxymetazoline (Nasal) *on page 1173*

◆ **Lonhala Magnair Refill Kit** *see* Glycopyrrolate (Oral Inhalation) *on page 743*

◆ **Lonhala Magnair Starter Kit** *see* Glycopyrrolate (Oral Inhalation) *on page 743*

◆ **Lonoctocog Alfa** *see* Antihemophilic Factor (Recombinant) *on page 153*

◆ **Lonsurf** *see* Trifluridine and Tipiracil *on page 1497*

◆ **Lo Ovral** *see* Ethinyl Estradiol and Norgestrel *on page 617*

Loperamide (loe PER a mide)

Brand Names: US Anti-Diarrheal [OTC]; Diamode [OTC]; Imodium A-D [OTC]; Loperamide A-D [OTC] [DSC]

Pharmacologic Category Antidiarrheal

Use

Diarrhea:

Rx labeling: Control and symptomatic relief of chronic diarrhea associated with inflammatory bowel disease in adults; acute nonspecific diarrhea in patients ≥2 years; to reduce volume of ileostomy discharge

OTC labeling: Control of symptoms of diarrhea, including Traveler's diarrhea

Local Anesthetic/Vasoconstrictor Precautions
No information available to require special precautions

Effects on Dental Treatment Key adverse event(s) related to dental treatment: Rare occurrences of erythema multiforme, Stevens-Johnson syndrome, and xerostomia (normal salivary flow resumes upon discontinuance) have been reported.

Effects on Bleeding No information available to require special precautions

Adverse Reactions 1% to 10%:

Central nervous system: Dizziness (1%)

Gastrointestinal: Constipation (2% to 5%), abdominal cramps (≤3%), nausea (≤3%)

<1%, postmarketing, and/or case reports: Abdominal discomfort, abdominal distention, abdominal pain, anaphylactic shock, anaphylactoid reaction, angioedema, bullous rash (rare), drowsiness, dyspepsia, erythema multiforme (rare), fatigue, flatulence, hypersensitivity reaction, megacolon, paralytic ileus, pruritus, skin rash, Stevens-Johnson syndrome (rare), toxic epidermal necrolysis (rare), toxic megacolon, urinary retention, urticaria, vomiting, xerostomia

Mechanism of Action Acts directly on circular and longitudinal intestinal muscles, through the opioid receptor, to inhibit peristalsis and prolong transit time; reduces fecal volume, increases viscosity, and diminishes fluid and electrolyte loss; demonstrates antisecretory activity. Loperamide increases tone on the anal sphincter

Pharmacodynamics/Kinetics

Half-life Elimination 9.4 to 14.4 hours

Time to Peak Liquid: 2.5 hours; Capsule: ~5 hours

Pregnancy Risk Factor C

Pregnancy Considerations Adverse effects have not been observed in animal reproduction studies. Information related to loperamide use in pregnancy is limited and data is conflicting (Einarson 2000; Källén 2008). For acute diarrhea in pregnant women, some clinicians recommend oral rehydration and dietary changes; loperamide in small amounts may be used only if symptoms are disabling (Wald 2003).

◆ **Loperamide A-D [OTC] [DSC]** *see* Loperamide *on page 928*

◆ **Loperamide HCl** *see* Loperamide *on page 928*

◆ **Loperamide Hydrochloride** *see* Loperamide *on page 928*
◆ **Lopid** *see* Gemfibrozil *on page 733*

Lopinavir and Ritonavir

(loe PIN a veer & ri TOE na vir)

Related Information

HIV Infection and AIDS *on page 1690*
Ritonavir *on page 1335*

Brand Names: US Kaletra

Brand Names: Canada Kaletra

Pharmacologic Category Antiretroviral, Protease Inhibitor (Anti-HIV)

Use

HIV-1 infection, treatment: Treatment of HIV-1 infection in adults and pediatric patients 14 days and older in combination with other antiretroviral agents.

Note: Lopinavir/ritonavir is not recommended as a component of initial therapy for the treatment of HIV (HHS [adults] 2019).

Local Anesthetic/Vasoconstrictor Precautions No information available to require special precautions

Effects on Dental Treatment Key adverse event(s) related to dental treatment: Dysphagia.

Effects on Bleeding Increased bleeding has been reported in HIV-infected patients with hemophilia (types A and B). Pediatric patients (4%) reported thrombocytopenia and less than 2% of adults reported anemia.

Adverse Reactions Data presented for short- and long-term combination antiretroviral therapy in both protease inhibitor experienced and naïve patients.

>10%:

Dermatologic: Skin rash (children 12%; adults ≤5%)

Endocrine & metabolic: Hypercholesterolemia (3% to 39%), increased serum triglycerides (3% to 36%), increased gamma-glutamyl transferase (10% to 29%)

Gastrointestinal: Diarrhea (7% to 28%; greater with once-daily dosing), dysgeusia (children 22%; adults <2%), vomiting (children 21%; adults 2% to 7%), nausea (5% to 16%), abdominal pain (1% to 11%)

Hepatic: Increased serum ALT (grade 3/4: 1% to 11%)

Respiratory: Upper respiratory tract infection (14%)

>2% to 10%:

Cardiovascular: Vasodilation (≤3%)

Central nervous system: Fatigue (8%, including weakness), headache (2% to 6%), anxiety (4%), insomnia (≤4%)

Dermatologic: Skin infection (3%, including cellulitis, folliculitis, furuncle)

Endocrine & metabolic: Hypertriglyceridemia (6%), hyperglycemia (≤5%), hyperuricemia (≤5%), alteration in sodium (children 3%), weight loss (≤3%)

Gastrointestinal: Increased serum amylase (3% to 8%), dyspepsia (≤6%), increased serum lipase (3% to 5%), flatulence (1% to 4%), gastroenteritis (3%)

Hematologic & oncologic: Thrombocytopenia (grade 3/4: 4% children), neutropenia (grade 3/4: 1% to 5%)

Hepatic: Increased serum AST (grade 3/4: 2% to 10%), hepatitis (4%, including increased AST, ALT, and gamma-glutamyl transferase), increased serum bilirubin (children 3%; adults 1%)

Hypersensitivity: Hypersensitivity (3%, including urticaria and angioedema)

Neuromuscular & skeletal: Weakness (≤9%), musculoskeletal pain (6%)

Respiratory: Lower respiratory tract infection (8%)

≤2%: Abdominal distension, abnormal dreams, abnormality in thinking, acne vulgaris, ageusia, agitation, alopecia, amenorrhea, amnesia, anemia, anorexia, apathy, arthralgia, asthma, ataxia, atherosclerotic disease, atrial fibrillation, atrioventricular block (second and third degree), atrophic striae, back pain, bacterial infection, benign neoplasm, bradycardia, brain disease, breast hypertrophy, bronchitis, cerebral infarction, cerebrovascular accident, change in appetite, chest pain, chills, cholangitis, cholecystitis, confusion, constipation, cough, Cushing's syndrome, cyst, decreased creatinine clearance, decreased glucose tolerance, decreased libido, deep vein thrombosis, dehydration, depression, dermal ulcer, diabetes mellitus, dizziness, drowsiness, duodenitis, dyskinesia, dysphagia, dyspnea, eczema, edema, ejaculatory disorder, emotional lability, enteritis, enterocolitis, erectile dysfunction, eructation, erythema multiforme, esophagitis, exfoliative dermatitis, extrapyramidal reaction, facial edema, facial paralysis, fecal incontinence, fever, first degree atrioventricular block, flu-like symptoms, gastritis, gastroesophageal reflux disease, gastrointestinal hemorrhage, gastrointestinal ulcer, gynecomastia, hematuria, hemorrhagic colitis, hemorrhoids, hepatic insufficiency, hepatomegaly, hyperacusis, hyperhidrosis, hypermenorrhea, hypersensitivity reaction, hypertension, hypertonia, hypogonadism (males), hypophosphatemia, hypothyroidism, immune reconstitution syndrome, impotence, jaundice, lactic acidosis, leukopenia, lipoma, liver steatosis, liver tenderness, lymphadenopathy, maculopapular rash, malaise, migraine, myalgia, myocardial infarction, neoplasm, nephritis, nervousness, neuropathy, night sweats, obesity, oral mucosa ulcer, orthostatic hypotension, osteonecrosis, otitis media, palpitations, pancreatitis, paresthesia, periodontitis, peripheral edema, peripheral neuropathy, pharyngitis, prolonged QT interval on ECG, propylene glycol toxicity (preterm neonates [includes cardiomyopathy, lactic acidosis, acute renal failure, respiratory complications]), pruritus, pulmonary edema, rectal hemorrhage, redistribution of body fat (including facial wasting), renal failure, rhabdomyolysis, rhinitis, seborrhea, seizure, sialadenitis, sinusitis, skin discoloration, splenomegaly, Stevens-Johnson syndrome, stomatitis, thrombophlebitis, tinnitus, torsades de pointes, tremor, tricuspid regurgitation, vasculitis, vertigo, viral infection, visual disturbance, vitamin deficiency, weight gain, xeroderma, xerostomia

Mechanism of Action A coformulation of lopinavir and ritonavir. The lopinavir component binds to the site of HIV-1 protease activity and inhibits the cleavage of viral Gag-Pol polyprotein precursors into individual functional proteins required for infectious HIV. This results in the formation of immature, noninfectious viral particles. The ritonavir component inhibits the CYP3A metabolism of lopinavir, allowing increased plasma levels of lopinavir.

Pharmacodynamics/Kinetics

Half-life Elimination Lopinavir: 5 to 6 hours

Time to Peak Lopinavir: ~4 hours

Reproductive Considerations

The Health and Human Services (HHS) perinatal HIV guidelines consider lopinavir combined with ritonavir an alternative protease inhibitor for females living with HIV who are not yet pregnant but are trying to conceive.

For males and females living with HIV and planning a pregnancy, maximum viral suppression below the limits of detection with antiretroviral therapy (ART), modification of therapy (if needed), optimization of the woman's health, and a discussion of the potential risks and benefits of ART therapy during pregnancy is recommended prior to conception (HHS [perinatal] 2019).

Pregnancy Considerations

Lopinavir has a low level of transfer across the human placenta; fetal exposure is increased with ritonavir.

Based on information collected by the Antiretroviral Pregnancy Registry, an increased risk of teratogenic effects has not been observed in humans. Maternal antiretroviral therapy (ART) may be associated with adverse pregnancy outcomes including preterm delivery, stillbirth, low birth weight, and small for gestational age infants. Actual risks may be influenced by maternal factors, such as disease severity, gestational age at initiation of therapy, and specific ART regimen, therefore close fetal monitoring is recommended. However, regimens containing lopinavir/ritonavir may be more closely associated with preterm delivery compared to others. Because there is clear benefit to appropriate treatment, maternal ART should not be withheld due to concerns for adverse neonatal outcomes. Long-term follow-up is recommended for all infants exposed to antiretroviral medications; children without HIV but who were exposed to ART in utero and develop significant organ system abnormalities of unknown etiology (particularly of the CNS or heart) should be evaluated for potential mitochondrial dysfunction. Hyperglycemia, new onset of diabetes mellitus, or diabetic ketoacidosis have been reported with protease inhibitors; it is not clear if pregnancy increases this risk. Consider performing the standard glucose screening test earlier in pregnancy in women who initiated protease inhibitor therapy prior to conception.

The Health and Human Services (HHS) perinatal HIV guidelines consider lopinavir combined with ritonavir an alternative protease inhibitor for pregnant females living with HIV who are antiretroviral-naive (initial therapy), who have had ART therapy in the past but are restarting, or who require a new ART regimen (due to poor tolerance or poor virologic response of current regimen). Females who become pregnant while taking lopinavir combined with ritonavir may continue if viral suppression is effective and the regimen is well tolerated. Pharmacokinetic studies suggest that standard dosing during pregnancy may provide decreased plasma concentrations; dose adjustments are required in women during the second and third trimesters of pregnancy. Although there is an abundance of data related to the use of lopinavir/ritonavir during pregnancy, the HHS perinatal HIV guidelines consider lopinavir/ritonavir to be an alternative protease inhibitor for initial therapy in antiretroviral-naive pregnant women due to the need for twice daily dosing, the increased incidence of diarrhea and nausea, and an association with preterm delivery. Lopinavir/ritonavir is not recommended for use in pregnant women with lopinavir-associated resistance substitutions. In addition, once-daily dosing is not recommended during pregnancy and use of the oral solution should be avoided (due to alcohol and propylene glycol content).

In general, ART is recommended for all pregnant females living with HIV to keep the viral load below the limit of detection and reduce the risk of perinatal transmission. Therapy should be individualized following a discussion of the potential risks and benefits of treatment during pregnancy. Monitoring of pregnant females is more frequent than in nonpregnant adults. ART should be continued postpartum for all females living with HIV and can be modified after delivery.

Lopinavir/ritonavir is under investigation for use in the treatment of COVID-19 (see http://www.ClinicalTrials.gov) and should only be given as part of a clinical trial for this indication (HHS 2020). The American College of Obstetricians and Gynecologists and the Society for Maternal-Fetal Medicine have developed an algorithm to aid practitioners in assessing and managing pregnant women with suspected or confirmed COVID-19 (https://www.acog.org/topics/covid-19; https://www.smfm.org/covid19). Interim guidance is also available from the CDC for pregnant women who are diagnosed with COVID-19 (https://www.cdc.gov/coronavirus/2019-ncov/hcp/inpatient-obstetric-healthcare-guidance.html).

Health care providers are encouraged to enroll pregnant females exposed to antiretroviral medications as early in pregnancy as possible in the Antiretroviral Pregnancy Registry (1-800-258-4263 or http://www.APRegistry.com). Health care providers caring for pregnant females living with HIV and their infants may contact the National Perinatal HIV Hotline (888-448-8765) for clinical consultation (HHS [perinatal] 2019).

Data collection to monitor maternal and infant outcomes following exposure to COVID-19 during pregnancy is ongoing. Health care providers are encouraged to enroll females exposed to COVID-19 during pregnancy in the Organization of Teratology Information Specialists pregnancy registry (877-311-8972; https://mothertobaby.org/join-study/) or the PRIORITY (**P**regnancy **C**o**R**onav**I**rus **O**utcomes **R**eg**I**s**T**r**Y**) (415-754-3729, https://priority.ucsf.edu/).

- **Lopinavir/Ritonavir** *see* Lopinavir and Ritonavir *on page 929*
- **Lopreeza** *see* Estradiol and Norethindrone *on page 598*
- **Lopressor** *see* Metoprolol *on page 1009*
- **Loprox** *see* Ciclopirox *on page 346*
- **Loradamed [OTC]** *see* Loratadine *on page 930*

Loratadine (lor AT a deen)

Related Information

Dentin Hypersensitivity, Acid Erosion, High Caries Index, Management of Alveolar Osteitis, and Xerostomia *on page 1762*

Brand Names: US Alavert [OTC]; Allergy Non-Drowsy [OTC] [DSC]; Allergy Relief Loratadine [OTC]; Allergy Relief [OTC]; Allergy [OTC] [DSC]; Childrens Loratadine [OTC]; Claritin Allergy Childrens [OTC]; Claritin Childrens [OTC]; Claritin Reditabs [OTC]; Claritin [OTC]; GoodSense Allergy Relief [OTC]; Loradamed [OTC]; Loratadine Childrens [OTC]; Loratadine Hives Relief [OTC] [DSC]; Triaminic Allerchews [OTC]

Pharmacologic Category Histamine H_1 Antagonist; Histamine H_1 Antagonist, Second Generation; Piperidine Derivative

Use

Allergic rhinitis or conjunctivitis: Relief of nasal and non-nasal symptoms of seasonal allergies.

OTC labeling: Patient-guided therapy for symptoms of hay fever or other upper respiratory allergies.

Urticaria: Treatment of itching due to hives (urticaria).

Local Anesthetic/Vasoconstrictor Precautions

No information available to require special precautions

Effects on Dental Treatment Key adverse event(s) related to dental treatment: Xerostomia (normal salivary flow resumes upon discontinuation) and stomatitis in children (2-5 years).

Effects on Bleeding No information available to require special precautions

Adverse Reactions

1% to 10%:

Central nervous system: Headache (adults: 8%), sedated state (adults: 8%), drowsiness (adults: 4%), fatigue (adults: 4%), nervousness (children: 4%)

Gastrointestinal: Xerostomia (adults: 2% to 4%), abdominal pain (children: 2%), vomiting (children: 2%), diarrhea (children: 1%)

Neuromuscular & skeletal: Hyperkinetic muscle activity (children: 3%)

Frequency not defined:

Dermatologic: Skin rash (adults)

Gastrointestinal: Gastritis (adults), nausea (adults)

Hypersensitivity: Hypersensitivity reaction (adults)

<1%, postmarketing, and/or case reports: Alopecia, anaphylaxis, cough, dizziness, dry nose, hepatic insufficiency, increased appetite, palpitations, seizure, tachycardia

Mechanism of Action Long-acting tricyclic antihistamine with selective peripheral histamine H_1-receptor antagonistic properties

Pharmacodynamics/Kinetics

Onset of Action 1-3 hours; Peak effect: 8-12 hours

Duration of Action >24 hours

Half-life Elimination 8.4 hours (range: 3 to 20 hours) (loratadine), 28 hours (range: 8.8 to 92 hours) (metabolite) (Claritin prescribing information 2000); hepatic impairment: 24 hours (loratadine), 37 hours (metabolite) (Claritin prescribing information 2000)

Time to Peak Loratadine: 1.3 hours (loratadine), 2.3 hours (metabolite) (Claritin prescribing information 2000)

Pregnancy Considerations

Guidelines for the use of antihistamines in the treatment of allergic rhinitis or urticaria in pregnancy are generally the same as in nonpregnant females. Loratadine may be used when a second generation antihistamine is needed. The lowest effective dose should be used (Powell 2015; Scadding 2017; Wallace 2008; Zuberbier 2018).

◆ **Loratadine-D 12 Hour [OTC]** *see* Loratadine and Pseudoephedrine *on page 931*

◆ **Loratadine-D 24 Hour [OTC]** *see* Loratadine and Pseudoephedrine *on page 931*

Loratadine and Pseudoephedrine

(lor AT a deen & soo doe e FED rin)

Related Information

Bacterial Infections *on page 1739*

Loratadine *on page 930*

Pseudoephedrine *on page 1291*

Brand Names: US Alavert Allergy and Sinus [OTC]; Allergy Relief-D [OTC]; Claritin-D 12 Hour Allergy & Congestion [OTC]; Claritin-D 24 Hour Allergy & Congestion [OTC]; Loratadine-D 12 Hour [OTC]; Loratadine-D 24 Hour [OTC]

Brand Names: Canada Chlor-Tripolon ND; Claritin Extra; Claritin Liberator

Pharmacologic Category Alpha/Beta Agonist; Decongestant; Histamine H_1 Antagonist; Histamine H_1 Antagonist, Second Generation; Piperidine Derivative

Use Cold, allergy symptoms: Temporary relief of sinus and nasal congestion, runny nose, sneezing, itching of nose or throat and itchy, watery eyes due to common cold, hay fever (allergic rhinitis), or other upper respiratory allergies or sinusitis

Local Anesthetic/Vasoconstrictor Precautions Use with caution since pseudoephedrine is a sympathomimetic amine which could interact with epinephrine to cause a pressor response

Effects on Dental Treatment Key adverse event(s) related to dental treatment: Pseudoephedrine: Xerostomia (normal salivary flow resumes upon discontinuation).

Effects on Bleeding No information available to require special precautions

Adverse Reactions See individual agents.

Pregnancy Considerations See individual agents.

◆ **Loratadine Childrens [OTC]** *see* Loratadine *on page 930*

◆ **Loratadine Hives Relief [OTC] [DSC]** *see* Loratadine *on page 930*

◆ **Loratadine/Pseudoephedrine** *see* Loratadine and Pseudoephedrine *on page 931*

LORazepam (lor A ze pam)

Related Information

Dentin Hypersensitivity, Acid Erosion, High Caries Index, Management of Alveolar Osteitis, and Xerostomia *on page 1762*

Management of the Patient With Anxiety or Depression *on page 1778*

Temporomandibular Dysfunction (TMD), Chronic Pain, and Fibromyalgia *on page 1773*

Related Sample Prescriptions

Sedation (Prior to Dental Treatment) - Sample Prescriptions *on page 45*

Brand Names: US Ativan; LORazepam Intensol

Brand Names: Canada APO-LORazepam; Ativan; DOM-LORazepam [DSC]; PMS-LORazepam; PRO-LORazepam; TEVA-LORazepam

Generic Availability (US) Yes

Pharmacologic Category Anticonvulsant, Benzodiazepine; Benzodiazepine

Dental Use Short-term relief of anxiety prior to dental appointment

Use

Anxiety (oral): Management of anxiety disorders or short-term (≤4 months) relief of anxiety.

Procedural anxiety, premedication (injection): Anesthesia premedication in adults to relieve anxiety or to produce amnesia (diminish recall) or sedation.

Status epilepticus (injection): Treatment of status epilepticus. May be used off label for acute seizures that have not yet progressed to status epilepticus.

Local Anesthetic/Vasoconstrictor Precautions No information available to require special precautions

Effects on Dental Treatment Key adverse event(s) related to dental treatment: Xerostomia (normal salivary flow resumes upon discontinuation) (see Dental Health Professional Considerations)

Effects on Bleeding No information available to require special precautions

Adverse Reactions

>10%:

Central nervous system: Drowsiness, sedation

Local: Pain at injection site (IM: 1% to 17%; IV: 2%)

Miscellaneous: Paradoxical reaction

1% to 10%:

Cardiovascular: Hypotension (≤2%)

Central nervous system: Dizziness (7%), unsteadiness (3%), hallucinations (1%), coma (≤1%), confusion (≤1%), delirium (≤1%), depression (≤1%), excessive crying (≤1%), headache (≤1%), restlessness (≤1%), stupor (≤1%)

Local: Erythema at injection site (2%)

Neuromuscular & skeletal: Asthenia (≤4%)

Respiratory: Respiratory failure (2%), apnea (1%), hypoventilation (≤1%)

Frequency not defined:

Central nervous system: Disinhibition, disorientation, drug dependence, dysarthria, dysautonomia, euphoria, extrapyramidal reaction, fatigue, hypothermia, memory impairment, sleep apnea (exacerbation), slurred speech, suicidal ideation, suicidal tendencies, vertigo, withdrawal syndrome

Dermatologic: Alopecia, skin rash

Endocrine & metabolic: Change in libido, hyponatremia, increased lactate dehydrogenase, SIADH

Gastrointestinal: Changes in appetite, constipation

Genitourinary: Impotence, orgasm disturbance

Hematologic & oncologic: Agranulocytosis, leukopenia, pancytopenia

Hepatic: Increased serum bilirubin, increased serum transaminases, jaundice

Hypersensitivity: Anaphylactoid reaction, anaphylaxis, hypersensitivity reaction

Ophthalmic: Visual disturbance

Respiratory: Exacerbation of chronic obstructive pulmonary disease), respiratory depression

<1%, postmarketing, and/or case reports: Abnormal gait, abnormal hepatic function tests, abnormality in thinking, acidosis, agitation, amnesia, ataxia, blurred vision, bradycardia, cardiac arrhythmia, cardiac failure, cerebral edema, chills, cystitis, diplopia, disorder of hemostatic components of blood, gastrointestinal hemorrhage, hearing loss, heart block, hepatotoxicity, hypertension, hyperventilation, increased serum alkaline phosphatase, infection, injection site reaction, myoclonus, nausea, nervousness, neuroleptic malignant syndrome, paralysis, pericardial effusion, pheochromocytoma (aggravation), pneumothorax, propylene glycol toxicity (IV), pulmonary edema, pulmonary hemorrhage, pulmonary hypertension, seizure, sialorrhea, tachycardia, thrombocytopenia, tremor, urinary incontinence, ventricular arrhythmia, vomiting

Dental Usual Dosage

Anxiety and sedation: Adults: Oral: 1 to 10 mg/day in 2 to 3 divided doses; usual dose: 2 to 6 mg/day in divided doses

Preoperative: Adults:

IM: 0.05 mg/kg administered 2 hours before surgery (maximum: 4 mg/dose)

IV: 0.044 mg/kg 15 to 20 minutes before surgery (usual maximum: 2 mg/dose)

Preprocedural anxiety: Adults: Oral: 1 to 2 mg 1 hour before procedure

Dosing

Adult Note: Avoid use in patients with, or at risk for, substance abuse disorders, except for acute or emergency situations (eg, acute agitation, status epilepticus).

Akathisia, antipsychotic-induced (alternative agent) (off-label use): IV, Oral: Initial: 0.5 to 1 mg twice daily; may increase dose based on response and tolerability up to 10 mg/day (Adler 1985; Bartels 1987; Marder 2019).

Anxiety:

Anxiety and agitation, acute/severe (monotherapy or adjunctive therapy): IM, IV, Oral: 0.5 to 2 mg every 4 to 6 hours as needed up to 10 mg/day; adjust dose based on response and tolerability. In severely agitated inpatients, some experts recommend doses up to 4 mg and repeat IM or IV doses as frequently as 10 to 30 minutes; may give alone or in combination with an antipsychotic (Moore 2019).

Anxiety disorder (monotherapy or adjunctive therapy) (alternative agent): Note: Most commonly used short-term for immediate symptom relief until concurrent therapy is effective (eg, ≤12 weeks). Long-term therapy may be considered for select patients only when other treatments are ineffective or poorly tolerated (Katzman 2014; WFSBP [Bandelow 2008]).

Oral: Initial: 0.5 to 1 mg 2 to 3 times daily; increase gradually based on response and tolerability up to 6 mg/day in 2 to 4 divided doses; some patients may require doses up to 10 mg/day for optimal response (Bystritsky 2019; manufacturer's labeling).

Advanced cancer and/or palliative care: IM, IV, Oral: 0.25 to 2 mg every 3 to 6 hours as needed (Irwin 2019; Roy-Byrne 2019). **Note:** The injectable solution may be administered rectally or subcutaneously, and the tablet and oral solution may be administered sublingually at the same doses when other routes are unavailable (Caillé 1983; Graves 1987; Greenblatt 1982; Harman 2019; Howard 2014; von Gunten 2019).

Performance- or phobia-related anxiety (monotherapy or adjunctive therapy): **Note**: Provide a test dose, at the same dose to be used for treatment, in advance of the stimulus to ensure tolerability (Stein 2019).

Oral: 0.5 to 2 mg once 30 to 60 minutes before the stimulus (Stein 2019; Swinson 2019).

Procedural anxiety (premedication):

Oral, Sublingual (off-label use): 0.5 to 2 mg once 30 to 90 minutes before procedure; if needed due to incomplete response, may repeat the dose (usually at 50% of the initial dose) after 30 to 60 minutes (Chang 2015; Choy 2019; Male 1984; Shih 2019).

IV: 1 to 4 mg **or** 0.02 to 0.04 mg/kg (maximum single dose: 4 mg) once 5 to 20 minutes before procedure; if needed based on incomplete response and/or duration of procedure, may repeat the dose (usually at 50% of the initial dose) after ≥5 minutes (Choy 2019; manufacturer's labeling). **Note:** In obese patients, non–weight-based dosing is preferred (Choy 2019).

Catatonia (off-label use):

Diagnosis: **Note:** Partial, temporary relief of signs following administration is consistent with the diagnosis; a negative response does not rule out catatonia (Coffey 2019a).

IV (preferred): 1 to 2 mg once; if no response in 5 to 10 minutes, repeat dose once (Coffey 2019a; Fink 2009; Rosebush 2010).

IM, Oral, Sublingual: 2 mg once; may administer up to 2 additional doses at 3-hour intervals if needed (Coffey 2019a; Rosebush 2010).

Treatment: **Note:** For patients with malignant catatonia, electroconvulsive therapy should begin immediately (WFSBP [Hasan 2012]).

IM, IV, Oral: Initial: 1 to 2 mg 3 times daily; IV preferred for initial dosing with switch to oral as patient improves. May increase dose based on response and tolerability in increments of 3 mg every 1 to 2 days to a usual dose of 6 to 21 mg/day. Doses up to 30 mg/day have been reported (Coffey 2019b; Daniels 2009; Fink 2009). For patients at risk of cardiorespiratory compromise or oversedation, some experts recommend initiating with 0.5 mg 3 times daily (Coffey 2019b; WFSBP [Hasan 2012]).

Duration of treatment: Remission is usually achieved in 4 to 10 days; maintenance therapy at the effective dose is usually continued for 3 to 6 months to maintain recovery, although longer courses may be needed (Coffey 2019b).

Chemotherapy-induced nausea and vomiting, prevention and treatment (adjunctive therapy) (off-label use):

Anticipatory or breakthrough nausea/vomiting, as an adjunct to conventional antiemetics: Oral, IV, Sublingual: 0.5 to 2 mg every 6 hours as needed (Lohr 2008).

Insomnia, sleep-onset or sleep-maintenance (alternative treatment) (off-label use): Note: Intended for short-term use (≤4 to 8 weeks), preferably in conjunction with nonpharmacologic therapies (ACP [Qaseem 2016]; Bonnet 2019; ESRS [Riemann 2017]). Chronic use should be limited to cases where nonpharmacologic treatments are not available or not effective and benefits are felt to outweigh risks (AASM [Sateia 2017]). Some experts advise against extended use of pharmacologic therapy for insomnia (ACP [Qaseem 2016]).

Oral: 0.5 to 2 mg at bedtime (Bonnet 2019; Winkelman 2015).

Intoxication: Cocaine, methamphetamine, and other sympathomimetics (off-label use): Based on limited data: IV: 2 to 4 mg every 3 to 10 minutes as needed for agitation, sedation, seizures, hypertension, and tachycardia until desired symptom control achieved. Large cumulative doses may be required for some patients; monitor for respiratory depression and hypotension (Arnold 2019; Boyer 2019b; Nelson 2019; Wodarz 2017). **Note:** Initiating treatment at 1 mg may be adequate in patients who are only mildly or moderately intoxicated, but doses should be repeated or increased as needed. Consider IM administration if IV access is not possible; however, effects will be delayed (Arnold 2019).

Neuroleptic malignant syndrome (adjunctive therapy) (off-label use): **Note**: For management of muscle rigidity or anxiety in patients with severe symptoms at presentation (hyperthermia, evidence of rhabdomyolysis) and for those not responding to initial withdrawal of medication and supportive care:

IM, IV: 0.5 to 2 mg every 4 to 6 hours until symptom resolution. Use higher doses (eg, 1 to 2 mg) for management of muscle rigidity (Wijdicks 2019).

Sedation/agitation, critical illness (alternative agent) (off-label use): Note: Titrate to light level of sedation (eg, Richmond Agitation-Sedation Scale 0 to −2). Intermittent as-needed therapy is preferred to avoid oversedation (SCCM [Devlin 2018]). For obese patients, fixed dosing is preferred; alternatively, some use IBW for weight-based dosing (Tietze 2019). Continuous infusions are not recommended for use in most ICU patients due to propylene glycol (PG) accumulation and subsequent complications (osmol gap metabolic acidosis, kidney failure); monitor PG accumulation with osmol gap; nonbenzodiazepine or midazolam continuous infusions are generally preferred (Arroliga 2004; Barnes 2006; Yahwak 2008).

Intermittent (preferred):

Fixed dose: IV: Initial dose: 1 to 4 mg; Maintenance: 1 to 4 mg every 2 to 6 hours as needed (Carson 2006; Tietze 2019).

Weight based: IV: Initial dose: 0.02 to 0.04 mg/kg (maximum single dose: 4 mg); Maintenance: 0.02 to 0.06 mg/kg every 2 to 6 hours as needed (maximum single dose: 4 mg) (Carson 2006; Cernaianu 1996; Rozendaal 2009; SCCM [Barr 2013]; Tietze 2019).

Continuous: IV: 0.01 to 0.1 mg/kg/hour continuous infusion (maximum dose: 10 mg/hour) (Rozendaal 2009; SCCM [Barr 2013]; Tietze 2019).

Seizures: Note: If IV access is not available, IM lorazepam is not recommended due to erratic absorption and a slow time to peak drug levels. May consider sublingual or subcutaneous lorazepam or IM midazolam (Drappatz 2019; Harman 2019; Leppik 2015).

Acute active seizures (non-status epilepticus) (off-label use): IV: 4 mg given at a maximum rate of 2 mg/minute; may repeat at 3 to 5 minutes if seizures continue (Drislane 2020; McKee 2015; O'Connor 2020; Schachter 2019).

Status epilepticus: IV: 4 mg given at a maximum rate of 2 mg/minute; may repeat at 3 to 5 minutes if seizures continue; a nonbenzodiazepine antiseizure agent should follow to prevent seizure recurrence, even if seizures have ceased (Drislane 2020; manufacturer's labeling).

Serotonin syndrome (serotonin toxicity) (off-label use): IV: 2 to 4 mg IV every 8 to 10 minutes based upon patient response (Boyer 2020).

Substance withdrawal:

Alcohol withdrawal syndrome (alternative agent) (off-label use): Note: Symptom-triggered regimens preferred over fixed-dose regimens. Dosage and frequency may vary based on institution-specific protocols. Although longer-acting benzodiazepines are preferred in general, shorter-acting benzodiazepines, including lorazepam, may be preferable in patients with impaired liver function. Some experts recommend avoiding IM administration due to variable absorption (Hoffman 2019; WFSBP [Soyka 2017]).

Symptom-triggered regimen: Oral, IV: 2 to 4 mg as needed; dose and frequency determined by withdrawal symptom severity using a validated severity-assessment scale such as the Clinical Institute Withdrawal Assessment for Alcohol, revised scale (CIWA-Ar) (Hoffman 2019; WFSBP [Soyka 2017]).

Fixed-dose regimen: Oral, IV: 6 to 8 mg/day in divided doses for 1 day, then gradually taper dose over 3 to 4 days; additional doses may be considered based on withdrawal symptoms and validated assessment scale scores (eg, CIWA-Ar) (Malcolm 2002; Myrick 2009; WFSBP [Soyka 2017]).

Opioid withdrawal (autonomic instability and agitation) (adjunctive therapy) (alternative agent) (off-label use): Based on limited data: IV: 1 to 2 mg every 10 minutes until hemodynamically stable and adequate sedation (Hanna 2018; Stolbach 2019; Wightman 2018).

Vertigo, acute episodes, treatment (alternative agent) (off-label use): IM, IV, Oral: 0.5 to 2 mg every 4 to 12 hours as needed for 24 to 48 hours (Furman 2019; Hain 2003; Swartz 2005).

Discontinuation of therapy: In patients receiving extended- or higher-dose benzodiazepine therapy, unless safety concerns require a more rapid withdrawal, gradually withdraw to detect reemerging symptoms and minimize rebound and withdrawal symptoms. Taper total daily dose by 10% to 20% every 1 to 2 weeks based on response and tolerability. The optimal taper rate and duration will vary; durations up to 6 months may be necessary for some patients on higher doses (Bystritsky 2019; Lader 2011; VA/DoD 2015). For patients on high doses, taper more rapidly in the beginning and slow the reduction rate as the taper progresses. For example, reduce the dose weekly by 25% until half of the dose remains. Thereafter, continue to reduce by ~12% every 4 to 7 days. For benzodiazepines with half-lives significantly less than 24 hours, including lorazepam, consider substituting an equivalent dose of a long-acting benzodiazepine to allow for a more gradual reduction in drug serum concentrations (VA/DoD 2015).

Geriatric Refer to adult dosing. Dose selection should generally be on the low end of the dosage range (initial dose not to exceed 2 mg).

Renal Impairment: Adult

Oral: No dosage adjustment necessary (Aronoff 2007).

Parenteral: Mild to severe impairment: No dosage adjustment necessary for acute doses; use repeated doses with caution; may increase the risk of propylene glycol toxicity. Monitor osmol gap closely, as a surrogate marker for propylene glycol accumulation, if using for prolonged periods of time or at high doses (Arroliga 2004; Barnes 2006; Yahwak 2008).

Hepatic Impairment: Adult

Oral:

Mild to moderate impairment: No dosage adjustment necessary.

Severe impairment and/or encephalopathy: Use with caution; may require lower doses.

Parenteral:

Mild to moderate impairment: No dosage adjustment necessary; use with caution.

Severe impairment or failure: Although manufacturer labeling suggests use is not recommended, clearance does not appear to be influenced by hepatic disease; use with caution (Kraus 1978; Peppers 1996).

Pediatric

Chemotherapy-induced nausea and vomiting, anticipatory: Limited data available: Infants, Children, and Adolescents: Oral: 0.04 to 0.08 mg/kg/dose; maximum dose: 2 mg/dose; administer a dose the night before chemotherapy and again the next day prior to chemotherapy administration (Dupuis 2014).

Chemotherapy-associated nausea and vomiting, breakthrough: Limited data available: Children and Adolescents: IV: 0.025 to 0.05 mg/kg/dose every 6 hours as needed; maximum dose: 2 mg/dose (Dupuis 2003).

Anxiety, acute:

Infants and Children <12 years: Limited data available: Oral, IV: Usual: 0.05 mg/kg/dose (maximum dose: 2 mg/dose) every 4 to 8 hours; range: 0.02 to 0.1 mg/kg/dose (Kliegman 2007).

Children ≥12 years and Adolescents: Oral: 0.25 to 2 mg/dose 2 or 3 times daily; maximum dose: 2 mg/dose (Kliegman 2011).

Sedation (preprocedure): Limited data available: Children and Adolescents: Oral: Usual: 0.05 mg/kg; range reported in literature: 0.02 to 0.09 mg/kg (Burtles 1983; Henry 1991; Mundeleer 1980; Peters 1982). **Note:** In adults, the maximum dose is 4 mg/dose.

Status epilepticus: Limited data available:

IV: Infants, Children, and Adolescents: 0.1 mg/kg slow IV; may repeat dose once in 5 to 10 minutes; maximum dose: 4 mg/dose (AES [Glauser 2016]; NCS [Brophy 2012]).

Intranasal: **Note:** Lorazepam is not the preferred agent for intranasal administration, guidelines recommend midazolam as the preferred agent (AES [Glauser 2016]).

Infants, Children, and Adolescents: 0.1 mg/kg/dose; maximum dose: 5 mg/dose (Ahmad 2006; Arya 2011; Kliegman 2020).

Dosage adjustment for concomitant therapy: Significant drug interactions exist, requiring dose/frequency adjustment or avoidance. Consult drug interactions database for more information.

Renal Impairment: Pediatric

Oral: Children ≥12 years and Adolescents: There are no dosage adjustments provided in the manufacturer's labeling; however, some clinicians recommend no dosage adjustments are necessary (Aronoff 2007).

IV: No dosage adjustment necessary for acute doses; use repeated doses with caution; may increase the risk of propylene glycol toxicity. Monitor closely if using for prolonged periods of time or at high doses. In adults, the osmolar gap has been shown to be a surrogate marker for propylene glycol accumulation (Arroliga 2004; Barnes 2006; Yahwak 2008).

Hepatic Impairment: Pediatric Children ≥12 years and Adolescents: No dosage adjustment necessary. For severe hepatic disease, use with caution; benzodiazepines may worsen hepatic encephalopathy.

Mechanism of Action Binds to stereospecific benzodiazepine receptors on the postsynaptic GABA neuron at several sites within the central nervous system, including the limbic system, reticular formation. Enhancement of the inhibitory effect of GABA on neuronal excitability results by increased neuronal membrane permeability to chloride ions. This shift in chloride ions results in hyperpolarization (a less excitable state) and stabilization. Benzodiazepine receptors and effects appear to be linked to the GABA-A receptors. Benzodiazepines do not bind to GABA-B receptors.

Contraindications

Hypersensitivity to lorazepam, any component of the formulation, or other benzodiazepines (cross-sensitivity with other benzodiazepines may exist); acute narrow-angle glaucoma; severe respiratory insufficiency (except during mechanical ventilation)

Parenteral: Additional contraindications: Hypersensitivity to polyethylene glycol, propylene glycol, or benzyl alcohol; sleep apnea; intra-arterial injection; use in premature infants

Canadian labeling: Additional contraindications (not in the US labeling): Myasthenia gravis

Warnings/Precautions [US Boxed Warning]: Concomitant use of benzodiazepines and opioids may result in profound sedation, respiratory depression, coma, and death. Reserve concomitant prescribing of these drugs for use in patients for whom alternative treatment options are inadequate. Limit dosages and durations to the minimum required. Follow patients for signs and symptoms of respiratory depression and sedation. In patients already receiving an opioid analgesic, prescribe a lower initial dose of lorazepam than indicated in the absence of an opioid and titrate based on clinical response. If an opioid is initiated in a patient already taking lorazepam, prescribe a lower initial dose of the opioid and titrate based upon clinical response.

Use with caution in elderly or debilitated patients, patients with hepatic disease (including alcoholics) or renal impairment. Elderly patients may be at an increased risk of death with use; risk has been found highest within the first 4 months of use in elderly dementia patients (Jennum 2015; Saarelainen 2018). Use with caution in patients with respiratory disease (chronic obstructive pulmonary disease or sleep apnea) or limited pulmonary reserve. Initial doses in elderly or debilitated patients should be at the lower end of the dosing range. May worsen hepatic encephalopathy. In pediatric and neonatal patients <3 years of age, the repeated or lengthy exposure to sedatives or anesthetics during surgery/procedures may have detrimental effects on the child's brain development and may contribute to various cognitive and behavioral problems. Epidemiological studies have reported various cognitive and behavioral problems, including neurodevelopmental delay (and related diagnoses), learning disabilities, and ADHD. Clinical data suggest that single, relatively short exposures are not likely to have similar negative effects. Further studies are needed to fully characterize findings and ensure that these findings are not related to underlying conditions or the procedure itself. No specific anesthetic/sedative has been found to be safer. For elective procedures, risk versus benefits should be evaluated and discussed with parents/caregivers/patients; critical surgeries should not be delayed (FDA 2016).

Causes CNS depression (dose-related) resulting in sedation, dizziness, confusion, or ataxia, which may impair physical and mental capabilities. Patients must be cautioned about performing tasks which require mental alertness (eg, operating machinery or driving). Potentially significant drug-drug interactions may exist, requiring dose or frequency adjustment, additional monitoring, and/or selection of alternative therapy. Hazardous sleep-related activities, such as sleep-driving, cooking and eating food, and making phone calls while asleep, have been noted with benzodiazepines (Dolder 2008). Benzodiazepines have been associated with falls and traumatic injury and should be used with extreme caution in patients who are at risk of these events (Nelson 1999). Lorazepam may cause anterograde amnesia (Nelson 1999). Paradoxical reactions, including hyperactive or aggressive behavior, have been reported with benzodiazepines; risk may be increased in adolescent/pediatric patients, geriatric patients, or patients with a history of alcohol use disorder or psychiatric/personality disorders (Mancuso 2004). Does not have analgesic, antidepressant, or antipsychotic properties.

Preexisting depression may worsen or emerge during therapy. Not recommended for use in primary depressive or psychotic disorders. Should not be used in patients at risk for suicide without adequate antidepressant treatment. Risk of dependence increases in patients with a history of alcohol or drug abuse and those with significant personality disorders; use with caution in these patients. Tolerance, psychological and physical dependence may also occur with higher dosages and prolonged use. The risk of dependence is decreased with short-term treatment (2 to 4 weeks); evaluate the need for continued treatment prior to extending therapy duration. Benzodiazepines have been associated with dependence and acute withdrawal symptoms on discontinuation or reduction in dose. Acute withdrawal, including seizures, may be precipitated after administration of flumazenil to patients receiving long-term benzodiazepine therapy. Lorazepam is a short half-life benzodiazepine. Tolerance develops to the sedative, hypnotic, and anticonvulsant effects. It does not develop to the anxiolytic effects (Vinkers 2012). Chronic use of this agent may increase the perioperative benzodiazepine dose needed to achieve desired effect.

As a hypnotic agent, should be used only after evaluation of potential causes of sleep disturbance. Failure of sleep disturbance to resolve after 7 to 10 days may indicate psychiatric or medical illness. A worsening of insomnia or the emergence of new abnormalities of thought or behavior may represent unrecognized psychiatric or medical illness and requires immediate and careful evaluation.

Status epilepticus should not be treated with injectable benzodiazepines alone; requires close observation and management and possibly ventilatory support. When used as a component of preanesthesia, monitor for heavy sedation and airway obstruction; equipment necessary to maintain airway and ventilatory support should be available. Parenteral formulation of lorazepam may contain polyethylene glycol, which has resulted in toxicity during high-dose and/or longer-term infusions. Parenteral formulation may also contain propylene glycol (PG); large amounts are potentially toxic and have been associated with hyperosmolality, lactic acidosis, seizures and respiratory depression; use caution (AAP 1997; Zar 2007). May consider using enteral delivery of lorazepam tablets to decrease the risk of PG toxicity (Lugo 1999).

Some dosage forms may contain benzyl alcohol; large amounts of benzyl alcohol (≥99 mg/kg/day) have been associated with a potentially fatal toxicity ("gasping syndrome") in neonates; the "gasping syndrome" consists of metabolic acidosis, respiratory distress, gasping respirations, CNS dysfunction (including convulsions, intracranial hemorrhage), hypotension, and cardiovascular collapse (AAP ["Inactive" 1997]; CDC 1982); some data suggests that benzoate displaces bilirubin from protein-binding sites (Ahlfors 2001); avoid or use dosage forms containing benzyl alcohol with caution in neonates. See manufacturer's labeling.

Warnings: Additional Pediatric Considerations In pediatric and neonatal patients <3 years of age and patients in third trimester of pregnancy (ie, times of rapid brain growth and synaptogenesis), the repeated or lengthy exposure to sedatives or anesthetics during surgery/procedures may have detrimental effects on the child's or fetus' brain development and may contribute to various cognitive and behavioral problems; the FDA is requiring warnings be included in the manufacturer's labeling for all general anesthetic/sedative drugs. Multiple animal species studies have shown adverse effects on brain maturation; in juvenile animals, drugs that potentiate GABA activity and/or block NMDA receptors for >3 hours demonstrated widespread neuronal and oligodendrocyte cell loss along with alteration in synaptic morphology and neurogenesis. Epidemiological studies in humans have reported various cognitive and behavioral problems including neurodevelopmental delay (and related diagnoses), learning disabilities, and ADHD. Human clinical data suggest that single, relatively short exposures are not likely to have similar negative effects. Further studies are needed to fully characterize findings and ensure that these findings are not related to underlying conditions or the procedure itself. No specific anesthetic/sedative has been found to be safer. For elective procedures, risk vs benefits should be evaluated and discussed with parents/caregivers/patients; critical surgeries should not be delayed (FDA 2016).

Use with caution in neonates, especially in preterm infants; several cases of neurotoxicity and myoclonus (rhythmic myoclonic jerking) have been reported. Paradoxical reactions, including hyperactive or aggressive behavior, have been reported with benzodiazepines, particularly in pediatric/adolescent or psychiatric patients; discontinue drug if this occurs.

Some dosage forms may contain propylene glycol; in neonates large amounts of propylene glycol delivered orally, intravenously (eg, >3,000 mg/day), or topically have been associated with potentially fatal toxicities which can include metabolic acidosis, seizures, renal failure, and CNS depression; toxicities have also been reported in children and adults including hyperosmolality, lactic acidosis, seizures, and respiratory depression; use caution (AAP 1997; Shehab 2009).

Drug Interactions

Metabolism/Transport Effects None known.

Avoid Concomitant Use

Avoid concomitant use of LORazepam with any of the following: Azelastine (Nasal); Bromperidol; Fexinidazole [INT]; MetroNIDAZOLE (Systemic); OLANZapine; Orphenadrine; Oxomemazine; Paraldehyde; Sodium Oxybate; Thalidomide

Increased Effect/Toxicity

LORazepam may increase the levels/effects of: Alcohol (Ethyl); Azelastine (Nasal); Blonanserin; Brexanolone; Buprenorphine; CloZAPine; CNS Depressants; Flunitrazepam; Fosphenytoin; Methadone; Methotrimeprazine; MetyroSINE; Opioid Agonists; Orphenadrine; OxyCODONE; Paraldehyde; Phenytoin; Piribedil; Pramipexole; Pyrimethamine; ROPINIRole; Rotigotine; Sodium Oxybate; Suvorexant; Thalidomide; Zolpidem

The levels/effects of LORazepam may be increased by: Alizapride; Brimonidine (Topical); Bromopride; Bromperidol; Cannabidiol; Cannabis; Chlormethiazole; Chlorphenesin Carbamate; Dimethindene (Topical); Doxylamine; Dronabinol; Droperidol; Esketamine; Fexinidazole [INT]; HydrOXYzine; Kava Kava; Lemborexant; Lisuride; Lofexidine; Loxapine; Magnesium Sulfate; Melatonin; Methotrimeprazine; Metoclopramide; MetroNIDAZOLE (Systemic); Minocycline (Systemic); Nabilone; OLANZapine; Oxomemazine; Perampanel; Probenecid; Rufinamide; Teduglutide; Tetrahydrocannabinol; Tetrahydrocannabinol and Cannabidiol; Trimeprazine; Valproate Products

Decreased Effect

The levels/effects of LORazepam may be decreased by: Theophylline Derivatives; Yohimbine

Pharmacodynamics/Kinetics

Onset of Action

Anticonvulsant: IV: Within 10 minutes

Hypnosis: IM: 20 to 30 minutes

Sedation: IV: Within 2 to 3 minutes (Greenblatt 1983)

Duration of Action Anesthesia premedication: Adults: IM, IV: ~6 to 8 hours

Half-life Elimination

Full-term neonates: IV: 40.2 ± 16.5 hours; range: 18 to 73 hours (McDermott 1992)

Pediatric patients (Chamberlain 2012): IV:

5 months to <3 years: 15.8 hours (range: 5.9 to 28.4 hours)

3 to <13 years: 16.9 hours (range: 7.5 to 40.6 hours)

13 to <18 years: 17.8 hours (range: 8.2 to 42 hours)

Adults: Oral: ~12 hours; IV: ~14 hours; IM: ~13 to 18 hours (Greenblatt 1983); End-stage renal disease (ESRD): ~18 hours

Time to Peak IM: ≤3 hours; Oral: ~2 hours; Sublingual tablet [Canadian product]: 1 hour

Pregnancy Considerations Lorazepam and its metabolite cross the human placenta. Teratogenic effects in humans have been observed with some benzodiazepines (including lorazepam); however, additional studies are needed. The incidence of premature birth and low birth weights may be increased following maternal use of benzodiazepines; hypoglycemia and respiratory problems in the neonate may occur following exposure late in pregnancy. Neonatal withdrawal symptoms may occur within days to weeks after birth and "floppy infant syndrome" (which also includes withdrawal symptoms) have been reported with some benzodiazepines (including lorazepam). Elimination of lorazepam in the newborn infant is slow; following in utero exposure, term infants may excrete lorazepam for up to 8 days (Bergman 1992; Iqbal 2002; Wikner 2007).

Breastfeeding Considerations Lorazepam is present in breast milk.

The relative infant dose (RID) of lorazepam is 2.4% to 4.7% when calculated using the highest breast milk concentration located following benzodiazepine monotherapy with lorazepam and compared to an infant therapeutic dose of 0.15 to 0.3 mg/kg/day (0.05 mg/kg/dose every 4 to 8 hours). In general, breastfeeding is considered acceptable when the RID is <10% (Anderson 2016; Ito 2000); however, some sources note breastfeeding should only be considered if the RID is <5% for psychotropic agents (Larsen 2015). Using the highest total milk concentration (12 mcg/L free lorazepam plus 35 mcg/L conjugated lorazepam), the estimated the daily infant dose via breast milk is 7.05 mcg/kg/day. These milk concentrations were obtained following maternal administration of oral lorazepam 2.5 mg twice daily for the first five days postpartum; the mother had begun treatment with lorazepam prior to delivery (route, dose, and duration not specified) (Whitelaw 1981). Higher milk concentrations were observed in one mother who received both oral lorazepam and lormetazepam, which is partially metabolized to lorazepam (Lemmer 2007).

In general, sedation, lethargy, irritability, poor weight gain, and apnea have been reported in breastfed infants exposed to benzodiazepines; however, these adverse effects were not observed in breastfed infants exposed to lorazepam (Kelly 2012). The manufacturer warns of the potential for sedation, irritability, and impaired suckling in the infant. Monitor breastfed infants for drowsiness (WHO 2002).

Although the manufacturer recommends that lorazepam should not be administered to breastfeeding women unless the expected benefit to the woman outweighs the potential risk to the infant, short-acting benzodiazepines, including lorazepam, are considered compatible with breastfeeding (Kelly 2012; WHO 2002). When possible, limit exposure to single doses (WHO 2002).

Controlled Substance C-IV

Dosage Forms: US

Concentrate, Oral:
- LORazepam Intensol: 2 mg/mL (30 mL)
- Generic: 2 mg/mL (30 mL)

Solution, Injection:
- Ativan: 2 mg/mL (1 mL, 10 mL); 4 mg/mL (1 mL, 10 mL)
- Generic: 2 mg/mL (1 mL, 10 mL); 4 mg/mL (1 mL, 10 mL)

Tablet, Oral:
- Ativan: 0.5 mg, 1 mg, 2 mg
- Generic: 0.5 mg, 1 mg, 2 mg

Dosage Forms: Canada

Solution, Injection:
- Generic: 2 mg/mL (1 mL); 4 mg/mL (1 mL)

Tablet, Oral:
- Ativan: 0.5 mg, 1 mg, 2 mg
- Generic: 0.5 mg, 1 mg, 2 mg

Tablet Sublingual, Sublingual:
- Ativan: 0.5 mg, 1 mg, 2 mg
- Generic: 0.5 mg, 1 mg, 2 mg

Dental Health Professional Considerations An adult companion should accompany the patient to and from dental office.

◆ **LORazepam Intensol** *see* LORazepam *on page 931*

◆ **Lorbrena** *see* Lorlatinib *on page 937*

◆ **Lorcet** *see* Hydrocodone and Acetaminophen *on page 764*

◆ **Lorcet HD** *see* Hydrocodone and Acetaminophen *on page 764*

◆ **Lorcet Plus** *see* Hydrocodone and Acetaminophen *on page 764*

Lorlatinib (lor LA ti nib)

Brand Names: US Lorbrena

Brand Names: Canada Lorbrena

Pharmacologic Category Antineoplastic Agent, Anaplastic Lymphoma Kinase Inhibitor; Antineoplastic Agent, Tyrosine Kinase Inhibitor

Use Non-small cell lung cancer, metastatic: Treatment of anaplastic lymphoma kinase (ALK)-positive metastatic non-small cell lung cancer (NSCLC) in patients whose disease has progressed on crizotinib and at least 1 other ALK inhibitor for metastatic disease; or progressed on alectinib as the first ALK inhibitor therapy for metastatic disease; or progressed on ceritinib as the first ALK inhibitor therapy for metastatic disease.

Local Anesthetic/Vasoconstrictor Precautions Lorlatinib is a lymphoma kinase inhibitor (LKI); while other LKIs have been reported to prolong the ECG QT interval (eg, ceritinib, crizotinib), so far there have been no reports with lorlatinib.

Effects on Dental Treatment No significant effects or complications reported

Effects on Bleeding

Bone marrow depression (eg, anemia, thrombocytopenia, lymphocytopenia) has been reported. In patients under active treatment with lorlatinib, medical consult is suggested.

Adverse Reactions

>10%:

Cardiovascular: Edema (57%)

Central nervous system: Peripheral neuropathy (47%; grade 3/4: 3%), cognitive dysfunction (27% to 29%), fatigue (26%), mood disorder (23% to 24%), headache (18%), dizziness (16%), speech disturbance (12% to 14%), sleep disorder (10%)

Dermatologic: Skin rash (14%)

Endocrine & metabolic: Hypercholesterolemia (96%), hypertriglyceridemia (90%), hyperglycemia (52%), hypoalbuminemia (33%), weight gain (24%), increased amylase (22%), hyperkalemia (21%), hypomagnesemia (21%), hypophosphatemia (21%)

Gastrointestinal: Increased serum lipase (24%), diarrhea (22%), nausea (18%), constipation (15%), vomiting (12%)

Hematologic & oncologic: Anemia (52%; grade 3/4: 5%), thrombocytopenia (23%; grade 3/4: <1%), lymphocytopenia (22%; grades 3/4: 3%)

Hepatic: Increased serum aspartate aminotransferase (37%), increased serum alanine aminotransferase (28%), increased serum alkaline phosphatase (24%)

Neuromuscular & skeletal: Arthralgia (23%), myalgia (17%), back pain (13%), limb pain (13%)

Ophthalmic: Visual disturbance (15%)

Respiratory: Dyspnea (27%), cough (18%), upper respiratory tract infection (12%)

Miscellaneous: Fever (12%)

1% to 10%:

Cardiovascular: Atrioventricular block (1%)

Central nervous system: Hallucination (7%), seizure (3%), mental status changes (2%)

Respiratory: Pneumonia (3%), interstitial pulmonary disease (≤2%), pneumonitis (≤2%), respiratory failure (1%)

Mechanism of Action Lorlatinib is a reversible potent third generation tyrosine kinase inhibitor that targets ALK and ROS1; it is highly selective, overcomes known ALK resistance mutations, and penetrates the blood brain barrier (Shaw 2017). Lorlatinib has antitumor activity against multiple mutant forms of the ALK enzyme, including some mutations detected in tumors at the time of disease progression on crizotinib and other ALK inhibitors. Antitumor activity of lorlatinib is dose-dependent and correlates with inhibition of ALK phosphorylation. Lorlatinib also exhibits activity against TYK1, FER, FPS, TRKA, TRKB, TRKC, FAK, FAK2, and ACK.

Pharmacodynamics/Kinetics

Half-life Elimination 24 hours

Time to Peak 1.2 hours (range: 0.5 to 4 hours) following a single dose; 2 hours (range: 0.5 to 23 hours) at steady state

Reproductive Considerations

Evaluate pregnancy status in females of reproductive potential prior to initiating therapy. Females of reproductive potential should avoid pregnancy and use an effective nonhormonal method of contraception during treatment and for at least 6 months after the final lorlatinib dose. Male patients with female partners of reproductive potential should use effective contraception during treatment and for at least 3 months after the last lorlatinib dose.

Pregnancy Considerations

Based on the mechanism of action and data from animal reproduction studies, lorlatinib may cause fetal harm if administered during pregnancy.

◆ **Lortab** *see* Hydrocodone and Acetaminophen *on page 764*

◆ **Loryna** *see* Ethinyl Estradiol and Drospirenone *on page 610*

◆ **Lorzone** *see* Chlorzoxazone *on page 344*

Losartan (loe SAR tan)

Related Information

Cardiovascular Diseases *on page 1654*

Brand Names: US Cozaar

Brand Names: Canada ACT Losartan [DSC]; AG-Losartan; APO-Losartan; Auro-Losartan; BIO-Losartan; Cozaar; JAMP-Losartan; MINT-Losartan; MYLAN-Losartan [DSC]; PMS-Losartan; Priva-Losartan; RAN-Losartan; SANDOZ Losartan; Septa-Losartan; TEVA-Losartan; VAN-Losartan [DSC]

Pharmacologic Category Angiotensin II Receptor Blocker; Antihypertensive

Use

Hypertension: Management of hypertension in adults and children ≥6 years of age

Proteinuric chronic kidney disease, diabetic: Treatment of diabetic nephropathy with an elevated serum creatinine and proteinuria (urinary albumin to creatinine ratio ≥300 mg/g) in patients with type 2 diabetes and a history of hypertension

Local Anesthetic/Vasoconstrictor Precautions

No information available to require special precautions

Effects on Dental Treatment Key adverse event(s) related to dental treatment: Patients may experience orthostatic hypotension as they stand up after treatment; especially if lying in dental chair for extended periods of time. Use caution with sudden changes in position during and after dental treatment.

Effects on Bleeding No information available to require special precautions

Adverse Reactions Incidences occurred with hypertensive patients unless otherwise specified.

1% to 10%:

Cardiovascular: Chest pain (type 2 diabetic nephropathy: ≥4%), hypotension (type 2 diabetic nephropathy: ≥4%), orthostatic hypotension (type 2 diabetic nephropathy: ≥4%), atrial fibrillation (<2%), cerebrovascular accident (<2%), edema (<2%), palpitations (<2%), syncope (<2%)

Central nervous system: Fatigue (type 2 diabetic nephropathy: ≥4%), myasthenia (type 2 diabetic nephropathy: ≥4%), dizziness (3%), depression (<2%), drowsiness (<2%), headache (<2%), migraine (<2%), paresthesia (<2%), sleep disorder (<2%), vertigo (<2%)

Dermatologic: Pruritus (<2%), skin photosensitivity (<2%), skin rash (<2%), urticaria (<2%)

Endocrine & metabolic: Hyperkalemia (type 2 diabetic nephropathy: ≥4%), hypoglycemia (type 2 diabetic nephropathy: ≥4%)

Gastrointestinal: Diarrhea (type 2 diabetic nephropathy: ≥4%), abdominal pain (<2%), constipation (<2%), nausea (<2%), vomiting (<2%)

Genitourinary: Urinary tract infection (type 2 diabetic nephropathy: ≥4%), impotence (<2%)

Hematologic & oncologic: Anemia (type 2 diabetic nephropathy: ≥4%; hypertension: <2%)

Neuromuscular & skeletal: Asthenia (type 2 diabetic nephropathy: ≥4%), back pain (hypertension and type 2 diabetic neuropathy: 2% to ≥4%), arthralgia (<2%), myalgia (<2%)

Otic: Tinnitus (<2%)

Respiratory: Upper respiratory tract infection (8%), cough (ARBs: 3%; Matchar 2008), nasal congestion (2%), dyspnea (<2%)

<1%, postmarketing, and/or case reports: Anaphylaxis, angioedema, dysgeusia, erythroderma, facial edema, glottis edema, Henoch-Schonlein purpura, hepatitis, hyponatremia, laryngeal edema, lip edema, malaise, pharyngeal edema, rhabdomyolysis, thrombocytopenia, tongue edema, vasculitis

Mechanism of Action As a selective and competitive, nonpeptide angiotensin II receptor antagonist, losartan blocks the vasoconstrictor and aldosterone-secreting effects of angiotensin II; losartan interacts reversibly at the AT1 and AT2 receptors of many tissues and has slow dissociation kinetics; its affinity for the AT1 receptor is 1000 times greater than the AT2 receptor. Angiotensin II receptor antagonists may induce a more complete inhibition of the renin-angiotensin system than ACE inhibitors, they do not affect the response to bradykinin, and are less likely to be associated with nonrenin-angiotensin effects (eg, cough and angioedema). Losartan increases urinary flow rate and in addition to being natriuretic and kaliuretic, increases excretion of chloride, magnesium, uric acid, calcium, and phosphate.

Pharmacodynamics/Kinetics

Onset of Action ~6 hours

Half-life Elimination

Losartan: Children 6 to 16 years: 2.3 ± 0.8 hours; Adults: 2.1 ± 0.7 hours

E-3174 (active metabolite): Children 6 to 16 years: 5.6 ± 1.2 hours; Adults: 7.4 ± 2.4 hours

Time to Peak Serum: Losartan: Children: 2 hours, Adults: 1 hour; E-3174 (active metabolite): Children: 4.1 hours, Adults: 3.5 hours

Reproductive Considerations

The use of angiotensin II receptor blockers should generally be avoided in women planning a pregnancy (ACOG 203 2019).

Pregnancy Risk Factor D

Pregnancy Considerations

[US Boxed Warning]: Drugs that act on the renin-angiotensin system can cause injury and death to the developing fetus. When pregnancy is detected, discontinue as soon as possible. The use of drugs which act on the renin-angiotensin system are associated with oligohydramnios. Oligohydramnios, due to decreased fetal renal function, may lead to fetal lung hypoplasia and skeletal malformations. Oligohydramnios may not appear until after irreversible fetal injury has occurred. Use during pregnancy is also associated with anuria, hypotension, renal failure, skull hypoplasia, and death in the fetus/neonate. The exposed fetus should be monitored for fetal growth, amniotic fluid volume, and organ formation. Infants exposed in utero should be monitored for hyperkalemia, hypotension, and oliguria (exchange transfusions or dialysis may be needed). These adverse events are generally associated with maternal use in the second and third trimesters.

Chronic maternal hypertension itself is also associated with adverse events in the fetus/infant. The risk of birth defects, low birth weight, premature delivery, stillbirth, and neonatal death may be increased with chronic hypertension in pregnancy. Actual risks may be related to duration and severity of maternal hypertension (ACOG 203 2019).

The use of angiotensin II receptor blockers is generally not recommended to treat chronic hypertension in pregnant women (ACOG 203 2019).

Losartan and Hydrochlorothiazide

(loe SAR tan & hye droe klor oh THYE a zide)

Related Information

HydroCHLOROthiazide *on page 762*

Losartan *on page 938*

Brand Names: US Hyzaar

Brand Names: Canada ACT Losartan/HCT; Apo-Losartan/HCTZ; Auro-Losartan HCT; Hyzaar; Hyzaar DS; JAMP-Losartan HCTZ; Losartan-HCT; Losartan-HCTZ; Mint-Losartan/HCTZ; Mint-Losartan/HCTZ DS; Mylan-Losartan/HCTZ; PMS-Losartan/HCTZ; Sandoz-Losartan HCT; Sandoz-Losartan HCT DS; Teva-Losartan/HCTZ

Pharmacologic Category Angiotensin II Receptor Blocker; Antihypertensive; Diuretic, Thiazide

Use

Hypertension: Management of hypertension.

Hypertension with left ventricular hypertrophy: To reduce the risk of stroke in patients with hypertension and left ventricular hypertrophy (LVH). Evidence suggests that this benefit does not apply to black patients.

Local Anesthetic/Vasoconstrictor Precautions

No information available to require special precautions

Effects on Dental Treatment Key adverse event(s) related to dental treatment: Patients may experience orthostatic hypotension as they stand up after treatment; especially if lying in dental chair for extended periods of time. Use caution with sudden changes in position during and after dental treatment.

Effects on Bleeding No information available to require special precautions

Adverse Reactions Based on clinical trials of the combination product in patients with primary hypertension. Also see individual agents.

1% to 10%:

Nervous system: Dizziness (6%)

Neuromuscular & skeletal: Back pain (2%)

Respiratory: Upper respiratory tract infection (6%)

Frequency not defined:

Cardiovascular: Chest pain, hypersensitivity angiitis, necrotizing angiitis, orthostatic syncope (dose-related), palpitations, tachycardia, vasculitis

Dermatologic: Cutaneous lupus erythematosus, pruritus, skin photosensitivity, skin rash, toxic epidermal necrolysis, urticaria

Endocrine & metabolic: Electrolyte disorder, glycosuria, hyperglycemia, hyperuricemia, hypokalemia, hyponatremia

Gastrointestinal: Abdominal pain, anorexia, dysgeusia, dyspepsia, gastric irritation, nausea, pancreatitis, sialadenitis, vomiting

Genitourinary: Erectile dysfunction, impotence

Hematologic & oncologic: Agranulocytosis, anemia, aplastic anemia, hemolytic anemia, leukopenia, purpuric disease

Hepatic: Hepatic insufficiency, intrahepatic cholestatic jaundice, jaundice

Nervous system: Headache, insomnia, malaise, migraine, paresthesia, restlessness

Neuromuscular & skeletal: Arthralgia, asthenia, muscle cramps, muscle spasm, myalgia

Ophthalmic: Blurred vision (transient), xanthopsia

Renal: Interstitial nephritis, renal failure syndrome, renal insufficiency

Respiratory: Nasal congestion

Postmarketing: Anaphylaxis, erythroderma, rhabdomyolysis, thrombocytopenia

Mechanism of Action

Losartan: As a selective and competitive, nonpeptide angiotensin II receptor antagonist, losartan blocks the vasoconstrictor and aldosterone-secreting effects of angiotensin II; losartan interacts reversibly at the AT1 and AT2 receptors of many tissues and has slow dissociation kinetics; its affinity for the AT1 receptor is 1000 times greater than the AT2 receptor. Angiotensin II receptor antagonists may induce a more complete inhibition of the renin-angiotensin system than ACE inhibitors, they do not affect the response to bradykinin, and are less likely to be associated with nonrenin-angiotensin effects (eg, cough and angioedema). Losartan increases urinary flow rate and in addition to being natriuretic and kaliuretic, increases excretion of chloride, magnesium, uric acid, calcium, and phosphate.

Hydrochlorothiazide: Inhibits sodium reabsorption in the distal tubules causing increased excretion of sodium and water as well as potassium and hydrogen ions.

Pregnancy Considerations

[US Boxed Warning]: Drugs that act directly on the renin-angiotensin system can cause injury and death to the developing fetus. When pregnancy is detected, discontinue therapy as soon as possible.

Refer to individual monographs for additional information.

◆ **Losartan/Hydrochlorothiazide** *see* Losartan and Hydrochlorothiazide *on page 939*

◆ **Losartan Potassium** *see* Losartan *on page 938*

◆ **LoSeasonique** *see* Ethinyl Estradiol and Levonorgestrel *on page 612*

◆ **Lotensin** *see* Benazepril *on page 225*

◆ **Lotrimin AF [OTC] [DSC]** *see* Clotrimazole (Topical) *on page 397*

◆ **Lotrimin AF [OTC]** *see* Miconazole (Topical) *on page 1019*

◆ **Lotrimin AF Deodorant Powder [OTC]** *see* Miconazole (Topical) *on page 1019*

◆ **Lotrimin AF For Her [OTC]** *see* Clotrimazole (Topical) *on page 397*

◆ **Lotrimin AF Jock Itch Powder [OTC]** *see* Miconazole (Topical) *on page 1019*

◆ **Lotrimin AF Powder [OTC]** *see* Miconazole (Topical) *on page 1019*

◆ **Lotronex** *see* Alosetron *on page 105*

Lovastatin (LOE va sta tin)

Related Information

Cardiovascular Diseases *on page 1654*

Brand Names: US Altoprev; Mevacor [DSC]

Brand Names: Canada ACT Lovastatin; APO-Lovastatin; DOM-Lovastatin; GMD-Lovastatin; MYLAN-Lovastatin [DSC]; PMS-Lovastatin; PRO-Lovastatin [DSC]; RIVA-Lovastatin [DSC]; SANDOZ Lovastatin [DSC]; TEVA-Lovastatin [DSC]

Pharmacologic Category Antilipemic Agent, HMG-CoA Reductase Inhibitor

Use

Adjunct to dietary therapy to decrease elevated serum total and LDL-cholesterol concentrations in primary hypercholesterolemia

Primary prevention of coronary artery disease (patients without symptomatic disease with average to moderately elevated total and LDL-cholesterol and below average HDL-cholesterol); slow progression of coronary atherosclerosis in patients with coronary heart disease and reduce the risk of myocardial infarction, unstable angina, and coronary revascularization procedures.

Adjunct to dietary therapy in adolescent patients (10 to 17 years of age, females >1 year postmenarche) with heterozygous familial hypercholesterolemia having LDL >189 mg/dL, **or** LDL >160 mg/dL with positive family history of premature cardiovascular disease (CVD), **or** LDL >160 mg/dL with the presence of at least two other CVD risk factors

Local Anesthetic/Vasoconstrictor Precautions

No information available to require special precautions

Effects on Dental Treatment Key adverse event(s) related to dental treatment: Assess unusual presentations of muscle weakness or myopathy resulting from lipid therapy such as patient having a difficult time brushing teeth or weakness with chewing. Refer patient back to their physician for evaluation and adjustment of lipid therapy.

Effects on Bleeding No information available to require special precautions

Adverse Reactions Percentages as reported with immediate release tablets; similar adverse reactions seen with extended release tablets.

>10%: Neuromuscular & skeletal: Increased creatine phosphokinase (>2x normal) (11%)

1% to 10%:

Central nervous system: Headache (2% to 3%), dizziness (≤1%)

Dermatologic: Skin rash (≤1%)

Gastrointestinal: Flatulence (4% to 5%), constipation (2% to 4%), abdominal pain (2% to 3%), diarrhea (2% to 3%), nausea (2% to 3%), dyspepsia (1% to 2%)

Neuromuscular & skeletal: Myalgia (2% to 3%), weakness (1% to 2%), muscle cramps (≤1%)

Ophthalmic: Blurred vision (≤1%)

<1%, postmarketing, and/or case reports: Acid regurgitation, alopecia, amnesia (reversible), arthralgia, chest pain, cognitive dysfunction (reversible), cystitis (interstitial; Huang 2015), dermatomyositis, diabetes mellitus (new-onset), elevated glycosylated hemoglobin (HbA_{1c}), eye irritation, increased blood glucose, insomnia, interstitial pulmonary disease, leg pain, memory impairment (reversible), paresthesia, pruritus, reversible confusional state, vomiting, xerostomia

Mechanism of Action Lovastatin acts by competitively inhibiting 3-hydroxyl-3-methylglutaryl-coenzyme A (HMG-CoA) reductase, the enzyme that catalyzes the rate-limiting step in cholesterol biosynthesis. In addition to the ability of HMG-CoA reductase inhibitors to decrease levels of high-sensitivity C-reactive protein (hsCRP), they also possess pleiotropic properties including improved endothelial function, reduced inflammation at the site of the coronary plaque, inhibition of platelet aggregation, and anticoagulant effects (de Denus 2002; Ray 2005).

Pharmacodynamics/Kinetics

Onset of Action LDL-cholesterol reductions: 3 days

Half-life Elimination 1.1-1.7 hours

Time to Peak Serum: Immediate release: 2-4 hours; extended release: 12-14 hours

Reproductive Considerations

Lovastatin is contraindicated in females who may become pregnant.

Adequate contraception is recommended if an HMG-CoA reductase inhibitor is required in females of reproductive potential. Females planning a pregnancy should discontinue the HMG-CoA reductase inhibitor 1 to 2 months prior to attempting to conceive (AHA/ACC [Grundy 2018]).

Pregnancy Considerations

Lovastatin is contraindicated in pregnant females.

There are reports of congenital anomalies following maternal use of HMG-CoA reductase inhibitors in pregnancy; however, maternal disease, differences in specific agents used, and the low rates of exposure limit the interpretation of the available data (Godfrey 2012; Lecarpentier 2012). Cholesterol biosynthesis may be important in fetal development; serum cholesterol and triglycerides increase normally during pregnancy. The discontinuation of lipid lowering medications temporarily during pregnancy is not expected to have significant impact on the long term outcomes of primary hypercholesterolemia treatment.

Lovastatin should be discontinued immediately if an unplanned pregnancy occurs during treatment.

◆ **Lovaza** *see* Omega-3 Fatty Acids *on page 1137*

◆ **Lovenox** *see* Enoxaparin *on page 566*

◆ **Low-Ogestrel** *see* Ethinyl Estradiol and Norgestrel *on page 617*

Loxapine (LOKS a peen)

Related Information

Dentin Hypersensitivity, Acid Erosion, High Caries Index, Management of Alveolar Osteitis, and Xerostomia *on page 1762*

Brand Names: US Adasuve

Brand Names: Canada APO-Loxapine; DOM-Loxapine; Loxapac; PHL-Loxapine [DSC]; Xylac

Pharmacologic Category First Generation (Typical) Antipsychotic

Use

Schizophrenia: IM, Oral: Treatment of schizophrenia.

Agitation associated with schizophrenia or bipolar I disorder: Inhalation: Acute treatment of agitation associated with schizophrenia or bipolar I disorder in adults. **Note**: As part of the Adasuve REMS program to mitigate the risk of bronchospasm, loxapine inhalation must be administered only in an enrolled health care facility.

Local Anesthetic/Vasoconstrictor Precautions No information available to require special precautions

Effects on Dental Treatment Key adverse event(s) related to dental treatment:

Xerostomia and changes in salivation (normal salivary flow resumes upon discontinuation).

Significant hypotension may occur, especially when the drug is administered parenterally; Patients may experience orthostatic hypotension as they stand up after treatment; especially if lying in dental chair for extended periods of time. Use caution with sudden changes in position during and after dental treatment. Orthostatic hypotension is due to alpha-receptor blockade, the elderly are at greater risk for orthostatic hypotension.

Tardive dyskinesia: Prevalence rate may be 40% in elderly; development of the syndrome and the irreversible nature are proportional to duration and total cumulative dose over time. Extrapyramidal reactions are more common in elderly with up to 50% developing these reactions after 60 years of age. Drug-induced Parkinson's syndrome occurs often; akathisia is the most common extrapyramidal reaction in elderly.

Increased confusion, memory loss, psychotic behavior, and agitation frequently occur as a consequence of anticholinergic effects. Antipsychotic associated sedation in nonpsychotic patients is extremely unpleasant due to feelings of depersonalization, derealization, and dysphoria.

Effects on Bleeding No information available to require special precautions

Adverse Reactions

Inhalation: Frequency not always defined.

Cardiovascular: Hypotension (3%), syncope (2%)

Central nervous system: Sedation (12%)

Gastrointestinal: Dysgeusia (14%)

Hypersensitivity: Hypersensitivity

Respiratory: Respiratory distress (includes bronchospasm, chest pain, cough, dyspnea, pharyngeal edema, wheezing; asthma patients: 54%; COPD patients: 19%), throat irritation (3%)

<1%: Extrapyramidal reaction

Oral: Frequency not defined.

Cardiovascular: ECG changes, edema, flushing (facial), hypertension, hypotension, orthostatic hypotension, syncope, tachycardia

Central nervous system: Agitation, confusion, disruption of body temperature regulation, dizziness, drowsiness, extrapyramidal reaction (akathisia, akinesia, dystonia, drug-induced parkinson's disease, tardive dyskinesia), headache, hyperpyrexia, insomnia, neuroleptic malignant syndrome (NMS), numbness, paresthesia, sedation, seizure, slurred speech, tension, unsteady gait

Dermatologic: Alopecia, dermatitis, pruritus, seborrhea, skin photosensitivity, skin rash

Endocrine & metabolic: Amenorrhea, galactorrhea, gynecomastia, hyperprolactinemia, menstrual disease, polydipsia, weight gain, weight loss

Gastrointestinal: Constipation, nausea, paralytic ileus, vomiting, xerostomia

Genitourinary: Impotence, priapism (rare), urinary retention

Hematologic & oncologic: Agranulocytosis, leukopenia, thrombocytopenia

Hepatic: Hepatitis, increased serum ALT, increased serum AST, jaundice

Neuromuscular & skeletal: Muscle twitching, weakness

Ophthalmic: Blepharoptosis, blurred vision

Respiratory: Dyspnea, nasal congestion

Mechanism of Action Loxapine is a dibenzoxazepine antipsychotic that blocks postsynaptic mesolimbic D_1 and D_2 receptors in the brain, and also possesses serotonin 5-HT_2-blocking activity.

Pharmacodynamics/Kinetics

Onset of Action

Oral, IM: Within 30 minutes; Peak effect: 1.5 to 3 hours

Inhalation: 2 minutes

Duration of Action Oral, IM: ~12 hours

Half-life Elimination Biphasic: Oral: Initial: 5 hours; Terminal: 19 hours; Inhalation: 6 to 8 hours

Pregnancy Risk Factor C

Pregnancy Considerations Adverse events have been observed in animal reproduction studies. Antipsychotic use during the third trimester of pregnancy has a risk for abnormal muscle movements (extrapyramidal symptoms [EPS]) and withdrawal symptoms in newborns following delivery. Symptoms in the newborn may include agitation, feeding disorder, hypertonia, hypotonia, respiratory distress, somnolence, and tremor; these effects may be self-limiting or require hospitalization.

- **Loxapine Succinate** *see* Loxapine *on page 940*
- **Loxitane** *see* Loxapine *on page 940*
- **LOXO-101** *see* Larotrectinib *on page 879*
- **LOXO-292** *see* Selpercatinib *on page 1364*
- **Lozi-Flur [DSC]** *see* Fluoride *on page 693*
- **Lo-Zumandimine** *see* Ethinyl Estradiol and Drospirenone *on page 610*
- **L-PAM** *see* Melphalan *on page 961*
- **L-Phenylalanine Mustard** *see* Melphalan *on page 961*
- **LP Lite Pak [DSC]** *see* Lidocaine and Prilocaine *on page 911*
- **LRH** *see* Gonadorelin *on page 746*
- **L-Sarcolysin** *see* Melphalan *on page 961*
- **LTG** *see* LamoTRIgine *on page 874*
- **L-Threo-Dihydroxyphenylserine** *see* Droxidopa *on page 535*
- ***L*-Thyroxine Sodium** *see* Levothyroxine *on page 900*
- **Lu-26-054** *see* Escitalopram *on page 590*
- **Lu AA21004** *see* Vortioxetine *on page 1555*

Lubiprostone (loo bi PROS tone)

Brand Names: US Amitiza

Pharmacologic Category Chloride Channel Activator; Gastrointestinal Agent, Miscellaneous

Use

Chronic idiopathic constipation: Treatment of chronic idiopathic constipation (CIC) in adults

Irritable bowel syndrome with constipation: Treatment of irritable bowel syndrome (IBS) with constipation in women ≥18 years of age

Opioid-induced constipation: Treatment of opioid-induced constipation (OIC) in adults with chronic noncancer pain, including patients with chronic pain related to prior cancer or its treatment who do not require frequent (eg, weekly) opioid dosage escalation.

Local Anesthetic/Vasoconstrictor Precautions No information available to require special precautions

Effects on Dental Treatment Key adverse event(s) related to dental treatment: Xerostomia (normal salivary flow resumes upon discontinuation).

Effects on Bleeding No information available to require special precautions

Adverse Reactions

>10%:

Central nervous system: Headache (2% to 11%)

Gastrointestinal: Nausea (8% to 29%; males: 8%; older adults: 19%), diarrhea (7% to 12%)

1% to 10%:

Cardiovascular: Edema (≤3%), chest discomfort (≤2%), chest pain (≤2%), peripheral edema (1%)

Central nervous system: Dizziness (3%), fatigue (≤2%)

Gastrointestinal: Abdominal pain (4% to 8%), flatulence (4% to 6%), abdominal distention (3% to 6%), abdominal distress (3%), loose stools (≤3%), vomiting (≤3%), dyspepsia (≤2%), xerostomia (≤1%)

Respiratory: Dyspnea (≤3%)

<1%, postmarketing, and/or case reports: Anorexia, anxiety, arthralgia (Anton 2017), asthenia, back pain (Anton 2017), bloody diarrhea (Anton 2017), bowel urgency, constipation, cough, decreased appetite, decreased serum potassium, depression, diaphoresis, dysgeusia, eructation, erythema, fecal impaction, fecal incontinence, fibromyalgia syndrome, frequent bowel movements, gastritis, gastroesophageal reflux disease, gastrointestinal disease, hyperhidrosis, hypersensitivity reaction (including skin rash, swelling, throat tightness), hypotension, increased serum alanine aminotransferase, increased serum aspartate aminotransferase, influenza, ischemic colitis, joint swelling, lethargy, malaise, muscle cramps, muscle spasm, myalgia, neck pain (Anton 2017), pain, palpitations, pharyngolaryngeal pain, pollakiuria, rectal hemorrhage, respiratory tract infection (Anton 2017), syncope, tachycardia, tremor, urinary tract infection, weight gain

Mechanism of Action A chloride channel activator that acts locally on the apical membrane of the gastrointestinal tract to increase intestinal fluid secretion and improve fecal transit. This action bypasses the antisecretory effects of opiates, which suppress secretomotor neuron excitability.

Pharmacodynamics/Kinetics

Half-life Elimination M3: 0.9 to 1.4 hours

Time to Peak Plasma: M3: ~1.1 hour

Pregnancy Considerations Adverse events have been observed in animal reproduction studies.

- ◆ **Lubricaine [OTC]** *see* Lidocaine (Topical) *on page 902*
- ◆ **Lucemyra** *see* Lofexidine *on page 926*
- ◆ **Lucentis** *see* Ranibizumab *on page 1309*
- ◆ **Ludiomil** *see* Maprotiline *on page 946*

Luliconazole (loo li KON a zole)

Brand Names: US Luzu

Pharmacologic Category Antifungal Agent, Topical

Use Fungal infections: Topical treatment of interdigital tinea pedis, tinea cruris, and tinea corporis caused by *Trichophyton rubrum* and *Epidermophyton floccosum*

Local Anesthetic/Vasoconstrictor Precautions No information available to require special precautions

Effects on Dental Treatment No significant effects or complications reported

Effects on Bleeding No information available to require special precautions

Adverse Reactions <1%, postmarketing, and/or case reports: Application site reaction, cellulitis, contact dermatitis

Mechanism of Action Azole antifungal that appears to inhibit ergosterol synthesis by inhibiting the enzyme lanosterol demethylase, resulting in decreased amounts of ergosterol and a corresponding accumulation of lanosterol.

Pregnancy Considerations Adverse events were observed in some animal reproduction studies. Small amounts of luliconazole are absorbed systemically.

Lumateperone (loo ma TE per one)

Brand Names: US Caplyta

Pharmacologic Category Second Generation (Atypical) Antipsychotic

Use Schizophrenia: Treatment of schizophrenia in adults.

Local Anesthetic/Vasoconstrictor Precautions No information available to require special precautions.

Effects on Dental Treatment Key adverse event(s) related to dental treatment: Infrequent occurrence of xerostomia (normal salivary flow resumes upon discontinuation); rare occurrence of orthostatic hypotension.

Effects on Bleeding No information available to require special precautions.

Adverse Reactions

>10%: Central nervous system: Drowsiness (≤24%), sedated state (≤24%)

1% to 10%:

Central nervous system: Extrapyramidal reaction (7%), dizziness (5%), fatigue (3%)

Gastrointestinal: Nausea (9%), xerostomia (6%), vomiting (3%), decreased appetite (2%)

Hepatic: Increased serum transaminases (2%)

Neuromuscular & skeletal: Increased creatine phosphokinase in blood specimen (4%)

<1%: Orthostatic hypotension

Frequency not defined:

Central nervous system: Dystonia

Endocrine & metabolic: Increased LDL cholesterol, increased serum cholesterol, increased serum triglyceride

Hematologic & oncologic: Elevated glycosylated hemoglobin

Postmarketing: Hyperglycemia, leukopenia, neutropenia

Mechanism of Action Lumateperone is a second-generation antipsychotic with antagonist activity at central serotonin 5-HT_{2A} receptors and postsynaptic antagonist activity at central dopamine D_2 receptors. Lumateperone has high binding affinity for serotonin 5-HT_{2A} receptors and moderate binding affinity for dopamine D_2 receptors. Lumateperone also has moderate binding affinity for dopamine D_1 and D_4 and adrenergic $alpha_{1A}$ and $alpha_{1B}$ receptors but has low binding affinity for muscarinic and histaminergic receptors.

Pharmacodynamics/Kinetics

Half-life Elimination ~18 hours after IV administration; following oral administration, steady state is reached in ~5 days.

Time to Peak 1 to 2 hours.

Reproductive Considerations

If treatment is needed in a woman planning a pregnancy, use of an agent other than lumateperone is preferred (Larsen 2015).

Pregnancy Considerations

Antipsychotic use during the third trimester of pregnancy has a risk for abnormal muscle movements (extrapyramidal symptoms) and/or withdrawal symptoms in newborns following delivery. Symptoms in the newborn may include agitation, feeding disorder, hypertonia, hypotonia, respiratory distress, somnolence, and tremor; these effects may be self-limiting or require hospitalization.

Safety data related to atypical antipsychotics during pregnancy are limited; as such, routine use is not recommended. However, if a woman is inadvertently exposed to an atypical antipsychotic while pregnant, continuing therapy may be preferable to switching to an agent that the fetus has not yet been exposed to; consider risk:benefit (ACOG 2008). If treatment is initiated during pregnancy, use of an agent other than lumateperone is preferred (Larsen 2015).

Data collection to monitor pregnancy and infant outcomes following exposure to lumateperone is ongoing. Health care providers are encouraged to enroll females exposed to lumateperone during pregnancy in the National Pregnancy Registry for Atypical Antipsychotics (1-866-961-2388 or http://womensmentalhealth.org/clinical-and-research-programs/pregnancyregistry).

- ◆ **Lumateperone Tosylate** *see* Lumateperone *on page 942*
- ◆ **Lumefantrine and Artemether** *see* Artemether and Lumefantrine *on page 168*
- ◆ **Luminal Sodium** *see* PHENobarbital *on page 1223*
- ◆ **Lumoxiti** *see* Moxetumomab Pasudotox *on page 1063*
- ◆ **Lunesta** *see* Eszopiclone *on page 606*
- ◆ **Lupron Depot (1-Month)** *see* Leuprolide *on page 890*
- ◆ **Lupron Depot (3-Month)** *see* Leuprolide *on page 890*
- ◆ **Lupron Depot (4-Month)** *see* Leuprolide *on page 890*
- ◆ **Lupron Depot (6-Month)** *see* Leuprolide *on page 890*
- ◆ **Lupron Depot-Ped (1-Month)** *see* Leuprolide *on page 890*
- ◆ **Lupron Depot-Ped (3-Month)** *see* Leuprolide *on page 890*

Lurasidone (loo RAS i done)

Brand Names: US Latuda

Brand Names: Canada Latuda

Pharmacologic Category Second Generation (Atypical) Antipsychotic

Use

Bipolar depression: Treatment of depressive episodes associated with bipolar I disorder, both as monotherapy (children ≥10 years of age, adolescents, and adults) and as an adjunct to lithium or divalproex (adults)

Schizophrenia: Treatment of adults and adolescents with schizophrenia

Local Anesthetic/Vasoconstrictor Precautions

No information available to require special precautions

Effects on Dental Treatment Key adverse event(s) related to dental treatment: Salivary hypersecretion has been reported (normal salivary flow resumes upon discontinuation)

Effects on Bleeding No information available to require special precautions

Adverse Reactions

>10%:

Endocrine & metabolic: Increased serum triglycerides (10% to 14%), increased serum cholesterol (6% to 14%), increased serum glucose (6% to 13%; fasting)

Gastrointestinal: Nausea (7% to 17%)

Infection: Viral infection (adolescents: 10% to 11%)

Nervous system: Extrapyramidal reaction (adults: 5% to 39%; children and adolescents: 6% to 14%), drowsiness (adults: 8% to 26%; children and adolescents: 11% to 15%), akathisia (adults: 6% to 22%; adolescents: 9%), parkinsonian-like syndrome (adults: 5% to 17%; adolescents: 4%), insomnia (5% to 11%)

1% to 10%:

Cardiovascular: Tachycardia (3%), orthostatic hypotension (≤3%), hypertension (adults: ≥1%)

Dermatologic: Pruritus (adults: ≥1%), skin rash (≥1%)

Endocrine & metabolic: Weight gain (2% to 7%), increased serum prolactin (≥5 x ULN: females: ≤6%; males: ≤2%)

Gastrointestinal: Dyspepsia (adults: 6% to 11%), vomiting (6% to 9%), xerostomia (adolescents and adults: 2% to 6%), diarrhea (3% to 5%), decreased appetite (children and adolescents: 4%; adults: ≥1%), sialorrhea (adults: 1% to 4%), abdominal pain (children and adolescents: 3%; adults: ≥1%), upper abdominal pain (children and adolescents: 3%)

Genitourinary: Urinary tract infection (adults: 1% to 2%)

Infection: Influenza (adults: 2%)

Nervous system: Agitation (adults: 5% to 10%), anxiety (adults: 4% to 7%), dystonia (adults: 2% to 7%; adolescents: ≤1%), dizziness (4% to 6%), fatigue (children and adolescents: 3%), restlessness (adults: 2% to 3%)

Neuromuscular & skeletal: Back pain (adults: 3% to 4%), increased creatine phosphokinase in blood specimen (adults: ≥1%), dyskinesia (adolescents: 1%)

Ophthalmic: Blurred vision (adults: ≥1%)

Renal: Increased serum creatinine (2% to 7%)

Respiratory: Rhinitis (adolescents: 8%), nasopharyngitis (adults: 4%), oropharyngeal pain (adolescents: ≤3%)

Frequency not defined: Nervous system: Suicidal ideation, suicidal tendencies, tardive dyskinesia

<1%, postmarketing, and/or case reports: Abnormal dreams, amenorrhea, anemia, angina pectoris, angioedema, bradycardia, breast hypertrophy, cerebrovascular accident, dysarthria, dysmenorrhea, dyspnea, dysuria, erectile dysfunction, first-degree atrioventricular block, galactorrhea, gastritis, hyponatremia, mastalgia, neuroleptic malignant syndrome, panic attack, pharyngeal edema, priapism, psychomotor agitation, renal failure syndrome, rhabdomyolysis, sleep disorder, syncope, tongue edema, urticaria, vertigo

Mechanism of Action Lurasidone is a benzoisothiazol-derivative atypical antipsychotic with mixed serotonin-dopamine antagonist activity. It exhibits high affinity for D_2, 5-HT_{2A}, and 5-HT_7 receptors; moderate affinity for alpha$_{2C}$-adrenergic receptors; and is a partial agonist for 5-HT_{1A} receptors. Lurasidone has no significant affinity for muscarinic M_1 and histamine H_1 receptors. The addition of serotonin antagonism to dopamine antagonism (classic neuroleptic mechanism) is thought to improve negative symptoms of psychoses and reduce the incidence of extrapyramidal side effects as compared to typical antipsychotics (Huttunen 1995).

Pharmacodynamics/Kinetics

Half-life Elimination 18 to 40 hours; Main active metabolite, ID-14283 (exo-hydroxy metabolite), exhibits a half-life of 7.5 to 10 hours (Citrome 2011)

Time to Peak 1 to 3 hours; steady state concentrations achieved within 7 days

Pregnancy Considerations

Antipsychotic use during the third trimester of pregnancy has a risk for abnormal muscle movements (extrapyramidal symptoms [EPS]) and/or withdrawal symptoms in newborns following delivery. Symptoms in the newborn may include agitation, feeding disorder, hypertonia, hypotonia, respiratory distress, somnolence, and tremor; these effects may be self-limiting or require hospitalization. Lurasidone may cause hyperprolactinemia, which may decrease reproductive function in both males and females.

The ACOG recommends that therapy during pregnancy be individualized; treatment with psychiatric medications during pregnancy should incorporate the clinical expertise of the mental health clinician, obstetrician, primary healthcare provider, and pediatrician. Safety data related to atypical antipsychotics during pregnancy is limited and routine use is not recommended. However, if a woman is inadvertently exposed to an atypical antipsychotic while pregnant, continuing therapy may be preferable to switching to a typical antipsychotic that the fetus has not yet been exposed to; consider risk: benefit (ACOG 2008).

Health care providers are encouraged to enroll women 18 to 45 years of age exposed to lurasidone during pregnancy in the Atypical Antipsychotics Pregnancy Registry (866-961-2388 or http://www.womensmentalhealth.org/clinical-and-research-programs/pregnancyregistry).

◆ **Lurasidone HCl** *see* Lurasidone *on page 943*

◆ **Lurasidone Hydrochloride** *see* Lurasidone *on page 943*

Lurbinectedin (LOOR bin EK te din)

Brand Names: US Zepzelca

Pharmacologic Category Antineoplastic Agent, Alkylating Agent

Use Small cell lung cancer, metastatic: Treatment of metastatic small cell lung cancer in adults with disease progression on or after platinum-based chemotherapy.

Local Anesthetic/Vasoconstrictor Precautions No information available to require special precautions.

Effects on Dental Treatment No significant effects or complications reported.

Effects on Bleeding Chemotherapy may result in significant myelosuppression, including thrombocytopenia. In patients under active treatment a medical consult is suggested.

Mechanism of Action Lurbinectedin is an alkylating agent and a selective inhibitor of oncogenic transcription which binds preferentially to guanine residues in the minor groove of DNA (Trigo 2020); this forms adducts and bends the DNA helix towards the major groove. Adduct formation affects the activities of DNA binding proteins, including some transcription factors and DNA repair pathways. Inhibition of oncogenic transcription results in tumor cell apoptosis (Trigo 2020).

Pharmacodynamics/Kinetics

Half-life Elimination 51 hours.

Reproductive Considerations

Evaluate pregnancy status prior to use in females of reproductive potential.

Females of reproductive potential should use effective contraception during therapy and for 6 months after the last lurbinectedin dose. Males with female partners of reproductive potential should use effective contraception during therapy and for 4 months after the last dose of lurbinectedin.

Pregnancy Considerations Based on the mechanism of action, and data from animal reproduction studies, in utero exposure to lurbinectedin may cause fetal harm.

◆ **Luteinizing Hormone Releasing Hormone** *see* Gonadorelin *on page 746*

◆ **Lutera** *see* Ethinyl Estradiol and Levonorgestrel *on page 612*

Lutropin Alfa (LOO troe pin AL fa)

Brand Names: Canada Luveris

Pharmacologic Category Gonadotropin; Ovulation Stimulator

Use Note: Not approved in the US

Infertility: Stimulation of follicular development in infertile hypogonadotropic hypogonadal (HH) women with profound luteinizing hormone (LH) deficiency (<1.2 units/L); to be used in combination with follitropin alfa

Local Anesthetic/Vasoconstrictor Precautions No information available to require special precautions

Effects on Dental Treatment No significant effects or complications reported

Effects on Bleeding No information available to require special precautions

Adverse Reactions

>10%:

Central nervous system: Headache (3% to 19%), pain (≤13%)

Endocrine & metabolic: Ovarian cyst (3% to 27%)

Gastrointestinal: Flatulence (≤16%), abdominal pain (7% to 15%)

Genitourinary: Dysmenorrhea (18%), mastalgia (7% to 18%)

1% to 10%:

Central nervous system: Fatigue (3% to 9%)

Endocrine & metabolic: Ovarian hyperstimulation (≤9%), ovarian disease (3% to 6%), increased serum cholesterol (4%)

Gastrointestinal: Nausea (3% to 9%), constipation (4% to 7%), diarrhea (≤6%)

Hepatic: Increased serum ALT (4%), increased serum AST (4%)

Local: Injection site reaction (≤7%)

Respiratory: Upper respiratory tract infection (≤3%)

<1%, postmarketing, and/or case reports: Accidental injury, acne vulgaris, anaphylaxis, anxiety, back pain, breast hypertrophy, conjunctivitis, cough, dental caries, depression, dizziness, drowsiness, dyspnea, dysuria, ectopic pregnancy, edema, endometrium disease, enlargement of abdomen, fever, flu like symptoms, genital edema, hemorrhage (in pregnancy), herpes simplex infection, hyperkinesia, hypersensitivity reaction, infection, insomnia, Klebsiella species, leg cramps, leg pain, leukorrhea, malaise, nail disease,

nervousness, ovarian hyperstimulation syndrome, ovary enlargement, pelvic congestion syndrome, pelvic pain, pharyngitis, porphyria, premenstrual syndrome, rhinitis, shock, skeletal pain, skin rash, spontaneous abortion, thromboembolism, urination disorder (change in frequency), uterine disease, uterine spasm, vaginal hemorrhage, vaginitis, vasodilation, vomiting, vulvovaginal candidiasis, weakness, xeroderma

Mechanism of Action Lutropin alfa is a recombinant luteinizing hormone prepared using Chinese hamster cell ovaries. Administration leads to increased follicular estradiol secretion needed for follicle stimulating hormone induced follicular development.

Pharmacodynamics/Kinetics

Half-life Elimination Terminal: 21 hours

Time to Peak Serum: 9 hours

Reproductive Considerations

Lutropin alfa is contraindicated for use in women who have medical conditions which are incompatible with a normal pregnancy.

Pregnancy Considerations

Use is contraindicated in women who are pregnant.

Ectopic pregnancy, miscarriage, spontaneous abortion, and multiple births have been reported. The incidence of congenital abnormality may be slightly higher after assisted reproductive techniques than with spontaneous conception; higher incidence may be related to parenteral characteristics (maternal age, sperm characteristics).

Product Availability Not available in the US

- **Luvox** *see* FluvoxaMINE *on page 708*
- **Luxiq** *see* Betamethasone (Topical) *on page 237*
- **Luzu** *see* Luliconazole *on page 942*
- **LY139603** *see* AtoMOXetine *on page 190*
- **LY146032** *see* DAPTOmycin *on page 437*
- **LY170053** *see* OLANZapine *on page 1127*
- **LY-188011** *see* Gemcitabine *on page 731*
- **LY231514** *see* PEMEtrexed *on page 1206*
- **LY246736** *see* Alvimopan *on page 112*
- **LY248686** *see* DULoxetine *on page 536*
- **LY303366** *see* Anidulafungin *on page 152*
- **LY333328** *see* Oritavancin *on page 1145*
- **LY-640315** *see* Prasugrel *on page 1252*
- **LY2148568** *see* Exenatide *on page 633*
- **LY3012207** *see* Olaratumab *on page 1131*
- **Lydexa** *see* Lidocaine (Topical) *on page 902*
- **LymePak** *see* Doxycycline *on page 522*
- **Lymphocyte Immune Globulin** *see* Antithymocyte Globulin (Equine) *on page 157*
- **Lymphocyte Mitogenic Factor** *see* Aldesleukin *on page 91*
- **Lynparza** *see* Olaparib *on page 1130*
- **Lyrica** *see* Pregabalin *on page 1268*
- **Lyrica CR** *see* Pregabalin *on page 1268*
- **Lysine4000 [OTC]** *see* L-Lysine *on page 925*
- **Lysodren** *see* Mitotane *on page 1041*
- **Lysteda** *see* Tranexamic Acid *on page 1478*
- **Lyumjev** *see* Insulin Lispro *on page 824*
- **Lyumjev KwikPen** *see* Insulin Lispro *on page 824*
- **Lyza** *see* Norethindrone *on page 1117*

Macitentan (ma si TEN tan)

Brand Names: US Opsumit

Brand Names: Canada Opsumit

Pharmacologic Category Endothelin Receptor Antagonist; Vasodilator

Use Pulmonary arterial hypertension: Treatment of pulmonary arterial hypertension (PAH) (WHO Group I) to reduce risks of disease progression and hospitalization

Local Anesthetic/Vasoconstrictor Precautions No information available to require special precautions

Effects on Dental Treatment No significant effects or complications reported

Effects on Bleeding No information available to require special precautions

Adverse Reactions

>10%:

Central nervous system: Headache (14%)

Hematologic & oncologic: Anemia (13%)

Respiratory: Nasopharyngitis (≤20%), pharyngitis (≤20%), bronchitis (12%)

1% to 10%:

Genitourinary: Urinary tract infection (9%)

Hematologic & oncologic: Decreased hemoglobin (9%)

Hepatic: Increased liver enzymes (>8 x ULN: 2%)

Infection: Influenza (6%)

<1%, postmarketing, and/or case reports: Angioedema, edema, fluid retention, hepatic insufficiency, hepatotoxicity, hypersensitivity reaction, increased serum ALT, increased serum AST, nasal congestion, pruritus, rash, symptomatic hypotension

Mechanism of Action Blocks endothelin (ET)-1 from binding to endothelin receptor subtypes ET_A and ET_B on vascular endothelium and smooth muscle. Stimulation of these receptors is associated with vasoconstriction, fibrosis, proliferation, hypertrophy, and inflammation.

Pharmacodynamics/Kinetics

Half-life Elimination ~16 hours (active metabolite: ~48 hours)

Time to Peak Plasma: 8 hours

Reproductive Considerations

[US Boxed Warnings]: For all female patients, macitentan is available only through a restricted program called the Opsumit Risk Evaluation and Mitigation Strategy (REMS). All females regardless of their reproductive potential must be enrolled in the REMS program; prescribers and pharmacies must also be enrolled in the program. Females of reproductive potential must be able to comply with pregnancy testing and contraception requirements of the program.

[US Boxed Warnings]: In female patients of reproductive potential, exclude pregnancy before the start of treatment, monthly during treatment, and 1 month after stopping treatment. Prevent pregnancy during treatment and for 1 month after stopping treatment by using acceptable methods of contraception. Women may use one highly effective form of contraception (intrauterine device, contraceptive implant, or tubal sterilization) or a combination of methods (hormonal contraceptive with a barrier method or two barrier methods). A hormonal contraceptive or barrier method must be used in addition to a partner's vasectomy, if that method is chosen. Females should be counseled on pregnancy prevention and planning and instructed to notify their prescriber immediately if a pregnancy should occur.

Sperm count may be reduced in men during treatment. Advise male patients of potential effects on fertility.

Pregnancy Considerations

[US Boxed Warnings]: Do not administer macitentan to a pregnant female because it may cause fetal harm. Based on data from animal reproduction studies, macitentan may cause harm if administered during pregnancy; therefore, use is contraindicated in pregnant women. Untreated maternal pulmonary arterial hypertension is also associated with an increased rate of maternal and fetal morbidity and mortality, including spontaneous abortion, intrauterine growth restriction and premature labor. Women with pulmonary arterial hypertension (PAH) are encouraged to avoid pregnancy (ESC [Regitz-Zagrosek 2018]; McLaughlin 2009; Taichman 2014).

[US Boxed Warnings]: For all female patients, macitentan is available only through a restricted program called the Opsumit Risk Evaluation and Mitigation Strategy (REMS).

- **MaC Patch [DSC]** *see* Capsaicin *on page 284*
- **Macrobid** *see* Nitrofurantoin *on page 1111*
- **Macrodantin** *see* Nitrofurantoin *on page 1111*
- **Macugen** *see* Pegaptanib *on page 1198*
- **Major-Prep Hemorrhoidal [OTC]** *see* Phenylephrine (Topical) *on page 1227*
- **Malarone** *see* Atovaquone and Proguanil *on page 193*
- **Mantoux** *see* Tuberculin Tests *on page 1503*
- **Mapap [OTC]** *see* Acetaminophen *on page 59*
- **Mapap Arthritis Pain [OTC]** *see* Acetaminophen *on page 59*
- **Mapap Children's [OTC]** *see* Acetaminophen *on page 59*
- **Mapap Extra Strength [OTC]** *see* Acetaminophen *on page 59*

Maprotiline (ma PROE ti leen)

Related Information

Dentin Hypersensitivity, Acid Erosion, High Caries Index, Management of Alveolar Osteitis, and Xerostomia *on page 1762*

Vasoconstrictor Interactions With Antidepressants *on page 1821*

Brand Names: Canada PMS-Maprotiline [DSC]; TEVA-Maprotiline [DSC]

Pharmacologic Category Antidepressant, Tetracyclic

Use

Depression: Treatment of major depressive disorder (MDD) and anxiety associated with depression

Local Anesthetic/Vasoconstrictor Precautions Although maprotiline is not a tricyclic antidepressant, it does block norepinephrine reuptake within CNS synapses as part of its mechanisms. It has been suggested that vasoconstrictor be administered with caution and to monitor vital signs in dental patients taking antidepressants that affect norepinephrine in this way, including maprotiline. Epinephrine and levonordefrin have been shown to have an increased pressor response in combination with TCAs. Maprotiline is one of the drugs confirmed to prolong the QT interval and is accepted as having a risk of causing torsade de pointes. The risk of drug-induced torsade de pointes is extremely low when a single QT interval prolonging drug is prescribed. In terms of epinephrine, it is not known what effect vasoconstrictors in the local anesthetic regimen will have in patients with a known history of congenital prolonged QT interval or in patients taking any medication that prolongs the QT interval. Until more information is obtained, it is suggested that the clinician consult with the physician prior to the use of a vasoconstrictor in suspected patients, and that the vasoconstrictor (epinephrine, mepivacaine and levonordefrin [Carbocaine® 2% with Neo-Cobefrin®]) be used with caution.

Effects on Dental Treatment Key adverse event(s) related to dental treatment: Xerostomia and changes in salivation (normal salivary flow resumes upon discontinuation).

Effects on Bleeding No information available to require special precautions

Adverse Reactions

>10%:

Central nervous system: Drowsiness (16%)

Gastrointestinal: Xerostomia (22%)

1% to 10%:

Central nervous system: Dizziness (8%), nervousness (6%), fatigue (4%), headache (4%), anxiety (3%), agitation (2%), insomnia (2%)

Gastrointestinal: Constipation (6%), nausea (2%)

Neuromuscular & skeletal: Weakness (4%), tremor (3%)

Ophthalmic: Blurred vision (4%)

<1%, postmarketing, and/or case reports: Abdominal cramps, abnormal liver function tests, accommodation disturbance, agranulocytosis, akathisia, alopecia, angle-closure glaucoma, ataxia, bitter taste, breast hypertrophy (female), cardiac arrhythmia, cerebrovascular accident, confusion, decreased libido, delusions, diaphoresis (excessive), diarrhea, disorientation, dysarthria, dysphagia, edema, EEG pattern changes, eosinophilia, epigastric distress, extrapyramidal reaction, feeling abnormal, fever, flushing, galactorrhea, gynecomastia (male), hallucination, heart block, hyperactivity, hyperglycemia, hypertension, hypoglycemia, hypomania, hypotension, impotence, increased libido, interstitial pneumonitis, jaundice, mania, melanoglossia, memory impairment, mydriasis, myocardial infarction, nasal congestion, nightmares, numbness, palpitations, paralytic ileus, peripheral neuropathy, petechia, pruritus, psychosis exacerbation, purpura, restlessness, sialorrhea, skin photosensitivity, skin rash, seizure, Stevens-Johnson syndrome, stomatitis, sublingual adenitis, syncope, tachycardia, testicle swelling, thrombocytopenia, tingling sensation, tinnitus, toxic epidermal necrolysis, urinary frequency, urinary hesitancy, urinary retention, vomiting, weight gain, weight loss

Mechanism of Action Increases the synaptic concentration of norepinephrine in the central nervous system by inhibition of its reuptake by the presynaptic neuronal membrane.

Pharmacodynamics/Kinetics

Onset of Action Depression: Initial effects may be observed within 1 to 2 weeks of treatment, with continued improvements through 4 to 6 weeks (Papakostas 2006; Posternak 2005; Szegedi 2009).

Half-life Elimination Serum: ~28 to 105 hours (Alkalay 1980)

Time to Peak Serum: 8 to 24 hours (Alkalay 1980; Pinder 1977)

Pregnancy Risk Factor B

Pregnancy Considerations Outcome information following maprotiline use in pregnancy is limited (Larsen 2015; McElhatton 1996).

The ACOG recommends that therapy for depression during pregnancy be individualized; treatment should incorporate the clinical expertise of the mental health clinician, obstetrician, primary health care provider, and pediatrician (ACOG 2008). According to the American Psychiatric Association (APA), the risks of medication treatment should be weighed against other treatment options and untreated depression. For women who discontinue antidepressant medications during pregnancy and who may be at high risk for postpartum depression, the medications can be restarted following delivery (APA 2010). Treatment algorithms have been developed by the ACOG and the APA for the management of depression in women prior to conception and during pregnancy (Yonkers 2009).

Pregnant women exposed to antidepressants during pregnancy are encouraged to enroll in the National Pregnancy Registry for Antidepressants (NPRAD). Women 18 to 45 years of age or their health care providers may contact the registry by calling 844-405-6185. Enrollment should be done as early in pregnancy as possible.

Dental Health Professional Considerations See Local Anesthetic/Vasoconstrictor Precautions

◆ **Maprotiline Hydrochloride** *see* Maprotiline *on page 946*

Maraviroc (mah RAV er rock)

Related Information

HIV Infection and AIDS *on page 1690*

Brand Names: US Selzentry

Brand Names: Canada Celsentri

Pharmacologic Category Antiretroviral, CCR5 Antagonist (Anti-HIV)

Use HIV-1 infection: Treatment of only CCR5-tropic HIV-1 infection in patients 2 years and older and weighing ≥10 kg, in combination with other antiretroviral agents

Local Anesthetic/Vasoconstrictor Precautions No information available to require special precautions

Effects on Dental Treatment Key adverse event(s) related to dental treatment: Stomatitis has been observed.

Effects on Bleeding No information available to require special precautions relative to hemostasis.

Adverse Reactions Includes data from both treatment-naive and treatment-experienced patients. Unless otherwise noted, frequency of adverse events is as reported in adults receiving combination antiretroviral therapy.

>10%:

Dermatologic: Skin rash (11%)

Gastrointestinal: Vomiting (children and adolescents: 12%; may be more common with oral solution)

Infection: Infection (55%)

Respiratory: Upper respiratory tract infection (23% to 32%), cough (14%)

Miscellaneous: Fever (13%)

1% to 10%:

Cardiovascular: Hypertension (3%), cardiac failure (<2%), cerebrovascular accident (<2%), coronary artery disease (<2%), coronary occlusion (<2%), endocarditis (<2%), myocardial infarction (<2%), portal vein thrombosis (<2%), septic shock (<2%), unstable angina pectoris (<2%)

Central nervous system: Dizziness (9%; children and adolescents: 3%; including postural dizziness), insomnia (8%), paresthesia (≤5%), dysesthesia (≤5%), anxiety (4%), impaired consciousness (4%), depression (4%), peripheral neuropathy (4%), malaise (≤4%), pain (≤4%), sensory disturbance (3% to 4%; includes body temperature perception disorder), memory impairment (3%), epilepsy (<2%), loss of consciousness (<2%), meningitis (<2%; includes viral), facial paralysis (<2%), seizure (<2%)

Dermatologic: Nail disease (6%; nail and nail bed disorder [excluding infection and infestation]), sweat gland disease (5%; apocrine and eccrine gland disorders), folliculitis (4%), pruritus (4%), tinea (4%), acne vulgaris (3%), alopecia (2%), erythema (2%), condyloma acuminatum (2%)

Endocrine & metabolic: Lipodystrophy (3% to 4%)

Gastrointestinal: Abdominal distension (≤10%), bloating (≤10%), flatulence (≤10%), decreased gastrointestinal motility (9%), change in appetite (8%), constipation (6%; may be more common with oral solution), abdominal pain (children and adolescents: 4%; may be more common with oral solution), diarrhea (children and adolescents: 4%; may be more common with oral solution), nausea (children and adolescents: 4%; may be more common with oral solution), carcinoma in situ of esophagus (<2%), colitis (*Clostridioides* [formerly *Clostridium*] *difficile*-associated: <2%)

Genitourinary: Genitourinary complaint (urinary tract/bladder symptoms, 3% to 5%), ejaculatory disorder (≤3%), erectile dysfunction (≤3%)

Hematologic & oncologic: Anemia (8%), neutropenia (4% to 6%), benign skin neoplasm (3%), basal cell carcinoma (<2%), bone marrow depression (<2%), Bowen disease (<2%), carcinoma (nasopharyngeal: <2%), hypoplastic anemia (<2%), liver metastases (<2%), malignant lymphoma (including diffuse large B-cell and anaplastic large cell lymphomas T- and null-cell types), malignant neoplasm (anal: <2%), malignant neoplasm of bile duct (cholangiocarcinoma; <2%), malignant neoplasm of tongue (<2%; malignant stage unspecified), neoplasm (<2%; includes abdominal and unspecified malignant endocrine neoplasm), squamous cell carcinoma (<2%), squamous cell carcinoma of skin (<2%)

Hepatic: Increased serum AST (>5 x ULN: 5%), cholestatic jaundice (<2%), hepatic cirrhosis (<2%), hepatic failure (<2%), jaundice (<2%)

Infection: Herpes virus infection (7% to 8%), bacterial infection (6%), herpes zoster (≤5%), varicella zoster infection (≤5%), meningococcal infection (3%) viral infection (3%), influenza (2%), bacterial infection (treponema <2%)

Neuromuscular & skeletal: Arthropathy (6% to 7%), myalgia (3%), increased creatine phosphokinase (<2%), myositis (<2%; may be infective), osteonecrosis (<2%), rhabdomyolysis (<2%), tremor (<2%; excluding congenital)

Ophthalmic: Conjunctivitis (2%), eye disease (2%; includes infection and inflammation), hemianopia (<2%), visual field defect (<2%)

Otic: Otitis media (2%)

Respiratory: Bronchitis (7% to 13%), upper respiratory complaint (6% to 9%), sinusitis (7%), irregular breathing (4%), nasal congestion (≤4%), rhinitis (≤4%), lower respiratory tract infection (≤3%), pulmonary infection (≤3%), paranasal sinus disease (3%), pneumonia (<2%)

Frequency not defined:

Hepatic: Hepatitis, hepatotoxicity

Immunologic: Immune reconstitution syndrome

<1%, postmarketing, and/or case reports: DRESS syndrome, ischemic heart disease, Stevens-Johnson syndrome, toxic epidermal necrolysis

Mechanism of Action Maraviroc, a CCR5 antagonist, selectively and reversibly binds to the chemokine (C-C motif receptor 5 [CCR5]) coreceptors located on human CD4 cells. CCR5 antagonism prevents interaction between the human CCR5 coreceptor and the gp120 subunit of the viral envelope glycoprotein, thereby inhibiting gp120 conformational change required for CCR5-tropic HIV-1 fusion with the CD4 cell and subsequent cell entry.

Pharmacodynamics/Kinetics

Half-life Elimination 14 to 18 hours

Time to Peak Plasma: 0.5 to 4 hours

Reproductive Considerations

The Health and Human Services perinatal HIV guidelines do not recommend maraviroc (except in special circumstances) for females living with HIV who are not yet pregnant but are trying to conceive.

For males and females living with HIV and planning a pregnancy, maximum viral suppression below the limits of detection with antiretroviral therapy (ART), modification of therapy (if needed), optimization of the woman's health, and a discussion of the potential risks and benefits of ART therapy during pregnancy is recommended prior to conception (HHS [perinatal] 2019).

Pregnancy Considerations

Maraviroc has moderate transfer across the human placenta.

Data collected by the antiretroviral pregnancy registry are insufficient to evaluate human teratogenic risk. Maternal antiretroviral therapy (ART) may be associated with adverse pregnancy outcomes including preterm delivery, stillbirth, low birth weight, and small for gestational age infants. Actual risks may be influenced by maternal factors, such as disease severity, gestational age at initiation of therapy, and specific ART regimen; therefore, close fetal monitoring is recommended. Because there is clear benefit to appropriate treatment, maternal ART should not be withheld due to concerns for adverse neonatal outcomes. Long-term follow-up is recommended for all infants exposed to antiretroviral medications; children without HIV but who were exposed to ART in utero and develop significant organ system abnormalities of unknown etiology (particularly of the CNS or heart) should be evaluated for potential mitochondrial dysfunction.

The Health and Human Services perinatal HIV guidelines do not recommend maraviroc for pregnant females living with HIV who are antiretroviral naive; maraviroc is not recommended (except in special circumstances) in pregnant females who have had ART therapy in the past but are restarting, or who require a new ART regimen (due to poor tolerance or poor virologic response of current regimen). Females who become pregnant while taking maraviroc may continue if viral suppression is effective and the regimen is well tolerated. Dose adjustments are not needed due to pregnancy.

In general, ART is recommended for all pregnant females living with HIV to keep the viral load below the limit of detection and reduce the risk of perinatal transmission. Therapy should be individualized following a discussion of the potential risks and benefits of treatment during pregnancy. Monitoring of pregnant females is more frequent than in nonpregnant adults. ART should be continued postpartum for all females living with HIV and can be modified after delivery.

Health care providers are encouraged to enroll pregnant females exposed to antiretroviral medications as early in pregnancy as possible in the Antiretroviral Pregnancy Registry (1-800-258-4263 or http://www.APRegistry.com). Health care providers caring for pregnant females living with HIV and their infants may contact the National Perinatal HIV Hotline (1-888-448-8765) for clinical consultation (HHS [perinatal] 2019).

◆ **Marcaine** *see* Bupivacaine *on page 256*

◆ **Marcaine/Epinephrine** *see* Bupivacaine and Epinephrine *on page 257*

◆ **Marcaine/Epinephrine PF** *see* Bupivacaine and Epinephrine *on page 257*

◆ **Marcaine Preservative Free** *see* Bupivacaine *on page 256*

◆ **Marcaine Spinal** *see* Bupivacaine *on page 256*

◆ **Marinol** *see* Dronabinol *on page 532*

◆ **Marlissa** *see* Ethinyl Estradiol and Levonorgestrel *on page 612*

◆ **Marqibo** *see* VinCRIStine (Liposomal) *on page 1546*

◆ **MAS Care-Pak** *see* DexAMETHasone (Systemic) *on page 463*

◆ **Matulane** *see* Procarbazine *on page 1278*

◆ **Matzim LA** *see* DilTIAZem *on page 499*

◆ **3M Avagard [OTC]** *see* Chlorhexidine Gluconate (Topical) *on page 335*

◆ **Mavenclad** *see* Cladribine *on page 359*

◆ **Mavenclad (4 Tabs)** *see* Cladribine *on page 359*

◆ **Mavenclad (5 Tabs)** *see* Cladribine *on page 359*

◆ **Mavenclad (6 Tabs)** *see* Cladribine *on page 359*

◆ **Mavenclad (7 Tabs)** *see* Cladribine *on page 359*

◆ **Mavenclad (8 Tabs)** *see* Cladribine *on page 359*

◆ **Mavenclad (9 Tabs)** *see* Cladribine *on page 359*

◆ **Mavenclad (10 Tabs)** *see* Cladribine *on page 359*

◆ **Mavik [DSC]** *see* Trandolapril *on page 1476*

◆ **Mavyret** *see* Glecaprevir and Pibrentasvir *on page 738*

◆ **Maxalt** *see* Rizatriptan *on page 1342*

◆ **Maxalt-MLT** *see* Rizatriptan *on page 1342*

◆ **Maxichlor PSE [OTC]** *see* Chlorpheniramine and Pseudoephedrine *on page 341*

◆ **Maximum Red Krill [OTC]** *see* Omega-3 Fatty Acids *on page 1137*

◆ **Maxipime [DSC]** *see* Cefepime *on page 307*

◆ **Maxzide** *see* Hydrochlorothiazide and Triamterene *on page 763*

◆ **Maxzide-25** *see* Hydrochlorothiazide and Triamterene *on page 763*

Measles, Mumps, and Rubella Virus Vaccine (MEE zels, mumpz & roo BEL a VYE rus vak SEEN)

Brand Names: US M-M-R II

Brand Names: Canada M-M-R II; Priorix

Pharmacologic Category Vaccine; Vaccine, Live (Viral)

Use Measles, mumps, and rubella prevention: Active immunization for simultaneous vaccination against measles, mumps, and rubella in patients ≥12 months of age

The Advisory Committee on Immunization Practices (ACIP) recommends routine vaccination for the following (CDC/ACIP [McLean 2013]):

- All children (first dose given at 12 to 15 months of age)
- Adults born in 1957 or later (without evidence of immunity or documentation of vaccination). Vaccine may be given to adults born prior to 1957 if they do not have contraindications to the MMR vaccine.
- Adults at higher risk for exposure to and transmission of measles, mumps, and rubella should receive special consideration for vaccination, unless an acceptable evidence of immunity exists. This includes international travelers, persons attending colleges and other post high school education, persons working in health care facilities.

Local Anesthetic/Vasoconstrictor Precautions No information available to require special precautions

Effects on Dental Treatment No significant effects or complications reported

Effects on Bleeding No information available to require special precautions

Adverse Reactions

Frequency not defined:

Cardiovascular: Syncope, vasculitis

Central nervous system: Acute disseminated encephalomyelitis, ataxia, dizziness, Guillain-Barré syndrome, headache, irritability, malaise, paresthesia, polyneuropathy, retrobulbar neuritis, seizure, sensorineural hearing loss, subacute sclerosing panencephalitis, transverse myelitis

Dermatologic: Erythema multiforme, IgA vasculitis (Henoch-Schnolein purpura/acute hemorrhagic edema of infancy), morbilliform rash, pruritus, rash, Stevens-Johnson syndrome, urticaria

Endocrine & metabolic: Diabetes mellitus

Gastrointestinal: Diarrhea, nausea, pancreatitis, parotitis, sore throat, vomiting

Genitourinary: Epididymitis, orchitis

Hematologic & oncologic: Leukocytosis, lymphadenopathy (regional), purpura, thrombocytopenia

Hypersensitivity: Anaphylactoid reaction, anaphylaxis, angioedema

Infection: Atypical measles

Local: Injection site reaction (including burning, induration, redness, stinging, swelling, tenderness, vesiculation, wheal and flare)

Neuromuscular & skeletal: Arthropathy (arthralgia/arthritis: Women 12% to 26%; children ≤3%), myalgia, panniculitis

Ophthalmic: Conjunctivitis, oculomotor nerve paralysis, optic neuritis, optic papillitis, retinitis

Otic: Otitis media

Respiratory: Bronchospasm, cough, pneumonia, rhinitis

Miscellaneous: Febrile seizures, fever

<1%, postmarketing, and/or case reports: Aseptic meningitis (associated with Urabe strain of mumps vaccine), brain disease, encephalitis

Mechanism of Action As a live, attenuated vaccine, MMR vaccine offers active immunity to disease caused by the measles, mumps, and rubella viruses.

Pharmacodynamics/Kinetics

Onset of Action The median seroconversion after 1 vaccine dose is 96% (measles), 99% (rubella), mumps (94%) (CDC/ACIP [McLean 2013]).

Duration of Action The median duration of immunity after 2 doses is ≥15 years for all components of the vaccine (CDC/ACIP [McLean 2013]).

Reproductive Considerations

This vaccine should not be administered to women who plan to become pregnant within 1 month of immunization.

Prenatal screening is recommended for all pregnant women who lack evidence of rubella immunity. Women of childbearing age without documentation of rubella vaccination or serologic evidence of immunity should be vaccinated (for women of childbearing potential, birth prior to 1957 is not acceptable evidence of immunity to rubella).

Sterility in males and infertility in prepubescent females may occur with natural mumps infection (CDC/ACIP [McLean 2013]).

Pregnancy Considerations

Based on information collected following inadvertent administration during pregnancy, adverse events have not been observed following use of rubella vaccine. However, theoretical risks cannot be ruled out; use of this vaccine is contraindicated in pregnant females. The risk of congenital rubella syndrome following vaccination is significantly less than the risk associated following infection; therefore, inadvertent administration of MMR during pregnancy is not considered an indication to terminate pregnancy.

Adverse consequences of natural infection in unvaccinated pregnant women have been reported. Measles infection during pregnancy may increase the risk of premature labor, preterm delivery, spontaneous abortion and low birth weights. Rubella infection during the first trimester may lead to miscarriages, stillbirths, and congenital rubella syndrome (includes auditory, ophthalmic, cardiac and neurologic defects; intrauterine and postnatal growth retardation); fetal rubella infection can occur during any trimester of pregnancy. Maternal mumps infection during the first trimester may increase the risk of spontaneous abortion or intrauterine fetal death.

Prenatal screening is recommended for all pregnant women who lack evidence of rubella immunity. Women of childbearing age without documentation of rubella vaccination or serologic evidence of immunity should be vaccinated (for women of childbearing potential, birth prior to 1957 is not acceptable evidence of immunity to rubella). Women who are pregnant should be vaccinated upon completion or termination of pregnancy, prior to discharge. Household contacts of pregnant women may be vaccinated (CDC/ACIP [McLean 2013]).

Measles, Mumps, Rubella, and Varicella Virus Vaccine

(MEE zels, mumpz, roo BEL a, & var i SEL a VYE rus vak SEEN)

Brand Names: US ProQuad

Brand Names: Canada Priorix-Tetra; ProQuad

Pharmacologic Category Vaccine; Vaccine, Live (Viral)

Use

Measles, mumps, rubella, and varicella vaccination: To provide active immunization for the prevention of measles, mumps, rubella, and varicella in children 12 months to 12 years of age.

The Advisory Committee on Immunization Practices (ACIP) recommends routine vaccination against measles, mumps, rubella, and varicella in healthy children; the first dose should be given at 12 to 15 months of age and the second dose at 4 to 6 years of age. For children receiving their first dose at 12 to 47 months of age, either the MMRV combination vaccine or separate MMR and varicella vaccines can be used. The ACIP prefers administration of separate MMR and varicella vaccines as the first dose in this age group unless the parent or caregiver expresses preference for the MMRV combination. For children receiving the first dose at ≥48 months or their second dose at any age, use of MMRV is preferred. For children with a personal or family history of seizures, the ACIP recommends vaccination with separate MMR and varicella vaccines, as opposed to the MMRV combination vaccine (CDC/ACIP [Marin 2010]).

Canadian labeling (not in US labeling): MMRV combination vaccine is approved for use in healthy children (Priorix-Tetra: 9 months to 6 years; ProQuad: 12 months to 6 years); may consider use in healthy children ≤12 years of age based upon prior experience with the separate component (live-attenuated MMR or live-attenuated varicella [OKA-strain]) vaccines.

Local Anesthetic/Vasoconstrictor Precautions No information available to require special precautions

Effects on Dental Treatment No significant effects or complications reported

Effects on Bleeding No information available to require special precautions

Adverse Reactions Also refer to Measles, Mumps, and Rubella Vaccine (M-M-R II) and Varicella Virus Vaccine (Varivax) monographs for additional adverse reactions reported with those agents.

>10%:

Local: Pain at injection site (≤41%), erythema at injection site (11% to 24%), local soreness/soreness at injection site (≤22%), tenderness at injection site (≤22%), swelling at injection site (8% to 16%)

Miscellaneous: Fever (8% to 22%; ≥38.9°C [≥102°F])

1% to 10%:

Central nervous system: Irritability (2% to 7%), drowsiness (1%)

Dermatologic: Morbilliform rash (≤5%), rubella-like rash (≤4%), varicella-like rash (≤2%), rash at injection site (2%), skin rash (≤2%), vesicular eruption (≤2%), injection site pruritus (1%), viral exanthem (1%)

Gastrointestinal: Vomiting (1%), diarrhea (≤1%)

Local: Bruising at injection site (1% to 2%)

Respiratory: Upper respiratory tract infection (1%), rhinorrhea (1%)

<1%, postmarketing, and/or case reports: Abdominal pain, acute disseminated encephalomyelitis, agitation, anaphylactoid shock, anaphylaxis, angioedema, apathy, aplastic anemia, arthralgia, arthritis, aseptic meningitis, ataxia, atypical measles, Bell palsy, bleeding at injection site, bronchitis, bronchospasm, burning sensation at injection site, candidiasis, cellulitis, cerebrovascular accident, dizziness, encephalitis, encephalopathy, epididymitis, epistaxis, erythema multiforme, eye irritation, eyelid edema, facial edema, febrile seizures, Guillain-Barré syndrome, headache, hematochezia, hematoma at injection site, hemorrhage, Henoch-Schonlein purpura (including acute hemorrhagic edema of infancy), herpes simplex infection, herpes zoster infection, hypersomnia, impetigo, induration at injection site, infection, inflammation, influenza, localized vesiculation, localized warm feeling (includes warmth to the touch), lower extremity pain, lymphadenitis, lymphadenopathy (regional), measles, measles inclusion body encephalitis, meningitis, musculoskeletal pain, myalgia, neck pain, necrotizing retinitis, nervousness, nonthrombocytopenic purpura, optic nerve palsy, optic neuritis, oral mucosa ulcer, orchitis, otalgia, pain (hip), panniculitis, paresthesia, parotitis, peripheral edema, pneumonia, polyneuropathy, pruritus, pulmonary congestion, residual mass at injection site, respiratory tract infection, retinitis, retrobulbar neuritis, rhinitis, seizure, sensorineural hearing loss, sinusitis, skin discoloration at injection site, skin infection, skin sclerosis, sore throat, Stevens-Johnson syndrome, stiffness, subacute sclerosing panencephalitis, syncope, thrombocytopenia, transverse myelitis, tremor, urticaria at injection site, varicella infection - chickenpox (vaccine strain), wheezing

Mechanism of Action A live, attenuated virus vaccine that induces active immunity to disease caused by the measles, mumps, rubella, and varicella-zoster viruses.

Pharmacodynamics/Kinetics

Onset of Action At 6 weeks postvaccination of a single dose, the antibody response rate in healthy children 12 to 23 months of age was ~91% to 99%. Following a second dose to children <3 years of age, the observed antibody response rate was ~98% to 99%.

Duration of Action Antibody levels persist 10 years or longer in most healthy recipients. Refer to the Varicella Virus Vaccine monograph and the Measles, Mumps, and Rubella Virus Vaccine monograph for details.

Reproductive Considerations

Pregnancy should be avoided for 3 months following vaccination (per manufacturer labeling).

Refer to the Varicella Virus Vaccine monograph and the Measles, Mumps, and Rubella Virus Vaccine monograph for additional information.

Pregnancy Considerations

Use is contraindicated in pregnant females.

Refer to the Varicella Virus Vaccine monograph and the Measles, Mumps, and Rubella Virus Vaccine monograph for additional information.

Mecamylamine (mek a MIL a meen)

Brand Names: US Vecamyl

Pharmacologic Category Ganglionic Blocking Agent

Use Hypertension: Management of moderately severe to severe hypertension and in uncomplicated malignant hypertension.

Local Anesthetic/Vasoconstrictor Precautions
No information available to require special precautions

Effects on Dental Treatment Key adverse event(s) related to dental treatment: Xerostomia (normal salivary flow resumes upon discontinuation). Patients may experience orthostatic (postural) hypotension as they stand up after treatment, especially if lying in dental chair for extended periods of time. Use caution with sudden changes in position during and after dental treatment.

Effects on Bleeding No information available to require special precautions

Adverse Reactions Frequency not defined.

- Cardiovascular: Orthostatic hypotension, syncope
- Central nervous system: Altered mental status, choreiform movements, convulsions, fatigue, orthostatic dizziness, paresthesia, sedation
- Endocrine & metabolic: Decreased libido
- Gastrointestinal: Anorexia, constipation (sometimes preceded by small, frequent stools), glossitis, intestinal obstruction, nausea, vomiting, xerostomia
- Genitourinary: Impotence, urinary retention
- Neuromuscular & skeletal: Tremor, weakness
- Ophthalmic: Blurred vision, mydriasis
- Respiratory: Pulmonary edema, pulmonary fibrosis

Mechanism of Action Mecamylamine inhibits acetylcholine at the autonomic ganglia, causing a decrease in blood pressure. The blood pressure lowering effect is predominantly orthostatic; the supine blood pressure is also significantly decreased.

Pharmacodynamics/Kinetics

Onset of Action 0.5 to 2 hours

Duration of Action 6 to ≥12 hours

Pregnancy Risk Factor C

Pregnancy Considerations

Mecamylamine crosses the placenta.

◆ **Mecamylamine HCl** *see* Mecamylamine *on page 951*

◆ **Mecamylamine Hydrochloride** *see* Mecamylamine *on page 951*

Mecasermin (mek a SER min)

Brand Names: US Increlex

Pharmacologic Category Growth Hormone

Use Primary insulin-like growth factor-1 deficiency: Treatment of growth failure in pediatric patients ≥2 years of age with severe primary insulin-like growth factor-1 (IGF-1) deficiency or with growth hormone (GH) gene deletion who have developed neutralizing antibodies to GH.

Local Anesthetic/Vasoconstrictor Precautions
No information available to require special precautions

Effects on Dental Treatment No significant effects or complications reported

Effects on Bleeding No information available to require special precautions

Adverse Reactions

>10%:

- Endocrine & metabolic: Hypoglycemia (42%)
- Immunologic: Antibody development
- Respiratory: Tonsillar hypertrophy (15%)

1% to 10%:

- Cardiovascular: Heart murmur (≥5%)
- Endocrine & metabolic: Severe hypoglycemia (7%), thymus hypertrophy (≥5%)
- Gastrointestinal: Vomiting (≥5%)
- Local: Bruising at injection site (≥5%), lipotrophy at injection site (≥5%)
- Nervous system: Hypoglycemic seizure (≤6%), loss of consciousness (≤6%), dizziness (≥5%), headache (≥5%), seizure (≥5%), intracranial hypertension (4%)
- Neuromuscular & skeletal: Arthralgia (≥5%), limb pain (≥5%)
- Otic: Abnormal tympanometry (≥5%), fluid in ear (≥5%; middle ear), hypoacusis (≥5%), otalgia (≥5%), otitis media (≥5%), serous otitis media (≥5%)
- Respiratory: Snoring (≥5%)

Frequency not defined:

- Cardiovascular: Cardiomegaly, heart valve disease
- Dermatologic: Thickening of the soft tissues of the face
- Endocrine & metabolic: Hypercholesterolemia, hypertriglyceridemia, increased lactate dehydrogenase
- Hepatic: Increased serum alanine aminotransferase, increased serum aspartate transaminase
- Neuromuscular & skeletal: Scoliosis progression

<1%, postmarketing, and/or case reports: Abnormal hair texture, alopecia, anaphylaxis, angioedema, avascular necrosis of bones, benign neoplasm, dyspnea, hypersensitivity reaction, injection site pruritus, injection site reaction, malignant neoplasm, osteonecrosis, slipped capital femoral epiphysis, urticaria, urticaria at injection site

Mechanism of Action Mecasermin is an insulin-like growth factor (IGF-1) produced using recombinant DNA technology to replace endogenous IGF-1. Endogenous IGF-1 circulates predominately bound to insulin-like growth factor-binding protein-3 (IGFBP-3) and a growth hormone-dependent acid-labile subunit (ALS). Acting at receptors in the liver and other tissues, endogenous growth hormone (GH) stimulates the synthesis and secretion of IGF-1. In patients with primary severe IGF-1 deficiency, growth hormone receptors in the liver are unresponsive to GH, leading to reduced endogenous IGF-I concentrations and decreased growth (skeletal, cell, and organ). Endogenous IGF-1 also suppresses liver glucose production, stimulates peripheral glucose utilization, and has an inhibitory effect on insulin secretion.

Pharmacodynamics/Kinetics

Half-life Elimination Severe primary IGFD: ~5.8 hours

Time to Peak Serum: 2 hours

Pregnancy Considerations Treatment is not recommended in for growth promotion in patients with closed epiphyses; use during pregnancy would not be expected.

- **Mecasermin (rDNA Origin)** *see* Mecasermin *on page 951*

Meclizine (MEK li zeen)

Brand Names: US Bonine [OTC]; Dramamine Less Drowsy [OTC]; Motion-Time [OTC]; Travel Sickness [OTC]; Travel-Ease [OTC]

Pharmacologic Category Antiemetic; Histamine H_1 Antagonist; Histamine H_1 Antagonist, First Generation; Piperazine Derivative

Use

Motion sickness: Prevention and treatment of nausea, vomiting, or dizziness associated with motion sickness.

Vertigo: Treatment of vertigo associated with diseases affecting vestibular system.

Local Anesthetic/Vasoconstrictor Precautions No information available to require special precautions

Effects on Dental Treatment Key adverse event(s) related to dental treatment: Slight to moderate drowsiness, thickening of bronchial secretions, significant xerostomia (normal salivary flow resumes upon discontinuation).

Effects on Bleeding No information available to require special precautions

Adverse Reactions Frequency not defined.

Central nervous system: Drowsiness, fatigue, headache

Gastrointestinal: Vomiting, xerostomia

Hypersensitivity: Anaphylactoid reaction

Ophthalmic: Blurred vision

Mechanism of Action Antihistamine that suppresses vestibular end-organ receptors and inhibits activation of central cholinergic pathways (Oosterveld 1985)

Pharmacodynamics/Kinetics

Onset of Action ~1 hour (Wang 2012)

Duration of Action ~24 hours (Wang 2012)

Half-life Elimination 5.2 ± 0.8 hours (Wang 2011; Wang 2012)

Time to Peak Plasma: 3.1 ± 1.4 hours (Wang 2011; Wang 2012)

Pregnancy Considerations

Based on epidemiologic studies, maternal meclizine use has generally not resulted in an increased risk of fetal abnormalities.

- **Meclizine HCl** *see* Meclizine *on page 952*
- **Meclizine Hydrochloride** *see* Meclizine *on page 952*

Meclofenamate (me kloe fen AM ate)

Related Information

Rheumatoid Arthritis, Osteoarthritis, and Osteoporosis *on page 1697*

Temporomandibular Dysfunction (TMD), Chronic Pain, and Fibromyalgia *on page 1773*

Pharmacologic Category Analgesic, Nonopioid; Nonsteroidal Anti-inflammatory Drug (NSAID), Oral

Use

Acute gouty arthritis: Acute and long-term use in the relief of signs and symptoms of acute gouty arthritis.

Ankylosing spondylitis: Acute and long-term use in the relief of signs and symptoms of ankylosing spondylitis.

Arthritis: Relief of signs and symptoms of juvenile arthritis, osteoarthritis, and rheumatoid arthritis.

Bursitis/tendinitis of the shoulder: Acute and long-term use in the relief of signs and symptoms of acute painful shoulder (acute subacromial bursitis/supraspinatus tendinitis).

Fever: Reduction of fever in adults.

Pain, mild to moderate: Relief of mild to moderate pain in adults.

Primary dysmenorrhea/excessive menstrual blood loss: Treatment of primary dysmenorrhea and idiopathic heavy menstrual blood loss.

Local Anesthetic/Vasoconstrictor Precautions No information available to require special precautions

Effects on Dental Treatment The dentist should be aware of the potential of abnormal coagulation. Caution should also be exercised in the use of NSAIDs in patients already on anticoagulant therapy with drugs such as warfarin (Coumadin®). Recovery of platelet function usually occurs 1-2 days after discontinuation of NSAIDs. See Effects on Bleeding.

Effects on Bleeding Nonselective NSAIDs such as meclofenamate inhibit platelet aggregation and prolong bleeding time in some patients. Unlike aspirin, the NSAID effect on platelet function is quantitatively less, of shorter duration, and reversible.

Adverse Reactions

>10%:

Central nervous system: Dizziness

Dermatologic: Skin rash

Gastrointestinal: Abdominal cramps, dyspepsia, heartburn, nausea

1% to 10%:

Central nervous system: Headache, nervousness

Dermatologic: Pruritus

Endocrine & metabolic: Fluid retention

Gastrointestinal: Vomiting

Otic: Tinnitus

<1%, postmarketing, and/or case reports: Acute renal failure, agranulocytosis, allergic rhinitis, anemia, angioedema, aseptic meningitis, auditory impairment, blurred vision, bone marrow depression, cardiac arrhythmia, cardiac failure, confusion, conjunctivitis, cystitis, depression, drowsiness, dyspnea, epistaxis, erythema multiforme, gastritis, gastrointestinal ulcer, hallucination, hemolytic anemia, hepatitis, hepatotoxicity (idiosyncratic; Chalasani 2014), hot flash, hypertension, insomnia, leukopenia, peripheral neuropathy, polydipsia, polyuria, Stevens-Johnson syndrome, tachycardia, thrombocytopenia, toxic amblyopia, toxic epidermal necrolysis, urticaria, xerophthalmia

Mechanism of Action Reversibly inhibits cyclooxygenase-1 and 2 (COX-1 and 2) enzymes, which results in decreased formation of prostaglandin precursors; has antipyretic, analgesic, and anti-inflammatory properties.

Other proposed mechanisms not fully elucidated (and possibly contributing to the anti-inflammatory effect to varying degrees) include inhibiting chemotaxis, altering lymphocyte activity, inhibiting neutrophil aggregation/activation, and decreasing proinflammatory cytokine levels.

Pharmacodynamics/Kinetics

Duration of Action 2 to 4 hours

Half-life Elimination Meclofenamate sodium: 0.8 to 2.1 hours; Metabolite I: ~15 hours

Time to Peak Serum: Meclofenamate sodium: 0.5 to 2 hours; Metabolite I: 0.5 to 4 hours

Reproductive Considerations

The chronic use of NSAIDs in women of reproductive age may be associated with infertility that is reversible upon discontinuation of the medication (Micu 2011).

Pregnancy Risk Factor C

Pregnancy Considerations

Birth defects have been observed following in utero NSAID exposure in some studies; however, data is conflicting (Bloor 2013). Nonteratogenic effects, including prenatal constriction of the ductus arteriosus, persistent pulmonary hypertension of the newborn, oligohydramnios, necrotizing enterocolitis, renal dysfunction or failure, and intracranial hemorrhage have been observed in the fetus/neonate following in utero NSAID exposure. In addition, non-closure of the ductus arteriosus postnatally may occur and be resistant to medical management (Bermas 2014; Bloor 2013). Because they may cause premature closure of the ductus arteriosus, the use of NSAIDs late in pregnancy should be avoided. Use of NSAIDs can be considered for the treatment of mild rheumatoid arthritis flares in pregnant women; however, use should be minimized or avoided early and late in pregnancy (Bermas 2014; Saavedra Salinas 2015).

The use of NSAIDs close to conception may be associated with an increased risk of miscarriage (Bermas 2014; Bloor 2013).

- ◆ **Meclofenamate Sodium** *see* Meclofenamate *on page 952*
- ◆ **Meclozine Hydrochloride** *see* Meclizine *on page 952*
- ◆ **Med-Derm Hydrocortisone [OTC] [DSC]** *see* Hydrocortisone (Topical) *on page 775*
- ◆ **MEDI-551** *see* Inebilizumab *on page 808*
- ◆ **MEDI4736** *see* Durvalumab *on page 538*
- ◆ **Medi-First Anti-Fungal [OTC] [DSC]** *see* Tolnaftate *on page 1462*
- ◆ **Medi-First Hydrocortisone [OTC] [DSC]** *see* Hydrocortisone (Topical) *on page 775*
- ◆ **Medi-Phenyl [OTC] [DSC]** *see* Phenylephrine (Systemic) *on page 1227*
- ◆ **Mediproxen [OTC]** *see* Naproxen *on page 1080*

Medium Chain Triglycerides

(mee DEE um chane trye GLIS er ides)

Brand Names: US Betaquik [OTC]; Liquigen [OTC]; MCT Oil [OTC]

Brand Names: Canada MCT Oil

Pharmacologic Category Nutritional Supplement

Use

Dietary supplement: An alternative source of energy used to replace or supplement long chain fats in the nutritional management of patients who cannot efficiently digest and absorb fats (Limketkai 2017).

Medical food: Used to manage many metabolic and digestive abnormalities such as pancreatic insufficiency, fat malabsorption, impaired lymphocyte chylomicron transport, and severe hyperchylomicronemia; component of adult and preterm infant formulas (Łoś-Rycharska 2016).

Local Anesthetic/Vasoconstrictor Precautions

No information available to require special precautions

Effects on Dental Treatment No significant effects or complications reported

Effects on Bleeding No information available to require special precautions

Adverse Reactions Frequency not defined.

Endocrine & metabolic: Decreased HDL cholesterol (>6 months daily use), increased serum triglycerides (>6 months daily use)

Gastrointestinal: Abdominal cramps, abdominal pain, bloating, diarrhea, nausea

Mechanism of Action MCTs are saturated fatty acids in chains of 6-12 carbon atoms. They are water soluble and can pass directly through intestinal cell membranes into portal venous blood. Unlike long chain fats, MCTs do not require the presence of bile acids and pancreatic lipase for absorption. MCTs provide a source of calories while reducing the amount of malabsorbed fat remaining in stool (Gracey, 1970; Ruppin, 1980).

Pharmacodynamics/Kinetics

Onset of Action Octanoic acid appeared in each subject by 30 minutes following ingestion; effect on seizures in children: Within 6 weeks

- ◆ **Medolor Pak** *see* Lidocaine and Prilocaine *on page 911*
- ◆ **Medrol** *see* MethylPREDNISolone *on page 999*
- ◆ **Medrol Dose Pack** *see* MethylPREDNISolone *on page 999*

MedroxyPROGESTERone

(me DROKS ee proe JES te rone)

Related Information

Endocrine Disorders and Pregnancy *on page 1684*

Brand Names: US Depo-Provera; Depo-SubQ Provera 104; Provera

Brand Names: Canada Depo-Provera; Provera

Pharmacologic Category Contraceptive; Progestin

Use

Abnormal uterine bleeding (tablet): Treatment of abnormal uterine bleeding due to hormonal imbalance in the absence of organic pathology, such as fibroids or uterine cancer.

Amenorrhea, secondary (tablet): Treatment of secondary amenorrhea due to hormonal imbalance in the absence of organic pathology, such as fibroids or uterine cancer.

Contraception (104 mg per 0.65 mL and 150 mg/mL injection): Prevention of pregnancy in females of reproductive potential.

Endometrial hyperplasia prevention (tablet): Prevention of endometrial hyperplasia in nonhysterectomized postmenopausal persons receiving daily oral conjugated estrogens 0.625 mg. **Note:** Due to safety considerations, when a progesterone is needed, use of micronized progesterone is preferred over medroxyprogesterone acetate (AACE [Goodman 2011]; AACE/ACE [Cobin 2017])

Endometrial carcinoma (400 mg/mL injection) (100 mg tablet [Canadian product]): Adjunctive therapy and/or palliative treatment of inoperable, recurrent, and/or metastatic endometrial carcinoma.

Endometriosis (104 mg/0.65 mL injection): Management of endometriosis-associated pain.

Local Anesthetic/Vasoconstrictor Precautions

No information available to require special precautions

Effects on Dental Treatment Progestins may predispose the patient to gingival bleeding.

Effects on Bleeding No information available to require special precautions

Adverse Reactions Adverse effects as reported with any dosage form.

>10%:

Endocrine & metabolic: Amenorrhea (6% to 68%), change in menstrual flow (18%; including irregular, increase or decrease flow, and spotting), hot flash (≤36%), menstrual disease (IM: 57% at 12 months;

32% at 24 months), weight gain (7% to 38%), weight loss (≤12%)
Gastrointestinal: Abdominal pain (4% to 11%)
Nervous system: Headache (9% to 17%), nervousness (11%)
1% to 10%:
Cardiovascular: Edema (2%)
Dermatologic: Acne vulgaris (1% to 4%), alopecia (1%), skin rash (1%)
Endocrine & metabolic: Decreased libido (3% to 6%)
Gastrointestinal: Abdominal distension (1% to <5%), bloating (2%), diarrhea (1% to <5%), nausea (1% to <5%)
Genitourinary: Bacterial vaginosis (≤5%), breast tenderness (≤2%), dysmenorrhea (≤2%), leukorrhea (3%), mastalgia (≤3%), urinary tract infection (4%), vaginitis (≤5%), vulvovaginal candidiasis (≤5%)
Local: Atrophy at injection site (≤1%), induration at injection site (≤1%), injection site reaction (5% to 6%)
Nervous system: Anxiety (1%), depression (2% to 3%), dizziness (1% to 6%), fatigue (≤4%), insomnia (1%), irritability (1%)
Neuromuscular & skeletal: Arthralgia (2%), asthenia (≤4%), back pain (2% to 3%), lower limb cramp (4%)
<1%:
Cardiovascular: Chest pain, syncope, tachycardia
Dermatologic: Pruritus, urticaria
Endocrine & metabolic: Fluid retention, galactorrhea not associated with childbirth
Gastrointestinal: Abdominal distension, diarrhea
Genitourinary: Dyspareunia, lump in breast
Hematologic & oncologic: Anemia
Hypersensitivity: Hypersensitivity reaction
Nervous system: Drowsiness, facial nerve paralysis, paresthesia
Respiratory: Asthma, dyspnea
Frequency not defined:
Cardiovascular: Acute myocardial infarction, cerebrovascular accident, retinal thrombosis
Dermatologic: Skin discoloration at injection site
Endocrine & metabolic: Decreased glucose tolerance, drug-induced Cushing's syndrome, hypercalcemia, lipodystrophy, spotty menstruation
Genitourinary: Change in cervical erosion, change in cervical secretions, nipple discharge
Hepatic: Cholestatic jaundice
Local: Injection site nodule, tenderness at injection site
Nervous system: Euphoria, malaise
Ophthalmic: Optic neuritis
Postmarketing:
Cardiovascular: Deep vein thrombosis, pulmonary embolism, thrombophlebitis, varicose veins
Dermatologic: Chloasma, diaphoresis, skin discoloration (melasma)
Endocrine & metabolic: Breast changes, hirsutism, increased libido, increased thirst
Gastrointestinal: Change in appetite
Genitourinary: Anovulation (prolonged), delayed return to fertility, genitourinary infection, lactation insufficiency, malignant neoplasm of cervix, nipple bleeding, uterine hyperplasia, vaginal cyst
Hematologic & oncologic: Malignant neoplasm of breast, rectal hemorrhage
Hepatic: Jaundice
Hypersensitivity: Anaphylaxis, angioedema, nonimmune anaphylaxis
Local: Residual mass at injection site, sterile abscess at injection site
Nervous system: Chills
Neuromuscular & skeletal: Axillary swelling, decreased bone mineral density, osteoporosis, pathological fracture due to osteoporosis, systemic sclerosis
Miscellaneous: Fever

Mechanism of Action Medroxyprogesterone acetate (MPA) transforms a proliferative endometrium into a secretory endometrium. When administered with conjugated estrogens, MPA reduces the incidence of endometrial hyperplasia and risk of adenocarcinoma. When used as an injection for contraception (doses of 150 mg IM or 104 mg SubQ), MPA inhibits secretion of pituitary gonadotropins, which prevents follicular maturation and ovulation and causes endometrial thinning. Progestogens, such as medroxyprogesterone when used for endometriosis, lead to atrophy of the endometrial tissue. They may also suppress new growth and implantation. Pain associated with endometriosis is decreased (ASRM 2014).

Pharmacodynamics/Kinetics

Onset of Action Time to ovulation (after last injection): 10 months (range: 6 to 12 months)

Half-life Elimination Oral: 12 to 17 hours; IM (Depo-Provera Contraceptive): ~50 days; SubQ: ~43 days

Time to Peak Oral: 2 to 4 hours; IM (Depo-Provera Contraceptive): ~3 weeks; SubQ: ~1 week

Reproductive Considerations

High doses impair fertility. **[US Boxed Warning]: Not recommended as a long-term (ie, longer than 2 years) birth control method unless other options are considered inadequate.**

Median time to conception/return to ovulation following discontinuation of MPA contraceptive injection is 10 months following the last injection and is unrelated to the duration of use.

Pregnancy Considerations

Most products are contraindicated in females who are pregnant, suspected to be pregnant or as a diagnostic test for pregnancy.

In general, there is not an increased risk of birth defects following inadvertent use of the injectable medroxyprogesterone acetate (MPA) contraceptives early in pregnancy. Hypospadias has been reported in male babies and clitoral enlargement and labial fusion have been reported in female babies exposed to MPA during the first trimester of pregnancy. Ectopic pregnancies have been reported with use of the MPA contraceptive injection.

◆ **Medroxyprogesterone Acetate** *see* MedroxyPROGESTERone *on page 953*

◆ **Medroxyprogesterone and Estrogens (Conjugated)** *see* Estrogens (Conjugated/Equine) and Medroxyprogesterone *on page 603*

◆ **Medroxyprogesterone and Oestrogens (Conjugated)** *see* Estrogens (Conjugated/Equine) and Medroxyprogesterone *on page 603*

Mefenamic Acid (me fe NAM ik AS id)

Related Information

Rheumatoid Arthritis, Osteoarthritis, and Osteoporosis *on page 1697*
Temporomandibular Dysfunction (TMD), Chronic Pain, and Fibromyalgia *on page 1773*

Brand Names: US Ponstel [DSC]

Brand Names: Canada DOM-Mefenamic Acid; PMS-Mefenamic Acid; Ponstan

Pharmacologic Category Analgesic, Nonopioid; Nonsteroidal Anti-inflammatory Drug (NSAID), Oral

Use

Pain, mild to moderate: Relief of mild to moderate pain in patients ≥14 years, when therapy will not exceed 1 week.

Primary dysmenorrhea: Treatment of primary dysmenorrhea.

Local Anesthetic/Vasoconstrictor Precautions No information available to require special precautions

Effects on Dental Treatment The dentist should be aware of the potential of abnormal coagulation. Caution should also be exercised in the use of NSAIDs in patients already on anticoagulant therapy with drugs such as warfarin (Coumadin®). Recovery of platelet function usually occurs 1-2 days after discontinuation of NSAIDs. See Effects on Bleeding.

Effects on Bleeding Nonselective NSAIDs such as mefenamic acid inhibit platelet aggregation and prolong bleeding time in some patients. Unlike aspirin, the NSAID effect on platelet function is quantitatively less, of shorter duration, and reversible.

Adverse Reactions

1% to 10%:

Central nervous system: Dizziness (3% to 9%), headache, nervousness

Dermatologic: Pruritus, skin rash

Endocrine & metabolic: Fluid retention

Gastrointestinal: Abdominal cramps, abdominal distress, abdominal pain, constipation, diarrhea, duodenal ulcer (with bleeding or perforation), dyspepsia, flatulence, gastric ulcer (with bleeding or perforation), gastritis, heartburn, nausea, vomiting

Hematologic & oncologic: Hemorrhage

Hepatic: Increased liver enzymes

Otic: Tinnitus

<1%, postmarketing, and/or case reports: Acute renal failure, agranulocytosis, allergic rhinitis, anemia, angioedema, aseptic meningitis, auditory impairment, blurred vision, bone marrow depression, cardiac arrhythmia, cardiac failure, confusion, conjunctivitis, cystitis, depression, drowsiness, dyspnea, epistaxis, erythema multiforme, gastrointestinal ulcer, hallucination, hemolytic anemia, hepatitis, hepatotoxicity (idiosyncratic; Chalasani 2014), hot flash, hypertension, insomnia, leukopenia, peripheral neuropathy, polydipsia, polyuria, Stevens-Johnson syndrome, stomatitis, tachycardia, thrombocytopenia, toxic amblyopia, toxic epidermal necrolysis, urticaria, xerophthalmia

Mechanism of Action Reversibly inhibits cyclooxygenase-1 and 2 (COX-1 and 2) enzymes, which results in decreased formation of prostaglandin precursors; has antipyretic, analgesic, and anti-inflammatory properties.

Other proposed mechanisms not fully elucidated (and possibly contributing to the anti-inflammatory effect to varying degrees) include inhibiting chemotaxis, altering lymphocyte activity, inhibiting neutrophil aggregation/activation, and decreasing proinflammatory cytokine levels.

Pharmacodynamics/Kinetics

Half-life Elimination ~2 hours

Time to Peak 2 to 4 hours

Reproductive Considerations

The chronic use of NSAIDs in women of reproductive age may be associated with infertility that is reversible upon discontinuation of the medication. Consider discontinuing use in women having difficulty conceiving or those undergoing investigation of fertility.

Pregnancy Considerations Mefenamic acid crosses the placenta (Mackenzie 1985). Birth defects have been observed following in utero NSAID exposure in some studies; however, data is conflicting (Bloor 2013). Nonteratogenic effects, including prenatal constriction of the ductus arteriosus, persistent pulmonary hypertension of the newborn, oligohydramnios, necrotizing enterocolitis, renal dysfunction or failure, and intracranial hemorrhage have been observed in the fetus/neonate following in utero NSAID exposure. In addition, nonclosure of the ductus arteriosus postnatally may occur and be resistant to medical management (Bermas 2014; Bloor 2013). Because NSAIDs may cause premature closure of the ductus arteriosus, product labeling for mefenamic acid specifically states use should be avoided starting at 30 weeks' gestation.

The use of NSAIDs close to conception may be associated with an increased risk of miscarriage (Bloor 2013; Bermas 2014).

Mefloquine (ME floe kwin)

Pharmacologic Category Antimalarial Agent

Use

Malaria, prophylaxis: Prophylaxis of *Plasmodium falciparum* and *Plasmodium vivax* malaria infections, including prophylaxis of chloroquine-resistant strains of *P. falciparum*.

Malaria, treatment: Treatment of uncomplicated malaria caused by mefloquine-susceptible strains of *P. falciparum* or by *P. vivax*. **Note:** The CDC guidelines also recommend use of mefloquine as an alternative agent for treatment of uncomplicated *Plasmodium ovale*, *Plasmodium malariae*, or *Plasmodium knowlesi* malaria (CDC 2020).

Note: Due to geographical resistance and cross-resistance, consult current CDC guidelines.

Local Anesthetic/Vasoconstrictor Precautions No information available to require special precautions

Effects on Dental Treatment No significant effects or complications reported

Effects on Bleeding No information available to require special precautions

Adverse Reactions

>10%: Central nervous system: Abnormal dreams (14%; Tickell-Painter 2017), insomnia (13%; Tickell-Painter 2017)

1% to 10%: Gastrointestinal: Vomiting (3%)

<1%, postmarketing, and/or case reports: Abdominal pain, abnormal sensory symptoms, abnormal T waves on ECG, aggressive behavior, agitation, agranulocytosis, alopecia, anaphylaxis, anorexia, aplastic anemia, arthralgia, asthenia, ataxia, atrioventricular block, auditory impairment, bradycardia, burning sensation, cardiac arrhythmia, cardiac conduction disturbance (transient), chest pain, chills, confusion, decreased hematocrit, depression, diarrhea, dizziness, drowsiness, dyspepsia, dyspnea, ECG changes, edema, emotional disturbance, emotional lability, encephalopathy, equilibrium disturbance, erythema, erythema multiforme, extrasystoles, fatigue, fever, first degree atrioventricular block, flushing, hallucination, headache, hepatic disease, hepatic failure, hyperhidrosis, hypersensitivity reaction, hypertension, hypotension, increased serum transaminases, insomnia, leukocytosis, leukopenia, loose stools, malaise, memory impairment, muscle cramps, myalgia, myasthenia, nausea, pain, palpitations, panic attack, paranoia, paresthesia,

pneumonitis (possibly allergic), polyneuropathy, prolonged QT interval on ECG, pruritus, psychotic reaction, restlessness, seizure, sensorimotor neuropathy, sinus arrhythmia, sinus bradycardia, skin rash, Stevens-Johnson syndrome, suicidal ideation (causal relationship not established), syncope, tachycardia, telogen effluvium, thrombocytopenia, tinnitus, tremor, urticaria, vertigo, vestibular disturbance, visual disturbance

Mechanism of Action Mefloquine is a quinoline-methanol compound structurally similar to quinine; mefloquine's effectiveness in the treatment and prophylaxis of malaria is due to the destruction of the asexual blood forms of the malarial pathogens that affect humans, *Plasmodium falciparum, P. vivax*

Pharmacodynamics/Kinetics

Half-life Elimination Children 4 to 10 years: Mean range: 11.6 to 13.6 days (range: 6.5 to 33 days) (Price 1999); Adults: ~3 weeks (range: 2 to 4 weeks); may be decreased during infection (2 weeks) (WHO 2010)

Time to Peak Plasma: ~17 hours (range: 6 to 24 hours)

Pregnancy Risk Factor B

Pregnancy Considerations

Mefloquine crosses the placenta; however, clinical experience with mefloquine has not shown an increased risk of adverse effects in pregnant women.

Malaria infection in pregnant women may be more severe than in nonpregnant women and has a high risk of maternal and perinatal morbidity and mortality. Malaria infection during pregnancy can lead to miscarriage, premature delivery, low birth weight, congenital infection, and/or perinatal death. Therefore, pregnant women and women who are likely to become pregnant are advised to avoid travel to malaria-risk areas. When travel is unavoidable, pregnant women should take precautions to avoid mosquito bites and use effective prophylactic medications (CDC 2020; CDC Yellow Book 2020).

When other treatment options are not available, mefloquine may be used for the treatment of chloroquine-resistant uncomplicated malaria in pregnancy. In pregnant patients with severe malaria, mefloquine may be used as interim oral therapy when the preferred IV agent is not readily available and other oral agents are not available (discontinue once IV treatment is initiated) (consult current CDC guidelines) (CDC 2020).

◆ **Mefloquine Hydrochloride** *see* Mefloquine *on page 955*

◆ **Megace ES [DSC]** *see* Megestrol *on page 956*

◆ **Megace Oral [DSC]** *see* Megestrol *on page 956*

◆ **Megadophilus [OTC]** *see Lactobacillus on page 869*

Megestrol (me JES trole)

Brand Names: US Megace ES [DSC]; Megace Oral [DSC]

Brand Names: Canada Megace [DSC]

Pharmacologic Category Antineoplastic Agent, Hormone; Appetite Stimulant; Progestin

Use

Anorexia or cachexia: *Suspension:* Treatment of anorexia, cachexia, or unexplained significant weight loss in patients with AIDS

Limitations of use: Treatment of AIDS-related weight loss should only be initiated after addressing the treatable causes (eg, malignancy, infection, malabsorption, endocrine disease, renal disease, psychiatric disorder) for weight loss. Megestrol is not intended to prevent weight loss.

Breast cancer: *Tablet:* Treatment (palliative) of advanced breast cancer

Endometrial cancer: *Tablet:* Treatment (palliative) of advanced endometrial carcinoma

Local Anesthetic/Vasoconstrictor Precautions No information available to require special precautions

Effects on Dental Treatment No significant effects or complications reported

Effects on Bleeding Thromboembolic events have been reported.

Adverse Reactions Frequency not always defined.

Cardiovascular: Hypertension (4% to 8%), cardiomyopathy (1% to 3%), chest pain (1% to 3%), edema (1% to 3%), palpitations (1% to 3%), peripheral edema (1% to 3%), cardiac failure

Central nervous system: Headache (3% to 10%), pain (4% to 6%, similar to placebo), insomnia (1% to 6%), abnormality in thinking (1% to 3%), confusion (1% to 3%), convulsions (1% to 3%), depression (1% to 3%), hypoesthesia (1% to 3%), neuropathy (1% to 3%), paresthesia (1% to 3%), carpal tunnel syndrome, lethargy, malaise, mood changes

Dermatologic: Skin rash (6% to 12%), alopecia (1% to 3%), dermatological disease (1% to 3%), diaphoresis (1% to 3%), pruritus (1% to 3%), vesicobullous dermatitis (1% to 3%)

Endocrine & metabolic: Hyperglycemia (6%), decreased libido (1% to 5%), albuminuria (1% to 3%), gynecomastia (1% to 3%), increased lactate dehydrogenase (1% to 3%), adrenocortical insufficiency, amenorrhea, Cushing's syndrome, diabetes mellitus, hot flash, HPA-axis suppression, hypercalcemia, weight gain (not attributed to edema or fluid retention)

Gastrointestinal: Diarrhea (10%, similar to placebo), flatulence (6% to 10%), vomiting (4% to 6%), nausea (4% to 5%), dyspepsia (2% to 3%), abdominal pain (1% to 3%), constipation (1% to 3%), oral moniliasis (1% to 3%), sialorrhea (1% to 3%), xerostomia (1% to 3%)

Genitourinary: Impotence (4% to 14%), urinary incontinence (1% to 3%), urinary tract infection (1% to 3%), urinary frequency (1% to 2%), breakthrough bleeding

Hematologic & oncologic: Leukopenia (1% to 3%), sarcoma (1% to 3%), tumor flare

Hepatic: Hepatomegaly (1% to 3%)

Infection: Candidiasis (1% to 3%), herpes virus infection (1% to 3%), infection (1% to 3%)

Neuromuscular & skeletal: Weakness (5% to 6%)

Ophthalmic: Amblyopia (1% to 3%)

Respiratory: Cough (1% to 3%), dyspnea (1% to 3%), pharyngitis (1% to 3%), pulmonary disorder (1% to 3%), pneumonia (1%), hyperventilation

Miscellaneous: Fever (1% to 6%)

Postmarketing and/or case reports: Decreased glucose tolerance, thromboembolic phenomena (including deep vein thrombosis, pulmonary embolism, thrombophlebitis)

Mechanism of Action A synthetic progestin with antiestrogenic properties which disrupt the estrogen receptor cycle. Megestrol interferes with the normal estrogen cycle and results in a lower LH titer. May also have a direct effect on the endometrium. Megestrol is an antineoplastic progestin thought to act through an antileutenizing effect mediated via the pituitary. May stimulate appetite by antagonizing the metabolic effects of catabolic cytokines.

Pharmacodynamics/Kinetics

Onset of Action Breast or endometrial cancer: At least 2 months of continuous therapy; Weight gain: 2 to 4 weeks

Half-life Elimination Suspension: 20 to 50 hours; Tablet: Mean: 34.2 hours (range: 13 to 105 hours)

Time to Peak Serum: Suspension: 5 hours; Tablet: 2.2 hours (range: 1 to 3 hours)

Reproductive Considerations

Evaluate pregnancy status prior to treatment in females of reproductive potential. Effective contraception should be used when treating anorexia or cachexia in females with HIV infection. In clinical studies, megestrol was shown to cause breakthrough vaginal bleeding in women.

Pregnancy Considerations

Use is contraindicated for the treatment of anorexia or cachexia in pregnant females with HIV infection.

Megestrol may cause fetal harm if administered during pregnancy.

- ◆ **Megestrol Acetate** *see* Megestrol *on page 956*
- ◆ **MEK162** *see* Binimetinib *on page 244*
- ◆ **Mekinist** *see* Trametinib *on page 1475*
- ◆ **Mektovi** *see* Binimetinib *on page 244*
- ◆ **Mellaril** *see* Thioridazine *on page 1438*
- ◆ **Melodetta 24 Fe** *see* Ethinyl Estradiol and Norethindrone *on page 614*

Meloxicam (mel OKS i kam)

Related Information

Rheumatoid Arthritis, Osteoarthritis, and Osteoporosis *on page 1697*

Brand Names: US Anjeso; Mobic; Qmiiz ODT; Vivlodex

Brand Names: Canada ACT Meloxicam; APO-Meloxicam; Auro-Meloxicam; DOM-Meloxicam; Mobicox [DSC]; MYLAN-Meloxicam [DSC]; PMS-Meloxicam; TEVA-Meloxicam

Generic Availability (US) May be product dependent

Pharmacologic Category Analgesic, Nonopioid; Nonsteroidal Anti-inflammatory Drug (NSAID), Oral; Nonsteroidal Anti-inflammatory Drug (NSAID), Parenteral

Use

IV:

Pain: Management of moderate to severe pain in adults, alone or in combination with non-nonsteroidal anti-inflammatory drug analgesics.

Limitation of use: Because of delayed onset of analgesia, meloxicam (injection) alone is not recommended for use when rapid onset of analgesia is required

Oral:

Osteoarthritis: Relief of the signs and symptoms of osteoarthritis (OA); management of OA pain.

Rheumatoid arthritis (orally disintegrating tablet [ODT], tablet, and suspension only): Relief of signs and symptoms of rheumatoid arthritis (RA); relief of the signs and symptoms of pauciarticular or polyarticular course juvenile RA in patients ≥2 years of age (suspension) and in patients weighing ≥60 kg (ODT, tablet).

Local Anesthetic/Vasoconstrictor Precautions

No information available to require special precautions

Effects on Dental Treatment Key adverse event(s) related to dental treatment: Taste perversion, ulcerative stomatitis, and xerostomia (normal salivary flow resumes upon discontinuation). The dentist should be aware of the potential of abnormal coagulation. Caution should also be exercised in the use of NSAIDs in patients already on anticoagulant therapy with drugs such as warfarin (Coumadin®). See Effects on Bleeding.

Effects on Bleeding Nonselective NSAIDs such as meloxicam inhibit platelet aggregation and prolong bleeding time in some patients. Unlike aspirin, the NSAID effect on platelet function is quantitatively less, of shorter duration, and reversible.

Adverse Reactions

1% to 10%:

Cardiovascular: Acute myocardial infarction (<2%), angina pectoris (<2%), cardiac arrhythmia (<2%), cardiac failure (<2%), edema (≤5%), facial edema (<2%), hypertension (<2%), hypotension (<2%), palpitations (<2%), presyncope (<2%), syncope (<2%), tachycardia (<2%), vasculitis (<2%)

Dermatologic: Alopecia (<2%), bullous rash (<2%), diaphoresis (<2%), ecchymoses (<2%), localized rash (IV only, infusion site: <2%), pruritus (<2%), skin photosensitivity (<2%), skin rash (<2%), urticaria (<2%)

Endocrine & metabolic: Albuminuria (<2%), dehydration (<2%), hot flash (<2%), hypokalemia (<2%), hypomagnesemia (<2%), increased gamma-glutamyl transferase (≤3%), weight gain (<2%), weight loss (<2%)

Gastrointestinal: Abdominal distention (<2%), abdominal distress (<2%), abdominal pain (≤3%), aphthous stomatitis (<2%), colitis (<2%), constipation (8%), diarrhea (≤8%), duodenal ulcer (<2%; duodenal ulcer with hemorrhage: <2%), dysgeusia (<2%), dyspepsia (6%), epigastric discomfort (<2%), eructation (<2%), esophagitis (<2%), flatulence (<2%), gastric ulcer (<2%; gastric ulcer with hemorrhage: <2%), gastritis (<2%), gastroenteritis (<2%), gastroesophageal reflux disease (<2%), gastrointestinal hemorrhage (<2%), gastrointestinal pain (<2%), gastrointestinal perforation (<2%; including duodenal, gastric), hematemesis (<2%), increased appetite (<2%), intestinal perforation (<2%), melena (<2%), nausea (2% to 4%), pancreatitis (<2%), xerostomia (<2%)

Genitourinary: Hematuria (<2%), pollakiuria (<2%), urinary retention (<2%)

Hematologic & oncologic: Anemia (2%), leukopenia (<2%), neutropenia (<2%), prolonged bleeding time (<2%), purpuric disease (<2%), rectal hemorrhage (<2%), thrombocythemia (<2%), thrombocytopenia (<2%), wound hematoma (IV only: <2%)

Hepatic: Abnormal hepatic function tests (<2%), hepatitis (<2%), hyperbilirubinemia (<2%), increased serum alanine aminotransferase (<2%), increased serum aspartate aminotransferase (<2%)

Hypersensitivity: Angioedema (<2%), hypersensitivity reaction (<2%)

Local: Incision site hemorrhage (IV only: <2%), infusion site reaction (IV only: <2%)

Nervous system: Abnormal dreams (<2%), anxiety (<2%), confusion (<2%), depression (<2%), disturbance in attention (<2%), dizziness (4%), drowsiness (<2%), falling (3%), fatigue (<2%), headache (2%), insomnia (<2%), malaise (<2%), migraine (<2%), nervousness (<2%), noncardiac chest pain (<2%), paresthesia (<2%), seizure (<2%), vertigo (<2%)

Neuromuscular & skeletal: Asthenia (<2%), back pain (<2%), muscle spasm (<2%), tremor (<2%)

Ophthalmic: Visual disturbance (<2%)

Otic: Tinnitus (<2%)

Renal: Increased blood urea nitrogen (<2%), increased serum creatinine (<2%), renal failure syndrome (<2%)

Respiratory: Asthma (<2%), bronchospasm (<2%), dyspnea (<2%), epistaxis (<2%), flu-like symptoms (3% to 6%), pharyngitis (3%), upper respiratory tract infection (3% to 7%)

Miscellaneous: Accidental injury (3% to 5%), fever (<2%), wound dehiscence (<2%)

Frequency not defined: Cardiovascular: Cerebrovascular accident, thrombosis

Postmarketing:

Dermatologic: Erythema multiforme, exfoliative dermatitis, Stevens-Johnson syndrome, toxic epidermal necrolysis

Hematologic & oncologic: Agranulocytosis

Hepatic: Hepatic failure, hepatotoxicity (idiosyncratic) (Chalasani 2014), jaundice

Hypersensitivity: Anaphylactic shock, anaphylaxis, nonimmune anaphylaxis

Nervous system: Mood changes

Renal: Interstitial nephritis, renal insufficiency, renal papillary necrosis

Dosing

Adult Note: Capsules and orally disintegrating tablets (ODT) are not interchangeable with other formulations of oral meloxicam even if the total milligram strength is the same. Do not substitute similar dose strengths of other meloxicam products.

Gout, acute flares (alternative agent) (off-label use): Oral: 15 mg once daily (Cheng 2004); initiate within 24 to 48 hours of flare onset preferably; discontinue 2 to 3 days after resolution of clinical signs; usual duration: 5 to 7 days (ACR [Khanna 2012]; Becker 2018).

Osteoarthritis: Capsule: Oral: Initial: 5 mg once daily; some patients may receive additional benefit from increasing dose to 10 mg once daily; maximum dose: 10 mg/day.

Osteoarthritis, rheumatoid arthritis: ODT/Tablet/Suspension: Oral: Initial: 7.5 mg once daily; some patients may receive additional benefit from increasing dose to 15 mg once daily; maximum dose: 15 mg/day.

Pain, moderate to severe: IV: 30 mg once daily. **Note:** Use for the shortest duration consistent with individual patient treatment goals; may be used as monotherapy or in combination with non-nonsteroidal anti-inflammatory drug analgesics.

Geriatric Refer to adult dosing. Use with caution; initiate oral dose at lower end of the dosing range.

Renal Impairment: Adult

IV:

eGFR ≥60 mL/minute/1.73 m^2: No dosage adjustment necessary.

eGFR <60 mL/minute/1.73 m^2: Use is not recommended; contraindicated in patients who are at risk for renal failure due to volume depletion.

Oral:

CrCl ≥20 mL/minute: No dosage adjustment necessary.

CrCl <20 mL/minute: There are no dosage adjustments provided in the manufacturer's labeling (has not been studied); use is not recommended.

Hemodialysis (not dialyzable): Use with caution and monitor closely. Maximum dose: 7.5 mg/day (orally disintegrating tablet/tablet/suspension); 5 mg/day (capsule). **Note:** Additional dose not necessary after hemodialysis.

KDIGO 2012 guidelines provide the following recommendations for nonsteroidal anti-inflammatory drugs:

eGFR 30 to <60 mL/minute/1.73 m^2: Temporarily discontinue in patients with intercurrent disease that increases risk of acute kidney injury.

eGFR <30 mL/minute/1.73 m^2: Avoid use.

Hepatic Impairment: Adult

IV: Mild to severe impairment: There are no dosage adjustments provided in the manufacturer's labeling (has not been studied).

Oral:

Mild to moderate impairment (Child-Pugh class A or B): No dosage adjustment necessary.

Severe impairment (Child-Pugh class C): There are no dosage adjustments provided in the manufacturer's labeling (has not been studied); use with caution.

Pediatric Note: Orally-disintegrating tablets (Qmiiz ODT) and capsules are not interchangeable with other formulations of oral meloxicam even if the total milligram strength is the same; do not substitute similar dose strengths of other meloxicam products.

Juvenile idiopathic arthritis (JIA): Note: To reduce the risk of adverse cardiovascular and GI effects, use the lowest effective dose for the shortest period of time; adjust dose to specific patient's clinical needs; higher doses (up to 0.375 mg/kg/**day** or 15 mg/**day**) have not demonstrated additional benefit in clinical trials (American Pain Society 2016). Oral:

Oral suspension, tablets (limited data available with tablets): Children ≥2 years and Adolescents: 0.125 mg/kg once daily; maximum daily dose: 7.5 mg/**day**.

Orally-disintegrating tablets (Qmiiz ODT): Children and Adolescents weighing ≥60 kg: 7.5 mg once daily.

Renal Impairment: Pediatric

Manufacturer's labeling:

Oral suspension: Children ≥2 years and Adolescents:

Mild to moderate impairment: No dosage adjustments are recommended.

Severe impairment (CrCl <20 mL/minute): Use is not recommended (has not been studied).

Hemodialysis: Not dialyzable; additional doses are not required after dialysis.

Orally-disintegrating tablet (Qmiiz ODT): Children and Adolescents weighing ≥60 kg:

Severe renal impairment: Use is not recommended.

Hemodialysis: In adults, lower daily doses are recommended (7.5 mg/day); however, in pediatric patients this is not possible due to available dosage forms and already reduced dose; consider alternate dosage forms.

KDIGO 2012 guidelines provide the following recommendations for NSAIDs (KDIGO 2013):

eGFR 30 to <60 mL/minute/1.73 m^2: Temporarily discontinue in patients with intercurrent disease that increases risk of acute kidney injury.

eGFR <30 mL/minute/1.73 m^2: Avoid use.

Hepatic Impairment: Pediatric

Children ≥2 years and Adolescents:

Mild to moderate impairment (Child-Pugh class A or B): No dosage adjustments are recommended.

Severe impairment: There are no dosage adjustments provided in the manufacturer's labeling (has not been studied); use with caution; meloxicam is significantly metabolized in the liver.

Mechanism of Action
Reversibly inhibits cyclooxygenase-1 and 2 (COX-1 and 2) enzymes, which results in decreased formation of prostaglandin precursors; has antipyretic, analgesic, and anti-inflammatory properties

Other proposed mechanisms not fully elucidated (and possibly contributing to the anti-inflammatory effect to varying degrees), include inhibiting chemotaxis, altering lymphocyte activity, inhibiting neutrophil aggregation/activation, and decreasing proinflammatory cytokine levels.

Contraindications
Hypersensitivity to meloxicam or any component of the formulation; history of asthma, urticaria, or other allergic-type reactions after taking aspirin or other nonsteroidal anti-inflammatory drugs; use in the setting of coronary artery bypass graft surgery; phenylketonuria (orally disintegrating tablet only); moderate to severe renal insufficiency patients who are at risk for renal failure due to volume depletion (injection only).

Canadian labeling: Additional contraindications (not in US labeling): Pregnancy (third trimester); breastfeeding; severe uncontrolled heart failure; active or recent GI/gastric/duodenal/peptic ulceration/perforation; active GI bleeding; cerebrovascular bleeding or other bleeding disorders; inflammatory bowel disease (Crohn disease or ulcerative colitis); severe liver impairment or active liver disease; severe renal impairment (creatinine clearance [CrCl] <30 mL/minute or 0.5 mL/second) or deteriorating renal disease; known hyperkalemia; pediatric patients <18 years; rare hereditary conditions that may be incompatible with an excipient of the product.

Warnings/Precautions **[US Boxed Warning]: Nonsteroidal anti-inflammatory drugs (NSAIDs) cause an increased risk of serious (and potentially fatal) adverse cardiovascular thrombotic events, including myocardial infarction [MI] and stroke. Risk may occur early during treatment and may increase with duration of use.** Relative risk appears to be similar in those with and without known cardiovascular disease or risk factors for cardiovascular disease; however, absolute incidence of serious cardiovascular thrombotic events (which may occur early during treatment) was higher in patients with known cardiovascular disease or risk factors. New onset hypertension or exacerbation of hypertension may occur (NSAIDs may also impair response to angiotensin-converting-enzyme [ACE] inhibitors, thiazide diuretics, or loop diuretics); may contribute to cardiovascular events; monitor BP; use with caution in patients with hypertension. May cause sodium and fluid retention, use with caution in patients with edema. Avoid use in patients with heart failure (ACCF/AHA [Yancy 2013]). Avoid use in patients with recent MI unless benefits outweigh risk of cardiovascular thrombotic events. Use the lowest effective dose for the shortest duration of time, consistent with individual patient goals, to reduce risk of cardiovascular events; alternate therapies should be considered for patients at high risk.

[US Boxed Warning]: Use is contraindicated in the setting of coronary artery bypass graft (CABG) surgery. Risk of MI and stroke may be increased with use within the first 10 to 14 days following CABG surgery.

Platelet adhesion and aggregation may be decreased; may prolong bleeding time; patients with coagulation disorders or who are receiving anticoagulants should be monitored closely. Anemia may occur; patients on long-term NSAID therapy should be monitored for anemia. Rarely, NSAID use may cause severe blood dyscrasias (eg, agranulocytosis, aplastic anemia, thrombocytopenia).

NSAID use may compromise existing renal function. Dose-dependent decreases in prostaglandin synthesis may result from NSAID use, causing a reduction in renal blood flow which may cause renal decompensation (usually reversible). Patients with impaired renal function, dehydration, hypovolemia, heart failure, hepatic impairment, those taking diuretics, ACE inhibitors, angiotensin II receptor blockers, and the elderly are at greater risk for renal toxicity. Rehydrate patient before starting therapy; monitor renal function closely. Avoid use in patients with advanced renal disease unless benefits are expected to outweigh risk of worsening renal function; monitor closely if therapy must be initiated. IV formulation is not recommended in patients with moderate to severe renal insufficiency and is contraindicated in patients with moderate to severe renal insufficiency who are at risk for renal failure due to volume depletion. Long-term NSAID use may result in renal papillary necrosis. NSAID use may increase the risk of hyperkalemia, particularly in the elderly, diabetics, renal disease, and with concomitant use of other agents capable of inducing hyperkalemia (eg, ACE inhibitors). Monitor potassium closely. Poor metabolizers of CYP2C9 may require dose reduction. Avoid chronic use of oral nonselective NSAIDs in patients who have undergone bariatric surgery; development of anastomotic ulcerations/perforations may occur.

[US Boxed Warning]: NSAIDs cause an increased risk of serious GI inflammation, ulceration, bleeding, and perforation (may be fatal); elderly patients and patients with history of peptic ulcer disease and/or GI bleeding are at greater risk for serious GI events. These events may occur at any time during therapy and without warning. Avoid use in patients with active GI bleeding. In patients with a history of acute lower GI bleeding, avoid use of non-aspirin NSAIDs, especially if due to angioectasia or diverticulosis (Strate 2016). Use caution with a history of GI ulcers, concurrent therapy known to increase the risk of GI bleeding (eg, aspirin, anticoagulants and/or corticosteroids, selective serotonin reuptake inhibitors), advanced hepatic disease, coagulopathy, smoking, use of alcohol, or in elderly or debilitated patients. Use the lowest effective dose for the shortest duration of time, consistent with individual patient goals, to reduce risk of GI adverse events; alternate therapies should be considered for patients at high risk. When used concomitantly with aspirin, a substantial increase in the risk of GI complications (eg, ulcer) occurs; concomitant gastroprotective therapy (eg, proton pump inhibitors) is recommended (Bhatt 2008).

NSAIDs may cause potentially fatal serious skin adverse events including exfoliative dermatitis, Stevens-Johnson syndrome and toxic epidermal necrolysis; may occur without warning; discontinue use at first appearance of skin rash (or any other sign of hypersensitivity). Anaphylactoid reactions may occur, even without prior exposure; patients with "aspirin triad" (bronchial asthma, aspirin intolerance, rhinitis) may be at increased risk. Contraindicated in patients who experience bronchospasm, asthma, rhinitis, or urticaria with

NSAID or aspirin therapy. Use caution in other forms of asthma. Use with caution in patients with hepatic impairment; patients with hepatic impairment may require reduced doses due to extensive hepatic metabolism. Patients with advanced hepatic disease are at an increased risk of GI bleeding with NSAIDs. Transaminase elevations have been reported with use; closely monitor patients with any abnormal LFT. Rare (sometimes fatal) severe hepatic reactions (eg, fulminant hepatitis, liver necrosis, hepatic failure) have occurred with NSAID use; discontinue immediately if signs or symptoms of hepatic disease develop or if systemic manifestations occur.

NSAIDs may cause drowsiness, dizziness, blurred vision, and other neurologic effects which may impair physical or mental abilities; patients must be cautioned about performing tasks that require mental alertness (eg, operating machinery, driving). Potentially significant drug-drug interactions may exist, requiring dose or frequency adjustment, additional monitoring, and/or selection of alternative therapy. Blurred and/or diminished vision has been reported; discontinue use and refer for ophthalmologic evaluation if such symptoms occur. Elderly patients are at greater risk for serious GI, cardiovascular, and/or renal adverse events. Use with caution; initiate dose at the lower end of the dosing range.

Injection is not indicated for long-term use. Onset of pain relief may be delayed up to several hours after administration; use of a non-NSAID analgesic with a rapid onset may be needed. Also, inadequate analgesia for the entire 24-hour dosing interval may be experienced; use of a short-acting, non-NSAID, immediate-release analgesic may be required. Orally disintegrating tablet may contain phenylalanine; use is contraindicated in patients with phenylketonuria. Oral suspension formulation may contain sorbitol. Concomitant use with sodium polystyrene sulfonate (Kayexalate) may cause intestinal necrosis (including fatal cases); combined use should be avoided. Withhold for at least 4 to 6 half-lives prior to surgical or dental procedures.

Clinical or population-based data regarding the risks of NSAIDs in the setting of coronavirus disease 2019 (COVID-19) are limited (FDA Safety Communication 2020; Kim 2020). Some experts recommend the use of acetaminophen as the preferred antipyretic agent, when possible, and if NSAIDs are needed, to use the lowest effective dose and shortest duration (EMA 2020; Kim 2020). In general, for patients already taking an NSAID for a comorbid condition, it is recommended to continue the NSAID as directed by their health care provider (EMA 2020; NIH 2020; WHO 2020).

Warnings: Additional Pediatric Considerations Pediatric patients ≥2 years may experience a higher frequency of some adverse effects than adults, including the following: Abdominal pain, diarrhea, fever, headache, and vomiting.

Drug Interactions

Metabolism/Transport Effects **Substrate** of CYP2C9 (major), CYP3A4 (minor); **Note:** Assignment of Major/Minor substrate status based on clinically relevant drug interaction potential

Avoid Concomitant Use

Avoid concomitant use of Meloxicam with any of the following: Acemetacin; Aminolevulinic Acid (Systemic); Calcium Polystyrene Sulfonate; Dexibuprofen; Dexketoprofen; Floctafenine; Ketorolac (Nasal); Ketorolac (Systemic); Macimorelin; Mifamurtide; Morniflumate; Nonsteroidal Anti-Inflammatory Agents (COX-2 Selective); Omacetaxine; Pelubiprofen; Phenylbutazone; Sodium Polystyrene Sulfonate; Talniflumate; Tenoxicam; Urokinase; Zaltoprofen

Increased Effect/Toxicity

Meloxicam may increase the levels/effects of: 5-Aminosalicylic Acid Derivatives; Agents with Antiplatelet Properties; Aliskiren; Aminoglycosides; Aminolevulinic Acid (Systemic); Aminolevulinic Acid (Topical); Anticoagulants; Apixaban; Bemiparin; Bisphosphonate Derivatives; Calcium Polystyrene Sulfonate; Cephalothin; Collagenase (Systemic); CycloSPORINE (Systemic); Dabigatran Etexilate; Deferasirox; Deoxycholic Acid; Desmopressin; Dexibuprofen; Digoxin; Drospirenone; Edoxaban; Enoxaparin; Eplerenone; Haloperidol; Heparin; Ibritumomab Tiuxetan; Lithium; MetFORMIN; Methotrexate; Nonsteroidal Anti-Inflammatory Agents (COX-2 Selective); Obinutuzumab; Omacetaxine; Porfimer; Potassium-Sparing Diuretics; PRALAtrexate; Quinolones; Rivaroxaban; Salicylates; Sodium Polystyrene Sulfonate; Tacrolimus (Systemic); Tenofovir Products; Thrombolytic Agents; Tolperisone; Urokinase; Vancomycin; Verteporfin; Vitamin K Antagonists

The levels/effects of Meloxicam may be increased by: Acalabrutinib; Acemetacin; Alcohol (Ethyl); Angiotensin II Receptor Blockers; Angiotensin-Converting Enzyme Inhibitors; Corticosteroids (Systemic); CycloSPORINE (Systemic); CYP2C9 Inhibitors (Moderate); Dasatinib; Dexketoprofen; Diclofenac (Systemic); Fat Emulsion (Fish Oil Based); Felbinac; Floctafenine; Glucosamine; Herbs (Anticoagulant/Antiplatelet Properties); Ibrutinib; Inotersen; Ketorolac (Nasal); Ketorolac (Systemic); Limaprost; Loop Diuretics; Lumacaftor and Ivacaftor; Morniflumate; Multivitamins/Fluoride (with ADE); Multivitamins/Minerals (with ADEK, Folate, Iron); Multivitamins/Minerals (with AE, No Iron); Naftazone; Omega-3 Fatty Acids; Pelubiprofen; Pentosan Polysulfate Sodium; Pentoxifylline; Phenylbutazone; Probenecid; Prostacyclin Analogues; Selective Serotonin Reuptake Inhibitors; Selumetinib; Serotonin/Norepinephrine Reuptake Inhibitors; Sodium Phosphates; Talniflumate; Tenoxicam; Thiazide and Thiazide-Like Diuretics; Tipranavir; Tolperisone; Tricyclic Antidepressants (Tertiary Amine); Vitamin E (Systemic); Voriconazole; Zaltoprofen; Zanubrutinib

Decreased Effect

Meloxicam may decrease the levels/effects of: Aliskiren; Angiotensin II Receptor Blockers; Angiotensin-Converting Enzyme Inhibitors; Beta-Blockers; Eplerenone; HydrALAZINE; Loop Diuretics; Macimorelin; Mifamurtide; Potassium-Sparing Diuretics; Prostaglandins (Ophthalmic); Salicylates; Selective Serotonin Reuptake Inhibitors; Sincalide; Thiazide and Thiazide-Like Diuretics

The levels/effects of Meloxicam may be decreased by: Bile Acid Sequestrants; Itraconazole; Lumacaftor and Ivacaftor; Salicylates

Dietary Considerations Oral: May be taken with food or milk to minimize GI irritation.

Pharmacodynamics/Kinetics

Half-life Elimination

Children 2 to 6 years (n=7): Oral: 13.4 hours (Burgos-Vargas 2004).

Children and Adolescents 7 to 16 years (n=11): Oral: 12.7 hours (Burgos-Vargas 2004).

Adults: IV: ~24 hours; Oral: ~15 to 22 hours.

Time to Peak

Children and Adolescents 2 to 16 years (n=18): Oral: Suspension: Initial: 1 to 3 hours; secondary: 6 to 12 hours (Burgos-Vargas 2004).

Adults:

IV: 0.12 ± 0.04 hours.

Oral: Initial: Within 2 hours (capsule); 4 to 5 hours (tablet); 4 to 12 hours (orally disintegrating tablet; prolonged with food); Secondary: ~8 hours (capsule); 12 to 14 hours (tablet).

Reproductive Considerations

The chronic use of NSAIDs in women of reproductive age may be associated with infertility that is reversible upon discontinuation of the medication. Consider discontinuing use in women having difficulty conceiving or those undergoing investigation of fertility (Bermas 2014; Bloor 2013).

Pregnancy Considerations

Birth defects have been observed following in utero NSAID exposure in some studies; however, data is conflicting (Bloor 2013). Nonteratogenic effects, including prenatal constriction of the ductus arteriosus, persistent pulmonary hypertension of the newborn, oligohydramnios, necrotizing enterocolitis, renal dysfunction or failure, and intracranial hemorrhage have been observed in the fetus/neonate following in utero NSAID exposure. In addition, non-closure of the ductus arteriosus postnatally may occur and be resistant to medical management (Bermas 2014; Bloor 2013). Because NSAIDs may cause premature closure of the ductus arteriosus, product labeling for meloxicam specifically states use should be avoided starting at 30-weeks gestation.

Use of NSAIDs can be considered for the treatment of mild rheumatoid arthritis flares in pregnant women; however, use should be minimized or avoided early and late in pregnancy (Bermas 2014; Saavedra Salinas 2015).

The use of NSAIDs close to conception may be associated with an increased risk of miscarriage (Bermas 2014; Bloor 2013).

Breastfeeding Considerations It is not known if meloxicam is present in breast milk.

In general, NSAIDs may be used in postpartum women who wish to breastfeed; however, agents other than meloxicam are preferred (Montgomery 2012) and use should be avoided in women breastfeeding infants with platelet dysfunction or thrombocytopenia (Bloor 2013; Sammaritano 2014). According to the manufacturer, the decision to continue or discontinue breastfeeding during therapy should consider the risk of infant exposure, the benefits of breastfeeding to the infant, and benefits of treatment to the mother.

Dosage Forms: US

Capsule, Oral:

Vivlodex: 5 mg, 10 mg

Injectable, Intravenous [preservative free]:

Anjeso: 30 mg/mL (1 mL)

Tablet, Oral:

Mobic: 7.5 mg, 15 mg

Generic: 7.5 mg, 15 mg, 15 mg

Tablet Disintegrating, Oral:

Qmiiz ODT: 7.5 mg, 15 mg

Dosage Forms: Canada

Tablet, Oral:

Generic: 7.5 mg, 15 mg

Melphalan (MEL fa lan)

Brand Names: US Alkeran; Evomela

Brand Names: Canada Alkeran

Pharmacologic Category Antineoplastic Agent, Alkylating Agent; Antineoplastic Agent, Alkylating Agent (Nitrogen Mustard)

Use

Multiple myeloma: Palliative treatment of multiple myeloma (injection [Alkeran and Evomela] and tablets); high-dose conditioning treatment prior to hematopoietic stem cell transplantation (HSCT) (Evomela only).

Ovarian cancer: Palliative treatment of nonresectable epithelial ovarian carcinoma (tablets)

Local Anesthetic/Vasoconstrictor Precautions

No information available to require special precautions

Effects on Dental Treatment Key adverse event(s) related to dental treatment: Stomatitis.

Effects on Bleeding Severe myelosuppression including anemia and thrombocytopenia occurs which may result in bleeding. Medical consult recommended.

Adverse Reactions

>10%:

Cardiovascular: Peripheral edema (conditioning: 33%)

Central nervous system: Fatigue (≥50%; conditioning: 77%), dizziness (conditioning: 38%)

Endocrine & metabolic: Hypokalemia (≥50% conditioning: 74%), hypophosphatemia (conditioning: 49%)

Gastrointestinal: Diarrhea (≥50%; conditioning: 93%), nausea (≥50%; conditioning: 90%), vomiting (≥50%; conditioning: 64%), decreased appetite (conditioning: 49%), constipation (conditioning: 48%), mucositis (conditioning: 38%), abdominal pain (conditioning: 28%), dysgeusia (conditioning: 28%), stomatitis (conditioning: 28%), dyspepsia (conditioning: 26%)

Hematologic & oncologic: Anemia (≥50%), decreased absolute lymphocyte count (≥50%), decreased neutrophils (≥50%), decreased platelet count (≥50%; nadir: 14 to 21 days; recovery: 28 to 35 days), decreased white blood cell count (≥50%; nadir: 14 to 21 days; recovery: 28 to 35 days), febrile neutropenia (conditioning: 41%; grades 3/4: 28%)

Miscellaneous: Fever (conditioning: 48%)

1% to 10%:

Gastrointestinal: Hematochezia

Genitourinary: Amenorrhea (9%)

Hypersensitivity: Hypersensitivity reaction (IV: 2%; less common in oral formula; includes bronchospasm, dyspnea, edema, hypotension, pruritus, skin rash, tachycardia, urticaria), anaphylaxis (≤2%)

Renal: Renal failure

Frequency not defined:

Cardiovascular: Vasculitis

Central nervous system: Flushing sensation, tingling sensation

Endocrine & metabolic: SIADH (dose related; Greenbaum-Lefkoe 1985)

Genitourinary: Infertility, inhibition of testicular function

Hematologic & oncologic: Bone marrow depression

Hepatic: Hepatic sinusoidal obstruction syndrome (formerly known as hepatic veno-occlusive disease), hepatitis, increased serum transaminases, jaundice

Renal: Increased blood urea nitrogen

Miscellaneous: Chromosomal abnormality

<1%, postmarketing, and/or case reports: Alopecia, bone marrow failure (irreversible), hemolytic anemia, interstitial pneumonitis, maculopapular rash, pulmonary fibrosis, skin ulceration at injection site, tissue necrosis at injection site (rarely requiring skin grafting)

Mechanism of Action Alkylating agent which is a derivative of mechlorethamine that inhibits DNA and RNA synthesis via formation of carbonium ions; cross-links strands of DNA; acts on both resting and rapidly dividing tumor cells.

Pharmacodynamics/Kinetics

Half-life Elimination Terminal: IV: ~75 minutes; Oral: 1.5 ± 0.83 hours

Time to Peak Serum: Oral: ~1 to 2 hours

Reproductive Considerations

Females of reproductive potential should be advised to avoid pregnancy. Treatment with melphalan may suppress ovarian function leading to amenorrhea. Reversible and irreversible testicular suppression has been reported in male patients after melphalan administration.

Pregnancy Considerations

May cause fetal harm if administered during pregnancy.

◆ **Melphalan HCl** *see* Melphalan *on page 961*

◆ **Melphalan Hydrochloride** *see* Melphalan *on page 961*

Memantine (me MAN teen)

Brand Names: US Namenda; Namenda Titration Pak; Namenda XR; Namenda XR Titration Pack

Brand Names: Canada ACT Memantine; APO-Memantine; Ebixa; MED-Memantine; MYLAN-Memantine [DSC]; PMS-Memantine; RAN-Memantine; RATIO-Memantine [DSC]; RIVA-Memantine; SANDOZ Memantine FCT; SANDOZ Memantine [DSC]

Pharmacologic Category N-Methyl-D-Aspartate (NMDA) Receptor Antagonist

Use Alzheimer disease, moderate to severe: Treatment of moderate to severe dementia of the Alzheimer type.

Local Anesthetic/Vasoconstrictor Precautions

No information available to require special precautions

Effects on Dental Treatment No significant effects or complications reported

Effects on Bleeding No information available to require special precautions

Adverse Reactions Adverse reactions similar in immediate and extended release formulations except as noted.

1% to 10%:

Cardiovascular: Hypertension (4%), hypotension (extended release: 2%)

Central nervous system: Dizziness (5% to 7%), confusion (6%), headache (6%), anxiety (extended release: 4%), depression (extended release: 3%), drowsiness (3%), hallucination (3%), pain (3%), aggressive behavior (2%), fatigue (2%)

Endocrine & metabolic: Weight gain (extended release: 3%)

Gastrointestinal: Diarrhea (5%), constipation (3% to 5%), vomiting (2% to 3%), abdominal pain (2%)

Genitourinary: Urinary incontinence (2%)

Infection: Influenza (4%)

Neuromuscular & skeletal: Back pain (3%)

Respiratory: Cough (4%), dyspnea (2%)

<1%, postmarketing, and/or case reports: Abnormal gait, abnormal hepatic function tests, acne vulgaris, agitation, agranulocytosis, anorexia, arthralgia, aspiration pneumonia, atrioventricular block, bone fracture, bradycardia, brain disease, bronchitis, cardiac failure, carpal tunnel syndrome, cerebral infarction, cerebrovascular accident, chest pain, cholelithiasis, claudication, colitis, coma, complete atrioventricular block, convulsions, decreased appetite, deep vein thrombosis, dehydration, delusions, dementia (Alzheimer type), disorientation, drug-induced Parkinson disease, dyskinesia, falling, fecal incontinence, fever, gastritis, gastroesophageal reflux disease, hepatic failure, hepatitis (including cytolytic and cholestatic), hyperglycemia, hyperlipidemia, hypoglycemia, impaired consciousness, impotence, increased INR, increased serum alkaline phosphatase, increased serum creatinine, insomnia, intracranial hemorrhage, irritability, lethargy, leukopenia, limb pain, loss of consciousness, malaise, myoclonus, nasopharyngitis, nausea, neuroleptic malignant syndrome, neutropenia, otitis media, pancreatitis, pancytopenia, peripheral edema, prolonged QT interval on ECG, psychotic reaction, renal failure, renal function test abnormality, renal insufficiency, restlessness, second degree atrioventricular block, sepsis, SIADH, Stevens-Johnson syndrome, suicidal ideation, suicidal tendencies, supraventricular tachycardia, tardive dyskinesia, thrombocytopenia, thrombotic thrombocytopenic purpura, tonic-clonic seizures, torsades de pointes, tremor, upper respiratory tract infection, urinary tract infection, weakness

Mechanism of Action Glutamate, the primary excitatory amino acid in the CNS, may contribute to the pathogenesis of Alzheimer's disease (AD) by overstimulating various glutamate receptors leading to excitotoxicity and neuronal cell death. Memantine is an uncompetitive antagonist of the N-methyl-D-aspartate (NMDA) type of glutamate receptors, located ubiquitously throughout the brain. Under normal physiologic conditions, the (unstimulated) NMDA receptor ion channel is blocked by magnesium ions, which are displaced after agonist-induced depolarization. Pathologic or excessive receptor activation, as postulated to occur during AD, prevents magnesium from reentering and blocking the channel pore resulting in a chronically open state and excessive calcium influx. Memantine binds to the intra-pore magnesium site, but with longer dwell time, and thus functions as an effective receptor blocker only under conditions of excessive stimulation; memantine does not affect normal neurotransmission.

Pharmacodynamics/Kinetics

Half-life Elimination Terminal: ~60 to 80 hours

Time to Peak Serum: Immediate release: 3 to 7 hours; Extended release: 9 to 12 hours

Pregnancy Considerations Adverse events have been observed in animal reproduction studies.

◆ **Memantine HCl** *see* Memantine *on page 962*

◆ **Memantine Hydrochloride** *see* Memantine *on page 962*

◆ **Menactra** *see* Meningococcal (Groups A / C / Y and W-135) Conjugate Vaccine *on page 964*

◆ **MenACWY** *see* Meningococcal (Groups A / C / Y and W-135) Conjugate Vaccine *on page 964*

◆ **MenACWY-D (Menactra)** *see* Meningococcal (Groups A / C / Y and W-135) Conjugate Vaccine *on page 964*

◆ **MenACWY-CRM197 (Menveo)** *see* Meningococcal (Groups A / C / Y and W-135) Conjugate Vaccine *on page 964*

Meningococcal Group B Vaccine

(me NIN joe kok al groop bee vak SEEN)

Brand Names: US Bexsero; Trumenba

Pharmacologic Category Vaccine; Vaccine, Inactivated (Bacterial)

Use Meningococcal group B disease prevention:

US labeling: Active immunization of children, adolescents, and adults aged 10 to 25 years against invasive meningococcal disease caused by *Neisseria meningitidis* serogroup B.

The Advisory Committee on Immunization Practices (ACIP) recommends routine vaccination of persons ≥10 years of age with increased risk of meningococcal disease related to the following indications (ACIP [Folaranmi 2015; Patton 2017]):

- Persons with persistent complement component deficiencies (including patients receiving complement inhibitors [eg, eculizumab, ravulizumab])
- Persons with anatomic or functional asplenia (including sickle cell disease)
- Microbiologists routinely exposed to isolates of *N. meningitidis*
- Persons identified to be at increased risk due to a serogroup B meningococcal disease outbreak

The ACIP states that a meningococcal group B vaccination series may be administered to adolescents and young adults aged 16 to 23 years as determined by shared clinical decision-making to provide short-term protection against most strains of serogroup B meningococcal disease. The preferred age for vaccination is 16 to 18 years (ACIP [MacNeil 2015; Patton 2017; Freedman 2020; Robinson 2020]).

Canadian labeling: Active immunization against invasive meningococcal disease caused by *N. meningitidis* serogroup B (Bexsero: patients 2 months through 25 years of age; Trumenba: patients 10 through 25 years of age).

The Canadian National Advisory Committee on Immunization (NACI) recommends use of Bexsero (patients ≥2 months of age) or Trumenba (patients ≥10 years of age) in patients at high risk for serogroup B meningococcal disease (including disease outbreaks) and may be considered on an individual basis in healthy patients (Bexsero: 2 months to 25 years of age; Trumenba: 10 to 25 years of age) (NACI/CATMAT 2015; NACI 2019).

Local Anesthetic/Vasoconstrictor Precautions No information available to require special precautions

Effects on Dental Treatment No significant effects or complications reported

Effects on Bleeding No information available to require special precautions

Adverse Reactions Frequencies reported may include concomitant administration with routine pediatric vaccines or other vaccines.

>10%:

Central nervous system: Irritability (infants and children: 43% to 79%), drowsiness (infants and children: 53% to 72%; children: 30% to 51%), excessive crying (infants and children: 56% to 69%; children: 27% to 33%), fatigue (children, adolescents, and adults: 35% to 62%), headache (10% to 55%), malaise (children and adolescents: 50% to 56%; adults: 14%), chills (children and adolescents: 16% to 29%)

Gastrointestinal: Change in appetite (infants and children: 21% to 51%), diarrhea (children: 2% to 37%; infants and children: 18% to 24%; children and adolescents: years 9% to 15%), nausea (children, adolescents, and adults: 16% to 19%), vomiting (infants, children, and adolescents: ≤13%)

Local: Pain at injection site (children, adolescents, and adults: 82% to 98%), erythema at injection site (children: 60% to 98%; infants and children: 60% to 64%; children, adolescents, and adults: 45% to 54%), tenderness at injection site (children: 81% to 89%; infants and children: 65% to 66%), swelling at injection site (children: 26% to 63%; children and adolescents: 18% to 39%; infants and children: 26% to 31%), induration at injection site (infants and children: 33% to 56%; children, adolescents, and adults: 28% to 40%)

Neuromuscular & skeletal: Myalgia (children, adolescents, and adults: 31% to 57%), arthralgia (children, adolescents, and adults: 13% to 33%)

Miscellaneous: Fever (infants and children: 69% to 79%, ≥40°C [104°F] ≤1%; children: 10% to 28%, ≥40°C [104°F] ≤3%; children, adolescents, and adults: 1% to 8%)

1% to 10%:

Dermatologic: Skin rash (children: ≤9%), urticaria (infants and children: 5% to 6%)

Respiratory: Upper respiratory tract infection (infants: 10%; mostly considered unrelated to vaccination), nasopharyngitis (children, adolescents, and adults: ≥2%)

<1% (postmarketing, and/or case reports): Eczema, febrile seizures, hypersensitivity reaction (includes anaphylaxis), injection site blister formation, injection site nodule, Kawasaki syndrome, pallor, seizure, swelling of eye, syncope, vasodepressor syncope

Mechanism of Action

Bexsero: Induces immunity against meningococcal disease caused by serogroup B *Neisseria meningitidis* (MenB) via the formation of antibodies directed toward the recombinant protein antigens combined together with outer membrane vesicles (OMV) from a group B strain.

Trumenba: Protection against invasive meningococcal disease is conferred mainly by complement-mediated antibody-dependent killing of *N. meningitidis*.

Efficacy:
 Bexsero: Composite hSBA titer response one month after the second dose: 63% to 88%
 Trumenba: 84% of adolescents had a ≥4-fold rise in hSBA titer and composite response after the third dose.

Pregnancy Considerations
Inactivated vaccines have not been shown to cause increased risks to the fetus (ACIP [Ezeanolue 2020]). However, the Advisory Committee on Immunization Practices (ACIP) recommends deferring meningococcal group B vaccination in pregnant women unless the woman is at increased risk for meningococcal disease and vaccination benefits outweigh the potential risks (ACIP [Patton 2017]).

Meningococcal (Groups A / C / Y and W-135) Conjugate Vaccine

(me NIN joe kok al groops aye, see, why & dubl yoo won thur tee fyve KON joo gate vak SEEN)

Brand Names: US Menactra; Menveo
Brand Names: Canada Menactra; Menveo; Nimenrix
Pharmacologic Category Vaccine; Vaccine, Inactivated (Bacterial)

Use

Meningococcal disease prevention: Active immunization against invasive meningococcal disease caused by *Neisseria meningitidis* serogroups A, C, Y, and W-135 in the following persons:
- ≥2 months to ≤55 years of age (Menveo)
- ≥9 months to ≤55 years of age (Menactra)
- ≥2 years of age (MenQuadfi)
- ≥6 weeks to ≤55 years of age (Nimenrix) [Canadian product]

The Advisory Committee on Immunization Practices (ACIP) (CDC/ACIP [Cohn 2013]; CDC/ACIP [MacNeil 2014]; CDC/ACIP [MacNeil 2016]):
ACIP recommends routine vaccination of the following:
- Children and adolescents 11 to 18 years of age
- Persons ≥2 months of age who are at increased risk of meningococcal disease
- Persons (in all recommended age groups) at increased risk who are part of outbreaks caused by vaccine preventable serogroups

Those at increased risk of meningococcal disease include the following:
- Persons ≥2 months of age with medical conditions such as anatomic or functional asplenia (including sickle cell disease), HIV, or persistent complement component deficiencies (eg, C_5-C_9, properdin, factor H, or factor D, persons receiving complement inhibitors [eg, eculizumab, ravulizumab])
- Persons ≥2 months of age who travel to or reside in countries where meningococcal disease is hyperendemic or epidemic, especially if contact with the local population will be prolonged
- Unvaccinated or incompletely vaccinated first year college students living in residence halls (CDC/ACIP [Bilukha 2005])
- Military recruits
- Microbiologists with occupational exposure

The Canadian National Advisory Committee on Immunization (NACI): NACI recommends a routine vaccination at ~12 years of age but no booster unless at a continued high risk of exposure. Either quadrivalent vaccine may be used; NACI does not have a preference. NACI recommends use of Menveo (off-label use) for high risk persons 2 months to 2 years of age if vaccination with a quadrivalent vaccine is needed; may also be considered for use in persons ≥56 years of age (NACI 39[1] 2013). Additional recommendations may be found at https://www.canada.ca/en/public-health/services/publications/healthy-living/canadian-immunization-guide-part-4-active-vaccines/page-13-meningococcal-vaccine.html.

Local Anesthetic/Vasoconstrictor Precautions No information available to require special precautions

Effects on Dental Treatment No significant effects or complications reported

Effects on Bleeding No information available to require special precautions

Adverse Reactions Actual percentages may vary by product and age group. Adverse reactions occur with children, adolescents, and adults unless otherwise specified.

>10%:
 Gastrointestinal: Anorexia (8% to 12%; infants: 30%), change in appetite (infants: 12% to 23%; children: 9% to 10%), diarrhea (infants, children, adolescents, & adults: 7% to 16%), nausea (5% to 12%), vomiting (2% to 3%; infants: 5% to 14%)
 Local: Pain at injection site (adolescents & adults: 36% to 59%; children: 33% to 45%), tenderness at injection site (infants: 10% to 37%), erythema at injection site (infants & children: 11% to 30%; adolescents & adults: 11% to 16%), induration at injection site (11% to 19%; infants: 7% to 8%), swelling at injection site (infants, children, adolescents, & adults: 11% to 17%)
 Nervous system: Pain (60%), irritability (infants: 27% to 57%; children: 12% to 22%), drowsiness (infants: 17% to 50%; children: 11% to 18%), headache (adolescents & adults: 22% to 41%; children: 5% to 18%), excessive crying (infants: 12% to 41%), fatigue (adolescents & adults: 17% to 38%), malaise (adolescents & adults: 10% to 24%; children: 11% to 14%)
 Neuromuscular & skeletal: Myalgia (10% to 43%), arthralgia (adolescents & adults: 6% to 20%; children: 3% to 7%)
 Miscellaneous: Crying (abnormal; infants: 33%), fever (infants, children, & adolescents: ≤12%; adults: 1% to 2%)

1% to 10%:
 Dermatologic: Skin rash (infants, children, & adolescents: 2% to 6%; adults: 1% to 2%)
 Nervous system: Chills (4% to 10%)

<1%, postmarketing, and/or case reports: Accidental injury, acute disseminated encephalomyelitis, anaphylaxis, angioedema, apnea (premature infants), appendicitis, auditory impairment, Bell palsy, blepharoptosis, cellulitis at injection site, Cushing syndrome, dehydration, dizziness, dyspnea, equilibrium disturbance, erythema of skin, exfoliation of skin, facial nerve paralysis, falling, febrile seizures, gastroenteritis, gastrointestinal disease (Vitello-intestinal duct remnant), Guillain-Barre syndrome, herniated disc, herpes zoster infection, hypersensitivity reaction, hypotension, increased serum alanine aminotransferase, inflammation, inguinal hernia, injection site pruritus, Kawasaki syndrome, lymphadenopathy, oropharyngeal pain, ostealgia, otalgia, paresthesia, pelvic inflammatory disease, pneumonia, pruritus, seizure, sepsis, staphylococcal infection, suicidal tendencies, swelling, swelling of injected limb, syncope, transverse myelitis, upper airway swelling, urticaria, vasopressor syncope, vertigo, vestibular disturbance, viral hepatitis, wheezing

Mechanism of Action Induces immunity against meningococcal disease via the formation of bactericidal antibodies directed toward the polysaccharide capsular components of *Neisseria meningitidis* serogroups A, C, Y and W-135.

Pregnancy Considerations

Based on available data, an increased risk of adverse pregnancy outcomes has not been observed following maternal vaccination with a meningococcal (Groups A / C / Y and W-135) diphtheria conjugate vaccine (Becerra-Culqui 2020; Myers 2017; Zheteyeva 2013).

Inactivated bacterial vaccines have not been shown to cause increased risks to the fetus. Use of meningococcal conjugate vaccines may be considered for use in pregnant women at increased risk of infection (ACIP [Ezeanolue 2020]). Pregnancy should not preclude vaccination if otherwise indicated (CDC/ACIP [Cohn 2013]).

Data collection to monitor pregnancy and infant outcomes following exposure to Menactra or MenQuadfi is ongoing. Health care providers are encouraged to enroll females exposed to Menactra or MedQuadfi during pregnancy in the Sanofi Pasteur Inc vaccine registry (1-800-822-2463).

Product Availability MenQuadfi: FDA approved April 2020; availability anticipated in 2021. Consult the prescribing information for additional information.

Meningococcal Polysaccharide (Groups C and Y) and *Haemophilus* b Tetanus Toxoid Conjugate Vaccine

(me NIN joe kok al pol i SAK a ride groops see & why & he MOF i lus bee TET a nus TOKS oyd KON joo gate vak SEEN)

Brand Names: US Menhibrix [DSC]

Pharmacologic Category Vaccine; Vaccine, Inactivated (Bacterial)

Use Meningococcal and *Haemophilus influenzae* type b disease prevention: To provide active immunity to prevent invasive disease caused by meningococcal serogroups C and Y and *Haemophilus influenzae* type b

The Advisory Committee on Immunization Practices (ACIP) (CDC/ACIP [Cohn 2013]) recommends vaccination only for infants 2-18 months of age who are at increased risk for meningococcal disease, including:

- Infants with persistent complement pathway deficiencies
- Infants with anatomic or functional asplenia, including sickle cell disease
- Infants in communities with serogroups C and Y meningococcal disease outbreaks

The ACIP does not recommend routine vaccination for infants not at increased risk for meningococcal disease. In addition, infants traveling to certain areas (eg, meningitis belt of sub-Saharan Africa) will require a meningococcal vaccine with serogroups A and W; vaccination with Hib-MenCY-TT will not be sufficient (CDC/ACIP [Cohn 2013])

Local Anesthetic/Vasoconstrictor Precautions

No information available to require special precautions

Effects on Dental Treatment No significant effects or complications reported

Effects on Bleeding No information available to require special precautions

Adverse Reactions

>10%:

Central nervous system: Irritability (62% to 71%), drowsiness (49% to 63%)

Gastrointestinal: Decreased appetite (30% to 34%)

Local: Pain at injection site (41% to 46%), erythema at injection site (21% to 36%), swelling at injection site (15% to 25%)

Miscellaneous: Fever ≥100.4°F/38°C (11% to 26%)

<1%, postmarketing, and/or case reports: Anaphylactoid reaction, anaphylaxis, angioedema, apnea, hypersensitivity reaction, hypotonic/hyporesponsive episode, induration at injection site, seizure (with or without fever), skin rash, swelling of injected limb (extensive), syncope, urticaria, vasodepressor syncope

Mechanism of Action Provides active immunity against meningococcal disease via the formation of bactericidal antibodies directed toward the polysaccharide capsular components of *Neisseria meningitidis* serogroups C and Y; stimulates production of anticapsular antibodies and to *Haemophilus influenzae* type b

Pharmacodynamics/Kinetics

Onset of Action Antibody response to the components of the vaccine occurs in ≥95% of children following the third dose and ≥98% following the fourth dose.

Pregnancy Risk Factor C

Pregnancy Considerations Animal reproduction studies have not been conducted.

Product Availability Menhibrix has been discontinued in the US for more than 1 year.

◆ **Meningococcal Vaccine** *see* Meningococcal Polysaccharide (Groups C and Y) and *Haemophilus* b Tetanus Toxoid Conjugate Vaccine *on page 965*

◆ **Menopur** *see* Menotropins *on page 965*

◆ **Menostar** *see* Estradiol (Systemic) *on page 596*

Menotropins (men oh TROE pins)

Brand Names: US Menopur

Brand Names: Canada Menopur

Pharmacologic Category Gonadotropin; Ovulation Stimulator

Use

For multiple follicle development and pregnancy in ovulatory women as part of an assisted reproductive technology cycle.

Limitations of use: Prior to therapy, preform a complete gynecologic exam and endocrinologic evaluation to diagnose the cause of infertility; exclude the possibility of pregnancy; evaluate the fertility status of the male partner; exclude a diagnosis of primary ovarian failure.

Local Anesthetic/Vasoconstrictor Precautions

No information available to require special precautions

Effects on Dental Treatment No significant effects or complications reported

Effects on Bleeding Has been associated with thrombotic events; however, no information available to require special precautions in dental procedures.

Adverse Reactions Adverse effects and incidences may vary according to specific product, indication, dosage, or route of administration.

>10%: Genitourinary: Multiple gestation (35%)

1% to 10%:

Central nervous system: Headache (5% to 6%)

Endocrine & metabolic: Ovarian disease (3% to 8%), ovarian hyperstimulation syndrome (2% to 7%)

Gastrointestinal: Abdominal pain (5% to 7%), nausea (4% to 7%), abdominal cramps (3% to 7%), enlargement of abdomen (2% to 6%), gastrointestinal fullness (≥5%), vomiting (3%), diarrhea (2%)
Genitourinary: Vaginal hemorrhage (3% to 8%), pelvic pain (1% to 3%), breast tenderness (2%), ectopic pregnancy (1%)
Infection: Infection (1%)
Local: Injection site reaction (2% to 8%), swelling at injection site (1% to 8%), pain at injection site (≤4%), inflammation at injection site (2%)
Respiratory: Dyspnea (1% to 2%)

Frequency not defined:
Cardiovascular: Tachycardia
Central nervous system: Dizziness
Dermatologic: Rash at injection site, skin rash
Endocrine & metabolic: Ovarian cyst, ovary enlargement
Hematologic & oncologic: Hemoperitoneum, ovarian neoplasm
Hypersensitivity: Anaphylaxis
Local: Irritation at injection site
Respiratory: Flu-like symptoms, tachypnea
Miscellaneous: Fetal abnormality, ovarian torsion

<1%, postmarketing, and/or case reports: Abdominal distention, abdominal distress, acne vulgaris, acute respiratory distress syndrome, angioedema, atelectasis, cerebrovascular accident, embolism, facial edema, fatigue, hot flash, hypersensitivity reaction, laryngeal edema, local tissue necrosis, lower abdominal pain, malaise, occlusion of cerebral arteries, occlusive arterial disease (may result in loss of limb), pulmonary complications, pulmonary embolism, pulmonary infarct, thromboembolism, thrombophlebitis (includes venous), thrombosis

Mechanism of Action Menotropins is a purified combination of follicle stimulating hormone (FSH) and luteinizing hormone (LH) extracted from the urine of postmenopausal women. Treatment provides ovarian follicular growth and maturation in females who do not have primary ovarian failure. Also stimulates spermatogenesis in males (off-label use)

Pharmacodynamics/Kinetics

Half-life Elimination Follicle-stimulating hormone (FSH) 11 to 13 hours (following multiple doses).

Time to Peak FSH (following a single dose): 18 hours (SubQ).

Reproductive Considerations

Menotropins are used for the induction of ovulation and assisted reproductive technology (ART). Pregnancy should be excluded prior to treatment.

Evaluate pregnancy status as well as the fertility of the male partner prior to ovulation induction.

Evaluate fertility status of the female partner prior to induction of spermatogenesis when treating males with hypogonadotropic hypogonadism (AACE [Petak 2002]).

Pregnancy Risk Factor X

Pregnancy Considerations

Menotropins are used for the induction of ovulation and with assisted reproductive technology (ART); use is contraindicated in women who are already pregnant.

Ectopic pregnancy, congenital abnormalities, spontaneous abortion, and multifetal gestations/ births have been reported. The incidence of congenital abnormality may be slightly higher after ART than with spontaneous conception; higher incidence may be related to parental characteristics (maternal age, genetics, sperm characteristics).

◆ **MenQuadfi** *see* Meningococcal (Groups A / C / Y and W-135) Conjugate Vaccine *on page 964*

◆ **Menveo** *see* Meningococcal (Groups A / C / Y and W-135) Conjugate Vaccine *on page 964*

Mepenzolate (me PEN zoe late)

Pharmacologic Category Anticholinergic Agent; Antispasmodic Agent, Gastrointestinal

Use Adjunctive treatment of peptic ulcer disease; has not been shown to be effective in contributing to the healing of peptic ulcer, preventing complications, or decreasing the rate of recurrence

Local Anesthetic/Vasoconstrictor Precautions No information available to require special precautions

Effects on Dental Treatment Key adverse event(s) related to dental treatment: Xerostomia (normal salivary flow resumes upon discontinuation), dry throat, dysphagia, and loss of taste.

Effects on Bleeding No information available to require special precautions

Adverse Reactions Frequency not defined.
Cardiovascular: Palpitations, tachycardia
Central nervous system: Confusion, dizziness, drowsiness, headache, insomnia, nervousness
Dermatologic: Hypohidrosis, urticaria
Gastrointestinal: Ageusia, bloating, constipation, delayed gastric emptying, nausea, vomiting, xerostomia
Genitourinary: Decreased lactation, impotence, urinary hesitancy, urinary retention
Hypersensitivity: Anaphylaxis
Neuromuscular & skeletal: Weakness
Ophthalmic: Blurred vision, cycloplegia, increased intraocular pressure, mydriasis

Mechanism of Action Mepenzolate is a postganglionic parasympathetic inhibitor. It decreases gastric acid and pepsin secretion and suppresses spontaneous contractions of the colon.

Pregnancy Risk Factor B

Pregnancy Considerations Adverse events were not observed in animal reproduction studies.

◆ **Mepenzolate Bromide** *see* Mepenzolate *on page 966*

Meperidine (me PER i deen)

Related Information

Management of the Patient With Anxiety or Depression *on page 1778*

Brand Names: US Demerol

Brand Names: Canada Demerol [DSC]

Generic Availability (US) Yes

Pharmacologic Category Analgesic, Opioid

Dental Use Adjunct in preoperative intravenous conscious sedation in patients undergoing dental surgery; alternate oral opioid in patients allergic to codeine to treat moderate to moderate-severe pain

Use

Pain management: Management of acute pain severe enough to require an opioid analgesic and for which alternative treatments are inadequate; obstetrical analgesia, preoperative medication (IV only).

Limitations of use: The American Pain Society and Institute for Safe Medication Practices do not recommend meperidine's use as an analgesic. If use in acute pain (in patients without renal or CNS disease) cannot be avoided, treatment should be limited to ≤48 hours and doses should not exceed 600 mg per 24 hours (APS 2016; ISMP 2007).

Local Anesthetic/Vasoconstrictor Precautions No information available to require special precautions

Effects on Dental Treatment Key adverse event(s) related to dental treatment: Xerostomia (normal salivary flow resumes upon discontinuation). See Dental Health Professional Considerations.

Effects on Bleeding No information available to require special precautions

Adverse Reactions Frequency not defined.

Cardiovascular: Bradycardia, cardiac arrest, circulatory depression, flushing, hypotension, palpitations, shock, syncope, tachycardia

Central nervous system: Agitation, confusion, delirium, disorientation, dizziness, drug dependence (physical dependence), habituation, hallucination, headache, increased intracranial pressure, involuntary muscle movements (including muscle twitching, myoclonus), mood changes (including euphoria, dysphoria), sedation, seizure (associated with metabolite accumulation), serotonin syndrome

Dermatologic: Diaphoresis, pruritus, skin rash, urticaria

Gastrointestinal: Biliary colic, constipation, nausea, spasm of sphincter of Oddi, vomiting, xerostomia

Genitourinary: Urinary retention

Hypersensitivity: Anaphylaxis, histamine release, hypersensitivity reaction

Local: Injection site reaction (including pain, wheal, and flare)

Neuromuscular & skeletal: Tremor, weakness

Ophthalmic: Visual disturbance

Respiratory: Dyspnea, respiratory arrest, respiratory depression

<1%, postmarketing, and/or case reports: Hypogonadism (Brennan 2013; Debono 2011)

Dental Usual Dosage Note: The American Pain Society (2008) and ISMP (2007) do not recommend meperidine's use as an analgesic. If use in acute pain (in patients without renal or CNS disease) cannot be avoided, treatment should be limited to ≤48 hours and doses should not exceed 600 mg/24 hours. Oral route is not recommended for treatment of acute or chronic pain. If IV route is required, consider a reduced dose. Patients with prior opioid exposure may require higher initial doses.

Pain (analgesic): Adults: Oral: Initial: Opioid-naive: 50 mg every 3 to 4 hours as needed; usual dosage range: 50 to 150 mg every 3 to 4 hours as needed (manufacturer's recommendation; oral route is not recommended for acute pain)

Dosing

Adult Note: The American Pain Society and ISMP do not recommend meperidine's use as an analgesic. If use in acute pain (in patients without renal or CNS disease) cannot be avoided, treatment should be limited to ≤48 hours and doses should not exceed 600 mg per 24 hours. Oral administration is not recommended for treatment of acute or chronic pain. If IV administration is required, consider a reduced dose. When treating pain, patients with prior opioid exposure may require higher initial doses (APS 2016; ISMP 2007).

Pain management:

Acute pain: IM, SubQ: 50 to 150 mg every 3 to 4 hours as needed.

Discontinuation of therapy: When discontinuing chronic opioid therapy, the dose should be gradually tapered down. An optimal universal tapering schedule for all patients has not been established (CDC [Dowell 2016]). Proposed schedules range from slow (eg, 10% reductions per week) to rapid (eg, 25% to 50% reduction every few days) (CDC 2015). Tapering schedules should be individualized to minimize opioid withdrawal while considering patient-specific goals and concerns as well as the pharmacokinetics of the opioid being tapered. An even slower taper may be appropriate in patients who have been receiving opioids for a long duration (eg, years), particularly in the final stage of tapering, whereas more rapid tapers may be appropriate in patients experiencing severe adverse events (CDC [Dowell 2016]). Monitor carefully for signs/symptoms of withdrawal. If the patient displays withdrawal symptoms, consider slowing the taper schedule; alterations may include increasing the interval between dose reductions, decreasing amount of daily dose reduction, pausing the taper and restarting when the patient is ready, and/or coadministration of an alpha-2 agonist (eg, clonidine) to blunt withdrawal symptoms (Berna 2015; CDC [Dowell 2016]). Continue to offer nonopioid analgesics as needed for pain management during the taper; consider nonopioid adjunctive treatments for withdrawal symptoms (eg, GI complaints, muscle spasm) as needed (Berna 2015; Sevarino 2018).

Obstetrical analgesia: IM, SubQ: 50 to 100 mg when pain becomes regular; may repeat at 1- to 3-hour intervals.

Preoperative: IM, SubQ: 50 to 100 mg administered 30 to 90 minutes before the beginning of anesthesia.

Postoperative shivering (off-label use): IV: 12.5 to 50 mg once (Crowley 2008; Kranke 2002; Mercandante 1994; Miller 2010; Wang 1999) **or** 0.2 mg/kg with adjunctive dexamethasone (Solhpour 2016)

Rigors from amphotericin B (conventional) (off-label use): IV: 25 to 50 mg once (Burks 1980; Ellis 1992; Nucci 1999)

Geriatric Avoid use as an analgesic (American Pain Society 2016; Beers Criteria [AGS 2019]; ISMP 2007).

Renal Impairment: Adult Avoid use as an analgesic in renal impairment (American Pain Society 2016; ISMP 2007).

Hepatic Impairment: Adult There are no dosage adjustments provided in the manufacturer's labeling; use with caution and titrate slowly; monitor closely for signs of CNS excitation (eg, seizure activity) and CNS and respiratory depression. In patients with severe impairment, consider a lower dose when initiating therapy; an increased opioid effect may be seen in patients with cirrhosis; dose reduction is more important for the oral (route not recommended [APS 2016]) than IV route (Tegeder 1999).

Pediatric Doses should be titrated to appropriate analgesic effect; when changing route of administration, note that oral doses are about half as effective as parenteral dose.

Note: The American Pain Society (2008) and ISMP (2007) do not recommend meperidine use as an analgesic. If use for acute pain (in patients without renal or CNS disease) cannot be avoided, treatment should be limited to ≤48 hours and doses should not exceed 600 mg/24 hours in adults. Oral route is not recommended for treatment of acute or chronic pain. If IV route is required, consider a reduced dose. Patients with prior opioid exposure may require higher initial doses.

Acute pain (analgesic) (Berde 2002): Initial:

Infants ≤6 months:

IM, IV, SubQ: 0.2 to 0.25 mg/kg/dose every 2 to 3 hours

Oral: 0.5 to 0.75 mg/kg/dose every 3 to 4 hours

Infants >6 months, Children, and Adolescents:

IM, IV, or SubQ; intermittent dosing:

Patient weight <50 kg: 0.8 to 1 mg/kg/dose every 2 to 3 hours as needed; maximum dose: 75 mg/dose

Patient weight ≥50 kg: 50 to 75 mg every 2 to 3 hours as needed

Oral:

Patient weight <50 kg: 2 to 3 mg/kg/dose every 3 to 4 hours as needed; maximum dose: 150 mg/dose

Patient weight ≥50 kg: 100 to 150 mg every 3 to 4 hours as needed

Analgesia for minor procedures/sedation; preoperative: Infants, Children, and Adolescents:

IM, IV, SubQ: 0.5 to 1 mg/kg given 30 to 90 minutes before the beginning of anesthesia; maximum dose: 2 mg/kg or 150 mg/dose (Zeltzer 1990)

Oral: 2 to 4 mg/kg given 30 to 90 minutes before the beginning of anesthesia; maximum dose: 150 mg/dose

Sickle cell disease, acute crisis; opioid naïve patients: (APS 1999): Infants ≥6 months, Children, and Adolescents: **Note:** Not recommended for use unless it is the only opioid effective for the patient (NHLBI 2014). Initial:

Patient weight <50 kg: IV: 0.75 to 1 mg/kg every 3 to 4 hours as needed; maximum dose: 1.75 mg/kg/dose or 100 mg/dose

Patient weight ≥50 kg: IV: 50 to 150 mg every 3 hours as needed

Renal Impairment: Pediatric The manufacturer recommends to use with caution and reduce dose; accumulation of meperidine and its active metabolite (normeperidine) may occur. The American Pain Society and ISMP recommend to avoid use in renal impairment. (American Pain Society 2008; ISMP 2007).

Hepatic Impairment: Pediatric Use with caution and reduce dose; accumulation of meperidine and its active metabolite (normeperidine) may occur.

Mechanism of Action Binds to opioid receptors in the CNS, causing inhibition of ascending pain pathways, altering the perception of and response to pain; produces generalized CNS depression

Contraindications

Hypersensitivity (eg, anaphylaxis) to meperidine or any component of the formulation; use with or within 14 days of MAO inhibitors; significant respiratory depression; acute or severe bronchial asthma in an unmonitored setting or in the absence of resuscitative equipment; GI obstruction, including paralytic ileus (known or suspected).

Canadian labeling: Additional contraindications (not in US labeling): Known or suspected mechanical GI obstruction (eg, bowel obstruction or strictures) or any diseases/conditions that affect bowel transit (eg, ileus of any type); suspected surgical abdomen (eg, acute appendicitis or pancreatitis); mild pain that can be managed with other pain medications; acute or severe bronchial asthma, chronic obstructive airway, status asthmaticus; acute respiratory depression; hypoxia; hypercapnia; cor pulmonale; acute alcoholism, delirium tremens, and convulsive disorders; severe CNS depression, increased cerebrospinal or intracranial pressure and head injury; concurrent use or use within 14 days of an MAOI

Documentation of allergenic cross-reactivity for opioids is limited. However, because of similarities in chemical structure and/or pharmacologic actions, the possibility of cross-sensitivity cannot be ruled out with certainty.

Warnings/Precautions [US Boxed Warning]: Serious, life-threatening, or fatal respiratory depression may occur. Monitor closely for respiratory depression, especially during initiation or dose escalation. Carbon dioxide retention from opioid-induced respiratory depression can exacerbate the sedating effects of opioids. Use with caution and monitor for respiratory depression in patients with significant chronic obstructive pulmonary disease or cor pulmonale, and those with a substantially decreased respiratory reserve, hypoxia, hypercapnia, or preexisting respiratory depression, particularly when initiating and titrating therapy; critical respiratory depression may occur, even at therapeutic dosages. Consider the use of alternative nonopioid analgesics in these patients.

[US Boxed Warning]: Concomitant use of opioids with benzodiazepines or other CNS depressants, including alcohol, may result in profound sedation, respiratory depression, coma, and death. Reserve concomitant prescribing of meperidine and benzodiazepines or other CNS depressants for use in patients for whom alternative treatment options are inadequate. Limit dosage and durations to the minimum required and follow patients for signs and symptoms of respiratory depression and sedation. [US Boxed Warning]: Use with all CYP3A4 inhibitors may result in an increase in meperidine plasma concentrations, which could increase or prolong adverse drug effects and may cause potentially fatal respiratory depression. In addition, discontinuation of a concomitant CYP3A4 inducer may result in increased meperidine concentrations. Monitor patients receiving meperidine and any CYP3A4 inhibitor or inducer. [US Boxed Warning]: Concomitant use of meperidine with monoamine oxidase inhibitors (MAOIs) can result in coma, severe respiratory depression, cyanosis, and hypotension. Use of meperidine with MAOIs within last 14 days is contraindicated. Potentially significant drug interactions may exist, requiring dose or frequency adjustment, additional monitoring, and/or selection of alternative therapy.

Meperidine offers no advantage over other opioids as an analgesic and has unique neurotoxicity. The use of meperidine in acute pain and/or cancer pain management should be avoided (APS 2016; ISMP 2007). Use is not recommended for the management of chronic pain. Normeperidine (an active metabolite and CNS stimulant) may accumulate and precipitate anxiety, tremors, or seizures; risk increases with CNS or renal dysfunction, prolonged use (>48 hours), and cumulative dose (>600 mg/24 hours in adults); oral meperidine should not be used since first-pass metabolism decreases efficacy while increasing normeperidine concentrations (APS 2016). Avoid in the elderly and in patients with renal impairment (APS 2016; ISMP 2007). Meperidine should be avoided in those older adults with, or at risk for, delirium because of the potential to cause or worsen delirium.

May cause CNS depression, which may impair physical or mental abilities; patients must be cautioned about performing tasks which require mental alertness (eg, operating machinery or driving). Use with extreme caution in patients with head injury, intracranial lesions, elevated intracranial pressure. Avoid use in patients with impaired consciousness or coma as these patients are susceptible to intracranial effects of carbon dioxide retention. Opioid use increases the risk for sleep-related disorders (eg, central sleep apnea, hypoxemia) in a dose-dependent fashion; use with caution. Use with caution in patients with hepatic disorders, supraventricular tachycardias (including atrial flutter), biliary tract dysfunction (including acute pancreatitis), delirium tremens, toxic psychosis, thyroid dysfunction, morbid obesity, adrenal insufficiency, Addison disease, seizure disorders, prostatic hyperplasia, urethral stricture, pheochromocytoma, and in cachectic or debilitated patients. May obscure diagnosis or clinical course of patients with acute abdominal conditions. May cause severe hypotension (including orthostatic hypotension and syncope); use with caution in patients with hypovolemia, cardiovascular disease (including acute myocardial infarction [MI]), or drugs which may exaggerate hypotensive effects (including phenothiazines or general anesthetics). Monitor for symptoms of hypotension following initiation or dose titration. Avoid use in patients with circulatory shock.

May cause constipation which may be problematic in patients with unstable angina and patients post-MI. Consider preventive measures (eg, stimulant laxative) to reduce the potential for constipation. Serotonin syndrome may occur with concomitant use of serotonergic agents (eg, selective serotonin reuptake inhibitors, serotonin-norepinephrine reuptake inhibitors, triptans, tricyclic antidepressants), lithium, St John's wort, agents that impair metabolism of serotonin (eg, MAO inhibitors), or agents that impair metabolism of tramadol (eg, CYP2D6 and 3A4 inhibitors). An opioid-containing analgesic regimen should be tailored to each patient's needs and based upon the route of administration, degree of tolerance for opioids (naive versus chronic user), age, weight, and medical condition. The optimal analgesic dose varies widely among patients; doses should be titrated to pain relief/prevention. Opioids decrease bowel motility; monitor for decrease bowel motility in postop patients receiving opioids. Use with caution in the perioperative setting; individualize treatment when transitioning from parenteral to oral analgesics. Abrupt discontinuation in patients who are physically dependent on opioids has been associated with serious withdrawal symptoms, uncontrolled pain, attempts to find other opioids (including illicit), and suicide. Use a collaborative, patient-specific taper schedule that minimizes the risk of withdrawal, considering factors such as current opioid dose, duration of use, type of pain, and physical and psychological factors. Monitor pain control, withdrawal symptoms, mood changes, suicidal ideation, and for use of other substances and provide care as needed. Concurrent use of mixed agonist/antagonist analgesics (eg, pentazocine, nalbuphine, butorphanol) or partial agonist (eg, buprenorphine) analgesics may also precipitate withdrawal symptoms and/or reduced analgesic efficacy in patients following prolonged therapy with mu opioid agonists.

In patients with sickle cell anemia, use with caution and decrease initial dose; normeperidine (active metabolite) may accumulate and induce seizures in these patients; **Note:** Meperidine recommended for use in sickle cell patients by the American Pain Society (APS 2016) and should only be used in sickle cell patients with a vaso-occlusive crisis if it is the only effective opioid for an individual patient (NHLBI 2014).

Some preparations may contain sulfites which may cause allergic reaction. **[US Boxed Warning]: Meperidine exposes patients and other users to the risks of addiction, abuse, and misuse, potentially leading to overdose and death. Assess each patient's risk prior to prescribing; monitor all patients regularly for development of these behaviors or conditions. [US Boxed Warning]: To ensure that the benefits of opioid analgesics outweigh the risks of addiction, abuse, and misuse, a REMS is required. Drug companies with approved opioid analgesic products must make REMS-compliant education programs available to health care providers. Health care providers are encouraged to complete a REMS-compliant education program; counsel patients and/or their caregivers, with every prescription, on safe use, serious risks, storage, and disposal of these products; emphasize to patients and their caregivers the importance of reading the Medication Guide every time it is provided by their pharmacist; and consider other tools to improve patient, household, and community safety.** Use with caution in patients with a history of drug abuse or acute alcoholism; potential for drug dependency exists. Other factors associated with increased risk for misuse include younger age, concomitant depression (major), and psychotropic medication use. **[US Boxed Warning]: Accidental ingestion of even one dose, especially in children, can result in a fatal overdose of meperidine.**

[US Boxed Warning]: Prolonged use of opioids during pregnancy can cause neonatal withdrawal syndrome, which may be life-threatening if not recognized and treated according to protocols developed by neonatology experts. If opioid use is required for a prolonged period in a pregnant woman, advise the patient of the risk of neonatal opioid withdrawal syndrome and ensure that appropriate treatment will be available. Signs and symptoms include irritability, hyperactivity and abnormal sleep pattern, high pitched cry, tremor, vomiting, diarrhea and failure to gain weight. Onset, duration and severity depend on the drug used, duration of use, maternal dose, and rate of drug elimination by the newborn.

[US Boxed Warning]: Ensure accuracy when prescribing, dispensing, and administering meperidine oral solution. Dosing errors due to confusion between mg and mL, and other meperidine solutions of different concentrations, can result in accidental overdose and death. Do not use a teaspoon or a tablespoon to measure a dose; use a calibrated measuring device. Use extreme caution in measuring the dosage.

Parenteral: Administer IV injections very slowly, preferably in the form of a diluted solution. Do not administer IV unless a opioid antagonist and the facilities for assisted or controlled respiration are immediately available. When meperidine is given parenterally, especially IV, the patient should be lying down.

Some dosage forms may contain sodium benzoate/ benzoic acid; benzoic acid (benzoate) is a metabolite of benzyl alcohol; large amounts of benzyl alcohol (≥99 mg/kg/day) have been associated with a potentially fatal toxicity ("gasping syndrome") in neonates; the "gasping syndrome" consists of metabolic acidosis, respiratory distress, gasping respirations, CNS dysfunction (including convulsions, intracranial hemorrhage), hypotension, and cardiovascular collapse (AAP ["Inactive" 1997]; CDC 1982); some data suggests that benzoate displaces bilirubin from protein binding sites (Ahlfors 2001); avoid or use dosage forms containing benzyl alcohol derivative with caution in neonates. See manufacturer's labeling.

Warnings: Additional Pediatric Considerations Due to decreased elimination rate, neonates and young infants may be at higher risk for adverse effects, especially respiratory depression; use with extreme caution and in reduced doses in this age group.

Drug Interactions

Metabolism/Transport Effects None known.

Avoid Concomitant Use

Avoid concomitant use of Meperidine with any of the following: Azelastine (Nasal); Bromperidol; Dapoxetine; Eluxadoline; Monoamine Oxidase Inhibitors (Antidepressant); Monoamine Oxidase Inhibitors (Type B); Opioids (Mixed Agonist / Antagonist); Orphenadrine; Oxomemazine; Paraldehyde; Thalidomide

Increased Effect/Toxicity

Meperidine may increase the levels/effects of: Alvimopan; Amifampridine; Azelastine (Nasal); Blonanserin; Desmopressin; Diuretics; Eluxadoline; FentaNYL; Flunitrazepam; Iohexol; Iomeprol; Iopamidol; Methotrimeprazine; MetyroSINE; Monoamine Oxidase Inhibitors (Antidepressant); Monoamine Oxidase Inhibitors (Type B); Opioid Agonists; Orphenadrine; Oxitriptan; OxyCODONE; Paraldehyde; Piribedil; Pramipexole; Ramosetron; ROPINIRole; Rotigotine; Selective Serotonin Reuptake Inhibitors; Serotonergic Agents (High Risk, Miscellaneous); Serotonin/Norepinephrine Reuptake Inhibitors; Suvorexant; Thalidomide; TraMADol; Tricyclic Antidepressants; Zolpidem

The levels/effects of Meperidine may be increased by: Alizapride; Almotriptan; Alosetron; Amphetamines; Anticholinergic Agents; Antiemetics (5HT3 Antagonists); Brimonidine (Topical); Bromopride; Bromperidol; BuPROPion; BusPIRone; Cannabidiol; Cannabis; Chlormethiazole; Chlorphenesin Carbamate; Cimetidine; CNS Depressants; CYP3A4 Inhibitors (Moderate); CYP3A4 Inhibitors (Strong); Dapoxetine; Dexmethylphenidate-Methylphenidate; Dextromethorphan; Dimethindene (Topical); Dronabinol; Droperidol; Eletriptan; Ergot Derivatives; HydrOXYzine; Kava Kava; Lemborexant; Linezolid; Lisuride; Lofexidine; Lorcaserin (Withdrawn From US Market); Magnesium Sulfate; Methotrimeprazine; Methylene Blue; Metoclopramide; Minocycline (Systemic); Nabilone; Nefazodone; Ondansetron; Oxomemazine; Ozanimod; Perampanel; Ramosetron; Rufinamide; Serotonergic Non-Opioid CNS Depressants; Serotonin 5-HT1D Receptor Agonists (Triptans); Sodium Oxybate; St John's Wort; Succinylcholine; Syrian Rue; Tetrahydrocannabinol; Tetrahydrocannabinol and Cannabidiol; Tricyclic Antidepressants

Decreased Effect

Meperidine may decrease the levels/effects of: Diuretics; Gastrointestinal Agents (Prokinetic); Pegvisomant; Sincalide

The levels/effects of Meperidine may be decreased by: CYP3A4 Inducers (Moderate); CYP3A4 Inducers (Strong); Fosphenytoin; Nalmefene; Naltrexone; Opioids (Mixed Agonist / Antagonist); Phenytoin; St John's Wort

Pharmacodynamics/Kinetics

Onset of Action Analgesic: Oral, IM, SubQ: 10 to 15 minutes; IV: ~5 minutes. Peak effect: IV: 5 to 7 minutes; IM, SubQ.: ~1 hour; Oral: 2 hours

Duration of Action Oral, IM, SubQ.: 2 to 4 hours; IV: 2 to 3 hours

Half-life Elimination

Parent drug: Terminal phase:

Preterm infants 3.6 to 65 days of age: 11.9 hours (range: 3.3 to 59.4 hours)

Term infants: 0.3 to 4 days of age: 10.7 hours (range: 4.9 to 16.8 hours); 26 to 73 days of age: 8.2 hours (range: 5.7 to 31.7 hours)

Neonates: 23 hours (range: 12 to 39 hours)

Infants 3 to 18 months: 2.3 hours

Children 5 to 8 years: 3 hours

Adults: 2.5 to 4 hours, Liver disease: 7 to 11 hours

Normeperidine (active metabolite): Neonates: 30 to 85 hours; Adults: 8 to 16 hours; normeperidine half-life is dependent on renal function and can accumulate with high doses or in patients with decreased renal function; normeperidine may precipitate tremors or seizures

Reproductive Considerations

Long-term opioid use may cause secondary hypogonadism, which may lead to sexual dysfunction or infertility in men and women (Brennan 2013).

Pregnancy Considerations Opioids cross the placenta.

According to some studies, maternal use of opioids may be associated with birth defects (including neural tube defects, congenital heart defects, and gastroschisis), poor fetal growth, stillbirth, and preterm delivery (CDC [Dowell 2016]).

[US Boxed Warning]: Prolonged use of meperidine during pregnancy can result in neonatal opioid withdrawal syndrome, which may be life-threatening if not recognized and treated, and requires management according to protocols developed by neonatology experts. If opioid use is required for a prolonged period in a pregnant woman, advise the patient of the risk of neonatal opioid withdrawal syndrome and ensure that appropriate treatment will be available. If chronic opioid exposure occurs in pregnancy, adverse events in the newborn (including withdrawal) may occur (Chou 2009). Symptoms of neonatal abstinence syndrome (NAS) following opioid exposure may be autonomic (eg, fever, temperature instability), gastrointestinal (eg, diarrhea, vomiting, poor feeding/weight gain), or neurologic (eg, high-pitched crying, hyperactivity, increased muscle tone, increased wakefulness/abnormal sleep pattern, irritability, sneezing, seizure, tremor, yawning) (Dow 2012; Hudak 2012). Mothers who are physically dependent on opioids may give birth to infants who are also physically dependent. Opioids may cause respiratory depression and psychophysiologic effects in the neonate; newborns of mothers receiving opioids during labor should be monitored.

Although approved for use in obstetrical analgesia, meperidine is not recommended for peripartum analgesia due to the prolonged half-life of the active metabolite in the mother and neonate (ACOG 209 2019), and it is not recommended to treat chronic noncancer pain in pregnant women or those who may become pregnant (CDC [Dowell 2016]; Chou 2009).

Breastfeeding Considerations Meperidine is present in breast milk.

Breast milk exposure to meperidine and normeperidine is consistently associated with neonatal sedation and may interfere with breastfeeding. Nonopioid analgesics are preferred for breastfeeding females who require pain control peripartum or for surgery outside of the postpartum period; meperidine is not recommended if an opioid is needed. Although a single dose is likely to be acceptable, close monitoring of the infant is required following multiple doses (ABM [Martin 2018]; ABM [Reece-Stremtan 2017]; Sachs 2013).

When opioids are needed in breastfeeding women, the lowest effective dose for the shortest duration of time should be used to limit adverse events in the mother and breastfeeding infant (ABM [Martin 2018]; ABM [Reece-Stremtan 2017]). Breastfeeding women using opioids for postpartum pain should monitor their infants for drowsiness, sedation, feeding difficulties, or limpness (ACOG 209 2019). Withdrawal symptoms may occur when maternal use is discontinued or breastfeeding is stopped. According to the manufacturer, the decision to breastfeed during therapy should consider the risk of infant exposure, the benefits of breastfeeding to the infant, and benefits of treatment to the mother.

Controlled Substance C-II

Dosage Forms: US

Solution, Injection:

Demerol: 50 mg/mL (30 mL); 100 mg/mL (20 mL)

Solution, Injection [preservative free]:

Demerol: 25 mg/mL (1 mL); 50 mg/mL (1 mL); 100 mg/2 mL (2 mL); 75 mg/mL (1 mL); 100 mg/mL (1 mL)

Generic: 25 mg/mL (1 mL); 50 mg/mL (1 mL); 100 mg/mL (1 mL)

Solution, Oral:

Generic: 50 mg/5 mL (500 mL)

Tablet, Oral:

Generic: 50 mg, 100 mg

Dosage Forms: Canada

Solution, Injection:

Generic: 50 mg/mL (1 mL); 75 mg/mL (1 mL); 100 mg/mL (1 mL)

Dental Health Professional Considerations

Meperidine is not to be used as the opioid drug of first choice. It is recommended only to be used in codeine-allergic patients when an opioid analgesic is indicated. Meperidine is not an anti-inflammatory agent. Meperidine, as with other opioid analgesics, is recommended only for limited acute dosing (ie, 3 days or less); common adverse effects in the dental patient are nausea, sedation, and constipation. Meperidine has a significant addiction liability, especially when given long-term.

Meperidine and Promethazine

(me PER i deen & proe METH a zeen)

Generic Availability (US) Yes

Pharmacologic Category Analgesic Combination (Opioid)

Use Pain: Possibly effective as analgesia for moderate to moderately severe pain.

Local Anesthetic/Vasoconstrictor Precautions No information available to require special precautions

Effects on Dental Treatment Key adverse event(s) related to dental treatment: Xerostomia (normal salivary flow resumes upon discontinuation).

Effects on Bleeding No information available to require special precautions

Adverse Reactions See individual agents.

Dosing

Adult Pain: Oral: One meperidine 50 mg/promethazine 25 mg capsule every 4 to 6 hours as needed.

Geriatric Avoid use (Beers Criteria [AGS 2019]).

Renal Impairment: Adult There are no dosage adjustments provided in the manufacturer's labeling. Use of meperidine should be avoided in renal impairment (ISMP, 2007).

Hepatic Impairment: Adult There are no dosage adjustments provided in the manufacturer's labeling; use with caution.

Mechanism of Action Meperidine is a opioid analgesic; promethazine is a phenothiazine derivative with sedative and anti-emetic activity. Also see individual agents.

Contraindications

Hypersensitivity to meperidine or promethazine or any component of the formulation; use with or within 14 days of MAO inhibitors; in comatose states; children <2 years of age.

Documentation of allergenic cross-reactivity for opioid analgesics is limited. However, because of similarities in chemical structure and/or pharmacologic actions, the possibility of cross-sensitivity cannot be ruled out with certainty.

Warnings/Precautions See individual agents.

Drug Interactions

Metabolism/Transport Effects Refer to individual components.

Avoid Concomitant Use

Avoid concomitant use of Meperidine and Promethazine with any of the following: Aclidinium; Aminolevulinic Acid (Systemic); Azelastine (Nasal); Bromopride; Bromperidol; Cimetropium; Dapoxetine; Eluxadoline; Glycopyrrolate (Oral Inhalation); Glycopyrronium (Topical); Ipratropium (Oral Inhalation); Levosulpiride; Metoclopramide; Monoamine Oxidase Inhibitors (Antidepressant); Monoamine Oxidase Inhibitors (Type B); Opioids (Mixed Agonist / Antagonist); Orphenadrine; Oxatomide; Oxomemazine; Paraldehyde; Potassium Chloride; Potassium Citrate; Pramlintide; Revefenacin; Thalidomide; Tiotropium; Umeclidinium

Increased Effect/Toxicity

Meperidine and Promethazine may increase the levels/effects of: Alvimopan; Amifampridine; Aminolevulinic Acid (Systemic); Aminolevulinic Acid (Topical); Anticholinergic Agents; Azelastine (Nasal); Blonanserin; Cimetropium; CloZAPine; Desmopressin; Diuretics; Eluxadoline; FentaNYL; Flunitrazepam; Glucagon; Glycopyrrolate (Oral Inhalation); Iohexol; Iomeprol; Iopamidol; Methotrimeprazine; Mirabegron; Monoamine Oxidase Inhibitors (Antidepressant); Monoamine Oxidase Inhibitors (Type B); Opioid Agonists; Orphenadrine; Oxitriptan; OxyCODONE; Paraldehyde; Piribedil; Porfimer; Potassium Chloride; Potassium Citrate; Pramipexole; Ramosetron; Revefenacin; ROPINIRole; Rotigotine; Selective Serotonin Reuptake Inhibitors; Serotonergic Agents (High Risk, Miscellaneous); Serotonin/Norepinephrine Reuptake

Inhibitors; Suvorexant; Thalidomide; Thiazide and Thiazide-Like Diuretics; Tiotropium; TraMADol; Tricyclic Antidepressants; Verteporfin; Zolpidem

The levels/effects of Meperidine and Promethazine may be increased by: Aclidinium; Alizapride; Almotriptan; Alosetron; Amantadine; Amphetamines; Anticholinergic Agents; Antiemetics (5HT3 Antagonists); Botulinum Toxin-Containing Products; Brimonidine (Topical); Bromopride; Bromperidol; BuPROPion; BusPIRone; Cannabidiol; Cannabis; Chlormethiazole; Chlorphenesin Carbamate; Cimetidine; CNS Depressants; CYP3A4 Inhibitors (Moderate); CYP3A4 Inhibitors (Strong); Dapoxetine; Dexmethylphenidate-Methylphenidate; Dextromethorphan; Dimethindene (Topical); Dronabinol; Droperidol; Eletriptan; Ergot Derivatives; Glycopyrronium (Topical); HydrOXYzine; Ipratropium (Oral Inhalation); Kava Kava; Lemborexant; Linezolid; Lisuride; Lofexidine; Lorcaserin (Withdrawn From US Market); Magnesium Sulfate; Methotrimeprazine; Methylene Blue; Metoclopramide; MetyroSINE; Minocycline (Systemic); Nabilone; Nefazodone; Ondansetron; Oxatomide; Oxomemazine; Ozanimod; Perampanel; Pramlintide; Ramosetron; Rufinamide; Serotonergic Non-Opioid CNS Depressants; Serotonin 5-HT1D Receptor Agonists (Triptans); Sodium Oxybate; St John's Wort; Succinylcholine; Syrian Rue; Tetrahydrocannabinol; Tetrahydrocannabinol and Cannabidiol; Tricyclic Antidepressants; Umeclidinium

Decreased Effect

Meperidine and Promethazine may decrease the levels/effects of: Acetylcholinesterase Inhibitors; Diuretics; EPINEPHrine (Nasal); EPINEPHrine (Oral Inhalation); Epinephrine (Racemic); EPINEPHrine (Systemic); Gastrointestinal Agents (Prokinetic); Itopride; Levosulpiride; Nitroglycerin; Pegvisomant; Secretin; Sincalide

The levels/effects of Meperidine and Promethazine may be decreased by: Acetylcholinesterase Inhibitors; CYP3A4 Inducers (Moderate); CYP3A4 Inducers (Strong); Fosphenytoin; Nalmefene; Naltrexone; Opioids (Mixed Agonist / Antagonist); Phenytoin; St John's Wort

Food Interactions

Ethanol: Avoid ethanol (may increase CNS depression).

Herb/Nutraceutical: Avoid valerian, St John's wort, kava kava, gotu kola (may increase CNS depression).

Pregnancy Considerations

[US Boxed Warnings]: Prolonged use of meperidine during pregnancy can result in neonatal opioid withdrawal syndrome, which may be life-threatening if not recognized and treated. If prolonged opioid use is required in a pregnant woman, advise the patient of the risk of neonatal opioid withdrawal syndrome and ensure that appropriate treatment will be available. Refer to individual monographs for additional information.

Breastfeeding Considerations

Meperidine is excreted into breastmilk (Spigset 2000); excretion of promethazine is not known. Due to the potential for serious adverse reactions in the nursing infant, the manufacturer recommends a decision be made whether to discontinue nursing or to discontinue the drug, taking into account the importance of treatment to the mother. Refer to individual monographs.

Controlled Substance C-II

◆ **Meperidine Hydrochloride** *see* Meperidine *on page 966*

◆ **Meperidine Hydrochloride and Promethazine Hydrochloride** *see* Meperidine and Promethazine *on page 971*

◆ **Mephyton** *see* Phytonadione *on page 1230*

Mepivacaine (me PIV a kane)

Related Information

Oral Pain *on page 1734*

Brand Names: US Carbocaine; Carbocaine Preservative-Free; Polocaine; Polocaine Dental; Polocaine-MPF; Scandonest 3% Plain

Brand Names: Canada Carbocaine; Polocaine

Generic Availability (US) Yes

Pharmacologic Category Local Anesthetic

Dental Use Amide-type anesthetic used for local infiltration anesthesia; injection near nerve trunks to produce nerve block

Use

Dental anesthesia: Production of local anesthesia for dental procedures by infiltration or nerve block in adult and pediatric patients.

Local or regional anesthesia (eg, epidural, caudal, or peripheral nerve blocks): Production of local or regional analgesia and anesthesia by local infiltration, peripheral and central neural techniques (epidural and caudal). **Not** for use in spinal anesthesia.

Local Anesthetic/Vasoconstrictor Precautions

No information available to require special precautions

Effects on Dental Treatment Key adverse event(s) related to dental treatment: Degree of adverse effects in the CNS and cardiovascular system is directly related to blood levels of mepivacaine (frequency not defined; more likely to occur after systemic administration rather than infiltration): Bradycardia, cardiovascular collapse, hypotension, myocardial depression, ventricular arrhythmias, nausea, vomiting, respiratory arrest, anaphylactoid reactions, blurred vision, heart block, transient stinging or burning at injection site

High blood levels: Anxiety, restlessness, disorientation, confusion, dizziness, and seizures, followed by CNS depression resulting in somnolence, unconsciousness, and possible respiratory arrest.

In some cases, symptoms of CNS stimulation may be absent and the primary CNS effects are somnolence and unconsciousness.

It is common to misinterpret psychogenic responses to local anesthetic injection as an allergic reaction. Intraoral injections are perceived by many patients as a stressful procedure in dentistry. Common symptoms to this stress are diaphoresis, palpitations, hyperventilation, generalized pallor, and a fainting feeling.

Effects on Bleeding No information available to require special precautions

Adverse Reactions Frequency not defined. Degree of adverse effects in the CNS and cardiovascular system is directly related to the blood levels of mepivacaine, route of administration, and physical status of the patient. The effects below are more likely to occur after systemic administration rather than infiltration.

Cardiovascular: Bradycardia, cardiac insufficiency, cardiovascular depression, cardiovascular stimulation, heart block, hypertension, hypotension, low cardiac output, syncope, tachycardia, ventricular arrhythmia

Central nervous system: Anxiety, chills, confusion, convulsions, dizziness, drowsiness, excitement, loss of consciousness, increased body temperature, nervousness, paralysis, persistent anesthesia, restlessness
Dermatologic: Diaphoresis, erythema, pruritus, urticaria
Gastrointestinal: Fecal incontinence, nausea, oral paresthesia (persistent; involving lips, tongue, and oral tissues), vomiting
Genitourinary: Urinary incontinence, urinary retention
Hematologic & oncologic: Methemoglobinemia
Hypersensitivity: Anaphylactoid reaction, angioedema, hypersensitivity reaction
Neuromuscular & skeletal: Chondrolysis (continuous intra-articular administration), tremor, weakness
Ophthalmic: Blurred vision, miosis
Otic: Tinnitus
Respiratory: Apnea, respiratory depression, sneezing

Dental Usual Dosage

Injectable local anesthetic: Dose varies with procedure, degree of anesthesia needed, vascularity of tissue, duration of anesthesia required, and physical condition of patient. The smallest dose and concentration required to produce the desired effect should be used.

Children: Injection: According to the manufacturer, a mepivacaine dose up to 6.6 mg/kg or 400 mg (whichever is less) may be administered during any single dental sitting. For most procedures, doses >180 mg are unnecessary. The American Academy of Pediatric Dentistry (AAPD) recommends a maximum mepivacaine dose of 4.4 mg/kg or a maximum total dose of 300 mg in any single dental sitting (AAPD 2015).

Adults: Maximum single or total dose given for one procedure: 400 mg; 500 mg if epinephrine has been added (Barash, 2009)

Cervical, brachial, intercostal, pudendal nerve block: 5-40 mL of a 1% solution (maximum: 400 mg) **or** 5-20 mL of a 2% solution (maximum: 400 mg). For pudendal block, inject one-half the total dose each side.

Transvaginal block (paracervical plus pudendal): Up to 30 mL (total for both sides) of a 1% solution (maximum: 300 mg). Inject one-half the total dose each side.

Paracervical block: Up to 20 mL (total for both sides) of a 1% solution (maximum: 200 mg). Inject one-half the total dose to each side. This is the maximum recommended dose per 90-minute procedure; inject slowly with 5 minutes between sides.

Caudal and epidural block (preservative free solutions only): 15-30 mL of a 1% solution (maximum: 300 mg) **or** 10-25 mL of a 1.5% solution (maximum: 375 mg) **or** 10-20 mL of a 2% solution (maximum: 400 mg)

Infiltration: Up to 40 mL of a 1% solution (maximum: 400 mg); up to 50 mL if epinephrine has been added (maximum: 500 mg) (Barash, 2009); an equivalent amount of a 0.5% solution (prepared by diluting the 1% solution with NS) may be used for large areas

Peripheral nerve block to provide a surgical level of anesthesia (Miller, 2010):

Major nerve block (blockade of two or more distinct nerves, a nerve plexus, or very large nerves at more proximal sites: 30-50 mL of a 1% or 1.5% solution (maximum: 500 mg)

Minor nerve block (blockade of a single nerve [eg, ulnar or radial]): 5-20 mL of a 1% solution (maximum: 200 mg)

Therapeutic block: 1-5 mL of 1% solution (maximum: 50 mg) **or** 1-5 mL of 2% solution (maximum: 100 mg)

Elderly: Decreased doses suggested by manufacturer's labeling; however, no dosing adjustments provided. Refer to adult dosing.

Dosage adjustment in renal impairment: No dosage adjustment provided in manufacturer's labeling; use with caution.

Dosage adjustment in hepatic impairment: No dosage adjustment provided in manufacturer's labeling; use with caution.

Dosing

Adult Note: Dose varies with procedure, degree of anesthesia needed, vascularity of tissue, duration of anesthesia required, and physical condition of patient. The smallest dose and concentration required to produce the desired effect should be used.

Local or regional anesthesia (eg, epidural, caudal, or peripheral nerve blocks):

Maximum single or total dose given for one procedure: 400 mg; 500 mg if epinephrine has been added (Barash 2009)

Maximum dose per 24 hours: 1,000 mg

Cervical, brachial, intercostal, pudendal nerve block: 5 to 40 mL of a 1% solution (maximum: 400 mg) **or** 5 to 20 mL of a 2% solution (maximum: 400 mg). For pudendal block, inject one-half the total dose each side.

Transvaginal block (paracervical plus pudendal): Up to 30 mL (total for both sides) of a 1% solution (maximum: 300 mg). Inject one-half the total dose each side.

Paracervical block: Up to 20 mL (total for both sides) of a 1% solution (maximum: 200 mg). Inject one-half the total dose to each side. This is the maximum recommended dose per 90-minute procedure; inject slowly with 5 minutes between sides.

Caudal and epidural block (preservative free solutions only): 15 to 30 mL of a 1% solution (maximum: 300 mg) **or** 10 to 25 mL of a 1.5% solution (maximum: 375 mg) **or** 10 to 20 mL of a 2% solution (maximum: 400 mg).

Infiltration: Up to 40 mL of a 1% solution (maximum: 400 mg); up to 50 mL if epinephrine has been added (maximum: 500 mg) (Barash 2009); an equivalent amount of a 0.5% solution (prepared by diluting the 1% solution with NS) may be used for large areas.

Peripheral nerve block to provide a surgical level of anesthesia (Miller 2010):

Major nerve block (blockade of two or more distinct nerves, a nerve plexus, or very large nerves at more proximal sites: 30 to 50 mL of a 1% or 1.5% solution (maximum: 500 mg)

Minor nerve block (blockade of a single nerve [eg, ulnar or radial]): 5 to 20 mL of a 1% solution (maximum: 200 mg)

Therapeutic block: 1 to 5 mL of 1% solution (maximum: 50 mg) **or** 1 to 5 mL of 2% solution (maximum: 100 mg)

Dental anesthesia:

Single site in upper or lower jaw: 51 mg as a 3% solution.

Infiltration and nerve block of entire oral cavity: 270 mg as a 3% solution, up to 6.6 mg/kg not to exceed 300 mg per appointment. Manufacturer's maximum recommended total dose: 400 mg.

The following number of dental cartridges (1.7 mL) provide the indicated amounts of mepivacaine dental anesthetic 3%. See table.

# of Cartridges (1.7 mL)	Mepivacaine mg (3%)
1	51
2	102
3	153
4	204
5	255
6	306
7	357
8	408

Geriatric Refer to adult dosing; reduce dose consistent with age and physical status.

Renal Impairment: Adult There are no dosage adjustments provided in the manufacturer's labeling; use with caution.

Hepatic Impairment: Adult There are no dosage adjustments provided in the manufacturer's labeling; use with caution. Patients with severe hepatic disease, because of their inability to metabolize local anesthetics normally, are at a greater risk of developing toxic plasma concentrations.

Pediatric Note: Dose varies with procedure, degree of anesthesia needed, vascularity of tissue, duration of anesthesia required, and physical condition of patient. The smallest dose and concentration required to produce the desired effect should be used. Consider incremental administration with negative aspiration prior to each injection; however, absence of blood in the syringe does not guarantee that intravascular injection has been avoided (Mulroy 2010). Should only be administered under the supervision of a qualified physician experienced in the use of anesthetics.

Dental anesthesia: Children and Adolescents: 3% solution: Injection:

Manufacturer's labeling: Maximum dose: 5 to 6 mg/kg; maximum total dose: 270 mg. In adults, the dose for single site in upper or lower jaw is 51 mg (one 1.7 mL cartridge)

Alternate dosing: American Academy Pediatric Dentistry (AAPD 2015): Maximum dose: 4.4 mg/kg; maximum total dose: 300 mg in any single dental sitting

Local or regional anesthesia (eg, epidural, caudal, or peripheral nerve blocks): Maximum single or total dose given for one procedure: 5 to 6 mg/kg (maximum adult dose per manufacturer: 400 mg); only concentrations <2% should be used in patients <3 years or <14 kg to ensure adequate drug volume for area and to decrease the potential for local anesthetic systemic toxicity

Renal Impairment: Pediatric There are no dosage adjustments provided in the manufacturer's labeling; use with caution.

Hepatic Impairment: Pediatric There are no dosage adjustments provided in the manufacturer's labeling; use with caution. Patients with severe hepatic disease, because of their inability to metabolize local anesthetics normally, are at a greater risk of developing toxic plasma concentrations.

Mechanism of Action Mepivacaine is an amide local anesthetic similar to lidocaine. Local anesthetics bind selectively to the intracellular surface of sodium channels to block influx of sodium into the axon. As a result, depolarization necessary for action potential propagation and subsequent nerve function is prevented. The block at the sodium channel is reversible. When drug diffuses away from the axon, sodium channel function is restored and nerve propagation returns.

Contraindications Hypersensitivity to mepivacaine, other amide-type local anesthetics, or any component of the formulation

Warnings/Precautions Careful and constant monitoring of the patient's state of consciousness should be done following each local anesthetic injection; at such times, restlessness, anxiety, tinnitus, dizziness, blurred vision, tremors, depression, or drowsiness may be early warning signs of CNS toxicity; treatment is primarily symptomatic and supportive. Continuous intra-articular Infusion of local anesthetics after arthroscopic or other surgical procedures is **not** an approved use; chondrolysis (primarily in the shoulder joint) has occurred following infusion, with some cases requiring arthroplasty or shoulder replacement. Mepivacaine may potentially trigger malignant hyperthermia; follow standard protocol for identification and treatment. Methemoglobinemia has been reported with local anesthetics; clinically significant methemoglobinemia requires immediate treatment along with discontinuation of the anesthetic and other oxidizing agents. Onset may be immediate or delayed (hours) after anesthetic exposure. Patients with glucose-6-phosphate dehydrogenase deficiency, congenital or idiopathic methemoglobinemia, cardiac or pulmonary compromise, exposure to oxidizing agents or their metabolites, or infants <6 months of age are more susceptible and should be closely monitored for signs and symptoms of methemoglobinemia (eg, cyanosis, headache, rapid pulse, shortness of breath, lightheadedness, fatigue). Use with caution in patients with cardiac disease, including rhythm disturbances, shock, heart block, and hypotension. Use with caution in patients with hepatic or renal disease; patients with severe hepatic disease, because of their inability to metabolize local anesthetics normally, are at a greater risk of developing, toxic plasma concentrations. Local anesthetics have been associated with rare occurrences of sudden respiratory arrest; convulsions due to systemic toxicity leading to cardiac arrest have been reported presumably due to intravascular injection. Intravascular injections should be avoided; aspiration should be performed prior to administration; the needle must be repositioned until no return of blood can be elicited by aspiration; however, absence of blood in the syringe does not guarantee that intravascular injection has been avoided. Use with caution when there is inflammation and/or sepsis in the region of the proposed injection. To avoid serious adverse effects and high plasma levels, the lowest dosage resulting in effective anesthesia should be administered. Repeated doses may cause significant increases in blood levels with each repeated dose due to the possibility of accumulation of the drug or its metabolites. Tolerance to elevated blood levels varies with patient status. A test dose is recommended prior to epidural administration and all reinforcing doses with continuous catheter technique. Do not use solutions containing preservatives for caudal or epidural block. Use caution in debilitated, elderly, children, or acutely-ill patients; reduce dose consistent with age and physical status. Resuscitative equipment, oxygen, and other resuscitative drugs should be available for immediate use. Potentially significant drug-drug interactions may exist, requiring dose or frequency adjustment, additional monitoring, and/or selection of alternative therapy.

Drug Interactions

Metabolism/Transport Effects None known.

Avoid Concomitant Use

Avoid concomitant use of Mepivacaine with any of the following: Bupivacaine (Liposomal)

Increased Effect/Toxicity

Mepivacaine may increase the levels/effects of: Bupivacaine (Liposomal); Neuromuscular-Blocking Agents

The levels/effects of Mepivacaine may be increased by: Beta-Blockers; Hyaluronidase; Methemoglobinemia Associated Agents

Decreased Effect

Mepivacaine may decrease the levels/effects of: Technetium Tc 99m Tilmanocept

Pharmacodynamics/Kinetics

Onset of Action Route and dose dependent: Range: 3 to 20 minutes; Dental: Upper jaw: 30 to 120 seconds; Lower jaw: 1 to 4 minutes

Duration of Action Route and dose dependent: 2 to 2.5 hours; Dental: Upper jaw: 20 minutes; Lower jaw: 40 minutes

Half-life Elimination Neonates: 8.7 to 9 hours; Adults: 1.9 to 3.2 hours

Pregnancy Considerations Animal reproduction studies have not been conducted. Mepivacaine has been used in obstetrical analgesia.

Breastfeeding Considerations It is not known if mepivacaine is present in breast milk. The manufacturer recommends that caution be exercised when administering mepivacaine to breastfeeding women. Usual infiltration doses of mepivacaine dental anesthetic given to breastfeeding mothers has not been shown to affect the health of the breastfeeding infant.

Dosage Forms: US

Solution, Injection:

Carbocaine: 1% (50 mL); 2% (50 mL)

Polocaine: 1% (50 mL); 2% (50 mL)

Solution, Injection [preservative free]:

Carbocaine Preservative-Free: 1% (30 mL); 1.5% (30 mL); 2% (20 mL)

Polocaine-MPF: 1% (30 mL); 1.5% (30 mL); 2% (20 mL)

Solution, Injection [dental use]:

Carbocaine: 3% (1.7 mL)

Polocaine Dental: 3% (1.7 mL)

Scandonest 3% Plain: 3% (1.7 mL)

Dental Health Professional Considerations Oral paresthesia: The occurrence of oral paresthesia associated with 4% solutions of prilocaine or articaine, although rare, continue to be slightly more frequent than other local anesthetics. From 1999 to 2008, there were 182 cases of nonsurgical paresthesia (Gaffen 2009). Of the cases, 172 involved mandibular block injection only.

A 2010 report, reviewed adverse events submitted voluntarily over a 10-year period involving the dental local anesthetics articaine, bupivacaine, lidocaine, mepivacaine, and prilocaine in the United States. Mepivacaine reported incidence: One case per 623,112,900 cartridges sold. The reported incidence of paresthesia was one case for 13,800,970 cartridges of all local anesthetics sold in the US (Garisto 2010).

Mepivacaine and Levonordefrin

(me PIV a kane & lee voe nor DEF rin)

Related Information

Mepivacaine *on page 972*

Oral Pain *on page 1734*

Brand Names: US Carbocaine 2% with Neo-Cobefrin; Polocaine Dental; Scandonest 2% L

Brand Names: Canada Carbocaine 2% with Neo-Cobefrin; Scandonest 2% with Levonordefrin

Generic Availability (US) No

Pharmacologic Category Local Anesthetic

Dental Use Amide-type anesthetic used for local infiltration anesthesia; injection near nerve trunks to produce nerve block

Use Dental anesthesia: Production of local anesthesia for dental procedures by infiltration or nerve block in adult and pediatric patients

Local Anesthetic/Vasoconstrictor Precautions No information available to require special precautions

Effects on Dental Treatment It is common to misinterpret psychogenic responses to local anesthetic injection as an allergic reaction. Intraoral injections are perceived by many patients as a stressful procedure in dentistry. Common symptoms to this stress are diaphoresis, palpitations, hyperventilation, generalized pallor and a fainting feeling. Patients may exhibit hypersensitivity to bisulfites contained in local anesthetic solution to prevent oxidation of levonordefrin. In general, patients reacting to bisulfites have a history of asthma and their airways are hyper-reactive to asthmatic syndrome.

Degree of adverse effects in the CNS and cardiovascular system is directly related to the blood levels of mepivacaine (frequency not defined; more likely to occur after systemic administration rather than infiltration): Bradycardia and reduction in cardiac output, nausea, vomiting, tremors, hypersensitivity reactions (extremely rare; may be manifest as dermatologic reactions and edema at injection site), asthmatic syndromes

High blood levels: Anxiety, restlessness, disorientation, confusion, dizziness, and seizures, followed by CNS depression resulting in somnolence, unconsciousness and possible respiratory arrest.

In some cases, symptoms of CNS stimulation may be absent and the primary CNS effects are somnolence and unconsciousness.

See Dental Health Professional Considerations.

Effects on Bleeding No information available to require special precautions

Adverse Reactions Degree of adverse effects in the CNS and cardiovascular system is directly related to the blood levels of mepivacaine. The effects below are more likely to occur after systemic administration rather than infiltration. Also see mepivacaine.

Frequency not defined:

Central nervous system: Disorientation, dizziness, drowsiness, excitement, loss of consciousness, nervousness, seizure

Hypersensitivity: Hypersensitivity reaction

Neuromuscular & skeletal: Tremor

Ophthalmic: Blurred vision

<1%, postmarketing, and/or case reports: Nonimmune anaphylaxis

Dental Usual Dosage Note: Dosage varies with the anesthetic procedure, degree of anesthesia needed, vascularity of tissue, duration of anesthesia required, and physical condition of patient. Always use the lowest effective dose along with careful aspiration.

Children: Calculate the weight-specific maximum mepivacaine dose; regardless of the patient's weight, the maximum pediatric **mepivacaine** dose is 5 to 6 mg/kg or 180 mg (whichever is less) during any single dental sitting (manufacturer labeling). Pediatric Weight-Specific Maximum Mepivacaine Dose (mg) = [Weight (lbs)/150] x 180 (manufacturer labeling). The American Academy of Pediatric Dentistry (AAPD) recommends a maximum dose of 4.4 mg/kg or a maximum total dose of 300 mg in any single dental sitting (AAPD, 2009).

Adults: Injection: Usual dose: Mepivacaine 34 mg (1.7 mL) per site or mepivacaine 180 mg (9 mL) for entire oral cavity; maximum cumulative **mepivacaine** dose: 6.6 mg/kg or 400 mg (whichever is less) during any single dental sitting

The following numbers of dental carpules (1.7 mL) provide the indicated amounts of mepivacaine hydrochloride 2% and levonordefrin 1:20,000. See table.

# of Cartridges (1.7 mL)	Mepivacaine (mg) (2%)	Vasoconstrictor (mg) (Levonordefrin 1:20,000)
1	34	0.085
2	68	0.170
3	102	0.255
4	136	0.340
5	170	0.425
6	204	0.510
7	238	0.595
8	272	0.680
9	306	0.765
10	340	0.850

Dosing

Adult Note: Dosage varies with the anesthetic procedure, degree of anesthesia needed, vascularity of tissue, duration of anesthesia required, and physical condition of patient. Always use the lowest effective dose along with careful aspiration.

Dental anesthesia, infiltration, or conduction block: Usual dose: Mepivacaine 34 mg (1.7 mL) per site or mepivacaine 180 mg (9 mL) for entire oral cavity; maximum cumulative **mepivacaine** dose: 6.6 mg/kg or 400 mg (whichever is less) during any single dental sitting

Geriatric Refer to adult dosing; reduce dose consistent with age and physical status.

Renal Impairment: Adult There are no dosage adjustments provided in the manufacturer's labeling; use with caution.

Hepatic Impairment: Adult There are no dosage adjustments provided in the manufacturer's labeling; use with caution. Patients with severe hepatic disease, because of their inability to metabolize local anesthetics normally, are at a greater risk of developing toxic plasma concentrations.

Pediatric Note: Dosage varies with the anesthetic procedure, degree of anesthesia needed, vascularity of tissue, duration of anesthesia required, and physical condition of patient. Always use the lowest effective dose along with careful aspiration.

Dental anesthesia, infiltration, or conduction block: Children and Adolescents: Maximum dosage must be carefully calculated on the basis of patient's weight. Manufacturer recommends a maximum mepivacaine dose of 6.6 mg/kg, but must not exceed 180 mg as a 2% solution. The American Academy of Pediatric Dentistry (AAPD) recommends a maximum mepivacaine dose of 4.4 mg/kg or a maximum total dose of 300 mg in any single dental sitting (AAPD 2015).

Renal Impairment: Pediatric There are no dosage adjustments provided in the manufacturer's labeling; use with caution.

Hepatic Impairment: Pediatric There are no dosage adjustments provided in the manufacturer's labeling; use with caution. Patients with severe hepatic disease, because of their inability to metabolize local anesthetics normally, are at a greater risk of developing toxic plasma concentrations.

Mechanism of Action

Mepivacaine: Local anesthetics bind selectively to the intracellular surface of sodium channels to block influx of sodium into the axon. As a result, depolarization necessary for action potential propagation and subsequent nerve function is prevented. The block at the sodium channel is reversible. When drug diffuses away from the axon, sodium channel function is restored and nerve propagation returns.

Levonordefrin: Prolongs the duration of the anesthetic actions of mepivacaine by causing vasoconstriction (alpha-adrenergic receptor agonist) of the vasculature surrounding the nerve axons. This prevents the diffusion of mepivacaine away from the nerves resulting in a longer retention in the axon.

Contraindications Hypersensitivity to mepivacaine, levonordefrin, local anesthetics of the amide-type, or any component of the formulation

Warnings/Precautions Local anesthetics have been associated with rare occurrences of sudden respiratory arrest. Careful and constant monitoring of the patient's state of consciousness should be done following each local anesthetic injection; at such times, restlessness, anxiety, tinnitus, dizziness, blurred vision, tremors, depression, or drowsiness may be early warning signs of CNS toxicity. Treatment is primarily symptomatic and supportive. Methemoglobinemia has been reported with local anesthetics; clinically significant methemoglobinemia requires immediate treatment along with discontinuation of the anesthetic and other oxidizing agents. Onset may be immediate or delayed (hours) after anesthetic exposure. Patients with glucose-6-phosphate dehydrogenase deficiency, congenital or idiopathic methemoglobinemia, cardiac or pulmonary compromise, exposure to oxidizing agents or their metabolites, or infants <6 months of age are more susceptible and should be closely monitored for signs and symptoms of methemoglobinemia (eg, cyanosis, headache, rapid pulse, shortness of breath, light-headedness, fatigue). Convulsions due to systemic toxicity leading to cardiac arrest have also been reported, presumably following unintentional intravascular injection. Methemoglobinemia has been reported with local anesthetics; clinically significant methemoglobinemia requires immediate treatment.

Use with caution in patients with arteriosclerotic heart disease, cerebral vascular insufficiency, heart block, hypertension, and ischemic heart disease; minimal amounts of vasoconstrictor should be used in this patient population. Use with caution in patients with diabetes, hepatic or renal impairment, and hyperthyroidism. Use with caution in pediatric or elderly patients or in patients who are acutely ill or debilitated; reduce dose consistent with age and physical status. Use caution in patients with asthma; some preparations may contain potassium metabisulfite which may cause severe hypersensitivity reactions (anaphylaxis) in some individuals. Potentially significant interactions may exist, requiring dose or frequency adjustment, additional monitoring, and/or selection of alternative therapy.

Intravascular injections should be avoided; aspiration should be performed prior to administration; the needle must be repositioned until no return of blood can be elicited by aspiration; however, absence of blood in the syringe does not guarantee that intravascular injection has been avoided. Use with caution when there is inflammation and/or sepsis in the region of the proposed injection. To avoid serious adverse effects and high plasma levels, the lowest dosage resulting in effective anesthesia should be administered. Repeated doses may cause significant increases in blood levels with each repeated dose due to the possibility of accumulation of the drug or its metabolites. Tolerance to elevated blood levels varies with patient status. Dental practitioners using local anesthetic agents should be well trained in diagnosis and management of emergencies that may arise from the use of these agents. Resuscitative equipment, oxygen, and other resuscitative drugs should be available for immediate use.

Drug Interactions

Metabolism/Transport Effects None known.

Avoid Concomitant Use

Avoid concomitant use of Mepivacaine and Levonordefrin with any of the following: Bupivacaine (Liposomal); Ergot Derivatives; Monoamine Oxidase Inhibitors

Increased Effect/Toxicity

Mepivacaine and Levonordefrin may increase the levels/effects of: Bupivacaine (Liposomal); Doxofylline; Neuromuscular-Blocking Agents; Solriamfetol; Sympathomimetics

The levels/effects of Mepivacaine and Levonordefrin may be increased by: AtoMOXetine; Beta-Blockers; Cannabinoid-Containing Products; Chloroprocaine; Cocaine (Topical); Ergot Derivatives; Guanethidine; Hyaluronidase; Methemoglobinemia Associated Agents; Monoamine Oxidase Inhibitors; Ozanimod; Procarbazine; Serotonin/Norepinephrine Reuptake Inhibitors; Tedizolid; Tricyclic Antidepressants

Decreased Effect

Mepivacaine and Levonordefrin may decrease the levels/effects of: Benzylpenicilloyl Polylysine; Technetium Tc 99m Tilmanocept

The levels/effects of Mepivacaine and Levonordefrin may be decreased by: Alpha1-Blockers; Spironolactone

Pharmacodynamics/Kinetics

Onset of Action Upper jaw: 30 to 120 seconds; Lower jaw: 1 to 4 minutes

Duration of Action Upper jaw: 1 to 2.5 hours; Lower jaw: 2.5 to 5.5 hours

Pregnancy Risk Factor C

Pregnancy Considerations Animal reproduction studies have not been conducted with this combination.

Breastfeeding Considerations It is not known if mepivacaine or levonordefrin is present in breast milk. The manufacturer recommends that caution be exercised when administering mepivacaine/levonordefrin to breastfeeding women. Usual infiltration doses of mepivacaine with levonordefrin given to breastfeeding mothers has not been shown to affect the health of the breastfed infant.

Dosage Forms: US

Injection, solution [for dental use]:

Carbocaine 2% with Neo-Cobefrin: Mepivacaine 2% and levonordefrin 1:20,000 (1.7 mL)

Scandonest 2% L: Mepivacaine 2% and levonordefrin 1:20,000 (1.7 mL)

Dental Health Professional Considerations Oral paresthesia: The occurrence of oral paresthesia associated with 4% solutions of prilocaine or articaine, although rare, continue to be slightly more frequent than other local anesthetics. From 1999-2008, there were 182 cases of nonsurgical paresthesia (Gaffen, 2009). Of the cases, 172 involved mandibular block injection only. A 2010 report, reviewed adverse events submitted voluntarily over a 10-year period involving the dental local anesthetics articaine, bupivacaine, lidocaine, mepivacaine, and prilocaine in the United States. Mepivacaine reported incidence: One case per 623,112,900 cartridges sold. The reported incidence of paresthesia was one case for 13,800,970 cartridges of all local anesthetics sold in the U.S. (Garisto, 2010). Levonordefrin may interact with medications such as beta-blockers, monoamine oxidase inhibitors, ergot derivatives, and tricyclic antidepressants to enhance vasopressor effects. Consult interaction analysis for full review.

◆ **Mepivacaine HCl** *see* Mepivacaine *on page 972*

◆ **Mepivacaine Hydrochloride** *see* Mepivacaine *on page 972*

Mepolizumab (me poe LIZ ue mab)

Brand Names: US Nucala

Brand Names: Canada Nucala

Pharmacologic Category Interleukin-5 Antagonist; Monoclonal Antibody, Anti-Asthmatic

Use

Asthma: Add-on maintenance treatment of severe asthma in adults and pediatric patients ≥6 years of age with an eosinophilic phenotype.

Limitations of use: Not indicated for treatment of other eosinophilic conditions or for the relief of acute bronchospasm or status asthmaticus.

Eosinophilic granulomatosis with polyangiitis: Treatment of adult patients with eosinophilic granulomatosis with polyangiitis.

Local Anesthetic/Vasoconstrictor Precautions No information available to require special precautions

Effects on Dental Treatment No significant effects or complications reported

Effects on Bleeding No information available to require special precautions

Adverse Reactions As reported in patients with severe asthma, unless otherwise noted.

>10%:

Central nervous system: Headache (19%)

Local: Injection site reaction (eosinophilic granulomatosis: 15%; asthma: 8%)

1% to 10%:
- Central nervous system: Fatigue (5%)
- Dermatologic: Eczema (3%), pruritus (3%)
- Gastrointestinal: Upper abdominal pain (3%)
- Genitourinary: Urinary tract infection (3%)
- Hypersensitivity: Hypersensitivity reaction (≤4%), angioedema (eosinophilic granulomatosis: 1%)
- Immunologic: Antibody development (asthma: 6%, eosinophilic granulomatosis: <2%; neutralizing: <1%)
- Infection: Influenza (3%)
- Neuromuscular & skeletal: Back pain (5%), muscle spasm (3%)

Frequency not defined:
- Hypersensitivity: Type IV hypersensitivity reaction
- Infection: Herpes zoster infection

Postmarketing: Anaphylaxis

Mechanism of Action Mepolizumab is an interleukin-5 antagonist (IgG1 kappa). IL-5 is the major cytokine responsible for the growth and differentiation, recruitment, activation, and survival of eosinophils (a cell type associated with inflammation and an important component of the pathogenesis of asthma). Mepolizumab, by inhibiting IL-5 signaling, reduces the production and survival of eosinophils; however, the mechanism of mepolizumab action in asthma has not been definitively established.

Pharmacodynamics/Kinetics

Half-life Elimination Terminal: 16 to 22 days

Pregnancy Considerations

Mepolizumab is a humanized monoclonal antibody (IgG1). Placental transfer of human IgG is dependent upon the IgG subclass, maternal serum concentrations, newborn birth weight, and gestational age, generally increasing as pregnancy progresses. The lowest exposure would be expected during the period of organogenesis (Palmeira 2012; Pentsuk 2009).

Uncontrolled asthma is associated with adverse events on pregnancy (increased risk of perinatal mortality, preeclampsia, preterm birth, low birth weight infants, cesarean delivery, and the development of gestational diabetes). Poorly controlled asthma or asthma exacerbations may have a greater fetal/maternal risk than what is associated with appropriately used asthma medications. Maternal treatment improves pregnancy outcomes by reducing the risk of some adverse events (eg, preterm birth and gestational diabetes). Maternal asthma symptoms should be monitored monthly during pregnancy (ERS/TSANZ [Middleton 2019]; GINA 2020).

Use of monoclonal antibodies for the treatment of asthma in pregnancy may be considered when conventional therapies are insufficient; use of an agent other than mepolizumab may be preferred (ERS/TSANZ [Middleton 2019]).

Data collection to monitor pregnancy and infant outcomes following exposure to mepolizumab is ongoing. Health care providers are encouraged to enroll exposed pregnant females in the MotherToBaby Pregnancy Studies conducted by the Organization of Teratology Information Specialists (OTIS) (877-311-8972 or http://mothertobaby.org). Patients may also enroll themselves.

◆ **Mepron** *see* Atovaquone *on page 192*

Mercaptopurine (mer kap toe PURE een)

Brand Names: US Purixan

Brand Names: Canada Purinethol

Pharmacologic Category Antineoplastic Agent, Antimetabolite; Antineoplastic Agent, Antimetabolite (Purine Analog); Immunosuppressant Agent

Use Acute lymphoblastic leukemia: Treatment of acute lymphoblastic leukemia (ALL), as part of a combination chemotherapy maintenance regimen.

Local Anesthetic/Vasoconstrictor Precautions No information available to require special precautions

Effects on Dental Treatment Key adverse event(s) related to dental treatment: Stomatitis and mucositis.

Effects on Bleeding Significant bleeding has been associated with drug-induced thrombocytopenia and altered hemostasis. Medical consult recommended.

Adverse Reactions Frequency not always defined.
- Central nervous system: Malaise (5% to 20%), drug fever
- Dermatologic: Skin rash (5% to 20%), hyperpigmentation (<5%), urticaria (<5%), alopecia
- Endocrine & metabolic: Hyperuricemia (<5%)
- Gastrointestinal: Anorexia (5% to 20%), diarrhea (5% to 20%), nausea (5% to 20%; minimal), vomiting (5% to 20%; minimal), oral lesion (<5%), pancreatitis (<5%), cholestasis, mucositis, sprue-like symptoms, stomach pain, ulcerative bowel lesion
- Genitourinary: Oligospermia, renal toxicity, uricosuria
- Hematologic & oncologic: Bone marrow depression (>20%; onset 7 to 10 days; nadir 14 days; recovery: 21 days), anemia, granulocytopenia, hemorrhage, hepatosplenic T-cell lymphomas, leukopenia, lymphocytopenia, metastases, neutropenia, thrombocytopenia
- Hepatic: Hyperbilirubinemia (<5%), increased serum transaminases (<5%), ascites, hepatic encephalopathy, hepatic fibrosis, hepatic injury, hepatic necrosis, hepatomegaly, hepatotoxicity, intrahepatic cholestasis, jaundice, toxic hepatitis
- Immunologic: Immunosuppression
- Infection: Infection
- Respiratory: Pulmonary fibrosis
- <1%, postmarketing, and/or case reports: Hypoglycemia, portal hypertension, skin photosensitivity

Mechanism of Action Mercaptopurine is a purine antagonist which inhibits DNA and RNA synthesis; acts as false metabolite and is incorporated into DNA and RNA, eventually inhibiting their synthesis; specific for the S phase of the cell cycle

Pharmacodynamics/Kinetics

Half-life Elimination Suspension: Median: 1.3 hours (range: 0.9 to 5.4 hours).

Time to Peak Serum: Suspension: Median: Children: 1 to 3 hours, Adults: 0.75 hours (range: 0.33 to 2.5 hours).

Reproductive Considerations

Verify pregnancy status in females of reproductive potential prior to initiating therapy.

Mercaptopurine is approved for use as part of combination maintenance therapy for acute lymphoblastic leukemia. Product labeling recommends females of reproductive potential use effective contraception during mercaptopurine treatment and for 6 months after the last mercaptopurine dose. Males with female partners of reproductive potential should be advised to use effective contraception during therapy and for 3 months after the last dose of mercaptopurine.

Mercaptopurine is also used (off label) for the treatment of ulcerative colitis and Crohn disease; monotherapy use for these indications may be continued in patients planning a pregnancy (Bermejo 2018). Mercaptopurine does not decrease fertility in patients with inflammatory bowel disease (AGA [Mahadevan 2019]; Bermejo 2018).

Pregnancy Considerations

Mercaptopurine may cause fetal harm if administered during pregnancy. An increased risk of miscarriage has been noted with mercaptopurine administration during the first trimester; adverse events, including miscarriage and stillbirth, have also been noted with second and third trimester use. Mercaptopurine is approved for use as part of combination therapy for acute lymphoblastic leukemia. Information is available following use for leukemia during pregnancy; outcomes may be influenced by concomitant medications (NTP 2013; Ticku 2013).

Mercaptopurine is also used (off label) for the treatment of ulcerative colitis and Crohn disease. The risk of adverse fetal events is decreased with monotherapy. In addition, maternal use to maintain remission may improve pregnancy outcomes. Females with inflammatory bowel disease who are on maintenance therapy with mercaptopurine monotherapy may continue treatment during pregnancy. Initiating treatment during pregnancy is not recommended. Combination therapy is also not recommended (AGA [Mahadevan 2019]; Puchner 2019; Restellini 2020).

The European Society for Medical Oncology has published guidelines for diagnosis, treatment, and follow-up of cancer during pregnancy; the guidelines recommend referral to a facility with expertise in cancer during pregnancy and encourage a multidisciplinary team (obstetrician, neonatologist, oncology team). In general, if chemotherapy is indicated, it should be avoided in the first trimester and there should be a 3-week time period between the last chemotherapy dose and anticipated delivery, and chemotherapy should not be administered beyond week 33 of gestation (Peccatori 2013).

Data collection to monitor outcomes following exposure to medications during pregnancy is ongoing. A pregnancy registry is available for all cancers diagnosed during pregnancy at Cooper Health (877-635-4499). Women exposed to medications during pregnancy for the treatment of an autoimmune disease (eg, Crohn disease) may contact the OTIS Autoimmune Diseases Study (877-311-8972).

◆ **6-Mercaptopurine (error-prone abbreviation)** *see* Mercaptopurine *on page 978*

Meropenem (mer oh PEN em)

Brand Names: US Merrem
Brand Names: Canada Merrem [DSC]
Pharmacologic Category Antibiotic, Carbapenem
Use

Intra-abdominal infections: Treatment of complicated appendicitis and peritonitis in adult and pediatric patients caused by viridans group streptococci, *Escherichia coli*, *Klebsiella pneumoniae*, *Pseudomonas aeruginosa*, *Bacteroides fragilis*, *Bacteroides thetaiotaomicron*, and *Peptostreptococcus* species.

Meningitis, bacterial: Treatment of bacterial meningitis in pediatric patients 3 months and older caused by *Haemophilus influenzae*, *Neisseria meningitidis*, and penicillin-susceptible isolates of *Streptococcus pneumoniae*.

Skin and skin structure infection, complicated: Treatment of complicated skin and skin structure infections in adults and pediatric patients 3 months and older caused by *Staphylococcus aureus* (methicillin-susceptible isolates only), *Streptococcus pyogenes*, *Streptococcus agalactiae*, viridans group streptococci, *Enterococcus faecalis* (vancomycin-susceptible isolates only), *P. aeruginosa*, *E. coli*, *Proteus mirabilis*, *B. fragilis*, and *Peptostreptococcus* species.

Local Anesthetic/Vasoconstrictor Precautions No information available to require special precautions

Effects on Dental Treatment Key adverse event(s) related to dental treatment: Infrequent occurrence of oral *Candida* infection and glossitis.

Effects on Bleeding Hematologic disorder including decreased prothrombin time, decreased hematocrit, and platelet disorder.

Adverse Reactions

1% to 10%:

Cardiovascular: Peripheral vascular disease (>1%), shock (1%), bradycardia (≤1%), cardiac arrest (≤1%), cardiac failure (≤1%), chest pain (≤1%), hypertension (≤1%), hypotension (≤1%), myocardial infarction (≤1%), peripheral edema (≤1%), pulmonary embolism (≤1%), syncope (≤1%), tachycardia (≤1%)

Central nervous system: Headache (2% to 8%), pain (≤5%), agitation (≤1%), anxiety (≤1%), chills (≤1%), confusion (≤1%), delirium (≤1%), depression (≤1%), dizziness (≤1%), drowsiness (≤1%), hallucination (≤1%), insomnia (≤1%), nervousness (≤1%), paresthesia (≤1%), seizure (≤1%)

Dermatologic: Skin rash (2% to 3%, includes diaper-area moniliasis in infants), pruritus (1%), dermal ulcer (≤1%), diaphoresis (≤1%), urticaria (≤1%)

Endocrine & metabolic: Hypoglycemia (>1%), hypervolemia (≤1%)

Gastrointestinal: Nausea (≤8%), diarrhea (4% to 7%), constipation (1% to 7%), vomiting (≤4%), oral candidiasis (≤2%), gastrointestinal disease (>1%), glossitis (1%), abdominal pain (≤1%), anorexia (≤1%), dyspepsia (≤1%), enlargement of abdomen (≤1%), flatulence (≤1%), intestinal obstruction (≤1%)

Genitourinary: Dysuria (≤1%), pelvic pain (≤1%), urinary incontinence (≤1%), vulvovaginal candidiasis (≤1%)

Hematologic & oncologic: Anemia (≤6%), hypochromic anemia (≤1%)

Hepatic: Cholestatic jaundice (≤1%), hepatic failure (≤1%), jaundice (≤1%)

Infection: Sepsis (2%)

Local: Inflammation at injection site (2%)

Neuromuscular & skeletal: Asthenia (≤1%), back pain (≤1%)

Renal: Renal failure (≤1%)

Respiratory: Pharyngitis (>1%), pneumonia (>1%), apnea (1%), asthma (≤1%), cough (≤1%), dyspnea (≤1%), hypoxia (≤1%), pleural effusion (≤1%), pulmonary edema (≤1%), respiratory tract disease (≤1%)

Miscellaneous: Accidental injury (>1%), fever (≤1%)

Frequency not defined:

Endocrine & metabolic: Hypokalemia, increased lactate dehydrogenase

Genitourinary: Hematuria

Hematologic & oncologic: Decreased hematocrit, decreased hemoglobin, decreased partial thromboplastin time, decreased prothrombin time, decreased white blood cell count, eosinophilia, leukocytosis, quantitative disorders of platelets

Hepatic: Increased serum alanine aminotransferase, increased serum alkaline phosphatase, increased serum aspartate aminotransferase, increased serum bilirubin

Renal: Increased blood urea nitrogen, increased serum creatinine

<1%, postmarketing, and/or case reports: Acute generalized exanthematous pustulosis, agranulocytosis, angioedema, *Clostridioides* (formerly *Clostridium*) *difficile*-associated diarrhea, DRESS syndrome, edema at insertion site, epistaxis, erythema multiforme, gastrointestinal hemorrhage, hemolytic anemia, hemoperitoneum, injection site reaction, leukopenia, localized phlebitis, local thrombophlebitis, melena, neutropenia, pain at injection site, positive direct Coombs test, positive indirect Coombs test, Stevens-Johnson syndrome, toxic epidermal necrolysis

Mechanism of Action Inhibits bacterial cell wall synthesis by binding to several of the penicillin-binding proteins, which in turn inhibit the final transpeptidation step of peptidoglycan synthesis in bacterial cell walls, thus inhibiting cell wall biosynthesis; bacteria eventually lyse due to ongoing activity of cell wall autolytic enzymes (autolysins and murein hydrolases) while cell wall assembly is arrested

Pharmacodynamics/Kinetics

Half-life Elimination

Neonates and Infants ≤3 months: Median: 2.7 hours; range: 1.6- 3.8 hours (Smith 2011)

Infants and Children 3 months to 2 years: 1.5 hours

Children 2-12 years and Adults: 1 hour

Time to Peak Tissue: ~1 hour following infusion except in bile, lung, and muscle; CSF: 2 to 3 hours with inflamed meninges

Pregnancy Considerations

Incomplete transplacental transfer of meropenem was found using an ex vivo human perfusion model (Hnat 2005).

Information related to the use of meropenem in pregnancy is limited (Yoshida 2013).

Meropenem and Vaborbactam

(mer oh PEN em & va bor BAK tam)

Brand Names: US Vabomere

Pharmacologic Category Antibiotic, Carbapenem; Beta-Lactamase Inhibitor

Use Urinary tract infections, complicated: Treatment of complicated urinary tract infections (cUTI), including pyelonephritis, caused by susceptible *Escherichia coli*, *Klebsiella pneumoniae*, and *Enterobacter cloacae* species complex in patients ≥18 years of age

Local Anesthetic/Vasoconstrictor Precautions No information available to require special precautions

Effects on Dental Treatment No significant effects or complications reported

Effects on Bleeding No information available to require special precautions

Adverse Reactions Note: Reactions may not be exclusive to meropenem and vaborbactam. Some patients in this study were switched to levofloxacin after 15 doses of meropenem and vaborbactam.

Also see Meropenem.

1% to 10%:

Cardiovascular: Phlebitis (≤4%)

Central nervous system: Headache (9%)

Endocrine & metabolic: Hypokalemia (1%)

Gastrointestinal: Diarrhea (3%), nausea (2%)

Hepatic: Increased serum ALT (2%), increased serum AST (2%)

Hypersensitivity: Hypersensitivity (2%)

Local: Infusion site reaction (≤4%)

Miscellaneous: Fever (2%)

Frequency not defined: Gastrointestinal: *Clostridioides* (formerly *Clostridium*) *difficile*-associated diarrhea

<1%, postmarketing, and/or case reports: Azotemia, chest discomfort, decreased appetite, deep vein thrombosis, dizziness, hallucination, hyperglycemia, hyperkalemia, hypoglycemia, hypotension, increased creatine phosphokinase, insomnia, lethargy, leukopenia, oral candidiasis, paresthesia, pharyngitis, renal impairment, tremor, vulvovaginal candidiasis

Mechanism of Action

Meropenem: Inhibits bacterial cell wall synthesis by binding to penicillin-binding proteins, which in turn inhibit the final transpeptidation step of peptidoglycan synthesis in bacterial cell walls, thus inhibiting cell wall biosynthesis; bacteria eventually lyse due to ongoing activity of cell wall autolytic enzymes (autolysins and murein hydrolases) while cell wall assembly is arrested

Vaborbactam is a beta-lactamase inhibitor that protects meropenem from degradation by certain serine beta-lactamases (eg, K. pneumonia carbapenemase [KPC]). Vaborbactam does not have antibacterial activity.

Pharmacodynamics/Kinetics

Half-life Elimination Meropenem: 1.22 hours; Vaborbactam: 1.68 hours

Pregnancy Considerations

Animal reproduction studies have not been conducted with this combination; adverse events were observed in animal reproduction studies following administration of the vaborbactam component.

Also refer to the meropenem monograph for additional information.

◆ **Merrem** *see* Meropenem *on page* 979

Mesalamine (me SAL a meen)

Brand Names: US Apriso; Asacol HD; Canasa; Delzicol; Lialda; Pentasa; Rowasa; SfRowasa

Brand Names: Canada Asacol; Asacol 800; Mesasal [DSC]; Mezavant; Mezera; Pentasa; Salofalk; TEVA-5 ASA

Pharmacologic Category 5-Aminosalicylic Acid Derivative

Use

US labeling:

Oral:

Apriso: Maintenance of remission of ulcerative colitis in patients ≥18 years

Asacol HD: Treatment of moderately active ulcerative colitis in adults

Delzicol: Treatment of mildly to moderately active ulcerative colitis in patients ≥5 years; maintenance of remission of ulcerative colitis in adults

Lialda: Treatment of mildly to moderately active ulcerative colitis in patients weighing ≥24 kg; treatment and maintenance of remission of mildly to moderately active ulcerative colitis in adults.

Pentasa: Treatment and maintenance of remission of mildly to moderately active ulcerative colitis

Rectal: Treatment of active mild to moderate distal ulcerative colitis (suspension only), proctosigmoiditis (suspension only), or proctitis (suspension and suppository)

Canadian labeling:

Oral:

Asacol, Mezavant: Treatment and maintenance of remission of mildly- to moderately-active ulcerative colitis

Asacol 800: Treatment of moderately active ulcerative colitis

Mesasal: Treatment and maintenance of remission of ulcerative colitis

Pentasa: Treatment and maintenance of remission of mildly to moderately active ulcerative colitis; treatment and maintenance of remission of mild to moderate Crohn disease

Rectal foam: Mezera: Treatment of mildly active ulcerative colitis of the sigmoid colon and rectum

Rectal suppository and suspension: Treatment and maintenance of remission of distal ulcerative colitis (extending to splenic flexure) and as adjunctive therapy in more extensive disease (suspension only); treatment and maintenance of ulcerative proctitis (suppository only)

Local Anesthetic/Vasoconstrictor Precautions No information available to require special precautions

Effects on Dental Treatment Key adverse event(s) related to dental treatment: Pharyngitis.

Effects on Bleeding No information available to require special precautions

Adverse Reactions Adverse effects vary depending upon dosage form; frequency similar in adult and pediatric patients unless otherwise noted. Incidence usually on lower end with enema and suppository dosage forms.

>10%:

Central nervous system: Headache (3% to 14%)

Gastrointestinal: Eructation (≤26%), abdominal pain (oral: 2% to 21%, children & adolescents: 10%; rectal: 5%), constipation (≤11%)

Respiratory: Nasopharyngitis (children and adolescents: 15%; adults: 1% to 4%)

1% to 10%:

Cardiovascular: Hypertension (≤1%)

Central nervous system: Dizziness (≤9%), fatigue (<3%), pain (<3%), vertigo (<3%), nervousness (≥2%), paresthesia (≥2%)

Dermatologic: Skin rash (≤6%), alopecia (<3%), acne vulgaris (≤1%)

Endocrine & metabolic: Increased serum triglycerides (<3%), weight loss (children and adolescents: 2%)

Gastrointestinal: Diarrhea (≤8%), exacerbation of ulcerative colitis (≤6%), flatulence (≤6%), upper abdominal pain (1% to 5%), dyspepsia (≤4%), nausea (≤4%), lower abdominal pain (<3%), gastroenteritis (≥2%), hemorrhoids (≥2%), tenesmus (≥2%), gastrointestinal hemorrhage (<1% to ≥2%), bloody diarrhea (children and adolescents: 2%), pancreatitis (children and adolescents: 2%), sclerosing cholangitis (children and adolescents: 2%), vomiting (≤2%), rectal pain (rectal: 1% to 2%), abdominal distention (≥1%), anorectal pain (rectal: 1%; includes pain on insertion of enema tip), nausea and vomiting (1%), colitis (≤1%)

Genitourinary: Hematuria (<3%), urinary frequency (<1% to ≥2%)

Hematologic & oncologic: Decreased hematocrit (<3%), decreased hemoglobin (<3%), rectal hemorrhage (<3%)

Hepatic: Cholestatic hepatitis (<3%), increased serum transaminases (<3%), hepatic insufficiency (2%)

Infection: Influenza (1% to 5%), infection (≥2%), viral infection (children and adolescents: 2%; adenovirus)

Neuromuscular & skeletal: Back pain (≤6%), arthralgia (<3%), arthropathy (≥2%), leg pain (rectal: ≤2%)

Ophthalmic: Visual disturbance (≥2%)

Otic: Tinnitus (<3%)

Renal: Decreased creatinine clearance (<3%)

Respiratory: Rhinitis (8%), sinusitis (children and adolescents: 7%; adults: <1%), cough (children & adolescents: 5%; adults: <1%), dyspnea (<3%)

Miscellaneous: Intolerance syndrome (3%), fever (≤3%)

<1%, postmarketing, and/or case reports: Abdominal cramps (rectal), abnormal stools, abnormal T waves on ECG, acute renal failure, agranulocytosis, albuminuria, amenorrhea, anaphylaxis, anemia, angioedema, anorectal pain (rectal; discomfort), anorexia, anxiety, aplastic anemia, arthritis, blurred vision, bronchitis, chest pain, chills, cholecystitis, cholestatic jaundice, chronic renal failure, confusion, conjunctivitis, decreased libido, depression, diaphoresis, DRESS syndrome, drowsiness, drug fever, duodenal ulcer, dysgeusia, dysmenorrhea, dysphagia, dysuria, ear disease, ecchymoses, eczema, edema, emotional lability, eosinophilia, eosinophilic pneumonitis, epididymitis, erythema, erythema nodosum, esophageal ulcer, Eustachian tube congestion, exacerbation of asthma, eye pain, facial edema, fecal discoloration (rectal), fecal incontinence, frequent bowel movements (rectal), gastritis, gout, granulocytopenia, Guillain-Barré syndrome, hepatic cirrhosis, hepatic failure, hepatic injury, hepatic necrosis, hepatitis, hepatotoxicity, hyperesthesia, hypermenorrhea, hypersensitivity pneumonitis, hypersensitivity reaction, hypertonia, hypomenorrhea, hypotension, idiopathic nephrotic syndrome, increased amylase, increased appetite, increased blood urea nitrogen, increased gamma-glutamyl transferase, increased lactate dehydrogenase, increased serum alkaline phosphatase, increased serum ALT, increased serum AST, increased serum bilirubin, increased serum creatinine, increased serum lipase, increased thirst, insomnia, interstitial nephritis, interstitial pneumonitis, interstitial pulmonary disease, intracranial hypertension, jaundice, Kawasaki-like syndrome, leg cramps, leukopenia, lichen planus, lupus-like syndrome, lymphadenopathy, malaise, male infertility (rectal), mastalgia, migraine, mucus stools (rectal), myalgia, myocarditis, nail disease, neck pain, nephrogenic diabetes insipidus, nephrotoxicity (rectal), neutropenia (rectal), oligospermia, oral candidiasis, oral mucosa ulcer, otalgia, painful defecation (rectal), palpitations, pancytopenia, perforated peptic ulcer, pericardial effusion, pericarditis, peripheral edema, peripheral neuropathy, pharyngitis, pharyngolaryngeal pain, pleurisy, pneumonitis, prurigo, pruritus, pruritus ani (rectal), psoriasis, pulmonary infiltrates, pulmonary fibrosis, pyoderma gangrenosum, rectal discharge (rectal), rectal polyp, renal disease (including minimal change nephropathy), renal insufficiency, renal failure, rheumatoid arthritis, skin photosensitivity, Stevens-Johnson syndrome, stomach discomfort

(rectal), stomatitis, swelling of eye, systemic lupus erythematosus, tachycardia, thrombocythemia, thrombocytopenia, transverse myelitis, tremor, ulcerative colitis (rectal; pancolitis), urinary urgency, urticaria, uterine hemorrhage, vasodilation, weakness, xeroderma, xerostomia

Mechanism of Action Mesalamine (5-aminosalicylic acid) is the active component of sulfasalazine; the specific mechanism of action is unknown; however, it is thought that mesalamine modulates local chemical mediators of the inflammatory response, especially leukotrienes, and is also postulated to be a free radical scavenger or an inhibitor of tumor necrosis factor (TNF); action appears topical rather than systemic

Pharmacodynamics/Kinetics

Half-life Elimination 5-ASA and N-acetyl-5-ASA: Variable; ~25 hours (range: 2 to 296 hours)

Time to Peak

Capsule: Apriso: ~4 hours; Delzicol: ~10 hours; Pentasa: 3 hours

Foam: Mezera [Canadian product]: ~1 hour

Rectal: Pentasa, Salofalk [Canadian products]: 2 to 6 hours

Tablet: Asacol HD (formulated with dibutyl phthalate [DBP]): 10 to 16 hours; Asacol HD (formulated without DBP): ~24 hours (mean); Lialda: 9 to 12 hours

Canadian products: Asacol: 7 hours; Asacol 800: 10 hours; Mesasal: ~7 hours; Mezavant: 8 hours (range: 4 to 34 hours)

Reproductive Considerations

Reversible oligospermia has been reported in males.

Pregnancy Considerations

Mesalamine is known to cross the placenta. An increased rate of congenital malformations has not been observed in human studies. Preterm birth, still birth, and decreased birth weight have been observed; however, these events may also be due to maternal disease.

Dibutyl phthalate (DBP) may be an inactive ingredient in the enteric coating of some products (eg, Asacol, Asacol HD); adverse effects in male rats were noted at doses greater than the recommended human dose. Refer to product labeling for current formulation.

When treatment for inflammatory bowel disease is needed during pregnancy, mesalamine may be used, although products with DBP should be avoided (Habal 2012; Mottet 2009; van der Woude 2015).

Product Availability

Asacol HD formulated **without** dibutyl phthalate (DBP) (NDC: 0023-5901-18) is available in the US as of May 2017.

Asacol HD formulated **with** DBP (NDC: 00430-0783-27) may still be available in the marketplace and on pharmacy shelves.

- **Mesalazine** *see* Mesalamine *on page 980*
- **Mestinon** *see* Pyridostigmine *on page 1293*
- **Metadate CD [DSC]** *see* Methylphenidate *on page 997*
- **Metadate ER** *see* Methylphenidate *on page 997*

Metaproterenol (met a proe TER e nol)

Related Information

Respiratory Diseases *on page 1680*

Pharmacologic Category $Beta_2$ Agonist

Use Asthma/Bronchospasm: Bronchial asthma and for reversible bronchospasm which may occur in association with bronchitis and emphysema.

Local Anesthetic/Vasoconstrictor Precautions No information available to require special precautions

Effects on Dental Treatment Key adverse event(s) related to dental treatment: Bad taste and xerostomia (normal salivary flow resumes upon discontinuation).

Effects on Bleeding No information available to require special precautions

Adverse Reactions

>10%:

Cardiovascular: Tachycardia (6% to 17%)

Central nervous system: Nervousness (5% to 20%)

Neuromuscular & skeletal: Tremor (2% to 17%)

1% to 10%:

Cardiovascular: Palpitations (4%)

Central nervous system: Headache (1% to 7%), dizziness (2%), insomnia (2%), fatigue (1%)

Gastrointestinal: Nausea (1% to 4%), diarrhea (1%)

Respiratory: Exacerbation of asthma (2%)

<1%, postmarketing, and/or case reports: Blurred vision, change in appetite, chest pain, chills, clonus, cough, diaphoresis, drowsiness, dry throat, edema, facial edema, fever, flu-like symptoms, hypertension, muscle spasm, pain, pruritus, sensory disturbance, swelling of fingers, syncope, unpleasant taste, urticaria, vomiting, weakness, xerostomia

Mechanism of Action Stimulates $beta_2$-receptors which increases the conversion of adenosine triphosphate (ATP) to 3'-5'-cyclic adenosine monophosphate (cAMP), resulting in bronchial smooth muscle relaxation

Pharmacodynamics/Kinetics

Onset of Action Bronchodilation: Oral: ~30 minutes; Peak effect: Oral: ~1 hour

Duration of Action ~2 to 6 hours, regardless of route administered

Pregnancy Risk Factor C

Pregnancy Considerations

Beta agonists, including metaproterenol, may interfere with uterine contractility if administered during labor; maternal and fetal tachycardia have been observed (Baillie 1970; Tyack 1971).

Uncontrolled asthma is associated with adverse events on pregnancy (increased risk of perinatal mortality, preeclampsia, preterm birth, low birth weight infants, cesarean delivery, and the development of gestational diabetes). Poorly controlled asthma or asthma exacerbations may have a greater fetal/maternal risk than what is associated with appropriately used asthma medications. Maternal treatment improves pregnancy outcomes by reducing the risk of some adverse events (eg, preterm birth and gestational diabetes). Maternal asthma symptoms should be monitored monthly during pregnancy. Agents other than metaproterenol are recommended to treat asthma during pregnancy (ERS/TSANZ [Middleton 2019]; GINA 2020).

- **Metaproterenol Sulfate** *see* Metaproterenol *on page 982*
- **Metaxall [DSC]** *see* Metaxalone *on page 982*

Metaxalone (me TAKS a lone)

Brand Names: US Metaxall [DSC]; Skelaxin

Pharmacologic Category Skeletal Muscle Relaxant

Use *Musculoskeletal conditions:* Relief of discomforts associated with acute, painful musculoskeletal conditions.

Local Anesthetic/Vasoconstrictor Precautions No information available to require special precautions

Effects on Dental Treatment No significant effects or complications reported

Effects on Bleeding No information available to require special precautions

Adverse Reactions Frequency not defined.

Central nervous system: Dizziness, drowsiness, headache, irritability, nervousness

Dermatologic: Skin rash (with or without pruritus)

Gastrointestinal: Gastrointestinal distress, nausea, vomiting

Hematologic & oncologic: Hemolytic anemia, leukopenia

Hepatic: Jaundice

Hypersensitivity: Anaphylactoid reaction (rare), anaphylaxis, hypersensitivity reaction

Mechanism of Action Precise mechanism has not been established; however, its clinical effect may be associated with general depression of the nervous system; has no direct effect on the contractile mechanism of striated muscle, the nerve fiber or the motor end plate.

Pharmacodynamics/Kinetics

Half-life Elimination 9 ± 4.8 hours

Time to Peak ~3 hours

Pregnancy Considerations Adverse events have not been observed in animal reproduction studies. Use during pregnancy (especially first trimester) only if benefits outweigh risks.

MetFORMIN (met FOR min)

Related Information

Endocrine Disorders and Pregnancy *on page 1684*

Brand Names: US D-Care DM2 [DSC]; Fortamet; Glucophage; Glucophage XR; Glumetza; Riomet; Riomet ER

Brand Names: Canada ACT MetFORMIN; APO-MetFORMIN; APO-MetFORMIN ER; Auro-Metformin; DOM-MetFORMIN; ECL-MetFORMIN [DSC]; Glucophage; Glumetza; Glycon; JAMP-MetFORMIN; JAMP-MetFORMIN Blackberry [DSC]; Mar-MetFORMIN [DSC]; MetFORMIN FC; MINT-MetFORMIN [DSC]; MYLAN-MetFORMIN [DSC]; PMS-MetFORMIN; PRO-MetFORMIN; RAN-MetFORMIN; RATIO-MetFORMIN; RIVA-MetFORMIN; SANDOZ MetFORMIN FC; Septa-MetFORMIN; TEVA-MetFORMIN [DSC]

Pharmacologic Category Antidiabetic Agent, Biguanide

Use

Diabetes mellitus, type 2: Management of type 2 diabetes mellitus when hyperglycemia cannot be managed with diet and exercise alone.

Note: If not contraindicated and if tolerated, metformin is the preferred initial pharmacologic agent for type 2 diabetes management (ADA 2020).

Local Anesthetic/Vasoconstrictor Precautions No information available to require special precautions

Effects on Dental Treatment Key adverse event(s) related to dental treatment: Taste disorder.

Metformin-dependent patients with diabetes (noninsulin dependent, Type 2) should be appointed for dental treatment in morning in order to minimize chance of stress-induced hypoglycemia.

Effects on Bleeding No information available to require special precautions

Adverse Reactions

>10%:

Gastrointestinal: Diarrhea (IR tablet: 12% to 53% [placebo: 12%]; ER tablet: 10% to 17% [placebo: 3%]), flatulence (4% to 12% [placebo: 6%]), nausea and vomiting (IR tablet: 26% [placebo 8%]; ER tablet: 7% [placebo: 2%])

Infection: Infection (21%)

1% to 10%:

Cardiovascular: Chest discomfort (1% to 5%), flushing (1% to 5%), palpitations (1% to 5%)

Dermatologic: Diaphoresis (1% to 5%)

Endocrine & metabolic: Cyanocobalamin deficiency (7%), hypoglycemia (1% to 5%)

Gastrointestinal: Abdominal distention (1% to 5%), abdominal distress (6%), abdominal pain (3% to 4%), abnormal stools (1% to 5%), dyspepsia (≤7% [placebo: 4%]), heartburn (1% to 5%)

Nervous system: Chills (1% to 5%), dizziness (1% to 5%), headache (5% to 6%), metallic taste (3%)

Neuromuscular & skeletal: Asthenia (9%), myalgia (1% to 5%)

Respiratory: Dyspnea (1% to 5%), flu-like symptoms (1% to 5%), rhinitis (4% to 6%), upper respiratory tract infection (1% to 5%)

Postmarketing:

Dermatologic: Lichen planus (Azzam 1997), nail disease (Lu 2013)

Endocrine & metabolic: Lactic acidosis (rare; DeFronzo 2016; Eppenga 2014; Salpeter 2010)

Hematologic & oncologic: Hemolytic anemia (Packer 2008)

Hepatic: Hepatic injury (cholestatic, hepatocellular, and mixed) (Babich 1998; Nammour 2003)

Hypersensitivity: Fixed drug eruption (Ramírez-Bellver 2017; Steber 2016)

Nervous system: Encephalopathy (Béjot 2015; Jung 2009; Kang 2013)

Mechanism of Action Decreases hepatic glucose production, decreases intestinal absorption of glucose and improves insulin sensitivity (increases peripheral glucose uptake and utilization)

Pharmacodynamics/Kinetics

Onset of Action Within days; maximum effects up to 2 weeks

Half-life Elimination Plasma: 4 to 9 hours; Blood ~17.6 hours

Time to Peak Serum: Immediate release: 2 to 3 hours; ER tablet: 7 hours (range: 4 to 8 hours); ER suspension: 4.5 hours (range: 3.5 to 6.5 hours).

Reproductive Considerations

Ovulation rates may increase in some anovulatory females; contraception should be discussed for women who do not wish to conceive (ACOG 194 2018). Females with diabetes mellitus who wish to conceive should use adequate contraception until glycemic control is achieved (ADA 2020).

Pregnancy Considerations

Metformin crosses the placenta; concentrations may be comparable to those found in the maternal plasma (Charles 2006; de Oliveira Baraldi 2011; Eyal 2010; Vanky 2005).

An increased risk of birth defects or adverse fetal/neonatal outcomes has not been observed following maternal use of metformin for gestational diabetes mellitus or type 2 diabetes mellitus when glycemic control is maintained (Balani 2009; Coetzee 1979; Coetzee 1984; Ekpebegh 2007; Niromanesh 2012; Rowan 2008; Rowan 2010; Tertti 2008). However, available guidelines note that long-term safety data are not available (ACOG 190 2018; ACOG 201 2018; ADA 2020).

Poorly controlled diabetes during pregnancy can be associated with an increased risk of adverse maternal and fetal outcomes, including diabetic ketoacidosis, preeclampsia, spontaneous abortion, preterm delivery, delivery complications, major birth defects, stillbirth, and macrosomia (ACOG 201 2018). To prevent adverse outcomes, prior to conception and throughout pregnancy, maternal blood glucose and HbA_{1c} should be kept as close to target goals as possible but without causing significant hypoglycemia (ADA 2020; Blumer 2013).

Agents other than metformin are currently recommended to treat diabetes mellitus in pregnancy (ADA 2020). However, metformin may be used as an alternative agent in some patients requiring therapy for gestational diabetes mellitus or type 2 diabetes mellitus (ACOG 190 2018; ACOG 201 2018). Pharmacokinetic studies suggest that clearance of metformin may increase during pregnancy and dosing may need adjusted in some women when used during the third trimester (Charles 2006; Eyal 2010; Gardiner 2003; Hughes 2006; Vanky 2005).

- ◆ **Metformin and Dapagliflozin** *see* Dapagliflozin and Metformin *on page 435*
- ◆ **Metformin and Ertugliflozin** *see* Ertugliflozin and Metformin *on page 588*
- ◆ **Metformin and Glyburide** *see* Glyburide and Metformin *on page 742*
- ◆ **Metformin and Linagliptin** *see* Linagliptin and Metformin *on page 917*
- ◆ **Metformin and Saxagliptin** *see* Saxagliptin and Metformin *on page 1360*
- ◆ **Metformin and Sitagliptin** *see* Sitagliptin and Metformin *on page 1376*
- ◆ **Metformin ER** *see* MetFORMIN *on page 983*
- ◆ **Metformin HCl** *see* MetFORMIN *on page 983*
- ◆ **Metformin HCl ER** *see* MetFORMIN *on page 983*
- ◆ **Metformin Hydrochloride** *see* MetFORMIN *on page 983*
- ◆ **Metformin Hydrochloride and Dapagliflozin** *see* Dapagliflozin and Metformin *on page 435*
- ◆ **Metformin Hydrochloride and Linagliptin** *see* Linagliptin and Metformin *on page 917*
- ◆ **Metformin Hydrochloride and Pioglitazone Hydrochloride** *see* Pioglitazone and Metformin *on page 1236*
- ◆ **Metformin Hydrochloride and Saxagliptin** *see* Saxagliptin and Metformin *on page 1360*
- ◆ **Metformin hydrochloride, empagliflozin, and linagliptin** *see* Empagliflozin, Linagliptin, and Metformin *on page 555*
- ◆ **Metformin hydrochloride, linagliptin, and empagliflozin** *see* Empagliflozin, Linagliptin, and Metformin *on page 555*
- ◆ **Metformin Hydrochloride, Saxagliptin, and Dapagliflozin** *see* Dapagliflozin, Saxagliptin, and Metformin *on page 436*

Methadone (METH a done)

Related Information

Clinical Risk Related to Drugs Prolonging QT Interval *on page 1675*

Brand Names: US Dolophine; Methadone HCl Intensol; Methadose; Methadose Sugar-Free

Brand Names: Canada Metadol; Metadol-D; Methadose; SANDOZ Methadone

Pharmacologic Category Analgesic, Opioid

Use

Opioid use disorder: Medically supervised withdrawal and maintenance treatment of opioid use disorder, in conjunction with appropriate social and medical services; injection is only for temporary treatment in patients unable to take oral medication.

Limitations of use: Injection: Not approved for outpatient treatment of opioid use disorder; only use in patients unable to take oral medication (eg, hospitalized patients).

Pain management:

Injection: Management of pain severe enough to require an opioid analgesic and for which alternative treatment options are inadequate.

Oral (Dolophine only): Management of pain severe enough to require daily, around-the-clock, long-term opioid treatment and for which alternative treatment options are inadequate.

Limitations of use: Reserve for use in patients for whom alternative treatment options (eg, nonopioid analgesics, opioid combination products) are ineffective, not tolerated, or would be otherwise inadequate to provide sufficient management of pain. Dolophine is not indicated for use as an as-needed analgesic.

Local Anesthetic/Vasoconstrictor Precautions

Methadone is one of the drugs confirmed to prolong the QT interval and is accepted as having a risk of causing torsades de pointes. The risk of drug-induced torsades de pointes is extremely low when a single QT interval prolonging drug is prescribed. In terms of epinephrine, it is not known what effect vasoconstrictors in the local anesthetic regimen will have in patients with a known history of congenital prolonged QT interval or in patients taking any medication that prolongs the QT interval. Until more information is obtained, it is suggested that the clinician consult with the physician prior to the use of a vasoconstrictor in suspected patients, and that the vasoconstrictor (epinephrine, levonordefrin [Neo-Cobefrin®]) be used with caution.

Effects on Dental Treatment Key adverse event(s) related to dental treatment: Significant xerostomia (normal salivary flow resumes upon discontinuation) and glossitis.

Effects on Bleeding No information available to require special precautions

Adverse Reactions

Frequency not defined:

Cardiovascular: Bigeminy, bradycardia, cardiac arrhythmia, cardiac failure, cardiomyopathy, ECG changes, edema, extrasystoles, flushing, hypotension, inversion T wave on ECG, palpitations, phlebitis, prolonged QT interval on ECG, shock, syncope, tachycardia, torsades de pointes, ventricular fibrillation, ventricular tachycardia

Central nervous system: Agitation, confusion, disorientation, dizziness, drug dependence (physical dependence), dysphoria, euphoria, hallucination, headache, insomnia, sedation, seizure

Dermatologic: Diaphoresis, hemorrhagic urticaria (rare), pruritus, skin rash, urticaria
Endocrine & metabolic: Adrenocortical insufficiency, altered hormone level (androgen deficiency; chronic opioid use), amenorrhea, antidiuretic effect, decreased libido, decreased plasma testosterone, hypokalemia, hypomagnesemia, weight gain
Gastrointestinal: Abdominal pain, anorexia, biliary tract spasm, constipation, glossitis, nausea, vomiting, xerostomia
Genitourinary: Asthenospermia, decreased ejaculate volume, male genital disease (reduced seminal vesicle secretions), prostatic disease (reduced prostate secretions), spermatozoa disorder (morphologic abnormalities), urinary hesitancy, urinary retention
Hematologic: Thrombocytopenia (reversible, reported in patients with chronic hepatitis)
Local: Erythema at injection site (intramuscular/subcutaneous), local pain (intramuscular/subcutaneous), local swelling (intramuscular/subcutaneous)
Neuromuscular & skeletal: Amyotrophy, bone fracture, osteoporosis, weakness
Ophthalmic: Visual disturbance
Respiratory: Pulmonary edema, respiratory depression

<1%, postmarketing, and/or case reports: Hypoglycemia (dosage >40 mg/day [Flory 2016]), hypogonadism, increased serum prolactin (transient increase with chronic use; Molitch 2008)

Mechanism of Action Binds to opiate receptors in the CNS, causing inhibition of ascending pain pathways, altering the perception of and response to pain; produces generalized CNS depression. Methadone has also been shown to have N-methyl-D-aspartate (NMDA) receptor antagonism.

Pharmacodynamics/Kinetics

Onset of Action Oral: Analgesic: 0.5 to 1 hour; Parenteral: 10 to 20 minutes; Peak effect: Parenteral: 1 to 2 hours; Oral: Continuous dosing: 3 to 5 days

Duration of Action Analgesia: Oral: 4 to 8 hours (single-dose studies), increases to 22 to 48 hours with repeated doses; slow release from the liver and other tissues may prolong duration of action

Half-life Elimination Terminal:
Children and Adolescents: 19.2 ± 13.6 hours (range: 3.8 to 62 hours) (Berde 1987)
Adults: 8 to 59 hours; may be prolonged with alkaline pH

Time to Peak 1 to 7.5 hours

Reproductive Considerations

Long-term opioid use may cause secondary hypogonadism, which may lead to sexual dysfunction or infertility in men and women (Brennan 2013). In males, reduced ejaculate volume, reduced seminal vesicle and prostate secretions, decreased serum testosterone, and abnormalities in sperm motility and morphology have been reported during treatment. Amenorrhea has been reported in females during treatment but may also develop secondary to substance abuse; pregnancy may occur following the initiation of methadone maintenance treatment. Contraception counseling is recommended to prevent unplanned pregnancies (Dow 2012).

Pregnancy Considerations

Methadone crosses the placenta and can be detected in cord blood, amniotic fluid, and newborn urine.

Data are available related to fetal/neonatal outcomes following maternal use of methadone during pregnancy. Information collected by the Teratogen Information System is complicated by maternal use of illicit drugs, nutrition, infection, and psychosocial circumstances. However, pregnant women in methadone treatment programs are reported to have improved fetal outcomes compared to pregnant women using illicit drugs. Fetal growth, birth weight, length, and/or head circumference may be decreased in infants born to mothers with opioid use disorder treated with methadone during pregnancy. Growth deficits do not appear to persist; however, decreased performance on psychometric and behavioral tests has been found to continue into childhood. Abnormal fetal nonstress tests have also been reported.

[US Boxed Warning]: Neonatal opioid withdrawal syndrome is an expected and treatable outcome of use of methadone during pregnancy. Neonatal opioid withdrawal syndrome may be life-threatening if not recognized and treated in the neonate. The balance between the risks of neonatal opioid withdrawal syndrome and the benefits of maternal methadone use may differ based on the risks associated with the mother's underlying condition, pain, or dependence. Advise the patient of the risk of neonatal opioid withdrawal syndrome so that appropriate planning for management of the neonate can occur. Symptoms following opioid exposure may present as autonomic (eg, fever, temperature instability), gastrointestinal (eg, diarrhea, vomiting, poor feeding/weight gain), or neurologic (eg, high-pitched crying, increased muscle tone, irritability, seizure, tremor) symptoms (Dow 2012; Hudak 2012). Monitoring is recommended for neonates born to mothers receiving methadone for neonatal abstinence syndrome (Chou 2014).

Opioid agonist pharmacotherapy using methadone is an option when treating opioid use disorder in pregnant women (ACOG 711 2017). Due to pregnancy-induced physiologic changes, some pharmacokinetic properties of methadone may be altered (clearance may be increased and half-life may be decreased); dosing adjustment may be required. Women receiving methadone for the treatment of opioid use disorder should also be maintained on their daily dose of methadone in addition to receiving the same pain management options during labor and delivery as opioid-naive women; maintenance doses of methadone will not provide adequate pain relief. Opioid agonist-antagonists should be avoided for the treatment of labor pain in women maintained on methadone due to the risk of precipitating acute withdrawal (ACOG 711 2017; Dow 2012).

Controlled Substance C-II

Prescribing and Access Restrictions When used for treatment of opioid addiction: May only be dispensed in accordance to guidelines established by the Substance Abuse and Mental Health Services Administration's (SAMHSA) Center for Substance Abuse Treatment (CSAT). Regulations regarding methadone use may vary by state and/or country. Obtain advice from appropriate regulatory agencies and/or consult with pain management/palliative care specialists.

Note: Regulatory Exceptions to the General Requirement to Provide Opioid Agonist Treatment (per manufacturer's labeling):

1. During inpatient care, when the patient was admitted for any condition other than concurrent opioid addiction, to facilitate the treatment of the primary admitting diagnosis.
2. During an emergency period of no longer than 3 days while definitive care for the addiction is being sought in an appropriately licensed facility.

Dental Health Professional Considerations See Local Anesthetic/Vasoconstrictor Precautions

◆ **Methadone HCl Intensol** *see* Methadone *on page 984*

◆ **Methadone Hydrochloride** *see* Methadone *on page 984*

◆ **Methadose** *see* Methadone *on page 984*

◆ **Methadose Sugar-Free** *see* Methadone *on page 984*

◆ **Methaminodiazepoxide Hydrochloride** *see* ChlordiazePOXIDE *on page 333*

Methamphetamine (meth am FET a meen)

Related Information

Management of the Chemically Dependent Patient *on page 1724*

Brand Names: US Desoxyn

Pharmacologic Category Anorexiant; Central Nervous System Stimulant; Sympathomimetic

Use Attention-deficit/hyperactivity disorder (ADHD): For a stabilizing effect in children >6 years with a behavioral syndrome characterized by the following group of developmentally inappropriate symptoms: Moderate to severe distractibility, short attention span, hyperactivity, emotional lability, and impulsivity

Local Anesthetic/Vasoconstrictor Precautions Use vasoconstrictor with caution in patients taking methamphetamine. Amphetamines enhance the sympathomimetic response of epinephrine and norepinephrine leading to potential hypertension and cardiotoxicity.

Effects on Dental Treatment Key adverse event(s) related to dental treatment: Methamphetamine causes tachycardia, increases in blood pressure, and palpitations. Consider monitoring blood pressure prior to using local anesthetic with a vasoconstrictor. Symptoms associated with bruxism have been observed in some patients.

Effects on Bleeding No information available to require special precautions

Adverse Reactions Frequency not defined.

Cardiovascular: Hypertension, increased blood pressure, palpitations, tachycardia

Central nervous system: Dizziness, drug dependence (prolonged use), dysphoria, euphoria, exacerbation of tics (motor, phonic, and Tourette's syndrome), headache, insomnia, overstimulation, psychotic symptoms, restlessness

Dermatologic: Alopecia, urticaria

Endocrine & metabolic: Change in libido, growth suppression (children)

Gastrointestinal: Constipation, diarrhea, gastrointestinal distress, unpleasant taste, xerostomia

Genitourinary: Frequent erections, impotence, prolonged erection

Neuromuscular & skeletal: Rhabdomyolysis, tremor

Mechanism of Action A sympathomimetic amine related to ephedrine and amphetamine with CNS stimulant activity; causes release of catecholamines (primarily dopamine and other catecholamines) from their storage sites in the presynaptic nerve terminals. Inhibits reuptake and metabolism of catecholamines through inhibition of monoamine transporters and oxidase.

Pharmacodynamics/Kinetics

Half-life Elimination 4 to 5 hours

Pregnancy Risk Factor C

Pregnancy Considerations

Methamphetamine and amphetamine were detected in newborn tissues following intermittent maternal use of Desoxyn during pregnancy (Garriott 1973). The majority of human data is based on illicit amphetamine/methamphetamine exposure and not from therapeutic maternal use (Golub 2005). Use of amphetamines during pregnancy may lead to an increased risk of premature birth and low birth weight; newborns may experience symptoms of withdrawal. Behavioral problems may also occur later in childhood (LaGasse 2012).

Controlled Substance C-II

◆ **Methamphetamine Hydrochloride** *see* Methamphetamine *on page 986*

MethazolAMIDE (meth a ZOE la mide)

Brand Names: US Neptazane [DSC]

Pharmacologic Category Carbonic Anhydrase Inhibitor; Diuretic, Carbonic Anhydrase Inhibitor; Ophthalmic Agent, Antiglaucoma

Use Glaucoma: Treatment of chronic open-angle or secondary glaucoma; short-term therapy of acute angle-closure glaucoma prior to surgery

Local Anesthetic/Vasoconstrictor Precautions No information available to require special precautions

Effects on Dental Treatment Key adverse event(s) related to dental treatment: Xerostomia (normal salivary flow resumes upon discontinuation) and metallic taste.

Effects on Bleeding No information available to require special precautions

Adverse Reactions Frequency not defined.

Central nervous system: Confusion, drowsiness, fatigue, flaccid paralysis, malaise, paresthesia, seizure

Dermatologic: Erythema multiforme, skin photosensitivity, skin rash, Stevens-Johnson syndrome, toxic epidermal necrolysis, urticaria

Endocrine & metabolic: Electrolyte disturbance, glycosuria, metabolic acidosis

Gastrointestinal: Decreased appetite, diarrhea, dysgeusia, melena, nausea, vomiting

Genitourinary: Crystalluria, hematuria

Hematologic & oncologic: Agranulocytosis, aplastic anemia, bone marrow depression, hemolytic anemia, immune thrombocytopenia, leukopenia, pancytopenia

Hepatic: Fulminant hepatic necrosis, hepatic insufficiency

Hypersensitivity: Anaphylaxis, hypersensitivity reaction

Ophthalmic: Myopia

Otic: Auditory disturbance, tinnitus

Renal: Nephrolithiasis, polyuria

Miscellaneous: Fever

Mechanism of Action Noncompetitive inhibition of the enzyme carbonic anhydrase; thought that carbonic anhydrase is located at the luminal border of cells of the proximal tubule. When the enzyme is inhibited, there is an increase in urine volume and a change to an alkaline pH with a subsequent decrease in the excretion of titratable acid and ammonia.

Pharmacodynamics/Kinetics

Onset of Action Slow in comparison with acetazolamide (2-4 hours); Peak effect: 6-8 hours

Duration of Action 10-18 hours

Half-life Elimination ~14 hours

Pregnancy Risk Factor C

Pregnancy Considerations Adverse events were observed in animal reproduction studies.

◆ **Methen/M-Blue/Sal/Na Phos/Hyos** *see* Methenamine, Sodium Phosphate Monobasic, Phenyl Salicylate, Methylene Blue, and Hyoscyamine *on page 987*

Methenamine (meth EN a meen)

Brand Names: US Hiprex

Brand Names: Canada Mandelamine

Pharmacologic Category Antibiotic, Miscellaneous

Use Urinary tract infection, prophylaxis/suppression: Prophylaxis or suppression of recurrent urinary tract infections when long-term therapy is indicated and infection has been eradicated by appropriate antimicrobial treatment

Local Anesthetic/Vasoconstrictor Precautions No information available to require special precautions

Effects on Dental Treatment No significant effects or complications reported

Effects on Bleeding No information available to require special precautions

Adverse Reactions Large doses (higher than recommended) have resulted in bladder irritation, frequent/painful micturition, albuminuria, and hematuria.

<4%:

Dermatologic: Pruritus, skin rash

Gastrointestinal: Dyspepsia, nausea, vomiting

<1%, postmarketing, and/or case reports: Increased serum ALT (reversible), increased serum AST (reversible)

Mechanism of Action Methenamine is hydrolyzed to formaldehyde and ammonia in acidic urine; formaldehyde has nonspecific bactericidal action. Other components, hippuric acid or mandelic acid, aid in maintaining urine acidity and may aid in suppressing bacteria.

Pharmacodynamics/Kinetics

Half-life Elimination ~4 hours (Allgén 1979)

Time to Peak 1 to 2 hours (Allgén 1979)

Pregnancy Risk Factor C (methenamine mandelate)

Pregnancy Considerations

Methenamine crosses the placenta and distributes to amniotic fluid (Allgén 1979). An increased risk of adverse fetal effects has not been observed in available studies (Furness 1975; Gordon 1972; Heinonen 1977). Methenamine use has been shown to interfere with urine estriol concentrations if measured via acid hydrolysis. Use of enzyme hydrolysis prevents this lab interference.

◆ **Methenamine Hippurate** *see* Methenamine *on page 987*

◆ **Methenamine Mandelate** *see* Methenamine *on page 987*

Methenamine, Phenyl Salicylate, Methylene Blue, Benzoic Acid, and Hyoscyamine

(meth EN a meen, fen nil sa LIS i late, METH i leen bloo, ben ZOE ik AS id & hye oh SYE a meen)

Brand Names: US Hyophen; Prosed/DS [DSC]; Urophen MB [DSC]

Pharmacologic Category Antibiotic, Miscellaneous

Use Urinary tract discomfort secondary to hypermotility resulting from infection or diagnostic procedures

Local Anesthetic/Vasoconstrictor Precautions No information available to require special precautions

Effects on Dental Treatment Key adverse event(s) related to dental treatment: Xerostomia (normal salivary flow resumes upon discontinuation).

Effects on Bleeding No information available to require special precautions

Adverse Reactions Frequency not defined.

Cardiovascular: Flushing, tachycardia

Central nervous system: Dizziness

Gastrointestinal: Fecal discoloration (blue), nausea, vomiting, xerostomia

Genitourinary: Difficulty in micturition, urinary retention (acute), urine discoloration (blue)

Ophthalmic: Blurred vision

Respiratory: Dyspnea

Pregnancy Risk Factor C

Pregnancy Considerations Reproduction studies have not been conducted with this combination. Methenamine and hyoscyamine cross the placenta.

Methenamine, Sodium Phosphate Monobasic, Phenyl Salicylate, Methylene Blue, and Hyoscyamine

(meth EN a meen, SOW dee um FOS fate mon oh BAY sik, fen nil sa LIS i late, METH i leen bloo, & hye oh SYE a meen)

Brand Names: US Azuphen MB [DSC]; Hyolev MB [DSC]; Phosphasal; Ur N-C [DSC]; Uramit MB [DSC]; Urelle; Uretron D/S; Uribel; Urimar-T; Urin DS; Uro-458; Uro-L [DSC]; Uro-MP; UroAv-81; UroAv-B; Ustell; Uticap; Utira-C; Utrona-C; Vilamit MB; Vilevev MB

Pharmacologic Category Antibiotic, Miscellaneous

Use Treatment of symptoms of irritative voiding; relief of local symptoms associated with urinary tract infections; relief of urinary tract symptoms caused by diagnostic procedures

Local Anesthetic/Vasoconstrictor Precautions No information available to require special precautions

Effects on Dental Treatment Key adverse event(s) related to dental treatment: Xerostomia (normal salivary flow resumes upon discontinuation).

Effects on Bleeding No information available to require special precautions

Adverse Reactions Frequency not defined.

Cardiovascular: Flushing, tachycardia

Central nervous system: Dizziness

Gastrointestinal: Nausea, vomiting, xerostomia

Genitourinary: Acute urinary retention, difficulty in micturition, urine discoloration (blue)

Ophthalmic: Blurred vision

Respiratory: Dyspnea

Pregnancy Risk Factor C

Pregnancy Considerations Reproduction studies have not been conducted with this combination. Methenamine and hyoscyamine cross the placenta.

◆ **Methergine** *see* Methylergonovine *on page 995*

MethIMAzole (meth IM a zole)

Related Information

Endocrine Disorders and Pregnancy *on page 1684*

Brand Names: US Tapazole

Brand Names: Canada APO-Methimazole; DOM-Methimazole [DSC]; Mar-Methimazole; PHL-Methimazole [DSC]; Tapazole

Pharmacologic Category Antithyroid Agent; Thioamide

Use Hyperthyroidism: Treatment of hyperthyroidism in patients with Graves disease or toxic multinodular goiter for whom surgery or radioactive iodine therapy is not appropriate; amelioration of hyperthyroid symptoms in preparation for thyroidectomy or radioactive iodine therapy.

Local Anesthetic/Vasoconstrictor Precautions No information available to require special precautions

Effects on Dental Treatment Key adverse event(s) related to dental treatment: Abnormal taste and salivary gland swelling.

Effects on Bleeding No information available to require special precautions

Adverse Reactions

Frequency not defined:

Cardiovascular: Edema, periarteritis

Central nervous system: Drowsiness, drug fever, headache, neuritis, paresthesia, vertigo

Dermatologic: Alopecia, pruritus, skin pigmentation, skin rash, urticaria

Endocrine & metabolic: Hypoglycemic coma, hypothyroidism, insulin autoimmune syndrome

Gastrointestinal: Ageusia, enlargement of salivary glands, epigastric distress, nausea, vomiting

Hematologic & oncologic: Agranulocytosis, aplastic anemia, granulocytopenia, hypoprothrombinemia, leukopenia, lymphadenopathy, thrombocytopenia

Hepatic: Hepatitis, jaundice

Neuromuscular & skeletal: Arthralgia, lupus-like syndrome, myalgia

Renal: Nephritis

Postmarketing: Acute hepatic failure, acute pancreatitis, acute renal injury, cerebral vasculitis, glomerulonephritis, hepatotoxicity, hypersensitivity angiitis, neuropathy, pulmonary alveolar hemorrhage, vasculitis (including ANCA positive)

Mechanism of Action Inhibits the synthesis of thyroid hormones by blocking the oxidation of iodine in the thyroid gland; blocks synthesis of thyroxine and triiodothyronine (T_3); does not inactivate circulating T_4 and T_3

Pharmacodynamics/Kinetics

Onset of Action Antithyroid: 12 to 18 hours (Clark 2006)

Duration of Action 36 to 72 hours (Clark 2006)

Half-life Elimination 4 to 6 hours (Clark 2006)

Time to Peak Serum: 1 to 2 hours (Clark 2006)

Reproductive Considerations

Females taking methimazole should notify their health care provider immediately once pregnancy is suspected (Alexander 2017).

Pregnancy Considerations Methimazole crosses the placenta.

Birth defects have been observed in neonates exposed to maternal methimazole in the first trimester of pregnancy and include anomalies of the upper gastrointestinal tract (esophageal atresia or tracheoesophageal fistula), respiratory tract (choanal atresia), skin (aplasia cutis), and facial dysmorphism. Additional abdominal wall defects (umbilicocele), ventricular septal defects, and defects of the eye and urinary system have also been reported (Alexander 2017). Hypothyroidism may occur in the newborn.

Uncontrolled maternal hyperthyroidism may result in adverse neonatal and maternal outcomes. Antithyroid drugs are the treatment of choice for the control of hyperthyroidism during pregnancy, although recommendations for specific agents vary by guideline (ACOG 2015; Alexander 2017; De Groot 2012). Dose requirements of methimazole may be decreased as pregnancy progresses. To prevent adverse pregnancy outcomes, maternal TT4/FT4 should be at or just above the pregnancy specific upper limit of normal (Alexander 2017).

◆ **Methitest** *see* MethylTESTOSTERone *on page 1006*

◆ **Meth/Meblue/Sod Phos/Psal/Hyos** *see* Methenamine, Sodium Phosphate Monobasic, Phenyl Salicylate, Methylene Blue, and Hyoscyamine *on page 987*

Methocarbamol (meth oh KAR ba mole)

Related Information

Temporomandibular Dysfunction (TMD), Chronic Pain, and Fibromyalgia *on page 1773*

Brand Names: US Robaxin; Robaxin-750

Brand Names: Canada Methocarbamol Omega; PMS-Methocarbamol [DSC]; Robaximol

Generic Availability (US) Yes

Pharmacologic Category Skeletal Muscle Relaxant

Dental Use Treatment of muscle spasm associated with acute temporomandibular joint pain (TMJ)

Use Muscle spasm: Adjunctive treatment of muscle spasm associated with acute painful musculoskeletal conditions.

Local Anesthetic/Vasoconstrictor Precautions No information available to require special precautions

Effects on Dental Treatment Key adverse event(s) related to dental treatment: Metallic taste.

Effects on Bleeding No information available to require special precautions

Adverse Reactions

Frequency not defined:

Cardiovascular: Bradycardia, flushing, hypotension, syncope, thrombophlebitis

Central nervous system: Amnesia, ataxia, confusion, dizziness, drowsiness, headache, insomnia, metallic taste, sedation, seizure, vertigo

Dermatologic: Pruritus, skin rash, urticaria

Gastrointestinal: Dyspepsia, nausea, vomiting

Hematologic & oncologic: Leukopenia

Hepatic: Cholestatic jaundice, jaundice

Hypersensitivity: Anaphylaxis, angioedema, hypersensitivity reaction

Local: Local skin exfoliation (injection), pain at injection site

Ophthalmic: Blurred vision, conjunctivitis, diplopia, nystagmus

Respiratory: Nasal congestion

Miscellaneous: Fever

Dental Usual Dosage Muscle spasm associated with acute TMJ pain: Children ≥16 years and Adults: Oral: 1.5 g 4 times/day for 2-3 days (up to 8 g/day may be given in severe conditions), then decrease to 4-4.5 g/day in 3-6 divided doses

Dosing

Adult

Muscle spasm:

Note: For skeletal muscle spasm and/or pain (eg, low back pain, neck pain) with muscle spasm, usually in combination with a nonsteroidal anti-inflammatory drug and/or acetaminophen (ACP [Chou 2017]; van Tulder 2003). In general, muscle relaxants should be used temporarily (eg, for a few days or intermittently for a few days when needed) (APS 2016).

Oral: 1.5 g 3 to 4 times daily for 2 to 3 days (up to 8 g/day may be given in severe conditions), then decrease to 750 mg to 1.5 g 3 to 4 times daily (up to 4.5 g/day) (Emrich 2015; Friedman 2018; manufacturer's labeling).

IM, IV: Initial: 1 g; may repeat every 8 hours; maximum dose: 3 g/day for no more than 3 consecutive days. If condition persists, may repeat course of therapy after a drug-free interval of 48 hours.

Geriatric Avoid use (Beers Criteria [AGS 2019]).

Renal Impairment: Adult No dosage adjustment provided in manufacturer's labeling. However, administration of the parenteral formulation is contraindicated in patients with renal dysfunction due to the presence of polyethylene glycol.

Hepatic Impairment: Adult No dosage adjustment provided in manufacturer's labeling. However, elimination may be reduced in patients with cirrhosis.

Pediatric

Muscle spasm: Adolescents ≥16 years: Oral: 1,500 mg 4 times daily for 2 to 3 days; maximum daily dose: 8 g/**day** (reserved for severe conditions); then decrease dose to 4,000 to 4,500 mg/day in 3 to 6 divided doses (ie, 1,000 mg 4 times daily or 750 mg every 4 hours or 1,500 mg 3 times/day)

Tetanus: Note: Use has generally been replaced by other agents (eg, benzodiazepines) (Hsu 2001): Infants, Children, and Adolescents: IV: 15 mg/kg/dose or 500 mg/$\mathbf{m^2}$/dose, may repeat every 6 hours as needed; usual adult dose: 1,000 to 2,000 mg/dose; maximum total dose: 1.8 g/$\mathbf{m^2}$ for 3 days; in adults, injection is not recommended for use longer than 3 days

Renal Impairment: Pediatric Children and Adolescents: There are no dosage adjustments provided in the manufacturer's labeling; however, administration of the parenteral formulation is contraindicated in patients with renal dysfunction due to the presence of polyethylene glycol.

Hepatic Impairment: Pediatric There are no dosage adjustments provided in the manufacturer's labeling; however, elimination may be reduced in patients with cirrhosis.

Mechanism of Action Causes skeletal muscle relaxation by general CNS depression

Contraindications Hypersensitivity to methocarbamol or any component of the formulation; renal impairment (injection formulation)

Warnings/Precautions May cause CNS depression, which may impair physical or mental abilities; patients must be cautioned about performing tasks which require mental alertness (eg, operating machinery or driving). Effects may be potentiated when used with other sedative drugs or ethanol. Plasma protein binding and clearance are decreased and the half-life is increased in patients with hepatic impairment. Injection: Contraindicated in renal impairment. Contains polyethylene glycol. Rate of injection should not exceed 3 mL/minute; solution is hypertonic; avoid extravasation. Use with caution in patients with a history of seizures. Use caution with hepatic impairment. Recommended only for the treatment of tetanus in pediatric patients.

Drug Interactions

Metabolism/Transport Effects None known.

Avoid Concomitant Use

Avoid concomitant use of Methocarbamol with any of the following: Azelastine (Nasal); Bromperidol; Orphenadrine; Oxomemazine; Paraldehyde; Thalidomide

Increased Effect/Toxicity

Methocarbamol may increase the levels/effects of: Alcohol (Ethyl); Azelastine (Nasal); Blonanserin; Botulinum Toxin-Containing Products; Brexanolone; Buprenorphine; CNS Depressants; Flunitrazepam; Methotrimeprazine; MetyroSINE; Opioid Agonists; Orphenadrine; OxyCODONE; Paraldehyde; Piribedil; Pramipexole; ROPINIRole; Rotigotine; Suvorexant; Thalidomide; Zolpidem

The levels/effects of Methocarbamol may be increased by: Alizapride; Brimonidine (Topical); Bromopride; Bromperidol; Cannabidiol; Cannabis; Chlormethiazole; Chlorphenesin Carbamate; Dimethindene (Topical); Doxylamine; Dronabinol; Droperidol; Eperisone; Esketamine; HydrOXYzine; Kava Kava; Lemborexant; Lisuride; Lofexidine; Magnesium Sulfate; Methotrimeprazine; Metoclopramide; Minocycline (Systemic); Nabilone; Oxomemazine; Perampanel; Rufinamide; Sodium Oxybate; Tetrahydrocannabinol; Tetrahydrocannabinol and Cannabidiol; Tolperisone; Trimeprazine

Decreased Effect

Methocarbamol may decrease the levels/effects of: Pyridostigmine

Pharmacodynamics/Kinetics

Onset of Action Muscle relaxation: Oral: ~30 minutes

Half-life Elimination 1 to 2 hours

Time to Peak Serum: Oral: 1 to 2 hours

Pregnancy Considerations Animal reproduction studies have not been conducted. The manufacturer notes that fetal and congenital abnormalities have been reported following in utero exposure (Hall 1982).

Breastfeeding Considerations It is not known if methocarbamol is present in breast milk. The manufacturer recommends that caution be exercised when administering methocarbamol to breastfeeding women.

Dosage Forms: US

Solution, Injection:

Robaxin: 1000 mg/10 mL (10 mL)
Generic: 1000 mg/10 mL (10 mL)

Solution, Injection [preservative free]:

Robaxin: 1000 mg/10 mL (10 mL)
Generic: 1000 mg/10 mL (10 mL)

Tablet, Oral:

Robaxin: 500 mg
Robaxin-750: 750 mg
Generic: 500 mg, 750 mg

Dosage Forms: Canada

Solution, Injection:

Robaximol: 100 mg/mL (10 mL)
Generic: 100 mg/mL (10 mL)

Methohexital (meth oh HEKS i tal)

Brand Names: US Brevital Sodium

Pharmacologic Category Barbiturate; General Anesthetic

Use

Induction of anesthesia: Induction of anesthesia prior to the use of other general anesthetic agents; to supplement other anesthetic agents for longer surgical procedures. **Note:** Use to maintain anesthesia using either the manufacturer recommended continuous infusion or intermittent dosing has fallen out of favor.

Procedural sedation: Short surgical, diagnostic, or therapeutic procedures associated with minimal painful stimuli.

Local Anesthetic/Vasoconstrictor Precautions No information available to require special precautions

Effects on Dental Treatment No significant effects or complications reported

Effects on Bleeding No information available to require special precautions

Adverse Reactions Frequency not defined.

Cardiovascular: Circulatory depression, circulatory shock, hypotension, local thrombophlebitis, tachycardia

Central nervous system: Anxiety, delirium (emergence), headache, involuntary muscle movements, neuropathy (adjacent to injection site), radial nerve palsy, restlessness, seizure, twitching

Dermatologic: Erythema, pruritus, urticaria

Gastrointestinal: Abdominal pain, hiccups, nausea, salivation, vomiting

Hepatic: Increased serum transaminases

Local: Pain at injection site

Neuromuscular & skeletal: Laryngospasm, muscle rigidity, tremor

Respiratory: Apnea, bronchospasm, cough, dyspnea, respiratory depression, rhinitis

<1%, postmarketing, and/or case reports: Anaphylaxis

Mechanism of Action Methohexital is an ultra short-acting IV barbiturate anesthetic. Barbiturates depress the sensory cortex, decrease motor activity, and alter cerebellar function producing drowsiness, sedation, and hypnosis.

Pharmacodynamics/Kinetics

Onset of Action IV: Immediate; IM (pediatrics): 2 to 10 minutes; Rectal (pediatrics): 5 to 15 minutes

Duration of Action Single dose:

IM: 1 to 1.5 hours

IV: Time to clinical recovery (ie, awake time, sitting and standing steadily, duration of amnesia): 5 to 15 minutes (psychomotor impairment may continue for up to 8 hours) (Barash 2009; Fredman 1994; Korttila 1975)

Rectal (pediatrics): 45 to 60 minutes (Cote 1994)

Half-life Elimination 1.6 to 3.9 hours (Ghoneim 1985)

Pregnancy Considerations Methohexital crosses the placenta.

Based on animal data, repeated or prolonged use of general anesthetic and sedation medications that block N-methyl-D-aspartate (NMDA) receptors and/or potentiate gamma-aminobutyric acid (GABA) activity may affect brain development. Evaluate benefits and potential risks of fetal exposure to methohexital when duration of surgery is expected to be >3 hours (Olutoye 2018).

Use of methohexital in obstetric anesthesia has been described (Holdcroft 1974; Lee 1966; Verma 1985). However, other agents are more commonly used (ACOG 209 2019; Devroe 2015).

The ACOG recommends that pregnant women should not be denied medically necessary surgery, regardless of trimester. If the procedure is elective, it should be delayed until after delivery (ACOG 775 2019).

Controlled Substance C-IV

◆ **Methohexital Sodium** *see* Methohexital *on page 989*

Methotrexate (meth oh TREKS ate)

Related Information

Rheumatoid Arthritis, Osteoarthritis, and Osteoporosis *on page 1697*

Brand Names: US Otrexup; Rasuvo; Rheumatrex [DSC]; Trexall; Xatmep

Brand Names: Canada JAMP-Methotrexate; Metoject; PMS-Methotrexate; RATIO-Methotrexate Sodium [DSC]

Pharmacologic Category Antineoplastic Agent, Antimetabolite (Antifolate); Antirheumatic, Disease Modifying; Immunosuppressant Agent

Use

Oncology uses: Acute lymphoblastic leukemia (ALL) maintenance treatment, ALL meningeal leukemia (preservative-free only; prophylaxis and treatment); treatment of trophoblastic neoplasms (gestational choriocarcinoma, chorioadenoma destruens and hydatidiform mole), breast cancer, head and neck cancer (epidermoid), cutaneous T-Cell lymphoma (advanced mycosis fungoides), lung cancer (squamous cell and small cell), relapsed/refractory or advanced non-Hodgkin lymphomas (NHL), osteosarcoma (preservative-free only).

Nononcology uses: Treatment of psoriasis (severe, recalcitrant, disabling) that is unresponsive to other therapies; severe, active rheumatoid arthritis (RA) that is unresponsive to or intolerant of first-line therapy including full dose nonsteroidal anti-inflammatory agents (NSAIDs); active polyarticular-course juvenile idiopathic arthritis (pJIA) that is unresponsive to or intolerant of first-line therapy including full dose NSAIDs.

Limitations of use: Otrexup and Rasuvo are not indicated for the treatment of neoplastic diseases.

Guideline recommendations: Rheumatoid arthritis: Treatment initiation with a disease-modifying antirheumatic drug (DMARD) is recommended in DMARD-naïve patients with either early rheumatoid arthritis (RA) (disease duration <6 months) or established RA (disease duration ≥6 months). Methotrexate is the preferred initial DMARD for most early or established RA patients (Singh [ACR 2016]).

Local Anesthetic/Vasoconstrictor Precautions No information available to require special precautions

Effects on Dental Treatment Key adverse event(s) related to dental treatment: Ulcerative stomatitis, gingivitis, glossitis, and mucositis (dose dependent; appears 3-7 days post-therapy and resolves within 2 weeks). Dental professionals should note before prescribing NSAIDS that concurrent administration with methotrexate may cause severe bone marrow suppression, aplastic anemia, and GI toxicity. Although the risk is lower at the methotrexate dosages used for rheumatoid conditions/psoriasis, the addition of an NSAID or salicylate may still lead to unexpected toxicities; caution is warranted.

Effects on Bleeding Suppression of hematopoiesis may cause myelosuppression including thrombocytopenia. Medical consult recommended.

Adverse Reactions Note: Adverse reactions vary by route and dosage. Frequency not always defined.

Cardiovascular: Arterial thrombosis, cerebral thrombosis, chest pain, deep vein thrombosis, hypotension, pericardial effusion, pericarditis, plaque erosion (psoriasis), pulmonary embolism, retinal thrombosis, thrombophlebitis, vasculitis

Dermatologic: Alopecia (≤10%), burning sensation of skin (psoriasis 3% to 10%), skin photosensitivity (3% to 10%), skin rash (≤3%), dermatitis (rheumatoid arthritis 1% to 3%), pruritus (rheumatoid arthritis 1% to 3%), acne vulgaris, dermal ulcer, diaphoresis, ecchymoses, erythema multiforme, erythematous rash, exfoliative dermatitis, furunculosis, hyperpigmentation, hypopigmentation, skin abnormalities related to radiation recall, skin necrosis, Stevens-Johnson syndrome, telangiectasia, toxic epidermal necrolysis, urticaria

Endocrine & metabolic: Decreased libido, decreased serum albumin, diabetes mellitus, gynecomastia, menstrual disease

Gastrointestinal: Diarrhea (≤11%), nausea and vomiting (≤11%), stomatitis (2% to 10%), abdominal distress, anorexia, aphthous stomatitis, enteritis, gastrointestinal hemorrhage, gingivitis, hematemesis, intestinal perforation, melena, pancreatitis

Genitourinary: Azotemia, cystitis, defective oogenesis, defective spermatogenesis, dysuria, hematuria, impotence, infertility, oligospermia, proteinuria, severe renal disease, vaginal discharge

Hematologic & oncologic: Thrombocytopenia (rheumatoid arthritis 3% to 10%; platelet count <100,000/mm^3), leukopenia (1% to 3%; WBC <3000/mm^3), pancytopenia (rheumatoid arthritis 1% to 3%), agranulocytosis, anemia, aplastic anemia, bone marrow depression (nadir: 7-10 days), decreased hematocrit, eosinophilia, gastric ulcer, hypogammaglobulinemia, lymphadenopathy, lymphoma, lymphoproliferative disorder, neutropenia, non-Hodgkin's lymphoma (in patients receiving low-dose oral methotrexate), tumor lysis syndrome

Hepatic: Increased liver enzymes (14% to 15%), cirrhosis (chronic therapy), hepatic failure, hepatic fibrosis (chronic therapy), hepatitis (acute), hepatotoxicity

Hypersensitivity: Anaphylactoid reaction

Infection: Cryptococcosis, cytomegalovirus disease (including cytomegaloviral pneumonia, sepsis, nocardiosis), herpes simplex infection, herpes zoster, histoplasmosis, infection, vaccinia (disseminated; following smallpox immunization)

Nervous system: Dizziness (≤3%), headache (pJIA 1%), abnormal cranial sensation, brain disease, chemical arachnoiditis (intrathecal; acute), chills, cognitive dysfunction (has been reported at low dosage), drowsiness, fatigue, leukoencephalopathy (intravenous administration after craniospinal irradiation or repeated high-dose therapy; may be chronic), malaise, mood changes (has been reported at low dosage), neurological signs and symptoms (at high dosages; including confusion, hemiparesis, transient blindness, seizures, and coma), severe neurotoxicity (reported with unexpectedly increased frequency among pediatric patients with acute lymphoblastic leukemia who were treated with intermediate-dose intravenous methotrexate), speech disturbance

Neuromuscular & skeletal: Arthralgia, myalgia, myelopathy (subacute), osteonecrosis (with radiotherapy), osteoporosis

Ophthalmic: Blurred vision, conjunctivitis, eye pain, visual disturbance

Otic: Tinnitus

Renal: Renal failure

Respiratory: Interstitial pneumonitis (rheumatoid arthritis 1%), chronic obstructive pulmonary disease, cough, epistaxis, pharyngitis, pneumonia (including *Pneumocystis jirovecii*), pulmonary alveolitis, pulmonary disease, pulmonary fibrosis, respiratory failure, upper respiratory tract infection

Miscellaneous: Fever, nodule, tissue necrosis

<1%, postmarketing, and/or case reports: Acute respiratory distress (Morgan 2011), bone fracture (stress), cerebrovascular accident (Morgan 2011), mesenteric ischemia (acute; Morgan 2011), skin carcinoma (Solomon 2020)

Mechanism of Action

Methotrexate is a folate antimetabolite that inhibits DNA synthesis, repair, and cellular replication. Methotrexate irreversibly binds to and inhibits dihydrofolate reductase, inhibiting the formation of reduced folates, and thymidylate synthetase, resulting in inhibition of purine and thymidylic acid synthesis, thus interfering with DNA synthesis, repair, and cellular replication. Methotrexate is cell cycle specific for the S phase of the cycle. Actively proliferative tissues are more susceptible to the effects of methotrexate.

The mechanism in the treatment of rheumatoid arthritis and polyarticular-course juvenile idiopathic arthritis is unknown, but may affect immune function. In psoriasis, methotrexate is thought to target rapidly proliferating epithelial cells in the skin.

In Crohn disease, it may have immune modulator and anti-inflammatory activity.

Pharmacodynamics/Kinetics

Onset of Action Antirheumatic: 3 to 6 weeks; additional improvement may continue longer than 12 weeks

Half-life Elimination

Children: ALL: 0.7 to 5.8 hours (dose range: 6.3 to 30 mg/m^2); pJIA: 0.9 to 2.3 hours (dose range: 3.75 to 26.2 mg/m^2)

Adults: Low dose: 3 to 10 hours; High dose: 8 to 15 hours

Time to Peak Serum: Oral: Children: 0.7 to 4 hours (reported for a 15 mg/m^2 dose); Adults: 0.75 to 6 hours; Children and Adults: IM: 30 to 60 minutes

Reproductive Considerations

[US Boxed Warning]: Use in rheumatoid arthritis, polyarticular-course juvenile idiopathic arthritis, and psoriasis is contraindicated in pregnancy. It is currently recommended that females with inflammatory bowel disease, psoriasis, or rheumatic and musculoskeletal diseases discontinue methotrexate 3 months prior to a planned pregnancy (ACR [Sammaritano 2020]; Mahadevan 2019; Rademaker 2018).

When methotrexate is used for the treatment of rheumatic and musculoskeletal diseases in women undergoing ovarian stimulation for oocyte retrieval or embryo cryopreservation, methotrexate may be continued in patients whose condition is stable and discontinuation of treatment may lead to uncontrolled disease (ACR [Sammaritano 2020]).

[US Boxed Warning]: Verify the pregnancy status of females of reproductive potential prior to initiating therapy. Advise females and males of reproductive potential to use effective contraception during and after treatment with methotrexate. Effective contraception is recommended for females of reproductive potential during therapy and for at least 6 months after the final dose. Effective contraception is recommended for males with female partners of reproductive potential during therapy and for at least 3 months after the final dose of methotrexate.

The use of methotrexate may impair fertility and cause menstrual irregularities or oligospermia during treatment and following therapy. It is not known if infertility may be reversed in all affected males or females.

Use of methotrexate may be considered for males with rheumatic and musculoskeletal diseases or psoriasis who are planning to father a child (recommendation based on limited human data) (ACR [Sammaritano 2020]; Lamb 2019; Rademaker 2018).

Pregnancy Considerations Methotrexate crosses the placenta (Schleuning 1987).

[US Boxed Warning]: Methotrexate can cause embryo-fetal toxicity, including fetal death. Following exposure during the first trimester, methotrexate may increase the risk of spontaneous abortion, skull anomalies, facial dysmorphism, CNS, limb and cardiac abnormalities; intellectual impairment may also occur. Intrauterine growth restriction and functional abnormalities may occur following second or third trimester exposure.

[US Boxed Warning]: Consider the benefits and risks of methotrexate and risks to the fetus when prescribing methotrexate to a pregnant patient with a neoplastic disease. Methotrexate is approved for the treatment of trophoblastic neoplasms (gestational choriocarcinoma, chorioadenoma destruens, and hydatidiform mole). Methotrexate is recommended for the medical management of ectopic pregnancy in appropriately selected patients (ACOG 193 2018; ASRM 2013). Methotrexate has been used for the medical termination of intrauterine pregnancy with a gestational age up to 49 days (ACOG 143 2014).

[US Boxed Warning]: Use in rheumatoid arthritis, polyarticular-course juvenile idiopathic arthritis, and psoriasis is contraindicated in pregnancy.

Product Availability RediTrex (methotrexate injection): FDA approved November 2019; anticipated availability is currently unknown. Information pertaining to this product within the monograph is pending revision. Consult the prescribing information for additional information.

◆ **Methotrexate Sodium** *see* Methotrexate *on page 990*

◆ **Methotrexatum** *see* Methotrexate *on page 990*

Methotrimeprazine (meth oh trye MEP ra zeen)

Brand Names: Canada Methoprazine; NOVO-Meprazine [DSC]; Nozinan; PMS-Methotrimeprazine [DSC]

Pharmacologic Category Analgesic, Nonopioid; Antimanic Agent; First Generation (Typical) Antipsychotic

Use Note: Not approved in the United States.

Anxiety/tension (tablet only): Treatment of conditions associated with anxiety and tension (eg, autonomic disturbances, personality disturbances, emotional disorders secondary to physical conditions).

Insomnia: Management of insomnia, sedation.

Nausea/vomiting: Management of nausea and vomiting.

Pain: Management of pain, including pain caused by neuralgia or cancer and as adjunct to general anesthesia (pre- and postoperatively).

Psychiatric disorders: Treatment of schizophrenia, senile psychosis, and manic-depressive syndromes.

Local Anesthetic/Vasoconstrictor Precautions Methotrimeprazine is one of the drugs confirmed to prolong the QT interval and is accepted as having a risk of causing torsade de pointes. The risk of drug-induced torsade de pointes is extremely low when a single QT interval prolonging drug is prescribed. In terms of epinephrine, it is not known what effect vasoconstrictors in the local anesthetic regimen will have in patients with a known history of congenital prolonged QT interval or in patients taking any medication that prolongs the QT interval. Until more information is obtained, it is suggested that the clinician consult with the physician prior to the use of a vasoconstrictor in suspected patients, and that the vasoconstrictor (epinephrine, mepivacaine and levonordefrin [Carbocaine® 2% with Neo-Cobefrin®]) be used with caution. See Dental Health Professional Considerations.

Effects on Dental Treatment Key adverse event(s) related to dental treatment: Anticholinergic side effects can cause a reduction of saliva production or secretion, contributing to discomfort and dental disease (ie, caries, oral candidiasis, and periodontal disease). Phenothiazines can cause extrapyramidal reactions which may appear as muscle twitching or increased motor activity of the face, neck, or head.

Effects on Bleeding No information available to require special precautions

Adverse Reactions Frequencies not defined; some reactions listed are based on reports for other agents in this same pharmacologic class, and may not be specifically reported for methotrimeprazine.

Cardiovascular: Orthostatic hypotension, prolonged QT interval on ECG, pulmonary embolism, tachycardia, venous thromboembolism

Dermatologic: Dermatological reaction (allergic skin reaction, skin photosensitivity)

Endocrine & metabolic: Decreased glucose tolerance, diabetic ketoacidosis, hyperglycemia, hyponatremia, SIADH, weight gain

Gastrointestinal: Constipation, necrotizing enterocolitis, xerostomia

Genitourinary: Priapism, urinary retention

Hematologic & oncologic: Agranulocytosis, granulocytopenia, neutropenia

Hepatic: Cholestatic jaundice, hepatic injury (cholestatic, hepatocellular, mixed)

Nervous system: Confusion, delirium, drowsiness, drug-induced extrapyramidal reaction (including akathisia, dystonia, parkinsonism), epilepsy, seizure, tardive dyskinesia

Postmarketing: Accommodation disturbance, antibody development, anxiety, apathy, deposits on or around the surface of the eye (brownish deposits due to accumulation of the drug), disruption of body temperature regulation, dyskinesia (early dyskinesia, including oculogyric crises, torticollis [spasmodic], trismus), ECG changes (depression of ST segment on ECG, U-wave changes, T-wave changes), hyperprolactinemia, leukopenia, mood changes, neuroleptic malignant syndrome, paralytic ileus, torsades de pointes

Mechanism of Action Aliphatic phenothiazine that antagonizes D1 and D2 dopamine receptor subtypes; also binds alpha-1, alpha-2, serotonin (5-HT_1 and 5-HT_2), and muscarinic (M_1 and M_2) receptors (Lal 1993)

Pharmacodynamics/Kinetics

Onset of Action Injection: 1 hour (Nozinan datasheet, Sanofi Aventis New Zealand limited 2010)

Duration of Action 2 to 4 hours (Nozinan datasheet, Sanofi Aventis New Zealand limited 2010)

Half-life Elimination 15 to 30 hours (Dahl 1976)

Time to Peak Serum: IM: 0.5 to 1.5 hours; Oral: 1 to 3 hours (Nozinan datasheet, Sanofi Aventis New Zealand limited 2010)

Reproductive Considerations

Hyperprolactinemia associated with methotrimeprazine may lead to impaired fertility in women. Limited data suggest that methotrimeprazine may also be associated with impaired fertility in men.

Pregnancy Considerations

Information related to use in pregnancy is limited (Callaghan 1966; DeKornfeld 1964). Antipsychotic use during the third trimester of pregnancy has a risk for abnormal muscle movements (extrapyramidal symptoms [EPS]) and withdrawal symptoms in newborns following delivery. Symptoms in the newborn may include agitation, feeding disorder, hypertonia, hypotonia, respiratory distress, somnolence, and tremor; these effects may be self-limiting or require hospitalization.

Product Availability Not available in the US

Dental Health Professional Considerations This drug is known to prolong the QT interval. The QT interval is measured as the time and distance between the Q point of the QRS complex and the end of the T wave in the ECG tracing. After adjustment for heart rate, the QT interval is defined as prolonged if it is more than 450 msec in men and 460 msec in women. A long QT syndrome was first described in the 1950s and 60s as a congenital syndrome involving QT interval prolongation and syncope and sudden death. Some of the congenital long QT syndromes were characterized by a peculiar electrocardiographic appearance of the QRS complex involving a premature atria beat followed by a pause, then a subsequent sinus beat showing marked QT prolongation and deformity. This type of cardiac arrhythmia was originally termed "torsade de pointes" (translated from the French as "twisting of the points").

Prolongation of the QT interval is thought to result from delayed ventricular repolarization. The repolarization process within the myocardial cell is due to the efflux of intracellular potassium. The channels associated with this current can be blocked by many drugs and predispose the electrical propagation cycle to torsade de pointes.

Methotrimeprazine is one of the drugs confirmed to prolong the QT interval and is accepted as having a risk of causing torsade de pointes. The risk of drug-induced torsade de pointes is extremely low when a single QT interval prolonging drug is prescribed. In terms of epinephrine, it is not known what effect vasoconstrictors in the local anesthetic regimen will have in patients with a known history of congenital prolonged QT interval or in patients taking any medication that prolongs the QT interval. Until more information is obtained, it is suggested that the clinician consult with the physician prior to the use of a vasoconstrictor in suspected patients, and that the vasoconstrictor (epinephrine, levonordefrin [Neo-Cobefrin®]) be used with caution.

◆ **Methotrimeprazine Hydrochloride** *see* Methotrimeprazine *on page 992*

◆ **Methoxy Peg-Epoetin Beta** *see* Methoxy Polyethylene Glycol-Epoetin Beta *on page 993*

Methoxy Polyethylene Glycol-Epoetin Beta (meth OX ee pol i ETH i leen GLY kol e POE e tin BAY ta)

Brand Names: US Mircera

Pharmacologic Category Colony Stimulating Factor; Erythropoiesis-Stimulating Agent (ESA); Hematopoietic Agent

Use

Anemia: Treatment of anemia associated with chronic kidney disease (CKD) in adult patients on dialysis, adult patients not on dialysis, and in pediatric patients 5 to 17 years of age on hemodialysis who are converting from another erythropoiesis-stimulating agent (ESA) after their hemoglobin level was stabilized with an ESA.

Limitations of use: Not indicated and is not recommended in the treatment of anemia due to cancer chemotherapy or as a substitute for RBC transfusions in patients who require immediate correction of anemia; has not been shown to improve symptoms, physical functioning or health-related quality of life.

Local Anesthetic/Vasoconstrictor Precautions

No information available to require special precautions

Effects on Dental Treatment No significant effects or complications reported

Effects on Bleeding Although erythropoiesis-stimulating agents have been associated with thromboembolic events, there is no information available to require special precautions for dental procedures.

Adverse Reactions

>10%:

Cardiovascular: Exacerbation of hypertension (27%), hypertension (13% to 19%)

Central nervous system: Headache (children and adolescents: 22%; adults: 9%)

Gastrointestinal: Diarrhea (adults: 11%), vomiting (6% to 11%)

Respiratory: Nasopharyngitis (children and adolescents: 22%; adults: 11%)

1% to 10%:

Cardiovascular: Procedural hypotension (adults: 8%), thrombosis of arteriovenous shunt used for hemodialysis (5% to 6%; arteriovenous fistula), arteriovenous fistula site complication (adults: 5%), hypotension (adults: 5%), thrombosis (children and adolescents: 5%; in device)

Endocrine & metabolic: Hypervolemia (adults: 7%), hyperkalemia (children and adolescents: 6%)

Gastrointestinal: Abdominal pain (children and adolescents: 8%), constipation (adults: 5%), gastrointestinal hemorrhage (adults: 1%; serious)

Genitourinary: Urinary tract infection (adults: 5%)

Hematologic & oncologic: Thrombocytopenia (children and adolescents: 6%), hemorrhage (adults: 5%; serious)

Infection: Infection (children and adolescents: 6%; device-related)

Neuromuscular & skeletal: Muscle spasm (adults: 8%), back pain (adults: 6%), limb pain (adults: 5%)

Respiratory: Bronchitis (children and adolescents: 9%), upper respiratory tract infection (adults: 9%), cough (6%), pharyngitis (children and adolescents: 6%)

Miscellaneous: Fever (children and adolescents: 6%)

<1%, postmarketing, and/or case reports: Anaphylaxis, angioedema, bronchospasm, erythema multiforme, hypertensive encephalopathy, pruritus, pure red cell aplasia, seizure, severe anemia, skin rash, Stevens-Johnson syndrome, tachycardia, toxic epidermal necrolysis, urticaria

Mechanism of Action Methoxy polyethylene glycol-epoetin beta is an erythropoietin receptor activator; erythropoietin is a primary growth factor for erythroid development and is produced in the kidney and released into the bloodstream in response to hypoxia. In response to hypoxia, erythropoietin interacts with erythroid progenitor cells to increase red blood cell production.

Pharmacodynamics/Kinetics

Onset of Action Hemoglobin increase (following a single initial dose): 7 to 15 days

Half-life Elimination

IV: 119 hours

SubQ: 124 hours

Time to Peak SubQ: 72 hours

Pregnancy Considerations Adverse events were observed in some animal reproduction studies. Information related to the use of methoxy polyethylene glycol-epoetin beta during pregnancy is limited.

Prescribing and Access Restrictions Distribution is restricted to certain dialysis centers.

Methscopolamine (meth skoe POL a meen)

Related Information

Dentin Hypersensitivity, Acid Erosion, High Caries Index, Management of Alveolar Osteitis, and Xerostomia *on page 1762*

Pharmacologic Category Anticholinergic Agent

Use

Peptic ulcer (adjunctive): Adjunctive therapy for the treatment of peptic ulcer

Limitations of use: Has not been shown to be effective in contributing to the healing of peptic ulcer, decreasing the rate of recurrence, or preventing complications

Local Anesthetic/Vasoconstrictor Precautions

No information available to require special precautions

Effects on Dental Treatment Key adverse event(s) related to dental treatment: Xerostomia and changes in salivation (normal salivary flow resumes upon discontinuation), and dry throat and nose. Anticholinergic side effects can cause a reduction of saliva production or secretion, contributing to discomfort and dental disease (ie, caries, oral candidiasis and periodontal disease).

Effects on Bleeding No information available to require special precautions

Adverse Reactions Frequency not defined.

Cardiovascular: Palpitation, tachycardia

Central nervous system: Headache, insomnia, flushing, nervousness, drowsiness, dizziness, confusion, fever, CNS stimulation may be produced with large doses

Dermatologic: Dry skin, urticaria

Endocrine & metabolic: Lactation suppressed

Gastrointestinal: Constipation, xerostomia, dry throat, dysphagia, nausea, vomiting, loss of taste

Genitourinary: Impotence, urinary hesitancy, urinary retention

Neuromuscular & skeletal: Weakness

Ocular: Blurred vision, cycloplegia, ocular tension increased, pupil dilation

Respiratory: Dry nose

Miscellaneous: Allergic reaction, diaphoresis decreased, hypersensitivity reactions, anaphylaxis

Mechanism of Action Methscopolamine is a quaternary ammonium derivative of scopolamine that exerts anticholinergic effects, which include reducing the volume and total acid content of gastric secretion, inhibiting gastrointestinal motility and salivary secretion, dilation of the pupil, and inhibition of accommodation that results in blurring of vision.

Pharmacodynamics/Kinetics

Onset of Action ~1 hour

Duration of Action 4 to 6 hours

Pregnancy Risk Factor C

Pregnancy Considerations Animal reproduction studies have not been conducted. Methscopolamine is a derivative of scopolamine. Scopolamine is reported to cross the placenta; fetal toxicity noted in case reports.

◆ **Methscopolamine Bromide, Pamine, Pamine Forte** *see* Methscopolamine *on page 994*

Methsuximide (meth SUKS i mide)

Brand Names: US Celontin

Pharmacologic Category Anticonvulsant, Succinimide

Use Absence (petit mal) seizures, refractory: Control of absence (petit mal) seizures that are refractory to other drugs

Local Anesthetic/Vasoconstrictor Precautions

No information available to require special precautions

Effects on Dental Treatment No significant effects or complications reported

Effects on Bleeding No information available to require special precautions

Adverse Reactions Frequency not defined.

Cardiovascular: Hyperemia

Central nervous system: Aggressiveness, ataxia, confusion, depression, dizziness, drowsiness, hallucinations (auditory), headache, hypochondriacal behavior, insomnia, irritability, mental instability, mental slowness, nervousness, psychosis, suicidal behavior

Dermatologic: Pruritus, rash, Stevens-Johnson syndrome, urticaria

Gastrointestinal: Abdominal pain, anorexia, constipation, diarrhea, epigastric pain, nausea, vomiting, weight loss

Genitourinary: Hematuria (microscopic), proteinuria

Hematologic: Eosinophilia, leukopenia, monocytosis, pancytopenia

Ocular: Blurred vision, periorbital edema, photophobia

Miscellaneous: Hiccups, systemic lupus erythematosus

Mechanism of Action Increases the seizure threshold and suppresses paroxysmal spike-and-wave pattern in absence seizures; depresses nerve transmission in the motor cortex

Pharmacodynamics/Kinetics

Half-life Elimination 2 to 4 hours

N-desmethylmethsuximide: Children: 26 hours; Adults: 28 to 80 hours

Time to Peak Serum: 1 to 3 hours

Reproductive Considerations

For women with epilepsy who are planning a pregnancy in advance, baseline serum concentrations should be measured once or twice prior to pregnancy during a period when seizure control is optimal (Patsalos 2008; Patsalos 2018).

Pregnancy Considerations

Epilepsy itself, the number of medications, genetic factors, or a combination of these may influence the teratogenicity of anticonvulsant therapy. In general, polytherapy may increase the risk of congenital malformations; monotherapy with the lowest effective dose is recommended (Harden 2009). For women with epilepsy who are planning a pregnancy in advance, baseline serum concentrations should be measured once or twice prior to pregnancy during a period when seizure control is optimal. Monitoring can then be continued up to once a month during pregnancy in women with stable seizure control (Patsalos 2008; Patsalos 2018).

Patients exposed to methsuximide during pregnancy are encouraged to enroll themselves into the NAAED Pregnancy Registry by calling 1-888-233-2334. Additional information is available at www.aedpregnancyregistry.org.

◆ **Methylacetoxyprogesterone** *see* MedroxyPROGESTERone *on page 953*

Methyldopa (meth il DOE pa)

Related Information
Cardiovascular Diseases *on page 1654*

Pharmacologic Category $Alpha_2$-Adrenergic Agonist; Antihypertensive

Use Hypertension: Management of hypertension. **Note: Not** recommended for the initial treatment of hypertension (ACC/AHA [Whelton 2017]).

Local Anesthetic/Vasoconstrictor Precautions No information available to require special precautions

Effects on Dental Treatment Key adverse event(s) related to dental treatment: Xerostomia (normal salivary flow resumes upon discontinuation). Anticholinergic side effects can cause a reduction of saliva production or secretion, contributing to discomfort and dental disease (ie, caries, oral candidiasis, and periodontal disease).

Effects on Bleeding No information available to require special precautions

Adverse Reactions
Frequency not defined:
Cardiovascular: Bradycardia, cardiac failure, exacerbation of angina pectoris, myocarditis, orthostatic hypotension, paradoxical pressor response (intravenous use), pericarditis, peripheral edema, prolonged carotid sinus syncope, vasculitis
Central nervous system: Bell's palsy, cerebrovascular insufficiency (symptoms), choreoathetosis, decreased mental acuity, depression, dizziness, drug fever, headache, nightmares, paresthesia, Parkinson's disease, sedation
Dermatologic: Skin rash, toxic epidermal necrolysis
Endocrine & metabolic: Amenorrhea, decreased libido, gynecomastia, hyperprolactinemia, weight gain
Gastrointestinal: Abdominal distention, colitis, constipation, diarrhea, flatulence, glossalgia, melanoglossia, nausea, pancreatitis, sialadenitis, vomiting, xerostomia
Genitourinary: Breast hypertrophy, impotence, lactation
Hematologic & oncologic: Bone marrow depression, eosinophilia, granulocytopenia, hemolytic anemia, leukopenia, positive ANA titer, positive direct Coombs test, thrombocytopenia
Hepatic: Abnormal hepatic function tests, hepatic disease (hepatitis), jaundice
Neuromuscular & skeletal: Arthralgia, lupus-like syndrome, myalgia, positive rheumatoid factor, weakness
Renal: Increased blood urea nitrogen
Respiratory: Nasal congestion
Miscellaneous: Positive LE cell preparation

Mechanism of Action Stimulation of central alpha-adrenergic receptors by a false neurotransmitter (alpha-methylnorepinephrine) that results in a decreased sympathetic outflow to the heart, kidneys, and peripheral vasculature

Pharmacodynamics/Kinetics

Onset of Action Peak effect: Hypotensive: Oral, IV: Single-dose: Within 3 to 6 hours; Multiple-dose: 48 to 72 hours

Duration of Action Oral: Single-dose: 12 to 24 hours, Multiple-dose: 24 to 48 hours; IV: 10 to 16 hours

Half-life Elimination Neonates: 10 to 20 hours; Adults:1.5 to 2 hours; End-stage renal disease: Prolonged (Myhre 1982)

Time to Peak Plasma: Oral: 2 to 4 hours (Myhre 1982)

Pregnancy Considerations Methyldopa crosses the placenta.

Available data show use during pregnancy does not cause fetal harm and improves fetal outcomes.

Chronic maternal hypertension may increase the risk of birth defects, low birth weight, preterm delivery, stillbirth, and neonatal death. Actual fetal/neonatal risks may be related to duration and severity of maternal hypertension. Untreated hypertension may also increase the risks of adverse maternal outcomes, including gestational diabetes, myocardial infarction, preeclampsia, stroke, and delivery complications (ACOG 203 2019).

If treatment for chronic hypertension during pregnancy is needed, oral methyldopa is an option; however, other agents may be preferred due to adverse events and decreased effectiveness when compared to other medications (ACOG 203 2019). Females with preexisting hypertension may continue their medication during pregnancy unless contraindications exist (Regitz-Zagrosek [ESC 2018]).

Product Availability Methyldopate injection is no longer available in the US.

◆ **Methyldopate Hydrochloride** *see* Methyldopa *on page 995*

◆ **Methylene Blue, Methenamine, Benzoic Acid, Phenyl Salicylate, and Hyoscyamine** *see* Methenamine, Phenyl Salicylate, Methylene Blue, Benzoic Acid, and Hyoscyamine *on page 987*

◆ **Methylene Blue, Methenamine, Sodium Phosphate Monobasic, Phenyl Salicylate, and Hyoscyamine** *see* Methenamine, Sodium Phosphate Monobasic, Phenyl Salicylate, Methylene Blue, and Hyoscyamine *on page 987*

◆ **Methylergometrine Maleate** *see* Methylergonovine *on page 995*

Methylergonovine (meth il er goe NOE veen)

Brand Names: US Methergine

Pharmacologic Category Ergot Derivative

Use Management of uterine atony, hemorrhage and subinvolution of the uterus following delivery of the placenta; control of uterine hemorrhage following delivery of the anterior shoulder in the second stage of labor

Local Anesthetic/Vasoconstrictor Precautions Use vasoconstrictor with caution in patients taking methylergonovine; this ergot alkaloid derivative causes constriction of peripheral blood vessels

Effects on Dental Treatment No significant effects or complications reported

Effects on Bleeding Thrombosis has been reported; however, there are no special precautions associated with bleeding related to dental procedures.

Adverse Reactions Frequency not defined.

Cardiovascular: Angina pectoris, atrioventricular block, bradycardia, cerebrovascular accident, chest pain, coronary artery vasospasm, hypertension, hypotension, local thrombophlebitis, myocardial infarction, palpitations, paresthesia, tachycardia, vasospasm, ventricular fibrillation

Central nervous system: Dizziness, hallucination, headache, seizure

Dermatologic: Diaphoresis, skin rash

Endocrine & metabolic: Water intoxication

Gastrointestinal: Abdominal pain, diarrhea, nausea, unpleasant taste, vomiting

Genitourinary: Hematuria

Hypersensitivity: Anaphylaxis

Neuromuscular & skeletal: Leg cramps

Otic: Tinnitus

Respiratory: Dyspnea, nasal congestion

Mechanism of Action Increases the tone, rate and amplitude of contractions on the smooth muscles of the uterus, producing sustained contractions which shortens the third stage of labor and reduces blood loss.

Pharmacodynamics/Kinetics

Onset of Action Oxytocic: Oral: 5-10 minutes; IM: 2-5 minutes; IV: Immediately

Duration of Action Oral: ~3 hours; IM: ~3 hours; IV: 45 minutes

Half-life Elimination ~3 hours (range: 1.5-12.7 hours)

Time to Peak Serum: Oral: 0.3-2 hours; IM: 0.2-0.6 hours

Pregnancy Risk Factor C

Pregnancy Considerations

Methylergonovine is intended for use after delivery of the anterior shoulder, after delivery of the placenta, or during the puerperium; use is contraindicated during pregnancy.

Methylergonovine is recommended when a supplemental uterotonic agent is needed; due to maternal side effects it is not preferred for initial use (ACOG 183 2017).

◆ **Methylergonovine Maleate** *see* Methylergonovine *on page 995*

Methylfolate (meth il FO late)

Brand Names: US Denovo [OTC]; Deplin 15; Deplin 7.5; Elfolate; L-Methylfolate Formula 15 [DSC]; L-Methylfolate Formula 7.5 [DSC]; L-Methylfolate Forte

Pharmacologic Category Medical Food

Use Medical food for the nutritional requirements of patients with suboptimal L-methylfolate and who have major depressive disorder or schizophrenia

Note: A medical food is formulated to be administered enterally under the supervision of a physician and is intended for the specific dietary management of a disease or condition for which distinctive nutritional requirements are established by medical evaluation. Medical foods are not drugs and, therefore, are not subject to any FDA regulatory requirements that specifically apply to drugs (eg, requirement for written/oral prescription prior to dispensing, premarket review or approval, proof of safety and efficacy).

Local Anesthetic/Vasoconstrictor Precautions No information available to require special precautions

Effects on Dental Treatment No significant effects or complications reported

Effects on Bleeding No information available to require special precautions

Mechanism of Action Methylfolate, or L-methylfolate, is the active form of folate in the body, which can be transported into peripheral tissues and across the blood-brain barrier. Folate is necessary for formation of numerous coenzymes in many metabolic systems, particularly for purine, pyrimidine, and nucleoprotein synthesis, and maintenance in erythropoiesis; stimulates WBC and platelet production in folate deficiency anemia.

◆ **Methylin** *see* Methylphenidate *on page 997*

◆ **Methylmorphine** *see* Codeine *on page 404*

Methylnaltrexone (meth il nal TREKS one)

Brand Names: US Relistor

Brand Names: Canada Relistor

Pharmacologic Category Gastrointestinal Agent, Miscellaneous; Opioid Antagonist, Peripherally-Acting

Use

Opioid-induced constipation with advanced illness (injection only): Treatment of opioid-induced constipation in adults with advanced illness or pain caused by active cancer who require opioid dosage escalation for palliative care.

Opioid-induced constipation with chronic non-cancer pain (tablets and injection): Treatment of opioid-induced constipation in adults with chronic non-cancer pain, including patients with chronic pain related to prior cancer or its treatment who do not require frequent (eg, weekly) opioid dosage escalation.

Local Anesthetic/Vasoconstrictor Precautions No information available to require special precautions

Effects on Dental Treatment No significant effects or complications reported

Effects on Bleeding No information available to require special precautions

Adverse Reactions

>10%: Gastrointestinal: Abdominal pain (14% to 29%), flatulence (13%), nausea (9% to 12%)

1% to 10%:

Central nervous system: Dizziness (7%), headache (4%), anxiety (2%), chills (1%)

Dermatologic: Hyperhidrosis (3% to 6%)

Endocrine & metabolic: Hot flash (3%)

Gastrointestinal: Diarrhea (5% to 6%), abdominal distention (4%), vomiting (2%)

Neuromuscular & skeletal: Muscle spasm (2%), tremor (1%)

Respiratory: Rhinorrhea (2%)

<1%, postmarketing, and/or case reports: Abdominal cramps, diaphoresis, flushing, gastrointestinal perforation, increased body temperature (Thomas 2008), malaise, opioid withdrawal syndrome, pain, syncope (Portenoy 2008)

Mechanism of Action An opioid receptor antagonist which blocks opioid binding at the mu receptor, methylnaltrexone is a quaternary derivative of naltrexone with restricted ability to cross the blood-brain barrier. It therefore functions as a peripheral acting opioid antagonist, including actions on the gastrointestinal tract to inhibit opioid-induced decreased gastrointestinal motility and delay in gastrointestinal transit time, thereby decreasing opioid-induced constipation. Does not affect opioid analgesic effects.

Pharmacodynamics/Kinetics

Half-life Elimination Terminal: ~15 hours (oral)

Time to Peak SubQ: 30 minutes; Oral: ~1.5 hours (delayed by 2 hours with high fat meal)

Pregnancy Considerations Adverse events have not been observed in animal reproduction studies. Maternal use of methylnaltrexone during pregnancy may precipitate opioid withdrawal effects in newborn.

◆ **Methylnaltrexone Bromide** *see* Methylnaltrexone *on page 996*

Methylphenidate (meth il FEN i date)

Brand Names: US Adhansia XR; Aptensio XR; Concerta; Cotempla XR-ODT; Daytrana; Jornay PM; Metadate CD [DSC]; Metadate ER; Methylin; QuilliChew ER; Quillivant XR; Relexxii; Ritalin; Ritalin LA

Brand Names: Canada ACT Methylphenidate ER; APO-Methylphenidate; APO-Methylphenidate ER; APO-Methylphenidate SR; Biphentin; Concerta; Foquest; PMS-Methylphenidate; PMS-Methylphenidate ER [DSC]; RATIO-Methylphenidate [DSC]; Ritalin; Ritalin SR; SANDOZ Methylphenidate SR; TEVA-Methylphenidate ER-C

Pharmacologic Category Central Nervous System Stimulant

Use

Attention-deficit/hyperactivity disorder: Treatment of attention-deficit/hyperactivity disorder (ADHD).

Narcolepsy (Methylin, Metadate ER, Ritalin, and Ritalin SR [Canadian product]): Symptomatic management of narcolepsy.

Local Anesthetic/Vasoconstrictor Precautions No information available to require special precautions

Effects on Dental Treatment Key adverse event(s) related to dental treatment: Frequent occurrences of xerostomia (normal salivary flow resumes upon discontinuance). Infrequent occurrences of bruxism, oropharyngeal pain, and sinusitis have been reported. Methylphenidate can cause tachycardia, increased blood pressure, and palpitations. Consider monitoring blood pressure prior to using local anesthetic with a vasoconstrictor. Rare occurrences of erythema multiforme have also been reported.

Effects on Bleeding No information available to require special precautions

Adverse Reactions

>10%:

Central nervous system: Insomnia (including initial insomnia; oral: 2% to 33%; transdermal: 6% to 13%), headache (2% to 22%), irritability (6% to 11%)

Endocrine & metabolic: Weight loss (2% to 13%)

Gastrointestinal: Decreased appetite (2% to 28%), xerostomia (oral: 4% to 14%), nausea (2% to 13%)

1% to 10%:

Cardiovascular: Tachycardia (oral: 5%; transdermal: ≤1%), palpitations (oral: 3%; transdermal: <1%), increased blood pressure (≥2%), increased heart rate (oral: ≥2%)

Central nervous system: Emotional lability (1% to 9%), anxiety (oral: 8%), jitteriness (oral: 3% to 8%), increased diastolic blood pressure (oral: 7%), tic disorder (transdermal: 7%; oral: 2%), dizziness (2% to 7%), psychomotor agitation (oral: 5%), depressed mood (oral: 4%), nervousness (oral: 3%; transdermal: <1%), restlessness (oral: 3%), aggressive behavior (oral: 2%), agitation (oral: 2%), depression (≤2%), hypertonia (oral: 2%), lack of emotion (oral: 2%), vertigo (oral: 2%), confusion (oral: 1%), sedated state (oral: 1%), tension (oral: 1%), tension headache (oral: 1%), paresthesia (≤1%)

Dermatologic: Hyperhidrosis (oral: 5%), excoriation of skin (oral: 4%), skin rash (oral: 2%)

Endocrine & metabolic: Decreased libido (oral: 2%)

Gastrointestinal: Vomiting (1% to 10%), abdominal pain (transdermal: 5% to 7%), diarrhea (oral: 3% to 7%), upper abdominal pain (oral: 4% to 6%), anorexia (2% to 5%), bruxism (oral: 2%), dyspepsia (oral: 2%), motion sickness (oral: 2%), constipation (oral: 1%)

Hematologic & oncologic: Bruise (oral: 3%)

Neuromuscular & skeletal: Back pain (oral: 3%), tremor (oral: 3%)

Ophthalmic: Blurred vision (≤2%), eye pain (oral: 2%)

Respiratory: Upper respiratory tract infection (oral: 2% to 4%), nasopharyngitis (oral: 3%), streptococcal pharyngitis (oral: 3%), cough (oral: 2%), oropharyngeal pain (oral: 1% to 2%)

Miscellaneous: Fever (oral: 2%)

Frequency not defined:

Cardiovascular: Cardiac arrhythmia, decreased blood pressure, decreased pulse, heart murmur, hypertension, increased pulse

Central nervous system: Delirium, drug abuse, drug dependence, Gilles de la Tourette syndrome (rare), hypervigilance, hypomania, mood changes, outbursts of anger, panic attack, sleep disorder, toxic psychosis

Dermatologic: Macular eruption

Endocrine & metabolic: Growth retardation, hot flash, increased thirst

Gastrointestinal: Abdominal distress, viral gastroenteritis

Genitourinary: Erectile dysfunction

Hematologic & oncologic: Anemia, leukopenia

Hepatic: Increased serum alanine aminotransferase

Infection: Viral infection

Neuromuscular & skeletal: Asthenia, muscle spasm

Ophthalmic: Dry eye syndrome

Respiratory: Bronchitis, dyspnea, sinusitis

<1%, postmarketing, and/or case reports: Accommodation disturbance, allergic contact dermatitis, alopecia, anaphylaxis, angina pectoris, angioedema, application site reaction, arthralgia, auditory hallucination, bradycardia, bullous skin disease, cerebral arteritis, cerebrovascular occlusion, change in libido, change in WBC count, chest discomfort, chest pain, contact hypersensitivity, diplopia, disorientation, drowsiness, drug tolerance, dyskinesia, erythema of skin, erythema multiforme, exfoliative dermatitis, extrasystoles, fatigue, hallucination, hepatic failure (acute), hepatic injury (severe), hyperpyrexia, hypersensitivity reaction, immune thrombocytopenia, increased liver enzymes, increased serum alkaline phosphatase, increased serum bilirubin, lethargy, leukoderma (chemical; FDA Safety Alert 2015), loss of scalp hair, mania, muscle twitching, myalgia, mydriasis, necrotizing angiitis, neuroleptic malignant syndrome, pancytopenia, peripheral vascular insufficiency, priapism, pruritus, Raynaud disease, rhabdomyolysis, seizure, supraventricular tachycardia, swelling of the ear, talkativeness, thrombocytopenia, urticaria, ventricular arrhythmia (Schelleman 2012), ventricular premature contractions, visual disturbance, visual hallucination, visual impairment

Mechanism of Action Mild CNS stimulant; blocks the reuptake of norepinephrine and dopamine into presynaptic neurons; appears to stimulate the cerebral cortex and subcortical structures similar to amphetamines

Pharmacodynamics/Kinetics

Onset of Action

Children (AAP 2011):

Oral:

ER formulations (capsule [Metadate CD, Ritalin LA], tablets (Concerta]): 20 to 60 minutes

IR formulations (chewable tablet, oral solution, tablet [Methylin, Ritalin]): 20 to 60 minutes

Sustained-release tablet (Ritalin SR [Canadian product]): 60 to 180 minutes

Transdermal (Daytrana): 60 minutes

Adults: Oral: Controlled-release capsule: Foquest [Canadian product]: Within 1 hour

Maximum effect: Oral: IR tablet: Within 2 hours; Sustained-release tablet (Ritalin SR [Canadian product]): Within 4 to 7 hours

Duration of Action

Oral:

Controlled-release capsule (Foquest [Canadian product]): 16 hours

ER capsule: Metadate CD, Ritalin LA: 6 to 8 hours (AAP 2011); Aptensio XR: ≤16 hours

ER tablet (Concerta): 8 to 12 hours (AAP 2011; Jain 2017)

ER tablet (Metadate ER): 8 hours

IR formulations (chewable tablet, oral solution, IR tablet [Methylin, Ritalin]): 3 to 5 hours (AAP 2011; Jain 2017)

Sustained-release tablet (Ritalin SR [Canadian product]): 2 to 8 hours (AAP 2011; Jain 2017)

Transdermal (Daytrana): 11 to 12 hours (AAP 2011)

Half-life Elimination

Controlled-release capsule: Biphentin [Canadian product]: Children: 2.4 hours; Adults: 2.1 hours; Foquest [Canadian product]: Adults: 6.95 ± 3.25 hours

ER capsule:

Adhansia XR:

Children 6 to 12 years of age: ~4 to 7 hours

Adolescents ≤17 years of age: ~5 hours

Adults: 7 hours

Aptensio XR: Adults: ~5 hours

Jornay PM: Adults: ~5.9 hours

Metadate CD: Adults: 6.8 hours

Ritalin LA: Children: 1.5 to 4 hours; Adults: 3 to 4.2 hours

ER chewable tablets: ~5.2 hours

ER orally disintegrating tablet: 4 to 4.5 hours

ER suspension: Quillivant XR: Children ≥9 years of age, Adolescents, and Adults: ~5 hours

ER tablet: Concerta: Adolescents and Adults: ~3.5 hours

IR chewable tablet: Methylin: Adults: 3 hours

IR solution: Methylin: Adults: 2.7 hours

IR tablet:

Children: 3.5 hours (1.5 to 5 hours)

Adults: 3.5 hours (1.3 to 7.7 hours)

Transdermal: Children and Adolescents 6 to 17 years of age: *d*-methylphenidate ~4 to 5 hours, *l*-methylphenidate 1.4 to 2.9 hours

Time to Peak

Controlled-release capsule:

Biphentin [Canadian product]: Children: Initial: ~2.5 hours; Adults: Initial: ~2 hours

Foquest [Canadian product]: Children: Initial peak between 1.5 to 2.0 hours followed by a second peak between 9 to 11 hours; Adults: Initial peak at ~1.6 hours followed by second peak at ~12.5 hours (range: 11 to 16 hours)

ER capsule:

Adhansia XR:

Children 6 to 12 years of age: Initial: 2 hours (range: 1 to 4 hours); Second peak: 10 hours (8 to 14 hours)

Adolescents ≤17 years of age: Initial: 2 hours (range: 1 to 4 hours); Second peak: 11 hours (8 to 14 hours)

Adults: Initial: 1.5 hours (range: 1 to 2.5 hours); Second peak: ~12 hours (range: 8.5 to 16 hours)

Aptensio XR: Adults: Initial: ~2 hours; Second peak: ~8 hours

Jornay PM: Adults: 14 hours

Metadate CD: Children: Initial: ~1.5 hours; Second peak: ~4.5 hours

Ritalin LA:

Children: Initial: 1 to 3 hours; Second peak: 5 to 11 hours

Adults: Initial: 1.3 to 4 hours; Second peak: 4.3 to 6.5 hours

ER chewable tablet: QuilliChew ER: Adults: 5 hours (median)

ER orally disintegrating tablet: Cotempla XR-ODT: ~5 hours

ER suspension: Quillivant XR: Children (9 to 12 years of age): 4.05 hours (range: 3.98 to 6 hours); Adolescents (13 to 15 years of age): 2 hours (range: 1.98 to 4 hours); Adults: 4 hours (range: 1.3 to 7.3 hours)

ER tablet: Concerta: Initial: ~1 hours, followed by gradually ascending concentrations over 5 to 9 hours; Mean peak: 6 to 10 hours

IR chewable tablet: Methylin: ~1 to 2 hours

IR solution: Methylin: 1 to 2 hours

IR tablet: Children: 1.9 hours (range: 0.3 to 4.4 hours); time to peak is faster after a high-fat meal as compared to without food (median T_{max}: 2.5 hours versus 3 hours, respectively).

Sustained-release tablet (Ritalin SR [Canadian product]): Children: 4.7 hours (range: 1.3 to 8.2 hours)

Transdermal: ~8 to 10 hours

Pregnancy Considerations

Information related to the use of methylphenidate in pregnant women with attention-deficit/hyperactivity disorder (Ornoy 2018) or narcolepsy (Calvo-Ferrandiz 2018; Maurovich-Horvat 2013; Thorpy 2013) is limited and outcome data is conflicting (Ornoy 2018). If treatment of ADHD in pregnancy is needed, methylphenidate may be considered (Larsen 2015; McAllister-Williams 2017).

Data collection to monitor pregnancy and infant outcomes following exposure to methylphenidate is ongoing. Health care providers are encouraged to enroll females exposed to methylphenidate during pregnancy in the National Pregnancy Registry for Psychostimulants at 1-866-961-2388.

Controlled Substance C-II

- ◆ **Methylphenidate HCl** *see* Methylphenidate *on page 997*
- ◆ **Methylphenidate Hydrochloride** *see* Methylphenidate *on page 997*
- ◆ **Methylphenoxy-Benzene Propanamine** *see* AtoMOXetine *on page 190*

- ◆ **Methylphenyl Isoxazolyl Penicillin** *see* Oxacillin *on page 1150*
- ◆ **Methylphytyl Napthoquinone** *see* Phytonadione *on page 1230*

MethylPREDNISolone (meth il pred NIS oh lone)

Related Information

Respiratory Diseases *on page 1680*

Related Sample Prescriptions

Ulcerative and Erosive Disorders - Sample Prescriptions *on page 46*

Brand Names: US DEPO-Medrol; Medrol; P-Care D40; P-Care D80; ReadySharp methylPREDNISolone [DSC]; SOLU-Medrol

Brand Names: Canada Depo-Medrol; Medrol; SOLU-medrol; Solu-MEDROL; Uni-Med

Generic Availability (US) Yes

Pharmacologic Category Corticosteroid, Systemic

Dental Use Treatment of a variety of oral diseases of allergic, inflammatory, or autoimmune origin

Use

Oral, IM (acetate or succinate), and IV (succinate only) administration: Anti-inflammatory or immunosuppressant agent in the treatment of a variety of diseases, including those of hematologic (eg, immune thrombocytopenia, warm autoimmune hemolytic anemia), allergic, gastrointestinal (eg, Crohn disease, ulcerative colitis), inflammatory, neoplastic, neurologic (eg, multiple sclerosis), rheumatic (eg, antineutrophil cytoplasmic antibody-associated vasculitis, dermatomyositis/polymyositis, giant-cell arteritis, gout [acute flare], giant cell arteritis, mixed cryoglobulinemia syndrome, polyarteritis nodosa, rheumatoid arthritis, systemic lupus erythematosus), and/or autoimmune origin.

Intra-articular or soft tissue administration (acetate only): Gout (acute flare), acute and subacute bursitis, acute nonspecific tenosynovitis, epicondylitis, rheumatoid arthritis, and/or synovitis of osteoarthritis.

Intralesional administration (acetate only): Alopecia areata; discoid lupus erythematosus; keloids; localized hypertrophic, infiltrated, inflammatory lesions of granuloma annulare, lichen planus, lichen simplex chronicus (neurodermatitis), and psoriatic plaques; and necrobiosis lipoidica diabeticorum. May be useful in cystic tumor of an aponeurosis or tendon (ganglia).

Local Anesthetic/Vasoconstrictor Precautions

No information available to require special precautions

Effects on Dental Treatment Key adverse event(s) related to dental treatment: Ulcerative esophagitis.

Effects on Bleeding No information available to require special precautions

Adverse Reactions

Frequency not defined:

Cardiovascular: Bradycardia, cardiac arrest, cardiac arrhythmia, cardiac failure, cardiomegaly, circulatory shock, edema, embolism (fat), hypertension, hypertrophic cardiomyopathy (in neonates), myocardial rupture (post MI), syncope, tachycardia, thromboembolism, thrombophlebitis, vasculitis

Central nervous system: Arachnoiditis, depression, emotional lability, euphoria, headache, increased intracranial pressure, insomnia, malaise, meningitis, myasthenia, neuritis, neuropathy, paraplegia, paresthesia, personality changes, psychic disorders, pseudotumor cerebri (usually following discontinuation), seizure, sensory disturbance, vertigo

Dermatologic: Acne vulgaris, allergic dermatitis, alopecia, atrophic striae, diaphoresis, ecchymoses, epidermal thinning, erythema, exfoliation of skin, facial erythema, hyperpigmentation, hypertrichosis, hypopigmentation, skin atrophy, skin rash, suppression of skin test reaction, thinning hair, urticaria, xeroderma

Endocrine & metabolic: Adrenal suppression, calcinosis, cushingoid state, Cushing syndrome, decreased glucose tolerance, diabetes mellitus, fluid retention, glycosuria, growth suppression (children), hirsutism, HPA-axis suppression, hyperglycemia, hyperlipidemia, hypokalemia, hypokalemic alkalosis, insulin resistance (increased requirements for insulin or oral hypoglycemic agents in diabetes), menstrual disease, moon face, negative nitrogen balance, protein catabolism, sodium retention, weight gain

Gastrointestinal: Abdominal distention, bladder dysfunction (after intrathecal administration, including bowel dysfunction), carbohydrate intolerance (increased), gastrointestinal hemorrhage, gastrointestinal perforation, hiccups, increased appetite, intestinal perforation (of both of the small and large intestines; especially in patients with inflammatory bowel disease), nausea, pancreatitis, peptic ulcer, spermatozoa disorder (decreased motility and number of spermatozoa), ulcerative esophagitis

Hematologic: Leukocytosis (transient), malignant neoplasm (secondary), petechia

Hepatic: Hepatomegaly, increased liver enzymes, increased serum transaminases

Hypersensitivity: Anaphylactoid reaction, anaphylaxis, angioedema, hypersensitivity reaction

Infection: Increased susceptibility to infection, infection (ophthalmic), sterile abscess

Local: Injection site infection

Neuromuscular & skeletal: Amyotrophy, arthropathy, aseptic necrosis of femoral head, aseptic necrosis of humoral head, bone fracture, Charcot-like arthropathy, lipotrophy, osteoporosis, rupture of tendon, steroid myopathy, vertebral compression fracture

Ophthalmic: Blindness, exophthalmoses, glaucoma, increased intraocular pressure, ophthalmic inflammation (ophthalmic), subcapsular posterior cataract, visual impairment

Respiratory: Pulmonary edema, rhinitis

Miscellaneous: Anaphylactoid reaction, anaphylaxis, angioedema, hypersensitivity reactions, tissue sloughing (residue or slough at injection site), wound healing impairment

<1%, postmarketing, and/or case reports: Venous thrombosis (Johannesdottir 2013)

Dental Usual Dosage Anti-inflammatory or immunosuppressive: Adults: Oral: 2 to 60 mg/day in 1 to 4 divided doses to start, followed by gradual reduction in dosage to the lowest possible level consistent with maintaining an adequate clinical response.

Dosing

Adult & Geriatric

Note:

Dosing: Evidence to support an optimal dose and duration are lacking for most indications; recommendations provided are general guidelines only and primarily based on expert opinion. In general, glucocorticoid dosing should be individualized and the minimum effective dose/duration should be used. For select indications with weight-based dosing, consider using ideal body weight in obese patients, especially with longer durations of therapy (Erstad 2004; Furst 2019a). **Hypothalamic-pituitary-adrenal suppression:** Although some patients may become hypothalamic-pituitary-adrenal (HPA) suppressed with lower doses or briefer exposure, some experts consider HPA-axis suppression likely in any adult receiving >16 mg/day (daytime dosing) or ≥4 mg per 24 hours (evening or night dosing) for >3 weeks, or with Cushingoid appearance (Furst 2019b; Joseph 2016); do not abruptly discontinue treatment in these patients; dose tapering may be necessary (Cooper 2003). **Safety:** Only the methylprednisolone **succinate** formulation (Solu-Medrol) may be given IV. Methylprednisolone **acetate** suspension (Depo-Medrol) is intended for IM or intra-articular administration only; do not administer the acetate preparation IV (Grissinger 2007; ISMP 2016).

Usual dosage range:

IV (succinate): 40 to 125 mg/day given in a single daily dose or in divided doses; rarely, for certain conditions, may go up to 1 to 2 mg/**kg**/day.

Initial high-dose "pulse" therapy for select indications (eg, severe systemic rheumatic disorders): 7 to 15 mg/kg/dose (or 500 mg to 1 g/dose) given once daily for 3 to 5 days.

Oral: 16 to 64 mg/day once daily or in divided doses.

The following dosing is from the commercially available tapered-dosage product (eg, dose-pack containing 21 × 4 mg tablets):

Day 1: 24 mg on day 1 administered as 8 mg (2 tablets) before breakfast, 4 mg (1 tablet) after lunch, 4 mg (1 tablet) after supper, and 8 mg (2 tablets) at bedtime **or** 24 mg (6 tablets) as a single dose or divided into 2 or 3 doses upon initiation (regardless of time of day).

Day 2: 20 mg on day 2 administered as 4 mg (1 tablet) before breakfast, 4 mg (1 tablet) after lunch, 4 mg (1 tablet) after supper, and 8 mg (2 tablets) at bedtime.

Day 3: 16 mg on day 3 administered as 4 mg (1 tablet) before breakfast, 4 mg (1 tablet) after lunch, 4 mg (1 tablet) after supper, and 4 mg (1 tablet) at bedtime.

Day 4: 12 mg on day 4 administered as 4 mg (1 tablet) before breakfast, 4 mg (1 tablet) after lunch, and 4 mg (1 tablet) at bedtime.

Day 5: 8 mg on day 5 administered as 4 mg (1 tablet) before breakfast and 4 mg (1 tablet) at bedtime.

Day 6: 4 mg on day 6 administered as 4 mg (1 tablet) before breakfast.

IM (acetate or succinate): 40 to 60 mg as a single dose.

Intra-articular (acetate suspension): **Note:** Dose ranges per manufacturer's labeling. Specific dose is determined based upon joint size, severity of inflammation, amount of articular fluid present, and clinician judgment.

Larger joint (eg, knee, shoulder, hip): 20 to 80 mg.

Medium joint (eg, wrist, ankle, elbow): 10 to 40 mg.

Small joint (eg, toe, finger): 4 to 10 mg.

Intralesional (acetate) (alternative agent): Note: Other agents (eg, triamcinolone acetonide) may be more commonly employed (Mathes 2020).

Usual dosage range: 20 to 60 mg; for large lesions, it may be necessary to distribute doses ranging from 20 to 40 mg by repeated local injections; 1 to 4 injections are usually employed with intervals between injections varying with the type of lesion being treated and clinical response.

Indication-specific dosing:

Acute respiratory distress syndrome, moderate to severe (off-label use): Note: May consider in most patients with persistent or refractory, moderate to severe acute respiratory distress syndrome, who are relatively early in the disease course (within 14 days) (Siegel 2020). Use ideal body weight to calculate dose. If patient is extubated between days 1 to 14, advance to day 15 of therapy and taper according to the following schedule. Do not abruptly discontinue since this may cause deterioration due to inflammatory response (Meduri 2007; SCCM/ESICM [Annane 2017]; Steinberg 2006).

IV (succinate): Loading dose of 1 mg/kg over 30 minutes, followed by a gradual taper:

Days 1 to 14: 1 mg/kg/day in divided doses or as a continuous infusion.

Days 15 to 21: 0.5 mg/kg/day in divided doses or as a continuous infusion.

Days 22 to 25: 0.25 mg/kg/day in divided doses or as a continuous infusion.

Days 26 to 28: 0.125 mg/kg/day in divided doses or as a continuous infusion.

Allergic conditions:

Anaphylaxis (adjunct to epinephrine for prevention of late-phase/biphasic reaction): **Note:** Do **not** use for initial or sole treatment of anaphylaxis because corticosteroids do not result in the prompt relief of upper or lower airway obstruction or shock (AAAAI [Lieberman 2015]; EAACI [Muraro 2014]; WAO [Simons 2011]; WAO [Simons 2015]). Some experts limit use to patients with severe or persistent steroid-responsive symptoms (eg, bronchospasm in patients with asthma) (Campbell 2020).

IV (succinate): 1 to 2 mg/kg (Campbell 2014) **or** 50 to 125 mg as a single dose (Campbell 2020; WAO [Simons 2011]).

Angioedema (acute allergic) and/or urticaria (acute): **Note:** For moderate to severe symptoms without signs of anaphylaxis. Use epinephrine if anaphylaxis symptoms (eg, risk of airway or cardiovascular compromise) are present (Cicardi 2014; Zuraw 2019). In patients with acute urticaria, consider reserving use for patients with significant angioedema or whose symptoms are unresponsive to antihistamines (Asero 2020; Barniol 2018; Bernstein 2014; EAACI [Zuberbier 2018]; Powell 2015). The optimal dosing strategy has not been defined (Bernstein 2014; EAACI [Zuberbier 2018]; James 2017; Powell 2015).

IV (succinate): Initial: 60 to 80 mg; switch to an oral corticosteroid as soon as possible, tapering the dose for a total treatment duration of ≤10 days (EAACI [Zuberbier 2018]; Zuraw 2019).

Oral: Initial: 16 to 32 mg/day in 1 to 2 divided doses for 3 to 4 days (Barniol 2018; Powell 2015; Zuraw 2019); may consider tapering the dose for a total treatment duration of ≤10 days (EAACI [Zuberbier 2018]; Zuraw 2019).

Asthma, acute exacerbation: Note: For moderate to severe exacerbations or in patients who do not respond promptly and completely to short-acting beta agonists; administer within 1 hour of presentation to emergency department (GINA 2020; NAEPP 2007).

Oral (preferred route), IV (succinate): 40 to 60 mg/day in 1 or 2 divided doses for 3 to 10 days (NAEPP 2007); doses up to 60 to 80 mg every 6 to 12 hours have been used in critically ill patients (Fanta 2019). If symptoms do not resolve and peak expiratory flow is not at least 70% of personal best, then longer treatment may be required (NAEPP 2007).

Chronic obstructive pulmonary disease, acute exacerbation (off-label use): Note: In patients with severe but not life-threatening exacerbations, oral regimens are recommended. Use IV route in patients who cannot tolerate oral therapy (eg, shock, mechanically ventilated) (GOLD 2019; Stoller 2019).

Oral; IV (succinate): 40 to 60 mg daily for 5 to 14 days (GOLD 2019; Stoller 2019). Doses up to 60 mg every 6 hours have been used in critically ill patients, although outcome data are limited. **Note:** Dose is based on an equivalent dose of prednisone; optimal dose has not been established. If patient improves with therapy, may discontinue without taper. If patient does not improve, a longer duration of therapy may be indicated (Stoller 2019).

Deceased organ donor management (hormonal resuscitation for the deceased organ donor) (off-label use): Note: Data supporting benefit are conflicting; if given, it should be administered after blood has been collected for tissue typing (Dupuis 2014; SCCM/ACCP/AOPO [Kotloff 2015]).

IV (succinate): Regimens include: 1 g (as an IV infusion) **or** 15 mg/kg (as an IV infusion) **or** 250 mg (as an IV bolus) followed by a continuous infusion at 100 mg/hour; usually given as part of combination hormone therapy (SCCM/ACCP/AOPO [Kotloff 2015]).

Giant cell arteritis, treatment: Note: Due to the rapidly progressive nature of the disease, start treatment **immediately** once diagnosis is highly suspected (Dasgupta 2010). In patients presenting **without** threatened/evolving vision loss, an oral glucocorticoid is suggested as initial therapy rather than IV methylprednisolone (Docken 2019).

Initial pulse therapy in patients presenting ***with*** *threatened/evolving vision loss:* IV (succinate): 500 mg to 1 g daily for 3 days, followed by an oral glucocorticoid (eg, prednisone) (Dasgupta 2010).

Gout, acute flare: Oral: 24 to 32 mg/day in 1 or 2 divided doses until symptom improvement, followed by a 7- to 10-day taper (or 14- to 21-day taper in patients with multiple prior flares) (Becker 2019). A tapered (6-day) dose pack may be sufficient in some patients (ACR [Khanna 2012]).

Unable to take orally, 1 to 2 joints affected, and no possibility of joint infection: **Note:** Clinicians must have sufficient expertise to perform arthrocentesis and injection.

Intra-articular (acetate): Usual dose: Larger joint (eg, knee): 40 mg; Medium joint (eg, wrist, ankle, elbow): 30 mg; Small joint (eg, toe, finger): 10 mg; a range of doses may be used based on patient factors and clinician judgment, see note at top of adult dosing section regarding intra-articular injection (ACR [Khanna 2012]; Becker 2019); may mix the glucocorticoid with an equal volume of local anesthetic (Cardone 2002; Roberts 2019).

Unable to take orally and/or not an appropriate candidate for intra-articular injection:

IM (acetate or succinate): Initial: 40 to 60 mg as a single dose; may repeat once or twice at ≥48-hour intervals if benefit fades or there is no flare resolution (ACR [Khanna 2012]; Becker 2019).

Hospitalized patients: IV (succinate): 20 mg twice daily until clinical improvement, followed by stepwise reduction in each dose by 50% until 5 mg twice daily; then maintain a dose of ≥4 mg (or oral equivalent) twice daily for 5 days (ACR [Khanna 2012]; Becker 2019).

Graft-vs-host disease, acute, treatment (off-label use): Note: For grade ≥2 acute graft-versus-host disease. An optimal regimen has not been identified; refer to institutional protocols as variations exist. Treatment is dependent on the severity and the rate of progression (ASBMT [Martin 2012]; EBMT/ELN [Ruutu 2014]).

IV (succinate): Initial: 2 mg/kg/day in 2 divided doses; dose may vary based on organ involvement and severity. Continue for several weeks, then taper over several months (ASBMT [Martin 2012]; Chao 2019; EBMT/ELN [Ruutu 2014]).

Immune thrombocytopenia (initial therapy): Note: Goal of therapy is to provide a safe platelet count to prevent clinically important bleeding rather than normalization of the platelet count (Arnold 2019).

Patients with severe bleeding (in combination with other treatments): IV (succinate): 1 g once daily for 3 doses (Arnold 2019; von dem Borne 1988). **Note:** Due to the short-term response, maintenance therapy with an oral glucocorticoid (eg, prednisone) may be required (Provan 2010).

Inflammatory bowel disease:

Crohn disease, acute (eg, severe/fulminant disease and/or unable to take oral) (adjunctive agent): **Note: Not** for long-term use (ACG [Lichtenstein 2018]). In patients with localized peritonitis, some experts recommend against initiating corticosteroids due to the potential of masking further clinical deterioration; however, if already receiving corticosteroids, continued use may be appropriate (Hashash 2019).

IV (succinate): 40 to 60 mg/day (ACG [Lichtenstein 2018]).

Note: For patients who have been receiving chronic treatment with a corticosteroid, a small increase in their daily dose may be required during an acute exacerbation (Hashash 2019). Steroid-sparing agents (eg, biologic agents, immunomodulators) should be introduced with a goal of discontinuing corticosteroid therapy as soon as possible (ACG [Lichtenstein 2018]).

Ulcerative colitis, acute (severe or fulminant): **Note: Not** for long-term use.

IV (succinate): 60 mg/day in 1 to 3 divided doses. If response to treatment is inadequate after 5 days (severe) or 3 days (fulminant), second-line therapy is initiated (ACG [Rubin 2019]; Peppercorn 2019).

Iodinated contrast media allergic-like reaction, prevention: Note: Generally for patients with a prior allergic-like or unknown-type iodinated contrast reaction who will be receiving another iodinated contrast agent. Nonurgent premedication with an oral corticosteroid is generally preferred when contrast administration is scheduled to begin in ≥12 hours; however, consider an urgent (accelerated) regimen with an IV corticosteroid for those requiring contrast in <12 hours (ACR 2018).

Nonurgent regimen:

Oral: 32 mg administered 12 hours and 2 hours before contrast medium administration in combination with oral diphenhydramine 50 mg (administered 1 hour prior to contrast) (ACR 2018; Davenport 2019).

Urgent (accelerated) regimen:

IV (succinate): 40 mg every 4 hours until contrast medium administration in combination with IV diphenhydramine 50 mg (administered 1 hour prior to contrast) (ACR 2018).

Multiple sclerosis, acute exacerbation: Note: For patients with an acute exacerbation resulting in neurologic symptoms and increased disability or impairments in vision, strength, or cerebellar function (Olek 2019).

Initial pulse therapy: IV (succinate): 500 mg to 1 g daily for 3 to 7 days (5 days typically), either alone or followed by an oral taper with prednisone (Goodin 2014; Le Page 2015; Myhr 2009; NICE 2014; Olek 2019).

Myopathies (dermatomyositis/polymyositis), treatment:

*Initial pulse therapy in patients presenting **with** severe systemic involvement or profound weakness:* IV (succinate): 1 g daily for 3 to 5 days, followed by oral prednisone (Dalakas 2011; Findlay 2015).

Nausea and vomiting of pregnancy, severe/ refractory (off-label use): Note: Reserve use as an add-on therapy when all other pharmacologic regimens have failed.

IV (succinate): 16 mg every 8 hours for 3 days. If no response within 3 days, discontinue treatment. If symptoms improve, complete 3-day course of treatment, then taper dose over 2 weeks (ACOG 189 2018; Safari 1998).

***Pneumocystis* pneumonia, adjunctive therapy for moderate to severe disease (off-label use): Note:** Recommended when on room air PaO_2 <70 mm Hg or PAO_2-PaO_2 ≥35 mm Hg. Dosing is based on an equivalent dose of prednisone.

IV (succinate): 30 mg twice daily on days 1 to 5 beginning as early as possible, followed by 30 mg once daily on days 6 to 10, then 15 mg once daily on days 11 to 21 (AST [Martin 2013]; HHS [OI adult 2019]; Sax 2020; Thomas 2019).

Prostate cancer, metastatic, castration-resistant (off-label use): Oral: 4 mg twice daily (in combination with ***micronized*** abiraterone acetate) (Stein 2018).

Systemic rheumatic disorders (eg, antineutrophil cytoplasmic antibody-associated vasculitis, mixed cryoglobulinemia syndrome, polyarteritis nodosa, rheumatoid arthritis, systemic lupus erythematosus), organ-threatening or life-threatening: Note: The following dosage ranges are for guidance only; dosing should be highly individualized, taking into account disease severity, the specific disorder, and disease manifestations.

Initial pulse therapy (optional): IV (succinate): 7 to 15 mg/kg/day (maximum dose: 500 mg to 1 g/ day) typically for up to 3 days, followed by an oral glucocorticoid (eg, prednisone); may be given as part of an appropriate combination regimen. Lower doses (eg, 250 mg/day) may be appropriate in some patients (eg, less severe manifestations) (Fervenza 2020; Forbess 2015; Merkel 2020; Merkel 2020; Muchtar 2017).

Warm autoimmune hemolytic anemia:

IV (succinate): 250 mg to 1 g daily for 1 to 3 days, followed by an oral glucocorticoid (eg, prednisone) (Barros 2010; Zanella 2014); a clinician experienced with the treatment of hemolytic anemia should be involved with therapy.

Renal Impairment: Adult There are no dosage adjustments provided in the manufacturer's labeling; use with caution.

Hepatic Impairment: Adult There are no dosage adjustments provided in the manufacturer's labeling; use with caution.

Pediatric Note: Adjust dose depending upon condition being treated and response of patient. The lowest possible dose should be used to control the condition; when dose reduction is possible, the dose should be reduced gradually. In life-threatening situations, parenteral doses larger than the oral dose may be needed. **Only sodium succinate salt may be given IV**

Asthma, exacerbation:

Acute, short-course "burst" (NAEPP 2007):

Infants and Children <12 years:

Oral: 1 to 2 mg/kg/day in divided doses once or twice daily for 3 to 10 days; maximum daily dose: 60 mg/**day**; **Note:** Burst should be continued until symptoms resolve or patient achieves peak expiratory flow 80% of personal best; usually requires 3 to 10 days of treatment (~5 days on average); longer treatment may be required

IM **(acetate)**: **Note:** This may be given in place of short-course "burst" of oral steroids in patients who are vomiting or if compliance is a problem.

Children ≤4 years: 7.5 mg/kg as a one-time dose; maximum dose: 240 mg

Children 5 to 11 years: 240 mg as a one-time dose

Children ≥12 years and Adolescents:

Oral: 40 to 60 mg/day in divided doses once or twice daily for 3 to 10 days; **Note:** Burst should be continued until symptoms resolve and peak expiratory flow is at least 80% of personal best; usually requires 3 to 10 days of treatment (~5 days on average); longer treatment may be required

IM **(acetate)**: 240 mg as a one-time dose; **Note:** This may be given in place of short-course "burst" of oral steroids in patients who are vomiting or if compliance is a problem

Hospital/emergency medical care doses:

Infants and Children <12 years: Oral, IV: 1 to 2 mg/kg/day in 2 divided doses; maximum daily dose: 60 mg/**day**; continue until peak expiratory flow is 70% of predicted or personal best

Children ≥12 years and Adolescents: Oral, IV: 40 to 80 mg/day in divided doses once or twice daily until peak expiratory flow is 70% of predicted or personal best

Status asthmaticus (previous NAEPP guidelines; still used by some clinicians): Children: IV: Loading dose: 2 mg/kg/dose, then 0.5 to 1 mg/kg/dose every 6 hours; **Note:** See NAEPP 2007 guidelines for asthma exacerbations (emergency medical care or hospital doses) listed above

Asthma, long-term treatment (maintenance) (NAEPP 2007):

Infants and Children <12 years: Oral: 0.25 to 2 mg/kg/day once daily in the morning or every other day as needed for asthma control; maximum daily dose: 60 mg/**day**

Children ≥12 years and Adolescents: Oral: 7.5 to 60 mg daily once daily in the morning or every other day as needed for asthma control

General dosing; anti-inflammatory or immunosuppressive: Infants, Children, and Adolescents: **Note:** Dosing range variable; individualize dose for disease state and patient response; Oral, IM (acetate or succinate), IV (succinate): Initial: 0.11 to 1.6 mg/kg/day or 3.2 to 48 mg/m^2/day; usual range: 0.5 to 1.7 mg/kg/day (Kliegman 2015); for oral, IM (succinate) and IV (succinate) administer in divided doses every 6 to 12 hours; for IM (acetate) administer as a single daily dose

"Pulse" therapy: IV (succinate): 15 to 30 mg/kg/dose once daily for 3 days; maximum dose: 1,000 mg

Long-acting: IM (acetate): 4 to 80 mg every 1 to 2 weeks

Kawasaki disease: Limited data available; optimal regimen not established; efficacy variable.

Primary treatment, patients at high risk for coronary artery aneurysms:

Pulse dosing: Infants and Children: IV: 30 mg/kg/dose as a single dose in combination with IVIG and aspirin (AHA [McCrindle 2017]; Ogata 2012; Okada 2009)

Taper dosing: Infants and Children: IV: 1.6 mg/kg/day in divided doses every 8 hours for 5 days or until afebrile, then transition to oral prednisolone; maximum daily dose: 48 mg/**day**; give in combination with aspirin and an additional dose of IVIG (AHA [McCrindle 2017]; Kobayashi 2012). **Note:** Dosing based on use of IV prednisolone product (2 mg/kg/day) which is not available in US; dosing converted to equivalent methylprednisolone dosing; however, clinical necessity of conversion is unknown.

Treatment, refractory/resistant disease: **Note:** Reserve use for patients who remain febrile after initial IVIG dose:

Pulse dosing: Infants and Children: IV: 30 mg/kg/dose once daily for 1 or 3 days; may be given in combination with additional IVIG dose (AHA [McCrindle 2017]; Ebato 2017; Miura 2008).

Taper dosing: Infants and Children: IV: 1.6 mg/kg/day in divided doses every 8 hours for 5 days or until afebrile, then transition to oral prednisolone; maximum daily dose: 48 mg/**day**; give in combination with aspirin and an additional dose of IVIG (AHA [McCrindle 2017]; Kobayashi 2012; Kobayashi 2013). **Note:** Dosing based on use of IV prednisolone product (2 mg/kg/day) which is not available in US; dosing converted to equivalent methylprednisolone dosing; however, clinical necessity of conversion is unknown.

Lupus nephritis: Children and Adolescents: IV (succinate): High-dose "pulse" therapy: 30 mg/kg/dose or 600 to 1,000 mg/**m**^{2}/dose once daily for 3 days; maximum dose: 1,000 mg (Adams 2006; Marks 2010)

Spinal cord injury, acute: Limited data available: Children and Adolescents: IV (succinate): 30 mg/kg over 15 minutes followed in 45 minutes by a continuous infusion of 5.4 mg/kg/hour for 23 hours (Bracken 1992; Jaffe 1991); **Note:** Due to insufficient evidence of clinical efficacy (ie, preserving or improving spinal cord function), the routine use of methylprednisolone in the treatment of acute spinal cord injury is no longer recommended. If used in this setting, methylprednisolone should not be initiated >8 hours after the injury; not effective in penetrating trauma (eg, gunshot) (Consortium for Spinal Cord Medicine 2008).

***Pneumocystis* pneumonia; moderate or severe infection: Note:** Initiate therapy within 72 hours of diagnosis, if possible.

Infants and Children: IV (succinate): 1 mg/kg/dose every 6 hours on days 1 to 7, then 1 mg/kg/dose twice daily on days 8 to 9, then 0.5 mg/kg/dose twice daily on days 10 and 11, and 1 mg/kg/dose once daily on days 12 to 16 (CDC 2009)

Adolescents: IV (succinate): 30 mg twice daily on days 1 to 5, then 30 mg once daily on days 6 to 10, then 15 mg once daily on days 11 to 21 (CDC 2009a)

Graft-versus-host disease, acute (GVHD): Infants, Children and Adolescents: IV (succinate): 1 to 2 mg/kg/dose once daily; if using low dose (1 mg/kg) and no improvement after 3 days, increase dose to 2 mg/kg. Continue therapy for 5 to 7 days; if improvement observed, may taper by 10% of starting dose every 4 days; if no improvement, then considered steroid-refractory GVHD and additional agents should be considered (Carpenter 2010)

Renal Impairment: Pediatric There are no dosage adjustments provided in the manufacturer's labeling; use with caution; slightly dialyzable (5% to 20%); administer dose posthemodialysis

Hepatic Impairment: Pediatric There are no dosage adjustments provided in the manufacturer's labeling.

Mechanism of Action In a tissue-specific manner, corticosteroids regulate gene expression subsequent to binding specific intracellular receptors and translocation into the nucleus. Corticosteroids exert a wide array of physiologic effects including modulation of carbohydrate, protein, and lipid metabolism and maintenance of fluid and electrolyte homeostasis. Moreover cardiovascular, immunologic, musculoskeletal, endocrine, and neurologic physiology are influenced by corticosteroids. Decreases inflammation by suppression of migration of polymorphonuclear leukocytes and reversal of increased capillary permeability.

Contraindications

Hypersensitivity to methylprednisolone or any component of the formulation; systemic fungal infection (except intra-articular injection for localized joint conditions); intrathecal administration; live or attenuated virus vaccines (with immunosuppressive doses of corticosteroids); use in premature infants (formulations containing benzyl alcohol preservative only); immune thrombocytopenia (formerly known as idiopathic thrombocytopenic purpura) (IM administration only)

Additional contraindication: Methylprednisolone sodium succinate 40 mg vial only: Hypersensitivity to cow's milk or its components or other dairy products which may contain trace amounts of milk ingredients (known or suspected).

Canadian labeling: Additional contraindications (not in US labeling):

Methylprednisolone tablets: Herpes simplex of the eye, vaccinia and varicella (except for short-term or emergency therapy)

Methylprednisolone acetate injection: Epidural or intravascular administration; intra-articular injections in unstable joints; herpes simplex of the eye, vaccinia and varicella (except for short-term or emergency therapy)

Methylprednisolone sodium succinate: Epidural administration; herpes simplex keratitis, vaccinia and varicella, arrested tuberculosis, acute psychoses, Cushing syndrome, peptic ulcer, markedly elevated serum creatinine (except for short-term or emergency therapy)

Documentation of allergenic cross-reactivity for corticosteroids is limited. However, because of similarities in chemical structure and/or pharmacologic actions, the possibility of cross-sensitivity cannot be ruled out with certainty.

Warnings/Precautions Corticosteroids are not approved for epidural injection. Serious neurologic events (eg, spinal cord infarction, paraplegia, quadriplegia, cortical blindness, stroke), some resulting in death, have been reported with epidural injection of corticosteroids, with and without use of fluoroscopy.

High doses of methylprednisolone IV (usually doses of 1 g/day in adults) may induce a toxic form of acute hepatitis (rare); serious hepatic injury may occur, resulting in acute liver failure and death. Time to onset can be several weeks or longer; resolution has been observed after discontinuation of therapy. Discontinue methylprednisolone if toxic hepatitis occurs. Avoid use of high doses in patients with a history of methylprednisone-induced toxic hepatitis.

Use with caution in patients with thyroid disease, hepatic impairment, renal impairment, cardiovascular disease, diabetes, glaucoma, cataracts, myasthenia gravis, osteoporosis, seizures, or GI diseases (diverticulitis, fresh intestinal anastomoses, active or latent peptic ulcer, ulcerative colitis, abscess or other pyogenic infection) due to perforation risk. Not recommended for the treatment of optic neuritis; may increase frequency of new episodes. Use with caution in patients with a history of ocular herpes simplex; corneal perforation has occurred; do not use in active ocular herpes simplex. Use caution following acute MI (corticosteroids have been associated with myocardial rupture). Use of higher dose corticosteroid therapy (in adults, ≥15 mg/day of prednisone or equivalent) in patients with systemic sclerosis may increase the risk of scleroderma renal crisis; avoid use when possible (Steen 1998; Trang 2012).

Use with caution in the elderly with the smallest possible effective dose for the shortest duration. May affect growth velocity; growth should be routinely monitored in pediatric patients. Withdraw therapy with gradual tapering of dose. Patients may require higher doses when subject to stress (ie, trauma, surgery, severe infection).

May cause hypercortisolism or suppression of hypothalamic-pituitary-adrenal (HPA) axis, particularly in younger children or in patients receiving high doses for prolonged periods. HPA axis suppression may lead to adrenal crisis. Withdrawal and discontinuation of a corticosteroid should be done slowly and carefully. Particular care is required when patients are transferred from systemic corticosteroids to inhaled products due to possible adrenal insufficiency or withdrawal from steroids, including an increase in allergic symptoms. Adult patients receiving >20 mg per day of prednisone (or equivalent) may be most susceptible. Fatalities have occurred due to adrenal insufficiency in asthmatic patients during and after transfer from systemic corticosteroids to aerosol steroids; aerosol steroids do not provide the systemic steroid needed to treat patients having trauma, surgery, or infections. Corticosteroids should not be administered for the treatment of sepsis in the absence of shock (SCCM/ESICM [Annane 2017]). Use in septic shock or sepsis syndrome may increase mortality in some populations (eg, patients with elevated serum creatinine, patients who develop secondary infections after use).

Acute myopathy has been reported with high dose corticosteroids, usually in patients with neuromuscular transmission disorders; may involve ocular and/or respiratory muscles; monitor creatine kinase; recovery may be delayed. Corticosteroid use may cause psychiatric disturbances, including euphoria, insomnia, mood swings, personality changes, severe depression, or psychotic manifestations. Preexisting psychiatric conditions may be exacerbated by corticosteroid use. Prolonged use of corticosteroids may increase the incidence of secondary infection, cause activation of latent infections, mask acute infection (including fungal infections), prolong or exacerbate viral or parasitic infections, or limit response to killed or inactivated vaccines. Exposure to chickenpox or measles should be avoided; corticosteroids should not be used to treat ocular herpes simplex. Corticosteroids should not be used for cerebral malaria, fungal infections, or viral hepatitis. Close observation is required in patients with latent tuberculosis and/or TB reactivity; restrict use in active TB (only fulminating or disseminated TB in conjunction with antituberculosis treatment). Amebiasis should be ruled out in any patient with recent travel to tropic climates or unexplained diarrhea prior to initiation of corticosteroids. Use with extreme caution in patients with *Strongyloides* infections; hyperinfection, dissemination and fatalities have occurred. Prolonged treatment with corticosteroids has been associated with the development of Kaposi sarcoma (case reports); discontinuation may result in clinical improvement (Goedert 2002).

High-dose corticosteroids should not be used to manage acute head injury. Rare cases of anaphylactoid reactions have been observed in patients receiving corticosteroids. Avoid injection or leakage into the dermis; dermal and/or subdermal skin depression may occur at the site of injection. Avoid deltoid muscle injection; subcutaneous atrophy may occur. Septic arthritis may occur as a complication to parenteral therapy; institute appropriate antimicrobial therapy as required. Potentially significant drug-drug interactions may exist, requiring dose or frequency adjustment, additional monitoring, and/or selection of alternative therapy.

Methylprednisolone **acetate** IM injection (multiple-dose vial) and the diluent for methylprednisolone **sodium succinate** injection may contain benzyl alcohol; large amounts of benzyl alcohol (≥99 mg/kg/day) have been associated with a potentially fatal toxicity ("gasping syndrome") in neonates; the "gasping syndrome" consists of metabolic acidosis, respiratory distress, gasping respirations, CNS dysfunction (including convulsions, intracranial hemorrhage), hypotension, and cardiovascular collapse (AAP ["Inactive" 1997]; CDC 1982); some data suggests that benzoate displaces bilirubin from protein binding sites (Ahlfors 2001); avoid or use dosage forms containing benzyl alcohol with caution in neonates. Additionally, benzyl alcohol may also be toxic to neural tissue when administered locally (eg, intra-articular, intralesional).

Some dosage forms may contain polysorbate 80 (also known as Tweens). Hypersensitivity reactions, usually a delayed reaction, have been reported following exposure to pharmaceutical products containing polysorbate 80 in certain individuals (Isaksson 2002; Lucente 2000; Shelley 1995). Thrombocytopenia, ascites, pulmonary deterioration, and renal and hepatic failure have been reported in premature neonates after receiving parenteral products containing polysorbate 80 (Alade 1986; CDC 1984). See manufacturer's labeling.

Warnings: Additional Pediatric Considerations May cause osteoporosis (at any age) or inhibition of bone growth in pediatric patients. Use with caution in patients with osteoporosis. In a population-based study of children, risk of fracture was shown to be increased with >4 courses of corticosteroids; underlying clinical condition may also impact bone health and osteoporotic effect of corticosteroids (Leonard, 2007). Increased IOP may occur, especially with prolonged use; in children, increased IOP has been shown to be dose dependent and produce a greater IOP in children <6 years than older children treated with ophthalmic dexamethasone (Lam, 2005). Hypertrophic cardiomyopathy has been reported in premature neonates.

Drug Interactions

Metabolism/Transport Effects **Substrate** of CYP3A4 (major); **Note:** Assignment of Major/Minor substrate status based on clinically relevant drug interaction potential

Avoid Concomitant Use

Avoid concomitant use of MethylPREDNISolone with any of the following: Abametapir; Aldesleukin; BCG (Intravesical); Cladribine; Conivaptan; Desmopressin; Fexinidazole [INT]; Fusidic Acid (Systemic); Idelalisib; Indium 111 Capromab Pendetide; Macimorelin; Mifamurtide; MiFEPRIStone; Natalizumab; Pimecrolimus; Tacrolimus (Topical)

Increased Effect/Toxicity

MethylPREDNISolone may increase the levels/effects of: Acetylcholinesterase Inhibitors; Amphotericin B; Androgens; Baricitinib; CycloSPORINE (Systemic); Deferasirox; Desirudin; Desmopressin; Fexinidazole [INT]; Fingolimod; Leflunomide; Loop Diuretics; Natalizumab; Nicorandil; Nonsteroidal Anti-Inflammatory Agents (COX-2 Selective); Nonsteroidal Anti-Inflammatory Agents (Nonselective); Ozanimod; Quinolones; Ritodrine; Sargramostim; Siponimod; Thiazide and Thiazide-Like Diuretics; Tofacitinib; Upadacitinib; Vaccines (Live); Vitamin K Antagonists

The levels/effects of MethylPREDNISolone may be increased by: Abametapir; Aprepitant; Cladribine; Clofazimine; Conivaptan; CycloSPORINE (Systemic); CYP3A4 Inhibitors (Moderate); CYP3A4 Inhibitors (Strong); Denosumab; DilTIAZem; Duvelisib; Erdafitinib; Estrogen Derivatives; Fosaprepitant; Fosnetupitant; Fusidic Acid (Systemic); Idelalisib; Indacaterol; Inebilizumab; Larotrectinib; MiFEPRIStone; Netupitant; Neuromuscular-Blocking Agents (Nondepolarizing); Ocrelizumab; Palbociclib; Pimecrolimus; Roflumilast; Salicylates; Simeprevir; Stiripentol; Tacrolimus (Topical); Trastuzumab

Decreased Effect

MethylPREDNISolone may decrease the levels/effects of: Aldesleukin; Antidiabetic Agents; Axicabtagene Ciloleucel; BCG (Intravesical); Calcitriol (Systemic); Coccidioides immitis Skin Test; Corticorelin; Cosyntropin; CycloSPORINE (Systemic); Hyaluronidase; Indium 111 Capromab Pendetide; Isoniazid; Macimorelin; Mifamurtide; Nivolumab; Pidotimod; Salicylates; Sipuleucel-T; Somatropin; Tacrolimus (Systemic); Tertomotide; Tisagenlecleucel; Urea Cycle Disorder Agents; Vaccines (Inactivated); Vaccines (Live)

The levels/effects of MethylPREDNISolone may be decreased by: Antacids; Bile Acid Sequestrants; CYP3A4 Inducers (Moderate); CYP3A4 Inducers (Strong); Dabrafenib; Deferasirox; Echinacea; Enzalutamide; Erdafitinib; Ivosidenib; MiFEPRIStone; Mitotane; Sarilumab; Siltuximab; Tocilizumab

Dietary Considerations Take tablets with meals to decrease GI upset; need diet rich in pyridoxine, vitamin C, vitamin D, folate, calcium, phosphorus, and protein.

Pharmacodynamics/Kinetics

Onset of Action IV (succinate): Within 1 hour; Intra-articular (acetate): 1 week

Duration of Action Intra-articular (acetate): 1 to 5 weeks

Half-life Elimination

Adolescents: IV: 1.9 ± 0.7 hours (age range: 12 to 20 years; Rouster-Stevens 2008)

Adults: Oral: 2.5 ± 1.2 hours (Czock 2005); IV (succinate): 0.25 ± 0.1 hour (Czock 2005)

Time to Peak

Oral: 2.1 ± 0.7 hours (Czock 2005)

IV (succinate): 0.8 hours (Czock 2005)

Pregnancy Considerations Methylprednisolone crosses the placenta (Anderson 1981). Some studies have shown an association between first trimester systemic corticosteroid use and oral clefts or decreased birth weight; however, information is conflicting and may be influenced by maternal dose/indication for use (Lunghi 2010; Park-Wyllie 2000; Pradat 2003). Hypoadrenalism may occur in newborns following maternal use of corticosteroids in pregnancy; monitor.

When systemic corticosteroids are needed in pregnancy for rheumatic disorders, it is generally recommended to use the lowest effective dose for the shortest duration of time, avoiding high doses during the first trimester (Götestam Skorpen 2016; Makol 2011; Østensen 2009).

For dermatologic disorders in pregnant women, systemic corticosteroids are generally not preferred for initial therapy; should be avoided during the first trimester; and used during the second or third trimester at the lowest effective dose (Bae 2012; Leachman 2006).

Uncontrolled asthma is associated with adverse events on pregnancy (increased risk of perinatal mortality, preeclampsia, preterm birth, low birth weight infants, cesarean delivery, and the development of gestational diabetes). Poorly controlled asthma or asthma exacerbations may have a greater fetal/maternal risk than what is associated with appropriately used asthma medications. Maternal treatment improves pregnancy outcomes by reducing the risk of some adverse events (eg, preterm birth, gestational diabetes). Maternal asthma symptoms should be monitored monthly during pregnancy. Inhaled corticosteroids are recommended for the treatment of asthma during pregnancy; however, systemic corticosteroids should be used to control acute exacerbations or treat severe persistent asthma (ERS/TSANZ [Middleton 2020]; GINA 2020).

Methylprednisolone may be considered for adjunctive treatment of severe nausea and vomiting in pregnant women. Due to risks of adverse fetal events associated with first trimester exposure, use is reserved for refractory cases in women with dehydration (ACOG 189 2018).

The Transplant Pregnancy Registry International (TPR) is a registry that follows pregnancies that occur in maternal transplant recipients or those fathered by male transplant recipients. The TPR encourages reporting of pregnancies following solid organ transplant by contacting them at 1-877-955-6877 or https://www.transplantpregnancyregistry.org.

Breastfeeding Considerations

Methylprednisolone is present in breast milk (Cooper 2015; Strijbos 2015).

The relative infant dose (RID) of methylprednisolone is 2.8% to 5.6% when calculated using the highest breast milk concentration located and compared to a weight-adjusted infant dose of 15 to 30 mg/kg/day.

In general, breastfeeding is considered acceptable when the RID is <10% (Anderson 2016; Ito 2000).

Using the highest milk concentration (5.55 mcg/mL), the estimated daily infant dose via breast milk is 0.8325 mg/kg/day. This milk concentration was obtained following maternal administration of methylprednisolone 1,000 mg IV infused over 2 hours. The maximum milk concentration occurred 1 hour after the maternal dose and methylprednisolone was below the limits of quantification 12 hours after the dose (Cooper 2015).

The manufacturer notes that when used systemically, maternal use of corticosteroids have the potential to cause adverse events in a breastfeeding infant (eg, growth suppression, interfere with endogenous corticosteroid production) and therefore recommends a decision be made whether to discontinue breastfeeding or to discontinue the drug, taking into account the importance of treatment to the mother.

Corticosteroids are generally considered acceptable in breastfeeding women when used in usual doses (Götestam Skorpen 2016; WHO 2002); however, monitoring of the nursing infant is recommended (WHO 2002). If there is concern about exposure to the infant, some guidelines recommend waiting 4 hours after the maternal dose of an oral systemic corticosteroid before breastfeeding in order to decrease potential exposure to the breastfeeding infant (based on a study using prednisolone) (Bae 2012; Butler 2014; Götestam Skorpen 2016; Leachman 2006; Makol 2011; Ost 1985).

Dosage Forms: US

Kit, Injection:

P-Care D40: 40 mg/mL

P-Care D80: 40 mg/mL

Solution Reconstituted, Injection:

SOLU-Medrol: 500 mg (1 ea)

Generic: 40 mg (1 ea); 125 mg (1 ea); 500 mg (1 ea); 1000 mg (1 ea)

Solution Reconstituted, Injection [preservative free]:

SOLU-Medrol: 40 mg (1 ea); 125 mg (1 ea); 500 mg (1 ea); 1000 mg (1 ea); 2 g (1 ea)

Suspension, Injection:

DEPO-Medrol: 20 mg/mL (5 mL); 40 mg/mL (1 mL, 5 mL, 10 mL); 80 mg/mL (1 mL, 5 mL)

Generic: 40 mg/mL (1 mL, 5 mL, 10 mL); 80 mg/mL (1 mL, 5 mL)

Suspension, Injection [preservative free]:

DEPO-Medrol: 40 mg/mL (1 mL)

Generic: 40 mg/mL (1 mL)

Tablet, Oral:

Medrol: 2 mg, 8 mg, 16 mg, 32 mg, 4 mg

Generic: 8 mg, 16 mg, 32 mg, 4 mg

Tablet Therapy Pack, Oral:

Medrol: 4 mg (21 ea)

Generic: 4 mg (21 ea)

Dosage Forms: Canada

Solution Reconstituted, Injection:

SOLU-medrol: 40 mg (1 ea)

Solu-MEDROL: 125 mg (1 ea); 500 mg (1 ea); 1000 mg (1 ea)

Generic: 40 mg (1 ea); 125 mg (1 ea); 500 mg (1 ea); 1000 mg (1 ea)

Suspension, Injection:

Depo-Medrol: 20 mg/mL (5 mL); 40 mg/mL (1 mL, 2 mL, 5 mL); 80 mg/mL (1 mL, 5 mL)

Generic: 40 mg/mL (1 mL, 2 mL, 5 mL); 80 mg/mL (1 mL, 5 mL)

Tablet, Oral:

Medrol: 16 mg, 4 mg

◆ **6-α-Methylprednisolone** *see* MethylPREDNISolone *on page 999*

◆ **Methylprednisolone Acetate** *see* MethylPREDNISolone *on page 999*

◆ **Methylprednisolone Sodium Succinate** *see* MethylPREDNISolone *on page 999*

◆ **4-Methylpyrazole** *see* Fomepizole *on page 710*

MethylTESTOSTERone (meth il tes TOS te rone)

Brand Names: US Android [DSC]; Methitest; Testred [DSC]

Pharmacologic Category Androgen

Use

Breast cancer, metastatic (females): Secondarily in women with advancing inoperable metastatic (skeletal) mammary cancer who are 1 to 5 years postmenopausal; has also been used in premenopausal women with breast cancer who have benefited from oophorectomy and are considered to have a hormone-responsive tumor.

Delayed puberty (males): To stimulate puberty in carefully selected males with clearly delayed puberty.

Local Anesthetic/Vasoconstrictor Precautions

No information available to require special precautions

Effects on Dental Treatment No significant effects or complications reported

Effects on Bleeding No information available to require special precautions

Adverse Reactions Frequency not defined.

Cardiovascular: Edema

Central nervous system: Anxiety, depression, headache, paresthesia

Dermatologic: Acne vulgaris, androgenetic alopecia

Endocrine & metabolic: Change in libido, gynecomastia (males), hirsutism (females), hypercalcemia, hypercholesterolemia, menstrual disease (includes amenorrhea)

Gastrointestinal: Nausea, vomiting

Genitourinary: Benign prostatic hypertrophy (males), impotence (males), mastalgia (females), oligospermia (males; at high doses), priapism (males), testicular atrophy (males), virilization (males and females)

Hematologic & oncologic: Clotting factors suppression, polycythemia, prostate carcinoma (males)

Hepatic: Abnormal liver function tests, cholestatic hepatitis, hepatic insufficiency, hepatic necrosis, jaundice, peliosis hepatitis

<1%, postmarketing, and/or case reports: Anaphylactoid reaction, hepatocellular neoplasm, hepatotoxicity (idiosyncratic; Chalasani 2014)

Mechanism of Action Endogenous androgen stimulates receptors in organs and tissues to promote growth and development of male sex organs and maintains secondary sex characteristics in androgen-deficient males

Pharmacodynamics/Kinetics

Half-life Elimination Variable: 10 to 100 minutes

Reproductive Considerations

Use is contraindicated in women who may become pregnant. Use of methyltestosterone may impair fertility; oligospermia may occur in males and amenorrhea may occur in females.

Pregnancy Risk Factor X

Pregnancy Considerations

Use is contraindicated in women who are pregnant. Exposure during pregnancy may cause virilization of the external genitalis of the female fetus, including clitoromegaly, abnormal vaginal development, and fusion of genital folds to form a scrotal-like structure. The degree of masculinization is dose related and most likely to occur when androgens are administered in the first trimester. If a patient becomes pregnant while taking androgens, she should be counseled on the potential hazard to the fetus.

Controlled Substance C-III

- **Methyltestosterone and Esterified Estrogen** *see* Estrogens (Esterified) and Methyltestosterone *on page 605*
- **Methyltestosterone and Oestrogen** *see* Estrogens (Esterified) and Methyltestosterone *on page 605*

Metipranolol (met i PRAN oh lol)

Pharmacologic Category Beta-Blocker, Nonselective; Ophthalmic Agent, Antiglaucoma

Use Elevated intraocular pressure: Treatment elevated intraocular pressure in patient with chronic open-angle glaucoma or ocular hypertension

Local Anesthetic/Vasoconstrictor Precautions

No information available to require special precautions

Effects on Dental Treatment Metipranolol is a nonselective beta-blocker and may enhance the pressor response to epinephrine, resulting in hypertension and bradycardia. Many nonsteroidal anti-inflammatory drugs, such as ibuprofen and indomethacin, can reduce the hypotensive effect of beta-blockers after 3 or more weeks of therapy with the NSAID. Short-term NSAID use (ie, 3 days) requires no special precautions in patients taking beta-blockers.

Effects on Bleeding No information available to require special precautions

Adverse Reactions Frequency not defined.

Cardiovascular: Angina, atrial fibrillation, bradycardia, hypertension, MI, palpitation

Central nervous system: Anxiety, depression, dizziness, headache, nervousness, somnolence

Dermatologic: Rash

Gastrointestinal: Nausea

Neuromuscular & skeletal: Arthritis, myalgia, weakness

Ocular: Abnormal vision, blepharitis, blurred vision, browache, conjunctivitis, discomfort, edema, eyelid dermatitis, photophobia, tearing, uveitis

Respiratory: Bronchitis, cough, dyspnea, epistaxis, rhinitis

Miscellaneous: Allergic reaction

Mechanism of Action Beta-adrenoceptor-blocking agent; lacks intrinsic sympathomimetic activity and membrane-stabilizing effects and possesses only slight local anesthetic activity; mechanism of action of metipranolol in reducing intraocular pressure appears to be via reduced production of aqueous humor. This effect may be related to a reduction in blood flow to the iris root-ciliary body. It remains unclear if the reduction in intraocular pressure observed with beta-blockers is actually secondary to beta-adrenoceptor blockade.

Pharmacodynamics/Kinetics

Onset of Action ≤30 minutes; Peak effect: Maximum: ~2 hours

Duration of Action Intraocular pressure reduction: Up to 24 hours

Half-life Elimination ~3 hours

Pregnancy Risk Factor C

Pregnancy Considerations Adverse events were observed in some animal reproduction studies. The same adverse effects observed with systemic administration of beta-blockers may occur following ophthalmic use of metipranolol. If ophthalmic agents are needed for the treatment of glaucoma during pregnancy, the minimum effective dose should be used in combination with punctal occlusion to decrease potential exposure to the fetus (Johnson 2001; Salim 2014; Samples 1988).

- **Metipranolol Hydrochloride** *see* Metipranolol *on page 1007*

Metoclopramide (met oh KLOE pra mide)

Brand Names: US Metozolv ODT [DSC]; Reglan

Brand Names: Canada APO-Metoclop; Metoclopramide Omega; Metonia

Pharmacologic Category Antiemetic; Dopamine Antagonist; Gastrointestinal Agent, Prokinetic; Serotonin 5-HT_4 Receptor Agonist

Use

Injection:

Chemotherapy-induced nausea and vomiting, prophylaxis: Prophylaxis of nausea and vomiting associated with emetogenic cancer chemotherapy. **Note:** Injectable metoclopramide prior to moderate- to high-emetic-risk chemotherapy is rarely indicated due to the potential for neurologic events and availability of more efficacious alternative agents.

Gastroparesis, diabetic: Relief of symptoms associated with acute and recurrent diabetic gastric stasis.

Oral:

Gastroesophageal reflux disease (GERD), refractory: Short-term (4 to 12 weeks) treatment in adults with documented symptomatic GERD who fail to respond to conventional therapy.

Note: May use metoclopramide as an adjunctive therapy **only** if gastroparesis is confirmed. The American College of Gastroenterology (ACG) guidelines for the treatment of GERD recommend that diagnostic evaluation to confirm underlying gastroparesis be performed **prior to** considering the use of prokinetic agents (ACG [Katz 2013]). Furthermore, American Gastroenterological Association (AGA) guidelines for the treatment of GERD recommend **against** the use of metoclopramide as monotherapy or adjunctive therapy in patients with GERD (AGA [Kahrilas 2008]).

Gastroparesis, diabetic: Relief of symptoms associated with acute and recurrent diabetic gastroparesis in adults.

Local Anesthetic/Vasoconstrictor Precautions

No information available to require special precautions

Effects on Dental Treatment Metoclopramide has relatively few adverse effects when used in low doses; however, extrapyramidal effects including akathisia (motor restlessness), acute dystonia (spasmodic contractures), pseudoparkinsonism, and tardive dyskinesia can occur. These effects are more likely in the elderly, patients taking other dopamine antagonists (including antipsychotic agents and some antiemetic agents), and patients with Parkinson's disease. Metoclopramide will increase gastric emptying which will aid in the absorption of orally administered anxiolytic or sedative agents used for minimal or moderate sedation as well as promote the emptying of the stomach following procedures during which blood may be swallowed causing GI upset.

Effects on Bleeding No information available to require special precautions

Adverse Reactions Frequency not always defined.

Cardiovascular: Atrioventricular block, bradycardia, cardiac failure, flushing (following high IV doses), hypertension, hypotension, supraventricular tachycardia

Central nervous system: Drowsiness (~10% to 70%; dose related), dystonic reaction (<1% to 25%; dose and age related), lassitude (~10%), restlessness (~10%), fatigue (2% to 10%), headache (4% to 5%), dizziness (1% to 4%), somnolence (2% to 3%), akathisia, confusion, depression, drug-induced Parkinson's disease, hallucination (rare), insomnia, neuroleptic malignant syndrome (rare), seizure, suicidal ideation, tardive dyskinesia

Dermatologic: Skin rash, urticaria

Endocrine & metabolic: Amenorrhea, fluid retention, galactorrhea, gynecomastia, hyperprolactinemia, porphyria

Gastrointestinal: Nausea (4% to 6%), vomiting (1% to 2%), diarrhea

Genitourinary: Impotence, urinary frequency, urinary incontinence

Hematologic & oncologic: Agranulocytosis, leukopenia, methemoglobinemia, neutropenia, sulfhemoglobinemia

Hepatic: Hepatotoxicity (rare)

Hypersensitivity: Angioedema (rare), hypersensitivity reaction

Neuromuscular & skeletal: Laryngospasm (rare)

Ophthalmic: Visual disturbance

Respiratory: Bronchospasm, laryngeal edema (rare)

Mechanism of Action Metoclopramide blocks dopamine receptors and (when given in higher doses) also blocks serotonin receptors in chemoreceptor trigger zone of the CNS; enhances the response to acetylcholine of tissue in upper GI tract causing enhanced motility and accelerated gastric emptying without stimulating gastric, biliary, or pancreatic secretions; increases lower esophageal sphincter tone

Pharmacodynamics/Kinetics

Onset of Action Oral: 30 to 60 minutes; IV: 1 to 3 minutes; IM: 10 to 15 minutes

Duration of Action Therapeutic: 1 to 2 hours, regardless of route

Half-life Elimination Normal renal function: Neonates, PMA 31 to 40 weeks: 5.4 hours (Kearns 1998); Infants: 4.15 hours (range: 2.23 to 10.3 hours) (Kearns 1988); Children: ~4 hours (range: 2 to 12.5 hours); half-life and clearance may be dose dependent; Adults: 5 to 6 hours (may be dose dependent)

Time to Peak Serum: Oral: Neonates, PMA 31 to 40 weeks: 2.45 hours (Kearns 1998); Infants: 2.2 hours; Adults: 1 to 2 hours

Reproductive Considerations

Metoclopramide may increase prolactin concentrations; hyperprolactinemia may suppress hypothalamic GnRH, resulting in reduced pituitary gonadotropin secretion which may inhibit reproductive function by impairing gonadal steroidogenesis. Amenorrhea and impotence have been reported.

Pregnancy Considerations

Metoclopramide crosses the placenta and can be detected in cord blood and amniotic fluid (Arvela 1983; Bylsma-Howell 1983). Available studies do not report an increased risk of adverse pregnancy-related outcomes following maternal use. Extrapyramidal symptoms or methemoglobinemia may potentially occur in the neonate.

Metoclopramide is one of the agents that may be considered for adjunctive treatment of nausea and vomiting in pregnant women when symptoms persist following initial pharmacologic therapy. Oral or IM therapy may be given in patients who are not dehydrated; IV therapy should be used when dehydration is present (ACOG 189 2018). Metoclopramide may be used for prophylaxis of nausea and vomiting associated with cesarean delivery (ASA 2016; Smith 2011).

Product Availability Gimoti nasal spray: FDA approved June 2020; availability anticipated in the 4th quarter of 2020. Information pertaining to this product within the monograph is pending revision. Gimoti is indicated for the relief of symptoms in adults with acute and recurrent diabetic gastroparesis. Consult the prescribing information for additional information.

◆ **Metoclopramide HCl** *see* Metoclopramide *on page 1007*

MetOLazone (me TOLE a zone)

Related Information

Cardiovascular Diseases *on page 1654*

Brand Names: Canada Zaroxolyn

Pharmacologic Category Diuretic, Thiazide-Related

Use Edema: Treatment of edema due to heart failure or renal diseases, including the nephrotic syndrome and states of diminished renal function.

Local Anesthetic/Vasoconstrictor Precautions

No information available to require special precautions

Effects on Dental Treatment Key adverse event(s) related to dental treatment: Xerostomia (normal salivary flow resumes upon discontinuation); Patients may experience orthostatic hypotension as they stand up after treatment; especially if lying in dental chair for extended periods of time. Use caution with sudden changes in position during and after dental treatment.

Effects on Bleeding No information available to require special precautions

Adverse Reactions Frequency not defined.

Cardiovascular: Chest discomfort, chest pain, necrotizing angiitis, orthostatic hypotension, palpitations, syncope, venous thrombosis

Central nervous system: Chills, depression, dizziness, drowsiness, fatigue, headache, neuropathy, paresthesia, restlessness, vertigo

Dermatologic: Pruritus, skin necrosis, skin photosensitivity, skin rash, Stevens-Johnson syndrome, toxic epidermal necrolysis, urticaria

Endocrine & metabolic: Glycosuria, gout, hypercalcemia, hyperglycemia, hyperuricemia, hypochloremia, hypochloremic alkalosis, hypokalemia, hypomagnesemia, hyponatremia, hypophosphatemia, hypovolemia
Gastrointestinal: Abdominal pain, anorexia, bloating, constipation, diarrhea, epigastric distress, nausea, pancreatitis, vomiting, xerostomia
Genitourinary: Impotence
Hematologic & oncologic: Agranulocytosis, aplastic anemia, hemoconcentration, hypoplastic anemia, leukopenia, petechia, purpura, thrombocytopenia
Hepatic: Cholestatic jaundice, hepatitis
Neuromuscular & skeletal: Arthralgia, muscle cramps, muscle spasm, weakness
Ophthalmic: Transient blurred vision
Renal: Increased blood urea nitrogen

Mechanism of Action Inhibits sodium reabsorption in the distal tubules causing increased excretion of sodium and water, as well as, potassium and hydrogen ions

Pharmacodynamics/Kinetics

Onset of Action Diuresis: ~60 minutes.

Duration of Action ≥24 hours.

Half-life Elimination 8 to 14 hours (Ernst 2009).

Pregnancy Considerations

Metolazone crosses the placenta and appears in cord blood.

Hypoglycemia, hypokalemia, hyponatremia, jaundice, and thrombocytopenia are reported as complications to the fetus or newborn following maternal use of thiazide diuretics.

Use to treat edema during normal pregnancies is not appropriate; use may be considered when edema is due to pathologic causes (as in the nonpregnant patient); monitor.

Metoprolol (me toe PROE lole)

Related Information

Cardiovascular Diseases *on page 1654*

Brand Names: US Kapspargo Sprinkle; Lopressor; Toprol XL

Brand Names: Canada AG-Metoprolol-L; APO-Metoprolol; APO-Metoprolol SR; APO-Metoprolol Type L; DOM-Metoprolol; DOM-Metoprolol-L; JAMP-Metoprolol-L; Lopresor SR; Lopresor [DSC]; Metoprolol-100; Metoprolol-25; Metoprolol-50; Metoprolol-L; MYLAN-Metoprolol [DSC]; PMS-Metoprolol-B; PMS-Metoprolol-L; RIVA-Metoprolol-L; SANDOZ Metoprolol (Type L) [DSC]; Sandoz Metoprolol SR; TEVA-Metoprolol

Pharmacologic Category Antianginal Agent; Antihypertensive; Beta-Blocker, Beta-1 Selective

Use

Angina: Long-term treatment of angina pectoris.

Heart failure with reduced ejection fraction (ER oral formulation): Treatment of stable, symptomatic (NYHA class II or III) heart failure of ischemic, hypertensive, or cardiomyopathic origin to reduce the rate of mortality plus hospitalization in patients already receiving angiotensin-converting enzyme inhibitors, diuretics, and/or digoxin.

Hypertension: Management of hypertension. **Note:** Beta-blockers are **not** recommended as first-line therapy (ACC/AHA [Whelton 2017]).

Myocardial infarction: Treatment of hemodynamically stable acute myocardial infarction to reduce cardiovascular mortality (injection to be used in combination with metoprolol oral maintenance therapy).

Local Anesthetic/Vasoconstrictor Precautions Metoprolol is a cardioselective beta-blocker. Local anesthetic with vasoconstrictor can be safely used in patients medicated with metoprolol. Nonselective beta-blockers (ie, propranolol, nadolol) enhance the pressor response to epinephrine, resulting in hypertension and bradycardia; this has not been reported for metoprolol. Many nonsteroidal anti-inflammatory drugs (NSAIDs), such as ibuprofen and indomethacin, can reduce the hypotensive effect of beta-blockers after 3 or more weeks of therapy with the NSAID. Short-term NSAID use (ie, 3 days) requires no special precautions in patients taking beta-blockers.

Effects on Dental Treatment Key adverse event(s) related to dental treatment: Infrequent occurrence of xerostomia has been reported. Rare occurrence of dysgeusia has also been reported.

Effects on Bleeding No information available to require special precautions

Adverse Reactions

>10%: Cardiovascular: Bradycardia (2% to 16% [placebo 6.7%]), hypotension (1% to 27%)

1% to 10%:
Cardiovascular: Arterial insufficiency (usually Raynaud type: 1%), cardiac failure (1%), cerebrovascular accident (1%), cold extremity (1%), first degree atrioventricular block (5% [placebo 1.9%]), palpitations (1%), peripheral edema (1%)
Dermatologic: Gangrene of skin and/or subcutaneous tissues (1%), pruritus (5%), skin rash (>2% to 5%)
Gastrointestinal: Constipation (1%), diarrhea (>2% to 5%), flatulence (1%), heartburn (1%), nausea (≤1%), stomach pain (1%), xerostomia (1%)
Nervous system: Depression (>2% to 5%), dizziness (2% to 10%), fatigue (1% to 10%), vertigo (≤2%)
Respiratory: Bronchospasm (1%), dyspnea (≤3%), wheezing (1%)
Miscellaneous: Accidental injury (1%)

<1%:
Dermatologic: Alopecia
Gastrointestinal: Abdominal pain
Genitourinary: Peyronie's disease
Nervous system: Anxiety
Neuromuscular & skeletal: Arthralgia, arthritis

Frequency not defined:
Cardiovascular: Claudication
Dermatologic: Exacerbation of psoriasis (Yilmaz 2002)
Endocrine & metabolic: Unstable diabetes, weight gain
Gastrointestinal: Vomiting
Genitourinary: Retroperitoneal fibrosis
Nervous system: Sleep disturbance, temporary amnesia
Ophthalmic: Visual disturbance
Otic: Tinnitus
Respiratory: Rhinitis

Postmarketing:
Cardiovascular: Chest pain, syncope
Dermatologic: Bullous pemphigoid (Perry 2005), diaphoresis, erythroderma (Doyon 2017), lichenoid dermatitis (Nguyen 2011), pemphigoid-like lesion (Patel 2019)
Endocrine & metabolic: Decreased HDL cholesterol (Day 1982: Rössner 1983), decreased libido (Ko 2002), increased serum triglycerides (Day 1982; Kim 2014)
Genitourinary: Erectile dysfunction (Cocco 2009), impotence (Ko 2002)

Hepatic: Hepatic insufficiency (Philips 2017), hepatitis (Larrey 1988), increased serum alkaline phosphatase (Larrey 1988), increased serum transaminases (Larrey 1988), jaundice (Hansen 2017; Phillis 2017)

Nervous system: Confusion (Fisher 2002), drowsiness, hallucination (Fisher 2002; Sirois 2006), headache (Nicpon 2006), insomnia, nervousness (Ahmed 2010), nightmares (Ahmed 2010), paresthesia

Neuromuscular & skeletal: Arthropathy (psoriatic) (Tatu 2017), musculoskeletal pain (Snyder 1991)

Mechanism of Action Selective inhibitor of $beta_1$-adrenergic receptors; competitively blocks $beta_1$-receptors, with little or no effect on $beta_2$-receptors at oral doses <100 mg (in adults); does not exhibit any membrane stabilizing or intrinsic sympathomimetic activity

Pharmacodynamics/Kinetics

Onset of Action Oral: Immediate release tablets: Within 1 hour; Peak effect: Oral: 1 to 2 hours (Regardh 1980); IV: 20 minutes (when infused over 10 minutes)

Duration of Action Oral: Immediate release: Variable (dose-related; 50% reduction in maximum heart rate after single doses of 20, 50, and 100 mg occurred at 3.3, 5, and 6.4 hours, respectively), Extended release: ~24 hours

Half-life Elimination Neonates: 5 to 10 hours (Morselli 1989); Adults: 3 to 4 hours (7 to 9 hours in poor CYP2D6 metabolizers or hepatic impairment)

Pregnancy Considerations

Metoprolol and the metabolite alpha-hydroxymetoprolol cross the placenta (Lindeberg 1987; Ryu 2016).

Exposure to beta-blockers during pregnancy may increase the risk for adverse events in the neonate. If maternal use of a beta-blocker is needed, fetal growth should be monitored during pregnancy and the newborn should be monitored for 48 hours after delivery for bradycardia, hypoglycemia, and respiratory depression (ESC [Regitz-Zagrosek 2018]).

Chronic maternal hypertension is also associated with adverse events in the fetus/infant. Chronic maternal hypertension may increase the risk of birth defects, low birth weight, premature delivery, stillbirth, and neonatal death. Actual fetal/neonatal risks may be related to duration and severity of maternal hypertension. Untreated chronic hypertension may also increase the risks of adverse maternal outcomes, including gestational diabetes, preeclampsia, delivery complications, stroke, and myocardial infarction (ACOG 203 2019).

The pharmacokinetics of metoprolol may be changed during pregnancy; the degree of changes may be dependent upon maternal CYP2D6 genotype (Ryu 2016).

When treatment of hypertension in pregnancy is indicated, beta-blockers may be used. Specific recommendations vary by guideline but use of metoprolol may be considered (ACOG 203 2019; ESC [Regitz-Zagrosek 2018]; Magee 2014). Females with preexisting hypertension may continue their medication during pregnancy unless contraindications exist (ESC [Regitz-Zagrosek 2018]). Metoprolol may be used for the treatment of maternal ventricular arrhythmias, atrial fibrillation/atrial flutter, or supraventricular tachycardia during pregnancy; consult current guidelines for specific recommendations (ACC/AHA/HRS [Page 2016]; ESC [Regitz-Zagrosek 2018]). Use of metoprolol may be considered if migraine prophylaxis is needed in a pregnant woman (Pringsheim 2012).

◆ **Metoprolol Succinate** *see* Metoprolol *on page 1009*

◆ **Metoprolol Tartrate** *see* Metoprolol *on page 1009*

◆ **Metozolv ODT [DSC]** *see* Metoclopramide *on page 1007*

Metreleptin (met re LEP tin)

Brand Names: US Myalept

Pharmacologic Category Leptin Analog

Use

Lipodystrophy: Replacement therapy to treat the complications of leptin deficiency, in addition to diet, in patients with congenital or acquired generalized lipodystrophy.

Limitations of use: Not indicated for use in patients with HIV-related lipodystrophy or for use in patients with metabolic disease (eg, diabetes mellitus, hypertriglyceridemia) without concurrent evidence of congenital or acquired generalized lipodystrophy.

Local Anesthetic/Vasoconstrictor Precautions No information available to require special precautions

Effects on Dental Treatment No significant effects or complications reported

Effects on Bleeding No information available to require special precautions

Adverse Reactions

>10%:

Endocrine & metabolic: Hypoglycemia (13% in patients with adjunctive insulin), weight loss (13%)

Immunologic: Antibody development (84%; neutralizing activity consistent with loss of endogenous leptin and/or loss of metreleptin efficacy: 6%)

Nervous system: Headache (13%)

1% to 10%:

Dermatologic: Urticaria at injection site (≤4%)

Endocrine & metabolic: Ovarian cyst (8%)

Gastrointestinal: Abdominal pain (10%), nausea (8%), diarrhea (6%), pancreatitis (4%; in patients with a history of pancreatitis)

Genitourinary: Proteinuria (6%)

Hematologic & oncologic: Anemia (6%)

Local: Erythema at injection site (≤4%)

Nervous system: Dizziness (8%), fatigue (8%), paresthesia (6%)

Neuromuscular & skeletal: Arthralgia (8%), back pain (6%)

Otic: Otic infection (8%)

Respiratory: Upper respiratory tract infection (8%)

Miscellaneous: Fever (6%)

<1%, postmarketing, and/or case reports: Anaphylaxis, anaplastic large cell lymphoma, autoimmune hepatitis (progression), hypersensitivity reaction, membranoproliferative glomerulonephritis (progression), T-cell lymphoma

Mechanism of Action Recombinant human leptin analog that binds to and activates the human leptin receptor (ObR) (which belongs to the class I cytokine family of receptors that signals through the JAK/STAT transduction pathway) to treat complications of leptin deficiency associated with generalized lipodystrophy.

Pharmacodynamics/Kinetics

Half-life Elimination 3.8-4.7 hours

Time to Peak 4 hours (range: 2-8 hours)

Reproductive Considerations

Because metreleptin can restore metabolic and endocrine function, normal menses may be restored in women with previous amenorrhea; fertility may be restored and pregnancies may occur (Chou 2011; Chou 2013; Maguire 2012).

Pregnancy Considerations

Reports of use of metreleptin during pregnancy are limited (Chou 2011; Chou 2013; Maguire 2012).

Adverse pregnancy outcomes are associated with lipodystrophy in pregnant women, including eclampsia, gestational diabetes, intrauterine growth retardation, intrauterine death, macrosomia, and miscarriage. Based on in vitro data, metreleptin may inhibit uterine contractility during labor. If use is needed during pregnancy, reconstitution with a preservative-free diluent is recommended; solutions containing benzyl alcohol should be avoided in pregnant women due to association with gasping syndrome in premature infants.

Data collection to monitor pregnancy and infant outcomes following exposure to metreleptin is ongoing. Pregnant women or their health care provider may enroll by calling 1-855-669-2537.

MetroNIDAZOLE (Systemic)

(met roe NYE da zole)

Related Information

Bacterial Infections *on page 1739*

Gastrointestinal Disorders *on page 1678*

Periodontal Diseases *on page 1748*

Ulcerative, Erosive, and Painful Oral Mucosal Disorders *on page 1758*

Related Sample Prescriptions

Bacterial Infections and Periodontal Diseases - Sample Prescriptions *on page 35*

Brand Names: US Flagyl

Brand Names: Canada APO-MetroNIDAZOLE; Auro-MetroNIDAZOLE; Flagyl; NOVO-Nidazol [DSC]; PMS-MetroNIDAZOLE

Generic Availability (US) Yes

Pharmacologic Category Amebicide; Antibiotic, Miscellaneous; Antiprotozoal, Nitroimidazole

Dental Use Treatment of oral soft tissue infections due to anaerobic bacteria including all anaerobic cocci, anaerobic gram-negative bacilli (*Bacteroides*), and gram-positive spore-forming bacilli (*Clostridium*). Useful as single agent or in combination with amoxicillin, amoxicillin/clavulanic acid, or ciprofloxacin in the treatment of periodontitis associated with presence of *Actinobacillus actinomycetemcomitans* (AA). In aggressive periodontitis, greatest benefit is seen after 3 months of therapy. No benefit was seen after 6 months of therapy (Varela 2011).

Use

Amebiasis: Treatment of acute intestinal amebiasis (amebic dysentery) and extraintestinal amebiasis (liver abscess)

Limitations of use: When used for amebic liver abscess, may be used concurrently with percutaneous needle aspiration when clinically indicated.

Anaerobic bacterial infections (caused by *Bacteroides* spp. , including the *B. fragilis* group):

Bacterial septicemia: Treatment of bacterial septicemia (also caused by *Clostridium* spp.)

Bone and joint infections: Treatment (adjunctive therapy) of bone and joint infections

CNS Infections: Treatment of CNS infections, including meningitis and brain abscess

Endocarditis: Treatment of endocarditis

Gynecologic infections: Treatment of gynecologic infections including endometritis, endomyometritis, tubo-ovarian abscess, and postsurgical vaginal cuff infection (also caused by *Clostridium* spp., *Peptococcus* spp., *Peptostreptococcus* spp., and *Fusobacterium* spp.)

Intra-abdominal infections: Treatment of intra-abdominal infections, including peritonitis, intra-abdominal abscess, and liver abscess (also caused by *Clostridium* spp., *Eubacterium* spp., *Peptococcus* spp., and *Peptostreptococcus* spp.)

Lower respiratory tract infections: Treatment of lower respiratory tract infections, including pneumonia, empyema, and lung abscess

Skin and skin structure infections: Treatment of skin and skin structure infections (also caused by *Clostridium* spp., *Peptococcus* spp., *Peptostreptococcus* spp., and *Fusobacterium* spp.)

Surgical prophylaxis (colorectal surgery): Injection: Preoperative, intraoperative, and postoperative prophylaxis to reduce the incidence of postoperative infection in patients undergoing elective colorectal surgery classified as contaminated or potentially contaminated

Trichomoniasis: Treatment of infections caused by *Trichomonas vaginalis*, including treatment of asymptomatic sexual partners

Local Anesthetic/Vasoconstrictor Precautions No information available to require special precautions

Effects on Dental Treatment Key adverse event(s) related to dental treatment: Unusual/metallic taste, xerostomia (normal salivary flow resumes upon discontinuation), dizziness, pharyngitis, sinusitis, bacterial infection, and candidiasis may occur; hairy tongue, dysgeusia, glossitis, and stomatitis have rarely occurred.

Effects on Bleeding No information available to require special precautions

Adverse Reactions

>10%:

- Central nervous system: Headache (18%)
- Gastrointestinal: Nausea (10% to 12%)
- Genitourinary: Vaginitis (15%)

1% to 10%:

- Central nervous system: Metallic taste (9%), dizziness (4%)
- Dermatologic: Genital pruritus (5%)
- Gastrointestinal: Abdominal pain (4%), diarrhea (4%), xerostomia (2%)
- Genitourinary: Dysmenorrhea (3%), urine abnormality (3%), urinary tract infection (2%)
- Infection: Bacterial infection (7%), candidiasis (3%)
- Respiratory: Flu-like symptoms (6%), upper respiratory tract infection (4%), pharyngitis (3%), sinusitis (3%)

Frequency not defined:

- Cardiovascular: Chest pain, facial edema, flattened T-wave on ECG, flushing, palpitations, peripheral edema, syncope, tachycardia
- Central nervous system: Aseptic meningitis, ataxia, brain disease, cerebral lesion (reversible), chills, confusion, convulsions, depression, disulfiram-like reaction (with alcohol), drowsiness, dysarthria, hypoesthesia, insomnia, irritability, malaise, numbness, paresthesia, peripheral neuropathy, psychosis, seizure, vertigo
- Dermatologic: Erythematous rash, hyperhidrosis, pruritus, Stevens-Johnson syndrome, toxic epidermal necrolysis, urticaria
- Endocrine & metabolic: Decreased libido

Gastrointestinal: Abdominal cramps, abdominal distress, anorexia, constipation, decreased appetite, dysgeusia, glossitis, hairy tongue, pancreatitis (rare), proctitis, stomatitis, vomiting

Genitourinary: Cystitis, dark urine (rare), dyspareunia, dysuria, urinary incontinence, urine discoloration, vaginal dryness, vulvovaginal candidiasis

Hematologic & oncologic: Agranulocytosis, eosinophilia, leukopenia, neutropenia (reversible), thrombocytopenia (reversible, rare)

Hepatic: Increased liver enzymes, jaundice, severe hepatotoxicity (patients with Cockayne syndrome)

Hypersensitivity: Anaphylaxis, hypersensitivity

Immunologic: DRESS syndrome, serum sickness-like reaction (joint pains)

Local: Inflammation at injection site (IV), injection site reaction

Neuromuscular & skeletal: Arthralgia, muscle spasm, myalgia, weakness

Ophthalmic: Abnormal eye movements (saccadic), nystagmus, optic neuropathy

Renal: Polyuria

Respiratory: Dyspnea, nasal congestion, rhinitis

Miscellaneous: Fever

Dental Usual Dosage

Anaerobic infections/abscess: Adults: Oral, IV: 500 mg every 6-8 hours, not to exceed 4 g/day

Periodontitis treatment (monotherapy or combination) associated with the presence of *Actinobacillus actinomycetemcomitans* (AA): Adults: Oral: 250-500 mg every 8 hours for 8-10 days used in addition to scaling and root planing (Varela 2011)

Dosing

Adult & Geriatric

Amebiasis, intestinal (acute dysentery) or extraintestinal (liver abscess): Oral: 500 to 750 mg every 8 hours for 7 to 10 days followed by an intraluminal agent (eg, paromomycin) (*Drugs for Parasitic Infections* 2013; Leder 2018a; Leder 2018b).

Bacterial vaginosis: Oral: 500 mg twice daily for 7 days (CDC [Workowski 2015]; SOGC [Yudin 2017]).

Balantidiasis (alternative agent) (off-label use): Oral: 750 mg 3 times daily for 5 days (CDC 2013; *Drugs for Parasitic Infections* 2013; Weller 2020).

Bite wound infection, prophylaxis or treatment, animal or human bite (alternative agent) (off-label use): Oral, IV: 500 mg every 8 hours (Baddour 2019a; Baddour 2019b; IDSA [Stevens 2014]). Duration is 3 to 5 days for prophylaxis; duration of treatment for established infection is typically 5 to 14 days and varies based on clinical response and patient-specific factors (Baddour 2019a; Baddour 2019b). **Note:** For animal bites, use in combination with an appropriate agent for *Pasteurella multocida*. For human bites, use in combination with an appropriate agent for *Eikenella corrodens* (IDSA [Stevens 2014]).

***Clostridioides* (formerly *Clostridium*) *difficile* infection (off-label use): Note**: Criteria for disease severity is based on expert opinion and should not replace clinical judgment (IDSA/SHEA [McDonald 2018]).

Nonsevere (supportive clinical data: WBC ≤15,000 cells/mm^3 and serum creatinine <1.5 mg/dL), initial episode (alternative agent if oral vancomycin or fidaxomicin unavailable or contraindicated): **Oral:** 500 mg 3 times daily for 10 days. **Note:** Treatment duration may be extended to 14 days if patient has improved but has not had symptom resolution (IDSA/SHEA [McDonald 2018]).

Fulminant infection (supportive clinical data: ileus, megacolon, and/or hypotension/shock): **IV:** 500 mg every 8 hours in combination with oral and/or rectal vancomycin (IDSA/SHEA [McDonald 2018]; Surawicz 2013).

Crohn disease, management after surgical resection (off-label use):

Monotherapy: **Oral:** 20 mg/kg/day (in 3 divided doses) **or** 1 to 2 g/day in divided doses for 3 months (ACG [Lichtenstein 2018]; Rutgeerts 1995); begin as soon as oral intake is resumed after surgery (Rutgeerts 1995).

Combination therapy: **Oral:** 250 mg 3 times daily (D'Haens 2008; Lopez-Sanromán 2017) **or** 1 to 2 g/day in divided doses for 3 months (ACG [Lichtenstein 2018]); begin as soon as oral intake is resumed after surgery and administer in combination with a thiopurine (azathioprine or mercaptopurine) or a TNF-alpha inhibitor (eg, adalimumab) (De Cruz 2015; D'Haens 2008).

Crohn disease, treatment of simple perianal fistulas (off-label use): Oral: 500 mg twice daily for 4 weeks initially; if clinical response (ie, cessation of drainage and closure of fistula), continue at 250 mg 3 times daily for an additional 4 weeks (Bitton 2019) **or** 10 to 20 mg/kg/day in divided doses for 4 to 8 weeks with or without ciprofloxacin (ACG [Lichtenstein 2018]).

***Dientamoeba fragilis* infection (off-label use): Oral:** 500 to 750 mg 3 times daily for 10 days (CDC 2012; Nagata 2012).

Giardiasis (alternative agent) (off-label use): Oral: 250 mg 3 times daily **or** 500 mg 2 times daily for 5 to 7 days (Bartelt 2020; *Drugs for Parasitic Infections* 2013; Ordonez-Mena 2017).

***Helicobacter pylori* eradication (off-label use):**

Clarithromycin triple regimen: **Oral:** Metronidazole 500 mg 3 times daily in combination with clarithromycin 500 mg twice daily and a standard-dose or double-dose proton pump inhibitor (PPI) twice daily; continue regimen for 14 days. **Note:** Avoid use of clarithromycin triple therapy in patients with risk factors for macrolide resistance (eg, prior macrolide exposure, local clarithromycin resistance rates ≥15%) (ACG [Chey 2017]; Fallone 2016).

Bismuth quadruple regimen: **Oral**: Metronidazole 250 mg 4 times daily or 500 mg 3 or 4 times daily in combination with either bismuth subsalicylate 300 to 524 mg or bismuth subcitrate 120 to 300 mg 4 times daily, tetracycline 500 mg 4 times daily, and a standard-dose PPI twice daily; continue regimen for 10 to 14 days (ACG [Chey 2017]; Fallone 2016).

Concomitant regimen: **Oral:** Metronidazole 500 mg twice daily in combination with clarithromycin 500 mg twice daily, amoxicillin 1 g twice daily, and a standard-dose PPI twice daily; continue regimen for 10 to 14 days (ACG [Chey 2017]; Fallone 2016).

Sequential regimen (alternative regimen): **Oral:** Amoxicillin 1 g twice daily plus a standard-dose PPI twice daily for 5 to 7 days; then follow with clarithromycin 500 mg twice daily, metronidazole 500 mg twice daily, and a standard-dose PPI twice daily for 5 to 7 days (ACG [Chey 2017]); some experts prefer the 10-day sequential regimen (amoxicillin for 5 days, followed by metronidazole and clarithromycin for 5 days) over the 14-day sequential regimen (amoxicillin for 7 days, followed by metronidazole and clarithromycin for 7 days) due to the lack of data showing superiority of the

14-day regimen over the 10-day regimen in North America (ACG [Chey 2017]; Crowe 2020).

Hybrid regimen (alternative regimen): **Oral:** Amoxicillin 1 g twice daily plus a standard-dose PPI twice daily for 7 days; then follow with amoxicillin 1 g twice daily, clarithromycin 500 mg twice daily, metronidazole 500 mg twice daily, and a standard-dose PPI twice daily for 7 days (ACG [Chey 2017]; Wang 2015).

Intra-abdominal infection: Oral, IV: 500 mg every 8 hours as part of an appropriate combination regimen. Duration of therapy is for 4 to 7 days following adequate source control (SIS/IDSA [Solomkin 2010]); for uncomplicated appendicitis and diverticulitis managed nonoperatively, a longer duration is necessary (Barshak 2018; Pemberton 2020). **Note:** Empiric oral regimens may be appropriate for patients with mild to moderate infection. Other patients may be switched from IV to oral therapy at the same dose when clinically improved and able to tolerate an oral diet (SIS/IDSA [Solomkin 2010]; SIS [Mazuski 2017]).

Intracranial abscess (brain abscess, intracranial epidural abscess): IV: 7.5 mg/kg (usually 500 mg) every 6 to 8 hours for 6 to 8 weeks in combination with other appropriate antimicrobial therapy (Bodilsen 2018; Sexton 2018b; Southwick 2020). **Note:** May switch IV metronidazole to oral metronidazole at the same dose to complete treatment course (Southwick 2020).

Pelvic inflammatory disease (PID):

Mild to moderate PID: **Oral:** 500 mg twice daily for 14 days (may be added to a combination of a second- or third-generation parenteral cephalosporin and doxycycline in select women) (CDC [Workowski 2015]).

PID with tubo-ovarian abscess, initial therapy (alternative regimen): **IV:** 500 mg every 8 hours as part of an appropriate combination regimen (Beigi 2018).

PID with tubo-ovarian abscess, oral therapy following clinical improvement on a parenteral regimen: **Oral:** 500 mg twice daily with doxycycline to complete at least 14 days of therapy (CDC [Workowski 2015]).

Periodontitis, severe (off-label use): Oral: 500 mg every 8 hours in combination with amoxicillin for 7 to 14 days; used in addition to periodontal debridement (Chow 2019; McGowan 2018; Wilder 2020).

Pneumonia, aspiration (alternative agent): Oral, IV: 500 mg 3 times daily in combination with an appropriate beta-lactam (eg, oral amoxicillin, IV penicillin, or an IV third-generation cephalosporin) for 7 days (Bartlett 2018).

Pouchitis (post ileal pouch-anal anastomosis) (off-label use):

Acute disease (alternative agent): **Oral:** 500 mg to 1 g every 12 hours for 14 days (Holubar 2010; Navaneethan 2009; Shen 2018; Wall 2011).

Chronic disease: **Oral:** 500 mg every 12 hours in combination with ciprofloxacin for at least 28 days (Mimura 2002; Shen 2018).

Skin and soft tissue infection:

Necrotizing infection (as a component of an appropriate combination regimen) (alternative agent): **IV:** 500 mg every 6 hours. Continue until further debridement is not necessary, patient has clinically improved, and patient is afebrile for 48 to 72 hours (IDSA [Stevens 2014]).

Surgical site infection, incisional (eg, intestinal or GU tract; axilla or perineum), warranting anaerobic coverage: **IV:** 500 mg every 8 hours in combination with other appropriate agents. Duration depends on severity, need for debridement, and clinical response (IDSA [Stevens 2014]).

Surgical prophylaxis:

IV: 500 mg within 60 minutes prior to surgical incision in combination with other antibiotics. Considered a recommended agent for select procedures involving the GI tract, urologic tract, or head and neck (Bratzler 2013).

Oral:

Colorectal surgical prophylaxis (off-label use): 1 g every 3 to 4 hours for 3 doses with additional oral antibiotics, starting after mechanical bowel preparation the evening before a morning surgery and followed by an appropriate IV antibiotic prophylaxis regimen (Bratzler 2013).

Uterine evacuation (induced abortion or pregnancy loss) (alternative agent) (off-label use): 500 mg as a single dose 1 hour prior to uterine aspiration; may be administered up to 12 hours before the procedure (ACOG 2018; Shih 2020). **Note:** The optimal dosing regimen has not been established; various protocols are in use (Achilles 2011).

Tetanus (*Clostridium tetani* infection) (off-label use): Oral, IV: 500 mg every 6 to 8 hours for 7 to 10 days in combination with supportive therapy (Ahmadsyah 1985; Sexton 2018a).

Trichomoniasis (index case and sex partner):

Initial treatment: **Oral:** 500 mg twice daily for 7 days. **Note:** Single 2 g dose is no longer preferred due to inferior efficacy (Howe 2017; Kissinger 2010; Kissinger 2018), but it can be used in patients unable to complete multiple dose treatment course (Sobel 2020). Coverage of trichomoniasis, along with other appropriate antimicrobials, is indicated in cases of recurrent or persistent urethritis in men who have sex with women and who live in regions where *T. vaginalis* is prevalent and for prophylaxis after sexual assault (CDC [Workowski 2015]).

Persistent or recurrent infection (ie, treatment failure of nitroimidazole [eg, metronidazole]): **Oral:** 500 mg twice daily for 7 days for failure of 2 g single-dose regimen. If this regimen fails, 2 g once daily for 7 days is recommended (CDC [Workowski 2015]).

Renal Impairment: Adult

Manufacturer's labeling:

Mild to moderate impairment: There are no dosage adjustments provided in the manufacturer's labeling; however, decreased renal function does not alter the single-dose pharmacokinetics.

Severe impairment: There are no dosage adjustments provided in the manufacturer's labeling; metronidazole metabolites may accumulate; monitor for adverse events.

ESRD requiring dialysis: Metronidazole metabolites may accumulate; monitor for adverse events. Accumulated metabolites may be rapidly removed by dialysis:

Intermittent hemodialysis (IHD): If administration cannot be separated from hemodialysis, consider supplemental dose following hemodialysis.

Peritoneal dialysis (PD): No dosage adjustment necessary.

Alternative dosing:

Intermittent hemodialysis (IHD) (administer after hemodialysis on dialysis days): Dialyzable (50% to 100%): 500 mg every 8 to 12 hours. **Note:** Dosing regimen highly dependent on clinical indication (trichomoniasis vs *C. difficile* colitis) (Heintz 2009). **Note:** Dosing dependent on the assumption of thrice-weekly, complete IHD sessions.

Continuous renal replacement therapy (CRRT) (Heintz 2009; Trotman 2005): Drug clearance is highly dependent on the method of renal replacement, filter type, and flow rate. Appropriate dosing requires close monitoring of pharmacologic response, signs of adverse reactions due to drug accumulation, as well as drug concentrations in relation to target trough (if appropriate). The following are general recommendations only (based on dialysate flow/ultrafiltration rates of 1 to 2 L/hour and minimal residual renal function) and should not supersede clinical judgment:

CVVH/CVVHD/CVVHDF: 500 mg every 6 to 12 hours (or per clinical indication; dosage reduction generally not necessary)

Hepatic Impairment: Adult

Manufacturer's labeling:

Mild or moderate impairment (Child-Pugh class A or B): No dosage adjustment necessary; use with caution and monitor for adverse events.

Severe impairment (Child-Pugh class C):

Capsules:

Amebiasis: 375 mg 3 times daily

Trichomoniasis: 375 mg once daily

Tablets, injection: Reduce dose by 50%

Alternative dosing: The pharmacokinetics of a single oral 500 mg dose were not altered in patients with cirrhosis; initial dose reduction is therefore not necessary (Daneshmend 1982). In one study of IV metronidazole, patients with alcoholic liver disease (with or without cirrhosis) demonstrated a prolonged elimination half-life (eg, ~18 hours). The authors recommended the dose be reduced accordingly (clearance was reduced by ~62%) and the frequency may be prolonged (eg, every 12 hours instead of every 6 hours) (Lau 1987). In another single IV dose study using metronidazole metabolism to predict hepatic function, patients classified as Child-Pugh class C demonstrated a half-life of ~21.5 hours (Muscara 1995).

Pediatric Note: Some clinicians recommend using adjusted body weight in obese children. Dosing weight = IBW + 0.45 (TBW-IBW)

General dosing, susceptible infection (*Red Book* [AAP 2018]): Infants, Children, and Adolescents:

Oral: 15 to 50 mg/kg/**day** in divided doses 3 times daily; maximum daily dose: 2,250 mg/**day**.

IV: 22.5 to 40 mg/kg/**day** in divided doses 3 or 4 times daily; maximum daily dose: 4,000 mg/**day**.

Amebiasis: Infants, Children, and Adolescents: Oral: 35 to 50 mg/kg/**day** in divided doses every 8 hours for 7 to 10 days; maximum dose: 750 mg/dose; for severe infection or extraintestinal disease, IV may be necessary (Bradley 2018; *Red Book* [AAP 2018]).

Appendicitis, perforated (divided dosing): Children and Adolescents: IV: 30 mg/kg/**day** in divided doses 3 times daily (Emil 2003).

Appendicitis, perforated (once-daily dosing): Limited data available: Children and Adolescents: IV: 30 mg/kg/dose once daily in combination with ceftriaxone; maximum reported daily dose: 1,500 mg/**day** (Yardeni 2013); however, other pediatric trials did not report a maximum; in adult patients, a maximum daily dose of 1,500 mg/day for once-daily dosing is suggested (IDSA [Solomkin 2010]); in pediatric patients, once-daily metronidazole in combination with ceftriaxone has been shown to have similar efficacy as triple-combination therapy with ampicillin, clindamycin, and gentamicin (Fraser 2010; St Peter 2006; St Peter 2008).

Balantidiasis: Infants, Children, and Adolescents: Oral: 35 to 50 mg/kg/**day** in divided doses every 8 hours for 5 days; maximum dose: 750 mg/dose (*Red Book* [AAP 2018]).

Catheter (peritoneal dialysis); exit-site or tunnel infection: Infants, Children, and Adolescents: Oral: 10 mg/kg/dose 3 times daily. Maximum dose: 500 mg/dose (ISPD [Warady 2012]).

***Clostridioides* (formerly *Clostridium*) *difficile* infection:**

Infants: *Mild to moderate infection*: Oral, IV: 7.5 mg/kg/dose every 6 hours for 10 days (*Red Book* [AAP 2018]).

Children and Adolescents:

Non-severe infection, initial or first recurrence: Oral: 7.5 mg/kg/dose 3 to 4 times daily for 10 days; maximum dose: 500 mg/dose (IDSA/SHEA [McDonald 2018]).

Severe/fulminant infection, initial: IV: 10 mg/kg/dose every 8 hours for 10 days; maximum dose: 500 mg/dose; use concomitantly with oral or rectal vancomycin (IDSA/SHEA [McDonald 2018]).

Dientamoeba fragilis: Infants, Children, and Adolescents: Oral: 35 to 50 mg/kg/**day** in divided doses every 8 hours for 10 days; maximum dose: 750 mg/dose (*Red Book* [AAP 2018]).

Giardiasis: Infants, Children, and Adolescents: Oral: 15 to 30 mg/kg/day in divided doses every 8 hours for 5 to 7 days; maximum dose: 250 mg/dose (Bradley 2018; Gardner 2001; Granados 2012; Ross 2013; *Red Book* [AAP 2018]).

***Helicobacter pylori* infection:** Children and Adolescents: Oral: 20 mg/kg/**day** in 2 divided doses for 10 to 14 days in combination with amoxicillin and proton pump inhibitor with or without clarithromycin; maximum daily dose: 1,000 mg/**day** (NASPGHAN/ESPGHAN [Koletzko 2011]).

Inflammatory bowel disease:

Crohn disease, perianal disease; induction: Children and Adolescents: Oral: 7.5 mg/kg/dose 3 times daily for 6 weeks with or without ciprofloxacin; maximum dose: 500 mg/dose (Sandhu 2010).

Ulcerative colitis, pouchitis, persistent: Children and Adolescents: Oral: 20 to 30 mg/kg/**day** in divided doses 3 times daily for 14 days with or without ciprofloxacin or oral budesonide; maximum dose: 500 mg/dose (Turner 2012).

Intra-abdominal infection: Infants, Children, and Adolescents: IV: 30 to 40 mg/kg/**day** in divided doses 3 times daily as part of combination therapy; maximum dose: 500 mg/dose (IDSA [Solomkin 2010]).

Pelvic inflammatory disease: Adolescents: Oral: 500 mg twice daily for 14 days; give with doxycycline plus a cephalosporin (CDC [Workowski 2015]).

Peritonitis (peritoneal dialysis) (ISPD [Warady 2012]):

Prophylaxis: Gastrointestinal or genitourinary procedures: Infants, Children, and Adolescents: IV: 10 mg/kg once prior to procedure in combination with cefazolin; Maximum dose: 1,000 mg/dose.

Treatment: Infants, Children, and Adolescents: Oral: 10 mg/kg/dose 3 times daily. Maximum daily dose: 1,200 mg/**day**.

Prophylaxis against sexually transmitted diseases following sexual assault (CDC [Workowski 2015]): Adolescents: Oral: 2,000 mg as a single dose in combination with azithromycin and ceftriaxone.

Surgical prophylaxis: Children and Adolescents: IV: 15 mg/kg as a single dose 30 to 60 minutes prior to procedure; maximum single dose: 500 mg (IDSA/ASHP [Bratzler 2013]).

Surgical prophylaxis, colorectal: Children and Adolescents: Oral: 15 mg/kg/dose every 3 to 4 hours for 3 doses, starting after mechanical bowel preparation the afternoon and evening before the procedure, with or without additional oral antibiotics and with an appropriate IV antibiotic prophylaxis regimen; maximum dose: 1,000 mg/dose (IDSA/ASHP [Bratzler 2013]).

Tetanus (Clostridium tetani infection): Infants, Children, and Adolescents: IV, Oral: 30 mg/kg/**day** in divided doses 4 times daily for 7 to 10 days; maximum daily dose: 4,000 mg/**day** (*Red Book* [AAP 2018]).

Trichomoniasis; treatment: Oral:

Children <45 kg: 45 mg/kg/**day** in divided doses 3 times daily for 7 days; maximum daily dose: 2,000 mg/**day** (*Red Book* [AAP 2018]).

Children ≥45 kg and Adolescents: 500 mg twice daily for 7 days **or** 2,000 mg as a single dose once (CDC [Workowski 2015]; *Red Book* [AAP 2018]). **Note:** 7-day-course has been shown to be more effective in adult women (Howe 2017; Kissinger 2010; Kissinger 2018).

Vaginosis, bacterial: Oral: Children >45 kg and Adolescents: 500 mg twice daily for 7 days (CDC [Workowski 2015]; *Red Book* [AAP 2018]).

Renal Impairment: Pediatric

Infants, Children, and Adolescents:

Manufacturer's labeling:

Mild, moderate, or severe impairment: There are no dosage adjustments provided in the manufacturer's labeling; however, decreased renal function does not alter the single-dose pharmacokinetics.

ESRD requiring dialysis: Metronidazole metabolites may accumulate; monitor for adverse events; accumulated metabolites may be rapidly removed by dialysis.

Intermittent hemodialysis (IHD): If administration cannot be separated from hemodialysis, consider supplemental dose following hemodialysis.

Peritoneal dialysis (PD): No dosage adjustment necessary

Alternate dosing: Others have used the following adjustments (Aronoff 2007). **Note:** Renally adjusted dose recommendations are based on doses of 15 to 30 mg/kg/**day** divided every 6 to 8 hours.

GFR ≥10 mL/minute/1.73 m^2: No adjustment required

GFR <10 mL/minute/1.73 m^2: 4 mg/kg/dose every 6 hours

Intermittent hemodialysis (IHD): Extensively removed by hemodialysis: 4 mg/kg/dose every 6 hours

Peritoneal dialysis (PD): Extensively removed by peritoneal dialysis: 4 mg/kg/dose every 6 hours

Continuous renal replacement therapy (CRRT): No adjustment required

Hepatic Impairment: Pediatric

Infants, Children, and Adolescents:

Manufacturer labeling:

Mild or moderate impairment (Child-Pugh class A or B): No dosage adjustment necessary; use with caution and monitor for adverse events

Severe impairment (Child-Pugh class C):

Immediate release tablets, injection: Reduce dose by 50%

Extended release tablets: Use is not recommended.

Alternate dosing: The pharmacokinetics of a single oral 500 mg dose were not altered in patients with cirrhosis; initial dose reduction is therefore not necessary (Daneshmend 1982). In one study of IV metronidazole, adult patients with alcoholic liver disease (with or without cirrhosis) demonstrated a prolonged elimination half-life (eg, ~18 hours). The authors recommended the dose be reduced accordingly (clearance was reduced by ~62%) and the frequency may be prolonged (eg, every 12 hours instead of every 6 hours) (Lau 1987). In another single IV dose study using metronidazole metabolism to predict hepatic function, patients classified as Child-Pugh class C demonstrated a half-life of ~21.5 hours (Muscara 1995).

Mechanism of Action

After diffusing into the organism, interacts with DNA to cause a loss of helical DNA structure and strand breakage resulting in inhibition of protein synthesis and cell death in susceptible organisms

Contraindications

Hypersensitivity to metronidazole, nitroimidazole derivatives, or any component of the formulation; pregnant patients (first trimester) with trichomoniasis; use of disulfiram within the past 2 weeks; use of alcohol or propylene glycol-containing products during therapy or within 3 days of therapy discontinuation

Canadian labeling: Additional contraindications (not in the US labeling): Active neurological disorders; history of blood dyscrasia; hypothyroidism; hypoadrenalism

Warnings/Precautions

[US Boxed Warning]: Possibly carcinogenic based on animal data. Reserve use for conditions described in Use; unnecessary use should be avoided. Use with caution in patients with hepatic impairment, severe renal impairment, and ESRD due to potential accumulation; dosage adjustment recommended in patients with severe hepatic impairment, and consider dosage reduction in patients with severe renal impairment (CrCl <10 mL/minute) who are receiving prolonged therapy. Dose should not specifically be reduced in anuric patients (accumulated metabolites may be rapidly removed by dialysis). Hemodialysis patients may need supplemental dosing. Use with caution in patients with blood; agranulocytosis, leukopenia, and neutropenia have occurred. Monitor CBC with differential at baseline, during and after treatment. Use with caution in patients with a history of seizure disorder.

Severe hepatotoxicity/acute hepatic failure (has been fatal) has been reported with systemic metronidazole in patients with Cockayne syndrome; onset is rapid after initiation of treatment. Use metronidazole only after risk vs benefit assessment and if there are no appropriate alternatives in patients with Cockayne syndrome. Obtain LFTs prior to treatment initiation, within the first 2 to 3 days of initiation, frequently during therapy, and after treatment is complete. Discontinue treatment if elevated LFTs occur and monitor until LFTs return to baseline.

Severe neurological disturbances, including aseptic meningitis (may occur within hours of a dose), cerebellar symptoms (ataxia, dizziness, dysarthria), convulsive seizures, encephalopathy, optic neuropathy, and peripheral neuropathy (usually of sensory type and characterized by numbness or paresthesia of an extremity) have been reported. CNS symptoms and CNS lesions are generally reversible within days to weeks of discontinuation of therapy; peripheral neuropathy symptoms may be prolonged after discontinuation. Avoid repeated or prolonged courses due to risk of cumulative neurotoxicity (IDSA/SHEA [McDonald 2018]). Monitor for neurologic symptoms and discontinue therapy if any abnormal neurologic symptoms occur. Prolonged use may result in fungal or bacterial superinfection, including *Clostridium difficile*-associated diarrhea (CDAD) and pseudomembranous colitis; CDAD has been observed >2 months postantibiotic treatment. Candidiasis infection (known or unknown) maybe more prominent during metronidazole treatment, antifungal treatment required.

Abdominal cramps, nausea, vomiting, headaches, and flushing have been reported with oral and injectable metronidazole and concomitant alcohol consumption; avoid alcoholic beverages or products containing propylene glycol during oral and injectable therapy and for at least 3 days after oral therapy. Use injection with caution in patients with heart failure, edema, or other sodium-retaining states, including corticosteroid treatment due to high sodium content. In patients receiving continuous nasogastric secretion aspiration, sufficient metronidazole may be removed in the aspirate to cause a reduction in serum levels. Potentially significant drug-drug interactions may exist, requiring dose or frequency adjustment, additional monitoring, and/or selection of alternative therapy.

Drug Interactions

Metabolism/Transport Effects **Substrate** of CYP2A6 (major); **Note:** Assignment of Major/Minor substrate status based on clinically relevant drug interaction potential; **Inhibits** CYP2C9 (weak)

Avoid Concomitant Use

Avoid concomitant use of MetroNIDAZOLE (Systemic) with any of the following: Alcohol (Ethyl); BCG (Intravesical); Carbocisteine; Cholera Vaccine; Disulfiram; Dronabinol; Mebendazole; Products Containing Propylene Glycol; Ritonavir

Increased Effect/Toxicity

MetroNIDAZOLE (Systemic) may increase the levels/effects of: Alcohol (Ethyl); Busulfan; Carbocisteine; Dronabinol; Fluorouracil Products; Fosphenytoin; Lithium; Lopinavir; Phenytoin; Products Containing Propylene Glycol; Tipranavir; TOLBUTamide; Vecuronium; Vitamin K Antagonists

The levels/effects of MetroNIDAZOLE (Systemic) may be increased by: Disulfiram; Mebendazole; Ritonavir

Decreased Effect

MetroNIDAZOLE (Systemic) may decrease the levels/effects of: BCG (Intravesical); BCG Vaccine (Immunization); Cholera Vaccine; Lactobacillus and Estriol; Mycophenolate; Sodium Picosulfate; Typhoid Vaccine

The levels/effects of MetroNIDAZOLE (Systemic) may be decreased by: Fosphenytoin; PHENobarbital; Phenytoin; Primidone

Food Interactions Peak antibiotic serum concentration lowered and delayed, but total drug absorbed not affected.

Dietary Considerations

Take with food to minimize stomach upset.

Sodium: Injectable dosage form may contain sodium.

Ethanol: Use of ethanol is contraindicated during therapy and for 3 days after therapy discontinuation.

Pharmacodynamics/Kinetics

Half-life Elimination

Neonates <7 days (Jager-Roman 1982): Within first week of life, more prolonged than with lower GA:

GA 28 to 30 weeks: 75.3 ± 16.9 hours

GA 32 to 35 weeks: 35.4 ± 1.5 hours

GA 36 to 40 weeks: 24.8 ± 1.6 hours

Neonates ≥7 days: ~22.5 hours (Upadhyaya 1988)

Children and Adolescents: 6 to 10 hours (Lamp 1999)

Adults: ~8 hours

Time to Peak Serum: Oral: 1 to 2 hours

Pregnancy Considerations Metronidazole crosses the placenta.

Cleft lip with or without cleft palate has been reported following first trimester exposure to metronidazole; however, most studies have not shown an increased risk of congenital anomalies or other adverse events to the fetus following maternal use during pregnancy. Because metronidazole was carcinogenic in some animal species, concern has been raised whether metronidazole should be used during pregnancy. Available studies have not shown an increased risk of infant cancer following metronidazole exposure during pregnancy; however, the ability to detect a signal for this may have been limited.

Metronidazole pharmacokinetics are similar between pregnant and nonpregnant patients (Amon 1981; Visser 1984; Wang 2011).

Bacterial vaginosis and vaginal trichomoniasis are associated with adverse pregnancy outcomes and metronidazole is recommended for the treatment of symptomatic pregnant patients. The dose of oral metronidazole for the treatment of bacterial vaginosis during pregnancy is the same as the CDC recommended twice daily dose in nonpregnant females. When treating vaginal trichomoniasis, the CDC recommends the single oral dose regimen in pregnancy. Although use of metronidazole for vaginal trichomoniasis during the first trimester is contraindicated by the manufacturer; available guidelines note treatment can be given at any stage of pregnancy (CDC [Workowski 2015]).

Metronidazole may also be used for the treatment of giardiasis in pregnant women (some sources recommend second and third trimester administration only) (Gardner 2001; HHS [OI adult 2020]) and symptomatic amebiasis during pregnancy (HHS [OI adult 2020]; Li 1996). Short courses may be used for the treatment of pouchitis or perianal disease in pregnant women with inflammatory bowel disease (avoid use in the first trimester) (van der Woude 2015).The use of other agents is preferred when treatment is needed during pregnancy for *Clostridioides* (formerly *Clostridium*) *difficile* (Surawicz 2013). Consult current recommendations for appropriate use in pregnant women.

Breastfeeding Considerations

Metronidazole and its active hydroxyl metabolite are present in breast milk at concentrations similar to maternal plasma concentrations.

The relative infant dose (RID) of metronidazole is 13.7% to 22.9% when calculated using the highest average breast milk concentration reported and compared to an oral infant therapeutic dose of 30 to 50 mg/kg/day. In general, breastfeeding is considered acceptable when the RID is <10%; when an RID is >25% breastfeeding should generally be avoided (Anderson 2016; Ito 2000). Using the highest average milk concentration (45.8 mcg/mL), the estimated daily infant dose via breast milk is 6.87 mg/kg/day. This milk concentration was obtained following a single maternal dose of oral metronidazole 2,000 mg; the authors estimated the infant would have been exposed to metronidazole 21.8 mg over the first 24 hours after the dose (Erickson 1981).

The highest average milk concentration occurred 2 to 4 hours after a single oral maternal dose; the half-life in breast milk was ~9 to 10 hours (Erickson 1981). Metronidazole and its active metabolite can be detected in the serum of breastfeeding infants (Gray 1961; Heisterberg 1983; Passmore 1988).

Loose stools, oral and perianal *Candida* growth, and oral thrush have been reported in breastfeeding infants exposed to metronidazole (Passmore 1988)

The manufacturer warns of the risk of carcinogenicity in patients exposed to metronidazole based on animal studies; theoretically, this risk is also present in breastfeeding infants exposed to metronidazole via breast milk. Therefore, the manufacturer recommends a decision be made whether to discontinue breastfeeding or to discontinue the drug, taking into account the importance of treatment to the mother. Some guidelines note if metronidazole is given, breastfeeding should be withheld for 12 to 24 hours after a single dose (CDC [Workowski 2015]; WHO 2002); alternatively, the mother may pump and discard breast milk for 24 hours after taking the last metronidazole dose. Breastfeeding should be avoided in women requiring treatment with metronidazole for inflammatory bowel disease (van der Woude 2015). Use of other agents is preferred when treating breastfeeding women for *Clostridioides* (formerly *Clostridium*) *difficile* infection (Surawicz 2013).

Dosage Forms Considerations

Parenteral solution contains 28 mEq of sodium/gram of metronidazole.

First-Metronidazole and MetroNIDAZOLE Benzo+Syr-Spend oral suspensions are a compounding kits. Refer to manufacturer's labeling for compounding instructions.

Dosage Forms: US

Capsule, Oral:
Flagyl: 375 mg
Generic: 375 mg

Solution, Intravenous:
Generic: 500 mg (100 mL)

Solution, Intravenous [preservative free]:
Generic: 500 mg (100 mL)

Tablet, Oral:
Flagyl: 250 mg, 500 mg
Generic: 250 mg, 500 mg

Dosage Forms: Canada

Capsule, Oral:
Flagyl: 500 mg
Generic: 500 mg

Solution, Intravenous:
Flagyl: 5 mg/mL (100 mL)
Generic: 5 mg/mL (100 mL)

Tablet, Oral:
Generic: 250 mg

- ◆ **Metronidazole Benzoate** *see* MetroNIDAZOLE (Systemic) *on page 1011*
- ◆ **Metronidazole, Bismuth Subcitrate Potassium, and Tetracycline** *see* Bismuth Subcitrate, Metronidazole, and Tetracycline *on page 245*
- ◆ **Metronidazole, Bismuth Subsalicylate, and Tetracycline** *see* Tetracycline, Bismuth Subsalicylate, and Metronidazole *on page 1433*
- ◆ **Metronidazole Hydrochloride** *see* MetroNIDAZOLE (Systemic) *on page 1011*
- ◆ **Metronidazole, Tetracycline, and Bismuth Subsalicylate** *see* Tetracycline, Bismuth Subsalicylate, and Metronidazole *on page 1433*
- ◆ **MET Tyrosine Kinase Inhibitor PF-02341066** *see* Crizotinib *on page 415*
- ◆ **Mevacor [DSC]** *see* Lovastatin *on page 940*
- ◆ **Mevinolin** *see* Lovastatin *on page 940*

Mexiletine (meks IL e teen)

Brand Names: Canada TEVA-Mexiletine

Pharmacologic Category Antiarrhythmic Agent, Class Ib

Use

Ventricular arrhythmias: Management of life-threatening ventricular arrhythmias

Note: The American Heart Association/American College of Cardiology/Heart Rhythm Society (AHA/ACC/HRS) states that mexiletine may be considered for those with long QT syndrome type 3 who present with torsades de pointes (ACC/AHA/HRS [Al-Khatib 2017]; Mazzanti 2016).

Local Anesthetic/Vasoconstrictor Precautions No information available to require special precautions

Effects on Dental Treatment Key adverse event(s) related to dental treatment: Xerostomia (normal salivary flow resumes upon discontinuation).

Effects on Bleeding No information available to require special precautions

Adverse Reactions

>10%:

Cardiovascular: Exacerbation of cardiac arrhythmia (10% to 15%; patients with malignant arrhythmia)

Central nervous system: Dizziness (11% to 25%), ataxia (10% to 20%), nervousness (5% to 10%), unsteady gait

Gastrointestinal: Gastrointestinal distress (41%), nausea (≤40%), vomiting (≤40%)

Neuromuscular & skeletal: Tremor (13%)

1% to 10%:

Cardiovascular: Palpitations (4% to 8%), chest pain (3% to 8%), angina pectoris (2%), ventricular premature contractions (1% to 2%)

Central nervous system: Insomnia (5% to 7%), numbness (fingers or toes: 2% to 4%), depression (2%), paresthesia (2%), confusion, headache

Dermatologic: Skin rash (4%)

Gastrointestinal: Constipation (≤5%), diarrhea (≤5%), xerostomia (3%), abdominal pain (1%)

Neuromuscular & skeletal: Weakness (5%), arthralgia (1%)

Ophthalmic: Blurred vision (5% to 7%), nystagmus (6%)

Otic: Tinnitus (2% to 3%)

Respiratory: Dyspnea (3%)

<1%, postmarketing, and/or case reports: Agranulocytosis, alopecia, amnesia (short-term), atrioventricular block, cardiac conduction disturbance, cardiac failure (patients with preexisting ventricular dysfunction), cardiogenic shock, decreased libido, diaphoresis, diplopia, dysphagia, edema, esophageal ulcer, exfoliative dermatitis, hallucination, hepatic necrosis, hepatitis, hot flash, hypertension, hypotension, impotence, increased liver enzymes, increased serum transaminases, leukopenia, lupus-like syndrome (drug-induced), malaise, myelofibrosis (patients with preexisting myeloid abnormalities), pancreatitis (rare), peptic ulcer, pharyngitis, positive ANA titer, psychological disorder, psychosis, pulmonary fibrosis, salivary gland disease, seizure, sinoatrial arrest, Stevens-Johnson syndrome, syncope, thrombocytopenia, torsades de pointes, upper gastrointestinal hemorrhage, urinary hesitancy, urinary retention, urticaria

Mechanism of Action Class IB antiarrhythmic, structurally related to lidocaine, which inhibits inward sodium current, decreases rate of rise of phase 0, increases effective refractory period/action potential duration ratio

Pharmacodynamics/Kinetics

Onset of Action 30 to 120 minutes (with loading regimen)

Half-life Elimination ~10 to 12 hours; ~15 hours in severe renal impairment (CrCl <10 mL/minute); ~25 hours in moderate to severe hepatic impairment

Time to Peak Serum: 2 to 3 hours

Pregnancy Considerations Adverse events have been observed in some animal reproduction studies. A few case reports have demonstrated safe use of mexiletine in pregnant women (Gregg 1988; Lownes 1987; Timmis 1980).

◆ **Mexiletine HCl** *see* Mexiletine *on page 1017*

◆ **M-Hist PD [OTC]** *see* Triprolidine *on page 1500*

◆ **Mibelas 24 Fe** *see* Ethinyl Estradiol and Norethindrone *on page 614*

◆ **Micaderm [OTC]** *see* Miconazole (Topical) *on page 1019*

Micafungin (mi ka FUN gin)

Related Information

Fungal Infections *on page 1752*

Brand Names: US Mycamine

Brand Names: Canada Mycamine

Pharmacologic Category Antifungal Agent, Parenteral; Echinocandin

Use

Candidemia, acute disseminated candidiasis, *Candida* peritonitis and abscesses: Treatment of candidemia, acute disseminated candidiasis, *Candida* peritonitis and abscesses in adults and pediatric patients ≥4 months of age or in pediatric patients ≤4 months of age without meningoencephalitis and/or ocular dissemination.

Esophageal candidiasis: Treatment of esophageal candidiasis in adults and pediatric patients ≥4 months of age.

Prophylaxis of *Candida* infections: Prophylaxis of *Candida* infections in adults and pediatric patients ≥4 months of age undergoing hematopoietic stem cell transplantation.

Local Anesthetic/Vasoconstrictor Precautions No information available to require special precautions

Effects on Dental Treatment No significant effects or complications reported

Effects on Bleeding May cause thrombocytopenia in ≤15% of patients.

Adverse Reactions

Candidiasis treatment:

>10%:

Cardiovascular: Phlebitis (19%)

Gastrointestinal: Diarrhea (7% to 11%), vomiting (7% to 18%)

Hematologic & oncologic: Anemia (infants, children, and adolescents: 18%)

Hepatic: Abnormal hepatic function tests (4%; infants, children, and adolescents: <15%), hyperbilirubinemia (infants, children, and adolescents: <15%)

Renal: Renal failure syndrome (infants, children, and adolescents: <15%)

Miscellaneous: Fever (9% to 13%)

1% to 10%:

Cardiovascular: Atrial fibrillation (adults: 3%), tachycardia (infants, children, and adolescents: 4%)

Dermatologic: Skin rash (2% to 5%)

Endocrine & metabolic: Abnormal aspartate transaminase (3%), hyperkalemia (adults: 5%), hypoglycemia (adults: 6%)

Gastrointestinal: Abdominal distention (infants, children, and adolescents: 2%), abdominal pain (infants, children, and adolescents: 4%), nausea (7% to 10%)

Hematologic & oncologic: Neutropenia (infants, children, and adolescents: 5%), thrombocytopenia (infants, children, and adolescents: 9%)

Hepatic: Increased serum alkaline phosphatase (3% to 6%)

Nervous system: Headache (adults: 9%)

Candidiasis prophylaxis in hematopoietic stem cell transplantation:

>10%:

Cardiovascular: Tachycardia (16% to 26%)

Dermatologic: Pruritus (infants, children, and adolescents: 33%), skin rash (25% to 30%), urticaria (<5%; infants, children, and adolescents: 19%)

Gastrointestinal: Abdominal distention (infants, children, and adolescents: 19%), abdominal pain (26% to 35%), diarrhea (77%; infants, children, and adolescents: 51%), nausea (70% to 71%), vomiting (65% to 66%)

Genitourinary: Decreased urine output (infants, children, and adolescents: 23%), hematuria (infants, children, and adolescents: 23%)

Hematologic & oncologic: Anemia (infants, children, and adolescents: 51%), febrile neutropenia (infants, children, and adolescents: 16%), neutropenia (75% to 77%), thrombocytopenia (72% to 75%)

Hepatic: Abnormal hepatic function tests (infants, children, and adolescents: <15%), hyperbilirubinemia (infants, children, and adolescents: <15%), increased serum alanine aminotransferase (16%)

Nervous system: Anxiety (22% to 23%), headache (adults: 44%), insomnia (adults: 37%)

Renal: Renal failure syndrome (infants, children, and adolescents: <15%)

Miscellaneous: Fever (infants, children, and adolescents: 61%), infusion-related reaction (infants, children, and adolescents: 16%)

1% to 10%:

Cardiovascular: Acute myocardial infarction (adults: <5%), pericardial effusion (adults: <5%)

Endocrine & metabolic: Hypernatremia (<5%), hypokalemia (<5%)

Hematologic & oncologic: Disorder of hemostatic components of blood (adults: <5%), pancytopenia (adults: <5%), thrombotic thrombocytopenic purpura (adults: <5%)
Hepatic: Hepatic failure (adults: <5%), hepatic injury (adults: <5%), hepatomegaly (adults: <5%), jaundice (adults: <5%)
Hypersensitivity: Anaphylaxis (adults: <5%), hypersensitivity reaction (adults: <5%)
Local: Infusion site reaction (adults: <5%), venous thrombosis at injection site (adults: <5%)
Nervous system: Encephalopathy (adults: <5%), delirium (adults: <5%), intracranial hemorrhage (adults: <5%), seizure (adults: <5%)
Respiratory: Epistaxis (infants, children, and adolescents: 9%)

Postmarketing (any indication):
Cardiovascular: Shock, vasodilation
Dermatologic: Facial swelling, Stevens-Johnson syndrome, toxic epidermal necrolysis
Hematologic & oncologic: Disseminated intravascular coagulation, hemolysis, hemolytic anemia
Hepatic: Hepatic disease
Hypersensitivity: Anaphylactic shock, anaphylaxis, nonimmune anaphylaxis, severe hypersensitivity reaction
Local: Injection site phlebitis, thrombophlebitis at injection site
Renal: Increased blood urea nitrogen, increased serum creatinine, renal insufficiency

Mechanism of Action Concentration-dependent inhibition of 1,3-beta-D-glucan synthase resulting in reduced formation of 1,3-beta-D-glucan, an essential polysaccharide comprising 30% to 60% of *Candida* cell walls (absent in mammalian cells); decreased glucan content leads to osmotic instability and cellular lysis

Pharmacodynamics/Kinetics

Half-life Elimination

Preterm infants:
PNA <1 week: 6.7 ± 2.2 hours (Kawada 2009).
PNA >3 weeks: Mean 8.3 hours (range: 5.6 to 11 hours) (Heresi 2006).
Term and preterm infants <4 months: Mean range: 11 to 13.6 hours (Benjamin 2010; Leroux 2018).
Infants ≥4 months and Children <2 years: 11.5 ± 2.17 hours (range: 7.9 to 16 hours) (Albano 2015).
Children 2 to 5 years: 11.1 ± 1.32 hours (range: 8.9 to 13.8 hours) (Albano 2015).
Children 6 to 11 years: 14.7 ± 6.98 hours (range: 9.8 to 28.4 hours) (Albano 2015).
Children ≥12 years and Adolescents ≤16 years: 13.1 ± 1.68 hours (range: 10.5 to 16.2 hours) (Albano 2015).
Healthy Adults: 11 to 21 hours.
Adults receiving bone marrow or peripheral stem-cell transplantation: 10.7 to 13.5 hours (Carver 2004).

Time to Peak

Serum:
Infants ≥4 months, Children, and Adolescents ≤16 years: 0.9 to 2 hours (Albano 2015; Benjamin 2013).

Pregnancy Considerations

Adverse events have been observed in animal reproduction studies.

Agents other than micafungin are preferred for the treatment of candidiasis in pregnancy (IDSA [Pappas 2016]).

◆ **Micafungin Sodium** *see* Micafungin *on page 1018*
◆ **Micardis** *see* Telmisartan *on page 1413*
◆ **Micatin [OTC]** *see* Miconazole (Topical) *on page 1019*
◆ **Miconazole 3** *see* Miconazole (Topical) *on page 1019*
◆ **Miconazole 3 Combo Pack [OTC]** *see* Miconazole (Topical) *on page 1019*
◆ **Miconazole 7 [OTC]** *see* Miconazole (Topical) *on page 1019*

Miconazole (Oral) (mi KON a zole)

Related Information

Fungal Infections *on page 1752*

Brand Names: US Oravig

Pharmacologic Category Antifungal Agent, Imidazole Derivative; Antifungal Agent, Oral Nonabsorbed

Use Treatment of oropharyngeal candidiasis

Local Anesthetic/Vasoconstrictor Precautions No information available to require special precautions

Effects on Dental Treatment Key adverse event(s) related to dental treatment: Application site reaction (including burning, discomfort, edema, glossodynia, pain, pruritus, toothache, ulceration), abnormal taste, oral discomfort, xerostomia and changes in salivation (normal salivary flow resumes upon discontinuation)

Effects on Bleeding No information available to require special precautions

Adverse Reactions

>10%: Local: Application site reaction (10% to 12%; including glossalgia, local discomfort, local pain, local pruritus, localized burning, localized edema, oral mucosa ulcer, toothache)

1% to 10%:
Central nervous system: Headache (5% to 8%), fatigue (3%), pain (1%)
Dermatologic: Pruritus (2%)
Endocrine & metabolic: Increased gamma-glutamyl transferase (1%)
Gastrointestinal: Diarrhea (6% to 9%), nausea (1% to 7%), dysgeusia (3% to 4%), vomiting (1% to 4%), oral discomfort (3%), xerostomia (3%), abdominal pain (1% to 3%), ageusia (2%), gastroenteritis (1%), sore throat (1%)
Hematologic & oncologic: Anemia (3%), lymphocytopenia (2%), neutropenia (1%)
Respiratory: Cough (3%), upper respiratory tract infection (2%)

Mechanism of Action Inhibits biosynthesis of ergosterol, damaging the fungal cell wall membrane, which increases permeability causing leaking of nutrients

Pharmacodynamics/Kinetics

Duration of Action Buccal adhesion: 15 hours

Pregnancy Considerations

There is minimal systemic absorption following buccal application. Topical treatment of oropharyngeal candidiasis in pregnancy is preferable to the use of systemic medications when possible (HHS [OI adult 2017]).

Miconazole (Topical) (mi KON a zole)

Related Information

Fungal Infections *on page 1752*

Brand Names: US Aloe Vesta Antifungal [OTC]; Aloe Vesta Clear Antifungal [OTC]; Antifungal [OTC]; Azolen Tincture [OTC]; Baza Antifungal [OTC] [DSC]; Carrington Antifungal [OTC]; Cavilon [OTC]; Critic-Aid Clear AF [OTC] [DSC]; Cruex Prescription Strength [OTC]; DermaFungal [OTC]; Desenex Jock Itch [OTC]; Desenex [OTC]; Fungoid Tincture [OTC]; GoodSense Miconazole 1 [OTC]; Lotrimin AF Deodorant Powder [OTC];

Lotrimin AF Jock Itch Powder [OTC]; Lotrimin AF Powder [OTC]; Lotrimin AF [OTC]; Micaderm [OTC]; Micatin [OTC]; Miconazole 3; Miconazole 3 Combo Pack [OTC]; Miconazole 7 [OTC]; Miconazole Antifungal [OTC]; Micro Guard [OTC] [DSC]; Podactin [OTC]; Remedy Antifungal Clear [OTC] [DSC]; Remedy Antifungal [OTC]; Remedy Phytoplex Antifungal [OTC]; Secura Antifungal Extra Thick [OTC] [DSC]; Secura Antifungal [OTC] [DSC]; Soothe & Cool INZO Antifungal [OTC]; Triple Paste AF [OTC]; Vagistat-3 [OTC] [DSC]; Zeasorb-AF [OTC]

Pharmacologic Category Antifungal Agent, Imidazole Derivative; Antifungal Agent, Oral Nonabsorbed/Partially Absorbed; Antifungal Agent, Topical; Antifungal Agent, Vaginal

Use Treatment of vulvovaginal candidiasis and a variety of skin and mucous membrane fungal infections

Local Anesthetic/Vasoconstrictor Precautions No information available to require special precautions

Effects on Dental Treatment No significant effects or complications reported

Effects on Bleeding No information available to require special precautions

Adverse Reactions Frequency not defined.

Topical:

Dermatologic: Allergic contact dermatitis, burning sensation of skin, maceration of skin

Vaginal:

Gastrointestinal: Abdominal cramps

Genitourinary: Vulvovaginal burning, vulvovaginal irritation, vulvovaginal pruritus

Mechanism of Action Inhibits biosynthesis of ergosterol, damaging the fungal cell wall membrane, which increases permeability causing leaking of nutrients

Pharmacodynamics/Kinetics

Half-life Elimination Multiphasic degradation: Alpha: 40 minutes; Beta: 126 minutes; Terminal: 24 hours

Reproductive Considerations

Vaginal products may weaken latex condoms and diaphragms (CDC [Workowski 2015]).

Pregnancy Considerations

Following vaginal administration, small amounts are absorbed systemically (Stevens 2002). Vaginal topical azole products (7-day therapies only) are the preferred treatment of vulvovaginal candidiasis in pregnant women (CDC [Workowski 2015]).

- **Miconazole Antifungal [OTC]** *see* Miconazole (Topical) *on page 1019*
- **Miconazole Nitrate** *see* Miconazole (Oral) *on page 1019*
- **Miconazole Nitrate** *see* Miconazole (Topical) *on page 1019*
- **MiCort-HC** *see* Hydrocortisone (Topical) *on page 775*
- **Microfibrillar Collagen Hemostat** *see* Collagen Hemostat *on page 410*
- **Microgestin 1.5/30** *see* Ethinyl Estradiol and Norethindrone *on page 614*
- **Microgestin 1/20** *see* Ethinyl Estradiol and Norethindrone *on page 614*
- **Microgestin 24 Fe [DSC]** *see* Ethinyl Estradiol and Norethindrone *on page 614*
- **Microgestin FE 1.5/30** *see* Ethinyl Estradiol and Norethindrone *on page 614*
- **Microgestin FE 1/20** *see* Ethinyl Estradiol and Norethindrone *on page 614*
- **Micro Guard [OTC] [DSC]** *see* Miconazole (Topical) *on page 1019*
- **Micro-K [DSC]** *see* Potassium Chloride *on page 1249*
- **Micronase** *see* GlyBURIDE *on page 741*
- **Microzide [DSC]** *see* HydroCHLOROthiazide *on page 762*
- **Midamor** *see* AMILoride *on page 116*

Midazolam (MID aye zoe lam)

Brand Names: US Nayzilam

Generic Availability (US) Yes

Pharmacologic Category Anticonvulsant, Benzodiazepine; Benzodiazepine

Dental Use Sedation component in IV conscious sedation in oral surgery patients; syrup formulation is used for children to help alleviate anxiety before a dental procedure

Use

Anesthesia: IV: Induction of general anesthesia before administration of other anesthetic agents; maintenance of anesthesia as a component of balanced anesthesia.

Sedation/anxiolysis/amnesia (preoperative/procedural):

IM: Preoperative sedation, anxiolysis, and amnesia.

IV: Sedation, anxiolysis, and amnesia prior to or during diagnostic, therapeutic, or endoscopic procedures, or prior to surgery.

Oral: Sedation, anxiolysis, and amnesia in children prior to diagnostic, therapeutic or endoscopic procedures or before induction of anesthesia.

Sedation for mechanically-ventilated patients: IV: Sedation of intubated and mechanically-ventilated patients as a component of anesthesia or during treatment in a critical care setting by continuous IV infusion.

Seizures, acute intermittent: Intranasal: Acute treatment of intermittent, stereotypic episodes of frequent seizure activity (ie, seizure clusters, acute repetitive seizures) that are distinct from a patient's usual seizure pattern in patients with epilepsy ≥12 years of age.

Local Anesthetic/Vasoconstrictor Precautions No information available to require special precautions

Effects on Dental Treatment No significant effects or complications reported (see Dental Health Professional Considerations)

Effects on Bleeding No information available to require special precautions

Adverse Reactions As reported in adults unless otherwise noted.

>10%: Respiratory: Bradypnea, decreased tidal volume

1% to 10%:

Cardiovascular: Hypotension (children: 3%)

Central nervous system: Drowsiness (1%), headache (1%), seizure-like activity (children: 1%), drug dependence (physical and psychological dependence with prolonged use), myoclonus (preterm infants), severe sedation

Gastrointestinal: Hiccups (adults: 4%; children: 1%), nausea (3%), vomiting (3%)

Local: Injection site reaction (IM: ≤4%, IV: ≤5%; severity less than diazepam), pain at injection site (IM: ≤4%, IV: ≤5%; severity less than diazepam)

Ophthalmic: Nystagmus (children: 1%)

Respiratory: Apnea (children: 3%), cough (1%)

Miscellaneous: Paradoxical reaction (children: 2%)

<1%, postmarketing, and/or case reports: Acidic taste, agitation, amnesia, bigeminy, bradycardia, bronchospasm, confusion, delirium (emergence), dyspnea, euphoria, hallucination, hyperventilation, laryngospasm, sialorrhea, skin rash, tachycardia, ventricular premature contractions, wheezing

Dental Usual Dosage Adults:

Preoperative sedation:

IM: 0.07 to 0.08 mg/kg 30 to 60 minutes prior to surgery/procedure; usual dose: 5 mg; **Note:** Reduce dose in patients with COPD, high-risk patients, patients ≥60 years of age, and patients receiving other opioids or CNS depressants

IV: 0.02 to 0.04 mg/kg; repeat every 5 minutes as needed to desired effect or up to 0.1 to 0.2 mg/kg

Intranasal (not an approved route): 0.2 mg/kg (up to 0.4 mg/kg in some studies); administer 30 to 45 minutes prior to surgery/procedure

Conscious sedation: IV: Initial: 0.5 to 2 mg slow IV over at least 2 minutes; slowly titrate to effect by repeating doses every 2 to 3 minutes if needed; usual total dose: 2.5 to 5 mg; use decreased doses in elderly.

Healthy Adults <60 years: Initial: Some patients respond to doses as low as 1 mg; no more than 2.5 mg should be administered over a period of 2 minutes. Additional doses of midazolam may be administered after a 2-minute waiting period and evaluation of sedation after each dose increment. A total dose >5 mg is generally not needed. If opioids or other CNS depressants are administered concomitantly, the midazolam dose should be reduced by 30%.

Dosing

Adult Note: The dose of midazolam needs to be individualized based on the patient's age, underlying diseases, and concurrent medications. Consider reducing dose by 20% to 50% in elderly, chronically ill, or debilitated patients and those receiving opioids or other CNS depressants (Miller 2010).

Anesthesia: IV:

Induction: Adults <55 years of age:

Unpremedicated patients: Initial: 0.3 to 0.35 mg/kg over 20 to 30 seconds; after 2 minutes, may repeat if necessary at ~25% of initial dose every 2 minutes, up to a total dose of 0.6 mg/kg in resistant cases.

Premedicated patients: Usual dosage range: 0.05 to 0.2 mg/kg (Barash 2009; Miller 2010). Use of 0.2 mg/kg administered over 5 to 10 seconds has been shown to safely produce anesthesia within 30 seconds (Samuelson 1981) and is recommended for ASA physical status P1 and P2 patients. When used with other anesthetic drugs (ie, coinduction), the dose is <0.1 mg/kg (Miller 2010).

ASA physical status >P3 or debilitation: Reduce dose by at least 20% (Miller 2010).

Maintenance: 0.05 mg/kg as needed (Miller 2010), or continuous infusion 0.015 to 0.06 mg/kg/**hour** (0.25 to 1 **mcg**/kg/minute) (Barash 2009; Miller 2010).

Palliative sedation (off-label use): Note: Use of midazolam in this setting should be done in close consult with or by an experienced palliative care provider. Ensure that flumazenil is readily available in the case of inadvertent overdose (ESMO [Cherney 2014]).

IV, SubQ: Continuous infusion: Initial: 0.5 to 1 mg/hour; may increase as needed. Usual dosage range: 1 to 20 mg/hour; may also intermittently administer 1 to 5 mg during infusion as needed (ESMO [Cherney 2014]). Some have recommended an initial bolus dose of 5 to 10 mg (size of dose depending on patient weight, age, and degree of debility) (Johanson 1993).

Sedation/anxiolysis/amnesia (preoperative/procedural):

Healthy adults <60 years of age:

Intranasal (solution, injection; off-label route): 0.1 mg/kg; administer 15 minutes prior to surgery/procedure (Uygur-Bayramiçli 2002). **Note:** Use 5 mg/mL injectable solution to deliver dose (Bailey 2017; Rech 2017).

IM: 0.07 to 0.08 mg/kg 30 to 60 minutes prior to surgery/procedure; usual dose: 5 mg.

IV: Initial: 0.5 to 2 mg over at least 2 minutes; slowly titrate to effect by repeating doses every 2 to 3 minutes if needed; usual total dose: 2.5 to 5 mg (ASGE [Waring 2003]).

Manufacturer's labeling: Dosing in the prescribing information may not reflect current clinical practice. Initial: Some patients respond to doses as low as 1 mg; no more than 2.5 mg should be administered over a period of at least 2 minutes. A total dose >5 mg is generally not needed.

Premedicated patients: Reduce initial dose by 30%.

Maintenance: 25% of dose used to reach sedative effect.

Adults ≥60 years of age, debilitated, or chronically ill: Refer to geriatric dosing.

Sedation in mechanically ventilated ICU patients: Note: Nonbenzodiazepine sedation may be preferred (SCCM [Devlin 2018]). IV: Initial: 0.01 to 0.05 mg/kg (~0.5 to 4 mg); may repeat at 10- to 15-minute intervals until adequate sedation achieved; maintenance infusion: 0.02 to 0.1 mg/kg/**hour** (0.3 to 1.7 **mcg**/kg/minute). Titrate to reach desired level of sedation (SCCM [Barr 2013]). Titration to maintain a light rather than a deep level of sedation is recommended unless clinically contraindicated (SCCM [Devlin 2018]). Consider a trial of daily awakening; if agitated after discontinuation of drip, then restart at 50% of the previous dose (Kress 2000).

Seizures, acute intermittent: Intranasal (nasal spray): 5 mg (one spray) as a single dose in one nostril; may repeat dose in 10 minutes in alternate nostril based on response and tolerability (do not repeat if the patient is having trouble breathing or excessive sedation). Maximum dose: 10 mg (2 sprays) per single episode. Maximum treatment frequency: Treatment of one episode every 3 days and treatment of 5 episodes in one month.

Status epilepticus (off-label use):

IM: 10 mg once (AES [Glauser 2016]) **or** 0.2 mg/kg once (maximum dose: 10 mg) (NCS [Brophy 2012]). **Note:** Midazolam IM is the preferred treatment in patients *without* IV access. Buccal and intranasal midazolam administration has also been used in patients without IV access, although these off-label routes are less well studied (AES [Glauser 2016]; Bailey 2017; deHaan 2010; NCS [Brophy 2012]; Scheepers 2000).

Prehospital status epilepticus: IM: 10 mg once; has been administered by paramedics when convulsions last >5 minutes **or** if convulsions are occurring after having intermittent seizures without regaining consciousness for >5 minutes (Silbergleit 2012).

Intranasal (solution, injection): Limited data available: 0.2 mg/kg (NCS [Brophy 2012]). **Note:** Use 5 mg/mL injectable concentrated solution to deliver dose (Bailey 2017; Rech 2017).

Buccal: Limited data available: 0.5 mg/kg (NCS [Brophy 2012]).

Status epilepticus, refractory (off-label use): IV: **Note:** Mechanical ventilation and cardiovascular monitoring required; titrate dose to cessation of electrographic seizures or burst suppression (NCS [Brophy 2012]).

Neurocritical Care Society recommendations:

Loading dose: 0.2 mg/kg followed by a continuous infusion (NCS [Brophy 2012]).

Continuous infusion: 0.05 to 2 mg/kg/**hour** (0.83 to 33.2 **mcg**/kg/minute) titrated to cessation of electrographic seizures or burst suppression. If patient experiences breakthrough status epilepticus while on the continuous infusion, administer a bolus of 0.1 to 0.2 mg/kg and increase infusion rate by 0.05 to 0.1 mg/kg/**hour** (0.83 to 1.66 **mcg**/kg/minute) every 3 to 4 hours (NCS [Brophy 2012]). Doses up to 2.9 mg/kg/**hour** have been described in the literature (Fernandez 2014). **Note:** A period of at least 24 to 48 hours of electrographic control is recommended prior to withdrawing the continuous infusion; withdraw gradually to prevent recurrent status epilepticus.

Geriatric

Intranasal (nasal spray): Refer to adult dosing; use with caution due to potential prolonged drug exposure.

Oral: Use is not recommended.

Parenteral: The dose of midazolam needs to be individualized based on the patient's age, underlying diseases, and concurrent medications. Consider reducing dose by 20% to 50% in elderly, chronically ill, or debilitated patients and those receiving opioids or other CNS depressants (Miller 2010). Titration of doses should also be slower (Strøm 2016).

Anesthesia: IV:

Induction: Adults ≥55 years of age:

Unpremedicated patients: Initial: 0.3 mg/kg.

Premedicated patients: Reduce dose by at least 20% (Miller 2010).

Maintenance: Refer to adult dosing.

Sedation/Anxiolysis/Amnesia (preoperative/procedural):

IM: 2 to 3 mg (or 0.02 to 0.05 mg/kg) 30 to 60 minutes prior to surgery/procedure; some may only require 1 mg if anticipated intensity and duration of sedation is less critical.

IV: Initial: 0.5 to 2 mg administered over at least 2 minutes (smaller doses may be used in the elderly); slowly titrate to effect by repeating doses every 2 to 3 minutes if needed; usual total dose: 2.5 to 5 mg (ASGE [Waring 2003]).

Manufacturer's labeling: Dosing in the prescribing information may not reflect current clinical practice. Initial: Some patients respond to doses as low as 1 mg; no more than 1.5 mg should be administered over a period of at least 2 minutes. A total dose of >3.5 mg is generally not needed.

Premedicated patients: Reduce initial dose by 50%.

Maintenance: 25% of dose used to reach sedative effect.

Renal Impairment: Adult There are no dosage adjustments provided in the manufacturer's labeling; use with caution; half-life of midazolam and metabolites may be prolonged. Patients with renal failure receiving a continuous infusion cannot adequately eliminate the active hydroxylated metabolites (eg, 1-hydroxymidazolam) contributing to prolonged sedation sometimes for days after discontinuation (Spina 2007).

Intermittent hemodialysis: Supplemental dose is not necessary.

Continuous venovenous hemofiltration: Unconjugated 1-hydroxymidazolam not effectively removed; 1-hydroxymidazolamglucuronide effectively removed; sieving coefficient = 0.45 (Swart 2005).

Peritoneal dialysis: Significant drug removal is unlikely based on physiochemical characteristics.

Intranasal (nasal spray):

Mild impairment: No dose adjustment necessary.

Moderate impairment: There are no dosage adjustments provided in the manufacturer's labeling; use with caution (not enough patients studied).

Severe impairment: There are no dosage adjustments provided in the manufacturer's labeling; use with caution (not studied).

Hepatic Impairment: Adult

There are no dosage adjustments provided in the manufacturer's labeling; use with caution.

IV:

Single dose (eg, induction): No dosage adjustment recommended; patients with hepatic impairment may be more sensitive compared to patients without hepatic impairment; anticipate longer duration of action (MacGilchrist 1986; Trouvin 1988).

Multiple dosing or continuous infusion: Expect longer duration of action and accumulation; based on patient response, dosage reduction likely to be necessary (Trouvin 1988).

Pediatric Dosage must be individualized and based on patient's age, underlying diseases, concurrent medications, and desired effect; decrease dose (by ~30%) if opioids or other CNS depressants are administered concomitantly; use multiple small doses and titrate to desired sedative effect; allow 3 to 5 minutes between doses to decrease the chance of oversedation. The nasal spray formulation delivers a fixed dose of 5 mg and is not appropriate for all pediatric patients; for smaller intranasal doses, parenteral solution for injection can be used; ensure appropriate product selection and administration technique.

Sedation, anxiolysis, and amnesia prior to procedure or before induction of anesthesia:

IM: Infants, Children, and Adolescents: Usual: 0.1 to 0.15 mg/kg 30 to 60 minutes before surgery or procedure; range: 0.05 to 0.15 mg/kg; doses up to 0.5 mg/kg have been used in more anxious patients; maximum total dose: 10 mg.

IV:

Infants 1 to 5 months: Limited data available in nonintubated infants; infants <6 months are at higher risk for airway obstruction and hypoventilation; titrate dose with small increments to desired clinical effect; monitor carefully.

Infants 6 months to Children 5 years: Initial: 0.05 to 0.1 mg/kg; titrate dose carefully; total dose of 0.6 mg/kg may be required; usual total dose maximum: 6 mg.

Children 6 to 12 years: Initial: 0.025 to 0.05 mg/kg; titrate dose carefully; total doses of 0.4 mg/kg may be required; usual total dose maximum: 10 mg.
Children 12 to 16 years: Dose as adults; usual total dose maximum: 10 mg.

Intranasal (parenteral solution for injection product): Limited data available: **Note:** Some investigators suggest premedication with intranasal lidocaine to decrease irritation and subsequent agitation (Chiaretti 2011; Lugo 1993):
Infants 1 to 5 months: 0.2 mg/kg (single dose) (Harcke 1995; Mittal 2006).
Infants ≥6 months, Children, and Adolescents: 0.2 to 0.3 mg/kg (maximum single dose: 10 mg); may repeat in 5 to 15 minutes to a maximum of 0.5 mg/kg (maximum total dose: 10 mg) (Acworth 2001; Chiaretti 2011; Harcke 1995; Lane 2008).

Oral: Infants >6 months, Children, and Adolescents <16 years: Single dose: 0.25 to 0.5 mg/kg once, depending on patient status and desired effect, usual: 0.5 mg/kg; maximum dose: 20 mg; **Note:** Younger patients (6 months to <6 years) and those less cooperative may require higher doses (up to 1 mg/kg); use lower initial doses (0.25 mg/kg) in older patients (6 to <16 years) and in patients with cardiac or respiratory compromise, concomitant CNS depressant, or high-risk surgical patients.

Rectal: Limited data available: Infants >6 months and Children: Usual: 0.25 to 0.5 mg/kg once (Krauss 2006); doses up to 1 mg/kg have been used in infants and young children (7 months to 5 years of age) but may be associated with a higher incidence of postprocedural agitation (Kanegaye 2003; Tanaka 2000).

Sedation, mechanically ventilated patient: Infants, Children, and Adolescents: IV: Loading dose: 0.05 to 0.2 mg/kg given slow IV over 2 to 3 minutes, then follow with initial continuous IV infusion: 0.06 to 0.12 mg/kg/**hour** (1 to 2 **mcg**/kg/minute); titrate to the desired effect; range: 0.024 to 0.36 mg/kg/**hour** (0.4 to 6 **mcg**/kg/minute).

Seizures, acute treatment:

Buccal: Limited data available: Reserve for patients without IV access (Ashrafi 2010; Kutlu 2003; McIntyre 2005; Mpimbaza 2008; Talukdar 2009):
Weight-based dosing: Infants ≥3 months, Children, and Adolescents: 0.2 to 0.5 mg/kg once; maximum dose: 10 mg/dose.
Age-based dosing (McIntyre 2005):
Infants 6 to 11 months: 2.5 mg.
Children 1 to 4 years: 5 mg.
Children 5 to 9 years: 7.5 mg.
Children and Adolescents ≥10 years: 10 mg.

IM: Limited data available: Infants, Children, and Adolescents: 0.2 mg/kg/dose; repeat every 10 to 15 minutes; maximum dose: 6 mg/dose (Hegenbarth 2008).

Intranasal:
Nasal spray (Nayzilam): Children ≥12 years and Adolescents: 5 mg administered as one spray into one nostril; may repeat dose in 10 minutes in alternate nostril based on response and tolerability; do not repeat dose if patient has difficulty breathing or excessive sedation; maximum dose: 10 mg/dose per episode (2 sprays); do not exceed maximum treatment frequency of one episode every 3 days and 5 episodes per month.
Parenteral solution for injection product: Limited data available (Bhattachyaryya 2006; Fişgin 2000; Fişgin 2002; Holsti 2007; Holsti 2010; Kutlu 2000): Reserve for patients without IV access; divide dose between nares:
Infants 1 to 5 months: 0.2 mg/kg once; maximum dose: 10 mg/dose.
Infants and Children ≥6 months: 0.2 mg/kg; one study used 0.3 mg/kg (n=9); maximum dose: 10 mg/dose; may repeat once to a total maximum of 0.4 mg/kg.

Status epilepticus:

Standard treatment: Infants, Children, and Adolescents: Limited data available:
IM:
Weight-based dosing: 0.2 mg/kg once; maximum dose: 10 mg/dose (NCS [Brophy 2012]).
Fixed dosing (AES [Glauser 2016]; NCS [Brophy 2012]):
13 to 40 kg: 5 mg once.
>40 kg: 10 mg once.
Intranasal: 0.2 mg/kg once; maximum dose: 10 mg/dose (AES [Glauser 2016]; NCS [Brophy 2012]).
Buccal: 0.5 mg/kg once; maximum dose: 10 mg/dose (AES [Glauser 2016]; McIntyre 2005; NCS [Brophy 2012]).

Refractory to standard treatment (NCS [Brophy 2012]): **Note:** Mechanical ventilation and cardiovascular monitoring required; titrate dose to cessation of electrographic seizures or burst suppression. Infants, Children, and Adolescents: Limited data available:
Loading dose: IV: 0.2 mg/kg followed by a continuous infusion.
Continuous IV infusion: 0.05 to 2 mg/kg/**hour** (0.83 to 33.3 **mcg**/kg/minute) titrated to cessation of electrographic seizures or burst suppression. If patient experiences breakthrough status epilepticus while on the continuous infusion, administer a bolus of 0.1 to 0.2 mg/kg and increase infusion rate by 0.05 to 0.1 mg/kg/**hour** (0.83 to 1.66 **mcg**/kg/minute) every 3 to 4 hours.

Renal Impairment: Pediatric There are no dosage adjustments provided in the manufacturer's labeling; use with caution; half-life of midazolam and metabolites may be prolonged. Adult patients with renal failure receiving a continuous infusion cannot adequately eliminate the active hydroxylated metabolites (eg, 1-hydroxymidazolam) contributing to prolonged sedation sometimes for days after discontinuation (Spina 2007).
Hemodialysis: Supplemental dose is not necessary.
Peritoneal dialysis: Significant drug removal is unlikely based on physiochemical characteristics

Hepatic Impairment: Pediatric There are no dosage adjustments provided in the manufacturer's labeling; use with caution. Based on experience in adult patients, the following have been suggested and may be considered in pediatric patients:
Single dose (eg, induction): No dosage adjustment recommended; patients with hepatic impairment may be more sensitive compared to patients without hepatic impairment; anticipate longer duration of action (MacGilchrist 1986; Trouvin 1988).
Multiple dosing or continuous infusion: Expect longer duration of action and accumulation; based on patient response, dosage reduction likely to be necessary (Trouvin 1988).

Mechanism of Action Binds to stereospecific benzodiazepine receptors on the postsynaptic GABA neuron at several sites within the central nervous system, including the limbic system, reticular formation. Enhancement of the inhibitory effect of GABA on neuronal excitability results by increased neuronal membrane permeability to chloride ions. This shift in chloride ions results in hyperpolarization (a less excitable state) and stabilization. Benzodiazepine receptors and effects appear to be linked to the GABA-A receptors. Benzodiazepines do not bind to GABA-B receptors (Brunton 2011).

Contraindications

Injection, oral: Hypersensitivity to midazolam or any component of the formulation; intrathecal or epidural injection of parenteral forms containing preservatives (ie, benzyl alcohol); use in premature infants for parenteral forms containing benzyl alcohol; acute narrow-angle glaucoma.

Concurrent use of oral midazolam with protease inhibitors (atazanavir, atazanavir-cobicistat, darunavir, indinavir, lopinavir-ritonavir, nelfinavir, ritonavir, saquinavir, tipranavir); concurrent use of oral or injectable midazolam with fosamprenavir.

Intranasal: Hypersensitivity to midazolam or any component of the formulation; acute narrow-angle glaucoma.

Documentation of allergenic cross-reactivity for benzodiazepines is limited. However, because of similarities in chemical structure and/or pharmacologic actions, the possibility of cross-sensitivity cannot be ruled out with certainty.

Canadian labeling: Additional contraindications (not in US labeling): Hypersensitivity to benzodiazepines; acute pulmonary insufficiency; severe chronic obstructive pulmonary disease.

Warnings/Precautions [US Boxed Warning]: Injection, oral: Has been associated with respiratory depression and respiratory arrest, especially when used for sedation in noncritical care settings; airway obstruction, desaturation, hypoxia, and apnea have also been reported, most often when used concomitantly with other CNS depressants (eg, opioids). In some cases, death or hypoxic encephalopathy resulted. Use only in hospital or ambulatory care settings that provide for continuous monitoring of respiratory and cardiac function (ie, pulse oximetry). Immediate availability of resuscitative drugs and age- and size-appropriate equipment for bag/valve/mask ventilation and intubation, and personnel trained in their use and skilled in airway management should be assured. For deeply sedated patients, a dedicated individual, other than the practitioner performing the procedure, should monitor the patient throughout the procedure. Risk of cardiorespiratory adverse events is increased in patients with abnormal airway anatomy, cyanotic congenital heart disease, sepsis or severe pulmonary disease. In patients with a risk of respiratory depression, consider administering the first dose of intranasal midazolam under health care supervision; this may be performed in the absence of a seizure episode. **[US Boxed Warning]: Concomitant use of benzodiazepines and opioids may result in profound sedation, respiratory depression, coma, and death. Reserve concomitant prescribing of these drugs for use in patients for whom alternative treatment options are inadequate. Limit dosages and durations to the minimum required. Follow patients for signs and symptoms of respiratory depression and sedation.** Benzodiazepines have been associated with anterograde amnesia (Nelson 1999). May cause CNS depression, which may impair physical or mental abilities; patients must be cautioned about performing tasks that require mental alertness (eg, operating machinery, driving). A minimum of one day should elapse after midazolam administration before attempting these tasks. Elapsed time to resume these tasks must be individualized, as pharmacologic effects are dependent on dose, route, duration of procedure, and presence of other medications. Paradoxical reactions, including hyperactive or aggressive behavior, have been reported with benzodiazepines; risk may be increased in adolescent/pediatric patients, geriatric patients, or patients with a history of alcohol use disorder or psychiatric/personality disorders (Mancuso 2004). Pooled analysis of trials involving various antiepileptics (regardless of indication) showed an increased risk of suicidal thoughts/behavior (incidence rate: 0.43% treated patients compared to 0.24% of patients receiving placebo); risk observed as early as one week after initiation and continued through duration of trials (most trials ≤24 weeks). Monitor all patients for notable changes in behavior that might indicate suicidal thoughts or depression; notify health care provider immediately if symptoms occur. May cause hypotension, particularly in pediatric patients or patients with hemodynamic instability. Use with caution in patients with glaucoma, heart failure, obesity, respiratory disease (eg, chronic obstructive pulmonary disease) or renal impairment. Use with caution in debilitated patients; decreased dosages recommended. Use with caution in the elderly; decreased dosages and slower titration is recommended due to an increased volume of distribution seen with lipophilic drugs in the elderly, resulting in slower distribution and lower clearance. Older patients can also take longer to recover completely after midazolam administration for the induction of anesthesia (Strøm 2016). Use of oral midazolam is not recommended in the elderly. Elderly patients may be at an increased risk of death with use; risk has been found highest within the first 4 months of use in elderly dementia patients (Jennum 2015; Saarelainen 2018). Pediatric patients with cardiac or respiratory compromise may be sensitive to the respiratory depressant effect of midazolam. Pediatric patients undergoing procedures involving the upper airway (eg, upper endoscopy, dental care) are vulnerable to episodes of desaturation and hypoventilation. In pediatric and neonatal patients <3 years of age and patients in third trimester of pregnancy (ie, times of rapid brain growth and synaptogenesis), the repeated or lengthy exposure to sedatives or anesthetics during surgery/procedures may have detrimental effects on child or fetal brain development and may contribute to various cognitive and behavioral problems. Epidemiological studies in humans have reported various cognitive and behavioral problems including neurodevelopmental delay (and related diagnoses), learning disabilities, and attention-deficit hyperactivity disorder. Human clinical data suggest that single, relatively short exposures are not likely to have similar negative effects. No specific anesthetic/sedative has been found to be safer. For elective procedures, risk vs benefits should be evaluated and discussed with parents/caregivers/patients; critical surgeries should not be delayed (US FDA Safety Communication 2017 Update). Use with extreme caution in patients who are at risk of falls; benzodiazepines have been associated with falls and traumatic injury (Nelson 1999).

Does not have analgesic, antidepressant, or antipsychotic properties. Does not protect against increases in intracranial pressure, heart rate, and/or blood pressure during intubation. Do not use in shock, coma, or acute alcohol intoxication with depression of vital signs. Avoid intra-arterial administration or extravasation of parenteral formulation. Use during upper airway procedures (ie, endoscopy, dental care) may increase risk of hypoventilation. Prolonged responses have been noted following extended administration by continuous infusion (possibly due to metabolite accumulation) or in the presence of drugs which inhibit midazolam metabolism. Oral midazolam is intended for use in monitored settings only and not for chronic or home use. Midazolam is a short half-life benzodiazepine and may be of benefit in patients where a rapidly and short-acting agent is desired (acute agitation). Duration of action after a single dose is determined by redistribution rather than metabolism. Tolerance develops to the sedative and anticonvulsant effects. It does not develop to the anxiolytic effects (Vinkers 2012). Withdrawal symptoms (convulsions, hallucinations, tremor, abdominal and muscle cramps, vomiting and sweating) may occur following abrupt discontinuation or large decreases in dose. Use caution when reducing dose or withdrawing therapy; decrease slowly and monitor for withdrawal symptoms. Potentially significant drug-drug interactions may exist, requiring dose or frequency adjustment, additional monitoring, and/or selection of alternative therapy.

Injection: **[US Boxed Warning]: Do not administer by rapid IV injection in neonates; severe hypotension and seizures have been reported following rapid IV administration, particularly with concomitant fentanyl use.** Neonates are also vulnerable to profound and/or prolonged respiratory effects of midazolam. **[US Boxed Warning]: Midazolam must never be used without individualization of dosage. The initial IV dose for sedation in adults may be as little as 1 mg, but should not exceed 2.5 mg in a healthy adult. Lower doses are necessary for older (>60 years of age) or debilitated patients and in patients receiving concomitant opioids or other CNS depressants. The initial dose and all subsequent doses should always be titrated slowly; administer over at least 2 minutes and allow an additional ≥2 minutes to fully evaluate the sedative effect. The use of the 1 mg/mL formulation or dilution of the 1 mg/mL or 5 mg/mL formulation is recommended to facilitate slower injection. Doses of sedative medications in pediatric patients must be calculated on a mg/kg basis, and initial doses and all subsequent doses should always be titrated slowly. The initial pediatric dose of midazolam for sedation/anxiolysis/amnesia is age, procedure, and route dependent.** Use IV midazolam with caution in patients with uncompensated acute illnesses, such as severe fluid or electrolyte disturbances. Avoid rapid IV administration in pediatric patients with cardiovascular instability.

Some dosage forms may contain benzyl alcohol; large amounts of benzyl alcohol (≥99 mg/kg/day) have been associated with a potentially fatal toxicity ("gasping syndrome") in neonates; the "gasping syndrome" consists of metabolic acidosis, respiratory distress, gasping respirations, CNS dysfunction (including convulsions, intracranial hemorrhage), hypotension, and cardiovascular collapse (AAP ["Inactive" 1997]; CDC 1982); some data suggest that benzoate displaces bilirubin from protein binding sites (Ahlfors 2001); avoid or use dosage forms containing benzyl alcohol with caution in neonates. See manufacturer's labeling.

Warnings: Additional Pediatric Considerations In pediatric and neonatal patients <3 years of age and patients in third trimester of pregnancy (ie, times of rapid brain growth and synaptogenesis), the repeated or lengthy exposure to sedatives or anesthetics during surgery/procedures may have detrimental effects on the child's or fetus' brain development and may contribute to various cognitive and behavioral problems; the FDA is requiring warnings be included in the manufacturer's labeling for all general anesthetic/sedative drugs. Multiple animal species studies have shown adverse effects on brain maturation; in juvenile animals, drugs that potentiate GABA activity and/or block NMDA receptors for >3 hours demonstrated widespread neuronal and oligodendrocyte cell loss along with alteration in synaptic morphology and neurogenesis. Epidemiological studies in humans have reported various cognitive and behavioral problems including neurodevelopmental delay (and related diagnoses), learning disabilities, and ADHD. Human clinical data suggest that single, relatively short exposures are not likely to have similar negative effects. Further studies are needed to fully characterize findings and ensure that these findings are not related to underlying conditions or the procedure itself. No specific anesthetic/sedative has been found to be safer. For elective procedures, risk vs benefits should be evaluated and discussed with parents/caregivers/patients; critical surgeries should not be delayed (FDA 2017).

In neonates, particularly premature neonates, several cases of myoclonus (rhythmic myoclonic jerking) have been reported (~8% incidence).

Drug Interactions

Metabolism/Transport Effects **Substrate** of CYP2B6 (minor), CYP3A4 (major); **Note:** Assignment of Major/Minor substrate status based on clinically relevant drug interaction potential

Avoid Concomitant Use

Avoid concomitant use of Midazolam with any of the following: Abametapir; Antihepaciviral Combination Products; Azelastine (Nasal); Bromperidol; Cobicistat; Conivaptan; Fusidic Acid (Systemic); Idelalisib; Itraconazole; Ketoconazole (Systemic); OLANZapine; Orphenadrine; Oxomemazine; Paraldehyde; Protease Inhibitors; Sodium Oxybate; Thalidomide

Increased Effect/Toxicity

Midazolam may increase the levels/effects of: Alcohol (Ethyl); Azelastine (Nasal); Blonanserin; Brexanolone; Buprenorphine; CloZAPine; CNS Depressants; Flunitrazepam; Methadone; Methotrimeprazine; MetyroSINE; Opioid Agonists; Orphenadrine; OxyCODONE; Paraldehyde; Piribedil; Pramipexole; Propofol; ROPINIRole; Rotigotine; Sodium Oxybate; Thalidomide; Zolpidem

The levels/effects of Midazolam may be increased by: Abametapir; Alizapride; Antihepaciviral Combination Products; Aprepitant; AtorvaSTATin; Brimonidine (Topical); Bromopride; Bromperidol; Cannabidiol; Cannabis; Chlormethiazole; Chlorphenesin Carbamate; Clofazimine; Cobicistat; Conivaptan; CYP3A4 Inhibitors (Moderate); CYP3A4 Inhibitors (Strong); Dimethindene (Topical); Doxylamine; Dronabinol; Droperidol; Duvelisib; Elagolix, Estradiol, and Norethindrone; Erdafitinib; Esketamine; Fosaprepitant; Fosnetupitant; Fusidic Acid (Systemic); HydrOXYzine; Idelalisib; Itraconazole; Kava Kava; Ketoconazole

(Systemic); Larotrectinib; Lemborexant; Lisuride; Lofexidine; Macrolide Antibiotics; Magnesium Sulfate; Melatonin; Methotrimeprazine; Metoclopramide; MiFEPRIStone; Minocycline (Systemic); Nabilone; Netupitant; OLANZapine; Oxomemazine; Palbociclib; Perampanel; Propofol; Protease Inhibitors; Roxithromycin; Rufinamide; Simeprevir; Stiripentol; Teduglutide; Tetrahydrocannabinol; Tetrahydrocannabinol and Cannabidiol; Tofisopam; Trimeprazine

Decreased Effect

The levels/effects of Midazolam may be decreased by: CYP3A4 Inducers (Moderate); CYP3A4 Inducers (Strong); Dabrafenib; Deferasirox; Elagolix; Enzalutamide; Erdafitinib; Ginkgo Biloba; Ivosidenib; Lumacaftor and Ivacaftor; Mitotane; Sarilumab; Siltuximab; Tecovirimat; Theophylline Derivatives; Tocilizumab; Yohimbine

Food Interactions Injection, oral: Grapefruit juice may increase serum concentrations of midazolam. Management: Avoid concurrent use of grapefruit juice with oral midazolam.

Dietary Considerations Avoid grapefruit juice with oral syrup.

Pharmacodynamics/Kinetics

Onset of Action

IM: Sedation: Children: Within 5 minutes; Adults: ~15 minutes; IV: 3 to 5 minutes; Oral: 10 to 20 minutes; Intranasal (nasal spray): Within 10 minutes; Intranasal (solution, injection): Children: 5.55 ± 2.22 minutes (Lee-Kim 2004); Adults: Within 5 minutes

Peak effect: IM: Children: 15 to 30 minutes; Adults: 30 to 60 minutes; IV: 3 to 5 minutes; Intranasal (nasal spray): 30 minutes; Intranasal (solution, injection): Children: 10 minutes (al-Rakaf 2001)

Duration of Action IM: Up to 6 hours; Mean: 2 hours; Intranasal (solution, injection): Children: 23.1 minutes (Chiaretti 2011); IV: Single dose: <2 hours (dose-dependent) (Fragen 1997)

Half-life Elimination

Prolonged in cirrhosis, congestive heart failure, obesity, renal failure, and elderly. **Note:** In patients with renal failure, reduced elimination of active hydroxylated metabolites leads to drug accumulation and prolonged sedation.

Preterm infants (n=24; GA: 26 to 34 weeks; PNA: 3 to 11 days): IV: Median: 6.3 hours (range: 2.6 to 17.7 hours) (de Wildt 2001)

Neonates: 4 to 12 hours; seriously ill neonates: 6.5 to 12 hours

Children: IV: 2.9 to 4.5 hours; Syrup: 2.2 to 6.8 hours

Adults: 3 hours (range: 1.8 to 6.4 hours); IM: 4.2 ± 1.87 hours; Intranasal (nasal spray): 2.1 to 6.2 hours

Time to Peak IM: 0.5 to 1 hour; Intranasal (nasal spray): median 17.3 minutes (7.8 to 28.2 minutes); Oral: 0.17 to 2.65 hours

Pregnancy Considerations

Midazolam crosses the placenta and can be detected in the serum of the umbilical vein and artery, as well as the amniotic fluid.

Teratogenic effects have been observed with some benzodiazepines; however, additional studies are needed. The incidence of premature birth and low birth weights may be increased following maternal use of benzodiazepines; hypoglycemia and respiratory problems in the neonate may occur following exposure late in pregnancy. Neonatal withdrawal symptoms may occur within days to weeks after birth and "floppy infant syndrome" (which also includes withdrawal symptoms) have been reported with some benzodiazepines (Bergman 1992; Iqbal 2002; Wikner 2007).

Based on animal data, repeated or prolonged use of general anesthetic and sedation medications that block N-methyl-D-aspartate (NMDA) receptors and/or potentiate gamma-aminobutyric acid (GABA) activity may affect brain development. Evaluate benefits and potential risks of fetal exposure to midazolam when duration of surgery is expected to be >3 hours (Olutoye 2018).

Due to pregnancy-induced physiologic changes, some pharmacokinetic properties of midazolam may be altered (Hebert 2008; Wilson 1987). Although use in obstetric procedures is not recommended by the manufacturer, midazolam use in obstetric anesthesia has been described (Frölich 2006; Heyman 1987; Kanto 1984; Neuman 2013; Senel 2014; Shergill 2012).

The ACOG recommends that pregnant women should not be denied medically necessary surgery regardless of trimester. If the procedure is elective, it should be delayed until after delivery (ACOG 775 2019).

Breastfeeding Considerations

Midazolam and hydroxymidazolam are present in breast milk.

The relative infant dose (RID) of midazolam is 0.35% when calculated using the highest breast milk concentration located and compared to a weight-adjusted maternal dose of 30 mg.

In general, breastfeeding is considered acceptable when an RID of a medication is <10% (Anderson 2016; Ito 2000).

The RID of midazolam was calculated using a milk concentration of 0.0001 mg/mL (30 nmol/L), providing an estimated daily infant dose via breast milk of 0.0015 mg/kg/day. This milk concentration was obtained following accidental maternal administration of two oral doses of midazolam 15 mg (total dose: 30 mg) (Matheson 1990). In most reports, midazolam and hydroxymidazolam concentrations in breast milk are below the limit of quantification 4 hours after a single dose (Koitabashi 1997; Matheson 1990).

CNS depression was reported in infants following exposure to benzodiazepines via breast milk (study included exposures to midazolam) (Kelly 2012). The manufacturer recommends that caution be exercised when administering midazolam to breastfeeding women. When used for sedation prior to a procedure, available guidelines suggest waiting for ≥4 hours after a maternal dose of midazolam to continue breastfeeding (Shergill 2012).

The Academy of Breast Feeding Medicine recommends postponing elective surgery until milk supply and breastfeeding are established. Milk should be expressed ahead of surgery when possible. In general, when the child is healthy and full term, breastfeeding may resume, or milk may be expressed once the mother is awake and in recovery. For children who are at risk for apnea, hypotension, or hypotonia, milk may be saved for later use when the child is at lower risk (ABM [Reece-Stremtan 2017]). Small supplemental doses of midazolam used during cesarean delivery should not prevent breastfeeding once the mother is stable and alert (ABM [Martin 2018]).

Product Availability

Seizalam (50 mg/10 mL injection): FDA approved October 2018; anticipated availability is currently unknown. Seizalam is indicated for the treatment of status epilepticus in adults. Information pertaining to this product within the monograph is pending revision. Consult the prescribing information for additional information.

Controlled Substance C-IV

Dosage Forms Considerations Midazolam+Syr-Spend SF PH4 oral suspension is a compounding kit. Refer to manufacturer's labeling for compounding instructions.

Dosage Forms: US

Solution, Injection:

Generic: 2 mg/2 mL (2 mL); 5 mg/5 mL (5 mL); 10 mg/10 mL (10 mL); 5 mg/mL (1 mL); 10 mg/2 mL (2 mL); 25 mg/5 mL (5 mL); 50 mg/10 mL (10 mL)

Solution, Injection [preservative free]:

Generic: 2 mg/2 mL (2 mL); 5 mg/5 mL (5 mL); 5 mg/mL (1 mL); 10 mg/2 mL (2 mL)

Solution, Intravenous:

Generic: 100 mg/100 mL in NaCl 0.8% (100 mL); 50 mg/50 mL in NaCl 0.8% (50 mL)

Solution, Nasal:

Nayzilam: 5 mg/0.1 mL (2 ea)

Syrup, Oral:

Generic: 2 mg/mL (118 mL)

Dosage Forms: Canada

Solution, Injection:

Generic: 1 mg/mL (2 mL, 5 mL, 10 mL); 5 mg/mL (1 mL, 2 mL, 3 mL, 5 mL, 10 mL, 50 mL); 50 mg/10 mL (10 mL)

Dental Health Professional Considerations An adult companion should accompany the patient to and from dental office.

Compared to oral sedation, intranasal (IN) sedation resulted in greater irritability during the first 10-15 minutes after administration, but a faster onset and shorter duration of sedation with improved behavior following onset of sedation. (Johnson 2010; Lee-Kim 2004). Monitor oxygen saturation with midazolam. If desaturation occurs, reposition airway (head tilt, chin lift).

◆ **Midazolam HCl** *see* Midazolam *on page 1020*

◆ **Midazolam Hydrochloride** *see* Midazolam *on page 1020*

Midodrine (MI doe dreen)

Brand Names: Canada Amatine; APO-Midodrine; MAR-Midodrine

Pharmacologic Category $Alpha_1$ Agonist

Use Hypotension, symptomatic orthostatic: Treatment of symptomatic orthostatic hypotension.

Local Anesthetic/Vasoconstrictor Precautions No information available to require special precautions

Effects on Dental Treatment Key adverse event(s) related to dental treatment: Xerostomia (normal salivary flow resumes upon discontinuation).

Effects on Bleeding No information available to require special precautions

Adverse Reactions

>10%:

Cardiovascular: Supine hypertension (7% to 13%)

Central nervous system: Paresthesia (18%)

Dermatologic: Piloerection (13%), pruritus (12%)

Genitourinary: Dysuria (≤13%), urinary retention, urinary urgency

Renal: Polyuria

1% to 10%:

Central nervous system: Chills (5%), pain (5%)

Dermatologic: Skin rash (2%)

Gastrointestinal: Abdominal pain

<1%, postmarketing, and/or case reports: Anxiety, aphthous stomatitis, back pain, confusion, dizziness, drowsiness, erythema multiforme, facial flushing, flatulence, flushing, gastrointestinal distress, headache, heartburn, hyperesthesia, increased intracranial pressure, insomnia, leg cramps, nausea, visual field defect, weakness, xeroderma, xerostomia

Mechanism of Action Midodrine forms an active metabolite, desglymidodrine, which is an $alpha_1$-agonist. This agent increases arteriolar and venous tone resulting in a rise in standing, sitting, and supine systolic and diastolic blood pressure in patients with orthostatic hypotension.

Pharmacodynamics/Kinetics

Onset of Action ~1 hour

Duration of Action 2 to 3 hours

Half-life Elimination Desglymidodrine: ~3 to 4 hours; Midodrine: 25 minutes

Time to Peak Desglymidodrine: 1 to 2 hours; Midodrine: 30 minutes

Pregnancy Considerations Adverse events were observed in animal reproduction studies. Information related to the use of midodrine in pregnancy is limited (Glatter 2005).

◆ **Midodrine HCl** *see* Midodrine *on page 1027*

◆ **Midodrine Hydrochloride** *see* Midodrine *on page 1027*

◆ **Midol Long Lasting Relief [OTC]** *see* Acetaminophen *on page 59*

Midostaurin (mye doe STAW rin)

Brand Names: US Rydapt

Brand Names: Canada Rydapt

Pharmacologic Category Antineoplastic Agent, FLT3 Inhibitor; Antineoplastic Agent, Tyrosine Kinase Inhibitor

Use

Acute myeloid leukemia, FLT3-positive: Treatment of adult patients with newly diagnosed FLT3 mutation-positive (as detected by an approved test) acute myeloid leukemia (AML), in combination with standard cytarabine and daunorubicin induction and cytarabine consolidation chemotherapy

Limitations of use: Not indicated as single-agent induction therapy for the treatment of patients with AML.

Mast cell leukemia: Treatment of adult patients with mast cell leukemia (MCL)

Systemic mastocytosis: Treatment of adult patients with aggressive systemic mastocytosis (ASM) or systemic mastocytosis with associated hematological neoplasm (SM-AHN)

Local Anesthetic/Vasoconstrictor Precautions Midostaurin is one of the drugs confirmed to prolong the QT interval and is accepted as having a risk of causing torsade de pointes. The risk of drug-induced torsade de pointes is extremely low when a single QT interval prolonging drug is prescribed. In terms of epinephrine, it is not known what effect vasoconstrictors in the local anesthetic regimen will have in patients with a known history of congenital prolonged QT interval or in patients taking any medication that prolongs the QT interval. Until more information is obtained, it is suggested that the clinician consult with the physician prior to the use of a vasoconstrictor in suspected patients, and that the vasoconstrictor (epinephrine, mepivacaine, and levonordefrin [Carbocaine® 2% with Neo-Cobefrin®]) be used with caution.

Effects on Dental Treatment Key adverse event(s) related to dental treatment: Mucositis has been reported

Effects on Bleeding Chemotherapy with midostaurin may result in significant myelosuppression, potentially including significant reduction in platelet counts (thrombocytopenia 50% grades ≥3: 27%) and altered hemostasis. In patients who are under active treatment with this agent, medical consult is suggested.

Adverse Reactions

>10%:

Cardiovascular: Edema (40%), prolonged QT interval on ECG (11%)

Central nervous system: Headache (26% to 46%), fatigue (34%), dizziness (13%), insomnia (11% to 12%)

Dermatologic: Hyperhidrosis (14%), skin rash (14%)

Endocrine & metabolic: Hyperglycemia (20% to 80%), hypocalcemia (39% to 74%), hyperuricemia (8% to 37%), increased gamma-glutamyl transferase (35%), hyponatremia (34%), hypoalbuminemia (27%), hypokalemia (25%), hyperkalemia (23%), hypophosphatemia (22%), hypernatremia (21%), hypomagnesemia (20%)

Gastrointestinal: Nausea (47% to 83%), vomiting (19% to 68%), mucositis (66%), diarrhea (54%), increased serum lipase (37%), abdominal pain (34%), constipation (29%), increased serum amylase (20%), hemorrhoids (15%), gastrointestinal hemorrhage (14%)

Genitourinary: Urinary tract infection (16%)

Hematologic & oncologic: Febrile neutropenia (8% to 83%; grades ≥3: 84%), lymphocytopenia (66%; grades ≥3: 42%), leukopenia (61%; grades ≥3: 19%), anemia (60%; grades ≥3: 38%), thrombocytopenia (50%; grades ≥3: 27%), neutropenia (49%; grades ≥3: 22%), petechia (36%), prolonged partial thromboplastin time (13%; grades ≥3: 3%)

Hepatic: Increased serum ALT (31% to 71%), increased serum alkaline phosphatase (39%), increased serum AST (32%), hyperbilirubinemia (29%)

Infection: Localized infection (24%; device related)

Neuromuscular & skeletal: Musculoskeletal pain (33% to 35%), arthralgia (14% to 19%)

Renal: Increased serum creatinine (25%), renal insufficiency (11% to 12%)

Respiratory: Upper respiratory tract infection (20% to 30%), epistaxis (12% to 28%), dyspnea (23%), cough (18%), pleural effusion (6% to 13%)

Miscellaneous: Fever (27%)

1% to 10%:

Cardiovascular: Hypotension (9%), hypertension (8%), cardiac failure (6%), thrombosis (5%), pericardial effusion (4%), ischemia (≤4%), myocardial infarction (≤4%)

Central nervous system: Disturbance in attention (7%), chills (5%), vertigo (5%), mental status changes (4%)

Dermatologic: Xeroderma (7%), cellulitis (≤7%), erysipelas (≤5%)

Endocrine & metabolic: Weight gain (6% to 7%), hypercalcemia (3%)

Gastrointestinal: Dyspepsia (6%), gastritis (3%)

Hematologic & oncologic: Bruise (6%), hematoma (6%)

Hypersensitivity: Hypersensitivity (4%)

Infection: Herpes virus infection (10%), sepsis (9%), fungal infection (7%)

Neuromuscular & skeletal: Tremor (4% to 6%)

Ophthalmic: Eyelid edema (3%)

Respiratory: Pneumonia (10%), bronchitis (6%), oropharyngeal pain (4%), pulmonary edema (3%), interstitial pulmonary disease (≤2%), pneumonitis (≤2%)

Mechanism of Action

Midostaurin is a tyrosine kinase inhibitor which inhibits multiple receptors, such as wild type FLT3, FLT3 mutant kinases ITD and TKD, KIT (wild type and D816V mutant), PDGFRα/β, and members of the serine/threonine protein kinase C (PKC) family.

Midostaurin inhibits FLT3 receptor signaling and cell proliferation, and induces apoptosis in ITD- and TKD-mutant expressing leukemic cells, as well as in cells overexpressing wild type FLT3 and PDGFR. It also may inhibit KIT signaling, cell proliferation, and histamine release (and induces apoptosis) in mast cells.

Pharmacodynamics/Kinetics

Half-life Elimination 19 hours (midostaurin); 32 hours (CGP62221); 482 hours (CGP52421)

Time to Peak 1 to 3 hours (fasted state); 2.5 to 3 hours (with standard or high-fat meal)

Reproductive Considerations

Pregnancy status should be verified within 7 days prior to therapy initiation. Females of reproductive potential and males with female partners of reproductive potential should use effective contraception during therapy and for at least 4 months after the last dose.

Pregnancy Considerations

Based on the mechanism of action and data from animal reproduction studies, in utero exposure to midostaurin may cause fetal harm.

Females who may have been exposed to midostaurin during pregnancy (directly or through a male partner receiving midostaurin) should contact the Novartis Pharmaceuticals Corporation at 1-888-669-6682 and/or at https://psi.novartis.com.

◆ **Mifeprex** *see* MiFEPRIStone *on page* *1028*

MiFEPRIStone (mi FE pris tone)

Related Information

Clinical Risk Related to Drugs Prolonging QT Interval *on page* *1675*

Brand Names: US Korlym; Mifeprex

Pharmacologic Category Abortifacient; Antiprogestin; Cortisol Receptor Blocker

Use

Korlym: To control hyperglycemia occurring secondary to hypercortisolism in adult patients with endogenous Cushing syndrome who have type 2 diabetes mellitus or glucose intolerance and who failed surgery or who are not surgical candidates.

Limitations of use: Should not be used in the treatment of patients with type 2 diabetes unless it is secondary to Cushing syndrome.

Mifeprex: Medical termination of intrauterine pregnancy through 70 days gestation, in combination with misoprostol.

Local Anesthetic/Vasoconstrictor Precautions

Mifepristone is one of the drugs confirmed to prolong the QT interval and is accepted as having a risk of causing torsade de pointes. The risk of drug-induced torsade de pointes is extremely low when a single QT interval prolonging drug is prescribed. In terms of epinephrine, it is not known what effect vasoconstrictors in the local anesthetic regimen will have in patients with a known history of congenital prolonged QT interval or in patients taking any medication that prolongs the QT interval. Until more information is obtained, it is suggested that the clinician consult with the physician prior to the use of a vasoconstrictor in suspected patients, and that the vasoconstrictor (epinephrine, mepivacaine and levonordefrin [Carbocaine® 2% with Neo-Cobefrin®]) be used with caution.

Effects on Dental Treatment No significant effects or complications reported

Effects on Bleeding No information available to require special precautions

Adverse Reactions Adverse reactions occur with treatment of hyperglycemia in patients with Cushing syndrome unless otherwise specified.

>10%:

Cardiovascular: Peripheral edema (26%), hypertension (24%)

Central nervous system: Fatigue (hyperglycemia: 48%; pregnancy termination: 10%), headache (hyperglycemia: 44%; pregnancy termination: 2% to 31%), dizziness (hyperglycemia: 22%; pregnancy termination: 1% to 12%), pain (14%)

Endocrine & metabolic: Hypokalemia (34% to 44%), abnormal thyroid function test (18%)

Gastrointestinal: Abdominal cramps (pregnancy termination: 96%), nausea (pregnancy termination: 43% to 61%; hyperglycemia: 48%), vomiting (hyperglycemia and pregnancy termination: 18% to 26%), decreased appetite (20%), diarrhea (hyperglycemia and pregnancy termination: 12% to 20%), xerostomia (18%)

Genitourinary: Uterine cramps (pregnancy termination: 83%), endometrium disease (hypertrophy: 38%), vaginal hemorrhage (14%; when used for pregnancy termination, vaginal bleeding for 9 to 16 days is expected, with the first 2 days being the heaviest; 8% of these patients experience bleeding for ≥30 days)

Neuromuscular & skeletal: Arthralgia (30%), back pain (hyperglycemia and pregnancy termination: 9% to 16%), myalgia (14%), limb pain (12%)

Respiratory: Dyspnea (16%), sinusitis (hyperglycemia: 14%; pregnancy termination: 2%), nasopharyngitis (12%)

1% to 10%:

Cardiovascular: Edema (5% to 10%), pitting edema (5% to 10%), syncope (pregnancy termination: 1% to 2%)

Central nervous system: Anxiety (hyperglycemia: 10%; pregnancy termination: 2%), drowsiness (10%), flank pain (5% to 10%), malaise (5% to 10%), insomnia (pregnancy termination: 3%), rigors (pregnancy termination: 3%)

Dermatologic: Pruritus (4%), skin rash (4%)

Endocrine & metabolic: Hypoglycemia (5% to 10%), increased serum triglycerides (5% to 10%), increased thirst (5% to 10%), adrenocortical insufficiency (4%)

Gastrointestinal: Anorexia (10%), constipation (10%), abdominal pain (5% to 10%), gastroesophageal reflux disease (5% to 10%), dyspepsia (pregnancy termination: 3%)

Genitourinary: Uterine hemorrhage (pregnancy termination: 5%), vaginitis (pregnancy termination: 3%), leukorrhea (pregnancy termination: 2%), pelvic pain (pregnancy termination: 2%), endometriosis (pregnancy termination: ≤1%), salpingitis (pregnancy termination: ≤1%), pelvic inflammatory disease (pregnancy termination: ≤1%)

Hematologic & oncologic: Decreased hemoglobin (pregnancy termination: 6%; >2 g/dL), anemia (pregnancy termination: 2%)

Infection: Viral infection (pregnancy termination: 4%)

Neuromuscular & skeletal: Musculoskeletal chest pain (5% to 10%), weakness (pregnancy termination: 2%), leg pain (pregnancy termination: 2%)

Miscellaneous: Fever (pregnancy termination: 4%)

Frequency not defined: Endocrine & metabolic: Decreased HDL cholesterol

<1%, postmarketing, and/or case reports: Acute pancreatitis, adult respiratory distress syndrome, bacterial infection (including an ectopic bacteria such as *Clostridium sordellii*), disseminated intravascular coagulopathy, dyspnea, ectopic pregnancy (rupture), exacerbation of Crohn's disease, hypersensitivity reaction (including urticaria), hypotension, infection (post-abortion), loss of consciousness, myocardial infarction, pelvic infection, prolonged QT interval on ECG, sepsis, septic shock, tachycardia, toxic shock syndrome

Mechanism of Action Mifepristone is a synthetic steroid. At low doses, it competitively binds to the intracellular progesterone receptor, blocking the effects of progesterone. When used for the termination of pregnancy, this leads to contraction-inducing activity in the myometrium. In the absence of progesterone, mifepristone acts as a partial progesterone agonist. At high doses used for the treatment of hyperglycemia in patients with Cushing's syndrome, mifepristone blocks the effect of cortisol at the glucocorticoid receptor (antagonizes the effects of cortisol on glucose metabolism) while at the same time increasing circulating cortisol concentrations.

Pharmacodynamics/Kinetics

Half-life Elimination Single dose: Terminal: 18 hours following a slower phase where 50% eliminated between 12-72 hours; Multiple doses (600 mg/day): 85 hours

Time to Peak Oral: 90 minutes; Range: Single dose: 1-2 hours, Multiple doses: 1-4 hours

Reproductive Considerations

Korlym: **[US Boxed Warning]:** When used to control hyperglycemia in women with Cushing syndrome, **pregnancy must be excluded before the initiation of treatment with mifepristone and prevented during treatment and for 1 month after stopping treatment by the use of a nonhormonal, medically acceptable method of contraception unless the patient has had a surgical sterilization, in which case, no additional contraception is needed. Pregnancy must also be excluded if treatment is interrupted for more than 14 days in females of reproductive potential.**

Mifeprex: This medication is used to terminate pregnancy. In sexually active women, pregnancy can occur prior to the first menstrual period following treatment. Appropriate contraception can be started as soon as termination of pregnancy is confirmed or before sexual intercourse is resumed.

Pregnancy Considerations

Mifepristone is contraindicated for use in pregnant women when used to control hyperglycemia in Cushing syndrome.

Korlym: **[US Boxed Warning]: Mifepristone is a potent antagonist of progesterone and cortisol via the progesterone and glucocorticoid (GR-II) receptors, respectively. The antiprogestational effects will result in the termination of pregnancy.**

Mifeprex: This medication is used to terminate pregnancy; there are no approved treatment indications for its use during pregnancy. If treatment fails, there is a risk of fetal malformation.

Prescribing and Access Restrictions Korlym is only available through a restricted access program. For prescriber registration and patient enrollment forms, please refer to https://www.korlym.com/hcp/access-support/support-program-access-reimbursement-korlym-spark/ or call 1-855-4Korlym (1-855-456-7596).

Dental Health Professional Considerations See Local Anesthetic/Vasoconstrictor Precautions

Migalastat (mi GAL a stat)

Brand Names: US Galafold

Brand Names: Canada Galafold

Pharmacologic Category Pharmacologic Chaperone

Use Fabry disease: Treatment of adults with a confirmed diagnosis of Fabry disease and an amenable galactosidase alpha gene (GLA) variant based on in vitro assay data.

Local Anesthetic/Vasoconstrictor Precautions No information available to require special precautions

Effects on Dental Treatment Key adverse event(s) related to dental treatment: Frequent occurrence of nasopharyngitis; frequent occurrence of cough; no oral soft tissue effects have been reported or observed in Fabry disease or with exposure to Migalastat.

Effects on Bleeding No information available to require special precautions

Adverse Reactions

>10%:

Central nervous system: Headache (35%)
Gastrointestinal: Nausea (12%)
Genitourinary: Urinary tract infection (15%)
Respiratory: Nasopharyngitis (18%)
Miscellaneous: Fever (12%)

1% to 10%:

Gastrointestinal: Abdominal pain (9%), diarrhea (9%)
Neuromuscular & skeletal: Back pain (9%)
Respiratory: Cough (9%), epistaxis (9%)

Mechanism of Action Migalastat is an oral pharmacological chaperone that stabilizes certain mutant variants of alpha-galactosidase to increase enzyme trafficking to lysosomes (Germain 2016). Migalastat reversibly binds to the active site of the alpha-galactosidase A (alpha-Gal A) protein (encoded by the galactosidase alpha gene, GLA), which is deficient in Fabry disease. Binding to the active site stabilizes alpha-Gal A allowing trafficking from the endoplasmic reticulum into the site of action, the lysosome.

Pharmacodynamics/Kinetics

Half-life Elimination ~4 hours

Time to Peak ~3 hours

Pregnancy Considerations

Information related to use in pregnancy is limited.

Data collection to monitor pregnancy and infant outcomes following exposure to migalastat is ongoing. Healthcare providers are encouraged to enroll females exposed to migalastat during pregnancy in the Fabry Pregnancy Registry (1-888-239-0758).

Product Availability Galafold: FDA approved August 2018; anticipated availability by August 17, 2018.

Dental Health Professional Considerations Fabry disease is an X-linked inborn error of glycosphingolipid catabolism resulting from deficient or absent activity of the lysosomal enzyme known as alpha-galactosidase A (GLA). This enzymatic defect is referred to as a mutant GLA. This enzymatic defect leads to the systemic accumulation of glycosphingolipids, most prominent of which is the ceramide known as globotriaoslyceramide (Gb3). Accumulation of Gb3 occurs in the plasma and cellular lysosomes of vessels, nerves, tissues, and organs throughout the body. The disorder is classified as a systemic disease, manifest as progressive renal failure, cardiac disease, cerebrovascular disease, small-fiber peripheral neuropathy, and skin lesions, among other abnormalities.

Migalastat, known in the literature as 1-deoxygalacyonojirimycin, is a first-in-class pharmacological chaperone treatment to facilitate the proper folding of mutant GLA by binding to its active site to result in improved enzyme stability and function. This results in significant increases in GLA activity in various organs with concomitant reductions in the accumulated globotriaoslyceramide (Gb3). Chaperone therapy is considered as a novel genotype-specific treatment for Fabry disease.

Migalastat is given as oral dosing every other day to adults with a confirmed diagnosis of Fabry disease and an amenable galactosidase alpha gene (GLA) variant based on in vitro assay data. To date, no oral soft tissue effects have been reported from exposure to Migalastat.

◆ **Migalastat Hydrochloride** *see* Migalastat *on page* 1030

◆ **Migergot** *see* Ergotamine and Caffeine *on page* 583

Miglitol (MIG li tol)

Related Information

Endocrine Disorders and Pregnancy *on page* 1684

Brand Names: US Glyset

Pharmacologic Category Antidiabetic Agent, Alpha-Glucosidase Inhibitor

Use Diabetes mellitus, type 2 (noninsulin-dependent, NIDDM): Adjunct to diet and exercise to improve glycemic control in adults with type 2 diabetes mellitus

Local Anesthetic/Vasoconstrictor Precautions No information available to require special precautions

Effects on Dental Treatment No significant effects or complications reported

Effects on Bleeding No information available to require special precautions

Adverse Reactions

>10%: Gastrointestinal: Flatulence (42%), diarrhea (29%), abdominal pain (12%)

1% to 10%: Dermatologic: Skin rash (4%)

<1%, postmarketing, and/or case reports: Abdominal distention, gastrointestinal pain, intestinal obstruction, nausea, paralytic ileus, pneumatosis cystoides intestinalis

Mechanism of Action In contrast to sulfonylureas, miglitol does not enhance insulin secretion; the antihyperglycemic action of miglitol results from a reversible inhibition of membrane-bound intestinal alpha-glucosidases which hydrolyze oligosaccharides and disaccharides to glucose and other monosaccharides in the brush border of the small intestine. In patients with diabetes, this enzyme inhibition results in delayed glucose absorption and lowering of postprandial hyperglycemia.

Pharmacodynamics/Kinetics

Half-life Elimination ~2 hours

Time to Peak 2-3 hours

Pregnancy Considerations

Poorly controlled diabetes during pregnancy can be associated with an increased risk of adverse maternal and fetal outcomes, including diabetic ketoacidosis, preeclampsia, spontaneous abortion, preterm delivery, delivery complications, major birth defects, stillbirth, and macrosomia (ACOG 201 2018). To prevent adverse outcomes, prior to conception and throughout pregnancy, maternal blood glucose and HbA_{1c} should be kept as close to target goals as possible but without causing significant hypoglycemia (ADA 2020; Blumer 2013).

Agents other than miglitol are currently recommended to treat diabetes mellitus in pregnancy (ADA 2020).

- ◆ **Migranal** *see* Dihydroergotamine *on page 499*
- ◆ **MIH Hydrochloride** *see* Procarbazine *on page 1278*
- ◆ **Mili** *see* Ethinyl Estradiol and Norgestimate *on page 616*
- ◆ **Millipred** *see* PrednisoLONE (Systemic) *on page 1255*
- ◆ **Millipred DP [DSC]** *see* PrednisoLONE (Systemic) *on page 1255*
- ◆ **Millipred DP 12-Day** *see* PrednisoLONE (Systemic) *on page 1255*

Milnacipran (mil NAY ci pran)

Related Information

Vasoconstrictor Interactions With Antidepressants *on page 1821*

Brand Names: US Savella; Savella Titration Pack

Pharmacologic Category Antidepressant, Serotonin/Norepinephrine Reuptake Inhibitor

Use Fibromyalgia: Management of fibromyalgia

Local Anesthetic/Vasoconstrictor Precautions

Although milnacipran is not a tricyclic antidepressant, it blocks norepinephrine reuptake within the CNS synapses as part of the mechanism of action. It has been suggested that vasoconstrictors be administered with caution and vial signs monitored in dental patients taking antidepressants that affect norepinephrine in this way.

Effects on Dental Treatment Key adverse event(s) related to dental treatment: Xerostomia and changes in salivation (normal salivary flow resumes upon discontinuation) and taste perversion.

Effects on Bleeding Serotonin/norepinephrine reuptake inhibitors (SNRIs) may impair platelet aggregation resulting in increased risk of bleeding events, particularly if used concomitantly with aspirin or NSAIDs.

Adverse Reactions

>10%:

Central nervous system: Headache (18%), insomnia (12%)

Endocrine & metabolic: Hot flash (12%)

Gastrointestinal: Nausea (37%), constipation (16%)

1% to 10%:

Cardiovascular: Palpitations (7%), increased heart rate (6%), hypertension (5%), flushing (3%), increased blood pressure (3%), tachycardia (2%), peripheral edema (≥1%)

Central nervous system: Dizziness (10%), migraine (5%), chills (2%), depression (≥1%), drowsiness (≥1%), falling (≥1%), fatigue (≥1%), irritability (≥1%)

Dermatologic: Hyperhidrosis (9%), skin rash (3%), night sweats (≥1%)

Endocrine & metabolic: Decreased libido (≥2%), hypercholesterolemia (≥1%), weight changes (≥1%)

Gastrointestinal: Vomiting (7%), xerostomia (5%), abdominal pain (3%), decreased appetite (2%), abdominal distension (≥1%), diarrhea (≥1%), dysgeusia (≥1%), dyspepsia (≥1%), flatulence (≥1%), gastroesophageal reflux disease (≥1%)

Genitourinary: Decreased urine output (≥2%), dysuria (≥2%), ejaculation failure (≥2%), ejaculatory disorder (≥2%), erectile dysfunction (≥2%), prostatitis (≥2%), scrotal pain (≥2%), testicular pain (≥2%), testicular swelling (≥2%), urethral pain (≥2%), urinary hesitancy (≥2%), urinary retention (≥2%), cystitis (≥1%), urinary tract infection (≥1%)

Neuromuscular & skeletal: Tremor (2%)

Ophthalmic: Blurred vision (2%)

Respiratory: Dyspnea (2%)

Miscellaneous: Fever (≥1%)

<1%, postmarketing, and/or case reports: Accommodation disturbance, acute pancreatitis, acute renal failure, aggressive behavior, angle-closure glaucoma, anorexia, cardiomyopathy (takotsubo), delirium, erythema multiforme, galactorrhea, hallucination, hepatitis, homicidal ideation, hyperprolactinemia, hypertensive crisis, hyponatremia, leukopenia, loss of consciousness, neuroleptic malignant syndrome (Stevens 2008), neutropenia, outbursts of anger, parkinsonian-like syndrome, Raynaud phenomenon (Khouri 2016; Peiró 2007), rhabdomyolysis, seizure, serotonin syndrome, Stevens-Johnson syndrome, supraventricular tachycardia, thrombocytopenia

Mechanism of Action Potent inhibitor of norepinephrine and serotonin reuptake (3:1). Milnacipran has no significant activity for serotonergic, alpha- and beta-adrenergic, muscarinic, histaminergic, dopaminergic, opiate, benzodiazepine, and GABA receptors. It does not possess MAO-inhibitory activity.

Pharmacodynamics/Kinetics

Half-life Elimination 6-8 hours

Time to Peak Plasma: Oral: 2-4 hours

Pregnancy Risk Factor C

Pregnancy Considerations

Adverse events were observed in some animal reproduction studies. Nonteratogenic effects in the newborn following SSRI/SNRI exposure late in the third trimester include respiratory distress, cyanosis, apnea, seizures, temperature instability, feeding difficulty, vomiting, hypoglycemia, hyper- or hypotonia, hyper-reflexia, jitteriness, irritability, constant crying, and tremor. Symptoms may be due to the toxicity of the SNRIs/SSRIs or a discontinuation syndrome and may be consistent with serotonin syndrome associated with SSRI treatment. The long-term effects of *in utero* SNRI/SSRI exposure on infant development and behavior are not known.

Women inadvertently exposed to milnacipran during pregnancy may be enrolled in the Savella Pregnancy Registry (877-643-3010 or http://www.savellapregnancyregistry.com).

- ◆ **Milnacipran HCl** *see* Milnacipran *on page 1031*

Milrinone (MIL ri none)

Pharmacologic Category Inotrope; Phosphodiesterase-3 Enzyme Inhibitor

Use

Heart failure with reduced ejection fraction: Short-term IV therapy for patients with acute decompensated heart failure with reduced ejection fraction in need of inotropic support.

Local Anesthetic/Vasoconstrictor Precautions No information available to require special precautions

Effects on Dental Treatment No significant effects or complications reported

Effects on Bleeding No information available to require special precautions

Adverse Reactions

>10%: Cardiovascular: Ventricular arrhythmia (ventricular ectopy: 9%, nonsustained ventricular tachycardia: 3%, ventricular tachycardia: 1%, ventricular fibrillation: <1%)

1% to 10%:

Cardiovascular: Supraventricular cardiac arrhythmia (4%), hypotension (3%), angina pectoris (≤1%), chest pain (≤1%)

Central nervous system: Headache (3%)

<1%, postmarketing, and/or case reports: Anaphylaxis, atrial fibrillation, bronchospasm, hepatic insufficiency, hypokalemia, injection site reaction, myocardial infarction, skin rash, thrombocytopenia, torsades de pointes, tremor

Mechanism of Action A selective phosphodiesterase inhibitor in cardiac and vascular tissue, resulting in vasodilation and inotropic effects with little chronotropic activity.

Pharmacodynamics/Kinetics

Onset of Action IV: 5 to 15 minutes

Half-life Elimination

Infants (after cardiac surgery): 3.15 ± 2 hours (Ramamoorthy 1998)

Children (after cardiac surgery): 1.86 ± 2 hours (Ramamoorthy 1998)

Adults:

Heart failure: 2.3 to 2.4 hours; renal impairment prolongs half-life (Rocci 1987)

Severe heart failure undergoing continuous venovenous hemofiltration (CVVH): 20.1 ± 3.3 hours (Taniguchi 2000)

Pregnancy Considerations Adverse events have not been observed in animal reproduction studies; however, increased resorption was reported in some studies.

- **Milrinone Lactate** *see* Milrinone *on page 1031*
- **Mimvey** *see* Estradiol and Norethindrone *on page 598*
- **Mimvey Lo [DSC]** *see* Estradiol and Norethindrone *on page 598*
- **Minastrin 24 Fe** *see* Ethinyl Estradiol and Norethindrone *on page 614*
- **Minipress** *see* Prazosin *on page 1254*
- **Minitran** *see* Nitroglycerin *on page 1112*
- **Minivelle** *see* Estradiol (Systemic) *on page 596*
- **Minocin** *see* Minocycline (Systemic) *on page 1032*

Minocycline (Systemic) (mi noe SYE kleen)

Brand Names: US CoreMino; Minocin; Minolira; Solodyn; Ximino

Brand Names: Canada CO Minocycline, DOM-Minocycline [DSC]; Minocycline-100 [DSC]; Minocycline-50 [DSC]; MYLAN-Minocycline [DSC]; PHL-Minocycline [DSC]; PMS-Minocycline [DSC]; SANDOZ MInocycline [DSC]; SANDOZ Minocycline [DSC]; TEVA-Minocycline

Generic Availability (US) May be product dependent

Pharmacologic Category Antibiotic, Tetracycline Derivative

Use

Acute intestinal amebiasis: Adjunctive therapy to amebicides in the treatment of acute intestinal amebiasis

Acne:

Oral (immediate release) and IV: Adjunctive therapy for the treatment of severe acne

Oral (extended-release): Treatment of only inflammatory lesions of non-nodular moderate to severe acne vulgaris in patients 12 years and older

Actinomycosis: Treatment of actinomycosis caused by *Actinomyces israelii* when penicillin is contraindicated

Anthrax: Treatment of anthrax caused by *Bacillus anthracis* when penicillin is contraindicated

Asymptomatic carriers of *Neisseria meningitidis*:

Oral (immediate-release): To eliminate the meningococci from the nasopharynx of asymptomatic carriers of *N. meningitidis*

Campylobacter: Treatment of infections caused by *Campylobacter fetus*

Cholera: Treatment of cholera caused by *Vibrio cholerae*

Clostridium: Treatment of infections caused by *Clostridium* spp when penicillin is contraindicated

Gram-negative infections: Treatment of infections caused by *Acinetobacter* spp, *Escherichia coli*, *Enterobacter aerogenes*, *Shigella* spp

Listeriosis: Treatment of listeriosis due to *Listeria monocytogenes* when penicillin is contraindicated

Meningitis: Treatment of meningitis due to *Neisseria meningitidis* when penicillin is contraindicated

Ophthalmic infections: Treatment of inclusion conjunctivitis or trachoma caused by *Chlamydia trachomatis*

Relapsing fever: Treatment of relapsing fever caused by *Borrelia recurrentis*

Respiratory tract infections: Treatment of respiratory tract infections caused by *Haemophilus influenzae*, *Klebsiella* spp, or *Mycoplasma pneumonia*. For the treatment of upper respiratory tract infections caused by *Streptococcus pneumoniae*.

Rickettsial infections: Treatment of Rocky Mountain spotted fever, typhus fever and the typhus group, Q fever, rickettsialpox, and tick fevers caused by *Rickettsiae*

Sexually transmitted infections: Treatment of lymphogranuloma venereum caused by *C. trachomatis*; nongonococcal urethritis, endocervical, or rectal infections in adults caused by *Ureaplasma urealyticum* or *C. trachomatis*; donovanosis (granuloma inguinale) caused by *Klebsiella granulomatis*; syphilis caused by *Treponema pallidum* subspecies *pallidum*, when penicillin is contraindicated

Skin and skin structure infections: Treatment of skin and skin structure infections caused by *Staphylococcus aureus* (not considered a first-line agent for any staphylococcal infection)

Urinary tract infections: Treatment of urinary tract infections caused by *Klebsiella* species

Vincent infection: Treatment of Vincent infection caused by *Fusobacterium fusiforme* when penicillin is contraindicated

Yaws: Treatment of yaws caused by *T. pallidum* subspecies *pertenue* when penicillin is contraindicated

Zoonotic infections: Treatment of psittacosis (ornithosis) due to *Chlamydia psittaci*; plague due to *Yersinia pestis*; tularemia due to *Francisella tularensis*; brucellosis due to *Brucella* spp (in conjunction with streptomycin); bartonellosis due to *Bartonella bacilliformis*

Local Anesthetic/Vasoconstrictor Precautions

No information available to require special precautions

Effects on Dental Treatment Key adverse event(s) related to dental treatment: Discoloration of teeth (children). Opportunistic "superinfection" with *Candida albicans*; tetracyclines are not recommended for use during pregnancy or in children ≤8 years of age since they have been reported to cause enamel hypoplasia and permanent teeth discoloration. The use of tetracyclines should only be used in these patients if other agents are contraindicated or alternative antimicrobials will not eradicate the organism. Long-term use associated with oral candidiasis.

Effects on Bleeding No information available to require special precautions

Adverse Reactions

1% to 10%:

- Dermatologic: Pruritus (5%), urticaria (2%)
- Nervous system: Dizziness (9%), fatigue (9%), malaise (4%), drowsiness (2%)
- Neuromuscular & skeletal: Arthralgia (1%)
- Otic: Tinnitus (2%)

Frequency not defined:

- Cardiovascular: Myocarditis, vasculitis
- Dermatologic: Skin photosensitivity, skin rash
- Gastrointestinal: Diarrhea, discoloration of permanent tooth, enamel hypoplasia
- Hematologic & oncologic: Lymphadenopathy
- Nervous system: Intracranial hypertension, vertigo
- Renal: Nephritis
- Miscellaneous: Fever

Postmarketing: Abnormal thyroid function test, acute renal failure, anaphylaxis, angioedema, autoimmune hepatitis, balanitis, bulging fontanel, *Clostridioides difficile* associated diarrhea, *Clostridioides difficile* colitis, drug reaction with eosinophilia and systemic symptoms, dysphagia, enterocolitis, eosinophilia, erythema multiforme, exacerbation of systemic lupus erythematosus, exfoliative dermatitis, fixed drug eruption, glossitis, hearing loss, hemolytic anemia, Henoch-Schonlein purpura, hepatic failure, hepatitis, hepatotoxicity (idiosyncratic) (Chalasani 2014), hypersensitivity reaction, intracranial hypertension (Tan 2019), lupus-like syndrome, malignant neoplasm of thyroid, microscopic thyroid discoloration (brown-black), mucous membrane hyperpigmentation, pancreatitis, pericarditis, pneumonitis, polyarthralgia, pseudotumor cerebri, pulmonary infiltrates (with eosinophilia), serum sickness, skin pigmentation, staining of tooth, Stevens-Johnson syndrome, thrombocytopenia

Dosing

Adult & Geriatric

Usual dosage range:

IV: Initial: 200 mg for 1 dose; Maintenance: 100 mg every 12 hours (maximum: 400 mg daily)

Oral: Initial: 200 mg for 1 dose; Maintenance: 100 mg every 12 hours; more frequent dosing intervals may be used (100 to 200 mg initially, followed by 50 mg 4 times daily)

Acne: Oral: Capsule or immediate-release tablet: 50 to 100 mg twice daily. **Note:** The shortest possible duration should be used to minimize development of bacterial resistance; re-evaluate at 3 to 4 months (AAD [Zaenglein 2016])

Acne (inflammatory, non-nodular, moderate to severe): Note: Therapy should be continued for 12 weeks. Safety of use beyond 12 weeks has not been established.

Extended-release capsule (Ximino): Oral: 1 mg/kg (rounded to the nearest capsule) once daily

Extended-release tablet: Oral:

Minolira:

- 45 to 59 kg: 52.5 mg (one-half of the 105 mg tablet) once daily
- 60 to 89 kg: 67.5 mg (one-half of the 135 mg tablet) once daily
- 90 to 125 kg: 105 mg once daily
- 126 to 136 kg: 135 mg once daily

CoreMino, Solodyn:

- 45 to 49 kg: 45 mg once daily
- 50 to 59 kg: 55 mg once daily
- 60 to 71 kg: 65 mg once daily
- 72 to 84 kg: 80 mg once daily
- 85 to 96 kg: 90 mg once daily
- 97 to 110 kg: 105 mg once daily
- 111 to 125 kg: 115 mg once daily
- 126 to 136 kg: 135 mg once daily

Cellulitis (purulent) due to community-acquired MRSA (off-label use): Oral: Initial: 200 mg; Maintenance: 100 mg twice daily for 5 to 10 days (Liu 2011)

Chlamydial or *Ureaplasma urealyticum* infection, uncomplicated: Oral, IV: Urethral, endocervical, or rectal: 100 mg every 12 hours for at least 7 days

Gonococcal infection, uncomplicated (males): Oral, IV:

Without urethritis or anorectal infection: Initial: 200 mg for 1 dose; Maintenance: 100 mg every 12 hours for at least 4 days (cultures 2 to 3 days post-therapy)

Urethritis: 100 mg every 12 hours for 5 days

Leprosy (alternative agent) (off-label use): Oral:

Lepromatous (multibacillary): 100 mg once daily for 24 months in combination with clofazimine and rifampin (NHDP [HRSA 2016])

Tuberculoid (paucibacillary): 100 mg once daily for 12 months in combination with rifampin (NHDP [HRSA 2016])

Meningococcal carrier state (manufacturer's labeling): Oral: 100 mg every 12 hours for 5 days. **Note:** CDC recommendations do not mention use of minocycline for eradicating nasopharyngeal carriage of meningococcal

Mycobacterium marinum: Oral: 100 mg every 12 hours for 6 to 8 weeks

Nocardiosis (off-label use): Oral: 100 to 200 mg every 12 hours, with or without other concomitant antimicrobials (Lerner 1996). Additional data may be necessary to further define the role of minocycline in this condition.

Prosthetic joint infection:

Staphylococci (oxacillin-sensitive or -resistant) oral phase treatment (after completion of pathogen-specific IV therapy) following 1-stage exchange:

Total ankle, elbow, hip, or shoulder arthroplasty: 100 mg twice daily for 3 months; **Note:** Must be used in combination with rifampin (Osmon 2013)

Total knee arthroplasty: 100 mg twice daily for 6 months; **Note:** Must be used in combination with rifampin (Osmon 2013)

Chronic oral antimicrobial suppression (off-label use): Oral:

Cutibacterium spp (alternative to penicillin or amoxicillin): 100 mg twice daily (Osmon 2013)

Staphylococci (oxacillin-resistant): 100 mg twice daily (Osmon 2013)

Rheumatoid arthritis (off-label use): Oral: 100 mg twice daily (Kloppenburg 1994; O'Dell 1997; O'Dell 2001; Stone 2003; Tilley 1995)

Syphilis: Oral, IV: Initial: 200 mg for 1 dose; Maintenance: 100 mg every 12 hours for 10 to 15 days

Renal Impairment: Adult

IV:

CrCl ≥80 mL/minute: No dosage adjustment necessary.

CrCl <80 mL/minute: Do not exceed 200 mg/day.

Oral:

Immediate release:

CrCl ≥80 mL/minute: No dosage adjustment necessary.

CrCl <80 mL/minute: Do not exceed 200 mg/day.

Extended release: There are no specific dosage adjustments provided in the manufacturer's labeling. Consider decreasing dose or increasing dosing interval.

Hepatic Impairment: Adult There are no dosage adjustments provided in the manufacturer's labeling; however, hepatotoxicity has been reported. Use with caution.

Pediatric

General dosing, susceptible infection: Children >8 years and Adolescents:

Oral: Immediate-release formulations: Initial: 4 mg/kg once (maximum dose: 200 mg), then 2 mg/kg/dose every 12 hours (maximum dose: 100 mg/dose).

IV: Initial: 4 mg/kg once (maximum dose: 200 mg), then 2 mg/kg/dose (maximum dose: 100 mg/dose) every 12 hours; maximum daily dose: 400 mg/**day**.

Acne, inflammatory, non-nodular, moderate to severe: Note: Higher doses do not confer greater efficacy and may be associated with more acute vestibular side effects. Due to emerging resistance patterns, should not typically be used as monotherapy for the management of acne vulgaris (AAD [Zaenglein 2016]; Eichenfield 2013).

Immediate-release formulations: Children ≥8 years and Adolescents: Oral: 50 to 100 mg 1 to 2 times daily in conjunction with topical therapy (eg, benzoyl peroxide); duration of 4 to 8 weeks of therapy usually necessary to evaluate initial clinical response with a longer duration for a maximum effect (3 to 6 months) (Eichenfield 2013).

Extended-release formulations: Children ≥12 years and Adolescents: Oral: ~1 mg/kg/dose once daily for 12 weeks.

Product-specific dosing:

Extended-release capsule: Ximino: Oral:

45 to 59 kg: 45 mg once daily.

60 to 90 kg: 90 mg once daily.

91 to 136 kg: 135 mg once daily.

Extended-release tablet:

Minolira: Oral:

45 to 59 kg: 52.5 mg (one-half of the 105 mg tablet) once daily.

60 to 89 kg: 67.5 mg (one-half of the 135 mg tablet) once daily.

90 to 125 kg: 105 mg once daily.

126 to 136 kg: 135 mg once daily.

CoreMino, Solodyn: Oral:

45 to 49 kg: 45 mg once daily.

50 to 59 kg: 55 mg once daily.

60 to 71 kg: 65 mg once daily.

72 to 84 kg: 80 mg once daily.

85 to 96 kg: 90 mg once daily.

97 to 110 kg: 105 mg once daily.

111 to 125 kg: 115 mg once daily.

126 to 136 kg: 135 mg once daily.

Skin and soft tissue infection (ie, purulent cellulitis), community-acquired MRSA: Note: Treatment duration based on clinical response; usual duration is 5 to 10 days for outpatient cellulitis (IDSA [Liu 2011]).

Children >8 years and Adolescents: Immediate-release formulations: Oral: Initial: 4 mg/kg (maximum dose: 200 mg), then 2 mg/kg/dose (maximum dose: 100 mg/dose) every 12 hours (IDSA [Liu 2011]; IDSA [Stevens 2014])

Renal Impairment: Pediatric

Immediate release: IV, Oral: There are no pediatric-specific recommendations; based on experience in adult patients; dosing adjustment suggested. Hemodialysis: Not dialyzable (Brogden 1975).

Extended-release formulations: Children ≥12 years and Adolescents: There are no specific dosage adjustments provided in the manufacturer's labeling. Consider decreasing dose or increasing dosing interval.

Hepatic Impairment: Pediatric There are no dosage adjustments provided in the manufacturer's labeling; however, hepatotoxicity has been reported. Use with caution.

Mechanism of Action Inhibits bacterial protein synthesis by binding with the 30S and possibly the 50S ribosomal subunit(s) of susceptible bacteria; cell wall synthesis is not affected.

Contraindications

Hypersensitivity to minocycline, other tetracyclines, or any component of the formulation

Canadian labeling: Additional contraindications (not in the US labeling): Severe liver disease; complete renal failure; myasthenia gravis; use in children <13 years of age; pregnancy; breastfeeding

Warnings/Precautions Anaphylaxis has been reported; discontinue drug immediately and institute supportive measures. May be associated with increases in BUN secondary to antianabolic effects; use caution in patients with renal impairment as this may lead to azotemia, hyperphosphatemia, acidosis, and possibly to drug accumulation and potential hepatotoxicity. Dosage adjustment recommended in patients with renal impairment (CrCl <80 mL/minute). Serious liver injury, including irreversible drug induced hepatitis and fulminant hepatic failure (sometimes fatal) have been reported with use for acne treatment; use caution in patients with hepatic insufficiency or in conjunction with other hepatotoxic drugs. Autoimmune syndromes (including serum sickness [eg, fever, arthralgia and malaise]) have been reported; discontinue if symptoms occur and assess liver function tests, ANA, and CBC. CNS effects (lightheadedness, dizziness, vertigo) may occur; patients must be cautioned about performing tasks which require mental alertness (eg, operating machinery or driving); symptoms usually disappear with continued therapy and when the drug is discontinued. Benign intracranial hypertension (pseudotumor cerebri [PTC]) (including headache, blurred vision, diplopia, vision loss, and/or papilledema) has been associated with use. Women of childbearing age who are overweight or have a history of intracranial hypertension are at greater risk. Concomitant use of isotretinoin (known to cause PTC) and minocycline should be avoided. Benign intracranial hypertension typically resolves after discontinuation of treatment; however, permanent visual loss is possible. If visual symptoms develop during treatment, prompt ophthalmologic evaluation is warranted. Intracranial pressure can remain elevated for weeks after drug discontinuation; monitor patients until they stabilize.

May cause photosensitivity; discontinue if skin erythema occurs. Use skin protection and avoid prolonged exposure to sunlight; avoid use of use tanning equipment or UVA/B treatment. Hyperpigmentation may occur in nails, bone, skin (including scar and injury sites), eyes, sclerae, thyroid, oral cavity, visceral tissue, and heart valves; skin and oral hyperpigmentation are independent of dose or administration duration. Prolonged use may result in fungal or bacterial superinfection, including *C. difficile*-associated diarrhea (CDAD) and pseudomembranous colitis; CDAD has been observed >2 months postantibiotic treatment. May cause tooth enamel hypoplasia, or permanent tooth discoloration; more common with long-term use, but observed with repeated, short courses; use of tetracyclines should be avoided during tooth development (infancy and children <8 years of age) unless other drugs are not likely to be effective or are contraindicated. Erythema multiforme, Stevens Johnson syndrome, or rash, along with eosinophilia, fever, and organ failure (Drug Rash with Eosinophilia and Systemic Symptoms [DRESS] syndrome) has been reported; discontinue treatment immediately if DRESS syndrome is suspected. Parenteral (IV) formulation contains magnesium; monitor serum magnesium in patients with renal impairment and signs of magnesium intoxication (eg, flushing, sweating, hypotension, depressed reflexes, flaccid paralysis, hypothermia, circulatory collapse, cardiac and CNS depression leading to respiratory paralysis). Also use with caution and closely monitor patients with heart block or myocardial damage. Potentially significant drug-drug interactions may exist, requiring dose or frequency adjustment, additional monitoring, and/or selection of alternative therapy.

Appropriate use: Acne: The American Academy of Dermatology acne guidelines recommends minocycline be used as adjunctive treatment for moderate and severe acne and forms of inflammatory acne that are resistant to topical treatments. Concomitant topical therapy with benzoyl peroxide or a retinoid is recommended should be administered with systemic antibiotic therapy (eg, minocycline) and continued for maintenance after the antibiotic course is completed (AAD [Zaenglein 2016]).

Warnings: Additional Pediatric Considerations Pseudotumor cerebri has been reported rarely in infants and adolescents; use with isotretinoin has been associated with cases of pseudotumor cerebri; avoid concomitant treatment with isotretinoin.

Drug Interactions

Metabolism/Transport Effects None known.

Avoid Concomitant Use

Avoid concomitant use of Minocycline (Systemic) with any of the following: Aminolevulinic Acid (Systemic); BCG (Intravesical); Cholera Vaccine; Mecamylamine; Methoxyflurane; Retinoic Acid Derivatives; Strontium Ranelate

Increased Effect/Toxicity

Minocycline (Systemic) may increase the levels/effects of: Aminolevulinic Acid (Systemic); Aminolevulinic Acid (Topical); CNS Depressants; Lithium; Mecamylamine; Methoxyflurane; Mipomersen; Neuromuscular-Blocking Agents; Porfimer; Retinoic Acid Derivatives; Verteporfin; Vitamin K Antagonists

Decreased Effect

Minocycline (Systemic) may decrease the levels/effects of: Atazanavir; BCG (Intravesical); BCG Vaccine (Immunization); Cholera Vaccine; Iron Preparations; Lactobacillus and Estriol; Penicillins; Sodium Picosulfate; Typhoid Vaccine

The levels/effects of Minocycline (Systemic) may be decreased by: Antacids; Bile Acid Sequestrants; Bismuth Subcitrate; Bismuth Subsalicylate; Calcium Salts; Iron Preparations; Lanthanum; Magnesium Salts; Multivitamins/Minerals (with ADEK, Folate, Iron); Multivitamins/Minerals (with AE, No Iron); Quinapril; Strontium Ranelate; Sucralfate; Sucroferric Oxyhydroxide; Zinc Salts

Food Interactions Minocycline serum concentrations are not significantly altered if taken with food or dairy products. Management: Administer without regard to food.

Pharmacodynamics/Kinetics

Half-life Elimination IV: 15 to 23 hours; 11 to 16 hours (hepatic impairment); 18 to 69 hours (renal impairment); Oral: 16 hours (range: 11 to 17 hours)

Time to Peak Capsule, pellet filled: 1 to 4 hours; Tablet: 1 to 3 hours; Extended release tablet: 3.5 to 4 hours

Reproductive Considerations

Minocycline is excreted in seminal fluid (Saivin 1988). Minocycline is not recommended for the treatment of acne in males or females attempting to conceive a child.

Pregnancy Considerations Minocycline crosses the placenta.

Tetracycline-class antibiotics may cause fetal harm following maternal use in pregnancy. Rare spontaneous reports of congenital anomalies, including limb reduction, have been reported following maternal minocycline use. Due to limited information, a causal association cannot be established. Tetracyclines accumulate in developing teeth and long tubular bones (Mylonas 2011). Permanent discoloration of teeth (yellow, gray, brown) can occur following in utero exposure and is more likely to occur following long-term or repeated exposure.

As a class, tetracyclines are generally considered second-line antibiotics in pregnant women and their use should be avoided (Mylonas 2011). Minocycline is not recommended for the treatment of Rocky Mountain Spotted Fever (Biggs 2016), Q fever (Anderson 2012), or anthrax infection (Meaney-Delman 2014) in pregnant women. Agents other than minocycline are recommended when systemic antibiotics are needed to treat acne during pregnancy (AAD [Zaenglein 2016]).

Breastfeeding Considerations

Minocycline is present in breast milk (Brogden 1975).

Oral absorption is not affected by dairy products; therefore, oral absorption of minocycline by the breastfed infant would not be expected to be diminished by the calcium in the maternal milk. There have been case reports of black discoloration of breast milk in women taking minocycline (Basler 1985; Hunt 1996).

According to the manufacturer, the decision to continue or discontinue breastfeeding during therapy should consider the risk of exposure to the infant and the benefits of treatment to the mother. As a class, tetracyclines have generally been avoided in breastfeeding women due to theoretical concerns that they may permanently stain the teeth of the breastfeeding infant (Chung 2002). Some sources note that breastfeeding can continue during tetracycline therapy (Chung 2002; WHO 2002) but recommend use of alternative medications when possible (WHO 2002). In general, antibiotics that are present in breast milk may cause nondose-related modification of bowel flora. Monitor infants for GI disturbances (Chung 2002; WHO 2002). Long-term use of tetracyclines (eg, for the treatment of acne) is not recommended in breastfeeding women (AAD [Zaenglein 2016]).

Dosage Forms Considerations

Minocin Kit contains minocycline oral capsules packaged with T3 Calming Wipes

Minocin for injection contains magnesium 2.2 mEq per vial

Dosage Forms: US

Capsule, Oral:

Generic: 50 mg, 75 mg, 100 mg

Capsule Extended Release 24 Hour, Oral:

Ximino: 45 mg, 90 mg, 135 mg

Generic: 135 mg, 45 mg, 90 mg

Solution Reconstituted, Intravenous [preservative free]:

Minocin: 100 mg (1 ea)

Tablet, Oral:

Generic: 50 mg, 75 mg, 100 mg

Tablet Extended Release 24 Hour, Oral:

CoreMino: 45 mg, 90 mg, 135 mg

Minolira: 105 mg, 135 mg

Solodyn: 55 mg, 65 mg, 80 mg, 105 mg, 115 mg

Generic: 45 mg, 55 mg, 65 mg, 80 mg, 90 mg, 105 mg, 115 mg, 135 mg

Dosage Forms: Canada

Capsule, Oral:

Generic: 50 mg, 100 mg

Minocycline (Topical) (mi noe SYE kleen)

Brand Names: US Amzeeq; Zilxi

Pharmacologic Category Acne Products; Antibiotic, Tetracycline Derivative; Tetracycline Derivative; Topical Skin Product, Acne

Use

Acne vulgaris: Topical treatment of inflammatory lesions of non-nodular moderate to severe acne vulgaris in adults and pediatric patients ≥9 years of age.

Note: The American Academy of Dermatology acne guidelines generally recommend topical antibiotics be used in conjunction with other therapies (not as monotherapy) due to the risk of bacterial resistance (AAD [Zaenglein 2016]).

Rosacea: Topical treatment of inflammatory lesions of rosacea in adults.

Local Anesthetic/Vasoconstrictor Precautions No information available to require special precautions.

Effects on Dental Treatment No significant effects or complications reported.

Effects on Bleeding No information available to require special precautions.

Adverse Reactions

>10%: Dermatologic: Erythema of skin (2% to 14%), hyperpigmentation (≤12%)

1% to 10%:

Central nervous system: Headache (3%)

Dermatologic: Xeroderma (≤7%), pruritus (≤5%), desquamation (≤3%)

Mechanism of Action The mechanism of action of minocycline for the treatment of acne or rosacea is unknown.

Pregnancy Considerations

Minocycline crosses the placenta and may cause fetal harm following oral administration. The amount of minocycline available systemically is less following topical application than with oral use. As a class, tetracyclines should be avoided during pregnancy.

Refer to the Minocycline (Systemic) monograph for additional information.

Product Availability Zilxi (minocycline 1.5% topical foam): FDA approved May 2020; anticipated availability in the fourth quarter of 2020.

◆ **Minocycline HCl** *see* Minocycline (Systemic) *on page 1032*

◆ **Minocycline Hydrochloride** *see* Minocycline (Systemic) *on page 1032*

◆ **Minocycline Hydrochloride** *see* Minocycline (Topical) *on page 1036*

Minocycline Hydrochloride (Periodontal)

(mi noe SYE kleen hye droe KLOR ide pair ee oh DON tol)

Related Information

Minocycline (Systemic) *on page 1032*

Periodontal Diseases *on page 1748*

Brand Names: US Arestin

Brand Names: Canada Arestin Microspheres

Pharmacologic Category Antibiotic, Tetracycline Derivative

Use Periodontitis: Adjunct to scaling and root planing procedures for reduction of pocket depth in patients with adult periodontitis. May be used as part of a periodontal maintenance program that includes good oral hygiene, scaling, and root planing.

Local Anesthetic/Vasoconstrictor Precautions No information available to require special precautions

Effects on Dental Treatment Key adverse event(s) related to dental treatment: Patients should avoid the following postadministration: Eating hard, crunchy, or sticky foods for 1 week; brushing for a 12-hour period; touching treated areas; use of interproximal cleaning devices for 10 days.

Effects on Bleeding No information available to require special precautions

Adverse Reactions

>10%: Gastrointestinal: Dental disease (12%)

1% to 10%:

Central nervous system: Headache (9%), pain (4%)

Gastrointestinal: Dental caries (10%), toothache (10%), gingivitis (9%), oral mucosa ulcer (5%), dyspepsia (4%), mucous membrane disease (3%)

Infection: Infection (8%)

Respiratory: Flu-like symptoms (5%), pharyngitis (4%)

<1%, postmarketing, and/or case reports: Anaphylaxis, angioedema, erythema multiforme (oral minocycline), facial swelling, pruritus, skin rash, Stevens-Johnson syndrome (oral minocycline), urticaria

Mechanism of Action Minocycline is bacteriostatic and exerts its antimicrobial activity by inhibiting protein synthesis.

Pregnancy Considerations

Tetracycline-class antibiotics may cause fetal harm following maternal use in pregnancy. Tetracyclines accumulate in developing teeth and long tubular bones (Mylonas 2011). Permanent discoloration of teeth (yellow, gray, brown) can occur following in utero exposure and is more likely to occur following long-term or repeated exposure.

As a class, tetracyclines are generally considered second-line antibiotics in pregnant women and their use should be avoided (Mylonas 2011).

Refer to the Minocycline (Systemic) monograph for additional information.

◆ **Minolira** *see* Minocycline (Systemic) *on page* 1032

Minoxidil (Systemic) (mi NOKS i dil)

Related Information

Cardiovascular Diseases *on page* 1654

Brand Names: Canada Loniten

Pharmacologic Category Antihypertensive; Vasodilator, Direct-Acting

Use Hypertension: Management of hypertension that is symptomatic or associated with target organ damage, and is not manageable with maximum therapeutic doses of a diuretic plus 2 other antihypertensives. Use in milder degrees of hypertension is not recommended because the benefit-risk ratio in such patients has not been defined. **Note: Not** recommended for the initial treatment of hypertension (ACC/AHA [Whelton 2018]).

Local Anesthetic/Vasoconstrictor Precautions No information available to require special precautions

Effects on Dental Treatment No significant effects or complications reported

Effects on Bleeding No information available to require special precautions

Adverse Reactions Frequency not always defined.

Cardiovascular: ECG changes (T-wave changes 60%), edema (reversible, 7% to 10%), pericardial effusion (occasionally with tamponade, 3%), angina pectoris, cardiac failure, pericarditis, tachycardia

Dermatologic: Hypertrichosis (80%), bullous rash (rare), skin rash, Stevens-Johnson syndrome (rare), toxic epidermal necrolysis

Endocrine & metabolic: Sodium retention, water retention, weight gain

Gastrointestinal: Nausea, vomiting

Hematologic & oncologic: Decreased hematocrit (transient, hemodilution), decreased red blood cells (transient, hemodilution), hemoglobin (transient, hemodilution), leukopenia (rare), thrombocytopenia (rare)

Hepatic: Ascites, increased serum alkaline phosphatase

Renal: Increased blood urea nitrogen (transient), increased serum creatinine (transient)

Respiratory: Pulmonary edema (Lee 2011)

<1%, postmarketing, and/or case reports: Breast tenderness (rare)

Mechanism of Action Produces vasodilation by directly relaxing arteriolar smooth muscle, with little effect on veins; effects may be mediated by cyclic AMP; stimulation of hair growth is secondary to vasodilation, increased cutaneous blood flow and stimulation of resting hair follicles

Pharmacodynamics/Kinetics

Onset of Action Hypotensive: ~30 minutes; Peak effect: 2 to 3 hours

Duration of Action Up to 2 to 5 days

Half-life Elimination 3.5 to 4.2 hours

Pregnancy Risk Factor C

Pregnancy Considerations Adverse events were observed in some animal studies. Neonatal hypertrichosis has been reported following exposure to minoxidil during pregnancy.

Mipomersen (mi poe MER sen)

Brand Names: US Kynamro

Pharmacologic Category Antihyperlipidemic Agent, Apolipoprotein B Antisense Oligonucleotide

Use

Homozygous familial hypercholesterolemia: Adjunct to dietary therapy and other lipid-lowering treatments to reduce low-density lipoprotein cholesterol (LDL-C), total cholesterol (TC), apolipoprotein B (apo B), and non-high-density lipoprotein cholesterol (non-HDL-C) in patients with homozygous familial hypercholesterolemia (HoFH)

Guideline recommendations: Mipomersen may be useful in patients with HoFH not responsive to PCSK9 inhibitor therapy (AACE [Jellinger 2017]). In addition, mipomersen may be considered in patients with ASCVD and baseline LDL-C ≥190 mg/dL who have an inadequate response to statins (with or without ezetimibe and PCSK9 inhibitors) (ACC [Lloyd-Jones 2016]).

Local Anesthetic/Vasoconstrictor Precautions No information available to require special precautions

Effects on Dental Treatment No significant effects or complications reported

Effects on Bleeding No information available to require special precautions

Adverse Reactions

>10%:

Central nervous system: Fatigue (15%), headache (12%)

Dermatologic: Skin discoloration at injection site (17%)

Gastrointestinal: Nausea (14%)

Hepatic: Increased serum ALT (≥3 x ULN to <5 x ULN: 12%; ≥5 x ULN to <10 x ULN: 3%; ≥10 x ULN: 1%)

Immunologic: Antibody development (38%)

Local: Injection site reaction (84%), erythema at injection site (59%), pain at injection site (56%), hematoma at injection site (32%), itching at injection site (29%), swelling at injection site (18%)

Respiratory: Flu-like symptoms (13% to 30%)

1% to 10%:

Cardiovascular: Hypertension (7%), peripheral edema (5%), angina pectoris (4%), palpitations (3%)

Central nervous system: Chills (6%), insomnia (3%)

Gastrointestinal: Vomiting (4%), abdominal pain (3%)

Genitourinary: Proteinuria (9%)

Hematologic & oncologic: Neoplasms (4%, benign and malignant)

Hepatic: Increased serum AST (≥3 x ULN to <5 x ULN: 7%; ≥5 x ULN to <10 x ULN: 3%), liver steatosis (7%), abnormal hepatic function tests (5%), increased liver enzymes (3%)

Hypersensitivity: Recall skin sensitization (8%, including local erythema, tenderness, and/or pruritus at previous injection sites)

Neuromuscular & skeletal: Limb pain (7%), musculoskeletal pain (4%)

Miscellaneous: Fever (8%)

<1%, postmarketing, and/or case reports: Angioedema, hypersensitivity reaction, immune thrombocytopenia, skin rash, urticaria

Mechanism of Action Mipomersen is an oligonucleotide inhibitor of apo B-100 synthesis. ApoB is the main component of LDL-C and very low density lipoprotein (VLDL), which is the precursor to LDL-C. Mipomersen binds to the messenger ribonucleic acid (mRNA) of apoB in a sequence-specific manner which results in degradation (RNase H-mediated) or disruption of the mRNA thereby reducing formation of apoB.

Pharmacodynamics/Kinetics

Half-life Elimination ~1 to 2 months

Time to Peak ~3 to 4 hours

Reproductive Considerations

Females of reproductive potential should use effective contraception during therapy.

Pregnancy Risk Factor B

Pregnancy Considerations

Adverse events have not been observed in animal reproduction studies.

◆ **Mipomersen Sodium** *see* Mipomersen *on page 1037*

Mirabegron (mir a BEG ron)

Brand Names: US Myrbetriq

Brand Names: Canada Myrbetriq

Pharmacologic Category $Beta_3$ Agonist

Use Overactive bladder: Treatment of overactive bladder (OAB) with symptoms of urinary frequency, urgency, or urge urinary incontinence as monotherapy or in combination with solifenacin

Local Anesthetic/Vasoconstrictor Precautions

No information available to require special precautions

Effects on Dental Treatment Key adverse event(s) related to dental treatment: Xerostomia (normal salivary flow resumes upon discontinuation)

Effects on Bleeding No information available to require special precautions

Adverse Reactions

>10%: Cardiovascular: Hypertension (9% to 11%)

1% to 10%:

Cardiovascular: Tachycardia (2%)

Central nervous system: Headache (2% to 4%), dizziness (1% to 3%)

Gastrointestinal: Constipation (1% to 3%), xerostomia (4%), diarrhea (2%), abdominal pain (1%)

Genitourinary: Urinary tract infection (3% to 6%), cystitis (2%)

Infection: Influenza (3%)

Neuromuscular & skeletal: Back pain (3%), arthralgia (2%)

Respiratory: Nasopharyngitis (4%), sinusitis (3%)

<1%, postmarketing, and/or case reports: Abdominal distension, angioedema, anxiety, atrial fibrillation, bladder pain, blurred vision, breast cancer, cerebrovascular accident, confusion, dry eye syndrome, dyspepsia, gastritis, elevated gamma-glutamyl transferase, genital pruritus, glaucoma, hallucination, hypersensitivity angiitis, increased lactate dehydrogenase, increased serum alanine aminotransferase, increased serum aspartate aminotransferase, insomnia, lip edema, malignant neoplasm of lung, malignant neoplasm of prostate, nausea, nephrolithiasis, nonthrombocytopenic purpura, osteoarthritis, palpitations, pruritus, rhinitis, skin rash, urinary retention, urticaria, vaginal infection

Mechanism of Action Mirabegron, a beta-3 adrenergic receptor agonist, activates beta-3 adrenergic receptors in the bladder resulting in relaxation of the detrusor smooth muscle during the urine storage phase, thus increasing bladder capacity. At usual doses, mirabegron is believed to display selectivity for the beta-3 adrenergic receptor subtype compared to its affinity for the beta-1 and -2 adrenoceptor subtypes. Data have shown that beta-adrenoceptors, predominately the beta-3 subtype, mediate detrusor smooth muscle tone and promote the storage function of the human bladder.

Pharmacodynamics/Kinetics

Onset of Action Efficacy is seen within 8 weeks; steady state achieved within 7 days

Half-life Elimination ~50 hours

Time to Peak ~3.5 hours

Pregnancy Considerations Adverse effects have been observed in some animal reproduction studies.

◆ **Mirapex** *see* Pramipexole *on page 1250*

◆ **Mirapex ER** *see* Pramipexole *on page 1250*

◆ **Mircera** *see* Methoxy Polyethylene Glycol-Epoetin Beta *on page 993*

◆ **Mircette** *see* Ethinyl Estradiol and Desogestrel *on page 609*

Mirtazapine (mir TAZ a peen)

Related Information

Vasoconstrictor Interactions With Antidepressants *on page 1821*

Brand Names: US Remeron; Remeron SolTab

Brand Names: Canada APO-Mirtazapine; Auro-Mirtazapine; Auro-Mirtazapine OD; DOM-Mirtazapine; JAMP-Mirtazapine; MYLAN-Mirtazapine; PMS-Mirtazapine; PRO-Mirtazapine; Remeron; Remeron RD; RIVA-Mirtazapine [DSC]; SANDOZ Mirtazapine; TEVA-Mirtazapine; TEVA-Mirtazapine OD [DSC]

Pharmacologic Category Antidepressant, Alpha-2 Antagonist

Use Major depressive disorder (unipolar): Treatment of unipolar major depressive disorder (MDD)

Local Anesthetic/Vasoconstrictor Precautions

Although mirtazapine is not a tricyclic antidepressant, it results in increased norepinephrine release as part of its mechanisms. It has been suggested that vasoconstrictor be administered with caution and to monitor vital signs in dental patients taking antidepressants that affect norepinephrine in this way, including mirtazapine.

Consider consult with patient's cardiologist prior to use of a vasoconstrictor. Closely monitor for additive/synergistic pharmacologic effects, and consider electrocardiographic monitoring when a local anesthetic is used in a patient receiving mirtazapine. Mirtazapine prolongs the QT interval and may cause torsade de pointes. The risk of drug-induced torsade de pointes may be small when a single QT interval prolonging drug is prescribed. In terms of epinephrine, it is not known what effect vasoconstrictors in the local anesthetic regimen will have in patients with a known history of congenital prolonged QT interval or in patients taking any medication that prolongs the QT interval.

Effects on Dental Treatment Key adverse event(s) related to dental treatment: Significant xerostomia (normal salivary flow resumes upon discontinuation); rare occurrence of aphthous stomatitis; gingival hemorrhage; facial, mouth, and tongue edema; glossitis; and tongue discoloration. Patient may experience an unpleasant metallic taste or have swallowing difficulty. Patients may rarely experience orthostatic hypotension as they stand up after treatment, especially if lying in dental chair for extended periods of time. Use caution with sudden changes in position during and after dental treatment.

Effects on Bleeding Rare occurrence of gingival hemorrhage.

Adverse Reactions

>10%:

Central nervous system: Drowsiness (54%)

Endocrine & metabolic: Weight gain (12%; weight gain of >7% reported in 8% of adults, 49% of pediatric patients), increased serum cholesterol (15%)

Gastrointestinal: Xerostomia (25%), increased appetite (17%), constipation (13%)

1% to 10%:

Cardiovascular: Peripheral edema (2%), edema (1%), hypertension, vasodilation

Central nervous system: Dizziness (7%), abnormal dreams (4%), abnormality in thinking (3%), confusion (2%), agitation, amnesia, anxiety, apathy, depression, hypoesthesia, malaise, myasthenia, paresthesia, twitching, vertigo

Dermatologic: Pruritus, skin rash

Endocrine & metabolic: Increased serum triglycerides (6%), increased thirst

Gastrointestinal: Abdominal pain, acute abdominal condition, anorexia, vomiting

Genitourinary: Urinary frequency (2%), urinary tract infection

Hepatic: Increased serum alanine aminotransferase (≥3 times ULN: 2%)

Neuromuscular & skeletal: Asthenia (8%), back pain (2%), myalgia (2%), tremor (2%), arthralgia, hyperkinetic muscle activity, hypokinesia

Respiratory: Flu-like symptoms (5%), dyspnea (1%), increased cough, sinusitis

Frequency not defined:

Cardiovascular: Orthostatic hypotension

<1%, postmarketing, and/or case reports: Abnormal accommodation, abnormal healing, abnormal hepatic function tests, abnormal lacrimation, acne vulgaris, acute myocardial infarction, ageusia, agranulocytosis, akathisia, alopecia, altered sense of smell, amenorrhea, anemia, angina pectoris, angle-closure glaucoma, aphasia, aphthous stomatitis, arthritis, asphyxia, asthma, ataxia, atrial arrhythmia, bigeminy, blepharitis, bone fracture, bradycardia, breast engorgement, breast hypertrophy, bronchitis, bullous dermatitis, bursitis, cardiomegaly, cellulitis, cerebral ischemia, chest pain, chills, cholecystitis, colitis, complex sleep-related disorder, conjunctivitis, cystitis, deafness, dehydration, delirium, delusion, dementia, depersonalization, dermal ulcer, diabetes mellitus, diplopia, drug dependence, dysarthria, dyskinesia, dysmenorrhea, dystonia, dysuria, ejaculatory disorder, emotional lability, enlargement of abdomen, enlargement of salivary glands, epistaxis, eructation, erythema multiforme, euphoria, exfoliative dermatitis, extrapyramidal reaction, eye pain, facial edema, fever, gastritis, gastroenteritis, gingival hemorrhage, glossitis, goiter, gout, hallucination, heavy menstrual bleeding, hematuria, hepatic cirrhosis, herpes simplex infection, herpes zoster infection, hiccups, hostility, hyperacusis, hyperprolactinemia, hyperreflexia, hypomania, hyponatremia, hypotension, hypothyroidism, hypotonia, impotence, increased acid phosphatase, increased libido, increased serum aspartate aminotransferase, increased serum creatine kinase, intestinal obstruction, keratoconjunctivitis, laryngitis, left ventricular failure, leukopenia, leukorrhea, lymphadenopathy, lymphocytosis, manic reaction, mastalgia, migraine, myoclonus, myositis, nausea, neck pain, neck stiffness, nephrolithiasis, nystagmus disorder, oral candidiasis, ostealgia, osteoarthritis, osteoporosis, otalgia, otitis media, pancreatitis, pancytopenia, paralysis, paranoid ideation, petechia, phlebitis, pneumonia, pneumothorax, polyuria, prolonged QT interval on ECG, psychomotor agitation, psychoneurosis, psychotic depression, pulmonary embolism, rhabdomyolysis, rupture of tendon, seborrhea, seizure, serotonin syndrome, severe neutropenia, sialorrhea, skin hypertrophy, skin photosensitivity, somnambulism, Stevens-Johnson syndrome, stomatitis, stupor, suicidal ideation, suicidal tendencies, syncope, tenosynovitis, thrombocytopenia, tongue discoloration, tongue edema, tonic clonic epilepsy, torsades de pointes, toxic epidermal necrolysis, ulcer, urethritis, urinary incontinence, urinary retention, urinary urgency, urticaria, uterine hemorrhage, vaginitis, vascular headache, ventricular premature contractions, ventricular tachycardia, weight loss, withdrawal syndrome, xeroderma

Mechanism of Action Mirtazapine is a tetracyclic antidepressant that works by its central presynaptic alpha$_2$-adrenergic antagonist effects, which results in increased release of norepinephrine and serotonin. It is also a potent antagonist of 5-HT$_2$ and 5-HT$_3$ serotonin receptors and H$_1$ histamine receptors and a moderate peripheral alpha$_1$-adrenergic and muscarinic antagonist; it does not inhibit the reuptake of norepinephrine or serotonin.

Pharmacodynamics/Kinetics

Onset of Action

Anxiety disorders (panic disorder): Initial effects may be observed within 2 weeks of treatment, with continued improvements through 4 to 6 weeks (WFSBP [Bandelow 2012]); some experts suggest up to 12 weeks of treatment may be necessary for response (BAP [Baldwin 2014]; Katzman 2014; WFSBP [Bandelow 2012]).

Depression: Initial effects may be observed within 1 to 2 weeks of treatment, with continued improvements through 4 to 6 weeks (Papakostas 2006; Posternak 2005; Szegedi 2009).

Half-life Elimination ~20 to 40 hours; increased with renal or hepatic impairment.

Time to Peak Serum: ~2 hours

Reproductive Considerations

If treatment for major depressive disorder is initiated for the first time in females planning a pregnancy, agents other than mirtazapine are preferred (use of mirtazapine is not preferred in pregnant women) (Larsen 2015).

The incidence of sexual dysfunction with mirtazapine is generally lower than with selective serotonin reuptake inhibitors (WFSBP [Bauer 2013]).

Pregnancy Considerations Mirtazapine crosses the placenta (Hatzidaki 2008).

A significant increase in major teratogenic effects has not been observed following exposure to mirtazapine during pregnancy; however, information is limited (CANMAT [MacQueen 2016]; Larsen 2015).

Untreated or inadequately treated psychiatric illness may lead to poor compliance with prenatal care. Therapy with antidepressants during pregnancy should be individualized (ACOG 92 2008; CANMAT [MacQueen 2016]). Psychotherapy or other nonmedication therapies may be considered for some women; however, antidepressant medication should be considered for pregnant women with moderate to severe major depressive disorder (MDD) (APA 2010). If treatment for MDD is initiated for the first time during pregnancy, mirtazapine is not recommended (CANMAT [MacQueen 2016]; Larsen 2015; WFSBP [Bauer 2013]); mirtazapine is considered a third-line agent for the treatment of mild to moderate depression during pregnancy (CANMAT [MacQueen 2016]).

Data collection to monitor pregnancy and infant outcomes following exposure to antidepressants is ongoing. Pregnant women exposed to antidepressants during pregnancy are encouraged to enroll in the National Pregnancy Registry for Antidepressants (NPRAD). Women 18 to 45 years of age or their health care providers may contact the registry by calling 844-405-6185. Enrollment should be done as early in pregnancy as possible.

MiSOPROStol (mye soe PROST ole)

Brand Names: US Cytotec

Brand Names: Canada NOVO-Misoprostol [DSC]; PMS-Misoprostol [DSC]

Pharmacologic Category Prostaglandin

Use

Nonsteroidal anti-inflammatory drug-induced gastric ulcers, prevention: To reduce the risk of nonsteroidal anti-inflammatory drug-induced gastric ulcers in patients at high risk of complications.

Termination of intrauterine pregnancy: Medical termination of intrauterine pregnancy through 70 days' gestation in combination with mifepristone (Mifeprex prescribing information April 2019).

Local Anesthetic/Vasoconstrictor Precautions No information available to require special precautions

Effects on Dental Treatment No significant effects or complications reported

Effects on Bleeding No information available to require special precautions

Adverse Reactions

>10%: Gastrointestinal: Diarrhea, abdominal pain

1% to 10%:

Central nervous system: Headache

Gastrointestinal: Constipation, dyspepsia, flatulence, nausea, vomiting

<1%, postmarketing, and/or case reports: Abnormal hepatobiliary function, alopecia, anaphylaxis, anemia, anxiety, arterial thrombosis, arthralgia, back pain, bronchitis, bronchospasm, cardiac arrhythmia, cerebrovascular accident, change in appetite, chest pain, chills, confusion, conjunctivitis, deafness, depression, dermatitis, diaphoresis, dizziness, drowsiness, dysgeusia, dysphagia, dyspnea, dysuria, edema, epistaxis, fatigue, fever, gastroesophageal reflux disease, gastrointestinal hemorrhage, GI inflammation, gingivitis, glycosuria, gout, gynecological disease (cramps, dysmenorrhea, hypermenorrhea, spotting, postmenopausal vaginal bleeding, and other menstrual disorders), hematuria, hypertension, hypotension, impotence, increased amylase, increased blood urea nitrogen, increased cardiac enzymes, increased erythrocyte sedimentation rate, increased serum alkaline phosphatase, increased thirst, loss of libido, mastalgia, muscle cramps, myalgia, myocardial infarction, neuropathy, otalgia, pallor, phlebitis, pneumonia, polyuria, psychoneurosis, pulmonary embolism, purpura, rigors, skin rash, stiffness, syncope, thrombocytopenia, tinnitus, upper respiratory tract infection, urinary tract infection, uterine rupture, visual disturbance, weakness, weight changes

Mechanism of Action Misoprostol is a synthetic prostaglandin E_1 analog that replaces the protective prostaglandins consumed with prostaglandin-inhibiting therapies (eg, NSAIDs); has been shown to induce uterine contractions

Pharmacodynamics/Kinetics

Onset of Action Inhibition of gastric acid secretion: 30 minutes

Duration of Action Inhibition of gastric acid secretion: 3 hours

Half-life Elimination Misoprostol acid: 20 to 40 minutes

Time to Peak Serum: Misoprostol acid: Fasting: 12 ± 3 minutes

Reproductive Considerations [US Boxed Warning]: Misoprostol should not be used for reducing the risk of nonsteroidal anti-inflammatory drug (NSAID)-induced ulcers in women of childbearing potential unless the patient is at high risk of complications from gastric ulcers associated with use of the NSAIDs, or is at high risk of developing gastric ulceration. In such patients, misoprostol may be prescribed if the patient has had a negative serum pregnancy test within 2 weeks prior to beginning therapy; is capable of complying with effective contraceptive measures; has received both oral and written warnings of the hazards of misoprostol, the risk of possible contraception failure, and the danger to other women of childbearing potential if the drug is taken by mistake; and will begin misoprostol only on the second or third day of the next normal menstrual period. Patients must be advised of the abortifacient property and warned not to give the drug to others.

Pregnancy Considerations

Use for the prevention of nonsteroidal anti-inflammatory drug (NSAID)-induced gastric ulcers is contraindicated in pregnant women.

[US Boxed Warning]: Misoprostol administration to women who are pregnant may cause birth defects, abortion, premature birth, or uterine rupture. Uterine rupture has been reported when misoprostol was administered in pregnant women to induce labor or to induce abortion. The risk of uterine rupture increases with advancing gestational ages and with prior uterine surgery, including cesarean delivery. Misoprostol should not be taken by pregnant women to reduce the risk of ulcers induced by NSAIDs.

Congenital anomalies following first trimester exposure have been reported, including skull defects, cranial nerve palsies, facial malformations, and limb defects. Misoprostol may produce uterine contractions; fetal death, uterine perforation, and abortion may occur.

Misoprostol is FDA approved for the medical termination of pregnancy of ≤70 days in conjunction with mifepristone.

Because misoprostol may induce or augment uterine contractions, it has been used off label as a cervical-ripening agent for induction of labor. Misoprostol should not be used for this purpose during the third trimester in conditions where a spontaneous labor and vaginal delivery would be contraindicated, including women who have had a prior cesarean delivery or major uterine surgery (because the risk of uterine rupture is increased) (ACOG 107 2009; ACOG 205 2019). It has also been used for the treatment of incomplete or missed abortion (ACOG 427 2009), early pregnancy loss (ACOG 200 2018), or severe postpartum hemorrhage (ACOG 183 2017; FIGO 2012a; FIGO 2012b). Misoprostol is effective for the management of postpartum hemorrhage. Misoprostol as adjunctive therapy with oxytocin has been used in high-risk patients; monotherapy is recommended in situations where oxytocin is not available (eg, resource-poor settings). The risk of adverse reactions may be associated with combination therapy (FIGO 2012a; FIGO 2012b; FIGO [Morris 2017]; Gallos 2018; Koch 2019; Leduc 2018; Morfaw 2019; Sweed 2018).

Various routes of administration have been used for postpartum hemorrhage. Sublingual administration has the most rapid onset, the oral route produces the most pronounced initial increase in tonus, and rectal and vaginal routes exhibit longer durations of action as compared to oral and sublingual routes (Leduc 2018). Buccal administration may be associated with lower plasma concentrations and a decreased risk of adverse reactions compared to sublingual administration (Schaff 2005).

Adverse events associated with off-label obstetric uses include uterine tachysystole (may impair placental blood flow), uterine rupture, amniotic fluid embolism, or adverse fetal heart changes. Chills, fever, and/or shivering are commonly associated with use of sublingual misoprostol when used for postpartum hemorrhage; incidence of adverse reactions may be dose related (FIGO 2012b).

[US Boxed Warning]: Patients must be advised of the abortifacient property and warned not to give the drug to others.

- **Misoprostol and Diclofenac** *see* Diclofenac and Misoprostol *on page 490*
- **MITC** *see* MitoMYcin (Systemic) *on page 1041*
- **Mitigare** *see* Colchicine *on page 405*
- **Mitigo** *see* Morphine (Systemic) *on page 1050*
- **MITO** *see* MitoMYcin (Systemic) *on page 1041*
- **MITO-C** *see* MitoMYcin (Systemic) *on page 1041*
- **Mitomycin-X** *see* MitoMYcin (Systemic) *on page 1041*
- **Mitomycin-C** *see* MitoMYcin (Systemic) *on page 1041*

MitoMYcin (Systemic) (mye toe MYE sin)

Brand Names: US Jelmyto; Mutamycin

Pharmacologic Category Antineoplastic Agent, Antibiotic

Use

Gastric cancer: Treatment of disseminated adenocarcinoma of the stomach (in combination with other chemotherapy agents) and as palliative treatment when other modalities have failed.

Pancreatic cancer: Treatment of disseminated adenocarcinoma of the pancreas (in combination with other chemotherapy agents) and as palliative treatment when other modalities have failed.

Limitations of use: Not recommended for single-agent primary therapy or to replace appropriate surgery and/or radiotherapy in the treatment of these conditions.

Local Anesthetic/Vasoconstrictor Precautions No information available to require special precautions

Effects on Dental Treatment Key adverse event(s) related to dental treatment: Stomatitis.

Effects on Bleeding Bone marrow toxicity (pancytopenia) including thrombocytopenia, leukopenia, and anemia has been reported in 64% of patients. Medical consult recommended.

Adverse Reactions

>10%:

Gastrointestinal: Anorexia (14%), nausea (14%), vomiting (14%)

Hematologic & oncologic: Bone marrow depression (64%; onset: 4 weeks; recovery: 8 to 10 weeks), hemolytic-uremic syndrome (HUS; ≤15%), thrombotic thrombocytopenic purpura (TTP; ≤15%)

Miscellaneous: Fever (14%)

1% to 10%:

Dermatologic: Alopecia (4%)

Gastrointestinal: Mucous membrane disease (toxicity: 4%), stomatitis (4%)

Renal: Increased serum creatinine (2%)

<1%, postmarketing, and/or case reports: Adult respiratory distress syndrome (ARDS), bladder spasm (intravesical administration), cardiac failure, dyspnea, extravasation reactions, fibrosis (bladder; intravesical administration), hepatic sinusoidal obstruction syndrome (formerly known as hepatic veno-occlusive disease), interstitial fibrosis, malaise, nonproductive cough, pulmonary infiltrates, renal failure (irreversible), skin rash, weakness

Mechanism of Action Mitomycin alkylates DNA to produce DNA cross-linking (primarily with guanine and cytosine pairs) and inhibits DNA and RNA synthesis. Mitomycin is not cell cycle specific but has its maximum effect against cells in late G and early S phases (Perry 2012).

Pharmacodynamics/Kinetics

Half-life Elimination 17 minutes (30 mg dose)

Pregnancy Considerations Adverse events have been observed in animal reproduction studies.

Mitotane (MYE toe tane)

Brand Names: US Lysodren

Brand Names: Canada Lysodren

Pharmacologic Category Antineoplastic Agent, Miscellaneous

Use Adrenocortical carcinoma: Treatment of inoperable (functional or nonfunctional) adrenocortical carcinoma

Local Anesthetic/Vasoconstrictor Precautions No information available to require special precautions

Effects on Dental Treatment No significant effects or complications reported

Effects on Bleeding No information available to require special precautions

Adverse Reactions

>10%:

Dermatologic: Skin rash (15%)

Gastrointestinal: Anorexia (≤80%), diarrhea (≤80%), nausea (≤80%), vomiting (≤80%)

Nervous system: Depression (≤40%), dizziness (≤40%), vertigo (≤40%)

Frequency not defined:

Cardiovascular: Flushing, hypertension, orthostatic hypotension

Endocrine & metabolic: Adrenocortical insufficiency, albuminuria, altered hormone level (decreased serum androstenedione), decreased plasma testosterone (males and females), growth retardation, gynecomastia, hypercholesterolemia, hypertriglyceridemia, hypothyroidism, increased sex hormone binding globulin, ovarian cyst (including bilateral, multiple)

Genitourinary: Hematuria, hemorrhagic cystitis

Hematologic & oncologic: Neutropenia, prolonged bleeding time

Hepatic: Hepatitis, increased liver enzymes

Nervous system: Ataxia, central nervous system toxicity, confusion, dysarthria, generalized ache or pain, headache, lethargy, mental deficiency, sedated state

Neuromuscular & skeletal: Asthenia

Ophthalmic: Blurred vision, cataract, diplopia, maculopathy, retinopathy

Miscellaneous: Fever

Postmarketing: Subacute cutaneous lupus erythematosus (Mayor-Ibarguren 2016)

Mechanism of Action Mitotane is an adrenolytic agent that suppresses (directly) the adrenal cortex and alters the peripheral metabolism of steroids

Pharmacodynamics/Kinetics

Onset of Action Antitumor response: Achieved at serum concentrations ≥14 mcg/mL; Pediatric patients: In experience with treatment of adenocarcinoma reported 1.5 to 12.5 months to reach 10 mcg/mL with subsequent rapid escalation of serum concentration, clinical response may be observed earlier (Rodriguez-Galindo 2005; Zancanella 2006).

Duration of Action Measurable serum levels may persist for months after discontinuation (Veytsman 2009).

Half-life Elimination 18 to 159 days (median: 53 days)

Reproductive Considerations

Mitotane has a long elimination half-life. Women of reproductive potential should use effective contraception during treatment and after treatment until plasma levels are no longer detected. When used to treat Cushing disease, available guidelines recommend avoiding pregnancy for years after stopping mitotane therapy (Nieman 2015).

Pregnancy Considerations

Mitotane crosses the placenta (Gerl 1992) and may cause fetal harm if administered during pregnancy. Although use in pregnancy is limited, preterm birth and early pregnancy loss have been reported (Baszko-Błaszyk 2011; Kojori 2011; Tripto-Shkolnik 2013).

MitoXANTRONE (mye toe ZAN trone)

Pharmacologic Category Antineoplastic Agent, Anthracenedione; Antineoplastic Agent, Topoisomerase II Inhibitor

Use

Acute myeloid leukemias: Initial treatment (in combination with other agents) of acute nonlymphocytic leukemia (ANLL [includes myelogenous, promyelocytic, monocytic and erythroid leukemias]).

Multiple sclerosis, relapsing or secondary progressive: Treatment of secondary (chronic) progressive, progressive relapsing, or worsening or relapsing-remitting multiple sclerosis (RRMS) to reduce neurologic disability and/or the frequency of clinical relapse.

Limitation of use: Mitoxantrone is not indicated for the treatment of primary progressive MS. Reserve use for rapidly-advancing, refractory multiple sclerosis (AAN [Rae-Grant 2018]; Olek 2019).

Prostate cancer: Treatment of advanced hormone-refractory prostate cancer (in combination with corticosteroids).

Local Anesthetic/Vasoconstrictor Precautions No information available to require special precautions

Effects on Dental Treatment Key adverse event(s) related to dental treatment: Mucositis and stomatitis.

Effects on Bleeding Myelosuppression is an extension of the pharmacologic effects; therefore, thrombocytopenia (grades 3/4: 3% to 4%) is expected. Anemia may also occur. Medical consult recommended.

Adverse Reactions Includes events reported with any indication; incidence varies based on treatment, dose, and/or concomitant medications.

>10%:

Cardiovascular: Edema (10% to 30%), cardiac disease (≤18%), cardiac arrhythmia (3% to 18%), ECG changes (≤11%)

Central nervous system: Pain (8% to 41%), fatigue (≤39%), headache (6% to 13%)

Dermatologic: Alopecia (20% to 61%), nail bed changes (≤11%)

Endocrine & metabolic: Menstrual disease (26% to 61%), amenorrhea (28% to 53%), hyperglycemia (10% to 31%), weight gain (≤17%), weight loss (≤17%), increased gamma-glutamyl transferase (3% to 15%)

Gastrointestinal: Nausea (26% to 76%), vomiting (6% to 72%), diarrhea (14% to 47%), mucositis (10% to 29%; onset: ≤1 week), stomatitis (8% to 29%; onset: ≤1 week), anorexia (22% to 25%), constipation (10% to 16%), gastrointestinal hemorrhage (2% to 16%), abdominal pain (9% to 15%), dyspepsia (5% to 14%)

Genitourinary: Urinary tract infection (7% to 32%), hematuria (≤11%), urine abnormality (5% to 11%)

Hematologic & oncologic: Neutropenia (79% to 100%; onset: ≤3 weeks; grade 4: 23% to 54%), leukopenia (9% to 100%), lymphocytopenia (72% to 95%), anemia (≤75%), decreased hemoglobin (≤75%), thrombocytopenia (33% to 39%; grades 3/4: 3% to 4%), bruise (≤11%), febrile neutropenia (≤11%), petechia (≤11%)

Hepatic: Increased serum alkaline phosphatase (≤37%), increased serum transaminases (5% to 20%)

Infection: Infection (4% to 60%), sepsis (≤34%), fungal infection (9% to 15%)

Neuromuscular & skeletal: Weakness (≤24%)

Renal: Increased blood urea nitrogen (≤22%), increased serum creatinine (≤13%)

Respiratory: Upper respiratory tract infection (7% to 53%), pharyngitis (≤19%), dyspnea (6% to 18%), cough (5% to 13%)

Miscellaneous: Fever (6% to 78%)

1% to 10%:

Cardiovascular: Cardiac failure (≤5%), ischemia (≤5%), decreased left ventricular ejection fraction (≤5%), hypertension (≤4%)

Central nervous system: Chills (≤5%), anxiety (5%), depression (5%), seizure (2% to 4%)

Dermatologic: Diaphoresis (≤9%), skin infection (≤5%)

Endocrine & metabolic: Hypocalcemia (10%), hypokalemia (7% to 10%), hyponatremia (9%), hypermenorrhea (7%)

Gastrointestinal: Aphthous stomatitis (≤10%)

Genitourinary: Impotence (≤7%), proteinuria (≤6%), sterility (≤5%)
Hematologic & oncologic: Granulocytopenia (6%), hemorrhage (5% to 6%), acute leukemia (≤3%; secondary; includes AML, APL)
Hepatic: Jaundice (3% to 7%)
Infection: Fungal infection (cutaneous: ≤10%)
Neuromuscular & skeletal: Back pain (6% to 8%), arthralgia (≤5%), myalgia (≤5%)
Ophthalmic: Conjunctivitis (≤5%), blurred vision (≤3%)
Renal: Renal failure (≤8%)
Respiratory: Rhinitis (10%), pneumonia (≤9%), sinusitis (≤6%)

<1%, postmarketing, and/or case reports: Anaphylactoid reaction, anaphylaxis, chest pain, dehydration, hypersensitivity reaction, interstitial pneumonitis (with combination chemotherapy), hyperuricemia, hypotension, ocular discoloration (blue discoloration of sclera), phlebitis (at infusion site), skin rash, tachycardia, urine discoloration (blue-green), urticaria

Mechanism of Action Mitoxantrone is an anthracenedione, which is related to the anthracyclines. Mitoxantrone intercalates into DNA resulting in cross-links and strand breaks; binds to nucleic acids and inhibits DNA and RNA synthesis by template disordering and steric obstruction; replication is decreased by binding to DNA topoisomerase II and may inhibit the incorporation of uridine into RNA and thymidine into DNA; mitoxantrone is active throughout entire cell cycle (cell-cycle nonspecific).

Pharmacodynamics/Kinetics

Half-life Elimination Terminal: 23 to 215 hours (median: ~75 hours)

Reproductive Considerations

Pregnancy status should be evaluated prior to treatment in females of reproductive potential. Mitoxantrone is associated with amenorrhea, ovarian failure, and male infertility (AAN [Rae-Grant 2018]).

In general, disease-modifying therapies for multiple sclerosis (MS) are stopped prior to a planned pregnancy except in females at high risk of MS activity (AAN [Rae-Grant 2018]). Consider use of agents other than mitoxantrone for females at high risk of disease reactivation who are planning a pregnancy. Delaying pregnancy is recommended for females with persistent high disease activity; when disease-modifying therapy is needed in these patients, other agents are preferred (ECTRIMS/EAN [Montalban 2018]).

Pregnancy Considerations

Based on the mechanism of action and adverse events observed in animal reproduction studies, mitoxantrone may cause fetal harm if administered during pregnancy. Information related to pregnancy outcomes following maternal use of mitoxantrone in pregnancy is limited (Amato 2015; Frau 2018; Houtchens 2013; NTP 2013).

In general, disease-modifying therapies for multiple sclerosis (MS) are not initiated during pregnancy, except in females at high risk of MS activity (AAN [Rae-Grant 2018]). When disease-modifying therapy is needed in these patients, other agents are preferred (ECTRIMS/EAN [Montalban 2018]).

The European Society for Medical Oncology has published guidelines for diagnosis, treatment, and follow-up of cancer during pregnancy. The guidelines recommend referral to a facility with expertise in cancer during pregnancy and encourage a multidisciplinary team (obstetrician, neonatologist, oncology team). In general, if chemotherapy is indicated, it should be avoided in the first trimester, there should be a 3-week time period between the last chemotherapy dose and anticipated delivery, and chemotherapy should not be administered beyond week 33 of gestation (Peccatori 2013).

◆ **Mitoxantrone Dihydrochloride** *see* MitoXANTRONE *on page 1042*

◆ **Mitoxantrone HCl** *see* MitoXANTRONE *on page 1042*

◆ **Mitoxantrone Hydrochloride** *see* MitoXANTRONE *on page 1042*

◆ **Mitozantrone** *see* MitoXANTRONE *on page 1042*

◆ **Mixed Amphetamine Salts** *see* Dextroamphetamine and Amphetamine *on page 475*

◆ **MK-217** *see* Alendronate *on page 95*

◆ **MK383** *see* Tirofiban *on page 1453*

◆ **MK-0431** *see* SITagliptin *on page 1376*

◆ **MK462** *see* Rizatriptan *on page 1342*

◆ **MK 0517** *see* Fosaprepitant *on page 713*

◆ **MK-0518** *see* Raltegravir *on page 1306*

◆ **MK594** *see* Losartan *on page 938*

◆ **MK0826** *see* Ertapenem *on page 586*

◆ **MK 869** *see* Aprepitant *on page 162*

◆ **MK-3222** *see* Tildrakizumab *on page 1448*

◆ **MK-3475** *see* Pembrolizumab *on page 1204*

◆ **MK4305** *see* Suvorexant *on page 1397*

◆ **MK4827** *see* Niraparib *on page 1109*

◆ **MLN341** *see* Bortezomib *on page 248*

◆ **MLN9708** *see* Ixazomib *on page 853*

◆ **MM-398** *see* Irinotecan (Liposomal) *on page 842*

◆ **MMC** *see* MitoMYcin (Systemic) *on page 1041*

◆ **MMF** *see* Mycophenolate *on page 1067*

◆ **MMI** *see* MethIMAzole *on page 988*

◆ **MMR** *see* Measles, Mumps, and Rubella Virus Vaccine *on page 949*

◆ **M-M-R II** *see* Measles, Mumps, and Rubella Virus Vaccine *on page 949*

◆ **MMRV** *see* Measles, Mumps, Rubella, and Varicella Virus Vaccine *on page 950*

◆ **MMR Vaccine** *see* Measles, Mumps, and Rubella Virus Vaccine *on page 949*

◆ **MOAB 2C4** *see* Pertuzumab *on page 1220*

◆ **MOAB ABX-EGF** *see* Panitumumab *on page 1187*

◆ **MOAB anti-Tac** *see* Daclizumab *on page 428*

◆ **MOAB C225** *see* Cetuximab *on page 329*

◆ **MoAb CD52** *see* Alemtuzumab *on page 93*

◆ **MOAB-CTLA-4** *see* Ipilimumab *on page 836*

◆ **MOAB HER2** *see* Trastuzumab *on page 1479*

◆ **Mobic** *see* Meloxicam *on page 957*

Modafinil (moe DAF i nil)

Brand Names: US Provigil

Brand Names: Canada Alertec; APO-Modafinil; Auro-Modafinil; BIO-Modafinil; Mar-Modafinil; TEVA-Modafinil

Pharmacologic Category Central Nervous System Stimulant

Use

Narcolepsy-related excessive daytime sleepiness: To improve wakefulness in adult patients with excessive sleepiness associated with narcolepsy.

Obstructive sleep apnea-related excessive daytime sleepiness: To improve wakefulness in adult patients with obstructive sleep apnea (OSA).

Shift work sleep disorder-related excessive daytime sleepiness: To improve wakefulness in adult patients with shift work sleep disorder (SWSD).

Local Anesthetic/Vasoconstrictor Precautions Use vasoconstrictor with caution. Patients may experience heart palpitations and increased heart rate when taking modafinil.

Effects on Dental Treatment Key adverse event(s) related to dental treatment: Modafinil causes tachycardia, increases in blood pressure, and palpitations. Consider monitoring blood pressure prior to using local anesthetic with a vasoconstrictor. Symptoms associated with bruxism have been observed in some patients.

Effects on Bleeding No information available to require special precautions

Adverse Reactions

>10%:

Central nervous system: Headache (adults: 34%; children: 20% [Biederman 2005])

Gastrointestinal: Decreased appetite (children: 16% [Biederman 2005]), abdominal pain (children: 12% [Greenhill 2006]), nausea (11%)

1% to 10%:

Cardiovascular: Chest pain (3%), hypertension (3%), palpitations (2%), tachycardia (2%), vasodilation (2%), edema (1%)

Central nervous system: Nervousness (7%), anxiety (5%), dizziness (5%), insomnia (5%), depression (2%), drowsiness (2%), paresthesia (2%), agitation (1%), chills (1%), confusion (1%), emotional lability (1%), hypertonia (1%), vertigo (1%)

Dermatologic: Diaphoresis (1%)

Endocrine & metabolic: Weight loss (children 5% [Greenhill 2006]), increased thirst (1%)

Gastrointestinal: Diarrhea (6%), dyspepsia (5%), xerostomia (4%), anorexia (4%), constipation (2%), dysgeusia (1%), flatulence (1%), oral mucosa ulcer (1%)

Genitourinary: Urine abnormality (1%)

Hematologic & oncologic: Eosinophilia (1%)

Hepatic: Hepatic insufficiency (2%)

Neuromuscular & skeletal: Back pain (6%), dyskinesia (1%), hyperkinesia (1%), tremor (1%)

Ophthalmic: Visual disturbance (1%)

Respiratory: Rhinitis (7%), pharyngitis (4%), asthma (1%), epistaxis (1%)

Frequency not defined:

Endocrine & metabolic: Increased gamma-glutamyl transferase

Hepatic: Increased serum alkaline phosphatase

<1%, postmarketing, and/or case reports: Aggressive behavior, agranulocytosis, anaphylaxis, angioedema, asystole, cerebrovascular accident, delusions, DRESS syndrome, erythema multiforme (pediatric patients), hallucination, hypersensitivity reaction, mania, multiorgan hypersensitivity, psychomotor agitation, psychosis, skin rash, Stevens-Johnson syndrome, suicidal ideation, toxic epidermal necrolysis

Mechanism of Action The exact mechanism of action is unclear. Modafinil has been shown to significantly increase dopamine in the brain by blocking dopamine transporters; however, has a lower affinity for dopamine receptors compared to amphetamines (Volkow 2009). EEG studies have shown modafinil increases high-frequency alpha waves while decreasing both delta and theta wave activity, effects consistent with generalized increases in mental alertness (James 2011). Studies also have demonstrated decreased GABA-mediated neurotransmission through increased turnover of serotonin and enhanced activity of 5-HT_2 receptors and that an intact central alpha-adrenergic system is required for modafinil's activity (Kumar 2008; Schwartz 2008).

Pharmacodynamics/Kinetics

Half-life Elimination Effective half-life: 15 hours

Time to Peak Serum: 2 to 4 hours; may be delayed ~1 hour with food.

Reproductive Considerations

Evaluate pregnancy status within a week prior to modafinil initiation. Efficacy of steroidal contraceptives (including depot and implantable contraceptives) may be decreased; alternate means of effective contraception should be used during modafinil therapy and for ≥1 month after modafinil is discontinued.

Pregnancy Risk Factor C

Pregnancy Considerations Outcome information following modafinil use in pregnancy is limited (Calvo-Ferrandiz 2018; Haervig 2014). Preliminary data from the Nuvigil/Provigil pregnancy registry suggest an increased risk of major fetal congenital malformations, including congenital cardiac anomalies (Alertec 2019). An increased risk of spontaneous abortion and intrauterine growth restriction has been reported with modafinil.

Health care providers are encouraged to register pregnant patients exposed to modafinil, or pregnant females may enroll themselves, by calling (866-404-4106).

Controlled Substance C-IV

- ◆ **Moderiba [DSC]** *see* Ribavirin (Systemic) *on page 1320*
- ◆ **Moderiba (600 MG Pack) [DSC]** *see* Ribavirin (Systemic) *on page 1320*
- ◆ **Moderiba 800 Dose Pack [DSC]** *see* Ribavirin (Systemic) *on page 1320*
- ◆ **Moderiba (800 MG Pack) [DSC]** *see* Ribavirin (Systemic) *on page 1320*
- ◆ **Moderiba (1000 MG Pack) [DSC]** *see* Ribavirin (Systemic) *on page 1320*
- ◆ **Moderiba 1200 Dose Pack [DSC]** *see* Ribavirin (Systemic) *on page 1320*
- ◆ **Moderiba (1200 MG Pack) [DSC]** *see* Ribavirin (Systemic) *on page 1320*
- ◆ **Modicon (28) [DSC]** *see* Ethinyl Estradiol and Norethindrone *on page 614*

Moexipril (mo EKS i pril)

Related Information

Cardiovascular Diseases *on page 1654*

Pharmacologic Category Angiotensin-Converting Enzyme (ACE) Inhibitor; Antihypertensive

Use

Hypertension: Management of hypertension

Guideline recommendations: The 2017 Guideline for the Prevention, Detection, Evaluation, and Management of High Blood Pressure in Adults recommends if monotherapy is warranted, in the absence of comorbidities (eg, cerebrovascular disease, chronic kidney disease, diabetes, heart failure, ischemic heart disease, etc.), that thiazide-like diuretics or dihydropyridine calcium channel blockers may be preferred options due to improved cardiovascular endpoints (eg, prevention of heart failure and stroke). ACE inhibitors and ARBs are also acceptable for monotherapy. Combination therapy may be required to achieve blood pressure goals and is initially preferred in patients at high risk (stage 2 hypertension or atherosclerotic cardiovascular disease [ASCVD] risk ≥10%) (ACC/AHA [Whelton 2017]).

Local Anesthetic/Vasoconstrictor Precautions No information available to require special precautions

Effects on Dental Treatment Key adverse event(s) related to dental treatment: Patients may experience orthostatic hypotension as they stand up after treatment; especially if lying in dental chair for extended periods of time. Use caution with sudden changes in position during and after dental treatment.

An angiotensin-converting enzyme (ACE) Inhibitor cough is a dry, hacking, nonproductive cough that can potentially interfere with longer dental procedures if patient has this side effect.

Effects on Bleeding No information available to require special precautions

Adverse Reactions

1% to 10%:

Cardiovascular: Flushing, hypotension, peripheral edema

Central nervous system: Dizziness, fatigue, headache

Dermatologic: Alopecia, skin rash

Endocrine & metabolic: Hyperkalemia, hyponatremia

Gastrointestinal: Diarrhea, heartburn, nausea

Neuromuscular & skeletal: Myalgia

Renal: Increased blood urea nitrogen (reversible), increased serum creatinine (reversible), polyuria

Respiratory: Cough, pharyngitis, sinusitis, upper respiratory tract infection

<1%, postmarketing, and/or case reports: Anemia, angioedema, bronchospasm, cardiac arrhythmia, cerebrovascular accident, chest pain, dyspnea, eosinophilic pneumonitis, hepatitis, hypercholesterolemia, increased liver enzymes, myocardial infarction, oliguria, orthostatic hypotension, palpitations, proteinuria, syncope

Mechanism of Action Competitive inhibitor of angiotensin-converting enzyme (ACE); prevents conversion of angiotensin I to angiotensin II, a potent vasoconstrictor; results in lower levels of angiotensin II which causes an increase in plasma renin activity and a reduction in aldosterone secretion

Pharmacodynamics/Kinetics

Onset of Action Within 2 hours; Peak effect: 3 to 6 hours

Duration of Action 24 hours

Half-life Elimination Moexipril: 1.3 hours; Moexiprilat: 2 to 9.8 hours

Time to Peak Moexiprilat: ~1.5 hours

Reproductive Considerations

Angiotensin-converting enzyme (ACE) inhibitors should be avoided in sexually active females of reproductive potential not using effective contraception (ADA 2020).

ACE inhibitors should generally be avoided for the treatment of hypertension in women planning a pregnancy; use should only be considered for cases of hypertension refractory to other medications (ACOG 203 2019).

Pregnancy Risk Factor D

Pregnancy Considerations

Exposure to an angiotensin-converting enzyme (ACE) inhibitor during the first trimester of pregnancy may be associated with an increased risk of fetal malformations (ACOG 203 2019; ESC [Regitz-Zagrosek 2018]); however, outcomes observed may also be influenced by maternal disease (ACC/AHA [Whelton 2017]).

[US Boxed Warning]: Drugs that act on the renin-angiotensin system can cause injury and death to the developing fetus. Discontinue as soon as possible once pregnancy is detected. Drugs that act on the renin-angiotensin system are associated with oligohydramnios. Oligohydramnios, due to decreased fetal renal function, may lead to fetal lung hypoplasia and skeletal malformations. The use of these drugs in pregnancy is also associated with anuria, hypotension, renal failure, skull hypoplasia, and death in the fetus/neonate. Infants exposed to an ACE inhibitor in utero should be monitored for hyperkalemia, hypotension, and oliguria. Oligohydramnios may not appear until after irreversible fetal injury has occurred. Exchange transfusions or dialysis may be required to reverse hypotension or improve renal function, although data related to the effectiveness in neonates is limited.

Chronic maternal hypertension is also associated with adverse events in the fetus/infant. Chronic maternal hypertension may increase the risk of birth defects, low birth weight, premature delivery, stillbirth, and neonatal death. Actual fetal/neonatal risks may be related to duration and severity of maternal hypertension. Untreated chronic hypertension may also increase the risks of adverse maternal outcomes, including gestational diabetes, pre-eclampsia, delivery complications, stroke and myocardial infarction (ACOG 203 2019).

When treatment of hypertension in pregnancy is indicated, ACE inhibitors should generally be avoided due to their adverse fetal events; use in pregnant women should only be considered for cases of hypertension refractory to other medications (ACOG 203 2019).

◆ **Moexipril Hydrochloride** *see* Moexipril *on page 1044*

◆ **Moi-Stir [OTC]** *see* Saliva Substitute *on page 1354*

Mometasone (Nasal) (moe MET a sone)

Brand Names: US Nasonex; Sinuva

Brand Names: Canada APO-Mometasone; Mosaspray [DSC]; Nasonex; SANDOZ Mometasone; TEVA-Mometasone

Pharmacologic Category Corticosteroid, Nasal

Use

Allergic rhinitis (seasonal and perennial) (spray only): Treatment of nasal symptoms of seasonal allergic and perennial allergic rhinitis in adults and pediatric patients ≥2 years.

Nasal congestion associated with seasonal rhinitis (spray only): Relief of nasal congestion associated with seasonal allergic rhinitis in adults and pediatric patients ≥2 years.

Nasal polyps: Treatment of nasal polyps in patients ≥18 years. **Note:** Implant is for patients who have had ethmoid sinus surgery.

Seasonal allergic rhinitis (prophylaxis) (spray only): Prophylaxis of nasal symptoms of seasonal allergic rhinitis in adults and pediatric patients ≥12 years.

Local Anesthetic/Vasoconstrictor Precautions No information available to require special precautions

Effects on Dental Treatment No significant effects or complications reported

Effects on Bleeding Shown to cause localized epistaxis (nosebleed) with prolonged use. The localized epistaxis is reversible following discontinuation of the drug. Impacts relating to the systemic circulation do not warrant special precautions.

Adverse Reactions

>10%:

Central nervous system: Headache (adolescents and adults, nasal spray: 26%; adults, sinus implant: 4%)

Infection: Viral infection (adolescents and adults, nasal spray: 14%)

Respiratory: Epistaxis (adolescents and adults, nasal spray: ≤13%; adults, sinus implant: 2%), pharyngitis (adolescents and adults, nasal spray: 12%), chronic sinusitis (adults, sinus implant: 11%), blood in nasal mucosa (adolescents and adults, nasal spray: ≤11%)

1% to 10%:

Cardiovascular: Chest pain (adolescents and adults, nasal spray: ≥2% to <5%)

Dermatologic: Skin changes (trauma; children, nasal spray: ≥2% to <5%)

Gastrointestinal: Vomiting (children, nasal spray: 5%), diarrhea (nasal spray: ≥2% to <5%), dyspepsia (adolescents and adults, nasal spray: ≥2% to <5%), nausea (adolescents and adults, nasal spray: ≥2% to <5%)

Genitourinary: Dysmenorrhea (adolescents and adults, nasal spray: 5%)

Hypersensitivity: Hypersensitivity reaction (adults, sinus implant: 4%)

Neuromuscular & skeletal: Musculoskeletal pain (adolescents and adults, nasal spray: 5%), arthralgia (adolescents and adults, nasal spray: ≥2% to <5%), myalgia (adolescents and adults, nasal spray: ≥2% to <5%)

Ophthalmic: Conjunctivitis (adolescents and adults, nasal spray: ≥2% to <5%)

Otic: Otalgia (adolescents and adults, nasal spray: ≥2% to <5%), otitis media (≥2% to <5%)

Respiratory: Upper respiratory tract infection (5% to 8%), cough (adolescents and adults, nasal spray: 7%), sinusitis (adolescents and adults, nasal spray: 5%), asthma (adolescents and adults: ≥2% to <5%), bronchitis (adolescents and adults: ≥2% to <5%), flu-like symptoms (adolescents and adults, nasal spray: ≥2% to <5%), nasal mucosa irritation (children, nasal spray: ≥2% to <5%), rhinitis (adolescents and adults, nasal spray: ≥2% to <5%), wheezing (children, nasal spray: ≥2% to <5%), nasopharyngitis (adults, sinus implant: 1%), sinus headache (adolescents and adults, nasal spray: 1%)

Frequency not defined: Respiratory: Nasal candidiasis, nasal mucosa ulcer, pharyngeal candidiasis

<1%, postmarketing, and/or case reports: Altered sense of smell, anaphylaxis, angioedema, blurred vision, burning sensation of the nose, dysgeusia, nasal septum perforation

Mechanism of Action May depress the formation, release, and activity of endogenous chemical mediators of inflammation (kinins, histamine, liposomal enzymes, prostaglandins). Leukocytes and macrophages may have to be present for the initiation of responses mediated by the above substances. Inhibits the margination and subsequent cell migration to the area of injury, and also reverses the dilatation and increased vessel permeability in the area resulting in decreased access of cells to the sites of injury.

Pharmacodynamics/Kinetics

Onset of Action Spray: Improvement in allergic rhinitis symptoms may be seen within 11 hours; Maximum effect: Within 1 to 2 weeks after starting therapy

Duration of Action Implant: ≤90 days

Half-life Elimination IV: ~5 to 6 hours

Pregnancy Risk Factor C

Pregnancy Considerations Maternal use of intranasal corticosteroids in usual doses are not associated with an increased risk of fetal malformations or preterm birth (ERS/TSANZ [Middleton 2020]). Although intranasal mometasone has limited systemic absorption and use in pregnancy is likely acceptable, other agents have more pregnancy data and may be preferred for the treatment of allergic rhinitis in pregnant women (Alhussien 2018; BSACI [Scadding 2017]; ERS/TSANZ [Middleton 2020]).

Mometasone (Oral Inhalation)

(moe MET a sone)

Related Information

Respiratory Diseases *on page 1680*

Brand Names: US Asmanex (120 Metered Doses); Asmanex (14 Metered Doses); Asmanex (30 Metered Doses); Asmanex (60 Metered Doses); Asmanex (7 Metered Doses); Asmanex HFA

Brand Names: Canada Asmanex Twisthaler

Pharmacologic Category Corticosteroid, Inhalant (Oral)

Use

Asthma: Maintenance treatment of asthma as prophylactic therapy in patients ≥4 years of age (Asmanex Twisthaler) and ≥5 years of age (Asmanex HFA).

Limitations of use: Not indicated for the relief of acute bronchospasm.

Local Anesthetic/Vasoconstrictor Precautions No information available to require special precautions

Effects on Dental Treatment Key adverse event(s) related to dental treatment: Localized infections with *Candida albicans* or *Aspergillus niger* occur frequently in the mouth and pharynx with repetitive use of an oral inhaler; may require treatment with appropriate antifungal therapy or discontinuance of inhaler use.

Effects on Bleeding No information available to require special precautions

Adverse Reactions

>10%:

Central nervous system: Headache (3% to 22%), fatigue (1% to 13%), depression (11%)

Gastrointestinal: Oral candidiasis (≤22%)

Neuromuscular & skeletal: Musculoskeletal pain (8% to 22%), arthralgia (13%)

Respiratory: Sinusitis (3% to 22%), allergic rhinitis (adolescents & adults 14% to 20%; children 4%), upper respiratory tract infection (8% to 15%), pharyngitis (8% to 13%)

1% to 10%:

Central nervous system: Pain (1% to <3%)

Gastrointestinal: Abdominal pain (3% to 6%), dyspepsia (5%), nausea (3%), vomiting (1% to ≤3%), anorexia (1% to <3%), gastroenteritis (1% to <3%)

Genitourinary: Dysmenorrhea (9%), urinary tract infection (children 2%)

Hematologic & oncologic: Bruise (children 2%)

Infection: Influenza (4%), infection (1% to <3%)

Neuromuscular & skeletal: Back pain (6%), myalgia (3%)

Ophthalmic: Increased intraocular pressure (3%)

Otic: Otalgia (1% to <3%)

Respiratory: Paranasal sinus congestion (9%), nasopharyngitis (5% to 8%), bronchitis (3%), dry throat (1% to <3%), epistaxis (1% to <3%), flu-like symptoms (1% to <3%), nasal discomfort (1% to <3%), voice disorder (1% to <3%)

Miscellaneous: Fever (children 7%)

Postmarketing and/or case reports: Anaphylaxis, angioedema, blurred vision, bronchospasm, cataract, cough, dyspnea, exacerbation of asthma, glaucoma, growth retardation, hypersensitivity reaction, pruritus, skin rash, wheezing

Mechanism of Action May depress the formation, release, and activity of endogenous chemical mediators of inflammation (kinins, histamine, liposomal enzymes, prostaglandins). Leukocytes and macrophages may have to be present for the initiation of responses mediated by the above substances. Inhibits the margination and subsequent cell migration to the area of injury, and also reverses the dilatation and increased vessel permeability in the area resulting in decreased access of cells to the sites of injury.

Pharmacodynamics/Kinetics

Onset of Action Maximum effects may not be evident for ≥1 to 2 weeks

Duration of Action Duration after discontinuation: Several days or more

Half-life Elimination Mean: 5 hours

Time to Peak Plasma: 0.5 to 2.5 hours

Pregnancy Considerations

Maternal use of inhaled corticosteroids (ICS) in usual doses is not associated with an increased risk of fetal malformations; a small risk of malformations was observed in one study following high maternal doses of an alternative inhaled corticosteroid. Uncontrolled asthma is associated with adverse events on pregnancy (increased risk of perinatal mortality, preeclampsia, preterm birth, low-birth-weight infants, cesarean delivery, and the development of gestational diabetes). Poorly controlled asthma or asthma exacerbations may have a greater fetal/maternal risk than what is associated with appropriately used asthma medications. Maternal treatment improves pregnancy outcomes by reducing the risk of some adverse events (eg, preterm birth, gestational diabetes) (ERS/TSANZ [Middleton 2020]; GINA 2020).

Inhaled corticosteroids are recommended for the treatment of asthma during pregnancy (GINA 2020). Mometasone oral inhalation is considered probably acceptable for use during pregnancy. Pregnant females adequately controlled on mometasone for asthma may continue therapy; if initiating treatment during pregnancy, use of an agent with more data in pregnant females may be preferred. The lowest dose that maintains asthma control should be used. Maternal asthma symptoms should be monitored monthly during pregnancy (ERS/TSANZ [Middleton 2020]).

Data collection to monitor pregnancy and infant outcomes associated with asthma and the medications used to treat asthma in pregnancy is ongoing. Health care providers are encouraged to enroll exposed pregnant females in the MotherToBaby Pregnancy Studies conducted by the Organization of Teratology Information Specialists (OTIS) (877-311-8972 or http://mothertobaby.org). Patients may also enroll themselves.

◆ **Mometasone and Eformoterol** *see* Mometasone and Formoterol *on page 1047*

Mometasone and Formoterol

(moe MET a sone & for MOH te rol)

Related Information

Formoterol *on page 711*

Mometasone (Oral Inhalation) *on page 1046*

Brand Names: US Dulera

Brand Names: Canada Zenhale

Pharmacologic Category $Beta_2$ Agonist, Long-Acting; $Beta_2$-Adrenergic Agonist, Long-Acting; Corticosteroid, Inhalant (Oral)

Use Asthma: Treatment of asthma in patients ≥5 years of age

Limitations of use: Not indicated for the relief of acute bronchospasm.

Local Anesthetic/Vasoconstrictor Precautions No information available to require special precautions

Effects on Dental Treatment Key adverse event(s) related to dental treatment: Formoterol: Xerostomia (normal salivary flow resumes upon discontinuation). Localized infections with *Candida albicans* or *Aspergillus niger* have occurred frequently in the mouth and pharynx with repetitive use of oral inhaler of corticosteroids. These infections may require treatment with appropriate antifungal therapy or discontinuance of treatment with corticosteroid inhaler.

Effects on Bleeding No information available to require special precautions

Adverse Reactions Also see individual agents.

1% to 10%:

Central nervous system: Voice disorder (adolescents and adults: 4% to 5%), headache (≥3%)

Infection: Influenza (children: ≥3%)

Respiratory: Nasopharyngitis (adolescents and adults: 5%), upper respiratory tract infection (children: ≥3%), sinusitis (adolescents and adults: 2% to 3%)

<1%, postmarketing, and/or case reports: Anaphylaxis, angina pectoris, angioedema, atrial fibrillation, blurred vision, cardiac arrhythmia, exacerbation of asthma, hyperglycemia, hypertension, hypokalemia, hypotension, oropharyngeal candidiasis, paradoxical bronchospasm, prolonged QT interval on ECG, pruritus, severe hypotension, skin rash, tachyarrhythmia, type I hypersensitivity reaction, type IV hypersensitivity reaction, ventricular premature contractions

Mechanism of Action

Formoterol: Relaxes bronchial smooth muscle by selective action on $beta_2$ receptors with little effect on heart rate. Formoterol has a long-acting effect.

Mometasone: A corticosteroid which controls the rate of protein synthesis, depresses the migration of polymorphonuclear leukocytes/fibroblasts, and reverses capillary permeability and lysosomal stabilization at the cellular level to prevent or control inflammation.

Pregnancy Considerations Animal reproduction studies have not been conducted with this combination. See individual agents.

◆ **Mometasone/Formoterol** *see* Mometasone and Formoterol *on page 1047*

◆ **Mometasone Furoate** *see* Mometasone (Nasal) *on page 1045*

◆ **Mometasone Furoate** *see* Mometasone (Oral Inhalation) *on page 1046*

◆ **Monacolin K** *see* Lovastatin *on page 940*

◆ **Mondoxyne NL** *see* Doxycycline *on page 522*

◆ **Monocaps [OTC]** *see* Vitamins (Multiple/Oral) *on page 1550*

- ◆ **Monoclate-P [DSC]** *see* Antihemophilic Factor (Human) *on page 152*
- ◆ **Monoclonal Antibody 2C4** *see* Pertuzumab *on page 1220*
- ◆ **Monoclonal Antibody ABX-EGF** *see* Panitumumab *on page 1187*
- ◆ **Monoclonal Antibody Campath-1H** *see* Alemtuzumab *on page 93*
- ◆ **Monoclonal Antibody CD52** *see* Alemtuzumab *on page 93*
- ◆ **Monodox [DSC]** *see* Doxycycline *on page 522*
- ◆ **Monoethanolamine** *see* Ethanolamine Oleate *on page 609*
- ◆ **Mono-Linyah** *see* Ethinyl Estradiol and Norgestimate *on page 616*

Monomethyl Fumarate

(MON oh METH il FUE ma rate)

Brand Names: US Bafiertam

Pharmacologic Category Fumaric Acid Derivative

Use Multiple sclerosis, relapsing: Treatment of relapsing forms of multiple sclerosis, including clinically isolated syndrome, relapsing-remitting disease, and active secondary progressive disease, in adults.

Local Anesthetic/Vasoconstrictor Precautions No information available to require special precautions.

Effects on Dental Treatment Key adverse event(s) related to dental treatment: Frequent occurrence of mild to moderate flushing (warmth, redness, itching, burning sensation) that generally resolves with subsequent dosing.

Effects on Bleeding No information available to require special precautions.

Adverse Reactions All adverse reactions are reported with dimethyl fumarate, the prodrug of monomethyl fumarate.

>10%:

Cardiovascular: Flushing (40%)

Gastrointestinal: Abdominal pain (18%), diarrhea (14%), nausea (12%)

Infection: Infection (60%)

1% to 10%:

Dermatologic: Erythema of skin (5%) pruritus (8%), skin rash (8%)

Endocrine & metabolic: Albuminuria (6%)

Gastrointestinal: Dyspepsia (5%), vomiting (9%)

Hematologic & oncologic: Lymphocytopenia (2% to 6%)

Hepatic: Increased serum aspartate aminotransferase (4%)

<1%: Nervous system: Progressive multifocal leukoencephalopathy

Frequency not defined:

Hematologic & oncologic: Eosinophilia

Hepatic: Increased liver enzymes, increased serum alanine aminotransferase

Hypersensitivity: Anaphylaxis, angioedema

Postmarketing:

Hepatic: Abnormal liver function, increased serum bilirubin, increased serum transaminases

Infection: Aspergillosis, cytomegalovirus disease, herpes simplex infection, herpes zoster infection (including disseminated, ophthalmicus, meningoencephalitis, and meningomyelitis), listeriosis, opportunistic infection, tuberculosis

Mechanism of Action Monomethyl fumarate (MMF) and its prodrug, dimethyl fumarate, have been shown to activate the nuclear factor (erythroid-derived 2)-like 2 (Nrf2) pathway, which is involved in cellular response to oxidative stress. The mechanism by which monomethyl fumarate exerts a therapeutic effect in multiple sclerosis is unknown, although it is believed to result from its anti-inflammatory and cytoprotective properties via activation of the Nrf2 pathway (Fox 2012; Gold 2012). MMF has also been identified as a nicotinic acid receptor agonist in vitro.

Pharmacodynamics/Kinetics

Half-life Elimination ~0.5 hour.

Time to Peak 4.03 hours; after high-fat meal: 11 hours.

Reproductive Considerations In general, disease-modifying therapies for multiple sclerosis (MS) are stopped prior to a planned pregnancy except in females at high risk of MS activity (AAN [Rae-Grant 2018]). Consider use of agents other than monomethylfumarate for females at high risk of disease reactivation who are planning a pregnancy. Delaying pregnancy is recommended for females with persistent high disease activity; when disease-modifying therapy is needed in these patients, other agents are preferred (ECTRIMS/EAN [Montalban 2018]).

Pregnancy Considerations In general, disease-modifying therapies for multiple sclerosis (MS) are not initiated during pregnancy, except in females at high risk of MS activity (AAN [Rae-Grant 2018]). When disease-modifying therapy is needed in these patients, other agents are preferred (ECTRIMS/ EAN [Montalban 2018]).

Product Availability Bafiertam: FDA approved April 2020; anticipated availability is currently unknown.

- ◆ **MonoNessa [DSC]** *see* Ethinyl Estradiol and Norgestimate *on page 616*
- ◆ **Monopril** *see* Fosinopril *on page 715*
- ◆ **Monovisc** *see* Hyaluronate and Derivatives *on page 761*

Montelukast (mon te LOO kast)

Related Information

Respiratory Diseases *on page 1680*

Brand Names: US Singulair

Brand Names: Canada ACH-Montelukast [DSC]; AG-Montelukast; APO-Montelukast; Auro-Montelukast; BIO-Montelukast; DOM-Montelukast; DOM-Montelukast FC; JAMP-Montelukast; M-Montelukast; Mar-Montelukast; MINT-Montelukast; MYLAN-Montelukast [DSC]; NRA-Montelukast; PMS-Montelukast; PRIVA-Montelukast; RAN-Montelukast; RIVA-Montelukast FC; SANDOZ Montelukast; Singulair; TEVA-Montelukast

Pharmacologic Category Leukotriene-Receptor Antagonist

Use

Allergic rhinitis (perennial or seasonal): Relief of symptoms of seasonal allergic rhinitis in adults and pediatric patients ≥2 years of age and perennial allergic rhinitis in adults and pediatric patients ≥6 months of age. Because the benefits may not outweigh the risk of neuropsychiatric symptoms in patients with allergic rhinitis, reserve use for patients who have had an inadequate response or intolerance to alternative therapies.

Asthma: Prophylaxis and chronic treatment of asthma.

Bronchoconstriction, exercise-induced (prevention): Prevention of exercise-induced bronchoconstriction.

Note: American Academy of Otolaryngology, Head and Neck Surgery (AAO-HNS) and American Academy of Allergy, Asthma, and Immunology (AAAAI) and American College of Allergy, Asthma, and Immunology (ACAAI) guidelines recommend *against* montelukast use as first-line therapy for allergic rhinitis (except in patients with concurrent asthma) (Dykewicz 2017; Seidman 2015). The Global Initiative for Asthma recommends montelukast in patients with concomitant allergic rhinitis or those who cannot take inhaled corticosteroids (GINA 2020).

Local Anesthetic/Vasoconstrictor Precautions No information available to require special precautions

Effects on Dental Treatment Key adverse event(s) related to dental treatment: Dental pain.

Effects on Bleeding Postmarket safety evaluation has identified increased bleeding tendency and thrombocytopenia.

Adverse Reactions

1% to 10%:

Central nervous system: Headache (children and adolescents: ≥2%), dizziness (adolescents and adults: 2%), fatigue (adolescents and adults: ≤2%)

Dermatologic: Atopic dermatitis (children: ≥2%), dermatitis (children: ≥2%), eczema (children: ≥2%), skin infection (children: ≥2%), urticaria (children: ≥2%), skin rash (2%)

Gastrointestinal: Abdominal pain (children: ≥2%), diarrhea (children and adolescents: ≥2%), nausea (children and adolescents: ≥2%), tooth infection (children: ≥2%), dyspepsia (2%), gastroenteritis (2%), toothache (adolescents and adults: 2%)

Genitourinary: Pyuria (adolescents and adults: 1%)

Hepatic: Increased serum aspartate aminotransferase (adolescents and adults: 2%), increased serum alanine aminotransferase (adolescents and adults: ≥1%)

Infection: Influenza (children and adolescents: ≥2%), varicella zoster infection (children: ≥2%), viral infection (children and adolescents: ≥2%)

Neuromuscular & skeletal: Asthenia (adolescents and adults: ≤2%)

Ophthalmic: Conjunctivitis (children: ≥2%), myopia (children: ≥2%)

Otic: Otalgia (children: ≥2%), otitis (children and adolescents: ≥2%), otitis media (children and adolescents: ≥2%)

Respiratory: Cough (3%), acute bronchitis (children: ≥2%), laryngitis (children and adolescents: ≥2%), pharyngitis (children: ≥2%), pneumonia (children: ≥2%), rhinitis (infective; children: ≥2%), rhinorrhea (children: ≥2%), nasal congestion (adolescents and adults: 2%), epistaxis (adolescents and adults: ≥1%), sinus headache (adolescents and adults: ≥1%), sinusitis (≥1%), upper respiratory tract infection (≥1%)

Miscellaneous: Fever (2%), trauma (adolescents and adults: 1%)

<1%, postmarketing and/or case reports: Abnormal dreams, aggressive behavior, agitation, anaphylaxis, angioedema, anxiety, arthralgia, behavioral changes, bleeding tendency disorder, bruise, depression, diarrhea, disorientation, drowsiness, edema, eosinophilia (systemic), eosinophilic granulomatosis with polyangiitis, eosinophilic pneumonitis, epistaxis, erythema multiforme, erythema nodosum, hallucination, hepatic eosinophilic infiltration, hepatitis (mixed pattern, hepatocellular, and cholestatic), hostility, hypersensitivity reaction, hypoesthesia, insomnia, irritability, lack of concentration, memory impairment, mood changes, muscle cramps, myalgia, nausea, obsessive compulsive disorder, palpitations, pancreatitis, paresthesia, pruritus, restlessness, seizure, somnambulism, Stevens-Johnson syndrome, stuttering, suicidal ideation, suicidal tendencies, thrombocytopenia, tic disorder, toxic epidermal necrolysis, tremor, urinary incontinence, urticaria, vasculitis, vomiting

Mechanism of Action Selective leukotriene receptor antagonist that inhibits the cysteinyl leukotriene receptor. Cysteinyl leukotrienes and leukotriene receptor occupation have been correlated with the pathophysiology of asthma, including airway edema, smooth muscle contraction, and altered cellular activity associated with the inflammatory process, which contribute to the signs and symptoms of asthma. Cysteinyl leukotrienes are also released from the nasal mucosa following allergen exposure leading to symptoms associated with allergic rhinitis (Jarvis, 2000).

Pharmacodynamics/Kinetics

Duration of Action >24 hours

Half-life Elimination 2.7-5.5 hours; Mild-to-moderate hepatic impairment: 7.4 hours

Time to Peak Tablet: 10 mg: 3 to 4 hours (fasting); Chewable tablet: 4 mg (children 2 to 5 years): 2 hours (fasting); Chewable tablet 5 mg: 2 to 2.5 hours (fasting); Granules: 2.3 ± 1 hours (fasting) and 6.4 ± 2.9 hours (with high-fat meal)

Pregnancy Considerations

Based on available data, an increased risk of teratogenic effects has not been observed with montelukast use in pregnancy (GINA 2020).

Uncontrolled asthma is associated with adverse events on pregnancy (increased risk of perinatal mortality, preeclampsia, preterm birth, low-birth-weight infants, cesarean delivery, and the development of gestational diabetes). Poorly controlled asthma or asthma exacerbations may have a greater fetal/maternal risk than what is associated with appropriately used asthma medications. Maternal treatment improves pregnancy outcomes by reducing the risk of some adverse events (eg, preterm birth, gestational diabetes). Maternal asthma symptoms should be monitored monthly during pregnancy. Montelukast should not be withheld during pregnancy when clinically indicated (ERS/TSANZ [Middleton 2020]; GINA 2020).

Data collection to monitor pregnancy and infant outcomes associated with asthma and the medications used to treat asthma in pregnancy is ongoing. Health care providers are encouraged to enroll exposed pregnant females in the MotherToBaby Pregnancy Studies conducted by the Organization of Teratology Information Specialists (OTIS) (877-311-8972 or http://mothertobaby.org). Patients may also enroll themselves.

- ◆ **Montelukast Sodium** *see* Montelukast *on page 1048*
- ◆ **Monurol** *see* Fosfomycin *on page 715*
- ◆ **MoreDophilus [OTC]** *see Lactobacillus on page 869*
- ◆ **Morgidox** *see* Doxycycline *on page 522*
- ◆ **Moroctocog Alfa** *see* Antihemophilic Factor (Recombinant) *on page 153*
- ◆ **MorphaBond ER [DSC]** *see* Morphine (Systemic) *on page 1050*

Morphine (Systemic) (MOR feen)

Related Information

Management of the Chemically Dependent Patient *on page 1724*

OxyMORphone *on page 1176*

Brand Names: US Arymo ER; Duramorph; Infumorph 200; Infumorph 500; Kadian; Mitigo; MorphaBond ER [DSC]; MS Contin

Brand Names: Canada BAR-Morphine SR; Doloral 1; Doloral 5; Kadian; Kadian SR; M-Ediat; M-Eslon; Morphine Extra Forte [DSC]; Morphine Forte [DSC]; Morphine HP; Morphine LP Epidural; Morphine SR; Morphine Sulfate SDZ; Morphine-Epd [DSC]; MS Contin; MS/IR; RATIO-Morphine [DSC]; Ratio-Morphine [DSC]; SANDOZ Morphine SR; Statex; TEVA-Morphine SR

Generic Availability (US) May be product dependent

Pharmacologic Category Analgesic, Opioid

Use

Pain management, acute and chronic pain:

Injection: Management of pain severe enough to require an opioid analgesic and for which alternative treatments are inadequate.

Preservative-free solutions only:

Duramorph: Epidural or intrathecal management of pain without attendant loss of motor, sensory, or sympathetic function. **Note:** Not for use in continuous microinfusion devices.

Infumorph, Mitigo: Used in continuous microinfusion devices for intrathecal or epidural administration in management of intractable chronic pain severe enough to require an opioid analgesic and for which less invasive means of controlling pain are inadequate. **Note:** Not for single-dose IV, IM, or subcutaneous administration or single-dose neuraxial injection.

Oral:

Extended release: Management of pain severe enough to require daily, around-the-clock, long-term opioid treatment and for which alternative treatment options are inadequate.

Immediate release: Management of acute and chronic pain severe enough to require an opioid analgesic and for which alternative treatments are inadequate. Oral solution 100 mg per 5 mL (20 mg/mL) is for opioid-tolerant patients.

Rectal: Management of acute and chronic pain severe enough to require an opioid analgesic and for which alternative treatments are inadequate.

Limitations of use: Reserve morphine for use in patients for whom alternative treatment options (eg, nonopioid analgesics, opioid combination products) are ineffective, not tolerated, or would be otherwise inadequate to provide sufficient management of pain. ER formulations are not indicated as as-needed analgesics.

Local Anesthetic/Vasoconstrictor Precautions No information available to require special precautions

Effects on Dental Treatment Key adverse event(s) related to dental treatment: Infrequent occurrence of xerostomia (normal salivary flow resumes upon discontinuation), GERD, and dysphagia have been reported. Anticholinergic side effects can cause a reduction of saliva production or secretion, contributing to discomfort and dental disease (ie, caries, oral candidiasis, and periodontal disease). Rare occurrence of dysgeusia has also been reported.

Effects on Bleeding No information available to require special precautions

Adverse Reactions

>10%:

Central nervous system: Drowsiness (oral: 9% to >10%), headache (<2% to >10%)

Gastrointestinal: Constipation (9% to >10%), nausea (7% to >10%), vomiting (2% to >10%)

Genitourinary: Urinary retention (<2%)

1% to 10%:

Cardiovascular: Peripheral edema (3% to 10%), chest pain (oral: 2%), atrial fibrillation (oral: <2%), bradycardia (oral, rectal: <2%), edema (oral, rectal: <2%), facial flushing (oral, rectal: <2%), flushing (oral: <2%), hypertension (oral: <2%), hypotension (oral: <2%), palpitations (oral, rectal: <2%), syncope (oral, rectal: <2%), tachycardia (oral: <2%), vasodilation (oral: <2%)

Central nervous system: Depression (oral: <2% to 10%), insomnia (oral, rectal: <2% to 10%), paresthesia (oral: <2% to 10%), dizziness (6%), anxiety (≤6%), abnormality in thinking (oral: <5%), confusion (<5%), seizure (<5%), pain (oral: 3%), abnormal dreams (oral: <2%), agitation (oral, rectal: <2%), amnesia (oral: <2%), apathy (oral: <2%), ataxia (oral: <2%), chills (oral: <2%), decreased cough reflex (<2%), euphoria (<2%), hallucination (oral: <2%), hypoesthesia (oral: <2%), lack of concentration (oral: <2%), lethargy (oral: <2%), malaise (oral: <2%), myoclonus (<2%), slurred speech (oral: <2%), vertigo (oral: <2%), voice disorder (oral: <2%), withdrawal syndrome (oral: <2%)

Dermatologic: Skin rash (oral, rectal: 3% to 10%), diaphoresis (oral, rectal: 2% to 10%), decubitus ulcer (oral: <2%), pallor (oral: <2%), pruritus (<2%)

Endocrine & metabolic: Amenorrhea (oral: <2%), decreased libido (oral, rectal: <2%), gynecomastia (oral: <2%), hyponatremia (oral: <2%), SIADH (oral: <2%)

Gastrointestinal: Abdominal pain (oral: 3% to 10%), anorexia (oral, rectal: 3% to 10%), diarrhea (3% to 10%), xerostomia (oral, rectal: 3% to 10%), biliary colic (oral: <2%), delayed gastric emptying (oral: <2%), dyspepsia (oral: <2%), dysphagia (oral: <2%), gastric atony (oral: <2%), gastroesophageal reflux disease (oral: <2%), hiccups (oral: <2%)

Genitourinary: Impotence (oral: <2%), urinary hesitancy (oral, rectal: <2%), urine abnormality (oral: <2%)

Hematologic & oncologic: Anemia (oral: 2% to <5%), thrombocytopenia (oral: <5%), leukopenia (oral: 2%)

Neuromuscular & skeletal: Back pain (oral: <2% to 10%), tremor (oral: 2%), asthenia (oral, rectal: ≤2%), arthralgia (oral: <2%), foot-drop (oral: <2%), ostealgia (oral: <2%)

Ophthalmic: Amblyopia (oral: <2%), blurred vision (oral: <2%), conjunctivitis (oral: <2%), diplopia (oral: <2%), miosis (oral, IV: <2%), nystagmus disorder (oral: <2%)

Respiratory: Dyspnea (3% to 10%), flu-like symptoms (oral: <2% to 10%), hypoventilation (<5%), asthma (oral: <2%), atelectasis (oral: <2%), hypoxia (oral: <2%), pulmonary edema (oral: <2%; includes non-cardiogenic), respiratory depression (IV, epidural, intrathecal: <2%), respiratory insufficiency (oral: <2%), rhinitis (oral: <2%)

Miscellaneous: Accidental injury (oral: 2% to 10%), fever (oral: 2% to 10%), increased severity of condition (oral: 3%)

Frequency not defined:

Cardiovascular: Circulatory depression (oral, IV), orthostatic hypotension (IM, IV), peripheral vascular insufficiency (IV), phlebitis (IV), presyncope (oral, rectal), shock

Central nervous system: Abnormal gait (oral), altered mental status (IV), coma (oral), delirium (oral), disorientation (oral, rectal), disruption of body temperature regulation (IV, epidural, intrathecal), dysphoria, dyssynergia (oral), fear (IV), feeling abnormal (oral), increased catecholamines (IV, epidural, intrathecal), increased intracranial pressure (oral), mood changes (oral), nervousness (oral), paradoxical central nervous system stimulation (IV, epidural, intrathecal), sedated state (oral, rectal), toxic psychosis (IM, IV, epidural, intrathecal)

Dermatologic: Hemorrhagic urticaria (IV, rectal), urticaria, xeroderma (oral)

Endocrine & metabolic: Antidiuretic effect (oral, rectal), increased thirst (oral), weight loss (oral)

Gastrointestinal: Biliary tract spasm (rectal), decreased appetite (IV), dysgeusia (oral), gastroenteritis (oral), gastrointestinal hypermotility (IV; in patients with chronic ulcerative colitis), rectal disease (oral), toxic megacolon (IV; patients with chronic ulcerative colitis)

Genitourinary: Dysuria (oral), ejaculatory disorder (oral), erectile dysfunction (IV), hypogonadism (oral), oliguria, ureteral spasm (IV)

Hematologic & oncologic: Granuloma (IV, epidural, intrathecal)

Hepatic: Increased liver enzymes (oral)

Hypersensitivity: Nonimmune anaphylaxis (IM)

Local: Erythema at injection site (IV), induration at injection site (SC), local irritation (IV, epidural, intrathecal), local swelling (IV, intrathecal, epidural; genital swelling in males following infusion device implant surgery), pain at injection site (SC), residual mass at injection site (inflammatory; IV, epidural, intrathecal)

Neuromuscular & skeletal: Decreased bone mineral density (oral), laryngospasm (oral), muscle rigidity (oral), muscle spasm (IV, epidural, intrathecal; myoclonic spasm of lower extremities), muscle twitching (oral), vesicle sphincter spasm (IV)

Ophthalmic: Eye pain (oral), visual disturbance (oral, rectal)

Respiratory: Apnea (oral, IV)

Miscellaneous: Impaired physical performance (IV)

<1%, postmarketing, and/or case reports: Anaphylaxis, bronchospasm, dehydration, difficulty thinking, fatigue, hyperalgesia, hypersensitivity reaction, hypertonia, increased serum prolactin (Molitch 2008; Vuong 2010), intestinal obstruction, sepsis

Dosing

Adult

Pain management, moderate to severe pain: Note: Opioids may be part of a comprehensive, multimodal, patient-specific treatment plan for pain. Maximize nonopioid analgesia, if appropriate, prior to initiation of opioid analgesia (CDC [Dowell 2016]; Hill 2018). Dosing provided is based on typical doses and some patients may require higher or lower doses. Individualize dosing and dosing intervals based on patient-specific factors (eg, comorbidities, severity of pain, concomitant medications, general condition, degree of opioid experience/tolerance) and titrate to patient-specific treatment goals (eg, improvement in function and quality of life, decrease in pain using a validated pain rating scale). Use the lowest effective dose for the shortest period of time. For acute non-cancer-related pain severe enough to require an opioid, utilize multimodal pain control, maximize nonopioid analgesics, and limit the quantity prescribed to the expected duration of acute pain; a quantity sufficient for ≤3 days is often adequate, whereas >7 days is rarely needed. Do not use long-acting preparations for treatment of acute pain in opioid-naive patients (APS 2016; CDC [Dowell 2016]). Before starting opioid therapy for chronic pain, establish realistic goals for pain and function, and consider how therapy will be discontinued if benefits do not outweigh risks (CDC [Dowell 2016]).

Acute pain:

General dosing: **Note:** Dosing presented in this section is for opioid-naive patients. Patients who are opioid-tolerant will likely require higher dosing; adjust doses accordingly (Arnold 2019).

Oral: Opioid-naive patients:

Immediate release: Oral solution, Tablet:

Note: Consider the use of other more commonly prescribed oral opioids (eg, oxycodone) instead of morphine (Pino 2019). The 100 mg/5 mL (or 20 mg/mL) concentrated oral solution is not intended for opioid-naive patients.

Initial: 10 mg every 4 hours as needed; if pain is not relieved, may increase dose as tolerated. May give up to 30 mg every 4 hours as needed for severe, acute pain in hospitalized patients at low risk for respiratory depression (APS 2016; Herzig 2019; Pharmacist's Letter [Cupp 2012]; manufacturer's labeling).

IV: Opioid-naive patients:

Intermittent: Initial: 1 to 4 mg every 1 to 4 hours as needed; if pain is not relieved, may increase dose as tolerated. May give up to 10 mg every 4 hours as needed for severe, acute pain in hospitalized patients at low risk for respiratory depression (APS 2016; Herzig 2019; Mariano 2019; SCCM [Barr 2013]; manufacturer's labeling). For some severe acute pain episodes (eg, trauma), may initially give more frequently (eg, every 5 to 15 minutes) if needed and titrate to pain relief; once pain relief is achieved, reduce frequency (eg, every 3 to 4 hours as needed) (Lvovschi 2008; Patanwala 2010). **Note:** When IV access is not available, SubQ administration using similar dosing may be considered; however, repeated intermittent SubQ injections cause local tissue irritation, pain, and induration and are not recommended (Mariano 2019).

Patient-controlled analgesia (Mariano 2019):

Example IV Patient-Controlled Analgesia Initial Dose Ranges for Opioid-Naive Patients[a]

Usual concentration	1 mg/mL
Demand dose	Usual range: 0.5 to 2 mg
Basal dose	In general, a continuous (basal) infusion is **not** recommended in an opioid-naive patient (ISMP 2009)[b]
Lockout interval	5 to 10 minutes
Maximum cumulative dose	7.5 mg within 1 hour (or 30 mg within a 4-hour period)

[a]For use to maintain pain control after initial pain control achieved. May adjust dosing and provide rescue bolus doses (eg, 0.5 to 2 mg) if analgesia is inadequate (Mariano 2019).

[b]The use of a continuous background infusion for patient-controlled analgesia is generally **not** recommended for most patients because of the risk of respiratory depression, and use should be limited to carefully selected patients who are opioid tolerant and/or receiving care in a critical care unit, or if required to maintain baseline opioid dosing during intervals when oral or transdermal opioid administration is not possible (Arnold 2019; Mariano 2019).

IM (not recommended for routine use): Opioid-naive patients: Initial: 5 to 10 mg every 3 to 4 hours as needed; if pain is not relieved, may increase dose as tolerated. **Note:** IM administration is generally not recommended due to pain associated with injection, variable absorption, and delayed time to peak effect (APS 2016; Mariano 2019).

Rectal (may be used as an alternative to IV or oral administration): Opioid-naive patients: Initial: 10 mg every 4 hours scheduled or as needed; may increase or decrease the dose as tolerated following the same precautions as oral dosing up to 30 mg every 4 hours scheduled or as needed.

Acute pain (specific indications):

Acute coronary syndrome, refractory ischemic chest pain:

Note: Use only in patients with continued ischemic chest pain despite maximally tolerated anti-ischemic medications (ACC/AHA [Amsterdam 2014]). Routine use in patients with acute coronary syndrome has been associated with worse clinical outcomes and concomitant use with oral P2Y12 inhibitors may diminish antiplatelet effects (Duarte 2019; Kubica 2016; Meine 2005).

IV: 2 to 4 mg initially, followed by 2 to 8 mg every 5 to 15 minutes as needed (ACCF/AHA [O'Gara 2013]; Reeder 2019; Simons 2019) **or** 1 to 5 mg initially, followed by 1 to 5 mg every 5 to 30 minutes as needed (ACC/AHA [Amsterdam 2014]).

Acute pain (eg, breakthrough cancer pain) in patients on chronic opioid therapy for pain: Oral, IV, SubQ: Usual dose: In conjunction with the scheduled long-acting opioid, administer 5% to 20% of the basal daily morphine milligram equivalents (MME) requirement given as needed using an IR formulation with subsequent dosage adjustments based upon response (Arnold 2019; Azhar 2019; Portenoy 2019).

Critically ill patients in the ICU (analgesia and sedation) (off-label use):

Note: Multimodal approaches (eg, a combination of analgesics and techniques) should typically be employed for pain control in this setting. Pain should be monitored using validated scales (eg, behavioral pain scale, critical-care observation tool) in medical, postoperative, or trauma (excluding brain injury) ICU patients who are unable to self-report (SCCM [Devlin 2018]).

IV:

Loading dose: 2 to 10 mg, followed by maintenance dosing (Tietze 2019). **Note:** More than 1 loading dose may be needed; onset of action following IV administration is 5 to 10 minutes. Reduce or omit initial loading dose in select patients (eg, older, hypovolemic, at-risk for hemodynamic compromise) (Tietze 2019).

Maintenance dosing: 2 to 4 mg every 1 to 2 hours **or** 4 to 8 mg every 3 to 4 hours (SCCM [Barr 2013]; Tietze 2019).

Postoperative pain:

Initial pain control in the post-anesthesia care unit: IV: 1 to 3 mg given as frequently as every 5 minutes until adequate pain relief or unwanted side effects (eg, respiratory depression, oxygen desaturation, hypotension) occur. **Note:** A maximum cumulative dose (eg, 20 mg) prompting reevaluation of continued morphine use and/or dose should be included as part of any medication order intended for short-term use (eg, *post-anesthesia care unit* orders); refer to institution-specific protocols as appropriate (Aubrun 2012; Casserly 2019; Mariano 2019).

Ongoing pain control: IV: 1 to 4 mg every 1 to 4 hours as needed; may give up to 10 mg every 2 to 4 hours as needed for severe, acute pain in patients at low risk for respiratory depression (APS 2016; Casserly 2019; Mariano 2019; SCCM [Barr 2013]). If patient-controlled analgesia is needed, refer to **Example IV Patient-Controlled Analgesia Initial Dose Ranges for Opioid-Naive Patients** table.

Sickle cell disease, vaso-occlusive pain:

Note: Dosing presented is for patients in emergency department and hospital settings (including day hospitals) whose previous opioid dose for prior episodes is unknown or who rarely require opioids for pain management. If opioid dose given for a prior episode is known, choose initial dose based on intensity of pain in comparison with previous episode and previous effective dose (DeBaun 2020).

IV: Initial: 0.1 to 0.15 mg/kg (maximum initial dose: 10 mg) given once within 30 minutes of presentation, reassess pain within 20 minutes; if continued severe pain, may repeat with doses of 0.02 to 0.05 mg/kg every 20 to 30 minutes to achieve pain relief (DeBaun 2020). If IV access is difficult, may administer SubQ (NIH 2014). If pain relief is not achieved after ≥3 doses, hospitalization for around-the-clock parenteral analgesics is generally indicated. Evaluate need for long-acting opioid; if patient usually requires a long-acting opioid at home, may convert to oral home regimen once IV dose is roughly equivalent to long-acting opioid dose (DeBaun 2020).

Chronic pain, including chronic cancer pain:

Note: Opioids, including morphine, are **not** the preferred therapy for chronic noncancer pain due to insufficient evidence of benefit and risk of serious harm; nonpharmacologic treatment and nonopioid analgesics are preferred, with the exception of chronic pain from sickle cell disease and end-of-life care. Opioids, including morphine, should **only** be considered in patients who experience clinically meaningful improvement in pain and function that outweighs patient safety risks (CDC [Dowell 2016; Dowell 2019]).

Opioid-naive patients: In general, for noncancer pain, morphine requirement should be established using IR formulations (CDC [Dowell 2016]). With cancer pain, may switch to a long-acting formulation earlier in the course of therapy (Portenoy 2019).

Oral: Immediate release: Oral solution, Tablet: **Note:** The 100 mg/5 mL (or 20 mg/mL) concentrated oral solution is not intended for opioid-naive patients.

Noncancer or cancer pain: Initial: 5 to 30 mg every 4 hours as needed or scheduled around the clock for some patients (eg, cancer pain) (Paice 2011; Pharmacist's Letter [Cupp 2012]; Portenoy 2019; Rosenquist 2019). For chronic noncancer pain, most patients will have pain control with initial doses <50 mg/day (Busse 2017).

Titration: For chronic noncancer pain, may increase the dose slowly in increments of no more than 25% to 50% of the total daily dose (Rosenquist 2019). For chronic cancer pain, may increase the fixed scheduled dose by 30% to 100% of the total dose taken in the prior 24-hour period, while taking into consideration the total amount of rescue medication used; if pain score decreased, continue current effective dosing (Paice 2011; Portenoy 2019). **Note:** In order to reduce risk of overdose, use caution when increasing opioid dosage to ≥50 MME/day and avoid increasing dosage to ≥90 MME/day or carefully justify a decision to titrate dosage to ≥90 MME/day (CDC [Dowell 2016]).

IV, SubQ: Note: Typically reserved for acute exacerbations or those who cannot tolerate oral administration. For progressive illnesses (eg, cancer), a continuous IV or SubQ infusion, with or without a patient-controlled analgesia option, can also be used as pain requirements increase. In general, SubQ dose is equivalent to IV dose (Anderson 2004). Individualize dose based on patient's previous opioid intake and appropriate opioid analgesic equivalents; titrate further, if needed, based on level of pain.

Noncancer or cancer pain: IV: Initial: 2 to 5 mg every 2 to 4 hours as needed (Portenoy 2019).

Cancer pain or palliative care: SubQ: Initial: 2 to 5 mg every 3 to 4 hours as needed (Portenoy 2019). If a continuous SubQ infusion is employed, refer to institutional protocols; reported dosing varies greatly and is based on practice and patient needs (Anderson 2004; Koshy 2005; Portenoy 2019; Walsh 2006).

*Opioid-tolerant patients (also refer to the section **Dose conversions for pain management**):*

Oral: Extended release:

Note: Although manufacturer's labeling contains directions for initiating ER morphine products in opioid-naive patients with chronic pain, these preparations should not be used as initial therapy. Instead, treatment should be initiated with an IR preparation to more accurately determine the daily opioid requirement and decrease the risk of overdose. Unless pain is associated with cancer, palliative care, or sickle cell disease, the Centers for Disease Control and Prevention recommends that ER opioids be reserved for patients who have received IR opioids daily for ≥1 week yet continue to experience severe, continuous pain (CDC [Dowell 2016]).

Capsules, extended release (Kadian): See **Dose conversions for pain management**: Calculated dose may be administered once daily or in 2 equally divided doses administered every 12 hours; may consider dose reduction with first several doses when converting from IR formulations. Example initial dose: 30 mg once daily or 15 mg every 12 hours. Dose adjustments may be made as frequently as every 1 to 2 days.

Tablets, extended release (Arymo ER, MorphaBond ER, MS Contin): See **Dose conversions for pain management**: Calculated dose may be administered in 2 equally divided doses (every 12 hours) or 3 equally divided doses (every 8 hours); may consider dose reduction with first several doses when converting from IR formulations. Example initial dose: 15 mg every 8 or 12 hours. Dose adjustments may be made as frequently as every 1 to 2 days.

Dose conversions for pain management: Note: Equianalgesic conversions serve only as a general guide to estimate opioid dose equivalents. Multiple factors must be considered for safely individualizing conversion of opioid analgesia. In general, for noncancer pain, the decision to convert from an IR to an ER formulation should be individualized and reserved for those with severe continuous pain who have been taking opioids for ≥1 week (Rosenquist 2019).

Converting from oral morphine to parenteral morphine:

Approximate equivalency: 30 mg (**oral** morphine): 10 mg (**IV/SubQ** morphine) (Pharmacist's Letter [Cupp 2012]).

Converting from oral IR morphine to oral ER morphine preparations:

Arymo ER, MorphaBond ER, MS Contin: Total daily oral morphine dose may be administered either in 2 divided doses (every 12 hours) **or** in 3 divided doses (every 8 hours).

Kadian: Total daily oral morphine dose administered once daily; in patients experiencing inadequate analgesia with once-daily dosing, total daily dose can be administered in 2 divided doses (every 12 hours).

Converting from oral morphine to rectal morphine:

Although the bioavailability of rectal morphine is believed to approximate oral morphine (ie, 1:1), absorption is variable and may be higher or lower than expected. Therefore, when switching from oral to rectal dosing, a reduction in rectal dose may be necessary (Brokjær 2015; Portenoy 2019).

Converting to/from morphine (parenteral or oral) to/from a different opioid (parenteral or oral):

Refer to published equianalgesic opioid conversion data for guidance (or refer to institutional protocols). Provided conversion ratios are only approximations and substantial interpatient variability exists; therefore, it is safer to underestimate a patient's daily oral requirement and provide breakthrough pain relief with IR formulations rather than risk overestimating daily requirements. **When switching to a new opioid (except to/from methadone), reduce the initial daily calculated equianalgesic dose of the new opioid by 25% to 50% to adjust for lack**

of complete mu receptor cross-tolerance (conversions to/from methadone are highly variable and require extreme caution) (Portenoy 2019).

Discontinuation of pain management therapy: When reducing the dose or discontinuing chronic opioid therapy, the dose should be gradually tapered. An optimal tapering schedule has not been established (CDC [Dowell 2016]). Proposed schedules range from slow (eg, 10% reduction per week) to rapid (eg, 25% to 50% reduction every few days) (CDC 2015). Individualize to minimize withdrawal while considering patient-specific goals and concerns as well as the opioid's pharmacokinetics. Slower tapers may be appropriate after long-term use (eg, years), particularly in the final stage of tapering, whereas more rapid tapers may be appropriate in patients experiencing severe adverse effects (CDC [Dowell 2016]). Monitor carefully for signs/symptoms of withdrawal. If the patient displays withdrawal symptoms, consider slowing the taper schedule; alterations may include increasing the interval between dose reductions, decreasing amount of daily dose reduction, pausing the taper and restarting when the patient is ready, and/or coadministration of an alpha-2 agonist (eg, clonidine) to blunt withdrawal symptoms (Berna 2015; CDC [Dowell 2016]). Continue to offer nonopioid analgesics as needed for pain management during the taper; consider nonopioid adjunctive treatments for withdrawal symptoms (eg, GI complaints, muscle spasm) as needed (Berna 2015; Sevarino 2019).

Neuraxial analgesia:

Epidural:

Note: Reserve use for severe pain (eg, after surgery, cancer pain). Must be administered by health care providers skilled in the care of patients receiving intraspinal opioids (APS [Chou 2016]). Use a **preservative-free (PF)** formulation intended for neuraxial use.

Single dose *(using 0.5 or 1 mg/mL PF solution):* Opioid-naive patients: Usual range: 2 to 3.75 mg (may depend upon patient comorbidities) (Bujedo 2012; Lanz 1985; Mariano 2019; Palmer 2000).

Continuous infusion *(using 0.5 or 1 mg/mL PF solution):* Opioid-naive patients: 0.2 to 0.4 mg/hour (Bujedo 2012). May be given alone or usually in combination with local anesthetics (eg, bupivacaine, ropivacaine); when combined with a local anesthetic, analgesic effect is increased due to synergy (Bujedo 2012; Manion 2011).

Continuous microinfusion *(using a device intended for continuous microinfusion):* **Note:** Must use a 10 mg/mL or 25 mg/mL PF solution (eg, Infumorph); dilution may be required.

Initial: 3.5 to 7.5 mg over 24 hours.

Intrathecal:

Note: Reserve use for severe pain (eg, after surgery, cancer pain). Must be administered by health care providers skilled in the care of patients receiving intraspinal opioids (APS [Chou 2016]). Use a **PF** formulation intended for neuraxial use. Intrathecal dose is usually $^{1}/_{10}$ (one-tenth) that of epidural dosage (APS 2016).

Single dose *(using 0.5 or 1 mg/mL PF solution):* Usual range: 0.1 to 0.2 mg coadministered with a local anesthetic; repeat doses are **not** recommended. If pain recurs within 24 hours of administration, use of an alternative route of administration is recommended (APS 2008; Mariano 2019). **Note:** Although product labeling recommends doses up to 1 mg, the risk of adverse effects (eg, nausea, respiratory depression) is higher with doses >0.3 mg; however, some patients with chronic intractable pain (eg, cancer pain) may require doses up to 0.5 mg (PACC [Deer 2017]; Rathmell 2005).

Continuous microinfusion *(using a device intended for continuous microinfusion):* **Note:** Must use a 10 mg/mL or 25 mg/mL PF solution (eg, Infumorph); dilution may be required.

Initial: 0.2 to 1 mg over 24 hours.

Dyspnea in palliative care patients (off-label use):

Opioid-naive patients:

Moderate dyspnea: Immediate release (may use 100 mg/5 mL [20 mg/mL] solution): Oral, Sublingual: Initial: 5 mg every 2 to 4 hours **with** 2.5 mg every 2 hours as needed or on an "offer, may refuse" basis (most patients will not need every dose) (Cancer Care Ontario 2010; Dudgeon 2020; Harman 2019). **Note:** Consider lower initial scheduled doses (eg, 2.5 mg every 2 hours) in patients who are older, frail, or with dyspnea in a setting of heart failure or chronic obstructive pulmonary disease (Harman 2019).

Severe dyspnea: SubQ, IV: Initial: 2.5 mg; if dyspnea persists and initial dose is well tolerated, may repeat every 30 to 60 minutes (SubQ) or every 15 to 30 minutes (IV). If 2 doses are well tolerated but fail to reduce dyspnea adequately, the dose may be doubled (Dudgeon 2020).

Opioid-tolerant patients: **Note:** Higher initial doses will likely be needed.

Moderate or severe dyspnea: Immediate release: Oral: Consider giving 10% to 15% of the basal daily opioid requirement (calculated in morphine equivalents) every 2 hours as needed or on an "offer, may refuse" basis. Consider increasing the regular daily dose by ~25% taking into consideration breakthrough doses used in the previous 24 hours (Dudgeon 2020; Harman 2019).

Severe dyspnea: SubQ, IV: Consider giving 5% of the oral basal daily opioid requirement (calculated in morphine equivalents) every 1 hour as needed or on an "offer, may refuse" basis. For breakthrough dyspnea, if already taking a parenteral opioid, may give ~10% of the current parenteral opioid daily dose (Dudgeon 2020; Harman 2019).

Geriatric Refer to adult dosing. Use with caution; may require reduced dosage.

Renal Impairment: Adult

The renal dosing recommendations are based upon the best available evidence and clinical expertise. Senior Editorial Team: Bruce Mueller, PharmD, FCCP, FASN, FNKF; Jason Roberts, PhD, BPharm (Hons), B App Sc, FSHP, FISAC; Michael Heung, MD, MS.

Note: Morphine clearance is similar in patients with altered and normal kidney function. However, glucuronide metabolites (M3G [inactive as an analgesic; may contribute to CNS stimulation and lower seizure threshold] and M6G [active analgesic]) significantly accumulate in patients with reduced kidney function (Osborne 1993). As kidney function deteriorates, M6G accounts for an increasing proportion of the analgesic effect and attainment of steady state is delayed; consequently, patients may experience CNS depression, sedation, and severe and prolonged respiratory depression, which may be delayed in presentation (Klimas 2014; Koncicki 2017; Lugo 2002; Niscola 2010).

Altered kidney function:

Oral, IM, IV, SubQ, Rectal:

Note: There are no specific dose adjustments provided in the manufacturer's labeling. ER formulations should preferably be avoided in patients with altered kidney function (Tawfic 2015). The following suggestions are based on expert opinion and selected references (Aronoff 2007; Golightly 2013):

CrCl ≥60 mL/minute: No dosage adjustment necessary.

CrCl 30 to <60 mL/minute: Consider use of an alternative opioid analgesic. If necessary, administer 50% to 75% of usual initial dose; may also consider extending dose interval. Titrate cautiously to response.

CrCl 15 to <30 mL/minute: Avoid use. If necessary, administer 25% to 50% of usual initial dose; may also consider extending dose interval. Titrate cautiously to response.

CrCl <15 mL/minute: Avoid use.

Epidural/intrathecal:

Moderate to severe impairment: There are no specific dose adjustments recommended; however, use with caution and monitor closely. Use of an alternative opioid analgesic may be preferred in patients with more severe impairment.

Hemodialysis, intermittent (thrice weekly): Morphine and M6G are dialyzable, although the extent of removal is not fully quantified (Angst 2000; Bastani 1997); slow distribution from CNS to plasma may result in prolonged CNS depression even after reduction in plasma levels following dialysis (Angst 2000).

Oral, IM, IV, SubQ, Rectal:

Note: There are no specific dose adjustments provided in the manufacturer's labeling. ER formulations should preferably be avoided in patients with altered kidney function (Tawfic 2015). The following suggestions are based on expert opinion and selected references (Aronoff 2007; Golightly 2013):

Avoid use; consider alternative opioid analgesic. If necessary, administer 25% to 50% of usual dose; may also consider extending dose interval. Titrate cautiously to response.

Epidural/intrathecal: There are no specific dose adjustments recommended; however, use with caution and monitor closely. Use of an alternative analgesic may be preferred.

Peritoneal dialysis: Avoid use; consider alternative opioid analgesic (Slater 2019). Morphine, M3G, and M6G are not significantly removed by peritoneal dialysis (Hanna 1993; Osborne 1993; Pauli-Magnus 1999).

CRRT: Other opioids are preferred (eg, hydromorphone, fentanyl) due to more reliable pharmacokinetic profiles (expert opinion). Morphine is not significantly removed by hemofiltration or hemodiafiltration (Jamal 1998), and the extent of M3G and M6G removal is unknown.

PIRRT (eg, sustained, low-efficiency diafiltration): Other opioids are preferred (eg, hydromorphone, fentanyl) due to more reliable pharmacokinetic profiles. The extent of morphine, M3G, and M6G removal is unknown (expert opinion).

Hepatic Impairment: Adult There are no dosage adjustments provided in the manufacturer's labeling. Pharmacokinetics unchanged in mild liver disease; substantial extrahepatic metabolism may occur. In cirrhosis, increases in half-life and AUC suggest dosage adjustment required.

Pediatric Doses should be titrated to appropriate effect; use lower doses in opioid naive patients; when changing routes of administration in chronically treated patients, please note that oral doses are approximately one-half as effective as parenteral dose.

Acute pain, moderate to severe: Note: Repeated SubQ administration causes local tissue irritation, pain, and induration. The use of IM injections is no longer recommended, especially for repeated administration due to painful administration, variable absorption, and lag time to peak effect; other routes are more reliable and less painful (American Pain Society 2016).

Infants ≤6 months, nonventilated: **Note:** Infants <3 months of age are more susceptible to respiratory depression; lower doses are recommended; consider frequent or continuous respiratory monitoring (eg, pulse oximetry) and be in a setting that permits rapid management of respiratory insufficiency (American Pain Society 2016; Berde 2002).

Oral: Oral solution (2 mg/mL or 4 mg/mL): 0.08 to 0.1 mg/kg/dose every 3 to 4 hours (American Pain Society 2008; Berde 2002).

IV or SubQ: 0.025 to 0.03 mg/kg/dose every 2 to 4 hours (American Pain Society 2008; Berde 2002).

Infants ≤6 months, ventilated: **Note:** Infants <3 months are more susceptible to respiratory depression. Patients should have continuous respiratory monitoring (eg, pulse oximetry) and be in a setting that permits rapid management of respiratory insufficiency.

IV; intermittent dosing: Infants ≥3 months: Initial: 0.05 mg/kg/dose every 2 to 4 hours; dosing based on experience in postoperative cardiothoracic patients (Penk 2018).

Continuous IV infusion: Initial: 0.008 to 0.02 mg/kg/**hour** (8 to 20 **mcg**/kg/**hour**); titrate carefully to effect (Berde 2002; Lynn 1998); reported dose range following titration: 0.015 to 0.04 mg/kg/**hour** (15 to 40 **mcg**/kg/**hour**); dosing based on studies in postoperative patients, most commonly following cardiac surgery (Koren 1985; Lynn 1998; Penk 2018; Valkenburg 2016). Lower initial doses have been reported in infants following cardiac surgery compared to non-cardiac surgical infants (Lynn 1998); infants with Down Syndrome have been shown to have similar morphine requirements postoperatively as patients without following cardiac surgery (Goot 2018; Valkenburg 2016).

Infants >6 months, Children, and Adolescents:

Oral: Immediate-release tablets, oral solution (2 mg/mL or 4 mg/mL):

Patient weight <50 kg: 0.2 to 0.5 mg/kg/dose every 3 to 4 hours as needed; some experts have recommended an initial dose of 0.3 mg/kg for severe pain; usual initial maximum dose: 15 to 20 mg (American Pain Society 2008; APA 2012; Berde 2002).

Patient weight ≥50 kg: 15 to 20 mg every 3 to 4 hours as needed (American Pain Society 2008; Berde 2002).

IM, IV, or SubQ; intermittent dosing:

Patient weight <50 kg: Opioid naïve: Initial: 0.05 mg/kg/dose; usual maximum initial dose: 1 to 2 mg/dose; higher doses may be required if pain not adequately controlled or if patient is opioid tolerant; usual range: 0.1 to 0.2 mg/kg/dose every 2 to 4 hours as needed; use lower doses in opioid naïve patients; usual maximum dose: Infants: 2 mg/dose; Children 1 to 6 years: 4 mg/dose; Children 7 to 12 years: 8 mg/dose; Adolescents: 10 mg/dose.

Patient weight ≥50 kg: Initial: 2 to 5 mg every 2 to 4 hours as needed; Use lower end of the dosing range in opioid naïve patients; higher doses have been recommended (5 to 8 mg every 2 to 4 hours as needed) and may be needed in tolerant patients (Berde 2002; Kliegman 2011).

Continuous IV infusion, SubQ continuous infusion: **Note:** Patients should have continuous respiratory monitoring (eg, pulse oximetry) and be in a setting that permits rapid management of respiratory insufficiency (American Pain Society 2016; Berde 2002).

Patient weight <50 kg: Initial: 0.01 mg/kg/**hour** (10 **mcg**/kg/**hour**); titrate carefully to effect; dosage range: 0.01 to 0.04 mg/kg/**hour** (10 to 40 **mcg**/kg/**hour**) (APA 2012; Friedrichsdorf 2007; Golianu 2000).

Patient weight ≥50 kg: 1.5 mg/**hour** (Berde 2002).

Conversion from intermittent IV morphine: Administer the patient's total daily IV morphine dose over 24 hours as a continuous infusion; titrate dose to appropriate effect.

Epidural: Astramorph/PF, Duramorph: Limited data available: **Note: Must use preservative-free formulation:**

Intermittent: Infants, Children, and Adolescents: 0.015 to 0.05 mg/kg (15 to 50 **mcg**/kg) (APA 2012; Henneberg 1993); a trial evaluating pain relief in pediatric patients after abdominal surgery (n=76; age: Newborn to 13 years; median age: 12 months) administered epidural morphine every 8 hours in combination with bupivacaine during the immediate postop period; most children achieved good pain relief with this regimen (Henneberg 1993). Maximum dose: 0.1 mg/kg (100 **mcg**/kg) or 5 mg/24 hours.

Continuous epidural infusion: Infants >6 months, Children, and Adolescents: 0.001 to 0.005 mg/kg/**hour** (1 to 5 **mcg**/kg/**hour**) (Suresh 2012).

Analgesia for minor procedures/sedation: Infants, Children, and Adolescents: IV: 0.05 to 0.1 mg/kg/dose; administer 5 minutes before the procedure; maximum dose: 4 mg; may repeat dose in 5 minutes if necessary (Cramton 2012; Zeltzer 1990).

Patient-controlled analgesia (PCA), opioid-naïve: Note: All patients should receive an initial loading dose of an analgesic (to attain adequate control of pain) before starting PCA for maintenance. Adjust doses, lockouts, and limits based on required loading dose, age, state of health, and presence of opioid tolerance. Use lower end of dosing range for opioid-naïve. Assess patient and pain control at regular intervals and adjust settings if needed (American Pain Society 2008): IV:

Children ≥5 years and Adolescents, weighing <50 kg: **Note:** PCA has been used in children as young as 5 years of age; however, clinicians need to assess children 5 to 8 years of age to determine if they are able to use the PCA device correctly (American Pain Society 2008).

Usual concentration: 1 mg/mL.

Demand dose: Usual initial: 0.02 mg/kg/dose; usual range: 0.01 to 0.03 mg/kg/dose.

Lockout: Usual initial: 5 doses/hour.

Lockout interval: Range: 6 to 8 minutes.

Usual basal rate: 0 to 0.03 mg/kg/hour.

Children ≥5 years and Adolescents, weighing ≥50 kg:

Usual concentration: 1 mg/mL.

Demand dose: Usual initial: 1 mg; usual range: 0.5 to 2.5 mg.

Lockout interval: Usual initial: 6 minutes; usual range: 5 to 10 minutes.

Chronic pain: Note: Patients taking opioids chronically may become tolerant and require doses higher than the usual dosage range to maintain the desired effect. Tolerance can be managed by appropriate dose titration. There is no optimal or maximal dose for morphine in chronic pain. The appropriate dose is one that relieves pain throughout its dosing interval without causing unmanageable side effects. Consider total daily dose, potency, prior opioid use, degree of opioid experience and tolerance, conversion from previous opioid (including opioid formulation), patient's general condition, concurrent medications, and type and severity of pain during prescribing process.

Oral: Extended-/controlled-release preparations: A patient's morphine requirement should be established using immediate-release formulations. Conversion to long acting products may be considered when chronic, continuous treatment is required. Higher dosages should be reserved for use only in opioid-tolerant patients.

Capsules, extended release (Kadian): Adolescents ≥18 years: **Note:** Not intended for use as an initial opioid in the management of pain; use immediate release formulations before initiation. Total daily oral morphine dose may be either administered once daily or in 2 divided doses daily (every 12 hours). The first dose of Kadian may be taken with the last dose of the immediate release morphine.

Tablets, controlled release (MS Contin): Children and Adolescent able to swallow tablets whole: Usually not used as an initial opioid in the management of pain; use immediate release formulations to titrate dose. Total daily morphine dose may be administered in 2 divided doses daily (every 12 hours) or in 3 divided doses daily (every 8 hours).

Weight-directed dosing: 0.3 to 0.6 mg/kg/dose every 12 hours (Berde 1990).

Alternate dosing; fixed dosing (Berde 2002):

Patient weight 20 to <35 kg: 10 to 15 mg every 8 to 12 hours; **Note:** 10 mg strength not available in US.

Patient weight 35 to <50 kg: 15 to 30 mg every 8 to 12 hours.

Patient weight ≥50 kg: 30 to 45 mg every 8 to 12 hours.

Discontinuation of extended-release formulations: In general, gradually titrate dose downward (eg, every 2 to 4 days). Do not discontinue abruptly.

Conversion from other oral morphine formulations to extended-release formulations:

Kadian: Adolescents ≥18 years: Total daily oral morphine dose may be either administered once daily or in 2 divided doses daily (every 12 hours).

MS Contin: Children and Adolescents: Total daily oral morphine dose may be administered either in 2 divided doses daily (every 12 hours) **or** in 3 divided doses (every 8 hours).

Conversion from parenteral morphine or other opioids to controlled/extended release formulations: Substantial interpatient variability exists in relative potency. Therefore, it is safer to underestimate a patient's daily oral morphine requirement and provide breakthrough pain relief with immediate-release morphine than to overestimate requirements. Consider the parenteral to oral morphine ratio or other oral or parenteral opioids to oral morphine conversions.

Continuous IV infusion, SubQ continuous infusion: Children and Adolescents: 0.01 to 0.04 mg/kg/**hour** (10 to 40 **mcg**/kg/**hour**) (APA 2012; Friedrichsdorf 2007; Golianu 2000); opioid-tolerate patients may require higher doses; in a small study of terminal pediatric oncology patients (n=8; age range: 3 to 16 years), the median required dose was 0.04 to 0.07 mg/kg/**hour** (40 to 70 **mcg**/kg/**hour**); range: 0.025 to 2.6 mg/kg/**hour** (Miser 1980); another study evaluating subcutaneous continuous infusion in children with cancer (n=17; age range: 22 months to 22 years) had similar findings; median dose: 0.06 mg/kg/**hour** (60 **mcg**/kg/**hour**); range: 0.025 to 1.79 mg/kg/**hour** (Miser 1983).

Conversion from intermittent IV morphine: Administer the patient's total daily IV morphine dose over 24 hours as a continuous infusion; titrate dose to appropriate effect.

Sickle cell disease, acute crisis; opioid naïve patients (APS 1999; NHLBI 2014): **Note:** Individualize dose; titrate to effect; Infants ≥6 months, Children, and Adolescents:

Patient weight <50 kg: Initial: IV: 0.1 to 0.15 mg/kg every 2 to 4 hours; maximum dose: 7.5 mg/dose.

Patient weight ≥50 kg: Initial: IV: 5 to 10 mg every 2 to 4 hours.

Tetralogy of fallot, hypercyanotic spell (infundibular spasm): Infants and Children: Limited data available: IM, IV, SubQ: 0.1 mg/kg has been used to decrease ventilatory drive and systemic venous return (Hegenbarth 2008).

Palliative care, dyspnea management: Limited data available: Children and Adolescents:

Inhalation (nebulization; preservative-free injection): Dose should be individualized and is dependent upon patient's previous or current systemic opioid exposure; doses not intended to provide analgesic activity; current systemic analgesia should be continued: Initial dose: Equivalent to patient's 4-hour systemic morphine requirement (eg, IV or oral dose); titrate to effect (Golianu 2000); every 4 to 6 hour administration has been suggested (Cohen 2002). In the only pediatric case report (end-stage CF, age: 10 years, weight: 20 kg), an initial dose of 2.5 mg was used and final dose was 10 mg every 4 to 6 hours (Cohen 2002); from experience in adult patients, an initial dose of 5 mg has been used and reported range 2.5 to 30 mg administered up to every 4 hours (Ferraresi 2005; Shirk 2006).

Continuous IV or SubQ infusion (when oral ineffective): Initial: 0.005 mg/kg/**hour** (5 **mcg**/kg/**hour**); titrate for comfort (Garcia-Salido 2015); dosing based on palliative management of terminal infants with spinal muscular atrophy (type 1); intermittent IV maximum doses of 0.4 mg/kg have been reported to control symptoms of dyspnea and pain (di Pede 2018).

Oral: 0.1 mg/kg/dose every 4 hours as needed (Garcia-Salido 2015); titrate for comfort; dosing based on palliative management of terminal infants with spinal muscular atrophy (type 1); maximum doses of 0.4 mg/kg have been reported to control symptoms of dyspnea and pain (di Pede 2018).

Renal Impairment: Pediatric Infants, Children and Adolescents: According to the manufacturers' labeling, no specific dosage adjustments are provided (all formulations). In general, the manufacturers recommend starting cautiously with lower doses; titrating slowly while carefully monitoring for side effects. However, the choice of an alternate opioid may be prudent in patients with baseline renal impairment or rapidly changing renal function especially since other analgesics may be safer and reduced initial morphine dosing may result in suboptimal analgesia. Although clearance of morphine is similar to patients with normal renal function, morphine glucuronide metabolites (M3G [inactive as an analgesic; may contribute to CNS stimulation] and M6G [active analgesic]) accumulate in renal impairment resulting in increased sensitivity; patients may experience severe and prolonged respiratory depression which may even be delayed (Lugo 2002; Niscola 2010).

Hepatic Impairment: Pediatric Infants, Children and Adolescents: There are no dosage adjustments provided in manufacturer's labeling. Pharmacokinetics are unchanged in mild liver disease; substantial extrahepatic metabolism may occur. In adults with cirrhosis, increases in half-life and AUC suggest dosage adjustment required.

Mechanism of Action Binds to opioid receptors in the CNS, causing inhibition of ascending pain pathways, altering the perception of and response to pain; produces generalized CNS depression

Contraindications

Hypersensitivity (eg, anaphylaxis) to morphine or any component of the formulation; significant respiratory depression; acute or severe bronchial asthma in an unmonitored setting or in the absence of resuscitative equipment; concurrent use of monoamine oxidase inhibitors (MAOIs) or use of MAOIs within the last 14 days; GI obstruction, including paralytic ileus (known or suspected).

Documentation of allergenic cross-reactivity for opioids is limited. However, because of similarities in chemical structure and/or pharmacologic actions, the possibility of cross-sensitivity cannot be ruled out with certainty.

Additional contraindications:

Epidural/intrathecal: Infection at infusion site; concomitant anticoagulant therapy; uncontrolled bleeding diathesis; presence of any other concomitant therapy or medical condition that would render administration hazardous; upper airway obstruction.

Canadian labeling: Additional contraindications (not in US labeling):

Contraindications may vary per product labeling; refer also to product labels: Suspected surgical abdomen (eg, acute appendicitis, pancreatitis); disease/condition that affects bowel transit (known or suspected); chronic obstructive airway; status asthmaticus; management of acute pain, including use in outpatient or day surgeries; mild, intermittent, or short-duration pain that can be managed with other pain medications; acute respiratory depression; hypercarbia; cor pulmonale; acute alcoholism; delirium tremens; convulsive disorders; severe CNS depression; increased cerebrospinal; intracranial pressure; brain tumor; head injury; cardiac arrhythmias; pregnancy; use during labor and delivery; breastfeeding; alcohol consumption or medications containing alcohol (Kadian, M-Eslon product monographs); toxic psychosis and severe kyphoscoliosis (Kadian product monograph); severe cirrhosis (M-Ediat product monograph); hypotension (M-Eslon product monograph), emotional instability and/or suicidal ideation (Statex product monograph); surgical anastomosis (morphine sulfate inj Sandoz product monograph)

Warnings/Precautions An opioid-containing analgesic regimen should be tailored to each patient's needs and based upon the type of pain being treated (acute versus chronic), the route of administration, degree of tolerance for opioids (naive versus chronic user), age, weight, and medical condition. The optimal analgesic dose varies widely among patients.

[US Boxed Warning]: To ensure that the benefits of opioid analgesics outweigh the risks of addiction, abuse, and misuse, the FDA has required a REMS for these products. Under the requirements of the REMS, drug companies with approved opioid analgesic products must make REMS compliant education programs available to health care providers. Health care providers are strongly encouraged to complete a REMS-compliant education program; counsel patients and/or their caregivers, with every prescription, on safe use, serious risks, storage, and disposal of these products; emphasize to patients and their caregivers the importance of reading the Medication Guide every time it is provided by their pharmacist; and consider other tools to improve patient, household, and community safety.

[US Boxed Warning]: Serious, life-threatening, or fatal respiratory depression may occur. Monitor closely for respiratory depression, especially during initiation or dose escalation. Swallow ER morphine formulations whole (or may sprinkle the contents of the capsule on applesauce and swallow without chewing); crushing, chewing, or dissolving the ER formulations can cause rapid release and absorption of a potentially fatal dose of morphine. Carbon dioxide retention from opioid-induced respiratory depression can exacerbate the sedating effects of opioids. Use with caution and monitor for respiratory depression in patients with significant chronic obstructive pulmonary disease or cor pulmonale and patients having a substantially decreased respiratory reserve, hypoxia, hypercarbia, or preexisting respiratory depression, particularly when initiating therapy and titrating with morphine; consider the use of alternative nonopioid analgesics in these patients. Opioid use increases the risk for sleep-related disorders (eg, central sleep apnea [CSA], hypoxemia) in a dose-dependent fashion. Use with caution for chronic pain and titrate dosage cautiously in patients with risk factors for sleep-disordered breathing (eg, heart failure, obesity). Consider dose reduction in patients presenting with CSA. Avoid opioids in patients with moderate to severe sleep-disordered breathing (CDC [Dowell 2016]). Infants <3 months of age are more susceptible to respiratory depression, use with caution and generally in reduced doses in this age group (APS 2008).

Use caution in patients with hypersensitivity reactions to other phenanthrene derivative opioid agonists (codeine, hydrocodone, hydromorphone, levorphanol, oxycodone, oxymorphone). Avoid use in patients with impaired consciousness or coma. May obscure diagnosis or clinical course of patients with acute abdominal conditions. May cause constipation, which may be problematic in patients with unstable angina and patients post-myocardial infarction. Some preparations contain sulfites, which may cause allergic reactions.

May cause CNS depression, which may impair physical or mental abilities; patients must be cautioned about performing tasks that require mental alertness (eg, operating machinery or driving). **[US Boxed Warning]: Concomitant use of opioids with benzodiazepines or other CNS depressants, including alcohol, may result in profound sedation, respiratory depression, coma, and death. Reserve concomitant prescribing of morphine and benzodiazepines or other CNS depressants for use in patients for whom alternative treatment options are inadequate. Limit dosage and durations to the minimum required and follow patients for signs and symptoms of respiratory depression and sedation. [US Boxed Warning]: Patients should not consume alcoholic beverages or medication containing ethanol while taking ER capsules; ethanol may increase morphine plasma levels, resulting in a potentially fatal overdose.** Potentially significant interactions may exist, requiring dose or frequency adjustment, additional monitoring, and/or selection of alternative therapy.

[US Boxed Warning]: Morphine exposes patients and other users to the risks of addiction, abuse, and misuse, potentially leading to overdose and death. Assess each patient's risk prior to prescribing; monitor all patients regularly for development of these behaviors or conditions. Use with caution in patients with a history of drug abuse or acute alcoholism; potential for drug dependency exists. Other factors associated with increased risk include younger age, concomitant depression (major), and psychotropic medication use. Consider offering naloxone prescriptions in patients with factors associated with an increased risk for overdose, such as history of overdose or substance use disorder, higher opioid dosages (≥50 morphine milligram equivalents/day orally), and concomitant benzodiazepine use (CDC [Dowell 2016]).

May cause severe hypotension (including orthostatic hypotension and syncope); use with caution in patients with hypovolemia, cardiovascular disease (including acute MI), circulatory shock, or drugs that may exaggerate hypotensive effects (including phenothiazines or general anesthetics). Monitor for symptoms of hypotension following initiation or dose titration. Avoid use in patients with circulatory shock. Use with extreme caution in patients with adrenal insufficiency, including Addison disease; biliary tract dysfunction or acute pancreatitis; head injury, intracranial lesions, or elevated intracranial pressure; delirium tremens; prostatic hyperplasia and/or urinary stricture; renal and/or hepatic impairment; seizure disorders; thyroid dysfunction; or toxic psychosis. Use opioids for chronic pain with caution in patients with mental health conditions (eg, depression, anxiety disorders, post-traumatic stress disorder) due to increased risk for opioid use disorder and overdose; more frequent monitoring is recommended (CDC [Dowell 2016]). Abrupt discontinuation in patients who are physically dependent on opioids has been associated with serious withdrawal symptoms, uncontrolled pain, attempts to find other opioids (including illicit), and suicide. Use a collaborative, patient-specific taper schedule that minimizes the risk of withdrawal, considering factors such as current opioid dose, duration of use, type of pain, and physical and psychological factors. Monitor pain control, withdrawal symptoms, mood changes, suicidal ideation, and for use of other substances; provide care as needed. Concurrent use of mixed agonist/antagonist analgesics (eg, pentazocine, nalbuphine, butorphanol) or partial agonist (eg, buprenorphine) analgesics may also precipitate withdrawal symptoms and/or reduced analgesic efficacy in patients following prolonged therapy with mu opioid agonists.

Use with caution in patients who are morbidly obese. Use with caution in cachectic or debilitated patients; there is a greater potential for critical respiratory depression, even at therapeutic dosages. Consider the use of alternative nonopioid analgesics in these patients. Use with caution in elderly patients; may be more sensitive to adverse effects, including life-threatening respiratory depression. Decrease initial dose. In the setting of chronic pain, monitor closely due to an increased potential for risks, including certain risks such as falls/fracture, cognitive impairment, and constipation. Clearance may also be reduced in older adults (with or without renal impairment) resulting in a narrow therapeutic window and increasing the risk for respiratory depression or overdose (CDC [Dowell 2016]). Consider the use of alternative nonopioid analgesics in these patients. Opioids decrease bowel motility; monitor for decreased bowel motility in postop patients receiving opioids. Use with caution in the perioperative setting; individualize treatment when transitioning from parenteral to oral analgesics. Some dosage forms may be contraindicated after biliary tract surgery, suspected surgical abdomen, or surgical anastomosis.

[US Boxed Warning]: Prolonged maternal use of opioids during pregnancy can cause neonatal withdrawal syndrome in the newborn, which may be life-threatening if not recognized and treated according to protocols developed by neonatology experts. If prolonged opioid therapy is required in a pregnant woman, ensure treatment is available and warn patient of risk to the neonate. Signs and symptoms include irritability, hyperactivity, abnormal sleep pattern, high-pitched cry, tremor, vomiting, diarrhea, and failure to gain weight. Onset, duration, and severity depend on the drug used, duration of use, maternal dose, and rate of drug elimination by the newborn. **[US Boxed Warning]: Accidental ingestion of even one dose, especially in children, can result in a fatal overdose of morphine.**

Oral solutions: **[US Boxed Warning]: Ensure accuracy when prescribing, dispensing, and administering morphine oral solution. Dosing errors due to confusion between mg and mL, and other morphine solutions of different concentrations, can result in accidental overdose and death.** The 100 mg per 5 mL (20 mg/mL) is for use in opioid-tolerant patients only.

Injections: **[US Boxed Warning]: Because of delay in maximum CNS effect with IV administration (30 minutes), rapid IV administration may result in overdosing. Observe patients in a fully equipped and staffed environment for at least 24 hours after each test dose of Infumorph or Mitigo and, as indicated, for the first several days after surgery.** Products are designed for administration by specific routes (ie, IV, intrathecal, epidural). Use caution when prescribing, dispensing, or administering to use formulations only by intended route(s). Rapid IV administration may result in chest wall rigidity. Use with caution when injecting IM into chilled areas or in patients with hypotension or shock (impaired perfusion may prevent complete absorption); if repeated injections are administered, an excessive amount may be suddenly absorbed if normal circulation is re-established.

Infumorph, Duramorph: Neuroaxial administration: **[US Boxed Warning]: Because of the risk of severe adverse effects when the epidural or intrathecal route of administration is employed, patients must be observed in a fully equipped and staffed environment for at least 24 hours after the initial dose. Single-dose Duramorph neuraxial administration may result in acute or delayed respiratory depression up to 24 hours. Monitor patients receiving Infumorph or Mitigo for the first several days after catheter implantation.** Naloxone injection should be immediately available. Thoracic epidural administration has been shown to dramatically increase the risk of early and late respiratory depression. High doses (>20 mg/day) of neuraxial morphine may produce myoclonic events. Patients with reduced circulating blood volume or impaired myocardial function, or on concomitant sympatholytic drugs should be monitored for orthostatic hypotension, a frequent complication in single-dose neuraxial morphine.

Infumorph: Should only be used in microinfusion devices; not for IV, IM, or SubQ administration or for single-dose administration. Administer intrathecal doses of 10 and 25 mg/mL to the lumbar area. Monitor closely, especially in the first 24 hours. Inflammatory masses (eg, granulomas), some resulting in severe neurologic impairment, have occurred when receiving Infumorph or Mitigo via indwelling intrathecal catheter; monitor carefully for new neurologic signs/symptoms. Improper or erroneous substitution of Infumorph or Mitigo for regular Duramorph is likely to result in serious overdosage, leading to seizures, respiratory depression, and possibly a fatal outcome.

ER formulations: Therapy should only be prescribed by health care providers familiar with the use of potent opioids for chronic pain. ER products are not interchangeable. When determining a generic equivalent or switching from one ER product to another, a thorough understanding of the pharmacokinetic properties is important in determining the proper generic equivalent or proper dose of the other extended-release product (review of the manufacturer's label may be necessary).

Arymo ER: Moistened tablets may become sticky, leading to difficulty in swallowing the tablets; choking, gagging, regurgitation, and tablets getting stuck in the throat may occur. Tablet stickiness and swelling may also predispose patients to intestinal obstruction and exacerbation of diverticulitis. Do not pre-soak, lick, or otherwise wet tablets prior to placing in the mouth; take one tablet at a time with enough water to ensure complete swallowing. Consider use of an alternative analgesic in patients who have difficulty swallowing and patients at risk for underlying GI disorders resulting in a small GI lumen (eg, esophageal cancer, colon cancer).

Chronic pain (outside of end-of-life or palliative care, active cancer treatment, sickle cell disease, or medication-assisted treatment for opioid use disorder) in outpatient setting in adults: Opioids should not be used as first-line therapy for chronic pain management (pain >3-month duration or beyond time of normal tissue healing) due to limited short-term benefits, undetermined long-term benefits, and association with serious risks (eg, overdose, MI, auto accidents, risk of developing opioid use disorder). Preferred management includes nonpharmacologic therapy and nonopioid therapy (eg, NSAIDS, acetaminophen, certain anticonvulsants and antidepressants). If opioid therapy is initiated, it should be combined with nonpharmacologic and nonopioid therapy, as appropriate. Prior to initiation, known risks of opioid therapy should be discussed and realistic treatment goals for pain/function should be established, including consideration for discontinuation if benefits do not outweigh risks. Therapy should be continued only if clinically meaningful improvement in pain/function outweighs risks. Therapy should be initiated at the lowest effective dosage using immediate-release opioids (instead of extended-release/long-acting opioids). Risk associated with use increases with higher opioid dosages. Risks and benefits should be re-evaluated when increasing dosage to ≥50 morphine milligram equivalents (MME)/day orally; dosages ≥90 MME/day orally should be avoided unless carefully justified (CDC [Dowell 2016]).

Some dosage forms may contain sodium benzoate/benzoic acid; benzoic acid (benzoate) is a metabolite of benzyl alcohol; large amounts of benzyl alcohol (≥99 mg/kg/day) have been associated with a potentially fatal toxicity ("gasping syndrome") in neonates; the "gasping syndrome" consists of metabolic acidosis, respiratory distress, gasping respirations, CNS dysfunction (including convulsions, intracranial hemorrhage), hypotension, and cardiovascular collapse (AAP ["Inactive" 1997]; CDC, 1982); some data suggests that benzoate displaces bilirubin from protein binding sites (Ahlfors 2001); avoid or use dosage forms containing benzyl alcohol derivative with caution in neonates. See manufacturer's labeling.

Warnings: Additional Pediatric Considerations

Prolonged use of any morphine product during pregnancy can result in neonatal opioid withdrawal syndrome, which may be life-threatening if not recognized and treated, and requires management according to protocols developed by neonatology experts.

For postoperative tonsillectomy (with/without adenoidectomy) pain management in pediatric patients, morphine has been shown to have a higher risk of adverse effects compared to other analgesics without additional analgesic benefit; patient-specific risk factors for these adverse events are not fully defined (Biesiade 2014; Jimenez 2012; Kelly 2015; Ragjavendran 2010; Sadhasivam 2012). Data is preliminary and large-scale population-based generalizations and recommendations for practice have not been made. However, racial differences in adverse effects have been observed. A statistically significant higher incidence of adverse effects (pruritus, emesis) was reported in Latino children and adolescents following perioperative morphine administration than the comparative non-Latino Caucasian cohort (Jimenez 2012). In another trial, Caucasian children and adolescents receiving peri/postoperative morphine showed a higher incidence of postoperative pruritus and emesis than African-American patients (Sadhasivam 2012). The observed risk for respiratory depression between racial groups has been variable, with some data showing no racial difference in risk between Latino and non-Latino Caucasians or between Caucasians and African-American patients, while other data shows a higher risk in African-American pediatric patients compared to Caucasians (Biesiada 2014; Jimenez 2012; Sadhasivam 2012). Regardless of race, an overall higher and clinically significant incidence of respiratory depression has been observed in patients with sleep disturbances requiring tonsillectomy procedure (eg, obstructive sleep apnea); a lower initial dose has been suggested in these patients (Ragjavendran 2010). Current guidelines recommend that children and adolescents receive intravenous dexamethasone intraoperatively and effective therapy for postoperative tonsillectomy pain; NSAIDs (except ketorolac) can be used safely (AAO-HNS [Baugh 2011]).

Drug Interactions

Metabolism/Transport Effects **Substrate** of P-glycoprotein/ABCB1, UGT1A1

Avoid Concomitant Use

Avoid concomitant use of Morphine (Systemic) with any of the following: Azelastine (Nasal); Bromperidol; Eluxadoline; Lasmiditan; Monoamine Oxidase Inhibitors; Opioids (Mixed Agonist / Antagonist); Orphenadrine; Oxomemazine; Paraldehyde; Thalidomide

Increased Effect/Toxicity

Morphine (Systemic) may increase the levels/effects of: Alvimopan; Amifostine; Azelastine (Nasal); Blonanserin; Bromperidol; Desmopressin; Diuretics; DULoxetine; Eluxadoline; Esmolol; Flunitrazepam; Gabapentin; Hypotension-Associated Agents; Levodopa-Containing Products; Methotrimeprazine; MetyroSINE; Nitroprusside; Opioid Agonists; Orphenadrine; OxyCODONE; Paraldehyde; Piribedil; Pramipexole; Ramosetron; ROPINIRole; Rotigotine; Serotonergic Agents (High Risk); Suvorexant; Thalidomide; Zolpidem

The levels/effects of Morphine (Systemic) may be increased by: Alfuzosin; Alizapride; Amphetamines; Anticholinergic Agents; Blood Pressure Lowering Agents; Brimonidine (Topical); Bromopride; Bromperidol; Cannabidiol; Cannabis; Chlormethiazole; Chlorphenesin Carbamate; CNS Depressants; Diazoxide; Dimethindene (Topical); Dronabinol; Droperidol; Erdafitinib; Gabapentin; Herbs (Hypotensive Properties); Kava Kava; Lasmiditan; Lemborexant; Lisuride; Lofexidine; Lumacaftor and Ivacaftor; Magnesium Sulfate; Methotrimeprazine; Metoclopramide; Minocycline (Systemic); Molsidomine; Monoamine Oxidase Inhibitors; Nabilone; Naftopidil; Nicergoline; Nicorandil; Obinutuzumab; Oxomemazine; Pentoxifylline; Perampanel; P-glycoprotein/ABCB1 Inhibitors; Phosphodiesterase 5 Inhibitors; Prostacyclin Analogues; Quinagolide; Rufinamide; Sodium Oxybate; Succinylcholine; Tetrahydrocannabinol; Tetrahydrocannabinol and Cannabidiol

Decreased Effect

Morphine (Systemic) may decrease the levels/effects of: Antiplatelet Agents (P2Y12 Inhibitors); Diuretics; Gastrointestinal Agents (Prokinetic); Pegvisomant; Sincalide

The levels/effects of Morphine (Systemic) may be decreased by: Bromperidol; Lumacaftor and Ivacaftor; Nalmefene; Naltrexone; Opioids (Mixed Agonist / Antagonist); P-glycoprotein/ABCB1 Inducers; RifAMPin

Food Interactions

Ethanol: Alcoholic beverages or ethanol-containing products may disrupt extended release formulation resulting in rapid release of entire morphine dose. Management: Avoid alcohol. **Do not administer Kadian with alcoholic beverages or ethanol-containing prescription or nonprescription products.**

Food: Administration of oral morphine solution with food may increase bioavailability (ie, a report of 34% increase in morphine AUC when morphine oral solution followed a high-fat meal). The bioavailability of MorphaBond, MS Contin, or Kadian does not appear to be affected by food. Management: Take consistently with or without meals.

Dietary Considerations Morphine may cause GI upset; take with food if GI upset occurs. Be consistent when taking morphine with or without meals.

Pharmacodynamics/Kinetics

Onset of Action Patient dependent; dosing must be individualized: Oral (immediate release): ~30 minutes; IV: 5 to 10 minutes

Duration of Action Patient dependent; dosing must be individualized: Pain relief:

Immediate-release formulations (tablet, oral solution, injection): 3 to 5 hours

Extended-release capsule and tablet: 8 to 24 hours (formulation dependent)

Epidural or intrathecal: Single dose: Up to 24 hours (Bujedo 2012)

Suppository: 3 to 7 hours

Half-life Elimination

Preterm: 10 to 20 hours

Neonates: 7.6 hours (range: 4.5 to 13.3 hours)

Infants 1 to 3 months: Median: 6.2 hours (range: 5 to 10 hours) (McRorie 1992)

Infants 3 to 6 months: Median: 4.5 hours (range: 3.8 to 7.3 hours) (McRorie 1992)

Infants 6 months to Children 2.5 years: Median: 2.9 hours (range: 1.4 to 7.8 hours) (McRorie 1992)

Preschool Children: 1 to 2 hours

Children with sickle cell disease (age: 6 to 19 years): ~1.3 hours (Dampier 1995)

Adults: Immediate-release forms: 2 to 4 hours; Kadian: 11 to 13 hours

Time to Peak

Plasma:

Tablets, oral solution, epidural: 1 hour

Extended release tablets: 3 to 4 hours; Kadian: ~10 hours

Suppository: 20 to 60 minutes

SubQ: 50 to 90 minutes

IM: 30 to 60 minutes

IV: 20 minutes

Cerebrospinal fluid: After an oral dose of controlled release morphine concentrations peak at 8 hours for both normal and reduced renal function; morphine-6-glucuronide (active analgesic) and morphine-3-glucuronide distribution into the CNS may be delayed peaking at 12 hours in patients with normal renal function or up to 24 hours in patients with ESRD (peak level of morphine-6-glucuronide is ~15 times higher than patients with normal renal function) (D'Honneur 1994).

Reproductive Considerations

Long-term opioid use may cause secondary hypogonadism, which may lead to sexual dysfunction or infertility in men and women (Brennan 2013).

Pregnancy Considerations Morphine crosses the placenta.

According to some studies, maternal use of opioids may be associated with birth defects (including neural tube defects, congenital heart defects, and gastroschisis), poor fetal growth, stillbirth, and preterm delivery (CDC [Dowell 2016]). Opioids used as part of obstetric analgesia/anesthesia during labor and delivery may temporarily affect the fetal heart rate (ACOG 209 2019).

[US Boxed Warning]: Prolonged use of morphine during pregnancy can result in neonatal opioid withdrawal syndrome, which may be life-threatening if not recognized and treated, and requires management according to protocols developed by neonatology experts. If opioid use is required for a prolonged period in a pregnant woman, advise the patient of the risk of neonatal opioid withdrawal syndrome and ensure that appropriate treatment will be available. If chronic opioid exposure occurs in pregnancy, adverse events in the newborn (including withdrawal) may occur (Chou 2009). Symptoms of neonatal abstinence syndrome (NAS) following opioid exposure may be autonomic (eg, fever, temperature instability), gastrointestinal (eg, diarrhea, vomiting, poor feeding/weight gain), or neurologic (eg, high-pitched crying, hyperactivity, increased muscle tone, increased wakefulness/abnormal sleep pattern, irritability, sneezing, seizure, tremor, yawning) (Dow 2012; Hudak 2012). Mothers who are physically dependent on opioids may give birth to infants who are also physically dependent. Opioids may cause respiratory depression and psychophysiologic effects in the neonate; newborns of mothers receiving opioids during labor should be monitored.

Morphine injection is commonly used for the treatment of pain during labor and immediately postpartum (ACOG 209 2019). Not all dosage forms are appropriate for this use. Agents other than morphine are used to treat chronic non-cancer pain in pregnant women or those who may become pregnant (CDC [Dowell 2016]; Chou 2009).

Breastfeeding Considerations

Morphine is present in breast milk. M6G, the active metabolite of morphine, can also be detected in breast milk (Baka 2002). Reported concentrations of morphine in breast milk are variable.

Morphine has been detected in the urine of a breastfeeding infant following maternal epidural dosing after cesarean delivery (Zakowski 1993) and the serum of an infant following chronic maternal oral use (Robieux 1990).

Nonopioid analgesics are preferred for breastfeeding females who require pain control peripartum or for surgery outside of the postpartum period. However, when a narcotic is needed to treat maternal pain, morphine is one of the preferred agents (ABM [Martin 2018]; ABM [Reece-Stremtan 2017]; Sachs 2013). Analgesics delivered by PCA or administered by the epidural route help limit infant exposure (Sachs 2013). **Note:** Not all formulations are indicated for intermittent pain control.

When opioids are needed in breastfeeding women, the lowest effective dose for the shortest duration of time should be used to limit adverse events in the mother and breastfeeding infant. In general, a single occasional dose of an opioid analgesic may be compatible with breastfeeding (WHO 2002). Breastfeeding women using opioids for postpartum pain or for the treatment of chronic maternal pain should monitor their infants for drowsiness, sedation, feeding difficulties, or limpness (ACOG 209 2019). Withdrawal symptoms may occur when maternal use is discontinued, or breastfeeding is stopped.

Controlled Substance C-II

Dosage Forms: US

Capsule Extended Release 24 Hour, Oral:
Kadian: 10 mg, 20 mg, 30 mg, 40 mg, 50 mg, 60 mg, 80 mg, 100 mg, 200 mg
Generic: 10 mg, 20 mg, 30 mg, 40 mg, 45 mg, 50 mg, 60 mg, 75 mg, 80 mg, 90 mg, 100 mg, 120 mg

Device, Intramuscular:
Generic: 10 mg/0.7 mL (0.7 mL)

Solution, Injection [preservative free]:
Duramorph: 0.5 mg/mL (10 mL); 1 mg/mL (10 mL)
Infumorph 200: 200 mg/20 mL (10 mg/mL) (20 mL)
Infumorph 500: 500 mg/20 mL (25 mg/mL) (20 mL)
Mitigo: 200 mg/20 mL (10 mg/mL) (20 mL); 500 mg/20 mL (25 mg/mL) (20 mL)
Generic: 0.5 mg/mL (10 mL); 1 mg/mL (10 mL); 2 mg/mL (1 mL); 4 mg/mL (1 mL); 5 mg/mL (1 mL); 8 mg/mL (1 mL); 10 mg/mL (1 mL)

Solution, Intravenous [preservative free]:
Generic: 1 mg/mL (30 mL); 2 mg/mL (1 mL); 4 mg/mL (1 mL); 8 mg/mL (1 mL); 10 mg/mL (1 mL); 25 mg/mL (10 mL); 50 mg/mL (20 mL, 50 mL)

Solution, Oral:
Generic: 10 mg/5 mL (5 mL, 15 mL, 100 mL, 500 mL); 20 mg/5 mL (5 mL, 100 mL, 500 mL); 20 mg/mL (30 mL, 118 mL, 120 mL); 100 mg/5 mL (15 mL, 30 mL, 120 mL, 240 mL)

Suppository, Rectal:
Generic: 5 mg (12 ea); 10 mg (12 ea); 20 mg (12 ea); 30 mg (12 ea)

Tablet, Oral:
Generic: 15 mg, 30 mg

Tablet Extended Release, Oral:
MS Contin: 15 mg, 30 mg, 60 mg, 100 mg, 200 mg
Generic: 15 mg, 30 mg, 60 mg, 100 mg, 200 mg

Tablet Extended Release Abuse-Deterrent, Oral:
Arymo ER: 15 mg (100 ea); 30 mg (100 ea); 60 mg (100 ea)

Dosage Forms: Canada

Capsule, Oral:
M-Ediat: 5 mg, 10 mg, 20 mg, 30 mg

Capsule Extended Release 12 Hour, Oral:
M-Eslon: 10 mg, 15 mg, 30 mg, 60 mg, 100 mg, 200 mg

Capsule Extended Release 24 Hour, Oral:
Kadian: 20 mg, 50 mg, 100 mg
Kadian SR: 10 mg

Solution, Injection:
Generic: 0.5 mg/mL (10 mL); 1 mg/mL (5 mL, 10 mL, 50 mL); 2 mg/mL (1 mL, 50 mL); 5 mg/mL (30 mL); 10 mg/mL (1 mL, 5 mL); 15 mg/ml (1 mL, 30 mL); 25 mg/ml (1 mL, 4 mL); 50 mg/mL (1 mL, 5 mL, 10 mL, 50 mL)

Suppository, Rectal:
Statex: 5 mg (10 ea); 10 mg (10 ea); 20 mg (10 ea); 30 mg (10 ea)

Syrup, Oral:
Doloral 1: 1 mg/mL (10 mL, 250 mL, 500 mL)
Doloral 5: 5 mg/mL (10 mL, 250 mL, 500 mL)

Tablet, Oral:
MS/IR: 5 mg, 10 mg, 20 mg, 30 mg
Statex: 5 mg, 10 mg, 25 mg, 50 mg

Tablet Extended Release, Oral:
MS Contin: 15 mg, 30 mg, 60 mg, 100 mg, 200 mg
Generic: 15 mg, 30 mg, 60 mg, 100 mg, 200 mg

◆ **Motegrity** *see* Prucalopride *on page 1291*

◆ **Motion Sickness [OTC] [DSC]** *see* DimenhyDRINATE *on page 501*

◆ **Motion-Time [OTC]** *see* Meclizine *on page 952*

◆ **Motrin Childrens [OTC]** *see* Ibuprofen *on page 786*

◆ **Motrin IB [OTC]** *see* Ibuprofen *on page 786*

◆ **Motrin Infants Drops [OTC]** *see* Ibuprofen *on page 786*

◆ **Mouth Kote [OTC]** *see* Saliva Substitute *on page 1354*

Mouthwash (Antiseptic) (MOUTH wosh)

Related Information

Bacterial Infections *on page 1739*
Dentin Hypersensitivity, Acid Erosion, High Caries Index, Management of Alveolar Osteitis, and Xerostomia *on page 1762*
Periodontal Diseases *on page 1748*
Ulcerative, Erosive, and Painful Oral Mucosal Disorders *on page 1758*

Related Sample Prescriptions

Antimicrobial Oral Rinse - Sample Prescriptions *on page 34*

Brand Names: US Crest Scope Outlast [OTC]; Crest Scope [OTC]; Listerine Antiseptic [OTC]; Listerine Naturals Antiseptic [OTC]; Listerine Ultraclean Antiseptic [OTC]

Generic Availability (US) Yes

Pharmacologic Category Antimicrobial Mouth Rinse; Antiplaque Agent; Mouthwash

Dental Use Aid in prevention and reduction of plaque and gingivitis; halitosis

Use Aid in prevention and reduction of plaque and gingivitis; halitosis

Local Anesthetic/Vasoconstrictor Precautions No information available to require special precautions

Effects on Dental Treatment No significant effects or complications reported (see Dental Health Professional Considerations)

Effects on Bleeding No information available to require special precautions

Adverse Reactions No data reported

Dental Usual Dosage Plaque/gingivitis prevention: Adults: Oral: Rinse full strength for 30 seconds with 20 mL morning and night

Dosing

Adult & Geriatric Plaque/gingivitis prevention: Oral: Rinse full strength for 30 seconds with 20 mL morning and night

Contraindications Hypersensitivity to any component of the formulation

Dental Health Professional Considerations Active ingredients:
Listerine® Antiseptic: Thymol 0.064%, eucalyptus 0.092%, methyl salicylate 0.060%, menthol 0.042%, alcohol 26.9%, water, benzoic acid, poloxamer 407, sodium benzoate, caramel

Fresh Burst Listerine® Antiseptic: Thymol 0.064%, eucalyptus 0.092%, methyl salicylate 0.060%, menthol 0.042%, alcohol 26.9%, water, benzoic acid, poloxamer 407, sodium benzoate, flavoring, sodium, saccharin, sodium citrate, citric acid, D&C yellow #10, FD&C green #3

Cool Mint Listerine® Antiseptic: Thymol 0.064%, eucalyptus 0.092%, methyl salicylate 0.060%, menthol 0.042%, alcohol 26.9%, water, benzoic acid, poloxamer 407, sodium benzoate, flavoring, sodium, saccharin, sodium citrate, citric acid, FD&C green #3

The following information is endorsed on the label of the Listerine® products by the Council on Scientific Affairs, American Dental Association: "Listerine® Antiseptic has been shown to help prevent and reduce supragingival plaque accumulation and gingivitis when used in a conscientiously applied program of oral hygiene and regular professional care. Its effect on periodontitis has not been determined."

◆ **Movantik** *see* Naloxegol *on page 1074*

◆ **Moxatag [DSC]** *see* Amoxicillin *on page 124*

Moxetumomab Pasudotox

(mox e TOOM oh mab pa SOO doe tox)

Brand Names: US Lumoxiti

Pharmacologic Category Antineoplastic Agent, Anti-CD22

Use

Hairy cell leukemia (relapsed or refractory): Treatment of relapsed or refractory hairy cell leukemia (HCL) in adult patients who have received at least 2 prior systemic therapies, including treatment with a purine nucleoside analog.

Limitations of use: Moxetumomab pasudotox is not recommended in patients with severe renal impairment (CrCl ≤29 mL/minute).

Local Anesthetic/Vasoconstrictor Precautions

No information available to require special precautions

Effects on Dental Treatment Key adverse event(s) related to dental treatment: Frequent occurrence of facial edema

Effects on Bleeding Chemotherapy may result in significant myelosuppression, potentially including significant reduction in platelet counts and altered hemostasis. In patients undergoing active treatment with these agents, medical consult is suggested.

Adverse Reactions

>10%:

Cardiovascular: Peripheral edema (5% to 39%), capillary leak syndrome (≤34%), facial edema (14%)

Central nervous system: Fatigue (34%), headache (33%)

Endocrine & metabolic: Hypoalbuminemia (64%), fluid retention (1% to 63%), electrolyte disorder (57%), hypocalcemia (25% to 54%), hypophosphatemia (53%), hyponatremia (41%), hypokalemia (25%), increased gamma-glutamyl transferase (25%), hypomagnesemia (23%), hyperuricemia (21%)

Gastrointestinal: Nausea (35%), constipation (23%), diarrhea (21%), abdominal distention (13%)

Genitourinary: Nephrotoxicity (26%)

Hematologic & oncologic: Decreased hemoglobin (43%; grade 3: 15%), neutropenia (41%; grade 3: 11%; grade 4: 20%), anemia (21%; grade 3: 10%), decreased platelet count (21%; grade 3: 11%; grade 4: 4%)

Hepatic: Increased serum alanine aminotransferase (65%), increased serum aspartate aminotransferase (55%), increased serum bilirubin (30%), increased serum alkaline phosphatase (20%)

Renal: Increased serum creatinine (17% to 96%)

Miscellaneous: Infusion-related reaction (9% to 50%), fever (31%)

1% to 10%:

Cardiovascular: Edema (5%), pericardial effusion (1%)

Endocrine & metabolic: Weight gain (8%), hypervolemia (1%)

Genitourinary: Proteinuria (8%)

Hematologic & oncologic: Hemolytic-uremic syndrome (7%; grade 3: 3%; grade 4: <1%), febrile neutropenia (grades 3/4: ≤5%)

Hepatic: Ascites (1%)

Local: Localized edema (4%)

Ophthalmic: Blurred vision (9%), xerophthalmia (8%), cataract (5%), eye discomfort (≤4%), eye pain (≤4%), ocular edema (≤4%), periorbital edema (≤4%), conjunctival hemorrhage (1%), conjunctivitis (1%), eye discharge (1%)

Renal: Acute renal failure (2%), renal insufficiency (2%)

Respiratory: Pleural effusion (6%)

Frequency not defined: Immunologic: Antibody development

<1%, postmarketing, and/or case reports: Hemoconcentration, hypotension

Mechanism of Action Moxetumomab pasudotox is a CD22-directed cytotoxin composed of a recombinant murine immunoglobulin genetically fused to truncated *Pseudomonas* exotoxin (PE38). Moxetumomab pasudotox binds CD22 on the cell surface of B-cells and is internalized. Moxetumomab pasudotox internalization results in ADP-ribosylation of elongation factor 2, inhibition of protein synthesis, and apoptotic cell death.

Pharmacodynamics/Kinetics

Onset of Action Achievement of hematologic remission: ~1 month (Kreitman 2018). Day 8 circulating CD19+ B cells (surrogate assay for CD22) were reduced 89% (from baseline) following the first 3 infusions.

Duration of Action Median duration of complete response (for patients with minimal residual disease): 5.9 months (Kreitman 2018). B cell reduction is sustained for at least 1 month after treatment.

Half-life Elimination 1.4 hours (range: 0.8 to 1.8 hours)

Reproductive Considerations

Evaluate pregnancy status prior to use. The manufacturer recommends females of reproductive potential use effective contraception during treatment and for at least 30 days after the last dose of moxetumomab pasudotox.

Pregnancy Considerations

Based on the mechanism of action and adverse events observed in nonpregnant animal studies, adverse maternal and fetal events may be expected if exposure occurs during pregnancy.

◆ **Moxetumomab Pasudotox-tdfk** *see* Moxetumomab Pasudotox *on page 1063*

Moxidectin (mox i DEK tin)

Pharmacologic Category Anthelmintic

Use

Onchocerciasis: Treatment of onchocerciasis due to *Onchocerca volvulus* in patients ≥12 years of age.

Limitations of use: Moxidectin does not kill adult *O. volvulus*; follow-up evaluation is advised. Safety and efficacy of repeat administration of moxidectin in patients with *O. volvulus* has not been studied.

Local Anesthetic/Vasoconstrictor Precautions
No information available to require special precautions

Effects on Dental Treatment Key adverse event(s) related to dental treatment: Patients may experience orthostatic hypotension as they stand up after treatment especially if lying in dental chair for extended period of time. Use caution with sudden changes in position during and after dental treatment.

Effects on Bleeding No information available to require special precautions

Adverse Reactions

>10%:

Cardiovascular: Tachycardia (39%), postural orthostatic tachycardia (34%), hypotension (30%), orthostatic hypotension (22%), peripheral edema (11%)

Central nervous system: Headache (58%), chills (≤27%), lymph node pain (13%), dizziness (12%)

Dermatologic: Pruritus (65%), skin rash (37%)

Endocrine & metabolic: Hyponatremia (12%)

Gastrointestinal: Abdominal pain (31%), diarrhea (≤15%), enteritis (≤15%), gastroenteritis (≤15%)

Hematologic & oncologic: Eosinophilia (18% to 74%; severe: 18%), lymphocytopenia (48%: grade 3: 23%), leukocytosis (25%), neutropenia (20%: grade 4: 7%)

Neuromuscular & skeletal: Musculoskeletal pain (64%)

Respiratory: Flu-like symptoms (23%), cough (17%)

Miscellaneous: Fever (≤27%)

1% to 10%:

Cardiovascular: Symptomatic orthostatic hypotension (5%)

Endocrine & metabolic: Increased gamma-glutamyl transferase (3%)

Hematologic & oncologic: Eosinopenia (5%)

Hepatic: Hyperbilirubinemia (3%), increased serum alanine aminotransferase (1%), increased serum aspartate aminotransferase (1%)

Ophthalmic: Eye pain (8%), eye pruritus (7%), visual impairment (3%; including blurred vision, low vision acuity), allergic conjunctivitis (2%), eyelid edema (2%), conjunctival hyperemia (≤2%), ocular hyperemia (≤2%), increased lacrimation (1%)

Frequency not defined: Dermatologic: Mazzotti reaction

Mechanism of Action Moxidectin, an anthelminthic agent, is active against the microfilariae of *O. volvulus*, but not effective in killing the adult worms. Studies with other nematodes suggest moxidectin binds to glutamate-gated chloride ions channels, gamma-aminobutyric acid (GABA) receptors, and/or APT-binding cassette transporters. This leads to increased permeability, influx of chloride ions, hyperpolarization, and muscle paralysis. There is also a reduction in motility of all stages of the parasite, excretion of immunomodulatory proteins, and the fertility of both male and female adult worms.

Pharmacodynamics/Kinetics

Half-life Elimination 23.3 days (559 hours)

Time to Peak 4 hours

Reproductive Considerations
Females of reproductive potential were required to use long acting contraception during clinical studies (Awadzi 2014; Korth-Bradley 2011) likely due to the long terminal half-life of moxidectin.

Pregnancy Considerations
Adverse events were observed in some animal reproduction studies.

Product Availability There are no plans for commercial distribution of moxidectin in the US. Product will be available for onchocerciasis endemic parts of the world.

Moxifloxacin (Systemic) (moxs i FLOKS a sin)

Related Information

Bacterial Infections *on page 1739*

Clinical Risk Related to Drugs Prolonging QT Interval *on page 1675*

Brand Names: US Avelox ABC Pack [DSC]; Avelox [DSC]

Brand Names: Canada AG-Moxifloxacin; APO-Moxifloxacin; Auro-Moxifloxacin; Avelox [DSC]; BIO-Moxifloxacin; JAMP-Moxifloxacin; M-Moxifloxacin; Mar-Moxifloxacin; Priva-Moxifloxacin [DSC]; RIVA-Moxifloxacin; SANDOZ Moxifloxacin; TEVA-Moxifloxacin

Pharmacologic Category Antibiotic, Fluoroquinolone; Antibiotic, Respiratory Fluoroquinolone

Use

Treatment of mild to moderate community-acquired pneumonia, including multidrug-resistant *Streptococcus pneumoniae* (MDRSP); acute bacterial exacerbation of chronic bronchitis; acute bacterial rhinosinusitis; complicated and uncomplicated skin and skin structure infections; complicated intra-abdominal infections; prophylaxis and treatment of plague, including pneumonic and septicemic plague, due to *Yersinia pestis*.

Limitations of use: Because fluoroquinolones have been associated with disabling and potentially irreversible serious adverse reactions (eg, tendinitis and tendon rupture, peripheral neuropathy, CNS effects), reserve moxifloxacin for use in patients who have no alternative treatment options for acute exacerbation of chronic bronchitis or acute sinusitis.

Local Anesthetic/Vasoconstrictor Precautions
Moxifloxacin is one of the drugs confirmed to prolong the QT interval and is accepted as having a risk of causing torsade de pointes. The risk of drug-induced torsade de pointes is extremely low when a single QT interval prolonging drug is prescribed. In terms of epinephrine, it is not known what effect vasoconstrictors in the local anesthetic regimen will have in patients with a known history of congenital prolonged QT interval or in patients taking any medication that prolongs the QT interval. Until more information is obtained, it is suggested that the clinician consult with the physician prior to the use of a vasoconstrictor in suspected patients, and that the vasoconstrictor (epinephrine, mepivacaine and levonordefrin [Carbocaine® 2% with Neo-Cobefrin®]) be used with caution.

Effects on Dental Treatment Key adverse event(s) related to dental treatment: Dry mouth, glossitis, stomatitis, and taste perversion.

Effects on Bleeding Anemia, prolonged prothrombin activation, prolonged activated partial thromboplastin time, increased platelet count, decreased hemoglobin, decreased hematocrit have been reported in a subset of all patients receiving systemic moxifloxacin at therapeutic concentrations. As a consequence, prothrombin time should be closely monitored during moxifloxacin therapy, especially if administered concomitantly with warfarin.

Adverse Reactions

1% to 10%:

Central nervous system: Headache (4%), dizziness (3%), insomnia (2%)

Endocrine & metabolic: Decreased serum glucose (≥2%), hyperchloremia (≥2%), increased serum albumin (≥2%), hypokalemia (1%)

Gastrointestinal: Nausea (7%), diarrhea (6%), decreased amylase (≥2%), constipation (2%), vomiting (2%), abdominal pain (1% to 2%), dyspepsia (1%)

Hematologic & oncologic: Decreased basophils (≥2%), decreased red blood cells (≥2%), eosinopenia (≥2%), increased MCH (≥2%), increased neutrophils (≥2%), leukocytosis (≥2%), prolonged prothrombin time (≥2%), anemia (1%)

Hepatic: Decreased serum bilirubin (≥2%), increased serum bilirubin (≥2%), increased serum alanine aminotransferase (1%)

Immunologic: Increased serum globulins (≥2%)

Renal: Increased ionized serum calcium (≥2%)

Respiratory: Hypoxia (≥2%)

Miscellaneous: Fever (1%)

<1%, postmarketing, and/or case reports: Abdominal distention, abdominal distress, abnormal gait, abnormal hepatic function tests, agitation, agranulocytosis, allergic dermatitis, anaphylactic shock, anaphylaxis, angina pectoris, angioedema, anorexia, anxiety, aplastic anemia, arthralgia, asthenia, asthma, ataxia, atrial fibrillation, auditory impairment, back pain, blurred vision, bradycardia, bronchospasm, candidiasis, cardiac failure, chest discomfort, chest pain, chills, cholestatic hepatitis, *Clostridioides difficile* associated diarrhea, *Clostridioides difficile* colitis, confusion, deafness, decreased appetite, dehydration, delirium, depression, disorientation, disturbance in attention, drowsiness, dysesthesia, dysgeusia, dyspnea, dysuria, edema, eosinophilia, erythema of skin, exacerbation of myasthenia gravis, facial edema, facial pain, fatigue, flatulence, fungal infection, gastritis, gastroenteritis, gastroesophageal reflux disease, hallucination, hemolytic anemia, hepatic failure, hepatic necrosis, hepatitis, hepatotoxicity (idiosyncratic) (Chalasani 2014), hyperglycemia, hyperhidrosis, hyperlipidemia, hypersensitivity pneumonitis, hypersensitivity reaction, hypertension, hypoesthesia, hypoglycemia, hypotension, idiopathic intracranial hypertension, increased amylase, increased blood urea nitrogen, increased gamma-glutamyl transferase, increased intracranial pressure, increased lactate dehydrogenase, increased serum alkaline phosphatase, increased serum aspartate aminotransferase, increased serum creatinine, increased serum lipase, increased serum triglycerides, increased uric acid, interstitial nephritis, jaundice, laryngeal edema, lethargy, leukopenia, limb pain, loss of consciousness, malaise, memory impairment, muscle spasm, musculoskeletal pain, myalgia, myasthenia, nervousness, neutropenia, nightmares, night sweats, pain, palpitations, pancytopenia, paranoid ideation, paresthesia, peripheral neuropathy (may be irreversible), pharyngeal edema, phlebitis, phototoxicity, polyneuropathy, prolonged partial thromboplastin time, prolonged QT interval on ECG, pruritus, renal failure syndrome, renal insufficiency, restlessness, rupture of tendon, seizure, serum sickness, skin photosensitivity, skin rash, Stevens-Johnson syndrome, suicidal ideation, suicidal tendencies, syncope, tachycardia, tendonitis, thrombocythemia, thrombocytopenia, thrombotic thrombocytopenic purpura, tingling sensation, tinnitus, torsades de pointes, toxic epidermal necrolysis, toxic psychosis, tremor, urticaria, vaginal infection, vasculitis, ventricular tachyarrhythmia, vertigo, vision loss, vulvovaginal pruritus, wheezing, xerostomia

Mechanism of Action Moxifloxacin is a DNA gyrase inhibitor, and also inhibits topoisomerase IV. DNA gyrase (topoisomerase II) is an essential bacterial enzyme that maintains the superhelical structure of DNA. DNA gyrase is required for DNA replication and transcription, DNA repair, recombination, and transposition; inhibition is bactericidal.

Pharmacodynamics/Kinetics

Half-life Elimination Single dose: Oral: 12-16 hours; IV: 8-15 hours

Pregnancy Considerations

Moxifloxacin crosses the placenta (Ozyüncü and Beksac 2010; Ozyüncü and Nemutlu 2010).

Due to pregnancy-induced physiologic changes, some pharmacokinetic properties of moxifloxacin may be altered (Nemutlu 2010; van Kampenhout 2017).

Dental Health Professional Considerations See Local Anesthetic/Vasoconstrictor Precautions

- **Moxifloxacin HCl** *see* Moxifloxacin (Systemic) *on page 1064*
- **Moxifloxacin Hydrochloride** *see* Moxifloxacin (Systemic) *on page 1064*
- **Mozobil** *see* Plerixafor *on page 1241*
- **4-MP** *see* Fomepizole *on page 710*
- **MPA** *see* MedroxyPROGESTERone *on page 953*
- **MPA** *see* Mycophenolate *on page 1067*
- **MPA and Estrogens (Conjugated)** *see* Estrogens (Conjugated/Equine) and Medroxyprogesterone *on page 603*
- **6-MP (error-prone abbreviation)** *see* Mercaptopurine *on page 978*
- **MPG-EPO** *see* Methoxy Polyethylene Glycol-Epoetin Beta *on page 993*
- **MRA** *see* Tocilizumab *on page 1457*
- **MSB0010718C** *see* Avelumab *on page 195*
- **MS Contin** *see* Morphine (Systemic) *on page 1050*
- **MS (error-prone abbreviation and should not be used)** *see* Morphine (Systemic) *on page 1050*
- **MSO_4 (error-prone abbreviation and should not be used)** *see* Morphine (Systemic) *on page 1050*
- **MTC** *see* MitoMYcin (Systemic) *on page 1041*
- **Mth/Me Blue/Sod Phos/Phen/Hyos** *see* Methenamine, Sodium Phosphate Monobasic, Phenyl Salicylate, Methylene Blue, and Hyoscyamine *on page 987*
- **MTX (error-prone abbreviation)** *see* Methotrexate *on page 990*
- **Mucinex Allergy [OTC] [DSC]** *see* Fexofenadine *on page 666*
- **Mucinex Nasal Spray Full Force [OTC] [DSC]** *see* Oxymetazoline (Nasal) *on page 1173*
- **Mucinex Nasal Spray Moisture [OTC] [DSC]** *see* Oxymetazoline (Nasal) *on page 1173*
- **Mucinex Sinus-Max Clear & Cool [OTC]** *see* Oxymetazoline (Nasal) *on page 1173*
- **Mucinex Sinus-Max Full Force [OTC] [DSC]** *see* Oxymetazoline (Nasal) *on page 1173*
- **Mucinex Sinus-Max Sinus/Allrgy [OTC]** *see* Oxymetazoline (Nasal) *on page 1173*

◆ **Mucosal Adherent Agent** *see* Mucosal Coating Agent *on page 1066*

◆ **Mucosal Barrier Agent** *see* Mucosal Coating Agent *on page 1066*

◆ **Mucosal Barrier Gel** *see* Mucosal Coating Agent *on page 1066*

◆ **Mucosal Bioadherent Agent** *see* Mucosal Coating Agent *on page 1066*

Mucosal Coating Agent
(myoo KOH sul KOH ting AY gent)

Brand Names: US Episil; Gelclair; Mucotrol; MuGard; Orafate; ProThelial

Pharmacologic Category Gastrointestinal Agent, Miscellaneous

Use Mucosal protection: Management of oral mucosal pain and protection from further irritation caused by oral mucositis/stomatitis (resulting from chemotherapy or radiation therapy); irritation; lesions, periodontal and gingival inflammation, tooth extractions, and wounds/lesions due to oral surgery; chafing; minor lesions; traumatic ulcers, and abrasions caused by braces/ill-fitting dentures or disease; diffuse aphthous ulcers (canker sores); sore throat/pharyngitis (Orafate only)

Local Anesthetic/Vasoconstrictor Precautions
No information available to require special precautions

Effects on Dental Treatment No significant effects or complications reported

Effects on Bleeding No information available to require special precautions

Adverse Reactions
<1%, postmarketing, and/or case reports: Burning sensation of mouth, mild stinging sensation (oral cavity), oral inflammation (mild)

Mechanism of Action Adheres to the mucosal surface of mouth forming a protective film or coating over the irritated areas and lesions, protecting the lesion from further irritation and pain.

◆ **Mucosal Protective Agent** *see* Mucosal Coating Agent *on page 1066*

◆ **Mucotrol** *see* Mucosal Coating Agent *on page 1066*

◆ **MuGard** *see* Mucosal Coating Agent *on page 1066*

◆ **Multaq** *see* Dronedarone *on page 533*

◆ **Multilex [OTC]** *see* Vitamins (Multiple/Oral) *on page 1550*

◆ **Multilex-T&M [OTC]** *see* Vitamins (Multiple/Oral) *on page 1550*

◆ **Multiple Vitamins** *see* Vitamins (Multiple/Oral) *on page 1550*

◆ **Multivitamins/Fluoride** *see* Vitamins (Fluoride) *on page 1550*

◆ **Mumps** *see* Measles, Mumps, and Rubella Virus Vaccine *on page 949*

◆ **Mumps** *see* Measles, Mumps, Rubella, and Varicella Virus Vaccine *on page 950*

◆ **Mumps, Measles, and Rubella Vaccine** *see* Measles, Mumps, and Rubella Virus Vaccine *on page 949*

◆ **Mumps, Rubella, Varicella, and Measles Vaccine** *see* Measles, Mumps, Rubella, and Varicella Virus Vaccine *on page 950*

Mupirocin (myoo PEER oh sin)

Brand Names: US Bactroban Nasal [DSC]; Bactroban [DSC]; Centany; Centany AT

Pharmacologic Category Antibiotic, Topical

Use

Impetigo: Treatment of impetigo due to *Staphylococcus aureus* and *Streptococcus pyogenes* (topical ointment).

Secondary skin infection: Treatment of secondarily infected traumatic skin lesions (up to 10 cm in length or 100 cm^2 in area) due to susceptible isolates of *S. aureus* and *S. pyogenes* (topical cream).

***S. aureus* (including methicillin-resistant) decolonization:** Eradication of nasal colonization with methicillin-resistant *S. aureus* (MRSA) in adult and pediatric patients ≥12 years of age and health care workers as part of a comprehensive infection control program to reduce the risk of infection among patients at high risk of MRSA infection during institutional outbreaks of infections with this microorganism (intranasal ointment).

Local Anesthetic/Vasoconstrictor Precautions
No information available to require special precautions

Effects on Dental Treatment Key adverse event(s) related to dental treatment: Xerostomia (normal salivary flow resumes upon discontinuation) and taste perversion.

Effects on Bleeding No information available to require special precautions

Adverse Reactions

1% to 10%:

Central nervous system: Headache (2% to 9%), localized burning (<4%), stinging sensation (<2%)
Dermatologic: Pruritus (≤2%), skin rash (≤1%)
Gastrointestinal: Nausea (1% to 5%), dysgeusia (3%)
Local: Local pain (<2%)
Respiratory: Rhinitis (6%), respiratory congestion (5%), pharyngitis (4%), cough (2%)

<1%, postmarketing, and/or case reports: Abdominal pain, aphthous stomatitis, blepharitis, cellulitis, *Clostridioides* (formerly *Clostridium*) *difficile*-associated diarrhea, contact dermatitis, dermatitis, diarrhea, dizziness, epistaxis, erythema, hypersensitivity reaction, increased wound secretion, localized edema, localized tenderness, otalgia, urticaria, wound infection (secondary), xeroderma, xerostomia

Mechanism of Action Binds to bacterial isoleucyl transfer-RNA synthetase resulting in the inhibition of protein synthesis

Pharmacodynamics/Kinetics

Half-life Elimination 17 to 36 minutes

Pregnancy Considerations Systemic absorption following topical application is minimal.

Product Availability Bactroban Nasal has been discontinued in the United States for more than 1 year.

◆ **Mupirocin Calcium** *see* Mupirocin *on page 1066*

◆ **Muse** *see* Alprostadil *on page 110*

◆ **Mutamycin** *see* MitoMYcin (Systemic) *on page 1041*

◆ **Mvasi** *see* Bevacizumab *on page 242*

◆ **Myadec [OTC]** *see* Vitamins (Multiple/Oral) *on page 1550*

◆ **Myalept** *see* Metreleptin *on page 1010*

◆ **Myambutol** *see* Ethambutol *on page 608*

◆ **Mycamine** *see* Micafungin *on page 1018*

◆ **Mycelex** *see* Clotrimazole (Oral) *on page 396*

◆ **Mycobutin** *see* Rifabutin *on page 1323*

◆ **Mycocide Clinical NS [OTC]** *see* Tolnaftate *on page 1462*

◆ **Mycolog-II** *see* Nystatin and Triamcinolone *on page 1123*

Mycophenolate (mye koe FEN oh late)

Brand Names: US CellCept; CellCept Intravenous; Myfortic

Brand Names: Canada ACH-Mycophenolate; APO-Mycophenolate; APO-Mycophenolic Acid; CellCept; CellCept IV; CO Mycophenolate [DSC]; JAMP-Mycophenolate; Myfortic; MYLAN-Mycophenolate [DSC]; SANDOZ Mycophenolate Mofetil; TEVA-Mycophenolate; VAN-Mycophenolate [DSC]

Pharmacologic Category Immunosuppressant Agent

Use Organ transplantation: Prophylaxis of organ rejection in patients receiving allogeneic renal (CellCept [mycophenolate mofetil], Myfortic [enteric-coated mycophenolate sodium]), cardiac (CellCept), or liver (CellCept) transplants, in combination with other immunosuppressants

Note: While traditionally used in combination with cyclosporine, mycophenolate is now used primarily in combination with tacrolimus and, to a lesser extent, with a mammalian target of rapamycin inhibitor (everolimus or sirolimus) for prophylaxis of rejection in renal, cardiac, and hepatic transplants (AASLD [Lucey 2013]; Aliabadi 2012; Eisen 2013; Groetzner 2009; Guethoff 2013; ISHLT [Costanzo 2010]; KDIGO [Chapman 2010]).

Myfortic may also be used to prevent organ rejection in patients receiving cardiac and hepatic transplantations although not labeled for these transplantations (Lehmkuhl 2008; Wang 2015).

Local Anesthetic/Vasoconstrictor Precautions No information available to require special precautions

Effects on Dental Treatment Key adverse event(s) related to dental treatment: Mouth ulceration, gum hyperplasia, gingivitis, dry mouth, dysphagia, oral *Candida* infection, and stomatitis (see Dental Health Professional Considerations)

Effects on Bleeding May be associated with hematologic effects, potentially including significant reduction in platelet counts with altered hemostasis. In patients who are under active treatment, medical consult is suggested.

Adverse Reactions Incidences include concomitant use with cyclosporine and corticosteroids. In general, lower doses used in renal rejection patients had less adverse effects than higher doses. Rates of adverse effects were similar for each indication, except for those unique to the specific organ involved.

>10%:

Cardiovascular: Hypertension (18% to 79%), edema (17% to 68%), hypotension (34%), tachycardia (22% to 23%), lower extremity edema (16%)

Central nervous system: Pain (25% to 79%), headache (11% to 59%), insomnia (24% to 52%), dizziness (34%), depression (20%), chills (3% to <20%), confusion (3% to <20%), drowsiness (3% to <20%), hypertonia (3% to <20%), malaise (3% to <20%), myasthenia (3% to <20%), paresthesia (3% to <20%)

Dermatologic: Skin rash (26%), ecchymoses (20%), cellulitis (3% to <20%)

Endocrine & metabolic: Hyperglycemia (44% to 48%), hypercholesterolemia (46%), hypomagnesemia (20% to 39%), hypokalemia (9% to 37%), hypocalcemia (11% to 30%), increased lactate dehydrogenase (24%), hyperkalemia (22%), acidosis (3% to <20%), weight loss (3% to <20%), hyperuricemia (13%), hyperlipidemia (10% to 12%), hypophosphatemia (9% to 11%)

Gastrointestinal: Abdominal pain (22% to 63%), nausea (27% to 56%), diarrhea (24% to 53%), constipation (38% to 44%), vomiting (20% to 39%), decreased appetite (25%), dyspepsia (19% to 23%), esophagitis (3% to <20%), gastric ulcer (3% to <20%), gastritis (3% to <20%), gastrointestinal hemorrhage (3% to <20%), hernia of abdominal cavity (3% to <20%), intestinal obstruction (3% to <20%), stomatitis (3% to <20%), upper abdominal pain (14%), flatulence (10% to 13%)

Genitourinary: Urinary tract infection (29% to 33%), hematuria (3% to <20%)

Hematologic & oncologic: Leukopenia (19% to 46%), anemia (20% to 45%), leukocytosis (22% to 43%), thrombocytopenia (24% to 38%), benign skin neoplasm (3% to <20%), disorder of hemostatic components of blood (3% to <20%), neoplasm (3% to <20%), pancytopenia (3% to <20%), skin carcinoma (3% to <20%; non-melanoma: 1% to 12%)

Hepatic: Increased liver enzymes (25%), hepatitis (3% to <20%), increased serum alkaline phosphatase (3% to <20%)

Infection: Bacterial infection (27% to 40%), viral infection (31%), cytomegalovirus disease (4% to 22%), fungal infection (11% to 12%)

Neuromuscular & skeletal: Asthenia (35% to 49%), tremor (12% to 34%), back pain (6% to 12%), arthralgia (7% to 11%)

Renal: Increased serum creatinine (10% to 42%), increased blood urea nitrogen (37%)

Respiratory: Dyspnea (31% to 44%), cough (41%), pleural effusion (34%)

Miscellaneous: Fever (13% to 56%)

1% to 10%:

Cardiovascular: Exacerbation of hypertension (<10%), peripheral edema (<10%), phlebitis (4%), thrombosis (4%)

Central nervous system: Anxiety (<10%), fatigue (<10%)

Dermatologic: Acne vulgaris (<10%), pruritus (<10%)

Endocrine & metabolic: Diabetes mellitus (<10%)

Gastrointestinal: Abdominal distension (<10%), gastroesophageal reflux disease (<10%), gingival hyperplasia (<10%), oral candidiasis (<10%)

Genitourinary: Urinary retention (<10%)

Hematologic & oncologic: Lymphocele (<10%), severe neutropenia (2% to 4%), malignant neoplasm (≤2%), malignant lymphoma (1%), lymphoproliferative disorder (≤1%)

Hepatic: Abnormal hepatic function tests (<10%)

Infection: Influenza (<10%), wound infection (<10%), herpes simplex infection (6% to 8%), herpes zoster infection (4% to 5%), sepsis (2% to 5%)

Neuromuscular & skeletal: Muscle cramps (<10%), myalgia (<10%), peripheral pain (<10%)

Ophthalmic: Blurred vision (<10%)

Renal: Renal insufficiency (<10%), renal tubular necrosis (<10%)

Respiratory: Dyspnea on exertion (<10%), nasopharyngitis (<10%), pneumonia (<10%), sinusitis (<10%), upper respiratory tract infection (<10%)

Frequency not defined:

Gastrointestinal: Mucocutaneous candidiasis

Infection: Protozoal infection

Respiratory: Pharyngitis, respiratory tract infection

<1%, postmarketing and/or case reports: Agranulocytosis, alopecia, anorexia, atypical mycobacterial infection, BK virus, bone marrow failure, bronchiectasis (Boddana 2011; Rook 2006), colitis, duodenal ulcer, endocarditis, esophageal ulcer, gastrointestinal perforation, hematemesis, hemorrhagic colitis, hemorrhagic gastritis, hypersensitivity reaction, hypogammaglobulinemia (Boddana 2011; Keven 2003; Robertson 2009), interstitial pulmonary disease, Kaposi sarcoma, lymphadenopathy, lymphopenia, melena, meningitis, osteomyelitis, pancreatitis, peritonitis, polyomavirus infection, progressive multifocal leukoencephalopathy, pulmonary edema, pulmonary fibrosis, pure red cell aplasia, reactivation of disease (HCV), reactivation of HBV, tuberculosis, venous thrombosis, wheezing, xerostomia

Mechanism of Action MPA exhibits a cytostatic effect on T and B lymphocytes. It is an inhibitor of inosine monophosphate dehydrogenase (IMPDH) which inhibits *de novo* guanosine nucleotide synthesis. T and B lymphocytes are dependent on this pathway for proliferation.

Pharmacodynamics/Kinetics

Onset of Action Peak effect: Correlation of toxicity or efficacy is still being developed; however, one study indicated that 12-hour AUCs >40 mcg/mL/hour were correlated with efficacy and decreased episodes of rejection.

Half-life Elimination

CellCept: MPA: Oral: 17.9 ± 6.5 hours; IV: 16.6 ± 5.8 hours

Myfortic: MPA: Oral: 8 to16 hours; MPAG: 13 to 17 hours

Time to Peak Plasma: Oral: MPA:

CellCept: 1 to 1.5 hours

Myfortic: 1.5 to 2.75 hours

Reproductive Considerations

[US Boxed Warning]: Females of reproductive potential must be counseled regarding pregnancy prevention and planning. Pregnancy testing, prevention, and planning must be discussed with all females of reproductive potential and male patients with female partners of reproductive potential. Alternative agents should be used whenever possible in patients planning a pregnancy.

Females of reproductive potential (girls who have entered puberty and women with a uterus who have not passed through clinically confirmed menopause) should have a negative pregnancy test with a sensitivity of ≥25 milliunits/mL immediately before mycophenolate therapy and the test should be repeated 8 to 10 days later. Pregnancy tests should then be repeated during routine follow-up visits. Acceptable forms of contraception should be used during treatment and for 6 weeks after therapy is discontinued. An intrauterine device, tubal sterilization, or vasectomy of the female patient's partner are acceptable contraceptive methods that can be used alone. If a hormonal contraceptive is used (eg, combination oral contraceptive pills, transdermal patches, vaginal rings, or progestin only products), then one barrier method must also be used (eg, diaphragm or cervical cap with spermicide, contraceptive sponge, male or female condom). Alternatively, the use of 2 barrier methods is also acceptable (eg, diaphragm or cervical cap with spermicide, or contraceptive sponge **PLUS** male or female condom). Refer to manufacturer's labeling for full details. The effectiveness of hormonal contraceptive agents may be affected by mycophenolate.

Mycophenolate has been used as an immunosuppressant in patients undergoing uterine transplant (limited data); mycophenolate is discontinued and changed to a different agent prior to embryo transfer (Jones 2019).

Mycophenolate should be discontinued, and therapy changed to an appropriate immunosuppressant prior to conception in kidney, liver, and heart transplant recipients who are planning a pregnancy (AASLD [Lucey 2013]); EBPG 2002; ISHLT [Costanzo 2010]; KDIGO 2009; López 2014). Mycophenolate should also be discontinued prior to conception in females treated for other indications who are planning a pregnancy. The Risk Evaluation and Mitigation Strategy (REMS) program recommends discontinuing mycophenolate in females at least 6 weeks before pregnancy is attempted. However, due to the potential for disease flare following discontinuation, women treated for rheumatic and musculoskeletal diseases should consider discontinuing mycophenolate 3 to 6 months prior to attempted pregnancy to allow for disease monitoring and potential change to another immunosuppressant (ACR [Sammaritano 2020]). Women taking mycophenolate for myasthenia gravis are recommended to discontinue therapy at least 4 months prior to planning a pregnancy (Sanders 2016).

When mycophenolate is used for the treatment of rheumatic and musculoskeletal diseases in women undergoing ovarian stimulation for oocyte retrieval or embryo cryopreservation, mycophenolate may be continued in patients whose condition is stable and discontinuation of treatment may lead to uncontrolled disease (ACR [Sammaritano 2020]).

Information related to the mycophenolate and male fertility or pregnancy outcomes following paternal use is limited; however, available data have not suggested safety concerns (Bermas 2019; Mouyis 2019). According to the manufacturer, sexually active male patients and/or their female partners should use effective contraception during treatment of the male patient and for at least 90 days after last dose. In addition, males should not donate semen during mycophenolate therapy and for 90 days following the last mycophenolate dose (recommendation based on animal data). However, use of mycophenolate may be considered for males with rheumatic and musculoskeletal diseases who are planning to father a child (recommendation based on limited human data) (ACR [Sammaritano 2020]; Midtvedt 2017).

Pregnancy Considerations

[US Boxed Warning]: Use during pregnancy is associated with increased risks of first trimester pregnancy loss and congenital malformations. Avoid if safer treatment options are available.

Congenital malformations have been reported in 23% to 27% of live births following exposure to mycophenolate during pregnancy. Birth defects include facial malformations (cleft lip, cleft palate, micrognathia, hypertelorism of the orbits); ear and eye abnormalities (abnormally formed or absent external/middle ear, coloboma, microphthalmos); finger malformations (brachydactyly, polydactyly, syndactyly); cardiac abnormalities (atrial and ventricular septal defects); esophageal malformations (esophageal atresia); and CNS malformations (spina bifida). The combination of ear, eye, and lip/palate abnormalities has been identified as mycophenolate embryopathy (Perez-Aytes 2017). The risk of first trimester pregnancy loss may be 45% to 49% following mycophenolate exposure.

Mycophenolate is not an acceptable immunosuppressant for use in patients who become pregnant following a kidney (EBPG 2002; KDIGO 2009; López 2014), liver (AASLD [Lucey 2013]), or heart (ISHLT [Costanzo 2010]) transplant. In addition, mycophenolate should not be used for the treatment of autoimmune hepatitis (AASLD [Mack 2019]), myasthenia gravis (Sanders 2016), lupus nephritis (ACR [Hahn 2012]; EULAR/ERA-EDTA [Bertsias 2012]) or rheumatic and musculoskeletal diseases (ACR [Sammaritano 2020]) during pregnancy.

Data collection to monitor pregnancy and infant outcomes following exposure to mycophenolate is ongoing. Health care providers should report female exposures to mycophenolate during pregnancy or within 6 weeks of discontinuing therapy to the Mycophenolate Pregnancy Registry (800-617-8191).

The Transplant Pregnancy Registry International (TPR) is a registry that follows pregnancies that occur in maternal transplant recipients or those fathered by male transplant recipients. The TPR encourages reporting of pregnancies following solid organ transplant by contacting them at 1-877-955-6877 or https://www.transplantpregnancyregistry.org.

Dental Health Professional Considerations Consider a medical consultation prior to any invasive dental procedure in patients who have received an organ transplant; delayed wound healing due to the immunosuppressive effects and an increased potential for postoperative infection may be of concern.

- **Mycophenolate Mofetil** *see* Mycophenolate *on page 1067*
- **Mycophenolate Sodium** *see* Mycophenolate *on page 1067*
- **Mycophenolic Acid** *see* Mycophenolate *on page 1067*
- **Mydayis** *see* Dextroamphetamine and Amphetamine *on page 475*
- **Mydriacyl** *see* Tropicamide *on page 1502*
- **Myfortic** *see* Mycophenolate *on page 1067*
- **Mylotarg** *see* Gemtuzumab Ozogamicin *on page 734*
- **Myobloc** *see* RimabotulinumtoxinB *on page 1328*
- **Myorisan** *see* ISOtretinoin (Systemic) *on page 846*
- **Myrbetriq** *see* Mirabegron *on page 1038*
- **Mysoline** *see* Primidone *on page 1276*
- **Mytotan** *see* Mitotane *on page 1041*
- **Myxredlin** *see* Insulin Regular *on page 829*
- **Myzilra [DSC]** *see* Ethinyl Estradiol and Levonorgestrel *on page 612*
- **N-0923** *see* Rotigotine *on page 1349*
- **Nabi-HB** *see* Hepatitis B Immune Globulin (Human) *on page 756*
- **Nabiximols** *see* Tetrahydrocannabinol and Cannabidiol *on page 1434*
- **nab-Paclitaxel** *see* PACLitaxel (Protein Bound) *on page 1179*

Nabumetone (na BYOO me tone)

Related Information

Rheumatoid Arthritis, Osteoarthritis, and Osteoporosis *on page 1697*

Temporomandibular Dysfunction (TMD), Chronic Pain, and Fibromyalgia *on page 1773*

Brand Names: US Relafen DS

Brand Names: Canada MYLAN-Nabumetone [DSC]; NU-Nabumetone [DSC]; PMS-Nabumetone [DSC]; TEVA-Nabumetone [DSC]

Pharmacologic Category Analgesic, Nonopioid; Nonsteroidal Anti-inflammatory Drug (NSAID), Oral

Use Arthritis: Relief of signs and symptoms of osteoarthritis and rheumatoid arthritis.

Local Anesthetic/Vasoconstrictor Precautions
No information available to require special precautions

Effects on Dental Treatment Key adverse event(s) related to dental treatment: Xerostomia (normal salivary flow resumes upon discontinuation) and stomatitis. The dentist should be aware of the potential of abnormal coagulation. Caution should also be exercised in the use of NSAIDs in patients already on anticoagulant therapy with drugs such as warfarin (Coumadin®). See Effects on Bleeding.

Effects on Bleeding Nonselective NSAIDs, such as nabumetone, inhibit platelet aggregation and prolong bleeding time in some patients. Unlike aspirin, the NSAID effect on platelet function is quantitatively less, of shorter duration, and reversible. Normal platelet function should occur in ~5 elimination half-lives or in <10 hours after discontinuation of nabumetone. Concomitant use of other NSAIDs should be avoided.

Adverse Reactions

>10%: Gastrointestinal: Diarrhea (14%), dyspepsia (13%), abdominal pain (12%)

1% to 10%:

Cardiovascular: Edema (3% to 9%)

Central nervous system: Dizziness (3% to 9%), headache (3% to 9%), drowsiness (1% to 3%), fatigue (1% to 3%), insomnia (1% to 3%), nervousness (1% to 3%)

Dermatologic: Pruritus (3% to 9%), skin rash (3% to 9%), diaphoresis (1% to 3%)

Gastrointestinal: Constipation (3% to 9%), flatulence (3% to 9%), nausea (3% to 9%), occult blood in stools (3% to 9%), gastritis (1% to 3%), stomatitis (1% to 3%), vomiting (1% to 3%), xerostomia (1% to 3%)

Otic: Tinnitus

<1%, postmarketing, and/or case reports: Acne vulgaris, agitation, albuminuria, alopecia, anaphylactoid reaction, anaphylaxis, anemia, angina pectoris, angioedema, anorexia, anxiety, asthma, azotemia, bullous rash, cardiac arrhythmia, cardiac failure, chills, cholelithiasis, confusion, cough, depression, duodenal ulcer, duodenitis, dysphagia, dyspnea, dysuria, eosinophilic pneumonitis, eructation, fever, erythema multiforme, gastric ulcer, gastroenteritis, gastrointestinal hemorrhage, gingivitis, glossitis, granulocytopenia, hematuria, hepatic failure, hepatic insufficiency, hepatotoxicity (idiosyncratic) (Chalasani, 2014), hyperbilirubinemia, hyperglycemia, hypersensitivity pneumonitis, hypertension, hyperuricemia, hypokalemia, impotence, interstitial nephritis, interstitial pneumonitis, jaundice, leukopenia, malaise, melena, myocardial infarction, nephrolithiasis, nephrotic syndrome, nightmares, palpitations, pancreatitis, paresthesia, pseudoporphyria (cutanea tarda), rectal

hemorrhage, renal failure, skin photosensitivity, Stevens-Johnson syndrome, syncope, taste disorder, thrombocytopenia, thrombophlebitis, toxic epidermal necrolysis, tremor, urticaria, vasculitis, vertigo, visual disturbance, weakness, weight gain, weight loss

Mechanism of Action Reversibly inhibits cyclooxygenase-1 and 2 (COX-1 and 2) enzymes, which results in decreased formation of prostaglandin precursors; has antipyretic, analgesic, and anti-inflammatory properties

Other proposed mechanisms not fully elucidated (and possibly contributing to the anti-inflammatory effect to varying degrees), include inhibiting chemotaxis, altering lymphocyte activity, inhibiting neutrophil aggregation/activation, and decreasing proinflammatory cytokine levels.

Pharmacodynamics/Kinetics

Half-life Elimination 6MNA: ~24 hours; terminal half-life was increased ~50% in patients with CrCl 30 to 49 mL/minute

Time to Peak Serum: 6MNA: Oral: Adults: 2.5 to 3 hours; Elderly: 4 hours

Reproductive Considerations

The chronic use of NSAIDs in women of reproductive age may be associated with infertility that is reversible upon discontinuation of the medication (Micu 2011).

Pregnancy Risk Factor C

Pregnancy Considerations Birth defects have been observed following in utero NSAID exposure in some studies; however, data is conflicting (Bloor 2013). Nonteratogenic effects, including prenatal constriction of the ductus arteriosus, persistent pulmonary hypertension of the newborn, oligohydramnios, necrotizing enterocolitis, renal dysfunction or failure, and intracranial hemorrhage have been observed in the fetus/neonate following in utero NSAID exposure. In addition, non-closure of the ductus arteriosus postnatally may occur and be resistant to medical management (Bermas 2014; Bloor 2013). Because they may cause premature closure of the ductus arteriosus, the use of NSAIDs late in pregnancy should be avoided. Use of NSAIDs can be considered for the treatment of mild rheumatoid arthritis flares in pregnant women; however, use should be minimized or avoided early and late in pregnancy (Bermas 2014; Saavedra Salinas 2015).

The use of NSAIDs close to conception may be associated with an increased risk of miscarriage (Bermas 2014; Bloor 2013).

- ◆ **N-acetylgalactosamine-6-sulfatase** *see* Elosulfase Alfa *on page 550*
- ◆ **N-Acetyl-P-Aminophenol** *see* Acetaminophen *on page 59*

Nadolol (NAY doe lol)

Related Information

Cardiovascular Diseases *on page 1654*

Brand Names: US Corgard

Brand Names: Canada TEVA-Nadolol [DSC]

Pharmacologic Category Antianginal Agent; Antihypertensive; Beta-Blocker, Nonselective

Use

Angina: Treatment of angina pectoris

Hypertension: Management of hypertension. **Note:** Beta-blockers are **not** recommended as first-line therapy (ACC/AHA [Whelton 2017]).

Local Anesthetic/Vasoconstrictor Precautions Use with caution; epinephrine has interacted with nonselective beta-blockers to result in initial hypertensive episode followed by bradycardia

Effects on Dental Treatment Nadolol is a nonselective beta-blocker and may enhance the pressor response to epinephrine, resulting in hypertension and bradycardia. Many nonsteroidal anti-inflammatory drugs, such as ibuprofen and indomethacin, can reduce the hypotensive effect of beta-blockers after 3 or more weeks of therapy with the NSAID. Short-term NSAID use (ie, 3 days) requires no special precautions in patients taking beta-blockers.

Effects on Bleeding No information available to require special precautions

Adverse Reactions

>10%: Central nervous system: Drowsiness, insomnia

1% to 10%:

Cardiovascular: Atrioventricular block, bradycardia, cardiac conduction disturbance, cardiac failure, cold extremities, edema, hypotension, palpitations, peripheral vascular insufficiency, Raynaud's phenomenon

Central nervous system: Depression, dizziness, fatigue, sedation

<1%, postmarketing, and/or case reports: Abdominal distress, anorexia, behavioral changes, bloating, blurred vision, bronchospasm, cardiac arrhythmia, chest pain, confusion (especially in the elderly), constipation, cough, decreased libido, diaphoresis, diarrhea, dyspepsia, dyspnea, facial edema, flatulence, hallucination, headache, impotence, nasal congestion, nausea, nervousness, paresthesia, pruritus, skin rash, slurred speech, thrombocytopenia, tinnitus, transient alopecia, vomiting, weight gain, xeroderma, xerophthalmia, xerostomia

Mechanism of Action Competitively blocks response to $beta_1$- and $beta_2$-adrenergic stimulation; does not exhibit any membrane stabilizing or intrinsic sympathomimetic activity. Nonselective beta-adrenergic blockers (propranolol, nadolol) reduce portal pressure by producing splanchnic vasoconstriction ($beta_2$ effect) thereby reducing portal blood flow.

Pharmacodynamics/Kinetics

Duration of Action 17 to 24 hours

Half-life Elimination

Infants 3 to 22 months (n=3): 3.2 to 4.3 hours (Mehta 1992)

Children 10 years (n=1): 15.7 hours (Mehta 1992)

Children ~15 years (n=1): 7.3 hours (Mehta 1992)

Adults: 20 to 24 hours; prolonged with renal impairment; (up to 45 hours in severe impairment) (Herrera 1979)

Time to Peak Serum: 3 to 4 hours

Pregnancy Considerations

Exposure to beta-blockers during pregnancy may increase the risk for adverse events in the neonate. If maternal use of a beta-blocker is needed, fetal growth should be monitored during pregnancy and the newborn should be monitored for 48 hours after delivery for bradycardia, hypoglycemia, and respiratory depression (ESC [Regitz-Zagrosek 2018]).

Chronic maternal hypertension is also associated with adverse events in the fetus/infant. Chronic maternal hypertension may increase the risk of birth defects, low birth weight, premature delivery, stillbirth, and neonatal death. Actual fetal/neonatal risks may be related to duration and severity of maternal hypertension. Untreated chronic hypertension may also increase the risks of adverse maternal outcomes, including gestational diabetes, preeclampsia, delivery complications, stroke, and myocardial infarction (ACOG 203 2019).

When treatment of chronic hypertension in pregnancy is indicated, agents other than nadolol are preferred (ACOG 203 2019; ESC [Regitz-Zagrosek 2018]; Magee 2014). Females with preexisting hypertension may continue their medication during pregnancy unless contraindications exist (ESC [Regitz-Zagrosek 2018])

Nadroparin (nad roe PA rin)

Related Information

Cardiovascular Diseases *on page* 1654

Brand Names: Canada Fraxiparine; Fraxiparine Forte

Pharmacologic Category Anticoagulant; Anticoagulant, Low Molecular Weight Heparin

Use

Note: Not approved in the US

Fraxiparine:

Acute coronary syndromes: Treatment of unstable angina and non-ST-elevation myocardial infarction (NSTEMI) myocardial infarction (ie, non-Q wave MI)

Anticoagulation during hemodialysis: Prevention of clotting during hemodialysis

Deep vein thrombosis: Treatment of deep vein thrombosis (DVT). **Note:** In patients with venous thromboembolism (VTE) (ie, DVT or PE) and *without* cancer, oral anticoagulants are preferred over LMWH (unless LMWH is used as initial parenteral anticoagulation prior to dabigatran, edoxaban, or while initiating warfarin). In patients with venous thromboembolism (VTE) (ie, DVT or PE) **and** cancer, ACCP recommends LMWH over oral anticoagulants for initial and long-term treatment (Kearon 2012; Kearon 2016).

Thromboprophylaxis: Prophylaxis of thromboembolic disorders (particularly DVT and pulmonary embolism [PE]) in general and orthopedic surgery, high-risk medical patients (respiratory failure and/or respiratory infection and/or cardiac failure) immobilized due to acute illness or hospitalized in ICU

Fraxiparine Forte: Treatment of deep vein thrombosis (DVT)

Local Anesthetic/Vasoconstrictor Precautions

No information available to require special precautions

Effects on Dental Treatment Key adverse event(s) related to dental treatment: Bleeding is the major adverse effect of nadroparin. See Effects on Bleeding.

Effects on Bleeding As with all anticoagulants, bleeding is the major adverse effect of nadroparin. Hemorrhage may occur at virtually any site; risk is dependent on multiple variables including the intensity of anticoagulation and patient susceptibility. At the recommended doses, LMWHS do not significantly influence platelet aggregation or affect global clotting time (ie, PT or aPTT). Medical consult is suggested.

Adverse Reactions As with all anticoagulants, bleeding is the major adverse effect of nadroparin. Hemorrhage may occur at virtually any site. Risk is dependent on multiple variables.

Frequency not defined:

Cardiovascular: Arterial thrombosis, thromboembolism, venous thrombosis

Dermatologic: Skin necrosis

Endocrine & metabolic: Calcinosis, hypoaldosteronism (causing hyperkalemia and/or hyponatremia)

Genitourinary: Priapism

Hematological & oncologic: Eosinophilia, hemorrhage, thrombocythemia, thrombocytopenia

Hepatic: Increased serum alanine aminotransferase, increased serum aspartate aminotransferase

Hypersensitivity: Angioedema, hypersensitivity reaction, nonimmune anaphylaxis

Local: Hematoma at injection site, injection site reaction

Neuromuscular & skeletal: Osteopenia

Postmarketing: Erythema of skin, headache, migraine, pruritus, skin rash, urticaria

Mechanism of Action Nadroparin is a low molecular weight heparin (LMWH) (average molecular weight is ~4,300 daltons, distributed as 2,000 to 8,000 daltons [75% to 85%]) that binds antithrombin III, enhancing the inhibition of several clotting factors, particularly factor Xa. Nadroparin anti-Xa activity (85 to 110 units/mg) is greater than anti-IIa activity (~27 units/mg) and it has a higher ratio of antifactor Xa to antifactor IIa activity compared to unfractionated heparin. LMWHs have a small effect on the activated partial thromboplastin time.

Pharmacodynamics/Kinetics

Duration of Action Anti-Xa activity: ≥18 hours

Half-life Elimination ~3.5 hours (prolonged in renal impairment)

Time to Peak Serum: SubQ: 3 to 6 hours

Reproductive Considerations

Prophylaxis with LMWH is not routinely recommended for women undergoing assisted reproduction therapy; however, LMWH therapy is recommended for women who develop severe ovarian hyperstimulation syndrome. For women who require long-term anticoagulation with warfarin and who are considering pregnancy, LMWH substitution should be done prior to conception when possible. When choosing therapy, fetal outcomes (ie, pregnancy loss, malformations), maternal outcomes (ie, VTE, hemorrhage), burden of therapy, and maternal preference should be considered (Bates 2012; Linnemann 2016).

Pregnancy Considerations Information related to placental transfer is limited.

Prosthetic valve thrombosis has been reported in patients receiving thromboprophylaxis therapy with low-molecular-weight heparins (LMWHs); pregnant women may be at increased risk. LMWH is recommended over unfractionated heparin for the treatment of acute venous thromboembolism (VTE) in pregnant women. LMWH is also recommended over unfractionated heparin for VTE prophylaxis in pregnant women with certain risk factors (eg, homozygous factor V Leiden, antiphospholipid antibody syndrome with ≥3 previous pregnancy losses). LMWH should be discontinued ≥24 hours prior to induction of labor or a planned cesarean delivery. For women undergoing cesarean section and who have additional risk factors for developing VTE, the prophylactic use of LMWH may be considered. When choosing LMWH therapy, fetal outcomes (ie, pregnancy loss, malformations), maternal outcomes (ie, VTE, hemorrhage), burden of therapy, and maternal preference should be considered (Bates 2012; Linnemann 2016).

Product Availability Not available in the US

◆ **Nadroparin Calcium** *see* Nadroparin *on page* 1071

Nafarelin (naf a REL in)

Brand Names: US Synarel

Brand Names: Canada Synarel

Pharmacologic Category Gonadotropin Releasing Hormone Agonist

Use

Central precocious puberty: Treatment of central precocious puberty (CPP) (gonadotropin-dependent precocious puberty) in children of both sexes.

Endometriosis: Management of endometriosis, including pain relief and reduction of endometriotic lesions.

Local Anesthetic/Vasoconstrictor Precautions No information available to require special precautions

Effects on Dental Treatment No significant effects or complications reported

Effects on Bleeding No information available to require special precautions

Adverse Reactions Adverse events may be more frequent in the first 6 weeks of treatment due to stimulation of the pituitary-gonadal axis.

CPP: 1% to 10%:

- Central nervous system: Emotional lability (6%)
- Dermatologic: Acne vulgaris (10%), hypertrichosis (transient, pubic region: 5%), body odor (4%), seborrhea (3%)
- Endocrine & metabolic: Breast hypertrophy (8%; transient), vaginal hemorrhage (8%), hot flashes (3%; transient), vaginal discharge (3%)
- Hypersensitivity: Hypersensitivity reaction (3%; including chest pain, pruritus, dyspnea, skin rash)
- Respiratory: Rhinitis (5%)

Endometriosis:

>10%:

- Central nervous system: Headache (18%), emotional lability (16%)
- Dermatologic: Acne vulgaris (14%)
- Endocrine & metabolic: Hot flash (90%), decreased libido (23%), hyperphosphatemia (10% to 15%), hypocalcemia (10% to 15%), hypertriglyceridemia (12%)
- Genitourinary: Vaginal dryness (19%)
- Hematologic & oncologic: Change in WBC count (10% to 15%; decreased), eosinophilia (10% to 15%)

1% to 10%:

- Cardiovascular: Edema (8%)
- Central nervous system: Insomnia (8%), depression (3%)
- Dermatologic: Hirsutism (3%)
- Endocrine & metabolic: Breast atrophy (10%), hypercholesterolemia (6%), increased libido (2%)
- Gastrointestinal: Weight gain (8%), weight loss (2%)
- Neuromuscular & skeletal: Myalgia (10%), decreased bone mineral density
- Respiratory: Nasal mucosa irritation (10%)

<1%, postmarketing, and/or case reports (any indication): Arterial thromboembolism, arthralgia, breast engorgement, chloasma, eye pain, hepatic injury, increased serum ALT, increased serum AST, lactation, maculopapular rash, palpitations, paresthesia, pituitary apoplexy, seizures, venous thromboembolism, weakness

Mechanism of Action Potent synthetic decapeptide analogue of gonadotropin-releasing hormone (GnRH; LHRH) which is approximately 200 times more potent than GnRH in terms of pituitary release of luteinizing hormone (LH) and follicle-stimulating hormone (FSH). Effects on the pituitary gland and sex hormones are dependent upon its length of administration. After acute administration, an initial stimulation of the release of LH and FSH from the pituitary is observed; an increase in androgens and estrogens subsequently follows. Continued administration of nafarelin, however, suppresses gonadotrope responsiveness to endogenous GnRH resulting in reduced secretion of LH and FSH and, secondarily, decreased ovarian and testicular steroid production.

Pharmacodynamics/Kinetics

Half-life Elimination ~3 hours; Metabolites: ~86 hours

Time to Peak Serum: 10 to 45 minutes

Reproductive Considerations

Use is contraindicated in women who may become pregnant during therapy and pregnancy should be excluded prior to initiating treatment.

Ovulation is inhibited and menstruation is stopped when used appropriately for the treatment of endometriosis, however contraception is not assured. Nonhormonal contraception is recommended. There is no evidence that pregnancy rates are enhanced or adversely affected by use.

Pregnancy Considerations Use is contraindicated in pregnant women.

◆ **Nafarelin Acetate** *see* Nafarelin *on page* 1071

Naftifine (NAF ti feen)

Brand Names: US Naftin

Pharmacologic Category Antifungal Agent, Topical

Use

Tinea infections: Cream 1% and 2%, Gel 1%: Topical treatment of tinea cruris (jock itch), tinea corporis (ringworm), and tinea pedis (athlete's foot).

Tinea pedis: Gel 2%: Topical treatment of tinea pedis (athlete's foot).

Local Anesthetic/Vasoconstrictor Precautions No information available to require special precautions

Effects on Dental Treatment No significant effects or complications reported

Effects on Bleeding No information available to require special precautions

Adverse Reactions

1% to 10%:

- Dermatologic: Burning sensation of skin (5% to 6%), xeroderma (3%), skin irritation (2%), erythema (≤2%), pruritus (1% to 2%)
- Local: Application site reaction (2%)

<1%, postmarketing, and/or case reports: Agranulocytosis, crusted skin, dizziness, headache, inflammation, leukopenia, maceration, pain, rash, serous drainage, skin blister, skin tenderness, swelling of skin

Mechanism of Action Synthetic, broad-spectrum antifungal agent in the allylamine class; appears to have both fungistatic and fungicidal activity. Exhibits antifungal activity by selectively inhibiting the enzyme squalene epoxidase in a dose-dependent manner which results in a reduced synthesis of ergosterol, the primary sterol within the fungal membrane, and increased squalene in cells.

Pharmacodynamics/Kinetics

Half-life Elimination 2 to 3 days

Pregnancy Considerations Naftifine is absorbed systemically (4% to 6%) following topical administration. Application over a limited area is considered likely acceptable during pregnancy (Patel 2017).

◆ **Naftifine HCl** *see* Naftifine *on page* 1072
◆ **Naftifine Hydrochloride** *see* Naftifine *on page* 1072
◆ **Naftin** *see* Naftifine *on page* 1072

Nalbuphine (NAL byoo feen)

Brand Names: Canada Nubain

Pharmacologic Category Analgesic, Opioid; Analgesic, Opioid Partial Agonist

Use

Pain management: Management of pain severe enough to require an opioid analgesic and for which alternative treatments are inadequate.

Limitations of use: Reserve nalbuphine for use in patients for whom alternative treatment options (eg, nonopioid analgesics) are ineffective, not tolerated, or would be otherwise inadequate to provide sufficient management of pain.

Surgical anesthesia supplement: Supplement to balanced anesthesia, for preoperative and postoperative analgesia, and for obstetrical analgesia during labor and delivery.

Local Anesthetic/Vasoconstrictor Precautions
No information available to require special precautions

Effects on Dental Treatment Key adverse event(s) related to dental treatment: Xerostomia and changes in salivation (normal salivary flow resumes upon discontinuation). Anticholinergic side effects can cause a reduction of saliva production or secretion, contributing to discomfort and dental disease (ie, caries, oral candidiasis, and periodontal disease).

Effects on Bleeding No information available to require special precautions

Adverse Reactions

>10%: Central nervous system: Sedation (36%)

1% to 10%:

Central nervous system: Dizziness (5%), headache (3%)

Dermatologic: Cold and clammy skin (9%)

Gastrointestinal: Nausea and vomiting (6%), xerostomia (4%)

<1%, postmarketing, and/or case reports: Abdominal pain, abnormal dreams, agitation, anaphylactoid reaction, anaphylaxis, anxiety, asthma, bitter taste, blurred vision, bradycardia, burning sensation, cardiac arrest, confusion, crying, delusions, depersonalization, depression, derealization, diaphoresis, drowsiness, dyspepsia, dysphoria, euphoria, fever, floating feeling, flushing, hallucination, hostility, hypersensitivity reaction, hypertension, hypogonadism (Brennan 2013; Debono 2011), hypotension, injection site reaction (pain, swelling, redness, burning), intestinal cramps, laryngeal edema, loss of consciousness, nervousness, numbness, pruritus, pulmonary edema, respiratory depression, respiratory distress, restlessness, seizure, skin rash, speech disturbance, stridor, tachycardia, tingling sensation, tremor, urinary urgency, urticaria

Mechanism of Action Agonist of kappa opiate receptors and partial antagonist of mu opiate receptors in the CNS, causing inhibition of ascending pain pathways, altering the perception of and response to pain; produces generalized CNS depression

Pharmacodynamics/Kinetics

Onset of Action Peak effect: SubQ, IM: <15 minutes; IV: 2 to 3 minutes

Duration of Action 3 to 6 hours

Half-life Elimination

Children: 0.9 to 3.5 hours; however, overall trend observed is longer half-life as age increases (Bressolle 2011; Jaillon 1989)

Adults: 5 hours

Reproductive Considerations
Long-term opioid use may cause secondary hypogonadism, which may lead to sexual dysfunction or infertility in men and women (Brennan 2013).

Pregnancy Considerations Nalbuphine crosses the placenta.

Nalbuphine concentrations in cord blood may be similar to or greater than the maternal serum concentrations. Elimination by the newborn may be delayed due to a longer half-life (Nicolle 1996; Wilson 1986).

Opioids used as part of obstetric analgesia/anesthesia during labor and delivery may temporarily affect the fetal heart rate (ACOG 209 2019). Severe bradycardia (which may be prolonged and result in neurologic damage), respiratory depression, apnea, cyanosis, and hypotonia have been reported in the fetus and newborn following exposure during labor. A sinusoidal fetal heart rate pattern has also been reported. Newborns should be monitored closely; naloxone may reverse some of these effects.

If chronic opioid exposure occurs in pregnancy, adverse events in the newborn (including withdrawal) may occur; monitoring of the neonate is recommended. The minimum effective dose should be used if opioids are needed (Chou 2009). Neonatal abstinence syndrome following opioid exposure may present with autonomic (eg, fever, temperature instability), gastrointestinal (eg, diarrhea, vomiting, poor feeding/weight gain), or neurologic (eg, high-pitched crying, increased muscle tone, irritability, seizure, tremor) symptoms (Dow 2012; Hudak 2012).

Nalbuphine is approved for use in obstetrical analgesia during labor and delivery. Nalbuphine has also been evaluated for the management of opioid-induced pruritus following neuraxial analgesia/anesthesia in women who have had cesarean deliveries (ACOG 209 2019; Jannuzzi 2016; Tubog 2019).

◆ **Nalbuphine HCl** *see* Nalbuphine *on page 1073*

◆ **Nalbuphine Hydrochloride** *see* Nalbuphine *on page 1073*

Naldemedine (nal DEM e deen)

Brand Names: US Symproic

Pharmacologic Category Gastrointestinal Agent, Miscellaneous; Opioid Antagonist, Peripherally-Acting

Use Opioid-induced constipation: Treatment of opioid-induced constipation (OIC) in adults with chronic noncancer pain, including patients with chronic pain related to prior cancer or its treatment who do not require frequent (eg, weekly) opioid dosage escalation.

Local Anesthetic/Vasoconstrictor Precautions
No information available to require special precautions

Effects on Dental Treatment No significant effects or complications reported

Effects on Bleeding No information available to require special precautions

Adverse Reactions

>10%:

Gastrointestinal: Abdominal pain (8%), diarrhea (7%)

1% to 10%:

Gastrointestinal: Nausea (4%), vomiting (3%), gastroenteritis (2%)

<1%, postmarketing, and/or case reports: Hypersensitivity reaction

Mechanism of Action Opioid antagonist that blocks opioid binding at the mu, delta, and kappa receptors; functions as a peripherally acting mu-opioid receptor antagonist, including actions on the GI tract to inhibit the delay in GI transit time, thereby decreasing the constipating effects of opioids.

Pharmacodynamics/Kinetics

Half-life Elimination 11 hours

Time to Peak 0.75 hours; 2.5 hours (with food)

Pregnancy Considerations Adverse events were observed in some animal reproduction studies. Based on animal data, naldemedine may cross the placenta and cause opioid withdrawal in the fetus if administered during pregnancy.

◆ **Naldemedine Tosylate** *see* Naldemedine *on page 1073*

◆ **Nalfon** *see* Fenoprofen *on page 642*

◆ ***N*-allylnoroxymorphine Hydrochloride** *see* Naloxone *on page 1074*

Naloxegol (nal OX ee gol)

Brand Names: US Movantik

Brand Names: Canada Movantik

Pharmacologic Category Gastrointestinal Agent, Miscellaneous; Opioid Antagonist, Peripherally-Acting

Use Opioid-induced constipation: Treatment of opioid-induced constipation (OIC) in adults with chronic noncancer pain, including patients with chronic pain related to prior cancer or its treatment who do not require frequent (eg, weekly) opioid dosage escalation.

Local Anesthetic/Vasoconstrictor Precautions No information available to require special precautions

Effects on Dental Treatment No significant effects or complications reported

Effects on Bleeding No information available to require special precautions

Adverse Reactions

>10%: Gastrointestinal: Abdominal pain (12% to 21%)

1% to 10%:

Central nervous system: Headache (4%), opioid withdrawal syndrome (1% to 3%)

Dermatologic: Hyperhidrosis (3%)

Gastrointestinal: Diarrhea (6% to 9%), nausea (7% to 8%), flatulence (6%), vomiting (5%)

<1%, postmarketing, and/or case reports: Angioedema, skin rash, urticaria

Mechanism of Action Naloxegol is a mu-opioid receptor antagonist. It is composed of naloxone conjugated with a polyethylene glycol polymer, which limits its ability to cross the blood-brain barrier. When administered at the recommended dose, naloxegol functions peripherally in tissues such as the GI tract, thereby decreasing the constipation associated with opioids (Webster, 2013).

Pharmacodynamics/Kinetics

Half-life Elimination 6 to 11 hours

Time to Peak <2 hours; in majority of subjects, a secondary C_{max} occurs ~0.4 to 3 hours after the first C_{max}

Pregnancy Considerations Adverse events were not observed in animal reproduction studies. However, exposure during pregnancy may potentiate opioid withdrawal in the fetus.

◆ **Naloxegol Oxalate** *see* Naloxegol *on page 1074*

Naloxone (nal OKS one)

Brand Names: US Evzio; Narcan

Brand Names: Canada Narcan; S.O.S. Naloxone Hydrochloride

Generic Availability (US) May be product dependent

Pharmacologic Category Antidote; Opioid Antagonist

Dental Use Reverse overdose effects of the two opioid agents, fentanyl and meperidine, used in the technique of IV conscious sedation

Use

Opioid overdose: For the complete or partial reversal of opioid depression (including respiratory depression) induced by natural and synthetic opioids (eg, propoxyphene, methadone, nalbuphine, butorphanol, pentazocine). Naloxone is also indicated for the diagnosis of suspected or known acute opioid overdosage.

Evzio (IM, SubQ), intranasal: For the emergency treatment of known or suspected opioid overdose as manifested by respiratory and/or CNS depression. Intended for immediate administration as emergency therapy in settings where opioids may be present. Not a substitute for emergency medical care.

Local Anesthetic/Vasoconstrictor Precautions No information available to require special precautions

Effects on Dental Treatment No significant effects or complications reported

Effects on Bleeding No information available to require special precautions

Adverse Reactions

Cardiovascular: Flushing (parenteral), hypertension, hypotension, tachycardia, ventricular fibrillation, ventricular tachycardia

Central nervous system: Agitation, body pain, brain disease, coma, confusion (parenteral), disorientation (parenteral), dizziness (parenteral), excessive crying (neonates), hallucination (parenteral), headache (nasal), hyperreflexia (neonates), irritability, nervousness, outbursts of anger (parenteral), paresthesia (parenteral), restlessness, seizure (neonates), shivering, tonic-clonic seizures (parenteral), withdrawal syndrome, yawning

Dermatologic: Diaphoresis, piloerection, xeroderma (nasal)

Endocrine & metabolic: Hot flash (parenteral)

Gastrointestinal: Abdominal cramps, constipation (nasal), diarrhea, nausea, toothache (nasal), vomiting

Local: Erythema at injection site (parenteral), injection site reaction

Neuromuscular & skeletal: Muscle spasm (nasal), musculoskeletal pain (nasal), tremor, weakness

Respiratory: Dry nose (nasal), dyspnea, hypoxia (parenteral), nasal congestion (nasal), nasal discomfort (pain; nasal), nasal mucosa swelling (nasal), pulmonary edema, respiratory depression (parenteral), rhinitis (nasal), rhinorrhea, sneezing

Miscellaneous: Fever

Dental Usual Dosage Opioid overdose: Adults: IV: 0.4 to 2 mg every 2 to 3 minutes as needed; may need to repeat doses every 20 to 60 minutes, if no response is observed after 10 mg, question the diagnosis. **Note:** Use 0.1 to 0.2 mg increments in patients who are opioid dependent and in postoperative patients to avoid large cardiovascular changes.

Dosing

Adult & Geriatric Note: Available routes of administration include IV (preferred), IM, SubQ, and intranasal; other available routes (off-label) include inhalation via nebulization (adults only), and intraosseous (IO). Endotracheal administration is the least desirable and is supported by only anecdotal evidence (case report) (AHA [Neumar 2010]):

Opioid overdose:

Note: For the initial treatment of an opioid-associated life-threatening emergency, the American Heart Association recommends, after initiation of CPR, the use of intranasal or IM naloxone with a repeat dose as needed. If there is an initial patient response (ie, purposeful movement, regular breathing, moan or other response) but the patient then stops responding, begin CPR and repeat naloxone dose. If no initial response, continue CPR and use AED as appropriate (AHA [Lavonas 2015]).

IV, IM, SubQ: Initial: 0.4 to 2 mg; may need to repeat doses every 2 to 3 minutes. A lower initial dose (0.1 to 0.2 mg) should be considered for patients with opioid dependence to avoid acute withdrawal or if there are concerns regarding concurrent stimulant overdose (Mokhlesi 2003). After reversal, may need to readminister dose(s) at a later interval (ie, 20 to 60 minutes) depending on type/duration of opioid. If no response is observed after 10 mg total, consider other causes of respiratory depression. **Note:** May be given endotracheally (off-label route) as 2 to 2.5 times the initial IV dose (ie, 0.8 to 5 mg) (AHA [Neumar 2010]).

IM, SubQ: Evzio: 2 mg (contents of 1 auto-injector) as a single dose; may repeat every 2 to 3 minutes until emergency medical assistance becomes available.

Continuous infusion (off-label dosing): IV: **Note:** For use with exposures to long-acting opioids (eg, methadone), sustained release product, and symptomatic body packers after initial naloxone response. Calculate dosage/hour based on effective intermittent dose used and duration of adequate response seen (Tenenbein 1984) **or** use two-thirds (2/3) of the initial effective naloxone bolus on an hourly basis (typically 0.25 to 6.25 mg/hour); one-half (1/2) of the initial bolus dose should be readministered 15 minutes after initiation of the continuous infusion to prevent a drop in naloxone levels; adjust infusion rate as needed to assure adequate ventilation and prevent withdrawal symptoms (Goldfrank 1986).

Inhalation via nebulization (off-label route): 2 mg; may repeat. Switch to IV or IM administration when possible (Weber 2012). **Note:** This administration method is not included in the AHA recommendations for initial management of opioid-associated life-threatening emergency (AHA [Lavonas 2015]).

Intranasal: **Note:** Onset of action is slightly delayed compared to IM or IV routes (Kelly 2005; Robertson 2009):

4 mg (contents of 1 nasal spray) as a single dose in one nostril; may repeat every 2 to 3 minutes in alternating nostrils until medical assistance becomes available **or** 2 mg (1 mg per nostril) using injectable solution (delivered with a mucosal atomization device); may repeat in 3 to 5 minutes if respiratory depression persists (AHA [Lavonas 2015]; AHA [Vanden Hoek 2010]; Kelly 2005; Robertson 2009; Walley 2013; manufacturer's labeling).

Reversal of respiratory depression with therapeutic opioid doses: IV: Initial: 0.02 to 0.2 mg; titrate to avoid profound withdrawal, seizures, arrhythmias, or severe pain (APS 2008; Doyon 2010; AHA [Lavonas 2015]). **Note:** May be given endotracheally (off-label route) as 2 to 2.5 times the initial recommended IV dose (ie, 0.04 to 0.5 mg) (AHA [Neumar 2010]).

Continuous infusion (off-label dosing): IV: **Note:** For use with exposures to long-acting opioids (eg, methadone) or sustained release products. Calculate dosage/hour based on effective intermittent dose used and duration of adequate response seen (Tenenbein 1984) **or** use two-thirds (2/3) of the initial effective naloxone bolus on an hourly basis (typically 0.2 to 0.6 mg/hour); one-half (1/2) of the initial bolus dose should be readministered 15 minutes after initiation of the continuous infusion to prevent a drop in naloxone levels; adjust infusion rate as needed to assure adequate ventilation and prevent withdrawal symptoms (Goldfrank 1986).

Opioid-dependent patients being treated for cancer pain (off-label dosing): IV: **Note:** May dilute 0.4 mg/mL (1 mL) ampule into 9 mL of normal saline for a total volume of 10 mL to achieve a 0.04 mg/mL (40 **mcg**/mL) concentration.

0.02 mg (20 **mcg**) IV push; administer every 2 minutes until improvement in symptoms (APS guidelines, v.6.2008) **or**

0.04 to 0.08 mg (40 to 80 **mcg**) slow IV push; administer every 30 to 60 seconds until improvement in symptoms; if no response is observed after total naloxone dose 1 mg, consider other causes of respiratory depression. If respiratory depression is due to long-acting opioids, may consider administering naloxone as a continuous infusion starting at 66% of the total bolus dose (or 0.2 mg per hour) to reverse the opioid toxicity (Howlett 2016).

Postoperative reversal: IV: 0.1 to 0.2 mg every 2 to 3 minutes until desired response (adequate ventilation and alertness without significant pain). **Note:** Repeat doses may be needed within 1 to 2 hour intervals depending on type, dose, and timing of the last dose of opioid administered.

Opioid-induced pruritus (off-label use): IV infusion: 0.25 **mcg/kg/hour** (Gan 1997). Doses up to ~3 **mcg/kg/hour** have been employed (Kendrick 1996). However, doses >2 **mcg/kg/hour** are more likely to lead to reversal of analgesia and are not recommended (Kjellberg 2001; Miller 2011). **Note:** Monitor pain control; verify that the naloxone is not reversing analgesia.

Renal Impairment: Adult There are no dosage adjustments provided in the manufacturer's labeling.

Hepatic Impairment: Adult There are no dosage adjustments provided in the manufacturer's labeling.

Pediatric

Opioid intoxication/overdose (full reversal):

IV (preferred), Intraosseous: **Note:** May be administered IM, SubQ, or E.T., but onset of action may be delayed, especially if patient has poor perfusion; E.T. preferred if IV/Intraosseous route not available; doses may need to be repeated (Hegenbarth 2008; PALS [Kleinman 2010]).

Infants and Children <5 years or ≤20 kg: 0.1 mg/kg/dose; repeat every 2 to 3 minutes if needed; monitor closely; may need to repeat doses (eg, every 20 to 60 minutes) if duration of action of opioid is longer than naloxone

Children ≥5 years or >20 kg and Adolescents: 2 mg/dose; if no response, repeat every 2 to 3 minutes; monitor closely; may need to repeat doses (eg, every 20 to 60 minutes) if duration of action of opioid is longer than naloxone

E.T.: Infants, Children, and Adolescents: Optimal endotracheal dose unknown; current expert recommendations are 2 to 3 times the IV dose (PALS [Kleinman 2010]).

IM, SubQ: **Note:** IM or SubQ absorption may be delayed or erratic.

Auto-injector: Evzio: Infants, Children, and Adolescents: 0.4 mg or 2 mg (contents of 1 auto-injector) as a single dose; may repeat every 2 to 3 minutes if needed until emergency medical assistance becomes available.

Parenteral formulation (Hegenbarth 2008): IM, SubQ:

Infants and Children <5 years or <20 kg: 0.1 mg/kg/dose; repeat every 2 to 3 minutes if needed; monitor closely; may need to repeat doses (eg, every 20 to 60 minutes) if duration of action of opioid is longer than naloxone

Children ≥5 years or ≥20 kg and Adolescents: 2 mg/dose; if no response, repeat every 2 to 3 minutes; monitor closely; may need to repeat doses (eg, every 20 to 60 minutes) if duration of action of opioid is longer than naloxone

Intranasal: **Note:** Onset of action is slightly delayed compared to IM or IV routes (Barton 2005; Kelly 2005).

Narcan Nasal Spray: Infants, Children, and Adolescents: 4 mg (contents of 1 nasal spray) as a single dose; may repeat every 2 to 3 minutes in alternating nostrils if needed until medical assistance becomes available

Alternate dosing: Parenteral formulation (1 mg/mL injection) for intranasal administration: Adolescents ≥13 years: 2 mg (1 mg per nostril) (Barton 2005; Kelly 2005)

Continuous IV infusion: Limited data available: Infants, Children, and Adolescents: 24 to 40 **mcg**/kg/**hour** has been reported (Gourlay 1983; Lewis 1984; Tenenbein 1984). Doses as low as 2.5 **mcg**/kg/**hour** have been reported in adults and a dose of 160 **mcg**/kg/**hour** was reported in one neonate (Tenenbein 1984). If continuous infusion is required, calculate the initial dosage/**hour** based on the effective intermittent dose used and duration of adequate response seen (Tenenbein 1984) **or** use two-thirds ($^2/_3$) of the initial effective naloxone bolus given as the hourly infusion (Perry 1996); titrate dose; **Note:** The infusion should be discontinued by reducing the infusion rate in decrements of 25%; closely monitor the patient (eg, pulse oximetry and respiratory rate) after each adjustment and after discontinuation of the infusion for recurrence of opioid-induced respiratory depression (Perry 1996).

Reversal of respiratory depression from therapeutic opioid dosing: Infants, Children, and Adolescents: IV: 0.001 to 0.005 mg/kg/dose; titrate to effect (PALS [Kleinman 2010]); AAP recommends a wider dosage range of 0.001 to 0.015 mg/kg/dose (Hegenbarth 2008); manufacturer's labeling suggests repeat doses may be given every 2 to 3 minutes as needed based on response

Opioid-induced pruritus: Limited data available:

Prevention: Children ≥6 years and Adolescents ≤17 years: Continuous IV infusion: 0.25 **mcg**/kg/**hour** was used in a double-blind, prospective, randomized, placebo-controlled study (n=20) which showed lower incidence and severity of opioid-induced side effects (ie, pruritus, nausea) without a loss of pain control (Maxwell 2005)

Treatment: Children ≥3 years and Adolescents: Continuous IV infusion: Initial: 2 **mcg**/kg/**hour**; if pruritus continues, may titrate by 0.5 **mcg**/kg/**hour** every few hours; dosing based on a retrospective study (n=30, age range: 3 to 20 years) with a reported mean (±SD) dose of 2.3 ± 0.68 **mcg**/kg/**hour**; monitor closely; doses ≥3 **mcg**/kg/**hour** may increase risk for loss of pain control and patients may require an increase in opioid dose (Vrchoticky 2000)

Renal Impairment: Pediatric There are no dosage adjustments provided in the manufacturer's labeling.

Hepatic Impairment: Pediatric There are no dosage adjustments provided in the manufacturer's labeling.

Mechanism of Action Pure opioid antagonist that competes and displaces opioids at opioid receptor sites

Contraindications Hypersensitivity to naloxone or any component of the formulation

Warnings/Precautions Use with caution in patients with cardiovascular disease or in patients receiving medications with potential adverse cardiovascular effects (eg, hypotension, pulmonary edema, or arrhythmias); pulmonary edema and cardiovascular instability, including ventricular fibrillation, have been reported in association with abrupt reversal when using opioid antagonists. Administration of naloxone causes the release of catecholamines, which may precipitate acute withdrawal or unmask pain in those who regularly take opioids. Symptoms of acute withdrawal in opioid-dependent patients may include pain, tachycardia, hypertension, fever, sweating, abdominal cramps, diarrhea, nausea, vomiting, agitation, and irritability. In neonates born to mothers with opioid dependence, opioid withdrawal may be life-threatening and symptoms may include excessive crying, shrill cry, failure to feed, seizures, and hyperactive reflexes. In settings other than acute opioid overdose (eg, postoperative patients), carefully titrate the dose to reverse hypoventilation; do not fully awaken patient or reverse analgesic effect (postoperative patient). The 2 mg nasal dose (off-label) is less likely to precipitate severe opioid withdrawal compared to the 4 mg dose; however, the 2 mg dose may not provide an adequate and timely reversal in patients who have been exposed to an overdose of a potent or very high dose of opioids. Excessive dosages should be avoided after use of opioids in surgery. Abrupt postoperative reversal may result in nausea, vomiting, sweating, tachycardia, hypertension, seizures, and other cardiovascular events (including pulmonary edema and arrhythmias). Reversal of partial opioid agonists or mixed opioid agonist/antagonists (eg, buprenorphine, pentazocine) may be incomplete and larger or repeat doses of naloxone may be required. Recurrence of respiratory and/or CNS depression is possible if the opioid involved is long-acting; continuously observe patients until there is no further risk of recurrent respiratory or CNS depression.

To prevent overdose deaths, there are initiatives to dispense naloxone for self- or buddy-administration to patients at risk of opioid overdose (eg, recipients of high-dose opioids, suspected or confirmed history of illicit opioid use) and individuals likely to be present in an overdose situation (eg, family members of illicit drug users) (Albert 2011; Bennett 2011). Clinical practice guidelines recommend patients being treated for opioid use disorder should be given prescriptions for naloxone. Patients and family members/significant others should be trained in the use of naloxone in overdose (Kampman [ASAM 2015]). Evzio is indicated for emergency treatment. Needleless administration via nebulization and the intranasal route by first responders and bystanders has also been described (Doe-Simkins 2009; Weber 2012). Needleless administration provides an alternative route of administration in patients with venous scarring due to illicit drug use (eg, heroin). There is a low incidence of death following naloxone reversal of opioid toxicity in patients who refuse transport to a healthcare facility (Wampler 2011). Nevertheless, patients who received naloxone in the out-of-hospital setting should seek immediate emergency medical assistance after the first dose due to the likelihood that respiratory and/or central nervous system depression will return.

When the auto-injector is administered to infants <1 year of age, monitor the injection site for residual needle parts and signs of infection.

Drug Interactions

Metabolism/Transport Effects None known.

Avoid Concomitant Use

Avoid concomitant use of Naloxone with any of the following: Methylnaltrexone; Naldemedine; Naloxegol

Increased Effect/Toxicity

Naloxone may increase the levels/effects of: Naldemedine; Naloxegol

The levels/effects of Naloxone may be increased by: Methylnaltrexone

Decreased Effect There are no known significant interactions involving a decrease in effect.

Pharmacodynamics/Kinetics

Onset of Action Endotracheal, IM, SubQ: 2 to 5 minutes; Inhalation via nebulization: ~5 minutes (Mycyk 2003); Intranasal: ~8 to 13 minutes (Kelly 2005; Robertson 2009); IV: ~2 minutes

Duration of Action Depending on route of administration, ~30 to 120 minutes; IV has a shorter duration of action than IM administration; since naloxone's action is shorter than that of most opioids, repeated doses are usually needed

Half-life Elimination Neonates: Mean 3.1 ± 0.5 hours; Adults: IM, IV, or SubQ: 0.5 to 1.5 hours; Intranasal: ~2 hours

Time to Peak IM, SubQ: 15 minutes; Intranasal: 19.8 to 30 minutes

Pregnancy Considerations Naloxone crosses the placenta.

Although naloxone may precipitate opioid withdrawal in the fetus in addition to the mother, treatment should not be withheld when needed in cases of maternal opioid overdose (ACOG 711 2017). When using the injection, starting at the low end of the dosing range is suggested to help avoid adverse fetal events but still provide treatment to the mother (Blandthorn 2018).

Naloxone is used off-label for the management of patients with opioid-induced pruritus, including women who received neuraxial opioids during labor and delivery (ACOG 209 2019; Kumar 2013; Miller 2011).

Breastfeeding Considerations

It is not known if naloxone is present in breast milk; however, systemic absorption following oral administration is minimal.

According to the manufacturer, the decision to continue or discontinue breastfeeding during therapy should consider the risk of infant exposure, the benefits of breastfeeding to the infant, and the benefits of treatment to the mother.

Dosage Forms: US

Liquid, Nasal:

Narcan: 4 mg/0.1 mL (2 ea)

Solution, Injection:

Generic: 0.4 mg/mL (1 mL); 4 mg/10 mL (10 mL)

Solution, Injection [preservative free]:

Generic: 0.4 mg/mL (1 mL)

Solution Auto-injector, Injection:

Evzio: 2 mg/0.4 mL (0.4 mL)

Solution Auto-injector, Injection [preservative free]:

Generic: 2 mg/0.4 mL (0.4 mL)

Solution Cartridge, Injection:

Generic: 0.4 mg/mL (1 mL)

Solution Prefilled Syringe, Injection [preservative free]:

Generic: 2 mg/2 mL (2 mL)

Dosage Forms: Canada

Liquid, Nasal:

Narcan: 4 mg/0.1 mL (0.1 mL)

Solution, Injection:

Generic: 0.4 mg/mL (1 mL, 10 mL); 1 mg/mL (2 mL)

◆ **Naloxone and Buprenorphine** *see* Buprenorphine and Naloxone *on page 270*

◆ **Naloxone and Oxycodone** *see* Oxycodone and Naloxone *on page 1169*

◆ **Naloxone HCl** *see* Naloxone *on page 1074*

◆ **Naloxone Hydrochloride** *see* Naloxone *on page 1074*

◆ **Naloxone Hydrochloride Dihydrate and Buprenorphine Hydrochloride** *see* Buprenorphine and Naloxone *on page 270*

Naltrexone (nal TREKS one)

Brand Names: US Vivitrol

Brand Names: Canada APO-Naltrexone; ReVia

Pharmacologic Category Antidote; Opioid Antagonist

Use

Alcohol use disorder: Treatment of alcohol use disorder.

Opioid use disorder: For the blockade of the effects of exogenously administered opioids.

Limitation of use: Oral naltrexone tablets have not been shown to be more effective than placebo for opioid use disorder due to poor patient adherence (SAMHSA 2018).

Local Anesthetic/Vasoconstrictor Precautions

No information available to require special precautions

Effects on Dental Treatment Key adverse event(s) related to dental treatment: Frequent occurrence of pharyngitis has been reported. Infrequent occurrence of xerostomia (normal salivary flow resumes upon discontinuance) and toothache have been reported. Rare occurrence of herpes labialis and sinusitis have been reported.

Effects on Bleeding No information available to require special precautions

Adverse Reactions

>10%:

Cardiovascular: Syncope (≤13%)

Central nervous system: Headache (25%), insomnia (≤14%), sleep disorder (≤14%), dizziness (≤13%), anxiety (12%)

Gastrointestinal: Nausea (33%), vomiting (14%), anorexia (≤14%), change in appetite (≤14%), decreased appetite (≤14%), diarrhea (13%), abdominal pain (11%)

Hepatic: Increased serum transaminases (20%), increased serum aspartate aminotransferase (2% to 14%)

Local: Injection site reaction (69%), tenderness at injection site (45%), induration at injection site (35%), pain at injection site (17%)

Neuromuscular & skeletal: Increased creatine phosphokinase in blood specimen (11% to 39%), asthenia (23%), arthralgia (≤12%), arthritis (≤12%), joint stiffness (≤12%)

Respiratory: Pharyngitis (11%)

1% to 10%:

Central nervous system: Depression (8% to 10%), drowsiness (≤4%), sedated state (≤4%), suicidal ideation (≤1%), suicidal tendencies (≤1%)

Dermatologic: Skin rash (6%)

Gastrointestinal: Xerostomia (5%)

Local: Itching at injection site (10%), bruising at injection site (7%)

Neuromuscular & skeletal: Muscle cramps (8%), back pain (≤6%), back stiffness (≤6%)

Frequency not defined:

Cardiovascular: Acute ischemic stroke, acute myocardial infarction, angina pectoris, atrial fibrillation, cardiac failure, cerebral aneurysm, chest pain, chest tightness, coronary arteriosclerosis, deep vein thrombosis, facial edema, palpitations, pulmonary embolism, unstable angina pectoris

Central nervous system: Abnormal dreams, agitation, alcohol withdrawal syndrome, chills, decreased mental acuity, delirium, disturbance in attention, euphoria, heat exhaustion, irritability, lethargy, migraine, paresthesia, peripheral pain, rigors, seizure

Dermatologic: Diaphoresis, night sweats, pruritus

Endocrine & metabolic: Decreased libido, dehydration, hot flash, hypercholesterolemia, weight gain, weight loss

Gastrointestinal: Abdominal discomfort, acute pancreatitis, cholecystitis, cholelithiasis, colitis, constipation, dysgeusia, flatulence, gastroenteritis, gastroesophageal reflux disease, gastrointestinal hemorrhage, hemorrhoids, increased appetite, paralytic ileus

Genitourinary: Abscess of rectum and/or peri-rectal area, urinary tract infection

Hematologic & oncologic: Decreased platelet count, eosinophilia, leukocytosis, lymphadenopathy

Hepatic: Increased serum alanine aminotransferase

Hypersensitivity: Seasonal allergy

Infection: Tooth abscess

Neuromuscular & skeletal: Muscle spasm, myalgia

Ophthalmic: Blurred vision, conjunctivitis

Respiratory: Bronchitis, chronic obstructive pulmonary disease, dyspnea, laryngitis, nasal congestion, pharyngolaryngeal pain, pneumonia, sinusitis, upper respiratory tract infection

Miscellaneous: Fever

Postmarketing: Anaphylaxis, angioedema, eosinophilic pneumonitis, hepatic insufficiency, hepatitis, hypersensitivity reaction, opioid withdrawal syndrome, retinal artery occlusion, urticaria

Mechanism of Action Naltrexone (a pure opioid antagonist) is a cyclopropyl derivative of oxymorphone similar in structure to naloxone and nalorphine (a morphine derivative); it acts as a competitive antagonist at opioid receptor sites, showing the highest affinity for mu receptors. Endogenous opioids are involved in modulating the expression of alcohol's reinforcing effects (Hemby 1997; Lee 2005). Naltrexone also modifies the hypothalamic-pituitary-adrenal axis to suppress alcohol consumption (Williams 2004).

Pharmacodynamics/Kinetics

Duration of Action Oral: 50 mg: 24 hours; 100 mg: 48 hours; 150 mg: 72 hours; IM: 4 weeks

Half-life Elimination Oral: 4 hours; 6-beta-naltrexol: 13 hours; IM: naltrexone and 6-beta-naltrexol: 5 to 10 days (dependent upon erosion of polymer)

Time to Peak Serum: Oral: ~60 minutes; IM: Biphasic: ~2 hours (first peak), ~2 to 3 days (second peak)

Reproductive Considerations Pregnancy testing is recommended prior to initiating naltrexone therapy for opioid use disorder (SAMHSA 2018).

Pregnancy Considerations

Naltrexone and the 6-beta-naltrexol metabolite cross the placenta (Towers 2020).

Alcohol use and opioid use disorder are associated with adverse fetal and obstetrical outcomes. Information related to the use of naltrexone during pregnancy is limited (ACOG 711 2017; Farid 2008; Towers 2020; Tran 2017).

Clinical practice guidelines recommend that if a woman being treated with naltrexone for the treatment of opioid use disorder becomes pregnant, naltrexone should be discontinued if the patient and physician agree that the risk of relapse if low. If patient is concerned about relapse and wishes to continue naltrexone, the patient should be informed of the potential risks of continuing treatment and consent for ongoing treatment should be obtained. If naltrexone is discontinued and the patient subsequently relapses, consideration should be given for treatment with methadone or buprenorphine (Kampman [ASAM 2015]). Pharmacological agents should not be used for the treatment of alcohol use disorder in pregnant women unless needed for the treatment of acute alcohol withdrawal or a coexisting disorder; agents other than naltrexone are recommended for acute alcohol withdrawal (APA [Reus 2018]).

Naltrexone and Bupropion

(nal TREKS one & byoo PROE pee on)

Brand Names: US Contrave

Brand Names: Canada Contrave

Pharmacologic Category Anorexiant; Antidepressant, Dopamine/Norepinephrine-Reuptake Inhibitor; Opioid Antagonist

Use

Weight management: Adjunct to a reduced-calorie diet and increased physical activity for chronic weight management in adults with an initial body mass index (BMI) of ≥30 kg/m^2 or ≥27 kg/m^2 in the presence of at least one weight-related comorbid condition (eg, hypertension, type 2 diabetes mellitus, and/or dyslipidemia)

Limitations of use: The effect of naltrexone/bupropion on cardiovascular morbidity and mortality has not been established. The safety and effectiveness of naltrexone/bupropion in combination with other products intended for weight loss, including prescription drugs, over-the-counter drugs, and herbal preparations, have not been established.

Local Anesthetic/Vasoconstrictor Precautions Part of the mechanism of buproprion is to block reuptake of norepinephrine along with dopamine. Because of the potential for norepinephrine elevation within CNS synapses, it is suggested that vasoconstrictor be administered with caution and to monitor vital signs in dental patients taking antidepressants that affect norepinephrine in this way.

Effects on Dental Treatment No significant effects or complications reported

Effects on Bleeding No information available to require special precautions

Adverse Reactions Also see individual agents.

>10%:

Central nervous system: Headache (18%), sleep disorder (14%)

Gastrointestinal: Nausea (33%), constipation (19%), vomiting (11%)

1% to 10%:

Cardiovascular: Hypertension (≤6%), increased blood pressure (≤6%), palpitations (2%), myocardial infarction (<2%), presyncope (<2%), tachycardia (<2%)

Central nervous system: Dizziness (10%), insomnia (9%; ≥65 years of age: 11%), depression (6%; ≥65 years of age: 7%), anxiety (4% to 6%), fatigue (4%), irritability (3%), disturbance in attention (<2% to 3%), abnormal dreams (<2%), agitation (<2%), altered mental status (<2%), amnesia (<2%), derealization (<2%), emotional lability (<2%), equilibrium disturbance (<2%), feeling abnormal (<2%), feeling hot (<2%), intention tremor (<2%), jitteriness (<2%), lethargy (<2%), memory impairment (<2%), nervousness (<2%), tension (<2%), vertigo (<2%)

Dermatologic: Hyperhidrosis (3%), alopecia (<2%)

Endocrine: Hot flash (4%), dehydration (<2%), increased thirst (<2%)

Gastrointestinal: Xerostomia (8%), diarrhea (7%), upper abdominal pain (4%), viral gastroenteritis (4%), abdominal pain (3%), dysgeusia (2%), cholecystitis (<2%), eructation (<2%), hematochezia (<2%), hernia (<2%), lower abdominal pain (<2%), motion sickness (<2%), swelling of lips (<2%)

Genitourinary: Urinary tract infection (3%), erectile dysfunction (<2%), irregular menses (<2%), urinary urgency (<2%), vaginal dryness (<2%), vaginal hemorrhage (<2%)

Hematologic & oncologic: Decreased hematocrit (<2%)

Hepatic: Increased liver enzymes (<2%)

Infection: Kidney infection (<2%), staphylococcal infection (<2%)

Neuromuscular & skeletal: Tremor (4%), strain (2%), herniated disk (<2%), jaw pain (<2%), weakness (<2%)

Otic: Tinnitus (3%)

Renal: Increased serum creatinine (<2%)

Respiratory: Pneumonia (<2%)

<1%, postmarketing, and/or case reports: Increased heart rate (resting), loss of consciousness, malaise, syncope

Mechanism of Action Naltrexone is a pure opioid antagonist, and bupropion is a relatively weak inhibitor of the neuronal reuptake of dopamine and norepinephrine. The exact neurochemical effects of naltrexone/bupropion leading to weight loss are not fully understood. Effects may result from action on areas of the brain involved in the regulation of food intake: the hypothalamus (appetite regulatory center) and the mesolimbic dopamine circuit (reward system).

Pregnancy Risk Factor X

Pregnancy Considerations

An increased risk of adverse maternal and fetal outcomes is associated with obesity. However, moderate weight gain based on prepregnancy BMI is required for positive fetal outcomes. Therefore, medications for weight loss therapy are not recommended at conception or during pregnancy (ACOG 156 2015; Stang 2016). Due to the lack of clinical benefit and potential for fetal harm, use of naltrexone/bupropion is contraindicated in pregnant females.

Also refer to individual monographs for additional information.

- **Naltrexone HCl/Bupropion HCl** *see* Naltrexone and Bupropion *on page 1078*
- **Naltrexone Hydrochloride** *see* Naltrexone *on page 1077*
- **Namenda** *see* Memantine *on page 962*
- **Namenda Titration Pak** *see* Memantine *on page 962*
- **Namenda XR** *see* Memantine *on page 962*
- **Namenda XR Titration Pack** *see* Memantine *on page 962*
- **Nanoliposomal Irinotecan** *see* Irinotecan (Liposomal) *on page 842*
- **Nanoparticle Albumin-Bound Paclitaxel** *see* PACLitaxel (Protein Bound) *on page 1179*

Naphazoline and Pheniramine

(naf AZ oh leen & fen NIR a meen)

Brand Names: US Naphcon-A [OTC]; Opcon-A [OTC]; Visine [OTC]; Visine-A [OTC]

Brand Names: Canada Naphcon-A; Visine Advanced Allergy

Pharmacologic Category Alkylamine Derivative; Alpha$_1$ Agonist; Histamine H$_1$ Antagonist; Histamine H$_1$ Antagonist, First Generation; Imidazoline Derivative; Ophthalmic Agent, Vasoconstrictor

Use Ocular itching/redness: Temporary relief of itching and redness of the eye(s) caused by grass, ragweed, pollen, animal dander and hair.

Local Anesthetic/Vasoconstrictor Precautions No information available to require special precautions

Effects on Dental Treatment No significant effects or complications reported

Effects on Bleeding No information available to require special precautions

Adverse Reactions Frequency not defined.

Central nervous system: Tingling sensation (eye)

Ophthalmic: Mydriasis

Mechanism of Action

Naphazoline: Stimulates alpha-adrenergic receptors in the arterioles of the conjunctiva to produce vasoconstriction.

Pheniramine: Inhibits the effect of histamine on conjunctival epithelial cells by preventing its release from mast cells.

◆ **Naphazoline HCl/Pheniramine** *see* Naphazoline and Pheniramine *on page 1079*

◆ **Naphcon-A [OTC]** *see* Naphazoline and Pheniramine *on page 1079*

◆ **Naprelan** *see* Naproxen *on page 1080*

◆ **Naprosyn** *see* Naproxen *on page 1080*

Naproxen (na PROKS en)

Related Information

Oral Pain *on page 1734*

Rheumatoid Arthritis, Osteoarthritis, and Osteoporosis *on page 1697*

Temporomandibular Dysfunction (TMD), Chronic Pain, and Fibromyalgia *on page 1773*

Related Sample Prescriptions

Oral Pain - Sample Prescriptions *on page 30*

Brand Names: US Aleve [OTC]; All Day Pain Relief [OTC]; All Day Relief [OTC]; Anaprox DS [DSC]; EC-Naprosyn; EC-Naproxen; Flanax Pain Relief; Flanax Pain Relief [OTC] [DSC]; GoodSense Naproxen Sodium [OTC]; Mediproxen [OTC]; Naprelan; Naprosyn; Naproxen Comfort Pac [DSC]; Naproxen DR

Brand Names: Canada Anaprox; Anaprox DS; APO-Napro-Na; APO-Naproxen; APO-Naproxen EC; APO-Naproxen SR; MYLAN-Naproxen EC [DSC]; MYLAN-Naproxen [DSC]; Naprelan [DSC]; Naprosyn; Naproxen-Na [DSC]; Naxen EC; Pediapharm Naproxen; PMS-Naproxen; PMS-Naproxen EC; PRO-Naproxen EC; TEVA-Naproxen; TEVA-Naproxen EC; TEVA-Naproxen Sodium; TEVA-Naproxen Sodium DS

Generic Availability (US) May be product dependent

Pharmacologic Category Analgesic, Nonopioid; Nonsteroidal Anti-inflammatory Drug (NSAID), Oral

Dental Use Management of pain and swelling

Use

Ankylosing spondylitis, bursitis, gout (acute flares), polyarticular juvenile idiopathic arthritis, osteoarthritis, rheumatoid arthritis, tendonitis (Rx products only): Relief of the signs and symptoms of acute flares of gout, ankylosing spondylitis, bursitis, polyarticular juvenile idiopathic arthritis (excluding ER tablets), osteoarthritis, rheumatoid arthritis, and tendonitis. Delayed-release naproxen is not recommended for initial treatment of acute pain.

Pain, primary dysmenorrhea (Rx and OTC products): Relief of mild to moderate pain and the treatment of primary dysmenorrhea. Delayed-release naproxen is not recommended for initial treatment of acute pain.

Local Anesthetic/Vasoconstrictor Precautions No information available to require special precautions

Effects on Dental Treatment Key adverse event(s) related to dental treatment: Occurrence of stomatitis has been reported. Rare occurrence of glossitis has also been reported.

Effects on Bleeding Nonselective NSAIDs, such as naproxen, inhibit platelet aggregation and prolong bleeding time in some patients. Unlike aspirin, the NSAID effect on platelet function is quantitatively less, of shorter duration, and reversible. Normal platelet function should occur in ~5 elimination half-lives or in <10 hours after discontinuation of naproxen. Concomitant use of other NSAIDs should be avoided.

Adverse Reactions

1% to 10%:

Cardiovascular: Edema (3% to 9%), palpitations (<3%)

Central nervous system: Dizziness (≤9%), drowsiness (3% to 9%), headache (3% to 9%), vertigo (<3%)

Dermatologic: Pruritus (3% to 9%), skin rash (3% to 9%), ecchymoses (3% to 9%), diaphoresis (<3%)

Endocrine & metabolic: Fluid retention (3% to 9%), increased thirst (<3%)

Gastrointestinal: Abdominal pain (3% to 9%), constipation (3% to 9%), nausea (3% to 9%), heartburn (3% to 9%), diarrhea (<3%), dyspepsia (<3%), stomatitis (<3%), flatulence, gastrointestinal hemorrhage, gastrointestinal perforation, gastrointestinal ulcer, vomiting

Hematologic & oncologic: Hemolysis (3% to 9%), purpura (<3%), anemia, prolonged bleeding time

Hepatic: Increased liver enzymes

Ophthalmic: Visual disturbance (<3%)

Otic: Tinnitus (3% to 9%), auditory disturbance (<3%)

Renal: Renal function abnormality

Respiratory: Dyspnea (3% to 9%)

<1%, postmarketing, and/or case reports: Abnormal dreams, agranulocytosis, alopecia, anaphylactoid reaction, anaphylaxis, angioedema, aphthous stomatitis, aseptic meningitis, asthma, blurred vision, cardiac arrhythmia, cardiac failure, cognitive dysfunction, colitis, coma, confusion, conjunctivitis, cystitis, depression, dysuria, eosinophilia, eosinophilic pneumonitis, erythema multiforme, exfoliative dermatitis, fever, glossitis, granulocytopenia, hallucination, hematemesis, hepatic failure, hepatitis, hepatotoxicity (idiosyncratic) (Chalasani, 2014), hyperglycemia, hypertension, hypoglycemia, hypotension, infection, interstitial nephritis, melena, jaundice, leukopenia, lymphadenopathy, menstrual disease, malaise, myalgia, myasthenia, myocardial infarction, oliguria, pancreatitis, pancytopenia, paresthesia, pneumonia, polyuria, proteinuria, rectal hemorrhage, renal failure, renal papillary necrosis, respiratory depression, sepsis, skin photosensitivity, Stevens-Johnson syndrome, tachycardia, seizure, syncope, thrombocytopenia, toxic epidermal necrolysis, vasculitis

Dental Usual Dosage

Mild-to-moderate pain: Adults: Initial: 500 mg, then 250 mg every 6 to 8 hours; maximum: 1250 mg/day naproxen base

Pain/fever (OTC labeling): Children ≥12 years and Adults: 200 mg naproxen base every 8 to 12 hours; if needed, may take 400 mg naproxen base for the initial dose; maximum: 400 mg naproxen base in any 8- to 12-hour period or 600 mg naproxen base/24 hours

Dosing

Adult Note: Dosage expressed as naproxen base; 200 mg naproxen base is equivalent to 220 mg naproxen sodium. For relief of acute pain, naproxen sodium may be preferred due to more rapid absorption and onset; naproxen base may also be used however EC-Naprosyn is not recommended.

Ankylosing spondylitis, osteoarthritis, rheumatoid arthritis: Oral: 500 to 1,000 mg daily in 2 divided doses; in patients who require higher level of anti-inflammatory/analgesic activity and have tolerated lower doses, may increase to 1,500 mg/day for limited time period (<6 months)

Naproxen extended-release tablets: Initial: 750 to 1,000 mg once daily; in patients who require higher level of anti-inflammatory/analgesic activity and have tolerated lower doses, may temporarily increase to 1,500 mg once daily

Rectal suppository [Canadian product]: Insert one 500 mg suppository into the rectum once daily (**Note:** Suppository may be used to substitute for one oral dose in patients receiving 1,000 mg naproxen daily).

Gout, acute flares (alternative agent): Oral: 500 mg twice daily (Janssens 2008); initiate within 24 to 48 hours of flare onset preferably; discontinue 2 to 3 days after resolution of clinical signs; usual duration: 5 to 7 days (ACR [Khanna 2012]; Becker 2018)

Manufacturer's labeling: Dosing in the prescribing information may not reflect current clinical practice.

Immediate release: Initial: 750 mg followed by 250 mg every 8 hours

Extended-release tablets: Initial: 1,000 to 1,500 mg once daily followed by 1,000 mg once daily. **Note:** Naproxen delayed-release tablets are not recommended because of the delay in absorption.

Pain (mild to moderate), dysmenorrhea, acute tendonitis, bursitis: Oral: Initial: 500 mg, followed by 500 mg every 12 hours or 250 mg every 6 to 8 hours; maximum daily dose: Day 1: 1,250 mg; subsequent daily doses should not exceed 1,000 mg

Naproxen extended-release tablets: Oral: Initial: 1,000 mg once daily; may temporarily increase to 1,500 mg once daily if greater pain relief is needed. Dose should be subsequently reduced to a maximum of 1,000 mg daily.

Episodic migraine prevention (off-label use): Oral: 250 to 500 mg twice daily (EFNS [Evers 2009]). Continue treatment for 2 to 3 months to assess clinical benefit; consider tapering or discontinuing dose if headaches are well-controlled after 3 to 6 months (AAN [Silberstein 2000]).

Migraine, acute (off label use): Initial: 750 mg; an additional 250 to 500 mg may be given if needed (maximum: 1,250 mg in 24 hours) (Andersson, 1989; Nestvold, 1985).

OTC labeling: Pain, fever: 200 mg every 8 to 12 hours; if needed, may take 400 mg for the initial dose; maximum: 400 mg in any 8- to 12-hour period or 600 mg/24 hours

Geriatric Use with caution; consider using a reduced dose. Refer to adult dosing.

Renal Impairment: Adult

CrCl ≥30 mL/minute: There are no specific dosage adjustments provided in the manufacturer's labeling; use with caution and consider using a reduced dose.

CrCl <30 mL/minute: Use is not recommended; avoid use in patients with advanced renal disease.

Hemodialysis: Not dialyzable (NCS/SCCM [Frontera 2016])

KDIGO 2012 guidelines provide the following recommendations for NSAIDs:

eGFR 30 to <60 mL/minute/1.73 m^2:Temporarily discontinue in patients with intercurrent disease that increases risk of acute kidney injury.

eGFR <30 mL/minute/1.73 m^2: Avoid use.

Hepatic Impairment: Adult There are no specific dosage adjustments provided in the manufacturer's labeling; use with caution and consider using a reduced dose.

Pediatric

Note: Dosage expressed as naproxen base; 200 mg naproxen base is equivalent to 220 mg naproxen sodium. In pediatric patients, all dosing is for the immediate release preparations.

Analgesia/pain, mild to moderate:

Children and Adolescents <60 kg: Limited data available: Oral: 5 to 6 mg/kg/dose every 12 hours; maximum daily dose: 1,000 mg/day (Berde 2002); doses as high as 10 mg/kg/dose have also been recommended (APS 2008)

Children and Adolescents ≥60 kg: Limited data available: Oral: 250 to 375 mg twice daily; maximum daily dose: 1,000 mg/day (Berde 2002)

OTC labeling: Children ≥12 years and Adolescents: Oral: 200 mg every 8 to 12 hours; if needed may take 400 mg for the initial dose; maximum daily dose: 600 mg/day

Fever: *OTC labeling:* Children ≥12 years and Adolescents: Oral: 200 mg every 8 to 12 hours; if needed may take 400 mg for the initial dose; maximum daily dose: 600 mg/day

Juvenile idiopathic arthritis: Children and Adolescents: Oral: 10 to 15 mg/kg/**day** in 2 divided doses; Maximum daily dose: 1,000 mg/day (Hollingsworth 1993; Kliegman 2016; Litalien 2001)

Ankylosing spondylitis: Limited data available: Children and Adolescents: Oral: 15 to 20 mg/kg/**day** in 2 divided doses; maximum daily dose: 1,500 mg/day; adult dosing suggests limiting this maximum daily dose to <6 months of therapy (APS 2008; Kliegman 2016)

Renal Impairment: Pediatric

Manufacturer's labeling: Children ≥2 years and Adolescents:

CrCl ≥30 mL/minute: There are no specific dosage adjustments provided in the manufacturer's labeling; use with caution and consider using a reduced dose. Use is not recommended in patients with moderate renal impairment.

CrCl <30 mL/minute: Use is not recommended; avoid use in patients with advanced renal disease.

KDIGO 2012 guidelines provide the following recommendations for NSAIDs (KDIGO 2013): Children and Adolescents:

eGFR 30 to <60 mL/minute/1.73 m^2: Temporarily discontinue in patients with intercurrent disease that increases risk of acute kidney injury

eGFR <30 mL/minute/1.73 m^2: Avoid use

Hepatic Impairment: Pediatric There are no specific dosage adjustments provided in the manufacturer's labeling; use with caution and consider using a reduced dose.

Mechanism of Action Reversibly inhibits cyclooxygenase-1 and 2 (COX-1 and 2) enzymes, which results in decreased formation of prostaglandin precursors; has antipyretic, analgesic, and anti-inflammatory properties

Other proposed mechanisms not fully elucidated (and possibly contributing to the anti-inflammatory effect to varying degrees), include inhibiting chemotaxis, altering lymphocyte activity, inhibiting neutrophil aggregation/activation, and decreasing proinflammatory cytokine levels.

Contraindications

Hypersensitivity to naproxen (eg, anaphylactic reactions, serious skin reactions) or any component of the formulation; history of asthma, urticaria, or allergic-type reactions after taking aspirin or other NSAIDs; use in the setting of coronary artery bypass graft (CABG) surgery

Canadian labeling: Additional contraindications (not in US labeling): Active gastric, duodenal, or peptic ulcers; active GI bleeding; cerebrovascular bleeding or other bleeding disorders; active GI inflammatory disease; severe liver impairment or active liver disease; severe renal impairment (CrCl <30 mL/minute) or deteriorating renal disease; severe uncontrolled heart failure; known hyperkalemia; third trimester of pregnancy; breastfeeding; inflammatory lesions or recent bleeding of the rectum or anus (suppository only); use in patients <16 years of age (suppository only); use in patients <18 years of age (naproxen enteric coated and sustained release tablets and naproxen sodium tablets); use in children <2 years (naproxen tablets and suspension).

Warnings/Precautions [US Boxed Warning]: NSAIDs cause an increased risk of serious (and potentially fatal) adverse cardiovascular thrombotic events, including MI and stroke. Risk may occur early during treatment and may increase with duration of use. Relative risk appears to be similar in those with and without known cardiovascular disease or risk factors for cardiovascular disease; however, absolute incidence of serious cardiovascular thrombotic events (which may occur early during treatment) was higher in patients with known cardiovascular disease or risk factors and in those receiving higher doses. New-onset hypertension or exacerbation of hypertension may occur (NSAIDs may also impair response to ACE inhibitors, thiazide diuretics, or loop diuretics); may contribute to cardiovascular events; monitor blood pressure; use with caution in patients with hypertension. May cause sodium and fluid retention, use with caution in patients with edema. Avoid use in heart failure (ACCF/AHA [Yancy 2013]). Avoid use in patients with a recent MI unless benefits outweigh risk of cardiovascular thrombotic events. Use the lowest effective dose for the shortest duration of time, consistent with individual patient goals, to reduce risk of cardiovascular events; alternate therapies should be considered for patients at high risk. **[US Boxed Warning]: Use is contraindicated in the setting of coronary artery bypass graft (CABG) surgery.** Risk of MI and stroke may be increased with use following CABG surgery.

NSAIDs cause increased risk of serious gastrointestinal inflammation, ulceration, bleeding, and perforation (may be fatal); elderly patients and patients with history of peptic ulcer disease and/or GI bleeding are at greater risk of serious GI events. These events may occur at any time during therapy and without warning. Avoid use in patients with active GI bleeding. Use caution with a history of GI ulcers, concurrent therapy known to increase the risk of GI bleeding (eg, aspirin, anticoagulants and/or corticosteroids, selective serotonin reuptake inhibitors), advanced hepatic disease, coagulopathy, smoking, use of alcohol, or in elderly or debilitated patients. Use the lowest effective dose for the shortest duration of time, consistent with individual patient goals, to reduce risk of GI adverse events; alternate therapies should be considered for patients at high risk. When used concomitantly with aspirin, a substantial increase in the risk of gastrointestinal complications (eg, ulcer) occurs; concomitant gastroprotective therapy (eg, proton pump inhibitors) is recommended (Bhatt 2008). Avoid chronic use of oral nonselective NSAIDs in patients who have undergone bariatric surgery; development of anastomotic ulcerations/perforations may occur.

May increase the risk of aseptic meningitis, especially in patients with systemic lupus erythematosus (SLE) and mixed connective tissue disorders. Platelet adhesion and aggregation may be decreased; may prolong bleeding time; patients with coagulation disorders or who are receiving anticoagulants should be monitored closely. Anemia may occur; patients on long-term NSAID therapy should be monitored for anemia. Rarely, NSAID use may cause severe blood dyscrasias (eg, agranulocytosis, aplastic anemia, thrombocytopenia).

NSAID use may compromise existing renal function; dose-dependent decreases in prostaglandin synthesis may result from NSAID use, reducing renal blood flow which may cause renal decompensation (usually reversible). Patients with impaired renal function, dehydration, hypovolemia, heart failure, hepatic impairment, those taking diuretics, and ACE inhibitors, and the elderly are at greater risk of renal toxicity. Rehydrate patient before starting therapy; monitor renal function closely. Long-term NSAID use may result in renal papillary necrosis and other renal injury. Avoid use in patients with advanced renal disease; discontinue use with persistent or worsening abnormal renal function tests.

NSAIDs may cause potentially fatal serious skin adverse events including exfoliative dermatitis, Stevens-Johnson Syndrome (SJS) and toxic epidermal necrolysis (TEN); may occur without warning; discontinue use at first sign of skin rash (or other hypersensitivity). Anaphylactoid reactions may occur, even without prior exposure; patients with "aspirin triad" (bronchial asthma, aspirin intolerance, rhinitis) may be at increased risk. Contraindicated in patients with aspirin-sensitive asthma; severe and potentially fatal bronchospasm may occur. Use caution in patients with other forms of asthma.

Transaminase elevations have been reported with use; closely monitor patients with any abnormal LFT. Rare (sometimes fatal) severe hepatic reactions (eg, fulminant hepatitis, hepatic necrosis, hepatic failure) have occurred with NSAID use; discontinue immediately if signs or symptoms of hepatic disease develop or if systemic manifestations occur. Use with caution in patients with hepatic impairment; patients with advanced hepatic disease are at an increased risk of GI bleeding with NSAIDs.

May cause drowsiness, dizziness, blurred vision and other neurologic effects which may impair physical or mental abilities; patients must be cautioned about performing tasks which require mental alertness (eg, operating machinery or driving). Discontinue use with blurred or diminished vision and perform ophthalmologic exam. Monitor vision with long-term therapy. Withhold for at least 4-6 half-lives prior to surgical or dental procedures.

Elderly patients are at greater risk for serious GI, cardiovascular, and/or renal adverse events; use with caution. Potentially significant interactions may exist, requiring dose or frequency adjustment, additional monitoring, and/or selection of alternative therapy.

OTC labeling: Prior to self-medication, patients should contact healthcare provider if they have had recurring stomach pain or upset, ulcers, bleeding problems, asthma, high blood pressure, heart or kidney disease, other serious medical problems, are currently taking a diuretic, anticoagulant, other NSAIDs, or are ≥60 years of age. Recommended dosages and duration should not be exceeded, due to an increased risk of GI bleeding, MI, and stroke. Patients should stop use and consult a healthcare provider if symptoms get worse, newly appear, or continue; if an allergic reaction occurs; if feeling faint, vomit blood or have bloody/black stools; if having difficulty swallowing or heartburn, or if fever lasts for >3 days or pain >10 days. Consuming ≥3 alcoholic beverages/day or taking longer than recommended may increase the risk of GI bleeding. Not for self-medication (OTC use) in children <12 years of age.

Warnings: Additional Pediatric Considerations Pseudoporphyria (ie, increased skin fragility and blistering with scarring in sun-exposed skin) has been reported in naproxen-treated children with JIA (reported incidence, 12%); discontinue therapy if this occurs (Lang 1994).

Drug Interactions

Metabolism/Transport Effects **Substrate** of CYP1A2 (minor), CYP2C9 (minor); **Note:** Assignment of Major/Minor substrate status based on clinically relevant drug interaction potential

Avoid Concomitant Use

Avoid concomitant use of Naproxen with any of the following: Acemetacin; Aminolevulinic Acid (Systemic); Dexibuprofen; Dexketoprofen; Floctafenine; Ketorolac (Nasal); Ketorolac (Systemic); Macimorelin; Mifamurtide; Morniflumate; Nonsteroidal Anti-Inflammatory Agents (COX-2 Selective); Omacetaxine; Pelubiprofen; Phenylbutazone; Talniflumate; Tenoxicam; Urokinase; Zaltoprofen

Increased Effect/Toxicity

Naproxen may increase the levels/effects of: 5-Aminosalicylic Acid Derivatives; Agents with Antiplatelet Properties; Aliskiren; Aminoglycosides; Aminolevulinic Acid (Systemic); Aminolevulinic Acid (Topical); Anticoagulants; Apixaban; Bemiparin; Bisphosphonate Derivatives; Cephalothin; Collagenase (Systemic); CycloSPORINE (Systemic); Dabigatran Etexilate; Deferasirox; Deoxycholic Acid; Desmopressin; Dexibuprofen; Digoxin; Drospirenone; Edoxaban; Enoxaparin; Eplerenone; Haloperidol; Heparin; Ibritumomab Tiuxetan; Lithium; MetFORMIN; Methotrexate; Nonsteroidal Anti-Inflammatory Agents (COX-2 Selective); Obinutuzumab; Omacetaxine; Porfimer; Potassium-Sparing Diuretics; PRALAtrexate; Quinolones; Rivaroxaban; Salicylates; Tacrolimus (Systemic); Tenofovir Products; Thrombolytic Agents; Tolperisone; Urokinase; Vancomycin; Verteporfin; Vitamin K Antagonists

The levels/effects of Naproxen may be increased by: Acalabrutinib; Acemetacin; Alcohol (Ethyl); Angiotensin II Receptor Blockers; Angiotensin-Converting Enzyme Inhibitors; Corticosteroids (Systemic); CycloSPORINE (Systemic); Dasatinib; Dexketoprofen; Diclofenac (Systemic); Fat Emulsion (Fish Oil Based); Felbinac; Floctafenine; Glucosamine; Herbs (Anticoagulant/Antiplatelet Properties); Ibrutinib; Inotersen; Ketorolac (Nasal); Ketorolac (Systemic); Limaprost; Loop Diuretics; Morniflumate; Multivitamins/Fluoride (with ADE); Multivitamins/Minerals (with ADEK, Folate, Iron); Multivitamins/Minerals (with AE, No Iron); Naftazone; Omega-3 Fatty Acids; Pelubiprofen; Pentosan Polysulfate Sodium; Pentoxifylline; Phenylbutazone; Probenecid; Prostacyclin Analogues; Selective Serotonin Reuptake Inhibitors; Selumetinib; Serotonin/Norepinephrine Reuptake Inhibitors; Sodium Phosphates; Talniflumate; Tenoxicam; Thiazide and Thiazide-Like Diuretics; Tipranavir; Tolperisone; Tricyclic Antidepressants (Tertiary Amine); Vitamin E (Systemic); Zaltoprofen; Zanubrutinib

Decreased Effect

Naproxen may decrease the levels/effects of: Aliskiren; Angiotensin II Receptor Blockers; Angiotensin-Converting Enzyme Inhibitors; Beta-Blockers; Eplerenone; HydrALAZINE; Loop Diuretics; Macimorelin; Mifamurtide; Potassium-Sparing Diuretics; Prostaglandins (Ophthalmic); Salicylates; Selective Serotonin Reuptake Inhibitors; Sincalide; Thiazide and Thiazide-Like Diuretics

The levels/effects of Naproxen may be decreased by: Bile Acid Sequestrants; Salicylates

Food Interactions Naproxen absorption rate/levels may be decreased if taken with food. Management: Administer with food, milk, or antacids to decrease GI adverse effects.

Dietary Considerations Sodium content: Naproxen sodium products contain about 50 mg (2 mEq) of sodium per 500 mg of naproxen. Naprosyn suspension contains 39 mg of sodium per 5 mL (125 mg). Consider this in patients whose overall intake of sodium must be severely restricted.

Pharmacodynamics/Kinetics

Onset of Action Analgesic: 30 to 60 minutes

Duration of Action Analgesic: <12 hours

Half-life Elimination

Children: Range: 8 to 17 hours

Children 8 to 14 years: 8 to 10 hours

Adults: Normal renal function: 12 to 17 hours; Moderate-to-severe renal impairment: ~15 to 21 hours (Anttila 1980)

Time to Peak Serum:

Tablets, naproxen: 2 to 4 hours

Tablets, naproxen sodium: 1 to 2 hours

Tablets, delayed-release (empty stomach): 4 to 6 hours; range: 2 to 12 hours

Tablets, delayed-release (with food): 12 hours; range: 4 to 24 hours

Suspension: 1 to 4 hours

Suppository [Canadian product]: 2 to 3 hours

Reproductive Considerations

The chronic use of NSAIDs in women of reproductive age may be associated with infertility that is reversible upon discontinuation of the medication. Consider discontinuing use in women having difficulty conceiving or those undergoing investigation of fertility.

Pregnancy Considerations Naproxen crosses the placenta (Brogden 1975). Birth defects have been observed following in utero NSAID exposure in some studies; however, data is conflicting (Bloor 2013). Nonteratogenic effects, including prenatal constriction of the ductus arteriosus, persistent pulmonary hypertension of the newborn, oligohydramnios, necrotizing enterocolitis, renal dysfunction or failure, and intracranial hemorrhage have been observed in the fetus/neonate following in utero NSAID exposure. In addition, nonclosure of the ductus arteriosus postnatally may occur and be resistant to medical management (Bermas 2014; Bloor 2013). Because NSAIDs may cause premature closure of the ductus arteriosus, product labeling for naproxen specifically states use should be avoided starting at 30-weeks gestation. Use of NSAIDs can be considered for the treatment of mild rheumatoid arthritis flares in pregnant women; however, use should be minimized or avoided early and late in pregnancy (Bermas 2014; Saavedra Salinas 2015).

The use of NSAIDs close to conception may be associated with an increased risk of miscarriage (Bloor 2013; Bermas 2014).

Breastfeeding Considerations Naproxen is present in breast milk.

The relative infant dose (RID) of naproxen is 3.3% when calculated using the highest breast milk concentration located and compared to a weight-adjusted maternal dose of 750 mg/day. In general, breastfeeding is considered acceptable when the RID is <10% (Anderson 2016; Ito 2000). Using the highest milk concentration (2.37 mcg/mL), the estimated daily infant dose via breast milk is 0.36 mg/kg/day. This milk concentration was obtained following maternal administration of oral naproxen 375 mg twice daily. Naproxen was detected in the urine of the breastfeeding infant (Jamali 1982; Jamali 1983).

In a study which included 20 mother-infant pairs, there were two cases of drowsiness and one case of vomiting in the breastfed infants (Ito 1993).

In general, NSAIDs may be used in postpartum women who wish to breastfeed; however, agents other than naproxen may be preferred (Montgomery 2012) and use should be avoided in women breastfeeding infants with platelet dysfunction or thrombocytopenia (Bloor 2013; Sammaritano 2014). When needed, naproxen may be considered for short-term use (<1 week) (Montgomery 2012). Other agents are preferred for treatment of migraine in a woman who is breastfeeding because the risk profile of naproxen is less certain (Amundsen 2015). According to the manufacturer, the decision to breastfeed during therapy should consider the risk of infant exposure, the benefits of breastfeeding to the infant, and benefits of treatment to the mother.

Dosage Forms Considerations

EnovaRX-Naproxen and Equipto-Naproxen creams are compounded from a kit. Refer to manufacturer's package insert for compounding instructions.

Naproxen Comfort Pac kit contains naproxen tablets and Duraflex Comfort Gel

Flanax Pain Relief kit contains naproxen tablets and Flanax Liniment

Dosage Forms: US

Capsule, Oral:
- Aleve [OTC]: 220 mg
- Generic: 220 mg

Kit, Combination:
- Flanax Pain Relief: 500 mg

Suspension, Oral:
- Naprosyn: 125 mg/5 mL (473 mL)
- Generic: 125 mg/5 mL (473 mL, 500 mL)

Tablet, Oral:
- Aleve [OTC]: 220 mg
- All Day Pain Relief [OTC]: 220 mg
- All Day Relief [OTC]: 220 mg
- GoodSense Naproxen Sodium [OTC]: 220 mg
- Mediproxen [OTC]: 220 mg
- Generic: 220 mg, 250 mg, 275 mg, 375 mg, 500 mg, 550 mg

Tablet Delayed Release, Oral:
- EC-Naprosyn: 375 mg
- EC-Naproxen: 375 mg, 500 mg
- Naproxen DR: 375 mg, 500 mg

Tablet Extended Release 24 Hour, Oral:
- Naprelan: 375 mg, 500 mg, 750 mg
- Generic: 375 mg, 500 mg

Dosage Forms: Canada

Suppository, Rectal:
- Generic: 500 mg (10 ea, 30 ea)

Suspension, Oral:
- Generic: 125 mg/5 mL (40 mL, 474 mL)

Tablet, Oral:
- Anaprox: 275 mg
- Anaprox DS: 550 mg
- Generic: 125 mg, 250 mg, 275 mg, 375 mg, 500 mg, 550 mg

Tablet Delayed Release, Oral:
- Naprosyn: 375 mg, 500 mg
- Naxen EC: 250 mg, 375 mg, 500 mg
- Generic: 250 mg, 375 mg, 500 mg

Tablet Extended Release 24 Hour, Oral:
- Naprosyn: 750 mg
- Generic: 750 mg

Dental Health Professional Considerations

Naproxen and naproxen sodium have the potential to interfere with the antiplatelet effect of low-dose aspirin. One study of naproxen and low-dose aspirin has suggested that naproxen may interfere with aspirin's antiplatelet activity when they are coadministered (Steinhubl 2005). However, naproxen 500 mg administered 2 hours before or after aspirin 100 mg did not interfere with aspirin's antiplatelet effect. The FDA stated that there is no data looking at doses of naproxen <500 mg. Naproxen over-the-counter strength is 220 mg tablets.

The FDA has warned that ibuprofen can interfere with the antiplatelet effect of low-dose aspirin (81 mg/day), potentially rendering aspirin less effective when used for cardioprotection and stroke protection. In situations where these drugs could be used concomitantly, the FDA has proved the following information: Patients who use immediate release aspirin (not enteric-coated aspirin) and take single doses of ibuprofen 400 mg, should dose the ibuprofen at least 30 minutes or longer after aspirin ingestion or more than 8 hours before aspirin ingestion to avoid attenuation of aspirin's effect. Similar recommendations may hold for concomitant may hold for concomitant naproxen and aspirin use. See Effects on Bleeding.

Naproxen and Esomeprazole

(na PROKS en & es oh ME pray zol)

Related Information

Esomeprazole *on page 594*
Naproxen *on page 1080*
Rheumatoid Arthritis, Osteoarthritis, and Osteoporosis *on page 1697*

Brand Names: US Vimovo

Brand Names: Canada MYLAN-Naproxen/Esomeprazole MR; Vimovo

Pharmacologic Category Analgesic, Nonopioid; Nonsteroidal Anti-inflammatory Drug (NSAID), Oral; Proton Pump Inhibitor; Substituted Benzimidazole

Use

Osteoarthritis, rheumatoid arthritis, ankylosing spondylitis: Reduction of the risk of NSAID-associated gastric ulcers in patients at risk of developing gastric ulcers who require an NSAID for the relief of signs and symptoms of osteoarthritis, rheumatoid arthritis, and ankylosing spondylitis in adults.

Juvenile idiopathic arthritis: Reduction of the risk of NSAID-associated gastric ulcers in patients at risk of developing gastric ulcers who require an NSAID for the relief of signs and symptoms of juvenile idiopathic arthritis (JIA) in pediatric patients ≥12 years weighing ≥38 kg.

Limitations of use: Not recommended for the initial treatment of pain; controlled studies do not extend beyond 6 months.

Local Anesthetic/Vasoconstrictor Precautions No information available to require special precautions

Effects on Dental Treatment Key adverse event(s) related to dental treatment: Esomeprazole: Xerostomia (normal salivary flow resumes upon discontinuation)

Effects on Bleeding Nonselective NSAIDs, such as naproxen and esomeprazole, inhibit platelet aggregation and prolong bleeding time in some patients. Unlike aspirin, the NSAID effect on platelet function is quantitatively less, of shorter duration, and reversible. Normal platelet function should occur in ~5 elimination half-lives or in <10 hours after discontinuation of naproxen and esomeprazole. Concomitant use of other NSAIDs should be avoided.

Adverse Reactions Also see individual agents.

>10%: Gastrointestinal: Gastritis (17%)

1% to 10%:

Cardiovascular: Peripheral edema (3%)

Central nervous system: Dizziness (3%), headache (3%)

Gastrointestinal: Diarrhea (6%), constipation (4%), flatulence (4%), upper abdominal pain (4%), dysgeusia (2%)

Genitourinary: Urinary tract infection (2%)

Respiratory: Upper respiratory tract infection (5%)

<1%, postmarketing and/or case reports: Abdominal distention, abdominal pain, abnormal gait, acute interstitial nephritis, bruise, falling, gastroesophageal reflux disease, hematochezia, joint swelling, muscle spasm, renal tubular necrosis

Mechanism of Action

Naproxen: Reversibly inhibits cyclooxygenase-1 and 2 (COX-1 and 2) enzymes, which result in decreased formation of prostaglandin precursors; has antipyretic, analgesic, and anti-inflammatory properties

Esomeprazole: Proton pump inhibitor which decreases acid secretion in gastric parietal cells

Pregnancy Considerations

Animal reproduction studies have not been conducted with this combination. Because they may cause premature closure of the ductus arteriosus, use of NSAIDs late in pregnancy should be avoided. Refer to individual monographs for additional information.

- ◆ **Naproxen Comfort Pac [DSC]** *see* Naproxen *on page 1080*
- ◆ **Naproxen DR** *see* Naproxen *on page 1080*
- ◆ **Naproxen Sodium** *see* Naproxen *on page 1080*
- ◆ **Naramin [OTC]** *see* DiphenhydrAMINE (Systemic) *on page 502*

Naratriptan (NAR a trip tan)

Related Information

Temporomandibular Dysfunction (TMD), Chronic Pain, and Fibromyalgia *on page 1773*

Brand Names: US Amerge

Brand Names: Canada Amerge; SANDOZ Naratriptan; TEVA-Naratriptan

Pharmacologic Category Antimigraine Agent; Serotonin 5-$HT_{1B, 1D}$ Receptor Agonist

Use Migraines: Acute treatment of migraine attacks with or without aura in adults.

Local Anesthetic/Vasoconstrictor Precautions No information available to require special precautions

Effects on Dental Treatment No significant effects or complications reported

Effects on Bleeding No information available to require special precautions

Adverse Reactions

1% to 10%:

Central nervous system: Pain (4%), fatigue (2%), dizziness (1% to 2%), drowsiness (1% to 2%), paresthesia (1% to 2%), hot and cold flashes (1%), sensation of pressure (1%; chest/neck/throat/jaw), vertigo (1%)

Gastrointestinal: Nausea (4% to 5%), vomiting (1%), xerostomia (1%)

Neuromuscular & skeletal: Neck pain (2%)

Ophthalmic: Photophobia (1%)

Respiratory: Constriction of the pharynx (2%), ENT infection (1%)

<1%, postmarketing, and/or case reports (limited to important or life-threatening): Abnormal bilirubin levels, abnormal hepatic function tests, anaphylactoid reaction, anaphylaxis, anemia, angina pectoris, angioedema, bradycardia, cerebral infarction, colonic ischemia, coronary artery vasospasm, depression, dyspnea, ECG changes (atrial fibrillation, atrial flutter, premature ventricular contractions, PR prolongation, or QT_c prolongation), glycosuria, hallucination, heart murmur, hypercholesterolemia, hyperglycemia, hyperlipidemia, hypersensitivity reaction (some cases severe, including circulatory collapse), hypertension, hypotension, hypothyroidism, ischemic heart disease, ketonuria, myocardial infarction, palpitations, panic, seizure, serotonin syndrome, skin rash, subarachnoid hemorrhage, subconjunctival hemorrhage, syncope, thrombocytopenia, transient ischemic attacks, ventricular fibrillation, ventricular tachycardia

Mechanism of Action Selective agonist for serotonin (5-HT_{1B} and 5-HT_{1D} receptors) in cranial arteries; causes vasoconstriction and reduces sterile inflammation associated with antidromic neuronal transmission correlating with relief of migraine

Pharmacodynamics/Kinetics

Onset of Action ~1 to 2 hours (Bomhof 1999; Tfelt-Hansen 2000)

Half-life Elimination 6 hours; Increased in renal impairment (moderate impairment; mean: 11 hours; range: 7 to 20 hours); Increased in hepatic impairment (moderate impairment: 8 to 16 hours)

Time to Peak 2 to 3 hours

Pregnancy Considerations

Pregnancy outcome information for naratriptan is available from a pregnancy registry sponsored by GlaxoSmithKline. As of September 2012, data were available for 57 infants/fetuses exposed to naratriptan, and seven exposed to both naratriptan and sumatriptan. Following naratriptan exposure, there was one infant born with a birth defect; this infant was also exposed to sumatriptan during the first trimester of pregnancy. The pregnancy registry was closed to enrollment in January 2012. Additional information related to the use of naratriptan in pregnancy is limited (Källén 2011; Nezvalová-Henriksen 2010; Nezvalová-Henriksen 2012). Until additional information is available, other agents are preferred for the initial treatment of migraine in pregnancy (Da Silva 2012; MacGregor 2012; Williams 2012).

- ◆ **NAratriptan HCl** *see* Naratriptan *on page 1085*
- ◆ **Naratriptan Hydrochloride** *see* Naratriptan *on page 1085*
- ◆ **Narcan** *see* Naloxone *on page 1074*
- ◆ **Naropin** *see* Ropivacaine *on page 1346*
- ◆ **Nasacort Allergy 24HR [OTC]** *see* Triamcinolone (Nasal) *on page 1489*

- **Nasacort Allergy 24HR Children [OTC]** *see* Triamcinolone (Nasal) *on page 1489*
- **Nasal Allergy 24 Hour [OTC]** *see* Triamcinolone (Nasal) *on page 1489*
- **Nasal Antiseptic [OTC] [DSC]** *see* Povidone-Iodine (Topical) *on page 1249*
- **Nasal Decongestant [OTC]** *see* Phenylephrine (Systemic) *on page 1227*
- **Nasal Decongestant [OTC]** *see* Pseudoephedrine *on page 1291*
- **Nasal Decongestant Spray [OTC]** *see* Oxymetazoline (Nasal) *on page 1173*
- **Nasal Spray 12 Hour [OTC]** *see* Oxymetazoline (Nasal) *on page 1173*
- **Nasal Spray Max Strength [OTC]** *see* Oxymetazoline (Nasal) *on page 1173*
- **Nascobal** *see* Cyanocobalamin *on page 417*
- **Nasonex** *see* Mometasone (Nasal) *on page 1045*
- **Natacyn** *see* Natamycin *on page 1087*

Natalizumab (na ta LIZ u mab)

Brand Names: US Tysabri

Brand Names: Canada Tysabri

Pharmacologic Category Gastrointestinal Agent, Miscellaneous; Monoclonal Antibody, Selective Adhesion-Molecule Inhibitor

Use

Crohn disease: Inducing and maintaining clinical response and remission in adults with moderately to severely active Crohn disease with evidence of inflammation who have had an inadequate response to, or are unable to tolerate, conventional Crohn disease therapies and inhibitors of tumor necrosis factor-alpha (TNF-alpha).

Multiple sclerosis, relapsing: As monotherapy for the treatment of patients with relapsing forms of multiple sclerosis, including clinically isolated syndrome, relapsing-remitting disease, and active secondary progressive disease. Natalizumab increases the risk of progressive multifocal leukoencephalopathy. When initiating and continuing treatment with natalizumab, consider whether the expected benefit of natalizumab is sufficient to offset this risk.

Canada labeling: Treatment of relapsing forms of multiple sclerosis in patients who have had an inadequate response to, or are unable to tolerate, other therapies for multiple sclerosis.

Local Anesthetic/Vasoconstrictor Precautions No information available to require special precautions

Effects on Dental Treatment No significant effects or complications reported

Effects on Bleeding No information available to require special precautions

Adverse Reactions

>10%:

Central nervous system: Headache (32% to 38%), fatigue (10% to 27%), depression (≤19%)

Dermatologic: Skin rash (6% to 12%)

Gastrointestinal: Nausea (≤17%), gastroenteritis (≤11%), abdominal distress (≤11%)

Genitourinary: Urinary tract infection (3% to 21%)

Infection: Influenza (≤12%)

Neuromuscular & skeletal: Arthralgia (8% to 19%), limb pain (16%), back pain (≤12%)

Respiratory: Upper respiratory tract infection (≤22%), lower respiratory tract infection (≤17%), flu-like symptoms (≤11%)

Miscellaneous: Infusion related reaction (11% to 24%)

1% to 10%:

Cardiovascular: Peripheral edema (5% to 6%), chest discomfort (≤5%), syncope (≤2%)

Central nervous system: Vertigo (≤6%), dysesthesia (3%), rigors (≤3%), drowsiness (≤2%)

Dermatologic: Dermatitis (≤7%), pruritus (≤4%), urticaria (≤2%), thermal injury (1%), night sweats (≤1%), xeroderma (≤1%)

Endocrine & metabolic: Menstrual disease (≤5%), amenorrhea (≤2%), ovarian cyst (≤2%), weight changes (≤2%)

Gastrointestinal: Diarrhea (10%), tooth infection (≤9%), dyspepsia (≤5%), abdominal pain (≤4%), constipation (≤4%), toothache (≤4%), flatulence (≤3%), aphthous stomatitis (≤2%), cholelithiasis (≤1%), gingival disease (infection: 1%)

Genitourinary: Vaginal infection (≤10%), vaginitis (≤10%), urinary frequency (≤9%), dysmenorrhea (2% to 6%), urinary incontinence (≤4%)

Hematologic & oncologic: Hematoma (1%)

Hepatic: Increased serum transaminases (≤5%)

Hypersensitivity: Hypersensitivity reaction (acute: 2% to 4%; serious acute: ≤1%; delayed: ≤5%)

Immunologic: Antibody development (9% to 10%)

Infection: Herpes virus infection (≤8%), viral infection (≤7%), serious infection (2% to 3%)

Local: Bleeding at injection site (≤3%)

Neuromuscular & skeletal: Muscle cramps (≤5%), tremor (1% to 3%), joint swelling (≤2%)

Respiratory: Sinusitis (≤8%), cough (≤7%), tonsillitis (≤7%), pharyngolaryngeal pain (≤6%), epistaxis (2%)

Miscellaneous: Limb injury (3%), laceration (2%)

<1%, postmarketing, and/or case reports: Acne vulgaris, agitation, anaphylactoid reaction, anaphylaxis, anemia, angina pectoris, appendicitis, aspergillosis (bronchopulmonary), decreased hemoglobin (mild, transient), dizziness, dyspnea, erythema, exacerbation of Crohn's disease, fever, flushing, gastroenteritis (cryptosporidial), hemolytic anemia, hepatic failure, hepatitis (cytomegalovirus), hepatotoxicity, herpes simplex encephalitis, hypotension, immune reconstitution syndrome, increased serum bilirubin, infection (*Burkholderia cepacia*), JC virus infection, joint stiffness, lethargy, leukocytosis, meningitis (herpes), nasopharyngitis, opportunistic infection (including bronchopulmonary infections, meningitis, and progressive multifocal leukoencephalopathy [PML]), muscle spasm, myasthenia, nail disease (onychorrhexis), paresis, pericarditis (case report), petechiae, pharyngitis, pneumonia (includes pneumonia caused by *Pneumocystis jirovecii* and varicella), psychomotor disturbance (hyperactivity), pulmonary infection (*Mycobacterium avium intracellulare*), suicidal ideation, tachycardia, thrombocytopenia, thrombophlebitis, vasodilation

Mechanism of Action Natalizumab is a monoclonal antibody against the alpha-4 subunit of integrin molecules. These molecules are important to adhesion and migration of cells from the vasculature into inflamed tissue. Natalizumab blocks integrin association with vascular receptors, limiting adhesion and transmigration of leukocytes. Efficacy in specific disorders may be related to reduction in specific inflammatory cell populations in target tissues. In multiple sclerosis, efficacy may be related to blockade of T-lymphocyte migration into the central nervous system; treatment results in a decreased frequency of relapse. In Crohn disease, natalizumab decreases inflammation by binding to alpha-4 integrin, blocking adhesion and migration of leukocytes in the gut.

Pharmacodynamics/Kinetics

Half-life Elimination Crohn disease: 3 to 17 days; Multiple sclerosis: 7 to 15 days

Reproductive Considerations

In general, disease-modifying therapies for multiple sclerosis (MS) are stopped prior to a planned pregnancy except in females at high risk of MS activity (AAN [Rae-Grant 2018]). Clinical rebound (new neurologic symptoms and increased lesions) has been reported when natalizumab was discontinued prior to pregnancy. Some studies suggest that continuing treatment until pregnancy is confirmed then restarting soon after delivery may prevent relapse in high-risk patients (De Giglio 2015; Kleerekooper 2017; Portaccio 2018b; Vukusic 2015). Consider use of agents other than natalizumab for females at high risk of disease reactivation who are planning a pregnancy (ECTRIMS/EAN [Montalban 2018]).

Delaying pregnancy is recommended for females with persistent high disease activity; however, when disease-modifying therapy is needed in these patients, natalizumab may be continued following a full discussion of potential risks (ECTRIMS/EAN [Montalban 2018]).

Inflammatory bowel disease is associated with adverse pregnancy outcomes; maternal disease and serum levels of biologic therapy should be optimized prior to conception (Mahadevan 2019).

Pregnancy Considerations

Natalizumab crosses the placenta (Haghikia 2014; Proschmann 2018).

Natalizumab is a humanized monoclonal antibody (IgG_4). Placental transfer of human IgG is dependent upon the IgG subclass, maternal serum concentrations, birth weight, and gestational age, generally increasing as pregnancy progresses. The lowest exposure would be expected during the period of organogenesis (Palmeira 2012; Pentsuk 2009).

Outcome information related to the use of natalizumab in pregnancy is available from pregnancy registries and systematic reviews in which most females discontinued use once pregnancy was detected. The risk of adverse outcomes (such as spontaneous abortion or birth defects) was not consistent between studies (Ebrahimi 2015; Friend 2016; Peng 2019; Portaccio 2018a). Hematological abnormalities in the newborn, such as anemia and thrombocytopenia, have been noted following maternal use during the third trimester (Haghikia 2014; Proschmann 2018).

In general, disease-modifying therapies for multiple sclerosis (MS) are not initiated during pregnancy, except in females at high risk of MS activity (AAN [Rae-Grant 2018]). Clinical rebound (new neurologic symptoms and increased lesions) has been reported when natalizumab was discontinued prior to or during pregnancy. Some studies suggest that continuing treatment until pregnancy is confirmed then restarting soon after delivery may prevent relapse in high-risk patients (De Giglio 2015; Kleerekooper 2017; Portaccio 2018b; Vukusic 2015). When disease-modifying therapy is needed in these patients, natalizumab may be continued during pregnancy following a full discussion of potential risks (ECTRIMS/ EAN [Montalban 2018]).

Inflammatory bowel disease is associated with adverse pregnancy outcomes including an increased risk of miscarriage, premature delivery, delivery of a low birth weight infant, and poor maternal weight gain. Treatment decreases disease flares, disease activity, and the incidence of adverse pregnancy outcomes. When treatment for inflammatory bowel disease is needed in pregnant women, appropriate biologic therapy can be continued without interruption. Serum levels should be evaluated prior to conception and optimized to avoid subtherapeutic concentrations or high levels which may increase placental transfer. Dosing can be adjusted so delivery occurs at the lowest serum concentration. For natalizumab, the final injection can be given 4 to 6 weeks prior to the estimated date of delivery, then continued 48 hours' postpartum (Mahadevan 2019).

Prescribing and Access Restrictions Canada: Natalizumab is only available through a controlled distribution program called Biogen ONE Support Program (855-676-6300 or http://www.BIOGENcareforMS.ca). This program is associated with the prescribing, administration, and monitoring of Canadian patients receiving natalizumab. Clinicians are educated on the appropriate use of natalizumab and are expected to discuss the benefits/risks of therapy. Clinicians should evaluate patients every 6 months during treatment. Under this program, only prescribers and pharmacies registered with the program are able to prescribe and dispense natalizumab. In addition, natalizumab can only be dispensed to patients who are registered and meet all the conditions of the Biogen ONE Support Program.

Natamycin (na ta MYE sin)

Brand Names: US Natacyn

Pharmacologic Category Antifungal Agent, Ophthalmic

Use Ocular fungal infections: Treatment of fungal blepharitis, conjunctivitis, and keratitis caused by susceptible organisms, including *Fusarium solani* keratitis.

Local Anesthetic/Vasoconstrictor Precautions No information available to require special precautions

Effects on Dental Treatment No significant effects or complications reported

Effects on Bleeding No information available to require special precautions

Adverse Reactions Postmarketing and/or case reports: Allergic reaction, chest pain, corneal opacity, dyspnea, eye discomfort, edema, hyperemia, irritation and/or pain, foreign body sensation, parasthesia, tearing, vision changes

Mechanism of Action Binds to sterol in fungal cell membrane and changes the cell wall permeability allowing for a reduction of cellular contents

Pregnancy Considerations Animal reproduction studies have not been conducted.

◆ **Natazia** *see* Estradiol and Dienogest *on page* 597

Nateglinide (na te GLYE nide)

Related Information

Endocrine Disorders and Pregnancy *on page* 1684

Brand Names: US Starlix

Pharmacologic Category Antidiabetic Agent, Meglitinide Analog

Use Diabetes mellitus, type 2: Treatment of adults with type 2 diabetes mellitus as an adjunct to diet and exercise to improve glycemic control

Local Anesthetic/Vasoconstrictor Precautions No information available to require special precautions

Effects on Dental Treatment No significant effects or complications reported

Effects on Bleeding May increase overall bleeding times

Adverse Reactions As reported with nateglinide monotherapy:

>10%: Respiratory: Upper respiratory infection (11%)

1% to 10%:

- Central nervous system: Dizziness (4%)
- Endocrine & metabolic: Hypoglycemia (2%), increased uric acid, weight gain
- Neuromuscular & skeletal: Arthropathy (3%)
- Respiratory: Flu-like symptoms (4%)
- Miscellaneous: Accidental injury (3%)

Postmarketing and/or case reports: Cholestatic hepatitis, hypersensitivity reaction (including pruritus, rash, urticaria), increased liver enzymes, jaundice

Mechanism of Action Nonsulfonylurea hypoglycemic agent which blocks ATP-dependent potassium channels, depolarizing the membrane and facilitating calcium entry through calcium channels. Increased intracellular calcium stimulates insulin release from the pancreatic beta cells. Nateglinide-induced insulin release is glucose-dependent.

Pharmacodynamics/Kinetics

Onset of Action Insulin secretion: ~20 minutes; Peak effect: 1 hour

Duration of Action 4 hours

Half-life Elimination 1.5 hours

Time to Peak ≤1 hour

Pregnancy Risk Factor C

Pregnancy Considerations

Information describing the effects of nateglinide on pregnancy outcomes is limited (Twaites 2007).

Poorly controlled diabetes during pregnancy can be associated with an increased risk of adverse maternal and fetal outcomes, including diabetic ketoacidosis, preeclampsia, spontaneous abortion, preterm delivery, delivery complications, major birth defects, stillbirth, and macrosomia (ACOG 201 2018). To prevent adverse outcomes, prior to conception and throughout pregnancy, maternal blood glucose and HbA_{1c} should be kept as close to target goals as possible but without causing significant hypoglycemia (ADA 2020; Blumer 2013).

Agents other than nateglinide are currently recommended to treat diabetes mellitus in pregnancy (ADA 2020).

- ◆ **Natesto** *see* Testosterone *on page* 1425
- ◆ **Natpara** *see* Parathyroid Hormone *on page* 1192
- ◆ **Natrecor [DSC]** *see* Nesiritide *on page* 1094
- ◆ **Natriuretic Peptide** *see* Nesiritide *on page* 1094
- ◆ **Natural Lung Surfactant** *see* Beractant *on page* 232
- ◆ **Natural Vitamin E [OTC]** *see* Vitamin E (Systemic) *on page* 1549
- ◆ **Nature-Throid** *see* Thyroid, Desiccated *on page* 1442
- ◆ **Navelbine** *see* Vinorelbine *on page* 1547
- ◆ **Nayzilam** *see* Midazolam *on page* 1020
- ◆ **N-benzoyl-staurosporine** *see* Midostaurin *on page* 1027
- ◆ **NBI-56418** *see* Elagolix *on page* 547
- ◆ ***n*-Docosanol** *see* Docosanol *on page* 508

Nebivolol (ne BIV oh lole)

Related Information

Cardiovascular Diseases *on page* 1654

Brand Names: US Bystolic

Brand Names: Canada Bystolic

Pharmacologic Category Antihypertensive; Beta-Blocker, Beta-1 Selective

Use Hypertension: Management of hypertension. **Note:** Beta-blockers are **not** recommended as first-line therapy (ACC/AHA [Whelton 2017]).

Local Anesthetic/Vasoconstrictor Precautions No information available to require special precautions

Effects on Dental Treatment Nebivolol is a cardioselective beta-blocker. Local anesthetic with vasoconstrictor can be safely used in patients medicated with nebivolol. Nonselective beta-blockers (ie, propranolol, nadolol) enhance the pressor response to epinephrine, resulting in hypertension and bradycardia; this has not been reported for nebivolol. Many nonsteroidal anti-inflammatory drugs, such as ibuprofen and indomethacin, can reduce the hypotensive effect of beta-blockers after 3 or more weeks of therapy with the NSAID. Short-term NSAID use (ie, 3 days) requires no special precautions in patients taking beta-blockers.

Effects on Bleeding No information available to require special precautions

Adverse Reactions

1% to 10%:

- Cardiovascular: Peripheral edema (1%), bradycardia (≤1%), chest pain (≤1%)
- Central nervous system: Headache (6% to 9%), fatigue (dose-related; 2% to 5%), dizziness (2% to 4%), insomnia (1%), paresthesia
- Dermatologic: Skin rash (≤1%)
- Endocrine & metabolic: Decreased HDL cholesterol, hypercholesterolemia, increased serum triglycerides, increased uric acid
- Gastrointestinal: Diarrhea (dose-related; 2% to 3%), nausea (1% to 3%), abdominal pain
- Hematologic & oncologic: Decreased platelet count
- Neuromuscular & skeletal: Weakness
- Renal: Increased blood urea nitrogen
- Respiratory: Dyspnea (≤1%)

<1%, postmarketing, and/or case reports: Acute pulmonary edema, acute renal failure, angioedema, atrioventricular block (second and third degree), bronchospasm, claudication, dermatological disease, drowsiness, erectile dysfunction, hepatic insufficiency, hypersensitivity angiitis, hypersensitivity reaction, increased serum ALT, increased serum AST, increased serum bilirubin, myocardial infarction, peripheral ischemia, pruritus, psoriasis, Raynaud's phenomenon, syncope, thrombocytopenia, urticaria, vertigo, vomiting

Mechanism of Action Highly-selective inhibitor of $beta_1$-adrenergic receptors; at doses ≤10 mg nebivolol preferentially blocks $beta_1$-receptors. Nebivolol, unlike other beta-blockers, also produces an endothelium-derived nitric oxide-dependent vasodilation resulting in a reduction of systemic vascular resistance.

Pharmacodynamics/Kinetics

Half-life Elimination Terminal: 12 hours (extensive metabolizers) or 19 hours (poor metabolizers); up to 32 hours has been reported in poor metabolizers (Mangrella 1998).

Time to Peak 1.5 to 4 hours

Pregnancy Considerations

Outcome information following maternal use of nebivolol in pregnancy is limited (Sullo 2015).

Exposure to beta-blockers during pregnancy may increase the risk for adverse events in the neonate. If maternal use of a beta-blocker is needed, fetal growth should be monitored during pregnancy and the newborn should be monitored for 48 hours after delivery for bradycardia, hypoglycemia, and respiratory depression (ESC [Regitz-Zagrosek 2018]).

Chronic maternal hypertension is also associated with adverse events in the fetus/infant. Chronic maternal hypertension may increase the risk of birth defects, low birth weight, premature delivery, stillbirth, and neonatal death. Actual fetal/neonatal risks may be related to duration and severity of maternal hypertension. Untreated chronic hypertension may also increase the risks of adverse maternal outcomes, including gestational diabetes, preeclampsia, delivery complications, stroke, and myocardial infarction (ACOG 203 2019).

When treatment of chronic hypertension in pregnancy is indicated, agents other than nebivolol are preferred (ACOG 203 2013; ESC [Regitz-Zagrosek 2018]; Magee 2014). Females with preexisting hypertension may continue their medication during pregnancy unless contraindications exist (ESC [Regitz-Zagrosek 2018]).

Nebivolol and Valsartan
(ne BIV oh lole & val SAR tan)

Brand Names: US Byvalson [DSC]

Pharmacologic Category Angiotensin II Receptor Blocker; Antihypertensive; Antihypertensive, Combination; Beta-Blocker, Beta-1 Selective

Use Hypertension: Management of hypertension.

Local Anesthetic/Vasoconstrictor Precautions No information available to require special precautions

Effects on Dental Treatment Key adverse events(s) related to dental treatment: Nebivolol component is a cardioselective beta-blocker. Local anesthetic with vasoconstrictor can be safely used in patients medicated with nebivolol. Nonselective beta-blockers (ie, propranolol, nadolol) enhance the pressor response to epinephrine, resulting in hypertension and bradycardia; this has not been reported for nebivolol. Many nonsteroidal anti-inflammatory drugs, such as ibuprofen and indomethacin, can reduce the hypotensive effect of beta-blockers after 3 or more weeks of therapy with the NSAID. Short-term NSAID use (ie, 3 days) requires no special precautions in patients taking beta-blockers.

Effects on Bleeding No information available to require special precautions

Adverse Reactions See individual agents for reactions.

Mechanism of Action

Nebivolol: Highly-selective inhibitor of $beta_1$-adrenergic receptors; at doses ≤10 mg nebivolol preferentially blocks $beta_1$-receptors. Nebivolol, unlike other beta-blockers, also produces an endothelium-derived nitric oxide-dependent vasodilation resulting in a reduction of systemic vascular resistance.

Valsartan: Produces direct antagonism of the angiotensin II (AT2) receptors, unlike the ACE inhibitors. It displaces angiotensin II from the AT1 receptor and produces its blood pressure-lowering effects by antagonizing AT1-induced vasoconstriction, aldosterone release, catecholamine release, arginine vasopressin release, water intake, and hypertrophic responses. This action results in more efficient blockade of the cardiovascular effects of angiotensin II and fewer side effects than the ACE inhibitors.

Pregnancy Considerations

[US Boxed Warning]: Drugs that act on the renin-angiotensin system can cause injury and death to the developing fetus. Discontinue as soon as possible once pregnancy is detected. Refer to individual monographs for additional information.

◆ **Nebivolol Hydrochloride** *see* Nebivolol *on page 1088*

Necitumumab (ne si TOOM oo mab)

Brand Names: US Portrazza

Pharmacologic Category Antineoplastic Agent, Epidermal Growth Factor Receptor (EGFR) Inhibitor; Antineoplastic Agent, Monoclonal Antibody

Use

Non-small cell lung cancer (squamous), metastatic: First-line treatment of metastatic squamous non-small cell lung cancer (NSCLC) in combination with gemcitabine and cisplatin

Limitations of use: Not indicated for treatment of non-squamous NSCLC.

Local Anesthetic/Vasoconstrictor Precautions No information available to require special precautions

Effects on Dental Treatment Key adverse event(s) related to dental treatment: Stomatitis (11%) has been reported

Effects on Bleeding No information available to require special precautions

Adverse Reactions Adverse reaction percentages reported as part of a combination regimen with gemcitabine and cisplatin.

>10%:

Central nervous system: Headache (11%)

Dermatologic: Skin toxicity (79%; grades 3/4: 8%), skin rash (44%; grades 3/4: 4%), acneiform eruption (15%; grades 3/4: 1%)

Endocrine & metabolic: Hypomagnesemia (43% to 83%; grades 3/4: 20%), hypocalcemia (45%; grades 3/4: 6%; with albumin corrected: 36%; grades 3/4: 4%), hypophosphatemia (31%; grades 3/4: 8%), hypokalemia (28%; grades 3/4: 5%), weight loss (13%)

Gastrointestinal: Vomiting (29%), diarrhea (16%), stomatitis (11%)

1% to 10%:

Cardiovascular: Venous thromboembolism (9%; grades 3/4: 5%), arterial thromboembolism (5%; grades 3/4: 4%), pulmonary embolism (5%), cardiorespiratory arrest (3%), deep vein thrombosis (2%), cerebrovascular accident (≤2%), ischemia (≤2%), myocardial infarction (1%)

Dermatologic: Acne vulgaris (9%), paronychia (7%), pruritus (7%), xeroderma (7%), skin fissure (5%)

Immunologic: Antibody development (4%; neutralizing: 1%)

Ophthalmic: Conjunctivitis (7%)

Respiratory: Hemoptysis (10%)

Miscellaneous: Infusion related reaction (2%; grade 3: <1%)

Mechanism of Action Necitumumab is a recombinant human IgG1 EGFR monoclonal antibody which binds (with a high affinity) to the ligand binding site of the EGFR receptor to prevent receptor activation and downstream signaling (Thatcher 2015).

Pharmacodynamics/Kinetics

Half-life Elimination ~14 days.

Reproductive Considerations

Females of reproductive potential should use effective contraception during therapy and for 3 months after the last necitumumab dose.

Pregnancy Considerations

Necitumumab is expected to cross the placenta. Based on the mechanism of action and data from animal reproduction studies, in utero exposure to necitumumab may cause fetal harm.

◆ **Necon 0.5/35 (28)** *see* Ethinyl Estradiol and Norethindrone *on page 614*

◆ **Necon 1/35 (28) [DSC]** *see* Ethinyl Estradiol and Norethindrone *on page 614*

◆ **Necon 7/7/7 [DSC]** *see* Ethinyl Estradiol and Norethindrone *on page 614*

◆ **Necon 10/11 (28) [DSC]** *see* Ethinyl Estradiol and Norethindrone *on page 614*

Nedocromil (Ophthalmic) (ne doe KROE mil)

Brand Names: US Alocril

Brand Names: Canada Alocril [DSC]

Pharmacologic Category Mast Cell Stabilizer

Use Allergic conjunctivitis: Treatment of itching associated with allergic conjunctivitis

Local Anesthetic/Vasoconstrictor Precautions

No information available to require special precautions

Effects on Dental Treatment Key adverse event(s) related to dental treatment: Unpleasant taste.

Effects on Bleeding No information available to require special precautions

Adverse Reactions

>10%:

- Central nervous system: Headache (40%)
- Gastrointestinal: Unpleasant taste
- Ophthalmic: Burning sensation of eyes, eye irritation, stinging of eyes
- Respiratory: Nasal congestion

1% to 10%:

- Ophthalmic: Conjunctivitis, eye redness, photophobia
- Respiratory: Asthma, rhinitis

Mechanism of Action Inhibits the activation of and mediator release from a variety of inflammatory cell types associated with hypersensitivity reactions including eosinophils, neutrophils, macrophages, mast cells, monocytes, and platelets; it inhibits the release of histamine, leukotrienes, and slow-reacting substance of anaphylaxis.

Pregnancy Considerations Nedocromil has minimal systemic absorption.

◆ **Nedocromil Sodium** *see* Nedocromil (Ophthalmic) *on page 1090*

Nefazodone (nef AY zoe done)

Related Information

Dentin Hypersensitivity, Acid Erosion, High Caries Index, Management of Alveolar Osteitis, and Xerostomia *on page 1762*

Vasoconstrictor Interactions With Antidepressants *on page 1821*

Pharmacologic Category Antidepressant, Serotonin Reuptake Inhibitor/Antagonist

Use Depression: Treatment of depression

Local Anesthetic/Vasoconstrictor Precautions

Nefazodone inhibits reuptake of both serotonin and norepinephrine and also blocks some serotonin receptors. No precautions with vasoconstrictors appear to be necessary.

Effects on Dental Treatment Key adverse event(s) related to dental treatment: Significant xerostomia (normal salivary flow resumes upon discontinuation) and taste perversion.

Effects on Bleeding No information available to require special precautions

Adverse Reactions

>10%:

- Central nervous system: Headache (36%), drowsiness (16% to 28%), dizziness (10% to 22%), insomnia (11%), agitation
- Gastrointestinal: Xerostomia (25%), nausea (22%), constipation (14%)
- Neuromuscular & skeletal: Weakness (11%)

1% to 10%:

- Cardiovascular: Orthostatic hypotension (4%), vasodilation (4%), peripheral edema (3%), hypotension (2%), bradycardia
- Central nervous system: Confusion (2% to 8%), memory impairment (4%), paresthesia (4%), abnormal dreams (3%), lack of concentration (3%), ataxia (2%), chills (2%), psychomotor retardation (2%), hypertonia (1%)
- Dermatologic: Pruritus (2%), skin rash (2%)
- Endocrine & metabolic: Decreased libido (1%), increased thirst (1%)
- Gastrointestinal: Dyspepsia (9%), diarrhea (8%), increased appetite (5%), dysgeusia (2%), vomiting (2%), gastroenteritis
- Genitourinary: Urinary frequency (2%), urinary retention (2%), mastalgia (1%), impotence
- Hematologic & oncologic: Decreased hematocrit (3%)
- Infection: Infection (8%)
- Neuromuscular & skeletal: Tremor (2%), arthralgia (1%), neck stiffness (1%)
- Ophthalmic: Visual disturbance (7% to 10%), blurred vision (3% to 9%), visual field defect (2%), eye pain
- Otic: Tinnitus (2% to 3%)
- Respiratory: pharyngitis (6%), cough (3%), flu-like symptoms (3%), bronchitis, dyspnea
- Miscellaneous: Fever (2%)

<1%, postmarketing, and/or case reports: Abnormal gait, abnormal hepatic function tests, abnormality in thinking, accommodation disturbance, acne vulgaris, ageusia, alopecia, amenorrhea, anemia, angina pectoris, angioedema, angle-closure glaucoma, anorgasmia, apathy, arthritis, asthma, atrioventricular block, attempted suicide, breast hypertrophy, bruise, bursitis, cardiac failure, cellulitis, cerebrovascular accident, colitis, conjunctivitis, convulsions, cystitis, deafness, dehydration, depersonalization, derealization, diplopia, disturbance in attention, dry eye syndrome, dysarthria, eczema, ejaculatory disorder, enlargement of abdomen, epistaxis, eructation, esophagitis, euphoria, facial edema, galactorrhea, gastritis, gingivitis, gout, gynecomastia, halitosis, hallucination, hangover effect, heavy eyelids, hematuria, hemorrhage, hepatic failure, hepatic necrosis, hepatitis, hernia, hiccups, hostility, hyperacusis, hypercholesterolemia, hyperesthesia, hyperkinesia, hypermenorrhea, hypersensitivity reaction, hypertension, hyperventilation, hypoglycemia, hyponatremia, hypotonia, increased lactate dehydrogenase, increased libido, increased serum alt, increased serum ast, increased serum prolactin, keratoconjunctivitis, laryngitis, leukopenia,

lymphadenopathy, maculopapular rash, malaise, muscle rigidity, mydriasis, myoclonus, nephrolithiasis, neuralgia, neuroleptic malignant syndrome, nocturia, nocturnal amblyopia, oliguria, oral candidiasis, oral mucosa ulcer, otalgia, pallor, paranoia, pelvic pain, peptic ulcer, periodontal abscess, photophobia, pneumonia, polyuria, priapism, rectal hemorrhage, rhabdomyolysis, seizure, serotonin syndrome (with lovastatin/simvastatin), sialorrhea, skin photosensitivity, stevens-johnson syndrome, stomatitis, suicidal ideation, syncope, tachycardia, tendinous contracture, tendonitis, tenosynovitis, thrombocytopenia, tonic-clonic seizures, twitching, ulcerative colitis, urinary incontinence, urinary urgency, urticaria, uterine fibroid enlargement, uterine hemorrhage, vaginal hemorrhage, varicose veins, ventricular premature contractions, vertigo, vesicobullous dermatitis, voice disorder, weight loss, xeroderma, yawning

Mechanism of Action Inhibits neuronal reuptake of serotonin and norepinephrine; also blocks 5-HT_2 and $alpha_1$ receptors; has no significant affinity for $alpha_2$, beta-adrenergic, 5-HT_{1A}, cholinergic, dopaminergic, or benzodiazepine receptors

Pharmacodynamics/Kinetics

Onset of Action Depression: Initial effects may be observed within 1 to 2 weeks of treatment, with continued improvements through 4 to 6 weeks (Papakostas 2006; Posternak 2005; Szegedi 2009).

Half-life Elimination Note: Active metabolites persist longer in all populations.

Children: 4.1 hours

Adolescents: 3.9 hours

Adults: Parent drug: 2 to 4 hours; active metabolites: 1.4 to 8 hours

Time to Peak Note: Prolonged in presence of food

Children and Adolescents: 0.5 to 1 hour

Adults: Serum: 1 hour

Pregnancy Risk Factor C

Pregnancy Considerations Adverse effects were observed in some animal reproduction studies.

The ACOG recommends that therapy with antidepressants during pregnancy be individualized; treatment of depression during pregnancy should incorporate the clinical expertise of the mental health clinician, obstetrician, primary health care provider, and pediatrician. According to the American Psychiatric Association (APA), the risks of medication treatment should be weighed against other treatment options and untreated depression. Consideration should be given to using agents with safety data in pregnancy. For women who discontinue antidepressant medications during pregnancy and who may be at high risk for postpartum depression, the medications can be restarted following delivery. Treatment algorithms have been developed by the ACOG and the APA for the management of depression in women prior to conception and during pregnancy (ACOG 2008; APA 2010; Yonkers 2009).

Pregnant women exposed to antidepressants during pregnancy are encouraged to enroll in the National Pregnancy Registry for Antidepressants (NPRAD). Women 18 to 45 years of age or their health care providers may contact the registry by calling 844-405-6185. Enrollment should be done as early in pregnancy as possible.

◆ **Nefazodone Hydrochloride** *see* Nefazodone *on page 1090*

Nelarabine (nel AY re been)

Brand Names: US Arranon

Brand Names: Canada Atriance

Pharmacologic Category Antineoplastic Agent, Antimetabolite; Antineoplastic Agent, Antimetabolite (Purine Analog)

Use T-cell acute lymphoblastic leukemia/lymphoma: Treatment of relapsed or refractory T-cell acute lymphoblastic leukemia/lymphoma in patients ≥1 year of age following at least 2 chemotherapy regimens

Local Anesthetic/Vasoconstrictor Precautions No information available to require special precautions

Effects on Dental Treatment Key adverse event(s) related to dental treatment: Taste perversion and stomatitis.

Effects on Bleeding Chemotherapy may result in significant myelosuppression. Thrombocytopenia has been reported in 86% to 88% (grade 4: 22% to 32%). Nosebleeds have occurred in 8% of patients. In patients who are under active treatment with these agents, medical consult is suggested.

Adverse Reactions

>10%:

Cardiovascular: Peripheral edema (adults: 15%), edema (adults: 11%)

Central nervous system: Fatigue (adults: 50%), drowsiness (adults: 23%; children and adolescents: 7%), dizziness (adults: 21%), hypoesthesia (adults: 17%; children and adolescents: 6%), headache (15% to 17%), paresthesia (adults: 15%; children and adolescents: 4%), peripheral sensory neuropathy (6% to 13%; children and adolescents, grade 3: 6%), pain (adults: 11%)

Endocrine & metabolic: Decreased serum potassium (children and adolescents: 11%)

Gastrointestinal: Nausea (adults: 41%), diarrhea (adults: 22%), vomiting (adults: 22%; children and adolescents: 10%), constipation (adults: 21%)

Hematologic & oncologic: Anemia (95% to 99%; children and adolescents, grade 3: 45%; adults, grade 3: 20%; grades ≥4: 10% to 14%), neutropenia (children and adolescents: 94%; adults: 81%; grade 3: 14% to 17%, children and adolescents, grades ≥4: 62%, adults, grades ≥4: 49%), thrombocytopenia (86% to 88%; adults, grade 3: 37%; children and adolescents, grade 3: 27%; children and adolescents, grades ≥4: 32%; adults, grades ≥4: 22%), leukopenia (children and adolescents: 38%; children and adolescents, grade 3: 14%; children and adolescents, grades ≥4: 7%), febrile neutropenia (adults: 12%; adults, grade 3: 9%; adults, grades ≥4: 1%), petechia (adults: 12%; adults, grade 3: 2%)

Hepatic: Increased serum transaminases (children and adolescents: 12%)

Neuromuscular & skeletal: Asthenia (adults: 17%; children and adolescents: 6%), myalgia (adults: 13%)

Respiratory: Cough (adults: 25%), dyspnea (adults: 20%)

Miscellaneous: Fever (adults: 23%)

1% to 10%:

Cardiovascular: Hypotension (adults: 8%), sinus tachycardia (adults: 8%), chest pain (adults: 5%)

Central nervous system: Ataxia (adults: 9%; children and adolescents: 2%), confusion (adults: 8%), myasthenia (adults: 8%), rigors (adults: 8%), insomnia (adults: 7%), peripheral motor neuropathy (4% to 7%; grade 3: 1% to 2%), abnormal gait (adults: 6%), depression (adults: 6%), impaired consciousness (adults: 6%), seizure (children and adolescents: 6%; adults, grade 3: 1%), peripheral neuropathy (5% to 6%; grade 3: 1% to 2%), noncardiac chest pain (adults: 5%), motor dysfunction (children and adolescents: 4%), neuropathy (adults: 4%), amnesia (adults: 3%), balance impairment (adults: 2%), abnormal sensory symptoms (1% to 2%), aphasia (adults, grade 3: 1%), burning sensation (adults: 1%), cerebral hemorrhage (adults, grade 4: 1%), cranial nerve palsy (third and sixth nerve, children and adolescents: 1%), coma (adults, grade 4: 1%), disturbance in attention (adults: 1%), dysarthria (1%), encephalopathy (children and adolescents, grade 4: 1%), hemiparesis (adults, grade 3: 1%), hydrocephalus (children and adolescents: 1%), hypertonia (children and adolescents, grade 3: 1%), hyporeflexia (1%), intracranial hemorrhage (adults, grade 4: 1%), lethargy (children and adolescents: 1%), leukoencephalopathy (adults, grade 4: 1%), loss of consciousness (adults, grade 3: 1%), mental status changes (children and adolescents: 1%), nerve palsy (adults: 1%), paralysis (children and adolescents: 1%), neuralgia (adults: 1%), sciatica (adults: 1%), speech disturbance (adults: 1%), status epilepticus (children and adolescents: 1%)

Endocrine & metabolic: Decreased serum albumin (children and adolescents: 10%), decreased serum calcium (children and adolescents: 8%), dehydration (adults: 7%), decreased serum glucose (children and adolescents: 6%), decreased serum magnesium (children and adolescents: 6%), hyperglycemia (adults: 6%)

Gastrointestinal: Abdominal pain (adults: 9%), anorexia (adults: 9%), stomatitis (adults: 8%; grade 3: 1%), abdominal distention (adults: 6%), dysgeusia (adults: 3%)

Hepatic: Increased serum bilirubin (children and adolescents: 10%), increased serum aspartate aminotransferase (adults: 6%)

Infection: Infection (5% to 9%)

Neuromuscular & skeletal: Arthralgia (adults: 9%), back pain (adults: 8%), limb pain (adults: 7%), tremor (4% to 5%)

Ophthalmic: Blurred vision (adults: 4%), nystagmus disorder (adults: 1%)

Renal: Increased serum creatinine (children and adolescents: 6%)

Respiratory: Pleural effusion (adults: 10%), epistaxis (adults: 8%), pneumonia (adults: 8%), dyspnea on exertion (adults: 7%), sinusitis (adults: 7%), wheezing (adults: 5%), sinus headache (adults: 1%)

Postmarketing: Demyelinating disease, increased creatine phosphokinase in blood specimen, opportunistic infection, progressive multifocal leukoencephalopathy, rhabdomyolysis, tumor lysis syndrome

Mechanism of Action Nelarabine, a prodrug of ara-G, is demethylated by adenosine deaminase to ara-G and then converted to ara-GTP. Ara-GTP is incorporated into the DNA of the leukemic blasts, leading to inhibition of DNA synthesis and inducing apoptosis. Ara-GTP appears to accumulate at higher levels in T-cells, which correlates to clinical response.

Pharmacodynamics/Kinetics

Half-life Elimination Pediatric patients: Nelarabine: 13 minutes, Ara-G: 2 hours; Adults: Nelarabine: 18 minutes, Ara-G: 3.2 hours

Time to Peak Adults: 3 to 25 hours (of day 1)

Reproductive Considerations

Verify pregnancy status in females of reproductive potential prior to therapy initiation. Females of reproductive potential should use effective contraception during nelarabine therapy. Male patients (including those who have had vasectomies) with female partners of reproductive potential should use condoms during nelarabine treatment and for 3 months after the last nelarabine dose.

Pregnancy Considerations

Based on its mechanism of action and findings in animal reproduction studies, nelarabine may cause fetal harm if administered during pregnancy.

The European Society for Medical Oncology has published guidelines for diagnosis, treatment, and follow-up of cancer during pregnancy. The guidelines recommend referral to a facility with expertise in cancer during pregnancy and encourage a multidisciplinary team (obstetrician, neonatologist, oncology team). In general, if chemotherapy is indicated, it should be avoided during the first trimester, there should be a 3-week time period between the last chemotherapy dose and anticipated delivery, and chemotherapy should not be administered beyond week 33 of gestation. Specific use of nelarabine is not discussed (Peccatori 2013).

Nelfinavir (nel FIN a veer)

Related Information

HIV Infection and AIDS *on page 1690*

Viral Infections *on page 1754*

Brand Names: US Viracept

Brand Names: Canada Viracept

Pharmacologic Category Antiretroviral, Protease Inhibitor (Anti-HIV)

Use

HIV-1 infection: In combination with other antiretroviral therapy in the treatment of HIV infection.

Note: Nelfinavir is no longer recommended for use in the treatment of HIV (HHS [adult] 2019).

Local Anesthetic/Vasoconstrictor Precautions No information available to require special precautions

Effects on Dental Treatment Key adverse event(s) related to dental treatment: Mouth ulcers.

Effects on Bleeding Increased bleeding has been noted with protease inhibitors in patients with hemophilia A or B. No information available to require routine special precautions relative to hemostasis in other patients.

Adverse Reactions

>10%: Gastrointestinal: Diarrhea (adults: 14% to 20%; children: 39% to 47%)

1% to 10%:

Central nervous system: Anxiety (<2%), depression (<2%), dizziness (<2%), drowsiness (<2%), emotional lability (<2%), headache (<2%), insomnia (<2%), malaise (<2%), migraine (<2%), myasthenia (<2%), pain (<2%), paresthesia (<2%), seizure (<2%), sleep disorder (<2%), suicidal ideation (<2%)

Dermatologic: Skin rash (adults: 1% to 3%), dermatitis (<2%), diaphoresis (<2%), folliculitis (<2%), fungal dermatitis (<2%), maculopapular rash (<2%), pruritus (<2%), urticaria (<2%)

Endocrine & metabolic: Dehydration (<2%), hyperglycemia (<2%), hyperlipidemia (<2%), hyperuricemia (<2%), hypoglycemia (<2%), increased amylase (<2%), increased gamma-glutamyl transferase (<2%), increased lactate dehydrogenase (<2%), lipodystrophy (<2%), redistribution of body fat (<2%)
Gastrointestinal: Nausea (adults: 3% to 7%), flatulence (adults: 1% to 5%), abdominal pain (<2%), anorexia (<2%), dyspepsia (<2%), epigastric pain (<2%), gastrointestinal hemorrhage (<2%), oral mucosa ulcer (<2%), pancreatitis (<2%), vomiting (<2%)
Genitourinary: Sexual disorder (<2%), urine abnormality (<2%)
Hematologic & oncologic: Lymphocytopenia (adults: 1% to 6%), decreased neutrophils (adults: 1% to 5%), anemia (<2%), leukopenia (<2%), thrombocytopenia (<2%)
Hepatic: Abnormal hepatic function tests (<2%), hepatitis (<2%), increased serum alkaline phosphatase (<2%), increased serum transaminases (<2%)
Hypersensitivity: Hypersensitivity reaction (<2%; including bronchospasm, edema, and skin rash)
Neuromuscular & skeletal: Arthralgia (<2%), arthritis (<2%), back pain (<2%), hyperkinesia (<2%), increased creatine phosphokinase (<2%), lipoatrophy (<2%), lipotrophy (<2%), muscle cramps (<2%), myalgia (<2%), myopathy (<2%), weakness (<2%)
Ophthalmic: Acute iritis (<2%), eye disease (<2%)
Renal: Nephrolithiasis (<2%)
Respiratory: Dyspnea (<2%), pharyngitis (<2%), rhinitis (<2%), sinusitis (<2%)
Miscellaneous: Fever (<2%)

<1%, postmarketing, and/or case reports: Hyperbilirubinemia, immune reconstitution syndrome, jaundice, metabolic acidosis, prolonged QT interval on ECG, torsades de pointes

Mechanism of Action Binds to the site of HIV-1 protease activity and inhibits cleavage of viral Gag-Pol polyprotein precursors into individual functional proteins required for infectious HIV. This results in the formation of immature, noninfectious viral particles.

Pharmacodynamics/Kinetics

Half-life Elimination 3.5 to 5 hours

Time to Peak Serum: 2 to 4 hours

Reproductive Considerations

Based on the Health and Humans Services (HHS) perinatal HIV guidelines, nelfinavir is not one of the recommended antiretroviral agents for use in females living with HIV who are trying to conceive.

Females living with HIV not planning a pregnancy may use any available type of contraception, considering possible drug interactions and contraindications of the specific method. Consult the drug interactions database for more detailed information specific to use of nelfinavir and specific contraceptives.

For males and females living with HIV and planning a pregnancy, maximum viral suppression below the limits of detection with antiretroviral therapy (ART), modification of therapy (if needed), optimization of the woman's health, and a discussion of the potential risks and benefits of ART therapy during pregnancy is recommended prior to conception (HHS [perinatal] 2019).

Pregnancy Considerations Nelfinavir crosses the human placenta.

Outcome information specific to nelfinavir use in pregnancy is no longer being reviewed and updated in the Health and Humans Services (HHS) perinatal guidelines. Maternal antiretroviral therapy (ART) may be associated with adverse pregnancy outcomes including preterm delivery, stillbirth, low birth weight, and small for gestational age infants. Actual risks may be influenced by maternal factors, such as disease severity, gestational age at initiation of therapy, and specific ART regimen; therefore, close fetal monitoring is recommended. Because there is clear benefit to appropriate treatment, maternal ART should not be withheld due to concerns for adverse neonatal outcomes. Long-term follow-up is recommended for all infants exposed to antiretroviral medications; children without HIV but who were exposed to ART in utero and develop significant organ system abnormalities of unknown etiology (particularly of the CNS or heart) should be evaluated for potential mitochondrial dysfunction. Hyperglycemia, new onset of diabetes mellitus, or diabetic ketoacidosis have been reported with protease inhibitors; it is not clear if pregnancy increases this risk. Consider performing the standard glucose screening test earlier in pregnancy in women who initiated protease inhibitor therapy prior to conception.

Based on the HHS perinatal HIV guidelines, nelfinavir is not one of the recommended antiretroviral agents for use during pregnancy.

In general, ART is recommended for all pregnant females living with HIV to keep the viral load below the limit of detection and reduce the risk of perinatal transmission. Therapy should be individualized following a discussion of the potential risks and benefits of treatment during pregnancy. Monitoring of pregnant females is more frequent than in nonpregnant adults. ART should be continued postpartum for all females living with HIV and can be modified after delivery.

Health care providers are encouraged to enroll pregnant females exposed to antiretroviral medications as early in pregnancy as possible in the Antiretroviral Pregnancy Registry (1-800-258-4263 or http://www.APRegistry.com). Health care providers caring for pregnant females living with HIV and their infants may contact the National Perinatal HIV Hotline (1-888-448-8765) for clinical consultation (HHS [perinatal] 2019).

◆ **Nembutal** *see* PENTobarbital *on page 1213*

◆ **NeoMultivite** *see* Vitamins (Multiple/Oral) *on page 1550*

◆ **NeoProfen** *see* Ibuprofen *on page 786*

◆ **Neoral** *see* CycloSPORINE (Systemic) *on page 421*

◆ **Neosar** *see* Cyclophosphamide *on page 420*

◆ **Neo-Synephrine 12 Hour Spray [OTC] [DSC]** *see* Oxymetazoline (Nasal) *on page 1173*

◆ **NEPA** *see* Netupitant and Palonosetron *on page 1095*

Nepafenac (ne pa FEN ak)

Brand Names: US Ilevro; Nevanac

Brand Names: Canada Ilevro; Nevanac

Pharmacologic Category Nonsteroidal Anti-inflammatory Drug (NSAID), Ophthalmic

Use Ocular pain and inflammation associated with cataract surgery: Treatment of pain and inflammation associated with cataract surgery

Local Anesthetic/Vasoconstrictor Precautions

No information available to require special precautions

Effects on Dental Treatment The dentist should be aware of the potential of abnormal coagulation. Caution should also be exercised in the use of NSAIDs in patients already on anticoagulant therapy with drugs such as warfarin (Coumadin®). See Effects on Bleeding.

Effects on Bleeding Nonselective NSAIDs, such as nepafenac, inhibit platelet aggregation and prolong bleeding time in some patients. Unlike aspirin, the NSAID effect on platelet function is quantitatively less, of shorter duration, and reversible. Normal platelet function should occur in ~5 elimination half-lives or in <10 hours after discontinuation of nepafenac. Concomitant use of other NSAIDs should be avoided.

Adverse Reactions

1% to 10%:

Cardiovascular: Hypertension (≤4%)

Central nervous system: Foreign body sensation of eye (≤10%), headache (≤4%)

Gastrointestinal: Nausea (≤4%), vomiting (≤4%)

Ophthalmic: Decreased visual acuity (≤10%), increased intraocular pressure (≤10%), sticky sensation of eye (≤10%), conjunctival edema (≤5%), corneal edema (≤5%), crusting of eyelid (≤5%), eye discomfort (≤5%), eye pain (≤5%), eye pruritus (≤5%), lacrimation (≤5%), ocular hyperemia (≤5%), photophobia (≤5%), vitreous detachment (≤5%), xerophthalmia (≤5%)

Respiratory: Sinusitis (≤4%)

Mechanism of Action Nepafenac is a prodrug which once converted to amfenac inhibits prostaglandin synthesis by decreasing the activity of the enzyme, cyclooxygenase, which results in decreased formation of prostaglandin precursors.

Pregnancy Risk Factor C

Pregnancy Considerations Teratogenic events were not observed in animal reproduction studies. Exposure to nonsteroidal anti-inflammatory drugs late in pregnancy may lead to premature closure of the ductus arteriosus.

◆ **Neptazane [DSC]** *see* MethazolAMIDE *on page* 986

Neratinib (ne RA ti nib)

Brand Names: US Nerlynx

Brand Names: Canada Nerlynx

Pharmacologic Category Antineoplastic Agent, Anti-HER2; Antineoplastic Agent, Epidermal Growth Factor Receptor (EGFR) Inhibitor; Antineoplastic Agent, Tyrosine Kinase Inhibitor

Use

Breast cancer:

Extended adjuvant treatment (as a single agent) of early-stage human epidermal growth receptor type 2 (HER2)-positive breast cancer (following adjuvant trastuzumab-based therapy).

Treatment of advanced or metastatic HER2-positive breast cancer (in combination with capecitabine) in patients who have received 2 or more prior anti-HER2 based regimens in the metastatic setting.

Local Anesthetic/Vasoconstrictor Precautions No information available to require special precautions

Effects on Dental Treatment Key adverse event(s) related to dental treatment: Stomatitis and xerostomia have been reported.

Effects on Bleeding No information available to require special precautions

Adverse Reactions

>10%:

Dermatologic: Skin rash (18%)

Gastrointestinal: Abdominal pain (36%; severe abdominal pain: <1%), decreased appetite (12%), diarrhea (95%; severe diarrhea: 2%), nausea (43%; severe nausea: <1%), stomatitis (14%; grade 3: <1%), vomiting (26%; severe vomiting: <1%)

Nervous system: Fatigue (27%; severe fatigue: <1%)

Neuromuscular & skeletal: Muscle spasm (11%)

1% to 10%:

Dermatologic: Nail disease (8%), skin fissure (2%), xeroderma (6%)

Endocrine & metabolic: Dehydration (4%; severe dehydration: <1%), weight loss (5%)

Gastrointestinal: Abdominal distension (5%), dyspepsia (10%), xerostomia (3%)

Genitourinary: Urinary tract infection (5%)

Hepatic: Increased serum alanine aminotransferase (9% to 10%; severely increased serum alanine aminotransferase: <1%), increased serum aspartate aminotransferase (5% to 7%; severely increased serum aspartate aminotransferase: <1%)

Respiratory: Epistaxis (5%)

<1%:

Dermatologic: Cellulitis, erysipelas

Renal: Renal failure syndrome

Frequency not defined: Hepatic: Hepatotoxicity

Mechanism of Action Neratinib is an irreversible tyrosine kinase inhibitor of human epidermal growth factor receptor 1, 2, and 4 (HER1, HER2, and HER4) (Chan 2016), as well as epidermal growth factor receptor (EGFR). Neratinib reduces EGFR and HER2 autophosphorylation and downstream MAPK and AKT signaling pathways and demonstrates antitumor activity in EGFR and/or HER2 expressing cancer cell lines.

Pharmacodynamics/Kinetics

Half-life Elimination 7 to 17 hours

Time to Peak 2 to 8 hours (parent drug and active metabolites M3, M6, and M7)

Reproductive Considerations

Women of reproductive potential should have a pregnancy test prior to treatment; effective contraception should be used during therapy and for at least 1 month after the last neratinib dose.

Male patients with female partners of reproductive potential should also use effective contraception during therapy and for 3 months after the last neratinib dose.

Pregnancy Considerations

Based on the mechanism of action and data from animal reproduction studies, use of neratinib in pregnancy may cause fetal harm.

Prescribing and Access Restrictions

Neratinib is available through select specialty pharmacies. Refer to http://www.nerlynx.com for further information.

◆ **Nerlynx** *see* Neratinib *on page* 1094

◆ **Nesacaine** *see* Chloroprocaine *on page* 337

◆ **Nesacaine-MPF** *see* Chloroprocaine *on page* 337

◆ **Nesina** *see* Alogliptin *on page* 105

Nesiritide (ni SIR i tide)

Brand Names: US Natrecor [DSC]

Pharmacologic Category Natriuretic Peptide, B-Type, Human

Use Acutely decompensated heart failure (HF): Treatment of acutely decompensated heart failure (HF) with dyspnea at rest or with minimal activity

Local Anesthetic/Vasoconstrictor Precautions No information available to require special precautions

Effects on Dental Treatment No significant effects or complications reported

Effects on Bleeding No information available to require special precautions

Adverse Reactions Note: Incidences of adverse reactions include unapproved dosing regimens as well as combination therapy data.

>10%:

Cardiovascular: Hypotension (4% to 12%)

Renal: Increased serum creatinine (28% with >0.5 mg/dL above baseline; 5% with 50% greater serum creatinine levels than at baseline), renal insufficiency (>25% decrease in glomerular filtration rate: 31%)

1% to 10%:

Central nervous system: Headache (7%)

Endocrine & metabolic: Hypoglycemia (≥2%)

Gastrointestinal: Nausea (3%)

Neuromuscular & skeletal: Back pain (3%)

<1%, postmarketing and/or case reports: Extravasation, hypersensitivity reactions, pruritus, skin rash

Mechanism of Action Binds to guanylate cyclase receptor on vascular smooth muscle and endothelial cells, increasing intracellular cyclic GMP, resulting in smooth muscle cell relaxation. Has been shown to produce dose-dependent reductions in pulmonary capillary wedge pressure (PCWP) and systemic arterial pressure.

Pharmacodynamics/Kinetics

Onset of Action PCWP reduction: 15 minutes (60% of 3-hour effect achieved within this time period); Peak effect: Within 1 hour

Duration of Action >60 minutes (up to several hours) for systolic blood pressure; hemodynamic effects persist longer than serum half-life would predict

Half-life Elimination Initial (distribution) ~2 minutes; Terminal: ~18 minutes

Pregnancy Considerations

Adverse events were not observed in an animal reproduction study.

Data in humans are inadequate to make recommendations for use in pregnancy (ESC [Regitz-Zagrosek 2018]).

Product Availability Natrecor is no longer available in the US.

- **NESP** *see* Darbepoetin Alfa *on page 440*
- **Nestorone and Ethinyl Estradiol** *see* Segesterone Acetate and Ethinyl Estradiol *on page 1362*

Netupitant and Palonosetron

(net UE pi tant & pal oh NOE se tron)

Brand Names: US Akynzeo

Brand Names: Canada Akynzeo

Pharmacologic Category Antiemetic; Selective 5-HT_3 Receptor Antagonist; Substance P/Neurokinin 1 Receptor Antagonist

Use Chemotherapy-induced nausea and vomiting: Prevention of acute and delayed nausea and vomiting associated with initial and repeat courses of cancer chemotherapy, including, but not limited to, highly emetogenic chemotherapy (in combination with dexamethasone).

Local Anesthetic/Vasoconstrictor Precautions No information available to require special precautions

Effects on Dental Treatment No significant effects or complications reported

Effects on Bleeding No information available to require special precautions

Adverse Reactions

1% to 10%:

Central nervous system: Headache (9%), fatigue (4% to 7%)

Dermatologic: Erythema (3%)

Gastrointestinal: Dyspepsia (4%), constipation (3%)

Neuromuscular & skeletal: Weakness (8%)

Mechanism of Action Netupitant is a selective substance P/neurokinin (NK_1) receptor antagonist, which augments the antiemetic activity of 5-HT_3 receptor antagonists and corticosteroids to inhibit acute and delayed chemotherapy-induced emesis. Palonosetron is a selective 5-HT_3 receptor antagonist, which blocks serotonin, both on vagal nerve terminals in the periphery and centrally in the chemoreceptor trigger zone. Palonosetron inhibits the cross-talk between the 5-HT_3 and NK_1 receptors. The combination of palonosetron and netupitant works synergistically to inhibit substance P response to a greater extent than either agent alone (Aapro 2014).

Pharmacodynamics/Kinetics

Half-life Elimination Netupitant: 80 ± 29 hours; Palonosetron: 50 ± 16 hours

Time to Peak Netupitant and palonosetron: ~4 to 5 hours

Pregnancy Considerations Adverse events were observed in some animal reproduction studies using the components of this combination product. Information related to the use of netupitant and palonosetron during pregnancy is limited.

- **Netupitant/Palonosetron HCl** *see* Netupitant and Palonosetron *on page 1095*
- **Neuac** *see* Clindamycin and Benzoyl Peroxide *on page 375*
- **Neulasta** *see* Pegfilgrastim *on page 1200*
- **Neulasta Onpro** *see* Pegfilgrastim *on page 1200*
- **Neulasta Onpro Kit** *see* Pegfilgrastim *on page 1200*
- **Neupogen** *see* Filgrastim *on page 668*
- **Neupro** *see* Rotigotine *on page 1349*
- **Neuro-K-50 [OTC]** *see* Pyridoxine *on page 1294*
- **Neuro-K-250 T.D. [OTC]** *see* Pyridoxine *on page 1294*
- **Neuro-K-250 Vitamin B6 [OTC]** *see* Pyridoxine *on page 1294*
- **Neuro-K-500 [OTC]** *see* Pyridoxine *on page 1294*
- **NeuroMed7 [OTC]** *see* Lidocaine (Topical) *on page 902*
- **Neurontin** *see* Gabapentin *on page 722*
- **NeutraCare** *see* Fluoride *on page 693*
- **NeutraGard Advanced [DSC]** *see* Fluoride *on page 693*
- **Neutrahist Pediatric [OTC] [DSC]** *see* Chlorpheniramine and Pseudoephedrine *on page 341*
- **NeutraSal** *see* Saliva Substitute *on page 1354*
- **Neuvaxin [DSC]** *see* Capsaicin *on page 284*
- **Nevanac** *see* Nepafenac *on page 1093*

Nevirapine (ne VYE ra peen)

Related Information

HIV Infection and AIDS *on page 1690*

Brand Names: US Viramune; Viramune XR

Brand Names: Canada APO-Nevirapine XR; Auro-Nevirapine; JAMP Nevirapine; MYLAN-Nevirapine; TEVA-Nevirapine [DSC]; Viramune XR [DSC]; Viramune [DSC]

Pharmacologic Category Antiretroviral, Reverse Transcriptase Inhibitor, Non-nucleoside (Anti-HIV)

Use

HIV-1 infection, treatment: Treatment of HIV-1, in combination therapy with other antiretroviral agents, in adults and pediatric patients ≥15 days of age (immediate release) and ≥6 years of age with a BSA of ≥1.17 m^2 (ER). **Note:** Nevirapine is not recommended as a component of initial therapy for the treatment of HIV (HHS [adults] 2019).

Limitations of use: Not recommended to be initiated, unless the benefit outweighs the risk, in adult females with $CD4^+$ cell counts >250 cells/mm^3 or adult males with $CD4^+$ cell counts >400 cells/mm^3.

Local Anesthetic/Vasoconstrictor Precautions No information available to require special precautions

Effects on Dental Treatment Key adverse event(s) related to dental treatment: Ulcerative stomatitis and oral lesions.

Effects on Bleeding No information available to require special precautions relative to hemostasis.

Adverse Reactions

>10%:

Endocrine & metabolic: Increased serum cholesterol (3% to 19%), increased LDL cholesterol (5% to 15%)

Hematologic & oncologic: Decreased serum phosphate (≤38%), neutropenia (1% to 13%)

Hepatic: Increased serum alanine aminotransferase (2% to 14%)

1% to 10%:

Central nervous system: Fatigue (2% to 5%), headache (1% to 4%)

Dermatologic: Skin rash (4% to 7%; children: 1%)

Endocrine & metabolic: Increased amylase (≤5%)

Gastrointestinal: Nausea (1% to 9%), abdominal pain (2% to 3%), diarrhea (2% to 4%)

Hematologic & oncologic: Granulocytopenia (≤2%)

Hepatic: Increased serum aspartate aminotransferase (2% to 9%), increased serum transaminases (asymptomatic; >5x ULN: 6%), hepatic disease (4%), hepatitis (2% to 4%; may be hypersensitivity related)

Neuromuscular & skeletal: Arthralgia (2%)

Miscellaneous: Fever (1% to 2%)

Frequency not defined:

Dermatologic: Erythematous maculopapular rash, pruritus

<1%, postmarketing, and/or case reports: Abnormal transaminase, anaphylaxis, anemia, angioedema, aphthous stomatitis, autoimmune disease, bullous rash, cholestatic hepatitis, conjunctivitis, DRESS syndrome, drowsiness, drug withdrawal, eosinophilia, facial edema, flu-like symptoms, fulminant hepatitis, Graves disease, Guillain-Barre syndrome, hepatic encephalopathy, hepatic failure, hepatic necrosis, hepatomegaly, hepatotoxicity, hyperbilirubinemia, hypersensitivity reaction, immune reconstitution syndrome, jaundice, lipotrophy, liver tenderness, lymphadenopathy, malaise, myalgia, oral lesion, paresthesia, polymyositis, prolonged partial thromboplastin time, redistribution of body fat, renal insufficiency, rhabdomyolysis, skin blister, Stevens-Johnson syndrome, toxic epidermal necrolysis, urticaria, vomiting

Mechanism of Action As a non-nucleoside reverse transcriptase inhibitor, nevirapine has activity against HIV-1 by binding to reverse transcriptase. It consequently blocks the RNA-dependent and DNA-dependent DNA polymerase activities including HIV-1 replication. It does not require intracellular phosphorylation for antiviral activity.

Pharmacodynamics/Kinetics

Half-life Elimination Decreases over 2- to 4-week time with chronic dosing due to autoinduction (ie, half-life = 45 hours initially [single dose] and decreases to 25 to 30 hours [multiple dosing])

Time to Peak Serum: Immediate release: 4 hours; Extended release:~24 hours

Reproductive Considerations

The Health and Human Services (HHS) perinatal HIV guidelines do not recommend nevirapine (except in special circumstances) in females living with HIV who are not yet pregnant but are trying to conceive.

For males and females living with HIV and planning a pregnancy, maximum viral suppression below the limits of detection with antiretroviral therapy (ART), modification of therapy (if needed), optimization of the woman's health, and a discussion of the potential risks and benefits of ART therapy during pregnancy is recommended prior to conception (HHS [perinatal] 2019).

Pregnancy Considerations

Nevirapine has a high level of transfer across the human placenta.

No increased risk of overall birth defects following first trimester exposure according to data collected by the antiretroviral pregnancy registry. Maternal antiretroviral therapy (ART) may be associated with adverse pregnancy outcomes including preterm delivery, stillbirth, low birth weight, and small for gestational age infants. Actual risks may be influenced by maternal factors such as disease severity, gestational age at initiation of therapy, and specific ART regimen, therefore close fetal monitoring is recommended. Because there is clear benefit to appropriate treatment, maternal ART should not be withheld due to concerns for adverse neonatal outcomes. Long-term follow-up is recommended for all infants exposed to antiretroviral medications; children without HIV but who were exposed to ART in utero and develop significant organ system abnormalities of unknown etiology (particularly of the CNS or heart) should be evaluated for potential mitochondrial dysfunction.

[US Boxed Warning]: Severe, life-threatening, and in some cases fatal hepatotoxicity, particularly in the first 18 weeks, has been reported in patients treated with nevirapine. Female gender and higher CD4+ cell counts at initiation of therapy place patients at increased risk; women with CD4+ cell counts greater than 250 cells/mm^3, including pregnant women receiving nevirapine in combination with other antiretrovirals for the treatment of HIV-1 infection, are at the greatest risk. Pregnancy itself does not appear to increase this risk. **Patients must be monitored intensively during the first 18 weeks of therapy. Extra vigilance is warranted during the first 6 weeks of therapy, which is the period of greatest risk of these events.**

The Health and Human Services (HHS) perinatal HIV guidelines do not recommend nevirapine as an initial non-nucleoside reverse transcriptase inhibitor for use in antiretroviral-naive pregnant patients because of the potential for adverse events, complex dosing, and low barrier to resistance. Use is not recommended (except in special circumstances) in pregnant females who have had ART therapy in the past but are restarting, or who require a new ART regimen (due to poor tolerance or poor virologic response of current regimen). Females who become pregnant while taking nevirapine may continue if viral suppression is effective and the regimen is well tolerated. Pharmacokinetics of the immediate-release formulation are not significantly altered during pregnancy; dose adjustment is not currently recommended (data not available for extended-release formulation).

In general, ART is recommended for all pregnant females living with HIV to keep the viral load below the limit of detection and reduce the risk of perinatal transmission. Therapy should be individualized following a discussion of the potential risks and benefits of treatment during pregnancy. Monitoring of pregnant females is more frequent than in nonpregnant adults. ART should be continued postpartum for all females living with HIV and can be modified after delivery.

Health care providers are encouraged to enroll pregnant females exposed to antiretroviral medications as early in pregnancy as possible in the Antiretroviral Pregnancy Registry (1-800-258-4263 or http://www.-APRegistry.com). Health care providers caring for pregnant females living with HIV and their infants may contact the National Perinatal HIV Hotline (1-888-448-8765) for clinical consultation (HHS [perinatal] 2019).

- **Nexafed [OTC]** *see* Pseudoephedrine *on page 1291*
- **NexAVAR** *see* SORAfenib *on page 1383*
- **NexIUM** *see* Esomeprazole *on page 594*
- **Nexium 24HR** *see* Esomeprazole *on page 594*
- **NexIUM 24HR [OTC]** *see* Esomeprazole *on page 594*
- **NexIUM 24HR Clear Minis [OTC]** *see* Esomeprazole *on page 594*
- **NexIUM I.V.** *see* Esomeprazole *on page 594*
- **Nexletol** *see* Bempedoic Acid *on page 224*
- **Nexlizet** *see* Bempedoic Acid and Ezetimibe *on page 224*
- **Nexplanon** *see* Etonogestrel *on page 625*
- **Nexterone** *see* Amiodarone *on page 118*
- **NFV** *see* Nelfinavir *on page 1092*
- **NGX-4010** *see* Capsaicin *on page 284*
- **NI-0501** *see* Emapalumab *on page 554*

Niacin (NYE a sin)

Related Information

Cardiovascular Diseases *on page 1654*

Brand Names: US Niacin-50 [OTC]; Niacor; Niaspan; Slo-Niacin [OTC]

Brand Names: Canada Niaspan FCT [DSC]; Niaspan [DSC]; Niodan

Generic Availability (US) Yes

Pharmacologic Category Antilipemic Agent, Miscellaneous; Vitamin, Water Soluble

Use

Dietary supplement: Use as a dietary supplement.

Dyslipidemias: Treatment of dyslipidemias (Fredrickson types IIa and IIb or primary hypercholesterolemia) as mono- or adjunctive therapy; to lower the risk of recurrent MI in patients with a history of MI and hyperlipidemia; to slow progression or promote regression of coronary artery disease; adjunctive therapy for severe hypertriglyceridemia in adults at risk of pancreatitis

Note: Niacin is no longer considered a primary or secondary agent for dyslipidemias. Although niacin consistently affects surrogate markers, especially LDL-C, it has not been shown to reduce cardiovascular disease outcomes beyond that achieved with statin use and may be associated with harm (ACC [Lloyd-Jones 2017]; Garg 2017; Wierzbicki 2014). In two large clinical trials, the addition of niacin to patients receiving simvastatin did not reduce cardiovascular morbidity or mortality (Boden 2011; Landray 2014). May consider use in patients with very high triglyceride levels (>500 mg/dL) or in dyslipidemia for patients who do not achieve the desired response or have intolerance to a statin or other alternative therapy (Boden 2014; Flink 2015).

Local Anesthetic/Vasoconstrictor Precautions No information available to require special precautions

Effects on Dental Treatment No significant effects or complications reported

Effects on Bleeding Sustained-release niacin has been shown to prolong blood clotting times, as observed by significant clotting factor synthesis deficiency and coagulopathy defined by prothrombin times 1.5 times greater than control. Caution is advised in patients with bleeding disorders or those using other anticoagulant medications. Mild leukopenia and increased eosinophil levels have also been reported.

Adverse Reactions Frequency not defined.

Cardiovascular: Atrial fibrillation, cardiac arrhythmia, edema, flushing, hypotension, orthostatic hypotension, palpitations, tachycardia

Central nervous system: Chills, dizziness, headache, insomnia, migraine, myasthenia, nervousness, pain, paresthesia

Dermatologic: Acanthosis nigricans, burning sensation of skin, diaphoresis, hyperpigmentation, maculopapular rash, pruritus, skin discoloration, skin rash, urticaria, xeroderma

Endocrine & metabolic: Decreased glucose tolerance, decreased serum phosphate, gout, hyperuricemia, increased amylase, increased lactate dehydrogenase

Gastrointestinal: Abdominal pain, diarrhea, dyspepsia, eructation, flatulence, nausea, peptic ulcer, vomiting

Hematologic & oncologic: Decreased platelet count, prolonged prothrombin time

Hepatic: Hepatitis, increased serum bilirubin, increased serum transaminases (dose-related), jaundice,

Neuromuscular & skeletal: Increased creatine phosphokinase, leg cramps, myalgia, myopathy (with concurrent HMG-CoA reductase inhibitor), weakness

Ophthalmic: Blurred vision, cystoid macular edema, toxic amblyopia

Respiratory: Cough, dyspnea

<1%, postmarketing, and/or case reports: Hepatic necrosis, hypersensitivity reaction (includes anaphylaxis, angioedema, laryngismus, vesiculobullous rash), rhabdomyolysis (with concurrent HMG-CoA reductase inhibitor), syncope

Dosing

Adult & Geriatric Note: Formulations of niacin (regular release versus extended release) are not interchangeable.

Dietary supplement (OTC labeling): Oral: 50 mg twice daily or 100 mg once daily. **Note:** Many over-the-counter formulations exist.

Dyslipidemia: Oral: **Note:** Niacin is no longer recommended, except in specific clinical situations (eg, high triglyceride levels [>500 mg/dL], if not able to achieve desired response, or intolerance to other therapies) (ACC [Lloyd-Jones 2017]; Boden 2014; Garg 2017; Landray 2014; Wierzbicki 2014).

Regular release formulation (Niacor): Initial: 250 mg once daily (with evening meal); increase frequency and/or dose every 4 to 7 days to desired response or first-level therapeutic dose (1.5 to 2 g daily in 2 to 3 divided doses); after 2 months, may increase at 2- to 4-week intervals to 3 g daily in 3 divided doses (maximum dose: 6 g daily in 3 divided doses). **Note:** Many over-the-counter formulations exist.

Sustained release (or controlled release) formulations: **Note:** Several over-the-counter formulations exist. Slo-Niacin: Usual dosage is 250 to 750 mg once daily, taken morning or evening, or as directed. Before using more than 500 mg daily, patient should consult health care provider.

Extended release formulation (Niaspan): Initial: 500 mg at bedtime for 4 weeks, then 1 g at bedtime for 4 weeks; adjust dose to response and tolerance; may increase daily dose every 4 weeks by not more than 500 mg daily to a maximum of 2 g daily. Recommended maintenance dose: 1,000 to 2,000 mg at bedtime.

Pellagra (off-label use): Oral: *Regular release formulation:* 50 to 100 mg 3 to 4 times daily; maximum: 500 mg daily (Prousky 2003; Delgado-Sanchez 2008; DesGroseilliers 1976; Oldham 2012). Some experts prefer niacinamide for treatment due to more favorable side effect profile (Hegyi 2004; Jen 2010).

Renal Impairment: Adult There are no dosage adjustments provided in the manufacturer's labeling (has not been studied); use with caution.

Hepatic Impairment: Adult There are no dosage adjustments provided in the manufacturer's labeling (has not been studied). Contraindicated in patients with significant or unexplained hepatic dysfunction, active liver disease or unexplained persistent transaminase elevations.

Adjustment for Toxicity: Adult Hepatic toxicity: Transaminases rise ≥3 times ULN, either persistent or if symptoms of nausea, fever, and/or malaise occur: Discontinue therapy.

Pediatric Note: Formulations of niacin (regular release [crystalline] versus extended release) are not interchangeable.

Dyslipidemias: Very limited data available (Miller 2015): **Note:** Niacin (nicotinic acid) is rarely used in pediatric patients for treatment of dyslipidemias and is not considered a primary agent nor a routine secondary, adjunctive agent for dyslipidemia management in pediatric patients (AAP [Daniels 2008]; AHA [McCrindle 2007]; NHLBI 2011)

Children ≥10 years and Adolescents (Miller 2015; NHLBI 2011): Oral:

Regular release: Initial: 100 to 250 mg/day in 3 divided doses with meals; maximum initial daily dose: 10 mg/kg/**day**; increase weekly by 100 mg/day or increase every 2 to 3 weeks by 250 mg/day as tolerated; evaluate efficacy and adverse effects with laboratory tests at 20 mg/kg/day or 1,000 mg/day (whichever is less); continue to increase if needed and as tolerated; re-evaluate at each 500 mg increment; daily doses up to 2,250 mg/**day** have been used (Colletti 1993)

Sustained release: Reported range: 500 to 1,500 mg/day; initiate at a low dose administered once daily (based on experience in adults); reported initial daily dose has not exceeded 10 mg/kg/**day;** titrate every 3 to 4 weeks (in adults, doses are titrated every 4 weeks) (AHA [McCrindle 2007]; Colletti 1993)

Pellagra; treatment: Children and Adolescents: Oral: Regular release: 50 to 300 mg/day in divided doses 3 times daily; usual treatment duration is 3 to 4 weeks (Kliegman 2016; WHO 2000)

Dosing adjustment for toxicity: Children ≥10 years and Adolescents: In a trial of pediatric patients, discontinuation of niacin therapy was reported for hepatotoxicity (eg, transaminases increases, either persistent or if symptoms of nausea, fever, and/or malaise), headache, abdominal pain and/or severe flushing (Colletti 1993)

Renal Impairment: Pediatric There are no dosage adjustments provided in the manufacturer's labeling (has not been studied); use with caution.

Hepatic Impairment: Pediatric All patients: There are no dosage adjustments provided in the manufacturer's labeling (has not been studied). Contraindicated in patients with significant or unexplained hepatic dysfunction, active liver disease, or unexplained persistent transaminase elevations.

Mechanism of Action Niacin (nicotinic acid) is bioconverted to nicotinamide which is further converted to nicotinamide adenine dinucleotide (NAD+) and the hydride equivalent (NADH) which are coenzymes necessary for tissue metabolism, lipid metabolism, and glycogenolysis (Belenky 2006; Sauve 2008). The mechanism by which niacin (in lipid-lowering doses) affects plasma lipoproteins is not fully understood. It may involve several actions including partial inhibition of release of free fatty acids from adipose tissue, and increased lipoprotein lipase activity, which may increase the rate of chylomicron triglyceride removal from plasma. Ultimately, niacin reduces total cholesterol, apolipoprotein (apo) B, triglycerides, VLDL, LDL, lipoprotein (a), and increases HDL and other important components and subfractions (eg, LPA-I) (Kamanna 2000)

Contraindications Hypersensitivity to niacin, niacinamide, or any component of the formulation; active hepatic disease or significant or unexplained persistent elevations in hepatic transaminases; active peptic ulcer; arterial hemorrhage

Warnings/Precautions Use with caution in patients with unstable angina or in the acute phase of an MI or renal disease. In patients with preexisting coronary artery disease, the incidence of atrial fibrillation was observed more frequently in those receiving immediate release (crystalline) niacin as compared to placebo (Coronary Drug Project Research Group 1975). Consider discontinuation if new-onset atrial fibrillation occurs during therapy. Use is associated with new-onset diabetes or worsening glucose tolerance in patients with preexisting diabetes (Garg 2017; Goldie 2016). Use with caution in patients with diabetes. Monitor glucose; adjustment of diet and/or hypoglycemic therapy may be necessary. Consider discontinuation if persistent hyperglycemia occurs during therapy. Use with caution in patients predisposed to gout. Consider discontinuation if acute gout occurs during therapy.

Use with caution in patients with a past history of hepatic impairment and/or who consume substantial amounts of ethanol; contraindicated with active liver disease or unexplained persistent transaminase elevation. Discontinue use if hepatic transaminase levels rise, particularly to 3 x ULN and are persistent, or if they are associated with symptoms of nausea, fever, and/or malaise. Rare cases of rhabdomyolysis have occurred during concomitant use with HMG-CoA reductase inhibitors. With concurrent use or if symptoms suggestive of myopathy occur, monitor creatine phosphokinase (CPK) and potassium; use with caution in patients with renal impairment, inadequately treated hypothyroidism, patients with diabetes or the elderly; risk for myopathy and rhabdomyolysis may be increased. May cause GI distress, vomiting, diarrhea, or aggravate peptic ulcer. GI distress may be attenuated with a gradual increase in dose and administration with food. Use is contraindicated in patients with active peptic ulcer disease; use with caution in patients with a past history of peptic ulcer. Consider discontinuation if unexplained abdominal pain/weight loss or other GI symptoms occur during therapy. Dose-related reductions in platelet count and increases of prothrombin time may occur. Has been associated with small but statistically significant dose-related reductions in phosphorus levels. Monitor phosphorus levels periodically in patients at risk for hypophosphatemia.

Formulations of niacin (immediate release versus extended release) are not interchangeable (bioavailability varies); cases of severe hepatotoxicity, including fulminant hepatic necrosis, have occurred in patients who have substituted niacin products at equivalent doses. Patients should be initiated with low doses (eg, niacin extended release 500 mg at bedtime) with titration to achieve desired response. Flushing and pruritus are common adverse effects of niacin; may be attenuated with a gradual increase in dose, administering with food, avoidance of concurrent ingestion of ethanol, hot or spicy foods/liquids, and/or by taking aspirin 30 minutes before dosing. May also use other NSAIDs according to the manufacturer. Flushing associated with extended-release preparation is significantly reduced (Guyton 2007). For immediate-release preparations, may administer in 2 to 3 divided doses to reduce the frequency and severity of flushing/pruritus. Consider discontinuation if persistent severe cutaneous symptoms occur during therapy.

Potentially significant interactions may exist, requiring dose or frequency adjustment, additional monitoring, and/or selection of alternative therapy.

Warnings: Additional Pediatric Considerations In pediatric patients, a high incidence of reversible adverse effects has been observed; in a dyslipidemia trial (n=21, age range: 4 to 14 years), flushing was most common (71%); increased liver enzymes were observed in 29% of patients; in the trial, dosage form (crystalline or sustained release) did not affect adverse effect incidence (Colletti 1993).

Drug Interactions

Metabolism/Transport Effects None known.

Avoid Concomitant Use There are no known interactions where it is recommended to avoid concomitant use.

Increased Effect/Toxicity

Niacin may increase the levels/effects of: HMG-CoA Reductase Inhibitors (Statins); Rosuvastatin; Simvastatin

The levels/effects of Niacin may be increased by: Alcohol (Ethyl)

Decreased Effect

Niacin may decrease the levels/effects of: Antidiabetic Agents

The levels/effects of Niacin may be decreased by: Bile Acid Sequestrants

Dietary Considerations Should be taken with meal; low-fat meal if treating dyslipidemia. Avoid alcohol, hot or spicy foods/liquids around the time of niacin dose.

Dietary adequate intake (National Academy of Sciences, 1998):

0 to 5 months: 2 mg daily
6 to 11 months: 3 mg daily

Dietary recommended daily allowances (National Academy of Sciences, 1998):

1 to 3 years: 6 mg daily
4 to 8 years: 8 mg daily
9 to 13 years: 12 mg daily
14 to 18 years: Females: 14 mg daily; Males: 16 mg daily
≥19 years: Females: 14 mg daily; Males: 16 mg daily
Pregnancy (all ages): 18 mg daily
Lactation (all ages): 17 mg daily

Pharmacodynamics/Kinetics

Half-life Elimination 25 to 48 minutes

Time to Peak Serum: Immediate release formulation: 30 to 60 minutes; extended release formulation: 4 to 5 hours

Pregnancy Risk Factor C

Pregnancy Considerations

Water soluble vitamins cross the placenta. When used as a dietary supplement, niacin requirements may be increased in pregnant women compared to nonpregnant women (IOM 1998). It is not known if niacin at lipid-lowering doses is harmful to the developing fetus. If a woman becomes pregnant while receiving niacin for primary hypercholesterolemia, niacin should be discontinued. If a woman becomes pregnant while receiving niacin for hypertriglyceridemia, the benefits and risks of continuing niacin should be assessed on an individual basis.

Breastfeeding Considerations Niacin is present in breast milk. When used as a dietary supplement, niacin requirements may be increased in breastfeeding women compared to non-breastfeeding women (IOM 1998). Due to the potential for serious adverse reactions in the breastfeeding infant, the manufacturer recommends a decision be made whether to discontinue breastfeeding or to discontinue the drug, taking into account the importance of treatment to the mother.

Dosage Forms: US

Capsule Extended Release, Oral:
Generic: 250 mg, 500 mg

Capsule Extended Release, Oral [preservative free]:
Generic: 250 mg, 500 mg

Powder, Oral:
Generic: (100 g, 500 g, 1000 g)

Tablet, Oral:
Niacin-50 [OTC]: 50 mg
Niacor: 500 mg
Generic: 50 mg, 100 mg, 250 mg, 500 mg

Tablet, Oral [preservative free]:
Generic: 500 mg

Tablet Extended Release, Oral:
Niaspan: 500 mg, 750 mg, 1000 mg
Slo-Niacin [OTC]: 250 mg, 500 mg, 750 mg
Generic: 500 mg, 750 mg, 1000 mg

Tablet Extended Release, Oral [preservative free]:
Generic: 250 mg, 500 mg, 1000 mg

Dosage Forms: Canada

Solution, Injection:
Generic: 100 mg/mL (30 mL)

Tablet Extended Release, Oral:
Niodan: 500 mg

◆ **Niacin-50 [OTC]** *see* Niacin *on page* 1097

Niacinamide (nye a SIN a mide)

Pharmacologic Category Vitamin, Water Soluble

Use Dietary supplement

Local Anesthetic/Vasoconstrictor Precautions No information available to require special precautions

Effects on Dental Treatment No significant effects or complications reported

Effects on Bleeding No information available to require special precautions

Mechanism of Action Used by the body as a source of niacin; is a component of two coenzymes which is necessary for tissue respiration, lipid metabolism, and glycogenolysis; does not have hypolipidemia or vasodilating effects.

Pharmacodynamics/Kinetics

Half-life Elimination 45 minutes

Time to Peak Serum: 20-70 minutes

Pregnancy Considerations Water-soluble vitamins cross the placenta (IOM 1998).

◆ **Niacor** *see* Niacin *on page* 1097

◆ **Niaspan** *see* Niacin *on page* 1097

◆ **Nicadan** *see* Vitamins (Multiple/Oral) *on page* 1550

NiCARdipine (nye KAR de peen)

Related Information

Calcium Channel Blockers and Gingival Hyperplasia *on page* 1816

Cardiovascular Diseases *on page* 1654

Brand Names: US Cardene IV

Pharmacologic Category Antianginal Agent; Antihypertensive; Calcium Channel Blocker; Calcium Channel Blocker, Dihydropyridine

Use

Angina: Management of chronic stable angina (oral only).

Hypertension: Management of hypertension (oral and IV); parenteral only for short-term use when oral treatment is not feasible or not desirable.

Local Anesthetic/Vasoconstrictor Precautions No information available to require special precautions

Effects on Dental Treatment Key adverse event(s) related to dental treatment: Xerostomia (normal salivary flow resumes upon discontinuation). Other drugs of this class can cause gingival hyperplasia (ie, nifedipine). The first case of nicardipine-induced gingival hyperplasia has been reported in a child taking 40-50 mg daily for 20 months.

Effects on Bleeding No information available to require special precautions

Adverse Reactions

1% to 10%:

Cardiovascular: Flushing (6% to 10%), pedal edema (dose related; 7% to 8%), exacerbation of angina pectoris (dose related; 6%), hypotension (IV 6%), palpitations (3% to 4%), tachycardia (1% to 4%), chest pain (IV 1%), extrasystoles (IV 1%), hemopericardium (IV 1%), hypertension (IV 1%), supraventricular tachycardia (IV 1%), edema (≤1%)

Central nervous system: Headache (6% to 15%), dizziness (4% to 7%), hypoesthesia (1%), intracranial hemorrhage (1%), pain (1%), somnolence (1%)

Dermatologic: Diaphoresis (1%), skin rash (≤1%)

Endocrine & metabolic: Hypokalemia (IV 1%)

Gastrointestinal: Nausea and vomiting (IV 5%), nausea (2%), dyspepsia (≤2%), abdominal pain (IV 1%), xerostomia (≤1%)

Genitourinary: Hematuria (1%)

Local: Injection site reaction (IV 1%), pain at injection site (IV 1%)

Neuromuscular & skeletal: Weakness (4% to 6%), myalgia (1%), paresthesia (1%)

<1%, postmarketing, and/or case reports: Abnormal dreams, abnormal hepatic function tests, abnormal vision, angina pectoris, anxiety, arthralgia, atrial fibrillation (not distinguishable from natural history of atherosclerotic vascular disease), atrioventricular block, atypical chest pain, blurred vision, cerebral ischemia (not distinguishable from natural history of atherosclerotic vascular disease), confusion, conjunctivitis, constipation, deep vein thrombophlebitis, depression, depression of ST segment on ECG, dyspnea, ear disease, ECG abnormal, fever, gingival hyperplasia, heart block (not distinguishable from natural history of atherosclerotic vascular disease), hot flash, hyperkinesia, hypersensitivity reaction, hypertonia, hypophosphatemia, impotence, infection, insomnia, inversion T wave on ECG, malaise, myocardial infarction (chronic therapy; may be due to disease progression), neck pain, nervousness, nocturia, orthostatic hypotension, oxygen saturation decreased (possible pulmonary shunting), parotitis, pericarditis (not distinguishable from natural history of atherosclerotic vascular disease), peripheral vascular disease, respiratory tract disease, rhinitis, sinus node dysfunction (chronic therapy; may be due to disease progression), sinusitis, sore throat, sustained tachycardia, syncope, thrombocytopenia, tinnitus, tremor, urinary frequency, ventricular extrasystoles, ventricular tachycardia, vertigo, vomiting

Mechanism of Action Inhibits calcium ion from entering the "slow channels" or select voltage-sensitive areas of vascular smooth muscle and myocardium during depolarization, producing a relaxation of coronary vascular smooth muscle and coronary vasodilation; increases myocardial oxygen delivery in patients with vasospastic angina

Pharmacodynamics/Kinetics

Onset of Action

IV: Within minutes (constant infusion); Oral: 0.5 to 2 hours.

Peak effect: Oral: 1 to 2 hours. IV continuous infusion: 50% of the maximum effect is seen by 45 minutes.

Duration of Action

IV: ≤8 hours. Upon discontinuation of continuous infusion, a 50% decrease in effect is seen in ~30 minutes with gradual discontinuing antihypertensive effects for ~50 hours.

Oral: ≤8 hours.

Half-life Elimination
Follows dose-dependent (nonlinear) pharmacokinetics; "apparent" or calculated half-life is dependent upon serum concentrations.
Oral: Half-life over the first 8 hours after oral dosing is 2 to 4 hours; terminal half-life: 8.6 hours.
IV: After IV infusion, serum concentrations decrease tri-exponentially; alpha half-life: 3 minutes; beta half-life: 45 minutes; terminal half-life: 14 hours (**Note:** Terminal half-life can only be seen after long-term infusions).
Time to Peak Serum: Oral: 30 to 120 minutes (mean: 1 hour).

Pregnancy Risk Factor C

Pregnancy Considerations
Nicardipine has limited placental transfer following maternal oral and IV administration (Bartels 2007; Carbonne 1993; Matsumura 2014).

Nicardipine has been shown to decrease maternal blood pressure without significant changes on placental perfusion or fetal hemodynamics (Cornette 2016). Although effective for the treatment of hypertension in pregnancy, nicardipine may have an increased risk of adverse maternal events (eg, headache, nausea, tachycardia) in comparison to other agents (Nooij 2014). Cases of acute pulmonary edema have been reported following use as a tocolytic (Melis 2015).

Chronic maternal hypertension may increase the risk of birth defects, low birth weight, preterm delivery, stillbirth, and neonatal death. Actual fetal/neonatal risks may be related to duration and severity of maternal hypertension. Untreated hypertension may also increase the risks of adverse maternal outcomes, including gestational diabetes, myocardial infarction, preeclampsia, stroke, and delivery complications (ACOG 203 2019).

Calcium channel blockers may be used to treat hypertension in pregnant women; however, agents other than nicardipine are more commonly used for chronic hypertension (ACOG 203 2019; ESC [Regitz-Zagrosek 2018]). Females with preexisting hypertension may continue their medication during pregnancy unless contraindications exist (ESC [Regitz-Zagrosek 2018]). Nicardipine may be used as an alternative agent for the treatment of acute onset, severe hypertension in pregnant females (ACOG 203 2019; ACOG 767 2019).

- ◆ **Nicardipine HCl** *see* NiCARdipine *on page 1100*
- ◆ **Nicardipine Hydrochloride** *see* NiCARdipine *on page 1100*
- ◆ **NicAzel Forte** *see* Vitamins (Multiple/Oral) *on page 1550*
- ◆ **Nicoderm CQ [OTC]** *see* Nicotine *on page 1101*
- ◆ **Nicomide-T** *see* Niacinamide *on page 1100*
- ◆ **Nicorelief [OTC]** *see* Nicotine *on page 1101*
- ◆ **Nicorette [OTC]** *see* Nicotine *on page 1101*
- ◆ **Nicorette Mini [OTC]** *see* Nicotine *on page 1101*
- ◆ **Nicorette Starter Kit [OTC]** *see* Nicotine *on page 1101*
- ◆ **Nicotinamide** *see* Niacinamide *on page 1100*

Nicotine (nik oh TEEN)

Related Information
Management of the Chemically Dependent Patient *on page 1724*

Brand Names: US GoodSense Nicotine [OTC]; Nicoderm CQ [OTC]; Nicorelief [OTC]; Nicorette Mini [OTC]; Nicorette Starter Kit [OTC]; Nicorette [OTC]; Nicotine Mini [OTC]; Nicotine Step 1 [OTC]; Nicotine Step 2 [OTC]; Nicotine Step 3 [OTC]; Nicotrol; Nicotrol NS; Thrive [OTC]

Generic Availability (US) May be product dependent

Pharmacologic Category Smoking Cessation Aid

Dental Use Treatment to aid smoking cessation for the relief of nicotine withdrawal symptoms (including nicotine craving)

Use Smoking cessation: Treatment to aid smoking cessation for the relief of nicotine withdrawal symptoms (including nicotine craving)

Local Anesthetic/Vasoconstrictor Precautions No information available to require special precautions

Effects on Dental Treatment Key adverse event(s) related to dental treatment: Chewing gum: Excessive salivation, mouth/throat soreness, jaw muscle ache, hiccups, tachycardia, headache (mild), vomiting, belching, nausea, xerostomia (normal salivary flow resumes upon discontinuation), dizziness, nervousness, GI distress, hoarseness, and muscle pain.

Effects on Bleeding No information available to require special precautions

Adverse Reactions
Nasal spray/inhaler:
>10%:
Central nervous system: Headache (18% to 26%)
Gastrointestinal: Oral irritation (≤66%), dyspepsia (18%)
Respiratory: Nasal discomfort (94%), throat irritation (≤66%), cough (32%), rhinitis (23%)
1% to 10%:
Central nervous system: Pain (>3%), paresthesia (>3%), withdrawal syndrome (>3%)
Dermatologic: Acne vulgaris (3%)
Gastrointestinal: Flatulence (4%), gingival disease (4%), diarrhea (>3%), dysgeusia (>3%), hiccups (>3%), nausea (>3%)
Genitourinary: Dysmenorrhea (3%)
Neuromuscular & skeletal: Back pain (6%), arthralgia (5%), jaw pain (>3%), neck pain (>3%)
Respiratory: Flu-like symptoms (>3%), sinusitis (>3%)
Miscellaneous: Fever (>3%)
<1%: Amnesia, aphasia, bronchospasm, hypersensitivity reaction, increased bronchial secretions, migraine, nonthrombocytopenic purpura, numbness, peripheral edema, skin rash, visual disturbance, xerostomia
Frequency not defined:
Central nervous system: Altered sense of smell, facial paresthesia
Dermatologic: Burning sensation of the nose, facial flushing
Gastrointestinal: Oral paresthesia
Ophthalmic: Burning sensation of eyes, eye irritation, watery eyes
Otic: Otalgia
Respiratory: Epistaxis, hoarseness, nasal congestion, nasal mucosa ulcer, pharyngitis, rhinorrhea, sneezing
Postmarketing: Anaphylaxis, chest pain, dysphagia

Adverse events reported for chewing gum, lozenge, and/or transdermal systems were reported in prescription labeling. Frequency not defined; may be product- or dose-specific:

Cardiovascular: Cardiac arrhythmia, increased blood pressure, palpitations

Central nervous system: Abnormal dreams, sleep disturbance

Dermatologic: Erythema of skin, skin rash

Gastrointestinal: Dyspepsia, heartburn, hiccups, oral irritation, sore throat

Hypersensitivity: Hypersensitivity reaction

Local: Application site reaction, localized edema

Neuromuscular & skeletal: Jaw pain

Dental Usual Dosage

Tobacco cessation (patients should be advised to completely stop smoking upon initiation of therapy): Adults:

Gum: Chew 1 piece of gum when urge to smoke, up to 24 pieces/day. Patients who smoke <25 cigarettes/day should start with 2-mg strength; patients smoking ≥25 cigarettes/day should start with the 4-mg strength. Use according to the following 12-week dosing schedule:

Weeks 1-6: Chew 1 piece of gum every 1-2 hours; to increase chances of quitting, chew at least 9 pieces/day during the first 6 weeks

Weeks 7-9: Chew 1 piece of gum every 2-4 hours

Weeks 10-12: Chew 1 piece of gum every 4-8 hours

Inhaler: Oral: Usually 6 to 16 cartridges per day; best effect was achieved by frequent continuous puffing (20 minutes); recommended duration of treatment is 3 months, after which patients may be weaned from the inhaler by gradual reduction of the daily dose over 6-12 weeks

Lozenge: Oral: Patients who smoke their first cigarette within 30 minutes of waking should use the 4 mg strength; otherwise the 2 mg strength is recommended. Use according to the following 12-week dosing schedule:

Weeks 1-6: One lozenge every 1-2 hours

Weeks 7-9: One lozenge every 2-4 hours

Weeks 10-12: One lozenge every 4-8 hours

Note: Use at least 9 lozenges/day during first 6 weeks to improve chances of quitting; do not use more than one lozenge at a time (maximum: 5 lozenges every 6 hours, 20 lozenges/day)

Spray: Nasal: 1-2 sprays/hour; do not exceed more than 5 doses (10 sprays) per hour [maximum: 40 doses/day (80 sprays); each dose (2 sprays) contains 1 mg of nicotine]

Transdermal patch: Topical: **Note:** Adjustment may be required during initial treatment (move to higher dose if experiencing withdrawal symptoms; lower dose if side effects are experienced).

NicoDerm CQ®:

Patients smoking >10 cigarettes/day: Begin with step 1 (21 mg/day) for 6 weeks, **followed by** step 2 (14 mg/day) for 2 weeks; **finish with** step 3 (7 mg/day) for 2 weeks

Patients smoking ≤10 cigarettes/day: Begin with step 2 (14 mg/day) for 6 weeks, **followed by** step 3 (7 mg/day) for 2 weeks

Dosing

Adult & Geriatric

Smoking cessation (patients should completely stop smoking upon initiation of therapy):

Gum: Chew 1 piece of gum when urge to smoke occurs. If strong or frequent cravings are present after 1 piece of gum, may use a second piece within the hour (do not continuously use one piece after the other). Patients who smoke their first cigarette within 30 minutes of waking should use the 4 mg strength; otherwise the 2 mg strength is recommended. Use according to the following 12-week dosing schedule:

Weeks 1 to 6: Chew 1 piece of gum every 1 to 2 hours (maximum: 24 pieces/day); to increase chances of quitting, chew at least 9 pieces/day during the first 6 weeks

Weeks 7 to 9: Chew 1 piece of gum every 2 to 4 hours (maximum: 24 pieces/day)

Weeks 10 to 12: Chew 1 piece of gum every 4 to 8 hours (maximum: 24 pieces/day)

Inhalation: Oral:

Initial treatment: 6 to 16 cartridges/day (at least 6 cartridges/day for the first 3 to 6 weeks) for up to 12 weeks; maximum: 16 cartridges/day. **Note:** Best effect achieved with frequent continuous puffing (20 minutes). Use beyond 6 months is not recommended (has not been studied). If patient is unable to stop smoking by the fourth week of therapy, consider discontinuation.

Discontinuation of therapy: After initial treatment, gradually reduce daily dose over 6 to 12 weeks. Some patients may not require gradual reduction of dosage and may stop treatment abruptly.

Lozenge: Oral: 1 lozenge when urge to smoke occurs; do not use more than 1 lozenge at a time. Patients who smoke their first cigarette within 30 minutes of waking should use the 4 mg strength; otherwise the 2 mg strength is recommended. Use according to the following 12-week dosing schedule:

Weeks 1 to 6: 1 lozenge every 1 to 2 hours (maximum: 5 lozenges every 6 hours; 20 lozenges/day); to increase chances of quitting, use at least 9 lozenges/day during the first 6 weeks

Weeks 7 to 9: 1 lozenge every 2 to 4 hours (maximum: 5 lozenges every 6 hours; 20 lozenges/day)

Weeks 10 to 12: 1 lozenge every 4 to 8 hours (maximum: 5 lozenges every 6 hours; 20 lozenges/day)

Nasal: Spray: Initial: 1 to 2 doses/hour (each dose [2 sprays, one in each nostril] contains 1 mg of nicotine); adjust dose as needed based on patient response; do not exceed more than 5 doses (10 sprays) per hour [maximum: 40 mg/day (80 sprays)] or 3 months of treatment. **Note:** For best results, use at least the recommended minimum of 8 doses per day (less is unlikely to be effective). Use beyond 6 months is not recommended (has not been studied). If patient is unable to stop smoking by the fourth week of therapy, consider discontinuation.

Discontinuation of therapy: Discontinue over 4 to 6 weeks. Some patients may not require gradual reduction of dosage and may stop treatment abruptly.

Transdermal patch: Topical: **Note:** Adjustment may be required during initial treatment (move to higher dose if experiencing withdrawal symptoms; lower dose if side effects are experienced).

Patients smoking >10 cigarettes/day: Begin with step 1 (21 mg/day) for 6 weeks, **followed by** step 2 (14 mg/day) for 2 weeks; **finish with** step 3 (7 mg/day) for 2 weeks

Patients smoking ≤10 cigarettes/day: Begin with step 2 (14 mg/day) for 6 weeks, **followed by** step 3 (7 mg/day) for 2 weeks

Renal Impairment: Adult There are no specific dosage adjustments provided in the manufacturer's labeling. However, nicotine clearance is decreased in moderate to severe renal impairment; consider dose reduction.

Hepatic Impairment: Adult There are no specific dosage adjustments provided in the manufacturer's labeling. However, nicotine clearance is decreased in moderate to severe hepatic impairment; consider dose reduction.

Mechanism of Action Nicotine, a naturally occurring alkaloid, binds stereo-selectively to nicotinic-cholinergic receptors at the autonomic ganglia, in the adrenal medulla, at neuromuscular junctions, and in the brain. Two types of CNS effects are believed to be the basis of nicotine's positively reinforcing properties; a stimulating effect is exerted mainly in the cortex via the locus ceruleus and a reward effect is exerted in the limbic system. At low doses the stimulant effects predominate while at high doses the reward effects predominate.

Contraindications

Hypersensitivity to nicotine or any component of the formulation.

OTC labeling: Nicorette lozenge: When used for self-medication, do not use if you are allergic to soya.

Warnings/Precautions Urge patients to stop smoking completely when initiating therapy. Nicotine can increase heart rate and blood pressure. The risk versus the benefits should be weighed in patients with cardiovascular or peripheral vascular diseases, specifically patients with a history of myocardial infarction and/or angina pectoris, serious cardiac arrhythmias, or vasospastic diseases (Buerger disease, Prinzmetal variant angina and Raynaud phenomena); use caution in patients with angina, hypertension, or recent MI. Discontinue use if irregular heartbeat or palpitations occur. Use caution in patients with accelerated hypertension due to the risk of malignant hypertension. Generally, avoid use during the immediate postmyocardial infarction period, in patients with serious arrhythmias, or with severe or worsening angina. Use with caution in patients with insulin-dependent diabetes; hyperthyroidism; pheochromocytoma. Use with caution in patients with esophagitis or active gastric or peptic ulcer disease; healing may be delayed. Nicotine clearance is decreased in patients with moderate to severe hepatic or renal impairment; use with caution. Monitor for adverse effects; consider dose reduction.

OTC labeling: When used for self-medication, discontinue use and contact a health care provider if symptoms of nicotine overdose (eg, nausea, vomiting, dizziness, diarrhea, weakness, rapid heartbeat) or an allergic reaction (eg, difficulty breathing, rash) occurs.

Chewing gum and lozenge: When used for self-medication, consult a health care provider before use in patients on a sodium-restricted diet and in patients with a history of seizures. Discontinue chewing gum and consult a health care provider if mouth, teeth or jaw problems occur. Discontinue lozenge and consult a health care provider if mouth problems, persistent indigestion, or severe sore throat occurs.

Inhaler: Use with caution in patients with bronchospastic disease (eg, asthma, chronic pulmonary disease); may cause bronchospasm due to potential airway irritation; other forms of nicotine replacement may be preferred in patients with severe bronchospastic airway disease. Sustained use (beyond 6 months) by patients who quit smoking is not recommended.

Nasal spray: Use of nasal product is not recommended with chronic nasal disorders (eg, allergy, rhinitis, nasal polyps, and sinusitis). Exacerbations of bronchospasm have been reported in patients with preexisting asthma; use in patients with severe reactive airway disease is not recommended. Nasal mucosa irritation may occur. Sustained use (beyond 6 months) by patients who quit smoking is not recommended.

Transdermal patch: May contain conducting metal (eg, aluminum); remove patch prior to MRI. When used for self-medication, consult a health care provider before use in patients who have an allergy to adhesive tape or who have skin problems. Discontinue use and contact a health care provider if skin redness caused by the patch does not resolve after 4 days or if inflammation or rash occurs. If vivid dreams or other sleep disturbances occur, remove the patch at bedtime and apply another patch in the morning.

Some products may contain phenylalanine.

Drug Interactions

Metabolism/Transport Effects Substrate of CYP1A2 (minor), CYP2A6 (minor), CYP2B6 (minor), CYP2C19 (minor), CYP2C9 (minor), CYP2D6 (minor), CYP2E1 (minor), CYP3A4 (minor); **Note:** Assignment of Major/Minor substrate status based on clinically relevant drug interaction potential

Avoid Concomitant Use There are no known interactions where it is recommended to avoid concomitant use.

Increased Effect/Toxicity

Nicotine may increase the levels/effects of: Adenosine

The levels/effects of Nicotine may be increased by: Cimetidine; Varenicline

Decreased Effect There are no known significant interactions involving a decrease in effect.

Food Interactions Lozenge: Acidic foods/beverages decrease absorption of nicotine.

Dietary Considerations Some products may contain phenylalanine and/or sodium.

Pharmacodynamics/Kinetics

Onset of Action Intranasal: More closely approximate the time course of plasma nicotine levels observed after cigarette smoking than other dosage forms (Svensson 1987)

Half-life Elimination Transdermal: ~4 hours (Bannon 1989); Nasal spray: 1 to 2 hours; Inhaler: 1 to 2 hours

Time to Peak Serum: Transdermal: ~2 to 8 hours (Bannon 1989; DeVeaugh-Geiss 2010); Intranasal: 10 to 20 minutes; Oral inhalation: ≤15 minutes; Gum: ~30 minutes (Svensson 1987)

Pregnancy Considerations Nicotine crosses the placenta (HHS 2014).

Multiple factors contribute to the toxicity of nicotine (eg, dose, route, and duration of exposure). Nicotine exposure via maternal smoking may increase the risk of orofacial clefts, ectopic pregnancy, preterm delivery, and stillbirth (HHS 2014). It is also associated with the development of intrauterine growth restriction, sudden infant death syndrome (SIDS), placenta previa, placental abruption, ectopic pregnancy, as well as adverse effects on fetal brain and lung tissue (ACOG 721 2017; HHS 2014). Smokeless tobacco and second-hand exposure are also associated with adverse pregnancy outcomes. (ACOG 721 2017; HHS 2014).

All pregnant females should be encouraged to stop smoking (ACOG 721 2017). Following smoking cessation, benefits to the mother and fetus occur at any time during pregnancy, with the most benefits observed when smoking is stopped <15 weeks gestation (ACOG 721 2017; Siu 2015). Although nicotine replacement products are effective in non-pregnant patients, only studies that also provided behavioral support showed effectiveness for smoking cessation during pregnancy (ACOG 721 2017; Coleman 2015; Siu 2015). Available guidelines also note that information related to the maternal and fetal benefits and risks of using nicotine replacement products in pregnancy is limited and often conflicting (ACOG 721 2017; Siu 2015). The benefits of smoking cessation and risks of nicotine exposure should be evaluated with each patient; use of nicotine replacement products during pregnancy should be done under close medical supervision (ACOG 721 2017; Siu 2015).

Breastfeeding Considerations

Nicotine from cigarette smoke is present in breast milk and can be detected in the serum of breastfed infants (Dahlström 2008).

The amount of nicotine in breast milk following maternal use of nicotine replacement products varies. In one study, breast milk concentrations of nicotine following either maternal use of the 21 mg/day patch or smoking ~17 cigarettes/day were similar; milk concentrations decreased when lower doses of the nicotine patch were used (Ilett 2003). Hepatic clearance of nicotine in the newborn is lowest at birth.

Nicotine replacement therapy is considered to be compatible with breastfeeding if the amount of nicotine is less than that received from smoking. Use of short-acting products (gum, lozenges) is preferred (Sachs 2013). The manufacturer recommends that caution be exercised when using nicotine replacement products in breastfeeding women.

Dosage Forms Considerations Nicotrol NS contains approximately 200 sprays.

Dosage Forms: US

Gum, Mouth/Throat:
GoodSense Nicotine [OTC]: 2 mg (20 ea); 4 mg (20 ea, 100 ea)
Nicorelief [OTC]: 2 mg (50 ea, 110 ea); 4 mg (50 ea, 110 ea)
Nicorette [OTC]: 2 mg (20 ea, 100 ea, 160 ea, 170 ea, 190 ea, 200 ea); 4 mg (20 ea, 100 ea, 160 ea, 170 ea, 200 ea)
Nicorette Starter Kit [OTC]: 2 mg (100 ea, 110 ea); 4 mg (110 ea)
Thrive [OTC]: 2 mg (100 ea)
Generic: 2 mg (20 ea, 40 ea, 50 ea, 100 ea, 110 ea); 4 mg (20 ea, 40 ea, 50 ea, 100 ea, 110 ea)

Inhaler, Inhalation:
Nicotrol: 10 mg (168 ea)

Kit, Transdermal:
Generic: 7 mg/24 hr (14s) & 14 mg/24 hr (14s) & 21 mg/24 hr (28s)

Lozenge, Mouth/Throat:
GoodSense Nicotine [OTC]: 2 mg (27 ea); 4 mg (24 ea, 27 ea, 72 ea)
Nicorette [OTC]: 2 mg (24 ea, 72 ea); 4 mg (24 ea, 72 ea)
Nicorette Mini [OTC]: 2 mg (20 ea, 81 ea, 135 ea); 4 mg (20 ea, 81 ea)
Nicotine Mini [OTC]: 2 mg (27 ea); 4 mg (27 ea)
Generic: 2 mg (24 ea, 27 ea, 72 ea); 4 mg (24 ea, 27 ea)

Patch 24 Hour, Transdermal:
Nicoderm CQ [OTC]: 7 mg/24 hr (14 ea); 14 mg/24 hr (14 ea, 21 ea); 21 mg/24 hr (7 ea, 14 ea, 21 ea)
Nicotine Step 3 [OTC]: 7 mg/24 hr (14 ea)
Nicotine Step 2 [OTC]: 14 mg/24 hr (14 ea)
Nicotine Step 1 [OTC]: 21 mg/24 hr (14 ea)
Generic: 7 mg/24 hr (1 ea, 7 ea, 14 ea); 14 mg/24 hr (1 ea, 7 ea, 14 ea, 28 ea); 21 mg/24 hr (1 ea, 7 ea, 14 ea, 28 ea)

Solution, Nasal:
Nicotrol NS: 10 mg/mL (10 mL)

- **Nicotine Mini [OTC]** *see* Nicotine *on page 1101*
- **Nicotine Patch** *see* Nicotine *on page 1101*
- **Nicotine Step 1 [OTC]** *see* Nicotine *on page 1101*
- **Nicotine Step 2 [OTC]** *see* Nicotine *on page 1101*
- **Nicotine Step 3 [OTC]** *see* Nicotine *on page 1101*
- **Nicotinic Acid** *see* Niacin *on page 1097*
- **Nicotinic Acid Amide** *see* Niacinamide *on page 1100*
- **Nicotrol** *see* Nicotine *on page 1101*
- **Nicotrol NS** *see* Nicotine *on page 1101*
- **Nifedical XL [DSC]** *see* NIFEdipine *on page 1104*

NIFEdipine (nye FED i peen)

Related Information

Calcium Channel Blockers and Gingival Hyperplasia *on page 1816*
Cardiovascular Diseases *on page 1654*

Brand Names: US Adalat CC [DSC]; Afeditab CR [DSC]; Nifedical XL [DSC]; Procardia; Procardia XL

Brand Names: Canada Adalat XL; APO-Nifed PA [DSC]; DOM-NIFEdipine; MYLAN-NIFEdipine; PMS-NIFEdipine; PMS-NIFEdipine ER

Pharmacologic Category Antianginal Agent; Antihypertensive; Calcium Channel Blocker; Calcium Channel Blocker, Dihydropyridine

Use

Angina: Management of chronic stable or vasospastic angina.

Hypertension: Management of hypertension (ER products only).

Local Anesthetic/Vasoconstrictor Precautions No information available to require special precautions

Effects on Dental Treatment Nifedipine has been reported to cause 10% incidence of gingival hyperplasia; effects from 30-100 mg/day have appeared after 1-9 months. Discontinuance results in complete disappearance or marked regression of symptoms; symptoms will reappear upon remedication. Marked regression occurs after 1 week and complete disappearance of symptoms has occurred within 15 days. If a gingivectomy is performed and use of the drug is continued or resumed, hyperplasia usually will recur. The success of the gingivectomy usually requires that the medication be discontinued or that a switch to a noncalcium channel blocker be made. If for some reason nifedipine cannot be discontinued, hyperplasia has not recurred after gingivectomy when extensive plaque control was performed. If nifedipine is changed to another class of cardiovascular agent, the gingival hyperplasia will probably regress and resolve. Switching to another calcium channel blocker may result in continued hyperplasia.

Effects on Bleeding No information available to require special precautions

Adverse Reactions

>10%:

Cardiovascular: Flushing (10% to 25%; extended release: 3% to 4%), peripheral edema (7% to 30%)

Central nervous system: Dizziness (10% to 27%), headache (10% to 23%)

Gastrointestinal: Heartburn (≤11%), nausea (≤11%)

1% to 10%:

Cardiovascular: Palpitations (≤7%), transient hypotension (5%), cardiac failure (2%)

Central nervous system: Mood changes (≤7%), nervousness (≤7%), fatigue (6%), chills (≤2%), disturbed sleep (≤2%), equilibrium disturbance (≤2%), jitteriness (≤2%), shakiness (≤2%)

Dermatologic: Dermatitis (≤2%), diaphoresis (≤2%), pruritus (≤2%), urticaria (≤2%)

Gastrointestinal: Gingival hyperplasia (≤10%), sore throat (≤6%), abdominal cramps (≤2%), constipation (≤2%), diarrhea (≤2%), flatulence (≤2%)

Genitourinary: Sexual difficulty (≤2%)

Neuromuscular & skeletal: Muscle cramps (≤8%), tremor (≤8%), weakness (<3%), joint stiffness (≤2%)

Ophthalmic: Blurred vision (≤2%)

Respiratory: Cough (≤6%), nasal congestion (≤6%), wheezing (≤6%), chest congestion (≤2%), dyspnea (≤2%)

Miscellaneous: Fever (≤2%), inflammation (≤2%)

<1%, postmarketing, and/or case reports: Acute generalized exanthematous pustulosis, agranulocytosis, alopecia, altered sense of smell, anemia, aplastic anemia, angina pectoris, angioedema, arthritis (with positive ANA), bezoar formation, cardiac arrhythmia, cerebral ischemia, depression, dysgeusia, epistaxis, extrapyramidal reaction, erectile dysfunction, erythema multiforme, erythromelalgia, exfoliative dermatitis, facial edema, gastroesophageal reflux disease, gastrointestinal obstruction, gastrointestinal ulcer, gynecomastia, hematuria, hepatitis (allergic), ischemia, leukopenia, malignant neoplasm of lip (Friedman 2012), memory impairment, migraine, myalgia, myoclonus, nocturia, paranoia, parotitis, periorbital edema, polyuria, purpura, skin photosensitivity, Stevens-Johnson syndrome, syncope, tachycardia, thrombocytopenia, tinnitus, toxic epidermal necrolysis, transient blindness, ventricular arrhythmia

Mechanism of Action Inhibits calcium ion from entering the "slow channels" or select voltage-sensitive areas of vascular smooth muscle and myocardium during depolarization, producing a relaxation of coronary vascular smooth muscle and coronary vasodilation; increases myocardial oxygen delivery in patients with vasospastic angina; also reduces peripheral vascular resistance, producing a reduction in arterial blood pressure.

Pharmacodynamics/Kinetics

Onset of Action Immediate release: ~20 minutes

Half-life Elimination Adults: Healthy: 2 to 5 hours; Cirrhosis: 7 hours; Elderly: 7 hours (extended release tablet)

Pregnancy Considerations

Nifedipine crosses the placenta (Manninen 1991; Silberschmidt 2008).

An increase in perinatal asphyxia, cesarean delivery, prematurity, and intrauterine growth retardation have been reported following maternal use.

Chronic maternal hypertension may increase the risk of birth defects, low birth weight, preterm delivery, stillbirth, and neonatal death. Actual fetal/neonatal risks may be related to duration and severity of maternal hypertension. Untreated hypertension may also increase the risks of adverse maternal outcomes, including gestational diabetes, MI, preeclampsia, stroke, and delivery complications (ACOG 203 2019).

If treatment for chronic hypertension during pregnancy is needed, oral nifedipine is one of the preferred agents (ACOG 203 2019; ESC [Regitz-Zagrosek 2018]). Oral immediate-release nifedipine is also recommended for the management of acute-onset, severe hypertension in pregnant and postpartum women, including those with preeclampsia or eclampsia (ACOG 767 2019; ESC [Regitz-Zagrosek 2018]).

Nifedipine has also been evaluated for the treatment of preterm labor. Tocolytics may be used for the short-term (48-hour) prolongation of pregnancy to allow for the administration of antenatal steroids and should not be used prior to fetal viability or when the risks of use to the fetus or mother are greater than the risk of preterm birth (ACOG 171 2016). Nifedipine is ineffective for maintenance tocolytic therapy (ACOG 171 2016; Aggarwal 2018; Roos 2013; Verspyck 2017).

- **Niftolid** *see* Flutamide *on page 702*
- **Nighttime Sleep Aid [OTC]** *see* DiphenhydrAMINE (Systemic) *on page 502*
- **Nikki** *see* Ethinyl Estradiol and Drospirenone *on page 610*
- **Nilandron** *see* Nilutamide *on page 1107*

Nilotinib (nye LOE ti nib)

Related Information

Clinical Risk Related to Drugs Prolonging QT Interval *on page 1675*

Brand Names: US Tasigna

Brand Names: Canada Tasigna

Pharmacologic Category Antineoplastic Agent, BCR-ABL Tyrosine Kinase Inhibitor; Antineoplastic Agent, Tyrosine Kinase Inhibitor

Use Chronic myelogenous leukemia:

Treatment of newly diagnosed Philadelphia chromosome-positive chronic myelogenous leukemia (CML) in chronic phase in pediatric patients ≥1 year and adults.

Treatment of chronic- and accelerated-phase Philadelphia chromosome-positive CML in adults resistant or intolerant to prior therapy that included imatinib.

Treatment of chronic phase Philadelphia chromosome-positive CML in pediatric patients ≥1 year with resistance or intolerance to prior tyrosine-kinase inhibitor therapy.

Local Anesthetic/Vasoconstrictor Precautions

Nilotinib is one of the drugs confirmed to prolong the QT interval and is accepted as having a risk of causing torsade de pointes. The risk of drug-induced torsade de pointes is extremely low when a single QT interval prolonging drug is prescribed. In terms of epinephrine, it is not known what effect vasoconstrictors in the local anesthetic regimen will have in patients with a known history of congenital prolonged QT interval or in patients taking any medication that prolongs the QT interval. Until more information is obtained, it is suggested that the clinician consult with the physician prior to the use of a vasoconstrictor in suspected patients, and that the vasoconstrictor (epinephrine, mepivacaine and levonordefrin [Carbocaine® 2% with Neo-Cobefrin®]) be used with caution.

Effects on Dental Treatment Key adverse event(s) related to dental treatment: Mouth ulcerations, stomatitis

Effects on Bleeding Chemotherapy may result in significant myelosuppression. Thrombocytopenia (grades 3/4) occurs in 10% to 37% of patients (median duration 22 days). In patients who are under active treatment with these agents, medical consult is suggested.

Adverse Reactions

>10%:

Cardiovascular: Prolonged QT interval on ECG (children and adolescents: >30 msec from baseline: 25%; adults: >60 msec from baseline: 4%; adults: >500 msec: <1%), occlusive arterial disease (9% to 15%), peripheral edema (9% to 15%), hypertension (10% to 11%)

Central nervous system: Headache (20% to 35%; children & adolescents: >20%), fatigue (23% to 32%), dizziness (12%), insomnia (7% to 12%)

Dermatologic: Skin rash (29% to 38%; children & adolescents: >20%), pruritus (20% to 32%), night sweats (12% to 27%), alopecia (11% to 13%), xeroderma (12%)

Endocrine & metabolic: Hyperglycemia (≤50%), hypophosphatemia (grade 3/4: 8% to 17%), increased HDL cholesterol, increased VLDL

Gastrointestinal: Nausea (22% to 37%; children & adolescents: >20%), vomiting (13% to 29%; children & adolescents: >20%), increased serum lipase (28%), diarrhea (19% to 28%), constipation (19% to 26%), upper abdominal pain (12% to 18%), decreased appetite (including anorexia; 15% to 17%), abdominal pain (15% to 16%)

Hematologic & oncologic: Neutropenia (15%; grades 3/4: 12% to 42%; children & adolescents: 41%), thrombocytopenia (18%; grades 3/4: 10% to 42%; children & adolescents: 44%), decreased absolute lymphocyte count (children & adolescents: 32%), anemia (8%; grades 3/4: 4% to 27%; children & adolescents: 30%)

Hepatic: Increased serum alanine aminotransferase (10% to 72%; children & adolescents: >20%), increased serum aspartate aminotransferase (10% to 47%; children & adolescents: >20%), hyperbilirubinemia (≥10%; children & adolescents: >20%)

Infection: Influenza (13%)

Neuromuscular & skeletal: Arthralgia (16% to 26%), limb pain (15% to 20%), myalgia (16% to 19%), back pain (15% to 19%), asthenia (14% to 16%), ostealgia (14% to 15%), muscle spasm (12% to 15%), musculoskeletal pain (11% to 12%)

Respiratory: Cough (17% to 27%), nasopharyngitis (15% to 27%), upper respiratory tract infection (10% to 17%; children & adolescents: >20%), dyspnea (9% to 15%), oropharyngeal pain (7% to 12%)

Miscellaneous: Fever (14% to 28%; children & adolescents: >20%)

1% to 10%:

Cardiovascular: Ischemic heart disease (≤9%), peripheral arterial disease (≤4%), cerebral ischemia (1% to 3%), pericardial effusion (≤2%), angina pectoris, cardiac arrhythmia (including AV block, atrial fibrillation, bradycardia, cardiac flutter, extrasystoles, and tachycardia), chest discomfort, chest pain (including noncardiac), flushing, palpitations

Central nervous system: Anxiety, depression, flank pain, hypoesthesia, malaise, myasthenia, pain, paresthesia, peripheral neuropathy, vertigo, voice disorder

Dermatologic: Acne vulgaris, dermatitis (including allergic, exfoliative, and acneiform), eczema, erythema of skin, folliculitis, hyperhidrosis, urticaria

Endocrine & metabolic: Decreased serum albumin (grade 3/4: 3% to 4%), fluid retention (grade 3/4: 3% to 4%), altered hormone level (growth hormone deficiency; children and adolescents: 2%), diabetes mellitus, electrolyte disorder, hypercalcemia, hypercholesterolemia, hyperkalemia, hyperlipidemia, hyperphosphatemia, hypertriglyceridemia, hypocalcemia, hypokalemia, hypomagnesemia, hyponatremia, increased gamma-glutamyl transferase, weight gain, weight loss

Gastrointestinal: Dyspepsia (4% to 10%), gastroenteritis (7%), gastrointestinal hemorrhage (≤5%), abdominal distension, abdominal distress, dysgeusia, flatulence, increased serum amylase, pancreatitis

Genitourinary: Pollakiuria

Hematologic & oncologic: Hemorrhage (grade 3/4: 1% to 2%), bruise, change in serum protein (decreased globulins), cutaneous papilloma, eosinophilia, febrile neutropenia, hemophthalmos, leukopenia, lymphocytopenia, pancytopenia

Hepatic: Ascites (≤2%), hepatic insufficiency, increased serum alkaline phosphatase

Neuromuscular & skeletal: Increased creatine phosphokinase in blood specimen, musculoskeletal chest pain, neck pain

Ophthalmic: Eyelid edema (1%), conjunctivitis, eye pruritus, xerophthalmia

Respiratory: Pleural effusion (≤2%), dyspnea on exertion, epistaxis

Frequency not defined:

Cardiovascular: Hypotension, pericarditis, reduced ejection fraction, shock (hemorrhagic), thrombosis, ventricular dysfunction

Central nervous system: Amnesia, breast induration, cerebral edema, confusion, disorientation, dysesthesia, dysphoria, lethargy, restless leg syndrome

Dermatologic: Cutaneous nodule (sebaceous hyperplasia), dermal ulcer, erythema multiforme, erythema nodosum, exfoliation of skin, furuncle, hyperkeratosis, palmar-plantar erythrodysesthesia, psoriasis, skin atrophy, skin blister, skin discoloration, skin hyperpigmentation, skin hypertrophy, skin photosensitivity, tinea pedis

Endocrine & metabolic: Altered hormone level (insulin C-peptide decreased), growth retardation, hyperparathyroidism (secondary), hyperuricemia, hypoglycemia, thyroiditis

Gastrointestinal: Cholestasis, enterocolitis, gastric ulcer (perforation possible), gingivitis, hematemesis, hemorrhoids, hiatal hernia, intestinal obstruction, oral lesion (papilloma), ulcerative esophagitis

Genitourinary: Dysmenorrhea, hematuria, urinary incontinence, urine discoloration

Hematologic & oncologic: Leukocytosis, paraproteinemia, petechia, rectal hemorrhage, retroperitoneal hemorrhage, thrombocythemia
Hepatic: Hepatomegaly
Hypersensitivity: Hypersensitivity
Infection: Abscess (subcutaneous), anal abscess, reactivation of HBV, sepsis
Local: Local swelling (nipple), localized edema
Neuromuscular & skeletal: Arthritis
Ophthalmic: Allergic conjunctivitis, blepharitis, diplopia, eye pain, optic neuritis, papilledema, photophobia, retinopathy (chorioretinopathy), swelling of eye
Otic: Auditory impairment, otalgia, tinnitus
Renal: Renal failure syndrome
Respiratory: Pulmonary hypertension, wheezing
Miscellaneous: Cyst (dermal), troponin increased in blood specimen

<1%, postmarketing, and/or case reports: Acute myocardial infarction, arteriosclerosis, ascorbic acid deficiency (Oak 2016), blurred vision, bronchitis, candidiasis, cardiac failure, cerebral infarction, chills, conjunctival hemorrhage, coronary artery disease, cyanosis, decreased visual acuity, dehydration, dental discomfort (sensitivity), dependent edema, disturbance in attention, dysuria, ecchymoses, erectile dysfunction, esophageal pain, exfoliative dermatitis, eye irritation, facial edema, fixed drug eruption, flu-like symptoms, gastritis, gastroesophageal reflux disease, gout, gynecomastia, heart murmur, hematoma, hepatotoxicity, hyperemia (scleral, conjunctival, ocular), hyperesthesia, hypertensive crisis, hyperthyroidism, hypothyroidism, increased appetite, increased blood urea nitrogen, increased lactate dehydrogenase, increased serum creatinine, intermittent claudication, interstitial pulmonary disease, intracranial hemorrhage, ischemic stroke, jaundice, joint swelling, local alterations in temperature sensations, loss of consciousness, mastalgia, melena, migraine, nocturia, oral mucosa ulcer, periorbital edema, pharyngolaryngeal pain, photopsia, pleurisy, pleuritic chest pain, pneumonia, pulmonary edema, skin pain, stiffness, stomatitis, syncope, throat irritation, thrombotic microangiopathy, toxic hepatitis, transient ischemic attacks, tremor, tumor lysis syndrome, urinary tract infection, urinary urgency, visual impairment, xerostomia

Mechanism of Action Nilotinib is a selective tyrosine kinase inhibitor that targets BCR-ABL kinase, c-KIT and platelet derived growth factor receptor (PDGFR); it does not have activity against the SRC family. Nilotinib inhibits BCR-ABL mediated proliferation of leukemic cell lines by binding to the ATP-binding site of BCR-ABL and inhibiting tyrosine kinase activity. Nilotinib has activity in imatinib-resistant BCR-ABL kinase mutations.

Pharmacodynamics/Kinetics

Half-life Elimination ~17 hours

Time to Peak 3 hours

Reproductive Considerations

Verify pregnancy status in females of reproductive potential prior to initiating therapy. Women of childbearing potential should be advised to use effective contraception during treatment and for at least 14 days after the last dose.

Pregnancy Considerations

Based on data from animal reproduction studies and the mechanism of action, nilotinib may cause fetal harm if administered during pregnancy.

Dental Health Professional Considerations See Local Anesthetic/Vasoconstrictor Precautions

◆ **Nilotinib HCl** *see* Nilotinib *on page 1105*

◆ **Nilotinib Hydrochloride Monohydrate** *see* Nilotinib *on page 1105*

Nilutamide (ni LOO ta mide)

Brand Names: US Nilandron

Brand Names: Canada Anandron

Pharmacologic Category Antineoplastic Agent, Antiandrogen

Use Prostate cancer, metastatic: Treatment of metastatic prostate cancer (in combination with surgical castration)

Local Anesthetic/Vasoconstrictor Precautions
No information available to require special precautions

Effects on Dental Treatment Key adverse event(s) related to dental treatment: Xerostomia (normal salivary flow resumes upon discontinuation).

Effects on Bleeding Although significant myelosuppression with associated altered hemostasis has been reported for many chemotherapeutic agents, myelosuppression is not common with nilutamide and no specific precautions appear to necessary.

Adverse Reactions Reactions reported from monotherapy and combination therapy.

>10%:
Endocrine & metabolic: Hot flash (28%)
Ophthalmic: Nocturnal amblyopia (13% to 57%)

1% to 10%:
Cardiovascular: Hypertension (5%), cardiac failure (3%), angina pectoris (2%), edema (2%), syncope (2%)
Central nervous system: Dizziness (7%), paresthesia (3%), malaise (2%), nervousness (2%)
Dermatologic: Pruritus (2%)
Endocrine & metabolic: Hyperglycemia (4%), increased haptoglobin (2%), weight loss (2%)
Gastrointestinal: Nausea (10%), constipation (7%), diarrhea (2%), gastrointestinal hemorrhage (2%), melena (2%), xerostomia (2%)
Hematologic & oncologic: Leukopenia (3%)
Hepatic: Increased serum ALT (8%), increased serum AST (8%), increased serum alkaline phosphatase (3%)
Neuromuscular & skeletal: Arthritis (2%)
Ophthalmic: Visual disturbance (7%), cataract (2%), photophobia (2%)
Renal: Increased blood urea nitrogen (2%), increased serum creatinine (2%)
Respiratory: Dyspnea (6%), cough (2%), interstitial pneumonitis (2%), rhinitis (2%)
Miscellaneous: Alcohol intolerance (5%)

<1%, postmarketing, and/or case reports: Anxiety, aplastic anemia, cold extremities, gynecomastia, headache, hepatic injury, hepatitis, maculopapular rash, palpitations, prolonged QT interval on ECG, urticaria, vomiting, weight gain

Mechanism of Action Nilutamide is a nonsteroidal antiandrogen which blocks testosterone effects at the androgen receptor level, preventing androgen response.

Pharmacodynamics/Kinetics

Half-life Elimination Terminal: 38 to 59 hours; Metabolites: 59 to 126 hours

Pregnancy Considerations Animal reproduction studies have not been conducted. Nilutamide is not indicated for use in women.

◆ **Nimenrix** *see* Meningococcal (Groups A / C / Y and W-135) Conjugate Vaccine *on page 964*

NiMODipine (nye MOE di peen)

Related Information

Calcium Channel Blockers and Gingival Hyperplasia *on page 1816*

Brand Names: US Nymalize

Brand Names: Canada Nimotop

Pharmacologic Category Calcium Channel Blocker; Calcium Channel Blocker, Dihydropyridine

Use Subarachnoid hemorrhage: For the improvement of neurological outcome by reducing the incidence and severity of ischemic deficits in adult patients with subarachnoid hemorrhage (SAH) from ruptured intracranial berry aneurysms regardless of their postictus neurological condition (ie, Hunt and Hess grades I to V)

Local Anesthetic/Vasoconstrictor Precautions No information available to require special precautions

Effects on Dental Treatment Other drugs of this class can cause gingival hyperplasia (ie, nifedipine) but there have been no reports for nimodipine.

Effects on Bleeding No information available to require special precautions

Adverse Reactions

1% to 10%:

Cardiovascular: Decreased blood pressure (4% to 5%), bradycardia (1%)

Central nervous system: Headache (1%)

Gastrointestinal: Nausea (1%)

<1%, postmarketing, and/or case reports: Anemia, decreased platelet count, diaphoresis, disseminated intravascular coagulation, dizziness, edema, flushing, gastrointestinal hemorrhage, gastrointestinal pseudo-obstruction, hematoma, hepatitis, hypertension, increased lactate dehydrogenase, increased serum alkaline phosphatase, increased serum ALT, increased serum glucose, intestinal obstruction, jaundice, muscle cramps, palpitations, pruritus, rebound vasospasm, thrombocytopenia, vomiting, wheezing

Mechanism of Action Nimodipine shares the pharmacology of other calcium channel blockers; animal studies indicate that nimodipine has a greater effect on cerebral arterials than other arterials; this increased specificity may be due to the drug's increased lipophilicity and cerebral distribution as compared to nifedipine; inhibits calcium ion from entering the "slow channels" or select voltage sensitive areas of vascular smooth muscle and myocardium during depolarization

Pharmacodynamics/Kinetics

Half-life Elimination 1 to 2 hours; prolonged with renal impairment

Time to Peak Serum: 0.25 to 1.05 hours.

Pregnancy Considerations Nimodipine crosses the placenta (Belfort 1994).

Nimodipine has been evaluated for the management of preeclampsia (Belfort 1994; Belfort 2003), but it is not one of the agents currently recommended for severe intrapartum or postpartum hypertension associated with preeclampsia or eclampsia (ACOG 767 2019).

◆ **Nimotop** *see* NiMODipine *on page 1108*

◆ **Ninlaro** *see* Ixazomib *on page 853*

Nintedanib (nin TED a nib)

Brand Names: US Ofev

Brand Names: Canada Ofev

Pharmacologic Category Tyrosine Kinase Inhibitor

Use

Chronic fibrosing interstitial lung diseases with a progressive phenotype: Treatment of chronic fibrosing interstitial lung diseases (ILD) with a progressive phenotype.

Idiopathic pulmonary fibrosis: Treatment of idiopathic pulmonary fibrosis.

Systemic sclerosis-associated interstitial lung disease: Indicated to slow the rate of decline in pulmonary function in patients with systemic sclerosis-associated ILD.

Local Anesthetic/Vasoconstrictor Precautions Nintedanib may cause hypertension; monitor blood pressure prior to vasoconstrictor use

Effects on Dental Treatment No significant effects or complications reported

Effects on Bleeding Altered hemostasis resulting in increased risk of bleeding. Medical consult is suggested prior to any dental surgical procedures.

Adverse Reactions

>10%:

Dermatologic: Dermal ulcer (18%)

Endocrine & metabolic: Weight loss (10% to 12%)

Gastrointestinal: Abdominal pain (15% to 18%), decreased appetite (9% to 11%), diarrhea (62% to 76%), nausea (24% to 32%), vomiting (12% to 25%)

Hepatic: Increased liver enzymes (13% to 14%)

Nervous system: Fatigue (10% to 11%)

Respiratory: Nasopharyngitis (13%)

1% to 10%:

Cardiovascular: Acute myocardial infarction (2%), arterial thrombosis (3%), hypertension (5%)

Endocrine & metabolic: Hypothyroidism (1%)

Genitourinary: Urinary tract infection (6%)

Hematologic & oncologic: Hemorrhage (10%; can be major hemorrhage)

Nervous system: Dizziness (6%), headache (8% to 9%)

Neuromuscular & skeletal: Back pain (6%)

Respiratory: Bronchitis (1%), pneumonia (4%), upper respiratory tract infection (7%)

Miscellaneous: Fever (6%)

<1%: Gastrointestinal: Gastrointestinal perforation

Postmarketing (any indication): Hepatotoxicity, pancreatitis, pruritus, skin rash, thrombocytopenia

Mechanism of Action Inhibits multiple receptor tyrosine kinases (RTKs) and nonreceptor tyrosine kinases (nRTKs), including platelet-derived growth factor (PDGFR alpha and PDGFR beta); fibroblast growth factor receptor (FGFR1, FGFR2, FGFR3); vascular endothelial growth factor (VEGFR1, VEGFR2, and VEGFR3); colony-stimulating factor 1 receptor (CSF1R); and Fms-like tyrosine kinase-3 (FLT3). Nintedanib binds competitively to the adenosine triphosphate (ATP) binding pocket of these receptors and blocks the intracellular signaling which is crucial for the proliferation, migration, and transformation of fibroblasts.

Pharmacodynamics/Kinetics

Half-life Elimination 9.5 hours

Time to Peak 2 hours (4 hours with food)

Reproductive Considerations

A pregnancy test is required prior to initiating treatment and periodically during treatment in women of reproductive potential. Women of reproductive potential should use highly effective contraception during therapy and for ≥3 months after the last dose; the addition of a barrier method is recommended if a hormonal contraceptive is used.

Pregnancy Considerations
Based on the mechanism of action and adverse events observed in animal reproduction studies, nintedanib may be expected to cause fetal harm if used during pregnancy.

◆ **Nintedanib Esylate** *see* Nintedanib *on page 1108*
◆ **Nipent** *see* Pentostatin *on page 1214*

Niraparib (nye RAP a rib)

Brand Names: US Zejula
Brand Names: Canada Zejula
Pharmacologic Category Antineoplastic Agent, PARP Inhibitor
Use
Ovarian, fallopian tube, or primary peritoneal cancer:
First-line maintenance treatment of advanced epithelial ovarian, fallopian tube, or primary peritoneal cancer in adults who are in a complete or partial response to first-line platinum-based chemotherapy.
Maintenance treatment of recurrent epithelial ovarian, fallopian tube, or primary peritoneal cancer in adults who are in a complete or partial response to platinum-based chemotherapy.
Treatment of advanced ovarian, fallopian tube, or primary peritoneal cancer in adults who have been treated with ≥3 prior chemotherapy regimens and whose cancer is associated with homologous recombination deficiency positive status, defined by either a deleterious or suspected deleterious BRCA mutation **or** genomic instability and progression >6 months after response to the last platinum-based chemotherapy. Select patients for therapy based on an approved companion diagnostic for niraparib.
Local Anesthetic/Vasoconstrictor Precautions Hypertension (20%), monitoring of blood pressure suggested, especially prior to using vasoconstrictor
Effects on Dental Treatment Key adverse event(s) related to dental treatment: Mucositis (≤20%), stomatitis (≤20%)
Effects on Bleeding Chemotherapy may result in significant myelosuppression, potentially including reduction in platelet counts (thrombocytopenia) and altered hemostasis. In patients under active treatment with this agent, medical consult is suggested.
Adverse Reactions
>10%:
Cardiovascular: Hypertension (20%)
Central nervous system: Fatigue (≤57%), insomnia (27%), headache (26%), dizziness (18%), anxiety (11%)
Dermatologic: Skin rash (21%)
Gastrointestinal: Nausea (74%), constipation (40%), vomiting (34%), decreased appetite (25%), stomatitis (≤20%), dyspepsia (18%)
Genitourinary: Urinary tract infection (13%)
Hematologic & oncologic: Thrombocytopenia (61%; grades 3/4: 29%), anemia (50%; grades 3/4: 25%), neutropenia (30%; grades 3/4: 20%), leukopenia (17%; grades 3/4: 5%)
Hepatic: Increased serum aspartate aminotransferase (≤36%), increased serum alanine aminotransferase (≤28%)
Neuromuscular & skeletal: Asthenia (≤57%), back pain (18%)
Respiratory: Nasopharyngitis (23%), dyspnea (20%), cough (16%)
1% to 10%:
Cardiovascular: Palpitations (10%), peripheral edema, tachycardia
Central nervous system: Depression
Endocrine & metabolic: Hypokalemia, increased gamma-glutamyl transferase, weight loss
Gastrointestinal: Dysgeusia (10%), xerostomia (10%)
Hepatic: Increased serum alkaline phosphatase
Ophthalmic: Conjunctivitis
Renal: Increased serum creatinine
Respiratory: Bronchitis, epistaxis
<1%: Acute myelocytic leukemia, myelodysplastic syndrome
Postmarketing: Anaphylaxis, confusion, disorientation, hallucination, hypersensitivity reaction, hypertensive crisis, pneumonia, reversible posterior leukoencephalopathy syndrome, skin photosensitivity
Mechanism of Action Niraparib is a poly (ADP-ribose) polymerase (PARP) enzyme inhibitor, which is highly selective for PARP-1 and PARP-2. PARP-1 and PARP-2 are involved in detecting DNA damage and promote repair (Mirza 2016). Inhibiting PARP enzymatic activity results in DNA damage, apoptosis and cell death. Niraparib induces cytotoxicity in tumor cell lines with and without BRCA1/2 deficiencies.
Pharmacodynamics/Kinetics
Half-life Elimination 36 hours
Time to Peak Within 3 hours
Reproductive Considerations Pregnancy testing should be conducted prior to treatment and effective contraception should be used during therapy and for at least 6 months after the last niraparib dose in females of reproductive potential.
Pregnancy Considerations
Animal reproduction studies have not been conducted, however based on the mechanism of action, niraparib may cause fetal harm if used during pregnancy.

◆ **Niraparib Tosylate** *see* Niraparib *on page 1109*

Nisoldipine (nye SOL di peen)

Related Information
Calcium Channel Blockers and Gingival Hyperplasia *on page 1816*
Cardiovascular Diseases *on page 1654*
Brand Names: US Sular
Pharmacologic Category Antihypertensive; Calcium Channel Blocker; Calcium Channel Blocker, Dihydropyridine
Use
Hypertension: Management of hypertension
Guideline recommendations: The 2017 Guideline for the Prevention, Detection, Evaluation, and Management of High Blood Pressure in Adults recommends if monotherapy is warranted, in the absence of comorbidities (eg, cerebrovascular disease, chronic kidney disease, diabetes, heart failure, ischemic heart disease, etc), that thiazide-like diuretics or dihydropyridine calcium channel blockers may be preferred options due to improved cardiovascular endpoints (eg, prevention of heart failure and stroke). ACE inhibitors and ARBs are also acceptable for monotherapy. Combination therapy may be required to achieve blood pressure goals and is initially preferred in patients at high risk (stage 2 hypertension or atherosclerotic cardiovascular disease [ASCVD] risk ≥10%) (ACC/AHA [Whelton 2017]).
Local Anesthetic/Vasoconstrictor Precautions No information available to require special precautions

Effects on Dental Treatment Key adverse event(s) related to dental treatment: Xerostomia (normal salivary flow resumes upon discontinuation).

Unlike other calcium channel blockers, information is sparse as to whether nisoldipine causes gingival hyperplasia. Consultation with physician is suggested if hyperplasia is observed in patients taking nisoldipine.

Effects on Bleeding No information available to require special precautions

Adverse Reactions

>10%:

Cardiovascular: Peripheral edema (7% to 29%; dose-related)

Central nervous system: Headache (22%)

1% to 10%:

Cardiovascular: Vasodilation (4%), palpitations (3%), exacerbation of angina pectoris (2%), chest pain (2%)

Central nervous system: Dizziness (3% to 10%)

Dermatologic: Skin rash (2%)

Gastrointestinal: Nausea (2%)

Respiratory: Pharyngitis (5%), sinusitis (3%)

<1%, postmarketing, and/or case reports: Abnormal dreams, abnormal hepatic function tests, abnormal T waves on ECG (flattening, inversion, non-specific changes), alopecia, amblyopia, amnesia, anemia, anorexia, anxiety, arthralgia, arthritis, asthma, ataxia, atrial fibrillation, blepharitis, bruise, cardiac failure (decompensated), cellulitis, cerebral ischemia, cerebrovascular accident, colitis, conjunctivitis, decreased libido, depression, dermal ulcer, diabetes mellitus, diaphoresis, diarrhea, drowsiness, dysgeusia, dyspepsia, dysphagia, dyspnea, dysuria, ejection murmur (systolic), epistaxis, exfoliative dermatitis, facial edema, fever, first degree atrioventricular block, flu-like symptoms, gastritis, gastrointestinal hemorrhage, gingival hyperplasia, glaucoma, glossitis, gout, gynecomastia, hematuria, hepatomegaly, herpes simplex infection, herpes zoster, hypersensitivity reaction (eg, angioedema, chest tightness, hypotension, shortness of breath, skin rash, tachycardia), hypertension, hypertonia, hypoesthesia, hypokalemia, hypotension, increased appetite, increased blood urea nitrogen, increased creatine phosphokinase, increased nonprotein nitrogen, increased serum creatinine, insomnia, jugular vein distention, keratoconjunctivitis, leukopenia, maculopapular rash, malaise, melena, migraine, myalgia, myasthenia, myocardial infarction, myositis, nocturia, oral mucosa ulcer, orthostatic hypotension, paresthesia, petechia, pleural effusion, pruritus, pustular rash, rales, retinal detachment, skin discoloration, skin photosensitivity, supraventricular tachycardia, syncope, tenosynovitis, thyroiditis, tremor, urinary frequency, urticaria, vaginal hemorrhage, venous insufficiency, ventricular premature contractions, vertigo, vision loss (temporary, unilateral), vitreous opacity, weight changes (gain/loss), wheezing (end inspiratory wheeze), xerostomia

Mechanism of Action As a dihydropyridine calcium channel blocker, structurally similar to nifedipine, nisoldipine impedes the movement of calcium ions into vascular smooth muscle and cardiac muscle. Dihydropyridines are potent vasodilators and are not as likely to suppress cardiac contractility and slow cardiac conduction as other calcium antagonists such as verapamil and diltiazem; nisoldipine is 5-10 times as potent a vasodilator as nifedipine.

Pharmacodynamics/Kinetics

Duration of Action >24 hours

Half-life Elimination 9-18 hours

Time to Peak 4-14 hours

Pregnancy Considerations

Chronic maternal hypertension may increase the risk of birth defects, low birth weight, preterm delivery, stillbirth, and neonatal death. Actual fetal/neonatal risks may be related to duration and severity of maternal hypertension. Untreated hypertension may also increase the risks of adverse maternal outcomes, including gestational diabetes, myocardial infarction, preeclampsia, stroke, and delivery complications (ACOG 203 2019).

Calcium channel blockers may be used to treat hypertension in pregnant women; however, agents other than nisoldipine are more commonly used (ACOG 203 2019; ESC [Regitz-Zagrosek 2018]). Females with preexisting hypertension may continue their medication during pregnancy unless contraindications exist (ESC [Regitz-Zagrosek 2018]).

◆ **Nitalapram** *see* Citalopram *on page 353*

Nitrazepam (nye TRA ze pam)

Brand Names: Canada APO-Nitrazepam; Mogadon; SANDOZ Nitrazepam [DSC]

Pharmacologic Category Benzodiazepine

Use Note: Not approved in the US

Insomnia: Short-term treatment and symptomatic relief of insomnia characterized by difficulty in falling asleep, frequent nocturnal awakenings, and/or early morning awakenings

Limitations of use: Restrict use to insomnia that impairs normal daytime functioning. Treatment should typically not exceed 7 to 10 consecutive days. Reevaluation of the patient is required if treatment continues for >2 to 3 consecutive weeks. Prescriptions should be written for short-term use (7 to 10 days) and limited to ≤1 month supply.

Seizures: Management of myoclonic seizures

Local Anesthetic/Vasoconstrictor Precautions No information available to require special precautions.

Effects on Dental Treatment Key adverse event(s) related to dental treatment: Excessive salivation has been reported. The mechanism of this effect is unknown, since many benzodiazepines cause xerostomia rather than salivation excess.

Effects on Bleeding No information available to require special precautions

Adverse Reactions Frequency not defined.

Cardiovascular: Hypotension, palpitations

Central nervous system: Aggressive behavior, agitation, amnesia, ataxia, confusion, delusions, depression, disorientation, dizziness, excitement, falling, fatigue, hallucination, hangover effect, headache, hyperactivity, irritability, lethargy, myasthenia, nervousness, nightmares, outbursts of anger, psychosis, restlessness, sedation, staggering, withdrawal syndrome (chronic use)

Dermatologic: Dermatological reaction

Endocrine & metabolic: Change in libido

Gastrointestinal: Constipation, diarrhea, heartburn, nausea, sialorrhea, vomiting

Hematologic & oncologic: Granulocytopenia, leukopenia

Hepatic: Abnormal hepatic function tests

Hypersensitivity: Anaphylaxis (or anaphylactoid reaction; angioedema, dyspnea, nausea, pharyngeal edema, vomiting)

Neuromuscular & skeletal: Muscle spasticity

Ophthalmic: Blurred vision
Respiratory: Aspiration, dyspnea, increased bronchial secretions

Mechanism of Action Binds to stereospecific benzodiazepine receptors on the postsynaptic GABA neuron at several sites within the CNS, including the limbic system, reticular formation. Enhancement of the inhibitory effect of GABA on neuronal excitability results by increased neuronal membrane permeability to chloride ions. This shift in chloride ions results in hyperpolarization (a less excitable state) and stabilization. Benzodiazepine receptors and effects appear to be linked to the GABA-A receptors. Benzodiazepines do not bind to GABA-B receptors.

Pharmacodynamics/Kinetics

Onset of Action 20 to 50 minutes

Half-life Elimination 30 hours (range: 18 to 57 hours), Elderly/ill patients: 40 hours

Time to Peak ~3 hours

Pregnancy Considerations Nitrazepam crosses the placenta.

Teratogenic effects have been observed with some benzodiazepines; however, additional studies are needed. The incidence of premature birth and low birth weights may be increased following maternal use of benzodiazepines; hypoglycemia and respiratory problems in the neonate may occur following exposure late in pregnancy. Neonatal withdrawal symptoms may occur within days to weeks after birth and "floppy infant syndrome" (which also includes withdrawal symptoms) have been reported with some benzodiazepines (Bergman 1992; Iqbal 2002; Wikner 2007). Symptoms may include hypoactivity, hypotonia, hypothermia, respiratory depression, apnea, feeding problems, and impaired metabolic response to cold stress. Use during pregnancy is not recommended.

Product Availability Not available in the US

Controlled Substance CDSA IV

◆ **Nitro-Bid** *see* Nitroglycerin *on page 1112*

◆ **Nitro-Dur** *see* Nitroglycerin *on page 1112*

Nitrofurantoin (nye troe fyoor AN toyn)

Brand Names: US Furadantin [DSC]; Macrobid; Macrodantin

Brand Names: Canada Auro-Nitrofurantoin; Macrobid; PMS-Nitrofurantoin; TEVA-Nitrofurantoin

Pharmacologic Category Antibiotic, Miscellaneous

Use

Cystitis, acute uncomplicated, treatment:

Nitrofurantoin monohydrate/macrocrystals (Macrobid): Treatment of acute uncomplicated cystitis caused by susceptible strains of *Escherichia coli* or *Staphylococcus saprophyticus* in patients ≥12 years of age.

Nitrofurantoin macrocrystals (Furadantin, Macrodantin): Treatment of acute uncomplicated cystitis when caused by susceptible strains of *E. coli*, enterococci, *Staphylococcus aureus*, and certain susceptible strains of *Klebsiella* and *Enterobacter* species.

Limitations of use: Not indicated for treatment of pyelonephritis or perinephric abscess.

Cystitis, uncomplicated, prophylaxis for recurrent infection: Nitrofurantoin macrocrystals (Furadantin, Macrodantin): Chronic suppression of recurrent urinary tract infections.

Local Anesthetic/Vasoconstrictor Precautions No information available to require special precautions

Effects on Dental Treatment No significant effects or complications reported

Effects on Bleeding No information available to require special precautions

Adverse Reactions

1% to 10%:

Central nervous system: Headache (6%)
Endocrine & metabolic: Increased serum phosphate (1% to 5%)
Gastrointestinal: Nausea (8%), flatulence (2%)
Hematologic & oncologic: Decreased hemoglobin (1% to 5%), eosinophilia (1% to 5%)
Hepatic: Increased serum alanine aminotransferase (1% to 5%), increased serum aspartate aminotransferase (1% to 5%)

Frequency not defined:

Cardiovascular: Bundle branch block, chest pain, ECG changes, nonspecific T wave on ECG, vasculitis
Central nervous system: Bulging fontanel (infants), confusion, depression, drug fever, peripheral neuropathy, pseudotumor cerebri, psychotic reaction, vertigo
Dermatologic: Eczematous rash, erythema multiforme, erythematous maculopapular rash, exfoliative dermatitis, maculopapular rash, skin rash, Stevens-Johnson syndrome
Gastrointestinal: Anorexia, clostridioides, *Clostridium difficile* colitis, pancreatitis, sialadenitis, vomiting
Genitourinary: Urine discoloration
Hematologic & oncologic: Agranulocytosis, aplastic anemia, glucose-6-phosphate dehydrogenase deficiency anemia, granulocytopenia, hemolytic anemia, leukopenia, megaloblastic anemia, methemoglobinemia, thrombocytopenia
Hepatic: Cholestatic jaundice, chronic active hepatitis, hepatic necrosis, hepatitis
Hypersensitivity: Anaphylaxis, angioedema, hypersensitivity reaction
Infection: Superinfection
Neuromuscular & skeletal: Arthralgia, asthenia, lupus-like syndrome, myalgia
Ophthalmic: Nystagmus
Respiratory: Acute pulmonary reaction, chronic pulmonary reaction, cough, cyanosis, dyspnea, dyspnea on exertion, interstitial pneumonitis, pleural effusion, pulmonary fibrosis, pulmonary infiltrates

<1%, postmarketing, and/or case reports: Abdominal pain, alopecia, amblyopia, chills, constipation, diarrhea, dizziness, drowsiness, dyspepsia, fever, hepatotoxicity, malaise, optic neuritis, pruritus, pulmonary hypersensitivity, urticaria

Mechanism of Action Nitrofurantoin is reduced by bacterial flavoproteins to reactive intermediates that inactivate or alter bacterial ribosomal proteins leading to inhibition of protein synthesis, aerobic energy metabolism, DNA, RNA, and cell wall synthesis. Nitrofurantoin is bactericidal in urine at therapeutic doses. The broad-based nature of this mode of action may explain the lack of acquired bacterial resistance to nitrofurantoin, as the necessary multiple and simultaneous mutations of the target macromolecules would likely be lethal to the bacteria.

Pharmacodynamics/Kinetics

Half-life Elimination 20 to 60 minutes; prolonged with renal impairment

Pregnancy Risk Factor B (contraindicated at term)

Pregnancy Considerations Nitrofurantoin crosses the placenta (Perry 1967).

Current studies evaluating maternal use of nitrofurantoin during pregnancy and the development of birth defects have had mixed results (ACOG 717 2017). An increased risk of neonatal jaundice was observed following maternal nitrofurantoin use during the last 30 days of pregnancy (Nordeng 2013).

Maternal serum concentrations of nitrofurantoin may be decreased in pregnancy (Philipson 1979). Use of nitrofurantoin may be considered for the treatment of asymptomatic bacteriuria in pregnancy (Nicolle [IDSA 2019]). Nitrofurantoin may be used to treat infections during pregnancy; use during the first trimester should be limited to situations where no alternative therapies are available. Prescriptions should be written when clinically appropriate and for the shortest effective duration for confirmed infections (ACOG 717 2017). Nitrofurantoin is contraindicated in pregnant patients at term (38 to 42 weeks' gestation), during labor and delivery, or when the onset of labor is imminent due to the possibility of hemolytic anemia in the neonate. Alternative antibiotics should be used in pregnant patients with G-6-PD deficiency (ACOG 717 2017; Nordeng 2013).

Nitroglycerin (nye troe GLI ser in)

Related Information

Cardiovascular Diseases *on page 1654*

Brand Names: US GoNitro; Minitran; Nitro-Bid; Nitro-Dur; Nitro-Time; Nitrolingual; NitroMist; Nitrostat; Rectiv

Brand Names: Canada APO-Nitroglycerin; Minitran; MYLAN-Nitro; Nitro-Dur; Nitroject; Nitrol [DSC]; Nitrolingual; RHO-Nitro; Transderm-Nitro; Trinipatch 0.2; Trinipatch 0.4; Trinipatch 0.6

Pharmacologic Category Antianginal Agent; Antidote, Extravasation; Vasodilator

Use

Oral administration: Treatment or prevention of angina pectoris.

IV administration: Treatment or prevention of angina pectoris; acute decompensated heart failure; perioperative hypertension; induction of intraoperative hypotension.

Intra-anal administration (Rectiv ointment): Treatment of moderate to severe pain associated with chronic anal fissure.

Local Anesthetic/Vasoconstrictor Precautions No information available to require special precautions

Effects on Dental Treatment Key adverse event(s) related to dental treatment: Xerostomia (normal salivary flow resumes upon discontinuation).

Effects on Bleeding No information available to require special precautions

Adverse Reactions

>10%: Central nervous system: Headache (patch, ointment: 50% to 64%; sublingual powder, lingual spray: >2%)

1% to 10%:

Cardiovascular: Hypotension (≤4%), syncope (≤4%), peripheral edema (lingual spray: ≤2%)

Central nervous system: Dizziness (>2% to 6%), paresthesia (>2%)

Gastrointestinal: Abdominal pain (lingual spray: ≤2%)

Neuromuscular & skeletal: Weakness (all sublingual forms: ≤2%)

Respiratory: Dyspnea (≤2%), pharyngitis (lingual spray: ≤2%), rhinitis (lingual spray: ≤2%)

Frequency not defined:

Cardiovascular: Bradycardia, exacerbation of angina pectoris, flushing, orthostatic hypotension

Dermatologic: Diaphoresis

Gastrointestinal: Vomiting

Miscellaneous: Drug tolerance

<1%, postmarketing, and/or case reports: Anaphylactoid reaction, application site irritation (patch), circulatory shock, contact dermatitis (ointment, patch), drowsiness, exfoliative dermatitis, fixed drug eruption (ointment, patch), hypersensitivity reaction, hypoxemia (transient), lactic acidosis (Smith 2019), methemoglobinemia, nausea, pallor, palpitations, rebound hypertension, restlessness, skin rash, tachycardia, vertigo, vomiting

Mechanism of Action Nitroglycerin forms free radical nitric oxide. In smooth muscle, nitric oxide activates guanylate cyclase which increases guanosine 3'5' monophosphate (cGMP) leading to dephosphorylation of myosin light chains and smooth muscle relaxation. Produces a vasodilator effect on the peripheral veins and arteries with more prominent effects on the veins. Primarily reduces cardiac oxygen demand by decreasing preload (left ventricular end-diastolic pressure); may modestly reduce afterload; dilates coronary arteries and improves collateral flow to ischemic regions. For use in rectal fissures, intra-anal administration results in decreased sphincter tone and intra-anal pressure.

Pharmacodynamics/Kinetics

Onset of Action Sublingual tablet: 1 to 3 minutes; Translingual spray: Similar to sublingual tablet; Extended release: ~60 minutes; Topical: 15 to 30 minutes; Transdermal: ~30 minutes; IV: Immediate

Peak effect: Sublingual powder: 7 minutes; Sublingual tablet: 5 minutes; Translingual spray: 4 to 15 minutes; Extended release: 2.5 to 4 hours; Topical: ~60 minutes; Transdermal: 120 minutes; IV: Immediate

Duration of Action Sublingual tablet: At least 25 minutes; Translingual spray: Similar to sublingual tablet; Extended release: 4 to 8 hours (Gibbons 2003); Topical: 7 hours; Transdermal: 10 to 12 hours; IV: 3 to 5 minutes

Half-life Elimination ~1 to 4 minutes

Pregnancy Considerations Nitroglycerin crosses the placenta (David 2000).

Following a single maternal IV bolus dose of nitroglycerin at the time of incision prior to cesarean delivery, concentrations in the umbilical cord at birth were significantly lower than the maternal plasma (~1 minute after dosing); a wide variation in maternal plasma concentrations was observed (David 2000). Following application of a transdermal patch 0.4 mg/hour to pregnant women 20 to 36 weeks gestation, concentrations of nitroglycerin were low but detectable in the fetal serum ~1 to 4 hours after the patch was applied (fetal/maternal ratio: 0.23) (Bustard 2003).

IV nitroglycerin is recommended for use in pregnant females with preeclampsia when severe hypertension is associated with pulmonary edema (ESC [Regitz-Zagrosek 2018]). Based on its ability to produce smooth muscle relaxation, nitroglycerin may be used in obstetrical procedures when immediate relaxation of the uterus is needed, such as: uterine inversion following delivery (ACOG 183 2017), uterine relaxation during removal of retained placental tissue (ASA 2016), and management of breech delivery (Caponas 2001; Cluver 2015). Additional data may be necessary to further define the role of nitroglycerin for preterm labor (ACOG 171 2016; Duckitt 2014).

◆ **Nitroglycerol** *see* Nitroglycerin *on page 1112*

◆ **Nitrolingual** *see* Nitroglycerin *on page 1112*

◆ **NitroMist** *see* Nitroglycerin *on page 1112*

◆ **Nitrostat** *see* Nitroglycerin *on page 1112*

◆ **Nitro-Time** *see* Nitroglycerin *on page 1112*

Nitrous Oxide (NYE trus OKS ide)

Related Information

Management of the Patient With Anxiety or Depression *on page 1778*

Generic Availability (US) Yes

Pharmacologic Category Dental Gases; General Anesthetic

Dental Use Induction of sedation and analgesia in anxious dental patients

Use Sedation, analgesia, and amnesia; principal adjunct to inhalation and intravenous general anesthesia

Local Anesthetic/Vasoconstrictor Precautions No information available to require special precautions

Effects on Dental Treatment No significant effects or complications reported

Effects on Bleeding No information available to require special precautions

Adverse Reactions Frequency not defined.

Cardiovascular: Hypotension

Central nervous system: Central nervous system stimulation, confusion, dizziness, headache

Gastrointestinal: Nausea and vomiting

Respiratory: Apnea

Dental Usual Dosage Sedation and analgesia: Children and Adults: Concentrations of 25% to 50% nitrous oxide with oxygen

Dosing

Adult & Geriatric

Surgical sedation and analgesia: Concentrations of 25% to 50% nitrous oxide with oxygen. For general anesthesia, concentrations of 40% to 70% via mask or endotracheal tube. Minimal alveolar concentration (MAC), which can be considered the ED_{50} of inhalational anesthetics, is 105%; therefore delivery in a hyperbaric chamber is necessary to use as a complete anesthetic. When administered at 70%, reduces the MAC of other anesthetics by half.

Dental: Sedation and analgesia: Concentrations of 25% to 50% nitrous oxide with oxygen

Pediatric Refer to adult dosing.

Mechanism of Action General CNS depressant action; may act similarly as inhalant general anesthetics by stabilizing axonal membranes to partially inhibit action potentials leading to sedation; may partially act on opiate receptor systems to cause mild analgesia; central sympathetic stimulating action supports blood pressure, systemic vascular resistance, and cardiac output; it does not depress carbon dioxide drive to breath. Nitrous oxide increases cerebral blood flow and intracranial pressure while decreasing hepatic and renal blood flow; has analgesic action similar to morphine.

Contraindications Hypersensitivity to nitrous oxide or any component of the formulation; nitrous oxide should not be administered without oxygen

Use is considered contraindicated in patients having undergone vitreoretinal surgery and presence of intraocular gas bubble (Lee, 2004; Fu, 2002).

Warnings/Precautions Nausea and vomiting occurs postoperatively in ~15% of patients. Prolonged use may produce bone marrow suppression and/or neurologic dysfunction. Oxygen should be briefly administered during emergence from prolonged anesthesia with nitrous oxide to prevent diffusion hypoxia. Patients with vitamin B_{12} deficiency (pernicious anemia) and those with other nutritional deficiencies (alcoholics) are at increased risk of developing neurologic disease and bone marrow suppression with exposure to nitrous oxide. May be associated with abuse and/or addiction.

Detached retina and other ocular disorders treated with vitreoretinal surgery where intraocular gas was used: Nitrous oxide can increase intraocular pressure which may result in retinal artery occlusion, ischemia, or optic nerve damage and vision loss in these patients. Nitrous oxide should not be used in patients who have had an intravitreal gas bubble unless it can be confirmed that the bubble has been completely resorbed (Fu, 2002; Lee, 2004). Avoid use in pneumothorax, pneumocephalus, middle ear surgery, or bowel obstruction (Miller 2010; Ohryn 1995; Sprehn 1992).

Drug Interactions

Metabolism/Transport Effects None known.

Avoid Concomitant Use

Avoid concomitant use of Nitrous Oxide with any of the following: Azelastine (Nasal); Bromperidol; Methotrexate; Orphenadrine; Oxomemazine; Paraldehyde; Thalidomide

Increased Effect/Toxicity

Nitrous Oxide may increase the levels/effects of: Alcohol (Ethyl); Azelastine (Nasal); Blonanserin; Brexanolone; Buprenorphine; CNS Depressants; Flunitrazepam; Methotrexate; Methotrimeprazine; MetyroSINE; Opioid Agonists; Orphenadrine; OxyCODONE; Paraldehyde; Piribedil; Pramipexole; ROPINIRole; Rotigotine; Suvorexant; Thalidomide; Zolpidem

The levels/effects of Nitrous Oxide may be increased by: Alizapride; Brimonidine (Topical); Bromopride; Bromperidol; Cannabidiol; Cannabis; Chlormethiazole; Chlorphenesin Carbamate; Dimethindene (Topical); Doxylamine; Dronabinol; Droperidol; Esketamine; HydrOXYzine; Kava Kava; Lemborexant; Lisuride; Lofexidine; Magnesium Sulfate; Methotrimeprazine; Metoclopramide; Minocycline (Systemic); Nabilone; Oxomemazine; Perampanel; Rufinamide; Sodium Oxybate; Tetrahydrocannabinol; Tetrahydrocannabinol and Cannabidiol; Trimeprazine

Decreased Effect There are no known significant interactions involving a decrease in effect.

Pharmacodynamics/Kinetics

Onset of Action Inhalation: 2-5 minutes

Reproductive Considerations

Infertility has been reported following prolonged occupational exposure. This risk is related to dose and duration of exposure and is decreased with proper administration procedures (Becker 2008; Rooks 2011; Zafirova 2018).

Pregnancy Considerations Nitrous oxide crosses the placenta.

Concentrations of nitrous oxide in the fetal circulation are ~80% of those in the maternal plasma. The half-life in the neonate is ~3 minutes and it is quickly eliminated from neonatal lungs with the onset of breathing (Rooks 2011).

Spontaneous abortion and congenital abnormalities have been reported in health care providers following prolonged occupational exposure (Becker 2008; Brodsky 1986; Rooks 2011). However, these adverse events are related to dose and duration of exposure and risks are decreased with proper administration procedures

(Rooks 2011; Zafirova 2018). Short duration of exposure to the pregnant women during obstetric procedural anesthesia is not associated with an increased risk of adverse events to the fetus (Neuman 2013).

Nitrous oxide is used in labor analgesia (ACOG 209 2019; Collins [AWHONN 2018]); Likis 2014; Rooks 2011; Rosen 2002) and may be used when needed for dental treatments that cannot be postponed during pregnancy (Becker 2008).

The ACOG recommends that pregnant women should not be denied medically necessary surgery, regardless of trimester. If the procedure is elective, it should be delayed until after delivery (ACOG 775 2019).

Breastfeeding Considerations

Nitrous oxide was not found to influence the initiation or continuation of breastfeeding when used during labor (Zanardo 2017).

The Academy of Breast Feeding Medicine recommends postponing elective surgery until milk supply and breastfeeding are established. Milk should be expressed ahead of surgery when possible. In general, when the child is healthy and full term, breastfeeding may resume, or milk may be expressed once the mother is awake and in recovery. For children who are at risk for apnea, hypotension, or hypotonia, milk may be saved for later use when the child is at lower risk (ABM [Reece-Stremtan 2017]).

Dosage Forms: US

Supplied in blue cylinders

◆ **Nitrozepamum** *see* Nitrazepam *on page 1110*

◆ **Nivestym** *see* Filgrastim *on page 668*

Nivolumab (nye VOL ue mab)

Brand Names: US Opdivo

Brand Names: Canada Opdivo

Pharmacologic Category Antineoplastic Agent, Anti-PD-1 Monoclonal Antibody; Antineoplastic Agent, Immune Checkpoint Inhibitor; Antineoplastic Agent, Monoclonal Antibody

Use

Colorectal cancer, metastatic (microsatellite instability high or mismatch repair deficient): Treatment (as a single agent or in combination with ipilimumab) of microsatellite instability-high or mismatch repair deficient metastatic colorectal cancer in adults and pediatric patients ≥12 years of age that has progressed following treatment with a fluoropyrimidine, oxaliplatin, and irinotecan.

Esophageal carcinoma, squamous cell (unresectable advanced, recurrent, or metastatic): Treatment of unresectable advanced, recurrent, or metastatic esophageal squamous cell carcinoma after prior fluoropyrimidine- and platinum-based chemotherapy.

Head and neck cancer, squamous cell (recurrent or metastatic): Treatment of recurrent or metastatic squamous cell carcinoma of the head and neck in patients with disease progression on or after platinum-based therapy.

Hepatocellular carcinoma: Treatment of hepatocellular carcinoma (either as a single agent or in combination with ipilimumab) in patients who have been previously treated with sorafenib.

Hodgkin lymphoma, classical: Treatment of classical Hodgkin lymphoma in adult patients that have relapsed or progressed following autologous hematopoietic stem cell transplant (HSCT) and brentuximab vedotin, or after ≥3 lines of systemic therapy that included autologous HSCT.

Melanoma:

Adjuvant treatment of melanoma with involvement of lymph nodes or metastatic disease following complete resection.

Treatment of unresectable or metastatic melanoma (either as a single agent or in combination with ipilimumab).

Non-small cell lung cancer, metastatic:

First-line treatment of metastatic non-small cell lung cancer (in combination with ipilimumab) in adults whose tumors express PD-L1 (≥1%) as determined by an approved test, and with no epidermal growth factor receptor (EGFR) or anaplastic lymphoma kinase (ALK) genomic tumor aberrations.

First-line treatment of metastatic or recurrent non-small cell lung cancer (in combination with ipilimumab and 2 cycles of platinum doublet chemotherapy) in adults with no EGFR or ALK genomic tumor aberrations.

Treatment of metastatic non-small cell lung cancer that has progressed on or after platinum-based chemotherapy. Patients with EGFR or ALK genomic tumor aberrations should have disease progression (on approved EGFR- or ALK-directed therapy) prior to receiving nivolumab.

Renal cell cancer, advanced:

Treatment (as a single agent) of advanced renal cell cancer (RCC) in patients who have received prior anti-angiogenic therapy

Treatment of intermediate or poor risk, previously untreated advanced RCC (in combination with ipilimumab)

Small cell lung cancer, metastatic: Treatment of metastatic small cell lung cancer in patients with progression after platinum-based chemotherapy and at least one other line of therapy.

Urothelial carcinoma, locally advanced or metastatic: Treatment of locally advanced or metastatic urothelial carcinoma in patients with disease progression during or following a platinum-containing therapy or disease progression within 12 months of neoadjuvant or adjuvant treatment with a platinum-containing therapy.

Local Anesthetic/Vasoconstrictor Precautions No information available to require special precautions

Effects on Dental Treatment No significant effects or complications reported

Effects on Bleeding Therapy with immune checkpoint inhibitors may result in significant myelosuppression, including thrombocytopenia. In patients under active treatment a medical consult is suggested.

Adverse Reactions Incidence of adverse reactions includes unapproved dosing regimens.

>10%:

Cardiovascular: Edema (≤13%), peripheral edema (≤13%), hypertension (11%)

Central nervous system: Fatigue (≤59%), malaise (<46%), headache (16% to 23%), dizziness (≤14%), peripheral neuropathy (≤14%; grade 3: <1%)

Dermatologic: Skin rash (1% to 40%; immune-mediated: 9% to 16%), pruritus (10% to 28%), vitiligo (≤11%)

Endocrine & metabolic: Hyperglycemia (19% to 46%), hyponatremia (19% to 41%), increased serum triglycerides (32%), hyperkalemia (11% to 30%), increased thyroid stimulating hormone level (≥10% to 26%), hypocalcemia (10% to 26%), increased serum cholesterol (21%), hypercalcemia (2% to 19%), thyroiditis (≤12% to 18%; including immune-mediated events), hypomagnesemia (14% to 17%), hypokalemia (14% to 16%), thyroid dysfunction (15%), hypothyroidism (≤12%; including immune-mediated events)

Gastrointestinal: Diarrhea (1% to 43%), nausea (20% to 34%), abdominal pain (13% to 34%), increased serum lipase (20% to 33%), decreased appetite (14% to 28%), vomiting (12% to 28%), constipation (10% to 23%), increased serum amylase (13% to 19%)

Genitourinary: Urinary tract infection (2% to 17%)

Hematologic & oncologic: Anemia (26% to 50%; grades 3/4: 3% to 8%), lymphocytopenia (27% to 42%; grades 3/4: ≤11%), leukopenia (11% to 38%; grades 3/4: ≤5%), thrombocytopenia (15% to 37%; grades 3/4: 1% to 3%), neutropenia (13% to 37%; grades 3/4: 4% to 5%)

Hepatic: Increased serum alkaline phosphatase (10% to 37%), increased serum aspartate aminotransferase (22% to 33%), increased serum alanine aminotransferase (23% to 32%), increased serum bilirubin (11% to 14%)

Immunologic: Graft versus host disease (20%; within 14 days of stem cell infusion), antibody development (11%; neutralizing: <1%)

Neuromuscular & skeletal: Asthenia (≤57%), musculoskeletal pain (20% to 42%), back pain (21%), arthralgia (10% to 21%)

Renal: Increased serum creatinine (12% to 42%)

Respiratory: Upper respiratory tract infection (2% to 44%), cough (≤36%), productive cough (≤36%), dyspnea (≤27%), dyspnea on exertion (≤27%), bronchopneumonia (≤13%), pneumonia (≤13%), nasal congestion (11%)

Miscellaneous: Febrile reaction (35%; events without an infectious cause that required steroids), fever (≤29%; may include tumor-associated fever), infusion-related reaction (≤14%)

1% to 10%:

Cardiovascular: Pulmonary embolism (2% to 3%)

Central nervous system: Neuritis (<10%), peripheral nerve palsy (peroneal: <10%), insomnia (9%)

Dermatologic: Erythema of skin (10%), xeroderma (7%)

Endocrine & metabolic: Weight loss (7% to 8%), hyperthyroidism (3% to 6%; including immune-mediated events), adrenocortical insufficiency (1%; including immune-mediated events), increased gamma-glutamyl transferase

Gastrointestinal: Intestinal perforation (<10%), stomatitis (<10%), colitis (including immune-mediated events: ≤6%)

Hepatic: Hepatitis (immune-mediated: 2% to 3%)

Immunologic: Sjogren's syndrome (<10%)

Infection: Sepsis (≥2%, systemic inflammatory response)

Neuromuscular & skeletal: Myopathy (<10%), rheumatism (spondyloarthropathy: <10%)

Renal: Acute renal failure (≥2%), nephritis (≤1%; immune-mediated), renal insufficiency (≤1%; immune-mediated)

Respiratory: Interstitial pulmonary disease (6%), pneumonitis (≤6%; including immune-mediated events), pleural effusion (1% to 5%), respiratory failure (≥2%)

Frequency not defined:

Central nervous system: Migraine

Dermatologic: Acneiform eruption, bullous dermatitis, dermatitis, erythematous rash, exfoliative dermatitis, maculopapular rash, morbilliform rash, palmar-plantar erythrodysesthesia, psoriasiform eruption, pustular rash, Stevens-Johnson syndrome, toxic epidermal necrolysis

Endocrine & metabolic: Dehydration

Gastrointestinal: Abdominal distress

Neuromuscular & skeletal: Limb pain

<1%, postmarketing, and/or case reports: Demyelinating disease (immune-mediated), diabetic ketoacidosis, duodenitis (immune-mediated), encephalitis (limbic/lymphocytic/viral; may be immune-mediated), facial nerve paralysis (immune-mediated), gastritis (immune-mediated), Guillain-Barré syndrome, hepatic sinusoidal obstruction syndrome, hypophysitis (including immune-mediated events), immunological signs and symptoms (hemophagocytic lymphohistiocytosis) (Hantel 2018), iritis (immune-mediated), lymphadenitis (immune-mediated; histiocytic necrotizing lymphadenitis [Kikuchi lymphadenitis]), motor dysfunction (immune-mediated), myasthenia (myasthenic syndrome), myocarditis (immune-mediated), myositis (immune-mediated), neuropathy (autoimmune; immune-mediated), pancreatitis (immune-mediated), pituitary insufficiency (immune-mediated), pneumonia due to *Pneumocystis jirovecii*, polymyalgia rheumatica (immune-mediated), rhabdomyolysis (immune-mediated), sarcoidosis (immune-mediated), sixth nerve palsy (abducens nerve palsy; immune-mediated), subacute cutaneous lupus erythematosus (Zitouni 2019), type I diabetes mellitus (immune-mediated event), uveitis (immune-mediated), vasculitis, Vogt-Koyanagi-Harada syndrome

Mechanism of Action

Nivolumab is a fully human immunoglobulin G4 (IgG4) monoclonal antibody that selectively inhibits programmed cell death-1 (PD-1) activity by binding to the PD-1 receptor to block the ligands PD-L1 and PD-L2 from binding. The negative PD-1 receptor signaling that regulates T-cell activation and proliferation is therefore disrupted (Robert 2015). This releases PD-1 pathway-mediated inhibition of the immune response, including the antitumor immune response.

Combining nivolumab (anti-PD-1) with ipilimumab (anti-CTLA-4) results in enhanced T-cell function that is greater than that of either antibody alone, resulting in improved anti-tumor responses in metastatic melanoma and advanced renal cell carcinoma.

Pharmacodynamics/Kinetics

Half-life Elimination ~25 days

Reproductive Considerations

Verify pregnancy status prior to treatment initiation in females of reproductive potential. Females of reproductive potential should use highly effective contraception during therapy and for at least 5 months after nivolumab treatment has been discontinued.

Pregnancy Considerations

Based on information from animal reproduction studies and the mechanism of action, nivolumab may cause fetal harm if administered during pregnancy. Nivolumab is a humanized monoclonal antibody (IgG_4). Potential placental transfer of human IgG is dependent upon the IgG subclass and gestational age, generally increasing as pregnancy progresses. The lowest exposure would be expected during the period of organogenesis (Palmeira 2012; Pentsuk 2009).

- **Nivolumab, inj** *see* Nivolumab *on page 1114*

Nizatidine (ni ZA ti deen)

Related Information
Gastrointestinal Disorders *on page 1678*

Brand Names: Canada APO-Nizatidine [DSC]; Axid; DOM-Nizatidine; NOVO-Nizatidine [DSC]; NU-Nizatidine [DSC]; PHL-Nizatidine [DSC]; PMS-Nizatidine

Pharmacologic Category Histamine H_2 Antagonist

Use

Duodenal ulcer: Treatment of active duodenal ulcer for up to 8 weeks and maintenance therapy after healing of active ulcer in adults.

Gastric ulcer, benign: Treatment of active benign gastric ulcer for up to 8 weeks in adults.

Gastroesophageal reflux disease: Treatment of endoscopically diagnosed esophagitis, including erosive and ulcerative esophagitis, and associated heartburn due to gastroesophageal reflux disease (GERD) for up to 12 weeks in adults (capsules and oral solution) and up to 8 weeks in children 12 years and older (oral solution only).

Local Anesthetic/Vasoconstrictor Precautions No information available to require special precautions

Effects on Dental Treatment Key adverse event(s) related to dental treatment: Xerostomia (normal salivary flow resumes upon discontinuation).

Effects on Bleeding No information available to require special precautions

Adverse Reactions

>10%: Central nervous system: Headache (16%)

1% to 10%:

Central nervous system: Anxiety, dizziness, drowsiness, insomnia, irritability (children), nervousness

Dermatologic: Pruritus, skin rash

Gastrointestinal: Abdominal pain, anorexia, constipation, diarrhea, flatulence, heartburn, nausea, vomiting, xerostomia

Respiratory: Cough (children), nasal congestion (children), nasopharyngitis (children)

Miscellaneous: Fever (children)

<1%, postmarketing, and/or case reports: Anaphylaxis, anemia, bronchospasm, confusion, eosinophilia, exfoliative dermatitis, gynecomastia, hepatitis, immune thrombocytopenia, increased serum alkaline phosphatase, increased serum ALT, increased serum AST, jaundice, laryngeal edema, serum sickness-like reaction, thrombocytopenia, vasculitis, ventricular tachycardia

Mechanism of Action Competitive inhibition of histamine at H_2-receptors of the gastric parietal cells, which inhibits gastric acid secretion, gastric volume, and hydrogen ion concentration are reduced. Does not affect pepsin secretion, pentagastrin-stimulated intrinsic factor secretion, or serum gastrin.

Pharmacodynamics/Kinetics

Half-life Elimination 1 to 2 hours; prolonged with moderate to severe renal impairment

Time to Peak Plasma: 0.5 to 3 hours

Pregnancy Risk Factor B

Pregnancy Considerations Adverse events have not been observed in animal reproduction studies. Nizatidine crosses the placenta (Dicke 1988). Information related to the use of nizatidine in pregnancy is limited; other agents may be preferred (Richter 2005).

- **Nizoral** *see* Ketoconazole (Systemic) *on page 856*
- **Nizoral [DSC]** *see* Ketoconazole (Topical) *on page 859*
- **Nizoral A-D [OTC]** *see* Ketoconazole (Topical) *on page 859*
- **NKTR-118** *see* Naloxegol *on page 1074*
- **N-Methylhydrazine** *see* Procarbazine *on page 1278*
- **N-methylnaltrexone Bromide** *see* Methylnaltrexone *on page 996*
- **NN2211** *see* Liraglutide *on page 920*
- **Nocdurna** *see* Desmopressin *on page 460*
- **Noctiva [DSC]** *see* Desmopressin *on page 460*
- **No Doz Maximum Strength [OTC] [DSC]** *see* Caffeine *on page 277*
- **Nolix** *see* Flurandrenolide *on page 700*
- **Nolvadex** *see* Tamoxifen *on page 1404*
- **Non-Aspirin Pain Reliever [OTC]** *see* Acetaminophen *on page 59*
- **Non-Pseudo Sinus Decongestant [OTC]** *see* Phenylephrine (Systemic) *on page 1227*
- **Non-Vitamin K Antagonist Oral Anticoagulant (NOAC) (error-prone acronym)** *see* Apixaban *on page 159*
- **Non-Vitamin K Antagonist Oral Anticoagulant (NOAC) (error-prone acronym)** *see* Dabigatran Etexilate *on page 426*
- **Non-Vitamin K Antagonist Oral Anticoagulant (NOAC) (error-prone acronym)** *see* Edoxaban *on page 542*
- **Non-Vitamin K Antagonist Oral Anticoagulant (NOAC) (error-prone acronym)** *see* Rivaroxaban *on page 1340*
- **Nora-BE** *see* Norethindrone *on page 1117*
- **Noradrenaline** *see* Norepinephrine *on page 1116*
- **Noradrenaline Acid Tartrate** *see* Norepinephrine *on page 1116*
- **Norco** *see* Hydrocodone and Acetaminophen *on page 764*
- **Nordeoxyguanosine** *see* Ganciclovir (Systemic) *on page 728*
- **Norditropin FlexPro** *see* Somatropin *on page 1381*
- **Norelgestromin and Ethinyl Estradiol** *see* Ethinyl Estradiol and Norelgestromin *on page 613*
- **Norelgestromin/Ethin.Estradiol** *see* Ethinyl Estradiol and Norelgestromin *on page 613*

Norepinephrine (nor ep i NEF rin)

Brand Names: US Levophed

Brand Names: Canada Levophed

Pharmacologic Category Alpha/Beta Agonist

Use

Hypotension/shock: Treatment of shock which persists after adequate fluid volume replacement; severe hypotension

Guideline recommendations:

Cardiogenic shock: The 2017 American Heart Association (AHA) scientific statement for the Contemporary Management of Cardiogenic Shock recommends norepinephrine as the vasopressor of choice for initial management in patients with hemodynamic instability (eg, systolic blood pressure <90 mm Hg or evidence of end organ hypoperfusion) or the following etiologies of cardiogenic shock: right ventricular failure, mitral regurgitation, ventricular septal defect after myocardial infarction, or pericardial tamponade (AHA [van Diepen 2017]).

Septic shock: The 2016 Surviving Sepsis Campaign: International Guidelines for Management of Sepsis and Septic Shock recommends norepinephrine as the first-choice vasopressor for management of septic shock (SCCM [Rhodes 2017]).

Local Anesthetic/Vasoconstrictor Precautions No information available to require special precautions

Effects on Dental Treatment No significant effects or complications reported

Effects on Bleeding Norepinephrine has been shown to cause platelet hyper-reactivity and enhance platelet-mediated coagulation associated with thrombotic risk.

Adverse Reactions

Frequency not defined:

Cardiovascular: Bradycardia, cardiac arrhythmia, cardiomyopathy (stress), peripheral vascular insufficiency

Central nervous system: Anxiety, transient headache

Respiratory: Dyspnea

<1%, postmarketing, and/or case reports: Peripheral gangrene, peripheral ischemia (digital [Daroca-Pérez 2017])

Mechanism of Action Stimulates beta$_1$-adrenergic receptors and alpha-adrenergic receptors causing increased contractility and heart rate as well as vasoconstriction, thereby increasing systemic blood pressure and coronary blood flow; clinically, alpha effects (vasoconstriction) are greater than beta effects (inotropic and chronotropic effects)

Pharmacodynamics/Kinetics

Onset of Action Very rapid acting.

Duration of Action Vasopressor: 1 to 2 minutes.

Half-life Elimination Mean: ~2.4 minutes.

Time to Peak Steady state: 5 minutes.

Pregnancy Considerations

Norepinephrine is an endogenous catecholamine and crosses the placenta (Minzter 2010; Wang 1999).

Medications used for the treatment of cardiac arrest in pregnancy are the same as in the non-pregnant woman. Appropriate medications should not be withheld due to concerns of fetal teratogenicity. Norepinephrine use during the post-resuscitation phase may be considered; however, the effects of vasoactive medications on the fetus should also be considered. Doses and indications should follow current Advanced Cardiovascular Life Support guidelines (Jeejeebhoy [AHA] 2015).

◆ **Norepinephrine Bitartrate** *see* Norepinephrine *on page 1116*

◆ **Norethind Ac/Ethinyl Estradiol** *see* Ethinyl Estradiol and Norethindrone *on page 614*

Norethindrone (nor ETH in drone)

Related Information

Endocrine Disorders and Pregnancy *on page 1684*

Brand Names: US Aygestin; Camila; Deblitane; Errin; Heather; Incassia; Jencycla; Jolivette [DSC]; Lyza; Nor-QD [DSC]; Nora-BE; Norlyda; Norlyroc; Ortho Micronor; Sharobel; Tulana

Brand Names: Canada Jencycla; Micronor [DSC]; Movisse; Norlutate

Pharmacologic Category Contraceptive; Progestin

Use

Abnormal uterine bleeding *(norethindrone acetate):* Treatment of abnormal uterine bleeding due to hormonal imbalance in absence of organic pathology, such as submucous fibroids or uterine cancer

Amenorrhea, secondary *(norethindrone acetate):* Treatment of secondary amenorrhea

Contraception *(norethindrone):* Prevention of pregnancy

Endometriosis *(norethindrone acetate):* Treatment of endometriosis

Limitations of use:

Norethindrone is not indicated for emergency contraception.

Norethindrone acetate is not indicated for use with estrogen therapy in postmenopausal women for endometrial protection.

Local Anesthetic/Vasoconstrictor Precautions No information available to require special precautions

Effects on Dental Treatment Until we know more about the mechanism of interaction, caution is required in prescribing antibiotics to female dental patients taking progestin-only hormonal contraceptives.

Effects on Bleeding Norethindrone has been shown to enhance the risk of thrombosis, as assessed by significant increases in prothrombin fragments 1+2, thrombin-antithrombin complex, and D-dimer. These increases were higher during the first 3 months of therapy and gradually declined following prolonged therapy (>3 months). Medical consult is suggested for patients who are under active norethindrone treatment.

Adverse Reactions Frequency not defined.

Cardiovascular: Cerebral embolism, cerebral thrombosis, deep vein thrombosis, edema, pulmonary embolism, retinal thrombosis

Central nervous system: Depression, dizziness, fatigue, headache, insomnia, migraine, emotional lability, nervousness

Dermatologic: Acne vulgaris, alopecia, chloasma, pruritus, skin rash, urticaria

Endocrine & metabolic: Amenorrhea, hirsutism, hypermenorrhea, menstrual disease, weight gain

Gastrointestinal: Abdominal pain, nausea, vomiting

Genitourinary: Breakthrough bleeding, breast hypertrophy, breast tenderness, cervical erosion, change in cervical secretions, decreased lactation, genital discharge, mastalgia, spotting, vaginal hemorrhage

Hypersensitivity: Anaphylaxis, hypersensitivity

Hepatic: Cholestatic jaundice, hepatitis, abnormal hepatic function tests

Neuromuscular & skeletal: Arm pain, leg pain

Ophthalmic: Optic neuritis (with or without vision loss)

Mechanism of Action Once absorbed, systemic disposition of norethindrone acetate (NETA) and norethindrone (NET) is the same.

NET is used in preparations for progestin-only contraception. NET suppresses ovulation, thickens cervical mucus (which inhibits sperm penetration), alters follicle-stimulating hormone (FSH) and luteinizing hormone (LH) concentrations, slows the movement of ovum through the fallopian tubes, and alters the endometrium.

Progestogens, such as NETA in the doses used for abnormal uterine bleeding, amenorrhea, and endometriosis, lead to atrophy of the endometrial tissue. They may also suppress new growth and implantation. Pain associated with endometriosis is decreased. When treating endometriosis, NETA may be used in combination with gonadotropin-releasing hormone agonists ▶

to decrease side effects from hypoestrogenism (ASRM 2014).

Pharmacodynamics/Kinetics

Half-life Elimination ~8 to 9 hours

Time to Peak ~2 hours (varies by dose and use of concomitant estrogen (Orme 1983)

Reproductive Considerations

Norethindrone: Progestin-only contraceptives may be started immediately postpartum (Curtis 2016a; Curtis 2016b). A rapid return to fertility occurs when progestin-only contraceptives are discontinued.

Norethindrone acetate: The contraceptive dose of norethindrone acetate is not known. Barrier contraception is recommended to prevent unintended pregnancy (eg, when treating endometriosis) (Kaser 2012).

Pregnancy Considerations

Use is contraindicated during pregnancy. First trimester exposure of progestins may cause genital abnormalities including hypospadias in male infants and mild virilization of external female genitalia. Changes in external genitalia have been reported in female infants exposed to norethindrone acetate (Fine 1963). Significant adverse events related to growth and development have not been observed following use of oral progestins in contraceptive doses (limited studies).

◆ **Norethindrone Acetate** *see* Norethindrone *on page 1117*

◆ **Norethindrone Acetate and Ethinyl Estradiol** *see* Ethinyl Estradiol and Norethindrone *on page 614*

◆ **Norethindrone and Estradiol** *see* Estradiol and Norethindrone *on page 598*

◆ **Norethindrone, elagolix, and estradiol** *see* Elagolix, Estradiol, and Norethindrone *on page 547*

◆ **Norethindrone, estradiol, and elagolix** *see* Elagolix, Estradiol, and Norethindrone *on page 547*

◆ **Norethisterone** *see* Norethindrone *on page 1117*

Norfloxacin (nor FLOKS a sin)

Brand Names: Canada ALTI-Norfloxacin; APO-Norfloxacin; CO Norfloxacin [DSC]; PMS-Norfloxacin [DSC]; TEVA-Norfloxacin [DSC]

Pharmacologic Category Antibiotic, Fluoroquinolone

Use

Uncomplicated and complicated urinary tract infections caused by susceptible gram-negative and gram-positive bacteria; sexually transmitted disease (eg, uncomplicated urethral and cervical gonorrhea) caused by *N. gonorrhoeae*; prostatitis due to *E. coli*

Note: As of April 2007, the CDC no longer recommends the use of fluoroquinolones for the treatment of gonococcal disease.

Limitations of use: Because fluoroquinolones have been associated with disabling and potentially irreversible serious adverse reactions (eg, tendinitis and tendon rupture, peripheral neuropathy, CNS effects), reserve norfloxacin for use in patients who have no alternative treatment options for acute uncomplicated urinary tract infections.

Local Anesthetic/Vasoconstrictor Precautions

Norfloxacin is one of the drugs confirmed to prolong the QT interval and is accepted as having a risk of causing torsade de pointes. The risk of drug-induced torsade de pointes is extremely low when a single QT interval prolonging drug is prescribed. In terms of epinephrine, it is not known what effect vasoconstrictors in the local anesthetic regimen will have in patients with a known history of congenital prolonged QT interval or in patients taking any medication that prolongs the QT interval. Until more information is obtained, it is suggested that the clinician consult with the physician prior to the use of a vasoconstrictor in suspected patients, and that the vasoconstrictor (epinephrine, mepivacaine and levonordefrin [Carbocaine® 2% with Neo-Cobefrin®]) be used with caution.

Effects on Dental Treatment No significant effects or complications reported

Effects on Bleeding Norfloxacin has been shown to alter leukocyte populations (reduce neutrophils and increase eosinophils). In more than 1 in 1000 patients, norfloxacin has been shown to reduce clotting ability through reduction in blood platelet concentrations. May also reduce the erythrocyte concentration following extended treatment.

Adverse Reactions

>1% to 10%:

Central nervous system: Dizziness (2% to 3%), headache (2% to 3%)

Gastrointestinal: Nausea (3% to 4%), abdominal cramping (2%)

Hematologic & oncologic: Eosinophilia (1% to 2%)

Hepatic: Liver enzymes increased (1% to 2%)

≥0.3% to 1%:

Central nervous system: Drowsiness

Dermatologic: Hyperhidrosis, pruritus, rash

Endocrine & metabolic: Decreased WBC count (1%), increased serum alkaline phosphatase (1%)

Gastrointestinal: Abdominal pain, anorectal pain, anorexia, constipation, diarrhea, dyspepsia, flatulence, loose stools, vomiting, xerostomia

Genitourinary: Proteinuria (1%)

Hematologic and oncologic: Decreased platelet count (1%), leukopenia (1%), thrombocytopenia (1%), decreased hematocrit, decreased hemoglobin

Neuromuscular & skeletal: Weakness (1%), back pain

Miscellaneous: Fever

<0.3%, postmarketing, and/or case reports: Abdominal swelling, acute renal failure, agranulocytosis, albuminuria, anaphylactoid reaction, anaphylaxis, angioedema, anxiety, arthralgia, arthritis, ataxia, bitter taste, blurred vision, bursitis, candiduria, casts in urine, chest pain, chills, cholestatic jaundice, *Clostridioides* (formerly *Clostridium*) *difficile*-associated diarrhea, confusion, crystalluria, depression, diplopia, DRESS syndrome, dysgeusia, dysmenorrhea, dyspnea, edema, erythema, erythema multiforme, exacerbation of myasthenia gravis, exfoliative dermatitis, gastrointestinal hemorrhage, glycosuria, Guillain-Barré syndrome, hearing loss, heartburn, hematuria, hemolytic anemia (sometimes associated with G6PD deficiency), hepatic failure, hepatic necrosis, hepatitis, hepatotoxicity (idiosyncratic) (Chalasani 2014), hypercholesterolemia, hyperglycemia, hyperkalemia, hypersensitivity angiitis, hypersensitivity reaction, hypertriglyceridemia, hypoesthesia, hypoglycemia, increased blood urea nitrogen, increased creatine phosphokinase, increased intracranial pressure, increased lactate dehydrogenase, increased serum creatinine, insomnia, interstitial nephritis, jaundice, muscle spasm, myalgia, myocardial infarction, myoclonus, neutropenia, nystagmus, oral mucosa ulcer, orthostatic hypotension, palpitations, pancreatitis (rare), paresthesia, peripheral edema, peripheral neuropathy (may be irreversible), phototoxicity, prolonged prothrombin time, prolonged QT interval on ECG, pruritus ani, pseudotumor cerebri, psychotic reaction, renal colic, rupture of tendon, seizure, skin

photosensitivity, Stevens-Johnson syndrome, stomatitis, tendonitis, tingling of the fingers, tinnitus, torsades de pointes, toxic epidermal necrolysis, tremor, urticaria, uveitis, vasculitis, ventricular arrhythmia, vulvovaginal candidiasis

Mechanism of Action Norfloxacin is a DNA gyrase inhibitor. DNA gyrase is an essential bacterial enzyme that maintains the superhelical structure of DNA. DNA gyrase is required for DNA replication and transcription, DNA repair, recombination, and transposition; bactericidal

Pharmacodynamics/Kinetics

Half-life Elimination 3 to 4 hours; Renal impairment (CrCl ≤30 mL/minute): 6.5 hours; Elderly: 4 hours

Time to Peak Serum: 1 to 2 hours

Pregnancy Risk Factor C

Pregnancy Considerations Adverse events have been observed in some animal reproduction studies. Norfloxacin crosses the placenta, distributing to cord blood and amniotic fluid (Wise 1984). Based on available data, an increased risk of teratogenic effects has not been observed following norfloxacin use during pregnancy (Bar-Oz 2009; Padberg 2014).

Product Availability Noroxin is no longer available in the US.

Dental Health Professional Considerations See Local Anesthetic/Vasoconstrictor Precautions

- ◆ **Norgesic** *see* Orphenadrine, Aspirin, and Caffeine *on page 1146*
- ◆ **Norgestimate and Estradiol** *see* Estradiol and Norgestimate *on page 599*
- ◆ **Norgestimate and Ethinyl Estradiol** *see* Ethinyl Estradiol and Norgestimate *on page 616*
- ◆ **Norgestrel and Ethinyl Estradiol** *see* Ethinyl Estradiol and Norgestrel *on page 617*
- ◆ **Norinyl 1+35 (28) [DSC]** *see* Ethinyl Estradiol and Norethindrone *on page 614*
- ◆ **Norlyda** *see* Norethindrone *on page 1117*
- ◆ **Norlyroc** *see* Norethindrone *on page 1117*
- ◆ **Normal Immunoglobulin** *see* Immune Globulin *on page 803*
- ◆ **Normodyne** *see* Labetalol *on page 867*
- ◆ **Norpace** *see* Disopyramide *on page 505*
- ◆ **Norpace CR** *see* Disopyramide *on page 505*
- ◆ **Norpramin** *see* Desipramine *on page 458*
- ◆ **Nor-QD [DSC]** *see* Norethindrone *on page 1117*
- ◆ **Nortemp Children's [OTC]** *see* Acetaminophen *on page 59*
- ◆ **Northera** *see* Droxidopa *on page 535*
- ◆ **Nortrel 0.5/35 (28)** *see* Ethinyl Estradiol and Norethindrone *on page 614*
- ◆ **Nortrel 1/35 (21)** *see* Ethinyl Estradiol and Norethindrone *on page 614*
- ◆ **Nortrel 1/35 (28)** *see* Ethinyl Estradiol and Norethindrone *on page 614*
- ◆ **Nortrel 7/7/7** *see* Ethinyl Estradiol and Norethindrone *on page 614*

Nortriptyline (nor TRIP ti leen)

Related Information

Vasoconstrictor Interactions With Antidepressants *on page 1821*

Brand Names: US Pamelor

Brand Names: Canada APO-Nortriptyline; Aventyl; PMS-Nortriptyline; TEVA-Nortriptyline [DSC]

Pharmacologic Category Antidepressant, Tricyclic (Secondary Amine)

Use Major depression, unipolar: Treatment of symptoms of unipolar major depression

Local Anesthetic/Vasoconstrictor Precautions Nortriptyline is one of the drugs confirmed to prolong the QT interval and is accepted as having a risk of causing torsade de pointes. In terms of epinephrine, it is not known what effect vasoconstrictors in the local anesthetic regimen will have in patients with a known history of congenital prolonged QT interval or in patients taking any medication that prolongs the QT interval. Until more information is obtained, it is suggested that the clinician consult with the physician prior to the use of a vasoconstrictor in suspected patients, and that the vasoconstrictor (epinephrine, mepivacaine and levonordefrin [Carbocaine® 2% with Neo-Cobefrin®]) be used with caution. See Dental Health Professional Considerations.

Effects on Dental Treatment Key adverse event(s) related to dental treatment: Xerostomia (normal salivary flow resumes upon discontinuation), black tongue, and unpleasant taste. Long-term treatment with TCAs, such as nortriptyline, increases the risk of caries by reducing salivation and salivary buffer capacity.

Effects on Bleeding No information available to require special precautions

Adverse Reactions Some reactions listed are based on reports for other agents in this same pharmacologic class and may not be specifically reported for nortriptyline.

Frequency not defined:

Cardiovascular: Acute myocardial infarction, cardiac arrhythmia, cerebrovascular accident, edema, flushing, heart block, hypertension, hypotension, palpitations, tachycardia

Central nervous system: Agitation, anxiety, ataxia, confusion, delusion, disorientation, dizziness, drowsiness, drug fever, EEG pattern changes, extrapyramidal reaction, fatigue, hallucination, headache, hypomania, insomnia, nightmares, numbness, panic, peripheral neuropathy, psychosis (exacerbation), restlessness, seizure, tingling of extremities, tingling sensation, withdrawal symptoms

Dermatologic: Alopecia, diaphoresis (excessive), pruritus, skin photosensitivity, skin rash, urticaria

Endocrine & metabolic: Decreased libido, decreased serum glucose, galactorrhea not associated with childbirth, gynecomastia, increased libido, increased serum glucose, SIADH, weight gain, weight loss

Gastrointestinal: Abdominal cramps, anorexia, constipation, diarrhea, epigastric distress, melanoglossia, nausea, paralytic ileus, parotid gland enlargement, stomatitis, sublingual adenitis, unpleasant taste, vomiting, xerostomia

Genitourinary: Breast hypertrophy, impotence, nocturia, testicular swelling, urinary hesitancy, urinary retention, urinary tract dilation

Hematologic & oncologic: Agranulocytosis, eosinophilia, petechia, purpuric disease, thrombocytopenia

Hepatic: Abnormal hepatic function tests, cholestatic jaundice

Neuromuscular & skeletal: Asthenia, tremor

Ophthalmic: Accommodation disturbance, blurred vision, eye pain, mydriasis

Otic: Tinnitus

Renal: Polyuria

<1%, postmarketing, and/or case reports: Angle-closure glaucoma, cardiac disorder (unmasking of Brugada syndrome), serotonin syndrome, suicidal ideation, suicidal tendencies

Mechanism of Action Traditionally believed to increase the synaptic concentration of serotonin and/or norepinephrine in the central nervous system by inhibition of their reuptake by the presynaptic neuronal membrane. Inhibits the activity of histamine, 5-hydroxytryptamine, and acetylcholine. It increases the pressor effect of norepinephrine but blocks the pressor response of phenethylamine. However, additional receptor effects have been found including desensitization of adenyl cyclase, down regulation of beta-adrenergic receptors, and down regulation of serotonin receptors.

Pharmacodynamics/Kinetics

Onset of Action Depression: Initial effects may be observed within 1 to 2 weeks of treatment, with continued improvements through 4 to 6 weeks (Papakostas 2006; Posternak 2005; Szegedi 2009).

Half-life Elimination

Adults: 14 to 51 hours (mean: 26 hours) (Dawling 1980)

Elderly: 23.5 to 79 hours (mean: 45 hours) (Dawling 1980)

Time to Peak Serum: 4 to 9 hours (Alexanderson 1972)

Pregnancy Considerations Nortriptyline and its metabolites cross the human placenta and can be detected in cord blood (Loughhead 2006). Tricyclic antidepressants may be associated with irritability, jitteriness, and convulsions (rare) in the neonate (Yonkers 2009).

The ACOG recommends that therapy for depression during pregnancy be individualized; treatment should incorporate the clinical expertise of the mental health clinician, obstetrician, primary health care provider, and pediatrician (ACOG 2008). According to the American Psychiatric Association (APA), the risks of medication treatment should be weighed against other treatment options and untreated depression. For women who discontinue antidepressant medications during pregnancy and who may be at high risk for postpartum depression, the medications can be restarted following delivery (APA 2010). Treatment algorithms have been developed by the ACOG and the APA for the management of depression in women prior to conception and during pregnancy (Yonkers 2009).

Pregnant women exposed to antidepressants during pregnancy are encouraged to enroll in the National Pregnancy Registry for Antidepressants (NPRAD). Women 18 to 45 years of age or their health care providers may contact the registry by calling 844-405-6185. Enrollment should be done as early in pregnancy as possible.

Dental Health Professional Considerations See Local Anesthetic/Vasoconstrictor Precautions

- ◆ **Nortriptyline HCl** *see* Nortriptyline *on page 1119*
- ◆ **Nortriptyline Hydrochloride** *see* Nortriptyline *on page 1119*
- ◆ **Norvasc** *see* AmLODIPine *on page 121*
- ◆ **Norvir** *see* Ritonavir *on page 1335*
- ◆ **Nourianz** *see* Istradefylline *on page 849*
- ◆ **Novantrone** *see* MitoXANTRONE *on page 1042*
- ◆ **Novel Erythropoiesis-Stimulating Protein** *see* Darbepoetin Alfa *on page 440*
- ◆ **Novoeight** *see* Antihemophilic Factor (Recombinant) *on page 153*
- ◆ **NovoLIN 70/30** *see* Insulin NPH and Insulin Regular *on page 828*
- ◆ **NovoLIN 70/30 FlexPen** *see* Insulin NPH and Insulin Regular *on page 828*
- ◆ **NovoLIN 70/30 FlexPen Relion** *see* Insulin NPH and Insulin Regular *on page 828*
- ◆ **NovoLIN N [OTC]** *see* Insulin NPH *on page 827*
- ◆ **NovoLIN N FlexPen [OTC]** *see* Insulin NPH *on page 827*
- ◆ **NovoLIN N FlexPen ReliOn [OTC]** *see* Insulin NPH *on page 827*
- ◆ **NovoLIN N ReliOn [OTC]** *see* Insulin NPH *on page 827*
- ◆ **NovoLIN R [OTC]** *see* Insulin Regular *on page 829*
- ◆ **NovoLIN R FlexPen [OTC]** *see* Insulin Regular *on page 829*
- ◆ **NovoLIN R FlexPen ReliOn [OTC]** *see* Insulin Regular *on page 829*
- ◆ **NovoLIN R ReliOn [OTC]** *see* Insulin Regular *on page 829*
- ◆ **NovoLOG** *see* Insulin Aspart *on page 817*
- ◆ **NovoLog 70/30** *see* Insulin Aspart Protamine and Insulin Aspart *on page 818*
- ◆ **NovoLOG FlexPen** *see* Insulin Aspart *on page 817*
- ◆ **NovoLOG Mix 70/30** *see* Insulin Aspart Protamine and Insulin Aspart *on page 818*
- ◆ **NovoLOG Mix 70/30 FlexPen** *see* Insulin Aspart Protamine and Insulin Aspart *on page 818*
- ◆ **NovoLOG PenFill** *see* Insulin Aspart *on page 817*
- ◆ **Noxafil** *see* Posaconazole *on page 1248*
- ◆ **NPH Insulin** *see* Insulin NPH *on page 827*
- ◆ **NPH Insulin and Regular Insulin** *see* Insulin NPH and Insulin Regular *on page 828*
- ◆ **NP Thyroid** *see* Thyroid, Desiccated *on page 1442*
- ◆ **NRP104** *see* Lisdexamfetamine *on page 921*
- ◆ **NRS Nasal Relief [OTC] [DSC]** *see* Oxymetazoline (Nasal) *on page 1173*
- ◆ **NS-304** *see* Selexipag *on page 1364*
- ◆ **NT 201** *see* IncobotulinumtoxinA *on page 806*
- ◆ **NTG** *see* Nitroglycerin *on page 1112*
- ◆ ***N*-trifluoroacetyladriamycin-14-valerate** *see* Valrubicin *on page 1520*
- ◆ **Nuartez** *see* Artesunate *on page 169*
- ◆ **Nubain** *see* Nalbuphine *on page 1073*
- ◆ **Nucala** *see* Mepolizumab *on page 977*
- ◆ **NuCort** *see* Hydrocortisone (Topical) *on page 775*
- ◆ **Nucynta** *see* Tapentadol *on page 1406*
- ◆ **Nucynta ER** *see* Tapentadol *on page 1406*
- ◆ **NuFera** *see* Vitamins (Multiple/Oral) *on page 1550*
- ◆ **Nulojix** *see* Belatacept *on page 221*
- ◆ **Numbonex [DSC]** *see* Lidocaine (Topical) *on page 902*
- ◆ **Numbrino** *see* Cocaine (Topical) *on page 403*
- ◆ **Numoisyn** *see* Saliva Substitute *on page 1354*
- ◆ **Nupercainal [OTC]** *see* Dibucaine *on page 483*
- ◆ **Nuplazid** *see* Pimavanserin *on page 1232*

Nystatin (Oral) (nye STAT in)

Related Information

Fungal Infections *on page 1752*

Related Sample Prescriptions

Fungal Infections - Sample Prescriptions *on page 38*

Brand Names: US Bio-Statin

Brand Names: Canada DOM-Nystatin; JAMP-Nystatin; Nyaderm; PMS-Nystatin; TEVA-Nystatin

Generic Availability (US) Yes

Pharmacologic Category Antifungal Agent, Oral Nonabsorbed/Partially Absorbed

Dental Use Treatment of susceptible cutaneous, mucocutaneous, and oral cavity fungal infections normally caused by the *Candida* species; treatment of removable intraoral appliances in patients who experience oral cavity fungal infections

Use Treatment of susceptible cutaneous, mucocutaneous, and oral cavity fungal infections normally caused by the *Candida* species

Local Anesthetic/Vasoconstrictor Precautions No information available to require special precautions

Effects on Dental Treatment No significant effects or complications reported

Effects on Bleeding No information available to require special precautions

Adverse Reactions

1% to 10%: Gastrointestinal: Diarrhea, nausea, stomach pain, vomiting

<1%, postmarketing, and/or case reports: Hypersensitivity reaction

Dental Usual Dosage Oral candidiasis: Suspension (swish and swallow orally):

Premature infants: 100,000 units 4 times/day; paint suspension into recesses of the mouth

Infants: 200,000 units 4 times/day or 100,000 units to each side of mouth 4 times/day; paint suspension into recesses of the mouth

Children and Adults: 400,000 to 600,000 units 4 times/day; swish in the mouth and retain for as long as possible (several minutes) before swallowing. For patients wearing a removable intraoral appliance, some experts recommend to also treat the oral appliance with the oral suspension overnight for 2 to 5 days.

Dosing

Adult & Geriatric

Intestinal infections: Oral tablets: 500,000-1,000,000 units every 8 hours

Oral candidiasis, mild disease (alternative agent): Suspension (swish and swallow): 400,000-600,000 units 4 times/day; swish in the mouth and retain for as long as possible (several minutes) before swallowing (HHS [adult OI] 2020; IDSA [Pappas 2016]).

Note: Powder for compounding: 1/8 teaspoon (500,000 units) to equal approximately 1/2 cup of water; give 4 times/day

Renal Impairment: Adult There are no dosage adjustments provided in the manufacturer's labeling.

Hepatic Impairment: Adult There are no dosage adjustments provided in the manufacturer's labeling.

Pediatric

Oral candidiasis: Oral suspension:

Infants: Oral: 200,000 to 400,000 units 4 times daily or 100,000 units to each side of mouth 4 times daily; one study of 14 patients (neonates and infants) found higher cure rates using 400,000 units/dose 4 times daily (Hoppe 1997)

Children and Adolescents: Oral: 400,000 to 600,000 units 4 times daily; administer half of dose to each side of mouth; swish and retain in the mouth for as long as possible before swallowing.

Peritonitis (Peritoneal dialysis), prophylaxis for high risk situations (eg, during antibiotic therapy or PEG placement): Oral Suspension: Infants, Children, and Adolescents: 10,000 units/kg once daily (Warady [ISPD] 2012)

Renal Impairment: Pediatric There are no dosage adjustments provided in the manufacturer's labeling.

Hepatic Impairment: Pediatric There are no dosage adjustments provided in the manufacturer's labeling.

Mechanism of Action Binds to sterols in fungal cell membrane, changing the cell wall permeability allowing for leakage of cellular contents

Contraindications Hypersensitivity to nystatin or any component of the formulation

Drug Interactions

Metabolism/Transport Effects None known.

Avoid Concomitant Use

Avoid concomitant use of Nystatin (Oral) with any of the following: Saccharomyces boulardii

Increased Effect/Toxicity There are no known significant interactions involving an increase in effect.

Decreased Effect

Nystatin (Oral) may decrease the levels/effects of: Saccharomyces boulardii

Pharmacodynamics/Kinetics

Onset of Action Symptomatic relief from candidiasis: 24-72 hours

Pregnancy Risk Factor C

Pregnancy Considerations Animal reproduction studies have not been conducted. Adverse events in the fetus or newborn have not been reported following maternal use of vaginal nystatin during pregnancy. Absorption following oral use is poor.

Breastfeeding Considerations Excretion into breast milk is not known; however, absorption following oral use is poor.

Dosage Forms: US

Capsule, Oral [preservative free]:

Bio-Statin: 500,000 units, 1,000,000 units

Powder, Oral:

Bio-Statin: (1 ea)

Suspension, Mouth/Throat:

Generic: 100,000 units/mL (5 mL, 60 mL, 473 mL, 480 mL)

Tablet, Oral:

Generic: 500,000 units

Dosage Forms: Canada

Suspension, Mouth/Throat:

Nyaderm: 100,000 units/mL (30 mL, 48 mL, 500 mL)

Generic: 100,000 units/mL (5 mL, 24 mL, 48 mL, 100 mL, 500 mL, 1000 mL)

Nystatin (Topical) (nye STAT in)

Related Information

Fungal Infections *on page 1752*

Related Sample Prescriptions

Fungal Infections - Sample Prescriptions *on page 38*

Brand Names: US Nyamyc; Nyata [DSC]; Nystop

Generic Availability (US) May be product dependent

Pharmacologic Category Antifungal Agent, Topical

Dental Use Treatment of cutaneous and mucocutaneous fungal infections caused by *Candida albicans* and other susceptible *Candida* species.

Use Fungal infections (cutaneous and mucocutaneous): Treatment of cutaneous and mucocutaneous fungal infections caused by *Candida albicans* and other susceptible *Candida* species.

Local Anesthetic/Vasoconstrictor Precautions No information available to require special precautions

Effects on Dental Treatment No significant effects or complications reported

Effects on Bleeding No information available to require special precautions

Adverse Reactions

Frequency not defined: Dermatologic: Contact dermatitis, Stevens-Johnson syndrome

<1%, postmarketing, and/or case reports: Hypersensitivity reaction

Dental Usual Dosage Mucocutaneous fungal infections: Children and Adults: Topical: Apply 2 to 3 times/day to affected areas

Dosing

Adult & Geriatric Fungal infections (cutaneous and mucocutaneous): Topical: **Note:** Cream is usually preferred to ointment for intertriginous areas; very moist lesions are best treated with topical powder

Cream, ointment: Apply to the affected areas twice daily or as indicated until healing is complete

Powder: Apply to the affected areas 2 to 3 times daily until healing is complete

Renal Impairment: Adult There are no dosage adjustments provided in the manufacturer's labeling. However, dosage adjustment unlikely due to low systemic absorption

Hepatic Impairment: Adult There are no dosage adjustments provided in the manufacturer's labeling. However, dosage adjustment unlikely due to low systemic absorption

Pediatric

Diaper dermatitis, candidal: Limited data available: Infants: Ointment, cream: Topical: Apply 2 to 4 times daily to affected area; most studies have used 4 times daily dosing (Hoppe, 1997; Munz 1982)

Mucocutaneous candidal infections: Infants, Children, and Adolescents:

Manufacturer's labeling:

Cream/ointment: Topical: Apply to affected area twice daily

Powder: Topical: Apply to affected area 2 to 3 times daily

Alternate dosing: Limited data available: Cream, ointment, powder: Topical: Apply to affected area 2 to 4 times daily (Bradley 2015)

Renal Impairment: Pediatric There are no dosage adjustments provided in the manufacturer's labeling; however, dosage adjustment unlikely due to low systemic absorption.

Hepatic Impairment: Pediatric There are no dosage adjustments provided in the manufacturer's labeling; however, dosage adjustment unlikely due to low systemic absorption.

Mechanism of Action Binds to sterols in fungal cell membrane, changing the cell wall permeability allowing for leakage of cellular contents

Contraindications Hypersensitivity to nystatin or any component of the formulation

Warnings/Precautions For topical use only; not for systemic, oral, intravaginal, or ophthalmic use. Hypersensitivity reactions may occur; immediately discontinue if signs of a hypersensitivity reaction occurs. Discontinue use if irritation occurs.

Warnings: Additional Pediatric Considerations Some dosage forms may contain propylene glycol; in neonates large amounts of propylene glycol delivered orally, intravenously (eg, >3,000 mg/day), or topically have been associated with potentially fatal toxicities which can include metabolic acidosis, seizures, renal failure, and CNS depression; toxicities have also been reported in children and adults including hyperosmolality, lactic acidosis, seizures, and respiratory depression; use caution (AAP, 1997; Shehab, 2009).

Drug Interactions

Metabolism/Transport Effects None known.

Avoid Concomitant Use

Avoid concomitant use of Nystatin (Topical) with any of the following: Progesterone

Increased Effect/Toxicity There are no known significant interactions involving an increase in effect.

Decreased Effect

Nystatin (Topical) may decrease the levels/effects of: Progesterone

Pharmacodynamics/Kinetics

Onset of Action Symptomatic relief from candidiasis: 24 to 72 hours

Pregnancy Risk Factor C

Pregnancy Considerations Animal reproduction studies have not been conducted. Absorption following oral use is poor and nystatin is not absorbed following application to mucous membranes or intact skin.

Breastfeeding Considerations It is not known if nystatin is excreted in breast milk; however, absorption following oral use is poor and nystatin is not absorbed following application to mucous membranes or intact skin. The manufacturer recommends that caution be exercised when administering nystatin to nursing women.

Dosage Forms Considerations

Nyata Kit contains nystatin powder and Curatin exfoliating serum.

Pediaderm AF Complete Kit contains nystatin cream and Pediaderm Diaper Defense cream.

Dosage Forms: US

Cream, External:

Generic: 100,000 units/g (15 g, 30 g)

Ointment, External:

Generic: 100,000 units/g (15 g, 30 g)

Powder, External:

Nyamyc: 100,000 units/g (15 g, 30 g, 60 g)
Nystop: 100,000 units/g (15 g, 30 g, 60 g)
Generic: 100,000 units/g (15 g, 30 g, 60 g)

Nystatin and Triamcinolone

(nye STAT in & trye am SIN oh lone)

Related Information

Fungal Infections *on page 1752*
Nystatin (Topical) *on page 1122*
Triamcinolone (Topical) *on page 1490*

Related Sample Prescriptions

Fungal Infections - Sample Prescriptions *on page 38*

Generic Availability (US) Yes

Pharmacologic Category Antifungal Agent, Topical; Corticosteroid, Topical

Dental Use Treatment of angular cheilitis (off-label use) and cutaneous candidiasis

Use Treatment of cutaneous candidiasis

Local Anesthetic/Vasoconstrictor Precautions No information available to require special precautions

Effects on Dental Treatment No significant effects or complications reported

Effects on Bleeding No information available to require special precautions

Adverse Reactions Frequency not defined.

Central nervous system: Localized burning

Dermatologic: Acne vulgaris, allergic dermatitis, atrophic striae, folliculitis, hypertrichosis, hypopigmentation, maceration of the skin, miliaria, perioral dermatitis, skin atrophy, xeroderma

Infection: Secondary infection

Local: Local irritation, local pruritus

Dental Usual Dosage Angular cheilitis (off-label use) and cutaneous candidiasis: Children and Adults: Topical: Apply sparingly 2 to 4 times/day. Therapy should be discontinued when control is achieved; if no improvement is seen, reassessment of diagnosis may be necessary.

Dosing

Adult & Geriatric Cutaneous *Candida*: Topical: Apply sparingly to affected area(s) twice daily. Therapy should be discontinued when control is achieved or if symptoms persist for >25 days of therapy.

Renal Impairment: Adult There are no dosage adjustments provided in the manufacturer's labeling.

Hepatic Impairment: Adult There are no dosage adjustments provided in the manufacturer's labeling.

Pediatric Refer to adult dosing.

Renal Impairment: Pediatric There are no dosage adjustments provided in the manufacturer's labeling.

Hepatic Impairment: Pediatric There are no dosage adjustments provided in the manufacturer's labeling.

Mechanism of Action See individual agents.

Contraindications Hypersensitivity to nystatin, triamcinolone, or any component of the formulation

Warnings/Precautions Avoid use of occlusive dressings; limit therapy to least amount necessary for effective therapy, pediatric patients may be more susceptible to HPA axis suppression due to larger BSA to weight ratio

Drug Interactions

Metabolism/Transport Effects None known.

Avoid Concomitant Use

Avoid concomitant use of Nystatin and Triamcinolone with any of the following: Aldesleukin; Progesterone

Increased Effect/Toxicity

Nystatin and Triamcinolone may increase the levels/effects of: Deferasirox; Ritodrine

Decreased Effect

Nystatin and Triamcinolone may decrease the levels/effects of: Aldesleukin; Corticorelin; Hyaluronidase; Progesterone

Pregnancy Considerations See individual agents.

Breastfeeding Considerations See individual agents.

Dosage Forms: US

Cream, External: Nystatin 100,000 units and triamcinolone 0.1% (15 g, 30 g, 60 g)

Ointment, External: Nystatin 100,000 units and triamcinolone 0.1% (15 g, 30 g, 60 g)

◆ **Nystatin/Triamcinolone** *see* Nystatin and Triamcinolone *on page 1123*

◆ **Nystop** *see* Nystatin (Topical) *on page 1122*

◆ **Nytol [OTC]** *see* DiphenhydrAMINE (Systemic) *on page 502*

◆ **Nytol Maximum Strength [OTC]** *see* DiphenhydrAMINE (Systemic) *on page 502*

◆ **Oasis** *see* Saliva Substitute *on page 1354*

Obeticholic Acid (oh bet i KOE lik AS id)

Brand Names: US Ocaliva

Brand Names: Canada Ocaliva

Pharmacologic Category Farnesoid X Receptor Agonist

Use Primary biliary cholangitis: Treatment of primary biliary cholangitis (PBC) in combination with ursodiol (ursodeoxycholic acid) in adults with an inadequate response to ursodiol, or as monotherapy in adults unable to tolerate ursodiol.

Local Anesthetic/Vasoconstrictor Precautions No information available to require special precautions

Effects on Dental Treatment Key adverse event(s) related to dental treatment: Oropharyngeal pain has been reported

Effects on Bleeding No information available to require special precautions

Adverse Reactions

>10%:

Central nervous system: Fatigue (19% to 25%)

Dermatologic: Pruritus (56% to 70%; severe: 19% to 23%)

Endocrine & metabolic: Decreased HDL cholesterol (9% to 20%)

Gastrointestinal: Abdominal pain (19%)

1% to 10%:
Cardiovascular: Peripheral edema (7%), palpitations (3% to 7%)
Central nervous system: Dizziness (7%)
Dermatologic: Skin rash (10%), eczema (3% to 6%)
Endocrine & metabolic: Thyroid dysfunction (4% to 6%)
Gastrointestinal: Constipation (7%)
Neuromuscular & skeletal: Arthralgia (6% to 10%)
Respiratory: Oropharyngeal pain (7% to 8%)
Miscellaneous: Fever (≤7%)

Frequency not defined: Gastrointestinal: Cholangitis (worsening)

<1%, postmarketing and/or case reports: Ascites, hepatic cirrhosis (new onset), hepatic encephalopathy (worsening), hepatic failure, hepatic insufficiency, increased direct serum bilirubin, increased serum bilirubin, jaundice (new onset and worsening), liver decompensation

Mechanism of Action Obeticholic acid is a farnesoid X receptor agonist; activation of FXR suppresses de novo synthesis of bile acids from cholesterol and increases transport of bile acids out of the hepatocytes, limiting the overall size of the circulating bile acid pool while promoting choleresis.

Pharmacodynamics/Kinetics

Time to Peak Plasma: Obeticholic acid: ~1.5 hours; glyco- and tauro-obeticholic acid: 10 hours

Pregnancy Considerations Adverse events have not been observed in animal reproduction studies.

Obinutuzumab (oh bi nue TOOZ ue mab)

Brand Names: US Gazyva

Brand Names: Canada Gazyva

Pharmacologic Category Antineoplastic Agent, Anti-CD20; Antineoplastic Agent, Monoclonal Antibody

Use

Chronic lymphocytic leukemia: Treatment of previously untreated chronic lymphocytic leukemia in combination with chlorambucil.

Follicular lymphoma:

Previously untreated: Treatment of previously untreated stage II bulky, stage III, or stage IV follicular lymphoma in combination with chemotherapy (followed by obinutuzumab monotherapy) in patients achieving at least a partial remission.

Relapsed/refractory: Treatment of follicular lymphoma (in combination with bendamustine followed by obinutuzumab monotherapy) in patients who relapsed after, or are refractory to, a rituximab-containing regimen.

Local Anesthetic/Vasoconstrictor Precautions No information available to require special precautions

Effects on Dental Treatment Key adverse event(s) related to dental treatment: Monoclonal antibodies used to treat chronic lymphocytic leukemia are known to cause stomatitis and mucositis.

Effects on Bleeding Chemotherapy may result in significant myelosuppression, including thrombocytopenia. In patients who are under active treatment, a medical consult is suggested.

Adverse Reactions Adverse reactions are reported in combination with chlorambucil or bendamustine unless incidence is identified as having occurred during the monotherapy phase.

>10%:
Dermatologic: Pruritus (11%), skin rash (monotherapy: ≥10%; combination therapy: 17%)
Endocrine & metabolic: Hyperkalemia (20% to 33%), hypernatremia (16%), hyperuricemia (28%), hypoalbuminemia (23% to 33%), hypocalcemia (32% to 39%), hypokalemia (14%), hyponatremia (26%), hypophosphatemia (36% to 41%)
Gastrointestinal: Constipation (8% to 32%) decreased appetite (14%), diarrhea (monotherapy: ≥10%; combination therapy: 10% to 30%)
Genitourinary: Urinary tract infection (monotherapy: ≥10%; combination therapy: 5% to 13%)
Hematologic & oncologic: Anemia (12% to 39%; grades 3/4: 5% to 10%), hemorrhage (12%; grades 3/4: 4%), hypoproteinemia (32%), leukopenia (84% to 92%; grades 3/4: 35% to 49%, grade 4: 17%), lymphocytopenia (monotherapy: grades 3/4: 23%, grade 4: 5%; combination therapy: 80% to 97%; grades 3/4: 39% to 92%; grade 4: 33%), neutropenia (monotherapy: 13% to 20%; grades 3/4: 21% to 25%, grade 4: 10%; combination therapy: 37% to 84%; grades 3/4: 33% to 59%; onset ≥28 days after completion of treatment: 4% to 16%; lasting ≥28 days: 1% to 3%), thrombocytopenia (14% to 68%; grades 3/4: 10% to 13%; onset within 24 hours of infusion: 4%)
Hepatic: Hyperbilirubinemia (21%), increased serum alanine aminotransferase (28% to 50%), increased serum alkaline phosphatase (18% to 27%), increased serum aspartate aminotransferase (27% to 44%)
Infection: Herpes virus infection (monotherapy: 13%; combination therapy: 18%), infection (38% to 82%)
Nervous system: Fatigue (monotherapy: ≥10%; combination therapy: 40%), headache (18%), insomnia (15%)
Neuromuscular & skeletal: Arthralgia (12% to 16%), musculoskeletal signs and symptoms (18% to 54%; including musculoskeletal pain: monotherapy: 20%; combination therapy: 28%)
Renal: Increased serum creatinine (30%)
Respiratory: Cough (monotherapy: 23%; combination therapy: 10% to 35%), pneumonia (14%), respiratory tract infection (monotherapy: ≥10%; combination therapy: 14%), upper respiratory tract infection (monotherapy: 40%; combination therapy: 36% to 50%)
Miscellaneous: Fever (19%), infusion related reaction (monotherapy: 8% to 9%; combination therapy: 66% to 72%, initial infusion: 37% to 65%, subsequent infusions and cycles: ≤23% [dependent on dose, cycle, and use of premeditations]; can be severe infusion related reaction)

1% to 10%:
Hematologic & oncologic: Febrile neutropenia (6%), tumor lysis syndrome (grades 3/4: ≤2%)
Hepatic: Increased liver enzymes (4%; may be secondary or exacerbated by premedications)
Immunologic: Antibody development (≤7%)
Infection: Sepsis (7%)
Neuromuscular & skeletal: Back pain (5%)
Respiratory: Nasopharyngitis (6%)

Frequency not defined:
Cardiovascular: Exacerbation of cardiac disease
Hepatic: Fulminant hepatitis, hepatic failure
Infection: JC virus infection, reactivation of HBV
Nervous system: Progressive multifocal leukoencephalopathy

Postmarketing:
Gastrointestinal: Gastrointestinal perforation
Hypersensitivity: Hypersensitivity reactions, serum sickness

Mechanism of Action Obinutuzumab is a glycoengineered type II anti-CD20 monoclonal antibody. The CD20 antigen is expressed on the surface of pre B- and mature B-lymphocytes; upon binding to CD20, obinutuzumab activates complement-dependent cytotoxicity, antibody-dependent cellular cytotoxicity and antibody-dependent cellular phagocytosis, resulting in cell death (Sehn 2012).

Pharmacodynamics/Kinetics

Half-life Elimination 25.5 to 35.3 days

Reproductive Considerations

Females of reproductive potential should use effective contraception during therapy and for 6 months after the last obinutuzumab dose.

Pregnancy Considerations

Obinutuzumab is a humanized monoclonal antibody (IgG_1). Potential placental transfer of human IgG is dependent upon the IgG subclass and gestational age, generally increasing as pregnancy progresses. The lowest exposure would be expected during the period of organogenesis (Palmeira 2012; Pentsuk 2009).

Based on the mechanism of action and on animal data, if exposure occurs during pregnancy, B-cell counts may be depleted and immunologic function may be affected in the neonate after birth. Administration of live vaccines to neonates and infants exposed in utero should be avoided until after B-cell recovery.

- ◆ **Ocaliva** *see* Obeticholic Acid *on page 1123*
- ◆ **OCBZ** *see* OXcarbazepine *on page 1154*
- ◆ **Ocean Blue MiniCaps Omega-3 [OTC]** *see* Omega-3 Fatty Acids *on page 1137*
- ◆ **Ocella** *see* Ethinyl Estradiol and Drospirenone *on page 610*

Ocrelizumab (ok re LIZ ue mab)

Brand Names: US Ocrevus

Brand Names: Canada Ocrevus

Pharmacologic Category Anti-CD20 Monoclonal Antibody; Monoclonal Antibody

Use Multiple sclerosis, relapsing or primary progressive: Treatment of primary progressive multiple sclerosis (MS) and relapsing forms of MS, including clinically isolated syndrome, relapsing remitting disease, and active secondary progressive disease.

Local Anesthetic/Vasoconstrictor Precautions No information available to require special precautions

Effects on Dental Treatment No significant effects or complications reported

Effects on Bleeding No information available to require special precautions

Adverse Reactions

>10%:

Dermatologic: Skin infection (14%)

Hematologic & oncologic: Decreased serum immunoglobulins (≤17%, IgM most affected), decreased neutrophils (13%)

Infection: Infection (58% to 70%)

Respiratory: Upper respiratory tract infection (40% to 49%)

Miscellaneous: Infusion related reaction (34% to 40%)

1% to 10%:

Cardiovascular: Peripheral edema (6%)

Central nervous system: Depression (8%)

Gastrointestinal: Diarrhea (6%)

Infection: Herpes virus infection (5% to 6%)

Neuromuscular & skeletal: Back pain (6%), limb pain (5%)

Respiratory: Lower respiratory tract infection (8% to 10%), cough (7%)

Frequency not defined:

Cardiovascular: Hypotension (infusion related)

Hypersensitivity: Anaphylaxis

Respiratory: Bronchospasm, laryngeal edema, pharyngeal edema

<1%, postmarketing, and/or case reports: Antibody development, malignant neoplasm of breast, severe infusion related reaction

Mechanism of Action Ocrelizumab is a recombinant humanized IgG monoclonal antibody directed against B-cells which express the cell surface antigen CD20; CD20 is present on pre-B and mature B lymphocytes. B-cells are thought to influence the course of multiple sclerosis through antigen presentation, autoantibody production, cytokine regulation, and formation of ectopic lymphoid aggregates in the meninges (Hauser 2017). Ocrelizumab selectively targets and binds with high affinity to the cell surface to deplete CD20 expressing B-cells through antibody-dependent cell-mediated phagocytosis and cytotoxicity, as well as complement-mediated cytolysis (Hauser 2017; Montalban 2017).

Pharmacodynamics/Kinetics

Onset of Action Serum CD-19+ B-cell counts (used as a marker for B-cell counts) are reduced within 14 days after infusion.

Duration of Action Median time for B-cell recovery (to baseline or the lower limit of normal): 72 weeks (range: 27 to 175 weeks).

Half-life Elimination 26 days

Reproductive Considerations

Females of reproductive potential should use effective contraception during therapy and for 6 months after the last ocrelizumab infusion.

In general, disease-modifying therapies for multiple sclerosis (MS) are stopped prior to a planned pregnancy except in females at high risk of MS activity (AAN [Rae-Grant 2018]). Consider use of agents other than ocrelizumab for females at high risk of disease reactivation who are planning a pregnancy. Delaying pregnancy is recommended for females with persistent high disease activity; when disease-modifying therapy is needed in these patients, other agents are preferred (ECTRIMS/EAN [Montalban 2018]).

Pregnancy Considerations

Ocrelizumab is a humanized monoclonal antibody (IgG_1). Potential placental transfer of human IgG is dependent upon the IgG subclass and gestational age, generally increasing as pregnancy progresses. The lowest exposure would be expected during the period of organogenesis (Palmeira 2012; Pentsuk 2009).

Information related to the use of ocrelizumab in pregnancy is limited (Fragoso 2018; Juanatey 2018). Transient peripheral B-cell depletion and lymphocytopenia have been observed in infants born to mothers who received similar agents; immune response to live or live-attenuated vaccines may be decreased in infants exposed to ocrelizumab in utero. Evaluate immune response by measuring $CD19^+$B-cells in exposed infants prior to the administration of live or live-attenuated vaccines.

In general, disease-modifying therapies for multiple sclerosis (MS) are not initiated during pregnancy, except in females at high risk of MS activity (AAN [Rae-Grant 2018]). When disease-modifying therapy is needed in these patients, other agents are preferred (ECTRIMS/EAN [Montalban 2018]).

- ◆ **Ocrevus** *see* Ocrelizumab *on page 1125*
- ◆ **Octagam** *see* Immune Globulin *on page 803*
- ◆ **Octocog Alfa** *see* Antihemophilic Factor (Recombinant) *on page 153*
- ◆ **Ocuvel** *see* Vitamins (Multiple/Oral) *on page 1550*
- ◆ **Ocuvite [OTC]** *see* Vitamins (Multiple/Oral) *on page 1550*
- ◆ **Ocuvite Adult 50+ [OTC]** *see* Vitamins (Multiple/Oral) *on page 1550*
- ◆ **Ocuvite Extra [OTC]** *see* Vitamins (Multiple/Oral) *on page 1550*
- ◆ **Ocuvite Lutein [OTC]** *see* Vitamins (Multiple/Oral) *on page 1550*
- ◆ **Odefsey** *see* Emtricitabine, Rilpivirine, and Tenofovir Alafenamide *on page 559*
- ◆ **O-desmethylvenlafaxine** *see* Desvenlafaxine *on page 462*
- ◆ **Odomzo** *see* Sonidegib *on page 1382*
- ◆ **Odorless Coated Fish Oil [OTC]** *see* Omega-3 Fatty Acids *on page 1137*
- ◆ **ODV** *see* Desvenlafaxine *on page 462*
- ◆ **Oestrogen and Methyltestosterone** *see* Estrogens (Esterified) and Methyltestosterone *on page 605*
- ◆ **Oestrogens** *see* Estrogens (Conjugated B/Synthetic) *on page 601*
- ◆ **Oestrogens and Bazedoxifene** *see* Estrogens (Conjugated/Equine) and Bazedoxifene *on page 603*
- ◆ **Oestrogens (Conjugated) and Medroxyprogesterone** *see* Estrogens (Conjugated/Equine) and Medroxyprogesterone *on page 603*
- ◆ **Oestrogens, Conjugated/Equine** *see* Estrogens (Conjugated/Equine, Systemic) *on page 601*
- ◆ **Oestrogens, Conjugated/Equine** *see* Estrogens (Conjugated/Equine, Topical) *on page 602*
- ◆ **Oestrogens Esterified** *see* Estrogens (Esterified) *on page 604*

Ofatumumab (oh fa TOOM yoo mab)

Brand Names: US Arzerra

Brand Names: Canada Arzerra [DSC]

Pharmacologic Category Antineoplastic Agent, Anti-CD20; Antineoplastic Agent, Monoclonal Antibody; Monoclonal Antibody

Use

Chronic lymphocytic leukemia, previously untreated: Treatment of previously untreated chronic lymphocytic leukemia (CLL) (in combination with chlorambucil) when fludarabine-based therapy is considered inappropriate

Chronic lymphocytic leukemia, relapsed : Treatment of relapsed CLL (in combination with fludarabine and cyclophosphamide).

Chronic lymphocytic leukemia, refractory: Treatment of CLL refractory to fludarabine and alemtuzumab

Chronic lymphocytic leukemia, extended treatment: Extended treatment of patients who are in complete or partial response after at least two lines of therapy for recurrent or progressive CLL

Local Anesthetic/Vasoconstrictor Precautions No information available to require special precautions

Effects on Dental Treatment No significant effects or complications reported

Effects on Bleeding Thrombocytopenia is not frequently observed (<1%) although it can rarely be seen. Neutropenia may be prolonged >2 weeks. In patients who are under active treatment with this agent, medical consult is suggested.

Adverse Reactions

>10%:

Central nervous system: Fatigue (15%)

Dermatologic: Skin rash (14%)

Gastrointestinal: Diarrhea (18%), nausea (11%)

Hematologic & oncologic: Neutropenia (24%; ≥grade 3: ≥22%; may be prolonged >2 weeks), anemia (16%; grades 3/4: 5%)

Infection: Infection (65% to 70%; includes bacterial, fungal, or viral), serious infection (20%)

Respiratory: Pneumonia (8% to 23%), cough (19%), upper respiratory tract infection (11% to 19%), dyspnea (14%), bronchitis (9% to 11%)

Miscellaneous: Infusion related reaction (46%; day 1 reactions: 25% to 44%; subsequent infusions: 2% to 29%), fever (20%)

1% to 10%:

Cardiovascular: Peripheral edema (9%), hypertension (5%), hypotension (5%), tachycardia (5%)

Central nervous system: Chills (8%), insomnia (5% to 7%), headache (6%)

Dermatologic: Urticaria (8%), hyperhidrosis (5%)

Hematologic & oncologic: Hypogammaglobulinemia (5%; grades 3/4: <1%)

Infection: Sepsis (8%), influenza (6%), herpes zoster (5% to 6%)

Neuromuscular & skeletal: Back pain (5% to 8%), muscle spasm (5%)

Respiratory: Nasopharyngitis (8%), sinusitis (5%)

<1%, postmarketing, and/or case reports: Antibody development, hepatitis B (new-onset or reactivation), porphyria cutanea tarda, progressive multifocal leukoencephalopathy, Stevens Johnson syndrome, tumor lysis syndrome

Mechanism of Action Ofatumumab is a monoclonal antibody which binds specifically the extracellular (large and small) loops of the CD20 molecule (which is expressed on normal B lymphocytes and in B-cell CLL) resulting in potent complement-dependent cell lysis and antibody-dependent cell-mediated toxicity in cells that overexpress CD20.

Pharmacodynamics/Kinetics

Half-life Elimination 17.6 days (following repeated infusions)

Pregnancy Considerations

Ofatumumab is a humanized monoclonal antibody (IgG_1). Potential placental transfer of human IgG is dependent upon the IgG subclass and gestational age, generally increasing as pregnancy progresses. The lowest exposure would be expected during the period of organogenesis (Palmeira 2012; Pentsuk 2009).

Based on animal data, prolonged depletion of circulating B cells may occur; avoid administering live vaccines to newborns exposed to ofatumumab in utero until B cell recovery occurs.

◆ **Ofev** *see* Nintedanib *on page 1108*

◆ **Ofirmev** *see* Acetaminophen *on page 59*

Ofloxacin (Systemic) (oh FLOKS a sin)

Related Information

Clinical Risk Related to Drugs Prolonging QT Interval *on page 1675*

Pharmacologic Category Antibiotic, Fluoroquinolone

Use

Treatment of acute exacerbations of chronic bronchitis, community-acquired pneumonia, skin and skin structure infections (uncomplicated), urethral and cervical gonorrhea (acute, uncomplicated), urethritis and cervicitis (nongonococcal) due to *Chlamydia trachomatis* infection, mixed infections of the urethra and cervix, pelvic inflammatory disease (acute), cystitis (uncomplicated), urinary tract infections (complicated), prostatitis

Note: As of April 2007, the CDC no longer recommends the use of fluoroquinolones for the treatment of gonococcal disease.

Local Anesthetic/Vasoconstrictor Precautions

Ofloxacin (Systemic) is one of the drugs confirmed to prolong the QT interval and is accepted as having a risk of causing torsade de pointes. The risk of drug-induced torsade de pointes is extremely low when a single QT interval prolonging drug is prescribed. In terms of epinephrine, it is not known what effect vasoconstrictors in the local anesthetic regimen will have in patients with a known history of congenital prolonged QT interval or in patients taking any medication that prolongs the QT interval. Until more information is obtained, it is suggested that the clinician consult with the physician prior to the use of a vasoconstrictor in suspected patients, and that the vasoconstrictor (epinephrine, mepivacaine and levonordefrin [Carbocaine® 2% with Neo-Cobefrin®]) be used with caution.

Effects on Dental Treatment Key adverse event(s) related to dental treatment: Xerostomia (normal salivary flow resumes upon discontinuation) and abnormal taste.

Effects on Bleeding Quinolone antibiotic administration has not been shown to independently effect bleeding; however, ofloxacin has been shown to potentiate the hypoprothrombinemic effect of warfarin and other coumarin anticoagulants. The hypoprothrombinemic mechanism may involve inhibition of coumarin metabolism and/or depletion of certain clotting factors due to suppression of vitamin K-producing intestinal flora.

Adverse Reactions

1% to 10%:

Cardiovascular: Chest pain (1% to 3%)

Central nervous system: Headache (1% to 9%), insomnia (3% to 7%), dizziness (1% to 5%), fatigue (1% to 3%), drowsiness (1% to 3%), sleep disorder (1% to 3%), nervousness (1% to 3%), pain (trunk)

Dermatologic: Pruritus (≤3%), skin rash (≤3%), genital pruritus (women: 1% to 3%)

Gastrointestinal: Nausea (3% to 10%), diarrhea (1% to 4%), vomiting (1% to 4%), abdominal cramps (1% to 3%), constipation (1% to 3%), decreased appetite (1% to 3%), dysgeusia (1% to 3%), flatulence (1% to 3%), gastrointestinal distress (1% to 3%), xerostomia (1% to 3%)

Genitourinary: Vaginitis (1% to 5%)

Ophthalmic: Visual disturbance (1% to 3%)

Respiratory: Pharyngitis (1% to 3%)

Miscellaneous: Fever (1% to 3%)

<1%, postmarketing, and/or case reports: Abnormal dreams, anaphylaxis, anxiety, auditory disturbance (decreased acuity), blurred vision, chills, cognitive dysfunction, cough, depression, ecchymosis, edema, erythema nodosum, euphoria, exacerbation of myasthenia gravis, Gilles de la Tourette's syndrome, hallucination, hepatic insufficiency, hepatic failure, hepatitis, hepatotoxicity (idiosyncratic; Chalasani 2014), hyperglycemia, hypoglycemia, hypertension, increased intracranial pressure, increased thirst, interstitial nephritis, limb pain, malaise, palpitations, paresthesia, peripheral neuropathy, photophobia, pneumonitis, pseudotumor cerebri, psychotic reaction, rhabdomyolysis, rupture of tendon, seizure, skin photosensitivity, Stevens-Johnson syndrome, syncope, tendonitis, tinnitus, torsades de pointes, toxic epidermal necrolysis, vasculitis, vasodilation, vertigo, weakness, weight loss

Mechanism of Action Ofloxacin is a DNA gyrase inhibitor. DNA gyrase is an essential bacterial enzyme that maintains the superhelical structure of DNA. DNA gyrase is required for DNA replication and transcription, DNA repair, recombination, and transposition; bactericidal

Pharmacodynamics/Kinetics

Half-life Elimination ~9 hours (biphasic: 4 to 5 hours [6.4 to 7.4 hours in elderly patients] and 20 to 25 hours [accounts for <5%]); prolonged with renal impairment

Time to Peak Serum: 1 to 2 hours

Pregnancy Risk Factor C

Pregnancy Considerations

Ofloxacin crosses the placenta and produces measurable concentrations in the amniotic fluid. Serum concentrations of ofloxacin may be lower during pregnancy than in nonpregnant patients (Giamarellou 1989). Based on available data, an increased risk of teratogenic effects has not been observed following ofloxacin use during pregnancy (Padberg 2014).

Dental Health Professional Considerations See Local Anesthetic/Vasoconstrictor Precautions

◆ **Ogestrel [DSC]** *see* Ethinyl Estradiol and Norgestrel *on page 617*

◆ **Ogivri** *see* Trastuzumab *on page 1479*

◆ **Okebo [DSC]** *see* Doxycycline *on page 522*

OLANZapine (oh LAN za peen)

Brand Names: US ZyPREXA; ZyPREXA Relprevv; ZyPREXA Zydis

Brand Names: Canada ACT OLANZapine ODT; ACT OLANZapine [DSC]; AG-Olanzapine FC; APO-OLANZapine; APO-OLANZapine ODT; Auro-Olanzapine ODT; JAMP OLANZapine FC; JAMP OLANZapine ODT; Mar-OLANZapine ODT; Mar-OLANZapine [DSC]; Mint-Olanzapine; MINT-OLANZapine ODT; MYLAN-OLANZapine ODT [DSC]; MYLAN-OLANZapine [DSC]; PHL-OLANZapine ODT [DSC]; PHL-OLANZapine [DSC]; PMS-OLANZapine; PMS-OLANZapine ODT; RAN-OLANZapine; RAN-OLANZapine ODT; RIVA-OLANZapine; RIVA-OLANZapine ODT [DSC]; SANDOZ OLANZapine; SANDOZ OLANZapine ODT; TEVA-OLANZapine; TEVA-OLANZapine ODT [DSC]; VAN-OLANZapine [DSC]; ZyPREXA; ZyPREXA Zydis

Pharmacologic Category Antimanic Agent; Second Generation (Atypical) Antipsychotic

Use

Agitation/Aggression (acute) associated with psychiatric disorders (short-acting IM): Treatment of acute agitation associated with schizophrenia and bipolar I mania.

Bipolar disorder (oral): Treatment of acute manic or mixed episodes of bipolar I disorder (as monotherapy or in combination with lithium or valproate) and maintenance treatment; treatment of bipolar depression in combination with fluoxetine.

Major depressive disorder (unipolar), treatment resistant (oral): Treatment of treatment-resistant depression in combination with fluoxetine.

Schizophrenia (oral, ER IM): Treatment of the manifestations of schizophrenia.

Local Anesthetic/Vasoconstrictor Precautions Olanzapine (IM) is one of the drugs confirmed to prolong the QT interval and is accepted as having a risk of causing torsade de pointes. The risk of drug-induced torsade de pointes is extremely low when a single QT interval prolonging drug is prescribed. In terms of epinephrine, it is not known what effect vasoconstrictors in the local anesthetic regimen will have in patients with a known history of congenital prolonged QT interval or in patients taking any medication that prolongs the QT interval. Until more information is obtained, it is suggested that the clinician consult with the physician prior to the use of a vasoconstrictor in suspected patients and that the vasoconstrictor (epinephrine, mepivacaine, and levonordefrin [Carbocaine 2% with Neo-Cobefrin]) be used with caution.

Effects on Dental Treatment Key adverse event(s) related to dental treatment:

Oral: Patients may experience orthostatic hypotension as they stand up after treatment, especially if lying in dental chair for extended period of time. Use caution with sudden changes in position during and after treatment.

IM: Rare occurrence of facial edema, tongue edema, and tardive dyskinesia have been reported. Occurrence of tooth infection/toothache have also been reported.

Effects on Bleeding IM: Rare occurrence of thrombocytopenia has been reported.

Adverse Reactions

Oral:

>10%:

Cardiovascular: Orthostatic hypotension (3% to ≥20%)

Endocrine & metabolic: Increased serum prolactin (adolescents: 47%; adults: 30%), weight gain (adults: 5% to 6%; has been reported as high as 40%; adolescents: 29% to 31%)

Gastrointestinal: Constipation (adolescents and adults: 4% to 11%), dyspepsia (adults: 7% to 11%; adolescents: 3%), increased appetite (adolescents: 17% to 29%; adults: 3% to 6%), xerostomia (dose dependent; adults: 3% to 22%; adolescents: 4% to 7%)

Hepatic: Decreased serum bilirubin (adolescents: 22%), increased serum alanine aminotransferase (≥3 x ULN; adolescents and adults: 5% to 12%), increased serum aspartate aminotransferase (adolescents: 28%)

Nervous system: Akathisia (adolescents and adults: 3% to 27%), dizziness (adults: 11% to 18%; adolescents: 7% to 8%), drowsiness (dose dependent; adolescents and adults: 20% to 39%), extrapyramidal reaction (dose dependent; adults: ≤32%; adolescents: ≤10%), fatigue (dose dependent; adolescents and adults: 2% to 14%), headache (adolescents: 17%), insomnia (12%), parkinsonian-like syndrome (14% to 20%; includes akinesia, cogwheel rigidity, extrapyramidal syndrome, hypertonia, hypokinesia, masked facies, and tremor)

Neuromuscular & skeletal: Asthenia (dose dependent; 8% to 20%)

Miscellaneous: Accidental injury (12%)

1% to 10%:

Cardiovascular: Chest pain (3%), hypertension (2%), peripheral edema (3%), tachycardia (3%)

Endocrine & metabolic: Breast changes (male and female adolescents: ≤2%; including discharge, enlargement, galactorrhea, gynecomastia, lactation disorder), increased gamma-glutamyl transferase (adolescents: 10%; adults: 2%), increased uric acid (4%), menstrual disease (2%; including amenorrhea, delayed menstruation, hypomenorrhea, oligomenorrhea)

Gastrointestinal: Abdominal pain (adolescents: 6%), diarrhea (adolescents: 3%), vomiting (≤4%)

Genitourinary: Sexual disorder (2%; adolescents: ≤1%; anorgasmia, delayed ejaculation, erectile dysfunction, changes in libido, abnormal orgasm, sexual dysfunction), urinary incontinence (adults and older adults: ≥2%), urinary tract infection (2%)

Hematologic & oncologic: Bruise (5%)

Hepatic: Increased liver enzymes (adolescents: ≤8%), increased serum alkaline phosphatase (≥1%)

Nervous system: Abnormal gait (6%), articulation impairment (2%), falling (older adults: ≥2%), hypertonia (3%), personality disorder (5% to 8%), restlessness (adolescents: 3%)

Neuromuscular & skeletal: Arthralgia (adults: 5%; adolescents: 2%), back pain (5%), dyskinesia (1%), limb pain (adolescents and adults: 5% to 6%), muscle rigidity (adolescents: 2%), tremor (4% to 7%; dose dependent)

Ophthalmic: Amblyopia (3%)

Respiratory: Cough (6%), epistaxis (adolescents: 3%), nasopharyngitis (adolescents: 4%), pharyngitis (4%), respiratory tract infection (adolescents: 3%), rhinitis (7%), sinusitis (adolescents: 3%)

Miscellaneous: Fever (≤6%)

Injection: Adverse events are reported for extended release injection unless otherwise indicated.

>10%: Nervous system: Headache (13% to 18%), parkinsonism (14% to 20%; short-acting solution for IM injection: 3%), sedated state (8% to 13%)

1% to 10%:

Cardiovascular: Hypertension (2% to 3%), hypotension (short-acting solution for IM injection: 2%), orthostatic hypotension (short-acting solution for IM injection: 1%), prolonged QT interval on ECG (2%)

Dermatologic: Acne vulgaris (2%)

Endocrine & metabolic: Weight gain (6% to 7%)

Gastrointestinal: Abdominal pain (3%), diarrhea (5% to 7%), flatulence (1% to 2%), increased appetite (1% to 6%), nausea (long-acting IM formula: 4% to 5%; short-acting solution for injection: <1%), vomiting (6%), xerostomia (2% to 6%)

Genitourinary: Vaginal discharge (4%)

Hepatic: Increased liver enzymes (3% to 4%)

Infection: Viral infection (2%)

Local: Pain at injection site (both IM injection formulations: 1% to 4%)

Nervous system: Abnormal dreams (2%), abnormality in thinking (3%), akathisia (short-acting solution for IM injection: 5%), auditory hallucination (3%), dizziness (both IM injection formulations: 4%), drowsiness (both IM injection formulations: 5% to 6%), dysarthria (1% to 2%), extrapyramidal reaction (solution for IM injection: 2% to 4%), fatigue (3% to 4%), pain (2% to 3%), restlessness (3%), sleep disorder (2%)

Neuromuscular & skeletal: Arthralgia (3%), back pain (5%), muscle spasm (1% to 3%), stiffness (4%), tremor (long-acting IM formula: 3%; short-acting solution for injection: 1%)

Otic: Otalgia (4%)

Respiratory: Cough (9%), nasal congestion (7%), nasopharyngitis (3% to 6%), pharyngolaryngeal pain (3%), sneezing (2%), upper respiratory tract infection (3% to 4%)

Miscellaneous: Fever (2%)

<1%, postmarketing, and/or case reports: Abdominal distension, abscess at injection site, accommodation disturbance, agranulocytosis, alopecia, anaphylactoid reaction, angioedema, ataxia, cerebrovascular accident, chills, coma, confusion, delirium, diabetes mellitus, diabetic ketoacidosis, diabetic coma, difficulty in micturition, DRESS syndrome, dry eye syndrome, dysarthria, facial edema, hangover effect, heavy menstrual bleeding, hepatic injury (cholestatic or mixed), hepatitis, hyperbilirubinemia, hypercholesterolemia, hyperglycemia, hyperlipidemia, hypertriglyceridemia, hypoproteinemia, impotence, increased creatine phosphokinase in blood specimen, intestinal obstruction, jaundice, ketosis, leukocytosis (eosinophilia), leukopenia, liver steatosis, mastalgia, mydriasis, myopathy, nausea, neuroleptic malignant syndrome, neutropenia, osteoporosis, pancreatitis, polyuria, postinjection delirium/sedation syndrome, priapism, pruritus, pulmonary edema, pulmonary embolism, respiratory depression (Cole 2007), restless legs syndrome, rhabdomyolysis, seizure, sialorrhea, skin photosensitivity, skin rash, sleep apnea syndrome (obstructive) (Health Canada 2016; Shirani 2011), speech disturbance, stupor, suicidal tendencies, syncope, tardive dyskinesia, thrombocytopenia, tongue edema, transient ischemic attacks, urinary frequency, urinary retention, urinary urgency, urticaria, vasodilation, venous thrombosis, withdrawal syndrome

Mechanism of Action Olanzapine is a second generation thienobenzodiazepine antipsychotic which displays potent antagonism of serotonin 5-HT_{2A} and 5-HT_{2C}, dopamine D_{1-4}, histamine H_1, and alpha$_1$-adrenergic receptors. Olanzapine shows moderate antagonism of 5-HT_3 and muscarinic M_{1-5} receptors, and weak binding to GABA-A, BZD, and beta-adrenergic receptors. Although the precise mechanism of action in schizophrenia and bipolar disorder is not known, the efficacy of olanzapine is thought to be mediated through combined antagonism of dopamine and serotonin type 2 receptor sites.

Pharmacodynamics/Kinetics

Onset of Action Within 1 to 2 weeks for control of aggression, agitation, insomnia; 3 to 6 weeks for control of mania and positive psychotic symptoms. Adequate trial: Typically 6 weeks at maximum tolerated doses

Half-life Elimination

Oral and IM (short-acting): Children: (10 to 18 years; n=8): 37.2 ± 5.1 hours (Grothe 2000); Adults: 30 hours [21 to 54 hours (5th to 95th percentile)]; approximately 1.5 times greater in elderly

Extended-release injection: ~30 days

Time to Peak Maximum plasma concentrations after IM administration are 5 times higher than maximum plasma concentrations produced by an oral dose.

Extended-release injection: ~7 days

Short-acting injection: 15 to 45 minutes

Oral: Children (10 to 18 years; n=8): 4.7 ± 3.7 hours (Grothe 2000); Adults: ~6 hours

Reproductive Considerations

Olanzapine may cause hyperprolactinemia, which may decrease reproductive function in both males and females.

Olanzapine may be used if treatment with an atypical antipsychotic is needed in a woman planning a pregnancy (Larsen 2015).

Pregnancy Considerations

Olanzapine crosses the placenta and can be detected in cord blood at birth (Newport 2007; Schoretsanitis 2019).

Based on available data, an increased risk of major birth defects, miscarriage, or adverse maternal or fetal outcomes has not been observed following maternal use of olanzapine (Brunner 2013; Damkier 2018; Huybrechts 2016). Antipsychotic use during the third trimester of pregnancy has a risk for abnormal muscle movements (extrapyramidal symptoms) and/or withdrawal symptoms in newborns following delivery. Symptoms in the newborn may include agitation, feeding disorder, hypertonia, hypotonia, respiratory distress, somnolence, and tremor; these effects may be self-limiting or require hospitalization.

The pharmacokinetic properties of olanzapine are not significantly altered by pregnancy (Westin 2018); however, serum levels may change, even at a stable dose, possibly due to decreased CYP1A2 activity during the second and third trimesters (Stiegler 2014; Westin 2018). The ACOG recommends that therapy during pregnancy be individualized; treatment with psychiatric medications during pregnancy should incorporate the clinical expertise of the mental health clinician, obstetrician, primary health care provider, and pediatrician. Safety data related to atypical antipsychotics during pregnancy are limited, as such, routine use is not recommended. However, if a woman is inadvertently exposed to an atypical antipsychotic while pregnant, continuing therapy may be preferable to switching to an agent that the fetus has not yet been exposed to; consider risk:benefit (ACOG 2008). If treatment is initiated during pregnancy, olanzapine may be used (Larsen 2015). The potential for excessive maternal weight gain and the development of gestational diabetes associated with olanzapine therapy should be considered (Damkier 2018).

Health care providers are encouraged to enroll women 18 to 45 years of age exposed to olanzapine during pregnancy in the Atypical Antipsychotics Pregnancy Registry (1-866-961-2388 or https://www.womensmentalhealth.org/pregnancyregistry).

◆ **Olanzapine Pamoate** *see* OLANZapine *on page* 1127

Olaparib (oh LAP a rib)

Brand Names: US Lynparza

Brand Names: Canada Lynparza

Pharmacologic Category Antineoplastic Agent, PARP Inhibitor

Use

Breast cancer, metastatic (BRCA-mutated, HER2-negative): Tablets: Treatment of deleterious or suspected deleterious germline BRCA-mutated (gBRCAm), HER2-negative metastatic breast cancer in adults who have been treated with chemotherapy in the neoadjuvant, adjuvant, or metastatic setting; patients with hormone receptor-positive disease should have received a prior endocrine therapy or be considered inappropriate for endocrine therapy (select patients for therapy based on an approved olaparib companion diagnostic test for gBRCA1m or gBRCA2m in blood specimen).

Ovarian cancer, advanced (BRCA-mutated): Tablets, capsules: Treatment of deleterious or suspected deleterious gBRCAm advanced ovarian cancer in adults who have been treated with 3 or more prior lines of chemotherapy (select patients for therapy based on an approved olaparib companion diagnostic test for gBRCA1m or gBRCA2m in blood specimen).

Ovarian cancer, advanced (BRCA-mutated), first-line maintenance therapy: Tablets: First-line maintenance treatment (as monotherapy) of deleterious or suspected deleterious germline or somatic BRCA-mutated advanced epithelial ovarian, fallopian tube, or primary peritoneal cancer in adults who are in complete or partial response to first-line, platinum-based chemotherapy (select patients for therapy based on an approved olaparib companion diagnostic test for BRCA1m or BRCA2m in tumor or blood specimen).

Ovarian cancer, advanced (homologous recombination deficient-positive), first-line maintenance therapy: Tablets: First-line maintenance treatment (in combination with bevacizumab) of advanced epithelial ovarian, fallopian tube, or primary peritoneal cancer in adults who are in complete or partial response to first-line, platinum-based chemotherapy and whose cancer is associated with homologous recombination deficiency (HRD)-positive status, defined by either a deleterious or suspected deleterious BRCA mutation and/or genomic instability (select patients for therapy based on an approved olaparib companion diagnostic test for BRCA1m, BRCA2m, and/or genomic instability in tumor specimen).

Ovarian cancer, recurrent (maintenance therapy): Tablets: Maintenance treatment of recurrent epithelial ovarian, fallopian tube, or primary peritoneal cancer in adults who are in complete or partial response to platinum-based chemotherapy.

Pancreatic cancer, metastatic (BRCA-mutated), first-line maintenance therapy: Tablets: First-line maintenance treatment of deleterious or suspected deleterious gBRCAm metastatic pancreatic adenocarcinoma in adults whose disease has not progressed on at least 16 weeks of a first-line, platinum-based chemotherapy regimen (select patients for therapy based on an approved olaparib companion diagnostic test for gBRCA1m or gBRCA2m in blood specimen).

Prostate cancer, metastatic, castration-resistant (homologous recombination repair gene-mutated): Tablets: Treatment of deleterious or suspected deleterious germline or somatic homologous recombination repair (HRR) gene-mutated metastatic castration-resistant prostate cancer in adults who have progressed following prior enzalutamide or abiraterone treatment (select patients for therapy based on an approved olaparib companion diagnostic test for ATMm, BRCA1m, BRCA2m, BARD1m, BRIP1m, CDK12m, CHEK1m, CHEK2m, FANCLm, PALB2m, RAD51Bm, RAD51Cm, RAD51Dm, or RAD54Lm in tumor specimen, or for gBRCA1m or gBRCA2m in blood specimen).

Local Anesthetic/Vasoconstrictor Precautions No information available to require special precautions

Effects on Dental Treatment No significant effects or complications reported

Effects on Bleeding Chemotherapy may result in significant myelosuppression, potentially including reduction in platelet counts (thrombocytopenia) and altered hemostasis. In patients who are under active treatment with this agent, medical consult is suggested.

Adverse Reactions

>10%:

Cardiovascular: Peripheral edema (14%)

Dermatologic: Skin rash (5% to 15%)

Endocrine & metabolic: Hypomagnesemia (5% to 14%)

Gastrointestinal: Nausea (45% to 77%), abdominal pain (45%), vomiting (20% to 43%), diarrhea (21% to 37%), constipation (16% to 28%), dysgeusia (9% to 27%), decreased appetite (16% to 25%), dyspepsia (5% to 25%), stomatitis (4% to 20%; grades 3/4: 1%)

Genitourinary: Urinary tract infection (13% to 14%)

Hematologic & oncologic: Increased MCV (57% to 89%), anemia (23% to 44%; grades 3/4: 7% to 21%), neutropenia (5% to 27%; grades 3/4: 4% to 9%), leukopenia (2% to 25%; grades 3/4: 3% to 5%), thrombocytopenia (4% to 14%; grades 3/4: 1% to 3%)

Infection: Influenza (≤36%)

Nervous system: Fatigue (≤67%), headache (7% to 26%), dizziness (7% to 20%)

Neuromuscular & skeletal: Asthenia (≤66%), arthralgia (≤30%), myalgia (≤30%), musculoskeletal pain (≤21%), back pain (14% to 19%)

Renal: Increased serum creatinine (3% to 99%)

Respiratory: Nasopharyngitis (≤36%), respiratory tract infection (≤36%), rhinitis (≤36%), sinusitis (≤36%), bronchitis (≤28%), cough (9% to 18%), dyspnea (13% to 15%)

1% to 10%:

Cardiovascular: Edema (8% to 9%), pulmonary embolism (≤1%), venous thrombosis (≤1%)

Dermatologic: Dermatitis (1%)

Gastrointestinal: Upper abdominal pain (7%)

Hematologic & oncologic: Myeloid leukemia (acute: 12%), lymphocytopenia (1% to 8%), myelodysplastic syndrome (≤1%)

Hypersensitivity: Hypersensitivity reaction (2%)

Nervous system: Peripheral neuropathy (5%), depression, insomnia

Miscellaneous: Fever (8% to 10%)

<1%, postmarketing, and/or case reports: Pneumonitis

Mechanism of Action Olaparib is a poly (ADP-ribose) polymerase (PARP) enzyme inhibitor, including PARP1, PARP2, and PARP3. PARP enzymes are involved in DNA transcription, cell cycle regulation, and DNA repair. Olaparib is a potent oral PARP inhibitor which induces synthetic lethality in BRCA1/2 deficient tumor cells through the formation of double-stranded DNA breaks which cannot be accurately repaired, which leads to disruption of cellular homeostasis and cell death (Ledermann 2012).

Pharmacodynamics/Kinetics

Half-life Elimination Tablet: 14.9 ± 8.2 hours; Capsule: Terminal: 11.9 ± 4.8 hours

Time to Peak Tablet: 1.5 hours; Capsule: 1 to 3 hours.

Reproductive Considerations

Pregnancy testing is recommended prior to treatment initiation in females of reproductive potential. Females of reproductive potential should use highly effective contraception during therapy and for at least 6 months after the last olaparib dose. Males with female partners of reproductive potential or female partners who are pregnant should use effective contraception during treatment and for 3 months after the last olaparib dose; male patients also should not donate sperm during therapy and for 3 months following the last olaparib dose.

Pregnancy Considerations

Based on the mechanism of action, and data from animal reproduction studies, in utero exposure to olaparib may cause fetal harm.

Product Availability Lynparza **capsules** are being permanently discontinued by the US manufacturer as of August 31, 2018. Lynparza **tablets** remain available.

Prescribing and Access Restrictions Olaparib is available through the authorized specialty pharmacy providers. For further information on patient assistance, product availability, and prescribing instructions, please refer to the following website: https://providerportal.-myaccess360.com or call 1-844-275-2360.

Olaratumab (oh lar AT ue mab)

Brand Names: US Lartruvo

Brand Names: Canada Lartruvo

Pharmacologic Category Antineoplastic Agent, Monoclonal Antibody; Antineoplastic Agent, PDGFR-alpha Blocker

Use

Soft tissue sarcoma: Treatment (in combination with doxorubicin) of adults with soft tissue sarcoma (STS) with a histologic subtype for which an anthracycline-containing regimen is appropriate and which is not amenable to curative treatment with radiotherapy or surgery.

Note: A confirmatory phase 3 randomized, blinded trial in patients with unresectable locally advanced or metastatic STS comparing olaratumab plus doxorubicin to placebo plus doxorubicin found no significant difference in overall survival due to the addition of olaratumab to doxorubicin (Tap 2020). Due to the trial results, the manufacturer has withdrawn olaratumab from the market.

Local Anesthetic/Vasoconstrictor Precautions

No information available to require special precautions

Effects on Dental Treatment Key adverse event(s) related to dental treatment: Mucositis

Effects on Bleeding Chemotherapy may result in significant myelosuppression. Higher incidence of grades 3 and 4 lymphopenia and neutropenia has been reported with olaratumab in combination with doxorubicin. Thrombocytopenia (all grades) also has a higher incidence.

Adverse Reactions

>10%:

Central nervous system: Fatigue (69%), neuropathy (22%), headache (20%), anxiety (11%)

Dermatologic: Alopecia (52%)

Endocrine & metabolic: Hyperglycemia (52%), hypokalemia (21%), hypophosphatemia (21%), hypomagnesemia (16%)

Gastrointestinal: Nausea (73%), mucositis (53%), vomiting (45%), diarrhea (34%), decreased appetite (31%), abdominal pain (23%)

Hematologic & oncologic: Lymphocytopenia (77%, grades 3/4: 44%), neutropenia (65%, grades 3/4: 48%), thrombocytopenia (63%, grades 3/4: 6%), prolonged partial thromboplastin time (33%, grades 3/4: 5%)

Hepatic: Increased serum alkaline phosphatase (16%)

Neuromuscular & skeletal: Musculoskeletal pain (64%)

Ophthalmic: Xerophthalmia (11%)

Miscellaneous: Infusion related reaction (13% to 14%)

1% to 10%: Immunologic: Development of IgG antibodies (4%; all patients had neutralizing antibodies; however, therapeutic effects of antibodies could not be assessed)

Mechanism of Action Olaratumab is a human (recombinant) IgG1 antibody which expressly binds to platelet-derived growth receptor alpha (PDGFR-α) to prevent binding of PDGF-AA, PDGF-BB, and PDGF-CC and block receptor activation and disrupt PDGF receptor signaling. The PDGF-alpha receptor has a role in cell differentiation, growth, and angiogenesis and has demonstrated antitumor activity in sarcomas (Tap 2016).

Pharmacodynamics/Kinetics

Half-life Elimination ~11 days (range: 6 to 24 days)

Reproductive Considerations

Females of reproductive potential should use effective contraception during therapy and for at least 3 months after the last olaratumab dose.

Pregnancy Considerations

Based on its mechanism of action, olaratumab would be expected to cause fetal harm if administered to a pregnant woman.

Prescribing and Access Restrictions Following the withdrawal of olaratumab from the global market in April 2019, patients receiving olaratumab prior to the market withdrawal may be eligible for continued access to therapy. For additional information, contact The Lilly Answers Center 1-800-LILLYRX (1-800-545-5979) or by emailing lartruvopatientaccessprogram@lilly.com (**Note:** May take up to 48 hours for a response).

◆ **Oleovitamin A** *see* Vitamin A *on page 1549*

Olmesartan (ole me SAR tan)

Related Information

Cardiovascular Diseases *on page 1654*

Brand Names: US Benicar

Brand Names: Canada ACH-Olmesartan; ACT Olmesartan; AG-Olmesartan; APO-Olmesartan; Auro-Olmesartan; GLN-Olmesartan; JAMP-Olmesartan; Olmetec; PMS-Olmesartan; RIVA-Olmesartan [DSC]; SANDOZ Olmesartan

Pharmacologic Category Angiotensin II Receptor Blocker; Antihypertensive

Use

Hypertension: Management of hypertension in adults and pediatric patients ≥6 years of age.

Local Anesthetic/Vasoconstrictor Precautions No information available to require special precautions

Effects on Dental Treatment Key adverse event(s) related to dental treatment: Patients may experience orthostatic hypotension as they stand up after treatment; especially if lying in dental chair for extended periods of time. Use caution with sudden changes in position during and after dental treatment.

Effects on Bleeding No information available to require special precautions

Adverse Reactions

1% to 10%:

Central nervous system: Dizziness (3%), headache (>1%)

Endocrine & metabolic: Hyperglycemia (>1%), hypertriglyceridemia (>1%)

Gastrointestinal: Diarrhea (>1%; may be severe and chronic)

Genitourinary: Hematuria (>1%)

Neuromuscular & skeletal: Back pain (>1%), increased creatine phosphokinase (>1%)

Respiratory: Bronchitis (>1%), flu-like symptoms (>1%), pharyngitis (>1%), rhinitis (>1%), sinusitis (>1%)

Frequency not defined: Hematologic & oncologic: Decreased hematocrit, decreased hemoglobin

<1%, postmarketing, and/or case reports: Abdominal pain, acute renal failure, alopecia, anaphylaxis, angioedema, arthralgia, arthritis, asthenia, chest pain, dyspepsia, facial edema, gastroenteritis, hypercholesterolemia, hyperkalemia, hyperlipidemia, hyperuricemia, increased liver enzymes, increased serum bilirubin, increased serum creatinine, myalgia, nausea, peripheral edema, pruritus, rhabdomyolysis, skin rash, sprue-like symptoms, tachycardia, urticaria, vertigo, vomiting

Mechanism of Action As a selective and competitive, nonpeptide angiotensin II receptor antagonist, olmesartan blocks the vasoconstrictor and aldosterone-secreting effects of angiotensin II; olmesartan interacts reversibly at the AT1 and AT2 receptors of many tissues and has slow dissociation kinetics; its affinity for the AT1 receptor is 12,500 times greater than the AT2 receptor. Angiotensin II receptor antagonists may induce a more complete inhibition of the renin-angiotensin system than ACE inhibitors, they do not affect the response to bradykinin, and are less likely to be associated with non-renin-angiotensin effects (eg, cough and angioedema). Olmesartan increases urinary flow rate and, in addition to being natriuretic and kaliuretic, increases excretion of chloride, magnesium, uric acid, calcium, and phosphate.

Pharmacodynamics/Kinetics

Half-life Elimination Terminal: 13 hours

Time to Peak 1 to 2 hours

Reproductive Considerations

The use of angiotensin II receptor blockers should generally be avoided in women planning a pregnancy (ACOG 203 2019).

Pregnancy Considerations

[US Boxed Warning]: Drugs that act on the renin-angiotensin system can cause injury and death to the developing fetus. When pregnancy is detected, discontinue as soon as possible. The use of drugs which act on the renin-angiotensin system are associated with oligohydramnios. Oligohydramnios, due to decreased fetal renal function, may lead to fetal lung hypoplasia and skeletal malformations. Oligohydramnios may not appear until after irreversible fetal injury has occurred. Use in pregnancy is also associated with anuria, hypotension, renal failure, skull hypoplasia, and death in the fetus/neonate. The exposed fetus should be monitored for fetal growth, amniotic fluid volume, and organ formation. Infants exposed in utero should be monitored for hyperkalemia, hypotension, and oliguria (exchange transfusions or dialysis may be needed). These adverse events are generally associated with maternal use in the second and third trimesters.

Chronic maternal hypertension itself is also associated with adverse events in the fetus/infant. The risk of birth defects, low birth weight, premature delivery, stillbirth, and neonatal death may be increased with chronic hypertension in pregnancy. Actual risks may be related to duration and severity of maternal hypertension (ACOG 203 2019).

The use of angiotensin II receptor blockers is generally not recommended to treat chronic hypertension in pregnant women (ACOG 203 2019).

- ◆ **Olmesartan and Amlodipine** *see* Amlodipine and Olmesartan *on page 122*
- ◆ **Olmesartan Medoxomil** *see* Olmesartan *on page 1131*
- ◆ **Olmesartan Medoxomil and Amlodipine Besylate** *see* Amlodipine and Olmesartan *on page 122*
- ◆ **Olodaterol and Tiotropium** *see* Tiotropium and Olodaterol *on page 1451*

Olopatadine (Nasal) (oh la PAT a deen)

Brand Names: US Patanase

Pharmacologic Category Histamine H_1 Antagonist; Histamine H_1 Antagonist, Second Generation; Piperidine Derivative

Use Treatment of the symptoms of seasonal allergic rhinitis

Local Anesthetic/Vasoconstrictor Precautions No information available to require special precautions

Effects on Dental Treatment Key adverse event(s) related to dental treatment: Taste perversion.

Effects on Bleeding No information available to require special precautions

Adverse Reactions

>10%:

Central nervous system: Bitter taste (13%; children: 1%)

Respiratory: Epistaxis (3% to 25%)

1% to 10%:

Central nervous system: Depression (2%), drowsiness (1%), fatigue (1%)

Dermatologic: Skin rash (children: 1%)

Endocrine & metabolic: Weight gain (1%)

Gastrointestinal: Xerostomia (1%)

Genitourinary: Urinary tract infection (1%)

Infection: Influenza (1%)

Neuromuscular & skeletal: Increased creatine phosphokinase (1%)

Respiratory: Nasal mucosa ulcer (9% to 10%), upper respiratory tract infection (children: 3%), pharyngolaryngeal pain (2%), post nasal drip (2%), cough (1%), throat irritation (1%)

<1%, postmarketing, and/or case reports: Altered sense of smell, anosmia, dizziness, dysgeusia, nasal discomfort, oropharyngeal pain

Mechanism of Action Selective histamine H_1-antagonist; inhibits release of histamine from mast cells.

Pharmacodynamics/Kinetics

Onset of Action 30 minutes in seasonal allergy patients

Half-life Elimination 8-12 hours

Time to Peak Serum: 15 minutes to 2 hours

Pregnancy Risk Factor C

Pregnancy Considerations

Other agents may be preferred for the treatment of allergic rhinitis in pregnant women (BSACI [Scadding 2017]).

- ◆ **Olopatadine HCl** *see* Olopatadine (Nasal) *on page 1132*
- ◆ **Olopatadine Hydrochloride** *see* Olopatadine (Nasal) *on page 1132*
- ◆ **Olumiant** *see* Baricitinib *on page 215*
- ◆ **Olux** *see* Clobetasol *on page 377*
- ◆ **Olux-E** *see* Clobetasol *on page 377*
- ◆ **Olysio [DSC]** *see* Simeprevir *on page 1372*

Omacetaxine (oh ma se TAX een)

Brand Names: US Synribo

Pharmacologic Category Antineoplastic Agent, Cephalotaxine; Antineoplastic Agent, Protein Synthesis Inhibitor

Use Chronic myeloid leukemia: Treatment of chronic or accelerated phase chronic myeloid leukemia (CML) in adult patients resistant and/or intolerant to 2 or more tyrosine kinase inhibitors

Local Anesthetic/Vasoconstrictor Precautions

Use vasoconstrictor with caution; patients may experience tachycardia and palpitations when taking omacetaxine

Effects on Dental Treatment Key adverse event(s) related to dental treatment: Abnormal taste, aphthous stomatitis, gingival bleeding, gingival pain, gingivitis, mouth ulceration, mouth hemorrhage, mucosal inflammation, oral pain, stomatitis, and xerostomia (normal salivary flow resumes upon discontinuation) have been reported.

Effects on Bleeding Chemotherapy may result in significant myelosuppression, potentially including significant reduction in platelet counts. Thrombocytopenia has been reported (grades 3/4: 49% to 88%). Gingival and GI bleeding have been reported. In patients who are under active treatment with these agents, medical consult is suggested.

Adverse Reactions

>10%:

Cardiovascular: Peripheral edema (16%)

Central nervous system: Fatigue (29% to 31%), headache (13% to 20%), chills (13%), insomnia (12%)

Dermatologic: Alopecia (15%), skin rash (11%)

Endocrine & metabolic: Increased uric acid (grades 3/4: 56% to 57%), hyperglycemia (grades 3/4: 10% to 15%; hyperosmolar nonketotic hyperglycemia <1%)

Gastrointestinal: Diarrhea (35% to 41%), nausea (29% to 35%), abdominal pain (16% to 23%), vomiting (12% to 15%), constipation (14%), anorexia (10% to 13%)

Hematologic & oncologic: Thrombocytopenia (58% to 76%; grades 3/4: 49% to 88%), neutropenia (20% to 53%; grades 3/4: 18% to 81%), anemia (51% to 61%; grades 3/4: 36% to 80%), leukocyte disorder (decreased: grades 3/4: 61% to 72%), febrile neutropenia (10% to 20%; grades 3/4: 10% to 16%), lymphocytopenia (17%; grades 3/4: 16%)

Infection: Infection (46% to 56%; grades 3/4: 11% to 20%)

Local: Injection site reaction (22% to 35%; includes edema, erythema, hematoma, hemorrhage, hypersensitivity, induration, inflammation, infusion related reaction, irritation, mass, pruritus, rash)

Neuromuscular & skeletal: Weakness (23% to 24%), arthralgia (19%), limb pain (11% to 13%), back pain (12%), myalgia (11%)

Renal: Increased serum creatinine (grades 3/4: 9% to 16%)

Respiratory: Epistaxis (11% to 17%), cough (≤16%), dyspnea (11%)

Miscellaneous: Fever (25% to 29%)

1% to 10%:

Cardiovascular: Acute coronary syndrome, angina pectoris, bradycardia, cardiac arrhythmia, chest pain, edema, hypertension, hypotension, palpitations, tachycardia, ventricular premature contractions

Central nervous system: Agitation, anxiety, cerebral hemorrhage, confusion, depression, dizziness, hyperthermia, hypoesthesia, lethargy, malaise, mental status changes, mouth pain, myasthenia, pain, paresthesia, sciatica, seizure, voice disorder

Dermatologic: Burning sensation of skin, dermal ulcer, desquamation, erythema, hyperhidrosis, hyperpigmentation, night sweats, pruritus, skin lesion, xeroderma

Endocrine & metabolic: Decreased serum glucose (grades 3/4: 6% to 8%), dehydration, diabetes mellitus, gout, hot flash

Gastrointestinal: Abdominal distention, anal fissure, aphthous stomatitis, decreased appetite, dysgeusia, dyspepsia, dysphagia, gastritis, gastroesophageal reflux disease, gastrointestinal hemorrhage, gingival hemorrhage, gingival pain, gingivitis, hemorrhoids, melena, mucosal inflammation, oral mucosa ulcer, stomatitis, xerostomia

Genitourinary: Dysuria

Hematologic & oncologic: Bone marrow failure (10%; grades 3/4: 10%), bruise, hematoma, hemorrhage (ear), oral hemorrhage, petechia, purpura

Hepatic: Increased serum bilirubin (grades 3/4: 6% to 9%), increased serum ALT (grades 3/4: 2% to 6%)

Hypersensitivity: Hypersensitivity reaction, transfusion reaction

Neuromuscular & skeletal: Muscle spasm, musculoskeletal chest pain, musculoskeletal pain (or discomfort), ostealgia, stiffness, tremor

Ophthalmic: Blurred vision, cataract, conjunctival hemorrhage, conjunctivitis, diplopia, eyelid edema, eye pain, increased lacrimation, xerophthalmia

Otic: Otalgia, tinnitus

Respiratory: Flu-like symptoms, hemoptysis, nasal congestion, pharyngolaryngeal pain, rales, rhinorrhea, sinus congestion

Mechanism of Action Omacetaxine is a reversible protein synthesis inhibitor which binds to the A-site cleft of the ribosomal subunit to interfere with chain elongation and inhibit protein synthesis. It acts independently of BCR-ABL1 kinase-binding activity, and has demonstrated activity against tyrosine kinase inhibitor-resistant BCR-ABL mutations.

Pharmacodynamics/Kinetics

Onset of Action

Chronic phase CML: Mean time to major cytogenetic response: 3.5 months

Accelerated phase CML: Mean time to response: 2.3 months

Duration of Action

Chronic phase CML: Median duration of major cytogenetic response: 12.5 months

Accelerated phase CML: Median duration of major hematologic response: 4.7 months

Half-life Elimination 14.6 hours

Time to Peak SubQ: ~30 minutes

Reproductive Considerations

Evaluate pregnancy status prior to use in females of reproductive potential. Females of reproductive potential should use effective contraception during therapy and for 6 months after the last omacetaxine dose. Males with female partners of reproductive potential should use effective contraception during therapy and for 3 months after the last dose of omacetaxine.

Pregnancy Considerations

Based on the mechanism of action and data from animal reproduction studies, omacetaxine may cause fetal harm if administered during pregnancy.

◆ **Omacetaxine Mepesuccinate** *see* Omacetaxine *on page 1133*

Omadacycline (oh MAD a SYE kleen)

Brand Names: US Nuzyra

Pharmacologic Category Antibiotic, Tetracycline Derivative

Use

Pneumonia, community-acquired: Treatment of community-acquired bacterial pneumonia (CABP) in adult patients caused by susceptible *Streptococcus pneumoniae*, *Staphylococcus aureus* (methicillin-susceptible isolates), *Haemophilus influenzae*, *H. parainfluenzae*, *Klebsiella pneumoniae*, *Legionella pneumophila*, *Mycoplasma pneumoniae*, and *Chlamydophila pneumoniae*.

Skin and skin structure infections: Treatment of acute bacterial skin and skin structure infections (ABSSSI) in adult patients caused by susceptible *Staphylococcus aureus* (methicillin-susceptible and -resistant isolates), *Staphylococcus lugdunensis*, *Streptococcus pyogenes*, *Streptococcus anginosus* grp. (includes *S. anginosus*, *S. intermedius*, and *S. constellatus*), *Enterococcus faecalis*, *Enterobacter cloacae*, and *Klebsiella pneumoniae*.

Local Anesthetic/Vasoconstrictor Precautions No information available to require special precautions

Effects on Dental Treatment Key adverse event(s) related to dental treatment: Although omadacycline is a member of the tetracyline family, there is no dental indication for it. Therefore, the concerns of tetracycline in dental patients relative to enamel incorporation in pediatrics are not applicable to omadacycline. Superinfection: Use may result in fungal or bacterial superinfection in the oral cavity.

Effects on Bleeding No information available to require special precautions

Adverse Reactions

>10%: Gastrointestinal: Nausea (2% to 22%), vomiting (3% to 11%)

1% to 10%:

Cardiovascular: Hypertension (3%), insomnia (3%), atrial fibrillation (<2%), tachycardia (<2%)

Central nervous system: Headache (2% to 3%), fatigue (<2%), lethargy (<2%), vertigo (<2%)

Dermatologic: Erythema (<2%), hyperhidrosis (<2%), pruritus (<2%), urticaria (<2%)

Endocrine & metabolic: Increased gamma-glutamyl transferase (3%)

Gastrointestinal: Diarrhea (3%), constipation (2%), abdominal pain (<2%), dysgeusia (<2%), dyspepsia (<2%), increased serum lipase (<2%), oral candidiasis (<2%)

Genitourinary: Vulvovaginal candidiasis (<2%)

Hematologic & oncologic: Anemia (<2%), thrombocythemia (<2%)

Hepatic: Increased serum alanine aminotransferase (4%), increased serum aspartate aminotransferase (2% to 4%), increased serum alkaline phosphatase (<2%), increased serum bilirubin (<2%)

Hypersensitivity: Hypersensitivity reaction (<2%)

Local: Infusion site reaction (5%)

Neuromuscular & skeletal: Increased creatine phosphokinase (<2%)

Respiratory: Oropharyngeal pain (<2%)

Mechanism of Action Omadacycline inhibits protein synthesis by binding with the 30S ribosomal subunit of susceptible bacteria.

Pharmacodynamics/Kinetics

Half-life Elimination IV: ~16 hours; Oral: 13.45 to 16.83 hours

Time to Peak IV: ~0.5 hours; Oral: 2.5 hours

Reproductive Considerations

Due to the potential for adverse pregnancy outcomes, the manufacturer recommends effective contraception for females of reproductive potential during omadacycline therapy.

Pregnancy Considerations

Tetracyclines accumulate in developing teeth and long tubular bones. Permanent discoloration of teeth (yellow, gray, brown) can occur following in utero exposure and is more likely to occur in the second or third trimesters and following long-term or repeated exposure. Reversible inhibition of bone growth may occur following maternal use of tetracyclines in the second and third trimesters.

◆ **Omadacycline Tosylate** *see* Omadacycline *on page 1134*

Omalizumab (oh mah lye ZOO mab)

Related Information

Respiratory Diseases *on page 1680*

Brand Names: US Xolair

Brand Names: Canada Xolair

Pharmacologic Category Monoclonal Antibody, Anti-Asthmatic

Use

Asthma: Treatment of moderate to severe persistent asthma in adults and patients 6 years and older who have a positive skin test or *in vitro* reactivity to a perennial aeroallergen and whose symptoms are inadequately controlled with inhaled corticosteroids.

Limitations of use: Not indicated for acute bronchospasm or status asthmaticus.

Chronic idiopathic urticaria: Treatment of chronic idiopathic urticaria in adults and adolescents 12 years and older who remain symptomatic despite H_1 antihistamine treatment.

Limitations of use: Not indicated for other allergic conditions or other forms of urticaria.

Local Anesthetic/Vasoconstrictor Precautions No information available to require special precautions

Effects on Dental Treatment No significant effects or complications reported

Effects on Bleeding No information available to require special precautions

Adverse Reactions Incidences reported in children and adults unless otherwise noted.

>10%:

Central nervous system: Headache (6% to 12%; children: ≥3%)

Local: Injection site reaction (asthma: 45%, severe 12%; chronic idiopathic urticaria: 3%; may include bleeding, bruising, burning, erythema, induration, inflammation, mass, pain, pruritus, stinging, swelling, warmth, urticaria)

1% to 10%:

Cardiovascular: Peripheral edema (≥2%)

Central nervous system: Pain (7%), dizziness (3%), fatigue (3%), anxiety (≥2%), migraine (≥2%)

Dermatologic: Alopecia (≥2%), urticaria (chronic idiopathic urticaria: ≥2%, asthma: <1%), dermatitis (2%), pruritus (2%)

Gastrointestinal: Upper abdominal pain (children: ≥3%), viral gastroenteritis (children: ≥3%), toothache (≥2%)

Genitourinary: Urinary tract infection (≥2%)

Infection: Fungal infection (≥2%)

Neuromuscular & skeletal: Arthralgia (3% to 8%), limb pain (2% to 4%), musculoskeletal pain (≥2%), myalgia (≥2%), bone fracture (2%)

Otic: Otitis media (children: ≥3%), otalgia (2%)

Respiratory: Nasopharyngitis (9%; children: ≥3%), sinusitis (5%), epistaxis (children: ≥3%), streptococcal pharyngitis (≥3%), upper respiratory tract infection (3%), asthma (≥2%), oropharyngeal pain (≥2%), sinus headache (≥2%), cough (2%), viral upper respiratory tract infection (≤2%)

Miscellaneous: Fever (≥2%)

<1%, postmarketing, and/or case reports: Anaphylaxis, angioedema, antibody development, arthritis, bronchospasm, chest tightness, decreased serum immunoglobulins (free IgE), dyspnea, eosinophilia, eosinophilic granulomatosis with polyangiitis, hypotension, increased serum immunoglobulin (total IgE), lymphadenopathy, malignant neoplasm, pharyngeal edema, serum sickness, severe thrombocytopenia, skin rash, swollen tongue, syncope, vasculitis

Mechanism of Action

Asthma: Omalizumab is an IgG monoclonal antibody (recombinant DNA derived) which inhibits IgE binding to the high-affinity IgE receptor on mast cells and basophils. By decreasing bound IgE, the activation and release of mediators in the allergic response (early and late phase) is limited. Serum free IgE levels and the number of high-affinity IgE receptors are decreased. Long-term treatment in patients with allergic asthma showed a decrease in asthma exacerbations and corticosteroid usage.

Chronic idiopathic urticaria: Omalizumab binds to IgE and lowers free IgE levels. Subsequently, IgE receptors (FcεRI) on cells down-regulate. The mechanism by which these effects of omalizumab result in an improvement of chronic idiopathic urticaria symptoms is unknown.

Pharmacodynamics/Kinetics

Onset of Action Response to therapy: ~12 to 16 weeks (87% of patients had measurable response in 12 weeks)

Half-life Elimination 26 days (asthma patients); 24 days (chronic idiopathic urticaria patients)

Time to Peak 7-8 days

Pregnancy Considerations

Omalizumab is a humanized monoclonal antibody (IgG_1). Placental transfer of human IgG is dependent upon the IgG subclass, maternal serum concentrations, newborn birth weight, and gestational age, generally increasing as pregnancy progresses. The lowest exposure would be expected during the period of organogenesis (Palmeira 2012; Pentsuk 2009).

Information related to the use of omalizumab in pregnancy is available from case reports of women with severe asthma (Kupryś-Lipińska 2014) or chronic idiopathic urticaria (some also with asthma) (Cuervo-Pardo 2016; Ensina 2017; Ghazanfar 2015; González-Medina 2017). In addition, information from the Xolair Pregnancy Registry (EXPECT) is available. Based on data collected from 250 women between 2006 and 2018, the incidence of major congenital malformations was not increased when compared to pregnant females with asthma not treated with omalizumab. The risk of low birth weight infants was increased; however, more severe asthma in the females taking omalizumab may also have contributed.

Uncontrolled asthma is associated with adverse events on pregnancy (increased risk of perinatal mortality, preeclampsia, preterm birth, low-birth-weight infants, cesarean delivery, and the development of gestational diabetes). Poorly controlled asthma or asthma exacerbations may have a greater fetal/maternal risk than what is associated with appropriately used asthma medications. Maternal treatment improves pregnancy outcomes by reducing the risk of some adverse events (eg, preterm birth, gestational diabetes). Maternal asthma symptoms should be monitored monthly during pregnancy (ERS/TSANZ [Middleton 2020]; GINA 2020).

Use of omalizumab in pregnancy may be considered when conventional therapies are insufficient (ERS/TSANZ [Middleton 2020]).

Data collection to monitor pregnancy and infant outcomes associated with asthma and the medications used to treat asthma in pregnancy is ongoing. Health care providers are encouraged to enroll exposed pregnant females in the MotherToBaby Pregnancy Studies conducted by the Organization of Teratology Information Specialists (OTIS) (877-311-8972 or http://mothertobaby.org). Patients may also enroll themselves.

Ombitasvir, Paritaprevir, and Ritonavir

(om BIT as vir, par i TA pre vir, & ri TOE na vir)

Brand Names: US Technivie

Brand Names: Canada Technivie [DSC]

Pharmacologic Category Antihepaciviral, NS3/4A Protease Inhibitor (Anti-HCV); Antihepaciviral, NS5A Inhibitor; Cytochrome P-450 Inhibitor; NS3/4A Inhibitor; NS5A Inhibitor

Use Chronic hepatitis C: Treatment of chronic hepatitis C virus (HCV) genotype 4 infection without cirrhosis or with compensated cirrhosis, in combination with ribavirin.

Local Anesthetic/Vasoconstrictor Precautions No information available to require special precautions

Effects on Dental Treatment No significant effects or complications reported

Effects on Bleeding No information available to require special precautions

Adverse Reactions

>10%: Neuromuscular & skeletal: Asthenia (25%)

1% to 10%:

Central nervous system: Fatigue (7%), insomnia (5%)

Dermatologic: Allergic skin reaction (5%), pruritus (5%)

Gastrointestinal: Nausea (9%)

Frequency not defined:

Hematologic & oncologic: Anemia, decreased hemoglobin

Hepatic: Increased serum alanine aminotransferase

<1%, postmarketing, and/or case reports: Anaphylaxis, erythema multiforme, hepatic failure (in patients with underlying cirrhosis; FDA Safety Alert, October 22, 2015), hypersensitivity reaction (including angioedema), liver decompensation (in patients with underlying cirrhosis; FDA Safety Alert, October 22, 2015), reactivation of HBV (FDA Safety Alert Dec. 8, 2016)

Mechanism of Action

Combines 2 direct-acting hepatitis C virus antiviral agents with distinct mechanisms of action. Ombitasvir inhibits HCV NS5A, and interferes with viral RNA replication and virion assembly. Paritaprevir inhibits HCV NS3/4A protease and interferes with HCV coded polyprotein cleavage necessary for viral replication.

Ritonavir is not active against HCV. Ritonavir is a potent CYP3A inhibitor that increases peak and trough plasma drug concentrations of paritaprevir and overall drug exposure (ie, AUC).

Pharmacodynamics/Kinetics

Half-life Elimination Ombitasvir: 21 to 25 hours; Paritaprevir: 5.5 hours; Ritonavir: 4 hours

Time to Peak Ombitasvir, paritaprevir, ritonavir: 4 to 5 hours

Reproductive Considerations

HCV-infected females of childbearing potential should consider postponing pregnancy until therapy is complete to reduce the risk of HCV transmission (AASLD/IDSA 2018).

Elevations of ALT (>5 × ULN) have been reported; women taking ethinyl estradiol products are at increased risk. Concurrent use of ethinyl estradiol-containing products such as contraceptives is contraindicated; these products may be restarted approximately 2 weeks following completion of HCV therapy. Alternative methods of contraception (eg, nonhormonal methods, progestin-only contraception) are recommended during therapy. Women using other estrogens (eg, estradiol, conjugated estrogens) had a rate of ALT elevation similar to patients not receiving any estrogens; coadminister with caution.

If used in combination with ribavirin, all warnings related to the use of ribavirin and contraception should be followed. Refer to the ribavirin monograph for additional information.

Pregnancy Considerations

Treatment of hepatitis C is not currently recommended to treat maternal infection or to decrease the risk of mother-to-child transmission during pregnancy (Tran 2016). When HCV infection is detected during pregnancy, treatment should be deferred until after delivery. Direct-acting antiviral medications should not be used in pregnant females outside of clinical trials until safety and efficacy information is available (SMFM [Hughes 2017]).

If used in combination with ribavirin, all warnings related to the use of ribavirin and pregnancy should be followed. Refer to the ribavirin monograph for additional information.

Product Availability Technivie has been discontinued by the manufacturer; estimated product availability until January 1, 2019.

Ombitasvir, Paritaprevir, Ritonavir, and Dasabuvir

(om BIT as vir, par i TA pre vir, ri TOE na vir, & da SA bue vir)

Brand Names: US Viekira Pak; Viekira XR

Brand Names: Canada Holkira Pak

Pharmacologic Category Antihepaciviral, NS3/4A Protease Inhibitor (Anti-HCV); Antihepaciviral, NS5A Inhibitor; Antihepaciviral, Polymerase Inhibitor (Anti-HCV); Cytochrome P-450 Inhibitor; NS3/4A Inhibitor; NS5A Inhibitor; NS5B RNA Polymerase Inhibitor

Use Chronic hepatitis C: Treatment of adults with chronic hepatitis C virus (HCV) infection genotype 1a without cirrhosis, in combination with ribavirin, and genotype 1b without cirrhosis or with compensated cirrhosis.

Local Anesthetic/Vasoconstrictor Precautions No information available to require special precautions

Effects on Dental Treatment No significant effects or complications reported

Effects on Bleeding No information available to require special precautions

Adverse Reactions Also see individual agents.

1% to 10%:

Central nervous system: Insomnia (5%)

Dermatologic: Pruritus (7%), skin rash (7%)

Gastrointestinal: Nausea (8%)

Hepatic: Increased serum bilirubin (≥2 x ULN; 2%), increased serum alanine aminotransferase (>5 x ULN; 1%)

Neuromuscular & skeletal: Asthenia (4%)

<1%, postmarketing, and/or case reports: Anaphylaxis, angioedema, erythema multiforme, hepatic failure, hypersensitivity reaction, liver decompensation, reactivation of HBV (FDA Safety Alert Dec. 8, 2016)

Mechanism of Action Combines 3 direct-acting hepatitis C virus antiviral agents with distinct mechanisms of action. Ombitasvir inhibits HCV NS5A, and interferes with viral RNA replication and virion assembly. Paritaprevir inhibits HCV NS3/4A protease and interferes with HCV coded polyprotein cleavage necessary for viral replication. Dasabuvir inhibits HCV RNA-dependent RNA polymerase (encoded by the NS5B gene) which is also necessary for viral replication.

Ritonavir is not active against HCV. Ritonavir is a potent CYP3A inhibitor that increases peak and trough plasma drug concentrations of paritaprevir and overall drug exposure (ie, AUC).

Pharmacodynamics/Kinetics

Half-life Elimination Ombitasvir: 21 to 25 hours; Paritaprevir: 5.5 hours; Ritonavir: 4 hours; Dasabuvir 5.5 to 6 hours

Time to Peak

Ombitasvir: ~5 hours

Paritaprevir: ~4 to 5 hours

Ritonavir: ~4 to 5 hours

Dasabuvir: ~4 hours (immediate release); 8 hours (ER)

Reproductive Considerations

Hepatitis C virus (HCV)-infected females of childbearing potential should consider postponing pregnancy until therapy is complete to reduce the risk of HCV transmission (AASLD/IDSA 2018).

Elevations of ALT (>5 times ULN) have been reported; women taking ethinyl estradiol products are at increased risk. Concurrent use of ethinyl estradiol-containing products such as contraceptives is contraindicated; these products may be restarted ~2 weeks following completion of HCV therapy. Alternative methods of contraception (eg, nonhormonal methods, progestin-only contraception) are recommended during therapy. Women using other estrogens (eg, estradiol, conjugated estrogens) had a rate of ALT elevation similar to patients not receiving any estrogens; coadminister with caution.

If used in combination with ribavirin, all warnings related to the use of ribavirin and contraception should be followed. Refer to the ribavirin monograph for additional information.

Pregnancy Considerations

Treatment of hepatitis C is not currently recommended to treat maternal infection or to decrease the risk of mother-to-child transmission during pregnancy (Tran 2016). When HCV infection is detected during pregnancy, treatment should be deferred until after delivery. Direct-acting antiviral medications should not be used in pregnant females outside of clinical trials until safety and efficacy information is available (SMFM [Hughes 2017]).

If used in combination with ribavirin, all warnings related to the use of ribavirin and pregnancy should be followed. Refer to the ribavirin monograph for additional information.

Product Availability Viekira XR has been discontinued by the manufacturer; estimated product availability until January 1, 2019.

- ◆ **Omeclamox-Pak®** *see* Omeprazole, Clarithromycin, and Amoxicillin *on page 1140*
- ◆ **Omega 3** *see* Omega-3 Fatty Acids *on page 1137*
- ◆ **Omega-3 2100 [OTC]** *see* Omega-3 Fatty Acids *on page 1137*
- ◆ **Omega-3-Acid Ethyl Esters** *see* Omega-3 Fatty Acids *on page 1137*
- ◆ **Omega-3 Fish Oil Ex St [OTC]** *see* Omega-3 Fatty Acids *on page 1137*
- ◆ **Omega-3 IQ [OTC] [DSC]** *see* Omega-3 Fatty Acids *on page 1137*

Omega-3 Fatty Acids

(oh MEG a three FAT tee AS ids)

Related Information

Cardiovascular Diseases *on page 1654*

Brand Names: US Dialyvite Omega-3 Concentrate [OTC]; Fish Oil Concentrate [OTC]; Lovaza; Maximum Red Krill [OTC]; Ocean Blue MiniCaps Omega-3 [OTC]; Odorless Coated Fish Oil [OTC]; Omega Power [OTC]; Omega-3 2100 [OTC]; Omega-3 Fish Oil Ex St [OTC]; Omega-3 IQ [OTC] [DSC]; Pro Nutrients Omega 3 [OTC]; Salmon Oil-1000 [OTC]; Sam-E.P.A. [OTC]; Sea-Omega [OTC]; Triklo [DSC]; Vascepa

Brand Names: Canada Vascepa

Generic Availability (US) May be product dependent

Pharmacologic Category Antilipemic Agent, Omega-3 Fatty Acids

Use

Cardiovascular risk reduction with mild hypertriglyceridemia (Vascepa): As an adjunct to maximally-tolerated statin therapy to reduce the risk of myocardial infarction, stroke, coronary revascularization, and unstable angina requiring hospitalization in adult patients with triglyceride levels ≥150 mg/dL and either established cardiovascular disease or type 2 diabetes mellitus with ≥2 risk factors for cardiovascular disease.

Dietary supplement: As dietary supplements for patients at early risk of coronary artery disease.

Note: Recommendations from the American Heart Association (AHA) state that patients without documented coronary heart disease (CHD) should eat a variety of fish, preferably oily fish (eg, salmon), at least twice a week, or daily in patients with documented CHD (AHA [Kris-Etherton 2002]).

Hypertriglyceridemia (Lovaza and Vascepa): As an adjunct to diet to reduce triglyceride levels in adults with severe (≥500 mg/dL) hypertriglyceridemia.

Note: The Endocrine Society recommends that omega-3 fatty acids may be considered for triglyceride levels >1,000 mg/dL and may be used alone or in combination with HMG-CoA reductase inhibitors (Berglund 2012). A number of OTC formulations containing omega-3 fatty acids are marketed as nutritional supplements; these do not have FDA-approved indications and may not contain the same amounts of the active ingredient.

Local Anesthetic/Vasoconstrictor Precautions No information available to require special precautions

Effects on Dental Treatment No significant effects or complications reported

Effects on Bleeding Prolongation of bleeding time has been observed in some clinical studies; however, there is no scientific evidence to warrant discontinuance prior to dental surgery. The clinician should anticipate the potential for slower clotting times.

Adverse Reactions

>10%: Hematologic & oncologic: Hemorrhage (12%)

1% to 10%:

Cardiovascular: Atrial fibrillation (≥3%), peripheral edema (≥3%), atrial flutter (≤3%)

Gastrointestinal: Dysgeusia (4%), eructation (4%), constipation (≥3%), gout (≥3%), dyspepsia (3%)

Hematologic & oncologic: Major hemorrhage (3%)

Neuromuscular & skeletal: Musculoskeletal pain (≥3%), arthralgia (≥1%)

Respiratory: Oropharyngeal pain (≥1%)

Frequency not defined:

Dermatologic: Pruritus, skin rash

Endocrine & metabolic: Increased LDL cholesterol

Gastrointestinal: Gastrointestinal disease, vomiting

Hepatic: Increased serum alanine aminotransferase, increased serum aspartate aminotransferase

<1%, postmarketing, and/or case reports: Abdominal distress, anaphylaxis, bleeding tendency disorder, diarrhea, increased serum triglycerides, limb pain, urticaria

Dosing

Adult & Geriatric

Cardiovascular risk reduction with mild hypertriglyceridemia (Vascepa) (adjunctive agent): Note: Consider in addition to maximally-tolerated statin therapy in patients with triglyceride levels ≥150 mg/dL and either established cardiovascular disease or type 2 diabetes mellitus with ≥2 risk factors for cardiovascular disease.

Oral: 2 g twice daily with meals (Bhatt 2019).

Hypertriglyceridemia: Oral:

Lovaza: 4 g (4 capsules) once daily or 2 g (2 capsules) twice daily.

Vascepa: 2 g (2 [1 g] capsules or 4 [0.5 g] capsules) twice daily with meals.

IgA nephropathy (off-label use): Oral: Lovaza: 4 g (4 capsules) once daily (Donadio 2001).

Renal Impairment: Adult There are no dosage adjustments provided in the manufacturer's labeling (has not been studied). EPA and DHA are not renally eliminated.

Hepatic Impairment: Adult There are no dosage adjustments provided in the manufacturer's labeling (has not been studied).

Mechanism of Action Reduction in the hepatic production of triglyceride-rich very low-density lipoproteins. Possible cellular mechanisms include inhibition of acyl CoA:1,2 diacylglycerol acyltransferase, increased hepatic mitochondrial and peroxisomal beta-oxidation, and a reduction in the hepatic synthesis of triglycerides. The mechanisms contributing to reduction of cardiovascular events are not completely understood but are likely multi-factorial (eg, increased eicosapentaenoic acid [EPA] composition from carotid plaques, increased circulating EPA/arachidonic acid ratio, inhibition of platelet aggregation).

Contraindications Hypersensitivity (eg, anaphylactic reaction) to omega-3 fatty acids or any component of formulation.

Warnings/Precautions Use with caution in patients with known allergy or sensitivity to fish and/or shellfish. Should be used as an adjunct to diet therapy and exercise. Secondary causes of hyperlipidemia should be ruled out prior to therapy. ALT may be increased without AST increasing. May increase LDL levels; periodically monitor LDL levels. Bleeding, including serious events, has been reported; risk may be increased with concomitant anticoagulant/antiplatelet use. Prolongation of bleeding time not exceeding normal limits has also been observed; use with caution in patients with coagulopathy. Monitor for signs and symptoms of bleeding. Atrial fibrillation (AF) or flutter requiring hospitalization may occur; risk increased in patients with a history of AF or flutter and within the first 2 to 3 months of therapy. The effect, if any, of omega-3 fatty acids on the risk of pancreatitis or cardiovascular mortality and morbidity in patients with severe hypertriglyceridemia is not known. Manage concurrent conditions (eg, diabetes, hypothyroidism, excessive alcohol intake) that may contribute to lipid abnormalities.

Drug Interactions

Metabolism/Transport Effects None known.

Avoid Concomitant Use There are no known interactions where it is recommended to avoid concomitant use.

Increased Effect/Toxicity

Omega-3 Fatty Acids may increase the levels/effects of: Agents with Antiplatelet Properties; Anticoagulants; Ibrutinib

Decreased Effect There are no known significant interactions involving a decrease in effect.

Dietary Considerations Dietary modification is important in the control of severe hypertriglyceridemia. Maintain standard cholesterol-lowering diet during therapy.

Pharmacodynamics/Kinetics

Half-life Elimination EPA: ~37 to 89 hours; DHA: ~46 hours

Time to Peak

Plasma:

Omega-3-carboxylic acids: Following repeat dosing with low-fat meals for ~2 weeks (steady state): EPA: 5 to 8 hours; DHA: 5 to 9 hours

Icosapent ethyl: EPA: ~5 hours

Pregnancy Considerations Adequate intake of omega-3 fatty acids is recommended during pregnancy (IOM 2005; Nordgren 2017). Maternal use of supplements or dietary consumption of omega-3 fatty acids (containing eicosapentaenoic acid and docosahexaenoic acid) influences fetal concentrations (Büyükuslu 2017; Coletta 2010; Miles 2011).

Triglyceride concentrations increase during pregnancy as required for normal fetal development. When increases are greater than expected, supervised dietary interventions that include omega-3 fatty acids may be initiated. In women who develop very severe hypertriglyceridemia and are at risk for pancreatitis, use of prescription omega-3 fatty acid products may be considered (Avis 2009; Berglund 2012; Jacobson 2015; Wong 2015).

Breastfeeding Considerations

Omega-3 fatty acids are present in breast milk and dietary supplementation may influence milk concentrations (IOM 2005).

According to the manufacturer, the decision to continue or discontinue breastfeeding during therapy should consider the risk of infant exposure, the benefits of breastfeeding to the infant, and benefits of treatment to the mother.

Dosage Forms Considerations

Lovaza: Each 1 g capsule contains the combination of EPA (~465 mg) and DHA (~375 mg) ethyl esters.

Vascepa: Icosapent ethyl contains ethyl esters of an omega-3 fatty acid, EPA, obtained from fish oil. It contains ≥96% EPA and does **not** contain DHA. Historically, mixtures containing both EPA and DHA have increased LDL cholesterol in patients with severe hypertriglyceridemia. However, studies have suggested that icosapent ethyl has not caused significant increases in LDL cholesterol while significantly decreasing triglyceride levels (Bays 2011; Miller 2011).

Dosage Forms: US

Capsule, Oral:

Dialyvite Omega-3 Concentrate [OTC]: 600 mg
Lovaza: 1 g
Ocean Blue MiniCaps Omega-3 [OTC]: 350 mg
Omega Power [OTC]: 1050 mg
Omega-3 2100 [OTC]: 1050 mg
Vascepa: 0.5 g, 1 g
Generic: 300 mg, 500 mg, 1000 mg, 1 g

Capsule, Oral [preservative free]:

Fish Oil Concentrate [OTC]: 1000 mg
Maximum Red Krill [OTC]: 300 mg
Omega-3 Fish Oil Ex St [OTC]: 880 mg
Salmon Oil-1000 [OTC]: 200 mg
Sam-E.P.A. [OTC]: 200-300 MG
Sea-Omega [OTC]: 1000 mg
Generic: 200 mg, 1000 mg, 1200 mg

Capsule Delayed Release, Oral:

Odorless Coated Fish Oil [OTC]: 1000 mg
Pro Nutrients Omega 3 [OTC]: 332.5 mg
Generic: 1000 mg

Dosage Forms: Canada

Capsule, Oral:

Vascepa: 1 g

◆ **Omega Power [OTC]** *see* Omega-3 Fatty Acids *on page 1137*

Omeprazole (oh MEP ra zole)

Related Information

Esomeprazole *on page 594*

Gastrointestinal Disorders *on page 1678*

Brand Names: US PriLOSEC; PriLOSEC OTC [OTC]

Brand Names: Canada APO-Omeprazole; BIO-Omeprazole; DOM-Omeprazole DR [DSC]; JAMP-Omeprazole DR; Losec; MYLAN-Omeprazole [DSC]; NAT-Omeprazole DR; Omeprazole-20; PMS-Omeprazole; PMS-Omeprazole DR; Priva-Omeprazole; RAN-Omeprazole; RATIO-Omeprazole [DSC]; RIVA-Omeprazole DR; SANDOZ Omeprazole; SANDOZ Omperazole; TEVA-Omeprazole; VAN-Omeprazole [DSC]

Pharmacologic Category Proton Pump Inhibitor; Substituted Benzimidazole

Use

Gastroesophageal reflux disease, erosive or nonerosive (Rx only):

Treatment of erosive esophagitis: Short-term treatment of erosive esophagitis (EE) due to acid-mediated gastroesophageal reflux disease (GERD) diagnosed by endoscopy in patients ≥1 year of age; short-term treatment (up to 6 weeks) of EE due to acid-mediated GERD in pediatric patients 1 month to <1 year of age.

Maintenance healing of erosive esophagitis: Maintenance healing of EE due to acid-mediated GERD in patients ≥1 year of age.

Symptomatic gastroesophageal reflux disease: Treatment of heartburn and other symptoms associated with GERD for up to 4 weeks in patients ≥1 year of age.

Heartburn (OTC only): Treatment of frequent, uncomplicated heartburn (occurring ≥2 or more days per week) in adults.

***Helicobacter pylori* eradication (Rx only):** Treatment of *H. pylori* infection and duodenal ulcer disease in adults as part of an appropriate combination regimen with antibiotics.

Peptic ulcer disease, treatment of duodenal or gastric ulcers (Rx only): Short-term treatment of active duodenal or gastric ulcers in adults.

Zollinger-Ellison syndrome (Rx only): Long-term treatment of pathological hypersecretory conditions, such as Zollinger-Ellison syndrome, in adults.

Local Anesthetic/Vasoconstrictor Precautions No information available to require special precautions

Effects on Dental Treatment Key adverse event(s) related to dental treatment: Rare occurrence of taste perversion, dry mouth, esophageal candidiasis, stomatitis, and mucosal atrophy (tongue).

Effects on Bleeding No information available to require special precautions

Adverse Reactions

1% to 10%:

Central nervous system: Headache (7%), dizziness (2%)

Dermatologic: Skin rash (2%)

Gastrointestinal: Abdominal pain (5%), diarrhea (4%), nausea (4%), flatulence (3%), vomiting (3%), acid regurgitation (2%), constipation (2%)

Neuromuscular & skeletal: Back pain (1%), weakness (1%)

Respiratory: Upper respiratory infection (2%), cough (1%)

<1%, postmarketing, and/or case reports (adverse event occurrence may vary based on formulation): Abdominal swelling, abnormal dreams, aggression, agitation, agranulocytosis, allergic reactions, alopecia, anaphylaxis, anemia, angina pectoris, angioedema, anorexia, anxiety, apathy, arthralgia, atrophic gastritis, blurred vision, bone fracture, bradycardia, bronchospasm, chest pain, cholestatic hepatitis, *Clostridioides* (formerly *Clostridium*) *difficile*-associated diarrhea (CDAD), colitis (microscopic), confusion, cutaneous lupus erythematosus, depression, dermatitis, diplopia, disturbed sleep, drowsiness, dysgeusia, epistaxis, erythema multiforme, esophageal candidiasis, fatigue, fecal discoloration, fever, gastric carcinoid tumor, gastric polyp (benign), glycosuria, gynecomastia, hallucination, hematuria, hemolytic anemia, hepatic disease (hepatocellular, cholestatic, mixed), hepatic encephalopathy, hepatic failure, hepatic necrosis, hepatitis, hepatocellular hepatitis, hepatotoxicity (idiosyncratic) (Chalasani 2014), hyperhidrosis, hypersensitivity reaction, hypertension, hypocalcemia, hypoglycemia, hypokalemia, hypomagnesemia, hyponatremia, increased gamma glutamyl transferase, increased serum alkaline phosphatase, increased serum ALT, increased serum AST, increased serum bilirubin, increased serum creatinine, insomnia, interstitial nephritis, irritable bowel syndrome, jaundice, leg pain, leukocytosis, leukopenia, malaise, microscopic pyuria, mucosal atrophy (tongue), muscle cramps, myalgia, myasthenia, nervousness, neutropenia, ocular irritation, optic atrophy, optic neuritis, optic neuropathy (anterior ischemic), osteoporosis-related fracture, pain, palpitation, pancreatitis, pancytopenia, paresthesia, peripheral edema, petechiae, photophobia, pneumonia, proteinuria, pruritus, psychiatric disturbance, purpura, renal disease (chronic; Lazarus 2016), skin photosensitivity, sore throat, Stevens-Johnson syndrome, stomatitis, systemic lupus erythematosus, tachycardia, testicular pain, thrombocytopenia, tinnitus, toxic epidermal necrolysis, tremor, urinary frequency, urinary tract infection, urticaria, vertigo, weight gain, xeroderma, xerophthalmia, xerostomia

Mechanism of Action Proton pump inhibitor; suppresses gastric basal and stimulated acid secretion by inhibiting the parietal cell H+/K+ ATP pump

Pharmacodynamics/Kinetics

Onset of Action Antisecretory: ~1 hour; Peak effect: Within 2 hours

Duration of Action Up to 72 hours; 50% of maximum effect at 24 hours; after stopping treatment, secretory activity gradually returns over 3 to 5 days; Maximum secretory inhibition: 4 days

Half-life Elimination 0.5 to 1 hour; hepatic impairment: ~3 hours

Time to Peak Plasma: 0.5 to 3.5 hours

Pregnancy Considerations Available data have not shown an increased risk of major birth defects following maternal use of omeprazole during pregnancy.

Recommendations for the treatment of GERD in pregnancy are available. As in nonpregnant patients, lifestyle modifications followed by other medications are the initial treatments (ACG [Katz 2013]; Body 2016; Huerta-Iga 2016; van der Woude 2014). Based on available data, PPIs may be used when clinically indicated (Body 2016; Matok 2012; Pasternak 2010; van der Woude 2014).

◆ **Omeprazole, Amoxicillin, and Clarithromycin** *see* Omeprazole, Clarithromycin, and Amoxicillin *on page 1140*

Omeprazole, Amoxicillin, and Rifabutin (oh MEP ra zole, a moks i SIL in, & rif a BYOO tin)

Brand Names: US Talicia

Pharmacologic Category Antibiotic, Penicillin; Gastrointestinal Agent, Miscellaneous; Proton Pump Inhibitor; Rifamycin; Substituted Benzimidazole

Use *Helicobacter pylori* infection: Treatment of *H. pylori* infection in adults.

Local Anesthetic/Vasoconstrictor Precautions No information available to require special precautions.

Effects on Dental Treatment Key adverse event(s) related to dental treatment: Omeprazole alone associated with rare occurrence of taste perversion, dry mouth, esophageal candidiasis, and mucosal atrophy (see omeprazole monograph); amoxicillin alone has caused oral candidiasis (frequency not reported, see amoxicillin monograph); rifabutin alone associated with occurrence of reddish-orange saliva; taste perversion. The reddish-orange color of the saliva may cause a unique coloration to plaque and calculus buildup. Some patients may want more regular cleanings to remove (see rifabutin monograph).

Effects on Bleeding No information available to require special precautions.

Adverse Reactions Also see individual agents.

>10%:

- Central nervous system: Headache (8% to 16%)
- Gastrointestinal: Diarrhea (10% to 14%)
- Genitourinary: Urine discoloration (13%)

1% to 10%:

- Dermatologic: Skin rash (3% to 5%)
- Gastrointestinal: Nausea (4% to 5%), abdominal pain (4%), vomiting (2%), dyspepsia (1% to 2%)
- Genitourinary: Vulvovaginal candidiasis (2%)
- Respiratory: Oropharyngeal pain (≤4%)

Mechanism of Action

Omeprazole: Suppresses gastric acid secretion by blocking the acid (proton) pump within gastric parietal cells.

Amoxicillin: Inhibits bacterial cell wall synthesis.

Rifabutin: Inhibits DNA-dependent RNA polymerase, preventing chain initiation.

Reproductive Considerations Amoxicillin and rifabutin may interact with hormonal contraceptives; therefore, a highly effective nonhormonal form of contraception is recommended by the manufacturer during therapy.

Pregnancy Considerations Amoxicillin and rifabutin cross the placenta.

Refer to individual monographs for additional information.

◆ **Omeprazole/Clarith/Amoxicillin** *see* Omeprazole, Clarithromycin, and Amoxicillin *on page* 1140

Omeprazole, Clarithromycin, and Amoxicillin
(oh MEP ra zole, kla RITH roe mye sin, & a moks i SIL in)

Related Information

Amoxicillin *on page* 124

Clarithromycin *on page* 361

Omeprazole *on page* 1139

Brand Names: US Omeclamox-Pak®

Pharmacologic Category Antibiotic, Macrolide Combination; Antibiotic, Penicillin; Gastrointestinal Agent, Miscellaneous; Proton Pump Inhibitor; Substituted Benzimidazole

Use *Helicobacter pylori* eradication: Eradication of *H. pylori* infection to reduce the risk of recurrent duodenal ulcer in adults with active or 1-year history of duodenal ulcer

Local Anesthetic/Vasoconstrictor Precautions Clarithromycin is one of the drugs confirmed to prolong the QT interval and is accepted as having a risk of causing torsade de pointes. In terms of epinephrine, it is not known what effect vasoconstrictors in the local anesthetic regimen will have in patients with a known history of congenital prolonged QT interval or in patients taking any medication that prolongs the QT interval. Until more information is obtained, it is suggested that the clinician consult with the physician prior to the use of a vasoconstrictor in suspected patients, and that the vasoconstrictor (epinephrine, mepivacaine and levonordefrin [Carbocaine® 2% with Neo-Cobefrin®]) be used with caution.

Effects on Dental Treatment No significant effects or complications reported

Effects on Bleeding No information available to require special precautions

Adverse Reactions Frequencies noted refer to experience with combination therapy. Also see individual agents.

>10%: Gastrointestinal: Diarrhea (14%)

1% to 10%:

- Central nervous system: Headache (7%)
- Gastrointestinal: Dysgeusia (10%)

<1%, postmarketing, and/or case reports: Hepatotoxicity (idiosyncratic) (Chalasani 2014)

Mechanism of Action

Omeprazole: A proton pump inhibitor, suppresses gastric acid secretion via inhibition of the parietal cell H+/K+ ATP pump.

Clarithromycin: An antibacterial agent, binds to the 50s ribosomal subunit of susceptible microorganisms resulting in inhibition of protein synthesis.

Amoxicillin: An antibacterial agent, inhibits bacterial cell wall synthesis.

Pregnancy Considerations Use of this combination for the eradication of *H. pylori* infection is not recommended during the first trimester of pregnancy (Nguyen 2019). Refer to individual monographs for additional information.

Dental Health Professional Considerations See Local Anesthetic/Vasoconstrictor Precautions

◆ **Omeprazole Magnesium, Amoxicillin, and Rifabutin** *see* Omeprazole, Amoxicillin, and Rifabutin *on page* 1140

◆ **Omeprazole, Rifabutin, and Amoxicillin** *see* Omeprazole, Amoxicillin, and Rifabutin *on page* 1140

◆ **Omnaris** *see* Ciclesonide (Nasal) *on page* 345

◆ **Omnicef** *see* Cefdinir *on page* 305

◆ **Omni Gel [OTC]** *see* Fluoride *on page* 693

◆ **Omnitarg** *see* Pertuzumab *on page* 1220

◆ **Omnitrope** *see* Somatropin *on page* 1381

OnabotulinumtoxinA
(oh nuh BOT yoo lin num TOKS in aye)

Brand Names: US Botox; Botox Cosmetic

Brand Names: Canada Botox; Botox Cosmetic

Pharmacologic Category Neuromuscular Blocker Agent, Toxin; Ophthalmic Agent, Toxin

Use

Axillary hyperhidrosis (Botox):

Treatment of severe primary axillary hyperhidrosis in adults not adequately managed with topical agents.

The safety and effectiveness for hyperhidrosis in other body areas have not been established. Weakness of hand muscles and blepharoptosis may occur in patients who receive onabotulinumtoxinA for palmar hyperhidrosis and facial hyperhidrosis, respectively. Patients should be evaluated for potential causes of secondary hyperhidrosis (eg, hyperthyroidism) to avoid symptomatic treatment of hyperhidrosis without the diagnosis and/or treatment of the underlying disease.

Cervical dystonia (Botox): Treatment of cervical dystonia in patients ≥16 years of age to reduce the severity of abnormal head position and neck pain.

Chronic migraine (Botox): Prophylaxis of chronic migraine headaches (≥15 days/month with headache lasting ≥4 hours/day) in adults.

Glabellar lines (Botox Cosmetic): Temporary improvement in the appearance of moderate to severe glabellar lines associated with corrugator and/or procerus muscle activity in adults.

Forehead lines (Botox Cosmetic): Temporary improvement in the appearance of moderate to severe forehead lines associated with frontalis muscle activity in adults.

Lateral canthal lines (Botox Cosmetic): Temporary improvement in the appearance of moderate to severe lateral canthal lines associated with orbicularis oculi activity in adults.

Overactive bladder (Botox): Treatment of overactive bladder with symptoms of urge urinary incontinence, urgency, and frequency in adults who have an inadequate response to or who are intolerant to an anticholinergic medication.

Spasticity (Botox): Treatment of spasticity in patients ≥2 years of age.

Limitations of use: Improvement in upper extremity functional abilities or range of motion at a joint affected by a fixed contracture has not been shown.

Strabismus and blepharospasm associated with dystonia (Botox): Treatment of strabismus and blepharospasm associated with dystonia, including benign essential blepharospasm or VII nerve disorders, in patients ≥12 years of age.

Urinary incontinence due to detrusor overactivity (Botox): Treatment of urinary incontinence due to detrusor overactivity associated with a neurologic condition (eg, spinal cord injury, multiple sclerosis) in adults who have an inadequate response to or are intolerant of an anticholinergic medication.

Canadian labeling: Additional use (not in US labeling): Dynamic equinus foot deformity in pediatric cerebral palsy patients

Local Anesthetic/Vasoconstrictor Precautions

No information available to require special precautions

Effects on Dental Treatment Key adverse event(s) related to dental treatment: Xerostomia (normal salivary flow resumes upon discontinuation), facial pain, and facial weakness. Effects occur in ~1 week and may last up to several months.

Effects on Bleeding No information available to require special precautions

Adverse Reactions As reported with adult patients, unless otherwise noted. Adverse effects usually occur in 1 week and may last up to several months.

>10%:

Bladder dysfunction: Genitourinary: Urinary tract infection (18% to 49%), bacteriuria (4% to 18%), urinary retention (6% to 17%), increased postvoid residual urine volume (not requiring catheterization: 3% to 17%)

Cervical dystonia:

Central nervous system: Headache (11%)

Gastrointestinal: Dysphagia (19%)

Neuromuscular & skeletal: Neck pain (11%)

Respiratory: Upper respiratory tract infection (12%)

Upper limb spasticity:

Respiratory: Upper respiratory tract infection (children and adolescents: 10% to 17%)

Other indications (blepharospasm, forehead lines, glabellar lines, lateral canthal lines, primary axillary hyperhidrosis, strabismus):

Central nervous system: Vertical strabismus (17%)

Ophthalmic: Blepharoptosis (strabismus: 1% to 38%; blepharospasm: 21%; forehead lines, glabellar lines: 2% to 3%)

1% to 10%:

Bladder dysfunction:

Central nervous system: Myasthenia (4%), abnormal gait (3%), falling (3%)

Gastrointestinal: Constipation (4%)

Genitourinary: Dysuria (4% to 9%), hematuria (4% to 5%)

Immunologic: Antibody development (neutralizing: 1%)

Neuromuscular & skeletal: Muscle spasm (2%)

Cervical dystonia:

Central nervous system: Dizziness (2% to 10%), drowsiness (2% to 10%), hypertonia (2% to 10%), numbness (2% to 10%), speech disturbance (2% to 10%)

Gastrointestinal: Nausea (2% to 10%), xerostomia (2% to 10%)

Immunologic: Antibody development (1%)

Local: Local soreness/soreness at injection site (2% to 10%)

Neuromuscular & skeletal: Back pain (2% to 10%), stiffness (2% to 10%), asthenia (2% to 10%)

Ophthalmic: Blepharoptosis (2% to 10%), diplopia (2% to 10%)

Respiratory: Cough (2% to 10%), dyspnea (2% to 10%), flu-like symptoms (2% to 10%), rhinitis (2% to 10%)

Miscellaneous: Fever (2% to 10%)

Chronic migraines:

Cardiovascular: Hypertension (2%)

Central nervous system: Headache (5%), exacerbation of migraine headache (4%), facial paresis (2%)

Local: Pain at injection site (3%)

Neuromuscular & skeletal: Neck pain (9%), myasthenia (4%), stiffness (4%), musculoskeletal pain (3%), myalgia (3%), muscle spasm (2%)

Ophthalmic: Blepharoptosis (4%)

Respiratory: Bronchitis (3%)

Lower limb spasticity:

Dermatologic: Excoriation of skin (children and adolescents: 2%)

Gastrointestinal: Decreased appetite (children and adolescents: 2%)

Local: Erythema at injection site (children and adolescents: 2%), pain at injection site (2%)

Neuromuscular & skeletal: Arthralgia (3%), back pain (3%), myalgia (2%), sprain (1% to 2%)

Respiratory: Oropharyngeal pain (children and adolescents: 2%), upper respiratory tract infection (2%)

Upper limb spasticity:

Central nervous system: Seizure (children and adolescents: 1% to 5%), fatigue (2% to 3%)

Gastrointestinal: Nausea (2% to 4%), constipation (children and adolescents: 3%)

Local: Pain at injection site (children and adolescents: 3% to 4%)

Neuromuscular & skeletal: Limb pain (5% to 9%), myasthenia (2% to 4%)

Respiratory: Rhinorrhea (children and adolescents: 4%), nasal congestion (children and adolescents: 3%), bronchitis (2% to 3%)

Other indications (blepharospasm, forehead lines, glabellar lines, lateral canthal lines, primary axillary hyperhidrosis, reduction of glabellar lines, strabismus):

Central nervous system: Anxiety (3% to 10%), pain (3% to 10%), headache (9%), facial pain (1%), facial paresis (1%)

Dermatologic: Diaphoresis (3% to 10%; nonaxillary), pruritus (3% to 10%), skin tightness (2%)

Immunologic: Antibody development (2%)

Infection: Infection (3% to 10%)

Local: Bleeding at injection site (3% to 10%), pain at injection site (3% to 10%)

Neuromuscular & skeletal: Back pain (3% to 10%), neck pain (3% to 10%), asthenia (1%)

Ophthalmic: Dry eye syndrome (6%), superficial punctate keratitis (6%), eyelid edema (1%)

Respiratory: Flu-like symptoms (3% to 10%), pharyngitis (3% to 10%)

Miscellaneous: Fever (3% to 10%)

Frequency not defined:

Other indications (blepharospasm, forehead lines, glabellar lines, lateral canthal lines, primary axillary hyperhidrosis, reduction of glabellar lines, strabismus):

Dermatologic: Skin rash

Ophthalmic: Diplopia, ectropion, eye irritation, eyelid entropion, keratitis, lacrimation, lagophthalmos

<1%, postmarketing, and/or case reports: *Any indication:* Abdominal pain, acute myocardial infarction, alopecia, amyotrophy, anaphylaxis, anorexia, antibody development (neutralizing), aspiration pneumonia, asthma, blurred vision, brachial plexopathy, cardiac arrhythmia, corneal perforation, corneal ulceration, denervation, dermatitis, diarrhea, drug toxicity (botulinum toxin effects), dysarthria, erythema of skin, erythema multiforme, exacerbation of myasthenia gravis, eye infection, focal facial paralysis, hyperhidrosis, hypersensitivity reaction, hypoacusis, hypoesthesia, inflammation at injection site, jaw pain, madarosis of the eyebrow, malaise, muscle twitching (localized), nerve root disorder, paresthesia, peripheral neuropathy, photophobia, pneumonia, psoriasiform eruption, reduced blinking, respiratory depression, respiratory failure, retinal vein occlusion, retrobulbar hemorrhage, serum sickness, syncope, tinnitus, urinary incontinence, urticaria, vertigo, visual disturbance, voice disorder, vomiting

Mechanism of Action OnabotulinumtoxinA (previously known as botulinum toxin type A) is a neurotoxin produced by *Clostridium botulinum*, spore-forming anaerobic bacillus, which appears to affect only the presynaptic membrane of the neuromuscular junction in humans, where it prevents calcium-dependent release of acetylcholine and produces a state of denervation. Muscle inactivation persists until new fibrils grow from the nerve and form junction plates on new areas of the muscle-cell walls. Intradetrusor injection affects efferent pathways of detrusor activity by inhibiting release of acetylcholine. Intradermal injection results in temporary sweat gland denervation, reducing local sweating.

Pharmacodynamics/Kinetics

Onset of Action Blepharospasm: ~3 to 4 days; Cervical dystonia: ~2 weeks; Detrusor overactivity associated with neurologic condition: ~2 weeks; Reduction of glabellar lines (Botox Cosmetic): 1 to 2 days, increasing in intensity during first week; Spasticity: Focal and cerebral palsy related: <2 weeks; Strabismus: ~1 to 2 days

Duration of Action Blepharospasm: ~3 to 4 months; Cervical dystonia: ≤3 to 4 months; Detrusor overactivity associated with neurologic condition: ~42 to 48 weeks; Reduction of glabellar lines (Botox Cosmetic): ~3 to 4 months; Spasticity: ~3 to 3.5 months; Strabismus: ~2 to 6 weeks; Primary axillary hyperhidrosis: 201 days (mean)

Time to Peak Blepharospasm: 1 to 2 weeks; Cervical dystonia: ~6 weeks; Spasticity (focal): 4 to 6 weeks; Strabismus: Within first week

Pregnancy Considerations

Information related to the use of onabotulinumtoxinA in pregnancy is limited to case reports for the treatment of cervical dystonia (Aranda 2012; Bodkin 2005; Krug 2015; Newman 2004), achalasia (Holliday 2016; Hooft 2015; Neubert 2019; Wataganara 2009), and migraine (Robinson 2014). In addition, case reports collected by the manufacturer include pregnancy outcome information following use for cosmetic procedures, movement disorders, pain disorders, and hyperhidrosis (Brin 2016).

Because information related to the use of onabotulinumtoxinA in pregnancy is limited, use for indications, such as cervical dystonia and cosmetic procedures, is not recommended (Contarino 2017; Trivedi 2017).

Dental Health Professional Considerations Cote and associates, published a paper describing all serious adverse reactions reported to the FDA (Cote, 2005). Included in the 217 serious effects reported, there were 28 deaths and 17 seizures. The deaths were attributed to heart attacks, cerebrovascular accident, pulmonary embolisms, pneumonia, or unknown causes. There were 1031 adverse effects reported after cosmetic use, 36 were of a serious nature. These included focal facial paralysis, muscle weakness, dysphagia, flu-like symptoms, and allergic reactions.

In contrast to the Cote study, the Naumann study reviewed the adverse reactions described and reported in randomized, controlled trials of onabotulinumtoxinA. They reviewed 36 studies involving 2309 subjects through the years 1966-2003. Of the 2309 subjects, 1425 received onabotulinumtoxinA treatment. No study reported severe adverse events. The only adverse event occurring significantly more often than with placebo was focal weakness.

◆ **Oncaspar** *see* Pegaspargase *on page 1199*

◆ **OncoVEX GM-CSF** *see* Talimogene Laherparepvec *on page 1403*

◆ **Oncovin** *see* VinCRIStine *on page 1546*

Ondansetron (on DAN se tron)

Related Information

Clinical Risk Related to Drugs Prolonging QT Interval *on page 1675*

Brand Names: US Zofran; Zofran ODT [DSC]; Zuplenz

Brand Names: Canada ACCEL-Ondansetron; ACT Ondansetron; APO-Ondansetron; CCP-Ondansetron; DOM-Ondansetron; JAMP Ondansetron; JAMP-Ondansetron; Mar-Ondansetron; MINT-Ondansetron; MINT-Ondansetron ODT; MYLAN-Ondansetron; NAT-Ondansetron; Ondansetron ODT; Ondansetron Omega; Ondissolve ODF; PMS-Ondansetron; RAN-Ondansetron; SANDOZ Ondansetron; Septa-Ondansetron; TEVA-Ondansetron [DSC]; VAN-Ondansetron [DSC]; VPI-Ondansetron ODT; Zofran; Zofran ODT

Pharmacologic Category Antiemetic; Selective 5-HT_3 Receptor Antagonist

Use

Cancer chemotherapy-induced nausea and vomiting:

IV: Prevention of nausea and vomiting associated with initial and repeat courses of emetogenic cancer chemotherapy (including high-dose cisplatin).

Oral:

Prevention of nausea and vomiting associated with highly emetogenic cancer chemotherapy (including cisplatin ≥50 mg/m^2).

Prevention of nausea and vomiting associated with initial and repeat courses of moderately emetogenic cancer chemotherapy.

Postoperative nausea and/or vomiting: IV, IM, Oral: Prevention of postoperative nausea and/or vomiting (PONV). If nausea/vomiting occur in a patient who had not received prophylactic ondansetron, IV ondansetron may be administered to prevent further episodes.

Limitations of use: Routine prophylaxis for PONV in patients with minimal expectation of nausea and/or vomiting is not recommended, although use is recommended in patients when nausea and vomiting must be avoided in the postoperative period, even if the incidence of PONV is low.

Radiotherapy-associated nausea and vomiting: Oral: Prevention of nausea and vomiting associated with radiotherapy in patients receiving either total body irradiation, single high-dose fraction to the abdomen, or daily fractions to the abdomen.

Local Anesthetic/Vasoconstrictor Precautions

Ondansetron is one of the drugs confirmed to prolong the QT interval and is accepted as having a risk of causing torsade de pointes. The risk of drug-induced torsade de pointes is extremely low when a single QT interval prolonging drug is prescribed. In terms of epinephrine, it is not known what effect vasoconstrictors in the local anesthetic regimen will have in patients with a known history of congenital prolonged QT interval or in patients taking any medication that prolongs the QT interval. Until more information is obtained, it is suggested that the clinician consult with the physician prior to the use of a vasoconstrictor in suspected patients, and that the vasoconstrictor (epinephrine, mepivacaine and levonordefrin [Carbocaine® 2% with Neo-Cobefrin®]) be used with caution.

Effects on Dental Treatment Ondansetron is an alternative to phenothiazines (ie, promethazine) for the treatment of moderate-to-severe postoperative nausea and vomiting. Ondansetron prolongs the QT interval in a dose-dependent manner. Avoid ondansetron in patients with congenital long QT syndrome.

Effects on Bleeding No information available to require special precautions

Adverse Reactions Note: Percentages reported in adult patients unless otherwise specified.

>10%:

Central nervous system: Headache (oral: 9% to 27%; IV: 17%), fatigue (oral: ≤9% to 13%), malaise (oral: ≤9% to 13%)

Gastrointestinal: Constipation (6% to 11%)

1% to 10%:

Central nervous system: Drowsiness (IV: ≤8%), sedation (IV: ≤8%), (dizziness (7%), agitation (oral: ≤6%), anxiety (oral: ≤6%), paresthesia (IV: 2%), sensation of cold (IV: 2%)

Dermatologic: Pruritus (2% to 5%), skin rash (1%)

Gastrointestinal: Diarrhea (oral: 6% to 7%; IV: Children 1 to 24 months of age: 2%)

Genitourinary: Gynecologic disease (oral: 7%), urinary retention (oral: 5%)

Hepatic: Increased serum ALT (>2 times ULN: 1% to 5%; transient), increased serum AST (>2 times ULN: 1% to 5%; transient)

Local: Injection site reaction (IV: 4%; includes burning sensation at injection site, erythema at injection site, injection site pain)

Respiratory: Hypoxia (oral: 9%)

Miscellaneous: Fever (2% to 8%)

<1%, postmarketing, and/or case reports: Abdominal pain, accommodation disturbance, anaphylactoid reaction, anaphylaxis, angina pectoris, angioedema, atrial fibrillation, bradycardia, bronchospasm, bullous skin disease, cardiac arrhythmia, cardiorespiratory arrest (IV), chest pain, chills, depression of ST segment on ECG, dyspnea, dystonic reaction, ECG changes, extrapyramidal reaction (IV), flushing, hepatic failure (when used with other hepatotoxic medications), hiccups, hypersensitivity reaction, hypokalemia, hypotension, ischemic heart disease, laryngeal edema, laryngospasm (IV), liver enzyme disorder, mucosal tissue reaction, myocardial infarction, neuroleptic malignant syndrome, oculogyric crisis, palpitations, positive lymphocyte transformation test, prolonged QT interval on ECG (dose dependent), second-degree atrioventricular block, serotonin syndrome, shock (IV), Stevens-Johnson syndrome, stridor, supraventricular tachycardia, syncope, tachycardia, tonic-clonic seizures, torsades de pointes, toxic epidermal necrolysis, transient blindness (lasted ≤48 hours), transient blurred vision (following infusion), urticaria, vascular occlusive events, ventricular premature contractions, ventricular tachycardia, weakness, xerostomia

Mechanism of Action Ondansetron is a selective 5-HT_3-receptor antagonist which blocks serotonin, both peripherally on vagal nerve terminals and centrally in the chemoreceptor trigger zone

Pharmacodynamics/Kinetics

Onset of Action ~30 minutes

Half-life Elimination

Children:

Cancer patients: Children and Adolescents: 4 to 18 years: 2.8 hours

Surgical patients: Infants 1 to 4 months: 6.7 hours; Infants and Children 5 months to 12 years: 2.9 hours

Adults: 3 to 6 hours; Mild-to-moderate hepatic impairment (Child-Pugh classes A and B): 12 hours; Severe hepatic impairment (Child-Pugh class C): 20 hours

Time to Peak Oral: ~2 hours; Oral soluble film: ~1 hour

Pregnancy Considerations

Ondansetron crosses the placenta (Elkomy 2014; Siu 2006).

Ondansetron can be detected in fetal tissue (Siu 2006). The risk of developing a major congenital malformation following first trimester exposure is under study. Risks related to specific birth defects (eg, cardiac anomalies, oral clefts) requires confirmation; human data are conflicting (ACOG 2018; Kaplan 2019; Lemon 2019; Lavecchia 2018; Picot 2020). Clearance is decreased immediately after birth in neonates exposed to ondansetron in utero (Elkomy 2014).

Due to pregnancy-induced physiologic changes, clearance of ondansetron may increase as pregnancy progresses (Lemon 2016). Dose adjustment is not needed when administered for the prevention of nausea and vomiting associated with cesarean delivery (Elkomy 2014).

Ondansetron may be considered for the treatment of severe or refractory nausea and vomiting of pregnancy (NVP) when preferred agents have failed (ACOG 2018; Campbell 2016). Until additional information related to fetal safety is available, current guidelines suggest use prior to 10 weeks gestation be individualized (ACOG 2018). Dose-dependent QT-interval prolongation can occur with use; therefore, ECG monitoring is recommended in patients with risk factors for arrhythmia (ACOG 2018); this may include patients with electrolyte abnormalities associated with some cases of NVP (Koren 2012).

Ondansetron may be considered as part of a multimodal approach to prevent nausea and vomiting associated with cesarean delivery. A combination of ≥2 antiemetics with different mechanisms of action is recommended to treat intraoperative and postoperative nausea and vomiting (Griffiths 2012; Habib 2013; Jetling 2017; Macones 2019; SOAP 2019; Zhou 2018). An international consensus panel recommends that 5-HT_3 antagonists (including ondansetron) can be used when necessary in pregnant patients receiving chemotherapy for the treatment of gynecologic cancers (Amant 2019).

Dental Health Professional Considerations

Ondansetron is a safer alternative than phenothiazines (ie, promethazine) for the treatment of moderate-to-severe postoperative nausea and vomiting. The cost can be a limitation.

Also see Local Anesthetic/Vasoconstrictor Precautions

- **Ondansetron HCl** *see* Ondansetron *on page 1143*
- **Ondansetron Hydrochloride** *see* Ondansetron *on page 1143*
- **One A Day Cholesterol Plus [OTC]** *see* Vitamins (Multiple/Oral) *on page 1550*
- **One A Day Energy [OTC]** *see* Vitamins (Multiple/Oral) *on page 1550*
- **One A Day Essential [OTC]** *see* Vitamins (Multiple/Oral) *on page 1550*
- **One A Day Maximum [OTC]** *see* Vitamins (Multiple/Oral) *on page 1550*
- **One A Day Men's 50+ Advantage [OTC]** *see* Vitamins (Multiple/Oral) *on page 1550*
- **One A Day Men's Health Formula [OTC]** *see* Vitamins (Multiple/Oral) *on page 1550*
- **One A Day Teen Advantage for Her [OTC]** *see* Vitamins (Multiple/Oral) *on page 1550*
- **One A Day Teen Advantage for Him [OTC]** *see* Vitamins (Multiple/Oral) *on page 1550*
- **One A Day Weight Smart Advanced [OTC]** *see* Vitamins (Multiple/Oral) *on page 1550*
- **One A Day® Women's 50+ Advantage [OTC]** *see* Vitamins (Multiple/Oral) *on page 1550*
- **One A Day Women's [OTC]** *see* Vitamins (Multiple/Oral) *on page 1550*
- **One A Day Women's Active Mind & Body [OTC]** *see* Vitamins (Multiple/Oral) *on page 1550*
- **One-Daily/Iron [OTC]** *see* Vitamins (Multiple/Oral) *on page 1550*
- **Onexton** *see* Clindamycin and Benzoyl Peroxide *on page 375*
- **Onfi** *see* CloBAZam *on page 376*
- **Ongentys** *see* Opicapone *on page 1144*
- **Onglyza** *see* SAXagliptin *on page 1360*
- **Onivyde** *see* Irinotecan (Liposomal) *on page 842*
- **Onmel [DSC]** *see* Itraconazole *on page 849*
- **ONO-4538** *see* Nivolumab *on page 1114*
- **ONT-380** *see* Tucatinib *on page 1503*
- **Ontruzant** *see* Trastuzumab *on page 1479*
- **Onxol** *see* PACLitaxel (Conventional) *on page 1178*
- **Onzetra Xsail** *see* SUMAtriptan *on page 1394*
- **Opana [DSC]** *see* OxyMORphone *on page 1176*
- **Opana ER [DSC]** *see* OxyMORphone *on page 1176*
- **OPC-13013** *see* Cilostazol *on page 349*
- **OPC-14597** *see* ARIPiprazole *on page 164*
- **OPC-41061** *see* Tolvaptan *on page 1463*
- **o,p'-DDD** *see* Mitotane *on page 1041*
- **Opcon-A [OTC]** *see* Naphazoline and Pheniramine *on page 1079*
- **Opdivo** *see* Nivolumab *on page 1114*

Opicapone (oh PIK a pone)

Pharmacologic Category Anti-Parkinson Agent, COMT Inhibitor

Use Parkinson disease: Adjunctive treatment to levodopa/carbidopa in patients with Parkinson disease experiencing "off" episodes.

Local Anesthetic/Vasoconstrictor Precautions No information available to require special precautions.

Effects on Dental Treatment Key adverse event(s) related to dental treatment: Occurrence of xerostomia; normal salivary flow upon discontinuance; patients may experience orthostatic hypotension as they stand up after treatment, especially if lying in dental chair for extended periods of time. Use caution with sudden changes in position during and after dental treatment. Occurrence of aggressive behavior and agitation.

Effects on Bleeding No information available to require special precautions.

Adverse Reactions

>10%: Neuromuscular & skeletal: Dyskinesia (20%)

1% to 10%:

Cardiovascular: Hypertension (3%), hypotension (including orthostatic hypotension: 5%), increased serum creatine kinase (5%), presyncope (5%), syncope (5%)

Endocrine & metabolic: Weight loss (4%)

Gastrointestinal: Constipation (6%), xerostomia (3%)
Nervous system: Aggressive behavior (1%), agitation (1%), delusion (1%), dizziness (3%), hallucination (3%), impulse control disorder (1%), insomnia (3%)
Frequency not defined: Nervous system: Sleep driving, sudden onset of sleep

Mechanism of Action Opicapone is a reversible and selective inhibitor of catechol-O-methyltransferase (COMT); COMT is the major degradation pathway for levodopa. When opicapone is taken with levodopa, the pharmacokinetics are altered, resulting in more sustained levodopa serum levels compared to levodopa taken alone. The resulting levels of levodopa provide for increased concentrations available for absorption across the blood-brain barrier, thereby providing for increased CNS levels of dopamine, the active metabolite of levodopa.

Pharmacodynamics/Kinetics

Half-life Elimination 1 to 2 hours.

Time to Peak 2 hours (range: 1 to 4 hours).

Pregnancy Considerations

Based on data from animal reproduction studies, in utero exposure to opicapone may cause fetal harm. Opicapone is used in combination with levodopa/carbidopa. Also refer to the Levodopa/Carbidopa monographs for additional information.

Product Availability Ongentys: FDA approved April 2020; anticipated availability in 2020.

- ◆ **Opsumit** *see* Macitentan *on page 945*
- ◆ **OPT-80** *see* Fidaxomicin *on page 668*
- ◆ **Optivite P.M.T. [OTC]** *see* Vitamins (Multiple/Oral) *on page 1550*
- ◆ **Orabloc** *see* Articaine and Epinephrine *on page 170*
- ◆ **Oracea** *see* Doxycycline *on page 522*
- ◆ **Orafate** *see* Mucosal Coating Agent *on page 1066*
- ◆ **Ora-film [OTC]** *see* Benzocaine *on page 228*
- ◆ **Oralone** *see* Triamcinolone (Topical) *on page 1490*
- ◆ **Oral Wound Care Products** *see* Mucosal Coating Agent *on page 1066*
- ◆ **Oramorph SR** *see* Morphine (Systemic) *on page 1050*
- ◆ **Orap [DSC]** *see* Pimozide *on page 1233*
- ◆ **Orapred ODT** *see* PrednisoLONE (Systemic) *on page 1255*
- ◆ **Oraqix** *see* Lidocaine and Prilocaine *on page 911*
- ◆ **OraVerse** *see* Phentolamine *on page 1226*
- ◆ **Oravig** *see* Miconazole (Oral) *on page 1019*
- ◆ **Orbactiv** *see* Oritavancin *on page 1145*
- ◆ **Orciprenaline Sulfate** *see* Metaproterenol *on page 982*
- ◆ **Orencia** *see* Abatacept *on page 53*
- ◆ **Orencia ClickJect** *see* Abatacept *on page 53*
- ◆ **Orenitram** *see* Treprostinil *on page 1482*
- ◆ **Oriahnn** *see* Elagolix, Estradiol, and Norethindrone *on page 547*
- ◆ **Oriahnn** *see* Elagolix, Estradiol, and Norethindrone *on page 547*
- ◆ **Orilissa** *see* Elagolix *on page 547*
- ◆ **Orinase** *see* TOLBUTamide *on page 1460*

Oritavancin (or it a VAN sin)

Brand Names: US Orbactiv

Pharmacologic Category Glycopeptide

Use Acute bacterial skin and skin structure infections: Treatment of adult patients with acute bacterial skin and skin structure infections (ABSSSI) caused by susceptible isolates of the following gram-positive microorganisms: *Staphylococcus aureus* (including methicillin-susceptible and methicillin-resistant isolates); *Streptococcus pyogenes; Streptococcus agalactiae; Streptococcus dysgalactiae, Streptococcus anginosus* group (including *S. anginosus, S. intermedius, S. constellatus*); and *Enterococcus faecalis* (vancomycin-susceptible isolates only)

Local Anesthetic/Vasoconstrictor Precautions No information available to require special precautions

Effects on Dental Treatment Key adverse event(s) related to dental treatment: Use may result in fungal or bacterial superinfection within the oral cavity

Effects on Bleeding No information available to require special precautions

Adverse Reactions

1% to 10%:
Cardiovascular: Tachycardia (3%), hypersensitivity angiitis (<2%; leucocytoclastic vasculitis), peripheral edema (<2%)
Central nervous system: Headache (7%), dizziness (3%)
Dermatologic: Erythema multiforme (<2%), pruritus (<2%), skin rash (<2%), urticaria (<2%)
Endocrine & metabolic: Hyperuricemia (<2%), hypoglycemia (<2%)
Gastrointestinal: Nausea (10%), vomiting (5%), diarrhea (4%)
Hematologic & oncologic: Anemia (<2%), eosinophilia (<2%)
Hepatic: Increased serum ALT (3%), increased serum AST (2%), increased total serum bilirubin (<2%)
Hypersensitivity: Angioedema (<2%), hypersensitivity reaction (<2%)
Infection: Abscess (subcutaneous and limb; 4%)
Local: Injection site phlebitis (3%), injection site reaction (2%), erythema at injection site (<2%), extravasation (<2%), induration at injection site (<2%)
Neuromuscular & skeletal: Myalgia (<2%), osteomyelitis (<2%), tenosynovitis (<2%)
Respiratory: Bronchospasm (<2%), wheezing (<2%)
<1%, postmarketing, and/or case reports: *Clostridioides* (formerly *Clostridium*) *difficile*-associated diarrhea

Mechanism of Action Oritavancin is a lipoglycopeptide with concentration-dependent bactericidal activity. It inhibits cell wall biosynthesis by inhibiting the polymerization step by binding to stem peptides of peptidoglycan precursors, by inhibiting crosslinking by binding to bridging segments, and by disrupting bacterial membrane integrity, leading to cell death.

Pharmacodynamics/Kinetics

Half-life Elimination ~245 hours

Pregnancy Considerations Adverse events were not observed in animal reproduction studies.

- ◆ **Oritavancin Diphosphate** *see* Oritavancin *on page 1145*

Orlistat (OR li stat)

Brand Names: US Alli [OTC]; Xenical

Brand Names: Canada Xenical

Pharmacologic Category Lipase Inhibitor

Use Obesity management:

OTC: Weight loss in overweight adults when used along with a reduced-calorie and low-fat diet.

Rx: Obesity management, including weight loss and weight maintenance, when used in conjunction with a reduced-calorie diet; to reduce the risk for weight regain after prior weight loss.

Limitations of use: Orlistat is indicated for obese patients with an initial body mass index of ≥30 kg/m^2 or ≥27 kg/m^2 in the presence of other risk factors (eg, hypertension, diabetes, dyslipidemia).

Local Anesthetic/Vasoconstrictor Precautions No information available to require special precautions

Effects on Dental Treatment No significant effects or complications reported

Effects on Bleeding No information available to require special precautions

Adverse Reactions The frequency of most adverse reactions (especially gastrointestinal effects) decreases over time. Frequency not always defined.

Cardiovascular: Pedal edema (≤3%)

Central nervous system: Headache (≤31%), fatigue (3% to 7%), anxiety (3% to 5%), sleep disorder (≤4%)

Dermatologic: Xeroderma (≤2%)

Endocrine & metabolic: Menstrual disease (≤10%), hypoglycemia (in patients with diabetes)

Gastrointestinal: Oily rectal leakage (4% to 27%), abdominal distress (≤26%), abdominal pain (≤26%), flatulence with discharge (2% to 24%), bowel urgency (3% to 22%), steatorrhea (6% to 20%), oily evacuation (2% to 12%), frequent bowel movements (3% to 11%), nausea (4% to 8%), fecal incontinence (2% to 8%), infectious diarrhea (≤5%), rectal pain (3% to 5%), gingival disease (4%), cholelithiasis (3%), abdominal distension (in patients with diabetes)

Genitourinary: Urinary tract infection (6% to 8%), vaginitis (3%)

Infection: Influenza (≤40%)

Neuromuscular & skeletal: Back pain (≤14%), leg pain (≤11%), myalgia (≤4%)

Otic: Otitis (4%)

Respiratory: Upper respiratory tract infection (38%), lower respiratory tract infection (≤8%)

<1%, postmarketing, and/or case reports: Acute renal failure, anaphylaxis, angioedema, bronchospasm, bullous skin disease, calcium oxalate nephrolithiasis, gastrointestinal hemorrhage (lower), hepatic failure, hepatitis, hypersensitivity, hypersensitivity angiitis, increased serum alkaline phosphatase, increased serum transaminases, pancreatitis, pruritus, renal disease (secondary to increased urinary oxalate excretion), skin rash, urticaria

Mechanism of Action A reversible inhibitor of gastric and pancreatic lipases, thus inhibiting absorption of dietary fats by 30%.

Pharmacodynamics/Kinetics

Onset of Action 24-48 hours

Duration of Action 48-72 hours

Half-life Elimination 1-2 hours

Time to Peak Serum: ~8 hours

Reproductive Considerations

Medications for weight loss therapy are not recommended at conception (ACOG 156 2015; Stang 2016).

Pregnancy Risk Factor X

Pregnancy Considerations

Outcome information following maternal use of orlistat during pregnancy is limited (Källén 2014; Perrio 2007).

An increased risk of adverse maternal and fetal outcomes is associated with obesity. However, moderate weight gain based on prepregnancy BMI is required for positive fetal outcomes. Therefore, medications for weight loss therapy are not recommended during pregnancy (ACOG 156 2015; Stang 2016). Due to the lack of clinical benefit and potential for fetal harm, use of orlistat is contraindicated in pregnant females.

◆ **Ormir [OTC]** *see* DiphenhydrAMINE (Systemic) *on page 502*

Orphenadrine (or FEN a dreen)

Related Information

Temporomandibular Dysfunction (TMD), Chronic Pain, and Fibromyalgia *on page 1773*

Pharmacologic Category Skeletal Muscle Relaxant

Use Treatment of muscle spasm associated with acute painful musculoskeletal conditions

Local Anesthetic/Vasoconstrictor Precautions No information available to require special precautions

Effects on Dental Treatment The peripheral anticholinergic effects of orphenadrine may decrease or inhibit salivary flow; normal salivation will return with cessation of drug therapy.

Effects on Bleeding No information available to require special precautions

Adverse Reactions Frequency not defined.

Cardiovascular: Palpitations, tachycardia

Central nervous system: Agitation, confusion, dizziness, drowsiness, euphoria, hallucination, headache

Dermatologic: Pruritus, urticaria

Gastrointestinal: Constipation, gastric irritation, nausea, vomiting, xerostomia

Genitourinary: Urinary retention, urination hesitancy

Hypersensitivity: Hypersensitivity reaction

Neuromuscular & skeletal: Tremor, weakness

Ophthalmic: Blurred vision, increased intraocular pressure, mydriasis, nystagmus

Respiratory: Nasal congestion

<1%, postmarketing, and/or case reports: Anaphylaxis (injection), aplastic anemia

Mechanism of Action Indirect skeletal muscle relaxant thought to work by central atropine-like effects; has some euphorigenic and analgesic properties

Pharmacodynamics/Kinetics

Onset of Action Peak effect: Oral: Within 2 to 4 hours

Duration of Action 4 to 6 hours

Half-life Elimination 14 to 16 hours

Pregnancy Risk Factor C

Pregnancy Considerations Animal reproduction studies have not been conducted.

Orphenadrine, Aspirin, and Caffeine

(or FEN a dreen, AS pir in, & KAF een)

Pharmacologic Category Skeletal Muscle Relaxant

Use Musculoskeletal pain: Relief of mild to moderate pain and discomfort associated with acute musculoskeletal disorders.

Local Anesthetic/Vasoconstrictor Precautions No information available to require special precautions

Effects on Dental Treatment Key adverse event(s) related to dental treatment: The peripheral anticholinergic effects of orphenadrine may decrease or inhibit salivary flow; normal salivation will return with cessation of drug therapy.

Aspirin: As with all drugs which may affect hemostasis, bleeding is associated with aspirin. Hemorrhage may occur at virtually any site; risk is dependent on multiple variables including dosage, concurrent use of multiple agents which alter hemostasis, and patient susceptibility. Many adverse effects of aspirin are dose related, and are rare at low dosages. Other serious reactions are idiosyncratic, related to allergy or individual sensitivity (see Dental Health Professional Considerations).

Aspirin as sole antiplatelet agent: Patients taking aspirin for ischemic stroke prevention are safe to continue it during dental procedures (Armstrong, 2013).

Concurrent aspirin use with other antiplatelet agents: Aspirin in combination with clopidogrel (Plavix®), prasugrel (Effient®), or ticagrelor (Brilinta™) is the primary prevention strategy against stent thrombosis after placement of drug-eluting metal stents in coronary patients. Premature discontinuation of combination antiplatelet therapy (ie, dual antiplatelet therapy) strongly increases the risk of a catastrophic event of stent thrombosis leading to myocardial infarction and/or death, so says a science advisory issued in January 2007 from the American Heart Association in collaboration with the American Dental Association and other professional healthcare organizations. The advisory stresses a 12-month therapy of dual antiplatelet therapy after placement of a drug-eluting stent in order to prevent thrombosis at the stent site. Any elective surgery should be postponed for 1 year after stent implantation, and if surgery must be performed, consideration should be given to continuing the antiplatelet therapy during the perioperative period in high-risk patients with drug-eluting stents.

This advisory was issued from a science panel made up of representatives from the American Heart Association (AHA), the American College of Cardiology, the Society for Cardiovascular Angiography and Interventions, the American College of Surgeons, the American Dental Association (ADA), and the American College of Physicians (Grines, 2007).

Effects on Bleeding Aspirin irreversibly inhibits platelet aggregation which can prolong bleeding. Upon discontinuation, normal platelet function returns only when new platelets are released (~7-10 days). However, in the case of dental surgery, there is no scientific evidence to support discontinuation of aspirin. This was recently supported by the American Academy of Neurology in patients with ischemic cerebrovascular disease (Armstrong, 2013). A recent study compared blood loss after a single tooth extraction in coronary artery disease patients who were either on aspirin (100 mg daily) or off aspirin for the extraction. The mean volume of bleeding was not statistically different between the groups. Local hemostatic measures were sufficient to control bleeding and there were no reported episodes of hemorrhaging intra- or postoperatively (Medeiros, 2011).

Adverse Reactions Also see individual agents.

Frequency not defined:

- Cardiovascular: Palpitations, syncope, tachycardia
- Dermatologic: Dermatologic disorder (rare), urticaria (rare)
- Gastrointestinal: Constipation, gastrointestinal hemorrhage (rare), nausea, vomiting, xerostomia
- Genitourinary: Urinary hesitancy, urinary retention
- Nervous system: Confusion (older adults), dizziness, drowsiness, hallucination, headache, mild central nervous system stimulation
- Neuromuscular & skeletal: Asthenia
- Ophthalmic: Blurred vision, increased intraocular pressure, mydriasis

Postmarketing: Hematologic & oncologic: Aplastic anemia

Mechanism of Action

Aspirin: Inhibits prostaglandin synthesis in the CNS and peripherally blocks pain impulse generation.

Caffeine: A CNS stimulant.

Orphenadrine: Indirect skeletal muscle relaxant thought to work by central atropine-like effects; has some euphorigenic and analgesic properties.

Pregnancy Considerations Refer to individual monographs.

Dental Health Professional Considerations There is no scientific evidence to warrant discontinuance of aspirin prior to dental surgery. Patients taking one aspirin tablet daily as an antithrombotic and who require dental surgery should be given special consideration in consultation with the physician before removal of the aspirin relative to prevention of postoperative bleeding.

◆ **Orphenadrine Citrate** *see* Orphenadrine *on page 1146*

◆ **Orsythia** *see* Ethinyl Estradiol and Levonorgestrel *on page 612*

◆ **Ortho Cept** *see* Ethinyl Estradiol and Desogestrel *on page 609*

◆ **Ortho Cyclen** *see* Ethinyl Estradiol and Norgestimate *on page 616*

◆ **Ortho-Cyclen (28) [DSC]** *see* Ethinyl Estradiol and Norgestimate *on page 616*

◆ **Ortho Est** *see* Estropipate *on page 605*

◆ **Ortho-Evra** *see* Ethinyl Estradiol and Norelgestromin *on page 613*

◆ **Ortho Micronor** *see* Norethindrone *on page 1117*

◆ **Ortho Novum** *see* Ethinyl Estradiol and Norethindrone *on page 614*

◆ **Ortho-Novum 1/35 (28) [DSC]** *see* Ethinyl Estradiol and Norethindrone *on page 614*

◆ **Ortho-Novum 7/7/7 (28) [DSC]** *see* Ethinyl Estradiol and Norethindrone *on page 614*

◆ **Ortho,para-DDD** *see* Mitotane *on page 1041*

◆ **Ortho Prefest** *see* Estradiol and Norgestimate *on page 599*

◆ **Ortho Tri Cyclen** *see* Ethinyl Estradiol and Norgestimate *on page 616*

◆ **Ortho Tri-Cyclen (28) [DSC]** *see* Ethinyl Estradiol and Norgestimate *on page 616*

◆ **Ortho Tri-Cyclen Lo [DSC]** *see* Ethinyl Estradiol and Norgestimate *on page 616*

◆ **Orthovisc** *see* Hyaluronate and Derivatives *on page 761*

◆ **OrthoWash** *see* Fluoride *on page 693*

◆ **Ortikos** *see* Budesonide (Systemic) *on page 252*

◆ **Orudis KT** *see* Ketoprofen *on page 860*

◆ **Oruvail** *see* Ketoprofen *on page 860*

◆ **Os-Cal [OTC]** *see* Calcium and Vitamin D *on page 280*

◆ **Os-Cal Calcium + D3 [OTC]** *see* Calcium and Vitamin D *on page 280*

◆ **Os-Cal Extra D3 [OTC]** *see* Calcium and Vitamin D *on page 280*

Oseltamivir (oh sel TAM i vir)

Related Information

Systemic Viral Diseases *on page 1709*

Brand Names: US Tamiflu

Brand Names: Canada MINT-Oseltamivir; NAT-Oseltamivir; Tamiflu

Pharmacologic Category Antiviral Agent; Neuraminidase Inhibitor

Use

Influenza, seasonal, prophylaxis: Prophylaxis of influenza (A or B) infection in patients ≥1 year of age.

Influenza, seasonal, treatment: Treatment of uncomplicated acute illness due to influenza (A or B) infection in patients ≥2 weeks of age who have been symptomatic for no more than 48 hours.

Note: The Advisory Committee on Immunization Practices (ACIP) recommends that treatment and prophylaxis be given to children <1 year of age when indicated (CDC 2018a).

Limitations of use: Not a substitute for annual influenza vaccination. Consider available information on influenza drug susceptibility patterns and treatment effects when deciding whether to use oseltamivir. Not recommended for patients with ESRD not undergoing dialysis.

Local Anesthetic/Vasoconstrictor Precautions No information available to require special precautions

Effects on Dental Treatment No significant effects or complications reported

Effects on Bleeding No information available to require special precautions

Adverse Reactions

>10%:

Gastrointestinal: Vomiting (2% to 16%)

Nervous system: Headache (adolescents and adults: 2% to 17%)

1% to 10%:

Gastrointestinal: Nausea (adolescents and adults: 8% to 10%)

Nervous system: Pain (adolescents and adults: 4%)

Postmarketing:

Cardiovascular: Cardiac arrhythmia

Dermatologic: Dermatitis, eczema, erythema multiforme, skin rash, Stevens-Johnson syndrome, toxic epidermal necrolysis, urticaria

Endocrine & metabolic: Exacerbation of diabetes mellitus

Gastrointestinal: Gastrointestinal hemorrhage, hemorrhagic colitis

Hepatic: Abnormal hepatic function tests, hepatitis

Hypersensitivity: Anaphylaxis, facial edema, hypersensitivity reaction, nonimmune anaphylaxis, swollen tongue

Nervous system: Abnormal behavior, agitation, anxiety, confusion, delirium, delusion, hallucination, hypothermia, impaired consciousness, nightmares, seizure

Mechanism of Action Oseltamivir, a prodrug, is hydrolyzed to the active form, oseltamivir carboxylate (OC). OC inhibits influenza virus neuraminidase, an enzyme known to cleave the budding viral progeny from its cellular envelope attachment point (neuraminic acid) just prior to release.

Pharmacodynamics/Kinetics

Half-life Elimination

Pediatric patients (Kimberlin 2013): Oseltamivir carboxylate:

≤2 months: Median: 6.64 hours; Range: 4.65 to 28.71 hours.

3 to 5 months: Median: 9.09 hours; Range: 6.25 to 19 hours.

6 to 8 months: Median:10.29 hours; Range: 1.02 to 78.26 hours.

9 to 11 months:

3 mg/kg: Median: 11.13 hours; Range: 5.4 to 51.86 hours.

3.5 mg/kg: Median: 14.56 hours; Range: 7.22 to 25.67 hours.

12 to 23 months:

3.5 mg/kg: Median: 14.82 hours; Range: 8.13 to 20.16 hours.

30 mg (fixed dose): Median: 7.98 hours; Range: 4.49 to 17.11 hours.

Adults: Oseltamivir: 1 to 3 hours; Oseltamivir carboxylate: 6 to 10 hours.

Pregnancy Considerations

Oseltamivir phosphate and its active metabolite oseltamivir carboxylate cross the placenta (Meijer 2012).

An increased risk of adverse neonatal or maternal outcomes has generally not been observed following maternal use of oseltamivir during pregnancy (CDC 2011).

Untreated influenza infection is associated with an increased risk of adverse events to the fetus and an increased risk of complications or death to the mother. Oseltamivir is currently recommended for the treatment or prophylaxis of influenza in pregnant women and women up to 2 weeks' postpartum (ACOG 2018; CDC 2011).

◆ **Oseltamivir Phosphate** *see* Oseltamivir *on page 1147*

◆ **OSI-774** *see* Erlotinib *on page 584*

Osilodrostat (oh SIL oh DROE stat)

Brand Names: US Isturisa

Pharmacologic Category Cortisol Synthesis Inhibitor

Use Cushing disease: Treatment of Cushing disease in adults for whom pituitary surgery is not an option or has not been curative.

Local Anesthetic/Vasoconstrictor Precautions Both hypertension and hypotension have been reported. Monitor for hypertension prior to using local anesthetic with vasoconstrictor; medical consult if necessary. Osilodrostat is one of the drugs confirmed to prolong the QT interval and is accepted as having a risk of causing torsades de pointes. The risk of drug-induced torsades de pointes is extremely low when a single QT interval prolonging drug is prescribed. In terms of epinephrine, it is not known what effect vasoconstrictors in the local anesthetic regimen will have in patients with a known history of congenital prolonged QT interval or in patients taking any medication that prolongs the QT interval. Until more information is obtained, it is suggested that the clinician consult with the physician prior to the use of a vasoconstrictor in suspected patients and that the vasoconstrictor (epinephrine, mepivacaine, and levonordefrin [Carbocaine 2% with Neo-Cobefrin]) be used with caution.

Effects on Dental Treatment Key adverse event(s) related to dental treatment: Frequent occurrence of nasopharyngitis.

Effects on Bleeding No information available to require special precautions.

Adverse Reactions

>10%:

Cardiovascular: Edema (7% to 21%), hypertension (10% to 14%), hypotension (12%)

Dermatologic: Acne vulgaris (9% to 11%), skin rash (15%)

Endocrine & metabolic: Adrenocortical insufficiency (43%), altered hormone level (12%; corticotrophin increased: 14%), decreased cortisol (18% to 31%), hirsutism (10% to 12%), hypokalemia (12% to 17%), increased testosterone level (11%)
Gastrointestinal: Abdominal pain (13%), decreased appetite (12%), diarrhea (15%), nausea (37%), vomiting (19%)
Genitourinary: Urinary tract infection (12%)
Hematologic & oncologic: Benign neoplasm (decrease in pituitary corticotroph tumor volume >20%: 18%), tumor growth (increase in pituitary corticotroph tumor volume >20%: 15%; no correlation between tumor volume and increase in adrenocorticotrophic hormone)
Nervous system: Dizziness (14%), fatigue (39%), headache (31%)
Neuromuscular & skeletal: Arthralgia (18%), back pain (15%), myalgia (12%)
Respiratory: Nasopharyngitis (20%)
Miscellaneous: Fever (11%)

1% to 10%:
Cardiovascular: Prolonged QT interval on ECG (4%), syncope (2%), tachycardia (7%)
Dermatologic: Alopecia (6%)
Gastrointestinal: Dyspepsia (8%), gastroenteritis (7%)
Hematologic & oncologic: Anemia (10%), neutropenia (1%)
Hepatic: Increased serum transaminases (4%)
Infection: Influenza (10%)
Nervous system: Anxiety (7%), depression (7%), insomnia (8%), malaise (7%)
Respiratory: Cough (10%)

Mechanism of Action Osilodrostat decreases cortisol synthesis via inhibition of 11beta-hydroxylase (CYP11B1), the enzyme responsible for the final step of cortisol biosynthesis in the adrenal gland.

Pharmacodynamics/Kinetics

Half-life Elimination ~4 hours.

Time to Peak ~1 hour.

Pregnancy Considerations Adverse events were not observed in animal reproduction studies.

◆ **Osilodrostat Phosphate** *see* Osilodrostat *on page 1148*

Osimertinib (oh si mer ti nib)

Brand Names: US Tagrisso

Brand Names: Canada Tagrisso

Pharmacologic Category Antineoplastic Agent, Epidermal Growth Factor Receptor (EGFR) Inhibitor; Antineoplastic Agent, Tyrosine Kinase Inhibitor

Use

Non-small cell lung cancer, metastatic:

First-line treatment of metastatic non-small cell lung cancer (NSCLC) in patients whose tumors have epidermal growth factor receptor (EGFR) exon 19 deletions or exon 21 L858R mutations as detected in tumor or plasma specimen by an approved test

Treatment of metastatic EGFR T790M mutation-positive (as detected in tumor or plasma specimen by an approved test) NSCLC in patients whose disease has progressed on or after EGFR tyrosine kinase inhibitor therapy

Local Anesthetic/Vasoconstrictor Precautions Osimertinib is one of the drugs confirmed to prolong the QT interval and is accepted as having a risk of causing torsade de points. In terms of epinephrine, it is not known what effect vasoconstrictors in the local anesthetic regimen will have in patients with a known history of congenital prolonged QT interval or in patients taking any medication that prolongs the QT interval. Until more information is obtained, it is suggested that the clinician consult with the physician prior to the use of a vasoconstrictor in suspected patients, and that the vasoconstrictor be used with caution.

Effects on Dental Treatment Key adverse event(s) related to dental treatment: Stomatitis has been reported

Effects on Bleeding Chemotherapy may result in significant myelosuppression, potentially including significant reduction in platelet counts (thrombocytopenia 54% grades 3/4: 1%) and altered hemostasis. In patients who are under active treatment with these agents, medical consult is suggested.

Adverse Reactions

>10%:
Dermatologic: Skin rash (58%), xeroderma (36%), nail disease (35%), pruritus (17%)
Endocrine & metabolic: Hypermagnesemia (30%), hypokalemia (16%)
Gastrointestinal: Diarrhea (58%), stomatitis (29%; grades 3/4: <1%), decreased appetite (20%), constipation (15%), nausea (14%), vomiting (11%)
Hematologic & oncologic: Lymphocytopenia (63%, grades 3/4: 6%), anemia (59%; grades 3/4: <1%), thrombocytopenia (51%, grades 3/4: <1%), neutropenia (41%, grades 3/4: 3%)
Hepatic: Increased serum aspartate aminotransferase (22%), increased serum alanine aminotransferase (21%), hyperbilirubinemia (14%)
Nervous system: Fatigue (21%), headache (12%)
Respiratory: Cough (17%), dyspnea (13%)

1% to 10%:
Cardiovascular: Prolonged QT interval on ECG (≤10%), decreased left ventricular ejection fraction (4%), cardiomyopathy (3%)
Respiratory: Upper respiratory tract infection (10%), interstitial pneumonitis (2% to 4%), pneumonia (3%), pulmonary embolism (2%)
Miscellaneous: Fever (10%)

<1%: Hyponatremia (Goss 2016), keratitis

Frequency not defined:
Dermatologic: Eczema, erythema of skin, leukonychia, nail bed changes, nail discoloration, nail hyperpigmentation, onychoclasis, onycholysis, onychomadesis, paronychia, skin erosion, skin fissure
Neuromuscular & skeletal: Asthenia
Ophthalmic: Eyelid pruritus

Postmarketing: Erythema multiforme, Stevens-Johnson syndrome

Mechanism of Action Osimertinib is an irreversible epidermal growth factor receptor (EGFR) tyrosine kinase inhibitor which binds to select mutant forms of EGFR, including T790M, L858R, and exon 19 deletion at lower concentrations than wild-type. Osimertinib exhibits less activity against wild-type EGFR (as compared to other EGFR inhibitors) and is selective for sensitizing mutations and the T790M resistance mutation, which is the most common mechanism of resistance to EGFR tyrosine kinase inhibitors (Janne 2015).

Pharmacodynamics/Kinetics

Half-life Elimination Mean (estimated): 48 hours

Time to Peak Median: 6 hours (range: 3 to 24 hours)

Reproductive Considerations
Verify pregnancy status in females of reproductive potential prior to initiating osimertinib. Females of reproductive potential should use effective contraception during therapy and for 6 weeks after the last osimertinib dose. Males with female partners of reproductive potential should also use effective contraception during therapy and for 4 months after the last osimertinib dose.

Pregnancy Considerations
Based on data from animal reproduction studies and the mechanism of action, use during pregnancy is expected to cause fetal harm.

Prescribing and Access Restrictions Available through specialty pharmacies and distributors. Further information may be obtained from the manufacturer, Astra Zeneca, at 1-844-275-2360 or at https://www.tagrisso.com.

◆ **Osmolex ER** *see* Amantadine *on page 112*

Ospemifene (os PEM i feen)

Brand Names: US Osphena

Pharmacologic Category Selective Estrogen Receptor Modulator (SERM)

Use

Dyspareunia: Treatment of moderate to severe dyspareunia, a symptom of vulvar and vaginal atrophy (VVA), due to menopause

Vaginal dryness: Treatment of moderate to severe vaginal dryness, symptoms of VVA, associated with menopause

Note: The International Society for the Study of Women's Sexual Health and The North American Menopause Society have endorsed the term genitourinary syndrome of menopause (GSM) as new terminology for vulvovaginal atrophy. The term GSM encompasses all genital and urinary signs and symptoms associated with a loss of estrogen due to menopause (Portman 2014).

Local Anesthetic/Vasoconstrictor Precautions
No information available to require special precautions

Effects on Dental Treatment No significant effects or complications reported

Effects on Bleeding Ospemifene has been associated with thromboembolic adverse events. There is no information available to require special precautions for dental procedures.

Adverse Reactions
>10%: Endocrine & metabolic: Hot flash (7% to 12%)

1% to 10%:

Central nervous system: Headache (3%)

Dermatologic: Hyperhidrosis (1% to 3%), night sweats (1%)

Genitourinary: Endometrial hyperplasia (10%), vaginal discharge (4% to 6%), endometrial polyps (2%), vaginal hemorrhage (1%)

Neuromuscular & skeletal: Muscle spasm (2% to 5%)

<1%, postmarketing, and/or case reports: Angioedema, benign neoplasm, cerebrovascular accident, cyst, deep vein thrombosis, endometrial carcinoma, erythematous rash, hypersensitivity reaction, malignant neoplasm, myocardial infarction, polyp, pruritus, pulmonary embolism, skin rash, thrombosis, urticaria

Mechanism of Action Ospemifene is a selective estrogen receptor modulator (SERM); it activates estrogen pathways in some tissues and blocks estrogen pathways in others, and specifically has agonistic effects on the endometrium. In women with VVA, ospemifene was shown to improve vaginal changes associated with the decrease in natural estrogen production associated with menopause (improves vaginal maturation index, decreases vaginal pH) and significantly decreased the most bothersome moderate-to-severe subjective findings reported by women (vaginal dryness and dyspareunia) after 12 weeks of therapy (Bachmann, 2010).

Pharmacodynamics/Kinetics

Onset of Action A significant decrease in vaginal dryness and dyspareunia were observed after 12 weeks of therapy (Bachmann, 2010).

Half-life Elimination ~26 hours

Time to Peak ~2 hours (range: 1-8 hours)

Reproductive Considerations
Use is contraindicated in women who may become pregnant.

Pregnancy Considerations
Use is contraindicated in women who are pregnant.

◆ **Osphena** *see* Ospemifene *on page 1150*

◆ **Otezla** *see* Apremilast *on page 161*

◆ **OTFC (Oral Transmucosal Fentanyl Citrate)** *see* FentaNYL *on page 642*

◆ **Otovel** *see* Ciprofloxacin and Fluocinolone *on page 351*

◆ **Otrexup** *see* Methotrexate *on page 990*

◆ **Ovcon-35 (28) [DSC]** *see* Ethinyl Estradiol and Norethindrone *on page 614*

◆ **Ovcon-50** *see* Ethinyl Estradiol and Norethindrone *on page 614*

◆ **Ovine Corticotrophin-Releasing Hormone (oCRH)** *see* Corticorelin *on page 411*

Oxacillin (oks a SIL in)

Pharmacologic Category Antibiotic, Penicillin

Use

Staphylococcal infections: Treatment of infections caused by penicillinase-producing staphylococci that have demonstrated susceptibility to the drug; empiric therapy in suspected cases of resistant staphylococcal infections.

Limitations of use: Oxacillin should not be used in infections caused by organisms susceptible to penicillin G.

Local Anesthetic/Vasoconstrictor Precautions
No information available to require special precautions

Effects on Dental Treatment Key adverse event(s) related to dental treatment: Prolonged use of penicillins may lead to development of oral candidiasis.

Effects on Bleeding No information available to require special precautions

Adverse Reactions
Frequency not defined.

Gastrointestinal: *Clostridioides difficile* associated diarrhea, *clostridioides difficile* colitis

Hepatic: Hepatotoxicity, increased serum aspartate aminotransferase

Renal: Acute interstitial nephritis, acute renal tubular disease

<1%, postmarketing, and/or case reports: Drug reaction with eosinophilia and systemic symptoms (Sharpe 2019)

Mechanism of Action Inhibits bacterial cell wall synthesis by binding to one or more of the penicillin-binding proteins (PBPs); which in turn inhibits the final transpeptidation step of peptidoglycan synthesis in bacterial cell walls, thus inhibiting cell wall biosynthesis. Bacteria eventually lyse due to ongoing activity of cell wall autolytic enzymes (autolysins and murein hydrolases) while cell wall assembly is arrested.

Pharmacodynamics/Kinetics

Half-life Elimination

Neonates (PNA: 8 to 15 days): 1.6 hours

Infants and Children ≤2 years: 0.9 to 1.8 hours

Adults: 20 to 30 minutes; prolonged with renal impairment

Time to Peak Serum: IM: 30 minutes; IV: 5 minutes

Pregnancy Considerations

Oxacillin is distributed into the amniotic fluid and is detected in cord blood. Maternal use of penicillins has generally not resulted in an increased risk of adverse fetal effects.

◆ **Oxacillin Sodium** *see* Oxacillin *on page 1150*

◆ **Oxalatoplatin** *see* Oxaliplatin *on page 1151*

◆ **Oxalatoplatinum** *see* Oxaliplatin *on page 1151*

Oxaliplatin (ox AL i pla tin)

Brand Names: Canada ACT Oxaliplatin [DSC]; Eloxatin [DSC]; PMS-Oxaliplatin; TARO-Oxaliplatin

Pharmacologic Category Antineoplastic Agent, Alkylating Agent; Antineoplastic Agent, Platinum Analog

Use

Colon cancer, stage III (adjuvant therapy): Adjuvant treatment of stage III colon cancer (in combination with infusional fluorouracil and leucovorin) after complete resection of primary tumor.

Colorectal cancer, advanced: Treatment of advanced colorectal cancer (in combination with infusional fluorouracil and leucovorin).

Local Anesthetic/Vasoconstrictor Precautions

No information available to require special precautions

Effects on Dental Treatment Key adverse event(s) related to dental treatment: Stomatitis, dysphagia, mucositis, and taste perversion.

Effects on Bleeding Chemotherapy may result in significant myelosuppression, potentially including significant reduction in platelet counts (infrequent, <1%) and altered hemostasis. In patients who are under active treatment with these agents, medical consult is suggested.

Adverse Reactions Percentages reported with monotherapy.

>10%:

Gastrointestinal: Abdominal pain (31%), anorexia (20%), constipation (31%), diarrhea (46%), nausea (64%), stomatitis (2% to 14%), vomiting (37%)

Hematologic & oncologic: Anemia (64%; grades 3/4: 1%), leukopenia (13%). thrombocytopenia (30%; grades 3/4: 3%)

Hepatic: Increased serum alanine aminotransferase (36%), increased serum aspartate aminotransferase (54%), increased serum bilirubin (13%)

Nervous system: Fatigue (61%), headache (13%), insomnia (11%), pain (14%), peripheral neuropathy (may be dose limiting; 76%, grades 3/4: 7%; acute 65%; grades 3/4: 5%; persistent 43%; grades 3/4: 3%)

Neuromuscular & skeletal: Back pain (11%)

Respiratory: Cough (11%), dyspnea (13%)

Miscellaneous: Fever (25%)

1% to 10%:

Cardiovascular: Chest pain (5%), edema (10%), flushing (3%), peripheral edema (5%), thromboembolism (2%)

Dermatologic: Alopecia (3%), palmar-plantar erythrodysesthesia (1%), skin rash (5%)

Endocrine & metabolic: Dehydration (5%), hypokalemia (3%)

Gastrointestinal: Dysgeusia (5%), dyspepsia (7%), dysphagia (acute 1% to 2%), flatulence (3%), gastroesophageal reflux disease (1%), hiccups (2%)

Genitourinary: Dysuria (1%)

Hematologic & oncologic: Neutropenia (7%)

Hypersensitivity: Hypersensitivity reaction (3%)

Local: Injection site reaction (9%)

Nervous system: Dizziness (7%), rigors (9%)

Neuromuscular & skeletal: Arthralgia (7%)

Ocular: Abnormal lacrimation (1%)

Renal: Increased serum creatinine (5% to 10%)

Respiratory: Epistaxis (2%), pharyngitis (2%), pharyngolaryngeal dysesthesia (grades 3/4: 1% to 2%), rhinitis (6%), upper respiratory tract infection (7%)

<1%, postmarketing, and/or case reports (reported with mono- and combination therapy): Abnormal gait, acute renal failure, anaphylaxis, anaphylactic shock, angioedema, aphonia, ataxia, blepharoptosis, cerebral hemorrhage, colitis, cranial nerve palsy, decreased deep tendon reflex, deafness, decreased visual acuity, diplopia, dysarthria, eosinophilic pneumonitis, fasciculations, febrile neutropenia, hematuria, hemolysis, hemolytic anemia (immuno-allergic), hemolytic-uremic syndrome, hemorrhage, hepatic failure, hepatic fibrosis (perisinusoidal), hepatic sinusoidal obstruction syndrome (SOS; veno-occlusive disease), hepatitis, hepatotoxicity, hypertension, hypomagnesemia, hypoxia, idiopathic noncirrhotic portal hypertension (nodular regenerative hyperplasia), increased INR, increased serum alkaline phosphatase, interstitial nephritis (acute), interstitial pulmonary disease, intestinal obstruction, lactic acidosis (Smith 2019), laryngospasm, leukemia, Lhermittes' sign, metabolic acidosis, muscle spasm, myoclonus, neutropenic enterocolitis, neutropenic infection (sepsis), nonimmune anaphylaxis, optic neuritis, pancreatitis, prolonged QT interval on ECG, prolonged prothrombin time, pulmonary fibrosis, purpura, rectal hemorrhage, renal tubular necrosis, reversible posterior leukoencephalopathy syndrome, rhabdomyolysis, seizure, sepsis, septic shock, temporary vision loss, thrombocytopenia (immuno-allergic), torsades de pointes, trigeminal neuralgia, ventricular arrhythmia, visual field loss, voice disorder

Mechanism of Action Oxaliplatin, a platinum derivative, is an alkylating agent. Following intracellular hydrolysis, the platinum compound binds to DNA forming cross-links which inhibit DNA replication and transcription, resulting in cell death. Cytotoxicity is cell-cycle nonspecific.

Pharmacodynamics/Kinetics

Half-life Elimination

Children: Oxaliplatin ultrafilterable platinum (terminal): Median: 293 hours; range: 187 to 662 hours (Beaty 2010).

Adults: Oxaliplatin ultrafilterable platinum: Distribution: Alpha phase: 0.43 hours; Beta phase: 16.8 hours; Terminal: 392 hours.

Reproductive Considerations Evaluate pregnancy status prior to treatment initiation in females of reproductive potential. Females of reproductive potential should use effective contraception during treatment and for at least 9 months after the last oxaliplatin dose. Males with female partners of reproductive potential should use effective contraception during treatment and for 6 months after the last oxaliplatin dose. Males and females of reproductive potential desiring children should consider fertility preservation prior to therapy (Levi 2015; O'Neil 2011).

Pregnancy Considerations

Based on findings from animal reproduction studies and the mechanism of action, in utero exposure to oxaliplatin may result in fetal harm. Reports of oxaliplatin for the treatment of advanced colorectal cancer in pregnancy are limited (Frydenberg 2020; Makoshi 2015; Robson 2017).

The European Society for Medical Oncology has published guidelines for diagnosis, treatment, and follow-up of cancer during pregnancy; the guidelines recommend referral to a facility with expertise in cancer during pregnancy and encourage a multidisciplinary team (obstetrician, neonatologist, oncology team). In general, if chemotherapy is indicated, it should be avoided in the first trimester, there should be a 3-week time period between the last chemotherapy dose and anticipated delivery, and chemotherapy should not be administered beyond week 33 of gestation (Peccatori 2013).

A pregnancy registry is available for all cancers diagnosed during pregnancy at Cooper Health (877-635-4499).

◆ **Oxandrin [DSC]** *see* Oxandrolone *on page 1152*

Oxandrolone (oks AN droe lone)

Brand Names: US Oxandrin [DSC]

Pharmacologic Category Androgen

Use

Weight gain (adjunctive therapy): Adjunctive therapy to promote weight gain after weight loss following extensive surgery, chronic infections, or severe trauma, and in some patients who, without definite pathophysiologic reasons, fail to gain or to maintain normal weight

Other indications included in manufacturer labeling: Adjunctive therapy to offset protein catabolism with prolonged corticosteroid administration; relief of bone pain associated with osteoporosis (current guidelines do not make recommendations regarding use of oxandrolone for osteoporosis related bone pain)

Local Anesthetic/Vasoconstrictor Precautions

No information available to require special precautions

Effects on Dental Treatment No significant effects or complications reported

Effects on Bleeding No information available to require special precautions

Adverse Reactions Frequency not defined.

Cardiovascular: Edema

Central nervous system: Deepening of the voice (females), depression, excitement, habituation, insomnia

Dermatologic: Acne vulgaris (females and prepubertal males), androgenetic alopecia (females)

Endocrine & metabolic: Changes in libido, decreased glucose tolerance, decreased HDL cholesterol, electrolyte disturbance, gynecomastia, hirsutism (females), increased LDL cholesterol, inhibition of gonadotropin secretion, menstrual disease (females)

Genitourinary: Clitoromegaly (females), epididymitis (postpubertal males), erectile dysfunction (prepubertal males; increased or persistent erections), impotence (postpubertal males), inhibition of testicular function (postpubertal males), irritable bladder (postpubertal males), oligospermia (postpubertal males), phallic enlargement (prepubertal males), priapism (chronic; postpubertal males), testicular atrophy (postpubertal males)

Hematologic & oncologic: Clotting factors suppression, prolonged prothrombin time

Hepatic: Cholestatic jaundice, hepatocellular neoplasm, increased serum alkaline phosphatase, increased serum ALT, increased serum AST, increased serum bilirubin, peliosis hepatitis (long-term therapy)

Neuromuscular & skeletal: Increased creatine phosphokinase, premature epiphyseal closure (children)

Renal: Increased creatinine clearance

<1%, postmarketing, and/or case reports: Hepatic necrosis, hepatotoxicity (idiosyncratic; Chalasani 2014)

Mechanism of Action Synthetic testosterone derivative with similar androgenic and anabolic actions

Pharmacodynamics/Kinetics

Half-life Elimination 10 to 13 hours

Time to Peak Concentration: ~1 hour (Orr 2004)

Pregnancy Risk Factor X

Pregnancy Considerations

Use is contraindicated in pregnant women; masculinization of the fetus has been reported.

Controlled Substance C-III

Oxaprozin (oks a PROE zin)

Related Information

Rheumatoid Arthritis, Osteoarthritis, and Osteoporosis *on page 1697*

Temporomandibular Dysfunction (TMD), Chronic Pain, and Fibromyalgia *on page 1773*

Brand Names: US Daypro

Brand Names: Canada APO-Oxaprozin [DSC]

Pharmacologic Category Analgesic, Nonopioid; Nonsteroidal Anti-inflammatory Drug (NSAID), Oral

Use

Juvenile rheumatoid arthritis: Relief of signs and symptoms of juvenile rheumatoid arthritis (JRA).

Osteoarthritis: Relief of signs and symptoms of osteoarthritis.

Rheumatoid arthritis: Relief of signs and symptoms of rheumatoid arthritis.

Local Anesthetic/Vasoconstrictor Precautions

No information available to require special precautions

Effects on Dental Treatment The dentist should be aware of the potential of abnormal coagulation. Caution should also be exercised in the use of NSAIDs in patients already on anticoagulant therapy with drugs such as warfarin (Coumadin®). See Effects on Bleeding.

Effects on Bleeding Nonselective NSAIDs, such as oxaprozin, inhibit platelet aggregation and prolong bleeding time in some patients. Unlike aspirin, the NSAID effect on platelet function is quantitatively less, of shorter duration, and reversible. Normal platelet function should occur in ~5 elimination half-lives or in <10 hours after discontinuation of oxaprozin. Concomitant use of other NSAIDs should be avoided.

Adverse Reactions

1% to 10%:

Cardiovascular: Edema

Central nervous system: Confusion, depression, disturbed sleep, dizziness, drowsiness, headache, sedation

Dermatologic: Pruritus, skin rash

Gastrointestinal: Abdominal distress, abdominal pain, anorexia, constipation, diarrhea, dyspepsia, flatulence, gastrointestinal perforation (with gross bleeding), gastrointestinal ulcer, heartburn, nausea, vomiting

Genitourinary: Dysuria, urinary frequency

Hematologic & oncologic: Anemia, prolonged bleeding time

Hepatic: Increased liver enzymes

Otic: Tinnitus

Renal: Renal insufficiency

<1%, postmarketing, and/or case reports: Hepatotoxicity (idiosyncratic; Chalasani 2014)

Mechanism of Action Reversibly inhibits cyclooxygenase-1 and 2 (COX-1 and 2) enzymes, which results in decreased formation of prostaglandin precursors; has antipyretic, analgesic, and anti-inflammatory properties.

Other proposed mechanisms not fully elucidated (and possibly contributing to the anti-inflammatory effect to varying degrees) include inhibiting chemotaxis, altering lymphocyte activity, inhibiting neutrophil aggregation/ activation, and decreasing proinflammatory cytokine levels.

Pharmacodynamics/Kinetics

Onset of Action Maximum effect: Due to its long half-life, several days of treatment are required for oxaprozin to reach its full effect

Half-life Elimination 41 to 55 hours

Time to Peak 2.4 to 3.1 hours

Reproductive Considerations

The chronic use of NSAIDs in women of reproductive age may be associated with infertility that is reversible upon discontinuation of the medication. Consider discontinuing use in women having difficulty conceiving or those undergoing investigation of fertility.

Pregnancy Considerations Birth defects have been observed following in utero NSAID exposure in some studies; however, data is conflicting (Bloor 2013). Nonteratogenic effects, including prenatal constriction of the ductus arteriosus, persistent pulmonary hypertension of the newborn, oligohydramnios, necrotizing enterocolitis, renal dysfunction or failure, and intracranial hemorrhage, have been observed in the fetus/neonate following in utero NSAID exposure. In addition, nonclosure of the ductus arteriosus postnatally may occur and be resistant to medical management (Bermas 2014; Bloor 2013). Because NSAIDs may cause premature closure of the ductus arteriosus, product labeling for oxaprozin specifically states use should be avoided starting at 30-weeks gestation.

Use of NSAIDs can be considered for the treatment of mild rheumatoid arthritis flares in pregnant women, however use should be minimized or avoided early and late in pregnancy (Bermas 2014; Saavedra Salinas 2015).

The use of NSAIDs close to conception may be associated with an increased risk of miscarriage (Bermas 2014; Bloor 2013).

◆ **Oxaydo** *see* OxyCODONE *on page 1157*

Oxazepam (oks A ze pam)

Related Information

Dentin Hypersensitivity, Acid Erosion, High Caries Index, Management of Alveolar Osteitis, and Xerostomia *on page 1762*

Brand Names: Canada APO-Oxazepam; BIO-Oxazepam; DOM-Oxazepam; Oxpam; PMS-Oxazepam [DSC]; RIVA-Oxazepam

Pharmacologic Category Benzodiazepine

Use

Alcohol withdrawal syndrome: Management of the symptoms associated with alcohol withdrawal, including tremor and anxiety.

Anxiety disorders: Treatment of anxiety disorders or short-term relief of the symptoms of anxiety, including anxiety associated with depression and anxiety, tension, agitation, and irritability in older patients.

Local Anesthetic/Vasoconstrictor Precautions

No information available to require special precautions

Effects on Dental Treatment Key adverse event(s) related to dental treatment: Xerostomia (normal salivary flow resumes upon discontinuation).

Effects on Bleeding No information available to require special precautions

Adverse Reactions Frequency not defined.

Cardiovascular: Edema, hypotension, syncope

Central nervous system: Amnesia, ataxia, dizziness, drowsiness, drug dependence, dysarthria, euphoria, headache, lethargy, memory impairment, slurred speech, vertigo

Dermatologic: Maculopapular rash, morbilliform rash, urticaria

Endocrine & metabolic: Decreased libido, menstrual disease

Gastrointestinal: Nausea

Genitourinary: Urinary incontinence

Hematologic & oncologic: Hematologic disease, leukopenia

Hepatic: Jaundice

Hypersensitivity: Fixed drug eruption

Neuromuscular & skeletal: Hyporeflexia, tremor

Ophthalmic: Blurred vision, diplopia

Miscellaneous: Paradoxical central nervous system stimulation, paradoxical excitation

Mechanism of Action Binds to stereospecific benzodiazepine receptors on the postsynaptic GABA neuron at several sites within the central nervous system, including the limbic system, reticular formation. Enhancement of the inhibitory effect of GABA on neuronal excitability results by increased neuronal membrane permeability to chloride ions. This shift in chloride ions results in hyperpolarization (a less excitable state) and stabilization. Benzodiazepine receptors and effects appear to be linked to the GABA-A receptors. Benzodiazepines do not bind to GABA-B receptors (Vinkers 2012).

Pharmacodynamics/Kinetics

Half-life Elimination ~8 hours (range: 6 to 11 hours)

Time to Peak Serum: ~3 hours

Pregnancy Considerations Oxazepam crosses the placenta. Teratogenic effects have been observed with some benzodiazepines; however, additional studies are needed. The incidence of premature birth and low birth weights may be increased following maternal use of benzodiazepines; hypoglycemia and respiratory problems in the neonate may occur following exposure late in pregnancy. Neonatal withdrawal symptoms may occur within days to weeks after birth and "floppy infant syndrome" (which also includes withdrawal symptoms) have been reported with some benzodiazepines (Bergman 1992; Iqbal 2002; Kangas 1980; Wikner 2007).

Controlled Substance C-IV

◆ **Oxbryta** *see* Voxelotor *on page 1556*

OXcarbazepine (ox car BAZ e peen)

Related Information

Temporomandibular Dysfunction (TMD), Chronic Pain, and Fibromyalgia *on page 1773*

Brand Names: US Oxtellar XR; Trileptal

Brand Names: Canada APO-OXcarbazepine; JAMP-OXcarbazepine; Trileptal

Pharmacologic Category Anticonvulsant, Miscellaneous

Use

Focal (partial) onset seizures:

Immediate release: Monotherapy or adjunctive therapy in the treatment of focal (partial) onset seizures in adults, as monotherapy in the treatment of focal (partial) onset seizures in children ≥4 years of age with epilepsy, and as adjunctive therapy in children ≥2 years of age with focal (partial) onset seizures.

Extended release: Treatment of focal (partial) onset seizures in adults and in children ≥6 years of age.

Local Anesthetic/Vasoconstrictor Precautions No information available to require special precautions

Effects on Dental Treatment No significant effects or complications reported

Effects on Bleeding No information available to require special precautions

Adverse Reactions Incidence of adverse effects is from monotherapy and adjunctive AED studies. Incidence in children was similar.

>10%:

Central nervous system: Dizziness (20% to 49%), drowsiness (12% to 36%), headache (8% to 32%), ataxia (2% to 31%), fatigue (3% to 21%), abnormal gait (3% to 17%), vertigo (2% to 15%)

Gastrointestinal: Vomiting (7% to 36%), nausea (15% to 29%), abdominal pain (5% to 13%)

Neuromuscular & skeletal: Tremor (4% to 16%)

Ophthalmic: Diplopia (10% to 40%), nystagmus (2% to 26%), visual disturbance (1% to 14%)

1% to 10%:

Cardiovascular: Chest pain (2%), edema (2%), lower extremity edema (2%), hypotension (1% to 2%)

Central nervous system: Emotional lability (3% to 8%), anxiety (7%), equilibrium disturbance (7%), confusion (2% to 7%), nervousness (2% to 7%), amnesia (4% to 5%), seizure (2% to 5%), falling (4%), abnormality in thinking (2% to 4%), insomnia (2% to 4%), hypoesthesia (3%), dysmetria (1% to 3%), speech disorder (1% to 3%), abnormal electroencephalogram (2%), agitation (2%), lack of concentration (2%), feeling abnormal (1% to 2%), myasthenia (1% to 2%)

Dermatologic: Skin rash (4%), diaphoresis (3%), acne vulgaris (1% to 2%)

Endocrine & metabolic: Hyponatremia (1% to 10%), hot flash (2%), increased thirst (2%), weight gain (2%)

Gastrointestinal: Diarrhea (7%), constipation (4% to 6%), dyspepsia (2% to 6%), anorexia (5%), dysgeusia (5%), upper abdominal pain (3%), xerostomia (3%), gastritis (2% to 3%), toothache (2%)

Genitourinary: Urinary tract infection (5%), urinary frequency (2%), vaginitis (2%)

Hematologic & oncologic: Bruise (2% to 4%), lymphadenopathy (2%), purpuric rash (2%), rectal hemorrhage (2%)

Hypersensitivity: Hypersensitivity reaction (2%)

Infection: Viral infection (7%), infection (2%)

Neuromuscular & skeletal: Asthenia (2% to 7%), back pain (4%), muscle spasm (2%), sprain (2%)

Ophthalmic: Blurred vision (4%), accommodation disturbance (2%)

Otic: Otalgia (2%), otic infection (2%)

Respiratory: Upper respiratory tract infection (7% to 10%), rhinitis (5% to 10%), cough (5%), epistaxis (4%), pulmonary infection (4%), sinusitis (3% to 4%), bronchitis (3%), nasopharyngitis (3%), pharyngitis (3%), pneumonia (2%)

Miscellaneous: Fever (3%), head trauma (2%)

Frequency not defined:

Cardiovascular: Bradycardia, cardiac failure, flushing, hypertension, orthostatic hypotension, palpitations, syncope, tachycardia

Central nervous system: Aggressive behavior, apathy, aphasia, aura, cerebral hemorrhage, delirium, delusions, dystonia, euphoria extrapyramidal reaction, hemiplegia, hyperkinesia, hyperreflexia, hypertonia, hypokinesia, hyporeflexia, hypotonia, hysteria, impaired consciousness, intoxicated feeling, malaise, manic behavior, migraine, neuralgia, nightmares, oculogyric crisis, panic disorder, paralysis, paranoia, personality disorder, precordial pain, psychomotor retardation, psychosis, rigors, speech disturbance, stupor, voice disorder

Dermatologic: Alopecia, contact dermatitis, eczema, erythematosus rash, facial rash, folliculitis, genital pruritus, maculopapular rash, miliaria, psoriasis, skin photosensitivity, urticaria, vitiligo

Endocrine & metabolic: Change in libido, decreased T4, heavy menstrual bleeding, hyperglycemia, hypocalcemia, hypoglycemia, hypokalemia, increased gamma-glutamyl transferase, intermenstrual bleeding, weight loss

Gastrointestinal: Aphthous stomatitis, biliary colic, bloody stools, cholelithiasis, colitis, duodenal ulcer, dysphagia, enteritis, eructation, esophagitis, flatulence, gastric ulcer, gingival hemorrhage, gingival hyperplasia, hematemesis, hemorrhoids, hiccups, increased appetite, retching, sialadenitis, stomatitis

Genitourinary: Dysuria, hematuria, leukorrhea, priapism, urinary tract pain

Hematologic & oncologic: Thrombocytopenia

Hepatic: Increased liver enzymes

Hypersensitivity: Angioedema

Neuromuscular & skeletal: Right hypochondrium pain, systemic lupus erythematosus, tetany

Ophthalmic: Blepharoptosis, cataract, conjunctival hemorrhage, hemianopia, mydriasis, ocular edema, photophobia, scotoma, xerophthalmia

Otic: Otitis externa, tinnitus

Renal: Nephrolithiasis, polyuria, renal pain

Respiratory: Asthma, dyspnea, laryngismus, pleurisy

<1%, postmarketing, and/or case reports: Acute generalized exanthematous pustulosis, agranulocytosis, anaphylaxis, aplastic anemia, atrioventricular block, bone fracture (long-term therapy), decreased bone mineral density (long-term therapy), DRESS syndrome, dysarthria, erythema multiforme, hepatitis (Hsu 2010), hypothyroidism, increased serum amylase, increased serum lipase, leukopenia, osteoporosis (long-term therapy), pancreatitis, pancytopenia, SIADH, Stevens-Johnson syndrome, suicidal ideation, suicidal tendencies, toxic epidermal necrolysis

Mechanism of Action Pharmacological activity results from both oxcarbazepine and its monohydroxy metabolite (MHD). Precise mechanism of anticonvulsant effect has not been defined. Oxcarbazepine and MHD block voltage-sensitive sodium channels, stabilizing hyperexcited neuronal membranes, inhibiting repetitive firing, and decreasing the propagation of synaptic impulses. These actions are believed to prevent the spread of seizures. Oxcarbazepine and MHD also increase potassium conductance and modulate the activity of high-voltage activated calcium channels.

Pharmacodynamics/Kinetics

Half-life Elimination

Children (Rey, 2004): 2 to 5 years: MHD: Single dose: Mean range: 4.8 to 6.7 hours; 6 to 12 years: MHD: Single dose: Mean range: 7.2 to 9.3 hours

Adults: Immediate release: Parent drug: 2 hours; MHD: 9 hours; renal impairment (CrCl 30 mL/minute): MHD: 19 hours; Extended release: Parent drug: 7 to 11 hours; MHD: 9 to 11 hours

Time to Peak

Children 2 to 12 years: Immediate release: Oxcarbazepine: 1 hour; MHD: 3 to 4 hours (Rey 2004)

Adults: Immediate release: MHD: Tablets: Median: 4.5 hours (range: 3 to 13 hours); Suspension: Median 6 hours; Extended release: MHD: 7 hours

Reproductive Considerations

Oxcarbazepine may decrease plasma concentrations of hormonal contraceptives. Use of an additional, nonhormonal contraceptive or alternative nonhormonal birth control is recommended.

Pregnancy Considerations

Oxcarbazepine, the active metabolite MHD and the inactive metabolite DHD, crosses the placenta and can be detected in the newborn (Myllynen 2001).

According to the manufacturer, limited data collected from pregnancy registries suggest congenital malformations may be associated with oxcarbazepine monotherapy, including craniofacial defects (such as oral clefts) and cardiac malformations (such as ventricular septal defects). However, use of oxcarbazepine in pregnancy is limited in comparison to other antiepileptic drugs and additional information may be needed to evaluate specific birth defects and other pregnancy outcomes (de Jong 2016; Martinez Ferri 2018; Tomson 2019; Weston 2016). In general, the risk of teratogenic effects is higher with AED polytherapy than monotherapy (Harden 2009). In case reports, symptoms similar to neonatal abstinence syndrome have been observed in newborns following in utero oxcarbazepine exposure (Chen 2017; Rolnitsky 2013).

Due to pregnancy-induced physiologic changes, plasma concentrations of the active metabolite, MHD, gradually decrease during pregnancy; patients should be monitored during pregnancy and postpartum.

Data collection to monitor pregnancy and infant outcomes following exposure to oxcarbazepine is ongoing. Patients exposed to oxcarbazepine during pregnancy are encouraged to enroll themselves into the NAAED Pregnancy Registry by calling 1-888-233-2334. Additional information is available at www.aedpregnancyregistry.org.

◆ **Oxecta** *see* OxyCODONE *on page 1157*

◆ **Oxervate** *see* Cenegermin *on page 321*

Oxiconazole (oks i KON a zole)

Brand Names: US Oxistat

Pharmacologic Category Antifungal Agent, Imidazole Derivative; Antifungal Agent, Topical

Use

Cream: Topical treatment of tinea pedis (athlete's foot); tinea cruris (jock itch); tinea corporis (ringworm) due to *Trichophyton rubrum*, *Trichophyton mentagrophytes*, or *Epidermophyton floccosum*; and tinea (pityriasis) versicolor due to *Malassezia furfur*

Lotion: Treatment of tinea pedis (athlete's foot); tinea cruris (jock itch); tinea corporis (ringworm) due to *Trichophyton rubrum, Trichophyton mentagrophytes*, or *Epidermophyton floccosum*

Local Anesthetic/Vasoconstrictor Precautions

No information available to require special precautions

Effects on Dental Treatment No significant effects or complications reported

Effects on Bleeding No information available to require special precautions

Adverse Reactions

1% to 10%:

Central nervous system: Localized burning (≤1%)

Dermatologic: Pruritus (<2%)

<1%, postmarketing, and/or case reports: Allergic contact dermatitis, dyshidrotic eczema, erythema, exfoliation of skin, folliculitis, maceration of the skin, nodule, pain, papule, skin fissure, skin irritation, skin rash, stinging of the skin, tingling of skin

Mechanism of Action The cytoplasmic membrane integrity of fungi is destroyed by oxiconazole which exerts a fungicidal activity through inhibition of ergosterol synthesis. Effective for treatment of tinea pedis, tinea cruris, tinea corporis, and tinea versicolor. Active against *Trichophyton rubrum*, *Trichophyton mentagrophytes*, *Trichophyton violaceum*, *Microsporum canis*, *Microsporum audouinii*, *Microsporum gypseum*, *Epidermophyton floccosum*, *Candida albicans*, and *Malassezia furfur*.

Pregnancy Risk Factor B

Pregnancy Considerations When administered orally, teratogenic effects were not observed in animal reproduction studies.

◆ **Oxiconazole Nitrate** *see* Oxiconazole *on page 1155*

◆ **Oxidized Regenerated Cellulose** *see* Cellulose (Oxidized/Regenerated) *on page 320*

◆ **Oxilapine Succinate** *see* Loxapine *on page 940*

◆ **Oxistat** *see* Oxiconazole *on page 1155*

◆ **Oxpentifylline** *see* Pentoxifylline *on page 1215*

◆ **Oxtellar XR** *see* OXcarbazepine *on page 1154*

◆ **Oxybate** *see* Sodium Oxybate *on page 1377*

Oxybutynin (oks i BYOO ti nin)

Related Information

Dentin Hypersensitivity, Acid Erosion, High Caries Index, Management of Alveolar Osteitis, and Xerostomia *on page 1762*

Brand Names: US Ditropan XL; Gelnique; Gelnique Pump [DSC]; Oxytrol; Oxytrol For Women [OTC]

Brand Names: Canada APO-Oxybutynin; Ditropan XL; DOM-Oxybutynin; Gelnique [DSC]; Oxytrol; PMS-Oxybutynin; RIVA-Oxybutynin; TEVA-Oxybutynin

Pharmacologic Category Antispasmodic Agent, Urinary

Use Overactive bladder: Treatment of symptoms associated with overactive bladder (eg, urge urinary incontinence, urgency, frequency, urinary leakage, dysuria); treatment of symptoms associated with overactive bladder due to a neurological condition (eg, spina bifida) in patients ≥6 years of age (extended-release tablet only).

Local Anesthetic/Vasoconstrictor Precautions

No information available to require special precautions

Effects on Dental Treatment Key adverse event(s) related to dental treatment: Frequent occurrences of xerostomia and changes in salivation (normal salivary flow resumes upon discontinuation). Infrequent occurrences of coated tongue, dysgeusia, fungal infection, sinus headache, and oropharyngeal pain have been reported.

Effects on Bleeding No information available to require special precautions

Adverse Reactions As reported with oral administration, unless otherwise noted.

>10%:

Central nervous system: Dizziness (oral: 5% to 17%; topical gel: 3%), drowsiness (6% to 14%)

Gastrointestinal: Xerostomia (oral: 35% to 72%; topical gel, transdermal: 4% to 10%), constipation (oral: 9% to 15%; transdermal: 3%; topical gel: 1%), nausea (5% to 12%)

Local: Application site pruritus (transdermal: 14% to 17%; topical gel: 2%)

1% to 10%:

Cardiovascular: Decreased blood pressure (1% to <5%), edema (1% to <5%), flushing (1% to <5%), increased blood pressure (1% to <5%), palpitations (1% to <5%), peripheral edema (1% to <5%), sinus arrhythmia (1% to <5%)

Central nervous system: Headache (oral: 8%; topical gel: 2%), nervousness (7%), insomnia (3% to 6%), confusion (1% to <5%), falling (1% to <5%), flank pain (1% to <5%), pain (1% to <5%), fatigue (oral, topical gel: 2% to 3%)

Dermatologic: Macular eruption (transdermal: 3%; application site), xeroderma (2% to 3%), pruritus (oral, topical gel: 1% to 2%)

Endocrine & metabolic: Fluid retention (<5%), increased thirst (<5%), increased serum glucose (1% to <5%)

Gastrointestinal: Diarrhea (3% to 8%), dyspepsia (5% to 6%), coated tongue (1% to <5%), eructation (1% to <5%), upper abdominal pain (1% to <5%), flatulence (1% to 3%), abdominal pain (2%), dysgeusia (2%), viral gastroenteritis (topical gel: 2%), vomiting (1% to 2%), gastroesophageal reflux disease (≤1%)

Genitourinary: Urinary hesitancy (2% to 9%), urinary tract infection (oral, topical gel: 7%), urinary retention (1% to 6%), cystitis (1% to <5%), pollakiuria (1% to <5%), increased post-void residual urine volume (2% to 4%), dysuria (oral, transdermal: 2%)

Infection: Fungal infection (1% to <5%)

Local: Application site erythema (transdermal: 6% to 8%), application site reaction (topical gel: 5%), application site rash (transdermal: 3%), application site vesicles (transdermal: 3%), application site dermatitis (topical gel: 2%)

Neuromuscular & skeletal: Arthralgia (1% to <5%), back pain (1% to <5%), limb pain (1% to <5%), asthenia (1% to <5%)

Ophthalmic: Blurred vision (4% to 10%), eye irritation (1% to <5%), keratoconjunctivitis sicca (1% to <5%), visual disturbance (transdermal: 3%), xerophthalmia (3%)

Respiratory: Dry nose (2% to 5%), upper respiratory tract infection (oral, topical gel: 1% to 5%), asthma (1% to <5%), bronchitis (1% to <5%), hoarseness (1% to <5%), nasal congestion (1% to <5%), nasopharyngitis (oral, topical gel: 1% to <5%), paranasal sinus congestion (1% to <5%), pharyngolaryngeal pain (1% to <5%), sinus headache (1% to <5%), cough (2% to 3%), dry throat (2% to 3%), oropharyngeal pain (2%)

<1%, postmarketing, and/or case reports: Abnormal behavior, agitation, anaphylaxis, angioedema, anorexia, cardiac arrhythmia, chest discomfort, confusion, cycloplegia, decreased gastrointestinal motility, delirium, dizziness, drowsiness, dysphagia, facial edema, frequent bowel movements, glaucoma, hallucination, headache, hot flash, hypersensitivity reaction, hypertension, hypohidrosis, impotence, lactation insufficiency, memory impairment, mydriasis, prolonged QT interval on ECG, psychotic reaction, seizure, skin rash, tachycardia, urticaria, voice disorder

Mechanism of Action Direct antispasmodic effect on smooth muscle, also inhibits the action of acetylcholine on smooth muscle (exhibits 1/5 the anticholinergic activity of atropine, but has 4-10 times the antispasmodic activity); does not block effects at skeletal muscle or at autonomic ganglia; increases bladder capacity, decreases uninhibited contractions, and delays desire to void, therefore, decreases urgency and frequency

Pharmacodynamics/Kinetics

Onset of Action Oral: Immediate release: 30 to 60 minutes; Peak effect: 3 to 6 hours; Extended release: Peak effect: 3 days

Duration of Action Oral: Immediate release: 6 to 10 hours; Extended release: Up to 24 hours; Transdermal 96 hours

Half-life Elimination IV: ~2 hours (parent drug), 7 to 8 hours (metabolites); Oral: Immediate release: ~2 to 3 hours; Extended release: ~13 hours; Transdermal: 64 hours

Time to Peak Serum: Oral: Immediate release: ~60 minutes; Extended release: 4 to 6 hours; Transdermal: 24 to 48 hours

Pregnancy Risk Factor B

Pregnancy Considerations

Adverse events were not observed in animal reproduction studies.

Information related to the use of oxybutynin in patients treated for neurogenic bladder during pregnancy is limited (Andretta 2018).

◆ **Oxybutynin Chloride** *see* Oxybutynin *on page 1156*

◆ **Oxybutynin Hydrochloride** *see* Oxybutynin *on page 1156*

OxyCODONE (oks i KOE done)

Related Information

Management of the Chemically Dependent Patient *on page 1724*

Oral Pain *on page 1734*

Brand Names: US Oxaydo; OxyCONTIN; Roxicodone; Xtampza ER

Brand Names: Canada ACT Oxycodone CR [DSC]; APO-Oxycodone CR; Oxy-IR; OxyNEO; PMS-OxyCODONE; PMS-OxyCODONE CR; Supeudol; Supeudol 10; Supeudol 20

Generic Availability (US) May be product dependent

Pharmacologic Category Analgesic, Opioid

Dental Use Treatment of postoperative pain

Use Pain management:

Immediate-release formulations: Management of acute or chronic moderate to severe pain where the use of an opioid analgesic is appropriate and for which alternative treatments are inadequate.

Extended-release formulations:

Capsules: Management of pain severe enough to require daily, around-the-clock, long-term opioid treatment and for which alternative treatment options are inadequate in adults

Tablets: Management of pain severe enough to require daily, around-the-clock, long-term opioid treatment and for which alternative treatment options are inadequate in adults and opioid-tolerant pediatric patients ≥11 years of age who are already receiving and tolerating a minimum daily opioid dose of at least 20 mg oxycodone orally or its equivalent.

Limitations of use: Reserve oxycodone for use in patients for whom alternative treatment options (eg, nonopioid analgesics, opioid combination products) are ineffective, not tolerated, or would be otherwise inadequate to provide sufficient management of pain. Oxycodone ER is not indicated as an as-needed analgesic.

Local Anesthetic/Vasoconstrictor Precautions No information available to require special precautions

Effects on Dental Treatment Key adverse event(s) related to dental treatment: Xerostomia (normal salivary flow resumes upon discontinuation).

Effects on Bleeding No information available to require special precautions

Adverse Reactions As reported with adult patients, unless otherwise noted.

>10%:

Central nervous system: Drowsiness (extended-release: 9% to 23%, extended-release, adolescents: 1% to <5%; immediate-release: ≥3%), headache (extended-release: 14%; immediate-release: ≥3%), dizziness (extended-release: 2% to 13%; immediate-release: ≥3%)

Dermatologic: Pruritus (extended-release: 3% to 13%; immediate-release: ≥3%)

Gastrointestinal: Nausea (extended-release: 11% to 23%; immediate-release: ≥3%), constipation (extended-release: 5% to 23%; extended-release, adolescents: 9%; immediate-release: ≥3%), vomiting (extended-release: 4% to 21%; immediate-release: 3%)

Miscellaneous: Fever (extended-release: 1% to 11%; immediate-release: ≥3%)

1% to 10%:

Cardiovascular: Flushing (extended-release: 1% to 5%), hypertension (extended-release: 1% to 5%), orthostatic hypotension (extended-release: 1% to 5%), oxygen saturation decreased (extended-release, adolescents: 1% to <5%), edema (immediate-release: ≤5%; extended-release: <1%), tachycardia (<5%), cardiac failure (immediate-release: <3%), deep vein thrombosis (immediate-release: <3%), hypotension (<3%), palpitations (<3%; may occur with withdrawal), peripheral edema (immediate-release: <3%; extended-release: <1%), thrombophlebitis (immediate-release: <3%), vasodilation (<3%)

Central nervous system: Abnormality in thinking (extended-release: 1% to 5%), dysphoria (extended-release: 1% to 5%), insomnia (1% to 5%), irritability (extended-release: 1% to 5%), twitching (extended-release: 1% to 5%), abnormal dreams (extended-release: ≤5%), anxiety (≤5%), chills (≤5%), confusion (≤5%), euphoria (extended-release: ≤5%), fatigue (extended-release: ≤5%), hypoesthesia (≤5%), migraine (≤5%), nervousness (≤5%), withdrawal syndrome (extended-release: ≤5%), agitation (<5%), pain (<5%), depression (extended-release, adolescents: 1% to <5%; extended-release, adults: <1%), lethargy (adolescents: 1% to <5%; extended-release, adults: <1%), paresthesia (extended-release, adolescents: 1% to <5%; extended-release, adults: <1%), procedural pain (extended-release, adolescents: 1% to <5%), hypertonia (<3%), neuralgia (<3%), personality disorder (immediate-release: <3%)

Dermatologic: Excoriation (extended-release: 1% to 5%), diaphoresis (≤5%), hyperhidrosis (≤5%), skin rash (≤5%), skin photosensitivity (immediate-release: <3%), urticaria (<3%)

Endocrine & metabolic: Hypochloremia (extended-release, adolescents: 1% to <5%), hyponatremia (extended-release: 1% to <5%), weight loss (extended-release, adolescents: 1% to <5%), hyperglycemia (≤5%), gout (immediate-release: <3%)

Gastrointestinal: Diarrhea (≤6%), xerostomia (≤6%), gastritis (extended-release: 1% to 5%), hiccups (extended-release: 1% to 5%), upper abdominal pain (extended-release: 1% to 5%), abdominal pain (≤5%), anorexia (≤5%), decreased appetite (≤5%), dyspepsia (≤5%), gastroesophageal reflux disease (extended-release: ≤5%), dysphagia (immediate-release: <3%; extended-release: <1%), gingivitis (immediate-release: <3%), glossitis (immediate-release: <3%)

Genitourinary: Dysuria (extended-release, adolescents: 1% to <5%; extended-release, adults: <1%), urinary retention (extended-release, adolescents: 1% to <5%; extended-release, adults: <1%), urinary tract infection (immediate-release: <3%)

Hematologic & oncologic: Decreased hemoglobin (extended-release, adolescents: 1% to <5%), decreased platelet count (extended-release, adolescents: 1% to <5%), decreased red blood cells (extended-release, adolescents: 1% to <5%), febrile neutropenia (extended-release, adolescents: 1% to <5%), neutropenia (extended-release, adolescents: 1% to <5%), anemia (immediate-release: <3%), hemorrhage (immediate-release: <3%), iron deficiency anemia (immediate-release: <3%), leukopenia (immediate-release: <3%)

Hepatic: Increased serum alanine aminotransferase (extended-release, adolescents: 1% to <5%)

Hypersensitivity: Hypersensitivity reaction (<3%)
Infection: Herpes simplex infection (immediate-release: <3%), infection (immediate-release: <3%), sepsis (immediate-release: <3%)
Neuromuscular & skeletal: Asthenia (1% to 6%), limb pain (extended-release, adolescents: 1% to <5%), arthralgia (≤5%), back pain (≤5%), musculoskeletal pain (extended release: ≤5%), myalgia (≤5%), tremor (≤5%), arthritis (immediate-release: <3%), laryngospasm (immediate-release: <3%), neck pain (immediate-release: <3%), ostealgia (immediate-release: <3%), pathological fracture (immediate-release: <3%)
Ophthalmic: Blurred vision (extended-release: 1% to 5%), amblyopia (immediate-release: <3%)
Respiratory: Cough (≤5%), dyspnea (≤5%), oropharyngeal pain (extended-release: ≤5%), bronchitis (immediate-release: <3%), epistaxis (immediate-release: <3%), flu-like symptoms (immediate-release: <3%), laryngismus (immediate-release: <3%), pharyngitis (immediate-release: <3%), pulmonary disease (immediate-release: <3%), rhinitis (immediate-release: <3%), sinusitis (immediate-release: <3%)
Miscellaneous: Seroma (extended-release, adolescents: 1% to <5%), accidental injury (<3%; extended-release: <1%)

Frequency not defined:
Cardiovascular: Circulatory depression, shock
Central nervous system: Depersonalization
Respiratory: Respiratory depression

<1%, postmarketing, and/or case reports: Abnormal gait, aggressive behavior, amenorrhea, amnesia, chest pain, choking sensation, cholestasis, dehydration, dental caries, depression of ST segment on ECG, diverticulitis of the gastrointestinal tract (exacerbation), drug abuse, drug dependence, drug overdose (may be intentional), dysgeusia, emotional lability, eructation, exfoliative dermatitis, facial edema, flatulence, gag reflex, gastrointestinal disease, hallucination, hematuria, hyperalgesia, hyperkinesia, hypogonadism, hypotonia, impotence, increased appetite, increased gamma-glutamyl transferase, increased heart rate, increased liver enzymes, increased thirst, intestinal obstruction, lymphadenopathy, malaise, memory impairment, mood changes, neonatal withdrawal, night sweats, pharyngeal edema, polyuria, restlessness, seizure, SIADH, sleep disturbance, speech disturbance, stomatitis, stupor, suicidal ideation, suicidal tendencies, syncope, tinnitus, vertigo, visual disturbance, voice disorder, xeroderma

Dental Usual Dosage Postoperative pain: Adults: Oral: 5 mg every 6 hours as needed

Dosing

Adult

Pain management: Note: All doses should be titrated to appropriate effect.

Immediate release:

Oral: Initial: 5 to 15 mg every 4 to 6 hours as needed; dosing range: 5 to 20 mg per dose (APS 2008). Start at the lower end of dosing range for opioid-naive patients; for acute pain use a low dose for ≤3 to 7 days (CDC [Dowell 2016]).

Rectal [Canadian product]: Initial: One suppository 3 to 4 times daily as needed.

Extended release: Oral:

Note: Oxycodone ER capsules are not bioequivalent to ER tablets. Dose of ER capsules is expressed as oxycodone base and the dose of ER tablets is expressed as oxycodone hydrochloride. Oxycodone ER 60 mg and 80 mg tablets are intended for use in opioid-tolerant patients only. Single doses >40 mg (ER tablets) or >36 mg (ER capsules), or a total dose of >80 mg daily (ER tablets) or >72 mg daily (ER capsules) are for use only in opioid-tolerant patients. Opioid tolerance is defined as: Patients already taking at least morphine 60 mg orally daily, oxymorphone 25 mg orally daily, transdermal fentanyl 25 mcg per hour, oxycodone 30 mg orally daily, hydromorphone 8 mg orally daily, hydrocodone 60 mg orally daily or an equivalent dose of another opioid for at least 1 week.

Opioid naive (use as the first opioid analgesic or use in patients who are not opioid tolerant): Initial:
ER tablet: 10 mg every 12 hours
ER capsules: 9 mg every 12 hours

Conversion from other oral oxycodone formulations to oxycodone ER: Initiate oxycodone ER with 50% of the total daily oral oxycodone daily dose (mg/day) administered every 12 hours.

Conversion from other opioids to oxycodone ER: Discontinue all other around-the-clock opioids when oxycodone ER is initiated. Initiate with 10 mg (ER tablets) or 9 mg (ER capsules) every 12 hours. Substantial interpatient variability exists due to patient specific factors, relative potency of different opioids, and dosage forms; therefore, it is preferable to underestimate the initial 24-hour oral oxycodone requirements and utilize rescue medication (immediate-release opioid).

Conversion from transdermal fentanyl patch to oxycodone ER: **Note:** Remove fentanyl patch at least 18 hours prior to starting oxycodone ER. The manufacturer suggests using the conservative conversion factor of oxycodone ER tablets 10 mg or oxycodone ER capsules 9 mg every 12 hours for each fentanyl 25 mcg/hour transdermal patch; systematic assessment of this suggested conversion has not been completed; monitor patients closely.

Conversion from methadone to oxycodone ER: Close monitoring is required when converting methadone to another opioid. Ratio between methadone and other opioid agonists varies widely according to previous dose exposure. Methadone has a long half-life and can accumulate in the plasma.

Maintenance dose: Dosage adjustment (titration): After initiation of oxycodone ER, adjust dose in increments (25% to 50%) no more frequently than every 1 to 2 days until desired pain control. Recommended maximum dose of ER capsules is 288 mg/day. Patients may require rescue doses of an immediate-release analgesic during dose titration. Observe for signs and symptoms of opioid withdrawal or signs of over sedation/toxicity; if unacceptable adverse reactions occur, the subsequent dose may be reduced. **Note:** Some clinicians have reported that in certain chronic pain patients, more frequent dosing (ie, every 8 hours) is required for effective pain relief (Gallagher 2007; Marcus 2004; Nicholson 2006), although dosing more frequently than every 12 hours is not recommended by the manufacturer, and safety and efficacy has not been established.

Discontinuation of therapy: When discontinuing chronic opioid therapy, the dose should be gradually tapered down. An optimal universal tapering schedule for all patients has not been established (CDC [Dowell 2016]). Proposed schedules range from slow (eg, 10% reductions per week) to rapid (eg, 25% to 50% reduction every few days) (CDC 2015). Tapering schedules should be individualized to minimize opioid withdrawal while considering patient-specific goals and concerns as well as the pharmacokinetics of the opioid being tapered. An even slower taper may be appropriate in patients who have been receiving opioids for a long duration (eg, years), particularly in the final stage of tapering, whereas more rapid tapers may be appropriate in patients experiencing severe adverse events (CDC [Dowell 2016]). Monitor carefully for signs/symptoms of withdrawal. If the patient displays withdrawal symptoms, consider slowing the taper schedule; alterations may include increasing the interval between dose reductions, decreasing amount of daily dose reduction, pausing the taper and restarting when the patient is ready, and/or coadministration of an alpha-2 agonist (eg, clonidine) to blunt withdrawal symptoms (Berna 2015; CDC [Dowell 2016]). Continue to offer nonopioid analgesics as needed for pain management during the taper; consider nonopioid adjunctive treatments for withdrawal symptoms (eg, GI complaints, muscle spasm) as needed (Berna 2015; Sevarino 2018).

Dosage adjustment in debilitated patients (non-opioid tolerant):

Immediate release: Oral, rectal [Canadian product]: Initial: There are no specific dosage adjustments provided in the manufacturer's labeling; use caution and with a reduced dose.

Extended release: Oral: Initial: Initiate oxycodone ER with 33% to 50% of the calculated recommended dose. If reduced dose is less than smallest available dosage form, consider alternative analgesic.

Geriatric Refer to adult dosing. Initiate therapy at low end of dosing range and use caution.

Renal Impairment: Adult

CrCl ≥60 mL/minute: There are no dosage adjustments provided in the manufacturer's labeling. Oxycodone clearance may decrease in patients with renal impairment; initiate therapy at low end of dosing range.

CrCl <60 mL/minute: Serum concentrations are increased ~50%. Initiate at the low end of the dosage range (use caution); adjust dose as clinically indicated. Alternatively, for both immediate- and extended-release forms, doses of 33% to 50% of usual initial dosing have been recommended (Oxy IR Canadian product labeling; OxyNeo Canadian product labeling; Supeudol Canadian product labeling). For ER tablets and capsules, if the reduced dose is less than smallest available dosage form, consider alternative analgesic.

Hepatic Impairment: Adult

Immediate release: Initiate therapy at 33% to 50% the usual dosage and titrate carefully.

Extended release tablets or *Extended release capsules*: Initial: Initiate oxycodone ER with 33% to 50% of the calculated recommended dose. If reduced dose is less than smallest available dosage form consider alternative analgesic.

Pediatric Note: Doses should be titrated to appropriate effect. Multiple concentrations of oral solution available (20 mg/mL and 1 mg/mL); the **highly concentrated formulation (20 mg/mL) should only be used in opioid tolerant patients (taking ≥30 mg/day of oxycodone or equivalent for ≥1 week)**. Orders for oxycodone oral solutions (20 mg/mL or 1 mg/mL) should be clearly written to include the intended dose (in mg not mL) and the intended product concentration to be dispensed to avoid potential dosing errors:

Analgesia, moderate to severe pain: *Immediate release:*

Infants ≤6 months: Limited data available: Oral: Initial dose: 0.025 to 0.05 mg/kg/dose every 4 to 6 hours as needed (Berde 2002)

Infants >6 months, Children, and Adolescents: Oral:

Patient weight <50 kg: Initial dose: 0.1 to 0.2 mg/kg/dose every 4 to 6 hours as needed; for severe pain some experts have recommended an initial dose of 0.2 mg/kg; usual maximum dose range: 5 to 10 mg (American Pain Society 2008; APA 2012; Berde 2002)

Patient weight ≥50 kg: Initial dose: 5 to 10 mg every 4 to 6 hours as needed; for severe pain an initial dose of 10 mg may be used; usual maximum dose: 20 mg/dose (American Pain Society 2008; Berde 2002)

Analgesia, severe pain requiring around-the-clock long-term opioid therapy: *Extended release tablets (eg, OxyContin):* **Note:** Use only in pediatric patients ≥11 years of age who are already receiving opioid therapy for at least 5 consecutive days, tolerating a minimum daily opioid dose of at least 20 mg of oxycodone orally or its equivalent at least for the 2 days immediately prior to starting extended release oxycodone tablets, and for which alternative treatment options are inadequate. Prior to initiation, all other around-the-clock opioid therapy must be discontinued.

Initial dose: Children ≥11 years and Adolescents: Oral: Initial dose based on current opioid regimen dose; use the following conversion factor table and equation to convert the current opioid(s) daily dose to the extended release oxycodone tablet daily dose. **Note:** Substantial interpatient variability exists due to patient specific factors, relative potency of different opioids, and dosage forms; therefore, it is preferable to underestimate the initial 24-hour oral oxycodone requirements and utilize rescue medication (immediate release opioid):

Initial dose of extended release oxycodone tablets administered every 12 hours = (mg/day of current opioid regimen X conversion factor)/2

Dose calculations or adjustments for specific clinical scenarios:

- If rounding is necessary, numerical value should be rounded **down** to the nearest tablet strength. If calculated **daily** dose is <20 mg, do not start extended release oxycodone tablet as there is no safe tablet strength available.
- If more than one opioid in the regimen, calculate the approximate extended release oxycodone tablet dose for each opioid and sum the totals for the approximate total **daily** extended release oxycodone tablet dose, then divide by 2 for the 12-hour extended release oxycodone dose.
- If current opioid regimen includes a fixed-dose opioid/nonopioid dosage form (eg, hydrocodone/acetaminophen), only the mg of opioid should be used in the conversion calculations.
- If patient receiving concomitant CNS depressants, reduce extended release oxycodone tablet starting dose by 1/3 to 1/2 the calculated initial dose.
- If asymmetric dosing, the higher dose should be scheduled as the morning dose, and the lower dose 12 hours later.

Note: The following conversion table should **ONLY** be used to convert opioid doses to extended release oxycodone tablet (not from extended release oxycodone tablet to other opioids; it is **NOT** a table of equianalgesic doses as it may overestimate initial dose).

Conversion Factor for Calculating Initial Extended Release Oxycodone Tablet Dose in Pediatric Patients ≥11 years

Current opioid regimen to be converted to extended release oxycodone tablet	Conversion Factor	
	Oral	Parenteral*
Oxycodone	1	–
Hydrocodone	0.9	–
Hydromorphone	4	20
Morphine	0.5	3
Tramadol	0.17	0.2

*For patients receiving high-dose parenteral opioids, a more conservative conversion factor should be applied (ie, lower numerical conversion factor); for example, for high-dose parenteral morphine, a conversion of 1.5 should be used for calculations instead of 3.

Conversion from fentanyl patch to extended release oxycodone tablet: Limited data available: Children ≥11 years and Adolescents: **Note:** Remove fentanyl patch at least 18 hours prior to starting extended release oxycodone. Initial dose based on current opioid regimen dose; the manufacturer suggests using the conservative conversion factor of 10 mg every 12 hours of extended release oxycodone tablet for each 25 mcg/hour fentanyl transdermal patch; systemic assessment of this suggested conversion has not been completed, monitor patients closely

Maintenance dose: Dosage adjustment (titration): After initiation of extended release oxycodone tablet, adjust dose in small increments (up to 25% of current total daily dosage) no more frequently than every 1 to 2 days until desired pain control; patients may require rescue doses of an immediate release analgesic during dose titration. Observe for signs and symptoms of opioid withdrawal or signs of oversedation/toxicity; if unacceptable adverse reactions occur, the subsequent dose may be reduced.

Renal Impairment: Pediatric In general, oxycodone clearance may be decreased in patients with renal impairment; initiate therapy at low end of dosing range.

Immediate release: Infants, Children, and Adolescents: There are no dosage adjustments provided in the manufacturer's labeling; however, the following adjustments have been recommended (Aronoff 2007):

GFR ≥50 mL/minute/1.73 m²: No dosage adjustment required

GFR 10 to 50 mL/minute/1.73 m²: Administer 75% of dose

GFR <10 mL/minute/1.73 m²: Administer 50% of dose

Hemodialysis: Administer 50% of dose posthemodialysis

Peritoneal dialysis: Administer 50% of dose

Extended release tablets (eg, Oxycontin): Children ≥11 years and Adolescents: CrCl <60 mL/minute: Serum concentrations are increased ~50%. Initiate at the low end of the dosage range (use caution); adjust dose as clinically indicated. Doses of 33% to 50% of usual initial dosing have been recommended; if the reduced dose is less than smallest available dosage form, consider alternative analgesic.

Hepatic Impairment: Pediatric

Immediate release: There are no dosage adjustments provided in the manufacturer's labeling; based on experience in adult patients, may consider a conservative approach of reduced initial doses; adjust dose based on clinical response.

Extended release tablets (eg, Oxycontin): Children ≥11 years and Adolescents: Initial: One-third (1/3) to one-half (1/2) of the usual starting dose; carefully titrate dose to appropriate effect. If reduced dose is less than smallest available dosage form, consider alternative analgesic.

Mechanism of Action Binds to opiate receptors in the CNS, causing inhibition of ascending pain pathways, altering the perception of and response to pain; produces generalized CNS depression

Contraindications

Hypersensitivity (eg, anaphylaxis, angioedema) to oxycodone or any component of the formulation; significant respiratory depression; hypercapnia; acute or severe bronchial asthma in an unmonitored setting or in the absence of resuscitative equipment; GI obstruction, including paralytic ileus (known or suspected).

Documentation of allergenic cross-reactivity for opioids is limited. However, because of similarities in chemical structure and/or pharmacologic actions, the possibility of cross-sensitivity cannot be ruled out with certainty.

Canadian labeling: Additional contraindications (not in US labeling): Hypersensitivity to other opioids; suspected surgical abdomen (eg, acute appendicitis or pancreatitis); any disease/condition that affects bowel transit; mild pain that can be managed with other pain medications (immediate release, suppository); mild, intermittent or short duration pain that can be managed with other pain medications or acute pain (extended release); chronic obstructive airway, status asthmaticus; cor pulmonale; acute alcoholism; delirium tremens; convulsive disorders; severe CNS depression; increased cerebrospinal or intracranial pressure; head injury; monoamine oxidase (MAO) inhibitors (concomitant use or within 14 days of therapy); pregnant women or during labor and delivery; breastfeeding.

Warnings/Precautions May cause CNS depression, which may impair physical or mental abilities; patients must be cautioned about performing tasks that require mental alertness (eg, operating machinery or driving). Potentially significant drug-drug interactions may exist, requiring dose or frequency adjustment, additional monitoring, and/or selection of alternative therapy. Use with caution in patients with hypersensitivity reactions to other phenanthrene-derivative opioid agonists (morphine, hydrocodone, hydromorphone, levorphanol, oxymorphone). Use with caution in pancreatitis or biliary tract disease, delirium tremens, morbid obesity, adrenocortical insufficiency (including Addison disease), history of seizure disorders, thyroid dysfunction, prostatic hyperplasia, urinary stricture, and toxic psychosis. Long-term opioid use may cause secondary hypogonadism, which may lead to mood disorders and osteoporosis (Brennan 2013). Use with caution and monitor for respiratory depression in patients with significant chronic obstructive pulmonary disease or cor pulmonale, and those with a substantially decreased respiratory reserve, hypoxia, hypercapnia, or preexisting respiratory depression, particularly when initiating and titrating therapy; critical respiratory depression may occur, even at therapeutic dosages. Consider the use of alternative nonopioid analgesics in these patients. Opioid use increases the risk for sleep-related disorders (eg, central sleep apnea [CSA], hypoxemia) in a dose-dependent fashion. Use with caution for chronic pain and titrate dosage cautiously in patients with risk factors for sleep-disordered breathing (eg, heart failure, obesity). Consider dose reduction in patients presenting with CSA. Avoid opioids in patients with moderate to severe sleep-disordered breathing (Dowell [CDC 2016]). May obscure diagnosis or clinical course of patients with acute abdominal conditions. Avoid use in patients with impaired consciousness or coma. Use with caution in patients with a history of drug abuse or acute alcoholism; potential for drug dependency exists. Other factors associated with increased risk for misuse include younger age, concomitant depression (major), and psychotropic medication use. Consider offering naloxone prescriptions in patients with factors associated with an increased risk for overdose, such as history of overdose or substance use disorder, higher opioid dosages (≥50 morphine milligram equivalents/day orally), and concomitant benzodiazepine use (Dowell [CDC 2016]). Use opioids with caution for chronic pain in patients with mental health conditions (eg, depression, anxiety disorders, post-traumatic stress disorder) due to increased risk for opioid use disorder and overdose; more frequent monitoring is recommended (Dowell [CDC 2016]).

Use with caution in cachectic or debilitated patients, and in hepatic or renal impairment. Use opioids for chronic pain with caution in older adults; monitor closely due to an increased potential for risks, including certain risks such as falls/fracture, cognitive impairment, and constipation. Clearance may also be reduced in older adults (with or without renal impairment) resulting in a narrow therapeutic window and increasing the risk for respiratory depression or overdose (Dowell [CDC 2016]). May cause severe hypotension (including orthostatic hypotension and syncope); use with caution in patients with hypovolemia, cardiovascular disease (including acute myocardial infarction [MI]), or drugs that may exaggerate hypotensive effects (including phenothiazines or general anesthetics). Monitor for symptoms of hypotension following initiation or dose titration. Avoid use in patients with circulatory shock. Use with extreme caution in patients with head injury, intracranial lesions, or elevated intracranial pressure (ICP); exaggerated elevation of ICP may occur. May cause constipation that may be problematic in patients with unstable angina and patients post-MI. Abrupt discontinuation in patients who are physically dependent on opioids has been associated with serious withdrawal symptoms, uncontrolled pain, attempts to find other opioids (including illicit), and suicide. Use a collaborative, patient-specific taper schedule that minimizes the risk of withdrawal, considering factors such as current opioid dose, duration of use, type of pain, and physical and psychological factors. Monitor pain control, withdrawal symptoms, mood changes, suicidal ideation, and for use of other substances and provide care as needed. Concurrent use of mixed agonist/antagonist analgesics (eg, pentazocine, nalbuphine, butorphanol) or partial agonist (eg, buprenorphine) analgesics may also precipitate withdrawal symptoms and/or reduced analgesic efficacy in patients following prolonged therapy with mu opioid agonists. Use with caution in the perioperative setting; individualize treatment when transitioning from parenteral to oral analgesics. Opioids decrease bowel motility; monitor for decreased bowel motility in postop patients receiving opioids. Use with caution in the perioperative setting; individualize treatment when transitioning from parenteral to oral analgesics. An opioid-containing analgesic regimen should be tailored to each patient's needs and based upon the type of pain being treated (acute versus chronic), the route of administration, degree of tolerance for opioids (naive versus chronic user), age, weight, and medical condition. The optimal analgesic dose varies widely among patients; doses should be titrated to pain relief/prevention.

Chronic pain: Opioids should **not** be used as first-line therapy for chronic pain management (pain >3-month duration or beyond time of normal tissue healing) due to limited short-term benefits, undetermined long-term benefits, and association with serious risks (eg, overdose, MI, auto accidents, risk of developing opioid use disorder). Preferred management includes nonpharmacologic therapy and nonopioid therapy (eg, nonsteroidal anti-inflammatory drugs, acetaminophen, certain anticonvulsants and antidepressants). If opioid therapy is initiated, it should be combined with nonpharmacologic and nonopioid therapy, as appropriate. Prior to initiation, known risks of opioid therapy should be discussed and realistic treatment goals for pain/function should be established, including consideration for discontinuation if benefits do not outweigh risks. Therapy should be continued only if clinically meaningful improvement in pain/function outweighs risks. Therapy should be initiated at the lowest effective dosage using immediate-release opioids (instead of extended-release/long-acting opioids). Risk associated with use increases with higher opioid dosages. Risks and benefits should be re-evaluated when increasing dosage to ≥50 morphine milligram equivalents (MME)/day orally; dosages ≥90 MME/day orally should be avoided unless carefully justified (Dowell [CDC 2016]).

[US Boxed Warning]: Serious, life-threatening, or fatal respiratory depression may occur. Monitor closely for respiratory depression, especially during initiation or dose escalation. Swallow ER tablets whole; crushing, chewing, or dissolving can cause rapid release and a potentially fatal dose. Carbon dioxide retention from opioid-induced respiratory depression can exacerbate the sedating effects of opioids. **[US Boxed Warning]: Use with all CYP3A4 inhibitors may result in an increase in oxycodone plasma concentrations, which could increase or prolong adverse drug effects and may cause potentially fatal respiratory depression. In addition, discontinuation of a concomitant CYP3A4 inducer may result in increased oxycodone concentrations. Monitor patients receiving oxycodone and any CYP3A4 inhibitor or inducer. [US Boxed Warning]: Concomitant use of opioids with benzodiazepines or other CNS depressants, including alcohol, may result in profound sedation, respiratory depression, coma, and death. Reserve concomitant prescribing of oxycodone and benzodiazepines or other CNS depressants for use in patients for whom alternative treatment options are inadequate. Limit dosage and durations to the minimum required and follow patients for signs and symptoms of respiratory depression and sedation. [US Boxed Warning]: Use exposes patients and other users to the risks of addiction, abuse, and misuse, potentially leading to overdose and death. Assess each patient's risk prior to prescribing; monitor all patients regularly for development of these behaviors or conditions. [US Boxed Warning]: Accidental ingestion of even one dose, especially in children, can result in a fatal overdose of oxycodone. [US Boxed Warning]: Prolonged use of opioids during pregnancy can cause neonatal withdrawal syndrome, which may be life-threatening if not recognized and treated according to protocols developed by neonatology experts. If opioid use is required for a prolonged period in a pregnant woman, advise the patient of the risk of neonatal opioid withdrawal syndrome and ensure that appropriate treatment will be available.** Signs and symptoms include irritability, hyperactivity and abnormal sleep pattern, high pitched cry, tremor, vomiting, diarrhea, and failure to gain weight. Onset, duration and severity depend on the drug used, duration of use, maternal dose, and rate of drug elimination by the newborn.

[US Boxed Warning]: Ensure accuracy when prescribing, dispensing, and administering oxycodone oral solution. Dosing errors due to confusion between mg and mL, and other oxycodone oral solutions of different concentrations can result in accidental overdose.

Extended-release tablets may be difficult to swallow and could become lodged in throat; patients with swallowing difficulties may be at increased risk. Cases of intestinal obstruction or diverticulitis exacerbation have also been reported, including cases requiring medical intervention to remove the tablet; patients with an underlying GI disease (eg, esophageal cancer, colon cancer) may be at increased risk.

Some dosage forms may contain sodium benzoate/benzoic acid; benzoic acid (benzoate) is a metabolite of benzyl alcohol; large amounts of benzyl alcohol (≥99 mg/kg/day) have been associated with a potentially fatal toxicity ("gasping syndrome") in neonates; the "gasping syndrome" consists of metabolic acidosis, respiratory distress, gasping respirations, CNS dysfunction (including convulsions, intracranial hemorrhage), hypotension, and cardiovascular collapse (AAP ["Inactive" 1997]; CDC 1982); some data suggests that benzoate displaces bilirubin from protein-binding sites (Ahlfors 2001); avoid or use dosage forms containing benzyl alcohol derivative with caution in neonates. See manufacturer's labeling.

[US Boxed Warning]: To ensure that the benefits of opioid analgesics outweigh the risks of addiction, abuse, and misuse, a REMS is required. Drug companies with approved opioid analgesic products must make REMS-compliant education programs available to health care providers. Health care providers are encouraged to complete a REMS-compliant education program; counsel patients and/or their caregivers, with every prescription, on safe use, serious risks, storage, and disposal of these products; emphasize to patients and their caregivers the importance of reading the Medication Guide every time it is provided by their pharmacist; and consider other tools to improve patient, household, and community safety.

Drug Interactions

Metabolism/Transport Effects **Substrate** of CYP2D6 (minor), CYP3A4 (major); **Note:** Assignment of Major/Minor substrate status based on clinically relevant drug interaction potential

Avoid Concomitant Use

Avoid concomitant use of OxyCODONE with any of the following: Abametapir; Azelastine (Nasal); Bromperidol; Conivaptan; Eluxadoline; Fusidic Acid (Systemic); Idelalisib; Monoamine Oxidase Inhibitors; Opioids (Mixed Agonist / Antagonist); Orphenadrine; Oxomemazine; Paraldehyde; Thalidomide

Increased Effect/Toxicity

OxyCODONE may increase the levels/effects of: Alvimopan; Azelastine (Nasal); Blonanserin; Desmopressin; Diuretics; Eluxadoline; Flunitrazepam; Methotrimeprazine; MetyroSINE; Monoamine Oxidase Inhibitors; Orphenadrine; Paraldehyde; Piribedil; Pramipexole; Ramosetron; ROPINIRole; Rotigotine; Serotonergic Agents (High Risk); Suvorexant; Thalidomide; Zolpidem

The levels/effects of OxyCODONE may be increased by: Abametapir; Alizapride; Amphetamines; Anticholinergic Agents; Aprepitant; Brimonidine (Topical); Bromopride; Bromperidol; Cannabidiol; Cannabis; Chlormethiazole; Chlorphenesin Carbamate; Clofazimine; CNS Depressants; Conivaptan; CYP3A4 Inhibitors (Moderate); CYP3A4 Inhibitors (Strong); Dimethindene (Topical); Dronabinol; Droperidol; Duvelisib; Erdafitinib; Fosaprepitant; Fosnetupitant; Fusidic Acid (Systemic); Idelalisib; Kava Kava; Larotrectinib; Lemborexant; Lisuride; Lofexidine; Magnesium Sulfate; Methotrimeprazine; Metoclopramide; MiFEPRIStone; Minocycline (Systemic); Nabilone; Netupitant; Oxomemazine; Palbociclib; Perampanel; PHENobarbital; Primidone; Rufinamide; Simeprevir; Sodium Oxybate; Stiripentol; Succinylcholine; Tetrahydrocannabinol; Tetrahydrocannabinol and Cannabidiol; Voriconazole

Decreased Effect

OxyCODONE may decrease the levels/effects of: Diuretics; Gastrointestinal Agents (Prokinetic); Pegvisomant; Sincalide

The levels/effects of OxyCODONE may be decreased by: CYP3A4 Inducers (Moderate); CYP3A4 Inducers (Strong); Dabrafenib; Deferasirox; Enzalutamide; Erdafitinib; Ivosidenib; Mitotane; Nalmefene; Naltrexone; Opioids (Mixed Agonist / Antagonist); PHENobarbital; Primidone; RifAMPin; Sarilumab; Siltuximab; St John's Wort; Tocilizumab

Dietary Considerations Instruct patient to avoid high-fat meals when taking some products (food has no effect on the reformulated OxyContin).

Pharmacodynamics/Kinetics

Onset of Action Pain relief: Immediate release: 10 to 15 minutes; Peak effect: Immediate release: 0.5 to 1 hour

Duration of Action Immediate release: 3 to 6 hours; Extended release: ≤12 hours

Half-life Elimination

Apparent: Immediate release: 3.2 to ~4 hours; Extended release tablet: 4.5 hours; Extended release capsule: 5.6 hours

Elimination: Children 2 to 10 years: 1.8 hours (range: 1.2 to 3 hours); Adults: 3.7 hours

Adults with CrCl <60 mL/minute: Half-life increases by 1 hour, but peak oxycodone concentrations increase by 50% and AUC increases by 60%

Adults with mild to moderate hepatic impairment: Half-life increases by 2.3 hours, peak oxycodone concentrations increase by 50%, and AUC increases by 95%

Time to Peak Plasma: Immediate release: 1.2 to 1.9 hours; Extended release: 4 to 5 hours

Reproductive Considerations

Long-term opioid use may cause secondary hypogonadism, which may lead to sexual dysfunction or infertility (Brennan 2013).

Pregnancy Considerations Oxycodone crosses the placenta (Kokki 2012).

According to some studies, maternal use of opioids may be associated with birth defects (including neural tube defects, congenital heart defects, and gastroschisis), poor fetal growth, stillbirth, and preterm delivery (CDC [Dowell 2016]).

[US Boxed Warning]: Prolonged use of oxycodone during pregnancy can result in neonatal opioid withdrawal syndrome, which may be life-threatening if not recognized and treated, and requires management according to protocols developed by neonatology experts. If opioid use is required for a prolonged period in a pregnant woman, advise the patient of the risk of neonatal opioid withdrawal syndrome and ensure that appropriate treatment will be available. If chronic opioid exposure occurs in pregnancy, adverse events in the newborn (including withdrawal) may occur (Chou 2009). Symptoms of neonatal abstinence syndrome (NAS) following opioid exposure may be autonomic (eg, fever, temperature instability), gastrointestinal (eg, diarrhea, vomiting, poor feeding/weight gain), or neurologic (eg, high-pitched crying, hyperactivity, increased muscle tone, increased wakefulness/abnormal sleep pattern, irritability, sneezing, seizure, tremor, yawning) (Dow 2012; Hudak 2012). Mothers who are physically dependent on opioids may give birth to infants who are also physically dependent. Opioids may cause respiratory depression and psychophysiologic effects in the neonate; newborns of mothers receiving opioids during labor should be monitored.

Oxycodone is not commonly used to treat pain during labor and immediately postpartum (ACOG 209 2019) or chronic noncancer pain in pregnant women or those who may become pregnant (CDC [Dowell 2016]; Chou 2009).

Breastfeeding Considerations

Oxycodone is present in breast milk in variable concentrations.

In one study, oxycodone was measurable in breast milk up to 37 hours after the last maternal dose and therapeutic concentrations were detected in the serum of a breastfeeding infant (Seaton 2007). Oxycodone was also detected in the urine of a breastfed infant (Sulton-Villavasso 2012).

CNS depression, constipation, decreased feeding, and respiratory distress/irregular breathing have been observed in infants exposed to oxycodone via breast milk (Lam 2012; Sulton-Villavasso 2012). Withdrawal symptoms may occur when maternal use is discontinued or breastfeeding is stopped.

Nonopioid analgesics are preferred for breastfeeding females who require pain control peripartum or for surgery outside of the postpartum period (ABM [Martin 2018]; ABM [Reece-Stremtan 2017]). When an opiate is needed, use of oxycodone in breastfeeding women is not recommended by some guidelines (Sachs 2013). Other guidelines note prolonged and frequent use may cause neonatal sedation (ABM [Martin 2018). Maternal doses greater than 30 mg/day are not recommended (ABM [Martin 2018; ACOG 209 2019).

When opioids are needed in breastfeeding women, the lowest effective dose for the shortest duration of time should be used to limit adverse events in the mother and breastfeeding infant. In general, a single occasional dose of an opioid analgesic may be compatible with breastfeeding (WHO 2002). Breastfeeding women using opioids for postpartum pain or for the treatment of chronic maternal pain should monitor their infants for drowsiness, sedation, feeding difficulties, or limpness (ACOG 209 2019).

Controlled Substance C-II

Dosage Forms Considerations

Xtampza ER: Strength is expressed in terms of oxycodone base.

9 mg equivalent to 10 mg oxycodone hydrochloride

13.5 mg equivalent to 15 mg oxycodone hydrochloride

18 mg equivalent to 20 mg oxycodone hydrochloride

36 mg equivalent to 40 mg oxycodone hydrochloride

Dosage Forms: US

Capsule, Oral:

Generic: 5 mg

Capsule ER 12 Hour Abuse-Deterrent, Oral:

Xtampza ER: 9 mg (100 ea); 13.5 mg (100 ea); 18 mg (100 ea); 27 mg (100 ea); 36 mg (100 ea)

Concentrate, Oral:

Generic: 100 mg/5 mL (15 mL, 30 mL)

Solution, Oral:

Generic: 5 mg/5 mL (5 mL, 15 mL, 473 mL, 500 mL)

Tablet, Oral:

Roxicodone: 5 mg, 15 mg, 30 mg

Generic: 5 mg, 10 mg, 15 mg, 20 mg, 30 mg

Tablet Abuse-Deterrent, Oral:

Oxaydo: 5 mg, 7.5 mg

Tablet ER 12 Hour Abuse-Deterrent, Oral:

OxyCONTIN: 10 mg, 15 mg, 20 mg, 30 mg, 40 mg, 60 mg, 80 mg

Generic: 10 mg, 15 mg, 20 mg, 30 mg, 40 mg, 60 mg, 80 mg

Dosage Forms: Canada

Suppository, Rectal:

Supeudol 10: 10 mg (12 ea)

Supeudol 20: 20 mg (12 ea)

Tablet, Oral:

Oxy-IR: 5 mg, 10 mg, 20 mg

Supeudol: 5 mg, 10 mg, 20 mg

Generic: 5 mg, 10 mg, 20 mg

Tablet ER 12 Hour Abuse-Deterrent, Oral:
OxyNEO: 10 mg, 15 mg, 20 mg, 30 mg, 40 mg, 60 mg, 80 mg

Tablet Extended Release 12 Hour, Oral:
Generic: 5 mg, 10 mg, 15 mg, 20 mg, 30 mg, 40 mg, 60 mg, 80 mg

◆ **Oxycodone/Acetaminophen** *see* Oxycodone and Acetaminophen *on page 1164*

Oxycodone and Acetaminophen

(oks i KOE done & a seet a MIN oh fen)

Related Information

Acetaminophen *on page 59*
Oral Pain *on page 1734*
OxyCODONE *on page 1157*

Related Sample Prescriptions

Oral Pain - Sample Prescriptions *on page 30*

Brand Names: US Endocet; Percocet; Primlev; Xartemis XR

Generic Availability (US) Yes: Excludes solution

Pharmacologic Category Analgesic Combination (Opioid); Analgesic, Opioid

Dental Use Treatment of moderate to moderately-severe postoperative dental pain

Use

Pain management

Extended release: Management of acute pain severe enough to require opioid treatment and for which alternative treatment options are inadequate.

Immediate release:

Endocet, Primlev: Management of moderate to moderately severe pain severe enough to require an opioid analgesic and for which alternative treatments are inadequate.

Percocet: Management of pain severe enough to require opioid treatment and for which alternative treatment options are inadequate.

Limitations of use: Reserve for use in patients for whom alternative treatment options (eg, nonopioid analgesics) are ineffective, not tolerated, or would be otherwise inadequate.

Local Anesthetic/Vasoconstrictor Precautions No information available to require special precautions

Effects on Dental Treatment Key adverse event(s) related to dental treatment: Nausea, sedation, constipation, and xerostomia (normal salivary flow resumes upon discontinuation) (see Dental Health Professional Considerations).

Effects on Bleeding As a single agent, acetaminophen does not appear to affect bleeding or platelet aggregation. Acetaminophen may prolong the INR and increase bleeding in patients taking warfarin (Coumadin). For patients taking warfarin, single acetaminophen doses or acetaminophen therapy of short duration should be safe, but if large (>1.3 g/day) doses are administered for longer than 10-14 days, then the INR should be monitored (see Dental Health Professional Considerations).

Adverse Reactions Also see individual agents.

>10%:

Central nervous system: Dizziness (13%)
Gastrointestinal: Nausea (31%)

1% to 10%:

Cardiovascular: Peripheral edema (1%)
Central nervous system: Headache (10%), drowsiness (4%), fatigue (≥1%), insomnia (≥1%)
Dermatologic: Skin rash (2%), erythema (1%), excoriation (1%), pruritus (1%), skin blister (1%)
Endocrine & metabolic: Hot flash (1%)
Gastrointestinal: Vomiting (9%), constipation (4%), diarrhea (≥1%), dyspepsia (≥1%), xerostomia (≥1%)
Genitourinary: Dysuria (1%)
Hepatic: Increased liver enzymes (≥1%)
Respiratory: Cough (≥1%)

Frequency not defined:

Cardiovascular: Circulatory depression, hypotension, shock
Central nervous system: Dysphoria
Dermatologic: Erythematous dermatitis
Hematologic & oncologic: Hemolytic anemia, neutropenia, pancytopenia, thrombocytopenia
Respiratory: Apnea, respiratory depression

<1%, postmarketing, and/or case reports: Abdominal distress, abdominal pain, abnormal hepatic function tests, acidosis, agitation, alkalosis, altered mental status, anaphylactoid reaction, anaphylaxis (acute), angioedema, anxiety, arthralgia, aspiration, asthma, blurred vision, bradycardia, bradypnea, bronchospasm, bruise, cardiac arrhythmia, cerebral edema, chest discomfort, chest pain, chills, cognitive dysfunction, confusion, decreased appetite, dehydration, depression, dermatitis, diaphoresis, disorientation, drug abuse, drug dependence, drug overdose (accidental and nonaccidental), dysgeusia, dyspnea, ecchymoses, emotional lability, esophageal spasm, euphoria, eye redness, falling, fever, flatulence, flushing, hallucination, hearing loss, hepatic disease, hepatic failure, hepatitis, hepatotoxicity, hiccups, hyperglycemia, hyperhidrosis, hyperkalemia, hypersensitivity, hypersensitivity reaction, hypertension, hypoesthesia, hypoglycemia, hypothermia, hypoventilation, impaired consciousness, increased blood pressure, increased gamma-glutamyl transferase, increased lactate dehydrogenase, increased serum ALT, increased serum AST, increased serum bilirubin, increased thirst, interstitial nephritis, intestinal obstruction, jaundice, jitteriness, laryngeal edema, lethargy, malaise, memory impairment, metabolic acidosis, migraine, miosis, myalgia, myoclonus, nervousness, noncardiac chest pain, oropharyngeal pain, orthostatic hypotension, palpitations, pancreatitis, paresthesia, proteinuria, pulmonary edema, renal failure, renal insufficiency, renal papillary necrosis, respiratory alkalosis, reduced urine flow, rhabdomyolysis, sedation, seizure, sleep disorder, stiffness, stupor, suicidal ideation, tachycardia, tachypnea, throat irritation, tinnitus, tremor, urinary retention, urticaria, visual disturbance, weakness, withdrawal syndrome

Dental Usual Dosage

Note: Initial dose is based on the **oxycodone** content; however, the maximum daily dose is based on the **acetaminophen** content.

Management of pain: Doses should be given every 4-6 hours as needed and titrated to appropriate analgesic effects.

Mild-to-moderate pain:

Children: Initial dose, **based on oxycodone content:** 0.05-0.1 mg/kg/dose

Maximum acetaminophen dose: Children <45 kg: 90 mg/kg/day; children >45 kg: 4 g/day

Adults: Initial dose, **based on oxycodone content:** 2.5-5 mg

Severe pain:

Children: Initial dose, **based on oxycodone content:** 0.3 mg/kg/dose

Adults: Initial dose, **based on oxycodone content:** 10-30 mg. Do not exceed acetaminophen 4 g/day.

Elderly: Doses should be titrated to appropriate analgesic effects: Initial dose, **based on oxycodone content:** 2.5-5 mg every 6 hours. Do not exceed acetaminophen 4 g/day.

Dosage adjustment in hepatic impairment: Dose should be reduced in patients with severe liver disease.

Dosing

Adult Note: Initial dose is based on the **oxycodone** content; however, the maximum daily dose is based on the **acetaminophen** content.

Pain management:

Extended release: Oral: Usual dose: 2 tablets every 12 hours; the second initial dose may be administered as early as 8 hours after the first initial dose if needed; subsequent doses are to be administered 2 tablets every 12 hours. Do not exceed acetaminophen 4 g/day. **NOTE:** Oxycodone/acetaminophen ER is not interchangeable with other oxycodone/acetaminophen products because of differing pharmacokinetic profiles that affect the frequency of administration.

Immediate release: Oral: Doses should be titrated to appropriate analgesic effects.

Initial dose, **based on oxycodone content**: 5 mg (moderate pain) or 10 to 20 mg (severe pain) (APS 2008) or 2.5 to 10 mg (manufacturer's labeling). Doses typically given every 4 to 6 hours as needed. Do not exceed acetaminophen 4 g/day (APS 2008).

Discontinuation of therapy: When discontinuing chronic opioid therapy, the dose should be gradually tapered down. An optimal universal tapering schedule for all patients has not been established (CDC [Dowell 2016]). Proposed schedules range from slow (eg, 10% reductions per week) to rapid (eg, 25% to 50% reduction every few days) (CDC 2015). Tapering schedules should be individualized to minimize opioid withdrawal while considering patient-specific goals and concerns as well as the pharmacokinetics of the opioid being tapered. An even slower taper may be appropriate in patients who have been receiving opioids for a long duration (eg, years), particularly in the final stage of tapering, whereas more rapid tapers may be appropriate in patients experiencing severe adverse events (CDC [Dowell 2016]). Monitor carefully for signs/symptoms of withdrawal. If the patient displays withdrawal symptoms, consider slowing the taper schedule; alterations may include increasing the interval between dose reductions, decreasing amount of daily dose reduction, pausing the taper and restarting when the patient is ready, and/or coadministration of an alpha-2 agonist (eg, clonidine) to blunt withdrawal symptoms (Berna 2015; CDC [Dowell 2016]). Continue to offer nonopioid analgesics as needed for pain management during the taper; consider nonopioid adjunctive treatments for withdrawal symptoms (eg, GI complaints, muscle spasm) as needed (Berna 2015; Sevarino 2018).

Geriatric

Refer to adult dosing. Use with caution and consider initiation at the low end of the dosing range; titrate slowly.

Immediate release: *Severe pain:* Elderly >70 years (off-label dosing): Consider decreasing the initial dose **(based on oxycodone content)** by 25% to 50%, then titrating the dose upward or downward as needed; monitor frequently during titration. Do not exceed acetaminophen 4 g/day (APS 2008).

Renal Impairment: Adult

Extended release: Initial dose: One tablet every 12 hours; adjust dose as needed.

Immediate release: There are no dosage adjustments provided in the manufacturer's labeling. Use with caution and initiate at the low end of the dosing range; titrate carefully and monitor closely.

Hepatic Impairment: Adult

Extended release: Initial dose: One tablet every 12 hours; adjust dose as needed.

Immediate release: There are no dosage adjustments provided in the manufacturer's labeling. Use with caution and initiate at the low end of the dosing range; titrate carefully and monitor closely.

Pediatric Note: Doses based on total oxycodone content; titrate dose to appropriate analgesic effects. All sources of acetaminophen (eg, prescription, OTC, combination products) should be considered when evaluating a patient's maximum daily acetaminophen dose. To lower the risk for hepatotoxicity, limit daily dose to ≤75 mg/kg/**day** (maximum of 5 daily doses), not to exceed 4,000 mg/**day**; while recommended doses are generally considered safe, hepatotoxicity has been reported (rarely) even with doses below recommendations (AAP [Sullivan 2011]; Heard 2014; Lavonas 2010).

Analgesic: Limited data available: Infants ≥6 months, Children, and Adolescents:

Patient weight:

<50 kg: Oral: Usual initial dose: Oxycodone 0.1 to 0.2 mg/kg/dose; doses typically given every 4 to 6 hours as needed; manufacturer's labeling recommends every 6 hours in adults (Berde 2002; Kliegman 2020; Thigpen 2019).

≥50 kg: Oral: Usual initial dose: Oxycodone 5 to 10 mg every 4 to 6 hours; manufacturer's labeling recommends every 6 hours in adults (Berde 2002; Thigpen 2019).

Discontinuation of therapy: Do not abruptly discontinue therapy in patients who are physically dependent; dose should be gradually tapered to avoid withdrawal. An optimal tapering schedule has not been established. The taper should be individualized to minimize withdrawal and should be based on total daily opioid dose, length of opioid exposure, and patient response. Monitor patients for signs and symptoms of opioid withdrawal (D'Souza 2018).

Renal Impairment: Pediatric There are no pediatric-specific recommendations. In general, oxycodone clearance may be decreased in patients with renal impairment. Based on experience in adult patients, use with caution and initiate at the low end of the dosing range; titrate carefully and monitor closely.

Hepatic Impairment: Pediatric There are no pediatric-specific recommendations; based on experience in adult patients, use with caution and initiate at the low end of the dosing range; titrate carefully and monitor closely. For acetaminophen, limited, low-dose therapy is usually well-tolerated in hepatic disease/cirrhosis; however, cases of hepatotoxicity at daily acetaminophen dosages <4,000 mg/day in adults have been reported. Avoid chronic use in hepatic impairment. See individual monographs.

Mechanism of Action

Oxycodone: Binds to opiate receptors in the CNS, causing inhibition of ascending pain pathways, altering the perception of and response to pain; produces generalized CNS depression.

Acetaminophen: Although not fully elucidated, the analgesic effects are believed to be due to activation of descending serotonergic inhibitory pathways in the CNS. Interactions with other nociceptive systems may be involved as well (Smith 2009). Antipyresis is produced from inhibition of the hypothalamic heat-regulating center.

Contraindications

Hypersensitivity (eg, anaphylaxis) to oxycodone, acetaminophen, or any component of the formulation; significant respiratory depression; acute or severe bronchial asthma (in an unmonitored setting or in the absence of resuscitative equipment); GI obstruction, including paralytic ileus (known or suspected)

Additional product-specific contraindications: *Endocet, Primlev*: Hypercarbia

Documentation of allergenic cross-reactivity for opioids is limited. However, because of similarities in chemical structure and/or pharmacologic actions, the possibility of cross-sensitivity cannot be ruled out with certainty.

Canadian labeling: Additional contraindications (not in US labeling): Severe hepatic insufficiency or active liver disease; suspected surgical abdomen (eg, acute appendicitis or pancreatitis); mild pain that can be managed with other pain medications; chronic obstructive airway; cor pulmonale; acute alcoholism, delirium tremens, or convulsive disorders; severe CNS depression, increased cerebrospinal or intracranial pressure, or head injury; concurrent use with or within 14 days following MAOI therapy; pregnant women or during labor and delivery; breastfeeding

Warnings/Precautions Hypersensitivity and anaphylactic reactions have been reported with acetaminophen use; discontinue immediately if symptoms of allergic or hypersensitivity reactions occur. Serious and potentially fatal skin reactions, including acute generalized exanthematous pustulosis (AGEP), Stevens-Johnson syndrome (SJS), and toxic epidermal necrolysis (TEN), have occurred rarely with acetaminophen use; discontinue therapy at the first appearance of skin rash. Use with caution in patients with hepatic or renal impairment; thyroid dysfunction; adrenal insufficiency, including Addison disease; seizure disorder; toxic psychosis; delirium tremens; morbid obesity; biliary tract impairment; acute pancreatitis; prostatic hyperplasia; or urethral stricture. Use with caution in patients with known G6PD deficiency. May obscure diagnosis or clinical course of patients with acute abdominal conditions. Avoid use in patients with impaired consciousness or coma. Some preparations contain sulfites, which may cause allergic reactions. May cause CNS depression, which may impair physical or mental abilities; caution must be used in performing tasks that require alertness (eg, operating machinery, driving). May cause severe hypotension (including orthostatic hypotension and syncope); use with caution in patients with hypovolemia, cardiovascular disease (including acute MI), or drugs that may exaggerate hypotensive effects (including phenothiazines or general anesthetics). Monitor for symptoms of hypotension following initiation or dose titration. Avoid use in patients with circulatory shock. Oxycodone decreases bowel motility; monitor for decreased bowel motility in postop patients receiving opioids. Abrupt discontinuation in patients who are physically dependent on opioids has been associated with serious withdrawal symptoms, uncontrolled pain, attempts to find other opioids (including illicit), and suicide. Use a collaborative, patient-specific taper schedule that minimizes the risk of withdrawal, considering factors such as current opioid dose, duration of use, type of pain, and physical and psychological factors. Monitor pain control, withdrawal symptoms, mood changes, suicidal ideation, and for use of other substances; provide care as needed. Concurrent use of mixed agonist/antagonist analgesics (eg, pentazocine, nalbuphine, butorphanol) or partial agonist (eg, buprenorphine) analgesics may also precipitate withdrawal symptoms and/or reduced analgesic efficacy in patients following prolonged therapy with mu opioid agonists. Use with caution in patients with hypersensitivity reactions to other phenanthrene-derivative opioid agonists (codeine, hydrocodone, hydromorphone, levorphanol, oxymorphone).

Use opioids with caution for chronic pain in patients with mental health conditions (eg, depression, anxiety disorders, post-traumatic stress disorder) due to increased risk for opioid use disorder and overdose; more frequent monitoring is recommended (Dowell [CDC 2016]). **[US Boxed Warning]: Serious, life-threatening, or fatal respiratory depression may occur. Monitor closely for respiratory depression, especially during initiation or dose escalation. Swallow oxycodone/acetaminophen ER whole; crushing, chewing, or dissolving oxycodone/acetaminophen ER can cause rapid release and absorption of a potentially fatal dose of oxycodone.** Carbon dioxide retention from opioid-induced respiratory depression can exacerbate the sedating effects of opioids. Use with caution and monitor for respiratory depression in patients with significant COPD or cor pulmonale, and those with a substantially decreased respiratory reserve, hypoxia, hypercapnia, or preexisting respiratory depression, particularly when initiating and titrating therapy; critical respiratory depression may occur, even at therapeutic dosages. Consider the use of alternative nonopioid analgesics in these patients. Opioid use increases the risk for sleep-related disorders (eg, central sleep apnea [CSA], hypoxemia) in a dose-dependent fashion. Use with caution for chronic pain and titrate dosage cautiously in patients with risk factors for sleep-disordered breathing (eg, heart failure, obesity). Consider dose reduction in patients presenting with CSA. Avoid opioids in patients with moderate to severe sleep-disordered breathing (Dowell [CDC 2016]). Use with extreme caution in patients with head injury, intracranial lesions, or increased intracranial pressure. Risk of respiratory depression is increased in elderly and cachectic or debilitated patients. Oxycodone clearance may be slightly reduced in elderly patients; use with caution and consider dosage adjustments or the use of alternative nonopioid analgesics in these patients. Use opioids for chronic pain with caution in older adults and monitor closely due to an increased potential for risks, including certain risks such as falls/fracture, cognitive impairment, and constipation (Dowell [CDC 2016]). Use with caution in patients with alcoholic liver disease; consuming ≥3 alcoholic drinks/day may increase the risk of liver damage. Limit acetaminophen dose from all sources (prescription and OTC) to <4 g/day in adults. Do not use oxycodone/acetaminophen concomitantly with other acetaminophen-containing products. Oxycodone may cause constipation which may be problematic in patients with unstable angina and patients post-MI.

[US Boxed Warning]: To ensure that the benefits of opioid analgesics outweigh the risks of addiction, abuse, and misuse, a REMS is required. Drug companies with approved opioid analgesic products must make REMS-compliant education programs

available to health care providers. Health care providers are encouraged to complete a REMS-compliant education program; counsel patients and/or their caregivers, with every prescription, on safe use, serious risks, storage, and disposal of these products; emphasize to patients and their caregivers the importance of reading the Medication Guide every time it is provided by their pharmacist; and consider other tools to improve patient, household, and community safety.

Potentially significant drug-drug interactions may exist, requiring dose or frequency adjustment, additional monitoring, and/or selection of alternative therapy. **[US Boxed Warning]: Concomitant use of opioids with benzodiazepines or other CNS depressants, including alcohol, may result in profound sedation, respiratory depression, coma, and death. Reserve concomitant prescribing of oxycodone/acetaminophen and benzodiazepines or other CNS depressants for use in patients for whom alternative treatment options are inadequate. Limit dosage and durations to the minimum required and follow patients for signs and symptoms of respiratory depression and sedation.**

[US Boxed Warning]: Prolonged use of opioids during pregnancy can cause neonatal withdrawal syndrome in the newborn, which may be life-threatening if not recognized and treated according to protocols developed by neonatology experts. If opioid use is required for a prolonged period in a pregnant woman, advise the patient of the risk of neonatal opioid withdrawal syndrome and ensure that appropriate treatment will be available. Signs and symptoms include irritability, hyperactivity and abnormal sleep pattern, high-pitched cry, tremor, vomiting, diarrhea, and failure to gain weight. Onset, duration, and severity depend on the drug used, duration of use, maternal dose, and rate of drug elimination by the newborn.

[US Boxed Warning]: Use exposes patients and other users to the risks of opioid addiction, abuse, and misuse, which can lead to overdose and death. Assess each patient's risk prior to prescribing oxycodone/acetaminophen, and monitor all patients regularly for the development of these behaviors or conditions. Use with caution in patients with a history of drug abuse or acute alcoholism; potential for drug dependency exists. Other factors associated with increased risk for misuse include younger age, concomitant depression (major), and psychotropic medication use. Consider offering naloxone prescriptions in patients with factors associated with an increased risk for overdose, such as history of overdose or substance use disorder, higher opioid dosages (≥50 morphine milligram equivalents/day orally), and concomitant benzodiazepine use (Dowell [CDC 2016]). Abuse or misuse of ER tablets by crushing, chewing, snorting, or injecting the dissolved product will result in the uncontrolled delivery of the oxycodone and can result in overdose and death.

Chronic pain: Opioids should **not** be used as first-line therapy for chronic pain management (pain >3-month duration or beyond time of normal tissue healing) due to limited short-term benefits, undetermined long-term benefits, and association with serious risks (eg, overdose, MI, auto accidents, risk of developing opioid use disorder). Preferred management includes nonpharmacologic therapy and nonopioid therapy (eg, NSAIDs, acetaminophen, certain anticonvulsants and antidepressants). If opioid therapy is initiated, it should be combined with nonpharmacologic and nonopioid therapy, as appropriate. Prior to initiation, known risks of opioid therapy should be discussed and realistic treatment goals for pain/function should be established, including consideration for discontinuation if benefits do not outweigh risks. Therapy should be continued only if clinically meaningful improvement in pain/function outweighs risks. Therapy should be initiated at the lowest effective dosage using immediate-release opioids (instead of extended-release/long-acting opioids). Risk associated with use increases with higher opioid dosages. Risks and benefits should be re-evaluated when increasing dosage to ≥50 morphine milligram equivalents (MME)/day orally; dosages ≥90 MME/day orally should be avoided unless carefully justified (Dowell [CDC 2016]).

[US Boxed Warning]: Acetaminophen has been associated with cases of acute liver failure, at times resulting in liver transplant and death. Most of the cases of liver injury are associated with the use of acetaminophen at doses that exceed 4 g/day in adults, and often involve more than 1 acetaminophen-containing product. Risk is increased with alcohol use, preexisting liver disease, and intake of more than one source of acetaminophen-containing medications. Chronic daily dosing in adults has also resulted in liver damage in some patients.

[US Boxed Warning]: Accidental ingestion of oxycodone/acetaminophen, especially in children, can result in a fatal overdose of oxycodone/acetaminophen. Do not to presoak, lick, or otherwise wet ER tablets prior to placing in the mouth; take one tablet at a time with enough water to ensure complete swallowing. Oxycodone/acetaminophen ER is not interchangeable with other oxycodone/acetaminophen products because of differing pharmacokinetic profiles that affect the frequency of administration. Do not abruptly stop ER tablets in patients who may be physically dependent; gradually decrease dose by 50% every 2 to 4 days to prevent signs and symptoms of withdrawal. Due to characteristics of the ER formulation that cause the tablets to swell and become sticky when wet, consider use of an alternative analgesic in patients who have difficulty swallowing and patients at risk for underlying GI disorders resulting in a small GI lumen.

[US Boxed Warning]: The concomitant use of oxycodone/acetaminophen with all cytochrome P450 3A4 inhibitors may result in an increase in oxycodone plasma concentrations, which could increase or prolong adverse reactions and may cause potentially fatal respiratory depression. In addition, discontinuation of a concomitantly used cytochrome P450 3A4 inducer may result in an increase in oxycodone plasma concentration. Monitor patients receiving oxycodone/acetaminophen and any CYP3A4 inhibitor or inducer.

An opioid-containing analgesic regimen should be tailored to each patient's needs and based upon the type of pain being treated (acute versus chronic), the route of administration, degree of tolerance for opioids (naive versus chronic user), age, weight, and medical condition. The optimal analgesic dose varies widely among patients; doses should be titrated to pain relief/prevention. Opioids decrease bowel motility; monitor for decrease bowel motility in postop patients receiving opioids. Use with caution in the perioperative setting;

individualize treatment when transitioning from parenteral to oral analgesics. Some dosage forms may contain sodium benzoate/benzoic acid; benzoic acid (benzoate) is a metabolite of benzyl alcohol; large amounts of benzyl alcohol (≥99 mg/kg/day) have been associated with a potentially fatal toxicity ("gasping syndrome") in neonates; the "gasping syndrome" consists of metabolic acidosis, respiratory distress, gasping respirations, CNS dysfunction (including convulsions, intracranial hemorrhage), hypotension, and cardiovascular collapse (AAP ["Inactive" 1997]; CDC 1982); some data suggest that benzoate displaces bilirubin from protein binding sites (Ahlfors 2001); avoid or use dosage forms containing benzyl alcohol derivative with caution in neonates. See manufacturer's labeling.

Some dosage forms may contain propylene glycol; large amounts are potentially toxic and have been associated with hyperosmolality, lactic acidosis, seizures, and respiratory depression; use caution (AAP 1997; Zar 2007).

Warnings: Additional Pediatric Considerations
Hepatotoxicity has been reported in patients using acetaminophen. In pediatric patients, this is most commonly associated with supratherapeutic dosing, more frequent administration than recommended, and use of multiple acetaminophen-containing products; however, hepatotoxicity has been rarely reported with recommended dosages (AAP [Sullivan 2011]; Heard 2014). All sources of acetaminophen (eg, prescription, OTC, combination) should be considered when evaluating a patient's maximum daily dose. To lower the risk for hepatotoxicity, the maximum daily acetaminophen dose should be limited to ≤75 mg/kg/day (maximum of 5 daily doses), not to exceed 4,000 mg/day (AAP [Sullivan 2011]; Heard 2014; Krenzelok 2012; Lavonas 2010). Acetaminophen avoidance or a lower total daily dose (2,000 to 3,000 mg/day) has been suggested for adults with increased risk for acetaminophen hepatotoxicity (eg, malnutrition, certain liver diseases, use of drugs that interact with acetaminophen metabolism); similar data are unavailable in pediatric patients (Hayward 2016; Larson 2007; Worriax 2007).

Infants born to women physically dependent on opioids will also be physically dependent and may experience respiratory difficulties or opioid withdrawal symptoms (neonatal abstinence syndrome [NAS]). Onset, duration, and severity of NAS depend upon the drug used (maternal), duration of use, maternal dose, and rate of drug elimination by the newborn. Symptoms of opioid withdrawal may include excessive crying, diarrhea, fever, hyper-reflexia, irritability, tremors, or vomiting or failure to gain weight. Opioid withdrawal syndrome in the neonate may be life-threatening and should be promptly treated.

Some dosage forms may contain propylene glycol; in neonates, large amounts of propylene glycol delivered orally, intravenously (eg, >3,000 mg/day), or topically have been associated with potentially fatal toxicities which can include metabolic acidosis, seizures, renal failure, and CNS depression; toxicities have also been reported in children and adults including hyperosmolality, lactic acidosis, seizures, and respiratory depression; use caution (AAP 1997; Shehab 2009).

Drug Interactions

Metabolism/Transport Effects Refer to individual components.

Avoid Concomitant Use

Avoid concomitant use of Oxycodone and Acetaminophen with any of the following: Abametapir; Azelastine (Nasal); Bromperidol; Conivaptan; Eluxadoline; Fusidic Acid (Systemic); Idelalisib; Monoamine Oxidase Inhibitors; Opioids (Mixed Agonist / Antagonist); Orphenadrine; Oxomemazine; Paraldehyde; Thalidomide

Increased Effect/Toxicity

Oxycodone and Acetaminophen may increase the levels/effects of: Alvimopan; Azelastine (Nasal); Blonanserin; Busulfan; Dasatinib; Desmopressin; Diuretics; Eluxadoline; Flunitrazepam; Imatinib; Local Anesthetics; Methotrimeprazine; MetyroSINE; Mipomersen; Monoamine Oxidase Inhibitors; Orphenadrine; Paraldehyde; Phenylephrine (Systemic); Piribedil; Pramipexole; Prilocaine; Ramosetron; ROPINIRole; Rotigotine; Serotonergic Agents (High Risk); Sodium Nitrite; SORAfenib; Suvorexant; Thalidomide; Vitamin K Antagonists; Zolpidem

The levels/effects of Oxycodone and Acetaminophen may be increased by: Abametapir; Alizapride; Amphetamines; Anticholinergic Agents; Aprepitant; Brimonidine (Topical); Bromopride; Bromperidol; Cannabidiol; Cannabis; Chlormethiazole; Chlorphenesin Carbamate; Clofazimine; CNS Depressants; Conivaptan; CYP3A4 Inhibitors (Moderate); CYP3A4 Inhibitors (Strong); Dapsone (Topical); Dasatinib; Dimethindene (Topical); Dronabinol; Droperidol; Duvelisib; Erdafitinib; Flucloxacillin; Fosaprepitant; Fosnetupitant; Fusidic Acid (Systemic); Idelalisib; Isoniazid; Kava Kava; Larotrectinib; Lemborexant; Lisuride; Lofexidine; Magnesium Sulfate; Methotrimeprazine; Metoclopramide; MetyraPONE; MiFEPRIStone; Minocycline (Systemic); Nabilone; Netupitant; Nitric Oxide; Oxomemazine; Palbociclib; Perampanel; PHENobarbital; Primidone; Probenecid; Rufinamide; Simeprevir; Sodium Oxybate; SORAfenib; Stiripentol; Succinylcholine; Tetrahydrocannabinol; Tetrahydrocannabinol and Cannabidiol; Voriconazole

Decreased Effect

Oxycodone and Acetaminophen may decrease the levels/effects of: Diuretics; Gastrointestinal Agents (Prokinetic); Pegvisomant; Sincalide

The levels/effects of Oxycodone and Acetaminophen may be decreased by: CYP3A4 Inducers (Moderate); CYP3A4 Inducers (Strong); Dabrafenib; Deferasirox; Enzalutamide; Erdafitinib; Isoniazid; Ivosidenib; Lorlatinib; Mitotane; Nalmefene; Naltrexone; Opioids (Mixed Agonist / Antagonist); PHENobarbital; Primidone; RifAMPin; Sarilumab; Siltuximab; St John's Wort; Tocilizumab

Reproductive Considerations
Long-term opioid use may cause secondary hypogonadism, which may lead to sexual dysfunction or infertility in men and women (Brennan 2013).

Pregnancy Risk Factor C

Pregnancy Considerations
[US Boxed Warning]: Prolonged use of opioids during pregnancy can result in neonatal opioid withdrawal syndrome, which may be life-threatening if not recognized and treated, and requires management according to protocols developed by neonatology experts. If opioid use is required for a prolonged period in a pregnant woman, advise the patient of the risk of neonatal opioid withdrawal syndrome and ensure appropriate treatment will be available. Refer to individual monographs for additional information.

Breastfeeding Considerations
Oxycodone and acetaminophen are present in breast milk. Due to the potential for serious adverse reactions in the breastfeeding infant, breastfeeding is not recommended by the manufacturer. Refer to individual monographs.

Controlled Substance C-II

Dosage Forms: US

Tablet, Oral:

Endocet 2.5/325: Oxycodone 2.5 mg and acetaminophen 325 mg

Endocet 5/325 [scored]: Oxycodone 5 mg and acetaminophen 325 mg

Endocet 7.5/325: Oxycodone 7.5 mg and acetaminophen 325 mg

Endocet 10/325: Oxycodone 10 mg and acetaminophen 325 mg

Percocet 2.5/325: Oxycodone 2.5 mg and acetaminophen 325 mg

Percocet 5/325 [scored]: Oxycodone 5 mg and acetaminophen 325 mg

Percocet 7.5/325: Oxycodone 7.5 mg and acetaminophen 325 mg

Percocet 10/325: Oxycodone 10 mg and acetaminophen 325 mg

Primlev 5/300: Oxycodone 5 mg and acetaminophen 300 mg

Primlev 7.5/300: Oxycodone 7.5 mg and acetaminophen 300 mg

Primlev 10/300: Oxycodone 10 mg and acetaminophen 300 mg

Generic: 2.5/325: Oxycodone hydrochloride 2.5 mg and acetaminophen 325 mg; 5/325: Oxycodone hydrochloride 5 mg and acetaminophen 325 mg; 7.5/325: Oxycodone hydrochloride 7.5 mg and acetaminophen 325 mg; 10/325: Oxycodone hydrochloride 10 mg and acetaminophen 325 mg

Tablet, Extended Release, Oral:

Xartemis XR: Oxycodone hydrochloride 7.5 mg and acetaminophen 325 mg

Dental Health Professional Considerations
Although the ***OTC product labeling*** for acetaminophen products state to limit the maximum dose to 3,000 mg daily (for extra strength) or 3,250 mg (for regular strength) (see this site for details: http://www.-tylenolprofessional.com/products-and-dosages.html), it is still appropriate for patients to take up to 4,000 mg daily "under the direction of a health care provider" (http://www.tylenolprofessional.com/dosage.html).

Oxycodone, as with other opioid analgesics, is recommended only for limited acute dosing (ie, 3 days or less). Oxycodone has an addictive liability, especially when given long-term. The acetaminophen component requires use with caution in patients who use alcohol, with preexisting liver disease, and those receiving more than one source of acetaminophen-containing medication.

Hepatotoxicity caused by acetaminophen is potentiated by chronic alcohol consumption. People who are taking acetaminophen, even at therapeutic doses, and consume alcohol are at risk of developing hepatotoxicity.

Acetaminophen may increase the levels and enhance the anticoagulant effects of vitamin K antagonists acenocoumarol and warfarin (Coumadin). Studies have reported that acetaminophen has increased the INR in warfarin treated patients with daily acetaminophen doses as low as 2 g, particularly when taking acetaminophen for >1 week (Antlitz, 1968; Boeijinga, 1982; Gebauer, 2003; Hylek, 1998; Rubin, 1984). In addition, case reports of bleeding as a result of increased INR have been published (Bagheri, 1999; Bartle, 1991). There is no known mechanism of the interaction; furthermore, some studies have failed to demonstrate this interaction (Gadisseur, 2003; Kwan, 1995; van den Bemt, 2002). In terms of risk, the data suggest that acetaminophen and warfarin could interact in some clinically significant manner but that the benefits of concomitant use of acetaminophen for pain control in dental patients taking warfarin usually outweigh the risks. An appropriate monitoring plan should be in place to identify potential negative effects and dosage adjustments may be necessary in a minority of patients. The interaction may be more likely to occur with daily acetaminophen doses of >1.3 g for >1 week.

There are no reports of acetaminophen interacting with antiplatelet drugs such as aspirin, clopidogrel (Plavix), or prasugrel (Effient). Also, there are no reports of acetaminophen in combination with hydrocodone, codeine, or oxycodone interacting with warfarin (Coumadin).

Oxycodone and Naloxone

(oks i KOE done & nal OKS one)

Related Information

Naloxone *on page 1074*
OxyCODONE *on page 1157*

Brand Names: Canada Targin

Generic Availability (US) No

Pharmacologic Category Analgesic, Opioid; Opioid Antagonist

Use

Note: Not approved in the US.

Pain management: Management of pain severe enough to require daily, around-the-clock, long-term opioid treatment and for which alternative treatment options are inadequate. **Note:** Naloxone included in the formulation for the relief of opioid-induced constipation.

Local Anesthetic/Vasoconstrictor Precautions
No information available to require special precautions

Effects on Dental Treatment Key adverse event(s) related to dental treatment: Nausea and xerostomia (normal salivary flow resumes upon discontinuation)

Effects on Bleeding No information available to require special precautions

Adverse Reactions

>10%: Hematologic & oncologic: Cancer pain (12%)

1% to 10%:

Central nervous system: Abdominal pain (8%), withdrawal syndrome (8%), weakness (7%), fatigue (5%), headache (5%), pain (3%), depression (≤2%), peripheral pain (2%), sciatica (2%), drowsiness (1%), migraine (1%), tremor (1%)

Dermatologic: Hyperhidrosis (7%), skin rash (≤1%)

Endocrine & metabolic: Peripheral edema (2% to 5%), increased serum glucose (2%), hyperglycemia (1%), hyperlipidemia (1%), hyperuricemia (1%)

Gastrointestinal: Anorexia (8%), nausea (8%), constipation (7%), vomiting (7%), xerostomia (3%), gastroenteritis (2%)

Genitourinary: Urinary tract infection (4%)

Hematologic & oncologic: Progression of cancer (9%), anemia (5%), decreased hemoglobin (≤5%)

Infection: Viral infection (2%), influenza (1%)

Neuromuscular & skeletal: Back pain (3%), lower extremity pain (2%), upper extremity pain (2%), osteoarthritis (1%)

Respiratory: Bronchitis (2%), sinusitis (1%)

<1%, postmarketing, and/or case reports: Abdominal distention, abnormal dreams, abnormal hepatic function tests, abnormality in thinking, anal fissure, angina pectoris, anorectal pain, antisocial behavior, anxiety, biliary obstruction, blurred vision, candidiasis, cellulitis, central nervous system dysfunction, chest pain, cholelithiasis, cold extremities, confusion, cough, deafness, decreased blood pressure, decreased hematocrit, decreased platelet count, decreased red blood cells, diarrhea, disorientation, diverticulitis of the gastrointestinal tract, drug dependence, drug overdose, dry eye syndrome, dysgeusia, dysmenorrhea, dyspnea, dyspnea on exertion, ECG abnormality, eczema, epistaxis, equilibrium disturbance, erectile dysfunction, eructation, euphoria, falling, first degree atrioventricular block, flu-like symptoms, furuncle, gastric disease, gastritis, gastroesophageal reflux disease, gastrointestinal hemorrhage, glossitis, gout, gouty arthritis, hallucination, hemoptysis, hypersensitivity, hypertensive crisis, hypogonadism (Brennan 2013; Debono 2011), hyponatremia, hypophosphatemia, hypotension, impacted cerumen, increased blood pressure, increased heart rate, increased lacrimation, increased lactate dehydrogenase, increased liver enzymes, increased serum ALT, increased serum bilirubin, increased thirst, irritability, joint swelling, laceration, lack of concentration, lethargy, lipoma, localized edema, loss of libido, lower abdominal pain, memory impairment, muscle injury, muscle spasm, muscle twitching, musculoskeletal chest pain, myalgia, neck pain, neuromuscular blockade, night sweats, nightmares, noncardiac chest pain, otitis externa, palpitations, panic attack, paresthesia, periodontitis, photopsia, pneumonia, pollakiuria, polyarthralgia, polyneuropathy, pruritic rash, pruritus, renal pain, respiratory depression, restless leg syndrome, restless sleep, rhinitis, right bundle branch block, sedation, sensation of cold, shoulder pain, speech disturbance, sprain, stasis dermatitis, stiffness, stupor, syncope, swelling, tenosynovitis, tension headache, thrombophlebitis, thrombosis, tinnitus, tonic-clonic seizures, urinary incontinence, urinary retention, urinary urgency, vaginal hemorrhage, visual disturbance, weight loss, yawning

Dosing

Adult Pain management: Oral:

Note: Oxycodone 5 mg/naloxone 2.5 mg tablets are intended only for use in titration or dosage adjustment. Multiple units of oxycodone 5 mg/naloxone 2.5 mg should not be substituted for other tablet strengths. Do not exceed single doses of oxycodone 40 mg/naloxone 20 mg or total daily doses of oxycodone 80 mg/naloxone 40 mg. Oxycodone 40 mg/naloxone 20 mg tablets are for use only in opioid-tolerant patients. Patients considered opioid tolerant are those already receiving opioid therapy for at least 1 week with doses exceeding 60 mg of oral morphine or its equivalent (American Pain Society 2016).

Opioid-naive patients: Initial dose: Oxycodone 10 mg/naloxone 5 mg every 12 hours

Opioid-experienced patients: Initial dose:

Currently on other oral oxycodone formulations: **Note:** Discontinue all other around-the-clock oxycodone medications prior to initiation of oxycodone/naloxone. Initiate oxycodone/naloxone at the same total daily oral oxycodone dosage, in 2 equally divided doses administered every 12 hours. Maximum single dose: Oxycodone 40 mg/naloxone 20 mg; Maximum daily dose: Oxycodone 80 mg/naloxone 40 mg/day.

Currently on other oral opioids: Discontinue all other around-the-clock opioids. Initiate oxycodone/naloxone at the lowest available strength; adequate rescue medication should be provided. Maximum single dose: Oxycodone 40 mg/naloxone 20 mg; Maximum daily dose: Oxycodone 80 mg/naloxone 40 mg/day.

Dose adjustment: Dose is individualized; titrate dose cautiously every 1 to 2 days until satisfactory response and acceptable adverse effects. Repeated pain at the end of the dosing interval may indicate the need for a dose adjustment rather than adjusting the dosing interval. Maximum single dose: Oxycodone 40 mg/naloxone 20 mg; Maximum daily dose: Oxycodone 80 mg/naloxone 40 mg/day.

Patients requiring rescue medication: Patients who experience breakthrough pain may require a rescue medication with an appropriate dose of an immediate-release analgesic. **Note:** Rescue medications used in clinical trials were immediate release oxycodone or combination products containing codeine.

Administer a single dose of an immediate release opioid that is approximately 16% of the equivalent daily dose of oxycodone. Patients requiring >2 doses daily of rescue medication should have oxycodone/naloxone dose titrated upward every 1 to 2 days until satisfactory response is achieved (not to exceed recommended maximum dosing). Dosing interval (every 12 hours) should not be adjusted.

Discontinuation of therapy: When discontinuing chronic opioid therapy, the dose should be gradually tapered down. An optimal universal tapering schedule for all patients has not been established (CDC [Dowell 2016]). Proposed schedules range from slow (eg, 10% reductions per week) to rapid (eg, 25% to 50% reduction every few days) (CDC 2015). Tapering schedules should be individualized to minimize opioid withdrawal while considering patient-specific goals and concerns as well as the pharmacokinetics of the opioid being tapered. An even slower taper may be appropriate in patients who have been receiving opioids for a long duration (eg, years), particularly in the final stage of tapering, whereas more rapid tapers may be appropriate in patients experiencing severe adverse events (CDC [Dowell 2016]). Monitor carefully for signs/symptoms of withdrawal. If the patient displays withdrawal symptoms, consider slowing the taper schedule; alterations may include increasing the interval between dose reductions, decreasing amount of daily dose reduction, pausing the taper and restarting when the patient is ready, and/or coadministration of an alpha-2 agonist (eg, clonidine) to blunt withdrawal symptoms (Berna 2015; CDC [Dowell 2016]). Continue to offer nonopioid analgesics as needed for pain management during the taper; consider nonopioid adjunctive treatments for withdrawal symptoms (eg, GI complaints, muscle spasm) as needed (Berna 2015; Sevarino 2018).

Geriatric Refer to adult dosing. Initiate therapy at low end of dosing range; titrate dose cautiously to lowest dose that provides adequate pain relief with acceptable side effects.

Renal Impairment: Adult

Mild or moderate impairment: Reduce dose to 33% to 50% of the usual starting dose; titrate cautiously; consider use of alternative treatments without naloxone in patients with severe renal impairment.

Severe impairment: Use is contraindicated.

Hepatic Impairment: Adult

Mild impairment: Initial: Reduce dose to 33% to 50% of the usual starting dose; titrate cautiously.

Moderate to severe impairment: Use is contraindicated.

Mechanism of Action

Oxycodone: Binds to opiate receptors in the CNS, causing inhibition of ascending pain pathways, altering the perception of and response to pain; produces generalized CNS depression; also binds to opiate receptors in peripheral organs including the gut to induce constipation.

Naloxone: Pure opioid antagonist that competes and displaces opioids at opioid receptor sites, including gut opioid receptors, which counteracts opioid-induced constipation.

Note: Compared to controlled release oxycodone, improved bowel function and similar efficacy in terms of pain relief have been observed with a controlled release formulation of oxycodone/naloxone (Ahmedzai 2012; Löwenstein 2010; Vondrackova 2008).

Contraindications

Hypersensitivity (eg, anaphylaxis) to oxycodone, naloxone, or any component of the formulation, hypersensitivity to other opioids; moderate to severe hepatic impairment (Child-Pugh classes B and C); severe renal impairment; known or suspected GI obstruction or any disease that affects bowel transit; suspected surgical abdomen (eg, acute appendicitis or pancreatitis); mild, intermittent, or short duration pain that can be managed with other pain medications; management of acute pain, including use in outpatient or day surgeries; management of perioperative pain; acute or severe bronchial asthma, chronic obstructive airway or status asthmaticus; acute respiratory depression; cor pulmonale; hypercapnia; acute alcoholism, delirium tremens, and convulsive disorders; severe CNS depression, increased cerebrospinal or intracranial pressure, and head injury; concurrent use or use within 14 days of MAOIs; opioid-dependent patients and for opioid withdrawal treatment; use in women who are breastfeeding, pregnant, or during labor and delivery; rectal administration

Documentation of allergenic cross-reactivity for opioids is limited. However, because of similarities in chemical structure and/or pharmacologic actions, the possibility of cross-sensitivity cannot be ruled out with certainty.

Warnings/Precautions **[Canadian Boxed Warning]: Due to the risks of addiction, abuse, and misuse with opioids, even at recommended doses, and because of the greater risks of overdose and death with controlled release opioid formulations, oxycodone/naloxone ER should only be used in patients for whom alternative treatment options (eg, nonopioid analgesics) are ineffective, not tolerated, or would otherwise be inadequate to provide appropriate pain management.** Not indicated as an as-needed analgesic; should not be used to treat nonopioid related constipation or for the management of addictive disorders. Patients with a history of addiction to drugs or alcohol may be at increased risk of addiction to oxycodone/naloxone ER. **Rectal administration is contraindicated due to the possible increased systemic availability of naloxone by this route and potential for occurrence of severe withdrawal effects.**

[Canadian Boxed Warning]: Serious, life-threatening, or fatal respiratory depression may occur with use of oxycodone/naloxone ER. Monitor closely for respiratory depression, especially during initiation of therapy or following a dose increase. Tablets must be swallowed whole; tablets that are broken, crushed, chewed, or dissolved may result in a rapid release and absorption of a potentially fatal dose of oxycodone. Patients should be instructed that opioid use is associated with hazards, including fatal overdose. In cases where pain suddenly subsides, respiratory depressant effects may rapidly become manifest. Careful dose titration is necessary to reduce the risk of respiratory depression. Limit use of oxycodone/naloxone 40 mg/20 mg tablets to patients with established tolerance to an opioid of comparable potency **(single doses >40 mg or daily doses >80 mg of oxycodone may cause fatal respiratory depression in patients who are not tolerant to the respiratory depressant effects of opioids).** Carbon dioxide retention from opioid-induced respiratory depression can exacerbate the sedating effects of opioids. Rare, but potentially life-threatening, serotonin syndrome has occurred with serotonergic agents (eg, SSRIs, SNRIs), particularly when used in combination with other serotonergic agents. Do not use in combination with MAOIs or serotonin precursors (eg, l-tryptophan, oxitriptan); use with caution in combination with other serotonergic agents (eg, triptans, TCAs, lithium, tramadol, St. John's wort). Discontinue treatment immediately if signs/symptoms arise. Use is contraindicated in patients with acute or severe bronchial asthma, chronic obstructive pulmonary disease, cor pulmonale, hypercapnia, or acute respiratory depression.

[Canadian Boxed Warning]: Accidental ingestion of even one dose of oxycodone/naloxone ER, especially in children, can result in a fatal overdose of oxycodone.

[Canadian Boxed Warning]: Use exposes patients and other users to the risks of opioid addiction, abuse, and misuse, which can lead to overdose and death. Assess each patient's risk prior to prescribing oxycodone/naloxone ER, and monitor all patients regularly for the development of these behaviors or conditions. Store securely to avoid theft or misuse. Tolerance, psychological, and physical dependence may occur with prolonged use. If abused parenterally, excipients in the tablet (eg, talc) may cause local tissue necrosis, infection, pulmonary granulomas, and increased risk of endocarditis and valvular heart injury. Marked withdrawal symptoms may occur if abused parenterally, intranasally, or rectally by those dependent on opioid agonists. Use with caution in patients with a history of drug or ethanol abuse, or with mental illness (eg, major depression); potential for drug dependency exists. Tolerance, psychological, and physical dependence may occur with prolonged use. Other factors associated with increased risk include younger age and psychotropic medication use. Consider offering naloxone prescriptions in patients with factors associated with an increased risk for overdose, such as history of overdose or substance use disorder, higher opioid dosages (≥50 morphine milligram equivalents/day orally), and concomitant benzodiazepine use (Dowell [CDC 2016]).

Chronic pain: Opioids should **not** be used as first-line therapy for chronic pain management (pain >3-month duration or beyond time of normal tissue healing) due to limited short-term benefits, undetermined long-term benefits, and association with serious risks (eg, overdose, MI, auto accidents, risk of developing opioid use disorder). Preferred management includes nonpharmacologic therapy and nonopioid therapy (eg, NSAIDs, acetaminophen, certain anticonvulsants and antidepressants). If opioid therapy is initiated, it should be combined with nonpharmacologic and nonopioid therapy, as appropriate. Prior to initiation, known risks of opioid therapy should be discussed and realistic treatment goals for pain/function should be established, including consideration for discontinuation if benefits do not outweigh risks. Therapy should be continued only if clinically meaningful improvement in pain/function outweighs risks. Therapy should be initiated at the lowest effective dosage using immediate-release opioids (instead of extended-release/long-acting opioids). Risk associated with use increases with higher opioid dosages. Risks and benefits should be re-evaluated when increasing dosage to ≥50 morphine milligram equivalents (MME)/day orally; dosages ≥90 MME/day orally should be avoided unless carefully justified (Dowell [CDC 2016]).

[Canadian Boxed Warning]: Prolonged use of opioids during pregnancy can result in neonatal opioid withdrawal syndrome, which may be life-threatening. Signs and symptoms include irritability, hyperactivity and abnormal sleep pattern, high pitched cry, tremor, vomiting, diarrhea and failure to gain weight. Onset, duration and severity depend on the drug used, duration of use, maternal dose, and rate of drug elimination by the newborn.

May cause CNS depression, which may impair physical or mental abilities; patients must be cautioned about performing tasks which require mental alertness (eg, operating machinery or driving). Avoid ethanol during therapy; may enhance CNS depression. Use is contraindicated in patients with severe CNS depression, head injury, or elevated cerebrospinal or intracranial pressure (ICP). Use is contraindicated in patients with convulsive disorders.

May cause severe hypotension (including orthostatic hypotension and syncope); use with caution in patients with hypovolemia, cardiovascular disease (including acute MI), or drugs which may exaggerate hypotensive effects (including phenothiazines or general anesthetics). Monitor for symptoms of hypotension following initiation or dose titration; dose adjustment may be warranted. Avoid use in patients with circulatory shock; vasodilatory effects of oxycodone may further reduce cardiac output and worsen hypotension.

Use opioids with caution for chronic pain in patients with mental health conditions (eg, depression, anxiety disorders, post-traumatic stress disorder) due to increased risk for opioid use disorder and overdose; more frequent monitoring is recommended (Dowell [CDC 2016]). Adrenocortical insufficiency has been reported with opioid use; usually occurs with use >1 month. Use with caution in patients with preexisting cardiovascular disease, adrenal insufficiency (including Addison disease), biliary tract dysfunction, acute pancreatitis, prostatic hyperplasia and/or urinary stricture, thyroid dysfunction, and toxic psychosis. Use opioids with caution for chronic pain and titrate dosage cautiously in patients with risk factors for sleep-disordered breathing, including HF and obesity. Avoid opioids in patients with moderate to severe sleep-disordered breathing (Dowell [CDC 2016]). Use with caution in cachectic, debilitated patients and in the elderly; consider the use of alternative nonopioid analgesics in these patients. Use opioids for chronic pain with caution in older adults; monitor closely due to an increased potential for risks, including certain risks such as falls/fracture, cognitive impairment, and constipation. Clearance may also be reduced in older adults (with or without renal impairment) resulting in a narrow therapeutic window and increasing the risk for respiratory depression or overdose (Dowell [CDC 2016]).

Use with caution in patients with mild hepatic impairment; use is contraindicated with moderate to severe hepatic impairment. Use with caution in patients with renal impairment; use is contraindicated in severe renal impairment. Not indicated in patients with cancer associated with peritoneal carcinomatosis; has not been studied. Oxycodone may cause constipation which may be problematic in patients with unstable angina and patients post-myocardial infarction. Consider preventive measures (eg, stool softener, increased fiber) to reduce the potential for constipation. Naloxone may cause diarrhea; patients should be instructed to report severe or persistent diarrhea lasting >3 days.

Use is contraindicated for perioperative use (ie, within 24 hours before or after procedure). Patients interrupting therapy to undergo pain-relieving procedures (eg, chordotomy) may require a dosage adjustment when resuming therapy after the postoperative recovery period.

An opioid-containing analgesic regimen should be tailored to each patient's needs and based upon the type of pain being treated (acute versus chronic), the route of administration, degree of tolerance for opioids (naive versus chronic user), age, weight, and medical condition. The optimal analgesic dose varies widely among patients; doses should be titrated to pain relief/prevention. Hyperalgesia may occur rarely with high doses of oxycodone; dose reduction or alternative opioid may be necessary. Concurrent use of agonist/antagonist (eg, pentazocine, nalbuphine, butorphanol) or partial agonist (eg, buprenorphine) analgesics may precipitate withdrawal symptoms and/or reduced analgesic efficacy in patients following prolonged therapy with mu opioid agonists. Taper dose gradually when discontinuing. Potentially significant drug-drug interactions may exist requiring dose or frequency adjustment, additional monitoring, and/or selection of alternative therapy. **[Canadian Boxed Warning]: Avoid concomitant use of alcohol with oxycodone/naloxone ER as it may result in dangerous addictive effects, resulting in serious injury or death.** Patients should be instructed not to consume alcohol during treatment. **[Canadian Boxed Warning]: Concomitant use of opioids with benzodiazepines or other CNS depressants may result in profound sedation, respiratory depression, coma, and death. Reserve concomitant prescribing of oxycodone/naloxone ER and benzodiazepines or other CNS depressants for use in patients for whom alternative treatment options are inadequate. Limit dosage and durations to the minimum required and follow patients for signs and symptoms of respiratory depression and sedation.**

Drug Interactions

Metabolism/Transport Effects Refer to individual components.

Avoid Concomitant Use

Avoid concomitant use of Oxycodone and Naloxone with any of the following: Abametapir; Azelastine (Nasal); Bromperidol; Conivaptan; Eluxadoline; Fusidic Acid (Systemic); Idelalisib; Methylnaltrexone; Monoamine Oxidase Inhibitors; Naldemedine; Naloxegol; Opioids (Mixed Agonist / Antagonist); Orphenadrine; Oxomemazine; Paraldehyde; Thalidomide

Increased Effect/Toxicity

Oxycodone and Naloxone may increase the levels/effects of: Alvimopan; Azelastine (Nasal); Blonanserin; Desmopressin; Diuretics; Eluxadoline; Flunitrazepam; Methotrimeprazine; MetyroSINE; Monoamine Oxidase Inhibitors; Naldemedine; Naloxegol; Orphenadrine; Paraldehyde; Piribedil; Pramipexole; Ramosetron; ROPINIRole; Rotigotine; Serotonergic Agents (High Risk); Suvorexant; Thalidomide; Zolpidem

The levels/effects of Oxycodone and Naloxone may be increased by: Abametapir; Alizapride; Amphetamines; Anticholinergic Agents; Aprepitant; Brimonidine (Topical); Bromopride; Bromperidol; Cannabidiol; Cannabis; Chlormethiazole; Chlorphenesin Carbamate; Clofazimine; CNS Depressants; Conivaptan; CYP3A4 Inhibitors (Moderate); CYP3A4 Inhibitors (Strong); Dimethindene (Topical); Dronabinol; Droperidol; Duvelisib; Erdafitinib; Fosaprepitant; Fosnetupitant; Fusidic Acid (Systemic); Idelalisib; Kava Kava; Larotrectinib; Lemborexant; Lisuride; Lofexidine; Magnesium Sulfate; Methotrimeprazine; Methylnaltrexone; Metoclopramide; MiFEPRIStone; Minocycline (Systemic); Nabilone; Netupitant; Oxomemazine; Palbociclib; Perampanel; PHENobarbital; Primidone; Rufinamide; Simeprevir; Sodium Oxybate; Stiripentol; Succinylcholine; Tetrahydrocannabinol; Tetrahydrocannabinol and Cannabidiol; Voriconazole

Decreased Effect

Oxycodone and Naloxone may decrease the levels/effects of: Diuretics; Gastrointestinal Agents (Prokinetic); Pegvisomant; Sincalide

The levels/effects of Oxycodone and Naloxone may be decreased by: CYP3A4 Inducers (Moderate); CYP3A4 Inducers (Strong); Dabrafenib; Deferasirox; Enzalutamide; Erdafitinib; Ivosidenib; Mitotane; Nalmefene; Naltrexone; Opioids (Mixed Agonist / Antagonist); PHENobarbital; Primidone; RifAMPin; Sarilumab; Siltuximab; St John's Wort; Tocilizumab

Pharmacodynamics/Kinetics

Duration of Action Oxycodone (controlled release): ≤12 hours

Half-life Elimination Oxycodone (controlled release): 4.5 hours (Oxycontin US product labeling 2016)

Time to Peak Oxycodone (controlled release): Plasma: ~4 to 5 hours (Oxycontin US product labeling 2016)

Reproductive Considerations

Long-term opioid use may cause secondary hypogonadism, which may lead to sexual dysfunction or infertility in men and women (Brennan 2013).

Pregnancy Considerations

Use is contraindicated during pregnancy and during labor and delivery.

[Canadian Boxed Warning]: Infants exposed to oxycodone in utero are at risk of life-threatening respiratory depression. Prolonged maternal use of opioids during pregnancy can cause neonatal withdrawal syndrome in the newborn which may be life-threatening.

Refer to individual monographs for additional information.

Breastfeeding Considerations

Use is contraindicated in breastfeeding women.

Oxycodone is present in breast milk; it is not known if naloxone is excreted in breast milk. **[Canadian Boxed Warning]: Infants exposed to oxycodone through breast milk are at risk of life-threatening respiratory depression.**

Refer to individual monographs for additional information.

Controlled Substance CDSA-I

Dosage Forms: Canada

Tablet Extended Release 12 Hour, Oral:

Targin: Oxycodone 10 mg and naloxone 5 mg, Oxycodone 20 mg and naloxone 10 mg, Oxycodone 40 mg and naloxone 20 mg, Oxycodone 5 mg and naloxone 2.5 mg

◆ **Oxycodone HCl** *see* OxyCODONE *on page 1157*

◆ **Oxycodone HCl/Acetaminophen** *see* Oxycodone and Acetaminophen *on page 1164*

◆ **Oxycodone Hydrochloride** *see* OxyCODONE *on page 1157*

◆ **Oxycodone Hydrochloride and Naloxone Hydrochloride** *see* Oxycodone and Naloxone *on page 1169*

◆ **OxyCONTIN** *see* OxyCODONE *on page 1157*

Oxymetazoline (Nasal) (oks i met AZ oh leen)

Related Information

Bacterial Infections *on page 1739*

Related Sample Prescriptions

Sinus Infection Treatment - Sample Prescriptions *on page 41*

Brand Names: US 12 Hour Decongestant [OTC]; 12 Hour Nasal Decongestant [OTC]; 12 Hour Nasal Relief Spray [OTC]; 12 Hour Nasal Spray [OTC]; Afrin 12 Hour [OTC]; Afrin Menthol Spray [OTC]; Afrin Nasal Spray [OTC]; Afrin NoDrip Extra Moisture [OTC]; Afrin NoDrip Original [OTC]; Afrin NoDrip Sinus [OTC]; Afrin Sinus [OTC]; Dristan Spray [OTC]; Long Lasting Nasal Spray [OTC]; Mucinex Nasal Spray Full Force [OTC] [DSC]; Mucinex Nasal Spray Moisture [OTC] [DSC]; Mucinex Sinus-Max Clear & Cool [OTC]; Mucinex Sinus-Max Full Force [OTC] [DSC]; Mucinex Sinus-Max Sinus/Allrgy [OTC]; Nasal Decongestant Spray [OTC]; Nasal Spray 12 Hour [OTC]; Nasal Spray Max Strength [OTC]; Neo-Synephrine 12 Hour Spray [OTC] [DSC]; NRS Nasal Relief [OTC] [DSC]; QlearQuil [OTC]; Sinus Nasal Spray [OTC]; Vicks Sinex 12 Hour Decongest [OTC]; Vicks Sinex Moisturizing [OTC]; Vicks Sinex Severe Decongest [OTC]; Vicks Sinex [OTC] [DSC]

Generic Availability (US) Yes

Pharmacologic Category Adrenergic Agonist Agent; Decongestant; Imidazoline Derivative

Use Nasal congestion: Temporary relief of nasal congestion (due to a cold, hay fever, or other upper respiratory allergies) and sinus congestion/pressure.

Local Anesthetic/Vasoconstrictor Precautions No information available to require special precautions

Effects on Dental Treatment No significant effects or complications reported

Effects on Bleeding No information available to require special precautions

Adverse Reactions Frequency not defined.

Respiratory: Dry nose, nasal congestion (rebound; chronic use), nasal mucosa irritation (temporary), sneezing

Dosing

Adult & Geriatric Nasal congestion: Intranasal: Instill 2 to 3 sprays into each nostril twice daily for ≤3 days (maximum dose: 2 doses/24 hours)

Renal Impairment: Adult There are no dosage adjustments provided in manufacturer's labeling.

Hepatic Impairment: Adult There are no dosage adjustments provided in manufacturer's labeling.

Pediatric Nasal congestion: Children ≥6 years and Adolescents: 0.05% solution: Intranasal: Instill 2 to 3 sprays into each nostril twice daily; doses should be separated by 10 to 12 hours; maximum daily dose: 2 doses/24 hours; therapy should not exceed 3 days. **Note:** Intranasal not recommended for use in children <6 years of age (especially in infants) due to CNS depression.

Renal Impairment: Pediatric There are no dosage adjustments provided in manufacturer's labeling.

Hepatic Impairment: Pediatric There are no dosage adjustments provided in manufacturer's labeling.

Mechanism of Action Stimulates alpha-adrenergic receptors in the arterioles of the nasal mucosa to produce vasoconstriction

Contraindications

OTC labeling: When used for self-medication, do not use for more than 3 days.

Documentation of allergenic cross-reactivity for ophthalmic sympathomimetics is limited. However, because of similarities in chemical structure and/or pharmacologic actions, the possibility of cross-sensitivity cannot be ruled out with certainty.

Warnings/Precautions Frequent or prolonged use may cause nasal congestion to recur or worsen Use with caution in the presence of hypertension, diabetes, hyperthyroidism, heart disease, or benign prostatic hyperplasia/urinary obstruction. Temporary discomfort such as burning, stinging, sneezing, or an increased nasal discharge may occur.

Accidental ingestion by children of over-the-counter (OTC) imidazoline-derivative eye drops and nasal sprays may result in serious harm. Serious adverse reactions (eg, coma, bradycardia, respiratory depression, sedation) requiring hospitalization have been reported in children ≤5 years of age who had ingested even small amounts (eg, 1 to 2 mL). Contact a poison control center and seek emergency medical care immediately for accidental ingestion (FDA Drug Safety Communication 2012).

Benzyl alcohol and derivatives: Some dosage forms may contain benzyl alcohol; large amounts of benzyl alcohol (≥99 mg/kg/day) have been associated with a potentially fatal toxicity ("gasping syndrome") in neonates; the "gasping syndrome" consists of metabolic acidosis, respiratory distress, gasping respirations, CNS dysfunction (including convulsions, intracranial hemorrhage), hypotension, and cardiovascular collapse (AAP ["Inactive" 1997]; CDC 1982); some data suggests that benzoate displaces bilirubin from protein binding sites (Ahlfors 2001); avoid or use dosage forms containing benzyl alcohol with caution in neonates. See manufacturer's labeling.

Some dosage forms may contain polysorbate 80 (also known as Tweens). Hypersensitivity reactions, usually a delayed reaction, have been reported following exposure to pharmaceutical products containing polysorbate 80 in certain individuals (Isaksson 2002; Lucente 2000; Shelley 1995). Thrombocytopenia, ascites, pulmonary deterioration, and renal and hepatic failure have been reported in premature neonates after receiving parenteral products containing polysorbate 80 (Alade 1986; CDC 1984). See manufacturer's labeling.

Potentially significant interactions may exist, requiring dose or frequency adjustment, additional monitoring, and/or selection of alternative therapy.

Warnings: Additional Pediatric Considerations

Some dosage forms may contain propylene glycol; in neonates large amounts of propylene glycol delivered orally, intravenously (eg, >3,000 mg/day), or topically have been associated with potentially fatal toxicities which can include metabolic acidosis, seizures, renal failure, and CNS depression; toxicities have also been reported in children and adults including hyperosmolality, lactic acidosis, seizures, and respiratory depression; use caution (AAP 1997; Shehab 2009).

Drug Interactions

Metabolism/Transport Effects None known.

Avoid Concomitant Use

Avoid concomitant use of Oxymetazoline (Nasal) with any of the following: Ergot Derivatives; Iobenguane Radiopharmaceutical Products; Monoamine Oxidase Inhibitors

Increased Effect/Toxicity

Oxymetazoline (Nasal) may increase the levels/effects of: Doxofylline; Solriamfetol; Sympathomimetics

The levels/effects of Oxymetazoline (Nasal) may be increased by: AtoMOXetine; Cannabinoid-Containing Products; Cocaine (Topical); Ergot Derivatives; Guanethidine; Linezolid; Monoamine Oxidase Inhibitors; Ozanimod; Procarbazine; Tedizolid; Tricyclic Antidepressants

Decreased Effect

Oxymetazoline (Nasal) may decrease the levels/effects of: Esketamine; FentaNYL; Iobenguane Radiopharmaceutical Products

The levels/effects of Oxymetazoline (Nasal) may be decreased by: Alpha1-Blockers; Tricyclic Antidepressants

Pharmacodynamics/Kinetics

Onset of Action Within 10 minutes (Chua 1989)

Duration of Action Up to 12 hours (Chua 1989)

Pregnancy Considerations

Adverse fetal/neonatal events have been noted in case reports following large doses or extended use of oxymetazoline nasal spray in the first trimester of pregnancy (Baxi 1985; Holm 1985; Menezes 2016). Fetal blood flow was not found to be affected by a one-time dose of oxymetazoline in noncomplicated, third trimester pregnancies (Rayburn 1990).

Decongestants are not recommended for the treatment of rhinitis during pregnancy (BSACI [Scadding 2017]). Use of oxymetazoline nasal spray can be considered if acute relief is needed (Mazzotta 1999).

Breastfeeding Considerations

If a decongestant is needed, nasal preparations may be preferred over systemic agents in nursing women (Anderson 2000).

Dosage Forms: US

Solution, Nasal:

12 Hour Decongestant [OTC]: 0.05% (30 mL)
12 Hour Nasal Decongestant [OTC]: 0.05% (30 mL)
12 Hour Nasal Relief Spray [OTC]: 0.05% (30 mL)
12 Hour Nasal Spray [OTC]: 0.05% (30 mL)
Afrin 12 Hour [OTC]: 0.05% (30 mL)
Afrin Menthol Spray [OTC]: 0.05% (15 mL)
Afrin Nasal Spray [OTC]: 0.05% (20 mL)
Afrin NoDrip Extra Moisture [OTC]: 0.05% (15 mL)
Afrin NoDrip Original [OTC]: 0.05% (15 mL)
Afrin NoDrip Sinus [OTC]: 0.05% (15 mL)
Afrin Sinus [OTC]: 0.05% (15 mL)
Dristan Spray [OTC]: 0.05% (15 mL)
Long Lasting Nasal Spray [OTC]: 0.05% (30 mL)
Mucinex Sinus-Max Clear & Cool [OTC]: 0.05% (22 mL)
Mucinex Sinus-Max Sinus/Allrgy [OTC]: 0.05% (22 mL)
Nasal Decongestant Spray [OTC]: 0.05% (15 mL, 30 mL)
Nasal Spray 12 Hour [OTC]: 0.05% (30 mL)
Nasal Spray Max Strength [OTC]: 0.05% (30 mL)
QlearQuil [OTC]: 0.05% (15 mL)
Sinus Nasal Spray [OTC]: 0.05% (30 mL)
Vicks Sinex 12 Hour Decongest [OTC]: 0.05% (15 mL)
Vicks Sinex Moisturizing [OTC]: 0.05% (15 mL)
Vicks Sinex Severe Decongest [OTC]: 0.05% (15 mL)
Generic: 0.05% (30 mL)

Oxymetazoline (Topical) (oks i met AZ oh leen)

Brand Names: US Rhofade

Pharmacologic Category Adrenergic Agonist Agent; Imidazoline Derivative

Use Rosacea: Treatment of persistent facial erythema associated with rosacea in adults

Local Anesthetic/Vasoconstrictor Precautions
No information available to require special precautions

Effects on Dental Treatment No significant effects or complications reported

Effects on Bleeding No information available to require special precautions

Adverse Reactions

1% to 10%:

Dermatologic: Exacerbation of acne rosacea (1%)
Local: Application site dermatitis (2%), application site erythema (1%), application site pain (1%)

Mechanism of Action Relatively selective $alpha_{1A}$-receptor agonist that when applied topically may decrease erythema through direct vasoconstriction.

Pregnancy Considerations Information related to topical use of oxymetazoline in pregnacy is limited. During clinical trials, two pregnancies were reported, resulting in one healthy baby and one spontaneous abortion (not considered related to treatment). Most available information is related to maternal use following nasal inhalation (see the oxymetazoline nasal monograph for additional information).

◆ **Oxymetazoline and Tetracaine** *see* Tetracaine and Oxymetazoline *on page 1429*

◆ **Oxymetazoline HCl** *see* Oxymetazoline (Nasal) *on page 1173*

◆ **Oxymetazoline Hydrochloride** *see* Oxymetazoline (Nasal) *on page 1173*

◆ **Oxymetazoline Hydrochloride** *see* Oxymetazoline (Topical) *on page 1175*

Oxymetholone (oks i METH oh lone)

Brand Names: US Anadrol-50

Pharmacologic Category Anabolic Steroid

Use Anemia: Treatment of anemias caused by deficient red cell production. **Note:** Androgen therapy (eg, oxymetholone) is generally not appropriate for the treatment of anemias except in certain rare situations (eg, Fanconi anemia).

Local Anesthetic/Vasoconstrictor Precautions
No information available to require special precautions

Effects on Dental Treatment No significant effects or complications reported

Effects on Bleeding No information available to require special precautions

Adverse Reactions

Frequency not defined:

Cardiovascular: Coronary artery disease, peripheral edema
Central nervous system: Chills, deepening of the voice (females), excitement, insomnia
Dermatologic: Acne vulgaris, androgenetic alopecia (postpubertal males, females), hyperpigmentation
Endocrine & metabolic: Amenorrhea, change in libido (decreased/increased), decreased glucose tolerance, decreased HDL cholesterol, gynecomastia, hirsutism (women), hypercalcemia, hyperchloremia, hyperkalemia, hypernatremia, hyperphosphatemia, increased LDL cholesterol, menstrual disease
Gastrointestinal: Diarrhea, nausea, vomiting
Genitourinary: Benign prostatic hypertrophy (elderly males), clitoromegaly, decreased ejaculate volume, epididymitis, erectile dysfunction (increased erections; prepubertal males), impotence, irritable bladder, oligospermia, phallic enlargement, priapism, testicular atrophy, testicular disease, virilization (females)
Hematologic & oncologic: Clotting factors suppression (II, V, VII, X), hemorrhage, increased INR, iron deficiency anemia, leukemia, malignant neoplasm of prostate, prolonged prothrombin time
Hepatic: Cholestatic hepatitis, cholestatic jaundice, hepatic failure, hepatic necrosis, hepatocellular neoplasm (including carcinoma), increased serum alkaline phosphatase, increased serum bilirubin, increased serum transaminases, peliosis hepatitis
Neuromuscular & skeletal: Increased creatine phosphokinase, premature epiphyseal closure (children)
Renal: Increased serum creatinine
Respiratory: Hoarseness (females)

<1%, postmarketing, and/or case reports: Hepatotoxicity (idiosyncratic; Chalasani 2014)

Mechanism of Action Enhances production of erythropoietin in patients with anemias which are due to bone marrow failure; stimulates erythropoiesis in anemias due to deficient red cell production

Pharmacodynamics/Kinetics

Onset of Action Response is not often immediate; a minimum trial of 3 to 6 months is recommended

Reproductive Considerations

Use is contraindicated in women who may become pregnant.

Oligospermia or amenorrhea may occur resulting in an impairment of fertility.

Pregnancy Risk Factor X

Pregnancy Considerations

Use is contraindicated in women who are pregnant.

Controlled Substance C-III

OxyMORphone (oks i MOR fone)

Related Information

Oral Pain *on page 1734*

Brand Names: US Opana ER [DSC]; Opana [DSC]

Pharmacologic Category Analgesic, Opioid

Use

Pain management:

Parenteral: Management of pain severe enough to require an opioid analgesic and for which alternative treatments are inadequate; obstetrical analgesia; preoperative medication; anesthesia support; relief of anxiety in patients with dyspnea associated with pulmonary edema secondary to acute left ventricular dysfunction.

Oral, immediate release: Management of acute pain severe enough to require an opioid analgesic and for which alternative treatments are inadequate.

Oral, extended release: Management of pain severe enough to require daily, around-the-clock, long-term opioid treatment and for which alternative treatment options are inadequate.

Limitations of use: Reserve oxymorphone for use in patients for whom alternative treatment options (eg, nonopioid analgesics, opioid combination products) are ineffective, not tolerated, or would be otherwise inadequate to provide sufficient pain management. Oxymorphone ER is not indicated as an as-needed analgesic.

Local Anesthetic/Vasoconstrictor Precautions No information available to require special precautions

Effects on Dental Treatment Key adverse event(s) related to dental treatment: Xerostomia (normal salivary flow resumes upon discontinuation). Anticholinergic side effects can cause a reduction of saliva production or secretion, contributing to discomfort and dental disease (ie, caries, oral candidiasis, and periodontal disease).

Effects on Bleeding No information available to require special precautions

Adverse Reactions Incidence usually on higher end with extended release (ER) tablet.

>10%:

Central nervous system: Dizziness (5% to 18%), drowsiness (2% to 17%), headache (3% to 12%)

Dermatologic: Pruritus (3% to 15%)

Gastrointestinal: Nausea (3% to 33%), constipation (4% to 28%), vomiting (9% to 16%)

Miscellaneous: Fever (1% to 14%)

1% to 10%:

Cardiovascular: Edema (oral), flushing, hypertension (oral), hypotension, tachycardia

Central nervous system: Fatigue (4%), insomnia (4%), confusion (3%), anxiety (oral), depression, disorientation (oral), lethargy (oral), nervousness, restlessness

Dermatologic: Diaphoresis

Endocrine & metabolic: Dehydration (oral), weight loss (oral)

Gastrointestinal: Xerostomia (6%), abdominal pain (3%), decreased appetite (oral: 3%), abdominal distention, diarrhea (oral), dyspepsia (oral), flatulence

Neuromuscular & skeletal: Asthenia

Ophthalmic: Blurred vision

Respiratory: Dyspnea, hypoxia

Frequency not defined:

Central nervous system: Agitation, cognitive dysfunction, drug abuse, opioid dependence, sedation

Dermatologic: Allergic dermatitis

Endocrine & metabolic: Adrenocortical insufficiency

Gastrointestinal: Anorexia, biliary colic, paralytic ileus

Genitourinary: Oliguria, ureteral spasm, urinary hesitancy

Local: Injection site reaction

Ophthalmic: Diplopia

Respiratory: Apnea, atelectasis, bronchospasm, laryngeal edema, laryngospasm

<1%, postmarketing, and/or case reports: Anaphylaxis, angioedema, bradycardia, bradypnea, central nervous system depression, choking sensation (tablets), cold and clammy skin, decreased oxygen saturation, dermatitis, difficulty in micturition, dysphagia, dysphoria, euphoria, facial edema, foreign body sensation (tablet stuck in throat), gag reflex (tablets; including regurgitation), hallucination, hand edema, hot flash, hypersensitivity reaction, hypogonadism (Brennan 2013; Debono 2011), impaired consciousness, increased serum prolactin (Molitch 2008; Vuong 2010), intestinal obstruction, lip edema, mental status changes, miosis, mouth edema, orthostatic hypotension, palpitations, periorbital edema, pharyngeal edema, respiratory depression, respiratory distress, skin rash, syncope, tongue edema, urinary retention, urticaria, visual disturbance

Mechanism of Action Oxymorphone is a potent opioid analgesic with uses similar to those of morphine. The drug is a semisynthetic derivative of morphine (phenanthrene derivative) and is closely related to hydromorphone chemically (Dilaudid).

Pharmacodynamics/Kinetics

Onset of Action Parenteral: 5 to 10 minutes

Duration of Action Analgesic: Parenteral: 3 to 6 hours

Half-life Elimination Oral: Immediate release: 7 to 9 hours; Extended release: 9 to 11 hours

Reproductive Considerations

Long-term opioid use may cause secondary hypogonadism, which may lead to sexual dysfunction or infertility in men and women (Brennan 2013).

Pregnancy Considerations Opioids cross the placenta.

According to some studies, maternal use of opioids may be associated with birth defects (including neural tube defects, congenital heart defects, and gastroschisis), poor fetal growth, stillbirth, and preterm delivery (CDC [Dowell 2016]).

[US Boxed Warning]: Prolonged use of oxymorphone during pregnancy can result in neonatal opioid withdrawal syndrome, which may be life-threatening if not recognized and treated, and requires management according to protocols developed by neonatology experts. If opioid use is required for a prolonged period in a pregnant woman, advise the patient of the risk of neonatal opioid withdrawal syndrome and ensure that appropriate treatment will be available. If chronic opioid exposure occurs in pregnancy, adverse events in the newborn (including withdrawal) may occur (Chou 2009). Symptoms of neonatal abstinence syndrome (NAS) following opioid exposure may be autonomic (eg, fever, temperature instability), gastrointestinal (eg, diarrhea, vomiting, poor feeding/weight gain), or neurologic (eg, high-pitched crying, hyperactivity, increased muscle tone, increased wakefulness/abnormal sleep pattern, irritability, sneezing, seizure, tremor, yawning) (Dow 2012; Hudak 2012). Mothers who are physically dependent on opioids may give birth to infants who are also physically dependent. Opioids may cause respiratory depression and psycho-physiologic effects in the neonate; newborns of mothers receiving opioids during labor should be monitored.

Oxymorphone is not commonly used to treat pain during labor and immediately postpartum (ACOG 209 2019) or chronic noncancer pain in pregnant women or those who may become pregnant (CDC [Dowell 2016]; Chou 2009).

Product Availability

Opana ER was withdrawn from the US market as of June 2017; however, generic oxymorphone extended-release tablets remain available.

Opana injection has been discontinued in the United States for more than 1 year.

Controlled Substance C-II

- **Oxymorphone HCl** *see* OxyMORphone *on page 1176*
- **Oxymorphone Hydrochloride** *see* OxyMORphone *on page 1176*

Oxytocin (oks i TOE sin)

Brand Names: US Pitocin

Pharmacologic Category Oxytocic Agent

Use

Antepartum: Induction of labor in patients with a medical indication (eg, Rh problems, maternal diabetes, preeclampsia, at or near term); stimulation or reinforcement of labor (as in selected cases of uterine inertia); adjunctive therapy in management of incomplete or inevitable abortion

Postpartum: To produce uterine contractions during the third stage of labor and to control postpartum bleeding or hemorrhage.

Local Anesthetic/Vasoconstrictor Precautions No information available to require special precautions

Effects on Dental Treatment No significant effects or complications reported

Effects on Bleeding No information available to require special precautions

Adverse Reactions

Frequency not defined:

Cardiovascular: Cardiac arrhythmia, hypertensive crisis, hypotension (Dyer 2011), subarachnoid hemorrhage, tachycardia (Dyer 2011), ventricular premature contractions

Endocrine & metabolic: Water intoxication (severe water intoxication with seizure and coma is associated with a slow oxytocin infusion over 24 hours)

Gastrointestinal: Nausea, vomiting

Genitourinary: Postpartum hemorrhage, uterine rupture

Hematologic & oncologic: Pelvic hematoma

Hypersensitivity: Anaphylaxis

Mechanism of Action Oxytocin stimulates uterine contraction by activating G-protein-coupled receptors that trigger increases in intracellular calcium levels in uterine myofibrils. Oxytocin also increases local prostaglandin production, further stimulating uterine contraction.

Pharmacodynamics/Kinetics

Onset of Action Uterine contractions: IM: 3 to 5 minutes; IV: ~1 minute

Duration of Action IM: 2 to 3 hours; IV: 1 hour

Half-life Elimination 1 to 6 minutes; decreased in late pregnancy and during lactation

Pregnancy Considerations

[US Boxed Warning]: To be used for medical rather than elective induction of labor.

Small amounts of exogenous oxytocin are expected to reach the fetal circulation. When used as indicated, teratogenic effects would not be expected. Nonteratogenic adverse reactions are reported in the neonate as well as the mother.

- **Oxytrol** *see* Oxybutynin *on page 1156*
- **Oxytrol For Women [OTC]** *see* Oxybutynin *on page 1156*
- **Oysco D [OTC] [DSC]** *see* Calcium and Vitamin D *on page 280*
- **Oysco 500+D [OTC]** *see* Calcium and Vitamin D *on page 280*

Ozanimod (oh ZAN i mod)

Brand Names: US Zeposia 7-Day Starter Pack; Zeposia Starter Kit

Pharmacologic Category Sphingosine 1-Phosphate (S1P) Receptor Modulator

Use Multiple sclerosis, relapsing: Treatment of relapsing forms of multiple sclerosis, including clinically isolated syndrome, relapsing-remitting disease, and active secondary progressive disease, in adults.

Local Anesthetic/Vasoconstrictor Precautions No information available to require special precautions.

Effects on Dental Treatment Key adverse event(s) related to dental treatment: Patients may experience orthostatic hypotension as they stand up after treatment, especially if lying in dental chair for extended periods of time. Use caution with sudden changes in position during and after dental treatment.

Effects on Bleeding No information available to require special precautions.

Adverse Reactions

>10%:

Infection: Infection (35%; serious: 1%)

Respiratory: Upper respiratory tract infection (26%)

1% to 10%:

Cardiovascular: Hypertension (4%), orthostatic hypotension (4%)

Gastrointestinal: Upper abdominal pain (2%)

Genitourinary: Urinary tract infection (4%)

Hematologic & oncologic: Lymphocytopenia (3%)

Hepatic: Increased serum alanine aminotransferase (3 x ULN: 6%; 5 x ULN: 2%), increased serum transaminases (10%)

Neuromuscular & skeletal: Back pain (4%)

<1%:

Cardiovascular: Bradycardia, hypertensive crisis

Infection: Herpes zoster infection

Ophthalmic: Macular edema (increased risk in patients with a history of uveitis or diabetes mellitus)

Nervous system: Reversible posterior leukoencephalopathy syndrome

Frequency not defined:

Hematologic & oncologic: Basal cell carcinoma of skin, malignant melanoma, malignant neoplasm (including seminoma), malignant neoplasm of breast

Hypersensitivity: Hypersensitivity reaction

Respiratory: Decrease in forced vital capacity, reduced forced expiratory volume

Mechanism of Action Ozanimod has a high affinity to sphingosine 1-phosphate receptors 1 and 5. Ozanimod blocks the lymphocytes' ability to emerge from lymph nodes; therefore, the amount of lymphocytes available to the CNS is decreased.

Pharmacodynamics/Kinetics

Half-life Elimination Ozanimod: ~21 hours; CC112273 and CC1084037 (active metabolites): 11 days.

Time to Peak ~6 to 8 hours.

Reproductive Considerations Evaluate pregnancy status prior to use in females of reproductive potential. Elimination of ozanimod takes ~3 months; to avoid potential fetal harm, females of childbearing potential should use effective contraception to avoid pregnancy during therapy and for 3 months after discontinuing treatment.

In general, disease-modifying therapies for multiple sclerosis (MS) are stopped prior to a planned pregnancy except in females at high risk of MS activity (AAN [Rae-Grant 2018]). Consider use other agents in females at high risk of disease reactivation who are planning a pregnancy. Delaying pregnancy is recommended for females with persistent high disease activity; when disease-modifying therapy is needed in these patients, other agents are preferred (ECTRIMS/EAN [Montalban 2018]).

Pregnancy Considerations Based on data from animal reproduction studies, in utero exposure to ozanimod may cause fetal harm.

In general, disease-modifying therapies for multiple sclerosis (MS) are not initiated during pregnancy, except in females at high risk of MS activity (AAN [Rae-Grant 2018]). When disease-modifying therapy is needed in these patients, other agents are preferred (ECTRIMS/EAN [Montalban 2018]).

◆ **Ozanimod hydrochloride** *see* Ozanimod *on page 1177*

◆ **Ozempic (0.25 or 0.5 MG/DOSE)** *see* Semaglutide *on page 1366*

◆ **Ozempic (1 MG/DOSE)** *see* Semaglutide *on page 1366*

Ozenoxacin (oz en OX a sin)

Brand Names: US Xepi

Brand Names: Canada Ozanex

Pharmacologic Category Antibiotic, Quinolone; Antibiotic, Topical

Use Impetigo: Treatment of impetigo due to *Staphylococcus aureus* or *Streptococcus pyogenes* in adult and pediatric patients ≥2 months of age

Local Anesthetic/Vasoconstrictor Precautions No information available to require special precautions

Effects on Dental Treatment No significant effects or complications reported

Effects on Bleeding No information available to require special precautions

Adverse Reactions <1%, postmarketing, and/or case reports: Rosacea-like face eruption, seborrheic dermatitis

Mechanism of Action Ozenoxacin is a quinolone antimicrobial that inhibits the bacterial DNA replication enzymes, DNA gyrase A, and topoisomerase IV.

Pregnancy Considerations Systemic absorption following topical application is negligible; exposure to the fetus is not expected.

◆ **Ozobax** *see* Baclofen *on page 213*

◆ **P01BE03** *see* Artesunate *on page 169*

◆ **P-071** *see* Cetirizine (Systemic) *on page 328*

◆ **PA-824** *see* Pretomanid *on page 1273*

◆ **Pacerone** *see* Amiodarone *on page 118*

PACLitaxel (Conventional)

(pac li TAKS el con VEN sha nal)

Brand Names: Canada APO-Paclitaxel

Pharmacologic Category Antineoplastic Agent, Antimicrotubular; Antineoplastic Agent, Taxane Derivative

Use

Breast cancer: Adjuvant treatment of node-positive breast cancer; treatment of metastatic breast cancer after failure of combination chemotherapy or relapse within 6 months of adjuvant chemotherapy (prior therapy should have included an anthracycline)

Kaposi sarcoma (AIDS-related): Second-line treatment of AIDS-related Kaposi sarcoma

Non-small cell lung cancer: First-line treatment of non-small cell lung cancer (in combination with cisplatin) in patients who are not candidates for potentially curative surgery and/or radiation therapy

Ovarian cancer: Subsequent therapy for treatment of advanced ovarian cancer; first-line therapy of ovarian cancer (in combination with cisplatin)

Local Anesthetic/Vasoconstrictor Precautions
No information available to require special precautions

Effects on Dental Treatment Key adverse event(s) related to dental treatment: Severe, potentially dose-limiting mucositis and stomatitis.

Effects on Bleeding Chemotherapy may result in significant myelosuppression, potentially including significant reduction in platelet counts (thrombocytopenia grades 3/4: 1% to 7%) and altered hemostasis. Bleeding in seen in ~14% of patients. In patients who are under active treatment with these agents, medical consult is suggested.

Adverse Reactions

>10%:

Cardiovascular: Flushing (28%), ECG abnormality (14% to 23%), edema (21%), hypotension (4% to 12%)

Dermatologic: Alopecia (87%), skin rash (12%)

Gastrointestinal: Nausea and vomiting (52%), diarrhea (38%), stomatitis (17% to 31%; grade 3/4: ≤3%)

Hematologic & oncologic: Neutropenia (78% to 98%; grade 4: 14% to 75%; median nadir: 11 days), leukopenia (90%; grade 4: 17%), anemia (47% to 90%; grades 3/4: 2% to 16%), thrombocytopenia (4% to 20%; grades 3/4: 1% to 7%), hemorrhage (14%)

Hepatic: Increased serum alkaline phosphatase (22%), increased serum aspartate aminotransferase (19%)

Hypersensitivity: Hypersensitivity reaction (31% to 45%)

Infection: Infection (15% to 30%)

Local: Injection site reaction (13%)

Nervous system: Peripheral neuropathy (42% to 70%; grades 3/4: ≤7%)

Neuromuscular & skeletal: Arthralgia (≤60%), myalgia (≤60%), asthenia (17%)

Miscellaneous: Fever (12%)

1% to 10%:

Cardiovascular: Bradycardia (3%), tachycardia (2%), hypertension (1%), cardiac arrhythmia (≤1%), syncope (≤1%), venous thrombosis (≤1%)

Dermatologic: Changes in nails (2%)

Hematologic & oncologic: Febrile neutropenia (2%)

Hepatic: Increased serum bilirubin (7%)
Hypersensitivity: Anaphylaxis (≤4%), severe hypersensitivity reaction (≤4%)
Respiratory: Dyspnea (2%)

Frequency not defined:
Dermatologic: Skin discoloration at injection site
Gastrointestinal: Abdominal pain, peritonitis
Hypersensitivity: Angioedema
Infection: Sepsis
Local: Erythema at injection site, swelling at injection site, tenderness at injection site
Respiratory: Pneumonia

<1%, postmarketing, and/or case reports: Acute myocardial infarction, anorexia, ascites, ataxia, atrial fibrillation, atrioventricular block, back pain, bigeminy, cardiac conduction disorder, cardiac failure, cellulitis, chills, confusion, conjunctivitis, constipation, dehydration, desquamation, dizziness, encephalopathy, esophagitis, exacerbation of scleroderma, fibrosis at injection site, headache, hearing loss, hepatic encephalopathy, hepatic necrosis, increased lacrimation, increased serum creatinine, induration at injection site, intestinal obstruction, intestinal perforation, interstitial pneumonitis, ischemic colitis, local skin exfoliation, maculopapular rash, malaise, neutropenic enterocolitis, optic nerve damage, ototoxicity, pancreatitis, paralytic ileus, phlebitis, photopsia, pruritus, pulmonary embolism, pulmonary fibrosis, radiation recall phenomenon, radiation pneumonitis, respiratory failure, seizure, shock, skin edema (diffuse), skin necrosis, skin sclerosis, Stevens-Johnson syndrome, subacute cutaneous lupus erythematosus (Sibaud 2016), supraventricular tachycardia, thickening of skin, tinnitus, tonic clonic epilepsy, toxic epidermal necrolysis, ventricular tachycardia (asymptomatic), vertigo, visual disturbance (scintillating scotomata)

Mechanism of Action Paclitaxel promotes microtubule assembly by enhancing the action of tubulin dimers, stabilizing existing microtubules, and inhibiting their disassembly, interfering with the late G_2 mitotic phase, and inhibiting cell replication. In addition, the drug can distort mitotic spindles, resulting in the breakage of chromosomes. Paclitaxel may also suppress cell proliferation and modulate immune response.

Pharmacodynamics/Kinetics

Half-life Elimination

Children: 4.6 to 17 hours (varies with dose and infusion duration)

Adults:

3-hour infusion: Mean (terminal): ~13 to 20 hours
24-hour infusion: Mean (terminal): ~16 to 53 hours

Reproductive Considerations

Females of reproductive potential should be advised to avoid becoming pregnant.

Pregnancy Risk Factor D

Pregnancy Considerations

Adverse events have been observed in animal reproduction. An ex vivo human placenta perfusion model illustrated that paclitaxel crossed the placenta at term. Placental transfer was low and affected by the presence of albumin; higher albumin concentrations resulted in lower paclitaxel placental transfer (Berveiller 2012). Some pharmacokinetic properties of paclitaxel may be altered in pregnant females (van Hasselt 2014).

A pregnancy registry is available for all cancers diagnosed during pregnancy at Cooper Health (877-635-4499).

PACLitaxel (Protein Bound)

(pac li TAKS el PROE teen bownd)

Brand Names: US Abraxane

Brand Names: Canada Abraxane

Pharmacologic Category Antineoplastic Agent, Antimicrotubular; Antineoplastic Agent, Taxane Derivative

Use

Breast cancer, metastatic: Treatment of breast cancer after failure of combination chemotherapy for metastatic disease or relapse within 6 months of adjuvant chemotherapy; prior therapy should have included an anthracycline unless clinically contraindicated.

Non-small cell lung cancer, locally advanced or metastatic: First-line treatment of locally advanced or metastatic non-small cell lung cancer (in combination with carboplatin) in patients who are not candidates for curative surgery or radiation therapy.

Pancreatic adenocarcinoma, metastatic: First-line treatment of metastatic adenocarcinoma of the pancreas (in combination with gemcitabine).

Guideline recommendations:

The American Society of Clinical Oncology (ASCO) guidelines for metastatic pancreatic cancer recommend paclitaxel (protein bound) (in combination with gemcitabine) as first-line therapy in patients with Eastern Cooperative Oncology Group (ECOG) performance status of 0 or 1, a relatively favorable comorbidity profile, a preference for relatively aggressive therapy, and a suitable support system. Paclitaxel (protein bound) (in combination with gemcitabine) may be utilized as second-line therapy in patients who received first-line FOLFIRINOX therapy, have an ECOG performance status of 0 or 1, have a relatively favorable comorbidity profile, a preference for aggressive therapy, and a suitable support system (ASCO [Sohal 2018]).

According to the ASCO guidelines for locally advanced, unresectable pancreatic cancer, induction with at least 6 months of initial systemic therapy (with a combination regimen) is generally recommended in patients with ECOG performance status of 0 or 1, a favorable comorbidity profile, a preference for aggressive therapy, and a suitable support system; there is no clear evidence to encourage one regimen over another. The paclitaxel (protein bound)-gemcitabine combination regimen (recommended in the metastatic setting) has not been evaluated in randomized, controlled studies for locally advanced, unresectable pancreatic cancer, but may be an option in patients with good performance status. If disease progression occurs, treatment according to guidelines for metastatic pancreatic cancer should be offered (ASCO [Balaban 2016]).

Local Anesthetic/Vasoconstrictor Precautions

No information available to require special precautions

Effects on Dental Treatment Key adverse event(s) related to dental treatment: Mucositis.

Effects on Bleeding Chemotherapy may result in significant myelosuppression, potentially including significant reduction in platelet counts (thrombocytopenia grades 3/4: <1%) and altered hemostasis. In patients who are under active treatment with these agents, medical consult is suggested.

Adverse Reactions Frequency may vary based on indication and/or concomitant therapy.

>10%:

Cardiovascular: ECG abnormality (60%; 35% in patients with a normal baseline), peripheral edema (10% to 46%)

Central nervous system: Peripheral sensory neuropathy (71%; grades 3/4: 10%; dose dependent; cumulative), fatigue (25% to 59%), peripheral neuropathy (48% to 54%; grade 3: 3% to 17%), headache (14%), depression (12%)

Dermatologic: Alopecia (50% to 90%), skin rash (10% to 30%)

Endocrine & metabolic: Dehydration (21%), increased gamma-glutamyl transferase (grades 3/4: 14%), hypokalemia (12%)

Gastrointestinal: Nausea (27% to 54%), diarrhea (15% to 44%), decreased appetite (17% to 36%), vomiting (12% to 36%), constipation (16%), dysgeusia (16%)

Genitourinary: Urinary tract infection (11%)

Hematologic & oncologic: Anemia (33% to 98%; grades 3/4: 1% to 28%), neutropenia (73% to 85%; grades 3/4: 34% to 47%), thrombocytopenia (2% to 74%; grades 3/4: ≤18%), bone marrow depression

Hepatic: Increased serum aspartate aminotransferase (39%), increased serum alkaline phosphatase (36%)

Infection: Infection (24%; including respiratory tract infection)

Neuromuscular & skeletal: Asthenia (16% to 47%), musculoskeletal pain (10% to 44%; myalgia/arthralgia), limb pain (11%)

Ophthalmic: Visual disturbance (13%; including blurred vision, keratitis)

Renal: Increased serum creatinine (11%)

Respiratory: Cough (7% to 17%), epistaxis (7% to 15%), dyspnea (1% to 12%)

Miscellaneous: Fever (41%)

1% to 10%:

Cardiovascular: Edema (10%), cardiac failure (<10%), hypertension (<10%), tachycardia (<10%), hypotension (≤5%), significant cardiovascular event (grades 3/4: 3%)

Gastrointestinal: Oral candidiasis (<10%), mucositis (7% to 10%)

Hematologic & oncologic: Hemorrhage (2%), febrile neutropenia (2%)

Hepatic: Increased serum bilirubin (7%)

Hypersensitivity: Hypersensitivity reaction (4%)

Infection: Sepsis (5%)

Ophthalmic: Cystoid macular edema (<10%)

Respiratory: Pneumonia (<10%), pneumonitis (4%)

Frequency not defined:

Cardiovascular: Ischemic heart disease, myocardial infarction, pulmonary thromboembolism, supraventricular tachycardia, thrombosis

<1%, postmarketing, and/or case reports: Anaphylaxis, atrioventricular block, autonomic neuropathy, bradycardia, cardiac arrhythmia, cerebrovascular accident, chest pain, cranial nerve palsy, decreased visual acuity, erythema, flushing, hepatic encephalopathy, hepatic necrosis, injection site reaction (mild), intestinal obstruction, intestinal perforation, ischemic colitis, left ventricular dysfunction, maculopapular rash, nail discoloration, neutropenic sepsis, optic nerve damage (rare), palmar-plantar erythrodysesthesia (in patients previously exposed to capecitabine), pancreatitis, pancytopenia, paralytic ileus, peripheral motor neuropathy, pneumothorax, pruritus, pulmonary embolism, radiation pneumonitis (with concurrent radiation therapy), radiation recall phenomenon, skin photosensitivity, Stevens-Johnson syndrome, toxic epidermal necrolysis, transient ischemic attacks, tumor lysis syndrome, vocal cord paralysis

Mechanism of Action Paclitaxel (protein bound) is an albumin-bound paclitaxel nanoparticle formulation; paclitaxel promotes microtubule assembly by enhancing the action of tubulin dimers, stabilizing existing microtubules, and inhibiting their disassembly, interfering with the late G_2 mitotic phase, and inhibiting cell replication. May also distort mitotic spindles, resulting in the breakage of chromosomes. Paclitaxel may also suppress cell proliferation and modulate immune response.

Pharmacodynamics/Kinetics

Half-life Elimination Terminal: 13 to 27 hours

Reproductive Considerations

Females of reproductive potential should have a pregnancy test prior to treatment initiation and use effective contraception during therapy and for at least 6 months after the last paclitaxel (protein bound) dose. Males with female partners of reproductive potential should use effective contraception during therapy and for at least 3 months after the last paclitaxel (protein bound) dose.

Pregnancy Considerations

Based on the mechanism of action and on findings in animal reproduction studies, paclitaxel (protein bound) may cause fetal harm if administered during pregnancy.

An ex vivo human placenta perfusion model illustrated that paclitaxel (non-protein bound preparation) crossed the placenta at term. Placental transfer was low and affected by the presence of albumin; higher albumin concentrations resulted in lower paclitaxel placental transfer (Berveiller 2012).

A pregnancy registry is available for all cancers diagnosed during pregnancy at Cooper Health (877-635-4499).

- **Paclitaxel, Albumin-Bound** *see* PACLitaxel (Protein Bound) *on page 1179*
- **Paclitaxel (Nanoparticle Albumin Bound)** *see* PACLitaxel (Protein Bound) *on page 1179*
- **Padcev** *see* Enfortumab Vedotin *on page 564*
- **Pain Eze [OTC]** *see* Acetaminophen *on page 59*
- **Pain & Fever Children's [OTC]** *see* Acetaminophen *on page 59*
- **Pain Relief Extra Strength [OTC]** *see* Acetaminophen *on page 59*
- **Pain Relief Maximum Strength [OTC]** *see* Lidocaine (Topical) *on page 902*
- **Pain Relieving [OTC]** *see* Lidocaine (Topical) *on page 902*

Palbociclib (pal boe SYE klib)

Brand Names: US Ibrance

Brand Names: Canada Ibrance

Pharmacologic Category Antineoplastic Agent, Cyclin-Dependent Kinase Inhibitor

Use

Breast cancer, advanced (initial endocrine-based therapy): Treatment of hormone receptor (HR)-positive, human epidermal growth factor receptor 2 (HER2)-negative advanced or metastatic breast cancer (in combination with an aromatase inhibitor) in postmenopausal females or in adult males as initial endocrine-based therapy.

Breast cancer, advanced (with disease progression following endocrine therapy): Treatment of HR-positive, HER2-negative advanced or metastatic breast cancer (in combination with fulvestrant) in adult patients with disease progression following endocrine therapy.

Local Anesthetic/Vasoconstrictor Precautions No information available to require special precautions

Effects on Dental Treatment Key adverse event(s) related to dental treatment: Stomatitis reported (25% incidence)

Effects on Bleeding Chemotherapy may result in significant myelosuppression, potentially including significant reduction in platelet counts (thrombocytopenia [17%; grade 3: 2%]); and altered hemostasis.

Adverse Reactions Percentages reported as part of combination therapy.

>10%:

Central nervous system: Fatigue (37% to 41%)

Dermatologic: Alopecia (18% to 33%), skin rash (17% to 18%), xeroderma (6% to 12%)

Gastrointestinal: Nausea (34% to 35%), stomatitis (28% to 30%; grade 3: 1%), diarrhea (24% to 26%), vomiting (16% to 19%), decreased appetite (15% to 16%)

Hematologic & oncologic: Neutropenia (80% to 83%; grade 3: 55% to 56%; grade 4: 10% to 11%), anemia (24% to 78%; grade 3: 3% to 6%; grade 4: <1%), leukopenia (39% to 53%; grade 3: 24% to 30%; grade 4: 1%), thrombocytopenia (16% to 23%; grade 3: 1% to 2%; grade 4: ≤1%)

Hepatic: Increased serum aspartate aminotransferase (8% to 52%), increased serum alanine aminotransferase (6% to 43%)

Infection: Infection (47% to 60%)

Neuromuscular & skeletal: Asthenia (8% to 17%)

Miscellaneous: Fever (12% to 13%)

1% to 10%:

Gastrointestinal: Dysgeusia (7% to 10%)

Hematologic & oncologic: Febrile neutropenia (≤3%)

Ophthalmic: Blurred vision (4% to 6%), increased lacrimation (6%), dry eye syndrome (4%)

Respiratory: Epistaxis (7% to 9%), interstitial pulmonary disease (≤1%), pneumonitis (≤1%)

Mechanism of Action Palbociclib is a reversible small molecule cyclin-dependent kinase (CDK) inhibitor which is selective for CDK 4 and 6. CDKs have a role in regulating progression through the cell cycle at the G1/S phase by blocking retinoblastoma (Rb) hyperphosphorylation (Finn 2015). Palbociclib reduces proliferation of breast cancer cell lines by preventing progression from the G1 to the S cell cycle phase. The combination of palbociclib with an antiestrogen provides for increased inhibition of Rb phosphorylation, downstream signaling, and tumor growth compared with each agent alone.

Pharmacodynamics/Kinetics

Half-life Elimination 29 ± 5 hours

Time to Peak Tablets: 4 to 12 hours; Capsules: 6 to 12 hours.

Reproductive Considerations

Evaluate pregnancy status prior to treatment in females of reproductive potential. Females of reproductive potential should use effective contraception during treatment and for at least 3 weeks after the last dose. Males with female partners of reproductive potential should use effective contraception during treatment and for 3 months after the last dose.

Adverse effects to male reproductive function and fertility were observed in animal toxicology studies; males of reproductive potential may want to consider sperm preservation prior to palbociclib therapy.

Pregnancy Considerations

Based on the mechanism of action and data from animal reproduction studies, palbociclib may be expected to cause fetal harm if used during pregnancy.

Prescribing and Access Restrictions Palbociclib is available through specialty pharmacies. For more information, refer to https://www.pfizeroncologytogether.com

◆ **Palbociclib Isethionate** *see* Palbociclib *on page 1180*

◆ **Palforzia** *see* Peanut Allergen Powder *on page 1198*

Palifermin (pal ee FER min)

Brand Names: US Kepivance

Pharmacologic Category Chemoprotective Agent; Keratinocyte Growth Factor

Use

Oral mucositis: To decrease the incidence and duration of severe oral mucositis associated with hematologic malignancies in patients receiving myelotoxic therapy in the setting of autologous hematopoietic stem cell support (when the preparative regimen is expected to result in mucositis ≥ grade 3 in most patients).

Limitations of use: Use (safety and efficacy) is not established for nonhematologic malignancies; use is not recommended with conditioning regimens containing melphalan 200 mg/m^2. Palifermin was not effective in decreasing the incidence of severe mucositis in patients with hematologic malignancies receiving myelotoxic therapy in the setting of allogeneic hematopoietic stem cell support.

Local Anesthetic/Vasoconstrictor Precautions No information available to require special precautions

Effects on Dental Treatment Key adverse event(s) related to dental treatment: Taste alteration, mouth/tongue discoloration or thickness. See Dental Health Professional Considerations.

Effects on Bleeding No information available to require special precautions

Adverse Reactions

>10%:

Cardiovascular: Edema (28%)

Central nervous system: Pain (16%), dysesthesia (12%; includes hypoesthesia, oral hyperesthesia, paresthesia)

Dermatologic: Skin rash (62%; grade 3: 3%), pruritus (35%), erythema (32%)

Gastrointestinal: Increased serum amylase (62%, grades 3/4: 38%), increased serum lipase (28%, grades 3/4: 11%), mouth discoloration (≤17%), swelling of mouth (≤17%), tongue discoloration (≤17%), tongue edema (≤17%), dysgeusia (16%)

Miscellaneous: Fever (39%)

1% to 10%:

Immunologic: Antibody development (2%)

Neuromuscular & skeletal: Arthralgia (10%)

<1%, postmarketing, and/or case reports: Cataract, cough, genital edema (vaginal), hyperpigmentation (flexural), palmar-plantar erythrodysesthesia (hand-foot syndrome), perineal pain, rhinitis, vaginal disease (erythema)

Mechanism of Action Palifermin is a recombinant keratinocyte growth factor (KGF) produced in *E. coli*. Endogenous KGF is produced by mesenchymal cells in response to epithelial tissue injury. KGF binds to the KGF receptor resulting in proliferation, differentiation and migration of epithelial cells in multiple tissues, including (but not limited to) the tongue, buccal mucosa, esophagus, and salivary gland.

Pharmacodynamics/Kinetics

Onset of Action Epithelial cell proliferation (dose-dependent): 48 hours

Half-life Elimination 4.5 hours (range: 3.3 to 5.7 hours)

Pregnancy Considerations Based on data from animal reproduction studies, in utero exposure to palifermin may cause fetal harm.

Dental Health Professional Considerations Palifermin works at the cellular level by protecting the epithelial cells lining the mouth and throat from damage caused by chemotherapy and radiation and by stimulating the growth and development of new epithelial cells to build up the mucosal barrier.

Paliperidone (pal ee PER i done)

Related Information

Clinical Risk Related to Drugs Prolonging QT Interval *on page 1675*

Brand Names: US Invega; Invega Sustenna; Invega Trinza

Brand Names: Canada Invega; Invega Sustenna; Invega Trinza

Pharmacologic Category Second Generation (Atypical) Antipsychotic

Use

Schizophrenia: Treatment of schizophrenia

Schizoaffective disorder (oral and monthly IM paliperidone): Treatment of schizoaffective disorder as monotherapy and as an adjunct to mood stabilizers or antidepressants

Local Anesthetic/Vasoconstrictor Precautions Paliperidone is one of the drugs confirmed to prolong the QT interval and is accepted as having a risk of causing torsade de pointes. The risk of drug-induced torsade de pointes is extremely low when a single QT interval prolonging drug is prescribed. In terms of epinephrine, it is not known what effect vasoconstrictors in the local anesthetic regimen will have in patients with a known history of congenital prolonged QT interval or in patients taking any medication that prolongs the QT interval. Until more information is obtained, it is suggested that the clinician consult with the physician prior to the use of a vasoconstrictor in suspected patients, and that the vasoconstrictor (epinephrine, mepivacaine and levonordefrin [Carbocaine® 2% with Neo-Cobefrin®]) be used with caution.

Effects on Dental Treatment Key adverse event(s) related to dental treatment: Significant xerostomia and changes in salivation (normal salivary flow resumes upon discontinuation).

Effects on Bleeding No information available to require special precautions

Adverse Reactions Unless otherwise noted, frequency of adverse effects is reported for the oral/IM formulation in adults.

>10%:

Cardiovascular: Tachycardia (adolescents and adults: 3% to 14%)

Central nervous system: Drowsiness (oral, adolescents: 13% to 26%; adults: 5% to 12%), extrapyramidal reaction (oral, adolescents and adults: 5% to 23%; IM: 2% to 5%), akathisia (adolescents and adults: 4% to 17%), headache (adolescents and adults: 4% to 15%), parkinsonian-like syndrome (adolescents and adults: 2% to 15%), dystonia (adolescents and adults: 1% to 14%)

Endocrine & metabolic: Increased serum prolactin (males: ≤56%; females: ≤44%), decreased HDL cholesterol (oral; adolescents and adults: 23% to 29%; IM: 14% to 16%), increased LDL cholesterol (adolescents and adults: 4% to 14%), weight gain (oral: adults: 3% to 9%, adolescents: 2% to 19%; IM: 6% to 13%), increased serum triglycerides (adolescents and adults: 6% to 13%), increased serum cholesterol (adolescents and adults: 4% to 11%), hyperglycemia (adolescents and adults: 3% to 11%)

Gastrointestinal: Vomiting (adolescents and adults: 5% to 11%)

Neuromuscular & skeletal: Hyperkinesia (oral, adolescents and adults: 6% to 17%; IM: 4% to 5%), tremor (oral, adolescents and adults: 4% to 12%; IM: 1%)

1% to 10%:

Cardiovascular: Orthostatic hypotension (oral: 2% to 4%; IM: <1%), bundle branch block (3%), first degree atrioventricular block (2%), hypertension (adolescents and adults: ≤2%), sinus arrhythmia (oral: ≤2%), bradycardia (adolescents and adults: <2%), edema (adolescents and adults: <2%), palpitations (adolescents and adults: <2%)

Central nervous system: Agitation (IM: 8% to 10%; oral: adolescents and adults: <2%), anxiety (adolescents and adults: 8% to 9%), sedation (IM: 5% to 7%), dizziness (adolescents and adults: 2% to 6%), dysarthria (1% to 4%), lethargy (adolescents: 3%), fatigue (adolescents and adults: 2% to 3%), sleep disorder (oral: 2% to 3%), nightmares (adolescents and adults: ≤2%), insomnia (adolescents and adults: <2%), opisthotonus (oral, adolescents and adults: <2%)

Dermatologic: Pruritus (adolescents and adults: <2%), skin rash (adolescents and adults: <2%)

Endocrine & metabolic: Amenorrhea (adolescents and adults: 2% to 6%), galactorrhea (IM, women: 1% to 4%), gynecomastia (adolescents and adults: 3%), decreased libido (IM: 1%)

Gastrointestinal: Nausea (4% to 8%), dyspepsia (5% to 6%), sialorrhea (adolescents and adults: 1% to 6%), constipation (4% to 5%), abdominal distress (≤4%), upper abdominal pain (≤4%), diarrhea (IM: 3%), swollen tongue (adolescents: 3%), increased appetite (2% to 3%), toothache (IM: 2% to 3%), xerostomia (adolescents and adults: 2% to 3%), stomach discomfort (oral: 2%), decreased appetite (1% to 2%), flatulence (adolescents and adults: <2%)

Genitourinary: Urinary tract infection (adolescents and adults: ≤3%), breast tenderness (adolescents and adults: <2%), irregular menses (adolescents and adults: <2%), retrograde ejaculation (adolescents and adults:<2%), erectile dysfunction (IM: ≤1%)

Hepatic: Increased serum ALT (adolescents and adults: <2%), increased serum AST (adolescents and adults: <2%)

Hypersensitivity: Anaphylaxis (adolescents and adults: <2%)

Local: Injection site reaction (IM: 3% to 10%), erythema at injection site (IM: ≤2%), swelling at injection site (IM: ≤2%)

Neuromuscular & skeletal: Dyskinesia (adolescents and adults: 2% to 9%), myalgia (1% to 4%), weakness (adolescents and adults: ≤4%), back pain (3%), tongue paralysis (oral, adolescents: 3%), limb pain (adolescents and adults: ≤3%), muscle rigidity (IM: 2%), arthralgia (adolescents and adults: <2%)

Ophthalmic: Blurred vision (adolescents and adults: 3%), abnormal eye movements (adolescents and adults: <2%; includes eye rolling)

Respiratory: Upper respiratory tract infection (2% to 10%), nasopharyngitis (adolescents and adults: 2% to 5%), cough (2% to 3%), rhinitis (oral: 1% to 3%), epistaxis (oral, adolescents: 2%), pharyngolaryngeal pain (oral: 1% to 2%), nasal congestion (adolescents and adults: <2%)

Frequency not defined:

Cardiovascular: Cerebrovascular accident (IM), ECG abnormality (IM), hypotension (oral), ischemia (oral), left bundle branch block (oral), peripheral edema (oral), postural orthostatic tachycardia (IM), transient ischemic attacks (oral)

Central nervous system: Abnormal gait (oral; parkinsonian gait), cogwheel rigidity (IM), drooling, hypertonia (IM), orthostatic dizziness (IM), psychomotor agitation (IM), restlessness (IM), seizure, tonic-clonic seizures (oral), trismus (oral), vertigo (IM)

Dermatologic: Fixed drug eruption (IM), papular rash (oral), urticaria (IM)

Endocrine & metabolic: Menstrual disease (IM)

Gastrointestinal: Abdominal pain (oral), hyperinsulinism (IM), oromandibular dystonia (IM)

Genitourinary: Breast engorgement (oral), breast hypertrophy (IM), breast swelling (IM), ejaculatory disorder (IM), mastalgia, nipple discharge (IM), sexual disorder (IM)

Hypersensitivity: Hypersensitivity (IM)

Neuromuscular & skeletal: Bradykinesia (IM), joint stiffness (IM), muscle spasm (IM), muscle twitching (IM), musculoskeletal pain (oral), neck stiffness (IM), torticollis (oral)

Ophthalmic: Oculogyric crisis (IM)

Respiratory: Aspiration pneumonia

<1%, postmarketing, and/or case reports: Agranulocytosis, angioedema, antiemetic effect, diabetes mellitus, intestinal obstruction (includes small intestine), leukopenia, motor dysfunction, neuroleptic malignant syndrome, neutropenia, priapism, prolonged QT interval on ECG, sensory disturbance (sensory instability), somnambulism, syncope, tardive dyskinesia, thrombotic thrombocytopenic purpura, urinary incontinence, urinary retention

Mechanism of Action Paliperidone is considered a benzisoxazole atypical antipsychotic as it is the primary active metabolite of risperidone. As with other atypical antipsychotics, its therapeutic efficacy is believed to result from mixed central serotonergic and dopaminergic antagonism. The addition of serotonin antagonism to dopamine antagonism (classic neuroleptic mechanism) is thought to improve negative symptoms of psychoses and reduce the incidence of extrapyramidal side effects (Huttunen 1995). Similar to risperidone, paliperidone demonstrates high affinity to α_1, α_2, D_2, H_1, and 5-HT_{2A} receptors and low affinity for muscarinic receptors. In contrast to risperidone, paliperidone displays nearly 10-fold lower affinity for α_2 and 5-HT_{2A} receptors, and nearly three- to fivefold less affinity for 5-HT_{1A} and 5-HT_{1D}, respectively.

Pharmacodynamics/Kinetics

Half-life Elimination

Oral: 23 hours; 24 to 51 hours with renal impairment (CrCl <80 mL/minute)

Monthly IM (following a single-dose administration): Range: 25 to 49 days

3-month IM: Deltoid injection range: 84 to 95 days; gluteal injection range: 118 to 139 days

Time to Peak Oral: ~24 hours; Monthly IM: 13 days; 3-month IM: 30 to 33 days

Reproductive Considerations

Paliperidone may cause hyperprolactinemia, which may cause a reversible decrease in fertility in females.

Pregnancy Considerations Information specific to paliperidone in pregnancy is limited (Onken 2018; Özdemir 2015; Zamora Rodriguez 2017).

Antipsychotic use during the third trimester of pregnancy has a risk for extrapyramidal symptoms (EPS) and/or withdrawal symptoms in newborns following delivery. Symptoms in the newborn may include agitation, feeding disorder, hypertonia, hypotonia, respiratory distress, somnolence, and tremor. These effects may be self-limiting and allow recovery within hours or days with no specific treatment, or they may be severe requiring prolonged hospitalization.

The ACOG recommends that therapy during pregnancy be individualized; treatment with psychiatric medications during pregnancy should incorporate the clinical expertise of the mental health clinician, obstetrician, primary healthcare provider, and pediatrician. Safety data related to atypical antipsychotics during pregnancy is limited and routine use is not recommended. However, if a woman is inadvertently exposed to an atypical antipsychotic while pregnant, continuing therapy may be preferable to switching to a typical antipsychotic that the fetus has not yet been exposed to; consider risk: benefit (ACOG 2008).

Paliperidone is the active metabolite of risperidone; refer to Risperidone monograph for additional information.

Health care providers are encouraged to enroll women 18 to 45 years of age exposed to paliperidone during pregnancy in the Atypical Antipsychotics Pregnancy Registry (1-866-961-2388 or http://www.womensmentalhealth.org/pregnancyregistry).

Dental Health Professional Considerations See Local Anesthetic/Vasoconstrictor Precautions

◆ **Paliperidone Palmitate** *see* Paliperidone *on page 1182*

Palivizumab (pah li VIZ u mab)

Brand Names: US Synagis

Brand Names: Canada Synagis

Pharmacologic Category Monoclonal Antibody

Use Respiratory syncytial virus prophylaxis: Prevention of serious lower respiratory tract disease caused by respiratory syncytial virus (RSV) in pediatric patients with a history of premature birth (≤35 weeks gestational age) and who are ≤6 months at the beginning of RSV season; pediatric patients with bronchopulmonary dysplasia (BPD) that required medical treatment within the previous 6 months and who are ≤24 months at the beginning of RSV season; or pediatric patients with hemodynamically significant congenital heart disease (CHD) and who are ≤24 months at the beginning of RSV season.

The American Academy of Pediatrics (AAP 2014) recommends RSV prophylaxis with palivizumab during RSV season for:

Infants born at ≤28 weeks 6 days gestational age and <12 months at the start of RSV season

Infants <12 months of age with chronic lung disease (CLD) of prematurity

Infants ≤12 months of age with hemodynamically significant CHD

Infants and children <24 months of age with CLD of prematurity necessitating medical therapy (eg, supplemental oxygen, bronchodilator, diuretic, or chronic steroid therapy) within 6 months prior to the beginning of RSV season

AAP also suggests that palivizumab prophylaxis may be considered in the following circumstances:

Infants <12 months of age with congenital airway abnormality or neuromuscular disorder that decreases the ability to manage airway secretions

Infants <12 months of age with cystic fibrosis with clinical evidence of CLD and/or nutritional compromise

Children <24 months with cystic fibrosis with severe lung disease (previous hospitalization for pulmonary exacerbation in the first year of life or abnormalities on chest radiography or chest computed tomography that persist when stable) or weight for length less than the 10th percentile

Infants and children <24 months who are profoundly immunocompromised

Infants and children <24 months undergoing cardiac transplantation during RSV season

Limitations of use: Safety and efficacy have not been established for treatment of RSV disease.

Local Anesthetic/Vasoconstrictor Precautions No information available to require special precautions

Effects on Dental Treatment No significant effects or complications reported

Effects on Bleeding No information available to require special precautions

Adverse Reactions

>10%:

Dermatologic: Skin rash (12%)

Miscellaneous: Fever (27%)

1% to 10%: Immunologic: Antibody development (1% to 2%)

<1%, postmarketing, and/or case reports: Anaphylaxis (very rare; includes angioedema, dyspnea, hypotonia, pruritus, respiratory failure, unresponsiveness, urticaria), hypersensitivity reaction, injection site reaction, thrombocytopenia

Mechanism of Action Exhibits neutralizing and fusion-inhibitory activity against RSV; these activities inhibit RSV replication in laboratory and clinical studies

Pharmacodynamics/Kinetics

Half-life Elimination Infants and Children <24 months without congenital heart disease: 20 to 24.5 days.

Time to Peak Serum: IM: Infants and Children <24 months: 3 to 5 days (Resch 2017); palivizumab concentrations sufficient to inhibit respiratory syncytial virus 2 days after administration (Sáez-Llorens 1998).

Pregnancy Considerations Not for adult use.

◆ **Palladone** *see* HYDROmorphone *on page* 776

Palonosetron (pal oh NOE se tron)

Brand Names: US Aloxi

Brand Names: Canada Aloxi

Pharmacologic Category Antiemetic; Selective 5-HT_3 Receptor Antagonist

Use

Chemotherapy-induced nausea and vomiting: Prevention of acute and delayed nausea and vomiting associated with initial and repeat courses in adults treated with moderately emetogenic cancer chemotherapy; prevention of acute nausea and vomiting associated with initial and repeat courses in adults treated with highly emetogenic cancer chemotherapy; prevention of acute nausea and vomiting associated with initial and repeat courses of emetogenic cancer chemotherapy (including highly emetogenic chemotherapy) in pediatric patients 1 month to <17 years of age.

Capsules [Canadian product]: Prevention of acute nausea and vomiting associated with moderately emetogenic cancer chemotherapy in adults.

Postoperative nausea and vomiting: Prevention of postoperative nausea and vomiting (PONV) for up to 24 hours following surgery in adults.

Limitations of use: Routine prophylaxis for PONV in patients with minimal expectation of nausea and/or vomiting is not recommended, although use is recommended in patients when nausea and vomiting must be avoided in the postoperative period, even if the incidence of PONV is low.

Local Anesthetic/Vasoconstrictor Precautions No information available to require special precautions

Effects on Dental Treatment No significant effects or complications reported

Effects on Bleeding No information available to require special precautions

Adverse Reactions

Frequencies reported for both indications (chemotherapy-associated nausea and vomiting and postoperative nausea and vomiting) and in adults unless otherwise noted.

1% to 10%:

Cardiovascular: Bradycardia (chemotherapy-associated: ≤1%; PONV: ≤1% to 4%), hypotension (≤1%), prolonged QT interval on ECG (chemotherapy-associated: ≤1%; PONV: ≤1% to 5%), sinus bradycardia (PONV: ≤1%), tachycardia (may be nonsustained; ≤1%)

Dermatologic: Pruritus (PONV: ≤1%)

Endocrine & metabolic: Hyperkalemia (chemotherapy-associated: ≤1%)

Gastrointestinal: Constipation (chemotherapy-associated: 5%; PONV: 2%), diarrhea (≤1%), flatulence (≤1%)

Genitourinary: Urinary retention (≤1%)

Hepatic: Increased serum alanine aminotransferase (≤1%; may be transient), increased serum aspartate aminotransferase (≤1%; may be transient)

Nervous system: Anxiety (chemotherapy-associated: ≤1%), dizziness (adults ≤1%; infants, children, adolescents <1%), headache (chemotherapy-associated: adults 3% to 9%; infants, children, and adolescents <1%)

Neuromuscular & skeletal: Asthenia (chemotherapy-associated: ≤1%)

<1%, postmarketing, and/or case reports: Abdominal pain, allergic dermatitis, amblyopia, anaphylactic shock, anaphylaxis, anemia, anorexia, arthralgia, cardiac arrhythmia, chills, decreased appetite, decreased gastrointestinal motility, decreased platelet count, dermatological disease (infants, children, and adolescents), distended vein, drowsiness, dyskinesia

(infants, children, and adolescents), dyspepsia, electrolyte disturbance, epistaxis, euphoria, extrasystoles, eye irritation, fatigue, fever, flattened T wave on ECG, flu-like symptoms, glycosuria, hiccups, hot flash, hyperglycemia, hypersensitivity reaction (including bronchospasm, dyspnea, edema, erythema of skin, swelling, urticaria), hypersomnia, hypertension, hypokalemia, hypoventilation, increased bilirubin (transient), increased liver enzymes, infusion site pain (infants, children, and adolescents), injection site reaction (includes burning sensation at injection site, discomfort at injection site, induration at injection site, pain at injection site), insomnia, ischemic heart disease, laryngospasm, limb pain, metabolic acidosis, motion sickness, paresthesia, serotonin syndrome, sialorrhea, sinoatrial nodal rhythm disorder, sinus tachycardia, skin rash, supraventricular extrasystole, tinnitus, vein discoloration, ventricular premature contractions, xerostomia

Mechanism of Action Palonosetron is a selective 5-HT_3 receptor antagonist, blocking serotonin, both on vagal nerve terminals in the periphery and centrally in the chemoreceptor trigger zone

Pharmacodynamics/Kinetics

Half-life Elimination IV: Children 1 month to 17 years: Median: 29.5 hours (range: 20 to 30 hours); Adults: ~40 hours

Time to Peak Plasma: Capsules [Canadian product]: 5.1 ± 5.9 hours

Pregnancy Considerations Information related to use of palonestron for the prevention of postoperative nausea and vomiting in women undergoing cesarean delivery has been evaluated (Swaro 2018).

◆ **Palonosetron and Fosnetupitant** *see* Fosnetupitant and Palonosetron *on page 717*

◆ **Palonosetron and Netupitant** *see* Netupitant and Palonosetron *on page 1095*

◆ **Palonosetron Hydrochloride** *see* Palonosetron *on page 1184*

◆ **Palonosetron Hydrochloride and Netupitant** *see* Netupitant and Palonosetron *on page 1095*

◆ **Palonosetron, inj** *see* Palonosetron *on page 1184*

◆ **Palonosetron/Pronetupitant** *see* Fosnetupitant and Palonosetron *on page 717*

◆ **Pamelor** *see* Nortriptyline *on page 1119*

Pamidronate (pa mi DROE nate)

Related Information

Osteonecrosis of the Jaw *on page 1699*

Brand Names: Canada Pamidronate Disodium Omega; PMS-Pamidronate

Pharmacologic Category Bisphosphonate Derivative

Use

Hypercalcemia of malignancy: Treatment of moderate or severe hypercalcemia associated with malignancy, with or without bone metastases, in conjunction with adequate hydration.

Osteolytic bone metastases of breast cancer and osteolytic lesions of multiple myeloma: Treatment of osteolytic bone metastases of breast cancer and osteolytic lesions of multiple myeloma in conjunction with standard antineoplastic therapy.

Paget disease: Treatment of patients with moderate to severe Paget disease of bone.

Note: Guidelines recommend IV zoledronic acid as the preferred treatment (Endocrine Society [Singer 2014]; Ralston 2019).

Local Anesthetic/Vasoconstrictor Precautions No information available to require special precautions

Effects on Dental Treatment Osteonecrosis of the jaw (ONJ), generally associated with local infection and/or tooth extraction and often with delayed healing, has been reported in patients taking bisphosphonates. Symptoms included nonhealing extraction socket or an exposed jawbone. Most reported cases of bisphosphonate-associated osteonecrosis have been in cancer patients treated with intravenous bisphosphonates. However, some have occurred in patients with postmenopausal osteoporosis taking oral bisphosphonates. Dental surgery, particularly tooth extraction, may increase the risk for ONJ. Patients who develop ONJ while on bisphosphonate therapy should receive care by an oral surgeon. See Dental Health Professional Considerations.

Effects on Bleeding No information available to require special precautions

Adverse Reactions

>10%:

Central nervous system: Fatigue (osteolytic bone metastases: 32% to 40%; hypercalcemia of malignancy: ≤12%), headache (24% to 27%; Paget disease: ≥10%), insomnia (osteolytic bone metastases: 25%; hypercalcemia of malignancy: ≤1%), anxiety (osteolytic bone metastases: 18%), pain (≤13%)

Endocrine & metabolic: Hypophosphatemia (9% to 18%), hypokalemia (4% to 18%), hypocalcemia (1% to 17%), hypomagnesemia (4% to 12%)

Gastrointestinal: Nausea (osteolytic bone metastases: 64%; hypercalcemia of malignancy: ≤18%; Paget disease: ≥5%), vomiting (osteolytic bone metastases: 36% to 46%; hypercalcemia of malignancy: ≤4%), anorexia (osteolytic bone metastases: 31%; hypercalcemia of malignancy: ≤12%), abdominal pain (osteolytic bone metastases: 20% to 24%; hypercalcemia of malignancy: ≤1%), dyspepsia (osteolytic bone metastases: 18%; hypercalcemia of malignancy: ≤4%)

Genitourinary: Urinary tract infection (16% to 20%)

Hematologic & oncologic: Anemia (osteolytic bone metastases: 40% to 48%; hypercalcemia of malignancy: ≤6%), metastases (osteolytic bone metastases: 31%), granulocytopenia (osteolytic bone metastases: 20%)

Local: Infusion site reaction (hypercalcemia of malignancy: ≤18%; includes erythema, induration, pain, and swelling)

Neuromuscular & skeletal: Myalgia (osteolytic bone metastases: 26%; hypercalcemia of malignancy: ≤1%), weakness (osteolytic bone metastases: 26%), ostealgia (5% to ≥15%), arthralgia (osteolytic bone metastases: 11% to 15%)

Renal: Increased serum creatinine (osteolytic bone metastases: 19%; mild)

Respiratory: Dyspnea (osteolytic bone metastases: 22% to 35%; other indications: <1%), upper respiratory tract infection (osteolytic bone metastases: 32%; hypercalcemia of malignancy: ≤3%), cough (osteolytic bone metastases: 25%), sinusitis (osteolytic bone metastases: 16%), pleural effusion (osteolytic bone metastases: 15%)

Miscellaneous: Fever (18% to 39%; may be transient, includes temperature increase of ≥1°C within 24 to 48 hours after treatment; Paget disease, includes temperature increase of ≥1°C within 48 hours after treatment, transient: ≤21%)

1% to 10%:

Cardiovascular: Atrial fibrillation (hypercalcemia of malignancy: ≤6%), hypertension (6%; Paget disease: ≥10%), syncope (hypercalcemia of malignancy: ≤6%), tachycardia (hypercalcemia of malignancy: ≤6%), atrial flutter (hypercalcemia of malignancy: ≤1%), cardiac failure (hypercalcemia of malignancy: ≤1%), edema (hypercalcemia of malignancy: ≤1%)

Central nervous system: Drowsiness (hypercalcemia of malignancy: ≤6%), psychosis (hypercalcemia of malignancy: ≤4%)

Endocrine & metabolic: Hypothyroidism (hypercalcemia of malignancy: ≤6%)

Gastrointestinal: Constipation (hypercalcemia of malignancy: ≤6%), gastrointestinal hemorrhage (hypercalcemia of malignancy: ≤6%), diarrhea (hypercalcemia of malignancy: ≤1%), stomatitis (hypercalcemia of malignancy: ≤1%)

Genitourinary: Uremia (hypercalcemia of malignancy: ≤4%)

Hematologic & oncologic: Leukopenia (hypercalcemia of malignancy: ≤4%), neutropenia (hypercalcemia of malignancy: ≤1%), thrombocytopenia (hypercalcemia of malignancy: ≤1%)

Infection: Candidiasis (hypercalcemia of malignancy: ≤6%)

Neuromuscular & skeletal: Arthropathy (Paget disease: ≥5%), back pain (Paget disease: ≥5%)

Renal: Renal insufficiency (osteolytic bone metastases, patients with normal baseline serum creatinine: 8%)

Respiratory: Rales (hypercalcemia of malignancy: ≤6%), rhinitis (hypercalcemia of malignancy: ≤6%)

Frequency not defined: Endocrine & metabolic: Hypervolemia (hypercalcemia of malignancy)

<1%, postmarketing, and/or case reports: Adult respiratory distress syndrome, anaphylactic shock, angioedema, confusion, conjunctivitis, electrolyte disturbance, episcleritis, femur fracture (subtrochanteric and diaphyseal), flu-like symptoms, focal segmental glomerulosclerosis (including collapsing variant), glomerulopathy, hematuria, herpes simplex infection (reactivation), herpes zoster (reactivation), hyperkalemia, hypernatremia, hypersensitivity reaction, hypotension, interstitial pulmonary disease, iritis, local inflammation (orbital), malaise, mineral abnormalities, nephrotic syndrome, osteonecrosis (primarily of the jaw), paresthesia, pruritus, renal failure, renal tubular disease, scleritis, skin rash, tetany, uveitis, visual hallucination

Mechanism of Action Pamidronate is a nitrogen-containing bisphosphonate; it inhibits bone resorption by disrupting osteoclast activity (Rogers 2011).

Pharmacodynamics/Kinetics

Onset of Action

Hypercalcemia of malignancy (HCM): Reduction of albumin-corrected serum calcium: Children: ~48 hours (Kerdudo 2005); Adults: ≤24 hours for decrease in albumin-corrected serum calcium; maximum effect: ≤7 days

Paget disease: ~1 month for ≥50% decrease in serum alkaline phosphatase

Maximum effect: Hypercalcemia of malignancy: ≤7 days

Duration of Action HCM: 7 to 14 days; Paget disease: 1 to 372 days

Half-life Elimination 28 ± 7 hours

Reproductive Considerations

Bisphosphonates are incorporated into the bone matrix and gradually released over time. Because exposure prior to pregnancy may theoretically increase the risk of fetal harm, most sources recommend discontinuing bisphosphonate therapy in females of reproductive potential as early as possible prior to a planned pregnancy. Use in premenopausal females should be reserved for special circumstances when rapid bone loss is occurring; a bisphosphonate with the shortest half-life should then be used (Bhalla 2010; Pereira 2012; Stathopoulos 2011).

Pregnancy Considerations

It is not known if bisphosphonates cross the placenta, but based on their lower molecular weight, fetal exposure is expected (Djokanovic 2008; Stathopoulos 2011).

Information related to the use of pamidronate in pregnancy is available from case reports and small retrospective studies (Baretić 2014; Green 2014; Koren 2018; Levy 2009; Stathopoulos 2011).

Bisphosphonates are incorporated into the bone matrix and gradually released over time. The amount available in the systemic circulation varies by drug, dose, and duration of therapy. Theoretically, there may be a risk of fetal harm when pregnancy follows the completion of therapy (hypocalcemia, low birth weight, and decreased gestation have been observed in some case reports); however, available data have not shown that exposure to bisphosphonates during pregnancy significantly increases the risk of adverse fetal events (Djokanovic 2008; Green 2014; Levy 2009; Machairiotis 2019; Sokal 2019; Stathopoulos 2011). Exposed infants should be monitored for hypocalcemia after birth (Djokanovic 2008; Stathopoulos 2011).

Dental Health Professional Considerations The American Association of Oral and Maxillofacial Surgeons position paper on bisphosphonate-related osteonecrosis of the jaws, 2009 update, stated that IV bisphosphonate exposure in the setting of managing malignancy remains the major risk factor for the development of ONJ. After reviewing case series, case-controlled studies, and cohort studies, the estimates of the cumulative incidence of IV bisphosphonate-associated ONJ ranges from 0.8% to 12%.

Two reports have attempted to assess more accurately the percent of cancer patients developing ONJ after bisphosphonate treatment. Maerevoet et al, reported that among 194 patients treated with Zometa® every 3-4 weeks, nine developed ONJ. Before receiving Zometa®, six had received Aredia® 90 mg every 3-4 weeks. The median duration of treatment with Aredia® was 39 months and for Zometa® 18 months. The incidence of ONJ in these patients was calculated to be 4.6%. Durie et al, described the results of a survey by the International Myeloma Foundation in 2004 to assess the risk factors of ONJ. Out of 1203 respondents, 904 had myeloma and 299 had breast cancer. Of the myeloma patients, 62 developed ONJ and 54 had suspicious findings. Of the breast cancer patients, 13 had ONJ and 23 had suspicious findings. The total number of cases of either ONJ or suspicious findings was 152. ONJ developed in 10% of 211 patients receiving Zometa® compared to 4% of 413 receiving Aredia®. The mean time to onset of ONJ among patients taking Zometa® was 18 months; the mean time to onset after

Aredia® was 6 years. It should be noted that an early report by authors from Novartis Pharmaceuticals Corporation stressed that Aredia® and Zometa® had been used in 2.5 million patients world wide and reports of ONJ during their extensive use had been rare (Tarassoff, 2003). In addition, these authors stated that review of the reported cases revealed multiple risk factors for avascular necrosis. McMahon et al, followed up with a report that, along with other factors, bisphosphonates are additional stressors of bone health that can tip the balance to osteonecrosis. They suggested that the prevention of ONJ should be stressed such as the elimination of chronic dental infections prior to chemotherapy and bisphosphonate use in cancer patients.

The most comprehensive review to date on osteonecrosis of the jaw bone (ONJ) has been published in the *Journal of Bone and Mineral Research* (Khan 2015), and written by an International Task Force of authors, totaling 34, from academe; industry; clinical medical and dental practice; oral and maxillofacial surgery; bone and mineral research; epidemiology; medical and dental oncology; orthopedic surgery; osteoporosis research; muscle and bone research; endocrinology and diagnostic sciences. The work provides a systematic review of the literature and international consensus on the classification, incidence, pathophysiology, diagnosis, and management of ONJ in both oncology and osteoporosis patient populations. This review of the literature from January 2003 to April 2014, with 299 references, offers recommendations for management of ONJ based on multidisciplinary international consensus.

Incidence of ONJ in oncology patients from the Task Force report:

The incidence of ONJ ranges from 1% to 15% in the oncology patient population where high doses of BPs are used at frequent intervals. The oncology patient with bone metastasis is exposed to more osteoclastic inhibition than those with osteoporosis, thus the incidence of ONJ is much higher.

- **Pamidronate Disodium** *see* Pamidronate *on page 1185*
- **p-Aminoclonidine** *see* Apraclonidine *on page 161*
- **Pandel** *see* Hydrocortisone (Topical) *on page 775*
- **Panglobulin** *see* Immune Globulin *on page 803*

Panitumumab (pan i TOOM yoo mab)

Brand Names: US Vectibix
Brand Names: Canada Vectibix
Pharmacologic Category Antineoplastic Agent, Epidermal Growth Factor Receptor (EGFR) Inhibitor; Antineoplastic Agent, Monoclonal Antibody

Use

Colorectal cancer (metastatic): Treatment of patients with wild-type *RAS* (defined as wild-type in both *KRAS* and *NRAS* as determined by an approved test) metastatic colorectal cancer (mCRC), either as first-line therapy in combination with FOLFOX (fluorouracil, leucovorin, and oxaliplatin) or as a single agent following disease progression after prior treatment with fluoropyrimidine-, oxaliplatin-, and irinotecan-containing chemotherapy

Limitations of use: Panitumumab is not indicated for the treatment of patients with *RAS*-mutant mCRC or for whom *RAS* mutation status is unknown.

Local Anesthetic/Vasoconstrictor Precautions No information available to require special precautions

Effects on Dental Treatment Key adverse event(s) related to dental treatment: Stomatitis and mucositis.

Effects on Bleeding Although significant myelosuppression with associated altered hemostasis has been reported for many chemotherapeutic agents, myelosuppression is not common with panitumumab and no specific precautions appear to necessary.

Adverse Reactions

Monotherapy:

>10%:

Central nervous system: Fatigue (26%)

Dermatologic: Skin toxicity (90%; grades 3/4: 15%), erythema (66%; grades 3/4: 6%), pruritus (58%; grades 3/4: 3%), acneiform eruption (57%; grades 3/4: 7%), paronychia (25%; grades 3/4: 2%), rash (22%; grades 3/4: 1%), skin fissure (20%; grades 3/4: 1%), exfoliative dermatitis (18%; grades 3/4: 2%), acne vulgaris (14%; grades 3/4: 1%)

Endocrine & metabolic: Hypomagnesemia (grades 3/4: 7%)

Gastrointestinal: Nausea (23%), diarrhea (21%; grades 3/4: 2%), vomiting (19%)

Ophthalmic: Ocular toxicity (16%)

Respiratory: Dyspnea (18%), cough (15%)

Miscellaneous: Fever (17%)

1% to 10%:

Cardiovascular: Pulmonary embolism (1%)

Central nervous system: Chills (3%)

Dermatologic: Nail toxicity (10%), xeroderma (10%), desquamation (9%; grades 3/4: <1%), dermal ulcer (6%; grades 3/4: <1%), pustular rash (4%), papular rash (2%)

Endocrine & metabolic: Dehydration (3%)

Gastrointestinal: Mucositis (7%), stomatitis (7%), xerostomia (5%)

Immunologic: Antibody formation (≤5%)

Ophthalmic: Abnormal eyelash growth (6%), conjunctivitis (5%)

Respiratory: Epistaxis (4%), interstitial pulmonary disease (1%)

Miscellaneous: Infusion related reaction (3%; grades 3/4: <1%)

<1%: Hypersensitivity reaction, pulmonary fibrosis

Combination therapy with FOLFOX:

>10%:

Dermatologic: Skin rash (56%; grades 3/4: 17% to 26%), acneiform eruption (32%; grades 3/4: 10%), pruritus (23%; grades 3/4: <1%), paronychia (21%; grades 3/4: 3%), xeroderma (21%; grades 3/4: 2%), erythema (16%; grades 3/4: 2%), skin fissure (16%; grades 3/4: <1%), alopecia (15%), acne vulgaris (14%; grades 3/4: 3%)

Endocrine & metabolic: Hypomagnesemia (30%), hypokalemia (21%), weight loss (18%)

Gastrointestinal: Diarrhea (62%), anorexia (36%), abdominal pain (28%), stomatitis (27%), mucosal inflammation (25%)

Neuromuscular & skeletal: Weakness (25%)

Ophthalmic: Conjunctivitis (18%)

Respiratory: Epistaxis (14%)

1% to 10%:

Cardiovascular: Deep vein thrombosis (5%)

Central nervous system: Fatigue (≥1%), paresthesia (≥1%)

Dermatologic: Nail disorder (10%; grades 3/4: 1%), palmar-plantar erythrodysesthesia (9%; grades 3/4: 1%), cellulitis (3%)

Endocrine & metabolic: Dehydration (8%), hypocalcemia (6%)
Hypersensitivity: Hypersensitivity (≥1%)
Local: Localized infection (4%)
<1%: Antibody development

Postmarketing and/or case reports (mono- and combination therapy): Abscess, angioedema, bullous skin disease (mucocutaneous), corneal ulcer, keratitis, necrotizing fasciitis, sepsis, skin necrosis, Stevens-Johnson syndrome, toxic epidermal necrolysis

Mechanism of Action Panitumumab is a recombinant human IgG2 monoclonal antibody which binds specifically to the epidermal growth factor receptor (EGFR, HER1, c-ErbB-1) and competitively inhibits the binding of epidermal growth factor (EGF) and other ligands. Binding to the EGFR blocks phosphorylation and activation of intracellular tyrosine kinases, resulting in inhibition of cell survival, growth, proliferation, and transformation. EGFR signal transduction may result in *KRAS* and *NRAS* wild-type activation; cells with *RAS* mutations appear to be unaffected by EGFR inhibition.

Pharmacodynamics/Kinetics

Half-life Elimination ~7.5 days (range: 4 to 11 days)

Reproductive Considerations

Females of reproductive potential should use effective contraception during treatment and for at least 2 months after treatment.

Pregnancy Considerations

Based on animal reproduction studies and on the mechanism of action, panitumumab may cause fetal harm if administered during pregnancy. Panitumumab is a humanized monoclonal antibody (IgG_2). Potential placental transfer of human IgG is dependent upon the IgG subclass and gestational age, generally increasing as pregnancy progresses. The lowest exposure would be expected during the period of organogenesis (Palmeira 2012; Pentsuk 2009).

Because panitumumab inhibits epidermal growth factor (EGF), a component of fetal development, adverse effects on pregnancy would be expected.

Panobinostat (pan oh BIN oh stat)

Brand Names: US Farydak

Pharmacologic Category Antineoplastic Agent, Histone Deacetylase (HDAC) Inhibitor

Use Multiple myeloma: Treatment of multiple myeloma (in combination with bortezomib and dexamethasone) in patients who have received at least 2 prior regimens, including bortezomib and an immunomodulatory agent.

Local Anesthetic/Vasoconstrictor Precautions Panobinostat is one of the drugs confirmed to prolong the QT interval and is accepted as having a risk of causing torsade de pointes. The risk of drug-induced torsade de pointes is extremely low when a single QT interval prolonging drug is prescribed. In terms of epinephrine, it is not known what effect vasoconstrictors in the local anesthetic regimen will have in patients with a known history of congenital prolonged QT interval or in patients taking any medication that prolongs the QT interval. Until more information is obtained, it is suggested that the clinician consult with the physician prior to the use of a vasoconstrictor in suspected patients, and that the vasoconstrictor (epinephrine, mepivacaine, and levonordefrin [Carbocaine 2% with Neo-Cobefrin]) be used with caution.

Effects on Dental Treatment No significant effects or complications reported

Effects on Bleeding Chemotherapy may result in significant myelosuppression, potentially including significant reduction in platelet counts (thrombocytopenia) and altered hemostasis. In patients who are under active treatment with these agents, medical consult is suggested.

Adverse Reactions Frequency not always defined.

>10%:
Cardiovascular: Abnormal T waves on ECG (40%), peripheral edema (29%; grades 3/4: 2%), depression of ST segment on ECG (22%), cardiac arrhythmia (12%; grades 3/4: 3%)
Central nervous system: Fatigue (≤60%, grades 3/4: ≤25%), lethargy (≤60%; grades 3/4: ≤25%), malaise (≤60%; grades 3/4: ≤25%)
Endocrine & metabolic: Hypocalcemia (67%; grades 3/4: 5%), hypoalbuminemia (63%; grades 3/4: 2%), hypophosphatemia (63%; grades 3/4: 20%), hypokalemia (52%; grades 3/4: 18%), hyponatremia (49%; grades 3/4: 13%), hyperphosphatemia (29%; grades 3/4: 2%), hypermagnesemia (27%; grades 3/4: 5%), weight loss (12%; grades 3/4: 2%)
Gastrointestinal: Diarrhea (68%; grades 3/4: 25%), nausea (36%; grades 3/4: 6%), decreased appetite (28%; grades 3/4: 3%), vomiting (26%; grades 3/4: 7%)
Hematologic & oncologic: Thrombocytopenia (97%; grades 3/4: 67%), lymphocytopenia (82%; grades 3/4: 53%), leukopenia (81%; grades 3/4: 23%), neutropenia (75%; grades 3/4: 34%), anemia (62%; grades 3/4: 18%)
Hepatic: Hyperbilirubinemia (21%; grades 3/4: 1%)
Infection: Severe infection (31%; includes bacterial, fungal, and viral infections)
Neuromuscular & skeletal: Weakness (≤60%; grades ≥3: ≤25%)
Renal: Increased serum creatinine (41%; grades 3/4: 1%)
Miscellaneous: Fever (26%)

1% to 10%:
Cardiovascular: Hypertension (>2% to <10%), hypotension (>2% to <10%), orthostatic hypotension (>2% to <10%), palpitations (>2% to <10%), syncope (>2% to <10%), ischemic heart disease (4%), ECG changes, prolonged QT interval on ECG
Central nervous system: Chills (>2% to <10%), dizziness (>2% to <10%), headache (>2% to <10%), insomnia (>2% to <10%)
Dermatologic: Cheilitis (>2% to <10%), erythema (>2% to <10%), skin lesion (>2% to <10%), skin rash (>2% to <10%)
Endocrine & metabolic: Dehydration (>2% to <10%), fluid retention (>2% to <10%), hyperglycemia (>2% to <10%), hyperuricemia (>2% to <10%), hypomagnesemia (>2% to <10%), hypothyroidism (>2% to <10%)
Gastrointestinal: Abdominal distention (>2% to <10%), abdominal pain (>2% to <10%), colitis (>2% to <10%), dysgeusia (>2% to <10%), dyspepsia (>2% to <10%), flatulence (>2% to <10%), gastritis (>2% to <10%), gastrointestinal pain (>2% to <10%), xerostomia (>2% to <10%), gastrointestinal toxicity
Genitourinary: Urinary incontinence (>2% to <10%)
Hematologic & oncologic: Hemorrhage (grades 3/4: 4%)
Hepatic: Hepatitis B (>2% to <10%), increased serum alkaline phosphatase (>2% to <10%), increased serum transaminases, increased serum bilirubin

Infection: Sepsis (6%)

Neuromuscular & skeletal: Joint swelling (>2% to <10%), tremor (>2% to <10%)

Renal: Increased blood urea nitrogen (>2% to <10%), mean glomerular filtration rate decreased (>2% to <10%), renal failure (>2% to <10%)

Respiratory: Cough (>2% to <10%), dyspnea (>2% to <10%), rales (>2% to <10%), respiratory failure (>2% to <10%), wheezing (>2% to <10%)

Mechanism of Action Panobinostat is a histone deacetylase (HDAC) inhibitor; inhibits enzymatic activity of HDACs resulting in increased acetylation of histone proteins. Accumulation of acetylated histones and other proteins induces cell cycle arrest and/or apoptosis of some transformed cells. Panobinostat has minimal activity in multiple myeloma as a single-agent; however, synergistic activity is demonstrated when combined with bortezomib and dexamethasone (San-Miguel 2014).

Pharmacodynamics/Kinetics

Half-life Elimination ~37 hours

Time to Peak Within 2 hours

Reproductive Considerations

Pregnancy should be ruled out prior to treatment. Women of reproductive potential should avoid pregnancy and use an effective contraceptive during therapy and for at least 3 months after the last panobinostat dose. Males should use condoms during therapy and for at least 6 months after the last dose of panobinostat.

Pregnancy Considerations

Adverse events were observed in animal reproduction studies. Pregnancy should be ruled out prior to treatment.

◆ **Panobinostat Lactate** *see* Panobinostat *on page 1188*

◆ **Panretin** *see* Alitretinoin (Topical) *on page 102*

Pantoprazole (pan TOE pra zole)

Related Information

Gastrointestinal Disorders *on page 1678*

Brand Names: US Protonix

Brand Names: Canada ACT Pantoprazole [DSC]; AG-Pantoprazole; AG-Pantoprazole Sodium; APO-Pantoprazole; Auro-Pantoprazole; BIO-Pantoprazole; DOM-Pantoprazole; JAMP-Pantoprazole; M-Pantoprazole; Mar-Pantoprazole; MINT-Pantoprazole; MYLAN-Pantoprazole T; MYLAN-Pantoprazole [DSC]; NRA-Pantoprazole; Panto IV [DSC]; Pantoloc; Pantoprazole; Pantoprazole T; Pantoprazole-20; Pantoprazole-40; PMS-Pantoprazole; Priva-Pantoprazole; RAN-Pantoprazole; RIVA-Pantoprazole; SANDOZ Pantoprazole; Tecta; TEVA-Pantoprazole; TEVA-Pantoprazole Magnesium; VAN-Pantoprazole [DSC]

Pharmacologic Category Proton Pump Inhibitor; Substituted Benzimidazole

Use

Oral:

Gastroesophageal reflux disease, erosive or nonerosive:

Treatment of erosive esophagitis: Short-term treatment in the healing and symptomatic relief of erosive esophagitis in adults and pediatric patients ≥5 years of age.

Maintenance healing of erosive esophagitis: Maintenance of healing of erosive esophagitis and reduction in relapse rates of daytime and nighttime heartburn symptoms in adult patients.

Zollinger-Ellison syndrome: Long-term treatment of pathological hypersecretory conditions, such as Zollinger-Ellison syndrome.

IV:

Gastroesophageal reflux disease associated with a history of erosive esophagitis: Short-term treatment of adult patients with gastroesophageal reflux disease and a history of erosive esophagitis.

Zollinger-Ellison syndrome: Treatment of adult patients with pathological hypersecretory conditions, such as Zollinger-Ellison syndrome.

Local Anesthetic/Vasoconstrictor Precautions

No information available to require special precautions

Effects on Dental Treatment Key adverse event(s) related to dental treatment: Occurrence of facial edema and xerostomia (normal salivation resumes upon discontinuation) have been reported. Rare occurrence of loss of taste (ageusia) or distortion of the sense of taste (dysgeusia) have also been reported.

Effects on Bleeding No information available to require special precautions

Adverse Reactions Incidences are associated with adults unless otherwise specified.

>10%: Central nervous system: Headache (adults 12%; children & adolescents: >4%)

1% to 10%:

Cardiovascular: Facial edema (children, adolescents, & adults: ≤4%), edema (≤2%), thrombophlebitis (IV: ≤2%)

Central nervous system: Dizziness (children, adolescents, & adults: ≤4%), vertigo (children, adolescents, & adults: ≤4%), depression (≤2%)

Dermatologic: Skin rash (adults: ≤2%; children & adolescents: >4%), urticaria (children, adolescents, & adults: ≤4%), pruritus (≤2%), skin photosensitivity (≤2%)

Endocrine & metabolic: Increased serum triglycerides (children, adolescents, & adults: ≤4%)

Gastrointestinal: Diarrhea (children, adolescents, & adults: 4% to 9%), abdominal pain (children & adolescents: >4%), vomiting (children, adolescents, & adults: ≥4%), constipation (children, adolescents, & adults: ≤4%), flatulence (children & adolescents: ≤4%), nausea (children & adolescents: ≤4%), xerostomia (≤2%)

Hematologic & oncologic: Leukopenia (≤2%), thrombocytopenia (≤2%)

Hepatic: Increased liver enzymes (children, adolescents, & adults: ≤4%), hepatitis (≤2%)

Hypersensitivity: Hypersensitivity reaction (children, adolescents, & adults: ≤4%)

Neuromuscular & skeletal: Arthralgia (children, adolescents, & adults: ≤4%), increased creatine phosphokinase (children, adolescents, & adults: ≤4%), myalgia (children, adolescents, & adults: ≤4%)

Ophthalmic: Blurred vision (≤2%)

Respiratory: Upper respiratory tract infection (children & adolescents: >4%)

Miscellaneous: Fever (adults: ≤2%; children & adolescents: >4%)

<1%, postmarketing, and/or case reports: Acute interstitial nephritis, ageusia, agranulocytosis, anaphylactic shock, anaphylaxis, angioedema, asthenia, bone fracture, *Clostridioides* (formerly *Clostridium*) *difficile*-associated diarrhea, confusion, cutaneous lupus erythematous, drowsiness, dysgeusia, erythema multiforme, fatigue, gastric polyp (fundic gland), hallucination, hepatic failure, hepatotoxicity, hypomagnesemia, hyponatremia, insomnia, jaundice, laboratory test abnormality (false-positive for THC),

malaise, pancytopenia, pneumonia (Eom 2011), renal disease (chronic; Lazarus 2016), rhabdomyolysis, severe dermatological reaction, Stevens-Johnson syndrome, systemic lupus erythematosus, toxic epidermal necrolysis, weight changes

Mechanism of Action Proton pump inhibitor, suppresses gastric acid secretion by inhibiting the parietal cell H^+/K^+ ATP pump

Pharmacodynamics/Kinetics

Onset of Action

Onset of action: Acid secretion: Oral: 2.5 hours; IV: 15 to 30 minutes

Maximum effect: IV: 2 hours

Duration of Action Oral, IV: 24 hours

Half-life Elimination

Neonates (PMA: 37 to 44 weeks): ~3 hours (Ward 2010)

Children and Adolescents (Kearns 2008): IV (2 to 16 years of age): 1.22 ± 0.68 hours; Oral (5 to 16 years of age): 1.27 ± 1.29 hours

Adults: 1 hour; increased to 3.5 to 10 hours with CYP2C19 deficiency

Time to Peak

Children and Adolescents (Kearns 2008): IV (2 to 16 years of age): 0.34 ± 0.12 hours; Oral (5 to 16 years of age): 2.54 ± 0.72 hours

Adults: Oral: 2.5 hours

Pregnancy Considerations Recommendations for the treatment of gastroesophageal reflux disease in pregnancy are available. As in nonpregnant patients, lifestyle modifications followed by other medications are the initial treatments (Body 2016; Huerta-Iga 2016; Katz 2013; van der Woude 2014). Based on available data, PPIs may be used when clinically indicated (Body 2016; Matok 2012; Pasternak 2010; van der Woude 2014).

◆ **Pantoprazole Magnesium** *see* Pantoprazole *on page 1189*

◆ **Pantoprazole Sodium** *see* Pantoprazole *on page 1189*

◆ **Panzyga** *see* Immune Globulin *on page 803*

Papillomavirus (Types 6, 11, 16, 18) Vaccine (Human, Recombinant)

(pap ih LO ma VYE rus typs six e LEV en SIX teen AYE teen vak SEEN YU man ree KOM be nant)

Brand Names: Canada Gardasil

Pharmacologic Category Vaccine; Vaccine, Inactivated (Viral)

Use

Prevention of human papillomavirus infection:

Females ≥9 years of age and ≤26 years of age: Prevention of anal cancer caused by HPV types 16 and 18; anal intraepithelial neoplasia caused by HPV types 6, 11, 16, and 18

Females ≥9 years of age and ≤45 years of age: Prevention of cervical, vulvar, and vaginal cancer caused by HPV types 16 and 18; genital warts caused by HPV types 6 and 11; cervical adenocarcinoma *in situ*, vulvar, vaginal, or cervical intraepithelial neoplasia caused by HPV types 6, 11, 16, and 18

Males ≥9 years of age and ≤26 years of age: Prevention of anal cancer caused by HPV types 16 and 18; anal intraepithelial neoplasia caused by HPV types 6, 11, 16, and 18; genital warts caused by HPV types 6 and 11

The Canadian National Advisory Committee on Immunization (NACI) recommends routine vaccination for females and males between 9 and 26 years of age. It should not be administered in patients <9 years of age but may be administered to patients >26 years of age who are at ongoing risk of exposure (NACI 2017).

Local Anesthetic/Vasoconstrictor Precautions No information available to require special precautions

Effects on Dental Treatment No significant effects or complications reported (see Dental Health Professional Considerations)

Effects on Bleeding No information available to require special precautions

Adverse Reactions

>10%:

Central nervous system: Headache (8% to 21%)

Local: Pain at injection site (females: 82%; males: 61%), swelling at injection site (females: 24%; males: 14%), erythema at injection site (17% to 22%)

Miscellaneous: Fever (6% to 13%)

1% to 10%:

Central nervous system: Dizziness (≤1%)

Dermatologic: Injection site pruritus (females: 3%)

Gastrointestinal: Nausea (2% to 4%), diarrhea (males: 3%), toothache (females: 2%), vomiting (≤1%)

Local: Hematoma at injection site (females: 3%)

Neuromuscular & skeletal: Limb pain (females: 2% to 3%), arthralgia (≤1%), myalgia (≤1%)

Respiratory: Oropharyngeal pain (males: 3%), upper respiratory tract infection (males: 2%)

<1%, postmarketing, and/or case reports: Acute disseminated encephalomyelitis, anaphylactoid reaction, anaphylaxis, arthropathy (impaired joint movement at injection site), asthma, autoimmune disease, autoimmune hemolytic anemia, bronchospasm, cellulitis, chills, fatigue, Guillain-Barré syndrome, hypersensitivity reaction, immune thrombocytopenia, lymphadenopathy, malaise, neuromuscular disease, pancreatitis, paralysis, pulmonary embolism, syncope (may result in falls or be associated with tonic-clonic movements), transverse myelitis, urticaria, weakness seizure, sepsis, syncope (may result in falls with injury or be associated with tonic-clonic movements), transverse myelitis, urticaria, weakness

Mechanism of Action

Contains inactive human papillomavirus (HPV) proteins HPV 6 L1, HPV 11 L1, HPV 16 L1, and HPV 18 L1 which produce neutralizing antibodies to prevent cervical cancer, cervical adenocarcinoma, cervical, vaginal and vulvar neoplasia, and genital warts caused by HPV. The vaccine has not been shown to provide cross-protective efficacy to HPV types not contained in the vaccine. Immunogenicity has been measured by the percentage of persons who became seropositive for antibodies contained in the vaccine; the minimum anti-HPV antibody concentration needed to protect against disease has not been determined. The population benefit to vaccination is influenced by the prevalence of HPV within the geographic area and subject characteristics (eg, lifetime sexual partners).

Efficacy: In females 16 to 26 years of age, HPV4 has shown to be ~100% effective against HPV types 16- and 18-related cervical disease and 95% to 99% effective against external genital lesions related to HPV types 6, 11, 16, or 18. In males 16 to 26 years of age, HPV4 vaccine has shown to be 84% to 100% effective against external genital lesions related to HPV types 6, 11, 16, or 18. In females 24 to 45 years of age, the vaccine was shown to be 91% effective against HPV 6, 11, 16, and 18 persistent infection and cervical or external genital disease and 83% effective against HPV types 16 and 18 only. In addition, vaccination against HPV types 16 and 18 may prevent ~70% of anogenital cancers and 60% of high-risk precancerous cervical lesions (NACI 2017).

Pharmacodynamics/Kinetics

Onset of Action Seroconversion was observed 1 month following the last dose of vaccine

Duration of Action Duration unknown. Clinical studies followed HPV4 vaccinated participants for 10 years and found no evidence of waning protection (NACI 2017).

Reproductive Considerations

The manufacturer recommends pregnancy be avoided during the vaccination series.

Pregnancy Considerations

Administration of the human papillomavirus vaccine during pregnancy is not recommended. Although exposure to human papillomavirus vaccine has not been causally associated with adverse pregnancy outcomes, until additional information is available the vaccine series (or completion of the series) should be delayed until pregnancy is completed (NACI 2017).

Exposures to quadrivalent human papillomavirus vaccine during pregnancy should be reported to the manufacturer (800-567-2594) or Vaccine Safety Section at Public Health Agency of Canada (866-844-0018 or http://www.phac-aspc.gc.ca/im/vssv/index-eng.php).

Dental Health Professional Considerations

Human papilloma virus is widespread and serotypes 16 and 18 have been associated with cervical cancer. Although most types that cause oral HPV lesions are not of these serotypes, the clinician should recommend appropriate surgical removal of all such lesions. Lesions in the posterior oral pharyngeal region are of particular concern. Pre-exposure vaccination is one of the most effective methods for preventing transmission of some serotypes of HPV. Quadrivalent HPV vaccine (Gardasil) and the bivalent HPV vaccine (Cervarix) are available. Gardasil is indicated for the prevention of a number of diseases caused by oncogenic human papillomavirus (HPV) types 16 and 18 and approved for use in girls and women 9-26 years of age. Gardasil is also indicated in boys and men 9-26 years of age for the prevention of a number of diseases caused by HPV types (see Use).

Details regarding HPV vaccination are available at www.cdc.gov/std/hpv. Vaccines for other STDs (eg, HIV and herpes simplex virus) are under development or undergoing clinical trials. Vaccines are not available for bacterial or fungal STDs.

Papillomavirus (Types 16, 18) Vaccine (Human, Recombinant)

(pap ih LO ma VYE rus typs SIX teen AYE teen vak SEEN YU man ree KOM be nant)

Brand Names: Canada Cervarix

Pharmacologic Category Vaccine; Vaccine, Inactivated (Viral)

Use

Prevention of human papillomavirus infection: Prevention in females 9 to 45 years of age of the following diseases caused by oncogenic HPV types 16 and 18: Cervical cancer, cervical intraepithelial neoplasia (CIN) grades 1 to 3 and cervical adenocarcinoma in situ

The Canadian National Advisory Committee on Immunization (NACI) recommends routine vaccination for females between 9 and 26 years of age. It should not be administered in females <9 years but may be administered to females >26 years who are at ongoing risk of exposure (NACI 2017).

Local Anesthetic/Vasoconstrictor Precautions

No information available to require special precautions

Effects on Dental Treatment No significant effects or complications reported (see Dental Health Professional Considerations)

Effects on Bleeding No information available to require special precautions

Adverse Reactions

>10%:

Central nervous system: Fatigue (55%)

Local: Pain at injection site (92%), erythema at injection site (48%), swelling at injection site (44%)

Neuromuscular & skeletal: Myalgia (49%), arthralgia (21%)

1% to 10%:

Dermatologic: Urticaria (7%), injection site pruritus (1%)

Genitourinary: Vaginal infection (1%)

Infection: Influenza (3%), infection (chlamydia: 2%)

Respiratory: Nasopharyngitis (4%), pharyngolaryngeal pain (3%), pharyngitis (2%)

<1%, postmarketing, and/or case reports: Anaphylactoid reaction, anaphylaxis, angioedema, erythema multiforme, hypersensitivity reaction, induration at injection site, lymphadenopathy, paresthesia (local), syncope (may be associated with tonic-clonic movements), vasodepressor syncope

Mechanism of Action Contains inactive human papillomavirus (HPV) proteins HPV 16 L1, and HPV 18 L1 which produce neutralizing antibodies to prevent cervical cancer, cervical adenocarcinoma, and cervical neoplasia cause by HPV.

Efficacy: HPV2 has shown to be 95% to 99% effective against HPV types 16 and 18-related cervical disease in females 15 to 25 years of age. In addition, vaccination against HPV types 16 and 18 may prevent ~70% of anogenital cancers and 60% of high-risk precancerous cervical lesions (NACI 2017).

Pharmacodynamics/Kinetics

Onset of Action Seroconversion was observed at month 7

Duration of Action Unknown. Clinical studies followed HPV2 vaccinated participants for 10 years and found no evidence of waning protection (NACI 2017).

Reproductive Considerations

The manufacturer recommends pregnancy be avoided for 2 months following vaccination.

Pregnancy Considerations

Administration of the human papillomavirus vaccine during pregnancy is not recommended. Although exposure to human papillomavirus vaccine has not been causally associated with adverse pregnancy outcomes, until additional information is available the vaccine series (or completion of the series) should be delayed until pregnancy is completed (NACI 2017).

Exposures to bivalent human papillomavirus vaccine during pregnancy should be reported to the manufacturer (800-387-7374).

Dental Health Professional Considerations

Human papilloma virus is widespread and serotypes 16 and 18 have been associated with cervical cancer. Although most types that cause oral HPV lesions are not of these serotypes, the clinician should recommend appropriate surgical removal of all such lesions. Lesions in the posterior oral pharyngeal region are of particular concern. Pre-exposure vaccination is one of the most effective methods for preventing transmission of some serotypes of HPV. Quadrivalent HPV vaccine (Gardasil) and the bivalent HPV vaccine (Cervarix) are available. Cervarix is indicated for the prevention of a number of diseases caused by oncogenic human papillomavirus (HPV) types 16 and 18 and approved for use in females 9-25 years of age (see Use).

Details regarding HPV vaccination are available at www.cdc.gov/std/hpv. Vaccines for other STDs (eg, HIV and herpes simplex virus) are under development or undergoing clinical trials. Vaccines are not available for bacterial or fungal STDs.

- **PAR-101** *see* Fidaxomicin *on page 668*
- **Para-Aminosalicylate Sodium** *see* Aminosalicylic Acid *on page 118*
- **Para-Aminosalicylic Acid** *see* Aminosalicylic Acid *on page 118*
- **Paracetamol** *see* Acetaminophen *on page 59*
- **Parafon Forte** *see* Chlorzoxazone *on page 344*
- **Parafon Forte DSC [DSC]** *see* Chlorzoxazone *on page 344*
- **Paragard Intrauterine Copper** *see* Copper IUD *on page 410*
- **Paraplatin** *see* CARBOplatin *on page 292*

Parathyroid Hormone (par a THYE roid HOR mone)

Brand Names: US Natpara

Pharmacologic Category Parathyroid Hormone Analog

Use

Hypoparathyroidism: Adjunct to calcium and vitamin D to control hypocalcemia in patients with hypoparathyroidism

Limitations of use: Because of the potential risk of osteosarcoma, recommended only for patients who cannot be well-controlled on calcium supplements and active forms of vitamin D alone; has not been studied in patients with hypoparathyroidism caused by calcium-sensing receptor mutations or in patients with acute postsurgical hypoparathyroidism

Local Anesthetic/Vasoconstrictor Precautions No information available to require special precautions

Effects on Dental Treatment No significant effects or complications reported

Effects on Bleeding No information available to require special precautions

Adverse Reactions

>10%:

Central nervous system: Paresthesia (31%), headache (25%), hypoesthesia (14%)

Endocrine & metabolic: Hypocalcemia (27%), hypercalcemia (19%)

Gastrointestinal: Diarrhea (12%), vomiting (12%)

Genitourinary: Hypercalciuria (11%)

Immunologic: Antibody development (9% to 16%)

Neuromuscular & skeletal: Arthralgia (11%)

1% to 10%:

Cardiovascular: Hypertension (6%)

Central nervous system: Peripheral pain (10%), facial hypoesthesia (6%)

Endocrine & metabolic: Inhibited conversion of vitamin D3 to 25-hydroxy-D3 (6%)

Gastrointestinal: Upper abdominal pain (7%)

Neuromuscular & skeletal: Neck pain (6%)

Respiratory: Upper respiratory tract infection (8%), sinusitis (7%)

<1%, postmarketing, and/or case reports: Anaphylaxis, angioedema, hypersensitivity reaction, seizure

Mechanism of Action Exogenous parathyroid hormone; parathyroid hormone raises serum calcium concentrations by increasing renal tubular calcium reabsorption, increasing intestinal calcium absorption, and by increasing bone turnover, which releases calcium into the circulation.

Pharmacodynamics/Kinetics

Onset of Action Peak effect: 10 to 12 hours

Duration of Action >24 hours

Half-life Elimination ~3 hours

Time to Peak 5 to 30 minutes

Pregnancy Risk Factor C

Pregnancy Considerations Adverse events were observed in animal reproduction studies.

- **Parathyroid Hormone (1-34)** *see* Teriparatide *on page 1424*
- **Parcopa** *see* Carbidopa and Levodopa *on page 290*

Paregoric (par e GOR ik)

Pharmacologic Category Analgesic, Opioid; Antidiarrheal

Use Diarrhea: Treatment of diarrhea

Local Anesthetic/Vasoconstrictor Precautions No information available to require special precautions

Effects on Dental Treatment No significant effects or complications reported

Effects on Bleeding No information available to require special precautions

Adverse Reactions Frequency not defined.

Cardiovascular: Hypotension, peripheral vasodilation

Central nervous system: Central nervous system depression, depression, dizziness, drowsiness, drug dependence (physical and psychological), dysphoria, euphoria, headache, increased intracranial pressure, insomnia, malaise, restlessness, sedation

Dermatologic: Pruritus

Gastrointestinal: Anorexia, biliary tract spasm, constipation, nausea, stomach cramps, vomiting

Genitourinary: Decreased urine output, ureteral spasm

Hepatic: Increased liver enzymes

Hypersensitivity: Histamine release

Neuromuscular & skeletal: Weakness

Ophthalmic: Miosis

Respiratory: Respiratory depression

Postmarketing and/or case reports: Hypogonadism (Brennan, 2013; Debono, 2011)

Mechanism of Action Increases smooth muscle tone in GI tract, decreases motility and peristalsis, diminishes digestive secretions

Reproductive Considerations Long-term opioid use may cause secondary hypogonadism, which may lead to sexual dysfunction and infertility (Brennan 2013).

Pregnancy Risk Factor C

Pregnancy Considerations Paregoric contains morphine 2 mg/5 mL and alcohol 45%. Morphine crosses the placenta and enters the fetal circulation. Maternal use of opioids may be associated with birth defects, poor fetal growth, stillbirth, and preterm delivery (CDC [Dowell 2016]). If chronic opioid exposure occurs in pregnancy, adverse events in the newborn (including withdrawal) may occur (Chou 2009). The alcohol content should also be taken into consideration in pregnant women. Paregoric is approved for the treatment of diarrhea in adults; however, agents other than paregoric should be used in pregnant women (Christie 2007; Zielinski 2015).

Refer to the Morphine (Systemic) monograph for additional information.

Controlled Substance C-III

Paricalcitol (pah ri KAL si tole)

Brand Names: US Zemplar
Brand Names: Canada Zemplar
Pharmacologic Category Vitamin D Analog
Use

IV: Prevention and treatment of secondary hyperparathyroidism in adults and pediatric patients 5 years and older with chronic kidney disease (CKD) on dialysis

Oral: Prevention and treatment in adults and pediatric patients 10 years and older with secondary hyperparathyroidism associated with stage 3 and 4 CKD and stage 5 CKD patients on hemodialysis or peritoneal dialysis

Local Anesthetic/Vasoconstrictor Precautions No information available to require special precautions

Effects on Dental Treatment Key adverse event(s) related to dental treatment: Xerostomia (normal salivary flow resumes upon discontinuation).

Effects on Bleeding No information available to require special precautions

Adverse Reactions As reported in adults, unless otherwise noted.

>10%:

Gastrointestinal: Nausea (children, adolescents, and adults: 5% to 13%), diarrhea (7% to 12%)
Infection: Infection (bacterial, fungal, viral: 3% to 15%)
Respiratory: Rhinitis (children and adolescents: 17%)

1% to 10%:

Cardiovascular: Hypertension (7%), edema (6% to 7%), hypotension (5%), palpitations (3%), chest pain (3%), peripheral edema (3%), syncope (3%), atrial flutter (<2%), cardiac arrhythmia (<2%), cerebrovascular accident (<2%), chest discomfort (<2%), ischemic bowel disease (<2%)
Central nervous system: Dizziness (5% to 7%), chills (5%), insomnia (5%), vertigo (5%), headache (3% to 5%), anxiety (3%), depression (3%), fatigue (3%), malaise (3%), abnormal gait (<2%), agitation (<2%), confusion (<2%), delirium (<2%), hypoesthesia (<2%), myoclonus (<2%), nervousness (<2%), paresthesia (<2%), restlessness (<2%)
Dermatologic: Skin rash (4% to 6%), dermal ulcer (3%), ecchymoses (3%), acne vulgaris (<2%), alopecia (<2%), burning sensation of skin (<2%), extravasation reactions (<2%), night sweats (<2%), pruritus (<2%), urticaria (<2%)
Endocrine & metabolic: Hypervolemia (5%), dehydration (3%), hypoglycemia (3%), hirsutism (<2%), hypercalcemia (<2%), hyperkalemia (<2%), hyperparathyroidism (<2%), hyperphosphatemia (<2%), hypocalcemia (<2%), hypoparathyroidism (<2%), increased thirst (<2%), weight loss (<2%)
Gastrointestinal: Vomiting (5% to 8%), gastrointestinal hemorrhage (5%), peritonitis (5%), constipation (4% to 5%), abdominal pain (4%), dyspepsia (3%), xerostomia (3%), decreased appetite (<2%), dysgeusia (<2%), dysphagia (<2%), gastritis (<2%), gastroesophageal reflux disease (<2%)
Genitourinary: Urinary urgency (children and adolescents: 6%), chronic renal failure (3%), uremia (3%), urinary tract infection (3%), erectile dysfunction (<2%), mastalgia (<2%), vaginal infection (<2%)
Hematologic & oncologic: Anemia (<2%), lymphadenopathy (<2%), malignant neoplasm of breast (<2%), prolonged bleeding time (<2%), rectal hemorrhage (<2%)
Hepatic: Abnormal hepatic function tests (<2%), increased serum AST (<2%)
Hypersensitivity: Hypersensitivity reaction (6%)
Infection: Influenza (5%), sepsis (5%)
Local: Pain at injection site (<2%)
Neuromuscular & skeletal: Arthralgia (5%), arthritis (5%), weakness (3% to 5%), back pain (3% to 4%), leg cramps (3%), muscle spasm (3%), joint stiffness (<2%), muscle twitching (<2%), myalgia (<2%)
Ophthalmic: Conjunctivitis (children and adolescents: 6%; adults: <2%), glaucoma (<2%), ocular hyperemia (<2%)
Otic: Otalgia (<2%)
Respiratory: Nasopharyngitis (8%), asthma (children and adolescents: 6%), pneumonia (5%), oropharyngeal pain (4%), bronchitis (3%), cough (3%), sinusitis (3%), dyspnea (<2%), orthopnea (<2%), pulmonary edema (<2%), upper respiratory tract infection (<2%), wheezing (<2%)
Miscellaneous: Fever (3% to 5%), laboratory test abnormality (<2%), swelling (<2%)

<1%, postmarketing, and/or case reports: Angioedema (including laryngeal edema), increased serum creatinine

Mechanism of Action Decreased renal conversion of vitamin D to its primary active metabolite (1,25-hydroxyvitamin D) in chronic renal failure leads to reduced activation of vitamin D receptor (VDR), which subsequently removes inhibitory suppression of parathyroid hormone (PTH) release; increased serum PTH (secondary hyperparathyroidism) reduces calcium excretion and enhances bone resorption. Paricalcitol is a synthetic vitamin D analog which binds to and activates the VDR in kidney, parathyroid gland, intestine and bone, thus reducing PTH levels and improving calcium and phosphate homeostasis.

Pharmacodynamics/Kinetics

Half-life Elimination

Healthy subjects: Oral: 4 to 6 hours; IV: 5 to 7 hours
Stage 3 and 4 CKD: Oral: 17 to 20 hours
Stage 5 CKD (on HD or PD): Oral: 14 to 18 hours; IV: 14 to 15 hours

Time to Peak Plasma: 3 hours: Delayed by food

Pregnancy Considerations Adverse events have been observed in some animal reproduction studies.

- **Pariprazole** *see* RABEprazole *on page 1302*
- **Paritaprevir, Ombitasvir, and Ritonavir** *see* Ombitasvir, Paritaprevir, and Ritonavir *on page 1135*
- **Paritaprevir, Ombitasvir, Ritonavir, and Dasabuvir** *see* Ombitasvir, Paritaprevir, Ritonavir, and Dasabuvir *on page 1136*
- **Parnate** *see* Tranylcypromine *on page 1479*
- **parodontax [OTC]** *see* Fluoride *on page 693*
- **Paroex** *see* Chlorhexidine Gluconate (Oral) *on page 334*

Paromomycin (par oh moe MYE sin)

Brand Names: Canada Humatin
Pharmacologic Category Amebicide

Use

Intestinal amebiasis: Treatment of acute and chronic intestinal amebiasis (not effective for extraintestinal amebiasis).

Hepatic coma: Management (adjunctive) of hepatic coma.

Local Anesthetic/Vasoconstrictor Precautions No information available to require special precautions

Effects on Dental Treatment No significant effects or complications reported

Effects on Bleeding No information available to require special precautions

Adverse Reactions

1% to 10%: Gastrointestinal: Abdominal cramps, diarrhea, heartburn, nausea, vomiting

<1%, postmarketing, and/or case reports: Enterocolitis (secondary), eosinophilia, headache, ototoxicity, pruritus, steatorrhea, vertigo

Mechanism of Action Acts directly on ameba; has antibacterial activity against normal and pathogenic organisms in the GI tract; interferes with bacterial protein synthesis by binding to 30S ribosomal subunits

Pregnancy Considerations Paromomycin is poorly absorbed when given orally. Information related to the use of paromomycin in pregnancy is limited (Kreutner 1981). Use may be considered for the treatment of giardiasis throughout pregnancy (Gardner 2001) or cryptosporidiosis after the first trimester (DHHS 2013) in pregnant women.

Product Availability Topical paromomycin is not commercially available in the US; IDSA/ASTMH guidelines for diagnosis and treatment of leishmaniasis suggest collaboration with a compounding pharmacy.

◆ **Paromomycin Sulfate** *see* Paromomycin *on page 1193*

PARoxetine (pa ROKS e teen)

Related Information

Dentin Hypersensitivity, Acid Erosion, High Caries Index, Management of Alveolar Osteitis, and Xerostomia *on page 1762*

Management of the Patient With Anxiety or Depression *on page 1778*

Vasoconstrictor Interactions With Antidepressants *on page 1821*

Brand Names: US Brisdelle; Paxil; Paxil CR; Pexeva

Brand Names: Canada ACT PARoxetine; AG-Paroxetine; APO-PARoxetine; Auro-PARoxetine; BIO-PARoxetine; DOM-PARoxetine; JAMP-PARoxetine; M-Paroxetine; Mar-PARoxetine; MINT-Paroxetine; MYLAN-PARoxetine [DSC]; NRA-Paroxetine; NU-PARoxetine [DSC]; PARoxetine-10; PARoxetine-20; PARoxetine-30; Paxil; Paxil CR; PMS-PARoxetine; Priva-PARoxetine; RIVA-PARoxetine; SANDOZ PARoxetine; TARO-PARoxetine; TEVA-PARoxetine

Pharmacologic Category Antidepressant, Selective Serotonin Reuptake Inhibitor

Use

Generalized anxiety disorder (immediate release): Treatment of generalized anxiety disorder.

Major depressive disorder (unipolar) (immediate and extended release): Treatment of unipolar major depressive disorder.

Obsessive-compulsive disorder (immediate release): Treatment of obsessions and compulsions in patients with obsessive-compulsive disorder.

Panic disorder (immediate and extended release): Treatment of panic disorder, with or without agoraphobia.

Posttraumatic stress disorder (immediate release): Treatment of posttraumatic stress disorder.

Premenstrual dysphoric disorder (extended release): Treatment of premenstrual dysphoric disorder.

Social anxiety disorder (immediate and extended release): Treatment of social anxiety disorder, also known as social phobia.

Vasomotor symptoms of menopause (immediate release; 7.5 mg capsule): Treatment of moderate to severe vasomotor symptoms associated with menopause.

Local Anesthetic/Vasoconstrictor Precautions Although caution should be used in patients taking tricyclic antidepressants, no interactions have been reported with vasoconstrictor and paroxetine, a nontricyclic antidepressant which acts to increase serotonin; no precautions appear to be needed

Effects on Dental Treatment Key adverse event(s) related to dental treatment: Xerostomia and changes in salivation (normal salivary flow resumes upon discontinuation), and abnormal taste. Patients may experience orthostatic hypotension as they stand up after treatment; especially if lying in dental chair for extended periods of time. Use caution with sudden changes in position during and after dental treatment. Problems with SSRI-induced bruxism have been reported and may preclude their use; clinicians attempting to evaluate any patient with bruxism or involuntary muscle movement, who is simultaneously being treated with an SSRI drug, should be aware of the potential association. Rare occurrence of aphthous stomatitis and tongue edema.

Effects on Bleeding May impair platelet aggregation resulting in increased risk of bleeding events, particularly if used concomitantly with aspirin, NSAIDs, warfarin, or other anticoagulants. Bleeding related to SSRI use has been reported to range from relatively minor bruising and epistaxis to life-threatening hemorrhage. Routine interruption of therapy for most dental procedures is not warranted. In medically complicated patients or extensive oral surgery, the decision to interrupt therapy must be based on the risk to benefit in an individual patient and a medical consult is suggested. If therapy is continued without interruption, the clinician should anticipate the potential for a prolonged bleeding time.

Adverse Reactions Incidence varies by dose and indication. Adverse reactions reported as a composite of all indications.

>10%:

Dermatologic: Diaphoresis (5% to 14%)

Endocrine & metabolic: Decreased libido (3% to 15% [placebo: 0% to 5%])

Gastrointestinal: Constipation (2% to 16%), decreased appetite (1% to 12%), diarrhea (6% to 18%), dyspepsia (2% to 13%), nausea (17% to 26%), xerostomia (3% to 18%)

Genitourinary: Ejaculatory disorder (13% to 28% [placebo: 0% to 2%])

Nervous system: Dizziness (6% to 14%), drowsiness (3% to 24%; less frequent in children and adolescents) (Safer 2006), headache (6% to 27%), insomnia (7% to 24%)

Neuromuscular & skeletal: Asthenia (12% to 22%), tremor (4% to 11%)

1% to 10%:

Cardiovascular: Chest pain (3%), hypertension (≥1%), palpitations (2% to 3%), tachycardia (≥1%), vasodilation (2% to 4%)

Dermatologic: Pruritus (≥1%), skin rash (2% to 3%)

Endocrine & metabolic: Weight gain (≥1%)

Gastrointestinal: Abdominal pain (4% to 7%), dysgeusia (2%), flatulence (4% to 6%), increased appetite (2% to 4%), nausea and vomiting (4%), vomiting (2% to 3%; more frequent in children [two- to threefold] and adolescents) (Safer 2006)

Genitourinary: Difficulty in micturition (3%), dysmenorrhea (5%), female genital tract disease (2% to 10% [placebo: 0% to 1%]), impotence (2% to 10% [placebo: 0% to 3%]), male genital disease (10% [placebo: 0%]), orgasm disturbance (2% to 10% [placebo: 0% to 1%]), urinary frequency (2% to 3%), urinary tract infection (2%), urination disorder (3%)

Infection: Infection (5% to 6%)

Nervous system: Abnormal dreams (3% to 4%), agitation (3% to 5%), amnesia (2%), anxiety (2% to 5%), chills (2%), confusion (1%), depersonalization (3%), drugged feeling (2%), emotional lability (≥1%), fatigue (5%), lack of concentration (3% to 4%), manic reaction (1% to 2%), myasthenia (1%), myoclonus (2% to 3%), nervousness (4% to 9%), paresthesia (4%), vertigo (≥1%), yawning (2% to 5%)

Neuromuscular & skeletal: Arthralgia (≥1%), back pain (3% to 5%), myalgia (2% to 5%), myopathy (2%)

Ophthalmic: Blurred vision (4%), visual disturbance (2% to 5%)

Otic: Tinnitus (≥1%)

Respiratory: Pharyngeal edema (2%), pharyngitis (4%), respiratory system disorder (7%), rhinitis (3%), sinusitis (≤8%)

Miscellaneous: Trauma (3% to 6%)

<1%:

Cardiovascular: Acute myocardial infarction, angina pectoris, bradycardia, bundle branch block, cardiac failure, cerebral ischemia, cerebrovascular accident, eclampsia, hypotension, ischemic heart disease, low cardiac output, phlebitis, pulmonary embolism, syncope, thrombophlebitis, thrombosis, torsades de pointes, vasculitis (Welsh 2006; Margolese 2001), ventricular arrhythmia

Dermatologic: Cellulitis, ecchymoses, erythema of skin, exfoliative dermatitis, fungal dermatitis, Stevens-Johnson syndrome, toxic epidermal necrolysis (Ahmed 2008)

Endocrine & metabolic: Dehydration, diabetes mellitus, goiter, hypercholesterolemia, hyperglycemia, hyperthyroidism, hypoglycemia, hypothyroidism, increased lactate dehydrogenase, ketosis

Gastrointestinal: Aphthous stomatitis, bloody diarrhea, cholelithiasis, colitis, dysphagia, esophageal achalasia, fecal impaction, gastroenteritis, hematemesis, intestinal obstruction, pancreatitis, peptic ulcer, peritonitis

Hematologic & oncologic: Anemia, hematoma, hemorrhage, hypergammaglobulinemia, lymphadenopathy, pancytopenia, prolonged bleeding time, quantitative disorders of platelets

Hepatic: Abnormal hepatic function tests, hepatic necrosis, hepatitis (Colakoglu 2005), hyperbilirubinemia, increased serum alkaline phosphatase, jaundice

Hypersensitivity: Anaphylaxis, angioedema (Mithani 1996), hypersensitivity reaction (Mera 2006), tongue edema (Mithani 1996)

Infection: Sepsis

Nervous system: Adrenergic syndrome, aphasia, behavioral problems, bulimia nervosa, delirium, drug dependence, dystonia, extrapyramidal reaction, Guillain-Barre syndrome, hallucination, meningitis, migraine, neuroleptic malignant syndrome (with drug interactions) (Tanii 2006; Uguz 2013), neuropathy, seizure, serotonin syndrome (Hudd 2020; Velez 2004), status epilepticus, suicidal ideation (Hammad 2006), suicidal tendencies (Hammad 2006)

Neuromuscular & skeletal: Akinesia, dyskinesia, increased creatine phosphokinase in blood specimen, myelitis, osteoarthritis, osteoporosis, tetany

Ophthalmic: Cataract

Otic: Deafness

Renal: Acute renal failure, increased blood urea nitrogen

Respiratory: Asthma, bronchitis, dyspnea, hemoptysis, pneumonia, pulmonary edema, pulmonary emphysema, pulmonary fibrosis, pulmonary hypertension

Postmarketing:

Cardiovascular: Atrial fibrillation, atrioventricular nodal arrhythmia (Kopp 2001), edema (Uguz 2014), orthostatic hypotension (Andrews 1998), ventricular fibrillation (Lee 2018), ventricular tachycardia

Dermatologic: Acute generalized exanthematous pustulosis (Mameli 2013), erythema multiforme (Rodriguez-Pazos 2011), hyperhidrosis, urticaria (Welsh 2006)

Endocrine & metabolic: Galactorrhea not associated with childbirth (Gonzales 2000; Morrison 2001), hyperprolactinemia (Evrensel 2016), hyponatremia (Gandhi 2017), porphyria, SIADH (Gandhi 2017), uncontrolled diabetes mellitus

Gastrointestinal: Acute pancreatitis, hemorrhagic pancreatitis, stomatitis (angular) (Verma 2012)

Genitourinary: Priapism (Ahmad 1995), urinary incontinence (Votolato 2000), urinary retention

Hematologic & oncologic: Abnormal erythrocytes, agranulocytosis, aplastic anemia, bone marrow aplasia, eosinophilia (Yasui-Furukori 2012), hemolytic anemia, Henoch-Schonlein purpura, immune thrombocytopenia, thrombocytopenia (Ono 2013)

Hepatic: Hepatic failure, hepatotoxicity (Azaz-Livshits 2002; Benbow 1997)

Hypersensitivity: Nonimmune anaphylaxis

Nervous system: Aggressive behavior (Nishida 2008; Sharma 2016), akathisia (Baldassano 1996), depression, disorientation (Wakeno 2007), homicidal ideation (Moore 2010), hyperactive behavior (agitation, hyperactivation, hyperkinesis, restlessness; more frequent in children [two- to threefold] and adolescents) (Safer 2006), hypertonia, malaise, restless leg syndrome (Rottach 2008; Sanz-Fuentenebro 1996), restlessness (Naslund 2017), tremor (Lai 2005), trismus, withdrawal syndrome (Fava 2015)

Ophthalmic: Acute angle-closure glaucoma (Eke 1997; Kirwan 1997; Lewis 1997), mydriasis (dose-dependent) (Nielsen 2010), optic neuritis

Respiratory: Hypersensitivity pneumonitis (Maia 2015), laryngismus

Mechanism of Action Paroxetine is a selective serotonin reuptake inhibitor, chemically unrelated to tricyclic, tetracyclic, or other antidepressants; presumably, the inhibition of serotonin reuptake from brain synapse stimulated serotonin activity in the brain

Pharmacodynamics/Kinetics

Onset of Action

Anxiety disorders (generalized anxiety, obsessive-compulsive, panic, and posttraumatic stress disorder): Initial effects may be observed within 2 weeks of treatment, with continued improvements through 4 to 6 weeks (Issari 2016; Varigonda 2016; WFSBP [Bandelow 2012]); some experts suggest up to 12 weeks of treatment may be necessary for response, particularly in patients with obsessive-compulsive disorder and posttraumatic stress disorder (BAP [Baldwin 2014]; Katzman 2014; WFSBP [Bandelow 2012]).

Body dysmorphic disorder: Initial effects may be observed within 2 weeks; some experts suggest up to 12 to 16 weeks of treatment may be necessary for response in some patients (Phillips 2008).

Depression: Initial effects may be observed within 1 to 2 weeks of treatment, with continued improvements through 4 to 6 weeks (Papakostas 2006; Posternak 2005; Szegedi 2009; Taylor 2006).

Premenstrual dysphoric disorder: Initial effects may be observed within the first few days of treatment, with response at the first menstrual cycle of treatment (ISPMD [Nevatte 2013]).

Half-life Elimination Paxil: 21 hours; Paxil CR: 15 to 20 hours; Pexeva: 33.2 hours

Time to Peak

Capsules: Median: 6 hours (range: 3 to 8 hours)

Tablets, oral suspension: Immediate release: Mean: 5.2 to 8.1 hours

Tablets: Controlled release: 6 to 10 hours

Pregnancy Risk Factor D/X (product specific)

Pregnancy Considerations

Paroxetine crosses the placenta (Hendrick 2003). An increased risk of teratogenic effects, including cardiovascular defects, may be associated with maternal use of paroxetine or other SSRIs; however, available information is conflicting. Nonteratogenic effects in the newborn following SSRI/SNRI exposure late in the third trimester include respiratory distress, cyanosis, apnea, seizures, temperature instability, feeding difficulty, vomiting, hypoglycemia, hypo- or hypertonia, hyper-reflexia, jitteriness, irritability, constant crying, and tremor. Symptoms may be due to the toxicity of the SSRIs/SNRIs or a discontinuation syndrome and may be consistent with serotonin syndrome associated with SSRI treatment. Persistent pulmonary hypertension of the newborn (PPHN) has also been reported with SSRI exposure. The long-term effects of in utero SSRI exposure on infant development and behavior are not known.

Due to pregnancy-induced physiologic changes, some pharmacokinetic parameters of paroxetine may be altered. The maternal CYP2D6 genotype also influences paroxetine plasma concentrations during pregnancy (Hostetter 2000; Ververs 2009).

The manufacturer suggests discontinuing paroxetine or switching to another antidepressant unless the benefits of therapy justify continuing treatment during pregnancy; consider other treatment options for women who are planning to become pregnant. The ACOG recommends that therapy with SSRIs or SNRIs during pregnancy be individualized; treatment of depression during pregnancy should incorporate the clinical expertise of the mental health clinician, obstetrician, primary health care provider, and pediatrician. The ACOG also recommends that therapy with paroxetine be avoided during pregnancy if possible and that fetuses exposed in early pregnancy be assessed with a fetal echocardiography (ACOG 2008). Other guidelines note that treatment with paroxetine should not be initiated in pregnant women (Bauer 2013). According to the American Psychiatric Association (APA), the risks of medication treatment should be weighed against other treatment options and untreated depression. The use of paroxetine is not recommended as first line therapy during pregnancy. For women who discontinue antidepressant medications during pregnancy and who may be at high risk for postpartum depression, the medications can be restarted following delivery (APA 2010). Treatment algorithms have been developed by the ACOG and the APA for the management of depression in women prior to conception and during pregnancy (Yonkers 2009).

Menopausal vasomotor symptoms do not occur during pregnancy; therefore, the use of paroxetine for the treatment of menopausal vasomotor symptoms is contraindicated in pregnant women.

Pregnant women exposed to antidepressants during pregnancy are encouraged to enroll in the National Pregnancy Registry for Antidepressants (NPRAD). Women 18 to 45 years of age or their health care providers may contact the registry by calling 844-405-6185. Enrollment should be done as early in pregnancy as possible.

- ◆ **Paroxetine HCl** *see* PARoxetine *on page 1194*
- ◆ **Paroxetine Hydrochloride** *see* PARoxetine *on page 1194*
- ◆ **Paroxetine Mesylate** *see* PARoxetine *on page 1194*
- ◆ **PARP Inhibitor AZD2281** *see* Olaparib *on page 1130*
- ◆ **PAS** *see* Aminosalicylic Acid *on page 118*
- ◆ **Paser** *see* Aminosalicylic Acid *on page 118*
- ◆ **Patanase** *see* Olopatadine (Nasal) *on page 1132*
- ◆ **Paxil** *see* PARoxetine *on page 1194*
- ◆ **Paxil CR** *see* PARoxetine *on page 1194*

PAZOPanib (paz OH pa nib)

Related Information

Clinical Risk Related to Drugs Prolonging QT Interval *on page 1675*

Brand Names: US Votrient

Brand Names: Canada Votrient

Pharmacologic Category Antineoplastic Agent, Tyrosine Kinase Inhibitor; Antineoplastic Agent, Vascular Endothelial Growth Factor (VEGF) Inhibitor

Use

Renal cell carcinoma, advanced: Treatment of advanced renal cell carcinoma

Soft tissue sarcoma, advanced: Treatment of advanced soft tissue sarcoma (in patients who have received prior chemotherapy)

Limitations of use: The efficacy of pazopanib for the treatment of adipocytic soft tissue sarcoma or gastrointestinal stromal tumors (GIST) has not been demonstrated.

Local Anesthetic/Vasoconstrictor Precautions

Hypertension can occur with the use of this drug, particularly early in the treatment course. Monitor for hypertension prior to using local anesthetic with vasoconstrictor; medical consult if necessary.

Pazopanib is one of the drugs confirmed to prolong the QT interval and is accepted as having a risk of causing torsade de pointes. The risk of drug-induced torsade de pointes is extremely low when a single QT interval prolonging drug is prescribed. In terms of epinephrine, it is not known what effect vasoconstrictors in the local anesthetic regimen will have in patients with a known history of congenital prolonged QT interval or in patients taking any medication that prolongs the QT interval. Until more information is obtained, it is suggested that the clinician consult with the physician prior to the use of a vasoconstrictor in suspected patients, and that the vasoconstrictor (epinephrine, mepivacaine and levonordefrin [Carbocaine® 2% with Neo-Cobefrin®]) be used with caution.

Effects on Dental Treatment Key adverse event(s) related to dental treatment: Taste alteration.

Effects on Bleeding Chemotherapy may result in significant myelosuppression, potentially including significant reduction in platelet counts (thrombocytopenia grades 3/4: <1%) and altered hemostasis. Hemorrhagic events have been reported. In patients who are under active treatment with these agents, medical consult is suggested.

Adverse Reactions

>10%:

Cardiovascular: Hypertension (40% to 42%; early in treatment), bradycardia (2% to 19%), peripheral edema (STS: 14%), cardiac insufficiency (11% to 13%)

Central nervous system: Fatigue (19%; STS: 65%), tumor pain (STS: 29%), headache (10%; STS: 23%), dizziness (11%)

Dermatologic: Hair discoloration (38% to 39%), exfoliative dermatitis (STS: 18%), alopecia (8% to 12%), dermatological disease (STS: 11%), hypopigmentation (STS, skin: 11%), palmar-plantar erythrodysesthesia (6% to 11%)

Endocrine & metabolic: Weight loss (9%, STS: 48%), increased serum glucose (41% to 45%), increased thyroid-stimulating hormone (TSH), decreased serum albumin (STS: 34%), decreased serum phosphate (34%), decreased serum sodium (31%), decreased serum magnesium (26%), decreased serum glucose (17%), increased serum potassium (STS: 16%)

Gastrointestinal: Diarrhea (52% to 59%), nausea (26%, STS: 56%), decreased appetite (STS: 40%), anorexia (22%), vomiting (21%, STS: 33%), dysgeusia (8%, STS: 28%), increased serum lipase (27%), gastrointestinal pain (STS: 23%), abdominal pain (11%), mucositis (STS: 12%), stomatitis (STS: 11%)

Hematologic & oncologic: Leukopenia (37% to 44%; STS, grade 3: 1%), lymphocytopenia (31%; grades 3/4: ≤4%; STS: 43%, grade 3: 10%), thrombocytopenia (32% to 36%; grades 3/4: ≤6%; grade 4: ≤1%), neutropenia (33% to 34%; grades 3/4 [in patients of East Asian descent]: 12%; grades 3/4 [in patients of non-East Asian descent]: ≤4%), hemorrhage (13% to 22%, including pulmonary, gastrointestinal, and genitourinary, grade 4: 1%, including intracranial, subarachnoid, and peritoneal)

Hepatic: Increased serum AST (51% to 53%), increased serum ALT (4% to 53%), increased serum bilirubin (29% to 36%), increased serum alkaline phosphatase (STS: 32%)

Neuromuscular & skeletal: Musculoskeletal pain (STS: 23%), myalgia (STS: 23%), weakness (14%)

Respiratory: Dyspnea (STS: 20%), cough (STS: 17%)

Miscellaneous: Tumor pain (29%)

1% to 10%:

Cardiovascular: Chest pain (5% to 10%; STS: grade 3: 2%), left ventricular systolic dysfunction (STS: 8%), venous thrombosis (STS: 5%), ischemia (≤2%), myocardial infarction (≤2%), prolonged QT interval on ECG (2%), facial edema (RCC: 1%), transient ischemic attacks (RCC: 1%)

Central nervous system: Insomnia (STS: 9%), voice disorder (4% to 8%), chills (STS: 5%)

Dermatologic: Skin rash (RCC: 8%), skin depigmentation (RCC: 3%), xeroderma (STS: 6%), nail disease (STS: 5%)

Endocrine & metabolic: Hypothyroidism (4% to 8%)

Gastrointestinal: Dyspepsia (5% to 7%), anal hemorrhage (STS: 2%), gastrointestinal fistula (≤1%), gastrointestinal perforation (≤1%)

Genitourinary: Proteinuria (1% to 9%), hematuria (RCC: 4%)

Hematologic & oncologic: Oral hemorrhage (STS: 3%), rectal hemorrhage (RCC: 1%)

Ophthalmic: Blurred vision (STS: 5%)

Respiratory: Epistaxis (2% to 8%), pneumothorax (≤3%), hemoptysis (RCC: 2%)

Frequency not defined:

Cardiovascular: Decreased left ventricular ejection fraction, hypertensive crisis

Central nervous system: Reversible posterior leukoencephalopathy syndrome

Hematologic & oncologic: Hemolytic-uremic syndrome, neutropenic infection, thrombotic thrombocytopenic purpura

Hepatic: Hepatotoxicity, severe hepatotoxicity

Infection: Serious infection

Neuromuscular & skeletal: Arthralgia (RCC), muscle spasm (RCC)

<1%, postmarketing, and/or case reports: Cardiac disease, cardiac failure, cerebral hemorrhage, cerebrovascular accident, interstitial pneumonitis, nephrotic syndrome, pancreatitis, polycythemia, retinal changes (tear), retinal detachment, torsades de pointes

Mechanism of Action Tyrosine kinase (multikinase) inhibitor; limits tumor growth via inhibition of angiogenesis by inhibiting cell surface vascular endothelial growth factor receptors (VEGFR-1, VEGFR-2, VEGFR-3), platelet-derived growth factor receptors (PDGFR-alpha and -beta), fibroblast growth factor receptor (FGFR-1 and -3), cytokine receptor (cKIT), interleukin-2 receptor inducible T-cell kinase, lymphocyte-specific protein tyrosine kinase (Lck), and transmembrane glycoprotein receptor tyrosine kinase (c-Fms)

Pharmacodynamics/Kinetics

Half-life Elimination ~31 hours

Time to Peak Plasma: 2 to 4 hours

Reproductive Considerations

Women of reproductive potential should avoid becoming pregnant during treatment and use effective contraception during therapy and for at least 2 weeks after the last pazopanib dose. Male patients (including vasectomized patients) with pregnant partners or with female partners of reproductive potential should use condoms during treatment and for at least 2 weeks after the last pazopanib dose.

Pregnancy Considerations

Based on its mechanism of action, pazopanib would be expected to cause fetal harm if administered to a pregnant woman.

Dental Health Professional Considerations See Local Anesthetic/Vasoconstrictor Precautions

◆ **Pazopanib HCl** *see* PAZOPanib *on page 1196*

◆ **Pazopanib Hydrochloride** *see* PAZOPanib *on page 1196*

◆ **PCA (error-prone abbreviation)** *see* Procainamide *on page 1277*

◆ **P-Care X** *see* Lidocaine (Systemic) *on page 901*

◆ **P-Care M** *see* Bupivacaine *on page 256*

◆ **P-Care D40** *see* MethylPREDNISolone *on page 999*

◆ **P-Care D80** *see* MethylPREDNISolone *on page 999*

◆ **P-Care K40** *see* Triamcinolone (Systemic) *on page 1485*

◆ **P-Care K80** *see* Triamcinolone (Systemic) *on page 1485*

◆ **PCB** *see* Procarbazine *on page 1278*

◆ **PCE [DSC]** *see* Erythromycin (Systemic) *on page 588*

◆ **PCEC** *see* Rabies Vaccine *on page 1303*

◆ **PCECV** *see* Rabies Vaccine *on page 1303*

◆ **PCI-32765** *see* Ibrutinib *on page 785*

◆ **PCV** *see* Pneumococcal Conjugate Vaccine (10-Valent) *on page 1241*

◆ **PCV** *see* Pneumococcal Conjugate Vaccine (13-Valent) *on page 1242*

◆ **PCV10** *see* Pneumococcal Conjugate Vaccine (10-Valent) *on page 1241*

◆ **PCV13** *see* Pneumococcal Conjugate Vaccine (13-Valent) *on page 1242*

◆ **PCZ** *see* Procarbazine *on page 1278*

◆ **PD 0332991** *see* Palbociclib *on page 1180*

◆ **PDGFR alpha/KIT mutant-specific inhibitor BLU-285** *see* Avapritinib *on page 194*

◆ **PDL-063** *see* Elotuzumab *on page 550*

◆ **PDX** *see* PRALAtrexate *on page 1250*

Peanut Allergen Powder
(pee nut AL er jen pow der)

Brand Names: US Palforzia

Pharmacologic Category Allergen-Specific Immunotherapy

Use

Peanut allergy: Oral immunotherapy for mitigation of allergic reactions, including anaphylaxis, that may occur with accidental exposure to peanut in patients with a confirmed diagnosis of peanut allergy. Initial dose escalation may be administered to patients 4 to 17 years of age. Up-dosing and maintenance may be continued in patients ≥4 years of age. Peanut allergen powder is to be used in conjunction with a peanut-avoidant diet.

Limitation of use: Not indicated for the emergency treatment of allergic reactions, including anaphylaxis.

Local Anesthetic/Vasoconstrictor Precautions No information available to require special precautions.

Effects on Dental Treatment Key adverse event(s) related to dental treatment: Frequent occurrence of oral paresthesia, throat irritation, pharyngeal edema

Effects on Bleeding No information available to require special precautions.

Adverse Reactions

>10%:

Dermatologic: Pruritus (8% to 33%), urticaria (4% to 28%)

Gastrointestinal: Abdominal pain (26% to 67% [placebo: 8% to 35%]), nausea (9% to 32% [placebo: 0.7% to 14%]), oral paresthesia (2% to 14% [placebo: 2% to 4%]), vomiting (3% to 37% [placebo: 0.7% to 16%])

Local: Local pruritus (oral: 9% to 31% [placebo: 3% to 10%])

Respiratory: Cough (3% to 32%), pharyngeal edema (3% to 14%), rhinorrhea (1% to 21%), sneezing (3% to 20%), throat irritation (9% to 40%), wheezing (≤12%)

1% to 10%:

Dermatologic: Pruritus of ear (≤6%)

Gastrointestinal: Eosinophilic esophagitis (1% [placebo: 0%])

Hypersensitivity: Anaphylaxis (≤9% [placebo: 0.3% to 4%])

Respiratory: Dyspnea (≤8%)

Mechanism of Action Not established.

Pregnancy Considerations Accidental exposure to peanuts in a peanut allergic woman may cause anaphylaxis, which may then decrease maternal BP and placental perfusion. Anaphylaxis may also occur following exposure to peanut allergen powder. Pregnant women were excluded from initial studies of peanut allergen powder as oral immunotherapy (PALISADE Group [Vickery 2018]). In general, immunotherapy should not be initiated during pregnancy (Pitsios 2019). Data collection to monitor pregnancy and infant outcomes following exposure to peanut allergen powder is ongoing. Health care providers are encouraged to enroll females exposed to peanut allergen powder during pregnancy in the pregnancy registry (1-833-246-2566).

◆ **Peanut (Arachis hypogaea) Allergen Powder-dnfp** *see* Peanut Allergen Powder *on page 1198*

◆ **PediaCare Childrens Allergy [OTC]** *see* DiphenhydrAMINE (Systemic) *on page 502*

◆ **PediaCare Childrens Long-Act [OTC]** *see* Dextromethorphan *on page 476*

◆ **Pedia-Lax [OTC]** *see* Docusate *on page 509*

◆ **Pedia-Lax Probiotic Yums [OTC]** *see Lactobacillus on page 869*

◆ **Pediapred** *see* PrednisoLONE (Systemic) *on page 1255*

◆ **PEG-L-asparaginase** *see* Pegaspargase *on page 1199*

◆ **Peganone** *see* Ethotoin *on page 619*

Pegaptanib (peg AP ta nib)

Brand Names: US Macugen

Pharmacologic Category Ophthalmic Agent; Vascular Endothelial Growth Factor (VEGF) Inhibitor

Use Macular degeneration (neovascular age-related): Treatment of neovascular (wet) age-related macular degeneration (AMD)

Local Anesthetic/Vasoconstrictor Precautions No information available to require special precautions

Effects on Dental Treatment No significant effects or complications reported

Effects on Bleeding No information available to require special precautions

Adverse Reactions

>10%:

Cardiovascular: Hypertension

Ophthalmic: Anterior chamber inflammation, blurred vision, cataract, conjunctival hemorrhage, corneal edema, decreased visual acuity, eye discharge, eye discomfort, eye irritation, eye pain, increased intraocular pressure, punctate keratitis, visual disturbance, vitreous opacity

1% to 10%:

Cardiovascular: Cerebrovascular accident (1% to 5%), chest pain (1% to 5%), occlusive arterial disease (carotid artery: 1% to 5%), transient ischemic attacks (1% to 5%)

Central nervous system: Dizziness (6% to 10%), headache (6% to 10%), vertigo (1% to 5%)

Dermatologic: Contact dermatitis (1% to 5%)

Endocrine & metabolic: Diabetes mellitus (1% to 5%)

Gastrointestinal: Diarrhea (6% to 10%), nausea (6% to 10%), dyspepsia (1% to 5%), vomiting (1% to 5%)

Genitourinary: Urinary tract infection (6% to 10%), urinary retention (1% to 5%)

Hematologic & oncologic: Bruise (1% to 5%), periorbital hematoma (1% to 5%), vitreous hemorrhage (1% to 5%)

Local: Local inflammation (eye: 1% to 5%), local irritation (eyelid: 1% to 5%)

Neuromuscular & skeletal: Arthritis (1% to 5%), bone spur (1% to 5%)

Ophthalmic: Blepharitis (6% to 10%), conjunctivitis (6% to 10%), photopsia (6% to 10%), vitreous disorder (6% to 10%; includes inflammation), allergic conjunctivitis (1% to 5%), conjunctival edema (1% to 5%), corneal abrasion (1% to 5%), corneal deposits (1% to 5%), epithelial keratopathy (1% to 5%), endophthalmitis (1% to 5%), meibomianitis (1% to 5%), mydriasis (1% to 5%), retinal edema (1% to 5%), swelling of eye (1% to 5%)

Otic: Auditory impairment (1% to 5%)

Respiratory: Bronchitis (6% to 10%), pleural effusion (1% to 5%)

<1%, postmarketing, and/or case reports: Accidental injury, anaphylactoid reaction, anaphylaxis, angioedema, arthropathy, blindness, choroidal detachment, colonic polyps, decreased white blood cell count, dysphagia, feeling abnormal, foreign body sensation of eye, giant-cell arteritis, hematochezia, hemoptysis, hemorrhage, iatrogenic traumatic cataracts, immune thrombocytopenia, increased heart rate, inflammation, intracranial hemorrhage, iridocyclitis, iritis, loss of consciousness, mass (pulmonary), musculoskeletal chest pain, myalgia, neuritis, non-small-cell lung carcinoma (adenocarcinoma), obstructive pulmonary disease, ocular hyperemia, pain, pain at injection site, prolonged partial thromboplastin time, pulmonary disease, pulmonary hemorrhage, retinal detachment, retinal hole without detachment, sclera disease, skin rash, sprue-like symptoms, subretinal neovascularization, syncope, tremor, urticaria, uveitis (intermediate)

Mechanism of Action Pegaptanib is an apatamer, an oligonucleotide covalently bound to polyethylene glycol, which can adopt a three-dimensional shape and bind to vascular endothelial growth factor (VEGF). Pegaptanib binds to extracellular VEGF, selectively inhibiting VEGF from binding to its receptors and thereby suppressing neovascularization and slowing vision loss.

Pharmacodynamics/Kinetics

Half-life Elimination Plasma: 10 ± 4 days

Reproductive Considerations

Evaluate pregnancy status prior to use in females of reproductive potential. Based on information from other VEGF inhibitors, women of reproductive potential should use effective contraception prior to initial dose, during treatment, and for at least 3 months after the last intravitreal injection (Peracha 2016).

Pregnancy Risk Factor B

Pregnancy Considerations

Pegaptanib is a vascular endothelial growth factor (VEGF) inhibitor; VEGF is required to achieve and maintain normal pregnancies. Reports of intravitreal VEGF inhibitor use in pregnancy are limited and information specific to use of pegaptanib has not been located (Peracha 2016). Based on studies in nonpregnant adults, VEGF inhibitors can alter systemic concentrations of VEGF and placental growth factor following intravitreal administration (Peracha 2016; Zehtner 2015). Until additional information is available, intravitreal use during the first trimester should be avoided and use later in pregnancy should be based on patient specific risks versus benefits (Peracha 2016; Polizzi 2015).

- ◆ **Pegaptanib Sodium** *see* Pegaptanib *on page 1198*
- ◆ **PEG-ASP** *see* Pegaspargase *on page 1199*
- ◆ **PEG-asparaginase** *see* Pegaspargase *on page 1199*

Pegaspargase (peg AS par jase)

Related Information

Asparaginase (*E. coli*) *on page 175*

Brand Names: US Oncaspar

Brand Names: Canada Oncaspar

Pharmacologic Category Antineoplastic Agent, Enzyme; Antineoplastic Agent, Miscellaneous

Use

Acute lymphoblastic leukemia and hypersensitivity to asparaginase: Treatment of acute lymphoblastic leukemia (ALL) in pediatric and adult patients with hypersensitivity to native forms of L-asparaginase (as a component of a multiagent chemotherapy regimen)

Acute lymphoblastic leukemia, first-line treatment: First-line treatment of ALL (as a component of a multiagent chemotherapy regimen) in pediatric and adult patients

Local Anesthetic/Vasoconstrictor Precautions

No information available to require special precautions

Effects on Dental Treatment No significant effects or complications reported

Effects on Bleeding Although significant myelosuppression with associated altered hemostasis has been reported for many chemotherapeutic agents, myelosuppression is not common with pegaspargase and no specific precautions appear to necessary.

Adverse Reactions

>10%:

Hepatic: Increased serum transaminases (grades 3/4: 3%)

Hypersensitivity: Hypersensitivity reaction (first-line treatment for acute lymphoblastic leukemia [ALL]: 3%, grades 3/4: 2%; relapsed ALL with no prior asparaginase hypersensitivity: 10%; relapsed ALL with prior asparaginase hypersensitivity: 32%)

Immunologic: Antibody development (induction: 2%; delayed intensification: 10% to 11%)

1% to 10%:
- Cardiovascular: Thromboembolic complications (grades 3/4: >5%)
- Endocrine & metabolic: Hyperglycemia (grades 3/4: 5%), hypertriglyceridemia (grades 3/4: >5%), hypoalbuminemia (grades 3/4: >5%)
- Gastrointestinal: Pancreatitis (grades 3/4: 2%)
- Hematologic & oncologic: Disorder of hemostatic components of blood (grades 3/4: 2%; includes prolonged prothrombin time or partial thromboplastin time or decreased serum fibrogen), febrile neutropenia (grades 3/4: >5%)
- Hepatic: Abnormal hepatic function tests (grades 3/4: 5%), hyperbilirubinemia (grades 3/4: 2%), increased serum transaminases (grades 3/4: 3%)
- Nervous system: Cerebral thrombosis (grades 3/4: 3%)

Postmarketing (any indication):
- Cardiovascular: Sagittal sinus thrombosis
- Endocrine & metabolic: Hyperammonemia, increased serum cholesterol
- Gastrointestinal: Hemorrhagic pancreatitis, necrotizing pancreatitis
- Hematologic & oncologic: Hemorrhage
- Hepatic: Hepatic insufficiency
- Hypersensitivity: Anaphylactic shock, anaphylaxis, angioedema
- Nervous system: Intracranial hemorrhage
- Miscellaneous: Cyst (pancreatic)

Mechanism of Action Pegaspargase is a modified version of L-asparaginase, conjugated with monomethoxypolyethylene glycol (mPEG). In leukemic cells, asparaginase hydrolyzes L-asparagine to ammonia and L-aspartic acid, leading to depletion of asparagine. Leukemia cells require exogenous asparagine; normal cells can synthesize asparagine. Asparagine depletion in leukemic cells leads to inhibition of protein synthesis and apoptosis.

Pharmacodynamics/Kinetics

Onset of Action Mean maximum asparaginase activity: On day 5 (following a single IM dose of 2,500 units/m^2)

Duration of Action Asparagine depletion: IV (in asparaginase-naive adults): 2 to 4 weeks (Douer 2007); IM: ~21 days

Half-life Elimination ~5.8 days (following a single IM dose of 2,500 units/m^2); ~5.3 days (following a single IV dose of 2,500 units/m^2); Asparaginase-naive adults: IV: 7 days (Douer 2007)

Reproductive Considerations

Evaluate pregnancy status prior to use in females of reproductive potential. Effective nonhormonal contraception should be used during therapy and for at least 3 months after the last pegaspargase dose. Hormonal contraceptives may not be effective and are not recommended as a form of contraception.

Pregnancy Considerations

Based on animal reproduction studies conducted with L-asparaginase, adverse effects to the fetus may be expected if exposure occurs during pregnancy.

◆ **Pegasys** *see* Peginterferon Alfa-2a *on page* 1201

◆ **Pegasys ProClick** *see* Peginterferon Alfa-2a *on page* 1201

Pegfilgrastim (peg fil GRA stim)

Brand Names: US Fulphila; Neulasta; Neulasta Onpro; Udenyca; Ziextenzo

Brand Names: Canada Fulphila; Lapelga; Neulasta; Ziextenzo

Pharmacologic Category Colony Stimulating Factor; Hematopoietic Agent

Use

Hematopoietic radiation injury syndrome, acute (Neulasta only): To increase survival in patients acutely exposed to myelosuppressive doses of radiation.

Prevention of chemotherapy-induced neutropenia (Neulasta and pegfilgrastim biosimilars): To decrease the incidence of infection (as manifested by febrile neutropenia), in patients with nonmyeloid malignancies receiving myelosuppressive cancer chemotherapy associated with a clinically significant incidence of febrile neutropenia.

Limitation of use: Pegfilgrastim products are not indicated for mobilization of peripheral blood progenitor cells for hematopoietic stem cell transplant.

Note: Fulphila (pegfilgrastim-jmdb), Udenyca (pegfilgrastim-cbqv), and Ziextenzo (pegfilgrastim-bmez) are approved as biosimilars to Neulasta (pegfilgrastim). In Canada, Fulphila and Lapelga are approved as biosimilars to Neulasta (pegfilgrastim).

Local Anesthetic/Vasoconstrictor Precautions
No information available to require special precautions

Effects on Dental Treatment No significant effects or complications reported

Effects on Bleeding No information available to require special precautions. Medical consultation may be necessary to confirm adequate platelet counts.

Adverse Reactions Adverse reaction incidences based on studies including concomitant docetaxel therapy.

>10%: Neuromuscular & skeletal: Ostealgia (31%)

1% to 10%: Neuromuscular & skeletal: Limb pain (9%)

<1%, postmarketing, and/or case reports: Acute respiratory distress syndrome, anaphylaxis, antibody development, capillary leak syndrome, erythema of skin, flushing, glomerulonephritis, hypersensitivity angiitis, injection site reaction, leukocytosis, local inflammation (aortitis), pulmonary alveolar hemorrhage, severe hypersensitivity, sickle cell crisis, skin rash, splenic rupture, splenomegaly, Sweet's syndrome, urticaria

Mechanism of Action Pegfilgrastim stimulates the production, maturation, and activation of neutrophils and activates neutrophils to increase both their migration and cytotoxicity. Pegfilgrastim has a prolonged duration of effect relative to filgrastim and a reduced renal clearance.

Pharmacodynamics/Kinetics

Half-life Elimination SubQ: Pediatrics (100 mcg/kg dose): 0 to 5 years: 30.1 ± 38.2 hours; 6 to 11 years: 20.2 ± 11.3 hours; 12 years and older: 21.2 ± 16 hours; Adults: 15 to 80 hours. Pharmacokinetics (in adults) were comparable between manual subcutaneous injection and the On-body injector system.

Pregnancy Considerations Adverse events were observed in some animal reproduction studies.

Product Availability Nyvepria: FDA approved June 2020; availability anticipated in 2020. Nyvepria is approved as a biosimilar to Neulasta.

◆ **Pegfilgrastim-bmez** *see* Pegfilgrastim *on page* 1200

◆ **Pegfilgrastim-cbqv** *see* Pegfilgrastim *on page* 1200

◆ **Pegfilgrastim-jmdb** *see* Pegfilgrastim *on page* 1200

◆ **PEG-IFN Alfa-2a** *see* Peginterferon Alfa-2a *on page* 1201

◆ **PEG-IFN Alfa-2b** *see* Peginterferon Alfa-2b *on page 1202*

Peginterferon Alfa-2a

(peg in ter FEER on AL fa too aye)

Related Information

Systemic Viral Diseases *on page 1709*

Brand Names: US Pegasys; Pegasys ProClick

Brand Names: Canada Pegasys

Pharmacologic Category Interferon

Use

Chronic hepatitis B: Treatment of adults with hepatitis B e antigen (HBeAg)-positive and HBeAg-negative chronic hepatitis B virus (HBV) infection who have compensated liver disease and evidence of viral replication and liver inflammation; treatment of pediatric patients ≥3 years of age with HBeAg-positive chronic HBV infection who are non-cirrhotic and have evidence of viral replication and elevations of serum alanine aminotransferase.

Local Anesthetic/Vasoconstrictor Precautions No information available to require special precautions

Effects on Dental Treatment Key adverse event(s) related to dental treatment: Xerostomia (normal salivary flow resumes upon discontinuation).

Effects on Bleeding Thrombocytopenia may occur in patients. Monitor for the potential for increased bleeding.

Adverse Reactions

>10%:

Central nervous system: Fatigue (adults: ≤56%; children and adolescents: 8%), headache (adults: 27% to 54%; children and adolescents: 21%), rigors (adults: 25% to 35%), insomnia (adults: 19%), anxiety (adults: ≤19%), irritability (adults: ≤19%), nervousness (adults: ≤19%), depression (adults: 18%), dizziness (adults: 16%; children and adolescents: 6%), pain (adults: 11%)

Dermatologic: Alopecia (adults: 18% to 23%; children and adolescents: 6%), pruritus (adults: 12%)

Endocrine & metabolic: Growth suppression (children and adolescents, percentile decrease (≥15 percentiles), weight: [11% to 43%], height: [6% to 25%])

Gastrointestinal: Nausea (adults: ≤24%; children and adolescents: 9%), vomiting (adults: ≤24%), anorexia (adults: 16% to 17%), abdominal pain (15% to 17%), diarrhea (adults: 16%)

Hematologic & oncologic: Neutropenia (adults: 21%)

Hepatic: Increased serum ALT (adults, hepatitis B: 25% to 27%; children and adolescents: 10%; adults, hepatitis C: 1%)

Local: Injection site reaction (adults: 22%)

Neuromuscular & skeletal: Weakness (adults: ≤56%; children and adolescents: 9%), myalgia (adults: 37%), arthralgia (adults: 28%)

Respiratory: Cough (children and adolescents: 15%; adults: 4%), flu-like symptoms (children and adolescents: 14%)

Miscellaneous: Fever (37% to 54%)

1% to 10%:

Central nervous system: Lack of concentration (adults: 8%), memory impairment (adults: 5%), mood changes (adults: 3%)

Dermatologic: Skin rash (5% to 10%), dermatitis (adults: 8%), diaphoresis (adults: 6%), xeroderma (adults: 4%), eczema (adults: 1%)

Endocrine & metabolic: Weight loss (adults: 4%), hypothyroidism (adults: 3% to 4%), hyperthyroidism (adults: ≤1%)

Gastrointestinal: Decreased appetite (children and adolescents: 6%), xerostomia (adults: 6%)

Hematologic & oncology: Thrombocytopenia (adults: 5%), lymphocytopenia (adults: 3%), anemia (adults: 2%)

Hepatic: Increased serum AST (children and adolescents: 10%), liver decompensation (in CHC/HIV patients; adults: 2%)

Infection: Bacterial infection (adults: ≤5%)

Neuromuscular & skeletal: Back pain (adults: 9%)

Ophthalmic: Blurred vision (adults: 4%)

Respiratory: Epistaxis (children and adolescents: 9%), upper respiratory tract infection (children and adolescents: 8%), nasopharyngitis (children and adolescents: 6%), dyspnea (adults: 4%)

≤1%, postmarketing, and/or case reports: Aggressive behavior, anaphylaxis, angina pectoris, angioedema, aplastic anemia, auditory impairment, autoimmune disorders, bipolar mood disorder, bronchiolitis obliterans, bronchoconstriction, cardiac arrhythmia, cerebral hemorrhage, chest pain, cholangitis, colitis, coma, corneal ulcer, dehydration, diabetes mellitus, dyspepsia, dyspnea on exertion, endocarditis, erythema multiforme major, exacerbation of hepatitis B, exfoliative dermatitis, gastrointestinal hemorrhage, graft rejection (hepatic, renal), hallucination, hearing loss, hematocrit decreased, hemoglobin decreased, hepatic insufficiency, hyperglycemia, hyperpigmentation, hypersensitivity reaction, hypertension, hypoglycemia, increased serum triglycerides, influenza, interstitial pneumonitis, limb abscess, liver steatosis, macular edema, mania, myocardial infarction, myositis, optic neuritis, pancreatitis, papilledema, peptic ulcer, peripheral neuropathy, pneumonia, psychiatric disturbance, psychosis, pulmonary embolism, pulmonary infiltrates, pure red cell aplasia, retinal cotton-wool spot, retinal detachment, retinal hemorrhage, retinal thrombosis (in artery or vein), retinopathy, rheumatoid arthritis, sarcoidosis, seizures, Stevens-Johnson syndrome, substance overdose, suicidal ideation, supraventricular arrhythmia, systemic lupus erythematosus, thrombotic thrombocytopenic purpura, tongue discoloration, urticaria, vesiculobullous reaction, vision loss

Mechanism of Action Alpha interferons are a family of proteins, produced by nucleated cells that have antiviral, antiproliferative, and immune-regulating activity. There are 16 known subtypes of alpha interferons. Interferons interact with cells through high affinity cell surface receptors. Following activation, multiple effects can be detected including induction of gene transcription. Interferons inhibit cellular growth, alter the state of cellular differentiation, interfere with oncogene expression, alter cell surface antigen expression, increase phagocytic activity of macrophages, and augment cytotoxicity of lymphocytes for target cells.

Pharmacodynamics/Kinetics

Half-life Elimination Terminal: 50-160 hours; increased with renal dysfunction

Time to Peak Serum: 72 to 96 hours

Reproductive Considerations

HCV-infected females of childbearing potential should consider postponing pregnancy until therapy is complete to reduce the risk of HCV transmission (AASLD/IDSA 2017).

Verify pregnancy status prior to administration in females of reproductive potential. Disruption of the normal menstrual cycle was observed in animal studies. Female patients of reproductive potential should use effective contraception during treatment.

If used in combination with ribavirin, all warnings related to the use of ribavirin and contraception should be followed. Refer to the ribavirin monograph for additional information.

Pregnancy Considerations

Alfa interferon is endogenous to normal amniotic fluid (Lebon 1982); however, placenta perfusion studies note exogenous interferon alfa does not cross the placenta (Waysbort 1993). The Health and Human Services (HHS) Perinatal HIV Guidelines recommend against the use of peginterferon-alfa during pregnancy because of its antigrowth and antiproliferative effects (HHS [perinatal] 2019). Animal reproduction studies have demonstrated abortifacient effects.

Treatment of hepatitis C is not currently recommended to treat maternal infection or to decrease the risk of mother-to-child transmission during pregnancy (Tran 2016).

Peginterferon alfa-2a in combination with ribavirin is contraindicated in pregnant females or males whose female partners are pregnant. Combination therapy with ribavirin may cause birth defects and death in an unborn child. All warnings related to the use of ribavirin and pregnancy should be followed. Refer to the ribavirin monograph for additional information.

Peginterferon Alfa-2b

(peg in ter FEER on AL fa too bee)

Related Information

Systemic Viral Diseases *on page 1709*

Brand Names: US Peg-Intron Redipen Pak 4 [DSC]; Peg-Intron Redipen [DSC]; PegIntron; Sylatron

Pharmacologic Category Antineoplastic Agent, Biological Response Modulator; Biological Response Modulator; Interferon

Use Melanoma (adjuvant therapy): Sylatron: Adjuvant treatment of melanoma (with microscopic or gross nodal involvement within 84 days of definitive surgical resection, including complete lymphadenectomy). **Note:** Indications in the manufacturer's labeling may not reflect current clinical practices.

Local Anesthetic/Vasoconstrictor Precautions
No information available to require special precautions

Effects on Dental Treatment Key adverse event(s) related to dental treatment: Xerostomia (normal salivary flow resumes upon discontinuation).

Effects on Bleeding Thrombocytopenia may occur in patients. Monitor for the potential for increased bleeding.

Adverse Reactions

Antiviral:

>10%:

Central nervous system: Headache (56%), fatigue (including asthenia; ≤52%), depression (29%), anxiety (≤28%), emotional lability (≤28%), irritability (≤28%), insomnia (23%), rigors (23%), dizziness (12%)

Dermatologic: Alopecia (22%), pruritus (12%)

Endocrine & metabolic: Weight loss (11%)

Gastrointestinal: Nausea (26%), anorexia (20%), diarrhea (18%), abdominal pain (15%)

Infection: Viral infection (11%)

Local: Inflammation at injection site (47%), injection site reaction (47%)

Neuromuscular & skeletal: Myalgia (54%), weakness (52%), musculoskeletal pain (28%), arthralgia (23%)

Miscellaneous: Fever (22%)

1% to 10%:

Cardiovascular: Chest pain (6%), flushing (6%)

Central nervous system: Lack of concentration (10%), right upper quadrant pain (8%), malaise (7%), nervousness (4%), agitation (2%), suicidal ideation (≤2%)

Dermatologic: Diaphoresis (6%), skin rash (6%)

Endocrine & metabolic: Hypothyroidism (5%), menstrual disease (4%), hyperthyroidism (3%)

Gastrointestinal: Vomiting (7%), dyspepsia (6%), xerostomia (6%), constipation (1%)

Hematologic & oncologic: Thrombocytopenia (7%), neutropenia (6%)

Hepatic: Increased serum alanine aminotransferase (10%), hepatomegaly (6%)

Immunologic: Antibody development (neutralizing: 2%)

Local: Pain at injection site (2% to 3%)

Ophthalmic: Conjunctivitis (4%), blurred vision (2%)

Respiratory: Pharyngitis (10%), cough (8%), sinusitis (7%), dyspnea (4%), rhinitis (2%)

Antineoplastic:

>10%:

Central nervous system: Fatigue (94%), headache (70%), chills (63%), depression (59%), dizziness (35%), neuropathy (olfactory) (23%), paresthesia (21%)

Dermatologic: Exfoliative dermatitis (36%), alopecia (34%)

Endocrine & metabolic: Weight loss (11%)

Gastrointestinal: Anorexia (69%), nausea (64%), dysgeusia (38%), diarrhea (37%), vomiting (26%)

Hepatic: Increased serum alanine aminotransferase (≤77%), increased serum aspartate aminotransferase (≤77%), increased serum alkaline phosphatase (23%)

Immunologic: Antibody development (binding antibodies: 35%)

Local: Injection site reaction (62%)

Neuromuscular & skeletal: Myalgia (68%), arthralgia (51%)

Miscellaneous: Fever (75%)

1% to 10%:

Cardiovascular: Bundle branch block (≤4%), myocardial infarction (≤4%), supraventricular cardiac arrhythmia (≤4%), ventricular tachycardia (≤4%)

Endocrine & metabolic: Increased gamma-glutamyl transferase (8%)

Genitourinary: Proteinuria (7%)

Hematologic & oncologic: Anemia (6%)

Respiratory: Dyspnea (6%), cough (5%)

<1%, postmarketing, and/or case reports: Aggressive behavior, amnesia, anaphylaxis, angina pectoris, angioedema, aphthous stomatitis, aplastic anemia, auditory impairment, bacterial infection, bipolar mood disorder, brain disease (including exacerbations), bronchiolitis obliterans, bronchoconstriction, cardiac arrest, cardiac arrhythmia, cardiomyopathy, cerebrovascular accident, colitis, cytopenia, dehydration, diabetes mellitus, diabetic ketoacidosis, drug dependence (including relapse), drug overdose, dysgeusia, erythema multiforme, exacerbation of autoimmune disease, fungal infection, hallucination, hearing loss, hemorrhagic colitis, homicidal ideation, hyperglycemia, hypersensitivity reaction, hypertension, hypertriglyceridemia, hypotension, immune thrombocytopenia, interstitial nephritis, interstitial pneumonitis, ischemic colitis, leukopenia, lupus-like syndrome, macular edema, mania, migraine, myositis, optic neuritis, palpitations, pancreatitis, papilledema,

paresthesia, pericarditis, peripheral neuropathy, pneumonia, psoriasis, pulmonary fibrosis, pulmonary hypertension, pulmonary infiltrates, pure red cell aplasia, reactivation of HBV, renal failure syndrome, renal insufficiency (includes increases in serum creatinine), retinal cotton-wool spot, retinal detachment, retinal hemorrhage, retinal thrombosis, retinopathy, rhabdomyolysis, rheumatoid arthritis, sarcoidosis, seizure, sepsis, Stevens-Johnson syndrome, systemic lupus erythematosus, tachycardia, thrombotic thrombocytopenic purpura, thyroiditis, tongue discoloration, toxic epidermal necrolysis, ulcerative colitis, urticaria, vertigo, vision loss, visual disturbance, Vogt-Koyanagi-Harada syndrome

Mechanism of Action Alpha interferons are a family of proteins, produced by nucleated cells, that have antiviral, antiproliferative, and immune-regulating activity. There are 16 known subtypes of alpha interferons. Interferons interact with cells through high affinity cell surface receptors. Following activation, multiple effects can be detected including induction of gene transcription. Inhibits cellular growth, alters the state of cellular differentiation, interferes with oncogene expression, alters cell surface antigen expression, increases phagocytic activity of macrophages, and augments cytotoxicity of lymphocytes for target cells.

Pharmacodynamics/Kinetics

Half-life Elimination CHC: ~40 hours (range: 22 to 60 hours); Melanoma: ~43 to 51 hours

Time to Peak CHC: 15 to 44 hours

Reproductive Considerations

HCV-infected females of childbearing potential should consider postponing pregnancy until therapy is complete to reduce the risk of HCV transmission (AASLD/IDSA 2017).

Verify pregnancy status prior to administration in females of reproductive potential. Disruption of the normal menstrual cycle was observed in animal studies. Female patients of reproductive potential should use effective contraception during treatment and for ≥10 days after the last peginterferon alfa-2b dose.

If used in combination with ribavirin, all warnings related to the use of ribavirin and contraception should be followed. Refer to the ribavirin monograph for additional information.

Pregnancy Considerations

Alfa interferon is endogenous to normal amniotic fluid (Lebon 1982); however, placenta perfusion studies note exogenous interferon alfa does not cross the placenta (Waysbort 1993). The Health and Human Services (HHS) perinatal HIV guidelines recommend against the use of peginterferon-alfa during pregnancy because of its antigrowth and antiproliferative effects (HHS [perinatal] 2019). Animal reproduction studies have demonstrated abortifacient effects.

Treatment of hepatitis C is not currently recommended to treat maternal infection or to decrease the risk of mother-to-child transmission during pregnancy (Tran 2016).

Peginterferon Alfa-2b in combination with ribavirin is contraindicated in pregnant females and males whose female partners are pregnant. Combination therapy with ribavirin may cause birth defects and death in an unborn child. If used in combination with ribavirin, all warnings related to the use of ribavirin and pregnancy should be followed. Refer to the ribavirin monograph for additional information.

Product Availability

PegIntron Redipen and PegIntron 80 mcg, 120 mcg, and 150 mcg vials have been discontinued in the US for more than 1 year. PegIntron 50 mcg vials remain available in limited quantities; based on current demand, Merck anticipates product should continue to be available through May 2021. Contact the Merck National Service Center for additional information: 800-672-6372.

Sylatron 600 mcg vials will be discontinued on or near December 2018. Sylatron 200 mcg and 300 mcg vials will be discontinued on or near December 2019. Contact the Merck National Service Center for additional information: 800-672-6372.

- ◆ **PegIntron** *see* Peginterferon Alfa-2b *on page 1202*
- ◆ **Peg-Intron Redipen [DSC]** *see* Peginterferon Alfa-2b *on page 1202*
- ◆ **Peg-Intron Redipen Pak 4 [DSC]** *see* Peginterferon Alfa-2b *on page 1202*
- ◆ **PEGLA** *see* Pegaspargase *on page 1199*

Pegloticase (peg LOE ti kase)

Brand Names: US Krystexxa

Pharmacologic Category Enzyme; Enzyme, Urate-Oxidase (Recombinant)

Use

Gout: Treatment of chronic gout in adults refractory to conventional therapy

Limitations of use: Not for the treatment of asymptomatic hyperuricemia

Local Anesthetic/Vasoconstrictor Precautions

No information available to require special precautions

Effects on Dental Treatment No significant effects or complications reported

Effects on Bleeding No information available to require special precautions

Adverse Reactions

>10%:

Dermatologic: Urticaria (11%)

Endocrine & metabolic: Gout (flare: 74%; within the first 3 months)

Gastrointestinal: Nausea (12%)

Hematologic & oncologic: Bruise (11%)

Immunologic: Antibody development (antipegloticase antibodies: 92%; anti-PEG antibodies: 42%)

Miscellaneous: Infusion-related reaction (26%)

1% to 10%:

Cardiovascular: Chest discomfort (10%), chest pain (6% to 10%), exacerbation of congestive heart failure (2%)

Dermatologic: Erythema (10%), pruritus (10%)

Gastrointestinal: Constipation (6%), vomiting (5%)

Hypersensitivity: Anaphylaxis (5% to 7%)

Respiratory: Dyspnea (7%), nasopharyngitis (7%)

<1%, postmarketing, and/or case reports: Asthenia, malaise, peripheral edema, type IV hypersensitivity reaction

Mechanism of Action Pegloticase is a pegylated recombinant form of urate-oxidase enzyme, also known as uricase (an enzyme normally absent in humans and high primates), which converts uric acid to allantoin (an inactive and water soluble metabolite of uric acid); it does not inhibit the formation of uric acid.

Pharmacodynamics/Kinetics

Onset of Action ~24 hours following the first dose, serum uric acid concentrations decreased

Duration of Action >300 hours (12.5 days)

Half-life Elimination Median: ~14 days

Pregnancy Considerations Adverse events have been observed in some animal reproduction studies.

◆ **PEG-Uricase** *see* Pegloticase *on page* 1203

◆ **Pegylated DOXOrubicin Liposomal** *see* DOXOrubicin (Liposomal) *on page* 521

◆ **Pegylated G-CSF** *see* Pegfilgrastim *on page* 1200

◆ **Pegylated Interferon Alfa-2a** *see* Peginterferon Alfa-2a *on page* 1201

◆ **Pegylated Interferon Alfa-2b** *see* Peginterferon Alfa-2b *on page* 1202

◆ **Pegylated Liposomal DOXOrubicin** *see* DOXOrubicin (Liposomal) *on page* 521

◆ **Pegylated Liposomal DOXOrubicin Hydrochloride (Doxil, Caelyx)** *see* DOXOrubicin (Liposomal) *on page* 521

◆ **Pegylated Urate Oxidase** *see* Pegloticase *on page* 1203

◆ **Pemazyre** *see* Pemigatinib *on page* 1207

Pembrolizumab (pem broe LIZ ue mab)

Brand Names: US Keytruda

Brand Names: Canada Keytruda

Pharmacologic Category Antineoplastic Agent, Anti-PD-1 Monoclonal Antibody; Antineoplastic Agent, Immune Checkpoint Inhibitor; Antineoplastic Agent, Monoclonal Antibody

Use

Cervical cancer (recurrent or metastatic): Treatment of recurrent or metastatic cervical cancer in patients whose tumors express PD-L1 (combined positive score [CPS] ≥1), as determined by an approved test, and with disease progression on or after chemotherapy.

Cutaneous squamous cell carcinoma (recurrent or metastatic): Treatment of recurrent or metastatic cutaneous squamous cell carcinoma not curable by surgery or radiation.

Endometrial carcinoma (advanced): Treatment of advanced endometrial carcinoma (in combination with lenvatinib) that is not microsatellite instability-high (MSI-H) or mismatch repair deficient (dMMR) in patients who have disease progression following prior systemic therapy and are not candidates for curative surgery or radiation.

Esophageal cancer (recurrent locally advanced or metastatic): Treatment of recurrent locally advanced or metastatic squamous cell carcinoma of the esophagus in patients whose tumors express PD-L1 (CPS ≥10) as determined by an approved test, with disease progression after one or more prior lines of systemic therapy.

Gastric cancer (recurrent locally advanced or metastatic): Treatment of recurrent locally advanced or metastatic gastric or gastroesophageal junction adenocarcinoma in patients whose tumors express PD-L1 (CPS ≥1), as determined by an approved test, with disease progression on or after two or more prior lines of therapy including fluoropyrimidine- and platinum-containing chemotherapy, and if appropriate, HER2/neu-targeted therapy.

Head and neck cancer, squamous cell (recurrent or metastatic):

First-line treatment (in combination with platinum and fluorouracil) of metastatic or unresectable recurrent head and neck squamous cell carcinoma (HNSCC).

First-line, single-agent treatment of metastatic or unresectable recurrent HNSCC in patients whose tumors express PD-L1 (CPS ≥1), as determined by an approved test.

Single-agent treatment of recurrent or metastatic HNSCC in patients with disease progression on or after platinum-containing chemotherapy.

Hepatocellular carcinoma (advanced): Treatment of hepatocellular carcinoma in patients who have been previously treated with sorafenib.

Hodgkin lymphoma, classical (relapsed or refractory): Treatment of adult and pediatric patients with refractory classical Hodgkin lymphoma or patients who have relapsed after 3 or more prior lines of therapy.

Melanoma:

Adjuvant treatment of melanoma with lymph node(s) involvement following complete resection.

Treatment of unresectable or metastatic melanoma.

Merkel cell carcinoma (recurrent or metastatic): Treatment of recurrent locally advanced or metastatic Merkel cell carcinoma in adult and pediatric patients.

Microsatellite instability-high or mismatch repair-deficient cancer (unresectable or metastatic):

Solid tumors: Treatment of unresectable or metastatic, microsatellite instability-high (MSI-H) or mismatch repair-deficient (dMMR) solid tumors in adult and pediatric patients that have progressed following prior treatment and have no satisfactory alternate treatment options.

Limitation of use: Safety and efficacy in pediatric patients with MSI-H central nervous system cancers have not been established.

Colorectal cancer: First-line treatment of unresectable or metastatic MSI-H of dMMR colorectal cancer; treatment of unresectable or metastatic, MSI-H or mismatch repair deficient colorectal cancer in adult and pediatric patients that have progressed following treatment with a fluoropyrimidine, oxaliplatin, and irinotecan.

Non-small cell lung cancer:

First-line, single-agent treatment of non-small cell lung cancer (NSCLC) in patients with stage III NSCLC (who are not candidates for surgical resection or definitive chemoradiation) or in patients with metastatic NSCLC, **and** with tumors with PD-L1 expression (tumor proportion score [TPS] ≥1%), as determined by an approved test, and with no epidermal growth factor receptor (EGFR) or anaplastic lymphoma kinase (ALK) genomic tumor aberrations.

First-line treatment (in combination with pemetrexed and platinum chemotherapy) of metastatic nonsquamous NSCLC in patients with no EGFR or ALK genomic tumor aberrations.

First-line treatment (in combination with carboplatin and either paclitaxel or paclitaxel [protein bound]) of metastatic squamous NSCLC.

Single-agent treatment of metastatic NSCLC in patients with tumors with PD-L1 expression (TPS ≥1%), as determined by an approved test, and with disease progression on or following platinum-containing chemotherapy. Patients with EGFR or ALK genomic tumor aberrations should have disease progression (on approved EGFR- or ALK-directed therapy) prior to receiving pembrolizumab.

Primary mediastinal large B-cell lymphoma (relapsed or refractory): Treatment of primary mediastinal large B-cell lymphoma (PMBCL) in adult and pediatric patients with refractory disease or who have relapsed after 2 or more prior lines of therapy.

Limitation of use: Not recommended for treatment of PMBCL in patients who require urgent cytoreductive therapy.

Renal cell carcinoma (advanced): First-line treatment of advanced renal cell carcinoma (in combination with axitinib).

Small cell lung cancer (metastatic): Treatment of metastatic small cell lung cancer in patients with disease progression on or after platinum-based chemotherapy and at least 1 other prior line of therapy.

Tumor mutational burden-high cancer (unresectable or metastatic): Treatment of unresectable or metastatic, tumor mutational burden-high solid tumors (TMB-H; ≥10 mutations/megabase [mut/Mb]; as determined by an approved test) in adult and pediatric patients who have progressed following prior treatment and have no satisfactory alternative treatment options.

Limitation of use: Safety and efficacy in pediatric patients with TMB-H CNS cancers have not been established.

Urothelial carcinoma:

Treatment of Bacillus Calmette-Guerin-unresponsive, high-risk, non-muscle invasive bladder cancer with carcinoma in situ with or without papillary tumors in patients who are ineligible for or have elected not to undergo cystectomy.

Treatment of locally advanced or metastatic urothelial cancer in patients who are not eligible for cisplatin-containing chemotherapy and whose tumors express PD-L1 (CPS ≥10) as determined by an approved test, or in patients who are not eligible for any platinum-containing chemotherapy regardless of PD-L1 status.

Treatment of locally advanced or metastatic urothelial cancer in patients with disease progression during or after platinum-containing chemotherapy or within 12 months of neoadjuvant or adjuvant platinum-containing chemotherapy.

Local Anesthetic/Vasoconstrictor Precautions No information available to require special precautions

Effects on Dental Treatment No significant effects or complications reported

Effects on Bleeding Therapy with immune checkpoint inhibitors may result in significant myelosuppression, including thrombocytopenia. In patients under active treatment a medical consult is suggested.

Adverse Reactions Incidence of adverse reactions include unapproved dosing regimens.

>10%:

Cardiovascular: Peripheral edema (11% to 15%), cardiac arrhythmia (11%)

Dermatologic: Pruritus (11% to 28%), skin rash (13% to 24%), vitiligo (13%)

Endocrine & metabolic: Hyperglycemia (19% to 59%), hyponatremia (10% to 46%), hypoalbuminemia (24% to 44%), hypertriglyceridemia (33% to 43%), hypophosphatemia (19% to 29%), hypocalcemia (15% to 27%), hyperkalemia (13% to 23%), decreased serum bicarbonate (22%), hypercalcemia (14% to 22%), hypercholesterolemia (20%), hypokalemia (15% to 20%), hypoglycemia (13% to 19%), hypothyroidism (9% to 18%), hypomagnesemia (16%), weight loss (10% to 15%)

Gastrointestinal: Diarrhea (12% to 28%), decreased appetite (15% to 25%), constipation (12% to 22%), abdominal pain (13% to 22%), nausea (11% to 22%), vomiting (11% to 19%)

Genitourinary: Hematuria (12% to 19%), urinary tract infection (12% to 19%)

Hematologic & oncologic: Lymphocytopenia (24% to 54%; grades 3/4: 1% to 25%), anemia (17% to 54%; grades 3/4: 1% to 24%), leukopenia (35%; grades 3/4: 9%), neutropenia (7% to 30%; grades 3/4: 1% to 11%), thrombocytopenia (12% to 27%; grades 3/4: 4%), increased INR (19% to 21%), hemorrhage (19%; grades 3/4: 5%), prolonged partial thromboplastin time (14%)

Hepatic: Increased serum alkaline phosphatase (17% to 42%), increased serum transaminases (27% to 34%), increased serum aspartate aminotransferase (20% to 34%), increased serum alanine aminotransferase (9% to 33%), increased liver enzymes (13%)

Immunologic: Graft versus host disease (followed by allogeneic hematopoietic stem cell transplantation: 26%)

Infection: Infection (16%)

Nervous system: Fatigue (23% to 43%), pain (22%), headache (11% to 14%)

Neuromuscular & skeletal: Musculoskeletal pain (19% to 32%), arthralgia (10% to 18%), myalgia (12%), back pain (11% to 12%), asthenia (10% to 11%)

Renal: Increased serum creatinine (11% to 35%)

Respiratory: Upper respiratory tract infection (13% to 28%), cough (14% to 26%), dyspnea (10% to 23%), pneumonia (12%), flu-like symptoms (11%)

Miscellaneous: Fever (10% to 28%)

1% to 10%:

Cardiovascular: Facial edema (10%), pericarditis (4%), pericardial effusion (2%)

Endocrine & metabolic: Hyperthyroidism (3% to 10%), thyroiditis (≤2%)

Gastrointestinal: Dysphagia (8%), stomatitis (3% to 4%; grades 3/4: 1%), colitis (2%)

Hepatic: Hyperbilirubinemia (10%), hepatic sinusoidal obstruction syndrome (followed by allogeneic hematopoietic stem cell transplantation: 9%), ascites (grades 3/4: 8%), hepatitis (≤3%)

Immunologic: Antibody development (2%; neutralizing: <1%)

Nervous system: Peripheral neuropathy (2% to 10%), insomnia (7%), dizziness (5%), peripheral sensory neuropathy (1%)

Neuromuscular & skeletal: Neck pain (6%), arthritis (2%), myositis (≤1%)

Ophthalmic: Uveitis (≤1%)

Renal: Acute renal failure (2%)

Respiratory: Nasopharyngitis (10%), pneumonitis (2% to 8%)

Miscellaneous: Infusion related reaction (≤9%)

Frequency not defined:

Cardiovascular: Acute myocardial infarction, cardiac failure, cardiac tamponade, edema, pulmonary embolism, septic shock

Dermatologic: Cellulitis, dermatitis, erythematous rash, follicular rash, maculopapular rash

Genitourinary: Uterine hemorrhage

Hematologic & oncologic: Rectal hemorrhage

Infection: Candidiasis, *Clostridioides difficile* associated diarrhea, herpes zoster infection, sepsis

Nervous system: Confusion, polyneuropathy

Neuromuscular & skeletal: Osteomyelitis

Respiratory: Epistaxis, hemoptysis, pleural effusion, respiratory failure

Miscellaneous: Fistula, physical health deterioration

<1%, postmarketing, and/or case reports: Adrenocortical insufficiency, anaphylaxis, chronic inflammatory demyelinating polyneuropathy (Maleissye 2016), diabetic ketoacidosis, encephalitis, Guillain-Barré syndrome, hemolytic anemia, hypersensitivity reaction, hypophysitis, myasthenia gravis, myelitis, myocarditis, nephritis, organ transplant rejection (solid), pancreatitis, sarcoidosis, subacute cutaneous lupus erythematosus (Blakeway 2019), type 1 diabetes mellitus, vasculitis

Mechanism of Action Pembrolizumab is a highly selective anti-PD-1 humanized monoclonal antibody which inhibits programmed cell death-1 (PD-1) activity by binding to the PD-1 receptor on T-cells to block PD-1 ligands (PD-L1 and PD-L2) from binding. Blocking the PD-1 pathway inhibits the negative immune regulation caused by PD-1 receptor signaling (Hamid 2013). Anti-PD-1 antibodies (including pembrolizumab) reverse T-cell suppression and induce antitumor responses (Robert 2014).

Pharmacodynamics/Kinetics

Half-life Elimination 22 days.

Reproductive Considerations

Verify pregnancy status prior to initiation of pembrolizumab treatment in females of reproductive potential. Females of reproductive potential should use effective contraception during therapy and for at least 4 months after treatment is complete.

Pregnancy Considerations

Pembrolizumab is a humanized monoclonal antibody (IgG_4). Potential placental transfer of human IgG is dependent upon the IgG subclass and gestational age, generally increasing as pregnancy progresses. The lowest exposure would be expected during the period of organogenesis (Palmeira 2012; Pentsuk 2009).

Based on the mechanism of action, pembrolizumab may cause fetal harm if administered during pregnancy; an alteration in the immune response or immune mediated disorders may develop following in utero exposure.

PEMEtrexed (pem e TREKS ed)

Brand Names: US Alimta

Brand Names: Canada Alimta; TARO-PEMEtrexed

Pharmacologic Category Antineoplastic Agent, Antimetabolite; Antineoplastic Agent, Antimetabolite (Antifolate)

Use

Mesothelioma: Initial treatment of malignant pleural mesothelioma (in combination with cisplatin) that is unresectable or in patients who are not otherwise candidates for curative surgery

Non-small cell lung cancer (NSCLC), nonsquamous:

Initial treatment of locally advanced or metastatic **non**squamous NSCLC (in combination with cisplatin)

Initial treatment of metastatic, **non**squamous NSCLC (in combination with platinum chemotherapy and pembrolizumab) in patients with no epidermal growth factor receptor (EGFR) or anaplastic lymphoma kinase (ALK) genomic tumor aberrations

Maintenance treatment (single-agent) of locally advanced or metastatic **non**squamous NSCLC if no progression after 4 cycles of platinum-based first-line therapy

Single-agent treatment (after prior chemotherapy) of recurrent/metastatic **non**squamous NSCLC

Limitation of use: Not indicated for the treatment of **squamous** cell NSCLC

Local Anesthetic/Vasoconstrictor Precautions No information available to require special precautions

Effects on Dental Treatment Key adverse event(s) related to dental treatment: Dysphagia, esophagitis, odynophagia, and stomatitis.

Effects on Bleeding Chemotherapy may result in significant myelosuppression, potentially including significant reduction in platelet counts (thrombocytopenia grades 3/4: 2%) and altered hemostasis. In patients who are under active treatment with these agents, medical consult is suggested.

Adverse Reactions

>10%:

Central nervous system: Fatigue (18% to 34%)

Dermatologic: Desquamation (≤14%), skin rash (≤14%)

Gastrointestinal: Nausea (12% to 31%), anorexia (19% to 22%), vomiting (6% to 16%), stomatitis (≤15%), diarrhea (5% to 13%)

Hematologic & oncologic: Anemia (15% to 19%; grades 3/4: 3% to 5%), neutropenia (6% to 11%; grades 3/4: 3% to 5%)

Respiratory: Pharyngitis (≤15%)

1% to 10%:

Cardiovascular: Edema (5%)

Central nervous system: Neuropathy (sensory: 9%; motor: ≤5%)

Dermatologic: Pruritus (7%), alopecia (6%), erythema multiforme (≤5%)

Gastrointestinal: Constipation (6%), abdominal pain (1% to <5%)

Hematologic & oncologic: Thrombocytopenia (8%; grades 3/4: 2%), febrile neutropenia (<5%)

Hepatic: Increased serum alanine aminotransferase (8% to 10%), increased serum aspartate aminotransferase (7% to 8%)

Hypersensitivity: Hypersensitivity reaction (<5%)

Infection: Infection (1% to <5%), sepsis (1%)

Ophthalmic: Conjunctivitis (≤5%), increased lacrimation (1% to <5%)

Miscellaneous: Fever (8%)

<1%, postmarketing, and/or case reports: Bullous rash, cardiac arrhythmia, colitis, depression, esophagitis, gastrointestinal obstruction, hemolytic anemia, interstitial pneumonitis, pain, pancreatitis, pulmonary embolism, radiation recall phenomenon, renal failure syndrome, Stevens-Johnson syndrome, supraventricular cardiac arrhythmia, syncope, toxic epidermal necrolysis, ventricular tachycardia

Mechanism of Action Pemetrexed is an antifolate; it disrupts folate-dependent metabolic processes essential for cell replication. Pemetrexed inhibits thymidylate synthase (TS), dihydrofolate reductase (DHFR), glycinamide ribonucleotide formyltransferase (GARFT), and aminoimidazole carboxamide ribonucleotide formyltransferase (AICARFT), the enzymes involved in folate metabolism and DNA synthesis, resulting in inhibition of purine and thymidine nucleotide and protein synthesis.

Pharmacodynamics/Kinetics

Half-life Elimination Normal renal function: 3.5 hours

Reproductive Considerations

Females of reproductive potential should use effective contraception during treatment and for at least 6 months after the last pemetrexed dose. Males with female partners of reproductive potential should use effective contraception during treatment and for 3 months after the last pemetrexed dose. Pemetrexed may impair fertility in males.

Pregnancy Considerations

Based on findings in animal reproduction studies and on the mechanism of action, pemetrexed may cause fetal harm if administered to a pregnant female.

Product Availability Pemfexy: FDA approved February 2020; availability anticipated in the first quarter of 2022. Information pertaining to this product within the monograph is pending revision. Pemfexy is a 25 mg/mL ready-to-dilute vial formulation. Consult the prescribing information for additional information.

◆ **Pemetrexed Disodium** *see* PEMEtrexed *on page 1206*

◆ **Pemfexy** *see* PEMEtrexed *on page 1206*

Pemigatinib (PEM i GA ti nib)

Brand Names: US Pemazyre

Pharmacologic Category Antineoplastic Agent, Fibroblast Growth Factor Receptor (FGFR) Inhibitor; Antineoplastic Agent, Tyrosine Kinase Inhibitor

Use Cholangiocarcinoma, unresectable, locally advanced or metastatic: Treatment of previously treated, unresectable locally advanced or metastatic cholangiocarcinoma in adults with a fibroblast growth factor receptor 2 fusion or other rearrangement (as detected by an approved test).

Local Anesthetic/Vasoconstrictor Precautions

No information available to require special precautions.

Effects on Dental Treatment Key adverse event(s) related to dental treatment: Frequent occurrence of taste alteration, stomatitis, xerostomia.

Effects on Bleeding Chemotherapy may result in significant myelosuppression including significant reduction in platelet counts (thrombocytopenia 28%) and altered hemostatsis. In patients undergoing active treatment with pemigatinib, medical consult is suggested.

Adverse Reactions

>10%:

Cardiovascular: Peripheral edema (18%)

Dermatologic: Alopecia (49%), changes in nails (43%), palmar-plantar erythrodysesthesia (15%), xeroderma (20%)

Endocrine & metabolic: Decreased serum albumin (34%), decreased serum calcium (17%), decreased serum glucose (11%), decreased serum potassium (26%), decreased serum sodium (39%), dehydration (15%), hyperphosphatemia (60% to 92%), hypophosphatemia (23%), increased serum calcium (43%), increased serum glucose (36%), increased serum potassium (12%), increased uric acid (30%), weight loss (16%)

Gastrointestinal: Abdominal pain (23%), constipation (35%), decreased appetite (33%), diarrhea (47%), dysgeusia (40%), nausea (40%), stomatitis (35%; grades ≥3: 5%), vomiting (27%), xerostomia (34%)

Genitourinary: Urinary tract infection (16%)

Hematologic & oncologic: Decreased hemoglobin (43%; grades ≥3: 6%), leukocytosis (27%; grades ≥3: <1%), leukopenia (18%; grades ≥3%: 1%), lymphocytopenia (36%; grades ≥3: 8%), thrombocytopenia (28%; grades ≥3: 3%)

Hepatic: Increased serum alanine aminotransferase (43%), increased serum alkaline phosphatase (41%), increased serum aspartate aminotransferase (43%), increased serum bilirubin (26%)

Nervous system: Fatigue (42%), headache (16%)

Neuromuscular & skeletal: Arthralgia (25%), back pain (20%), limb pain (19%)

Ophthalmic: Dry eye syndrome (27% to 35%)

Renal: Increased serum creatinine (41%)

1% to 10%:

Gastrointestinal: Cholangitis (≥2%, including infective), intestinal obstruction (≥2%)

Neuromuscular & skeletal: Bone fracture (2%), pathological fracture (1%)

Ophthalmic: Retinal pigment epithelium detachment (6%)

Renal: Acute renal failure (≥2%)

Respiratory: Pleural effusion (≥2%)

Miscellaneous: Fever (≥2%)

Frequency not defined:

Dermatologic: Nail bed changes, nail discoloration, onychoclasis, onycholysis, onychomadesis, onychomycosis, paronychia

Ophthalmic: Conjunctival abnormalities, increased lacrimation, keratitis, punctate keratitis

Mechanism of Action Pemigatinib is a fibroblast growth factor receptor (FGFR) kinase inhibitor that binds to and inhibits FGFR1, FGFR2, and FGFR3 enzyme activity. FGFR phosphorylation inhibition results in decreased FGFR-related signaling and decreased cell viability in cell lines expressing FGFR genetic alterations, leading to decreased proliferation and survival of malignant cells.

Pharmacodynamics/Kinetics

Half-life Elimination 15.4 hours.

Time to Peak ~1 hour (range: 0.5 to 6 hours).

Reproductive Considerations

Evaluate pregnancy status prior to use in females of reproductive potential.

Females of reproductive potential should use effective contraception during pemigatinib therapy and for 1 week after the last dose. Males with female partners of reproductive potential should use effective contraception during therapy and for 1 week after the last pemigatinib dose.

Pregnancy Considerations Based on the mechanism of action and data from animal reproduction studies, in utero exposure to pemigatinib may cause fetal harm.

Penciclovir (pen SYE kloe veer)

Related Information

Systemic Viral Diseases *on page 1709*

Viral Infections *on page 1754*

Related Sample Prescriptions

Viral Infections - Sample Prescriptions *on page 43*

Brand Names: US Denavir

Generic Availability (US) No

Pharmacologic Category Antiviral Agent

Dental Use Topical treatment of recurrent herpes simplex labialis (cold sores)

Use Herpes labialis (cold sores): Topical treatment of recurrent herpes labialis (cold sores) adults and children ≥12 years of age

Local Anesthetic/Vasoconstrictor Precautions

No information available to require special precautions

Effects on Dental Treatment No significant effects or complications reported

Effects on Bleeding No information available to require special precautions

Adverse Reactions

>10%: Dermatologic: Erythema (50%; mild)

1% to 10%:

Central nervous system: Headache (5%)

Local: Application site reaction (1%)

<1%, postmarketing, and/or case reports: Altered sense of smell, erythematous rash, local anesthesia, localized edema, oropharyngeal edema, pain, paresthesia, pruritus, skin discoloration, urticaria

Dental Usual Dosage Treatment of herpes simplex labialis (cold sores): Children ≥12 years and Adults: Topical: Apply cream at the first sign or symptom of cold sore (eg, tingling, swelling); apply every 2 hours during waking hours for 4 days

Dosing

Adult & Geriatric Herpes labialis (cold sores): Topical: Apply cream at the first sign or symptom of cold sore (eg, tingling, swelling) or appearance of lesion; apply every 2 hours during waking hours for 4 days.

Renal Impairment: Adult There are no dosage adjustments provided in the manufacturer's labeling. However, dosage adjustment unlikely due to low systemic absorption.

Hepatic Impairment: Adult There are no dosage adjustments provided in the manufacturer's labeling. However, dosage adjustment unlikely due to low systemic absorption.

Pediatric Herpes labialis (cold sores): Children ≥12 years and Adolescents: Topical: Cream: Apply every 2 hours during waking hours for 4 days; start at the first sign or symptom of cold sore (eg, tingling, redness, itching, swelling) or appearance of lesion

Renal Impairment: Pediatric All patients: There are no dosage adjustments provided in the manufacturer's labeling; however, dosage adjustment unlikely due to low systemic absorption.

Hepatic Impairment: Pediatric All patients: There are no dosage adjustments provided in the manufacturer's labeling; however, dosage adjustment unlikely due to low systemic absorption.

Mechanism of Action In cells infected with HSV-1 or HSV-2, viral thymidine kinase phosphorylates penciclovir to a monophosphate form which, in turn, is converted to penciclovir triphosphate by cellular kinases. Penciclovir triphosphate inhibits HSV polymerase competitively with deoxyguanosine triphosphate. Consequently, herpes viral DNA synthesis and, therefore, replication are selectively inhibited

Contraindications Hypersensitivity to the penciclovir or any component of the formulation

Warnings/Precautions Penciclovir should only be used on herpes labialis on the lips and face; because no data are available, application to mucous membranes is not recommended. Avoid application in or near eyes since it may cause irritation. The effect of penciclovir has not been established in immunocompromised patients.

Warnings: Additional Pediatric Considerations Some dosage forms may contain propylene glycol; in neonates large amounts of propylene glycol delivered orally, intravenously (eg, >3,000 mg/day), or topically have been associated with potentially fatal toxicities which can include metabolic acidosis, seizures, renal failure, and CNS depression; toxicities have also been reported in children and adults including hyperosmolality, lactic acidosis, seizures, and respiratory depression; use caution (AAP 1997; Shehab 2009).

Drug Interactions

Metabolism/Transport Effects None known.

Avoid Concomitant Use There are no known interactions where it is recommended to avoid concomitant use.

Increased Effect/Toxicity There are no known significant interactions involving an increase in effect.

Decreased Effect

Penciclovir may decrease the levels/effects of: Talimogene Laherparepvec

Pharmacodynamics/Kinetics

Onset of Action Resolution of pain: Adults: 3.5 days (Spruance 1997); Cutaneous healing: Adults: 4.8 days (Spruance 1997)

Pregnancy Considerations Penciclovir is not absorbed systemically following topical administration; exposure to the fetus is not expected.

Breastfeeding Considerations Penciclovir is not absorbed systemically following topical administration; exposure to an infant via breast milk is not expected.

Dosage Forms: US

Cream, External:

Denavir: 1% (5 g)

◆ **Pen G Benz/Pen G Procaine** *see* Penicillin G Benzathine and Penicillin G Procaine *on page 1209*

Penicillin G Benzathine

(pen i SIL in jee BENZ a theen)

Related Information

Sexually-Transmitted Diseases *on page 1707*

Brand Names: US Bicillin L-A

Brand Names: Canada Bicillin L-A

Pharmacologic Category Antibiotic, Penicillin

Use

Acute glomerulonephritis: Prophylaxis (secondary) in patients with a history of acute glomerulonephritis

Respiratory tract infections: Treatment of mild to moderate upper respiratory tract infections (including pharyngitis) caused by streptococci susceptible to low, prolonged serum concentrations of penicillin G

Rheumatic fever and chorea: Prophylaxis (secondary) of rheumatic fever and/or chorea

Rheumatic heart disease: Prophylaxis (secondary) in patients with rheumatic heart disease

Syphilis and other venereal diseases: Treatment of syphilis, yaws, bejel, and pinta

Local Anesthetic/Vasoconstrictor Precautions No information available to require special precautions

Effects on Dental Treatment No significant effects or complications reported

Effects on Bleeding No information available to require special precautions

Adverse Reactions

Frequency not defined:

Cardiovascular: Cerebrovascular accident, hypersensitivity angiitis, hypotension, palpitations, pulmonary embolism, syncope, tachycardia, vasodilation, vasospasm, vasodepressor syncope

Central nervous system: Anxiety, coma, confusion, dizziness, drowsiness, euphoria, fatigue, headache, localized warm feeling, nervousness, neurologic abnormality (neurogenic bladder), numbness of extremities, pain, seizure, transverse myelitis

Dermatologic: Diaphoresis, gangrene of skin and/or other subcutaneous tissues, pallor, pruritus, skin mottling, skin or other tissue necrosis (Nicolau syndrome), skin ulceration at injection site

Gastrointestinal: Blood in stool, *Clostridioides difficile* associated diarrhea, intestinal necrosis, nausea, vomiting

Genitourinary: Hematuria, impotence, priapism, proteinuria

Hematologic & oncologic: Lymphadenopathy

Hepatic: Increased serum aspartate aminotransferase

Hypersensitivity: Anaphylaxis, hypersensitivity reaction

Immunologic: Jarisch-Herxheimer reaction

Local: Abscess at injection site, atrophy at injection site, bleeding at injection site, bruising at injection site, cellulitis at injection site, localized edema (at injection site), inflammation at injection site, injection site reaction (neurovascular damage), pain at injection site, residual mass at injection site, tissue necrosis at injection site

Neuromuscular & skeletal: Arthropathy, asthenia, exacerbation of arthritis, periosteal disease, rhabdomyolysis, tremor

Ophthalmic: Blindness, blurred vision

Renal: Increased blood urea nitrogen, increased serum creatinine, myoglobinuria, renal failure syndrome

Respiratory: Apnea, cyanotic extremities, dyspnea, hypoxia, pulmonary hypertension

Mechanism of Action Interferes with bacterial cell wall synthesis during active multiplication, causing cell wall death and resultant bactericidal activity against susceptible bacteria

Pharmacodynamics/Kinetics

Duration of Action Dose dependent: 1 to 4 weeks; larger doses result in more sustained levels

Time to Peak Serum: Within 12 to 24 hours; serum levels are usually detectable for 1 to 4 weeks depending on the dose; larger doses result in more sustained levels rather than higher levels

Pregnancy Considerations

Penicillin G benzathine crosses the placenta (Nathan 1993; Weeks 1997).

Maternal use of penicillins has generally not resulted in an increased risk of adverse fetal effects. Penicillin G is the drug of choice for treatment of syphilis during pregnancy (CDC [Workowski 2015]).

Penicillin G Benzathine and Penicillin G Procaine

(pen i SIL in jee BENZ a theen & pen i SIL in jee PROE kane)

Related Information

Penicillin G Benzathine *on page 1208*

Penicillin G Procaine *on page 1210*

Brand Names: US Bicillin C-R; Bicillin C-R 900/300

Pharmacologic Category Antibiotic, Penicillin

Use

Pneumococcal infections: Treatment of moderately severe pneumonia and otitis media due to susceptible *Pneumococcus* spp. (eg, *Streptococcus pneumoniae*)

Streptococcal infections, group A: Treatment of moderately severe to severe infections, without associated bacteremia, of the upper respiratory tract, scarlet fever, erysipelas, and skin and soft tissue infections due to group A streptococci

Note: Bicillin C-R 900/300 is only indicated in pediatric patients.

Limitations of use: Not considered appropriate for the treatment of sexually transmitted diseases, including syphilis, gonorrhea, yaws, bejel, and pinta. When high, sustained serum levels are required, use alternative penicillin preparations.

Local Anesthetic/Vasoconstrictor Precautions No information available to require special precautions

Effects on Dental Treatment No significant effects or complications reported

Effects on Bleeding No information available to require special precautions

Adverse Reactions Also see individual agents.

<1%, postmarketing, and/or case reports: Central nervous system disease (Hoigne syndrome), *Clostridioides difficile* associated diarrhea

Mechanism of Action Inhibits bacterial cell wall synthesis by binding to one or more of the penicillin-binding proteins (PBPs); which in turn inhibits the final transpeptidation step of peptidoglycan synthesis in bacterial cell walls, thus inhibiting cell wall biosynthesis. Bacteria eventually lyse due to ongoing activity of cell wall autolytic enzymes (autolysins and murein hydrolases) while cell wall assembly is arrested.

Pharmacodynamics/Kinetics

Time to Peak Serum: IM: Within 3 hours

Pregnancy Considerations Adverse events have not been observed in animal reproduction studies. Maternal use of penicillins has generally not resulted in an increased risk of adverse fetal effects. See individual agents

Penicillin G (Parenteral/Aqueous)

(pen i SIL in jee, pa REN ter al, AYE kwee us)

Related Information

Sexually-Transmitted Diseases *on page 1707*

Brand Names: US Pfizerpen

Brand Names: Canada Crystapen [DSC]

Pharmacologic Category Antibiotic, Penicillin

Use

Anthrax: Treatment of anthrax caused by *Bacillus anthracis*

Actinomycosis: Treatment of actinomycosis (cervicofacial disease and thoracic and abdominal disease) caused by *Actinomyces israelii*

Clostridial infections: Treatment of botulism (adjunctive therapy to antitoxin), gas gangrene, and tetanus (adjunctive therapy to human tetanus immune globulin) caused by *Clostridium* spp.

Diphtheria: Treatment of diphtheria (adjunctive therapy to antitoxin and prevention of the carrier state) caused by *Corynebacterium diphtheriae*

Erysipelothrix endocarditis: Treatment of erysipelothrix endocarditis caused by *Erysipelothrix rhusiopathiae*

Fusospirochetosis: Treatment of fusospirochetosis, including severe infections of the oropharynx [Vincent], lower respiratory tract and genital area, caused by *Fusobacterium* spp. and spirochetes

Listeria infections: Treatment of listeria infections, including meningitis and endocarditis, caused by *Listeria monocytogenes*

Meningococcal infection: Treatment of meningococcal meningitis and/or septicemia caused by *Neisseria meningitidis*

Pasteurella infections: Treatment of pasteurella infections, including bacteremia and meningitis, caused by *Pasteurella multocida*

Rat bite fever: Treatment of rat bite fever (including Haverhill fever) caused by *Spirillum minus* or *S. moniliformis*

Serious gram-positive infections: Treatment of septicemia, empyema, pneumonia, pericarditis, endocarditis, and meningitis caused by *Streptococcus pyogenes* (group A beta-hemolytic streptococcus), other beta-hemolytic streptococci including groups C, H, G, L and M, *Streptococcus pneumoniae* and *Staphylococcus* species (nonpenicillinase-producing strains)

Syphilis: Treatment of syphilis (congenital and neurosyphilis) caused by *Treponema pallidum*

Local Anesthetic/Vasoconstrictor Precautions No information available to require special precautions

Effects on Dental Treatment No significant effects or complications reported

Effects on Bleeding No information available to require special precautions

Adverse Reactions

Frequency not defined:

- Cardiovascular: Local thrombophlebitis, localized phlebitis
- Central nervous system: Coma (high doses), hyperreflexia (high doses), myoclonus (high doses), seizure (high doses)
- Dermatologic: Exfoliative dermatitis, maculopapular rash, skin rash
- Endocrine & metabolic: Electrolyte disorder (high doses)
- Gastrointestinal: *Clostridioides difficile* associated diarrhea, *Clostridioides difficile* colitis
- Hematologic & oncologic: Neutropenia, positive direct Coombs test (rare, high doses)
- Hypersensitivity: Anaphylaxis, angioedema, hypersensitivity reaction (immediate and delayed), serum sickness-like reaction
- Immunologic: Jarisch-Herxheimer reaction
- Local: Pain at injection site
- Renal: Acute interstitial nephritis (high doses), renal tubular disease (high doses)

Mechanism of Action Interferes with bacterial cell wall synthesis during active multiplication, causing cell wall death and resultant bactericidal activity against susceptible bacteria

Pharmacodynamics/Kinetics

Half-life Elimination

Neonates: <6 days of age: 3.2 hours; ≥14 days of age: 1.4 hours

Adults: Normal renal function: 31 to 50 minutes

End-stage renal disease (ESRD): 6 to 20 hours (Aronoff 2007)

Time to Peak Serum: IV: Immediately after infusion

Pregnancy Considerations Penicillin G crosses the placenta.

Maternal use of penicillins has generally not resulted in an increased risk of adverse fetal effects.

Penicillin G is the drug of choice for treatment of syphilis during pregnancy and penicillin G (parenteral/aqueous) is the drug of choice for the prevention of early-onset Group B Streptococcal (GBS) disease in newborns (ACOG 797 2020; CDC [Workowski 2015]). When IV therapy is required for anthrax infection in pregnant and postpartum women, penicillin G may be used as an alternative agent (Meaney-Delman 2014).

◆ **Penicillin G Potassium** *see* Penicillin G (Parenteral/Aqueous) *on page 1209*

Penicillin G Procaine (pen i SIL in jee PROE kane)

Brand Names: Canada Penpro [DSC]

Pharmacologic Category Antibiotic, Penicillin

Use

Anthrax, prophylaxis: To reduce the incidence of the disease following exposure to aerosolized *Bacillus anthracis*.

Anthrax, treatment: Treatment of anthrax, including post-exposure inhalational disease due to aerosolized *B. anthracis*.

Diphtheria: As an adjunct to antitoxin for prevention of the carrier stage of diphtheria caused by susceptible *Corynebacterium diphtheriae*.

Endocarditis, subacute: Treatment of subacute bacterial endocarditis, only in extremely sensitive infections, caused by susceptible group A streptococci.

Erysipeloid: Treatment of erysipeloid caused by susceptible *Erysipelothrix rhusiopathiae*.

Fusospirochetosis: Treatment of fusospirochetosis (Vincent gingivitis and pharyngitis) in conjunction with dental care, and moderately severe infections of the oropharynx caused by susceptible fusiform bacilli and spirochetes.

Pneumococcal infection: Treatment of moderately severe infections of the respiratory tract caused by susceptible pneumococci.

Limitations of use: Severe pneumonia, empyema, bacteremia, pericarditis, meningitis, peritonitis, and arthritis of pneumococcal etiology are better treated with aqueous penicillin G during the acute stage.

Rat bite fever: Treatment of rat bite fever caused by susceptible *Streptobacillus moniliformis* and *Spirillum minus* organisms.

Skin and soft tissue infection: Treatment of moderately severe infections of the skin and soft tissues caused by susceptible staphylococci (penicillin G-susceptible).

Streptococcal infections: Treatment of moderately severe to severe infections of the upper respiratory tract, skin and soft tissue infections, scarlet fever, and erysipelas caused by susceptible streptococci (group A, without bacteremia).

Limitations of use: Some streptococcal groups, including group D (enterococcus), are resistant. Aqueous penicillin is recommended for streptococcal infections with bacteremia.

Syphilis: Treatment of syphilis (all stages) caused by susceptible *Treponema pallidum*.

Yaws, bejel, and pinta: Treatment of yaws, bejel, and pinta caused by susceptible organisms.

Limitations of use: When high, sustained serum levels are required, use aqueous penicillin G, either intramuscularly (IM) or intravenously (IV). Do not use in the treatment of beta-lactamase-producing organisms, which includes most strains of *Neisseria gonorrhea*.

Local Anesthetic/Vasoconstrictor Precautions No information available to require special precautions

Effects on Dental Treatment No significant effects or complications reported

Effects on Bleeding No information available to require special precautions

Adverse Reactions Frequency not defined.

<1%, postmarketing, and/or case reports: Anaphylaxis, central nervous system toxicity, *Clostridioides difficile* colitis, exfoliative dermatitis, hypersensitivity reaction, Jarisch-Herxheimer reaction, maculopapular rash, serum sickness-like reaction, skin rash, urticaria

Mechanism of Action Inhibits bacterial cell wall synthesis by binding to one or more of the penicillin-binding proteins (PBPs); which in turn inhibits the final transpeptidation step of peptidoglycan synthesis in bacterial cell walls, thus inhibiting cell wall biosynthesis. Bacteria eventually lyse due to ongoing activity of cell wall autolytic enzymes (autolysins and murein hydrolases) while cell wall assembly is arrested.

Pharmacodynamics/Kinetics

Duration of Action Therapeutic: 15 to 24 hours

Time to Peak Serum: Within 1 to 4 hours and can persist within the therapeutic range for 15 to 24 hours

Pregnancy Considerations Penicillin G crosses the placenta.

Maternal use of penicillins has generally not resulted in an increased risk of adverse fetal effects. Penicillin G procaine may be used in the treatment of syphilis during pregnancy (consult current guidelines) (CDC [Workowski 2015]). Penicillin G procaine is also approved for the management of *Bacillus anthracis*; however, other agents are preferred for use in pregnant women (Meaney-Delman 2014).

◆ **Penicillin G Procaine and Benzathine Combined** *see* Penicillin G Benzathine and Penicillin G Procaine *on page 1209*

◆ **Penicillin G Procaine/Benzath** *see* Penicillin G Benzathine and Penicillin G Procaine *on page 1209*

◆ **Penicillin G Sodium** *see* Penicillin G (Parenteral/Aqueous) *on page 1209*

Penicillin V Potassium

(pen i SIL in vee poe TASS ee um)

Related Information

Bacterial Infections *on page 1739*

Viral Infections *on page 1754*

Related Sample Prescriptions

Bacterial Infections and Periodontal Diseases - Sample Prescriptions *on page 35*

Brand Names: Canada APO-Pen VK; NOVO-Pen VK [DSC]; Pen-VK

Generic Availability (US) Yes

Pharmacologic Category Antibiotic, Penicillin

Dental Use Treatment of common orofacial infections caused by aerobic gram-positive cocci and anaerobes. These orofacial infections include cellulitis, periapical abscess, periodontal abscess, acute suppurative pulpitis, oronasal fistula, pericoronitis, osteitis, osteomyelitis, postsurgical and post-traumatic infection.

Use

Fusospirochetosis (Vincent gingivitis and pharyngitis): Treatment of fusospirochetosis (Vincent gingivitis and pharyngitis), in conjunction with dental care for infections involving gum tissue.

Pneumococcal infections: Treatment of mild to moderately severe pneumococcal respiratory tract infections, including otitis media.

Rheumatic fever and/or chorea prophylaxis: Prophylaxis (chronic, secondary) of rheumatic fever and/or chorea.

Staphylococcal infections (penicillin G-sensitive): Treatment of mild infections of the skin and soft tissues.

Streptococcal infections (without bacteremia): Treatment of mild to moderate streptococcal infections of the upper respiratory tract, scarlet fever, and mild erysipelas.

Local Anesthetic/Vasoconstrictor Precautions No information available to require special precautions

Effects on Dental Treatment Key adverse event(s) related to dental treatment: Oral candidiasis (prolonged use).

Effects on Bleeding No information available to require special precautions

Adverse Reactions

>10%: Gastrointestinal: Melanoglossia, mild diarrhea, nausea, oral candidiasis, vomiting

<1%: Acute interstitial nephritis, anaphylaxis, convulsions, exfoliative dermatitis, fever, hemolytic anemia, hypersensitivity reaction, positive direct Coombs test, serum-sickness like reaction

Dental Usual Dosage

Orofacial infections: Oral:

Children <12 years: 25 to 50 mg/kg/day in divided doses every 6 to 8 hours (maximum dose: 3,000 mg daily)

Children ≥12 years and Adults: 125 to 500 mg every 6 to 8 hours

Dosing

Adult & Geriatric

Usual dosage range: Oral: 125 to 500 mg every 6 to 8 hours

Actinomycosis (off-label use): Oral: **Note:** Duration is dependent upon disease location and patient-specific factors; complicated infections requiring surgical intervention usually initiate IV therapy with penicillin G until disease subsidence followed by long term oral therapy (Hsieh 1993; Sudhakar 2004):

2 to 4 g/day in divided doses every 6 hours (Smego 1998)

Anthrax (off-label use): Note: Consult public health officials for event-specific recommendations.

Inhalational exposure (postexposure prophylaxis [PEP]): Oral: 500 mg every 6 hours for 42 to 60 days (CDC [Hendricks 2014]).

Note: Anthrax vaccine should also be administered to exposed individuals (CDC [Bower 2019]; CDC [Hendricks 2014]).

Duration of therapy: If the PEP anthrax vaccine series is administered on schedule (for all regimens), antibiotics may be discontinued in immunocompetent adults aged 18 to 65 years at 42 days after initiation of vaccine or 2 weeks after the last dose of the vaccine (whichever comes last and not to exceed 60 days); if the vaccination series cannot be completed, antibiotics should continue for 60 days (CDC [Bower 2019]). In addition, adults with immunocompromising conditions or receiving immunosuppressive therapy, patients >65 years of age, and patients who are pregnant or breastfeeding should receive antibiotics for 60 days (CDC [Bower 2019]).

Cutaneous (without systemic involvement), treatment: Oral: 500 mg 4 times daily.

Duration of therapy: For community-acquired cutaneous anthrax, treatment should continue for 7 to 10 days (IDSA [Stevens 2014]); for bioterrorism-related cases, treatment should continue for 60 days (CDC [Hendricks 2014]).

Bite wounds (animal) (off-label use): Oral: 500 mg 4 times daily in combination with dicloxacillin (IDSA [Stevens 2014])

Cutaneous erysipeloid (off-label use): Oral: 500 mg 4 times daily for 7 to 10 days (IDSA [Stevens 2014])

Erysipelas: Oral:

500 mg 4 times daily (IDSA [Stevens 2014])

Manufacturer's labeling: Dosing in the prescribing information may not reflect current clinical practice. 125 to 250 mg every 6 to 8 hours.

Fusospirochetosis (Vincent infection): Oral: 250 to 500 mg every 6 to 8 hours

Pneumococcal prophylaxis in hematopoietic cell transplant (off-label use): Oral: 250 to 500 mg twice daily. **Note:** Use only in areas where incidence of penicillin-resistant *S. pneumoniae* is low (Tomblyn 2009).

Prosthetic joint infection (off-label use): *Chronic oral antimicrobial suppression (Enterococcus spp [penicillin-susceptible], streptococci [beta-hemolytic], Cutibacterium spp):* Oral: 500 mg 2 to 4 times daily (Osmon 2013)

Streptococcal skin infection (off-label dose): Oral: 250 to 500 mg every 6 hours (IDSA [Stevens 2014])

Streptococcus (group A): Oral:

Pharyngitis, acute treatment: 500 mg 2 to 3 times daily for 10 days (AHA [Gerber 2009]); **or** 250 mg 4 times daily or 500 mg twice daily for 10 days (IDSA [Shulman 2012])

Secondary prophylaxis for rheumatic fever (prevention of recurrent attacks) (alternative agent): 250 mg twice daily. Duration depends on risk factors and presence of valvular disease (AHA [Gerber 2009]).

Chronic carriage (off-label use): 500 mg 4 times daily for 10 days in combination with oral rifampin. **Note:** Most individuals with chronic carriage do not require antibiotics (IDSA [Shulman 2012])

Renal Impairment: Adult There are no dosage adjustments provided in manufacturer's labeling. Use with caution; excretion is prolonged in patients with renal impairment.

Hepatic Impairment: Adult There are no dosage adjustments provided in manufacturer's labeling.

Pediatric

General dosing: Infants, Children, and Adolescents: Mild to moderate infection: Oral: 25 to 50 mg/kg/day in divided doses every 6 hours; maximum daily dose: 2,000 mg/**day** (Bradley 2019; *Red Book* [AAP 2018]).

Anthrax (penicillin-susceptible strains) (alternative agent) (AAP [Bradley 2014]): Infants, Children, and Adolescents:

Postexposure prophylaxis, exposure to aerosolized spores: Oral: 50 to 75 mg/kg/day in divided doses every 6 to 8 hours for 60 days.

Cutaneous, without systemic involvement: Oral: 50 to 75 mg/kg/day in divided doses every 6 to 8 hours. Duration: 7 to 10 days for naturally acquired infection, up to 60 days for biological weapon-related event/exposure to aerosolized spore.

Systemic, oral step-down therapy: Oral: 50 to 75 mg/kg/day in divided doses every 6 to 8 hours to complete 60-day course; should be used as a component of combination therapy.

Fusospirochetosis (Vincent infection), mild to moderately severe infections: Children ≥12 years and Adolescents: Oral: 250 to 500 mg every 6 to 8 hours.

Group A streptococcal infection:

Pharyngitis, acute treatment (primary prevention of rheumatic fever) (AHA [Gerber 2009]; IDSA [Shulman 2012]; *Red Book* [AAP 2018]; WHO 2004):

Children <27 kg: Oral: 250 mg 2 to 3 times daily for 10 days.

Children ≥27 kg and Adolescents: Oral: 500 mg 2 to 3 times daily for 10 days; in adolescents, 250 mg 4 times daily has also been suggested.

Rheumatic fever, secondary prevention: Children and Adolescents: Oral: 250 mg twice daily (AHA [Gerber 2009]).

Chronic carriers of Group A Streptococcus, treatment: **Note:** Antibiotic therapy is generally not recommended for chronic *Streptococcus pyogenes* carriage; however, it may be considered in certain cases (IDSA [Shulman 2012]; *Red Book* [AAP 2018]).

Children and Adolescents: Oral: 50 mg/kg/day in 4 divided doses for 10 days in combination with oral rifampin for the last 4 days; maximum daily dose: 2,000 mg/**day** (IDSA [Shulman 2012]).

Pneumonia, community-acquired; Group A *Streptococcus*, mild infection or step-down therapy: Infants, Children, and Adolescents: Oral: 50 to 75 mg/kg/day in divided doses 4 times daily (Bradley 2019; *Red Book* [AAP 2018]); **Note:** Usual adult maximum daily dose is 2,000 mg/**day**.

Pneumococcal infection prophylaxis, anatomic or functional asplenia (eg, sickle cell disease [SCD]) (AAP 2000; Gaston 1986; NHLBI 2014):

Infants (as soon as SCD diagnosed or asplenic) and Children <3 years: Oral: 125 mg twice daily.

Children ≥3 years: Oral: 250 mg twice daily.

Note: Current guidelines recommend discontinuation of prophylaxis at 5 years of age unless the patient has experienced invasive pneumococcal infection or splenectomy; data regarding when to discontinue are limited and practice varies; decision should be made on a case-by-case basis (McCavit 2013; *Red Book* [AAP 2018]).

Pneumococcal infection prophylaxis, patients post-hematopoietic cell transplant with chronic graft-versus-host disease or low IgG levels (Tomblyn 2009): **Note:** Use only in areas where incidence of penicillin-resistant *Streptococcus pneumoniae* is low.

Infants ≥2 months and Children ≤3 years: Oral: 125 mg twice daily.

Children >3 years: Oral: 250 mg twice daily.

Adolescents: Oral: 250 to 500 mg twice daily or 500 to 1,000 mg once daily.

Renal Impairment: Pediatric There are no dosage adjustments provided in the manufacturer's labeling. Use with caution; excretion is prolonged in patients with kidney impairment.

Hepatic Impairment: Pediatric There are no dosage adjustments provided in the manufacturer's labeling.

Mechanism of Action Inhibits bacterial cell wall synthesis by binding to one or more of the penicillin-binding proteins (PBPs); which in turn inhibits the final transpeptidation step of peptidoglycan synthesis in bacterial cell walls, thus inhibiting cell wall biosynthesis. Bacteria eventually lyse due to ongoing activity of cell wall autolytic enzymes (autolysins and murein hydrolases) while cell wall assembly is arrested.

Contraindications Hypersensitivity to penicillin or any component of the formulation

Warnings/Precautions Use with caution in patients with severe renal impairment or history of seizures. Serious and occasionally severe or fatal hypersensitivity (anaphylactic) reactions have been reported in patients on penicillin therapy, especially with a history of beta-lactam hypersensitivity or history of sensitivity to multiple allergens. Use with caution in asthmatic patients. If a serious reaction occurs, treatment with supportive care measures and airway protection should be instituted immediately. Extended duration of therapy or use associated with high serum concentrations may be associated with an increased risk for some adverse reactions. Prolonged use may result in fungal or bacterial superinfection, including *C. difficile*-associated diarrhea (CDAD) and pseudomembranous colitis; CDAD has been observed >2 months postantibiotic treatment. Potentially significant interactions may exist, requiring dose or frequency adjustment, additional monitoring, and/or selection of alternative therapy.

Benzyl alcohol and derivatives: Some dosage forms may contain sodium benzoate/benzoic acid; benzoic acid (benzoate) is a metabolite of benzyl alcohol; large amounts of benzyl alcohol (≥99 mg/kg/day) have been associated with a potentially fatal toxicity ("gasping syndrome") in neonates; the "gasping syndrome" consists of metabolic acidosis, respiratory distress, gasping respirations, CNS dysfunction (including convulsions, intracranial hemorrhage), hypotension, and cardiovascular collapse (AAP ["Inactive" 1997]; CDC, 1982); some data suggests that benzoate displaces bilirubin from protein binding sites (Ahlfors 2001); avoid or use dosage forms containing benzyl alcohol derivative with caution in neonates. See manufacturer's labeling.

Drug Interactions

Metabolism/Transport Effects **Substrate** of OAT1/3

Avoid Concomitant Use

Avoid concomitant use of Penicillin V Potassium with any of the following: BCG (Intravesical); Cholera Vaccine

Increased Effect/Toxicity

Penicillin V Potassium may increase the levels/effects of: Dichlorphenamide; Methotrexate; Vitamin K Antagonists

The levels/effects of Penicillin V Potassium may be increased by: Acemetacin; Nitisinone; Pretomanid; Probenecid; Teriflunomide; Tolvaptan

Decreased Effect

Penicillin V Potassium may decrease the levels/effects of: Aminoglycosides; BCG (Intravesical); BCG Vaccine (Immunization); Cholera Vaccine; Lactobacillus and Estriol; Mycophenolate; Sodium Picosulfate; Typhoid Vaccine

The levels/effects of Penicillin V Potassium may be decreased by: Tetracyclines

Food Interactions Food decreases drug absorption rate; decreases drug serum concentration. Management: Take on an empty stomach 1 hour before or 2 hours after meals around-the-clock to promote less variation in peak and trough serum levels.

Pregnancy Considerations Penicillin crosses the placenta.

Maternal use of penicillins has generally not resulted in an increased risk of adverse fetal effects. Due to pregnancy-induced physiologic changes, some pharmacokinetic parameters of penicillin V may be altered in the second and third trimester (Heikkilä 1993). If treatment for the management of *Bacillus anthracis* is needed in pregnant women, other agents are preferred (Meaney-Delman 2014)

Breastfeeding Considerations Penicillin V is present in breast milk (Matheson 1988).

The relative infant dose (RID) of penicillin V is 0.6% when calculated using the highest breast milk concentration located and compared to a weight-adjusted maternal daily dose of 2,640 mg.

In general, breastfeeding is considered acceptable when the RID is <10 (Anderson 2016; Ito 2000).

Using the highest milk concentration located (1.55 mg/L), the estimated daily infant dose via breast milk is 0.23 mg/kg/day. This milk concentration was obtained following a maternal administration of oral penicillin V regimen consisting of an initial dose of 1,320 mg followed by daily administration of three doses at 8-hour intervals of 660 mg, 660 mg, and 1,320 mg, respectively. Milk concentrations reached a peak 2 to 8 hours after a 1,320 mg dose; the half-life in breast milk ranged from 1 to 3.8 hours in women with mastitis (Matheson 1988).

Penicillin V may be detected in the urine of some breastfeeding infants (Matheson 1988).

Loose stools and rash have been reported in breastfeeding infants exposed to penicillin V (Matheson 1988). In general, antibiotics that are present in breast milk may cause nondose-related modification of bowel flora. Monitor infants for GI disturbances (WHO 2002).

Penicillin V is considered compatible with breastfeeding when used in usual recommended doses (WHO 2002).

Dosage Forms: US

Solution Reconstituted, Oral:

Generic: 125 mg/5 mL (100 mL, 200 mL); 250 mg/5 mL (100 mL, 200 mL)

Tablet, Oral:

Generic: 250 mg, 500 mg

Dosage Forms: Canada

Solution Reconstituted, Oral:

Generic: 125 mg/5 mL (100 mL); 300 mg/5 mL (100 mL)

Tablet, Oral:

Generic: 300 mg

◆ **Penlac [DSC]** *see* Ciclopirox *on page* *346*

◆ **Pennsaid** *see* Diclofenac (Topical) *on page* *489*

◆ **Pentasa** *see* Mesalamine *on page* *980*

◆ **Pentasodium Colistin Methanesulfonate** *see* Colistimethate *on page* *408*

◆ **Pentavalent Human-Bovine Reassortant Rotavirus Vaccine (PRV)** *see* Rotavirus Vaccine *on page* *1349*

PENTobarbital (pen toe BAR bi tal)

Brand Names: US Nembutal

Pharmacologic Category Anticonvulsant, Barbiturate; Barbiturate

Use

Sedative/hypnotic/preanesthesia: Short-term (<2 weeks) treatment of insomnia or as preanesthesia.

Seizures: Emergency control of certain anticonvulsive episodes (eg, status epilepticus, cholera, eclampsia, meningitis, tetanus, toxic reactions to strychnine or local anesthetics).

Local Anesthetic/Vasoconstrictor Precautions No information available to require special precautions

Effects on Dental Treatment No significant effects or complications reported

Effects on Bleeding No information available to require special precautions

Adverse Reactions Frequency not defined.

Cardiovascular: Bradycardia, hypotension, syncope

Central nervous system: Abnormality in thinking, agitation, anxiety, ataxia, central nervous system stimulation, confusion, depression, dizziness, drowsiness, hallucination, headache, insomnia, nervousness, nightmares, psychiatric disturbance

Dermatologic: Exfoliative dermatitis, skin rash

Gastrointestinal: Constipation, nausea, vomiting

Hematologic & oncologic: Megaloblastic anemia

Hepatic: Hepatotoxicity

Hypersensitivity: Angioedema, hypersensitivity reaction

Local: Injection site reaction

Neuromuscular & skeletal: Hyperkinesia, laryngospasm

Respiratory: Apnea (especially with rapid IV use), hypoventilation, respiratory depression

Miscellaneous: Fever

Mechanism of Action Barbiturate with sedative, hypnotic, and anticonvulsant properties. Barbiturates depress the sensory cortex, decrease motor activity, alter cerebellar function, and produce drowsiness, sedation, and hypnosis. In high doses, barbiturates exhibit anticonvulsant activity; barbiturates produce dose-dependent respiratory depression; reduce brain metabolism and cerebral blood flow in order to decrease intracranial pressure

Pharmacodynamics/Kinetics

Onset of Action Krauss 2006: Children and Adults: Sedation: IM: 10 to 15 minutes; IV: Almost immediate, within 3 to 5 minutes; Oral, Rectal: 15 to 60 minutes

Duration of Action Krauss 2006: Children and Adults: Sedation: IM: 1 to 2 hours; IV: 15 to 45 minutes; Oral, Rectal: 1 to 4 hours

Half-life Elimination Terminal: Children: 26 ± 16 hours (Schaible 1982); Adults: Healthy: 22 hours (average) (Ehrnebo 1974); Range: 15 to 50 hours; dose dependent

Pregnancy Risk Factor D

Pregnancy Considerations Barbiturates can be detected in the placenta, fetal liver and fetal brain. Fetal and maternal blood concentrations may be similar following parenteral administration. An increased incidence of fetal abnormalities may occur following maternal use. When used during the third trimester of pregnancy, withdrawal symptoms may occur in the neonate including seizures and hyperirritability; symptoms may be delayed up to 14 days. Use of hypnotic doses during labor does not impair uterine activity; however, use of full anesthetic doses decrease the force and frequency of uterine contractions. Respiratory depression may occur in the newborn when sedative-hypnotic barbiturates are administered to the mother during labor; resuscitation equipment should be available, especially for premature infants.

Controlled Substance C-II

◆ **Pentobarbital Sodium** *see* PENTobarbital *on page 1213*

Pentosan Polysulfate Sodium

(PEN toe san pol i SUL fate SOW dee um)

Brand Names: US Elmiron

Brand Names: Canada Elmiron

Pharmacologic Category Analgesic, Urinary

Use Interstitial cystitis: Relief of bladder pain or discomfort due to interstitial cystitis

Local Anesthetic/Vasoconstrictor Precautions

No information available to require special precautions

Effects on Dental Treatment No significant effects or complications reported

Effects on Bleeding Pentosan polysulfate sodium is a low-molecular weight heparin-like compound with anticoagulant and fibrinolytic effects. Medical consult is suggested.

Adverse Reactions

1% to 10%:

Central nervous system: Headache (3%), dizziness (1%)

Dermatologic: Alopecia (4%), skin rash (3%)

Gastrointestinal: Diarrhea (4%), nausea (4%), abdominal pain (2%), dyspepsia (2%)

Hematologic & oncologic: Rectal hemorrhage (6%)

Hepatic: Abnormal hepatic function tests (1%; dose-related)

<1%, postmarketing, and/or case reports: Amblyopia, anemia, anorexia, colitis, conjunctivitis, constipation, dehydration, depression, diaphoresis, dyspnea, ecchymoses, emotional lability, epistaxis, esophagitis, flatulence, gastritis, gingival hemorrhage, hyperkinetic muscle activity, hypersensitivity reaction, insomnia, leukopenia, maculopathy (Hanif 2019), optic neuritis, oral mucosa ulcer, pharyngitis, prolonged partial thromboplastin time, prolonged prothrombin time, pruritus, retinal hemorrhage, rhinitis, skin photosensitivity, thrombocytopenia, tinnitus, urticaria, vomiting

Mechanism of Action Although pentosan polysulfate sodium is a low-molecular weight heparinoid, it is not known whether these properties play a role in its mechanism of action in treating interstitial cystitis; the drug appears to adhere to the bladder wall mucosa where it may act as a buffer to protect the tissues from irritating substances in the urine.

Pharmacodynamics/Kinetics

Half-life Elimination 20-27 hours

Time to Peak Serum: 2 hours (range: 0.6-120 hours)

Pregnancy Considerations

No adverse events were noted in animal reproduction studies; however, reversible limb bud abnormalities were noted during in vitro animal studies. Use with caution and only if clearly needed during pregnancy. Based on limited data, pentosan polysulfate does not appear to cross the placenta.

Pentostatin (pen toe STAT in)

Brand Names: US Nipent

Pharmacologic Category Antineoplastic Agent, Antimetabolite; Antineoplastic Agent, Antimetabolite (Purine Analog)

Use Hairy cell leukemia: Treatment (as a single agent) of untreated and interferon alfa-refractory hairy cell leukemia in patients with active disease (clinically significant anemia, neutropenia, thrombocytopenia, or disease-related symptoms).

Local Anesthetic/Vasoconstrictor Precautions

No information available to require special precautions

Effects on Dental Treatment Key adverse event(s) related to dental treatment: Stomatitis.

Effects on Bleeding Chemotherapy may result in significant myelosuppression, potentially including significant reduction in platelet counts (thrombocytopenia: 6% to 32%) and altered hemostasis. In patients who are under active treatment with these agents, medical consult is suggested.

Adverse Reactions

>10%:

Central nervous system: Fatigue (29% to 42%), pain (8% to 20%), chills (11% to 19%), headache (13% to 17%), central nervous system toxicity (1% to 11%)

Dermatologic: Skin rash (26% to 43%), pruritus (10% to 21%), skin changes (4% to 17%)

Gastrointestinal: Nausea (≤63%), vomiting (≤63%), diarrhea (15% to 17%), anorexia (13% to 16%), abdominal pain (4% to 16%), stomatitis (5% to 12%)

Hematologic & oncologic: Leukopenia (22% to 60%), anemia (8% to 35%), thrombocytopenia (6% to 32%)

Hepatic: Increased serum transaminases (2% to 19%)

Hypersensitivity: Hypersensitivity reaction (2% to 11%)

Infection: Infection (7% to 38%)

Neuromuscular & skeletal: Myalgia (11% to 19%), asthenia (10% to 12%)

Respiratory: Cough (17% to 20%), upper respiratory tract infection (13% to 16%), rhinitis (10% to 11%), dyspnea (8% to 11%)

Miscellaneous: Fever (42% to 46%)

1% to 10%:

Cardiovascular: Chest pain (3% to 10%), facial edema (3% to 10%), hypotension (3% to 10%), peripheral edema (3% to 10%), angina pectoris (<3%), atrioventricular block (<3%), bradycardia (<3%), cardiac arrhythmia (<3%), cardiac failure (<3%), deep vein thrombophlebitis (<3%), hypertension (<3%), pericardial effusion (<3%), phlebitis (<3%), pulmonary embolism (<3%), sinoatrial arrest (<3%), syncope (<3%), tachycardia (<3%), vasculitis (<3%), ventricular premature contractions (<3%)

Central nervous system: Anxiety (3% to 10%), confusion (3% to 10%), depression (3% to 10%), dizziness (3% to 10%), drowsiness (3% to 10%), insomnia (3% to 10%), nervousness (3% to 10%), paresthesia (3% to 10%), abnormal dreams (<3%), abnormality in thinking (<3%), amnesia (<3%), ataxia (<3%), dysarthria (<3%), emotional lability (<3%), encephalitis (<3%), hallucination (<3%), hangover effect (<3%), hostility (<3%), meningism (<3%), neuralgia (<3%), neuritis (<3%), neuropathy (<3%), neurosis (<3%), paralysis (<3%), seizure (<3%), twitching (<3%), vertigo (<3%)

Dermatologic: Diaphoresis (8% to 10%), urticaria (3% to 10%), xeroderma (3% to 10%), cellulitis (6%), furunculosis (4%), acne vulgaris (<3%), alopecia (<3%), eczema (<3%), skin photosensitivity (<3%)

Endocrine & metabolic: Amenorrhea (<3%), decreased libido (<3%), hypercalcemia (<3%), hyponatremia (<3%), gout (<3%), loss of libido (<3%)

Gastrointestinal: Dyspepsia (3% to 10%), flatulence (3% to 10%), gingivitis (3% to 10%), constipation (<3%), dysgeusia (<3%), dysphagia (<3%), glossitis (<3%), intestinal obstruction (<3%), oral candidiasis (2%)

Genitourinary: Urinary tract infection (3%), impotence (<3%), lump in breast (<3%)

Hematologic & oncologic: Agranulocytosis (3% to 10%), hemorrhage (3% to 10%), acute leukemia (<3%), aplastic anemia (<3%), hemolytic anemia (<3%), neoplasm (<3%), petechial rash (<3%)

Infection: Herpes zoster infection (8%), viral infection (8%), bacterial infection (5%), herpes simplex infection (4%), sepsis (3%), abscess (2%)

Neuromuscular & skeletal: Arthralgia (3% to 6%), arthritis (<3%), hyperkinetic muscle activity (<3%), osteomyelitis (1%)

Ophthalmic: Conjunctivitis (4%), amblyopia (<3%), disease of the lacrimal apparatus (<3%), nonreactive pupils (<3%), photophobia (<3%), retinopathy (<3%), visual disturbance (<3%), watery eyes (<3%), xerophthalmia (<3%)

Otic: Deafness (<3%), labyrinthitis (<3%), otalgia (<3%), tinnitus (<3%)

Renal: Increased serum creatinine (3% to 10%), nephrolithiasis (<3%), renal disease (<3%), renal failure syndrome (<3%), renal function abnormality (<3%), renal insufficiency (<3%)

Respiratory: Pharyngitis (8% to 10%), sinusitis (6%), pneumonia (5%), asthma (3% to 10%), bronchitis (3%), bronchospasm (<3%), flu-like symptoms (<3%), laryngeal edema (<3%)

<1%: Fungal skin infection, uveitis, vision loss

Frequency not defined:

Hematologic & oncologic: Bone marrow depression, neutropenia

Hepatic: Hepatotoxicity

Renal: Nephrotoxicity

Respiratory: Pulmonary toxicity

Postmarketing: Acute respiratory failure, autoimmune thrombocytopenia, exfoliative dermatitis, febrile neutropenia, hemolytic-uremic syndrome, pulmonary edema, thrombotic thrombocytopenic purpura

Mechanism of Action Pentostatin is a purine antimetabolite that inhibits adenosine deaminase, preventing the deamination of adenosine to inosine. Accumulation of deoxyadenosine (dAdo) and deoxyadenosine 5′-triphosphate (dATP) results in a reduction of purine metabolism which blocks DNA synthesis and leads to cell death.

Pharmacodynamics/Kinetics

Half-life Elimination Terminal: 5.7 hours; Renal impairment (CrCl <50 mL/minute): 18 hours (range: 11 to 23 hours [Lathia 2002]).

Reproductive Considerations

Females of reproductive potential should avoid becoming pregnant during treatment.

Pregnancy Considerations

Based on the mechanism of action and on findings from animal reproduction studies, in utero exposure to pentostatin may cause fetal harm.

Pentoxifylline (pen toks IF i lin)

Pharmacologic Category Blood Viscosity Reducer Agent

Use

Intermittent claudication: Treatment of intermittent claudication on the basis of chronic occlusive arterial disease of the limbs.

Limitations of use: May improve function and symptoms, but not intended to replace more definitive therapy. **Note:** The American College of Chest Physicians (ACCP) discourages the use of pentoxifylline for the treatment of intermittent claudication refractory to exercise therapy (and smoking cessation) (Guyatt, 2012).

Local Anesthetic/Vasoconstrictor Precautions

No information available to require special precautions

Effects on Dental Treatment No significant effects or complications reported

Effects on Bleeding Pentoxifylline is a methylxanthine derivative with potent hemorrheologic properties. Pentoxifylline has been shown to decrease platelet aggregation and adhesion, and enhances plasminogen activator while decreasing fibrinogen and alpha$_2$-antiplasmin.

Adverse Reactions

1% to 10%: Gastrointestinal: Nausea (2%), vomiting (1%)

<1%, postmarketing, and/or case reports: Anaphylactic shock, anaphylactoid reaction, anaphylaxis, angioedema, angina pectoris, anorexia, anxiety, aplastic anemia, aseptic meningitis, bloating, blurred vision, cardiac arrhythmia, chest pain, cholecystitis, confusion, conjunctivitis, constipation, decreased serum fibrinogen, depression, dysgeusia, dyspnea, edema, epistaxis, eructation, flatulence, flu-like symptoms, hallucination, hepatitis, hypotension, increased liver enzymes, jaundice, laryngitis, leukemia, leukopenia, malaise, nail disease (brittle fingernails), nasal congestion, otalgia, pancytopenia, pruritus, purpura, scotoma, seizure, sialorrhea, skin rash, sore throat, tachycardia, thrombocytopenia, tremor, urticaria, weight changes, xerostomia

Mechanism of Action Pentoxifylline increases blood flow to the affected microcirculation. Although the precise mechanism of action is not well-defined, blood viscosity is lowered, erythrocyte flexibility is increased, leukocyte deformability is increased, and neutrophil adhesion and activation are decreased. Overall, tissue oxygenation is significantly increased.

Pharmacodynamics/Kinetics

Onset of Action 2 to 4 weeks with multiple doses

Half-life Elimination Parent drug: 24 to 48 minutes; Metabolites: 60 to 96 minutes

Time to Peak Serum: 2 to 4 hours

Reproductive Considerations

Pentoxifylline may be used to test sperm viability when evaluating nonfertile males (ASRM 2015). It has also been evaluated for the treatment of infertility due to endometriosis, but use for this purpose is not currently recommended (Lu 2012).

Pregnancy Considerations

Adverse events have been observed in animal reproduction studies.

◆ **Pen VK** *see* Penicillin V Potassium *on page 1211*

◆ **Pepcid** *see* Famotidine *on page 635*

◆ **Pepcid AC Maximum Strength [OTC]** *see* Famotidine *on page 635*

◆ **P-Ephed HCl/Cod/Chlorphenir** *see* Chlorpheniramine, Pseudoephedrine, and Codeine *on page 341*

◆ **P-Ephed Sul/Loratadine** *see* Loratadine and Pseudoephedrine *on page 931*

Peramivir (pe RA mi veer)

Brand Names: US Rapivab

Brand Names: Canada Rapivab

Pharmacologic Category Antiviral Agent; Neuraminidase Inhibitor

Use

Influenza: Treatment of acute, uncomplicated influenza in patients ≥2 years of age who have been symptomatic ≤2 days.

Limitations of use: Efficacy is based on clinical trials in which influenza A was the predominant virus; a limited number of subjects with influenza B have been studied.

Local Anesthetic/Vasoconstrictor Precautions

No information available to require special precautions

Effects on Dental Treatment No significant effects or complications reported

Effects on Bleeding No information available to require special precautions

Adverse Reactions

As reported with adult patients, unless otherwise noted.

1% to 10%:

Cardiovascular: Hypertension (2%)

Endocrine: Increased serum glucose (>160 mg/dL: 5%)

Gastrointestinal: Constipation (4%), diarrhea (8%), vomiting (children & adolescents: 3%)

Genitourinary: Proteinuria (children & adolescents: 3%)

Hematologic and oncologic: Neutropenia (<1 x 10^9/L: 8%)

Hepatic: Increased serum alanine aminotransferase (>2.5 x ULN: 3%), increased serum aspartate aminotransferase (3%)

Nervous system: Insomnia (3%)

Neuromuscular & skeletal: Increased creatine phosphokinase in blood specimen (≥6 x ULN: 4%)

Postmarketing:

Dermatologic: Erythema multiforme, exfoliative dermatitis, skin rash, Stevens-Johnson syndrome

Hypersensitivity: Anaphylaxis, nonimmune anaphylaxis

Nervous system: Abnormal behavior, delirium, hallucination

Mechanism of Action Peramivir, a cyclopentane analogue, selectively inhibits the influenza virus neuraminidase enzyme, preventing the release of viral particles from infected cells.

Pharmacodynamics/Kinetics

Half-life Elimination ~20 hours

Pregnancy Considerations Information related to the use of peramivir in pregnancy is limited (Hernandez 2011; Sorbello 2012). Based on information from one case, the pharmacokinetics of peramivir may be changed with pregnancy (Clay 2011).

Untreated influenza infection is associated with an increased risk of adverse events to the fetus and an increased risk of complications or death to the mother. Neuraminidase inhibitors are currently recommended for the treatment or prophylaxis of influenza in pregnant women and women up to 2 weeks' postpartum, however agents other than peramivir are preferred (ACOG 2018; CDC 60[1], 2011).

Perampanel (per AM pa nel)

Brand Names: US Fycompa

Brand Names: Canada Fycompa

Pharmacologic Category AMPA Glutamate Receptor Antagonist; Anticonvulsant, Miscellaneous

Use

Partial-onset seizures: Treatment of partial-onset seizures with or without secondarily generalized seizures as adjunct or monotherapy in patients with epilepsy who are ≥4 years of age.

Primary generalized tonic-clonic seizures: Treatment of primary generalized tonic-clonic seizures as adjunct therapy in patients with epilepsy who are ≥12 years of age.

Local Anesthetic/Vasoconstrictor Precautions

No information available to require special precautions

Effects on Dental Treatment Key adverse event(s) related to dental treatment: Cough, upper respiratory tract infection, and oropharyngeal pain

Effects on Bleeding No information available to require special precautions

Adverse Reactions Many adverse effects are dose-related. Frequency not always defined.

Cardiovascular: Peripheral edema (2%)

Central nervous system: Dizziness (16% to ≤47%), vertigo (3% to ≤47%), hostility (≤12% to ≤20%), aggressive behavior (2% to ≤20%), drowsiness (9% to 18%), abnormal gait (4% to 16%), fatigue (8% to 15%), headache (12% to 13%), irritability (2% to 12%), falling (5% to 10%), ataxia (≤8%), equilibrium disturbance (3% to 5%), anxiety (2% to 5%), dysarthria (1% to 4%), hypoesthesia (3%), hypersomnia (1% to 3%), anger (1% to 3%), memory impaired (2%), paresthesia (2%), confusion (1% to 2%), euphoria (≤2%), mood changes (1% to 2%), agitation, altered mental status, delusion, disorientation, emotional lability, homicidal ideation, paranoia, psychiatric disturbance (worsening)

Dermatologic: Skin rash (4%)

Endocrine & metabolic: Weight gain (4% to 9%), hyponatremia (2%)
Gastrointestinal: Vomiting (4% to 9%), nausea (6% to 8%), abdominal pain (5%), constipation (3%)
Genitourinary: Urinary tract infection (4%)
Hematologic & oncologic: Bruise (2% to 6%)
Neuromuscular & skeletal: Back pain (5%), sprain (4%), myalgia (3%), arthralgia (2% to 3%), limb pain (2% to 3%), musculoskeletal pain (2%), weakness (2%)
Ophthalmic: Blurred vision (3% to 4%), diplopia (3%)
Respiratory: Cough (4%), upper respiratory tract infection (4%), oropharyngeal pain (2%)
Miscellaneous: Head trauma (3%), laceration (2%), limb injury (1% to 2%)
<1%, postmarketing, and/or case reports: Acute psychosis, delirium, DRESS syndrome, hallucination, increased serum triglycerides, suicidal ideation

Mechanism of Action The exact mechanism by which perampanel exerts antiseizure activity is not definitively known; it is a noncompetitive antagonist of the ionotropic alpha-amino-3-hydroxy-5-methyl-4-isoxazolepropionic acid (AMPA) glutamate receptor on postsynaptic neurons. Glutamate is a primary excitatory neurotransmitter in the central nervous center causing many neurological disorders from neuronal over excitation.

Pharmacodynamics/Kinetics

Half-life Elimination ~105 hours

Time to Peak 0.5 to 2.5 hours; delayed ~1 to 3 hours with food

Reproductive Considerations

Contraceptives containing levonorgestrel may be less effective; additional nonhormonal forms of contraception are recommended during perampanel therapy and for 1 month after discontinuation of therapy.

Pregnancy Considerations

Adverse events have been observed in animal reproduction studies at doses equivalent to the human dose (based on BSA).

Patients exposed to perampanel during pregnancy are encouraged to enroll in the North American Antiepileptic Drug (NAAED) Pregnancy Registry by calling 1-888-233-2334. Additional information is available at www.aedpregnancyregistry.org.

Controlled Substance C-III

◆ **Percocet** *see* Oxycodone and Acetaminophen *on page 1164*

◆ **Perforomist** *see* Formoterol *on page 711*

◆ **Periactin** *see* Cyproheptadine *on page 424*

Periciazine (per ee CYE ah zeen)

Brand Names: Canada Neuleptil; RHO-Pericyazine [DSC]

Pharmacologic Category First Generation (Typical) Antipsychotic

Use Note: Not approved in the US

Psychosis: Adjunctive therapy in select psychotic patients to control prevailing hostility, impulsivity, or aggression

Local Anesthetic/Vasoconstrictor Precautions Periciazine is one of the drugs confirmed to prolong the QT interval and is accepted as having a risk of causing torsade de pointes. The risk of drug-induced torsade de pointes is extremely low when a single QT interval prolonging drug is prescribed. In terms of epinephrine, it is not known what effect vasoconstrictors in the local anesthetic regimen will have in patients with a known history of congenital prolonged QT interval or in patients taking any medication that prolongs the QT interval. Until more information is obtained, it is suggested that the clinician consult with the physician prior to the use of a vasoconstrictor in suspected patients, and that the vasoconstrictor (epinephrine, mepivacaine and levonordefrin [Carbocaine 2% with Neo-Cobefrin]) be used with caution.

Effects on Dental Treatment Key adverse event(s) related to dental treatment:

Significant hypotension may occur, especially when the drug is administered parenterally. Patients may experience orthostatic hypotension as they stand up after treatment; especially if lying in dental chair for extended periods of time. Use caution with sudden changes in position during and after dental treatment. Orthostatic hypotension is due to alpha-receptor blockade; elderly are at greater risk.

Tardive dyskinesia: Prevalence rate may be 40% in elderly; development of the syndrome and the irreversible nature are proportional to duration and total cumulative dose over time. Extrapyramidal reactions are more common in elderly with up to 50% developing these reactions after 60 years of age. Drug-induced Parkinson's syndrome occurs often; akathisia is the most common extrapyramidal reaction in elderly.

Increased confusion, memory loss, psychotic behavior, and agitation frequently occur as a consequence of anticholinergic effects. Antipsychotic-associated sedation in nonpsychotic patients is extremely unpleasant due to feelings of depersonalization, derealization, and dysphoria.

Effects on Bleeding No information available to require special precautions

Adverse Reactions Frequency not defined; listing includes adverse reactions reported with other agents from the phenothiazine class.

Cardiovascular: Atrioventricular block, cardiac arrhythmias, ECG changes, edema, hypotension, orthostatic hypotension, prolonged QT interval on ECG, pulmonary embolism, sinus tachycardia, tachycardia, venous thromboembolism, ventricular fibrillation
Central nervous system: Aggressive behavior, agitation, disruption of body temperature regulation, disturbed sleep, dizziness, drowsiness, EEG pattern changes, extrapyramidal reaction (tremor, akathisia, dystonia, dyskinesia, oculogyric, opisthotonos, hyper-reflexia, pseudo-Parkinsonism, rigidity, sialorrhea), headache, hyperpyrexia, insomnia, neuroleptic malignant syndrome, psychomotor retardation, psychosis (paradoxical), seizure, tardive dyskinesia, temperature regulation impaired
Dermatologic: Diaphoresis, skin photosensitivity, skin pigmentation (prolonged therapy)
Endocrine & metabolic: Change in libido, diabetic ketoacidosis, galactorrhea, gynecomastia, hyperglycemia, menstrual disease (including delayed ovulation), weight changes
Gastrointestinal: Cholestasis, constipation, diarrhea, fecal impaction, increased appetite, nausea, paralytic ileus, vomiting, xerostomia
Genitourinary: Ejaculatory disorder, false positive pregnancy test, priapism, urinary incontinence
Hematologic & oncologic: Agranulocytosis
Hepatic: Cholestatic jaundice
Hypersensitivity: Angioedema
Ophthalmic: Blurred vision, corneal deposits (prolonged therapy), glaucoma, pigment deposits on lens
Respiratory: Asthma, laryngeal edema, nasal congestion, pneumonia, pneumonitis

Mechanism of Action Phenothiazine of the piperidine group with sedative and weak antipsychotic properties; blocks subcortical dopamine receptors in the brain; depresses the release of hypothalamic and hypophyseal hormones

Pregnancy Considerations Use of antipsychotic agents during the third trimester may increase the risk of extrapyramidal and/or withdrawal symptoms (eg, agitation, feeding disorder, hypertonia, hypotonia, respiratory distress, somnolence, and tremor) in newborns. Reported adverse events have ranged from self-limiting to severe.

Product Availability Not available in the US

Dental Health Professional Considerations This drug is known to prolong the QT interval. The QT interval is measured as the time and distance between the Q point of the QRS complex and the end of the T wave in the ECG tracing. After adjustment for heart rate, the QT interval is defined as prolonged if it is more than 450 msec in men and 460 msec in women. A long QT syndrome was first described in the 1950s and 60s as a congenital syndrome involving QT interval prolongation and syncope and sudden death. Some of the congenital long QT syndromes were characterized by a peculiar electrocardiographic appearance of the QRS complex involving a premature atria beat followed by a pause, then a subsequent sinus beat showing marked QT prolongation and deformity. This type of cardiac arrhythmia was originally termed "torsade de pointes" (translated from the French as "twisting of the points").

Prolongation of the QT interval is thought to result from delayed ventricular repolarization. The repolarization process within the myocardial cell is due to the efflux of intracellular potassium. The channels associated with this current can be blocked by many drugs and predispose the electrical propagation cycle to torsade de pointes.

Periciazine is one of the drugs confirmed to prolong the QT interval and is accepted as having a risk of causing torsade de pointes. The risk of drug-induced torsade de pointes is extremely low when a single QT interval prolonging drug is prescribed. In terms of epinephrine, it is not known what effect vasoconstrictors in the local anesthetic regimen will have in patients with a known history of congenital prolonged QT interval or in patients taking any medication that prolongs the QT interval. Until more information is obtained, it is suggested that the clinician consult with the physician prior to the use of a vasoconstrictor in suspected patients, and that the vasoconstrictor (epinephrine, levonordefrin [Neo-Cobefrin®]) be used with caution.

◆ **Pericyazine** *see* Periciazine *on page* 1217

◆ **Peridex** *see* Chlorhexidine Gluconate (Oral) *on page* 334

Perindopril (per IN doe pril)

Related Information

Cardiovascular Diseases *on page* 1654

Brand Names: US Aceon [DSC]

Brand Names: Canada AG-Perindopril; APO-Perindopril; Auro-Perindopril; Coversyl; JAMP-Perindopril; M-Perindopril Erbumine; MAR-Perindopril; MINT-Perindopril; NRA-Perindopril; PMS-Perindopril; Priva-Perindopril Erbumine; RIVA-Perindopril; SANDOZ Perindopril Erbumine; TEVA-Perindopril

Pharmacologic Category Angiotensin-Converting Enzyme (ACE) Inhibitor; Antihypertensive

Use

Hypertension: Management of hypertension

Guideline recommendations: The 2017 Guideline for the Prevention, Detection, Evaluation, and Management of High Blood Pressure in Adults recommends if monotherapy is warranted, in the absence of comorbidities (eg, cerebrovascular disease, chronic kidney disease, diabetes, heart failure, ischemic heart disease, etc.), that thiazide-like diuretics or dihydropyridine calcium channel blockers may be preferred options due to improved cardiovascular endpoints (eg, prevention of heart failure and stroke). ACE inhibitors and ARBs are also acceptable for monotherapy. Combination therapy may be required to achieve blood pressure goals and is initially preferred in patients at high risk (stage 2 hypertension or atherosclerotic cardiovascular disease [ASCVD] risk ≥10%) (ACC/AHA [Whelton 2017]).

Stable coronary artery disease: To reduce the risk of cardiovascular mortality or nonfatal myocardial infarction in patients with stable coronary artery disease (CAD)

Guideline recommendations: Based on the American College of Cardiology/American Heart Association guideline for the diagnosis and management of patients with stable ischemic heart disease, an ACE inhibitor or ARB should be prescribed in all patients with stable ischemic heart disease who also have hypertension, diabetes mellitus, LVEF <40%, or CKD unless contraindicated.

Local Anesthetic/Vasoconstrictor Precautions No information available to require special precautions

Effects on Dental Treatment Key adverse event(s) related to dental treatment: Patients may experience orthostatic hypotension as they stand up after treatment; especially if lying in dental chair for extended periods of time. Use caution with sudden changes in position during and after dental treatment.

An angiotensin-converting enzyme (ACE) Inhibitor cough is a dry, hacking, nonproductive cough that can potentially interfere with longer dental procedures if patient has this side effect.

Effects on Bleeding No information available to require special precautions

Adverse Reactions

Some reactions occurred at an incidence of >1% but ≤ placebo.

>10%:

Central nervous system: Headache (24%)

Respiratory: Cough (12%; incidence higher in women, 3:1)

1% to 10%:

Cardiovascular: Edema (4%), chest pain (2%), ECG abnormality (2%), palpitations (1%)

Central nervous system: Hypertonia (3%), sleep disorder (3%), depression (2%), paresthesia (2%), drowsiness (1%), nervousness (1%)

Dermatologic: Skin rash (2%)

Endocrine & metabolic: Increased serum triglycerides (1%), menstrual disease (1%)

Gastrointestinal: Diarrhea (4%), abdominal pain (3%), dyspepsia (2%), nausea (2%), vomiting (2%), flatulence (1%)

Genitourinary: Urinary tract infection (3%), proteinuria (2%), sexual disorder (male: 1%)

Hepatic: Increased serum ALT (2%)

Hypersensitivity: Seasonal allergy (2%)

Infection: Viral infection (3%)
Neuromuscular & skeletal: Weakness (8%), back pain (6%), leg pain (5%), arm pain (3%), arthralgia (1%), arthritis (1%), myalgia (1%), neck pain (1%)
Otic: Tinnitus (2%), otic infection (1%)
Respiratory: Upper respiratory tract infection (9%), sinusitis (5%), rhinitis (5%), pharyngitis (3%)
Miscellaneous: Fever (2%)

<1%, postmarketing, and/or case reports: Amnesia, anaphylaxis, angioedema, anxiety, arthralgia, bronchitis, bruise, cardiac conduction disturbance, cerebrovascular accident, chills, conjunctivitis, constipation, diaphoresis, dyspnea, epistaxis, erythema, facial edema, flank pain, fluid retention, gastroenteritis, gout, heart murmur, hematoma, hematuria, hyperglycemia, hypokalemia, hypotension, increased appetite, increased serum alkaline phosphatase, increased serum AST, increased serum cholesterol, increased serum creatinine, increased uric acid, leukopenia, malaise, migraine, myocardial infarction, nephrolithiasis, neutropenia, orthostatic hypotension, otalgia, pain, pruritus, psychological disorder (psychosexual disorder), pulmonary fibrosis, purpura, rhinorrhea, sneezing, syncope, tinea, urinary frequency, urinary retention, vaginitis, vasodilation, ventricular premature contractions, vertigo, visual hallucination (Doane 2013), xeroderma, xerostomia

Mechanism of Action Perindopril is a prodrug for perindoprilat, which acts as a competitive inhibitor of ACE; prevents conversion of angiotensin I to angiotensin II, a potent vasoconstrictor; results in lower levels of angiotensin II which, in turn, causes an increase in plasma renin activity and a reduction in aldosterone secretion.

Pharmacodynamics/Kinetics

Onset of Action Peak effect: 1 to 2 hours

Half-life Elimination Parent drug: 1.5 to 3 hours; Metabolite: Effective: 3 to 10 hours, Terminal: 30 to 120 hours

Time to Peak Chronic therapy: Perindopril: ~1 hour; Perindoprilat: 3 to 7 hours (maximum perindoprilat serum levels are 2 to 3 times higher and T_{max} is shorter following chronic therapy); CHF: Perindoprilat: 6 hours

Reproductive Considerations

Angiotensin-converting enzyme (ACE) inhibitors should be avoided in sexually active females of reproductive potential not using effective contraception (ADA 2020).

ACE inhibitors should generally be avoided for the treatment of hypertension in women planning a pregnancy; use should only be considered for cases of hypertension refractory to other medications (ACOG 203 2019).

Pregnancy Risk Factor D

Pregnancy Considerations

Exposure to an angiotensin-converting enzyme (ACE) inhibitor during the first trimester of pregnancy may be associated with an increased risk of fetal malformations (ACOG 203 2019; ESC [Regitz-Zagrosek 2018]); however, outcomes observed may also be influenced by maternal disease (ACC/AHA [Whelton 2017]).

[US Boxed Warning]: Drugs that act directly on the renin-angiotensin system can cause injury and death to the developing fetus. Discontinue as soon as possible once pregnancy is detected. Drugs that act on the renin-angiotensin system are associated with oligohydramnios. Oligohydramnios, due to decreased fetal renal function, may lead to fetal lung hypoplasia and skeletal malformations. Their use in pregnancy is also associated with anuria, hypotension, renal failure, skull hypoplasia, and death in the fetus/neonate. Infants exposed to an ACE inhibitor in utero should be monitored for hyperkalemia, hypotension, and oliguria. Oligohydramnios may not appear until after irreversible fetal injury has occurred. Exchange transfusions or dialysis may be required to reverse hypotension or improve renal function, although data related to the effectiveness in neonates is limited.

Chronic maternal hypertension is also associated with adverse events in the fetus/infant. Chronic maternal hypertension may increase the risk of birth defects, low birth weight, premature delivery, stillbirth, and neonatal death. Actual fetal/neonatal risks may be related to duration and severity of maternal hypertension. Untreated chronic hypertension may also increase the risks of adverse maternal outcomes, including gestational diabetes, preeclampsia, delivery complications, stroke, and myocardial infarction (ACOG 203 2019).

When treatment of hypertension in pregnancy is indicated, ACE inhibitors should generally be avoided due to their adverse fetal events; use in pregnant women should only be considered for cases of hypertension refractory to other medications (ACOG 203 2019). ACE inhibitors are not recommended for the treatment of heart failure in pregnancy (Regitz-Zagrosek [ESC 2018]).

- **Perindopril Erbumine** *see* Perindopril *on page 1218*
- **Periogard** *see* Chlorhexidine Gluconate (Oral) *on page 334*
- **PerioMed** *see* Fluoride *on page 693*
- **Perjeta** *see* Pertuzumab *on page 1220*
- **Perlane [DSC]** *see* Hyaluronate and Derivatives *on page 761*
- **Perlane-L [DSC]** *see* Hyaluronate and Derivatives *on page 761*
- **Perox-A-Mint [OTC]** *see* Hydrogen Peroxide *on page 776*
- **Peroxide** *see* Hydrogen Peroxide *on page 776*
- **Peroxyl Spot Treatment [OTC]** *see* Hydrogen Peroxide *on page 776*

Perphenazine (per FEN a zeen)

Brand Names: Canada PMS-Perphenazine

Pharmacologic Category Antiemetic; First Generation (Typical) Antipsychotic; Phenothiazine Derivative

Use

Nausea/vomiting: Control of severe nausea and vomiting in adults

Schizophrenia: Treatment of schizophrenia

Local Anesthetic/Vasoconstrictor Precautions

No information available to require special precautions

Effects on Dental Treatment Key adverse event(s) related to dental treatment:

Significant hypotension may occur, especially when the drug is administered parenterally; Patients may experience orthostatic hypotension as they stand up after treatment; especially if lying in dental chair for extended periods of time. Use caution with sudden changes in position during and after dental treatment. Orthostatic hypotension is due to alpha-receptor blockade, the elderly are at greater risk for orthostatic hypotension.

Tardive dyskinesia: Prevalence rate may be 40% in elderly; development of the syndrome and the irreversible nature are proportional to duration and total cumulative dose over time. Extrapyramidal reactions are more common in elderly with up to 50% developing these reactions after 60 years of age. Drug-induced Parkinson's syndrome occurs often; akathisia is the most common extrapyramidal reaction in elderly.

Effects on Bleeding No information available to require special precautions

Adverse Reactions Frequency not defined.

Cardiovascular: Bradycardia, ECG changes, hypertension, hypotension, orthostatic hypotension, peripheral edema, tachycardia

Central nervous system: Bizarre dream, catatonic-like state, cerebral edema, confusion (nocturnal), disruption of body temperature regulation, dizziness, drowsiness, extrapyramidal reaction (akathisia, dystonia, Parkinsonian-like syndrome, tardive dyskinesia), headache, hyperactivity, hyperpyrexia, insomnia, lethargy, myasthenia, neuroleptic malignant syndrome (NMS), paradoxical excitation, paranoia, restlessness, seizure

Dermatologic: Diaphoresis, pallor, skin discoloration (blue-gray), skin photosensitivity

Endocrine & metabolic: Amenorrhea, change in libido, galactorrhea, glycosuria, gynecomastia, hyperglycemia, hypoglycemia, menstrual disease, SIADH (syndrome of inappropriate antidiuretic hormone secretion), weight gain

Gastrointestinal: Anorexia, constipation, diarrhea, fecal impaction, increased appetite, nausea, obstipation, paralytic ileus, salivation, vomiting, xerostomia

Genitourinary: Bladder paralysis, breast hypertrophy, ejaculatory disorder, lactation, urinary incontinence, urinary retention

Hematologic & oncologic: Agranulocytosis, eosinophilia, hemolytic anemia, immune thrombocytopenia (formerly known as immune thrombocytopenic purpura), leukopenia, pancytopenia

Hepatic: Hepatotoxicity, jaundice

Hypersensitivity: Hypersensitivity reaction

Neuromuscular & skeletal: Lupus-like syndrome

Ophthalmic: Blurred vision, corneal changes, epithelial keratopathy, glaucoma, lens disease, miosis, mydriasis, photophobia, retinitis pigmentosa

Renal: Polyuria

Respiratory: Nasal congestion

<1%, postmarketing, and/or case reports: Parotid gland enlargement

Mechanism of Action Perphenazine is a piperazine phenothiazine antipsychotic which blocks dopamine, subtype 2 (D_2), receptors in mesolimbocortical and nigrostriatal areas of the brain (APA [Lehman, 2004]).

Pharmacodynamics/Kinetics

Onset of Action 2 to 4 weeks for control of psychotic symptoms (hallucinations, disorganized thinking or behavior, delusions); adequate trial: 6 weeks at moderate to high dose based on tolerability (APA [Lehman 2004])

Half-life Elimination Perphenazine: 9 to 12 hours; 7-hydroxyperphenazine: 10 to 19 hours

Time to Peak Serum: Perphenazine: 1 to 3 hours; 7-hydroxyperphenazine: 2 to 4 hours

Pregnancy Considerations Jaundice or hyper- or hyporeflexia have been reported in newborn infants following maternal use of phenothiazines. Antipsychotic use during the third trimester of pregnancy has a risk for abnormal muscle movements (extrapyramidal symptoms [EPS]) and withdrawal symptoms in newborns following delivery. Symptoms in the newborn may include agitation, feeding disorder, hypertonia, hypotonia, respiratory distress, somnolence, and tremor; these effects may be self-limiting or require hospitalization. If needed, the minimum effective maternal dose should be used in order to decrease the risk of EPS (ACOG 2008).

◆ **Perseris** *see* RisperiDONE *on page 1333*

Pertuzumab (per TU zoo mab)

Brand Names: US Perjeta

Brand Names: Canada Perjeta

Pharmacologic Category Antineoplastic Agent, Anti-HER2; Antineoplastic Agent, Monoclonal Antibody

Use

Breast cancer, metastatic: Treatment of human epidermal growth factor receptor 2 (HER2)-positive metastatic breast cancer (in combination with trastuzumab and docetaxel) in patients who have not received prior anti-HER2 therapy or chemotherapy to treat metastatic disease.

Breast cancer, early (adjuvant): Adjuvant treatment of HER2-positive early breast cancer at high risk of recurrence (in combination with trastuzumab and chemotherapy).

Breast cancer, early (neoadjuvant): Neoadjuvant treatment of locally advanced, inflammatory, or early stage HER2-positive, breast cancer (either greater than 2 cm in diameter or node positive) in combination with trastuzumab and chemotherapy (as part of a complete treatment regimen for early breast cancer).

Local Anesthetic/Vasoconstrictor Precautions No information available to require special precautions

Effects on Dental Treatment Key adverse event(s) related to dental treatment: A significant number of patients have experienced mucosal inflammation (28%), stomatitis (19%), or abnormal taste (18%)

Effects on Bleeding Although significant myelosuppression with associated altered hemostasis has been reported for many chemotherapeutic agents, myelosuppression is not common with pertuzumab and no specific precautions appear necessary.

Adverse Reactions Reactions reported in combination therapy with trastuzumab and docetaxel unless otherwise noted.

>10%:

Central nervous system: Fatigue (26% to 36%), headache (11% to 21%), decreased left ventricular ejection fraction (8% to 16%), insomnia (8% to 13%), dizziness (3% to 13%)

Dermatologic: Alopecia (52% to 65%), skin rash (11% to 34%), pruritus (4% to 14%), palmar-plantar erythrodysesthesia (11%), xeroderma (9% to 11%)

Gastrointestinal: Diarrhea (46% to 67%), nausea (39% to 53%), vomiting (13% to 36%), decreased appetite (11% to 29%), mucositis (20% to 28%), constipation (23%), stomatitis (17% to 19%; grades 3/4: <1%), dysgeusia (13% to 18%)

Hematologic & oncologic: Neutropenia (47% to 53%; grades 3/4: 43% to 49%), anemia (3% to 23%; grades 3/4: 2% to 4%), leukopenia (9% to 16%; grades 3/4: 5% to 12%), febrile neutropenia (8% to 14%; grades 3/4: 9% to 13%)

Hypersensitivity: Hypersensitivity (1% to 11%)

Neuromuscular & skeletal: Asthenia (15% to 26%), myalgia (11% to 22%), arthralgia (10% to 12%)

Respiratory: Upper respiratory tract infection (4% to 17%), epistaxis (11%)

Miscellaneous: Fever (9% to 19%), infusion reactions (13%)

1% to 10%:

Cardiovascular: Left ventricular dysfunction (3% to 4%), peripheral edema (3% to 4%)

Central nervous system: Peripheral sensory neuropathy (8%; grades 3/4: <1%), peripheral neuropathy (1%)

Dermatologic: Nail disease (7%), paronychia (1% to 7%)

Gastrointestinal: Dyspepsia (8%)

Hematologic & oncologic: Thrombocytopenia (1%)

Hepatic: Increased serum alanine aminotransferase (3%)

Ophthalmic: Increased lacrimation (4% to 5%)

Respiratory: Dyspnea (8%), nasopharyngitis (7%), oropharyngeal pain (7%), cough (5%)

<1%, postmarketing, and/or case reports: Left systolic heart failure, pleural effusion, sepsis, tumor lysis syndrome

Mechanism of Action Pertuzumab is a recombinant humanized monoclonal antibody which targets the extracellular human epidermal growth factor receptor 2 protein (HER2) dimerization domain. Inhibits HER2 dimerization and blocks HER downstream signaling halting cell growth and initiating apoptosis. Pertuzumab binds to a different HER2 epitope than trastuzumab so that when pertuzumab is combined with trastuzumab, a more complete inhibition of HER2 signaling occurs (Baselga 2012).

Pharmacodynamics/Kinetics

Half-life Elimination Terminal: 18 days

Reproductive Considerations

[US Boxed Warning]: Exposure to pertuzumab can result in embryo-fetal death and birth defects. Advise patients of these risks and the need for effective contraception.

Evaluate pregnancy status prior to treatment in females of reproductive potential; effective contraception should be used during therapy and for 7 months after the last dose of pertuzumab in combination with trastuzumab (or trastuzumab/hyaluronidase).

Pregnancy Considerations

[US Boxed Warning]: Exposure to pertuzumab can result in embryo-fetal death and birth defects. Advise patients of these risks.

Based on the mechanism of action of pertuzumab and data from similar agents, oligohydramnios or oligohydramnios sequence may occur resulting in pulmonary hypoplasia, skeletal anomalies, and neonatal death. Monitor for oligohydramnios if exposure occurs during pregnancy or within 7 months prior to conception; conduct appropriate fetal testing if oligohydramnios occurs. Information related to inadvertent exposure to pertuzumab in combination with trastuzumab in pregnancy is limited (Yildirim 2018).

European Society for Medical Oncology (ESMO) guidelines for cancer during pregnancy recommend delaying treatment with HER2-targeted agents until after delivery in pregnant patients with HER2-positive disease (Peccatori 2013).

Advise patients to immediately report to health care provider if pregnancy is suspected during treatment. If pertuzumab exposure occurs during pregnancy or exposure to pertuzumab in combination with trastuzumab (or trastuzumab/hyaluronidase) occurs within 7 months following the last dose of pertuzumab, report the exposure to Genentech (888-835-2555).

◆ **Pertuzumab, hyaluronidase, and trastuzumab** *see* Pertuzumab, Trastuzumab, and Hyaluronidase *on page 1221*

Pertuzumab, Trastuzumab, and Hyaluronidase

(per TU zoo mab, tras TU zoo mab, & hye al yoor ON i dase)

Brand Names: US Phesgo

Pharmacologic Category Antineoplastic Agent, Anti-HER2; Antineoplastic Agent, Monoclonal Antibody

Use

Breast cancer, early (adjuvant or neoadjuvant): Neoadjuvant treatment of HER2-positive, locally advanced, inflammatory, or early stage breast cancer (either >2 cm in diameter or node positive), in combination with chemotherapy, as part of a complete treatment regimen for early breast cancer in adults; adjuvant treatment of HER2-positive early breast cancer, in combination with chemotherapy, in adults at high risk of recurrence.

Breast cancer, metastatic: Treatment of HER2-positive metastatic breast cancer (in combination with docetaxel) in adults who have not received prior anti-HER2 therapy or chemotherapy for metastatic disease.

Local Anesthetic/Vasoconstrictor Precautions No information available to require special precautions.

Effects on Dental Treatment Key adverse event(s) related to dental treatment: Frequent occurrence of altered taste (dysgeusia) and stomatitis. Occurrence of nasopharyngitis, rhinorrhea.

Effects on Bleeding Bone marrow depression has been reported (eg, anemia, thrombocytopenia, lymphocytopenia). In patients under active treatment with this drug, medical consult is suggested.

Adverse Reactions Adverse reactions include neoadjuvant chemotherapy. Also see individual agents.

>10%:

Dermatologic: Alopecia (77%), skin rash (16%), xeroderma (15%)

Endocrine & metabolic: Decreased serum albumin (16%), decreased serum sodium (13%), hot flash (12%), increased serum potassium (13%), weight loss (11%)

Gastrointestinal: Constipation (22%), decreased appetite (17%), diarrhea (60%), dysgeusia (17%), dyspepsia (14%), nausea (60%), stomatitis (15% to 25%; grades 3/4: ≤1%), vomiting (20%)

Hematologic & oncologic: Anemia (36% to 90%; grades 3/4: 2% to 3%), decreased absolute lymphocyte count (89%; grade 3/4: 37%), neutropenia (22%; grades 3/4: 14%), thrombocytopenia (27%)

Hepatic: Increased serum alanine aminotransferase (58%), increased serum aspartate aminotransferase (50%)

Local: Injection site reaction (15%)

Nervous system: Dizziness (13%), fatigue (29%), headache (17%), insomnia (17%), peripheral neuropathy (12%; grades 3/4: ≤1%), peripheral sensory neuropathy (16%), procedural pain (13%)

Neuromuscular & skeletal: Arthralgia (24%), asthenia (31%), myalgia (25%)

Renal: Increased serum creatinine (84%)

Respiratory: Cough (15%), epistaxis (12%), upper respiratory tract infection (11%)

Miscellaneous: Fever (13%), radiation injury (19%, skin)

1% to 10%:

Cardiovascular: Cardiac failure (≤1%), peripheral edema (8%), reduced ejection fraction (4%)

Dermatologic: Dermatitis (7%), erythema of skin (9%), nail discoloration (9%), nail disease (7%), palmar-plantar erythrodysesthesia (6%), paronychia (7%), pruritus (3%)

Endocrine & metabolic: Decreased serum glucose (9%), hypokalemia (7%), increased serum sodium (7%)

Gastrointestinal: Abdominal pain (9%), hemorrhoids (9%), upper abdominal pain (8%)

Genitourinary: Urinary tract infection (7%)

Hematologic & oncologic: Febrile neutropenia (7%; grades 3/4: 7%; serious febrile neutropenia: 4%), leukopenia (9%; grades 3/4: 2%)

Hepatic: Increased serum bilirubin (9%)

Hypersensitivity: Hypersensitivity reaction (1%)

Immunologic: Antibody development (1% to 5%)

Infection: Neutropenic sepsis (1%)

Local: Pain at injection site (2%)

Nervous system: Malaise (7%), paresthesia (10%)

Neuromuscular & skeletal: Back pain (10%), limb pain (6%), muscle spasm (6%), musculoskeletal pain (6%), ostealgia (7%)

Ophthalmic: Dry eye syndrome (5%), increased lacrimation (5%)

Respiratory: Dyspnea (10%), flu-like symptoms (5%), nasopharyngitis (9%), rhinorrhea (7%)

Miscellaneous: Infusion related reaction (4%)

Frequency not defined:

Cardiovascular: Cardiac arrhythmia, cardiomyopathy, hypertension, left ventricular dysfunction

Respiratory: Pulmonary toxicity

Mechanism of Action

Pertuzumab is a recombinant humanized monoclonal antibody that targets the extracellular HER2 protein dimerization domain. It inhibits HER2 dimerization and blocks HER downstream, signaling halting cell growth and initiating apoptosis. Pertuzumab binds to a different HER2 epitope than trastuzumab so that when pertuzumab is combined with trastuzumab, a more complete inhibition of HER2 signaling occurs (Baselga 2012).

Trastuzumab is a monoclonal antibody that binds to the extracellular domain of HER2; it mediates antibody-dependent cellular cytotoxicity by inhibiting proliferation of cells that overexpress HER2 protein.

Hyaluronidase increases the dispersion and absorption rate of SubQ trastuzumab-containing products by increasing permeability of SubQ tissue through temporary depolymerization of hyaluronan; at the recommended doses, hyaluronidase acts transiently and locally; permeability of the SubQ tissue is restored within 24 to 48 hours.

Pharmacodynamics/Kinetics

Time to Peak SubQ: Pertuzumab and Trastuzumab: 4 days.

Reproductive Considerations

Evaluate pregnancy status prior to use in females of reproductive potential.

[US Boxed Warning]: Exposure to pertuzumab/trastuzumab/hyaluronidase can result in embryo-fetal death and birth defects. Advise patients of these risks and the need for effective contraception. Exposure within 7 months prior to pregnancy can cause fetal harm.

Females of reproductive potential should use effective contraception during therapy and for 7 months after the last pertuzumab/trastuzumab/hyaluronidase dose.

Refer to the Pertuzumab and Trastuzumab monographs for additional information.

Pregnancy Considerations

[US Boxed Warning]: Exposure to pertuzumab/trastuzumab/hyaluronidase can result in embryo-fetal death and birth defects. Exposure during therapy or within 7 months prior to pregnancy can cause fetal harm. Monitor for oligohydramnios and conduct gestational age-appropriate fetal testing if exposure occurs.

Refer to the Pertuzumab and Trastuzumab monographs for additional information.

Data collection to monitor pregnancy and infant outcomes following exposure to pertuzumab/trastuzumab/hyaluronidase is ongoing. Healthcare providers are encouraged to enroll females exposed during pregnancy or within 7 months after the last pertuzumab/trastuzumab/hyaluronidase dose in the Pregnancy Registry (1-888-835-2555).

◆ **Pertuzumab, trastuzumab, and hyaluronidase-zzxf** *see* Pertuzumab, Trastuzumab, and Hyaluronidase *on page 1221*

◆ **Pertuzumab/trastuzumab/hyaluronidase** *see* Pertuzumab, Trastuzumab, and Hyaluronidase *on page 1221*

◆ **Pethidine Hydrochloride** *see* Meperidine *on page 966*

◆ **Pexeva** *see* PARoxetine *on page 1194*

◆ **PF-00299804** *see* Dacomitinib *on page 429*

◆ **PF-00299804-03** *see* Dacomitinib *on page 429*

◆ **PF-02341066** *see* Crizotinib *on page 415*

◆ **PF-04449913** *see* Glasdegib *on page 737*

◆ **PF-06463922** *see* Lorlatinib *on page 937*

◆ **PFA** *see* Foscarnet *on page 713*

◆ **Pfizerpen** *see* Penicillin G (Parenteral/Aqueous) *on page 1209*

◆ **PGE_1** *see* Alprostadil *on page 110*

◆ **PGI_2** *see* Epoprostenol *on page 578*

◆ **PGX** *see* Epoprostenol *on page 578*

◆ **Pharbechlor [OTC]** *see* Chlorpheniramine *on page 340*

◆ **Pharbedryl [OTC]** *see* DiphenhydrAMINE (Systemic) *on page 502*

◆ **Pharbetol [OTC]** *see* Acetaminophen *on page 59*

◆ **Pharbetol Extra Strength [OTC]** *see* Acetaminophen *on page 59*

◆ **Phenadoz [DSC]** *see* Promethazine *on page 1282*

Phenazopyridine (fen az oh PEER i deen)

Brand Names: US AZO Urinary Pain Relief [OTC]; Baridium [OTC] [DSC]; Pyridium; Urinary Pain Relief [OTC]

Brand Names: Canada Phenazo; Pyridium

Pharmacologic Category Analgesic, Urinary

Use Dysuria, symptomatic relief: Symptomatic relief of pain, burning, urgency, frequency, and other discomforts arising from irritation of the lower urinary tract mucosa caused by infection, trauma, surgery, endoscopic procedures, or the passage of sounds or catheters.

Local Anesthetic/Vasoconstrictor Precautions No information available to require special precautions

Effects on Dental Treatment No significant effects or complications reported

Effects on Bleeding No information available to require special precautions

Adverse Reactions

1% to 10%:

Central nervous system: Headache, dizziness

Gastrointestinal: Stomach cramps

<1%, postmarketing, and/or case reports: Acute renal failure, hemolytic anemia, hepatitis, methemoglobinemia, skin pigmentation, skin rash, vertigo

Mechanism of Action An azo dye which exerts local anesthetic or analgesic action on urinary tract mucosa through an unknown mechanism

Pregnancy Risk Factor B

Pregnancy Considerations Adverse events have not been observed in animal reproduction studies. Phenazopyridine crosses the placenta and can be detected in amniotic fluid (Meyer 1991).

◆ **Phenazopyridine HCl** *see* Phenazopyridine *on page 1222*

◆ **Phenazopyridine Hydrochloride** *see* Phenazopyridine *on page 1222*

Phendimetrazine (fen dye ME tra zeen)

Pharmacologic Category Anorexiant; Sympathomimetic

Use Obesity (short-term adjunct): Short-term (eg, ≤12 weeks) adjunct in a regimen of weight reduction based on exercise, behavioral modification, and caloric restriction in the management of exogenous obesity in patients with an initial BMI ≥30 kg/m^2 or a BMI ≥27 kg/m^2 with at least one weight-related comorbidity (eg, controlled hypertension, diabetes, hyperlipidemia) who have not responded to lifestyle modifications alone.

Local Anesthetic/Vasoconstrictor Precautions Use vasoconstrictor with caution in patients taking phendimetrazine. Phendimetrazine can enhance the sympathomimetic response to epinephrine leading to potential hypertension and cardiotoxicity.

Effects on Dental Treatment Key adverse event(s) related to dental treatment: Xerostomia (normal salivary flow resumes upon discontinuation).

Effects on Bleeding No information available to require special precautions

Adverse Reactions Frequency not defined.

Cardiovascular: Flushing, hypertension, ischemic events, palpitations, tachycardia, valvular disease (regurgitant)

Central nervous system: Agitation, dizziness, headache, insomnia, overstimulation, psychosis, restlessness

Endocrine & metabolic: Changes in libido

Gastrointestinal: Constipation, diarrhea, nausea, stomach pain, xerostomia

Genitourinary: Dysuria, urinary frequency

Neuromuscular & skeletal: Tremor

Ocular: Blurred vision, mydriasis

Respiratory: Primary pulmonary hypertension

Miscellaneous: Diaphoresis, tachyphylaxis

<1%, postmarketing, and/or case reports: Dilated cardiomyopathy, retinal vein occlusion (Cho 2016)

Mechanism of Action Phendimetrazine is a sympathomimetic amine with pharmacologic properties similar to the amphetamines. The mechanism of action in reducing appetite appears to be secondary to CNS effects, including stimulation of the hypothalamus to release norepinephrine.

Pharmacodynamics/Kinetics

Half-life Elimination ~3.7 hours

Reproductive Considerations

Medications for weight loss therapy are not recommended at conception (ACOG 156 2015).

Pregnancy Risk Factor X/C (product dependent)

Pregnancy Considerations

Animal reproduction studies have not been conducted. Use is contraindicated by some manufacturers in pregnant women (lack of potential benefit and possible fetal harm). An increased risk of adverse maternal and fetal outcomes is associated with obesity; however, medications for weight loss therapy are not recommended during pregnancy (ACOG 156 2015).

Controlled Substance C-III

◆ **Phendimetrazine Tartrate** *see* Phendimetrazine *on page 1223*

◆ **Phenergan** *see* Promethazine *on page 1282*

◆ **Pheniramine and Naphazoline** *see* Naphazoline and Pheniramine *on page 1079*

PHENobarbital (fee noe BAR bi tal)

Pharmacologic Category Anticonvulsant, Barbiturate; Barbiturate

Use

Sedation: Use as a sedative

Seizures: Management of generalized tonic-clonic, status epilepticus, and partial seizures

Local Anesthetic/Vasoconstrictor Precautions No information available to require special precautions

Effects on Dental Treatment No significant effects or complications reported

Effects on Bleeding No information available to require special precautions

Adverse Reactions Frequency not defined.

Cardiovascular: Bradycardia, hypotension, syncope, thrombophlebitis (IV)

Central nervous system: Agitation, anxiety, ataxia, central nervous system stimulation, central nervous system depression, confusion, dizziness, drowsiness, hallucination, hangover effect, headache, impaired judgement, insomnia, lethargy, nervousness, nightmares

Dermatologic: Exfoliative dermatitis, skin rash, Stevens-Johnson syndrome

Gastrointestinal: Constipation, nausea, vomiting

Genitourinary: Oliguria

Hematologic & oncologic: Agranulocytosis, thrombocytopenia, megaloblastic anemia

Local: Pain at injection site

Neuromuscular & skeletal: Hyperkinesia, laryngospasm

Respiratory: Apnea (especially with rapid IV use), hypoventilation, respiratory depression

Mechanism of Action Long-acting barbiturate with sedative, hypnotic, and anticonvulsant properties. Barbiturates depress the sensory cortex, decrease motor activity, alter cerebellar function, and produce drowsiness, sedation, and hypnosis. In high doses, barbiturates exhibit anticonvulsant activity; barbiturates produce dose-dependent respiratory depression.

Pharmacodynamics/Kinetics

Onset of Action Oral: ≥60 minutes; IV: 5 minutes; Peak effect: IV: CNS depression: ≥15 minutes.

Duration of Action Oral: 10 to 12 hours; IV: >6 hours.

Half-life Elimination

≤10 days of life: 114.2 ± 43 hours (Alonso Gonzales 1993; Patsalos 2008).

11 to 30 days of life: 73.19 ± 24.17 hours (Alonso Gonzales 1993; Patsalos 2008).

2 to 3 months: 62.9 ± 5.2 hours (Heimann 1977).

4 to 12 months: 63.2 ± 4.2 hours (Heimann 1977).

1 to 5 years: 68.5 ± 3.2 hours (Heimann 1977).

Adults: ~79 hours (range: 53 to 118 hours).

Time to Peak

Serum: Oral:

Newborns: 1.5 to 6 hours (Patsalos 2008).

Adults: 2 to 4 hours (Patsalos 2018).

Pregnancy Risk Factor D

Pregnancy Considerations

Phenobarbital crosses the placenta (Harden 2009b). Barbiturates can be detected in the placenta, fetal liver, and fetal brain. Fetal and maternal blood concentrations may be similar following parenteral administration. An increased incidence of fetal abnormalities may occur following maternal use. When used during the third trimester of pregnancy, withdrawal symptoms may occur in the neonate, including seizures and hyperirritability; symptoms of withdrawal may be delayed in the neonate up to 14 days after birth. Use during labor does not impair uterine activity; however, respiratory depression may occur in the newborn; resuscitation equipment should be available, especially for premature infants. Use for the treatment of epilepsy should be avoided during pregnancy (Harden 2009a).

A registry is available for women exposed to phenobarbital during pregnancy: Pregnant women may enroll themselves into the North American Antiepileptic Drug (AED) Pregnancy Registry (888-233-2334 or http://www.aedpregnancyregistry.org).

Controlled Substance C-IV

- **Phenobarbital Sodium** *see* PHENobarbital *on page 1223*
- **Phenobarbitone** *see* PHENobarbital *on page 1223*
- **Phenoxymethyl Penicillin** *see* Penicillin V Potassium *on page 1211*

Phentermine (FEN ter meen)

Brand Names: US Adipex-P; Lomaira

Brand Names: Canada RHO-Phentermine

Pharmacologic Category Anorexiant; Central Nervous System Stimulant; Sympathomimetic

Use Obesity (short-term adjunct): Short-term (few weeks) adjunct in a regimen of weight reduction based on exercise, behavioral modification and caloric restriction in the management of exogenous obesity with an initial body mass index (BMI) ≥30 kg/m^2 or ≥27 kg/m^2 in the presence of other risk factors (eg, diabetes, hyperlipidemia, controlled hypertension).

Local Anesthetic/Vasoconstrictor Precautions Use vasoconstrictor with caution in patients taking phentermine. Amphetamines enhance the sympathomimetic response of epinephrine and norepinephrine leading to potential hypertension and cardiotoxicity.

Effects on Dental Treatment Key adverse event(s) related to dental treatment: Phentermine causes tachycardia, increases in blood pressure, and palpitations. Consider monitoring blood pressure prior to using local anesthetic with a vasoconstrictor. Symptoms associated with bruxism have been observed in some patients.

Effects on Bleeding No information available to require special precautions

Adverse Reactions Frequency not defined.

Cardiovascular: Hypertension, ischemia, palpitations, tachycardia

Central nervous system: Dizziness, dysphoria, euphoria, headache, insomnia, overstimulation, psychosis, restlessness

Dermatologic: Urticaria

Endocrine & metabolic: Change in libido

Gastrointestinal: Constipation, diarrhea, gastrointestinal distress, unpleasant taste, xerostomia

Genitourinary: Impotence

Neuromuscular & skeletal: Tremor

<1%, postmarketing, and/or case reports: Acquired valvular heart disease (regurgitant), primary pulmonary hypertension

Mechanism of Action Phentermine is a sympathomimetic amine with pharmacologic properties similar to the amphetamines. The mechanism of action in reducing appetite appears to be secondary to CNS effects, including stimulation of the hypothalamus to release norepinephrine.

Pharmacodynamics/Kinetics

Half-life Elimination ~20 hours

Time to Peak 3 to 4.4 hours

Reproductive Considerations

Medications for weight loss therapy are not recommended at conception (ACOG 156 2015).

Pregnancy Risk Factor X

Pregnancy Considerations

Use of phentermine is contraindicated during pregnancy (lack of potential benefit and possible fetal harm). Limited information is available about the use of phentermine in pregnancy (Jones 2002; McElhatton 2006). An increased risk of adverse maternal and fetal outcomes is associated with obesity; however, medications for weight loss therapy are not recommended during pregnancy (ACOG 156 2015).

Product Availability Suprenza has been discontinued in the US for more than 1 year.

Controlled Substance C-IV

Dental Health Professional Considerations Many diet physicians have prescribed fenfluramine ("fen") and phentermine ("phen"). When taken together the combination is known as "fen-phen". The diet drug dexfenfluramine (Redux®) is chemically similar to fenfluramine (Pondimin®) and was also used in combination with phentermine called "Redux-phen". While each of the three drugs alone had approval from the FDA for sale in the treatment of obesity, neither combination had an official approval. The use of the combinations in the treatment of obesity was considered an "off-label" use. Reports in medical literature have been accumulating for some years about significant side effects associated with fenfluramine and dexfenfluramine. In 1997, the manufacturers, at the urging of the FDA, agreed to voluntarily withdraw the drugs from the market. The action was based on findings from physicians who evaluated patients taking fenfluramine and dexfenfluramine with echocardiograms. The findings indicated that approximately 30% of patients had abnormal echocardiograms, even though they had no symptoms. This was a much higher than expected percentage of abnormal test results. This conclusion was based on a sample of 291 patients examined by five different physicians. Under normal conditions, fewer than 1%

of patients would be expected to show signs of heart valve disease. The findings suggested that fenfluramine and dexfenfluramine were the likely cause of heart valve problems of the type that promoted FDA's earlier warnings concerning "fen-phen". The earlier warning included the following: The mitral valve and other valves in the heart are damaged by a strange white coating and allow blood to flow back, causing heart muscle damage. In several cases, valve replacement surgery has been done. As a rule, the person must, thereafter for life, be on a blood thinner to prevent clots from the mechanical valve. This type of valve damage had only been seen before in persons who were exposed to large amounts of serotonin. The fenfluramine increases the availability of serotonin.

Phentermine and Topiramate

(FEN ter meen & toe PYRE a mate)

Related Information

Phentermine *on page 1224*

Topiramate *on page 1464*

Brand Names: US Qsymia

Pharmacologic Category Anorexiant; Anticonvulsant, Miscellaneous; Sympathomimetic

Use Weight management: Adjunct to a reduced-calorie diet and increased physical activity, in patients with either an initial body mass index (BMI) of ≥30 kg/m^2 **or** an initial BMI of ≥27 kg/m^2 and at least one weight-related comorbid condition (eg, hypertension, dyslipidemia, type 2 diabetes)

Local Anesthetic/Vasoconstrictor Precautions Use vasoconstrictor with caution in patients taking phentermine and topiramate. Phentermine is a sympathomimetic amine with pharmacologic properties similar to amphetamines. The phentermine component may enhance the sympathomimetic response of epinephrine and levonordefrin leading to potential hypertension and cardiotoxicity.

Effects on Dental Treatment Key adverse event(s) related to dental treatment: The following effects were reported more frequently than placebo during 1 year of treatment (n=1580): Paresthesia (experienced by ≤20% of patients), dysgeusia (metallic taste, experienced by ≤9% of patients), and dry mouth (experienced by ≤19% of patients). The paresthesia was characterized as tingling in hands, feet, or face.

Effects on Bleeding No information available to require special precautions

Adverse Reactions As reported with combination product (also see individual agents):

>10%:

Cardiovascular: Increased heart rate (>5 bpm: 70% to 78%; >10 bpm: 50% to 56%; >15 bpm: 33% to 37%; >20 bpm: 14% to 20%)

Central nervous system: Paresthesia (4% to 20%), headache (10% to 11%), insomnia (6% to 11%)

Endocrine & metabolic: Decreased serum bicarbonate (6% to 13%; marked reductions [to <17 mEq/L] ≤1%)

Gastrointestinal: Xerostomia (7% to 19%), constipation (8% to 16%)

Respiratory: Upper respiratory tract infection (14% to 16%), nasopharyngitis (9% to 13%)

1% to 10%:

Cardiovascular: Palpitations (≤2%), chest discomfort (≤2%)

Central nervous system: Dizziness (3% to 9%), depression (3% to 8%), anxiety (2% to 8%), cognitive dysfunction (including problems with concentration, memory, and language [word finding]; 2% to 8%), fatigue (4% to 6%), hypoesthesia (4%), disturbance in attention (2% to 4%), irritability (2% to 4%), oral paresthesia (≤2%)

Dermatologic: Alopecia (2% to 4%), skin rash (2% to 3%)

Endocrine & metabolic: Decreased serum potassium (<3.5 mEq/L: 4% to 5%; <3 mEq/L: <1%), hypokalemia (≤3%), increased thirst (2%)

Gastrointestinal: Dysgeusia (metallic taste; 1% to 9%), nausea (4% to 7%), diarrhea (5% to 6%), gastroesophageal reflux disease (3%), dyspepsia (2% to 3%), gastroenteritis (2% to 3%), decreased appetite (2%)

Genitourinary: Urinary tract infection (5%), dysmenorrhea (≤2%)

Infection: Influenza (4% to 8%)

Neuromuscular & skeletal: Back pain (5% to 7%), muscle spasm (3%), musculoskeletal pain (2% to 3%), neck pain (1% to 2%)

Ophthalmic: Blurred vision (4% to 6%), dry eye syndrome (≤3%), eye pain (2%)

Renal: Increased serum creatinine (≥0.3 mg/dL: 2% to 8%; ≥50% over baseline: ≤3%), nephrolithiasis (≤1%)

Respiratory: Sinusitis (7% to 8%), bronchitis (4% to 7%), cough (4% to 5%), pharyngolaryngeal pain (2% to 3%), sinus congestion (2% to 3%), nasal congestion (1% to 2%)

Postmarketing and/or case reports: Acute angle-closure glaucoma, suicidal ideation

Mechanism of Action

Phentermine: A sympathomimetic amine with pharmacologic properties similar to amphetamines. The mechanism of action in reducing appetite appears to be secondary to CNS effects, including stimulation of the hypothalamus to release norepinephrine.

Topiramate: Effect on weight management may be due to its effects on appetite suppression and satiety enhancement and based on a combination of potential mechanisms: blocks neuronal voltage-dependent sodium channels, enhances GABA(A) activity, antagonizes AMPA/kainite glutamate receptors, and weakly inhibits carbonic anhydrase.

Reproductive Considerations

Females of reproductive potential should have a negative pregnancy test prior to and monthly during therapy. Effective contraception should be used during treatment. Medications for weight loss therapy are not recommended at conception (ACOG 156 2015).

Pregnancy Risk Factor X

Pregnancy Considerations

Use of this combination product is contraindicated in pregnant women. An increased risk in oral clefts (cleft lip with or without cleft palate) has been reported with first trimester exposure. Refer to individual monographs for additional information. An increased risk of adverse maternal and fetal outcomes is associated with obesity; however, medications for weight loss therapy are not recommended during pregnancy (ACOG 156 2015).

Health care providers are encouraged to enroll women exposed to Qsymia during pregnancy in the Qsymia Pregnancy Surveillance Program (888-998-4887).

Controlled Substance C-IV

Dental Health Professional Considerations According to product labeling, phentermine and topiramate can cause an increase in resting heart rate. A higher percentage of overweight and obese adults taking phentermine and topiramate experienced heart rate increases from baseline of more than 5, 10, 15, and 20 beats per minute compared to placebo-treated overweight and obese adults. The clinical significance of a heart rate elevation with treatment is presently unclear. Regular measurement of resting heart rate is recommended for all patients taking phentermine and topiramate. Product labeling states that patients should inform healthcare provider of palpitations or feelings of a racing heartbeat while at rest during treatment.

◆ **Phentermine HCl** *see* Phentermine *on page 1224*

◆ **Phentermine Hydrochloride** *see* Phentermine *on page 1224*

◆ **Phentermine/Topiramate** *see* Phentermine and Topiramate *on page 1225*

Phentolamine (fen TOLE a meen)

Related Information

Oral Pain *on page 1734*

Brand Names: US OraVerse

Brand Names: Canada OraVerse; Rogitine

Pharmacologic Category Alpha$_1$ Blocker; Antidote, Extravasation; Antihypertensive

Use

Pheochromocytoma: Diagnosis of pheochromocytoma via the phentolamine-blocking test (see **"Note"**); prevention and management of hypertensive episodes associated with pheochromocytoma resulting from stress or manipulation during the perioperative period

Extravasation management: Prevention and treatment of dermal necrosis/sloughing after extravasation of norepinephrine

Local anesthesia reversal (OraVerse): Reversal of soft tissue (lip, tongue) anesthesia and the associated functional deficits resulting from an intraoral submucosal injection of a local anesthetic containing a vasoconstrictor in adult and pediatric patients ≥3 years.

Note: The phentolamine-blocking test for the diagnosis of pheochromocytoma has largely been supplanted by the measurement of catecholamine concentrations and catecholamine metabolites (eg, metanephrine) in the plasma and urine; reserve phentolamine for cases when additional confirmation is necessary to determine diagnosis.

Local Anesthetic/Vasoconstrictor Precautions Although the alpha-adrenergic blocking effects could antagonize epinephrine, there is no information available to require special precautions

Effects on Dental Treatment Key adverse event(s) related to dental treatment: The most common reaction that was greater than controls was injection site pain (~4% to 6%). A few incidences of paresthesia associated with OraVerse have been reported. These incidences were mild and transient, and resolved during the same time period. Patients may experience orthostatic hypotension as they stand up after treatment; especially if lying in dental chair for extended periods of time. Use caution with sudden changes in position during and after dental treatment.

Effects on Bleeding No information available to require special precautions

Adverse Reactions Frequency not always defined.

Cardiovascular: Bradycardia (OraVerse 2% to 4%), hypertension (OraVerse <3%), cerebrovascular occlusion, hypotension, myocardial infarction

Central nervous system: Mouth pain (OraVerse ≤19%), headache (OraVerse 6%), paresthesia (OraVerse <3%; mild, transient), cerebrovascular spasm

Dermatologic: Facial swelling (OraVerse <3%), pruritus (OraVerse <3%)

Gastrointestinal: Diarrhea (OraVerse <3%), upper abdominal pain (OraVerse <3%), vomiting (OraVerse <3%), nausea

Local: Pain at injection site (OraVerse 6%)

Neuromuscular & skeletal: Jaw pain (OraVerse <3%)

Miscellaneous: Postinjection pain (10%)

Postmarketing and/or case reports: Cardiac arrhythmia, dizziness, flushing, nasal congestion, orthostatic hypotension, weakness

Mechanism of Action Competitively blocks alpha-adrenergic receptors (nonselective) to produce brief antagonism of circulating epinephrine and norepinephrine to reduce hypertension caused by alpha effects of these catecholamines and minimizes tissue injury due to extravasation of these and other sympathomimetic vasoconstrictors (eg, dopamine, phenylephrine); also has a positive inotropic and chronotropic effect on the heart thought to be due to presynaptic alpha-2 receptor blockade which results in release of presynaptic norepinephrine (Hoffman 1980)

OraVerse: Causes vasodilation and increased blood flow in injection area via alpha-adrenergic blockade to accelerate reversal of soft tissue anesthesia

Pharmacodynamics/Kinetics

Onset of Action IM: 15 to 20 minutes; IV: 1 to 2 minutes (Chobanian 2003)

Peak effect: OraVerse: 10 to 20 minutes

Duration of Action IM: 30 to 45 minutes; IV: 10 to 30 minutes (Chobanian 2003)

Half-life Elimination IV: 19 minutes; Submucosal injection: ~2 to 3 hours

Pregnancy Risk Factor C

Pregnancy Considerations Adverse events have been observed in some oral animal reproduction studies. Diagnosing and treating pheochromocytoma is critical for favorable maternal and fetal outcomes (Schenker 1971; Schenker 1982).

Dental Health Professional Considerations OraVerse (solution for injection/dental cartridge) is administered as a submucosal injection and is not to be confused with phentolamine used as an intramuscular or intravenous injection for the treatment of hypertension associated with pheochromocytoma.

In adolescents >12 years and adults, OraVerse reduced the median time to recovery of normal sensation in the lower lip by 85 minutes compared to control. OraVerse reduced the median time to recovery of normal sensation in the upper lip by 83 minutes. Within 1 hour after administration, 41% of patients reported normal lower lip sensation as compared to 7% in the control group and 59% of patients given OraVerse reported normal upper lip sensation as compared to 12% in the control group.

In children 6 to 11 years of age, the median time to normal sensation was reduced by 75 minutes after OraVerse administration, a 56% acceleration of the time to normal sensation.

While dental treatment is attainable using local anesthesia without the use of this reversal agent phentolamine, research suggests its use prevents self-inflicted soft tissue trauma in pediatric patients visiting a portable dental clinic. Such post-procedural soft tissue injuries are more likely in pediatric patients receiving local anesthesia with one or more of the following factors: Attention deficit disorder, obesity and/or the use of an inferior alveolar nerve block (Boynes 2013).

- ◆ **Phentolamine Mesylate** *see* Phentolamine *on page 1226*
- ◆ **Phenylalanine Mustard** *see* Melphalan *on page 961*
- ◆ **Phenylazo Diamino Pyridine Hydrochloride** *see* Phenazopyridine *on page 1222*

Phenylephrine (Systemic) (fen il EF rin)

Brand Names: US Biorphen; Little Colds Decongestant [OTC]; Medi-Phenyl [OTC] [DSC]; Nasal Decongestant [OTC]; Non-Pseudo Sinus Decongestant [OTC]; Sudafed PE Childrens [OTC]; Sudafed PE Sinus Congestion [OTC]; Sudogest PE [OTC]; Vazculep

Brand Names: Canada Neo-Synephrine

Pharmacologic Category Alpha-Adrenergic Agonist

Use

Hypotension/shock: Treatment of hypotension, vascular failure in shock. **Note:** Not recommended for routine use in the treatment of septic shock; use should be limited until more evidence demonstrating positive clinical outcomes becomes available (Rhodes 2017).

Guideline recommendations:

Cardiogenic shock: The 2017 American Heart Association (AHA) scientific statement for the Contemporary Management of Cardiogenic Shock recommends phenylephrine, if needed, be considered for initial vasoactive management of cardiogenic shock due to aortic stenosis, mitral stenosis, or dynamic left ventricular outflow tract (LVOT) obstruction (AHA [van Diepen 2017]).

Hypotension during anesthesia: As a vasoconstrictor in regional analgesia

Nasal congestion: As a decongestant [OTC]

Local Anesthetic/Vasoconstrictor Precautions

Use with caution since phenylephrine is a sympathomimetic amine which could interact with epinephrine to cause a pressor response

Effects on Dental Treatment Key adverse event(s) related to dental treatment: Tachycardia, palpitations (use vasoconstrictor with caution), and xerostomia (normal salivary flow resumes upon discontinuation).

Effects on Bleeding No information available to require special precautions

Adverse Reactions Frequency not defined.

Injection:

Cardiovascular: Cardiac arrhythmia (rare), exacerbation of angina, hypertension, hypertensive crisis, ischemia, localized blanching, low cardiac output, peripheral vasoconstriction (severe), reflex bradycardia, visceral vasoconstriction (severe), worsening of heart failure

Central nervous system: Anxiety, dizziness, excitability, headache, insomnia, nervousness, paresthesia, precordial pain (or discomfort), restlessness

Dermatologic: Pallor, piloerection, pruritus

Endocrine & metabolic: Metabolic acidosis

Gastrointestinal: Epigastric pain, gastric irritation, nausea, vomiting

Genitourinary: Decreased renal blood flow, decreased urine output

Hypersensitivity: Hypersensitivity reaction (including skin rash, urticaria, leukopenia, agranulocytosis, thrombocytopenia)

Neuromuscular & skeletal: Neck pain, tremor, weakness

Ophthalmic: Blurred vision

Respiratory: Dyspnea, respiratory distress

Oral: Central nervous system: Anxiety, dizziness, excitability, headache, insomnia, nervousness, restlessness

Mechanism of Action Potent, direct-acting alpha-adrenergic agonist with virtually no beta-adrenergic activity; produces systemic arterial vasoconstriction. Such increases in systemic vascular resistance may result in dose-dependent increases in systolic and diastolic blood pressure and reductions in heart rate and cardiac output (most noticeable in patients with preexisting cardiac dysfunction).

Pharmacodynamics/Kinetics

Onset of Action

Blood pressure increase/vasoconstriction: IM, SubQ: 10 to 15 minutes; IV: Immediate

Nasal decongestant: Oral: 15 to 30 minutes (Kollar 2007)

Duration of Action

Blood pressure increase/vasoconstriction: IM: 1 to 2 hours; IV: ~15 to 20 minutes; SubQ: 50 minutes

Nasal decongestant: Oral: ≤4 hours (Kollar 2007)

Half-life Elimination Alpha phase: ~5 minutes; Terminal phase: 2 to 3 hours (Hengstmann 1982; Kanfer 1993)

Time to Peak Oral: 0.75 to 2 hours (Kanfer 1993)

Pregnancy Considerations Phenylephrine crosses the placenta at term.

Maternal use of phenylephrine during the first trimester of pregnancy is not strongly associated with an increased risk of fetal malformations; maternal dose and duration of therapy were not reported in available publications. Phenylephrine is available over-the-counter for the symptomatic relief of nasal congestion. Decongestants are not the preferred agents for the treatment of rhinitis during pregnancy. Oral phenylephrine should be avoided during the first trimester of pregnancy; short-term use (<3 days) of intranasal phenylephrine may be beneficial to some patients although its safety during pregnancy has not been studied. Phenylephrine injection is used at delivery for the prevention and/or treatment of maternal hypotension associated with spinal anesthesia in women undergoing cesarean section. Phenylephrine may be associated with a more favorable fetal acid base status than ephedrine; however, overall fetal outcomes appear to be similar. Nausea or vomiting may be less with phenylephrine than ephedrine but is also dependent upon blood pressure control. Phenylephrine may be preferred in the absence of maternal bradycardia.

Phenylephrine (Topical) (fen il EF rin)

Brand Names: US Anu-Med [OTC] [DSC]; GoodSense Hemorrhoidal [OTC]; GRX Hemorrhoidal [OTC]; Hemorrhoidal Cooling [OTC]; Hemorrhoidal [OTC]; Major-Prep Hemorrhoidal [OTC]; Preparation H Totables [OTC] [DSC]; Preparation H [OTC]; Rectacaine [OTC]

Brand Names: Canada Rectogel HC

Pharmacologic Category Alpha-Adrenergic Agonist; Antihemorrhoidal Agent

Use For OTC use as treatment of hemorrhoids

Local Anesthetic/Vasoconstrictor Precautions No information available to require special precautions

Effects on Dental Treatment No significant effects or complications reported

Effects on Bleeding No information available to require special precautions

Adverse Reactions Rare systemic effects may occur.

Mechanism of Action Potent, direct-acting alpha-adrenergic agonist with virtually no beta-adrenergic activity; produces local vasoconstriction.

Pregnancy Considerations When administered intravenously, phenylephrine crosses the placenta. Refer to the Phenylephrine (Systemic) monograph for details. There is limited information available supporting the use of topical agents for the treatment of hemorrhoids. Products containing phenylephrine should be used with caution in pregnant women, especially patients with hypertension or diabetes.

- ◆ **Phenylephrine HCl** *see* Phenylephrine (Systemic) *on page* 1227
- ◆ **Phenylephrine HCl** *see* Phenylephrine (Topical) *on page* 1227
- ◆ **Phenylephrine Hydrochloride** *see* Phenylephrine (Systemic) *on page* 1227
- ◆ **Phenylephrine Hydrochloride** *see* Phenylephrine (Topical) *on page* 1227
- ◆ **Phenylethylmalonylurea** *see* PHENobarbital *on page* 1223
- ◆ **Phenylhistine DH [OTC] [DSC]** *see* Chlorpheniramine, Pseudoephedrine, and Codeine *on page* 341
- ◆ **Phenyl Salicylate, Methenamine, Methylene Blue, Benzoic Acid, and Hyoscyamine** *see* Methenamine, Phenyl Salicylate, Methylene Blue, Benzoic Acid, and Hyoscyamine *on page* 987
- ◆ **Phenyl Salicylate, Methenamine, Methylene Blue, Sodium Biphosphate, and Hyoscyamine** *see* Methenamine, Sodium Phosphate Monobasic, Phenyl Salicylate, Methylene Blue, and Hyoscyamine *on page* 987
- ◆ **Phenyltoloxamine Citrate and Hydrocodone Bitartrate** *see* Hydrocodone and Phenyltoloxamine *on page* 773
- ◆ **Phenytek** *see* Phenytoin *on page* 1228

Phenytoin (FEN i toyn)

Related Information

Fosphenytoin *on page* 717

Brand Names: US Dilantin; Dilantin Infatabs; Phenytek; Phenytoin Infatabs

Brand Names: Canada APO-Phenytoin Sodium; Dilantin; Dilantin Infatabs; Dilantin-125; Dilantin-30; NOVO-Phenytoin [DSC]; TARO-Phenytoin; Tremytoine

Pharmacologic Category Anticonvulsant, Hydantoin

Use

Focal (partial) onset seizures and generalized onset seizures: Treatment of patients with focal and generalized onset seizures and prevention of seizures following craniotomy. May be used off-label for other seizure types.

Status epilepticus: Treatment of patients with convulsive and nonconvulsive status epilepticus.

Local Anesthetic/Vasoconstrictor Precautions No information available to require special precautions

Effects on Dental Treatment Gingival hyperplasia is a common problem observed during the first 6 months of phenytoin therapy appearing as gingivitis or gum inflammation. To minimize severity and growth rate of gingival tissue begin a program of professional cleaning and patient plaque control within 10 days of starting anticonvulsant therapy.

Effects on Bleeding No information available to require special precautions

Adverse Reactions

Frequency not defined:

Cardiovascular: Cardiac arrhythmia, cardiac conduction disturbance (depression), circulatory shock, hypotension, ventricular fibrillation

Central nervous system: Ataxia, cerebral atrophy (elevated serum levels and/or long-term use), cerebral dysfunction (elevated serum levels and/or long-term use), confusion, dizziness, drowsiness, headache, insomnia, nervousness, paresthesia, peripheral neuropathy (associated with chronic treatment), slurred speech, suicidal ideation, suicidal tendencies, twitching, vertigo

Dermatologic: Bullous dermatitis, exfoliative dermatitis, morbilliform rash, scarlatiniform rash, skin or other tissue necrosis, skin rash

Endocrine & metabolic: Decreased T4, increased gamma-glutamyl transferase, vitamin D deficiency (associated with chronic treatment)

Gastrointestinal: Constipation, dysgeusia, gingival hyperplasia, nausea, swelling of lips, vomiting

Genitourinary: Peyronie's disease

Hematologic & oncologic: Macrocytosis, megaloblastic anemia, pseudolymphoma, purpuric dermatitis

Hepatic: Acute hepatic failure, hepatic injury, hepatitis, increased serum alkaline phosphatase, toxic hepatitis

Local: Injection site reaction ("purple glove syndrome;" edema, discoloration, and pain distal to injection site), local inflammation, local irritation, localized tenderness, local tissue necrosis

Neuromuscular & skeletal: Osteomalacia

Ophthalmic: Nystagmus

Miscellaneous: Fever, tissue sloughing

<1%, postmarketing, and/or case reports: Acute generalized exanthematous pustulosis, agranulocytosis, anaphylaxis, angioedema, asterixis, bone fracture, bone marrow depression, bradycardia, chorea, decreased bone mineral density, DRESS syndrome, dyskinesia, dystonia, enlargement of facial features, granulocytopenia, hepatotoxicity, Hodgkin lymphoma, hyperglycemia, hypertrichosis, immunoglobulin abnormality, leukopenia, lymphadenopathy, malignant lymphoma, osteoporosis, pancytopenia, polyarteritis nodosa, Stevens-Johnson syndrome, systemic lupus erythematosus, thrombocytopenia, toxic epidermal necrolysis, tremor, urticaria

Mechanism of Action Stabilizes neuronal membranes and decreases seizure activity by increasing efflux or decreasing influx of sodium ions across cell membranes in the motor cortex during generation of nerve impulses; prolongs effective refractory period and suppresses ventricular pacemaker automaticity, shortens action potential in the heart

Pharmacodynamics/Kinetics

Onset of Action IV: ~0.5 to 1 hour

Half-life Elimination Note: Elimination is not first-order (ie, follows Michaelis-Menten pharmacokinetics); half-life increases with increasing phenytoin concentrations; best described using parameters such as V_{max} and K_m (Patsalos 2008).

IV: 10 to 12 hours.
Oral:
Capsule, oral suspension: Average 22 hours (range: 7 to 42 hours).
Chewable tablet: Average 14 hours (range: 7 to 29 hours).

Time to Peak Serum (formulation dependent): Oral: Extended-release capsule: 4 to 12 hours; Immediate-release preparation: 1.5 to 3 hours

Reproductive Considerations

Effective contraception is recommended for females of reproductive potential who are not planning a pregnancy. Phenytoin may decrease the efficacy of hormonal contraceptives; consult drug interactions database for more detailed information.

Females with epilepsy who are planning a pregnancy should have baseline serum concentrations measured once or twice prior to pregnancy during a period when seizure control is optimal (Patsalos 2008).

Pregnancy Considerations

Phenytoin crosses the placenta (Harden 2009a). An increased risk of congenital malformations and adverse outcomes may occur following in utero phenytoin exposure. Reported malformations include orofacial clefts, cardiac defects, dysmorphic facial features, nail/digit hypoplasia, growth abnormalities including microcephaly, and mental deficiency. Isolated cases of malignancies (including neuroblastoma) and coagulation defects in the neonate (may be life threatening) following delivery have also been reported. Maternal use of phenytoin should be avoided when possible to decrease the risk of cleft palate and poor cognitive outcomes. Polytherapy may also increase the risk of congenital malformations; monotherapy is recommended (Harden 2009b). The maternal use of folic acid throughout pregnancy is recommended to reduce the risk of major congenital malformations (Harden 2009a). Potentially life-threatening bleeding disorders in the newborn may also occur due to decreased concentrations of vitamin K-dependent clotting factors following phenytoin exposure in utero; vitamin K administration to the mother prior to delivery and the newborn after birth is recommended.

Total plasma concentrations of phenytoin are decreased in the mother during pregnancy; unbound plasma (free) concentrations are also decreased and plasma clearance is increased. Due to pregnancy-induced physiologic changes, women who are pregnant may require dose adjustments of phenytoin in order to maintain clinical response; monitoring during pregnancy should be considered (Harden 2009a). For women with epilepsy who are planning a pregnancy in advance, baseline serum concentrations should be measured once or twice prior to pregnancy during a period when seizure control is optimal. Monitoring can then be continued once each trimester during pregnancy and postpartum; more frequent monitoring may be needed in some patients. Monitoring of unbound plasma concentrations is recommended (Patsalos 2008; Patsalos 2018).

Patients exposed to phenytoin during pregnancy are encouraged to enroll themselves in the North American Antiepileptic Drug Pregnancy Registry by calling 1-888-233-2334. Additional information is available at http://aedpregnancyregistry.org.

- ◆ **Phenytoin Infatabs** *see* Phenytoin *on page 1228*
- ◆ **Phenytoin Sodium** *see* Phenytoin *on page 1228*
- ◆ **Phenytoin Sodium, Extended** *see* Phenytoin *on page 1228*
- ◆ **Phenytoin Sodium, Prompt** *see* Phenytoin *on page 1228*
- ◆ **Phesgo** *see* Pertuzumab, Trastuzumab, and Hyaluronidase *on page 1221*
- ◆ **PHiD-CV** *see* Pneumococcal Conjugate Vaccine (10-Valent) *on page 1241*
- ◆ **Philith** *see* Ethinyl Estradiol and Norethindrone *on page 614*
- ◆ **Phos-Flur [DSC]** *see* Fluoride *on page 693*
- ◆ **Phos-Flur Rinse [OTC]** *see* Fluoride *on page 693*
- ◆ **Phosphasal** *see* Methenamine, Sodium Phosphate Monobasic, Phenyl Salicylate, Methylene Blue, and Hyoscyamine *on page 987*
- ◆ **Phosphonoformate** *see* Foscarnet *on page 713*
- ◆ **Phosphonoformic Acid** *see* Foscarnet *on page 713*
- ◆ **Photofrin** *see* Porfimer *on page 1247*
- ◆ **Photrexa** *see* Riboflavin 5'-Phosphate *on page 1323*
- ◆ **Photrexa-Photrexa Viscous Kit** *see* Riboflavin 5'-Phosphate *on page 1323*
- ◆ **Photrexa Viscous** *see* Riboflavin 5'-Phosphate *on page 1323*
- ◆ ***p*-Hydroxyampicillin** *see* Amoxicillin *on page 124*
- ◆ **Phylloquinone** *see* Phytonadione *on page 1230*
- ◆ **Physicians EZ Use B-12** *see* Cyanocobalamin *on page 417*

Physostigmine (fye zoe STIG meen)

Pharmacologic Category Acetylcholinesterase Inhibitor; Antidote

Use

Reversal of central nervous system anticholinergic syndrome

Note: Consultation with a clinical toxicologist or poison control center may be prudent if physostigmine administration is being considered. Physostigmine is most efficacious for delirium resulting from drugs with predominant anticholinergic properties (eg, atropine, benztropine, scopolamine, dimenhydrinate, diphenhydramine, *Atropa belladonna* [deadly nightshade], jimson weed [*Datura* spp]), but may also be beneficial for other medications with anticholinergic effects (eg, atypical antipsychotics, cyclobenzaprine, hydroxyzine [Cole 2012; Grenga 2018; Rasimas 2014; Weizberg 2006]). Risk:benefit should always be considered. When indicated and used properly by a clinical toxicologist, physostigmine is safe and effective (Arens 2018; Watkins 2015).

Local Anesthetic/Vasoconstrictor Precautions

No information available to require special precautions

Effects on Dental Treatment Key adverse event(s) related to dental treatment: Salivation.

Effects on Bleeding No information available to require special precautions

Adverse Reactions

Frequency not defined:
Cardiovascular: Bradycardia
Gastrointestinal: Nausea, salivation, vomiting
Nervous system: Seizures

Mechanism of Action Physostigmine is a carbamate which inhibits the enzyme acetylcholinesterase and prolongs the central and peripheral effects of acetylcholine

Pharmacodynamics/Kinetics
Onset of Action Within 3 to 8 minutes
Duration of Action 45 to 60 minutes
Half-life Elimination 1 to 2 hours
Pregnancy Considerations In general, medications used as antidotes should take into consideration the health and prognosis of the mother; antidotes should be administered to pregnant women if there is a clear indication for use and should not be withheld because of fears of teratogenicity (Bailey 2003).

- ◆ **Physostigmine Salicylate** *see* Physostigmine *on page 1229*
- ◆ **Physostigmine Sulfate** *see* Physostigmine *on page 1229*
- ◆ **Phytomenadione** *see* Phytonadione *on page 1230*

Phytonadione (fye toe na DYE one)

Brand Names: US Mephyton
Brand Names: Canada AquaMEPHYTON; Konakion; Mephyton
Pharmacologic Category Vitamin, Fat Soluble
Use
Anticoagulant-induced prothrombin deficiency: Treatment of anticoagulant-induced prothrombin deficiency caused by coumarin or indandione derivatives
Vitamin K deficiency bleeding (formerly known as hemorrhagic disease) of the newborn: Prophylaxis and therapy of vitamin K deficiency bleeding (formerly known as hemorrhagic disease) of the newborn (injection only)
Hypoprothrombinemia: Hypoprothrombinemia secondary to factors limiting absorption or synthesis of vitamin K (eg, obstructive jaundice, biliary fistula, sprue, ulcerative colitis, celiac disease, intestinal resection, cystic fibrosis of the pancreas, regional enteritis), and other drug-induced hypoprothrombinemia where it is definitely shown that the result is due to interference with vitamin K metabolism (eg, salicylates, antibacterial therapy)
Local Anesthetic/Vasoconstrictor Precautions
No information available to require special precautions
Effects on Dental Treatment Key adverse event(s) related to dental treatment: Abnormal taste.
Effects on Bleeding Phytonadione is a synthetic form of vitamin K and has been used as an antidote to reverse warfarin-induced bleeding complications or endogenous vitamin K deficiencies.
Adverse Reactions
Frequency not defined:
Cardiovascular: Chest pain, flushing, hypotension, tachycardia, weak pulse
Central nervous system: Dizziness
Dermatologic: Diaphoresis, eczematous rash, erythema, erythematous rash, pruritic plaques of the skin, urticaria
Gastrointestinal: Dysgeusia
Hepatic: Hyperbilirubinemia
Hypersensitivity: Anaphylactoid reaction, anaphylaxis, hypersensitivity reaction
Local: Injection site reaction (including pain, swelling, tenderness)
Respiratory: Cyanosis, dyspnea
Miscellaneous: Lesion (scleroderma-like)
Mechanism of Action Promotes liver synthesis of clotting factors (II, VII, IX, X); however, the exact mechanism as to this stimulation is unknown. Menadiol is a water soluble form of vitamin K; phytonadione has a more rapid and prolonged effect than menadione; menadiol sodium diphosphate (K_4) is half as potent as menadione (K_3).
Pharmacodynamics/Kinetics
Onset of Action
Onset of action: Increased coagulation factors: Oral: 6 to 10 hours; IV: 1 to 2 hours
Peak effect: INR values return to normal: Oral: 24 to 48 hours; IV: 12 to 14 hours
Pregnancy Considerations
Phytonadione crosses the placenta in limited concentrations (Kazzi 1990).

The dietary requirements of vitamin K are the same in pregnant and nonpregnant women (IOM 2000). In general, medications used as antidotes should take into consideration the health and prognosis of the mother; antidotes should be administered to pregnant women if there is a clear indication for use and should not be withheld because of fears of teratogenicity (Bailey 2003). Use of preservative free solutions are preferred when the injection is needed during pregnancy.

- ◆ **PI_3K Delta Inhibitor CAL-101** *see* Idelalisib *on page 795*
- ◆ **Pibrentasvir and Glecaprevir** *see* Glecaprevir and Pibrentasvir *on page 738*
- ◆ **Pidorubicin** *see* EpiRUBicin *on page 576*
- ◆ **Pidorubicin Hydrochloride** *see* EpiRUBicin *on page 576*
- ◆ **Pifeltro** *see* Doravirine *on page 513*

Pilocarpine (Systemic) (pye loe KAR peen)

Related Information
Dentin Hypersensitivity, Acid Erosion, High Caries Index, Management of Alveolar Osteitis, and Xerostomia *on page 1762*
Perioral Premalignant Lesions and Management of Patients Undergoing Cancer Therapy *on page 1781*
Brand Names: US Salagen
Brand Names: Canada ACCEL-Pilocarpine; Salagen
Generic Availability (US) Yes
Pharmacologic Category Cholinergic Agonist
Dental Use Treatment of xerostomia caused by radiation therapy in patients with head and neck cancer and from Sjögren's syndrome
Use Xerostomia: Treatment of symptoms of dry mouth from salivary gland hypofunction caused by radiotherapy for cancer of the head and neck; treatment of symptoms of dry mouth in patients with Sjögren syndrome.
Local Anesthetic/Vasoconstrictor Precautions
No information available to require special precautions
Effects on Dental Treatment Key adverse event(s) related to dental treatment: Increased salivation (therapeutic effect) (see Dental Health Professional Considerations)
Effects on Bleeding No information available to require special precautions
Adverse Reactions
>10%:
Cardiovascular: Flushing (8% to 13%)
Central nervous system: Chills (3% to 15%), dizziness (5% to 12%), headache (11%)
Gastrointestinal: Nausea (6% to 15%)
Genitourinary: Urinary frequency (9% to 12%)
Neuromuscular & skeletal: Weakness (2% to 12%)
Respiratory: Rhinitis (5% to 14%)

Miscellaneous: Diaphoresis (29% to 68%)

1% to 10%:

Cardiovascular: Edema (<1% to 5%), facial edema, hypertension (3%), palpitation, tachycardia

Central nervous system: Pain (4%), fever, somnolence

Dermatologic: Pruritus, rash

Gastrointestinal: Diarrhea (4% to 7%), dyspepsia (7%), vomiting (3% to 4%), constipation, flatulence, glossitis, salivation increased, stomatitis, taste perversion

Genitourinary: Vaginitis, urinary incontinence

Neuromuscular & skeletal: Myalgias, tremor

Ocular: Lacrimation (6%), amblyopia (4%), abnormal vision, blurred vision, conjunctivitis

Otic: Tinnitus

Respiratory: Cough increased, dysphagia, epistaxis, sinusitis

Miscellaneous: Allergic reaction, voice alteration

<1%: Abnormal dreams, abnormal thinking, alopecia, angina pectoris, anorexia, anxiety, aphasia, appetite increased, arrhythmia, arthralgia, arthritis, bilirubinemia, body odor, bone disorder, bradycardia, breast pain, bronchitis, cataract, cholelithiasis, colitis, confusion, contact dermatitis, cyst, deafness, depression, dry eyes, dry mouth, dry skin, dyspnea, dysuria, ear pain, ECG abnormality, eczema, emotional lability, eructation, erythema nodosum, esophagitis, exfoliative dermatitis, eye hemorrhage, eye pain, gastritis, gastroenteritis, gastrointestinal disorder, gingivitis, glaucoma, hematuria, hepatitis, herpes simplex, hiccup, hyperkinesias, hypoesthesia, hypoglycemia, hypotension, hypothermia, insomnia, intracranial hemorrhage, laryngismus, laryngitis, leg cramps, leukopenia, liver function test abnormal, lymphadenopathy, mastitis, melena, menorrhagia, metrorrhagia, migraine, moniliasis, myasthenia, MI, neck pain, photosensitivity reaction, nervousness, ovarian disorder, pancreatitis, paresthesia, parotid gland enlargement, peripheral edema, platelet abnormality, pneumonia, pyuria, salivary gland enlargement, salpingitis, seborrhea, skin ulcer, speech disorder, sputum increased, stridor, syncope, taste loss, tendon disorder, tenosynovitis, thrombocythemia, thrombocytopenia, thrombosis, tongue disorder, twitching, urethral pain, urinary impairment, urinary urgency, vaginal hemorrhage, vaginal moniliasis, vesiculobullous rash, WBC abnormality, yawning

Dental Usual Dosage Treatment of xerostomia: Adults: Oral: Following head and neck cancer: 5 mg 3 times daily, titration up to 10 mg 3 times daily may be considered for patients who have not responded adequately; do not exceed 2 tablets per dose

Sjögren's syndrome: 5 mg 3 to 4 times daily

Dosing

Adult & Geriatric

Xerostomia: Oral:

Associated with head and neck cancer: Initial: 5 mg 3 times daily; may titrate dose based on response and tolerability; usual dosage range: 15 to 30 mg/day; maximum: 10 mg/dose

Sjögren syndrome: 5 mg 4 times daily

Renal Impairment: Adult There are no dosage adjustments provided in the manufacturer's labeling.

Hepatic Impairment: Adult

Mild impairment (Child-Pugh score 5 to 6): No dosage adjustment necessary.

Moderate impairment (Child-Pugh score 7 to 9): Initial: 5 mg twice daily; adjust dose based on response and tolerability.

Severe impairment (Child-Pugh score 10 to 15): Use is not recommended.

Mechanism of Action Binds to muscarinic (cholinergic) receptors, causing an increase in secretion of exocrine glands (such as salivary and sweat glands) and increase tone of smooth muscle in gastrointestinal and urinary tracts

Contraindications Hypersensitivity to pilocarpine or any component of the formulation; uncontrolled asthma; when miosis is undesirable (eg, acute iritis, angle-closure glaucoma)

Warnings/Precautions Use caution with significant cardiovascular disease; patients may have difficulty compensating for transient changes in hemodynamics or rhythm induced by pilocarpine. Use with caution in patients with controlled asthma, chronic bronchitis, or COPD; may increase airway resistance, bronchial smooth muscle tone, and bronchial secretions. Use with caution in patients with cholelithiasis, biliary tract disease, and nephrolithiasis; may induce smooth muscle spasms, precipitating renal colic or ureteral reflux in patients with nephrolithiasis. Use with caution in patients with moderate hepatic impairment; dosage adjustment recommended; use is not recommended in patients with severe hepatic impairment.

Drug Interactions

Metabolism/Transport Effects None known.

Avoid Concomitant Use There are no known interactions where it is recommended to avoid concomitant use.

Increased Effect/Toxicity

The levels/effects of Pilocarpine (Systemic) may be increased by: Acetylcholinesterase Inhibitors; Beta-Blockers

Decreased Effect

Pilocarpine (Systemic) may decrease the levels/effects of: Cimetropium; Sincalide

Food Interactions Fat decreases the rate of absorption, maximum concentration and increases the time it takes to reach maximum concentration. Management: Avoid administering with a high-fat meal.

Pharmacodynamics/Kinetics

Onset of Action 20 minutes; Maximum effect: 1 hour

Duration of Action 3 to 5 hours

Half-life Elimination 0.76 to 1.35 hours; Mild to moderate hepatic impairment: 2.1 hours

Time to Peak Serum: 0.85 to 1.25 hours (increased to 1.47 hours with a high-fat meal)

Pregnancy Considerations Adverse events have been observed in some animal reproduction studies.

Breastfeeding Considerations It is not known if pilocarpine is excreted in breast milk. Due to the potential for serious adverse reactions in the nursing infant, the manufacturer recommends a decision be made to discontinue nursing or to discontinue the drug, taking into account the importance of treatment to the mother.

Dosage Forms: US

Tablet, Oral:

Salagen: 5 mg, 7.5 mg

Generic: 5 mg, 7.5 mg

Dosage Forms: Canada

Tablet, Oral:

Salagen: 5 mg

Generic: 5 mg

Dental Health Professional Considerations Pilocarpine may have potential as a salivary stimulant in individuals suffering from xerostomia induced by antidepressants and other medications. At the present time however, the FDA has not approved pilocarpine for use in drug-induced xerostomia (clinical studies required). In an attempt to discern the efficacy of pilocarpine as a salivary stimulant in patients suffering from Sjögren's syndrome (SS), Rhodus and Schuh studied 9 patients with SS given daily doses of pilocarpine over a 6-week period. A dose of 5 mg daily produced a significant overall increase in both whole unstimulated salivary flow and parotid stimulated salivary flow. These results support the use of pilocarpine to increase salivary flow in patients with SS.

- **Pilocarpine HCl** *see* Pilocarpine (Systemic) *on page 1230*
- **Pilocarpine Hydrochloride** *see* Pilocarpine (Systemic) *on page 1230*
- **Pimaricin** *see* Natamycin *on page 1087*

Pimavanserin (pim a VAN ser in)

Brand Names: US Nuplazid

Pharmacologic Category Second Generation (Atypical) Antipsychotic

Use Parkinson disease psychosis: Treatment of hallucinations and delusions associated with Parkinson disease psychosis

Local Anesthetic/Vasoconstrictor Precautions Pimavanserin is one of the drugs confirmed to prolong the QT interval and is accepted as having a risk of causing torsades de pointes. The risk of drug-induced torsades de pointes is extremely low when a single QT interval prolonging drug is prescribed. In terms of epinephrine, it is not known what effect vasoconstrictors in the local anesthetic regimen will have in patients with a known history of congenital prolonged QT interval or in patients taking any medication that prolongs the QT interval. Until more information is obtained, it is suggested that the clinician consult with the physician prior to the use of a vasoconstrictor in suspected patients, and that the vasoconstrictor (epinephrine, mepivacaine, and levonordefrin [Carbocaine 2% with Neo-Cobefrin]) be used with caution.

Effects on Dental Treatment Key adverse event(s) related to dental treatment: May cause orthostatic hypotension; monitor patient rising from dental chair for signs of dizziness.

Effects on Bleeding No information available to require special precautions

Adverse Reactions

1% to 10%:

Cardiovascular: Peripheral edema (7%)

Central nervous system: Confusion (6%), hallucination (5%), abnormal gait (2%)

Gastrointestinal: Nausea (7%), constipation (4%)

Frequency not defined: Cardiovascular: Prolonged QT interval on ECG

<1%, postmarketing, and/or case reports: Aggressive behavior, agitation, angioedema, drowsiness, falling, skin rash, urticaria

Mechanism of Action Pimavanserin acts as an inverse agonist and antagonist with high affinity for 5-HT_{2A} receptors and low affinity for 5-HT_{2C} and sigma 1 receptors; no affinity for 5-HT_{2B}, dopaminergic (including D_2), muscarinic, histaminergic, or adrenergic receptors, or to calcium channels.

Pharmacodynamics/Kinetics

Half-life Elimination Pimavanserin: ~57 hours; N-desmethylated metabolite: ~200 hours

Time to Peak 6 hours (median: 4 to 24 hours)

Pregnancy Considerations Adverse events were observed in some animal reproduction studies.

- **Pimavanserin Tartrate** *see* Pimavanserin *on page 1232*

Pimecrolimus (pim e KROE li mus)

Brand Names: US Elidel

Brand Names: Canada Elidel

Pharmacologic Category Calcineurin Inhibitor; Immunosuppressant Agent; Topical Skin Product

Use Atopic dermatitis: Second-line therapy for short-term and noncontinuous long-term treatment of mild to moderate atopic dermatitis in nonimmunocompromised patients 2 years and older who have failed to respond adequately to other topical prescription treatments, or when those treatments are not advisable.

Local Anesthetic/Vasoconstrictor Precautions No information available to require special precautions

Effects on Dental Treatment No significant effects or complications reported

Effects on Bleeding No information available to require special precautions

Adverse Reactions

>10%:

Central nervous system: Headache (children and adolescents 11% to 25%; adults 7%), fever (children and adolescents 13%; adults 1%)

Infection: Influenza (3% to 13%)

Local: Local burning (adults 26%; children and adolescents 2% to 8%; tends to resolve/improve as lesions resolve), application site reaction (adults 15%; children and adolescents 2%)

Respiratory: Nasopharyngitis (infants, children, and adolescents 10% to 27%; adults 8%), upper respiratory tract infection (children and adolescents 14% to 19%; adults 4%), cough (children and adolescents 9% to 16%; adults 2%), bronchitis (children and adolescents ≤11%; adults ≤2%)

1% to 10%:

Dermatologic: Folliculitis (adults 6%; children and adolescents 1%), skin infection (5% to 6%), impetigo (4%), warts (children and adolescents ≤3%), acne vulgaris (≤2%), herpes simplex dermatitis (≤2%), molluscum contagiosum (children and adolescents ≤2%), urticaria (≤1%)

Gastrointestinal: Diarrhea (children and adolescents 1% to 8%; adults ≤2%), gastroenteritis (children and adolescents ≤7%; adults 2%), vomiting (1% to 4%), constipation (children and adolescents ≤4%), abdominal pain (≤3%), toothache (≤3%), nausea (1% to 2%)

Genitourinary: Dysmenorrhea (1% to 2%)

Hypersensitivity: Hypersensitivity (3% to 5%)

Infection: Viral infection (children and adolescents ≤7%), herpes simplex infection (≤4%), bacterial infection (1% to 2%), staphylococcal infection (1% to 2%), varicella (≤1%)

Local: Local irritation (adults ≤6%; children and adolescents ≤1%), local pruritus (1% to 6%), localized erythema (≤2%)

Neuromuscular & skeletal: Arthralgia (≤2%), back pain (≤2%)

Ocular: Conjunctivitis (≤2% to 3%), eye infection (≤1%)

Otic: Otic infection (1% to 6%), otitis media (1% to 3%)

Respiratory: Sore throat (4% to 8%), pharyngitis (children and adolescents 1% to 8%; adults 1%), tonsillitis (children and adolescents ≤6%; adults <1%), asthma (3% to 4%), asthma aggravated (children and adolescents ≤4%), streptococcal pharyngitis (children and adolescents 3%), nasal congestion (1% to 3%), sinusitis (1% to 3%), epistaxis (≤3%), dyspnea (≤2%), flu-like symptoms (≤2%), pneumonia (≤2%), rhinitis (≤2%), rhinorrhea (children and adolescents ≤2%), viral upper respiratory tract infection (≤2%), wheezing (children and adolescents ≤1%)

Miscellaneous: Laceration (children and adolescents ≤2%)

<1%, postmarketing, and/or case reports: Anaphylaxis, angioedema, eczema (herpeticum), eye irritation (following application near eyes), facial edema, flushing (ethanol-associated), lymphadenopathy, malignant neoplasm (basal cell carcinoma, squamous cell carcinoma, malignant melanoma, malignant lymphoma), skin discoloration

Mechanism of Action Penetrates inflamed epidermis to inhibit T cell activation by blocking transcription of proinflammatory cytokine genes such as interleukin-2, interferon gamma (Th1-type), interleukin-4, and interleukin-10 (Th2-type). Pimecrolimus binds to the intracellular protein FKBP-12, inhibiting calcineurin, which blocks cytokine transcription and inhibits T-cell activation. Prevents release of inflammatory cytokines and mediators from mast cells *in vitro* after stimulation by antigen/IgE.

Pharmacodynamics/Kinetics

Onset of Action Time to significant improvement: 8 days (Wellington 2001)

Half-life Elimination Terminal: Oral: 30 to 40 hours

Time to Peak Serum: Topical: 2 to 6 hours

Pregnancy Risk Factor C

Pregnancy Considerations Adverse events were not observed in animal reproduction studies following topical application.

Pimozide (PI moe zide)

Related Information

Clinical Risk Related to Drugs Prolonging QT Interval *on page 1675*

Brand Names: US Orap [DSC]

Brand Names: Canada Orap; PMS-Pimozide

Pharmacologic Category First Generation (Typical) Antipsychotic

Use Tourette disorder: Suppression of severe motor and phonic tics in patients with Tourette disorder who have failed to respond satisfactorily to standard treatment. **Note:** The American Academy of Neurology comprehensive systematic review of the treatment of tics in people with Tourette syndrome and chronic tic disorders concluded there is low confidence that pimozide is superior to placebo at reducing tics (AAN [Pringsheim 2019]).

Local Anesthetic/Vasoconstrictor Precautions Pimozide is one of the drugs confirmed to prolong the QT interval and is accepted as having a risk of causing torsade de pointes. The risk of drug-induced torsade de pointes is extremely low when a single QT interval prolonging drug is prescribed. In terms of epinephrine, it is not known what effect vasoconstrictors in the local anesthetic regimen will have in patients with a known history of congenital prolonged QT interval or in patients taking any medication that prolongs the QT interval. Until more information is obtained, it is suggested that the clinician consult with the physician prior to the use of a vasoconstrictor in suspected patients, and that the vasoconstrictor (epinephrine, mepivacaine and levonordefrin [Carbocaine® 2% with Neo-Cobefrin®]) be used with caution.

Effects on Dental Treatment Key adverse event(s) related to dental treatment: Tourette's disorder: Xerostomia and increased salivation (normal salivary flow resumes upon discontinuation), taste disturbance, and dysphagia.

Effects on Bleeding No information available to require special precautions

Adverse Reactions Frequencies as reported in adults (limited data) and/or children with Tourette's disorder.

>10%:

Central nervous system: Sedation (70%), akathisia (40%), drowsiness (35%; children: ≤25%), behavioral changes (22% to 25%), hypertonia (15%)

Gastrointestinal: Xerostomia (25%), constipation (20%)

Genitourinary: Impotence (15%)

Neuromuscular & skeletal: Akinesia (40%), weakness (14%)

Ophthalmic: Decreased accommodation (20%), visual disturbance (3% to 20%)

1% to 10%:

Cardiovascular: ECG abnormality (3%)

Central nervous system: Depression (10%), insomnia (10%), speech disturbance (10%), nervousness (5% to 6%), writing difficulty (handwriting change: 5%), headache (3% to 5%), abnormal dreams (3%)

Dermatologic: Skin rash (3%)

Endocrine & metabolic: Increased thirst (5%)

Gastrointestinal: Sialorrhea (6%), diarrhea (5%), dysgeusia (5%), increased appetite (5%), dysphagia (3%)

Neuromuscular & skeletal: Muscle rigidity (10%), stooped posture (10%), hyperkinesia (3%), myalgia (3%), torticollis (3%), tremor (3%)

Ophthalmic: Photophobia (5%)

Frequency not defined (some reported for disorders other than Tourette's disorder):

Cardiovascular: Chest pain, hypertension, hypotension, orthostatic hypotension, prolonged QT interval on ECG, syncope, tachycardia, ventricular arrhythmia

Central nervous system: Dizziness, excitement, drug-induced extrapyramidal reaction (dystonia, pseudoparkinsonism, tardive dyskinesia), neuroleptic malignant syndrome, palpitations, seizure

Dermatologic: Diaphoresis, skin irritation

Endocrine & metabolic: Decreased libido, hyponatremia, weight changes (gain/loss)

Gastrointestinal: Anorexia, gastrointestinal distress, nausea, vomiting

Genitourinary: Nocturia

Hematologic & oncologic: Hemolytic anemia

Ophthalmic: Blurred vision, cataract, periorbital edema

Renal: Polyuria

<1%, postmarketing, and/or case reports: Gingival hyperplasia

Mechanism of Action Pimozide, a diphenylbutylperidine conventional antipsychotic, is a potent centrally-acting dopamine-receptor antagonist resulting in its characteristic neuroleptic effects

Pharmacodynamics/Kinetics

Onset of Action Within 1 week; Maximum effect: 4 to 6 weeks

Duration of Action Variable

Half-life Elimination Children 6 to 13 years (n=4): Mean ± SD: 66 ± 49 hours; Adults 23 to 39 years (n=7): Mean ± SD: 111 ± 57 hours (Sallee 1987)

Time to Peak Serum: 6 to 8 hours (range: 4 to 12 hours)

Pregnancy Risk Factor C

Pregnancy Considerations Adverse events were observed in some animal reproduction studies. Antipsychotic use during the third trimester of pregnancy has a risk for abnormal muscle movements (extrapyramidal symptoms [EPS]) and withdrawal symptoms in newborns following delivery. Symptoms in the newborn may include agitation, feeding disorder, hypertonia, hypotonia, respiratory distress, somnolence, and tremor; these effects may be self-limiting or require hospitalization.

Dental Health Professional Considerations See Local Anesthetic/Vasoconstrictor Precautions

◆ **Pimtrea** *see* Ethinyl Estradiol and Desogestrel *on page 609*

Pindolol (PIN doe lole)

Related Information

Cardiovascular Diseases *on page 1654*

Brand Names: Canada APO-Pindol; DOM-Pindolol; PMS-Pindolol; SANDOZ Pindolol [DSC]; TEVA-Pindolol; Visken

Pharmacologic Category Antihypertensive; Beta-Blocker With Intrinsic Sympathomimetic Activity

Use Hypertension: Management of hypertension. **Note:** Beta-blockers are **not** recommended as first-line therapy (ACC/AHA [Whelton 2017]).

Local Anesthetic/Vasoconstrictor Precautions Use with caution; epinephrine has interacted with nonselective beta-blockers to result in initial hypertensive episode followed by bradycardia

Effects on Dental Treatment Pindolol is a nonselective beta-blocker and may enhance the pressor response to epinephrine, resulting in hypertension and bradycardia. Many nonsteroidal anti-inflammatory drugs, such as ibuprofen and indomethacin, can reduce the hypotensive effect of beta-blockers after 3 or more weeks of therapy with the NSAID. Short-term NSAID use (ie, 3 days) requires no special precautions in patients taking beta-blockers.

Effects on Bleeding No information available to require special precautions

Adverse Reactions

>10%: Cardiovascular: Edema (6% to 16%)

1% to 10%:

Cardiovascular: Bradycardia (≤2%), claudication (≤2%), cold extremities (≤2%), heart block (≤2%), hypotension (≤2%), syncope (≤2%), tachycardia (≤2%), palpitations (≤1%)

Central nervous system: Insomnia (10%), dizziness (9%), fatigue (8%), nervousness (7%), abnormal dreams (5%), anxiety (≤2%), lethargy (≤2%)

Dermatologic: Hyperhidrosis (≤2%), pruritus (1%)

Endocrine & metabolic: Weight gain (≤2%)

Gastrointestinal: Nausea (5%), diarrhea (≤2%), vomiting (≤2%)

Genitourinary: Impotence (≤2%), pollakiuria (≤2%)

Hepatic: Increased serum ALT (7%), increased serum AST (7%)

Neuromuscular & skeletal: Myalgia (10%), arthralgia (7%), weakness (4%), muscle cramps (3%)

Ophthalmic: Burning sensation of eyes (≤2%), eye discomfort (≤2%), visual disturbance (≤2%)

Renal: Polyuria (≤2%)

Respiratory: Dyspnea (5%), wheezing (≤2%)

<1%, postmarketing, and/or case reports: Cardiac failure, hallucination, hyperuricemia, increased lactic acid dehydrogenase, increased serum alkaline phosphatase

Mechanism of Action Blocks both $beta_1$- and $beta_2$-receptors and has mild intrinsic sympathomimetic activity; pindolol has negative inotropic and chronotropic effects and can significantly slow AV nodal conduction. Augmentive action of antidepressants thought to be mediated via a serotonin 1A autoreceptor antagonism.

Pharmacodynamics/Kinetics

Half-life Elimination 3 to 4 hours; prolonged in the elderly (average 7 hours; up to 15 hours reported), and cirrhosis (range: 2.5 to 30 hours)

Time to Peak Serum: ~1 hour

Pregnancy Risk Factor B

Pregnancy Considerations Pindolol crosses the placenta (Gonçalves 2007).

Exposure to beta-blockers during pregnancy may increase the risk for adverse events in the neonate. If maternal use of a beta-blocker is needed, fetal growth should be monitored during pregnancy and the newborn should be monitored for 48 hours after delivery for bradycardia, hypoglycemia, and respiratory depression (ESC [Regitz-Zagrosek 2018]).

Chronic maternal hypertension is also associated with adverse events in the fetus/infant. Chronic maternal hypertension may increase the risk of birth defects, low birth weight, premature delivery, stillbirth, and neonatal death. Actual fetal/neonatal risks may be related to duration and severity of maternal hypertension. Untreated chronic hypertension may also increase the risks of adverse maternal outcomes, including gestational diabetes, preeclampsia, delivery complications, stroke, and myocardial infarction (ACOG 203 2019).

Due to pregnancy-induced physiologic changes, some pharmacokinetic properties of pindolol may be altered (Gonçalves 2002). When treatment of hypertension in pregnancy is indicated, specific recommendations vary by guideline. Although other agents are preferred, use of pindolol may be considered (ACOG 203 2019; ESC [Regitz-Zagrosek 2018]; Magee 2014). Females with preexisting hypertension may continue their medication during pregnancy unless contraindications exist (ESC [Regitz-Zagrosek 2018]).

Pioglitazone (pye oh GLI ta zone)

Related Information

Endocrine Disorders and Pregnancy *on page 1684*

Brand Names: US Actos

Brand Names: Canada ACCEL Pioglitazone [DSC]; ACH-Pioglitazone; ACT Pioglitazone; Actos [DSC]; APO-Pioglitazone; DOM-Pioglitazone [DSC]; JAMP-Pioglitazone; MINT-Pioglitazone; MYLAN-Pioglitazone [DSC]; PMS-Pioglitazone; PRO-Pioglitazone; RAN-Pioglitazone; SANDOZ Pioglitazone; TEVA-Pioglitazone [DSC]; VAN-Pioglitazone [DSC]

Pharmacologic Category Antidiabetic Agent, Thiazolidinedione

Use Diabetes mellitus, type 2, treatment: As an adjunct to diet and exercise, to improve glycemic control in adults with type 2 diabetes mellitus

Local Anesthetic/Vasoconstrictor Precautions No information available to require special precautions

Effects on Dental Treatment Key adverse event(s) related to dental treatment: Pioglitazone-dependent diabetics should be appointed for dental treatment in morning in order to minimize chance of stress-induced hypoglycemia.

Effects on Bleeding No information available to require special precautions

Adverse Reactions Adverse reactions and incidences reported are associated with monotherapy unless otherwise stated.

>10%:

Cardiovascular: Edema (combination trials: ≤27%)

Endocrine and metabolic: Hypoglycemia (combination trials: ≤27%)

Respiratory: Upper respiratory tract infection (13%)

1% to 10%:

Cardiovascular: Cardiac failure (combination trials: ≤8%)

Central nervous system: Headache (9%)

Neuromuscular & skeletal: Bone fracture (females: ≤5%), myalgia (5%)

Respiratory: Sinusitis (6%), pharyngitis (5%)

Frequency not defined:

Endocrine & metabolic: Decreased serum triglycerides, increased HDL-cholesterol, weight gain, weight loss

Hematologic & oncologic: Decreased hematocrit, decreased hemoglobin

<1%, postmarketing, and/or case reports: Bladder carcinoma, blurred vision, decreased visual acuity, dyspnea (associated with weight gain and/or edema), hepatic failure (very rare), hepatitis, increased creatine phosphokinase, increased serum transaminases, macular edema (new-onset or worsening), pulmonary edema, rhabdomyolysis

Mechanism of Action Thiazolidinedione antidiabetic agent that lowers blood glucose by improving target cell response to insulin, without increasing pancreatic insulin secretion. It has a mechanism of action that is dependent on the presence of insulin for activity. Pioglitazone is a potent and selective agonist for peroxisome proliferator-activated receptor-gamma (PPARgamma). Activation of nuclear PPARgamma receptors influences the production of a number of gene products involved in glucose and lipid metabolism. PPARgamma is abundant in the cells within the renal collecting tubules; fluid retention results from stimulation by thiazolidinediones which increases sodium reabsorption.

Pharmacodynamics/Kinetics

Onset of Action Delayed; Peak effect: Glucose control: Several weeks

Half-life Elimination Parent drug: 3 to 7 hours; M-III and M-IV metabolites: 16 to 24 hours

Time to Peak ~2 hours; delayed with food

Reproductive Considerations

Thiazolidinediones may cause ovulation in anovulatory premenopausal females, increasing the risk of unintended pregnancy. Due to long-term safety concerns associated with their use, thiazolidinediones should be avoided in females of reproductive age (Fauser 2012).

Pregnancy Considerations

Information related to the use of pioglitazone in pregnancy is limited (Glueck 2003; Ortega-Gonzalez 2005; Ota 2008).

Poorly controlled diabetes during pregnancy can be associated with an increased risk of adverse maternal and fetal outcomes, including diabetic ketoacidosis, preeclampsia, spontaneous abortion, preterm delivery, delivery complications, major birth defects, stillbirth, and macrosomia. To prevent adverse outcomes, prior to conception and throughout pregnancy, maternal blood glucose and HbA_{1c} should be kept as close to target goals as possible but without causing significant hypoglycemia (ADA 2020; Blumer 2013).

Agents other than pioglitazone are currently recommended to treat diabetes mellitus in pregnancy (ADA 2020).

Pioglitazone and Glimepiride

(pye oh GLI ta zone & GLYE me pye ride)

Related Information

Glimepiride *on page 740*

Pioglitazone *on page 1234*

Brand Names: US Duetact

Pharmacologic Category Antidiabetic Agent, Sulfonylurea; Antidiabetic Agent, Thiazolidinedione

Use Diabetes mellitus, type 2, treatment: As an adjunct to diet and exercise to improve glycemic control in adults with type 2 diabetes mellitus when treatment with both pioglitazone and glimepiride is appropriate.

Local Anesthetic/Vasoconstrictor Precautions No information available to require special precautions

Effects on Dental Treatment Key adverse event(s) related to dental treatment: Patients with diabetes should be questioned by the dental professional at each dental visit to assess their risk for stress-induced hypoglycemia. The dental professional should inquire about the patient's routine (ie, work, sleep schedule, eating patterns), history of hypoglycemia, time of last medication dose, last meal, and most recent blood sugar assessment. Keep a supply of glucose tablets and other carbohydrates in the office to prepare for a hypoglycemic event. Seek medical attention when necessary (American Diabetes Association, 2018).

Effects on Bleeding No information available to require special precautions

Adverse Reactions Also see individual agents.

>10%:

Cardiovascular: Peripheral edema (6% to 12%)

Endocrine & metabolic: Hypoglycemia (13% to 16%), weight gain (9% to 13%)

Respiratory: Upper respiratory tract infection (12% to 15%)

1% to 10%:

Central nervous system: Headache (4% to 7%)

Gastrointestinal: Diarrhea (4% to 6%), nausea (4% to 5%)

Genitourinary: Urinary tract infection (6% to 7%)

Hematologic & oncologic: Anemia (≤2%)

Neuromuscular & skeletal: Limb pain (4% to 5%)

<1%, postmarketing, and/or case reports: Bladder carcinoma (FDA Safety Alert, Dec. 19, 2016)

Mechanism of Action

Pioglitazone: A thiazolidinedione that lowers blood glucose by improving target cell response to insulin, without increasing pancreatic insulin secretion. It has a mechanism of action that is dependent on the presence of insulin for activity.

Glimepiride: A sulfonylurea that stimulates insulin release from the pancreatic beta cells; reduces glucose output from the liver; insulin sensitivity is increased at peripheral target sites.

Reproductive Considerations

Refer to individual monographs.

Pregnancy Considerations

Refer to individual monographs.

Pioglitazone and Metformin

(pye oh GLI ta zone & met FOR min)

Related Information

MetFORMIN *on page 983*
Pioglitazone *on page 1234*

Brand Names: US Actoplus Met; Actoplus Met XR [DSC]

Pharmacologic Category Antidiabetic Agent, Biguanide; Antidiabetic Agent, Thiazolidinedione

Use Diabetes mellitus, type 2: As an adjunct to diet and exercise to improve glycemic control in adults with type 2 diabetes mellitus when treatment with both pioglitazone and metformin is appropriate.

Local Anesthetic/Vasoconstrictor Precautions No information available to require special precautions

Effects on Dental Treatment Pioglitazone-dependent patients with diabetes (noninsulin dependent, type 2) or metformin-dependent patients with diabetes (noninsulin dependent, type 2) should be appointed for dental treatment in morning in order to minimize chance of stress-induced hypoglycemia.

Effects on Bleeding No information available to require special precautions

Adverse Reactions Percentages of adverse effects as reported with the combination product. Also see individual agents.

>10%:

Cardiovascular: Lower extremity edema (3% to 11%)

Respiratory: Upper respiratory tract infection (12% to 16%)

1% to 10%:

Central nervous system: Headache (2% to 6%), dizziness (5%)

Endocrine & metabolic: Weight gain (3% to 7%)

Gastrointestinal: Diarrhea (5% to 6%), nausea (4% to 6%)

Genitourinary: Urinary tract infection (5% to 6%)

Hematologic & oncologic: Anemia (≤2%)

Respiratory: Sinusitis (4% to 5%)

<1%, postmarketing, and/or case reports: Bladder carcinoma (FDA Safety Alert, Dec. 19, 2016)

Mechanism of Action

Pioglitazone is a thiazolidinedione antidiabetic agent that lowers blood glucose by improving target cell response to insulin, without increasing pancreatic insulin secretion. It has a mechanism of action that is dependent on the presence of insulin for activity.

Metformin decreases hepatic glucose production, decreasing intestinal absorption of glucose, and improves insulin sensitivity (increases peripheral glucose uptake and utilization).

Reproductive Considerations

Refer to individual monographs.

Pregnancy Considerations

Metformin crosses the placenta (ADA 2020). Refer to individual monographs for additional information.

◆ **Pioglitazone HCl** *see* Pioglitazone *on page 1234*

◆ **Pioglitazone HCl/Glimepiride** *see* Pioglitazone and Glimepiride *on page 1235*

◆ **Pioglitazone HCl/Metformin HCl** *see* Pioglitazone and Metformin *on page 1236*

Piperacillin and Tazobactam

(pi PER a sil in & ta zoe BAK tam)

Brand Names: US Zosyn

Pharmacologic Category Antibiotic, Penicillin

Use

Intra-abdominal infections: Treatment of appendicitis complicated by rupture or abscess and peritonitis in adults and pediatric patients ≥2 months of age caused by beta-lactamase-producing strains of *Escherichia coli*, *Bacteroides fragilis*, *Bacteroides ovatus*, *Bacteroides thetaiotaomicron*, or *Bacteroides vulgatus*.

Pelvic infections: Treatment of postpartum endometritis or pelvic inflammatory disease in adults caused by beta-lactamase-producing strains of *E. coli*.

Pneumonia, community-acquired: Treatment of moderate severity community-acquired pneumonia in adults caused by beta-lactamase-producing strains of *Haemophilus influenzae*.

Pneumonia, hospital-acquired (nosocomial): Treatment of moderate to severe hospital-acquired (nosocomial) pneumonia in adults and pediatric patients ≥2 months of age caused by beta-lactamase-producing strains of *Staphylococcus aureus* and by piperacillin/tazobactam-susceptible *Acinetobacter baumannii*, *H. influenzae*, *Klebsiella pneumoniae*, and *Pseudomonas aeruginosa*.

Skin and skin structure infections: Treatment of skin and skin structure infections, including cellulitis, cutaneous abscesses, and ischemic/diabetic foot infections in adults caused by beta-lactamase-producing strains of *S. aureus*.

Local Anesthetic/Vasoconstrictor Precautions No information available to require special precautions

Effects on Dental Treatment Key adverse event(s) related to dental treatment: Prolonged use of penicillins may lead to development of oral candidiasis.

Effects on Bleeding May inhibit platelet aggregation (dose related). The clinical significance may be greater with those penicillins that are combined with a beta-lactamase inhibitor and/or with agents that have greater activity against specific enteric bacterial species.

Adverse Reactions

>10%: Gastrointestinal: Diarrhea (11%)

1% to 10%:

Cardiovascular: Flushing (≤1%), hypotension (≤1%), phlebitis (1%), thrombophlebitis (≤1%)

Dermatologic: Pruritus (3%), skin rash (4%)

Endocrine & metabolic: Hypoglycemia (≤1%)

Gastrointestinal: Abdominal pain (1%), *Clostridioides difficile* colitis (≤1%), constipation (8%), dyspepsia (3%), nausea (7%), vomiting (3%)

Hematologic & oncologic: Purpuric disease (≤1%)

Hypersensitivity: Anaphylaxis (≤1%)

Infection: Candidiasis (2%)

Local: Injection site reaction (≤1%)

Nervous system: Headache (8%), insomnia (7%), rigors (≤1%)

Neuromuscular & skeletal: Arthralgia (≤1%), myalgia (≤1%)

Respiratory: Epistaxis (≤1%)

Miscellaneous: Fever (2%)

Frequency not defined:

Endocrine & metabolic: Decreased serum albumin, decreased serum glucose, decreased serum total protein, electrolyte disorder (increases and decreases in sodium, potassium, and calcium), hyperglycemia, hypokalemia, increased gamma-glutamyl transferase

Hematologic & oncologic: Decreased hematocrit, decreased hemoglobin, eosinophilia, leukopenia (Reichardt 1999), positive direct Coombs test, prolonged bleeding time, prolonged partial thromboplastin time, prolonged prothrombin time, thrombocythemia

Hepatic: Increased serum alanine aminotransferase, increased serum alkaline phosphatase, increased serum aspartate aminotransferase, increased serum bilirubin

Renal: Increased blood urea nitrogen, increased serum creatinine, renal failure syndrome

Postmarketing:

Cardiovascular: Shock

Dermatologic: Acute generalized exanthematous pustulosis (Peermohamed 2011), dermatologic disorder (linear IgA bullous dermatosis) (Ho 2018), erythema multiforme, exfoliative dermatitis, Stevens-Johnson syndrome (Lin 2014), toxic epidermal necrolysis (Copaescu 2020)

Gastrointestinal: *Clostridioides difficile* associated diarrhea (Watson 2018)

Hematologic & oncologic: Agranulocytosis (He 2013), bone marrow depression (He 2013), hemolytic anemia (Bollotte 2014; McDonald 2019), immune thrombocytopenia (Boyce 2016), neutropenia (Darwiche 2017), pancytopenia (Lee 2009), thrombocytopenia (Kumar 2003)

Hepatic: Hepatic insufficiency (He 2013), hepatitis, jaundice

Hypersensitivity: Nonimmune anaphylaxis

Immunologic: Drug reaction with eosinophilia and systemic symptoms (Cabanas 2014), serum sickness like reaction (Linares 2011)

Nervous system: Delirium (Tong 2004), encephalopathy (Grill 2011), intracranial hemorrhage (periprocedural) (Bower 2018), tonic-clonic epilepsy (Lin 2007)

Renal: Acute renal failure (Kadomura 2019), interstitial nephritis (Lui 2012), nephrotoxicity (Kadomura 2019)

Respiratory: Eosinophilic pneumonitis (García-Moguel 2019)

Miscellaneous: Drug fever (Linares 2011)

Mechanism of Action Piperacillin inhibits bacterial cell wall synthesis by binding to one or more of the penicillin-binding proteins (PBPs); which in turn inhibits the final transpeptidation step of peptidoglycan synthesis in bacterial cell walls, thus inhibiting cell wall biosynthesis. Bacteria eventually lyse due to ongoing activity of cell wall autolytic enzymes (autolysins and murein hydrolases) while cell wall assembly is arrested. Piperacillin exhibits time-dependent killing. Tazobactam inhibits many beta-lactamases, including staphylococcal penicillinase and Richmond-Sykes types 2, 3, 4, and 5, including extended spectrum enzymes; it has only limited activity against class 1 beta-lactamases other than class 1C types.

Pharmacodynamics/Kinetics

Half-life Elimination

Piperacillin:

Neonates and Infants <2 months: Median: 3.5 hours; range: 1.7 to 8.9 hours (Cohen-Wolkowiez 2014)

Infants 2 to 5 months: 1.4 ± 0.5 hours (Reed 1994)

Infants and Children 6 to 23 months: 0.9 ± 0.3 hours (Reed 1994)

Children 2 to 5 years: 0.7 ± 0.1 hours (Reed 1994)

Children 6 to 12 years: 0.7 ± 0.2 hours (Reed 1994)

Adults: 0.7 to 1.2 hours

Metabolite: 1 to 1.5 hours

Tazobactam:

Infants 2 to 5 months: 1.6 ± 0.5 hours (Reed 1994)

Infants and Children 6 to 23 months: 1 ± 0.4 hours (Reed 1994)

Children 2 to 5 years: 0.8 ± 0.2 hours (Reed 1994)

Children 6 to 12 years: 0.9 ± 0.4 hours (Reed 1994)

Adults: 0.7 to 0.9 hour

Time to Peak Immediately following completion of 30-minute infusion

Pregnancy Considerations Piperacillin and tazobactam cross the placenta.

Due to pregnancy-induced physiologic changes, some pharmacokinetic properties of piperacillin/tazobactam may be altered (Bourget 1998). Piperacillin/tazobactam is approved for the treatment of postpartum gynecologic infections, including endometritis or pelvic inflammatory disease, caused by susceptible organisms.

- ◆ **Piperacillin and Tazobactam Sodium** *see* Piperacillin and Tazobactam *on page 1236*
- ◆ **Piperacillin Sodium and Tazobactam Sodium** *see* Piperacillin and Tazobactam *on page 1236*
- ◆ **Piperacillin Sodium/Tazobactam** *see* Piperacillin and Tazobactam *on page 1236*
- ◆ **Piperacillin/Tazobactam Sod** *see* Piperacillin and Tazobactam *on page 1236*
- ◆ **Piperazine Estrone Sulfate** *see* Estropipate *on page 605*
- ◆ **Piperonyl Butoxide and Pyrethrins** *see* Pyrethrins and Piperonyl Butoxide *on page 1293*
- ◆ **Pirmella 1/35** *see* Ethinyl Estradiol and Norethindrone *on page 614*
- ◆ **Pirmella 7/7/7** *see* Ethinyl Estradiol and Norethindrone *on page 614*

Piroxicam (Systemic) (peer OKS i kam)

Related Information

Rheumatoid Arthritis, Osteoarthritis, and Osteoporosis *on page 1697*

Temporomandibular Dysfunction (TMD), Chronic Pain, and Fibromyalgia *on page 1773*

Brand Names: US Feldene

Brand Names: Canada APO-Piroxicam; DOM-Piroxicam [DSC]; PMS-Piroxicam [DSC]; TEVA-Piroxicam

Pharmacologic Category Analgesic, Nonopioid; Nonsteroidal Anti-inflammatory Drug (NSAID), Oral

Use Arthritis: Relief of signs and symptoms of osteoarthritis and rheumatoid arthritis.

Local Anesthetic/Vasoconstrictor Precautions No information available to require special precautions

Effects on Dental Treatment The dentist should be aware of the potential of abnormal coagulation. Caution should also be exercised in the use of NSAIDs in patients already on anticoagulant therapy with drugs such as warfarin (Coumadin®). See Effects on Bleeding.

Effects on Bleeding Nonselective NSAIDs, such as piroxicam, inhibit platelet aggregation and prolong bleeding time in some patients. Unlike aspirin, the NSAID effect on platelet function is quantitatively less, of shorter duration, and reversible. Normal platelet function should occur in ~5 elimination half-lives or in <10 hours after discontinuation of piroxicam. Concomitant use of other NSAIDs should be avoided.

Adverse Reactions

1% to 10%:

Cardiovascular: Edema

Central nervous system: Dizziness, headache

Dermatologic: Pruritus, skin rash

Gastrointestinal: Abdominal pain, anorexia, constipation, diarrhea, dyspepsia, flatulence, gastrointestinal hemorrhage, gastrointestinal perforation, heartburn, nausea, ulcer (gastric, duodenal), vomiting

Hematologic & oncologic: Anemia, prolonged bleeding time
Hepatic: Increased liver enzymes
Otic: Tinnitus
Renal: Renal function abnormality

<1%, postmarketing, and/or case reports: Abnormal dreams, agranulocytosis, akathisia, alopecia, anaphylactoid reactions, anaphylaxis, angioedema, anxiety, aplastic anemia, aseptic meningitis, asthma, blurred vision, bone marrow depression, bruise, cardiac arrhythmia, cardiac failure, change in appetite, colic, coma, confusion, conjunctivitis, cystitis, depression, desquamation, diaphoresis, drowsiness, dyspnea, dysuria, ecchymoses, eosinophilia, epistaxis, eructation, erythema, erythema multiforme, esophagitis, exacerbation of angina pectoris, exfoliative dermatitis, fever, fluid retention, flu-like symptoms, gastritis, GI inflammation, glomerulonephritis, glossitis, hallucination, hearing loss, hematemesis, hematuria, hemolytic anemia, hepatic failure, hepatitis, hepatotoxicity (idiosyncratic) (Chalasani 2014), hyperglycemia, hyperkalemia, hypertension, hypoglycemia, hypotension, infection, insomnia, interstitial nephritis, jaundice, leukopenia, lymphadenopathy, malaise, melena, meningitis, mood changes, myocardial infarction, nephrotic syndrome, nervousness, oliguria, onycholysis, palpitations, pancreatitis, pancytopenia, paresthesia, petechial rash, pneumonia, polydipsia, polyuria, positive ANA titer, proteinuria, purpura, rectal hemorrhage, reduced fertility (female), renal failure, respiratory depression, seizure, sepsis, serum sickness, skin photosensitivity, Stevens-Johnson syndrome, stomatitis, swelling of eye, syncope, tachycardia, thrombocytopenia, toxic epidermal necrolysis, tremor, urticaria, vasculitis, vertigo, vesiculobullous reaction, weakness, weight changes, xerostomia

Mechanism of Action Reversibly inhibits cyclooxygenase-1 and 2 (COX-1 and 2) enzymes, which results in decreased formation of prostaglandin precursors; has antipyretic, analgesic, and anti-inflammatory properties

Other proposed mechanisms not fully elucidated (and possibly contributing to the anti-inflammatory effect to varying degrees), include inhibiting chemotaxis, altering lymphocyte activity, inhibiting neutrophil aggregation/activation, and decreasing proinflammatory cytokine levels.

Pharmacodynamics/Kinetics

Onset of Action Analgesia: Oral: Within 1 hour; Maximum effect: 3 to 5 hours

Half-life Elimination

Children and Adolescents 7 to 16 years: 32.6 hours; Range: 22 to 40 hours (Mäkelä 1991)
Adults: 50 hours

Time to Peak 3 to 5 hours

Reproductive Considerations

The chronic use of nonsteroidal anti-inflammatory drugs (NSAIDs) in women of reproductive age may be associated with infertility. Rupture of ovarian follicles may be delayed or prevented; some studies have also shown a reversible delay in ovulation. Consider discontinuing use in women having difficulty conceiving or those undergoing investigation of fertility.

Use of NSAIDs may be continued in males with rheumatic and musculoskeletal diseases who are planning to father a child (ACR [Sammaritano 2020]).

Pregnancy Considerations The use of nonsteroidal anti-inflammatory drugs (NSAIDs) close to conception may be associated with an increased risk of miscarriage (Bermas 2014; Bloor 2013).

Birth defects have been observed following in utero NSAID exposure in some studies; however, data is conflicting (Bloor 2013). Nonteratogenic effects, including prenatal constriction of the ductus arteriosus, persistent pulmonary hypertension of the newborn, oligohydramnios, necrotizing enterocolitis, renal dysfunction or failure, and intracranial hemorrhage, have been observed in the fetus/neonate following in utero NSAID exposure. In addition, nonclosure of the ductus arteriosus postnatally may occur and be resistant to medical management (Bermas 2014; Bloor 2013). Because NSAIDs may cause premature closure of the ductus arteriosus, product labeling for piroxicam specifically states use should be avoided starting at 30 weeks' gestation.

Use of NSAIDs may be considered during the first two trimesters of pregnancy for the treatment of rheumatic and musculoskeletal diseases (ACR [Sammaritano 2020]).

◆ ***p*-Isobutylhydratropic Acid** *see* Ibuprofen *on page 786*

◆ **Pit** *see* Oxytocin *on page 1177*

Pitavastatin (pi TA va sta tin)

Related Information

Cardiovascular Diseases *on page 1654*

Brand Names: US Livalo; Zypitamag

Pharmacologic Category Antilipemic Agent, HMG-CoA Reductase Inhibitor

Use

Primary hyperlipidemia and mixed dyslipidemia: As an adjunctive therapy to diet to reduce elevated total cholesterol, low-density lipoprotein cholesterol (LDL-C), apolipoprotein B (apo B), and triglycerides (TG), and to increase high-density lipoprotein cholesterol (HDL-C) in adults with primary hyperlipidemia or mixed dyslipidemia.

Heterozygous familial hypercholesterolemia: As an adjunctive therapy to diet to reduce elevated total cholesterol, LDL-C, and apo B in children and adolescents ≥8 years of age.

Local Anesthetic/Vasoconstrictor Precautions No information available to require special precautions

Effects on Dental Treatment Key adverse event(s) related to dental treatment: Assess unusual presentations of muscle weakness or myopathy resulting from lipid therapy such as patient having a difficult time brushing teeth or weakness with chewing. Refer patient back to their physician for evaluation and adjustment of lipid therapy.

Effects on Bleeding No information available to require special precautions

Adverse Reactions

1% to 10%:

Gastrointestinal: Constipation (4%), diarrhea (3%)
Neuromuscular & skeletal: Back pain (4%), myalgia (2% to 3%)

Frequency not defined:

Central nervous system: Headache
Dermatologic: Pruritus, skin rash, urticaria
Endocrine & metabolic: Increased serum glucose
Hepatic: Increased serum alkaline phosphatase, increased serum bilirubin, increased serum transaminases
Hypersensitivity: Hypersensitivity reaction
Infection: Influenza

Neuromuscular & skeletal: Arthralgia, increased creatine phosphokinase in blood specimen
Respiratory: Nasopharyngitis

<1%, postmarketing, and/or case reports: Abdominal distress, abdominal pain, amnesia, angioedema, asthenia, cognitive dysfunction, confusion, depression, dizziness, dyspepsia, elevated glycosylated hemoglobin, erectile dysfunction, fatigue, forgetfulness, hepatic failure, hepatitis, hypoesthesia, immune-mediated necrotizing myopathy, insomnia, interstitial pulmonary disease, jaundice, malaise, memory impairment, muscle spasm, myopathy, nausea, peripheral neuropathy, rhabdomyolysis

Mechanism of Action Inhibitor of 3-hydroxy-3-methylglutaryl coenzyme A (HMG-CoA) reductase, the rate-limiting enzyme in cholesterol synthesis (reduces the production of mevalonic acid from HMG-CoA); this then results in a compensatory increase in the expression of LDL receptors on hepatocyte membranes and a stimulation of LDL catabolism. In addition to the ability of HMG-CoA reductase inhibitors to decrease levels of high-sensitivity C-reactive protein (hsCRP), they also possess pleiotropic properties including improved endothelial function, reduced inflammation at the site of the coronary plaque, inhibition of platelet aggregation, and anticoagulant effects (de Denus 2002; Ray 2005).

Pharmacodynamics/Kinetics

Half-life Elimination ~12 hours

Time to Peak ~1 hour

Reproductive Considerations

Adequate contraception is recommended if an HMG-CoA reductase inhibitor is required in females of reproductive potential. Females planning a pregnancy should discontinue the HMG-CoA reductase inhibitor 1 to 2 months prior to attempting to conceive (AHA/ACC [Grundy 2018]).

Pregnancy Considerations Pitavastatin is contraindicated in pregnant females.

There are reports of congenital anomalies following maternal use of HMG-CoA reductase inhibitors in pregnancy; however, maternal disease, differences in specific agents used, and the low rates of exposure limit the interpretation of the available data (Godfrey 2012; Lecarpentier 2012). Cholesterol biosynthesis may be important in fetal development; serum cholesterol and triglycerides increase normally during pregnancy. The discontinuation of lipid lowering medications temporarily during pregnancy is not expected to have significant impact on the long term outcomes of primary hypercholesterolemia treatment.

Pitavastatin should be discontinued immediately if an unplanned pregnancy occurs during treatment.

◆ **Pitavastatin Calcium** *see* Pitavastatin *on page 1238*

◆ **Pitocin** *see* Oxytocin *on page 1177*

Pitolisant (pi TOL i sant)

Brand Names: US Wakix

Pharmacologic Category Central Nervous System Stimulant; Histamine-3 (H3) Receptor Antagonist/ Inverse Agonist

Use Narcolepsy: To improve wakefulness in adult patients with excessive daytime sleepiness associated with narcolepsy

Local Anesthetic/Vasoconstrictor Precautions Occurrence of prolonged QT interval has been reported for pitolisant. The risk of drug-induced torsades de pointes (arrhythmias) is low when a single QT interval-prolonging drug is prescribed. In terms of epinephrine, it is not known what effect vasoconstrictors in the local anesthetic regimen will have in patients with a known history of congenital prolonged QT interval or in patients taking any medication that prolongs the QT interval. Until more information is obtained, it is suggested that the clinician consult with the physician prior to the use of a vasoconstrictor in suspected patients, and that the vasoconstrictor (epinephrine, levonordefrin [Neo-Cobefrin]) be used with caution.

Effects on Dental Treatment Occurrence of xerostomia; normal salivary flow resumes upon discontinuation.

Effects on Bleeding No information available to require special precautions

Adverse Reactions

>10%: Central nervous system: Headache (18%)

1% to 10%:
Cardiovascular: Increased heart rate (3%)
Central nervous system: Insomnia (6%), anxiety (5%), hallucination (3%), irritability (3%), sleep disturbance (3%), cataplexy (2%)
Dermatologic: Skin rash (2%)
Gastrointestinal: Nausea (6%), abdominal pain (3%), decreased appetite (3%), xerostomia (2%)
Neuromuscular & skeletal: Musculoskeletal pain (5%)
Respiratory: Upper respiratory tract infection (5%)

Frequency not defined:
Cardiovascular: Prolonged QT interval on ECG, tachycardia
Central nervous system: Migraine, sleep paralysis, sleep talking

Postmarketing: Abnormal behavior, abnormal dreams, bipolar mood disorder, depressed mood, depression, epilepsy, fatigue, lack of emotion (anhedonia), nightmares, pruritus, sleep disorder, suicidal ideation, suicidal tendencies, weight gain

Mechanism of Action The mechanism of action of pitolisant is unclear, but may be mediated through its activity as an antagonist/inverse agonist at histamine-3 receptors.

Pharmacodynamics/Kinetics

Onset of Action In the treatment of narcolepsy, it may take up to 8 weeks for patients to achieve a clinical response.

Half-life Elimination
~20 hours (7.5 to 24.2 hours)

Time to Peak T_{max}: 3.5 hours (2 to 5 hours)

Reproductive Considerations

Pitolisant may reduce the effectiveness of hormonal contraceptives. Females of reproductive potential should be advised to use an alternative nonhormonal contraceptive method during treatment and for ≥21 days after the last dose of pitolisant.

Pregnancy Considerations

Adverse events were observed in some animal reproduction studies.

Data collection to monitor pregnancy and infant outcomes following exposure to pitolisant is ongoing. Patients exposed to pitolisant during pregnancy are encouraged to enroll in the Pregnancy Registry (1-800-833-7460).

◆ **Pitolisant Hydrochloride** *see* Pitolisant *on page 1239*

Pivmecillinam (piv meh SIL li nam)

Pharmacologic Category Antibiotic, Penicillin

Use Note: Not approved in the US

Urinary tract infections: Treatment of acute uncomplicated cystitis and chronic/recurrent urinary tract infection (UTI) caused by susceptible strains of *Escherichia coli*, *Klebsiella* species, *Enterobacter* species, and *Proteus* species in adults and children >6 years of age and >40 kg.

Local Anesthetic/Vasoconstrictor Precautions No information available to require special precautions

Effects on Dental Treatment Key adverse event(s) related to dental treatment: Oral mucosal ulcers have been reported; prolonged use may result in oral opportunistic fungal infections

Effects on Bleeding No information available to require special precautions

Adverse Reactions

1% to 10%:

Gastrointestinal: Diarrhea, nausea

Genitourinary: Vulvovaginal candidiasis

<1%, postmarketing, and/or case reports: Abdominal pain, abnormal hepatic function tests, acute porphyria, anaphylaxis, *Clostridioides* (formerly *Clostridium*) *difficile* colitis, decreased plasma carnitine concentrations, dizziness, dyspepsia, erythematous rash, esophageal ulcer, esophagitis, fatigue, headache, hypersensitivity reaction, macular eruption, maculopapular rash, oral mucosa ulcer, pruritus, skin rash, thrombocytopenia, urticaria, vertigo, vomiting

Mechanism of Action Pivmecillinam is a 6-aminopenicillanic acid derivative that is metabolized to the active form of the drug, mecillinam. Mecillinam interferes with the bacterial cell wall and has a mode of action different from other penicillins by exerting high specificity against penicillin-binding protein 2 (PBP-2) in the gram-negative cell wall.

Pharmacodynamics/Kinetics

Half-life Elimination ~1 hour

Time to Peak 1 to 1.5 hours (mecillinam)

Pregnancy Considerations

Mecillinam, the active metabolite of pivmecillinam, crosses the placenta.

Information related to the use of pivmecillinam in pregnancy is available (Guinto 2010; Kjer 1986; Larsen 2001; Nørgaard 2008; Vinther Skriver 2004). Based on available data, an increased risk of adverse fetal/neonatal outcomes has not been observed.

Product Availability Selexid: Health Canada approved July 2016; anticipated availability is unknown.

- **Pivmecillinam Hydrochloride** *see* Pivmecillinam *on page 1240*
- **Pizensy** *see* Lactitol *on page 869*
- **PKC 412** *see* Midostaurin *on page 1027*
- **Plaquenil** *see* Hydroxychloroquine *on page 778*
- **Platinol** *see* CISplatin *on page 352*
- **Platinol-AQ** *see* CISplatin *on page 352*
- **Plavix** *see* Clopidogrel *on page 390*

Plazomicin (pla zoe MYE sin)

Brand Names: US Zemdri

Pharmacologic Category Antibiotic, Aminoglycoside

Use Urinary tract infection, complicated (including pyelonephritis): Treatment of complicated urinary tract infections (UTI), including pyelonephritis caused by *Escherichia coli*, *Klebsiella pneumoniae*, *Proteus mirabilis*, and *Enterobacter cloacae* in patients ≥18 years. **Note:** Reserve for use in complicated UTI patients who have limited or no alternative treatment options.

Local Anesthetic/Vasoconstrictor Precautions No information available to require special precautions

Effects on Dental Treatment No significant effects or complications reported

Effects on Bleeding No information available to require special precautions

Adverse Reactions

1% to 10%:

Cardiovascular: Hypertension (2%), hypotension (1%)

Central nervous system: Headache (1%)

Gastrointestinal: Diarrhea (2%), nausea (1%), vomiting (1%)

Genitourinary: Nephrotoxicity (4%)

Otic: Ototoxicity (2%)

Renal: Increased serum creatinine (4%; CrCl: 30 to 90 mL/minute: ≤10%), acute renal failure (≤4%), decreased creatinine clearance (≤4%), renal disease (≤4%), renal failure syndrome (≤4%), renal insufficiency (≤4%)

Frequency not defined:

Central nervous system: Dizziness

Endocrine & metabolic: Hypokalemia

Gastrointestinal: Constipation, gastritis

Genitourinary: Hematuria

Hepatic: Increased serum alanine aminotransferase

Respiratory: Dyspnea

<1%, postmarketing, and/or case reports: Hypoacusis (reversible), tinnitus (irreversible), vertigo

Mechanism of Action Interferes with bacterial protein synthesis by binding to 30S ribosomal subunit resulting in a defective bacterial cell membrane.

Pharmacodynamics/Kinetics

Half-life Elimination 3 to 4 hours (Cass 2011)

Time to Peak IV: At the end of or just after infusion (Cass 2011)

Pregnancy Considerations

[US Boxed Warning]: Aminoglycosides may cause fetal harm if administered to a pregnant woman.

There are several reports of total irreversible bilateral congenital deafness in children whose mothers received another aminoglycoside (streptomycin) during pregnancy. Although serious side effects to the fetus/infant have not been reported following maternal use of all aminoglycosides, a potential for harm exists.

Plecanatide (ple KAN a tide)

Brand Names: US Trulance

Pharmacologic Category Gastrointestinal Agent, Miscellaneous; Guanylate Cyclase-C (GC-C) Agonist

Use

Chronic idiopathic constipation: Treatment of chronic idiopathic constipation (CIC) in adults

Irritable bowel syndrome with constipation: Treatment of irritable bowel syndrome with constipation (IBS-C) in adults

Local Anesthetic/Vasoconstrictor Precautions No information available to require special precautions

Effects on Dental Treatment No significant effects or complications reported

Effects on Bleeding No information available to require special precautions

Adverse Reactions

1% to 10%:

Central nervous system: Dizziness (1% to <2%)

Gastrointestinal: Diarrhea (4% to 5%), abdominal distension (<2%), abdominal tenderness (<2%), flatulence (<2%), nausea (1% to <2%), severe diarrhea (≤1%)

Genitourinary: Urinary tract infection (1% to <2%)

Hepatic: Increased serum ALT (<2%), increased serum AST (<2%)

Respiratory: Sinusitis (<2%), upper respiratory tract infection (<2%), nasopharyngitis (1% to <2%)

Mechanism of Action Plecanatide and its active metabolite bind and agonize guanylate cyclase-C on the luminal surface of intestinal epithelium. Intracellular and extracellular cyclic guanosine monophosphate (cGMP) concentrations are subsequently increased resulting in chloride and bicarbonate secretion into the intestinal lumen. Intestinal fluid increases and GI transit time is accelerated.

Pregnancy Considerations Plecanatide and its metabolite are not measurable in plasma when used at recommended doses. Maternal use is not expected to result in fetal exposure.

◆ **Plendil** *see* Felodipine *on page 639*

Plerixafor (pler IX a fore)

Brand Names: US Mozobil

Brand Names: Canada Mozobil

Pharmacologic Category Hematopoietic Agent; Hematopoietic Stem Cell Mobilizer

Use Peripheral stem cell mobilization: Mobilization of hematopoietic stem cells (HSCs) for collection and subsequent autologous transplantation (in combination with filgrastim) in patients with non-Hodgkin lymphoma (NHL) and multiple myeloma (MM)

Local Anesthetic/Vasoconstrictor Precautions No information available to require special precautions

Effects on Dental Treatment Key adverse event(s) related to dental treatment: Xerostomia (normal salivary flow resumes upon discontinuation).

Effects on Bleeding No information available to require special precautions

Adverse Reactions Adverse reactions reported with filgrastim combination therapy.

>10%:

Central nervous system: Fatigue (27%), headache (22%), dizziness (11%)

Gastrointestinal: Diarrhea (37%), nausea (34%)

Local: Injection site reaction (34%, including edema, erythema, hematoma, hemorrhage, induration, inflammation, irritation, pain, paresthesia, pruritus, skin rash, urticaria)

Neuromuscular & skeletal: Arthralgia (13%)

1% to 10%:

Central nervous system: Insomnia (7%), malaise (<5%)

Dermatologic: Erythema (<5%), hyperhidrosis (<5%)

Gastrointestinal: Vomiting (10%), flatulence (7%), abdominal distension (<5%), abdominal distress (<5%), abdominal pain (<5%), constipation (<5%), dyspepsia (<5%), oral hypoesthesia (<5%), xerostomia (<5%)

Hematologic & oncologic: Hyperleukocytosis (7%)

Neuromuscular & skeletal: Musculoskeletal pain (<5%)

<1%, postmarketing, and/or case reports: Abnormal dreams, anaphylaxis, diaphoresis, dyspnea, hypersensitivity reaction, hypoxia, leukocytosis, nightmares, orthostatic hypotension, periorbital swelling, syncope, thrombocytopenia

Mechanism of Action Plerixafor reversibly inhibits binding of stromal cell-derived factor-1-alpha (SDF-1α), expressed on bone marrow stromal cells, to the CXC chemokine receptor 4 (CXCR4), resulting in mobilization of hematopoietic stem and progenitor cells from bone marrow into peripheral blood. Plerixafor used in combination with filgrastim results in synergistic increase in CD34+ cell mobilization. Mobilized CD34+ cells are capable of engrafting with extended repopulating capacity.

Pharmacodynamics/Kinetics

Onset of Action Peak CD34+ mobilization (healthy volunteers): Plerixafor monotherapy: 6 to 9 hours after administration; Plerixafor + filgrastim: 10 to14 hours

Duration of Action Sustained elevation in CD34+ cells (healthy volunteers): 4 to 18 hours after administration

Half-life Elimination Terminal: 3 to 5 hours

Time to Peak Plasma: SubQ: 30 to 60 minutes

Reproductive Considerations

Evaluate pregnancy status prior to use in females of repro- ductive potential. Pregnancy should be avoided during therapy. Females of reproductive potential should use adequate contraception during treatment and for 1 week after the final plerixafor dose.

Pregnancy Considerations

Based on data from animal reproduction studies, in utero exposure to plerixafor may cause fetal harm.

◆ **Pliaglis** *see* Lidocaine and Tetracaine *on page 914*

◆ **PLX4032** *see* Vemurafenib *on page 1537*

◆ **PM-01183** *see* Lurbinectedin *on page 944*

◆ **PMPA** *see* Tenofovir Disoproxil Fumarate *on page 1419*

◆ **Pneumo-C-10** *see* Pneumococcal Conjugate Vaccine (10-Valent) *on page 1241*

◆ **Pneumococcal 10-Valent Conjugate Vaccine** *see* Pneumococcal Conjugate Vaccine (10-Valent) *on page 1241*

Pneumococcal Conjugate Vaccine (10-Valent) (noo moe KOK al KON ju gate vak SEEN, ten vay lent)

Brand Names: Canada Synflorix

Pharmacologic Category Vaccine; Vaccine, Inactivated (Bacterial)

Use Note: Not approved in the US.

Pneumococcal disease prevention: Immunization of infants ≥6 weeks and children through 5 years of age against *Streptococcus pneumoniae* invasive diseases, pneumonia, and acute otitis media caused by serotypes included in the vaccine.

Local Anesthetic/Vasoconstrictor Precautions No information available to require special precautions

Effects on Dental Treatment No significant effects or complications reported

Effects on Bleeding No information available to require special precautions

Adverse Reactions

>10%:

Gastrointestinal: Anorexia (17% to 31%)

Local: Pain at injection site (23% to 57%), erythema at injection site (24% to 52%) swelling at injection site (16% to 44%)

Nervous system: Irritability (32% to 66%), drowsiness (33% to 58%)

Miscellaneous: Fever (rectal; ≥38° C: 26% to 37%; >39° C: 1% to 7%)

1% to 10%: Local: Induration at injection site

<1%, postmarketing, and/or case reports: Allergic dermatitis, anaphylaxis, angioedema, apnea (in premature infants ≤28 weeks' gestation), atopic dermatitis, bleeding at injection site, crying, diarrhea, eczema, febrile seizure, headache, hematoma at injection site, hypersensitivity reaction, hypotonic/hyporesponsive episode, injection site nodule, injection site pruritus, Kawasaki syndrome, nausea, seizure, skin rash, swelling of injected limb (may involve adjacent joint), urticaria, vomiting

Mechanism of Action Promotes active immunization against invasive disease caused by *S. pneumoniae* capsular serotypes 1, 4, 5, 6B, 7F, 9V, 14, 18C, 19F, and 23F, all which are individually conjugated to a carrier protein (protein D, tetanus toxoid, or diphtheria toxoid); the aluminum salt, a mineral adjuvant, enhances the antibody response.

Pregnancy Considerations Animal reproduction studies have not been conducted. Inactivated vaccines have not been shown to cause increased risks to the fetus (ACIP [Ezeanolue 2020]). This product is indicated for use in infants and children.

Product Availability Not available in the US

◆ **Pneumococcal 13-Valent Conjugate Vaccine** *see* Pneumococcal Conjugate Vaccine (13-Valent) *on page 1242*

Pneumococcal Conjugate Vaccine (13-Valent)

(noo moe KOK al KON ju gate vak SEEN, thur TEEN vay lent)

Brand Names: US Prevnar 13

Brand Names: Canada Prevnar 13

Pharmacologic Category Vaccine; Vaccine, Inactivated (Bacterial)

Use

Pneumococcal disease prevention:

- Active immunization of infants ≥6 weeks of age, children, adolescents, and adults for prevention of invasive disease caused by *Streptococcus pneumoniae* serotypes contained in the vaccine
- Active immunization of infants ≥6 weeks of age and children <6 years of age for the prevention of otitis media caused by *S. pneumoniae* serotypes 4, 6B, 9V, 14, 18C, 19F, and 23F
- Active immunization of adolescents ≥18 years of age and adults for the prevention of pneumonia caused by *S. pneumoniae* serotypes contained in the vaccine

Advisory Committee on Immunization Practices recommendations:

The Advisory Committee on Immunization Practices (ACIP) recommends routine vaccination for the following (ACIP [Kobayashi 2015]; CDC/ACIP [Nuorti 2010]):

- All infants and children 2 to 59 months of age
- Children 60 to 71 months of age with underlying medical conditions including immunocompetent children with chronic heart disease (particularly cyanotic congenital heart disease and heart failure), chronic lung disease (including asthma if treated with high dose corticosteroids), diabetes, cerebrospinal fluid leaks, or cochlear implants; children with functional or anatomic asplenia, including sickle cell disease or other hemoglobinopathies, congenital or acquired asplenia, or splenic dysfunction; children with immunocompromising conditions including congenital immunodeficiency (includes B or T cell deficiency, complement deficiencies and phagocytic disorders; excludes chronic granulomatous disease), HIV infection, chronic renal failure, nephrotic syndrome, leukemia, lymphoma, Hodgkin disease, generalized malignancies, solid organ transplant, or other diseases requiring immunosuppressive drugs (including long term systemic corticosteroids and radiation therapy)
- Children ≥6 years of age and Adolescents ≤18 years of age (CDC/ACIP, 62[25] 2013), and Adults ≥19 years (CDC/ACIP, 61[40] 2012): The ACIP also recommends routine vaccination for persons with the following underlying medical conditions: Immunocompetent persons with cerebrospinal fluid leaks or cochlear implants; persons with functional or anatomic asplenia, including sickle cell disease or other hemoglobinopathies, congenital or acquired asplenia; persons with immunocompromising conditions including congenital or acquired immunodeficiency (includes B or T cell deficiency, complement deficiencies and phagocytic disorders; excludes chronic granulomatous disease), HIV infection, chronic renal failure, nephrotic syndrome, leukemia, lymphoma, Hodgkin disease, generalized malignancies, solid organ transplant, multiple myeloma, or other diseases requiring immunosuppressive drugs (including long term systemic corticosteroids and radiation therapy)
- Adults ≥65 years of age (CDC/ACIP [Matanock 2019]): Routine vaccination for all individuals is not recommended. For persons who are immunocompetent, do not have a cerebrospinal fluid leak or cochlear implant, and who have not previously received pneumococcal conjugate vaccine, 13-valent (PCV13), ACIP recommends shared clinical decision-making to determine if PCV13 vaccination is appropriate for a particular person; consideration should be given to potential increased risk for exposure to PCV13 serotypes and risk for developing pneumococcal disease as a result of underlying conditions. Those at potentially increased risk for exposure to PCV13 serotypes include: Nursing home or long-term care residents; those residing in setting with low pediatric PCV13 uptake; and those traveling to setting with no pediatric PCV13 immunization program.

Local Anesthetic/Vasoconstrictor Precautions No information available to require special precautions

Effects on Dental Treatment No significant effects or complications reported

Effects on Bleeding No information available to require special precautions

Adverse Reactions

>10%:

Central nervous system: Chills (adults), drowsiness, fatigue (adults), headache (adults), insomnia, irritability (infants and children)

Dermatologic: Skin rash (adults: >10%; children and infants: >1%; including urticaria-like rash)

Gastrointestinal: Decreased appetite

Local: Erythema at injection site, pain at injection site (adults), swelling at injection site, tenderness at injection site

Neuromuscular & skeletal: Arthralgia (adults), decreased range of motion (arm), myalgia (adults)
Miscellaneous: Fever
1% to 10%:
Dermatologic: Urticaria
Gastrointestinal: Diarrhea, vomiting
<1%, postmarketing, and/or case reports: Anaphylactic shock, anaphylactoid reaction, anaphylaxis, angioedema, apnea, injection site inflammation (dermatitis), injection-site pruritus, crying (abnormal), cyanosis, erythema multiforme, febrile seizures, hypersensitivity reaction (bronchospasm, dyspnea, facial edema), hypotonia, lymphadenopathy (injection site), pallor, seizure, urticaria at injection site

Mechanism of Action Promotes active immunization against invasive disease caused by *S. pneumoniae* capsular serotypes 1, 3, 4, 5, 6A, 6B, 7F, 9V, 14, 18C, 19A, 19F, and 23F, all which are individually conjugated to CRM197 protein

Pregnancy Considerations Animal reproduction studies have not shown adverse fetal effects. Inactivated vaccines have not been shown to cause increased risks to the fetus (ACIP [Ezeanolue 2020]).

◆ **Pneumococcal Conjugate Vaccine (Nontypeable *Haemophilus influenzae* [NTHi] Protein D, Diphtheria or Tetanus Toxoid Conjugates) Adsorbed** *see* Pneumococcal Conjugate Vaccine (10-Valent) *on page 1241*

◆ **PNU-140690E** *see* Tipranavir *on page 1452*

◆ **Podactin [OTC]** *see* Miconazole (Topical) *on page 1019*

◆ **Podactin [OTC]** *see* Tolnaftate *on page 1462*

◆ **Pod-Care 100C** *see* Betamethasone (Systemic) *on page 233*

◆ **Pod-Care 100K** *see* Triamcinolone (Systemic) *on page 1485*

Poliovirus Vaccine (Inactivated)

(POE lee oh VYE rus vak SEEN, in ak ti VAY ted)

Brand Names: US IPOL

Brand Names: Canada Imovax Polio

Pharmacologic Category Vaccine; Vaccine, Inactivated (Viral)

Use Poliovirus prevention:

Active immunization of infants (≥6 weeks [US labeling]; ≥2 months [Canadian labeling]), children, adolescents, and adults for prevention of poliomyelitis caused by poliovirus types 1, 2, and 3.

US labeling: Infants (as young as 6 weeks), children, adolescents, and adults

Canadian labeling: Infants (as young as 2 months), children, adolescents, and adults

The Advisory Committee on Immunization Practices (ACIP) recommends routine vaccination for the following:

- All infants and children (first dose given at 2 months of age) (CDC/ACIP, 58[30] 2009)

Routine immunization of adults in the United States is generally not recommended. Adults with previous wild poliovirus disease, who have never been immunized, or those who are incompletely immunized may receive inactivated poliovirus vaccine if they fall into one of the following categories (CDC/ACIP [Prevots 2000]):

- Travelers to regions or countries where poliomyelitis is endemic or epidemic
- Healthcare workers in close contact with patients who may be excreting poliovirus
- Laboratory workers handling specimens that may contain poliovirus
- Members of communities or specific population groups with diseases caused by wild poliovirus
- Incompletely vaccinated or unvaccinated adults in a household or with other close contact with children receiving oral poliovirus (may be at increased risk of vaccine associated paralytic poliomyelitis)

Local Anesthetic/Vasoconstrictor Precautions No information available to require special precautions

Effects on Dental Treatment No significant effects or complications reported

Effects on Bleeding No information available to require special precautions

Adverse Reactions

Percentages noted with concomitant administration of DTP or DTaP vaccine and observed within 48 hours of injection.

>10%:
Central nervous system: Irritability (7% to 65%; most common in infants 2 months of age), fatigue (4% to 61%)
Gastrointestinal: Anorexia (1% to 17%)
Local: Tenderness at injection site (≤29%), swelling at injection site (≤11%)

1% to 10%:
Central nervous system: Excessive crying (≤1%; reported within 72 hours)
Gastrointestinal: Vomiting (1% to 3%)
Local: Erythema at injection site (≤3%)
Miscellaneous: Fever (>39°C: ≤4%)

<1%, postmarketing, and/or case reports: Agitation, anaphylactic shock, anaphylaxis, arthralgia, drowsiness, febrile seizures, headache, hypersensitivity reaction, lymphadenopathy, myalgia, paresthesia, seizure, skin rash, urticaria

Mechanism of Action As an inactivated virus vaccine, poliovirus vaccine induces active immunity against poliovirus types 1, 2, and 3 infection

Pregnancy Considerations Animal reproduction studies have not been conducted. Although adverse effects of IPV have not been documented in pregnant women or their fetuses, vaccination of pregnant women should be avoided on theoretical grounds. Pregnant women at increased risk for infection and requiring immediate protection against polio may be administered the vaccine (CDC/ACIP [Prevots 2000]).

◆ **Polocaine** *see* Mepivacaine *on page 972*

◆ **Polocaine Dental** *see* Mepivacaine *on page 972*

◆ **Polocaine Dental** *see* Mepivacaine and Levonordefrin *on page 975*

◆ **Polocaine-MPF** *see* Mepivacaine *on page 972*

◆ **Polydeoxyribonucleotide** *see* Defibrotide *on page 449*

◆ **Polyethylene Glycol-L-asparaginase** *see* Pegaspargase *on page 1199*

◆ **Polyethylene Glycol-Conjugated Uricase** *see* Pegloticase *on page 1203*

◆ **Polyethylene Glycol Interferon Alfa-2b** *see* Peginterferon Alfa-2b *on page 1202*

◆ **Polygam** *see* Immune Globulin *on page 803*

Polymyxin B (pol i MIKS in bee)

Pharmacologic Category Antibiotic, Irrigation; Antibiotic, Miscellaneous

Use

Infections, acute:

Pseudomonal infections: Treatment of infections of the urinary tract, meninges, and bloodstream caused by susceptible strains of *Pseudomonas aeruginosa*

Serious infections: Treatment of serious infections caused by susceptible strains of the following organisms, when less potentially toxic drugs are ineffective or contraindicated: *H. influenzae*, specifically meningeal infections; *Escherichia coli*, specifically urinary tract infections; *Aerobacter aerogenes*, specifically bacteremia; *Klebsiella pneumoniae*, specifically bacteremia

In meningeal infections, polymyxin B sulfate should be administered only by the intrathecal route.

Local Anesthetic/Vasoconstrictor Precautions
No information available to require special precautions

Effects on Dental Treatment No significant effects or complications reported

Effects on Bleeding No information available to require special precautions

Adverse Reactions Frequency not defined.

Cardiovascular: Facial flushing

Central nervous system: Neurotoxicity (includes ataxia, blurred vision, drowsiness, irritability, numbness of extremities oral paresthesia), dizziness, drug fever, meningitis (intrathecal administration)

Dermatologic: Urticaria

Endocrine & metabolic: Hypocalcemia, hypochloremia, hypokalemia, hyponatremia

Genitourinary: Nephrotoxicity

Hypersensitivity: Anaphylactoid reaction

Local: Pain at injection site

Neuromuscular & skeletal: Neuromuscular blockade, weakness

Mechanism of Action Binds to phospholipids, alters permeability, and damages the bacterial cytoplasmic membrane permitting leakage of intracellular constituents

Pharmacodynamics/Kinetics

Half-life Elimination 6 hours, increased with reduced renal function (Evans 1999)

Time to Peak Serum: IM: Within 2 hours (Hoeprich 1970)

Pregnancy Considerations

[US Boxed Warning]: Safety in pregnancy has not been established.

Limited data related to systemic use in pregnancy are available (Heinonen 1977; Kazy 2005). Based on the relative toxicity compared to other antibiotics, systemic use in pregnancy is not recommended (Knothe 1985). Due to poor tissue diffusion, topical use would be expected to have only minimal risk to the mother or fetus (Leachman 2006).

◆ **Polymyxin B Sulfate** *see* Polymyxin B *on page 1244*

◆ **Polymyxin E** *see* Colictimethate *on page 408*

◆ **Poly-Vi-Flor®** *see* Vitamins (Fluoride) *on page 1550*

◆ **Poly-Vi-Flor® With Iron** *see* Vitamins (Fluoride) *on page 1550*

Polyvinylpyrrolidone and Sodium Hyaluronate

(pol e VI nil pi ROL i don & SOW dee um hye al yoor ON ate)

Brand Names: US Ameseal™

Pharmacologic Category Protectant, Topical

Local Anesthetic/Vasoconstrictor Precautions
No information available to require special precautions

Effects on Dental Treatment No significant effects or complications reported

Effects on Bleeding No information available to require special precautions

Mechanism of Action Polyvinylpyrrolidone (PVP) sets up a barrier at application site to protect ulcer from irritants and irritation

◆ **Polyvinylpyrrolidone with Iodine** *see* Povidone-Iodine (Topical) *on page 1249*

◆ **P-OM3** *see* Omega-3 Fatty Acids *on page 1137*

Pomalidomide (poe ma LID oh mide)

Brand Names: US Pomalyst

Brand Names: Canada Pomalyst

Pharmacologic Category Angiogenesis Inhibitor; Antineoplastic Agent

Use

Kaposi sarcoma: Treatment of AIDS-related Kaposi sarcoma in adults after failure of highly active antiretroviral therapy (HAART); treatment of Kaposi sarcoma in HIV-negative adults.

Multiple myeloma, relapsed/refractory: Treatment of multiple myeloma (in combination with dexamethasone) in adults who have received at least 2 prior therapies, including lenalidomide and a proteasome inhibitor, and have demonstrated disease progression on or within 60 days of completion of the last therapy.

Local Anesthetic/Vasoconstrictor Precautions
No information available to require special precautions

Effects on Dental Treatment No significant effects or complications reported

Effects on Bleeding Chemotherapy may result in significant myelosuppression, neutropenia (50% to 52%; grades 3/4: 43% to 47%), anemia (38%; grades 3/4: 22%), thrombocytopenia (25%; grades 3/4: 22%), leukopenia (11%; grades 3/4: 6%). In patients who are under active treatment with these agents, medical consult is suggested.

Adverse Reactions

>10%:

Cardiovascular: Peripheral edema (25%)

Central nervous system: Fatigue (≤58%), dizziness (22%), peripheral neuropathy (22%), neuropathy (18%), headache (15%), anxiety (13%), confusion (12%)

Dermatologic: Skin rash (21%), pruritus (15%)

Endocrine & metabolic: Hypercalcemia (22%), weight loss (15%), hypokalemia (12%), hyperglycemia (11%), hyponatremia (11%)

Gastrointestinal: Constipation (36%), nausea (36%), diarrhea (35%), decreased appetite (23%), vomiting (14%)

Hematologic & oncologic: Neutropenia (53%; grades 3/4: 48%), anemia (38%; grades 3/4: 23%), thrombocytopenia (26%; grades 3/4: 22%), leukopenia (13%; grades 3/4: 7%)

Neuromuscular & skeletal: Asthenia (≤58%), back pain (35%), musculoskeletal chest pain (23%), muscle spasm (22%), arthralgia (17%), myasthenia (14%), musculoskeletal pain (12%), ostealgia (12%)
Renal: Increased serum creatinine (19%), renal failure syndrome (15%)
Respiratory: Upper respiratory tract infection (37%), dyspnea (36%), pneumonia (28%; includes streptococcal pneumonia), cough (17%), epistaxis (17%)
Miscellaneous: Fever (23%)

1% to 10%:
Central nervous system: Chills (10%), insomnia (7%)
Dermatologic: Xeroderma (9%), hyperhidrosis (8%)
Endocrine & metabolic: Dehydration (<10%), hypocalcemia (6%)
Genitourinary: Urinary tract infection (10%)
Hematologic & oncologic: Febrile neutropenia (<10%), lymphocytopenia (4%; grades 3/4: 2%)
Infection: Sepsis (<10%)
Neuromuscular & skeletal: Tremor (10%), limb pain (8%)
Respiratory: Productive cough (9%), oropharyngeal pain (6%)
Miscellaneous: Night sweats (5%)

Frequency not defined:
Cardiovascular: Acute myocardial infarction, angina pectoris, atrial fibrillation, cardiac failure, hypotension, septic shock, syncope
Central nervous system: Altered mental status, falling, impaired consciousness, noncardiac chest pain, vertigo
Dermatologic: Cellulitis
Endocrine & metabolic: Hyperkalemia
Gastrointestinal: Abdominal pain, *Clostridioides difficile* associated diarrhea
Genitourinary: Pelvic pain, urinary retention, urinary tract infection with sepsis
Hepatic: Hyperbilirubinemia, increased serum alanine aminotransferase
Infection: Bacteremia, neutropenic sepsis, viral infection
Neuromuscular & skeletal: Bone fracture, vertebral compression fracture
Respiratory: Bronchospasm, interstitial pulmonary disease, lobar pneumonia, pneumonia due to *Pneumocystis jirovecii*, respiratory syncytial virus infection
Miscellaneous: Failure to thrive, multiorgan failure, physical health deterioration

<1%, postmarketing, and/or case reports: Acute hepatoxicity, acute myelocytic leukemia, anaphylaxis, angioedema, basal cell carcinoma of skin, cerebrovascular accident, deep vein thrombosis, drug reaction with eosinophilia and systemic symptoms, gastrointestinal hemorrhage, hepatic failure, herpes zoster infection, hypersensitivity reaction, hyperthyroidism, hypothyroidism, increased liver enzymes, organ transplant rejection, pancytopenia, pulmonary embolism, reactivation of HBV, squamous cell carcinoma of skin, Stevens-Johnson syndrome, toxic epidermal necrolysis, tumor lysis syndrome, weight gain

Mechanism of Action Pomalidomide induces cell cycle arrest and apoptosis directly in multiple myeloma cells. It enhances T cell- and natural killer (NK) cell-mediated cytotoxicity, inhibits production of proinflammatory cytokines tumor necrosis factor-α (TNF-α), IL-1, IL-6, and IL-12, and inhibits angiogenesis (Zhu 2013).

Pharmacodynamics/Kinetics

Half-life Elimination ~7.5 hours.

Time to Peak 2 to 3 hours

Reproductive Considerations

[US Boxed Warning]: In females of reproductive potential, obtain two negative pregnancy tests before starting pomalidomide treatment. Females of reproductive potential must use two forms of contraception or continuously abstain from heterosexual sex during and for 4 weeks after stopping pomalidomide. Women of childbearing potential should be treated only if they are able to comply with the conditions of the Pomalyst REMS Program. Pregnancy must be avoided for ≥4 weeks prior to beginning therapy. Contraception should be used in females of reproductive potential during treatment, during treatment interruptions, and for ≥4 weeks after pomalidomide is discontinued. Two forms of effective/reliable contraception or total abstinence from heterosexual intercourse must be used by women of reproductive potential even with a history of infertility (unless due to hysterectomy). Reliable methods of birth control include one highly effective method (eg, tubal ligation, IUD, hormonal [birth control pills, injections, hormonal patches, vaginal rings, or implants], or partner's vasectomy) and one additional effective method (eg, male latex or synthetic condom, diaphragm, or cervical cap). Pregnancy tests should be performed 10 to 14 days and 24 hours prior to beginning therapy; weekly for the first 4 weeks and then every 4 weeks (every 2 weeks if menstrual cycle irregular) thereafter and during therapy interruptions for at least 4 weeks after discontinuation. Pomalidomide must be immediately discontinued for a missed period, abnormal pregnancy test, or abnormal menstrual bleeding; refer patient to a reproductive toxicity specialist if pregnancy occurs during treatment.

Pomalidomide is present in the semen of males taking this medication. Males (including those vasectomized) should use a latex or synthetic condom during any sexual contact with women of childbearing age during treatment, during treatment interruptions, and for 4 weeks after discontinuation. Male patients should not donate sperm.

Pregnancy Considerations

[US Boxed Warning]: Pomalidomide is contraindicated in pregnancy. Pomalidomide is a thalidomide analogue. Thalidomide is a known human teratogen that causes severe birth defects or embryo-fetal death. Anomalies observed in humans following exposure to thalidomide include amelia, phocomelia, bone defects, ear and eye abnormalities, facial palsy, congenital heart defects, urinary and genital tract malformations; mortality in ~40% of infants at or shortly after birth has also been reported. Discontinue immediately if a pregnancy occurs during pomalidomide therapy.

Data collection to monitor pregnancy and infant outcomes following exposure to pomalidomide is ongoing. Any suspected fetal exposure should be reported to the FDA via the MedWatch program (1-800-332-1088) and to Celgene Corporation (1-888-423-5436).

Prescribing and Access Restrictions In Canada, pomalidomide is only available through a restricted distribution program called RevAid. Only physicians and pharmacists registered with the program are authorized to prescribe or dispense pomalidomide. Patients must also be registered and meet all conditions of the program. Two negative pregnancy tests with a sensitivity of at least 25 milliunits/mL are required prior to initiating therapy in women of childbearing potential. Further information is available at 1-888-738-2431 or www.RevAid.ca.

◆ **Pomalyst** *see* Pomalidomide *on page 1244*

PONATinib (poe NA ti nib)

Brand Names: US Iclusig

Brand Names: Canada Iclusig

Pharmacologic Category Antineoplastic Agent, BCR-ABL Tyrosine Kinase Inhibitor; Antineoplastic Agent, Tyrosine Kinase Inhibitor

Use

Acute lymphoblastic leukemia: Treatment of Philadelphia chromosome-positive acute lymphoblastic leukemia (Ph+ ALL) in patients for whom no other tyrosine kinase inhibitor therapy is indicated or who are T315I-positive.

Chronic myeloid leukemia: Treatment of chronic myeloid leukemia (CML) in chronic, accelerated, or blast phase in patients for whom no other tyrosine kinase inhibitor therapy is indicated or who are T315I-positive.

Limitations of use: Ponatinib is not indicated and not recommended for treatment of newly diagnosed chronic phase CML.

Local Anesthetic/Vasoconstrictor Precautions Ponatinib may cause hypertension; monitor blood pressure prior to vasoconstrictor use

Effects on Dental Treatment Key adverse event(s) related to dental treatment: Oral mucositis

Effects on Bleeding Chemotherapy may result in significant myelosuppression, potentially including significant reduction in platelet counts (thrombocytopenia grades 3/4: 36% to 57%) and altered hemostasis. In patients who are under active treatment with these agents, medical consult is suggested.

Adverse Reactions

>10%:

Cardiovascular: Hypertension (53% to 74%), arterial ischemia (11% to 42%), acute myocardial infarction (≤35%), cerebrovascular accident (≤35%), occlusive arterial disease (≤35%), peripheral vascular disease (≤35%), peripheral edema (15% to 25%), coronary occlusion (21%), cardiac arrhythmia (19%), cardiac failure (≤15%), mesenteric artery occlusion (≤12%), peripheral arterial disease (≤12%)

Dermatologic: Skin rash (28% to 63%), xeroderma (25% to 42%), pruritus (≤13%), cellulitis (≤11%), alopecia (6% to 11%)

Endocrine & metabolic: Increased serum glucose (54%), decreased serum phosphate (33%), fluid retention (31%), decreased serum calcium (30%), decreased serum albumin (27%), decreased serum sodium (27%), decreased serum bicarbonate (19%), increased serum potassium (19%), decreased serum potassium (18%), decreased serum glucose (13%), weight loss (5% to 13%), increased serum calcium (12%)

Gastrointestinal: Constipation (27% to 53%), abdominal pain (34% to 48%), increased serum lipase (38% to 42%), nausea (22% to 34%), decreased appetite (8% to 31%), diarrhea (13% to 29%), vomiting (18% to 27%), stomatitis (9% to 23%; grades 3/4: ≤3%), increased serum amylase (18%)

Genitourinary: Urinary tract infection (2% to 14%)

Hematologic & oncologic: Leukopenia (grades 3/4: 12% to 63%), bone marrow depression (59%; grade 3/4: 50%), neutropenia (grades 3/4: 23% to 59%), anemia (grades 3/4: 8% to 52%), thrombocytopenia (grades 3/4: 35% to 49%), lymphocytopenia (grades 3/4: 10% to 32%), hemorrhage (28%), febrile neutropenia (1% to 25%)

Hepatic: Increased serum alanine aminotransferase (41%), increased serum alkaline phosphatase (40%), increased serum aspartate aminotransferase (35%), hepatotoxicity (29%), increased serum bilirubin (13%)

Infection: Sepsis (2% to 13%)

Nervous system: Fatigue (≤49%), headache (25% to 43%), peripheral neuropathy (4% to 24% grades 3/4: ≤3%), pain (6% to 16%), dizziness (3% to 16%), insomnia (11% to 13%), chills (8% to 13%)

Neuromuscular & skeletal: Asthenia (≤49%), arthralgia (13% to 33%), myalgia (6% to 24%), limb pain (13% to 23%), back pain (13% to 21%), ostealgia (9% to 14%), muscle spasm (5% to 14%), musculoskeletal pain (6% to 11%)

Ophthalmic: Conjunctival edema (≤14%), conjunctival hemorrhage (≤14%), conjunctival hyperemia (≤14%), conjunctival irritation (≤14%), conjunctivitis (≤14%), corneal abrasion (≤14%), corneal erosion (≤14%), dry eye syndrome (≤14%), eye pain (≤14%)

Renal: Increased serum creatinine (21%)

Respiratory: Cough (6% to 22%), dyspnea (6% to 20%), pleural effusion (5% to 19%), nasopharyngitis (3% to 18%), pneumonia (6% to 16%), upper respiratory tract infection (3% to 14%)

Miscellaneous: Fever (25% to 40%)

1% to 10%:

Cardiovascular: Cerebrovascular occlusion (9%), left ventricular dysfunction (≤9%), venous thromboembolism (6% to 9%), atrial fibrillation (7%), venous thromboembolism (6%), pericardial effusion (4%), reduced ejection fraction (3%), severe hypertension (3%), deep vein thrombosis (2%), pulmonary embolism (2%), syncope (2%), retinal vein occlusion (≤2%), subdural hematoma (1%)

Dermatologic: Erythema of skin (6% to 10%)

Endocrine & metabolic: Increased serum sodium (10%), hyperuricemia (7%), increased serum triglycerides (3%)

Gastrointestinal: Gastrointestinal hemorrhage (1% to 9%), pancreatitis (7%), dysgeusia (2%)

Hematologic & oncologic: Major hemorrhage (6%)

Hepatic: Ascites (≤3%)

Nervous system: Paresthesia (5%), hypoesthesia (3%), cranial nerve palsy (2%), myasthenia (2%), cerebral hemorrhage (1%), hyperesthesia (1%)

Neuromuscular & skeletal: Swelling of the extremities (3%)

Ophthalmic: Blurred vision (6%), macular edema (≤2%), retinal hemorrhage (≤2%)

Frequency not defined:

Cardiovascular: Hypertensive crisis

Hepatic: Hepatic failure

Ophthalmic: Blepharitis, cataract, corneal ulcer, eyelid edema, glaucoma, iridocyclitis, iritis, ocular hyperemia, periorbital edema

Postmarketing: Atrial flutter, atrial tachycardia, bradycardia, complete atrioventricular block, dehydration, erythema multiforme, gastrointestinal fistula, gastrointestinal perforation, loss of consciousness, prolonged QT interval on ECG, reversible posterior leukoencephalopathy syndrome, severe dermatological reaction, sinus node dysfunction, Stevens-Johnson syndrome, superficial thrombophlebitis, supraventricular tachycardia, tachycardia, thrombotic microangiopathy, tumor lysis syndrome, ventricular arrhythmia, ventricular tachycardia, wound healing impairment

Mechanism of Action Ponatinib is a pan-BCR-ABL tyrosine kinase inhibitor with *in vitro* activity against cells expressing native or mutant BCR-ABL (including T315I); it also inhibits VEGFR, FGFR, PDGFR, EPH, and SRC kinases, as well as KIT, RET, TIE2, and FLT3.

Pharmacodynamics/Kinetics

Half-life Elimination ~24 hours (range: 12 to 66 hours)

Time to Peak ≤6 hours

Reproductive Considerations

Verify pregnancy status prior to initiating ponatinib treatment. Women of childbearing potential should use effective contraception during treatment and for 3 weeks after the last dose.

Pregnancy Considerations

Based on animal data and its mechanism of action, ponatinib is expected to cause fetal harm if used during pregnancy.

Prescribing and Access Restrictions Patient access and support is available through the ARIAD PASS program. Information regarding program enrollment may be found at http://www.ariadpass.com or by calling 1-855-447-PASS (7277). In Canada, ponatinib is available through the Iclusig Controlled Distribution Program; information about the program may be found at www.iclusigcdp.ca or by calling 1-888-867-7426.

◆ **Ponatinib HCl** *see* PONATinib *on page 1246*

◆ **Ponatinib Hydrochloride** *see* PONATinib *on page 1246*

◆ **Ponstel [DSC]** *see* Mefenamic Acid *on page 954*

Poractant Alfa (por AKT ant AL fa)

Brand Names: US Curosurf

Brand Names: Canada Curosurf

Pharmacologic Category Lung Surfactant

Use Respiratory distress syndrome (RDS): Treatment (rescue) of respiratory distress syndrome (RDS) in premature infants; reduces mortality and pneumothoraces associated with RDS.

Local Anesthetic/Vasoconstrictor Precautions No information available to require special precautions

Effects on Dental Treatment No significant effects or complications reported

Effects on Bleeding No information available to require special precautions

Adverse Reactions All reported adverse reactions occurred in premature neonates as safety and efficacy has not been established in full term neonates and older pediatric patients with respiratory failure. Frequency not always defined.

Cardiovascular: Patent ductus arteriosus (60%), bradycardia, hypotension

Hematologic & oncologic: Oxygen desaturation

Miscellaneous: Obstruction of endotracheal tube

<1%, postmarketing, and/or case reports: Pulmonary hemorrhage

Mechanism of Action Endogenous pulmonary surfactant reduces surface tension at the air-liquid interface of the alveoli during ventilation and stabilizes the alveoli against collapse at resting transpulmonary pressures. A deficiency of pulmonary surfactant in preterm infants results in respiratory distress syndrome characterized by poor lung expansion, inadequate gas exchange, and atelectasis. Poractant alfa compensates for the surfactant deficiency and restores surface activity to the infant's lungs. It reduces mortality and pneumothoraces associated with RDS.

Pregnancy Considerations This drug is not indicated for use in adults.

◆ **Porcine Lung Surfactant** *see* Poractant Alfa *on page 1247*

Porfimer (POR fi mer)

Brand Names: US Photofrin

Brand Names: Canada Photofrin [DSC]

Pharmacologic Category Antineoplastic Agent, Miscellaneous

Use

Barrett esophagus dysplasia (photodynamic therapy): Ablation of high-grade dysplasia in Barrett esophagus (in patients who do not undergo esophagectomy)

Endobronchial cancer (photodynamic therapy): Treatment of microinvasive endobronchial non-small cell lung cancer (NSCLC) in patients for whom surgery and radiation therapy are not indicated; reduction of obstruction and symptom palliation in patients with obstructing (partial or complete) endobronchial NSCLC

Esophageal cancer (photodynamic therapy): Palliation of completely obstructing esophageal cancer, or partially obstructing esophageal cancer in patients who cannot be treated satisfactorily with Nd:YAG laser therapy.

Local Anesthetic/Vasoconstrictor Precautions No information available to require special precautions

Effects on Dental Treatment Key adverse event(s) related to dental treatment: Dysphagia.

Effects on Bleeding No information available to require special precautions

Adverse Reactions

>10%:

Cardiovascular: Chest pain (8% to 22%), edema (5% to 18%)

Dermatologic: Skin photosensitivity (19% to 69%)

Gastrointestinal: Esophageal stenosis (6% to 38%), nausea (24%), constipation (5% to 24%), abdominal pain (20%), vomiting (17%), dysphagia (10%)

Hematologic & oncologic: Anemia (esophageal cancer: 32%)

Nervous system: Pain (5% to 22%), insomnia (5% to 14%)

Neuromuscular & skeletal: Back pain (3% to 11%)

Respiratory: Pleural effusion (5% to 32%), dyspnea (7% to 30%), bronchial obstruction (≤21%), bronchial plugs (≤21%), pneumonia (12% to 18%), hemoptysis (16%), cough (7% to 15%), bronchoconstriction (bronchostenosis: 11%), pharyngitis (11%)

Miscellaneous: Fever (16% to 31%), serous drainage (22%)

1% to 10%:

Cardiovascular: Atrial fibrillation (10%), hypotension (7%), peripheral edema (5% to 7%), cardiac failure (≤7%), hypertension (6%), tachycardia (6%), substernal pain (5%), acute myocardial infarction (<5%), angina pectoris (<5%), bradycardia (<5%), pulmonary embolism (<5%), sick sinus syndrome (<5%), supraventricular tachycardia (<5%)

Endocrine & metabolic: Weight loss (9%), dehydration (7%)

Gastrointestinal: Anorexia (8%), disease of esophagus (esophageal edema: 8%), hematemesis (8%), tracheoesophageal fistula (6%), dyspepsia (2% to 6%), diarrhea (5%), eructation (5%), esophagitis (5%), melena (5%), esophageal perforation (<5%), gastric ulcer (<5%), intestinal obstruction (<5%), peritonitis (<5%)

Genitourinary: Urinary tract infection (7%)

Hematologic & oncologic: Tumor hemorrhage (8%), pulmonary hemorrhage (<5%)

Hepatic: Jaundice (<5%)

Infection: Candidiasis (9%), abscess (lung: <5%)

Nervous system: Confusion (8%), anxiety (6% to 7%), voice disorder (5%)

Neuromuscular & skeletal: Asthenia (6%)

Ophthalmic: Diplopia (<5%), eye pain (<5%), photophobia (<5%), visual disturbance (<5%)

Respiratory: Bronchitis (≤10%), respiratory insufficiency (6% to 10%), bronchospasm (<5%), laryngeal edema (<5%), pneumonitis (<5%), productive cough (8%), pulmonary edema (<5%), respiratory failure (<5%), stridor (<5%)

Miscellaneous: Ulcer (bronchial: 9%), postoperative complication (5%)

<1%, postmarketing, and/or case reports: Cataract, cerebrovascular accident, cutaneous nodule, fluid volume disorder, fragile skin, gastrointestinal necrosis, gastrointestinal perforation, hemorrhage, hypertrichosis, infusion related reaction (including dizziness and urticaria), local tissue necrosis (esophageal), pseudoporphyria, sepsis, skin discoloration, thromboembolism, wrinkling of skin

Mechanism of Action Porfimer's cytotoxic activity is dependent on light and oxygen. Following administration, the drug is selectively retained in neoplastic tissues. Exposure of the drug to laser light at wavelengths >630 nm results in the production of oxygen free-radicals. Release of thromboxane A_2, leading to vascular occlusion and ischemic necrosis, may also occur.

Pharmacodynamics/Kinetics

Half-life Elimination First dose: 17 days; Second dose: 30 days

Reproductive Considerations Evaluate pregnancy status prior to use in females of reproductive potential. Females of reproductive potential should use effective contraception during treatment and for 5 months after the last porfimer dose. Males with female partners of reproductive potential should use condoms during treatment and for 5 months after the last porfimer dose.

Pregnancy Considerations

Based on the mechanism of action and data from animal reproduction studies, in utero exposure to porfimer may cause fetal harm.

◆ **Porfimer Sodium** *see* Porfimer *on page 1247*

◆ **Portia-28** *see* Ethinyl Estradiol and Levonorgestrel *on page 612*

◆ **Portrazza** *see* Necitumumab *on page 1089*

Posaconazole (poe sa KON a zole)

Related Information

Fungal Infections *on page 1752*

Brand Names: US Noxafil

Brand Names: Canada Posanol

Pharmacologic Category Antifungal Agent, Oral

Use

Candidiasis, oropharyngeal: Suspension (≥13 years of age): Treatment of oropharyngeal candidiasis (including patients refractory to itraconazole and/or fluconazole)

Invasive fungal infections, prophylaxis: Suspension and delayed-release tablets (≥13 years of age) and injection (≥18 years of age): Prophylaxis of invasive *Aspergillus* and *Candida* infections in patients who are at high risk of developing these infections due to being severely immunocompromised (eg, hematopoietic stem cell transplant [HSCT] recipients with graft-versus-host disease [GVHD] or those with prolonged neutropenia secondary to chemotherapy for hematologic malignancies).

Local Anesthetic/Vasoconstrictor Precautions

No information available to require special precautions

Effects on Dental Treatment Key adverse event(s) related to dental treatment: Xerostomia (normal salivary flow resumes upon discontinuation), abnormal taste, mucositis.

Effects on Bleeding No information available to require special precautions

Adverse Reactions

>10%:

Cardiovascular: Thrombophlebitis (intravenous via peripheral venous catheter: 60%), hypertension (8% to 18%), peripheral edema (12% to 16%), lower extremity edema (oral: 15%), hypotension (oral: 14%), tachycardia (oral: 12%)

Central nervous system: Headache (8% to 28%), rigors (oral: ≤20%), fatigue (3% to 17%), insomnia (oral: 1% to 17%), chills (10% to 16%), dizziness (oral: 11%)

Dermatologic: Skin rash (3% to 24%), pruritus (oral: 11%)

Endocrine & metabolic: Hypokalemia (oral: ≤30%), hypomagnesemia (10% to 18%), hyperglycemia (oral: 11%)

Gastrointestinal: Diarrhea (10% to 42%), nausea (9% to 38%), vomiting (7% to 29%), abdominal pain (5% to 27%), constipation (8% to 21%), anorexia (oral: 2% to 15%), stomatitis (oral: 14%), decreased appetite (10% to 12%), upper abdominal pain (6% to 11%)

Hematologic & oncologic: Thrombocytopenia (≤29%), anemia (2% to 25%), neutropenia (oral: 4% to 23%), petechia (8% to 11%)

Hepatic: Increased serum alanine aminotransferase (oral: ≤17%)

Neuromuscular & skeletal: Musculoskeletal pain (oral: 16%), arthralgia (oral: 11%)

Respiratory: Cough (3% to 24%), dyspnea (1% to 20%), epistaxis (14% to 17%), pharyngitis (oral: 12%)

Miscellaneous: Fever (21% to 45%)

1% to 10%:

Cardiovascular: Edema (oral: 9%), pulmonary embolism (<5%), torsades de pointes (<5%)

Central nervous system: Paresthesia (<5%), pain (oral: 1%)

Dermatologic: Diaphoresis (oral: 2%)

Endocrine & metabolic: Hypocalcemia (9%), adrenocortical insufficiency (<5%), dehydration (oral: 1%), weight loss (oral: 1%)

Gastrointestinal: Dyspepsia (10%), pancreatitis (<5%), oral candidiasis (oral: 1%)

Genitourinary: Vaginal hemorrhage (oral: 10%)

Hematologic & oncologic: Hemolytic-uremic syndrome (<5%), thrombotic thrombocytopenic purpura (<5%)

Hepatic: Hyperbilirubinemia (≤10%), hepatic insufficiency (<5%), hepatitis (<5%), hepatomegaly (<5%), increased liver enzymes (<5%), jaundice (<5%), increased serum aspartate aminotransferase (≤4%), increased serum alkaline phosphatase (oral: ≤3%)

Hypersensitivity: Hypersensitivity reaction (<5%)

Infection: Herpes simplex infection (oral: 3%)

Neuromuscular & skeletal: Back pain (oral: 10%), asthenia (oral: 2% to 10%)
Renal: Acute renal failure (<5%)
Respiratory: Pneumonia (oral: 3%)
<1%, postmarketing, and/or case reports: Cholestasis, prolonged QT interval on ECG, pseudoaldosteronism

Mechanism of Action Interferes with fungal cytochrome P450 (lanosterol-14α-demethylase) activity, decreasing ergosterol synthesis (principal sterol in fungal cell membrane) and inhibiting fungal cell membrane formation.

Pharmacodynamics/Kinetics

Half-life Elimination Suspension: 35 hours (range: 20 to 66 hours); Tablets: 26 to 31 hours; Injection: ~27 hours

Time to Peak Plasma: Suspension: ~3 to 5 hours; Tablets: ~4 to 5 hours

Pregnancy Considerations Adverse events have been observed in animal reproduction studies.

Dental Health Professional Considerations This drug is known to prolong the QT interval. The QT interval is measured as the time and distance between the Q point of the QRS complex and the end of the T wave in the ECG tracing. After adjustment for heart rate, the QT interval is defined as prolonged if it is more than 450 msec in men and 460 msec in women. A long QT syndrome was first described in the 1950s and 60s as a congenital syndrome involving QT interval prolongation and syncope and sudden death. Some of the congenital long QT syndromes were characterized by a peculiar electrocardiographic appearance of the QRS complex involving a premature atria beat followed by a pause, then a subsequent sinus beat showing marked QT prolongation and deformity. This type of cardiac arrhythmia was originally termed "torsade de pointes" (translated from the French as "twisting of the points").

Prolongation of the QT interval is thought to result from delayed ventricular repolarization. The repolarization process within the myocardial cell is due to the efflux of intracellular potassium. The channels associated with this current can be blocked by many drugs and predispose the electrical propagation cycle to torsade de pointes.

Posaconazole is one of the drugs confirmed to prolong the QT interval and is accepted as having a risk of causing torsade de pointes. The risk of drug-induced torsade de pointes is extremely low when a single QT interval prolonging drug is prescribed. In terms of epinephrine, it is not known what effect vasoconstrictors in the local anesthetic regimen will have in patients with a known history of congenital prolonged QT interval or in patients taking any medication that prolongs the QT interval. Until more information is obtained, it is suggested that the clinician consult with the physician prior to the use of a vasoconstrictor in suspected patients, and that the vasoconstrictor (epinephrine, levonordefrin [Neo-Cobefrin®]) be used with caution.

Potassium Chloride (poe TASS ee um KLOR ide)

Brand Names: US K-Tab; Klor-Con; Klor-Con 10; Klor-Con M10; Klor-Con M15; Klor-Con M20; Klor-Con Sprinkle; Micro-K [DSC]; Potassium Chloride PROAMP [DSC]

Brand Names: Canada APO-K; Micro-K; Slo-Pot 600

Pharmacologic Category Electrolyte Supplement, Oral; Electrolyte Supplement, Parenteral

Use Hypokalemia: Treatment or prevention of hypokalemia.

Local Anesthetic/Vasoconstrictor Precautions No information available to require special precautions

Effects on Dental Treatment No significant effects or complications reported

Effects on Bleeding No information available to require special precautions

Adverse Reactions

Frequency not defined:
Cardiovascular: Cardiac arrhythmia, cardiac conduction disturbance, edema, peripheral edema
Endocrine & metabolic: Fluid and electrolyte disturbance, hypervolemia
Gastrointestinal: Abdominal cramps, abdominal distress, abdominal pain, diarrhea, flatulence, gastrointestinal hemorrhage, gastrointestinal irritation, gastrointestinal obstruction, gastrointestinal perforation, gastrointestinal ulcer, nausea, vomiting
Respiratory: Pulmonary edema

Postmarketing: Angioedema, asystole (with rapid administration or hyperkalemia), bradycardia, burning sensation at injection site, chest pain, dyspnea, encephalopathy (hyponatremic), erythema at injection site, hyperkalemia, hypersensitivity reaction, hyponatremia, infusion-site pain, injection site phlebitis, irritation at injection site, skin rash, swelling at injection site, venous thrombosis at injection site, ventricular fibrillation (with rapid administration or hyperkalemia)

Mechanism of Action Potassium is the major cation of intracellular fluid and is essential for the conduction of nerve impulses in heart, brain, and skeletal muscle; contraction of cardiac, skeletal and smooth muscles; maintenance of normal renal function, acid-base balance, carbohydrate metabolism, and gastric secretion

Pregnancy Considerations Potassium requirements are the same in pregnant and nonpregnant women. Adverse events have not been observed following use of potassium supplements in healthy women with normal pregnancies. Use caution in pregnant women with other medical conditions (eg, preeclampsia; may be more likely to develop hyperkalemia) (IOM 2004). Potassium supplementation (that does not cause maternal hyperkalemia) would not be expected to cause adverse fetal events.

◆ **Potassium Chloride PROAMP [DSC]** *see* Potassium Chloride *on page 1249*

◆ **Potassium Clorazepate** *see* Clorazepate *on page 395*

Povidone-Iodine (Topical)

(POE vi done EYE oh dyne)

Related Information

Perioral Premalignant Lesions and Management of Patients Undergoing Cancer Therapy *on page 1781*

Brand Names: US Aplicare Povidone-Iodine Scrub [OTC]; Aplicare Povidone-Iodine [OTC]; Betadine Skin Cleanser [OTC] [DSC]; Betadine Surgical Scrub [OTC]; Betadine Swab Aid [OTC] [DSC]; Betadine Swabsticks [OTC]; Betadine [OTC]; Clorox Nasal Antiseptic [OTC] [DSC]; ExCel AP [OTC] [DSC]; Nasal Antiseptic [OTC] [DSC]; NuPrep 5% Povidone-Iodine [OTC] [DSC]; PVP Prep [OTC]; PVP Scrub [OTC]; Scrub Care Povidone-iodine [OTC]; Summers Eve Disp Medicated [OTC]

Pharmacologic Category Antiseptic, Topical; Antiseptic, Vaginal; Topical Skin Product

Use External antiseptic with broad microbicidal spectrum for the prevention or treatment of topical infections associated with surgery, burns, minor cuts/scrapes; relief of minor vaginal irritation

Local Anesthetic/Vasoconstrictor Precautions No information available to require special precautions

Effects on Dental Treatment No significant effects or complications reported

Effects on Bleeding No information available to require special precautions

Adverse Reactions Frequency not defined.

Local: Edema, irritation, pruritus, rash

Mechanism of Action Povidone-iodine is known to be a powerful broad spectrum germicidal agent effective against a wide range of bacteria, viruses, fungi, protozoa, and spores.

Pregnancy Considerations Vaginal products should not be used during pregnancy. Povidine-iodine is absorbed systemically as iodine following topical administration to the vaginal mucosa (Velasco 2009; Vorherr 1980). Following vaginal administration as a douche, iodine concentrations are increased in the maternal urine, amniotic fluid, cord blood and fetal thyroid (Bachrach 1984; Mahillon 1989). Transient hypothyroidism in the newborn has been reported following topical use prior to delivery (Danziger 1987).

- ◆ **PPD** *see* Tuberculin Tests *on page* 1503
- ◆ **PPI-0903** *see* Ceftaroline Fosamil *on page* 312
- ◆ **PPI-0903M** *see* Ceftaroline Fosamil *on page* 312
- ◆ **PPS** *see* Pentosan Polysulfate Sodium *on page* 1214
- ◆ **Pradaxa** *see* Dabigatran Etexilate *on page* 426

PRALAtrexate (pral a TREX ate)

Brand Names: US Folotyn

Brand Names: Canada Folotyn

Pharmacologic Category Antineoplastic Agent, Antimetabolite; Antineoplastic Agent, Antimetabolite (Antifolate)

Use Peripheral T-cell lymphoma: Treatment of relapsed or refractory peripheral T-cell lymphoma (PTCL)

Local Anesthetic/Vasoconstrictor Precautions No information available to require special precautions

Effects on Dental Treatment Key adverse event(s) related to dental treatment: Mucositis and stomatitis

Effects on Bleeding No information available to require special precautions

Adverse Reactions

>10%:

Cardiovascular: Edema (30%)

Central nervous system: Fatigue (36%)

Dermatologic: Skin rash (15%), pruritus (14%; grade 3: 2%), night sweats (11%)

Endocrine & metabolic: Hypokalemia (15%)

Gastrointestinal: Mucositis (70%; grade 3: 17%; grade 4: 4%), nausea (40%), constipation (33%), vomiting (25%), diarrhea (21%), anorexia (15%), abdominal pain (12%)

Hematologic & oncologic: Thrombocytopenia (41%; grade 3: 14%; grade 4: 19%), anemia (34%; grade 3: 15%; grade 4: 2%), neutropenia (24%; grade 3: 13%; grade 4: 7%), leukopenia (11%; grade 3: 3%; grade 4: 4%)

Hepatic: Increased serum transaminases (13%; grade 3: 5%)

Infection: Infection

Neuromuscular & skeletal: Limb pain (12%), back pain (11%)

Respiratory: Cough (28%), epistaxis (26%), dyspnea (19%), pharyngolaryngeal pain (14%)

Miscellaneous: Fever (32%)

1% to 10%:

Cardiovascular: Tachycardia (10%)

Endocrine & metabolic: Severe dehydration (>3%)

Hematologic & oncologic: Febrile neutropenia (serious: >3%)

Infection: Sepsis (serious: >3%)

Neuromuscular & skeletal: Weakness (10%)

Respiratory: Upper respiratory tract infection (10%)

<1%, postmarketing, and/or case reports: Dermal ulcer, desquamation, intestinal obstruction, lymphocytopenia, odynophagia, pancytopenia, toxic epidermal necrolysis, tumor lysis syndrome

Mechanism of Action Pralatrexate is an antifolate analog; inhibits DNA, RNA, and protein synthesis by selectively entering cells expressing reduced folate carrier (RFC-1), is polyglutamylated by folylpolyglutamate synthetase (FPGS) and then competes for the DHFR-folate binding site to inhibit dihydrofolate reductase (DHFR).

Pharmacodynamics/Kinetics

Half-life Elimination 12 to 18 hours

Reproductive Considerations

Evaluate pregnancy status prior to use in females of reproductive potential.

Females of reproductive potential should use effective contraception during therapy and for 6 months after the last pralatrexate dose. Males with female partners of reproductive potential should use effective contraception during therapy and for 3 months after the last dose of pralatrexate.

Pregnancy Considerations

Based on the mechanism of action and data from animal reproduction studies, in utero exposure to pralatrexate may cause fetal harm.

- ◆ **Praluent** *see* Alirocumab *on page* 101
- ◆ **PrameGel [OTC]** *see* Pramoxine *on page* 1252

Pramipexole (pra mi PEKS ole)

Brand Names: US Mirapex; Mirapex ER

Brand Names: Canada ACT Pramipexole; APO-Pramipexole; Auro-Pramipexole; DOM-Pramipexole [DSC]; Mirapex; MYLAN-Pramipexole [DSC]; PMS-Pramipexole [DSC]; RATIO-Pramipexole; SANDOZ Pramipexole; TEVA-Pramipexole [DSC]

Pharmacologic Category Anti-Parkinson Agent, Dopamine Agonist

Use

Parkinson disease: Treatment of Parkinson disease.

Restless legs syndrome (immediate release only): Treatment of moderate to severe primary restless legs syndrome.

Local Anesthetic/Vasoconstrictor Precautions No information available to require special precautions

Effects on Dental Treatment Key adverse event(s) related to dental treatment: Xerostomia (normal salivary flow resumes upon discontinuation) and dysphagia.

Effects on Bleeding No information available to require special precautions

Adverse Reactions Actual frequency may be dependent on dose, formulation, and/or concomitant levodopa. All adverse reactions are as reported for Parkinson disease (PD) unless otherwise noted.

>10%:
Cardiovascular: Orthostatic hypotension (3% to 53%)
Central nervous system: Drowsiness (PD: 9% to 36%; RLS: 6%), extrapyramidal reaction (28%), insomnia (PD: 4% to 27%; RLS: 13%), dizziness (2% to 26%), hallucination (5% to 17%; includes auditory, visual, and mixed hallucinations), headache (RLS: 16%; PD: 4% to 7%), restless leg syndrome (10% to 12%; includes augmentation, rebound, worsening), abnormal dreams (PD and RLS: 8% to 11%)
Gastrointestinal: Nausea (PD and RLS: 11% to 28%), constipation (PD: 6% to 14%; RLS: 4%)
Neuromuscular & skeletal: Dyskinesia (17% to 47%), asthenia (3% to 14%)
Miscellaneous: Accidental injury (17%)

1% to 10%:
Cardiovascular: Peripheral edema (2% to 8%), edema (4% to 5%), chest pain (3%)
Central nervous system: Confusion (4% to 10%), fatigue (PD and RLS: 6% to 9%), dystonia (2% to 8%), abnormal gait (7%), hypertonia (7%), amnesia (4% to 6%), sleep disorder (1% to 6%; includes sleep attacks), falling (4%), impulse control disorder (3% to 4%; eg, binge eating, compulsive shopping, hypersexuality, pathological gambling), vertigo (2% to 4%), hypoesthesia (3%), abnormality in thinking (2% to 3%), akathisia (2% to 3%), malaise (2% to 3%), depression (2%), equilibrium disturbance (2%), paranoia (2%), delusions (1%), myasthenia (1%), myoclonus (1%)
Dermatologic: Dermatologic disorders (2%)
Endocrine & metabolic: Weight loss (2%), decreased libido (1%)
Gastrointestinal: Xerostomia (PD and RLS: 3% to 7%), diarrhea (RLS: 1% to 7%; PD: 2%), anorexia (4% to 5%), vomiting (4%), upper abdominal pain (3% to 4%), dyspepsia (3%), increased appetite (2% to 3%), dysphagia (2%), sialorrhea (2%), abdominal distress (1% to 2%)
Genitourinary: Urinary frequency (6%), urinary tract infection (4%), impotence (2%), urinary incontinence (2%)
Infection: Influenza (RLS: 3% to 7%)
Neuromuscular & skeletal: Limb pain (RLS: 3% to 7%), muscle spasm (5%), arthritis (3%), tremor (3%), back pain (2% to 3%), bursitis (2%), twitching (2%), increased creatine phosphokinase (1%)
Ophthalmic: Accommodation disturbance (4%), visual disturbance (3%), diplopia (1%)
Respiratory: Nasal congestion (RLS: 3% to 6%), dyspnea (4%), cough (3%), rhinitis (3%), pneumonia (2%)
Miscellaneous: Fever (1%)

<1%, postmarketing, and/or case reports: Abnormal stools (ER tablet residue; may be associated with worsening of PD symptoms), abnormal posture (postural deformities including antecollis, captocormia [Bent Spine syndrome], pleurothonus [Pisa syndrome]), aggressive behavior, agitation, altered mental status, behavioral changes, cardiac failure, delirium, disorientation, erythema, pruritus, psychotic symptoms, pulmonary fibrosis, retroperitoneal fibrosis, rhabdomyolysis, SIADH, skin rash, syncope, urticaria, weight gain

Mechanism of Action Pramipexole is a nonergot dopamine agonist with specificity for the D_2 subfamily dopamine receptor, and has also been shown to bind to D_3 and D_4 receptors. By binding to these receptors, it is thought that pramipexole can stimulate dopamine activity on the nerves of the striatum and substantia nigra.

Pharmacodynamics/Kinetics

Half-life Elimination 8.5 hours; Elderly: 12 hours

Time to Peak Serum: Immediate release: ~2 hours; Extended release: 6 hours

Pregnancy Considerations Information related to the use of pramipexole for the treatment of Parkinson disease (Benbir 2014; Lamichhane 2014; Mucchiut 2004; Tüfekçioglu 2018) or restless legs syndrome (RLS) (Dostal 2013) in pregnant women is limited. Current guidelines note that the available information is insufficient to make a recommendation for the treatment of RLS in pregnant women (Aurora 2012).

◆ **Pramipexole Dihydrochloride Monohydrate** *see* Pramipexole *on page 1250*

Pramlintide (PRAM lin tide)

Related Information

Endocrine Disorders and Pregnancy *on page 1684*

Brand Names: US SymlinPen 120; SymlinPen 60

Pharmacologic Category Amylinomimetic; Antidiabetic Agent

Use Diabetes mellitus, type 1 and type 2: Adjunct treatment in patients with type 1 or type 2 diabetes who use mealtime insulin therapy and who have failed to achieve desired glucose control despite optimal insulin therapy.

Local Anesthetic/Vasoconstrictor Precautions No information available to require special precautions

Effects on Dental Treatment No significant effects or complications reported

Effects on Bleeding No information available to require special precautions

Adverse Reactions

>10%:
Central nervous system: Headache (5% to 13%)
Endocrine & metabolic: Severe hypoglycemia (type 1 diabetes ≤17%)
Gastrointestinal: Nausea (28% to 48%), anorexia (≤17%), vomiting (7% to 11%)
Miscellaneous: Accidental injury (8% to 14%)

1% to 10%:
Central nervous system: Fatigue (3% to 7%), dizziness (2% to 6%)
Endocrine & metabolic: Severe hypoglycemia (type 2 diabetes ≤8%)
Gastrointestinal: Abdominal pain (2% to 8%)
Hypersensitivity: Hypersensitivity reaction (≤6%)
Neuromuscular & skeletal: Arthralgia (2% to 7%)
Respiratory: Cough (2% to 6%), pharyngitis (3% to 5%)

Postmarketing and/or case reports: Injection site reaction, pancreatitis

Mechanism of Action Synthetic analog of human amylin cosecreted with insulin by pancreatic beta cells; reduces postprandial glucose increases via the following mechanisms: 1) prolongation of gastric emptying time, 2) reduction of postprandial glucagon secretion, and 3) reduction of caloric intake through centrally-mediated appetite suppression

Pharmacodynamics/Kinetics

Duration of Action ~3 hours

Half-life Elimination ~48 minutes

Time to Peak 20 minutes

Pregnancy Considerations

Based on in vitro data, pramlintide has a low potential to cross the placenta.

Poorly controlled diabetes during pregnancy can be associated with an increased risk of adverse maternal and fetal outcomes, including diabetic ketoacidosis, preeclampsia, spontaneous abortion, preterm delivery, delivery complications, major birth defects, stillbirth, and macrosomia (ACOG 201 2018). To prevent adverse outcomes, prior to conception and throughout pregnancy, maternal blood glucose and HbA_{1c} should be kept as close to target goals as possible but without causing significant hypoglycemia (ADA 2020; Blumer 2013).

Agents other than pramlintide are currently recommended to treat diabetes mellitus in pregnancy (ADA 2020).

◆ **Pramlintide Acetate** *see* Pramlintide *on page 1251*

◆ **Pramox** *see* Pramoxine *on page 1252*

Pramoxine (pra MOKS een)

Brand Names: US Calaclear [OTC]; Caladryl Clear [OTC]; Caldyphen Clear [OTC]; Callergy Clear [OTC]; CeraVe Itch Relief [OTC] [DSC]; GoodSense Clear Anti-Itch [OTC]; Itch-X [OTC]; Ivy Wash Poison Ivy Cleanser [OTC]; PrameGel [OTC]; Pramox; Prax [OTC]; Proctofoam [OTC]; Sarna Sensitive [OTC]

Pharmacologic Category Antihemorrhoidal Agent; Local Anesthetic

Use Temporary relief of pain and itching associated with hemorrhoids, burns, minor cuts, scrapes, or minor skin irritations

Local Anesthetic/Vasoconstrictor Precautions No information available to require special precautions

Effects on Dental Treatment No significant effects or complications reported

Effects on Bleeding No information available to require special precautions

Mechanism of Action Pramoxine, like other anesthetics, decreases the neuronal membrane's permeability to sodium ions; both initiation and conduction of nerve impulses are blocked, thus depolarization of the neuron is inhibited

Pharmacodynamics/Kinetics

Onset of Action 3-5 minutes

◆ **Pramoxine HCl** *see* Pramoxine *on page 1252*

◆ **Pramoxine Hydrochloride** *see* Pramoxine *on page 1252*

◆ **Prandin [DSC]** *see* Repaglinide *on page 1317*

Prasugrel (PRA soo grel)

Related Information

Antiplatelet and Anticoagulation Considerations in Dentistry *on page 1666*

Cardiovascular Diseases *on page 1654*

Brand Names: US Effient

Brand Names: Canada Effient [DSC]

Pharmacologic Category Antiplatelet Agent; Antiplatelet Agent, Thienopyridine; P2Y12 Antagonist

Use Acute coronary syndrome managed by percutaneous coronary intervention: To reduce the rate of thrombotic cardiovascular events (including stent thrombosis) in patients with acute coronary syndrome who are to be managed with percutaneous coronary intervention for unstable angina, non-ST-elevation myocardial infarction (MI), or ST-elevation MI.

Local Anesthetic/Vasoconstrictor Precautions No information available to require special precautions

Effects on Dental Treatment Key adverse event(s) related to dental treatment: May cause bleeding during invasive dental procedures and medical consultation is suggested prior to any consideration of discontinuation. If possible, manage bleeding without discontinuing therapy; premature discontinuation of treatment may increase the risk for cardiac adverse effects.

Aspirin in combination with clopidogrel (Plavix®), prasugrel (Effient®), or ticagrelor (Brilinta™) is the primary prevention strategy against stent thrombosis after placement of drug-eluting metal stents in coronary patients. Premature discontinuation of combination antiplatelet therapy (ie, dual antiplatelet therapy) strongly increases the risk of a catastrophic event of stent thrombosis leading to myocardial infarction and/or death, so says a science advisory issued in January 2007 from the American Heart Association in collaboration with the American Dental Association and other professional healthcare organizations. The advisory stresses a 12-month therapy of dual antiplatelet therapy after placement of a drug-eluting stent in order to prevent thrombosis at the stent site. Any elective surgery should be postponed for 1 year after stent implantation, and if surgery must be performed, consideration should be given to continuing the antiplatelet therapy during the perioperative period in high-risk patients with drug-eluting stents.

This advisory was issued from a science panel made up of representatives from the American Heart Association (AHA), the American College of Cardiology, the Society for Cardiovascular Angiography and Interventions, the American College of Surgeons, the American Dental Association (ADA), and the American College of Physicians (Grines, 2007).

Effects on Bleeding Prasugrel blocks platelet aggregation and may prolong bleeding time. Inhibition is irreversible; on discontinuation of prasugrel, normal platelet function returns only when new platelets are released from the bone marrow. Normal platelet function will occur within 5-9 days of discontinuation. There is no scientific evidence to warrant the discontinuance of prasugrel prior to dental surgery.

Dual antiplatelet therapy: Aspirin irreversibly inhibits platelet aggregation which can prolong bleeding. Upon discontinuation, normal platelet function returns only when new platelets are released (~7-10 days). However, in the case of dental surgery, there is no scientific evidence to support discontinuation of aspirin. The discontinuation of aspirin may place the patient at risk for a thrombotic event or other cardiovascular complication. In particular, aspirin should **not** be discontinued in patients with cardiac stents that have not completed their full course of dual antiplatelet therapy (eg, aspirin and clopidogrel [prasugrel or ticagrelor]); patient-specific situations need to be discussed with cardiologist. When feasible, postponement of dental surgery until the completion of dual antiplatelet therapy should be considered. Any modification of aspirin therapy should be discussed with the prescribing physician.

Adverse Reactions

1% to 10%:

Cardiovascular: Hypertension (8%), hypotension (4%), atrial fibrillation (3%), bradycardia (3%), peripheral edema (3%)

Central nervous system: Headache (6%), dizziness (4%), fatigue (4%), noncardiac chest pain (3%)
Dermatologic: Skin rash (3%)
Endocrine & metabolic: Hypercholesterolemia (≤7%), hyperlipidemia (≤7%)
Gastrointestinal: Nausea (5%), diarrhea (2%), gastrointestinal hemorrhage (2%)
Hematologic & oncologic: Leukopenia (3%), anemia (2%), major hemorrhage (2%), minor hemorrhage (2%), major hemmorhage (life-threatening: 1%)
Neuromuscular & skeletal: Back pain (5%), limb pain (3%)
Respiratory: Epistaxis (6%), dyspnea (5%), cough (4%)
Miscellaneous: Fever (3%)

<1%, postmarketing, and/or case reports: Abnormal hepatic function tests, anaphylaxis, angioedema, hematoma, hemoptysis, hemorrhage (requiring inotropes or transfusion), hypersensitivity reaction, intracranial hemorrhage (symptomatic), re-operation due to bleeding, thrombocytopenia, thrombotic thrombocytopenic purpura

Mechanism of Action Prasugrel, an inhibitor of platelet activation and aggregation, is a prodrug that is metabolized to both active (R-138727) and inactive metabolites. The active metabolite irreversibly blocks the $P2Y_{12}$ component of ADP receptors on the platelet, which prevents activation of the GPIIb/IIIa receptor complex, thereby reducing platelet activation and aggregation

Pharmacodynamics/Kinetics

Onset of Action Inhibition of platelet aggregation (IPA): Dose dependent: 60 mg loading dose: <30 minutes; median time to reach ≥20% IPA: 30 minutes (Brandt 2007).

Peak effect: Time to maximal IPA: Dose-dependent: **Note:** Degree of IPA based on adenosine diphosphate (ADP) concentration used during light aggregometry: 60 mg loading dose: Occurs ~4 hours post administration; Mean IPA (ADP 5 micromol/L): ~84.1%; Mean IPA (ADP 20 micromole/L): ~78.8% (Brandt 2007).

Duration of Action Duration of effect: Platelet aggregation gradually returns to baseline values over 5 to 9 days after discontinuation; reflective of new platelet production.

Half-life Elimination Half-life elimination: Active metabolite: ~7 hours (range: 2 to 15 hours).

Time to Peak Active metabolite: ~30 minutes; With high-fat/high-calorie meal: 1.5 hours.

Pregnancy Considerations Adverse events have not been observed in animal reproduction studies. Information related to use during pregnancy is limited (Tello-Montoliu 2013).

Dental Health Professional Considerations There is no scientific evidence to warrant the discontinuance of prasugrel prior to dental surgery. Patients requiring dental surgery who are taking 1 tablet daily as an antithrombotic or taking 1 tablet daily in combination with aspirin should be given special consideration in consultation with their healthcare provider.

◆ **Prasugrel Hydrochloride** *see* Prasugrel *on page 1252*

◆ **Pravachol** *see* Pravastatin *on page 1253*

Pravastatin (prav a STAT in)

Related Information

Cardiovascular Diseases *on page 1654*

Brand Names: US Pravachol

Brand Names: Canada ACH-Pravastatin; ACT Pravastatin [DSC]; AG-Pravastatin; APO-Pravastatin; AURO-Pravastatin; BIO-Pravastatin; DOM-Pravastatin; JAMP-Pravastatin; M-Pravastatin; MAR-Pravastatin; MINT-Pravastatin; MYLAN-Pravastin [DSC]; PMS-Pravastatin; Pravachol; Priva-Pravastatin; RAN-Pravastatin; RIVA-Pravastatin [DSC]; SANDOZ Pravastatin; TEVA-Pravastatin

Pharmacologic Category Antilipemic Agent, HMG-CoA Reductase Inhibitor

Use

Hyperlipidemia

Dysbetalipoproteinemia: Treatment of primary dysbetalipoproteinemia (Fredrickson type III) in patients who do not respond adequately to diet.

Heterozygous familial hypercholesterolemia: Adjunct to diet in children ≥8 years and adolescents with heterozygous familial hypercholesterolemia (HeFH) if after an adequate trial of diet therapy the following findings are present: LDL-C ≥190 mg/dL or LDL ≥160 mg/dL with positive family history of premature cardiovascular disease (CVD), or with 2 or more other CVD risk factors.

Hypercholesterolemia and mixed dyslipidemia: Adjunct to diet to reduce elevated total cholesterol, LDL-C, apo B, and triglyceride (TG) levels and to increase HDL-C in patients with primary hypercholesterolemia and mixed dyslipidemia (Fredrickson Types IIa and IIb).

Limitations of use: Has not been studied in conditions where the major lipid abnormality is elevation of chylomicrons (Fredrickson types I and V).

Prevention of cardiovascular disease

Primary prevention of cardiovascular disease: To reduce the risk of myocardial infarction, revascularization procedures and cardiovascular mortality in hypercholesterolemic patients without established coronary heart disease (CHD).

Secondary prevention of cardiovascular disease: To slow the progression of coronary atherosclerosis; to reduce the risk of myocardial infarction, revascularization procedures, and total mortality; and to reduce the risk of stroke and transient ischemic attacks (TIA) in patients with established CHD.

Local Anesthetic/Vasoconstrictor Precautions No information available to require special precautions

Effects on Dental Treatment Key adverse event(s) related to dental treatment: Assess unusual presentations of muscle weakness or myopathy resulting from lipid therapy such as patient having a difficult time brushing teeth or weakness with chewing. Refer patient back to their physician for evaluation and adjustment of lipid therapy.

Effects on Bleeding No information available to require special precautions

Adverse Reactions As reported in short-term trials; safety and tolerability with long-term use were similar to placebo.

1% to 10%:

Cardiovascular: Chest pain (4%)
Central nervous system: Headache (2% to 6%), fatigue (4%), dizziness (1% to 3%)
Dermatologic: Skin rash (4%)

Gastrointestinal: Nausea (≤7%), vomiting (≤7%), diarrhea (6%), heartburn (3%)
Genitourinary: Cystitis (interstitial; Huang 2015)
Hepatic: Increased serum transaminases (>3x normal on 2 occasions: 1%)
Infection: Influenza (2%)
Neuromuscular & skeletal: Myalgia (2%)
Respiratory: Cough (3%)

<1%, postmarketing, and/or case reports: Alopecia, amnesia (reversible), anaphylaxis, angioedema, cataract, change in libido, cholestatic jaundice, cognitive dysfunction (reversible), confusion (reversible), cranial nerve dysfunction, decreased appetite, dermatitis, dermatomyositis, dysgeusia, edema, erythema multiforme, fever, flushing, fulminant hepatic necrosis, gynecomastia, hemolytic anemia, hepatic cirrhosis, hepatic neoplasm, hepatitis, hypersensitivity reaction, increased erythrocyte sedimentation rate, insomnia, lupus-like syndrome, memory impairment (reversible), myasthenia, myopathy, neuropathy, pancreatitis, paresthesia, peripheral nerve palsy, polymyalgia rheumatica, positive ANA titer, pruritus, purpura, rhabdomyolysis, sexual disorder, Stevens-Johnson syndrome, tremor, urticaria, vasculitis, vertigo, xeroderma

Mechanism of Action Pravastatin is a competitive inhibitor of 3-hydroxy-3-methylglutaryl coenzyme A (HMG-CoA) reductase, which is the rate-limiting enzyme involved in *de novo* cholesterol synthesis. In addition to the ability of HMG-CoA reductase inhibitors to decrease levels of high-sensitivity C-reactive protein (hsCRP), they also possess pleiotropic properties including improved endothelial function, reduced inflammation at the site of the coronary plaque, inhibition of platelet aggregation, and anticoagulant effects (de Denus 2002; Ray 2005).

Pharmacodynamics/Kinetics

Onset of Action Several days; Peak effect: 4 weeks; LDL-reduction: 40 mg/day: 34% (for each doubling of this dose, LDL-C is lowered by ~6%)

Half-life Elimination

Children and Adolescents (4.9-15.6 years): 1.6 hours; range: 0.85 to 4.2 hours (Hedman 2003)
Adults: 77 hours (including all metabolites); Pravastatin: ~2 to 3 hours (Pan 1990); 3 alpha hydroxy-isopravastatin: ~1.5 hours (Gustavson 2005)

Time to Peak Serum: 1-1.5 hours

Reproductive Considerations

Pravastatin is contraindicated in females who may become pregnant.

Adequate contraception is recommended if an HMG-CoA reductase inhibitor is required in females of reproductive potential. Females planning a pregnancy should discontinue the HMG-CoA reductase inhibitor 1 to 2 months prior to attempting to conceive (AHA/ACC [Grundy 2018]).

Pregnancy Considerations

Pravastatin is contraindicated in pregnant females.

Pravastatin was found to cross the placenta in an ex vivo study using term human placentas (Nanovskaya 2013). There are reports of congenital anomalies following maternal use of HMG-CoA reductase inhibitors in pregnancy; however, maternal disease, differences in specific agents used, and the low rates of exposure limit the interpretation of the available data (Godfrey 2012; Lecarpentier 2012). Cholesterol biosynthesis may be important in fetal development; serum cholesterol and triglycerides increase normally during pregnancy. The discontinuation of lipid lowering medications temporarily during pregnancy is not expected to have significant impact on the long term outcomes of primary hypercholesterolemia treatment.

Pravastatin should be discontinued immediately if an unplanned pregnancy occurs during treatment.

◆ **Pravastatin Sodium** *see* Pravastatin *on page 1253*
◆ **Prax [OTC]** *see* Pramoxine *on page 1252*
◆ **Praxbind** *see* IdaruCIZUmab *on page 795*

Prazosin (PRAZ oh sin)

Related Information

Cardiovascular Diseases *on page 1654*

Brand Names: US Minipress

Brand Names: Canada APO-Prazo; Minipress; TEVA-Prazosin

Pharmacologic Category Alpha$_1$ Blocker; Antihypertensive

Use Hypertension: Management of hypertension. **Note:** Alpha blockers are not recommended as first-line therapy (ACC/AHA [Whelton 2017]).

Local Anesthetic/Vasoconstrictor Precautions No information available to require special precautions

Effects on Dental Treatment Key adverse event(s) related to dental treatment: Significant xerostomia (normal salivary flow resumes upon discontinuation); Patients may experience orthostatic hypotension as they stand up after treatment; especially if lying in dental chair for extended periods of time. Use caution with sudden changes in position during and after dental treatment.

Effects on Bleeding No information available to require special precautions

Adverse Reactions

>4%:

Cardiovascular: Palpitations (5%)
Central nervous system: Dizziness (10%), drowsiness (8%), headache (8%), fatigue (7%)
Gastrointestinal: Nausea (5%)
Neuromuscular & skeletal: Weakness (7%)

1% to 4%:

Cardiovascular: Edema, orthostatic hypotension, syncope
Central nervous system: Depression, nervousness, vertigo
Dermatologic: Skin rash
Gastrointestinal: Constipation, diarrhea, vomiting, xerostomia
Genitourinary: Urinary frequency
Ophthalmic: Blurred vision, injected sclera
Respiratory: Dyspnea, epistaxis, nasal congestion

<1%, postmarketing, and/or case reports: Abdominal distress, abnormal hepatic function tests, alopecia, angina pectoris, arthralgia, bradycardia, cataplexy, cataract (both development of cataract and disappearance have been reported), diaphoresis, eye pain, fever, flushing, gynecomastia, hallucination, hypersensitivity reaction, impotence, insomnia, leukopenia, lichen planus, malaise, myocardial infarction, narcolepsy (worsened), pain, pancreatitis, paresthesia, positive ANA titer, priapism, pruritus, retinal pigment changes (mottled), retinopathy (serous), systemic lupus erythematosus, tachycardia, tinnitus, urinary incontinence, urticaria, vasculitis

Mechanism of Action Competitively inhibits postsynaptic alpha-adrenergic receptors which results in vasodilation of veins and arterioles and a decrease in total peripheral resistance and blood pressure

Pharmacodynamics/Kinetics

Onset of Action Antihypertensive: Within 2 hours; Peak effect: 2 to 4 hours

Duration of Action 10 to 24 hours

Half-life Elimination 2 to 3 hours, prolonged with CHF

Time to Peak Plasma: ~3 hours

Pregnancy Considerations

Prazosin crosses the placenta and its pharmacokinetics may be slightly altered during pregnancy (Bourget 1995; Rubin 1983); bioavailability was increased, time to peak serum concentration, and elimination rates were longer in women during the third trimester (Rubin 1983). Limited use in pregnant women has not demonstrated any fetal abnormalities or adverse effects (maternal treatment started after the first trimester) (Dommisse 1983; Lubbe 1981).

Chronic maternal hypertension may increase the risk of birth defects, low birth weight, preterm delivery, stillbirth, and neonatal death. Actual fetal/neonatal risks may be related to duration and severity of maternal hypertension. Untreated hypertension may also increase the risks of adverse maternal outcomes, including gestational diabetes, myocardial infarction, preeclampsia, stroke, and delivery complications (ACOG 203 2019).

Agents other than prazosin are more commonly used to treat hypertension in pregnancy (ACOG 203 2019; ESC [Regitz-Zagrosek 2018]); use of prazosin should be considered in consult with subspecialists (ACOG 203 2019). Females with preexisting hypertension may continue their medication during pregnancy unless contraindications exist (ESC [Regitz-Zagrosek 2018]). Although rare, use of prazosin for the treatment of hypertension due to a pheochromocytoma during pregnancy has been described (Mazza 2014).

- ◆ **Prazosin HCl** *see* Prazosin *on page 1254*
- ◆ **Prazosin Hydrochloride** *see* Prazosin *on page 1254*
- ◆ **Precedex** *see* DexMEDEtomidine *on page 472*
- ◆ **Precose** *see* Acarbose *on page 57*
- ◆ **Predator [OTC]** *see* Lidocaine (Topical) *on page 902*

Prednicarbate (pred ni KAR bate)

Brand Names: US Dermatop [DSC]

Brand Names: Canada Dermatop

Pharmacologic Category Corticosteroid, Topical

Use Dermatoses: Relief of the inflammatory and pruritic manifestations of corticosteroid-responsive dermatoses (medium potency topical corticosteroid)

Local Anesthetic/Vasoconstrictor Precautions No information available to require special precautions

Effects on Dental Treatment No significant effects or complications reported

Effects on Bleeding No information available to require special precautions

Adverse Reactions

1% to 10%: Dermatologic: Skin atrophy (children: 3% to 8%; adults: 1%), telangiectasia (mild; children: 5%), taut and shiny skin (children: 3%)

<1%, postmarketing, and/or case reports: Acneiform eruption, allergic contact dermatitis, atrophic striae, burning sensation of skin, edema, folliculitis, hypopigmentation, miliaria, paresthesia, perioral dermatitis, pruritus, secondary infection, skin rash, urticaria

Mechanism of Action Topical corticosteroids have anti-inflammatory, antipruritic, and vasoconstrictive properties. May depress the formation, release, and activity of endogenous chemical mediators of inflammation (kinins, histamine, liposomal enzymes, prostaglandins) through the induction of phospholipase A_2 inhibitory proteins (lipocortins) and sequential inhibition of the release of arachidonic acid. Prednicarbate has intermediate range potency.

Pregnancy Risk Factor C

Pregnancy Considerations Adverse events have been observed in animal reproduction studies. Topical corticosteroids are not recommended for extensive use, in large quantities, or for long periods of time in pregnant women (Koutroulis, 2011; Leachman, 2006).

PrednisoLONE (Systemic) (pred NISS oh lone)

Related Information

PredniSONE *on page 1260*

Respiratory Diseases *on page 1680*

Brand Names: US Millipred; Millipred DP 12-Day; Millipred DP [DSC]; Orapred ODT; Pediapred; Veripred 20 [DSC]

Brand Names: Canada Pediapred; PMS-Prednisolone

Generic Availability (US) May be product dependent

Pharmacologic Category Corticosteroid, Systemic

Use

Allergic states: Control of severe or incapacitating allergic conditions intractable to adequate trials of conventional treatment in asthma, atopic dermatitis, drug hypersensitivity reactions, seasonal or perennial allergic rhinitis, and serum sickness.

Dermatologic diseases: Bullous dermatitis herpetiformis; contact dermatitis; exfoliative erythroderma; exfoliative dermatitis; mycosis fungoides; pemphigus; severe erythema multiforme (Stevens-Johnson syndrome); severe psoriasis; severe seborrheic dermatitis.

Endocrine disorders: Congenital adrenal hyperplasia; hypercalcemia associated with cancer; nonsuppurative thyroiditis; primary or secondary adrenocortical insufficiency (hydrocortisone or cortisone is the first choice; synthetic analogs may be used in conjunction with mineralocorticoids where applicable).

GI diseases: During acute episodes of Crohn disease or ulcerative colitis.

Hematologic disorders: Acquired (autoimmune) hemolytic anemia; congenital (erythroid) hypoplastic anemia (Diamond-Blackfan anemia); erythroblastopenia (RBC anemia); immune thrombocytopenia (formerly known as idiopathic thrombocytopenic purpura), pure red cell aplasia; secondary thrombocytopenia.

Neoplastic diseases: Treatment of acute leukemia and aggressive lymphomas.

Nervous system: Acute exacerbations of multiple sclerosis; cerebral edema associated with primary or metastatic brain tumor, craniotomy, or head injury. **Note**: Treatment guidelines recommend the use of high dose IV or oral methylprednisolone for acute exacerbations of multiple sclerosis (AAN [Scott 2011]; NICE 2014).

Ophthalmic diseases: Allergic conjunctivitis; allergic corneal marginal ulcers; anterior segment inflammation; chorioretinitis; diffuse posterior uveitis and choroiditis; herpes zoster ophthalmicus; iritis and iridocyclitises; keratitis; optic neuritis; sympathetic ophthalmia; uveitis and other ocular inflammatory conditions unresponsive to topical corticosteroids.

Renal disorders: To induce diuresis or remission of proteinuria in nephrotic syndrome, without uremia, of the idiopathic type or that due to lupus erythematosus.

Respiratory diseases: Acute exacerbations of chronic obstructive pulmonary disease (COPD); allergic bronchopulmonary aspergillosis; aspiration pneumonitis; asthma; berylliosis; fulminating or disseminated pulmonary tuberculosis when used concurrently with appropriate antituberculous chemotherapy; hypersensitivity pneumonitis; idiopathic bronchiolitis obliterans with organizing pneumonia; idiopathic eosinophilic pneumonias; idiopathic pulmonary fibrosis; Loeffler syndrome (not manageable by other means); *Pneumocystis carinii* pneumonia (PCP) associated with hypoxemia occurring in an HIV-positive individual who is also under treatment with appropriate anti-PCP antibiotics; symptomatic sarcoidosis.

Rheumatic disorders: As adjunctive therapy for short-term administration in acute and subacute bursitis, acute gout flares, acute nonspecific tenosynovitis, ankylosing spondylitis, epicondylitis, polymyalgia rheumatica/temporal arteritis, posttraumatic osteoarthritis, psoriatic arthritis, relapsing polychondritis, rheumatoid arthritis (including juvenile rheumatoid arthritis), synovitis of osteoarthritis, acute rheumatic carditis, systemic lupus erythematosus, dermatomyositis/polymyositis, Sjogren syndrome, and certain cases of vasculitis.

Miscellaneous: Acute or chronic solid organ rejection; trichinosis with neurologic or myocardial involvement; tuberculous meningitis with subarachnoid block or impending block, tuberculosis with enlarged mediastinal lymph nodes causing respiratory difficulty, tuberculosis with pleural or pericardial effusion (use appropriate antituberculous chemotherapy concurrently when treating any tuberculosis complications).

Local Anesthetic/Vasoconstrictor Precautions No information available to require special precautions

Effects on Dental Treatment Key adverse event(s) related to dental treatment: Ulcerative esophagitis.

Effects on Bleeding No information available to require special precautions

Adverse Reactions Frequency not defined.

Cardiovascular: Cardiac failure, cardiomyopathy, edema, facial edema, hypertension

Central nervous system: Headache, insomnia, malaise, myasthenia, nervousness, pseudotumor cerebri, psychological disorder, seizure, vertigo

Dermatologic: Diaphoresis, facial erythema, skin atrophy, suppression of skin test reaction, urticaria

Endocrine & metabolic: Cushing's syndrome, diabetes mellitus, growth suppression, hirsutism, HPA-axis suppression, hyperglycemia, hypernatremia, hypokalemia, hypokalemic alkalosis, menstrual disease, negative nitrogen balance, weight gain

Gastrointestinal: Abdominal distention, carbohydrate intolerance, dyspepsia, increased appetite, nausea, pancreatitis, peptic ulcer, ulcerative esophagitis

Hematologic & oncologic: Bruise, petechia

Hepatic: Increased liver enzymes (usually reversible)

Neuromuscular & skeletal: Amyotrophy, arthralgia, aseptic necrosis of bones (humeral/femoral heads), bone fracture, rupture of tendon, weakness

Ophthalmic: Cataract, exophthalmos, eye irritation, eyelid edema, glaucoma, increased intraocular pressure

Respiratory: Epistaxis

Miscellaneous: Wound healing impairment

<1%, postmarketing, and/or case reports: Venous thrombosis (Johannesdottir 2013)

Dosing

Adult Dose depends upon condition being treated and response of patient. Consider alternate day therapy for long-term therapy. Discontinuation of long-term therapy requires gradual withdrawal by tapering the dose.

Usual dose (range): Oral: 5 to 60 mg/day

Adrenal insufficiency, chronic (primary, classic congenital adrenal hyperplasia) (off-label dose; alternative agent): Oral: 3 to 6 mg daily in 1 to 2 divided doses; use of a liquid dosage form may be preferable to allow for better dose titration (Endocrine Society [Bornstein 2016]; Endocrine Society [Speiser 2018]).

Alcoholic hepatitis (severe) (Maddrey Discriminant Function [MDF] score ≥32) (off-label use): Oral: 40 mg daily for 28 days, followed by a 2 to 4 week taper (AASLD [O'Shea 2010]; ACG [Singal 2018]).

Asthma exacerbations: Oral:

Global Initiative for Asthma guidelines (GINA 2020): Management in primary care or acute care facility: 40 to 50 mg/day as a single daily dose usually given for 5 to 7 days.

National Asthma Education and Prevention Program guidelines (NAEPP 2007):

Asthma exacerbations (emergency care or hospital doses): 40 to 80 mg/day in a single dose or in 2 divided doses until peak expiratory flow is 70% of predicted or personal best.

Short-course outpatient "burst" (acute asthma): 40 to 60 mg/day in a single dose or in 2 divided doses for 5 to 10 days. **Note:** Burst should be continued until symptoms resolve and peak expiratory flow is at least 80% of personal best; usually requires 3 to 10 days of treatment; longer treatment may be required.

Long-term treatment: 7.5 to 60 mg daily given as a single dose in the morning or every other day as needed for asthma control.

Bell's palsy (off-label use): Oral: 60 mg once daily for 5 days, then taper dose downward by 10 mg daily for 5 days (total treatment duration: 10 days) (Berg 2012; Engstrom 2008) **or** 50 mg daily (in 1 or 2 divided doses) for 10 days (begin within 72 hours of onset of symptoms) (Baugh 2013; Sullivan 2007).

Chronic obstructive pulmonary disease (acute exacerbation) (off-label use): Oral: 40 mg daily for 5 to 7 days (GOLD 2019).

Gout, acute flares: Oral: 0.5 mg/kg/day for 5 to 10 days followed by discontinuation (ACR [Khanna 2012]) **or** 30 to 40 mg/day given once daily or in 2 divided doses until symptom improvement, followed by a 7- to 10-day taper (or 14- to 21-day taper in patients with multiple prior flares) (Becker 2018).

Multiple sclerosis:

Note: Treatment guidelines recommend the use of high dose IV or oral methylprednisolone for acute exacerbations of multiple sclerosis (AAN [Scott 2011]; NICE 2014).

Oral: 200 mg daily for 1 week followed by 80 mg every other day for 1 month.

Geriatric Refer to adult dosing; use lowest effective dose.

Renal Impairment: Adult There are no dosage adjustments provided in the manufacturer's labeling. Use with caution.

Hemodialysis: Slightly dialyzable (7% to 17.5%) (Frey 1990).

Intermittent hemodialysis: Supplemental dose necessary (Aronoff 2007).

Peritoneal dialysis: Supplemental dose is not necessary (Aronoff 2007).

Hepatic Impairment: Adult There are no dosage adjustments provided in the manufacturer's labeling. Use with caution.

Pediatric Note: Dose depends upon condition being treated and response of patient; dosage for infants and children should be based on disease severity and patient response, rather than by rigid adherence to dosage guidelines by age, weight, or body surface area. Consider alternate day therapy for long-term therapy. Discontinuation of long-term therapy requires gradual withdrawal by tapering the dose.

Bronchopulmonary dysplasia, treatment: Infants: Oral: 2 mg/kg/day divided twice daily for 5 days, followed by 1 mg/kg/day once daily for 3 days, followed by 1 mg/kg/dose every other day for 3 doses was used in 131 former premature neonates (postmenstrual age: ≥36 weeks) with BPD; results showed weaning of supplemental oxygen was facilitated in patients with capillary pCO_2 <48.5 mm Hg and pulmonary acuity score <0.5 (Bhandari 2008)

Asthma: NIH Asthma Guidelines (NAEPP 2007):

Infants and Children <12 years: Oral:

Asthma exacerbations (emergency care or hospital doses): 1 to 2 mg/kg/day in 2 divided doses (maximum: 60 mg/day) until peak expiratory flow is 70% of predicted or personal best

Short-course "burst" (acute asthma): 1 to 2 mg/kg/day in divided doses 1 to 2 times/day for 3 to 10 days; maximum dose: 60 mg/day; **Note:** Burst should be continued until symptoms resolve or patient achieves peak expiratory flow 80% of personal best; usually requires 3 to 10 days of treatment (~5 days on average); longer treatment may be required

Long-term treatment: 0.25 to 2 mg/kg/day given as a single dose in the morning or every other day as needed for asthma control; maximum dose: 60 mg/day

Children ≥12 years and Adolescents: Oral:

Asthma exacerbations (emergency care or hospital doses): 40 to 80 mg/day in divided doses 1 to 2 times/day until peak expiratory flow is 70% of predicted or personal best

Short-course "burst" (acute asthma): 40 to 60 mg/day in divided doses 1 to 2 times/day for 3 to 10 days; **Note:** Burst should be continued until symptoms resolve and peak expiratory flow is at least 80% of personal best; usually requires 3 to 10 days of treatment (~5 days on average); longer treatment may be required

Long-term treatment: 7.5 to 60 mg daily given as a single dose in the morning or every other day as needed for asthma control

Anti-inflammatory or immunosuppressive dose: Infants, Children, and Adolescents: Oral: 0.1 to 2 mg/kg/day in divided doses 1 to 4 times/day

Kawasaki disease (KD), treatment: Limited data available: **Note:** Use to transition patients receiving IV corticosteroids for treatment of KD (in combination with IVIG and aspirin). Infants and Children: Oral: 2 mg/kg/day in divided doses every 8 hours until CRP normalizes; maximum daily dose: 60 mg/**day**; once CRP normalized, decrease dose every 5 days using the following taper: 2 mg/kg/day for 5 days (maximum daily dose: 60 mg/**day**), then 1 mg/kg/day for 5 days (maximum daily dose: 30 mg/**day**), then 0.5 mg/kg/day for 5 days (maximum daily dose: 15 mg/**day**), then discontinue; a longer course, tapering over 2 to 3 weeks, may be considered (AHA [McCrindle 2017]; Kobayashi 2012; Kobayashi 2013)

Nephrotic syndrome; steroid-sensitive (SSNS): Children and Adolescents: **Note:** Obese patients should be dosed based on ideal body weight: Oral:

Initial episode: 2 mg/kg/day or 60 mg/m^2/day once daily, maximum daily dose: 60 mg/**day** for 4 to 6 weeks; then adjust to an alternate-day schedule of 1.5 mg/kg/dose or 40 mg/m^2/dose on alternate days as a single dose, maximum dose: 40 mg/dose (Gipson 2009; KDIGO 2012; KDOQI 2013); duration of therapy based on patient response.

Relapse: 2 mg/kg/day or 60 mg/m^2/day once daily, maximum daily dose: 60 mg/**day**; continue until complete remission for at least 3 days; then adjust to an alternate-day schedule of 1.5 mg/kg/dose or 40 mg/m^2/dose on alternate days as a single dose, maximum dose: 40 mg/dose, recommended duration of alternate day dosing is variable: may continue for at least 4 weeks then taper. Longer duration of treatment may be necessary in patients who relapse frequently, some patients may require up to 3 months of treatment (Gipson 2009; KDIGO 2012; KDOQI 2013).

Maintenance therapy for frequently relapsing SSNS: Taper previous dose down to lowest effective dose which maintains remission using an alternate day schedule; usual effective range: 0.1 to 0.5 mg/kg/dose on alternating days; other patients may require doses up to 0.7 mg/kg/dose every other day (KDIGO 2012; KDOQI 2013)

Renal Impairment: Pediatric There are no dosage adjustments provided in the manufacturer's labeling. Use with caution.

Hepatic Impairment: Pediatric There are no dosage adjustments provided in the manufacturer's labeling. Use with caution.

Mechanism of Action Decreases inflammation by suppression of migration of polymorphonuclear leukocytes and reversal of increased capillary permeability; suppresses the immune system by reducing activity and volume of the lymphatic system

Contraindications

Hypersensitivity to prednisolone or any component of the formulation; live or attenuated virus vaccines (with immunosuppressive doses of corticosteroids); systemic fungal infections.

Canadian labeling: Additional contraindications (not in US labeling): Chicken pox; measles; uncontrolled active infections.

Documentation of allergenic cross-reactivity for corticosteroids is limited. However, because of similarities in chemical structure and/or pharmacologic actions, the possibility of cross-sensitivity cannot be ruled out with certainty.

Warnings/Precautions May cause hypercortisolism or suppression of hypothalamic-pituitary-adrenal (HPA) axis, particularly in younger children or in patients receiving high doses for prolonged periods. HPA axis suppression may lead to adrenal crisis. Withdrawal and discontinuation of a corticosteroid should be done slowly and carefully. Particular care is required when patients are transferred from systemic corticosteroids to inhaled products due to possible adrenal insufficiency or withdrawal from steroids, including an increase in allergic symptoms. Adult patients receiving >20 mg per day of prednisone (or equivalent) may be most susceptible. Fatalities have occurred due to adrenal insufficiency in asthmatic patients during and after transfer from systemic corticosteroids to aerosol steroids; aerosol steroids do **not** provide the systemic steroid needed to treat patients having trauma, surgery, or infections. Use with caution in patients with systemic sclerosis; an increase in scleroderma renal crisis incidence has been observed with corticosteroid use. Monitor BP and renal function in patients with systemic sclerosis treated with corticosteroids (EULAR [Kowal-Bielecka 2017]).

Acute myopathy has been reported with high dose corticosteroids, usually in patients with neuromuscular transmission disorders; may involve ocular and/or respiratory muscles; monitor creatine kinase; recovery may be delayed. Corticosteroid use may cause psychiatric disturbances, including severe depression, euphoria, insomnia, mood swings, and personality changes to frank psychotic manifestations. Preexisting psychiatric conditions may be exacerbated by corticosteroid use. Prolonged use of corticosteroids may also increase the incidence of secondary infection, mask acute infection (including fungal infections) or prolong or exacerbate viral infections or limit response to killed or inactivated vaccines. Exposure to chickenpox or measles should be avoided; corticosteroids should not be used to treat ocular herpes simplex. Corticosteroids should not be used for cerebral malaria or viral hepatitis. Close observation is required in patients with latent tuberculosis and/or TB reactivity; restrict use in active TB (only fulminating or disseminated TB in conjunction with antituberculosis treatment). Amebiasis should be ruled out in any patient with recent travel to tropic climates or unexplained diarrhea prior to initiation of corticosteroids. Use with extreme caution in patients with *Strongyloides* infections; hyperinfection, dissemination and fatalities have occurred. Increased intraocular pressure, open-angle glaucoma, and cataracts have occurred with prolonged use. Use with caution in patients with a history of ocular herpes simplex; corneal perforation has occurred; do not use in active ocular herpes simplex. Not recommended for the treatment of optic neuritis; may increase frequency of new episodes. Consider routine eye exams in chronic users. Prolonged treatment with corticosteroids has been associated with the development of Kaposi sarcoma (case reports); if noted, discontinuation of therapy should be considered (Goedert 2002). Rare cases of anaphylactoid reactions have been observed in patients receiving corticosteroids.

Use with caution in patients with thyroid disease, hepatic impairment, renal impairment, heart failure, hypertension, diabetes, glaucoma, cataracts, myasthenia gravis, patients at risk for osteoporosis, patients at risk for seizures, or GI diseases (diverticulitis, fresh intestinal anastomoses, active or latent peptic ulcer, ulcerative colitis, abscess or other pyogenic infection). Use caution following acute MI (corticosteroids have been associated with myocardial rupture). Use cautiously in the elderly with the smallest possible effective dose for the shortest duration. Withdraw therapy with gradual tapering of dose. May affect growth velocity; growth should be routinely monitored in pediatric patients. Patients may require higher doses when subject to stress (ie, trauma, surgery, severe infection). Potentially significant drug-drug interactions may exist, requiring dose or frequency adjustment, additional monitoring, and/or selection of alternative therapy.

Benzyl alcohol and derivatives: Some dosage forms may contain sodium benzoate/benzoic acid; benzoic acid (benzoate) is a metabolite of benzyl alcohol; large amounts of benzyl alcohol (≥99 mg/kg/day) have been associated with a potentially fatal toxicity ("gasping syndrome") in neonates; the "gasping syndrome" consists of metabolic acidosis, respiratory distress, gasping respirations, CNS dysfunction (including convulsions, intracranial hemorrhage), hypotension, and cardiovascular collapse (AAP ["Inactive" 1997]; CDC 1982); some data suggests that benzoate displaces bilirubin from protein binding sites (Ahlfors 2001); avoid or use dosage forms containing benzyl alcohol derivative with caution in neonates. See manufacturer's labeling.

Propylene glycol: Some dosage forms may contain propylene glycol; large amounts are potentially toxic and have been associated hyperosmolality, lactic acidosis, seizures, and respiratory depression; use caution (AAP 1997; Zar 2007).

Warnings: Additional Pediatric Considerations May cause osteoporosis (at any age) or inhibition of bone growth in pediatric patients. Use with caution in patients with osteoporosis. In a population-based study of children, risk of fracture was shown to be increased with >4 courses of corticosteroids; underlying clinical condition may also impact bone health and osteoporotic effect of corticosteroids (Leonard, 2007). Increased IOP may occur, especially with prolonged use; in children, increased IOP has been shown to be dose dependent and produce a greater IOP in children <6 years than older children treated with ophthalmic dexamethasone (Lam, 2005). Corticosteroids have been associated with myocardial rupture; hypertrophic cardiomyopathy has been reported in premature neonates.

Some dosage forms may contain propylene glycol; in neonates large amounts of propylene glycol delivered orally, intravenously (eg, >3,000 mg/day), or topically have been associated with potentially fatal toxicities which can include metabolic acidosis, seizures, renal failure, and CNS depression; toxicities have also been reported in children and adults including hyperosmolality, lactic acidosis, seizures, and respiratory depression; use caution (AAP, 1997; Shehab, 2009).

Drug Interactions

Metabolism/Transport Effects **Substrate** of CYP3A4 (minor); **Note:** Assignment of Major/Minor substrate status based on clinically relevant drug interaction potential

Avoid Concomitant Use

Avoid concomitant use of PrednisoLONE (Systemic) with any of the following: Aldesleukin; BCG (Intravesical); Cladribine; Desmopressin; Fexinidazole [INT]; Indium 111 Capromab Pendetide; Macimorelin; Mifamurtide; MiFEPRIStone; Natalizumab; Pimecrolimus; Tacrolimus (Topical)

Increased Effect/Toxicity

PrednisoLONE (Systemic) may increase the levels/effects of: Acetylcholinesterase Inhibitors;

Amphotericin B; Androgens; Baricitinib; CycloSPORINE (Systemic); Deferasirox; Desirudin; Desmopressin; Fexinidazole [INT]; Fingolimod; Leflunomide; Loop Diuretics; Natalizumab; Nicorandil; Nonsteroidal Anti-Inflammatory Agents (COX-2 Selective); Nonsteroidal Anti-Inflammatory Agents (Nonselective); Ozanimod; Quinolones; Ritodrine; Sargramostim; Siponimod; Thiazide and Thiazide-Like Diuretics; Tofacitinib; Upadacitinib; Vaccines (Live); Vitamin K Antagonists

The levels/effects of PrednisoLONE (Systemic) may be increased by: Aprepitant; Cladribine; CycloSPORINE (Systemic); CYP3A4 Inhibitors (Strong); Denosumab; DilTIAZem; Estrogen Derivatives; Fosaprepitant; Indacaterol; Inebilizumab; MiFEPRIStone; Neuromuscular-Blocking Agents (Nondepolarizing); Ocrelizumab; Pimecrolimus; Ritonavir; Roflumilast; Salicylates; Tacrolimus (Topical); Trastuzumab

Decreased Effect

PrednisoLONE (Systemic) may decrease the levels/effects of: Aldesleukin; Antidiabetic Agents; Axicabtagene Ciloleucel; BCG (Intravesical); Calcitriol (Systemic); Coccidioides immitis Skin Test; Corticorelin; Cosyntropin; CycloSPORINE (Systemic); Hyaluronidase; Indium 111 Capromab Pendetide; Isoniazid; Macimorelin; Mifamurtide; Nivolumab; Pidotimod; Salicylates; Sipuleucel-T; Somatropin; Tacrolimus (Systemic); Tertomotide; Tisagenlecleucel; Urea Cycle Disorder Agents; Vaccines (Inactivated); Vaccines (Live)

The levels/effects of PrednisoLONE (Systemic) may be decreased by: Antacids; Bile Acid Sequestrants; Carbimazole; CYP3A4 Inducers (Strong); Echinacea; MethIMAzole; MiFEPRIStone; Mitotane

Dietary Considerations Should be taken after meals or with food or milk to decrease GI upset; increase dietary intake of pyridoxine, vitamin C, vitamin D, folate, calcium, and phosphorus.

Pharmacodynamics/Kinetics

Duration of Action 18 to 36 hours (Pickup 1979)

Half-life Elimination 2 to 4 hours; reduced in children and prolonged in hepatic disease (Pickup 1979)

Time to Peak Plasma: 1 to 2 hours; prolonged with food

Pregnancy Considerations

Prednisolone crosses the placenta; prior to reaching the fetus, prednisolone is converted by placental enzymes to prednisone. As a result, the amount of prednisolone reaching the fetus is ~8 to 10 times lower than the maternal serum concentration (healthy women at term; similar results observed with preterm pregnancies complicated by HELLP syndrome) (Beitins 1972; van Runnard Heimel 2005). Some studies have shown an association between first trimester systemic corticosteroid use and oral clefts or decreased birth weight; however, information is conflicting and may be influenced by maternal dose/indication for use (Lunghi 2010; Park-Wyllie 2000; Pradat 2003). Hypoadrenalism may occur in newborns following maternal use of corticosteroids in pregnancy; monitor.

Prednisolone may be used (alternative agent) to treat primary adrenal insufficiency (PAI) in pregnant women. Pregnant females with PAI should be monitored at least once each trimester (Endocrine Society [Bornstein 2016]). Prednisolone may be used to treat females during pregnancy who require therapy for congenital adrenal hyperplasia (Endocrine Society [Speiser 2018]).

When systemic corticosteroids are needed in pregnancy for rheumatic disorders, it is generally recommended to use the lowest effective dose for the shortest duration of time, avoiding high doses during the first trimester (Götestam Skorpen 2016; Makol 2011; Østensen 2009).

For dermatologic disorders in pregnant females, systemic corticosteroids are generally not preferred for initial therapy; should be avoided during the first trimester; and used during the second or third trimester at the lowest effective dose (Bae 2012; Leachman 2006). Topical agents are preferred for managing atopic dermatitis in pregnancy; for severe symptomatic or recalcitrant atopic dermatitis, a short course of prednisolone may be used during the third trimester (Koutroulis 2011).

Uncontrolled asthma is associated with adverse events in pregnancy (increased risk of perinatal mortality, preeclampsia, preterm birth, low birth weight infants, cesarean delivery, and the development of gestational diabetes). Poorly controlled asthma or asthma exacerbations may have a greater fetal/maternal risk than what is associated with appropriately used asthma medications. Maternal treatment improves pregnancy outcomes by reducing the risk of some adverse events (eg, preterm birth, gestational diabetes). Inhaled corticosteroids are recommended for the treatment of asthma during pregnancy; however, systemic corticosteroids should be used to control acute exacerbations or treat severe persistent asthma. Maternal asthma symptoms should be monitored monthly during pregnancy (ERS/TSANZ [Middleton 2020]; GINA 2020).

Breastfeeding Considerations Prednisolone is present in breast milk.

The relative infant dose (RID) of prednisolone is 4% when calculated using the highest breast milk concentration located and compared to a weight-adjusted maternal dose of 80 mg/day.

In general, breastfeeding is considered acceptable when the RID of a medication is <10% (Anderson 2016; Ito 2000).

The RID of prednisolone was calculated using a milk concentration of 317 ng/mL, providing an estimated daily infant dose via breast milk of 0.05 mg/kg/day. This milk concentration was obtained following maternal administration oral prednisolone 80 mg/day to a woman 53 days' postpartum. Using data from all women in this study, (n=6), milk concentrations were 5% to 25% of the maternal serum concentration with peak concentrations occurring ~1 hour after the maternal dose. The milk/plasma ratio was found to be 0.2 with doses ≥30 mg/day and 0.1 with doses <30 mg/day (Ost 1985).

One manufacturer notes that when used systemically, maternal use of corticosteroids have the potential to cause adverse events in a breastfeeding infant (eg, growth suppression, interfere with endogenous corticosteroid production). Therefore, the decision to breastfeed during therapy should consider the risk of infant exposure, the benefits of breastfeeding to the infant, and benefits of treatment to the mother.

Corticosteroids are generally considered acceptable in breastfeeding females when used in usual doses (Götestam Skorpen 2016; WHO 2002); however, monitoring of the infant is recommended (WHO 2002). If there is concern about exposure to the infant, some guidelines recommend waiting 4 hours after the maternal dose of an oral systemic corticosteroid before breastfeeding in order to decrease potential exposure to the breastfed infant (Bae 2012; Butler 2014; ERS/TSANZ [Middleton 2020]; Götestam Skorpen 2016; Leachman 2006; Makol 2011; Ost 1985).

Dosage Forms Considerations

Orapred oral solution contains fructose.

Orapred ODT dispersible tablets contain sucrose.

Dosage Forms: US

Solution, Oral:

Pediapred: 5 mg/5 mL (120 mL)

Generic: 10 mg/5 mL (237 mL); 15 mg/5 mL (237 mL, 240 mL, 480 mL); 20 mg/5 mL (237 mL); 25 mg/5 mL (30 mL, 237 mL); 5 mg/5 mL (120 mL)

Tablet, Oral:

Millipred: 5 mg

Millipred DP 12-Day: 5 mg

Tablet Disintegrating, Oral:

Orapred ODT: 10 mg, 15 mg, 30 mg

Generic: 10 mg, 15 mg, 30 mg

Dosage Forms: Canada

Solution, Oral:

Pediapred: 5 mg/5 mL (120 mL)

Generic: 5 mg/5 mL (120 mL)

◆ **Prednisolone Sodium Phosphate** *see* PredniSOLONE (Systemic) *on page 1255*

◆ **Prednisolone Sod Phosphate** *see* PredniSOLONE (Systemic) *on page 1255*

PredniSONE (PRED ni sone)

Related Information

PredniSOLONE (Systemic) *on page 1255*

Respiratory Diseases *on page 1680*

Rheumatoid Arthritis, Osteoarthritis, and Osteoporosis *on page 1697*

Ulcerative, Erosive, and Painful Oral Mucosal Disorders *on page 1758*

Related Sample Prescriptions

Ulcerative and Erosive Disorders - Sample Prescriptions *on page 46*

Brand Names: US Deltasone; predniSONE Intensol; Rayos

Brand Names: Canada APO-PredniSONE; TEVA-PredniSONE; Winpred

Generic Availability (US) May be product dependent

Pharmacologic Category Corticosteroid, Systemic

Use

Anti-inflammatory or immunosuppressant agent in the treatment of a variety of diseases, including allergic, hematologic (eg, immune thrombocytopenia, warm autoimmune hemolytic anemia), dermatologic, GI, inflammatory, ophthalmic, neoplastic, rheumatic (eg, acute gout flare, vasculitis, dermatomyositis, mixed cryoglobulinemia syndrome, polyarteritis nodosa, polymyositis, polymyalgia rheumatica, rheumatoid arthritis, systemic lupus erythematosus), autoimmune, nervous system (eg, acute exacerbations of multiple sclerosis), renal, respiratory (eg, asthma), and endocrine (eg, primary or secondary adrenocorticoid deficiency); solid organ rejection (acute/chronic).

Local Anesthetic/Vasoconstrictor Precautions

No information available to require special precautions

Effects on Dental Treatment No significant effects or complications reported (see Dental Health Professional Considerations)

Effects on Bleeding No information available to require special precautions

Adverse Reactions Frequency not defined.

Cardiovascular: Cardiac failure (in susceptible patients), hypertension

Central nervous system: Emotional lability, headache, increased intracranial pressure (with papilledema), myasthenia, psychiatric disturbance (including euphoria, insomnia, mood swings, personality changes, severe depression), seizure, vertigo

Dermatologic: Diaphoresis, facial erythema, skin atrophy, urticaria

Endocrine & metabolic: Cushing's syndrome, decreased serum potassium, diabetes mellitus, fluid retention, growth suppression (children), hypokalemic alkalosis, hypothyroidism (enhanced), menstrual disease, negative nitrogen balance (due to protein catabolism), sodium retention

Gastrointestinal: Abdominal distention, carbohydrate intolerance, pancreatitis, peptic ulcer (with possible perforation and hemorrhage), ulcerative esophagitis

Hematologic & oncologic: Bruise, Kaposi's sarcoma, petechia

Hepatic: Increased serum alkaline phosphatase, increased serum ALT, increased serum AST

Hypersensitivity: Anaphylaxis, hypersensitivity reaction

Infection: Infection

Neuromuscular & skeletal: Amyotrophy, aseptic necrosis of bones (femoral and humeral heads), osteoporosis, pathological fracture (long bones), rupture of tendon (particularly Achilles tendon), steroid myopathy, vertebral compression fracture

Ophthalmic: Exophthalmos, glaucoma, increased intraocular pressure, subcapsular posterior cataract

Miscellaneous: Wound healing impairment

<1%, postmarketing, and/or case reports: Venous thrombosis (Johannesdottir 2013)

Dosing

Adult Note: Dosing: Evidence to support an optimal dose and duration is lacking for most indications; recommendations provided are general guidelines only and primarily based on expert opinion. In general, glucocorticoid dosing should be individualized and the minimum effective dose/duration should be used. For select indications with weight-based dosing, consider using ideal body weight in obese patients, especially with longer durations of therapy (Erstad 2004; Furst 2019a). **Hypothalamic-pituitary-adrenal (HPA) suppression:** Although some patients may become HPA suppressed with lower doses or briefer exposure, some experts consider HPA-axis suppression likely in any adult receiving >20 mg/day (daytime dosing) or ≥5 mg per 24 hours (evening or night dosing) for >3 weeks or with cushingoid appearance (Furst 2019b; Joseph 2016); do not abruptly discontinue treatment in these patients; dose tapering may be necessary (Cooper 2003).

Usual dosage range:

Oral: 10 to 60 mg/day given in a single daily dose or in 2 to 4 divided doses; *Low dose:* 2.5 to 10 mg/day; *High dose:* 1 to 1.5 mg/**kg**/day (usually not to exceed 80 to 100 mg/day).

The following dosing is from the commercially available tapered-dosage product (eg, dose pack containing 21 x 5 mg tablets):

Day 1: 30 mg on day 1 administered as 10 mg (2 tablets) at breakfast, 5 mg (1 tablet) at lunch, 5 mg (1 tablet) at dinner, and 10 mg (2 tablets) at bedtime.

Day 2: 25 mg on day 2 administered as 5 mg (1 tablet) at breakfast, 5 mg (1 tablet) at lunch, 5 mg (1 tablet) at dinner, and 10 mg (2 tablets) at bedtime.

Day 3: 20 mg on day 3 administered as 5 mg (1 tablet) at breakfast, 5 mg (1 tablet) at lunch, 5 mg (1 tablet) at dinner, and 5 mg (1 tablet) at bedtime.

Day 4: 15 mg on day 4 administered as 5 mg (1 tablet) at breakfast, 5 mg (1 tablet) at lunch, and 5 mg (1 tablet) at bedtime.

Day 5: 10 mg on day 5 administered as 5 mg (1 tablet) at breakfast and 5 mg (1 tablet) at bedtime.

Day 6: 5 mg on day 6 administered as 5 mg (1 tablet) at breakfast.

Indication-specific dosing:

Adrenal insufficiency, primary chronic (alternative agent): Note: In general, hydrocortisone is preferred. Use in conjunction with fludrocortisone. Dose is based on prednisolone equivalency.

Oral: 2.5 to 7.5 mg once daily (Bornstein 2016; Nieman 2019).

Allergic conditions:

Angioedema (acute allergic) and/or urticaria (acute): **Note:** For moderate to severe symptoms without signs of anaphylaxis. Use epinephrine if anaphylaxis symptoms (eg, risk of airway or cardiovascular compromise) are present (Cicardi 2014; Zuraw 2019). In patients with acute urticaria, consider reserving use for patients with significant angioedema or whose symptoms are unresponsive to antihistamines (Asero 2020; Bernstein 2014; EAACI [Zuberbier 2018]; Powell 2015). The optimal dosing strategy has not been defined (Bernstein 2014; EAACI [Zuberbier 2018]; James 2017; Powell 2015).

Oral: Initial: 20 to 40 mg daily in 1 to 2 divided doses for 3 to 4 days (EAACI [Zuberbier 2018]; Powell 2015; Zuraw 2019). May consider tapering the dose for a total treatment duration of ≤10 days (EAACI [Zuberbier 2018]; Zuraw 2019).

Asthma, acute exacerbation: Note: For moderate to severe exacerbations or in patients who do not respond promptly and completely to short-acting beta agonists; administer within 1 hour of presentation to emergency department (GINA 2020; NAEPP 2007).

Oral: 40 to 60 mg daily for 3 to 10 days; administer in 1 or 2 divided doses. If symptoms do not resolve and peak expiratory flow is not at least 70% of personal best, then longer treatment may be required (NAEPP 2007).

Bell palsy, new onset (off-label use): Oral: 60 to 80 mg daily for 5 to 7 days; administer in 1 or 2 divided doses; may be followed by a 5-day taper. Treatment should begin within 72 hours of onset of symptoms; a concomitant antiviral agent may be indicated in select patients (Austin 1993; de Almeida 2014; Engström 2008; OHNS [Baugh 2013]; Ronthal 2020).

Chronic obstructive pulmonary disease, acute exacerbation (off-label use): Note: In patients with severe but not life-threatening exacerbations, oral regimens are recommended. In patients who cannot tolerate oral therapy (eg, shock, mechanically ventilated), use IV methylprednisolone (GOLD 2019; Stoller 2019).

Oral: 40 to 60 mg once daily for 5 to 14 days (GOLD 2019; Stoller 2019). **Note:** The optimal dose has not been established. If patient improves with therapy, may discontinue without taper. If patient does not improve, a longer duration of therapy may be indicated (Stoller 2019).

Chronic spontaneous urticaria, acute exacerbation (off-label use): Note: For the temporary control of severe exacerbations (Bernstein 2014; EAACI [Zuberbier 2018]; Powell 2015).

Oral: 35 to 40 mg once daily until symptoms are controlled (usually occurs after 2 to 3 days of therapy) (Bernstein 2014; Khan 2020; Powell 2015); then taper by 5 to 10 mg/day over a period of 2 to 3 weeks followed by discontinuation (Khan 2020).

Duchenne muscular dystrophy (off-label use):

Oral: 0.75 mg/kg/day (AAN [Gloss 2016]; Escolar 2011). Some experts use a maximum dose of 40 mg/day due to potential for greater adverse effects and decreased benefit at higher doses (Darras 2020).

Note: In patients who experience intolerable adverse effects, may decrease the dose by 25% to 33% (Birnkrant 2018). If adverse effects persist, continue to gradually taper to as low as 0.3 mg/kg/day, which may provide benefit (AAN [Gloss 2016]; Darras 2020). Doses as high as 1.5 mg/kg/day have been studied, but there is no evidence that doses >0.75 mg/kg/day provide greater efficacy (AAN [Gloss 2016]; Matthews 2016).

Giant cell arteritis, treatment (off-label use):

Note: To reduce the risk of visual loss, start treatment **immediately** once diagnosis is highly suspected (BSR/BHPR [Dasgupta 2010]; Loddenkemper 2007). In patients presenting **with** threatened/evolving vision loss, pulse IV methylprednisolone is suggested as initial therapy prior to an oral glucocorticoid (eg, prednisone) (Docken 2019a).

*Initial therapy in patients presenting **without** vision loss (or following initial therapy with pulse IV methylprednisolone in patients **with** threatened/evolving vision loss):* **Oral:** High-dose: 1 mg/kg (maximum: 60 mg/day) once daily for 2 to 4 weeks; once signs/symptoms have declined and laboratory values have returned to normal or near normal, begin to taper until discontinuation over the next 6 to 12 months (BSR/BHPR [Dasgupta 2010]; Docken 2019a; González-Gay 2018).

Gout, acute flare: Oral: 0.5 mg/kg/day for 5 to 10 days followed by discontinuation (ACR [Khanna 2012]) **or** 30 to 40 mg/day given once daily or in 2 divided doses until symptom improvement, followed by a 7- to 10-day taper (or 14- to 21-day taper in patients with multiple prior flares) (Becker 2019). If unable to take orally, consider intra-articular or parenteral methylprednisolone.

Graft-versus-host disease, acute, treatment (off-label use): Note: For grade II or higher acute graft-versus-host disease. An optimal regimen has not been identified; refer to institutional protocols as variations exist. Treatment is dependent on the severity and the rate of progression (Martin 2012; Ruutu 2014).

Oral: Initial: 2 to 2.5 mg/kg/day in divided doses; dose may vary based on organ involvement and severity. Continue for several weeks then taper over several months (Chao 2019; Martin 2012).

Hepatitis, autoimmune (off-label use): Note: Approach to treatment should be patient specific and guided by response to treatment. Monotherapy induction regimen included below; other induction regimens (eg, combination therapy with a glucocorticoid-sparing agent) may be used in select patients (AASLD [Manns 2010]; EASL 2015; Heneghan 2020).

Induction: Initial: **Oral:** 60 mg once daily for 1 week, followed by a taper (eg, reduce daily dose by 5 to 10 mg at weekly intervals) based on symptoms and laboratory values until 20 mg once daily is reached for maintenance of remission (AASLD [Manns 2010]). Some experts initiate therapy at 20 to 40 mg once daily depending on severity of disease (Heneghan 2020).

Maintenance: Further taper dose to one that maintains remission (eg, taper the dose by 2.5 to 5 mg/day at weekly intervals to reach 5 mg/day). Specific maintenance approach will depend on patient response to initial treatment and tapering (AASLD [Manns 2010]).

Immune thrombocytopenia: Note: Goal of therapy is to provide a safe platelet count to prevent clinically important bleeding rather than normalization of the platelet count (Arnold 2019).

Initial therapy: **Oral:** 1 mg/kg/day for 1 to 2 weeks, followed by a gradual taper (Arnold 2019) **or** 0.5 to 2 mg/kg/day for several days to several weeks until platelet count increases (Provan 2010).

Pregnancy associated: **Oral:** Initial: 10 to 20 mg once daily (ACOG 207 2019). Adjust to the minimum effective dose to achieve response; generally, continue for at least 21 days, then taper to the minimum effective dose required to maintain platelet count to prevent major bleeding (ACOG 207 2019; ASH [Neunert 2011]) **or** 1 mg/kg/day for 2 weeks, followed by a gradual taper (George 2019).

Fetal alloimmune thrombocytopenia (maternal administration): **Oral:** 0.5 to 1 mg/kg/day. Dose is dependent upon gestational age and risk of fetal/neonatal intracranial hemorrhage and is administered in addition to immune globulin IV (ACOG 207 2019; Pacheco 2011).

Inflammatory bowel disease:

Crohn disease (moderate to severe or select patients with mild disease), induction: **Note: Not** for long-term use (ACG [Lichtenstein 2018]).

Oral: 40 to 60 mg once daily for 7 to 14 days, followed by a taper of up to 3 months (eg, reduce dose by 5 mg/day at weekly intervals until 20 mg/day is reached, then further reduce by 2.5 to 5 mg/day at weekly intervals) (ACG [Lichtenstein 2018]). Tapering regimens vary; some experts recommend a more rapid taper with a goal of discontinuing therapy within 1 to 2 months; if symptoms return, may resume therapy and taper more slowly (Regueiro 2019). Steroid-sparing agents (eg, biologic agents, immunomodulators) should be introduced with a goal of discontinuing corticosteroid therapy as soon as possible (ACG [Lichtenstein 2018]).

Ulcerative colitis (moderate to severe), induction: **Note: Not** for long-term use (ACG [Rubin 2019]).

Oral: 40 to 60 mg/day in 1 to 2 divided doses. Clinical improvement is expected within 7 days; pace of tapering (usually over 1 to 3 months) should be guided by symptoms, cumulative steroid exposure, and onset of action of additional therapies (ACG [Rubin 2019]; al Hashash 2019; Cohen 2020).

Iodinated contrast media allergic-like reaction, prevention: Note: Generally reserved for patients with a prior allergic-like or unknown-type iodinated contrast reaction who will be receiving another iodinated contrast agent. Nonurgent premedication with an oral corticosteroid is generally preferred when contrast administration is scheduled to begin in ≥12 hours; however, consider an urgent (accelerated) regimen with an IV corticosteroid (eg, methylprednisolone) for those requiring contrast in <12 hours (ACR 2018).

Nonurgent regimen: **Oral:** 50 mg administered 13 hours, 7 hours, and 1 hour before contrast medium administration in combination with oral diphenhydramine 50 mg (administered 1 hour prior to contrast) (ACR 2018).

Minimal change disease, treatment (off-label use): Initial therapy: **Oral:** 1 mg/kg/day (maximum: 80 mg/day) once daily **or** 2 mg/kg every other day (maximum: 120 mg every other day) for 8 to 16 weeks (most patients experience remission by 16 weeks); after achieving remission, gradually taper (eg, decrease by 5 to 10 mg/week over a period of up to 6 months); the duration of initial pulse therapy and tapering schedule can vary (Hogan 2013; Meyrier 2019; Vivarelli 2017).

Multiple myeloma (previously untreated; transplant ineligible) (off-label use):

≥65 years of age or <65 years of age and transplant ineligible: **Oral:** 60 mg/m^2/day for 4 days (days 1 to 4) every 6 weeks for 9 cycles (dexamethasone at a dose of 20 mg was substituted for prednisone on day 1 of each cycle) in combination with daratumumab, bortezomib, and melphalan; after cycle 9, daratumumab is continued as a single agent (Mateos 2018) **or** 60 mg/m^2/day for 4 days (days 1 to 4) every 6 weeks (in combination with bortezomib and melphalan) for 9 cycles (San Miguel 2008) **or** 2 mg/kg/day for 4 days (days 1 to 4) every 6 weeks (in combination with melphalan and thalidomide) for 12 cycles (Facon 2007).

≥65 years of age: **Oral:** 2 mg/kg/day for 4 days (days 1 to 4) every 6 weeks (in combination with melphalan) for 12 cycles (Facon 2006).

Multiple sclerosis, acute exacerbation: Note: For patients with an acute exacerbation resulting in neurologic symptoms and increased disability or impairments in vision, strength, or cerebellar function (Olek 2019).

Initial pulse therapy using an oral glucocorticoid (alternative agent to IV methylprednisolone pulse therapy): **Oral:** 625 mg to 1.25 g daily for 3 to 7 days (5 days typically), either alone or followed by a taper (Morrow 2004; Olek 2019).

Taper following IV methylprednisolone or prednisone pulse therapy: **Oral:** 1 mg/kg/day (maximum: 80 mg/day), followed by a taper; total duration of oral therapy is usually 11 to 14 days (Goodin 2014; Murray 2006; Myhr 2009). Tapering schedules vary and some experts prefer to omit taper following initial pulse glucocorticoid therapy (Olek 2019).

Myasthenia gravis, crisis (adjunctive therapy) (off-label use): Note: Used in conjunction with immune globulin IV or plasma exchange (Bird 2019).

Oral: 1 mg/kg/day (usual dose range: 60 to 80 mg daily), followed by a taper (Bird 2019; Lacomis 2005).

Myopathies (dermatomyositis/polymyositis), treatment:

Initial therapy (or following initial therapy with pulse IV methylprednisolone in select patients): **Oral:** 1 mg/kg/day (maximum: 80 mg/day) as a single daily dose until improvement (usually for 4 to 6 weeks); then gradually tapered (total duration usually 9 to 12 months) (Dalakas 2011; Findlay 2015; Miller 2019). **Note:** Continuing high dose (1 mg/kg/day) for more than 6 weeks may increase risk of developing glucocorticoid-associated myopathy (Miller 2019).

Pericarditis, acute (alternative agent) (off-label use): Note: May be used for patients with contraindications (eg, renal failure) or incomplete response to aspirin/nonsteroidal anti-inflammatory drugs (NSAIDs) and colchicine (ESC [Adler 2015]). Glucocorticoid therapy early in the course of pericarditis is more likely to be associated with recurrent episodes (Imazio 2020).

Oral: 0.2 to 0.5 mg/kg/day until resolution of symptoms and normalization of CRP (2 to 4 weeks); then taper dose over 3 months (ESC [Adler 2015]; Imazio 2020).

***Pneumocystis* pneumonia, adjunctive therapy for moderate to severe disease (off-label use): Note:** Recommended when on room air PaO_2 <70 mm Hg or PAO_2-PaO_2 ≥35 mm Hg.

Oral: 40 mg twice daily on days 1 to 5 beginning as early as possible, followed by 40 mg once daily on days 6 to 10, then 20 mg once daily on days 11 to 21 (HHS [OI adult 2019]; Martin 2013; Sax 2020; Thomas 2019).

Polymyalgia rheumatica: Note: Goal of therapy is to alleviate symptoms; therapy has not been shown to improve prognosis or prevent progression to giant cell arteritis (Docken 2019b).

Oral: Initial: Usual dose: 15 mg/day in a single daily dose or in divided doses; some experts consider lower initial doses of 7.5 to 10 mg/day for smaller patients with mild symptoms or at high risk for side effects (eg, labile diabetes) and higher initial doses of 20 mg/day (or 25 mg/daily [rarely]) for patients with more severe symptoms. Divided doses may help with pain and stiffness in evenings and following morning. Once symptoms are controlled, maintain dose for 2 to 4 weeks and gradually taper (generally over a 1- to 2-year period); some patients may require longer treatment (Castañeda 2019; EULAR/ACR [Dejaco 2015]; Docken 2019b).

Prostate cancer, metastatic, castration resistant (off-label use): Oral: 5 mg twice daily (in combination with abiraterone) until disease progression or unacceptable toxicity (de Bono 2011; Ryan 2015) **or** 10 mg once daily (in combination with cabazitaxel) for up to 10 cycles (de Bono 2010) **or** 5 mg twice daily (in combination with docetaxel) for up to 10 cycles (Berthold 2008; Tannock 2004).

Systemic rheumatic disorders (eg, antineutrophil cytoplasmic antibody-associated vasculitis, mixed cryoglobulinemia syndrome, polyarteritis nodosa, rheumatoid arthritis, systemic lupus erythematosus): Note: The following dosage ranges are for guidance only; dosing should be highly individualized, taking into account disease severity, the specific disorder, and disease manifestations:

Mild to moderate disease: **Oral:** Initial: 5 to 30 mg/day in a single daily dose or in divided doses, then taper to the minimum effective dose, depending on response (ACR 2002; Cohen 2019a; Fervenza 2020; O'Dell 2019; Wallace 2019).

Severe disease: Initial therapy (or following initial therapy with pulse IV methylprednisolone in select patients):

Oral: Usual dose: Initial: 1 mg/kg/day (maximum: 60 to 80 mg/day) in a single daily dose or in divided doses; typically given for several weeks, then tapered gradually; may be given as part of an appropriate combination regimen; for severe systemic lupus erythematosus, up to 2 mg/kg/day may be given initially (Merkel 2020; Fervenza 2020; Muchtar 2017; Pietrogrande 2011; Wallace 2019).

Takayasu arteritis (off-label use): Oral: Initial: 40 to 60 mg daily in combination with appropriate steroid-sparing agent; gradually taper to lowest effective dose (ACCF/AHA [Hiratzka 2010]; EULAR [Hellmich 2020]); some experts initiate treatment with 1 mg/kg/day (maximum: 60 to 80 mg/day) (Merkel 2020). **Note:** Long-term therapy may be required to prevent progression (ACCF/AHA [Hiratzka 2010]; Merkel 2020).

Thyroiditis, subacute (off-label use): Note: For use in patients whose pain does not respond to full dose of NSAIDs over several days **or** patients who present initially with moderate to severe pain (ATA [Ross 2016]).

Oral: Initial: 40 mg/day for 1 to 2 weeks; gradually taper (eg, by 5 to 10 mg/day every 5 to 7 days) based on clinical response. If pain recurs, increase to the lowest dose that controlled the pain; maintain that dose for ~2 weeks and attempt to taper again (ATA [Ross 2016]; Burman 2020).

Tuberculosis, pulmonary (prevention of immune reconstitution inflammatory syndrome in HIV-infected patients) (off-label use): Note: For use in antiretroviral-naive patients with CD4 count ≤100 cells/mm^3 who start antiretroviral therapy within 30 days of antituberculosis therapy initiation (Meintjes 2018).

Oral: 40 mg once daily for 14 days, followed by 20 mg once daily for 14 days, during the first 4 weeks after initiation of antiretroviral therapy (Meintjes 2018).

Warm autoimmune hemolytic anemia: Oral: 1 to 2 mg/kg/day until a hemoglobin response has occurred (typically within 1 to 3 weeks). After hemoglobin stabilization, begin tapering to the lowest dose to maintain remission followed by gradual tapering with an eventual goal of discontinuation (total duration of therapy: 3 to 12 months); a clinician experienced with the treatment of hemolytic anemia should be involved with therapy (Barros 2010; Brodsky 2019; Roumier 2014; Zanella 2014).

Geriatric Refer to adult dosing; use the lowest effective dose.

Renal Impairment: Adult There are no dosage adjustments provided in the manufacturer's labeling. Hemodialysis: Supplemental dose is not necessary.

Hepatic Impairment: Adult There are no dosage adjustments provided in the manufacturer's labeling.

Pediatric

Note: All pediatric dosing based on immediate release products. Dose depends upon condition being treated and response of patient; dosage for infants and children should be based on disease severity and patient response rather than by rigid adherence to dosage guidelines by age, weight, or body surface area. Consider alternate day therapy for long-term therapy. Discontinuation of long-term therapy requires gradual withdrawal by tapering the dose.

General dosing; anti-inflammatory or immunosuppressive: Infants, Children, and Adolescents: Oral 0.05 to 2 mg/kg/day divided every 6 to 24 hours (Bertsias 2012; Kliegman 2007)

Asthma, acute exacerbation:

NAEPP 2007:

Infants and Children <12 years: Oral:

Emergency care or hospital doses: 1 to 2 mg/kg/day in 2 divided doses; maximum daily dose: 60 mg/**day**; continue until peak expiratory flow is 70% of predicted or personal best

Short-course "burst" (Outpatient): 1 to 2 mg/kg/day in divided doses 1 to 2 times daily for 3 to 10 days; maximum daily dose: 60 mg/**day**; **Note:** Burst should be continued until symptoms resolve or patient achieves peak expiratory flow 80% of personal best; usually requires 3 to 10 days of treatment (~5 days on average); longer treatment may be required

Children ≥12 years and Adolescents: Oral:

Emergency care or hospital doses: 40 to 80 mg/day in divided doses 1 to 2 times daily until peak expiratory flow is 70% of predicted or personal best

Short-course "burst" (Outpatient): 40 to 60 mg/day in divided doses 1 to 2 times daily for 3 to 10 days; **Note:** Burst should be continued until symptoms resolve and peak expiratory flow is at least 80% of personal best; usually requires 3 to 10 days of treatment (~5 days on average); longer treatment may be required

GINA 2014:

Infants and Children <12 years: Oral: 1 to 2 mg/kg/day for 3 to 5 days

Maximum daily dose age-dependent:

Infants and Children <2 years: 20 mg/**day**

Children 2 to 5 years: 30 mg/**day**

Children 6 to 11 years: 40 mg/**day**

Children ≥12 years and Adolescents: Oral: 1 mg/kg/day for 5 to 7 days; maximum daily dose 50 mg/**day**

Asthma, maintenance therapy (nonacute) (NAEPP 2007):

Infants and Children <12 year: Oral: 0.25 to 2 mg/kg/day administered as a single dose in the morning or every other day as needed for asthma control; maximum daily dose: 60 mg/**day**

Children ≥12 years and Adolescents: Oral: 7.5 to 60 mg daily administered as a single dose in the morning or every other day as needed for asthma control

Autoimmune hepatitis (monotherapy or in combination with azathioprine): Limited data available: Infants, Children, and Adolescents: Oral: Initial: 1 to 2 mg/kg/day for 2 weeks; maximum daily dose: 60 mg/**day**; taper upon response over 6 to 8 weeks to a dose of 0.1 to 0.2 mg/kg/day or 2.5 to 5 mg daily; an alternate day schedule to decrease risk of adverse effect has been used; however, a higher incidence of relapse has been observed in some cases and use is not suggested (AASLD [Manns 2010]; Della Corte 2012).

Bell palsy: Limited data available:

Infants, Children, and Adolescents <16 years: Oral: 1 mg/kg/day for 1 week, then taper over 1 week; ideally start within the 72 hours of onset of symptoms; maximum daily dose: 60 mg/**day** (Kliegman 2011)

Adolescents ≥16 years: Oral: 60 mg daily for 5 days, followed by a 5-day taper. Treatment should begin within 72 hours of onset of symptoms (OHNS [Baugh 2013]).

Congenital adrenal hyperplasia: Note: Individualize dose by monitoring growth, hormone levels, and bone age; mineralocorticoid (eg, fludrocortisone) and sodium supplement may be required in salt losers (AAP 2000; Endocrine Society [Speiser] 2010):

Infants, Children and Adolescents (actively growing): Not recommended because impedes statural growth more so than shorter-acting systemic glucocorticoid (ie, hydrocortisone) (Endocrine Society [Speiser] 2010)

Adolescents (fully grown): Oral: 5 to 7.5 mg daily in divided doses 2 times daily (Endocrine Society [Speiser] 2010)

Crohn disease: Children and Adolescents: Oral: 1 to 2 mg/kg/day; maximum daily dose: 60 mg/**day**; continue for 2 to 4 weeks until remission, then gradually taper (Kliegman 2011; Rufo 2012; Sandhu 2010)

Dermatomyositis, moderately severe; initial treatment: Limited data available: Children and Adolescents: Oral: Initial: 2 mg/kg/day divided once or twice daily; maximum daily dose: 60 mg/**day**; continue for 4 weeks then if adequate patient response, begin taper; most recommend an initial 20% reduction in dose with subsequent wean based upon response; use in combination with other immunosuppressants (eg, methotrexate) (CARRA [Huber 2010])

Immune thrombocytopenia (ITP): Infants, Children, and Adolescents: Oral: 1 to 2 mg/kg/day; titrate dose according to platelet count; when and if able, a rapid taper is recommended; a maximum duration of therapy of 14 days has been suggested; others have used a higher dose with shorter course of 4 mg/kg/day for 3 to 4 days (Neunert 2011; Provan 2010)

Juvenile idiopathic arthritis: Infants ≥6 months, Children and Adolescents: Oral: Initial: 1 mg/kg/day administered once daily (maximum daily dose: 60 mg/**day**); may be used in combination with methylprednisolone pulse therapy; evaluate initial response at 1 to 2 weeks and then at 1 month of therapy; if patient improves then taper prednisone, if unchanged then continue current prednisone therapy and if worsened then increase dose to 2 mg/kg/day (maximum daily dose: 100 mg/day). After 1 month, if improvement, begin taper; if condition worsens or unchanged then increase or continue prednisone dose at 2 mg/kg/day (maximum daily dose: 100 mg/day) and/or may add or repeat methylprednisolone pulse therapy. After 3 months of glucocorticoid therapy, if improvement (prednisone dose <50% starting dose), continue taper and reassess monthly; if patient remains unchanged (prednisone dose >50% of starting dose) or worsened, additional therapy should be considered (CARRA [Dewitt 2012])

Lupus nephritis: Children and Adolescents: Oral: Initial therapy:

With concurrent methylprednisolone pulse therapy: Prednisone: 0.5 to 1.5 mg/kg/day; maximum daily dose: 60 mg/**day**, taper usually over 6 months to a dose ≤10 mg/day according to clinical response; use in combination with cyclophosphamide or mycophenolate (Bertsias 2012; KDIGO 2012; KDOQI 2013; Mina 2012)

Without concurrent methylprednisolone pulse therapy: Prednisone: 2 mg/kg/day for 6 weeks, maximum daily dose variable: for weeks 1 to 4: maximum daily dose: 80 mg/**day** and for weeks 5 and 6: 60 mg/**day**; taper over 6 months; use in combination with cyclophosphamide or mycophenolate (Mina 2012)

Malignancy (antineoplastic): Note: Used for various types of malignancy and neoplasm; see specific protocols for details concerning dosing in combination regimens.

Hodgkin lymphoma (BEACOPP regimen): Children and Adolescents: Oral: 40 mg/m^2/day in 2 divided doses on days 0 to 13; in combination with bleomycin, etoposide, doxorubicin, cyclophosphamide, vincristine, and procarbazine (Kelly 2002; Kelly 2011)

Nephrotic syndrome; steroid-sensitive (SSNS): Children and Adolescents: **Note:** Obese patients should be dosed based on ideal body weight: Oral:

Initial episode: 2 mg/kg/day or 60 mg/m^2/day once daily, maximum daily dose: 60 mg/**day** for 4 to 6 weeks; then adjust to an alternate-day schedule of 1.5 mg/kg/dose or 40 mg/m^2/dose on alternate days as a single dose, maximum dose: 40 mg/dose (Gipson 2009; KDIGO 2012; KDOQI 2013); duration of therapy based on patient response.

Relapse: 2 mg/kg/day or 60 mg/m^2/day once daily, maximum daily dose: 60 mg/**day** continue until complete remission for at least 3 days; then adjust to an alternate-day schedule of 1.5 mg/kg/dose or 40 mg/m^2/dose on alternate days as a single dose, maximum dose: 40 mg/dose, recommended duration of alternate day dosing is variable: may continue for at least 4 weeks then taper. Longer duration of treatment may be necessary in patients who relapse frequently, some patients may require up to 3 months of treatment (Gipson 2009; KDIGO 2012; KDOQI 2013).

Maintenance therapy for frequently relapsing SSNS: Taper previous dose down to lowest effective dose which maintains remission using an alternate day schedule; usual effective range: 0.1 to 0.5 mg/kg/dose on alternating days; other patients may require doses up to 0.7 mg/kg/dose every other day (KDIGO 2012, KDOQI 2013)

Physiologic replacement: Children and Adolescents: Oral: 2 to 2.5 mg/m^2/day (Ahmet 2011; Gupta 2008). **Note:** Hydrocortisone is generally preferred in growing children and adolescents due to its lower growth suppressant effects compared to prednisone (Gupta 2008).

***Pneumocystis jirovecii* pneumonia (PCP), treatment; HIV-exposed/-positive: Note:** Begin as soon as possible after diagnosis and within 72 hours of PCP therapy initiation.

Infants and Children: Oral: 1 mg/kg/dose twice daily on days 1 to 5, then 0.5 to 1 mg/kg/dose twice daily on days 6 to 10, then 0.5 mg/kg/dose once daily for days 11 to 21 (DHHS [pediatric] 2013)

Adolescents: Oral: 40 mg twice daily on days 1 to 5, followed by 40 mg once daily on days 6 to 10, followed by 20 mg once daily on days 11 to 21 or until antimicrobial regimen is completed (DHHS [adult] 2014).

Ulcerative colitis: Children and Adolescents: Oral: 1 to 2 mg/kg/day administered in the morning; maximum daily dose: 60 mg/**day**; if no response after 7 to 14 days optimal dosing and compliance should be assessed (Kliegman 2011; Rufo 2012; Turner 2012)

Renal Impairment: Pediatric There are no dosage adjustments provided in the manufacturer's labeling; use with caution.

Hepatic Impairment: Pediatric There are no dosage adjustments provided in the manufacturer's labeling. Prednisone is inactive and must be metabolized by the liver to prednisolone. This conversion may be impaired in patients with liver disease; however, prednisolone levels are observed to be higher in patients with severe liver failure than in normal patients. Therefore, compensation for the inadequate conversion of prednisone to prednisolone occurs.

Mechanism of Action Decreases inflammation by suppression of migration of polymorphonuclear leukocytes and reversal of increased capillary permeability; suppresses the immune system by reducing activity and volume of the lymphatic system; suppresses adrenal function at high doses. Antitumor effects may be related to inhibition of glucose transport, phosphorylation, or induction of cell death in immature lymphocytes. Antiemetic effects are thought to occur due to blockade of cerebral innervation of the emetic center via inhibition of prostaglandin synthesis.

Contraindications Hypersensitivity to prednisone or any component of the formulation; administration of live or live attenuated vaccines with immunosuppressive doses of prednisone; systemic fungal infections

Canadian labeling: Additional contraindications (not in US labeling): Herpes simplex of the eye, measles, or chickenpox (except when being used for short-term or emergency therapy); peptic ulcer; nonspecific ulcerative colitis; diverticulitis; viral or bacterial infection not controlled by anti-infectives

Documentation of allergenic cross-reactivity for corticosteroids is limited. However, because of similarities in chemical structure and/or pharmacologic actions, the possibility of cross-sensitivity cannot be ruled out with certainty.

Warnings/Precautions May cause hypercortisolism or suppression of hypothalamic-pituitary-adrenal (HPA) axis, particularly in younger children or in patients receiving high doses for prolonged periods. HPA axis suppression may lead to adrenal crisis. Withdrawal and discontinuation of a corticosteroid should be done slowly and carefully. Particular care is required when patients are transferred from systemic corticosteroids to inhaled products due to possible adrenal insufficiency or withdrawal from steroids, including an increase in allergic symptoms. Adult patients receiving >20 mg per day of prednisone (or equivalent) may be most susceptible. Fatalities have occurred due to adrenal insufficiency in asthmatic patients during and after transfer from systemic corticosteroids to aerosol steroids; aerosol steroids do **not** provide the systemic steroid needed to treat patients having trauma, surgery, or infections.

Acute myopathy has been reported with high dose corticosteroids, usually in patients with neuromuscular transmission disorders; may involve ocular and/or respiratory muscles; monitor creatine kinase; recovery may be delayed. Prolonged use of corticosteroids may increase the incidence of secondary infection, mask acute infection (including fungal infections), prolong or exacerbate viral infections, or limit response to killed or inactivated vaccines. Exposure to chickenpox or measles should be avoided. Corticosteroids should not be used to treat viral hepatitis or cerebral malaria. Close observation is required in patients with latent tuberculosis (TB) and/or TB reactivity; restrict use in active TB (only fulminating or disseminated TB in conjunction with antituberculosis treatment). Latent or active amebiasis should be ruled out in any patient with recent travel to tropic climates or unexplained diarrhea prior to corticosteroid initiation. Use with extreme caution in patients with Strongyloides infections; hyperinfection, dissemination and fatalities have occurred. Prolonged treatment with corticosteroids has been associated with the development of Kaposi sarcoma (case reports); if noted, discontinuation of therapy should be considered (Goedert 2002). Use with caution in patients with cataracts and/or glaucoma; increased intraocular pressure, open-angle glaucoma, and cataracts have occurred with prolonged use. Use with caution in patients with a history of ocular herpes simplex; corneal perforation has occurred; do not use in active ocular herpes simplex. Consider routine eye exams in chronic users. Corticosteroid use may cause psychiatric disturbances, including euphoria, insomnia, mood swings, personality changes, severe depression or frank psychotic manifestations. Preexisting psychiatric conditions may be exacerbated by corticosteroid use. Rare cases of anaphylactoid reactions have been observed in patients receiving corticosteroids.

Use with caution in patients with heart failure, hypertension, diabetes, GI diseases (diverticulitis, fresh intestinal anastomoses, active or latent peptic ulcer, ulcerative colitis [nonspecific]), hepatic impairment, myasthenia gravis, myocardial infarction, patients with or who are at risk for osteoporosis, renal impairment, seizure disorders, or thyroid disease. Use with caution in patients with systemic sclerosis; an increase in scleroderma renal crisis incidence has been observed with corticosteroid use. Monitor BP and renal function in patients with systemic sclerosis treated with corticosteroids (EULAR [Kowal-Bielecka 2017]). May affect growth velocity; growth and development should be routinely monitored in pediatric patients. Use with caution in elderly patients in the smallest possible effective dose for the shortest duration.

Withdraw therapy with gradual tapering of dose. Increased mortality was observed in patients receiving high-dose IV methylprednisolone; high-dose corticosteroids should not be used for the management of head injury. Patients may require higher doses when subject to stress (ie, trauma, surgery, severe infection). Potentially significant drug-drug interactions may exist, requiring dose or frequency adjustment, additional monitoring, and/or selection of alternative therapy.

Some dosage forms may contain sodium benzoate/benzoic acid; benzoic acid (benzoate) is a metabolite of benzyl alcohol; large amounts of benzyl alcohol (≥99 mg/kg/day) have been associated with a potentially fatal toxicity ("gasping syndrome") in neonates; the "gasping syndrome" consists of metabolic acidosis, respiratory distress, gasping respirations, CNS dysfunction (including convulsions, intracranial hemorrhage), hypotension, and cardiovascular collapse (AAP ["Inactive" 1997]; CDC 1982); some data suggests that benzoate displaces bilirubin from protein binding sites (Ahlfors 2001); avoid or use dosage forms containing benzyl alcohol derivative with caution in neonates. See manufacturer's labeling.

Some dosage forms may contain propylene glycol; large amounts are potentially toxic and have been associated hyperosmolality, lactic acidosis, seizures, and respiratory depression; use caution (AAP ["Inactive" 1997]; Zar 2007).

Warnings: Additional Pediatric Considerations May cause osteoporosis (at any age) or inhibition of bone growth in pediatric patients. Use with caution in patients with osteoporosis. In a population-based study of children, risk of fracture was shown to be increased with >4 courses of corticosteroids; underlying clinical condition may also impact bone health and osteoporotic effect of corticosteroids (Leonard 2007). Increased IOP may occur, especially with prolonged use; in children, increased IOP has been shown to be dose dependent and produce a greater IOP in children <6 years than older children treated with ophthalmic dexamethasone (Lam 2005). Corticosteroids have been associated with myocardial rupture; hypertrophic cardiomyopathy has been reported in premature neonates.

Drug Interactions

Metabolism/Transport Effects **Substrate** of CYP3A4 (minor); **Note:** Assignment of Major/Minor substrate status based on clinically relevant drug interaction potential

Avoid Concomitant Use

Avoid concomitant use of PredniSONE with any of the following: Aldesleukin; BCG (Intravesical); Cladribine; Desmopressin; Disulfiram; Fexinidazole [INT]; Indium 111 Capromab Pendetide; Macimorelin; Methotrimeprazine; Mifamurtide; MiFEPRIStone; Natalizumab; Pimecrolimus; Tacrolimus (Topical)

Increased Effect/Toxicity

PredniSONE may increase the levels/effects of: Acetylcholinesterase Inhibitors; Amphotericin B; Androgens; Baricitinib; CycloSPORINE (Systemic); Deferasirox; Desirudin; Desmopressin; Fexinidazole [INT]; Fingolimod; Leflunomide; Loop Diuretics; Methotrimeprazine; Natalizumab; Nicorandil; Nonsteroidal Anti-Inflammatory Agents (COX-2 Selective); Nonsteroidal Anti-Inflammatory Agents (Nonselective); Ozanimod; Quinolones; Ritodrine; Sargramostim; Siponimod; Somatropin; Thiazide and Thiazide-Like Diuretics; Tofacitinib; Upadacitinib; Vaccines (Live); Vitamin K Antagonists

The levels/effects of PredniSONE may be increased by: Aprepitant; Cladribine; CycloSPORINE (Systemic); CYP3A4 Inhibitors (Strong); Denosumab; DilTIAZem; Disulfiram; Estrogen Derivatives; Fluconazole; Fosaprepitant; Indacaterol; Inebilizumab; MiFEPRIStone; Neuromuscular-Blocking Agents (Nondepolarizing); Ocrelizumab; Pimecrolimus; Ritonavir; Roflumilast; Salicylates; Tacrolimus (Topical); Trastuzumab

Decreased Effect

PredniSONE may decrease the levels/effects of: Aldesleukin; Antidiabetic Agents; Axicabtagene Ciloleucel; BCG (Intravesical); Calcitriol (Systemic); Coccidioides immitis Skin Test; Corticorelin; Cosyntropin; CycloSPORINE (Systemic); Hyaluronidase; Indium 111 Capromab Pendetide; Isoniazid; Macimorelin; Mifamurtide; Nivolumab; Pidotimod; Salicylates; Sipuleucel-T; Tacrolimus (Systemic); Tertomotide; Tisagenlecleucel; Urea Cycle Disorder Agents; Vaccines (Inactivated); Vaccines (Live)

The levels/effects of PredniSONE may be decreased by: Antacids; Bile Acid Sequestrants; CYP3A4 Inducers (Strong); Echinacea; MiFEPRIStone; Mitotane; Somatropin; Tesamorelin

Dietary Considerations May require increased dietary intake of pyridoxine, vitamin C, vitamin D, folate, calcium, and phosphorus; may require decreased dietary intake of sodium and potassium supplementation

Pharmacodynamics/Kinetics

Half-life Elimination 2 to 3 hours

Time to Peak Oral: Immediate-release tablet: 2 hours; Delayed-release tablet: 6 to 6.5 hours

Pregnancy Considerations

Prednisone and its metabolite, prednisolone, cross the placenta.

In the mother, prednisone is converted to the active metabolite prednisolone by the liver. Prior to reaching the fetus, prednisolone is converted by placental enzymes back to prednisone. As a result, the level of prednisone remaining in the maternal serum and reaching the fetus are similar; however, the amount of prednisolone reaching the fetus is ~8 to 10 times lower than the maternal serum concentration (healthy women at term) (Beitins 1972).

Some studies have shown an association between first trimester systemic corticosteroid use and oral clefts or decreased birth weight; however, information is conflicting and may be influenced by maternal dose, duration/frequency of exposure, and indication for use (Lunghi 2010; Park-Wyllie 2000; Pradat 2003). Hypoadrenalism may occur in newborns following maternal use of corticosteroids in pregnancy; monitor. An increased risk of adverse maternal outcomes, including gestational diabetes, may be associated with use of high doses over extended periods (Murase 2014; Rademaker 2018).

When systemic corticosteroids are needed in pregnancy for rheumatic disorders, it is generally recommended to use the lowest effective dose for the shortest duration of time, avoiding high doses during the first trimester (Götestam Skorpen 2016; Makol 2011; Østensen 2009).

For dermatologic disorders in pregnant women, systemic corticosteroids are generally not preferred for initial therapy; should be avoided during the first trimester; and used during the second or third trimester at the lowest effective dose (Leachman 2006). Prednisone is preferred by some guidelines when an oral corticosteroid is needed because placental enzymes limit passage to the embryo (Murase 2014; Rademaker 2018).

Uncontrolled asthma is associated with adverse events in pregnancy (increased risk of perinatal mortality, preeclampsia, preterm birth, low birth weight infants, cesarean delivery, and the development of gestational diabetes). Poorly controlled asthma or asthma exacerbations may have a greater fetal/maternal risk than what is associated with appropriately used asthma medications. Maternal treatment improves pregnancy outcomes by reducing the risk of some adverse events. Inhaled corticosteroids are recommended for the treatment of asthma during pregnancy; however, systemic corticosteroids, including prednisone, should be used to control acute exacerbations or treat severe persistent asthma. Maternal asthma symptoms should be monitored monthly during pregnancy (ERS/TSANZ [Middleton 2020]; GINA 2020).

Prednisone may be used to treat lupus nephritis in pregnant women who have active nephritis or substantial extrarenal disease activity (Hahn 2012). Prednisone is recommended for use in fetal-neonatal alloimmune thrombocytopenia and pregnancy-associated immune thrombocytopenia (ACOG 207 2019). Prednisone is the preferred immunosuppressant for the treatment of myasthenia gravis in pregnancy (Sanders 2016).

The Transplant Pregnancy Registry International (TPR) is a registry that follows pregnancies that occur in maternal transplant recipients or those fathered by male transplant recipients. The TPR encourages reporting of pregnancies following solid organ transplant by contacting them at 1-877-955-6877 or https://www.transplantpregnancyregistry.org.

Breastfeeding Considerations

Prednisone and its metabolite, prednisolone, are present in breast milk. Actual concentrations are dependent upon maternal dose (Berlin 1979; Katz 1975; Sagraves 1981). Peak concentrations of prednisone and prednisolone in breast milk occur ~2 hours after an oral maternal dose (Berlin 1979; Sagraves 1981); the half-life in breast milk is 1.9 hours (prednisone) and 4.2 hours (prednisolone) (Sagraves 1981).

In a study which included six mother-infant pairs, adverse events were not observed in breastfeeding infants (maternal prednisone dose not provided) (Ito 1993).

The manufacturer notes that maternal use of high doses of systemic corticosteroids have the potential to cause adverse events in a breastfeeding infant (eg, growth suppression, interfere with endogenous corticosteroid production); therefore, the decision to breastfeed during therapy should consider the risk of infant exposure, the benefits of breastfeeding to the infant, and the benefits of treatment to the mother. The lowest effective dose should be used to minimize potential infant exposure via breast milk.

Corticosteroids are generally considered acceptable in breastfeeding women when used in usual doses (Götestam Skorpen 2016; WHO 2002); however, monitoring of the breastfeeding infant is recommended (WHO 2002). Prednisone is one of the oral corticosteroids preferred for use in breastfeeding women (Butler 2014). If there is concern about exposure to the infant, some guidelines recommend waiting 4 hours after the maternal dose of an oral systemic corticosteroid before breastfeeding in order to decrease potential exposure to the breastfeeding infant (based on a study using prednisolone) (Butler 2014; ERS/TSANZ [Middleton 2020]; Götestam Skorpen 2016; Leachman 2006; Makol 2011; Ost 1985; Rademaker 2018).

Dosage Forms: US

Concentrate, Oral:

predniSONE Intensol: 5 mg/mL (30 mL)

Solution, Oral:

Generic: 5 mg/5 mL (120 mL, 500 mL)

Tablet, Oral:
Deltasone: 20 mg
Generic: 1 mg, 2.5 mg, 5 mg, 10 mg, 20 mg, 50 mg
Tablet Delayed Release, Oral:
Rayos: 1 mg, 2 mg, 5 mg
Tablet Therapy Pack, Oral:
Generic: 10 mg (21 ea, 48 ea); 5 mg (21 ea, 48 ea)

Dosage Forms: Canada
Tablet, Oral:
Winpred: 1 mg
Generic: 1 mg, 5 mg, 50 mg

Dental Health Professional Considerations Preoperative steroid use, particularly in patient on longer term corticosteroids (>2 weeks), increases the risk of infection and delays wound healing.

◆ **predniSONE Intensol** *see* PredniSONE *on page 1260*

◆ **Prefest** *see* Estradiol and Norgestimate *on page 599*

Pregabalin (pre GAB a lin)

Brand Names: US Lyrica; Lyrica CR
Brand Names: Canada ACT Pregabalin [DSC]; AG-Pregabalin; APO-Pregabalin; Auro-Pregabalin; DOM-Pregabalin; JAMP-Pregabalin; Lyrica; M-Pregabalin; Mar-Pregabalin; MINT-Pregabalin; MYLAN-Pregabalin [DSC]; NAT-Pregabalin; NRA-Pregabalin; PMS-Pregabalin; RIVA-Pregabalin; SANDOZ Pregabalin; TARO-Pregabalin; TEVA-Pregabalin
Generic Availability (US) May be product dependent
Pharmacologic Category Anticonvulsant, Miscellaneous; GABA Analog
Use
Fibromyalgia (immediate release only): Management of fibromyalgia
Neuropathic pain associated with diabetic peripheral neuropathy (immediate release and extended release): Management of neuropathic pain associated with diabetic peripheral neuropathy
Neuropathic pain associated with spinal cord injury (immediate release only): Management of neuropathic pain associated with spinal cord injury
Postherpetic neuralgia (immediate release and extended release): Management of postherpetic neuralgia
Seizures, focal (partial) onset (immediate release only): Adjunctive therapy in patients ≥1 month of age with focal onset (partial-onset) seizures

Local Anesthetic/Vasoconstrictor Precautions No information available to require special precautions

Effects on Dental Treatment Key adverse event(s) related to dental treatment: Xerostomia and changes in salivation (normal salivary flow resumes upon discontinuation).

Effects on Bleeding May be associated with thrombocytopenia (3%). No information available to require routine special precautions

Adverse Reactions As reported with adult patients, unless otherwise noted.
>10%:
Cardiovascular: Peripheral edema (1% to 16% [placebo: 2% to 4%])
Endocrine & metabolic: Weight gain (2% to 14% [placebo: 1% to 2%])
Gastrointestinal: Xerostomia (≤15%)
Nervous system: Dizziness (3% to 45% [placebo: 0.5% to 9%]), drowsiness (≤36% [placebo: 0% to 12%]; infants, children, and adolescents: 13% to 26% [placebo: 9% to 14%]), fatigue (4% to 11%), headache (2% to 14%)
Ophthalmic: Blurred vision (≤12% [placebo: 2% to 3%]), visual field loss (13% [placebo: 12%])
1% to 10%:
Cardiovascular: Chest pain (2%), edema (≤8%), facial edema (1% to 3%), hypertension (2%), hypotension (2%)
Dermatologic: Contact dermatitis (1%), ecchymoses (≥1%), pressure ulcer (3%)
Endocrine & metabolic: Decreased libido (≥1%), fluid retention (2% to 3%), hypoglycemia (2% to 3%)
Gastrointestinal: Abdominal distension (2%), abdominal pain (≥1%), constipation (3% to 10%), diarrhea (1%), flatulence (2% to 3%), gastroenteritis (≥1%), increased appetite (3% to 10%), nausea (3% to 5%), sialorrhea (children and adolescents: 1% to 4%), viral gastroenteritis (≤1%), vomiting (1% to 3%)
Genitourinary: Erectile dysfunction (≤1%), impotence (≥1%), urinary frequency (≥1%), urinary incontinence (1% to 3%), urinary tract infection (1%)
Hematologic & oncologic: Thrombocytopenia (3%, including severe thrombocytopenia)
Hepatic: Increased serum alanine aminotransferase (≤1%), increased serum aspartate aminotransferase (≤1%)
Hypersensitivity: Hypersensitivity reaction (≥1%)
Infection: Infection (6% to 8%), viral infection (infants and children: 6%)
Nervous system: Abnormal gait (1% to 8%), abnormality in thinking (1% to 6%), amnesia (1% to 4%), anorgasmia (≥1%), ataxia (2% to 9%), balance impairment (2% to 9%), confusion (1% to 7%), depersonalization (≥1%), disorientation (1% to 2%), disturbance in attention (4% to 6%), euphoria (2% to 7%), feeling abnormal (1% to 3%), hypertonia (≥1%), hypoesthesia (2% to 3%), insomnia (4%), intoxicated feeling (1% to 2%), lethargy (1% to 2%), memory impairment (1% to 4%), myasthenia (1% to 5%), nervousness (1%), neuropathy (5%), pain (3% to 5%), paresthesia (2%), sedated state (≥1%), speech disturbance (1% to 3%), stupor (≥1%), twitching (≥1%; includes myokymia), vertigo (1% to 4%)
Neuromuscular & skeletal: Arthralgia (1% to 6%), asthenia (4% to 7%), increased creatine phosphokinase in blood specimen (2% to 3% [placebo: <1%]), joint swelling (≤2%), lower limb cramp (≥1%), muscle spasm (4%), tremor (1% to 3%)
Ophthalmic: Conjunctivitis (≥1%), decreased visual acuity (7% [placebo: 5%]), diplopia (≤4% [placebo: 0%]), eye disease (1% to 2%), nystagmus disorder (≥1%), visual disturbance (1% to 5%)
Otic: Otitis media (≥1%), tinnitus (≥1%)
Respiratory: Bronchitis (3%), dyspnea (2%), flu-like symptoms (2%), nasopharyngitis (1% to 8%), pharyngolaryngeal pain (3%), pneumonia (infants and children: 1% to 9%; adults: <1%), respiratory tract infection (1%), sinusitis (≤7%)
Miscellaneous: Accidental injury (3% to 6% [placebo: 2% to 3%]), fever (≥1%)
<1%:
Cardiovascular: Cardiac failure, depression of ST segment on ECG, orthostatic hypotension, palpitations, retinal vascular disease, shock, syncope, tachycardia, thrombophlebitis, ventricular fibrillation

Dermatologic: Alopecia, cellulitis, cutaneous nodule, dermal ulcer, eczema, erythema of skin, exfoliative dermatitis, lichenoid dermatitis, nail disease, pustular rash, skin atrophy, skin blister, skin necrosis, skin photosensitivity, skin rash, Stevens-Johnson syndrome, subcutaneous nodule, urticaria, vesiculobullous dermatitis, xeroderma

Endocrine & metabolic: Albuminuria, decreased glucose tolerance, glycosuria, increased libido

Gastrointestinal: Ageusia, aphthous stomatitis, cholecystitis, cholelithiasis, colitis, dry mucous membranes, dysgeusia, dysphagia, esophageal ulcer, esophagitis, gastritis, gastrointestinal hemorrhage, hiccups, increased serum lipase, melena, oral mucosa ulcer, oral paresthesia, pancreatitis, periodontal abscess

Genitourinary: Ejaculatory disorder, oliguria, pelvic pain, proteinuria, retroperitoneal fibrosis, urate crystalluria, urinary retention, urine abnormality, uterine hemorrhage

Hematologic & oncologic: Anemia, eosinophilia, granuloma, hemophthalmos, hypochromic anemia, hypoprothrombinemia, increased neutrophils, leukocytosis, leukopenia, lymphadenopathy, myelofibrosis, nonthrombocytopenic purpura, petechial rash, polycythemia, purpuric rash, rectal hemorrhage, thrombocythemia

Hepatic: Ascites

Hypersensitivity: Angioedema (Ortega-Camarero 2012)

Infection: Abscess

Local: Local inflammation (coccydynia)

Nervous system: Abnormal dreams, agitation, apathy, aphasia, cerebellar syndrome, chills, cognitive dysfunction, cogwheel rigidity, delirium, delusion, drug dependence, dysarthria, dysautonomia, dystonia, encephalopathy, extraocular palsy, extrapyramidal reaction, hallucination, hangover effect, hostility, hypalgesia, hyperalgesia, hyperesthesia, hypotonia, impaired consciousness, irritability, malaise, myoclonus, neuralgia, psychomotor disturbance, sciatica, self-inflicted intentional injury, sleep disorder, trismus, yawning

Neuromuscular & skeletal: Bradykinesia, dyskinesia, hyperkinetic muscle activity, hypokinesia, joint stiffness, neck stiffness

Ophthalmic: Accommodation disturbance, blindness, iritis, miosis, mydriasis, night blindness, periorbital edema, photophobia

Renal: Acute renal failure, glomerulonephritis, nephritis, nephrolithiasis, pyelonephritis

Respiratory: Apnea, pulmonary edema

Frequency not defined:

Cardiovascular: Prolongation P-R interval on ECG (Schiavo 2017)

Neuromuscular & skeletal: Rhabdomyolysis (Gunathilake 2013; Kato 2016; Kaufman 2012)

Postmarketing:

Dermatologic: Toxic epidermal necrolysis (Frey 2017)

Endocrine & metabolic: Gynecomastia (Málaga 2006)

Immunologic: Drug reaction with eosinophilia and systemic symptoms (Thein 2019)

Respiratory: Respiratory depression (FDA Safety Alert, Dec 19, 2019)

Dosing

Adult Note: For patients with respiratory disease, initiate therapy at the lowest dose (FDA 2019).

Cough, chronic refractory (alternative agent) (off-label use): Immediate release: Oral: Initial: 75 mg once daily; may increase gradually over the first week in increments of 75 mg/day based on response and tolerability up to a maximum of 300 mg/day in 3 divided doses (eg, 75 mg in morning and midday with 150 mg in the evening) (Vertigan 2016).

Fibromyalgia (alternative agent): Note: For patients who do not respond to or tolerate preferred agents (Goldenberg 2018).

Immediate release: Oral: Initial: 75 mg twice daily; may increase to 150 mg twice daily within 1 week based on response and tolerability; maximum dose: 450 mg/day (manufacturer's labeling). **Note:** Some experts suggest lower initial doses of 25 to 50 mg at bedtime; some patients may respond to maintenance doses <300 mg/day (Goldenberg 2018).

Generalized anxiety disorder (alternative agent) (off-label use): Note: Monotherapy or adjunctive therapy for patients who do not tolerate or respond to preferred agents (BAP [Baldwin 2014]; Craske 2018).

Immediate release: Oral: Initial: 150 mg/day in 2 to 3 divided doses; may increase based on response and tolerability at weekly intervals in increments of 150 mg/day up to a usual dose of 300 mg/day. May further increase up to 600 mg/day (Kasper 2014; WFSBP [Bandelow 2008]); however, additional benefit of doses >300 mg/day is uncertain (Lydiard 2010). **Note:** Some experts suggest a lower initial dose of 50 mg/day (Bystritsky 2018).

Neuropathic pain:

General dosing recommendations: Immediate release: Oral: Initial: 25 to 150 mg/day in 2 to 3 divided doses; may increase in increments of 25 to 150 mg/day at weekly intervals based on response and tolerability up to a usual dose of 300 to 600 mg/day in 2 to 3 divided doses (CPS [Moulin 2014]; IASP [Finnerup 2015]; manufacturer's labeling).

Critically ill ICU patients (off-label use): Oral: Initial: 75 mg once or twice daily in combination with opioids; maintenance dose: 150 to 300 mg twice daily (SCCM [Devlin 2018]; Tietze 2019).

Diabetic neuropathy:

Immediate release: Oral: Initial: 75 to 150 mg/day in 2 to 3 divided doses; may increase daily dose in 75 mg increments every ≥3 days based on response and tolerability up to a maximum dose of 300 to 450 mg/day (ADA [Pop-Busui 2017]; Feldman 2020; manufacturer's labeling). Higher doses up to 600 mg/day may have greater adverse effects without additional benefit (Arnold 2017).

Extended release: Oral: Initial: 165 mg once daily; may increase within 1 week based on response and tolerability up to maximum dose of 330 mg once daily.

Postherpetic neuralgia:

Immediate release: Oral: Initial: 150 mg/day in divided doses (75 mg twice daily or 50 mg 3 times daily); may increase to 300 mg/day within 1 week based on response and tolerability; after 2 to 4 weeks, may further increase up to the maximum dose of 600 mg/day.

Extended release: Oral: Initial: 165 mg once daily; may increase to 330 mg once daily within 1 week based on response and tolerability; after 2 to 4 weeks, may further increase up to the maximum dose of 660 mg/day.

Spinal cord injury-associated neuropathic pain: Immediate release: Oral: Initial: 75 mg twice daily; may increase within 1 week based on response and tolerability to 150 mg twice daily; after 2 to 3 weeks, may further increase up to a maximum of 600 mg/day.

Postoperative pain (off-label use): Immediate release: Oral: 75 to 300 mg as a single dose, 1 to 2 hours prior to surgery as part of a multimodal analgesia regimen. The use of multiple doses has not been found to provide additional benefit (APS [Chou 2016]; Mishriky 2015).

Pruritus, chronic (alternative agent) (off-label use): Note: For patients with pruritus resistant to preferred therapies (Matsuda 2016; Weisshaar 2012).

Neuropathic (eg, brachioradial pruritus, notalgia paresthetica) or malignancy related: Based on limited data: Immediate release: Oral: Initial: 75 mg twice daily; may increase based on response and tolerability up to 150 to 300 mg/day in 2 to 3 divided doses (Atis 2017; Fazio 2018; Matsuda 2016; Vestita 2016). Higher doses up to 600 mg/day have been used in oncology populations (Dalal 2018).

Uremic: Immediate release: Oral: Variable dosing has been used and includes: 50 mg every other day given after dialysis on hemodialysis days (Foroutan 2017) or 25 mg daily (Kobrin 2018), each increased based on response and tolerability to 50 or 75 mg daily; 75 mg twice weekly given after dialysis on hemodialysis days also appears effective (Yue 2015).

Restless legs syndrome (off-label use): Immediate release: Oral: Initial: 50 to 75 mg once daily, 1 to 3 hours before bedtime; gradually increase (eg, in increments of 75 to 150 mg) every 5 to 7 days based on response and tolerability to a usual effective dose of 150 to 450 mg/day (Allen 2010; Allen 2014; Garcia-Borreguero 2014).

Seizures, focal (partial) onset (adjunctive therapy with other anticonvulsants): Immediate release: Oral: Initial: 150 mg/day in 2 or 3 divided doses; may increase based on response and tolerability at weekly intervals up to a maximum dose of 600 mg/day.

Social anxiety disorder (alternative agent) (off-label use): Note: Monotherapy or adjunctive therapy for patients who do not tolerate or respond to preferred agents (Stein 2018). Immediate release: Oral: Initial: 100 mg 3 times daily; may increase over 1 week in increments of 150 mg/day based on response and tolerability up to 600 mg/day (Feltner 2011; Greist 2011; Pande 2004).

Vasomotor symptoms associated with menopause (alternative agent) (off-label use): Note: Used as a nonhormonal alternative in patients unable or unwilling to take preferred agents (Stuenkel 2015). Some experts prefer gabapentin over pregabalin as an alternative agent because of greater available evidence (Santen 2018).

Immediate release: Oral: Initial: 50 mg once daily at bedtime; may increase at weekly intervals based on response and tolerability to 50 mg twice daily, and then up to 75 mg twice daily; may further increase up to 150 mg twice daily (Loprinzi 2010).

***Dosing conversion from immediate-release oral formulations to extended-release oral formulation:* Note:** On the day of the switch, administer morning dose of immediate-release product as prescribed, and initiate extended-release therapy after the evening meal.

Immediate-release total daily dose of 75 mg is equivalent to extended-release dose of 82.5 mg once daily

Immediate-release total daily dose of 150 mg is equivalent to extended-release dose of 165 mg once daily

Immediate-release total daily dose of 225 mg is equivalent to extended-release dose of 247.5 mg once daily

Immediate-release total daily dose of 300 mg is equivalent to extended-release dose of 330 mg once daily

Immediate-release total daily dose of 450 mg is equivalent to extended-release dose of 495 mg once daily

Immediate-release total daily dose of 600 mg is equivalent to extended-release dose of 660 mg once daily

Discontinuation of therapy: In patients receiving pregabalin chronically, unless safety concerns require a more rapid withdrawal, pregabalin should be withdrawn gradually over ≥1 week to minimize the potential of increased seizure frequency (in patients with epilepsy) or other withdrawal symptoms (eg, agitation, confusion, delirium, delusions, GI symptoms, mood changes, sweating, withdrawal seizures) (Bonnet 2017; "Gabapentin and Pregabalin" 2012).

Geriatric Initiate therapy at the lowest dose (FDA 2019). Refer to adult dosing; use with caution. In the management of restless legs syndrome, a starting dose of 50 mg once daily in patients >65 years has been recommended (Garcia-Borreguero 2016).

Renal Impairment: Adult Immediate release: Renal function may be estimated using the Cockcroft-Gault formula. Then determine recommended dosage regimen based on the indication-specific total daily dose for normal renal function (CrCl ≥60 mL/minute). For example, if the indication-specific daily dose is 450 mg daily for normal renal function, the daily dose should be reduced to 225 mg daily (in 2 to 3 divided doses) for a creatinine clearance of 30 to 60 mL/minute (see table).

Immediate-Release Pregabalin Renal Impairment Dosing

CrCl (mL/minute)	Total Pregabalin Daily Dose (mg/day)				Dosing Frequency
≥60 (normal renal function)	150	300	450	600	2 to 3 divided doses
30 to 60	75	150	225	300	2 to 3 divided doses
15 to 30	25 to 50	75	100 to 150	150	1 to 2 divided doses
<15	25	25 to 50	50 to 75	75	Single daily dose

Hemodialysis: Dialyzable (~50%); supplementary dosage posthemodialysis (as a single additional dose):

25 mg/day schedule: Single supplementary dose of 25 mg **or** 50 mg
25 to 50 mg/day schedule: Single supplementary dose of 50 mg **or** 75 mg
50 to 75 mg/day schedule: Single supplementary dose of 75 mg **or** 100 mg
75 mg/day schedule: Single supplementary dose of 100 mg **or** 150 mg

Extended release: Renal function may be estimated using the Cockcroft-Gault formula. Then determine recommended dosage regimen based on the indication-specific total daily dose for normal renal function (CrCl ≥60 mL/minute). For example, if the indication-specific daily dose is 495 mg once daily for normal renal function, the daily dose should be reduced to 247.5 mg once daily for a creatinine clearance of 30 to 60 mL/minute (see table).

Extended-Release Pregabalin Renal Impairment Dosing

CrCl (mL/minute)	Total Pregabalin Daily Dose (mg/day)				Dosing Frequency
≥60 (normal renal function)	165	330	495	660	Once daily
30 to 60	82.5	165	247.5	330	Once daily
<30	Extended-release product not recommended; use immediate-release product				
Hemodialysis					

Hepatic Impairment: Adult There are no dosage adjustments provided in the manufacturer's labeling. However, no adjustment is expected since undergoes minimal hepatic metabolism.

Pediatric Note: When discontinuing, taper off gradually over at least 1 week.

Seizures, partial onset; adjunctive therapy: Immediate release:

Infants and Children <4 years weighing <30 kg: Oral: Initial dose: 3.5 mg/kg/day in 3 divided doses; dose may be increased weekly based on clinical response and tolerability; maximum daily dose: 14 mg/kg/**day**.

Children ≥4 years and Adolescents <17 years:

<30 kg: Oral: Initial dose: 3.5 mg/kg/day in 2 or 3 divided doses; dose may be increased weekly based on clinical response and tolerability; maximum daily dose: 14 mg/kg/**day**.

≥30 kg: Oral: Initial dose: 2.5 mg/kg/day in 2 or 3 divided doses; dose may be increased weekly based on clinical response and tolerability; maximum daily dose: 10 mg/kg/**day** not to exceed 600 mg/**day**.

Adolescents ≥17 years: Oral: Initial dose: 150 mg daily in 2 or 3 divided doses; may be increased weekly based on tolerability and effect; maximum daily dose: 600 mg/**day**.

Fibromyalgia: Limited data available: Immediate release: Children ≥12 years and Adolescents: Oral: Initial: 37.5 mg twice daily for 1 week, then titrate based on clinical response and tolerability to 150 to 450 mg/day in 2 divided doses; maximum daily dose: 450 mg/**day**. Dosing based on a multi-center, double-blind, placebo-controlled trial (15 weeks) and secondary open-label continuation trial (6 months) (n=107; pregabalin n=54; age range: 12 to 17 years); total daily doses were titrated weekly to an individually optimized dose of 150 mg/day, 300 mg/day, or 450 mg/day; maximum daily dose: 450 mg/**day**; mean dose during maintenance phase of double-blind study was 244.5 mg/day and in the open label trial it was 254.3 mg/day. Although the primary endpoint of change in mean pain scores from baseline to week 15 was not statistically significant, there was a trend toward improvement in the pregabalin group. Change in weekly mean pain scores was significantly greater with pregabalin compared to placebo for 10 of the 15 weeks; the patient global impression of change was also significantly improved in patients receiving pregabalin (53.1%) compared to placebo (29.5%). The authors reported a large placebo effect, particularly at non-US study centers; however, significance of this is unknown (Arnold 2016).

Renal Impairment: Pediatric Immediate release: There are no pediatric-specific dosage adjustments provided in manufacturer's labeling (has not been studied); based on experience in adult patients, dosing adjustment may be necessary.

Hepatic Impairment: Pediatric Immediate release: There are no dosage adjustments provided in the manufacturer's labeling; however, no adjustment is expected since pregabalin undergoes minimal hepatic metabolism.

Mechanism of Action Binds to alpha-2-delta subunit of voltage-gated calcium channels within the CNS and modulates calcium influx at the nerve terminals, thereby inhibiting excitatory neurotransmitter release including glutamate, norepinephrine (noradrenaline), serotonin, dopamine, substance P, and calcitonin gene-related peptide (Gajraj 2007; McKeage 2009). Although structurally related to GABA, it does not bind to GABA or benzodiazepine receptors. Exerts antinociceptive and anticonvulsant activity. Pregabalin may also affect descending noradrenergic and serotonergic pain transmission pathways from the brainstem to the spinal cord.

Contraindications Hypersensitivity (eg, angioedema) to pregabalin or any component of the formulation

Warnings/Precautions Pooled analysis if trials involving various antiepileptics (regardless of indication) showed an increased risk of suicidal thoughts/behavior (incidence rate: 0.43% treated patients compared to 0.24% patients receiving placebo); risk observed as early as one week after initiation and continued through duration of trials (most trials ≤24 weeks). Monitor all patients for notable changes in behavior that might indicate suicidal thoughts or depression; notify healthcare provider immediately if symptoms occur. Angioedema has been reported during initial and chronic treatment; may be life threatening. Symptoms reported include facial, mouth (tongue, lips, and gums), and neck (throat and larynx) swelling. Use with caution in patients with a history of angioedema episodes. Concurrent use with other drugs known to cause angioedema (eg, ACE inhibitors) may increase risk. Discontinue treatment immediately if angioedema occurs. Hypersensitivity reactions, including skin redness, blistering, hives, rash, dyspnea, and wheezing have been reported shortly after initiation of treatment; discontinue treatment if hypersensitivity occurs. Dizziness and somnolence are commonly reported; effects generally occur shortly after initiation and occur more frequently at higher doses. Patients must be cautioned about performing tasks which require mental alertness (eg, operating machinery or driving). Visual disturbances (blurred vision, decreased acuity and visual field changes) have been associated with pregabalin therapy; patients should be instructed to notify their physician if these effects are noted.

Pregabalin has been associated with increases in creatine kinase and rare cases of rhabdomyolysis. Patients should be instructed to notify their prescriber if unexplained muscle pain, tenderness, or weakness, particularly if fever and/or malaise are associated with these symptoms. Discontinue treatment if myopathy is suspected or diagnosed or if markedly elevated creatine kinase levels occur. Use may cause weight gain; weight gain generally associated with dose and duration (average weight gain was 5.2 kg for diabetic patients receiving pregabalin for ≥2 years); weight gain was not limited to patients with edema and did not appear to be associated with baseline BMI, gender, age, or loss of glycemic control in diabetic patients. Use may cause peripheral edema; use with caution in patients with heart failure (NYHA Class III or IV) due to limited data in this patient population. In addition, effect on weight gain/edema may be additive with the thiazolidinedione class of antidiabetic agents; use caution when coadministering these agents, particularly in patients with prior cardiovascular disease. In a scientific statement from the American Heart Association, pregabalin has been determined to be an agent that may exacerbate underlying myocardial dysfunction (magnitude: minor to moderate) (AHA [Page 2016]). May decrease platelet count (extremely rare) or prolong PR interval (clinical significance unknown). Serious, life-threatening, and fatal respiratory depression may occur in patients taking pregabalin; risk may be increased with conditions such as chronic obstructive pulmonary disease, in elderly patients, and with the concomitant use of opioids and other CNS depressants. Initiate at the lowest dose and monitor patients for symptoms of respiratory depression and sedation in patients with underlying respiratory disease (FDA 2019). Pregabalin may cause respiratory depression; use caution and initiate with the lowest recommended dose in patients with respiratory compromise and in elderly patients (FDA 2019).

Has been noted to be tumorigenic (increased incidence of hemangiosarcoma) in animal studies; significance of these findings in humans is unknown. Anticonvulsants should not be discontinued abruptly because of the possibility of increasing seizure frequency; therapy should be withdrawal gradually unless safety concerns require a more rapid withdrawal. Tapering over at least 1 week is recommended. Abrupt discontinued with pregabalin has been associated with anxiety, diarrhea, headache, hyperhidrosis, insomnia and nausea. Use caution in renal impairment; dosage adjustment required. Use with caution in patients with a history of substance abuse; potential for behavioral dependence in this population exists (Bonnet 2017). Potentially significant drug-drug interactions may exist, requiring dose or frequency adjustment, additional monitoring, and/or selection of alternative therapy.

Drug Interactions

Metabolism/Transport Effects None known.

Avoid Concomitant Use

Avoid concomitant use of Pregabalin with any of the following: Azelastine (Nasal); Bromperidol; Orphenadrine; Oxomemazine; Paraldehyde; Thalidomide

Increased Effect/Toxicity

Pregabalin may increase the levels/effects of: Alcohol (Ethyl); Azelastine (Nasal); Blonanserin; Brexanolone; Buprenorphine; CNS Depressants; Flunitrazepam; Methotrimeprazine; MetyroSINE; Opioid Agonists; Orphenadrine; OxyCODONE; Paraldehyde; Piribedil; Pramipexole; ROPINIRole; Rotigotine; Suvorexant; Thalidomide; Thiazolidinediones; Zolpidem

The levels/effects of Pregabalin may be increased by: Alizapride; Angiotensin-Converting Enzyme Inhibitors; Brimonidine (Topical); Bromopride; Bromperidol; Cannabidiol; Cannabis; Chlormethiazole; Chlorphenesin Carbamate; Dimethindene (Topical); Doxylamine; Dronabinol; Droperidol; Esketamine; HydrOXYzine; Kava Kava; Lemborexant; Lisuride; Lofexidine; Magnesium Sulfate; Methotrimeprazine; Metoclopramide; Minocycline (Systemic); Nabilone; Oxomemazine; Perampanel; Rufinamide; Sodium Oxybate; Tetrahydrocannabinol; Tetrahydrocannabinol and Cannabidiol; Trimeprazine

Decreased Effect

The levels/effects of Pregabalin may be decreased by: Mefloquine; Mianserin; Orlistat

Food Interactions Extended release: Bioavailability is reduced if taken on an empty stomach. The AUC is approximately 30% lower when fasting relative to following an evening meal. Management: Administer after evening meal.

Pharmacodynamics/Kinetics

Onset of Action Pain management: Effects may be noted as early as the first week of therapy

Half-life Elimination

Children ≤6 years: 3 to 4 hours

Children 7 to <17 years: 4 to 6 hours

Adult: 6.3 hours

Time to Peak

Extended release: Median: 8 hours with food (range: 5 to 12 hours)

Immediate release:

Infants ≥3 months, Children, and Adolescents <17 years: 0.5 to 2 hours fasting

Adults: Within 1.5 hours fasting; ~3 hours with food

Reproductive Considerations

In a study conducted in males, pregabalin was found to temporarily decrease mean sperm concentrations; no effects on sperm morphology or motility were observed. Concentrations increased after pregabalin was discontinued. The clinical relevance of this is not known.

Pregnancy Considerations

Pregabalin crosses the placenta (Ohman 2011). Studies which evaluated neonatal outcomes following pregabalin exposure during pregnancy are limited (Mostacci 2017; Patorno 2017; Veiby 2014; Winterfeld 2016). Pregabalin has been evaluated as an adjuvant pain medication following cesarean section and pregnancy termination (El Kenany 2016; Lavand'homme 2010).

Data collection to monitor pregnancy and infant outcomes following exposure to pregabalin is ongoing. Patients exposed to pregabalin during pregnancy are encouraged to enroll themselves into the North American Antiepileptic Drug (NAAED) Pregnancy Registry by calling 1-888-233-2334. Additional information is available at www.aedpregnancyregistry.org.

Breastfeeding Considerations Pregabalin is present in breast milk.

The relative infant dose (RID) of pregabalin is ~7% when calculated using an average breast milk concentration compared to a weight-adjusted maternal dose of 300 mg/day.

In general, breastfeeding is considered acceptable when the RID of a medication is <10% (Anderson 2016; Ito 2000).

The RID of pregabalin was calculated using an average milk concentration of 2.05 mcg/mL, providing an estimated daily infant dose via breast milk of 0.31 mg/kg/day. This milk concentration was obtained following maternal administration of pregabalin 150 mg orally twice daily for 4 doses. The study included 10 women who were ~37 weeks' postpartum (range: 15 to 81 weeks). Infants were not breastfed during the study period. Peak concentrations in breast milk were generally lower than those in the maternal plasma (Lockwood 2016). A slightly higher RID of ~8% was noted in a case report (Ohman 2011). Poor latching on, lasting ~8 hours, was observed in three infants immediately postpartum following a single maternal dose of pregabalin for pain during cesarean delivery (El Kenany 2016). Breastfeeding is not recommended by the manufacturer.

Controlled Substance C-V

Dosage Forms: US

Capsule, Oral:

Lyrica: 25 mg, 50 mg, 75 mg, 100 mg, 150 mg, 200 mg, 225 mg, 300 mg

Generic: 25 mg, 50 mg, 75 mg, 100 mg, 150 mg, 200 mg, 225 mg, 300 mg

Solution, Oral:

Lyrica: 20 mg/mL (473 mL)

Generic: 20 mg/mL (473 mL)

Tablet Extended Release 24 Hour, Oral:

Lyrica CR: 82.5 mg, 165 mg, 330 mg

Dosage Forms: Canada

Capsule, Oral:

Lyrica: 25 mg, 50 mg, 75 mg, 150 mg, 225 mg, 300 mg

Generic: 25 mg, 50 mg, 75 mg, 150 mg, 225 mg, 300 mg

- ◆ **Pregnenedione** *see* Progesterone *on page 1280*
- ◆ **Prelone** *see* PrednisoLONE (Systemic) *on page 1255*
- ◆ **Premarin** *see* Estrogens (Conjugated/Equine, Systemic) *on page 601*
- ◆ **Premarin** *see* Estrogens (Conjugated/Equine, Topical) *on page 602*
- ◆ **Premium Lidocaine** *see* Lidocaine (Topical) *on page 902*
- ◆ **Premphase** *see* Estrogens (Conjugated/Equine) and Medroxyprogesterone *on page 603*
- ◆ **Prempro** *see* Estrogens (Conjugated/Equine) and Medroxyprogesterone *on page 603*
- ◆ **Preparation H [OTC]** *see* Hydrocortisone (Topical) *on page 775*
- ◆ **Preparation H [OTC]** *see* Phenylephrine (Topical) *on page 1227*
- ◆ **Preparation H Totables [OTC] [DSC]** *see* Phenylephrine (Topical) *on page 1227*
- ◆ **PreserVision AREDS [OTC]** *see* Vitamins (Multiple/Oral) *on page 1550*
- ◆ **PreserVision AREDS 2 Formula + Multivitamin [OTC]** *see* Vitamins (Multiple/Oral) *on page 1550*
- ◆ **PreserVision Lutein [OTC]** *see* Vitamins (Multiple/Oral) *on page 1550*

Pretomanid (pre TOE ma nid)

Pharmacologic Category Antimycobacterial, Nitroimidazole; Antitubercular Agent

Use

Tuberculosis: Treatment of pulmonary extensively drug resistant or treatment-intolerant or nonresponsive multidrug-resistant tuberculosis (TB), as part of a combination regimen with bedaquiline and linezolid, in adult patients.

Limitations of use: Not indicated for drug-sensitive tuberculosis, latent infection due to *Mycobacterium tuberculosis*, or multidrug-resistant TB that is not treatment-intolerant or nonresponsive to standard therapy. Safety and efficacy have not been established for use in combination with drugs other than bedaquiline and linezolid.

Local Anesthetic/Vasoconstrictor Precautions Pretomanid is one of the drugs confirmed to prolong the QT interval and is accepted as having a risk of causing torsade de pointes. The risk of drug-induced torsade de pointes is extremely low when a single QT interval prolonging drug is prescribed. In terms of epinephrine, it is not known what effect vasoconstrictors in the local anesthetic regimen will have in patients with a known history of congenital prolonged QT interval or in patients taking any medication that prolongs the QT interval. Until more information is obtained, it is suggested that the clinician consult with the physician prior to the use of a vasoconstrictor in suspected patients, and that the vasoconstrictor (epinephrine, mepivacaine and levonordefrin [Carbocaine 2% with Neo-Cobefrin]) be used with caution.

Effects on Dental Treatment Key adverse event(s) related to dental treatment: Occurrence of altered taste sensation.

Effects on Bleeding Occurrence of neutropenia, leukopenia, and thrombocytopenia. Medical consult suggested.

Adverse Reactions As reported in combination with bedaquiline and linezolid. Also see bedaquiline and linezolid monographs.

>10%:

Central nervous system: Peripheral neuropathy (81%), headache (28%), severe peripheral neuropathy (22%)

Dermatologic: Acne vulgaris (39%), skin rash (21%), pruritus (20%)

Endocrine & metabolic: Increased gamma-glutamyl transferase (17%), hypoglycemia (11%)

Gastrointestinal: Nausea (37%), vomiting (34%), dyspepsia (24%), decreased appetite (22%), abdominal pain (19%), increased serum amylase (14%)

Hematologic & oncologic: Anemia (37%)

Hepatic: Increased serum transaminases (28%), increased serum alanine aminotransferase (11%)

Neuromuscular & skeletal: Musculoskeletal pain (29%)

Ophthalmic: Visual impairment (12%)

Respiratory: Pleuritic chest pain (19%), lower respiratory tract infection (15%), hemoptysis (13%), cough (12%)

1% to 10%:

Cardiovascular: Hypertension (7%), prolonged QT interval on ECG (6%)

Central nervous system: Insomnia (6%), dizziness (<5%), seizure (<5%)

Dermatologic: Xeroderma (7%)

Endocrine & metabolic: Weight loss (10%), hyperglycemia (<5%), hyperkalemia (<5%), hypokalemia (<5%), hypomagnesemia (<5%), hyponatremia (<5%)

Gastrointestinal: Diarrhea (10%), constipation (8%), gastritis (8%), increased serum lipase (5% to 6%), dysgeusia (<5%), pancreatitis (<5%)

Hematologic & oncologic: Neutropenia (8%), thrombocytopenia (6%), leukopenia (<5%)

Hepatic: Increased serum aspartate aminotransferase (8%), increased serum bilirubin (7%), increased serum alkaline phosphatase (<5%)

Neuromuscular & skeletal: Increased creatine phosphokinase in blood specimen (<5%)

Ophthalmic: Optic neuropathy (2%)

Renal: Increased serum creatinine (<5%)

Frequency not defined:

Endocrine & metabolic: Lactic acidosis

Hematologic & oncologic: Pancytopenia

Hepatic: Hepatotoxicity

Mechanism of Action Pretomanid is an antimycobacterial drug that kills actively replicating *Mycobacterium tuberculosis* by inhibiting mycolic acid biosynthesis, blocking cell wall production. Against nonreplicating bacteria, under anaerobic conditions, pretomanid acts as a respiratory poison following nitric oxide release.

Pharmacodynamics/Kinetics

Half-life Elimination 16 hours.

Time to Peak 4.5 hours (median).

Pregnancy Considerations Adverse events were observed in some animal reproduction studies. Pretomanid is used in combination with bedaquiline and linezolid.

Product Availability Pretomanid tablets: FDA approved August 2019; anticipated availability in 2019.

- **Prevacid** *see* Lansoprazole *on page 876*
- **Prevacid 24HR [OTC]** *see* Lansoprazole *on page 876*
- **Prevacid SoluTab** *see* Lansoprazole *on page 876*
- **Prevalite** *see* Cholestyramine Resin *on page 345*
- **PreviDent** *see* Fluoride *on page 693*
- **PreviDent 5000 Booster [DSC]** *see* Fluoride *on page 693*
- **PreviDent 5000 Booster Plus** *see* Fluoride *on page 693*
- **PreviDent 5000 Dry Mouth** *see* Fluoride *on page 693*
- **PreviDent 5000 Plus** *see* Fluoride *on page 693*
- **Previfem** *see* Ethinyl Estradiol and Norgestimate *on page 616*
- **Prevnar 13** *see* Pneumococcal Conjugate Vaccine (13-Valent) *on page 1242*
- **Prevpac** *see* Lansoprazole, Amoxicillin, and Clarithromycin *on page 877*
- **Prevymis** *see* Letermovir *on page 888*
- **Prexxartan** *see* Valsartan *on page 1521*
- **Prezista** *see* Darunavir *on page 441*
- **Prialt** *see* Ziconotide *on page 1569*
- **Priftin** *see* Rifapentine *on page 1325*
- **Prikaan** *see* Lidocaine and Prilocaine *on page 911*
- **Prikaan Lite** *see* Lidocaine and Prilocaine *on page 911*

Prilocaine (PRIL oh kane)

Related Information

Oral Pain *on page 1734*

Brand Names: US Citanest Plain Dental

Brand Names: Canada 4% Citanest Plain Dental

Generic Availability (US) No

Pharmacologic Category Local Anesthetic

Dental Use Amide-type anesthetic used for local infiltration anesthesia; injection near nerve trunks to produce nerve block

Use

Local anesthesia: Production of local anesthesia in dentistry by nerve block or infiltration techniques.

Local Anesthetic/Vasoconstrictor Precautions No information available to require special precautions

Effects on Dental Treatment It is common to misinterpret psychogenic responses to local anesthetic injection as an allergic reaction. Intraoral injections are perceived by many patients as a stressful procedure in dentistry. Common symptoms to this stress are diaphoresis, palpitations, hyperventilation, generalized pallor and a fainting feeling.

Degree of adverse effects in the CNS and cardiovascular system is directly related to blood levels of prilocaine (frequency not defined; more likely to occur after systemic administration rather than infiltration): Bradycardia and reduction in cardiac output, hypersensitivity reactions (may be manifest as dermatologic reactions and edema at injection site), asthmatic syndromes

High blood levels: Anxiety, restlessness, disorientation, confusion, dizziness, tremors, and seizures, followed by CNS depression, resulting in somnolence, unconsciousness and possible respiratory arrest; nausea and vomiting

In some cases, symptoms of CNS stimulation may be absent and the primary CNS effects are somnolence and unconsciousness.

Effects on Bleeding No information available to require special precautions

Adverse Reactions Degree of adverse effects in the central nervous system and cardiovascular system are directly related to the blood levels of local anesthetic. The effects below are more likely to occur after systemic administration rather than infiltration.

Frequency not defined.

Cardiovascular: Bradycardia, cardiac arrest, cardiovascular signs and symptoms (stimulation/depression), circulatory shock, edema, hypotension

Central nervous system: Apprehension, confusion, convulsions, dizziness, drowsiness, euphoria, localized warm feeling, loss of consciousness, nervousness, numbness, oral paresthesia (may be persistent), sensation of cold, twitching

Dermatologic: Dermal ulcer, urticaria

Gastrointestinal: Vomiting

Hematologic & oncologic: Methemoglobinemia

Hypersensitivity: Anaphylactoid reaction, hypersensitivity reaction

Neuromuscular & skeletal: Tremor

Ophthalmic: Blurred vision, diplopia

Otic: Tinnitus

Respiratory: Respiratory arrest, respiratory depression

Dental Usual Dosage Dental anesthesia: Infiltration or conduction block:

Children <10 years: Doses >40 mg (1 mL) as a 4% solution per procedure rarely needed for procedures involving a single tooth, in a maxillary infiltration for 2 to 3 teeth, or for an entire quadrant with a mandibular block.

Children ≥10 years, Adolescents, and Adults: Initial: 40 to 80 mg (1 to 2 mL) as a 4% solution. AAPD guidelines, 2009 maximum recommended dose within a 2-hour period:

<70 kg: 6 mg/kg (400 mg)

≥70 kg: 400 mg or 5 to 6 cartridges

Note: The effective anesthetic dose varies with procedure, intensity of anesthesia needed, duration of anesthesia required and physical condition of the patient. Always use the lowest effective dose along with careful aspiration.

The following numbers of dental carpules (1.8 mL) provide the indicated amounts of prilocaine hydrochloride 4%. See table.

Prilocaine

# of Cartridges (1.8 mL)	mg Prilocaine (4%)
1	72
2	144
3	216
4	288
5	360
6	432
7	504
8	576

Note: Adult and children doses of prilocaine hydrochloride cited from http://www.aapd.org/media/Policies_Guidelines/G_LocalAnesthesia.pdf.

Dosing

Adult & Geriatric Dental anesthesia: Infiltration or conduction block: Initial: 40 to 80 mg (1 to 2 mL) as a 4% solution. AAPD guidelines, 2009 maximum recommended dose within a 2-hour period:

<70 kg: 6 mg/kg (400 mg)

≥70 kg: 400 mg or 5 to 6 cartridges

Note: The effective anesthetic dose varies with procedure, intensity of anesthesia needed, duration of anesthesia required and physical condition of the patient. Always use the lowest effective dose along with careful aspiration.

Renal Impairment: Adult There are no dosage adjustments provided in the manufacturer's labeling. Undergoes renal metabolism; use with caution.

Hepatic Impairment: Adult There are no dosage adjustments provided in the manufacturer's labeling. Undergoes hepatic metabolism; use with caution.

Pediatric

Dental anesthesia: Infiltration or conduction block:

Children <10 years: Doses >40 mg (1 mL) as a 4% solution per procedure rarely needed for procedures involving a single tooth, in a maxillary infiltration for 2 to 3 teeth, or for an entire quadrant with a mandibular block.

Children ≥10 years and Adolescents: Refer to adult dosing.

Renal Impairment: Pediatric There are no dosage adjustments provided in the manufacturer's labeling. Undergoes renal metabolism; use with caution.

Hepatic Impairment: Pediatric There are no dosage adjustments provided in the manufacturer's labeling. Undergoes hepatic metabolism; use with caution.

Mechanism of Action Local anesthetics bind selectively to the intracellular surface of sodium channels to block influx of sodium into the axon. As a result, depolarization necessary for action potential propagation and subsequent nerve function is prevented. The block at the sodium channel is reversible. When drug diffuses away from the axon, sodium channel function is restored and nerve propagation returns.

Contraindications

Hypersensitivity to local anesthetics of the amide type or any component of the formulation; patients with congenital or idiopathic methemoglobinemia

Canadian labeling: Additional contraindications (not in US labeling): Citanest Plain Dental: Severe shock or heart block; inflammation or sepsis in the region of proposed injection

Warnings/Precautions Methemoglobinemia been reported with local anesthetics; clinically significant methemoglobinemia requires immediate treatment along with discontinuation of the anesthetic and other oxidizing agents. Onset may be immediate or delayed (hours) after anesthetic exposure. Patients with glucose-6-phosphate dehydrogenase deficiency, congenital or idiopathic methemoglobinemia, cardiac or pulmonary compromise, exposure to oxidizing agents or their metabolites, or infants <6 months of age are more susceptible and should be closely monitored for signs and symptoms of methemoglobinemia (eg, cyanosis, headache, rapid pulse, shortness of breath, lightheadedness, fatigue). Use is contraindicated in patients with congenital or idiopathic methemoglobinemia. Careful and constant monitoring of the patient's state of consciousness should be done following each local anesthetic injection; at such times, restlessness, anxiety, tinnitus, dizziness, blurred vision, tremors, depression, or drowsiness may be early warning signs of CNS toxicity. Treatment is primarily symptomatic and supportive. Intravascular injections should be avoided. Prilocaine may potentially trigger malignant hyperthermia; follow standard protocol for identification and treatment. Local anesthetics have also been associated with rare occurrences of sudden respiratory arrest, seizures, and cardiac arrest. Use with caution in patients with cardiovascular disease, severe shock, or heart block. Use with caution in patients with hepatic impairment; amide-type anesthetics are metabolized hepatically. Use with caution in acutely ill, debilitated, pediatric or elderly patients. Aspirate the syringe after tissue penetration and before injection to minimize chance of direct vascular injection. Resuscitative equipment, oxygen, and other resuscitative drugs should be available for immediate use. Potentially significant drug-drug interactions may exist, requiring dose or frequency adjustment, additional monitoring, and/or selection of alternative therapy.

Drug Interactions

Metabolism/Transport Effects None known.

Avoid Concomitant Use

Avoid concomitant use of Prilocaine with any of the following: Bupivacaine (Liposomal)

Increased Effect/Toxicity

Prilocaine may increase the levels/effects of: Bupivacaine (Liposomal); Local Anesthetics; Neuromuscular-Blocking Agents; Sodium Nitrite

The levels/effects of Prilocaine may be increased by: Dapsone (Topical); Hyaluronidase; Methemoglobinemia Associated Agents; Nitric Oxide

Decreased Effect

Prilocaine may decrease the levels/effects of: Technetium Tc 99m Tilmanocept

Pharmacodynamics/Kinetics

Onset of Action Infiltration: <2 minutes; Inferior alveolar nerve block: <3 minutes

Duration of Action Infiltration: Complete anesthesia for procedures lasting 20 minutes; Inferior alveolar nerve block: ~2.5 hours

Half-life Elimination 1.6 hours; may be prolonged with hepatic or renal impairment

Pregnancy Risk Factor B

Pregnancy Considerations Adverse events have not been observed in animal reproduction studies. Prilocaine crosses the placenta.

Breastfeeding Considerations It is not known if prilocaine is excreted in breast milk. The manufacturer recommends that caution be exercised when administering prilocaine to nursing women.

Dosage Forms: US

Solution, Injection:

Citanest Plain Dental: 4% (1.8 mL)

Dosage Forms: Canada

Solution, Injection:

4% Citanest Plain Dental: 4% (1.8 mL)

- ◆ **Prilocaine and Lidocaine** *see* Lidocaine and Prilocaine *on page 911*
- ◆ **Prilocaine and Lignocaine** *see* Lidocaine and Prilocaine *on page 911*
- ◆ **Prilocaine HCl** *see* Prilocaine *on page 1274*
- ◆ **Prilolid** *see* Lidocaine and Prilocaine *on page 911*
- ◆ **PriLOSEC** *see* Omeprazole *on page 1139*
- ◆ **PriLOSEC OTC [OTC]** *see* Omeprazole *on page 1139*
- ◆ **Prilovix** *see* Lidocaine and Prilocaine *on page 911*
- ◆ **Priloxx LP [DSC]** *see* Lidocaine and Prilocaine *on page 911*
- ◆ **Primaclone** *see* Primidone *on page 1276*
- ◆ **Primacor** *see* Milrinone *on page 1031*

Primaquine (PRIM a kwin)

Pharmacologic Category Aminoquinoline (Antimalarial); Antimalarial Agent

Use Malaria, treatment: Radical cure (prevention of relapse) malaria caused by *Plasmodium vivax*. **Note:** CDC guidelines also recommend primaquine for radical cure (prevention of relapse) of malaria caused by *Plasmodium ovale* (CDC 2020).

Local Anesthetic/Vasoconstrictor Precautions No information available to require special precautions

Effects on Dental Treatment No significant effects or complications reported

Effects on Bleeding No information available to require special precautions.

Adverse Reactions Frequency not defined.

Cardiovascular: Cardiac arrhythmia, dizziness, prolonged QT interval on ECG

Dermatologic: Pruritus, skin rash

Gastrointestinal: Abdominal cramps, epigastric distress, nausea, vomiting

Hematologic & oncologic: Anemia, hemolytic anemia (in patients with G6PD deficiency), leukopenia, methemoglobinemia (in NADH-methemoglobin reductase-deficient individuals)

Mechanism of Action Primaquine is an antiprotozoal agent active against exoerythrocytic stages of *Plasmodium ovale* and *P. vivax*, also active against the primary exoerythrocytic stages of *P. falciparum* and gametocytes of *Plasmodia*; disrupts mitochondria and binds to DNA

Pharmacodynamics/Kinetics

Half-life Elimination 7 hours; reported range: 3.7 to 9.6 hours

Time to Peak Serum: 1 to 3 hours

Reproductive Considerations

Sexually active females should have a pregnancy test prior to treatment with primaquine. Females of reproductive potential should use effective contraception during therapy and until the next menses following discontinuation of treatment. Males with female partners of reproductive potential should use condoms during therapy and for 3 months after treatment is discontinued.

Pregnancy Considerations Primaquine is contraindicated in pregnant women.

Malaria infection in pregnant women may be more severe than in nonpregnant women and has a high risk of maternal and perinatal morbidity and mortality. Malaria infection during pregnancy can lead to miscarriage, premature delivery, low birth weight, congenital infection, and/or perinatal death. Therefore, pregnant women and women who are likely to become pregnant are advised to avoid travel to malaria-risk areas. When travel is unavoidable, pregnant women should take precautions to avoid mosquito bites and use effective prophylactic medications (CDC 2020; CDC Yellow Book 2020).

Because primaquine may cause acute hemolytic anemia in a fetus with glucose-6-phosphate dehydrogenase deficiency, use is contraindicated in pregnancy. When treatment is needed, other agents are preferred (CDC 2020; CDC Yellow Book 2020). Consult current CDC guidelines for the treatment of malaria during pregnancy.

- ◆ **Primaquine Phosphate** *see* Primaquine *on page 1276*
- ◆ **Primatene Mist** *see* EPINEPHrine (Oral Inhalation) *on page 573*
- ◆ **Primaxin I.M. [DSC]** *see* Imipenem and Cilastatin *on page 799*
- ◆ **Primaxin I.V.** *see* Imipenem and Cilastatin *on page 799*

Primidone (PRI mi done)

Brand Names: US Mysoline

Pharmacologic Category Anticonvulsant, Miscellaneous; Barbiturate

Use Management of grand mal, psychomotor, and focal seizures

Local Anesthetic/Vasoconstrictor Precautions No information available to require special precautions

Effects on Dental Treatment No significant effects or complications reported

Effects on Bleeding Primidone has been associated with clotting factor defects in children, including elevated prothrombin time, elevated partial thromboplastin time, and diminished factors V, VII, or X. These defects are reversible; clotting factors return to normal after discontinuation of primidone.

Adverse Reactions Frequency not defined.

Central nervous system: Ataxia, drowsiness, emotional disturbance, fatigue, hyperirritability, suicidal ideation, vertigo

Dermatologic: Morbilliform rash

Gastrointestinal: Anorexia, nausea, vomiting

Genitourinary: Impotence

Hematologic & oncologic: Agranulocytosis, granulocytopenia, megaloblastic anemia (idiosyncratic), pure red cell aplasia, red cell hypoplasia

Ophthalmic: Diplopia, nystagmus

Mechanism of Action Decreases neuron excitability, raises seizure threshold similar to phenobarbital; primidone has two active metabolites, phenobarbital and phenylethylmalonamide (PEMA); PEMA may enhance the activity of phenobarbital

Pharmacodynamics/Kinetics

Half-life Elimination Primidone: 5 to16 hours (variable); PEMA: 16 to 50 hours (variable); Phenobarbital: 50 to 150 hours (Bourgeois 2000, Neels 2004)

Time to Peak Serum: 0.5 to 9 hours (variable) (Neels 2004)

Pregnancy Considerations Primidone and its metabolites (PEMA, phenobarbital, and p-hydroxyphenobarbital) cross the placenta; neonatal serum concentrations at birth are similar to those in the mother. Withdrawal symptoms may occur in the neonate and may be delayed due to the long half-life of primidone and its metabolites. Use may be associated with birth defects and adverse events; the use of folic acid throughout pregnancy and vitamin K during the last month of pregnancy is recommended. Epilepsy itself, number of medications, genetic factors, or a combination of these probably influence the teratogenicity of anticonvulsant therapy.

Patients exposed to primidone during pregnancy are encouraged to enroll themselves into the NAAED Pregnancy Registry by calling 1-888-233-2334. Additional information is available at www.aedpregnancyregistry.org.

- **Primlev** *see* Oxycodone and Acetaminophen *on page 1164*
- **Primsol** *see* Trimethoprim *on page 1498*
- **Principen** *see* Ampicillin *on page 140*
- **Prinivil** *see* Lisinopril *on page 922*
- **Pristiq** *see* Desvenlafaxine *on page 462*
- **Privigen** *see* Immune Globulin *on page 803*
- **Prizotral II** *see* Lidocaine and Prilocaine *on page 911*
- **Pro-C-Dure 5** *see* Triamcinolone (Systemic) *on page 1485*
- **Pro-C-Dure 6** *see* Triamcinolone (Systemic) *on page 1485*
- **ProAir Digihaler** *see* Albuterol *on page 90*
- **ProAir HFA** *see* Albuterol *on page 90*
- **ProAir RespiClick** *see* Albuterol *on page 90*
- **ProAmatine** *see* Midodrine *on page 1027*

Probenecid (proe BEN e sid)

Pharmacologic Category Uricosuric Agent

Use

Treatment of hyperuricemia associated with gout or gouty arthritis; prolongation and elevation of beta-lactam plasma levels

Guideline recommendations:

Gout: Uricosurics, such as probenecid, are recommended alone or in combination with allopurinol in patients without proper control with allopurinol alone (EULAR [Richette 2016]).

Local Anesthetic/Vasoconstrictor Precautions No information available to require special precautions

Effects on Dental Treatment Key adverse event(s) related to dental treatment: Sore gums.

Effects on Bleeding No information available to require special precautions

Adverse Reactions Frequency not defined.

Cardiovascular: Flushing

Central nervous system: Dizziness, headache, pain (costovertebral)

Dermatologic: Alopecia, dermatitis, pruritus, skin rash

Endocrine & metabolic: Gouty arthritis (acute)

Gastrointestinal: Anorexia, dyspepsia, gastroesophageal reflux disease, gingival pain, nausea, vomiting

Genitourinary: Hematuria, nephrotic syndrome

Hematologic & oncologic: Anemia, aplastic anemia, hemolytic anemia (in G6PD deficiency), leukopenia

Hepatic: Hepatic necrosis

Hypersensitivity: Anaphylaxis, hypersensitivity reaction

Renal: Polyuria, renal colic

Miscellaneous: Fever

Mechanism of Action Competitively inhibits the reabsorption of uric acid at the proximal convoluted tubule, thereby promoting its excretion and reducing serum uric acid levels; increases plasma levels of weak organic acids (penicillins, cephalosporins, or other beta-lactam antibiotics) by competitively inhibiting their renal tubular secretion

Pharmacodynamics/Kinetics

Onset of Action Effect on penicillin levels: 2 hours; Uric acid renal clearance: 30 minutes

Half-life Elimination Dose dependent: Normal renal function: 6 to 12 hours

Time to Peak Serum: 2 to 4 hours

Pregnancy Considerations Probenecid crosses the placenta. Based on available data, an increased risk of adverse fetal events have not been reported (Gutman, 2012).

- **Probenecid and Colchicine** *see* Colchicine and Probenecid *on page 406*
- **Probuphine Implant Kit** *see* Buprenorphine *on page 260*

Procainamide (pro KANE a mide)

Related Information

Clinical Risk Related to Drugs Prolonging QT Interval *on page 1675*

Brand Names: Canada APO-Procainamide; Procan SR

Pharmacologic Category Antiarrhythmic Agent, Class Ia

Use

Ventricular arrhythmias: Intravenous: Treatment of life-threatening ventricular arrhythmias

Supraventricular arrhythmias: Oral [Canadian product]: Treatment of supraventricular arrhythmias. **Note:** In the treatment of atrial fibrillation, use only when preferred treatment is ineffective or cannot be used. Use in paroxysmal atrial tachycardia when reflex stimulation or other measures are ineffective.

Local Anesthetic/Vasoconstrictor Precautions Procainamide is one of the drugs confirmed to prolong the QT interval and is accepted as having a risk of causing torsade de pointes. The risk of drug-induced torsade de pointes is extremely low when a single QT interval prolonging drug is prescribed. In terms of epinephrine, it is not known what effect vasoconstrictors in the local anesthetic regimen will have in patients with a known history of congenital prolonged QT interval or in patients taking any medication that prolongs the QT interval. Until more information is obtained, it is suggested that the clinician consult with the physician prior to the use of a vasoconstrictor in suspected patients, and that the vasoconstrictor (epinephrine, mepivacaine and levonordefrin [Carbocaine® 2% with Neo-Cobefrin®]) be used with caution.

Effects on Dental Treatment Key adverse event(s) related to dental treatment: Taste disorder.

Effects on Bleeding Patients may develop procainamide-induced syndrome, which causes prolonged thrombin and Reptilase® clotting times of plasma. Clinical manifestations of procainamide-induced syndrome subside following procainamide cessation.

Adverse Reactions

>10%:

Hematologic & oncologic: Positive ANA titer (≤50%)

Neuromuscular & skeletal: Lupus-like syndrome (≤30%, increased incidence with long-term therapy or slow acetylators; syndrome may include abdominal pain, arthralgia, arthritis, chills, fever, hepatomegaly, myalgia, pericarditis, pleural effusion, pulmonary infiltrates, skin rash)

1% to 10%:

Cardiovascular: Hypotension (intravenous: ≤5%)

Dermatologic: Skin rash

Gastrointestinal: Diarrhea (oral: 3% to 4%), dysgeusia (oral: 3% to 4%), nausea (oral: 3% to 4%), vomiting (oral: 3% to 4%)

<1%, postmarketing, and/or case reports: Agranulocytosis, angioedema, anorexia, aplastic anemia, arthralgia, asystole, bone marrow depression, cerebellar ataxia, confusion, demyelinating disease (demyelinating polyradiculoneuropathy), depression, depression of myocardial contractility, disorientation, dizziness, drug fever, exacerbation of cardiac arrhythmia, exacerbation of myasthenia gravis, fever, first degree atrioventricular block, flushing, gastrointestinal pseudo-obstruction, granulomatous hepatitis, hallucination, hemolytic anemia, hepatic failure, hyperbilirubinemia, hypoplastic anemia, increased serum alkaline phosphatase, increased serum transaminases, intrahepatic cholestasis, leukopenia, maculopapular rash, mania, myocarditis, myopathy, neuromuscular blockade, neutropenia, pancreatitis, pancytopenia, peripheral neuropathy, pleural effusion, polyneuropathy, positive direct Coombs test, prolonged QT interval on ECG, psychosis, pruritus, pulmonary embolism, second degree atrioventricular block, tachycardia, thrombocytopenia, torsades de pointes, urticaria, vasculitis, ventricular fibrillation, ventricular tachycardia (paradoxical; in atrial fibrillation/flutter), weakness

Mechanism of Action Decreases myocardial excitability and conduction velocity and may depress myocardial contractility, by increasing the electrical stimulation threshold of ventricle, His-Purkinje system and through direct cardiac effects

Pharmacodynamics/Kinetics

Onset of Action IM 10 to 30 minutes

Half-life Elimination

Procainamide (hepatic acetylator, phenotype, cardiac and renal function dependent): Children: 1.7 hours; Adults: 2.5 to 4.7 hours; Anephric: 11 hours

NAPA (renal function dependent): Children: 6 hours; Adults: 6 to 8 hours; Anephric: 42 hours

Time to Peak Serum: IM: 15 to 60 minutes

Pregnancy Considerations

Procainamide crosses the placenta (Dumesic 1982; Oudijk 2002); procainamide and its active metabolite (N-acetyl procainamide) can be detected in the cord blood and neonatal serum (Pittard 1983). Intravenous procainamide may be considered for the acute treatment of SVT in pregnant women. Due to adverse events (lupus-like syndrome), long-term therapy should be avoided unless other options are not available (Page [ACC/AHA/HRS 2015]).

Dental Health Professional Considerations See Local Anesthetic/Vasoconstrictor Precautions

◆ **Procainamide Hydrochloride** *see* Procainamide *on page 1277*

◆ **Procaine Amide Hydrochloride** *see* Procainamide *on page 1277*

◆ **Procaine Benzylpenicillin** *see* Penicillin G Procaine *on page 1210*

◆ **Procaine Penicillin G** *see* Penicillin G Procaine *on page 1210*

◆ **Procanbid** *see* Procainamide *on page 1277*

Procarbazine (proe KAR ba zeen)

Brand Names: US Matulane

Brand Names: Canada Matulane

Pharmacologic Category Antineoplastic Agent, Alkylating Agent

Use Hodgkin lymphoma: Treatment of stage III or IV Hodgkin lymphoma (in combination with other chemotherapy agents)

Local Anesthetic/Vasoconstrictor Precautions No information available to require special precautions

Effects on Dental Treatment Key adverse event(s) related to dental treatment: Xerostomia (normal salivary flow resumes upon discontinuation), stomatitis, and dysphagia.

Effects on Bleeding Chemotherapy may result in significant myelosuppression, potentially including significant reduction in platelet counts and altered hemostasis. In patients who are under active treatment with these agents, medical consult is suggested.

Adverse Reactions Frequency not always defined.

Cardiovascular: Edema, flushing, hypotension, syncope, tachycardia

Central nervous system: Apprehension, ataxia, chills, coma, confusion, depression, dizziness, drowsiness, falling, fatigue, hallucination, headache, hyporeflexia, insomnia, lethargy, nervousness, neuropathy, nightmares, pain, paresthesia, seizure, slurred speech, unsteadiness

Dermatologic: Alopecia, dermatitis, diaphoresis, hyperpigmentation, pruritus, skin rash, urticaria

Endocrine & metabolic: Gynecomastia (in prepubertal and early pubertal males)

Gastrointestinal: Nausea and vomiting (60% to 90%; increasing the dose in a stepwise fashion over several days may minimize), abdominal pain, anorexia, constipation, diarrhea, dysphagia, hematemesis, melena, stomatitis, xerostomia

Genitourinary: Reduced fertility (>10%), azoospermia (reported with combination chemotherapy), hematuria, nocturia

Hematologic & oncologic: Malignant neoplasm (2% to 15%; secondary; nonlymphoid; reported with combination therapy), anemia, bone marrow depression, eosinophilia, hemolysis (in patients with G6PD deficiency), hemolytic anemia, pancytopenia, petechia, purpura, thrombocytopenia

Hepatic: Hepatic insufficiency, jaundice

Hypersensitivity: Hypersensitivity reaction

Infection: Herpes virus infection, increased susceptibility to infection

Neuromuscular & skeletal: Arthralgia, foot-drop, myalgia, tremor, weakness

Ophthalmic: Accommodation disturbance, diplopia, nystagmus, papilledema, photophobia, retinal hemorrhage

Otic: Hearing loss

Renal: Polyuria

Respiratory: Cough, epistaxis, hemoptysis, hoarseness, pleural effusion, pneumonitis, pulmonary toxicity (<1%)

Miscellaneous: Fever

Mechanism of Action Procarbazine inhibits DNA, RNA, and protein synthesis by inhibiting transmethylation of methionine into transfer RNA; may also damage DNA directly through alkylation.

Pharmacodynamics/Kinetics

Half-life Elimination ~1 hour

Time to Peak ≤1 hour

Reproductive Considerations

Females of reproductive potential should avoid becoming pregnant during treatment.

Azoospermia and infertility have been reported with procarbazine when used in combination with other chemotherapy agents.

Pregnancy Considerations

Procarbazine may cause fetal harm if administered to a pregnant female. There are case reports of fetal malformations in the offspring of pregnant women exposed to procarbazine as part of a combination chemotherapy regimen.

◆ **Procarbazine HCl** *see* Procarbazine *on page 1278*

◆ **Procarbazine Hydrochloride** *see* Procarbazine *on page 1278*

◆ **Procardia** *see* NIFEdipine *on page 1104*

◆ **Procardia XL** *see* NIFEdipine *on page 1104*

◆ **ProCentra** *see* Dextroamphetamine *on page 474*

◆ **Procetofene** *see* Fenofibrate and Derivatives *on page 640*

◆ **Prochieve** *see* Progesterone *on page 1280*

Prochlorperazine (proe klor PER a zeen)

Related Information

Dentin Hypersensitivity, Acid Erosion, High Caries Index, Management of Alveolar Osteitis, and Xerostomia *on page 1762*

Management of the Patient With Anxiety or Depression *on page 1778*

Brand Names: US Compro

Brand Names: Canada PMS-Prochlorperazine; Prochlorazine; SANDOZ Prochlorperazine

Pharmacologic Category Antiemetic; First Generation (Typical) Antipsychotic; Phenothiazine Derivative

Use Nausea/vomiting: Management of severe nausea and vomiting

Local Anesthetic/Vasoconstrictor Precautions

May lower seizure threshold; use caution when administering prochlorperazine in combination with other agents that reduce seizure threshold (ie, local anesthetics). Due to prochlorperazine induced alpha-adrenergic blockade, administration of local anesthetics containing vasoconstrictors (epinephrine or levonordefrin), causes unopposed stimulation of beta-adrenergic receptors in heart and peripheral blood vessels that may result in tachycardia, peripheral vasodilation, or hypotension. Effects on blood pressure are greater in combination with epinephrine than levonordefrin.

Effects on Dental Treatment Key adverse event(s) related to dental treatment: All reactions listed are based on reports for other agents in this same pharmacologic class and may not be specifically reported for prochlorperazine. Frequent occurrence of xerostomia and changes in salivation (normal salivary flow resumes upon discontinuation).

Considerations for dental care: Significant hypotension may occur, especially when the drug is administered parenterally or following administration of local anesthetics containing vasoconstrictors (ie, epinephrine or levonordefrin); patients may experience orthostatic hypotension as they stand up after treatment, especially if lying in dental chair for extended periods of time. Use caution with sudden changes in position during and after dental treatment. Orthostatic hypotension is due to alpha-receptor blockade; the elderly are at greater risk for orthostatic hypotension.

Significant sedation can occur and may be increased in the elderly and in patients taking other CNS depressants (ie, opioid analgesics or benzodiazepines).

Extrapyramidal effects including akathisia (motor restlessness), acute dystonia (spasmodic contractures), pseudoparkinsonism, and tardive dyskinesia can occur with 1 dose. These effects are more likely in the elderly, patients taking other dopamine antagonists (including antipsychotic agents and some antiemetic agents), and patients with Parkinson disease.

Due to increased risk of adverse effects and drug interactions especially with opioid analgesics, reserve use for patients with moderate to severe postoperative nausea and vomiting, who cannot afford ondansetron, and for whom promethazine did not provide adequate control.

Effects on Bleeding No information available to require special precautions

Adverse Reactions Frequency not defined. Reactions listed are based on reports for other agents in this same pharmacologic class and may not be specifically reported for prochlorperazine.

Cardiovascular: ECG abnormality (Q wave and T wave distortions), hypotension, peripheral edema

Central nervous system: Agitation, altered cerebrospinal proteins, catatonia, cerebral edema, coma, decreased cough reflex, disruption of body temperature regulation, dizziness, drowsiness, dystonia (carpopedal spasm, protrusion of tongue, torticollis, trismus), extrapyramidal reaction (akathisia, dystonias, hyperreflexia, pseudoparkinsonism, tardive dyskinesia), headache, hyperpyrexia, insomnia, jitteriness, neuroleptic malignant syndrome (NMS), opisthotonos, restlessness, seizure

Dermatologic: Contact dermatitis, diaphoresis, erythema, eczema, exfoliative dermatitis, pruritus, skin photosensitivity, skin changes, skin pigmentation, urticaria

Endocrine & metabolic: Amenorrhea, change in libido, galactorrhea, gynecomastia, glycosuria, hyperglycemia, hypoglycemia, menstrual disease, weight gain

Gastrointestinal: Atony of colon, cholestasis, increased appetite, constipation, intestinal obstruction, nausea, obstipation, vomiting, xerostomia

Genitourinary: Ejaculatory disorder, impotence, lactation, priapism, urinary retention

Hematologic & oncologic: Agranulocytosis, aplastic anemia, eosinophilia, hemolytic anemia, immune thrombocytopenia, leukopenia, pancytopenia

Hepatic: Cholestatic jaundice, hepatotoxicity

Hypersensitivity: Anaphylactoid reaction, angioedema, hypersensitivity reaction
Infection: Infection
Neuromuscular & skeletal: Lupus-like syndrome, tremor
Ophthalmic: Blurred vision, cataract, epithelial keratopathy, corneal deposits, miosis, mydriasis, oculogyric crisis, retinitis pigmentosa
Respiratory: Asphyxia, asthma, laryngeal edema, nasal congestion
Miscellaneous: Fever (mild; intramuscular administration)

Mechanism of Action Prochlorperazine is a piperazine phenothiazine antipsychotic which blocks postsynaptic mesolimbic dopaminergic D_1 and D_2 receptors in the brain, including the chemoreceptor trigger zone; exhibits a strong alpha-adrenergic and anticholinergic blocking effect and depresses the release of hypothalamic and hypophyseal hormones; believed to depress the reticular activating system, thus affecting basal metabolism, body temperature, wakefulness, vasomotor tone and emesis

Pharmacodynamics/Kinetics

Onset of Action Oral: 30 to 40 minutes; IM: 10 to 20 minutes; Rectal: ~60 minutes; Peak antiemetic effect: IV: 30 to 60 minutes

Duration of Action Rectal: 3 to 12 hours; IM, Oral: 3 to 4 hours

Half-life Elimination Oral: 6 to 10 hours (single dose), 14 to 22 hours (repeated dosing) (Isah 1991); IV: 6 to 10 hours (Isah 1991; Taylor 1987)

Reproductive Considerations
Use may interfere with pregnancy tests, causing false positive results.

Pregnancy Considerations Jaundice or hyper- or hyporeflexia have been reported in newborn infants following maternal use of phenothiazines. Antipsychotic use during the third trimester of pregnancy has a risk for abnormal muscle movements (extrapyramidal symptoms [EPS]) and withdrawal symptoms in newborns following delivery. Symptoms in the newborn may include agitation, feeding disorder, hypertonia, hypotonia, respiratory distress, somnolence, and tremor; these effects may be self-limiting or require hospitalization.

The use of prochlorperazine may be considered for adjunctive treatment of nausea and vomiting in pregnant patients when symptoms persist following initial pharmacologic therapy (ACOG 189 2018).

- ◆ **Prochlorperazine Edisylate** *see* Prochlorperazine *on page 1279*
- ◆ **Prochlorperazine Maleate** *see* Prochlorperazine *on page 1279*
- ◆ **Prochlorperazine Mesylate** *see* Prochlorperazine *on page 1279*
- ◆ **Prociclide** *see* Defibrotide *on page 449*
- ◆ **Procrit** *see* Epoetin Alfa *on page 577*
- ◆ **Proctocort** *see* Hydrocortisone (Topical) *on page 775*
- ◆ **Proctofene** *see* Fenofibrate and Derivatives *on page 640*
- ◆ **Proctofoam [OTC]** *see* Pramoxine *on page 1252*
- ◆ **Procto-Med HC** *see* Hydrocortisone (Topical) *on page 775*
- ◆ **Procto-Pak** *see* Hydrocortisone (Topical) *on page 775*
- ◆ **Proctosol HC** *see* Hydrocortisone (Topical) *on page 775*
- ◆ **Proctozone-HC** *see* Hydrocortisone (Topical) *on page 775*

Procyclidine (proe SYE kli deen)

Brand Names: Canada PDP-Procyclidine

Pharmacologic Category Anti-Parkinson Agent, Anticholinergic; Anticholinergic Agent

Use Note: Not available in the US

Parkinson disease: Treatment of parkinsonism, including postencephalitic, arteriosclerotic, and idiopathic types.

Extrapyramidal side effects: Relieves symptoms (eg, dystonia, dyskinesia, akathisia, and parkinsonism) induced by phenothiazine or rauwolfia compounds during treatment of mental depression.

Local Anesthetic/Vasoconstrictor Precautions
No information available to require special precautions

Effects on Dental Treatment Key adverse event(s) related to dental treatment: Xerostomia (normal salivary flow resumes upon discontinuation) and dry throat and nose. Prolonged use of antidyskinetics may decrease or inhibit salivary flow, contributing to discomfort and dental disease (ie, caries, oral candidiasis, and periodontal disease).

Effects on Bleeding No information available to require special precautions

Adverse Reactions Frequency not defined.
Central nervous system: Dizziness
Dermatologic: Skin rash
Gastrointestinal: Constipation, epigastric distress, nausea, vomiting, xerostomia
Hypersensitivity: Hypersensitivity reaction
Neuromuscular & skeletal: Weakness
Ophthalmic: Blurred vision, mydriasis
<1%, postmarketing, and/or case reports: Suppurative parotitis (acute)

Mechanism of Action Thought to act by blocking excess acetylcholine at cerebral synapses; many of its effects are due to its pharmacologic similarities with atropine; it exerts an antispasmodic effect on smooth muscle, is a potent mydriatic; inhibits salivation

Pharmacodynamics/Kinetics

Onset of Action 45 to 60 minutes (Whiteman 1985)

Duration of Action Significant autonomic effects have been observed up to 12 hours (Whiteman 1985)

Half-life Elimination ~12.6 hours (Whiteman 1985)

Time to Peak ~1.1 hour (Whiteman 1985)

Pregnancy Considerations
Safe use during pregnancy has not been established.

Product Availability Not available in the US

- ◆ **Procyclidine Hydrochloride** *see* Procyclidine *on page 1280*
- ◆ **Prodigen** *see Lactobacillus on page 869*
- ◆ **Pro-Ex Antifungal [OTC]** *see* Clotrimazole (Topical) *on page 397*
- ◆ **ProFeno [DSC]** *see* Fenoprofen *on page 642*

Progesterone (proe JES ter one)

Brand Names: US Crinone; Endometrin; Prometrium

Brand Names: Canada ACT Progesterone; AURO-Progesterone; Crinone; Endometrin; PMS-Progesterone; Prometrium; REDDY-Progesterone; TEVA-Progesterone

Pharmacologic Category Progestin

Use

Oral: Prevention of endometrial hyperplasia in nonhysterectomized, postmenopausal women who are receiving conjugated estrogens; treatment of secondary amenorrhea

IM: Treatment of amenorrhea or abnormal uterine bleeding due to hormonal imbalance in the absence of organic pathology, such as submucous fibroids or uterine cancer

Intravaginal gel: Part of assisted reproductive technology (ART) for infertile women with progesterone deficiency; treatment of secondary amenorrhea

Vaginal insert: To support embryo implantation and early pregnancy by supplementation of corpus luteal function as part of ART for infertile women

Local Anesthetic/Vasoconstrictor Precautions
No information available to require special precautions

Effects on Dental Treatment Key adverse event(s) related to dental treatment: Progestins may predispose the patient to gingival bleeding.

Effects on Bleeding No information available to require special precautions

Adverse Reactions

Intramuscular injection: Frequency not defined:

Cardiovascular: Edema

Central nervous system: Depression, drowsiness, insomnia

Dermatologic: Acne vulgaris, allergic skin rash, alopecia, hirsutism, pruritus, skin rash, urticaria

Endocrine & metabolic: Amenorrhea, change in menstrual flow, galactorrhea not associated with childbirth, weight gain, weight loss

Gastrointestinal: Nausea

Genitourinary: Breakthrough bleeding, breast tenderness, cervical erosion, change in cervical secretions, spotting

Hepatic: Cholestatic jaundice

Hypersensitivity: Anaphylactoid shock

Local: Erythema at injection site, irritation at injection site, pain at injection site

Miscellaneous: Fever

Oral (percentages reported when used in combination with or cycled with conjugated estrogens):

>10%:

Central nervous system: Headache (16% to 31%), dizziness (15% to 24%), depression (19%)

Endocrine & metabolic: Breast tenderness (27%), mastalgia (6% to 16%)

Gastrointestinal: Abdominal pain (20%), bloating (12%)

Genitourinary: Urinary tract abnormality (11%)

Infection: Viral infection (12%)

Neuromuscular & skeletal: Musculoskeletal pain (12%)

1% to 10%:

Cardiovascular: Chest pain (7%)

Central nervous system: Anxiety (8%), fatigue (8%), irritability (8%)

Gastrointestinal: Nausea and vomiting (≤8%), diarrhea (7% to 8%), constipation (3% to <5%), cholecystectomy (2% to <5%)

Genitourinary: Vaginal discharge (10%)

Hematologic & oncologic: Malignant neoplasm of breast (2% to <5%)

Respiratory: Cough (8%)

Frequency not defined:

Cardiovascular: Cerebrovascular accident, deep vein thrombosis, myocardial infarction, pulmonary embolism

Central nervous system: Dementia

<1%, postmarketing and/or case reports: Abnormal gait, abnormal uterine bleeding, acute pancreatitis, aggressive behavior, alopecia, anaphylaxis, arthralgia, asthma, blurred vision, choking sensation, cholestasis, cholestatic hepatitis, circulatory shock, cleft lip, cleft palate, confusion, congenital heart disease, depersonalization, diplopia, disorientation, drowsiness, dysarthria, dysphagia, dyspnea, endometrial carcinoma, facial edema, feeling abnormal, heavy menstrual bleeding, hepatic failure, hepatic necrosis, hepatitis, hypersensitivity reaction, hypertension, hypospadias, hypotension, impaired consciousness, increased liver enzymes, increased serum glucose, intoxicated feeling, jaundice, loss of consciousness, menstrual disease, muscle cramps, ovarian cyst, paresthesia, pruritus, sedation, seizure, slurred speech, spontaneous abortion, stupor, suicidal ideation, syncope, tachycardia, tinnitus, tongue edema, transient ischemic attacks, urticaria, vertigo, visual disturbance, weight gain, weight loss

Vaginal gel (percentages reported with Assisted Reproductive Technology):

>10%:

Central nervous system: Drowsiness (27%), headache (13% to 17%), nervousness (16%), depression (11%)

Gastrointestinal: Constipation (27%), nausea (7% to 22%), muscle cramps (15%), abdominal pain (12%)

Genitourinary: Breast hypertrophy (40%), perineal pain (17%), mastalgia (13%), nocturia (13%)

1% to 10%:

Central nervous system: Pain (8%), dizziness (5%)

Dermatologic: Genital pruritus (5%)

Endocrine & metabolic: Decreased libido (10%)

Gastrointestinal: Diarrhea (8%), bloating (7%), vomiting (5%)

Genitourinary: Vaginal discharge (7%), dyspareunia (6%), genital candidiasis (5%)

Neuromuscular & skeletal: Arthralgia (8%)

Vaginal insert (percentages reported with Assisted Reproductive Technology):

>10%: Gastrointestinal: Abdominal pain (12%)

1% to 10%:

Central nervous system: Headache (3% to 4%), fatigue (2% to 3%)

Endocrine & metabolic: Ovarian hyperstimulation syndrome (7%)

Gastrointestinal: Nausea (7% to 8%), abdominal distention (4%), constipation (2% to 3%), vomiting (2% to 3%)

Genitourinary: Uterine spasm (3% to 4%), vaginal hemorrhage (3%), urinary tract infection (1% to 2%)

<1%, postmarketing, and/or case reports: Peripheral edema, urticaria, vaginal discomfort, vulvovaginal burning, vulvovaginal irritation, vulvovaginal pruritus

Mechanism of Action Natural steroid hormone that induces secretory changes in the endometrium, promotes mammary gland development, relaxes uterine smooth muscle, blocks follicular maturation and ovulation, and maintains pregnancy. When used as part of an ART program in the luteal phase, progesterone supports embryo implantation.

Pharmacodynamics/Kinetics

Half-life Elimination Vaginal gel: 5 to 20 minutes

Time to Peak Oral: Within 3 hours; IM: ~8 hours; Intravaginal gel: 3.55 ± 2.48 to 7 ± 2.88 hours; Vaginal insert: 17.3 to 24 hours

Reproductive Considerations
The vaginal gel and insert are indicated for use in assisted reproductive technology (ART).

Pregnancy Risk Factor B (oral)

Pregnancy Considerations
The oral capsules are contraindicated for use during pregnancy.

Adverse events following maternal use in pregnancy (eg, hypospadias, congenital heart disease, cleft lip/palate) have been noted in postmarketing data; however, a causal relationship has not been clearly established. Use of vaginal progesterone may be considered to decrease the risk of recurrent spontaneous preterm birth in women with a singleton pregnancy and prior spontaneous preterm singleton birth (therapy may begin at 16 to 24 weeks, regardless of cervical length). It may also be used to prevent spontaneous preterm birth in women with a singleton pregnancy who have a cervix <20 mm before or at 24 weeks' gestation. Use is not recommended as an intervention for women with multiple gestations (ACOG 2012).

Product Availability Milprosa: FDA approved April 2020; anticipated availability is currently unknown. Milprosa is indicated to support embryo implantation and early pregnancy (up to 10 weeks post-embryo transfer) by supplementation of corpus luteal function as part of an Assisted Reproductive Technology (ART) treatment program for infertile women up to and including 34 years of age. Information pertaining to this product within the monograph is pending revision. Consult the prescribing information for additional information.

- **Progestin** *see* Progesterone *on page 1280*
- **Prograf** *see* Tacrolimus (Systemic) *on page 1398*
- **Proguanil and Atovaquone** *see* Atovaquone and Proguanil *on page 193*
- **Proguanil Hydrochloride and Atovaquone** *see* Atovaquone and Proguanil *on page 193*
- **Prokine** *see* Sargramostim *on page 1358*
- **Proleukin** *see* Aldesleukin *on page 91*
- **Prolia** *see* Denosumab *on page 453*
- **Prolixin** *see* FluPHENAZine *on page 699*
- **Promacta** *see* Eltrombopag *on page 551*
- **Promella in Prebiotic** *see Lactobacillus on page 869*

Promethazine (proe METH a zeen)

Brand Names: US Phenadoz [DSC]; Phenergan; Promethegan

Pharmacologic Category Antiemetic; Histamine H_1 Antagonist; Histamine H_1 Antagonist, First Generation; Phenothiazine Derivative

Use

Allergic conditions, treatment: Perennial and seasonal allergic rhinitis; vasomotor rhinitis; allergic conjunctivitis due to inhalant allergens and foods; mild, uncomplicated allergic skin manifestations of urticaria and angioedema; amelioration of allergic reactions to blood or plasma; dermographism; anaphylactic reactions, as adjunctive therapy to epinephrine and other standard measures, after the acute manifestations have been controlled

Nausea and vomiting: Prevention and control of nausea and vomiting associated with certain types of anesthesia and surgery; antiemetic therapy in postoperative patients

Motion sickness: Active and prophylactic treatment of motion sickness

Surgical analgesia/hypnotic; pre-/postoperative adjunct: Adjunctive therapy with analgesics and/or anesthesia

Sedation: Preoperative, postoperative, and obstetric sedation; for sedation, relief of apprehension, and production of light sleep from which the patient can be easily aroused

Local Anesthetic/Vasoconstrictor Precautions
Due to promethazine-induced alpha-adrenergic blockade, administration of local anesthetics containing the vasoconstrictors epinephrine or levonordefrin, causes unopposed stimulation of beta-adrenergic receptors in heart and peripheral blood vessels that may result in tachycardia and peripheral vasodilation causing hypotension. Effects on blood pressure are greater in combination with epinephrine than levonordefrin.

Effects on Dental Treatment Key adverse event(s) related to dental treatment: Unreported frequency of xerostomia (normal salivary flow resumes upon discontinuation) has been observed.

Erratic changes in blood pressure have also been observed. Significant hypotension may occur, especially when the drug is administered parenterally or following administration of local anesthetics containing vasoconstrictors (ie, epinephrine or levonordefrin); Patients may experience orthostatic hypotension as they stand up after treatment; especially if lying in dental chair for extended periods of time. Use caution with sudden changes in position during and after dental treatment. Orthostatic hypotension is due to alpha-receptor blockade, the elderly are at greater risk for orthostatic hypotension.

Note: Significant sedation can occur and may be increased in the elderly and in patients taking or administered other CNS depressants (ie, opioid analgesics or benzodiazepines).

Extrapyramidal effects including akathisia (motor restlessness), acute dystonia (spasmodic contractures), pseudoparkinsonism, and tardive dyskinesia can occur with a single dose. These effects are more likely in the elderly, patients taking other dopamine antagonists (including antipsychotic agents and some antiemetic agents), and patients with Parkinson's disease.

Promethazine is a less expensive alternative for moderate-to-severe postoperative nausea than ondansetron but with a greater chance of adverse effects and drug interactions especially with opioid analgesics.

Effects on Bleeding No information available to require special precautions

Adverse Reactions
Frequency not defined.

Cardiovascular: Bradycardia, decreased blood pressure, increased blood pressure, local thrombophlebitis (injection), localized phlebitis (injection), peripheral vasospasm (injection), tachycardia, venous thrombosis (injection)

Central nervous system: Abnormal sensory symptoms (injection), agitation, catatonia, confusion, delirium, disorientation, dizziness, drowsiness, euphoria, excitement, extrapyramidal reaction, fatigue, hallucination, hyperexcitability, hysteria, insomnia, lassitude, movement disorder, paralysis (injection), nervousness, neuroleptic malignant syndrome, nightmares, sedated state, seizure

Dermatologic: Dermatitis, gangrene of skin and/or other subcutaneous tissues (injection), skin photosensitivity, urticaria

Gastrointestinal: Nausea, vomiting, xerostomia

Hematologic & oncologic: Agranulocytosis, immune thrombocytopenia, leukopenia, thrombocytopenia

Hepatic: Cholestatic jaundice, jaundice

Hypersensitivity: Angioedema

Local: Abscess at injection site, burning sensation at injection site, erythema at injection site, local tissue necrosis (injection), pain at injection site, swelling at injection site

Neuromuscular & skeletal: Tremor

Ophthalmic: Blurred vision, diplopia

Otic: Tinnitus

Respiratory: Apnea, asthma, nasal congestion

<1%, postmarketing, and/or case reports: Respiratory depression

Mechanism of Action Phenothiazine derivative; blocks postsynaptic mesolimbic dopaminergic receptors in the brain; exhibits a strong alpha-adrenergic blocking effect and depresses the release of hypothalamic and hypophyseal hormones; competes with histamine for the H_1-receptor; muscarinic-blocking effect may be responsible for antiemetic activity; reduces stimuli to the brainstem reticular system

Pharmacodynamics/Kinetics

Onset of Action Oral, IM: ~20 minutes; IV: ~5 minutes

Duration of Action Usually 4 to 6 hours (up to 12 hours)

Half-life Elimination IM: ~10 hours; IV: 9 to 16 hours; Suppositories, syrup: 16 to 19 hours (range: 4 to 34 hours) (Strenkoski-Nix 2000)

Time to Peak Maximum serum concentration (Brunton 2011): Oral (syrup): 2.8 ± 1.4 hours; Rectal: 8.2 ± 3.4 hours

Pregnancy Risk Factor C

Pregnancy Considerations

Promethazine crosses the placenta (Potts 1961). Platelet aggregation may be inhibited in newborns following maternal use of promethazine within 2 weeks of delivery.

Promethazine is indicated for use during labor for obstetric sedation and may be used alone or as an adjunct to opioid analgesics. Promethazine may be used as adjunctive therapy in the management of nausea and vomiting of pregnancy when the preferred agents do not provide initial symptom improvement or when symptoms persist despite other therapies (ACOG 189 2018). Although promethazine is approved for the treatment of allergic conditions (eg, allergic rhinitis, urticaria), other agents are preferred for use in pregnancy (Scadding 2017; Wallace 2008; Zuberbier 2014).

Dental Health Professional Considerations **Sedation:** When used alone as a sedative agent the degree of sedation is often mild. As a sedative agent, promethazine is effective in managing pediatric patients that require mild anxiety control. It is ineffective when used alone in children with extreme apprehension or for the disruptive, unmanageable child. A more profound sedation will occur if promethazine is administered in combination with an opioid or benzodiazepine. If promethazine is combined with an opioid, the dose of the opioid should be decreased by 25% to 50%.

Promethazine and Codeine

(proe METH a zeen & KOE deen)

Related Information

Codeine *on page 404*

Promethazine *on page 1282*

Pharmacologic Category Analgesic, Opioid; Antitussive; Histamine H_1 Antagonist; Histamine H_1 Antagonist, First Generation; Phenothiazine Derivative

Use Cough and upper respiratory symptoms: Temporary relief of coughs and upper respiratory symptoms associated with allergy or the common cold.

Local Anesthetic/Vasoconstrictor Precautions

No information available to require special precautions

Effects on Dental Treatment Although promethazine is a phenothiazine derivative, extrapyramidal reactions or tardive dyskinesias are not seen with the use of this drug.

Effects on Bleeding No information available to require special precautions

Adverse Reactions Also see individual agents.

Postmarketing and/or case reports: Hypogonadism (Brennan 2013; Debono 2011)

Mechanism of Action

Codeine: Binds to opioid receptors in the CNS, causing inhibition of ascending pain pathways, altering the perception of and response to pain; causes cough suppression by direct central action in the medulla; produces generalized CNS depression.

Promethazine: Phenothiazine derivative; blocks postsynaptic mesolimbic dopaminergic receptors in the brain; exhibits a strong alpha-adrenergic blocking effect and depresses the release of hypothalamic and hypophyseal hormones; competes with histamine for the H1-receptor; muscarinic-blocking effect may be responsible for antiemetic activity; reduces stimuli to the brainstem reticular system.

Reproductive Considerations

Long-term opioid use may cause secondary hypogonadism, which may lead to sexual dysfunction or infertility in men and women (Brennan 2013).

Pregnancy Risk Factor C

Pregnancy Considerations

Animal reproduction studies have not been conducted with this combination. See individual monographs for additional information.

Controlled Substance C-V

- **Promethazine and Meperidine** *see* Meperidine and Promethazine *on page 971*
- **Promethazine/Codeine** *see* Promethazine and Codeine *on page 1283*
- **Promethazine HCl** *see* Promethazine *on page 1282*
- **Promethazine HCl/Codeine** *see* Promethazine and Codeine *on page 1283*
- **Promethazine Hydrochloride** *see* Promethazine *on page 1282*
- **Promethegan** *see* Promethazine *on page 1282*
- **Prometrium** *see* Progesterone *on page 1280*
- **Promolaxin [OTC]** *see* Docusate *on page 509*
- **Pronestyl** *see* Procainamide *on page 1277*
- **Pronetupitant and Palonosetron** *see* Fosnetupitant and Palonosetron *on page 717*
- **Pronetupitant/Palonosetron** *see* Fosnetupitant and Palonosetron *on page 717*

- ◆ **Pronto Plus Complete Lice Removal System [OTC]** *see* Pyrethrins and Piperonyl Butoxide *on page 1293*
- ◆ **Pro Nutrients Omega 3 [OTC]** *see* Omega-3 Fatty Acids *on page 1137*
- ◆ **Pronutrients Vitamin D3 [OTC]** *see* Cholecalciferol *on page 344*

Propafenone (pro PAF en one)

Related Information

Cardiovascular Diseases *on page 1654*

Clinical Risk Related to Drugs Prolonging QT Interval *on page 1675*

Dentin Hypersensitivity, Acid Erosion, High Caries Index, Management of Alveolar Osteitis, and Xerostomia *on page 1762*

Brand Names: US Rythmol SR; Rythmol [DSC]

Brand Names: Canada APO-Propafenone; MYL-Propafenone [DSC]; MYLAN-Propafenone; NU-Propafenone [DSC]; PMS-Propafenone; Rythmol

Pharmacologic Category Antiarrhythmic Agent, Class Ic

Use

Treatment of life-threatening ventricular arrhythmias; to prolong the time to recurrence of paroxysmal atrial fibrillation/flutter (PAF) or paroxysmal supraventricular tachycardia (PSVT) in patients with disabling symptoms without structural heart disease

Guideline recommendations: Due to safety risks, propafenone should be reserved for use in patients without structural or ischemic heart disease who are not candidates for, or prefer not to undergo catheter ablation and in whom other therapies have failed or are contraindicated (ACC/AHA/HRS [Page 2015]; AHA/ACC/HRS [Al-Khatib 2017]).

Extended-release capsule: Prolong the time to recurrence of symptomatic atrial fibrillation in patients without structural heart disease

Local Anesthetic/Vasoconstrictor Precautions In some patients, propafenone has been reported to induce new or worsened arrhythmias (proarrhythmic effect). It is suggested that vasoconstrictors be used with caution since epinephrine has the potential to stimulate the heart rate when given in the anesthetic regimen. The manufacturer notes that propafenone may increase the QT interval; however, due to QRS prolongation; changes in the QT interval are difficult to interpret. Cases of torsade de pointes have been reported. The risk of drug-induced torsade de pointes is extremely low when a single QT interval prolonging drug is prescribed. In terms of epinephrine, it is not known what effect vasoconstrictors in the local anesthetic regimen will have in patients with a known history of congenital prolonged QT interval or in patients taking any medication that prolongs the QT interval. Until more information is obtained, it is suggested that the clinician consult with the physician prior to the use of a vasoconstrictor in suspected patients, and that the vasoconstrictor (epinephrine, mepivacaine and levonordefrin [Carbocaine® 2% with Neo-Cobefrin®]) be used with caution.

Effects on Dental Treatment Key adverse event(s) related to dental treatment: Unusual taste and significant xerostomia (normal salivary flow resumes upon discontinuation).

Effects on Bleeding No information available to require special precautions

Adverse Reactions

>10%:

Central nervous system: Unusual taste (3% to 23%), dizziness (4% to 15%)

Gastrointestinal: Nausea (≤11%), vomiting (≤11%)

1% to 10%:

Cardiovascular: Cardiac arrhythmia (2% to 10%; new or worsened; proarrhythmic effect), angina pectoris (2% to 5%), cardiac failure (1% to 4%), first degree atrioventricular block (1% to 3%), palpitations (1% to 3%), ventricular tachycardia (1% to 3%), bradycardia (1% to 2%), chest pain (1% to 2%), widened QRS complex on ECG (1% to 2%), syncope (1% to 2%), ventricular premature contractions (1% to 2%), atrial fibrillation (1%), bundle branch block (≤1%), edema (≤1%), cardiac conduction delay (≤1%; intraventricular), hypotension (≤1%)

Central nervous system: Fatigue (2% to 6%), headache (2% to 5%), ataxia (≤2%), insomnia (≤2%), anxiety (1% to 2%), drowsiness (1%)

Dermatologic: Skin rash (1% to 3%), diaphoresis (1%)

Gastrointestinal: Constipation (2% to 7%), diarrhea (1% to 3%), dyspepsia (1% to 3%), abdominal pain (1% to 2%), anorexia (1% to 2%), xerostomia (1% to 2%), flatulence (≤1%)

Neuromuscular & skeletal: Weakness (1% to 2%), arthralgia (≤1%), tremor (≤1%)

Ophthalmic: Blurred vision (1% to 6%)

Respiratory: Dyspnea (2% to 5%)

<1%, postmarketing, and/or case reports: Abnormal dreams, agranulocytosis, alopecia, altered sense of smell, amnesia, anemia, apnea, asystole, atrioventricular block (second or third degree), atrioventricular dissociation, cardiac failure, cholestasis, coma, confusion, depression, eye irritation, flushing, gastroenteritis, granulocytopenia, hepatitis, hyperglycemia, hyponatremia, impotence, increased serum transaminases, leukopenia, lupus erythematosus, mania, muscle cramps, myasthenia, nephrotic syndrome, numbness, pain, paresthesia, peripheral neuropathy, positive ANA titer, prolongation P-R interval on ECG, prolonged bleeding time, pruritus, psychosis, purpura, renal failure, seizure, SIADH (syndrome of inappropriate antidiuretic hormone secretion), sinoatrial arrest, sinus node dysfunction, speech disturbance, thrombocytopenia, tinnitus, torsades de pointes, ventricular fibrillation, vertigo, visual disturbance

Mechanism of Action Propafenone is a class 1c antiarrhythmic agent which possesses local anesthetic properties, blocks the fast inward sodium current, and slows the rate of increase of the action potential. Prolongs conduction and refractoriness in all areas of the myocardium, with a slightly more pronounced effect on intraventricular conduction; it prolongs effective refractory period, reduces spontaneous automaticity and exhibits some beta-blockade activity.

Pharmacodynamics/Kinetics

Half-life Elimination Extensive metabolizers: 2-10 hours; Poor metabolizers: 10-32 hours

Time to Peak Serum: IR: 3.5 hours; ER: 3-8 hours

Reproductive Considerations

When used in males, reversible impairment of spermatogenesis may occur.

Pregnancy Considerations

Propafenone and the 5-hydroxypropafenone metabolite cross the placenta and can be detected in the newborn (Libardoni 1991).

Due to pregnancy-induced physiologic changes, some pharmacokinetic properties of propafenone may be altered (Libardoni 1991).

Untreated maternal arrhythmias may cause adverse events in the mother and fetus; guidelines are available for the management of arrhythmias during pregnancy (ESC [Regitz-Zagrosek 2018]). Propafenone may be used for the ongoing management of pregnant women with highly symptomatic supraventricular tachycardia (SVT). The lowest effective dose is recommended; avoid use during the first trimester if possible (ACC/AHA/HRS [Page 2015]). Use is also recommended for the prevention of SVT in patients with Wolff-Parkinson-White (WPW) syndrome. Until more information is available, when prevention of SVT in patients without WPW syndrome, atrial tachycardia, or atrial fibrillation is needed in pregnant women, propafenone is generally reserved for use when other agents are not effective (ESC [Regitz-Zagrosek 2018]).

Dental Health Professional Considerations See Local Anesthetic/Vasoconstrictor Precautions

- ◆ **Propafenone HCl** *see* Propafenone *on page 1284*
- ◆ **Propafenone Hydrochloride** *see* Propafenone *on page 1284*

Propantheline (proe PAN the leen)

Generic Availability (US) Yes

Pharmacologic Category Anticholinergic Agent

Dental Use Induce dry field (xerostomia) in oral cavity

Use Peptic ulcer: Adjunctive therapy in the treatment of peptic ulcer

Local Anesthetic/Vasoconstrictor Precautions No information available to require special precautions

Effects on Dental Treatment Key adverse event(s) related to dental treatment: Significant xerostomia (therapeutic effect; normal salivary flow resumes upon discontinuation), dry throat, nasal dryness, and dysphagia.

Effects on Bleeding No information available to require special precautions

Adverse Reactions Frequency not defined.

Cardiovascular: Palpitations, tachycardia

Central nervous system: Confusion, dizziness, drowsiness, headache, insomnia, nervousness

Dermatologic: Hypohidrosis

Gastrointestinal: Ageusia, bloating, constipation, nausea, vomiting, xerostomia

Genitourinary: Decreased lactation, impotence, urinary hesitancy, urinary retention

Hypersensitivity: Anaphylaxis, hypersensitivity reaction

Neuromuscular & skeletal: Weakness

Ophthalmic: Blurred vision, cycloplegia, increased intraocular pressure, mydriasis

Dental Usual Dosage Antisecretory (off-label use); Treatment of Salivary Hypersecretion/Sialorrhea: Oral:

Children: 1-2 mg/kg/day in 3-4 divided doses

Adults: 15 mg 3 times/day before meals or food and 30 mg at bedtime

Elderly: 7.5 mg 3 times/day before meals and at bedtime

Dosing

Adult Peptic ulcer: Oral: 15 mg 3 times daily before meals or food and 30 mg at bedtime; adjust dosage according to patient response and tolerance.

Geriatric Avoid use (Beers Criteria [AGS 2019]).

Renal Impairment: Adult There are no dosage adjustments provided in the manufacturer's labeling; use with caution

Hepatic Impairment: Adult There are no dosage adjustments provided in the manufacturer's labeling; use with caution

Pediatric GI or bladder spasm, irritable bowel syndrome: Limited data available: Children and Adolescents: Oral: 1.5 to 3 mg/kg/day in divided doses every 4 to 6 hours (Kliegman 2007; Rudolph 1996); maximum daily dose: 75 mg/**day**

Renal Impairment: Pediatric There are no dosage adjustments provided in the manufacturer's labeling.

Hepatic Impairment: Pediatric There are no dosage adjustments provided in the manufacturer's labeling.

Mechanism of Action Competitively blocks the action of acetylcholine at postganglionic parasympathetic receptor sites and inhibits gastrointestinal motility

Contraindications Glaucoma; obstructive disease of the gastrointestinal tract (eg, pyloroduodenal stenosis, achalasia, paralytic ileus); obstructive uropathy (eg, bladder-neck obstruction due to prostatic hypertrophy); intestinal atony of elderly or debilitated patients; severe ulcerative colitis or toxic megacolon complicating ulcerative colitis; unstable cardiovascular adjustment in acute hemorrhage; myasthenia gravis.

Warnings/Precautions May cause drowsiness and/or blurred vision, which may impair physical or mental abilities; patients must be cautioned about performing tasks which require mental alertness (eg, operating machinery or driving). Use with caution in patients with hyperthyroidism, hiatal hernia with reflux esophagitis, autonomic neuropathy, hepatic, or renal disease. Use with caution in patients with coronary artery disease, tachyarrhythmias, heart failure, or hypertension. Heat prostration may occur in the presence of increased environmental temperature; use caution in hot weather and/or exercise. Use with caution in patients with ulcerative colitis; large doses may suppress intestinal motility. Diarrhea may be a sign of incomplete intestinal obstruction, discontinue treatment if this occurs. Use with caution in elderly patients. Potentially significant interactions may exist, requiring dose or frequency adjustment, additional monitoring, and/or selection of alternative therapy.

Polysorbate 80: Some dosage forms may contain polysorbate 80 (also known as Tweens). Hypersensitivity reactions, usually a delayed reaction, have been reported following exposure to pharmaceutical products containing polysorbate 80 in certain individuals (Isaksson 2002; Lucente 2000; Shelley 1995). Thrombocytopenia, ascites, pulmonary deterioration, and renal and hepatic failure have been reported in premature neonates after receiving parenteral products containing polysorbate 80 (Alade 1986; CDC 1984). See manufacturer's labeling.

Propylene glycol: Some dosage forms may contain propylene glycol; large amounts are potentially toxic and have been associated with hyperosmolality, lactic acidosis, seizures and respiratory depression; use caution (AAP 1997; Zar 2007). See manufacturer's labeling.

Warnings: Additional Pediatric Considerations Infants, patients with Down syndrome, and children with spastic paralysis or brain damage may be hypersensitive to antimuscarinic effects.

Some dosage forms may contain propylene glycol; in neonates large amounts of propylene glycol delivered orally, intravenously (eg, >3,000 mg/day), or topically have been associated with potentially fatal toxicities which can include metabolic acidosis, seizures, renal failure, and CNS depression; toxicities have also been reported in children and adults including hyperosmolality, lactic acidosis, seizures, and respiratory depression; use caution (AAP 1997; Shehab 2009).

Drug Interactions

Metabolism/Transport Effects None known.

Avoid Concomitant Use

Avoid concomitant use of Propantheline with any of the following: Aclidinium; Cimetropium; Eluxadoline; Glycopyrrolate (Oral Inhalation); Glycopyrronium (Topical); Ipratropium (Oral Inhalation); Levosulpiride; Oxatomide; Potassium Chloride; Potassium Citrate; Pramlintide; Revefenacin; Tiotropium; Umeclidinium

Increased Effect/Toxicity

Propantheline may increase the levels/effects of: Anticholinergic Agents; Cannabinoid-Containing Products; Cimetropium; CloZAPine; Eluxadoline; Glucagon; Glycopyrrolate (Oral Inhalation); Mirabegron; Opioid Agonists; Potassium Chloride; Potassium Citrate; Ramosetron; Revefenacin; Thiazide and Thiazide-Like Diuretics; Tiotropium; Topiramate

The levels/effects of Propantheline may be increased by: Aclidinium; Amantadine; Botulinum Toxin-Containing Products; Chloral Betaine; Glycopyrronium (Topical); Ipratropium (Oral Inhalation); Mianserin; Oxatomide; Pramlintide; Umeclidinium

Decreased Effect

Propantheline may decrease the levels/effects of: Acetylcholinesterase Inhibitors; Gastrointestinal Agents (Prokinetic); Itopride; Levosulpiride; Nitroglycerin; Secretin

The levels/effects of Propantheline may be decreased by: Acetylcholinesterase Inhibitors

Dietary Considerations Some products may contain lactose.

Pharmacodynamics/Kinetics

Duration of Action 6 hours

Half-life Elimination Serum: ~1.6 hours

Time to Peak Plasma: ~1 hour

Pregnancy Risk Factor C

Pregnancy Considerations Animal reproduction studies have not been conducted.

Breastfeeding Considerations It is not known if propantheline is excreted in breast milk. Suppression of lactation may occur with anticholinergics. The manufacturer recommends that caution be exercised when administering propantheline to nursing women.

Dosage Forms: US

Tablet, Oral:

Generic: 15 mg

◆ **Propantheline Bromide** *see* Propantheline *on page 1285*

Proparacaine (proe PAR a kane)

Brand Names: US Alcaine

Pharmacologic Category Local Anesthetic, Ophthalmic

Use Anesthesia, ocular: Topical anesthesia for tonometry, gonioscopy; suture removal from cornea; removal of corneal foreign body; short operative procedure involving the cornea and conjunctiva

Local Anesthetic/Vasoconstrictor Precautions No information available to require special precautions

Effects on Dental Treatment No significant effects or complications reported

Effects on Bleeding No information available to require special precautions

Adverse Reactions Frequency not defined.

Dermatologic: Allergic contact dermatitis

Hypersensitivity: Hypersensitivity reaction (corneal; characterized by acute, intense, and diffuse epithelial keratitis; gray, ground glass appearance; exfoliation of skin; corneal filaments; and can include iritis with descemetitis)

Ophthalmic: Burning sensation of eyes, conjunctival hemorrhage, conjunctival hyperemia, corneal erosion, cycloplegia, eye redness, mydriasis, stinging of eyes

Mechanism of Action Prevents initiation and transmission of impulse at the nerve cell membrane by decreasing ion permeability through stabilizing

Pharmacodynamics/Kinetics

Onset of Action Within 20 seconds of instillation

Duration of Action ~10 to 20 minutes

Pregnancy Considerations Animal reproduction studies have not been conducted.

◆ **Proparacaine HCl** *see* Proparacaine *on page 1286*

◆ **Proparacaine Hydrochloride** *see* Proparacaine *on page 1286*

◆ **Propecia** *see* Finasteride *on page 669*

◆ **Propericiazine** *see* Periciazine *on page 1217*

◆ **Propitocaine Hydrochloride** *see* Prilocaine *on page 1274*

Propofol (PROE po fole)

Brand Names: US Diprivan; Fresenius Propoven

Brand Names: Canada Diprivan; Propofol-II [DSC]; TEVA-Propofol

Pharmacologic Category General Anesthetic

Use Induction of anesthesia in patients ≥3 years of age; maintenance of anesthesia in patients >2 months of age; in adults, for monitored anesthesia care sedation during procedures; in adults, for sedation in intubated, mechanically-ventilated ICU patients

Note: Consult local regulations and individual institutional policies and procedures.

Local Anesthetic/Vasoconstrictor Precautions No information available to require special precautions

Effects on Dental Treatment No significant effects or complications reported

Effects on Bleeding No information available to require special precautions

Adverse Reactions

>10%:

Cardiovascular: Hypotension (adults: 3% to 26%; children: 17%)

Central nervous system: Involuntary body movements (children: 17%; adults: 3% to 10%)

Local: Burning sensation at injection site (adults: ≤18%; children: ≤10%), pain at injection site (includes stinging; adults: ≤18%; children: ≤10%)

Respiratory: Apnea (30 to 60 seconds duration: adults: 24%, children: 10%; >60 seconds duration: adults: 12%, children: 5%)

1% to 10%:

Cardiovascular: Hypertension (children: 8%), bradycardia (1% to 3%), cardiac arrhythmia (1% to 3%), low cardiac output (1% to 3%; concurrent opioid use increases incidence), tachycardia (1% to 3%)

Dermatologic: Skin rash (children: 5%; adults: 1% to 3%), pruritus (1% to 3%)

Endocrine & metabolic: Hypertriglyceridemia (3% to 10%), respiratory acidosis (during weaning; 3% to 10%)

<1%, postmarketing, and/or case reports: Agitation, amblyopia, anaphylaxis, anaphylactoid reaction, anticholinergic syndrome, asystole, atrial arrhythmia, atrial premature contractions, bigeminy, chills, cloudy urine, cough, decreased lung function, delirium, dizziness, drowsiness, fever, flushing, hair discoloration (green), hemorrhage, hypertonia, hypomagnesemia, hypoxia, infusion-related reaction (propofol-related infusion syndrome), infusion site reaction (including pain, swelling, blisters and/or tissue necrosis following accidental extravasation), laryngospasm, leukocytosis, limb pain, loss of consciousness (postoperative; with or without increased muscle tone), myalgia, myoclonus (rarely including seizure and opisthotonos), nail discoloration (nailbeds green), nausea, pancreatitis, paresthesia, phlebitis, pulmonary edema, rhabdomyolysis, sialorrhea, syncope, thrombosis, urine discoloration (green), ventricular premature contractions, visual disturbance, wheezing

Mechanism of Action Propofol is a short-acting, lipophilic intravenous general anesthetic. The drug is unrelated to any of the currently used barbiturate, opioid, benzodiazepine, arylcyclohexylamine, or imidazole intravenous anesthetic agents. Propofol causes global CNS depression, presumably through agonism of $GABA_A$ receptors and perhaps reduced glutamatergic activity through NMDA receptor blockade.

Pharmacodynamics/Kinetics

Onset of Action Anesthetic: Bolus infusion (dose dependent): 9 to 51 seconds (average: 30 seconds)

Duration of Action 3 to 10 minutes depending on the dose, rate and duration of administration; with prolonged use (eg, 10 days ICU sedation), propofol accumulates in tissues and redistributes into plasma when the drug is discontinued, so that the time to awakening (duration of action) is increased; however, if dose is titrated on a daily basis, so that the minimum effective dose is utilized, time to awakening may be within 10 to 15 minutes even after prolonged use

Half-life Elimination Biphasic: Initial: 40 minutes; Terminal: 4 to 7 hours (after 10-day infusion, may be up to 1 to 3 days)

Pregnancy Considerations

Propofol crosses the placenta and may be associated with neonatal CNS and respiratory depression.

Based on animal data, repeated or prolonged use of general anesthetic and sedation medications that block N-methyl-D-aspartate (NMDA) receptors and/or potentiate gamma-aminobutyric acid (GABA) activity may affect brain development. Evaluate benefits and potential risks of fetal exposure to propofol when duration of surgery is expected to be >3 hours (Olutoye 2018).

Propofol is not recommended by the manufacturer for obstetrical use, including cesarean section deliveries. However, in cases where general anesthesia is needed for cesarean delivery, propofol has been used as an induction agent (ACOG 209 2019; Devroe 2015).

The ACOG recommends that pregnant women should not be denied medically necessary surgery, regardless of trimester. If the procedure is elective, it should be delayed until after delivery (ACOG 775 2019).

Note: A propofol 2% emulsion, Fresenius Propoven, was approved for emergency use during the coronavirus disease 2019 (COVID-19) pandemic. This formulation is double the concentration of FDA-approved products. It should not be used in pregnant women unless no other FDA-approved products are available to maintain sedation in patients who require mechanical ventilation in an ICU setting.

Prescribing and Access Restrictions

The FDA has issued an emergency use authorization (EUA) during the coronavirus disease 2019 (COVID-19) pandemic to permit the emergency use of the unapproved product Fresenius Propoven 2% (propofol 20 mg/mL) emulsion. As part of the EUA, fact sheets pertaining to emergency use of Fresenius Propoven 2% are required to be available for health care providers and patients/caregivers and certain mandatory requirements for administration under the EUA must be met as outlined in the FDA EUA letter; the fact sheets and EUA letter may be accessed at:

EUA Letter: https://www.fda.gov/media/137888/download

Fact Sheet tor Health Care Providers: https://www.fda.gov/media/137889/download

Fact Sheet for Patients And Parent/Caregivers: https://www.fda.gov/media/137890/download

Additionally, health care providers must track and report all medication errors and serious adverse events potentially associated with Fresenius Propoven 2% use by either submitting a MedWatch form (https://www.fda.gov/medwatch/report.htm) or FDA Form 3500 (health professional) by fax (1-800-FDA-0178).

Propranolol (proe PRAN oh lole)

Related Information

Cardiovascular Diseases *on page 1654*

Endocrine Disorders and Pregnancy *on page 1684*

Brand Names: US Hemangeol; Inderal LA; Inderal XL; InnoPran XL

Brand Names: Canada APO-Propranolol; DOM-Propranolol HCl [DSC]; DOM-Propranolol [DSC]; Hemangiol; Inderal LA; PMS-Propranolol; TEVA-Propranolol

Pharmacologic Category Antianginal Agent; Antiarrhythmic Agent, Class II; Antihypertensive; Beta-Adrenergic Blocker, Nonselective

Use

Angina, chronic stable: To decrease angina frequency and increase exercise tolerance in patients with angina pectoris.

Cardiac arrhythmias: Control of supraventricular arrhythmias (eg, atrial fibrillation and flutter, atrioventricular nodal reentrant tachycardia) and ventricular tachycardias (eg, catecholamine-induced arrhythmias, digoxin toxicity).

Essential tremor: Management of familial or hereditary essential tremor.

Hypertension: Management of hypertension. **Note:** Beta-blockers are **not** recommended as first-line therapy (ACC/AHA [Whelton 2018]).

Migraine headache prophylaxis: Prophylaxis of common migraine headache.

Myocardial infarction, early treatment and secondary prevention: To reduce cardiovascular mortality in patients who have survived the acute phase of myocardial infarction and are clinically stable.

Obstructive hypertrophic cardiomyopathy: Symptomatic treatment of obstructive hypertrophic cardiomyopathy (formerly known as hypertrophic subaortic stenosis).

Pheochromocytoma: As an adjunct to alpha-adrenergic blockade to control blood pressure and reduce symptoms of catecholamine-secreting tumors.

Proliferating infantile hemangioma (Hemangeol): Treatment of proliferating infantile hemangioma requiring systemic therapy.

Local Anesthetic/Vasoconstrictor Precautions Use with caution; epinephrine has interacted with nonselective beta-blockers to result in initial hypertensive episode followed by bradycardia

Effects on Dental Treatment Propranolol is a nonselective beta-blocker and may enhance the pressor response to epinephrine, resulting in hypertension and bradycardia. Many nonsteroidal anti-inflammatory drugs, such as ibuprofen and indomethacin, can reduce the hypotensive effect of beta-blockers after 3 or more weeks of therapy with the NSAID. Short-term NSAID use (ie, 3 days) requires no special precautions in patients taking beta-blockers.

Effects on Bleeding No information available to require special precautions

Adverse Reactions Frequency not always defined.

Cardiovascular: Cold extremities (infants: 7% to 8%), angina pectoris, atrioventricular conduction disturbance, bradycardia, cardiac failure, cardiogenic shock, hypotension, ineffective myocardial contractions, syncope

Central nervous system: Sleep disorder (infants: 16% to 18%), agitation (infants: 5% to 9%), fatigue (5% to 7%), dizziness (4% to 7%), nightmares (infants: 2% to 6%), irritability (infants: 1% to 6%), drowsiness (infants: 1% to 5%), amnesia, carpal tunnel syndrome (rare), catatonia, cognitive dysfunction, confusion, hypersomnia, lethargy, paresthesia, psychosis, vertigo

Dermatologic: Changes in nails, contact dermatitis, dermal ulcer, eczematous rash, erosive lichen planus, hyperkeratosis, pruritus, skin rash

Endocrine & metabolic: Hyperglycemia, hyperkalemia, hyperlipidemia, hypoglycemia

Gastrointestinal: Diarrhea (infants: 5% to 6%), abdominal pain (infants: ≤4%), decreased appetite (infants: 3% to 4%), constipation (1% to 3%), anorexia, stomach discomfort

Genitourinary: Oliguria (rare), proteinuria (rare)

Hematologic & oncologic: Immune thrombocytopenia, thrombocytopenia

Hepatic: Increased serum alkaline phosphatase, increased serum transaminases

Neuromuscular & skeletal: Arthropathy, oculomucocutaneous syndrome, polyarthritis

Ophthalmic: Conjunctival hyperemia, decreased visual acuity, mydriasis

Renal: Increased blood urea nitrogen, interstitial nephritis (rare)

Respiratory: Bronchitis (infants: 8% to 13%; associated with cough, fever, diarrhea, and vomiting), bronchiolitis (infants; associated with cough, fever, diarrhea, and vomiting), bronchospasm, dyspnea, pulmonary edema, wheezing

Miscellaneous: Ulcer

<1%, postmarketing, and/or case reports: Abdominal cramps, agranulocytosis, alopecia, altered mental status, arterial insufficiency, arterial mesenteric thrombosis, decreased heart rate (infants), decreased serum glucose (infants), depression, emotional lability, epigastric distress, erythema multiforme, erythematous rash, exfoliative dermatitis, fever combined with generalized ache, sore throat, laryngospasm, and respiratory distress), hallucination, hypersensitivity reaction (including anaphylaxis, anaphylactoid reaction), impotence, insomnia, ischemic colitis, lassitude, lupus-like syndrome, myotonia, myopathy, nausea, nonthrombocytopenic purpura, peripheral arterial disease (exacerbation), Peyronie's disease, pharyngitis, psoriasiform eruption, purpura, Raynaud's phenomenon, second degree atrioventricular block (infants; in a patient with an underlying conduction disorder), Stevens-Johnson syndrome, systemic lupus erythematosus, temporary amnesia, tingling of extremities (hands), toxic epidermal necrolysis, urticaria, visual disturbance, vivid dream, vomiting, weakness, xerophthalmia

Mechanism of Action Nonselective beta-adrenergic blocker (class II antiarrhythmic); competitively blocks response to beta$_1$- and beta$_2$-adrenergic stimulation which results in decreases in heart rate, myocardial contractility, blood pressure, and myocardial oxygen demand. Nonselective beta-adrenergic blockers (propranolol, nadolol) reduce portal pressure by producing splanchnic vasoconstriction (beta$_2$ effect) thereby reducing portal blood flow.

Pharmacodynamics/Kinetics

Onset of Action Beta-blockade: Oral: 1 to 2 hours; IV: ≤5 minutes; Peak effect: Hypertension: A few days to several weeks.

Duration of Action Immediate release: 6 to 12 hours; Extended-release formulations: ~24 to 27 hours

Half-life Elimination Neonates: Possible increased half-life; Infants (35 to 150 days of age): Median 3.5 hours; Children: 3.9 to 6.4 hours; Adults: Immediate release formulation: 3 to 6 hours; Extended-release formulations: 8 to 10 hours

Time to Peak Immediate release: Adults: 1 to 4 hours; Infants: ≤2 hours (Hemangeol); Extended release capsule (Inderal XL, InnoPran XL): 12 to 14 hours; Long acting capsule (Inderal LA): 6 hours

Pregnancy Considerations Propranolol crosses the placenta.

According to the manufacturer, congenital abnormalities have been reported following maternal use of propranolol. Exposure to propranolol during pregnancy may also increase the risk for other adverse events in the neonate. If maternal use of a beta-blocker is needed, fetal growth should be monitored during pregnancy and the newborn should be monitored for 48 hours after delivery for bradycardia, hypoglycemia, and respiratory depression (ESC [Regitz-Zagrosek 2018]).

Chronic maternal hypertension is also associated with adverse events in the fetus/infant. Chronic maternal hypertension may increase the risk of birth defects, low birth weight, premature delivery, stillbirth, and neonatal death. Actual fetal/neonatal risks may be related to duration and severity of maternal hypertension. Untreated chronic hypertension may also increase the risks of adverse maternal outcomes, including gestational diabetes, preeclampsia, delivery complications, stroke, and myocardial infarction (ACOG 203 2019).

The pharmacokinetics of propranolol are not significantly changed by pregnancy (Livingstone 1983; O'Hare 1984; Rubin 1987; Smith 1983).

When treatment of chronic hypertension in pregnancy is indicated, agents other than propranolol are preferred (ACOG 203 2019; ESC [Regitz-Zagrosek 2018]); however, use of propranolol may be considered (Magee 2014). Females with preexisting hypertension may continue their medication during pregnancy unless contraindications exist (ESC [Regitz-Zagrosek 2018]).

Propranolol may be used for the treatment of maternal ventricular arrhythmias, atrial fibrillation/atrial flutter, or supraventricular tachycardia during pregnancy; consult current guidelines for specific recommendations (ACC/AHA/HRS [Page 2016]; ESC [Regitz-Zagrosek 2018]).

Propranolol is recommended for use in controlling hypermetabolic symptoms of thyrotoxicosis in pregnancy (Alexander 2017).

Propranolol may be used if prophylaxis of migraine is needed in pregnant women; it should be discontinued 2 to 3 days prior to delivery to decrease the risk of adverse events to the fetus/neonate and potential reductions in uterine contraction (Pringsheim 2012).

Prescribing and Access Restrictions Prescriptions for Hemangeol may be obtained via the Hemangeol Patient Access program. Visit http://www.hemangeol.com/hcp/hemangeol-direct/ or call 855-618-4950 for ordering information.

◆ **Propranolol HCl** *see* Propranolol *on page 1287*

◆ **Propranolol Hydrochloride** *see* Propranolol *on page 1287*

◆ **Propulsid®** *see* Cisapride *on page 352*

◆ **2-Propylpentanoic Acid** *see* Valproic Acid and Derivatives *on page 1518*

Propylthiouracil (proe pil thye oh YOOR a sil)

Related Information

Endocrine Disorders and Pregnancy *on page 1684*

Brand Names: Canada Propyl-Thyracil [DSC]

Pharmacologic Category Antithyroid Agent; Thioamide

Use Hyperthyroidism: Treatment of hyperthyroidism in patients with Graves' disease or toxic multinodular goiter who are intolerant of methimazole and for whom surgery or radioactive iodine therapy is not an appropriate treatment regimen; amelioration of hyperthyroid symptoms in preparation for thyroidectomy or radioactive iodine therapy (in patients who are intolerant of methimazole).

Local Anesthetic/Vasoconstrictor Precautions

No information available to require special precautions

Effects on Dental Treatment Key adverse event(s) related to dental treatment: Loss of taste perception.

Effects on Bleeding Propylthiouracil administration may cause a bishydroxycoumarin-like hypocoagulable condition that is clinically observed by hemorrhagic diathesis. The syndrome is usually responsive to vitamin K therapy. It is suggested that all patients receiving propylthiouracil have their prothrombin times evaluated.

Adverse Reactions Frequency not defined.

Cardiovascular: Edema, periarteritis, vasculitis (ANCA-positive, cutaneous, leukocytoclastic)

Central nervous system: Drowsiness, drug fever, headache, neuritis, paresthesia, vertigo

Dermatologic: Alopecia, dermal ulcer, erythema nodosum, exfoliative dermatitis, pruritus, skin pigmentation, skin rash, Stevens-Johnson syndrome, toxic epidermal necrolysis, urticaria

Gastrointestinal: Ageusia, dysgeusia, nausea, salivary gland disease, stomach pain, vomiting

Hematologic & oncologic: Agranulocytosis, aplastic anemia, granulocytopenia, hemorrhage, hypoprothrombinemia, leukopenia, lymphadenopathy, splenomegaly, thrombocytopenia

Hepatic: Acute hepatic failure, hepatitis, hepatotoxicity (idiosyncratic) (Chalasani 2014), jaundice

Neuromuscular & skeletal: Arthralgia, lupus-like syndrome, myalgia

Renal: Acute renal failure, glomerulonephritis, nephritis

Respiratory: Interstitial pneumonitis, pulmonary alveolar hemorrhage

Miscellaneous: Fever

Mechanism of Action Inhibits the synthesis of thyroid hormones by interfering with thyroid peroxidase (TPO) which oxidizes iodide, subsequently catalyzes formation of mono- and di-iodotyrosines (MIT and DIT) on thyroglobulin, and catalyzes coupling reactions between MIT and DIT to form thyroxine (T_4) and triiodothyronine (T_3) (Burch 2015); also blocks conversion of T_4 to T_3 in peripheral tissues (does not inactivate existing T_4 and T_3 stores in circulating blood and the thyroid and does not interfere with replacement thyroid hormones).

Pharmacodynamics/Kinetics

Onset of Action For significant therapeutic effects 24 to 36 hours are required; remission of hyperthyroidism usually does not occur before 4 months of continued therapy

Duration of Action 12 to 24 hours (Clark 2006)

Half-life Elimination ~1 hour (Clark 2006)

Time to Peak 1 to 2 hours (Clark 2006)

Reproductive Considerations

[US Boxed Warning]: Propylthiouracil may be the treatment of choice when an antithyroid drug is indicated just prior to the first trimester of pregnancy. Females taking propylthiouracil should notify their health care provider immediately once pregnancy is suspected (Alexander 2017).

Pregnancy Risk Factor D

Pregnancy Considerations Propylthiouracil crosses the placenta.

Nonteratogenic adverse effects, including fetal and neonatal hypothyroidism, goiter, and hyperthyroidism, have been reported following maternal propylthiouracil use.

Uncontrolled maternal hyperthyroidism may result in adverse neonatal outcomes (eg, prematurity, low birth weight) and adverse maternal outcomes (eg, preeclampsia, congestive heart failure, stillbirth, and abortion).

The pharmacokinetic properties of propylthiouracil are not significantly changed by pregnancy; however, the severity of hyperthyroidism may fluctuate throughout pregnancy (De Groot 2012; Sitar 1979; Sitar 1982). Doses of propylthiouracil may be decreased as pregnancy progresses and discontinued weeks to months prior to delivery.

Antithyroid drugs are the treatment of choice for the control of hyperthyroidism during pregnancy (ACOG 148 2015; Alexander 2017; De Groot 2012). **[US Boxed Warning]: Propylthiouracil may be the treatment of choice when an antithyroid drug is indicated during the first trimester of pregnancy.** Due to adverse maternal events, other antithyroid medications should be considered after the first trimester. To prevent adverse outcomes, maternal TT4/FT4 should be at or just above the pregnancy specific upper limit of normal (Alexander 2017). Propylthiouracil may be used for the treatment of thyroid storm in pregnant females (ACOG 148 2015).

Females taking propylthiouracil should notify their health care provider immediately once pregnancy is suspected (Alexander 2017).

◆ **2-Propylvaleric Acid** *see* Valproic Acid and Derivatives *on page 1518*

◆ **ProQuad** *see* Measles, Mumps, Rubella, and Varicella Virus Vaccine *on page 950*

◆ **Proquin XR** *see* Ciprofloxacin (Systemic) *on page 350*

◆ **Proscar** *see* Finasteride *on page 669*

◆ **Prosed/DS [DSC]** *see* Methenamine, Phenyl Salicylate, Methylene Blue, Benzoic Acid, and Hyoscyamine *on page 987*

◆ **ProSom** *see* Estazolam *on page 595*

◆ **Prostacyclin** *see* Epoprostenol *on page 578*

◆ **Prostaglandin E_1** *see* Alprostadil *on page 110*

◆ **Prostate Cancer Vaccine, Cell-Based** *see* Sipuleucel-T *on page 1374*

◆ **Prostin VR** *see* Alprostadil *on page 110*

◆ **Proteasome Inhibitor MLN9708** *see* Ixazomib *on page 853*

◆ **Protein-Bound Paclitaxel** *see* PACLitaxel (Protein Bound) *on page 1179*

◆ **ProThelial** *see* Mucosal Coating Agent *on page 1066*

◆ **Protonix** *see* Pantoprazole *on page 1189*

◆ **Protopic** *see* Tacrolimus (Topical) *on page 1400*

Protriptyline (proe TRIP ti leen)

Related Information

Dentin Hypersensitivity, Acid Erosion, High Caries Index, Management of Alveolar Osteitis, and Xerostomia *on page 1762*

Vasoconstrictor Interactions With Antidepressants *on page 1821*

Pharmacologic Category Antidepressant, Tricyclic (Secondary Amine)

Use Depression: Treatment of depression

Local Anesthetic/Vasoconstrictor Precautions Use with caution; epinephrine and levonordefrin have been shown to have an increased pressor response in combination with TCAs. Protriptyline is one of the drugs confirmed to prolong the QT interval and is accepted as having a risk of causing torsade de pointes. The risk of drug-induced torsade de pointes is extremely low when a single QT interval prolonging drug is prescribed. In terms of epinephrine, it is not known what effect vasoconstrictors in the local anesthetic regimen will have in patients with a known history of congenital prolonged QT interval or in patients taking any medication that prolongs the QT interval. Until more information is obtained, it is suggested that the clinician consult with the physician prior to the use of a vasoconstrictor in suspected patients, and that the vasoconstrictor (epinephrine, mepivacaine and levonordefrin [Carbocaine® 2% with Neo-Cobefrin®]) be used with caution.

Effects on Dental Treatment Key adverse event(s) related to dental treatment: Xerostomia and changes in salivation (normal salivary flow resumes upon discontinuation), unpleasant taste, and trouble with gums. Long-term treatment with TCAs, such as protriptyline, increases the risk of caries by reducing salivation and salivary buffer capacity.

Effects on Bleeding No information available to require special precautions

Adverse Reactions Frequency not defined. Some reactions listed are based on reports for other agents in this same pharmacologic class and may not be specifically reported for protriptyline.

Cardiovascular: Cardiac arrhythmia, cerebrovascular accident, edema, flushing, heart block, hypertension, hypotension, myocardial infarction, orthostatic hypotension, palpitations, tachycardia

Central nervous system: Agitation, anxiety, ataxia, confusion, delusions, disorientation, dizziness, drowsiness, drug fever, EEG pattern changes, extrapyramidal reaction, fatigue, hallucination, headache, hyperpyrexia, hypomania, insomnia, nightmares, numbness, panic, peripheral neuropathy, psychosis (exacerbation), restlessness, seizure, tingling of extremities, tingling sensation, withdrawal syndrome

Dermatologic: Alopecia, diaphoresis (excessive), pruritus, skin photosensitivity, skin rash, urticaria

Endocrine & metabolic: Decreased libido, decreased serum glucose, galactorrhea, gynecomastia, increased libido, increased serum glucose, SIADH, weight gain, weight loss

Gastrointestinal: Abdominal cramps, anorexia, constipation, diarrhea, epigastric distress, melanoglossia, nausea, paralytic ileus, parotid gland enlargement, stomatitis, sublingual adenitis, unpleasant taste, vomiting, xerostomia

Genitourinary: Breast hypertrophy, impotence, nocturia, testicular swelling, urinary hesitancy, urinary retention, urinary tract dilation

Hematologic & oncologic: Agranulocytosis, eosinophilia, leukopenia, petechia, purpura, thrombocytopenia

Hepatic: Abnormal hepatic function tests, cholestatic jaundice

Neuromuscular & skeletal: Tremor, weakness

Ophthalmic: Accommodation disturbance, blurred vision, eye pain, increased intraocular pressure

Otic: Tinnitus

Renal: Polyuria

Postmarketing and/or case reports: Angle-closure glaucoma, suicidal ideation, suicidal tendencies

Mechanism of Action Increases the synaptic concentration of serotonin and/or norepinephrine in the central nervous system by inhibition of their reuptake by the presynaptic neuronal membrane

Pharmacodynamics/Kinetics

Onset of Action Depression: Initial effects may be observed within 1 to 2 weeks of treatment, with continued improvements through 4 to 6 weeks (Papakostas 2006; Posternak 2005; Szegedi 2009).

Duration of Action 1 to 2 days

Half-life Elimination 54 to 92 hours (average: 74 hours) (Ziegler 1978)

Time to Peak Serum: ~6 to 12 hours (Ziegler 1978)

Pregnancy Considerations Adverse events have not been observed in animal reproduction studies. Tricyclic antidepressants may be associated with irritability, jitteriness, and convulsions (rare) in the neonate (Yonkers 2009).

The ACOG recommends that therapy for depression during pregnancy be individualized; treatment should incorporate the clinical expertise of the mental health clinician, obstetrician, primary health care provider, and pediatrician (ACOG 2008). According to the American Psychiatric Association (APA), the risks of medication treatment should be weighed against other treatment options and untreated depression. For women who discontinue antidepressant medications during pregnancy and who may be at high risk for postpartum depression, the medications can be restarted following delivery (APA 2010). Treatment algorithms have been developed by the ACOG and the APA for the management of depression in women prior to conception and during pregnancy (Yonkers 2009).

Pregnant women exposed to antidepressants during pregnancy are encouraged to enroll in the National Pregnancy Registry for Antidepressants (NPRAD). Women 18 to 45 years of age or their health care providers may contact the registry by calling 844-405-6185. Enrollment should be done as early in pregnancy as possible.

Dental Health Professional Considerations See Local Anesthetic/Vasoconstrictor Precautions

- ◆ **Protriptyline HCl** *see* Protriptyline *on page 1290*
- ◆ **Protriptyline Hydrochloride** *see* Protriptyline *on page 1290*
- ◆ **Provenge** *see* Sipuleucel-T *on page 1374*
- ◆ **Proventil HFA** *see* Albuterol *on page 90*
- ◆ **Provera** *see* MedroxyPROGESTERone *on page 953*
- ◆ **Provigil** *see* Modafinil *on page 1043*
- ◆ **Provil [OTC]** *see* Ibuprofen *on page 786*
- ◆ **Provisc** *see* Hyaluronate and Derivatives *on page 761*
- ◆ **Proxymetacaine** *see* Proparacaine *on page 1286*
- ◆ **PROzac** *see* FLUoxetine *on page 697*
- ◆ **PROzac Weekly [DSC]** *see* FLUoxetine *on page 697*
- ◆ **PRT064445** *see* Andexanet Alfa *on page 151*

Prucalopride (proo KAL oh pride)

Brand Names: US Motegrity

Brand Names: Canada APO-Prucalopride; Resotran

Pharmacologic Category Gastrointestinal Agent, Prokinetic; Serotonin 5-HT_4 Receptor Agonist

Use Chronic idiopathic constipation: Treatment of chronic idiopathic constipation in adults

Local Anesthetic/Vasoconstrictor Precautions No information available to require special precautions

Effects on Dental Treatment No significant effects or complications reported

Effects on Bleeding No information available to require special precautions

Adverse Reactions

>10%:

Central nervous system: Headache (19%)

Gastrointestinal: Abdominal pain (16%), nausea (14%), diarrhea (13%)

1% to 10%:

Central nervous system: Dizziness (4%), fatigue (2%), migraine (<2%)

Genitourinary: Pollakiuria (<2%)

Gastrointestinal: Abdominal distension (5%), flatulence (3%), vomiting (3%), severe diarrhea (2%), abnormal bowel sounds (<2%), decreased appetite (<2%)

<1%, postmarketing, and/or case reports: Amnesia (Anton 2017), dyspnea, facial edema, loss of balance (Anton 2017), palpitations (Anton 2017), pruritus, skin rash, suicidal ideation, suicidal tendencies, urticaria, vaginal hemorrhage, visual hallucination (Anton 2017)

Mechanism of Action Prucalopride is a selective, high affinity 5-HT_4 receptor agonist whose action at the receptor site promotes cholinergic and nonadrenergic, noncholinergic neurotransmission by enteric neurons leading to stimulation of the peristaltic reflex, intestinal secretions, and gastrointestinal motility.

Pharmacodynamics/Kinetics

Half-life Elimination ~24 hours; terminal half-life increases to 34, 43, and 47 hours in mild, moderate, and severe renal impairment, respectively (Resotran Canadian product labeling)

Time to Peak 2 to 3 hours

Reproductive Considerations

Consider use of appropriate contraception in females of reproductive potential.

Pregnancy Considerations

Information related to use in pregnancy is limited; spontaneous abortions were observed in clinical trials; however, available data is insufficient to evaluate the risk of adverse maternal or fetal outcomes.

- ◆ **Prucalopride Succinate** *see* Prucalopride *on page 1291*
- ◆ **Prudoxin** *see* Doxepin (Topical) *on page 519*
- ◆ **Prymaccone** *see* Primaquine *on page 1276*
- ◆ **PS-341** *see* Bortezomib *on page 248*

Pseudoephedrine (soo doe e FED rin)

Related Information

Bacterial Infections *on page 1739*

Brand Names: US Childrens Silfedrine [OTC]; Decongestant 12Hour Max St [OTC]; Genaphed [OTC]; Nasal Decongestant [OTC]; Nexafed [OTC]; Shopko Nasal Decongestant Max [OTC]; Shopko Nasal Decongestant [OTC]; Simply Stuffy [OTC]; Sudafed 12 Hour [OTC] [DSC]; Sudafed Childrens [OTC]; Sudafed Congestion [OTC]; Sudafed Sinus Congestion 12HR [OTC]; Sudafed Sinus Congestion 24HR [OTC]; Sudafed Sinus Congestion [OTC]; Sudafed [OTC]; SudoGest 12 Hour [OTC]; SudoGest Maximum Strength [OTC]; SudoGest [OTC]; Zephrex-D [OTC]

Pharmacologic Category Alpha/Beta Agonist; Decongestant

Use Nasal congestion: Temporary symptomatic relief of nasal congestion due to common cold, hay fever, or upper respiratory allergies; temporary relief of sinus congestion and pressure; promotes nasal or sinus drainage; temporarily restores freer breathing through the nose

Local Anesthetic/Vasoconstrictor Precautions Use with caution since pseudoephedrine is a sympathomimetic amine which could interact with epinephrine to cause a pressor response

Effects on Dental Treatment Key adverse event(s) related to dental treatment: Xerostomia (normal salivary flow resumes upon discontinuation).

Effects on Bleeding No information available to require special precautions

Adverse Reactions Frequency not defined.

Cardiovascular: Cardiac arrhythmia, chest tightness, circulatory shock (with hypotension), hypertension, palpitations, tachycardia

Central nervous system: Ataxia, central nervous system stimulation (transient), chills, confusion, dizziness, drowsiness, excitability, fatigue, hallucination, headache, insomnia, nervousness, neuritis, restlessness, seizure, vertigo

Dermatologic: Diaphoresis, skin photosensitivity, skin rash, urticaria

Gastrointestinal: Anorexia, constipation, diarrhea, dry throat, ischemic colitis, nausea, vomiting, xerostomia

Genitourinary: Difficulty in micturition, dysuria, urinary retention
Hematologic & oncologic: Agranulocytosis, hemolytic anemia, thrombocytopenia
Hypersensitivity: Anaphylaxis
Neuromuscular & skeletal: Tremor, weakness
Ophthalmic: Blurred vision, diplopia
Otic: Tinnitus
Renal: Polyuria
Respiratory: Dry nose, dyspnea, nasal congestion, pharyngeal edema, thickening of bronchial secretions, wheezing

Mechanism of Action Directly stimulates alpha-adrenergic receptors of respiratory mucosa causing vasoconstriction; directly stimulates beta-adrenergic receptors causing bronchial relaxation, increased heart rate and contractility

Pharmacodynamics/Kinetics

Onset of Action Decongestant: Oral: 30 minutes (Chua, 1989); Peak effect: Decongestant: Oral: ~1-2 hours (Chua, 1989)

Duration of Action Immediate release tablet: 3-8 hours (Chua, 1989)

Half-life Elimination Varies by urine pH and flow rate; alkaline urine decreases renal elimination of pseudoephedrine (Kanfer, 1993)
Children: ~3 hours (urine pH ~6.5) (Simons, 1996)
Adults: 9-16 hours (pH 8); 3-6 hours (pH 5) (Chua, 1989)

Time to Peak
Children (immediate release) ~2 hours (Simons, 1996)
Adults (immediate release): 1-3 hours (dose dependent) (Kanfer, 1993)

Pregnancy Considerations Use of pseudoephedrine during the first trimester may be associated with a possible risk of gastroschisis, small intestinal atresia, and hemifacial microsomia due to pseudoephedrine's vasoconstrictive effects; additional studies are needed to define the magnitude of risk. Single doses of pseudoephedrine were not found to adversely affect the fetus during the third trimester of pregnancy (limited data); however, fetal tachycardia was noted in a case report following maternal use of an extended release product for multiple days. Decongestants are not the preferred agents for the treatment of rhinitis during pregnancy. Oral pseudoephedrine should be avoided during the first trimester.

◆ **Pseudoephedrine and Chlorpheniramine** *see* Chlorpheniramine and Pseudoephedrine *on page 341*

Pseudoephedrine and Ibuprofen

(soo doe e FED rin & eye byoo PROE fen)

Related Information

Ibuprofen *on page 786*
Pseudoephedrine *on page 1291*

Brand Names: US Advil Cold & Sinus [OTC]

Brand Names: Canada Advil Cold & Sinus; Advil Cold & Sinus Daytime; Children's Advil Cold; Sudafed Sinus Advance

Pharmacologic Category Analgesic, Nonopioid; Decongestant/Analgesic

Use Common cold/flu symptoms: Temporary relief of symptoms (headache, fever, sinus pressure, nasal congestion, minor aches and pains) associated with the common cold or flu.

Local Anesthetic/Vasoconstrictor Precautions Use with caution since pseudoephedrine is a sympathomimetic amine which could interact with epinephrine to cause a pressor response

Effects on Dental Treatment Key adverse event(s) related to dental treatment: Pseudoephedrine: Xerostomia (normal salivary flow resumes upon discontinuation).

The dentist should be aware of the potential of abnormal coagulation. Caution should also be exercised in the use of NSAIDs in patients already on anticoagulant therapy with drugs such as warfarin (Coumadin®). See Effects on Bleeding.

Effects on Bleeding Nonselective NSAIDs, such as pseudoephedrine and ibuprofen, inhibit platelet aggregation and prolong bleeding time in some patients. Unlike aspirin, the NSAID effect on platelet function is quantitatively less, of shorter duration, and reversible. Normal platelet function should occur in ~5 elimination half-lives or in <10 hours after discontinuation of pseudoephedrine and ibuprofen. Concomitant use of other NSAIDs should be avoided.

Adverse Reactions See individual agents.

Mechanism of Action
Ibuprofen: Reversibly inhibits cyclooxygenase-1 and 2 (COX-1 and 2) enzymes, which results in decreased formation of prostaglandin precursors; has antipyretic, analgesic, and anti-inflammatory properties.
Pseudoephedrine: Directly stimulates alpha-adrenergic receptors of respiratory mucosa causing vasoconstriction; directly stimulates beta-adrenergic receptors causing bronchial relaxation, increased heart rate and contractility.

Pregnancy Considerations Refer to individual agents.

◆ **Pseudoephedrine and Loratadine** *see* Loratadine and Pseudoephedrine *on page 931*
◆ **Pseudoephedrine, Chlophedianol, and Dexbrompheniramine** *see* Chlophedianol, Dexbrompheniramine, and Pseudoephedrine *on page 332*
◆ **Pseudoephedrine, Chlorpheniramine, and Codeine** *see* Chlorpheniramine, Pseudoephedrine, and Codeine *on page 341*
◆ **Pseudoephedrine, Dexbrompheniramine, and Chlophedianol** *see* Chlophedianol, Dexbrompheniramine, and Pseudoephedrine *on page 332*
◆ **Pseudoephedrine HCl** *see* Pseudoephedrine *on page 1291*
◆ **Pseudoephedrine Hydrochloride** *see* Pseudoephedrine *on page 1291*
◆ **Pseudoephedrine Sulfate** *see* Pseudoephedrine *on page 1291*
◆ **Pseudomonic Acid A** *see* Mupirocin *on page 1066*
◆ **Psorcon** *see* Diflorasone *on page 494*
◆ **Pteroylglutamic Acid** *see* Folic Acid *on page 709*
◆ **PTG** *see* Teniposide *on page 1417*
◆ **PTH(1-84)** *see* Parathyroid Hormone *on page 1192*
◆ **PTU (error-prone abbreviation)** *see* Propylthiouracil *on page 1289*
◆ **Pulmicort** *see* Budesonide (Oral Inhalation) *on page 254*
◆ **Pulmicort Flexhaler** *see* Budesonide (Oral Inhalation) *on page 254*
◆ **Pulmozyme** *see* Dornase Alfa *on page 515*

◆ **Purified Chick Embryo Cell** *see* Rabies Vaccine *on page 1303*

◆ **Purinethol** *see* Mercaptopurine *on page 978*

◆ **Purixan** *see* Mercaptopurine *on page 978*

◆ **PVP-I** *see* Povidone-Iodine (Topical) *on page 1249*

◆ **PVP Prep [OTC]** *see* Povidone-Iodine (Topical) *on page 1249*

◆ **PVP Scrub [OTC]** *see* Povidone-Iodine (Topical) *on page 1249*

◆ **PXD101** *see* Belinostat *on page 223*

◆ **Pylera** *see* Bismuth Subcitrate, Metronidazole, and Tetracycline *on page 245*

Pyrazinamide (peer a ZIN a mide)

Brand Names: Canada PDP-Pyrazinamide; Tebrazid

Pharmacologic Category Antitubercular Agent

Use Tuberculosis: Adjunctive treatment of tuberculosis (TB) in combination with other antituberculosis agents

Local Anesthetic/Vasoconstrictor Precautions No information available to require special precautions

Effects on Dental Treatment No significant effects or complications reported

Effects on Bleeding No information available to require special precautions

Adverse Reactions

1% to 10%:

Central nervous system: Malaise

Gastrointestinal: Anorexia, nausea, vomiting

Neuromuscular & skeletal: Arthralgia, myalgia

<1%, postmarketing, and/or case reports: Acne vulgaris, acquired blood coagulation disorder (anticoagulant effect), angioedema (rare), dysuria, fever, gout, hepatotoxicity, interstitial nephritis, porphyria, pruritus, sideroblastic anemia, skin photosensitivity, skin rash, thrombocytopenia, urticaria

Mechanism of Action Converted to pyrazinoic acid in susceptible strains of *Mycobacterium* which lowers the pH of the environment; exact mechanism of action has not been elucidated

Pharmacodynamics/Kinetics

Half-life Elimination 9 to 10 hours, prolonged with reduced renal or hepatic function

Time to Peak Serum: Within 2 hours

Pregnancy Risk Factor C

Pregnancy Considerations Adverse events have not been observed in animal reproduction studies. Due to the risk of tuberculosis to the fetus, treatment is recommended when the probability of maternal disease is moderate to high. Drug-susceptible TB guidelines recommend pyrazinamide as part of the initial treatment regimen; however, risks and benefits of use during pregnancy should be considered for each individual patient (Nahid 2016).

◆ **Pyrazinoic Acid Amide** *see* Pyrazinamide *on page 1293*

Pyrethrins and Piperonyl Butoxide
(pye RE thrins & pi PER oh nil byo TOKS ide)

Brand Names: US A-200 Lice Treatment Kit [OTC]; A-200 Maximum Strength [OTC]; LiceMD Complete [OTC]; LiceMD Treatment [OTC]; Licide [OTC]; Pronto Plus Complete Lice Removal System [OTC]; RID Lice Elimination Essentials [OTC] [DSC]; RID Lice Killing [OTC]; RID Lice Treatment Complete [OTC]

Brand Names: Canada Pronto Lice Control; R & C II; R & C Shampoo/Conditioner; RID Mousse

Pharmacologic Category Antiparasitic Agent, Topical; Pediculocide; Shampoo, Pediculocide

Use *Pediculus humanus* infestations: Treatment of *Pediculus humanus* infestations (head lice, body lice, pubic lice, and their eggs)

Local Anesthetic/Vasoconstrictor Precautions No information available to require special precautions

Effects on Dental Treatment No significant effects or complications reported

Effects on Bleeding No information available to require special precautions

Adverse Reactions Frequency not defined.

Central nervous system: Localized burning

Dermatologic: Burning sensation of skin, pruritus, skin irritation (with repeat use), stinging of the skin

Mechanism of Action Pyrethrins are derived from flowers that belong to the chrysanthemum family. The mechanism of action on the neuronal membranes of lice is similar to that of DDT. Piperonyl butoxide is usually added to pyrethrin to enhance the product's activity by decreasing the metabolism of pyrethrins in arthropods.

Pregnancy Considerations Pregnant women may be treated with pyrethrins and piperonyl butoxide (CDC [Workowski 2015]).

◆ **Pyri 500 [OTC]** *see* Pyridoxine *on page 1294*

◆ **Pyridium** *see* Phenazopyridine *on page 1222*

Pyridostigmine (peer id oh STIG meen)

Brand Names: US Mestinon; Regonol

Brand Names: Canada Mestinon; Mestinon SR

Pharmacologic Category Acetylcholinesterase Inhibitor

Use

Myasthenia gravis (oral only): Treatment of myasthenia gravis.

Reversal of nondepolarizing muscle relaxants (injection only): Reversal agent or antagonist to the neuromuscular blocking effects of nondepolarizing muscle relaxants.

Military use: Pretreatment for Soman nerve gas exposure

Local Anesthetic/Vasoconstrictor Precautions No information available to require special precautions

Effects on Dental Treatment Key adverse event(s) related to dental treatment: Dysphagia.

Effects on Bleeding No information available to require special precautions

Adverse Reactions

1% to 10%:

Central nervous system: Twitching (3%), hyperesthesia (2%)

Dermatologic: Xeroderma (2%)

Gastrointestinal: Abdominal pain (7%), diarrhea (7%)

Genitourinary: Dysmenorrhea (5%), urinary frequency (2%)

Neuromuscular & skeletal: Myalgia (2%), neck pain (2%)

Ophthalmic: Amblyopia (2%)

Respiratory: Epistaxis (2%)

Frequency not defined:

Cardiovascular: Bradycardia (transient), chest tightness, decreased heart rate, increased blood pressure

Central nervous system: Confusion, depressed mood, disturbed sleep, drowsiness, headache, hypertonia, lack of concentration, lethargy, localized warm feeling, numbness of tongue, tingling of extremities, vertigo
Dermatologic: Alopecia, diaphoresis, skin rash
Gastrointestinal: Abdominal cramps, bloating, borborygmi, flatulence, increased peristalsis, nausea, salivation, vomiting
Hypersensitivity: Hypersensitivity reaction
Neuromuscular & skeletal: Fasciculations, muscle cramps, weakness
Ophthalmic: Eye pain, lacrimation, miosis, visual disturbance
Respiratory: Acute bronchitis (exacerbation), exacerbation of asthma, increased bronchial secretions

<1%, postmarketing, and/or case reports: Fecal incontinence, loss of consciousness, pallor (postsyncopal), stiffness (arms or upper torso), thrombophlebitis, urinary incontinence

Mechanism of Action Inhibits destruction of acetylcholine by acetylcholinesterase which facilitates transmission of impulses across neuromuscular junction

Pharmacodynamics/Kinetics

Onset of Action

Recovery from vincristine neurotoxicity: Onset of action: 1 to 2 weeks (Akbayram 2010)
Myasthenia gravis: Oral: Within 30 minutes (Maggi 2011); IM: 15 to 30 minutes; IV: Within 2 to 5 minutes

Duration of Action Oral: 3 to 4 hours in the daytime (Maggi 2011); IM, IV: 2 to 3 hours

Half-life Elimination

Oral: 1 to 2 hours; renal failure: ~6 hours (Aquilonius 1986)
IV: ~1.5 hours (Aquilonius 1980)

Time to Peak Oral: 1 to 2 hours (Aquilonius 1986)

Pregnancy Considerations Pyridostigmine may cross the placenta (Buckley 1968).

Oral pyridostigmine is the agent of choice for treating myasthenia gravis during pregnancy; the IV route may cause uterine contractions and is not recommended (Sanders 2016). Use should be continued during labor (Norwood 2014). Transient neonatal myasthenia gravis may occur in neonates due to placental transfer of maternal antibodies (Norwood 2014; Sanders 2016).

In general, medications used as antidotes should take into consideration the health and prognosis of the mother; antidotes should be administered to pregnant women if there is a clear indication for use and should not be withheld because of fears of teratogenicity (Bailey 2003).

◆ **Pyridostigmine Bromide** *see* Pyridostigmine *on page 1293*

Pyridoxine (peer i DOKS een)

Brand Names: US Neuro-K-250 T.D. [OTC]; Neuro-K-250 Vitamin B6 [OTC]; Neuro-K-50 [OTC]; Neuro-K-500 [OTC]; Pyri 500 [OTC]

Pharmacologic Category Vitamin, Water Soluble

Use Pyridoxine deficiency: Treatment and prevention of pyridoxine (vitamin B_6) deficiency.

Local Anesthetic/Vasoconstrictor Precautions No information available to require special precautions

Effects on Dental Treatment No significant effects or complications reported

Effects on Bleeding No information available to require special precautions

Adverse Reactions Frequency not defined.

Central nervous system: Ataxia, drowsiness, headache, neuropathy, paresthesia, seizure (following very large IV doses)
Endocrine & metabolic: Acidosis, folate deficiency
Gastrointestinal: Nausea
Hepatic: Increased serum AST
Hypersensitivity: Hypersensitivity reaction

Mechanism of Action Precursor to pyridoxal, which functions in the metabolism of proteins, carbohydrates, and fats; pyridoxal also aids in the release of liver and muscle-stored glycogen and in the synthesis of GABA (within the central nervous system) and heme

When used for the treatment of ethylene glycol poisoning, pyridoxine is theorized to increase the formation of glycine, a nontoxic metabolite (Barceloux 1999).

Pharmacodynamics/Kinetics

Half-life Elimination Biologic: 15 to 20 days

Pregnancy Risk Factor A

Pregnancy Considerations Water soluble vitamins cross the placenta. Maternal pyridoxine plasma concentrations may decrease as pregnancy progresses and requirements may be increased in pregnant women (IOM 1998). Pyridoxine is used to treat nausea and vomiting of pregnancy (ACOG 189 2018; Neibyl 2010; Campbell [SOGC] 2016).

◆ **Pyridoxine HCl** *see* Pyridoxine *on page 1294*

◆ **Pyridoxine Hydrochloride** *see* Pyridoxine *on page 1294*

Pyrimethamine (peer i METH a meen)

Brand Names: US Daraprim

Pharmacologic Category Antimalarial Agent

Use Toxoplasmosis: Treatment of toxoplasmosis (in combination with a sulfonamide).

Local Anesthetic/Vasoconstrictor Precautions No information available to require special precautions

Effects on Dental Treatment Key adverse event(s) related to dental treatment: Xerostomia (normal salivary flow resumes upon discontinuation). Atrophic glossitis has been reported.

Effects on Bleeding No information available to require special precautions

Adverse Reactions Frequency not defined.

Cardiovascular: Cardiac arrhythmia (large doses)
Dermatologic: Erythema multiforme, skin rash, Stevens-Johnson syndrome, toxic epidermal necrolysis
Gastrointestinal: Anorexia, glossitis (atrophic), vomiting
Hematologic & oncologic: Leukopenia, megaloblastic anemia, pancytopenia, thrombocytopenia
Genitourinary: Hematuria
Hypersensitivity: Anaphylaxis
Respiratory: Eosinophilic pneumonitis

Mechanism of Action Inhibits parasitic dihydrofolate reductase, resulting in inhibition of vital tetrahydrofolic acid synthesis

Pharmacodynamics/Kinetics

Half-life Elimination 80 to 95 hours (White 1985)

Time to Peak Serum: 2 to 6 hours

Reproductive Considerations

Pregnancy should be avoided during therapy.

Pregnancy Risk Factor C

Pregnancy Considerations

Pyrimethamine should be used with caution in patients with possible folate deficiency, including pregnant women. If administered during pregnancy (ie, for toxoplasmosis), supplementation of folate is strongly recommended.

Pyrimethamine is recommended for treatment of *T. gondii* in pregnant women living with HIV, including those with a strong suspicion of fetal infection. Pyrimethamine should not be used in the first trimester (HHS [OI adult 2019]).

Prescribing and Access Restrictions As of June 2015, pyrimethamine is no longer available in retail pharmacies in the United States. It is available through a special pharmacy program (https://www.-daraprimdirect.com/Home/HCP).

- ◆ **QAB149** *see* Indacaterol *on page 807*
- ◆ **Qbrelis** *see* Lisinopril *on page 922*
- ◆ **Q-Dryl [OTC] [DSC]** *see* DiphenhydrAMINE (Systemic) *on page 502*
- ◆ **Qinghao Derivative** *see* Artesunate *on page 169*
- ◆ **Qinghaosu Derivative** *see* Artesunate *on page 169*
- ◆ **Qinlock** *see* Ripretinib *on page 1330*
- ◆ **QIV (Quadrivalent Inactivated Influenza Vaccine)** *see* Influenza Virus Vaccine (Inactivated) *on page 812*
- ◆ **QlearQuil [OTC]** *see* Oxymetazoline (Nasal) *on page 1173*
- ◆ **Qmiiz ODT** *see* Meloxicam *on page 957*
- ◆ **Qnasl** *see* Beclomethasone (Nasal) *on page 217*
- ◆ **Qnasl Childrens** *see* Beclomethasone (Nasal) *on page 217*
- ◆ **Qnexa** *see* Phentermine and Topiramate *on page 1225*
- ◆ **Q-Pan H5N1 Influenza Vaccine** *see* Influenza A Virus Vaccine (H5N1) *on page 811*
- ◆ **Q-Pap [OTC] [DSC]** *see* Acetaminophen *on page 59*
- ◆ **Q-Pap Children's [OTC] [DSC]** *see* Acetaminophen *on page 59*
- ◆ **Q-Pap Extra Strength [OTC] [DSC]** *see* Acetaminophen *on page 59*
- ◆ **Q-Pap Infants' [OTC] [DSC]** *see* Acetaminophen *on page 59*
- ◆ **Qsymia** *see* Phentermine and Topiramate *on page 1225*
- ◆ **Qternmet XR** *see* Dapagliflozin, Saxagliptin, and Metformin *on page 436*
- ◆ **Quad Pill** *see* Elvitegravir, Cobicistat, Emtricitabine, and Tenofovir Disoproxil Fumarate *on page 553*
- ◆ **Quadrivalent Human Papillomavirus Vaccine** *see* Papillomavirus (Types 6, 11, 16, 18) Vaccine (Human, Recombinant) *on page 1190*
- ◆ **Quadrivalent Recombinant Hemagglutinin (rHA) Vaccine** *see* Influenza Virus Vaccine (Recombinant) *on page 815*
- ◆ **Qualaquin** *see* QuiNINE *on page 1300*
- ◆ **Quartette** *see* Ethinyl Estradiol and Levonorgestrel *on page 612*
- ◆ **Quasense [DSC]** *see* Ethinyl Estradiol and Levonorgestrel *on page 612*

Quazepam (KWAZ e pam)

Related Information

Dentin Hypersensitivity, Acid Erosion, High Caries Index, Management of Alveolar Osteitis, and Xerostomia *on page 1762*

Brand Names: US Doral

Pharmacologic Category Benzodiazepine

Use Insomnia: For the treatment of insomnia characterized by difficulty in falling asleep, frequent nocturnal awakenings, and/or early morning

Local Anesthetic/Vasoconstrictor Precautions

No information available to require special precautions

Effects on Dental Treatment Key adverse event(s) related to dental treatment: Xerostomia (normal salivary flow resumes upon discontinuation) and abnormal taste perception.

Effects on Bleeding No information available to require special precautions

Adverse Reactions

>10%: Central nervous system: Daytime sedation (12%)

<10%:

Central nervous system: Headache (5%), dizziness (2%), fatigue (2%)

Gastrointestinal: Xerostomia (2%), dyspepsia (1%)

Frequency not defined.

Cardiovascular: Palpitations

Central nervous system: Abnormality in thinking, agitation, amnesia, anxiety, apathy, ataxia, confusion, depression, drug dependence, euphoria, malaise, nervousness, nightmares, paranoia, speech disturbance

Dermatologic: Pruritus, skin rash

Endocrine & metabolic: Decreased libido

Gastrointestinal: Abdominal pain, anorexia, constipation, diarrhea, dysgeusia, nausea

Genitourinary: Impotence, urinary incontinence

Neuromuscular & skeletal: Hyperkinesia, hypokinesia, tremor, weakness

Ophthalmic: Cataract, visual disturbance

<1%, postmarketing, and/or case reports: Anaphylaxis, angioedema, sleep disorder (complex sleep-related behavior, eg, cooking while sleeping, eating food while sleeping, making phone calls while sleeping, sleep driving)

Mechanism of Action Binds to stereospecific benzodiazepine receptors on the postsynaptic GABA neuron at several sites within the central nervous system, including the limbic system, reticular formation. Enhancement of the inhibitory effect of GABA on neuronal excitability results by increased neuronal membrane permeability to chloride ions. This shift in chloride ions results in hyperpolarization (a less excitable state) and stabilization. Benzodiazepine receptors and effects appear to be linked to the GABA-A receptors. Benzodiazepines do not bind to GABA-B receptors (Vinkers 2012).

Pharmacodynamics/Kinetics

Half-life Elimination Serum: Quazepam, 2-oxoquazepam: 39 hours; N-desalkyl-2-oxoquazepam: 73 hours

Time to Peak ~2 hours

Pregnancy Considerations Although information specific to the use of quazepam has not been located, all benzodiazepines are assumed to cross the placenta. Teratogenic effects have been observed with some benzodiazepines; hypoglycemia and respiratory problems in the neonate may occur following exposure late in pregnancy. Maternal use of quazepam later in pregnancy may also be associated with difficulty feeding, hypothermia, hypotonia, and respiratory depression in neonates. Neonatal withdrawal symptoms may occur within days to weeks after birth and "floppy infant syndrome" (which also includes withdrawal symptoms) has been reported with some benzodiazepines (Bergman 1992; Iqbal 2002; Wikner 2007).

Controlled Substance C-IV

- **Qudexy XR** *see* Topiramate *on page 1464*
- **Quenalin [OTC] [DSC]** *see* DiphenhydrAMINE (Systemic) *on page 502*
- **Questran** *see* Cholestyramine Resin *on page 345*
- **Questran Light** *see* Cholestyramine Resin *on page 345*

QUEtiapine (kwe TYE a peen)

Related Information

Clinical Risk Related to Drugs Prolonging QT Interval *on page 1675*

Brand Names: US SEROquel; SEROquel XR

Brand Names: Canada ACCEL-QUEtiapine [DSC]; ACT QUEtiapine; AG-Quetiapine; APO-QUEtiapine; APO-QUEtiapine XR; Auro-QUEtiapine; BIO-QUEtiapine; DOM-QUEtiapine; JAMP-QUEtiapine; Mar-QUEtiapine; MINT-QUEtiapine; MYLAN-QUEtiapine [DSC]; NAT-QUEtiapine; NRA-Quetiapine; PHL-QUEtiapine [DSC]; PMS-QUEtiapine; Priva-QUEtiapine; PRO-QUEtiapine; RAN-QUEtiapine; RIVA-QUEtiapine; SANDOZ QUEtiapine; SANDOZ QUEtiapine XRT; SEROquel; SEROquel XR; TEVA-QUEtiapine; TEVA-QUEtiapine XR; VAN-QUEtiapine [DSC]

Pharmacologic Category Second Generation (Atypical) Antipsychotic

Use

Bipolar disorder: Acute treatment of manic (both immediate release and ER) or mixed (ER only) episodes and acute hypomanic episodes (off-label) associated with bipolar I disorder, both as monotherapy and as an adjunct to antimanic therapy; maintenance treatment of bipolar I disorder, as monotherapy (off-label) or as an adjunct to antimanic therapy; acute treatment of bipolar major depression, as monotherapy.

Major depressive disorder (unipolar) (ER only): Adjunctive therapy in patients with an inadequate response to antidepressants for the treatment of major depressive disorder.

Schizophrenia: Treatment of schizophrenia.

Local Anesthetic/Vasoconstrictor Precautions Quetiapine is one of the drugs confirmed to prolong the QT interval and is accepted as having a risk of causing torsade de pointes. The risk of drug-induced torsade de pointes is extremely low when a single QT interval prolonging drug is prescribed. In terms of epinephrine, it is not known what effect vasoconstrictors in the local anesthetic regimen will have in patients with a known history of congenital prolonged QT interval or in patients taking any medication that prolongs the QT interval. Until more information is obtained, it is suggested that the clinician consult with the physician prior to the use of a vasoconstrictor in suspected patients, and that the vasoconstrictor (epinephrine, mepivacaine and levonordefrin [Carbocaine 2% with Neo-Cobefrin]) be used with caution.

Effects on Dental Treatment Key adverse event(s) related to dental treatment: Xerostomia (normal salivary flow resumes upon discontinuation).

Effects on Bleeding No information available to require special precautions

Adverse Reactions Actual frequency may be dependent upon dose and/or indication. Unless otherwise noted, frequency of adverse effects is reported for adult patients; spectrum and incidence of adverse effects similar in children (with significant exceptions noted).

>10%:

Cardiovascular: Increased diastolic blood pressure (≥10 mm Hg; children and adolescents: 41% to 47%), increased systolic blood pressure (≥20 mm Hg; children and adolescents: 7% to 15%), tachycardia (1% to 11%)

Endocrine & metabolic: Decreased HDL cholesterol (≤40 mg/dL: 9% to 20%), hyperglycemia (≥200 mg/dL post glucose challenge or fasting glucose ≥126 mg/dL: 2% to 3%), increased LDL cholesterol (≥160 mg/dL: 4% to 8%), increased serum triglycerides (≥200 mg/dL: 8% to 22%), total cholesterol increased (≥240 mg/dL: 7% to 18%), weight gain (dose related; 4% to 28%)

Gastrointestinal: Constipation (2% to 11%), increased appetite (2% to 12%), xerostomia (adults: 9% to 44%; children and adolescents: 4% to 10%)

Hematologic & oncologic: Decreased hemoglobin (8% to 11%)

Nervous system: Agitation (6% to 20%), dizziness (7% to 19%), drowsiness (16% to 57%), extrapyramidal reaction (1% to 13%), fatigue (3% to 14%), headache (17% to 21%), withdrawal syndrome (12%)

1% to 10%:

Cardiovascular: Hypertension (2%), hypotension (3%), increased heart rate (1% to 9%), orthostatic hypotension (adults: 2% to 7%; children and adolescents: <1%), palpitations (4%), peripheral edema (4%), syncope (1% to 2%)

Dermatologic: Acne vulgaris (children and adolescents: 2% to 3%), diaphoresis (2%), hyperhidrosis (2%), pallor (children and adolescents: 1% to 2%), skin rash (4%)

Endocrine & metabolic: Decreased libido (≤2%), hyperprolactinemia (4%), hypothyroidism (≤2%), increased thirst (children and adolescents: 2%)

Gastrointestinal: Abdominal pain (1% to 7%), anorexia (1% to 3%), decreased appetite (2%), diarrhea (children and adolescents: 5%), dyspepsia (2% to 7%), dysphagia (2%), gastroenteritis (2%), gastroesophageal reflux disease (2%), nausea (5% to 10%), periodontal abscess (adolescents: 1% to 3%), toothache (2% to 3%), viral gastroenteritis (4%), vomiting (3% to 8%)

Genitourinary: Pollakiuria (2%), urinary tract infection (2%)

Hematologic & oncologic: Leukopenia (≥1%), neutropenia (≤2%)

Hepatic: Increased serum alanine aminotransferase (5%), increased serum aspartate aminotransferase (3%), increased serum transaminases (1% to 6%)

Hypersensitivity: Seasonal allergy (2%)

Infection: Influenza (1% to 2%)

Nervous system: Abnormal dreams (2% to 3%), abnormality in thinking (2%), aggressive behavior (children and adolescents: 1% to 3%), akathisia (1% to 5%), anxiety (2% to 4%), ataxia (2%), confusion (2%), decreased mental acuity (2%), depression (2% to 3%), disorientation (2%), disturbance in attention (2%), drug-induced Parkinson's disease

(≤6%), dysarthria (2% to 5%), dystonic reaction (1% to 3%), falling (2%), hypersomnia (2% to 3%), hypertonia (4%), hypoesthesia (2%), irritability (3% to 5%), lack of concentration (2%), lethargy (2% to 5%), migraine (2%), pain (7%), paresthesia (2% to 3%), restless leg syndrome (2%), restlessness (2%), twitching (4%), vertigo (2%)

Neuromuscular & skeletal: Arthralgia (1% to 4%), asthenia (1% to 10%), back pain (1% to 5%), dyskinesia (3% to 4%), limb pain (2%), muscle rigidity (3%), muscle spasm (2% to 3%), myalgia (2%), neck pain (2%), stiffness (children and adolescents: 3%), tremor (2% to 8%)

Ophthalmic: Amblyopia (2% to 3%), blurred vision (2% to 4%)

Otic: Otalgia (2%)

Respiratory: Cough (1% to 3%), dyspnea (1% to 3%), epistaxis (adolescents: 3%), nasal congestion (3% to 6%), paranasal sinus congestion (2% to 3%), pharyngitis (4% to 6%), rhinitis (3% to 4%), sinus headache (2%), sinusitis (2%), upper respiratory tract infection (3%)

Miscellaneous: Fever (2% to 4%)

<1%: Cardiovascular: Hypertensive crisis

Frequency not defined: Nervous system: Suicidal ideation, suicidal tendencies

Postmarketing:

Cardiovascular: Cardiomyopathy, colonic ischemia, myocarditis, prolonged QT interval on ECG

Dermatologic: Acute generalized exanthematous pustulosis, Stevens-Johnson syndrome, toxic epidermal necrolysis

Endocrine & metabolic: Hyponatremia, ketoacidosis, SIADH

Gastrointestinal: Intestinal obstruction, pancreatitis

Genitourinary: Nocturia, urinary retention

Hematologic & oncologic: Agranulocytosis, decreased platelet count

Hepatic: Hepatic failure, hepatic necrosis, hepatitis

Hypersensitivity: Anaphylaxis

Immunologic: Drug reaction with eosinophilia and systemic symptoms

Nervous system: Diabetes mellitus with hyperosmolar coma, neuroleptic malignant syndrome, retrograde amnesia, sleep apnea, tardive dyskinesia

Neuromuscular & skeletal: Rhabdomyolysis

Respiratory: Obstructive sleep apnea syndrome (Health Canada 2016; Shirani 2011)

Mechanism of Action Quetiapine is a dibenzothiazepine atypical antipsychotic. It has been proposed that this drug's antipsychotic activity is mediated through a combination of dopamine type 2 (D_2) and serotonin type 2 (5-HT_2) antagonism. It is an antagonist at multiple neurotransmitter receptors in the brain: Serotonin 5-HT_{1A} and 5-HT_2, dopamine D_1 and D_2, histamine H_1, and adrenergic alpha$_1$- and alpha$_2$-receptors; but appears to have no appreciable affinity at cholinergic muscarinic and benzodiazepine receptors. Norquetiapine, an active metabolite, differs from its parent molecule by exhibiting high affinity for muscarinic M1 receptors.

Antagonism at receptors other than dopamine and 5-HT_2 with similar receptor affinities may explain some of the other effects of quetiapine. The drug's antagonism of histamine H_1-receptors may explain the somnolence observed. The drug's antagonism of adrenergic alpha$_1$-receptors may explain the orthostatic hypotension observed.

Pharmacodynamics/Kinetics

Half-life Elimination

Children and Adolescents 12 to 17 years: Quetiapine: 5.3 hours (McConville 2000)

Adults: Mean: Terminal: Quetiapine: ~6 hours; Extended release: ~7 hours

Metabolite: N-desalkyl quetiapine: 12 hours

Time to Peak

Children and Adolescents 12 to 17 years: Immediate release: 0.5-3 hours (McConville 2000)

Adults: Plasma: Immediate release: 1.5 hours; Extended release: 6 hours

Reproductive Considerations

Quetiapine may cause hyperprolactinemia, which may decrease reproductive function in both males and females.

If treatment with atypical antipsychotic is needed in a woman planning a pregnancy, use of quetiapine may be considered (Larsen 2015).

Pregnancy Considerations

Quetiapine crosses the placenta and can be detected in cord blood (Newport 2007). Congenital malformations have not been observed in humans (based on available data). Antipsychotic use during the third trimester of pregnancy has a risk for abnormal muscle movements (extrapyramidal symptoms) and/or withdrawal symptoms in newborns following delivery. Symptoms in the newborn may include agitation, feeding disorder, hypertonia, hypotonia, respiratory distress, somnolence, and tremor; these effects may be self-limiting or require hospitalization.

Treatment algorithms have been developed by the American College of Obstetricians and Gynecologists (ACOG) and the American Psychiatric Association (APA) for the management of depression in women prior to conception and during pregnancy (Yonkers 2009). The ACOG recommends that therapy during pregnancy be individualized; treatment with psychiatric medications during pregnancy should incorporate the clinical expertise of the mental health clinician, obstetrician, primary health care provider, and pediatrician. Safety data related to atypical antipsychotics during pregnancy are limited; as such, routine use is not recommended. However, if a woman is inadvertently exposed to an atypical antipsychotic while pregnant, continuing therapy may be preferable to switching to an agent that the fetus has not yet been exposed to; consider risk:benefit (ACOG 2008). If treatment is initiated during pregnancy, use of quetiapine may be considered (Larsen 2015).

Health care providers are encouraged to enroll women 18 to 45 years of age exposed to quetiapine during pregnancy in the Atypical Antipsychotics Pregnancy Registry (1-866-961-2388 or http://www.womensmentalhealth.org/pregnancyregistry).

Dental Health Professional Considerations See Local Anesthetic/Vasoconstrictor Precautions

- ◆ **Quetiapine Fumarate** *see* QUEtiapine *on page 1296*
- ◆ **Quflora FE** *see* Vitamins (Multiple/Oral) *on page 1550*
- ◆ **QuilliChew ER** *see* Methylphenidate *on page 997*
- ◆ **Quillivant XR** *see* Methylphenidate *on page 997*

Quinapril (KWIN a pril)

Related Information

Cardiovascular Diseases *on page 1654*

Brand Names: US Accupril

Brand Names: Canada Accupril; APO-Quinapril; GD-Quinapril [DSC]; PMS-Quinapril

Pharmacologic Category Angiotensin-Converting Enzyme (ACE) Inhibitor; Antihypertensive

Use

Heart failure: Adjunctive treatment of heart failure (HF)

Guideline recommendations: The American College of Cardiology/American Heart Association (ACC/AHA) 2013 Heart Failure Guidelines recommend the use of ACE inhibitors, along with other guideline-directed medical therapies, to prevent progression of HF and reduced ejection fraction in asymptomatic patients with or without a history of myocardial infarction (Stage B HF), or to treat those with symptomatic HF and reduced ejection fraction to reduce morbidity and mortality (Stage C HFrEF).

Hypertension: Management of hypertension

Guideline recommendations: The 2017 Guideline for the Prevention, Detection, Evaluation, and Management of High Blood Pressure in Adults recommends if monotherapy is warranted, in the absence of comorbidities (eg, cerebrovascular disease, chronic kidney disease, diabetes, heart failure, ischemic heart disease, etc.), that thiazide-like diuretics or dihydropyridine calcium channel blockers may be preferred options due to improved cardiovascular endpoints (eg, prevention of heart failure and stroke). ACE inhibitors and ARBs are also acceptable for monotherapy. Combination therapy may be required to achieve blood pressure goals and is initially preferred in patients at high risk (stage 2 hypertension or atherosclerotic cardiovascular disease [ASCVD] risk ≥10%) (ACC/AHA [Whelton 2017]).

Local Anesthetic/Vasoconstrictor Precautions

No information available to require special precautions

Effects on Dental Treatment Key adverse event(s) related to dental treatment: Patients may experience orthostatic hypotension as they stand up after treatment; especially if lying in dental chair for extended periods of time. Use caution with sudden changes in position during and after dental treatment.

An angiotensin-converting enzyme (ACE) Inhibitor cough is a dry, hacking, nonproductive cough that can potentially interfere with longer dental procedures if patient has this side effect.

Effects on Bleeding No information available to require special precautions

Adverse Reactions Frequency ranges include data from hypertension and heart failure trials. Higher rates of adverse reactions have generally been noted in patients with CHF. However, the frequency of adverse effects associated with placebo is also increased in this population.

1% to 10%:

- Cardiovascular: Hypotension (3%), chest pain (2%)
- Central nervous system: Dizziness (4% to 8%), headache (2% to 6%), fatigue (3%)
- Endocrine & metabolic: Hyperkalemia (≤2%)
- Gastrointestinal: Nausea (≤2%), vomiting (≤2%), diarrhea (2%), abdominal pain (1%)
- Neuromuscular & skeletal: Back pain (≤1%)
- Renal: Increased blood urea nitrogen (≤2%), increased serum creatinine (≤2%)
- Respiratory: Cough (2% to 4%)

<1%, postmarketing, and/or case reports: Abnormal hepatic function tests, acute renal failure, agranulocytosis, alopecia, amblyopia, anaphylactoid reaction, angina pectoris, angioedema, arthralgia, cardiac arrhythmia, cardiac failure, cardiogenic shock, cerebrovascular accident, constipation, depression, diaphoresis, drowsiness, dry throat, dyspepsia, edema, eosinophilic pneumonitis, exacerbation of renal failure, exfoliative dermatitis, flatulence, gastrointestinal hemorrhage, hemolytic anemia, hepatitis, hypertensive crisis, hyponatremia, impotence, insomnia, malaise, myocardial infarction, nervousness, orthostatic hypotension, palpitations, pancreatitis, paresthesia, pemphigus, pharyngitis, polymyositis (dermatopolymyositis), pruritus, skin photosensitivity, syncope, tachycardia, thrombocytopenia, urinary tract infection, vasodilation, vertigo, viral infection, visual hallucination (Doane 2013), xerostomia

Mechanism of Action Competitive inhibitor of angiotensin-converting enzyme (ACE); prevents conversion of angiotensin I to angiotensin II, a potent vasoconstrictor; results in lower levels of angiotensin II which causes an increase in plasma renin activity and a reduction in aldosterone secretion; a CNS mechanism may also be involved in hypotensive effect as angiotensin II increases adrenergic outflow from CNS; vasoactive kallikreins may be decreased in conversion to active hormones by ACE inhibitors, thus reducing blood pressure

Pharmacodynamics/Kinetics

Onset of Action 1 hour; Peak effect: Antihypertensive: 2 to 4 hours postdose

Duration of Action 24 hours (chronic dosing)

Half-life Elimination

Infants and Children <7 years: Quinaprilat: 2.3 hours (Blumer 2003)

Adults: Quinapril: 0.8 hours; Quinaprilat: 3 hours; increases as CrCl decreases

Time to Peak

Infants and Children <7 years: 1.7 hours (range: 1 to 4 hours) (Blumer 2003)

Adults: Serum: Quinapril: 1 hour; Quinaprilat: ~2 hours

Reproductive Considerations

Angiotensin-converting enzyme (ACE) inhibitors should be avoided in sexually active females of reproductive potential not using effective contraception (ADA 2020).

ACE inhibitors should generally be avoided for the treatment of hypertension in women planning a pregnancy; use should only be considered for cases of hypertension refractory to other medications (ACOG 203 2019).

Pregnancy Risk Factor D

Pregnancy Considerations Quinapril crosses the placenta.

Exposure to an angiotensin-converting enzyme (ACE) inhibitor during the first trimester of pregnancy may be associated with an increased risk of fetal malformations (ACOG 203 2019; ESC [Regitz-Zagrosek 2018]); however, outcomes observed may also be influenced by maternal disease (ACC/AHA [Whelton 2017]).

[US Boxed Warning]: Drugs that act on the renin-angiotensin system can cause injury and death to the developing fetus. Discontinue as soon as possible once pregnancy is detected. Drugs that act on the renin-angiotensin system are associated with oligohydramnios. Oligohydramnios, due to decreased fetal renal function, may lead to fetal lung hypoplasia and skeletal malformations. The use of these drugs in pregnancy is also associated with anuria, hypotension, renal failure, skull hypoplasia, and death in the fetus/neonate. Infants exposed to an ACE inhibitor in utero should be monitored for hyperkalemia, hypotension, and oliguria. Oligohydramnios may not appear until after irreversible fetal injury has occurred. Exchange transfusions or dialysis may be required to reverse hypotension or improve renal function, although data related to the effectiveness in neonates is limited.

Chronic maternal hypertension is also associated with adverse events in the fetus/infant. Chronic maternal hypertension may increase the risk of birth defects, low birth weight, premature delivery, stillbirth, and neonatal death. Actual fetal/neonatal risks may be related to duration and severity of maternal hypertension. Untreated chronic hypertension may also increase the risks of adverse maternal outcomes, including gestational diabetes, preeclampsia, delivery complications, stroke and myocardial infarction (ACOG 203 2019).

When treatment of hypertension in pregnancy is indicated, ACE inhibitors should generally be avoided due to their adverse fetal events; use in pregnant women should only be considered for cases of hypertension refractory to other medications (ACOG 203 2019). ACE inhibitors are not recommended for the treatment of heart failure in pregnancy (Regitz-Zagrosek [ESC 2018]).

- ◆ **Quinapril HCl** *see* Quinapril *on page 1298*
- ◆ **Quinapril Hydrochloride** *see* Quinapril *on page 1298*
- ◆ **Quinidex** *see* QuiNIDine *on page 1299*

QuiNIDine (KWIN i deen)

Related Information

Clinical Risk Related to Drugs Prolonging QT Interval *on page 1675*

Pharmacologic Category Antiarrhythmic Agent, Class Ia; Antimalarial Agent

Use

Quinidine gluconate and sulfate salts: Conversion and prevention of relapse into atrial fibrillation and/or flutter; suppression of ventricular arrhythmias. **Note:** Due to proarrhythmic effects, use should be reserved for life-threatening arrhythmias. Moreover, the use of quinidine has largely been replaced by more effective/safer antiarrhythmic agents and/or nonpharmacologic therapies (eg, radiofrequency ablation).

Quinidine gluconate (IV formulation): Conversion of atrial fibrillation/flutter and ventricular tachycardia. **Note:** The use of IV quinidine gluconate for these indications has been replaced by more effective/safer antiarrhythmic agents (eg, amiodarone and procainamide).

Guideline recommendation: **Ventricular arrhythmias:** Based on the American Heart Association/American College of Cardiology/Heart Rhythm Society (AHA/ACC/HRS) patients with Brugada syndrome with or without an implantable cardioverter-defibrillator (ICD) experiencing symptomatic ventricular arrhythmias are recommended to receive intensification of therapy with quinidine or catheter ablation (AHA/ACC/HRS [Al-Khatib 2017]; Belhassen 2015). Patients with short QT syndrome and recurrent sustained ventricular arrhythmias may benefit from treatment with quinidine (AHA/ACC/HRS [Al-Khatib 2017]).

Quinidine gluconate (IV formulation): Treatment of malaria (*Plasmodium falciparum*)

Local Anesthetic/Vasoconstrictor Precautions Quinidine is one of the drugs confirmed to prolong the QT interval and is accepted as having a risk of causing torsade de pointes. The risk of drug-induced torsade de pointes is extremely low when a single QT interval prolonging drug is prescribed. In terms of epinephrine, it is not known what effect vasoconstrictors in the local anesthetic regimen will have in patients with a known history of congenital prolonged QT interval or in patients taking any medication that prolongs the QT interval. Until more information is obtained, it is suggested that the clinician consult with the physician prior to the use of a vasoconstrictor in suspected patients, and that the vasoconstrictor (epinephrine, mepivacaine and levonordefrin [Carbocaine® 2% with Neo-Cobefrin®]) be used with caution.

Effects on Dental Treatment When taken over a long period of time, the anticholinergic side effects from quinidine can cause a reduction of saliva production or secretion contributing to discomfort and dental disease (ie, caries, oral candidiasis, and periodontal disease).

Effects on Bleeding Quinidine has been shown to induce thrombocytopenia through the generation of both drug-dependent and drug-independent antibodies. In general, quinidine-induced thrombocytopenia is reversible following 9 days of discontinuation.

Adverse Reactions Frequency not always defined.

Cardiovascular: Palpitations (7%), angina pectoris (6%), cardiac arrhythmia (3%; new or worsened; proarrhythmic effect), ECG abnormality (3%), cerebral ischemia (2%), prolonged QT interval on ECG (modest prolongation is common; however, excessive prolongation is rare and indicates toxicity), syncope

Central nervous system: Dizziness (3% to 15%), fatigue (7%), headache (3% to 7%), disturbed sleep (3%), nervousness (2%), ataxia (1%)

Dermatologic: Skin rash (5% to 6%)

Gastrointestinal: Diarrhea (24% to 35%), gastrointestinal distress (upper; 22%), nausea and vomiting (3%), esophagitis

Neuromuscular & skeletal: Weakness (2% to 5%), tremor (2%)

Ophthalmic: Visual disturbance (3%)

Miscellaneous: Fever (6%)

<1%, postmarketing, and/or case reports: Acute psychosis, agranulocytosis, angioedema, arthralgia, bradycardia (exacerbated, in sick sinus syndrome), bronchospasm, cerebrovascular insufficiency (possibly resulting in ataxia, apprehension, and seizure), cinchonism (may include tinnitus, high-frequency hearing loss, deafness, vertigo, blurred vision, diplopia, photophobia, headache, confusion, and delirium; usually associated with chronic toxicity but may occur after brief exposure to a moderate dose), depression, dyschromia, exfoliative dermatitis, flushing, granulomatous hepatitis, hemolytic anemia, hepatotoxicity (rare), hypotension, immune thrombocytopenia, increased creatine phosphokinase, lupus-like syndrome, lymphadenopathy, myalgia, mydriasis, nocturnal amblyopia, optic neuritis, pneumonitis, pruritus, psoriasiform eruption, scotoma, skin photosensitivity, Sjogren's syndrome, thrombocytopenia, torsades de pointes, urticaria, uveitis, vasculitis, ventricular fibrillation, ventricular tachycardia (including paradoxical, during atrial fibrillation/flutter), visual field loss, vision color changes

Mechanism of Action Class Ia antiarrhythmic agent; depresses phase 0 of the action potential; decreases myocardial excitability and conduction velocity, and myocardial contractility by decreasing sodium influx during depolarization and potassium efflux in repolarization; also reduces calcium transport across cell membrane

Pharmacodynamics/Kinetics

Half-life Elimination Plasma: Children: 3 to 4 hours; Adults: 6 to 8 hours; prolonged with elderly, cirrhosis, and congestive heart failure

Time to Peak Serum: Oral: Sulfate: Immediate release: 2 hours; Gluconate: Extended release: 3 to 5 hours

Pregnancy Risk Factor C

Pregnancy Considerations Quinidine crosses the placenta and can be detected in the amniotic fluid and neonatal serum.

Product Availability Quinidine injection has been discontinued in the United States for more than 1 year.

Dental Health Professional Considerations See Local Anesthetic/Vasoconstrictor Precautions

- **Quinidine Gluconate** *see* QuiNIDine *on page 1299*
- **Quinidine Polygalacturonate** *see* QuiNIDine *on page 1299*
- **Quinidine Sulfate** *see* QuiNIDine *on page 1299*

QuiNINE (KWYE nine)

Related Information

Clinical Risk Related to Drugs Prolonging QT Interval *on page 1675*

Brand Names: US Qualaquin

Brand Names: Canada APO-QuiNINE; JAMP-QuiNINE; PRO-QuiNINE-200; QuiNINE-Odan; TEVA-QuiNINE

Pharmacologic Category Antimalarial Agent

Use Malaria, treatment: Treatment of uncomplicated, chloroquine-resistant *Plasmodium falciparum* malaria, in combination with other antimalarial agents. **Note:** Centers for Disease Control and Prevention guidelines also recommend quinine, in combination with other antimalarial agents, as an alternative agent for treatment of malaria due to other chloroquine-sensitive or chloroquine-resistant *Plasmodium* species, and as oral treatment for severe malaria after completion of IV therapy or as interim oral therapy pending IV therapy (CDC 2020).

Local Anesthetic/Vasoconstrictor Precautions Quinine is one of the drugs confirmed to prolong the QT interval and is accepted as having a risk of causing torsade de pointes. The risk of drug-induced torsade de pointes is extremely low when a single QT interval prolonging drug is prescribed. In terms of epinephrine, it is not known what effect vasoconstrictors in the local anesthetic regimen will have in patients with a known history of congenital prolonged QT interval or in patients taking any medication that prolongs the QT interval. Until more information is obtained, it is suggested that the clinician consult with the physician prior to the use of a vasoconstrictor in suspected patients, and that the vasoconstrictor (epinephrine, mepivacaine and levonordefrin [Carbocaine® 2% with Neo-Cobefrin®]) be used with caution.

Effects on Dental Treatment No significant effects or complications reported

Effects on Bleeding Quinine has been shown to induce platelet-reactive monoclonal antibodies responsible for immune thrombocytopenia, leading to prolonged bleeding times. This drug-dependent antibody generation leads to the destruction of endogenous platelets. Quinine-induced thrombocytopenia can be treated through the discontinuation of the drug. Severe cases require a platelet transfusion.

Adverse Reactions Frequency not defined.

Cardiovascular: Appearance of U waves on ECG, atrial fibrillation, atrioventricular block, bradycardia, cardiac arrhythmia, chest pain, flushing, hypersensitivity angiitis, hypotension, nodal rhythm disorder (nodal escape beats), orthostatic hypotension, palpitations, prolonged QT interval on ECG, syncope, tachycardia, torsades de pointes, unifocal premature ventricular contractions, vasodilation, ventricular fibrillation, ventricular tachycardia

Central nervous system: Altered mental status, aphasia, ataxia, chills, coma, confusion, disorientation, dizziness, dystonic reaction, headache, restlessness, seizure, vertigo

Dermatologic: Allergic contact dermatitis, bullous dermatitis, diaphoresis, exfoliative dermatitis, erythema multiforme, pruritus, skin necrosis (acral), skin photosensitivity, skin rash (papular rash, scarlatiniform rash, urticaria), Stevens-Johnson syndrome, toxic epidermal necrolysis

Endocrine & metabolic: Hypoglycemia

Gastrointestinal: Abdominal pain, anorexia, diarrhea, esophagitis, gastric irritation, nausea, vomiting

Genitourinary: Hemoglobinuria

Hematologic & oncologic: Agranulocytosis, aplastic anemia, blood coagulation disorder, bruise, disseminated intravascular coagulation, hemolysis (blackwater fever), hemolytic anemia, hemolytic-uremic syndrome, hemorrhage, hypoprothrombinemia, immune thrombocytopenia (ITP), leukopenia, neutropenia, pancytopenia, petechia, thrombocytopenia, thrombotic thrombocytopenic purpura

Hepatic: Abnormal hepatic function tests, granulomatous hepatitis, hepatitis, jaundice

Hypersensitivity: Hypersensitivity reaction

Immunologic: Antibody development (lupus anticoagulant syndrome)

Neuromuscular & skeletal: Lupus-like syndrome, myalgia, tremor, weakness

Ophthalmic: Blindness, blurred vision (with or without scotomata), diplopia, mydriasis, nocturnal amblyopia, optic neuritis, photophobia, vision color changes, vision loss (sudden), visual field loss

Otic: Auditory impairment, deafness, tinnitus

Renal: Acute interstitial nephritis, renal failure, renal insufficiency

Respiratory: Asthma, dyspnea, pulmonary edema

Miscellaneous: Fever

Mechanism of Action Depresses oxygen uptake and carbohydrate metabolism; intercalates into DNA, disrupting the parasite's replication and transcription; cardiovascular effects similar to quinidine

Pharmacodynamics/Kinetics

Half-life Elimination

Children: ~3 hours in healthy subjects; ~12 hours with malaria

Healthy adults: 10 to 13 hours

Healthy elderly subjects: 18 hours

Time to Peak

Children: Serum: 2 hours in healthy subjects; 4 hours with malaria

Adults: Serum: 2 to 4 hours in healthy subjects; 1 to 11 hours with malaria

Reproductive Considerations
A decrease in sperm motility and an increase in abnormal sperm morphology was observed in men receiving quinine.

Pregnancy Considerations Quinine crosses the placenta.

Cord plasma to maternal plasma quinine ratios have been reported as 0.18 to 0.46 and should not be considered therapeutic to the infant. Based on available data, therapeutic doses used for malaria are not associated with an increased risk of adverse fetal events.

Quinine may cause significant maternal hypoglycemia and an increased risk of other adverse maternal events, including dizziness, nausea, tinnitus, and vomiting. Pregnant women may also be at risk for a rare triad of complications which includes massive hemolysis, hemoglobinemia, and hemoglobinuria.

Malaria infection in pregnant women may be more severe than in nonpregnant women and has a high risk of maternal and perinatal morbidity and mortality. Malaria infection during pregnancy can lead to miscarriage, premature delivery, low birth weight, congenital infection, and/or perinatal death. Therefore, pregnant women and women who are likely to become pregnant are advised to avoid travel to malaria-risk areas. When travel is unavoidable, pregnant women should take precautions to avoid mosquito bites and use effective prophylactic medications (CDC 2020; CDC Yellow Book 2020).

Quinine may be used to treat chloroquine-resistant uncomplicated malaria during all trimesters of pregnancy. In pregnant patients with severe malaria, quinine may be used as interim oral therapy when the preferred IV agent is not readily available (discontinue once IV treatment is initiated) (CDC 2020; WHO 2015); consult current CDC guidelines.

Dental Health Professional Considerations See Local Anesthetic/Vasoconstrictor Precautions

- ◆ **Quinine Sulfate** *see* QuiNINE *on page 1300*
- ◆ **Quintabs [OTC]** *see* Vitamins (Multiple/Oral) *on page 1550*
- ◆ **Quintabs-M [OTC]** *see* Vitamins (Multiple/Oral) *on page 1550*
- ◆ **Quintabs-M Iron-Free [OTC]** *see* Vitamins (Multiple/Oral) *on page 1550*

Quinupristin and Dalfopristin

(kwi NYOO pris tin & dal FOE pris tin)

Brand Names: US Synercid

Brand Names: Canada Synercid

Pharmacologic Category Antibiotic, Streptogramin

Use Skin and skin structure infections, complicated: Treatment of complicated skin and skin structure infections caused by methicillin-susceptible *Staphylococcus aureus* or *Streptococcus pyogenes*

Local Anesthetic/Vasoconstrictor Precautions No information available to require special precautions

Effects on Dental Treatment No significant effects or complications reported

Effects on Bleeding No information available to require special precautions

Adverse Reactions

>10%:

Hepatic: Hyperbilirubinemia (3% to 35%)

Local: Local pain (40% to 44%), local inflammation (at infusion site: 38% to 42%), localized edema (17% to 18%), infusion site reaction (12% to 13%)

Neuromuscular & skeletal: Arthralgia (≤47%), myalgia (≤47%)

1% to 10%:

Cardiovascular: Thrombophlebitis (2%)

Central nervous system: Pain (2% to 3%), headache (2%)

Dermatologic: Skin rash (3%), pruritus (2%)

Endocrine & metabolic: Increased lactate dehydrogenase (3%), increased gamma-glutamyl transferase (2%), hyperglycemia (1%)

Gastrointestinal: Nausea (3% to 5%), vomiting (3% to 4%), diarrhea (3%)

Hematologic & oncologic: Anemia (3%)

Neuromuscular & skeletal: Increased creatine phosphokinase (2%)

<1%, postmarketing, and/or case reports: Abdominal pain, anaphylactoid reaction, anxiety, apnea, blood coagulation disorder, brain disease, cardiac arrhythmia, chest pain, confusion, constipation, dermal ulcer, diaphoresis, dizziness, dysautonomia, dyspepsia, dyspnea, fever, gastrointestinal hemorrhage, gout, hematuria, hemolysis, hemolytic anemia, hepatitis, hyperkalemia, hypersensitivity reaction, hypertonia, hypoglycemia, hyponatremia, hypotension, hypoventilation, hypovolemia, increased blood urea nitrogen, increased serum creatinine, increased serum transaminases, infection, insomnia, leg cramps, maculopapular rash, mesenteric artery occlusion, myasthenia, neck stiffness, neuropathy, oral candidiasis, ostealgia, palpitations, pancreatitis, pancytopenia, paraplegia, paresthesia, pericarditis, peripheral edema, phlebitis, pleural effusion, pseudomembranous colitis, respiratory distress, seizure, shock, stomatitis, syncope, thrombocytopenia, tremor, urticaria, vaginitis, vasodilation

Mechanism of Action Quinupristin/dalfopristin inhibits bacterial protein synthesis by binding to different sites on the 50S bacterial ribosomal subunit thereby inhibiting protein synthesis

Pharmacodynamics/Kinetics

Half-life Elimination Quinupristin: 0.85 hour; Dalfopristin: 0.7 hour (mean elimination half-lives, including metabolites: 3 and 1 hours, respectively)

Pregnancy Considerations Adverse events have not been observed in animal reproduction studies.

- ◆ **Quinupristin/Dalfopristin** *see* Quinupristin and Dalfopristin *on page 1301*
- ◆ **Qutenza** *see* Capsaicin *on page 284*
- ◆ **Quzyttir** *see* Cetirizine (Systemic) *on page 328*
- ◆ **Qvar [DSC]** *see* Beclomethasone (Oral Inhalation) *on page 218*
- ◆ **Qvar RediHaler** *see* Beclomethasone (Oral Inhalation) *on page 218*
- ◆ **R788** *see* Fostamatinib *on page 718*
- ◆ **R-1569** *see* Tocilizumab *on page 1457*
- ◆ **R7159** *see* Obinutuzumab *on page 1124*
- ◆ **R093877** *see* Prucalopride *on page 1291*
- ◆ **R108512** *see* Prucalopride *on page 1291*
- ◆ **R935788** *see* Fostamatinib *on page 718*
- ◆ **R05072759** *see* Obinutuzumab *on page 1124*
- ◆ **RabAvert** *see* Rabies Vaccine *on page 1303*

RABEprazole (ra BEP ra zole)

Related Information

Gastrointestinal Disorders *on page 1678*

Brand Names: US Aciphex; AcipHex Sprinkle

Brand Names: Canada APO-Rabeprazole; DOM-Rabeprazole EC; MYLAN-Rabeprazole [DSC]; Pariet; PMS-Rabeprazole EC; PRO-Rabeprazole; RAN-Rabeprazole; RIVA-Rabeprazole EC [DSC]; SANDOZ Rabeprazole; TEVA-Rabeprazole EC

Pharmacologic Category Proton Pump Inhibitor; Substituted Benzimidazole

Use

Duodenal ulcers (tablets only): Short-term (4 weeks or fewer) treatment in the healing and symptomatic relief of duodenal ulcers in adults.

Gastroesophageal reflux disease:

Erosive or ulcerative (tablets only): Short-term (4 to 8 weeks) treatment in the healing and symptomatic relief of erosive or ulcerative gastroesophageal reflux disease (GERD) in adults; for maintaining healing and reduction in relapse rates of heartburn symptoms in adults with erosive or ulcerative GERD.

Symptomatic (nonerosive): Treatment of symptomatic GERD for up to 4 weeks in adults (tablets only), up to 8 weeks in children ≥12 years and adolescents (tablets only), and up to 12 weeks in children 1 to 11 years of age (capsules only).

***Helicobacter pylori* eradication (tablets only):** In combination with amoxicillin and clarithromycin as a 3-drug regimen for the treatment of adults with *H. pylori* infection and duodenal ulcer disease (active or history of within the past 5 years) to eradicate *H. pylori*.

Pathological hypersecretory conditions (tablets only): Long-term treatment of pathological hypersecretory conditions, including Zollinger-Ellison syndrome in adults.

Local Anesthetic/Vasoconstrictor Precautions No information available to require special precautions

Effects on Dental Treatment No significant effects or complications reported

Effects on Bleeding No information available to require special precautions

Adverse Reactions

>10%: Gastrointestinal: Diarrhea (children and adolescents: 5% to 21%; adults: <2%), abdominal pain (children: 16%; adolescents and adults: ≤4%), vomiting (children: 10% to 14%; adolescents: 4%)

1% to 10%:

Cardiovascular: Peripheral edema (adults: <2%)

Central nervous system: Headache (children and adolescents: 5% to 10% adults: <2%), pain (adults: 3%), dizziness (adults: <2%)

Gastrointestinal: Nausea (children and adolescents: 2% to 9%), flatulence (adults: 3%), constipation (adults: 2%), xerostomia (<2%)

Hepatic: Hepatic encephalopathy (adults: <2%), hepatitis (adults: <2%), increased liver enzymes (adults: <2%)

Infection: Infection (adults: 2%)

Neuromuscular & skeletal: Arthralgia (adults: <2%), myalgia (adults: <2%)

Respiratory: Pharyngitis (adults: 3%)

<1%, postmarketing, and/or case reports: Agranulocytosis, anaphylaxis, angioedema, blurred vision, bone fracture, bullous rash, *Clostridioides* (formerly *Clostridium*) *difficile*-associated diarrhea, coma, cutaneous lupus erythematous, delirium, disorientation, erythema multiforme, hemolytic anemia, hepatotoxicity (idiosyncratic) (Chalasani 2014), hyperammonemia, hypomagnesemia, increased thyroid stimulating hormone level, interstitial nephritis, jaundice, leukopenia, pancytopenia, pneumonia (interstitial), polyp (fundic gland), renal disease (chronic; Lazarus 2016), rhabdomyolysis, severe dermatological reaction, Stevens-Johnson syndrome, systemic lupus erythematosus, thrombocytopenia, toxic epidermal necrolysis, vertigo

Mechanism of Action Potent proton pump inhibitor; suppresses gastric acid secretion by inhibiting the parietal cell H+/K+ ATP pump

Pharmacodynamics/Kinetics

Onset of Action Within 1 hour

Duration of Action 24 hours

Half-life Elimination Dose dependent:

Children ≤11 years: 2.5 hours

Children ≥12 years and Adolescents: 20 mg tablet: 0.97 ± 0.19 hours (James 2007)

Adults: 1 to 2 hours

Time to Peak Plasma:

Children ≤11 years: Sprinkle capsule: 2 to 4 hours

Children ≥12 years and Adolescents: 20 mg tablet: 4.1 ± 0.45 hours (James 2007)

Adults: Tablet: 2 to 5 hours; Sprinkle capsule: 1 to 6.5 hours

Pregnancy Considerations Recommendations for the treatment of GERD in pregnancy are available. As in nonpregnant patients, lifestyle modifications followed by other medications are the initial treatments (Body 2016; Huerta-Iga 2016; Katz 2013; van der Woude 2014). Based on available data, PPIs may be used when clinically indicated (use of agents with more data in pregnancy may be preferred) (Body 2016; Matok 2012; Pasternak 2010; van der Woude 2014).

◆ **Rabeprazole Sodium** *see* RABEprazole *on page 1302*

Rabies Immune Globulin (Human)

(RAY beez i MYUN GLOB yoo lin, HYU man)

Brand Names: US HyperRAB; HyperRAB S/D; Imogam Rabies-HT; Kedrab

Brand Names: Canada HyperRAB; HyperRAB S/D; Imogam Rabies Pasteurized; Kamrab

Pharmacologic Category Blood Product Derivative; Immune Globulin

Use

Rabies, postexposure prophylaxis: Component of postexposure prophylaxis for patients with suspected rabies exposure. Provides passive immunity until active immunity with rabies vaccine is established. Not for use in patients with a history of complete vaccination (preexposure or postexposure prophylaxis) and documentation of antibody response, as these patients require only the vaccination. Each exposure to possible rabies infection should be individually evaluated.

Factors to consider include: species of biting animal, circumstances of biting incident (provoked vs unprovoked bite), type of exposure to rabies infection (bite vs nonbite), vaccination status of biting animal, presence of rabies in the region. See product information for additional details.

Local Anesthetic/Vasoconstrictor Precautions No information available to require special precautions

Effects on Dental Treatment No significant effects or complications reported

Effects on Bleeding No information available to require special precautions

Adverse Reactions

>10%:

Central nervous system: Headache (8% to 15%)

Local: Pain at injection site (31% to 33%)

1% to 10%:

Central nervous system: Fatigue (2% to 6%), dizziness (1% to 6%)

Dermatologic: Sunburn (≤3%)

Gastrointestinal: Diarrhea (8%), flatulence (8%), nausea (4%), abdominal pain (1% to 4%)

Genitourinary: Leukocyturia (3% to 5%), hematuria (2% to 4%)

Hematologic & oncologic: Bruise (1% to 3%)

Local: Injection site nodule (8%)

Neuromuscular & skeletal: Myalgia (7% to 9%), arthralgia (≤6%)

Respiratory: Upper respiratory tract infection (9% to 10%), nasal congestion (8%), oropharyngeal pain (8%)

Frequency not defined:

Central nervous system: Malaise

Dermatologic: Skin rash

Genitourinary: Nephrotic syndrome

Hypersensitivity: Anaphylaxis, angioedema

Local: Local soreness/soreness at injection site, tenderness at injection site

Neuromuscular & skeletal: Stiffness (at injection site)

Miscellaneous: Fever (mild)

<1%, postmarketing, and/or case reports: Hypersensitivity reaction, hypoesthesia, limb pain

Mechanism of Action Rabies immune globulin is a solution of globulins dried from the plasma or serum of selected adult human donors who have been immunized with rabies vaccine and have developed high titers of rabies antibody.

Pregnancy Risk Factor C

Pregnancy Considerations Animal reproduction studies have not been conducted. Pregnancy is not a contraindication to postexposure prophylaxis. Preexposure prophylaxis may be indicated during pregnancy if the risk for exposure to rabies is significant (CDC 2011).

Rabies Vaccine (RAY beez vak SEEN)

Brand Names: US Imovax Rabies; RabAvert

Brand Names: Canada Imovax Rabies

Pharmacologic Category Vaccine; Vaccine, Inactivated (Viral)

Use Rabies disease prevention: Preexposure and postexposure vaccination against rabies

Factors to consider include: species of biting animal, circumstances of biting incident (provoked vs unprovoked bite), type of exposure to rabies infection (bite vs nonbite), vaccination status of biting animal, and presence of rabies in the region. Refer to local/state health department and CDC for more information.

The Advisory Committee on Immunization Practices (ACIP) recommends a primary course of prophylactic immunization (preexposure vaccination) for the following (ACIP [Manning 2008]):

- Persons with continuous risk of infection, including rabies research laboratory and biologics production workers
- Persons with frequent risk of infection, including rabies diagnostic laboratory workers, cavers, veterinarians and their staff, and animal control and wildlife workers in areas where rabies is enzootic; persons who frequently handle bats
- Persons with infrequent risk of infection, including veterinarians and animal control staff working with terrestrial animals in areas where rabies infection is rare, veterinary students, and travelers visiting areas where rabies is enzootic and immediate access to medical care and biologicals is limited

The ACIP recommends the use of postexposure vaccination for a particular person be assessed by the severity and likelihood versus the actual risk of acquiring rabies. Consideration should include the type of exposure, epidemiology of rabies in the area, species of the animal, circumstances of the incident, and the availability of the exposing animal for observation or rabies testing. Postexposure vaccination is used in both previously vaccinated and previously unvaccinated individuals (ACIP [Manning 2008]; ACIP [Rupprecht 2010]).

Local Anesthetic/Vasoconstrictor Precautions No information available to require special precautions

Effects on Dental Treatment No significant effects or complications reported

Effects on Bleeding No information available to require special precautions

Adverse Reactions

>10%:

Central nervous system: Dizziness, headache, malaise

Dermatologic: Injection site pruritus

Gastrointestinal: Abdominal pain, nausea

Hematologic & oncologic: Lymphadenopathy

Local: Erythema at injection site, pain at injection site, swelling at injection site

Neuromuscular & skeletal: Myalgia

Frequency not defined:

Cardiovascular: Cardiovascular toxicity, edema, palpitations, swelling of injected limb (extensive)

Central nervous system: Chills, encephalitis, fatigue, Guillain-Barre syndrome, meningitis, neuropathy, paralysis (may be transient; includes neuroparalysis), paresthesia (transient), retrobulbar neuritis, seizure, vertigo

Dermatologic: Pruritus, urticaria (including urticaria pigmentosa)

Endocrine & metabolic: Hot flash

Gastrointestinal: Diarrhea, vomiting

Hematologic & oncologic: Adenopathy

Hypersensitivity: Anaphylaxis, hypersensitivity reaction, serum sickness

Local: Hematoma at injection site

Neuromuscular & skeletal: Arthralgia, arthritis (one joint), limb pain, multiple sclerosis, myelitis, weakness

Ophthalmic: Visual disturbance

Respiratory: Bronchospasm, dyspnea, wheezing

Miscellaneous: Fever >38°C (100°F)

Mechanism of Action Rabies vaccine is an inactivated virus vaccine which promotes immunity by inducing an active immune response. The production of specific antibodies requires about 7-10 days to develop. Rabies immune globulin or antirabies serum, equine (ARS) is given in conjunction with rabies vaccine to provide immune protection until an antibody response can occur.

Pharmacodynamics/Kinetics

Onset of Action IM: Rabies antibody: ~7 to 10 days; Peak effect: ~30 to 60 days

Duration of Action ≥1 year

Pregnancy Considerations Animal reproduction studies have not been conducted. Pregnancy is not a contraindication to postexposure prophylaxis. Pre-exposure prophylaxis during pregnancy may also be considered if risk of rabies is great. Inactivated vaccines have not been shown to cause increased risks to the fetus (ACIP [Ezeanolue 2020]).

- ◆ **Racemic Amphetamine Sulfate** *see* Amphetamine *on page 135*
- ◆ **Racemic Epinephrine** *see* EPINEPHrine (Oral Inhalation) *on page 573*
- ◆ **Racepinephrine** *see* EPINEPHrine (Oral Inhalation) *on page 573*
- ◆ **Racepinephrine HCL** *see* EPINEPHrine (Oral Inhalation) *on page 573*
- ◆ **RAD001** *see* Everolimus *on page 628*
- ◆ **Radicava** *see* Edaravone *on page 542*
- ◆ **rAHF** *see* Antihemophilic Factor (Recombinant) *on page 153*
- ◆ **rAHF (Fc Fusion Protein)** *see* Antihemophilic Factor (Recombinant [Fc Fusion Protein]) *on page 154*
- ◆ **Rajani [DSC]** *see* Ethinyl Estradiol, Drospirenone, and Levomefolate *on page 618*
- ◆ **RAL** *see* Raltegravir *on page 1306*
- ◆ **R-albuterol** *see* Levalbuterol *on page 892*

Raloxifene (ral OKS i feen)

Related Information

Endocrine Disorders and Pregnancy *on page 1684*

Rheumatoid Arthritis, Osteoarthritis, and Osteoporosis *on page 1697*

Brand Names: US Evista

Brand Names: Canada ACT Raloxifene; APO-Raloxifene; Evista; PMS-Raloxifene [DSC]; TEVA-Raloxifene [DSC]

Generic Availability (US) Yes

Pharmacologic Category Selective Estrogen Receptor Modulator (SERM)

Use

Osteoporosis: Treatment and prevention of osteoporosis in postmenopausal females.

Risk reduction for invasive breast cancer: Risk reduction of invasive breast cancer in postmenopausal females with osteoporosis; risk reduction of invasive breast cancer in postmenopausal females with high risk for invasive breast cancer (high risk is defined as at least 1 breast biopsy showing lobular carcinoma in situ or atypical hyperplasia, one or more first-degree relatives with breast cancer, or a 5-year predicted risk of breast cancer 1.66% or more [based on the modified Gail model]; factors included in the modified Gail model include current age, number of first-degree relatives with breast cancer, number of breast biopsies, age at menarche, nulliparity, or age of first live birth).

Limitations of use: Raloxifene does not eliminate the risk of breast cancer; patients should have a breast exam and mammogram prior to initiating raloxifene and continue regular breast exams and mammograms as per current guideline recommendations. Raloxifene is not indicated for the treatment of invasive breast cancer or reduction of the risk of recurrence. Raloxifene is not indicated for the reduction of the risk of noninvasive breast cancer. There are no data available regarding the effect of raloxifene on invasive breast cancer incidence in females with inherited mutations BRCA1, BRCA2 to be able to make specific recommendations on the effectiveness of raloxifene.

Local Anesthetic/Vasoconstrictor Precautions No information available to require special precautions

Effects on Dental Treatment No significant effects or complications reported

Effects on Bleeding Has been associated with thromboembolic adverse events. No information available to require routine special precautions for dental procedures.

Adverse Reactions

>10%:

Cardiovascular: Peripheral edema (3% to 14%)

Endocrine & metabolic: Hot flash (8% to 29%)

Infection: Infection (11%)

Neuromuscular & skeletal: Arthralgia (11% to 16%), leg cramps (≤12%), muscle spasm (≤12%)

Respiratory: Flu-like symptoms (14% to 15%)

1% to 10%:

Cardiovascular: Chest pain (3%), syncope (<2%), venous thromboembolism (1% to 2%; includes deep vein thrombosis, pulmonary embolism, retinal vein thrombosis)

Central nervous system: Insomnia (6%), hypoesthesia (<2%), neuralgia (<2%)

Dermatologic: Skin rash (6%), diaphoresis (3%)

Endocrine & metabolic: Weight gain (9%)

Gastrointestinal: Abdominal pain (7%), vomiting (5%), gastrointestinal disease (3%), flatulence (2% to 3%), gastroenteritis (≤3%)

Genitourinary: Vaginal hemorrhage (3% to 6%), mastalgia (4%), leukorrhea (3%), urinary tract abnormality (3%), uterine disease (3%), endometrium disease (≤3%)

Neuromuscular & skeletal: Myalgia (8%), tendon disease (4%)

Respiratory: Bronchitis (10%), sinusitis (10%), pharyngitis (8%), pneumonia (3%), laryngitis (≤2%)

<1%, postmarketing, and/or case reports: Cerebrovascular accident, decreased LDL cholesterol (Delmas 1997; Walsh 1998), decreased serum cholesterol (Delmas 1997; Walsh 1998), decreased serum fibrinogen (Walsh 1998), hypertriglyceridemia (in women with a history of increased triglycerides in response to oral estrogens), retinal vein occlusion, superficial thrombophlebitis

Dosing

Adult & Geriatric Note: Patients with osteoporosis should receive supplemental calcium and vitamin D if dietary intake is inadequate.

Osteoporosis (postmenopausal females):

Treatment (alternative agent) and prevention: **Note:** May be considered as an alternative treatment option to reduce the risk of vertebral fractures in patients for whom bisphosphonates and denosumab are unsuitable, or in patients with a high risk of fracture and a high risk of invasive breast cancer, if they also have a low risk of deep vein thrombosis (AACE [Camacho 2016]; ES [Eastell 2019]).

Oral: 60 mg once daily.

Duration of therapy: Continued raloxifene therapy is necessary to maintain increases in bone mineral density (BMD). In 1 study, BMD increases were maintained during 7 years of therapy in postmenopausal females with osteoporosis (Siris 2005). Effects on BMD diminish relatively quickly (eg, within 1 to 2 years) when raloxifene is discontinued (AACE [Camacho 2016]; Siris 2005).

Risk reduction for invasive breast cancer in postmenopausal females: Oral: 60 mg once daily.

Duration of therapy for breast cancer risk reduction: 5 years; may be used longer than 5 years in females with osteoporosis where breast cancer risk reduction is a secondary benefit (Visvanathan 2013).

Renal Impairment: Adult CrCl ≤50 mL/minute: There are no dosage adjustments provided in the manufacturer's labeling; use with caution.

Hepatic Impairment: Adult There are no dosage adjustments provided in the manufacturer's labeling (has not been studied); use with caution.

Mechanism of Action Raloxifene is an estrogen agonist/antagonist (a selective estrogen receptor modulator [SERM]); selective binding activates estrogenic pathways in some tissues and antagonizes estrogenic pathways in other tissues. Raloxifene acts like an estrogen agonist in the bone to prevent bone loss and has estrogen antagonist activity to block some estrogen effects in the breast and uterine tissues. Raloxifene decreases bone resorption, increasing bone mineral density and decreasing fracture incidence.

Contraindications History of or current venous thromboembolic disorders (including DVT, PE, and retinal vein thrombosis); pregnancy

Warnings/Precautions [US Boxed Warning]: Raloxifene may increase the risk for deep vein thrombosis (DVT) and pulmonary embolism (PE); use is contraindicated in patients with history of or current venous thromboembolic disorders (including DVT, PE, or retinal vein thrombosis). Consider risks versus benefits in females at risk for thromboembolism (HF, superficial thrombophlebitis, active malignancy). The risk for DVT and PE are higher during the first 4 months of treatment. Superficial thrombophlebitis has also been reported. Discontinue raloxifene at least 72 hours prior to and during prolonged immobilization (postoperative recovery or prolonged bed rest); restart only once patient fully ambulatory. Advise patients to move periodically during prolonged travel.

[US Boxed Warning]: The risk of death due to stroke is increased in postmenopausal females with coronary heart disease or at increased risk for major coronary events; consider risks versus benefits in females at risk for stroke. Do not use for primary or secondary prevention of cardiovascular disease. Assess risks versus benefits in females at risk for stroke (eg, prior stroke, transient ischemic attack, atrial fibrillation, hypertension, smokers). Females with a history of marked elevated triglycerides (>5.6 mmol/L or >500 mg/dL) in response to treatment with oral estrogens (or estrogen/progestin) may also develop elevated triglycerides when treated with raloxifene; monitor triglycerides.

The use of raloxifene has not been adequately studied in females with a prior history of breast cancer. Safety has not been established in premenopausal females; use is not indicated and not recommended. Raloxifene does not eliminate the risk of breast cancer; investigate unexplained breast abnormality that occurs during treatment. Raloxifene is not indicated for treatment of invasive breast cancer, to reduce the risk of recurrence of invasive breast cancer, or to reduce the risk of noninvasive breast cancer. The efficacy (for breast cancer risk reduction) in females with inherited BRCA1 and BRCA1 mutations has not been established. The American Society of Clinical Oncology (ASCO) guidelines for breast cancer risk reduction (Visvanathan 2013) recommend raloxifene (for 5 years) as an option to reduce the risk of ER-positive invasive breast cancer in postmenopausal females with a 5-year projected risk (based on NCI trial model) of ≥1.66%, or with lobular carcinoma in situ. Raloxifene should not be used in premenopausal females. Females with osteoporosis may use raloxifene beyond 5 years of treatment. Investigate unexplained uterine bleeding.

Use with caution in patients with hepatic or renal impairment; safety and efficacy have not been established. Safety and efficacy have not been established in men; raloxifene is not indicated for use in men. Potentially significant drug-drug interactions may exist, requiring dose or frequency adjustment, additional monitoring, and/or selection of alternative therapy. Concurrent use with systemic estrogen therapy is not recommended; safety has not been established.

Drug Interactions

Metabolism/Transport Effects None known.

Avoid Concomitant Use

Avoid concomitant use of Raloxifene with any of the following: Ospemifene

Increased Effect/Toxicity

Raloxifene may increase the levels/effects of: Ospemifene

Decreased Effect

Raloxifene may decrease the levels/effects of: Fluoroestradiol F18; Levothyroxine; Ospemifene

The levels/effects of Raloxifene may be decreased by: Bile Acid Sequestrants

Dietary Considerations Osteoporosis prevention or treatment: Ensure adequate calcium and vitamin D intake; if dietary intake is inadequate, dietary supplementation is recommended. Females and males should consume:

Calcium: 1,000 mg/day (males: 50 to 70 years) **or** 1,200 mg/day (females ≥51 years and males ≥71 years) (IOM 2011; NOF [Cosman 2014]).

Vitamin D: 800 to 1,000 int. units daily (males and females ≥50 years) (NOF [Cosman 2014]). Recommended Dietary Allowance (RDA): 600 int. units daily (males and females ≤70 years) **or** 800 int. units daily (males and females ≥71 years) (IOM 2011).

Pharmacodynamics/Kinetics

Half-life Elimination 27.7 hours (following a single dose); 32.5 hours (following multiple doses)

Reproductive Considerations Raloxifene is not indicated for use in females of reproductive potential.

Pregnancy Considerations Raloxifene is contraindicated during pregnancy.

Breastfeeding Considerations It is not known if raloxifene is present in breast milk.

Raloxifene is not indicated for use in females of reproductive potential.

Dosage Forms: US

Tablet, Oral:

Evista: 60 mg

Generic: 60 mg

Dosage Forms: Canada

Tablet, Oral:

Evista: 60 mg

Generic: 60 mg

◆ **Raloxifene HCl** *see* Raloxifene *on page 1304*

◆ **Raloxifene Hydrochloride** *see* Raloxifene *on page 1304*

Raltegravir (ral TEG ra vir)

Related Information

HIV Infection and AIDS *on page 1690*

Brand Names: US Isentress; Isentress HD

Brand Names: Canada Isentress; Isentress HD

Pharmacologic Category Antiretroviral, Integrase Inhibitor (Anti-HIV)

Use HIV-1 infection, treatment: Treatment of HIV-1 infection in combination with other antiretroviral agents

Local Anesthetic/Vasoconstrictor Precautions No information available to require special precautions

Effects on Dental Treatment No significant effects or complications reported

Effects on Bleeding No information available to require special precautions related to hemostasis.

Adverse Reactions

>10%: Hepatic: Increased serum ALT (1% to 11%; incidence higher with hepatitis B and/or C coinfection)

1% to 10%:

Central nervous system: Headache (≤4%), insomnia (≤4%), abnormal dreams (≥2%), nightmares (≥2%), dizziness (≤2%), fatigue (≤2%), depression (<2%; particularly in subjects with a preexisting history of psychiatric illness), suicidal ideation (<2%), suicidal tendencies (<2%), psychomotor agitation (children and adolescents), abnormal behavior (children and adolescents)

Dermatologic: Allergic rash (children and adolescents: 1%)

Endocrine & metabolic: Increased serum glucose (126 to 250 mg/dL: 7% to 10%; 251 to 500 mg/dL: 2% to 3%)

Gastrointestinal: Increased serum lipase (≤5%), increased serum amylase (≤4%), nausea (≤3%), decreased appetite (≥2%), diarrhea (≥2%), flatulence (≥2%), abdominal pain (<2%), dyspepsia (<2%), gastritis (<2%), vomiting (<2%)

Genitourinary: Herpes genitalis (<2%)

Hematologic & oncologic: Decrease in absolute neutrophil count (1% to 4%), thrombocytopenia (≤3%), decreased hemoglobin (≤1%)

Hepatic: Increased serum AST (≤9%; incidence higher with hepatitis B and/or C coinfection), hyperbilirubinemia (≤6%; incidence slightly higher with hepatitis B and/or C coinfection), increased serum alkaline phosphatase (≤2%), hepatitis (<2%)

Hypersensitivity: Hypersensitivity reaction (<2%)

Infection: Herpes zoster (<2%)

Neuromuscular & skeletal: Increased creatine phosphokinase (1% to 4%), weakness (<2%)

Renal: Nephrolithiasis (<2%), renal failure (<2%), increased serum creatinine (≤1%)

Frequency not defined:

Hematologic & oncologic: Malignant neoplasm

Neuromuscular & skeletal: Myopathy, rhabdomyolysis

<1%, postmarketing, and/or case reports: Anxiety, cerebellar ataxia, DRESS syndrome (Perry 2013), hepatic failure, immune reconstitution syndrome, paranoia, skin rash, Stevens-Johnson syndrome, toxic epidermal necrolysis

Mechanism of Action Incorporation of viral DNA into the host cell's genome is required to produce a self-replicating provirus and propagation of infectious virion particles. The viral cDNA strand produced by reverse transcriptase is subsequently processed and inserted into the human genome by the enzyme HIV-1 integrase (encoded by the pol gene of HIV). Raltegravir inhibits the catalytic activity of integrase, thus preventing integration of the proviral gene into human DNA.

Pharmacodynamics/Kinetics

Half-life Elimination ~9 hours

Time to Peak Film-coated tablet (400 mg formulation): ~3 hours; film-coated tablet (600 mg formulation): ~1.5 to 2 hours

Reproductive Considerations

The Health and Human Services (HHS) Perinatal HIV Guidelines consider raltegravir a preferred integrase strand transfer inhibitor for females living with HIV who are not yet pregnant but are trying to conceive.

For males and females living with HIV and planning a pregnancy, maximum viral suppression below the limits of detection with antiretroviral therapy (ART), modification of therapy (if needed), optimization of the woman's health, and a discussion of the potential risks and benefits of ART therapy during pregnancy is recommended prior to conception (HHS [perinatal] 2019).

Pregnancy Considerations

Raltegravir has high transfer across the human placenta.

No increased risk of overall birth defects has been observed following first trimester exposure according to data collected by the antiretroviral pregnancy registry. Maternal antiretroviral therapy (ART) may be associated with adverse pregnancy outcomes including preterm delivery, stillbirth, low birth weight, and small for gestational age infants. Actual risks may be influenced by maternal factors such as disease severity, gestational age at initiation of therapy, and specific ART regimen; therefore, close fetal monitoring is recommended. Because there is clear benefit to appropriate treatment, maternal ART should not be withheld due to concerns for adverse neonatal outcomes. Long-term follow-up is recommended for all infants exposed to antiretroviral medications; children without HIV but who were exposed to ART in utero and develop significant organ system abnormalities of unknown etiology (particularly of the CNS or heart) should be evaluated for potential mitochondrial dysfunction.

The Health and Human Services (HHS) Perinatal HIV Guidelines consider raltegravir a preferred integrase strand transfer inhibitor (INSTI) for pregnant females living with HIV who are antiretroviral-naive, who have had ART therapy in the past but are restarting, or who require a new ART regimen (due to poor tolerance or poor virologic response of current regimen). In addition, females who become pregnant while taking raltegravir may continue if viral suppression is effective and the regimen is well tolerated. Raltegravir is an alternative component of a regimen when acute HIV infection is detected during pregnancy. INSTIs can rapidly suppress viral load. A regimen with raltegravir may be useful when drug interactions or the potential for preterm delivery with protease inhibitors are a concern. In addition, use of raltegravir, may be beneficial in women with HIV who are not on ART and present for care late in pregnancy, as a fourth drug in women with high viral loads, or as part of a new regimen for a woman experiencing virologic failure on ART.

The pharmacokinetics of raltegravir are variable. Dose adjustments are not required in pregnant patients; however, once daily dosing is not recommended until more data in pregnancy are available.

In general, ART is recommended for all pregnant females living with HIV to keep the viral load below the limit of detection and reduce the risk of perinatal transmission. Therapy should be individualized following a discussion of the potential risks and benefits of treatment during pregnancy. Monitoring of pregnant females is more frequent than in nonpregnant adults. ART should be continued postpartum for all females living with HIV and can be modified after delivery.

Health care providers are encouraged to enroll pregnant females exposed to antiretroviral medications as early in pregnancy as possible in the Antiretroviral Pregnancy Registry (1-800-258-4263 or http://www.-APRegistry.com). Health care providers caring for females living with HIV and their infants may contact the National Perinatal HIV Hotline (1-888-448-8765) for clinical consultation (HHS [perinatal] 2019).

◆ **Raltegravir Potassium** *see* Raltegravir *on page 1306*

Ramelteon (ra MEL tee on)

Brand Names: US Rozerem

Pharmacologic Category Hypnotic, Miscellaneous; Melatonin Receptor Agonist

Use Insomnia: Treatment of insomnia characterized by difficulty with sleep onset

Local Anesthetic/Vasoconstrictor Precautions No information available to require special precautions

Effects on Dental Treatment Key adverse event(s) related to dental treatment: Taste perversion.

Effects on Bleeding No information available to require special precautions

Adverse Reactions

1% to 10%:

Central nervous system: Dizziness (4% to 5%), somnolence (3% to 5%), fatigue (3% to 4%), insomnia worsened (3%), depression (2%)

Endocrine & metabolic: Serum cortisol decreased (1%)

Gastrointestinal: Nausea (3%), taste perversion (2%)

Neuromuscular & skeletal: Myalgia (2%), arthralgia (2%)

Respiratory: Upper respiratory infection (3%)

Miscellaneous: Influenza (1%)

Postmarketing and/or case reports: Anaphylaxis, angioedema, complex sleep-related behavior (sleep-driving, cooking or eating food, making phone calls), prolactin levels increased, testosterone levels decreased

Mechanism of Action Potent, selective agonist of melatonin receptors MT_1 and MT_2 (with little affinity for MT_3) within the suprachiasmic nucleus of the hypothalamus, an area responsible for determination of circadian rhythms and synchronization of the sleep-wake cycle. Agonism of MT_1 is thought to preferentially induce sleepiness, while MT_2 receptor activation preferentially influences regulation of circadian rhythms. Ramelteon is eightfold more selective for MT_1 than MT_2 and exhibits nearly sixfold higher affinity for MT_1 than melatonin, presumably allowing for enhanced effects on sleep induction (Hatta 2014).

Pharmacodynamics/Kinetics

Onset of Action 30 minutes

Half-life Elimination Ramelteon: 1 to 2.6 hours; M-II: 2 to 5 hours

Time to Peak Median: 0.5 to 1.5 hours

Reproductive Considerations

May cause disturbances of reproductive hormonal regulation (eg, disruption of menses or decreased libido).

Pregnancy Considerations

Adverse events were observed in some animal reproduction studies.

Ramipril (RA mi pril)

Related Information

Cardiovascular Diseases *on page 1654*

Brand Names: US Altace

Brand Names: Canada ACT Ramipril [DSC]; AG-Ramipril; Altace; APO-Ramipril; Auro-Ramipril; DOM-Ramipril; JAMP-Ramipril; Mar-Ramipril; MINT-Ramipril; MYLAN-Ramipril [DSC]; NRA-Ramipril; Pharma-Ramipril; PMS-Ramipril; PRIVA-Ramipril; PRO-Ramipril-1.25; PRO-Ramipril-10; PRO-Ramipril-2.5; PRO-Ramipril-5; Ramace [DSC]; RAN-Ramipril; SANDOZ Ramipril; TARO-Ramipril; TEVA-Ramipril; VAN-Ramipril [DSC]

Pharmacologic Category Angiotensin-Converting Enzyme (ACE) Inhibitor; Antihypertensive

Use

Heart failure post-myocardial infarction: Treatment of heart failure (HF) after myocardial infarction (MI)

Guideline recommendations: The American College of Cardiology/American Heart Association (ACC/AHA) 2013 Heart Failure Guidelines recommend the use of ACE inhibitors, along with other guideline-directed medical therapies, to prevent progression of HF and reduced ejection fraction in asymptomatic patients with or without a history of myocardial infarction (Stage B HF), or to treat those with symptomatic HF and reduced ejection fraction to reduce morbidity and mortality (Stage C HFrEF).

Hypertension: Management of hypertension

Guideline recommendations: The 2017 Guideline for the Prevention, Detection, Evaluation, and Management of High Blood Pressure in Adults recommends if monotherapy is warranted, in the absence of comorbidities (eg, cerebrovascular disease, chronic kidney disease, diabetes, HF, ischemic heart disease, etc.), that thiazide-like diuretics or dihydropyridine calcium channel blockers may be preferred options due to improved cardiovascular endpoints (eg, prevention of HF and stroke). ACE inhibitors and ARBs are also acceptable for monotherapy. Combination therapy may be required to achieve blood pressure goals and is initially preferred in patients at high risk (stage 2 hypertension or atherosclerotic cardiovascular disease [ASCVD] risk ≥10%) (ACC/AHA [Whelton 2017]).

Reduction in risk of MI, stroke, and death from cardiovascular causes: To reduce the risk of MI, stroke, and death in patients ≥55 years of age at high risk of developing major cardiovascular events.

Local Anesthetic/Vasoconstrictor Precautions

No information available to require special precautions

Effects on Dental Treatment Key adverse event(s) related to dental treatment: Patients may experience orthostatic hypotension as they stand up after treatment; especially if lying in dental chair for extended periods of time. Use caution with sudden changes in position during and after dental treatment.

An angiotensin-converting enzyme (ACE) Inhibitor cough is a dry, hacking, nonproductive cough that can potentially interfere with longer dental procedures if patient has this side effect.

Effects on Bleeding No information available to require special precautions

Adverse Reactions Frequency ranges include data from hypertension and heart failure trials. Higher rates of adverse reactions have generally been noted in patients with cardiac failure. However, the frequency of adverse effects associated with placebo is also increased in this population.

>10%:

Cardiovascular: Hypotension (11%)

Respiratory: Increased cough (7% to 12%)

1% to 10%:

Cardiovascular: Angina pectoris (≤3%), orthostatic hypotension (2%), syncope (≤2%)

Central nervous system: Headache (1% to 5%), dizziness (2% to 4%), fatigue (2%), vertigo (≤2%), noncardiac chest pain (1%)

Endocrine & metabolic: Hyperkalemia (1% to 10%)

Gastrointestinal: Nausea (≤2%), vomiting (≤2%)

Renal: Increased blood urea nitrogen (≤3%; transient increases may occur more frequently), increased serum creatinine (1% to 2%; transient increases may occur more frequently), renal insufficiency (1%)

Respiratory: Cough (1% to 10%)

<1%, postmarketing, and/or case reports: Abdominal pain, agitation, agranulocytosis, amnesia, anaphylactoid reaction, angioedema, anorexia, anxiety, arthralgia, arthritis, auditory impairment, bone marrow depression, cardiac arrhythmia, cerebrovascular disease, constipation, decreased hematocrit, decreased hemoglobin, depression, diaphoresis, diarrhea, drowsiness, dysgeusia, dyspepsia, dysphagia, dyspnea, edema, eosinophilia, epistaxis, erythema multiforme, gastroenteritis, hemolytic anemia, hepatitis, hypersensitivity reaction (fever, skin rash, urticaria), hyponatremia, impotence, increased serum transaminases, insomnia, malaise, myalgia, myocardial infarction, nervousness, neuralgia, neuropathy, onycholysis, palpitations, pancreatitis, pancytopenia, paresthesia, pemphigoid, pemphigus, proteinuria, purpura, seizure, sialorrhea, skin photosensitivity, Stevens-Johnson syndrome, symptomatic hypotension, thrombocytopenia, tinnitus, toxic epidermal necrolysis, tremor, visual disturbance, visual hallucination (Doane 2013), weight gain, xerostomia

Mechanism of Action Ramipril is an ACE inhibitor which prevents the formation of angiotensin II from angiotensin I and exhibits pharmacologic effects that are similar to captopril. Ramipril must undergo enzymatic saponification by esterases in the liver to its biologically active metabolite, ramiprilat. The pharmacodynamic effects of ramipril result from the high-affinity, competitive, reversible binding of ramiprilat to angiotensin-converting enzyme, thus preventing the formation of the potent vasoconstrictor angiotensin II. This isomerized enzyme-inhibitor complex has a slow rate of dissociation, which results in high potency and a long duration of action; a CNS mechanism may also be involved in the hypotensive effect as angiotensin II increases adrenergic outflow from CNS; vasoactive kallikreins may be decreased in conversion to active hormones by ACE inhibitors, thus reducing blood pressure

Pharmacodynamics/Kinetics

Onset of Action 1-2 hours

Duration of Action 24 hours

Half-life Elimination Ramiprilat: Effective: 13-17 hours; Terminal: >50 hours

Time to Peak Serum: Ramipril: ~1 hour; Ramiprilat: 2-4 hours

Reproductive Considerations

Angiotensin-converting enzyme (ACE) inhibitors should be avoided in sexually active females of reproductive potential not using effective contraception (ADA 2020).

ACE inhibitors should generally be avoided for the treatment of hypertension in women planning a pregnancy; use should only be considered for cases of hypertension refractory to other medications (ACOG 203 2019).

Pregnancy Considerations Ramipril crosses the placenta.

Exposure to an angiotensin-converting enzyme (ACE) inhibitor during the first trimester of pregnancy may be associated with an increased risk of fetal malformations (ACOG 203 2019; ESC [Regitz-Zagrosek 2018]); however, outcomes observed may also be influenced by maternal disease (ACC/AHA [Whelton 2017]).

[US Boxed Warning]: Drugs that act on the renin-angiotensin system can cause injury and death to the developing fetus. Discontinue as soon as possible once pregnancy is detected. Drugs that act on the renin-angiotensin system are associated with oligohydramnios. Oligohydramnios, due to decreased fetal renal function, may lead to fetal lung hypoplasia and skeletal malformations. The use of these drugs in pregnancy is also associated with anuria, hypotension, renal failure, skull hypoplasia, and death in the fetus/neonate. Infants exposed to an ACE inhibitor in utero should be monitored for hyperkalemia, hypotension, and oliguria. Oligohydramnios may not appear until after irreversible fetal injury has occurred. Exchange transfusions or dialysis may be required to reverse hypotension or improve renal function, although data related to the effectiveness in neonates is limited.

Chronic maternal hypertension is also associated with adverse events in the fetus/infant. Chronic maternal hypertension may increase the risk of birth defects, low birth weight, premature delivery, stillbirth, and neonatal death. Actual fetal/neonatal risks may be related to duration and severity of maternal hypertension. Untreated chronic hypertension may also increase the risks of adverse maternal outcomes, including gestational diabetes, preeclampsia, delivery complications, stroke, and myocardial infarction (ACOG 203 2019).

When treatment of hypertension in pregnancy is indicated, ACE inhibitors should generally be avoided due to their adverse fetal events; use in pregnant women should only be considered for cases of hypertension refractory to other medications (ACOG 203 2019). ACE inhibitors are not recommended for the treatment heart failure in pregnancy (Regitz-Zagrosek [ESC 2018]).

Ramucirumab (ra mue SIR ue mab)

Brand Names: US Cyramza

Brand Names: Canada Cyramza

Pharmacologic Category Antineoplastic Agent, Monoclonal Antibody; Antineoplastic Agent, Vascular Endothelial Growth Factor (VEGF) Inhibitor; Antineoplastic Agent, Vascular Endothelial Growth Factor Receptor 2 (VEGFR2) Inhibitor

Use

Colorectal cancer, metastatic: Treatment (in combination with FOLFIRI [irinotecan, leucovorin, and fluorouracil]) of metastatic colorectal cancer in patients with disease progression on or after prior therapy with bevacizumab, oxaliplatin, and a fluoropyrimidine.

Gastric cancer, advanced or metastatic: Treatment (single agent or in combination with paclitaxel) of advanced or metastatic gastric or gastroesophageal junction adenocarcinoma in patients with disease progression on or following fluoropyrimidine- or platinum-containing chemotherapy.

Hepatocellular carcinoma, advanced or relapsed/refractory: Treatment (as a single agent) of hepatocellular carcinoma in patients who have an alpha fetoprotein of ≥400 ng/mL and have been treated with sorafenib.

Non-small cell lung cancer, metastatic:

First-line treatment (in combination with erlotinib) of metastatic non-small cell lung cancer in patients whose tumors have epidermal growth factor receptor (EGFR) exon 19 deletions or exon 21 (L858R) substitution mutations.

Treatment (in combination with docetaxel) of metastatic non-small cell lung cancer in patients with disease progression on or after platinum-based chemotherapy. Patients with epidermal growth factor receptor or anaplastic lymphoma kinase genomic tumor aberrations should have disease progression on approved therapy for these aberrations prior to receiving ramucirumab.

Local Anesthetic/Vasoconstrictor Precautions No information available to require special precautions

Effects on Dental Treatment Key adverse event(s) related to dental treatment: Ramucirumab impairs wound healing; medical consultation advised prior to dental surgery.

Effects on Bleeding Ramucirumab associated with an increased risk of hemorrhage, which may be severe and sometimes fatal.

Adverse Reactions As reported with monotherapy.

>10%:

Cardiovascular: Hypertension (16% to 25%, severe hypertension: 6% to 15%), peripheral edema (25%)

Endocrine & metabolic: Hypoalbuminemia (33%), hypocalcemia (16%), hyponatremia (6% to 32%)

Gastrointestinal: Abdominal pain (25%), decreased appetite (23%), diarrhea (14%), nausea (19%)

Genitourinary: Proteinuria (3% to 20%)

Hematologic & oncologic: Neutropenia (5% to 24%; grade ≥3: 8%), thrombocytopenia (46%; grade ≥3: 8%)

Hepatic: Ascites (3% to 18%)

Nervous system: Fatigue (36%), headache (9% to 14%), insomnia (11%)

Respiratory: Epistaxis (5% to 14%)

1% to 10%:

Cardiovascular: Arterial thromboembolism (2%)

Dermatologic: Skin rash (4%)

Gastrointestinal: Intestinal obstruction (2%), vomiting (10%)

Hematologic & oncologic: Anemia (4%)

Hepatic: Hepatic encephalopathy (5% to 6%), hepatorenal syndrome (2% to 6%)

Immunologic: Antibody development (3%; neutralizing: <1%)

Neuromuscular & skeletal: Back pain (10%)

Respiratory: Pneumonia (3%)

Miscellaneous: Fever (10%), infusion related reaction (≤9%; reactions minimized with premedications)

<1%: Gastrointestinal: Gastrointestinal perforation

Frequency not defined:

Cardiovascular: Acute myocardial infarction, cerebral ischemia, cerebrovascular accident

Endocrine & metabolic: Hypothyroidism

Gastrointestinal: Gastrointestinal hemorrhage

Genitourinary: Nephrotic syndrome

Hematologic & oncologic: Major hemorrhage

Nervous system: Reversible posterior leukoencephalopathy syndrome

Postmarketing:

Hematologic & oncologic: Hemangioma, thrombotic microangiopathy

Nervous system: Voice disorder

Mechanism of Action Ramucirumab is a recombinant monoclonal antibody which inhibits vascular endothelial growth factor receptor 2 (VEGFR2). Ramucirumab has a high affinity for VEGFR2 (Spratlin 2010), binding to it and blocking binding of VEGFR ligands, VEGF-A, VEGF-C, and VEGF-D to inhibit activation of VEGFR2, thereby inhibiting ligand-induced proliferation and migration of endothelial cells. VEGFR2 inhibition results in reduced tumor vascularity and growth (Fuchs 2014).

Pharmacodynamics/Kinetics

Half-life Elimination 14 days

Reproductive Considerations

Verify pregnancy status prior to treatment initiation in females of reproductive potential. Females of reproductive potential should use effective contraception during and for 3 months after the last ramucirumab dose.

Pregnancy Considerations

Based on the mechanism of action, ramucirumab may cause fetal harm if administered during pregnancy.

◆ **Ramucirumab** *see* Ramucirumab *on page 1308*

◆ **Ranexa** *see* Ranolazine *on page 1310*

Ranibizumab (ra nib i ZUE mab)

Brand Names: US Lucentis

Brand Names: Canada Lucentis

Pharmacologic Category Angiogenesis Inhibitor; Monoclonal Antibody; Ophthalmic Agent; Vascular Endothelial Growth Factor (VEGF) Inhibitor

Use

Diabetic macular edema: Treatment of diabetic macular edema (DME).

Diabetic retinopathy: Treatment of diabetic retinopathy

Macular degeneration: Treatment of neovascular (wet) age-related macular degeneration (AMD)

Macular edema: Treatment of macular edema following retinal vein occlusion (RVO)

Myopic choroidal neovascularization: Treatment of myopic choroidal neovascularization (mCNV).

Local Anesthetic/Vasoconstrictor Precautions No information available to require special precautions

Effects on Dental Treatment No significant effects or complications reported

Effects on Bleeding No information available to require special precautions in dental procedures.

Adverse Reactions As reported with AMD, RVO, and DME studies:

>10%:

Cardiovascular: Arterial thromboembolism (AMD trials during first year: 2%; DME trials at 3 years: 11%)

Central nervous system: Foreign body sensation of eye (7% to 16%), headache (6% to 12%)

Hematologic & oncologic: Anemia (4% to 11%)

Neuromuscular & skeletal: Arthralgia (2% to 11%)

Ophthalmic: Conjunctival hemorrhage (47% to 74%), eye pain (17% to 35%), vitreous opacity (7% to 27%), increased intraocular pressure (7% to 24%), blurred vision (5% to 18%), intraocular inflammation (1% to 18%)

Note: Cataract, blepharitis, dry eye syndrome, eye irritation, increased lacrimation, maculopathy, ocular hyperemia, eye pruritus, and vitreous detachment occurred in >10% of patients, but also occurred either in similar percentages to the control or more often in the control in some studies.

Respiratory: Nasopharyngitis (5% to 16%), bronchitis (6% to 11%)

1% to 10%:

Cardiovascular: Peripheral edema (6%), atrial fibrillation (1% to 5%), cerebrovascular accident (AMD trials during 2 years: 3%; DME trials at 3 years: 2%)

Central nervous system: Peripheral neuropathy (1% to 5%)

Endocrine & metabolic: Hypercholesterolemia (3% to 7%)

Gastrointestinal: Nausea (9% to 10%), constipation (8%), gastroesophageal reflux disease (1% to 6%)

Genitourinary: Chronic renal failure (6%)

Immunologic: Antibody formation (1% to 9%), seasonal allergy (8%)

Infection: Influenza (3% to 7%)

Local: Bleeding at injection site (1% to 5%)

Ophthalmic: Retinal degeneration (1% to 8%)

Note: Conjunctival hyperemia, eye discomfort, posterior capsule opacification, and retinopathy occurred in 1% to 10% of patients, but also occurred in similar percentages to the control or more often in the control in some of the studies.

Renal: Renal failure (7%)

Respiratory: Upper respiratory tract infection (9%), cough (5% to 9%), sinusitis (3% to 8%), chronic obstructive pulmonary disease (3% to 6%)

Miscellaneous: Wound healing impairment (1%)

All indications: <1%, postmarketing, and/or case reports: Anterior chamber inflammation, anxiety, back pain, corneal edema, corneal erosion, coronary artery occlusion, decreased visual acuity, dizziness, endophthalmitis, epithelial keratopathy, eye discharge (lid margin), eyelid pain, hypoglycemia, iatrogenic traumatic cataracts, intestinal obstruction, photophobia, retinal pigment epithelium tear, rhegmatogenous retinal detachment, rhinorrhea, urticaria

As reported with choroidal neovascularization secondary to pathologic myopia (not in US labeling):

>10%:

Ophthalmic: Conjunctival hemorrhage (11%)

Respiratory: Nasopharyngitis (11%)

1% to 10%:

Cardiovascular: Hypertension (3%)

Central nervous system: Headache (8%), migraine (2%)

Endocrine & metabolic: Diabetes mellitus (2%)

Gastrointestinal: Abdominal pain (3%), nausea (2%), toothache (2%), vomiting (2%)

Genitourinary: Urinary tract infection (3%), bacteriuria (2%)

Infection: Influenza (2%)

Local: Bleeding at injection site (4%)

Neuromuscular & skeletal: Back pain (2%), herniated disk (2%), limb pain (2%), osteoporosis (2%)

Ophthalmic: Punctate keratitis (8%), vitreous opacity (5%), dry eye syndrome (4%), eye pain (4%), increased intraocular pressure (3%), blepharitis (2%), conjunctivitis (2%), eyelid edema (2%), retinal hole without detachment (2%)

Respiratory: Upper respiratory tract infection (3%), pharyngitis (2%)

<1%: Allergic conjunctivitis, arthralgia, bronchitis, cataract, conjunctival edema, corneal erosion, cough, eye irritation, hepatic insufficiency, hypercholesterolemia, hypersensitivity, increased intracranial pressure, iridocyclitis, ocular hyperemia, pain at injection site, retinal hemorrhage, sciatica, tendonitis, uveitis, viral conjunctivitis (adenovirus), vitreous detachment

Mechanism of Action Ranibizumab is a recombinant humanized monoclonal antibody fragment which binds to and inhibits human vascular endothelial growth factor A (VEGF-A). Ranibizumab inhibits VEGF from binding to its receptors and thereby suppressing neovascularization and slowing vision loss.

Pharmacodynamics/Kinetics

Half-life Elimination Vitreous: ~9 days

Reproductive Considerations

Evaluate pregnancy status prior to use in females of reproductive potential. Women of reproductive potential should use effective contraception prior to initial dose, during treatment, and for at least 3 months after the last intravitreal injection (Peracha 2016).

Pregnancy Considerations

Ranibizumab is a vascular endothelial growth factor (VEGF) inhibitor; VEGF is required to achieve and maintain normal pregnancies. Reports of intravitreal VEGF inhibitor use in pregnancy (Peracha 2016), and information specific to use of ranibizumab in pregnancy, are limited (Fossum 2018; Jouve 2015; Sarhianaki 2012). Based on studies in nonpregnant adults, VEGF inhibitors can alter systemic concentrations of VEGF and placental growth factor following intravitreal administration (Peracha 2016; Zehtner 2015). Until additional information is available, use during the first trimester should be avoided and use later in pregnancy should be based on patient specific risks versus benefits (Peracha 2016; Polizzi 2015).

◆ **Raniclor** *see* Cefaclor *on page 297*

Ranolazine (ra NOE la zeen)

Related Information

Clinical Risk Related to Drugs Prolonging QT Interval *on page 1675*

Brand Names: US Ranexa

Pharmacologic Category Antianginal Agent; Cardiovascular Agent, Miscellaneous

Use Chronic angina: Treatment of chronic angina

Note: According to the 2012 ACCF/AHA/ACP/AATS/PCNA/SCAI/STS guidelines for patients with stable ischemic heart disease, ranolazine may be useful when prescribed as a substitute for beta blockers for relief of symptoms if initial treatment with beta blockers leads to unacceptable side effects, is less effective, or if initial treatment with beta-blockers is contraindicated. May also be used in combination with beta-blockers, for relief of symptoms when initial treatment with beta-blockers is not successful (Fihn 2012).

Local Anesthetic/Vasoconstrictor Precautions Ranolazine is one of the drugs confirmed to prolong the QT interval and is accepted as having a risk of causing torsade de pointes. The risk of drug-induced torsade de pointes is extremely low when a single QT interval prolonging drug is prescribed. In terms of epinephrine, it is not known what effect vasoconstrictors in the local anesthetic regimen will have in patients with a known history of congenital prolonged QT interval or in patients taking any medication that prolongs the QT interval. Until more information is obtained, it is suggested that the clinician consult with the physician prior to the use of a vasoconstrictor in suspected patients, and that the vasoconstrictor (epinephrine, mepivacaine and levonordefrin [Carbocaine® 2% with Neo-Cobefrin®]) be used with caution.

Effects on Dental Treatment Key adverse event(s) related to dental treatment: Xerostomia (normal salivary flow resumes upon discontinuation).

Effects on Bleeding No information available to require special precautions

Adverse Reactions

>0.5% to 10%:

Cardiovascular: Bradycardia (≤4%), hypotension (≤4%), orthostatic hypotension (≤4%), palpitation (≤4%), peripheral edema (≤4%), prolonged QT interval on ECG (>500 msec: ≤1%)

Central nervous system: Dizziness (6%; may be dose-related), headache (≤6%), confusion (≤4%), syncope (≤4%), vertigo (≤4%)

Dermatologic: Hyperhidrosis (≤4%)

Gastrointestinal: Constipation (5%), abdominal pain (≤4%), anorexia (≤4%), dyspepsia (≤4%), nausea (≤4%; dose-related), vomiting (≤4%), xerostomia (≤4%)

Genitourinary: Hematuria (≤4%)

Neuromuscular: Weakness (≤4%)

Ophthalmic: Blurred vision (≤4%)

Otic: Tinnitus (≤4%)

Respiratory: Dyspnea (≤4%)

≤0.5%, postmarketing, and/or case reports: Angioedema, ataxia, decreased glycosylated hemoglobin, decreased T-wave amplitude, dysuria, eosinophilia, hallucination, hypoesthesia, hypoglycemia (diabetic patients), increased blood urea nitrogen, increased serum creatinine, leukopenia, pancytopenia, paresthesia, pruritus, pulmonary fibrosis, renal failure, skin rash, thrombocytopenia, torsade de pointes (Morrow 2007), tremor, T-wave changes (notched), urinary retention, urine discoloration

Mechanism of Action Ranolazine exerts antianginal and anti-ischemic effects without changing hemodynamic parameters (heart rate or blood pressure). At therapeutic levels, ranolazine inhibits the late phase of the inward sodium channel (late I_{Na}) in ischemic cardiac myocytes during cardiac repolarization reducing intracellular sodium concentrations and thereby reducing calcium influx via Na^+-Ca^{2+} exchange. Decreased intracellular calcium reduces ventricular tension and myocardial oxygen consumption. It is thought that ranolazine produces myocardial relaxation and reduces anginal symptoms through this mechanism although this is uncertain. At higher concentrations, ranolazine inhibits the rapid delayed rectifier potassium current (I_{Kr}) thus prolonging the ventricular action potential duration and subsequent prolongation of the QT interval.

Pharmacodynamics/Kinetics

Half-life Elimination Ranolazine: Terminal: 7 hours; Metabolites (activity undefined): 6 to 22 hours

Time to Peak 2 to 5 hours

Pregnancy Considerations Adverse events have been observed in animal reproduction studies.

Dental Health Professional Considerations See Local Anesthetic/Vasoconstrictor Precautions

- **Rapaflo** *see* Silodosin *on page 1370*
- **Rapamune** *see* Sirolimus *on page 1374*
- **Rapamycin** *see* Sirolimus *on page 1374*
- **Rapivab** *see* Peramivir *on page 1216*
- **Raplixa [DSC]** *see* Fibrin Sealant *on page 667*

Rasagiline (ra SA ji leen)

Brand Names: US Azilect

Brand Names: Canada APO-Rasagiline; Azilect; TEVA-Rasagiline

Pharmacologic Category Anti-Parkinson Agent, MAO Type B Inhibitor

Use Parkinson disease: Treatment of Parkinson disease

Local Anesthetic/Vasoconstrictor Precautions Rasagiline in approved doses of 0.5-1 mg daily should not inhibit type-A MAO; however, the possibility exists of nonselective MAO inhibition at higher doses and/or in certain sensitive individuals. Therefore, attempts should be made to avoid use of vasoconstrictors due to possibility of hypertensive episodes.

Effects on Dental Treatment Key adverse event(s) related to dental treatment: Xerostomia and changes in salivation (normal salivary flow resumes upon discontinuation). Anticholinergic side effects can cause a reduction of saliva production or secretion, contributing to discomfort and dental disease (ie, caries, oral candidiasis, and periodontal disease). Patients may experience orthostatic hypotension as they stand up after treatment; especially if lying in dental chair for extended periods of time. Use caution with sudden changes in position during and after dental treatment.

Effects on Bleeding No information available to require special precautions

Adverse Reactions Unless otherwise noted, the following adverse reactions are as reported for monotherapy. Spectrum of adverse events was generally similar with adjunctive therapy, though the incidence tended to be higher. Frequency not always defined.

>10%:

Cardiovascular: Orthostatic hypotension (adjunctive therapy 3% to 13%, adjunctive therapy dose-related 6% to 9%; adjunctive therapy, 1 mg dose 3%; mild to moderate systolic blood pressure decrease [≥20 mmHg], 1 mg dose 44%; mild to moderate diastolic blood pressure decrease [≥10 mmHg], 1 mg dose 40%; severe diastolic blood pressure decrease [≥20 mmHg], 1 mg dose 9%; severe systolic blood pressure decrease [≥40 mmHg], 1 mg dose 7%), hypotension (3% post-treatment [systolic <90 mmHg or diastolic <50 mmHg combined with significant decrease from baseline, systolic >30 mmHg or diastolic >20 mmHg])

Central nervous system: Headache (14%; adjunctive therapy 6% to 11%)

Gastrointestinal: Nausea (adjunctive therapy 6% to 12%)

Neuromuscular & skeletal: Dyskinesia (adjunctive therapy 18%)

Miscellaneous: Trauma (adjunctive therapy 8% to 12%)

1% to 10%:

Cardiovascular: Peripheral edema (7%), increased blood pressure (adjunctive therapy, significant increase, >180 mmHg systolic or >100 mmHg diastolic 4%; adjunctive therapy, post-treatment [>180 mmHg systolic or >100 mmHg diastolic combined with significant increase from baseline >30 mmHg systolic or >20 mmHg diastolic] 2%), angina, bundle branch block, chest pain

Central nervous system: Dizziness (7%), drowsiness (adjunctive therapy 4% to 6%), ataxia (adjunctive therapy 3% to 6%), depression (5%), falling (5%; adjunctive therapy 6% to 12%), abnormal dreams (adjunctive therapy 1% to 4%), dystonia (adjunctive therapy 2% to 3%), malaise (2%), paresthesia (2%; adjunctive therapy 2% to 5%), insomnia (adjunctive therapy 4%), hallucinations (1%; adjunctive therapy 4% to 5%), myasthenia (adjunctive therapy 2%), vertigo (2%), anxiety

Dermatologic: Skin rash (adjunctive therapy 3% to 6%), ecchymosis (2%; adjunctive therapy 2% to 5%), diaphoresis (adjunctive therapy 2% to 3%), alopecia, skin carcinoma, vesiculobullous rash

Endocrine & metabolic: Weight loss (adjunctive therapy, dose-related 2% to 9%), impotence, libido decreased

Gastrointestinal: Constipation (adjunctive therapy 4% to 9%), dyspepsia (7%; adjunctive therapy 4% to 5%), diarrhea (adjunctive therapy 5% to 7%), vomiting (adjunctive therapy 4% to 7%), xerostomia (adjunctive therapy, dose-related 2% to 6%), abdominal pain (adjunctive therapy 2% to 5%), anorexia (adjunctive therapy 2% to 5%), gastroenteritis (3%), gingivitis (adjunctive therapy 1% to 2%), hernia (adjunctive therapy 1% to 2%), gastrointestinal hemorrhage

Genitourinary: Hematuria, urinary incontinence

Hematologic and oncologic: Hemorrhage (adjunctive therapy 1% to 2%), leukopenia

Hepatic: Liver function tests increased

Infection: Infection (adjunctive therapy 2% to 3%)

Neuromuscular & skeletal: Arthralgia (7%; adjunctive therapy 5% to 8%), back pain (adjunctive therapy 4%), neck pain (2%; adjunctive therapy 1% to 3%), tenosynovitis (adjunctive therapy 1% to 3%), arthritis (2%), abnormal gait, hyperkinesias, hypertonia, neuropathy, weakness

Ophthalmic: Conjunctivitis (3%)

Renal: Albuminuria

Respiratory: Flu-like symptoms (5%), dyspnea (adjunctive therapy 3% to 5%), cough (adjunctive therapy 4%), upper respiratory tract infection (adjunctive therapy 4%), rhinitis (3%), asthma

Miscellaneous: Fever (3%), allergic reaction

<1%, postmarketing, case reports and/or frequency not defined: Abnormal behavior, abnormality in thinking, acute kidney failure, aggressive behavior, agitation, altered sense of smell, amyotrophy, aphasia, apnea, arterial thrombosis, atrial arrhythmia, atrioventricular block, bigeminy, blepharitis, blepharoptosis, blindness, cardiac failure, cerebral hemorrhage, cerebral ischemia, confusion, deafness, deep vein thrombophlebitis, delirium, delusions, diplopia, disorientation, dysautonomia, dysesthesia, emphysema, esophageal ulcer, exacerbation of hypertension, excessive daytime sleepiness (including during operation of motor vehicles), exfoliative dermatitis, facial paralysis, gastric ulcer, genitourinary disorders, glaucoma, gynecomastia, hematemesis, hemiplegia, hostility, hypocalcemia, hypotension (while supine), impulse control disorder (pathological gambling, hypersexuality, intense urges to spend money, binge eating, and/or other intense urges and the inability to control the urges), interstitial pneumonitis, intestinal obstruction, intestinal perforation, intestinal stenosis, jaundice, keratitis, large intestine perforation, laryngeal edema, laryngismus, leukoderma, leukorrhea, macrocytic anemia, manic depressive reaction, mania, megacolon, menstrual abnormalities, myelitis, myocardial infarction, nephrolithiasis, neuralgia, neuritis, (a complex resembling) neuroleptic malignant syndrome (associated with rapid dose reduction, withdrawal of or changes in medication; includes autonomic insufficiency, hyperthermia, impaired consciousness, muscle rigidity), nocturia, oral paresthesia, osteonecrosis, paranoia, personality disorder, pleural effusion, pneumothorax, polyuria, psychiatric disturbance (new or worsening mental status and behavioral changes that may be severe, including psychotic-like behavior during or after starting or increasing doses), psychoneurosis, psychotic symptoms, psychotic depression, pulmonary fibrosis, purpura, retinal degeneration, retinal detachment, seizure, strabismus, stupor, thrombocythemia, tongue edema, ventricular fibrillation, ventricular tachycardia, vestibular disturbance, visual field defect, vulvovaginal candidiasis

Mechanism of Action Potent, irreversible and selective inhibitor of brain monoamine oxidase (MAO) type B, which plays a major role in the catabolism of dopamine. Inhibition of dopamine depletion in the striatal region of the brain reduces the symptomatic motor deficits of Parkinson's disease. There is also experimental evidence of rasagiline conferring neuroprotective effects (antioxidant, antiapoptotic), which may delay onset of symptoms and progression of neuronal deterioration.

Pharmacodynamics/Kinetics

Duration of Action ~1 week (irreversible inhibition)

Half-life Elimination ~3 hours (no correlation with biologic effect due to irreversible inhibition)

Time to Peak ~1 hour

Pregnancy Considerations Adverse effects have been observed in animal reproduction studies. Information related to rasagiline use in pregnancy is limited (Seier 2017; Tüfekçioğlu 2018).

◆ **Rasagiline Mesylate** *see* Rasagiline *on page 1311*

Rasburicase (ras BYOOR i kayse)

Brand Names: US Elitek

Brand Names: Canada Fasturtec

Pharmacologic Category Enzyme; Enzyme, Urate-Oxidase (Recombinant)

Use

Hyperuricemia associated with malignancy: Initial management of plasma uric acid levels in pediatric and adult patients with leukemia, lymphoma, and solid tumor malignancies receiving chemotherapy expected to result in tumor lysis and elevation of plasma uric acid

Limitations of use: Indicated only for a single course of treatment

Local Anesthetic/Vasoconstrictor Precautions No information available to require special precautions

Effects on Dental Treatment Key adverse event(s) related to dental treatment: Mucositis.

Effects on Bleeding No information available to require special precautions

Adverse Reactions

>10%:

Cardiovascular: Peripheral edema (50%)

Central nervous system: Headache (26%), anxiety (24%)

Dermatologic: Rash (13%; serious: <1%)

Endocrine & metabolic: Hypophosphatemia (17%), hypervolemia (12%)

Gastrointestinal: Nausea (27% to 58%), vomiting (38% to 50%), abdominal pain (20% to 22%), constipation (20%), diarrhea (20%), mucositis (15%)

Hepatic: Hyperbilirubinemia (16%), increased serum ALT (11%)

Immunologic: Antibody development (children: 11%; IgE: 6%), development of IgG antibodies (18%; neutralizing 8%)

Infection: Sepsis (12%; serious: 5%)

Respiratory: Pharyngolaryngeal pain (14%)

Miscellaneous: Fever (46%)

1% to 10%:

Cardiovascular: Ischemic heart disease (≥2%), supraventricular arrhythmia (≥2%)

Endocrine & metabolic: Hyperphosphatemia (10%)

Gastrointestinal: Gastrointestinal infection (≥2%)

Hematologic & oncologic: Pulmonary hemorrhage (≥2%)

Hypersensitivity: Hypersensitivity (4%)

Infection: Infection (abdominal, ≥2%)

Respiratory: Respiratory failure (≥2%)

<1%, postmarketing, and/or case reports: Anaphylaxis, hemolysis, methemoglobinemia, muscle spasm, seizure

Mechanism of Action Rasburicase is a recombinant urate-oxidase enzyme, which converts uric acid to allantoin (an inactive and soluble metabolite of uric acid); it does not inhibit the formation of uric acid.

Pharmacodynamics/Kinetics

Onset of Action Uric acid levels decrease within 4 hours of initial administration

Half-life Elimination ~16 to 23 hours

Pregnancy Considerations Based on data from animal reproduction studies, in utero exposure to rasburicase may cause fetal harm. Information related to the use of rasburicase in pregnancy is limited (Middeke 2014).

◆ **Rasuvo** *see* Methotrexate *on page 990*

Ravulizumab (rav ue LIZ ue mab)

Brand Names: US Ultomiris

Pharmacologic Category Monoclonal Antibody; Monoclonal Antibody, Complement Inhibitor

Use

Atypical hemolytic uremic syndrome: Treatment of atypical hemolytic uremic syndrome to inhibit complement-mediated thrombotic microangiopathy in adult and pediatric patients ≥1 month of age.

Limitations of use: Not indicated for the treatment of Shiga toxin *Escherichia coli*-related hemolytic uremic syndrome.

Paroxysmal nocturnal hemoglobinuria: Treatment of paroxysmal nocturnal hemoglobinuria in adults.

Local Anesthetic/Vasoconstrictor Precautions No information available to require special precautions

Effects on Dental Treatment No significant effects or complications reported

Effects on Bleeding No information available to require special precautions

Adverse Reactions

>10%:

Central nervous system: Headache (32%)

Respiratory: Upper respiratory tract infection (39%)

1% to 10%:

Central nervous system: Dizziness (5%)

Gastrointestinal: Diarrhea (9%), nausea (9%), abdominal pain (6%)

Neuromuscular & skeletal: Limb pain (6%), arthralgia (5%)

Miscellaneous: Fever (7%), infusion related reaction (2%)

<1%, postmarketing, and/or case reports: Antibody development, hyperthermia, meningococcal infection, sepsis

Mechanism of Action Ravulizumab is a humanized monoclonal antibody which is a terminal complement inhibitor that specifically binds to the complement protein C5 (with high affinity), inhibiting its cleavage to C5a (the proinflammatory anaphylatoxin) and C5b (the initiating subunit of the terminal complement complex [C5b-9]) and preventing generation of the terminal complement complex C5b9. Ravulizumab inhibits terminal complement-mediated intravascular hemolysis in paroxysmal nocturnal hemoglobinuria (PNH) and complement-mediated thrombotic microangiopathy in atypical hemolytic uremic syndrome. The C5 inhibition of complement-mediated hemolysis achieved by ravulizumab in patients with PNH is immediate, thorough, and sustained (Lee 2019).

Pharmacodynamics/Kinetics

Onset of Action Lactate dehydrogenase (LDH) reduction: Rapid and sustained, beginning as early as day 8 (Roth 2018). LDH normalization: By week 4 (in complement-inhibitor naive patients with paroxysmal nocturnal hemoglobinuria).

Half-life Elimination Terminal: 51.8 days (atypical hemolytic uremic syndrome patients); 49.7 days (paroxysmal nocturnal hemoglobinuria patients).

Pregnancy Considerations

Ravulizumab is a humanized monoclonal antibody (IgG_2). Placental transfer of human IgG is dependent upon the IgG subclass, maternal serum concentrations, birth weight, and gestational age, generally increasing as pregnancy progresses. The lowest exposure would be expected during the period of organogenesis (Palmeira 2012; Pentsuk 2009). Females who were pregnant or planning to become pregnant were excluded from initial clinical studies (Kulasekararaj 2019; Lee 2019).

Adverse pregnancy outcomes are associated with untreated paroxysmal nocturnal hemoglobinuria (PNH) and atypical hemolytic uremic syndrome (aHUS). Adverse maternal outcomes associated with PNH may include worsening cytopenias, thrombotic events, infections, bleeding, fetal loss, and increased maternal mortality; increased fetal death and premature delivery is also reported. Women with aHUS may have an increased risk of preeclampsia and preterm delivery; intrauterine growth restriction/low birth weight and fetal death may also occur.

◆ **Ravulizumab-cwvz** *see* Ravulizumab *on page 1313*

◆ **Rayaldee** *see* Calcifediol *on page 279*

◆ **Rayos** *see* PredniSONE *on page 1260*

◆ **ReadySharp Betamethasone** *see* Betamethasone (Systemic) *on page 233*

◆ **ReadySharp Bupivacaine [DSC]** *see* Bupivacaine *on page 256*

- ◆ **ReadySharp Dexamethasone** *see* DexAMETHasone (Systemic) *on page 463*
- ◆ **ReadySharp Ketorolac** *see* Ketorolac (Systemic) *on page 861*
- ◆ **ReadySharp Lidocaine** *see* Lidocaine (Systemic) *on page 901*
- ◆ **ReadySharp methylPREDNISolone [DSC]** *see* MethylPREDNISolone *on page 999*
- ◆ **ReadySharp Triamcinolone [DSC]** *see* Triamcinolone (Systemic) *on page 1485*
- ◆ **Rebetol [DSC]** *see* Ribavirin (Systemic) *on page 1320*
- ◆ **Rebif** *see* Interferon Beta-1a *on page 833*
- ◆ **Rebif Rebidose** *see* Interferon Beta-1a *on page 833*
- ◆ **Rebif Rebidose Titration Pack** *see* Interferon Beta-1a *on page 833*
- ◆ **Rebif Titration Pack** *see* Interferon Beta-1a *on page 833*
- ◆ **Recarbrio** *see* Imipenem, Cilastatin, and Relebactam *on page 800*
- ◆ **Reclast** *see* Zoledronic Acid *on page 1574*
- ◆ **Reclipsen** *see* Ethinyl Estradiol and Desogestrel *on page 609*
- ◆ **Recombinant α-L-Iduronidase (Glycosaminoglycan α-L-Iduronohydrolase)** *see* Laronidase *on page 878*
- ◆ **Recombinant Desulfatohirudin** *see* Desirudin *on page 459*
- ◆ **Recombinant Granulocyte-Macrophage Colony Stimulating Factor** *see* Sargramostim *on page 1358*
- ◆ **Recombinant Hirudin** *see* Desirudin *on page 459*
- ◆ **Recombinant Human Deoxyribonuclease** *see* Dornase Alfa *on page 515*
- ◆ **Recombinant human hyaluronidase mixed with daratumumab** *see* Daratumumab and Hyaluronidase *on page 439*
- ◆ **Recombinant Human Interleukin-2** *see* Aldesleukin *on page 91*
- ◆ **Recombinant Human Luteinizing Hormone** *see* Lutropin Alfa *on page 944*
- ◆ **Recombinant Human Parathyroid Hormone (1-34)** *see* Teriparatide *on page 1424*
- ◆ **Recombinant Human Parathyroid Hormone (1-84)** *see* Parathyroid Hormone *on page 1192*
- ◆ **Recombinant Human Platelet-Derived Growth Factor B** *see* Becaplermin *on page 217*
- ◆ **Recombinant Human Thyrotropin** *see* Thyrotropin Alpha *on page 1442*
- ◆ **Recombinant Influenza Vaccine, Quadrivalent** *see* Influenza Virus Vaccine (Recombinant) *on page 815*
- ◆ **Recombinant Insulin-Like Growth Factor-1** *see* Mecasermin *on page 951*
- ◆ **Recombinant Methionyl-Human Leptin** *see* Metreleptin *on page 1010*
- ◆ **Recombinant Plasminogen Activator** *see* Reteplase *on page 1318*
- ◆ **Recombinant Urate Oxidase** *see* Rasburicase *on page 1312*
- ◆ **Recombinant Urate Oxidase, Pegylated** *see* Pegloticase *on page 1203*
- ◆ **Recombinant zoster vaccine** *see* Zoster Vaccine (Recombinant) *on page 1586*
- ◆ **Recombinate** *see* Antihemophilic Factor (Recombinant) *on page 153*
- ◆ **Recombivax HB** *see* Hepatitis B Vaccine (Recombinant) *on page 757*
- ◆ **Recort Plus [OTC]** *see* Hydrocortisone (Topical) *on page 775*
- ◆ **Recothrom** *see* Thrombin (Topical) *on page 1440*
- ◆ **Recothrom Spray Kit** *see* Thrombin (Topical) *on page 1440*
- ◆ **Rectacaine [OTC]** *see* Phenylephrine (Topical) *on page 1227*
- ◆ **RectaSmoothe [OTC]** *see* Lidocaine (Topical) *on page 902*
- ◆ **RectiCare [OTC]** *see* Lidocaine (Topical) *on page 902*
- ◆ **Rectiv** *see* Nitroglycerin *on page 1112*
- ◆ **Rederm [OTC] [DSC]** *see* Hydrocortisone (Topical) *on page 775*
- ◆ **Refissa** *see* Tretinoin (Topical) *on page 1484*
- ◆ **Regitine [DSC]** *see* Phentolamine *on page 1226*
- ◆ **Reglan** *see* Metoclopramide *on page 1007*
- ◆ **REGN88** *see* Sarilumab *on page 1359*
- ◆ **REGN727** *see* Alirocumab *on page 101*
- ◆ **REGN2810** *see* Cemiplimab *on page 320*
- ◆ **Regonol** *see* Pyridostigmine *on page 1293*

Regorafenib (re goe RAF e nib)

Brand Names: US Stivarga

Brand Names: Canada Stivarga

Pharmacologic Category Antineoplastic Agent, Tyrosine Kinase Inhibitor; Antineoplastic Agent, Vascular Endothelial Growth Factor (VEGF) Inhibitor

Use

Colorectal cancer, metastatic: Treatment of metastatic colorectal cancer in patients previously treated with fluoropyrimidine-, oxaliplatin-, and irinotecan-based chemotherapy, an anti-VEGF therapy, and an anti-EGFR therapy (if *RAS* wild type).

GI stromal tumors: Treatment of locally advanced, unresectable, or metastatic GI stromal tumor in patients previously treated with imatinib and sunitinib.

Hepatocellular carcinoma: Treatment of hepatocellular carcinoma in patients previously treated with sorafenib.

Local Anesthetic/Vasoconstrictor Precautions Use vasoconstrictor with caution; patients may experience significant hypertension when taking regorafenib

Effects on Dental Treatment Key adverse event(s) related to dental treatment: Mucositis, xerostomia (normal salivary flow resumes upon discontinuation), and taste disturbance

Effects on Bleeding Chemotherapy may result in significant myelosuppression, potentially including significant reduction in platelet counts and altered hemostasis. Thrombocytopenia has been reported (41%; grade 3: 2%; grade 4: <1%). Bleeding has been reported in 21% in patients. In patients who are under active treatment with these agents, medical consult is suggested.

Adverse Reactions

>10%:

Cardiovascular: Hypertension (30% to 59%)

Central nervous system: Fatigue (≤64%), pain (55% to 59%), voice disorder (18% to 39%), headache (10% to 16%)

Dermatologic: Palmar-plantar erythrodysesthesia (45% to 67%), skin rash (26% to 30%), alopecia (7% to 24%)

Endocrine & metabolic: Hypophosphatemia (55% to 70%), hypocalcemia (17% to 59%), weight loss (13% to 32%), hypokalemia (21% to 31%), hyponatremia (30%), increased amylase (23% to 26%), hypothyroidism (6% to 18%)
Gastrointestinal: Gastrointestinal pain (60%), diarrhea (41% to 47%), decreased appetite (31% to 47%), increased serum lipase (14% to 46%), stomatitis (13% to 40%; grade ≥3: 1% to 4%), nausea (17% to 20%), vomiting (13% to 17%)
Hematologic & oncologic: Anemia (79%; grade 3: 5%; grade 4: 1%), lymphocytopenia (30% to 68%; grade 3: 8% to 16%; grade 4: 2%), thrombocytopenia (13% to 63%; grade 3: 1% to 5%; grade 4: <1%), increased INR (24% to 44%; grade 3: 4%), hemorrhage (11% to 21%; grade ≥3: 2% to 5%), neutropenia (3% to 16%; grade 3: 1% to 3%; grade 4: 1%)
Hepatic: Increased serum aspartate aminotransferase (58% to 93%), hyperbilirubinemia (33% to 78%), increased serum alanine aminotransferase (45% to 70%)
Infection: Infection (31% to 32%)
Neuromuscular & skeletal: Asthenia (≤64%), muscle spasm (10% to 14%)
Renal: Proteinuria (51% to 84%)
Miscellaneous: Fever (20% to 28%)

1% to 10%:
Dermatologic: Exfoliative dermatitis (1%)
Gastrointestinal: Mucocutaneous candidiasis (≤3%), pancreatitis (2%)
Genitourinary: Urinary tract infection (6%)
Hepatic: Hepatic failure (≤2%)
Infection: Fungal infection (≤3%)
Neuromuscular & skeletal: Tremor (1%)
Respiratory: Nasopharyngitis (4%), pneumonia (3%)

Frequency not defined: Hepatic: Hepatotoxicity

<1%, postmarketing, and/or case reports: Acute myocardial infarction, cardiac failure, erythema multiforme, gastrointestinal fistula, gastrointestinal perforation, hepatic injury, hypersensitivity reaction, hypertensive crisis, ischemic heart disease, nephrotic syndrome, reversible posterior leukoencephalopathy syndrome, Stevens-Johnson syndrome, toxic epidermal necrolysis

Mechanism of Action Regorafenib is a multikinase inhibitor; it targets kinases involved with tumor angiogenesis, oncogenesis, and maintenance of the tumor microenvironment which results in inhibition of tumor growth. Specifically, it inhibits VEGF receptors 1-3, KIT, PDGFR-alpha, PDGFR-beta, RET, FGFR1 and 2, TIE2, DDR2, TrkA, Eph2A, RAF-1. BRAF, $BRAF^{V600E}$, SAPK2, PTK5, and Abl.

Pharmacodynamics/Kinetics

Half-life Elimination Regorafenib: 28 hours (range: 14 to 58 hours); M-2 metabolite: 25 hours (range: 14 to 32 hours); M-5 metabolite: 51 hours (range: 32 to 70 hours)

Time to Peak 4 hours

Reproductive Considerations

Women of reproductive potential and men with female partners of reproductive potential should use effective contraception during therapy and for at least 2 months following treatment.

Pregnancy Considerations

Based on animal reproduction studies and on the mechanism of action, regorafenib may cause fetal harm if administered during pregnancy.

◆ **Regranex** *see* Becaplermin *on page 217*
◆ **Regular Insulin** *see* Insulin Regular *on page 829*
◆ **Regular Insulin and NPH Insulin** *see* Insulin NPH and Insulin Regular *on page 828*
◆ **Relador Pak** *see* Lidocaine and Prilocaine *on page 911*
◆ **Relafen** *see* Nabumetone *on page 1069*
◆ **Relafen DS** *see* Nabumetone *on page 1069*
◆ **Relebactam, Cilastatin, and Imipenem** *see* Imipenem, Cilastatin, and Relebactam *on page 800*
◆ **Relebactam, Imipenem, and Cilastatin** *see* Imipenem, Cilastatin, and Relebactam *on page 800*
◆ **Relebactam Monohydrate, Cilastatin Sodium, and Imipenem Monohydrate** *see* Imipenem, Cilastatin, and Relebactam *on page 800*
◆ **Releevia [DSC]** *see* Capsaicin *on page 284*
◆ **Releevia MC [DSC]** *see* Capsaicin *on page 284*
◆ **Relenza Diskhaler** *see* Zanamivir *on page 1567*
◆ **Relexxii** *see* Methylphenidate *on page 997*
◆ **Re-Lieved Maximum Strength [OTC]** *see* Lidocaine (Topical) *on page 902*
◆ **Relistor** *see* Methylnaltrexone *on page 996*
◆ **Relpax** *see* Eletriptan *on page 549*
◆ **Remedy Antifungal [OTC]** *see* Miconazole (Topical) *on page 1019*
◆ **Remedy Antifungal Clear [OTC] [DSC]** *see* Miconazole (Topical) *on page 1019*
◆ **Remedy Phytoplex Antifungal [OTC]** *see* Miconazole (Topical) *on page 1019*
◆ **Remeron** *see* Mirtazapine *on page 1038*
◆ **Remeron SolTab** *see* Mirtazapine *on page 1038*
◆ **Remicade** *see* InFLIXimab *on page 809*

Remifentanil (rem i FEN ta nil)

Brand Names: US Ultiva

Pharmacologic Category Analgesic, Opioid; Anilidopiperidine Opioid

Use Anesthesia: Analgesic for use during the induction and maintenance of general anesthesia; continued analgesia into the immediate postoperative period in adults; analgesic component of monitored anesthesia in adults

Local Anesthetic/Vasoconstrictor Precautions No information available to require special precautions

Effects on Dental Treatment No significant effects or complications reported

Effects on Bleeding No information available to require special precautions

Adverse Reactions Frequency of adverse events may vary based on surgical procedures and rate of infusion.

>10%:
Cardiovascular: Hypotension (2% to 19%)
Central nervous system: Headache (<2% to 18%)
Dermatologic: Pruritus (<2% to 18%)
Gastrointestinal: Nausea (<36% to 44%), vomiting (<16% to 22%)
Neuromuscular & skeletal: Muscle rigidity (≤11%; includes chest wall rigidity)

1% to 10%:
Cardiovascular: Bradycardia (1% to 7%; dose-dependent), shivering (<5%), hypertension (1% to 2%; dose-dependent), flushing (1%), flushing sensation (1%), tachycardia (≤1%; dose-dependent)
Central nervous system: Dizziness (<5%), chills (1%), agitation (≤1%)
Dermatologic: Diaphoresis (6%)

Local: Pain at injection site (1%)
Respiratory: Respiratory depression (<7%), apnea (<3%), hypoxia (≤1%)
Miscellaneous: Fever (<5%), postoperative pain (<2%)

<1%, postmarketing, and/or case reports: Abdominal distress, amnesia, anaphylaxis, anxiety, awareness under anesthesia without pain, bronchitis, bronchospasm, cardiac arrhythmia, chest pain, confusion, constipation, cough, diarrhea, disorientation, disruption of body temperature regulation, dysphagia, dysphoria, dyspnea, dysuria, ECG changes, electrolyte disturbance, erythema, gastroesophageal reflux disease, hallucination, heart block, heartburn, hepatic insufficiency, hiccups, hyperglycemia, increased creatine phosphokinase, intestinal obstruction, involuntary body movements, laryngospasm, leukocytosis, lymphocytopenia, nasal congestion, nightmares, nystagmus, oliguria, paresthesia, pharyngitis, pleural effusion, prolonged emergence from anesthesia, pulmonary edema, rales, rapid awakening from anesthesia, rhinorrhea, rhonchi, seizure, skin rash, sleep disorder, stridor, syncope, thrombocytopenia, tremor, twitching, urinary incontinence, urinary retention, urticaria, xerostomia

Mechanism of Action Binds with stereospecific mu-opioid receptors at many sites within the CNS, increases pain threshold, alters pain reception, inhibits ascending pain pathways

Pharmacodynamics/Kinetics

Onset of Action IV: 1 to 3 minutes; Peak effect: 3 to 5 minutes

Duration of Action 3 to 10 minutes (Scott 2005)

Half-life Elimination Dose dependent:

Pediatric patients (Ross 2001): Effective:
Neonates ≤2 months: 5.4 minutes (range: 3 to 8 minutes)
Infants and Children >2 months to <2 years: 3.4 minutes (range: 2 to 6 minutes)
Children 2 to 6 years: 3.6 minutes (range: 1 to 6 minutes)
Children 7 to 12 years: 5.3 minutes (range: 3 to 7 minutes)
Adolescents: 13 to <16 years: 3.7 minutes (range: 2 to 5 minutes)
Adolescents 16 to 18 years: 5.7 minutes (range: 5 to 6 minutes)

Adults: Terminal: 10 to 20 minutes; Effective: 3 to 10 minutes

Time to Peak Intranasal: Children ≤7 years: ~3.5 minutes (Verghese 2008)

Pregnancy Considerations

Remifentanil crosses the placenta; fetal and maternal concentrations may be similar.

Prolonged use of opioids during pregnancy can cause neonatal withdrawal syndrome, which may be life-threatening if not recognized and treated according to protocols developed by neonatology experts. Opioids used as part of obstetric analgesia/anesthesia during labor and delivery may temporarily affect the fetal heart rate (ACOG 209 2019). Opioids may cause respiratory depression and psychophysiologic effects in the neonate; newborns of mothers receiving remifentanil during labor should be closely monitored (Devroe 2015; Noskova 2015).

Pharmacokinetic properties of remifentanil are not significantly altered by pregnancy; dosing adjustment is not required for maternal indications (Smith 2017). Remifentanil is used to treat maternal pain during labor and immediately postpartum (ACOG 209 2019; Devroe 2015; Weibel 2017).

The ACOG recommends that pregnant women should not be denied medically necessary surgery, regardless of trimester. If the procedure is elective, it should be delayed until after delivery (ACOG 775 2019).

Controlled Substance C-II

Remimazolam

Pharmacologic Category Benzodiazepine

Use Sedation: Induction and maintenance of procedural sedation in adults undergoing procedures lasting ≤30 minutes.

Local Anesthetic/Vasoconstrictor Precautions No information available to require special precautions.

Effects on Dental Treatment See Dental Health Professional Considerations.

Effects on Bleeding No information available to require special precautions.

Adverse Reactions

>10%:
Cardiovascular: Bradycardia (4% to 11%), decreased diastolic blood pressure (8% to 14%), hypertension (20% to 28%), hypotension (33% to 39%; increased diastolic blood pressure 10% to 25%), systolic hypertension (5% to 22%)
Respiratory: Hypoxia (22%), tachypnea (14%)

1% to 10%:
Cardiovascular: Tachycardia (8%)
Gastrointestinal: Nausea (4%)
Nervous system: Headache (3%)
Miscellaneous: Fever (4%)

Mechanism of Action Binds to brain benzodiazepine sites (GABA-A receptors) while its carboxylic acid metabolite (CNS7054) has a 300 times lower affinity for the receptor. Remimazolam does not show a clear selectivity between subtypes of the GABA-A receptor

Pharmacodynamics/Kinetics

Duration of Action 11 to 14 minutes after last dose.

Half-life Elimination 37 to 53 minutes.

Time to Peak Sedation: 3 to 3.5 minutes (single dose); 11 to 14 minutes (multiple dose).

Pregnancy Considerations Benzodiazepines cross the placenta.

Teratogenic effects have been observed with some benzodiazepines; however, data are inconsistent and additional studies are needed. Based on data from other benzodiazepines, neonatal hypotonia, lethargy, respiratory depression, sedation, and withdrawal symptoms may occur following in utero exposure to remimazolam.

Based on animal data, repeated or prolonged use of general anesthetic and sedation medications that block N-methyl-D-aspartate receptors and/or potentiate GABA activity may affect brain development.

The American College of Obstetricians and Gynecologists recommends that pregnant women should not be denied medically necessary surgery regardless of trimester. If the procedure is elective, it should be delayed until after delivery (ACOG 775 2019).

Product Availability Byfavo: FDA approved July 2020; anticipated availability in 2nd half of 2020.

Dental Health Professional Considerations [US Boxed Warning]: Only personnel trained in the administration of procedural sedation should administer remimazolam and must be trained in the detection and management of airway obstruction, hypoventilation, and apnea, including the maintenance of a patent airway, supportive ventilation, and cardiovascular resuscitation. Remimazolam has been associated with hypoxia, bradycardia, and hypotension; continuously monitor vital signs during sedation and during the recovery period. Resuscitative drugs and age- and size-appropriate equipment for bag/valve/mask assisted ventilation must be immediately available during administration.

- **Remimazolam besylate** *see* Remimazolam *on page 1316*
- **Remodulin** *see* Treprostinil *on page 1482*
- **Renflexis** *see* InFLIXimab *on page 809*
- **Renova** *see* Tretinoin (Topical) *on page 1484*
- **Renova Pump** *see* Tretinoin (Topical) *on page 1484*
- **Renovo** *see* Capsaicin *on page 284*

Repaglinide (re PAG li nide)

Related Information

Endocrine Disorders and Pregnancy *on page 1684*

Brand Names: US Prandin [DSC]

Brand Names: Canada ACT Repaglinide; APO-Repaglinide; Auro-Repaglinide; GlucoNorm; JAMP Repaglinide; SANDOZ Repaglinide

Pharmacologic Category Antidiabetic Agent, Meglitinide Analog

Use Diabetes mellitus, type 2: To improve glycemic control in adults with type 2 diabetes mellitus as an adjunct to diet and exercise

Local Anesthetic/Vasoconstrictor Precautions No information available to require special precautions

Effects on Dental Treatment No significant effects or complications reported

Effects on Bleeding No information available to require special precautions

Adverse Reactions

>10%:

Central nervous system: Headache (9% to 11%)

Endocrine & metabolic: Hypoglycemia (16% to 31%)

Respiratory: Upper respiratory tract infection (10% to 16%)

1% to 10%:

Cardiovascular: Ischemia (4%), chest pain (2% to 3%)

Gastrointestinal: Diarrhea (4% to 5%), constipation (2% to 3%)

Genitourinary: Urinary tract infection (2% to 3%)

Hypersensitivity: Hypersensitivity reaction (1% to 2%)

Neuromuscular & skeletal: Back pain (5% to 6%), arthralgia (3% to 6%)

Respiratory: Sinusitis (3% to 6%), bronchitis (2% to 6%)

<1%, postmarketing, and/or case reports: Alopecia, anaphylactoid reaction, blurred vision (transient), cardiac arrhythmia, ECG abnormality, hemolytic anemia, hepatic insufficiency (severe), hepatitis, hypertension, increased liver enzymes, jaundice, leukopenia, myocardial infarction, palpitations, pancreatitis, Stevens-Johnson syndrome, thrombocytopenia, visual disturbance (transient)

Mechanism of Action Nonsulfonylurea hypoglycemic agent which blocks ATP-dependent potassium channels, depolarizing the membrane and facilitating calcium entry through calcium channels. Increased intracellular calcium stimulates insulin release from the pancreatic beta cells. Repaglinide-induced insulin release is glucose-dependent.

Pharmacodynamics/Kinetics

Half-life Elimination ~1 hour

Time to Peak Plasma: 1 hour

Pregnancy Considerations

Repaglinide was shown to have a low potential to cross the placenta using an ex vivo perfusion model (Tertti 2011). Information describing the effects of repaglinide on pregnancy outcomes is limited.

Poorly controlled diabetes during pregnancy can be associated with an increased risk of adverse maternal and fetal outcomes, including diabetic ketoacidosis, preeclampsia, spontaneous abortion, preterm delivery, delivery complications, major birth defects, stillbirth, and macrosomia. To prevent adverse outcomes, prior to conception and throughout pregnancy, maternal blood glucose and HbA_{1c} should be kept as close to target goals as possible but without causing significant hypoglycemia (ADA 2020; Blumer 2013).

Agents other than repaglinide are currently recommended to treat diabetes mellitus in pregnancy (ADA 2020).

- **Repatha** *see* Evolocumab *on page 631*
- **Repatha Pushtronex System** *see* Evolocumab *on page 631*
- **Repatha SureClick** *see* Evolocumab *on page 631*
- **Replace [OTC]** *see* Vitamins (Multiple/Oral) *on page 1550*
- **Replace Without Iron [OTC]** *see* Vitamins (Multiple/Oral) *on page 1550*
- **Repliva 21/7** *see* Vitamins (Multiple/Oral) *on page 1550*
- **Repository Corticotropin** *see* Corticotropin *on page 412*
- **Reprexain [DSC]** *see* Hydrocodone and Ibuprofen *on page 769*
- **Requip [DSC]** *see* ROPINIRole *on page 1345*
- **Requip XL** *see* ROPINIRole *on page 1345*
- **Rescriptor [DSC]** *see* Delavirdine *on page 451*

Reslizumab (res LIZ ue mab)

Brand Names: US Cinqair

Brand Names: Canada Cinqair

Pharmacologic Category Interleukin-5 Antagonist; Monoclonal Antibody, Anti-Asthmatic

Use

Asthma: Add-on maintenance treatment of severe asthma in adults with an eosinophilic phenotype

Limitations of use: Not indicated for treatment of other eosinophilic conditions or for the relief of acute bronchospasm or status asthmaticus.

Local Anesthetic/Vasoconstrictor Precautions No information available to require special precautions

Effects on Dental Treatment Key adverse event(s) related to dental treatment: Oropharyngeal pain has been reported

Effects on Bleeding No information available to require special precautions

Adverse Reactions

Immunologic: Antibody development (5%)

Neuromuscular & skeletal: Increased creatine phosphokinase (20%; transient), myalgia (1%)

Respiratory: Oropharyngeal pain (3%)

<1%, postmarketing, and/or case reports: Anaphylaxis

Mechanism of Action Reslizumab is an interleukin-5 antagonist (IgG4 kappa). IL-5 is the major cytokine responsible for the growth and differentiation, recruitment, activation, and survival of eosinophils (a cell type associated with inflammation and an important component in the pathogenesis of asthma). Reslizumab, by inhibiting IL-5 signaling, reduces the production and survival of eosinophils; however, the mechanism of reslizumab action in asthma has not been definitively established.

Pharmacodynamics/Kinetics

Half-life Elimination ~24 days

Pregnancy Considerations

Reslizumab is a humanized monoclonal antibody (IgG_4). Potential placental transfer of human IgG is dependent upon the IgG subclass and gestational age, generally increasing as pregnancy progresses. The lowest exposure would be expected during the period of organogenesis (Palmeira 2012; Pentsuk 2009).

Uncontrolled asthma is associated with adverse events in pregnancy (increased risk of perinatal mortality, preeclampsia, preterm birth, low-birth-weight infants, cesarean delivery, and the development of gestational diabetes). Poorly controlled asthma or asthma exacerbations may have a greater fetal/maternal risk than what is associated with appropriately used asthma medications. Maternal treatment improves pregnancy outcomes by reducing the risk of some adverse events (eg, preterm birth, gestational diabetes) (ERS/TSANZ [Middleton 2020]; GINA 2020).

Use of monoclonal antibodies for the treatment of asthma in pregnancy may be considered when conventional therapies are insufficient; use of an agent other than reslizumab may be preferred (ERS/TSANZ [Middleton 2020]). The long half-life of reslizumab should be considered if required for a pregnant woman.

Data collection to monitor pregnancy and infant outcomes associated with asthma and the medications used to treat asthma in pregnancy is ongoing. Health care providers are encouraged to enroll exposed pregnant females in the MotherToBaby Pregnancy Studies conducted by the Organization of Teratology Information Specialists (877-311-8972 or https://mothertobaby.org). Patients may also enroll themselves.

- **Respa-BR [DSC]** *see* Brompheniramine *on page 252*
- **Restasis** *see* CycloSPORINE (Ophthalmic) *on page 423*
- **Restasis MultiDose** *see* CycloSPORINE (Ophthalmic) *on page 423*
- **Restoril** *see* Temazepam *on page 1415*
- **Restylane [DSC]** *see* Hyaluronate and Derivatives *on page 761*
- **Restylane-L [DSC]** *see* Hyaluronate and Derivatives *on page 761*
- **Restylane Kysse** *see* Hyaluronate and Derivatives *on page 761*
- **Restylane Lyft** *see* Hyaluronate and Derivatives *on page 761*
- **Restylane Silk** *see* Hyaluronate and Derivatives *on page 761*
- **Retacrit** *see* Epoetin Alfa *on page 577*

Retapamulin (re te PAM ue lin)

Brand Names: US Altabax

Brand Names: Canada Altargo [DSC]

Pharmacologic Category Antibiotic, Pleuromutilin; Antibiotic, Topical

Use Impetigo: Treatment of impetigo due to *Staphylococcus aureus* (methicillin-susceptible isolates only) or *Streptococcus pyogenes* in adults and pediatric patients 9 months and older.

Local Anesthetic/Vasoconstrictor Precautions

No information available to require special precautions

Effects on Dental Treatment No significant effects or complications reported

Effects on Bleeding No information available to require special precautions

Adverse Reactions

1% to 10%:

Central nervous system: Headache (1% to 2%)

Dermatologic: Eczema (infants, children & adolescents: 1%)

Gastrointestinal: Diarrhea (1% to 2%), nausea (1%)

Local: Application site irritation (adults: 2%), application site pruritus (infants, children & adolescents: 2%)

Respiratory: Nasopharyngitis (1% to 2%)

<1%, postmarketing, and/or case reports: Angioedema, application site burning, application site pain, contact dermatitis, epistaxis, erythema, hypersensitivity reaction, increased creatine phosphokinase

Mechanism of Action Primarily bacteriostatic; inhibits normal bacterial protein biosynthesis by binding at a unique site (protein L3) on the ribosomal 50S subunit; prevents formation of active 50S ribosomal subunits by inhibiting peptidyl transfer and blocking P-site interactions at this site

Pregnancy Considerations Retapamulin has limited systemic absorption following topical administration. Use during pregnancy is not expected to result in significant exposure to the fetus.

- **Retavase** *see* Reteplase *on page 1318*
- **Retavase Half-Kit** *see* Reteplase *on page 1318*

Reteplase (RE ta plase)

Related Information

Cardiovascular Diseases *on page 1654*

Brand Names: US Retavase; Retavase Half-Kit

Pharmacologic Category Thrombolytic Agent

Use

ST-elevation myocardial infarction, acute: Use in acute ST-elevation myocardial infarction (STEMI) to reduce the risk of death and heart failure

Limitation of use: The risk of stroke may outweigh the benefit produced by thrombolytic therapy in patients whose STEMI puts them at low risk for death or heart failure.

Local Anesthetic/Vasoconstrictor Precautions

No information available to require special precautions

Effects on Dental Treatment Key adverse event(s) related to dental treatment: Bleeding is the most frequent adverse effect of reteplase. See Effects on Bleeding.

Effects on Bleeding Bleeding is the most frequent adverse effect associated with reteplase. It is unlikely that ambulatory patients presenting for dental treatment will be taking intravenous anticoagulant therapy.

Adverse Reactions
>10%: Local: Bleeding at injection site (49%)
1% to 10%:
Gastrointestinal: Gastrointestinal hemorrhage (9%)
Hematologic & oncologic: Hemorrhage (genitourinary: 10%), anemia (1%)
<1%, postmarketing, and/or case reports: Anaphylactoid shock, hypersensitivity reaction, intracranial hemorrhage

Mechanism of Action Reteplase is a recombinant plasminogen activator which catalyzes the cleavage of endogenous plasminogen to generate plasmin. Plasmin in turn degrades the fibrin matrix of the thrombus, thereby exerting its thrombolytic action.

Pharmacodynamics/Kinetics
Onset of Action Thrombolysis: 30 to 90 minutes
Half-life Elimination 13 to 16 minutes

Pregnancy Considerations Adverse events have been observed in some animal reproduction studies. The risk of bleeding may be increased in pregnant women.

- **Retevmo** *see* Selpercatinib *on page 1364*
- **Retin-A** *see* Tretinoin (Topical) *on page 1484*
- **Retin-A Micro** *see* Tretinoin (Topical) *on page 1484*
- **Retin-A Micro Pump** *see* Tretinoin (Topical) *on page 1484*
- **RET Inhibitor LOXO-292** *see* Selpercatinib *on page 1364*
- **Retinoic Acid** *see* Tretinoin (Topical) *on page 1484*
- **Retinol** *see* Vitamin A *on page 1549*
- **RET Kinase Inhibitor LOXO-292** *see* Selpercatinib *on page 1364*
- **Retrovir** *see* Zidovudine *on page 1569*
- **Revatio** *see* Sildenafil *on page 1369*

Revefenacin (REV e FEN a sin)

Brand Names: US Yupelri

Pharmacologic Category Anticholinergic Agent; Anticholinergic Agent, Long-Acting

Use Chronic obstructive pulmonary disease: Maintenance treatment of chronic obstructive pulmonary disease (COPD)

Local Anesthetic/Vasoconstrictor Precautions No information available to require special precautions

Effects on Dental Treatment Key adverse event(s) related to dental treatment: Nasopharyngitis, upper respiratory tract infection, bronchitis, and oropharyngeal pain have been observed.

Effects on Bleeding No information available to require special precautions

Adverse Reactions
1% to 10%:
Cardiovascular: Hypertension (1% to <2%)
Central nervous system: Headache (4%), dizziness (1% to <2%)
Neuromuscular & skeletal: Back pain (2%)
Respiratory: Nasopharyngitis (4%), upper respiratory tract infection (3%), bronchitis (1% to <2%), oropharyngeal pain (1% to <2%)
<1%, postmarketing, and/or case reports: Paradoxical bronchospasm

Mechanism of Action Revefenacin is a long-acting muscarinic antagonist which competitively and reversibly inhibits the action of acetylcholine at type 3 muscarinic (M_3) receptors in bronchial smooth muscle causing bronchodilation.

Pharmacodynamics/Kinetics
Onset of Action Bronchodilation onset is within 45 minutes after a single dose and peak FEV_1 effect is 2 to 3 hours following a single dose (Quinn 2018)
Duration of Action Bronchodilation: Up to 24 hours (Quinn 2018)
Half-life Elimination 22 to 70 hours (revefenacin and active metabolite)
Time to Peak 14 to 41 minutes (after start of nebulization)

Reproductive Considerations
Females of reproductive potential were not included in original studies (Pudi 2017; Quinn 2017).

Pregnancy Considerations
Adverse events were not observed in animal reproduction studies.

- **Revlimid** *see* Lenalidomide *on page 883*
- **Revolade** *see* Eltrombopag *on page 551*
- **Revonto** *see* Dantrolene *on page 434*
- **Rexaphenac** *see* Diclofenac (Topical) *on page 489*
- **Reyataz** *see* Atazanavir *on page 186*
- **Reyvow** *see* Lasmiditan *on page 880*
- **ReZyst IM [DSC]** *see Lactobacillus on page 869*
- **RG7204** *see* Vemurafenib *on page 1537*
- **RG7601** *see* Venetoclax *on page 1538*
- **RG7853** *see* Alectinib *on page 92*
- **rhAT** *see* Antithrombin *on page 156*
- **rhATIII** *see* Antithrombin *on page 156*
- **rhDNase** *see* Dornase Alfa *on page 515*
- **Rheumatrex [DSC]** *see* Methotrexate *on page 990*
- **rhIGF-1 (Mecasermin [Increlex])** *see* Mecasermin *on page 951*
- **Rhinocort Allergy [OTC]** *see* Budesonide (Nasal) *on page 253*
- **Rhinocort Allergy OTC** *see* Budesonide (Nasal) *on page 253*
- **Rhinocort Aqua [DSC]** *see* Budesonide (Nasal) *on page 253*
- **r-Hirudin** *see* Desirudin *on page 459*
- **rhKGF** *see* Palifermin *on page 1181*
- **r-hLH** *see* Lutropin Alfa *on page 944*
- **Rhofade** *see* Oxymetazoline (Topical) *on page 1175*
- **rhPTH(1-34)** *see* Teriparatide *on page 1424*
- **rhPTH(1-84)** *see* Parathyroid Hormone *on page 1192*
- **rh-TSH** *see* Thyrotropin Alpha *on page 1442*
- ***r*HuEPO** *see* Epoetin Alfa *on page 577*
- ***r*HuEPO-Beta** *see* Methoxy Polyethylene Glycol-Epoetin Beta *on page 993*
- **rhuFabV2** *see* Ranibizumab *on page 1309*
- **rhuGM-CSF** *see* Sargramostim *on page 1358*
- **rhu Keratinocyte Growth Factor** *see* Palifermin *on page 1181*
- **rHu-KGF** *see* Palifermin *on page 1181*
- **rhuMAb-2C4** *see* Pertuzumab *on page 1220*
- **rhuMAb-E25** *see* Omalizumab *on page 1134*

- **rHuMAb-EGFr** *see* Panitumumab *on page* 1187
- **rhuMAb HER2** *see* Trastuzumab *on page* 1479
- **rhuMAb-VEGF** *see* Bevacizumab *on page* 242
- **RiaSTAP** *see* Fibrinogen Concentrate (Human) *on page* 666
- **Ribasphere [DSC]** *see* Ribavirin (Systemic) *on page* 1320
- **Ribasphere RibaPak (600 Pack) [DSC]** *see* Ribavirin (Systemic) *on page* 1320
- **Ribasphere RibaPak (800 Pack) [DSC]** *see* Ribavirin (Systemic) *on page* 1320
- **Ribasphere RibaPak (1000 Pack) [DSC]** *see* Ribavirin (Systemic) *on page* 1320
- **Ribasphere Ribapak (1200 Pack) [DSC]** *see* Ribavirin (Systemic) *on page* 1320

Ribavirin (Systemic) (rye ba VYE rin)

Brand Names: US Copegus [DSC]; Moderiba (1000 MG Pack) [DSC]; Moderiba (1200 MG Pack) [DSC]; Moderiba (600 MG Pack) [DSC]; Moderiba (800 MG Pack) [DSC]; Moderiba 1200 Dose Pack [DSC]; Moderiba 800 Dose Pack [DSC]; Moderiba [DSC]; Rebetol [DSC]; Ribasphere RibaPak (1000 Pack) [DSC]; Ribasphere Ribapak (1200 Pack) [DSC]; Ribasphere RibaPak (600 Pack) [DSC]; Ribasphere RibaPak (800 Pack) [DSC]; Ribasphere [DSC]

Brand Names: Canada Ibavyr; Moderiba [DSC]

Pharmacologic Category Antihepaciviral, Nucleoside (Anti-HCV)

Use Hepatitis C virus infection, chronic: Ribavirin, in combination with direct-acting antivirals, is recommended in the AASLD/IDSA guidelines as part of an alternative regimen for certain clinical scenarios. Hepatitis C treatment guidelines are constantly changing with the advent of new treatment therapies and information; consult current clinical practice guidelines for the most recent treatment recommendations. The combination of peginterferon and ribavirin, even with additional preferred HCV antiviral agent(s), is **not** recommended for hepatitis C virus (HCV) (regardless of genotype) in HCV adult treatment guidelines (treatment-naive or treatment-experienced). Peginterferon and ribavirin-based regimens, however, may remain in use in resource-limited settings where interferon-free regimens are inaccessible or unavailable (AASLD/IDSA 2018).

Local Anesthetic/Vasoconstrictor Precautions No information available to require special precautions

Effects on Dental Treatment Key adverse event(s) related to dental treatment: Xerostomia (normal salivary flow resumes upon discontinuation) and taste perversion.

Effects on Bleeding No information available to require special precautions

Adverse Reactions Clinical trials were conducted in patients receiving peginterferon alfa-2a, peginterferon alfa-2b, and interferon alfa-2b and it is not possible to correlate frequency of adverse events with ribavirin alone. Moreover, ribavirin monotherapy is not an effective treatment for chronic hepatitis.

>10%:

Dermatologic: Alopecia (17% to 36%; children and adolescents: 17% to 23%), dermatitis (13% to 16%), dermatologic disorder (children and adolescents: 47%), diaphoresis (4% to 11%), pruritus (13% to 29%; children and adolescents: 11% to 12%), skin rash (5% to 34%; children and adolescents: 15% to 17%), xeroderma (10% to 24%)

Endocrine & metabolic: Growth retardation (children and adolescents: <3rd percentile height decrease: 70%, >15 percentile height or weight decrease: 11% to 43%, >30 percentile height decrease: ≤13%), hyperuricemia (33% to 38%), weight loss (10% to 29%; children and adolescents: 19%)

Gastrointestinal: Abdominal pain (8% to 21%), anorexia (21% to 32%; children and adolescents: 29% to 51%), decreased appetite (children and adolescents: 11% to 22%), diarrhea (10% to 22%), dyspepsia (5% to 16%; children and adolescents: <1%), gastrointestinal disease (children and adolescents: 49% to 56%), nausea (≤47%; children and adolescents: 18% to 33%), upper abdominal pain (children and adolescents: 12%), vomiting (≤29%; children and adolescents: 27% to 42%), xerostomia (4% to 12%)

Hematologic & oncologic: Anemia (11% to 35%), hemolytic anemia (10% to 13%), lymphocytopenia (12% to 14%), neutropenia (8% to 40%; severe neutropenia (children and adolescents: 1%)

Hepatic: Hyperbilirubinemia (10% to 14%)

Infection: Viral infection (12%)

Local: Erythema at injection site (children and adolescents: 29%), inflammation at injection site (13% to 25%; children and adolescents: 14%), injection site reaction (5% to 58%; children and adolescents: 19% to 45%)

Nervous system: Anxiety (≤47%), chills (23% to 39%; children and adolescents: 21%), depression (≤40%, severe depression: <1%; children and adolescents: 1% to 13%), dizziness (13% to 26%), emotional lability (≤47%; children and adolescents: 16%), fatigue (≤68%; children and adolescents: 25% to 58%), headache (41% to 69%; severe headache: children and adolescents: 1%), insomnia (26% to 41%; children and adolescents: 9% to 14%), irritability (≤47%; children and adolescents: 10% to 24%), lack of concentration (10% to 21%; children and adolescents: 5%), nervousness (≤38%; children and adolescents: 3% to 7%), pain (9% to 13%), right upper quadrant pain (6% to 12%), rigors (25% to 48%; children and adolescents: 25%)

Neuromuscular & skeletal: Arthralgia (21% to 34%; children and adolescents: 15% to 17%), asthenia (≤68%; children and adolescents: 5% to 15%), musculoskeletal pain (19% to 21%; children and adolescents: 21% to 35%), myalgia (22% to 64%; children and adolescents: 17% to 32%)

Respiratory: Cough (7% to 23%), dyspnea (13% to 26%; children and adolescents: 5%), flu-like symptoms (15% to 16%; children and adolescents: 31% to 91%), pharyngitis (12% to 13%), sinusitis (5% to 12%; children and adolescents: <1%), upper respiratory tract infection (children and adolescents: 60%)

Miscellaneous: Fever (21% to 55%; children and adolescents: 61% to 80%; high fever: children and adolescents: 4%)

1% to 10%:

Cardiovascular: Chest pain (5% to 9%), flushing (3% to 4%)

Dermatologic: Eczema (4% to 5%)

Endocrine & metabolic: Hypothyroidism (4% to 5%), menstrual disease (6% to 7%)
Gastrointestinal: Constipation (5%), decompensated liver disease (2%), dysgeusia (4% to 9%; children and adolescents: <1%)
Hematologic & oncologic: Leukopenia (5% to 10%), thrombocytopenia (≤8%)
Hepatic: Hepatomegaly (4%), increased serum alanine aminotransferase (2.1 to 5 x baseline: 1% to 5%; 5.1 x 10 x baseline: 3%; 2 x baseline: ≤1%)
Infection: Bacterial infection (3% to 5%), fungal infection (1% to 6%)
Local: Pain at injection site (children and adolescents: 1%; severe)
Nervous system: Aggressive behavior (children and adolescents: 3%), agitation (5% to 8%), hostility (children and adolescents: 2%), malaise (4% to 6%), memory impairment (5% to 6%), mood changes (5% to 9%), suicidal ideation (≤2%)
Neuromuscular & skeletal: Back pain (5%), limb pain (children and adolescents: 1%; severe)
Ophthalmic: Blurred vision (2% to 6%), conjunctivitis (4% to 5%)
Respiratory: Dyspnea on exertion (4% to 7%), rhinitis (6% to 8%)

<1%:
Cardiovascular: Angina pectoris, cardiac arrhythmia
Endocrine & metabolic: Gout
Gastrointestinal: Cholangitis, gastrointestinal hemorrhage, peptic ulcer
Hematologic & oncologic: Thrombotic thrombocytopenic purpura
Hepatic: Liver steatosis
Nervous system: Hallucination, peripheral neuropathy
Neuromuscular & skeletal: Myositis

Frequency not defined: Hematologic & oncologic: Hemolysis

Postmarketing:
Dermatologic: Exfoliative dermatitis, Stevens-Johnson syndrome, toxic epidermal necrolysis
Endocrine & metabolic: Dehydration, diabetes mellitus, lactic acidosis (Smith 2019)
Gastrointestinal: Colitis
Hematologic & oncologic: Aplastic anemia, bone marrow depression, pure red cell aplasia, sarcoidosis
Hypersensitivity: Anaphylaxis, angioedema, hypersensitivity reaction
Immunologic: Autoimmune disease, exacerbation of sarcoidosis
Nervous system: Cerebrovascular disease, homicidal ideation, vertigo
Ophthalmic: Retinal detachment (serous)
Otic: Auditory disturbance, hearing loss
Respiratory: Bronchoconstriction, pneumonia, pneumonitis, pulmonary disease, pulmonary hypertension, pulmonary infiltrates

Mechanism of Action Inhibits replication of RNA and DNA viruses; inhibits influenza virus RNA polymerase activity and inhibits the initiation and elongation of RNA fragments resulting in inhibition of viral protein synthesis

Pharmacodynamics/Kinetics

Half-life Elimination Plasma: Adults:
Capsule, single dose: 24 hours in healthy adults, 44 hours with chronic hepatitis C infection (increases to ~298 hours at steady state)
Tablet, single dose: ~120 to 170 hours

Time to Peak Serum: Oral capsule: Multiple doses: Children and Adolescents 3 to 16 years: ~2 hours; Adults: 3 hours; Tablet: 2 hours

Reproductive Considerations

Use is contraindicated in females who may become pregnant. **[US Boxed Warning]: Avoid pregnancy during therapy and for 6 months after completion of treatment in both female patients and female partners of male patients who are taking ribavirin therapy. Effective contraception must be utilized during treatment and during the 6-month post-treatment follow-up period.**

Evaluate pregnancy status prior to use in females of reproductive potential. A negative pregnancy test is required immediately before initiation, and periodically during therapy, and during the 6 months after treatment is discontinued. If patient or female partner becomes pregnant during treatment, she should be counseled about potential risks of exposure.

Concentrations of ribavirin are higher in seminal fluid than serum in male patients treated for HCV infection; in addition, alterations in spermatogenesis have been noted (Sinclair 2017).

HCV-infected females of childbearing potential should consider postponing pregnancy until therapy is complete to reduce the risk of HCV transmission (AASLD/IDSA 2018).

Pregnancy Considerations

[US Boxed Warning]: Significant teratogenic and embryocidal effects have been demonstrated in all animal species exposed to ribavirin. In addition, ribavirin has a multiple dose half-life of 12 days, and may persist in non-plasma compartments for as long as 6 months. Therefore, ribavirin therapy is contraindicated in women who are pregnant and in the male partners of women who are pregnant. Preliminary data from the Ribavirin Pregnancy Registry is available but given slow enrollment insufficient to draw conclusions related to teratogenic effects in humans (Sinclair 2017).

Treatment of hepatitis C is not currently recommended to treat maternal infection or to decrease the risk of mother-to-child transmission during pregnancy (Tran 2016).

[US Boxed Warning]: Avoid pregnancy during therapy and for 6 months after completion of treatment in both female patients and female partners of male patients who are taking ribavirin therapy.

Health care providers and patients are encouraged to enroll females exposed to ribavirin during pregnancy or within 6 months after treatment in the Ribavirin Pregnancy Registry (800-593-2214).

Ribavirin (Oral Inhalation) (rye ba VYE rin)

Brand Names: US Virazole

Brand Names: Canada Virazole

Pharmacologic Category Antiviral Agent

Use Respiratory syncytial virus: Treatment of hospitalized infants and young children with respiratory syncytial virus (RSV) infections with efficacy possibly increased in early course therapy; treatment of severe lower respiratory tract RSV infections in patients with an underlying compromising condition (prematurity, cardiopulmonary disease, or immunosuppression)

Local Anesthetic/Vasoconstrictor Precautions No information available to require special precautions

Effects on Dental Treatment Key adverse event(s) related to dental treatment: Xerostomia (normal salivary flow resumes upon discontinuation) and taste perversion.

Effects on Bleeding No information available to require special precautions

Adverse Reactions

Frequency not defined:

Cardiovascular: Bigeminy, bradycardia, chest pain, hypotension, tachycardia

Dermatologic: Skin rash

Ophthalmic: Conjunctivitis

Respiratory: Apnea, atelectasis, bacterial pneumonia, bronchospasm, cyanosis, dyspnea, hypoventilation, pneumothorax, pulmonary complications (ventilator dependence), pulmonary edema, severe dyspnea (worsening of respiratory status)

<1%, postmarketing, and/or case reports: Anemia, hemolytic anemia, reticulocytosis

Mechanism of Action Inhibits replication of RNA and DNA viruses; inhibits influenza virus RNA polymerase activity and inhibits the initiation and elongation of RNA fragments resulting in inhibition of viral protein synthesis

Pharmacodynamics/Kinetics

Half-life Elimination

Respiratory tract secretions: Infants and Children 6 weeks to 7 years: ~2 hours (Englund 1990)

Plasma: Infants and Children: Inhalation: 9.5 hours

Time to Peak Serum: Inhalation: At end of inhalation period

Reproductive Considerations

Use is contraindicated in females who may become pregnant.

Pregnancy Considerations

Use is contraindicated in females who are pregnant. **[US Boxed Warning]: Aerosolized ribavirin is not indicated for use in adults. Be aware that ribavirin has been shown to produce testicular lesions in rodents and to be teratogenic in all animal species in which adequate studies have been conducted (rodents and rabbits).** The manufacturer recommends that pregnant health care workers take precautions to limit exposure to ribavirin aerosol; potential occupational exposure may be greatest if administration is via oxygen tent or hood, and lower if administered via mechanical ventilation. The minimum interval following exposure to ribavirin inhalation prior to pregnancy is not known.

Ribociclib (rye boe SYE klib)

Brand Names: US Kisqali (200 MG Dose); Kisqali (400 MG Dose); Kisqali (600 MG Dose)

Brand Names: Canada Kisqali

Pharmacologic Category Antineoplastic Agent, Cyclin-Dependent Kinase Inhibitor

Use

Breast cancer, advanced or metastatic:

Treatment of hormone receptor (HR)-positive, human epidermal growth factor receptor 2 (HER2)-negative advanced or metastatic breast cancer (in combination with an aromatase inhibitor) in pre-/perimenopausal or postmenopausal females as initial endocrine-based therapy.

Treatment of HR-positive, HER2-negative advanced or metastatic breast cancer (in combination with fulvestrant) in postmenopausal females as initial endocrine-based therapy or following disease progression on endocrine therapy.

Local Anesthetic/Vasoconstrictor Precautions Ribociclib is one of the drugs confirmed to prolong the QT interval and is accepted as having a risk of causing torsades de pointes. The risk of drug-induced torsades de pointes is extremely low when a single QT interval prolonging drug is prescribed. In terms of epinephrine, it is not known what effect vasoconstrictors in the local anesthetic regimen will have in patients with a known history of congenital prolonged QT interval or in patients taking any medication that prolongs the QT interval. Until more information is obtained, it is suggested that the clinician consult with the physician prior to the use of a vasoconstrictor in suspected patients, and that the vasoconstrictor (epinephrine, levonordefrin [Neo-Cobefrin®]) be used with caution.

Effects on Dental Treatment No significant effects or complications reported

Effects on Bleeding Chemotherapy may result in significant reduction in platelet counts (thrombocytopenia) and altered hemostasis.

Adverse Reactions As reported with combination therapy.

>10%:

Cardiovascular: Peripheral edema (12% to 15%)

Central nervous system: Fatigue (37%), headache (22%), dizziness (13%), insomnia (12%)

Dermatologic: Alopecia (19% to 33%), skin rash (17% to 23%), pruritus (10% to 20%)

Endocrine & metabolic: Increased gamma-glutamyl transferase (42% to 52%), decreased serum glucose (10% to 23%), decreased serum albumin (12%), decreased serum potassium (11%)

Gastrointestinal: Nausea (31% to 52%), diarrhea (29% to 35%), vomiting (27% to 29%), constipation (16% to 25%), decreased appetite (16% to 19%), abdominal pain (11% to 17%), stomatitis (10% to 12%; grade 3: <1%)

Genitourinary: Urinary tract infection (11%)

Hematologic & oncologic: Neutropenia (69% to 78%; grade 3: 46% to 55%; grade 4: 7% to 10%), leukopenia (27% to 33%; grade 3: 12% to 20%; grade 4: ≤1%), anemia (17% to 19%; grade 3: 1% to 3%; grade 4: <1%), abnormal serum phosphorus level (decreased; 13% to 18%; grade 3: 2% to 5%; grade 4: 1%), lymphocytopenia (11%; grade 3: 6%; grade 4: 1%)

Hepatic: Increased serum aspartate aminotransferase (13% to 49%), increased serum alanine aminotransferase (13% to 46%), abnormal hepatic function tests (18%)

Infection: Infection (35% to 42%)

Neuromuscular & skeletal: Arthralgia (33%), back pain (20%), asthenia (12% to 14%)

Renal: Increased serum creatinine (20% to 65%)

Respiratory: Cough (15% to 22%), dyspnea (12% to 15%)

Miscellaneous: Fever (11% to 17%)

1% to 10%:

Cardiovascular: Prolonged QT interval on ECG (1% to 6%), syncope (≤3%)

Central nervous system: Vertigo (5%)

Dermatologic: Xeroderma (8%), erythema of skin (4%), vitiligo (3%)

Endocrine & metabolic: Hypocalcemia (2% to 4%)

Gastrointestinal: Dyspepsia (5% to 10%), dysgeusia (7%), xerostomia (5%)
Hematologic & oncologic: Thrombocytopenia (9%), febrile neutropenia (1%)
Hepatic: Increased serum bilirubin (1%)
Neuromuscular & skeletal: Limb pain (10%)
Ophthalmic: Dry eye syndrome (4% to 5%), increased lacrimation (4%)
Respiratory: Oropharyngeal pain (7%), interstitial pulmonary disease (≤1%), pneumonitis (≤1%)

<1%: Acute respiratory distress syndrome, gastroenteritis, hypersensitivity pneumonitis, pulmonary fibrosis, pulmonary infiltrates, sepsis

Mechanism of Action Ribociclib is a small molecule cyclin-dependent kinase (CDK) inhibitor which is selective for CDK 4 and 6; it blocks retinoblastoma protein phosphorylation and prevents progression through the cell cycle, resulting in arrest at the G1 phase (Hortobagyi 2016). The combination of ribociclib and an aromatase inhibitor causes increased inhibition of tumor growth compared with each agent alone. The combination of ribociclib and fulvestrant resulted in tumor growth inhibition in estrogen receptor-positive breast cancer models.

Pharmacodynamics/Kinetics

Half-life Elimination Terminal: ~30 to 55 hours

Time to Peak 1 to 4 hours

Reproductive Considerations

Women of reproductive potential should have a pregnancy test prior to treatment and use effective contraception during treatment and for at least 3 weeks after the last ribociclib dose.

Pregnancy Considerations

Based on the mechanism of action and data from animal reproduction studies, ribociclib may be expected to cause fetal harm if used during pregnancy.

Riboflavin (RYE boe flay vin)

Brand Names: US B-2-400 [OTC]

Pharmacologic Category Vitamin, Water Soluble

Use Dietary supplement

Local Anesthetic/Vasoconstrictor Precautions

No information available to require special precautions

Effects on Dental Treatment No significant effects or complications reported

Effects on Bleeding No information available to require special precautions

Adverse Reactions Frequency not defined: Genitourinary: Urine discoloration (yellow-orange)

Mechanism of Action Component of flavoprotein enzymes that work together, which are necessary for normal tissue respiration; also needed for activation of pyridoxine and conversion of tryptophan to niacin

Pharmacodynamics/Kinetics

Half-life Elimination Biologic: 66 to 84 minutes

Pregnancy Considerations Water-soluble vitamins cross the placenta. Riboflavin requirements may be increased in pregnant women compared to nonpregnant women (IOM 1998).

Riboflavin 5'-Phosphate

(RYE boe flay vin five FOS fate)

Brand Names: US Photrexa Viscous; Photrexa-Photrexa Viscous Kit

Pharmacologic Category Corneal Collagen Cross-Linking Agent, Ophthalmic; Ophthalmic Agent

Use

Corneal ectasia following refractive surgery: Treatment of corneal ectasia following refractive surgery with the KXL System in corneal collagen cross-linking.

Keratoconus, progressive: Treatment of progressive keratoconus with the KXL System in corneal collagen cross-linking.

Local Anesthetic/Vasoconstrictor Precautions

No information available to require special precautions

Effects on Dental Treatment No significant effects or complications reported

Effects on Bleeding No information available to require special precautions

Adverse Reactions

>10%:

Central nervous system: Foreign body sensation of eye (14% to 15%)
Ophthalmic: Corneal opacity (haze) (64% to 71%), corneal disease (3% to 28%), eye pain (17% to 26%), punctate keratitis (20% to 25%), corneal edema (in progressive keratoconus patients: 24%; all other patients: 3% to 9%), photophobia (2% to 19%), blurred vision (16% to 17%), ocular hyperemia (8% to 14%), dry eye syndrome (6% to 14%), decreased visual acuity (10% to 11%)

1% to 10%:

Central nervous system: Headache (4% to 8%)
Ophthalmic: Increased lacrimation (5% to 10%), eye discomfort (9%), conjunctival edema (7%), eyelid edema (5% to 6%), anterior chamber inflammation (2% to 6%), visual impairment (3% to 4%), blepharitis (3%), keratitis (1% to 3%), asthenopia (2%), diplopia (2%), eye discharge (2%), eye pruritus (2%), vitreous detachment (2%), eye injury (associated with device; 1% to 2%), visual halos around lights (1% to 2%)

Mechanism of Action Photo enhancer that generates singlet oxygen in corneal collagen cross-linking.

Pregnancy Considerations Animal reproduction studies have not been conducted with riboflavin 5'-phosphate. The manufacturer recommends that the corneal collagen cross-linking procedure not be done during pregnancy. Pregnancy may be a risk factor for the progression of keratoconus (Bilgihan 2011).

- ◆ **RID Lice Elimination Essentials [OTC] [DSC]** *see* Pyrethrins and Piperonyl Butoxide *on page 1293*
- ◆ **RID Lice Killing [OTC]** *see* Pyrethrins and Piperonyl Butoxide *on page 1293*
- ◆ **RID Lice Treatment Complete [OTC]** *see* Pyrethrins and Piperonyl Butoxide *on page 1293*

Rifabutin (rif a BYOO tin)

Related Information

Systemic Viral Diseases *on page 1709*

Brand Names: US Mycobutin

Brand Names: Canada Mycobutin

Pharmacologic Category Antitubercular Agent; Rifamycin

Use *Mycobacterium avium* complex (MAC), prophylaxis: Prevention of disseminated MAC disease in patients with advanced human immunodeficiency virus (HIV) infection

Local Anesthetic/Vasoconstrictor Precautions

No information available to require special precautions

Effects on Dental Treatment Key adverse event(s) related to dental treatment: Saliva (reddish orange). The reddish-orange color of the saliva may cause a unique coloration to plaque and calculus buildup. Some patients may want more regular cleanings to remove.

Effects on Bleeding No information available to require special precautions

Adverse Reactions

>10%:

Dermatologic: Skin rash (11%)

Genitourinary: Discoloration of urine (30%)

Hematologic & oncologic: Neutropenia (25%), leukopenia (10% to 17%)

1% to 10%:

Gastrointestinal: Nausea (≤6%), abdominal pain (4%), dysgeusia (3%), dyspepsia (3%), eructation (3%), vomiting (≤3%), flatulence (2%)

Hematologic & oncologic: Thrombocytopenia (5%)

Neuromuscular & skeletal: Myalgia (2%)

Miscellaneous: Fever (2%)

<1%, postmarketing, and/or case reports: Abnormal T waves on ECG, agranulocytosis, aphasia, arthralgia, bronchospasm, chest pain, *Clostridioides* (formerly *Clostridium*) *difficile*-associated diarrhea, confusion, corneal deposits, dyspnea, flu-like symptoms, granulocytopenia, hemolysis, hepatitis, hypersensitivity, jaundice, lymphocytopenia, myositis, pancytopenia, paresthesia, pseudomembranous colitis, seizure, skin discoloration, thrombotic thrombocytopenic purpura, uveitis

Mechanism of Action Inhibits DNA-dependent RNA polymerase at the beta subunit which prevents chain initiation

Pharmacodynamics/Kinetics

Half-life Elimination Terminal: 45 hours (range: 16 to 69 hours)

Time to Peak Serum: 2 to 4 hours

Pregnancy Considerations Based on human placenta perfusion studies, rifabutin crosses the placenta (Magee 1996).

◆ **Rifadin** *see* RifAMPin *on page 1324*

◆ **Rifamate [DSC]** *see* Rifampin and Isoniazid *on page 1325*

◆ **Rifampicin** *see* RifAMPin *on page 1324*

RifAMPin (rif AM pin)

Related Information

Rifapentine *on page 1325*

Brand Names: US Rifadin

Brand Names: Canada Rifadin; Rofact

Pharmacologic Category Antitubercular Agent; Rifamycin

Use

Meningococcal prophylaxis: Treatment of asymptomatic carriers of *Neisseria meningitidis* to eliminate meningococci from the nasopharynx.

Tuberculosis: Treatment of tuberculosis in combination with other agents.

Local Anesthetic/Vasoconstrictor Precautions No information available to require special precautions

Effects on Dental Treatment Key adverse event(s) related to dental treatment: Saliva (reddish orange). The reddish-orange color of the saliva may cause a unique coloration to plaque and calculus buildup. Some patients may want more regular cleanings to remove.

Effects on Bleeding Rifampin doses >600 mg may be associated with more adverse events including hemolytic anemia and thrombocytopenia.

Adverse Reactions

Frequency not defined:

Cardiovascular: Decreased blood pressure, flushing, shock, vasculitis

Central nervous system: Ataxia, behavioral changes, confusion, dizziness, drowsiness, fatigue, headache, lack of concentration, myasthenia, numbness, peripheral pain, sore mouth

Dermatologic: Erythema multiforme, pemphigoid reaction, pruritus, skin rash, urticaria

Endocrine & metabolic: Adrenocortical insufficiency, menstrual disease

Gastrointestinal: Abdominal cramps, anorexia, diarrhea, epigastric discomfort, flatulence, glossalgia, heartburn, nausea, staining of tooth, vomiting

Genitourinary: Hemoglobinuria, hematuria

Hematologic & oncologic: Decreased hemoglobin, disorder of hemostatic components of blood (vitamin K-dependent), disseminated intravascular coagulation, eosinophilia, hemolysis, hemolytic anemia, hemorrhage, leukopenia, thrombocytopenia (especially with high-dose therapy)

Hepatic: Abnormal hepatic function tests, hepatic insufficiency, hyperbilirubinemia, jaundice

Hypersensitivity: Hypersensitivity reaction

Neuromuscular & skeletal: Myopathy

Ophthalmic: Conjunctivitis, visual disturbance

Renal: Acute renal failure, interstitial nephritis, renal insufficiency, renal tubular necrosis

Respiratory: Dyspnea, flu-like symptoms, wheezing

Miscellaneous: Fever

<1%, postmarketing, and/or case reports: Acute generalized exanthematous pustulosis, agranulocytosis, anaphylaxis, cerebral hemorrhage, cholestasis, *Clostridioides difficile* colitis, cutaneous lupus erythematosus (Patel 2001), drug reaction with eosinophilia and systemic symptoms, facial edema, hepatitis (including shock-like syndrome with hepatic involvement), increased blood urea nitrogen, increased uric acid, peripheral edema, psychosis, severe dermatological reaction, Stevens-Johnson syndrome, toxic epidermal necrolysis

Mechanism of Action Inhibits bacterial RNA synthesis by binding to the beta subunit of DNA-dependent RNA polymerase, blocking RNA transcription

Pharmacodynamics/Kinetics

Duration of Action ≤24 hours

Half-life Elimination 3 to 4 hours, prolonged with hepatic impairment; End-stage renal disease: 1.8 to 11 hours

Time to Peak Serum: Oral: 2 to 4 hours

Pregnancy Considerations

Rifampin crosses the human placenta. Postnatal hemorrhages have been reported in the infant and mother with administration during the last few weeks of pregnancy.

Maternal treatment of tuberculosis is recommended when the probability of maternal disease is moderate to high due to the risk of infection to the fetus (ATC/CDC 2003). Rifampin may be considered for use as an alternative agent in pregnant women for the treatment of mild illness due to human anaplasmosis (also known as human granulocytic anaplasmosis [HGA]); case reports have shown favorable maternal and pregnancy outcomes in small numbers of rifampin-treated pregnant women (CDC [Biggs 2016]).

Rifampin and Isoniazid

(rif AM pin & eye soe NYE a zid)

Related Information

Isoniazid *on page 844*

RifAMPin *on page 1324*

Brand Names: US Rifamate [DSC]

Brand Names: Canada Rifamate

Pharmacologic Category Antibiotic, Miscellaneous

Use Management of active tuberculosis; see individual agents for additional information

Local Anesthetic/Vasoconstrictor Precautions No information available to require special precautions

Effects on Dental Treatment No significant effects or complications reported

Effects on Bleeding Rifampin doses >600 mg may be associated with more adverse events including hemolytic anemia and thrombocytopenia.

Adverse Reactions See individual agents.

Mechanism of Action

Rifampin inhibits bacterial RNA synthesis by binding to the beta subunit of DNA-dependent RNA polymerase, blocking transcription

Isoniazid inhibits mycolic acid synthesis resulting in disruption of the bacterial cell wall

Pregnancy Considerations Animal reproduction studies have not been conducted with this combination. Refer to individual agents.

◆ **Rifampin/Isoniazid** *see* Rifampin and Isoniazid *on page 1325*

Rifamycin

(RIF a MYE sin)

Brand Names: US Aemcolo

Pharmacologic Category Rifamycin

Use

Travelers' diarrhea: Treatment of travelers' diarrhea (TD) caused by noninvasive strains of *Escherichia coli* in adults

Limitations of use: Rifamycin is not indicated in patients with diarrhea complicated by fever or bloody stool or due to pathogens other than noninvasive strains of *E. coli.*

Local Anesthetic/Vasoconstrictor Precautions No information available to require special precautions

Effects on Dental Treatment Key adverse event(s) related to dental treatment: Superinfection: Prolonged use may result in bacterial superinfection.

Effects on Bleeding No information available to require special precautions

Adverse Reactions

1% to 10%:

Central nervous system: Headache (3%)

Gastrointestinal: Constipation (4%), dyspepsia (<2%)

Frequency not defined:

Gastrointestinal: Abdominal pain

Miscellaneous: Fever

Mechanism of Action Rifamycin inhibits bacterial synthesis by inhibiting the beta-subunit of the bacterial DNA-dependent RNA polymerase.

Pregnancy Considerations Maternal systemic absorption is limited following oral administration, therefore exposure to the fetus is not expected.

◆ **Rifamycin sodium** *see* Rifamycin *on page 1325*

Rifapentine

(rif a PEN teen)

Related Information

RifAMPin *on page 1324*

Brand Names: US Priftin

Pharmacologic Category Antitubercular Agent; Rifamycin

Use

Tuberculosis, active: Treatment of active pulmonary tuberculosis caused by *Mycobacterium tuberculosis* in adults and children 12 years and older; must be used in combination with one or more antituberculosis drugs to which the isolate is susceptible.

Limitations of use: Rifapentine should not be used once weekly in the continuation phase regimen in combination with isoniazid in HIV-infected patients with active pulmonary tuberculosis because of a higher rate of failure and/or relapse with rifampin-resistant organisms. Rifapentine has not been studied as part of the initial phase treatment regimen in HIV-infected patients with active pulmonary tuberculosis.

Tuberculosis, latent infection: Treatment of latent tuberculosis infection caused by *Mycobacterium tuberculosis*, in combination with isoniazid, in adults and children 2 years and older at high risk of progression to tuberculosis disease. To identify candidates for latent tuberculosis infection treatment, refer to Centers for Disease Control and Prevention (CDC) guidelines for current recommendations.

Limitations of use: Rifapentine in combination with isoniazid is not recommended for individuals presumed to be exposed to rifamycin- or isoniazid-resistant *M. tuberculosis.*

Local Anesthetic/Vasoconstrictor Precautions No information available to require special precautions

Effects on Dental Treatment No significant effects or complications reported

Effects on Bleeding No information available to require special precautions

Adverse Reactions Frequency may vary based on treatment phase; adverse reaction data is based on rifapentine combination therapy.

>10%:

Endocrine & metabolic: Hyperuricemia (≤32%; most likely due to pyrazinamide from initiation phase)

Genitourinary: Pyuria (11% to 22%), hematuria (10% to 18%), urinary tract infection (7% to 13%)

Hematologic & oncologic: Neutropenia (6% to 13%), lymphocytopenia (3% to 13%), anemia (2% to 11%)

1% to 10%:

Cardiovascular: Chest pain (3% to 6%), edema (1%)

Central nervous system: Pain (3% to 6%), headache (≤3%), dizziness (≤1%), fatigue (≤1%)

Dermatologic: Diaphoresis (2% to 5%), skin rash (3% to 4%), acne vulgaris (≤3%), pruritus (≤3%), maculopapular rash (≤2%)

Endocrine & metabolic: Hypoglycemia (5% to 10%), hyperglycemia (1% to 4%), increased nonprotein nitrogen (1% to 3%), gout (1%), hyperphosphatemia (1%)

Gastrointestinal: Anorexia (3% to 4%), nausea (≤3%), constipation (1% to 2%), dyspepsia (1% to 2%), abdominal pain (≤2%), diarrhea (≤2%), vomiting (≤2%), hemorrhoids (1%)

Genitourinary: Casts in urine (4% to 8%), cystitis (1%)

Hematologic & oncologic: Leukopenia (4% to 7%), thrombocytosis (≤6%), leukocytosis (2% to 3%), neutrophilia (1% to 3%), thrombocythemia (1% to 3%), polycythemia (≤2%), lymphadenopathy (≤1%)
Hepatic: Increased serum ALT (2% to 7%), increased serum AST (2% to 6%), hepatotoxicity (≤2%)
Hypersensitivity: Hypersensitivity reaction (≤4%; children & adolescents 1%)
Infection: Influenza (3% to 8%), herpes zoster (1%), infection (1%)
Neuromuscular & skeletal: Back pain (4% to 7%), arthralgia (≤4%), osteoarthrosis (1%), tremor (1%)
Ophthalmic: Conjunctivitis (≤3%)
Respiratory: Hemoptysis (2% to 8%), cough (3% to 6%), bronchitis (3%), pharyngitis (1% to 2%), epistaxis (1%), pleurisy (1%)
Miscellaneous: Accidental injury (1% to 5%), fever (≤1%)

<1%, postmarketing, and/or case reports: Ageusia, allergic skin reaction, alopecia, anaphylaxis, anxiety, asthma, azotemia, bronchial hyperactivity, bronchospasm, chills, confusion, convulsions, decreased appetite, depression, diabetes mellitus, disorientation, drowsiness, dyspnea, dysuria, enlargement of salivary glands, erythematous rash, esophagitis, facial edema, fungal infection, gastritis, hematoma, hepatitis, hepatomegaly, hyperbilirubinemia, hypercalcemia, hyperhidrosis, hyperkalemia, hyperlipidemia, increased blood urea nitrogen, increased serum alkaline phosphatase, jaundice, jitteriness, laryngeal edema, laryngitis, leukorrhea, lymphocytosis, myalgia, myasthenia, myositis, oropharyngeal pain, orthostatic hypotension, palpitations, pancreatitis, paresthesia, pericarditis, peripheral neuropathy, pneumonitis, pulmonary fibrosis, pulmonary tuberculosis (exacerbation), purpura, pyelonephritis, rhabdomyolysis, seizure, skin discoloration, suicidal ideation, syncope, tachycardia, thrombosis, urinary incontinence, urticaria, vaginal hemorrhage, vaginitis, viral infection, voice disorder, vulvovaginal candidiasis, vulvovaginal pruritus, weakness, weight gain, weight loss, xerostomia

Mechanism of Action Inhibits DNA-dependent RNA polymerase in susceptible strains of *Mycobacterium tuberculosis* (MTB) (but not in mammalian cells). Rifapentine is bactericidal against both intracellular and extracellular MTB organisms.

Pharmacodynamics/Kinetics

Half-life Elimination Rifapentine: ~17 hours; 25-desacetyl rifapentine: ~24 hours

Time to Peak Serum: 3 to 10 hours

Reproductive Considerations The efficacy of hormonal contraceptives may be decreased during treatment with rifapentine. A nonhormonal contraceptive or the addition of a barrier contraceptive is recommended during therapy.

Pregnancy Considerations

Information related to the use of rifapentine in pregnant women is limited. Rifapentine may increase the risk of maternal postpartum hemorrhage and neonatal bleeding when exposure occurs near delivery. Monitoring of the prothrombin time in the mother and neonate is recommended following exposure late in pregnancy; treatment with vitamin K may be needed.

Agents other than rifapentine are recommended for the treatment and prophylaxis of tuberculosis in pregnant women (CDC [Borisov 2018]; HHS [OI 2019]; Nahid 2019).

RifAXIMin (rif AX i min)

Brand Names: US Xifaxan

Brand Names: Canada Zaxine

Pharmacologic Category Rifamycin

Use

Hepatic encephalopathy: Reduction in the risk of overt hepatic encephalopathy recurrence in adults.

Irritable bowel syndrome without constipation: Treatment of moderate to severe irritable bowel syndrome without constipation in adults.

Travelers' diarrhea: Treatment of travelers' diarrhea caused by noninvasive strains of *Escherichia coli* in adults and pediatric patients ≥12 years of age.

Limitations of use: Rifaximin should not be used in patients with diarrhea complicated by fever or blood in the stool or diarrhea caused by pathogens other than *E. coli*.

Local Anesthetic/Vasoconstrictor Precautions No information available to require special precautions

Effects on Dental Treatment No significant effects or complications reported

Effects on Bleeding No information available to require special precautions

Adverse Reactions Frequency of adverse events generally higher following treatment for hepatic encephalopathy (HE). Percentages are presented for HE unless otherwise stated.

>10%:
Cardiovascular: Peripheral edema (15%)
Central nervous system: Dizziness (13%), fatigue (12%)
Hepatic: Ascites (11%)
Gastrointestinal: Nausea (14%; irritable bowel syndrome with diarrhea 2% to 3%)

2% to 10%:
Central nervous system: Headache (travelers' diarrhea 10%), depression (7%)
Dermatological: Pruritus (9%), skin rash (5%)
Gastrointestinal: Abdominal pain (>2% to 9%), pseudomembranous colitis (<5%; travelers' diarrhea or irritable bowel syndrome with diarrhea <2%)
Hematologic & oncologic: Anemia (8%)
Hepatic: Increased serum ALT (irritable bowel syndrome with diarrhea 2%)
Neuromuscular & skeletal: Muscle spasm (9%), arthralgia (6%), increased creatine phosphokinase (<5%; travelers' diarrhea or irritable bowel syndrome with diarrhea <2%)
Respiratory: Nasopharyngitis (7%), dyspnea (6%), epistaxis (>2% to 5%)
Miscellaneous: Fever (6%)

All indications: <2%, postmarketing, and/or case reports: Anaphylaxis, angioedema, *Clostridioides* (formerly *Clostridium*) *difficile*-associated diarrhea, exfoliative dermatitis, flushing, hypersensitivity reaction, urticaria

Mechanism of Action Rifaximin inhibits bacterial RNA synthesis by binding to bacterial DNA-dependent RNA polymerase.

Pharmacodynamics/Kinetics

Half-life Elimination Healthy subjects: 5.6 hours; IBS without constipation: 6 hours

Time to Peak Healthy subjects and patients with IBS without constipation: ~1 hour

Pregnancy Considerations Adverse events have been observed in some animal reproduction studies. Due to the limited oral absorption of rifaximin in patients with normal hepatic function, exposure to the fetus is expected to be low.

- **rIFN beta-1a** *see* Interferon Beta-1a *on page 833*
- **rIFN beta-1b** *see* Interferon Beta-1b *on page 835*
- **RIG** *see* Rabies Immune Globulin (Human) *on page 1302*

Rilpivirine (ril pi VIR een)

Related Information

Clinical Risk Related to Drugs Prolonging QT Interval *on page 1675*

HIV Infection and AIDS *on page 1690*

Brand Names: US Edurant

Brand Names: Canada Edurant

Pharmacologic Category Antiretroviral, Reverse Transcriptase Inhibitor, Non-nucleoside (Anti-HIV)

Use HIV-1 infection: Treatment of HIV-1 infections in antiretroviral treatment-naive patients ≥12 years of age and weighing ≥35 kg, with HIV-1 RNA ≤100,000 copies/mL at the start of therapy in combination with other antiretroviral agents

Local Anesthetic/Vasoconstrictor Precautions Rilpivirine is one of the drugs confirmed to prolong the QT interval and is accepted as having a risk of causing torsade de pointes. The risk of drug-induced torsade de pointes is extremely low when a single QT interval prolonging drug is prescribed. In terms of epinephrine, it is not known what effect vasoconstrictors in the local anesthetic regimen will have in patients with a known history of congenital prolonged QT interval or in patients taking any medication that prolongs the QT interval. Until more information is obtained, it is suggested that the clinician consult with the physician prior to the use of a vasoconstrictor in suspected patients, and that the vasoconstrictor (epinephrine, mepivacaine and levonordefrin [Carbocaine® 2% with Neo-Cobefrin®]) be used with caution.

Effects on Dental Treatment No significant effects or complications reported

Effects on Bleeding No information available to require special precautions

Adverse Reactions

>10%:

Central nervous system: Depression (5% to 9%; children and adolescents: 19%), headache (3%; children and adolescents: 19%), drowsiness (children and adolescents: 14%)

Endocrine & metabolic: Decreased plasma cortisol (7%; children and adolescents: 20%; decrease from baseline via ACTH stimulation test; clinical significance is unknown), increased serum cholesterol (7% to 17%), increased LDL cholesterol (5% to 14%)

Gastrointestinal: Nausea (1%; children and adolescents: 11%)

Hepatic: Increased serum ALT (1% to 18%), increased serum AST (1% to 16%)

1% to 10%:

Central nervous system: Dizziness (1%; children and adolescents: 8%), insomnia (3%), abnormal dreams (2%), fatigue (2%)

Dermatologic: Skin rash (3% to 6%)

Endocrine & metabolic: Increased serum triglycerides (2%)

Gastrointestinal: Abdominal pain (2%; children and adolescents: 8%), vomiting (1%; children and adolescents: 6%)

Hepatic: Increased serum bilirubin (1% to 5%)

Renal: Increased serum creatinine (1% to 6%)

<1%, postmarketing, and/or case reports (Limited to important or life-threatening): Angioedema, conjunctivitis, DRESS syndrome, facial edema, fever, hepatitis, hypersensitivity reaction, localized vesiculation, nephrotic syndrome, suicidal ideation

Mechanism of Action As a non-nucleoside reverse transcriptase inhibitor, rilpivirine has activity against HIV-1 by binding to reverse transcriptase. It consequently blocks the RNA-dependent and DNA-dependent DNA polymerase activities, including HIV-1 replication. It does not require intracellular phosphorylation for antiviral activity.

Pharmacodynamics/Kinetics

Half-life Elimination ~50 hours

Time to Peak Plasma: 4 to 5 hours

Reproductive Considerations

The Health and Human Services perinatal HIV guidelines consider rilpivirine an alternative component of antiretroviral therapy for females living with HIV who are not yet pregnant but are trying to conceive.

For males and females living with HIV and planning a pregnancy, maximum viral suppression below the limits of detection with antiretroviral therapy (ART), modification of therapy (if needed), optimization of the woman's health, and a discussion of the potential risks and benefits of ART therapy during pregnancy is recommended prior to conception (HHS [perinatal] 2019).

Pregnancy Considerations

Rilpivirine has moderate to high placental transfer.

No increased risk of overall birth defects has been observed following first trimester exposure according to data collected by the antiretroviral pregnancy registry. Maternal antiretroviral therapy (ART) may be associated with adverse pregnancy outcomes including preterm delivery, stillbirth, low birth weight, and small for gestational age infants. Actual risks may be influenced by maternal factors, such as disease severity, gestational age at initiation of therapy, and specific ART regimen; therefore, close fetal monitoring is recommended. Because there is clear benefit to appropriate treatment, maternal ART should not be withheld due to concerns for adverse neonatal outcomes. Long-term follow-up is recommended for all infants exposed to antiretroviral medications; children without HIV but who were exposed to ART in utero and develop significant organ system abnormalities of unknown etiology (particularly of the CNS or heart) should be evaluated for potential mitochondrial dysfunction. Hypersensitivity reactions (including hepatic toxicity and rash) are more common in women on nonneucleoside reverse transcriptase inhibitor therapy; it is not known if pregnancy increases this risk.

The Health and Human Services (HHS) perinatal HIV guidelines consider rilpivirine an alternative ART for pregnant females living with HIV who are antiretroviral naive, who have had ART therapy in the past but are restarting, or who require a new ART regimen (due to poor tolerance or poor virologic response of current regimen). Females who become pregnant while taking rilpivirine may continue if viral suppression is effective and the regimen is well tolerated. The pharmacokinetics are highly variable in pregnancy; data are insufficient to recommend pregnancy-specific dosing; however, viral loads should be monitored more frequently when standard doses are used in pregnant females.

The HHS perinatal HIV guidelines recommend rilpivirine as a component in alternative regimens for initial use in antiretroviral-naive pregnant females with a pretreatment HIV RNA ≤100,000 copies/mL and CD4 cell count ≥200 cells/mm^3.

In general, ART is recommended for all pregnant females living with HIV to keep the viral load below the limit of detection and reduce the risk of perinatal transmission. Therapy should be individualized following a discussion of the potential risks and benefits of treatment during pregnancy. Monitoring of pregnant females is more frequent than in nonpregnant adults. ART should be continued postpartum for all females living with HIV and can be modified after delivery.

Health care providers are encouraged to enroll pregnant females exposed to antiretroviral medications as early in pregnancy as possible in the Antiretroviral Pregnancy Registry (1-800-258-4263 or http://www.-APRegistry.com). Health care providers caring for pregnant females living with HIV and their infants may contact the National Perinatal HIV Hotline (1-888-448-8765) for clinical consultation (HHS [perinatal] 2019).

Dental Health Professional Considerations See Local Anesthetic/Vasoconstrictor Precautions

- **Rilpivirine and Dolutegravir** *see* Dolutegravir and Rilpivirine *on page 512*
- **Rilpivirine, Emtricitabine, and Tenofovir Alafenamide** *see* Emtricitabine, Rilpivirine, and Tenofovir Alafenamide *on page 559*
- **Rilpivirine, Emtricitabine, and Tenofovir Disoproxil Fumarate** *see* Emtricitabine, Rilpivirine, and Tenofovir Disoproxil Fumarate *on page 559*
- **Rilpivirine HCl** *see* Rilpivirine *on page 1327*
- **Rilutek** *see* Riluzole *on page 1328*

Riluzole (RIL yoo zole)

Brand Names: US Rilutek; Tiglutik

Brand Names: Canada APO-Riluzole; MYLAN-Riluzole; Rilutek

Pharmacologic Category Glutamate Inhibitor

Use Amyotrophic lateral sclerosis: Treatment of patients with amyotrophic lateral sclerosis (ALS); may extend survival and/or time to tracheostomy

Local Anesthetic/Vasoconstrictor Precautions No information available to require special precautions

Effects on Dental Treatment Key adverse event(s) related to dental treatment: Oral *Candida* infection and stomatitis.

Effects on Bleeding No information available to require special precautions

Adverse Reactions

>10%:

Gastrointestinal: Nausea (16%), oral hypoesthesia (oral film: 38%)

Hepatic: Increased serum alanine aminotransferase (>ULN: 50%; >3 x ULN: 8%; >5 x ULN: 2%)

Nervous system: Dizziness (females 11%; males. 4%)

Neuromuscular & skeletal: Asthenia (19%)

1% to 10%:

Cardiovascular: Hypertension (5%), peripheral edema (3%), tachycardia (3%)

Dermatologic: Eczema (2%), pruritus (4%)

Gastrointestinal: Abdominal pain (5%), flatulence (3%), oral paresthesia (2%), vomiting (4%), xerostomia (4%)

Genitourinary: Urinary tract infection (3%)

Nervous system: Drowsiness (2%), insomnia (4%), vertigo (2%)

Neuromuscular & skeletal: Arthralgia (4%)

Respiratory: Decreased lung function (10%), increased cough (3%)

Frequency not defined:

Gastrointestinal: Constipation

Hematologic & oncologic: Severe neutropenia

Hepatic: Hepatic injury, increased serum transaminases

Respiratory: Interstitial pulmonary disease (including hypersensitivity pneumonitis)

Postmarketing:

Gastrointestinal: Pancreatitis

Hepatic: Hepatitis (acute), toxic hepatitis (icteric)

Renal: Renal tubular disease

Mechanism of Action Mechanism of action is not known. Pharmacologic properties include inhibitory effect on glutamate release, inactivation of voltage-dependent sodium channels; and ability to interfere with intracellular events that follow transmitter binding at excitatory amino acid receptors

Pharmacodynamics/Kinetics

Half-life Elimination 12 hours

Time to Peak Suspension: 0.8 hours

Pregnancy Considerations Adverse events have been observed in animal reproduction studies.

Product Availability Exservan (riluzole oral film): FDA approved November 2019; anticipated availability is currently unknown. Consult the prescribing information for additional information.

RimabotulinumtoxinB

(rime uh BOT yoo lin num TOKS in bee)

Related Information

Dentin Hypersensitivity, Acid Erosion, High Caries Index, Management of Alveolar Osteitis, and Xerostomia *on page 1762*

Brand Names: US Myobloc

Pharmacologic Category Neuromuscular Blocker Agent, Toxin

Use

Cervical dystonia: Treatment of cervical dystonia (spasmodic torticollis)

Sialorrhea: Treatment of chronic sialorrhea in adults

Local Anesthetic/Vasoconstrictor Precautions No information available to require special precautions

Effects on Dental Treatment Key adverse event(s) related to dental treatment: Xerostomia (normal salivary flow resumes upon discontinuation), stomatitis, and abnormal taste.

Effects on Bleeding No information available to require special precautions

Adverse Reactions

>10%:

Central nervous system: Headache (10% to 16%), pain (13%)

Gastrointestinal: Xerostomia (12% to 39%; severe: 6%), dysphagia (4% to 25%; severe: 3%)

Immunologic: Antibody development (20% to 50%; neutralizing: 10% to 18%)

Local: Pain at injection site (12% to 16%)

1% to 10%:

Cardiovascular: Chest pain (≥2%), edema (≥2%), vasodilation (≥2%)

Central nervous system: Dizziness (3% to 6%), anxiety (≥2%), chills (≥2%), hyperesthesia (≥2%), malaise (≥2%), migraine (≥2%), vertigo (≥2%)

Dermatologic: Pruritus (≥2%)

Gastrointestinal: Dyspepsia (10%), dental caries (5% to 7%), gastrointestinal disease (≥2%), hernia of abdominal cavity (≥2%)

Genitourinary: Cystitis (≥2%), urinary tract infection (≥2%)

Hematologic & oncologic: Bruise (≥2%)

Infection: Abscess (≥2%), viral infection (≥2%)

Neuromuscular & skeletal: Arthralgia (7%), back pain (4% to 7%), asthenia (6%)

Ophthalmic: Amblyopia (≥2%), visual disturbance (≥2%)

Respiratory: Flu-like symptoms (6% to 9%), increased cough (6% to 7%), dyspnea (≥2%), pneumonia (≥2%)

Miscellaneous: Cyst (≥2%)

Postmarketing: Angioedema, constipation, hypersensitivity reaction, respiratory failure, skin rash, urticaria

Mechanism of Action RimabotulinumtoxinB (previously known as botulinum toxin type B) is a neurotoxin produced by *Clostridium botulinum*, spore-forming anaerobic bacillus. It cleaves synaptic Vesicle Association Membrane Protein (VAMP; synaptobrevin) which is a component of the protein complex responsible for docking and fusion of the synaptic vesicle to the presynaptic membrane. By blocking neurotransmitter release, rimabotulinumtoxinB paralyzes the muscle.

Pharmacodynamics/Kinetics

Duration of Action 12-16 weeks

Pregnancy Considerations

Animal reproduction studies have not been conducted.

RiMANTAdine (ri MAN ta deen)

Related Information

Systemic Viral Diseases *on page 1709*

Brand Names: US Flumadine [DSC]

Pharmacologic Category Antiviral Agent; Antiviral Agent, Adamantane

Use

Influenza A virus, prophylaxis: Prophylaxis against influenza A virus in adults and children 1 year and older.

Influenza A virus, treatment: Treatment of illness caused by influenza A virus in adults.

Note: Due to high resistance rates, rimantadine is no longer recommended for the treatment or prophylaxis of influenza A (CDC 2018; IDSA [Uyeki 2019]). Please refer to the current CDC recommendations.

Local Anesthetic/Vasoconstrictor Precautions No information available to require special precautions

Effects on Dental Treatment Key adverse event(s) related to dental treatment: Xerostomia (normal salivary flow resumes upon discontinuation).

Effects on Bleeding No information available to require special precautions

Adverse Reactions

1% to 10%:

Central nervous system: Insomnia (2% to 3%), lack of concentration (≤2%), dizziness (1% to 2%), nervousness (1% to 2%), fatigue (1%), headache (1%)

Gastrointestinal: Nausea (3%), anorexia (2%), vomiting (2%), xerostomia (2%), abdominal pain (1%)

Neuromuscular & skeletal: Weakness (1%)

<1%, postmarketing, and/or case reports: Abnormal gait, agitation, altered sense of smell, ataxia, bronchospasm, cardiac failure, confusion, cough, depression, diarrhea, drowsiness, dysgeusia, dyspepsia, dyspnea, euphoria, hallucination, heart block, hyperkinesia, hypertension, lactation, palpitations, pallor, pedal edema, seizure, skin rash, syncope, tachycardia, tinnitus, tremor

Mechanism of Action Exerts its inhibitory effect on three antigenic subtypes of influenza A virus (H1N1, H2N2, H3N2) early in the viral replicative cycle, possibly inhibiting the uncoating process; it has no activity against influenza B virus and is two- to eightfold more active than amantadine

Pharmacodynamics/Kinetics

Onset of Action Antiviral activity: No data exist establishing a correlation between plasma concentration and antiviral effect

Half-life Elimination

Children 5 to 8 years: 24.8 ± 9.4 hours (Anderson 1987)

Adults: 25.4 hours (range: 13 to 65 hours); Elderly (71 to 79 years of age): 32 hours (range: 20 to 65 hours)

Time to Peak 6 hours

Pregnancy Risk Factor C

Pregnancy Considerations Adverse events have been observed in animal reproduction studies. Untreated influenza infection is associated with an increased risk of adverse events to the fetus and an increased risk of complications or death to the mother. Neuraminidase inhibitors are currently recommended for the treatment or prophylaxis influenza in pregnant women and women up to 2 weeks postpartum. Appropriate antiviral agents are currently recommended as an adjunct to vaccination and should not be used as a substitute for vaccination in pregnant women (CDC 60 [1] 2011; CDC March 13, 2014; CDC January 2015).

Health care providers are encouraged to refer women exposed to influenza vaccine, or who have taken an antiviral medication during pregnancy to the Vaccines and Medications in Pregnancy Surveillance System (VAMPSS) by contacting The Organization of Teratology Information Specialists (OTIS) at 1-877-311-8972.

◆ **Rimantadine Hydrochloride** *see* RiMANTAdine *on page 1329*

Rimegepant (ri ME je pant)

Brand Names: US Nurtec

Pharmacologic Category Antimigraine Agent; Calcitonin Gene-Related Peptide (CGRP) Receptor Antagonist

Use

Migraine, treatment: Acute treatment of migraine with or without aura in adults.

Limitations of use: Not indicated for the preventive treatment of migraine.

Local Anesthetic/Vasoconstrictor Precautions No information available to require special precautions.

Effects on Dental Treatment No significant effects or complications reported.

Effects on Bleeding No information available to require special precautions.

Adverse Reactions

1% to 10%: Gastrointestinal: Nausea (2%)

<1%:

Dermatologic: Skin rash

Hypersensitivity: Hypersensitivity reaction

Respiratory: Dyspnea

Frequency not defined: Hypersensitivity: Type IV hypersensitivity reaction

Mechanism of Action Rimegepant is a calcitonin gene-related peptide receptor antagonist.

Pharmacodynamics/Kinetics

Onset of Action ≤2 hours (Croop 2019).

Duration of Action Up to 48 hours (Croop 2019).

Half-life Elimination ~11 hours.

Time to Peak 1.5 hours; delayed 1 hour following a high fat meal.

Pregnancy Considerations

Adverse events were observed in some animal reproduction studies at doses that also caused maternal toxicity.

Agents other than rimegepant are preferred for the management of acute migraine in pregnant women (Burch 2019).

◆ **Rimegepant sulfate** *see* Rimegepant *on page* 1329

Rimexolone (ri MEKS oh lone)

Brand Names: US Vexol [DSC]

Pharmacologic Category Corticosteroid, Ophthalmic

Use Ophthalmic inflammatory conditions: Treatment of postoperative inflammation following ocular surgery; treatment of anterior uveitis

Local Anesthetic/Vasoconstrictor Precautions No information available to require special precautions

Effects on Dental Treatment No significant effects or complications reported

Effects on Bleeding No information available to require special precautions

Adverse Reactions

1% to 5%:

Central nervous system: Foreign body sensation of eye

Ophthalmic: Blurred vision, eye discharge, eye discomfort, eye pain, eye pruritus, increased intraocular pressure, ocular hyperemia

<2%:

Cardiovascular: Hypotension

Central nervous system: Headache

Gastrointestinal: Dysgeusia

Respiratory: Pharyngitis, rhinitis

Frequency not defined:

Infection: Secondary ocular infection

Ophthalmic: Cataract, eye disease (defects in visual activity), eye perforation, optic nerve damage

<1%, postmarketing, and/or case reports: Anterior chamber fibrin deposition, brow ache, conjunctival edema, corneal edema, corneal erosion, corneal infiltrates, corneal staining, corneal ulcer, crusting of eyelid, eye irritation, keratitis, lacrimation, ocular edema, photophobia, sticky sensation of eye, xerophthalmia

Mechanism of Action Suppresses the inflammatory response by inhibiting edema, capillary dilation, leukocyte migration and scar formation.

Pharmacodynamics/Kinetics

Half-life Elimination 1 to 2 hours

Pregnancy Risk Factor C

Pregnancy Considerations Adverse events have been observed in animal reproduction studies following subcutaneous administration. The amount of rimexolone absorbed systemically following ophthalmic administration is low (<80 to 470 pg/mL).

Product Availability Vexol has been discontinued in the United States for more than 1 year.

◆ **Rinvoq** *see* Upadacitinib *on page* 1508

◆ **Riomet** *see* MetFORMIN *on page* 983

◆ **Riomet ER** *see* MetFORMIN *on page* 983

Ripretinib (rip RE ti nib)

Brand Names: US Qinlock

Pharmacologic Category Antineoplastic Agent, KIT Inhibitor; Antineoplastic Agent, PDGFR-alpha Blocker; Antineoplastic Agent, Tyrosine Kinase Inhibitor

Use Gastrointestinal stromal tumor, advanced: Treatment of advanced gastrointestinal stromal tumor (GIST) in adults who have previously received treatment with ≥3 kinase inhibitors, including imatinib.

Local Anesthetic/Vasoconstrictor Precautions Hypertension can occur with this drug; monitor for hypertension prior to using local anesthetic with vasoconstrictor; medical consult if necessary.

Effects on Dental Treatment Key adverse event(s) related to dental treatment: Frequent occurrence of stomatitis.

Effects on Bleeding Increased INR, prolonged partial thromboplastin time; unanticipated bleeding may be possible.

Adverse Reactions

>10%:

Cardiovascular: Hypertension (14%), peripheral edema (17%)

Dermatologic: Alopecia (52%), palmar-plantar erythrodysesthesia (21%), pruritus (11%), xeroderma (13%)

Endocrine & metabolic: Decreased serum calcium (23%), decreased serum phosphate (26%), decreased serum sodium (17%), increased serum triglycerides (26%), weight loss (19%)

Gastrointestinal: Abdominal pain (36%), constipation (34%), decreased appetite (27%), diarrhea (28%), increased serum amylase (13%), increased serum lipase (32%), nausea (39%), stomatitis (11%), vomiting (21%)

Hematologic & oncologic: Increased INR (21%; grades 3/4: 4%), prolonged partial thromboplastin time (35%)

Hepatic: Increased serum alanine aminotransferase (12%), increased serum bilirubin (22%)

Nervous system: Fatigue (42%), headache (19%)

Neuromuscular & skeletal: Arthralgia (18%), increased creatine phosphokinase in blood specimen (21%), muscle spasm (15%), myalgia (32%)

Respiratory: Dyspnea (13%)

1% to 10%:

Cardiovascular: Cardiac disorder (2%; including left ventricular failure, ventricular hypertrophy), cardiac failure (1%), ischemic heart disease (1%; including acute coronary syndrome, acute myocardial infarction), reduced ejection fraction (grade 3: 3%)

Hematologic & oncologic: Anemia (4%), keratoacanthoma (2%), malignant melanoma (≤2%), neutropenia (10%), squamous cell carcinoma of skin (5% to 7%)

Frequency not defined:
Dermatologic: Dermatologic disorder
Nervous system: Agitation, hyperesthesia
Neuromuscular & skeletal: Arthritis
Miscellaneous: Physical health deterioration

Mechanism of Action Ripretinib is a switch control tyrosine kinase inhibitor that inhibits KIT proto-oncogene receptor tyrosine kinase (KIT) and platelet derived growth factor receptor A (PDGFRA) kinase signaling (George 2020). It binds to both wild type and mutant forms (including primary and secondary mutations) of KIT and PDGRA, preventing the switch from inactive to active conformations of these kinases. Ripretinib also inhibits other kinases, including PDGFRB, TIE2, VEGFR2, and BRAF.

Pharmacodynamics/Kinetics

Half-life Elimination Ripretinib: 14.8 hours; DP-5439: 17.8 hours.

Time to Peak Ripretinib: 4 hours; DP-5439: 15.6 hours.

Reproductive Considerations Evaluate pregnancy status prior to use in females of reproductive potential.

Females of reproductive potential should use effective contraception during therapy and for at least 1 week after the last ripretinib dose. Males with female partners of reproductive potential should use effective contraception during therapy and for at least 1 week after the last dose of ripretinib.

Pregnancy Considerations Based on the mechanism of action and data from animal reproduction studies, in utero exposure to ripretinib may cause fetal harm.

Prescribing and Access Restrictions Ripretinib is available through a specialty pharmacy network and specialty distributors; information may be found at QinlockHCP.com/resources or at 1.888.724.3274.

◆ **Risa-Bid [OTC]** *see Lactobacillus on page 869*
◆ **RisaQuad [OTC]** *see Lactobacillus on page 869*
◆ **RisaQuad-2 [OTC]** *see Lactobacillus on page 869*

Risedronate (ris ED roe nate)

Related Information

Osteonecrosis of the Jaw *on page 1699*
Rheumatoid Arthritis, Osteoarthritis, and Osteoporosis *on page 1697*

Brand Names: US Actonel; Atelvia

Brand Names: Canada Actonel; Actonel DR; APO-Risedronate; Auro-Risedronate; DOM-Risedronate; JAMP-Risedronate; MYLAN-Risedronate [DSC]; PMS-Risedronate; Risedronate-35; RIVA-Risedronate; SANDOZ Risedronate; TEVA-Risedronate

Pharmacologic Category Bisphosphonate Derivative

Use

Osteoporosis:

Actonel: Treatment and prevention of osteoporosis in postmenopausal females; treatment of osteoporosis in males; treatment and prevention of glucocorticoid-induced osteoporosis (daily dosage of ≥7.5 mg prednisone or equivalent).

Atelvia, Actonel DR [Canadian product]: Treatment of osteoporosis in postmenopausal females.

Paget disease: *Actonel*: Treatment of Paget disease of the bone.

Local Anesthetic/Vasoconstrictor Precautions No information available to require special precautions

Effects on Dental Treatment Osteonecrosis of the jaw (ONJ), generally associated with local infection and/or tooth extraction and often with delayed healing, has been reported in patients taking bisphosphonates. Symptoms included nonhealing extraction socket or an exposed jawbone. Most reported cases of bisphosphonate-associated osteonecrosis have been in cancer patients treated with intravenous bisphosphonates. However, some have occurred in patients with postmenopausal osteoporosis taking oral bisphosphonates. Dental surgery, particularly tooth extraction, may increase the risk for ONJ. Patients who develop ONJ while on bisphosphonate therapy should receive care by an oral surgeon. See Dental Health Professional Considerations.

Effects on Bleeding No information available to require special precautions

Adverse Reactions Frequency may vary with product, dose, and indication.

>10%:
Cardiovascular: Hypertension (11%)
Central nervous system: Headache (3% to 18%)
Dermatologic: Skin rash (8% to 12%)
Gastrointestinal: Gastrointestinal disease (perforations, ulcers, or bleeding; 51%), diarrhea (5% to 20%), nausea (4% to 13%), abdominal pain (2% to 12%)
Genitourinary: Urinary tract infection (11%)
Infection: Infection (31%)
Neuromuscular & skeletal: Arthralgia (7% to 33%), back pain (6% to 28%)

1% to 10%:
Cardiovascular: Peripheral edema (8%), chest pain (7%), cardiac arrhythmia (2%)
Central nervous system: Depression (7%), dizziness (3% to 7%)
Endocrine & metabolic: Increased parathyroid hormone (8% to 9%; >1.5 x ULN: ≤2%), hypocalcemia (≤5%), hypophosphatemia (<3% decrease from baseline)
Gastrointestinal: Dyspepsia (4% to 8%), constipation (3% to 7%), vomiting (2% to 5%), gastritis (1% to 3%), gastroesophageal reflux disease (1% to 2%), duodenitis (≤1%), glossitis (≤1%)
Genitourinary: Benign prostatic hyperplasia (5%), nephrolithiasis (3%)
Hypersensitivity: Acute phase reaction-like symptoms (≤8%; includes fever, influenza-like illness)
Infection: Influenza (6% to 7%)
Neuromuscular & skeletal: Arthropathy (7%), myalgia (1% to 7%), limb pain (2% to 4%), musculoskeletal pain (2%), muscle spasm (1% to 2%)
Ophthalmic: Cataract (7%)
Respiratory: Flu-like symptoms (10%), pharyngitis (6%), rhinitis (6%), bronchitis (4%), upper respiratory tract infection (3% to 4%)

<1%, postmarketing, and/or case reports: Abnormal hepatic function tests, angioedema, bullous skin reaction, cough, esophageal ulcer, esophagitis, exacerbation of asthma, femur fracture, gastric ulcer, hypersensitivity reaction, iritis, ostealgia, osteonecrosis (primarily of the jaw), Stevens-Johnson syndrome, toxic epidermal necrolysis, uveitis

Mechanism of Action A bisphosphonate which inhibits bone resorption via actions on osteoclasts or on osteoclast precursors; decreases the rate of bone resorption, leading to an indirect increase in bone mineral density. In Paget's disease, characterized by disordered resorption and formation of bone, inhibition of resorption leads to an indirect decrease in bone formation; but the newly-formed bone has a more normal architecture.

Pharmacodynamics/Kinetics

Onset of Action May require weeks

Half-life Elimination Initial: 1.5 hours; Terminal: 480 to 561 hours

Time to Peak Serum: 1 to 3 hours

Reproductive Considerations

Underlying causes of osteoporosis should be evaluated and treated prior to considering bisphosphonate therapy in premenopausal women; effective contraception is recommended when bisphosphonate therapy is required (Pepe 2020). Bisphosphonates are incorporated into the bone matrix and gradually released over time. Because exposure prior to pregnancy may theoretically increase the risk of fetal harm, most sources recommend discontinuing bisphosphonate therapy in females of reproductive potential as early as possible prior to a planned pregnancy. Use in premenopausal females should be reserved for special circumstances when rapid bone loss is occurring; a bisphosphonate with the shortest half-life should then be used (Bhalla 2010; Pereira 2012; Stathopoulos 2011). When bisphosphonate therapy is needed in a premenopausal woman, risedronate may be preferred based on its shorter half-life compared to other agents. Treatment should be discontinued 6 to 12 months prior to a planned conception (Machairiotis 2019).

Oral bisphosphonates can be considered for the prevention of glucocorticoid-induced osteoporosis in premenopausal females with moderate to high risk of fracture who do not plan to become pregnant during the treatment period and who are using effective birth control (or are not sexually active); intravenous therapy should be reserved for high risk patients only (Buckley [ACR 2017]).

Pregnancy Considerations

It is not known if bisphosphonates cross the placenta, but fetal exposure is expected (Djokanovic 2008; Stathopoulos 2011).

Information related to the use of risedronate in pregnancy is available from small retrospective studies (Levy 2009; Sokal 2019).

Bisphosphonates are incorporated into the bone matrix and gradually released over time. The amount available in the systemic circulation varies by drug, dose, and duration of therapy. Theoretically, there may be a risk of fetal harm when pregnancy follows the completion of therapy (hypocalcemia, low birth weight, and decreased gestation have been observed in some case reports); however, available data have not shown that exposure to bisphosphonates during pregnancy significantly increases the risk of adverse fetal events (Djokanovic 2008; Green 2014; Levy 2009; Machairiotis 2019; Sokal 2019; Stathopoulos 2011). Exposed infants should be monitored for hypocalcemia after birth (Djokanovic 2008; Stathopoulos 2011).

Dental Health Professional Considerations A review of 2,408 published cases of bisphosphonate-associated osteonecrosis of the jaw bone (BP-associated ONJ) was done by Filleul 2010. BP therapy was associated with 89% of the cases to treat malignancies and 11% of the cases to treat nonmalignant conditions. Information on the specific bisphosphonate used was available for 1,694 of the patients. Intravenous therapy (primarily zoledronic acid) was received by 88% of the patients and 12% received oral treatment (primarily alendronate). Of all the cases of BP-associated ONJ, 67% were preceded by tooth extraction and for 26% of patients, there was no predisposing factor identified.

A 2010 retrospective case review reported the prevalence of BP-associated ONJ in patients using alendronate-type drugs was one out of 952 patients or ~0.1% (Lo 2010). Of the 8,572 respondents, nine cases of ONJ were identified; five had developed ONJ spontaneously and four developed ONJ after tooth extraction. When extrapolated to patient-years of bisphosphonate exposure, this prevalence rate of 0.1% equates to a frequency of 28 cases per 100,000 person-years of oral bisphosphonate treatment. An Australian group (Mavrokokki 2007), identified the frequency of BP-associated ONJ in osteoporotic patients, mainly taking weekly oral alendronate, was 1 in 8,470 to 1 in 2,260 (0.01% to 0.04%) patients. If extractions were carried out, the calculated frequency was 1 in 1,130 to 1 in 296 (0.09% to 0.34%) patients. The median time to onset of ONJ in alendronate patients was 24 months.

According to the 2011 report by the American Dental Association (ADA), the incidence of BP-associated ONJ remains low and the benefits of using oral bisphosphonates significantly outweighs the risk of developing BP-associated ONJ for treatment and prevention of osteoporosis and cancer treatment (Hellstein 2011). The full 47-page report can be accessed at http://www.ada.org/~/media/ADA/Member%20Center/FIles/topics_ARONJ_report.ashx.

The ADA review of 2011 stated the incidence of oral BP-associated ONJ was one case for every 1,000 individuals exposed to oral bisphosphonates (0.1%) (Hellstein 2011).

The most comprehensive review to date on osteonecrosis of the jaw bone (ONJ) has been published in the *Journal of Bone and Mineral Research* (Khan 2015), and written by an International Task Force of authors, totaling 34, from academe; industry; clinical medical and dental practice; oral and maxillofacial surgery; bone and mineral research; epidemiology; medical and dental oncology; orthopedic surgery; osteoporosis research; muscle and bone research; endocrinology and diagnostic sciences. The work provides a systematic review of the literature and international consensus on the classification, incidence, pathophysiology, diagnosis, and management of ONJ in both oncology and osteoporosis patient populations. This review of the literature from January 2003 to April 2014, with 299 references, offers recommendations for management of ONJ based on multidisciplinary international consensus.

Prevalence and incidence of ONJ in osteoporosis patients from the Task Force report:

Prevalence – the percent of osteoporotic population affected with ONJ

After reviewing all literature reports on this subject, the Task Force concluded that the prevalence of ONJ in patients prescribed oral BPs for the treatment of osteoporosis ranges from 0% to 0.04% with the majority being below 0.001%. However, the Task Force does cite the study of (Lo et al) that evaluated the Kaiser Permanente database and found the prevalence of ONJ in those receiving BPs for more than 2 years to range from 0.05% to 0.21% and appeared to be related to duration of exposure. As mentioned above, the American Dental Association has previously reported that the prevalence of ONJ in osteoporosis patients using oral BPs to be 1 out of 1,000 or 0.1% (Hellstein 2011).

Incidence - the rate at which ONJ occurs or the number of times it happens

From currently available data, the incidence of ONJ in the osteoporosis patient population appears to be low ranging from 0.15% to less than 0.001% person-years drug exposure. In terms of the osteoporosis patient population taking oral BPs, the incidence ranges from 1.04 to 69 per 100,000 patient years of drug exposure.

- ◆ **Risedronate Sodium** *see* Risedronate *on page 1331*
- ◆ **RisperDAL** *see* RisperiDONE *on page 1333*
- ◆ **Risperdal M-Tab** *see* RisperiDONE *on page 1333*
- ◆ **RisperDAL M-TAB [DSC]** *see* RisperiDONE *on page 1333*
- ◆ **RisperDAL Consta** *see* RisperiDONE *on page 1333*

RisperiDONE (ris PER i done)

Related Information

Clinical Risk Related to Drugs Prolonging QT Interval *on page 1675*

Brand Names: US Perseris; RisperDAL; RisperDAL Consta; RisperDAL M-TAB [DSC]; risperiDONE M-TAB [DSC]

Brand Names: Canada ACT Risperidone [DSC]; AG-Risperidone; APO-Risperidone; DOM-Risperidone; JAMP-Risperidone; JOI-Risperidone; Mar-Risperidone; MINT-Risperidon; MYLAN-Risperidone ODT; MYLAN-Risperidone [DSC]; PMS-Risperidone; PMS-Risperidone ODT [DSC]; PRO-Risperidone; RAN-Risperidone; RisperDAL; RisperDAL Consta; RisperDAL M-TAB [DSC]; RIVA-Risperidone; SANDOZ Risperidone; TEVA-Risperidone

Pharmacologic Category Antimanic Agent; Second Generation (Atypical) Antipsychotic

Use

Long-acting IM injection:

Bipolar disorder: As monotherapy or as adjunctive therapy to lithium or valproate for the maintenance treatment of bipolar I disorder.

Schizophrenia: Treatment of schizophrenia.

Oral:

Bipolar mania: As monotherapy or as adjunctive therapy to lithium or valproate for the treatment of acute manic or mixed episodes associated with bipolar disorder in adults or as monotherapy for the treatment of acute manic or mixed episodes associated with bipolar disorder in children and adolescents 10 to 17 years of age.

Irritability associated with autistic disorder: For the treatment of irritability associated with autistic disorder in children and adolescents 5 to 17 years of age, including symptoms of aggression toward others, deliberate self-injuriousness, temper tantrums, and quickly changing moods.

Schizophrenia: For the treatment of schizophrenia in adults and adolescents 13 to 17 years of age.

Local Anesthetic/Vasoconstrictor Precautions RisperiDONE is one of the drugs confirmed to prolong the QT interval and is accepted as having a risk of causing torsades de pointes. The risk of drug-induced torsades de pointes is extremely low when a single QT interval prolonging drug is prescribed. In terms of epinephrine, it is not known what effect vasoconstrictors in the local anesthetic regimen will have in patients with a known history of congenital prolonged QT interval or in patients taking any medication that prolongs the QT interval. Until more information is obtained, it is suggested that the clinician consult with the physician prior to the use of a vasoconstrictor in suspected patients, and that the vasoconstrictor (epinephrine, mepivacaine, and levonordefrin [Carbocaine 2% with Neo-Cobefrin]) be used with caution.

Effects on Dental Treatment Key adverse event(s) related to dental treatment: Frequent occurrence of drooling has been reported. Infrequent occurrence of xerostomia (normal salivary flow resumes upon discontinuation), orthostatic hypotension (use caution with sudden changes in position during and after dental treatment), tardive dyskinesia, sinusitis/congestion, and toothache have been reported. Rare occurrence of dysgeusia, tongue paralysis/spasm, and trismus have also been reported.

Effects on Bleeding No information available to require special precautions

Adverse Reactions

>10%:

Endocrine & metabolic: Hyperprolactinemia (children and adolescents: 49% to 87%; adults: <4%), weight gain (≥7% kg increase from baseline: adults: 8% to 42%; children: 8% to 33%)

Gastrointestinal: Increased appetite (children and adolescents: 4% to 44%; adults: 2% to 4%), vomiting (children and adolescents: 10% to 20%; adults <4%), constipation (5% to 17%), upper abdominal pain (adolescents: 13% to 16%), nausea (3% to 16%)

Genitourinary: Urinary incontinence (children: 16%; adults <4%)

Nervous system: Sedated state (children and adolescents: 12% to 63%; adults: 5% to 11%), drowsiness (adults: 5% to 41%), drug-induced extrapyramidal reaction (2% to 35%), insomnia (≤32%), fatigue (children and adolescents: 18% to 31%; adults: 1% to 9%), parkinsonism (children and adolescents: 6% to 28%; adults: 8% to 25%), headache (12% to 21%), anxiety (adults ≤16%; children and adolescents: 6% to 8%), dizziness (3% to 16%), drooling (children: 12%; adults: <4%), akathisia (3% to 11%)

Neuromuscular & skeletal: Tremor (adults: ≤24%; children and adolescents: ≤11%; including head titubation)

Respiratory: Nasopharyngitis (children: 19%; adults: ≤4%), cough (children: ≤17%; adults: ≤4%), rhinorrhea (children: 12%; adults: <4%)

Miscellaneous: Fever (children: 16%; adults: 1% to 2%)

1% to 10%:

Cardiovascular: Bradycardia (<4%), bundle branch block (<4%), chest discomfort (<4%), chest pain (<4%), ECG changes (<4%), facial edema (<4%), first-degree atrioventricular block (<4%), hypotension (<4%), orthostatic hypotension (<4%), palpitations (<4%), prolonged QT interval on ECG (<4%), tachycardia (adults: <4%), hypertension (≤3%), peripheral edema (≤3%), syncope (1% to 2%)

Dermatologic: Skin rash (≤8%), eczema (<4%), pruritus (<4%), xeroderma (≤3%), acne vulgaris (≤2%)

Endocrine & metabolic: Decrease in HDL cholesterol (10%), increased thirst (children: ≤7%), increased serum cholesterol (4% to 6%), amenorrhea (4%), weight loss (≤4%), decreased libido (<4%), delayed ejaculation (<4%), galactorrhea not associated with childbirth (<4%), glycosuria (<4%), gynecomastia (<4%), hyperglycemia (<4%), increased gamma-glutamyl transferase (<4%), infrequent uterine bleeding (<4%), menstrual disease (<4%), increased serum triglycerides (3%)

Gastrointestinal: Xerostomia (≤10%), dyspepsia (3% to 10%), sialorrhea (1% to 10%), diarrhea (≤8%), decreased appetite (≤6%), stomach discomfort (<6%), abdominal pain (adults: <4%), anorexia (<4%), gastritis (<4%), gastroenteritis (<4%), abdominal distress (1% to 3%), toothache (≤3%)

Genitourinary: Menstruation (≤4%; delayed), cystitis (<4%), erectile dysfunction (<4%), irregular menses (<4%), mastalgia (<4%), sexual disorder (<4%), urinary tract infection (<4%)

Hematologic & oncologic: Anemia (<4%), neutropenia (<4%)

Hepatic: Increased liver enzymes (<4%), increased serum alanine aminotransferase (<4%), increased serum aspartate aminotransferase (<4%)

Hypersensitivity: Hypersensitivity reaction (<4%)

Infection: Abscess at injection site (<4%), infection (<4%), influenza (<4%), localized infection (<4%), viral infection (<4%)

Local: Induration at injection site (<4%), injection site reaction (<4%), local pain (buttock: <4%), pain at injection site (<4%), swelling at injection site (<4%)

Nervous system: Dystonia (2% to 6%), abnormal gait (4%), procedural pain (4%), pain (1% to 4%), disturbance in attention (≤4%), agitation (<4%), ataxia (<4%), depression (<4%), dysarthria (<4%), falling (<4%), lethargy (<4%), malaise (<4%), nervousness (<4%), orthostatic dizziness (<4%), paresthesia (<4%), seizure (<4%), sleep disturbance (<4%), tardive dyskinesia (<4%), vertigo (<4%), hypoesthesia (≤2%)

Neuromuscular & skeletal: Limb pain (≤8%), back pain (≤7%), dyskinesia (adults: ≤6%), musculoskeletal pain (5%), arthralgia (2% to 4%), abnormal posture (<4%), akinesia (<4%), hypokinesia (<4%), musculoskeletal chest pain (<4%), myalgia (<4%), myasthenia (<4%), neck pain (<4%), muscle spasm (3%), muscle rigidity (≤3%), asthenia (1% to 2%), increased creatine phosphokinase in blood specimen (≤2%)

Ophthalmic: Blurred vision (2% to 7%), conjunctivitis (<4%), decreased visual acuity (<4%)

Otic: Otalgia (≤4%), otic infection (<4%)

Respiratory: Nasal congestion (≤10%), pharyngolaryngeal pain (3% to 10%), rhinitis (≤9%), respiratory tract infection (≤8%), bronchitis (<4%), dyspnea (<4%), flu-like symptoms (<4%), pharyngitis (<4%), pneumonia (<4%), sinusitis (<4%), epistaxis (≤2%), paranasal sinus congestion (≤2%)

<1%, postmarketing, and/or case reports: Abnormal eye movements (eye rolling), agranulocytosis, alopecia, anaphylaxis, angioedema, anorgasmia, aspiration pneumonia, atrial fibrillation, blepharospasm, blunted affect, breast engorgement, breast hypertrophy, breast secretion, breast tenderness, bronchopneumonia, bruxism, cellulitis, cerebral ischemia, cerebrovascular accident, cerebrovascular disease, cheilitis, chills, cogwheel rigidity, cold extremity, coma, confusion, crusting of eyelid, cutaneous nodule, cyst, decreased serum glucose, dermal ulcer, dermatitis (acarodermatitis), dermatologic disorders, diabetes mellitus, diabetic coma, diabetic ketoacidosis, disruption of body temperature regulation, drug-induced hypersensitivity reaction, drug withdrawal, dry eye syndrome, dysgeusia, dysphagia, dysuria, edema, eosinophilia, erythema of skin, esophageal motility disorder, eye discharge, eye infection, eyelid edema, fecal incontinence, fecaloma, feeling abnormal, flushing, glaucoma, granulocytopenia, hematoma, hyperkeratosis, hyperthermia, hypertonia, hypertriglyceridemia, hyperventilation, hypoglycemia, hypomenorrhea, hypothermia, impaired consciousness, increased serum transaminases, intestinal obstruction, jaundice, joint stiffness, joint swelling, lacrimation, leukopenia, lip edema, loss of balance, lower respiratory tract infection, maculopapular rash, mania, mask-like face, movement disorder, muscle twitching, nasal mucosa swelling, neuroleptic malignant syndrome, night sweats, ocular hyperemia, onychomycosis, oral hypoesthesia, oromandibular dystonia, otitis media (including chronic), pancreatitis, papular rash, photophobia, pitting edema, pituitary neoplasm, pollakiuria, polydipsia, precocious puberty, priapism, pulmonary congestion, pulmonary embolism, rales, respiratory congestion, respiratory distress, restlessness, retinal artery occlusion, retrograde ejaculation, rhabdomyolysis, seborrheic dermatitis of scalp, SIADH, skin discoloration, skin lesion, sleep apnea, somnambulism, speech disturbance, Stevens-Johnson syndrome, swelling of eye, thrombocytopenia, thrombotic thrombocytopenic purpura, tinnitus, tissue necrosis, tongue paralysis, tongue spasm, tonsillitis, torticollis, toxic epidermal necrolysis, tracheobronchitis, transient ischemic attacks, trismus, unresponsive to stimuli, urinary retention, vaginal discharge, ventricular tachycardia, visual disturbance, voice disorder, water intoxication, wheezing

Mechanism of Action Risperidone is a benzisoxazole atypical antipsychotic with high 5-HT_2 and dopamine-D_2 receptor antagonist activity. $Alpha_1$, $alpha_2$ adrenergic, and histaminergic receptors are also antagonized with high affinity. Risperidone has low to moderate affinity for 5-HT_{1C}, 5-HT_{1D}, and 5-HT_{1A} receptors, weak affinity for D_1 and no affinity for muscarinics or $beta_1$ and $beta_2$ receptors.

Pharmacodynamics/Kinetics

Half-life Elimination

Active moiety (risperidone and its active metabolite 9-hydroxyrisperidone):

Oral: 20 hours (mean); prolonged in elderly patients

Extensive metabolizers: Risperidone: 3 hours; 9-hydroxyrisperidone: 21 hours

Poor metabolizers: Risperidone: 20 hours; 9-hydroxyrisperidone: 30 hours

IM: 3 to 6 days; related to microsphere erosion and subsequent absorption of risperidone

Risperidone: SubQ: 9 to 11 days

Time to Peak

Oral: Risperidone: Within 1 hour; 9-hydroxyrisperidone: Extensive metabolizers: 3 hours; Poor metabolizers: 17 hours

SubQ: Risperidone: First peak: 4 to 6 hours; Second peak: 10 to 14 days

Reproductive Considerations

Risperidone may cause hyperprolactinemia, which may cause a reversible decrease in reproductive function in females.

If treatment with an atypical antipsychotic is needed in a woman planning a pregnancy, use of an agent other than risperidone is preferred (Larsen 2015). When using the IM injection, patients should notify health care provider if they intend to become pregnant during therapy or within 12 weeks of last injection.

Pregnancy Considerations

Risperidone and its metabolite cross the placenta (Newport 2007). Agenesis of the corpus callosum has been noted in one case report of an infant exposed to risperidone in utero; relationship to risperidone exposure is not known. Antipsychotic use during the third trimester of pregnancy has a risk for extrapyramidal symptoms (EPS) and/or withdrawal symptoms in newborns following delivery. Symptoms in the newborn may include agitation, feeding disorder, hypertonia, hypotonia, respiratory distress, somnolence, and tremor. These effects may be self-limiting and allow recovery within hours or days with no specific treatment, or they may be severe requiring prolonged hospitalization.

When using the IM injection, patients should notify health care provider if they become pregnant during therapy or within 12 weeks of last injection.

The ACOG recommends that therapy during pregnancy be individualized; treatment with psychiatric medications during pregnancy should incorporate the clinical expertise of the mental health clinician, obstetrician, primary health care provider, and pediatrician. Safety data related to atypical antipsychotics during pregnancy is limited. As a result, routine use is not recommended. However, if a woman is inadvertently exposed to an atypical antipsychotic while pregnant, continuing therapy may be preferable to switching to an agent that the fetus has not yet been exposed to; consider risk:benefit (ACOG 2008). If treatment is initiated during pregnancy, use of an agent other than risperidone is preferred (Larsen 2015).

Health care providers are encouraged to enroll women 18 to 45 years of age exposed to risperidone during pregnancy in the Atypical Antipsychotics Pregnancy Registry (1-866-961-2388 or http://www.womensmentalhealth.org/pregnancyregistry).

Dental Health Professional Considerations See Local Anesthetic/Vasoconstrictor Precautions

◆ **risperiDONE M-TAB [DSC]** *see* RisperiDONE *on page 1333*

◆ **Ritalin** *see* Methylphenidate *on page 997*

◆ **Ritalin LA** *see* Methylphenidate *on page 997*

Ritonavir (ri TOE na veer)

Related Information

HIV Infection and AIDS *on page 1690*

Brand Names: US Norvir

Brand Names: Canada Norvir

Pharmacologic Category Antiretroviral, Protease Inhibitor (Anti-HIV)

Local Anesthetic/Vasoconstrictor Precautions

No information available to require special precautions

Effects on Dental Treatment Key adverse event(s) related to dental treatment: Xerostomia (normal salivary flow resumes upon discontinuation) and taste perversion.

Effects on Bleeding Increased bleeding has been noted with protease inhibitors in patients with hemophilia A or B. No information available to require routine special precautions relative to hemostasis in other patients.

Adverse Reactions Incidences as reported for combined experiences in both treatment-naive and experienced adults unless otherwise noted:

>10%:

Cardiovascular: Flushing (13%)

Dermatologic: Pruritus (12%), skin rash (27%)

Endocrine & metabolic: Hypercholesterolemia (3%; >240 mg/dL: 37% to 45%), increased serum triglycerides (9%; >800 mg/dL: 17% to 34%; >1500 mg/dL: 1% to 13%)

Gastrointestinal: Abdominal pain (26%), diarrhea (68%), dysgeusia (16%), dyspepsia (12%), nausea (57%), vomiting (32%)

Hepatic: Increased gamma-glutamyl transferase (5% to 20%)

Nervous system: Dizziness (16%), fatigue (46%; including asthenia), paresthesia (51%; including oral paresthesia)

Neuromuscular & skeletal: Arthralgia (≤19%), back pain (≤19%), increased creatine phosphokinase in blood specimen (4% to 12%)

Respiratory: Cough (22%), oropharyngeal pain (16%)

1% to 10%:

Cardiovascular: Cold extremity (1%), edema (≤6%), hypertension (3%), hypotension (2%; including orthostatic hypotension), peripheral edema (≤6%), syncope (3%)

Dermatologic: Acne vulgaris (4%)

Endocrine & metabolic: Increased uric acid (≤4%), lipodystrophy (acquired, 3%)

Gastrointestinal: Flatulence (8%), gastroesophageal reflux disease (1%), gastrointestinal hemorrhage (2%), gout (1%), increased serum amylase (grades 3/4; infants, children, and adolescents: 7%)

Genitourinary: Urinary frequency (4%)

Hematologic & oncologic: Anemia (grades 3/4; infants, children, and adolescents: 4%), neutropenia (grades 3/4; infants, children, and adolescents: 9%), thrombocytopenia (grades 3/4; infants, children, and adolescents: 5%)

Hepatic: Hepatitis (9%), increased serum alanine aminotransferase (8% to 9%), increased serum aspartate aminotransferase (6% to 10%; infants, children, and adolescents: 3%), increased serum bilirubin (1%)

Hypersensitivity: Hypersensitivity reaction (8%)

Nervous system: Confusion (3%), disturbance in attention (3%), peripheral neuropathy (10%)

Neuromuscular & skeletal: Myalgia (9%), myopathy (≤4%)

Ophthalmic: Blurred vision (6%)

Frequency not defined:

Gastrointestinal: Pancreatitis

Postmarketing:
- Cardiovascular: Atrioventricular block (first, second, or third degree), prolongation P-R interval on ECG, right bundle branch block
- Dermatologic: Stevens-Johnson syndrome, toxic epidermal necrolysis
- Endocrine & metabolic: Dehydration
- Hypersensitivity: Angioedema
- Immunologic: Immune reconstitution syndrome
- Nervous system: Seizure
- Renal: Renal insufficiency
- Respiratory: Bronchospasm

Mechanism of Action Binds to the site of HIV-1 protease activity and inhibits cleavage of viral Gag-Pol polyprotein precursors into individual functional proteins required for infectious HIV. This results in the formation of immature, noninfectious viral particles.

Pharmacodynamics/Kinetics

Half-life Elimination Children: 2 to 4 hours; Adults: 3 to 5 hours

Time to Peak Oral solution: 2 hours (fasted); 4 hours (nonfasted)

Reproductive Considerations

The Health and Human Services (HHS) perinatal HIV guidelines consider ritonavir, when used as a booster for other protease inhibitors, to be a preferred or alternate component of regimens for females living with HIV who are not yet pregnant but are trying to conceive.

For males and females living with HIV and planning a pregnancy, maximum viral suppression below the limits of detection with antiretroviral therapy (ART), modification of therapy (if needed), optimization of the woman's health, and a discussion of the potential risks and benefits of ART therapy during pregnancy is recommended prior to conception (HHS [perinatal] 2019).

Pregnancy Considerations

Ritonavir has a low level of transfer across the human placenta.

No increased risk of overall birth defects has been observed following first trimester exposure according to data collected by the antiretroviral pregnancy registry. Maternal antiretroviral therapy (ART) may be associated with adverse pregnancy outcomes including preterm delivery, stillbirth, low birth weight, and small for gestational age infants. Actual risks may be influenced by maternal factors, such as disease severity, gestational age at initiation of therapy, and specific ART regimen; therefore, close fetal monitoring is recommended. Because there is clear benefit to appropriate treatment, maternal ART should not be withheld due to concerns for adverse neonatal outcomes. Long-term follow-up is recommended for all infants exposed to antiretroviral medications; children without HIV but who were exposed to ART in utero and develop significant organ system abnormalities of unknown etiology (particularly of the CNS or heart) should be evaluated for potential mitochondrial dysfunction.

Hyperglycemia, new onset of diabetes mellitus, or diabetic ketoacidosis have been reported with protease inhibitors (PI); it is not clear if pregnancy increases this risk. Consider performing the standard glucose screening test earlier in pregnancy in women who initiated PI therapy prior to conception.

The Health and Human Services (HHS) perinatal HIV guidelines do not recommend treatment doses of ritonavir in pregnant women. Ritonavir should only be used as a low-dose booster; when used as a pharmacologic booster for other PIs, ritonavir is the preferred pharmacologic booster for use in pregnancy.

The HHS perinatal HIV guidelines consider ritonavir, when used as a booster for other PIs, to be a preferred or alternate component of regimens for pregnant females living with HIV who are antiretroviral naive, who have had ART therapy in the past but are restarting, or who require a new ART regimen (due to poor tolerance or poor virologic response of current regimen). In addition, females who become pregnant while taking ritonavir (used as a booster) may continue if viral suppression is effective and the regimen is well tolerated. A ritonavir-boosted PI regimen is also recommended when acute HIV infection is detected during pregnancy. Plasma levels are lower during pregnancy compared to postpartum; however, dosage adjustment is not needed when used as a low-dose booster in pregnant females. The oral solution contains alcohol and, therefore, is not recommended for use in pregnant patients.

In general, ART is recommended for all pregnant females living with HIV to keep the viral load below the limit of detection and reduce the risk of perinatal transmission. Therapy should be individualized following a discussion of the potential risks and benefits of treatment during pregnancy. Monitoring of pregnant females is more frequent than in nonpregnant adults. ART should be continued postpartum for all females living with HIV and can be modified after delivery.

Health care providers are encouraged to enroll pregnant females exposed to antiretroviral medications as early in pregnancy as possible in the Antiretroviral Pregnancy Registry (1-800-258-4263 or http://www.APRegistry.com). Health care providers caring for pregnant females living with HIV and their infants may contact the National Perinatal HIV Hotline (1-888-448-8765) for clinical consultation (HHS [perinatal] 2019).

Product Availability Norvir **capsules** have been discontinued in the United States for more than 1 year.

◆ **Ritonavir and Lopinavir** *see* Lopinavir and Ritonavir *on page 929*

◆ **Ritonavir, Ombitasvir, and Paritaprevir** *see* Ombitasvir, Paritaprevir, and Ritonavir *on page 1135*

◆ **Ritonavir, Ombitasvir, Paritaprevir, and Dasabuvir** *see* Ombitasvir, Paritaprevir, Ritonavir, and Dasabuvir *on page 1136*

◆ **Rituxan** *see* RiTUXimab *on page 1336*

◆ **Rituxan Hycela** *see* Rituximab and Hyaluronidase *on page 1338*

RiTUXimab (ri TUK si mab)

Brand Names: US Rituxan; Ruxience; Truxima

Brand Names: Canada Rituxan; Ruxience; Truxima

Pharmacologic Category Antineoplastic Agent, Anti-CD20; Antineoplastic Agent, Monoclonal Antibody; Antirheumatic Miscellaneous; Immunosuppressant Agent; Monoclonal Antibody

Use

Chronic lymphocytic leukemia (Rituxan and rituximab biosimilars): Treatment of previously untreated or previously treated CD20-positive chronic lymphocytic leukemia (CLL) in adults (in combination with fludarabine and cyclophosphamide).

Note: Other medications have approval for use in combination with rituximab (eg, idelalisib, venetoclax, ibrutinib) for the treatment of relapsed or refractory CLL.

Granulomatosis with polyangiitis (Rituxan and rituximab biosimilars): Treatment of granulomatosis with polyangiitis (Wegener granulomatosis) (in combination with glucocorticoids) in adults (Rituxan and rituximab biosimilars) and pediatric patients ≥2 years of age (Rituxan only).

Microscopic polyangiitis (Rituxan and rituximab biosimilars): Treatment of microscopic polyangiitis (in combination with glucocorticoids) in adults (Rituxan and rituximab biosimilars) and pediatric patients ≥2 years of age (Rituxan only).

Non-Hodgkin lymphomas (Rituxan and rituximab biosimilars): Treatment of CD20-positive non-Hodgkin lymphomas (NHL) in adults with:

Relapsed or refractory, low-grade or follicular B-cell NHL (as a single agent).

Follicular B-cell NHL, previously untreated (in combination with first-line chemotherapy, and as single-agent maintenance therapy if complete or partial response to rituximab with chemotherapy).

Nonprogressing (including stable disease), low-grade B-cell NHL (as a single agent after first-line cyclophosphamide, vincristine, and prednisone [CVP] treatment).

Diffuse large B-cell NHL, previously untreated (in combination with cyclophosphamide, doxorubicin, vincristine, and prednisone [CHOP] chemotherapy, or other anthracycline-based regimen).

Pemphigus vulgaris (Rituxan only): Treatment of moderate to severe pemphigus vulgaris in adults.

Rheumatoid arthritis (Rituxan and Truxima [rituximab biosimilar] only): Treatment of moderately to severely active rheumatoid arthritis (in combination with methotrexate) in adults with inadequate response to one or more tumor necrosis factor-antagonist therapies.

Note: Ruxience (rituximab-pvvr) and Truxima (rituximab-abbs) have been approved as biosimilars to Rituxan (rituximab).

Local Anesthetic/Vasoconstrictor Precautions No information available to require special precautions

Effects on Dental Treatment No significant effects or complications reported

Effects on Bleeding Chemotherapy may result in significant myelosuppression, potentially including significant reduction in platelet counts (thrombocytopenia grades 3/4: 2% to 11%) and altered hemostasis. In patients who are under active treatment with these agents, medical consult is suggested.

Adverse Reactions Patients treated with rituximab for rheumatoid arthritis (RA) may experience fewer adverse reactions. Most reported adverse reactions are from studies in which rituximab was given concomitantly with chemotherapeutic agents, glucocorticoid steroids, or methotrexate.

>10%:

Cardiovascular: Cardiac disorder (5% to 29%), flushing (5% to 14%), hypertension (6% to 12%), peripheral edema (8% to 16%)

Dermatologic: Night sweats (15%), pruritus (≤17%), skin rash (≤17%)

Endocrine & metabolic: Hypophosphatemia (12% to 21%), weight gain (11%)

Gastrointestinal: Abdominal pain (14%), diarrhea (10% to 17%), nausea (8% to 23%)

Genitourinary: Urinary tract infection

Hematologic & oncologic: Anemia (8% to 35%; grades 3/4: 3%), febrile neutropenia (grades 3/4: 9% to 15%), hypogammaglobulinemia (27% to 58%), leukopenia (10% to 23%; grades 3/4: 4% to 23%), lymphocytopenia (48%; grades 3/4: 40%; median duration: 14 days), neutropenia (8% to 49%; grades 3/4: 4% to 49%; prolonged lasting up to 42 days: 25%; late-onset occurring >42 days after last dose: 15% to 39%), thrombocytopenia (12%; grades 3/4: 2% to 11%)

Hepatic: Hepatobiliary disease (17%), increased serum alanine aminotransferase (13%)

Hypersensitivity: Angioedema (11%)

Immunologic: Antibody development (1% to 23%)

Infection: Bacterial infection (19%), infection (19% to 62%), serious infection (2% to 11%)

Nervous system: Chills (3% to 33%), fatigue (13% to 39%), headache (17% to 19%), insomnia (14%), pain (12%), peripheral sensory neuropathy (30%)

Neuromuscular & skeletal: Arthralgia (6% to 13%), asthenia (2% to 26%), muscle spasm (17%)

Respiratory: Bronchitis, cough (13% to 15%), epistaxis (11%), nasopharyngitis, pulmonary disease (31%), pulmonary toxicity (18%), rhinitis (3% to 12%)

Miscellaneous: Fever (5% to 56%), infusion related reaction (first dose: 12% to 77%; decreases with subsequent infusions)

1% to 10%:

Cardiovascular: Chest tightness (7%), hypotension (10%), significant cardiovascular event (2%)

Dermatologic: Urticaria (2% to 8%)

Endocrine & metabolic: Hyperglycemia (9%), hyperuricemia (2%), increased lactate dehydrogenase (7%)

Gastrointestinal: Dyspepsia (3%), upper abdominal pain (2%), vomiting (10%)

Hematologic & oncologic: Pancytopenia (grades 3/4: 3%)

Hepatic: Hepatitis B (grades 3/4: 2%)

Infection: Fungal infection (1%), viral infection (10%)

Nervous system: Anxiety (2% to 5%), dizziness (10%), migraine (2%), paresthesia (2%), rigors (10%)

Neuromuscular & skeletal: Back pain (10%), myalgia (10%)

Respiratory: Bronchospasm (8%), dyspnea (7% to 10%), sinusitis (6%), throat irritation (2% to 9%), upper respiratory tract infection (7%)

<1%:

Hematologic & oncologic: Hemolytic anemia, pure red cell aplasia

Frequency not defined:

Cardiovascular: Acute myocardial infarction, cardiogenic shock, supraventricular cardiac arrhythmia, ventricular fibrillation, ventricular tachycardia

Dermatologic: Cellulitis

Gastrointestinal: Acute mucocutaneous toxicity

Hepatic: Fulminant hepatitis, hepatic failure, hepatitis

Hypersensitivity: Nonimmune anaphylaxis

Infection: Influenza, lower respiratory tract infection

Respiratory: Acute respiratory distress syndrome, hypoxia, pneumonia, pneumonitis, pulmonary infiltrates

Postmarketing:

Cardiovascular: Cardiac failure, vasculitis (systemic; with rash)

Dermatologic: Lichenoid dermatitis, pemphigus (paraneoplastic), pyoderma gangrenosum (including genital presentation), Stevens-Johnson syndrome, toxic epidermal necrolysis, vesiculobullous dermatitis

Gastrointestinal: Gastrointestinal perforation, intestinal obstruction, intestinal perforation
Hematologic & oncologic: Bone marrow depression, increased serum immunoglobulins (hyperviscosity syndrome in Waldenstrom's macroglobulinemia), Kaposi sarcoma (progression), tumor lysis syndrome
Hypersensitivity: Serum sickness
Infection: Reactivation of HBV
Nervous system: Progressive multifocal leukoencephalopathy, reversible posterior leukoencephalopathy syndrome
Neuromuscular & skeletal: Arthritis (polyarticular), lupus-like syndrome
Ophthalmic: Optic neuritis, uveitis
Renal: Nephrotoxicity
Respiratory: Bronchiolitis obliterans, interstitial pulmonary disease, pleurisy

Mechanism of Action Rituximab is a monoclonal antibody directed against the CD20 antigen on the surface of B-lymphocytes. CD20 regulates cell cycle initiation; and, possibly, functions as a calcium channel. Rituximab binds to the antigen on the cell surface, activating complement-dependent B-cell cytotoxicity; and to human Fc receptors, mediating cell killing through an antibody-dependent cellular toxicity. B-cells are believed to play a role in the development and progression of rheumatoid arthritis. Signs and symptoms of rheumatoid arthritis are reduced by targeting B-cells and the progression of structural damage is delayed.

Pharmacodynamics/Kinetics

Onset of Action

Immune thrombocytopenia: Initial response: 7 to 56 days; Peak response: 14 to 180 days (Neunert 2011)
NHL: B-cell depletion: Within 3 weeks.
Rheumatoid arthritis (RA): B-cell depletion: Within 2 weeks.

Duration of Action

NHL: Detectable in serum 3 to 6 months after completion of treatment; B-cell depletion is sustained for up to 6 to 9 months and B-cell recovery begins ~6 months following completion of treatment; median B-cell levels return to normal by 12 months following completion of treatment
RA: B-cell depletion persists for at least 6 months.

Half-life Elimination

Chronic lymphocytic leukemia: Median terminal half-life: 32 days (range: 14 to 62 days).
Non-Hodgkin lymphomas: Median terminal half-life: 22 days (range: 6 to 52 days).
Rheumatoid arthritis: Mean terminal half-life: 18 days (range: 5 to 78 days).
Granulomatosis with polyangiitis/microscopic polyangiitis:
Children ≥6 years and Adolescents ≤17 years: Median: 22 days (range: 11 to 42 days).
Adults: Median: 25 days (range: 11 to 52 days).

Reproductive Considerations

Effective contraception should be used in women of reproductive potential during therapy and for at least 12 months following the last rituximab dose.

When treating rheumatoid arthritis, it is recommended to discontinue use and switch to a safer medication prior to conception unless no other pregnancy compatible medication is able to control maternal disease (Götestam Skorpen 2016).

Pregnancy Considerations Rituximab crosses the placenta and can be detected in the newborn. In one infant born at 41 weeks' gestation, in utero exposure occurred from week 16 to 37; rituximab concentrations were higher in the neonate at birth (32,095 ng/mL) than the mother (9,750 ng/mL) and still measurable at 18 weeks of age (700 ng/mL infant; 500 ng/mL mother) (Friedrichs 2006).

B-cell lymphocytopenia lasting <6 months may occur in exposed infants. Retrospective case reports of inadvertent pregnancy during rituximab treatment collected by the manufacturer (often combined with concomitant teratogenic therapies) describe premature births and infant hematologic abnormalities and infections; no specific pattern of birth defects has been observed (limited data) (Chakravarty 2011). Similar information from a British pregnancy registry and a case series has also been published (Das 2018; De Cock 2017).

The European Society for Medical Oncology has published guidelines for diagnosis, treatment, and follow-up of cancer during pregnancy. The guidelines recommend referral to a facility with expertise in cancer during pregnancy and encourage a multidisciplinary team (obstetrician, neonatologist, oncology team). Based on limited data, if pregnancy occurs during rituximab treatment, the pregnancy may continue provided rituximab treatment is withheld. In general, although the risk of B-cell depletion in the newborn is increased, if postponing rituximab treatment would significantly compromise maternal outcome in patients diagnosed with B-cell lymphoma during pregnancy, rituximab use is not discouraged during the pregnancy (Peccatori 2013). An international consensus panel has published guidelines for hematologic malignancies during pregnancy. In patients with aggressive lymphomas, rituximab (as a component of the R-CHOP chemotherapy regimen) may be administered in the second and third trimesters, however, the cytotoxic portion of the regimen should not be administered within 3 weeks prior to anticipated delivery (Lishner 2016).

Other agents are preferred for treating lupus nephritis in pregnant women (Hahn 2012). When treating rheumatoid arthritis, it is recommended to discontinue use and switch to a safer medication prior to conception unless no other pregnancy compatible medication is able to control maternal disease (Götestam Skorpen 2016).

Data collection to monitor pregnancy and infant outcomes following exposure to rituximab is ongoing. A pregnancy registry is available for all cancers diagnosed during pregnancy at Cooper Health (877-635-4499).

◆ **Rituximab, IV** *see* RiTUXimab *on page 1336*
◆ **Rituximab-abbs** *see* RiTUXimab *on page 1336*

Rituximab and Hyaluronidase

(ri TUK si mab & hye al yoor ON i dase)

Brand Names: US Rituxan Hycela
Brand Names: Canada Rituxan SC
Pharmacologic Category Antineoplastic Agent, Anti-CD20; Antineoplastic Agent, Monoclonal Antibody

Use

Chronic lymphocytic leukemia: Treatment of adult patients with previously untreated and previously treated chronic lymphocytic leukemia (CLL) (in combination with fludarabine and cyclophosphamide)
Diffuse large B-cell lymphoma: Treatment of adult patients with previously untreated diffuse large B-cell lymphoma (DLBCL) in combination with cyclophosphamide, doxorubicin, vincristine, prednisone (CHOP) or other anthracycline-based chemotherapy regimens

Follicular lymphoma: Treatment of adult patients with:
- Relapsed or refractory follicular lymphoma (FL) as a single agent;
- Previously untreated FL (in combination with first-line chemotherapy) and, in patients achieving a complete or partial response to rituximab in combination with chemotherapy (as single-agent maintenance therapy);
- Non-progressing (including stable disease) FL as a single agent after first-line cyclophosphamide, vincristine, and prednisone (CVP) chemotherapy

Limitations of use: Initiate treatment with rituximab/hyaluronidase only after patients have received at least 1 full dose of a rituximab product by intravenous infusion; rituximab/hyaluronidase is not indicated for the treatment of non-malignant conditions.

Local Anesthetic/Vasoconstrictor Precautions No information available to require special precautions

Effects on Dental Treatment No significant effects or complications reported

Effects on Bleeding Chemotherapy may result in significant myelosuppression, potentially including significant reduction in platelet counts (thrombocytopenia grades 3/4: 2% to 11%) and altered hemostasis. In patients who are under active treatment with these agents, medical consult is suggested.

Adverse Reactions Also see individual agents. All incidences are from combination therapy regimens.

>10%:
- Dermatologic: Alopecia (14% to 24%), dermatological reaction (16%), erythema of skin (9% to 15%), skin rash (10% to 12%; including severe mucocutaneous reactions)
- Gastrointestinal: Nausea (22% to 38%), constipation (8% to 25%), vomiting (11% to 21%), diarrhea (14% to 18%), abdominal pain (7% to 14%)
- Hematologic & oncologic: Neutropenia (31% to 65%; grades 3/4: 25% to 56%), anemia (15% to 23%; grades 3/4: 5%), leukopenia (6% to 19%; grades 3/4: 3% to 4%), febrile neutropenia (8% to 14%; grades 3/4: 7% to 14%)
- Immunologic: Antibody development (anti-hyaluronidase antibodies: 11% to 13%; anti-rituximab antibodies: 2%)
- Infection: Serious infection (46% to 56%)
- Local: Erythema at injection site (13% to 26%)
- Nervous system: Fatigue (11% to 20%), paresthesia (9% to 16%), chills (8% to 13%), headache (6% to 13%), peripheral neuropathy (12%; grades 3/4: ≤2%)
- Neuromuscular & skeletal: Asthenia (8% to 17%), arthralgia (9% to 13%)
- Respiratory: Cough (11% to 23%), upper respiratory tract infection (13% to 15%), dyspnea (4% to 11%), pneumonia (2% to 11%)
- Miscellaneous: Fever (13% to 32%)

1% to 10%:
- Cardiovascular: Peripheral edema (5% to 8%), chest pain (6%), hypertension (6%), hypotension (1%)
- Dermatologic: Pruritus (8% to 10%)
- Endocrine & metabolic: Weight loss (8%)
- Gastrointestinal: Decreased appetite (8%), dyspepsia (5% to 8%), stomatitis (5% to 8%; grades 3/4: ≤1%), upper abdominal pain (5%)
- Genitourinary: Urinary tract infection (2% to 8%)
- Hematologic & oncologic: Lymphocytopenia (5%; grades 3/4: 1%)
- Infection: Influenza (4%)
- Local: Pain at injection site (8% to 16%)
- Nervous system: Insomnia (1% to 9%), dizziness (7%)
- Neuromuscular & skeletal: Limb pain (7% to 10%), ostealgia (6% to 10%), back pain (9%), muscle spasm (8%), myalgia (8%)
- Ophthalmic: Conjunctivitis (5%)
- Respiratory: Nasopharyngitis (10%), oropharyngeal pain (6% to 9%), bronchitis (7% to 8%), sinusitis (7%), flu-like symptoms (3%)

Frequency not defined:
- Hepatic: Fulminant hepatitis, hepatic failure
- Hypersensitivity: Hypersensitivity reaction
- Infection: JC virus infection, reactivation of HBV
- Local: Infusion site reaction (≤7% monotherapy in maintenance setting; higher with combination therapy and initial infusions)

<1%, postmarketing, and/or case reports: Bone marrow depression, bronchiolitis obliterans, hypogammaglobulinemia (prolonged), inflammatory polyarthropathy, interstitial pulmonary disease, intestinal obstruction, intestinal perforation, Kaposi sarcoma (disease progression), lichenoid dermatitis, lupus-like syndrome, optic neuritis, pancytopenia (prolonged), pemphigoid reaction, pleurisy, progressive multifocal leukoencephalopathy, pyoderma gangrenosum (including genital presentation), serum sickness, severe dermatological reaction, Stevens-Johnson syndrome, toxic epidermal necrolysis, uveitis, vasculitis (systemic; with rash), vesiculobullous dermatitis, viral infection

Mechanism of Action

Rituximab is a monoclonal antibody directed against the CD20 antigen on the surface of pre-B and mature B-lymphocytes. CD20 regulates cell cycle initiation; and, possibly, functions as a calcium channel. Rituximab binds to the antigen on the cell surface, activating complement-dependent B-cell cytotoxicity; and to human Fc receptors, mediating cell killing through an antibody-dependent cellular toxicity.

Hyaluronidase increases the absorption rate of rituximab-containing products by increasing permeability of subcutaneous tissue through temporary depolymerization of hyaluronan; at the recommended doses, hyaluronidase acts locally and the effects are reversible. Permeability of the subcutaneous tissue is restored within 24 to 48 hours.

Pharmacodynamics/Kinetics

Onset of Action

CLL: B-cells begin to deplete following the first cycle of rituximab, with 28% of patients B-cell depleted prior to the dose in cycle 2; by cycle 6, 96% of patients were B-cell depleted.

FL: Peripheral B-cell counts decrease to levels below normal following the first cycle of rituximab and are maintained during treatment with rituximab/hyaluronidase.

Duration of Action

CLL: Patients remained B-cell depleted until month 9, where signs of repletion were seen.

FL: After discontinuing rituximab/hyaluronidase, B-cell repletion begins after 6 months (may be longer in some patients)

Half-life Elimination Terminal: 32 days (CLL); 34.1 days (FL)

Reproductive Considerations

Verify pregnancy status prior to treatment initiation in females of reproductive potential.

Effective contraception should be used in females of reproductive potential during therapy and for 12 months following the last rituximab/hyaluronidase dose.

Rituximab/hyaluronidase may be used as monotherapy or in combination with other chemotherapy agents (eg, cyclophosphamide, doxorubicin, fludarabine, vincristine); refer to the rituximab, hyaluronidase, and other individual monographs for additional information.

Pregnancy Considerations

Rituximab crosses the placenta. Based on human data, rituximab-containing products may cause adverse outcomes in infants following in utero exposure.

Rituximab/hyaluronidase may be used as monotherapy or in combination with other chemotherapy agents (eg, cyclophosphamide, doxorubicin, fludarabine, vincristine); refer to the rituximab, hyaluronidase, and other individual monographs for additional information.

- **Rituximab Conventional** *see* RiTUXimab *on page 1336*
- **Rituximab Intravenous** *see* RiTUXimab *on page 1336*
- **Rituximab-pvvr** *see* RiTUXimab *on page 1336*
- **Rituximab Subcutaneous** *see* Rituximab and Hyaluronidase *on page 1338*
- **RIV** *see* Influenza Virus Vaccine (Recombinant) *on page 815*
- **RIV4** *see* Influenza Virus Vaccine (Recombinant) *on page 815*

Rivaroxaban (riv a ROX a ban)

Related Information

Antiplatelet and Anticoagulation Considerations in Dentistry *on page 1666*

Brand Names: US Xarelto; Xarelto Starter Pack

Brand Names: Canada Xarelto; Xarelto Starter Pack [DSC]

Pharmacologic Category Anticoagulant; Anticoagulant, Factor Xa Inhibitor; Direct Oral Anticoagulant (DOAC)

Use

Atrial fibrillation, nonvalvular: Prevention of stroke and systemic embolism in patients with nonvalvular atrial fibrillation.

Coronary artery disease (stable) or peripheral artery disease: Reduction of risk of major cardiovascular (CV) events (CV death, myocardial infarction, and stroke) in patients with coronary artery disease (chronic) or peripheral artery disease.

Indefinite anticoagulation (reduced intensity dosing against venous thromboembolism recurrence): Reduction in the risk of recurrence of deep vein thrombosis (DVT) and pulmonary embolism (PE) in patients at continued risk of DVT and PE following ≥6 months of initial full therapeutic anticoagulant treatment for DVT and/or PE.

Venous thromboembolism (deep vein thrombosis or pulmonary embolism): Treatment of DVT or PE.

Venous thromboembolism prophylaxis in acutely ill medical patients: Prophylaxis of venous thromboembolism (VTE) and VTE-related death during hospitalization and posthospital discharge in adults admitted for an acute medical illness who are at risk for thromboembolic complications due to moderate or severe restricted mobility and other risk factors for VTE and not at high risk of bleeding.

Venous thromboembolism prophylaxis in total hip or knee arthroplasty: Postoperative thromboprophylaxis of DVT, which may lead to PE in patients undergoing total hip arthroplasty or total knee arthroplasty.

Local Anesthetic/Vasoconstrictor Precautions No information available to require special precautions

Effects on Dental Treatment Key adverse event(s) related to dental treatment: Bleeding. See Effects on Bleeding.

Effects on Bleeding Rivaroxaban inhibits platelet activation and fibrin clot formation via direct, selective, and reversible inhibition of factor Xa. As with all anticoagulants, bleeding is the major adverse effect of rivaroxaban. Hemorrhage may occur at virtually any site; risk is dependent on multiple variables including the intensity of anticoagulation and patient susceptibility. Medical consult is suggested.

Adverse Reactions

>10%: Hematologic & oncologic: Hemorrhage (5% to 28%; major: ≤4%)

1% to 10%:

Cardiovascular: Syncope (1%)

Dermatologic: Pruritus (2%), skin blister (1%), wound secretion (3%)

Gastrointestinal: Abdominal pain (3%), gastrointestinal hemorrhage (2%)

Hepatic: Increased serum transaminases (>3 x ULN: 2% [Watkins 2011])

Nervous system: Anxiety (1%), depression (1%), dizziness (2%), fatigue (1%), insomnia (2%)

Neuromuscular & skeletal: Back pain (3%), limb pain (2%), muscle spasm (1%)

<1%:

Hematologic & oncologic: Hemophthalmos, surgical bleeding

Nervous system: Intracranial hemorrhage

Postmarketing:

Cardiovascular: Cardiac tamponade (Oladiran 2018), hemopericardium (Basnet 2017), hypersensitivity angiitis (Lee 2019), thrombosis (with premature discontinuation) (Nagasayi 2017; Shaw 2020)

Dermatologic: Bullous pemphigoid (Ferreira 2018), Stevens-Johnson syndrome

Endocrine & metabolic: Adrenal hemorrhage (bilateral) (Alidoost 2019)

Gastrointestinal: Cholestasis (Aslan 2016)

Hematologic & oncologic: Agranulocytosis, pulmonary hemorrhage (Ciofoaia 2018; Hammar 2015), retroperitoneal hemorrhage (Borekci 2019a; Börekci 2019b), spinal hematoma (Goldfine 2018; Madhisetti 2015), splenic rupture (Nagaraja 2018), thrombocytopenia (Mima 2014), vitreous hemorrhage (spontaneous) (Jun 2015)

Hepatic: Hepatic failure (Baig 2015), hepatic injury (Glenn 2017; Licata 2018), hepatitis (Russmann 2014), jaundice (Glenn 2017)

Hypersensitivity: Anaphylactic shock, anaphylaxis, angioedema (Patil 2019)

Immunologic: Drug reaction with eosinophilia and systemic symptoms (Chiasson 2017)

Nervous system: Cerebral hemorrhage (Hagii 2014; Wilson 2016), epidural intracranial hemorrhage (Burjorjee 2018; Jaeger 2012)

Respiratory: Bronchiectasis

Mechanism of Action Inhibits platelet activation and fibrin clot formation via direct, selective and reversible inhibition of factor Xa (FXa) in both the intrinsic and extrinsic coagulation pathways. FXa, as part of the prothrombinase complex consisting also of factor Va, calcium ions, factor II and phospholipid, catalyzes the conversion of prothrombin to thrombin. Thrombin both activates platelets and catalyzes the conversion of fibrinogen to fibrin.

Pharmacodynamics/Kinetics

Half-life Elimination Terminal: 5 to 9 hours; Elderly: 11 to 13 hours

Time to Peak Plasma: 2 to 4 hours

Reproductive Considerations

Information related to the use of direct acting oral anticoagulants in pregnancy is limited; until safety data are available, adequate contraception is recommended during therapy for females of childbearing potential. Females planning a pregnancy should be switched to alternative anticoagulants prior to conception (Cohen 2016).

Pregnancy Considerations

Based on ex vivo data, rivaroxaban crosses the placenta (Bapat 2015).

Information related to the use of rivaroxaban during pregnancy (Beyer-Westendorf 2016; Hoeltzenbein 2015; Königsbrügge 2014; Lameijer 2018; Myers 2016) and postpartum (Rudd 2015) is limited. Use of direct acting oral anticoagulants increases the risk of bleeding in all patients. When used in pregnancy, there is also the potential for fetal bleeding or subclinical placental bleeding which may increase the risk of miscarriage, preterm delivery, fetal compromise, or stillbirth (Cohen 2016).

Data are insufficient to evaluate the safety of direct acting oral anticoagulants during pregnancy (Bates 2012) and use in pregnant females is not recommended (Regitz-Zagrosek [ESC 2018]). Agents other than rivaroxaban are preferred for the treatment of AF or VTE in pregnant patients (Kearon 2016; Lip 2018; Regitz-Zagrosek [ESC 2018]). Patients should be switched to an alternative anticoagulant if pregnancy occurs during therapy. Fetal monitoring that includes evaluations for fetal bleeding and assessments for risk of preterm delivery are recommended if the direct acting oral anticoagulant is continued (Cohen 2016).

Dental Health Professional Considerations Medical consult is suggested prior to dental invasive procedures. At this time there are no coagulation parameters for rivaroxaban to predict the extent of bleeding. Increased bleeding may occur during invasive dental procedures in patients taking rivaroxaban. Currently, postsurgical treatment with rivaroxaban is ~12 days for knee replacement patients and ~35 days for hip replacement patients. There are no reports of interactions between the anticoagulant and amoxicillin, cephalexin, cefazolin, ampicillin, or clindamycin; therefore, any of these preprocedural antibiotics can safely be used in patients taking rivaroxaban. Routine coagulation testing (INR) is not required, or necessary, for Direct-Acting Oral Anticoagulants (DOAC).

Rivastigmine (ri va STIG meen)

Brand Names: US Exelon

Brand Names: Canada APO-Rivastigmine; Auro-Rivastigmine; Exelon; JAMP Rivastigmine; MED-Rivastigmine; MINT-Rivastigmine [DSC]; MYLAN-Rivastigmine; NOVO-Rivastigmine [DSC]; PMS-Rivastigmine; RATIO-Rivastigmine [DSC]; SANDOZ Rivastigmine

Pharmacologic Category Acetylcholinesterase Inhibitor (Central)

Use

Alzheimer dementia:

Oral: Treatment of mild to moderate dementia of the Alzheimer type.

Transdermal: Treatment of mild, moderate, and severe dementia of the Alzheimer type.

Parkinson disease dementia: Treatment of mild to moderate dementia associated with Parkinson disease.

Local Anesthetic/Vasoconstrictor Precautions No information available to require special precautions

Effects on Dental Treatment No significant effects or complications reported

Effects on Bleeding No information available to require special precautions

Adverse Reactions

>10%:

Central nervous system: Dizziness (oral: 6% to 21%; transdermal: ≤6%), headache (oral: 4% to 17%; transdermal ≤4%), agitation (transdermal: 1% to 14%), falling (6% to 12%)

Endocrine & metabolic: Weight loss (3% to 26%)

Gastrointestinal: Nausea (oral: 17% to 47%; transdermal: 2% to 10%), vomiting (oral: 13% to 31%; transdermal: 3% to 9%), diarrhea (oral: 5% to 19%; transdermal: ≤7%), anorexia (oral: ≤17%; transdermal: ≤3%), abdominal pain (oral: 13%; transdermal: 2%)

Local: Application site erythema (transdermal: 1% to 13%)

Neuromuscular & skeletal: Tremor (oral: 4% to 23%; transdermal: 7%)

1% to 10%:

Cardiovascular: Hypertension (1% to 3%), syncope (oral: 3%)

Central nervous system: Fatigue (oral: 4% to 9%; transdermal: 2% to 4%), insomnia (1% to 9%), confusion (oral: 8%), depression (2% to 6%), drowsiness (4% to 6%), malaise (oral: 5%), anxiety (1% to 5%), hallucination (2% to 5%), abnormal gait (transdermal: 4%), psychomotor agitation (transdermal: 1% to 3%), aggressive behavior (1% to 3%), exacerbation of Parkinson disease (oral: 1% to 3%), cogwheel rigidity (oral: 1% to 3%), restlessness (oral: 1% to 3%), drug-induced Parkinson disease (oral: 2%)

Dermatologic: Diaphoresis (oral: 2% to 4%)

Endocrine & metabolic: Dehydration (1% to 2%)

Gastrointestinal: Dyspepsia (oral: 9%), decreased appetite (≤9%), upper abdominal pain (≤4%), sialorrhea (oral: 1% to 2%)

Genitourinary: Urinary tract infection (1% to 10%), urinary incontinence (≤3%)

Local: Application site pruritus (transdermal: ≤5%), application site irritation (transdermal: ≤3%), application site rash (transdermal: 2%)

Neuromuscular & skeletal: Weakness (2% to 6%;), bradykinesia (3% to 4%), hypokinesia (1% to 4%), dyskinesia (3%)

<1%, postmarketing, and/or case reports: Abnormal hepatic function tests, allergic dermatitis, atrial fibrillation, atrioventricular block, bradycardia, dermatitis (transdermal patch), dystonia, edema, extrapyramidal reaction, gastrointestinal hemorrhage, hepatic failure, hepatitis, hyperacidity, hypersensitivity reaction, nightmares, pancreatitis, seizure, severe vomiting (with esophageal rupture; following inappropriate reinitiation of dose), sick-sinus syndrome, skin blister, Stevens-Johnson syndrome, tachycardia, urticaria

Mechanism of Action A deficiency of cortical acetylcholine is thought to account for some of the symptoms of Alzheimer disease and the dementia of Parkinson disease; rivastigmine increases acetylcholine in the central nervous system through reversible inhibition of its hydrolysis by cholinesterase

Pharmacodynamics/Kinetics

Duration of Action Anticholinesterase activity (CSF): ~10 hours (6 mg oral dose)

Half-life Elimination Oral: 1.5 hours; Transdermal patch: ~3 hours (after removal)

Time to Peak Oral: 1 hour; Transdermal patch: 8 to 16 hours following first dose

Pregnancy Considerations Adverse events have not been observed in animal reproduction studies.

- **Rivastigmine Tartrate** *see* Rivastigmine *on page 1341*
- **Rivelsa** *see* Ethinyl Estradiol and Levonorgestrel *on page 612*

Rizatriptan (rye za TRIP tan)

Brand Names: US Maxalt; Maxalt-MLT

Brand Names: Canada ACCEL-Rizatriptan ODT; ACT Rizatriptan; ACT Rizatriptan ODT [DSC]; AG-Rizatriptan ODT; APO-Rizatriptan; APO-Rizatriptan RPD; Auro-Rizatriptan; CCP-Rizatriptan ODT; DOM-Rizatriptan RDT; JAMP-Rizatriptan; JAMP-Rizatriptan IR; JAMP-Rizatriptan ODT; MAR-Rizatriptan; MAR-Rizatriptan ODT; Maxalt; Maxalt RPD; MINT-Rizatriptan ODT [DSC]; MYLAN-Rizatriptan ODT; NAT-Rizatriptan ODT; NRA-Rizatriptan ODT; PMS-Rizatriptan RDT; RIVA-Rizatriptan ODT [DSC]; SANDOZ Rizatriptan ODT; TEVA-Rizatriptan ODT; VAN-Rizatriptan ODT [DSC]; VAN-Rizatriptan [DSC]

Pharmacologic Category Antimigraine Agent; Serotonin 5-$HT_{1B, 1D}$ Receptor Agonist

Use Migraine: Acute treatment of migraine with or without aura

Local Anesthetic/Vasoconstrictor Precautions No information available to require special precautions

Effects on Dental Treatment Key adverse event(s) related to dental treatment: Xerostomia (normal salivary flow resumes upon discontinuation).

Effects on Bleeding No information available to require special precautions

Adverse Reactions

1% to 10%:

Cardiovascular: Chest pain (≤3%), flushing (>1%), palpitations (>1%), flushing

Central nervous system: Dizziness (4% to 9%), drowsiness (4% to 8%), fatigue (adults: 4% to 7%; children: >1%), paresthesia (3% to 4%), pain (3%), feeling of heaviness (≤2%), headache (≤2%), euphoria (>1%), hypoesthesia (>1%)

Gastrointestinal: Nausea (4% to 6%), xerostomia (3%), sore throat (≤2%), abdominal distress (children: >1%), diarrhea (>1%), vomiting (>1%)

Neuromuscular & skeletal: Weakness (4% to 7%), jaw pain (≤2%), jaw pressure (≤2%), jaw tightness (≤2%), neck pain (≤2%), neck pressure (≤2%), neck tightness (≤2%), tremor (>1%)

Respiratory: Pharyngeal edema (≤2%), pressure on pharynx (≤2%), dyspnea (>1%)

<1%, postmarketing, and/or case reports: Abdominal distention, abnormal gait, agitation, anaphylaxis, anaphylactoid reaction, angina pectoris, angioedema, ataxia (children), auditory impairment (children), blurred vision, bradycardia, cardiac arrhythmia, cold extremities, confusion, diaphoresis, dysgeusia, dyspepsia, edema, erythema, facial edema, hallucination (children), hot flash, hypertensive crisis, increased blood pressure (diastolic/systolic), insomnia, ischemic heart disease, lack of concentration (children), memory impairment, muscle rigidity, muscle spasm, myalgia, myocardial infarction, pharyngeal edema, pruritus, seizure, skin rash, swelling of eye, syncope, tachycardia, tinnitus, tongue edema, toxic epidermal necrolysis, urticaria, vasospasm, vertigo, wheezing

Mechanism of Action Selective agonist for serotonin (5-HT_{1B} and 5-HT_{1D} receptors) in cranial arteries; causes vasoconstriction and reduces sterile inflammation associated with antidromic neuronal transmission correlating with relief of migraine

Pharmacodynamics/Kinetics

Onset of Action Most patients have response to treatment within 2 hours

Half-life Elimination 2-3 hours

Time to Peak Maxalt: 1 to 1.5 hours; Maxalt-MLT: 1.6 to 2.5 hours

Pregnancy Considerations

A registry has been established to monitor outcomes of women exposed to rizatriptan during pregnancy. Preliminary data from the pregnancy registry (prospectively collected from 65 live births 1998-2004) does not show an increased risk of congenital malformations in comparison to the general population (Fiore 2005). Additional information collected through 2018 has not shown a pattern of birth defects or other adverse outcomes; however, data is limited and loss to follow-up is significant. Information related to rizatriptan use in pregnancy is limited in comparison to other medications in this class (Källén 2011; Nezvalová-Henriksen 2010; Nezvalová-Henriksen 2012; Nezvalová-Henriksen 2013; Spielmann 2018).

Until additional information is available, other agents are preferred for the initial treatment of migraine in pregnancy (MacGregor 2014; Worthington 2013).

- **Rizatriptan Benzoate** *see* Rizatriptan *on page 1342*
- **rLFN-α2** *see* Interferon Alfa-2b *on page 831*
- **rLP2086** *see* Meningococcal Group B Vaccine *on page 963*
- **R-modafinil** *see* Armodafinil *on page 167*
- **Ro 5488** *see* Tretinoin (Systemic) *on page 1483*
- **RO5185426** *see* Vemurafenib *on page 1537*
- **RO5424802** *see* Alectinib *on page 92*
- **RoActemra** *see* Tocilizumab *on page 1457*
- **Robafen Cough [OTC]** *see* Dextromethorphan *on page 476*
- **Robaxin** *see* Methocarbamol *on page 988*
- **Robaxin-750** *see* Methocarbamol *on page 988*
- **Robinul [DSC]** *see* Glycopyrrolate (Systemic) *on page 742*
- **Robinul-Forte [DSC]** *see* Glycopyrrolate (Systemic) *on page 742*
- **Robitussin 12 Hour Cough [OTC]** *see* Dextromethorphan *on page 476*
- **Robitussin 12 Hour Cough Child [OTC]** *see* Dextromethorphan *on page 476*
- **Robitussin Childrens Cough LA [OTC]** *see* Dextromethorphan *on page 476*
- **Robitussin Lingering CoughGels [OTC]** *see* Dextromethorphan *on page 476*
- **Robitussin Lingering LA Cough [OTC] [DSC]** *see* Dextromethorphan *on page 476*
- **Rocaltrol** *see* Calcitriol (Systemic) *on page 279*

◆ **Rocephin** *see* CefTRIAXone *on page 316*

Roflumilast (roe FLUE mi last)

Brand Names: US Daliresp
Brand Names: Canada Daxas
Pharmacologic Category Phosphodiesterase-4 Enzyme Inhibitor
Use
COPD: To reduce the risk of COPD exacerbations in patients with severe COPD associated with chronic bronchitis and a history of exacerbations
Limitations of use: Not indicated for the relief of acute bronchospasm
Local Anesthetic/Vasoconstrictor Precautions No information available to require special precautions
Effects on Dental Treatment No significant effects or complications reported
Effects on Bleeding No information available to require special precautions
Adverse Reactions
2% to 10%:
Central nervous system: Headache (4%), dizziness (2%), insomnia (2%)
Endocrine & metabolic: Weight loss (5% to 10% of body weight: 8% to 20%; >10% loss: 7%)
Gastrointestinal: Diarrhea (10%), nausea (5%), decreased appetite (2%)
Infection: Influenza (3%)
Neuromuscular & skeletal: Back pain (3%)
<2%, postmarketing, and/or case reports: Abdominal pain, anemia, anxiety, arthralgia, arthritis, atrial fibrillation, constipation, depression, dysgeusia, dyspepsia, epistaxis, fatigue, gastritis, gastroesophageal reflux disease, gynecomastia, hematochezia, hypersensitivity, hypersensitivity reaction (including angioedema, urticaria, and rash), increased gamma-glutamyl transferase, increased lactate dehydrogenase, increased serum AST, limb pain, lung carcinoma, malaise, muscle spasm, myalgia, myasthenia, nervousness, pancreatitis, paresthesia, prostate carcinoma, renal failure, respiratory tract infection, rhinitis, sinusitis, suicidal ideation, suicidal tendencies, suicide, supraventricular cardiac arrhythmia, tremor, urinary tract infection, vertigo, vomiting, weakness
Mechanism of Action Roflumilast and its active N-oxide metabolite selectively inhibit phosphodiesterase-4 (PDE4) leading to an accumulation of cyclic AMP (cAMP) within inflammatory and structural cells important in the pathogenesis of COPD. Anti-inflammatory effects include suppression of cytokine release and inhibition of lung infiltration by neutrophils and other leukocytes. Pulmonary remodeling and mucociliary malfunction are also attenuated.
Pharmacodynamics/Kinetics
Half-life Elimination 17 hours; N-oxide metabolite: 30 hours
Time to Peak ~1 hour (delayed by food); N-oxide metabolite: ~8 hours
Pregnancy Considerations Adverse events were observed in some animal reproduction studies.

Rolapitant (roe LA pi tant)

Brand Names: US Varubi (180 MG Dose); Varubi [DSC]
Pharmacologic Category Antiemetic; Substance P/ Neurokinin 1 Receptor Antagonist
Use Chemotherapy-induced nausea and vomiting (CINV), prevention: Prevention of delayed nausea and vomiting associated with initial and repeat courses of emetogenic cancer chemotherapy, including, but not limited to highly emetogenic chemotherapy (in combination with other antiemetic agents).
Local Anesthetic/Vasoconstrictor Precautions No information available to require special precautions
Effects on Dental Treatment Key adverse event(s) related to dental treatment: Stomatitis has been reported from clinical trials receiving combination therapy with dexamethasone and 5-HT3 receptor antagonist
Effects on Bleeding No information available to require special precautions
Adverse Reactions Percentages reported as part of combination regimens.
1% to 10%:
Central nervous system: Dizziness (6%)
Gastrointestinal: Decreased appetite (9%), hiccups (5%), dyspepsia (4%), stomatitis (4%), abdominal pain (3%)
Genitourinary: Urinary tract infection (4%)
Hematologic & oncologic: Neutropenia (7% to 9%), anemia (3%)
Miscellaneous: Infusion-related reactions (3%)
<1%, postmarketing, and/or case reports: Anaphylactic shock (FDA Safety Alert, Jan 16, 2018), anaphylaxis (FDA Safety Alert, Jan 16, 2018)
Mechanism of Action Rolapitant prevents delayed nausea and vomiting associated with emetogenic chemotherapy by selectively and competitively inhibiting the substance P/neurokinin 1 (NK_1) receptor.
Pharmacodynamics/Kinetics
Half-life Elimination Oral: ~7 days (range: 169 to 183 hours); IV: 7.6 days (range: 138 to 205 hours)
Time to Peak Oral: ~4 hours
Pregnancy Considerations Adverse events were observed in some animal reproduction studies.

◆ **Rolapitant Hydrochloride** *see* Rolapitant *on page 1343*

◆ **Rolapitant Monohydrate Hydrochloride** *see* Rolapitant *on page 1343*

◆ **Romazicon** *see* Flumazenil *on page 685*

RomiDEPsin (roe mi DEP sin)

Related Information
Clinical Risk Related to Drugs Prolonging QT Interval *on page 1675*
Brand Names: US Istodax (Overfill); Istodax [DSC]
Brand Names: Canada Istodax
Pharmacologic Category Antineoplastic Agent, Histone Deacetylase (HDAC) Inhibitor
Use
Cutaneous T-cell lymphoma: Treatment of cutaneous T-cell lymphoma (CTCL) in adult patients who have received at least one prior systemic therapy
Peripheral T-cell lymphoma: Treatment of peripheral T-cell lymphoma (PTCL) in adult patients who have received at least one prior therapy
Local Anesthetic/Vasoconstrictor Precautions Romidepsin is one of the drugs confirmed to prolong the QT interval and is accepted as having a risk of causing torsade de pointes. The risk of drug-induced torsade de pointes is extremely low when a single QT interval prolonging drug is prescribed. In terms of epinephrine, it is not known what effect vasoconstrictors in

the local anesthetic regimen will have in patients with a known history of congenital prolonged QT interval or in patients taking any medication that prolongs the QT interval. Until more information is obtained, it is suggested that the clinician consult with the physician prior to the use of a vasoconstrictor in suspected patients, and that the vasoconstrictor (epinephrine, mepivacaine and levonordefrin [Carbocaine® 2% with Neo-Cobefrin®]) be used with caution.

Effects on Dental Treatment Key adverse event(s) related to dental treatment: Taste alteration.

Effects on Bleeding Chemotherapy may result in significant myelosuppression, potentially including significant reduction in platelet counts (thrombocytopenia grades 3/4: ≤36%) and altered hemostasis. In patients who are under active treatment with these agents, medical consult is suggested.

Adverse Reactions

>10%:

Cardiovascular: ECG changes (ST-T wave changes: 2% to 63%), hypotension (7% to 23%)

Central nervous system: Fatigue (53% to 77%), headache (15% to 34%), chills (11% to 17%)

Dermatologic: Pruritus (7% to 31%), dermatitis (≤27%), exfoliative dermatitis (≤27%)

Endocrine & metabolic: Hypocalcemia (4% to 52%), hyperglycemia (2% to 51%), hypoalbuminemia (3% to 48%), hyperuricemia (≤33%), hypomagnesemia (22% to 28%), hypermagnesemia (≤27%), hypophosphatemia (≤27%), hyponatremia (≤20%), hypokalemia (6% to 20%), weight loss (10% to 15%)

Gastrointestinal: Nausea (56% to 86%), anorexia (23% to 54%), vomiting (34% to 52%), dysgeusia (15% to 40%), constipation (12% to 40%), diarrhea (20% to 36%), abdominal pain (13% to 14%)

Hematologic & oncologic: Anemia (19% to 72%; grades 3/4: 3% to 28%), thrombocytopenia (17% to 72%; grades 3/4: ≤36%), neutropenia (11% to 66%; grades 3/4: 4% to 47%), lymphocytopenia (4% to 57%; grades 3/4: ≤37%), leukopenia (4% to 55%; grades 3/4: ≤45%)

Hepatic: Increased serum AST (3% to 28%), increased serum ALT (3% to 22%)

Infection: Infection (46% to 54%; including infection of central line)

Neuromuscular & skeletal: Weakness (53% to 77%)

Respiratory: Cough (18% to 21%), dyspnea (13% to 21%)

Miscellaneous: Fever (20% to 47%)

1% to 10%:

Cardiovascular: Tachycardia (≤10%), peripheral edema (6% to 10%), chest pain, deep vein thrombosis, edema, prolonged QT interval on ECG, pulmonary embolism, supraventricular cardiac arrhythmia, syncope, ventricular arrhythmia

Dermatologic: Cellulitis

Endocrine & metabolic: Dehydration

Gastrointestinal: Stomatitis (6% to 10%)

Hematologic & oncologic: Tumor lysis syndrome (1% to 2%), febrile neutropenia

Hepatic: Hyperbilirubinemia

Hypersensitivity: Hypersensitivity reaction

Infection: Sepsis

Respiratory: Hypoxia, pneumonia, pneumonitis

<1%, postmarketing, and/or case reports: Acute renal failure, acute respiratory distress, atrial fibrillation, bacteremia, candidiasis, cardiac failure, cardiogenic shock, ischemic heart disease, multi-organ failure, reactivation of latent Epstein-Barr virus, respiratory failure, septic shock

Mechanism of Action Romidepsin is a histone deacetylase (HDAC) inhibitor; HDACs catalyze acetyl group removal from protein lysine residues (including histone and transcription factors). Inhibition of HDAC results in accumulation of acetyl groups, leading to alterations in chromatin structure and transcription factor activation causing termination of cell growth (induces arrest in cell cycle at G1 and G2/M phases) leading to cell death.

Pharmacodynamics/Kinetics

Half-life Elimination ~3 hours

Reproductive Considerations

Evaluate pregnancy status in females of reproductive potential within 7 days prior to initiating treatment with romidepsin. Females of reproductive potential should use an effective non-hormonal method of contraception during treatment and for at least 1 month after the final romidepsin dose. Males with female partners of reproductive potential should use effective contraception during treatment and for at least 1 month after the last romidepsin dose.

Pregnancy Considerations

Based on the mechanism of action and findings from animal reproduction studies, romidepsin may cause fetal harm if administered to a pregnant female.

Dental Health Professional Considerations See Local Anesthetic/Vasoconstrictor Precautions

Romosozumab (ROE moe SOZ ue mab)

Brand Names: US Evenity

Brand Names: Canada Evenity

Pharmacologic Category Monoclonal Antibody; Sclerostin Inhibitor

Use

Osteoporosis: Treatment of osteoporosis in postmenopausal females at high risk for fracture (defined as a history of osteoporotic fracture or multiple risk factors for fracture), or patients who have failed or are intolerant to other available osteoporosis therapy.

Limitations of use: The anabolic effect of romosozumab wanes after 12 monthly doses of therapy. Therefore, the duration of romosozumab use should be limited to 12 monthly doses. If osteoporosis therapy remains warranted, continued therapy with an anti-resorptive agent should be considered.

Local Anesthetic/Vasoconstrictor Precautions

No information available to require special precautions

Effects on Dental Treatment Key adverse event(s) related to dental treatment: Osteonecrosis of the jaw (ONJ), also referred to as medication-related osteonecrosis of the jaw (MRONJ), has been reported in patients receiving romosozumab. Known risk factors for MRONJ include tooth extraction or other invasive dental procedures, cancer diagnosis, radiotherapy, concomitant therapy (eg, angiogenesis inhibitors, bisphosphonates, chemotherapy, corticosteroids, denosumab), poor oral hygiene, and comorbid disorders (anemia, coagulopathy, infection, preexisting dental or periodontal disease). Routine oral exam is recommended prior to initiation of therapy; patients should maintain good oral hygiene during treatment. Consider risk/benefits of therapy in patients requiring invasive dental procedures. Patients developing ONJ during therapy should receive care by an oral surgeon or dentist; consider discontinuation of therapy based on risk/benefit assessment.

Effects on Bleeding No information available to require special precautions

Adverse Reactions

>10%: Neuromuscular & skeletal: Arthralgia (8% to 13%)

1% to 10%:

Cardiovascular: Cardiac disorder (2%), peripheral edema (2%)

Central nervous system: Headache (5% to 7%), insomnia (2%), paresthesia (1%)

Dermatologic: Skin rash (1%)

Hypersensitivity: Hypersensitivity reaction (7%)

Local: Injection site reaction (5%), pain at injection site (2%), erythema at injection site (1%)

Neuromuscular & skeletal: Muscle spasm (3% to 5%), asthenia (3%), neck pain (2%)

<1%, postmarketing, and/or case reports: Acute myocardial infarction, angioedema, cerebrovascular accident, dermatitis, erythema multiforme, femur fracture, hypocalcemia, osteonecrosis of the jaw, urticaria

Mechanism of Action Romosozumab inhibits sclerostin, a regulatory factor in bone metabolism that inhibits Wnt/Beta-catenin signaling pathway regulating bone growth (MacDonald 2009; McClung 2018); romosozumab increases bone formation and to a lesser extent, decreases bone resorption.

Pharmacodynamics/Kinetics

Onset of Action Peak increase in bone formation marker procollagen type 1 N-telopeptide (P1NP) and peak decrease in bone resorption marker type 1 collagen C-telopeptide (CTX) observed 2 weeks after initiation. Increased histomorphometric indices of bone formation observed 2 months after therapy initiation.

Duration of Action CTX decrease persists throughout 12 months of therapy; P1NP returns to baseline by 9 months and declines at 12 months; anabolic effect wanes after 12 months of treatment. After discontinuation of therapy, an increase in CTX above baseline value occurs within 3 months. CTX, P1NP, and bone mineral density (BMD) return to baseline within ~12 months of discontinuing therapy.

Half-life Elimination 12.8 days after 3 doses over 12-week period (ie, 1 dose every 4 weeks)

Time to Peak Median: 5 days (range: 2 to 7 days)

Reproductive Considerations

Romosozumab is not indicated for use in females of reproductive potential.

Pregnancy Considerations

Romosozumab is a humanized monoclonal antibody (IgG_2). Potential placental transfer of human IgG is dependent upon the IgG subclass and gestational age, generally increasing as pregnancy progresses. The lowest exposure would be expected during the period of organogenesis (Palmeira 2012; Pentsuk 2009).

Romosozumab is not indicated for use in females of reproductive potential.

◆ **Romosozumab-aqqg** *see* Romosozumab *on page 1344*

ROPINIRole (roe PIN i role)

Brand Names: US Requip XL; Requip [DSC]

Brand Names: Canada JAMP-Ropinirole; PMS-Ropinirole; RAN-Ropinirole; Requip [DSC]; TEVA-Ropinirole

Pharmacologic Category Anti-Parkinson Agent, Dopamine Agonist

Use

Parkinson disease: Treatment of Parkinson disease.

Restless legs syndrome (immediate release only): Treatment of moderate to severe primary restless legs syndrome.

Local Anesthetic/Vasoconstrictor Precautions No information available to require special precautions

Effects on Dental Treatment Key adverse event(s) related to dental treatment: Xerostomia and dysphagia occur with use. Normal salivary flow resumes upon discontinuation of treatment.

Effects on Bleeding No information available to require special precautions

Adverse Reactions Data inclusive of trials in early Parkinson disease (PD) without levodopa and restless legs syndrome (RLS). Extended-release data from trials in early PD without levodopa. As reported with immediate-release formulation, unless otherwise noted.

>10%:

Cardiovascular: Hypotension (RLS: ≤25%; PD: 2%), orthostatic hypotension (RLS: ≤25%; PD: 6%; extended release: 14%), hypertension (PD: 5%; extended release: 3% to 15%), syncope (PD: ≤12%; RLS: 1% to 2%; sometimes associated with bradycardia)

Central nervous system: Drowsiness (PD: ≤40%; extended release: 8% to 15%; RLS: 12%), dizziness (PD: 40%; extended release: 6% to 10%; RLS: 11%), headache (PD, extended release: 5% to 15%)

Gastrointestinal: Nausea (PD: 60%; RLS: 40%; extended release: 10% to 33%), vomiting (PD: 12%; extended release: 10%; RLS: 11%)

Infection: Viral infection (PD: 11%)

Neuromuscular & skeletal: Asthenia (PD: 16%; RLS: 9%), back pain (PD, extended release: 5% to 15%)

1% to 10%:

Cardiovascular: Lower extremity edema (PD: 7%), dependent edema (PD: 6%), chest pain (PD: 4%), flushing (PD: 3%), palpitations (PD: 3%), peripheral ischemia (PD: 3%), atrial fibrillation (PD: 2%), extrasystoles (PD: 2%), peripheral edema (RLS: 2%), tachycardia (PD: 2%)

Central nervous system: Pain (PD: 8%), confusion (PD: 5%), hallucination (PD: 5%), narcolepsy (PD, extended release: 5% to 10%), hypoesthesia (PD: 4%), amnesia (PD: 3%), paresthesia (RLS: 3%), yawning (PD: 3%), lack of concentration (PD: 2%), vertigo (2%)

Dermatologic: Diaphoresis (PD: 6%), hyperhidrosis (RLS: 3%)

Gastrointestinal: Dyspepsia (PD: 10%; RLS: 4%), abdominal pain (PD: 6% to 7%; includes immediate release and extended release), constipation (PD, extended release: 5%), diarrhea (RLS: 5%), xerostomia (PD: 5%; RLS: 3%), anorexia (PD: 4%), flatulence (PD: 3%), upper abdominal pain (RLS: 3%)

Genitourinary: Urinary tract infection (PD: 5%), impotence (PD: 3%)

Hepatic: Increased serum alkaline phosphatase (PD: 3%)

Infection: Influenza (RLS: 3%)

Neuromuscular & skeletal: Increased creatine phosphokinase in blood specimen (PD, extended release: 10%), arthralgia (RLS: 4%), limb pain (RLS: 3%), muscle cramps (RLS: 3%), hyperkinetic muscle activity (PD: 2%)

Ophthalmic: Visual disturbance (PD: 6%), eye disease (PD: 3%), xerophthalmia (PD: 2%)

Respiratory: Nasopharyngitis (RLS: 9%), pharyngitis (PD: 6%), rhinitis (PD: 4%), sinusitis (PD: 4%), bronchitis (PD: 3%), cough (RLS: 3%), dyspnea (PD: 3%), nasal congestion (RLS: 2%)

<1%: Pleural effusion

Postmarketing: Aggressive behavior, agitation, behavioral problems, delirium, delusion, disorientation, heart valve disease, impulse control disorder (Bastiaens 2013; Corvol 2018), interstitial pulmonary disease, mental status changes, paranoid ideation, pleuropulmonary fibrosis, psychiatric disturbance, psychosis

Mechanism of Action Ropinirole has a high relative *in vitro* specificity and full intrinsic activity at the D_2 and D_3 dopamine receptor subtypes, binding with higher affinity to D_3 than to D_2 or D_4 receptor subtypes; relevance of D_3 receptor binding in Parkinson disease is unknown. Ropinirole has moderate *in vitro* affinity for opioid receptors. Ropinirole and its metabolites have negligible *in vitro* affinity for dopamine D_1, 5-HT_1, 5-HT_2, benzodiazepine, GABA, muscarinic, $alpha_1$-, $alpha_2$-, and beta-adrenoreceptors. Although precise mechanism of action of ropinirole is unknown, it is believed to be due to stimulation of postsynaptic dopamine D_2-type receptors within the caudate putamen in the brain. Ropinirole caused decreases in systolic and diastolic blood pressure at doses >0.25 mg. The mechanism of ropinirole-induced postural hypotension is believed to be due to D_2-mediated blunting of the noradrenergic response to standing and subsequent decrease in peripheral vascular resistance.

Pharmacodynamics/Kinetics

Half-life Elimination ~6 hours

Time to Peak Immediate release: ~1-2 hours; Extended release: 6-10 hours; T_{max} increased by 2.5-3 hours when taken with a high-fat meal

Pregnancy Considerations

Information related to the use of ropinirole for the treatment of restless legs syndrome in pregnant women is limited. Current guidelines note that the available information is insufficient to make a recommendation for use in pregnant women (Aurora 2012; Dostal 2013; Tüfekçioğlu 2018).

◆ **Ropinirole HCl** *see* ROPINIRole *on page 1345*

◆ **Ropinirole Hydrochloride** *see* ROPINIRole *on page 1345*

Ropivacaine (roe PIV a kane)

Related Information

Oral Pain *on page 1734*

Brand Names: US Naropin

Brand Names: Canada Naropin

Pharmacologic Category Local Anesthetic

Use

Acute pain management: For acute pain management administered as an epidural continuous infusion, intermittent bolus (eg, postoperative or labor), or local infiltration.

Surgical anesthesia: For the production of local or regional anesthesia for surgery administered as an epidural block, including cesarean section, major nerve block, or local infiltration.

Local Anesthetic/Vasoconstrictor Precautions No information available to require special precautions (see Dental Health Professional Considerations)

Effects on Dental Treatment No significant effects or complications reported

Effects on Bleeding No information available to require special precautions

Adverse Reactions

>10%:

Cardiovascular: Hypotension (32% to 69%), bradycardia (6% to 20%)

Gastrointestinal: Nausea (13% to 25%), vomiting (7% to 12%)

Neuromuscular & skeletal: Back pain (4% to 16%)

1% to 10%:

Cardiovascular: Chest pain (1% to 5%), hypertension (1% to 5%), tachycardia (1% to 5%)

Central nervous system: Headache (5% to 8%), pain (4% to 8%), paresthesia (2% to 6%), dizziness (3%), chills (≤3%), rigors (≤3%), hypoesthesia (2%), anxiety (1%)

Dermatologic: Pruritus (1% to 5%)

Endocrine & metabolic: Hypokalemia (1% to 5%)

Genitourinary: Oliguria (1% to 5%), urinary retention (1% to 5%), urinary tract infection (1% to 5%), disorder of breast milk secretion (1%), poor progression of labor (1%)

Hematologic & oncologic: Anemia (6%)

Neuromuscular & skeletal: Muscle cramps (1% to 5%)

Respiratory: Dyspnea (1% to 5%), rhinitis (1%)

Miscellaneous: Fever (2% to 9%), postoperative complication (3% to 7%)

<1%, postmarketing, and/or case reports: Accidental injury, agitation, amnesia, angioedema, asthenia, atrial fibrillation, auditory disturbance, blepharoptosis, bronchospasm, cardiac arrhythmia, coma, confusion, cough, deep vein thrombosis, drowsiness, dyskinesia, ECG abnormality, emotional lability, extrasystoles, fecal incontinence, hallucination, Horner's syndrome, hypersensitivity reaction, hypokinesia, hypomagnesemia, hypothermia, hypotonia, insomnia, jaundice, malaise, myalgia, myocardial infarction, nervousness, neuropathy, nightmares, orthostatic hypotension, pain at injection site, paresis, phlebitis, pulmonary embolism, seizure, skin rash, ST segment changes on ECG, stupor, syncope, tenesmus, tinnitus, tremor, urinary incontinence, urination disorder, urticaria, uterine atony, vertigo, visual disturbance

Mechanism of Action Blocks both the initiation and conduction of nerve impulses by decreasing the neuronal membrane's permeability to sodium ions, which results in inhibition of depolarization with resultant blockade of conduction

Pharmacodynamics/Kinetics

Onset of Action Anesthesia (route dependent): 3 to 15 minutes

Duration of Action Dose and route dependent: 3 to 15 hours

Half-life Elimination

Children: Epidural: Terminal phase:4.9 hours (range: 3 to 6.7 hours) (Hansen 2000)

Adults: Epidural: 5 to 7 hours; IV: Terminal: 111 ± 62 minutes (Lee 1989)

Time to Peak Serum (dose and route dependent): Caudal:

Infants: Median: 60 minutes (range: 15 to 90 minutes) (Wulf 2000)

Children: Mean: 60 minutes (range: 12 to 249 minutes (Lonnqvist 2000)

Pregnancy Risk Factor B

Pregnancy Considerations
When used for epidural block during labor and delivery, systemically absorbed ropivacaine may cross the placenta, resulting in varying degrees of fetal or neonatal effects (eg, CNS or cardiovascular depression). Fetal or neonatal adverse events include fetal bradycardia (12%), neonatal jaundice (8%), low Apgar scores (3%), fetal distress (2%), neonatal respiratory disorder (3%). Maternal hypotension may also result from systemic absorption. In cases of hypotension, position pregnant woman in left lateral decubitus position to prevent aortocaval compression by the gravid uterus. Epidural anesthesia may prolong the second stage of labor.

Dental Health Professional Considerations Not available with vasoconstrictor (epinephrine) and not available in dental (1.8 mL) carpules

◆ **Ropivacaine Hydrochloride** *see* Ropivacaine *on page 1346*

Rosiglitazone (roh si GLI ta zone)

Related Information
Endocrine Disorders and Pregnancy *on page 1684*

Brand Names: US Avandia

Brand Names: Canada Avandia

Pharmacologic Category Antidiabetic Agent, Thiazolidinedione

Use Diabetes mellitus, type 2, treatment: Adjunct to diet and exercise to improve glycemic control in adults with type 2 diabetes mellitus.

Local Anesthetic/Vasoconstrictor Precautions
No information available to require special precautions

Effects on Dental Treatment Rosiglitazone-dependent patients with diabetes should be appointed for dental treatment in morning in order to minimize chance of stress-induced hypoglycemia.

Effects on Bleeding Rosiglitazone has been demonstrated to induce severe thrombocytopenia (rare). Analysis of the patient's serum shows rosiglitazone-induced antibody, responsible for thrombocytopenia, confirming an immune-mediated platelet depletion.

Adverse Reactions Note: As reported in monotherapy studies; the rate of certain adverse reactions (eg, anemia, edema, hypoglycemia) may be higher with some combination therapies. Rare cases of hepatocellular injury have been reported in men in their 60s within 2 to 3 weeks after initiation of rosiglitazone therapy. LFTs in these patients revealed severe hepatocellular injury which responded with rapid improvement of liver function and resolution of symptoms upon discontinuation of rosiglitazone. Patients were also receiving other potentially hepatotoxic medications (Al-Salman 2000; Freid 2000).

>10%: Endocrine & metabolic: Increased HDL cholesterol, increased LDL cholesterol, increased serum cholesterol (total), weight gain

1% to 10%:

Cardiovascular: Edema (5%), hypertension (4%); cardiac failure (≤3% in patients receiving insulin; incidence likely higher in patients with preexisting cardiac failure), ischemic heart disease (3%; incidence likely higher in patients with preexisting CAD)

Central nervous system: Headache (6%)

Endocrine & metabolic: Hypoglycemia (1% to 3%; combination therapy with insulin: 12% to 14%)

Gastrointestinal: Diarrhea (3%)

Hematologic & oncologic: Anemia (2%)

Neuromuscular & skeletal: Bone fracture (≤9%; incidence greater in females; usually upper arm, hand, or foot), arthralgia (5%), back pain (4% to 5%)

Respiratory: Upper respiratory tract infection (4% to 10%), nasopharyngitis (6%)

Miscellaneous: Trauma (8%)

<1%, postmarketing, and/or case reports: Anaphylaxis, angina pectoris, angioedema, blurred vision, cardiac arrest, coronary artery disease, coronary thrombosis, decreased HDL cholesterol, decreased hematocrit, decreased hemoglobin, decreased visual acuity, decreased white blood cell count, dyspnea, hepatic failure, hepatitis, increased serum bilirubin, increased serum transaminases, jaundice (reversible), macular edema, myocardial infarction, pleural effusion, pruritus, pulmonary edema, skin rash, Stevens-Johnson syndrome, thrombocytopenia, urticaria, weight gain (rapid, excessive; usually due to fluid accumulation)

Mechanism of Action Thiazolidinedione antidiabetic agent that lowers blood glucose by improving target cell response to insulin, without increasing pancreatic insulin secretion. It has a mechanism of action that is dependent on the presence of insulin for activity. Rosiglitazone is an agonist for peroxisome proliferator-activated receptor-gamma (PPARgamma). Activation of nuclear PPARgamma receptors influences the production of a number of gene products involved in glucose and lipid metabolism. PPARgamma is abundant in the cells within the renal collecting tubules; fluid retention results from stimulation by thiazolidinediones which increases sodium reabsorption.

Pharmacodynamics/Kinetics

Onset of Action Delayed; Maximum effect: Up to 12 weeks

Half-life Elimination 3 to 4 hours; prolonged by approximately 2 hours in patients with moderate-to-severe hepatic impairment

Time to Peak 1 hour; delayed with food

Reproductive Considerations
Thiazolidinediones may cause ovulation in anovulatory premenopausal females, increasing the risk of unintended pregnancy. Due to long-term safety concerns associated with their use, thiazolidinediones should be avoided in females of reproductive age (Fauser 2012).

Pregnancy Considerations Rosiglitazone crosses the placenta (Chan 2005).

Inadvertent use early in pregnancy has been reported, although in the majority of cases, the medication was stopped as soon as pregnancy was detected (Chan 2005; Kalyoncu 2005; Yaris 2004).

Poorly controlled diabetes during pregnancy can be associated with an increased risk of adverse maternal and fetal outcomes, including diabetic ketoacidosis, preeclampsia, spontaneous abortion, preterm delivery, delivery complications, major birth defects, stillbirth, and macrosomia. To prevent adverse outcomes, prior to conception and throughout pregnancy, maternal blood glucose and HbA_{1c} should be kept as close to target goals as possible but without causing significant hypoglycemia (ADA 2020; Blumer 2013).

Agents other than rosiglitazone are currently recommended to treat diabetes mellitus in pregnancy (ADA 2020).

Prescribing and Access Restrictions Health Canada requires written informed consent for new and current patients receiving rosiglitazone.

Rosuvastatin (roe soo va STAT in)

Related Information

Cardiovascular Diseases *on page 1654*

Brand Names: US Crestor; Ezallor Sprinkle

Brand Names: Canada ACH-Rosuvastatin; ACT Rosuvastatin [DSC]; AG-Rosuvastatin; APO-Rosuvastatin; Auro-Rosuvastatin; BIO-Rosuvastatin; Crestor; DOM-Rosuvastatin; JAMP-Rosuvastatin; Mar-Rosuvastatin; MED-Rosuvastatin; MINT-Rosuvastatin [DSC]; MYLAN-Rosuvastatin [DSC]; NRA-Rosuvastatin; PMS-Rosuvastatin; Priva-Rosuvastatin; RIVA-Rosuvastatin; SANDOZ Rosuvastatin; TARO-Rosuvastatin; TEVA-Rosuvastatin

Pharmacologic Category Antilipemic Agent, HMG-CoA Reductase Inhibitor

Use

Familial hypercholesterolemia:

Pediatric (excluding Ezallor): Adjunct to diet to reduce total cholesterol, LDL-C, and apoB levels in children and adolescents 8 to 17 years of age with heterozygous familial hypercholesterolemia (HeFH) if after an adequate trial of diet therapy the following findings are present: LDL-C greater than 190 mg/dL or greater than 160 mg/dL and there is a positive family history of premature cardiovascular disease or 2 or more other cardiovascular disease risk factors; adjunct to diet to reduce LDL-C, total cholesterol, nonHDL-C, and apoB in children and adolescents 7 to 17 years of age with homozygous familial hypercholesterolemia (HoFH), either alone or with other lipid-lowering treatments (eg, LDL apheresis).

Adult: To reduce LDL-C, total cholesterol, and apoB in adults with familial hypercholesterolemia as an adjunct to other lipid-lowering treatments (eg, LDL apheresis) or alone if such treatments are unavailable.

Prevention of cardiovascular disease (Crestor only):

Primary prevention of atherosclerotic cardiovascular disease: To reduce the risk of myocardial infarction (MI), stroke, revascularization procedures, and angina in adults without a history of coronary heart disease (CHD) but who have multiple CHD risk factors.

Secondary prevention in patients with established atherosclerotic cardiovascular disease: To reduce the risk of MI, stroke, revascularization procedures, and angina in adults with a history of CHD.

Local Anesthetic/Vasoconstrictor Precautions

No information available to require special precautions

Effects on Dental Treatment Key adverse event(s) related to dental treatment: Assess unusual presentations of muscle weakness or myopathy resulting from lipid therapy such as patient having a difficult time brushing teeth or weakness with chewing. Refer patient back to their physician for evaluation and adjustment of lipid therapy.

Effects on Bleeding No information available to require special precautions

Adverse Reactions

>10%: Neuromuscular & skeletal: Myalgia (2% to 13%)

1% to 10%:

Central nervous system: Headache (6% to 9%), dizziness (4%)

Endocrine & metabolic: Diabetes mellitus (new onset: 3%)

Gastrointestinal: Nausea (4% to 6%), constipation (3% to 5%)

Genitourinary: Cystitis (interstitial; Huang 2015)

Hepatic: Increased serum ALT (2%; >3 times ULN)

Neuromuscular & skeletal: Arthralgia (4% to 10%), increased creatine phosphokinase (3%; >10 x ULN: Children 3%), weakness (5%)

<1%, postmarketing, and/or case reports: Abnormal thyroid function test, cognitive dysfunction (reversible; includes amnesia, confusion, memory impairment), depression, elevated glycosylated hemoglobin (HbA_{1c}), gynecomastia, hematuria (microscopic), hepatic failure, hepatitis, hypersensitivity reaction (including angioedema, pruritus, skin rash, urticaria), immune-mediated necrotizing myopathy, increased gamma-glutamyl transferase, increased serum alkaline phosphatase, increased serum bilirubin, increased serum glucose, increased serum transaminases, interstitial pulmonary disease, jaundice, myoglobinuria, myopathy, myositis, pancreatitis, peripheral neuropathy, proteinuria (dose related), renal failure, rhabdomyolysis, sleep disorder (including insomnia and nightmares), thrombocytopenia

Mechanism of Action Inhibitor of 3-hydroxy-3-methylglutaryl coenzyme A (HMG-CoA) reductase, the rate-limiting enzyme in cholesterol synthesis (reduces the production of mevalonic acid from HMG-CoA); this then results in a compensatory increase in the expression of LDL receptors on hepatocyte membranes and a stimulation of LDL catabolism. In addition to the ability of HMG-CoA reductase inhibitors to decrease levels of high-sensitivity C-reactive protein (hsCRP), they also possess pleiotropic properties including improved endothelial function, reduced inflammation at the site of the coronary plaque, inhibition of platelet aggregation, and anticoagulant effects (de Denus 2002; Ray 2005).

Pharmacodynamics/Kinetics

Onset of Action Within 1 week; maximal at 4 weeks

Half-life Elimination 19 hours

Time to Peak Plasma: 3 to 5 hours

Reproductive Considerations

Rosuvastatin is contraindicated in females who may become pregnant.

Adequate contraception is recommended if an HMG-CoA reductase inhibitor is required in females of reproductive potential. Females planning a pregnancy should discontinue the HMG-CoA reductase inhibitor 1 to 2 months prior to attempting to conceive (AHA/ACC [Grundy 2019]).

Pregnancy Considerations Rosuvastatin is contraindicated in pregnant females.

Adverse events have been observed in some animal reproduction studies. There are reports of congenital anomalies following maternal use of HMG-CoA reductase inhibitors in pregnancy; however, maternal disease, differences in specific agents used, and the low rates of exposure limit the interpretation of the available data (Godfrey 2012; Lecarpentier 2012). Cholesterol biosynthesis may be important in fetal development; serum cholesterol and triglycerides increase normally during pregnancy. The discontinuation of lipid lowering medications temporarily during pregnancy is not expected to have significant impact on the long term outcomes of primary hypercholesterolemia treatment.

Rosuvastatin should be discontinued immediately if an unplanned pregnancy occurs during treatment.

◆ **Rosuvastatin Calcium** *see* Rosuvastatin *on page 1348*

◆ **Rotarix** *see* Rotavirus Vaccine *on page 1349*

◆ **RotaTeq** *see* Rotavirus Vaccine *on page* 1349

Rotavirus Vaccine (ROE ta vye rus vak SEEN)

Brand Names: US Rotarix; RotaTeq

Brand Names: Canada Rotarix; RotaTeq

Pharmacologic Category Vaccine; Vaccine, Live (Viral)

Use

Rotavirus gastroenteritis prevention:

Rotarix: Prevention of rotavirus gastroenteritis in infants 6 to 24 weeks of age caused by the serotypes G1, G3, G4, and G9 when administered as a 2-dose series.

RotaTeq: Prevention of rotavirus gastroenteritis in infants 6 to 32 weeks of age caused by the serotypes G1, G2, G3, G4, and G9 when administered as a 3-dose series.

The Advisory Committee on Immunization Practices (ACIP) recommends routine vaccination of all infants (CDC/ACIP [Cortese 2009]).

Local Anesthetic/Vasoconstrictor Precautions No information available to require special precautions

Effects on Dental Treatment No significant effects or complications reported

Effects on Bleeding No information available to require special precautions

Adverse Reactions Ranges reported; actual percentage may vary between products.

>10%:

Central nervous system: Irritability (≤52%)

Gastrointestinal: Diarrhea (4% to 24%), vomiting (3% to 15%)

Otic: Otitis media (15%)

Miscellaneous: Fussiness (≤52%)

1% to 10%:

Gastrointestinal: Flatulence (2%)

Respiratory: Nasopharyngitis (7%), bronchospasm (1%)

<1%, postmarketing, and/or case reports: Anaphylaxis, angioedema, gastroenteritis (with severe diarrhea and prolonged vaccine viral shedding in infants with SCID), hematochezia, immune thrombocytopenia (ITP), intussusception, Kawasaki syndrome, secondary infection (transmission of vaccine virus from recipient to nonvaccinated contacts), seizure, urticaria

Mechanism of Action A live vaccine; replicates in the small intestine and promotes active immunity to rotavirus gastroenteritis. Rotarix is specifically indicated for prevention of rotavirus gastroenteritis caused by serotypes G1, G3, G4, and G9 and RotaTeq is specifically indicated for prevention of rotavirus gastroenteritis caused by serotypes G1, G2, G3, G4, and G9. However, these vaccines may provide immunity to other rotavirus serotypes.

Pharmacodynamics/Kinetics

Onset of Action Seroconversion:

Rotarix: Antirotavirus IgA antibodies were noted 1 to 2 months following completion of the 2-dose series in 77% to 87% of infants.

RotaTeq: A threefold increase in antirotavirus IgA was noted following completion of the 3-dose regimen in 93% to 100% of infants.

Duration of Action Following administration of rotavirus vaccine, efficacy of protecting against any grade of rotavirus gastroenteritis through two seasons was 71% to 79%.

Pregnancy Considerations Rotavirus vaccine is not indicated for use in women of reproductive age. Infants living in households with pregnant women may be vaccinated (CDC/ACIP [Cortese 2009]).

◆ **Rotavirus Vaccine, Pentavalent** *see* Rotavirus Vaccine *on page* 1349

Rotigotine (roe TIG oh teen)

Brand Names: US Neupro

Brand Names: Canada Neupro

Pharmacologic Category Anti-Parkinson's Agent, Dopamine Agonist

Use

Parkinson disease: For the treatment of Parkinson disease.

Restless legs syndrome: For the treatment of moderate to severe primary restless legs syndrome.

Local Anesthetic/Vasoconstrictor Precautions No information available to require special precautions

Effects on Dental Treatment Key adverse event(s) related to dental treatment: Xerostomia and changes in salivation (normal salivary flow resumes upon discontinuation). Dopamine agonists may cause syncope. Patients may experience orthostatic hypotension as they stand up after treatment; especially if lying in dental chair for extended periods of time. Use caution with sudden changes in position during and after dental treatment. Parkinson's disease patients should be carefully assisted from the chair and observed for signs of orthostatic hypotension.

Effects on Bleeding No information available to require special precautions

Adverse Reactions

>10%:

Cardiovascular: Systolic hypotension (13% to 32%), orthostatic hypotension (8% to 29%), peripheral edema (3% to 14%)

Central nervous system: Drowsiness (5% to 32%), dizziness (5% to 23%), headache (10% to 21%), fatigue (6% to 18%), malaise (≤14%), sleep disorder (disturbance in initiating/maintaining sleep; 2% to 14%), hallucination (3% to 13%)

Dermatologic: Hyperhidrosis (1% to 11%)

Endocrine & metabolic: Decreased serum glucose (1% to 15%)

Gastrointestinal: Nausea (15% to 48%), vomiting (2% to 20%)

Hematologic & oncologic: Decreased hematocrit (8% to 17%), decreased hemoglobin (8% to 15%)

Local: Application site reaction (21% to 46%)

Neuromuscular & skeletal: Dyskinesia (14% to 17%), asthenia (≤14%), arthralgia (8% to 11%)

1% to 10%:

Cardiovascular: Increased diastolic blood pressure (4% to 8%), systolic hypertension (5%), hypertension (1% to 5%), atrioventricular block (3%), hypoesthesia (3%), abnormal T waves on ECG (2% to 3%)

Central nervous system: Abnormal dreams (1% to 7%), nightmares (3% to 5%), paresthesia (3% to 4%), vertigo (3% to 4%), depression (2% to 3%), equilibrium disturbance (2% to 3%), irritability (1% to 3%), sudden onset of sleep (1% to 2%)

Dermatologic: Pruritus (4% to 9%), erythema (2% to 6%)

Endocrine & metabolic: Weight gain (2% to 9%), change in libido (4% to 6%), hot flash (3% to 4%), low serum ferritin (2%), menstrual disease (1% to 2%)

Gastrointestinal: Constipation (5% to 9%), anorexia (2% to 9%), xerostomia (7%), diarrhea (5% to 7%), dyspepsia (2% to 3%), viral gastroenteritis (1% to 2%)
Hematologic & oncologic: Basal cell carcinoma (3%), leukocyturia (3%)
Infection: Herpes simplex infection (3%), influenza (1% to 3%)
Neuromuscular & skeletal: Tremor (4%), muscle spasm (3% to 4%)
Ophthalmic: Visual disturbance (3% to 5%)
Otic: Tinnitus (2% to 3%)
Renal: Increased blood urea nitrogen (3% to 11%)
Respiratory: Nasopharyngitis (8% to 10%), cough (3%), nasal congestion (3%), paranasal sinus congestion (2% to 3%), sinusitis (2% to 3%)

<1%, postmarketing, and/or case reports: Aggressive behavior, agitation, confusion, delirium, delusions, disorientation, heavy headedness (dropped head syndrome), impulse control disorder, increased creatine phosphokinase, increased pulse, neuroleptic malignant syndrome (resembling), paranoia, psychotic symptoms, skin rash

Mechanism of Action Rotigotine is a nonergot dopamine agonist with specificity for D_3-, D_2-, and D_1-dopamine receptors. Although the precise mechanism of action of rotigotine is unknown, it is believed to be due to stimulation of postsynaptic dopamine D_2-type auto receptors within the substantia nigra in the brain, leading to improved dopaminergic transmission in the motor areas of the basal ganglia, notably the caudate nucleus/putamen regions.

Pharmacodynamics/Kinetics

Half-life Elimination After removal of patch: 5 to 7 hours.

Time to Peak 15 to 18 hours; can occur 4 to 27 hours post application

Pregnancy Considerations

Information related to the use of rotigotine in pregnancy is limited (Dostal 2013).

Available guidelines note there is insufficient evidence to recommend rotigotine for use in pregnant females with restless leg syndrome (Picchietti 2015) or Parkinson disease (Seier 2017)

- **Rowasa** *see* Mesalamine *on page 980*
- **Roweepra** *see* LevETIRAcetam *on page 894*
- **Roweepra XR** *see* LevETIRAcetam *on page 894*
- **Roxanol** *see* Morphine (Systemic) *on page 1050*
- **Roxicet** *see* Oxycodone and Acetaminophen *on page 1164*
- **Roxicodone** *see* OxyCODONE *on page 1157*
- **Rozerem** *see* Ramelteon *on page 1307*
- **RP-6976** *see* DOCEtaxel *on page 507*
- **RP-46161** *see* Temozolomide *on page 1415*
- **RP-54274** *see* Riluzole *on page 1328*
- **RP-59500** *see* Quinupristin and Dalfopristin *on page 1301*
- **r-PA** *see* Reteplase *on page 1318*
- **rPDGF-BB** *see* Becaplermin *on page 217*
- **(R,R)-Formoterol L-Tartrate** *see* Arformoterol *on page 163*
- **RS7-SN38** *see* Sacituzumab Govitecan *on page 1352*
- **RS-25259** *see* Palonosetron *on page 1184*
- **RS-25259-197** *see* Palonosetron *on page 1184*
- **RTCA** *see* Ribavirin (Oral Inhalation) *on page 1321*
- **RTCA** *see* Ribavirin (Systemic) *on page 1320*
- **RU 0211** *see* Lubiprostone *on page 941*
- **RU-486** *see* MiFEPRIStone *on page 1028*
- **RU-23908** *see* Nilutamide *on page 1107*
- **RU-38486** *see* MiFEPRIStone *on page 1028*
- **Rubella** *see* Measles, Mumps, and Rubella Virus Vaccine *on page 949*
- **Rubella** *see* Measles, Mumps, Rubella, and Varicella Virus Vaccine *on page 950*
- **Rubella, Measles, and Mumps Vaccine** *see* Measles, Mumps, and Rubella Virus Vaccine *on page 949*
- **Rubella, Varicella, Measles, and Mumps Vaccine** *see* Measles, Mumps, Rubella, and Varicella Virus Vaccine *on page 950*
- **Rubidomycin Hydrochloride** *see* DAUNOrubicin (Conventional) *on page 445*
- **RUF 331** *see* Rufinamide *on page 1350*

Rufinamide (roo FIN a mide)

Brand Names: US Banzel

Brand Names: Canada Banzel

Pharmacologic Category Anticonvulsant, Triazole Derivative

Use Lennox-Gastaut syndrome: Adjunctive treatment of seizures associated with Lennox-Gastaut syndrome in adults and children 1 year and older

Local Anesthetic/Vasoconstrictor Precautions
No information available to require special precautions

Effects on Dental Treatment No significant effects or complications reported

Effects on Bleeding No information available to require special precautions

Adverse Reactions

>10%:

Cardiovascular: Shortened QT interval (46% to 65%; dose related)
Central nervous system: Headache (adults 27%, children 16%), drowsiness (11% to 24%), dizziness (3% to 19%), fatigue (9% to 16%)
Gastrointestinal: Vomiting (children 17%, adults 5%), nausea (7% to 12%)

1% to 10%:

Central nervous system: Ataxia (4% to 5%), status epilepticus (≤4%), aggressive behavior (children 3%), anxiety (adults 3%), disturbance in attention (children 3%), hyperactivity (children 3%), vertigo (adults 3%), abnormal gait (1% to 3%), convulsions (children 2%)
Dermatologic: Skin rash (children 4%), pruritus (children 3%)
Gastrointestinal: Decreased appetite (children 5%), constipation (adults 3%), dyspepsia (adults 3%), upper abdominal pain (3%), increased appetite (≥1%)
Hematologic & oncologic: Leukopenia (4%), anemia (1%)
Infection: Influenza (children 5%)
Neuromuscular & skeletal: Tremor (adults 6%), back pain (adults 3%)
Ophthalmic: Diplopia (4% to 9%), blurred vision (adults 6%), nystagmus (adults 6%)
Otic: Otic infection (children 3%), pollakiuria (1%)
Respiratory: Nasopharyngitis (children 5%), bronchitis (children 3%), sinusitis (children 3%)

<1%, postmarketing, and/or case reports: Atrioventricular block (first degree), bundle branch block (right), dysuria, hematuria, hypersensitivity (multiorgan), iron-deficiency anemia, lymphadenopathy, nephrolithiasis, neutropenia, nocturia, polyuria, Stevens-Johnson syndrome, suicidal ideation, thrombocytopenia, urinary incontinence

Mechanism of Action A triazole-derivative antiepileptic whose exact mechanism is unknown. *In vitro*, it prolongs the inactive state of the sodium channels, thereby limiting repetitive firing of sodium-dependent action potentials mediating anticonvulsant effects.

Pharmacodynamics/Kinetics

Half-life Elimination ~6 to 10 hours

Time to Peak 4 to 6 hours

Reproductive Considerations

Some hormonal contraceptives may be less effective with concurrent rufinamide use; additional forms of nonhormonal contraceptives should be used.

Pregnancy Considerations

Adverse effects were seen in animal reproduction studies.

Patients exposed to rufinamide during pregnancy are encouraged to enroll themselves into the AED Pregnancy Registry by calling 1-888-233-2334. Additional information is available at www.aedpregnancyregistry.org.

◆ **Rukobia** *see* Fostemsavir *on page 719*

◆ **Ruxience** *see* RiTUXimab *on page 1336*

Ruxolitinib (rux oh LI ti nib)

Brand Names: US Jakafi

Brand Names: Canada Jakavi

Pharmacologic Category Antineoplastic Agent, Janus Associated Kinase Inhibitor; Antineoplastic Agent, Tyrosine Kinase Inhibitor; Janus Associated Kinase Inhibitor

Use

Graft-versus-host disease, acute: Treatment of steroid-refractory acute graft-versus-host disease (GVHD) in adult and pediatric patients ≥12 years

Myelofibrosis: Treatment of intermediate or high-risk myelofibrosis in adults, including primary myelofibrosis, post-polycythemia vera myelofibrosis and post-essential thrombocythemia myelofibrosis

Polycythemia vera: Treatment of polycythemia vera in adults with an inadequate response to or intolerance to hydroxyurea

Local Anesthetic/Vasoconstrictor Precautions

No information available to require special precautions

Effects on Dental Treatment No significant effects or complications reported

Effects on Bleeding Chemotherapy may result in significant myelosuppression, potentially including significant reduction in platelet counts and altered hemostasis. In patients who are under active treatment with these agents, medical consult is suggested.

Adverse Reactions

>10%:

Dermatologic: Bruise (23%)

Endocrine & metabolic: Increased serum cholesterol (17% to 35%), hypertriglyceridemia (15%)

Gastrointestinal: Diarrhea (15%)

Hematologic & oncologic: Anemia (72% to 96%; grade 3: ≤34%; grade 4: ≤11%), thrombocytopenia (27% to 70%; grade 3: 5% to 9%; grade 4: ≤4%), neutropenia (3% to 19%; grade 3: 5%; grade 4: ≤2%)

Hepatic: Increased serum alanine aminotransferase (25%), increased serum aspartate aminotransferase (17% to 23%)

Nervous system: Dizziness (15% to 18%), headache (15%), insomnia (12%) (Verstovsek 2012)

Neuromuscular & skeletal: Muscle spasm (12%)

Respiratory: Dyspnea (13%)

1% to 10%:

Cardiovascular: Hypertension (5%)

Endocrine & metabolic: Weight gain (6% to 7%)

Gastrointestinal: Constipation (8%), nausea (6%), flatulence (5%)

Genitourinary: Urinary tract infection (6% to 9%)

Infection: Herpes zoster infection (2% to 6%)

Frequency not defined:

Endocrine & metabolic: Increased LDL cholesterol

Hematologic & oncologic: Basal cell carcinoma of skin, Merkel cell carcinoma, skin carcinoma, squamous cell carcinoma of skin

Infection: Serious infection

<1%, postmarketing, and/or case reports: Exacerbation of hepatitis B, progressive multifocal leukoencephalopathy, tuberculosis

Mechanism of Action Ruxolitinib is a kinase inhibitor which selectively inhibits Janus Associated Kinases (JAKs), JAK1 and JAK2. JAK1 and JAK2 mediate signaling of cytokine and growth factors responsible for hematopoiesis and immune function; JAK mediated signaling involves recruitment of STATs (signal transducers and activators of transcription) to cytokine receptors which leads to modulation of gene expression. In myelofibrosis and polycythemia vera, JAK1/2 activity is dysregulated; ruxolitinib modulates the affected JAK1/2 activity. JAK-STAT signaling is involved with the regulation of the development, proliferation, and activation of immune cell types important to GVHD pathogenesis; an animal model suggests that ruxolitinib may lead to decreased expression of inflammatory cytokines in colon homogenates and decreased immune cell infiltration in the colon.

Pharmacodynamics/Kinetics

Onset of Action

Acute graft-versus-host disease (GVHD): Median time to response: 1.5 weeks (range: 1 to 11 weeks) (Zeiser 2015)

Chronic GVHD: Median time to response: 3 weeks (range: 1 to 25 weeks) (Zeiser 2015); responses were observed within 2 weeks of ruxolitinib initiation in another study (Khoury 2018)

Half-life Elimination Ruxolitinib: ~3 hours (hepatic impairment: 4.1 to 5 hours); Ruxolitinib + metabolites: ~5.8 hours

Pregnancy Considerations Adverse events have been observed in animal reproduction studies. Use of ruxolitinib in pregnant females is not recommended; other agents are preferred for management of polycythemia vera and myeloproliferative disease (Gerds 2017; Kiladjian 2015).

Prescribing and Access Restrictions Available through specialty/network pharmacies. Further information may be obtained from the manufacturer, Incyte, at 1-855-452-5234 or at www.Jakafi.com.

◆ **Ruxolitinib Phosphate** *see* Ruxolitinib *on page 1351*

◆ **Ruzurgi** *see* Amifampridine *on page 114*

◆ **RV1 (Rotarix)** *see* Rotavirus Vaccine *on page 1349*

◆ **RV5 (RotaTeq)** *see* Rotavirus Vaccine *on page 1349*

◆ **rVWF** *see* von Willebrand Factor (Recombinant) *on page 1551*

- **RWJ-270201** *see* Peramivir *on page* 1216
- **Ryanodex** *see* Dantrolene *on page* 434
- **Rybelsus** *see* Semaglutide *on page* 1366
- **RyClora** *see* Dexchlorpheniramine *on page* 471
- **Rydapt** *see* Midostaurin *on page* 1027
- **Rytary** *see* Carbidopa and Levodopa *on page* 290
- **Rythmol [DSC]** *see* Propafenone *on page* 1284
- **Rythmol SR** *see* Propafenone *on page* 1284
- **RyVent** *see* Carbinoxamine *on page* 292
- **Ryzolt** *see* TraMADol *on page* 1468
- **RZV** *see* Zoster Vaccine (Recombinant) *on page* 1586
- **S2 (Racepinephrine) [OTC]** *see* EPINEPHrine (Oral Inhalation) *on page* 573
- **S-(+)-3-isobutylgaba** *see* Pregabalin *on page* 1268
- **6(S)-5-methyltetrahydrofolate** *see* Methylfolate *on page* 996
- **6(S)-5-MTHF** *see* Methylfolate *on page* 996
- **S-4661** *see* Doripenem *on page* 515
- **S-033188** *see* Baloxavir Marboxil *on page* 214
- **S-649266** *see* Cefiderocol *on page* 308
- **Sabril** *see* Vigabatrin *on page* 1542

Sacituzumab Govitecan

(SAK i TOOZ ue mab GOE vi TEE kan)

Brand Names: US Trodelvy

Pharmacologic Category Antineoplastic Agent, Anti-Trop-2; Antineoplastic Agent, Antibody Drug Conjugate; Antineoplastic Agent, Monoclonal Antibody; Antineoplastic Agent, Topoisomerase I Inhibitor

Use Breast cancer (triple negative), metastatic, refractory: Treatment of metastatic triple-negative breast cancer in adults who have received ≥2 prior therapies for metastatic disease.

Local Anesthetic/Vasoconstrictor Precautions No information available to require special precautions.

Effects on Dental Treatment Key adverse event(s) related to dental treatment: Frequent occurrence of altered taste, stomatitis.

Effects on Bleeding Chemotherapy may result in significant myelosuppression including reduction in platelet counts (thrombocytopenia 14%; grade ¾: 3%) and altered hemostatsis. In patients undergoing active treatment with sacituzumab govitecan, medical consult is suggested.

Adverse Reactions

>10%:

Cardiovascular: Edema (19%)

Dermatologic: Alopecia (38%), pruritus (17%), skin rash (31%), xeroderma (15%)

Endocrine & metabolic: Decreased serum albumin (39%), decreased serum calcium (49%), decreased serum glucose (19%), decreased serum sodium (25%), dehydration (13%), hyperglycemia (24%), hypermagnesemia (24%), hypokalemia (19%), hypomagnesemia (21%), hypophosphatemia (16%)

Gastrointestinal: Abdominal pain (26%), constipation (34%), decreased appetite (30%), diarrhea (62% to 63%; severe diarrhea: 4%), dysgeusia (11%), nausea (69%; severe nausea: 3%), stomatitis (14%; grade 3/4: 1%), vomiting (45% to 49%; severe vomiting: 5%)

Genitourinary: Urinary tract infection (21%)

Hematologic & oncologic: Anemia (52%; grade 3/4: 12%), prolonged prothrombin time (60%; grades 3/4: 12%), leukopenia (91%, grades 3/4: 26%), neutropenia (including severe neutropenia: 54% to 64%; grades 3/4: 43%; grade 4: 13%), thrombocytopenia (14%; grade 3/4: 3%)

Hepatic: Increased serum alanine aminotransferase (35%), increased serum alkaline phosphatase (57%), increased serum aspartate aminotransferase (45%)

Hypersensitivity: Hypersensitivity reaction (37%)

Nervous system: Dizziness (22%), fatigue (57%), headache (23%), insomnia (13%), neuropathy (24%)

Neuromuscular & skeletal: Arthralgia (17%), back pain (23%), limb pain (11%)

Respiratory: Cough (22%), dyspnea (21%), pneumonia (2%), respiratory tract infection (26%)

Miscellaneous: Fever (14%)

1% to 10%:

Gastrointestinal: Neutropenic enterocolitis (1% to 2%)

Hematologic & oncologic: Febrile neutropenia (6%)

Immunologic: Antibody development (2%)

Respiratory: Pleural effusion (2%)

Frequency not defined:

Gastrointestinal: Esophagitis

Hypersensitivity: Anaphylaxis

Infection: Influenza

Neuromuscular & skeletal: Asthenia

Ophthalmic: Periorbital edema

Mechanism of Action Sacituzumab govitecan is an antibody drug conjugate that consists of a humanized antitrophoblast cell-surface antigen 2 (Trop-2) monoclonal antibody coupled to the topoisomerase 1 inhibitor SN-38 via a cleavable linker (Bardia 2019). Trop-2 is overexpressed in many epithelial cancers and is associated with cancer cell growth; it has been detected in breast cancer cells (including triple-negative breast cancer cells). Sacituzumab govitecan binds to Trop-2 and is internalized; SN-38 is released in tumors both intracellularly and in the tumor microenvironment, leading to DNA damage, apoptosis, and cell death (Bardia 2019).

Pharmacodynamics/Kinetics

Half-life Elimination Sacituzumab govitecan: 16 hours; free SN-38: 18 hours.

Reproductive Considerations Evaluate pregnancy status prior to use in females of reproductive potential. Females of reproductive potential should use effective contraception during therapy and for 6 months after the last sacituzumab govitecan dose. Males with female partners of reproductive potential should use effective contraception during therapy and for 3 months after the last dose of sacituzumab govitecan.

Pregnancy Considerations

Based on the mechanism of action, in utero exposure to sacituzumab govitecan may cause fetal harm.

Sacituzumab govitecan is composed of sacituzumab linked to SN-38. Sacituzumab is a humanized monoclonal antibody (IgG_1). Placental transfer of human IgG is dependent upon the IgG subclass, maternal serum concentrations, newborn birth weight, and gestational age, generally increasing as pregnancy progresses. The lowest fetal IgG exposure would be expected during the period of organogenesis (Palmeira 2012; Pentsuk 2009). SN-38 is the genotoxic component.

- **Sacituzumab Govitecan-hziy** *see* Sacituzumab Govitecan *on page* 1352

Sacubitril and Valsartan

(sak UE bi tril & val SAR tan)

Brand Names: US Entresto

Brand Names: Canada Entresto

Pharmacologic Category Angiotensin II Receptor Blocker; Neprilysin Inhibitor

Use

Heart failure:

Adult: Reduce the risk of cardiovascular death and hospitalization for heart failure (HF) in patients with chronic HF (New York Heart Association Class II-IV) and reduced ejection fraction; usually administered in conjunction with other HF therapies, in place of an angiotensin-converting enzyme inhibitor or other angiotensin II receptor blocker.

Pediatric: Treatment of symptomatic HF with systemic left ventricular systolic dysfunction in pediatric patients ≥1 year of age.

Local Anesthetic/Vasoconstrictor Precautions No information available to require special precautions

Effects on Dental Treatment Key adverse event(s) related to dental treatment: Hypotension in general and orthostatic hypotension has been reported; Patients may experience orthostatic hypotension as they stand up after treatment; especially if lying in dental chair for extended periods of time. Use caution with sudden changes in position during and after dental treatment.

Effects on Bleeding No information available to require special precautions

Adverse Reactions Also see individual agents.

>10%:

Cardiovascular: Hypotension (18%)

Endocrine & metabolic: Increased serum potassium (4% to 16%), hyperkalemia (12%)

Renal: Increased serum creatinine (2% to 16%)

1% to 10%:

Cardiovascular: Orthostatic hypotension (2%)

Central nervous system: Dizziness (6%), falling (2%)

Hematologic & oncologic: Decreased hematocrit (≤5%), decreased hemoglobin (≤5%)

Hypersensitivity: Angioedema (black patients: 2%; others: <1%)

Renal: Renal failure (5%)

Respiratory: Cough (9%)

<1%, postmarketing and/or case reports: Anaphylaxis, hypersensitivity, pruritus, skin rash

Mechanism of Action

Sacubitril: Prodrug that inhibits neprilysin (neutral endopeptidase) through the active metabolite LBQ657, leading to increased levels of peptides, including natriuretic peptides; induces vasodilation and natriuresis (Hubers 2016).

Valsartan: Produces direct antagonism of the angiotensin II (AT2) receptors. Displaces angiotensin II from the AT1 receptor; antagonizes AT1-induced vasoconstriction, aldosterone release, catecholamine release, arginine vasopressin release, water intake, and hypertrophic responses.

Pharmacodynamics/Kinetics

Half-life Elimination Sacubitril: 1.4 hours; LBQ657: 11.5 hours; Valsartan: 9.9 hours

Time to Peak Sacubitril: 0.5 hours; LBQ657: 2 hours; Valsartan: 1.5 hours

Pregnancy Considerations [US Boxed Warning]: Drugs that act directly on the renin-angiotensin system can cause injury and death to the developing fetus. When pregnancy is detected, discontinue sacubitril/valsartan as soon as possible. Refer to the valsartan monograph for additional information.

◆ **Sacubitril/Valsartan** *see* Sacubitril and Valsartan *on page 1353*

Safinamide (sa FIN a mide)

Brand Names: US Xadago

Brand Names: Canada Onstryv

Pharmacologic Category Anti-Parkinson Agent, MAO Type B Inhibitor

Use Parkinson disease: Adjunctive treatment to levodopa/carbidopa in patients with Parkinson disease experiencing "off" episodes.

Local Anesthetic/Vasoconstrictor Precautions Safinamide inhibits MAO-type B, not MAO-type A. Therefore, there should not be any potential for interaction with vasoconstrictor. As a precautionary measure however, monitoring of the patient for signs of interaction is suggested.

Effects on Dental Treatment No significant effects or complications reported

Effects on Bleeding No information available to require special precautions

Adverse Reactions

>10%: Neuromuscular & skeletal: Dyskinesia (17% to 21%)

1% to 10%:

Cardiovascular: Hypertension (including exacerbation of hypertension: 5% to 7%), orthostatic hypotension (2%)

Central nervous system: Falling (6%), insomnia (4%), anxiety (2%)

Gastrointestinal: Nausea (6%), dyspepsia (2%)

Hepatic: Increased serum ALT (5% to 7%), increased serum AST (6% to 7%)

Respiratory: Cough (2%)

Frequency not defined: Central nervous system: Impulse control disorder

<1%, postmarketing, and/or case reports: Sudden onset of sleep (high dose)

Mechanism of Action Inhibitor of MAO-B. Plasma concentrations achieved via administration in recommended doses (≤100 mg/day) confer selective inhibition of MAO-B activity, blocking the catabolism of dopamine, resulting in an increase in dopamine levels and a subsequent increase in dopaminergic activity in the brain. The precise mechanism by which safinamide exerts its effect in Parkinson disease is unknown.

Pharmacodynamics/Kinetics

Half-life Elimination 20 to 26 hours

Time to Peak 2 to 3 hours

Pregnancy Considerations

Adverse events were observed in animal reproduction studies.

The incidence of Parkinson disease in pregnancy is relatively rare. When treatment for Parkinson disease is needed, agents other than safinamide may be preferred in pregnant women (Seier 2017).

◆ **Safinamide Mesylate** *see* Safinamide *on page 1353*

◆ **Safyral** *see* Ethinyl Estradiol, Drospirenone, and Levomefolate *on page 618*

◆ **SAHA** *see* Vorinostat *on page 1554*

◆ **Saizen** *see* Somatropin *on page 1381*
◆ **Saizen Click.Easy [DSC]** *see* Somatropin *on page 1381*
◆ **Saizenprep** *see* Somatropin *on page 1381*
◆ **Salagen** *see* Pilocarpine (Systemic) *on page 1230*
◆ **Salazosulfapyridine** *see* SulfaSALAzine *on page 1392*
◆ **Salbutamol** *see* Albuterol *on page 90*
◆ **Salbutamol and Ipratropium** *see* Ipratropium and Albuterol *on page 839*
◆ **Salbutamol Sulphate** *see* Albuterol *on page 90*
◆ **Salicylazosulfapyridine** *see* SulfaSALAzine *on page 1392*
◆ **Salicylsalicylic Acid** *see* Salsalate *on page 1356*
◆ **SalivaMAX** *see* Saliva Substitute *on page 1354*

Saliva Substitute (sa LYE va SUB stee tute)

Related Information

Dentin Hypersensitivity, Acid Erosion, High Caries Index, Management of Alveolar Osteitis, and Xerostomia *on page 1762*

Perioral Premalignant Lesions and Management of Patients Undergoing Cancer Therapy *on page 1781*

Brand Names: US Aquoral; Biotene Dry Mouth Gentle [OTC]; Biotene Moisturizing Mouth Spray [OTC]; Biotene Oral Balance [OTC]; BocaSal; Caphosol; Entertainer's Secret [OTC]; Moi-Stir [OTC]; Mouth Kote [OTC]; NeutraSal; Numoisyn; Oasis; SalivaMAX; SalivaSure [OTC]; Salivate Rx [DSC]; Xerostomia Relief Spray

Generic Availability (US) No

Pharmacologic Category Gastrointestinal Agent, Miscellaneous

Dental Use Relief of dry mouth and throat in xerostomia

Use

Mucositis (due to high-dose chemotherapy or radiation therapy): Adjunct to standard oral care in relief of symptoms associated with chemotherapy or radiation therapy-induced mucositis

Xerostomia: Relief of dry mouth and throat in xerostomia or hyposalivation

Local Anesthetic/Vasoconstrictor Precautions No information available to require special precautions

Effects on Dental Treatment No significant effects or complications reported

Effects on Bleeding No information available to require special precautions

Adverse Reactions Frequency not defined.

Central nervous system: Speech disturbance

Gastrointestinal: Dysgeusia, dysphagia, gastrointestinal disease (minor)

Dosing

Adult & Geriatric

Mucositis (due to high-dose chemotherapy or radiation therapy): Oral:

Caphosol (dispersible tablet and solution), NeutraSal: Swish and spit 4 to 10 doses daily (use for the duration of chemo- or radiation therapy).

SalivaMax, SalivateRx: Swish and spit 2 to 10 doses daily

Xerostomia: Oral: Use as needed, or product-specific dosing:

Aquoral: Two sprays 3 to 4 times daily

Biotene Dry Mouth Gentle oral rinse: Swish and spit 15 mL up to 3 times daily

Biotene Oral Balance gel: Apply one-half inch length onto tongue and spread evenly; repeat as often as needed

Caphosol (dispersible tablet and solution), NeutraSal, SalivaMax, SalivateRx: Swish and spit 2 to 10 doses daily.

Entertainer's Secret: Spray as often as needed.

Mouth Kote spray: Spray 3 to 5 times, swish for 8 to 10 seconds, then spit or swallow; use as often as needed.

Numoisyn liquid: Use 2 mL as needed.

Numoisyn lozenges: Dissolve 1 lozenge slowly; maximum 16 lozenges/day.

Oasis mouthwash: Rinse mouth with ~30 mL twice daily or as needed; do not swallow.

Oasis spray: 1 to 2 sprays as needed; maximum 60 sprays/day.

SalivaSure: Dissolve 1 lozenge slowly as needed; for severe symptoms, 1 lozenge per hour is recommended.

Renal Impairment: Adult There are no dosage adjustments provided in the manufacturer's labeling.

Hepatic Impairment: Adult There are no dosage adjustments provided in the manufacturer's labeling.

Pediatric Xerostomia: Oral: Children ≥12 years of age and Adolescents: Biotene Dry Mouth Gentle oral rinse: Refer to adult dosing.

Mechanism of Action Protein or electrolyte mixtures which restore/replace saliva, lubricate, moisten, clean, and/or provide a coating on oral mucosa

Contraindications Hypersensitivity to saliva substitute or any component of the formulation; fructose intolerance (Numoisyn lozenges only)

Drug Interactions

Metabolism/Transport Effects None known.

Avoid Concomitant Use There are no known interactions where it is recommended to avoid concomitant use.

Increased Effect/Toxicity There are no known significant interactions involving an increase in effect.

Decreased Effect There are no known significant interactions involving a decrease in effect.

Dietary Considerations

Caphosol: Dispersible tablet formulation contains sodium 1 g/50 mL dose and solution formulation contains sodium 71 mg/30 mL dose

Moi-Stir: Contains sodium: 6.47 mEq/120 mL, potassium: 1.93 mEq/120 mL, magnesium: 0.128 mEq/120 mL

Dosage Forms: US

Gel, oral:

Biotene Oral Balance [OTC]: Glycerin, water, sorbitol, xylitol, carbomer, hydroxyethylcellulose, sodium hydroxide

Liquid, oral:

Biotene Dry Mouth Gentle [OTC]: Water, glycerin, xylitol, sorbitol, propylene glycol, poloxamer 407, potassium sorbate, hydroxyethylcellulose, sodium phosphate, cetylpyridinium chloride, disodium phosphate

Numoisyn: Water, sorbitol, linseed extract, *Chondrus crispus*, methylparaben, sodium benzoate, potassium sorbate, dipotassium phosphate, propylparaben

Lozenge, oral:

Numoisyn: Sorbitol 0.3 g/lozenge, polyethylene glycol, malic acid, sodium citrate, calcium phosphate dibasic, hydrogenated cottonseed oil, citric acid, magnesium stearate, silicon dioxide

SalivaSure [OTC]: Xylitol, citric acid, apple acid, sodium citrate dihydrate, sodium carboxymethylcellulose, dibasic calcium phosphate, silica colloidal, magnesium stearate, stearic acid

Powder, for reconstitution, oral:

BocaSal: Calcium chloride, sodium bicarbonate, sodium chloride, and sodium phosphates

NeutraSal: Calcium chloride, sodium bicarbonate, sodium chloride, and sodium phosphates

SalivaMAX: Calcium chloride, sodium bicarbonate, sodium chloride, and sodium phosphates

Solution, oral:

Caphosol: Dibasic sodium phosphate 0.032%, monobasic sodium phosphate 0.009%, calcium chloride 0.052%, sodium chloride 0.569%, purified water

Entertainer's Secret [OTC]: Sodium carboxymethylcellulose, aloe vera gel, glycerin (60 mL)

Solution, oral [mouthwash/gargle]:

Oasis: Water, glycerin, sorbitol, poloxamer 338, PEG-60, hydrogenated castor oil, copovidone, sodium benzoate, carboxymethylcellulose

Solution, oral [spray]:

Aquoral: Oxidized glycerol triesters and silicon dioxide

Biotene Moisturizing Mouth Spray [OTC]: Water, polyglycitol, propylene glycol, sunflower oil, xylitol, milk protein extract, potassium sorbate, acesulfame K, potassium thiocyanate, lysozyme, lactoferrin, lactoperoxidase

Moi-Stir [OTC]: Water, sorbitol, sodium carboxymethylcellulose, methylparaben, propylparaben, potassium chloride, dibasic sodium phosphate, calcium chloride, magnesium chloride, sodium chloride

Mouth Kote [OTC]: Water, xylitol, sorbitol, yerba santa, citric acid, ascorbic acid, sodium saccharin, sodium benzoate

Oasis: Glycerin, cetylpyridinium, copovidone

Xerostomia Relief: Oxidized glycerol triesters and silicon dioxide

◆ **SalivaSure [OTC]** *see* Saliva Substitute *on page 1354*

◆ **Salivate Rx [DSC]** *see* Saliva Substitute *on page 1354*

◆ **Salk Vaccine** *see* Poliovirus Vaccine (Inactivated) *on page 1243*

Salmeterol (sal ME te role)

Related Information

Respiratory Diseases *on page 1680*

Brand Names: US Serevent Diskus

Brand Names: Canada Serevent Diskhaler Disks [DSC]; Serevent Diskus

Pharmacologic Category $Beta_2$ Agonist; $Beta_2$-Adrenergic Agonist, Long-Acting

Use

Asthma/Bronchospasm: Treatment of asthma and the prevention of bronchospasm (as concomitant therapy with an inhaled corticosteroid [ICS]) in patients ≥4 years of age with reversible obstructive airway disease, including patients with symptoms of nocturnal asthma.

Chronic obstructive pulmonary disease: Maintenance treatment of bronchospasm associated with chronic obstructive pulmonary disease (COPD) (including emphysema and chronic bronchitis).

Exercise-induced bronchospasm: Prevention of exercise-induced bronchospasm (EIB) in patients ≥4 years of age (use in combination with an ICS in patients with persistent asthma).

Note: Not indicated for the relief of acute bronchospasm.

Local Anesthetic/Vasoconstrictor Precautions No information available to require special precautions

Effects on Dental Treatment Key adverse event(s) related to dental treatment: Xerostomia (normal salivary flow resumes upon discontinuation), dental pain, and oropharyngeal candidiasis.

Effects on Bleeding No information available to require special precautions

Adverse Reactions

>10%: Central nervous system: Headache (13% to 17%), pain (1% to 12%)

1% to 10%:

Cardiovascular: Hypertension (4%), edema (1% to 3%)

Central nervous system: Dizziness (4%), sleep disorder (1% to 3%), anxiety (1% to 3%), migraine (1% to 3%), paresthesia (1% to 3%)

Dermatologic: Skin rash (1% to 4%), contact dermatitis (1% to 3%), eczema (1% to 3%), urticaria (3%), photodermatitis (1% to 2%), pallor

Endocrine & metabolic: Hyperglycemia (1% to 3%)

Gastrointestinal: Dyspepsia (1% to 3%), gastrointestinal infection (1% to 3%), nausea (1% to 3%), oropharyngeal candidiasis (1% to 3%), toothache (1% to 3%), xerostomia (1% to 3%)

Hepatic: Increased liver enzymes

Infection: Influenza (5%)

Neuromuscular & skeletal: Muscle cramps (≤3%), muscle spasm (≤3%), arthritis (1% to 3%), arthralgia (1% to 3%), muscle rigidity (1% to 3%)

Ophthalmic: Conjunctivitis (≤3%), keratitis (≤3%)

Respiratory: Nasal congestion (4% to 9%), bronchitis (≤7%), throat irritation (7%), tracheitis (≤7%; may be paradoxical), pharyngitis (≤6%), cough (5%), viral respiratory tract infection (5%), sinusitis (4% to 5%), rhinitis (4% to 5%), asthma (3% to 4%)

Miscellaneous: Fever (1% to 3%)

<1%, postmarketing, and/or case reports: Abdominal pain, agitation, aggressive behavior, anaphylaxis (some in patients with severe milk allergy), angioedema, aphonia, atrial fibrillation, bruise, cardiac arrhythmia, cataract, chest congestion, chest tightness, choking sensation, eosinophilic granulomatosis with polyangiitis (formerly known as Churg-Strauss), Cushing's syndrome, Cushingoid appearance, decreased linear skeletal growth rate (children and adolescents), depression, dysmenorrhea, dyspnea, ecchymoses, edema (facial, oropharyngeal), eosinophilia, glaucoma, hypercorticoidism, hypersensitivity reaction (immediate and delayed), hypokalemia, hypothyroidism, increased intraocular pressure, irregular menses, laryngospasm, local irritation (larynx), myositis, oropharyngeal irritation, osteoporosis, otalgia, paradoxical bronchospasm, pelvic inflammatory disease, prolonged QT interval on ECG, restlessness, sinus pain (paranasal), stridor, supraventricular tachycardia, syncope, tremor, vaginitis, vulvovaginal candidiasis, vulvovaginitis, ventricular tachycardia, weight gain

Mechanism of Action Relaxes bronchial smooth muscle by selective action on beta-2 receptors with little effect on heart rate; salmeterol acts locally in the lung.

Pharmacodynamics/Kinetics

Onset of Action Asthma: 30 to 48 minutes, COPD: 2 hours; Peak effect: Asthma: 3 hours, COPD: 2 to 5 hours

Duration of Action 12 hours

Half-life Elimination 5.5 hours

Time to Peak Serum: ~20 minutes

Pregnancy Considerations

Maternal use of beta-2 agonists are not associated with an increased risk of fetal malformations (GINA 2020).

Uncontrolled asthma is associated with adverse events in pregnancy (increased risk of perinatal mortality, pre-eclampsia, preterm birth, low-birth-weight infants, cesarean delivery, and the development of gestational diabetes). Poorly controlled asthma or asthma exacerbations may have a greater fetal/maternal risk than what is associated with appropriately used asthma medications. Maternal treatment improves pregnancy outcomes by reducing the risk of some adverse events (eg, preterm birth, gestational diabetes) (ERS/TSANZ [Middleton 2020]; GINA 2020).

Short-acting beta-2 agonists are preferred over long acting agents when treatment for asthma is needed during pregnancy. Pregnant females adequately controlled on salmeterol for asthma may continue therapy; if initiating treatment during pregnancy, salmeterol is the preferred long acting beta-2 agonist. Maternal asthma symptoms should be monitored monthly during pregnancy (ERS/TSANZ [Middleton 2020]).

Beta-agonists have the potential to affect uterine contractility if administered during labor.

Data collection to monitor pregnancy and infant outcomes associated with asthma and the medications used to treat asthma in pregnancy is ongoing. Health care providers are encouraged to enroll exposed pregnant females in the MotherToBaby Pregnancy Studies conducted by the Organization of Teratology Information Specialists (877-311-8972 or https://mothertobaby.org). Patients may also enroll themselves.

◆ **Salmeterol and Fluticasone** *see* Fluticasone and Salmeterol *on page 705*

◆ **Salmeterol Xinafoate** *see* Salmeterol *on page 1355*

◆ **Salmon Oil-1000 [OTC]** *see* Omega-3 Fatty Acids *on page 1137*

◆ **Salonpas Gel-Patch Hot [OTC]** *see* Capsaicin *on page 284*

◆ **Salonpas Hot [OTC] [DSC]** *see* Capsaicin *on page 284*

◆ **Salonpas Pain Relieving [OTC]** *see* Lidocaine (Topical) *on page 902*

◆ **Salonpas Pain Relieving Gel-Patch** *see* Lidocaine (Topical) *on page 902*

Salsalate (SAL sa late)

Related Information

Temporomandibular Dysfunction (TMD), Chronic Pain, and Fibromyalgia *on page 1773*

Brand Names: US Disalcid [DSC]

Pharmacologic Category Salicylate

Use Rheumatic disorders: Treatment of signs and symptoms of osteoarthritis, rheumatoid arthritis, and related rheumatic disorders

Local Anesthetic/Vasoconstrictor Precautions
No information available to require special precautions

Effects on Dental Treatment The dentist should be aware of the potential of abnormal coagulation. Caution should also be exercised in the use of NSAIDs in patients already on anticoagulant therapy with drugs such as warfarin (Coumadin®). See Effects on Bleeding.

Effects on Bleeding Nonacetylated salicylate formulations are known to reversibly decrease platelet aggregation via mechanisms different than observed with aspirin. Caution should also be exercised in the use of NSAIDs in patients already on anticoagulant therapy with drugs such as warfarin (Coumadin®). Unlike most salicylates/NSAIDs, salsalate does not interfere with platelet aggregation and presumably carries less risk of bleeding and/or effect on concurrent warfarin therapy.

With respect to surgery, dental practitioners should note that recommendations differ between general surgery (eg, appendectomy, hip replacement) and dental surgery. NSAIDs should be avoided (if possible) in general surgery patients for 3-5 half-lives of the drug (usually 1-3 days) prior to surgery to reduce the risk of excessive bleeding. However, there is no scientific evidence to warrant discontinuance of NSAIDs prior to dental surgery. In medically complicated patients or extensive oral surgery, the decision to interrupt therapy must be based on the risk to benefit in an individual patient and a medical consult is suggested. Routine interruption of NSAID therapy for most dental procedures is not warranted. If therapy is continued without interruption, the clinician should anticipate the potential for slower clotting times.

Adverse Reactions Frequency not defined.

Cardiovascular: Hypotension

Central nervous system: Vertigo

Dermatologic: Skin rash, Stevens-Johnson syndrome, toxic epidermal necrolysis, urticaria

Gastrointestinal: Abdominal pain, diarrhea, gastrointestinal hemorrhage, gastrointestinal perforation, gastrointestinal ulcer, nausea

Hematologic & oncologic: Anemia

Hepatic: Abnormal hepatic function tests, hepatitis

Hypersensitivity: Anaphylactic shock, angioedema

Otic: Auditory impairment, tinnitus

Renal: Decreased creatinine clearance, nephritis

Respiratory: Bronchospasm

Mechanism of Action Salsalate inhibits prostaglandin synthesis providing, anti-inflammatory effects with less inhibition of platelet aggregation than aspirin

Pharmacodynamics/Kinetics

Onset of Action Therapeutic: 3 to 4 days of continuous dosing

Half-life Elimination Salsalate: ~1 hour; Salicylic acid 3.5 to ≥16 hours (due to capacity limited biotransformation)

Pregnancy Risk Factor C

Pregnancy Considerations Adverse events have not been observed in animal reproduction studies. Due to the known effects of salicylates (closure of ductus arteriosus), use during late pregnancy should be avoided.

◆ **Sam-E.P.A. [OTC]** *see* Omega-3 Fatty Acids *on page 1137*

◆ **Samsca** *see* Tolvaptan *on page 1463*

- **Sancuso** *see* Granisetron *on page 748*
- **SandIMMUNE** *see* CycloSPORINE (Systemic) *on page 421*
- **Sandoglobulin** *see* Immune Globulin *on page 803*
- **Sanilvudine** *see* Stavudine *on page 1387*
- **Santyl** *see* Collagenase (Topical) *on page 409*
- **Saphris** *see* Asenapine *on page 174*

Saquinavir (sa KWIN a veer)

Related Information

Clinical Risk Related to Drugs Prolonging QT Interval *on page 1675*

HIV Infection and AIDS *on page 1690*

Brand Names: US Invirase

Brand Names: Canada Invirase

Pharmacologic Category Antiretroviral, Protease Inhibitor (Anti-HIV)

Use HIV-1 infection, treatment: Treatment of HIV-1 infection in adults (>16 years of age) in combination with ritonavir and other antiretroviral agents. **Note:** Saquinavir is not recommended as a component of initial therapy for the treatment of HIV (HHS [adult] 2019).

Local Anesthetic/Vasoconstrictor Precautions Saquinavir is one of the drugs confirmed to prolong the QT interval and is accepted as having a risk of causing torsade de pointes. The risk of drug-induced torsade de pointes is extremely low when a single QT interval prolonging drug is prescribed. In terms of epinephrine, it is not known what effect vasoconstrictors in the local anesthetic regimen will have in patients with a known history of congenital prolonged QT interval or in patients taking any medication that prolongs the QT interval. Until more information is obtained, it is suggested that the clinician consult with the physician prior to the use of a vasoconstrictor in suspected patients, and that the vasoconstrictor (epinephrine, mepivacaine and levonordefrin [Carbocaine® 2% with Neo-Cobefrin®]) be used with caution.

Effects on Dental Treatment Key adverse event(s) related to dental treatment: Buccal mucosa ulceration and taste alteration.

Effects on Bleeding Increased bleeding has been noted with protease inhibitors in patients with hemophilia A or B. No information available to require routine special precautions relative to hemostasis in other patients.

Adverse Reactions

Incidence data for saquinavir soft gel capsule formulation (no longer available) in combination with ritonavir:

10%: Gastrointestinal: Nausea (11%)

1% to 10%:

Cardiovascular: Chest pain

Central nervous system: Fatigue (6%), anxiety, depression, headache, insomnia, pain, paresthesia

Dermatologic: Pruritus (3%), skin rash (3%), eczema (2%), cheilosis (≤2%), xeroderma (≤2%), warts

Endocrine & metabolic: Lipodystrophy (5%), hyperglycemia (3%), change in libido, hypoglycemia, hyperkalemia

Gastrointestinal: Diarrhea (8%), vomiting (7%), abdominal pain (6%), constipation (2%), abdominal distress, decreased appetite, dysgeusia, dyspepsia, flatulence, increased serum amylase, oral mucosa ulcer

Hepatic: Increased serum ALT, increased serum AST, increased serum bilirubin

Infection: Influenza (3%)

Neuromuscular & skeletal: Back pain (2%), increased creatine phosphokinase, weakness

Respiratory: Pneumonia (5%), bronchitis (3%), sinusitis (3%)

Miscellaneous: Fever (3%)

Frequency not defined; reported for hard or soft gel capsule with/without ritonavir:

Cardiovascular: Heart valve disease (including murmur), hypertension, hypotension, peripheral vasoconstriction, prolongation P-R interval on ECG, prolonged QT interval on ECG, syncope, thrombophlebitis

Central nervous system: Agitation, amnesia, ataxia, colic, confusion, drowsiness, hallucination, hyperreflexia, hyporeflexia, neuropathy, poliomyelitis, progressive multifocal leukoencephalopathy, psychosis, seizure, speech disturbance

Dermatologic: Alopecia, bullous dermatitis, dermal ulcer, dermatitis, erythema, maculopapular rash, skin photosensitivity, Stevens-Johnson syndrome, urticaria

Endocrine & metabolic: Dehydration, diabetes mellitus, electrolyte disturbance, increased gamma-glutamyl transferase, increased lactate dehydrogenase, increased thyroid stimulating hormone level

Gastrointestinal: Bloody stools, dysphagia, esophagitis, gastritis, intestinal obstruction, pancreatitis, stomatitis

Genitourinary: Benign prostatic hypertrophy, hematuria, impotence, urinary tract infection

Hematologic & oncologic: Acute myelocytic leukemia, anemia (including hemolytic), leukopenia, neutropenia, pancytopenia, rectal hemorrhage, splenomegaly, thrombocytopenia

Hepatic: Ascites, hepatic disease (exacerbation), hepatitis, hepatomegaly, hepatosplenomegaly, increased serum alkaline phosphatase, jaundice

Immunologic: Immune reconstitution syndrome

Infection: Infection (bacterial, fungal, viral)

Neuromuscular & skeletal: Arthritis

Ophthalmic: Blepharitis, visual disturbance

Otic: Auditory impairment, otitis, tinnitus

Renal: Nephrolithiasis

Respiratory: Cyanosis, dyspnea, hemoptysis, pharyngitis, upper respiratory tract infection

<1%, postmarketing, and/or case reports: Atrioventricular block (second or third degree), autoimmune disease, torsades de pointes

Mechanism of Action Binds to the site of HIV-1 protease activity and inhibits cleavage of viral Gag-Pol polyprotein precursors into individual functional proteins required for infectious HIV. This results in the formation of immature, noninfectious viral particles.

Pharmacodynamics/Kinetics

Half-life Elimination Serum: 1 to 2 hours

Reproductive Considerations

Based on the Health and Humans Services (HHS) perinatal HIV guidelines, saquinavir is not one of the recommended antiretroviral agents for use in females living with HIV who are trying to conceive.

Females living with HIV not planning a pregnancy may use any available type of contraception, considering possible drug interactions and contraindications of the specific method. Consult the drug interactions database for more detailed information specific to use of saquinavir and specific contraceptives.

For males and females living with HIV and planning a pregnancy, maximum viral suppression below the limits of detection with antiretroviral therapy (ART), modification of therapy (if needed), optimization of the woman's health, and a discussion of the potential risks and benefits of ART therapy during pregnancy is recommended prior to conception (HHS [perinatal] 2019).

Pregnancy Considerations Saquinavir crosses the human placenta.

Outcome information specific to saquinavir use in pregnancy is no longer being reviewed and updated in the Health and Humans Services (HHS) perinatal guidelines. Maternal antiretroviral therapy (ART) may be associated with adverse pregnancy outcomes including preterm delivery, stillbirth, low birth weight, and small for gestational age infants. Actual risks may be influenced by maternal factors, such as disease severity, gestational age at initiation of therapy, and specific ART regimen; therefore, close fetal monitoring is recommended. Because there is clear benefit to appropriate treatment, maternal ART should not be withheld due to concerns for adverse neonatal outcomes. Long-term follow-up is recommended for all infants exposed to antiretroviral medications; children without HIV but who were exposed to ART in utero and develop significant organ system abnormalities of unknown etiology (particularly of the CNS or heart) should be evaluated for potential mitochondrial dysfunction. Hyperglycemia, new onset of diabetes mellitus, or diabetic ketoacidosis have been reported with protease inhibitors (PI); it is not clear if pregnancy increases this risk. Consider performing the standard glucose screening test earlier in pregnancy in women who initiated PI therapy prior to conception.

Based on the HHS perinatal HIV guidelines, saquinavir is not one of the recommended antiretroviral agents for use during pregnancy.

In general, ART is recommended for all pregnant females living with HIV to keep the viral load below the limit of detection and reduce the risk of perinatal transmission. Therapy should be individualized following a discussion of the potential risks and benefits of treatment during pregnancy. Monitoring of pregnant females is more frequent than in nonpregnant adults. ART should be continued postpartum for all females living with HIV and can be modified after delivery.

Health care providers are encouraged to enroll pregnant females exposed to antiretroviral medications as early in pregnancy as possible in the Antiretroviral Pregnancy Registry (1-800-258-4263 or http://www.APRegistry.com). Health care providers caring for pregnant females living with HIV and their infants may contact the National Perinatal HIV Hotline (1-888-448-8765) for clinical consultation (HHS [perinatal] 2019).

Product Availability Invirase 200 mg capsules have been discontinued in the United States for more than 1 year.

Dental Health Professional Considerations See Local Anesthetic/Vasoconstrictor Precautions

◆ **Saquinavir Mesylate** *see* Saquinavir *on page* 1357

◆ **SAR153191** *see* Sarilumab *on page* 1359

◆ **SAR236553** *see* Alirocumab *on page* 101

◆ **SAR650984** *see* Isatuximab *on page* 842

◆ **Sarafem** *see* FLUoxetine *on page* 697

◆ **Sarclisa** *see* Isatuximab *on page* 842

Sarecycline (sar e SYE kleen)

Brand Names: US Seysara

Pharmacologic Category Antibiotic, Tetracycline Derivative

Use Acne vulgaris, non-nodular, moderate to severe: Treatment of inflammatory lesions of non-nodular moderate to severe acne vulgaris in patients ≥9 years.

Local Anesthetic/Vasoconstrictor Precautions No information available to require special precautions

Effects on Dental Treatment Key adverse event(s) related to dental treatment: Although sarecycline is a member of the tetracyline family, there is no dental indication for it. Therefore the concerns of tetracycline in dental patients relative to enamel incorporation in pediatrics are not applicable to sarecycline. Superinfection: use may result in fungal or bacterial superinfection.

Effects on Bleeding No information available to require special precautions

Adverse Reactions

1% to 10%: Gastrointestinal: Nausea (3%)

<1%, postmarketing, and/or case reports: Vulvovaginal candidiasis, vulvovaginal infection

Mechanism of Action Tetracyclines inhibit protein synthesis by binding with the 30S and possibly the 50S ribosomal subunit(s) of susceptible bacteria (Griffin 2010).

Pharmacodynamics/Kinetics

Half-life Elimination 21 to 22 hours

Time to Peak 1.5 to 2 hours; delayed by ~0.53 hour when administered with high-fat, high-calorie meal that included milk

Pregnancy Considerations Tetracycline-class antibiotics may cause fetal harm following maternal use in pregnancy. Tetracyclines accumulate in developing teeth and long tubular bones. Permanent discoloration of teeth (yellow, gray, brown) can occur following in utero exposure and is more likely to occur following long-term or repeated exposure. Reversible inhibition of bone growth may occur following maternal use of tetracyclines in the second and third trimesters. Sarecycline should be discontinued immediately if pregnancy occurs during treatment.

◆ **Sarecycline Hydrochloride** *see* Sarecycline *on page* 1358

Sargramostim (sar GRAM oh stim)

Brand Names: US Leukine

Pharmacologic Category Colony Stimulating Factor; Hematopoietic Agent

Use

Acute myeloid leukemia (following induction chemotherapy): To shorten time to neutrophil recovery and to reduce the incidence of severe, life-threatening, or fatal infections following induction chemotherapy in adults 55 years of age and older with acute myeloid leukemia (AML).

Allogeneic bone marrow transplantation (myeloid reconstitution): Acceleration of myeloid reconstitution in pediatric patients 2 years of age and older and adults undergoing allogeneic bone marrow transplantation from HLA-matched related donors.

Allogeneic or autologous bone marrow transplantation (treatment of delayed neutrophil recovery or graft failure): Treatment of delayed or failed neutrophil recovery in pediatric patients 2 years of age and older and adults who have undergone allogeneic or autologous bone marrow transplantation.

Autologous peripheral blood progenitor cell mobilization and collection: Mobilization of hematopoietic progenitor cells into peripheral blood for collection by leukapheresis in adults with cancer undergoing autologous hematopoietic stem cell transplantation.

Autologous peripheral blood progenitor cell and bone marrow transplantation: To accelerate myeloid reconstitution following autologous peripheral blood progenitor cell transplantation or bone marrow transplantation in pediatric patients 2 years of age and older and adults with acute lymphoblastic leukemia (ALL), Hodgkin lymphoma (HL), and non-Hodgkin lymphoma (NHL).

Hematopoietic radiation injury syndrome (acute): Treatment to increase survival due to acute exposure to myelosuppressive radiation doses (hematopoietic syndrome of acute radiation syndrome [H-ARS]) in infants, children, adolescents, and adults.

Local Anesthetic/Vasoconstrictor Precautions No information available to require special precautions

Effects on Dental Treatment Key adverse event(s) related to dental treatment: Dysphagia.

Effects on Bleeding No information available to require special precautions. Medical consultation may be considered to confirm adequate platelet counts.

Adverse Reactions

>10%:

Cardiovascular: Hypertension (34%), edema (13% to 25%), pericardial effusion (4% to 25%), chest pain (15%), peripheral edema (11%), tachycardia (11%)

Central nervous system: Malaise (57%), headache (26%), chills (25%), anxiety (11%), insomnia (11%)

Dermatologic: Skin changes (77%), skin rash (44%), pruritus (23%)

Endocrine & metabolic: Elevated serum glucose (49%), weight loss (37%), decreased serum albumin (36%), hyperglycemia (25%), hypomagnesemia (15%)

Gastrointestinal: Diarrhea (81% to 89%), nausea (58% to 70%), vomiting (46% to 70%), abdominal pain (38%), anorexia (13%), hematemesis (13%), dysphagia (11%), gastrointestinal hemorrhage (11%)

Genitourinary: Urinary tract infection (14%)

Hepatic: Hyperbilirubinemia (30%)

Neuromuscular & skeletal: Asthenia (66%), ostealgia (21%), arthralgia (11% to 21%), myalgia (18%)

Ophthalmic: Retinal hemorrhage (11%)

Renal: Increased serum creatinine (15%)

Respiratory: Pharyngitis (23%), epistaxis (17%), dyspnea (15%)

Miscellaneous: Fever (81%), laboratory test abnormality (58%, metabolic)

1% to 10%:

Immunologic: Antibody development (2%)

Respiratory: Pleural effusion (1%)

<1%, postmarketing, and/or case reports: Anaphylaxis, bone marrow dysplasia, capillary leak syndrome, cardiac disease, decreased serum total protein, eosinophilia, erythema, flushing, hemorrhage (neurocortical events), hypersensitivity reaction, hypotension, hypoxia, increased monocytes, infusion related reaction, injection site reaction, leukocytosis, liver function impairment, pain, prolonged prothrombin time, respiratory distress, supraventricular cardiac arrhythmia, syncope, thromboembolic complications, urticaria, weight gain

Mechanism of Action Sargramostim is a colony stimulating growth factor which stimulates proliferation, differentiation, and functional activity of neutrophils, eosinophils, monocytes, and macrophages.

Pharmacodynamics/Kinetics

Onset of Action Increase in WBC in 7 to 14 days

Duration of Action WBCs return to baseline within 1 to 2 weeks of discontinuing drug

Half-life Elimination

Children 6 months to 15 years: IV: Median: 1.6 hours; range: 0.9 to 2.5 hours; SubQ: Median: 2.3 hours (0.3 to 3.8 hours) (Stute 1995)

Adults: IV: 3.84 hours; SubQ: 1.4 hours

Time to Peak Serum: IV: During or immediately after infusion; SubQ: 2.4 to 4 hours

Pregnancy Considerations

Data regarding use in pregnant females is limited. Some dosage forms may contain benzyl alcohol (avoid in pregnant women due to association with gasping syndrome in premature infants); if use is necessary during pregnancy, lyophilized powder reconstituted with preservative-free sterile water for injection is recommended.

Sarilumab (sar IL ue mab)

Brand Names: US Kevzara

Brand Names: Canada Kevzara

Pharmacologic Category Antirheumatic, Disease Modifying; Interleukin-6 Receptor Antagonist; Monoclonal Antibody

Use Rheumatoid arthritis: Treatment of moderate to severe active rheumatoid arthritis in adults who have had an inadequate response or intolerance to one or more disease-modifying antirheumatic drugs.

Local Anesthetic/Vasoconstrictor Precautions No information available to require special precautions

Effects on Dental Treatment Key adverse event(s) related to dental treatment: Oral herpes has been reported

Effects on Bleeding No information available to require special precautions

Adverse Reactions

Incidence as reported for combination therapy unless otherwise noted. Combination therapy refers to use in rheumatoid arthritis with nonbiological disease-modifying antirheumatic drugs.

>10%: Hepatic: Increased serum alanine aminotransferase (≤3 X ULN: 5% to 43%), increased serum aspartate aminotransferase (≤3 X ULN: 30%)

1% to 10%:

Dermatologic: Injection site pruritus (2%)

Endocrine & metabolic: Hypertriglyceridemia (1%)

Gastrointestinal: Oral herpes simplex infection (<2%)

Genitourinary: Urinary tract infection (3%)

Hematologic & oncologic: Decreased platelet count (1%), leukopenia (2%), neutropenia (10%)

Immunologic: Antibody development (monotherapy) (9%; neutralizing: 7%)

Local: Erythema at injection site (4%), injection site reaction (7%)

Respiratory: Nasopharyngitis (≤4%), upper respiratory tract infection (3%)

<1%:

Gastrointestinal: Gastrointestinal perforation

Hypersensitivity: Hypersensitivity reaction

Frequency not defined:
Dermatologic: Cellulitis
Endocrine & metabolic: Increased HDL cholesterol, increased LDL cholesterol
Hematologic & oncologic: Malignant neoplasm
Respiratory: Pneumonia
Postmarketing:
Infection: Candidiasis, opportunistic infection, serious infection
Respiratory: Infection due to an organism in genus *Pneumocystis*, tuberculosis

Mechanism of Action Sarilumab is an interleukin-6 (IL-6) receptor antagonist which binds to both soluble and membrane-bound IL-6 receptors. Endogenous IL-6 is induced by inflammatory stimuli and mediates a variety of immunological responses. IL-6 produced by synovial and endothelial cells leads to local production of IL-6 in joints affected by inflammatory processes such as rheumatoid arthritis. Inhibition of IL-6 receptors by sarilumab leads to a reduction in CRP levels.

Pharmacodynamics/Kinetics

Half-life Elimination
Concentration dependent:
200 mg every 2 weeks: Up to 10 days
150 mg every 2 weeks: Up to 8 days

Time to Peak 2 to 4 days

Reproductive Considerations
The effectiveness of oral contraceptives may be decreased during therapy and for several weeks after sarilumab is discontinued.

Pregnancy Considerations
Sarilumab is a humanized monoclonal antibody (IgG_1). Potential placental transfer of human IgG is dependent upon the IgG subclass and gestational age, generally increasing as pregnancy progresses. The lowest exposure would be expected during the period of organogenesis (Palmeira 2012; Pentsuk 2009).

Based on animal data and the mechanism of action, maternal use of sarilumab may delay parturition.

Immune response in infants exposed to sarilumab in utero may be affected. Consider risks/benefits prior to administering live or live-attenuated vaccines to infants exposed to sarilumab during pregnancy.

A pregnancy registry has been established to monitor outcomes of women exposed to sarilumab during pregnancy. Health care providers or pregnant patients are encouraged to register (877-311-8972).

◆ **Sarna Sensitive [OTC]** *see* Pramoxine *on page* 1252

◆ **Sarnol-HC [OTC]** *see* Hydrocortisone (Topical) *on page* 775

◆ **Savaysa** *see* Edoxaban *on page* 542

◆ **Savella** *see* Milnacipran *on page* 1031

◆ **Savella Titration Pack** *see* Milnacipran *on page* 1031

SAXagliptin (sax a GLIP tin)

Related Information
Endocrine Disorders and Pregnancy *on page* 1684

Brand Names: US Onglyza

Brand Names: Canada Onglyza

Pharmacologic Category Antidiabetic Agent, Dipeptidyl Peptidase 4 (DPP-4) Inhibitor

Use Diabetes mellitus, type 2, treatment: As an adjunct to diet and exercise to improve glycemic control in adults with type 2 diabetes mellitus as monotherapy or combination therapy.

Local Anesthetic/Vasoconstrictor Precautions
No information available to require special precautions

Effects on Dental Treatment Key adverse event(s) related to dental treatment: Saxagliptin dependent patients with diabetes should be appointed for dental treatment in the morning in order to minimize chance of stress-induced hypoglycemia.

Effects on Bleeding No information available to require special precautions

Adverse Reactions
1% to 10%:
Cardiovascular: Peripheral edema (4%)
Central nervous system: Headache (7%)
Endocrine & metabolic: Hypoglycemia (6%)
Genitourinary: Urinary tract infection (7%)
Hematologic & oncologic: Lymphocytopenia (2%)
Hypersensitivity: Hypersensitivity reaction (2%; including facial edema and urticaria)
Frequency not defined: Cardiovascular: Thrombocytopenia
<1%, postmarketing, and/or case reports: Acute pancreatitis, anaphylaxis, angioedema, bullous pemphigoid, exfoliative dermatitis, immune thrombocytopenia, increased creatine phosphokinase in blood specimen, increased serum creatinine, pancreatitis, rhabdomyolysis, severe arthralgia

Mechanism of Action Saxagliptin inhibits dipeptidyl peptidase 4 (DPP-4) enzyme resulting in prolonged active incretin levels. Incretin hormones (eg, glucagon-like peptide-1, glucose-dependent insulinotropic polypeptide) regulate glucose homeostasis by increasing insulin synthesis and release from pancreatic beta cells and decreasing glucagon secretion from pancreatic alpha cells. Decreased glucagon secretion results in decreased hepatic glucose production. Under normal physiologic circumstances, incretin hormones are released by the intestine throughout the day and levels are increased in response to a meal; incretin hormones are rapidly inactivated by the DPP-4 enzyme.

Pharmacodynamics/Kinetics

Duration of Action 24 hours

Half-life Elimination Saxagliptin: 2.5 hours; 5-hydroxy saxagliptin: 3.1 hours

Time to Peak Plasma: Saxagliptin: 2 hours; 5-hydroxy saxagliptin: 4 hours

Pregnancy Considerations
Poorly controlled diabetes during pregnancy can be associated with an increased risk of adverse maternal and fetal outcomes, including diabetic ketoacidosis, preeclampsia, spontaneous abortion, preterm delivery, delivery complications, major birth defects, stillbirth, and macrosomia. To prevent adverse outcomes, prior to conception and throughout pregnancy, maternal blood glucose and HbA_{1c} should be kept as close to target goals as possible but without causing significant hypoglycemia (ADA 2020; Blumer 2013).

Agents other than saxagliptin are currently recommended to treat diabetes mellitus in pregnancy (ADA 2020).

Saxagliptin and Metformin
(sax a GLIP tin & met FOR min)

Related Information
MetFORMIN *on page* 983
SAXagliptin *on page* 1360

Brand Names: US Kombiglyze XR

Brand Names: Canada Komboglyze

Pharmacologic Category Antidiabetic Agent, Biguanide; Antidiabetic Agent, Dipeptidyl Peptidase 4 (DPP-4) Inhibitor

Use Diabetes mellitus, type 2, treatment: Adjunct to diet and exercise to improve glycemic control in adults with type 2 diabetes mellitus.

Local Anesthetic/Vasoconstrictor Precautions No information available to require special precautions

Effects on Dental Treatment Key adverse event(s) related to dental treatment: Saxagliptin- and metformin-dependent patients with diabetes should be appointed for dental treatment in the morning in order to minimize chance of stress-induced hypoglycemia.

Effects on Bleeding No information available to require special precautions

Adverse Reactions See individual agents.

Mechanism of Action

Saxagliptin inhibits dipeptidyl peptidase IV (DPP-IV) enzyme resulting in prolonged active incretin levels. Incretin hormones (eg, glucagon-like peptide-1 [GLP-1] and glucose-dependent insulinotropic polypeptide [GIP]) regulate glucose homeostasis by increasing insulin synthesis and release from pancreatic beta cells and decreasing glucagon secretion from pancreatic alpha cells. Decreased glucagon secretion results in decreased hepatic glucose production. Under normal physiologic circumstances, incretin hormones are released by the intestine throughout the day and levels are increased in response to a meal; incretin hormones are rapidly inactivated by the DPP-IV enzyme.

Metformin decreases hepatic glucose production, decreasing intestinal absorption of glucose and improves insulin sensitivity (increases peripheral glucose uptake and utilization).

Pregnancy Considerations Metformin crosses the placenta (ADA 2020). Refer to individual monographs.

- ◆ **Saxagliptin and Metformin Hydrochloride** *see* Saxagliptin and Metformin *on page 1360*
- ◆ **Saxagliptin, Dapagliflozin, and Metformin Hydrochloride** *see* Dapagliflozin, Saxagliptin, and Metformin *on page 436*
- ◆ **Saxagliptin HCl** *see* SAXagliptin *on page 1360*
- ◆ **Saxagliptin HCl/Metformin HCl** *see* Saxagliptin and Metformin *on page 1360*
- ◆ **Saxagliptin, Metformin, and Dapagliflozin** *see* Dapagliflozin, Saxagliptin, and Metformin *on page 436*
- ◆ **Saxenda** *see* Liraglutide *on page 920*
- ◆ **SB-265805** *see* Gemifloxacin *on page 733*
- ◆ **SB-497115** *see* Eltrombopag *on page 551*
- ◆ **SB-497115-GR** *see* Eltrombopag *on page 551*
- ◆ **SB659746-A** *see* Vilazodone *on page 1544*
- ◆ **Scalacort [DSC]** *see* Hydrocortisone (Topical) *on page 775*
- ◆ **Scalacort DK** *see* Hydrocortisone (Topical) *on page 775*
- ◆ **Scalpicin Maximum Strength [OTC]** *see* Hydrocortisone (Topical) *on page 775*
- ◆ **Scandonest 2% L** *see* Mepivacaine and Levonordefrin *on page 975*
- ◆ **Scandonest 3% Plain** *see* Mepivacaine *on page 972*
- ◆ **Scenesse** *see* Afamelanotide *on page 88*
- ◆ **SCH 13521** *see* Flutamide *on page 702*
- ◆ **SCH 52365** *see* Temozolomide *on page 1415*
- ◆ **SCH 56592** *see* Posaconazole *on page 1248*
- ◆ **SCH 90045** *see* Pembrolizumab *on page 1204*
- ◆ **SCH530348** *see* Vorapaxar *on page 1551*
- ◆ **SCH-619734** *see* Rolapitant *on page 1343*
- ◆ **SCIG** *see* Immune Globulin *on page 803*
- ◆ **Scot-Tussin Allergy Relief [OTC] [DSC]** *see* DiphenhydrAMINE (Systemic) *on page 502*
- ◆ **Scot-Tussin Diabetes CF [OTC] [DSC]** *see* Dextromethorphan *on page 476*
- ◆ **SC-PEG** *see* Calaspargase Pegol *on page 278*
- ◆ **Scrub Care Povidone-iodine [OTC]** *see* Povidone-Iodine (Topical) *on page 1249*
- ◆ **SD/01** *see* Pegfilgrastim *on page 1200*
- ◆ **SDX-105** *see* Bendamustine *on page 226*
- ◆ **SDZ ENA 713** *see* Rivastigmine *on page 1341*
- ◆ **Sea-Omega [OTC]** *see* Omega-3 Fatty Acids *on page 1137*
- ◆ **Seasonique** *see* Ethinyl Estradiol and Levonorgestrel *on page 612*
- ◆ **Sectral [DSC]** *see* Acebutolol *on page 58*
- ◆ **Secuado** *see* Asenapine *on page 174*

Secukinumab (sek ue KIN ue mab)

Brand Names: US Cosentyx; Cosentyx (300 MG Dose); Cosentyx Sensoready (300 MG); Cosentyx Sensoready Pen

Brand Names: Canada Cosentyx

Pharmacologic Category Anti-interleukin 17A Monoclonal Antibody; Antipsoriatic Agent; Monoclonal Antibody

Use

Ankylosing spondylitis: Treatment of active ankylosing spondylitis in adults.

Axial spondyloarthritis (nonradiographic): Treatment of active nonradiographic axial spondyloarthritis in adults with objective signs of inflammation.

Plaque psoriasis: Treatment of moderate to severe plaque psoriasis in adults who are candidates for systemic therapy or phototherapy.

Psoriatic arthritis: Treatment of active psoriatic arthritis in adults.

Local Anesthetic/Vasoconstrictor Precautions No information available to require special precautions

Effects on Dental Treatment Key adverse event(s) related to dental treatment: Mucocutaneous candidiasis, oral herpes, and pharyngitis have been reported.

Effects on Bleeding No information available to require special precautions

Adverse Reactions

>10%:

Infection: Infection (29% to 48%; serious infection: ≤1%)

Respiratory: Nasopharyngitis (11% to 12%)

1% to 10%:

Dermatologic: Urticaria (≤1%)

Endocrine & metabolic: Hypercholesterolemia (≥2%)

Gastrointestinal: Diarrhea (3% to 4%), inflammatory bowel disease (≤1%; Crohn's disease, exacerbation of Crohn's disease, exacerbation of ulcerative colitis, ulcerative colitis: <1%), mucocutaneous candidiasis (1%), nausea (≥2%), oral herpes simplex infection (≤1%)

Nervous system: Headache (≥2%)

Respiratory: Pharyngitis (1%), rhinitis (1%), rhinorrhea (≤1%), upper respiratory tract infection (3%)

Frequency not defined:

Gastrointestinal: Colitis, gastritis, hematochezia, lower abdominal pain

Genitourinary: Urinary tract infection

Hypersensitivity: Anaphylaxis, hypersensitivity reaction

Infection: Candidiasis, herpes virus infection, staphylococcal infection

<1%, postmarketing, and/or case reports: Antibody development (including neutralizing; neutralizing antibodies not associated with drug efficacy), conjunctivitis, impetigo, increased serum transaminases, neutropenia, oral candidiasis, otitis externa, otitis media, sinusitis, tinea pedis, tonsillitis

Mechanism of Action Secukinumab is a human IgG1 monoclonal antibody that selectively binds to the interleukin-17A (IL-17A) cytokine and inhibits its interaction with the IL-17 receptor. IL-17A is a naturally occurring cytokine involved in normal inflammatory and immune responses. Secukinumab inhibits the release of proinflammatory cytokines and chemokines.

Pharmacodynamics/Kinetics

Half-life Elimination 22 to 31 days

Time to Peak ~6 days

Reproductive Considerations

The American Academy of Dermatology considers secukinumab for the treatment of psoriasis to be likely compatible for use in male patients planning to father a child (AAD-NPF [Menter 2019]).

Women and men with well-controlled psoriasis who are planning a pregnancy and wish to avoid fetal exposure can consider discontinuing secukinumab 19 weeks prior to attempting pregnancy (Rademaker 2018).

Possible failure of tubal sterilization following placement of an implantable birth control device (Essure) was observed in a female treated with secukinumab (Nardin 2018). **Note:** Distribution of Essure in the United States was stopped in December 2018.

Pregnancy Considerations

Secukinumab is a humanized monoclonal antibody (IgG_1). Placental transfer of human IgG is dependent upon the IgG subclass, maternal serum concentrations, birth weight, and gestational age, generally increasing as pregnancy progresses. The lowest exposure would be expected during the period of organogenesis (Palmeira 2012; Pentsuk 2009).

Outcome information following exposure to secukinumab in pregnancy is limited (Nardin 2018; Warren 2018).

- ◆ **Secura Antifungal [OTC] [DSC]** *see* Miconazole (Topical) *on page 1019*
- ◆ **Secura Antifungal Extra Thick [OTC] [DSC]** *see* Miconazole (Topical) *on page 1019*
- ◆ **Seebri Neohaler** *see* Glycopyrrolate (Oral Inhalation) *on page 743*
- ◆ **SEG101** *see* Crizanlizumab *on page 414*

Segesterone Acetate and Ethinyl Estradiol

(se JES ter one AS e tate & ETH in il es tra DYE ole)

Brand Names: US Annovera

Pharmacologic Category Contraceptive; Estrogen and Progestin Combination

Use Contraceptive: To prevent pregnancy in females of reproductive potential

Local Anesthetic/Vasoconstrictor Precautions No information available to require special precautions

Effects on Dental Treatment Key adverse event(s) related to dental treatment: When prescribing antibiotics, patient must be warned to use additional methods of birth control if taking contraceptives containing estrogen derivatives.

Effects on Bleeding No information available to require special precautions

Adverse Reactions

>10%:

Central nervous system: Headache (≤39%), migraine (≤39%)

Gastrointestinal: Nausea (≤25%), vomiting (≤25%), abdominal pain (≤13%), lower abdominal pain (≤13%), upper abdominal pain (≤13%)

Genitourinary: Vulvovaginal candidiasis (15%), dysmenorrhea (13%), vaginal discharge (12%)

1% to 10%:

Cardiovascular: Cerebral thrombosis (≥2%), deep vein thrombosis (≥2%), pulmonary embolism (≥2%)

Central nervous system: Psychiatric disturbance (≥2%)

Dermatologic: Genital pruritus (6%)

Endocrine & metabolic: Heavy menstrual bleeding (≤8%), menstrual disease (≤8%), amenorrhea (≤5%)

Gastrointestinal: Diarrhea (7%)

Genitourinary: Breakthrough bleeding (≤10%), breast tenderness (≤10%), cystitis (≤10%), genitourinary infection (≤10%), mastalgia (≤10%), spotting (≤10%), urinary tract infection (≤10%), spontaneous abortion (≥2%)

Hypersensitivity: Drug-induced hypersensitivity (≥2%)

Renal: Pyelonephritis (≤10%)

Mechanism of Action Combination hormonal contraceptives lower the risk of pregnancy primarily by suppressing ovulation.

Pharmacodynamics/Kinetics

Onset of Action Effective on the day of insertion when inserted between days 2 and 5 of menstrual period

Half-life Elimination

Ethinyl estradiol: 15.1 ± 7.5 hours

Segesterone acetate: 4.5 ± 3.4 hours

Time to Peak Ethinyl estradiol and segesterone acetate: 2 hours (median) following cycle 1; peak concentrations decline over subsequent dosing cycles

Reproductive Considerations

Information related to concomitant use with diaphragms, cervical caps and female condoms is not available. Use is compatible with male condoms made with natural rubber latex, polyisoprene, and polyurethane. Fertility is expected to return within 6 months after discontinuing use.

Due to the increased risk of venous thromboembolism (VTE) postpartum, combination hormonal contraceptives should not be started in females <4 weeks following delivery who are not breastfeeding. The risk decreases to baseline by postpartum day 42. Use of combination hormonal contraceptives in females between 21 and 42 days after delivery should take into consideration the individual woman's risk factors for VTE (eg, age ≥35 years, previous VTE, thrombophilia, immobility, preeclampsia, transfusion at delivery, cesarean delivery, peripartum cardiomyopathy, BMI, postpartum hemorrhage, or smoking) (Curtis 2016b).

Pregnancy Considerations

Combination hormonal contraceptives are used to prevent pregnancy; treatment should be discontinued if pregnancy occurs. In general, the use of combination hormonal contraceptives, when inadvertently used early in pregnancy, have not been associated with adverse fetal or maternal effects (Curtis 2016b).

◆ **Segluromet** *see* Ertugliflozin and Metformin *on page 588*

Selegiline (se LE ji leen)

Related Information

Dentin Hypersensitivity, Acid Erosion, High Caries Index, Management of Alveolar Osteitis, and Xerostomia *on page 1762*

Brand Names: US Eldepryl [DSC]; Emsam; Zelapar

Brand Names: Canada APO-Selegiline; DOM-Selegiline [DSC]; MYLAN-Selegiline [DSC]; PMS-Selegiline [DSC]; TEVA-Selegiline

Pharmacologic Category Anti-Parkinson Agent, MAO Type B Inhibitor; Antidepressant, Monoamine Oxidase Inhibitor

Use

Parkinson disease: Adjunct in the management of patients with Parkinson disease being treated with levodopa/carbidopa who exhibit deterioration in the quality of their response to this therapy (oral products).

Major depressive disorder: Treatment of major depressive disorder (MDD) in adults (transdermal patch)

Local Anesthetic/Vasoconstrictor Precautions Selegiline in doses of 10 mg a day or less does not inhibit type-A MAO. Therefore, there are no precautions with the use of vasoconstrictors.

Effects on Dental Treatment Key adverse event(s) related to dental treatment: Xerostomia and changes in salivation (normal salivary flow resumes upon discontinuation). Anticholinergic side effects can cause a reduction of saliva production or secretion, contributing to discomfort and dental disease (ie, caries, oral candidiasis, and periodontal disease).

Orally disintegrating tablet: Dysphagia, stomatitis, and taste perversion.

Effects on Bleeding No information available to require special precautions

Adverse Reactions Unless otherwise noted, the percentage of adverse events is reported for the transdermal patch (ODT = orally disintegrating tablet, Oral = capsule/tablet)

>10%:

Central nervous system: Headache (18%; ODT: 7%; oral: 4%), dizziness (oral: 14%; ODT: 11%), insomnia (12%; ODT: 7%)

Gastrointestinal: Nausea (oral: 20%; ODT: 11%)

Local: Application site reaction (24%)

1% to 10%:

Cardiovascular: Hypotension (3% to 10%; including orthostatic hypotension), hypertension (≥1%; ODT: 3%), chest pain (≥1%; ODT: 2%), palpitations (oral: 2%), peripheral edema (≥1%)

Central nervous system: Pain (ODT: 8%; oral: 2%), confusion (oral: 6%; ODT: 4%), hallucination (oral: 6%; ODT: 4%), vivid dream (oral: 4%), ataxia (<1%; ODT: 3%), drowsiness (ODT: 3%), depression (<1%; ODT: 2%), lethargy (oral: 2%), abnormality in thinking (≥1%), agitation (≥1%), amnesia (≥1%), paresthesia (≥1%)

Dermatologic: Skin rash (4%), acne vulgaris (≥1%), diaphoresis (≥1%), pruritus (≥1%)

Endocrine & metabolic: Weight loss (5%; oral: 2%), hypokalemia (ODT: 2%)

Gastrointestinal: Diarrhea (9%; ODT: 2%; oral: 2%), xerostomia (8%; oral: 6%; ODT: 4%), abdominal pain (oral: 8%), dyspepsia (4%; ODT: 5%), stomatitis (ODT: 5%), constipation (≥1%; ODT: 4%), vomiting (≥1%; ODT: 3%), dental caries (ODT: 2%), dysgeusia (≥1%; ODT: 2%), dysphagia (ODT: 2%), flatulence (≥1%; ODT: 2%), anorexia (≥1%), gastroenteritis (≥1%)

Genitourinary: Urinary retention (oral: 2%), dysmenorrhea (≥1%), sexual disorder (≥1%), urinary frequency (≥1%), urinary tract infection (≥1%), uterine hemorrhage (≥1%)

Hematologic & oncologic: Bruise (≥1%; ODT: 2%)

Neuromuscular & skeletal: Dyskinesia (ODT: 6%), back pain (ODT: 5%; oral: 2%), leg cramps (ODT: 3%; oral: 2%), myalgia (≥1%; ODT: 3%), tremor (<1%; ODT: 3%), neck pain (≥1%)

Otic: Tinnitus (≥1%)

Respiratory: Rhinitis (ODT: 7%), pharyngitis (3%; ODT: 4%), dyspnea (<1%; ODT: 3%), sinusitis (3%), bronchitis (≥1%), cough (≥1%)

Frequency not defined:

Cardiovascular: Atrial fibrillation, bradycardia, cardiac arrhythmia, facial edema, myocardial infarction, peripheral vascular disease, syncope, tachycardia, vasodilation

Central nervous system: Altered sense of smell, behavioral changes, chorea, delusions, depersonalization, emotional lability, euphoria, heatstroke, hostility, hyperesthesia, hypertonia, impulse control disorder (including binge eating, hypersexuality, pathological gambling), loss of balance, mania, migraine, mood changes, myasthenia, myoclonus, oral paresthesia, paranoia, psychoneurosis, twitching, vertigo

Dermatologic: Maculopapular rash, skin hypertrophy, urticaria, vesiculobullous dermatitis

Endocrine & metabolic: Dehydration, hypercholesterolemia, hyperglycemia, hypoglycemia, hyponatremia, increased lactate dehydrogenase, increased libido

Gastrointestinal: Colitis, eructation, gastritis, glossitis, increased appetite, melena, periodontal abscess, sialorrhea

Genitourinary: Benign prostatic hypertrophy, hematuria (females), hernia, mastalgia, pelvic pain, urinary urgency, urination disorder (males; impairment), vaginal hemorrhage, vaginitis, vulvovaginal candidiasis

Hematologic & oncologic: Benign skin neoplasm, breast neoplasm (female), leukocytosis, leukopenia, lymphadenopathy, neoplasm, rectal hemorrhage

Hepatic: Abnormal hepatic function tests, hyperbilirubinemia, increased serum alkaline phosphatase

Hypersensitivity: Tongue edema

Infection: Bacterial infection, candidiasis, fungal infection, parasitic infection, viral infection

Neuromuscular & skeletal: Bradykinesia, hyperkinesia, muscle spasm (generalized), osteoporosis, tenosynovitis

Ophthalmic: Visual field defect

Otic: Otitis externa

Renal: Nephrolithiasis (females), polyuria (females)

Respiratory: Asthma, epistaxis, laryngismus, pneumonia

Miscellaneous: Fever

Mechanism of Action Potent, irreversible inhibitor of monoamine oxidase (MAO). Selegiline has a greater affinity for MAO-B compared to MAO-A (intestinal MAO is predominantly type A; in the brain, both isoenzymes exist). In the CNS, MAO plays a major role in the catabolism of dopamine, serotonin, norepinephrine, and epinephrine. At lower doses, selegiline can serve as a selective inhibitor of MAO-B; however, as selegiline concentrations increase, MAO-B selectivity is lost. Selegiline may increase dopaminergic activity by interfering with dopamine reuptake at the synapse. Effects may also be mediated through its metabolites, including amphetamine and methamphetamine, which interfere with neuronal uptake and enhance release of several neurotransmitters (eg, norepinephrine, dopamine, serotonin). The extent to which these metabolites contribute to the effects of selegiline are unknown. Plasma concentrations achieved via administration of oral dosage forms in recommended doses confer selective inhibition of MAO type B. When administered transdermally, selegiline achieves higher blood levels with significantly lower exposure for all metabolites when compared with oral dosing. Attention to the dose-dependent nature of selegiline's selectivity is necessary if it is to be used without diet and concomitant drug restrictions.

Pharmacodynamics/Kinetics

Onset of Action Depression: Initial effects may be observed within 1 to 2 weeks of treatment, with continued improvements through 4 to 6 weeks (Papakostas 2006; Posternak 2005; Szegedi 2009).

Half-life Elimination Oral: 10 hours

Pregnancy Risk Factor C

Pregnancy Considerations Adverse events have been observed in some animal reproduction studies. Information related to the use of selegiline in pregnant women for the treatment of depression (Bauer 2017) or Parkinson disease (Seier 2017) is limited.

◆ **Selegiline HCl** *see* Selegiline *on page 1363*

◆ **Selegiline Hydrochloride** *see* Selegiline *on page 1363*

Selexipag (se LEX i pag)

Brand Names: US Uptravi

Brand Names: Canada Uptravi

Pharmacologic Category Prostacyclin; Prostacyclin IP Receptor Agonist; Vasodilator

Use Pulmonary arterial hypertension: Treatment of pulmonary arterial hypertension (PAH) (WHO Group I) to delay disease progression and reduce the risk of hospitalization for PAH.

Local Anesthetic/Vasoconstrictor Precautions No information available to require special precautions

Effects on Dental Treatment Key adverse event(s) related to dental treatment: Jaw pain reported in significant numbers of subjects (26%)

Effects on Bleeding No information available to require special precautions

Adverse Reactions

>10%:

Cardiovascular: Flushing (12%)

Central nervous system: Headache (65%)

Dermatologic: Skin rash (11%)

Gastrointestinal: Diarrhea (42%), nausea (33%), vomiting (18%)

Neuromuscular & skeletal: Jaw pain (26%), limb pain (17%), myalgia (16%), arthralgia (11%)

1% to 10%:

Endocrine & metabolic: Hyperthyroidism (1%)

Gastrointestinal: Decreased appetite (6%)

Hematologic & oncologic: Decreased hemoglobin (below 10 g/dL: 9%), anemia (8%)

<1%, postmarketing, and/or case reports: Symptomatic hypotension

Mechanism of Action Selexipag is a selective prostacyclin IP receptor agonist. Prostacyclin is produced in the endothelial cells and induces vasodilation; also inhibits platelet aggregation. Patients with pulmonary arterial hypertension appear to have a dysregulation in the prostacyclin metabolic pathways (Galie 2013).

Pharmacodynamics/Kinetics

Half-life Elimination Terminal: Selexipag: 0.8 to 2.5 hours; Active metabolite: 6.2 to 13.5 hours

Time to Peak Selexipag: 1 to 3 hours; Active metabolite: 3 to 4 hours; Delayed with food

Pregnancy Considerations Adverse events have not been observed in animal reproduction studies. Women with pulmonary arterial hypertension (PAH) are encouraged to avoid pregnancy (McLaughlin 2009).

◆ **SelG1** *see* Crizanlizumab *on page 414*

Selpercatinib (SEL per KA tih nib)

Brand Names: US Retevmo

Pharmacologic Category Antineoplastic Agent, RET Kinase Inhibitor; Antineoplastic Agent, Tyrosine Kinase Inhibitor

Use

Non-small cell lung cancer, metastatic, RET fusion-positive: Treatment of metastatic RET fusion-positive non-small cell lung cancer (NSCLC) in adults.

Thyroid cancer, medullary, RET-mutant: Treatment of advanced or metastatic RET-mutant medullary thyroid cancer (MTC) in adults and pediatric patients ≥12 years of age who require systemic therapy.

Thyroid cancer, RET fusion-positive: Treatment of advanced or metastatic RET fusion-positive thyroid cancer in adults and pediatric patients ≥12 years of age who require systemic therapy and who are refractory to radioactive iodine (if radioactive iodine is appropriate).

Local Anesthetic/Vasoconstrictor Precautions Hypertension can occur with the use of this drug. Monitor for hypertension prior to using local anesthetic with vasoconstrictor; medical consult if necessary. Selpercatinib is one of the drugs confirmed to prolong the QT interval and is accepted as having a risk of causing torsades de pointes. The risk of drug-induced torsades de pointes is extremely low when a single QT interval prolonging drug is prescribed. In terms of epinephrine, it is not known what effect vasoconstrictors in the local anesthetic regimen will have in patients with a known history of congenital prolonged QT interval or in patients taking any medication that prolongs the QT interval. Until more information is obtained, it is suggested that the clinician consult with the physician prior to the use of a vasoconstrictor in suspected patients and that the vasoconstrictor (epinephrine, mepivacaine, and levonordefrin [Carbocaine 2% with Neo-Cobefrin]) be used with caution.

Effects on Dental Treatment Key adverse event(s) related to dental treatment: Frequent occurrence of xerostomia. Normal salivary flow resumes with drug discontinuance.

Effects on Bleeding Chemotherapy may result in significant myelosuppression including significant reduction in platelet counts (thrombocytopenia 33%; grades 3/4: 3%) and altered hemostasis. In patients undergoing active treatment with selpercatinib, medical consult is suggested.

Adverse Reactions

>10%:

Cardiovascular: Edema (33%), hypertension (35%), prolonged QT interval on ECG (17%)

Dermatologic: Skin rash (27%)

Endocrine & metabolic: Decreased serum albumin (42%), decreased serum calcium (41%), decreased serum glucose (22%), decreased serum magnesium (24%), decreased serum sodium (27%), increased serum cholesterol (31%), increased serum glucose (44%), increased serum potassium (24%)

Gastrointestinal: Abdominal pain (23%), constipation (25%), diarrhea (37%), nausea (23%), vomiting (15%), xerostomia (39%)

Hematologic & oncologic: Hemorrhage (15%; grades 3/4: 2%), leukopenia (43%; grades 3/4: 2%), thrombocytopenia (33%; grades 3/4: 3%)

Hepatic: Increased serum alanine aminotransferase (45%), increased serum alkaline phosphatase (36%), increased serum aspartate aminotransferase (51%), increased serum bilirubin (23%)

Nervous system: Fatigue (35%), headache (23%)

Renal: Increased serum creatinine (37%)

Respiratory: Cough (18%), dyspnea (16%)

1% to 10%:

Endocrine & metabolic: Hypothyroidism (9%)

Hepatic: Severe hepatic disease (3%)

Hypersensitivity: Hypersensitivity reaction (4%)

Respiratory: Pneumonia (≥2%)

Mechanism of Action Selpercatinib is a highly selective anti-RET (REarranged during Transfection) kinase inhibitor (Solomon 2020). Selpercatinib inhibits wild-type RET, multiple mutated RET isoforms, vascular endothelial growth factor receptors 1 and 3 (VEGFR1 and VEGFR3), and fibroblast growth factor receptor (FGFR) 1, 2, and 3. Certain point mutations in RET or chromosomal rearrangements involving in-frame fusions of RET can result in constitutively activated chimeric RET fusion proteins, which may act as oncogenic drivers, promoting tumor cell line proliferation. Selpercatinib has demonstrated anti-tumor activity in cells harboring constitutive activation of RET protein resulting from gene fusions and mutations (including CCDC6-RET, KIF5B-RET, RET V804M, and RET M918T).

Pharmacodynamics/Kinetics

Half-life Elimination 32 hours.

Time to Peak 2 hours.

Reproductive Considerations

Evaluate pregnancy status prior to use in females of reproductive potential.

Females of reproductive potential should use effective contraception during therapy and for at least 1 week after the last selpercatinib dose. Males with female partners of reproductive potential should use effective contraception during therapy and for 1 week after the last selpercatinib dose.

Pregnancy Considerations Based on the mechanism of action and data from animal reproduction studies, in utero exposure to selpercatinib may cause fetal harm.

Selumetinib (SEL ue ME ti nib)

Brand Names: US Koselugo

Pharmacologic Category Antineoplastic Agent, MEK Inhibitor

Use Neurofibromatosis type 1: Treatment of neurofibromatosis type 1 in pediatric patients ≥2 years of age who have symptomatic, inoperable plexiform neurofibromas.

Local Anesthetic/Vasoconstrictor Precautions Hypertension and tachycardia can occur with the use of this drug; monitor for hypertension prior to using local anesthetic with vasoconstrictor; medical consult if necessary.

Effects on Dental Treatment Key adverse event(s) related to dental treatment: Frequent occurrence of stomatitis and xerostomia.

Effects on Bleeding Selumetinib presents a bleeding risk since the selumetinib capsules contain up to 36 mg vitamin E. Vitamin E can inhibit platelet aggregation. Monitor for any unanticipated bleeding with medical consult if necessary.

Adverse Reactions

>10%:

Cardiovascular: Cardiomyopathy (23%), edema (20%), facial edema (<20%), hypertension (<20%), reduced ejection fraction (22%), sinus tachycardia (20%)

Dermatologic: Acneiform eruption (50% to 54%), changes of hair (32%), dermatitis (36%), eczema (28%), maculopapular rash (39%), paronychia (48%), pruritus (46%), skin infection (20%), skin rash (80% to 91%), xeroderma (60%)

Endocrine & metabolic: Decreased serum albumin (51%), decreased serum potassium (18%), decreased serum sodium (16%), increased amylase (18%), increased serum potassium (27%), increased serum sodium (18%), weight gain (<20%)

Gastrointestinal: Abdominal pain (76%), constipation (34%), decreased appetite (22%), diarrhea (70% to 77%; severe diarrhea: 24%), increased serum lipase (32%), nausea (66%), stomatitis (50%), vomiting (82%), xerostomia (<20%)

Genitourinary: Hematuria (22%), proteinuria (22%)

Hematologic & oncologic: Anemia (24%), decreased neutrophils (33%, grades ≥3: 4%), lymphocytopenia (20%, grades ≥3: 2%)

Hepatic: Increased serum alanine aminotransferase (35%), increased serum alkaline phosphatase (18%), increased serum aspartate aminotransferase (41%)

Nervous system: Fatigue (56%), headache (48%)

Neuromuscular & skeletal: Increased creatine phosphokinase in blood specimen (76% to 79%), musculoskeletal pain (58%)

Ophthalmic: Blurred vision (≤15%), cataract (≤15%), ocular hypertension (≤15%), periorbital edema (<20%), photophobia (≤15%), visual impairment (<20%)

Renal: Acute renal failure (<20%)

Respiratory: Dyspnea (<20%), epistaxis (28%), hypoxia (24%)

Miscellaneous: Fever (56%)

Mechanism of Action Selumetinib is a selective mitogen-activated extracellular kinase (MEK) inhibitor which inhibits MEK protein kinases 1 and 2 (Dombi 2016). MEK1/2 proteins are upstream regulators of the extracellular signal-related kinase (ERK) pathway. Both MEK and ERK are critical components of the RAS-regulated RAF-MEK-ERK pathway, which is often activated in different cancer types. In mouse neurofibromatosis type 1 (NF1) models genetically modified to mirror human NF1 genotype and phenotype, selumetinib inhibited ERK phosphorylation, and reduced neurofibroma numbers, volume, and proliferation.

Pharmacodynamics/Kinetics

Half-life Elimination Children ≥2 years and Adolescents: 6.2 hours.

Time to Peak Children ≥2 years and Adolescents: 1 to 1.5 hours.

Reproductive Considerations

Evaluate pregnancy status prior to use in females of reproductive potential.

Females of reproductive potential should use effective contraception during therapy and for 1 week after the last selumetinib dose. Males with female partners of reproductive potential should use effective contraception during therapy and for 1 week after the last dose of selumetinib.

Pregnancy Considerations

Based on the mechanism of action and data from animal reproduction studies, in utero exposure to selumetinib may cause fetal harm.

◆ **Selumetinib Sulfate** *see* Selumetinib *on page 1365*

◆ **Selzentry** *see* Maraviroc *on page 947*

Semaglutide (sem a GLOO tide)

Brand Names: US Ozempic (0.25 or 0.5 MG/DOSE); Ozempic (1 MG/DOSE); Rybelsus

Brand Names: Canada Ozempic (0.25 or 0.5 MG/DOSE); Ozempic (1 MG/DOSE); Rybelsus

Pharmacologic Category Antidiabetic Agent, Glucagon-Like Peptide-1 (GLP-1) Receptor Agonist

Use Diabetes mellitus, type 2, treatment: Glycemic control: As an adjunct to diet and exercise to improve glycemic control in adults with type 2 diabetes mellitus; risk reduction of major cardiovascular events (cardiovascular death, nonfatal myocardial infarction, nonfatal stroke) in adults with type 2 diabetes mellitus and established cardiovascular disease (Ozempic only).

Local Anesthetic/Vasoconstrictor Precautions No information available to require special precautions

Effects on Dental Treatment Key adverse event(s) related to dental treatment: Schedule type 1 and type 2 diabetic patients for dental treatment in the morning in order to minimize chance of stress-induced hypoglycemia.

Effects on Bleeding No information available to require special precautions

Adverse Reactions

>10%:

Endocrine & metabolic: Increased amylase (10% to 13%)

Gastrointestinal: GI adverse effects (32% to 41%), increased serum lipase (oral: 30% to 34%; SubQ: 22%), nausea (11% to 20%), abdominal pain (6% to 11%)

1% to 10%:

Endocrine & metabolic: Hypoglycemia (2% to 4%), severe hypoglycemia (oral: 1%)

Gastrointestinal: Diarrhea (9% to 10%), decreased appetite (oral: 6% to 9%), vomiting (5% to 9%), constipation (3% to 6%), dyspepsia (3% to 4%), eructation (≤3%), abdominal distension (oral: 2% to 3%), flatulence (1% to 2%), gastritis (oral: 2%), gastroesophageal reflux disease (2%), cholelithiasis (≤2%)

Immunologic: Antibody development (≤1%)

<1%: Acute pancreatitis, discomfort at injection site, dizziness, dysgeusia, erythema at injection site, fatigue

Frequency not defined:

Cardiovascular: Increased heart rate

Hypersensitivity: Anaphylaxis, angioedema, hypersensitivity reaction

Postmarketing: Acute renal failure, chronic renal failure

Mechanism of Action Semaglutide is selective glucagon-like peptide-1 (GLP-1) receptor agonist. Acting on the same receptor as the endogenous hormone incretin, semaglutide increases glucose-dependent insulin secretion, decreases inappropriate glucagon secretion, and slows gastric emptying. Increases first- and second-phase insulin secretion.

Pharmacodynamics/Kinetics

Half-life Elimination ~1 week

Time to Peak Plasma: Oral: 1 hour; SubQ: 1 to 3 days

Reproductive Considerations

In females of reproductive potential, semaglutide should be discontinued for ≥2 months prior to a planned pregnancy.

Pregnancy Considerations

Poorly controlled diabetes during pregnancy can be associated with an increased risk of adverse maternal and fetal outcomes, including diabetic ketoacidosis, preeclampsia, spontaneous abortion, preterm delivery, delivery complications, major birth defects, stillbirth, and macrosomia (ACOG 201 2018). To prevent adverse outcomes, prior to conception and throughout pregnancy, maternal blood glucose and HbA_{1c} should be kept as close to target goals as possible but without causing significant hypoglycemia (ADA 2020; Blumer 2013).

Agents other than semaglutide are currently recommended to treat diabetes mellitus in pregnancy (ADA 2020).

◆ **Sensodyne Repair** & **Protect [OTC]** *see* Fluoride *on page 693*

◆ **Sensorcaine** *see* Bupivacaine *on page 256*

◆ **Sensorcaine/EPINEPHrine** *see* Bupivacaine and Epinephrine *on page 257*

◆ **Sensorcaine-MPF** *see* Bupivacaine *on page 256*

◆ **Sensorcaine-MPF/EPINEPHrine** *see* Bupivacaine and Epinephrine *on page 257*

◆ **Sensorcaine-MPF Spinal [DSC]** *see* Bupivacaine *on page 256*

◆ **Septocaine with Epinephrine 1:100,000** *see* Articaine and Epinephrine *on page 170*

◆ **Septocaine with Epinephrine 1:200,000** *see* Articaine and Epinephrine *on page 170*

◆ **Septra** *see* Sulfamethoxazole and Trimethoprim *on page 1391*

◆ **Serax** *see* Oxazepam *on page 1153*

◆ **Serevent Diskus** *see* Salmeterol *on page 1355*

◆ **Sernivo** *see* Betamethasone (Topical) *on page 237*

◆ **SEROquel** *see* QUEtiapine *on page 1296*

◆ **SEROquel XR** *see* QUEtiapine *on page 1296*

◆ **Serostim** *see* Somatropin *on page 1381*

Sertaconazole (ser ta KOE na zole)

Brand Names: US Ertaczo

Pharmacologic Category Antifungal Agent, Imidazole Derivative; Antifungal Agent, Topical

Use Tinea pedis: Topical treatment of interdigital tinea pedis in immunocompetent patients 12 years of age and older, caused by *Trichophyton rubrum*, *Trichophyton mentagrophytes*, and *Epidermophyton floccosum*.

Local Anesthetic/Vasoconstrictor Precautions No information available to require special precautions

Effects on Dental Treatment No significant effects or complications reported

Effects on Bleeding No information available to require special precautions

Adverse Reactions

1% to 10%: Dermatologic: Burning sensation of skin, contact dermatitis, skin tenderness, xeroderma

<1%, postmarketing and/or case reports: Desquamation, erythema, hyperpigmentation, pruritus, skin vesicle

Mechanism of Action Alters fungal cell wall membrane permeability; inhibits the CYP450-dependent synthesis of ergosterol

Pregnancy Risk Factor C

Pregnancy Considerations Adverse events were not observed in animal reproduction studies following oral administration.

◆ **Sertaconazole Nitrate** *see* Sertaconazole *on page 1367*

Sertraline (SER tra leen)

Related Information

Management of the Patient With Anxiety or Depression *on page 1778*

Vasoconstrictor Interactions With Antidepressants *on page 1821*

Brand Names: US Zoloft

Brand Names: Canada ACT Sertraline [DSC]; AG-Sertraline; APO-Sertraline; Auro-Sertraline; BIO-Sertraline; DOM-Sertraline; JAMP-Sertraline; Mar-Sertraline; MINT-Sertraline; MYLAN-Sertraline [DSC]; NRA-Sertraline; PMS-Sertraline; Priva-Sertraline; RAN-Sertraline; RIVA-Sertraline; SANDOZ Sertraline; TEVA-Sertraline; VAN-Sertraline [DSC]; Zoloft

Pharmacologic Category Antidepressant, Selective Serotonin Reuptake Inhibitor

Use

Major depressive disorder (unipolar): Treatment of unipolar major depressive disorder (MDD) in adults.

Obsessive-compulsive disorder: Treatment of obsessions and compulsions in patients with obsessive-compulsive disorder (OCD).

Panic disorder: Treatment of panic disorder in adults with or without agoraphobia.

Posttraumatic stress disorder: Treatment of posttraumatic stress disorder (PTSD) in adults.

Premenstrual dysphoric disorder: Treatment of premenstrual dysphoric disorder (PMDD) in adults.

Social anxiety disorder: Treatment of social anxiety disorder (social phobia) in adults.

Local Anesthetic/Vasoconstrictor Precautions Although caution should be used in patients taking tricyclic antidepressants, no interactions have been reported with vasoconstrictor and sertraline, a nontricyclic antidepressant which acts to increase serotonin; no precautions appear to be needed

Effects on Dental Treatment Key adverse event(s) related to dental treatment: Xerostomia (normal salivary flow resumes upon discontinuation) (see Effects on Bleeding and Dental Health Professional Considerations).

Effects on Bleeding May impair platelet aggregation resulting in increased risk of bleeding events, particularly if used concomitantly with aspirin, NSAIDs, warfarin, or other anticoagulants. Bleeding related to SSRI use has been reported to range from relatively minor bruising and epistaxis to life-threatening hemorrhage. Routine interruption of therapy for most dental procedures is not warranted. In medically complicated patients or extensive oral surgery, the decision to interrupt therapy must be based on the risk to benefit in an individual patient and a medical consult is suggested. If therapy is continued without interruption, the clinician should anticipate the potential for a prolonged bleeding time.

Adverse Reactions

>10%:

Gastrointestinal: Diarrhea (20%), nausea (26%), xerostomia (14%)

Nervous system: Dizziness (12%), drowsiness (adults: 11%; literature suggests incidence occurs less frequently in children and adolescents compared to adults [Safer 2006]), fatigue (12%), insomnia (20%)

1% to 10%:

Cardiovascular: Edema (<2%), hypertension (<2%), palpitations (4%), syncope (<2%), tachycardia (<2%), vasodilation (<2%)

Dermatologic: Alopecia (<2%), bullous dermatitis (<2%), dermatitis (<2%), diaphoresis (<2%), erythematous rash (<2%), follicular rash (<2%), hyperhidrosis (7%), maculopapular rash (<2%), pruritus (<2%), urticaria (<2%)

Endocrine & metabolic: Decreased libido (4% to 7% [placebo: 2%]), diabetes mellitus (<2%), galactorrhea not associated with childbirth (<2%), hypercholesterolemia (<2%), hypoglycemia (<2%), hypothyroidism (<2%), weight loss (>7% of body weight; children: 7%; adolescents: 2%)

Gastrointestinal: Abdominal pain (≥5%), bruxism (<2%), constipation (6%), decreased appetite (7%), dyspepsia (8%), hematochezia (<2%), increased appetite (<2%), melena (<2%), vomiting (adults: 4%; literature suggests incidence is higher in adolescents compared to adults, and is two- to threefold higher in children compared to adults [Safer 2006])

Genitourinary: Ejaculation failure (8% [placebo: 1%]), ejaculatory disorder (3% [placebo: 0%]), erectile dysfunction (4% [placebo: 1%]), hematuria (<2%), priapism (<2%), sexual disorder (males: 2% [placebo: 0%]), urinary incontinence (≥2%), vaginal hemorrhage (<2%)

Hematologic & oncologic: Hemorrhage (<2%), rectal hemorrhage (<2%)

Hepatic: Increased liver enzymes (<2%)

Hypersensitivity: Anaphylaxis (<2%)

Nervous system: Abnormal gait (<2%), agitation (8%), anxiety (children and adolescents: ≥2%), ataxia (<2%), coma (<2%), confusion (<2%), euphoria (<2%), hallucination (<2%), hypertonia (<2%), hypoesthesia (<2%), impaired consciousness (<2%), irritability (<2%), lethargy (<2%), malaise (≥5%), psychomotor agitation (<2%), seizure (<2%), yawning (<2%)

Neuromuscular & skeletal: Hyperkinetic muscle activity (children and adolescents: ≥2%), muscle spasm (<2%), tremor (9%)

Ophthalmic: Blurred vision (<2%), mydriasis (<2%), visual disturbance (4%)

Otic: Tinnitus (<2%)

Respiratory: Bronchospasm (<2%)

Frequency not defined:

Nervous system: Aggressive behavior

Neuromuscular & skeletal: Arthralgia, muscle twitching

Respiratory: Epistaxis

Miscellaneous: Fever

Postmarketing:

Cardiovascular: Atrial arrhythmia, atrioventricular block, bradycardia, prolonged QT interval on ECG (Beach 2014; Funk 2013), torsades de pointes (Danielsson 2015), vasculitis, ventricular tachycardia (Patel 2013)

Dermatologic: Erythema multiforme (Khan 2012), skin photosensitivity, Stevens-Johnson syndrome (Jan 1999), toxic epidermal necrolysis

Endocrine & metabolic: Gynecomastia (Kaufman 2013), hyperglycemia (Khoza 2011), hyperprolactinemia, hyponatremia (Pinon 2017), menstrual disease, secondary amenorrhea (Ekinci 2019), SIADH (Jacob 2006), weight gain (slight increase, primarily in adults with long-term therapy) (Fava 2000)

Gastrointestinal: Pancreatitis (Malbergier 2004)

Genitourinary: Decreased penile sensation (Bolton 2006), orgasm disturbance (Jing 2016)

Hematologic & oncologic: Agranulocytosis (Trescoli-Serrano 1996), aplastic anemia, coagulation time increased (altered platelet function) (Apseleoff 1997), immune thrombocytopenia (Krivy 1995), leukopenia, pancytopenia, neutropenia (Ozcanli 2005), purpuric disease (periorbital) (Kayhan 2015)

Hepatic: Hepatic failure, hepatitis (Persky 2003), hepatotoxicity (Persky 2003), jaundice (Verrico 2000)

Hypersensitivity: Angioedema (Gales 1994), hypersensitivity reaction (Dadic-Hero 2011), serum sickness

Nervous system: Akathisia (Madusoodanan 2010), dystonia (Madusoodanan 2010), hyperactive behavior (agitation, hyperactivation, hyperkinesis, restlessness occurring in children at a two- to threefold higher incidence compared to adolescents [Safer 2006]), hypomania (Kumar 2000), intracranial hemorrhage (Douros 2018), mania (Ghaziuddin 1994), neuroleptic malignant syndrome (Stevens 2008), nightmares, psychosis (Popli 1997), reversible cerebral vasoconstriction syndrome (Bain 2013), serotonin syndrome (Duignan 2019), suicidal ideation (children and adolescents) (Hammad 2006), suicidal tendencies (children and adolescents) (Hammad 2006), trismus (Holmberg 2018), withdrawal syndrome (Fava 2015)

Neuromuscular & skeletal: Bone fracture (Rabenda 2013), lupus-like syndrome (Hussain 2008), rhabdomyolysis (Gareri 2009)

Ophthalmic: Acute angle-closure glaucoma (Kirkam 2016), blindness, cataract (Erie 2014), maculopathy (Dang 2016), oculogyric crisis, optic neuritis

Renal: Acute renal failure

Respiratory: Hypersensitivity pneumonitis (Virdee 2019), pulmonary hypertension

Mechanism of Action Antidepressant with selective inhibitory effects on presynaptic serotonin (5-HT) reuptake and only very weak effects on norepinephrine and dopamine neuronal uptake. In vitro studies demonstrate no significant affinity for adrenergic, cholinergic, GABA, dopaminergic, histaminergic, serotonergic, or benzodiazepine receptors.

Pharmacodynamics/Kinetics

Onset of Action

Anxiety disorders (generalized anxiety, obsessive-compulsive, panic, and posttraumatic stress disorder): Initial effects may be observed within 2 weeks of treatment, with continued improvements through 4 to 6 weeks (Issari 2016; Varigonda 2016; WFSBP [Bandelow 2012]); some experts suggest up to 12 weeks of treatment may be necessary for response, particularly in patients with obsessive-compulsive disorder and posttraumatic stress disorder (BAP [Baldwin 2014]; Katzman 2014; WFSBP [Bandelow 2012]).

Body dysmorphic disorder: Initial effects may be observed within 2 weeks; some experts suggest up to 12 to 16 weeks of treatment may be necessary for response in some patients (Phillips 2008).

Depression: Initial effects may be observed within 1 to 2 weeks of treatment, with continued improvements through 4 to 6 weeks (Papakostas 2006; Posternak 2005; Szegedi 2009; Taylor 2006).

Premenstrual dysphoric disorder: Initial effects may be observed within the first few days of treatment, with response at the first menstrual cycle of treatment (ISPMD [Nevatte 2013]).

Half-life Elimination

Sertraline: Mean: 26 hours; N-desmethylsertraline: 62 to 104 hours

Children 6 to 12 years: Mean: 26.2 hours (Alderman 1998)

Children 13 to 17 years: Mean: 27.8 hours (Alderman 1998)

Adults 18 to 45 years: Mean: 27.2 hours (Alderman 1998)

Time to Peak Plasma: Sertraline: 4.5 to 8.4 hours

Pregnancy Considerations Sertraline crosses the human placenta.

Available studies evaluating teratogenic effects following maternal use of sertraline in the first trimester have not shown an overall increased risk of major birth defects. Studies evaluating specific birth defects have provided inconsistent results. Nonteratogenic effects in the newborn following SSRI/SNRI exposure late in the third trimester include respiratory distress, cyanosis, apnea, seizures, temperature instability, feeding difficulty, vomiting, hypoglycemia, hypo- or hypertonia, hyper-reflexia, jitteriness, irritability, constant crying, and tremor. Symptoms may be due to the toxicity of the SSRIs/SNRIs or a discontinuation syndrome and may be consistent with serotonin syndrome associated with SSRI treatment. Persistent pulmonary hypertension of the newborn (PPHN) has also been reported with SSRI exposure. The long-term effects of in utero SSRI exposure on infant development and behavior are not known.

Due to pregnancy-induced physiologic changes, women who are pregnant may require adjusted doses of sertraline to achieve euthymia. The ACOG recommends that therapy with SSRIs or SNRIs during pregnancy be individualized; treatment of depression during pregnancy should incorporate the clinical expertise of the mental health clinician, obstetrician, primary health care provider, and pediatrician. According to the American Psychiatric Association (APA), the risks of medication treatment should be weighed against other treatment options and untreated depression. For women who discontinue antidepressant medications during pregnancy and who may be at high risk for postpartum depression, the medications can be restarted following delivery. Treatment algorithms have been developed by the ACOG and the APA for the management of depression in women prior to conception and during pregnancy (ACOG 2008; APA 2010; Yonkers 2009).

Pregnant women exposed to antidepressants during pregnancy are encouraged to enroll in the National Pregnancy Registry for Antidepressants (NPRAD). Women 18 to 45 years of age or their health care providers may contact the registry by calling 844-405-6185. Enrollment should be done as early in pregnancy as possible.

Dental Health Professional Considerations Problems with SSRI-induced bruxism have been reported and may preclude their use; clinicians attempting to evaluate any patient with bruxism or involuntary muscle movement, who is simultaneously being treated with an SSRI drug, should be aware of the potential association.

- ◆ **Sertraline HCl** *see* Sertraline *on page 1367*
- ◆ **Sertraline Hydrochloride** *see* Sertraline *on page 1367*
- ◆ **Serzone** *see* Nefazodone *on page 1090*
- ◆ **Setlakin** *see* Ethinyl Estradiol and Levonorgestrel *on page 612*
- ◆ **Seysara** *see* Sarecycline *on page 1358*
- ◆ **SfRowasa** *see* Mesalamine *on page 980*
- ◆ **S/GSK1349572** *see* Dolutegravir *on page 511*
- ◆ **Sharobel** *see* Norethindrone *on page 1117*
- ◆ **Shingles Vaccine** *see* Zoster Vaccine (Live/Attenuated) *on page 1585*
- ◆ **Shingles Vaccine** *see* Zoster Vaccine (Recombinant) *on page 1586*
- ◆ **Shingrix** *see* Zoster Vaccine (Recombinant) *on page 1586*
- ◆ **Shopko Athletes Foot [OTC]** *see* Clotrimazole (Topical) *on page 397*
- ◆ **Shopko Nasal Decongestant [OTC]** *see* Pseudoephedrine *on page 1291*
- ◆ **Shopko Nasal Decongestant Max [OTC]** *see* Pseudoephedrine *on page 1291*
- ◆ **Sila III** *see* Triamcinolone (Topical) *on page 1490*
- ◆ **Silace [OTC]** *see* Docusate *on page 509*
- ◆ **Siladryl Allergy [OTC]** *see* DiphenhydrAMINE (Systemic) *on page 502*
- ◆ **SilaLite Pak [DSC]** *see* Triamcinolone (Topical) *on page 1490*
- ◆ **Silapap Children's [OTC]** *see* Acetaminophen *on page 59*

Sildenafil (sil DEN a fil)

Brand Names: US Revatio; Viagra

Brand Names: Canada ACCEL-Sildenafil; ACT Sildenafil [DSC]; AG-Sildenafil; APO-Sildenafil; APO-Sildenafil R; AURO-Sildenafil; BIO-Sildenafil; GD-Sildenafil [DSC]; JAMP-Sildenafil; M-Sildenafil; Mar-Sildenafil; MINT-Sildenafil; MYL-Sildenafil [DSC]; NRA-Sildenafil; PMS-Sildenafil; PMS-Sildenafil R; Priva-Sildenafil; PRZ-Sildenafil; RAN-Sildenafil; Revatio; RIVA-Sildenafil; SANDOZ Sildenafil [DSC]; TEVA-Sildenafil; TEVA-Sildenafil R; VAN-Sildenafil [DSC]; Viagra

Pharmacologic Category Phosphodiesterase-5 Enzyme Inhibitor

Use

Erectile dysfunction: Viagra: Treatment of erectile dysfunction.

Pulmonary arterial hypertension: Revatio: Treatment of pulmonary arterial hypertension (WHO group I) in adults to improve exercise ability and delay clinical worsening; efficacy established predominately in patients with NYHA functional class II and III symptoms.

Local Anesthetic/Vasoconstrictor Precautions No information available to require special precautions

Effects on Dental Treatment Key adverse event(s) related to dental treatment: Occurrence of stomatitis has been reported. Rare occurrence of gingivitis, glossitis, stomatitis, xerostomia (normal salivary flow resumes upon discontinuation), and orthostatic hypotension have also been reported; use caution with sudden changes in position during and after dental treatment.

Effects on Bleeding No information available to require special precautions

Adverse Reactions Based upon normal doses for either indication or route. (Adverse effects such as flushing, diarrhea, myalgia, and visual disturbances may be increased with adult doses >100 mg/24 hours.)

>10%:

Cardiovascular: Flushing (10% to 19%)

Central nervous system: Headache (16% to 46%)

Gastrointestinal: Dyspepsia (3% to 17%; dose-related)

Ophthalmic: Visual disturbance (2% to 11%; including vision color changes, blurred vision, and photophobia; dose-related)

Respiratory: Epistaxis (9% to 13%)

2% to 10%:

Central nervous system: Insomnia (≤7%), dizziness (2% to 4%), paresthesia (≤3%)

Dermatologic: Erythema (6%), skin rash (1% to 3%)

Gastrointestinal: Diarrhea (3% to 9%), gastritis (≤3%), nausea (2% to 3%)

Genitourinary: Urinary tract infection (3%)

Hepatic: Increased liver enzymes (2% to 10%)

Neuromuscular & skeletal: Myalgia (2% to 7%), back pain (3% to 4%)

Respiratory: Nasal congestion (4% to 9%), exacerbation of dyspnea (≤7%), nasal congestion (4%), rhinitis (4%), sinusitis (3%)

Miscellaneous: Fever (6%)

<2%, postmarketing, and/or case reports (limited to important or life-threatening): Abdominal pain, abnormal dreams, abnormal hepatic function tests, absent reflexes, accidental injury, amnesia (transient global), anemia, angina pectoris, anorgasmia, anterior chamber eye hemorrhage, anterior ischemic optic neuropathy, anxiety, arthritis, asthma, ataxia, atrioventricular block, auditory impairment, basal cell carcinoma (Loeb ▶

2015), bone pain, breast hypertrophy, bronchitis, burning sensation of eyes, cardiac arrest, cardiac failure, cardiomyopathy, cataract, cerebral hemorrhage, cerebral thrombosis, cerebrovascular hemorrhage, chest pain, chills, colitis, conjunctivitis, contact dermatitis, cystitis, depression, dermal ulcer, diaphoresis, diplopia, drowsiness, dry eye syndrome, dysphagia, ECG abnormality, edema, ejaculatory disorder, esophagitis, exfoliative dermatitis, eye pain, eye redness, facial edema, falling, gastroenteritis, genital edema, gingivitis, glossitis, gout, hearing loss, hematuria, hemorrhage, herpes simplex infection, hyperglycemia, hypernatremia, hypersensitivity reaction, hypertension, hypertonia, hyperuricemia, hypoesthesia, hypoglycemia, hypotension, increased bronchial secretions, increased cough, increased intraocular pressure, increased thirst, ischemic heart disease, leukopenia, laryngitis, malignant melanoma (Li 2014; Loeb 2015), migraine, myasthenia, mydriasis, myocardial infarction, neuralgia, neuropathy, nocturia, orthostatic hypotension, ostealgia, osteoarthritis, otalgia, pain, palpitations, peripheral edema, pharyngitis, photophobia, priapism, prolonged erection, pruritus, pulmonary hemorrhage, rectal hemorrhage, retinal edema, retinal hemorrhage, retinal vascular disease, rupture of tendon, seizure, severe sickle cell crisis (vaso-occlusive crisis in patients with pulmonary hypertension associated with sickle cell disease), shock, skin photosensitivity, stomatitis, subarachnoid hemorrhage, swelling of eye, syncope, synovitis, tachycardia, temporary vision loss, tenosynovitis, tinnitus, transient ischemic attacks, tremor, unstable diabetes, urinary frequency, urinary incontinence, urticaria, ventricular arrhythmia, vertigo, visual field loss, vitreous detachment, vitreous traction, vomiting, weakness, xerostomia

Mechanism of Action

Erectile dysfunction: Does not directly cause penile erections but affects the response to sexual stimulation. The physiologic mechanism of erection of the penis involves release of nitric oxide (NO) in the corpus cavernosum during sexual stimulation. NO then activates the enzyme guanylate cyclase, which results in increased levels of cyclic guanosine monophosphate (cGMP), producing smooth muscle relaxation and inflow of blood to the corpus cavernosum. Sildenafil enhances the effect of NO by inhibiting phosphodiesterase type 5 (PDE-5), which is responsible for degradation of cGMP in the corpus cavernosum; when sexual stimulation causes local release of NO, inhibition of PDE-5 by sildenafil causes increased levels of cGMP in the corpus cavernosum, resulting in smooth muscle relaxation and inflow of blood to the corpus cavernosum; at recommended doses, it has no effect in the absence of sexual stimulation.

Pulmonary arterial hypertension (PAH): Inhibits phosphodiesterase type 5 (PDE-5) in smooth muscle of pulmonary vasculature where PDE-5 is responsible for the degradation of cyclic guanosine monophosphate (cGMP). Increased cGMP concentration results in pulmonary vasculature relaxation; vasodilation in the pulmonary bed and the systemic circulation (to a lesser degree) may occur.

Pharmacodynamics/Kinetics

Onset of Action Onset: Erectile dysfunction: ~60 minutes; Peak effect: Decrease blood pressure: Oral: 1 to 2 hours

Duration of Action Erectile dysfunction: 2 to 4 hours; Decrease blood pressure: <8 hours

Half-life Elimination

Sildenafil: Terminal:

Neonates: PNA 1 day: 55.9 hours (Mukherjee 2009)
Neonates: PNA 7 days: 47.7 hours (Mukherjee 2009)
Adults: 4 hours

Active N-desmethyl metabolite: Terminal:

Neonates: 11.9 hours (Mukherjee 2009)
Adults: 4 hours

Time to Peak Oral: Fasting: 30 to 120 minutes (median 60 minutes); delayed by 60 minutes with a high-fat meal

Pregnancy Considerations

Sildenafil was shown to cross the placenta in an ex vivo placenta perfusion study (Russo 2018).

Because sildenafil causes vasodilation in the uterus, it is currently under study for various obstetric uses (Dunn 2016; Dunn 2017; Groom 2019; Maged 2018; Maher 2019; Pels 2017; Sharp 2018). However, due to adverse events in the newborn observed using preliminary data from a study evaluating sildenafil for fetal growth restriction, use of sildenafil in pregnant women outside of a controlled clinical study is not currently recommended (Groom 2018; Levin 2019).

Information related to the use of sildenafil for the treatment of pulmonary arterial hypertension (PAH) in pregnant women is limited (Cartago 2014; Hsu 2011; Lim 2019; Wollein 2016). Untreated PAH in pregnancy increases the risk for heart failure, stroke, preterm delivery, and maternal/fetal death. Women with PAH are encouraged to avoid pregnancy (McLaughlin 2009; Taichman 2014).

◆ **Sildenafil Citrate** *see* Sildenafil *on page* 1369

◆ **Silenor** *see* Doxepin (Systemic) *on page* 518

Silodosin (SI lo doe sin)

Brand Names: US Rapaflo

Brand Names: Canada Rapaflo

Pharmacologic Category Alpha$_1$ Blocker

Use Treatment of signs and symptoms of benign prostatic hyperplasia (BPH)

Local Anesthetic/Vasoconstrictor Precautions
No information available to require special precautions

Effects on Dental Treatment Key adverse event(s) related to dental treatment: Dizziness; nasal congestion or rhinitis; Patients may experience orthostatic hypotension as they stand up after treatment; especially if lying in dental chair for extended periods of time. Use caution with sudden changes in position during and after dental treatment.

Effects on Bleeding No information available to require special precautions

Adverse Reactions

>10%: Genitourinary: Retrograde ejaculation (28%)

1% to 10%:

Cardiovascular: Orthostatic hypotension (3%; increased in elderly ≥65 years up to 5%)

Central nervous system: Dizziness (3%), headache (2%), insomnia (1% to 2%)

Gastrointestinal: Diarrhea (3%), abdominal pain (1% to 2%)

Genitourinary: Prostate specific antigen increased (1% to 2%)

Neuromuscular & skeletal: Weakness (1% to 2%)

Respiratory: Nasal congestion (2%), rhinorrhea (1% to 2%), sinusitis (1% to 2%)

<1%, postmarketing, and/or case reports: Hepatic insufficiency, hypersensitivity reaction, increased serum transaminases, intraoperative floppy iris syndrome, jaundice, pharyngeal edema, priapism, pruritus, purpura, skin rash (including toxic), swollen tongue, syncope, urticaria

Mechanism of Action Silodosin is a selective antagonist of alpha$_{1A}$-adrenoreceptors in the prostate and bladder. Smooth muscle tone in the prostate is mediated by alpha$_{1A}$-adrenoreceptors; blocking them leads to relaxation of smooth muscle in the bladder neck and prostate causing an improvement of urine flow and decreased symptoms of BPH. Approximately 75% of the alpha1-receptors in the prostate are of the alpha$_{1A}$ subtype.

Pharmacodynamics/Kinetics

Half-life Elimination Healthy volunteers: Silodosin: ~13 hours (mean); KMD-3213G: ~24 hours

Time to Peak Silodosin: ~3 hours; KMD-3213G: ~5.5 hours (Lepor 2010)

Pregnancy Risk Factor B

Pregnancy Considerations Teratogenic effects were not observed in animal studies; however, silodosin is not approved for use in women.

- **Silphen Cough [OTC] [DSC]** *see* DiphenhydrAMINE (Systemic) *on page 502*
- **Silphen DM Cough [OTC]** *see* Dextromethorphan *on page 476*

Siltuximab (sil TUX i mab)

Brand Names: US Sylvant

Brand Names: Canada Sylvant

Pharmacologic Category Antineoplastic Agent, Monoclonal Antibody; Interleukin-6 Inhibitor

Use Castleman disease: Treatment of multicentric Castleman disease (MCD) in patients who are human immunodeficiency virus (HIV) negative and human herpesvirus-8 (HHV-8) negative

Limitations of use: Siltuximab has not been studied in patients with MCD who are HIV positive or HHV-8 positive because in a nonclinical study, siltuximab did not bind to virally produced IL-6

Local Anesthetic/Vasoconstrictor Precautions
No information available to require special precautions

Effects on Dental Treatment Key adverse event(s) related to dental treatment: Oropharyngeal pain and hypotension have been reported; Patients may experience orthostatic hypotension as they stand up after treatment; especially if lying in dental chair for extended periods of time. Use caution with sudden changes in position during and after dental treatment.

Effects on Bleeding No information available to require special precautions

Adverse Reactions

>10%:

Cardiovascular: Edema (≤26%)
Dermatologic: Pruritus (28%), skin rash (28%)
Endocrine & metabolic: Weight gain (19%), hyperuricemia (11%)
Local: Localized edema (≤26%)
Respiratory: Upper respiratory tract infection (26%)

1% to 10%:

Cardiovascular: Hypotension (4%)
Central nervous system: Headache (8%)
Dermatologic: Eczema (4%), psoriasis (4%), skin hyperpigmentation (4%), xeroderma (4%)
Endocrine & metabolic: Hypertriglyceridemia (8%), hypercholesterolemia (4%)
Gastrointestinal: Constipation (8%)
Hematologic & oncologic: Thrombocytopenia (9%)
Hypersensitivity: Hypersensitivity reaction (≤6.3%)
Immunologic: Antibody development (2%, non-neutralizing)
Renal: Renal insufficiency (8%)
Respiratory: Lower respiratory tract infection (8%), oropharyngeal pain (8%)
Miscellaneous: Infusion related reaction (≤6.3%)

Frequency not defined:

Cardiovascular: Hypertension
Central nervous system: Dizziness
Gastrointestinal: Abdominal pain, diarrhea, gastroesophageal reflux disease, nausea, oral mucosa ulcer, vomiting
Genitourinary: Urinary tract infection
Hematologic & oncologic: Neutropenia
Respiratory: Nasopharyngitis

<1%: Anaphylaxis

Mechanism of Action Chimeric monoclonal antibody which binds with high affinity and specificity to IL-6; prevents IL-6 from binding to both soluble and membrane-bound IL-6 receptors. Overproduction of IL-6 may lead to systemic manifestations in multicentric Castleman disease (MCD) patients by inducing C-reactive protein (CRP) synthesis (Kurzrock 2013). Lowering serum IL-6 levels may improve systemic symptoms of Castleman disease.

Pharmacodynamics/Kinetics

Onset of Action Response is usually evident after 3 to 4 doses; lymphadenopathy resolves at a median of 5 months (van Rhee 2018)

Half-life Elimination ~21 days (range: 14.2 to 29.7 days)

Reproductive Considerations
Females of reproductive potential should use effective contraception during treatment and for 3 months after the last dose of siltuximab.

Pregnancy Considerations
Siltuximab is a humanized monoclonal antibody; monoclonal antibodies are expected to cross the placenta, generally increasing as pregnancy progresses. Infants born to pregnant females treated with siltuximab may be at increased risk for infection.

Silver Nitrate (SIL ver NYE trate)

Pharmacologic Category Antibiotic, Topical; Cauterizing Agent, Topical; Topical Skin Product, Antibacterial

Use Astringent, cauterization of wounds, germicidal, removal of granulation tissue, corns, and warts

Local Anesthetic/Vasoconstrictor Precautions
No information available to require special precautions

Effects on Dental Treatment No significant effects or complications reported

Effects on Bleeding No information available to require special precautions

Adverse Reactions Frequency not defined.

Dermatologic: Burning sensation of skin, skin discoloration, skin irritation
Hematologic & oncologic: Methemoglobinemia

Mechanism of Action Free silver ions precipitate bacterial proteins by combining with chloride in tissue forming silver chloride; coagulates cellular protein to form an eschar; silver ions or salts or colloidal silver preparations can inhibit the growth of both gram-positive and gram-negative bacteria. This germicidal action is attributed to the precipitation of bacterial proteins by liberated silver ions. Silver nitrate coagulates cellular protein to form an eschar, and this mode of action is the postulated mechanism for control of benign hematuria, rhinitis, and recurrent pneumothorax.

Simeprevir (sim E pre vir)

Related Information

Systemic Viral Diseases *on page 1709*

Brand Names: US Olysio [DSC]

Brand Names: Canada Galexos [DSC]

Pharmacologic Category Antihepaciviral, NS3/4A Protease Inhibitor (Anti-HCV); NS3/4A Inhibitor

Use

Chronic hepatitis C: Treatment of genotype 1 chronic hepatitis C in combination with sofosbuvir in adults without cirrhosis

Limitations of use: Not recommended for use in patients who have previously failed a simeprevir-containing regimen or another regimen containing HCV protease inhibitors.

Local Anesthetic/Vasoconstrictor Precautions No information available to require special precautions

Effects on Dental Treatment No significant effects or complications reported

Effects on Bleeding No information available to require special precautions

Adverse Reactions Percentages reported for combination therapy with peginterferon alfa and ribavirin (Peg-IFN-alfa and RBV) unless otherwise noted.

>10%:

Central nervous system: Headache (with sofosbuvir 7% to 49%), fatigue (with sofosbuvir 10% to 47%), insomnia (with sofosbuvir 14%), dizziness (with sofosbuvir 5% to 10%)

Dermatologic: Skin photosensitivity (with sofosbuvir ≤5% to ≤34%; grade 3: ≤1%; with Peg-IFN-alfa and RBV ≤28%; grade 3: <1%), skin rash (with sofosbuvir ≤5% to ≤34%; grade 3: ≤1%; with Peg-IFN-alfa and RBV ≤28%; including erythema, eczema, maculopapular rash, urticaria, toxic skin eruption, dermatitis exfoliative, cutaneous vasculitis; grade 3: ≤1%), pruritus (with Peg-IFN-alfa and RBV 22%; with sofosbuvir 11%)

Endocrine & metabolic: Increased amylase (with sofosbuvir)

Gastrointestinal: Nausea (with sofosbuvir 4% to 40%; with Peg-IFN-alfa and RBV 22%), diarrhea (with sofosbuvir 5% to 18%)

Hepatic: Increased serum bilirubin (<66%), hyperbilirubinemia (with sofosbuvir)

Neuromuscular & skeletal: Myalgia (16%)

Respiratory: Dyspnea (12%)

1% to 10%:

Gastrointestinal: Increased serum lipase (with sofosbuvir)

Hepatic: Increased serum alkaline phosphatase

<1%, postmarketing, and/or case reports: Hepatic failure, liver decompensation, reactivation of HBV (FDA Safety Alert Dec. 8, 2016)

Mechanism of Action Simeprevir is an inhibitor of HCV NS3/4A protease, a protease that is essential for viral replication. It is considered a direct-acting antiviral treatment for HCV, also called a specifically targeted antiviral therapy for HCV (STAT-C).

Pharmacodynamics/Kinetics

Half-life Elimination Plasma: 10 to 13 hours (healthy volunteers); 41 hours (HCV-infected patients)

Time to Peak Serum: 4 to 6 hours

Reproductive Considerations

HCV-infected females of childbearing potential should consider postponing pregnancy until therapy is complete to reduce the risk of HCV transmission (AASLD/IDSA 2018).

Simeprevir is not used as monotherapy; when used in combination with ribavirin, all warnings related to the use of ribavirin and contraception should be followed. Also refer to the ribavirin monograph for additional information.

Pregnancy Considerations

Simeprevir is not used as monotherapy; combination therapy with ribavirin is contraindicated in pregnant females and males whose female partners are pregnant. If used in combination with ribavirin, all warnings related to the use of ribavirin and pregnancy should be followed. Also refer to the ribavirin monograph for additional information.

Treatment of hepatitis C is not currently recommended to treat maternal infection or to decrease the risk of mother-to-child transmission during pregnancy (Tran 2016). When HCV infection is detected during pregnancy, treatment should be deferred until after delivery. Direct-acting antiviral medications should not be used in pregnant females outside of clinical trials until safety and efficacy information is available (SMFM [Hughes 2017]).

Product Availability Olysio tablets have been discontinued in the US for more than 1 year.

- ◆ **Simeprevir Sodium** *see* Simeprevir *on page 1372*
- ◆ **Simliya** *see* Ethinyl Estradiol and Desogestrel *on page 609*
- ◆ **Simoctocog Alfa** *see* Antihemophilic Factor (Recombinant) *on page 153*
- ◆ **Simpesse** *see* Ethinyl Estradiol and Levonorgestrel *on page 612*
- ◆ **Simply Sleep [OTC]** *see* DiphenhydrAMINE (Systemic) *on page 502*
- ◆ **Simply Stuffy [OTC]** *see* Pseudoephedrine *on page 1291*
- ◆ **Simponi** *see* Golimumab *on page 744*
- ◆ **Simponi Aria** *see* Golimumab *on page 744*
- ◆ **Simulect** *see* Basiliximab *on page 216*

Simvastatin (sim va STAT in)

Related Information

Cardiovascular Diseases *on page 1654*

Brand Names: US FloLipid; Zocor

Brand Names: Canada ACT Simvastatin [DSC]; AG-Simvastatin; APO-Simvastatin; Auro-Simvastatin; BCI Simvastatin [DSC]; BIO-Simvastatin; DOM-Simvastatin; JAMP-Simvastatin; Mar-Simvastatin; MINT-Simvastatin; MYLAN-Simvastatin [DSC]; PHARMA-Simvastatin; PMS-Simvastatin; PRIVA-Simvastatin; RIVA-Simvastatin [DSC]; SANDOZ Simvastatin; Simvastatin-10; Simvastatin-20; Simvastatin-40; Simvastatin-80; TARO-Simvastatin; TEVA-Simvastatin; Zocor

Pharmacologic Category Antilipemic Agent, HMG-CoA Reductase Inhibitor

Use

Hyperlipidemias:

Dysbetalipoproteinemia: Reduce elevated triglycerides (TG) and very low-density lipoprotein cholesterol (VLDL-C) in patients with primary dysbetalipoproteinemia (Fredrickson type III)

Heterozygous familial and nonfamilial hypercholesterolemia and mixed dyslipidemia: To reduce elevated total cholesterol (total-C), low-density lipoprotein cholesterol (LDL-C), apolipoprotein B (apo B), and TG, and to increase high-density lipoprotein cholesterol (HDL-C) in patients with primary hyperlipidemia (Fredrickson type IIa, heterozygous familial and nonfamilial) or mixed dyslipidemia (Fredrickson type IIb)

Heterozygous familial hypercholesterolemia (HeFH) in adolescents: To reduce total-C, LDL-C, and apo B levels in boys and postmenarche girls 10 to 17 years of age with heterozygous familial hypercholesterolemia with either LDL-C ≥190 mg/dL, LDL-C ≥160 mg/dL with positive family history of premature cardiovascular disease (CVD), or LDL-C ≥160 mg/dL with two or more other CVD risk factors

Homozygous familial hypercholesterolemia: To reduce total-C and LDL-C in patients with homozygous familial hypercholesterolemia as an adjunct to other lipid-lowering treatments (eg, LDL apheresis) or if such treatments are unavailable

Hypertriglyceridemia: To reduce elevated serum triglyceride levels in patients with hypertriglyceridemia (Fredrickson type IV)

Limitations of use: Has not been studied in conditions where the major lipid abnormality is elevation of chylomicrons (Fredrickson types I and V)

Prevention of cardiovascular events: To reduce the risk of nonfatal MI, stroke, and total mortality; and to reduce the need for coronary/non-coronary revascularization procedures in patients at high risk of coronary events (eg, patients with coronary heart disease, diabetes, PVD, history of stroke or other cerebrovascular disease)

Local Anesthetic/Vasoconstrictor Precautions
No information available to require special precautions

Effects on Dental Treatment Key adverse event(s) related to dental treatment: Assess unusual presentations of muscle weakness or myopathy resulting from lipid therapy such as patient having a difficult time brushing teeth or weakness with chewing. Refer patient back to their physician for evaluation and adjustment of lipid therapy.

Effects on Bleeding No information available to require special precautions

Adverse Reactions

1% to 10%:

Cardiovascular: Atrial fibrillation (6%), edema (3%)

Central nervous system: Headache (3% to 7%), vertigo (5%)

Dermatologic: Eczema (5%)

Gastrointestinal: Abdominal pain (7%), constipation (7%), gastritis (5%), nausea (5%)

Genitourinary: Cystitis (interstitial; Huang 2015)

Hepatic: Increased serum transaminases (≤2%)

Neuromuscular & skeletal: Increased creatine phosphokinase in blood specimen (>3 x normal; 5%), myalgia (4%)

Respiratory: Upper respiratory infection (9%), bronchitis (7%)

Frequency not defined:

Dermatologic: Skin rash

Endocrine & metabolic: Increased gamma-glutamyl transferase

Gastrointestinal: Diarrhea, dyspepsia, flatulence, gastrointestinal disease

Hepatic: Increased serum alkaline phosphatase

Neuromuscular & skeletal: Asthenia

<1%, postmarketing, and/or case reports: Alopecia, amnesia, anaphylaxis, anemia, angioedema, arthralgia, arthritis, changes in nails, changes of hair, chills, cognitive dysfunction, confusion, depression, dermatomyositis, dizziness, dry mucous membranes, dysgeusia (Tuccori 2011), dyspnea, elevated glycosylated hemoglobin, eosinophilia, erectile dysfunction, erythema multiforme, fever, flushing, forgetfulness, hemolytic anemia, hepatic failure, hepatitis, hypersensitivity reaction, immune-mediated necrotizing myopathy, increase in fasting plasma glucose, increased erythrocyte sedimentation rate, interstitial pulmonary disease, jaundice, leukopenia, lupus-like syndrome, malaise, memory impairment, muscle cramps, myopathy, nodule, nonthrombocytopenic purpura, pancreatitis, paresthesia, peripheral neuropathy, polymyalgia rheumatica, positive ANA titer, pruritus, rhabdomyolysis, skin changes, skin discoloration, skin photosensitivity, Stevens-Johnson syndrome, thrombocytopenia, toxic epidermal necrolysis, urticaria, vasculitis, vomiting, xeroderma

Mechanism of Action Simvastatin is a methylated derivative of lovastatin that acts by competitively inhibiting 3-hydroxy-3-methylglutaryl-coenzyme A (HMG-CoA) reductase, the enzyme that catalyzes the rate-limiting step in cholesterol biosynthesis. In addition to the ability of HMG-CoA reductase inhibitors to decrease levels of high-sensitivity C-reactive protein (hsCRP), they also possess pleiotropic properties including improved endothelial function, reduced inflammation at the site of the coronary plaque, inhibition of platelet aggregation, and anticoagulant effects (de Denus 2002; Ray 2005).

Pharmacodynamics/Kinetics

Onset of Action

Onset of action: >3 days; Peak effect: 2 weeks

LDL-C reduction: 20 to 40 mg/day: 35% to 41% (for each doubling of this dose, LDL-C is lowered ~6%)

Average HDL-C increase: 5% to 15%

Average triglyceride reduction: 7% to 30%

Half-life Elimination Unknown

Time to Peak 1.3 to 2.4 hours

Reproductive Considerations

Simvastatin is contraindicated in females who may become pregnant.

Adequate contraception is recommended if an HMG-CoA reductase inhibitor is required in females of reproductive potential. Females planning a pregnancy should discontinue the HMG-CoA reductase inhibitor 1 to 2 months prior to attempting to conceive (AHA/ACC [Grundy 2018]).

Pregnancy Risk Factor X

Pregnancy Considerations Simvastatin is contraindicated in pregnant females.

There are reports of congenital anomalies following maternal use of HMG-CoA reductase inhibitors in pregnancy; however, maternal disease, differences in specific agents used, and the low rates of exposure limit the interpretation of the available data (Godfrey 2012; Lecarpentier 2012). Cholesterol biosynthesis may be important in fetal development; serum cholesterol and triglycerides increase normally during pregnancy. The discontinuation of lipid lowering medications temporarily during pregnancy is not expected to have significant impact on the long-term outcomes of primary hypercholesterolemia treatment.

Simvastatin should be discontinued immediately if an unplanned pregnancy occurs during treatment.

- ◆ **Simvastatin and Ezetimibe** *see* Ezetimibe and Simvastatin *on page 634*
- ◆ **Simvastatin/Ezetimibe** *see* Ezetimibe and Simvastatin *on page 634*
- ◆ **Sinelee [DSC]** *see* Capsaicin *on page 284*
- ◆ **Sinemet** *see* Carbidopa and Levodopa *on page 290*
- ◆ **Sinemet CR [DSC]** *see* Carbidopa and Levodopa *on page 290*
- ◆ **Sinequan** *see* Doxepin (Systemic) *on page 518*
- ◆ **Singulair** *see* Montelukast *on page 1048*
- ◆ **Sinus Nasal Spray [OTC]** *see* Oxymetazoline (Nasal) *on page 1173*
- ◆ **Sinuva** *see* Mometasone (Nasal) *on page 1045*

Sipuleucel-T (si pu LOO sel tee)

Brand Names: US Provenge

Pharmacologic Category Cellular Immunotherapy, Autologous

Use Prostate cancer, metastatic: Treatment of asymptomatic or minimally symptomatic metastatic castrate-resistant (hormone-refractory) prostate cancer.

Local Anesthetic/Vasoconstrictor Precautions No information available to require special precautions

Effects on Dental Treatment No significant effects or complications reported

Effects on Bleeding No information available to require special precautions

Adverse Reactions Note: Initial infusion-related events usually present within the first 24 hours after administration.

>10%:

Central nervous system: Chills (53%; grades ≥3: 2%), fatigue (41%; grades ≥3: 1%), headache (18%; grades ≥3: <1%), dizziness (12%; grades ≥3: <1%), pain (12%)

Gastrointestinal: Nausea (22%; grades ≥3: <1%), vomiting (13% grades ≥3: <1%), constipation (12%; grades ≥3: <1%)

Hematologic: Anemia (13%)

Hypersensitivity: Severe infusion related reaction (71%; grade 3: 4%)

Neuromuscular & skeletal: Back pain (30%; grades ≥3: 3%), myalgia (12%; grades ≥3: <1%), weakness (11%; grades ≥3: 1%)

Miscellaneous: Fever (31%; grades ≥3: 1%), citrate toxicity (15%)

1% to 10%:

Cardiovascular: Hypertension (8% grades ≥3: <1%), hemorrhagic stroke (4%)

Dermatologic: Diaphoresis (5%; grades ≥3: <1%), skin rash (5%)

Gastrointestinal: Anorexia (7%), acute ischemic stroke (4%)

Genitourinary: Hematuria (8%)

Neuromuscular & skeletal: Musculoskeletal pain (9%; grades ≥3: <1%), muscle spasm (8%; grades ≥3: <1%), neck pain (6%), tremor (5%)

Renal: Hematuria (8%)

Respiratory: Flu-like symptoms (10%), dyspnea (9%; grades ≥3: 2%)

<1%, postmarketing, and/or case reports: Cerebrovascular accident, eosinophilia, hypotension, myasthenia gravis, myocardial infarction, myositis, paresthesia (grades ≥3), pulmonary embolism, rhabdomyolysis, sepsis, syncope, transient ischemic attacks, tumor flare, venous thrombosis

Mechanism of Action Sipuleucel-T is an autologous cellular immunotherapy that stimulates an immune response against an antigen (prostatic acid phosphatase [PAP]) expressed in most prostate cancer tissues. Peripheral blood is collected (~3 days prior to infusion) from the patient via leukapheresis, from which peripheral blood mononuclear cells (PBMCs) are isolated. Antigen presenting cell (APC) precursors, consisting of CD54-positive cells that include dendritic cells, are isolated from the PBMCs. The APCs are then activated (in vitro) with a recombinant human fusion protein, PAP-GM-CSF (also termed PA2024), composed of an antigen specific for prostate cancer, PAP linked to granulocyte-macrophage colony-stimulating factor and cultured for ~40 hours. The final product, sipuleucel-T, is reinfused into the patient, inducing T-cell immunity to tumors that express PAP.

Pregnancy Considerations Animal reproduction studies have not been conducted. Not indicated for use in women.

Prescribing and Access Restrictions Patients may receive Sipuleucel-T at a participating site. Physicians must go through an inservice and register to prescribe the treatment; patients must also complete an enrollment form. Information on registration and enrollment is available at 1-877-336-3736 or at DendreonONCall.-com.

- ◆ **Sirdalud** *see* TiZANidine *on page 1455*

Sirolimus (sir OH li mus)

Brand Names: US Rapamune

Brand Names: Canada Rapamune

Pharmacologic Category Immunosuppressant Agent; mTOR Kinase Inhibitor

Use

Lymphangioleiomyomatosis: Treatment of lymphangioleiomyomatosis. Therapeutic drug monitoring is recommended for all patients receiving sirolimus.

Renal transplantation (rejection prophylaxis): Prophylaxis of organ rejection in patients receiving renal transplants (in low-to-moderate immunologic risk patients in combination with cyclosporine and corticosteroids with cyclosporine withdrawn 2 to 4 months after transplant, and in high immunologic risk patients in combination with cyclosporine and corticosteroids for the first year after transplant). Therapeutic drug monitoring is recommended for all patients receiving sirolimus. High immunologic risk renal transplant patients are defined (per the manufacturer's labeling) as Black transplant recipients and/or repeat renal transplant recipients who lost a previous allograft based on an immunologic process and/or patients with high PRA (panel-reactive antibodies; peak PRA level >80%).

Limitations of use (renal transplantation): Cyclosporine withdrawal has not been studied in patients with Banff grade 3 acute rejection or vascular rejection prior to cyclosporine withdrawal, patients who are dialysis-dependent, patients with serum creatinine >4.5 mg/dL, Black patients, patients with multiorgan transplants or secondary transplants, or those with high levels of PRA. In patients at high immunologic risk, the safety and efficacy of sirolimus used in combination with cyclosporine and corticosteroids have not been studied beyond 1 year; therefore, after the first 12 months following transplantation, consider any adjustments to the immunosuppressive regimen on the basis of the clinical status of the patient. The safety and efficacy of sirolimus have not been established in patients younger than 13 years or in pediatric renal transplant patients younger than 18 years who are considered at high immunologic risk. The Kidney Disease: Improving Global Outcomes (KDIGO) guidelines for the care of renal transplant recipients recommend not initiating sirolimus until graft function has been established and surgical wounds have healed (KDIGO 2009). Avoid the use of sirolimus in combination with calcineurin inhibitors, particularly in the early posttransplant period due to an increased risk of nephrotoxicity (KDIGO 2009; Webster 2006).

Local Anesthetic/Vasoconstrictor Precautions No information available to require special precautions

Effects on Dental Treatment Key adverse event(s) related to dental treatment: Mouth ulceration, oral candida infection, stomatitis, gingival hyperplasia, gingivitis, and dysphagia (see Dental Health Professional Considerations)

Effects on Bleeding Thrombocytopenia (15% to 30%) has been associated with use; severe thrombocytopenia (rare) may be associated with delayed coagulation. Consultation to ensure adequate platelet counts may be considered in patients with signs/symptoms or a history of thrombocytopenia.

Adverse Reactions Incidence of many adverse effects is dose related. Reported events exclusive to renal transplant patients unless otherwise noted. Frequency not always defined.

Cardiovascular: Peripheral edema (≥20% to 58%, LAM and renal transplants), hypertension (49%), edema (18% to 20%), chest pain (LAM), deep vein thrombosis, pulmonary embolism, tachycardia

Central nervous system: Headache (≥20% to 34%, LAM and renal transplants), pain (29% to 33%), dizziness (LAM)

Dermatologic: Acne vulgaris (≥20% to 22%, LAM and renal transplants), skin rash (10% to 20%)

Endocrine & metabolic: Hypertriglyceridemia (45% to 57%), hypercholesterolemia (≥20% to 46%, LAM and renal transplants), amenorrhea, diabetes mellitus, hypermenorrhea, hypervolemia, hypokalemia, increased lactate dehydrogenase, menstrual disease, ovarian cyst

Gastrointestinal: Constipation (36% to 38%), abdominal pain (≥20% to 36%, LAM and renal transplants), diarrhea (≥20% to 35%, LAM and renal transplants), nausea (≥20% to 31%, LAM and renal transplants), stomatitis (3% to >20%)

Genitourinary: Urinary tract infection (33%)

Hematologic & oncologic: Anemia (23% to 33%), thrombocytopenia (14% to 30%), lymphoproliferative disorder (≤3%; including lymphoma), skin carcinoma (≤3%; includes basal cell carcinoma, squamous cell carcinoma, melanoma), hemolytic-uremic syndrome, leukopenia, lymphocele, thrombotic thrombocytopenic purpura

Infection: Herpes simplex infection, herpes zoster, sepsis

Neuromuscular & skeletal: Arthralgia (25% to 31%), myalgia (LAM), osteonecrosis

Renal: Increased serum creatinine (39% to 40%), pyelonephritis

Respiratory: Nasopharyngitis (LAM), epistaxis, pneumonia, upper respiratory tract infection (LAM)

Miscellaneous: Wound healing impairment

<3%, postmarketing, and/or case reports: Abnormal hepatic function tests, anaphylactoid reaction, anaphylaxis, angioedema, ascites, azoospermia, cardiac tamponade, cytomegalovirus, dehiscence (fascial), Epstein-Barr infection, exfoliative dermatitis, fluid retention, focal segmental glomerulosclerosis, gingival hyperplasia, hepatic necrosis, hepatotoxicity, hyperglycemia, hypersensitivity angiitis, hypersensitivity reaction, hypophosphatemia, incisional hernia, increased serum ALT, increased serum AST, increased susceptibility to infection (including opportunistic), interstitial pulmonary disease (dose related; includes pneumonitis, pulmonary fibrosis, and bronchiolitis obliterans organizing pneumonia with no identified infectious etiology), joint disorders, lymphedema, Merkel cell carcinoma, mycobacterium infection, nephrotic syndrome, neutropenia, pancreatitis, pancytopenia, pericardial effusion, pleural effusion, pneumonia due to *Pneumocystis carinii*, progressive multifocal leukoencephalopathy, proteinuria, pseudomembranous colitis, pulmonary alveolitis, pulmonary hemorrhage, renal disease (BK virus-associated), reversible posterior leukoencephalopathy syndrome, tuberculosis, weight loss, wound dehiscence

Mechanism of Action Sirolimus inhibits T-lymphocyte activation and proliferation in response to antigenic and cytokine stimulation and inhibits antibody production. Its mechanism differs from other immunosuppressants. Sirolimus binds to FKBP-12, an intracellular protein, to form an immunosuppressive complex which inhibits the regulatory kinase, mTOR (mechanistic target of rapamycin). This inhibition suppresses cytokine mediated T-cell proliferation, halting progression from the G1 to the S phase of the cell cycle. It inhibits acute rejection of allografts and prolongs graft survival.

In lymphangioleiomyomatosis, the mTOR signaling pathway is activated through the loss of the tuberous sclerosis complex (TSC) gene function (resulting in cellular proliferation and release of lymphangiogenic growth factors). By inhibiting the mTOR pathway, sirolimus prevents the proliferation of lymphangioleiomyomatosis cells.

Pharmacodynamics/Kinetics

Half-life Elimination

Children: 13.7 ± 6.2 hours

Adults: Mean: 62 hours (range; 46 to 78 hours); extended in hepatic impairment (Child-Pugh class A or B) to 113 hours

Time to Peak Oral solution: 1 to 3 hours; Tablet: 1 to 6 hours

Reproductive Considerations

Female patients of reproductive potential should initiate highly effective contraception before therapy with sirolimus, during treatment, and for 12 weeks after sirolimus is discontinued.

Male and female fertility may be impaired during treatment. Amenorrhea and menorrhagia have been reported in females; azoospermia (which may be reversible) has been reported in males.

Pregnancy Considerations

Based on the mechanism of action and data from animal reproduction studies, in utero exposure to sirolimus may cause fetal harm. Information related to the use of sirolimus in pregnancy is limited (Chu 2008; Framarino dei Malatesta 2011; Sifontis 2006).

The Transplant Pregnancy Registry International (TPR) is a registry that follows pregnancies that occur in maternal transplant recipients or those fathered by male transplant recipients. The TPR encourages reporting of pregnancies following solid organ transplant by contacting them at 1-877-955-6877 or https://www.transplant-pregnancyregistry.org.

Dental Health Professional Considerations Consider a medical consultation prior to any invasive dental procedure in patients who have received an organ transplant; delayed wound healing due to the immunosuppressive effects and an increased potential for post-operative infection may be of concern.

SITagliptin (sit a GLIP tin)

Related Information

Endocrine Disorders and Pregnancy *on page 1684*

Brand Names: US Januvia

Brand Names: Canada Januvia

Pharmacologic Category Antidiabetic Agent, Dipeptidyl Peptidase 4 (DPP-4) Inhibitor

Use Diabetes mellitus, type 2, treatment: As an adjunct to diet and exercise to improve glycemic control in adults with type 2 diabetes mellitus, as monotherapy or combination therapy.

Local Anesthetic/Vasoconstrictor Precautions No information available to require special precautions

Effects on Dental Treatment Key adverse event(s) related to dental treatment: Rare occurrence of oral mucosal ulcers, stomatitis. Sitagliptin-dependent patients with diabetes should be appointed for dental treatment in the morning in order to minimize chance of stress-induced hypoglycemia.

Effects on Bleeding No information available to require special precautions

Adverse Reactions

1% to 10%:

Endocrine & metabolic: Hypoglycemia (1%)

Respiratory: Nasopharyngitis (5%)

Frequency not defined: Gastrointestinal: Diarrhea, nausea

Postmarketing:

Dermatologic: Bullous pemphigoid (García-Díez 2018; Tanaka 2019), skin rash (Nakai 2014), Stevens-Johnson syndrome (Desai 2010), toxic epidermal necrolysis (Desai 2010)

Gastrointestinal: Acute pancreatitis (including hemorrhagic or necrotizing forms) (Butler 2013; Elashoff 2011; Scheen 2018), constipation (Williams-Herman 2010), oral mucosa ulcer (Jinbu 2013), stomatitis, vomiting

Hepatic: Increased liver enzymes (Shahbaz 2018)

Hypersensitivity: Anaphylaxis (Desai 2010), angioedema (Arcani 2017; Gosmanov 2012; Skalli 2010), drug reaction with eosinophilia and systemic symptoms (Sin 2012)

Nervous system: Headache (Zaghloul 2018)

Neuromuscular & skeletal: Arthralgia (FDA safety alert; Mascolo 2016), myalgia (Tarapues 2013)

Renal: Acute renal failure (possibly requiring dialysis) (Shih 2016)

Mechanism of Action Sitagliptin inhibits dipeptidyl peptidase-4 (DPP-4) enzyme resulting in prolonged active incretin levels. Incretin hormones (eg, glucagon-like peptide-1 [GLP-1] and glucose-dependent insulinotropic polypeptide [GIP]) regulate glucose homeostasis by increasing insulin synthesis and release from pancreatic beta cells and decreasing glucagon secretion from pancreatic alpha cells. Decreased glucagon secretion results in decreased hepatic glucose production. Under normal physiologic circumstances, incretin hormones are released by the intestine throughout the day and levels are increased in response to a meal; incretin hormones are rapidly inactivated by the DPP-4 enzyme.

Pharmacodynamics/Kinetics

Half-life Elimination 12.4 hours

Time to Peak 1 to 4 hours

Pregnancy Considerations

Information related to the use of sitagliptin in pregnancy is limited (Sun 2017).

Poorly controlled diabetes during pregnancy can be associated with an increased risk of adverse maternal and fetal outcomes, including diabetic ketoacidosis, preeclampsia, spontaneous abortion, preterm delivery, delivery complications, major birth defects, stillbirth, and macrosomia. To prevent adverse outcomes, prior to conception and throughout pregnancy, maternal blood glucose and HbA_{1c} should be kept as close to target goals as possible but without causing significant hypoglycemia (ADA 2020; Blumer 2013).

Agents other than sitagliptin are currently recommended to treat diabetes mellitus in pregnancy (ADA 2020).

Health care providers are encouraged to enroll women exposed to sitagliptin during pregnancy in the registry (1-800-986-8999).

◆ **Sitagliptin and Ertugliflozin** *see* Ertugliflozin and Sitagliptin *on page 588*

Sitagliptin and Metformin
(sit a GLIP tin & met FOR min)

Related Information

MetFORMIN *on page 983*

SITagliptin *on page 1376*

Brand Names: US Janumet; Janumet XR

Brand Names: Canada Janumet; Janumet XR

Pharmacologic Category Antidiabetic Agent, Biguanide; Antidiabetic Agent, Dipeptidyl Peptidase 4 (DPP-4) Inhibitor

Use Diabetes mellitus, type 2, treatment: Adjunct to diet and exercise to improve glycemic control in adults with type 2 diabetes mellitus.

Local Anesthetic/Vasoconstrictor Precautions No information available to require special precautions

Effects on Dental Treatment Sitagliptin- and metformin-dependent patients with diabetes (noninsulin dependent, Type 2) should be appointed for dental treatment in morning in order to minimize chance of stress-induced hypoglycemia.

Effects on Bleeding No information available to require special precautions

Adverse Reactions Also see individual agents.

1% to 10%:

Central nervous system: Headache (6%)

Gastrointestinal: Diarrhea (8%), nausea (5%), abdominal pain (3%), vomiting (2%)

Respiratory: Upper respiratory tract infection (6%)

<1%, postmarketing and/or case reports: Arthralgia, back pain, constipation, hypersensitivity reaction (including anaphylaxis, angioedema, skin rash, urticaria, hypersensitivity angiitis, exfoliative skin conditions

[including Stevens-Johnson syndrome]), increased liver enzymes, lactic acidosis, limb pain, myalgia, oral mucosa ulcer, pancreatitis (including hemorrhagic or necrotizing), pemphigoid, pruritus, renal failure, renal insufficiency, severe arthralgia (FDA Safety Alert, Aug 28, 2015), stomatitis

Mechanism of Action Sitagliptin inhibits dipeptidyl peptidase IV (DPP-IV) enzymes resulting in prolonged active incretin levels. Incretin hormones [eg, glucagon-like peptide-1 (GLP-1) and glucose-dependent insulinotropic polypeptide (GIP)] regulate glucose homeostasis by increasing insulin synthesis and release from pancreatic beta cells and decreasing glucagon secretion from pancreatic alpha cells. Decreased glucagon secretion results in decreased hepatic glucose production. Under normal physiologic circumstances, incretin hormones are released by the intestine throughout the day and levels are increased in response to a meal; incretin hormones are rapidly inactivated by DPP-IV enzymes.

Metformin decreases hepatic glucose production, decreasing intestinal absorption of glucose, and improves insulin sensitivity (increases peripheral glucose uptake and utilization).

Pregnancy Considerations

Metformin crosses the placenta (ADA 2020). See individual monographs for additional information.

Health professionals are encouraged to report any prenatal exposure to sitagliptin/metformin combination by contacting Merck's pregnancy registry (1-800-986-8999).

- ◆ **Sitagliptin Phos/Metformin HCl** *see* Sitagliptin and Metformin *on page 1376*
- ◆ **Sitagliptin Phosphate** *see* SITagliptin *on page 1376*
- ◆ **Sitagliptin Phosphate and Metformin Hydrochloride** *see* Sitagliptin and Metformin *on page 1376*
- ◆ **Sitavig** *see* Acyclovir (Topical) *on page 82*
- ◆ **Sivextro** *see* Tedizolid *on page 1409*
- ◆ **Skelaxin** *see* Metaxalone *on page 982*
- ◆ **SKF 104864** *see* Topotecan *on page 1465*
- ◆ **SKF 104864-A** *see* Topotecan *on page 1465*
- ◆ **Sleep Aid [OTC]** *see* Doxylamine *on page 532*
- ◆ **Sleep Tabs [OTC]** *see* DiphenhydrAMINE (Systemic) *on page 502*
- ◆ **S-leucovorin** *see* LEVOleucovorin *on page 899*
- ◆ **6S-leucovorin** *see* LEVOleucovorin *on page 899*
- ◆ **Slo-Niacin [OTC]** *see* Niacin *on page 1097*
- ◆ **Slow FE** *see* Ferrous Sulfate *on page 664*
- ◆ **Slow Fe [OTC]** *see* Ferrous Sulfate *on page 664*
- ◆ **Slow Iron [OTC]** *see* Ferrous Sulfate *on page 664*
- ◆ **Slynd** *see* Drospirenone *on page 534*
- ◆ **SM-5688** *see* Droxidopa *on page 535*
- ◆ **SM-13496** *see* Lurasidone *on page 943*
- ◆ **SMX-TMP** *see* Sulfamethoxazole and Trimethoprim *on page 1391*
- ◆ **SMZ-TMP** *see* Sulfamethoxazole and Trimethoprim *on page 1391*
- ◆ **(+)-(*S*)-*N*-Methyl-γ-(1-naphthyloxy)-2-thiophenepropylamine Hydrochloride** *see* DULoxetine *on page 536*
- ◆ **Sodium 4-Hydroxybutyrate** *see* Sodium Oxybate *on page 1377*
- ◆ **Sodium *L*-Triiodothyronine** *see* Liothyronine *on page 919*
- ◆ **Sodium Artesunate** *see* Artesunate *on page 169*
- ◆ **Sodium Benzoate and Caffeine** *see* Caffeine *on page 277*
- ◆ **Sodium Cromoglicate** *see* Cromolyn (Oral Inhalation) *on page 416*
- ◆ **Sodium Cromoglicate** *see* Cromolyn (Systemic) *on page 416*
- ◆ **Sodium Cromoglycate** *see* Cromolyn (Oral Inhalation) *on page 416*
- ◆ **Sodium Cromoglycate** *see* Cromolyn (Systemic) *on page 416*
- ◆ **Sodium Diuril** *see* Chlorothiazide *on page 339*
- ◆ **Sodium Edecrin** *see* Ethacrynic Acid *on page 608*
- ◆ **Sodium Etidronate** *see* Etidronate *on page 620*
- ◆ **Sodium Fluoride** *see* Fluoride *on page 693*
- ◆ **Sodium Hyaluronate** *see* Hyaluronate and Derivatives *on page 761*

Sodium Oxybate (SOW dee um ox i BATE)

Brand Names: US Xyrem

Brand Names: Canada Xyrem

Pharmacologic Category Central Nervous System Depressant

Use Narcolepsy: Treatment of cataplexy or excessive daytime sleepiness in patients ≥7 years of age with narcolepsy

Local Anesthetic/Vasoconstrictor Precautions No information available to require special precautions

Effects on Dental Treatment Key adverse event(s) related to dental treatment: Tooth ache (see Dental Health Professional Considerations).

Effects on Bleeding No information available to require special precautions

Adverse Reactions

>10%:

Central nervous system: Confusion (adults: 3% to 17%), headache (≤16%), dizziness (6% to 15%)

Endocrine & metabolic: Weight loss (≤12%)

Gastrointestinal: Nausea (8% to 20%), vomiting (2% to 16%)

Genitourinary: Urinary incontinence (children and adolescents: 18%; adults: 3% to 7%)

1% to 10%:

Cardiovascular: Peripheral edema (adults: 3%)

Central nervous system: Drowsiness (adults: 8%), depression (adults: 3% to 7%), somnambulism (adults: 3% to 6%), anxiety (adults: 2% to 6%), disturbance in attention (adults: 1% to 4%), intoxicated feeling (adults: 3%), irritability (adults: 3%), pain (adults: 3%), sleep paralysis (adults: 3%), disorientation (adults: 2% to 3%), paresthesia (adults: 2% to 3%), severe central nervous system depression (adults: 2%)

Dermatologic: Hyperhidrosis (adults: 1% to 3%)

Gastrointestinal: Decreased appetite (≤8%), diarrhea (adults: 3% to 4%), upper abdominal pain (adults: 3%)

Neuromuscular & skeletal: Tremor (adults: 2% to 5%), limb pain (adults: 3%), cataplexy (adults: 2%)

Frequency not defined:

Central nervous system: Central nervous system depression, obtundation, sleep apnea

Hematologic & oncologic: Oxygen desaturation

Respiratory: Respiratory depression

<1%, postmarketing, and/or case reports: Acute psychosis, aggressive behavior, agitation, arthralgia, blurred vision, falling, fluid retention, hallucination, hangover effect, hypersensitivity reaction, hypertension, increased libido, memory impairment, nocturia, panic attack, paranoia, psychosis, suicidal ideation

Mechanism of Action Sodium oxybate is derived from gamma aminobutyric acid (GABA) and acts as an inhibitory chemical transmitter in the brain. May function through specific receptors for gamma hydroxybutyrate (GHB) and GABA (B).

Pharmacodynamics/Kinetics

Half-life Elimination 30 to 60 minutes

Time to Peak 30 to 75 minutes

Pregnancy Considerations The injection formulation, when used as an anesthetic during labor and delivery, was shown to cross the placenta; a slight decrease in Apgar scores due to sleepiness in the neonate was observed.

Controlled Substance C-I (illicit use); C-III (medical use)

Prescribing and Access Restrictions In Canada, access to sodium oxybate is restricted under the Xyrem Success Program. The program is intended to educate prescribers, pharmacists, and patients on the safe use, storage, and handling of the drug, to maintain a registry of trained physicians, pharmacies, and patients, and to limit distribution through a single wholesaler to pharmacies on an as-needed basis after a prescription is received by the pharmacy. Initial dispensing of prescriptions should occur only after the prescriber, pharmacist, and patient have received and read the educational materials. Further information regarding the program may be obtained at 1-866-599-7365.

Dental Health Professional Considerations Sodium oxybate is a known substance of abuse. When used illegally, it has been referred to as a "date-rape drug". The dentist should be aware of patients showing signs of CNS depression, as with all other drugs in this class.

◆ **Sodium PAS** *see* Aminosalicylic Acid *on page* 118

Sodium Phenylbutyrate

(SOW dee um fen il BYOO ti rate)

Brand Names: US Buphenyl

Brand Names: Canada Pheburane

Pharmacologic Category Urea Cycle Disorder (UCD) Treatment Agent

Use Urea cycle disorders: Adjunctive therapy in the chronic management of patients with urea cycle disorder involving deficiencies of carbamoylphosphate synthetase, ornithine transcarbamylase, or argininosuccinic acid synthetase; neonatal-onset deficiency (complete enzymatic deficiency, presenting within the first 28 days of life); late-onset disease (partial enzymatic deficiency, presenting after the first month of life) who have a history of hyperammonemic encephalopathy

Local Anesthetic/Vasoconstrictor Precautions No information available to require special precautions

Effects on Dental Treatment Key adverse event(s) related to dental treatment: Abnormal taste.

Effects on Bleeding No information available to require special precautions

Adverse Reactions

>10%: Endocrine & metabolic: Amenorrhea (≤23%), menstrual disease (≤23%), acidosis (14%), hypoalbuminemia (11%)

1% to 10%:

Cardiovascular: Syncope (≤2%)

Central nervous system: Depression (≤2%), headache (≤2%)

Dermatologic: Body odor (3%), skin rash (≤2%)

Endocrine & metabolic: Alkalosis (7%), hyperchloremia (7%), hypophosphatemia (6%), decreased serum total protein (3%), hyperuricemia (2%), hyperphosphatemia (2%), hypernatremia (1%), hypokalemia (1%)

Gastrointestinal: Anorexia (4%), dysgeusia (3%), abdominal pain (≤2%), gastritis (≤2%), nausea (≤2%), vomiting (≤2%)

Hematologic & oncologic: Anemia (9%), leukocytosis (4%), leukopenia (4%), thrombocytopenia (3%), thrombocythemia (1%)

Hepatic: Increased serum alkaline phosphatase (6%), increased serum transaminases (4%), hyperbilirubinemia (1%)

Renal: Renal tubular acidosis (≤2%)

<1%, postmarketing, and/or case reports: Aplastic anemia, bruise, cardiac arrhythmia, constipation, dizziness, drowsiness, edema, fatigue, memory impairment, neuropathy (exacerbation), pancreatitis, peptic ulcer, rectal hemorrhage

Mechanism of Action Sodium phenylbutyrate is a prodrug which is rapidly converted to phenylacetate, followed by conjugation with glutamine to form phenylacetylglutamine; phenylacetylglutamine serves as a substitute for urea as it is clears nitrogenous waste from the body when excreted in the urine.

Pharmacodynamics/Kinetics

Half-life Elimination Phenylbutyrate (tablets and powder): 0.76 to 0.77 hours; Phenylacetate (tablets and powder): 1.15 to 1.29 hours

Time to Peak Plasma: Phenylbutyrate (tablets and powder): 1 to 1.35 hours; Phenylacetate (tablets and powder): 3.55 to 3.74 hours

Pregnancy Considerations

Animal reproduction studies have not been conducted.

◆ **Sodium Phosphate Monobasic, Methenamine, Methylene Blue, Phenyl Salicylate, and Hyoscyamine** *see* Methenamine, Sodium Phosphate Monobasic, Phenyl Salicylate, Methylene Blue, and Hyoscyamine *on page* 987

◆ **Sof-Lax [OTC] [DSC]** *see* Docusate *on page* 509

Sofosbuvir

(soe FOS bue vir)

Related Information

Systemic Viral Diseases *on page* 1709

Brand Names: US Sovaldi

Brand Names: Canada Sovaldi

Pharmacologic Category Antihepaciviral, Polymerase Inhibitor (Anti-HCV); NS5B RNA Polymerase Inhibitor

Use Chronic hepatitis C: Treatment of genotype 1, 2, 3, or 4 chronic hepatitis C virus (HCV) infection in adults and genotype 2 or 3 chronic HCV infection in pediatric patients ≥3 years of age, without cirrhosis or with compensated cirrhosis, as a component of a combination antiviral treatment regimen.

Local Anesthetic/Vasoconstrictor Precautions No information available to require special precautions

Effects on Dental Treatment No significant effects or complications reported

Effects on Bleeding No information available to require special precautions

Adverse Reactions Adverse reactions reported with combination therapy.

>10%:

Central nervous system: Fatigue (30% to 59%), headache (24% to 36%), insomnia (15% to 25%), chills (2% to 17%), irritability (10% to 13%)

Dermatologic: Pruritus (11% to 27%), skin rash (8% to 18%)

Gastrointestinal: Nausea (22% to 34%), decreased appetite (18%), diarrhea (9% to 12%)

Hematologic & oncologic: Anemia (6% to 21%), neutropenia (<1% [interferon-free regimen] to 17% [interferon-containing regimen])

Neuromuscular & skeletal: Asthenia (5% to 21%), myalgia (6% to 14%)

Respiratory: Flu-like symptoms (6% to 16%)

Miscellaneous: Fever (4% to 18%)

1% to 10%:

Gastrointestinal: Increased serum lipase (>3 times ULN: ≤2%)

Hematologic & oncologic: Thrombocytopenia (≤1%)

Hepatic: Increased serum bilirubin (>2.5 times ULN: 3%)

Renal: Increased creatine phosphokinase (≥10 times ULN: 1% to 2%)

<1%, postmarketing, and/or case reports: Angioedema, bradycardia, lactic acidosis (Smith 2019), pancytopenia, reactivation of HBV, severe depression, suicidal ideation

Mechanism of Action Sofosbuvir, a direct-acting antiviral agent against the hepatitis C virus, is a prodrug converted to its pharmacologically active form (GS-461203) via intracellular metabolism. It inhibits HCV NS5B RNA-dependent RNA polymerase, essential for viral replication, and acts as a chain terminator.

Pharmacodynamics/Kinetics

Half-life Elimination 0.4 hours

Time to Peak ~0.5 to 2 hours

Reproductive Considerations

HCV-infected females of childbearing potential should consider postponing pregnancy until therapy is complete to reduce the risk of HCV transmission (AASLD/IDSA 2018).

Sofosbuvir is not used as monotherapy; if used in combination with ribavirin or peginterferon, all warnings related to the use of ribavirin or peginterferon and contraception should be followed. Refer to the ribavirin and peginterferon monographs for additional information.

Pregnancy Considerations

Sofosbuvir is not used as monotherapy; combination therapy with ribavirin is contraindicated in pregnant females and males whose female partners are pregnant. If used in combination with ribavirin or peginterferon, all warnings related to the use of ribavirin or peginterferon and pregnancy should be followed. Refer to the ribavirin and peginterferon monographs for additional information.

Treatment of hepatitis C is not currently recommended to treat maternal infection or to decrease the risk of mother-to-child transmission during pregnancy (Tran 2016). When HCV infection is detected during pregnancy, treatment should be deferred until after delivery. Direct-acting antiviral medications should not be used in pregnant females outside of clinical trials until safety and efficacy information is available (SMFM [Hughes 2017]).

Product Availability Sovaldi oral pellets: FDA approved August 2019; anticipated availability is currently unknown. Consult the prescribing information for additional information.

Sofosbuvir and Velpatasvir

(soe FOS bue vir & vel PAT as vir)

Brand Names: US Epclusa

Brand Names: Canada Epclusa

Pharmacologic Category Antihepaciviral, NS5A Inhibitor; Antihepaciviral, Polymerase Inhibitor (Anti-HCV); NS5A Inhibitor; NS5B RNA Polymerase Inhibitor

Use Chronic hepatitis C: Treatment of chronic hepatitis C virus (HCV) genotype 1, 2, 3, 4, 5, or 6 infection in adults and pediatric patients ≥6 years of age or weighing ≥17 kg without cirrhosis or with compensated cirrhosis or in combination with ribavirin in patients with decompensated cirrhosis.

Local Anesthetic/Vasoconstrictor Precautions No information available to require special precautions

Effects on Dental Treatment No significant effects or complications reported

Effects on Bleeding No information available to require special precautions

Adverse Reactions Also see Sofosbuvir monograph.

>10%: Nervous system: Fatigue (15%), headache (22%)

1% to 10%:

Dermatologic: Skin rash (2%)

Gastrointestinal: Increased serum lipase (>3X ULN: 3% to 6%), nausea (9%)

Nervous system: Depression (1%), insomnia (5%), irritability (≥5%)

Neuromuscular & skeletal: Asthenia (5%), increased serum creatine kinase (≥10X ULN: 1% to 2%)

Postmarketing: Infection: Reactivation of HBV

Mechanism of Action Velpatasvir inhibits the HCV NS5A protein necessary for viral replication; sofosbuvir is a prodrug converted to its pharmacologically active form (GS-461203), which inhibits NS5B RNA-dependent RNA polymerase, also essential for viral replication, and acts as a chain terminator.

Pharmacodynamics/Kinetics

Half-life Elimination Velpatasvir: 15 hours; Sofosbuvir: 0.5 hours

Time to Peak Velpatasvir: 3 hours; Sofosbuvir: 0.5 to 1 hour

Reproductive Considerations

HCV-infected females of childbearing potential should consider postponing pregnancy until therapy is complete to reduce the risk of HCV transmission (AASLD/IDSA 2018).

If used in combination with ribavirin, all warnings related to the use of ribavirin and contraception should be followed. Refer to the ribavirin monograph for additional information.

Pregnancy Considerations

Use in combination with ribavirin is contraindicated in pregnancy. If used in combination with ribavirin, all warnings related to the use of ribavirin and pregnancy should be followed. Refer to the ribavirin monograph for additional information.

Treatment of hepatitis C is not currently recommended to treat maternal infection or to decrease the risk of mother-to-child transmission during pregnancy (Tran 2016). When HCV infection is detected during pregnancy, treatment should be deferred until after delivery.

Direct-acting antiviral medications should not be used in pregnant females outside of clinical trials until safety and efficacy information is available (SMFM [Hughes 2017]).

Product Availability

Epclusa (sofosbuvir 200 mg/velpatasvir 50 mg) tablets: FDA approved March 2020; availability anticipated in the fall of 2020. Sofosbuvir 200 mg/velpatasvir 50 mg tablets are indicated for use in pediatric patients. Consult the prescribing information for additional information.

Sofosbuvir, Velpatasvir, and Voxilaprevir

(soe FOS bue vir, vel PAT as vir, & vox i LA pre vir)

Brand Names: US Vosevi

Brand Names: Canada Vosevi

Pharmacologic Category Antihepaciviral, NS5A Inhibitor; Antihepaciviral, Polymerase Inhibitor (Anti-HCV); NS3/4A Inhibitor; NS5A Inhibitor; NS5B RNA Polymerase Inhibitor

Use **Chronic hepatitis C:** Treatment of adults with chronic hepatitis C virus (HCV) infection without cirrhosis or with compensated cirrhosis (Child-Pugh class A) who have genotype 1, 2, 3, 4, 5, or 6 infection and have previously been treated with an HCV regimen containing an NS5A inhibitor or who have genotype 1a or 3 infection and have previously been treated with an HCV regimen containing sofosbuvir without an NS5A inhibitor

Local Anesthetic/Vasoconstrictor Precautions No information available to require special precautions

Effects on Dental Treatment No significant effects or complications reported

Effects on Bleeding No information available to require special precautions

Adverse Reactions Also see Sofosbuvir monograph.

>10%:

Central nervous system: Headache (21% to 23%), fatigue (17% to 19%)

Gastrointestinal: Diarrhea (13% to 14%), nausea (10% to 13%)

Hepatic: Increased serum bilirubin (4% to 13%)

1% to 10%:

Central nervous system: Insomnia (3% to 6%), depression (≤1%)

Dermatologic: Skin rash (2%)

Gastrointestinal: Increased serum lipase (2%)

Neuromuscular & skeletal: Asthenia (4% to 6%)

Frequency not defined: Infection: Reactivation of HBV

<1%, postmarketing, and/or case reports: Acute hepatic failure, increased serum creatine kinase, liver decompensation, severe hepatic disease

Mechanism of Action

Sofosbuvir is an inhibitor of the HCV NS5B RNA-dependent RNA polymerase, which is required for viral replication and acts a s a chain terminator.

Velpatasvir is an inhibitor of the HCV NS5A protein, which is also required for viral replication.

Voxilaprevir is a noncovalent, reversible inhibitor of the NS3/4A protease, which is necessary for the proteolytic cleavage of the HCV-encoded polyprotein (into mature forms of the NS3, NS4A, NS4B, NS5A, and NS5B proteins) and is essential for viral replication.

Reproductive Considerations

HCV-infected females of childbearing potential should consider postponing pregnancy until therapy is complete to reduce the risk of HCV transmission (AASLD/IDSA 2018).

Pregnancy Considerations

Adverse events were not observed in animal reproduction studies using individual components of this combination. Refer to the sofosbuvir monograph for additional information.

Treatment of hepatitis C is not currently recommended to treat maternal infection or to decrease the risk of mother-to-child transmission during pregnancy (Tran 2016). When HCV infection is detected during pregnancy, treatment should be deferred until after delivery. Direct-acting antiviral medications should not be used in pregnant females outside of clinical trials until safety and efficacy information is available (SMFM [Hughes 2017]).

◆ **Solaraze [DSC]** *see* Diclofenac (Topical) *on page 489*

Solifenacin (sol i FEN a sin)

Brand Names: US VESIcare

Brand Names: Canada ACT Solifenacin [DSC]; APO-Solifenacin; Auro-Solifenacin; JAMP-Solifenacin; MED-Solifenacin; MINT-Solifenacin [DSC]; PMS-Solifenacin; SANDOZ Solifenacin; TARO-Solifenacin; TEVA-Solifenacin; VESIcare

Pharmacologic Category Anticholinergic Agent

Use

Neurogenic detrusor overactivity (oral suspension): Treatment of neurogenic detrusor overactivity in pediatric patients ≥2 years of age.

Overactive bladder (tablet): Treatment of overactive bladder with symptoms of urinary frequency, urgency, or urge incontinence in adults.

Local Anesthetic/Vasoconstrictor Precautions No information available to require special precautions

Effects on Dental Treatment Key adverse event(s) related to dental treatment: Xerostomia (normal salivary flow resumes upon discontinuation). Prolonged xerostomia may contribute to discomfort and dental disease (eg, caries, periodontal disease, and oral candidiasis).

Effects on Bleeding No information available to require special precautions

Adverse Reactions

>10%: Gastrointestinal: Constipation (5% to 13%, dose-dependent), xerostomia (11% to 28%, dose-dependent; children and adolescents: 3%)

1% to 10%:

Cardiovascular: Hypertension (1%), lower extremity edema (1%)

Gastrointestinal: Abdominal pain (1%), dyspepsia (4%), nausea (3%), upper abdominal pain (2%), vomiting (1%)

Genitourinary: Urinary retention (1%), urinary tract infection (2% to 5%)

Infection: Influenza (2%)

Nervous system: Depression (1%), drowsiness (1%), fatigue (2%)

Ophthalmic: Blurred vision (4% to 5%), dry eye syndrome (2%)

Respiratory: Cough (1%)

<1%, postmarketing, and/or case reports: Abnormal hepatic function tests, anaphylaxis, angioedema, atrial fibrillation, confusion, decreased appetite, delirium, dizziness, dry nose, dysgeusia, erythema multiforme, exfoliative dermatitis, fecal impaction, gastroesophageal reflux disease, gastrointestinal obstruction, glaucoma, hallucination, headache, hepatic disease, hyperkalemia, hypersensitivity reaction, increased gamma-glutamyl transferase, increased serum alanine aminotransferase, increased serum aspartate aminotransferase, intestinal obstruction, myasthenia, palpitations, peripheral edema, pharyngitis, prolonged QT interval on ECG, renal insufficiency, sialadenitis, tachycardia, torsades de pointes, voice disorder, xeroderma

Mechanism of Action Inhibits muscarinic receptors resulting in decreased urinary bladder contraction, increased residual urine volume, and decreased detrusor muscle pressure.

Pharmacodynamics/Kinetics

Half-life Elimination

Children ≥2 years and Adolescents ≤17 years: Oral suspension: Median: 26 hours; prolonged in severe kidney impairment (CrCl <30 mL/minute/1.73 m^2) or moderate hepatic impairment.

Adults: 45 to 68 hours following chronic dosing; prolonged in severe renal (CrCl <30 mL/minute) or moderate hepatic (Child-Pugh class B) impairment.

Time to Peak Plasma:

Children ≥2 years and Adolescents ≤17 years: Oral suspension: 2 to 6 hours.

Adults: Tablets: 3 to 8 hours.

Pregnancy Considerations Adverse events were observed in some animal reproduction studies.

Product Availability

Vesicare LS 5 mg/5 mL oral suspension: FDA approved May 2020; availability anticipated in late 2020.

◆ **Solifenacin Succinate** *see* Solifenacin *on page 1380*

◆ **Soliqua** *see* Insulin Glargine and Lixisenatide *on page 823*

◆ **Solodyn** *see* Minocycline (Systemic) *on page 1032*

◆ **Soloxide** *see* Doxycycline *on page 522*

◆ **Soltamox** *see* Tamoxifen *on page 1404*

◆ **Soluble Ferric Pyrophosphate (SFP)** *see* Ferric Pyrophosphate Citrate *on page 664*

◆ **Solu-CORTEF** *see* Hydrocortisone (Systemic) *on page 773*

◆ **Solumedrol** *see* MethylPREDNISolone *on page 999*

◆ **SOLU-Medrol** *see* MethylPREDNISolone *on page 999*

◆ **SoluVita E [OTC]** *see* Vitamin E (Systemic) *on page 1549*

◆ **Soluvite-F** *see* Vitamins (Fluoride) *on page 1550*

◆ **Solzira** *see* Gabapentin Enacarbil *on page 727*

◆ **Soma** *see* Carisoprodol *on page 293*

Somatropin (soe ma TROE pin)

Brand Names: US Genotropin; Genotropin MiniQuick; Humatrope; Norditropin FlexPro; Nutropin AQ NuSpin 10; Nutropin AQ NuSpin 20; Nutropin AQ NuSpin 5; Omnitrope; Saizen; Saizen Click.Easy [DSC]; Saizenprep; Serostim; Zomacton; Zomacton (for Zoma-Jet 10); Zorbtive

Brand Names: Canada Genotropin GoQuick; Genotropin MiniQuick; Humatrope; Norditropin NordiFlex Pen; Nutropin AQ NuSpin 10; Nutropin AQ NuSpin 20; Nutropin AQ NuSpin 5; Nutropin AQ Pen [DSC]; Omnitrope; Saizen; Serostim

Pharmacologic Category Growth Hormone

Use

Growth failure (pediatric patients):

Treatment of growth failure due to inadequate endogenous growth hormone secretion (Genotropin, Humatrope, Norditropin, Nutropin, Nutropin AQ, Omnitrope, Saizen, Tev-Tropin, Zomacton).

Treatment of short stature associated with Turner syndrome (Genotropin, Humatrope, Norditropin, Nutropin, Nutropin AQ, Omnitrope, Zomacton).

Treatment of Prader-Willi syndrome (Genotropin, Norditropin, Omnitrope).

Treatment of growth failure associated with chronic kidney disease up until the time of renal transplantation (Nutropin, Nutropin AQ).

Treatment of growth failure in children born small for gestational age who fail to manifest catch-up growth by 2 years of age (Genotropin, Omnitrope) or by 2 to 4 years of age (Humatrope, Norditropin, Zomacton)

Treatment of idiopathic short stature (nongrowth hormone-deficient short stature), defined by height standard deviation score (SDS) ≤-2.25 and growth rate not likely to attain adult height in the normal range, in pediatric patients whose epiphyses are not closed and for whom other causes associated with short stature have been excluded (Genotropin, Humatrope, Norditropin, Nutropin, Nutropin AQ, Omnitrope, Zomacton).

Treatment of short stature or growth failure associated with short stature homeobox gene (SHOX) deficiency (Humatrope, Zomacton).

Treatment of short stature associated with Noonan syndrome (Norditropin)

Growth hormone deficiency (adults): Replacement of endogenous growth hormone in adults with growth hormone deficiency who meet either of the following criteria (Genotropin, Humatrope, Norditropin, Nutropin, Nutropin AQ, Omnitrope, Saizen, Zomacton):

Adult-onset: Patients who have adult growth hormone deficiency whether alone or with multiple hormone deficiencies (hypopituitarism) as a result of pituitary disease, hypothalamic disease, surgery, radiation therapy, or trauma

or

Childhood-onset: Patients who were growth hormone deficient during childhood as a result of congenital, genetic, acquired, or idiopathic causes, confirmed as an adult before replacement therapy is initiated

HIV-associated wasting, cachexia: Treatment of HIV patients with wasting or cachexia (Serostim).

Short bowel syndrome: Treatment of short-bowel syndrome in patients receiving specialized nutritional support (Zorbtive).

Local Anesthetic/Vasoconstrictor Precautions No information available to require special precautions

Effects on Dental Treatment No significant effects or complications reported

Effects on Bleeding No information available to require special precautions

Adverse Reactions

>10%:

Cardiovascular: Peripheral edema (≤69%), facial edema (≤50%), edema (adults: ≤41%; children: ≤3%), lower extremity edema (adults: ≤15%)

Central nervous system: Pain (≤19%), hypoesthesia (≤15%), headache (adults: ≤18%; children: ≤7%), paresthesia (≤13%)

Endocrine & metabolic: Hypothyroidism (children: ≤16%; adults: ≤5%), elevated glycosylated hemoglobin (children: ≤14%), eosinophilia (children: ≤12%)
Gastrointestinal: Nausea (≤13%), flatulence (≤25%), abdominal pain (≤25%), vomiting (≤19%)
Immunologic: Antibody development (children: ≤24%; binding capacity ≥0.02 mg/mL: 2%; binding capacity >2 mg/mL: <1%)
Infection: Infection (adults: ≤13%)
Local: Pain at injection site (≤31%), injection site reaction (≤19%)
Neuromuscular & skeletal: Arthralgia (≤44%), arthropathy (adults: ≤27%; children: 11%), myalgia (≤30%), scoliosis (children: ≤19%; exacerbation or new), limb pain (4% to 19%), swelling of extremities (18%), ostealgia (adults: ≤11%)
Otic: Otitis media (children: ≤16%)
Respiratory: Upper respiratory tract infection (≤16%)

1% to 10%:
Cardiovascular: Chest pain (adults: ≤5%), hypertension (≤8%)
Central nervous system: Fatigue (6% to 9%), nipple pain (≤6%), depression (adults: ≤5%), insomnia (adults: ≤5%), carpal tunnel syndrome (1% to <5%), sleep apnea (adults)
Dermatologic: Diaphoresis (≤8%), melanocytic nevus (≤2%)
Endocrine & metabolic: Impaired glucose tolerance/prediabetes (10%), hyperglycemia (1% to 9%), hyperlipidemia (children: ≤8%), gynecomastia (≤6%), dependent edema (adults: ≤5%), diabetes mellitus (≤5%; includes exacerbation and new-onset), hypertriglyceridemia (≤5%), fluid retention (3% to 5%)
Genitourinary: Breast hypertrophy (≤6%), breast neoplasm (≤6%), breast swelling (≤6%), breast tenderness (≤6%), mastalgia (≤6%), urinary tract infection (children: ≤3%)
Hematologic & oncologic: Hematoma (children: ≤9%)
Infection: Influenza (children: ≤3%)
Neuromuscular & skeletal: Stiffness (adults: ≤8%; includes extremities and musculoskeletal), joint stiffness (4% to 8%), joint swelling (5% to 6%), lower extremity pain (children: ≤5%), arthralgia of hip (children: ≤3%), tonsillitis (children: ≤3%), abnormal bone growth (children: ≤2%; including disproportional growth of lower jaw)
Ophthalmic: Periorbital edema (1% to <5%)
Otic: Otitis (children: ≤3%)
Respiratory: Bronchitis (9%), flu-like symptoms (≤8%), sinusitis (children: ≤3%), dyspnea (adults)

Frequency not defined:
Central nervous system: Aggressive behavior (children), seizure (children)
Dermatologic: Alopecia (children), exacerbation of psoriasis (children), rash at injection site (children)
Endocrine & metabolic: Fluid volume disorder (children), glycosuria (adults), hypoglycemia (children)
Gastrointestinal: Gastroenteritis (children)
Genitourinary: Hematuria (children)
Hematologic & oncologic: Meningioma (children)
Local: Bleeding at injection site (children), burning sensation at injection site (children), erythema at injection site (children), fibrosis at injection site (children), inflammation at injection site (children), injection site nodule (children), injection site numbness (children), local skin hyperpigmentation (children; injection site), swelling at injection site (children)
Neuromuscular & skeletal: Asthenia (adults), lipoatrophy (children), musculoskeletal disease (discomfort)
Respiratory: Pharyngitis (children)

<1%, postmarketing, and/or case reports: Anaphylaxis, angioedema, arthritis, avascular necrosis of femoral head (Legg-Calve-Perthes disease), benign neoplasm (children; new or recurring), bone fracture, brain neoplasm, cardiac disease, CNS neoplasm (children), decreased T4, diabetic coma, diabetic ketoacidosis, diabetic retinopathy, hypersensitivity reaction, illness (acute critical), increased serum alkaline phosphatase, intracranial hypertension (includes benign intracranial hypertension in children), leukemia, malignant neoplasm (includes new or recurring), nerve compression, pancreatitis, papilledema, precocious puberty, slipped capital femoral epiphysis, visual disturbance

Mechanism of Action Somatropin is a purified polypeptide hormones of recombinant DNA origin; somatropin contains the identical sequence of amino acids found in human growth hormone; human growth hormone assists growth of linear bone, skeletal muscle, and organs by stimulating chondrocyte proliferation and differentiation, lipolysis, protein synthesis, and hepatic glucose output; stimulates erythropoietin which increases red blood cell mass; exerts both insulin-like and diabetogenic effects; enhances the transmucosal transport of water, electrolytes, and nutrients across the gut

Pharmacodynamics/Kinetics

Half-life Elimination
Genotropin: SubQ: 3 hours
Humatrope: SubQ: 3.8 hours
Norditropin: SubQ: ~7 to 10 hours
Nutropin, Nutropin AQ: SubQ: 2.1 ± 0.43 hours
Omnitrope: SubQ: 2.5 to 2.8 hours
Saizen: SubQ: ~2 hours
Serostim: SubQ: 4.28 ± 2.15 hours
Zomacton: SubQ: ~2.7 hours
Zorbtive: SubQ: 4 ± 2 hours

Reproductive Considerations Adequate somatropin use prior to conception may improve fertility in women with hypopituitarism (Vila 2019).

Pregnancy Considerations During normal pregnancy, maternal production of endogenous growth hormone decreases as placental growth hormone production increases. Data with somatropin use during pregnancy in women with hypopituitarism is limited; however, adequate replacement prior to conception may improve fertility (Vila 2019). The Endocrine Society guidelines for hormonal replacement in hypopituitarism suggest discontinuation of somatropin during pregnancy (ES [Fleseriu 2016]).

Product Availability Nutropin (lyophilized powder) has been discontinued in the US for more than 1 year.

◆ **Sominex [OTC] [DSC]** *see* DiphenhydrAMINE (Systemic) *on page 502*

◆ **Sonata [DSC]** *see* Zaleplon *on page 1566*

Sonidegib (soe ni DEG ib)

Brand Names: US Odomzo

Pharmacologic Category Antineoplastic Agent, Hedgehog Pathway Inhibitor

Use Basal cell carcinoma, locally advanced: Treatment of adult patients with locally advanced basal cell carcinoma (BCC) that has recurred following surgery or radiation therapy, or those who are not candidates for surgery or radiation therapy.

Local Anesthetic/Vasoconstrictor Precautions No information available to require special precautions

Effects on Dental Treatment No significant effects or complications reported

Effects on Bleeding No information available to require special precautions

Adverse Reactions

>10%:

Central nervous system: Fatigue (41%), headache (15%), pain (14%)

Dermatologic: Alopecia (53%)

Endocrine & metabolic: Hyperglycemia (51%), weight loss (30%), increased serum ALT (19%), increased serum AST (19%), increased amylase (16%)

Gastrointestinal: Dysgeusia (46%), increased serum lipase (43%), nausea (39%), diarrhea (32%), decreased appetite (23%), abdominal pain (18%), vomiting (11%)

Hematologic & oncologic: Anemia (32%), lymphocytopenia (28%, grades 3/4: 3%)

Neuromuscular & skeletal: Increased creatine phosphokinase (61%, grades 3/4: 8%), muscle spasm (54%; grade 3: 3%), musculoskeletal pain (32%, grade 3: 1%), myalgia (19%)

Renal: Increased serum creatinine (92%)

1% to 10%:

Dermatologic: Pruritus (10%)

<1%, postmarketing, and/or case reports: Amenorrhea, rhabdomyolysis

Mechanism of Action Basal cell cancer is associated with mutations in Hedgehog pathway components. Hedgehog regulates cell growth and differentiation in embryogenesis; while generally not active in adult tissue, Hedgehog mutations associated with basal cell cancer can activate the pathway resulting in unrestricted proliferation of skin basal cells (Von Hoff, 2009). Sonidegib is a selective Hedgehog pathway inhibitor which binds to and inhibits Smoothened homologue (SMO), the transmembrane protein involved in Hedgehog signal transduction.

Pharmacodynamics/Kinetics

Half-life Elimination ~28 days

Time to Peak 2 to 4 hours

Reproductive Considerations

[US Boxed Warning]: Verify the pregnancy status of females of reproductive potential prior to initiating therapy. Advise females of reproductive potential to use effective contraception during treatment with sonidegib and for at least 20 months after the last dose. Advise males of the potential risk of exposure through semen and to use condoms with a pregnant partner or a female partner of reproductive potential during treatment with sonidegib and for at least 8 months after the last dose.

Amenorrhea lasting for at least 18 months was observed in women of reproductive potential.

It is not known if sonidegib is present in semen. Males with female partners of reproductive potential should use condoms even following a vasectomy. Advise male patients not to donate sperm during sonidegib treatment and for at least 8 months after the last sonidegib dose.

Pregnancy Considerations

[US Boxed Warning]: Sonidegib can cause embryo-fetal death or severe birth defects when administered to a pregnant woman. Sonidegib is embryotoxic, fetotoxic, and teratogenic in animals. Based on the mechanism of action and data from animal reproduction studies, in utero exposure to sonidegib may cause fetal harm.

Data collection to monitor pregnancy and infant outcomes following exposure to sonidegib is ongoing. Health care providers should notify the manufacturer of pregnancies which may occur following exposure to sonidegib (800-406-7984).

◆ **Sonidegib Phosphate** *see* Sonidegib *on page 1382*

◆ **Soothe & Cool INZO Antifungal [OTC]** *see* Miconazole (Topical) *on page 1019*

SORAfenib (sor AF e nib)

Related Information

Osteonecrosis of the Jaw *on page 1699*

Brand Names: US NexAVAR

Brand Names: Canada NexAVAR

Pharmacologic Category Antineoplastic Agent, Tyrosine Kinase Inhibitor; Antineoplastic Agent, Vascular Endothelial Growth Factor (VEGF) Inhibitor

Use

Hepatocellular carcinoma: Treatment of unresectable hepatocellular carcinoma (HCC).

Renal cell carcinoma, advanced: Treatment of advanced renal cell carcinoma (RCC).

Thyroid carcinoma, differentiated: Treatment of locally recurrent or metastatic, progressive, differentiated thyroid carcinoma (refractory to radioactive iodine treatment).

Local Anesthetic/Vasoconstrictor Precautions Sorafenib may cause hypertension; monitor blood pressure prior to vasoconstrictor use

Effects on Dental Treatment Key adverse event(s) related to dental treatment: Mouth pain, mucositis, stomatitis, xerostomia (normal salivary flow resumes upon discontinuation), and dysphagia.

Effects on Bleeding Chemotherapy may result in significant myelosuppression, potentially including significant reduction in platelet counts (thrombocytopenia grades 3/4: 1% to 4%) and altered hemostasis. In patients who are under active treatment with these agents, medical consult is suggested.

Adverse Reactions

>10%:

Cardiovascular: Hypertension (9% to 41%; grade 3: 3% to 4%; grade 4: <1%; grades 3/4: 10%, onset: ~3 weeks)

Central nervous system: Fatigue (37% to 46%), headache (≤10% to 17%), mouth pain (14%), voice disorder (13%), peripheral sensory neuropathy (≤13%), pain (11%)

Dermatologic: Palmar-plantar erythrodysesthesia (21% to 69%; grade 3: 6% to 8%; grades 3/4: 19%), alopecia (14% to 67%), skin rash (including desquamation; 19% to 40%; grade 3: ≤1%; grades 3/4: 5%), pruritus (14% to 20%), xeroderma (10% to 13%), erythema (≥10%)

Endocrine & metabolic: Hypoalbuminemia (≤59%), weight loss (10% to 49%), hypophosphatemia (35% to 45%; grade 3: 11% to 13%; grade 4: <1%), increased thyroid stimulating hormone level (>0.5 mU/L: 41%; due to impairment of exogenous thyroid suppression), hypocalcemia (12% to 36%), increased amylase (30% to 34% [usually transient])

Gastrointestinal: Diarrhea (43% to 68%; grade 3: 2% to 10%; grade 4: <1%), increased serum lipase (40% to 41% [usually transient]), abdominal pain (11% to 31%), decreased appetite (30%), anorexia (16% to 29%), stomatitis (24%), nausea (21% to 24%), constipation (14% to 16%), vomiting (11% to 16%)

Hematologic & oncologic: Lymphocytopenia (23% to 47%; grades 3/4: ≤13%), thrombocytopenia (12% to 46%; grades 3/4: 1% to 4%), increased INR (≤42%), neutropenia (≤18%; grades 3/4: ≤5%), hemorrhage (15% to 17%; grade 3: 2%), leukopenia

Hepatic: Increased serum ALT (59%; grades 3/4: 4%), increased serum AST (54%; grades 3/4: 2%), hepatic insufficiency (≤11%; grade 3: 2%; grade 4: 1%)

Infection: Infection

Neuromuscular & skeletal: Limb pain (15%), weakness (12%), myalgia

Respiratory: Dyspnea (≤14%), cough (≤13%)

Miscellaneous: Fever (11%)

1% to 10%:

Cardiovascular: Ischemic heart disease (including myocardial infarction; ≤3%), cardiac failure (2%, congestive), flushing

Central nervous system: Depression, glossalgia

Dermatologic: Hyperkeratosis (7%), acne vulgaris, exfoliative dermatitis, folliculitis

Endocrine & metabolic: Hypokalemia (5% to 10%), hyponatremia, hypothyroidism

Gastrointestinal: Dysgeusia (6%), dyspepsia, dysphagia, gastroesophageal reflux disease, mucositis, xerostomia

Genitourinary: Erectile dysfunction, proteinuria

Hematologic & oncologic: Squamous cell carcinoma of skin (3%; grades 3/4: 3%), anemia

Hepatic: Increased serum transaminases (transient)

Neuromuscular & skeletal: Muscle spasm (10%), arthralgia (≤10%), myalgia

Renal: Renal failure

Respiratory: Epistaxis (7%), flu-like symptoms, hoarseness, rhinorrhea

<1%, postmarketing, and/or case reports: Acute renal failure, anaphylaxis, angioedema, aortic dissection, amyotrophy, cardiac arrhythmia, cardiac failure, cerebral hemorrhage, cholangitis, cholecystitis, dehydration, eczema, erythema multiforme, gastritis, gastrointestinal hemorrhage, gastrointestinal perforation, gynecomastia, hepatic failure, hepatitis, hypersensitivity reaction (skin reaction, urticaria), hypertensive crisis, hyperthyroidism, increased serum alkaline phosphatase, increased serum bilirubin, interstitial pulmonary disease (acute respiratory distress, interstitial pneumonia, lung inflammation, pneumonitis, pulmonitis, radiation pneumonitis), jaundice, malignant neoplasm of skin (keratoacanthomas), nephrotic syndrome, ostealgia, osteonecrosis of the jaw, pancreatitis, pleural effusion, prolonged QT interval on ECG, respiratory tract hemorrhage, reversible posterior leukoencephalopathy syndrome, rhabdomyolysis, Stevens-Johnson syndrome, thromboembolism, tinnitus, toxic epidermal necrolysis, transient ischemic attacks, tumor lysis syndrome, tumor pain

Mechanism of Action Sorafenib is a multikinase inhibitor that inhibits tumor growth and angiogenesis by inhibiting intracellular Raf kinases (CRAF, BRAF, and mutant BRAF), and cell surface kinase receptors (VEGFR-1, VEGFR-2, VEGFR-3, PDGFR-beta, cKIT, FLT-3, RET, and RET/PTC)

Pharmacodynamics/Kinetics

Half-life Elimination 25 to 48 hours

Time to Peak ~3 hours

Reproductive Considerations

Evaluate pregnancy status in females of reproductive potential prior to initiating sorafenib treatment. Females of reproductive potential should use effective contraception during treatment and for 6 months after the final sorafenib dose. Males with female partners of reproductive potential should use effective contraception during treatment and for 3 months after the last sorafenib dose.

Pregnancy Considerations

Information related to sorafenib use in pregnancy is limited (Mahdi 2018). Based on the mechanism of action and findings from animal reproduction studies, in utero exposure to sorafenib may cause fetal harm. Sorafenib inhibits angiogenesis, which is a critical component of fetal development.

Prescribing and Access Restrictions Available from specialty pharmacies. Further information may be obtained at 1-866-639-2827 or www.nexavar-us.-com.

◆ **Sorafenib Tosylate** *see* SORAfenib *on page 1383*

◆ **Sore Throat Relief [OTC] [DSC]** *see* Benzocaine *on page 228*

◆ **Sorine** *see* Sotalol *on page 1384*

Sotalol (SOE ta lole)

Related Information

Cardiovascular Diseases *on page 1654*

Clinical Risk Related to Drugs Prolonging QT Interval *on page 1675*

Brand Names: US Betapace; Betapace AF; Sorine; Sotylize

Brand Names: Canada APO-Sotalol; CO Sotalol [DSC]; DOM-Sotalol; JAMP-Sotalol; MED Sotalol; MYLAN-Sotalol [DSC]; PMS-Sotalol; PRO-Sotalol; RATIO-Sotalol; RIVA-Sotalol; SANDOZ Sotalol [DSC]

Pharmacologic Category Antiarrhythmic Agent, Class II; Antiarrhythmic Agent, Class III; Beta-Adrenergic Blocker, Nonselective

Use

Atrial fibrillation/flutter, symptomatic: Maintenance of normal sinus rhythm (delay in time to recurrence of atrial fibrillation/atrial flutter) in patients with symptomatic atrial fibrillation/atrial flutter who are currently in sinus rhythm.

According to the American Heart Association/American College of Cardiology/Heart Rhythm Society (AHA/ACC/HRS), sotalol is not effective for conversion of atrial fibrillation to sinus rhythm but may be used to prevent atrial fibrillation (AHA/ACC/HRS [January 2014])

Ventricular arrhythmias: Treatment of documented, life-threatening ventricular arrhythmias (ie, sustained ventricular tachycardia)

Local Anesthetic/Vasoconstrictor Precautions Use with caution; epinephrine has interacted with nonselective beta-blockers to result in initial hypertensive episode followed by bradycardia. Sotalol is one of the drugs confirmed to prolong the QT interval and is accepted as having a risk of causing torsade de pointes. The risk of drug-induced torsade de pointes is extremely low when a single QT interval prolonging drug is prescribed. In terms of epinephrine, it is not known what effect vasoconstrictors in the local anesthetic regimen will have in patients with a known history of congenital prolonged QT interval or in patients taking any medication that prolongs the QT interval. Until more information is obtained, it is suggested that the clinician consult with the physician prior to the use of a vasoconstrictor in suspected patients, and that the vasoconstrictor (epinephrine, mepivacaine and levonordefrin [Carbocaine 2% with Neo-Cobefrin]) be used with caution.

Effects on Dental Treatment Sotalol is a nonselective beta-blocker and may enhance the pressor response to epinephrine, resulting in hypertension and bradycardia. Many nonsteroidal anti-inflammatory drugs, such as ibuprofen and indomethacin, can reduce the hypotensive effect of beta-blockers after 3 or more weeks of therapy with the NSAID. Short-term NSAID use (ie, 3 days) requires no special precautions in patients taking beta-blockers.

Adverse Reactions There is minimal clinical experience with IV sotalol; however, since exposure is similar between IV and oral sotalol, adverse reactions are expected to be similar.

>10%:
- Cardiovascular: Bradycardia (dose related; 8% to 13%), chest pain (8%), palpitations (8%)
- Nervous system: Dizziness (13% to 16%), fatigue (dose related; 19% to 26%), headache (12%)
- Neuromuscular & skeletal: Asthenia (5% to 11%)
- Respiratory: Dyspnea (dose related; 9% to 18%)

1% to 10%:
- Cardiovascular: Complete atrioventricular block (1%), second degree atrioventricular block (1%), torsades de pointes (dose related; ≤4%), ventricular tachycardia (new or worsened: ≤1%)
- Dermatologic: Diaphoresis (5%)
- Gastrointestinal: Abdominal pain (4%), diarrhea (5% to 6%), nausea and vomiting (6% to 8%)
- Neuromuscular & skeletal: Musculoskeletal pain (4%)
- Ophthalmic: Visual disturbance (5%)

<1%:
- Cardiovascular: Sinoatrial arrest, sinus node dysfunction, sinus pause
- Nervous system: Peripheral neuropathy

Frequency not defined: Cardiovascular: Cardiac failure, hypotension, prolonged QT interval on ECG, sinus bradycardia

Postmarketing:
- Dermatologic: Alopecia, pruritus, skin photosensitivity
- Endocrine & metabolic: Hyperlipidemia
- Hematologic & oncologic: Eosinophilia, leukopenia, thrombocytopenia
- Nervous system: Altered mental status, ataxia, emotional lability, paralysis, vertigo
- Neuromuscular & skeletal: Myalgia
- Respiratory: Pulmonary edema
- Miscellaneous: Fever

Mechanism of Action

Beta-blocker which contains both beta-adrenoreceptor-blocking (Vaughan Williams Class II) and cardiac action potential duration prolongation (Vaughan Williams Class III) properties

Class II effects: Increased sinus cycle length, slowed heart rate, decreased AV nodal conduction, and increased AV nodal refractoriness Sotalol has both $beta_1$- and $beta_2$-receptor blocking activity. The beta-blocking effect of sotalol is a noncardioselective (half maximal at about 80 mg/day and maximal at doses of 320 to 640 mg/day). Significant beta-blockade occurs at oral doses as low as 25 mg/day.

Class III effects: Prolongation of the atrial and ventricular monophasic action potentials, and effective refractory prolongation of atrial muscle, ventricular muscle, and atrioventricular accessory pathways in both the antegrade and retrograde directions. Sotalol is a racemic mixture of *d*- and *l*-sotalol; both isomers have similar Class III antiarrhythmic effects while the *l*-isomer is responsible for virtually all of the beta-blocking activity. The Class III effects are seen only at oral doses ≥160 mg/day.

Pharmacodynamics/Kinetics

Onset of Action

Oral: Rapid; at 1 to 2 hours post dosing (steady-state), reductions in heart rate and cardiac index seen (Winters 1993)

IV: When administered IV over 5 minutes for ongoing VT, onset of action is ~5 to 10 minutes (Ho 1994)

Half-life Elimination

Oral:
- Neonates ≤1 month: 8.4 hours (Saul 2001b)
- Infants and Children >1 month to 24 months: 7.4 hours (Saul 2001b)
- Children >2 years to <7 years: 9.1 hours (Saul 2001b)
- Children 7 to 12 years: 9.2 hours (Saul 2001b)
- Adults: 12 hours
- Adults with renal failure (anuric): Up to 69 hours

IV: Pharmacokinetics of the IV formulation (administered over 5 hours) are similar to the oral formulations (Somberg 2010).

Time to Peak Serum: Oral: Infants and Children 3 days to 12 years: Mean range: 2 to 3 hours; Adults: 2.5 to 4 hours

Reproductive Considerations Beta-blockers, including sotalol, may cause erectile dysfunction.

Pregnancy Considerations Sotalol crosses the placenta.

Adverse fetal/neonatal events have been reported with beta-blockers as a class. If maternal use of a beta-blocker is needed, fetal growth should be monitored during pregnancy and the newborn should be monitored for 48 hours after delivery for bradycardia, hypoglycemia, and respiratory depression (ESC [Regitz-Zagrosek 2018]).

Because sotalol crosses the placenta in concentrations similar to the maternal serum, it has been studied for the treatment of fetal atrial flutter or fetal supraventricular tachycardia (SVT). Sotalol may be considered for the in utero management of fetal SVT or atrial flutter with hydrops or ventricular dysfunction. Sotalol may also be considered for SVT without hydrops or ventricular dysfunction if heart rate is ≥200 bpm, atrial flutter, or other rare tachycardias with an average heart rate of ≥200 bpm. In addition, sotalol may be considered fetal ventricular tachycardia (VT) with normal QTc with or without hydrops but is contraindicated for the treatment of fetal VT when long QT syndrome is suspected or confirmed (AHA [Donofrio 2014]).

The pharmacokinetic properties of sotalol are not significantly altered by pregnancy (O'Hare 1983). Sotalol may be used for the treatment of maternal ventricular arrhythmias, atrial fibrillation/atrial flutter, or supraventricular tachycardia during pregnancy; consult current guidelines for specific recommendations (ACC/AHA/HRS [Page 2015]; ESC [Regitz-Zagrosek 2018]).

Dental Health Professional Considerations See Local Anesthetic/Vasoconstrictor Precautions

◆ **Sotalol HCl** *see* Sotalol *on page* 1384

◆ **Sotalol Hydrochloride** *see* Sotalol *on page* 1384

◆ **Sotylize** *see* Sotalol *on page* 1384

◆ **Sovaldi** *see* Sofosbuvir *on page* 1378

◆ **SPD417** *see* CarBAMazepine *on page* 288

◆ **Spectazole** *see* Econazole *on page* 542

◆ **Spectracef** *see* Cefditoren *on page* 306

◆ **SPI 0211** *see* Lubiprostone *on page* 941

Spiramycin (speer a MYE sin)

Brand Names: Canada Rovamycine 250; Rovamycine 500

Pharmacologic Category Antibiotic, Macrolide

Use Note: Not approved in the US

Treatment of infections of the respiratory tract, buccal cavity, skin and soft tissues due to susceptible organisms. *N. gonorrhoeae*: as an alternate choice of treatment for gonorrhea in patients allergic to the penicillins. Before treatment of gonorrhea, the possibility of concomitant infection due to *T. pallidum* should be excluded

Local Anesthetic/Vasoconstrictor Precautions No information available to require special precautions

Effects on Dental Treatment No significant effects or complications reported

Effects on Bleeding No information available to require special precautions

Adverse Reactions

Frequency not defined.

Central nervous system: Paresthesia (transient)

Dermatologic: Pruritus, skin rash, urticaria

Gastrointestinal: Diarrhea, nausea, vomiting

<1%, postmarketing, and/or case reports: Abnormal hepatic function tests, anaphylactic shock, angioedema, *Clostridioides* (formerly *Clostridium*) *difficile* colitis, hemolysis (acute), Henoch-Schonlein purpura, hepatotoxicity (idiosyncratic; Chalasani 2014), vasculitis

Mechanism of Action Inhibits growth of susceptible organisms; mechanism not established.

Pregnancy Considerations Spiramycin concentrates in the placenta but does not transfer in sufficient quantities to treat fetal infection. Spiramycin is recommended for the treatment of acute toxoplasmosis infection in pregnant women to decrease placental parasitic transfer. Treatment should continue until delivery. Agents other than spiramycin are recommended if fetal infection has occurred or when maternal infection is acquired ≥18 weeks gestation (ACOG 151 2015; HHS [OI adult 2020]; Mandelbrot 2018; Montoya 2008; SOGC [Paquet 285 2018]).

Product Availability Not available in the US

Prescribing and Access Restrictions Spiramycin is not commercially available in the US; it is available for treatment of toxoplasmosis in pregnant women through the US Food and Drug Administration (301-796-1400).

◆ **Spiriva HandiHaler** *see* Tiotropium *on page* 1450

◆ **Spiriva Respimat** *see* Tiotropium *on page* 1450

Spironolactone (speer on oh LAK tone)

Related Information

Cardiovascular Diseases *on page* 1654

Brand Names: US Aldactone; CaroSpir

Brand Names: Canada Aldactone; MINT-Spironolactone; TEVA-Spironolactone

Pharmacologic Category Antihypertensive; Diuretic, Potassium-Sparing; Mineralocorticoid (Aldosterone) Receptor Antagonists

Use

Ascites due to cirrhosis: Management of edema in cirrhosis of the liver unresponsive to fluid and sodium restriction.

Heart failure with reduced ejection fraction: To increase survival, manage edema, and reduce need for hospitalization in patients with heart failure with reduced ejection fraction and New York Heart Association class III to IV symptoms; usually administered in conjunction with other heart failure therapies.

Hypertension: Management of hypertension unresponsive to other therapies.

Primary hyperaldosteronism (tablet only): Short-term preoperative treatment of primary hyperaldosteronism; long-term maintenance therapy for patients with discrete aldosterone-producing adrenal adenomas who are not candidates for surgery; long-term maintenance therapy for bilateral micro- or macronodular adrenal hyperplasia (idiopathic hyperaldosteronism).

Local Anesthetic/Vasoconstrictor Precautions No information available to require special precautions

Effects on Dental Treatment No significant effects or complications reported

Effects on Bleeding No information available to require special precautions

Adverse Reactions

1% to 10%: Endocrine & metabolic: Gynecomastia (9%; dose and duration related)

Frequency not defined:

Cardiovascular: Vasculitis

Dermatologic: Chloasma, erythematous maculopapular rash, pruritus, Stevens-Johnson syndrome, toxic epidermal necrolysis, urticaria

Endocrine & metabolic: Amenorrhea (Levitt 1970), decreased libido, gout, hyperglycemia, hyperkalemia, hyperuricemia, hypocalcemia, hypomagnesemia, hyponatremia, hypovolemia

Gastrointestinal: Abdominal cramps, diarrhea, gastritis, gastrointestinal hemorrhage, gastrointestinal ulcer, nausea, vomiting

Genitourinary: Erectile dysfunction, irregular menses, mastalgia, postmenopausal bleeding

Hematologic & oncologic: Agranulocytosis (Whitling 1997), leukopenia, thrombocytopenia

Hepatic: Hepatotoxicity

Hypersensitivity: Anaphylaxis

Immunologic: Drug reaction with eosinophilia and systemic symptoms

Nervous system: Ataxia, confusion, dizziness, drowsiness, headache, lethargy, nipple pain

Neuromuscular & skeletal: Lower limb cramp

Renal: Renal failure syndrome, renal insufficiency

Miscellaneous: Fever

Postmarketing: Metabolic acidosis (in patients with cirrhosis) (Feinfeld 1978; Gabow 1979)

Mechanism of Action Competes with aldosterone for receptor sites in the distal renal tubules, increasing sodium chloride and water excretion while conserving potassium and hydrogen ions; may block the effect of aldosterone on arteriolar smooth muscle as well

Pharmacodynamics/Kinetics

Duration of Action Tablet: 2 to 3 days

Half-life Elimination

Tablet: Spironolactone: 1.4 hours; Canrenone: 16.5 hours (terminal); 7-alpha-spirolactone: 13.8 hours (terminal)

Suspension: Spironolactone: 1 to 2 hours; Canrenone, 7-alpha-spirolactone, and 6-beta-hydroxy-7-alpha: 10 to 35 hours

Time to Peak Serum:

Tablet: 2.6 to 4.3 hours (primarily as active metabolites)

Suspension: Spironolactone: 0.5 to 1.5 hours; Canrenone: 2.5 to 5 hours

Reproductive Considerations

Use of spironolactone is associated with menstrual irregularities (dose dependent); contraception is recommended when used in premenopausal women for the treatment of conditions such as hirsutism and acne (AAD [Zaenglein 2016]; Endocrine Society [Martin 2018]).

Women who require use of spironolactone for the treatment of primary hyperaldosteronism should use the lowest effective dose prior to a planned pregnancy, then stop treatment once the pregnancy is confirmed (Riester 2015).

Pregnancy Considerations

Spironolactone crosses the placenta (Regitz-Zagrosek [ESC 2018]).

Based on the mechanism of action and data from animal reproduction studies, in utero exposure to spironolactone may cause feminization of a male fetus (limited human data; Liszewski 2019).

Chronic maternal hypertension is associated with adverse events in the fetus/infant. The risk of birth defects, low birth weight, premature delivery, stillbirth, and neonatal death may be increased with chronic hypertension in pregnancy. Actual risks may be related to duration and severity of maternal hypertension. The use of mineralocorticoid receptor antagonists for the treatment of hypertension in pregnancy is generally not recommended (ACOG 203 2019).

The treatment of edema associated with chronic heart failure during pregnancy is similar to that of nonpregnant patients. However, the use of mineralocorticoid receptor antagonists is not recommended. Patients diagnosed after delivery can be treated according to heart failure guidelines (ESC [Bauersachs 2016]; ESC [Regitz-Zagrosek 2018]).

Information related to the use of mineralocorticoid receptor antagonists for the treatment of primary hyperaldosteronism in pregnancy is limited. Women who require use of spironolactone for the treatment of primary hyperaldosteronism should stop treatment during the first trimester once the pregnancy is confirmed. Use of a mineralocorticoid receptor antagonist can be considered again in the second and third trimesters if necessary; high doses have been associated with intrauterine growth restriction (monitor) (Riester 2015).

- ◆ **SPM 927** *see* Lacosamide *on page 868*
- ◆ **Sporanox** *see* Itraconazole *on page 849*
- ◆ **Sporanox Pulsepak** *see* Itraconazole *on page 849*
- ◆ **SPP100** *see* Aliskiren *on page 102*
- ◆ **Spravato** *see* Esketamine *on page 591*
- ◆ **Spravato (56 MG Dose)** *see* Esketamine *on page 591*
- ◆ **Spravato (84 MG Dose)** *see* Esketamine *on page 591*
- ◆ **Sprintec 28** *see* Ethinyl Estradiol and Norgestimate *on page 616*
- ◆ **Spritam** *see* LevETIRAcetam *on page 894*
- ◆ **Sprycel** *see* Dasatinib *on page 443*
- ◆ **SQV** *see* Saquinavir *on page 1357*
- ◆ **SR33589** *see* Dronedarone *on page 533*
- ◆ **Sronyx** *see* Ethinyl Estradiol and Levonorgestrel *on page 612*
- ◆ **SS734** *see* Besifloxacin *on page 232*
- ◆ **ST 1435** *see* Segesterone Acetate and Ethinyl Estradiol *on page 1362*
- ◆ **Stadol** *see* Butorphanol *on page 275*
- ◆ **Stalevo** *see* Levodopa, Carbidopa, and Entacapone *on page 897*
- ◆ **StanGard Perio** *see* Fluoride *on page 693*
- ◆ **Stannous Fluoride** *see* Fluoride *on page 693*
- ◆ **Starlix** *see* Nateglinide *on page 1087*

Stavudine (STAV yoo deen)

Related Information

HIV Infection and AIDS *on page 1690*

Brand Names: US Zerit [DSC]

Brand Names: Canada Zerit XR [DSC]; Zerit [DSC]

Pharmacologic Category Antiretroviral, Reverse Transcriptase Inhibitor, Nucleoside (Anti-HIV)

Use HIV-1: Treatment of HIV-1 infection in combination with other antiretroviral agents. **Note:** Stavudine is no longer recommended for use in the treatment of HIV (HHS [adult] 2019).

Local Anesthetic/Vasoconstrictor Precautions

No information available to require special precautions

Effects on Dental Treatment No significant effects or complications reported

Effects on Bleeding No information available to require special precautions relative to hemostasis.

Adverse Reactions Adverse reactions reported below represent experience with combination therapy with other nucleoside analogues and protease inhibitors.

>10%:

Central nervous system: Headache (25% to 46%), peripheral neuropathy (8% to 21%)

Dermatologic: Skin rash (18% to 30%)

Endocrine & metabolic: Increased amylase (21% to 31%; grades 3/4: 4% to 8%), increased gamma-glutamyl transferase (15% to 28%; grades 3/4: 2% to 5%)

Gastrointestinal: Nausea (43% to 53%), diarrhea (34% to 45%), vomiting (18% to 30%), increased serum lipase (27%; grades 3/4: 5% to 6%)

Hepatic: Hyperbilirubinemia (65% to 68%; grades 3/4: 7% to 16%), increased serum AST (42% to 53%; grades 3/4: 5% to 7%), increased serum ALT (40% to 50%; grades 3/4: 6% to 8%)

<1%, postmarketing, and/or case reports: Abdominal pain, anemia, anorexia, chills, diabetes mellitus, fever, hepatic failure, hepatitis, hepatomegaly with steatosis (some fatal), hyperglycemia, hyperlipidemia, hypersensitivity reaction, immune reconstitution syndrome, insomnia, insulin resistance, lactic acidosis (some

fatal), leukopenia, lipoatrophy, lipotrophy, macrocytosis, myalgia, neutropenia, pancreatitis (some fatal), redistribution of body fat, severe weakness (severe neuromuscular weakness resembling Guillain-Barré), thrombocytopenia

Mechanism of Action Stavudine is a thymidine analog which interferes with HIV viral DNA dependent DNA polymerase resulting in inhibition of viral replication; nucleoside reverse transcriptase inhibitor

Pharmacodynamics/Kinetics

Half-life Elimination

Note: Half-life is prolonged with renal dysfunction
Newborns (at birth): 5.3 ± 2 hours
Neonates 14 to 28 days old: 1.6 ± 0.3 hours
Children 5 weeks to 15 years: 0.9 ± 0.3 hours
Adults: 1.6 ± 0.2 hours
Intracellular: Adults: 3.5 to 7 hours

Time to Peak Serum: 1 hour

Reproductive Considerations

Based on the Health and Humans Services perinatal HIV guidelines, stavudine is not one of the recommended antiretroviral agents for use in females living with HIV who are trying to conceive (HHS [perinatal] 2019).

For males and females living with HIV and planning a pregnancy, maximum viral suppression below the limits of detection with antiretroviral therapy (ART), modification of therapy (if needed), optimization of the woman's health, and a discussion of the potential risks and benefits of ART therapy during pregnancy is recommended prior to conception (HHS [perinatal] 2019).

Pregnancy Considerations Stavudine crosses the human placenta.

[US Boxed Warning]: Fatal lactic acidosis has been reported in pregnant individuals using didanosine and stavudine in combination with other antiretroviral agents; coadministration of stavudine and didanosine is contraindicated.

Outcome information specific to stavudine use in pregnancy is no longer being reviewed and updated in the Health and Humans Services (HHS) perinatal guidelines. Maternal antiretroviral therapy (ART) may be associated with adverse pregnancy outcomes, including preterm delivery, stillbirth, low birth weight, and small-for-gestational-age infants. Actual risks may be influenced by maternal factors such as disease severity, gestational age at initiation of therapy, and specific ART regimen; therefore, close fetal monitoring is recommended. Because there is clear benefit to appropriate treatment, maternal ART should not be withheld due to concerns for adverse neonatal outcomes. Long-term follow-up is recommended for all infants exposed to antiretroviral medications; children without HIV but who were exposed to ART in utero and develop significant organ system abnormalities of unknown etiology (particularly of the CNS or heart) should be evaluated for potential mitochondrial dysfunction.

Based on the HHS perinatal HIV guidelines, stavudine is not one of the recommended antiretroviral agents for use during pregnancy.

In general, ART is recommended for all pregnant females living with HIV to keep the viral load below the limit of detection and reduce the risk of perinatal transmission. Therapy should be individualized following a discussion of the potential risks and benefits of treatment during pregnancy. Monitoring of pregnant females is more frequent than in nonpregnant adults. ART should be continued postpartum for all females living with HIV and can be modified after delivery.

Health care providers are encouraged to enroll pregnant females exposed to antiretroviral medications as early in pregnancy as possible in the Antiretroviral Pregnancy Registry (1-800-258-4263 or http://www.APRegistry.com). Health care providers caring for pregnant females living with HIV and their infants may contact the National Perinatal HIV Hotline (888-448-8765) for clinical consultation (HHS [perinatal] 2019).

- ◆ **Staxyn** *see* Vardenafil *on page 1532*
- ◆ **Stay Awake [OTC]** *see* Caffeine *on page 277*
- ◆ **Stay Awake Maximum Strength [OTC]** *see* Caffeine *on page 277*
- ◆ **Steglatro** *see* Ertugliflozin *on page 587*
- ◆ **Steglujan** *see* Ertugliflozin and Sitagliptin *on page 588*
- ◆ **Stelara** *see* Ustekinumab *on page 1510*
- ◆ **Stelazine** *see* Trifluoperazine *on page 1496*
- ◆ **Stendra** *see* Avanafil *on page 194*
- ◆ **STI-571** *see* Imatinib *on page 797*
- ◆ **Stimate** *see* Desmopressin *on page 460*
- ◆ **Stiolto Respimat** *see* Tiotropium and Olodaterol *on page 1451*

Stiripentol (stir i PEN tol)

Brand Names: US Diacomit

Brand Names: Canada Diacomit

Pharmacologic Category Anticonvulsant, Miscellaneous

Use Dravet syndrome: Adjunctive treatment of refractory generalized tonic-clonic seizures in conjunction with clobazam and valproic acid (off-label) in patients ≥2 years with Dravet syndrome (previously known as severe myoclonic epilepsy in infancy) (Chiron 2000; Wirrell 2016).

Local Anesthetic/Vasoconstrictor Precautions No information available to require special precautions

Effects on Dental Treatment No significant effects or complications reported

Effects on Bleeding No information available to require special precautions

Adverse Reactions Note: Adverse reactions reported with combination (clobazam) therapy.

>10%:

Central nervous system: Drowsiness (67%), agitation (27%), ataxia (27%), hypotonia (18% to 24%), dysarthria (12%), insomnia (12%)
Endocrine & metabolic: Weight loss (27%)
Gastrointestinal: Decreased appetite (45% to 46%), nausea (15%)
Hematologic & oncologic: Decreased platelet count (13%), neutropenia (13%)
Neuromuscular & skeletal: Tremor (15%)

1% to 10%:

Central nervous system: Aggressive behavior (9%), fatigue (9%)
Endocrine & metabolic: Weight gain (6%)
Gastrointestinal: Vomiting (9%), sialorrhea (6%)
Respiratory: Bronchitis (6%), nasopharyngitis (6%)
Miscellaneous: Fever (6%)

Mechanism of Action Precise mechanism behind anticonvulsant effects is unknown. May enhance GABAergic inhibitory neurotransmission by weak partial agonism and/or positive allosteric modulation of gamma-aminobutyric acid (GABA)-A receptors (Fisher 2009). Also inhibits multiple cytochrome P450 isoenzymes involved in the metabolism of other anticonvulsants; concurrent use may increase their systemic exposure and efficacy.

Pharmacodynamics/Kinetics

Half-life Elimination Adults: 4.5 to 13 hours (dose-dependent)

Time to Peak Median: 2 to 3 hours

Pregnancy Considerations

Adverse events have been observed in animal reproduction studies. Information related to the use of stiripentol in pregnancy has not been located (de Jong 2016).

Stiripentol is used in combination with clobazam or valproic acid (off-label); refer to individual monographs for additional information.

Data collection to monitor pregnancy and infant outcomes following exposure to stiripentol is ongoing. Patients may enroll themselves in the North American Antiepileptic Drug (NAAED) Pregnancy Registry (1-888-233-2334 or http://www.aedpregnancyregistry.org).

- **Stivarga** *see* Regorafenib *on page 1314*
- **St Joseph Adult Aspirin [OTC]** *see* Aspirin *on page 177*
- **Stool Softener [OTC]** *see* Docusate *on page 509*
- **Strattera** *see* AtoMOXetine *on page 190*

Streptozocin (strep toe ZOE sin)

Brand Names: US Zanosar

Brand Names: Canada Zanosar [DSC]

Pharmacologic Category Antineoplastic Agent, Alkylating Agent; Antineoplastic Agent, Alkylating Agent (Nitrosourea)

Use Pancreatic neuroendocrine tumors: Treatment of metastatic islet cell carcinoma of the pancreas (symptomatic or progressive disease)

Local Anesthetic/Vasoconstrictor Precautions No information available to require special precautions

Effects on Dental Treatment No significant effects or complications reported

Effects on Bleeding Chemotherapy may result in significant myelosuppression, potentially including significant reduction in platelet counts and altered hemostasis. In patients who are under active treatment with these agents, medical consult is suggested.

Adverse Reactions Frequency not defined.

Endocrine & metabolic: Decreased glucose tolerance, glycosuria, hyperglycemia, hypoalbuminemia, hypoglycemia, hypophosphatemia, increased lactate dehydrogenase

Gastrointestinal: Diarrhea, nausea, vomiting

Genitourinary: Anuria, azotemia, nephrotoxicity, proteinuria

Hepatic: Increased serum transaminases

Local: Injection site reaction (includes burning sensation at injection site, erythema at injection site, inflammation at injection site, irritation at injection site, swelling at injection site, tenderness at injection site)

Renal: Increased blood urea nitrogen, increased serum creatinine, renal insufficiency, renal tubular acidosis

<1%, postmarketing, and/or case reports: Anemia, bone marrow depression (nadir: 2 to 3 weeks), confusion, depression, diabetes insipidus, hepatic insufficiency, lethargy, leukopenia, metastases, thrombocytopenia

Mechanism of Action Streptozocin inhibits DNA synthesis by alkylation and cross-linking the strands of DNA, and by possible protein modification; cell cycle nonspecific

Pharmacodynamics/Kinetics

Onset of Action 1,500 mg/m^2 once weekly: Onset of response: 17 days; median time to maximum response: 35 days

Half-life Elimination <1 hour (Perry 2012)

Pregnancy Considerations Adverse events have been observed in animal reproduction studies.

- **Streptozotocin** *see* Streptozocin *on page 1389*
- **Striant [DSC]** *see* Testosterone *on page 1425*
- **Stribild** *see* Elvitegravir, Cobicistat, Emtricitabine, and Tenofovir Disoproxil Fumarate *on page 553*
- **Strovite** *see* Vitamins (Multiple/Oral) *on page 1550*
- **Strovite Forte** *see* Vitamins (Multiple/Oral) *on page 1550*
- **Strovite Plus [DSC]** *see* Vitamins (Multiple/Oral) *on page 1550*
- **SU011248** *see* SUNItinib *on page 1396*
- **Suberoylanilide Hydroxamic Acid** *see* Vorinostat *on page 1554*
- **Sublimaze** *see* FentaNYL *on page 642*
- **Sublocade** *see* Buprenorphine *on page 260*
- **Suboxone** *see* Buprenorphine and Naloxone *on page 270*
- **Subsys** *see* FentaNYL *on page 642*
- **Subutex** *see* Buprenorphine *on page 260*
- **Subvenite** *see* LamoTRIgine *on page 874*
- **Subvenite Starter Kit-Blue** *see* LamoTRIgine *on page 874*
- **Subvenite Starter Kit-Green** *see* LamoTRIgine *on page 874*
- **Subvenite Starter Kit-Orange** *see* LamoTRIgine *on page 874*
- **Succinimidyl Carbonate Monomethoxypolyethylene Glycol E. coli L-asparaginase** *see* Calaspargase Pegol *on page 278*
- **Succinimidyl Carbonate-PEG E. coli L-asparaginase** *see* Calaspargase Pegol *on page 278*

Sucralfate (soo KRAL fate)

Related Information

Perioral Premalignant Lesions and Management of Patients Undergoing Cancer Therapy *on page 1781*

Brand Names: US Carafate

Brand Names: Canada APO-Sucralfate; Cytogard; DOM-Sucralfate [DSC]; PMS-Sucralfate; Sulcrate; Sulcrate Plus; TEVA-Sucralfate

Pharmacologic Category Gastrointestinal Agent, Miscellaneous

Use Duodenal ulcer: Short-term (≤8 weeks) treatment of active duodenal ulcers; maintenance therapy for duodenal ulcers (tablets only)

Local Anesthetic/Vasoconstrictor Precautions No information available to require special precautions

Effects on Dental Treatment No significant effects or complications reported

Effects on Bleeding No information available to require special precautions

Adverse Reactions

1% to 10%: Gastrointestinal: Constipation (2%)

<1%, postmarketing, and/or case reports: Anaphylaxis, back pain, bezoar formation, bronchospasm, diarrhea, dizziness, drowsiness, dyspepsia, facial edema, flatulence, gastric distress, headache, hyperglycemia, hypersensitivity reaction, insomnia, laryngeal edema, mouth edema, nausea, pharyngeal edema, pruritus, pulmonary edema, skin rash, vertigo, vomiting, xerostomia

Mechanism of Action Forms a complex by binding with positively charged proteins in exudates, forming a viscous paste-like, adhesive substance. This selectively forms a protective coating that acts locally to protect the gastric lining against peptic acid, pepsin, and bile salts.

Pharmacodynamics/Kinetics

Onset of Action Paste formation and ulcer adhesion: 1 to 2 hours; acid neutralizing capacity: ~14 to 16 mEq/1 g dose of sucralfate

Pregnancy Considerations

Sucralfate is only minimally absorbed following oral administration. Based on available data, sucralfate does not appear to increase the risk of adverse fetal events when used during the first trimester. Sucralfate is considered acceptable for use in pregnancy (Dağlı 2017; Gomes 2018; Thélin 2020).

◆ **Sucralfate Paste (Orafate, ProThelial)** *see* Mucosal Coating Agent *on page 1066*

◆ **Sudafed** *see* Pseudoephedrine *on page 1291*

◆ **Sudafed [OTC]** *see* Pseudoephedrine *on page 1291*

◆ **Sudafed 12 Hour [OTC] [DSC]** *see* Pseudoephedrine *on page 1291*

◆ **Sudafed Childrens [OTC]** *see* Pseudoephedrine *on page 1291*

◆ **Sudafed Congestion [OTC]** *see* Pseudoephedrine *on page 1291*

◆ **Sudafed PE Childrens [OTC]** *see* Phenylephrine (Systemic) *on page 1227*

◆ **Sudafed PE Sinus Congestion [OTC]** *see* Phenylephrine (Systemic) *on page 1227*

◆ **Sudafed Sinus Congestion [OTC]** *see* Pseudoephedrine *on page 1291*

◆ **Sudafed Sinus Congestion 12HR [OTC]** *see* Pseudoephedrine *on page 1291*

◆ **Sudafed Sinus Congestion 24HR [OTC]** *see* Pseudoephedrine *on page 1291*

◆ **SudoGest [OTC]** *see* Pseudoephedrine *on page 1291*

◆ **SudoGest 12 Hour [OTC]** *see* Pseudoephedrine *on page 1291*

◆ **SudoGest Maximum Strength [OTC]** *see* Pseudoephedrine *on page 1291*

◆ **Sudogest PE [OTC]** *see* Phenylephrine (Systemic) *on page 1227*

◆ **SudoGest Sinus & Allergy [OTC]** *see* Chlorpheniramine and Pseudoephedrine *on page 341*

SUFentanil (soo FEN ta nil)

Brand Names: US Dsuvia

Pharmacologic Category Analgesic, Opioid; Anilidopiperidine Opioid; General Anesthetic

Use

Acute pain management (sublingual tablet): Management of acute pain severe enough to require an opioid analgesic and for which alternative treatments are inadequate

Limitations of use: Reserve for use in patients for whom alternative treatment options (eg, nonopioid analgesics, opioid combination products) are ineffective, not tolerated, or would be otherwise inadequate to provide sufficient management of pain. Administer by health care provider in a health care setting (eg, hospital, surgical center, emergency department) only; not for home use. Do not administer >72 hours (has not been studied).

Epidural analgesia (injection): For epidural administration as an analgesic combined with low-dose bupivacaine during labor and vaginal delivery.

Surgical analgesia (injection): Analgesic adjunct for the maintenance of balanced general anesthesia in patients who are intubated and ventilated.

Surgical anesthesia (injection): As a primary anesthetic agent for the induction and maintenance of anesthesia with 100% oxygen in patients undergoing major surgical procedures; in patients who are intubated and ventilated, such as cardiovascular surgery or neurosurgical procedures in the sitting position; to provide favorable myocardial and cerebral oxygen balance or when extended postoperative ventilation is anticipated.

Local Anesthetic/Vasoconstrictor Precautions

No information available to require special precautions

Effects on Dental Treatment Key adverse event(s) related to dental treatment: Patients may experience orthostatic hypotension as they stand up after treatment; especially if lying in dental chair for extended periods of time. Use caution with sudden changes in position during and after dental treatment.

Effects on Bleeding No information available to require special precautions

Adverse Reactions

>10%:

Central nervous system: Headache (12%)

Dermatologic: Pruritus (epidural administration with bupivacaine: 25%)

Gastrointestinal: Nausea (29%)

1% to 10%:

Cardiovascular: Hypotension (5%)

Central nervous system: Dizziness (6%)

Gastrointestinal: Vomiting (6%)

Frequency not defined:

Cardiovascular: Bradycardia, ECG abnormality, flushing, hypertension, orthostatic hypotension, oxygen saturation decreased, peripheral vasodilation, presyncope, sinus tachycardia, syncope

Central nervous system: Agitation, anxiety, confusion, disorientation, drowsiness, drug abuse, drug dependence, euphoria, hallucination, insomnia, lethargy, memory impairment, mental status changes, sedation

Dermatologic: Hyperhidrosis, skin rash

Gastrointestinal: Abdominal distension, abdominal distress, constipation, decreased gastrointestinal motility, diarrhea, dyspepsia, eructation, flatulence, gastritis, hiccups, intestinal obstruction (postoperative), oral hypoesthesia, retching, upper abdominal pain, xerostomia

Genitourinary: Decreased urine output, oliguria, urinary hesitancy, urinary retention

Hepatic: Increased liver enzymes, increased serum aspartate aminotransferase

Neuromuscular & skeletal: Muscle rigidity, muscle spasm
Ophthalmic: Miosis
Renal: Renal failure syndrome
Respiratory: Apnea, atelectasis, bradypnea, hypoventilation, hypoxia, respiratory depression, respiratory distress, respiratory failure

<1%, postmarketing, and/or case reports: Anaphylaxis

Mechanism of Action Binds to opioid receptors throughout the CNS. Once receptor binding occurs, effects are exerted by opening K+ channels and inhibiting Ca++ channels. These mechanisms increase pain threshold, alter pain perception, inhibit ascending pain pathways; short-acting opioid; dose-related inhibition of catecholamine release (up to 30 mcg/kg) controls sympathetic response to surgical stress.

Pharmacodynamics/Kinetics

Onset of Action Analgesia: IV: 1 to 3 minutes; Epidural: 10 minutes; Sublingual tablets: ~30 minutes (Fisher 2018)

Duration of Action

Dose dependent: Anesthesia adjunct doses:

IV: Context-sensitive half-time and recovery varies depending on dose, duration of administration, concomitant anesthesia, and other clinical factors (Miller 2015).

Epidural: 10 to 15 mcg with bupivacaine 0.125%: 1.7 hours.

Sublingual tablets: ~3 hours (Fisher 2018).

Half-life Elimination

IV: Neonates: 7.2 ± 2.7 hours; Infants and Children (2 to 8 years): 97 ± 42 minutes; Adolescents 10 to 15 years: 76 ± 33 minutes; Adults: 164 minutes

Sublingual tablet: 2.5 ± 0.85 hours (Fisher 2018)

Time to Peak Sublingual tablet: 1 hour

Reproductive Considerations

Long-term opioid use may cause secondary hypogonadism, which may lead to sexual dysfunction or infertility in men and women (Brennan 2013).

Pregnancy Considerations

Sufentanil crosses the placenta (Cuypers 1995; Loftus 1995).

According to some studies, maternal use of opioids may be associated with birth defects (including neural tube defects, congenital heart defects, and gastroschisis), poor fetal growth, stillbirth, and preterm delivery (CDC [Dowell 2016]). Opioids used as part of obstetric analgesia/anesthesia during labor and delivery may temporarily affect the fetal heart rate (ACOG 209 2019).

Prolonged use of opioids during pregnancy can cause neonatal withdrawal syndrome, which may be life-threatening if not recognized and treated according to protocols developed by neonatology experts. If opioid use is required for a prolonged period in a pregnant woman, advise the patient of the risk of neonatal opioid withdrawal syndrome and ensure that appropriate treatment will be available. If chronic opioid exposure occurs in pregnancy, adverse events in the newborn (including withdrawal) may occur (Chou 2009). Symptoms of neonatal abstinence syndrome (NAS) following opioid exposure may be autonomic (eg, fever, temperature instability), gastrointestinal (eg, diarrhea, vomiting, poor feeding/weight gain), or neurologic (eg, high-pitched crying, hyperactivity, increased muscle tone, increased wakefulness/abnormal sleep pattern, irritability, sneezing, seizure, tremor, yawning) (Dow 2012; Hudak 2012). Opioids may cause respiratory depression and psychophysiologic effects in the neonate; newborns of mothers receiving opioids during labor should be monitored.

Sufentanil injection is commonly used to treat maternal pain during labor and immediately postpartum (ACOG 209 2019). Administration of epidural sufentanil with bupivacaine with or without epinephrine is indicated for use in labor and delivery. Sufentanil tablets are not recommended for use during or immediately before labor.

The ACOG recommends that pregnant women should not be denied medically necessary surgery, regardless of trimester. If the procedure is elective, it should be delayed until after delivery (ACOG 775 2019).

Controlled Substance C-II

- **Sufentanil Citrate** *see* SUFentanil *on page 1390*
- **Sular** *see* Nisoldipine *on page 1109*
- **Sulbactam and Ampicillin** *see* Ampicillin and Sulbactam *on page 144*

Sulconazole (sul KON a zole)

Brand Names: US Exelderm

Pharmacologic Category Antifungal Agent, Imidazole Derivative; Antifungal Agent, Topical

Use Fungal infections:

Cream: Treatment of tinea pedis (athlete's foot), tinea cruris, and tinea corporis caused by *Trichophyton rubrum*, *Trichophyton mentagrophytes*, *Epidermophyton floccosum*, and *Microsporum canis*; treatment of tinea versicolor

Solution: Treatment of tinea cruris and tinea corporis caused by *Trichophyton rubrum*, *Trichophyton mentagrophytes*, *Epidermophyton floccosum*, and *Microsporum canis*; treatment of tinea versicolor

Limitations of use: Effectiveness has not been proven in tinea pedis (athlete's foot).

Local Anesthetic/Vasoconstrictor Precautions No information available to require special precautions

Effects on Dental Treatment No significant effects or complications reported

Effects on Bleeding No information available to require special precautions

Adverse Reactions 1% to 10%:

Central nervous system: Localized burning

Dermatologic: Localized erythema, pruritus, stinging of the skin

Mechanism of Action Substituted imidazole derivative which inhibits metabolic reactions necessary for the synthesis of ergosterol, an essential membrane component. The end result is usually fungistatic; however, sulconazole may act as a fungicide in *Candida albicans* and *Candida parapsilosis* during certain growth phases.

Pregnancy Risk Factor C

Pregnancy Considerations Adverse events have been observed in animal reproduction studies with large doses administered orally. Systemic absorption is limited following topical administration.

- **Sulconazole Nitrate** *see* Sulconazole *on page 1391*

Sulfamethoxazole and Trimethoprim

(sul fa meth OKS a zole & trye METH oh prim)

Related Information

Trimethoprim *on page 1498*

Brand Names: US Bactrim; Bactrim DS; Sulfatrim Pediatric

Brand Names: Canada APO-Sulfatrim; Protrin DF [DSC]; Septra; Sulfatrim; Sulfatrim DS; Sulfatrim Pediatric; TEVA-Trimel; TEVA-Trimel DS

Pharmacologic Category Antibiotic, Miscellaneous; Antibiotic, Sulfonamide Derivative

Use

Oral: Treatment of urinary tract infections (UTIs) due to *Escherichia coli, Klebsiella* and *Enterobacter* spp, *Morganella morganii, Proteus mirabilis,* and *Proteus vulgaris*; acute otitis media; acute exacerbations of chronic obstructive pulmonary disease due to susceptible strains of *Haemophilus influenzae* or *Streptococcus pneumoniae*; treatment and prophylaxis of *Pneumocystis* pneumonia (PCP); traveler's diarrhea due to enterotoxigenic *E. coli*; treatment of shigellosis caused by *Shigella flexneri* or *Shigella sonnei.*

IV: Treatment of PCP; treatment of shigellosis caused by *S. flexneri* or *S. sonnei*; treatment of severe or complicated UTIs due to *E. coli, Klebsiella* and *Enterobacter* spp, *M. morganii, P. mirabilis,* and *P. vulgaris.*

Local Anesthetic/Vasoconstrictor Precautions No information available to require special precautions

Effects on Dental Treatment Key adverse event(s) related to dental treatment: Stomatitis.

Effects on Bleeding No information available to require special precautions

Adverse Reactions Frequency not defined:

Cardiovascular: Allergic myocarditis, periarteritis nodosa (rare)

Central nervous system: Apathy, aseptic meningitis, ataxia, chills, depression, fatigue, hallucination, headache, insomnia, nervousness, peripheral neuritis, seizure, vertigo

Dermatologic: Erythema multiforme (rare), exfoliative dermatitis (rare), pruritus, skin photosensitivity, skin rash, Stevens-Johnson syndrome (rare), toxic epidermal necrolysis (rare), urticaria

Endocrine & metabolic: Hyperkalemia (generally at high dosages), hypoglycemia (rare), hyponatremia

Gastrointestinal: Abdominal pain, anorexia, diarrhea, glottis edema, kernicterus (in neonates), nausea, pancreatitis, pseudomembranous colitis, stomatitis, vomiting

Genitourinary: Crystalluria, diuresis (rare), nephrotoxicity (in association with cyclosporine), toxic nephrosis (with anuria and oliguria)

Hematologic & oncologic: Agranulocytosis, anaphylactoid purpura (IgA vasculitis; rare), aplastic anemia, eosinophilia, hemolysis (with G6PD deficiency), hemolytic anemia, hypoprothrombinemia, leukopenia, megaloblastic anemia, methemoglobinemia, neutropenia, thrombocytopenia

Hepatic: Cholestatic jaundice, hepatotoxicity (including hepatitis, cholestasis, and hepatic necrosis), hyperbilirubinemia, increased transaminases

Hypersensitivity: Anaphylaxis, angioedema, hypersensitivity reaction, serum sickness

Neuromuscular & skeletal: Arthralgia, myalgia, rhabdomyolysis (mainly in AIDS patients), systemic lupus erythematosus (rare), weakness

Ophthalmic: Conjunctival injection, injected sclera, uveitis

Otic: Tinnitus

Renal: Increased blood urea nitrogen, increased serum creatinine, interstitial nephritis, renal failure

Respiratory: Cough, dyspnea, pulmonary infiltrates

Miscellaneous: Fever

<1%, postmarketing, and/or case reports: Acute respiratory distress syndrome (Miller 2019), dysgeusia (Syed 2016), immune thrombocytopenia (formerly known as idiopathic thrombocytopenic purpura), metabolic acidosis, prolonged QT interval on ECG, thrombotic thrombocytopenic purpura

Mechanism of Action Sulfamethoxazole interferes with bacterial folic acid synthesis and growth via inhibition of dihydrofolic acid formation from para-aminobenzoic acid; trimethoprim inhibits dihydrofolic acid reduction to tetrahydrofolate resulting in sequential inhibition of enzymes of the folic acid pathway

Pharmacodynamics/Kinetics

Half-life Elimination

TMP: Prolonged in renal failure

Newborns: ~19 hours; range: 11 to 27 hours (Springer 1982)

Infants 2 months to 1 year: ~4.6 hours; range: 3 to 6 hours (Hoppu 1989)

Children 1 to 10 years: 3.7 to 5.5 hours (Hoppu 1987)

Children and Adolescents >10 years: 8.19 hours

Adults: 6 to 11 hours

SMX: 9 to 12 hours, prolonged in renal failure

Time to Peak Serum: Oral: 1 to 4 hours

Pregnancy Considerations

Sulfamethoxazole and trimethoprim cross the placenta. An increased risk of congenital malformations (neural tube defects, cardiovascular malformations, urinary tract defects, oral clefts, club foot) following maternal use of sulfamethoxazole and trimethoprim during pregnancy has been observed in some studies. Folic acid supplementation may decrease this risk (Crider 2009; Czeizel 2001; Hernandez-Diaz 2000; Hernandez-Diaz 2001; Matok 2009). Due to theoretical concerns that sulfonamides pass the placenta and may cause kernicterus in the newborn, neonatal health care providers should be informed if maternal sulfonamide therapy is used near the time of delivery (HHS [OI adult 2020]).

The pharmacokinetics of sulfamethoxazole and trimethoprim are similar to nonpregnant values in early pregnancy (Ylikorkala 1973). Sulfamethoxazole and trimethoprim are recommended for the prophylaxis or treatment of *Pneumocystis jirovecii* pneumonia (PCP), prophylaxis of *Toxoplasmic gondii* encephalitis (TE), and for the acute and chronic treatment of Q fever in pregnancy (Anderson [CDC 2013]; HHS [OI adult 2020]). Sulfonamides may also be used to treat other infections in pregnant women when clinically appropriate; use during the first trimester should be limited to situations where no alternative therapies are available (ACOG 717 2017).

◆ **Sulfamethoxazole-Trimethoprim** *see* Sulfamethoxazole and Trimethoprim *on page 1391*

SulfaSALAzine (sul fa SAL a zeen)

Brand Names: US Azulfidine; Azulfidine EN-tabs

Brand Names: Canada APO-Sulfasalazine; PMS-Sulfasalazine; Salazopyrin

Pharmacologic Category 5-Aminosalicylic Acid Derivative

Use

Juvenile rheumatoid arthritis: Delayed release: Treatment of pediatric patients with polyarticular-course juvenile rheumatoid arthritis who have responded inadequately to salicylates or other NSAIDs.

Rheumatoid arthritis: Delayed release: Treatment of rheumatoid arthritis in patients who have responded inadequately to salicylates or other NSAIDs. **Note:** Treatment initiation with a DMARD is recommended in DMARD-naive patients with either early rheumatoid arthritis (RA) (disease duration <6 months) or established RA (disease duration ≥6 months) (Singh [ACR 2016]).

Ulcerative colitis: Immediate and delayed release: Treatment of mild to moderate ulcerative colitis; adjunctive therapy in severe ulcerative colitis; prolongation of the remission period between acute attacks of ulcerative colitis.

Local Anesthetic/Vasoconstrictor Precautions No information available to require special precautions

Effects on Dental Treatment No significant effects or complications reported

Effects on Bleeding Sulfasalazine has been shown to induce a rare but potentially serious autoimmune thrombocytopenia, as detected by a significant decrease in platelet counts. Sulfasalazine-induced thrombocytopenia can be resolved by discontinuation of the drug.

Adverse Reactions

>10%:

Dermatologic: Skin rash (RA 13%)

Gastrointestinal: Nausea (RA 19%), dyspepsia (RA 13%), anorexia, gastric distress, vomiting

Genitourinary: Oligospermia (reversible)

Nervous system: Headache (RA 9%)

1% to 10%:

Dermatologic: Pruritus (RA 4%), urticaria

Gastrointestinal: Abdominal pain (RA 8%), stomatitis (RA 4%)

Hematologic & oncologic: Leukopenia (RA 3%), thrombocytopenia (RA 1%), acquired Heinz body anemia, hemolytic anemia

Hepatic: Abnormal hepatic function tests (RA 4%)

Nervous system: Dizziness

Respiratory: Cyanosis

Miscellaneous: Fever

<1%, postmarketing, and/or case reports (includes reactions reported with mesalamine or other sulfonamides): Agranulocytosis, alopecia, anaphylaxis, angioedema, aplastic anemia, arthralgia, ataxia, cauda equina syndrome, cholestasis, cholestatic hepatitis, cholestatic jaundice, conjunctival injection, crystalluria, depression, diarrhea, drowsiness, drug reaction with eosinophilia and systemic symptoms, eosinophilia, exfoliative dermatitis, folate deficiency, fulminant hepatitis, Guillain-Barre syndrome, hallucination, hearing loss, hematologic abnormality, hematologic disease (pseudomononucleosis), hematuria, hemolytic-uremic syndrome, hepatic cirrhosis, hepatic failure, hepatic necrosis, hepatitis, hepatotoxicity (idiosyncratic) (Chalasani, 2014), hypoglycemia, hypoprothrombinemia, injected sclera, insomnia, interstitial nephritis, interstitial pulmonary disease, intracranial hypertension (Tan 2019), jaundice, Kawasaki syndrome (single case report), lupus-like syndrome, megaloblastic anemia, meningitis, methemoglobinemia, myelitis, myelodysplastic syndrome, myocarditis (allergic), nephritis, nephrolithiasis, nephrotic syndrome, neutropenia (congenital), neutropenic enterocolitis, oropharyngeal pain, pallor, pancreatitis, parapsoriasis varioliformis acuta, periarteritis nodosa, pericarditis, periorbital edema, peripheral neuropathy, pleurisy, pneumonia, pneumonitis, proteinuria, pulmonary alveolitis, purpuric rash, renal disease (acute), rhabdomyolysis, seizure, sepsis, serum sickness-like reaction (children with JRA have frequent and severe reaction), skin discoloration, skin photosensitivity, Stevens-Johnson syndrome, thyroid function impairment, tinnitus, toxic epidermal necrolysis, toxic nephrosis, urinary tract infection, urine discoloration, vasculitis, vertigo

Mechanism of Action 5-aminosalicylic acid (5-ASA) is the active component of sulfasalazine; the specific mechanism of action of 5-ASA is unknown; however, it is thought that it modulates local chemical mediators of the inflammatory response, especially leukotrienes, and is also postulated to be a free radical scavenger or an inhibitor of tumor necrosis factor (TNF); action appears topical rather than systemic

Pharmacodynamics/Kinetics

Onset of Action Rheumatoid arthritis: >4 weeks; Ulcerative colitis: >3 to 4 weeks

Half-life Elimination Sulfasalazine: 7.6 ± 3.4 hours (prolonged in elderly patients); Sulfapyridine: 14.8 hours (slow acetylators) and 10.4 hours (fast acetylators)

Time to Peak Sulfasalazine: 3 to 12 hours (mean: 6 hours); Sulfapyridine and 5-aminosalicylic acid (5-ASA): ~10 hours

Reproductive Considerations

Sulfasalazine maintenance doses for the management of inflammatory bowel disease may be continued in women planning a pregnancy. A 3- to 6-month remission prior to conception reduces the risk of flare-up during pregnancy (AGA [Mahadevan 2019]). Based on available information, sulfasalazine can be continued in females with rheumatic and musculoskeletal diseases who are planning a pregnancy. Conception should be planned during a period of quiescent/low disease activity (ACR [Sammaritano 2020]). Supplementation with folic acid is recommended (ACR [Sammaritano 2020]; AGA [Mahadevan 2019]).

Sulfasalazine may cause oligospermia and reversible infertility in males; however, there is no data which suggest it would be teratogenic. Based on available information, sulfasalazine can be continued in males with rheumatic and musculoskeletal diseases who are planning to father a child. A semen analysis should be considered if conception does not occur (ACR [Sammaritano 2020]).

Pregnancy Considerations Sulfasalazine and sulfapyridine cross the placenta.

Based on available data, an increase in fetal malformations has not been observed following maternal use of sulfasalazine for the treatment of inflammatory bowel disease. Cases of neural tube defects have been reported (causation undetermined). Agranulocytosis was noted in an infant following maternal use of sulfasalazine during pregnancy. Although sulfapyridine has poor bilirubin-displacing ability, a potential for kernicterus in the newborn exists.

Aminosalicylates may be continued at prepregnancy maintenance doses for the management of inflammatory bowel disease; however, sulfasalazine is not the preferred drug in this class for use in pregnant women (AGA [Mahadevan 2019]). Based on available information, sulfasalazine can be continued during pregnancy in females with rheumatic and musculoskeletal diseases (ACR [Sammaritano 2020]). Sulfasalazine is known to inhibit the absorption and metabolism of folic acid and may diminish the effects of folic acid supplementation. Supplementation with folic acid is recommended (ACR [Sammaritano 2020]; AGA [Mahadevan 2019]).

- ◆ **Sulfatrim** *see* Sulfamethoxazole and Trimethoprim *on page 1391*
- ◆ **Sulfatrim Pediatric** *see* Sulfamethoxazole and Trimethoprim *on page 1391*

Sulindac (SUL in dak)

Related Information

Rheumatoid Arthritis, Osteoarthritis, and Osteoporosis *on page 1697*

Temporomandibular Dysfunction (TMD), Chronic Pain, and Fibromyalgia *on page 1773*

Brand Names: Canada ALTI-Sulindac; APO-Sulin [DSC]; TEVA-Sulindac

Pharmacologic Category Analgesic, Nonopioid; Nonsteroidal Anti-inflammatory Drug (NSAID), Oral

Use

Acute gouty arthritis: Relief of signs and symptoms of acute gouty arthritis.

Ankylosing spondylitis: Relief of signs and symptoms of ankylosing spondylitis.

Arthritis: Relief of signs and symptoms of osteoarthritis and rheumatoid arthritis (RA).

Bursitis/tendinitis of the shoulder: Relief of signs and symptoms of acute painful shoulder (acute subacromial bursitis/supraspinatus tendinitis).

Local Anesthetic/Vasoconstrictor Precautions

No information available to require special precautions

Effects on Dental Treatment The dentist should be aware of the potential of abnormal coagulation. Caution should also be exercised in the use of NSAIDs in patients already on anticoagulant therapy with drugs such as warfarin (Coumadin®). See Effects on Bleeding.

Effects on Bleeding Nonselective NSAIDs, such as sulindac, inhibit platelet aggregation and prolong bleeding time in some patients. Unlike aspirin, the NSAID effect on platelet function is quantitatively less, of shorter duration, and reversible. Normal platelet function should occur in ~5 elimination half-lives or in <10 hours after discontinuation of sulindac. Concomitant use of other NSAIDs should be avoided.

Adverse Reactions

1% to 10%:

Cardiovascular: Edema (1% to 3%)

Central nervous system: Dizziness (3% to 9%), headache (3% to 9%), nervousness (1% to 3%)

Dermatologic: Skin rash (3% to 9%), pruritus (1% to 3%)

Gastrointestinal: Gastrointestinal pain (10%), constipation (3% to 9%), diarrhea (3% to 9%), dyspepsia (3% to 9%), nausea (3% to 9%), abdominal cramps (1% to 3%), anorexia (1% to 3%), flatulence (1% to 3%), vomiting (1% to 3%)

Otic: Tinnitus (1% to 3%)

<1%, postmarketing, and/or case reports: Agranulocytosis, ageusia, alopecia, anaphylaxis, angioedema, aplastic anemia, aseptic meningitis, auditory impairment, bitter taste, blurred vision, bone marrow depression, bowel stricture, bronchospasm, bruise, cardiac arrhythmia, cardiac failure, cholestasis, colitis, conjunctivitis, crystalluria, depression, drowsiness, dry mucous membranes, dyspnea, dysuria, epistaxis, erythema multiforme, exfoliative dermatitis, fever, gastritis, gastrointestinal hemorrhage, gastrointestinal perforation, glossitis, gynecomastia, hematuria, hemolytic anemia, hepatic failure, hepatic insufficiency, hepatitis, hepatotoxicity (idiosyncratic; Chalasani 2014), hyperglycemia, hyperkalemia, hypersensitivity angiitis, hypersensitivity reaction (including hypersensitivity syndrome with chills, diaphoresis, fever, flushing), hypertension, insomnia, interstitial nephritis, jaundice, leukopenia, metallic taste, necrotizing fasciitis, nephrolithiasis, nephrotic syndrome, neuritis, neutropenia, palpitations, pancreatitis, paresthesia, peptic ulcer, proteinuria, psychosis, purpura, renal failure, renal insufficiency, retinopathy, seizure, skin photosensitivity, Stevens-Johnson syndrome, stomatitis, syncope, thrombocytopenia, toxic epidermal necrolysis, urine discoloration, urticaria, vaginal hemorrhage, vertigo, visual disturbance, weakness

Mechanism of Action

Reversibly inhibits cyclooxygenase-1 and 2 (COX-1 and 2) enzymes, which results in decreased formation of prostaglandin precursors; has antipyretic, analgesic, and anti-inflammatory properties.

Other proposed mechanisms not fully elucidated (and possibly contributing to the anti-inflammatory effect to varying degrees), include inhibiting chemotaxis, altering lymphocyte activity, inhibiting neutrophil aggregation/activation, and decreasing proinflammatory cytokine levels.

Pharmacodynamics/Kinetics

Onset of Action

Therapeutic response: Within 1 week

Half-life Elimination Sulindac: 7.8 hours; Sulfide metabolite: 16.4 hours

Time to Peak Sulindac: ~3 to 4 hours; Sulfide and sulfone metabolites: ~5 to 6 hours

Reproductive Considerations

The chronic use of NSAIDs in women of reproductive age may be associated with infertility that is reversible upon discontinuation of the medication (Micu 2011).

Pregnancy Risk Factor C

Pregnancy Considerations Sulindac crosses the placenta.

Birth defects have been observed following in utero NSAID exposure in some studies; however, data is conflicting (Bloor 2013). Nonteratogenic effects, including prenatal constriction of the ductus arteriosus, persistent pulmonary hypertension of the newborn, oligohydramnios, necrotizing enterocolitis, renal dysfunction or failure, and intracranial hemorrhage have been observed in the fetus/neonate following in utero NSAID exposure. In addition, nonclosure of the ductus arteriosus postnatally may occur and be resistant to medical management (Bermas 2014; Bloor 2013). Because they may cause premature closure of the ductus arteriosus, the use of NSAIDs in pregnancy should be avoided. Use of NSAIDs can be considered for the treatment of mild rheumatoid arthritis flares in pregnant women; however, use should be minimized or avoided early and late in pregnancy (Bermas 2014; Saavedra Salinas 2015).

The use of NSAIDs close to conception may be associated with an increased risk of miscarriage (Bloor 2013; Bermas 2014).

SUMAtriptan (soo ma TRIP tan)

Related Information

Temporomandibular Dysfunction (TMD), Chronic Pain, and Fibromyalgia *on page 1773*

Brand Names: US Imitrex; Imitrex STATdose Refill; Imitrex STATdose System; Onzetra Xsail; Sumavel DosePro; Tosymra; Zembrace SymTouch

Brand Names: Canada ACT SUMAtriptan; APO-SUMAtriptan; DOM-SUMAtriptan; Imitrex; Imitrex DF; MYLAN-SUMAtriptan; PMS-SUMAtriptan; RATIO-SUMAtriptan; SANDOZ SUMAtriptan; SUMAtriptan DF; TARO-SUMAtriptan; TEVA-SUMAtriptan; TEVA-SUMAtriptan DF

Pharmacologic Category Antimigraine Agent; Serotonin 5-$HT_{1B, 1D}$ Receptor Agonist

Use

Cluster headache, acute: SubQ (excluding Zembrace): Acute treatment of cluster headache episodes in adults as monotherapy or in combination with 100% oxygen (May 2020)

Migraine, moderate to severe, acute: Intranasal, Oral, SubQ: Acute treatment of migraine with or without aura in adults

Local Anesthetic/Vasoconstrictor Precautions No information available to require special precautions

Effects on Dental Treatment Key adverse event(s) related to dental treatment: Bad taste, dysphagia, hyposalivation (tablet), mouth/tongue discomfort (injection).

Effects on Bleeding No information available to require special precautions

Adverse Reactions

Injection:

>10%:

Central nervous system: Tingling sensation (14%), dizziness (≤12%), vertigo (≤12%), feeling hot (≤11%)

Local: Injection site reaction (30% to 59%), warm sensation at injection site (≤11%)

1% to 10%:

Cardiovascular: Flushing (7%), chest discomfort (5%), chest tightness (3%), chest pressure (2%)

Central nervous system: Burning sensation (7%), feeling of heaviness (7%), sensation of pressure (7%), numbness (5%), paresthesia (5%), sensation of tightness (5%), drowsiness (≤3%), sedated state (≤3%), local discomfort (jaw or throat: 2% to 3%), headache (2%), strange feeling (2%), tight feeling in the head (2%)

Dermatologic: Diaphoresis (2%)

Gastrointestinal: Nausea and vomiting (4%)

Neuromuscular & skeletal: Asthenia (5%), neck pain (≤5%), neck stiffness (≤5%), myalgia (2%)

Respiratory: Nasal discomfort (nasal cavity: ≤2%), sinus discomfort (≤2%), bronchospasm (1%)

Nasal:

>10%:

Gastrointestinal: Dysgeusia (≤25%), unusual taste (≤25%), nausea (≤14%), vomiting (≤14%)

Respiratory: Nasal discomfort (≤11%)

1% to 10%:

Central nervous system: Localized numbness (≤5%), nasal cavity pain (≤5%), paresthesia (≤5%), dizziness (≤2%), vertigo (≤2%), localized burning (1%)

Local: Local irritation (≤5%)

Respiratory: Rhinorrhea (≤5%), sore nose (≤5%), nasal signs and symptoms (≤4%), sinus discomfort (≤4%), rhinitis (2%)

Tablet:

1% to 10%:

Cardiovascular: Hot and cold flashes (3%), chest pain (≤2%), chest pressure (≤2%), chest tightness (≤2%)

Central nervous system: Pain (≤8%), sensation of pressure (≤8%), paresthesia (3% to 5%), fatigue (≤3%), feeling of heaviness (≤3%), malaise (≤3%), sensation of tightness (≤3%), heaviness of chest (≤2%), vertigo (2%)

Gastrointestinal: Sore throat (≤3%)

Local: Local pain (2%)

Neuromuscular & skeletal: Jaw pain (≤3%), jaw pressure (≤3%), jaw tightness (≤3%), neck pain (≤3%)

Respiratory: Pharyngeal edema (≤3%)

Route unspecified:

Frequency not defined:

Cardiovascular: Ischemia, Raynaud's disease

Hematologic & oncologic: Splenic infarction

<1%, postmarketing, and/or case reports: Acute myocardial infarction, anaphylaxis, angioedema, blindness, cerebral hemorrhage, cerebrovascular accident, dystonia, epistaxis, heaviness in neck (includes jaw or throat), hypersensitivity reaction, hypotension, neck pressure, neck tightness, nonimmune anaphylaxis, palpitations, seizure, significant cardiovascular event, subarachnoid hemorrhage, tremor, vision loss (partial)

Mechanism of Action Selective agonist for serotonin (5-HT_{1B} and 5-HT_{1D} receptors) on intracranial blood vessels and sensory nerves of the trigeminal system; causes vasoconstriction and reduces neurogenic inflammation associated with antidromic neuronal transmission correlating with relief of migraine

Pharmacodynamics/Kinetics

Onset of Action Oral: ~30 minutes; Intranasal: Solution: ~15 to 30 minutes; SubQ: ~10 minutes; Peak effect: Oral: 2 to 4 hours

Half-life Elimination Distribution: 15 minutes; Terminal: 2 hours; range: 1 to 4 hours

Time to Peak Oral: 2 to 2.5 hours; Intranasal: Powder: ~45 minutes; Spray: Median 10 minutes (range: 5 to 23 minutes); SubQ: 12 minutes (range: 4 to 20 minutes)

Pregnancy Considerations

In a study using full-term, healthy human placentas, limited amounts of sumatriptan were found to cross the placenta (Schenker 1995).

Pregnancy outcome information for sumatriptan is available from a pregnancy registry sponsored by GlaxoSmithKline. As of September 2012, data were available for 617 pregnancies (626 infants/fetuses) exposed to sumatriptan (including 7 pregnancies also exposed to naratriptan). Following sumatriptan exposure, the risk of major birth defects following first trimester exposure was 4.2% and no consistent pattern of birth defects was observed. The pregnancy registry was closed to enrollment in January 2012 (Ephross 2014).

An analysis of data collected between 1995 and 2008 using the Swedish Medical Birth Register reported pregnancy outcomes following 5-HT1B/1D agonist exposure. An increased risk of major congenital malformations was not observed following sumatriptan exposure (2,229 exposed during the first trimester) (Källén 2011). An increased risk of major congenital malformations was also not observed using data collected from a Norwegian pregnancy registry study. This study included 415 women who used sumatriptan during the first trimester of pregnancy between 2004 and 2007 (Nezvalová-Henriksen 2013).

If acute treatment for cluster headaches is needed during pregnancy, use of sumatriptan may be considered (Jürgens 2009; VanderPluym 2016). Other agents are preferred for the initial treatment of migraine in pregnancy; however, sumatriptan may be considered if first-line agents fail (CHS [Worthington 2013]; MacGregor 2014).

◆ **Sumatriptan Succinate** *see* SUMAtriptan *on page 1394*

◆ **Sumavel DosePro** *see* SUMAtriptan *on page 1394*

◆ **Summers Eve Disp Medicated [OTC]** *see* Povidone-Iodine (Topical) *on page 1249*

SUNItinib (su NIT e nib)

Related Information

Clinical Risk Related to Drugs Prolonging QT Interval *on page 1675*

Osteonecrosis of the Jaw *on page 1699*

Brand Names: US Sutent

Brand Names: Canada Sutent

Pharmacologic Category Antineoplastic Agent, Tyrosine Kinase Inhibitor; Antineoplastic Agent, Vascular Endothelial Growth Factor (VEGF) Inhibitor; Vascular Endothelial Growth Factor (VEGF) Inhibitor

Use

Gastrointestinal stromal tumor: Treatment of gastrointestinal stromal tumor (GIST) after disease progression on or intolerance to imatinib

Pancreatic neuroendocrine tumors, advanced: Treatment of progressive, well-differentiated pancreatic neuroendocrine tumors in patients with unresectable locally advanced or metastatic disease

Renal cell carcinoma: Adjuvant treatment of adult patients at high risk of recurrent renal cell carcinoma (RCC) following nephrectomy; treatment of advanced RCC

Local Anesthetic/Vasoconstrictor Precautions Hypertension can occur with the use of this drug, particularly early in the treatment course. Monitor for hypertension prior to using local anesthetic with vasoconstrictor; medical consult if necessary.

Sunitinib is one of the drugs confirmed to prolong the QT interval and is accepted as having a risk of causing torsade de pointes. The risk of drug-induced torsade de pointes is extremely low when a single QT interval prolonging drug is prescribed. In terms of epinephrine, it is not known what effect vasoconstrictors in the local anesthetic regimen will have in patients with a known history of congenital prolonged QT interval or in patients taking any medication that prolongs the QT interval. Until more information is obtained, it is suggested that the clinician consult with the physician prior to the use of a vasoconstrictor in suspected patients, and that the vasoconstrictor (epinephrine, mepivacaine and levonordefrin [Carbocaine® 2% with Neo-Cobefrin®]) be used with caution.

Effects on Dental Treatment Key adverse event(s) related to dental treatment: Xerostomia (normal salivary flow resumes upon discontinuation), mucositis/stomatitis, taste perversion, and oral pain.

Effects on Bleeding Chemotherapy may result in significant myelosuppression, potentially including significant reduction in platelet counts (thrombocytopenia grades 3/4: 5% to 9%) and altered hemostasis. Bleeding has been reported in 18% to 37% of patients. In patients who are under active treatment with these agents, medical consult is suggested.

Adverse Reactions

>10%:

Cardiovascular: Increased serum creatine kinase (49%), hypertension (15% to 39%), peripheral edema (≤24%), decreased left ventricular ejection fraction (11% to 16%), chest pain (13%)

Central nervous system: Fatigue (≤62%), headache (18% to 23%), insomnia (15% to 18%), chills (14%), mouth pain (6% to 14%), depression (11%), dizziness (11%)

Dermatologic: Palmar-plantar erythrodysesthesia (14% to 50%), skin discoloration (18% to 30%; yellow color), skin rash (14% to 29%), hair discoloration (7% to 29%), xeroderma (14% to 23%), alopecia (5% to 14%), erythema of skin (12%), pruritus (12%)

Endocrine & metabolic: Increased uric acid (46%), decreased serum calcium (34% to 42%), decreased serum albumin (28% to 41%), decreased serum phosphate (31% to 36%), hypothyroidism (≤24%), increased thyroid stimulating hormone level (≤24%), decreased serum potassium (12% to 21%), decreased serum sodium (20%), decreased serum magnesium (19%), weight loss (16%), increased serum calcium (13%), increased serum sodium (10% to 13%)

Gastrointestinal: Diarrhea (40% to 66%), stomatitis (29% to 61%; grades 3/4: 3% to 6%; grade 4: <1%), nausea (34% to 58%), increased serum lipase (17% to 56%), anorexia (≤48%), dysgeusia (21% to 47%), abdominal pain (25% to 39%), vomiting (19% to 39%), increased serum amylase (17% to 35%), dyspepsia (15% to 34%), constipation (12% to 23%), decreased appetite (≤19%), flatulence (14%), xerostomia (13%), gastroesophageal reflux disease (12%), glossalgia (11%)

Hematologic & oncologic: Decreased hemoglobin (26% to 79%; grades 3/4: 3% to 8%; grade 4: 2%), lymphocytopenia (38% to 68%; grades 3/4: 3% to 18%, grade 4: 2%), hemorrhage (22% to 37%; grades 3/4: ≤4%), neutropenia (grades 3/4: 13%)

Hepatic: Increased serum aspartate aminotransferase (≤72%), increased serum alanine aminotransferase (≤61%), increased serum alkaline phosphatase (24% to 46%), increased serum bilirubin (16% to 37%), increased indirect serum bilirubin (10% to 13%)

Local: Localized edema (18%)

Neuromuscular & skeletal: Asthenia (≤57%), limb pain (≤40%), arthralgia (11% to 30%), back pain (28%), myalgia (≤14%)

Renal: Increased serum creatinine (12% to 70%)

Respiratory: Cough (27%), dyspnea (26%), epistaxis (21%), nasopharyngitis (14%), oropharyngeal pain (14%), upper respiratory tract infection (11%)

Miscellaneous: Fever (12% to 22%)

1% to 10%:

Cardiovascular: Edema (≤10%), venous thromboembolism (4%), cardiac failure (3%)

Endocrine & metabolic: Hypoglycemia (2% to 10%), hyperglycemia (grades 3/4: 2%), hyperkalemia (grades 3/4: 2%)

Gastrointestinal: Hemorrhoids (10%), pancreatitis (1%)

Hematologic & oncologic: Thrombocytopenia (grades 3/4: 5%), leukopenia (grades 3/4: 3%)

Respiratory: Flu-like symptoms (5%)

Frequency not defined:

Gastrointestinal: Aphthous stomatitis, dry mucous membranes, gingival pain, gingivitis, glossitis, hematemesis, hematochezia, melena, oral discomfort, oral mucosal ulcer, tongue ulcer

Genitourinary: Abnormal uterine bleeding

Hematologic & oncologic: Hematoma

Respiratory: Hemoptysis

<1%, postmarketing, and/or case reports: Acute renal failure, angioedema, arterial thrombosis, cardiac failure, cardiomyopathy, cerebral hemorrhage, cerebral infarction, cerebrovascular accident, cholecystitis (particularly acalculous), erythema multiforme, esophagitis, fistula (sometimes associated with tumor

necrosis and/or regression), necrotizing fasciitis (including of the perineum), gastrointestinal hemorrhage, gastrointestinal perforation, hemolytic-uremic syndrome, hepatic failure, hepatotoxicity, hypersensitivity reaction, hyperthyroidism, ischemic heart disease, myocardial infarction, myopathy, nephrotic syndrome, neutropenic infection, osteonecrosis of the jaw, pleural effusion, preeclampsia (like syndrome with proteinuria and reversible hypertension) (Gallucci 2013; Patel 2008), prolonged QT interval on ECG, proteinuria, pulmonary embolism, pulmonary hemorrhage, pyoderma gangrenosum (including positive dechallenges), renal insufficiency, respiratory tract hemorrhage, respiratory tract infection, reversible posterior leukoencephalopathy syndrome, rhabdomyolysis, seizure, sepsis, septic shock, serious infection, skin infection, Stevens-Johnson syndrome, thrombotic microangiopathy, thrombotic thrombocytopenic purpura, thyroiditis (Feldt 2012), torsades de pointes, toxic epidermal necrolysis, transient ischemic attacks, tumor hemorrhage, tumor lysis syndrome, urinary tract hemorrhage, urinary tract infection, ventricular arrhythmia, wound healing impairment

Mechanism of Action Sunitinib exhibits antitumor and antiangiogenic properties by inhibiting multiple receptor tyrosine kinases, including platelet-derived growth factors (PDGFRα and PDGFRβ), vascular endothelial growth factors (VEGFR1, VEGFR2, and VEGFR3), FMS-like tyrosine kinase-3 (FLT3), colony-stimulating factor type 1 (CSF-1R), and glial cell-line-derived neurotrophic factor receptor (RET).

Pharmacodynamics/Kinetics

Half-life Elimination Terminal: Sunitinib: 40 to 60 hours; SU12662: 80 to 110 hours

Time to Peak 6 to 12 hours

Reproductive Considerations

Obtain a pregnancy test prior to treatment initiation in women of reproductive potential; effective contraception should be used during treatment and for at least 4 weeks after the last sunitinib dose. Male patients with female partners of reproductive potential should use effective contraception during treatment and for 7 weeks after the last sunitinib dose. Male and female fertility may be affected.

Pregnancy Considerations

Based on animal reproduction studies and its mechanism of action, sunitinib may cause fetal harm if administered to a pregnant woman. Because sunitinib inhibits angiogenesis, a critical component of fetal development, adverse effects on pregnancy would be expected.

Dental Health Professional Considerations See Local Anesthetic/Vasoconstrictor Precautions

- **Sunitinib Malate** *see* SUNItinib *on page 1396*
- **Supartz [DSC]** *see* Hyaluronate and Derivatives *on page 761*
- **Supartz FX** *see* Hyaluronate and Derivatives *on page 761*
- **Superdophilus [OTC]** *see Lactobacillus on page 869*
- **Supprelin LA** *see* Histrelin *on page 759*
- **Suprax** *see* Cefixime *on page 308*
- **Sure Result SR Relief [OTC]** *see* Capsaicin *on page 284*
- **Surgicel SNoW 1"x2" [DSC]** *see* Cellulose (Oxidized/Regenerated) *on page 320*
- **Surgicel SNoW 2"x4" [DSC]** *see* Cellulose (Oxidized/Regenerated) *on page 320*
- **Surgicel SNoW 4"x4" [DSC]** *see* Cellulose (Oxidized/Regenerated) *on page 320*
- **Surgifoam** *see* Gelatin (Absorbable) *on page 731*
- **Surgifoam Hermorrhoidectomy** *see* Gelatin (Absorbable) *on page 731*
- **Surmontil [DSC]** *see* Trimipramine *on page 1499*
- **Survanta** *see* Beractant *on page 232*
- **Sustiva** *see* Efavirenz *on page 543*
- **Sustol** *see* Granisetron *on page 748*
- **Sutent** *see* SUNItinib *on page 1396*

Suvorexant (soo voe REX ant)

Brand Names: US Belsomra

Brand Names: Canada Belsomra [DSC]

Pharmacologic Category Hypnotic, Miscellaneous; Orexin Receptor Antagonist

Use Insomnia: Treatment of insomnia characterized by difficulties with sleep onset and/or sleep maintenance.

Local Anesthetic/Vasoconstrictor Precautions No information available to require special precautions

Effects on Dental Treatment Key adverse event(s) related to dental treatment: Xerostomia (normal salivary flow resumes after discontinuation)

Effects on Bleeding No information available to require special precautions

Adverse Reactions

1% to 10%:

Gastrointestinal: Diarrhea (2%), xerostomia (2%; more common in females)

Nervous system: Headache (7%; more common in females), drowsiness (2% to 7%; more common in females), dizziness (3%), abnormal dreams (2%; more common in females)

Respiratory: Cough (2%; more common in females), upper respiratory tract infection (2%; more common in females)

Frequency not defined:

Endocrine & metabolic: Increased serum cholesterol

Nervous system: Central nervous system depression, daytime sedation, exacerbation of depression, hypnogenic hallucination, sleep paralysis, suicidal ideation

Neuromuscular & skeletal: Lower extremity weakness (cataplexy-like symptoms)

Postmarketing:

Cardiovascular: Palpitations, tachycardia

Dermatologic: Pruritus

Nervous system: Anxiety, complex sleep-related disorder, psychomotor agitation

Mechanism of Action Suvorexant blocks the binding of wake-promoting neuropeptides orexin A and orexin B to receptors OX1R and OX2R, which is thought to suppress wake drive. Antagonism of orexin receptors may also underlie potential adverse effects such as signs of narcolepsy/cataplexy.

Pharmacodynamics/Kinetics

Onset of Action ~30 minutes

Half-life Elimination ~12 hours; Half-life terminal: ~15 hours (healthy subjects, range: 10 to 22 hours), ~19 hours (moderate hepatic disease, range: 11 to 49 hours)

Time to Peak 2 hours (range: 30 minutes to 6 hours); Delayed approximately 1.5 hours when administered with a meal.

Pregnancy Considerations Adverse events have been observed in some animal reproduction studies.

Controlled Substance C-IV

- ◆ **Syeda** *see* Ethinyl Estradiol and Drospirenone *on page 610*
- ◆ **Syk Kinase Inhibitor R935788** *see* Fostamatinib *on page 718*
- ◆ **Sylatron** *see* Peginterferon Alfa-2b *on page 1202*
- ◆ **Sylvant** *see* Siltuximab *on page 1371*
- ◆ **Symbicort** *see* Budesonide and Formoterol *on page 255*
- ◆ **Symfi** *see* Efavirenz, Lamivudine, and Tenofovir Disoproxil Fumarate *on page 545*
- ◆ **Symfi Lo** *see* Efavirenz, Lamivudine, and Tenofovir Disoproxil Fumarate *on page 545*
- ◆ **Symjepi** *see* EPINEPHrine (Systemic) *on page 569*
- ◆ **SymlinPen 60** *see* Pramlintide *on page 1251*
- ◆ **SymlinPen 120** *see* Pramlintide *on page 1251*
- ◆ **Symmetrel** *see* Amantadine *on page 112*
- ◆ **Sympazan** *see* CloBAZam *on page 376*
- ◆ **Symproic** *see* Naldemedine *on page 1073*
- ◆ **Symtuza** *see* Darunavir, Cobicistat, Emtricitabine, and Tenofovir Alafenamide *on page 442*
- ◆ **Synagis** *see* Palivizumab *on page 1183*
- ◆ **Synalar** *see* Fluocinolone (Topical) *on page 689*
- ◆ **Synalar (Cream)** *see* Fluocinolone (Topical) *on page 689*
- ◆ **Synalar (Ointment)** *see* Fluocinolone (Topical) *on page 689*
- ◆ **Synalar TS** *see* Fluocinolone (Topical) *on page 689*
- ◆ **Synarel** *see* Nafarelin *on page 1071*
- ◆ **Syndros** *see* Dronabinol *on page 532*
- ◆ **Synera** *see* Lidocaine and Tetracaine *on page 914*
- ◆ **Synercid** *see* Quinupristin and Dalfopristin *on page 1301*
- ◆ **Synribo** *see* Omacetaxine *on page 1133*
- ◆ **Synthroid** *see* Levothyroxine *on page 900*
- ◆ **Synvisc** *see* Hyaluronate and Derivatives *on page 761*
- ◆ **Synvisc-One** *see* Hyaluronate and Derivatives *on page 761*
- ◆ **Syringe Avitene** *see* Collagen Hemostat *on page 410*
- ◆ **T_3 Sodium (error-prone abbreviation)** *see* Liothyronine *on page 919*
- ◆ **T_3/T_4 Liotrix** *see* Liotrix *on page 919*
- ◆ **T_4** *see* Levothyroxine *on page 900*
- ◆ **T-20** *see* Enfuvirtide *on page 564*
- ◆ **T-91825** *see* Ceftaroline Fosamil *on page 312*
- ◆ **Tabloid** *see* Thioguanine *on page 1438*
- ◆ **Tabrecta** *see* Capmatinib *on page 283*
- ◆ **TachoSil** *see* Fibrin Sealant *on page 667*

Tacrolimus (Systemic) (ta KROE li mus)

Brand Names: US Astagraf XL; Envarsus XR; Prograf

Brand Names: Canada Advagraf; Envarsus PA; Prograf; SANDOZ Tacrolimus

Pharmacologic Category Calcineurin Inhibitor; Immunosuppressant Agent

Use Organ rejection prophylaxis:

Advagraf [Canadian product]: Prevention of organ rejection in allogeneic kidney or liver transplant adult patients in combination with other immunosuppressants.

Astagraf XL: Prevention of organ rejection in kidney transplant recipients in combination with other immunosuppressants.

Envarsus PA [Canadian product]: Prevention of organ rejection in allogeneic kidney or liver transplant adult patients in combination with other immunosuppressants.

Envarsus XR: Prevention of organ rejection in kidney transplant recipients in combination with other immunosuppressants.

Prograf: Prevention of organ rejection in heart, kidney, and liver transplant recipients in combination with other immunosuppressants.

Note: ER products (Advagraf [Canadian product], Astagraf XL, Envarsus PA [Canadian product], and Envarsus XR) are not interchangeable or substitutable with immediate release tacrolimus. In addition, the once-daily formulations (Advagraf [Canadian product], Astagraf XL, Envarsus PA [Canadian product], and Envarsus XR) are not interchangeable with each other due to significantly different pharmacokinetic properties.

Local Anesthetic/Vasoconstrictor Precautions No information available to require special precautions

Effects on Dental Treatment Key adverse event(s) related to dental treatment: Stomatitis, oral candida infection, dysphagia, and esophagitis (including ulcerative) (see Dental Health Professional Considerations)

Effects on Bleeding Thrombocytopenia (14% to 24%) has been associated with use; severe thrombocytopenia (rare) may be associated with delayed coagulation. Consultation to ensure adequate platelet counts may be considered in patients with signs/symptoms or a history of thrombocytopenia.

Adverse Reactions Adverse reactions reported with combination therapy.

>10%:

Cardiovascular: Acute cardiorespiratory failure, angina pectoris, atrial fibrillation, atrial flutter, bradycardia, cardiac arrhythmia, cardiac failure, cardiac fibrillation, chest pain, deep vein thrombophlebitis, deep vein thrombosis, ECG abnormality (including abnormal QRS complex), edema, flushing, hemorrhagic stroke, hypertension, hypotension, orthostatic hypotension, peripheral edema, phlebitis, ST segment changes on ECG, syncope, tachycardia, thrombosis, vasodilation

Central nervous system: Abnormal dreams, abnormality in thinking, agitation, amnesia, anxiety, ataxia, chills, confusion, depression, dizziness, drowsiness, emotional lability, encephalopathy, falling, fatigue, flaccid paralysis, hallucination, headache, hypertonia, hypoesthesia, insomnia, intolerance to temperature, mobility disorder, mood elevation, myoclonus, nerve compression, nervousness, neuralgia, neuropathy, neurotoxicity, nightmares, pain, paralysis (monoparesis, quadriparesis, quadriplegia), paresthesia, peripheral neuropathy, psychomotor disturbance, psychosis, seizure, vertigo, voice disorder, writing difficulty

Dermatologic: Acne vulgaris, alopecia, cellulitis, condyloma acuminatum, dermal ulcer, dermatitis, diaphoresis, ecchymoses, exfoliative dermatitis, fungal dermatitis, hyperhidrosis, hypotrichosis, pityriasis versicolor, pruritus, skin discoloration, skin photosensitivity, skin rash

Endocrine & metabolic: Acidosis, albuminuria, alkalosis, anasarca, cushingoid appearance, Cushing syndrome, decreased serum bicarbonate, decreased serum iron, dehydration, diabetes mellitus (including new-onset), gout, hirsutism, hypercalcemia, hypercholesterolemia, hyperkalemia, hyperlipidemia, hyperphosphatemia, hypertriglyceridemia, hyperuricemia, hypervolemia, hypocalcemia, hypoglycemia, hypokalemia, hypomagnesemia, hyponatremia, hypophosphatemia, increased gamma-glutamyl transferase, increased lactate dehydrogenase, metabolic acidosis, weight gain

Gastrointestinal: Abdominal distention, abdominal pain, anorexia, aphthous stomatitis, biliary tract disease, cholangitis, cholestasis, constipation, diarrhea, duodenitis, dyspepsia, dysphagia, esophagitis, flatulence, gastritis, gastroenteritis, gastroesophageal reflux disease, gastrointestinal disease, gastrointestinal hemorrhage, gastrointestinal perforation, hernia of abdominal cavity, hiccups, increased appetite, intestinal obstruction, nausea, oral candidiasis, pancreatic pseudocyst, peritonitis, stomatitis, ulcerative esophagitis, vomiting

Genitourinary: Anuria, bladder spasm, cystitis, dysuria, hematuria, nephrotoxicity, nocturia, oliguria, proteinuria, pyuria, toxic nephrosis, urinary frequency, urinary incontinence, urinary retention, urinary tract infection, urinary urgency, vaginitis

Hematologic & oncologic: Anemia, benign skin neoplasm, decreased platelet count, decreased white blood cell count, disorder of hemostatic components of blood, hemolytic anemia, hemorrhage, hypochromic anemia, hypoproteinemia, hypoprothrombinemia, increased hematocrit, Kaposi sarcoma, leukocytosis, leukopenia, neutropenia, polycythemia, thrombocytopenia, thrombotic microangiopathy

Hepatic: Abnormal hepatic function tests, ascites, cholestatic jaundice, granulomatous hepatitis, hepatitis (including acute and chronic), hepatotoxicity, hyperbilirubinemia, increased liver enzymes, increased serum alanine aminotransferase, increased serum alkaline phosphatase, increased serum aspartate aminotransferase, jaundice

Hypersensitivity: Hypersensitivity reaction

Immunologic: CMV viremia, graft complications

Infection: Abscess, bacterial infection (may be serious), BK virus (including nephropathy), candidiasis, cytomegalovirus disease, Epstein-Barr infection, herpes simplex infection, herpes zoster infection, infection, opportunistic infection, polyomavirus infection, sepsis (children & adolescents), serious infection

Neuromuscular & skeletal: Arthralgia, asthenia, back pain, lower limb cramp, muscle cramps, muscle spasm, myalgia, myasthenia, osteoporosis, tremor

Ophthalmic: Amblyopia, blurred vision, conjunctivitis, visual disturbance

Otic: Otalgia, otitis media, tinnitus

Renal: Acute renal failure, hydronephrosis, increased blood urea nitrogen, increased serum creatinine, renal insufficiency, renal failure syndrome, renal tubular necrosis

Respiratory: Acute respiratory distress syndrome, asthma, atelectasis, bronchitis, decreased lung function, dyspnea, flu-like symptoms, increased cough, nasopharyngitis, pharyngitis, pleural effusion, pneumonia, pneumothorax, productive cough, pulmonary edema, pulmonary emphysema, respiratory tract infection, rhinitis, sinusitis

Miscellaneous: Abnormal healing, accidental injury, crying, fever, postoperative pain, postoperative wound complication, ulcer, wound healing impairment

1% to 10%:

Gastrointestinal: Gastrointestinal infection

Infection: Fungal infection

Respiratory: Upper respiratory tract infection

<1%, postmarketing, and/or case reports: Abnormal T waves on ECG, acute myocardial infarction, agranulocytosis, allergic rhinitis, aphasia, biliary obstruction, blindness, carpal tunnel syndrome, cerebral infarction, colitis, coma, cortical blindness, deafness, decreased serum fibrinogen, delayed gastric emptying, disseminated intravascular coagulation, dysarthria, enterocolitis, Epstein-Barr-associated lymphoproliferative disorder, febrile neutropenia, gastric ulcer, glycosuria, graft versus host disease, hearing loss, hemiparesis, hemolytic-uremic syndrome, hemorrhagic cystitis, hemorrhagic pancreatitis, hepatic cirrhosis, hepatic cytolysis, hepatic failure, hepatic necrosis, hepatic sinusoidal obstruction syndrome, hepatosplenic T-cell lymphomas, hot and cold flashes, hot flash, hyperpigmentation, hypertrophic cardiomyopathy, immune thrombocytopenia, increased amylase, increased INR, inflammatory polyarthropathy, interstitial pulmonary disease, ischemic heart disease, jitteriness, leukemia, leukoencephalopathy, limb pain (including calcineurin-inhibitor induced pain syndrome), liver steatosis, lymphoproliferative disorder, malignant lymphoma, malignant melanoma, mental status changes, multi-organ failure, mutism, necrotizing pancreatitis, optic atrophy, optic neuropathy, oral mucosa ulcer, pancreatitis, pancytopenia, pericardial effusion, photophobia, progressive multifocal leukoencephalopathy, prolonged partial thromboplastin time, prolonged QT interval on ECG, pulmonary hypertension, pulmonary infiltrates, pure red cell aplasia, respiratory distress, respiratory failure, reversible posterior leukoencephalopathy syndrome, rhabdomyolysis, speech disturbance, status epilepticus, Stevens-Johnson syndrome, supraventricular extrasystole, supraventricular tachycardia, thrombotic thrombocytopenic purpura, torsades de pointes, toxic epidermal necrolysis, urticaria, ventricular fibrillation, ventricular premature contractions, weight loss

Mechanism of Action Suppresses cellular immunity (inhibits T-lymphocyte activation), by binding to an intracellular protein, FKBP-12 and complexes with calcineurin dependent proteins to inhibit calcineurin phosphatase activity

Pharmacodynamics/Kinetics

Half-life Elimination

Children: Kidney transplant: 10.2 ± 5 hours; Infants and Children: Liver transplant: 11.5 ± 3.8 hours

Adults:

Immediate release: Variable, 23 to 46 hours in healthy volunteers; 2.1 to 36 hours in transplant patients; prolonged in patients with severe impairment

Extended release: 38 ± 3 hours; prolonged in patients with severe impairment

Time to Peak Oral: 0.5 to 6 hours

Reproductive Considerations

Family planning and contraceptive options for males and females of reproductive potential should be evaluated prior to starting treatment.

Pregnancy Considerations

Tacrolimus crosses the human placenta and is measurable in the cord blood, amniotic fluid, and newborn serum. Tacrolimus concentrations in the placenta may be higher than the maternal serum (Jain 1997). Infants with lower birth weights have been found to have higher tacrolimus concentrations (Bramham 2013).

Miscarriage, preterm delivery, low birth weight, birth defects (including cardiac, craniofacial, neurologic, renal/urogenital, and skeletal abnormalities), renal dysfunction, transient neonatal hyperkalemia, and fetal distress have been reported following in utero exposure to tacrolimus in infants of organ transplant recipients. However, mothers were also taking a concomitant medication known to cause adverse pregnancy outcomes.

Tacrolimus pharmacokinetics are altered during pregnancy. Whole blood concentrations decrease as pregnancy progresses; however, unbound concentrations increase. Measuring unbound concentrations may be preferred, especially in females with anemia or hypoalbuminemia. If unbound concentration measurement is not available, interpretation of whole blood concentrations should account for RBC count and serum albumin concentration (Hebert 2013; Zheng 2012).

Tacrolimus may be used as an immunosuppressant during pregnancy. The risk of infection, hypertension, and pre-eclampsia may be increased in pregnant females who have had a kidney transplant (EBPG 2002). Hypertension and diabetes during pregnancy have been reported in both kidney and liver transplant patients receiving tacrolimus.

The Transplant Pregnancy Registry International (TPRI) is a registry that follows pregnancies that occur in maternal transplant recipients or those fathered by male transplant recipients. The TPRI encourages reporting of pregnancies following solid organ transplant by contacting them at 1-877-955-6877 or https://www.transplantpregnancyregistry.org.

Dental Health Professional Considerations Consider a medical consultation prior to any invasive dental procedure in patients who have received an organ transplant; delayed wound healing due to the immunosuppressive effects and an increased potential for postoperative infection may be of concern.

Tacrolimus (Topical) (ta KROE li mus)

Brand Names: US Protopic

Brand Names: Canada Protopic

Pharmacologic Category Calcineurin Inhibitor; Immunosuppressant Agent; Topical Skin Product

Use Moderate to severe atopic dermatitis: Treatment of moderate to severe atopic dermatitis in immunocompetent patients not responsive to conventional therapy or when conventional therapy is not appropriate

Local Anesthetic/Vasoconstrictor Precautions No information available to require special precautions

Effects on Dental Treatment No significant effects or complications reported

Effects on Bleeding No information available to require special precautions

Adverse Reactions As reported in children and adults, unless otherwise noted. Frequency not always defined.

Cardiovascular: Peripheral edema (adults 3% to 4%), hypertension (adults 1%)

Central nervous system: Headache (adults 19% to 20%), tingling of skin (2% to 8%), hyperesthesia (adults 3% to 7%), insomnia (adults 4%), paresthesia (adults 3%), depression (adults 2%), pain (1% to 2%)

Dermatologic: Burning sensation of skin (43% to 58%), pruritus (41% to 46%), erythema (25% to 28%), skin infection (adults 12%), acne vulgaris (adults 4% to 7%), urticaria (adults 3% to 6%), folliculitis (2% to 6%), skin rash (adults 2% to 5%), dermatological disease (children 4%), vesiculobullous dermatitis (children 4%), contact dermatitis (3% to 4%), pustular rash (adults 2% to 4%), contact eczema herpeticum (children 2%), fungal dermatitis (adults 1% to 2%), sunburn (adults 1% to 2%), alopecia (adults 1%), xeroderma (children 1%)

Gastrointestinal: Diarrhea (3% to 5%), dyspepsia (adults 1% to 4%), abdominal pain (children 3%), gastroenteritis (adults 2%), vomiting (adults 1%), nausea (children 1%)

Genitourinary: Dysmenorrhea (adults 4%), urinary tract infection (adults 1%)

Hematologic & oncologic: Lymphadenopathy (children 3%), malignant lymphoma, malignant neoplasm of skin

Hypersensitivity: Hypersensitivity reaction (adults 6% to 12%)

Infection: Herpes zoster (1% to 5%), varicella zoster infection (1% to 5%), infection (adults 1% to 2%)

Neuromuscular & skeletal: Myalgia (adults 2% to 3%), weakness (adults 2% to 3%), arthralgia (adults 1% to 3%), back pain (adults 2%)

Ocular: Conjunctivitis (adults 2%)

Otic: Otitis media (children 12%), otalgia (children 1%)

Respiratory: Flu-like symptoms (23% to 31%), increased cough (children 18%), asthma (adults 6%), rhinitis (children 6%), pharyngitis (adults 4%), sinusitis (adults 2% to 4%), bronchitis (adults 2%), pneumonia (adults 1%)

Miscellaneous: Fever (children 21%), allergic reaction (4% to 12%), alcohol intolerance (adults 3% to 7%), accidental injury (6%), cyst (adults 1% to 3%)

<1%, postmarketing, and/or case reports (Limited to important or life-threatening): Abnormality in thinking, abscess, acne rosacea, acute renal failure, aggravated tooth caries, anaphylactoid reaction, anemia, anorexia, anxiety, application site edema, arthritis, arthropathy, basal cell carcinoma, benign neoplasm (breast), blepharitis, bone disease, bursitis, candidiasis, cataract, chest pain, chills, colitis, conjunctival edema, constipation, cutaneous candidiasis, cystitis, dehydration, dermal ulcer, diaphoresis, dizziness, dry nose, dysgeusia, dyspnea, ear disease, ecchymoses, edema, epistaxis, eye pain, furunculosis, gastritis, gastrointestinal disease, heart valve disease, hernia, hyperbilirubinemia, hypercholesterolemia, hypertonia, hypothyroidism, impetigo (bullous), laryngitis, leukoderma, malaise, malignant lymphoma, malignant melanoma, migraine, muscle cramps, nail disease, neck pain, neoplasm (benign), oral candidiasis, oral mucosa ulcer, osteoarthritis, osteomyelitis, otitis externa, pulmonary disease, rectal disease, renal insufficiency, seborrhea, seizure, septicemia, skin carcinoma, skin discoloration, skin hypertrophy, skin photosensitivity, squamous cell carcinoma, stomatitis, syncope, tachycardia, tendon disease, unintended pregnancy, vaginitis, vasodilation, vertigo, visual

disturbance, vulvovaginal candidiasis, xerophthalmia, xerostomia

Mechanism of Action Suppresses cellular immunity (inhibits T-lymphocyte activation), by binding to an intracellular protein, FKBP-12 and complexes with calcineurin dependent proteins to inhibit calcineurin phosphatase activity

Pregnancy Considerations

Tacrolimus(Topical) crosses the human placenta and is measurable in the cord blood, amniotic fluid, and newborn serum following systemic use. Refer to the Tacrolimus (Systemic) monograph for additional information.

Tadalafil (tah DA la fil)

Brand Names: US Adcirca; Alyq; Cialis

Brand Names: Canada ACT Tadalafil [DSC]; Adcirca; APO-Tadalafil; APO-Tadalafil PAH; Auro-Tadalafil; Cialis; JAMP-Tadalafil; Mar-Tadalafil; MINT-Tadalafil; MYLAN-Tadalafil; PMS-Tadalafil; Priva-Tadalafil; RAN-Tadalafil; RIVA-Tadalafil; TEVA-Tadalafil

Pharmacologic Category Phosphodiesterase-5 Enzyme Inhibitor

Use

Benign prostatic hyperplasia (Cialis only): Treatment of the signs and symptoms of benign prostatic hyperplasia (BPH).

Erectile dysfunction (Cialis only): Treatment of erectile dysfunction.

Erectile dysfunction and benign prostatic hyperplasia (Cialis only): Treatment of erectile dysfunction and the signs and symptoms of BPH.

Pulmonary arterial hypertension (Adcirca only): Treatment of pulmonary arterial hypertension (World Health Organization group 1) to improve exercise ability. Studies establishing effectiveness included predominately patients with New York Heart Association (NYHA) functional class II to III symptoms and etiologies of idiopathic or heritable pulmonary arterial hypertension (61%) or pulmonary arterial hypertension associated with connective tissue diseases (23%).

Local Anesthetic/Vasoconstrictor Precautions

No information available to require special precautions

Effects on Dental Treatment No significant effects or complications reported

Effects on Bleeding No information available to require special precautions

Adverse Reactions

>10%:

Cardiovascular: Flushing (2% to 13%)

Central nervous system: Headache (4% to 42%)

Gastrointestinal: Nausea (≤11%)

Neuromuscular & skeletal: Myalgia (1% to 14%), limb pain (1% to 11%)

Respiratory: Respiratory tract infection (13%), nasopharyngitis (6% to 13%)

1% to 10%:

Cardiovascular: Hypertension (1% to 3%), angina pectoris (<2%), chest pain (<2%), facial edema (<2%), hypotension (<2%), myocardial infarction (<2%), orthostatic hypotension (<2%), palpitations (<2%), peripheral edema (<2%), syncope (<2%), tachycardia (<2%)

Central nervous system: Dizziness (<2%), drowsiness (<2%), fatigue (<2%), hypoesthesia (<2%), insomnia (<2%), pain (<2%), paresthesia (<2%), vertigo (<2%)

Dermatologic: Diaphoresis (<2%), pruritus (<2%), skin rash (<2%)

Endocrine & metabolic: Increased gamma-glutamyl transferase (<2%)

Gastrointestinal: Dyspepsia (2% to 10%), gastroenteritis (3% to 5%), gastroesophageal reflux disease (≤3%), diarrhea (1% to 3%), abdominal pain (1% to 2%), dysphagia (<2%), esophagitis (<2%), gastritis (<2%), hemorrhoidal bleeding (<2%), loose stools (<2%), upper abdominal pain (<2%), vomiting (<2%), xerostomia (<2%)

Genitourinary: Urinary tract infection (2%), prolonged erection (<2%), spontaneous erections (<2%)

Hematologic & oncologic: Rectal hemorrhage (<2%)

Hepatic: Abnormal hepatic function tests (<2%)

Neuromuscular & skeletal: Back pain (2% to 10%), arthralgia (<2%), asthenia (<2%), neck pain (<2%)

Ophthalmic: Blurred vision (<2%), conjunctival hyperemia (<2%), conjunctivitis (<2%), eyelid edema (<2%), eye pain (<2%), increased lacrimation (<2%), vision color changes (<2%)

Otic: Hearing loss (<2%), tinnitus (<2%)

Renal: Renal insufficiency (<2%)

Respiratory: Nasal congestion (≤9%), paranasal sinus congestion (≤9%), upper respiratory tract infection (3% to 4%), cough (2% to 4%), dyspnea (<2%), epistaxis (<2%), pharyngitis (<2%)

<1%, postmarketing, and/or case reports: Amnesia (transient global), anterior ischemic optic neuropathy (nonarteritic), basal cell carcinoma (Loeb 2015), cardiovascular toxicity, cerebrovascular accident, hypersensitivity reaction, malignant melanoma (Loeb 2015), migraine, muscle spasm, permanent vision loss, priapism, retinal artery occlusion, retinal vein occlusion, seizure, Stevens-Johnson syndrome, vision loss, visual field loss

Mechanism of Action

BPH: Exact mechanism unknown; effects likely due to PDE-5 mediated reduction in smooth muscle and endothelial cell proliferation, decreased nerve activity, and increased smooth muscle relaxation and tissue perfusion of the prostate and bladder

Erectile dysfunction: Does not directly cause penile erections, but affects the response to sexual stimulation. The physiologic mechanism of erection of the penis involves release of nitric oxide (NO) in the corpus cavernosum during sexual stimulation. NO then activates the enzyme guanylate cyclase, which results in increased levels of cyclic guanosine monophosphate (cGMP), producing smooth muscle relaxation and inflow of blood to the corpus cavernosum. Tadalafil enhances the effect of NO by inhibiting phosphodiesterase type 5 (PDE-5), which is responsible for degradation of cGMP in the corpus cavernosum; when sexual stimulation causes local release of NO, inhibition of PDE-5 by tadalafil causes increased levels of cGMP in the corpus cavernosum, resulting in smooth muscle relaxation and inflow of blood to the corpus cavernosum. At recommended doses, it has no effect in the absence of sexual stimulation.

PAH: Inhibits phosphodiesterase type 5 (PDE-5) in smooth muscle of pulmonary vasculature where PDE-5 is responsible for the degradation of cyclic guanosine monophosphate (cGMP). Increased cGMP concentration results in pulmonary vasculature relaxation; vasodilation in the pulmonary bed and the systemic circulation (to a lesser degree) may occur.

Pharmacodynamics/Kinetics

Onset of Action Within 1 hour; Peak effect: Pulmonary artery vasodilation: 75 to 90 minutes (Ghofrani 2004)

Duration of Action Erectile dysfunction: Up to 36 hours

Half-life Elimination 15 to 17.5 hours; Pulmonary hypertension (not receiving bosentan): 35 hours

Time to Peak Plasma: ~2 hours (range: 30 minutes to 6 hours)

Reproductive Considerations

Less than 0.0005% is found in the semen of healthy males.

Pregnancy Considerations

Tadalafil likely crosses the placenta (Sakamoto 2016). Women with pulmonary arterial hypertension are encouraged to avoid pregnancy (McLaughlin 2009; Taichman 2014).

Tafenoquine (ta FEN oh kwin)

Brand Names: US Arakoda; Krintafel

Pharmacologic Category Aminoquinoline (Antimalarial); Antimalarial Agent

Use

Malaria, primary prophylaxis (Arakoda): Prophylaxis of malaria in patients ≥18 years of age.

Malaria, treatment (prevention of relapse) (Krintafel): Radical cure (prevention of relapse) of *Plasmodium vivax* malaria in patients ≥16 years of age who are receiving appropriate antimalarial therapy for acute *P. vivax* infection. **Note:** Centers for Disease Control and Prevention guidelines also recommend tafenoquine for radical cure (prevention of relapse) of malaria caused by *Plasmodium ovale* (CDC 2020).

Limitation of use: Not indicated for the treatment of acute *P. vivax* malaria; must be used in combination with appropriate antimalarial therapy.

Local Anesthetic/Vasoconstrictor Precautions

No information available to require special precautions

Effects on Dental Treatment No significant effects or complications reported

Effects on Bleeding Hemolytic anemia may occur in patients with G6PD deficiency; decreased hemoglobin levels were also reported in some G6PD-normal patients. Patients should have been screened for G6PD deficiency prior to initiation of therapy. Use of the drug is contraindicated in patients with G6PD deficiency or unknown G6PD status.

Methemoglobinemia: Asymptomatic elevations in methemoglobin have been reported in patients taking tafenoquine. Main symptoms include cyanosis, especially the lips and fingers. If observed, physician consult suggested.

Adverse Reactions

>10%:

Central nervous system: Headache (15%)

Gastrointestinal: Diarrhea (5% to 18%)

Hematologic & oncologic: Methemoglobinemia (13%)

Neuromuscular & skeletal: Back pain (14%)

Ophthalmic: Epithelial keratopathy (21% to 93%)

1% to 10%:

Central nervous system: Dizziness (1% to 5%), sleep disorder (3% to 4%), drowsiness (≤3%), abnormal dreams (2%), insomnia (2%), anxiety (≤1%), depressed mood (≤1%), depression (≤1%)

Gastrointestinal: Nausea (5% to 7%), motion sickness (5%), vomiting (5%)

Hematologic & oncologic: Decreased hemoglobin (2%)

Hepatic: Increased serum alanine aminotransferase (4%)

Hypersensitivity: Hypersensitivity reaction (≤3%)

Ophthalmic: Photophobia (≤3%)

Renal: Increased serum creatinine (≤3%)

<1%, postmarketing and/or case reports: Agitation, amnesia, anemia, ataxia, blurred vision, cholestatic jaundice, corneal disease, decreased estimated GFR (eGFR), decreased visual acuity, hemolytic anemia, hyperacusis, hyperbilirubinemia, hyperesthesia, hypoesthesia, Meniere disease, nocturnal amblyopia, psychoneurosis, retinopathy, suicidal ideation, syncope, thrombocytopenia, tremor, urticaria, visual field defect, visual impairment, vitreous opacity

Mechanism of Action Tafenoquine is an 8-aminoquinoline antimalarial drug active against pre-erythrocytic (liver) forms (including hypnozoite [dormant stage]) and erythrocytic (asexual) forms, as well as gametocytes, of *Plasmodium* species, including *P. falciparum* and *P. vivax*. Activity against the pre-erythrocytic liver stage prevents development of the erythrocytic forms of the parasite, which are responsible for relapses in *P. vivax* malaria. Also causes red blood cell shrinkage in vitro.

Pharmacodynamics/Kinetics

Half-life Elimination 15 to 16.5 days

Time to Peak 12 to 15 hours

Reproductive Considerations

Pregnancy status should be evaluated prior to therapy. When tafenoquine is used in females of reproductive potential, effective contraception should be used during therapy and for 3 months after the last dose.

Pregnancy Considerations

Malaria infection in pregnant women may be more severe than in nonpregnant women and has a high risk of maternal and perinatal morbidity and mortality. Malaria infection during pregnancy can lead to miscarriage, premature delivery, low birth weight, congenital infection, and/or perinatal death. Therefore, pregnant women and women who are likely to become pregnant are advised to avoid travel to malaria-risk areas. When travel is unavoidable, pregnant women should take precautions to avoid mosquito bites and use effective prophylactic medications (CDC 2020; CDC Yellow Book 2020).

Because tafenoquine may cause acute hemolytic anemia in a fetus with G6PD deficiency, tafenoquine should not be used in pregnant women. When treatment is needed, other agents are preferred (CDC 2020; CDC Yellow Book 2020). Consult current Centers for Disease Control and Prevention guidelines for the treatment of malaria during pregnancy.

◆ **Tafenoquine Succinate** *see* Tafenoquine *on page 1402*

◆ **Tagrisso** *see* Osimertinib *on page 1149*

◆ **TAK-375** *see* Ramelteon *on page 1307*

◆ **TAK-390MR** *see* Dexlansoprazole *on page 471*

◆ **TAK-599** *see* Ceftaroline Fosamil *on page 312*

Talazoparib (tal a ZOE pa rib)

Brand Names: US Talzenna

Pharmacologic Category Antineoplastic Agent, PARP Inhibitor

Use Breast cancer, locally advanced or metastatic (BRCA-mutated, HER2-negative): Treatment of deleterious or suspected deleterious germline breast cancer susceptibility gene (BRCA)-mutated (gBRCAm) human epidermal growth factor receptor 2 (HER2)-negative locally advanced or metastatic breast cancer in adults (as detected by an approved test).

Local Anesthetic/Vasoconstrictor Precautions No information available to require special precautions

Effects on Dental Treatment Key adverse event(s) related to dental treatment: Stomatitis has been reported

Effects on Bleeding Chemotherapy may result in significant myelosuppression, potentially including reduction in platelet counts (thrombocytopenia) and altered hemostasis. In patients under active treatment with this agent, medical consult is suggested.

Adverse Reactions

>10%:

Central nervous system: Fatigue (62%), headache (33%), dizziness (17%)

Dermatologic: Alopecia (25%)

Endocrine & metabolic: Increased serum glucose (54%), decreased serum calcium (28%)

Gastrointestinal: Nausea (49%), vomiting (25%), diarrhea (22%), decreased appetite (21%), abdominal pain (19%)

Hematologic & oncologic: Decreased hemoglobin (90%; grade 3: 39%), anemia (53%; grade 3: 38%; grade 4: 1%), neutropenia (35%; grade 3: 18%; grade 4: 3%), thrombocytopenia (27%; grade 3: 11%; grade 4: 4%), leukopenia (17%)

Hepatic: Increased serum aspartate aminotransferase (37%), increased serum alkaline phosphatase (36%), increased serum alanine aminotransferase (33%)

1% to 10%:

Gastrointestinal: Dysgeusia (10%), dyspepsia (10%), stomatitis (8%)

Hematologic & oncologic: Lymphocytopenia (7%)

Frequency not defined: Hematologic & oncologic: Bone marrow depression

<1%, postmarketing, and/or case reports: Acute myelocytic leukemia, myelodysplastic syndrome

Mechanism of Action Talazoparib is a poly (ADP-ribose) polymerase (PARP) enzyme inhibitor, including PARP1 and PARP2. PARP enzymes are involved in DNA transcription, cell cycle regulation, and DNA repair. Talazoparib is a potent PARP inhibitor, with both strong catalytic inhibition and a PARP-trapping potential that is significantly greater than other PARP inhibitors (Litton 2018). Catalytic inhibition causes cell death due to accumulation of irreparable DNA damage; talazoparib also traps PARP-DNA complexes, which may be more effective in cell death than enzymatic inhibition alone (Litton 2018).

Pharmacodynamics/Kinetics

Half-life Elimination 90 (±58) hours

Time to Peak 1 to 2 hours

Reproductive Considerations

Pregnancy testing is recommended prior to therapy in females of reproductive potential. Females of reproductive potential should use effective contraception during therapy and for at least 7 months after the last talazoparib dose. Males with female partners of reproductive potential or female partners who are pregnant should also use effective contraception during therapy and for at least 4 months after the last talazoparib dose.

Pregnancy Considerations

Based on the mechanism of action and information from animal reproduction studies, talazoparib may cause fetal harm if administered during pregnancy.

◆ **Talazoparib Tosylate** *see* Talazoparib *on page 1402*

◆ **Talicia** *see* Omeprazole, Amoxicillin, and Rifabutin *on page 1140*

Talimogene Laherparepvec

(tal IM oh jeen la her pa REP vek)

Brand Names: US Imlygic

Pharmacologic Category Antineoplastic Agent, Oncolytic Virus

Use

Melanoma, unresectable: Treatment (local) of unresectable cutaneous, subcutaneous, and nodal lesions in patients with melanoma recurrent after initial surgery

Limitations of use: Has not been shown to improve overall survival or have an effect on visceral metastases.

Local Anesthetic/Vasoconstrictor Precautions No information available to require special precautions

Effects on Dental Treatment Key adverse event(s) related to dental treatment: Oral herpes has been reported as an adverse effect (frequency not defined)

Effects on Bleeding No information available to require special precautions

Adverse Reactions Most reactions resolved within 72 hours.

>10%:

Central nervous system: Fatigue (50%), chills (49%), headache (19%)

Gastrointestinal: Nausea (36%), vomiting (21%), diarrhea (19%), constipation (12%)

Local: Pain at injection site (28%)

Neuromuscular & skeletal: Myalgia (18%), arthralgia (17%), limb pain (16%)

Respiratory: Flu-like symptoms (31%)

Miscellaneous: Fever (43%)

1% to 10%:

Central nervous system: Dizziness (10%)

Endocrine & metabolic: Weight loss (6%)

Gastrointestinal: Abdominal pain (9%)

Respiratory: Oropharyngeal pain (6%)

Frequency not defined:

Cardiovascular: Deep vein thrombosis, vasculitis

Dermatologic: Cellulitis, dermatitis, exacerbation of psoriasis, skin rash, vitiligo

Gastrointestinal: Oral herpes

Infection: Bacterial infection (systemic), herpes virus infection

Ophthalmic: Herpes simplex keratitis

Renal: Glomerulonephritis

Respiratory: Acute asthma, pneumonitis

Mechanism of Action Talimogene laherparepvec is a genetically modified attenuated herpes simplex virus 1 (HSV) oncolytic virus which selectively replicates in and lyses tumor cells (Andtbacka 2015). Talimogene laherparepvec is modified through deletion of two nonessential viral genes. Deletion of the herpes virus neurovirulence factor gene ICP34.5 diminishes viral pathogenicity and increases tumor-selective replication; deletion of the ICP47 gene reduces virally mediated suppression of antigen presentation and increases the expression of the HSV US11 gene (Andtbacka 2015). Virally derived GM-CSF recruits and activates antigen-presenting cells, leading to an antitumor immune response.

Pharmacodynamics/Kinetics

Time to Peak Peak levels of talimogene laherparepvec were detected in the urine on the day of treatment

Reproductive Considerations

Women of reproductive potential should use effective contraception during therapy.

Pregnancy Considerations Use is contraindicated in pregnant women.

Talimogene laherparepvec is a live, attenuated, genetically modified herpes simplex virus type 1 (HSV-1). HSV-1 is known to cross the placenta, can be transmitted during birth, and produce infections in the fetus or neonate. It is not known if this can occur following exposure to talimogene laherparepvec. Pregnant women should not prepare or administer this medication. Pregnant women who are in close contact of patients treated with talimogene laherparepvec should not change dressings or clean injection sites, and should avoid direct contact with the injection site, dressings, or body fluids of patients.

- **Talminogene Laherparepvec** *see* Talimogene Laherparepvec *on page 1403*
- **Taltz** *see* Ixekizumab *on page 854*
- **Talzenna** *see* Talazoparib *on page 1402*
- **Tambocor** *see* Flecainide *on page 671*
- **Tamiflu** *see* Oseltamivir *on page 1147*

Tamoxifen (ta MOKS i fen)

Brand Names: US Soltamox

Brand Names: Canada APO-Tamox; DOM-Tamoxifen [DSC]; MYLAN-Tamoxifen [DSC]; Nolvadex D; PMS-Tamoxifen [DSC]; TEVA-Tamoxifen

Pharmacologic Category Antineoplastic Agent, Estrogen Receptor Antagonist; Selective Estrogen Receptor Modulator (SERM)

Use

Breast cancer, risk reduction: *Risk reduction in females at high risk:* To reduce the incidence of breast cancer in adult females at high risk for breast cancer

Breast cancer, treatment:

Adjuvant treatment: Adjuvant treatment of adult patients with early stage estrogen receptor-positive breast cancer; to reduce the incidence of contralateral breast cancer in adult patients when used as adjuvant therapy for the treatment of breast cancer

Ductal carcinoma in situ: To reduce the risk of invasive breast cancer in adult females with ductal carcinoma in situ (following breast surgery and radiation)

Metastatic breast cancer: Treatment of adult patients with estrogen receptor-positive metastatic breast cancer

Local Anesthetic/Vasoconstrictor Precautions No information available to require special precautions

Effects on Dental Treatment No significant effects or complications reported

Effects on Bleeding Although significant myelosuppression with associated altered hemostasis has been reported for many chemotherapeutic agents, myelosuppression is not common with tamoxifen and no specific precautions appear to necessary.

Adverse Reactions

>10%:

Cardiovascular: Flushing (33%), hypertension (11%), peripheral edema (11%), vasodilation (41%)

Dermatologic: Skin changes (6% to 19%), skin rash (13%)

Endocrine & metabolic: Amenorrhea (16%), fluid retention (32%), hot flash (3% to 80% [placebo 0.2% to 68%]), weight loss (23%)

Gastrointestinal: Nausea (5% to 26%), nausea and vomiting (12%)

Genitourinary: Irregular menses (13% to 25%), vaginal discharge (12% to 55%), vaginal hemorrhage (2% to 23%)

Hematologic & oncologic: Lymphedema (11%)

Nervous system: Depression (2% to 12%), fatigue (≤18%), mood changes (12% to 18%), pain (3% to 16%)

Neuromuscular & skeletal: Arthralgia (11%), arthritis (14%), asthenia (≤18%)

Respiratory: Pharyngitis (14%)

1% to 10%:

Cardiovascular: Chest pain (5%), edema (4%), ischemic heart disease (3%), venous thrombosis (5%)

Dermatologic: Alopecia (≤5%), diaphoresis (6%)

Endocrine & metabolic: Hypercholesterolemia (3%), infrequent uterine bleeding (9%), menstrual disease (6%), ovarian cyst (3%), weight gain (9%)

Gastrointestinal: Abdominal cramps (1%), abdominal pain (9%), anorexia (1%), constipation (4% to 8%), diarrhea (7%), dyspepsia (6%)

Genitourinary: Leukorrhea (9%), mastalgia (6%), urinary tract infection (10%), vaginitis (5%), vulvovaginitis (5%)

Hematologic & oncologic: Anemia (5%), neoplasm (5%; second primary), thrombocytopenia (2% to 10%)

Hepatic: Increased serum aspartate aminotransferase (5%), increased serum bilirubin (2%)

Hypersensitivity: Hypersensitivity reaction (3%)

Infection: Infection (≤9%), sepsis (≤6%)

Nervous system: Anxiety (6%), dizziness (8%), headache (8%), insomnia (9%), paresthesia (5%)

Neuromuscular & skeletal: Arthropathy (5%), back pain (10%), bone fracture (7%), musculoskeletal pain (3%), myalgia (5%), ostealgia (6%), osteoporosis (7%)

Ophthalmic: Cataract (8% [placebo 7%])

Renal: Increased serum creatinine (2%)

Respiratory: Bronchitis (5%), cough (4% to 9%), dyspnea (8%), flu-like symptoms (6%), sinusitis (5%), throat irritation (oral solution: 5%)

Miscellaneous: Cyst (5%)

<1%:

Cardiovascular: Deep vein thrombosis (placebo 0.2%), pulmonary embolism (placebo 0.2%), superficial thrombophlebitis

Hepatic: Hepatic neoplasm

Frequency not defined:

Cardiovascular: Cerebrovascular accident (Fisher 2005; Lai 2017)

Dermatologic: Pruritus vulvae (Day 2001)

Endocrine & metabolic: Hypercalcemia (Legha 1981; Nikolic-Tomasevic 2001)

Gastrointestinal: Cholestasis (Blackburn 1984), dysgeusia (Schiffman 2018)

Genitourinary: Vaginal dryness (Mortimer 1999; Mourits 2002)

Hematologic & oncologic: Tumor flare (during treatment of metastatic breast cancer; generally resolves with continuation; includes increased lesion size and erythema) (Mulvenna 1999; Plotkin 1978)

Hepatic: Hepatic necrosis (Ching 1992; Storen 2000), hepatitis (Oien 1999; Pinto 1995), liver steatosis (Roy 2019; Saphner 2009)

Nervous system: Tumor pain (during treatment of metastatic breast cancer; generally resolves with continuation) (Mulvenna 1999)

Postmarketing:

Cardiovascular: Portal vein thrombosis (Hsu 2015), retinal thrombosis (Demirci 2019; Onder 2013)

Dermatologic: Bullous pemphigoid, cutaneous lupus erythematosus (Andrew 2014), erythema multiforme, night sweats (Day 2001; Moon 2017), Stevens-Johnson syndrome, toxic epidermal necrolysis (Madabhavi 2015)

Endocrine & metabolic: Decreased libido (Morales 2004; Mourits 2002), hyperglycemia (Hozumi 1997; Kim 2014), hypertriglyceridemia (Liu 2003; Singh 2016), loss of libido (males) (Pemmaraju 2012; Wibowo 2016)

Gastrointestinal: Pancreatitis (Singh 2016; Tey 2019)

Genitourinary: Dyspareunia (Mourits 2002), endometrial hyperplasia (Cheng 1997; Lindahl 2008), endometrial polyps (Cohen 1996; Neven 1998), endometriosis (Kraft 2006), impotence (Pemmaraju 2012)

Hematologic & oncologic: Agranulocytosis (Ching 1992; Herrscher 2020), endometrial carcinoma (Cohen 1996; Fisher 2004), leukopenia, malignant neoplasm of ovary (Cohen 1996; Ohara 2002), malignant neoplasm of uterus (Kloos 2002; Yildirim 2005), neutropenia (Herrscher 2020), pancytopenia (Mitani 2006), tumor lysis syndrome (Cech 1986), uterine carcinoma, uterine fibroids (Polin 2008)

Hypersensitivity: Angioedema (Bork 2017; Rousset-Jablonski 2009)

Neuromuscular & skeletal: Subacute cutaneous lupus erythematosus (Andrew 2014)

Ophthalmic: Corneal deposits (Muftuoglu 2006; Tarafdar 2012), epithelial keratopathy (Noureddin 1999; Pavlidis 1992), macular edema (Murray 1998; Zafeiropoulos 2014), maculopathy (Bommireddy 2016; Srikantia 2010), optic neuritis (Colley 2004; Noureddin 1999), retinal hole without detachment (macula hole) (Cronin 2005), retinal pigment changes (Noureddin 1999), retinopathy (Georgalas 2013; Wang 2015), vision color changes (Eisner 2011; Salomao 2007)

Respiratory: Eosinophilic pneumonitis (Kwon 2019), interstitial pneumonitis (Ahmed 2016), pulmonary fibrosis (Bentzen 1996), pulmonary injury (Etori 2017)

Mechanism of Action Tamoxifen is a selective estrogen receptor modulator (SERM) that competitively binds to estrogen receptors on tumors and other tissue targets, producing a nuclear complex that decreases DNA synthesis and inhibits estrogen effects; nonsteroidal agent with potent antiestrogenic properties which compete with estrogen for binding sites in breast and other tissues; cells accumulate in the G_0 and G_1 phases; therefore, tamoxifen is cytostatic rather than cytocidal.

Pharmacodynamics/Kinetics

Half-life Elimination Tamoxifen: ~5 to 7 days; N-desmethyl tamoxifen: ~14 days

Time to Peak Serum: Children 2 to 10 years (female): ~8 hours; Adults: ~5 hours

Reproductive Considerations

Tamoxifen may induce ovulation (Steiner 2005) or cause menstrual cycle irregularities. Based on animal data, tamoxifen may impair embryo implantation in females of reproductive potential, but may not reliably cause infertility, even if menstrual cycles are irregular.

Confirm a negative pregnancy test in females of reproductive potential prior to initiating tamoxifen therapy. Females of reproductive potential should use effective nonhormonal contraception during tamoxifen therapy and for 2 months following the last tamoxifen dose.

Pregnancy Considerations

Based on the mechanism of action, and data from animal reproduction studies, in utero exposure to tamoxifen may cause fetal harm. However, available data are insufficient to establish a causal relationship; no pattern of birth defects has been observed, and the long term effects of tamoxifen on development are not known (Braems 2011; Schuurman 2019). There have been reports of vaginal bleeding, birth defects, spontaneous abortions and fetal death following use in pregnancy. Tamoxifen use during pregnancy may have a potential long-term risk to the fetus of a diethylstilbestrol (DES)-like syndrome (based on animal data).

◆ **Tamoxifen Citras** *see* Tamoxifen *on page 1404*

◆ **Tamoxifen Citrate** *see* Tamoxifen *on page 1404*

Tamsulosin (tam SOO loe sin)

Brand Names: US Flomax

Brand Names: Canada APO-Tamsulosin CR; Flomax CR; MYLAN-Tamsulosin [DSC]; RATIO-Tamsulosin; SANDOZ Tamsulosin; SANDOZ Tamsulosin CR; TEVA-Tamsulosin; TEVA-Tamsulosin CR

Pharmacologic Category $Alpha_1$ Blocker

Use

Benign prostatic hyperplasia: Treatment of signs and symptoms of benign prostatic hyperplasia (BPH)

Limitations of use: Not indicated for the treatment of hypertension.

Local Anesthetic/Vasoconstrictor Precautions

No information available to require special precautions

Effects on Dental Treatment Key adverse event(s) related to dental treatment: Rare occurrence of xerostomia; normal salivary flow resumes upon discontinuation; infrequent occurrence of pharyngitis. Patients may experience orthostatic hypotension as they stand up after treatment; especially if lying in dental chair for extended periods of time. Use caution with sudden changes in position during and after dental treatment.

Effects on Bleeding No information available to require special precautions

Adverse Reactions
>10%:
Cardiovascular: Orthostatic hypotension (first dose: 6% to 19%; symptomatic orthostatic hypotension (chronic therapy) <1%)
Central nervous system: Headache (19% to 21%), dizziness (15% to 17%)
Genitourinary: Ejaculation failure (8% to 18%)
Infection: Infection (9% to 11%)
Respiratory: Rhinitis (13% to 18%)
1% to 10%:
Central nervous system: Drowsiness (3% to 4%), insomnia (1% to 2%), vertigo (≤1%)
Endocrine & metabolic: Loss of libido (2%)
Gastrointestinal: Diarrhea (6%), nausea (4%)
Neuromuscular & skeletal: Weakness (8% to 9%), back pain (7% to 8%)
Ophthalmic: Blurred vision (≤2%)
Respiratory: Pharyngitis (6%), cough (3% to 5%), sinusitis (4%)
<1%, postmarketing, and/or case reports: Constipation, decreased visual acuity, epistaxis, erythema multiforme, exfoliation of skin, exfoliative dermatitis, hypersensitivity reaction, hypotension, intraoperative floppy iris syndrome, palpitations, priapism, syncope, vomiting, xerostomia

Mechanism of Action Tamsulosin is an antagonist of alpha$_{1A}$-adrenoreceptors in the prostate. Smooth muscle tone in the prostate is mediated by alpha$_{1A}$-adrenoreceptors; blocking them leads to relaxation of smooth muscle in the bladder neck and prostate causing an improvement of urine flow and decreased symptoms of BPH. Approximately 75% of the alpha$_1$-receptors in the prostate are of the alpha$_{1A}$ subtype.

Pharmacodynamics/Kinetics

Half-life Elimination Healthy volunteers: 9 to 13 hours; Target population: 14 to15 hours

Time to Peak
Fasting: 4 to 5 hours; With food: 6 to 7 hours
Steady-state: By the fifth day of once-daily dosing

Pregnancy Considerations Information related to the use of tamsulosin for treating ureteral calculi in pregnancy is limited (Bailey 2016). Other treatments such as stents or ureteroscopy, are currently recommended if stone removal is needed (Assimos 2016; Lloyd 2016).

◆ **Tamsulosin and Dutasteride** *see* Dutasteride and Tamsulosin *on page* 540

◆ **Tamsulosin HCl** *see* Tamsulosin *on page* 1405

◆ **Tamsulosin Hydrochloride** *see* Tamsulosin *on page* 1405

◆ **Tamsulosin Hydrochloride and Dutasteride** *see* Dutasteride and Tamsulosin *on page* 540

◆ **Tanzeum** *see* Albiglutide *on page* 89

◆ **Tanzeum [DSC]** *see* Albiglutide *on page* 89

◆ **TAP-144** *see* Leuprolide *on page* 890

◆ **Tapazole** *see* MethIMAzole *on page* 988

Tapentadol (ta PEN ta dol)

Related Information
Oral Pain *on page* 1734

Brand Names: US Nucynta; Nucynta ER

Brand Names: Canada Nucynta ER; Nucynta IR

Pharmacologic Category Analgesic, Opioid

Use

Neuropathic pain associated with diabetic peripheral neuropathy: Extended-release: Management of neuropathic pain associated with diabetic peripheral neuropathy (DPN) severe enough to require daily, around-the-clock, long-term opioid treatment and for which alternative treatment options are inadequate. **Note:** Tapentadol ER is generally not recommended as first or second line therapy due to a high risk for addiction and safety concerns compared to modest pain reduction (Pop-Busui 2017).

Pain management:
Immediate release: Management of acute pain severe enough to require an opioid analgesic and for which alternative treatments are inadequate in adults.
Extended release: Management of pain severe enough to require daily, around-the-clock, long-term opioid treatment and for which alternative treatments are inadequate.

Limitations of use: Reserve tapentadol for use in patients for whom alternative treatment options (eg, nonopioid analgesics, opioid combination products) are ineffective, not tolerated, or would be otherwise inadequate to provide sufficient management of pain. Tapentadol ER is not indicated as an as-needed analgesic.

Local Anesthetic/Vasoconstrictor Precautions Although part of the mechanism of tapentadol inhibits the reuptake of norepinephrine, there is no information available to require any special precautions.

Effects on Dental Treatment Key adverse effect(s) related to dental treatment: Xerostomia (normal salivary flow resumes upon discontinuation)

Effects on Bleeding No information available to require special precautions

Adverse Reactions
>10%:
Gastrointestinal: Nausea (21% to 30%), vomiting (8% to 18%), constipation (8% to 17%)
Nervous system: Dizziness (17% to 24%), drowsiness (12% to 15%), headache (ER: 10% to 15%)
1% to 10%:
Cardiovascular: Hypotension (ER: 1%)
Dermatologic: Pruritus (1% to 8%), hyperhidrosis (3% to 5%), skin rash (1%)
Endocrine & metabolic: Hot flash (ER: 2% to 3%; IR: 1%)
Gastrointestinal: Diarrhea (ER: 7%), xerostomia (4% to 7%), decreased appetite (ER: 2% to 6%; IR: 2%), dyspepsia (1% to 3%), abdominal distress (≤1%)
Genitourinary: Erectile dysfunction (ER: 1%), urinary tract infection (IR: 1%)
Nervous system: Fatigue (ER: 9%: IR: 3%), anxiety (ER: 2% to 5%; IR: 1%), insomnia (2% to 4%), irritability (≤2%), abnormal dreams (1% to 2%), lethargy (1% to 2%), vertigo (ER: 1% to 2%), chills (ER: 1%), depression (ER: 1%), feeling hot (IR: 1%), confusion (≤1%), disturbance in attention (≤1%), hypoesthesia (≤1%), lack of concentration (≤1%), nervousness (≤1%), sedated state (≤1%), withdrawal syndrome (≤1%)
Neuromuscular & skeletal: Tremor (ER: 1% to 3%; IR: 1%), asthenia (ER: 2%)
Ophthalmic: Blurred vision (ER: 1%)
Respiratory: Nasopharyngitis (IR: 1%), upper respiratory tract infection (IR: 1%), dyspnea (≤1%)

<1%: Abnormality in thinking, agitation, altered mental status, ataxia, balance impairment, cough, decreased blood pressure, decreased heart rate, delayed gastric emptying, disorientation, drug dependence, dysarthria, edema, euphoria, feeling abnormal, feeling of heaviness, hallucination, hypersensitivity reaction, hypogonadism (Brennan 2013; Debono 2011), illusion, impaired consciousness, increased gamma-glutamyl transferase, increased heart rate, increased serum alanine aminotransferase, increased serum aspartate aminotransferase, intoxicated feeling, left bundle branch block, memory impairment, muscle spasm, nightmares, oxygen desaturation, palpitations, paresthesia, pollakiuria, presyncope, respiratory depression, restlessness, seizure, sexual difficulty, syncope, urinary hesitancy, urticaria, visual disturbance, weight loss

Frequency not defined:

Nervous system: Drug abuse, neonatal withdrawal

Postmarketing: Anaphylaxis, panic attack, suicidal ideation

Mechanism of Action Binds to μ-opiate receptors in the CNS causing inhibition of ascending pain pathways, altering the perception of and response to pain; also inhibits the reuptake of norepinephrine, which also modifies the ascending pain pathway

Pharmacodynamics/Kinetics

Half-life Elimination Immediate release: ~4 hours; Long acting formulations: ~5-6 hours

Time to Peak Plasma: Immediate release: 1.25 hours; Long acting formulations: 3-6 hours

Reproductive Considerations

Long-term opioid use may cause secondary hypogonadism, which may lead to sexual dysfunction or infertility in men and women (Brennan 2013).

Pregnancy Considerations Opioids cross the placenta.

According to some studies, maternal use of opioids may be associated with birth defects (including neural tube defects, congenital heart defects, and gastroschisis), poor fetal growth, stillbirth, and preterm delivery (CDC [Dowell 2016]). Information related to tapentadol exposure in pregnancy is limited (Stollenwerk 2018).

[US Boxed Warning]: Prolonged use of tapentadol during pregnancy can result in neonatal opioid withdrawal syndrome, which may be life-threatening if not recognized and treated, and requires management according to protocols developed by neonatology experts. If opioid use is required for a prolonged period in a pregnant woman, advise the patient of the risk of neonatal opioid withdrawal syndrome and ensure that appropriate treatment will be available. If chronic opioid exposure occurs in pregnancy, adverse events in the newborn (including withdrawal) may occur (Chou 2009). Symptoms of neonatal abstinence syndrome (NAS) following opioid exposure may be autonomic (eg, fever, temperature instability), gastrointestinal (eg, diarrhea, vomiting, poor feeding/weight gain), or neurologic (eg, high-pitched crying, hyperactivity, increased muscle tone, increased wakefulness/abnormal sleep pattern, irritability, sneezing, seizure, tremor, yawning) (Dow 2012; Hudak 2012). Mothers who are physically dependent on opioids may give birth to infants who are also physically dependent. Opioids may cause respiratory depression and psychophysiologic effects in the neonate; newborns of mothers receiving opioids during labor should be monitored.

Tapentadol is not commonly used to treat pain during labor (ACOG 209 2019) or chronic noncancer pain in pregnant women or those who may become pregnant (CDC [Dowell 2016]; Chou 2009).

Controlled Substance C-II

Dental Health Professional Considerations

Tapentadol is classified as an opioid analgesic having a unique ability to bind to μ-opiate receptors and to also inhibit the reuptake of norepinephrine. It shares many properties of the traditional opioid drugs including addiction liability. A report by Kleinert et al, showed that single doses of tapentadol ≥75 mg effectively reduced moderate-to-severe postoperative dental pain in a dose related fashion and were well tolerated compared to 60 mg morphine. The study showed that tapentadol was a highly effective, centrally acting analgesic with a favorable side effect profile with rapid onset of action.

- **Tapentadol HCl** *see* Tapentadol *on page 1406*
- **Tapentadol Hydrochloride** *see* Tapentadol *on page 1406*
- **TaperDex 6-Day** *see* DexAMETHasone (Systemic) *on page 463*
- **TaperDex 7-Day** *see* DexAMETHasone (Systemic) *on page 463*
- **TaperDex 12-Day** *see* DexAMETHasone (Systemic) *on page 463*
- **Tarceva** *see* Erlotinib *on page 584*
- **TargaDOX** *see* Doxycycline *on page 522*
- **Targiniq ER** *see* Oxycodone and Naloxone *on page 1169*
- **Tarina 24 Fe** *see* Ethinyl Estradiol and Norethindrone *on page 614*
- **Tarina FE 1/20** *see* Ethinyl Estradiol and Norethindrone *on page 614*
- **Tarina FE 1/20 EQ** *see* Ethinyl Estradiol and Norethindrone *on page 614*
- **TAS-102** *see* Trifluridine and Tipiracil *on page 1497*
- **Tasigna** *see* Nilotinib *on page 1105*

Tasimelteon (tas i MEL tee on)

Brand Names: US Hetlioz

Pharmacologic Category Hypnotic, Miscellaneous; Melatonin Receptor Agonist

Use Non-24-hour sleep-wake disorder: Treatment of non-24-hour sleep-wake disorder (non-24). **Note:** Efficacy was established in totally blind patients with non-24-hour sleep-wake disorder.

Local Anesthetic/Vasoconstrictor Precautions

No information available to require special precautions

Effects on Dental Treatment No significant effects or complications reported

Effects on Bleeding No information available to require special precautions

Adverse Reactions

>10%: Central nervous system: Headache (17%)

1% to 10%:

Central nervous system: Abnormal dreams (10%)

Genitourinary: Urinary tract infection (7%)

Hepatic: Increased serum ALT (10%)

Respiratory: Upper respiratory tract infection (7%)

Mechanism of Action Agonist of melatonin receptors MT_1 and MT_2 (greater affinity for the MT_2 receptor than the MT_1 receptor). Agonism of MT_1 is thought to preferentially induce sleepiness, while MT_2 receptor activation preferentially influences regulation of circadian rhythms.

Pharmacodynamics/Kinetics

Onset of Action Effect may take weeks or months (due to individual differences in circadian rhythms)

Half-life Elimination ~1 to 2 hours

Time to Peak Fasting: ~0.5 to 3 hours (increased by ~1.75 hours with a high-fat meal)

Pregnancy Considerations Adverse events were observed in some animal reproduction studies.

- **Tasmar** *see* Tolcapone *on page 1461*
- **Tasoprol** *see* Clobetasol *on page 377*
- **Tavalisse** *see* Fostamatinib *on page 718*
- **Tavist Allergy [OTC] [DSC]** *see* Clemastine *on page 367*
- **Tavist ND** *see* Loratadine *on page 930*
- **Taxol** *see* PACLitaxel (Conventional) *on page 1178*
- **Taxotere** *see* DOCEtaxel *on page 507*
- **Taytulla** *see* Ethinyl Estradiol and Norethindrone *on page 614*

Tazarotene (taz AR oh teen)

Brand Names: US Arazlo; Avage [DSC]; Fabior; Tazorac

Brand Names: Canada Tazorac

Pharmacologic Category Acne Products; Keratolytic Agent; Retinoic Acid Derivative; Topical Skin Product, Acne

Use

Acne (Arazlo 0.045% lotion, Fabior, Tazorac 0.1% cream, Tazorac 0.1% gel): Topical treatment of acne vulgaris in patients ≥9 years of age (Arazlo) or ≥12 years of age.

Palliation of fine facial wrinkles, facial mottled hyper-/hypopigmentation, benign facial lentigines (Avage): Adjunctive agent for use in the mitigation (palliation) of facial fine wrinkling, facial mottled hyper- and hypopigmentation, and benign facial lentigines in patients ≥17 years of age who use comprehensive skin care and sunlight avoidance programs.

Psoriasis:

Tazorac 0.05% and 0.1% cream: Topical treatment of plaque psoriasis in patients ≥18 years of age.

Tazorac 0.05% and 0.1% gel: Topical treatment of stable plaque psoriasis of up to 20% body surface area involvement in patients ≥12 years of age.

Limitations of use: Does not eliminate or prevent wrinkles, repair sun-damaged skin, reverse photoaging, or restore more youthful or younger skin. Has not demonstrated a mitigating effect on significant signs of chronic sunlight exposure such as coarse or deep wrinkling, tactile roughness, telangiectasia, skin laxity, keratinocytic atypia, melanocytic atypia, or dermal elastosis. Safety and effectiveness for the prevention or treatment of actinic keratoses, skin neoplasms, or lentigo maligna has not been established. Safe and effective daily use >52 weeks is not known. Safety of gel use on more than 20% body surface area has not been established.

Local Anesthetic/Vasoconstrictor Precautions No information available to require special precautions

Effects on Dental Treatment No significant effects or complications reported

Effects on Bleeding No information available to require special precautions

Adverse Reactions Percentage of incidence varies with formulation and/or strength:

>10%: Dermatologic: Desquamation (0.1% cream 40%; foam 6%), erythema (0.1% cream 34%; foam 6%), burning sensation of skin (26%), xeroderma (7% to 16%), skin irritation (10% to 14%), exacerbation of psoriasis, skin pain

1% to 10%:

Cardiovascular: Peripheral edema

Dermatologic: Pruritus (0.1% cream 10%; foam 1%), contact dermatitis (8%), stinging of the skin (3%), skin rash (≤3%), cheilitis (1%), dermatitis (1%), skin photosensitivity (1%), eczema, skin discoloration, skin fissure

Endocrine & metabolic: Hypertriglyceridemia

Local: Application site pain (1%), local hemorrhage

Ophthalmic: Ocular irritation (including edema, irritation, and inflammation of the eye or eyelid; 4%)

Frequency not defined: Hypersensitivity: Hypersensitivity reaction, local hypersensitivity reaction

<1%, postmarketing, and/or case reports: Application site edema, exfoliation of skin, impetigo, pain, skin blister

Mechanism of Action Synthetic, acetylenic retinoid which modulates differentiation and proliferation of epithelial tissue and exerts some degree of anti-inflammatory and immunological activity

Pharmacodynamics/Kinetics

Onset of Action Psoriasis: 1 week

Duration of Action Therapeutic: Psoriasis: Effects have been observed for up to 3 months after a 3-month course of topical treatment

Half-life Elimination Cream, gel: ~81 hours (tazarotenic acid); Foam: 8.1 ± 3.7 hours

Reproductive Considerations

Evaluate pregnancy status prior to use in females of reproductive potential. A negative pregnancy test should be obtained within 2 weeks prior to treatment; treatment should begin during a normal menstrual period. Adequate contraception should be used in females of reproductive potential.

Pregnancy Considerations Use in pregnancy is contraindicated.

Inadvertent exposure to a limited number of pregnant women occurred during premarketing studies; however, the available data are inadequate to evaluate outcomes. Based on data from animal reproduction studies, retinoid pharmacology, and the potential for systemic absorption, in utero exposure to tazarotene may cause fetal harm.

Topical products are recommended as initial therapy for the treatment of acne or psoriasis in pregnant women. Because the safety of tazarotene is uncertain, use during pregnancy is contraindicated (Bae 2012; Chien 2016; Kong 2013).

Tazemetostat (TAZ e MET oh stat)

Brand Names: US Tazverik

Pharmacologic Category Antineoplastic Agent, EZH2-Inhibitor; Antineoplastic Agent, Histone Methyltransferase (HMT) Inhibitor

Use

Epithelioid sarcoma, metastatic or locally advanced: Treatment of metastatic or locally advanced epithelioid sarcoma not eligible for complete resection in adults and adolescents ≥16 years of age.

Follicular lymphoma, relapsed/refractory:

Treatment of relapsed or refractory follicular lymphoma in adults whose tumors are positive for an EZH2 mutation (as detected by an approved test) and who have received at least 2 prior systemic therapies.

Treatment of relapsed or refractory follicular lymphoma in adults who have no satisfactory alternative treatment options.

Local Anesthetic/Vasoconstrictor Precautions No information available to require special precautions.

Effects on Dental Treatment No significant effects or complications reported.

Effects on Bleeding Frequent occurrence of hemorrhage, prolonged partial thromboplastin time; medical consult suggested.

Adverse Reactions

>10%:

Endocrine & metabolic: Decreased serum albumin, decreased serum calcium, decreased serum glucose, decreased serum phosphate, decreased serum potassium, decreased serum sodium, increased serum glucose, increased serum potassium, increased serum triglycerides, weight loss

Gastrointestinal: Abdominal pain, constipation, decreased appetite, diarrhea, nausea, vomiting

Hematologic & oncologic: Anemia, decreased white blood cell count, hemorrhage, lymphocytopenia, prolonged partial thromboplastin time

Hepatic: Increased serum alanine aminotransferase, increased serum alkaline phosphatase, increased serum aspartate aminotransferase

Nervous system: Fatigue, headache, pain

Renal: Increased serum creatinine

Respiratory: Cough, dyspnea

<1%: Myelodysplastic syndrome, myeloid leukemia, T-cell lymphoma

Frequency not defined:

Dermatologic: Skin infection

Hematologic & oncologic: Pulmonary hemorrhage, rectal hemorrhage, wound hemorrhage

Nervous system: Cerebral hemorrhage, intracranial hemorrhage

Respiratory: Hemoptysis, pleural effusion, respiratory distress

Mechanism of Action Tazemetostat is a potent and selective inhibitor of histone methyltransferase EZH2 (enhancer of zeste homolog 2); it also inhibits some EZH2 gain-of-function mutations (including Y646X and A687V), as well as EZH1. EZH2 is overexpressed or mutated in many cancer types and plays a role in tumor proliferation. SWItch/Sucrose Non-Fermentable (SWI/SNF) complex aids in facilitating gene expression and terminal differentiation; altered EZH2 upregulation and loss-of-function mutations in SWI/SNF are oncogenic in many human cancers; tazemetostat has antitumor activity in EZH2-mutant cell lines (Italiano 2018). Tazemetostat suppressed B-cell lymphoma cell lines proliferation in vitro, and showed antitumor activity in an animal model of B-cell lymphoma with or without EZH2 gain-of-function mutations; tazemetostat demonstrated increased inhibition of lymphoma cell line proliferation with mutant EZH2.

Pharmacodynamics/Kinetics

Half-life Elimination 3.1 hours.

Time to Peak 1 to 2 hours.

Reproductive Considerations

Evaluate pregnancy status prior to use in females of reproductive potential. Females of reproductive potential should use effective nonhormonal contraception during therapy and for 6 months after the last tazemetostat dose. Males with female partners of reproductive potential should use effective contraception during therapy and for at least 3 months after the last dose of tazemetostat.

Pregnancy Considerations

Based on the mechanism of action, and data from animal reproduction studies, in utero exposure to tazemetostat may cause fetal harm.

Product Availability Tazverik: FDA approved January 2020; anticipated availability by February 2020.

Prescribing and Access Restrictions

Tazemetostat is available through a specialty pharmacy and specialty distributors. For further information, contact 833-437-4669 or https://www.tazverik.com/Content/pdf/ordering-and-distribution-sheet.pdf.

- ◆ **Tazemetostat hydrobromide** *see* Tazemetostat *on page 1408*
- ◆ **Tazicef** *see* CefTAZidime *on page 313*
- ◆ **Tazidime** *see* CefTAZidime *on page 313*
- ◆ **Tazobactam and Ceftolozane** *see* Ceftolozane and Tazobactam *on page 315*
- ◆ **Tazobactam and Piperacillin** *see* Piperacillin and Tazobactam *on page 1236*
- ◆ **Tazorac** *see* Tazarotene *on page 1408*
- ◆ **Taztia XT** *see* DilTIAZem *on page 499*
- ◆ **Tazverik** *see* Tazemetostat *on page 1408*
- ◆ **Tbo-Filgrastim** *see* Filgrastim *on page 668*
- ◆ **TB Skin Test** *see* Tuberculin Tests *on page 1503*
- ◆ **3TC** *see* LamiVUDine *on page 872*
- ◆ **3TC, Abacavir, and Zidovudine** *see* Abacavir, Lamivudine, and Zidovudine *on page 52*
- ◆ **T-Cell Growth Factor** *see* Aldesleukin *on page 91*
- ◆ **TCGF** *see* Aldesleukin *on page 91*
- ◆ **TCN** *see* Tetracycline (Systemic) *on page 1431*
- ◆ **TD-4208** *see* Revefenacin *on page 1319*
- ◆ **TD-6424** *see* Telavancin *on page 1411*
- ◆ **TDF** *see* Tenofovir Disoproxil Fumarate *on page 1419*
- ◆ **T-DM1** *see* Ado-Trastuzumab Emtansine *on page 86*
- ◆ **Tecfidera** *see* Dimethyl Fumarate *on page 501*
- ◆ **Technivie** *see* Ombitasvir, Paritaprevir, and Ritonavir *on page 1135*
- ◆ **Technosphere Insulin (TI)** *see* Insulin (Oral Inhalation) *on page 828*

Tedizolid (ted eye ZOE lid)

Brand Names: US Sivextro

Pharmacologic Category Antibiotic, Oxazolidinone

Use Skin and skin structure infections: Treatment of adults and pediatric patients ≥12 years of age with acute bacterial skin and skin structure infections caused by susceptible isolates of the following gram-positive microorganisms: *Staphylococcus aureus* (including methicillin-resistant and methicillin-susceptible isolates), *Streptococcus pyogenes, Streptococcus* agalactiae, *Streptococcus anginosus* group (including *Streptococcus anginosus, Streptococcus intermedius,* and *Streptococcus constellatus*), and *Enterococcus faecalis*

Local Anesthetic/Vasoconstrictor Precautions No information available to require special precautions.

Effects on Dental Treatment Key adverse event(s) related to dental treatment: Oral candidiasis, facial paralysis, and paresthesia have all been reported with prolonged use of tedizolid.

Effects on Bleeding No information available to require special precautions

Adverse Reactions

1% to 10%:

Cardiovascular: Flushing (<2%), hypertension (<2%), palpitations (<2%), tachycardia (<2%)

Central nervous system: Headache (5%), dizziness (2%), facial nerve paralysis (<2%), hypoesthesia (<2%), insomnia (<2%), paresthesia (<2%), peripheral neuropathy (1%)

Dermatologic: Dermatitis (<2%), pruritus (<2%), urticaria (<2%)

Endocrine & metabolic: Increased gamma-glutamyl transferase (<2%)

Gastrointestinal: Nausea (7%), diarrhea (4%), vomiting (3%), *Clostridioides difficile* colitis (<2%), oral candidiasis (<2%)

Hematologic & oncologic: Decreased hemoglobin (males <10.1 g/dL; females <9 g/dL: 3%), decreased platelet count (<112,000/mm^3: 2%), anemia (<2%), decreased white blood cell count (<2%)

Hepatic: Increased serum alanine aminotransferase (<2%), increased serum aspartate transaminase (<2%), increased serum transaminases (<2%)

Hypersensitivity: Hypersensitivity (<2%)

Infection: Fungal infection (vulvovaginal: <2%)

Local: Injection site reaction (≤4%)

Ophthalmic: Asthenopia (<2%), blurred vision (<2%), visual impairment (<2%), vitreous opacity (<2%)

Miscellaneous: Infusion related reaction (≤4%)

<1%, postmarketing, and/or case reports: *Clostridioides difficile* associated diarrhea, decrease in absolute neutrophil count (<800/mm^3), optic neuropathy

Mechanism of Action After conversion from the prodrug, tedizolid phosphate, tedizolid binds to the 50S bacterial ribosomal subunit. This prevents the formation of a functional 70S initiation complex that is essential for the bacterial translation process and subsequently inhibits protein synthesis. Tedizolid is bacteriostatic against enterococci, staphylococci, and streptococci (Kisgen 2014).

Pharmacodynamics/Kinetics

Half-life Elimination ~12 hours

Time to Peak Oral: ~3 hours; IV: 1 to 1.5 hours

Pregnancy Considerations Adverse events were observed in animal reproduction studies.

◆ **Tedizolid Phosphate** *see* Tedizolid *on page 1409*

Teduglutide (te due GLOO tide)

Brand Names: US Gattex

Brand Names: Canada Revestive

Pharmacologic Category Glucagon-Like Peptide-2 (GLP-2) Analog

Use Short bowel syndrome: Treatment of short bowel syndrome in adults and pediatric patients ≥1 year of age who are dependent on parenteral support.

Local Anesthetic/Vasoconstrictor Precautions No information available to require special precautions

Effects on Dental Treatment No significant effects or complications reported

Effects on Bleeding No information available to require special precautions

Adverse Reactions

>10%:

Endocrine & metabolic: Fluid retention (1% to 12%)

Gastrointestinal: Abdominal pain (30%), nausea (23%), abdominal distension (20%), vomiting (12%)

Immunologic: Antibody development (3% to 54%; incidence increased with prolonged use)

Local: Injection site reaction (13%)

Respiratory: Upper respiratory tract infection (21%)

Miscellaneous: Intestinal stoma complication (42%)

1% to 10%:

Cardiovascular: Peripheral edema (10%), cardiac failure (3%)

Central nervous system: Sleep disturbance (5%)

Dermatologic: Dermal hemorrhage (5%)

Gastrointestinal: Flatulence (9%), decreased appetite (7%), intestinal stenosis (<5%; including colonic), pancreatic disease (<5%; duct stenosis), cholecystitis (4%), intestinal obstruction (≤4%), gallbladder perforation (1%)

Hypersensitivity: Hypersensitivity reaction (10%)

Infection: Influenza (7%)

Respiratory: Cough (5%), dyspnea (<5%)

Frequency not defined:

Cardiovascular: Edema, flushing, jugular vein distention

Dermatologic: Erythema of skin, pruritus, skin rash

Gastrointestinal: Cholelithiasis, cholestasis, colonic polyp, pancreatic pseudocyst, pancreatitis, rectal polyp

Hematologic & oncologic: Hematoma

Ophthalmic: Eyelid edema

<1%, postmarketing, and/or case reports: Cholangitis, malignant neoplasm

Mechanism of Action Teduglutide is an analog of glucagon-like peptide-2 (GLP-2), which is secreted in the distal intestine. Endogenous GLP-2 increases intestinal and portal blood flow while inhibiting gastric acid secretion, thereby reducing intestinal losses and improving intestinal absorption. Teduglutide binds and activates GLP-2 receptors, resulting in release of mediators including insulin-like growth factor (IGF)-1, nitric oxide and keratinocyte growth factor (KGF).

Pharmacodynamics/Kinetics

Half-life Elimination

Children 1 to 11 years: 0.7 ± 0.2 hours

Children 12 to 17 years: 1 ± 0.01 hours

Adults: 1.3 hours

Time to Peak Plasma: SubQ: 3 to 5 hours

Pregnancy Considerations

Information related to use of teduglutide in pregnancy is limited.

Short bowel syndrome may cause maternal malnutrition, which is associated with adverse fetal effects, including congenital malformations, intrauterine growth restriction, low birth weight, perinatal mortality and preterm birth.

◆ **Teduglutide [rDNA origin]** *see* Teduglutide *on page 1410*

◆ **Teduglutide Recombinant** *see* Teduglutide *on page 1410*

◆ **Teflaro** *see* Ceftaroline Fosamil *on page 312*

◆ **Tegaderm CHG Dressing [OTC]** *see* Chlorhexidine Gluconate (Topical) *on page 335*

Tegaserod (teg a SER od)

Brand Names: US Zelnorm

Pharmacologic Category Gastrointestinal Agent, Prokinetic; Serotonin 5-HT_4 Receptor Agonist

Use Irritable bowel syndrome with constipation: Treatment of irritable bowel syndrome with constipation in women (<65 years of age)

Local Anesthetic/Vasoconstrictor Precautions No information available to require special precautions

Effects on Dental Treatment No significant effects or complications reported

Effects on Bleeding No information available to require special precautions

Adverse Reactions

>10%:

Central nervous system: Headache (14%)

Gastrointestinal: Abdominal pain (11%)

1% to 10%:

Central nervous system: Dizziness (4%), migraine (≤2%), vertigo (≤2%)

Gastrointestinal: Diarrhea (8%), nausea (8%), flatulence (6%), dyspepsia (4%), increased appetite (≤2%)

Hematologic & oncologic: Anemia (≤2%), rectal hemorrhage (≤2%)

Neuromuscular & skeletal: Arthropathy (≤2%), asthenia (≤2%), increased creatine phosphokinase in blood specimen (≤2%), tendonitis (≤2%)

<1%: Suicidal ideation, suicidal tendencies

Postmarketing: Acute myocardial infarction, alopecia, anaphylaxis, cerebrovascular accident, cholecystitis, choledocholithiasis, hepatitis, hypersensitivity reaction, increased serum alanine aminotransferase, increased serum aspartate transaminase, increased serum bilirubin, intestinal necrosis (gangrenous bowel), ischemic colitis, mesenteric ischemia, severe diarrhea, spasm of sphincter of Oddi

Mechanism of Action Tegaserod is a partial neuronal 5-HT_4 receptor agonist. Its action at the receptor site leads to stimulation of the peristaltic reflex and intestinal secretion, and moderation of visceral sensitivity.

Pharmacodynamics/Kinetics

Half-life Elimination Terminal: 4.6 to 8.1 hours

Time to Peak ~1 hour

Pregnancy Considerations Adverse events were observed in some animal reproduction studies. Pregnant women were excluded from clinical trials and outcome information following inadvertent pregnancy exposure is limited (Appel-Dingemanse 2002).

- ◆ **Tegaserod Maleate** *see* Tegaserod *on page 1411*
- ◆ **TEGretol** *see* CarBAMazepine *on page 288*
- ◆ **TEGretol-XR** *see* CarBAMazepine *on page 288*
- ◆ **Tegsedi** *see* Inotersen *on page 816*
- ◆ **TEI-6720** *see* Febuxostat *on page 637*
- ◆ **Tekturna** *see* Aliskiren *on page 102*

Telavancin (tel a VAN sin)

Brand Names: US Vibativ

Brand Names: Canada Vibativ

Pharmacologic Category Glycopeptide

Use

Complicated skin and skin structure infections: Treatment of complicated skin and skin structure infections caused by susceptible gram-positive organisms including methicillin-susceptible or -resistant *Staphylococcus aureus*, vancomycin-susceptible *Enterococcus faecalis*, and *Streptococcus pyogenes*, *Streptococcus agalactiae*, or *Streptococcus anginosus* group

Hospital-acquired and ventilator-associated bacterial pneumonia (HABP/VABP): Treatment of HABP/VABP caused by susceptible isolates of *Staphylococcus aureus* when alternative treatments are not appropriate

Local Anesthetic/Vasoconstrictor Precautions Telavancin is one of the drugs confirmed to prolong the QT interval and is accepted as having a risk of causing torsade de pointes. The risk of drug-induced torsade de pointes is extremely low when a single QT interval prolonging drug is prescribed. In terms of epinephrine, it is not known what effect vasoconstrictors in the local anesthetic regimen will have in patients with a known history of congenital prolonged QT interval or in patients taking any medication that prolongs the QT interval. Until more information is obtained, it is suggested that the clinician consult with the physician prior to the use of a vasoconstrictor in suspected patients, and that the vasoconstrictor (epinephrine, mepivacaine and levonordefrin [Carbocaine® 2% with Neo-Cobefrin®]) be used with caution.

Effects on Dental Treatment Key adverse event(s) related to dental treatment: Metallic or abnormal taste

Effects on Bleeding Although there are no reports of enhanced bleeding, telavancin may interfere with tests used to monitor coagulation (eg, prothrombin time, INR, activated partial thromboplastin time, activated clotting time, and coagulation-based factor Xa tests). Thrombocytopenia occurs in 7% of patients.

Adverse Reactions

>10%:

Central nervous system: Metallic taste (33%)

Gastrointestinal: Nausea (5% to 27%), vomiting (5% to 14%)

Renal: Increased serum creatinine (8% to 16%; ≥65 years of age: 11%; <65 years of age: 8%), foamy urine (13%)

1% to 10%:

Central nervous system: Dizziness (6%), infusion site pain (4%), rigors (4%)

Dermatologic: Pruritus (3% to 6%), skin rash (4%), localized erythema (3%)

Gastrointestinal: Diarrhea (7%), decreased appetite (3%), abdominal pain (2%)

Local: Infusion site reaction (3%)

Renal: Renal insufficiency (3%; ≥65 years of age: 9%; <65 years of age: 2%), acute renal failure (5%)

<1%, postmarketing, and/or case reports: *Clostridioides* (formerly *Clostridium*) *difficile*-associated diarrhea, flushing, hypersensitivity reaction (including anaphylaxis), nephrotoxicity, prolonged QT interval on ECG, transient flushing of upper body, urticaria

Mechanism of Action Exerts concentration-dependent bactericidal activity; inhibits bacterial cell wall synthesis by blocking polymerization and cross-linking of peptidoglycan by binding to D-Ala-D-Ala portion of cell wall. Unlike vancomycin, additional mechanism involves disruption of membrane potential and changes cell permeability due to presence of lipophilic side chain moiety.

Pharmacodynamics/Kinetics

Half-life Elimination 6.6 to 9.6 hours

Reproductive Considerations
[US Boxed Warning]: Verify pregnancy status in females of reproductive potential prior to initiating telavancin. Advise females of reproductive potential to use effective contraception during treatment with telavancin and for 2 days after the final dose.

Pregnancy Considerations
Telavancin crosses the placenta (Nanovskaya 2012). **[US Boxed Warning]: Telavancin may cause fetal harm. In animal reproduction studies, adverse developmental outcomes were observed in 3 animal species at clinically relevant doses. Advise pregnant women of the potential risk to a fetus.**

Data collection to monitor pregnancy and infant outcomes following exposure to telavancin is ongoing. Health care providers are encouraged to enroll females exposed to telavancin during pregnancy in the Vibativ Pregnancy Registry (1-877-484-2700). Pregnant females may also enroll themselves.

Dental Health Professional Considerations See Local Anesthetic/Vasoconstrictor Precautions

◆ **Telavancin HCl** *see* Telavancin *on page 1411*

◆ **Telavancin Hydrochloride** *see* Telavancin *on page 1411*

Telbivudine (tel BI vyoo deen)

Related Information
HIV Infection and AIDS *on page 1690*
Systemic Viral Diseases *on page 1709*

Brand Names: US Tyzeka [DSC]

Brand Names: Canada Sebivo [DSC]

Pharmacologic Category Antihepadnaviral, Reverse Transcriptase Inhibitor, Nucleoside (Anti-HBV)

Use Treatment of chronic hepatitis B with evidence of viral replication and either persistent transaminase elevations or histologically-active disease

Local Anesthetic/Vasoconstrictor Precautions
No information available to require special precautions

Effects on Dental Treatment No significant effects or complications reported

Effects on Bleeding No information available to require special precautions regarding hemostasis.

Adverse Reactions
>10%:
Central nervous system: Fatigue (13%)
Neuromuscular & skeletal: Increased creatine phosphokinase (79%; grades 3/4: 16%, most asymptomatic and transient)

1% to 10%:
Central nervous system: Headache (10%), dizziness (4%), fever (4%), insomnia (3%)
Dermatologic: Skin rash (4%), pruritus (2%)
Endocrine & metabolic: Increased serum lipase (grades 3/4: 2%)
Gastrointestinal: Diarrhea (6%), abdominal pain (3% to 6%), nausea (5%), abdominal distension (3%), dyspepsia (3%)
Hematologic & oncologic: Neutropenia (grades 3/4: 2%)
Hepatic: Increased serum ALT (grades 3/4: 5% to 7%), increased serum AST (grades 3/4: 6%)
Infection: Exacerbation of hepatitis B (2%)
Neuromuscular & skeletal: Arthralgia (4%), back pain (4%), myalgia (3%)
Respiratory: Cough (6%), pharyngolaryngeal pain (5%)

<1%, postmarketing, and/or case reports: Hepatomegaly, hyperbilirubinemia, hypoesthesia, increased amylase, lactic acidosis, liver steatosis, myopathy, myositis, paresthesia, peripheral neuropathy, rhabdomyolysis, thrombocytopenia

Mechanism of Action Telbivudine, a synthetic thymidine nucleoside analogue (L-enantiomer of thymidine), is intracellularly phosphorylated to the active triphosphate form, which competes with the natural substrate, thymidine 5'-triphosphate, to inhibit hepatitis B viral DNA polymerase; enzyme inhibition blocks reverse transcriptase activity thereby reducing viral DNA replication.

Pharmacodynamics/Kinetics
Half-life Elimination Terminal: 40-49 hours
Time to Peak 1-4 hours

Pregnancy Considerations
In hepatitis B-infected women (not coinfected with HIV), the AASLD chronic hepatitis B treatment guidelines suggest antiviral therapy to reduce the risk of perinatal transmission of hepatitis B in HBsAg-positive pregnant women with an HBV DNA >200,000 units/mL. There are limited data on the level of HBV DNA for when antiviral therapy is routinely recommended (>200,000 units/mL is a conservative recommendation); however, the AASLD recommends against antiviral therapy to reduce the risk of perinatal transmission in HBsAg-positive pregnant women with an HBV DNA ≤200,000 units/mL. Telbivudine is one of the antivirals that has been studied in pregnant women, with most studies initiating antiviral therapy at 28 to 32 weeks gestation and discontinuing antiviral therapy between birth to 3 months postpartum (monitor for ALT flares every 3 months for 6 months following discontinuation). There is insufficient long-term safety data in infants born to mothers who took antiviral agents during pregnancy (AASLD [Terrault 2016]).

Health professionals are encouraged to contact the antiretroviral pregnancy registry to monitor outcomes of pregnant women exposed to antiretroviral medications (1-800-258-4263).

Product Availability Tyzeka has been discontinued in the US for more than 1 year.

Telithromycin (tel ith roe MYE sin)

Related Information
Clinical Risk Related to Drugs Prolonging QT Interval *on page 1675*

Brand Names: US Ketek [DSC]

Pharmacologic Category Antibiotic, Ketolide

Use Community-acquired pneumonia: Treatment of mild to moderate community-acquired pneumonia (CAP) due to *Streptococcus pneumoniae* (including multidrug-resistant isolates), *Haemophilus influenzae*, *Moraxella catarrhalis*, *Chlamydophila* (also known as *Chlamydia*) *pneumoniae*, or *Mycoplasma pneumoniae* in patients 18 years and older.

Local Anesthetic/Vasoconstrictor Precautions
Telithromycin is one of the drugs confirmed to prolong the QT interval and is accepted as having a risk of causing torsade de pointes. The risk of drug-induced torsade de pointes is extremely low when a single QT interval prolonging drug is prescribed. In terms of epinephrine, it is not known what effect vasoconstrictors in the local anesthetic regimen will have in patients with a known history of congenital prolonged QT interval or in patients taking any medication that prolongs the QT interval. Until more information is obtained, it is

suggested that the clinician consult with the physician prior to the use of a vasoconstrictor in suspected patients, and that the vasoconstrictor (epinephrine, mepivacaine and levonordefrin [Carbocaine® 2% with Neo-Cobefrin®]) be used with caution.

Effects on Dental Treatment Key adverse event(s) related to dental treatment: Xerostomia (normal salivary flow resumes upon discontinuation), glossitis, stomatitis, and tooth discoloration.

Effects on Bleeding No information available to require special precautions

Adverse Reactions

>10%: Gastrointestinal: Diarrhea (10% to 11%)

2% to 10%:

Central nervous system: Headache (2% to 6%), dizziness (3% to 4%)

Gastrointestinal: Nausea (7% to 8%), vomiting (2% to 3%), dysgeusia (2%), loose stools (2%)

≥0.2% to <2%:

Central nervous system: Drowsiness, fatigue, insomnia, vertigo

Dermatologic: Diaphoresis, skin rash

Gastrointestinal: Abdominal distension, abdominal pain, anorexia, constipation, dyspepsia, flatulence, gastric distress, gastritis, gastroenteritis, glossitis, oral candidiasis, stomatitis, xerostomia

Genitourinary: Fungal vaginosis, vaginitis, vulvovaginal candidiasis

Hematologic & oncologic: Thrombocythemia

Hepatic: Abnormal hepatic function tests, increased serum transaminases

Ophthalmic: Accommodation disturbance, blurred vision, diplopia

<0.2%, postmarketing, and/or case reports: Ageusia, altered sense of smell, anaphylaxis, angioedema, anosmia, anxiety, arthralgia, atrial arrhythmia, bradycardia, cardiac arrhythmia, confusion, convulsions, dyspnea, eczema, eosinophilia, erythema multiforme, exacerbation of myasthenia gravis, facial edema, flushing, hallucination, hepatic failure, hepatic injury (including necrosis), hepatitis, hypersensitivity reaction, hypotension, increased serum alkaline phosphatase, increased serum bilirubin, ischemic heart disease, jaundice, loss of consciousness (may be vagal-related), muscle cramps, myalgia, palpitations, pancreatitis, paresthesia, prolonged QT interval on ECG, pruritus, pseudomembranous colitis, respiratory failure, syncope, torsades de pointes, tremor, urticaria, urine discoloration, ventricular arrhythmia, ventricular tachycardia

Mechanism of Action Inhibits bacterial protein synthesis by binding to two sites on the 50S ribosomal subunit. Telithromycin has also been demonstrated to alter secretion of IL-1alpha and TNF-alpha; the clinical significance of this immunomodulatory effect has not been evaluated.

Pharmacodynamics/Kinetics

Half-life Elimination 10 hours

Time to Peak Plasma: 1 hour

Pregnancy Risk Factor C

Pregnancy Considerations Adverse events have been observed in animal reproduction studies

Product Availability Ketek has been discontinued in the United States for more than 1 year.

Dental Health Professional Considerations See Local Anesthetic/Vasoconstrictor Precautions

Telmisartan (tel mi SAR tan)

Related Information

Cardiovascular Diseases *on page 1654*

Brand Names: US Micardis

Brand Names: Canada ACT Telmisartan [DSC]; APO-Telmisartan; Auro-Telmisartan; Micardis; MINT-Telmisartan; MYLAN-Telmisartan [DSC]; PMS-Telmisartan; RAN-Telmisartan; SANDOZ Telmisartan; TEVA-Telmisartan; VAN-Telmisartan [DSC]

Pharmacologic Category Angiotensin II Receptor Blocker; Antihypertensive

Use

Cardiovascular risk reduction: Cardiovascular risk reduction in patients ≥55 years of age unable to take ACE inhibitors and who are at high risk of major cardiovascular events (eg, MI, stroke, death)

Hypertension: Management of hypertension

Guideline recommendations: The 2017 Guideline for the Prevention, Detection, Evaluation, and Management of High Blood Pressure in Adults recommends if monotherapy is warranted, in the absence of comorbidities (eg, cerebrovascular disease, chronic kidney disease, diabetes, heart failure, ischemic heart disease, etc.), that thiazide-like diuretics or dihydropyridine calcium channel blockers may be preferred options due to improved cardiovascular endpoints (eg, prevention of heart failure and stroke). ACE inhibitors and ARBs are also acceptable for monotherapy. Combination therapy may be required to achieve blood pressure goals and is initially preferred in patients at high risk (stage 2 hypertension or atherosclerotic cardiovascular disease [ASCVD] risk ≥10%) (ACC/AHA [Whelton 2017]).

Local Anesthetic/Vasoconstrictor Precautions No information available to require special precautions

Effects on Dental Treatment Key adverse event(s) related to dental treatment: Patients may experience orthostatic hypotension as they stand up after treatment; especially if lying in dental chair for extended periods of time. Use caution with sudden changes in position during and after dental treatment.

Effects on Bleeding No information available to require special precautions

Adverse Reactions

1% to 10%:

Cardiovascular: Intermittent claudication (7%), chest pain (≥1%), hypertension (≥1%), peripheral edema (≥1%)

Central nervous system: Dizziness (≥1%), fatigue (≥1%), headache (≥1%), pain (≥1%)

Dermatologic: Dermal ulcer (3%)

Gastrointestinal: Diarrhea (3%), abdominal pain (≥1%), dyspepsia (≥1%), nausea (≥1%)

Genitourinary: Urinary tract infection (≥1%)

Neuromuscular & skeletal: Back pain (3%), myalgia (≥1%)

Respiratory: Upper respiratory tract infection (7%), sinusitis (3%), cough (≥1%), flu-like symptoms (≥1%), pharyngitis (1%)

<1%, postmarketing, and/or case reports: Abscess, acute renal failure, anaphylaxis, anemia, angina pectoris, angioedema, anxiety, arthralgia, arthritis, asthenia, asthma, atrial fibrillation, bradycardia, bronchitis, cardiac failure, cerebrovascular disease, conjunctivitis, constipation, cystitis, dependent edema, depression, dermatitis, diabetes mellitus, diaphoresis, drowsiness, dyspnea, ECG abnormality, eczema, edema, enteritis, eosinophilia, epistaxis, erectile

dysfunction, erythema, exacerbation of hypertension, facial edema, fever, fixed drug eruption, flatulence, flushing, fungal infection, gastritis, gastroenteritis, gastroesophageal reflux disease, gastrointestinal disease, gout, hemorrhoids, hepatic disease, hepatic insufficiency, hypercholesterolemia, hyperkalemia, hypersensitivity reaction, hypoesthesia, hypoglycemia (diabetic patients), hypotension, impotence, increased creatine phosphokinase, increased uric acid, infection, insomnia, lower extremity edema, lower extremity pain, lower limb cramp, malaise, migraine, muscle cramps, muscle spasm, myocardial infarction, nervousness, orthostatic hypotension, otalgia, otitis media, palpitations, paresthesia, pruritus, renal insufficiency, rhabdomyolysis, rhinitis, skin rash, skin toxicity, syncope, tachycardia, tendonitis, tendon pain, tenosynovitis, thrombocytopenia, tinnitus, toothache, urinary frequency, urticaria, vertigo, visual disturbance, vomiting, xerostomia

Mechanism of Action Angiotensin II acts as a vasoconstrictor. In addition to causing direct vasoconstriction, angiotensin II also stimulates the release of aldosterone. Once aldosterone is released, sodium as well as water is reabsorbed. The end result is an elevation in blood pressure. Telmisartan is a nonpeptide AT1 angiotensin II receptor antagonist. This binding prevents angiotensin II from binding to the receptor thereby blocking the vasoconstriction and the aldosterone secreting effects of angiotensin II.

Pharmacodynamics/Kinetics

Onset of Action 1 to 2 hours; Peak effect: 0.5 to 1 hours

Duration of Action Up to 24 hours

Half-life Elimination Terminal: 24 hours

Time to Peak Plasma: 0.5 to 1 hours

Reproductive Considerations

The use of angiotensin II receptor blockers should generally be avoided in women planning a pregnancy (ACOG 203 2019).

Pregnancy Considerations

[US Boxed Warning]: Drugs that act on the renin-angiotensin system can cause injury and death to the developing fetus. When pregnancy is detected, discontinue as soon as possible. The use of drugs which act on the renin-angiotensin system are associated with oligohydramnios. Oligohydramnios, due to decreased fetal renal function, may lead to fetal lung hypoplasia and skeletal malformations. Oligohydramnios may not appear until after irreversible fetal injury has occurred. Use in pregnancy is also associated with anuria, hypotension, renal failure, skull hypoplasia, and death in the fetus/neonate. The exposed fetus should be monitored for fetal growth, amniotic fluid volume, and organ formation. Infants exposed in utero should be monitored for hyperkalemia, hypotension, and oliguria (exchange transfusions or dialysis may be needed). These adverse events are generally associated with maternal use in the second and third trimesters.

Chronic maternal hypertension itself is also associated with adverse events in the fetus/infant. The risk of birth defects, low birth weight, premature delivery, stillbirth, and neonatal death may be increased with chronic hypertension in pregnancy. Actual risks may be related to duration and severity of maternal hypertension (ACOG 203 2019).

The use of angiotensin II receptor blockers is generally not recommended to treat chronic hypertension in pregnant women (ACOG 203 2019).

◆ **Telmisartan/Amlodipine** *see* Telmisartan and Amlodipine *on page 1414*

Telmisartan and Amlodipine

(tel mi SAR tan & am LOE di peen)

Related Information

AmLODIPine *on page 121*

Telmisartan *on page 1413*

Brand Names: US Twynsta

Brand Names: Canada Twynsta

Pharmacologic Category Angiotensin II Receptor Blocker; Antianginal Agent; Antihypertensive; Calcium Channel Blocker; Calcium Channel Blocker, Dihydropyridine

Use Hypertension: Treatment of hypertension, including initial treatment in patients who will require multiple antihypertensives for adequate control

Local Anesthetic/Vasoconstrictor Precautions

No information available to require special precautions

Effects on Dental Treatment Key adverse event(s) related to dental treatment: Patients may experience orthostatic hypotension as they stand up after treatment; especially if lying in dental chair for extended periods of time. Use caution with sudden changes in position during and after dental treatment.

Fewer reports of gingival hyperplasia reported with amlodipine use than with other calcium channel blockers (usually resolves upon discontinuation); consult with healthcare provider.

Effects on Bleeding No information available to require special precautions

Adverse Reactions Reactions/percentages reported with combination product; also see individual agents.

>10%: Cardiovascular: Peripheral edema (dose related: 1% to 11%)

1% to 10%:

Cardiovascular: Orthostatic hypotension (6%), edema (<2%), hypotension (<2%), syncope (<2%)

Central nervous system: Dizziness (3%)

Neuromuscular & skeletal: Back pain (2%)

Mechanism of Action

Telmisartan is a nonpeptide AT1 (angiotensin II type 1) receptor antagonist. Angiotensin II acts as a vasoconstrictor. In addition to causing direct vasoconstriction, angiotensin II also stimulates the release of aldosterone. Once aldosterone is released, sodium and water are reabsorbed. The end result is an elevation in blood pressure. Telmisartan binding to AT1 prevents angiotensin II from binding to the receptor thereby blocking the vasoconstriction and the aldosterone secreting effects of angiotensin II.

Amlodipine inhibits calcium ion from entering the "slow channels" or select voltage-sensitive areas of vascular smooth muscle and myocardium during depolarization, producing a relaxation of coronary vascular smooth muscle and coronary vasodilation; increases myocardial oxygen delivery in patients with vasospastic angina. Amlodipine directly acts on vascular smooth muscle to produce peripheral arterial vasodilation reducing peripheral vascular resistance and blood pressure.

Pregnancy Considerations [US Boxed Warning]: Drugs that act on the renin-angiotensin system can cause injury and death to the developing fetus. Discontinue as soon as possible once pregnancy is detected. Also see individual agents.

Temazepam (te MAZ e pam)

Related Information

Dentin Hypersensitivity, Acid Erosion, High Caries Index, Management of Alveolar Osteitis, and Xerostomia *on page 1762*

Brand Names: US Restoril

Brand Names: Canada DOM-Temazepam [DSC]; PHL-Temazepam [DSC]; PMS-Temazepam; Restoril; Temazepam-15 [DSC]; Temazepam-30 [DSC]; TEVA-Temazepam [DSC]

Pharmacologic Category Benzodiazepine

Use Insomnia: Short-term treatment of insomnia

Local Anesthetic/Vasoconstrictor Precautions

No information available to require special precautions

Effects on Dental Treatment Key adverse event(s) related to dental treatment: Significant xerostomia (normal salivary flow resumes upon discontinuation).

Effects on Bleeding No information available to require special precautions

Adverse Reactions

1% to 10%:

Central nervous system: Drowsiness (9%), dizziness (5%), lethargy (5%), hangover effect (3%), euphoria (2%), anxiety, confusion, dysarthria, fatigue, headache, vertigo

Dermatologic: Diaphoresis, skin rash

Endocrine & metabolic: Decreased libido

Gastrointestinal: Diarrhea (2%)

Neuromuscular & skeletal: Weakness

Ophthalmic: Blurred vision

<1%, postmarketing, and/or case reports: Abnormal behavior, aggressive behavior, agitation, amnesia, anaphylaxis, angioedema, anorexia, ataxia, back pain, burning sensation of eyes, depersonalization, drug dependence, dyspnea, equilibrium disturbance, extroversion, hallucination, hematologic disease, hyperhidrosis, hyporeflexia, increased dream activity, menstrual disease, nausea, nystagmus, palpitations, paradoxical reaction, pharyngeal edema, sleep disorder (sleep-driving, cooking or eating food, making phone calls), tremor, vomiting

Mechanism of Action Binds to stereospecific benzodiazepine receptors on the postsynaptic GABA neuron at several sites within the central nervous system, including the limbic system, reticular formation. Enhancement of the inhibitory effect of GABA on neuronal excitability results by increased neuronal membrane permeability to chloride ions. This shift in chloride ions results in hyperpolarization (a less excitable state) and stabilization. Benzodiazepine receptors and effects appear to be linked to the GABA-A receptors. Benzodiazepines do not bind to GABA-B receptors.

Pharmacodynamics/Kinetics

Half-life Elimination 3.5-18.4 hours

Time to Peak Serum: 1.2-1.6 hours

Pregnancy Risk Factor X

Pregnancy Considerations

Adverse events were observed in animal reproduction studies. All benzodiazepines are assumed to cross the placenta. Teratogenic effects have been observed with some benzodiazepines; however, additional studies are needed. The incidence of premature birth and low birth weights may be increased following maternal use of benzodiazepines; hypoglycemia and respiratory problems in the neonate may occur following exposure late in pregnancy. Neonatal withdrawal symptoms may occur within days to weeks after birth and "floppy infant syndrome" (which also includes withdrawal symptoms) have been reported with some benzodiazepines (Bergman 1992; Iqbal 2002; Wikner 2007). Use during pregnancy is contraindicated.

Controlled Substance C-IV

- **Temixys** *see* Lamivudine and Tenofovir Disoproxil Fumarate *on page 873*
- **Temodar** *see* Temozolomide *on page 1415*
- **Temovate** *see* Clobetasol *on page 377*
- **Temovate E [DSC]** *see* Clobetasol *on page 377*

Temozolomide (te moe ZOE loe mide)

Brand Names: US Temodar

Brand Names: Canada ACH-Temozolomide; ACT Temozolomide; TARO-Temozolomide; Temodal

Pharmacologic Category Antineoplastic Agent, Alkylating Agent (Triazene)

Use

Anaplastic astrocytoma (refractory): Treatment of refractory anaplastic astrocytoma in adults who have experienced disease progression on a regimen containing a nitrosourea and procarbazine.

Glioblastoma (newly diagnosed): Treatment of newly diagnosed glioblastoma in adults (initially in combination with radiotherapy, then as maintenance treatment).

Local Anesthetic/Vasoconstrictor Precautions

No information available to require special precautions

Effects on Dental Treatment Key adverse event(s) related to dental treatment: Stomatitis, dysphagia, and taste perversion.

Effects on Bleeding Chemotherapy may result in significant myelosuppression, potentially including significant reduction in platelet counts and altered hemostasis. In patients who are under active treatment with these agents, medical consult is suggested.

Adverse Reactions With CNS malignancies, it may be difficult to distinguish between CNS adverse events caused by temozolomide versus the effects of progressive disease.

>10%:

Cardiovascular: Peripheral edema (11%)

Dermatologic: Alopecia (55%), skin rash (8% to 13%)

Gastrointestinal: Nausea (49% to 53%), vomiting (29% to 42%), constipation (22% to 33%), anorexia (9% to 27%), diarrhea (10% to 16%)

Hematologic & oncologic: Lymphocytopenia (grades 3/4: 55%), thrombocytopenia (8%; grades 3/4: 4% to 19%), decreased neutrophils (grades 3/4: 14%), leukopenia (grades 3/4: 11%)

Infection: Viral infection (11%)

Nervous system: Fatigue (34% to 61%), headache (23% to 41%), seizure (6% to 23%), hemiparesis (18%), dizziness (5% to 12%), ataxia (8% to 11%)

Neuromuscular & skeletal: Asthenia (7% to 13%)

Miscellaneous: Fever (13%)

1% to 10%:

Dermatologic: Pruritus (5% to 8%), xeroderma (5%), erythema of skin (1%)

Endocrine & metabolic: Hypercorticoidism (8%), weight gain (5%)

Gastrointestinal: Stomatitis (9%; grades ≥3: 1%), abdominal pain (5% to 9%), dysphagia (7%), dysgeusia (5%)

Genitourinary: Urinary incontinence (8%), urinary tract infection (8%), mastalgia (females: 6%), urinary frequency (6%)

Hematologic & oncologic: Decreased hemoglobin (grades 3/4: 4%)
Hypersensitivity: Hypersensitivity reaction (3%)
Nervous system: Amnesia (10%), insomnia (4% to 10%), drowsiness (9%), paresthesia (9%), paresis (8%), anxiety (7%), memory impairment (7%), abnormal gait (6%), depression (6%), confusion (5%)
Neuromuscular & skeletal: Back pain (8%), arthralgia (6%), myalgia (5%)
Ophthalmic: Blurred vision (5% to 8%), diplopia (5%), visual disturbance (visual deficit/vision changes: 5%)
Respiratory: Pharyngitis (8%), upper respiratory tract infection (8%), cough (5% to 8%), sinusitis (6%), dyspnea (5%)

Frequency not defined:
Hematologic & oncologic: Anemia, myelodysplastic syndrome, secondary acute myelocytic leukemia
Respiratory: Pneumonia due to *Pneumocystis jirovecii*

<1%, postmarketing, and/or case reports: Anaphylaxis, aplastic anemia, cholestasis, diabetes insipidus, erythema multiforme, hematoma, hepatitis, hepatotoxicity, hyperbilirubinemia, increased liver enzymes, injection site reaction (erythema, irritation, pain, pruritus, swelling, warmth), interstitial pneumonitis, opportunistic infection, pancytopenia (may be prolonged), petechia, pneumonitis, pulmonary alveolitis, pulmonary fibrosis, Stevens-Johnson syndrome, toxic epidermal necrolysis

Mechanism of Action Temozolomide is a prodrug which is rapidly and nonenzymatically converted to the active alkylating metabolite MTIC [(methyl-triazene-1-yl)-imidazole-4-carboxamide]; this conversion is spontaneous, nonenzymatic, and occurs under physiologic conditions in all tissues to which it distributes (Marchesi 2007; Villano 2009). The cytotoxic effects of MTIC are manifested through alkylation (methylation) of DNA at the O^6, N^7 guanine positions which lead to DNA double strand breaks and apoptosis (Villano 2009). Temozolomide is noncell cycle specific (Marchesi 2007).

Pharmacodynamics/Kinetics

Half-life Elimination Mean: Parent drug: Children: 1.7 hours; Adults: 1.8 hours

Time to Peak Oral: Median: 1 hour; with food (high-fat meal): 2.25 hours.

Reproductive Considerations

Evaluate pregnancy status prior to use in females of reproductive potential. Females of reproductive potential should use effective contraception during treatment and for at least 6 months after the last temozolomide dose. Males with pregnant partners or with female partners of reproductive potential should use condoms during treatment and for at least 3 months after the last temozolomide dose.

Males should not donate semen during treatment and for at least 3 months after the last temozolomide dose.

Temozolomide may impair fertility; limited data indicate changes in sperm parameters during temozolomide treatment; however, there is no information in duration or reversibility of sperm changes.

Pregnancy Considerations

Based on the mechanism of action and findings in animal reproduction studies, in utero exposure to temozolomide may cause fetal harm.

Temsirolimus (tem sir OH li mus)

Brand Names: US Torisel
Brand Names: Canada Torisel

Pharmacologic Category Antineoplastic Agent, mTOR Kinase Inhibitor

Use Renal cell carcinoma, advanced: Treatment of advanced renal cell carcinoma (RCC)

Local Anesthetic/Vasoconstrictor Precautions No information available to require special precautions

Effects on Dental Treatment Key adverse event(s) related to dental treatment: Effects on oral cavity including mucositis, stomatitis, and taste disturbances.

Effects on Bleeding Thrombocytopenia has been associated with use; severe thrombocytopenia (grades 3/4: 1%) may be associated with delayed coagulation. Consultation to ensure adequate platelet counts may be considered in patients with signs/symptoms or a history of thrombocytopenia.

Adverse Reactions

>10%:
Cardiovascular: Edema (35%), chest pain (16%)
Central nervous system: Pain (28%), headache (15%), insomnia (12%)
Dermatologic: Skin rash (47%), pruritus (19%), nail disease (14%), xeroderma (11%)
Endocrine & metabolic: Increased serum glucose (89%; grades 3/4: 16%), increased serum cholesterol (87%; grades 3/4: 2%), hypertriglyceridemia (83%; grades 3/4: 44%), hypophosphatemia (49%; grades 3/4: 18%), hyperglycemia (26%), hyperlipidemia (≥30%), hypokalemia (21%; grades 3/4: 5%), weight loss (19%)
Gastrointestinal: Mucositis (41%), nausea (37%), anorexia (32%), diarrhea (27%), abdominal pain (21%; grades 3/4: 4%), constipation (20%), dysgeusia (20%), stomatitis (20%), vomiting (19%)
Genitourinary: Urinary tract infection (15%)
Hematologic & oncologic: Decreased hemoglobin (94%; grades 3/4: 20%), lymphocytopenia (53%; grades 3/4: 16%), thrombocytopenia (40%; grades 3/4: 1%; dose-limiting toxicity), decreased white blood cell count (32%; grades 3/4: 1%), anemia (≥30%), decreased neutrophils (19%; grades 3/4: 5%)
Hepatic: Increased serum alkaline phosphatase (68%; grades 3/4: 3%), increased serum AST (38%; grades 3/4: 2%)
Infection: Infection (20%; grades 3/4: 3%; includes abscess, bronchitis, cellulitis, herpes simplex, herpes zoster)
Neuromuscular & skeletal: Weakness (51%), back pain (20%), arthralgia (18%)
Renal: Increased serum creatinine (57%; grades 3/4: 3%)
Respiratory: Dyspnea (28%), cough (26%), epistaxis (12%), pharyngitis (12%)
Miscellaneous: Fever (24%; grades 3/4: 1%)

1% to 10%:
Cardiovascular: Hypertension (7%), venous thromboembolism (2%; includes deep vein thrombosis and pulmonary embolism), pericardial effusion (1%), thrombophlebitis (1%)
Central nervous system: Chills (8%), depression (4%), convulsions (1%)
Dermatologic: Acne vulgaris (10%)
Endocrine & metabolic: Diabetes mellitus (5%)
Gastrointestinal: Gastrointestinal hemorrhage (1%)
Hematologic & oncologic: Rectal hemorrhage (1%)
Hepatic: Hyperbilirubinemia (8%)
Infection: Sepsis (1%), wound infection (1%)
Neuromuscular & skeletal: Myalgia (8%)
Ophthalmic: Conjunctivitis (8%; including lacrimation disorder)

Respiratory: Rhinitis (10%), pneumonia (8%), upper respiratory tract infection (7%), pleural effusion (4%)
Miscellaneous: Wound healing impairment (1%)
<1%, postmarketing, and/or case reports: Acute renal failure, angioedema, causalgia, cholecystitis, cholelithiasis, decreased glucose tolerance, extravasation reactions (with pain, swelling, warmth, erythema), hypersensitivity reaction, interstitial pulmonary disease, intestinal perforation, pancreatitis, pneumonitis, rhabdomyolysis, seizure, Stevens-Johnson syndrome

Mechanism of Action Temsirolimus and its active metabolite, sirolimus, are targeted inhibitors of mTOR (mechanistic target of rapamycin) kinase activity. Temsirolimus (and sirolimus) bind to FKBP-12, an intracellular protein, to form a complex which inhibits mTOR signaling, halting the cell cycle at the G1 phase in tumor cells. Inhibition of mTOR blocks downstream phosphorylation of p70S6k and S6 ribosomal proteins. In renal cell carcinoma, mTOR inhibition also exhibits anti-angiogenesis activity by reducing levels of HIF-1 and HIF-2 alpha (hypoxia inducible factors) and vascular endothelial growth factor (VEGF).

Pharmacodynamics/Kinetics

Half-life Elimination Temsirolimus: ~17 hours; Sirolimus: ~55 hours

Time to Peak Temsirolimus: At end of infusion; Sirolimus: 0.5 to 2 hours after temsirolimus infusion

Reproductive Considerations

Females of reproductive potential should be advised to avoid pregnancy and use effective contraception during treatment and for 3 months after the last temsirolimus dose. Male patients with female partners of reproductive potential should also use effective birth control during treatment and for 3 months after the last temsirolimus dose.

Pregnancy Considerations

Based on findings in animal reproduction studies and on the mechanism of action, temsirolimus may cause fetal harm if administered to a pregnant woman.

Tenapanor (ten A pa nor)

Pharmacologic Category Sodium/Hydrogen Exchanger 3 (NHE3) Inhibitor

Use Irritable bowel syndrome with constipation: Treatment of irritable bowel syndrome with constipation in adults.

Local Anesthetic/Vasoconstrictor Precautions No information available to require special precautions.

Effects on Dental Treatment No significant effects or complications reported.

Effects on Bleeding No information available to require special precautions.

Adverse Reactions

>10%: Gastrointestinal: Diarrhea (15% to 16%)
1% to 10%:
Central nervous system: Dizziness (2%)
Gastrointestinal: Flatulence (3%), severe diarrhea (3%), abdominal distension (2% to 3%), abnormal bowel sounds (<2%)
Hematologic & oncologic: Rectal hemorrhage (<2%)

Mechanism of Action Tenapanor is a sodium/hydrogen exchanger 3 inhibitor, which acts locally to reduce sodium absorption from the small intestine and colon. Reduced sodium absorption results in increased intestinal lumen water secretion, accelerating intestinal transit time, and softening stool consistency. Tenapanor also decreases intestinal permeability and visceral hypersensitivity in animal models, which may reduce abdominal pain.

Pregnancy Considerations Tenapanor has limited systemic absorption following oral administration. Use during pregnancy is not expected to result in significant exposure to the fetus.

Product Availability Ibsrela: FDA approved September 2019; anticipated availability is currently unknown.

◆ **Tenapanor Hydrochloride** *see* Tenapanor *on page 1417*

◆ **Tenex [DSC]** *see* GuanFACINE *on page 749*

Teniposide (ten i POE side)

Brand Names: Canada Vumon [DSC]

Pharmacologic Category Antineoplastic Agent, Podophyllotoxin Derivative; Antineoplastic Agent, Topoisomerase II Inhibitor

Use Acute lymphoblastic leukemia, refractory: Treatment of refractory childhood acute lymphoblastic leukemia (ALL) in combination with other chemotherapy

Local Anesthetic/Vasoconstrictor Precautions No information available to require special precautions

Effects on Dental Treatment Key adverse event(s) related to dental treatment: Mucositis.

Effects on Bleeding Chemotherapy may result in significant myelosuppression, including significant thrombocytopenia (85%), and altered hemostasis. In patients who are under active treatment with these agents, medical consult is suggested.

Adverse Reactions

>10%:
Gastrointestinal: Mucositis (76%), diarrhea (33%), nausea and vomiting (29%; mild to moderate)
Hematologic & oncologic: Neutropenia (95%), leukopenia (89%), anemia (88%), thrombocytopenia (85%), bone marrow depression (75%)
Infection: Infection (12%)
1% to 10%:
Cardiovascular: Hypotension (2%; may be intractable; associated with rapid [<30 minutes] infusions)
Dermatologic: Alopecia (9%; usually reversible), skin rash (3%)
Hematologic & oncologic: Hemorrhage (5%)
Hypersensitivity: Hypersensitivity reaction (5%; includes bronchospasm, chills, dyspnea, fever, flushing, hypertension, hypotension, tachycardia, or urticaria)
Miscellaneous: Fever (3%)
<1%, postmarketing, and/or case reports: Cardiac arrhythmia, central nervous system depression, confusion, fluid and electrolyte disturbance, headache, hepatic insufficiency, metabolic acidosis, neuropathy (severe), neurotoxicity, renal insufficiency, thrombophlebitis, weakness

Mechanism of Action Teniposide does not inhibit microtubular assembly; it has been shown to delay transit of cells through the S phase and arrest cells in late S or early G_2 phase, preventing cells from entering mitosis. Teniposide is a topoisomerase II inhibitor, and appears to cause DNA strand breaks by inhibition of strand-passing and DNA ligase action.

Pharmacodynamics/Kinetics

Half-life Elimination Children: 5 hours

Reproductive Considerations

Females of reproductive potential should avoid becoming pregnant during teniposide treatment.

Pregnancy Risk Factor D

Pregnancy Considerations

Adverse effects were observed in animal reproduction studies. May cause fetal harm if administered during pregnancy.

Tenofovir Alafenamide

(ten OF oh vir al a FEN a mide)

Brand Names: US Vemlidy

Brand Names: Canada Vemlidy

Pharmacologic Category Antihepadnaviral, Reverse Transcriptase Inhibitor, Nucleotide (Anti-HBV)

Use Chronic hepatitis B: Treatment of chronic hepatitis B virus (HBV) infection in adults with compensated liver disease

Local Anesthetic/Vasoconstrictor Precautions No information available to require special precautions

Effects on Dental Treatment No significant effects or complications reported

Effects on Bleeding No information available to require special precautions

Adverse Reactions

>10%:

Central nervous system: Headache (12%)

Neuromuscular & skeletal: Decreased bone mineral density (5% to 11%)

1% to 10%:

Cardiovascular: Increased serum creatine kinase (grades 3/4: 3%)

Central nervous system: Fatigue (6%)

Dermatologic: Skin rash (<5%)

Endocrine & metabolic: Increased LDL cholesterol (grades 3/4: 6%), glycosuria (grades 3/4: 5%), increased amylase (grades 3/4: 3%)

Gastrointestinal: Abdominal pain (9%), nausea (6%), diarrhea (5%), dyspepsia (5%), flatulence (<5%), vomiting (<5%)

Hepatic: Increased serum alanine aminotransferase (grades 3/4: 8%), increased serum aspartate aminotransferase (grades 3/4: 3%)

Neuromuscular & skeletal: Back pain (6%), arthralgia (5%)

Respiratory: Cough (8%)

<1%, postmarketing, and/or case reports: Angioedema, urticaria

Mechanism of Action Tenofovir alafenamide, an analog of adenosine 5'-monophosphate, is converted intracellularly by hydrolysis to tenofovir and subsequently phosphorylated to the active tenofovir diphosphate. The active moiety inhibits replication of HBV by inhibiting HBV polymerase.

Pharmacodynamics/Kinetics

Half-life Elimination Serum: 0.51 hours

Time to Peak Serum: 0.48 hours

Reproductive Considerations

The Health and Human Services perinatal HIV guidelines note there are insufficient data to recommend tenofovir alafenamide in females living with HIV who are not yet pregnant but are trying to conceive (HHS [perinatal] 2019).

For males and females living with HIV and planning a pregnancy, maximum viral suppression below the limits of detection with antiretroviral therapy (ART), modification of therapy (if needed), optimization of the woman's health, and a discussion of the potential risks and benefits of ART therapy during pregnancy are recommended prior to conception (HHS [perinatal] 2019).

Pregnancy Considerations

Tenofovir alafenamide has a low level of transfer across the human placenta.

Data collected by the antiretroviral registry related to the use of tenofovir alafenamide in pregnancy are insufficient to evaluate teratogenicity.

Maternal antiretroviral therapy (ART) may be associated with adverse pregnancy outcomes, including preterm delivery, stillbirth, low birth weight, and small-for-gestational-age infants. Actual risks may be influenced by maternal factors such as disease severity, gestational age at initiation of therapy, and specific ART regimen; therefore, close fetal monitoring is recommended. Because there is clear benefit to appropriate treatment, maternal ART should not be withheld due to concerns for adverse neonatal outcomes. Long-term follow-up is recommended for all infants exposed to antiretroviral medications; children without HIV but who were exposed to ART in utero and develop significant organ system abnormalities of unknown etiology (particularly of the CNS or heart) should be evaluated for potential mitochondrial dysfunction. Cases of lactic acidosis and hepatic steatosis have been reported in pregnant women with use of nucleoside reverse transcriptase inhibitors.

The Health and Human Services perinatal HIV guidelines note the safety and pharmacokinetic data of tenofovir alafenamide are insufficient to recommend initiation in pregnant females living with HIV who are antiretroviral naive, who have had ART therapy in the past but are restarting, or who require a new ART regimen (due to poor tolerance or poor virologic response of current regimen). However, females who become pregnant while taking tenofovir alafenamide may continue if viral suppression is effective and the regimen is well tolerated. Pharmacokinetics of tenofovir alafenamide are not significantly altered during pregnancy; dose adjustments are not needed.

Females coinfected with HIV and hepatitis B virus who are taking tenofovir alafenamide prior to pregnancy and are virally suppressed should be offered a choice to switch to tenofovir disoproxil fumarate or continue with the current regimen.

In general, ART is recommended for all pregnant females living with HIV to keep the viral load below the limit of detection and reduce the risk of perinatal transmission. Therapy should be individualized following a discussion of the potential risks and benefits of treatment during pregnancy. Monitoring of pregnant females is more frequent than in nonpregnant adults. ART should be continued postpartum for all females living with HIV and can be modified after delivery.

Health care providers are encouraged to enroll pregnant females exposed to antiretroviral medications as early in pregnancy as possible in the Antiretroviral Pregnancy Registry (1-800-258-4263 or www.APRegistry.com). Health care providers caring for pregnant females living with HIV and their infants may contact the National Perinatal HIV Hotline (888-448-8765) for clinical consultation (HHS [perinatal] 2019).

◆ **Tenofovir Alafenamide and Emtricitabine** *see* Emtricitabine and Tenofovir Alafenamide *on page 557*

◆ **Tenofovir Alafenamide, Darunavir, Cobicistat, and Emtricitabine** *see* Darunavir, Cobicistat, Emtricitabine, and Tenofovir Alafenamide *on page 442*

◆ **Tenofovir Alafenamide, Elvitegravir, Cobicistat, and Emtricitabine** *see* Elvitegravir, Cobicistat, Emtricitabine, and Tenofovir Alafenamide *on page 553*

◆ **Tenofovir Alafenamide, Emtricitabine, and Rilpivirine** *see* Emtricitabine, Rilpivirine, and Tenofovir Alafenamide *on page 559*

◆ **Tenofovir Alafenamide Fumarate** *see* Tenofovir Alafenamide *on page 1418*

◆ **Tenofovir Alafenamide, Rilpivirine, and Emtricitabine** *see* Emtricitabine, Rilpivirine, and Tenofovir Alafenamide *on page 559*

Tenofovir Disoproxil Fumarate

(ten OF oh vir dye soe PROX il FUE ma rate)

Related Information

HIV Infection and AIDS *on page 1690*

Systemic Viral Diseases *on page 1709*

Brand Names: US Viread

Brand Names: Canada APO-Tenofovir; Auro-Tenofovir; JAMP-Tenofovir; MYLAN-Tenofovir Disoproxil; NAT-Tenofovir; PMS-Tenofovir; TEVA-Tenofovir; Viread

Pharmacologic Category Antihepadnaviral, Reverse Transcriptase Inhibitor, Nucleotide (Anti-HBV); Antiretroviral, Reverse Transcriptase Inhibitor, Nucleotide (Anti-HIV)

Use

Chronic hepatitis B: Treatment of chronic hepatitis B virus (HBV) in patients ≥2 years of age weighing ≥10 kg

HIV-1 infection, treatment: Treatment of HIV-1 infection in patients ≥2 years of age weighing ≥10 kg, in combination with other antiretroviral agents.

Local Anesthetic/Vasoconstrictor Precautions

No information available to require special precautions

Effects on Dental Treatment No significant effects or complications reported

Effects on Bleeding No information available to require special precautions regarding hemostasis.

Adverse Reactions Includes data from both treatment-naive and treatment-experienced HIV patients and in chronic hepatitis B.

>10%:

Central nervous system: Insomnia (3% to 18%), headache (5% to 14%), pain (12% to 13%), dizziness (8% to 13%), depression (4% to 11%)

Dermatologic: Skin rash (includes maculopapular, pustular, or vesiculobullous rash; pruritus; or urticaria: 5% to 18%), pruritus (16%)

Endocrine & metabolic: Hypercholesterolemia (19% to 22%), increased serum triglycerides (1% to 4%)

Gastrointestinal: Abdominal pain (4% to 22%), nausea (8% to 20%), diarrhea (9% to 16%), vomiting (2% to 13%)

Neuromuscular & skeletal: Decreased bone mineral density (28%; ≥5% at spine or ≥7% at hip), increased creatine phosphokinase (2% to 12%), weakness (6% to 11%)

Miscellaneous: Fever (4% to 11%)

1% to 10%:

Cardiovascular: Chest pain (3%)

Central nervous system: Fatigue (9%), anxiety (6%), peripheral neuropathy (1% to 5%)

Dermatologic: Diaphoresis (3%)

Endocrine & metabolic: Weight loss (2% to 4%), glycosuria (grades 3/4: ≤3%), hyperglycemia (grades 3/4: 2% to 3%), lipodystrophy (1%)

Gastrointestinal: Increased serum amylase (grades 3/4: 4% to 9%), anorexia (3% to 4%), dyspepsia (3% to 4%), flatulence (3% to 4%)

Genitourinary: Hematuria (≤ grades 3/4: 3% to 7%)

Hematologic & oncologic: Neutropenia (3%)

Hepatic: Increased serum ALT (2% to 10%), increased serum AST (3% to 5%), increased serum transaminases (2% to 5%), increased serum alkaline phosphatase (1%)

Neuromuscular & skeletal: Back pain (4% to 9%), arthralgia (5%), myalgia (4%)

Renal: Increased serum creatinine (9%), renal failure (7%)

Respiratory: Sinusitis (8%), upper respiratory tract infection (8%), nasopharyngitis (5%), pneumonia (2% to 5%)

Postmarketing and/or case reports: Angioedema, dyspnea, exacerbation of hepatitis B (following discontinuation), Fanconi's syndrome, hepatitis, hypersensitivity reaction, hypokalemia, hypophosphatemia, immune reconstitution syndrome, increased gamma-glutamyl transferase, interstitial nephritis, lactic acidosis, myasthenia, myopathy, nephrogenic diabetes insipidus, nephrotoxicity, osteomalacia, pancreatitis, polyuria, proteinuria, proximal tubular nephropathy, renal insufficiency, renal tubular necrosis, rhabdomyolysis, severe hepatomegaly with steatosis

Mechanism of Action Tenofovir disoproxil fumarate (TDF), a nucleotide reverse transcriptase inhibitor, is an analog of adenosine 5'-monophosphate; it interferes with the HIV viral RNA dependent DNA polymerase resulting in inhibition of viral replication. TDF is first converted intracellularly by hydrolysis to tenofovir and subsequently phosphorylated to the active tenofovir diphosphate. Tenofovir inhibits replication of HBV by inhibiting HBV polymerase.

Pharmacodynamics/Kinetics

Half-life Elimination Serum: 17 hours; intracellular: 10 to 50 hours

Time to Peak Serum: Fasting: 36 to 84 minutes; With high-fat meal: 96 to 144 minutes

Reproductive Considerations

The Health and Human Services perinatal HIV guidelines consider tenofovir disoproxil fumarate a preferred nucleoside reverse transcriptase inhibitor for females living with HIV who are not yet pregnant but are trying to conceive.

Tenofovir disoproxil fumarate is one of the agents recommended for pre-exposure prophylaxis in couples with differing HIV status who are planning a pregnancy. The partner without HIV should begin therapy 1 month prior to attempting conception and continue therapy for 1 month after attempting conception.

For males and females living with HIV and planning a pregnancy, maximum viral suppression below the limits of detection with antiretroviral therapy (ART), modification of therapy (if needed), optimization of the woman's health, and a discussion of the potential risks and benefits of ART therapy during pregnancy are recommended prior to conception (HHS [perinatal] 2019).

Pregnancy Considerations

Tenofovir has a high level of transfer across the human placenta following maternal use of tenofovir disoproxil fumarate.

No increased risk of overall birth defects has been observed following first trimester exposure according to data collected by the antiretroviral pregnancy registry. Maternal antiretroviral therapy (ART) may be associated with adverse pregnancy outcomes, including preterm delivery, stillbirth, low birth weight, and small-for-gestational-age infants. Actual risks may be influenced by maternal factors such as disease severity, gestational age at initiation of therapy, and specific ART regimen; therefore, close fetal monitoring is recommended. Because there is clear benefit to appropriate treatment, maternal ART should not be withheld due to concerns for adverse neonatal outcomes. Long-term follow-up is recommended for all infants exposed to antiretroviral medications; children without HIV but who were exposed to ART in utero and develop significant organ system abnormalities of unknown etiology (particularly of the CNS or heart) should be evaluated for potential mitochondrial dysfunction. Cases of lactic acidosis and hepatic steatosis have been reported in pregnant women with use of nucleoside reverse transcriptase inhibitors (NRTIs).

The Health and Human Services (HHS) perinatal HIV guidelines consider tenofovir disoproxil fumarate a preferred NRTI for pregnant females living with HIV who are antiretroviral naive, who have had ART therapy in the past but are restarting, or who require a new ART regimen (due to poor tolerance or poor virologic response of current regimen). In addition, females who become pregnant while taking tenofovir disoproxil fumarate may continue if viral suppression is effective and the regimen is well tolerated. Maternal exposure is modestly decreased during the third trimester; dose adjustments are not needed.

The HHS perinatal HIV guidelines consider tenofovir disoproxil fumarate in combination with emtricitabine or lamivudine to be preferred dual NRTI backbone for initial therapy in antiretroviral-naive pregnant females. The guidelines also consider tenofovir disoproxil fumarate plus emtricitabine or lamivudine as recommended dual NRTI backbone for HIV/hepatitis B virus coinfected pregnant females. Hepatitis B flare may occur if tenofovir disoproxil fumarate is discontinued. Tenofovir disoproxil fumarate is also a preferred component of a regimen when acute HIV infection is detected during pregnancy.

In general, ART is recommended for all pregnant females living with HIV to keep the viral load below the limit of detection and reduce the risk of perinatal transmission. Therapy should be individualized following a discussion of the potential risks and benefits of treatment during pregnancy. Monitoring of pregnant females is more frequent than in nonpregnant adults. ART should be continued postpartum for all females living with HIV and can be modified after delivery.

In hepatitis B-infected women (not coinfected with HIV), the American Association for the Study of Liver Disease (AASLD) chronic hepatitis B treatment guidelines suggest antiviral therapy to reduce the risk of perinatal transmission of hepatitis B in HBsAg-positive pregnant women with an HBV DNA >200,000 units/mL. There are limited data on the level of HBV DNA for when antiviral therapy is routinely recommended (>200,000 units/mL is a conservative recommendation); however, the AASLD recommends against antiviral therapy to reduce the risk of perinatal transmission in HBsAg-positive pregnant women with an HBV DNA ≤200,000 units/mL. Tenofovir is one of the antivirals that has been studied in pregnant women (and may be the preferred agent); with most studies initiating antiviral therapy at 28 to 32 weeks' gestation and discontinuing antiviral therapy between birth to 3 months postpartum (monitor for ALT flares every 3 months for 6 months following discontinuation). There are insufficient long-term safety data in infants born to mothers who took antiviral agents during pregnancy (AASLD [Terrault 2016]). The safety profile of tenofovir disoproxil fumarate, when administered during the third trimester to females with chronic hepatitis B infection, is similar to nonpregnant adults.

Health care providers are encouraged to enroll pregnant females exposed to antiretroviral medications as early in pregnancy as possible in the Antiretroviral Pregnancy Registry (1-800-258-4263 or http://www.APRegistry.com). Health care providers caring for pregnant females living with HIV and their infants may contact the National Perinatal HIV Hotline (888-448-8765) for clinical consultation (HHS [perinatal] 2019).

- ◆ **Tenofovir Disoproxil Fumarate and Emtricitabine** *see* Emtricitabine and Tenofovir Disoproxil Fumarate *on page 558*
- ◆ **Tenofovir Disoproxil Fumarate and Lamivudine** *see* Lamivudine and Tenofovir Disoproxil Fumarate *on page 873*
- ◆ **Tenofovir Disoproxil Fumarate, Doravirine, and Lamivudine** *see* Doravirine, Lamivudine, and Tenofovir Disoproxil Fumarate *on page 514*
- ◆ **Tenofovir Disoproxil Fumarate, Efavirenz, and Emtricitabine** *see* Efavirenz, Emtricitabine, and Tenofovir Disoproxil Fumarate *on page 545*
- ◆ **Tenofovir Disoproxil Fumarate, Elvitegravir, Cobicistat, and Emtricitabine** *see* Elvitegravir, Cobicistat, Emtricitabine, and Tenofovir Disoproxil Fumarate *on page 553*
- ◆ **Tenofovir Disoproxil Fumarate, Emtricitabine, and Rilpivirine** *see* Emtricitabine, Rilpivirine, and Tenofovir Disoproxil Fumarate *on page 559*
- ◆ **Tenofovir Disoproxil Fumarate, Lamivudine, and Doravirine** *see* Doravirine, Lamivudine, and Tenofovir Disoproxil Fumarate *on page 514*
- ◆ **Tenofovir Disoproxil Fumarate, Lamivudine, and Efavirenz** *see* Efavirenz, Lamivudine, and Tenofovir Disoproxil Fumarate *on page 545*
- ◆ **Tenofovir Disoproxil Fumarate, Rilpivirine, and Emtricitabine** *see* Emtricitabine, Rilpivirine, and Tenofovir Disoproxil Fumarate *on page 559*
- ◆ **Tenoretic** *see* Atenolol and Chlorthalidone *on page 190*
- ◆ **Tenormin** *see* Atenolol *on page 189*
- ◆ **Tenuate** *see* Diethylpropion *on page 494*
- ◆ **Tenuate Dospan** *see* Diethylpropion *on page 494*
- ◆ **Tepadina** *see* Thiotepa *on page 1439*
- ◆ **Tepezza** *see* Teprotumumab *on page 1420*

Teprotumumab (TEP roe TOOM ue mab)

Brand Names: US Tepezza

Pharmacologic Category Insulin-Like Growth Factor-1 Receptor (IGF-1R) Antagonist; Monoclonal Antibody

Use Thyroid eye disease: Treatment of thyroid eye disease.

Local Anesthetic/Vasoconstrictor Precautions No information available to require special precautions.

Effects on Dental Treatment Key adverse event(s) related to dental treatment: Occurrence of distorted sense of taste (dysgeusia).

Effects on Bleeding No information available to require special precautions.

Adverse Reactions

>10%:

Dermatologic: Alopecia (13%)

Gastrointestinal: Nausea (17%), diarrhea (12%)

Nervous system: Fatigue (12%)

Neuromuscular & skeletal: Muscle spasm (25%)

1% to 10%:

Dermatologic: Xeroderma (8%)

Endocrine & metabolic: Hyperglycemia (10%)

Gastrointestinal: Dysgeusia (8%)

Nervous system: Headache (8%)

Otic: Auditory impairment (10%)

Miscellaneous: Infusion related reaction (4%)

Mechanism of Action Teprotumumab's mechanism of action in patients with thyroid eye disease has not been fully characterized. Teprotumumab binds to insulin-like growth factor-1 receptor inhibitor and blocks its activation and signaling.

Pharmacodynamics/Kinetics

Half-life Elimination 20 ± 5 days.

Reproductive Considerations Females of reproductive potential should use effective contraception prior to treatment, during therapy and for 6 months after the last dose of teprotumumab.

Pregnancy Considerations

Teprotumumab is a humanized monoclonal antibody (IgG1). Placental transfer of human IgG is dependent upon the IgG subclass, maternal serum concentrations, birth weight, and gestational age, generally increasing as pregnancy progresses. The lowest exposure would be expected during the period of organogenesis (Palmeira 2012; Pentsuk 2009).

Based on the mechanism of action, and data from animal reproduction studies, in utero exposure to teprotumumab may cause fetal harm.

◆ **Teprotumumab-trbw** *see* Teprotumumab *on page 1420*

◆ **Terazol 3 [DSC]** *see* Terconazole *on page 1423*

◆ **Terazol 7 [DSC]** *see* Terconazole *on page 1423*

Terazosin (ter AY zoe sin)

Related Information

Cardiovascular Diseases *on page 1654*

Brand Names: Canada APO-Terazosin; DOM-Terazosin; Hytrin [DSC]; PMS-Terazosin; TEVA-Terazosin

Pharmacologic Category $Alpha_1$ Blocker; Antihypertensive

Use

Benign prostatic hyperplasia: Treatment of symptomatic benign prostatic hyperplasia (BPH)

Hypertension: Management of hypertension. **Note:** Alpha blockers are not recommended as first line therapy (ACC/AHA [Whelton 2017]).

Local Anesthetic/Vasoconstrictor Precautions No information available to require special precautions

Effects on Dental Treatment Key adverse event(s) related to dental treatment: Xerostomia (normal salivary flow resumes upon discontinuation); Patients may experience orthostatic hypotension as they stand up after treatment; especially if lying in dental chair for extended periods of time. Use caution with sudden changes in position during and after dental treatment.

Effects on Bleeding No information available to require special precautions

Adverse Reactions

>10%:

Central nervous system: Dizziness (9% to 19%), myasthenia (7% to 11%)

1% to 10%:

Cardiovascular: Peripheral edema (1% to 6%), orthostatic hypotension (1% to 4%), palpitations (≤4%), tachycardia (≤2%), syncope (≤1%)

Central nervous system: Drowsiness (4% to 5%), paresthesia (≤3%), vertigo (1%)

Endocrine & metabolic: Decreased libido (≤1%), weight gain (≤1%)

Gastrointestinal: Nausea (2% to 4%)

Genitourinary: Impotence (≤2%)

Neuromuscular & skeletal: Limb pain (≤4%), back pain (≤2%)

Ophthalmic: Blurred vision (≤2%)

Respiratory: Nasal congestion (2% to 6%), dyspnea (2% to 3%), sinusitis (≤3%)

<1%, postmarketing, and/or case reports: Abdominal pain, anaphylaxis, anxiety, arthralgia, arthritis, arthropathy, atrial fibrillation, bronchitis, cardiac arrhythmia, chest pain, conjunctivitis, constipation, cough, diaphoresis, diarrhea, dyspepsia, epistaxis, facial edema, fever, flatulence, flu-like symptoms, gout, hypersensitivity reaction, insomnia, intraoperative floppy iris syndrome (IFIS), myalgia, neck pain, pharyngitis, polyuria, priapism, pruritus, rhinitis, shoulder pain, skin rash, thrombocytopenia, tinnitus, urinary incontinence, urinary tract infection, vasodilation, visual disturbance, vomiting, xerostomia

Mechanism of Action $Alpha_1$-specific blocking agent with minimal $alpha_2$ effects; this allows peripheral postsynaptic blockade, with the resultant decrease in arterial tone, while preserving the negative feedback loop which is mediated by the peripheral presynaptic $alpha_2$-receptors; terazosin relaxes the smooth muscle of the bladder neck, thus reducing bladder outlet obstruction

Pharmacodynamics/Kinetics

Onset of Action Antihypertensive effect: 15 minutes; Peak effect: Antihypertensive effect: 2 to 3 hours

Duration of Action Antihypertensive effect: 24 hours

Half-life Elimination ~12 hours

Time to Peak Plasma: ~1 hour; delayed ~40 minutes with food

Pregnancy Risk Factor C

Pregnancy Considerations

Adverse events have been observed in some animal reproduction studies.

Chronic maternal hypertension may increase the risk of birth defects, low birth weight, preterm delivery, stillbirth, and neonatal death. Actual fetal/neonatal risks may be related to duration and severity of maternal hypertension. Untreated hypertension may also increase the risks of adverse maternal outcomes, including gestational diabetes, myocardial infarction, preeclampsia, stroke, and delivery complications (ACOG 203 2019).

Agents other than terazosin are more commonly used to treat hypertension in pregnancy (ACOG 203 2019; ESC [Regitz-Zagrosek 2018]). Females with preexisting hypertension may continue their medication during pregnancy unless contraindications exist (ESC [Regitz-Zagrosek 2018]).

Terbinafine (Systemic) (TER bin a feen)

Brand Names: US LamISIL [DSC]

Brand Names: Canada ACT Terbinafine; APO-Terbinafine; Auro-Terbinafine; DOM-Terbinafine; JAMP-Terbinafine; LamISIL; MYLAN-Terbinafine [DSC]; PHL-Terbinafine [DSC]; PMS-Terbinafine; RIVA-Terbinafine; SANDOZ Terbinafine [DSC]; Terbinafine-250; TEVA-Terbinafine [DSC]

Pharmacologic Category Antifungal Agent, Oral

Use

Onychomycosis (tablets only): Treatment of onychomycosis of the toenail or fingernail caused by dermatophytes (tinea unguium).

Tinea capitis (granules only): Treatment of tinea capitis in patients 4 years and older.

Local Anesthetic/Vasoconstrictor Precautions No information available to require special precautions

Effects on Dental Treatment Key adverse event(s) related to dental treatment: Taste disturbance.

Effects on Bleeding No information available to require special precautions

Adverse Reactions

>10%: Central nervous system: Headache (7% to 13%)

1% to 10%:

Dermatologic: Skin rash (6%; children: 2%), pruritus (1% to 3%), urticaria (1%)

Gastrointestinal: Diarrhea (3% to 6%), vomiting (<1%; children: 5%), dyspepsia (4%), upper abdominal pain (children: 4%), dysgeusia (3%; may be severe and result in weight loss, anxiety, and depression), nausea (2% to 3%), abdominal pain (children: 2%), pharyngolaryngeal pain (children: 2%), toothache (children: 1%)

Hepatic: Liver enzyme disorder (3%)

Infection: Influenza (children: 2%)

Ophthalmic: Vision color changes (children: 5%; color confusion), decreased visual acuity (children: 1% to 2%)

Respiratory: Nasopharyngitis (children: 10%), cough (children: 6%), upper respiratory tract infection (children: 5%), nasal congestion (children: 2%), rhinorrhea (children: 2%)

Miscellaneous: Fever (<1%; children: 7%)

<1%, postmarketing, and/or case reports: Acute generalized exanthematous pustulosis, ageusia, agranulocytosis, alopecia, altered sense of smell, anaphylaxis, anemia, angioedema, anosmia, anxiety, arthralgia, auditory impairment, bullous dermatitis, cholestasis, cutaneous lupus erythematosus, depression, DRESS syndrome, erythema multiforme, exacerbation of psoriasis, exacerbation of systemic lupus erythematosus, exfoliative dermatitis, fatigue, flu-like symptoms, hemolytic-uremic syndrome, hepatic insufficiency, hepatic failure, hepatitis, hypersensitivity reaction, hypoesthesia, increased creatine phosphokinase, lens disease, malaise, myalgia, pancreatitis, pancytopenia, paresthesia, psoriasiform eruption, retinopathy, rhabdomyolysis, serum sickness-like reaction, severe neutropenia, skin photosensitivity, Stevens-Johnson syndrome, systemic lupus erythematosus, thrombocytopenia, thrombotic thrombocytopenic purpura, tinnitus, toxic epidermal necrolysis, vasculitis, vertigo, visual field defect

Mechanism of Action Synthetic allylamine derivative that inhibits squalene epoxidase, a key enzyme in sterol biosynthesis in fungi. This results in a deficiency in ergosterol within the fungal cell membrane and results in fungal cell death.

Pharmacodynamics/Kinetics

Half-life Elimination Terminal half-life: 200 to 400 hours; very slow release of drug from skin and adipose tissues occurs; effective half-life: Children: 27 to 31 hours; Adults: ~36 hours

Time to Peak Plasma: Children and Adults: Within 2 hours

Pregnancy Considerations

Published information related to the use of systemic terbinafine in pregnancy is limited (Gupta 1997; Sarkar 2003).

Systemic therapy for the treatment of onychomycosis or tinea capitis is not recommended during pregnancy (Kaul 2017; Murase 2014).

Product Availability Lamisil granules have been discontinued in the United States for more than 1 year.

◆ **Terbinafine HCl** *see* Terbinafine (Systemic) *on page 1421*

◆ **Terbinafine Hydrochloride** *see* Terbinafine (Systemic) *on page 1421*

Terbutaline (ter BYOO ta leen)

Brand Names: Canada Bricanyl Turbuhaler

Pharmacologic Category Antidote, Extravasation; $Beta_2$ Agonist

Use Asthma/Bronchospasm: Prevention and reversal of bronchospasm in patients ≥12 years of age with asthma and reversible bronchospasm associated with bronchitis and emphysema

Local Anesthetic/Vasoconstrictor Precautions No information available to require special precautions

Effects on Dental Treatment Key adverse event(s) related to dental treatment: Xerostomia (normal salivary flow resumes upon discontinuation) and bad taste in mouth.

Effects on Bleeding No information available to require special precautions

Adverse Reactions

>10%:

Central nervous system: Nervousness, restlessness

Endocrine & metabolic: Decreased serum potassium, increased serum glucose

Neuromuscular & skeletal: Tremor

1% to 10%:

Cardiovascular: Hypertension, tachycardia

Central nervous system: Dizziness, drowsiness, headache, insomnia

Dermatologic: Diaphoresis

Gastrointestinal: Dysgeusia, nausea, vomiting, xerostomia

Neuromuscular & skeletal: Muscle cramps, weakness

<1%, postmarketing, and/or case reports: Cardiac arrhythmia, chest pain, hyperglycemia (preterm labor), hypokalemia (preterm labor), hypotension (preterm labor), ischemic heart disease (preterm labor), lactic acidosis (Smith 2019), myocardial infarction (preterm labor), paradoxical bronchospasm, pulmonary edema (preterm labor)

Mechanism of Action Relaxes bronchial and uterine smooth muscle by action on $beta_2$-receptors with less effect on heart rate

Pharmacodynamics/Kinetics

Onset of Action Oral: 30 to 45 minutes; SubQ: 6 to 15 minutes; Inhalation: 5 minutes (maximum effect: 15 to 60 minutes)

Duration of Action Oral: 4 to 8 hours; Oral inhalation: 3 to 6 hours; SubQ: 1.5 to 4 hours

Half-life Elimination 5.7 hours (range: 2.9 to 14 hours)

Time to Peak Serum: SubQ: 0.5 hours

Pregnancy Considerations

Terbutaline crosses the placenta; umbilical cord concentrations are ~11% to 48% of maternal blood levels.

Terbutaline may affect uterine contractility; use caution if needed to control bronchospasm in pregnant women. Uncontrolled asthma is associated with adverse events in pregnancy (increased risk of perinatal mortality, preeclampsia, preterm birth, low-birth-weight infants, cesarean delivery, and the development of gestational diabetes). Poorly controlled asthma or asthma exacerbations may have a greater fetal/maternal risk than what is associated with appropriately used asthma medications. Maternal treatment improves pregnancy outcomes by reducing the risk of some adverse events (eg, preterm birth, gestational diabetes). Although short acting beta-2 agonists should be used to treat acute asthma exacerbations in pregnant women, agents other than terbutaline are preferred (ERS/TSANZ [Middleton 2020]; GINA 2020)

[US Boxed Warning]: Terbutaline injection has not been approved for and should not be used for prolonged tocolysis (beyond 48 to 72 hours). Oral terbutaline sulfate has not been approved and should not be used for acute or maintenance tocolysis. In particular, terbutaline should not be used for maintenance tocolysis in the outpatient or home setting. Serious adverse reactions, including death, have been reported after administration of terbutaline to pregnant women. In mothers, these adverse reactions include increased heart rate, transient hyperglycemia, hypokalemia, cardiac arrhythmias, pulmonary edema, and myocardial ischemia. Increased fetal heart rate and neonatal hypoglycemia may occur as a result of maternal administration. Terbutaline has been used in the management of preterm labor. Tocolytics may be used for the short-term (48 hour) prolongation of pregnancy to allow for the administration of antenatal steroids and should not be used prior to fetal viability or when the risks of use to the fetus or mother are greater than the risk of preterm birth (ACOG 171 2016).

◆ **Terbutaline Sulfate** *see* Terbutaline *on page* 1422

Terconazole (ter KONE a zole)

Brand Names: US Terazol 3 [DSC]; Terazol 7 [DSC]; Zazole [DSC]

Brand Names: Canada TARO-Terconazole; Terazol 7 [DSC]

Pharmacologic Category Antifungal Agent, Azole Derivative; Antifungal Agent, Vaginal

Use Candidiasis, vulvovaginal: For the local treatment of vulvovaginal candidiasis (moniliasis). As terconazole is effective only for vulvovaginitis caused by the genus *Candida*, the diagnosis should be confirmed by KOH smears or cultures.

Local Anesthetic/Vasoconstrictor Precautions No information available to require special precautions

Effects on Dental Treatment No significant effects or complications reported

Effects on Bleeding No information available to require special precautions

Adverse Reactions

>10%: Central nervous system: Headache

1% to 10%:

- Central nervous system: Chills, pain
- Gastrointestinal: Abdominal pain
- Genitourinary: Dysmenorrhea, vaginal discomfort (burning, irritation, or itching)
- Miscellaneous: Fever

<1%, postmarketing, and/or case reports: Anaphylaxis, asthenia, bronchospasm, burning sensation of the penis, dizziness, facial edema, flu-like symptoms (including nausea, vomiting, myalgia, arthralgia, malaise), hypersensitivity, skin rash, toxic epidermal necrolysis, urticaria

Mechanism of Action Terconazole is a triazole ketal antifungal agent; involves inhibition of fungal cytochrome P450. Specifically, terconazole inhibits cytochrome P450-dependent 14-alpha-demethylase which results in accumulation of membrane disturbing 14-alpha-demethylsterols and ergosterol depletion.

Pharmacodynamics/Kinetics

Half-life Elimination 6.4 to 8.5 hours

Time to Peak ~5 to 10 hours

Reproductive Considerations

This product may weaken latex condoms and diaphragms (CDC [Workowski 2015]).

Pregnancy Considerations

The rate and extent of absorption are similar in pregnant and nonpregnant patients with vulvovaginal candidiasis. Although the manufacturer recommends that use should be avoided during the first trimester of pregnancy (due to systemic absorption) and that use may be considered in the second or third trimesters if the benefits outweigh risks to the fetus, guidelines state that 7-day topical azole vaginal products are the preferred treatment of vulvovaginal candidiasis in pregnant women (CDC [Workowski 2015].

Teriflunomide (ter i FLOO noh mide)

Brand Names: US Aubagio

Brand Names: Canada Aubagio

Pharmacologic Category Pyrimidine Synthesis Inhibitor

Use Multiple sclerosis, relapsing: Treatment of relapsing forms of multiple sclerosis, including clinically isolated syndrome, relapsing-remitting disease, and active secondary progressive disease in adults.

Local Anesthetic/Vasoconstrictor Precautions Use vasoconstrictor with caution; patients may experience significant hypertension and palpitations when taking teriflunomide

Effects on Dental Treatment Key adverse event(s) related to dental treatment: Abnormal taste, aphthous stomatitis, and toothache have been reported.

Effects on Bleeding Thrombocytopenia has been reported.

Adverse Reactions

>10%:

- Central nervous system: Headache (16% to 18%)
- Dermatologic: Alopecia (10% to 13%)
- Endocrine & metabolic: Hypophosphatemia (18%)
- Gastrointestinal: Diarrhea (13% to 14%), nausea (8% to 11%)
- Hematologic & oncologic: Lymphocytopenia (10% to 12%)
- Hepatic: Increased serum alanine aminotransferase (13% to 15%)

1% to 10%:

- Cardiovascular: Hypertension (3% to 4%)
- Central nervous system: Paresthesia (8% to 9%)

Hematologic & oncologic: Neutropenia (4% to 6%)
Neuromuscular & skeletal: Arthralgia (6% to 8%), peripheral neuropathy (including carpal tunnel syndrome; 1% to 2%)

<1%, postmarketing, and/or case reports: Anaphylaxis, angioedema, cytomegalovirus disease (reactivation), hypersensitivity reaction, increased serum creatinine, interstitial pulmonary disease, jaundice, pancreatitis, Stevens-Johnson syndrome, thrombocytopenia, toxic epidermal necrolysis, uric acid nephropathy

Mechanism of Action Teriflunomide is an immunomodulatory agent that inhibits pyrimidine synthesis, resulting in antiproliferative and anti-inflammatory effects. It may reduce the number of activated lymphocytes in the CNS.

Pharmacodynamics/Kinetics

Half-life Elimination Median: 18-19 days; enterohepatic recycling appears to contribute to the long half-life of this agent, since activated charcoal and cholestyramine substantially reduce plasma half-life

Time to Peak Plasma: 1-4 hours

Reproductive Considerations

[US Boxed Warning]: Teriflunomide is contraindicated in females of reproductive potential who are not using effective contraception. Exclude pregnancy before the start of treatment with teriflunomide in females of reproductive potential. Women of childbearing potential should not receive therapy until pregnancy has been excluded, they have been counseled concerning fetal risk, and reliable contraceptive measures have been confirmed.

[US Boxed Warning]: Advise females of reproductive potential to use effective contraception during teriflunomide treatment and during an accelerated drug elimination procedure after teriflunomide treatment. Women who wish to become pregnant, as well as all females of reproductive potential, should undergo the accelerated drug elimination procedure when teriflunomide is discontinued. Pregnancy should be avoided until undetectable serum concentrations (<0.02 mg/L) are verified.

Teriflunomide is found in semen. Males and their female partners should use reliable contraception during therapy. Males who wish to father a child should discontinue teriflunomide and undergo the accelerated drug elimination procedure or wait until plasma teriflunomide concentrations are <0.02 mg/L.

In general, disease-modifying therapies for multiple sclerosis (MS) are stopped prior to a planned pregnancy except in females at high risk of MS activity (AAN [Rae-Grant 2018]). Consider use of agents other than teriflunomide for females at high risk of disease reactivation who are planning a pregnancy. Delaying pregnancy is recommended for females with persistent high disease activity; when disease-modifying therapy is needed in these patients, other agents are preferred (ECTRIMS/EAN [Montalban 2018]).

Pregnancy Considerations

[US Boxed Warning]: Teriflunomide is contraindicated in pregnant women because of the potential for fetal harm. Teratogenicity and embryolethality occurred in animals at plasma teriflunomide exposures lower than that in humans. Stop teriflunomide and use an accelerated drug elimination procedure if the patient becomes pregnant. Pregnancy outcome information following maternal use during pregnancy or following use in male patients who fathered a child are limited (Andersen 2018; Kieseier 2014).

In general, disease-modifying therapies for multiple sclerosis (MS) are not initiated during pregnancy, except in females at high risk of MS activity (AAN [Rae-Grant 2018]). When disease-modifying therapy is needed in these patients, other agents are preferred (ECTRIMS/EAN [Montalban 2018]).

Data collection to monitor pregnancy and infant outcomes following exposure to teriflunomide is ongoing. Health care providers are encouraged to enroll females exposed to teriflunomide during pregnancy in the pregnancy registry (800-745-4447, option 2).

Teriparatide (ter i PAR a tide)

Related Information

Rheumatoid Arthritis, Osteoarthritis, and Osteoporosis *on page 1697*

Brand Names: US Forteo

Brand Names: Canada Forteo; TEVA-Teriparatide

Pharmacologic Category Parathyroid Hormone Analog

Use

Osteoporosis: Treatment of osteoporosis in postmenopausal females who are at high risk for fracture (defined as history of osteoporotic fracture or multiple risk factors for fracture); treatment to increase bone mass in males with primary or hypogonadal osteoporosis who are high risk for fracture; treatment of males and females with glucocorticoid-induced osteoporosis associated with chronic systemic glucocorticoids with a prednisone dosage of ≥5 mg/day (or equivalent) at a high risk for fracture. May also be used in patients who have failed or are intolerant to other available osteoporosis therapy.

Limitations of use: Cumulative lifetime duration of teriparatide and any other parathyroid hormone therapy (eg, abaloparatide) should not exceed 2 years.

Local Anesthetic/Vasoconstrictor Precautions No information available to require special precautions

Effects on Dental Treatment Key adverse event(s) related to dental treatment: May have beneficial effects for treatment of osteoporosis in patients with osteonecrosis of the jaw due to bisphosphonates; however, teriparatide may have cost constraints.

Effects on Bleeding No information available to require special precautions

Adverse Reactions

>10%: Endocrine & metabolic: Hypercalcemia (transient increases noted 4 to 6 hours postdose [women 11%; men 6%])

1% to 10%:

Cardiovascular: Orthostatic hypotension (5%; transient), angina pectoris (3%), syncope (3%)
Central nervous system: Dizziness (8%), headache (8%), insomnia (5%), anxiety (4%), depression (4%), vertigo (4%)
Endocrine & metabolic: Hyperuricemia (3%)
Gastrointestinal: Nausea (9% to 14%), gastritis (7%), dyspepsia (5%), vomiting (3%)
Immunologic: Antibody development (3% of women in long-term treatment; hypersensitivity reactions or decreased efficacy were not associated in preclinical trials)
Infection: Herpes zoster (3%)
Neuromuscular & skeletal: Arthralgia (10%), weakness (9%), leg cramps (3%)
Respiratory: Rhinitis (10%), pharyngitis (6%), dyspnea (4% to 6%), pneumonia (3% to 6%)

<1%, postmarketing and/or case reports: Anaphylaxis, angioedema, chest pain, dyspnea (acute), facial edema, hypercalcemia (>13 mg/dL), hypersensitivity reaction, injection site reactions (bruising, pain, swelling), mouth edema, muscle spasm, osteosarcoma, urticaria

Mechanism of Action Teriparatide is a recombinant formulation of endogenous parathyroid hormone (PTH), containing a 34-amino-acid sequence which is identical to the N-terminal portion of this hormone. The pharmacologic activity of teriparatide, which is similar to the physiologic activity of PTH, includes stimulating osteoblast function, increasing gastrointestinal calcium absorption, and increasing renal tubular reabsorption of calcium. Treatment with teriparatide results in increased bone mineral density, bone mass, and strength. In postmenopausal females, teriparatide has been shown to decrease osteoporosis-related fractures.

Pharmacodynamics/Kinetics

Half-life Elimination IV: 5 minutes; SubQ: ~1 hour

Time to Peak Serum: ~30 minutes

Pregnancy Considerations Adverse events were observed in animal reproduction studies; consider discontinuing treatment once pregnancy is recognized.

Product Availability Bonsity: FDA approved October 2019; anticipated availability is currently unknown. Consult the prescribing information for additional information.

◆ **TESPA** *see* Thiotepa *on page* 1439

◆ **Tessalon Perles** *see* Benzonatate *on page* 231

◆ **Testim** *see* Testosterone *on page* 1425

◆ **Testopel** *see* Testosterone *on page* 1425

Testosterone (tes TOS ter one)

Brand Names: US Androderm; AndroGel; AndroGel Pump; Aveed; Axiron [DSC]; Depo-Testosterone; Fortesta; Jatenzo; Natesto; Striant [DSC]; Testim; Testopel; Vogelxo; Vogelxo Pump; Xyosted

Brand Names: Canada Andriol [DSC]; Androderm; AndroGel; Axiron [DSC]; Delatestryl; Depo-Testosterone; Natesto; PMS-Testosterone Enhanthate [DSC]; PMS-Testosterone Undecanoate; TARO-Testosterone; Testim

Pharmacologic Category Androgen

Use

Breast cancer, metastatic: IM injection (enanthate): Secondary treatment in women with advancing inoperable metastatic (skeletal) mammary cancer who are 1 to 5 years postmenopausal. Use may be considered in premenopausal women with breast cancer who have benefited from oophorectomy and have a hormone-responsive tumor.

Delayed puberty: IM injection (enanthate); pellet: To stimulate puberty in carefully selected males with delayed puberty.

Hypogonadism, hypogonadotropic (congenital or acquired): Buccal; Capsule (oral); Gel (nasal, transdermal); IM injection (cypionate, enanthate, undecanoate); Patch (transdermal); Pellet; Solution (transdermal); SubQ injection (enanthate): Gonadotropin or luteinizing hormone-releasing hormone deficiency, or pituitary-hypothalamic injury from tumors, trauma, or radiation.

Hypogonadism, primary (congenital or acquired): Buccal; Capsule (oral); Gel (nasal, transdermal); IM injection (cypionate, enanthate, undecanoate); Patch (transdermal); Pellet; Solution (transdermal); SubQ injection (enanthate): Treatment of testicular failure due to cryptorchidism, bilateral torsion, orchitis, vanishing testis syndrome, orchiectomy, Klinefelter syndrome, chemotherapy, or toxic damage from alcohol or heavy metals.

Limitations of use: Safety and efficacy in men with age-related hypogonadism (or late-onset hypogonadism) has not been established (manufacturer's labeling). However, the Endocrine Society recommends offering testosterone therapy to patients with symptoms of testosterone deficiency and consistently and unequivocally low morning testosterone concentrations. In men >65 years of age, treatment should only be initiated on an individual basis and after consultation with the patient regarding risks and benefits (Endocrine Society [Bhasin 2018]).

Local Anesthetic/Vasoconstrictor Precautions No information available to require special precautions

Effects on Dental Treatment Key adverse event(s) related to dental treatment: Buccal administration: Bitter taste, gum edema, gum or mouth irritation, gum tenderness, and taste perversion.

Effects on Bleeding No information available to require special precautions

Adverse Reactions

>10%:

Cardiovascular: Hypertension (≤13%; intranasal: >6%)

Dermatologic: Skin blister (application site; transdermal: 12%)

Genitourinary: Prostate specific antigen increase (≤18%; buccal, oral: 2%), benign prostatic hypertrophy (12%)

Hematologic & oncologic: Increased hematocrit (subcutaneous: 8% to 14%; topical, oral: ≤6%; buccal, intramuscular: 1%)

Local: Application-site pruritus (transdermal: 17% to 37%)

1% to 10%:

Cardiovascular: Peripheral edema (<1%; subcutaneous: 3%), peripheral vascular disease (transdermal: <3%)

Central nervous system: Emotional lability (buccal: ≤8%; intramuscular, topical: ≤3%), altered sense of smell (intranasal: 5% to >6%; topical: 1%), anosmia (intranasal: 6%; buccal: 1%), headache (≤5%), procedural pain (intramuscular, intranasal: 4%), depression (≤3%), nervousness (≤3%), abnormality in thinking (transdermal: <3%), anxiety (<3%), body pain (transdermal: <3%), chills (transdermal: <3%), confusion (transdermal: <3%), fatigue (<3%), paresthesia (<3%), vertigo (transdermal: <3%), irritability (intramuscular: 2%), sleep apnea (2%), insomnia (intramuscular, subcutaneous, topical: 1% to 2%), aggressive behavior (buccal, intramuscular: 1%), stinging sensation (lips; buccal: 1%)

Dermatologic: Acne vulgaris (≤8%), crusted skin (nasal scab; intranasal: 4% to 6%), excoriation of skin (nasal; intranasal: ≤6%), contact dermatitis (topical, transdermal: 2% to 4%), bulla (application site; transdermal: <3%), skin rash (<3%), pruritus (≤2%), xeroderma (topical: ≤2%), erythema (topical: ≥1%), hyperhidrosis (intramuscular: 1%), alopecia (topical: ≤1%)

Endocrine & metabolic: Decreased HDL cholesterol (topical, oral: ≤6%), hyperlipidemia (≤6%), hypokalemia (topical: ≤6%), increased serum triglycerides (≤6%), increased thyroid stimulating hormone level (intranasal: ≤6%), increased plasma estradiol concentration (intramuscular: 3%), decreased libido (≤3%), gynecomastia (≤3%), hot flash (intramuscular, topical: 1%), weight gain (intramuscular: 1%)

Gastrointestinal: Gingivitis (buccal: ≤9%), oral irritation (buccal: ≤9%), decreased appetite (intranasal: ≤6%), nausea (≤6%; oral, subcutaneous: 2%), diarrhea (≤4%), gingival pain (buccal: 3%; includes gingival tenderness), dysgeusia (<3%), gastroesophageal reflux disease (transdermal: <3%), gastrointestinal hemorrhage (transdermal: <3%), increased appetite (topical, transdermal: <3%), abdominal pain (buccal, subcutaneous: 2%), gingival swelling (buccal: 2%), toothache (buccal: ≤1%), oral mucosa changes (buccal; includes buccal mucosa roughening and gum blister)

Genitourinary: Testicular atrophy (intranasal, topical: ≤6%), prostatic disease (topical, transdermal: 3% to 5%), hypogonadism (intramuscular: 3%), mastalgia (topical: ≤3%; buccal: 1%), prostatitis (intramuscular, subcutaneous, transdermal: ≤3%), urinary tract infection (subcutaneous, transdermal: ≤3%), dysuria (intramuscular, transdermal: <3%), hematuria (subcutaneous, transdermal: <3%), impotence (transdermal: <3%), pelvic pain (transdermal: <3%), urinary incontinence (transdermal: <3%), testicular disease (including testicular tenderness and non-palpable testes: topical: 2%), urinary frequency (topical: ≤2%), breast hypertrophy (buccal: 1%), difficulty in micturition (buccal, topical: 1%), ejaculatory disorder (intramuscular: 1%), prostate induration (intramuscular: 1%), spontaneous erections (topical: 1%)

Hematologic & oncologic: Anemia (topical: 3%), polycythemia (≤3%), prostate carcinoma (topical, transdermal: <3%), increased hemoglobin (intramuscular, topical: ≤2%)

Hepatic: Increased serum bilirubin (topical: ≤6%), abnormal hepatic function tests (1%)

Local: Bruising at injection site (subcutaneous: 4% to 7%), application-site erythema (topical, transdermal: ≤7%), application-site vesicles (transdermal: 6%), bleeding at injection site (subcutaneous: 3% to 6%), application-site reaction (topical: ≤6%), pain at injection site (intramuscular: 5%), application-site induration (transdermal: 3%), erythema at injection site (subcutaneous: 3%; intramuscular: 1%), application-site irritation (transdermal: <3%), application-site rash (transdermal: <3%), local skin exfoliation (transdermal; application site: <3%), application-site burning (topical, transdermal: 1% to 3%), application-site edema (topical: ≥1%)

Neuromuscular & skeletal: Back pain (subcutaneous, transdermal: 3% to 6%), myalgia (intramuscular, intranasal: ≤6%), limb pain (intranasal, topical: ≤4%), increased creatine phosphokinase in blood specimen (subcutaneous: 3% to 4%), asthenia (topical: ≤3%), abnormal bone growth (accelerated; transdermal: <3%), hemarthrosis (transdermal: <3%), arthralgia (subcutaneous: 2%)

Renal: Increased serum creatinine (topical: ≤6%), polyuria (transdermal: <3%)

Respiratory: Nasopharyngitis (intranasal: 4% to 9%; topical: ≥1%), rhinorrhea (intranasal: 4% to 8%), epistaxis (intranasal: 4% to 7%), nasal discomfort (intranasal: 4% to 6%), bronchitis (intranasal: 4%), upper respiratory tract infection (intranasal: 4%), dry nose (intranasal: ≤4%), nasal congestion (intranasal: ≤4%), sinusitis (intramuscular, intranasal: ≤4%), cough (intramuscular, intranasal, subcutaneous: ≤3%), nasal mucosa swelling (buccal: 1%)

Frequency not defined:

Cardiovascular: Exacerbation of hypertension (buccal)

Central nervous system: Hostility (topical)

Gastrointestinal: Gingival recession (buccal)

Hepatic: Hepatic adenoma (intramuscular; long-term testosterone enanthate therapy)

Local: Induration at injection site (subcutaneous)

<1%, postmarketing, and/or case reports: Abscess at injection site, acute myocardial infarction, allergic dermatitis, altered hormone level (fluctuating testosterone levels), amnesia, anaphylactic shock, anaphylaxis, androgenetic alopecia, angina pectoris, angioedema, asthma, azoospermia, bitter taste, breast induration, calcium retention, cardiac failure, cerebral infarction, cerebrovascular accident, cerebrovascular insufficiency, change in HDL, chest pain, cholestatic jaundice, chronic obstructive pulmonary disease, circulatory shock, clotting factors suppression (factors II, V, VII, X), coronary artery disease, coronary occlusion, decreased plasma testosterone, decreased thyroxine binding globulin, deep vein thrombosis, diabetes mellitus, diaphoresis, discomfort at injection site, dizziness, drug abuse, dyspnea, edema, electrolyte disorder (calcium, nitrogen, phosphorus, potassium, sodium), erectile dysfunction, fluid retention, flu-like symptoms, frequent erections, genitourinary infection (prostate), gingival erythema, hair discoloration, hearing loss (sudden), hematoma at injection site, hepatic neoplasm, hepatocellular neoplasm, hepatotoxicity (idiosyncratic; Chalasani 2014), hirsutism, hyperchloremia, hypernatremia, hyperparathyroidism, hypersensitivity angiitis, hypersensitivity reaction, hyperventilation, increased gamma-glutamyl transferase, increased intraocular pressure, increased libido, increased serum alanine aminotransferase, increased serum aspartate aminotransferase, increased serum prolactin, increased serum transaminases, increased testosterone level, infection, injection site reaction, inorganic phosphate retention, irritation at injection site, Korsakoff syndrome (nonalcoholic), lip edema, localized infection (abscess, cellulitis), malaise, malignant neoplasm of prostate, migraine, musculoskeletal chest pain, musculoskeletal pain, nephrolithiasis, nipple tenderness (sensitivity), nonimmune anaphylaxis, oligospermia (may occur at high dosages), oral inflammation, oral mucosa ulcer, orgasm disturbance (male), osteoporosis, papular rash, peliosis hepatitis, peripheral venous insufficiency, pharyngeal edema, pharyngolaryngeal pain, pollakiuria, potassium retention, priapism, prolonged partial thromboplastin time, prolonged prothrombin time, prostatic intraepithelial neoplasia, pulmonary embolism (including pulmonary oil microembolism), renal colic, renal function abnormality, renal pain, respiratory distress, restlessness, reversible ischemic neurological deficit, rhinitis, sleep disorder, snoring, sodium retention, spermatocele, stomatitis, suicidal ideation, syncope, systemic lupus erythematosus, tachycardia, testicular pain, thrombocytopenia, thromboembolism, thrombosis, tinnitus, transient ischemic attacks, upper abdominal pain, urination disorder, vasodilation, venous thromboembolism, vitreous detachment, voice disorder, xerostomia

Mechanism of Action Principal endogenous androgen responsible for promoting the growth and development of the male sex organs and maintaining secondary sex characteristics in androgen-deficient males

Pharmacodynamics/Kinetics

Duration of Action Route and ester dependent; IM: Cypionate and enanthate esters: 2 to 4 weeks; Undecanoate: 10 weeks; Transdermal gel: 24 hours

Half-life Elimination Variable: 10 to 100 minutes; Testosterone cypionate: ~8 days

Time to Peak IM (undecanoate): 7 days (median; range: 4 to 42 days); Intranasal: ~40 minutes; Transdermal system: 8 hours (range: 4 to 12 hours); Buccal system: 10 to 12 hours; Oral capsule: Jatenzo: ~2 to 4 hours; 40 mg capsule [Canadian product]: 4 to 5 hours; SubQ (enanthate): 11.9 hours (median; range: 5.8 to 168.7 hours) following weekly administration for 12 weeks

Reproductive Considerations

Use is contraindicated in persons who may become pregnant.

Large doses of testosterone may suppress spermatogenesis; the impact on fertility may be irreversible. Treatment of hypogonadotropic hypogonadism is not recommended for men desiring fertility (Endocrine Society [Bhasin 2018]).

Pregnancy Considerations Use is contraindicated during pregnancy.

Exposure to a fetus may cause virilization of varying degrees. Because of the potential for secondary exposure, all children and women should avoid skin-to-skin contact to areas where testosterone has been applied topically on another person.

Some products contain benzyl alcohol, which can cross the placenta.

Controlled Substance C-III

◆ **Testosterone Cypionate** *see* Testosterone *on page 1425*

◆ **Testosterone Enanthate** *see* Testosterone *on page 1425*

◆ **Testosterone Undecanoate** *see* Testosterone *on page 1425*

◆ **Testred [DSC]** *see* MethylTESTOSTERone *on page 1006*

◆ **Tetanus** *see* Meningococcal Polysaccharide (Groups C and Y) and *Haemophilus* b Tetanus Toxoid Conjugate Vaccine *on page 965*

Tetanus Immune Globulin (Human)

(TET a nus i MYUN GLOB yoo lin HYU man)

Brand Names: US HyperTET S/D

Brand Names: Canada HyperTET S/D

Pharmacologic Category Blood Product Derivative; Immune Globulin

Use

Tetanus, prophylaxis: Prophylaxis against tetanus following injury in patients whose immunization is incomplete or uncertain

Tetanus, treatment: Treatment of active tetanus

The Advisory Committee on Immunization Practices (ACIP) recommends passive immunization with TIG for the following:

- Persons with a wound that is not clean or minor and who have received ≤2 or an unknown number of adsorbed tetanus toxoid doses (CDC 55[RR3] 2006; CDC 55[RR17] 2006).
- Persons who are wounded in bombings or similar mass casualty events if no reliable history of completed primary vaccination with tetanus exists. In case of shortage, use should be reserved for persons ≥60 years of age and immigrants from regions other than Europe or North America (CDC 57 [RR6] 2008).

Local Anesthetic/Vasoconstrictor Precautions No information available to require special precautions

Effects on Dental Treatment No significant effects or complications reported

Effects on Bleeding No information available to require special precautions

Adverse Reactions Frequency not defined.

Central nervous system: Increased body temperature

Local: Local soreness/soreness at injection site, pain at injection site, tenderness at injection site

<1%, postmarketing, and/or case reports: Anaphylactic shock, angioedema, nephrotic syndrome

Mechanism of Action Provides passive immunity towards tetanus by supplying antibodies to neutralize the free form of toxins produced by *Clostridium tetani*.

Pharmacodynamics/Kinetics

Half-life Elimination Individuals with normal IgG concentration: ~23 days

Time to Peak Plasma: IgG concentration: IM: ~2 days

Pregnancy Risk Factor C

Pregnancy Considerations Animal reproduction studies have not been conducted. Tetanus immune globulin and a tetanus toxoid containing vaccine are recommended by the ACIP as part of the standard wound management to prevent tetanus in pregnant women (CDC 57[RR6], 2008; CDC 62[7], 2013).

Tetracaine (Systemic) (TET ra kane)

Brand Names: Canada Pontocaine [DSC]

Generic Availability (US) Yes

Pharmacologic Category Local Anesthetic

Dental Use Ester-type local anesthetic

Use Spinal anesthesia: For the production of spinal anesthesia for procedures requiring 2 to 3 hours

Local Anesthetic/Vasoconstrictor Precautions No information available to require special precautions

Effects on Dental Treatment No significant effects or complications reported

Effects on Bleeding No information available to require special precautions

Adverse Reactions Frequency not defined. Adverse effects listed are those characteristics of local anesthetics. Systemic adverse effects are generally associated with excessive doses or rapid absorption.

Cardiovascular: Hypotension

Central nervous system: Chills, dizziness, drowsiness, loss of consciousness, nervousness, seizure

Dermatologic: Urticaria

Gastrointestinal: Nausea, vomiting

Hematologic & oncologic: Methemoglobinemia

Hypersensitivity: Anaphylaxis, hypersensitivity reaction

Neuromuscular & skeletal: Tremor

Ophthalmic: Blurred vision, miosis

Otic: Tinnitus

Dosing

Adult & Geriatric Spinal anesthesia: Injection: **Note:** Dosage varies with the anesthetic procedure, the degree of anesthesia required, and the individual patient response; it is administered by subarachnoid injection for spinal anesthesia.

Perineal anesthesia: 5 mg

Perineal and lower extremities: 10 mg

Anesthesia extending up to costal margin: 15 mg; doses up to 20 mg may be given, but are reserved for exceptional cases

Low spinal anesthesia (saddle block): 2-5 mg

Renal Impairment: Adult No dosage adjustment provided in manufacturer's labeling.

Hepatic Impairment: Adult No dosage adjustment provided in manufacturer's labeling.

Pediatric Note: Dosage varies with the anesthetic procedure, the degree of anesthesia required, and the individual patient response; it is administered by subarachnoid injection for spinal anesthesia.

Spinal anesthesia: Limited data available (Coté 2013; Miller 2009): **Note:** The dose required to produce spinal anesthesia decreases with increasing age; doses presented are a reference point; isobaric or hyperbaric 1% solution has been used (Coté 2013; Miller 2009); Infants, Children, and Adolescents: Subarachnoid injection:

Patient weight:

5 to 15 kg: 0.3 to 0.4 mg/kg

>15 kg: 0.2 to 0.3 mg/kg

Maximum dose: Should not exceed usual procedure-specific adult doses:

Perineal anesthesia: 5 mg

Perineal and lower extremities: 10 mg

Anesthesia extending up to the costal margin: 15 mg; doses up to 20 mg may be given, but are reserved for exceptional cases

Low spinal anesthesia (saddle block): 2 to 5 mg

Renal Impairment: Pediatric There are no dosage adjustments provided in the manufacturer's labeling.

Hepatic Impairment: Pediatric There are no dosage adjustments provided in the manufacturer's labeling.

Mechanism of Action Ester local anesthetic blocks both the initiation and conduction of nerve impulses by decreasing the neuronal membrane's permeability to sodium ions, which results in inhibition of depolarization with resultant blockade of conduction

Contraindications Hypersensitivity to tetracaine, ester-type anesthetics, aminobenzoic acid, or any component of the formulation; injection should not be used when spinal anesthesia is contraindicated

Warnings/Precautions Methemoglobinemia has been reported with local anesthetics; clinically significant methemoglobinemia requires immediate treatment along with discontinuation of the anesthetic and other oxidizing agents. Onset may be immediate or delayed (hours) after anesthetic exposure. Patients with G6PD deficiency, congenital or idiopathic methemoglobinemia, cardiac or pulmonary compromise, exposure to oxidizing agents or their metabolites, or infants <6 months of age are more susceptible and should be closely monitored for signs and symptoms of methemoglobinemia (eg, cyanosis, headache, rapid pulse, shortness of breath, lightheadedness, fatigue). Use with caution in patients with cardiac disease (especially rhythm disturbances, heart block, or shock), hyperthyroidism, and abnormal or decreased levels of plasma esterases. Use of the lowest effective dose is recommended. Acutely ill, elderly, debilitated, obstetric patients, or patients with increased intra-abdominal pressure may require decreased doses. Dental practitioners and/or clinicians using local anesthetic agents should be well-trained in diagnosis and management of emergencies that may arise from the use of these agents. Resuscitative equipment, oxygen, and other resuscitative drugs should be available for immediate use.

Drug Interactions

Metabolism/Transport Effects None known.

Avoid Concomitant Use

Avoid concomitant use of Tetracaine (Systemic) with any of the following: Bupivacaine (Liposomal)

Increased Effect/Toxicity

Tetracaine (Systemic) may increase the levels/effects of: Bupivacaine (Liposomal); Neuromuscular-Blocking Agents

The levels/effects of Tetracaine (Systemic) may be increased by: Hyaluronidase; Methemoglobinemia Associated Agents

Decreased Effect

Tetracaine (Systemic) may decrease the levels/effects of: Technetium Tc 99m Tilmanocept

Pharmacodynamics/Kinetics

Duration of Action 1.5 to 3 hours

Pregnancy Risk Factor C

Pregnancy Considerations Animal reproduction studies have not been conducted.

Breastfeeding Considerations It is not known if tetracaine (systemic) is excreted in breast milk. The manufacturer recommends that caution be exercised when administering tetracaine (systemic) to nursing women.

Dosage Forms: US

Solution, Injection [preservative free]:

Generic: 1% (2 mL)

Tetracaine (Topical) (TET ra kane)

Related Information

Oral Pain *on page 1734*

Ulcerative, Erosive, and Painful Oral Mucosal Disorders *on page 1758*

Brand Names: Canada Ametop

Pharmacologic Category Local Anesthetic

Dental Use Ester-type local anesthetic; applied to throat for various diagnostic procedures and on cold sores and fever blisters for pain

Use Topical anesthetic: To produce anesthesia of the skin prior to venipuncture or venous cannulation, including intravenous injections of medications.

Local Anesthetic/Vasoconstrictor Precautions No information available to require special precautions

Effects on Dental Treatment No significant effects or complications reported

Effects on Bleeding No information available to require special precautions

Adverse Reactions <1%, postmarketing, and/or case reports: Application site edema (severe), application site erythema (severe), application site pruritus (severe), skin blister (application site)

Dental Usual Dosage Topical mucous membranes (rhinolaryngology): Adults: Used as a 0.25% or 0.5% solution by direct application or nebulization; total dose should not exceed 20 mg

Dosing

Adult & Geriatric

Anesthesia, local: Topical: Apply up to ~1 g (1 tube) per venipuncture or venous cannulation site; maximum of 5 sites may be anesthetized per course of treatment not to exceed a cumulative dose of ~7 g (7 tubes) in 24 hours.

Renal Impairment: Adult There are no dosage adjustments provided in the manufacturer's labeling.

Hepatic Impairment: Adult There are no dosage adjustments provided in the manufacturer's labeling.

Pediatric

Anesthesia, local: Infants ≥1 month of age, Children, and Adolescents: Topical: Apply up to ~1 g (1 tube) per venipuncture or venous cannulation site not to exceed a cumulative dose of ~2 g (2 tubes) in 24 hours.

Renal Impairment: Pediatric There are no dosage adjustments provided in the manufacturer's labeling.

Hepatic Impairment: Pediatric There are no dosage adjustments provided in the manufacturer's labeling.

Mechanism of Action Ester local anesthetic blocks both the initiation and conduction of nerve impulses by decreasing the neuronal membrane's permeability to sodium ions, which results in inhibition of depolarization with resultant blockade of conduction

Contraindications Hypersensitivity to tetracaine, other ester-type anesthetic agents, or any component of the formulation; use in premature infants and full-term infants <1 month of age; application to broken skin, mucous membranes, eyes, or ears

Warnings/Precautions Use with caution; may lower seizure threshold. Should not be used to provide anesthesia prior to immunization. Methemoglobinemia has been reported with local anesthetics; clinically significant methemoglobinemia requires immediate treatment along with discontinuation of the anesthetic and other oxidizing agents. Onset may be immediate or delayed (hours) after anesthetic exposure. Patients with glucose-6-phosphate dehydrogenase deficiency, congenital or idiopathic methemoglobinemia, cardiac or pulmonary compromise, exposure to oxidizing agents or their metabolites, or infants <6 months of age are more susceptible and should be closely monitored for signs and symptoms of methemoglobinemia (eg, cyanosis, headache, rapid pulse, shortness of breath, lightheadedness, fatigue).

Drug Interactions

Metabolism/Transport Effects None known.

Avoid Concomitant Use There are no known interactions where it is recommended to avoid concomitant use.

Increased Effect/Toxicity

Tetracaine (Topical) may increase the levels/effects of: Local Anesthetics; Prilocaine; Sodium Nitrite

The levels/effects of Tetracaine (Topical) may be increased by: Dapsone (Topical); Methemoglobinemia Associated Agents; Nitric Oxide

Decreased Effect There are no known significant interactions involving a decrease in effect.

Pregnancy Considerations Animal reproduction studies have not been conducted.

Breastfeeding Considerations It is not known if tetracaine is present in breast milk. Breastfeeding is not recommended by the manufacturer.

Product Availability Not available in the US

Dosage Forms: Canada

Gel, External:

Ametop: 4% (1.5 g) [delivers ~1 g]

- **Tetracaine and Lidocaine** *see* Lidocaine and Tetracaine *on page 914*
- **Tetracaine and Lignocaine** *see* Lidocaine and Tetracaine *on page 914*

Tetracaine and Oxymetazoline

(TET ra kane & oks i met AZ oh leen)

Pharmacologic Category Adrenergic Agonist Agent; Imidazoline Derivative; Local Anesthetic

Use Anesthesia, dental: Regional anesthesia when performing a restorative procedure on teeth 4-13 and A-J in adults and children who weigh 40 kg or more.

Local Anesthetic/Vasoconstrictor Precautions No information available to require special precautions

Effects on Dental Treatment Key adverse event(s) related to dental treatment: Nasal congestion, nasal discomfort, oropharyngeal pain, oral discomfort, and rhinorrhea have been observed; the oxymetazoline component is a sympathomimetic and hypertension may occur. Monitor patients for increased blood pressure. Not recommended in patients with uncontrolled hypertension. Tetracaine component may cause methemoglobinemia; use is not recommended in patients with a history of congenital or idiopathic methemoglobinemia. See Warnings/Precautions "Concerns related to adverse effects".

Effects on Bleeding No information available to require special precautions

Adverse Reactions Also see individual agents.

>10%:

Ophthalmic: Increased lacrimation (13%)

Respiratory: Rhinorrhea (52%), nasal congestion (32%), nasal discomfort (26%), oropharyngeal pain (14%)

1% to 10%:

Cardiovascular: Increased systolic blood pressure (5%), bradycardia (3%), hypertension (3%), increased diastolic blood pressure (3%)

Central nervous system: Headache (10%), hypoesthesia (intranasal: 10%; pharyngeal: 10%), nasal cavity pain (6%), dizziness (3%), abnormal sensory symptoms (2%)

Gastrointestinal: Dysgeusia (8%), oral discomfort (2%), dysphagia (1%)

Respiratory: Throat irritation (9%), sneezing (4%), nasal mucosa ulcer (3%), sinus headache (3%), dry nose (2%), epistaxis (2%)

Dosing

Adult & Geriatric Anesthesia, dental: Intranasal: 2 sprays administered 4 to 5 minutes apart in the nostril ipsilateral (same side) to the maxillary tooth on which the dental procedure will be performed. Initiate the dental procedure 10 minutes after the second spray. May administer 1 additional spray 10 minutes after the second initial spray if inadequate anesthesia.

Renal Impairment: Adult There are no dosage adjustments provided in the manufacturer's labeling (has not been studied).

Hepatic Impairment: Adult There are no dosage adjustments provided in the manufacturer's labeling (has not been studied); use with caution in patients with severe impairment.

Pediatric

Anesthesia, dental: Children and Adolescents ≥3 years and ≥40 kg: Intranasal: 2 sprays administered 4 to 5 minutes apart in the nostril ipsilateral (same side) to the maxillary tooth on which the dental procedure will be performed. Initiate the dental procedure 10 minutes after the second spray.

Renal Impairment: Pediatric There are no dosage adjustments provided in the manufacturer's labeling (has not been studied).

Hepatic Impairment: Pediatric There are no dosage adjustments provided in the manufacturer's labeling (has not been studied); use with caution in patients with severe impairment.

Mechanism of Action

Tetracaine: Local ester anesthetic that blocks both the initiation and conduction of nerve impulses by decreasing the neuronal membrane's permeability to sodium ions, which results in inhibition of depolarization with resultant blockade of conduction.

Oxymetazoline: Imidazoline derivative with sympathomimetic activity that stimulates alpha-adrenergic receptors in the arterioles of the nasal mucosa to produce vasoconstriction.

Contraindications Hypersensitivity to or intolerance of tetracaine, benzyl alcohol, other ester local anesthetics, *p*-aminobenzoic acid (PABA), oxymetazoline, or any component of the formulation.

Warnings/Precautions Methemoglobinemia has been reported with local anesthetics; clinically significant methemoglobinemia requires immediate treatment along with discontinuation of the anesthetic and other oxidizing agents. Onset may be immediate or delayed (hours) after anesthetic exposure. Patients with glucose-6-phosphate dehydrogenase deficiency, congenital or idiopathic methemoglobinemia, cardiac or pulmonary compromise, exposure to oxidizing agents or their metabolites, or infants <6 months of age are more susceptible and should be closely monitored for signs and symptoms of methemoglobinemia (eg, cyanosis, headache, rapid pulse, shortness of breath, lightheadedness, fatigue). Allergic or anaphylactoid reactions, including urticaria, angioedema, bronchospasm, and shock may occur. Dysphagia, epistaxis, and hypertension have been reported. Avoid use in patients with a history of frequent nose bleeds (≥5 per month). Use is not recommended in patients with uncontrolled hypertension. Patients with severe hepatic impairment or pseudocholinesterase deficiency may be at a greater risk of developing toxic plasma concentrations of tetracaine; monitor these patients for signs of local anesthetic toxicity. Use is not recommended in patients with inadequately controlled active thyroid disease.

Potentially significant drug-drug interactions may exist, requiring dose or frequency adjustment, additional monitoring, and/or selection of alternative therapy. Avoid use with other intranasal products, including other oxymetazoline-containing nasal sprays. Discontinue oxymetazoline-containing products 24 hours prior to administration of tetracaine/oxymetazoline.

Some dosage forms may contain benzyl alcohol; large amounts of benzyl alcohol (≥99 mg/kg/day) have been associated with a potentially fatal toxicity ("gasping syndrome") in neonates; the "gasping syndrome" consists of metabolic acidosis, respiratory distress, gasping respirations, CNS dysfunction (including convulsions, intracranial hemorrhage), hypotension and cardiovascular collapse (AAP 1997; CDC 1982); some data suggests that benzoate displaces bilirubin from protein binding sites (Ahlfors 2001); avoid or use dosage forms containing benzyl alcohol with caution in neonates. See manufacturer's labeling.

Drug Interactions

Metabolism/Transport Effects None known.

Avoid Concomitant Use

Avoid concomitant use of Tetracaine and Oxymetazoline with any of the following: Ergot Derivatives; Iobenguane Radiopharmaceutical Products; Monoamine Oxidase Inhibitors

Increased Effect/Toxicity

Tetracaine and Oxymetazoline may increase the levels/effects of: Doxofylline; Local Anesthetics; Prilocaine; Sodium Nitrite; Solriamfetol; Sympathomimetics

The levels/effects of Tetracaine and Oxymetazoline may be increased by: AtoMOXetine; Cannabinoid-Containing Products; Cocaine (Topical); Dapsone (Topical); Ergot Derivatives; Guanethidine; Linezolid; Methemoglobinemia Associated Agents; Monoamine Oxidase Inhibitors; Nitric Oxide; Ozanimod; Procarbazine; Tedizolid; Tricyclic Antidepressants

Decreased Effect

Tetracaine and Oxymetazoline may decrease the levels/effects of: Esketamine; FentaNYL; Iobenguane Radiopharmaceutical Products

The levels/effects of Tetracaine and Oxymetazoline may be decreased by: Alpha1-Blockers; Tricyclic Antidepressants

Pharmacodynamics/Kinetics

Half-life Elimination

Pediatric patients 4 to 15 years of age: Oxymetazoline: ~1.6 to 4.3 hours; Tetracaine metabolite *p*-butylaminobenzoic acid (PBBA): ~1.6 to 2.8 hours.

Adults: Oxymetazoline: ~5.2 hours; Tetracaine metabolite (PBBA): ~2.6 hours.

Time to Peak Median:

Pediatric patients 4 to 15 years of age: Oxymetazoline: ~10 to 30 minutes; Tetracaine metabolite (PBBA): ~20 to 30 minutes.

Adults: Oxymetazoline: 5 minutes; Tetracaine metabolite (PBBA): 20 minutes.

Pregnancy Considerations Adverse events have been observed in some animal reproduction studies using this combination subcutaneously. See individual monographs.

Breastfeeding Considerations It is not known if tetracaine or oxymetazoline are excreted in breast milk following nasal administration. According to the manufacturer, the decision to continue or discontinue breastfeeding during therapy should take into account the risk of infant exposure, the benefits of breastfeeding to the infant, and benefits of treatment to the mother.

Product Availability Kovanaze: FDA approved July 2016; anticipated availability is currently undetermined.

◆ **Tetracaine HCl** *see* Tetracaine (Systemic) *on page 1427*

◆ **Tetracaine HCl** *see* Tetracaine (Topical) *on page 1428*

◆ **Tetracaine Hydrochloride** *see* Tetracaine (Systemic) *on page 1427*

◆ **Tetracaine Hydrochloride** *see* Tetracaine (Topical) *on page 1428*

◆ **Tetracaine Hydrochloride and Oxymetazoline Hydrochloride** *see* Tetracaine and Oxymetazoline *on page 1429*

Tetracycline (Systemic) (tet ra SYE kleen)

Related Information

Bacterial Infections *on page 1739*
Gastrointestinal Disorders *on page 1678*
Periodontal Diseases *on page 1748*
Ulcerative, Erosive, and Painful Oral Mucosal Disorders *on page 1758*

Generic Availability (US) Yes

Pharmacologic Category Antibiotic, Tetracycline Derivative

Dental Use Treatment of periodontitis associated with presence of *Actinobacillus actinomycetemcomitans* (AA); as adjunctive therapy in recurrent aphthous ulcers

Use

Acute intestinal amebiasis: Adjunctive therapy in acute intestinal amebiasis caused by *Entamoeba histolytica.*

Acne: Adjunctive therapy for the treatment of severe acne.

Actinomycosis: Treatment of actinomycosis caused by *Actinomyces* species when penicillin is contraindicated.

Anthrax: Treatment of anthrax due to *Bacillus anthracis* when penicillin is contraindicated.

Campylobacter: Treatment of infections caused by *Campylobacter fetus.*

Cholera: Treatment of cholera caused by *Vibrio cholerae.*

Clostridium: Treatment of infections caused by *Clostridium* spp. when penicillin is contraindicated.

Gram-negative infections: Treatment of infections caused by *Escherichia coli, Enterobacter aerogenes, Shigella* spp., *Acinetobacter* spp., *Klebsiella* spp., and *Bacteroides* spp.

Listeriosis: Treatment of listeriosis due to *Listeria monocytogenes* when penicillin is contraindicated.

Ophthalmic infections: Treatment of inclusion conjunctivitis or trachoma caused by *Chlamydia trachomatis.*

Relapsing fever: Treatment of relapsing fever due to *Borrelia* spp.

Respiratory tract infection: Treatment of respiratory tract infections caused by *Haemophilus influenzae* (upper respiratory tract only), *Klebsiella* spp. (lower respiratory tract only), *Mycoplasma pneumoniae* (lower respiratory tract only), *Streptococcus pneumoniae*, or *Streptococcus pyogenes.*

Rickettsial infections: Treatment of Rocky Mountain spotted fever, typhus group infections, Q fever, and rickettsialpox caused by *Rickettsiae.*

Sexually transmitted diseases: Treatment of lymphogranuloma venereum or uncomplicated urethral, endocervical, or rectal infections caused by *C. trachomatis*; chancroid caused by *Haemophilus ducreyi*; granuloma inguinale (donovanosis) caused by *Klebsiella granulomatis*; syphilis caused by *Treponema pallidum*, when penicillin is contraindicated.

Limitations of use: Tetracycline is **not** a recommended alternative for uncomplicated gonorrhea according to the Centers for Disease Control and Prevention (CDC) sexually transmitted diseases guidelines (CDC [Workowski 2015]).

Skin and skin structure infections: Treatment of skin and skin structure infections caused by *Staphylococcus aureus* or *S. pyogenes.*

Urinary tract infections: Treatment of urinary tract infections caused by susceptible gram-negative organisms (eg, *E. coli, Klebsiella* spp.).

Vincent infection: Treatment of Vincent infection caused by *Fusobacterium fusiforme* when penicillin is contraindicated.

Yaws: Treatment of yaws caused by *Treponema pertenue* when penicillin is contraindicated.

Zoonotic infections: Treatment of psittacosis (ornithosis) due to *Chlamydophila psittaci*; plague due to *Yersinia pestis*; tularemia due to *Francisella tularensis*; brucellosis due to *Brucella* spp. (in conjunction with an aminoglycoside); bartonellosis due to *Bartonella bacilliformis.*

Local Anesthetic/Vasoconstrictor Precautions No information available to require special precautions

Effects on Dental Treatment Key adverse event(s) related to dental treatment: Esophagitis, superinfections, and candidal superinfection. Opportunistic "superinfection" with *Candida albicans*; tetracyclines are not recommended for use during pregnancy or in children ≤8 years of age since they have been reported to cause enamel hypoplasia and permanent teeth discoloration. The use of tetracyclines should only be used in these patients if other agents are contraindicated or alternative antimicrobials will not eradicate the organism. Long-term use associated with oral candidiasis.

Effects on Bleeding No information available to require special precautions

Adverse Reactions

Frequency not defined:

Cardiovascular: Pericarditis

Central nervous system: Bulging fontanel, idiopathic intracranial hypertension

Dermatologic: Erythematous rash, maculopapular rash, skin photosensitivity, urticaria

Endocrine & metabolic: Growth retardation (fibula)

Gastrointestinal: Anorexia, diarrhea, dysphagia, enterocolitis, epigastric distress, glossitis, melanoglossia, nausea, vomiting

Genitourinary: Inflammatory anogenital lesion (with monilial overgrowth)

Hematologic & oncologic: Henoch-Schonlein purpura

Hepatic: Hepatic failure, hepatotoxicity

Hypersensitivity: Anaphylaxis, angioedema, hypersensitivity reaction

Immunologic: Serum sickness-like reaction

Neuromuscular & skeletal: Exacerbation of systemic lupus erythematosus

Postmarketing: Discoloration of permanent tooth, dysgeusia (Syed 2016), enamel hypoplasia (infants, young children), eosinophilia, esophageal ulcer, esophagitis, exfoliative dermatitis, hemolytic anemia, immune thrombocytopenia, increased blood urea nitrogen, lupus-like syndrome (Lee 2013), microscopic thyroid discoloration, nail discoloration, neutropenia, onycholysis, staining of tooth (infants, young children), thrombocytopenia

Dental Usual Dosage Periodontitis: Adults: Oral: 250 mg every 6 hours until improvement (usually 10 days)

Dosing

Adult & Geriatric

Usual dosage range: Oral: 250 to 500 mg every 6 to 12 hours.

Acne: Oral: Initial dose: 1 g daily in divided doses; reduce gradually to 125 to 500 mg/day once improvement is noted (alternate day or intermittent therapy may be adequate in some patients). **Note:** The shortest possible duration should be used to minimize development of bacterial resistance; reevaluate at 3 to 4 months (AAD [Zaenglein 2016]).

***Helicobacter pylori* eradication (off-label use): Oral:**
American College of Gastroenterology guidelines (Chey 2007; Chey 2017):
Bismuth quadruple regimen : 500 mg 4 times daily, in combination with standard-dose proton pump inhibitor twice daily, metronidazole 250 mg 4 times daily or 500 mg 3 or 4 times daily, and either bismuth subcitrate 120 to 300 mg 4 times daily or bismuth subsalicylate 300 mg 4 times daily; continue regimen for 10 to 14 days.

Malaria, treatment, uncomplicated (alternative agent) (off-label use): Oral: 250 mg 4 times daily for 7 days with quinine sulfate (quinine sulfate duration is region specific). **Note:** If used for *Plasmodium vivax* or *Plasmodium ovale*, use in combination with primaquine (CDC 2020).

Periodontitis (off-label use): Oral: 250 mg every 6 hours until improvement (usually 10 days).

Syphilis, penicillin-allergic patients: Note: Data to support the use of alternatives to penicillin are limited in primary and secondary syphilis and are not well documented in the treatment of latent syphilis (CDC [Workowski 2015]).
Early syphilis (primary or secondary infection): 500 mg 4 times daily for 14 days.
Latent syphilis (late or of unknown duration): 500 mg 4 times daily for 28 days.

Tularemia (mild to moderate): Oral: 500 mg 4 times daily for at least 14 days (IDSA [Stevens 2014]).

***Vibrio cholerae:* Oral:** 500 mg 4 times daily for 3 days (Seas 1996).

Renal Impairment: Adult
Manufacturer's labeling: There are no specific dosage adjustments provided in the manufacturer's labeling; decrease dose and/or extend dosing interval.
Alternative dosing (Aronoff 2007): **Note:** Renally adjusted dose recommendations are based on doses of 250 mg to 500 mg twice daily to 4 times daily.
GFR >50 mL/minute: Administer recommended dose based on indication every 8 to 12 hours.
GFR 10 to 50 mL/minute: Administer recommended dose based on indication every 12 to 24 hours.
GFR <10 mL/minute: Administer recommended dose based on indication every 24 hours.

Hepatic Impairment: Adult There are no dosage adjustments provided in the manufacturer's labeling.

Pediatric

General dosing, susceptible infection: Children ≥8 years and Adolescents: Oral: 25 to 50 mg/kg/**day** in divided doses every 6 hours

Acne: Children ≥8 years and Adolescents: Oral: 500 mg/dose twice daily (Eichenfield 2013)

Malaria, treatment: Note: Use in combination with other antimalarial agents:
Uncomplicated infection (P. falciparum, P. vivax or unknown species), chloroquine-resistant or unknown resistance: Children ≥8 years and Adolescents:
Non-HIV-exposed/-positive: Oral: 6.25 mg/kg/dose every 6 hours for 7 days; maximum dose: 250 mg/dose (CDC 2013)
HIV-exposed/-positive: Oral: 6 to 12.5 mg/kg/dose every 6 hours for 7 days; maximum dose: 500 mg/dose (HHS [OI pediatric 2013])
Severe infection: **Note:** Use in combination with other antimalarial agents; Children ≥8 years and Adolescents:
Non-HIV-exposed/-positive: Oral: 6.25 mg/kg/dose every 6 hours for 7 days; maximum dose: 250 mg/dose (CDC 2013)
HIV-exposed/-positive: Oral: 6 to 12.5 mg/kg/dose every 6 hours for 7 days; maximum dose: 500 mg/dose (HHS [OI pediatric 2013])

Syphilis, penicillin-allergic patients: Note: Data to support the use of alternatives to penicillin are limited in primary and secondary syphilis and are not well documented in the treatment of latent syphilis (CDC [Workowski 2015]): Adolescents: Oral:
Early syphilis (primary or secondary infection): 500 mg/dose 4 times daily for 14 days
Latent syphilis (late or of unknown duration): 500 mg/dose 4 times daily for 28 days

Renal Impairment: Pediatric Children ≥8 years and Adolescents: Decrease dose and/or extend dosing interval.

Hepatic Impairment: Pediatric There are no dosage adjustments provided in the manufacturer's labeling.

Mechanism of Action Inhibits bacterial protein synthesis by binding with the 30S and possibly the 50S ribosomal subunit(s) of susceptible bacteria; may also cause alterations in the cytoplasmic membrane

Contraindications
Hypersensitivity to any of the tetracyclines or any component of the formulation.
Canadian labeling: Additional contraindications (not in US labeling): Severe liver disease; severe renal disease; use in children <12 years of age for therapy of common infections or conditions where bactericidal effect is essential (bacterial endocarditis); surgical prophylaxis; pregnancy; breastfeeding.

Warnings/Precautions Use with caution in patients with renal or hepatic impairment; dosage modification required in patients with renal impairment. May be associated with increases in serum urea nitrogen (BUN) secondary to antianabolic effects. Hepatotoxicity has been reported rarely; risk may be increased in patients with preexisting hepatic or renal impairment. Intracranial hypertension (headache, blurred vision, diplopia, vision loss, and/or papilledema) has been associated with use. Women of childbearing age who are overweight or have a history of intracranial hypertension are at greater risk. Concomitant use of isotretinoin (known to cause pseudotumor cerebri) and tetracycline should be avoided. Intracranial hypertension typically resolves after discontinuation of treatment; however, permanent visual loss is possible. If visual symptoms develop during treatment, prompt ophthalmologic evaluation is warranted. Intracranial pressure can remain elevated for weeks after drug discontinuation; monitor patients until they stabilize. May cause photosensitivity; discontinue if skin erythema occurs. Use skin protection and avoid prolonged exposure to sunlight; do not use tanning equipment. Prolonged use may result in fungal or bacterial superinfection, including *Clostridioides* (formerly *Clostridium*) *difficile*-associated diarrhea (CDAD) and pseudomembranous colitis; CDAD has been observed >2 months postantibiotic treatment. May cause tissue hyperpigmentation, enamel hypoplasia, or permanent tooth discoloration; use of tetracyclines should be avoided during tooth development (children <8 years of age) unless other drugs are not likely to be effective or are contraindicated.

Appropriate use: Acne: The American Academy of Dermatology acne guidelines recommend tetracycline as adjunctive treatment for moderate and severe acne and forms of inflammatory acne that are resistant to topical treatments. Concomitant topical therapy with benzoyl peroxide or a retinoid should be administered with systemic antibiotic therapy (eg, tetracycline) and continued for maintenance after antibiotic course is completed (AAD [Zaenglein 2016])

Warnings: Additional Pediatric Considerations Do not administer to children <8 years of age (except for treatment of Anthrax when there is a contraindication to penicillin) due to permanent discoloration of teeth and retardation of skeletal development and bone growth; more common with long-term use, but may be observed with repeated, short courses). Tetracyclines have been associated with increases in BUN secondary to antianabolic effects. Pseudotumor cerebri has been reported rarely in infants and adolescents; use with isotretinoin has been associated with cases of pseudotumor cerebri; avoid concomitant treatment with isotretinoin.

Drug Interactions

Metabolism/Transport Effects **Substrate** of CYP3A4 (major); **Note:** Assignment of Major/Minor substrate status based on clinically relevant drug interaction potential

Avoid Concomitant Use

Avoid concomitant use of Tetracycline (Systemic) with any of the following: Aminolevulinic Acid (Systemic); BCG (Intravesical); Cholera Vaccine; Mecamylamine; Methoxyflurane; Retinoic Acid Derivatives; Strontium Ranelate

Increased Effect/Toxicity

Tetracycline (Systemic) may increase the levels/effects of: Aminolevulinic Acid (Systemic); Aminolevulinic Acid (Topical); Lithium; Mecamylamine; Methoxyflurane; Mipomersen; Neuromuscular-Blocking Agents; Porfimer; QuiNINE; Retinoic Acid Derivatives; Verteporfin; Vitamin K Antagonists

Decreased Effect

Tetracycline (Systemic) may decrease the levels/effects of: Atovaquone; BCG (Intravesical); BCG Vaccine (Immunization); Cholera Vaccine; Iron Preparations; Lactobacillus and Estriol; Penicillins; Sodium Picosulfate; Typhoid Vaccine

The levels/effects of Tetracycline (Systemic) may be decreased by: Antacids; Bile Acid Sequestrants; Bismuth Subcitrate; Bismuth Subsalicylate; Calcium Salts; CYP3A4 Inducers (Moderate); CYP3A4 Inducers (Strong); Dabrafenib; Deferasirox; Enzalutamide; Erdafitinib; Iron Preparations; Ivosidenib; Lanthanum; Magnesium Salts; Mitotane; Multivitamins/Minerals (with ADEK, Folate, Iron); Multivitamins/Minerals (with AE, No Iron); Quinapril; Sarilumab; Siltuximab; Strontium Ranelate; Sucralfate; Sucroferric Oxyhydroxide; Tocilizumab; Zinc Salts

Food Interactions Serum concentrations may be decreased if taken with dairy products. Management: Take on an empty stomach 1 hour before or 2 hours after meals to increase total absorption. Administer around-the-clock to promote less variation in peak and trough serum levels.

Dietary Considerations Take on an empty stomach (ie, 1 hour prior to, or 2 hours after meals). Take at least 1-2 hours prior to, or 4 hours after antacid.

Pharmacodynamics/Kinetics

Half-life Elimination 6 to 11 hours (Agwuh 2006)

Time to Peak Serum: Oral: 2 to 4 hours (Agwuh 2006)

Pregnancy Risk Factor D

Pregnancy Considerations

Tetracycline crosses the placenta (Leblanc 1967). Tetracyclines accumulate in developing teeth and long tubular bones (Mylonas 2011). Permanent discoloration of teeth (yellow, gray, brown) can occur following in utero exposure and is more likely to occur following long-term or repeated exposure. The pharmacokinetics of tetracycline are not altered in pregnant patients with normal renal function (Whalley 1966; Whalley 1970). Hepatic toxicity during pregnancy, potentially associated with tetracycline use, has been reported. Pregnant women with renal disease may be more likely to develop hepatic failure with tetracycline use.

As a class, tetracyclines are generally considered second-line antibiotics in pregnant women and their use should be avoided (Mylonas 2011). Many guidelines consider use of tetracycline to be contraindicated during pregnancy, or to be a relative contraindication in pregnant women if other agents are available and appropriate for use (CDC 2020; CDC [Anderson 2013]; CDC [Workowski 2015]; HHS [OI adult 2020]; IDSA [Stevens 2014]). When systemic antibiotics are needed for acne or dermatologic conditions in pregnant women, other agents are preferred (AAD [Zaenglein 2016]; Murase 2014).

Breastfeeding Considerations

Tetracycline is excreted into breast milk (Knowles 1965; Matsuda 1984).

According to the manufacturer, the decision to continue or discontinue breastfeeding during therapy should consider the risk of exposure to the infant and the benefits of treatment to the mother. The calcium in the maternal milk is expected to decrease the amount of tetracycline absorbed by the breastfeeding infant (Chung 2002).

As a class, tetracyclines have generally been avoided in nursing women due to theoretical concerns that they may permanently stain the teeth of the breastfeeding infant (Chung 2002). Some sources note that breastfeeding can continue during tetracycline therapy (Chung 2002; WHO 2002) but recommend use of alternative medications when possible (WHO 2002). Breastfeeding is not recommended when tetracycline is being used for maternal treatment of acne (AAD [Zaenglein 2016]. In general, antibiotics that are present in breast milk may cause nondose-related modification of bowel flora. Monitor infants for GI disturbances (Chung 2002; WHO 2002).

Dosage Forms: US

Capsule, Oral:

Generic: 250 mg, 500 mg

Dosage Forms: Canada

Capsule, Oral:

Generic: 250 mg

Tetracycline, Bismuth Subsalicylate, and Metronidazole

(TET ra SYE kleen, BIZ muth SUB sa LIS i late, & MET roe NID a zole)

Brand Names: US Helidac Therapy

Pharmacologic Category Antibiotic, Miscellaneous; Antibiotic, Tetracycline Derivative; Antidiarrheal; Gastrointestinal Agent, Miscellaneous

Use *Helicobacter pylori* infection: Treatment of patients with *H. pylori* infection and duodenal ulcer disease (active or a history of duodenal ulcer), in combination with an H_2 antagonist. **Note:** Although combination therapy with an H_2 antagonist is recommended in the product labeling, proton pump inhibitors are preferred (ACG [Chey 2017]).

Local Anesthetic/Vasoconstrictor Precautions No information available to require special precautions.

Effects on Dental Treatment Key adverse event(s) related to dental treatment: Occurrence of darkening of tongue, metallic taste; rare occurrence of glossitis, stomatitis, xerostomia (normal salivary flow resumes upon discontinuation.

Effects on Bleeding No information available to require special precautions.

Adverse Reactions Also see individual agents.

>10%: Gastrointestinal: Nausea (12%)

1% to 10%:

Gastrointestinal: Abdominal pain (7%), anorectal pain (1%), anorexia (2%), constipation (2%), darkening of stools (1%), diarrhea (7%), duodenal ulcer (1%), dyspepsia (2%), flatulence (1%), gastrointestinal hemorrhage (1%), melena (3%), tongue discoloration (darkening: 2%), vomiting (2%)

Nervous system: Dizziness (2%), headache (2%), insomnia (1%), metallic taste (1%), pain (1%), paresthesia (1%)

Neuromuscular & skeletal: Asthenia (2%)

Respiratory: Sinusitis (1%), upper respiratory tract infection (2%)

<1%:

Cardiovascular: Acute myocardial infarction, cerebral ischemia, chest pain, hypertension, syncope

Dermatologic: Acne vulgaris, ecchymoses, pruritus, skin photosensitivity, skin rash

Gastrointestinal: Dysphagia, eructation, gastrointestinal candidiasis, glossitis, intestinal obstruction, stomatitis, xerostomia

Genitourinary: Urinary tract infection

Hematologic & oncologic: Neoplasm, rectal hemorrhage

Hepatic: Increased serum alanine aminotransferase, increased serum aspartate aminotransferase

Infection: Infection

Nervous system: Drowsiness, malaise, nervousness

Neuromuscular & skeletal: Arthritis, rheumatoid arthritis, tendonitis

Ophthalmic: Conjunctivitis

Respiratory: Flu-like symptoms, rhinitis

Mechanism of Action

Bismuth: Has both antisecretory and antimicrobial action; may provide some anti-inflammatory action as well.

Metronidazole: After diffusing into the organism, interacts with DNA to cause a loss of helical DNA structure and strand breakage, resulting in inhibition of protein synthesis and cell death in susceptible organisms.

Tetracycline: Inhibits bacterial protein synthesis by binding with the 30S and possibly the 50S ribosomal subunit(s) of susceptible bacteria; may also cause alterations in the cytoplasmic membrane.

Bismuth, metronidazole, and tetracycline individually have demonstrated in vitro activity against most susceptible strains of *H. pylori* isolated from patients with duodenal ulcers.

Pregnancy Risk Factor D

Pregnancy Considerations

Tetracyclines, metronidazole, and salicylates cross the placenta. Use of this combination during pregnancy may cause adverse maternal and fetal outcomes. The combination of tetracycline, bismuth subsalicylate, and metronidazole should not be used in pregnant women; other agents are recommended for the treatment of *H. pylori* infection in pregnancy (Nguyen 2019).

Refer to individual monographs for additional information

◆ **Tetracycline HCl** *see* Tetracycline (Systemic) *on page 1431*

◆ **Tetracycline Hydrochloride** *see* Tetracycline (Systemic) *on page 1431*

◆ **Tetracycline, Metronidazole, and Bismuth Subcitrate Potassium** *see* Bismuth Subcitrate, Metronidazole, and Tetracycline *on page 245*

◆ **Tetracycline, Metronidazole, and Bismuth Subsalicylate** *see* Tetracycline, Bismuth Subsalicylate, and Metronidazole *on page 1433*

◆ **Tetra-Formula Nighttime Sleep [OTC]** *see* DiphenhydrAMINE (Systemic) *on page 502*

◆ **Tetrahydrocannabinol** *see* Dronabinol *on page 532*

Tetrahydrocannabinol and Cannabidiol

(TET ra hye droe can NAB e nol & can nab e DYE ol)

Brand Names: Canada Sativex

Pharmacologic Category Cannabinoid; Skeletal Muscle Relaxant

Use Note: Not approved in the United States.

Multiple sclerosis: Adjunctive treatment in adults with multiple sclerosis for the symptomatic relief of spasticity that is nonresponsive to other therapy.

Local Anesthetic/Vasoconstrictor Precautions No information available to require special precautions

Effects on Dental Treatment Key adverse event(s) related to dental treatment: Xerostomia and changes in salivation (normal salivary flow resumes upon discontinuation), abnormal taste, oral pain; administered as buccal spray, associated with irritation to the buccal (oral) mucosa. Patients may experience orthostatic hypotension as they stand up after treatment; especially if lying in dental chair for extended periods of time. Use caution with sudden changes in position during and after dental treatment.

Effects on Bleeding No information available to require special precautions

Adverse Reactions Also see Cannabidiol monograph.

>10%: Nervous system: Dizziness (25%), fatigue (13%)

1% to 10%:

Cardiovascular: Palpitations (1%), tachycardia (1%)

Gastrointestinal: Anorexia (2%), constipation (2%), diarrhea (6%), dysgeusia (3%), increased appetite (1%), nausea (10%), oral mucosa changes (≤2%; including mucosal exfoliation), oral mucosa ulcer (2%), staining of tooth (2%), upper abdominal pain (1%), vomiting (4%), xerostomia (6%)

Nervous system: Amnesia (1%), balance impairment (3%), confusion (≤4%), depersonalization (2%), depression (3%), disorientation (≤4%), disturbance in attention (4%), drowsiness (8%), dysarthria (2%), euphoria (2%), falling (2%), feeling abnormal (2%), intoxicated feeling (3%), lethargy (2%), malaise (1%), memory impairment (1%), vertigo (7%)

Neuromuscular & skeletal: Asthenia (6%)

Ophthalmic: Blurred vision (2%)
<1%:
Cardiovascular: Hypertension, syncope
Gastrointestinal: Oral mucosa hyperpigmentation, stomatitis
Nervous system: Auditory hallucination, delusion, illusion, visual hallucination
Frequency not defined:
Cardiovascular: Orthostatic hypotension, variable blood pressure (transient)
Nervous system: Drug withdrawal
Miscellaneous: Drug tolerance
Postmarketing:
Gastrointestinal: Oral leukoplakia
Nervous system: Suicidal ideation

Mechanism of Action Stimulates cannabinoid receptors CB1 and CB2 in the CNS and dorsal root ganglia as well as other sites in the body. Cannabinoid receptors in the pain pathways of the brain and spinal cord mediate cannabinoid-induced analgesia. Peripheral CB2 receptors modulate immune function through cytokine release.

Pharmacodynamics/Kinetics

Half-life Elimination Biphasic:
Initial (plasma; prolonged with higher doses): CBD: ~5 to 9 hours; THC: ~2 to 5 hours.
Terminal: 24 to 36 hours (or longer) secondary to redistribution from fatty tissue.

Time to Peak 45 to 120 minutes.

Reproductive Considerations

Use is contraindicated in women of childbearing potential and men not using reliable contraception.

Cannabinoids have been associated with reproductive toxicity. Animal studies indicate possible effects on fetal development and spermatogenesis. Women of childbearing potential and males who are capable of causing pregnancy should use a reliable form of contraception for the duration of treatment and for 3 months following discontinuation.

Pregnancy Considerations Use is contraindicated during pregnancy.

Product Availability Not available in the US

Controlled Substance CDSA-II

Tetrahydrozoline (Nasal)

(tet ra hye DROZ a leen)

Brand Names: US Tyzine [DSC]

Pharmacologic Category Adrenergic Agonist Agent; Decongestant; Imidazoline Derivative

Use Symptomatic relief of nasal congestion

Local Anesthetic/Vasoconstrictor Precautions No information available to require special precautions

Effects on Dental Treatment No significant effects or complications reported

Effects on Bleeding No information available to require special precautions

Adverse Reactions
>10%: Respiratory: Sneezing, stinging sensation of the nose
1% to 10%:
Cardiovascular: Hypertension, palpitations, tachycardia
Central nervous system: Headache
Neuromuscular & skeletal: Tremor
Ophthalmic: Blurred vision

Mechanism of Action Stimulates alpha-adrenergic receptors in the arterioles of the nasal mucosa to produce vasoconstriction

Pharmacodynamics/Kinetics

Onset of Action Decongestant: 4-8 hours

Pregnancy Risk Factor C

Pregnancy Considerations Animal reproduction studies have not been conducted.

- **Tetrahydrozoline HCl** *see* Tetrahydrozoline (Nasal) *on page 1435*
- **Tetrahydrozoline Hydrochloride** *see* Tetrahydrozoline (Nasal) *on page 1435*
- **Tetraiodothyronine and Triiodothyronine** *see* Thyroid, Desiccated *on page 1442*
- **Tetryzoline** *see* Tetrahydrozoline (Nasal) *on page 1435*
- **Tevagrastim** *see* Filgrastim *on page 668*
- **Teveten** *see* Eprosartan *on page 579*
- **Texacort** *see* Hydrocortisone (Topical) *on page 775*
- **TG** *see* Thioguanine *on page 1438*
- **6-TG (error-prone abbreviation)** *see* Thioguanine *on page 1438*

Thalidomide (tha LI doe mide)

Related Information

HIV Infection and AIDS *on page 1690*
Ulcerative, Erosive, and Painful Oral Mucosal Disorders *on page 1758*

Brand Names: US Thalomid

Brand Names: Canada Thalomid

Pharmacologic Category Angiogenesis Inhibitor; Antineoplastic Agent

Use

Erythema nodosum leprosum: Acute treatment of cutaneous manifestations of moderate to severe erythema nodosum leprosum; maintenance treatment for prevention and suppression of cutaneous manifestations of erythema nodosum leprosum recurrence
Limitation of use: Thalidomide is not indicated as monotherapy for erythema nodosum leprosum treatment in the presence of moderate to severe neuritis.

Multiple myeloma: Treatment of newly diagnosed multiple myeloma (in combination with dexamethasone)

Local Anesthetic/Vasoconstrictor Precautions No information available to require special precautions

Effects on Dental Treatment Key adverse event(s) related to dental treatment: Oral *Candida* infection (HIV-seropositive patients), toothache, xerostomia (normal salivary flow resumes upon discontinuation), and aphthous stomatitis.

Effects on Bleeding No information available to require special precautions

Adverse Reactions Incidences of adverse reactions may include combination therapy.
>10%: Central nervous system: Drowsiness (≤38%), headache (≤13%), peripheral neuropathy (≥10%)
1% to 10%:
Cardiovascular: Facial edema (≤4%), peripheral edema (≤4%)
Central nervous system: Malaise (≤8%), pain (≤8%), vertigo (≤8%), dizziness (≤4%)
Dermatologic: Pruritus (≤8%), fungal dermatitis (≤4%), maculopapular rash (≤4%), nail disease (≤4%)
Gastrointestinal: Constipation (≤4%), nausea (≤4%), oral candidiasis (≤4%), toothache (≤4%)
Genitourinary: Impotence (≤8%)

Neuromuscular & skeletal: Weakness (≤8%), back pain (≤4%), neck pain (≤4%), neck stiffness (≤4%), tremor (≤4%)

Miscellaneous: Accidental injury (≤4%)

<1%, postmarketing, and/or case reports: Acute renal failure, amenorrhea, aphthous stomatitis, auditory impairment, biliary obstruction, bradycardia, carpal tunnel syndrome, cerebrovascular accident, change in prothrombin time, chronic myelocytic leukemia, cytomegalovirus disease, diplopia, ECG abnormality, erythema multiforme, erythema nodosum, erythroleukemia, febrile neutropenia, foot-drop, galactorrhea, gastric ulcer, gynecomastia, hangover effect, Hodgkin lymphoma, hypercalcemia, hypersensitivity reaction, hypomagnesemia, hyponatremia, hypothyroidism, increased serum alkaline phosphatase, interstitial pulmonary disease, intestinal perforation, lethargy, loss of consciousness, lymphedema, lymphocytopenia, mental status changes, migraine, myocardial infarction, myxedema, neutropenia, nystagmus, oliguria, orthostatic hypotension, pancytopenia, Parkinson disease, petechia, pleural effusion, pulmonary embolism, pulmonary hypertension, purpura, Raynaud phenomenon, reactivation of HBV, renal failure, seizure, sepsis, septic shock, sexual disorder, sick sinus syndrome, status epilepticus, Stevens-Johnson syndrome, stupor, suicidal tendencies, syncope, thrombocytopenia, tonic-clonic seizures, toxic epidermal necrolysis, tumor lysis syndrome, urinary incontinence, uterine hemorrhage, varicella zoster infection

Mechanism of Action Thalidomide exhibits immunomodulatory and antiangiogenic characteristics; immunologic effects may vary based on conditions. Thalidomide may suppress excessive tumor necrosis factor-alpha production in patients with erythema nodosum leprosum, yet may increase plasma tumor necrosis factor-alpha levels in HIV-positive patients. In multiple myeloma, thalidomide is associated with an increase in natural killer cells and increased levels of interleukin-2 and interferon gamma. Other proposed mechanisms of action include suppression of angiogenesis, prevention of free-radical-mediated DNA damage, increased cell mediated cytotoxic effects, and altered expression of cellular adhesion molecules.

Pharmacodynamics/Kinetics

Half-life Elimination 5.5 to 7.3 hours

Time to Peak Plasma: ~2 to 5 hours

Reproductive Considerations

[US Boxed Warning]: Thalidomide should never be used by females who could become pregnant while taking thalidomide. When alternative treatments are not available, females of reproductive potential may be treated when adequate precautions are taken to avoid pregnancy. **[US Boxed Warning]: In an effort to make the chance of embryo-fetal exposure to thalidomide as negligible as possible, thalidomide is approved for marketing only through a special restricted distribution program: Thalomid REMS program, approved by the Food and Drug Administration. Information about Thalomid and the Thalomid REMS program is available at https://www.-celgeneriskmanagement.com or by calling the manufacturer's toll-free number 1-888-423-5436.**

Females of reproductive potential must avoid pregnancy beginning 4 weeks prior to therapy, during therapy, during therapy interruptions, and for ≥4 weeks after therapy is discontinued. A negative pregnancy test (sensitivity of ≥50 milliunits/mL) 10 to 14 days prior to therapy, within 24 hours prior to beginning therapy, weekly during the first 4 weeks, and every 4 weeks (every 2 weeks for females with irregular menstrual cycles) thereafter is required for women of childbearing potential. Two forms of reliable contraception must be used simultaneously in females of reproductive potential (unless they commit to total abstinence from heterosexual intercourse): One highly effective method (eg, tubal ligation, IUD, hormonal birth control methods) or partners vasectomy; plus one additional effective method (eg, male latex or synthetic condom, diaphragm, or cervical cap). Contraception is required even in cases of infertility (unless due to hysterectomy). Thalidomide must be immediately discontinued for a missed period, abnormal pregnancy test, or abnormal menstrual bleeding. Some forms of contraception may not be appropriate in certain patients. An intrauterine device or implantable contraceptive may increase the risk of infection or bleeding; estrogen-containing products may increase the risk of thromboembolism.

Females of reproductive potential (including health care workers and caregivers) must also avoid contact with thalidomide capsules.

Thalidomide is also present in the semen of males. Males taking thalidomide (even those vasectomized) must use a latex or synthetic condom during any sexual contact with women of childbearing potential and for up to 28 days following discontinuation of therapy. Males taking thalidomide must not donate sperm.

Pregnancy Considerations

Use is contraindicated in pregnant females. **[US Boxed Warning]: If thalidomide is taken during pregnancy, it can cause severe birth defects or embryo-fetal death. Thalidomide should never be used by females who are pregnant or who could become pregnant while taking thalidomide. Even a single dose (1 capsule [regardless of strength]) taken by a pregnant woman during pregnancy may cause severe birth defects.** Thalidomide induces a high frequency of severe and life-threatening birth defects. Anomalies observed in humans include amelia, phocomelia, bone defects, ear and eye abnormalities, facial palsy, congenital heart defects, urinary and genital tract malformations; mortality in ~40% of infants at or shortly after birth has also been reported. Discontinue thalidomide immediately if pregnancy occurs during treatment and refer patient to a reproductive toxicity specialist.

A pregnancy exposure registry has been created to monitor outcomes in females exposed to thalidomide during pregnancy and female partners of male patients and to understand the root cause for the pregnancy. The pregnancy exposure registry may be contacted at 1-888-423-5436. If pregnancy occurs during treatment, thalidomide must be immediately discontinued and the patient referred to a reproductive toxicity specialist. Any suspected fetal exposure to thalidomide must be reported to the FDA via the MedWatch program (1-800-FDA-1088) and to Celgene Corporation (1-888-423-5436).

Prescribing and Access Restrictions **Canada:** Access to thalidomide is restricted through a controlled distribution program called RevAid. Only physicians and pharmacists enrolled in this program are authorized to prescribe or dispense thalidomide. Patients must be enrolled in the program by their physicians. Further information is available at www.RevAid.ca or by calling 1-888-738-2431.

◆ **Thalomid** *see* Thalidomide *on page* 1435

◆ **Tham** *see* Tromethamine *on page* 1502

- ◆ **THC** *see* Dronabinol *on page 532*
- ◆ **THC and CBD** *see* Tetrahydrocannabinol and Cannabidiol *on page 1434*
- ◆ **Theo-24** *see* Theophylline *on page 1437*
- ◆ **Theobid Duracaps** *see* Theophylline *on page 1437*
- ◆ **TheoCap** *see* Theophylline *on page 1437*
- ◆ **Theochron** *see* Theophylline *on page 1437*
- ◆ **Theo-Dur** *see* Theophylline *on page 1437*

Theophylline (thee OFF i lin)

Related Information

Aminophylline *on page 117*

Respiratory Diseases *on page 1680*

Brand Names: US Elixophyllin; Theo-24; Theochron

Brand Names: Canada AA-Theo LA; PMS-Theophylline [DSC]; Pulmophylline; TEVA-Theophylline SR [DSC]; Theo ER; Theolair; Uniphyl

Pharmacologic Category Phosphodiesterase Enzyme Inhibitor, Nonselective

Use

Reversible airflow obstruction:

Oral: Treatment of symptoms and reversible airflow obstruction associated with chronic asthma, or other chronic lung diseases (eg, emphysema, chronic bronchitis).

Injection: Treatment of acute exacerbations of the symptoms and reversible airflow obstruction associated with asthma and other chronic lung diseases (eg, chronic bronchitis, emphysema) as an adjunct to inhaled beta-2 selective agonists and systemically administered corticosteroids. Guideline recommendations:

Guideline recommendations:

Asthma: The 2020 Global Initiative for Asthma Guidelines (GINA) and the 2007 National Heart, Lung and Blood Institute Asthma Guidelines recommend against theophylline for the treatment of asthma exacerbations due to poor efficacy and safety concerns (GINA 2020; NAEPP 2007). Theophylline is not recommended for routine use as a long-term control medication in asthma due to weak efficacy. Oral theophylline is a potential alternative option (not preferred) in adolescents and adults as a long-term control medication in mild asthma or as an add-on long-term control medication in moderate to severe asthma; however, a stepwise approach using inhaled corticosteroids (+/- inhaled long-acting beta agonists depending on asthma severity) is preferred to theophylline due to efficacy concerns and potential for adverse events (GINA 2020).

COPD: Based on the Global Initiative for Chronic Obstructive Lung Disease Guidelines (2019), use of theophylline in patients with COPD is controversial and lacks data. Theophylline may favorably impact functional impairment in COPD patients, but exact effects are unclear. Studies that demonstrated improvement were done with slow-release preparations. Theophylline is not a preferred agent for COPD exacerbations due to its potential for toxicity.

Local Anesthetic/Vasoconstrictor Precautions No information available to require special precautions

Effects on Dental Treatment Prescribe erythromycin products with caution to patients taking theophylline products. Erythromycin will delay the normal metabolic inactivation of theophyllines leading to increased blood levels; this has resulted in nausea, vomiting, and CNS restlessness. Azithromycin does not cause these effects in combination with theophylline products.

Effects on Bleeding No information available to require special precautions

Adverse Reactions Frequency not defined. Adverse events observed at therapeutic serum levels.

Cardiovascular: Cardiac flutter, tachycardia

Central nervous system: Headache, hyperactivity (children), insomnia, restlessness, seizure, status epilepticus (nonconvulsive)

Endocrine & metabolic: Hypercalcemia (with concomitant hyperthyroid disease)

Gastrointestinal: Gastroesophageal reflux (aggravation), gastrointestinal ulcer (aggravation), nausea, vomiting

Genitourinary: Difficulty in micturition (elderly males with prostatism), diuresis (transient)

Neuromuscular & skeletal: Tremor

Mechanism of Action Theophylline has two distinct actions; smooth muscle relaxation (ie, bronchodilation) and suppression of the response of the airways to stimuli (ie, non-bronchodilator prophylactic effects). Bronchodilation is mediated by inhibition of two isoenzymes, phosphodiesterase (PDE III and, to a lesser extent, PDE IV) while non-bronchodilation effects are mediated through other molecular mechanisms. Theophylline increases the force of contraction of diaphragmatic muscles through enhancement of calcium uptake through adenosine-mediated channels.

Pharmacodynamics/Kinetics

Onset of Action IV: <30 minutes

Half-life Elimination Highly variable and dependent upon age, hepatic function, cardiac function, lung disease, and smoking history (Hendeles 1995):

Premature infants, postnatal age 3 to 15 days: 30 hours (range: 17 to 43 hours)

Premature infants, postnatal age 25 to 57 days: 20 hours (range: 9.4 to 30.6 hours)

Term infants, postnatal age 1 to 2 days: 25.7 hours (range: 25 to 26.5 hours)

Term infants, postnatal age 3 to 30 weeks: 11 hours (range: 6 to 29 hours)

Children 1 to 4 years: 3.4 hours (range: 1.2 to 5.6 hours)

Children and Adolescents 6 to 17 years: 3.7 hours (range: 1.5 to 5.9 hours)

Adults ≥18 years to ≤60 years (nonsmoking, asthmatic, otherwise healthy): 8.7 hours (range: 6.1 to 12.8 hours)

Elderly >60 years (nonsmoking, healthy): 9.8 hours (range: 1.6 to 18 hours)

Time to Peak Serum: Oral (solution and immediate release): 1 to 2 hours; IV: Within 30 minutes

Pregnancy Risk Factor C

Pregnancy Considerations Theophylline crosses the placenta.

Maternal use of theophylline is not associated with an increased risk of fetal malformations (ERS/TSANZ [Middleton 2020]; GINA 2020). Infants exposed to theophylline during the third trimester should be monitored for adverse events (irritability, tachycardia, vomiting) (ERS/TSANZ [Middleton 2020]).

Uncontrolled asthma is associated with adverse events in pregnancy (increased risk of perinatal mortality, preeclampsia, preterm birth, low birth weight infants, cesarean delivery, and the development of gestational diabetes). Poorly controlled asthma or asthma exacerbations may have a greater fetal/maternal risk than what is associated with appropriately used asthma ▶

medications. Maternal treatment improves pregnancy outcomes by reducing the risk of some adverse events (eg, preterm birth, gestational diabetes) (ERS/TSANZ [Middleton 2020]; GINA 2020).

Theophylline is considered compatible for use during pregnancy (ERS/TSANZ [Middleton 2020]). Due to pregnancy-induced physiologic changes, some pharmacokinetic properties of theophylline are altered. The half-life is similar to that observed in otherwise healthy, nonsmoking adults with asthma during the first and second trimesters (~8.7 hours) but may increase to 13 hours (range: 8 to 18 hours) during the third trimester. The volume of distribution is also increased during the third trimester. Monitor serum levels. In addition, maternal asthma symptoms should be monitored monthly during pregnancy. Use at term may inhibit uterine contractions (ERS/TSANZ [Middleton 2020]).

- ◆ **Theophylline Anhydrous** *see* Theophylline *on page 1437*
- ◆ **Theophylline Ethylenediamine** *see* Aminophylline *on page 117*
- ◆ **TheraCare Pain Relief [OTC]** *see* Lidocaine (Topical) *on page 902*
- ◆ **Theragran** *see* Vitamins (Multiple/Oral) *on page 1550*
- ◆ **Theramill Forte [OTC]** *see* Vitamins (Multiple/Oral) *on page 1550*
- ◆ **Therapeutic Multivitamins** *see* Vitamins (Multiple/Oral) *on page 1550*
- ◆ **Therapevo [DSC]** *see* Hyaluronate and Derivatives *on page 761*
- ◆ **Thera-Tabs M [OTC]** *see* Vitamins (Multiple/Oral) *on page 1550*
- ◆ **The Treatment Formula 3 [OTC] [DSC]** *see* Tolnaftate *on page 1462*
- ◆ **Thiamazole** *see* MethIMAzole *on page 988*

Thioguanine (thye oh GWAH neen)

Brand Names: US Tabloid

Brand Names: Canada Lanvis

Pharmacologic Category Antineoplastic Agent, Antimetabolite; Antineoplastic Agent, Antimetabolite (Purine Analog)

Use

Acute myeloid leukemia: Treatment (remission induction and consolidation) of acute myeloid (nonlymphocytic) leukemia (AML)

Limitations of use: The use of thioguanine for AML maintenance therapy or other similar long-term continuous treatments is not recommended due to the high risk of hepatotoxicity.

Local Anesthetic/Vasoconstrictor Precautions

No information available to require special precautions

Effects on Dental Treatment Key adverse event(s) related to dental treatment: Stomatitis.

Effects on Bleeding Chemotherapy may result in significant myelosuppression, potentially including significant reduction in platelet counts and altered hemostasis. In patients who are under active treatment with these agents, medical consult is suggested.

Adverse Reactions

Frequency not defined:

Cardiovascular: Esophageal varices, portal hypertension

Endocrine & metabolic: Fluid retention, hyperuricemia (common), increased gamma-glutamyl transferase, weight gain

Gastrointestinal: Anorexia, intestinal necrosis, intestinal perforation, nausea, stomatitis, vomiting

Hematologic & oncologic: Anemia (may be delayed), bone marrow depression, granulocytopenia, hemorrhage, leukopenia (common; may be delayed), pancytopenia, splenomegaly, thrombocytopenia (common; may be delayed)

Hepatic: Ascites, hepatic disease (hepatoportal sclerosis), hepatic focal nodular hyperplasia (regenerative), hepatic necrosis (centrilobular), hepatic sinusoidal obstruction syndrome, hepatomegaly (tender), hepatotoxicity, hyperbilirubinemia, increased liver enzymes, increased serum alkaline phosphatase, jaundice, peliosis hepatitis, periportal fibrosis

Infection: Infection

Neuromuscular & skeletal: Bone hypoplasia

Mechanism of Action Thioguanine is a purine analog of guanine that is incorporated into DNA and RNA resulting in the blockage of synthesis and metabolism of purine nucleotides.

Pharmacodynamics/Kinetics

Half-life Elimination Terminal: 5 to 9 hours

Time to Peak Serum: Within 8 hours; predominantly metabolite(s)

Reproductive Considerations

Females of reproductive potential should avoid becoming pregnant during treatment.

Pregnancy Risk Factor D

Pregnancy Considerations

Adverse effects have been observed in animal reproduction studies. May cause fetal harm if administered during pregnancy.

- ◆ **6-Thioguanine (error-prone abbreviation)** *see* Thioguanine *on page 1438*
- ◆ **Thiophosphoramide** *see* Thiotepa *on page 1439*
- ◆ **Thioplex** *see* Thiotepa *on page 1439*

Thioridazine (thye oh RID a zeen)

Related Information

Clinical Risk Related to Drugs Prolonging QT Interval *on page 1675*

Pharmacologic Category First Generation (Typical) Antipsychotic; Phenothiazine Derivative

Use Schizophrenia: Treatment of patients with schizophrenia who fail to respond adequately to treatment with other antipsychotic drugs, either because of insufficient effectiveness or the inability to achieve an effective dose because of intolerable adverse effects from those medications. Before initiating treatment with thioridazine, it is strongly recommended that a patient be given at least 2 trials, each with a different antipsychotic drug product, at an adequate dose and for an adequate duration.

Local Anesthetic/Vasoconstrictor Precautions

Thioridazine is one of the drugs confirmed to prolong the QT interval and is accepted as having a risk of causing torsade de pointes. The risk of drug-induced torsade de pointes is extremely low when a single QT interval prolonging drug is prescribed. In terms of epinephrine, it is not known what effect vasoconstrictors in the local anesthetic regimen will have in patients with a known history of congenital prolonged QT interval or in patients taking any medication that prolongs the QT interval. Until more information is obtained, it is suggested that the clinician consult with the physician prior to the use of a vasoconstrictor in suspected patients, and that the vasoconstrictor (epinephrine, mepivacaine and levonordefrin [Carbocaine® 2% with Neo-Cobefrin®]) be used with caution.

Effects on Dental Treatment Key adverse event(s) related to dental treatment: Xerostomia and changes in salivation (normal salivary flow resumes upon discontinuation). Significant hypotension may occur, especially when the drug is administered parenterally; orthostatic hypotension is due to alpha-receptor blockade, the elderly are at greater risk for orthostatic hypotension.

Tardive dyskinesia; Prevalence rate may be 40% in elderly; development of the syndrome and the irreversible nature are proportional to duration and total cumulative dose over time. Extrapyramidal reactions are more common in elderly with up to 50% developing these reactions after 60 years of age. Drug-induced Parkinson's syndrome occurs often; akathisia is the most common extrapyramidal reaction in elderly.

Effects on Bleeding No information available to require special precautions

Adverse Reactions Frequency not defined.

Cardiovascular: ECG changes, hypotension, orthostatic hypotension, peripheral edema, prolonged QT Interval on ECG, torsades de pointes

Central nervous system: Confusion (sundowning), disruption of temperature regulation (Martinez 2002), drowsiness, drug-induced Parkinson disease, extrapyramidal reaction, headache, hyperactive behavior, lethargy, psychotic reaction, restlessness, seizure, tardive dyskinesia (Lehman 2004)

Dermatologic: Dermatitis, hyperpigmentation (Lehman 2004), pallor, skin photosensitivity, skin rash, urticaria

Endocrine & metabolic: Amenorrhea, galactorrhea not associated with childbirth, weight gain (Lehman 2004)

Gastrointestinal: Constipation, diarrhea, nausea, parotid gland enlargement, vomiting, xerostomia

Genitourinary: Breast engorgement, inhibited ejaculation, priapism, sexual difficulty (La Torre 2013), sexual disorder (La Torre 2013)

Hematologic & oncologic: Agranulocytosis, leukopenia

Ophthalmic: Blurred vision, corneal opacity (Lehman 2004), retinitis pigmentosa

Respiratory: Nasal congestion

Mechanism of Action Thioridazine is a piperidine phenothiazine which blocks postsynaptic mesolimbic dopaminergic receptors in the brain; also has activity at serotonin, noradrenaline, and histamine receptors (Fenton, 2007).

Pharmacodynamics/Kinetics

Half-life Elimination 5 to 27 hours (Mårtensson 1973; Muusze 1977; Vanderheeren 1977)

Time to Peak Serum: ~1 to 4 hours (Mårtensson 1973)

Reproductive Considerations

Because thioridazine increases prolactin concentrations, amenorrhea in women and impotence in men have been reported. False pregnancy tests may also occur with thioridazine use.

Pregnancy Considerations

Although outcome information has been published in case reports following maternal use of thioridazine in pregnancy, most information is available for phenothiazines as a class (Erkkola 1983; Heinonen 1977; Scanlan 1972; Slone 1977; Vince 1969). Jaundice or hyper- or hyporeflexia have been reported in newborn infants following maternal use of phenothiazines. Antipsychotic use during the third trimester of pregnancy has a risk for abnormal muscle movements (extrapyramidal symptoms [EPS]) and withdrawal symptoms in newborns following delivery. Symptoms in the newborn may include agitation, feeding disorder, hypertonia, hypotonia, respiratory distress, somnolence, and tremor; these effects may be self-limiting or require hospitalization.

When use in pregnancy is needed, the minimum effective maternal dose should be used to decrease the risk of EPS (ACOG 2008).

Dental Health Professional Considerations See Local Anesthetic/Vasoconstrictor Precautions

- **Thioridazine HCl** *see* Thioridazine *on page 1438*
- **Thioridazine Hydrochloride** *see* Thioridazine *on page 1438*

Thiotepa (thye oh TEP a)

Brand Names: US Tepadina

Brand Names: Canada Tepadina

Pharmacologic Category Antineoplastic Agent, Alkylating Agent

Use Beta-thalassemia, class 3: To reduce the risk of graft rejection when used in conjunction with high-dose busulfan and cyclophosphamide as a preparative regimen for allogeneic hematopoietic progenitor (stem) cell transplantation in pediatric patients with class 3 beta-thalassemia.

Local Anesthetic/Vasoconstrictor Precautions No information available to require special precautions

Effects on Dental Treatment No significant effects or complications reported

Effects on Bleeding Chemotherapy may result in significant myelosuppression, potentially including significant reduction in platelet counts and altered hemostasis. In patients who are under active treatment with these agents, medical consult is suggested.

Adverse Reactions

As a preparative regimen prior to allogeneic or autologous hemtopoietic progenitor cell transplantation:

Frequency not defined:

Central nervous system: Intracranial hemorrhage, seizure

Dermatologic: Skin rash

Gastrointestinal: Mucositis

Hematologic & oncologic: Anemia, hemorrhage, neutropenia, thrombocytopenia

Hepatic: Increased serum ALT, increased serum AST, increased serum bilirubin

Infection: Cytomegalovirus disease

Respiratory: Pneumonia

Other approved/nonapproved uses:

Frequency not defined:

Dermatologic: Alopecia, contact dermatitis, dermatitis, skin depigmentation, skin rash, urticaria

Central nervous system: Dizziness, fatigue, headache

Endocrine & metabolic: Amenorrhea

Gastrointestinal: Abdominal pain, anorexia, nausea, vomiting

Genitourinary: Cystitis, dysuria, hemorrhagic cystitis, inhibition of Spermatogenesis, urinary retention
Hypersensitivity: Anaphylactic shock, hypersensitivity reaction
Infection: Infection
Local: Pain at injection site
Neuromuscular & skeletal: Weakness
Ophthalmic: Blurred vision, conjunctivitis
Respiratory: Asthma, laryngeal edema, wheezing
Miscellaneous: Febrile reaction

<1%, postmarketing, and/or case reports: Abnormal gait, acute myelocytic leukemia, acute respiratory distress, acute sinusitis, amnesia, apathy, aphasia, arteriosclerosis (pulmonary arteriopathy), ascites, aspiration, ataxia, behavioral problems, blepharoptosis, blindness, blood coagulation disorder, blood platelet disorder (refractoriness to transfusion), bone marrow aplasia, bone marrow depression (bone marrow transplant rejection), bradycardia, brain disease, candidiasis, capillary leak syndrome, cardiac failure, cerebrovascular accident, cognitive dysfunction, coma, confusion, cranial nerve palsy, deafness, delirium, depression, diarrhea, disorientation, drowsiness, dysphagia, dyspnea on exertion, encephalitis, enterocolitis, epstein-barr infection, fever, forgetfulness, fungal infection, gastritis, gastroenteritis, gastrointestinal hemorrhage, hallucination, hematuria, hemiplegia, hepatomegaly, hyponatremia, hypotonia, immunosuppression, infection due to enterococcus, interstitial pulmonary disease, klebsiella species, lesion (including central nervous system and white matter), leukemia (recurrent), leukoencephalopathy, lower respiratory tract infection (viral), lymphoproliferative disorder (posttransplant), malaise, malignant lymphoma (including central nervous system lymphoma), malignant neoplasm (recurrence), malignant neoplasm of breast (metastatic), memory impairment, motor dysfunction, mouth disease (palatal disorder), myelodysplastic syndrome, neoplasm (metastatic), neurotoxicity, pain, papilledema, paralysis (retrobulbar), paresis (quadriparesis), pericardial effusion, pericarditis, pneumonitis, pseudomonas infection, psychomotor retardation, pulmonary aspergillosis, pulmonary disease, pulmonary hypertension, pulmonary veno-occlusive disease, pure red cell aplasia, renal failure, respiratory distress, respiratory tract infection, sepsis, septic shock, speech disturbance, staphylococcal bacteremia, staphylococcal infection, Stevens-Johnson Syndrome, strabismus, subarachnoid hemorrhage, subdural hematoma, suicidal ideation, thrombotic thrombocytopenic purpura (cerebral), toxic epidermal necrolysis, toxic nephrosis, tremor, urinary tract infection, vasodilation (cerebral ventricle), ventricular hypertrophy, weight gain

Mechanism of Action Thiotepa is an alkylating agent which produces cross-linking of DNA strands leading to inhibition of DNA, RNA, and protein synthesis; thiotepa is cell-cycle independent (Perry 2012)

Pharmacodynamics/Kinetics

Half-life Elimination Terminal:

Pediatrics (5 mg/kg IV dose): Thiotepa: 1.7 hours; TEPA: 4 hours

Adults (20 mg to 250 mg/m^2 IV dose): Thiotepa: 1.4 to 3.7 hours; TEPA: 4.9 to 17.6 hours

Reproductive Considerations

Verify pregnancy status in females of reproductive potential prior to therapy initiation. Effective contraception should be used during treatment and for at least 6 months after the final dose. Males with female partners of reproductive potential should use effective contraception during therapy and for at least 1 year after the final dose.

Pregnancy Risk Factor D

Pregnancy Considerations

Based on the mechanism of action, and data from animal reproduction studies, in utero exposure to thiotepa may cause fetal harm.

- ◆ **Thorazine** *see* ChlorproMAZINE *on page 341*
- ◆ **Thrive [OTC]** *see* Nicotine *on page 1101*
- ◆ **Thrombate III** *see* Antithrombin *on page 156*
- ◆ **Thrombi-Gel** *see* Thrombin (Topical) *on page 1440*
- ◆ **Thrombin alfa** *see* Thrombin (Topical) *on page 1440*
- ◆ **Thrombin-JMI** *see* Thrombin (Topical) *on page 1440*
- ◆ **Thrombin-JMI Epistaxis Kit** *see* Thrombin (Topical) *on page 1440*
- ◆ **Thrombin-JMI Pump Spray Kit** *see* Thrombin (Topical) *on page 1440*
- ◆ **Thrombin-JMI Syringe Spray Kit** *see* Thrombin (Topical) *on page 1440*

Thrombin (Topical) (THROM bin, TOP i kal)

Related Information

Antiplatelet and Anticoagulation Considerations in Dentistry *on page 1666*

Cardiovascular Diseases *on page 1654*

Brand Names: US Evithrom [DSC]; Recothrom; Recothrom Spray Kit; Thrombi-Gel; Thrombi-Pad; Thrombin-JMI; Thrombin-JMI Epistaxis Kit; Thrombin-JMI Pump Spray Kit; Thrombin-JMI Syringe Spray Kit

Brand Names: Canada Recothrom

Generic Availability (US) No

Pharmacologic Category Blood Product Derivative; Hemostatic Agent

Dental Use Hemostasis whenever minor bleeding from capillaries and small venules is accessible

Use

Hemostasis aid:

Evithrom, Recothrom, Thrombin-JMI only: As an aid to hemostasis whenever oozing blood and minor bleeding from capillaries and small venules is accessible and control of bleeding by standard surgical techniques is ineffective or impractical.

Thrombi-Gel, Thrombi-Pad only: As a trauma dressing for temporary control of moderate to severe bleeding wounds; control of surface bleeding from vascular access sites and percutaneous catheters and tubes.

Local Anesthetic/Vasoconstrictor Precautions
No information available to require special precautions

Effects on Dental Treatment No significant effects or complications reported

Effects on Bleeding General dental procedures and simple restorative procedures are not associated with bleeding; therefore, there is no contraindication to general dental treatment for most patients with bleeding disorders. However, after dental extractions and other dental surgeries including deep scaling, block anesthesia, and large fillings, in patients with homophilia, drugs such as topical thrombin may be useful in controlling bleeding. A carefully coordinated strategy between the dental and medical team may be required to ensure adequate procedures for hemostasis.

Adverse Reactions Frequency not always defined.

Cardiovascular: Thromboembolism (1% to 9%)
Dermatologic: Pruritus

Gastrointestinal: Nausea, vomiting
Hematologic & oncologic: Increased INR, increased neutrophils, lymphocytopenia, prolonged partial thromboplastin time, prolonged prothrombin time
Hypersensitivity: Hypersensitivity reaction
Immunologic: Antibody development (≤2%)
Local: Postoperative wound complication

Dental Usual Dosage Topical: Hemostasis: **Note:** For topical use only; do not administer intravenously or intra-arterially:

Evithrom: Children and Adults: Dose depends on area to be treated; up to 10 mL was used with absorbable gelatin sponge in clinical studies

Recothrom: Adults: Dose depends on area to be treated

Thrombi-Gel 10, 40, 100: Adults: Wet product with up to 3 mL, 10 mL, or 20 mL, respectively, of 0.9% sodium chloride or SWFI; apply directly over source of the bleeding with manual pressure

Thrombi-Pad: Adults: Apply pad directly over source of bleeding; may apply dry or wetted with up to 10 mL of 0.9% sodium chloride. If desired, product may be left in place for up to 24 hours; do not leave in the body.

Thrombin-JMI: Adults:

Solution: Use 1000-2000 units/mL of solution where bleeding is profuse; use 100 units/mL for bleeding from skin or mucosal surfaces

Powder: May apply powder directly to the site of bleeding or on oozing surfaces

Dosing

Adult & Geriatric Hemostasis aid: Topical: **Note:** For topical use only; do not administer intravenously or intra-arterially:

Evithrom: Dose depends on area to be treated; for direct application, flood treatment area; up to 10 mL was used with absorbable gelatin sponge in clinical studies.

Recothrom: Dose depends on area to be treated. Apply to the bleeding site directly or in conjunction with absorbable gelatin sponge.

Thrombi-Gel: Apply directly over source of the bleeding with adjunct manual pressure until hemostasis is achieved.

Thrombin-JMI:

Solution: Apply 1,000 to 2,000 units/mL of solution where bleeding is profuse. Apply 100 units/mL for bleeding from skin or mucosal surfaces (eg, skin grafting, dental extractions, plastic surgery).

Powder: May apply dry powder directly to the site on oozing surfaces.

Thrombi-Pad: Apply dry or wetted pad directly over source of bleeding with adjunct manual pressure. If desired, product may be left in place for up to 24 hours; do not leave in the body.

Renal Impairment: Adult There are no dosage adjustments provided in the manufacturer's labeling.

Hepatic Impairment: Adult There are no dosage adjustments provided in the manufacturer's labeling.

Pediatric

Hemostasis: Topical: **Note:** For topical use only; do not administer intravenously or intra-arterially:

Evithrom: Infants, Children, and Adolescents: Dose depends on area to be treated; may apply directly or in conjunction with an absorbable gelatin sponge; up to 10 mL was used with absorbable gelatin sponge in clinical studies

Recothrom: Infants ≥1 month, Children, and Adolescents: Dose depends on area to be treated including size of and number of bleeding sites; may apply directly or in conjunction with an absorbable gelatin sponge

Renal Impairment: Pediatric There are no dosage adjustments provided in the manufacturer's labeling.

Hepatic Impairment: Pediatric There are no dosage adjustments provided in the manufacturer's labeling.

Mechanism of Action Activates platelets and catalyzes the conversion of fibrinogen to fibrin to promote hemostasis.

Contraindications Known hypersensitivity to any component of the formulation.

Evithrom: Additional contraindications: Known anaphylactic or severe systemic reactions to blood products; treatment of severe or brisk arterial bleeding

Recothrom: Additional contraindications: Known hypersensitivity to hamster proteins; injection directly into the circulatory system; treatment of massive or brisk arterial bleeding.

Thrombi-Gel: Additional contraindications: Use in the closure of skin incisions.

Thrombin-JMI: Additional contraindications: Known sensitivity to material of bovine origin; injection directly into the circulatory system; re-exposure if there are known or suspected antibodies to bovine thrombin and/or factor V; treatment of severe or brisk arterial bleeding.

Thrombi-Pad: Additional contraindications: Known sensitivity to bovine-derived materials.

Warnings/Precautions For topical use only. Do not inject intravenously or intra-arterially. Intravascular clotting, possibly leading to death, may occur following injection. Powder and solution formulations may be used in combination with absorbable gelatin sponges; The 5,000 unit syringe spray kit may be used in conjunction with Gel-Flow NT. Hypersensitivity reactions, including anaphylaxis, may occur. Institute supportive measures and treat individual symptoms immediately.

[US Boxed Warning]: Thrombin topical (bovine) can cause fatal severe bleeding or thrombosis. Thrombosis may result from the development of antibodies against bovine thrombin. Bleeding may result from the development of antibodies against factor V. These may cross-react with human factor V and lead to its deficiency. Do not re-expose patients to thrombin topical (bovine) if there are known or suspected antibodies to bovine thrombin and/or factor V. Monitor patients for abnormal coagulation laboratory values, bleeding, or thrombosis.

Evithrom is a product of human plasma; may potentially contain infectious agents, such as viruses and, theoretically the Creutzfeldt-Jacob disease agent, or an unknown infectious agent. Screening of donors, as well as testing and/or inactivation or removal of certain viruses, reduces the risk. Infections thought to be transmitted by this product should be reported to the manufacturer. Recothrom should be used with caution in patients with known hypersensitivity to snake or hamster proteins (manufacturing process uses a genetically modified hamster cell line and snake proteins); the potential for allergic reaction theoretically exists.

Do not use Thrombi-Gel or Thrombi-Pad in the presence of infection; use caution in areas of contamination. Thrombi-Pad is nonabsorbable and should not be used as a replacement for absorbable hemostats; do not leave in the body.

Drug Interactions

Metabolism/Transport Effects None known.

Avoid Concomitant Use There are no known interactions where it is recommended to avoid concomitant use.

Increased Effect/Toxicity There are no known significant interactions involving an increase in effect.

Decreased Effect There are no known significant interactions involving a decrease in effect.

Pregnancy Considerations Animal reproduction studies have not been conducted. Reproduction studies conducted with the solvent/detergent used in processing the human-derived product (Evithrom) showed adverse events in animals. Only residual levels of the solvent/detergent would be expected to remain in the finished product.

Breastfeeding Considerations

It is not known if thrombin topical is present in breast milk.

According to the manufacturer, the decision to breastfeed during therapy should consider the risk of infant exposure, the benefits of breastfeeding to the infant, and the benefits of treatment to the mother.

Dosage Forms: US

Pad, topical [preservative free]:
Thrombi-Pad 3x3: ≥200 units

Powder for reconstitution, topical:
Thrombin-JMI: 5000 units, 20,000 units
Thrombin-JMI Epistaxis kit: 5000 units
Thrombin-JMI Pump Spray Kit: 20,000 units
Thrombin-JMI Syringe Spray Kit: 5000 units; 20,000 units

Powder for reconstitution, topical [preservative free]:
Recothrom: 5000 units; 20,000 units
Recothrom Spray Kit: 20,000 units

Sponge, topical [preservative free]:
Thrombi-Gel10: ≥1000 units (10s)
Thrombi-Gel 40: ≥1000 units (5s)
Thrombi-Gel 100: ≥2000 units (5s)

◆ **Thrombi-Pad** *see* Thrombin (Topical) *on page 1440*

◆ **Thymocyte Stimulating Factor** *see* Aldesleukin *on page 91*

◆ **Thyrogen** *see* Thyrotropin Alpha *on page 1442*

Thyroid, Desiccated (THYE roid DES i kay tid)

Related Information

Endocrine Disorders and Pregnancy *on page 1684*

Brand Names: US Armour Thyroid; Nature-Throid; NP Thyroid; Westhroid; WP Thyroid

Pharmacologic Category Thyroid Product

Use Hypothyroidism: Replacement or supplemental therapy in hypothyroidism

Local Anesthetic/Vasoconstrictor Precautions No precautions with vasoconstrictor are necessary if patient is well controlled with thyroid preparations

Effects on Dental Treatment No significant effects or complications reported

Effects on Bleeding No information available to require special precautions

Adverse Reactions Adverse reactions are often indicative of excess thyroid replacement and/or hyperthyroidism.

<1%, postmarketing, and/or case reports: Abdominal cramps, alopecia, ataxia, cardiac arrhythmia, chest pain, constipation, diaphoresis, diarrhea, dyspnea, fever, headache, heat intolerance, increased appetite, insomnia, menstrual disease, myalgia, nervousness, palpitations, tachycardia, tremor, tremor of hands, vomiting, weight loss

Mechanism of Action The primary active compound is T_3 (triiodothyronine), which may be converted from T_4 (thyroxine) and then circulates throughout the body to influence growth and maturation of various tissues; exact mechanism of action is unknown; however, it is believed the thyroid hormone exerts its many metabolic effects through control of DNA transcription and protein synthesis; involved in normal metabolism, growth, and development; promotes gluconeogenesis, increases utilization and mobilization of glycogen stores and stimulates protein synthesis, increases basal metabolic rate

Pharmacodynamics/Kinetics

Onset of Action Liothyronine (T_3): ~3 hours

Half-life Elimination

T_4: Euthyroid: 6 to 7 days; Hyperthyroid: 3 to 4 days; Hypothyroid: 9 to 10 days
T_3: 0.75 days (Brent, 2011)

Time to Peak Serum: T_4: 2 to 4 hours; T_3: 2 to 3 days

Reproductive Considerations

Desiccated thyroid is not the preferred treatment for hypothyroidism in pregnant women. Women treated with desiccated thyroid who are planning to conceive should be transitioned to a preferred therapy and TSH should be monitored (ACOG 2015; ATA/AACE [Garber 2012]).

Pregnancy Risk Factor A

Pregnancy Considerations

Endogenous thyroid hormones minimally cross the placenta. Desiccated thyroid has not been found to adversely affect the fetus following maternal use during pregnancy.

Uncontrolled maternal hypothyroidism may result in adverse neonatal and maternal outcomes (ACOG 2015). Subnormal intellectual development may occur in infants of mothers with serum thyroxine concentrations in the lowest tenth percentile at the end of the first trimester (ATA/AACE [Garber 2012]). To prevent adverse events, normal maternal thyroid function should be maintained prior to conception and throughout pregnancy and thyroid replacement should not be discontinued during pregnancy (ACOG 2015). However, desiccated thyroid is not the preferred treatment for hypothyroidism in pregnant women because use may result in lowering serum thyroxine concentrations. Women treated with desiccated thyroid who become pregnant should be transitioned to a preferred therapy and TSH should be monitored (ACOG 2015; ATA/AACE [Garber 2012]).

◆ **Thyroid Extract** *see* Thyroid, Desiccated *on page 1442*

◆ **Thyroid USP** *see* Thyroid, Desiccated *on page 1442*

◆ **Thyrolar** *see* Liotrix *on page 919*

Thyrotropin Alpha (thye roe TROH pin AL fa)

Brand Names: US Thyrogen

Brand Names: Canada Thyrogen

Pharmacologic Category Diagnostic Agent

Use

Diagnostic imaging: Adjunctive diagnostic tool for serum thyroglobulin (Tg) testing (with or without radioiodine imaging) in follow-up of patients with well-differentiated thyroid cancer (DTC) who have previously undergone thyroidectomy.

Limitations of use: Thyrotropin alfa-stimulated Tg levels are generally lower than and do not correlate with Tg levels after thyroid hormone withdrawal; even when thyrotropin alfa-stimulated Tg testing is performed in combination with radioiodine imaging, there is a risk of missing a thyroid cancer diagnosis or of underestimating disease extent. Anti-Tg antibodies may confound Tg assay and render Tg levels uninterpretable; in such cases, even with a negative or low-stage thyrotropin alfa radioiodine scan, consider further patient evaluation.

Thyroid tissue remnant ablation: Adjunctive treatment for radioiodine ablation of thyroid tissue remnants after total or near-total thyroidectomy in patients with well-differentiated thyroid cancer without evidence of metastatic disease.

Limitations of use: The effect of thyrotropin alfa on thyroid cancer recurrence >5 years postremnant ablation has not been evaluated.

Guideline recommendations: The American Thyroid Association guidelines recommend thyrotropin alfa as a reasonable alternative to thyroid hormone withdrawal prior to remnant ablation or adjuvant therapy in patients with low- or intermediate-risk DTC without extensive lymph node involvement. Thyrotropin alfa may also be considered in intermediate-risk DTC with extensive lymph node disease (but without distance metastases), though the evidence is of lower quality (ATA [Haugen 2016).

Local Anesthetic/Vasoconstrictor Precautions No information available to require special precautions

Effects on Dental Treatment No significant effects or complications reported

Effects on Bleeding No information available to require special precautions

Adverse Reactions

>10%: Gastrointestinal: Nausea (11%)

1% to 10%:

Central nervous system: Headache (6%), dizziness (2%), fatigue (2%)

Gastrointestinal: Vomiting (2%)

Neuromuscular & skeletal: Weakness (1%)

Frequency not defined: Endocrine & metabolic: Altered thyroid hormone levels (increased)

<1%, postmarketing, and/or case reports: Cerebrovascular accident (with and without physiologic symptoms like unilateral weakness), flu-like symptoms (transient; including arthralgia, chills, fever, malaise, myalgia, shivering), hypersensitivity reaction (including dyspnea, flushing, pruritus, skin rash, urticaria), injection site reaction (including bruising, erythema, pain, and pruritus)

Mechanism of Action Thyrotropin alfa, derived from a recombinant DNA source, has the identical amino acid sequence as endogenous human thyroid stimulating hormone (TSH). As a diagnostic tool in conjunction with serum thyroglobulin (Tg) testing, thyrotropin alfa stimulates the secretion of Tg from any remaining thyroid tissues (remnants). Under conditions of successful thyroidectomy and complete ablation, very little serum Tg should be detected under TSH stimulatory conditions; conversely, elevated Tg levels suggest the presence of remnant thyroid tissues. Since the source of TSH is exogenous, stimulation of Tg synthesis can be achieved in euthyroid patients, avoiding the need for thyroid hormone withdrawal.

As an adjunctive agent for radioiodine ablation treatment of thyroid cancer tissue remnants, thyrotropin alfa binds to TSH receptors on these tissues, stimulating the uptake and organification of iodine, including radiolabeled iodine (I^{131}). Cancerous tissue is destroyed via gamma emission from the radioiodine concentrated in these tissues.

Pharmacodynamics/Kinetics

Half-life Elimination 25 ± 10 hours

Time to Peak Median: 10 hours (range: 3 to 24 hours)

Reproductive Considerations

Evaluate pregnancy status prior to use in females of reproductive potential when thyrotropin alfa is administered with radioiodine (ATA [Haugen 2016]).

Pregnancy Considerations Use of thyrotropin alfa administered with radioiodine is contraindicated during pregnancy.

◆ **Thyrotropin Alpha** *see* Thyrotropin Alpha *on page 1442*

◆ **Tiacumicin B** *see* Fidaxomicin *on page 668*

◆ **Tiadylt ER** *see* DilTIAZem *on page 499*

TiaGABine (tye AG a been)

Brand Names: US Gabitril

Pharmacologic Category Anticonvulsant, Miscellaneous

Use Partial seizures: Adjunctive therapy in adults and children ≥12 years in the treatment of partial seizures

Local Anesthetic/Vasoconstrictor Precautions No information available to require special precautions

Effects on Dental Treatment Key adverse event(s) related to dental treatment: Stomatitis, gingivitis, and mouth ulceration.

Effects on Bleeding No information available to require special precautions

Adverse Reactions

>10%:

Central nervous system: Dizziness (27% to 31%), drowsiness (18% to 21%), nervousness (10% to 14%), lack of concentration (7% to 14%)

Gastrointestinal: Nausea (11%)

Infection: Infection (19%)

Neuromuscular & skeletal: Weakness (18% to 23%), tremor (9% to 21%)

Miscellaneous: Accidental injury (21%)

1% to 10%:

Cardiovascular: Vasodilation (2%), chest pain (≥1%), edema (≥1%), hypertension (≥1%), palpitations (≥1%), peripheral edema (≥1%), syncope (≥1%), tachycardia (≥1%)

Central nervous system: Ataxia (5% to 9%), pain (5% to 7%), depression (1% to 7%), insomnia (5% to 6%), confusion (5%), status epilepticus (5%), abnormal gait (3% to 5%), hostility (2% to 5%), memory impairment (4%), paresthesia (4%), speech disturbance (4%), emotional lability (3%), chills (≥1%), depersonalization (≥1%), dysarthria (≥1%), euphoria (≥1%), hallucination (≥1%), hypertonia (≥1%), hypoesthesia (≥1%), hyporeflexia (≥1%), hypotonia (≥1%), malaise (≥1%), migraine (≥1%), myoclonus (≥1%), paranoia (≥1%), personality disorder (≥1%), stupor (≥1%), twitching (≥1%), vertigo (≥1%), agitation (1%), myasthenia (1%)

Dermatologic: Bruise (6%), skin rash (5%), pruritus (2%), alopecia (≥1%), xeroderma (≥1%)

Gastrointestinal: Diarrhea (7% to 10%), vomiting (7%), abdominal pain (5% to 7%), increased appetite (2%), gingivitis (≥1%), stomatitis (≥1%), oral mucosa ulcer (1%)

Endocrine & metabolic: Weight gain (≥1%), weight loss (≥1%)

Genitourinary: Urinary tract infection (5%), abnormal uterine bleeding (≥1%), dysmenorrhea (≥1%), dysuria (≥1%), urinary incontinence (≥1%), vaginitis (≥1%)
Hematologic & oncologic: Lymphadenopathy (≥1%)
Hypersensitivity: Hypersensitivity reaction (≥1%)
Neuromuscular & skeletal: Myalgia (5%), arthralgia (≥1%), hyperkinesia (≥1%), hypokinesia (≥1%), neck pain (≥1%)
Ophthalmic: Amblyopia (9%), nystagmus (2%), visual disturbance (≥1%)
Otic: Otalgia (≥1%), otitis media (≥1%), tinnitus (≥1%)
Respiratory: Flu-like symptoms (6% to 9%), pharyngitis (7% to 8%), increased cough (4%), bronchitis (≥1%), dyspnea (≥1%), epistaxis (≥1%), pneumonia (≥1%)
Miscellaneous: Language problems (2%), cyst (≥1%), diaphoresis (≥1%)

<1%, postmarketing, and/or case reports: Abnormal dreams, abnormal electroencephalogram, abnormal erythrocytes, abnormal hepatic function tests, abnormal pap smear, abnormal stools, abscess, ageusia, altered sense of smell, amenorrhea, anemia, angina pectoris, apathy, aphthous stomatitis, apnea, arthritis, asthma, benign skin neoplasm, blepharitis, blindness, blurred vision, brain disease, breast hypertrophy, bullous dermatitis, bursitis, cellulitis, cerebral ischemia, cholecystitis, cholelithiasis, CNS neoplasm, coma, contact dermatitis, cutaneous nodule, cystitis, deafness, dehydration, delusions, dental caries, dermal ulcer, dysgeusia, dysphagia, dystonia, ECG abnormality, eczema, eructation, esophagitis, exfoliative dermatitis, eye pain, facial edema, fecal incontinence, fibrocystic breast disease, furunculosis, gastritis, gastrointestinal hemorrhage, gingival hyperplasia, glossitis, goiter, halitosis, hematuria, hemiplegia, hemoptysis, hemorrhage, hepatomegaly, hernia, herpes simplex infection, herpes zoster, hiccups, hirsutism, hyperacusis, hypercholesteremia, hyperglycemia, hyperlipemia, hypermenorrhea, hyperreflexia, hyperventilation, hypoglycemia, hypokalemia, hyponatremia, hypotension, hypothyroidism, impotence, increased libido, increased thirst, keratoconjunctivitis, laryngitis, leg cramps, leukopenia, maculopapular rash, mastalgia, melena, movement disorder, muscle spasm, myocardial infarction, neck stiffness, neoplasm, neuritis, nocturia, oral paresthesia, orthostatic hypotension, osteoarthrosis, otitis externa, pallor, paralysis, pelvic pain, periodontal abscess, peripheral neuritis, peripheral vascular disease, petechia, phlebitis, photophobia, polyuria, psoriasis, psychoneurosis, psychosis, pyelonephritis, rectal hemorrhage, renal failure, salpingitis, seizure (in patients with or without underlying seizure disorder), sepsis, sialorrhea, skin carcinoma, skin discoloration, skin photosensitivity, status epilepticus, Stevens-Johnson syndrome, subcutaneous nodule, suicidal ideation, suicidal tendencies, tendinous contracture, thrombocytopenia, thrombophlebitis, urethritis, urinary retention, urinary urgency, urticaria, vaginal hemorrhage, vesiculobullous dermatitis, visual field defect, voice disorder, withdrawal syndrome (seizures with abrupt withdrawal), xerostomia

Mechanism of Action The exact mechanism by which tiagabine exerts antiseizure activity is not definitively known; however, *in vitro* experiments demonstrate that it enhances the activity of gamma aminobutyric acid (GABA). It is thought that the binding of tiagabine to the GABA uptake carrier inhibits the uptake of GABA into presynaptic neurons, allowing an increased amount of GABA to be available to postsynaptic neurons; based on *in vitro* studies, tiagabine does not inhibit the uptake of dopamine, norepinephrine, serotonin, glutamate, or choline

Pharmacodynamics/Kinetics

Half-life Elimination

Children 3 to 10 years: Mean: 5.7 hours (range: 2 to 10 hours); receiving enzyme-inducing AEDs: Mean: 3.2 hours (range: 2 to 7.8 hours)
Adults: 7 to 9 hours; receiving enzyme-inducing AEDs: 2 to 5 hours

Time to Peak Plasma: Fasting state: 45 minutes

Pregnancy Considerations

Adverse events were observed in animal reproduction studies. Information specific to the use of tiagabine in pregnancy is limited (Leppik 1999; Neppe 2000).

Patients exposed to tiagabine during pregnancy are encouraged to enroll themselves into the North American Antiepileptic Drug (NAAED) Pregnancy Registry by calling 1-888-233-2334. Additional information is available at www.aedpregnancyregistry.org.

◆ **Tiagabine HCl** *see* TiaGABine *on page 1443*

◆ **Tiagabine Hydrochloride** *see* TiaGABine *on page 1443*

◆ **Tiazac** *see* DilTIAZem *on page 499*

◆ **Tibsovo** *see* Ivosidenib *on page 851*

Ticagrelor (tye KA grel or)

Related Information

Antiplatelet and Anticoagulation Considerations in Dentistry *on page 1666*
Cardiovascular Diseases *on page 1654*

Brand Names: US Brilinta

Brand Names: Canada Brilinta

Pharmacologic Category Antiplatelet Agent; Antiplatelet Agent, Non-thienopyridine; P2Y12 Antagonist

Use

Acute coronary syndrome: To reduce the risk of cardiovascular death, myocardial infarction (MI), and stroke in patients with acute coronary syndrome (ACS) or a history of MI. Ticagrelor also reduces the risk of stent thrombosis in patients who have been stented for treatment of ACS.

Coronary artery disease (stable) and high risk for ischemic cardiovascular events, primary prevention: To reduce the risk of first MI or stroke in patients with coronary artery disease at high risk for such events. **Note:** Efficacy was established in patients with type 2 diabetes mellitus (Steg 2019), but the manufacturer does not limit use to this setting.

Local Anesthetic/Vasoconstrictor Precautions No information available to require special precautions

Effects on Dental Treatment No significant effects or complications reported (see Dental Health Professional Considerations)

Aspirin in combination with clopidogrel (Plavix), prasugrel (Effient), or ticagrelor (Brilinta) is the primary prevention strategy against stent thrombosis after placement of drug-eluting metal stents in coronary patients. Premature discontinuation of combination antiplatelet therapy (ie, dual antiplatelet therapy) strongly increases the risk of a catastrophic event of stent thrombosis leading to myocardial infarction and/or death, so says a science advisory issued in January 2007 from the American Heart Association in collaboration with the American Dental Association and other professional healthcare organizations. The advisory stresses a 12-month therapy of dual antiplatelet therapy after placement of a drug-eluting stent in order to prevent thrombosis at the stent site. Any elective surgery should be postponed for 1 year after stent implantation, and if surgery must be performed, consideration should be given to continuing the antiplatelet therapy during the perioperative period in high-risk patients with drug-eluting stents.

This advisory was issued from a science panel made up of representatives from the American Heart Association (AHA), the American College of Cardiology, the Society for Cardiovascular Angiography and Interventions, the American College of Surgeons, the American Dental Association (ADA), and the American College of Physicians (Grines, 2007).

Effects on Bleeding Ticagrelor is an antiplatelet agent similar in actions to clopidogrel. Major bleeding has been reported with a frequency of 12% of individuals (as composite of major fatal or life-threatening and other major bleeding events). Minor bleeding has occurred in ~5% of patients; also reported have been anemia, hematoma, and postprocedural hemorrhage (2%).

Dual antiplatelet therapy: Aspirin irreversibly inhibits platelet aggregation which can prolong bleeding. Upon discontinuation, normal platelet function returns only when new platelets are released (~7-10 days). However, in the case of dental surgery, there is no scientific evidence to support discontinuation of aspirin. The discontinuation of aspirin may place the patient at risk for a thrombotic event or other cardiovascular complication. In particular, aspirin should **not** be discontinued in patients with cardiac stents that have not completed their full course of dual antiplatelet therapy (eg, aspirin and clopidogrel [prasugrel or ticagrelor]); patient-specific situations need to be discussed with cardiologist. When feasible, postponement of dental surgery until the completion of dual antiplatelet therapy should be considered. Any modification of aspirin therapy should be discussed with the prescribing physician.

Adverse Reactions As with all drugs which may affect hemostasis, bleeding is associated with ticagrelor. Hemorrhage may occur at virtually any site. Risk is dependent on multiple variables, including the concurrent use of multiple agents which alter hemostasis and patient susceptibility.

>10%: Respiratory: Dyspnea (14%)

1% to 10%:

Cardiovascular: ECG abnormality (ventricular pause; 2% to 6%), presyncope (≤2%), syncope (≤2%)

Central nervous system: Dizziness (5%), loss of consciousness (≤2%)

Gastrointestinal: Nausea (4%)

Hematologic & oncologic: Major hemorrhage (4%), minor hemorrhage (4%)

Renal: Increased serum creatinine (7%; transient; mechanism undetermined)

Frequency not defined: Endocrine & metabolic: Increased uric acid

<1%, postmarketing, and/or case reports: Angioedema, atrioventricular block, bradycardia, gout, hypersensitivity reaction, skin rash, thrombotic thrombocytopenic purpura (Wang 2018)

Mechanism of Action Reversibly and noncompetitively binds the adenosine diphosphate (ADP) $P2Y_{12}$ receptor on the platelet surface which prevents ADP-mediated activation of the GPIIb/IIIa receptor complex thereby reducing platelet aggregation. Due to the reversible antagonism of the $P2Y_{12}$ receptor, recovery of platelet function is likely to depend on serum concentrations of ticagrelor and its active metabolite.

Pharmacodynamics/Kinetics

Onset of Action Inhibition of platelet aggregation (IPA): 180 mg loading dose: ~41% within 30 minutes (similar to clopidogrel 600 mg at 8 hours); Peak effect: Time to maximal IPA: 180 mg loading dose: IPA ~88% at 2 hours post administration

Duration of Action

IPA: 180 mg loading dose: 87% to 89% maintained from 2 to 8 hours; 24 hours after the last maintenance dose, IPA is 58% (similar to maintenance dosing for clopidogrel)

Time after discontinuation when IPA is 30%: ~56 hours; IPA 10%: ~110 hours (Gurbel 2009). Mean IPA observed with ticagrelor at 3 days post-discontinuation was comparable to that observed with clopidogrel at 5 days post discontinuation.

Half-life Elimination Parent drug: ~7 hours; active metabolite: ~9 hours

Time to Peak

Whole tablets: Parent drug: 1.5 hours (median; range: 1 to 4 hours); Active metabolite (AR-C124910XX): 2.5 hours (median; range: 1.5 to 5 hours)

Crushed tablets: Oral or nasogastric tube administration: Parent drug: ~1 hour (median; range: 1 to 4 hours); Active metabolite (AR-C124910XX): 2 hours (median; range: 1 to 8 hours). **Note:** Significantly higher concentrations of both ticagrelor and AR-C124910XX may appear at earlier time points (0.5 and 1 hour, respectively) when administered as crushed tablets (Teng 2015).

Pregnancy Considerations

Information related to the use of ticagrelor in pregnancy is limited (Verbruggen 2015).

Due to lack of data, use in pregnancy is not recommended (ESC [Regitz-Zagrosek 2018]).

Dental Health Professional Considerations Premature discontinuation of ticagrelor therapy may increase the risk of cardiac events (eg, stent thrombosis with subsequent fatal or nonfatal myocardial infarction). Duration of therapy, in general, is determined by the type of stent placed (bare metal or drug eluting) and whether an acute coronary syndrome event was ongoing at the time of placement. Patient-specific situations need to be discussed with healthcare provider.

Patients taking ticagrelor may have shortness of breath.

If patient is taking aspirin along with ticagrelor, aspirin dose should not exceed 100 mg/day. Patient should also avoid taking any other medicine containing aspirin.

Ticarcillin and Clavulanate Potassium

(tye kar SIL in & klav yoo LAN ate poe TASS ee um)

Brand Names: US Timentin [DSC]

Pharmacologic Category Antibiotic, Penicillin

Use

Bone and joint infections: Treatment of bone and joint infections caused by beta-lactamase-producing isolates of *Staphylococcus aureus*.

Endometritis: Treatment of endometritis caused by beta-lactamase-producing isolates of *Prevotella melaninogenicus*, *Enterobacter* species (including *E. cloacae*), *Klebsiella pneumoniae*, *Escherichia coli*, *S. aureus*, or *Staphylococcus epidermidis*.

Lower respiratory tract infections: Treatment of lower respiratory tract infections caused by beta-lactamase-producing isolates of *S. aureus*, *Haemophilus influenzae*, or *Klebsiella* species.

Peritonitis: Treatment of peritonitis caused by beta-lactamase-producing isolates of *E. coli*, *K. pneumonia*, or *Bacteroides fragilis* group.

Septicemia: Treatment of septicemia (including bacteremia) caused by beta-lactamase-producing isolates of *Klebsiella* species, *E. coli*, *S. aureus*, or *Pseudomonas aeruginosa* (or other *Pseudomonas* species).

Skin and skin structure infections: Treatment of skin and skin structure infections caused by beta-lactamase-producing isolates of *S. aureus*, *Klebsiella* species, or *E. coli*.

Urinary tract infections: Treatment of complicated and uncomplicated urinary tract infections caused by beta-lactamase-producing isolates of *E. coli*, *Klebsiella* species, *P. aeruginosa* (and other *Pseudomonas* species), *Citrobacter* species, *Enterobacter cloacae*, *Serratia marcescens*, or *S. aureus*.

Local Anesthetic/Vasoconstrictor Precautions
No information available to require special precautions

Effects on Dental Treatment Key adverse event(s) related to dental treatment: Prolonged use of penicillins may lead to development of oral candidiasis.

Effects on Bleeding May inhibit platelet aggregation (dose related). No information available to require special precautions

Adverse Reactions Frequency not defined.

Cardiovascular: Local thrombophlebitis (with IV injection)

Central nervous system: Confusion, drowsiness, headache, seizure

Dermatologic: Skin rash

Endocrine & metabolic: Electrolyte disturbance, hypernatremia, hypokalemia

Gastrointestinal: *Clostridioides* (formerly *Clostridium*) *difficile*-diarrhea, diarrhea, nausea

Genitourinary: Proteinuria (false positive)

Hematologic & oncologic: Bleeding complication, eosinophilia, hemolytic anemia, positive direct Coombs' test (false positive)

Hepatic: Hepatotoxicity, increased serum ALT, increased serum AST, jaundice

Immunologic: Jarisch Herxheimer reaction

Infection: Superinfection (fungal or bacterial)

Renal: Interstitial nephritis (acute)

Miscellaneous: Anaphylaxis

Postmarketing and/or case reports: Abdominal pain, altered sense of smell, arthralgia, chest discomfort, chills, decreased hematocrit, decreased hemoglobin, decreased serum potassium, dizziness, dysgeusia, erythema multiforme, fever, flatulence, headache, hemorrhagic cystitis, hypersensitivity reaction, hypouricemia, increased blood urea nitrogen, increased lactate dehydrogenase, increased serum alkaline phosphatase, increased serum bilirubin, increased serum creatinine, injection site reaction (burning, induration, pain, swelling), leukopenia, myalgia, myclonus, neutropenia, prolonged prothrombin time, pruritus, pseudomembranous colitis (during or after antibacterial treatment), Stevens-Johnson syndrome, stomatitis, thrombocytopenia, toxic epidermal necrolysis, urticaria, vomiting

Mechanism of Action Inhibits bacterial cell wall synthesis by binding to one or more of the penicillin-binding proteins (PBPs), which in turn inhibits the final transpeptidation step of peptidoglycan synthesis in bacterial cell walls, thus inhibiting cell wall biosynthesis. Bacteria eventually lyse due to ongoing activity of cell wall autolytic enzymes (autolysins and murein hydrolases) while cell wall assembly is arrested.

Pharmacodynamics/Kinetics

Half-life Elimination

Neonates: Ticarcillin: 4.4 hours; Clavulanic acid: 1.9 hours

Children (1 month to 9.3 years): Ticarcillin: 66 minutes; Clavulanic acid: 54 minutes

Adults: Ticarcillin: 66 to 72 minutes; 13 hours (in patients with renal failure); Clavulanic acid: 66 to 90 minutes; clavulanic acid does not affect the clearance of ticarcillin

Time to Peak Immediately following completion of 30-minute infusion

Pregnancy Risk Factor B

Pregnancy Considerations
Ticarcillin and clavulanate cross the placenta (Maberry, 1992). Maternal use of penicillins has generally not resulted in an increased risk of adverse fetal effects (Crider 2009; Santos 2011). Ticarcillin/clavulanate is approved for the treatment of postpartum gynecologic infections, including endometritis, caused by susceptible organisms.

Product Availability Not available in the US

- **Ticarcillin and Clavulanic Acid** *see* Ticarcillin and Clavulanate Potassium *on page 1445*
- **Ticarcillin/K Clavulanate** *see* Ticarcillin and Clavulanate Potassium *on page 1445*
- **Ticaspray [DSC]** *see* Fluticasone (Nasal) *on page 703*

Ticlopidine (tye KLOE pi deen)

Related Information
Antiplatelet and Anticoagulation Considerations in Dentistry *on page 1666*

Brand Names: Canada Apo-Ticlopidine; Teva-Ticlopidine

Pharmacologic Category Antiplatelet Agent; Antiplatelet Agent, Thienopyridine; P2Y12 Antagonist

Use Platelet aggregation inhibitor that reduces the risk of thrombotic stroke in patients who have had a stroke or stroke precursors (**Note:** Due to its association with life-threatening hematologic disorders, ticlopidine should be reserved for patients who are intolerant to aspirin, who have failed aspirin therapy, or who are not eligible to receive other antiplatelet therapy.)

Local Anesthetic/Vasoconstrictor Precautions
No information available to require special precautions

Effects on Dental Treatment No significant effects or complications reported; if a patient is to undergo elective surgery and an antiplatelet effect is not desired, ticlopidine should be discontinued at least 7 days prior to surgery.

Effects on Bleeding Ticlopidine blocks platelet aggregation and may prolong bleeding time. Inhibition is irreversible; on discontinuation, normal platelet function returns only when new platelets are released from the bone marrow. Dental practitioners should note that recommendations differ between general surgery (eg, appendectomy, hip replacement) and dental surgery. Prior to elective general surgery, it may be temporarily discontinued (usually for 5-10 days) to restore platelet function. However, routine interruption of therapy for noninvasive dental procedures is NOT warranted and there is no scientific evidence to warrant the discontinuance of ticlopidine prior to dental surgery. In particular, ticlopidine should NOT be discontinued in patients with cardiac stents that have not completed their full course of dual antiplatelet therapy (aspirin, clopidogrel/ticlopidine); patient specific situations need to be discussed with cardiologist. When feasible, postponement of dental surgery until the completion of dual antiplatelet therapy should be considered.

Adverse Reactions As with all drugs which may affect hemostasis, bleeding is associated with ticlopidine. Hemorrhage may occur at virtually any site. Risk is dependent on multiple variables, including the use of multiple agents which alter hemostasis and patient susceptibility.

>10%:

Endocrine & metabolic: Hyperlipidemia (8% to 10%; within 1 month of therapy), increased serum triglycerides

Gastrointestinal: Diarrhea (13%; may be chronic)

1% to 10%:

Central nervous system: Dizziness (1%)

Dermatologic: Skin rash (5%), pruritus (1%)

Gastrointestinal: Dyspepsia (7%), nausea (7%), gastrointestinal pain (4%), flatulence (2%), vomiting (2%), anorexia (1%)

Hematologic & oncologic: Neutropenia (2%), purpura (2%)

Hepatic: Increased serum alkaline phosphatase (>2 x upper limit of normal: 8%), abnormal hepatic function tests (1%)

<1%, postmarketing, and/or case reports: Agranulocytosis, anaphylaxis, angioedema, aplastic anemia, arthropathy, bone marrow depression, bronchiolitis obliterans organizing pneumonia, conjunctival hemorrhage, ecchymosis, eosinophilia, epistaxis, erythema multiforme, erythema nodosum, exfoliative dermatitis, gastrointestinal hemorrhage, headache, hematuria, hemolytic anemia, hepatic necrosis, hepatitis, hypermenorrhea, hypersensitivity pneumonitis, hyponatremia, increased serum bilirubin, intracranial hemorrhage, immune thrombocytopenia, increased serum creatinine, jaundice, maculopapular rash, myositis, nephrotic syndrome, pain, pancytopenia, peptic ulcer, peripheral neuropathy, positive ANA titer, renal failure, sepsis, serum sickness, Stevens-Johnson syndrome, systemic lupus erythematosus, thrombocythemia, thrombotic thrombocytopenic purpura (TTP), tinnitus, urticaria, vasculitis, weakness

Mechanism of Action Ticlopidine requires *in vivo* biotransformation to an unidentified active metabolite. This active metabolite irreversibly blocks the P2Y12 component of ADP receptors, which prevents activation of the GPIIb/IIIa receptor complex, thereby reducing platelet aggregation. Platelets blocked by ticlopidine are affected for the remainder of their lifespan.

Pharmacodynamics/Kinetics

Onset of Action ~6 hours; Peak effect: 3-5 days; serum levels do not correlate with clinical antiplatelet activity

Half-life Elimination 13 hours

Time to Peak ~2 hours

Pregnancy Risk Factor B

Pregnancy Considerations

Teratogenic effects have not been observed in animal reproduction studies. Information related to ticlopidine use in a pregnant woman has been noted in a case report (Ueno 2001).

Product Availability Ticlopidine is no longer available in the US.

◆ **Ticlopidine HCl** *see* Ticlopidine *on page 1446*

◆ **Ticlopidine Hydrochloride** *see* Ticlopidine *on page 1446*

◆ **TIG** *see* Tetanus Immune Globulin (Human) *on page 1427*

Tigecycline (tye ge SYE kleen)

Brand Names: US Tygacil

Brand Names: Canada Tygacil

Pharmacologic Category Antibiotic, Glycylcycline

Use

Intra-abdominal infections, complicated: Treatment of complicated intra-abdominal infections in patients ≥18 years of age caused by *Citrobacter freundii*, *Enterobacter cloacae*, *Escherichia coli*, *Klebsiella oxytoca*, *Klebsiella pneumoniae*, *Enterococcus faecalis* (vancomycin-susceptible isolates), *Staphylococcus aureus* (methicillin-susceptible and methicillin-resistant isolates), *Streptococcus anginosus* group (includes *S. anginosus*, *Streptococcus intermedius*, and *Streptococcus constellatus*), *Bacteroides fragilis*, *Bacteroides thetaiotaomicron*, *Bacteroides uniformis*, *Bacteroides vulgatus*, *Clostridium perfringens*, and *Peptostreptococcus micros*.

Pneumonia, community acquired: Treatment of community-acquired bacterial pneumonia in patients ≥18 years of age caused by *Streptococcus pneumoniae* (penicillin-susceptible isolates), including cases with concurrent bacteremia, *Haemophilus influenzae*, and *Legionella pneumophila*.

Skin and skin structure infections, complicated: Treatment of complicated skin and skin structure infections in patients ≥18 years of age caused by *E. coli*, *E. faecalis* (vancomycin-susceptible isolates), *S. aureus* (methicillin-susceptible and methicillin-resistant isolates), *Streptococcus agalactiae*, *S. anginosus* group (includes *S. anginosus*, *S. intermedius*, and *S. constellatus*), *Streptococcus pyogenes*, *E. cloacae*, *K. pneumoniae*, and *B. fragilis*.

Local Anesthetic/Vasoconstrictor Precautions

No information available to require special precautions

Effects on Dental Treatment Key adverse events(s) related to dental treatment: Tigecycline is structurally similar to tetracycline. Therefore, tigecycline is not recommended for use in pregnancy or in children ≤8 years of age. Permanent discoloration of the teeth may occur if used during tooth development.

Effects on Bleeding No information available to require special precautions

Adverse Reactions

>10%: Gastrointestinal: Nausea (24% to 35%), vomiting (16% to 20%), diarrhea (12%)

1% to 10%:

Cardiovascular: Localized phlebitis (≤3%), septic shock (<2%), thrombophlebitis (<2%)

Central nervous system: Headache (6%), dizziness (3%), chills (<2%)

Dermatologic: Skin rash (3%), pruritus (<2%)

Endocrine & metabolic: Increased amylase (3%), hyponatremia (2%), hypocalcemia (<2%), hypoglycemia (<2%)

Gastrointestinal: Abdominal pain (6%), dyspepsia (2%), abnormal stools (<2%), anorexia (<2%), dysgeusia (<2%)

Genitourinary: Leukorrhea (<2%), vaginitis (<2%), vulvovaginal candidiasis (<2%)

Hematologic & oncologic: Anemia (5%), hypoproteinemia (5%), eosinophilia (<2%), increased INR (<2%), prolonged partial thromboplastin time (<2%), prolonged prothrombin time (<2%), thrombocytopenia (<2%)
Hepatic: Increased serum ALT (5%), increased serum AST (4%), increased serum alkaline phosphatase (3%), hyperbilirubinemia (2%), jaundice (<2%)
Hypersensitivity: Hypersensitivity reaction (<2%)
Infection: Infection (7%), abscess (2%)
Local: Inflammation at injection site (<2%), injection site reaction (<2%), pain at injection site (<2%), swelling at injection site (<2%)
Neuromuscular & skeletal: Weakness (3%)
Renal: Increased blood urea nitrogen (3%), increased serum creatinine (<2%)
Respiratory: Pneumonia (2%)

<1%, postmarketing, and/or case reports: Acute pancreatitis, allergic skin reaction, anaphylactoid reaction, anaphylaxis, *Clostridioides* (formerly *Clostridium*) *difficile*-associated diarrhea, hepatic dysfunction, hepatic failure, hypersensitivity reaction, hypoglycemia signs and symptoms (diabetic and nondiabetic patients), intrahepatic cholestasis, Stevens-Johnson syndrome

Mechanism of Action A glycylcycline antibiotic that binds to the 30S ribosomal subunit of susceptible bacteria, thereby, inhibiting protein synthesis. Generally considered bacteriostatic; however, bactericidal activity has been demonstrated against isolates of *S. pneumoniae* and *L. pneumophila*. Tigecycline is a derivative of minocycline (9-t-butylglycylamido minocycline), and while not classified as a tetracycline, it may share some class-associated adverse effects. Tigecycline has demonstrated activity against a variety of gram-positive and -negative bacterial pathogens including methicillin-resistant staphylococci.

Pharmacodynamics/Kinetics

Half-life Elimination Single dose: 27 hours; following multiple doses: 42 hours; increased by 23% in moderate hepatic impairment and 43% in severe hepatic impairment

Pregnancy Considerations Tigecycline crosses the placenta.

Tetracyclines accumulate in developing teeth and long tubular bones (Mylonas 2011). Permanent discoloration of teeth (yellow, gray, brown) can occur following in utero exposure and is more likely to occur following long-term use or short-term repeated exposure. In addition, tetracycline use has been associated with reversible retardation of skeletal development and reduced bone growth.

- **Tiglutik** *see* Riluzole *on page 1328*
- **Tikosyn** *see* Dofetilide *on page 509*

Tildrakizumab (til dra KIZ ue mab)

Brand Names: US Ilumya

Pharmacologic Category Antipsoriatic Agent; Interleukin-23 Inhibitor; Monoclonal Antibody

Use Plaque psoriasis: Treatment of adults with moderate to severe plaque psoriasis who are candidates for systemic therapy or phototherapy.

Local Anesthetic/Vasoconstrictor Precautions No information available to require special precautions

Effects on Dental Treatment No significant effects or complications reported

Effects on Bleeding No information available to require special precautions

Adverse Reactions

>10%:
Infection: Infection (23%)
Respiratory: Upper respiratory tract infection (14%)

1% to 10%:
Gastrointestinal: Diarrhea (2%)
Immunologic: Antibody development (7%; neutralizing: 3%)
Local: Injection site reaction (3%)

Frequency not defined:
Dermatologic: Urticaria
Hypersensitivity: Angioedema
Respiratory: Tuberculosis

<1%, postmarketing, and/or case reports: Dizziness, limb pain, severe infection

Mechanism of Action Human IgG1/k monoclonal antibody which selectively binds to the p19 subunit of interleukin (IL)-23, thereby inhibiting its interaction with the IL-23 receptor, resulting in inhibition of the proinflammatory cytokines and chemokines associated the binding of naturally occurring IL-23.

Pharmacodynamics/Kinetics

Half-life Elimination ~23 days

Time to Peak ~6 days; steady state concentrations reached by week 16

Reproductive Considerations Contraception was required of females of reproductive potential and males with female partners of reproductive potential during the initial studies of tildrakizumab (Haycraft 2020).

Pregnancy Considerations

Tildrakizumab is a humanized monoclonal antibody (IgG_1). Placental transfer of human IgG is dependent upon the IgG subclass, maternal serum concentrations, birth weight, and gestational age, generally increasing as pregnancy progresses. The lowest exposure would be expected during the period of organogenesis (Palmeira 2012; Pentsuk 2009).

Outcome information following inadvertent exposure to tildrakizumab during pregnancy is limited. During the initial studies, tildrakizumab was discontinued in all cases (n=14) once pregnancy was confirmed (Haycraft 2020).

- **Tildrakizumab-asmn** *see* Tildrakizumab *on page 1448*
- **Tilia Fe** *see* Ethinyl Estradiol and Norethindrone *on page 614*
- **Timentin [DSC]** *see* Ticarcillin and Clavulanate Potassium *on page 1445*
- **Timolol and Dorzolamide** *see* Dorzolamide and Timolol *on page 516*
- **Tinactin [OTC]** *see* Tolnaftate *on page 1462*
- **Tinactin Deodorant [OTC]** *see* Tolnaftate *on page 1462*
- **Tinactin Jock Itch [OTC] [DSC]** *see* Tolnaftate *on page 1462*
- **Tinaspore [OTC]** *see* Tolnaftate *on page 1462*
- **Tindamax** *see* Tinidazole *on page 1448*
- **Tindamax [DSC]** *see* Tinidazole *on page 1448*

Tinidazole (tye NI da zole)

Brand Names: US Tindamax [DSC]

Pharmacologic Category Amebicide; Antibiotic, Miscellaneous; Antiprotozoal, Nitroimidazole

Use

Amebiasis: Treatment of intestinal amebiasis and amebic liver abscess caused by *Entamoeba histolytica* in adults and pediatric patients older than 3 years.

Limitations of use: Not indicated for the treatment of asymptomatic cyst passage.

Bacterial vaginosis: Treatment of bacterial vaginosis (formerly referred to as *Haemophilus* vaginitis, *Gardnerella vaginitis*, nonspecific vaginitis, or anaerobic vaginosis) in adult women.

Giardiasis: Treatment of giardiasis caused by *Giardia duodenalis* (also termed *Giardia lamblia*) in adults and pediatric patients older than 3 years.

Trichomoniasis: Treatment of trichomoniasis caused by *Trichomonas vaginalis*; treat partners of infected patients simultaneously to prevent reinfection.

Local Anesthetic/Vasoconstrictor Precautions
No information available to require special precautions

Effects on Dental Treatment Key adverse event(s) related to dental treatment: Xerostomia and changes in salivation (normal salivary flow resumes upon discontinuation), metallic/bitter taste, oral candidiasis, tongue discoloration, stomatitis, furry tongue. See Dental Health Professional Considerations.

Effects on Bleeding No information available to require special precautions

Adverse Reactions

1% to 10%:

- Central nervous system: Fatigue (≤2%), malaise (≤2%), dizziness (≤1%), headache (≤1%)
- Dermatologic: Body odor (vaginal: >2%)
- Endocrine & metabolic: Hypermenorrhea (>2%)
- Gastrointestinal: Dysgeusia (bitter taste, metallic taste: 4% to 6%), nausea (3% to 5%), anorexia (2% to 3%), decreased appetite (>2%), flatulence (>2%), dyspepsia (≤2%), abdominal cramps (≤2%), epigastric distress (≤2%), vomiting (1% to 2%), constipation (≤1%)
- Genitourinary: Vulvovaginal candidiasis (5%), dysuria (>2%), pelvic pain (>2%), urine abnormality (>2%), vulvovaginal disease (discomfort) (>2%)
- Neuromuscular & skeletal: Weakness (1% to 2%)
- Renal: Urinary tract infection (>2%)
- Respiratory: Upper respiratory tract infection (>2%)

Frequency not defined:

- Cardiovascular: Flushing, palpitations
- Central nervous system: Ataxia, burning sensation, drowsiness, insomnia, peripheral neuropathy (transient; includes numbness and paresthesia), seizure, vertigo
- Dermatologic: Diaphoresis, pruritus, skin rash, urticaria
- Endocrine & metabolic: Increased thirst
- Gastrointestinal: Abdominal pain, diarrhea, oral candidiasis, salivation, stomatitis, tongue discoloration, xerostomia
- Genitourinary: Dark urine, vaginal discharge
- Hematologic & oncologic: Leukopenia (transient), neutropenia (transient)
- Hepatic: Increased serum transaminases
- Hypersensitivity: Angioedema
- Infection: Candidiasis (overgrowth)
- Neuromuscular & skeletal: Arthralgia, arthritis, myalgia
- Miscellaneous: Fever

<1%, postmarketing, and/or case reports: Bronchospasm, coma, confusion, depression, dyspnea, erythema multiforme, hairy tongue, hypersensitivity reaction (acute, severe), pharyngitis, Stevens-Johnson syndrome, thrombocytopenia (reversible)

Mechanism of Action After diffusing into the organism, it is proposed that tinidazole causes cytotoxicity by damaging DNA and preventing further DNA synthesis.

Pharmacodynamics/Kinetics

Half-life Elimination 13.2 hours

Time to Peak 1.6 hours (fasting, delayed ~2 hours when given with food)

Pregnancy Considerations

Tinidazole crosses the human placenta and enters the fetal circulation (Karhunen 1984).

The safety of tinidazole for the treatment of bacterial vaginosis or trichomoniasis in pregnant women has not been well evaluated. Other agents are preferred for use during pregnancy (CDC [Workowski 2015]).

Dental Health Professional Considerations
Although this drug is a member of the metronidazole family, there is no specific dental indication for its use. Just as with metronidazole, alcohol in any form is contraindicated while the patient is on this medication because of the danger of a disulfiram-type reaction.

Tinzaparin (tin ZA pa rin)

Related Information

Cardiovascular Diseases *on page 1654*

Brand Names: Canada Innohep

Pharmacologic Category Anticoagulant; Anticoagulant, Low Molecular Weight Heparin

Use Note: Not available in the United States.

Anticoagulation in extracorporeal circuit during hemodialysis: Prevention of clotting in indwelling intravenous lines and extracorporeal circuit during hemodialysis (in patients without high bleeding risk).

Deep vein thrombosis/pulmonary embolus (treatment): Treatment of deep vein thrombosis (DVT) and/or pulmonary embolism (PE). **Note:** In patients with venous thromboembolism (VTE) (ie, DVT or PE) and *without* cancer, oral anticoagulants are preferred over low molecular weight heparin (LMWH) (unless LMWH is used as initial parenteral anticoagulation prior to dabigatran, edoxaban, or while initiating warfarin). In patients with venous thromboembolism (VTE) (ie, DVT or PE) **and** cancer, ACCP recommends LMWH over oral anticoagulants for initial and long-term treatment (Kearon 2012; Kearon 2016).

Postoperative thromboprophylaxis: Prevention of VTE following orthopedic surgery or following general surgery in patients at high risk of VTE.

Local Anesthetic/Vasoconstrictor Precautions
No information available to require special precautions

Effects on Dental Treatment Key adverse event(s) related to dental treatment: Bleeding is the major adverse effect of tinzaparin. See Effects on Bleeding.

Effects on Bleeding As with all anticoagulants, bleeding is the major adverse effect of tinzaparin. Hemorrhage may occur at virtually any site; risk is dependent on multiple variables including the intensity of anticoagulation and patient susceptibility. At the recommended doses, LMWHS do not significantly influence platelet aggregation or affect global clotting time (ie, PT or aPTT). Medical consult is suggested.

Adverse Reactions As with all anticoagulants, bleeding is the major adverse effect of tinzaparin. Hemorrhage may occur at virtually any site. Risk is dependent on multiple variables.

>10%:

- Hepatic: Increased serum ALT (≤13%)
- Local: Hematoma at injection site

1% to 10%:

Cardiovascular: Chest pain (2%), angina pectoris (≥1%), cardiac arrhythmia (≥1%), coronary thrombosis (≥1%), myocardial infarction (≥1%), thromboembolism (≥1%)

Central nervous system: Headache (2%), pain (2%)

Dermatologic: Bullous rash (≥1%), erythematous rash (≥1%), maculopapular rash (≥1%), skin necrosis (≥1%)

Endocrine & metabolic: Dependent edema (≥1%)

Gastrointestinal: Nausea (2%), abdominal pain (1%), constipation (1%), diarrhea (1%), vomiting (1%)

Genitourinary: Urinary tract infection (4%)

Hematologic & oncologic: Granulocytopenia (≥1%), hemorrhage (≥1%, including anorectal bleeding, gastrointestinal hemorrhage, hemarthrosis, hematemesis, hematuria, hemopericardium, injection site bleeding, melena, purpura, intra-abdominal bleeding, vaginal bleeding, wound hemorrhage; major: ≤3%, including intracranial, retroperitoneal, or bleeding into a major prosthetic joint), neoplasm (≥1%), thrombocytopenia (≥1%)

Hepatic: Increased serum AST (9%)

Hypersensitivity: Hypersensitivity reaction (≥1%)

Local: Cellulitis at injection site (≥1%)

Neuromuscular & skeletal: Back pain (2%)

Respiratory: Epistaxis (2%), dyspnea (1%)

Miscellaneous: Fever (2%)

<1%, postmarketing, and/or case reports: Agranulocytosis, angioedema, anaphylactoid reaction, epidural hematoma (spinal), hemophthalmos, hemoptysis, hyperkalemia, increased gamma-glutamyl transferase, increased, lactate dehydrogenase, increased serum lipase, metabolic acidosis, osteoporosis, priapism, pruritus, skin rash, Stevens-Johnson syndrome, suppression of aldosterone synthesis, thrombocythemia, toxic epidermal necrolysis, urticaria

Mechanism of Action Tinzaparin is a low molecular weight heparin (average molecular weight ranges between 5,500 and 7,500 daltons, distributed as <2,000 daltons [<10%], 2,000 to 8,000 daltons [60% to 72%], and >8,000 daltons [22% to 36%]) that binds antithrombin III, enhancing the inhibition of several clotting factors, particularly factor Xa. Tinzaparin anti-Xa activity (70 to 120 units/mg) is greater than anti-IIa activity (~55 units/mg) and it has a higher ratio of antifactor Xa to antifactor IIa activity compared to unfractionated heparin. Low molecular weight heparins have a small effect on the activated partial thromboplastin time.

Pharmacodynamics/Kinetics

Duration of Action Detectable anti-Xa activity persists for 24 hours

Half-life Elimination 82 minutes; prolonged in renal impairment

Time to Peak 4 to 6 hours

Pregnancy Considerations

Use is contraindicated in conditions involving increased risks of hemorrhage, including women with imminent abortion.

Tinzaparin does not cross the human placenta; increased risks of fetal bleeding or teratogenic effects have not been reported (Bates 2012). Low molecular weight heparin (LMWH) is recommended over unfractionated heparin for the treatment of acute venous thromboembolism (VTE) in pregnant women. LMWH is also recommended over unfractionated heparin for VTE prophylaxis in pregnant women with certain risk factors. LMWH should be discontinued prior to induction of labor or a planned cesarean delivery. For women undergoing cesarean section and who have additional risk factors for developing VTE, the prophylactic use of LMWH may be considered (Bates 2012). When choosing therapy, fetal outcomes (ie, pregnancy loss, malformations), maternal outcomes (ie, VTE, hemorrhage), burden of therapy, and maternal preference should be considered (Bates 2012).

Multiple-dose vials contain benzyl alcohol (avoid use in pregnant women due to association with gasping syndrome in premature infants); use of preservative-free formulation is recommended.

◆ **Tinzaparin Sodium** *see* Tinzaparin *on page 1449*

Tioconazole (tye oh KONE a zole)

Brand Names: US Vagistat-1 [OTC] [DSC]

Pharmacologic Category Antifungal Agent, Imidazole Derivative; Antifungal Agent, Vaginal

Use Candidiasis, vulvovaginal: Local treatment of vulvovaginal candidiasis

Local Anesthetic/Vasoconstrictor Precautions No information available to require special precautions

Effects on Dental Treatment No significant effects or complications reported

Effects on Bleeding No information available to require special precautions

Adverse Reactions Frequency not defined.

Central nervous system: Headache

Gastrointestinal: Abdominal pain

Dermatologic: Burning sensation of skin, exfoliation of skin

Genitourinary: Dyspareunia, dysuria, nocturia, vaginal discharge, vaginal pain, vaginitis, vulvar swelling, vulvovaginal irritation, vulvovaginal pruritus

Mechanism of Action A 1-substituted imidazole derivative with a broad antifungal spectrum against a wide variety of dermatophytes and yeasts, including *Trichophyton mentagrophytes*, *T. rubrum*, *T. erinacei*, *T. tonsurans*, *Microsporum canis*, *Microsporum gypseum*, and *Candida albicans*. Both agents appear to be similarly effective against *Epidermophyton floccosum*.

Pharmacodynamics/Kinetics

Onset of Action Onset of action: Some improvement: Within 24 hours; Complete relief: Within 7 days

Reproductive Considerations

This product may weaken latex condoms and diaphragms (CDC [Workowski 2015]).

Pregnancy Considerations

Following vaginal administration, small amounts of imidazoles are absorbed systemically. Single dose, topical azole regimens are not recommended for the treatment of vulvovaginal candidiasis; only topical azole products with 7-day regimens are recommended in pregnant women with vulvovaginal candidiasis.

◆ **Tioguanine** *see* Thioguanine *on page 1438*

Tiotropium (ty oh TRO pee um)

Related Information

Dentin Hypersensitivity, Acid Erosion, High Caries Index, Management of Alveolar Osteitis, and Xerostomia *on page 1762*

Respiratory Diseases *on page 1680*

Brand Names: US Spiriva HandiHaler; Spiriva Respimat

Brand Names: Canada Spiriva; Spiriva Respimat

Pharmacologic Category Anticholinergic Agent; Anticholinergic Agent, Long-Acting

Use

Asthma (Spiriva Respimat only): Maintenance treatment of asthma in patients ≥6 years.

Chronic obstructive pulmonary disease: Maintenance treatment of bronchospasm associated with chronic obstructive pulmonary disease (COPD), including chronic bronchitis and emphysema; reduction of COPD exacerbations.

Limitations of use: Not indicated for the relief of acute bronchospasm.

Local Anesthetic/Vasoconstrictor Precautions No information available to require special precautions

Effects on Dental Treatment Key adverse event(s) related to dental treatment: Xerostomia (normal salivary flow resumes upon discontinuation) and ulcerative stomatitis.

Effects on Bleeding No information available to require special precautions

Adverse Reactions Non-postmarketing incidences listed are for powder for inhalation unless otherwise specified.

>10%:

Gastrointestinal: Xerostomia (powder and solution: 4% to 16%)

Respiratory: Upper respiratory tract infection (41% to 43%), pharyngitis (powder and solution: 7% to 16%), sinusitis (powder and solution: 3% to 11%)

1% to 10%:

Cardiovascular: Chest pain (powder and solution: ≤7%), edema (dependent, 3% to 5%), angina pectoris (1% to 3%; includes exacerbation of angina pectoris), palpitations (powder and solution: ≤3%), hypertension (solution: 1% to 2%)

Central nervous system: Headache (powder and solution: 4% to 6%), depression (≤4%), insomnia (powder and solution: ≤4%), paresthesia (1% to 3%), dizziness (powder and solution: ≤3%), voice disorder (powder and solution: ≤3%)

Dermatologic: Skin rash (powder and solution: 1% to 4%), pruritus (powder and solution: ≤3%)

Endocrine & metabolic: Hypercholesterolemia (1% to 3%), hyperglycemia (1% to 3%)

Gastrointestinal: Abdominal pain (5% to 6%), dyspepsia (1% to 6%), constipation (powder and solution: 1% to 5%), vomiting (1% to 4%), gastrointestinal disease (not otherwise specified; 1% to 3%), gastroesophageal reflux disease (powder and solution: ≤3%), oropharyngeal candidiasis (powder and solution: ≤3%), stomatitis (includes ulcerative stomatitis; powder and solution: ≤3%), diarrhea (solution: 1% to 2%)

Genitourinary: Urinary tract infection (powder and solution: 1% to 7%)

Hypersensitivity: Hypersensitivity reaction (powder and solution: ≤3%)

Infection: Candidiasis (3% to 4%), infection (1% to 4%), herpes zoster (powder and solution: ≤3%)

Neuromuscular & skeletal: Arthralgia (powder and solution: ≤4%), myalgia (4%), arthritis (≥3%), leg pain (1% to 3%), skeletal pain (1% to 3%)

Ophthalmic: Cataract (1% to 3%)

Respiratory: Rhinitis (powder and solution: ≤6%), epistaxis (powder and solution: ≤4%), cough (powder: ≥3%; solution: 1% to 2%), flu-like symptoms (≥3%), bronchitis (solution: 3%), laryngitis (powder and solution: ≤3%), allergic rhinitis (solution: 1% to 2%)

Miscellaneous: Fever (solution: 1% to 2%)

<1%, postmarketing, and/or case reports: Abnormal hepatic function tests, anaphylaxis, angioedema, application site irritation (powder; includes glossitis, oral mucosa ulcer, pharyngolaryngeal pain), atrial fibrillation, blurred vision, bronchospasm, dehydration, dermal ulcer, dysphagia, dysuria, gingivitis, glaucoma, glossitis, hepatic insufficiency, hoarseness, increased intraocular pressure, intestinal obstruction (includes paralytic ileus), joint swelling, limb pain, muscle spasm, mydriasis (if powder comes in contact with eyes), oropharyngeal pain, paradoxical bronchospasm, skin infection, supraventricular tachycardia, tachycardia, throat irritation, tonsillitis, urinary retention, urticaria, xeroderma

Mechanism of Action Competitively and reversibly inhibits the action of acetylcholine at type 3 muscarinic (M_3) receptors in bronchial smooth muscle causing bronchodilation

Pharmacodynamics/Kinetics

Half-life Elimination

Dry powder inhaler: COPD: ~25 hours

Soft-mist inhaler: Asthma: 44 hours; COPD: 25 hours

Time to Peak

Dry powder inhaler: Plasma: 7 minutes (following inhalation)

Soft-mist inhaler: Plasma: 5 to 7 minutes (following inhalation)

Pregnancy Considerations

Uncontrolled asthma is associated with adverse events in pregnancy (increased risk of perinatal mortality, preeclampsia, preterm birth, low birth weight infants, cesarean delivery, and the development of gestational diabetes). Poorly controlled asthma or asthma exacerbations may have a greater fetal/maternal risk than what is associated with appropriately used asthma medications. Maternal treatment improves pregnancy outcomes by reducing the risk of some adverse events (eg, preterm birth, gestational diabetes) (ERS/TSANZ [Middleton 2020]; GINA 2020).

Although information related to tiotropium use in pregnancy is limited, use is likely acceptable. Maternal asthma symptoms should be monitored monthly during pregnancy (ERS/TSANZ [Middleton 2020]).

Data collection to monitor pregnancy and infant outcomes associated with asthma and the medications used to treat asthma in pregnancy is ongoing. Health care providers are encouraged to enroll exposed pregnant females in the MotherToBaby Pregnancy Studies conducted by the Organization of Teratology Information Specialists (1-877-311-8972 or https://mothertobaby.org). Patients may also enroll themselves.

Tiotropium and Olodaterol

(ty oh TRO pee um & oh loe DA ter ol)

Brand Names: US Stiolto Respimat

Brand Names: Canada Inspiolto Respimat

Pharmacologic Category Anticholinergic Agent; Anticholinergic Agent, Long-Acting; $Beta_2$ Agonist; $Beta_2$ Agonist, Long-Acting

Use COPD: Maintenance treatment of patients with COPD, including chronic bronchitis and/or emphysema.

Local Anesthetic/Vasoconstrictor Precautions No information available to require special precautions

Effects on Dental Treatment Key adverse event(s) related to dental treatment: The anticholinrgic effect of tiopropium resulting in xerostomia should be anticipated. Normal salivary flow should resume upon discontinuation.

Effects on Bleeding No information available to require special precautions

Adverse Reactions

>10%:

Respiratory: Nasopharyngitis (12%)

1% to 10%:

Neuromuscular & skeletal: Back pain (4%)

Respiratory: Cough (4%)

≤3%, postmarketing, and/or case reports: Angioedema, arthralgia, atrial fibrillation, blurred vision, bronchospasm, constipation, dehydration, dermal ulcer, dizziness, dysphagia, dysuria, epistaxis, gastroesophageal reflux disease, gingivitis, glaucoma, glossitis, hypersensitivity (including immediate reactions), hypertension, increased intraocular pressure, insomnia, intestinal obstruction (including paralytic ileus), joint swelling, laryngitis, oropharyngeal candidiasis, palpitations, pharyngitis, pruritus, sinusitis, skin infection, skin rash, stomatitis, supraventricular tachycardia, tachycardia, urinary retention, urinary tract infection, urticaria, voice disorder, xeroderma, xerostomia

Mechanism of Action

Tiotropium: Competitively and reversibly inhibits the action of acetylcholine at type 3 muscarinic (M3) receptors in bronchial smooth muscle causing bronchodilation.

Olodaterol: Long acting beta$_2$-receptor agonist; activates beta$_2$ airway receptors, resulting in the stimulation of intracellular adenyl cyclase and a subsequent increase in the synthesis of cyclic-3',5' adenosine monophosphate (cAMP). Elevated cAMP levels induce bronchodilation by relaxation of airway smooth muscle cells. Has much greater affinity for beta$_2$-receptors than for beta$_1$- or beta$_3$-receptors.

Pregnancy Considerations Animal reproduction studies have not been conducted with this combination. Beta-agonists have the potential to affect uterine contractility if administered during labor. See individual monographs.

◆ **Tiotropium Br/Olodaterol HCl** *see* Tiotropium and Olodaterol *on page 1451*

◆ **Tiotropium Bromide and Olodaterol** *see* Tiotropium and Olodaterol *on page 1451*

◆ **Tiotropium Bromide Monohydrate** *see* Tiotropium *on page 1450*

◆ **Tipiracil and Trifluridine** *see* Trifluridine and Tipiracil *on page 1497*

Tipranavir (tip RA na veer)

Related Information

HIV Infection and AIDS *on page 1690*

Brand Names: US Aptivus

Brand Names: Canada Aptivus

Pharmacologic Category Antiretroviral, Protease Inhibitor (Anti-HIV)

Use HIV-1 infection, treatment: Treatment of HIV-1 infection in combination with ritonavir and other antiretroviral agents; limited to treatment-experienced, multi-protease inhibitor-resistant patients. **Note:** Tipranavir is no longer recommended for use in the initial treatment of HIV (HHS [adult] 2019).

Local Anesthetic/Vasoconstrictor Precautions No information available to require special precautions

Effects on Dental Treatment No significant effects or complications reported

Effects on Bleeding Increased bleeding has been noted with protease inhibitors in patients with hemophilia A or B. No information available to require routine special precautions relative to hemostasis in other patients.

Adverse Reactions

>10%:

Dermatologic: Skin rash (children: 21%; adults: 3% to 10%)

Endocrine & metabolic: Hypertriglyceridemia (>400 mg/dL: 61%), hypercholesterolemia (>300 mg/dL: 22%)

Gastrointestinal: Diarrhea (15%; children: 4%)

Hepatic: Increased serum transaminases (>2.5 x ULN: 26% to 32%; grades 3/4: 10% to 20%)

Neuromuscular & skeletal: Increased creatine phosphokinase (children, grades 3/4: 11%)

1% to 10%:

Central nervous system: Fatigue (6%), headache (5%), dizziness, drowsiness, insomnia, intracranial hemorrhage, malaise, peripheral neuropathy, sleep disorder

Dermatologic: Pruritus

Endocrine & metabolic: Increased amylase (grade 3: 6% to 8%), weight loss (3%), dehydration (2%), increased gamma-glutamyl transferase (2%), diabetes mellitus, hyperglycemia, lipodystrophy (acquired), lipohypertrophy

Gastrointestinal: Nausea (5% to 9%), vomiting (6%), abdominal pain (4%), abdominal distension, anorexia, decreased appetite, dyspepsia, flatulence, gastroesophageal reflux disease, increased serum lipase, pancreatitis

Hematologic & oncologic: Hemorrhage (children: 8%), decreased white blood cell count (grade 3: 5%), anemia (3%), neutropenia (2%), thrombocytopenia

Hepatic: Increased serum ALT (2%, grades 3/4: 10%), increased serum AST (grades 3/4: 6%), hepatic failure, hepatitis, hyperbilirubinemia, liver steatosis

Hypersensitivity: Hypersensitivity reaction

Immunologic: Immune reconstitution syndrome

Neuromuscular & skeletal: Myalgia (2%), amyotrophy (facial), lipoatrophy, muscle cramps

Renal: Renal insufficiency

Respiratory: Cough (children: 6%), dyspnea (2%), epistaxis (children: 4%), flu-like symptoms

Miscellaneous: Fever (6% to 8%), drug toxicity (mitochondrial damage)

Mechanism of Action Binds to the site of HIV-1 protease activity and inhibits cleavage of viral Gag-Pol polyprotein precursors into individual functional proteins required for infectious HIV. This results in the formation of immature, noninfectious viral particles.

Pharmacodynamics/Kinetics

Half-life Elimination Children 2 to <6 years of age: ~8 hours, 6 to <12 years of age: ~7 hours, 12 to 18 years: ~5 hours; Adults: Males: 6 hours; Females: 5.5 hours

Time to Peak Children and Adolescents 2 to 18 years: 2.5 to 2.7 hours; Adults: 3 hours

Reproductive Considerations

Based on the Health and Humans Services perinatal HIV guidelines, tipranavir is not one of the recommended antiretroviral agents for use in females who are trying to conceive.

Females living with HIV not planning a pregnancy may use any available type of contraception, considering possible drug interactions and contraindications of the specific method. Consult drug interactions database for more detailed information specific to use of tipranavir and specific contraceptives.

For males and females living with HIV and planning a pregnancy, maximum viral suppression below the limits of detection with antiretroviral therapy (ART), modification of therapy (if needed), optimization of the woman's health, and a discussion of the potential risks and benefits of ART therapy during pregnancy are recommended prior to conception (HHS [perinatal] 2019).

Pregnancy Considerations Tipranavir crosses the placenta.

Outcome information specific to tipranavir use in pregnancy is no longer being reviewed and updated in the Health and Human Services (HHS) perinatal guidelines. Maternal antiretroviral therapy (ART) may be associated with adverse pregnancy outcomes, including preterm delivery, stillbirth, low birth weight, and small-for-gestational-age infants. Actual risks may be influenced by maternal factors such as disease severity, gestational age at initiation of therapy, and specific ART regimen, therefore close fetal monitoring is recommended. Because there is clear benefit to appropriate treatment, maternal ART should not be withheld due to concerns for adverse neonatal outcomes. Long-term follow-up is recommended for all infants exposed to antiretroviral medications; children without HIV but who were exposed to ART in utero and develop significant organ system abnormalities of unknown etiology (particularly of the CNS or heart) should be evaluated for potential mitochondrial dysfunction. Hyperglycemia, new onset of diabetes mellitus, or diabetic ketoacidosis have been reported with protease inhibitors; it is not clear if pregnancy increases this risk. Consider performing the standard glucose screening test earlier in pregnancy in women who initiated protease inhibitor therapy prior to conception.

Based on the HHS perinatal HIV guidelines, tipranavir is not one of the recommended antiretroviral agents for use during pregnancy.

In general, ART is recommended for all pregnant females living with HIV to keep the viral load below the limit of detection and reduce the risk of perinatal transmission. Therapy should be individualized following a discussion of the potential risks and benefits of treatment during pregnancy. Monitoring of pregnant females is more frequent than in nonpregnant adults. ART should be continued postpartum for all females living with HIV and can be modified after delivery.

Health care providers are encouraged to enroll pregnant females exposed to antiretroviral medications as early in pregnancy as possible in the Antiretroviral Pregnancy Registry (1-800-258-4263 or http://www.APRegistry.com). Health care providers caring for pregnant females living with HIV and their infants may contact the National Perinatal HIV Hotline (888-448-8765) for clinical consultation (HHS [perinatal] 2019).

Tirofiban (tye roe FYE ban)

Related Information

Cardiovascular Diseases *on page 1654*

Brand Names: US Aggrastat

Brand Names: Canada Aggrastat

Pharmacologic Category Antiplatelet Agent, Glycoprotein IIb/IIIa Inhibitor

Use Unstable angina/non-ST-elevation myocardial infarction: To decrease the rate of thrombotic cardiovascular events (combined end point of death, MI, or refractory ischemia/repeat cardiac procedure) in patients with non-ST-elevation acute coronary syndrome (unstable angina/non-ST-elevation myocardial infarction [UA/NSTEMI]).

Local Anesthetic/Vasoconstrictor Precautions No information available to require special precautions

Effects on Dental Treatment Key adverse event(s) related to dental treatment: Bleeding is a potential adverse effect of tirofiban. See Effects on Bleeding.

Effects on Bleeding As with all anticoagulants, bleeding is a potential adverse effect of tirofiban during dental surgery; risk is dependent on multiple variables, including the intensity of anticoagulation and patient susceptibility. Medical consult is suggested. It is unlikely that ambulatory patients presenting for dental treatment will be taking intravenous anticoagulant therapy.

Adverse Reactions Bleeding is the major drug-related adverse effect. Patients received background treatment with aspirin and heparin. Adverse reactions reported are derived from both the high-dose bolus regimen **and** the dosing regimen used in studies that established the effectiveness of tirofiban. Frequency not always defined.

>10%: Hematologic & oncologic: Minor hemorrhage (TIMI criteria minor bleeding; 10.5% to 12%; transfusion required: 4% to 4.3%)

1% to 10%:

- Cardiovascular: Coronary artery dissection (5%), bradycardia (4%), edema (2%), vasodepressor syncope (2%)
- Central nervous system: Dizziness (3%), headache (>1%)
- Dermatologic: Diaphoresis (2%)
- Gastrointestinal: Nausea (>1%)
- Genitourinary: Pelvic pain (6%)
- Hematologic & oncologic: Major hemorrhage (TIMI criteria major bleeding: 1.4% to 2.2%; including hematoma [femoral]: 2% [Valgimigli 2005], intracranial bleeding, GI bleeding, retroperitoneal bleeding [Aydin 2003], GU bleeding, pulmonary alveolar hemorrhage [Guo 2012], spinal-epidural hematoma), thrombocytopenia: <90,000/mm^3 (1.5% to 1.9%), <50,000/mm^3 (0.3% to 0.5%)
- Neuromuscular & skeletal: Leg pain (3%)
- Miscellaneous: Fever (>1%)

<1%, postmarketing, and/or case reports: Anaphylaxis, hemopericardium, hypersensitivity, skin rash, urticaria

Mechanism of Action A reversible antagonist of fibrinogen binding to the glycoprotein (GP) IIb/IIIa receptor, the major platelet surface receptor involved in platelet aggregation. When administered intravenously, it inhibits *ex vivo* platelet aggregation in a dose- and concentration-dependent manner. When given according to the recommended regimen, >90% inhibition is attained within 10 minutes after initiation. Platelet aggregation inhibition is reversible following cessation of the infusion.

Pharmacodynamics/Kinetics

Onset of Action >90% inhibition of platelet aggregation (reversible after discontinuation) seen within 10 minutes

Half-life Elimination 2 hours; **Note:** In ~90% of patients, *ex vivo* platelet aggregation returns to near baseline in 4 to 8 hours after discontinuation.

Pregnancy Considerations Information related to use in pregnancy is limited (Boztosun 2008; Hajj-Chahine 2010).

- ◆ **Tirofiban Hydrochloride** *see* Tirofiban *on page 1453*
- ◆ **Tirosint** *see* Levothyroxine *on page 900*
- ◆ **Tirosint-Sol** *see* Levothyroxine *on page 900*
- ◆ **Tirosint-SOL** *see* Levothyroxine *on page 900*

Tisagenlecleucel (tis a jen lek LOO sel)

Brand Names: US Kymriah

Pharmacologic Category Antineoplastic Agent, Anti-CD19; Antineoplastic Agent, CAR-T Immunotherapy; CAR-T Cell Immunotherapy; Cellular Immunotherapy, Autologous; Chimeric Antigen Receptor T-Cell Immunotherapy

Use

Acute lymphoblastic leukemia (relapsed or refractory): Treatment of B-cell precursor acute lymphoblastic leukemia (ALL) that is refractory or in second or later relapse in patients up to 25 years of age.

Diffuse large B-cell lymphoma (relapsed or refractory): Treatment of relapsed or refractory large B-cell lymphoma in adults (after 2 or more lines of systemic therapy), including diffuse large B-cell lymphoma (DLBCL) not otherwise specified, high-grade B-cell lymphoma, and DLBCL arising from follicular lymphoma.

Limitation of use: Not indicated for treatment of primary CNS lymphoma.

Local Anesthetic/Vasoconstrictor Precautions No information available to require special precautions

Effects on Dental Treatment No significant effects or complications reported

Effects on Bleeding Chemotherapy may result in significant myelosuppression; anemia, neutropenia, and thrombocytopenia are significant (See adverse reactions); In patients under active treatment with tisagenlecleucel, medical consult is suggested.

Adverse Reactions

>10%:

Cardiovascular: Hypotension (26% to 31%), tachycardia (children, adolescents, and adults: 26%; adults: 13%), edema (21% to 23%), hypertension (children, adolescents, and adults: 19%; adults: 2%)

Central nervous system: Headache (children, adolescents, and adults: 37%; adults: 21%), encephalopathy (children, adolescents, and adults: 34%; adults: 16%), fatigue (25% to 26%), delirium (children, adolescents, and adults: 21%; adults: 6%), pain (15% to 18%), chills (10% to 13%), anxiety (9% to 13%), dizziness (6% to 11%)

Dermatologic: Skin rash (8% to 16%)

Endocrine & metabolic: Hypokalemia (children, adolescents, and adults; grades 3/4: 27%; adults, grades 3/4: 12%), hypophosphatemia (grades 3/4: 19% to 24%), hyponatremia (adults, grades 3/4: 11%), weight loss (adults: 11%)

Gastrointestinal: Decreased appetite (children, adolescents, and adults: 37%; adults: 12%), vomiting (children, adolescents, and adults: 26%; adults: 9%), diarrhea (26% to 31%), nausea (26% to 27), constipation (16% to 18%), abdominal pain (9% to 16%)

Hematologic & oncologic: Anemia (children, adolescents, and adults: 100%; adults, grades 3/4: 58%), neutropenia (children, adolescents, and adults: 100%; grades 3/4: 17% to 40%; adults, grades 3/4: 81%), thrombocytopenia (children, adolescents, and adults: 100%; grades 3/4: 12% to 27%; adults, grades 3/4: 54%), lymphocytopenia (adults, grades 3/4: 94%), leukopenia (adults, grades 3/4: 77%), hypogammaglobulinemia (children, adolescents, and adults: 43%; adults: 14%; grades ≥3: 4% to 7%), febrile neutropenia (children, adolescents, and adults: 37%; grades ≥3: 37%; adults: 17%; grades ≥3: 17%), hypofibrinogenemia (children, adolescents, and adults; grades 3/4: 16%; with cytokine release syndrome), increased INR (children, adolescents, and adults: 13%)

Hepatic: Increased serum aspartate aminotransferase (children, adolescents, and adults; grades 3/4: 28%), increased serum alanine aminotransferase (children, adolescents, and adults; grades 3/4: 21%), increased serum bilirubin (children, adolescents, and adults; grades 3/4: 21%)

Hypersensitivity: Cytokine release syndrome (74% to 79%)

Infection: Infection (41% to 55%; unknown pathogen), viral infection (children, adolescents, and adults: 26%; adults: 9%), bacterial infection (children, adolescents, and adults: 19%; adults: 9%), fungal infection (9% to 13%)

Neuromuscular & skeletal: Myalgia (7% to 15%), arthralgia (10% to 12%)

Renal: Acute renal failure (17% to 24%)

Respiratory: Hypoxia (children, adolescents, and adults: 24%; adults: 8%), cough (19% to 21%), dyspnea (16% to 18%), pulmonary edema (children, adolescents, and adults: 16%; adults: 3%), tachypnea (children, adolescents, and adults: 12%)

Miscellaneous: Fever (34% to 40%)

1% to 10%:

Cardiovascular: Cardiac failure (children, adolescents, and adults: 7%), thrombosis (3% to 7%), cardiac arrhythmia (adults: 6%), capillary leak syndrome (1% to 3%), cerebral infarction (adults: 1%)

Central nervous system: Sleep disorder (9% to 10%), peripheral neuropathy (4% to 8%), motor dysfunction (adults: 6%; children, adolescents, and adults: 1%), seizure (3%), speech disturbance (3%), ataxia (adults: 2%)

Dermatologic: Dermatitis (adults: 4%)

Endocrine & metabolic: Fluid retention (children, adolescents, and adults: 10%; adults: 3%)

Gastrointestinal: Abdominal distress (abdominal compartment syndrome; children, adolescents, and adults: 1%), fecal incontinence (adults: 1%)

Hematologic & oncologic: Disseminated intravascular coagulation (children, adolescents, and adults: 9%; adults: 3%), lymphocytosis (histiocytosis lymphoticytic hemophagocytosis; children, adolescents, and adults: 7%; adults: 1%), disorder of hemostatic components of blood (children, adolescents, and adults: 6%), prolonged partial thromboplastin time (children, adolescents, and adults: 6%), tumor lysis syndrome (children, adolescents, and adults: 6%; adults: 1%), pancytopenia (adults: 2%),

Immunologic: Antibody development (adults: 5%), graft versus host disease (children, adolescents, and adults: 1%)

Neuromuscular & skeletal: Back pain (6% to 10%), tremor (7% to 9%), asthenia (adults: 7%)

Ophthalmic: Visual impairment (3% to 7%)

Respiratory: Nasal congestion (children, adolescents, and adults: 10%), pleural effusion (5% to 10%), oropharyngeal pain (6% to 8%), respiratory distress (children, adolescents, and adults: 6%), respiratory failure (children, adolescents, and adults: 6%), acute respiratory distress (children, adolescents, and adults: 4%)

Miscellaneous: Multi-organ failure (3%)

Frequency not defined: Central nervous system: Aphasia, mutism

Mechanism of Action Tisagenlecleucel is a CD19-directed genetically modified autologous T cell immunotherapy (containing human cells modified with a lentivirus) in which a patient's T cells are reprogrammed with a transgene encoding a chimeric antigen receptor (CAR) to identify and eliminate CD19-expressing malignant and normal cells. The CAR is comprised of a murine single-chain antibody fragment which recognizes CD19 and is fused to intracellular signaling domains from 4-1BB (CD137) and CD3 zeta. CD3 zeta is a critical component for initiating T-cell activation and antitumor activity, while 4-1BB enhances expansion and persistence of tisagenlecleucel. After binding to CD19-expressing cells, the CAR transmits a signal to promote T-cell expansion, activation, target cell elimination, and persistence of the tisagenlecleucel cells. Tisagenlecleucel is prepared from the patient's peripheral blood cells obtained via leukapheresis.

Pharmacodynamics/Kinetics

Half-life Elimination ALL: ~17 days (in responding patients); DLBCL: ~45 days (in responding patients)

Time to Peak ~10 days (in responding patients)

Reproductive Considerations

Evaluate pregnancy status prior to use in females of reproductive potential. The duration of contraception needed following tisagenlecleucel administration is not known.

Pregnancy Considerations

Based on the mechanism of action, if placental transfer were to occur, fetal toxicity, including B-cell lymphocytopenia, may occur. Pregnant women who have received tisagenlecleucel may have hypogammaglobulinemia; assess immunoglobulin levels in newborns of mothers treated with tisagenlecleucel.

Data collection to monitor pregnancy and infant outcomes following exposure to tisagenlecleucel is ongoing. Pregnancies that may occur during treatment should be reported to Novartis Pharmaceuticals Corporation (888-669-6682).

- **Tisseel** *see* Fibrin Sealant *on page 667*
- **Tisseel VH S/D** *see* Fibrin Sealant *on page 667*
- **Tivicay** *see* Dolutegravir *on page 511*
- **Tivicay PD** *see* Dolutegravir *on page 511*
- **TIV (Trivalent Inactivated Influenza Vaccine)** *see* Influenza Virus Vaccine (Inactivated) *on page 812*

TiZANidine (tye ZAN i deen)

Related Information

Dentin Hypersensitivity, Acid Erosion, High Caries Index, Management of Alveolar Osteitis, and Xerostomia *on page 1762*

Brand Names: US Zanaflex

Brand Names: Canada GEN-TiZANidine; MYLAN-TiZANidine [DSC]; PAL-TiZANidine

Pharmacologic Category Alpha$_2$-Adrenergic Agonist

Use Spasticity: Management of spasticity; reserve treatment with tizanidine for daily activities and times when relief of spasticity is most important.

Local Anesthetic/Vasoconstrictor Precautions No information available to require special precautions

Effects on Dental Treatment Key adverse event(s) related to dental treatment: Frequent occurrence of xerostomia (normal salivary flow resumes upon discontinuation) has been reported. Rare occurrence of Stevens-Johnson syndrome has also been reported.

Effects on Bleeding No information available to require special precautions

Adverse Reactions

>10%:

Cardiovascular: Hypotension (16% to 33%)

Central nervous system: Drowsiness (48% to 92%), dizziness (16% to 45%)

Gastrointestinal: Xerostomia (49% to 88%)

Neuromuscular & skeletal: Asthenia (41% to 78%)

1% to 10%:

Cardiovascular: Bradycardia (2% to 10%)

Central nervous system: Nervousness (3%), speech disturbance (3%), delusion (≤3%), visual hallucination (≤3%)

Gastrointestinal: Constipation (4%), vomiting (3%)

Genitourinary: Urinary tract infection (10%), urinary frequency (3%)

Hepatic: Abnormal hepatic function tests (6%)

Infection: Infection (6%)

Neuromuscular & skeletal: Dyskinesia (3%)

Ophthalmic: Blurred vision (3%)

Respiratory: Flu-like symptoms (3%), pharyngitis (3%), rhinitis (3%)

Frequency not defined:

Central nervous system: Drug withdrawal, sedated state

Hypersensitivity: Hypersensitivity reaction

<1%, postmarketing, and/or case reports: Anaphylaxis, arthralgia, depression, exfoliative dermatitis, fatigue, hepatitis, hepatotoxicity, muscle spasm, paresthesia, seizure, skin rash, Stevens-Johnson syndrome, syncope, tremor, ventricular tachycardia

Mechanism of Action An alpha$_2$-adrenergic agonist agent which decreases spasticity by increasing presynaptic inhibition; effects are greatest on polysynaptic pathways; overall effect is to reduce facilitation of spinal motor neurons.

Pharmacodynamics/Kinetics

Onset of Action Single dose (8 mg): Peak effect: 1 to 2 hours

Duration of Action Single dose (8 mg): 3 to 6 hours

Half-life Elimination ~2.5 hours

Time to Peak

Fasting state: Capsule, tablet: 1 hour

Fed state: Capsule: 3 to 4 hours, Tablet: 1.5 hours

Pregnancy Risk Factor C

Pregnancy Considerations Adverse events were observed in some animal reproduction studies.

- **Tizanidine HCl** *see* TiZANidine *on page 1455*
- **TL-HEM 150** *see* Vitamins (Multiple/Oral) *on page 1550*
- **7T Lido** *see* Lidocaine (Topical) *on page 902*
- **TMC-114** *see* Darunavir *on page 441*
- **TMC125** *see* Etravirine *on page 627*
- **TMC278** *see* Rilpivirine *on page 1327*
- **TMC435** *see* Simeprevir *on page 1372*
- **TMP** *see* Trimethoprim *on page 1498*

- ◆ **TMP-SMX** *see* Sulfamethoxazole and Trimethoprim *on page 1391*
- ◆ **TMP-SMZ** *see* Sulfamethoxazole and Trimethoprim *on page 1391*
- ◆ **TMX-67** *see* Febuxostat *on page 637*
- ◆ **TMZ** *see* Temozolomide *on page 1415*
- ◆ **TNG** *see* Nitroglycerin *on page 1112*
- ◆ **Tobi** *see* Tobramycin (Oral Inhalation) *on page 1456*
- ◆ **Tobi Podhaler** *see* Tobramycin (Oral Inhalation) *on page 1456*

Tobramycin (Systemic) (toe bra MYE sin)

Brand Names: Canada JAMP-Tobramycin

Pharmacologic Category Antibiotic, Aminoglycoside

Use

Bloodstream infection: Treatment of bloodstream infection caused by *Pseudomonas aeruginosa*, *Escherichia coli*, and *Klebsiella* spp., in adult and pediatric patients.

Bone infections: Treatment of bone infections caused by *P. aeruginosa*, *Proteus* spp., *E. coli*, *Klebsiella* spp., *Enterobacter* spp., and *Staphylococcus aureus* in adult and pediatric patients.

Intra-abdominal infections: Treatment of intra-abdominal infections, including peritonitis, caused by *E. coli*, *Klebsiella* spp., and *Enterobacter* spp. in adult and pediatric patients.

Meningitis, bacterial: Treatment of bacterial meningitis caused by susceptible bacteria in adult and pediatric patients.

Pneumonia: Treatment of pneumonia caused by *P. aeruginosa*, *Klebsiella* spp., *Enterobacter* spp., *Serratia* spp., *E. coli*, and *Staphylococcus aureus* in adult and pediatric patients.

Skin and skin structure infections: Treatment of skin and skin structure infections caused by *P. aeruginosa*, *Proteus* spp., *E. coli*, *Klebsiella* spp., *Enterobacter* spp., and *S. aureus* in adult and pediatric patients.

Urinary tract infections: Treatment of complicated urinary tract infections caused by *P. aeruginosa*, *Proteus* spp., (indole-positive and indole-negative), *E. coli*, *Klebsiella* spp., *Enterobacter* spp., *Serratia* spp., *S. aureus*, *Providencia* spp., and *Citrobacter* spp. in adult and pediatric patients.

Local Anesthetic/Vasoconstrictor Precautions No information available to require special precautions

Effects on Dental Treatment No significant effects or complications reported

Effects on Bleeding No information available to require special precautions

Adverse Reactions Frequency not defined.

Central nervous system: Confusion, disorientation, dizziness, headache, lethargy, vertigo

Dermatologic: Exfoliative dermatitis, pruritus, skin rash, urticaria

Endocrine & metabolic: Decreased serum calcium, decreased serum magnesium, decreased serum potassium, decreased serum sodium, increased lactate dehydrogenase, increased nonprotein nitrogen

Gastrointestinal: Diarrhea, nausea, vomiting

Genitourinary: Casts in urine, oliguria, proteinuria

Hematologic & oncologic: Anemia, eosinophilia, granulocytopenia, leukocytosis, leukopenia, thrombocytopenia

Hepatic: Increased serum ALT, increased serum AST, increased serum bilirubin

Local: Pain at injection site

Otic: Auditory ototoxicity, hearing loss, tinnitus, vestibular ototoxicity

Renal: Increased blood urea nitrogen, increased serum creatinine

Miscellaneous: Fever

<1%, postmarketing, and/or case reports: Anaphylaxis, *Clostridioides* (formerly *Clostridium*) *difficile*-associated diarrhea, erythema multiforme, Stevens-Johnson syndrome, toxic epidermal necrolysis

Mechanism of Action Interferes with bacterial protein synthesis by binding to 30S ribosomal subunit, resulting in a defective bacterial cell membrane

Pharmacodynamics/Kinetics

Half-life Elimination

Neonates: ≤1,200 g: 11 hours; >1,200 g: 2 to 9 hours

Infants: 4 ± 1 hour

Children: 2 ± 1 hour

Adolescents: 1.5 ± 1 hour

Adults: IV: 2 to 3 hours; directly dependent upon glomerular filtration rate

Adults with impaired renal function: 5 to 70 hours

Time to Peak

Serum: IM: 30 to 60 minutes; IV: ~30 minutes.

Note: Distribution is prolonged after larger doses (≥60 minutes after 60-minute infusion of 10 mg/kg [Aminimanizani 2002]; ≥90 minutes after 60-minute infusion of a high-dose aminoglycoside [gentamicin 7 mg/kg] [Demczar 1997]).

Pregnancy Considerations Tobramycin crosses the placenta.

[US Boxed Warning]: Tobramycin and other aminoglycosides can cause fetal harm when administered to a pregnant woman. If tobramycin is used during pregnancy or if the patient becomes pregnant while taking tobramycin, apprise the patient of the potential hazard to the fetus.

There are several reports of total irreversible bilateral congenital deafness in children whose mothers received another aminoglycoside (streptomycin) during pregnancy. Although serious side effects to the fetus/infant have not been reported following maternal use of all aminoglycosides, a potential for harm exists.

Due to pregnancy-induced physiologic changes, some pharmacokinetic parameters of tobramycin may be altered (Bourget 1991). Tobramycin injection may be used for the management of cystic fibrosis in pregnant patients with *P. aeruginosa* (inhalation is preferred unless risk of infection is great) (Edenborough 2008) and as an alternative antibiotic for prophylactic use prior to cesarean delivery (Bratzler 2013).

Tobramycin (Oral Inhalation)
(toe bra MYE sin)

Brand Names: US Bethkis; Kitabis Pak; Tobi; Tobi Podhaler

Brand Names: Canada TEVA-Tobramycin; Tobi; Tobi Podhaler

Pharmacologic Category Antibiotic, Aminoglycoside

Use

Cystic fibrosis: Management of cystic fibrosis in adults and pediatric patients ≥6 years of age with *Pseudomonas aeruginosa*.

Limitations of use: Safety and efficacy have not been demonstrated in patients with FEV_1 <40% or >80% predicted (Bethkis) or FEV_1 <25% or >80% predicted (TOBI Podhaler) or FEV_1 <25% or >75% predicted (Kitabis Pak; TOBI), or in patients colonized with *Burkholderia cepacia*.

Local Anesthetic/Vasoconstrictor Precautions No information available to require special precautions

Effects on Dental Treatment No significant effects or complications reported

Effects on Bleeding No information available to require special precautions

Adverse Reactions

>10%:

Central nervous system: Voice disorder (4% to 14%), headache (11% to 12%)

Respiratory: Cough (powder: 10% to 48%, solution: 31%), rhinitis (solution: 11% to 35%), pulmonary disease (30% to 34%; includes pulmonary or cystic fibrosis exacerbations), reduced forced expiratory volume (solution: 1% to 31%, powder: 4%), discoloration of sputum (21%), productive cough (18% to 20%), rales (solution: 6% to 19%, powder: 7%), dyspnea (12% to 16%), decreased lung function (7% to 16%), oropharyngeal pain (11% to 14%), hemoptysis (12% to 13%), pharyngolaryngeal pain (powder: 11%, solution: 3%)

Miscellaneous: Fever (12% to 16%)

1% to 10%:

Cardiovascular: Chest discomfort (3% to 7%)

Central nervous system: Malaise (6%)

Dermatologic: Skin rash (2%)

Endocrine: Increased serum glucose (powder: 3%, solution: <1%)

Gastrointestinal: Nausea (8% to 10%), dysgeusia (powder: 4% to 7%, solution: <1%), vomiting (6%), diarrhea (2% to 4%)

Hematologic & oncologic: Increased erythrocyte sedimentation rate (solution: 8%), eosinophilia (solution: 2%), increased serum immunoglobulins (solution: 2%)

Neuromuscular & skeletal: Musculoskeletal chest pain (<1% to 5%), myalgia (solution: ≤5%)

Otic: Hypoacusis (powder: 10%), tinnitus (2% to 3%), deafness (≤1%; including unilateral deafness, reported as mild to moderate hearing loss or increased hearing loss)

Respiratory: Upper respiratory tract infection (7% to 9%), nasal congestion (7% to 8%), wheezing (5% to 7%), throat irritation (2% to 5%), bronchospasm (≤1% to 5%), laryngitis (solution: ≤5%) bronchitis (solution: 3%), epistaxis (2% to 3%), tonsillitis (solution: 2%)

<1%, postmarketing, and/or case reports: Aphonia, decreased appetite, hypersensitivity reaction, increased bronchial secretions, pneumonitis, pruritus, pulmonary congestion, urticaria

Mechanism of Action Interferes with bacterial protein synthesis by binding to 30S ribosomal subunit, resulting in a defective bacterial cell membrane

Pharmacodynamics/Kinetics

Half-life Elimination

Solution for inhalation: ~4.4 hours (Bethkis); ~3 hours (TOBI)

Powder for inhalation: ~3 hours (after a single 112 mg dose)

Time to Peak Serum: Powder for inhalation: 60 minutes

Pregnancy Considerations

Aminoglycosides may cause fetal harm if administered to a pregnant woman. Systemic absorption of tobramycin following oral inhalation is expected to be low compared to intravenous administration; however, systemic exposure was associated with total irreversible bilateral congenital deafness in children whose mothers received another aminoglycoside during pregnancy.

Tobramycin inhalation may be used for the management of cystic fibrosis in pregnant patients with *Pseudomonas aeruginosa* (Edenborough 2008).

- **Tobramycin Sulfate** *see* Tobramycin (Oral Inhalation) *on page 1456*
- **Tobramycin Sulfate** *see* Tobramycin (Systemic) *on page 1456*

Tocilizumab (toe si LIZ oo mab)

Related Information

Rheumatoid Arthritis, Osteoarthritis, and Osteoporosis *on page 1697*

Brand Names: US Actemra; Actemra ACTPen

Brand Names: Canada Actemra

Pharmacologic Category Antirheumatic, Disease Modifying; Interleukin-6 Receptor Antagonist

Use

Cytokine release syndrome, severe or life-threatening: Treatment of chimeric antigen receptor (CAR) T-cell induced severe or life-threatening cytokine release syndrome in patients ≥2 years of age

Giant cell arteritis: Treatment of giant cell arteritis (GCA) in adult patients

Polyarticular juvenile idiopathic arthritis: Treatment of active polyarticular juvenile idiopathic arthritis (pJIA) in patients ≥2 years of age

Rheumatoid arthritis: Treatment of adults with moderately to severely active rheumatoid arthritis (RA) who have had an inadequate response to one or more disease-modifying antirheumatic drugs (DMARDs)

Systemic juvenile idiopathic arthritis: Treatment of active systemic juvenile idiopathic arthritis (SJIA) in patients ≥2 years of age

Local Anesthetic/Vasoconstrictor Precautions No information available to require special precautions

Effects on Dental Treatment Key adverse event(s) related to dental treatment: Tocilizumab belongs to the class of disease-modifying antirheumatic drugs and, as such, has immunosuppressive properties. Consider a medical consult prior to any invasive treatment for patients under active treatment with tocilizumab. Delayed wound healing due to the immunosuppressive effects and increased potential for postsurgical infection may be of concern.

Effects on Bleeding No information available to require special precautions

Adverse Reactions Incidence as reported for adults unless otherwise noted. Incidence as reported for monotherapy and combination therapy. Combination therapy refers to use in rheumatoid arthritis with nonbiological disease-modifying antirheumatic drugs or use in systemic juvenile idiopathic arthritis or polyarticular juvenile idiopathic arthritis in trials where most patients (~70% to 80%) were taking methotrexate at baseline.

>10%:

Endocrine & metabolic: Increased serum cholesterol (19% to 20%; children and adolescents: ≤2%)

Hepatic: Increased serum alanine aminotransferase (≤36%), increased serum aspartate aminotransferase (≤22%)
Local: Injection site reaction (SubQ: Children and adolescents: 15% to 44% [higher incidence occurred in weight ≥30 kg]; adults: 7% to 10%)
Miscellaneous: Infusion-related reaction (4% to 20%)
1% to 10%:
Cardiovascular: Hypertension (6%), peripheral edema (<2%)
Dermatologic: Skin rash (2%)
Endocrine & metabolic: Hypothyroidism (<2%), increased LDL cholesterol (9% to 10%; children and adolescents: ≤2%)
Gastrointestinal: Diarrhea (children and adolescents: ≥5%), gastric ulcer (<2%), gastritis (1%), oral mucosa ulcer (2%), stomatitis (<2%), upper abdominal pain (2%), weight gain (<2%)
Hematologic & oncologic: Leukopenia (<2%), neutropenia (children and adolescents <30 kg, grade 3: 26%; children and adolescents ≥30 kg, grade 3: 4%; adults, grade 3: 3% to 4%), thrombocytopenia (1%)
Hepatic: Increased serum bilirubin (<2%)
Immunologic: Antibody development (children and adolescents: ≤6%; adults: <2%; neutralizing, adults: ≤1%)
Infection: Herpes simplex infection (<2%)
Nervous system: Dizziness (3%), headache (7%)
Ophthalmic: Conjunctivitis (<2%)
Renal: Nephrolithiasis (<2%)
Respiratory: Bronchitis (3%), cough (<2%), dyspnea (<2%), nasopharyngitis (7%), upper respiratory tract infection (7%)
Frequency not defined:
Cardiovascular: Hypotension
Endocrine & metabolic: Increased HDL cholesterol
Gastrointestinal: Nausea
Hematologic & oncologic: Malignant neoplasm
Hypersensitivity: Angioedema
Otic: Otitis media
Postmarketing:
Dermatologic: Cellulitis, Stevens-Johnson syndrome
Gastrointestinal: Diverticulitis of the gastrointestinal tract, gastroenteritis, gastrointestinal perforation, pancreatitis
Genitourinary: Urinary tract infection
Hepatic: Hepatic failure, hepatic injury (Genovese 2017), hepatitis, hepatotoxicity, jaundice
Hypersensitivity: Anaphylaxis, hypersensitivity reaction
Infection: Aspergillosis, candidiasis, cryptococcosis, sepsis, serious infection, varicella zoster infection, viral infection
Nervous system: Chronic inflammatory demyelinating polyneuropathy
Neuromuscular & skeletal: Multiple sclerosis, septic arthritis
Respiratory: Active tuberculosis, infection due to an organism in genus *Pneumocystis*, pneumonia

Mechanism of Action Tocilizumab is an antagonist of the interleukin-6 (IL-6) receptor. Endogenous IL-6 is induced by inflammatory stimuli and mediates a variety of immunological responses. Inhibition of IL-6 receptors by tocilizumab leads to a reduction in cytokine and acute phase reactant production.

Pharmacodynamics/Kinetics

Onset of Action Cytokine release syndrome (CRS): Median time to defervescence: 4 hours (Fitzgerald 2017); Fever and hypotension typically resolve within a few hours (Lee 2014); Blood pressure stabilization: 1 to 3 days (Abboud 2016; Maude 2014b). A median of 1 dose (range: 1 to 4) was required for management of CRS due to chimeric antigen receptor T-cell therapy.

Half-life Elimination
IV: Concentration dependent: Steady state: Children and Adolescents: SJIA: Up to 16 days; PJIA: Up to 17 days; Adults: RA: Up to 11 to 13 days
SubQ: Concentration dependent: Children and Adolescents: SJIA: Up to 14 days; PJIA: Up to 10 days; Adults: RA: Up to 5 days (every-other-week dosing) or up to 13 days (every-week dosing); GCA: 4.2 to 7.9 days (every other week dosing) or 18.3 to 18.9 days (every-week dosing)

Time to Peak SubQ: ~3 days (for every-week dosing); ~4.5 days (for every-2-week dosing)

Reproductive Considerations

Based on limited data, tocilizumab may be considered for use in women with rheumatic and musculoskeletal diseases who are planning a pregnancy; however, treatment should be discontinued once pregnancy is confirmed. Conception should be planned during a period of quiescent/low disease activity (ACR [Sammaritano 2020]).

Information related to paternal use of tocilizumab is limited (Hoeltzenbein 2016). Therefore, recommendations are not available for use in males with rheumatic and musculoskeletal diseases who are planning to father a child (ACR [Sammaritano 2020]).

Pregnancy Considerations

Tocilizumab crosses the placenta (Saito 2018; Saito 2019a; Tada 2019). Tocilizumab is a humanized monoclonal antibody (IgG_1). Potential placental transfer of human IgG is dependent upon the IgG subclass, maternal serum concentrations, newborn birth weight, and gestational age, generally increasing as pregnancy progresses. The lowest exposure would be expected during the period of organogenesis (Palmeira 2012; Pentsuk 2009).

Postmarketing data reviewed through 2014 have not shown an increased rate of congenital malformations or a pattern of specific malformations following in utero exposure to tocilizumab. The review included pregnancy outcome data from 399 women who received tocilizumab for rheumatic disorders; the majority received a dose during the first trimester or within 6 weeks of conception. Using this data, the incidence of preterm birth and spontaneous abortion may be increased when compared to the background rate, but these outcomes may also be influenced by maternal disease and concomitant medications (Hoeltzenbein 2016). Outcome data are limited when maternal use continues throughout pregnancy (Dalkilic 2019; Hoeltzenbein 2016; Kaneko 2016; Nakajima 2016; Saito 2018; Saito 2019a; Tada 2019).

Until additional information is available, tocilizumab is not currently recommended for the treatment of rheumatic and musculoskeletal diseases during pregnancy. Tocilizumab should be discontinued once pregnancy is confirmed (ACR [Sammaritano 2020]).

Data collection to monitor pregnancy and infant outcomes following exposure to tocilizumab is ongoing. Health care providers or pregnant patients are encouraged to enroll exposed pregnancies in the Genentech Actemra registry (877-311-8972).

Tocilizumab is currently under investigation for use in the treatment of coronavirus disease 2019 (COVID-19)-associated pulmonary complications with elevated IL-6 levels (see ClinicalTrials.gov). At this time, safety and efficacy have not been established and information specific to pregnancy has not been located. However, data collection to monitor maternal and infant outcomes following exposure to COVID-19 during pregnancy is ongoing. Health care providers are encouraged to enroll females exposed to COVID-19 during pregnancy in the Organization of Teratology Information Specialists pregnancy registry (877-311-8972; https://mothertobaby.org/join-study/) or the PRIORITY (**P**regnancy **C**o**R**onav**I**rus **O**utcomes **R**eg**I**s**T**r**Y**) (415-754-3729, https://priority.-ucsf.edu/). The American College of Obstetricians and Gynecologists and the Society for Maternal-Fetal Medicine have developed an algorithm to aid practitioners in assessing and managing pregnant women with suspected or confirmed COVID-19 (https://www.acog.org/topics/covid-19; https://www.smfm.org/covid19). Interim guidance is also available from the Centers for Disease Control and Prevention for pregnant women who are diagnosed with COVID-19 (https://www.cdc.gov/coronavirus/2019-ncov/hcp/inpatient-obstetric-healthcare-guidance.html).

Tofacitinib (toe fa SYE ti nib)

Related Information

Rheumatoid Arthritis, Osteoarthritis, and Osteoporosis *on page 1697*

Brand Names: US Xeljanz; Xeljanz XR

Brand Names: Canada Xeljanz; Xeljanz XR

Pharmacologic Category Antirheumatic Miscellaneous; Antirheumatic, Disease Modifying; Janus Associated Kinase Inhibitor

Use

Psoriatic arthritis: Treatment of active psoriatic arthritis in adults who have had an inadequate response or intolerance to methotrexate or other disease-modifying antirheumatic drugs (DMARDs)

Rheumatoid arthritis: Treatment of moderately to severely active rheumatoid arthritis (as monotherapy or in combination with methotrexate or other nonbiologic DMARDs) in adults who have had an inadequate response to, or are intolerant of, methotrexate

Ulcerative colitis: Treatment of moderately to severely active ulcerative colitis in adults who have had an inadequate response or intolerance to tumor necrosis factor blockers

Limitations of use: The use of tofacitinib in combination with biologic DMARDs or with potent immunosuppressants (eg, azathioprine, cyclosporine) is not recommended.

Local Anesthetic/Vasoconstrictor Precautions No information available to require special precautions

Effects on Dental Treatment Key adverse event(s) related to dental treatment: Tofacitinib belongs to the class of disease-modifying antirheumatic drugs and, as such, has immunosuppressive properties. Consider a medical consult prior to any invasive treatment for patients under active treatment with tofacitinib. Delayed wound healing due to the immunosuppressive effects and increased potential for postsurgical infection may be of concern.

Effects on Bleeding Active therapy with tofacitinib may result in significant myelosuppression; medical consult is suggested.

Adverse Reactions Incidences of adverse reactions may include unapproved dosing regimens and combination therapy.

>10%:

- Infection: Infection (20% to 22%)
- Respiratory: Nasopharyngitis (3% to 14%)

1% to 10%:

- Cardiovascular: Hypertension (2%)
- Central nervous system: Headache (3% to 9%)
- Dermatologic: Skin rash (6%), acne vulgaris (≥2%)
- Endocrine & metabolic: Increased serum cholesterol (5% to 9%)
- Gastrointestinal: Diarrhea (3% to 5%), gastroenteritis (4%), nausea (4%)
- Genitourinary: Urinary tract infection (2%)
- Hematologic & oncologic: Anemia (4%)
- Infection: Herpes zoster infection (5%; including disseminated cutaneous, meningoencephalitis, ophthalmologic)
- Neuromuscular & skeletal: Increased creatine phosphokinase (3% to 7%)
- Renal: Increased serum creatinine (<2%)
- Respiratory: Upper respiratory tract infection (4% to 7%)
- Miscellaneous: Fever (≥2%)

Frequency not defined:

- Cardiovascular: Peripheral edema
- Central nervous system: Fatigue, insomnia, paresthesia
- Dermatologic: Erythema, pruritus
- Endocrine & metabolic: Dehydration
- Gastrointestinal: Abdominal pain, diverticulitis of the gastrointestinal tract, dyspepsia, gastritis, vomiting
- Hematologic & oncologic: Malignant lymphoma, skin carcinoma (nonmelanoma)
- Hepatic: Increased liver enzymes, liver steatosis
- Infection: Bacterial infection, fungal infection, opportunistic infection, serious infection, viral infection
- Neuromuscular & skeletal: Arthralgia, joint swelling, musculoskeletal pain, tendonitis
- Respiratory: Cough, dyspnea, interstitial pulmonary disease, paranasal sinus congestion

<1%, postmarketing, and/or case reports: Angioedema, appendicitis, arterial thrombosis, BK virus, cellulitis, cryptococcosis, cytomegalovirus disease, deep vein thrombosis, esophageal candidiasis, gastric carcinoma, gastrointestinal perforation, hepatotoxicity, histoplasmosis, hypersensitivity reaction, infection due to an organism in genus pneumocystis, listeriosis, lung carcinoma, lymphocytopenia, lymphocytosis, malignant melanoma, malignant neoplasm, malignant neoplasm of breast, malignant neoplasm of colon or rectum, mycobacterium infection, neutropenia, pancreatic adenocarcinoma, pneumonia, prostate carcinoma, pulmonary embolism, reactivation of HBV, renal cell carcinoma, thrombosis (FDA Safety Alert, Aug 5, 2019), tuberculosis, urticaria

Mechanism of Action Tofacitinib inhibits Janus kinase (JAK) enzymes, which are intracellular enzymes involved in stimulating hematopoiesis and immune cell function through a signaling pathway. In response to extracellular cytokine or growth factor signaling, JAKs activate signal transducers and activators of transcription (STATs), which regulate gene expression and intracellular activity. Inhibition of JAKs prevents cytokine- or growth factor-mediated gene expression and intracellular activity of immune cells, reduces circulating CD16/56+ natural killer cells, serum IgG, IgM, IgA, and C-reactive protein, and increases B cells.

Pharmacodynamics/Kinetics

Half-life Elimination ~3 hours (immediate release); ~6 to 8 hours (extended release).

Time to Peak 0.5 to 1 hour (immediate release); 4 hours (extended release)

Pregnancy Considerations

Outcome information following tofacitinib for rheumatoid arthritis or psoriasis in pregnancy is limited (Clowse 2016). Some guidelines recommend avoiding use in pregnant women until additional information is available (Götestam Skorpen 2016).

Data collection to monitor pregnancy and infant outcomes following exposure to tofacitinib is ongoing. Patients may enroll themselves in the Xeljanz Pregnancy Registry (877-311-8972).

Prescribing and Access Restrictions Available through specialty/network pharmacies. Further information may be obtained from the manufacturer, Pfizer Inc, at 1-855-493-5526 or at http://www.xeljanz.com/.

◆ **Tofacitinib Citrate** *see* Tofacitinib *on page 1459*

◆ **Tofranil [DSC]** *see* Imipramine *on page 801*

TOLAZamide (tole AZ a mide)

Related Information

Endocrine Disorders and Pregnancy *on page 1684*

Pharmacologic Category Antidiabetic Agent, Sulfonylurea

Use

Adjunct to diet for the management of mild-to-moderately severe, stable, type 2 diabetes mellitus

Guideline recommendations: First-generation sulfonylureas (eg, tolazamide) are not recommended treatment options for type 2 diabetes; later-generation sulfonylureas with lower hypoglycemic risks (eg, glipizide) are preferred (ADA 2020).

Local Anesthetic/Vasoconstrictor Precautions No information available to require special precautions

Effects on Dental Treatment Key adverse event(s) related to dental treatment: Patients with diabetes should be questioned by the dental professional at each dental visit to assess their risk for stress-induced hypoglycemia. The dental professional should inquire about the patient's routine (ie, work, sleep schedule, eating patterns), history of hypoglycemia, time of last medication dose, last meal, and most recent blood sugar assessment. Keep a supply of glucose tablets and other carbohydrates in the office to prepare for a hypoglycemic event. Seek medical attention when necessary (American Diabetes Association, 2018).

Effects on Bleeding No information available to require special precautions

Adverse Reactions Frequency not defined.

Central nervous system: Disulfiram-like reaction, dizziness, fatigue, headache, malaise, vertigo

Dermatologic: Maculopapular rash, morbilliform rash, pruritus, skin photosensitivity, skin rash, urticaria

Endocrine & metabolic: Hepatic porphyria, hypoglycemia, hyponatremia, porphyria cutanea tarda, SIADH (syndrome of inappropriate antidiuretic hormone secretion)

Gastrointestinal: Anorexia, constipation, diarrhea, epigastric fullness, heartburn, nausea, vomiting

Genitourinary: Diuretic effect

Hematologic & oncologic: Agranulocytosis, aplastic anemia, hemolytic anemia, leukopenia, pancytopenia, thrombocytopenia

Hepatic: Cholestatic jaundice

Neuromuscular & skeletal: Weakness

Mechanism of Action Stimulates insulin release from the pancreatic beta cells; reduces glucose output from the liver; insulin sensitivity is increased at peripheral target sites

Pharmacodynamics/Kinetics

Onset of Action Hypoglycemic effect: 20 minutes; Peak hypoglycemic effect: 4-6 hours

Duration of Action 10-24 hours

Half-life Elimination 7 hours

Time to Peak Serum: 3-4 hours

Pregnancy Risk Factor C

Pregnancy Considerations

Severe hypoglycemia lasting 4 to 10 days has been noted in infants born to mothers taking a sulfonylurea at the time of delivery. Additional adverse events have been reported and may be influenced by maternal glycemic control (Piacquadio 1991). The manufacturer recommends if tolazamide is used during pregnancy, it should be discontinued at least 2 weeks before the expected delivery date.

Poorly controlled diabetes during pregnancy can be associated with an increased risk of adverse maternal and fetal outcomes, including diabetic ketoacidosis, preeclampsia, spontaneous abortion, preterm delivery, delivery complications, major birth defects, stillbirth, and macrosomia (ACOG 201 2018). To prevent adverse outcomes, prior to conception and throughout pregnancy, maternal blood glucose and HbA_{1c} should be kept as close to target goals as possible but without causing significant hypoglycemia (ADA 2020; Blumer 2013).

Agents other than tolazamide are currently recommended to treat diabetes mellitus in pregnancy (ADA 2020).

TOLBUTamide (tole BYOO ta mide)

Related Information

Endocrine Disorders and Pregnancy *on page 1684*

Pharmacologic Category Antidiabetic Agent, Sulfonylurea

Use Diabetes mellitus, type 2: Adjunct to diet for the management of type 2 diabetes mellitus

Guideline recommendations: First-generation sulfonylureas (eg, tolbutamide) are not recommended treatment options for type 2 diabetes; later-generation sulfonylureas with lower hypoglycemic risks (eg, glipizide) are preferred (ADA 2020).

Local Anesthetic/Vasoconstrictor Precautions No information available to require special precautions

Effects on Dental Treatment Key adverse event(s) related to dental treatment: Patients with diabetes should be questioned by the dental professional at each dental visit to assess their risk for stress-induced hypoglycemia. The dental professional should inquire about the patient's routine (ie, work, sleep schedule, eating patterns), history of hypoglycemia, time of last medication dose, last meal, and most recent blood sugar assessment. Keep a supply of glucose tablets and other carbohydrates in the office to prepare for a hypoglycemic event. Seek medical attention when necessary (American Diabetes Association, 2018).

Effects on Bleeding No information available to require special precautions

Adverse Reactions Frequency not defined.

Central nervous system: Disulfiram-like reaction, headache

Dermatologic: Erythema, maculopapular rash, morbilliform rash, pruritus, skin photosensitivity, urticaria

Endocrine & metabolic: Hepatic porphyria, hypoglycemia, hyponatremia, porphyria cutanea tarda, SIADH (syndrome of inappropriate antidiuretic hormone secretion)

Gastrointestinal: Dysgeusia, epigastric fullness, heartburn, nausea

Hematologic & oncologic: Agranulocytosis, aplastic anemia, hemolytic anemia, leukopenia, pancytopenia, thrombocytopenia

Hepatic: Cholestatic jaundice

Hypersensitivity: Hypersensitivity reaction

Mechanism of Action Stimulates insulin release from the pancreatic beta cells; reduces glucose output from the liver; insulin sensitivity is increased at peripheral target sites, suppression of glucagon may also contribute

Pharmacodynamics/Kinetics

Onset of Action 1 hour

Duration of Action Oral: 6-24 hours

Half-life Elimination 4.5-6.5 hours (range: 4-25 hours)

Time to Peak Serum: 3-4 hours

Pregnancy Risk Factor C

Pregnancy Considerations

Tolbutamide crosses the placenta and can be measured in the serum of newborn infants following maternal use during pregnancy (Miller 1962).

Severe hypoglycemia lasting 4 to 10 days has been noted in infants born to mothers taking a sulfonylurea at the time of delivery. Additional adverse events have been reported and may be influenced by maternal glycemic control (Larsson 1960; Saili 1991; Schiff 1970). The manufacturer recommends if tolbutamide is used during pregnancy, it should be discontinued at least 2 weeks before the expected delivery date.

Poorly controlled diabetes during pregnancy can be associated with an increased risk of adverse maternal and fetal outcomes, including diabetic ketoacidosis, preeclampsia, spontaneous abortion, preterm delivery, delivery complications, major birth defects, stillbirth, and macrosomia (ACOG 201 2018). To prevent adverse outcomes, prior to conception and throughout pregnancy, maternal blood glucose and HbA_{1c} should be kept as close to target goals as possible but without causing significant hypoglycemia (ADA 2020; Blumer 2013).

Agents other than tolbutamide are currently recommended to treat diabetes mellitus in pregnancy (ADA 2020).

◆ **Tolbutamide Sodium** *see* TOLBUTamide *on page 1460*

Tolcapone (TOLE ka pone)

Brand Names: US Tasmar

Pharmacologic Category Anti-Parkinson Agent, COMT Inhibitor

Use Adjunct to levodopa and carbidopa for the treatment of signs and symptoms of idiopathic Parkinson disease in patients with motor fluctuations not responsive to other therapies

Local Anesthetic/Vasoconstrictor Precautions No information available to require special precautions

Effects on Dental Treatment Key adverse event(s) related to dental treatment: Significant xerostomia (normal salivary flow resumes upon discontinuation).

Dopaminergic therapy in Parkinson's disease (ie, treatment with levodopa) is associated with orthostatic hypotension. Tolcapone enhances levodopa bioavailability and may increase the occurrence of hypotension/syncope in the dental patient. The patient should be carefully assisted from the chair and observed for signs of orthostatic hypotension.

Effects on Bleeding No information available to require special precautions

Adverse Reactions

>10%:

Cardiovascular: Orthostatic hypotension (17%)

Central nervous system: Drowsiness (14% to 32%), sleep disorder (24% to 25%), hallucination (8% to 24%), dystonia (19% to 22%), increased dream activity (16% to 21%), dizziness (6% to 13%), confusion (10% to 11%), headache (10% to 11%)

Gastrointestinal: Nausea (28% to 50%), diarrhea (16% to 34%; severe: 3% to 4%), anorexia (19% to 23%)

Neuromuscular & skeletal: Dyskinesia (42% to 51%), muscle cramps (17% to 18%)

1% to 10%:

Cardiovascular: Syncope (4% to 5%), chest pain (1% to 3%), hypotension (2%), palpitations

Central nervous system: Fatigue (3% to 7%), loss of balance (2% to 3%), paresthesia (1% to 3%), burning sensation (1% to 2%), agitation (1%), euphoria (1%), hyperactivity (1%), malaise (1%), panic (1%), irritability (1%), mental deficiency (1%), depression, emotional lability, flank pain, hypoesthesia, speech disturbance, vertigo

Dermatologic: Diaphoresis (4% to 7%), alopecia (1%), skin rash

Gastrointestinal: Vomiting (8% to 10%), constipation (6% to 8%), abdominal pain (5% to 6%), xerostomia (5% to 6%), dyspepsia (3% to 4%), flatulence (2% to 4%)

Genitourinary: Urinary tract infection (5%), hematuria (4% to 5%), urine discoloration (2% to 3%), urination disorder (1% to 2%), impotence, urinary incontinence

Hematologic & oncologic: Hemorrhage (1%), skin neoplasm (1%), uterine neoplasm (1%)

Hepatic: Increased serum transaminases (1% to 3%; 3 x ULN, usually with first 6 months of therapy)

Infection: Influenza (3% to 4%), infection

Neuromuscular & skeletal: Hyperkinesia (≤3%), hypokinesia (≤3%), muscle rigidity (2%), neck pain (2%), arthritis (1% to 2%), myalgia, rhabdomyolysis, tremor

Ophthalmic: Cataract (1%), ophthalmic inflammation (1%)

Otic: Tinnitus

Respiratory: Upper respiratory tract infection (5% to 7%), dyspnea (3%), sinus congestion (1% to 2%), bronchitis, pharyngitis

Miscellaneous: Fever (1%), accidental injury

<1%, postmarketing, and/or case reports: Abnormal stools, abnormality in thinking, abscess, altered sense of smell, amnesia, anemia, antisocial behavior, apathy, apnea, arteriosclerosis, arthropathy, asthma, bacterial infection, bladder calculus, brain disease, breast neoplasm, carcinoma, cardiovascular signs and symptoms, cellulitis, cerebral ischemia, cerebrovascular accident, change in libido, chills, cholecystitis, cholelithiasis, choreoathetosis, colitis, cough, dehydration, delirium, delusions, dermatological disease, diabetes mellitus, diplopia, disease of the lacrimal apparatus, duodenal ulcer, dysphagia, dysuria, eczema, edema, epistaxis, erythema multiforme, esophagitis, extrapyramidal reaction, eye pain, facial edema, fungal infection, furunculosis, gastric atony, gastroenteritis, gastrointestinal carcinoma, gastrointestinal hemorrhage, genitourinary disease, glaucoma, hemiplegia, hemophthalmos, hernia, herpes simplex infection, herpes zoster, hiccups, hostility, hypercholesteremia, hypersensitivity reaction, hyperventilation, hypoxia, increased thirst, laryngitis, leukemia, manic reaction, meningitis, myoclonus, neoplasm, nephrolithiasis, nervousness, neuralgia, neuropathy, nocturia, oliguria, oral mucosa ulcer, otalgia, otitis media, ovarian carcinoma, pain, paranoia, pericardial effusion, polyuria, prostate carcinoma, prostatic disease, pruritus, psychosis, pulmonary edema, rectal disease, rhinitis, seborrhea, sialorrhea, skin discoloration, surgery, tenosynovitis, thrombocytopenia, thrombosis, tongue disease, twitching, urinary retention, urticaria, uterine atony, uterine disease, uterine hemorrhage, vaginitis, viral infection

Mechanism of Action Tolcapone is a selective and reversible inhibitor of catechol-o-methyltransferase (COMT). In the presence of a decarboxylase inhibitor (eg, carbidopa), COMT is the major degradation pathway for levodopa. Inhibition of COMT leads to more sustained plasma levels of levodopa and enhanced central dopaminergic activity.

Pharmacodynamics/Kinetics

Half-life Elimination 2 to 3 hours

Time to Peak ~2 hours

Pregnancy Considerations Adverse events were observed in animal reproduction studies.

Prescribing and Access Restrictions A patient signed consent form acknowledging the risks of hepatic injury should be obtained by the treating physician.

Tolnaftate (tole NAF tate)

Brand Names: US Anti-Fungal [OTC]; Antifungal [OTC]; Athletes Foot Spray [OTC]; Dr Gs Clear Nail [OTC]; Fungi-Guard [OTC]; Fungoid-D [OTC] [DSC]; Jock Itch Spray [OTC]; LamISIL AF Defense [OTC] [DSC]; Medi-First Anti-Fungal [OTC] [DSC]; Mycocide Clinical NS [OTC]; Podactin [OTC]; The Treatment Formula 3 [OTC] [DSC]; Tinactin Deodorant [OTC]; Tinactin Jock Itch [OTC] [DSC]; Tinactin [OTC]; Tinaspore [OTC]; Tolnaftate Antifungal [OTC] [DSC]

Pharmacologic Category Antifungal Agent, Topical

Use Treatment of tinea pedis, tinea cruris, tinea corporis; prevention of tinea pedis

Local Anesthetic/Vasoconstrictor Precautions No information available to require special precautions

Effects on Dental Treatment No significant effects or complications reported

Effects on Bleeding No information available to require special precautions

Adverse Reactions Frequency not defined.

Dermatologic: Contact dermatitis, pruritus, stinging of the skin

Local: Irritation

Mechanism of Action Distorts the hyphae and stunts mycelial growth in susceptible fungi

Pharmacodynamics/Kinetics

Onset of Action 24 to 72 hours

- **Tolnaftate Antifungal [OTC] [DSC]** *see* Tolnaftate *on page 1462*
- **Tolsura** *see* Itraconazole *on page 849*

Tolterodine (tole TER oh deen)

Brand Names: US Detrol; Detrol LA

Brand Names: Canada APO-Tolterodine; Detrol; Detrol LA; MINT-Tolterodine; MYLAN-Tolterodine ER; SANDOZ Tolterodine LA; TEVA-Tolterodine; TEVA-Tolterodine LA

Pharmacologic Category Anticholinergic Agent

Use Treatment of patients with an overactive bladder with symptoms of urge urinary incontinence, urgency, or frequency

Local Anesthetic/Vasoconstrictor Precautions No information available to require special precautions

Effects on Dental Treatment The anticholinergic effects of tolterodine are selective for the urinary bladder rather than salivary glands; xerostomia and changes in salivation (normal salivary flow resumes upon discontinuation).

Effects on Bleeding No information available to require special precautions

Adverse Reactions As reported with immediate release tablet, unless otherwise specified.

>10%: Gastrointestinal: Xerostomia (35%; extended release capsules: 23%)

1% to 10%:

Cardiovascular: Chest pain (2%)

Central nervous system: Headache (7%; extended release capsules: 6%), dizziness (5%; extended release capsules: 2%), fatigue (4%; extended release capsules: 2%), drowsiness (immediate and extended release: 3%), anxiety (extended release capsules: 1%)

Dermatologic: Xeroderma (1%)

Endocrine & metabolic: Weight gain (1%)

Gastrointestinal: Constipation (7%; extended release capsules: 6%), abdominal pain (5%; extended release capsules: 4%), diarrhea (4%), dyspepsia (4%; extended release capsules: 3%)

Genitourinary: Dysuria (2%; extended-release capsules: 1%)

Infection: Infection (1%)

Neuromuscular & skeletal: Arthralgia (2%)

Ophthalmic: Xerophthalmia (immediate and extended release: 3%), visual disturbance (2%; extended release capsules: 1%)

Respiratory: Flu-like symptoms (3%), bronchitis (2%), sinusitis (extended release capsules: 2%)

<1%, postmarketing, and/or case reports: Anaphylaxis, angioedema, confusion, dementia (aggravated), disorientation, hallucination, memory impairment, palpitations, peripheral edema, prolonged QT interval on ECG, tachycardia

Mechanism of Action Tolterodine is a competitive antagonist of muscarinic receptors. In animal models, tolterodine demonstrates selectivity for urinary bladder receptors over salivary receptors. Urinary bladder contraction is mediated by muscarinic receptors. Tolterodine increases residual urine volume and decreases detrusor muscle pressure.

Pharmacodynamics/Kinetics

Half-life Elimination

Immediate release tablet: Extensive metabolizers: ~2 hours; Poor metabolizers: ~10 hours

Extended release capsule: Extensive metabolizers: ~7 hours; Poor metabolizers: ~18 hours

Time to Peak Immediate release tablet: 1-2 hours; Extended release capsule: 2-6 hours

Pregnancy Considerations Adverse events were observed in some animal reproduction studies.

◆ **Tolterodine Tartrate** *see* Tolterodine *on page* 1462

Tolvaptan (tol VAP tan)

Brand Names: US Jynarque; Samsca

Brand Names: Canada Jinarc; Samsca

Pharmacologic Category Vasopressin Antagonist

Use

Autosomal dominant polycystic kidney disease: Jynarque, Jinarc [Canadian product]: Slow the progression of kidney function decline in adults at risk of rapidly progressing autosomal dominant polycystic kidney disease (ADPKD)

Hypervolemic or euvolemic hyponatremia: Samsca: Treatment of clinically significant hypervolemic or euvolemic hyponatremia (serum sodium <125 mEq/L or less marked hyponatremia that is symptomatic and resistant to fluid restriction), including patients with heart failure and syndrome of inappropriate antidiuretic hormone (SIADH).

Limitations of use: Not indicated for use when urgent treatment of hyponatremia is required to prevent or treat serious neurological symptoms. It has not been established that raising serum sodium with tolvaptan provides symptomatic benefit.

Local Anesthetic/Vasoconstrictor Precautions No information available to require special precautions

Effects on Dental Treatment No significant effects or complications reported

Effects on Bleeding No information available to require special precautions

Adverse Reactions

>10%:

Central nervous system: Fatigue (14%), dizziness (11%)

Endocrine & metabolic: Increased thirst (12% to 64%)

Gastrointestinal: Nausea (21%), xerostomia (7% to 16%), diarrhea (13%)

Renal: Polyuria (including pollakiuria, 4% to 70%)

1% to 10%:

Cardiovascular: Palpitations (4%), cerebrovascular accident (<2%), deep vein thrombosis (<2%), intracardiac thrombus (<2%), pulmonary embolism (<2%), ventricular fibrillation (<2%)

Dermatologic: Xeroderma (5%), skin rash (4%)

Endocrine & metabolic: Increased serum sodium (2% to 7%), hyperglycemia (6%), hyperuricemia (4%), hypernatremia (≤4%), dehydration (2% to 3%), hypovolemia (2%), diabetic ketoacidosis (<2%)

Gastrointestinal: Gastrointestinal hemorrhage (cirrhosis patients, 10%), dyspepsia (8%), constipation (7%), decreased appetite (7%), abdominal distention (5%), anorexia (4%), ischemic colitis (<2%)

Genitourinary: Urethral bleeding (<2%), vaginal hemorrhage (<2%)

Hematologic & oncologic: Disseminated intravascular coagulation (<2%), prolonged prothrombin time (<2%)

Hepatic: Increased serum alanine aminotransferase (5%)

Neuromuscular & skeletal: Asthenia (9%), rhabdomyolysis (<2%)

Respiratory: Respiratory failure (<2%)

Miscellaneous: Fever (4%)

<1%, postmarketing, and/or case reports: Anaphylactic shock, anaphylaxis, hepatic failure, hepatotoxicity, hyperkalemia, hypersensitivity reaction, increased serum bilirubin, osmotic demyelination syndrome, skin rash

Mechanism of Action An arginine vasopressin (AVP) receptor antagonist with affinity for AVP receptor subtypes V_2 and V_{1a} in a ratio of 29:1. Antagonism of the V_2 receptor by tolvaptan promotes the excretion of free water (without loss of serum electrolytes) resulting in net fluid loss, increased urine output, decreased urine osmolality, and subsequent restoration of normal serum sodium levels.

Pharmacodynamics/Kinetics

Onset of Action Aquaretic and sodium increasing effects (Samsca): 2 to 4 hours

Peak effect: Aquaretic and sodium increasing effects (Samsca): 4 to 8 hours

Duration of Action Aquaretic and sodium increasing effects (Samsca): 60% peak serum sodium elevation is retained at 24 hours; urinary excretion of free water is no longer elevated

Half-life Elimination 15 mg doses: 3 hours; ≥120 mg doses: ~12 hours. **Note:** Half-life increases with higher doses due to a more prolonged absorption.

Time to Peak Plasma: 2 to 4 hours

Pregnancy Risk Factor C

Pregnancy Considerations Adverse events were observed in animal reproduction studies.

Prescribing and Access Restrictions Jinarc [Canadian product]: Only physicians experienced in the diagnosis and treatment of polycystic kidney disease should prescribe Jinarc. Prior to initiating therapy, a patient-prescriber agreement (PPAF) is required outlining relevant patient selection criteria for consideration, expected benefits and risks of treatment, and the need for mandatory hepatic function monitoring. Jinarc is available only through a hepatic safety monitoring and distribution program conducted and maintained by Otsuka Canada Pharmaceuticals Incorporated. All patients initiating therapy should be offered participation in the Canadian Jinarc patient outcomes registry.

◆ **Tomoxetine** *see* AtoMOXetine *on page* 190

◆ **Topamax** *see* Topiramate *on page* 1464

◆ **Topamax Sprinkle** *see* Topiramate *on page* 1464

◆ **Topex Topical Anesthetic** *see* Benzocaine *on page* 228

◆ **Topicaine [OTC]** *see* Lidocaine (Topical) *on page* 902

◆ **Topicaine 5 [OTC]** *see* Lidocaine (Topical) *on page* 902

◆ **TopiDex** *see* DexAMETHasone (Systemic) *on page* 463

Topiramate (toe PYRE a mate)

Brand Names: US Qudexy XR; Topamax; Topamax Sprinkle; Trokendi XR

Brand Names: Canada ACCEL-Topiramate [DSC]; ACH-Topiramate; AG-Topiramate; APO-Topiramate; Auro-Topiramate; DOM-Topiramate; GLN-Topiramate; JAMP-Topiramate; Mar-Topiramate; MINT-Topiramate; MYLAN-Topiramate; PMS-Topiramate; PRO-Topiramate; RAN-Topiramate; SANDOZ Topiramate; TEVA-Topiramate; Topamax; Topamax Sprinkle

Pharmacologic Category Anticonvulsant, Miscellaneous

Use

Migraine (prevention): Prophylaxis of migraine headache in patients ≥12 years of age

Seizures: Monotherapy or adjunctive therapy in patients ≥2 years of age (immediate release and Qudexy XR) or ≥6 years of age (Trokendi XR) with focal (partial) onset or primary generalized tonic-clonic seizures; adjunctive therapy in patients ≥2 years of age (immediate release and Qudexy XR) or ≥6 years of age (Trokendi XR only) with seizures associated with Lennox-Gastaut syndrome

Local Anesthetic/Vasoconstrictor Precautions No information available to require special precautions

Effects on Dental Treatment Key adverse event(s) related to dental treatment: Frequent occurrence of distorted sense of taste (dysgeusia); occurrence of loss of taste (ageusia), xerostomia (normal salivary flow resumes upon discontinuance); gingival hemorrhage has been reported.

Effects on Bleeding No information available to require special precautions

Adverse Reactions Adverse events are reported for adult and pediatric patients for various indications and regimens. A wide range of dosages were studied. Incidence of adverse events was frequently lower in the pediatric population studied.

>10%:

Central nervous system: Paresthesia (adolescents and adults: 19% to 51%; children and adolescents: 3% to 12%), fatigue (8% to 15%), drowsiness (adolescents and adults: 6% to 15%), dizziness (adolescents and adults: 6% to 14%), memory impairment (1% to 11%)

Endocrine & metabolic: Decreased serum bicarbonate (adolescents and adults: 14% to 77%; children and adolescents: 9% to 25%; >5 mEq/L to <17 mEq/L: 1% to 11%), hyperammonemia (adolescents: 14% to 26%; ≥50% above ULN [adolescents]: 9%), weight loss (4% to 17%)

Gastrointestinal: Abdominal pain (adolescents and adults: 6% to 15%), anorexia (adolescents and adults: 4% to 15%), dysgeusia (adolescents and adults: 3% to 15%), nausea (adolescents and adults: 8% to 13%), diarrhea (2% to 11%)

Respiratory: Upper respiratory tract infection (13% to 26%)

Miscellaneous: Fever (1% to 12%)

1% to 10%:

Cardiovascular: Flushing (children and adolescents: ≤5%), chest pain (adults: 1% to 2%)

Central nervous system: Disturbance in attention (≤10%), lack of concentration (≤10%), depression (adults: 7% to 9%; children and adolescents: ≤3%), insomnia (adolescents and adults: 6% to 9%), mood disorder (1% to 8%), hypoesthesia (adolescents and adults 4% to 7%), anxiety (adolescents and adults: 4% to 6%), cognitive dysfunction (1% to 6%), psychomotor impairment (adolescents and adults: 2% to 5%), headache (children and adolescents: 4%), nervousness (adolescents and adults: 4%), ataxia (adolescents and adults: 1% to 4%), behavioral problems (children and adolescents: ≤3%), confusion (≤3%), hypertonia (adults: ≤3%), vertigo (children and adolescents: ≤3%), agitation (adolescents and adults: 2%), exacerbation of depression (adolescents and adults: 2%), speech disturbance (adolescents and adults: 1%)

Dermatologic: Alopecia (1% to 4%), pruritus (adolescents and adults: 1% to 4%), skin rash (1% to 4%), acne vulgaris (adults: 2% to 3%)

Endocrine & metabolic: Menstrual disease (adolescents and adults: 3%), intermenstrual bleeding (children and adolescents: ≤3%), increased gamma-glutamyl transferase (adults: 1% to 3%), increased thirst (adolescents and adults: 2%)

Gastrointestinal: Dyspepsia (adolescents and adults: 4% to 5%), constipation (adolescents and adults: 1% to 4%), gastroenteritis (adolescents and adults: 3%), gastritis (adults: ≤3%), xerostomia (adolescents and adults: 1% to 3%), gastroesophageal reflux disease (adults: 1% to 2%), ageusia (adolescents and adults: 1%)

Genitourinary: Urinary tract infection (adolescents and adults: 1% to 4%), premature ejaculation (adolescents and adults: 3%), decreased libido (adults: ≤3%), urinary frequency (≤3%), vaginal hemorrhage (adults: ≤3%), cystitis (adults: 1% to 3%), urinary incontinence (children and adolescents: 1% to 3%), dysuria (adults: ≤2%)

Hematologic & oncologic: Hemorrhage (4% to 5%), anemia (children and adolescents: 1% to 3%), neoplasm (adolescents and adults: 2%)

Hypersensitivity: Hypersensitivity reaction (adolescents and adults: 2% to 4%)

Infection: Viral infection (3% to 8%), infection (2% to 8%)

Neuromuscular & skeletal: Arthralgia (adolescents and adults: 3% to 7%), asthenia (≤6%), muscle spasm (≤3%), lower extremity pain (adolescents and adults: 2% to 3%)

Ophthalmic: Conjunctivitis (adolescents and adults: 2% to 7%), blurred vision (adolescents and adults: 4%), visual disturbance (adolescents and adults: 1% to 2%)

Otic: Otitis media (adolescents and adults: 1% to 2%)

Renal: Nephrolithiasis (adolescents and adults: ≤3%)

Respiratory: Sinusitis (1% to 10%), cough (adolescents and adults: 2% to 7%), rhinitis (2% to 7%), pharyngitis (adolescents and adults: 5% to 6%), bronchitis (1% to 5%), epistaxis (children and adolescents: ≤4%), dyspnea (adolescents and adults: 1% to 3%)

Miscellaneous: Accidental injury (adolescents and adults: 9%), language problems (adolescents and adults: 6% to 7%)

Frequency not defined:

Cardiovascular: Hypotension, orthostatic hypotension, syncope

Central nervous system: Suicidal ideation, suicidal tendencies

Endocrine & metabolic: Hyperchloremia, increased serum total protein, increased uric acid
Gastrointestinal: Gingival hemorrhage, hematuria
Hematologic & oncologic: Abnormal serum phosphorus level (decreased), decreased neutrophils, decreased white blood cell count, eosinophilia, quantitative disorders of platelets (increased)
Hepatic: Increased serum alkaline phosphatase
Neuromuscular & skeletal: Myalgia
Ophthalmic: Myopia, scotoma, visual field defect
Renal: Increased blood urea nitrogen, increased serum creatinine

<1%, postmarketing, and/or case reports: Acute myopia with secondary angle-closure glaucoma, bullous rash, calcium nephrolithiasis, erythema multiforme, hepatic failure, hepatitis, hyperammonemic encephalopathy, hyperchloremic metabolic acidosis (nonanion gap), hyperthermia, hypohidrosis, maculopathy, major hemorrhage (children), pancreatitis, pemphigus, Stevens-Johnson syndrome, toxic epidermal necrolysis

Mechanism of Action Anticonvulsant activity may be due to a combination of potential mechanisms: Blocks neuronal voltage-dependent sodium channels, enhances GABA(A) activity, antagonizes AMPA/kainate glutamate receptors, and weakly inhibits carbonic anhydrase.

Pharmacodynamics/Kinetics

Half-life Elimination

Immediate release:
Not receiving concomitant enzyme inducers or valproic acid:
Neonates (full-term) with hypothermia: ~43 hours (Filippi 2009)
Infants and Children 9 months to <4 years: 10.4 hours (range: 8.5 to 15.3 hours) (Mikaeloff 2004)
Children 4 to 7 years: Mean range: 7.7 to 8 hours (Rosenfeld 1999)
Children 8 to 11 years: Mean range: 11.3 to 11.7 hours (Rosenfeld 1999)
Children and Adolescents 12 to 17 years: Mean range: 12.3 to 12.8 hours (Rosenfeld 1999)
Receiving concomitant enzyme inducers (eg, carbamazepine, phenytoin, phenobarbital):
Neonates (full-term) with hypothermia: 26.5 hours (Filippi 2009)
Infants and Children 9 months to <4 years: 6.5 hours (range: 3.75 to 10.2 hours) (Mikaeloff 2004)
Children and Adolescents 4 to 17 years: 7.5 hours (Rosenfeld 1999)
Receiving valproic acid: Infants and Children 9 months to 4 years: 9.2 hours (range: 7.23 to 12 hours) (Mikaeloff 2004)
Adults: 19 to 23 hours (mean: 21 hours)
Adults with renal impairment: 59 ± 11 hours
Extended release: Qudexy XR: ~56 hours; Trokendi XR: ~31 hours

Time to Peak

Immediate release:
Neonates (full-term) with hypothermia: 3.8 hours (Filippi 2009)
Infants and Children 9 months to <4 years: 3.7 hours (range: 1.5 to 10.2 hours) (Mikaeloff 2004)
Children 4 to 17 years: Mean range: 1 to 2.8 hours (Rosenfeld 1999)
Adults: 2 hours; range: 1.4 to 4.3 hours
Extended release: Qudexy XR: ~20 hours; Trokendi XR: ~24 hours

Reproductive Considerations

Effective contraception should be used in females of reproductive potential who are not planning a pregnancy; consider use of alternative medications in women who wish to become pregnant.

Pregnancy Considerations

Based on limited data (n=5), topiramate was found to cross the placenta and could be detected in neonatal serum (Ohman 2002).

Topiramate may cause fetal harm if administered to a pregnant woman. An increased risk of oral clefts (cleft lip and/or palate) and for being small for gestational age (SGA) has been observed following in utero exposure. Data from the North American Antiepileptic Drug (NAAED) Pregnancy Registry reported that the prevalence of oral clefts was 1.1% for infants exposed to topiramate during the first trimester of pregnancy, versus 0.36% for infants exposed to a reference antiepileptic drug, and 0.12% for infants with no exposure born to mothers without epilepsy; the relative risk of oral clefts in infants exposed to topiramate was calculated to be 9.6 (95% CI: 4 to 23). Data from the NAAED Pregnancy Registry reported that the prevalence of small for gestational age newborns was 19.7% for newborns exposed to topiramate in utero, versus 7.9% for newborns exposed to a reference antiepileptic drug, and 5.4% for newborns with no exposure born to mothers without epilepsy. Although not evaluated during pregnancy, metabolic acidosis may be induced by topiramate. Metabolic acidosis during pregnancy may result in adverse effects and fetal death. Pregnant women and their newborns should be monitored for metabolic acidosis. In general, maternal polytherapy with antiepileptic drugs may increase the risk of congenital malformations; monotherapy with the lowest effective dose is recommended. Newborns of women taking antiepileptic medications may be at an increased risk of a 1 minute Apgar score <7 (Harden 2009).

Maternal serum concentrations may decrease during the second and third trimesters of pregnancy; therefore, therapeutic drug monitoring should be considered during pregnancy and postpartum in patients who require therapy (Ohman 2009; Westin 2009).

Data collection to monitor pregnancy and infant outcomes following exposure to topiramate is ongoing. Patients may enroll themselves into the NAAED Pregnancy Registry by calling 1-888-233-2334. Additional information is available at www.aedpregnancyregistry.org.

◆ **Topiramate and Phentermine** *see* Phentermine and Topiramate *on page 1225*

◆ **Toposar** *see* Etoposide *on page 626*

Topotecan (toe poe TEE kan)

Brand Names: US Hycamtin

Brand Names: Canada ACT Topotecan; Hycamtin [DSC]; PMS-Topotecan

Pharmacologic Category Antineoplastic Agent, Camptothecin; Antineoplastic Agent, Topoisomerase I Inhibitor

Use

Cervical cancer, recurrent or persistent: Injection: Treatment (in combination with cisplatin) of stage IVB, recurrent or persistent cervical cancer that is not amenable to curative treatment

Ovarian cancer, metastatic: Injection: Treatment of metastatic ovarian cancer (as a single agent) after disease progression on or after initial or subsequent chemotherapy

Small cell lung cancer, relapsed or progressive:

Injection: Treatment of small cell lung cancer (as a single agent) in patients with platinum-sensitive disease which has progressed at least 60 days after initiation of first-line chemotherapy

Oral: Treatment of relapsed small cell lung cancer in patients with a prior complete or partial response and who are at least 45 days from the end of first-line chemotherapy

Local Anesthetic/Vasoconstrictor Precautions No information available to require special precautions

Effects on Dental Treatment Key adverse event(s) related to dental treatment: Stomatitis.

Effects on Bleeding Chemotherapy may result in significant myelosuppression, potentially including significant thrombocytopenia (grade 4: 6% to 27%, nadir 15 days, duration 3-5 days) and altered hemostasis. In patients who are under active treatment with these agents, medical consult is suggested.

Adverse Reactions

>10%:

Central nervous system: Fatigue (oral: 11% to 19%; intravenous: grades 3/4: 6% to 7%)

Dermatologic: Alopecia (oral: 10% to 20%)

Gastrointestinal: Nausea (oral: 27% to 33%; intravenous: grades 3/4: 8% to 10%), diarrhea (oral: 14% to 22%; intravenous: grades 3/4: 6%), vomiting (oral: 19% to 21%; intravenous: grades 3/4: 10%), anorexia (oral: 7% to 14%)

Hematologic & oncologic: Anemia (oral: 94% to 98%; grades 3/4: 25%; grade 3: 15% to 18%; grade 4: 7% to 10%; intravenous: grades 3/4: 37% to 42%), neutropenia (oral: 83% to 91%; grade 3: 24% to 28%; grade 4: 32% to 33%; intravenous: grade 4: 70% to 80%; nadir 12 to 15 days; duration: 7 days), thrombocytopenia (oral: 81%; grade 3: 29% to 30%; grade 4: 6% to 7%; intravenous: grade 4: 27% to 29%; nadir: 15 days; duration: 3 to 5 days), febrile neutropenia (intravenous: grade 3/4: 23% to 28%; grade 4: 5%; oral: grade 4: 4%), neutropenic infection (13% to 17%)

1% to 10%:

Central nervous system: Pain (intravenous: grades 3/4: 5%)

Gastrointestinal: Abdominal pain (intravenous: grades 3/4: 5% to 6%), constipation (intravenous: grades 3/4: 5%), intestinal obstruction (intravenous: grades 3/4: 5%)

Hepatic: Increased serum alanine aminotransferase (intravenous: grades 3/4: ≤4%). increased serum aspartate aminotransferase (intravenous: grades 3/4: ≤4%), increased serum bilirubin (intravenous: grades 3/4: <2%)

Neuromuscular & skeletal: Asthenia (intravenous: grades 3/4: 5% to 9%; oral: 3% to 7%)

Respiratory: Dyspnea (intravenous: grades 3/4: 6% to 9%), pneumonia (intravenous: grades 3/4: 8%)

Miscellaneous: Fever (oral: 5% to 7%), sepsis (2% to 4%)

Frequency not defined:

Hematologic & oncologic: Bone marrow depression

<1%, postmarketing, and/or case reports: Angioedema, arthralgia, chest pain, dermatitis (severe), gastrointestinal perforation, headache, hemorrhage (severe, associated with thrombocytopenia), hypersensitivity reaction, interstitial pulmonary disease, leukopenia, myalgia, neutropenic enterocolitis, nonimmune anaphylaxis, pancytopenia, pruritus (severe), stomatitis, typhlitis

Mechanism of Action Topotecan binds to topoisomerase I and stabilizes the cleavable complex so that religation of the cleaved DNA strand cannot occur. This results in the accumulation of cleavable complexes and single-strand DNA breaks. Topotecan acts in S phase of the cell cycle.

Pharmacodynamics/Kinetics

Half-life Elimination

Pediatric patients (0 to 18 years of age): Lactone moiety: 2.58 hours ± 0.15 (range: 0.2 to 7.1 hours) (Santana 2005)

Adults: IV: 2 to 3 hours; Oral: 3 to 6 hours

Time to Peak

Pediatric patients (1 to 18 years of age): Parenteral formulation (reconstituted lyophilized formulation): 0.75 to 2 hours (Zamboni 1999)

Adults: Oral: 1 to 2 hours; delayed with high-fat meal (1.5 to 4 hours)

Reproductive Considerations

Verify pregnancy status in females of reproductive potential prior to treatment initiation. Females of reproductive potential should use effective contraception during treatment and for at least 6 months after the last topotecan dose. Males with female partners of reproductive potential should use effective contraception during treatment and for 3 months after the last topotecan dose.

Pregnancy Considerations

Based on the mechanism of action and data from animal reproduction studies, in utero exposure to topotecan may cause fetal harm.

◆ **Topotecan HCl** *see* Topotecan *on page 1465*

◆ **Topotecan Hydrochloride** *see* Topotecan *on page 1465*

◆ **Toprol XL** *see* Metoprolol *on page 1009*

◆ **Toradol** *see* Ketorolac (Systemic) *on page 861*

◆ **Torasemide** *see* Torsemide *on page 1467*

Toremifene (tore EM i feen)

Related Information

Clinical Risk Related to Drugs Prolonging QT Interval *on page 1675*

Brand Names: US Fareston

Pharmacologic Category Antineoplastic Agent, Estrogen Receptor Antagonist; Selective Estrogen Receptor Modulator (SERM)

Use Breast cancer, metastatic: Treatment of metastatic breast cancer in postmenopausal women with estrogen receptor-positive or unknown tumors

Local Anesthetic/Vasoconstrictor Precautions Toremifene is one of the drugs confirmed to prolong the QT interval and is accepted as having a risk of causing torsade de pointes. The risk of drug-induced torsade de pointes is extremely low when a single QT interval prolonging drug is prescribed. In terms of epinephrine, it is not known what effect vasoconstrictors in the local anesthetic regimen will have in patients with a known history of congenital prolonged QT interval or in patients taking any medication that prolongs the QT interval. Until more information is obtained, it is suggested that the clinician consult with the physician prior to the use of a vasoconstrictor in suspected patients, and that the vasoconstrictor (epinephrine, mepivacaine and levonordefrin [Carbocaine® 2% with Neo-Cobefrin®]) be used with caution.

Effects on Dental Treatment No significant effects or complications reported

Effects on Bleeding Although significant myelosuppression with associated altered hemostasis has been reported for many chemotherapeutic agents, myelosuppression is not common with toremifene and no specific precautions appear to necessary.

Adverse Reactions

>10%:

Dermatologic: Diaphoresis (20%)

Endocrine & metabolic: Hot flash (35%)

Gastrointestinal: Nausea (14%)

Genitourinary: Vaginal discharge (13%)

Hepatic: Increased serum alkaline phosphatase (8% to 19%), increased serum AST (5% to 19%)

1% to 10%:

Cardiovascular: Edema (5%), cardiac arrhythmia (≤2%), cerebrovascular accident (≤2%), local thrombophlebitis (≤2%), pulmonary embolism (≤2%), thrombosis (≤2%), transient ischemic attacks (≤2%), cardiac failure (≤1%), myocardial infarction (≤1%)

Central nervous system: Dizziness (9%)

Endocrine & metabolic: Hypercalcemia (≤3%)

Gastrointestinal: Vomiting (4%)

Genitourinary: Vaginal hemorrhage (2%)

Hepatic: Increased serum bilirubin (1% to 2%)

Ophthalmic: Cataract (≤10%), xerophthalmia (≤9%), visual field defect (≤4%), corneal disease (≤2%), glaucoma (≤2%), visual disturbance (≤2%), diplopia (≤2%)

<1%, postmarketing, and/or case reports: Alopecia, angina pectoris, anorexia, arthritis, ataxia, blurred vision, constipation, corneal opacity (reversible; including corneal verticulata), depression, dermatitis, dyspnea, endometrial carcinoma, endometrial hyperplasia, fatigue, hepatotoxicity (including hepatitis, nonalcoholic fatty liver disease), jaundice, lethargy, leukopenia, paresis, polyp (uterine), prolonged QT interval on ECG, pruritus, rigors, skin discoloration, thrombocytopenia, toxic hepatitis, tremor, tumor flare, vertigo, weakness

Mechanism of Action Nonsteroidal, triphenylethylene derivative with potent antiestrogenic properties (also has estrogenic effects). Competitively binds to estrogen receptors on tumors and inhibits the growth stimulating effects of estrogen.

Pharmacodynamics/Kinetics

Half-life Elimination Toremifene: ~5 days, ~7 days (females >60 years); N-demethyltoremifene: 6 days

Time to Peak Serum: ≤3 hours

Reproductive Considerations

Toremifene is only approved for use in postmenopausal women; however, if prescribed in premenopausal women, effective nonhormonal contraception should be used.

Pregnancy Risk Factor D

Pregnancy Considerations

Based on the mechanism of action and data from animal reproduction studies, in utero exposure to toremifene may cause fetal harm.

Dental Health Professional Considerations See Local Anesthetic/Vasoconstrictor Precautions

- **Toremifene Citrate** *see* Toremifene *on page 1466*
- **Torezolid** *see* Tedizolid *on page 1409*
- **Torisel** *see* Temsirolimus *on page 1416*

Torsemide (TORE se mide)

Related Information

Cardiovascular Diseases *on page 1654*

Brand Names: US Demadex [DSC]

Pharmacologic Category Antihypertensive; Diuretic, Loop

Use

Edema: Treatment of edema associated with heart failure and hepatic or renal disease.

Hypertension: Management of hypertension.

Note: Not recommended for the initial treatment of hypertension (ACC/AHA [Whelton 2017]).

Local Anesthetic/Vasoconstrictor Precautions No information available to require special precautions

Effects on Dental Treatment No significant effects or complications reported

Effects on Bleeding No information available to require special precautions

Adverse Reactions

1% to 10%:

Cardiovascular: ECG abnormality (2%), chest pain (1%)

Central nervous system: Nervousness (1%)

Gastrointestinal: Constipation (2%), diarrhea (2%), dyspepsia (2%), nausea (2%), sore throat (2%)

Neuromuscular & skeletal: Arthralgia (2%), myalgia (2%), weakness (2%)

Renal: Polyuria (7%)

Respiratory: Rhinitis (3%), cough (2%)

<1%, postmarketing, and/or case reports: Angioedema, arthritis, atrial fibrillation, esophageal hemorrhage, gastrointestinal hemorrhage, hyperglycemia, hyperuricemia, hypokalemia, hyponatremia, hypotension, hypovolemia, impotence, increased thirst, leukopenia, pancreatitis, rectal hemorrhage, shunt thrombosis, skin rash, Stevens-Johnson syndrome, syncope, thrombocytopenia, toxic epidermal necrolysis, ventricular tachycardia, vomiting

Mechanism of Action Inhibits reabsorption of sodium and chloride in the ascending loop of Henle and distal renal tubule, interfering with the chloride-binding cotransport system, thus causing increased excretion of water, sodium, chloride, magnesium, and calcium; does not alter GFR, renal plasma flow, or acid-base balance

Pharmacodynamics/Kinetics

Onset of Action Diuresis: Within 1 hour; Peak effect: Diuresis: 1 to 2 hours; Antihypertensive: 4 to 6 weeks (up to 12 weeks)

Duration of Action Diuresis: ~6 to 8 hours

Half-life Elimination ~3.5 hours

Time to Peak Plasma: Within 1 hour; delayed ~30 minutes when administered with food

Pregnancy Considerations Adverse events have been observed in animal reproduction studies.

- **Tosymra** *see* SUMAtriptan *on page 1394*
- **Total Allergy [OTC]** *see* DiphenhydrAMINE (Systemic) *on page 502*
- **Total Allergy Medicine [OTC]** *see* DiphenhydrAMINE (Systemic) *on page 502*

◆ **Toujeo Max SoloStar** *see* Insulin Glargine *on page* *822*

◆ **Toujeo SoloStar** *see* Insulin Glargine *on page* *822*

◆ **Tovet** *see* Clobetasol *on page* *377*

◆ **Toviaz** *see* Fesoterodine *on page* *665*

◆ **tPA** *see* Alteplase *on page* *111*

◆ **TPV** *see* Tipranavir *on page* *1452*

◆ **TR-700** *see* Tedizolid *on page* *1409*

◆ **TR-701 FA** *see* Tedizolid *on page* *1409*

◆ **tRA** *see* Tretinoin (Systemic) *on page* *1483*

◆ **Tracleer** *see* Bosentan *on page* *249*

◆ **Tradjenta** *see* LinaGLIPtin *on page* *917*

◆ **Trajenta** *see* LinaGLIPtin *on page* *917*

TraMADol (TRA ma dole)

Related Sample Prescriptions

Oral Pain - Sample Prescriptions *on page* *30*

Brand Names: US ConZip; Ultram; Ultram ER [DSC]

Brand Names: Canada APO-Tramadol; AURO-Tramadol; Durela; MAR-Tramadol; Ralivia; TARO-Tramadol ER; Tridural; Ultram; Zytram XL

Generic Availability (US) Yes

Pharmacologic Category Analgesic, Opioid

Dental Use Relief of moderate to moderately-severe dental pain

Use

Pain management:

Extended release: Management of pain severe enough to require daily, around-the-clock, long-term opioid treatment and for which alternative treatment options are inadequate.

Immediate release: Management of pain severe enough to require an opioid analgesic and for which alternative treatments are inadequate.

Limitations of use: Reserve tramadol for use in patients for whom alternative treatment options (eg, nonopioid analgesics) are ineffective, not tolerated, or would be otherwise inadequate to provide sufficient management of pain. Tramadol ER is not indicated as an as-needed analgesic.

Local Anesthetic/Vasoconstrictor Precautions No information available to require special precautions

Effects on Dental Treatment Key adverse event(s) related to dental treatment: Xerostomia and changes in salivation (normal salivary flow resumes upon discontinuation). See Dental Health Professional Considerations.

Effects on Bleeding No information available to require special precautions

Adverse Reactions

>10%:

Gastrointestinal: Constipation (9% to 46%), nausea (16% to 40%), vomiting (5% to 17%), xerostomia (5% to 13%), dyspepsia (1% to 13%)

Nervous system: Dizziness (≤33%), vertigo (≤33%), headache (12% to 32%), drowsiness (7% to 25%), central nervous system stimulation (7% to 14%)

Neuromuscular & skeletal: Asthenia (≤12%)

1% to 10%:

Cardiovascular: Flushing (8%), chest pain (1% to <5%), hypertension (1% to <5%), vasodilation (1% to <5%), peripheral edema (<5%), orthostatic hypotension (≤4%)

Dermatologic: Diaphoresis (1% to 9%), dermatitis (1% to <5%), skin rash (1% to <5%), pruritus (3%)

Endocrine & metabolic: Hot flash (1% to <5%), hyperglycemia (1% to <5%), weight loss (1% to <5%)

Gastrointestinal: Diarrhea (5% to 10%), anorexia (1% to 6%), abdominal pain (1% to <5%), decreased appetite (1% to <5%), sore throat (1% to <5%), viral gastroenteritis (1% to <5%), flatulence (<1% to <5%)

Genitourinary: Menopausal symptoms (1% to <5%), pelvic pain (1% to <5%), prostatic disease (1% to <5%), urine abnormality (1% to <5%), urinary tract infection (1% to <5%), urinary frequency (<5%), urinary retention (<5%)

Infection: Influenza (1% to <5%)

Nervous system: Anxiety (1% to <5%), apathy (1% to <5%), ataxia (1% to <5%), chills (1% to <5%), confusion (1% to <5%), depersonalization (1% to <5%), depression (1% to <5%), falling (1% to <5%), feeling hot (1% to <5%), hypoesthesia (1% to <5%), lethargy (1% to <5%), nervousness (1% to <5%), pain (1% to <5%), paresthesia (1% to <5%), restlessness (1% to <5%), rigors (1% to <5%), agitation (<5%), euphoria (<5%), hypertonia (<5%), malaise (<5%), sleep disorder (<5%), withdrawal syndrome (<5%), insomnia (2%)

Neuromuscular & skeletal: Arthralgia (≤5%), back pain (1% to <5%), increased creatine phosphokinase in blood specimen (1% to <5%), limb pain (1% to <5%), myalgia (<5%), neck pain (1% to <5%), tremor (<5%)

Ophthalmic: Blurred vision (1% to <5%), miosis (1% to <5%), visual disturbance (1% to <5%)

Respiratory: Bronchitis (1% to <5%), cough (1% to <5%), nasal congestion (1% to <5%), nasopharyngitis (1% to <5%), pharyngitis (1% to <5%), rhinitis (1% to <5%), rhinorrhea (1% to <5%), sinus congestion (1% to <5%), sinusitis (1% to <5%), sneezing (1% to <5%), upper respiratory tract infection (1% to <5%)

Miscellaneous: Fever (1% to <5%), flu-like syndrome (1% to <5%), accidental injury (<5%)

<1%, postmarketing, and/or case reports: Abnormal dreams, abnormal gait, abnormality in thinking, acute myocardial infarction, adrenocortical insufficiency, amnesia, anaphylactoid reaction, anaphylaxis, anemia, angioedema, appendicitis, arthritis, bronchospasm, cataract, cellulitis, cholecystitis, cholelithiasis, cognitive dysfunction, cold and clammy skin, deafness, decreased hemoglobin, decreased libido, delirium, difficulty in micturition, disorientation, diverticulitis of the gastrointestinal tract, dysgeusia, dyspnea, dysuria, ecchymoses, ECG abnormality, emotional lability, eye disease, femoral neck fracture (Wei 2020), gastroenteritis, gastrointestinal hemorrhage, gout, hair disease, hallucination, hematuria, hepatic failure, hepatitis, hyperkinesia, hypersensitivity reaction, hypoglycemia, hypotension, increased blood urea nitrogen, increased gamma-glutamyl transferase, increased liver enzymes, increased serum ALT, increased serum AST, increased serum creatinine, irritability, ischemic heart disease, jitteriness, joint stiffness, lack of concentration, lacrimal dysfunction, lower extremity edema, menstrual disease, migraine, movement disorder, muscle cramps, muscle injury, muscle spasm, muscle twitching, mydriasis, neck stiffness, night sweats, osteoarthritis, otitis, palpitations, pancreatitis, peripheral ischemia, piloerection, pneumonia, prolonged QT interval on ECG, proteinuria, pulmonary edema, pulmonary embolism, sedated state, seizure, serotonin syndrome, sexual difficulty, skin vesicle, speech disturbance, Stevens-Johnson

syndrome, stomatitis, suicidal tendencies, syncope, tachycardia, tinnitus, toothache, torsades de pointes, urticaria viral infection, yawning

Dental Usual Dosage Moderate-to-severe chronic pain: Oral:

Adults:

Immediate release formulation: 50 to 100 mg every 4 to 6 hours (not to exceed 400 mg/day)

For patients not requiring rapid onset of effect, tolerability may be improved by starting dose at 25 mg/day and titrating dose by 25 mg every 3 days, until reaching 25 mg 4 times/day. The total daily dose may then be increased by 50 mg every 3 days as tolerated, to reach dose of 50 mg 4 times/day. After titration, 50 to 100 mg may be given every 4 to 6 hours as needed up to a maximum 400 mg/day.

Extended release formulations:

Ultram ER:

Patients not currently on immediate-release: 100 mg once daily; titrate every 5 days (maximum: 300 mg/day)

Patients currently on immediate-release: Calculate 24-hour immediate release total and initiate total daily dose (round dose to the next lowest 100 mg increment); titrate (maximum: 300 mg/day)

Ralivia (Canadian labeling, not available in US): 100 mg once daily; titrate every 5 days as needed based on clinical response and severity of pain (maximum: 300 mg/day)

Tridural (Canadian labeling, not available in US): 100 mg once daily; titrate by 100 mg/day every 2 days as needed based on clinical response and severity of pain (maximum: 300 mg/day)

Zytram XL (Canadian labeling, not available in US): 150 mg once daily; if pain relief is not achieved may titrate by increasing dosage incrementally, with sufficient time to evaluate effect of increased dosage; generally not more often than every 7 days (maximum: 400 mg/day)

Elderly >75 years:

Immediate release: 50 mg every 6 hours (not to exceed 300 mg/day); see dosing adjustments for renal and hepatic impairment.

Extended release formulation: Use with great caution. See adult dosing.

Dosing

Adult

Pain management, moderate to severe:

Note: In general, opioids may be considered a potential component of a comprehensive, multimodal, patient-specific treatment plan for pain. Nonopioid analgesia should be maximized, if appropriate, prior to initiation of opioid analgesia; combination therapy with analgesics with differing mechanisms of action may improve efficacy and reduce the doses and/or frequency required for each agent (APS 2016; Hill 2018). Tramadol doses should be titrated to appropriate analgesic effect; use the lowest effective dose for the shortest period of time. Tramadol is used for a variety of moderate to moderately severe painful conditions and may be of particular benefit for patients with mixed nociceptive and neuropathic pain due to its dual mechanism of action (APS 2016).

Acute pain (eg, postoperative):

Note: In patients who are experiencing acute pain severe enough to require opioids (in addition to appropriate nonopioid analgesia), limit the quantity prescribed to the expected duration of acute pain; a quantity sufficient for ≤3 days is often adequate, whereas >7 days is rarely needed (CDC [Dowell 2016]). Long-acting preparations are **not** recommended for treatment of acute pain in opioid-naive patients (CDC [Dowell 2016]).

Immediate release: **Oral:** Initial: 50 mg every 4 to 6 hours as needed (APS 2016); some experts suggest that 25 to 50 mg 3 times per day may be sufficient for patients with moderate acute pain (Isaac 2019; Pino 2018). The dose may be increased as needed and tolerated to 50 to 100 mg every 4 to 6 hours (maximum: 400 mg/day) (APS 2016; manufacturer's labeling).

Chronic pain (alternative agent):

Note: Opioids, including tramadol, are **not** the preferred therapy for chronic noncancer pain due to insufficient evidence of benefit and risk of serious harm; nonpharmacologic treatment and nonopioid analgesics are preferred with the exception of pain from sickle cell disease and in end-of-life care (CDC [Dowell 2016]; CDC [Dowell 2019]). Opioids, including tramadol, should **only** be considered in patients who experience clinically meaningful improvement in pain and function that outweighs patient safety risks (CDC [Dowell 2016]). The utility of tramadol in patients with chronic pain due to cancer is questionable, especially considering its dual mechanism of action and dose ceiling (Bandieri 2016; Wiffen 2017).

*Opioid-naive patients **not** currently on tramadol immediate release:*

Immediate release: **Oral:** The ideal dosing regimen has not been established; consider restricting the initial dose to <300 mg tramadol per day (ie, <50 mg *morphine equivalents daily*) (Busse 2017). An example initial dose is 25 to 50 mg every 6 hours as needed (Rosenquist 2018). The dose may be increased as needed and tolerated to 50 to 100 mg every 4 to 6 hours (maximum: 400 mg/day) (APS 2016; manufacturer's labeling).

Extended release:

Note: Although manufacturer's labeling contains the following directions for initiating extended-release tramadol products in opioid-naive patients with chronic pain, it is recommended that when starting opioid therapy, treatment be initiated with an immediate-release preparation to more accurately determine the daily opioid requirement and decrease the risk of overdose (CDC [Dowell 2016]). The CDC recommends that extended-release opioids be reserved for patients who have received immediate-release opioids daily for ≥1 week yet continue to experience severe, continuous pain (CDC [Dowell 2016]).

Initial: **Oral:** 100 mg once daily; titrate by 100 mg/day increments every 5 days as needed (maximum: 300 mg/day)

Tridural [Canadian product]: Initial: **Oral:** 100 mg once daily; titrate by 100 mg/day increments every 2 days as needed (maximum: 300 mg/day)

Zytram XL [Canadian product]: **Oral:** 150 mg once daily; if pain relief is not achieved, may titrate by increasing dosage incrementally with sufficient time to evaluate effect of increased dosage, generally not more often than every 7 days (maximum: 400 mg/day).

Patients currently on tramadol immediate release for ≥1 week: Calculate 24-hour tramadol immediate-release total dose and initiate total extended-release daily dose (round dose to the next lowest 100 mg increment); titrate as needed and tolerated to desired effect (maximum: 300 mg/day). In patients who experience breakthrough pain, clinicians may consider the addition of an immediate-release rescue analgesic (eg, NSAID or short-acting weak opioid).

Discontinuation of therapy: When discontinuing chronic opioid therapy, the dose should be gradually tapered down. An optimal universal tapering schedule for all patients has not been established (CDC [Dowell 2016]). Proposed schedules range from slow (eg, 10% reductions per week) to rapid (eg, 25% to 50% reduction every few days) (CDC 2015). Tapering schedules should be individualized to minimize opioid withdrawal while considering patient-specific goals and concerns as well as the pharmacokinetics of the opioid being tapered. An even slower taper may be appropriate in patients who have been receiving opioids for a long duration (eg, years), particularly in the final stage of tapering, whereas more rapid tapers may be appropriate in patients experiencing severe adverse events (CDC [Dowell 2016]). Monitor carefully for signs/symptoms of withdrawal. If the patient displays withdrawal symptoms, consider slowing the taper schedule; alterations may include increasing the interval between dose reductions, decreasing amount of daily dose reduction, pausing the taper and restarting when the patient is ready, and/or coadministration of an alpha-2 agonist (eg, clonidine) to blunt withdrawal symptoms (Berna 2015; CDC [Dowell 2016]; manufacturer's labeling). Continue to offer nonopioid analgesics as needed for pain management during the taper; consider nonopioid adjunctive treatments for withdrawal symptoms (eg, GI complaints, muscle spasm) as needed (Berna 2015; Sevarino 2018).

Premature ejaculation (alternative agent) (off-label use):

Note: Tramadol may be considered in patients who have failed other therapies (eg, SSRIs, topical anesthetics). Consideration should be given to the risk of addiction and adverse effects associated with opioids (ISSM [Althof 2014]); to promote safe use, regular follow-up to monitor for response, toxicity, and misuse is recommended.

Immediate release: **Oral:** The ideal dosing regimen has not been established; dosage range studied: 25 to 50 mg administered on demand 1 to 3 hours prior to intercourse (Alghobary 2010; Eassa 2013; Gameel 2013; Kaynar 2012; Safarinejad 2006; Salem 2008).

Restless legs syndrome, refractory (alternative agent) (off-label use):

Note: Use of opioids for restless legs syndrome (RLS) is typically restricted to patients with severe symptoms refractory to first-line agents for RLS (Silber 2018). Consideration should be given to the risk of addiction and adverse effects associated with opioids; to promote safe use, regular follow-up to monitor for response, toxicity, and misuse is recommended. Clinicians should note that the adverse effect of RLS augmentation (ie, worsening of symptoms) has been reported with tramadol use (Earley 2006; Vetrugno 2007).

Immediate release: **Oral:** Initial: 50 mg once daily at bedtime or during the night; titrate to the lowest effective dose (Silber 2018). Usual effective dosage range: 50 to 100 mg/day (Silber 2013).

Extended release: **Oral:** Initial: 100 mg once daily at bedtime or during the night; titrate to the lowest effective dose. Usual effective dosage range: 100 to 200 mg/day (Silber 2018). **Note:** Extended-release formulations may be preferred to decrease end-of-dose rebound; consider conversion to an extended-release formulation after establishment of efficacy and tolerability (≥7 days based on chronic pain recommendations [CDC (Dowell 2016)]) with an immediate-release formulation (Silber 2018).

Geriatric Elderly >65 years to ≤75 years: Refer to adult dosing; use with caution and initiate at the low end of the dosing range.

Elderly >75 years:

Immediate release: Maximum: 300 mg/day.

Extended release: Use with extreme caution.

Renal Impairment: Adult

Immediate release:

CrCl ≥30 mL/minute: There are no dosage adjustments provided in the manufacturer's labeling; use with caution.

CrCl <30 mL/minute: Increase dosing interval to every 12 hours (maximum: 200 mg/day).

Dialysis: Dialyzable (7%); increase dosing interval to every 12 hours; (maximum: 200 mg/day); administer regular dose on the day of dialysis.

Extended release:

CrCl ≥30 mL/minute: There are no dosage adjustments provided in the manufacturer's labeling; use with caution.

CrCl <30 mL/minute: Avoid use.

Hepatic Impairment: Adult

Immediate release:

Mild to moderate impairment: There are no dosage adjustments provided in the manufacturer's labeling.

Severe impairment: 50 mg every 12 hours.

Extended release:

Mild to moderate impairment (Child-Pugh class A and B): There are no dosage adjustments provided in the manufacturer's labeling; use with caution.

Severe impairment (Child-Pugh class C): Avoid use.

Pediatric Note: Doses should be titrated to appropriate analgesic effect; use the lowest effective dose for the shortest period of time:

Pain management, moderate to severe pain (excluding postoperative tonsillectomy/adenoidectomy pain): Note: The FDA has recommended that tramadol not be used in pediatric patients <12 years of age and all pediatric patients undergoing tonsillectomy and/or adenoidectomy due to increased risk of breathing problems (sometimes fatal). Slowed or difficult breathing has been reported in pediatric patients <18 years of age; risk may be increased in pediatric patients who are obese or have conditions such as obstructive sleep apnea or severe lung disease, or who are ultrarapid metabolizers of the drug (FDA 2015; FDA 2017).

Acute pain: *Immediate-release formulations*:

Children and Adolescents 4 to ≤16 years: Limited data available: Oral: 1 to 2 mg/kg/dose every 4 to 6 hours; maximum single dose: 100 mg (usual adult starting dose: 50 to 100 mg); maximum daily dose is the lesser of 8 mg/kg/**day or** 400 mg/**day** (Finkel 2002; Payne 2002; Rose 2003). **Note:** Due to potential respiratory complications, tramadol should be avoided in patients <12 years of age and all pediatric patients undergoing tonsillectomy and/or adenoidectomy (FDA 2017).

Adolescents ≥17 years: Oral: 50 to 100 mg every 4 to 6 hours; maximum daily dose: 400 mg/**day**. For patients not requiring rapid onset of effect, tolerability to adverse effects may be improved by initiating therapy at 25 mg/day and titrating dose by 25 mg every 3 days until 25 mg 4 times daily is reached. Dose may then be increased by 50 mg every 3 days as tolerated to reach 50 mg 4 times daily.

Chronic pain: *Extended-release formulations*: Adolescents ≥18 years: Oral: **Note:** For patients requiring around-the-clock pain management for an extended period of time. Opioids, including tramadol, are **not** the preferred therapy for chronic noncancer pain due to insufficient evidence of benefit and risk of serious harm; nonpharmacologic treatment and nonopioid analgesics are preferred with the exception of pain from sickle cell disease and in end-of-life care (CDC [Dowell 2016]; CDC [Dowell 2019]). Opioids, including tramadol, should **only** be considered in patients who experience clinically meaningful improvement in pain and function that outweighs patient safety risks (CDC [Dowell 2016]).

Patients not currently on immediate-release tramadol: 100 mg once daily; titrate every 5 days; maximum daily dose: 300 mg/**day**.

Patients currently on immediate-release tramadol: Calculate 24-hour total immediate-release tramadol dose and initiate total extended-release daily dose (round dose to the next lowest 100 mg increment) once daily; titrate as tolerated to desired effect; maximum daily dose: 300 mg/**day**.

Renal Impairment: Pediatric

Immediate release: Adolescents ≥17 years:

CrCl ≥30 mL/minute: There are no dosage adjustments provided in the manufacturer's labeling; use with caution.

CrCl <30 mL/minute: Increase dosing interval to every 12 hours; maximum daily dose: 200 mg/**day.**

Dialysis: Dialyzable (7%); increase dosing interval to every 12 hours; maximum daily dose: 200 mg/**day**; administer regular dose on the day of dialysis.

Extended release: Adolescents ≥18 years:

CrCl ≥30 mL/minute: There are no dosage adjustments provided in the manufacturer's labeling; use with caution.

CrCl <30 mL/minute: Avoid use.

Hepatic Impairment: Pediatric

Immediate release: Adolescents ≥17 years: There are no dosage adjustments provided in the manufacturer's labeling. In patients with cirrhosis, recommended dose is 50 mg every 12 hours.

Extended release: Adolescents ≥18 years:

Mild to moderate impairment (Child-Pugh class A and B): There are no dosage adjustments provided in the manufacturer's labeling; use with caution.

Severe impairment (Child-Pugh class C): Avoid use.

Mechanism of Action Tramadol and its active metabolite (M1) binds to μ-opiate receptors in the CNS causing inhibition of ascending pain pathways, altering the perception of and response to pain; also inhibits the reuptake of norepinephrine and serotonin, which are neurotransmitters involved in the descending inhibitory pain pathway responsible for pain relief (Grond 2004)

Contraindications

Hypersensitivity (eg, anaphylaxis) to tramadol, opioids, or any component of the formulation; pediatric patients <12 years; postoperative management in pediatric patients <18 years who have undergone tonsillectomy and/or adenoidectomy; significant respiratory depression; acute or severe bronchial asthma in the absence of appropriately monitored settings and/or resuscitative equipment; GI obstruction, including paralytic ileus (known or suspected); concomitant use with or within 14 days following MAO inhibitor therapy.

Canadian products: Additional contraindications (not in US labeling): (**Note:** Contraindications may differ between product labeling; refer also to product labeling): Severe renal impairment (CrCl <30 mL/minute), severe hepatic impairment (Child-Pugh class C); mild, intermittent or short-duration pain that can be managed with other pain medication; management of perioperative pain; status asthmaticus, chronic obstructive airway, acute respiratory depression, hypercapnia, cor pulmonale, delirium tremens, seizure disorder, severe CNS depression, increased cerebrospinal or intracranial pressure, head injury, suspected surgical abdomen (eg, acute appendicitis or pancreatitis); acute intoxication with ethanol, hypnotics, centrally acting analgesics, opioids, or psychotropic drugs; breastfeeding, pregnancy; use during labor and delivery.

Warnings/Precautions [US Boxed Warning]: Serious, life-threatening, or fatal respiratory depression may occur. Monitor closely for respiratory depression, especially during initiation or dose escalation. Swallow ER tablets whole; crushing, chewing, or dissolving can cause rapid release and a potentially fatal dose. Carbon dioxide retention from opioid-induced respiratory depression can exacerbate the sedating effects of opioids. Use with caution and monitor for respiratory depression in patients with significant chronic obstructive pulmonary disease or cor pulmonale, and those with a substantially decreased respiratory reserve, hypoxia, hypercapnia, or preexisting respiratory depression, particularly when initiating and titrating therapy; critical respiratory depression may occur, even at therapeutic dosages. Consider the use of alternative nonopioid analgesics in these patients.

[US Boxed Warning]: Life-threatening respiratory depression and death have occurred in children who received tramadol. Some of the reported cases occurred following tonsillectomy and/or adenoidectomy; in at least 1 case, the child had evidence of being an ultra-rapid metabolizer of tramadol due to a CYP450 2D6 polymorphism. Tramadol is contraindicated in pediatric patients <12 years and in pediatric patients <18 years following tonsillectomy and/or adenoidectomy. Avoid the use of tramadol in pediatric patients 12 to 18 years of age who have other risk factors that may increase their sensitivity to the respiratory depressant effects of tramadol. Risk factors include conditions associated with hypoventilation, such as postoperative status, obstructive sleep apnea, obesity, severe pulmonary disease, neuromuscular disease, and concomitant use of other medications that cause respiratory depression. Deaths have also occurred in breastfeeding infants after being exposed to high concentrations of morphine because the mothers were ultra-rapid metabolizers of codeine. **[US Boxed Warning]: Use exposes patients and other users to the risks of addiction, abuse, and misuse, potentially leading to overdose and death. Assess each patient's risk prior to prescribing; monitor all patients regularly for development of these behaviors or conditions.** Use with caution in patients with a history of drug abuse or acute alcoholism; potential for drug dependency exists. Other risk factors associated with increased risk include a personal or family history of substance use disorder or mental illness (eg, major depression). Consider offering naloxone prescriptions in patients with factors associated with an increased risk for overdose, such as history of overdose or substance use disorder, higher opioid dosages (≥50 morphine milligram equivalents/day orally), and concomitant benzodiazepine use (CDC [Dowell 2016]). **[US Boxed Warning]: Accidental ingestion of even one dose of tramadol, especially in children, can result in a fatal overdose of tramadol.**

[US Boxed Warning]: Concomitant use of opioids with benzodiazepines or other CNS depressants, including alcohol, may result in profound sedation, respiratory depression, coma, and death. Reserve concomitant prescribing of tramadol and benzodiazepines or other CNS depressants for use in patients for whom alternative treatment options are inadequate. Limit dosage and durations to the minimum required and follow patients for signs and symptoms of respiratory depression and sedation. [US Boxed Warning]: Use with all CYP3A4 inhibitors may result in an increase in tramadol plasma concentrations, which could increase or prolong adverse drug effects and may cause potentially fatal respiratory depression. In addition, discontinuation of a concomitant CYP3A4 inducer may result in increased tramadol concentrations. Monitor patients receiving tramadol and any CYP3A4 inhibitor or inducer. Potentially significant interactions may exist, requiring dose or frequency adjustment, additional monitoring, and/or selection of alternative therapy.

Even when taken within the recommended dosage seizures may occur; risk is increased in patients receiving serotonin reuptake inhibitors (SSRIs), serotonin norepinephrine reuptake inhibitors (SNRIs), anorectics, other opioids, tricyclic antidepressants and other tricyclic compounds (eg, cyclobenzaprine, promethazine), neuroleptics, MAO inhibitors, other drugs which may lower seizure threshold, or drugs which impair metabolism of tramadol (eg, CYP2D6 and 3A4 inhibitors). Patients with a history of seizures, or with a risk of seizures (head trauma, metabolic disorders, CNS infection, malignancy, or during alcohol/drug withdrawal) are also at increased risk. Serious anaphylactoid reactions (including rare fatalities) often following initial dosing have been reported. Pruritus, hives, bronchospasm, angioedema, toxic epidermal necrolysis (TEN), and Stevens-Johnson syndrome have also been reported. Previous anaphylactoid reactions to opioids may increase risks for similar reactions to tramadol; avoid use in these patients. If anaphylaxis or other hypersensitivity occurs, discontinue permanently; do not rechallenge. May cause CNS depression, which may impair physical or mental abilities; patients must be cautioned about performing tasks which require mental alertness (eg, operating machinery or driving).

Hypoglycemia (including severe cases) has been reported (rare) particularly within the first 30 days of tramadol initiation (Fournier 2015). May cause severe hypotension (including orthostatic hypotension and syncope); use with caution in patients with hypovolemia, cardiovascular disease (including acute MI), or drugs which may exaggerate hypotensive effects (including phenothiazines or general anesthetics). Monitor for symptoms of hypotension following initiation or dose titration. Avoid use in patients with circulatory shock. Serotonin syndrome may occur with concomitant use of serotonergic agents (eg, SSRIs, SNRIs, triptans, TCAs), lithium, St John's wort, agents that impair metabolism of serotonin (eg, MAO inhibitors), or agents that impair metabolism of tramadol (eg, CYP2D6 and 3A4 inhibitors). May obscure diagnosis or clinical course of patients with acute abdominal conditions. Avoid use in patients with impaired consciousness or coma as these patients are susceptible to intracranial effects of CO2 retention. Use with caution in patients who are morbidly obese. Use with caution in patients with adrenal insufficiency (including Addison disease); biliary tract dysfunction or acute pancreatitis; delirium tremens; head injury, intracranial lesions, or elevated intracranial pressure; prostatic hyperplasia and/or urinary stricture; toxic psychosis; and/or thyroid dysfunction.

Use with caution; extended-release formulations should not be used in severe hepatic impairment (Child-Pugh class C). Reduce dosage of immediate-release formulations in patients with severe renal impairment; extended-release formulations should be avoided in severe renal impairment. Use opioids with caution for chronic pain in patients with mental health conditions (eg, depression, anxiety disorders, post-traumatic stress disorder) due to increased risk for opioid use disorder and overdose; more frequent monitoring is recommended. Opioid use increases the risk for sleep-related disorders (eg, central sleep apnea [CSA], hypoxemia) in a dose-dependent fashion. Use with caution for chronic pain and titrate dosage cautiously in patients with risk factors for sleep-disordered breathing (eg, heart failure, obesity). Consider dose reduction in patients presenting with CSA. Avoid opioids in patients with moderate to severe sleep-disordered breathing (CDC [Dowell 2016]). Avoid use in patients who are suicidal; use with caution in patients taking tranquilizers and/or antidepressants, or those with an emotional disturbance including depression. Consider the use of alternative nonopioid analgesics in these patients. Avoid use in patients who are ultra-rapid metabolizers because of a specific CYP2D6 genotype (gene duplications donated as *1/*1xN or *1/*2xN); these patients may have extensive conversion to its active metabolite and thus increased opioid-mediated effects. The occurrence of this phenotype is seen in approximately 1% to 2% of East Asians (Chinese, Japanese, Korean), 1% to 10% of Caucasians, 3% to 4% of African-Americans, and may be >10% in certain racial/ethnic groups (ie, Oceanian, Northern African, Middle Eastern, Ashkenazi Jews, Puerto Rican). Use with caution in cachectic or debilitated patients; there is a greater potential for critical respiratory depression, even at therapeutic dosages; consider the use of alternative nonopioid analgesics in these patients.

Use opioids for chronic pain with caution in older adults; monitor closely due to an increased potential for risks, including certain risks such as falls/fracture, cognitive impairment, and constipation. Clearance may also be reduced in older adults (with or without renal impairment) resulting in a narrow therapeutic window and increasing the risk for respiratory depression or overdose (CDC [Dowell 2016]). Consider the use of alternative nonopioid analgesics in these patients.

[US Boxed Warning]: Prolonged use of opioids during pregnancy can cause neonatal withdrawal syndrome in the newborn which may be life-threatening if not recognized and treated according to protocols developed by neonatology experts. If opioid use is required for a prolonged period in a pregnant woman, advise the patient of the risk of neonatal opioid withdrawal syndrome and ensure that appropriate treatment will be available. Signs and symptoms include irritability, hyperactivity and abnormal sleep pattern, high pitched cry, tremor, vomiting, diarrhea and failure to gain weight. Onset, duration and severity depend on the drug used, duration of use, maternal dose, and rate of drug elimination by the newborn.

[US Boxed Warning]: To ensure that the benefits of opioid analgesics outweigh the risks of addiction, abuse, and misuse, a REMS is required. Drug companies with approved opioid analgesic products must make REMS-compliant education programs available to health care providers. Health care providers are encouraged to complete a REMS-compliant education program; counsel patients and/or their caregivers, with every prescription, on safe use, serious risks, storage, and disposal of these products; emphasize to patients and their caregivers the importance of reading the Medication Guide every time it is provided by their pharmacist; and consider other tools to improve patient, household, and community safety. An opioid-containing analgesic regimen should be tailored to each patient's needs and based upon the type of pain being treated (acute versus chronic), the route of administration, degree of tolerance for opioids (naive versus chronic user), age, weight, and medical condition. The optimal analgesic dose varies widely among patients; doses should be titrated to pain relief/prevention. Opioids decrease bowel motility; monitor for decrease bowel motility in postop patients receiving opioids. Use with caution in the perioperative setting; individualize treatment when transitioning from parenteral to oral analgesics. Abrupt discontinuation in patients who are physically dependent on opioids has been associated with serious withdrawal symptoms, uncontrolled pain, attempts to find other opioids (including illicit), and suicide. Use a collaborative, patient-specific taper schedule that minimizes the risk of withdrawal, considering factors such as current opioid dose, duration of use, type of pain, and physical and psychological factors. Monitor pain control, withdrawal symptoms, mood changes, suicidal ideation, and for use of other substances and provide care as needed. Concurrent use of mixed agonist/antagonist (eg, pentazocine, nalbuphine, butorphanol) or partial agonist (eg, buprenorphine) analgesics may also precipitate withdrawal symptoms and/or reduced analgesic efficacy in patients following prolonged therapy with mu opioid agonists.

Chronic pain: Opioids should **not** be used as first-line therapy for chronic pain management (pain >3-month duration or beyond time of normal tissue healing) due to limited short-term benefits, undetermined long-term benefits, and association with serious risks (eg, overdose, MI, auto accidents, risk of developing opioid use disorder). Preferred management includes nonpharmacologic therapy and nonopioid therapy (eg, NSAIDs, acetaminophen, certain anticonvulsants and antidepressants). If opioid therapy is initiated, it should be combined with nonpharmacologic and nonopioid therapy, as appropriate. Prior to initiation, known risks of opioid therapy should be discussed and realistic treatment goals for pain/function should be established, including consideration for discontinuation if benefits do not outweigh risks. Therapy should be continued only if clinically meaningful improvement in pain/function outweighs risks. Therapy should be initiated at the lowest effective dosage using immediate-release opioids (instead of extended-release/long-acting opioids). Risk associated with use increases with higher opioid dosages. Risks and benefits should be re-evaluated when increasing dosage to ≥50 morphine milligram equivalents (MME)/day orally; dosages ≥90 MME/day orally should be avoided unless carefully justified (CDC [Dowell 2016]).

Warnings: Additional Pediatric Considerations

Tramadol may cause slowed or difficult breathing, including fatal respiratory depression. In April 2017, the FDA announced tramadol use should be avoided in all pediatric patients less than 12 years and all pediatric patients undergoing tonsillectomy or adenoidectomy. Additionally, tramadol should be avoided in pediatric patients 12 to 18 years who are obese or have conditions such as obstructive sleep apnea or severe lung disease, which may increase the risk of serious breathing problems. The FDA is requiring updated manufacturer labeling to include in the following contraindications: Use in patients <12 years to treat pain and use in patients <18 years to treat postoperative tonsillectomy/adenoidectomy pain (FDA 2017). Patients who are ultrarapid metabolizers of CYP2D6 are thought to produce more active opioid metabolites, potentially increasing risk for adverse effects. A case report describes a 5-year old who underwent adenotonsillectomy for obstructive sleep apnea syndrome (OSAS) who experienced severe respiratory depression after taking a single dose of tramadol; the patient was found to be an ultrarapid metabolizer of CYP2D6 which potentially added to the inherent increased risk for opioid-induced respiratory depression that patients with OSAS have (Orliaguet 2015).

Drug Interactions

Metabolism/Transport Effects Substrate of CYP2B6 (minor), CYP2D6 (major), CYP3A4 (major); **Note:** Assignment of Major/Minor substrate status based on clinically relevant drug interaction potential

Avoid Concomitant Use

Avoid concomitant use of TraMADol with any of the following: Azelastine (Nasal); Bromperidol; CarBAMazepine; Dapoxetine; Eluxadoline; Iobenguane Radiopharmaceutical Products; Monoamine Oxidase Inhibitors (Antidepressant); Monoamine Oxidase Inhibitors (Type B); Opioids (Mixed Agonist / Antagonist); Orphenadrine; Oxomemazine; Paraldehyde; Thalidomide

Increased Effect/Toxicity

TraMADol may increase the levels/effects of: Alvimopan; Amifampridine; Azelastine (Nasal); Blonanserin; CarBAMazepine; Desmopressin; Diuretics; Eluxadoline; Flunitrazepam; Hypoglycemia-Associated Agents; Iohexol; Iomeprol; Iopamidol; Methotrimeprazine; MetyroSINE; Monoamine Oxidase Inhibitors (Type B); Orphenadrine; Oxitriptan; OxyCODONE; Paraldehyde; Piribedil; Pramipexole; Ramosetron; ROPINIRole; Rotigotine; Selective Serotonin Reuptake Inhibitors; Serotonergic Agents (High Risk, Miscellaneous); Suvorexant; Thalidomide; Tricyclic Antidepressants; Vitamin K Antagonists; Zolpidem

The levels/effects of TraMADol may be increased by: Ajmaline; Alizapride; Almotriptan; Amphetamines; Androgens; Anticholinergic Agents; Antidiabetic Agents; Antiemetics (5HT3 Antagonists); Brimonidine (Topical); Bromopride; Bromperidol; BuPROPion; BusPIRone; Cannabidiol; Cannabis; Chlormethiazole; Chlorphenesin Carbamate; CNS Depressants; Cobicistat; CYP2D6 Inhibitors (Moderate); CYP2D6 Inhibitors (Strong); CYP3A4 Inhibitors (Strong); Dapoxetine; Dexmethylphenidate-Methylphenidate; Dextromethorphan; Dimethindene (Topical); Dronabinol; Droperidol; DULoxetine; Eletriptan; Ergot Derivatives; Herbs (Hypoglycemic Properties); Kava Kava; Lemborexant; Linezolid; Lisuride; Lofexidine; Lorcaserin (Withdrawn From US Market); Lumefantrine; Magnesium Sulfate; Maitake; Methotrimeprazine; Methylene Blue; Metoclopramide; Minocycline (Systemic); Monoamine Oxidase Inhibitors (Antidepressant); Nabilone; Nefazodone; Ondansetron; Oxomemazine; Ozanimod; Peginterferon Alfa-2b; Pegvisomant; Perampanel; PHENobarbital; Primidone; Prothionamide; Quinolones; Ritonavir; Rufinamide; Salicylates; Selective Serotonin Reuptake Inhibitors (Strong CYP2D6 Inhibitors); Serotonergic Non-Opioid CNS Depressants; Serotonergic Opioids (High Risk); Serotonin 5-HT1D Receptor Agonists (Triptans); Serotonin/Norepinephrine Reuptake Inhibitors; Sodium Oxybate; St John's Wort; Succinylcholine; Syrian Rue; Tetrahydrocannabinol; Tetrahydrocannabinol and Cannabidiol; Tricyclic Antidepressants

Decreased Effect

TraMADol may decrease the levels/effects of: CarBAMazepine; Diuretics; Gastrointestinal Agents (Prokinetic); Iobenguane Radiopharmaceutical Products; Pegvisomant; Sincalide

The levels/effects of TraMADol may be decreased by: CarBAMazepine; CYP2D6 Inhibitors (Moderate); CYP2D6 Inhibitors (Strong); CYP3A4 Inducers (Moderate); CYP3A4 Inducers (Strong); Dabrafenib; Deferasirox; DULoxetine; Enzalutamide; Erdafitinib; Ivosidenib; Mitotane; Nalmefene; Naltrexone; Ondansetron; Opioids (Mixed Agonist / Antagonist); Peginterferon Alfa-2b; PHENobarbital; Primidone; Quinolones; Ritonavir; Sarilumab; Selective Serotonin Reuptake Inhibitors (Strong CYP2D6 Inhibitors); Siltuximab; St John's Wort; Tocilizumab

Pharmacodynamics/Kinetics

Onset of Action Immediate release: Within 1 hour; Peak effect: 2 to 3 hours

Half-life Elimination

Immediate release: 6.3 ± 1.4 hours; active metabolite (M1): 7.4 ± 1.4 hours; prolonged in elderly

Extended release:

Capsules: ~10 hours; active metabolite (M1): ~11 hours

Tablets: ~7.9 hours; active metabolite (M1): 8.8 hours

Time to Peak

Immediate release: ~2 hours; active metabolite (M1): 3 hours

Extended release: ~4 to 12 hours; active metabolite (M1): ~5 to 15 hours

Reproductive Considerations

Long-term opioid use may cause secondary hypogonadism, which may lead to sexual dysfunction or infertility in men and women (Brennan 2013).

Premature ejaculation may contribute to male infertility. Tramadol may be an alternative treatment for this condition; however, due to the risk of addiction and adverse effects associated with opioid use, it should only be used in patients who have experienced treatment failure with other therapies (ISSM [Althof 2014]; Martyn-St. James 2015).

Pregnancy Considerations Tramadol crosses the placenta.

According to some studies, maternal use of opioids may be associated with birth defects (including neural tube defects, congenital heart defects, and gastroschisis), poor fetal growth, stillbirth, and preterm delivery (CDC [Dowell 2016]).

[US Boxed Warning]: Prolonged use of tramadol during pregnancy can result in neonatal opioid withdrawal syndrome, which may be life-threatening if not recognized and treated, and requires management according to protocols developed by neonatology experts. If opioid use is required for a prolonged period in a pregnant woman, advise the patient of the risk of neonatal opioid withdrawal syndrome and ensure that appropriate treatment will be available. If chronic opioid exposure occurs in pregnancy, adverse events in the newborn (including withdrawal) may occur (Chou 2009). Symptoms of neonatal abstinence syndrome (NAS) following opioid exposure may be autonomic (eg, fever, temperature instability), gastrointestinal (eg, diarrhea, vomiting, poor feeding/weight gain), or neurologic (eg, high-pitched crying, hyperactivity, increased muscle tone, increased wakefulness/abnormal sleep pattern, irritability, sneezing, seizure, tremor, yawning) (Dow 2012; Hudak 2012). Mothers who are physically dependent on opioids may give birth to infants who are also physically dependent. Opioids may cause respiratory depression and psychophysiologic effects in the neonate; newborns of mothers receiving opioids during labor should be monitored.

Tramadol is not commonly used to treat pain during labor and immediately postpartum (ACOG 209 2019) or chronic noncancer pain in pregnant women or those who may become pregnant (CDC [Dowell 2016]; Chou 2009).

Breastfeeding Considerations

Tramadol and the active M1 metabolite are present in breast milk. M1 has stronger opioid activity than tramadol. Actual exposure to a breastfeeding infant may depend on the mothers CYP2D6 metabolism (Salman 2011).

Tramadol is not recommended for use in breastfeeding women. Due to the potential for serious adverse events in the breastfed infant (including excess sedation and respiratory depression), use during breastfeeding is not recommended by the manufacturer. Nonopioid analgesics are preferred for breastfeeding females who require pain control peripartum or for surgery outside of the postpartum period (ABM [Martin 2018]; ABM [Reece-Stremtan 2017]). When opioids are needed in breastfeeding women, the lowest effective dose for the shortest duration of time should be used to limit adverse events in the mother and breastfeeding infant. In general, a single occasional dose of an opioid analgesic may be compatible with breastfeeding (WHO 2002). Breastfeeding women using opioids for postpartum pain or for the treatment of chronic maternal pain should monitor their infants for drowsiness, sedation, feeding difficulties, or limpness (ACOG 209 2019). Withdrawal symptoms may occur when maternal use is discontinued or breastfeeding is stopped.

Controlled Substance C-IV

Dosage Forms Considerations

ConZip extended release capsules are formulated as a biphasic product, providing immediate and extended release components:

100 mg: 25 mg (immediate release) and 75 mg (extended release)

200 mg: 50 mg (immediate release) and 150 mg (extended release)

300 mg: 50 mg (immediate release) and 250 mg (extended release)

EnovaRX-Tramadol and Active-Tramadol creams are compounded from kits. Refer to manufacturer's labeling for compounding instructions.

Synapryn FusePaq is a compounding kit for the preparation of an oral suspension. Refer to manufacturer's labeling for compounding instructions.

Dosage Forms: US

Capsule Extended Release 24 Hour, Oral:

ConZip: 100 mg, 200 mg, 300 mg

Generic: 100 mg, 150 mg, 200 mg, 300 mg

Tablet, Oral:

Ultram: 50 mg

Generic: 50 mg, 100 mg

Tablet Extended Release 24 Hour, Oral:

Generic: 100 mg, 200 mg, 300 mg

Dosage Forms: Canada

Capsule Extended Release 24 Hour, Oral:

Durela: 100 mg, 200 mg, 300 mg

Tablet, Oral:

Ultram: 50 mg

Generic: 50 mg

Tablet Extended Release 24 Hour, Oral:

Ralivia: 100 mg, 200 mg, 300 mg

Tridural: 100 mg, 200 mg, 300 mg

Zytram XL: 75 mg, 100 mg, 150 mg, 200 mg, 300 mg, 400 mg

Generic: 100 mg, 200 mg, 300 mg

Dental Health Professional Considerations Based on systematic reviews evaluating benefits and harms of analgesics for acute dental pain, opioids or medication combinations containing opioids were associated with greater adverse effects. Adverse effects associated with opioid use include drowsiness, respiratory depression, dizziness, nausea, vomiting, and constipation (Moore 2018). Evidence-based recommendations for analgesic efficacy for dental pain recommend NSAIDS as the drug of choice unless contraindicated or ineffective (ADA 2016; Aminoshariae 2016). The ADA has adopted policy consistent with CDC guidelines regarding pain management; opioid prescriptions should be limited to <7 days for the treatment of acute pain (ADA 2018).

Studies have been conducted in adult patients evaluating efficacy of tramadol in the treatment of dental pain. The combination of tramadol and flurbiprofen may be more beneficial than either drug alone when given for the management of endodontic pain. Doses evaluated were flurbiprofen 100 mg loading dose, followed by 50 mg every 6 hours and tramadol 100 mg loading dose, followed by 100 mg every 6 hours (Doroschak 1999). In a comparison of tramadol/acetaminophen (total dose: 75 mg/650 mg) versus tramadol monotherapy (total dose: 100 mg) for postoperative dental pain, tramadol/acetaminophen had superior analgesic efficacy (Fricke 2004). One study showed that naproxen 500 mg was more effective than tramadol 100 mg when given as a single dose following a root canal (Mehrvarzfar 2012). In a study comparing efficacy of tramadol 100 mg and ketorolac 20 mg for the relief of pain after molar extraction, tramadol was equally effective to ketorolac (Mishra 2012).

◆ **Tramadol HCl** *see* TraMADol *on page 1468*

◆ **Tramadol Hydrochloride** *see* TraMADol *on page 1468*

◆ **Tramadol Hydrochloride and Acetaminophen** *see* Acetaminophen and Tramadol *on page 71*

Trametinib (tra ME ti nib)

Brand Names: US Mekinist

Brand Names: Canada Mekinist

Pharmacologic Category Antineoplastic Agent, MEK Inhibitor

Use

Melanoma:

Adjuvant treatment of melanoma (in combination with dabrafenib) in patients with BRAF V600E or BRAF V600K mutations (as detected by an approved test), and lymph node involvement, following complete resection.

Treatment of unresectable or metastatic melanoma in patients with BRAF V600E or BRAF V600K mutations (as detected by an approved test), either as a single-agent (in BRAF inhibitor treatment-naive patients) or in combination with dabrafenib.

Non-small cell lung cancer (metastatic): Treatment of metastatic non-small cell lung cancer in patients with BRAF V600E mutation as detected by an approved test (in combination with dabrafenib).

Thyroid cancer, anaplastic, locally advanced or metastatic: Treatment of locally advanced or metastatic anaplastic thyroid cancer (in combination with dabrafenib) in patients with BRAF V600E mutation and with no satisfactory locoregional treatment options.

Local Anesthetic/Vasoconstrictor Precautions No information available to require special precautions

Effects on Dental Treatment No significant effects or complications reported

Effects on Bleeding No information available to require special precautions

Adverse Reactions

Adverse reactions reported with monotherapy:

>10%:

Cardiovascular: Hypertension (15%), cardiomyopathy (7% to 11%)

Dermatologic: Skin toxicity (87%, most commonly dermatitis acneiform rash, palmar-plantar erythrodysesthesia, erythema, skin rash; severe: 12%; severe toxicity and secondary skin infection requiring hospitalization: 6%), skin rash (57%), acneiform eruption (19%), xeroderma (11%)
Endocrine & metabolic: Hypoalbuminemia (42%)
Gastrointestinal: Diarrhea (43%), stomatitis (15%), abdominal pain (13%)
Hematologic & oncologic: Anemia (38%), lymphedema (32%), hemorrhage (13%; grades 3/4: <1%)
Hepatic: Increased serum aspartate aminotransferase (60%), increased serum alanine aminotransferase (39%), increased serum alkaline phosphatase (24%)

1% to 10%:
Cardiovascular: Decreased left ventricular ejection fraction (5%, ≥20% below baseline), bradycardia
Central nervous system: Dizziness
Dermatologic: Paronychia (10%), pruritus (10%), cellulitis, folliculitis, pustular rash
Gastrointestinal: Dysgeusia, xerostomia
Neuromuscular & skeletal: Rhabdomyolysis
Ophthalmic: Blurred vision, dry eye syndrome
Respiratory: Interstitial pulmonary disease (≤2%), pneumonitis (≤2%)

<1%, postmarketing, and/or case reports: Retinal detachment, retinal vein occlusion

Adverse reactions reported with dual therapy (trametinib plus dabrafenib):

>10%:
Cardiovascular: Hypertension (25% to 26%), peripheral edema (21% to 25%; includes edema and lymphedema; grades 3/4: ≤1%), prolonged QT Interval on ECG (4% QTcF increased >60 msec; <1% QTcF prolongation to >500 msec)
Central nervous system: Fatigue (51% to 59%), headache (30% to 39%), chills (23% to 37%), dizziness (11% to 14%)
Dermatologic: Skin toxicity (55%; severe toxicity: <1%), skin rash (28% to 42%), xeroderma (10% to 31%)
Endocrine & metabolic: Hyperglycemia (60% to 71%), hyponatremia (24% to 57%), hypoalbuminemia (25% to 53%), hypophosphatemia (36% to 42%), exacerbation of diabetes mellitus (27%)
Gastrointestinal: Nausea (34% to 45%), vomiting (25% to 33%), diarrhea (30% to 33%), decreased appetite (29%), abdominal pain (18% to 26%), constipation (13%)
Hematologic & oncologic: Neutropenia (44% to 50%; grades 3/4: 6% to 8%), leukopenia (48%; grades 3/4: 8%), anemia (25% to 46%; grades 3/4: ≤10%), lymphocytopenia (26% to 42%; grades 3/4: 5% to 14%), hemorrhage (18% to 23%; grades 3/4: 2% to 3%; includes hepatic hematoma, duodenal ulcer hemorrhage), thrombocytopenia (19% to 21%; grades 3/4: <1%), malignant neoplasm (1%)
Hepatic: Increased serum alkaline phosphatase (38% to 64%), increased serum aspartate aminotransferase (57% to 61%), increased serum alanine aminotransferase (32% to 48%)
Neuromuscular & skeletal: Arthralgia (25% to 28%), myalgia (13% to 20%)
Renal: Increased serum creatinine (21%)
Respiratory: Cough (20% to 22%), dyspnea (20%)
Miscellaneous: Fever (54% to 63%), febrile reaction (complicated with dehydration: 2%, complicated with severe chills/rigors: <1%, complicated with renal failure: <1%, complicated with syncope: <1%)

1% to 10%:
Cardiovascular: Bradycardia (<10%), cardiomyopathy (6%), reduced ejection fraction (5%), venous thromboembolism (3%; deep vein thrombosis, pulmonary embolism), hypertension
Central nervous system: Intracranial hemorrhage (1%)
Gastrointestinal: Gastrointestinal hemorrhage (6%), pancreatitis
Hematologic & oncologic: Basal cell carcinoma (3%), squamous cell carcinoma of skin (3%; including keratoacanthoma)
Neuromuscular & skeletal: Rhabdomyolysis (<10%)
Ophthalmic: Blurred vision (6%)
Respiratory: Pneumonitis (≤2%)

<1%, postmarketing, and/or case reports: Malignant melanoma

Mechanism of Action Trametinib reversibly and selectively inhibits mitogen-activated extracellular kinase (MEK) 1 and 2 activation and kinase activity. MEK is a downstream effector of the protein kinase B-raf (BRAF); BRAF V600 mutations result in constitutive activation of the BRAF pathway (including MEK1 and MEK2). Through inhibition of MEK 1 and 2 kinase activity, trametinib causes decreased cellular proliferation, cell cycle arrest, and increased apoptosis (Kim 2013). The combination of trametinib and dabrafenib allows for greater inhibition of the MAPK pathway, resulting in BRAF V600 melanoma cell death (Flaherty 2012a). Trametinib plus dabrafenib has been reported to synergistically inhibit cell growth in lung cancer cell lines which are BRAF V600E-mutant (Planchard 2016).

Pharmacodynamics/Kinetics

Half-life Elimination ~4 to 5 days

Time to Peak 1.5 hours; delayed with a high-fat, high-calorie meal (~1,000 calories)

Reproductive Considerations

Verify pregnancy status in females of reproductive potential prior to treatment initiation. Females of reproductive potential should use effective contraceptive during trametinib therapy and for 4 months after the last trametinib dose. Males (including those with vasectomies) with pregnant partners or female partners of reproductive potential should use condoms during trametinib treatment and for ≥4 months after the last trametinib dose.

Pregnancy Considerations

Based on its mechanism of action and on findings in animal reproduction studies, in utero exposure to trametinib may cause fetal harm.

◆ **Trametinib Dimethyl Sulfoxide** *see* Trametinib *on page 1475*

◆ **Trandate** *see* Labetalol *on page 867*

Trandolapril (tran DOE la pril)

Related Information

Cardiovascular Diseases *on page 1654*

Brand Names: US Mavik [DSC]

Brand Names: Canada AURO-Trandolapril; Mavik; Odrik; PMS-Trandolapril; SANDOZ Trandolapril; TEVA-Trandolapril

Pharmacologic Category Angiotensin-Converting Enzyme (ACE) Inhibitor; Antihypertensive

Use

Hypertension: Management of hypertension

Guideline recommendations: The 2017 Guideline for the Prevention, Detection, Evaluation, and Management of High Blood Pressure in Adults recommends if monotherapy is warranted, in the absence of comorbidities (eg, cerebrovascular disease, chronic kidney disease, diabetes, heart failure [HF], ischemic heart disease, etc.), that thiazide-like diuretics or dihydropyridine calcium channel blockers may be preferred options due to improved cardiovascular endpoints (eg, prevention of HF and stroke). ACE inhibitors and ARBs are also acceptable for monotherapy. Combination therapy may be required to achieve blood pressure goals and is initially preferred in patients at high risk (stage 2 hypertension or atherosclerotic cardiovascular disease [ASCVD] risk ≥10%) (ACC/AHA [Whelton 2017]).

Post-myocardial infarction (MI) heart failure or left-ventricular dysfunction: Treatment of post-MI HF in patients who are symptomatic from HF within the first few days after sustaining acute MI or post-MI left ventricular dysfunction in stable patients who have evidence of left ventricular systolic dysfunction (identified by wall motion abnormalities)

Local Anesthetic/Vasoconstrictor Precautions
No information available to require special precautions

Effects on Dental Treatment Key adverse event(s) related to dental treatment: Patient may experience orthostatic hypotension as they stand up after treatment; especially if lying in the dental chair for an extended period of time. Use caution with sudden changes in position during and after dental treatment.

An angiotensin-converting enzyme (ACE) Inhibitor cough is a dry, hacking, nonproductive cough that can potentially interfere with longer dental procedures if patient has this side effect.

Effects on Bleeding No information available to require special precautions

Adverse Reactions Frequency ranges include data from hypertension and heart failure trials. Higher rates of adverse reactions have generally been noted in patients with heart failure. However, the frequency of adverse effects associated with placebo is also increased in this population.

>10%:

- Cardiovascular: Hypotension (≤11%)
- Central nervous system: Dizziness (1% to 23%)
- Endocrine & metabolic: Increased uric acid (15%)
- Respiratory: Cough (2% to 35%)

1% to 10%:

- Cardiovascular: Syncope (6%), bradycardia (≤5%), cardiogenic shock (4%), intermittent claudication (4%), cerebrovascular accident (3%)
- Endocrine & metabolic: Hyperkalemia (5%), hypocalcemia (5%)
- Gastrointestinal: Gastritis (4%), diarrhea (1%)
- Neuromuscular & skeletal: Myalgia (5%), weakness (3%)
- Renal: Increased blood urea nitrogen (9%), increased serum creatinine (1% to 5%)

<1%, postmarketing, and/or case reports: Abdominal distention, abdominal pain, agranulocytosis, alopecia, angina pectoris, angioedema, anxiety, bronchitis, bronchospasm, cardiac arrhythmia, cardiac failure, cerebral hemorrhage, chest pain, cholestasis, constipation, decreased libido, depression, dermatitis, diaphoresis, drowsiness, dyspepsia, dyspnea, edema, epistaxis, equilibrium disturbance, fever, first degree atrioventricular block, flushing, gout, hallucination, hepatitis, hypersensitivity angiitis, hyponatremia, impotence, increased serum ALT, increased serum AST, increased serum bilirubin, increased serum transaminases, insomnia, intestinal angioedema, intestinal obstruction, ischemic heart disease, jaundice, laryngeal edema, leukopenia, limb pain, malaise, myalgia, myocardial infarction, nausea, neutropenia, palpitations, pancreatitis, pancytopenia, paresthesia, pemphigus, pharyngitis, pruritus, renal failure, skin rash, Stevens-Johnson syndrome, symptomatic hypotension, tachycardia, thrombocytopenia, toxic epidermal necrolysis, transient ischemic attacks, upper respiratory tract infection, urticaria, ventricular tachycardia, vertigo, visual impairment, vomiting, xerostomia

Mechanism of Action Trandolapril is an ACE inhibitor which prevents the formation of angiotensin II from angiotensin I. Trandolapril must undergo enzymatic hydrolysis, mainly in liver, to its biologically active metabolite, trandolaprilat. A CNS mechanism may also be involved in the hypotensive effect as angiotensin II increases adrenergic outflow from the CNS. Vasoactive kallikreins may be decreased in conversion to active hormones by ACE inhibitors, thus reducing blood pressure.

Pharmacodynamics/Kinetics

Half-life Elimination Trandolapril: ~6 hours; Trandolaprilat: Effective: 22.5 hours

Time to Peak Trandolapril: ~1 hour; Trandolaprilat: 4 to 10 hours

Reproductive Considerations

Angiotensin-converting enzyme (ACE) inhibitors should be avoided in sexually active females of reproductive potential not using effective contraception (ADA 2020).

ACE inhibitors should generally be avoided for the treatment of hypertension in women planning a pregnancy; use should only be considered for cases of hypertension refractory to other medications (ACOG 203 2019).

Pregnancy Risk Factor D

Pregnancy Considerations

Exposure to an angiotensin-converting enzyme (ACE) inhibitor during the first trimester of pregnancy may be associated with an increased risk of fetal malformations (ACOG 203 2019; ESC [Regitz-Zagrosek 2018]); however, outcomes observed may also be influenced by maternal disease (ACC/AHA [Whelton 2017]).

[US Boxed Warning]: Drugs that act on the renin-angiotensin system can cause injury and death to the developing fetus. Discontinue as soon as possible once pregnancy is detected. Drugs that act on the renin-angiotensin system are associated with oligohydramnios. Oligohydramnios, due to decreased fetal renal function, may lead to fetal lung hypoplasia and skeletal malformations. The use of these drugs in pregnancy is also associated with anuria, hypotension, renal failure, skull hypoplasia, and death in the fetus/neonate. Infants exposed to an ACE inhibitor in utero should be monitored for hyperkalemia, hypotension, and oliguria. Oligohydramnios may not appear until after irreversible fetal injury has occurred. Exchange transfusions or dialysis may be required to reverse hypotension or improve renal function, although data related to the effectiveness in neonates is limited.

Chronic maternal hypertension is also associated with adverse events in the fetus/infant. Chronic maternal hypertension may increase the risk of birth defects, low birth weight, premature delivery, stillbirth, and neonatal death. Actual fetal/neonatal risks may be related to duration and severity of maternal hypertension. Untreated chronic hypertension may also increase the risks of adverse maternal outcomes, including gestational diabetes, preeclampsia, delivery complications, stroke, and myocardial infarction (ACOG 203 2019).

When treatment of hypertension in pregnancy is indicated, ACE inhibitors should generally be avoided due to their adverse fetal events; use in pregnant women should only be considered for cases of hypertension refractory to other medications (ACOG 203 2019). ACE inhibitors are not recommended for the treatment of heart failure in pregnancy (Regitz-Zagrosek [ESC 2018]).

Tranexamic Acid (tran eks AM ik AS id)

Related Information

Antiplatelet and Anticoagulation Considerations in Dentistry *on page 1666*

Brand Names: US Cyklokapron; Lysteda

Brand Names: Canada Cyklokapron; Erfa-Tranexamic; GD-Tranexamic Acid; MAR-Tranexamic Acid

Pharmacologic Category Antifibrinolytic Agent; Antihemophilic Agent; Hemostatic Agent; Lysine Analog

Use

Menstrual bleeding, heavy (oral): Treatment of cyclic heavy menstrual bleeding.

Tooth extraction in patients with hemostatic defects (injection, oral [Cyklokapron; Canadian product]): Short-term use in hemophilia patients to reduce or prevent hemorrhage and reduce need for replacement therapy during and following tooth extraction.

Local Anesthetic/Vasoconstrictor Precautions No information available to require special precautions

Effects on Dental Treatment No significant effects or complications reported. See Effects on Bleeding and Dental Health Professional Considerations.

Effects on Bleeding General dental procedures and simple restorative procedures are not associated with bleeding; therefore, there is no contraindication to general dental treatment for most patients with bleeding disorders. However, after dental extractions and other dental surgeries including deep scaling, block anesthesia, and large fillings, in patients with hemophilia, antifibrinolytic drugs such as tranexamic acid are useful in controlling bleeding. A carefully coordinated strategy between the dental and medical team may be required to ensure adequate procedures for hemostasis. As preparation for selected dental procedures tranexamic acid may be required.

Immediately before dental extraction in hemophilic patients, administer 10 mg/kg tranexamic acid IV together with replacement therapy.

Adverse Reactions

>10%:

Gastrointestinal: Abdominal pain (oral: 20%)

Nervous system: Headache (oral: 50%)

Neuromuscular & skeletal: Back pain (oral: 21%), musculoskeletal pain (oral: 11%)

Respiratory: Nasal signs and symptoms (oral: 25%; including sinus symptoms)

1% to 10%:

Hematologic & oncologic: Anemia (oral: 6%)

Nervous system: Fatigue (oral: 5%)

Neuromuscular & skeletal: Arthralgia (oral: 7%), muscle cramps (oral: ≤7%), muscle spasm (oral: ≤7%)

Postmarketing:

Cardiovascular: Cerebral thrombosis, deep vein thrombosis, hypotension (with rapid IV injection), pulmonary embolism

Dermatologic: Allergic dermatitis, allergic skin reaction

Gastrointestinal: Diarrhea, nausea, vomiting

Genitourinary: Ureteral obstruction

Hypersensitivity: Anaphylactic shock, anaphylaxis, hypersensitivity reaction, nonimmune anaphylaxis, severe hypersensitivity reaction

Nervous system: Dizziness, seizure (Lecker 2016)

Ophthalmic: Chromatopsia, conjunctivitis (ligneous), retinal artery occlusion, retinal vein occlusion, visual disturbance

Renal: Renal cortical necrosis

Mechanism of Action Forms a reversible complex that displaces plasminogen from fibrin resulting in inhibition of fibrinolysis; it also inhibits the proteolytic activity of plasmin

With reduction in plasmin activity, tranexamic acid also reduces activation of complement and consumption of C1 esterase inhibitor (C1-INH), thereby decreasing inflammation associated with hereditary angioedema.

Pharmacodynamics/Kinetics

Half-life Elimination IV: ~2 hours; Oral: ~11 hours.

Time to Peak Oral:

Single dose: Mean: 2.5 hours (range: 1 to 5 hours).

Multiple dose: Mean: 2.5 hours (range: 2 to 3.5 hours).

Reproductive Considerations

Tranexamic acid is an alternative agent for the treatment of heavy menstrual bleeding and one option for females who desire future fertility (ACOG 785 2019). The manufacturer recommends non-hormonal contraception during treatment, as hormonal contraceptives may increase the risk of thromboembolic events. However, tranexamic acid in combination with oral contraceptives may be considered for the treatment of heavy menstrual bleeding when monotherapy is ineffective and other treatment options have failed (ACOG 557 2013; ACOG 785 2019).

Pregnancy Considerations

Tranexamic acid crosses the placenta; concentrations within cord blood are similar to maternal serum.

Oral tranexamic acid is used off label for the long-term prophylaxis of hereditary angioedema (HAE) and use for this indication in pregnant females has been reported (González-Quevedo 2016; Machado 2017; Milingos 2009). Tranexamic acid may be considered for long-term prophylaxis of HAE during pregnancy when preferred treatment is not available (WAO/EEACI [Maurer 2018]).

IV tranexamic acid is used off label for the treatment of postpartum hemorrhage (Ducloy-Bouthors 2011; WOMAN Trial Collaborators 2017). A significant reduction in risk of death due to bleeding was observed when treatment was started within 3 hours of vaginal birth or cesarean section (WOMAN Trial Collaborators 2017). Tranexamic acid is recommended for the treatment of obstetric hemorrhage when initial therapy fails (ACOG 183 2017; WHO 2017).

IV tranexamic acid has also been studied for prophylaxis of postpartum hemorrhage in females prior to vaginal or cesarean delivery (Novikova 2015; Saccone 2019; Sentilhes 2018; Simonazzi 2016; Xia 2020).

Tranexamic acid may be considered as adjunctive therapy in women at high risk for postpartum hemorrhage. However, available data related to prophylactic use is insufficient and use for routine prophylaxis against postpartum hemorrhage is not currently recommended outside of the context of clinical research (ACOG 183 2017; Muñoz 2019).

Dental Health Professional Considerations Antifibrinolytic drugs are useful for the control of bleeding after dental extractions in patients with hemophilia because the oral mucosa and saliva are rich in plasminogen activators.

- ◆ **Transamine Sulphate** *see* Tranylcypromine *on page 1479*
- ◆ **trans-Retinoic Acid** *see* Tretinoin (Systemic) *on page 1483*
- ◆ **trans-Retinoic Acid** *see* Tretinoin (Topical) *on page 1484*
- ◆ **trans Vitamin A Acid** *see* Tretinoin (Systemic) *on page 1483*
- ◆ **Tranxene-T** *see* Clorazepate *on page 395*
- ◆ **Tranxene T-Tab** *see* Clorazepate *on page 395*

Tranylcypromine (tran il SIP roe meen)

Related Information

Vasoconstrictor Interactions With Antidepressants *on page 1821*

Brand Names: US Parnate

Brand Names: Canada Parnate

Pharmacologic Category Antidepressant, Monoamine Oxidase Inhibitor

Use Major depressive disorder (unipolar): Treatment of major depressive disorder in adult patients who have not responded adequately to other antidepressants.

Local Anesthetic/Vasoconstrictor Precautions Attempts should be made to avoid use of vasoconstrictor due to possibility of hypertensive episodes with monoamine oxidase inhibitors

Effects on Dental Treatment Key adverse event(s) related to dental treatment: Orthostatic hypotension. Avoid use as an analgesic due to toxic reactions with MAO inhibitors. Xerostomia (normal salivary flow resumes upon discontinuation).

Effects on Bleeding No information available to require special precautions

Adverse Reactions Frequency not defined.

Cardiovascular: Edema, orthostatic hypotension, palpitations, tachycardia

Central nervous system: Agitation, anxiety, chills, dizziness, drowsiness, headache, insomnia, mania, myoclonus, numbness, paresthesia, restlessness

Dermatologic: Diaphoresis, urticaria

Endocrine & metabolic: SIADH (syndrome of inappropriate antidiuretic hormone secretion)

Gastrointestinal: Abdominal pain, anorexia, constipation, diarrhea, nausea, xerostomia

Genitourinary: Sexual disorder (anorgasmia, ejaculatory disturbance, impotence), urinary retention

Hematologic & oncologic: Agranulocytosis, anemia, leukopenia, thrombocytopenia

Neuromuscular & skeletal: Muscle spasm, tremor, weakness

Ophthalmic: Blurred vision

Otic: Tinnitus

<1%, postmarketing, and/or case reports: Acne vulgaris (cystic acne), akinesia, alopecia, amnesia, ataxia, cheilitis (angular), confusion, disorientation, hepatitis, polyuria, scleroderma (localized), skin rash, urinary incontinence, withdrawal syndrome

Mechanism of Action Tranylcypromine is a nonhydrazine monoamine oxidase inhibitor. It increases endogenous concentrations of epinephrine, norepinephrine, and serotonin through inhibition of the enzyme (monoamine oxidase) responsible for the breakdown of these neurotransmitters.

Pharmacodynamics/Kinetics

Onset of Action Depression: Initial effects may be observed within 1 to 2 weeks of treatment, with continued improvements through 4 to 6 weeks (Papakostas 2006; Posternak 2005; Szegedi 2009).

Duration of Action MAO inhibition may persist for up to 10 days following discontinuation.

Half-life Elimination 2.5 hours (Mallinger 1990)

Time to Peak Serum: 1.5 hours (Mallinger 1990)

Pregnancy Considerations

Information related to the use of tranylcypromine in pregnancy is limited (Kennedy 2017).

Pregnant women exposed to antidepressants during pregnancy are encouraged to enroll in the National Pregnancy Registry for Antidepressants (NPRAD). Women 18 to 45 years of age or their health care providers may contact the registry by calling 844-405-6185. Enrollment should be done as early in pregnancy as possible.

- ◆ **Tranylcypromine Sulfate** *see* Tranylcypromine *on page 1479*
- ◆ **Tranzarel [DSC]** *see* Lidocaine (Topical) *on page 902*

Trastuzumab (tras TU zoo mab)

Brand Names: US Herceptin; Herzuma; Kanjinti; Ogivri; Ontruzant; Trazimera

Brand Names: Canada Herceptin; Herzuma; Kanjinti; Ogivri; Trazimera

Pharmacologic Category Antineoplastic Agent, Anti-HER2; Antineoplastic Agent, Monoclonal Antibody

Use

Breast cancer, adjuvant treatment: Treatment (adjuvant) of HER2-overexpressing node positive or node negative (estrogen receptor/progesterone receptor negative or with 1 high-risk feature) breast cancer as part of a treatment regimen consisting of doxorubicin, cyclophosphamide, and either paclitaxel or docetaxel; as part of a treatment regimen with docetaxel and carboplatin; or as a single agent following multimodality anthracycline-based therapy.

Breast cancer, metastatic: First-line treatment of HER2-overexpressing metastatic breast cancer (in combination with paclitaxel); single agent treatment of HER2-overexpressing breast cancer in patients who have received 1 or more chemotherapy regimens for metastatic disease.

Gastric cancer, metastatic: Treatment of HER2-overexpressing metastatic gastric or gastroesophageal junction adenocarcinoma (in combination with cisplatin and either capecitabine or 5-fluorouracil) in patients who have not received prior treatment for metastatic disease.

Limitations of use: Patients should be selected for breast and gastric cancer therapy based on an approved companion diagnostic test for tumor specimen for HER2 overexpression or HER2 gene amplification. Due to differences in disease histopathology (eg, incomplete membrane staining, more frequent heterogeneous HER2 expression in gastric cancer), tests appropriate for the specific tumor type (breast or gastric) should be used to assess HER2 status.

Note: Herzuma (trastuzumab-pkrb), Kanjinti (trastuzumab-anns), Ogivri (trastuzumab-dkst), Ontruzant (trastuzumab-dttb), and Trazimera (trastuzumab-qyyp) are approved as biosimilars to Herceptin (trastuzumab). In Canada, Herzuma, Ogivri, and Trazimera are biosimilars to Herceptin (trastuzumab).

Local Anesthetic/Vasoconstrictor Precautions No information available to require special precautions

Effects on Dental Treatment No significant effects or complications reported

Effects on Bleeding Although significant myelosuppression with associated altered hemostasis has been reported for many chemotherapeutic agents, myelosuppression is not common with trastuzumab and no specific precautions appear to necessary.

Adverse Reactions Percentages reported with single-agent therapy.

>10%:

Cardiovascular: Decreased left ventricular ejection fraction (4% to 22%)

Central nervous system: Pain (47%), chills (5% to 32%), headache (10% to 26%), insomnia (14%), dizziness (4% to 13%)

Dermatologic: Skin rash (4% to 18%)

Gastrointestinal: Nausea (6% to 33%), diarrhea (7% to 25%), vomiting (4% to 23%), abdominal pain (2% to 22%), anorexia (14%)

Infection: Infection (20%)

Neuromuscular & skeletal: Weakness (4% to 42%), back pain (5% to 22%)

Respiratory: Cough (5% to 26%), dyspnea (3% to 22%), rhinitis (2% to 14%), pharyngitis (12%)

Miscellaneous: Infusion related reaction (21% to 40%, chills and fever most common; severe: 1%), fever (6% to 36%)

1% to 10%:

Cardiovascular: Peripheral edema (5% to 10%), edema (8%), cardiac failure (2% to 7%; severe: <1%), tachycardia (5%), hypertension (4%), arrhythmia (3%), palpitations (3%)

Central nervous system: Paresthesia (2% to 9%), depression (6%), peripheral neuritis (2%), neuropathy (1%)

Dermatologic: Acne vulgaris (2%), nail disease (2%), pruritus (2%)

Gastrointestinal: Constipation (2%), dyspepsia (2%)

Genitourinary: Urinary tract infection (3% to 5%)

Hematologic & oncologic: Anemia (4%; grade 3: <1%), leukopenia (3%)

Hypersensitivity: Hypersensitivity reaction (3%)

Infection: Influenza (4%), herpes simplex infection (2%)

Neuromuscular & skeletal: Arthralgia (6% to 8%), ostealgia (3% to 7%), myalgia (4%), muscle spasm (3%)

Respiratory: Flu-like symptoms (2% to 10%), sinusitis (2% to 9%), nasopharyngitis (8%), upper respiratory tract infection (3%), epistaxis (2%), pharyngolaryngeal pain (2%)

Miscellaneous: Accidental injury (6%)

<1%, postmarketing, and/or case reports (as a single-agent or with combination chemotherapy): Abnormality in thinking, adult respiratory distress syndrome, amblyopia, anaphylactic shock, anaphylactoid reaction, anaphylaxis, angioedema, apnea, ascites, asthma, ataxia, blood coagulation disorder, bradycardia, bronchitis, bronchospasm, cardiogenic shock, cardiomyopathy, cellulitis, cerebral edema, cerebrovascular accident, cerebrovascular disease, chest discomfort, colitis, coma, confusion, cystitis, deafness, dermal ulcer, dermatitis, dyspnea on exertion, dysuria, erysipelas, esophageal ulcer, febrile neutropenia, focal segmental glomerulosclerosis, gastritis, gastroenteritis, glomerulonephritis (membraneous, focal and fibrillary), glomerulopathy, hematemesis, hemorrhage, hemorrhagic cystitis, hepatic failure, hepatic injury, hepatitis, herpes zoster, hiccups, hydrocephalus, hydronephrosis, hypercalcemia, hypervolemia, hypoprothrombinemia, hypotension, hypothyroidism, hypoxia, immune thrombocytopenia, intestinal obstruction, interstitial pneumonitis, interstitial pulmonary disease, jaundice, laryngeal edema, laryngitis, lethargy, leukemia (acute), limb pain, lymphangitis, madarosis, mania, mastalgia, meningitis, musculoskeletal pain, myopathy, nephrotic syndrome, neutropenia, neutropenic sepsis, oligohydramnios, onychoclasis, osteonecrosis, oxygen desaturation, pancreatitis, pancytopenia, paresis, paroxysmal nocturnal dyspnea, pathological fracture, pericardial effusion, pericarditis, pleural effusion, pneumonitis, pneumothorax, pulmonary edema (noncardiogenic), pulmonary fibrosis, pulmonary hypertension, pulmonary infiltrates, pyelonephritis, radiation injury, renal failure, respiratory distress, respiratory failure, seizure, sepsis, shock, syncope, stomatitis, thrombosis (including mural), thyroiditis (autoimmune), urticaria, vertigo, ventricular dysfunction, wheezing

Mechanism of Action Trastuzumab is a monoclonal antibody which binds to the extracellular domain of the human epidermal growth factor receptor 2 protein (HER-2); it mediates antibody-dependent cellular cytotoxicity by inhibiting proliferation of cells which overexpress HER-2 protein.

Reproductive Considerations

[US Boxed Warning]: Advise patients of the risks of trastuzumab exposure in pregnancy and the need for effective contraception. Verify pregnancy status in females of reproductive potential prior to initiation of therapy. Females of reproductive potential should use effective contraception during treatment and for at least 7 months after the last trastuzumab dose.

Pregnancy Considerations

Trastuzumab inhibits human epidermal growth receptor 2 (HER2) protein, which has a role in embryonic development. **[US Boxed Warning]: Trastuzumab exposure during pregnancy may result in oligohydramnios and oligohydramnios sequence (pulmonary hypoplasia, skeletal malformations, and neonatal death). Advise patients of these risks.** Oligohydramnios (reversible in some cases) has been reported with trastuzumab use alone or with combination chemotherapy. Monitor for oligohydramnios if trastuzumab exposure occurs during pregnancy or within 7 months prior to conception; conduct appropriate fetal testing if oligohydramnios occurs.

Herceptin: If Herceptin is administered during pregnancy, or if a patient becomes pregnant during or within 7 months after treatment, report exposure to Genentech Adverse Events at 1-888-835-2555.

European Society for Medical Oncology guidelines for cancer during pregnancy recommend delaying treatment with trastuzumab (and other HER2-targeted agents) until after delivery in pregnant patients with HER2-positive disease (Peccatori 2013).

- **Trastuzumab-MCC-DM1** *see* Ado-Trastuzumab Emtansine *on page 86*
- **Trastuzumab-anns** *see* Trastuzumab *on page 1479*
- **Trastuzumab (Conventional)** *see* Trastuzumab *on page 1479*
- **Trastuzumab Deruxtecan** *see* Fam-Trastuzumab Deruxtecan *on page 636*
- **Trastuzumab-dkst** *see* Trastuzumab *on page 1479*
- **Trastuzumab-DM1** *see* Ado-Trastuzumab Emtansine *on page 86*
- **Trastuzumab-dttb** *see* Trastuzumab *on page 1479*
- **Trastuzumab Emtansine** *see* Ado-Trastuzumab Emtansine *on page 86*
- **Trastuzumab, hyaluronidase, and pertuzumab** *see* Pertuzumab, Trastuzumab, and Hyaluronidase *on page 1221*
- **Trastuzumab, pertuzumab, and hyaluronidase** *see* Pertuzumab, Trastuzumab, and Hyaluronidase *on page 1221*
- **Trastuzumab-pkrb** *see* Trastuzumab *on page 1479*
- **Trastuzumab-qyyp** *see* Trastuzumab *on page 1479*
- **Travel-Ease [OTC]** *see* Meclizine *on page 952*
- **Travel Sickness [OTC]** *see* Meclizine *on page 952*
- **Trazimera** *see* Trastuzumab *on page 1479*

TraZODone (TRAZ oh done)

Related Information

Clinical Risk Related to Drugs Prolonging QT Interval *on page 1675*

Management of the Patient With Anxiety or Depression *on page 1778*

Vasoconstrictor Interactions With Antidepressants *on page 1821*

Brand Names: Canada APO-TraZODone; APO-TraZODone D; DOM-TraZODone; Oleptro; PMS-TraZODone; RATIO-TraZODone [DSC]; TEVA-TraZODone; TraZODone-100; TraZODone-150; TraZODone-50

Pharmacologic Category Antidepressant, Serotonin Reuptake Inhibitor/Antagonist

Use Major depressive disorder (unipolar): Treatment of unipolar major depressive disorder

Local Anesthetic/Vasoconstrictor Precautions Trazodone inhibits reuptake of both serotonin and norepinephrine and also blocks some serotonin receptors. No precautions with vasoconstrictors appear to be necessary.

Trazodone is one of the drugs confirmed to prolong the QT interval and is accepted as having a risk of causing torsade de pointes. The risk of drug-induced torsade de pointes is extremely low when a single QT interval prolonging drug is prescribed. In terms of epinephrine, it is not known what effect vasoconstrictors in the local anesthetic regimen will have in patients with a known history of congenital prolonged QT interval or in patients taking any medication that prolongs the QT interval. Until more information is obtained, it is suggested that the clinician consult with the physician prior to the use of a vasoconstrictor in suspected patients, and that the vasoconstrictor (epinephrine, mepivacaine and levonordefrin [Carbocaine® 2% with Neo-Cobefrin®]) be used with caution.

Effects on Dental Treatment Key adverse event(s) related to dental treatment: Significant xerostomia (normal salivary flow resumes upon discontinuation).

Effects on Bleeding No information available to require special precautions

Adverse Reactions

>10%:

Gastrointestinal: Nausea and vomiting (10% to 13%), xerostomia (15% to 34%)

Nervous system: Dizziness (20% to 28%), drowsiness (24% to 41%), fatigue (6% to 11%), headache (10% to 20%), nervousness (15%)

Ophthalmic: Blurred vision (6% to 15%)

1% to 10%:

Cardiovascular: Chest pain (<2%), hypotension (4% to 7% [placebo: 0% to 1%]), palpitations (<2%), sinus bradycardia (<2%), syncope (3% to 5% [placebo: 1% to 2%]), tachycardia (<2%; may include syncope)

Endocrine & metabolic: Change in menstrual flow (<2%), increased libido (<2%), weight gain (1% to 5%), weight loss (6%)

Gastrointestinal: Constipation (7% to 8%), diarrhea (5%), flatulence (<2%), gastrointestinal disease (6%), increased appetite (<2%), sialorrhea (<2%)

Genitourinary: Early menses (<2%), hematuria (<2%), impotence (<2%), retrograde ejaculation (<2%), urinary frequency (<2%), urinary hesitancy (<2%)

Hematologic & oncologic: Anemia (<2%)

Hypersensitivity: Angioedema (3% to 7%), hypersensitivity reaction (<2%)

Nervous system: Akathisia (<2%), ataxia (2% to 5%), confusion (5%), delusion (<2%), disorientation (2%), hallucination (<2%), heavy headedness (3%), hypomania (<2%), lack of concentration (1% to 3%), malaise (3%), memory impairment (<2%), numbness (<2%), paresthesia (<2%), speech disturbance (<2%)

Neuromuscular & skeletal: Muscle twitching (<2%), myalgia (5% to 6%), tremor (3% to 5%)

Ophthalmic: Asthenopia (≤3%), eye pruritus (≤3%), eye redness (≤3%)

Respiratory: Dyspnea (<2%), nasal congestion (≤6%), paranasal sinus congestion (≤6%)

Frequency not defined:

Cardiovascular: Hypertension, ventricular premature contractions

Nervous system: Suicidal ideation, suicidal tendencies

Postmarketing:

Cardiovascular: Acute myocardial infarction, atrial fibrillation (White 1985), bradycardia (Li 2011), cardiac arrhythmia, cardiac conduction disorder, cardiac failure, cerebrovascular accident, complete atrioventricular block (Rausch 1984), edema (Barnett 1985), first-degree atrioventricular block (Winkler 2006), orthostatic hypotension (Asayesh 1986; Spivak 1987), prolonged QT interval on ECG (de Meester 2001; Levenson 1999), torsades de pointes (de Meester 2001; Levenson 1999), ventricular ectopy, ventricular tachycardia (Aronson 1986, Vittulo 1990)

Dermatologic: Alopecia, leukonychia (Longstreth 1985), psoriasis (Barth 1986), skin rash, urticaria

Endocrine & metabolic: Hirsutism, SIADH

Gastrointestinal: Cholestasis (Sheikh 1983), esophageal achalasia

Genitourinary: Breast engorgement, breast hypertrophy, lactation, priapism (Raskin 1985; Scher 1983), urinary incontinence, urinary retention

Hematologic & oncologic: Hemolytic anemia, leukocytosis, methemoglobinemia

Hepatic: Hepatotoxicity (Fernandes 2000; Rettman 2001)

Nervous system: Abnormal dreams, anxiety, aphasia, delirium (Lennkh 1998), extrapyramidal reaction (Sotto 2015), female sexual disorder (Battaglia 2009; Purcell 1995), insomnia, mania (Hu 2017), paranoid ideation, psychosis (Mizoguchi 2005), seizure (Vanpee 1999), stupor, tardive dyskinesia (Lin 2008), vertigo

Ophthalmic: Diplopia

Respiratory: Apnea

Mechanism of Action Inhibits reuptake of serotonin, causes adrenoreceptor subsensitivity, acts as a $5HT_{2a}$ receptor antagonist and induces significant changes in 5-HT presynaptic receptor adrenoreceptors. Trazodone also significantly blocks histamine (H_1) and alpha1-adrenergic receptors.

Pharmacodynamics/Kinetics

Onset of Action Depression: Initial effects may be observed within 1 to 2 weeks of treatment, with continued improvements through 4 to 6 weeks (Papakostas 2006; Posternak 2005; Szegedi 2009).

Half-life Elimination 5 to 9 hours, prolonged in obese patients

Time to Peak

Immediate release: 30 to 100 minutes; delayed with food (up to 2.5 hours)

Extended release: 9 hours; not significantly affected by food

Pregnancy Considerations

The ACOG recommends that therapy with antidepressants during pregnancy be individualized; treatment of depression during pregnancy should incorporate the clinical expertise of the mental health clinician, obstetrician, primary health care provider, and pediatrician. According to the American Psychiatric Association (APA), the risks of medication treatment should be weighed against other treatment options and untreated depression. Consideration should be given to using agents with safety data in pregnancy. For women who discontinue antidepressant medications during pregnancy and who may be at high risk for postpartum depression, the medications can be restarted following delivery. Treatment algorithms have been developed by the ACOG and the APA for the management of depression in women prior to conception and during pregnancy (ACOG 2008; APA 2010; Yonkers 2009).

Pregnant women exposed to antidepressants during pregnancy are encouraged to enroll in the National Pregnancy Registry for Antidepressants (NPRAD). Women 18 to 45 years of age or their health care providers may contact the registry by calling 844-405-6185. Enrollment should be done as early in pregnancy as possible.

Product Availability Oleptro has been discontinued in the United States for more than 1 year.

Dental Health Professional Considerations See Local Anesthetic/Vasoconstrictor Precautions

◆ **Trazodone Hydrochloride** *see* TraZODone *on page 1481*

◆ **Treanda** *see* Bendamustine *on page 226*

◆ **Trelstar [DSC]** *see* Triptorelin *on page 1500*

◆ **Trelstar Mixject** *see* Triptorelin *on page 1500*

◆ **Tremfya** *see* Guselkumab *on page 750*

◆ **Trental** *see* Pentoxifylline *on page 1215*

Treprostinil (tre PROST in il)

Brand Names: US Orenitram; Remodulin; Tyvaso; Tyvaso Refill; Tyvaso Starter

Brand Names: Canada Remodulin

Pharmacologic Category Prostacyclin; Prostaglandin; Vasodilator

Use Pulmonary arterial hypertension:

Injection: Treatment of pulmonary arterial hypertension (PAH) (World Health Organization [WHO] Group I) in patients with New York Heart Association (NYHA) Class II to IV symptoms to decrease exercise-associated symptoms; to diminish clinical deterioration when transitioning from epoprostenol.

Inhalation: Treatment of PAH (WHO Group I) in patients with NYHA Class III symptoms to improve exercise ability.

Oral: Treatment of PAH (WHO Group 1) in patients with WHO Functional Class II to III symptoms to delay disease progression and to delay disease progression and to improve exercise capacity or PAH associated with connective tissue disease.

Local Anesthetic/Vasoconstrictor Precautions No information available to require special precautions

Effects on Dental Treatment No significant effects or complications reported. Treprostinil may enhance the risk of bleeding associated with other antiplatelet agents (aspirin or NSAIDs).

Effects on Bleeding Treprostinil is an inhibitor of platelet aggregation and may prolong bleeding times.

Adverse Reactions

>10%:

Cardiovascular: Flushing (oral: 15% to 45%; oral inhalation: 15%), vasodilation (SubQ: 11%)

Central nervous system: Infusion-site pain (SubQ: 85%, severe: 39%), headache (oral: 63% to 75%; oral inhalation: 41%; SubQ: 27%)

Dermatologic: Skin rash (SubQ: 14%)

Gastrointestinal: Diarrhea (oral: 30% to 69%; SubQ: 25%), nausea (19% to 40%), vomiting (oral: 17% to 36%), upper abdominal pain (oral: 5% to 12%)

Local: Infusion site reaction (SubQ: 83%, severe: 38%, including erythema, induration, skin rash)

Neuromuscular & skeletal: Limb pain (oral: 14% to 18%), jaw pain (11% to 18%)

Respiratory: Cough (inhalation: 54%), pharyngolaryngeal pain (inhalation: ≤25%), throat irritation (inhalation: ≤25%)

1% to 10%:

Cardiovascular: Edema (SubQ: 9%), syncope (inhalation: 6%), hypotension (SubQ: 4%)

Endocrine & metabolic: Hypokalemia (oral: 4% to 9%)

Gastrointestinal: Abdominal distress (oral: 6% to 8%)

Frequency not defined:

Central nervous system: Pain, paresthesia

Gastrointestinal: Sore throat

Hematologic & oncologic: Bleeding tendency disorder, decreased platelet aggregation, hematoma

Neuromuscular & skeletal: Swelling of extremities (arm)

Respiratory: Epistaxis (long-term therapy), hemoptysis (long-term therapy), nasal discomfort (long-term therapy), pneumonia (long-term therapy), wheezing (long-term therapy)

<1%, postmarketing, and/or case reports: Angioedema, arthralgia, catheter infection (central venous), cellulitis, dizziness, dyspepsia, maculopapular rash, muscle spasm, myalgia, ostealgia, papular rash, pruritus, thrombocytopenia, thrombophlebitis

Mechanism of Action Treprostinil is a direct vasodilator of both pulmonary and systemic arterial vascular beds; also inhibits platelet aggregation.

Pharmacodynamics/Kinetics

Half-life Elimination Terminal: ~4 hours

Time to Peak Oral: 4 to 6 hours

Pregnancy Considerations

Information related to the use of treprostinil for the treatment of pulmonary arterial hypertension (PAH) in pregnant women is limited (Lim 2019; Rosengarten 2015; Smith 2012; Xiang 2018; Zhang 2018).

Untreated PAH in pregnancy increases the risk for maternal heart failure, stroke, preterm delivery, low birth weight, and maternal/fetal death. Women with PAH are encouraged to avoid pregnancy. When treatment is needed, agents with more information may be preferred for use in pregnant women (ESC [Regitz-Zagrosek 2018]).

◆ **Treprostinil Sodium** *see* Treprostinil *on page 1482*

◆ **Tresiba** *see* Insulin Degludec *on page 819*

◆ **Tresiba FlexTouch** *see* Insulin Degludec *on page 819*

◆ **Tretin-X [DSC]** *see* Tretinoin (Topical) *on page 1484*

Tretinoin (Systemic) (TRET i noyn)

Brand Names: Canada Vesanoid

Pharmacologic Category Antineoplastic Agent, Retinoic Acid Derivative; Retinoic Acid Derivative

Use Acute promyelocytic leukemia (remission induction): Induction of remission in patients with acute promyelocytic leukemia, French American British (FAB) classification M3 (including the M3 variant) characterized by t(15;17) translocation and/or PML/RARα gene presence

Local Anesthetic/Vasoconstrictor Precautions

No information available to require special precautions

Effects on Dental Treatment Key adverse event(s) related to dental treatment: Xerostomia (normal salivary flow resumes upon discontinuation).

Effects on Bleeding Although significant myelosuppression with associated altered hemostasis has been reported for many chemotherapeutic agents, myelosuppression is not common with tretinoin and no specific precautions appear to necessary.

Adverse Reactions Most patients will experience drug-related toxicity, especially headache, fever, weakness and fatigue. These are seldom permanent or irreversible and do not typically require therapy interruption.

>10%:

Cardiovascular: Peripheral edema (52%), chest discomfort (32%), edema (29%), cardiac arrhythmia (23%), flushing (23%), hypotension (14%), hypertension (11%), localized phlebitis (11%)

Central nervous system: Headache (86%), malaise (66%), shivering (63%), pain (37%), dizziness (20%), anxiety (17%), paresthesia (17%), depression (14%), insomnia (14%), confusion (11%)

Dermatologic: Xeroderma (≤77%), skin rash (54%), diaphoresis (20%), pruritus (20%), alopecia (14%), skin changes (14%)

Endocrine & metabolic: Hypercholesterolemia (≤60%), hypertriglyceridemia (≤60%), weight gain (23%), weight loss (17%)

Gastrointestinal: Dry mucous membranes (≤77%), nausea (≤57%), vomiting (≤57%), gastrointestinal hemorrhage (34%), abdominal pain (31%), mucositis (26%), diarrhea (23%), anorexia (17%), constipation (17%), dyspepsia (14%), abdominal distention (11%)

Hematologic & oncologic: Hemorrhage (60%), leukocytosis (40%), disseminated intravascular coagulation (26%)

Hepatic: Increased liver enzymes (50% to 60%)

Infection: Infection (58%)

Neuromuscular & skeletal: Ostealgia (77%), APL differentiation syndrome (≤25%), myalgia (14%)

Ophthalmic: Eye disease (17%), visual disturbance (17%)

Otic: Otalgia (23%; ear fullness)

Renal: Renal insufficiency (11%)

Respiratory: Upper respiratory complaint (63%), dyspnea (60%), respiratory insufficiency (26%), pleural effusion (20%), pneumonia (14%), rales (14%), wheezing (expiratory: 14%)

Miscellaneous: Fever (83%)

1% to 10%:

Cardiovascular: Cardiac failure (6%), facial edema (6%), cardiomegaly (3%), cardiomyopathy (3%), cerebrovascular accident (3%), heart murmur (3%), ischemia (3%), myocardial infarction (3%), myocarditis (3%), pericarditis (3%)

Central nervous system: Agitation (9%), cerebral hemorrhage (9%), flank pain (9%), intracranial hypertension (9%), hallucination (6%), abnormal gait (3%), agnosia (3%), aphasia (3%), asterixis (3%), ataxia (3%), brain disease (3%), cerebral edema (cerebellar: 3%), central nervous system depression (3%), coma (3%), dementia (3%), drowsiness (3%), dysarthria (3%), facial paralysis (3%), forgetfulness (3%), hemiplegia (3%), hyporeflexia (3%), hypothermia (3%), loss of consciousness (3%), seizure (3%), speech disturbance (3%)

Dermatologic: Cellulitis (8%), pallor (6%)

Endocrine & metabolic: Disturbance in fluid balance (6%), acidosis (3%)

Gastrointestinal: Gastrointestinal ulcer (3%)

Genitourinary: Dysuria (9%), benign prostatic hypertrophy (3%), urinary frequency (3%)

Hematologic & oncologic: Lymphatic disease (6%)

Hepatic: Hepatosplenomegaly (9%), ascites (3%), hepatitis (3%)

Local: Local inflammation (bone: 3%)

Neuromuscular & skeletal: Lower extremity weakness (3%), myelopathy (3%), tremor (3%)

Ophthalmic: Decreased visual acuity (6%), decreased pupillary reflex (3%), visual field defect (3%)

Otic: Hearing loss (6%; may be irreversible)

Renal: Acute renal failure (3%), renal tubular necrosis (3%)

Respiratory: Lower respiratory signs and symptoms (9%), pulmonary infiltrates (6%), asthma (3%), laryngeal edema (3%), pulmonary hypertension (3%)

<1%, postmarketing, and/or case reports: Arterial thrombosis, basophilia, erythema nodosum, histamine release (hyperhistaminemia), hypercalcemia, hypersensitivity angiitis, myositis, pancreatitis, pseudotumor cerebri, renal infarction, Sweet's syndrome, thrombocythemia, ulcer (genital), venous thrombosis

Mechanism of Action Tretinoin appears to bind one or more nuclear receptors and decreases proliferation and induces differentiation of APL cells; initially produces maturation of primitive promyelocytes and repopulates the marrow and peripheral blood with normal hematopoietic cells to achieve complete remission

Pharmacodynamics/Kinetics

Half-life Elimination Terminal: Parent drug: 0.5 to 2 hours

Time to Peak Serum: 1 to 2 hours

Reproductive Considerations

[US Boxed Warning]: There is a high risk that a severely deformed infant will result if tretinoin capsules are administered during pregnancy. If, nonetheless, it is determined that tretinoin capsules represent the best available treatment for a woman of childbearing potential, it must be assured that the patient has received full information and warnings of the risk to the fetus if she were to be pregnant and of the risk of possible contraception failure and has been instructed in the need to use two reliable forms of contraception simultaneously during therapy and for 1 month following discontinuation of therapy, and has acknowledged her understanding of the need for using dual contraception, unless abstinence is the chosen method. Within 1 week prior to the institution of tretinoin capsules therapy, the patient should have blood or urine collected for a serum or urine pregnancy test with a sensitivity of at least 50 mIU/mL. When possible, tretinoin capsules therapy should be delayed until a negative result from this test is obtained. When a delay is not possible, the patient should be placed on two reliable forms of contraception. Pregnancy testing and contraception counseling should be repeated monthly throughout the period of tretinoin capsules treatment. Contraception must be used even when there is a history of infertility or menopause, unless a hysterectomy has been performed. Microdosed progesterone products ("minipill") may provide inadequate pregnancy protection.

Pregnancy Risk Factor D

Pregnancy Considerations

[US Boxed Warning]: There is a high risk that a severely deformed infant will result if tretinoin capsules are administered during pregnancy. Tretinoin was detected in the serum of a neonate at birth following maternal use of standard doses during pregnancy (Takitani 2005). Major fetal abnormalities and spontaneous abortions have been reported with other retinoids; some of these abnormalities were fatal. Birth defects associated with exposure to retinoids include facial dysmorphia, cleft palate, eye abnormalities and abnormalities of the central nervous system, cardiovascular system, musculoskeletal system, and parathyroid hormone deficiencies. All exposed fetuses have the potential to be affected.

Use in humans for the treatment of acute promyelocytic leukemia (APL) is limited and exposure occurred after the first trimester in most cases (Valappil 2007). If the clinical condition of a patient presenting with APL during pregnancy warrants immediate treatment, tretinoin use should be avoided in the first trimester; treatment with tretinoin may be considered in the second and third trimester with careful fetal monitoring, including cardiac monitoring (Sanz 2009).

Tretinoin (Topical) (TRET i noyn)

Brand Names: US Altreno; Atralin; Avita; Refissa; Renova; Renova Pump; Retin-A; Retin-A Micro; Retin-A Micro Pump; Tretin-X [DSC]

Brand Names: Canada Retin-A; Retin-A Micro; Stieva-A

Pharmacologic Category Acne Products; Retinoic Acid Derivative; Topical Skin Product, Acne

Use

Acne vulgaris: Altreno, Atralin, Avita, Retin-A, Retin-A Micro, Stieva-A [Canadian product], Tretin-X, Vitamin-A Acid [Canadian product]: Treatment of acne vulgaris.

Palliation of fine wrinkles: Renova: Adjunctive treatment for mitigation (palliation) of fine wrinkles in patients who use comprehensive skin care and sun avoidance programs.

Palliation of fine wrinkles, mottled hyperpigmentation, and facial skin roughness: Refissa: Adjunctive treatment for mitigation (palliation) of fine wrinkles, mottled hyperpigmentation, and tactile roughness of facial skin in patients who do not achieve such palliation using comprehensive skin care and sun avoidance programs alone.

Local Anesthetic/Vasoconstrictor Precautions No information available to require special precautions

Effects on Dental Treatment No significant effects or complications reported

Effects on Bleeding No information available to require special precautions

Adverse Reactions

>10%:

Dermatologic: Stinging of the skin (21%), local dryness (4% to 16%), hypopigmentation (≤12%)

Local: Application site erythema (2% to 51%), application site irritation (1% to 50%; severe: ≤3%), local skin exfoliation (1% to 49%), application site pruritus (2% to 35%), application site burning (8% to 30%), local desquamation (12%)

1% to 10%:

Dermatologic: Hyperpigmentation (≤2%)

Local: Application site dermatitis (4%), application site pain (1% to 3%)

Frequency not defined: Dermatologic: Skin photosensitivity

<1%, postmarketing, and/or case reports: Contact dermatitis, skin changes (atypical changes in melanocytes and keratinocytes, increased dermal elastosis; treatment lasting >48 weeks)

Mechanism of Action Tretinoin is a derivative of vitamin A. When used topically, it modifies epithelial growth and differentiation. In patients with acne, it decreases the cohesiveness of follicular epithelial cells and decreases micromedo formation. Additionally, tretinoin stimulates mitotic activity and increased turnover of follicular epithelial cells causing extrusion of the comedones.

Pharmacodynamics/Kinetics

Onset of Action Acne: ≥2 weeks, may take ≥7 weeks; Facial wrinkles: Up to 6 months

Reproductive Considerations

These products should not be used in women who are attempting to conceive or at high risk for pregnancy.

Pregnancy Considerations

Adverse events were observed in some animal reproduction studies following topical application of tretinoin. Teratogenic effects were also observed in pregnant women following topical use; however, a causal association has not been established.

When treatment for acne is needed during pregnancy, other agents are preferred (Chien 2016; Kong 2013; Leachman 2006). These products should not be used in women who are pregnant.

- ◆ **Tretinoinum** *see* Tretinoin (Systemic) *on page 1483*
- ◆ **Trexall** *see* Methotrexate *on page 990*
- ◆ **Triaconazole** *see* Terconazole *on page 1423*

Triamcinolone (Systemic) (trye am SIN oh lone)

Related Information

Respiratory Diseases *on page 1680*

Brand Names: US Arze-Ject-A [DSC]; Kenalog; Kenalog-80; P-Care K40; P-Care K80; Pod-Care 100K; Pro-C-Dure 5; Pro-C-Dure 6; ReadySharp Triamcinolone [DSC]; Zilretta

Brand Names: Canada Aristospan [DSC]; Kenalog-10; Kenalog-40

Generic Availability (US) May be product dependent

Pharmacologic Category Corticosteroid, Systemic

Dental Use Adjunctive treatment and temporary relief of symptoms associated with oral inflammatory lesions and ulcerative lesions resulting from trauma

Use

Intra-articular or soft tissue administration (triamcinolone hexacetonide [Canadian product]): Symptomatic treatment of subacute and chronic inflammatory joint diseases including: synovitis, tendinitis, bursitis, epicondylitis, rheumatoid arthritis (RA), juvenile idiopathic arthritis (JIA), osteoarthritis, or post-traumatic arthritis.

Intralesional administration (triamcinolone acetonide [Kenalog-10 only]): Alopecia areata; discoid lupus erythematosus; keloids; localized hypertrophic, infiltrated, inflammatory lesions of granuloma annulare, lichen planus, lichen simplex chronicus (neurodermatitis), and psoriatic plaques; necrobiosis lipoidica diabeticorum; cystic tumors of an aponeurosis or tendon (ganglia).

Intramuscular administration (triamcinolone acetonide [Kenalog-40] only):

Allergic states: Control of severe or incapacitating allergic conditions intractable to adequate trials of conventional treatment in asthma, drug hypersensitivity reactions, perennial or seasonal allergic rhinitis, serum sickness, or transfusion reactions.

Dermatologic diseases: Atopic dermatitis, bullous dermatitis herpetiformis, contact dermatitis, exfoliative erythroderma, mycosis fungoides, pemphigus, or severe erythema multiforme (Stevens-Johnson syndrome).

Endocrine disorders: Primary or secondary adrenocortical insufficiency (hydrocortisone or cortisone is the drug of choice), congenital adrenal hyperplasia, hypercalcemia associated with cancer, or nonsuppurative thyroiditis.

GI diseases: To tide the patient over a critical period of disease in Crohn disease or ulcerative colitis.

Hematologic disorders: Acquired (autoimmune) hemolytic anemia, Diamond-Blackfan anemia, pure red cell aplasia, select cases of secondary thrombocytopenia.

Neoplastic diseases: Palliative management of leukemias and lymphomas.

Nervous system: Acute exacerbations of multiple sclerosis; cerebral edema associated with primary or metastatic brain tumor or craniotomy. **Note**: Treatment guidelines recommend the use of high dose IV or oral methylprednisolone for acute exacerbations of multiple sclerosis (AAN [Scott 2011]; NICE 2014).

Ophthalmic diseases: Sympathetic ophthalmia, temporal arteritis, uveitis, and ocular inflammatory conditions unresponsive to topical corticosteroids.

Renal diseases: To induce diuresis or remission of proteinuria in idiopathic nephrotic syndrome or that is caused by lupus erythematosus.

Respiratory diseases: Berylliosis, fulminating or disseminated pulmonary tuberculosis when used concurrently with appropriate antituberculous chemotherapy, idiopathic eosinophilic pneumonias, symptomatic sarcoidosis.

Rheumatic disorders: As adjunctive therapy for short-term administration in acute gout flares; acute rheumatic carditis; ankylosing spondylitis; psoriatic arthritis; RA, including juvenile RA; treatment of dermatomyositis, polymyositis, and systemic lupus erythematosus.

Miscellaneous: Trichinosis with neurologic or myocardial involvement; tuberculous meningitis with subarachnoid block or impending block when used with appropriate antituberculous chemotherapy.

Local Anesthetic/Vasoconstrictor Precautions No information available to require special precautions

Effects on Dental Treatment Key adverse event(s) related to dental treatment: Ulcerative esophagitis, perioral dermatitis, atrophy of oral mucosa, burning, irritation, and oral monilia (oral inhaler).

Effects on Bleeding No information available to require special precautions

Adverse Reactions Most reactions listed are based on reports for other agents in this same pharmacologic class and may not be specifically reported for systemic triamcinolone.

1% to 10%:

Hematologic & oncologic: Bruise (extended release: 2%)

Neuromuscular & skeletal: Joint swelling (extended release: 3%)

Respiratory: Cough (extended release: 2%), sinusitis (extended release: 2%)

Frequency not defined:

Cardiovascular: Bradycardia, cardiac arrhythmia, cardiac failure, cardiomegaly, cerebrovascular accident, circulatory shock, edema, embolism (fat), hypertension, hypertrophic cardiomyopathy (premature infants), myocardial rupture (following recent myocardial infarction), syncope, tachycardia, thromboembolism, thrombophlebitis, vasculitis

Dermatologic: Acne vulgaris, allergic dermatitis, atrophic striae, diaphoresis, ecchymoses, epidermal thinning, erythema of skin, exfoliation of skin, hyperpigmentation, hypertrichosis, hypopigmentation, inadvertent suppression of skin test reaction, skin atrophy, skin rash, subcutaneous atrophy, thinning hair, urticaria, xeroderma

Endocrine & metabolic: Calcinosis, decreased glucose tolerance, decreased serum potassium, diabetes mellitus, drug-induced Cushing's syndrome, fluid retention, glycosuria, growth retardation, hirsutism, impaired glucose tolerance/prediabetes, insulin resistance, menstrual disease, moon face, negative nitrogen balance, redistribution of body fat, secondary adrenocortical insufficiency, sodium retention, weight gain

Gastrointestinal: Abdominal distention, change in bowel habits, gastrointestinal hemorrhage, gastrointestinal perforation, hiccups, increased appetite, nausea, pancreatitis, peptic ulcer, ulcerative esophagitis

Genitourinary: Bladder dysfunction, postmenopausal bleeding, spermatozoa disorder

Hematologic & oncologic: Nonthrombocytopenic purpura, petechia

Hepatic: Hepatomegaly, increased liver enzymes

Hypersensitivity: Anaphylaxis, angioedema

Infection: Increased susceptibility to infection, infection, sterile abscess

Local: Postinjection flare

Nervous system: Abnormal sensory symptoms, arachnoiditis, depression, emotional lability, euphoria, headache, idiopathic intracranial hypertension (upon discontinuation), increased intracranial pressure, insomnia, malaise, meningitis, mood changes, myasthenia, neuritis, neuropathy, paraplegia, paresthesia, personality changes, psychiatric disturbance, quadriplegia, seizure, spinal cord infarction, vertigo

Neuromuscular & skeletal: Amyotrophy, aseptic necrosis of femoral head, aseptic necrosis of humeral head, bone fracture, Charcot arthropathy, lupus erythematous-like rash, osteoporosis, rupture of tendon, steroid myopathy, vertebral compression fracture

Ophthalmic: Blindness (periocular; rare), cataract, cortical blindness, exophthalmos, glaucoma, increased intraocular pressure, papilledema

Renal: Increased urine calcium excretion

Respiratory: Pulmonary edema

Miscellaneous: Wound healing impairment

Dosing

Adult & Geriatric Note: Adjust dose depending upon condition being treated and response of patient. The lowest possible dose should be used to control the condition; when dose reduction is possible, the dose should be reduced gradually.

Dermatoses (steroid-responsive): Acetonide (Kenalog-10): 1 mg Intralesional: Initial dose varies depending on the specific disease and lesion being treated; may be repeated at weekly or less frequent intervals; multiple sites may be injected if they are ≥1 cm apart.

Gout, acute flares (alternative agent): Note: Do not use if there is suspicion for infectious involvement.

Patients whose gout flare is limited to 1 to 2 joints and/or who are unable to take oral medications: Intra-articular: Acetonide (Kenalog-10): Larger joint (eg, knee): 40 mg; Medium joint (eg, wrist, ankle, elbow): 30 mg; Small joint: 10 mg (Becker 2020).

Patients with polyarticular involvement unable to take oral medications and who are not candidates for intra-articular injection: IM: Acetonide (Kenalog-40): Initial: 40 to 60 mg as a single dose; may repeat once or twice at ≥48-hour intervals if benefit fades or there is no flare resolution (Alloway 1993; Becker 2020; Siegal 1994).

Inflammatory/allergic conditions/other steroid-responsive systemic conditions: Acetonide (Kenalog-40): IM: Initial: 60 mg; adjust dose to a range of 40 to 80 mg. For patients with hay fever or pollen asthma who are not responding to pollen administration and other conventional therapy, a single injection of 40 to 100 mg per season may be given.

Multiple sclerosis (acute exacerbation):

Note: Treatment guidelines recommend the use of high dose IV or oral methylprednisolone for acute exacerbations of multiple sclerosis (AAN [Scott 2011]; NICE 2014).

Acetonide (Kenalog-40): IM: 160 mg daily for 1 week, followed by 64 mg every other day for 1 month.

Rheumatic conditions (excluding acute gout flares):

Intra-articular (or similar injection as designated): **Note:** Dose ranges per manufacturer's labeling. Specific dose is determined based upon joint size, severity of inflammation, amount of articular fluid present, and clinician judgment.

Acetonide: Intra-articular, intrabursal, tendon sheaths: Initial: Smaller joints: 2.5 to 5 mg, larger joints: 5 to 15 mg; may require up to 10 mg for small joints and up to 40 mg for large joints; maximum dose/treatment (several joints at one time): 80 mg.

Zilretta only: Intra-articular: Single dose: 32 mg. **Note:** For osteoarthritis (OA) pain of the knee only (use for OA pain of shoulder and hip have not been evaluated); use is not suitable for small joints (eg, hand). Safety and efficacy of repeat administration has not been studied.

Hexacetonide [Canadian product]: Intra-articular: Average dose: 2 to 20 mg; smaller joints (interphalangeal, metacarpophalangeal): 2 to 6 mg; large joints (knee, hip, shoulder): 10 to 20 mg. Frequency of injection into a single joint is every 3 to 4 weeks as necessary; to avoid possible joint destruction use as infrequently as possible.

IM: Acetonide (Kenalog-40): Initial: 60 mg; range: 2.5 to 100 mg/day.

Renal Impairment: Adult There are no dosage adjustments provided in the manufacturer's labeling; use with caution.

Hepatic Impairment: Adult There are no dosage adjustments provided in the manufacturer's labeling; use with caution.

Pediatric Note: Adjust dose depending upon condition being treated and response of patient. The lowest possible dose should be used to control the condition; when dose reduction is possible, the dose should be reduced gradually.

General dosing, treatment of inflammatory and allergic conditions:

Children and Adolescents: Triamcinolone acetonide (Kenalog-40): IM: Initial: 0.11 to 1.6 mg/kg/day (or 3.2 to 48 mg/m^2/day) in 3 to 4 divided doses.

Juvenile idiopathic arthritis (JIA), other rheumatic conditions:

Triamcinolone acetonide (Kenalog-10, -40, or -80): Children and Adolescents: Intra-articular: Initial: Smaller joints: 2.5 to 5 mg, larger joints: 5 to 15 mg; maximum dose/treatment (several joints at one time): 20 to 80 mg.

Canadian labeling: Triamcinolone hexacetonide (Canadian product; not available in the US):

Children 3 to 12 years: Intra-articular:

Large joints (knees, hips, shoulders): 1 mg/kg/dose.

Small joints (ankles, wrists, elbows): 0.5 mg/kg/dose.

Hands and feet:

Metacarpophalangeal/metatarsophalangeal joints: 1 to 2 mg/**dose**.

Proximal interphalangeal joints: 0.6 to 1 mg/**dose**.

Adolescents: Intra-articular: Average dose: 2 to 20 mg/**dose** every 3 to 4 weeks as necessary; to avoid possible joint destruction use as infrequently as possible. Dose dependent upon degree of inflammation and joint involved:

Large joints (knee, hip, shoulder): 10 to 20 mg/**dose**.

Smaller joints (interphalangeal, metacarpophalangeal): 2 to 6 mg/**dose**.

Infantile hemangioma, severe: Limited data available: Infants and Children ≤49 months: Triamcinolone acetonide (Kenalog-10 or -40): Intralesional: Dosage dependent upon size of lesion: Commonly reported: 1 to 2 mg/kg/dose administered in divided doses along the lesion perimeter ~monthly (4 to 5 weeks most frequently reported interval); a maximum dose up to 30 mg/dose has been used; others have reported: 1 to 30 mg of the 10 mg/mL acetonide injection divided into multiple injections along the lesion; has also been used in combination with betamethasone intralesional injections (AAP [Darrow 2015]; Chen 2000; Maguiness 2012; Pandey 2009; Prasetyono 2011). From the largest reported experience (n=1,514; age range: 1 to 49 months), triamcinolone (1 to 2 mg/kg once every month) alone or in combination with oral corticosteroid (if no response after 6 injections of monotherapy) showed lesion size decrease of 50% or more in 90.3% of infants (age <1 year) and 80% in those >1 year (Pandey 2009). Another trial (n=155; age range at first injection: 2 to 12 months) which used 1 to 30 mg of a 10 mg/mL concentration administered approximately once monthly (mean interval: 5 weeks) for 3 to 6 months showed lesion size decreased by at least 50% in 85% of the patients (Chen 2000).

Dermatoses (steroid-responsive, including contact/atopic dermatitis):

Triamcinolone acetonide (Kenalog-10): Intradermal: Adolescents: Up to 1 mg per injection site and may be repeated 1 or more times weekly; multiple sites may be injected if they are 1 cm or more apart, not to exceed 30 mg.

Renal Impairment: Pediatric There are no dosage adjustments provided in the manufacturer's labeling.

Hepatic Impairment: Pediatric There are no dosage adjustments provided in the manufacturer's labeling.

Mechanism of Action A long acting corticosteroid with minimal sodium-retaining potential. Decreases inflammation by suppression of migration of polymorphonuclear leukocytes and reversal of increased capillary permeability; suppresses the immune system by reducing activity and volume of the lymphatic system; suppresses adrenal function at high doses

Contraindications

Triamcinolone acetonide: Hypersensitivity to triamcinolone or any component of the formulation; immune thrombocytopenia (formerly known as idiopathic thrombocytopenic purpura) (IM administration only)

Canadian labeling: Additional contraindications (not in US labeling): Systemic infections; injection into infected areas

Triamcinolone hexacetonide [Canadian product]: Hypersensitivity to triamcinolone or any component of the formulation; acute psychoses; active tuberculosis; herpes simplex keratitis; systemic mycoses; parasitosis (strongyloides infections); children <3 years of age (due to benzyl alcohol); epidural or intrathecal administration

Documentation of allergenic cross-reactivity for corticosteroids is limited. However, because of similarities in chemical structure and/or pharmacologic actions, the possibility of cross-sensitivity cannot be ruled out with certainty.

Warnings/Precautions May cause hypercortisolism or suppression of hypothalamic-pituitary-adrenal (HPA) axis, particularly in younger children or in patients receiving high doses for prolonged periods. HPA axis suppression may lead to adrenal crisis. Withdrawal and discontinuation of a corticosteroid should be done slowly and carefully. Particular care is required when patients are transferred from systemic corticosteroids to inhaled products due to possible adrenal insufficiency or withdrawal from steroids, including an increase in allergic symptoms. Adult patients receiving >20 mg per day of prednisone (or equivalent) may be most susceptible. Fatalities have occurred due to adrenal insufficiency in asthmatic patients during and after transfer from systemic corticosteroids to aerosol steroids; aerosol steroids do not provide the systemic steroid needed to treat patients having trauma, surgery, or infections.

Acute myopathy has been reported with high-dose corticosteroids, usually in patients with neuromuscular transmission disorders or when given concomitantly with neuromuscular blocking agents; may involve ocular and/or respiratory muscles; monitor creatine kinase; recovery may be delayed. Corticosteroid use may cause psychiatric disturbances, including euphoria, insomnia, mood swings, and personality changes to severe depression and frank psychotic manifestations. Preexisting psychiatric conditions may be exacerbated by corticosteroid use. Prolonged use of corticosteroids may also increase the incidence of secondary infection, cause activation of latent infections, mask acute infection (including fungal infections), prolong or exacerbate viral infections, or limit response to killed or inactivated vaccines. Exposure to chickenpox or measles should be avoided; corticosteroids should not be used to treat ocular herpes simplex, cerebral malaria, fungal infections, or viral hepatitis. Close observation is required in patients with latent tuberculosis and/or TB reactivity; restrict use in active TB (only fulminating or disseminated TB in conjunction with antituberculosis treatment). Amebiasis should be ruled out in any patient with recent travel to tropic climates or unexplained diarrhea prior to initiation of corticosteroids. Use with extreme caution in patients with *Strongyloides* infections; hyperinfection, dissemination, and fatalities have occurred. Prolonged treatment with corticosteroids has been associated with the development of Kaposi sarcoma (case reports); if noted, discontinuation of therapy should be considered (Goedert 2002). Increased mortality was observed in patients receiving high-dose IV methylprednisolone; high-dose corticosteroids should not be used for the management of head injury.

Use with caution in patients with thyroid disease, hepatic impairment, renal impairment, cardiovascular disease, diabetes, myasthenia gravis, osteoporosis, and patients at risk for seizures. Use with caution or avoid use in patients with GI diseases (diverticulosis, diverticulitis, fresh intestinal anastomoses, active or latent peptic ulcer, ulcerative colitis, abscess or other pyogenic infection). Use cautiously in the elderly with the smallest possible effective dose for the shortest duration. Use with caution in patients with cataracts and/or glaucoma; increased intraocular pressure, open-angle glaucoma, and cataracts have occurred with prolonged use. Use with caution in patients with a history of ocular herpes simplex; corneal perforation has occurred; do not use in active ocular herpes simplex. Not recommended for the treatment of optic neuritis; may increase frequency of new episodes. Consider routine eye exams in chronic users.

Withdraw therapy with gradual tapering of dose. Administer products only via recommended route (depending on product used). Do **not** administer any triamcinolone product via the intrathecal route; serious adverse events, including fatalities, have been reported. Corticosteroids are not approved for epidural injection. Serious neurologic events (eg, spinal cord infarction, paraplegia, quadriplegia, cortical blindness, stroke), some resulting in death, have been reported with epidural injection of corticosteroids, with and without use of fluoroscopy. Intra-articular injection may result in damage to joint tissues. Avoid injection into an infected site; injection into a previously infected joint is not usually recommended. Injection into unstable joints is generally not recommended. Examine any joint fluid present to exclude a septic process. Septic arthritis may occur as a complication to intra-articular or soft tissue administration; institute appropriate antimicrobial therapy as required. Atrophy at the injection site has been reported. Avoid IM deltoid injection; subcutaneous atrophy may occur.

Rare cases of anaphylactoid reactions have been observed in patients receiving corticosteroids. Cases of serious anaphylaxis, including death, have been reported with triamcinolone acetonide. Use may affect growth velocity; growth should be routinely monitored in pediatric patients. Patients may require higher doses when subject to stress (ie, trauma, surgery, severe infection). Use with caution in patients with systemic sclerosis; an increase in scleroderma renal crisis incidence has been observed with corticosteroid use. Monitor BP and renal function in patients with systemic sclerosis treated with corticosteroids (EULAR [Kowal-Bielecka 2017]). Potentially significant drug-drug interactions may exist, requiring dose or frequency adjustment, additional monitoring, and/or selection of alternative therapy.

Benzyl alcohol and derivatives: Some dosage forms may contain benzyl alcohol; large amounts of benzyl alcohol (≥99 mg/kg/day) have been associated with a potentially fatal toxicity ("gasping syndrome") in neonates; the "gasping syndrome" consists of metabolic acidosis, respiratory distress, gasping respirations, CNS dysfunction (including convulsions, intracranial hemorrhage), hypotension, and cardiovascular collapse (AAP ["Inactive" 1997], CDC 1982); some data suggests that benzoate displaces bilirubin from protein binding sites (Ahlfors 2001); avoid or use dosage forms containing benzyl alcohol with caution in neonates. See manufacturer's labeling.

Polysorbate 80: Some dosage forms may contain polysorbate 80 (also known as Tweens). Hypersensitivity reactions, usually a delayed reaction, have been reported following exposure to pharmaceutical products containing polysorbate 80 in certain individuals (Isaksson 2002, Lucente 2000, Shelley 1995). Thrombocytopenia, ascites, pulmonary deterioration, and renal and hepatic failure have been reported in premature neonates after receiving parenteral products containing polysorbate 80 (Alade 1986, CDC 1984). See manufacturer's labeling.

Warnings: Additional Pediatric Considerations Adrenal suppression with failure to thrive has been reported in infants and young children receiving intralesional corticosteroid injections for the treatment of infantile hemangioma; failure to gain weight may persist until HPA axis recovers; time to recovery of adrenal function may be prolonged (mean: 19.5 weeks; range 4 to 65 weeks) (DeBoer 2008; Morkane 2011). May cause osteoporosis (at any age) or inhibition of bone growth in pediatric patients. Use with caution in patients with osteoporosis. In a population-based study of children, risk of fracture was shown to be increased with >4 courses of corticosteroids; underlying clinical condition may also impact bone health and osteoporotic effect of corticosteroids (Leonard 2007). Tissue atrophy at the site of IM injection has been reported; avoid intramuscular injections into the deltoid area. Cutaneous atrophy was reported in 2.5% of pediatric patients when given intra-articularly (Bloom 2011). Prevention of periarticular subcutaneous atrophy via injecting small amounts of saline into the joint and applying pressure following the injection has been recommended (Hashkes 2005).

Drug Interactions

Metabolism/Transport Effects **Substrate** of CYP3A4 (minor); **Note:** Assignment of Major/Minor substrate status based on clinically relevant drug interaction potential

Avoid Concomitant Use

Avoid concomitant use of Triamcinolone (Systemic) with any of the following: Aldesleukin; BCG (Intravesical); Cladribine; Desmopressin; Fexinidazole [INT]; Indium 111 Capromab Pendetide; Loxapine; Macimorelin; Mifamurtide; MiFEPRIStone; Natalizumab; Pimecrolimus; Tacrolimus (Topical)

Increased Effect/Toxicity

Triamcinolone (Systemic) may increase the levels/effects of: Acetylcholinesterase Inhibitors; Amphotericin B; Androgens; Baricitinib; Deferasirox; Desirudin; Desmopressin; Fexinidazole [INT]; Fingolimod; Leflunomide; Loop Diuretics; Loxapine; Natalizumab; Nicorandil; Nonsteroidal Anti-Inflammatory Agents (COX-2 Selective); Nonsteroidal Anti-Inflammatory Agents (Nonselective); Ozanimod; Quinolones; Ritodrine; Sargramostim; Siponimod; Thiazide and Thiazide-Like Diuretics; Tofacitinib; Upadacitinib; Vaccines (Live); Vitamin K Antagonists

The levels/effects of Triamcinolone (Systemic) may be increased by: Antihepaciviral Combination Products; Aprepitant; Cladribine; CYP3A4 Inhibitors (Strong); Denosumab; DilTIAZem; Estrogen Derivatives; Fosaprepitant; Indacaterol; Inebilizumab; MiFEPRIStone; Neuromuscular-Blocking Agents (Nondepolarizing); Ocrelizumab; Pimecrolimus; Ritonavir; Roflumilast; Salicylates; Tacrolimus (Topical); Trastuzumab

Decreased Effect

Triamcinolone (Systemic) may decrease the levels/effects of: Aldesleukin; Antidiabetic Agents; Axicabtagene Ciloleucel; BCG (Intravesical); Calcitriol (Systemic); Coccidioides immitis Skin Test; Corticorelin; Cosyntropin; Hyaluronidase; Indium 111 Capromab Pendetide; Isoniazid; Macimorelin; Mifamurtide; Nivolumab; Pidotimod; Salicylates; Sipuleucel-T; Somatropin; Tacrolimus (Systemic); Tertomotide;

Tisagenlecleucel; Urea Cycle Disorder Agents; Vaccines (Inactivated); Vaccines (Live)

The levels/effects of Triamcinolone (Systemic) may be decreased by: CYP3A4 Inducers (Strong); Echinacea; MiFEPRIStone; Mitotane; Tobacco (Smoked)

Dietary Considerations Ensure adequate intake of calcium and vitamins (or consider supplementation) in patients on medium-to-high doses of systemic corticosteroids.

Pharmacodynamics/Kinetics

Onset of Action Adrenal suppression: IM (acetonide): 24 to 48 hours; Intra-articular: >24 hours

Duration of Action Adrenal suppression: IM (acetonide): 30 to 40 days; Intra-articular: 28 to 42 days

Half-life Elimination Plasma: 300 minutes (Asare 2007)

Pregnancy Considerations

Adverse events have been observed with corticosteroids in animal reproduction studies.

Some studies have shown an association between first trimester systemic corticosteroid use and oral clefts or decreased birth weight; however, information is conflicting and may be influenced by maternal dose/indication for use (Lunghi 2010; Park-Wyllie 2000; Pradat 2003). Hypoadrenalism may occur in newborns following maternal use of corticosteroids in pregnancy; monitor.

When systemic corticosteroids are needed in pregnancy for rheumatic disorders, it is generally recommended to use the lowest effective dose for the shortest duration of time, avoiding high doses during the first trimester. Intra-articular dosing may be used (Götestam Skorpen 2016; Makol 2011; Østensen 2009).

For dermatologic disorders in pregnant females, systemic corticosteroids are generally not preferred for initial therapy; should be avoided during the first trimester; and used during the second or third trimester at the lowest effective dose (Bae 2012; Leachman 2006).

Breastfeeding Considerations Corticosteroids are present in breast milk.

The manufacturer notes that when used systemically, maternal use of corticosteroids have the potential to cause adverse events in a breastfeeding infant (eg, growth suppression, interfere with endogenous corticosteroid production); therefore, caution should be used if administered to a breastfeeding female. A case report notes a decrease in milk production following a high-dose triamcinolone injection in a breastfeeding mother with a previously abundant milk supply (McGuire 2012).

Corticosteroids are generally considered acceptable in breastfeeding females when used in usual doses (Götestam Skorpen 2016; WHO 2002); however, monitoring of the breastfeeding infant is recommended (WHO 2002). If there is concern about exposure to the infant, some guidelines recommend waiting 4 hours after the maternal dose of an oral systemic corticosteroid before breastfeeding in order to decrease potential exposure to the breastfeeding infant (based on a study using prednisolone) (Bae 2012; Butler 2014; Götestam Skorpen 2016; Leachman 2006; Makol 2011; Ost 1985).

Dosage Forms: US

Kit, Injection:

P-Care K40: 40 mg/mL (1 x 1 mL)
P-Care K80: 40 mg/mL (2 x 1 mL)
Pod-Care 100K: 40 mg/mL (1 x 1 mL)
Pro-C-Dure 5: 40 mg/mL (2 x 1 mL)
Pro-C-Dure 6: 40 mg/mL (3 x 1 mL)

Suspension, Injection:

Kenalog: 10 mg/mL (5 mL); 40 mg/mL (1 mL, 5 mL, 10 mL)
Kenalog-80: 80 mg/mL (1 mL, 5 mL)
Generic: 40 mg/mL (1 mL, 5 mL, 10 mL)

Suspension Reconstituted ER, Intra-articular:

Zilretta: 32 mg (1 ea)

Dosage Forms: Canada

Suspension, Injection:

Kenalog-10: 10 mg/mL (5 mL)
Kenalog-40: 40 mg/mL (1 mL, 5 mL)
Generic: 10 mg/mL (5 mL); 20 mg/mL (1 mL); 40 mg/mL (1 mL, 5 mL)

Triamcinolone (Nasal) (trye am SIN oh lone)

Brand Names: US GoodSense Nasal Allergy Spray [OTC]; Nasacort Allergy 24HR Children [OTC]; Nasacort Allergy 24HR [OTC]; Nasal Allergy 24 Hour [OTC]

Brand Names: Canada APO-Triamcinolone AQ; Nasacort AQ

Pharmacologic Category Corticosteroid, Nasal

Use

Allergic rhinitis (Rx products): Management of seasonal and perennial allergic rhinitis in adults and children 2 years and older

Upper respiratory allergies (OTC products): Relief of hay fever and other upper respiratory allergies (eg, nasal congestion, runny nose, sneezing, itchy nose) in adults and children 2 years and older

Local Anesthetic/Vasoconstrictor Precautions No information available to require special precautions

Effects on Dental Treatment No significant effects or complications reported

Effects on Bleeding No information available to require special precautions

Adverse Reactions

>10%:

Central nervous system: Headache (2% to 51%)
Respiratory: Pharyngitis (5% to 25%)

1% to 10%:

Cardiovascular: Facial edema (1% to 3%)
Central nervous system: Pain (1% to 3%), voice disorder (1% to 3%)
Dermatologic: Skin photosensitivity (1% to 3%), skin rash (1% to 3%), burning sensation of the nose (≥2%; transient)
Endocrine & metabolic: Weight gain (1% to 3%), dysmenorrhea (≥2%)
Gastrointestinal: Dysgeusia (5% to 8%), dyspepsia (3% to 5%), abdominal pain (1% to 5%), nausea (2% to 3%), diarrhea (1% to 3%), oral candidiasis (1% to 3%), toothache (1% to 3%), vomiting (1% to 3%), xerostomia (1% to 3%)
Genitourinary: Cystitis (1% to 3%), urinary tract infection (1% to 3%), vulvovaginal candidiasis (1% to 3%)
Hypersensitivity: Hypersensitivity reaction (≥2%)
Infection: Infection (≥2%)
Neuromuscular & skeletal: Back pain (2% to 8%), bursitis (1% to 3%), myalgia (1% to 3%), tenosynovitis (1% to 3%)
Ophthalmic: Conjunctivitis (1% to 4%)
Otic: Otitis media (≥2%)
Respiratory: Flu-like symptoms (2% to 9%), sinusitis (2% to 9%), cough (≤8%), epistaxis (≤5%), bronchitis (children: 3%), chest congestion (1% to 3%), asthma (≥2%), rhinitis (≥2%), stinging sensation of the nose (≥2%; transient)

<1%, postmarketing, and/or case reports: Anaphylaxis, cataract, decreased bone mineral density (prolonged use), decreased plasma cortisol, dizziness, dry throat, dyspnea, fatigue, glaucoma, growth suppression, hoarseness, increased intraocular pressure, insomnia, nasal septum perforation, osteoporosis (prolonged use), pruritus, sneezing, throat irritation, urticaria, wheezing, wound healing impairment

Mechanism of Action Controls the rate of protein synthesis, depresses the migration of polymorphonuclear leukocytes and fibroblasts, reverses capillary permeability, and stabilizes lysosomal membranes at the cellular level to prevent or control inflammation

Pharmacodynamics/Kinetics

Half-life Elimination Biologic: 18-36 hours; Terminal (intranasal): 3.1 hours

Pregnancy Considerations

Information related to the use of intranasal triamcinolone in pregnant women is limited (Bérard 2016).

Maternal use of intranasal corticosteroids in usual doses are generally not associated with an increased risk of fetal malformations or preterm birth (ERS/TSANZ [Middleton 2020]). However, intranasal triamcinolone has a high systemic bioavailability, and adverse fetal events have been reported. Agents other than intranasal triamcinolone may be preferred for the treatment of allergic rhinitis during pregnancy (Alhussien 2018; BSACI [Scadding 2017]).

Triamcinolone (Topical) (trye am SIN oh lone)

Related Information

Ulcerative, Erosive, and Painful Oral Mucosal Disorders *on page 1758*

Related Sample Prescriptions

Ulcerative and Erosive Disorders - Sample Prescriptions *on page 46*

Brand Names: US Dermasorb TA [DSC]; Dermazone [DSC]; Kenalog; Oralone; Sila III; SilaLite Pak [DSC]; Trianex; Triderm

Brand Names: Canada Aristocort C; Aristocort R; Oracort; Triaderm

Generic Availability (US) May be product dependent

Pharmacologic Category Corticosteroid, Topical

Dental Use Oral topical: Adjunctive treatment and temporary relief of symptoms associated with oral inflammatory lesions and ulcerative lesions resulting from trauma

Use

Aphthous stomatitis: Oral/dental paste: Adjunctive treatment and temporary relief of symptoms associated with oral inflammatory and ulcerative lesions resulting from trauma.

Corticosteroid-responsive dermatoses (eg, atopic dermatitis, contact dermatitis, vulvar dermatitis, psoriasis, seborrheic dermatitis): Topical: Relief of inflammatory and pruritic manifestations of corticosteroid-responsive dermatoses.

Local Anesthetic/Vasoconstrictor Precautions No information available to require special precautions

Effects on Dental Treatment Key adverse event(s) related to dental treatment: Ulcerative esophagitis, perioral dermatitis, atrophy of oral mucosa, burning, and irritation.

Effects on Bleeding No information available to require special precautions

Adverse Reactions Reactions listed are based on reports for other agents in this same pharmacologic class and may not be specifically reported for topical triamcinolone.

Frequency not defined:

Dermatologic: Acneiform eruption, allergic contact dermatitis, atrophic striae, desquamation, folliculitis, hypertrichosis, hypopigmentation, local dryness, maceration of the skin, miliaria, perioral dermatitis, skin atrophy, skin blister

Endocrine & metabolic: Cushing syndrome, glycosuria, HPA-axis suppression, hyperglycemia

Gastrointestinal: Oral mucosa changes (paste; atrophy or maceration)

Infection: Secondary infection

Local: Application site burning, application site irritation, application site pruritus

Dental Usual Dosage Oral inflammatory lesions/ulcers: Adults: Oral topical: Press a small dab (about 1/4 inch) to the lesion until a thin film develops; a larger quantity may be required for coverage of some lesions. For optimal results, use only enough to coat the lesion with a thin film; do not rub in.

Dosing

Adult

Note:

Potency: The potency classifications of topical triamcinolone products are provided in the table. In general, start with the lowest-potency agent appropriate for the condition severity and application site. Vehicle, concentration, site of application, use of occlusive dressings, and other factors can alter potency:

Potency of Topical Triamcinolone Products[1]

Vehicle	Strength	Potency (According to the US Classification System)
Cream, Ointment	0.5%	High (group 3)
Aerosol spray	(delivering ~0.2 mg per 2-second spray)	Medium (group 4)
Cream, Ointment, Oral/ Dental Paste	0.1%	Medium (group 4)
Ointment	0.05%	Medium (group 4)
Lotion	0.1%	Lower-mid (group 5)
Ointment	0.025%	Lower-mid (group 5)
Cream, Lotion	0.025%	Low (group 6)

[1]Goldstein 2019; Tadicherla 2009

In the management of corticosteroid-responsive dermatoses, lower-potency agents are often preferred for sites at increased risk for corticosteroid-induced skin atrophy (eg, face, intertriginous areas). However, use of higher-potency agents in these areas can be appropriate for certain indications when prescribed under the guidance of a dermatologist.

Vehicle: Optimal response depends on choosing a vehicle that is appropriate for body location and lesion characteristics, as well as consideration of patient preference.

Frequency of application: Corticosteroid-responsive dermatoses: Usual: Once or twice daily.

Duration of therapy: Corticosteroid-responsive dermatoses: Topical corticosteroids are generally well tolerated when used appropriately. Treatment courses of ~2 weeks are common; however, longer courses of treatment or repeated intermittent courses can be appropriate, particularly when prescribed under the guidance of a dermatologist. Conversely, a shorter course may be sufficient depending upon response and when used for minor self-limiting skin conditions (Drake 1996; Goldstein 2019; Tadicherla 2009).

Indication-specific dosing:

Aphthous stomatitis (recurrent), mild to moderate: Note: Initiate at first indication of an outbreak.

Triamcinolone 0.1% (oral/dental paste): Topical: Apply a small amount to the lesion 2 to 4 times daily until healed; do not rinse afterwards and avoid eating or drinking for 30 minutes after application (Altenburg 2014; McBride 2000; Taylor 2014).

Atopic dermatitis (eczema): Note: Concurrent use of emollients (applied liberally) is recommended.

Mild disease: Triamcinolone 0.025% (ointment, cream, lotion) or 0.1% (lotion): Topical: Apply once or twice daily to affected areas for 2 to 4 weeks (Buys 2007; Weston 2019).

Moderate to severe disease: Triamcinolone 0.05% (ointment), 0.1% (ointment, cream), ~0.2 mg/spray (aerosol spray), or 0.5% (ointment, cream): Topical: Apply once or twice daily to affected areas for 2 to 4 weeks (Hoare 2000; Weston 2019); in patients with improvement, maintenance therapy is suggested with an intermittent application once daily for 2 consecutive days per week (eg, weekends) or 2 to 3 times per week to previously affected areas for up to 16 weeks. **Note:** For areas affecting the face, groin, or other areas with skin folds, lower-potency preparations are generally recommended (unless limited to short-term use [5 to 7 days] and then switched to lower potency) (Eichenfield 2014; Weston 2019).

Contact dermatitis: Note: If condition does not show prompt improvement (eg, within 1 to 2 weeks), reassess diagnosis and choice of treatment; consider evaluation by an experienced specialist (AAAAI/ACAAI 2006).

Allergic contact dermatitis (localized), mild to moderate:

Face and/or flexural areas: Triamcinolone: 0.025% (cream, lotion, ointment), 0.05% (ointment), 0.1% (cream, lotion, ointment): Topical: Apply once or twice daily to affected areas for 1 to 2 weeks (Brod 2020).

Hands, feet, or nonflexural areas: Triamcinolone 0.5% (cream, ointment): Topical: Apply once or twice daily to affected areas for 2 to 4 weeks, or until resolution of symptoms (Brod 2020).

Irritant contact dermatitis (localized), mild to moderate, acute or chronic: Note: In general, ointments are the preferred vehicle.

Face and/or flexural areas: Triamcinolone 0.025% (cream, lotion, ointment) or 0.1% (lotion): Topical: Apply once or twice daily to affected areas for 1 to 2 weeks (Brod 2020).

Nonfacial and/or nonflexural areas: Triamcinolone 0.5% (cream, ointment): Topical: Apply once or twice daily to affected areas for 2 to 4 weeks (Brod 2020).

Genital pruritus (due to dermatitis) (adjunct): Note: Use with conservative measures (eg, keeping area clean and dry, removal of offending agents). An evaluation for the underlying cause is essential as the etiology may be due to an infectious, neoplastic, systemic, or other process requiring definitive management.

Vulvar dermatitis, mild: Triamcinolone 0.025% (cream, ointment, lotion), 0.05% (ointment), or 0.1% (cream, ointment, lotion): Topical: Apply to affected area once or twice daily for 2 to 4 weeks; therapy can be continued indefinitely at the minimum frequency for effective control of pruritus (goal <14 days per month). Ointments are preferred (Johnson 2019; Savas 2018; van der Meijden 2017).

Psoriasis, plaque (limited disease):

Face and/or intertriginous areas: Triamcinolone 0.025% (cream, lotion): Topical: Apply twice daily until lesions resolve; a common treatment course is 2 weeks (Feldman 2019; Samarasekera 2013).

Seborrheic dermatitis: Note: Administer alone or in combination with a topical antifungal.

Face, trunk, and/or intertriginous areas: Triamcinolone 0.025% (cream, lotion): Topical: Apply once or twice daily until symptoms subside (usually 1 to 2 weeks) (Sasseville 2019).

Chest or upper back: Triamcinolone 0.05% (ointment), 0.1% (cream, ointment), or ~0.2 mg/spray (aerosol spray): Topical: Apply once or twice daily until symptoms subside (usually 1 to 2 weeks) (Sasseville 2019).

Stasis dermatitis (off-label use): Triamcinolone 0.1% (ointment) or 0.5% (ointment): Topical: Apply once or twice daily for 1 to 2 weeks; due to risk of skin atrophy and ulceration, avoid prolonged use (Fransway 2019).

Geriatric Refer to adult dosing. Use the lowest effective dose.

Renal Impairment: Adult There are no dosage adjustments provided in the manufacturer's labeling.

Hepatic Impairment: Adult There are no dosage adjustments provided in the manufacturer's labeling.

Pediatric Note: Dosage should be based on severity of disease and patient response; use smallest amount for shortest period of time to avoid HPA axis suppression. Therapy should be discontinued when control is achieved.

Dermatoses (corticosteroid-responsive, including contact/atopic dermatitis): Infants, Children, and Adolescents: Topical:

Cream, Ointment:

0.025% or 0.05%: Apply thin film to affected areas 2 to 4 times daily

0.1% or 0.5%: Apply thin film to affected areas 2 to 3 times daily

Lotion: 0.025% or 0.1%: Apply 3 to 4 times daily

Spray: Apply to affected area up to 3 to 4 times daily

Renal Impairment: Pediatric There are no dosage adjustments provided in the manufacturer's labeling.

Hepatic Impairment: Pediatric There are no dosage adjustments provided in the manufacturer's labeling.

Mechanism of Action Topical corticosteroids have anti-inflammatory, antipruritic, and vasoconstrictive properties. May depress the formation, release, and activity of endogenous chemical mediators of inflammation (kinins, histamine, liposomal enzymes, prostaglandins) through the induction of phospholipase A_2 inhibitory proteins (lipocortins) and sequential inhibition of the release of arachidonic acid. Triamcinolone has intermediate to high range potency (dosage-form dependent).

Contraindications

Hypersensitivity to triamcinolone or any component of the formulation

Oral topical formulations only: Fungal, viral, or bacterial infections of the mouth or throat

Warnings/Precautions For external use only; avoid contact with eyes. Do not apply oral paste to skin or eyes. Topical corticosteroids may be absorbed percutaneously. Absorption may cause manifestations of Cushing syndrome, hyperglycemia, or glycosuria. Absorption is increased by the use of occlusive dressings, application to denuded skin, or application to large surface areas. Do not use occlusive dressings on weeping or exudative lesions and general caution with occlusive dressings should be observed; discontinue if skin irritation or contact dermatitis should occur; do not use in patients with decreased skin circulation. May cause hypercortisolism or suppression of hypothalamic-pituitary-adrenal (HPA) axis, particularly in younger children or in patients receiving high doses for prolonged periods. HPA axis suppression may lead to adrenal crisis.

Prolonged use may result in fungal or bacterial superinfection; discontinue if dermatological infection persists despite appropriate antimicrobial therapy. Topical use has been associated with local sensitization (redness, irritation); discontinue if sensitization is noted. When used as a topical agent in the oral cavity, if significant regeneration or repair of oral tissues has not occurred in seven days, re-evaluation of the etiology of the oral lesion is advised.

Because of the risk of adverse effects associated with systemic absorption, topical corticosteroids should be used cautiously in the elderly in the smallest possible effective dose for the shortest duration. Children may absorb proportionally larger amounts after topical application and may be more prone to systemic effects. HPA axis suppression, intracranial hypertension, and Cushing syndrome have been reported in children receiving topical corticosteroids. Prolonged use may affect growth velocity; growth should be routinely monitored in pediatric patients. Some dosage forms may contain polysorbate 80 (also known as Tweens). Hypersensitivity reactions, usually a delayed reaction, have been reported following exposure to pharmaceutical products containing polysorbate 80 in certain individuals (Isaksson 2002; Lucente 2000; Shelley 1995). Thrombocytopenia, ascites, pulmonary deterioration, and renal and hepatic failure have been reported in premature neonates after receiving parenteral products containing polysorbate 80 (Alade 1986; CDC 1984). See manufacturer's labeling. Do not apply aerosol solution to underarms or groin unless directed by a health care professional; if improvement is not seen within 2 weeks, contact prescriber. Aerosol solution is flammable; avoid heat, smoking, or flames when applying. Potentially significant interactions may exist, requiring dose or frequency adjustment, additional monitoring, and/or selection of alternative therapy.

Warnings: Additional Pediatric Considerations Topical corticosteroids may be absorbed percutaneously. The extent of absorption is dependent on several factors, including epidermal integrity (intact vs abraded skin), formulation, age of the patient, prolonged duration of use, and the use of occlusive dressings. Percutaneous absorption of topical steroids is increased in neonates (especially preterm neonates), infants, and young children. Hypothalamic-pituitary-adrenal (HPA) suppression may occur, particularly in younger children or in patients receiving high doses for prolonged periods; acute adrenal insufficiency (adrenal crisis) may occur with abrupt withdrawal after long-term therapy or with stress. Infants and small children may be more susceptible to HPA axis suppression or other systemic toxicities due to larger skin surface area to body mass ratio; use with caution in pediatric patients.

Some dosage forms may contain propylene glycol; in neonates large amounts of propylene glycol delivered orally, intravenously (eg, >3,000 mg/day), or topically have been associated with potentially fatal toxicities which can include metabolic acidosis, seizures, renal failure, and CNS depression; toxicities have also been reported in children and adults including hyperosmolality, lactic acidosis, seizures and respiratory depression; use caution (AAP 1997; Shehab 2009).

Drug Interactions

Metabolism/Transport Effects None known.

Avoid Concomitant Use

Avoid concomitant use of Triamcinolone (Topical) with any of the following: Aldesleukin

Increased Effect/Toxicity

Triamcinolone (Topical) may increase the levels/effects of: Deferasirox; Ritodrine

Decreased Effect

Triamcinolone (Topical) may decrease the levels/effects of: Aldesleukin; Corticorelin; Hyaluronidase

Pharmacodynamics/Kinetics

Half-life Elimination Biologic: 18 to 36 hours

Pregnancy Risk Factor C

Pregnancy Considerations

Adverse events have been observed in some animal reproduction studies. Systemic bioavailability of topical corticosteroids is variable (integrity of skin, use of occlusion, etc.) and may be further influenced by trimester of pregnancy (Chi 2017). In general, the use of topical corticosteroids is not associated with a significant risk of adverse pregnancy outcomes. However, there may be an increased risk of low birth weight infants following maternal use of potent or very potent topical products, especially in high doses. Use of mild to moderate potency topical corticosteroids is preferred in pregnant females and the use of large amounts or use for prolonged periods of time should be avoided (Chi 2016; Chi 2017; Murase 2014). Also avoid areas of high percutaneous absorption (Chi 2017). The risk of stretch marks may be increased with use of topical corticosteroids (Murase 2014).

Breastfeeding Considerations

It is not known if sufficient quantities of triamcinolone are absorbed following topical administration to produce detectable amounts in breast milk.

Systemic corticosteroids are present in breast milk. Although the manufacturer recommends that caution be used, topical corticosteroids are generally considered acceptable for use in breastfeeding females (Butler 2014; WHO 2002). Do not apply topical corticosteroids to breast until breastfeeding ceases (Leachman 2006); hypertension was noted in a breastfed infant when a high potency topical corticosteroid was applied to the nipple (Butler 2014; Leachman 2006).

Dosage Forms Considerations Dermazone therapy pack is a kit containing triamcinolone acetonide cream 0.1% (80 g) and silicone gel sheets.

Dosage Forms: US

Aerosol Solution, External:

Kenalog: 0.147 mg/g (63 g, 100 g)

Generic: 0.147 mg/g (63 g, 100 g)

Cream, External:

Triderm: 0.1% (28.4 g, 85.2 g); 0.5% (454 g)

Generic: 0.025% (15 g, 80 g, 453.6 g, 454 g); 0.1% (15 g, 30 g, 80 g, 453.6 g, 454 g); 0.5% (15 g)

Lotion, External:
Generic: 0.025% (60 mL); 0.1% (60 mL)
Ointment, External:
Trianex: 0.05% (430 g)
Generic: 0.025% (15 g, 80 g, 454 g); 0.05% (430 g); 0.1% (15 g, 30 g, 80 g, 453.6 g, 454 g); 0.5% (15 g)
Paste, Mouth/Throat:
Oralone: 0.1% (5 g)
Generic: 0.1% (5 g)
Therapy Pack, External:
Sila III: 0.1% (1 ea)

Dosage Forms: Canada
Cream, External:
Aristocort C: 0.5% (15 g, 50 g)
Aristocort R: 0.1% (15 g, 30 g, 500 g)
Triaderm: 0.025% (15 g, 500 g); 0.1% (15 g, 500 g)
Ointment, External:
Aristocort R: 0.1% (30 g)
Triaderm: 0.1% (15 g, 454 g)
Paste, Mouth/Throat:
Generic: 0.1% (7.5 g)

- ◆ **Triamcinolone Acetonide** *see* Triamcinolone (Nasal) *on page 1489*
- ◆ **Triamcinolone Acetonide** *see* Triamcinolone (Systemic) *on page 1485*
- ◆ **Triamcinolone Acetonide** *see* Triamcinolone (Topical) *on page 1490*
- ◆ **Triamcinolone Acetonide, Parenteral** *see* Triamcinolone (Systemic) *on page 1485*
- ◆ **Triamcinolone and Nystatin** *see* Nystatin and Triamcinolone *on page 1123*
- ◆ **Triamcinolone Hexacetonide** *see* Triamcinolone (Systemic) *on page 1485*
- ◆ **Triaminic Allerchews [OTC]** *see* Loratadine *on page 930*
- ◆ **Triaminic Children's Fever Reducer Pain Reliever [OTC]** *see* Acetaminophen *on page 59*
- ◆ **Triaminic Cough/Runny Nose [OTC] [DSC]** *see* DiphenhydrAMINE (Systemic) *on page 502*
- ◆ **Triaminic Long Acting Cough [OTC]** *see* Dextromethorphan *on page 476*

Triamterene (trye AM ter een)

Related Information
Cardiovascular Diseases *on page 1654*
Brand Names: US Dyrenium
Pharmacologic Category Antihypertensive; Diuretic, Potassium-Sparing
Use Edema: Treatment of edema associated with congestive heart failure, cirrhosis of the liver and the nephrotic syndrome; also in steroid-induced edema, idiopathic edema and edema due to secondary hyperaldosteronism.
Local Anesthetic/Vasoconstrictor Precautions
No information available to require special precautions
Effects on Dental Treatment No significant effects or complications reported
Effects on Bleeding No information available to require special precautions
Adverse Reactions Frequency not defined.
Central nervous system: Dizziness, fatigue, headache
Dermatologic: Skin photosensitivity, skin rash
Endocrine & metabolic: Hyperkalemia, hypokalemia, increased uric acid, metabolic acidosis
Gastrointestinal: Diarrhea, nausea, vomiting, xerostomia
Genitourinary: Azotemia
Hematologic & oncologic: Hematologic abnormality, megaloblastic anemia, thrombocytopenia
Hepatic: Jaundice, liver enzyme disorder
Hypersensitivity: Anaphylaxis
Neuromuscular & skeletal: Weakness
Renal: Acute interstitial nephritis (rare), acute renal failure (rare), increased blood urea nitrogen, increased serum creatinine, nephrolithiasis
Mechanism of Action Blocks epithelial sodium channels in the late distal convoluted tubule (DCT) and collecting duct which inhibits sodium reabsorption from the lumen. This effectively reduces intracellular sodium, decreasing the function of Na+/K+ ATPase, leading to potassium retention and decreased calcium, magnesium, and hydrogen excretion. As sodium uptake capacity in the DCT/collecting duct is limited, the natriuretic, diuretic, and antihypertensive effects are generally considered weak.
Pharmacodynamics/Kinetics
Onset of Action Diuresis: 2 to 4 hours; **Note:** Maximum therapeutic effect may not occur until after several days of therapy
Duration of Action Diuresis: 7 to 9 hours
Time to Peak Plasma: ~3 hours
Pregnancy Considerations Triamterene crosses the placenta and is found in cord blood. Use of triamterene to treat edema during normal pregnancies is not appropriate; use may be considered when edema is due to pathologic causes (as in the nonpregnant patient); monitor.

- ◆ **Triamterene and Hydrochlorothiazide** *see* Hydrochlorothiazide and Triamterene *on page 763*
- ◆ **Trianex** *see* Triamcinolone (Topical) *on page 1490*

Triazolam (trye AY zoe lam)

Related Information
Management of the Patient With Anxiety or Depression *on page 1778*
Related Sample Prescriptions
Sedation (Prior to Dental Treatment) - Sample Prescriptions *on page 45*
Brand Names: US Halcion
Generic Availability (US) Yes
Pharmacologic Category Benzodiazepine
Dental Use Oral premedication before dental procedures
Use Insomnia: Short-term (generally 7 to 10 days) treatment of insomnia
Local Anesthetic/Vasoconstrictor Precautions
No information available to require special precautions
Effects on Dental Treatment No significant effects or complications reported (see Dental Health Professional Considerations)
Effects on Bleeding No information available to require special precautions
Adverse Reactions
>10%: Nervous system: Drowsiness (14%)
1% to 10%:
Gastrointestinal: Nausea and vomiting (5%)
Nervous system: Ataxia (5%), dizziness (5% to 8%), headache (10%)
<1%:
Cardiovascular: Tachycardia
Dermatologic: Dermatitis

Gastrointestinal: Constipation, diarrhea, dysgeusia, xerostomia
Nervous system: Abnormal dreams, confusion, depression, dysesthesia, euphoria, insomnia, memory impairment, nightmares, pain, paresthesia
Neuromuscular & skeletal: Asthenia, muscle cramps
Ophthalmic: Visual disturbance
Otic: Tinnitus
Respiratory: Paranasal sinus congestion
Postmarketing:
Cardiovascular: Chest pain, syncope
Dermatologic: Pruritus
Endocrine & metabolic: Change in libido, menstrual disease
Gastrointestinal: Anorexia, glossalgia, glossitis, stomatitis
Genitourinary: Urinary incontinence, urinary retention
Hepatic: Jaundice
Nervous system: Abnormal behavior, aggressive behavior, agitation, anterograde amnesia, anxiety, central nervous system depression, complex sleep-related disorder, delusion, depersonalization, drug habituation, dysarthria, dystonia, falling, fatigue, hallucination, impaired consciousness, irritability, mania, rebound insomnia, restlessness, sedated state, somnambulism, withdrawal syndrome
Neuromuscular & skeletal: Muscle spasticity
Miscellaneous: Paradoxical reaction

Dental Usual Dosage Preprocedure sedation (off-label use): Adults: Oral: 0.25 mg 1 hour before procedure; 0.125 mg used for elderly patients or patients sensitive to sedative effects of medications (Dionne, 2006)

Dosing

Adult

Insomnia (short-term use): Usual dose: 0.25 mg at bedtime; 0.125 mg at bedtime may be sufficient in some patients, such as those with low body weight; maximum dose: 0.5 mg/day.

Dental preprocedure oral sedation (off-label use): 0.25 mg 1 hour before procedure; 0.125 mg used for elderly patients or patients sensitive to sedative effects (Dionne 2006).

Geriatric Elderly and/or debilitated patients: Insomnia (short-term use): Oral: Initial: 0.125 mg at bedtime; maximum dose: 0.25 mg/day.

Renal Impairment: Adult There are no dosage adjustments provided in the manufacturer's labeling; use with caution.

Hepatic Impairment: Adult There are no dosage adjustments provided in the manufacturer's labeling; use with caution.

Pediatric Insomnia (short-term use): Adolescents ≥18 years: Oral: 0.125 to 0.25 mg at bedtime; the lower dose of 0.125 mg at bedtime may be sufficient in some patients, such as those with low body weight; maximum daily dose: 0.5 mg/day

Renal Impairment: Pediatric There are no dosage adjustments provided in the manufacturer's labeling; use with caution.

Hepatic Impairment: Pediatric There are no dosage adjustments provided in the manufacturer's labeling; use with caution.

Mechanism of Action Binds to stereospecific benzodiazepine receptors on the postsynaptic GABA neuron at several sites within the central nervous system, including the limbic system and reticular formation. Enhancement of the inhibitory effect of GABA on neuronal excitability results by increased neuronal membrane permeability to chloride ions. This shift in chloride ions results in hyperpolarization (a less excitable state) and stabilization. Benzodiazepine receptors and effects appear to be linked to the GABA-A receptors. Benzodiazepines do not bind to GABA-B receptors (Vinkers 2012).

Contraindications Hypersensitivity to triazolam, other benzodiazepines, or any component of the formulation; concurrent therapy with strong cytochrome P450 3A (CYP 3A) inhibitors (eg, itraconazole, ketoconazole, nefazodone, lopinavir, ritonavir).

Warnings/Precautions As a hypnotic, should be used only after evaluation of potential causes of sleep disturbance. Failure of sleep disturbance to resolve after 7 to 10 days may indicate psychiatric or medical illness. Use for >21 days requires complete reevaluation of patient. A worsening of insomnia or the emergence of new abnormalities of thought or behavior may represent unrecognized psychiatric or medical illness and requires immediate and careful evaluation. Prescription should be written for a maximum of 7 to 10 days and should not be prescribed in quantities exceeding a 1-month supply. Use lowest effective dose; adverse reactions of triazolam are dose related. Rebound insomnia or withdrawal symptoms may occur following abrupt discontinuation or large decreases in dose. Use caution when reducing dose or withdrawing therapy; decrease slowly and monitor for withdrawal symptoms. Flumazenil may cause withdrawal in patients receiving long-term benzodiazepine therapy. An increase in daytime anxiety may occur after as few as 10 days of continuous use, which may be related to withdrawal reaction in some patients.

Use with caution in elderly or debilitated patients, patients with hepatic disease (including alcoholics), or renal impairment. Use with caution in patients with respiratory compromise, COPD, or sleep apnea. Elderly patients experience greater sedation and increased psychomotor impairment (Greenblatt 1991). Elderly patients may be at an increased risk of death with use; risk has been found highest within the first 4 months of use in elderly dementia patients (Jennum 2015; Saarelainen 2018). In debilitated patients, benzodiazepines increase the risk for oversedation, impaired coordination, and dizziness with use. Reports of hypersensitivity reactions, including anaphylaxis and angioedema, have been reported with triazolam.

Causes CNS depression (dose-related) resulting in sedation, dizziness, confusion, or ataxia which may impair physical and mental capabilities. Patients must be cautioned about performing tasks which require mental alertness (eg, operating machinery or driving). Benzodiazepines have been associated with anterograde amnesia (Nelson 1999). Traveler's amnesia (if taken to induce sleep while traveling) due to insufficient time for sleep prior to awakening and initiating activity has also been reported. Anterograde amnesia may occur at a higher rate with triazolam than with other benzodiazepines. Hazardous sleep-related activities such as sleep-driving, cooking and eating food, and making phone calls while asleep have been noted with benzodiazepines (Dolder 2008). Benzodiazepines have been associated with falls and traumatic injury and should be used with extreme caution in patients who are at risk of these events (especially the elderly) (Nelson 1999).

Use caution in patients with suicidal risk. Minimize risks of overdose by prescribing the least amount of drug that is feasible in suicidal patients. Worsening of depressive symptoms has also been reported with use of benzodiazepines. Use with caution in patients with a history of drug dependence. Paradoxical reactions, including hyperactive or aggressive behavior have been reported with benzodiazepines; risk may be increased in adolescent/pediatric patients, geriatric patients, or patients with a history of alcohol use disorder or psychiatric/personality disorders (Mancuso 2004). Triazolam is a short half-life benzodiazepine. Tolerance develops to the hypnotic effects (Vinkers 2012). Chronic use of this agent may increase the perioperative benzodiazepine dose needed to achieve desired effect. Does not have analgesic, antidepressant, or antipsychotic properties. Potentially significant drug-drug interactions may exist, requiring dose or frequency adjustment, additional monitoring, and/or selection of alternative therapy. **[US Boxed warning]: Concomitant use of benzodiazepines and opioids may result in profound sedation, respiratory depression, coma, and death. Reserve concomitant prescribing of these drugs for use in patients for whom alternative treatment options are inadequate. Limit dosages and durations to the minimum required. Follow patients for signs and symptoms of respiratory depression and sedation.**

Drug Interactions

Metabolism/Transport Effects **Substrate** of CYP3A4 (major); **Note:** Assignment of Major/Minor substrate status based on clinically relevant drug interaction potential

Avoid Concomitant Use

Avoid concomitant use of Triazolam with any of the following: Abametapir; Azelastine (Nasal); Bromperidol; Conivaptan; CYP3A4 Inhibitors (Strong); Fusidic Acid (Systemic); Idelalisib; OLANZapine; Orphenadrine; Oxomemazine; Paraldehyde; Sodium Oxybate; Thalidomide; Tipranavir

Increased Effect/Toxicity

Triazolam may increase the levels/effects of: Alcohol (Ethyl); Azelastine (Nasal); Blonanserin; Brexanolone; Buprenorphine; CloZAPine; CNS Depressants; Flunitrazepam; Methadone; Methotrimeprazine; MetyroSINE; Opioid Agonists; Orphenadrine; OxyCODONE; Paraldehyde; Piribedil; Pramipexole; ROPINIRole; Rotigotine; Sodium Oxybate; Suvorexant; Thalidomide; Zolpidem

The levels/effects of Triazolam may be increased by: Abametapir; Alizapride; Brimonidine (Topical); Bromopride; Bromperidol; Cannabidiol; Cannabis; Chlormethiazole; Chlorphenesin Carbamate; Clofazimine; Conivaptan; CYP3A4 Inhibitors (Moderate); CYP3A4 Inhibitors (Strong); CYP3A4 Inhibitors (Weak); Dimethindene (Topical); Doxylamine; Dronabinol; Droperidol; Erdafitinib; Esketamine; Fusidic Acid (Systemic); Hormonal Contraceptives; HydrOXYzine; Idelalisib; Kava Kava; Lemborexant; Lisuride; Lofexidine; Magnesium Sulfate; Melatonin; Methotrimeprazine; Metoclopramide; Minocycline (Systemic); Nabilone; OLANZapine; Oxomemazine; Perampanel; RaNITIdine (Withdrawn from US Market); Rufinamide; Simeprevir; Stiripentol; Teduglutide; Tetrahydrocannabinol; Tetrahydrocannabinol and Cannabidiol; Tipranavir; Trimeprazine

Decreased Effect

The levels/effects of Triazolam may be decreased by: CYP3A4 Inducers (Moderate); CYP3A4 Inducers (Strong); Dabrafenib; Deferasirox; DexAMETHasone (Systemic); Enzalutamide; Erdafitinib; Ivosidenib; Lumacaftor and Ivacaftor; Mitotane; Sarilumab; Siltuximab; Theophylline Derivatives; Tocilizumab; Yohimbine

Food Interactions Benzodiazepine serum concentrations may be increased by grapefruit juice. Management: Limit or avoid grapefruit juice (Sugimoto 2006).

Pharmacodynamics/Kinetics

Onset of Action Hypnotic: 15 to 30 minutes (Pakes 1981)

Duration of Action Hypnotic: 6 to 7 hours

Half-life Elimination 1.5 to 5.5 hours

Time to Peak Oral: Within 2 hours

Pregnancy Considerations

A case report describes placental transfer of triazolam following a maternal overdose (Sakai 1996).

Teratogenic effects have been observed with some benzodiazepines; however, additional studies are needed. The incidence of premature birth and low birth weights may be increased following maternal use of benzodiazepines; hypoglycemia and respiratory problems in the neonate may occur following exposure late in pregnancy. Neonatal withdrawal symptoms may occur within days to weeks after birth and "floppy infant syndrome" (which also includes withdrawal symptoms) have been reported with some benzodiazepines (Bergman 1992; Iqbal 2002; Wikner 2007). Infants exposed to triazolam during pregnancy should be monitored for respiratory depression, sedation, withdrawal, or feeding problems.

Data collection to monitor pregnancy and infant outcomes following exposure to triazolam is ongoing. Health care providers are encouraged to enroll females exposed to triazolam during pregnancy in the National Pregnancy Registry for Other Psychiatric Medications (866-961-2388 or https://womensmentalhealth.org/research/pregnancyregistry/othermedications/).

Breastfeeding Considerations It is not known if triazolam is present in breast milk.

Although information specific to triazolam has not been located, all benzodiazepines are expected to be present in breast milk. Drowsiness, lethargy, or weight loss in breastfed infants have been observed in case reports following maternal use of some benzodiazepines (Iqbal 2002). According to the manufacturer, the decision to continue or discontinue breastfeeding during therapy should consider the risk of infant exposure, the benefits of breastfeeding to the infant, and the benefits of treatment to the mother. Infants exposed to triazolam via breast milk should be monitored for respiratory depression, sedation, withdrawal, or feeding problems. Breastfeeding women may express and discard milk during therapy and for 28 hours after the last triazolam dose to minimize possible exposure to the infant.

Controlled Substance C-IV

Dosage Forms: US

Tablet, Oral:

Halcion: 0.25 mg

Generic: 0.125 mg, 0.25 mg

Dosage Forms: Canada

Tablet, Oral:

Generic: 0.25 mg

Dental Health Professional Considerations An adult companion should accompany the patient to and from dental office.

Triazolam (0.25 mg) 1 hour prior to dental procedure has been used as an oral preop sedative. There has been recent interest in its use as an orally titratable sedative to render anxious patients at ease during difficult dental procedures. This technique has been referred to as enteral conscious sedation (ECS) and oral conscious sedation (OCS).

Triazolam has the shortest half-life of all the orally administered benzodiazepines. Although midazolam is shorter, it is used parenterally, not orally. The relatively fast onset of action (15 to 30 minutes) of triazolam offers an advantage in its use as an oral sedative. The clinician is reminded that no kinetic data has been reported with multiple titration doses of triazolam, a technique often used in the ECS/OCS regimen.

◆ **Tribasic Calcium Phosphate and Vitamin D** *see* Calcium and Vitamin D *on page 280*

◆ **Tribavirin** *see* Ribavirin (Oral Inhalation) *on page 1321*

◆ **Tribavirin** *see* Ribavirin (Systemic) *on page 1320*

◆ **Tri-Buffered Aspirin [OTC]** *see* Aspirin *on page 177*

◆ **Tricode AR [DSC]** *see* Chlorpheniramine, Pseudoephedrine, and Codeine *on page 341*

◆ **Tricor** *see* Fenofibrate and Derivatives *on page 640*

◆ **Triderm** *see* Triamcinolone (Topical) *on page 1490*

◆ **Tridesilon** *see* Desonide *on page 461*

◆ **Tridil** *see* Nitroglycerin *on page 1112*

◆ **Tri-Estarylla** *see* Ethinyl Estradiol and Norgestimate *on page 616*

◆ **Triethylenethiophosphoramide** *see* Thiotepa *on page 1439*

Trifarotene (trye FAR oh teen)

Brand Names: US Aklief

Brand Names: Canada Aklief

Pharmacologic Category Acne Products; Retinoic Acid Derivative; Topical Skin Product, Acne

Use Acne vulgaris: Topical treatment of acne vulgaris in patients ≥9 years of age.

Local Anesthetic/Vasoconstrictor Precautions No information available to require special precautions

Effects on Dental Treatment No significant effects or complications reported

Effects on Bleeding No information available to require special precautions

Adverse Reactions

1% to 10%:

- Dermatologic: Sunburn (3%)
- Local: Application site irritation (8%), application-site pruritus (2%)

<1%: Acne vulgaris, allergic dermatitis, application site pain, application site rash, application-site edema, erythema of skin, local dryness of skin, local skin discoloration, skin erosion

Mechanism of Action Trifarotene is a retinoic acid receptor (RAR) agonist, with greater selectivity at the gamma subtype. RAR stimulation results in modulation of target genes which are associated with cell differentiation and mediation of inflammation.

Pharmacodynamics/Kinetics

Half-life Elimination Terminal: 2 to 9 hours.

Pregnancy Considerations In general, topical products are recommended for the treatment of acne in pregnancy due to lower systemic exposure. However, because trifarotene may share the characteristic of teratogenicity with other retinoids, other agents may be preferred. Avoid applying large amounts over prolonged periods of time to decrease the potential for systemic absorption (Kong 2013).

◆ **Tri Femynor** *see* Ethinyl Estradiol and Norgestimate *on page 616*

◆ **Triferic** *see* Ferric Pyrophosphate Citrate *on page 664*

Trifluoperazine (trye floo oh PER a zeen)

Pharmacologic Category First Generation (Typical) Antipsychotic; Phenothiazine Derivative

Use

Nonpsychotic anxiety: Short-term treatment of generalized nonpsychotic anxiety.

Schizophrenia: Management of schizophrenia.

Local Anesthetic/Vasoconstrictor Precautions No information available to require special precautions

Effects on Dental Treatment Key adverse event(s) related to dental treatment: Significant hypotension may occur, especially when the drug is administered parenterally; orthostatic hypotension is due to alpha-receptor blockade, the elderly are at greater risk for orthostatic hypotension. Xerostomia (normal salivary flow resumes upon discontinuation).

Tardive dyskinesia: Prevalence rate may be 40% in elderly; development of the syndrome and the irreversible nature are proportional to duration and total cumulative dose over time. Extrapyramidal reactions are more common in elderly with up to 50% developing these reactions after 60 years of age. Drug-induced Parkinson's syndrome occurs often; akathisia is the most common extrapyramidal reaction in elderly.

Effects on Bleeding No information available to require special precautions

Adverse Reactions Frequency not defined.

- Cardiovascular: Hypotension, orthostatic hypotension
- Central nervous system: Decreased seizure threshold, dizziness, disruption of body temperature regulation, extrapyramidal reaction (akathisia, dystonia, Parkinsonian-like syndrome, tardive dyskinesia), headache, neuroleptic malignant syndrome (NMS)
- Dermatologic: Skin discoloration (blue-gray), skin photosensitivity (includes increased sensitivity to sun), skin rash
- Endocrine & metabolic: Change in libido, change in menstrual flow, galactorrhea, gynecomastia, hyperglycemia, hypoglycemia, weight gain
- Gastrointestinal: Constipation, nausea, stomach pain, vomiting, xerostomia
- Genitourinary: Difficulty in micturition, ejaculatory disorder, lactation, mastalgia, priapism, urinary retention
- Hematologic & oncologic: Agranulocytosis, aplastic anemia, eosinophilia, hemolytic anemia, immune thrombocytopenia, leukopenia, pancytopenia
- Hepatic: Cholestatic jaundice, hepatotoxicity
- Neuromuscular & skeletal: Tremor
- Ophthalmic: Corneal changes, lens disease, retinitis pigmentosa
- Respiratory: Nasal congestion

Mechanism of Action Trifluoperazine is a piperazine phenothiazine antipsychotic which blocks dopamine, subtype 2 (D_2), receptors in mesolimbocortical and nigrostriatal areas of the brain (APA [Lehman, 2004]).

Pharmacodynamics/Kinetics

Onset of Action For control of agitation, aggression, hostility: 2 to 4 weeks; For control of psychotic symptoms (hallucinations, disorganized thinking or behavior, delusions): Within 1 week; Adequate trial: 6 weeks at moderate to high dose based on tolerability

Duration of Action Variable

Half-life Elimination 3 to 12 hours (Midha 1984)

Time to Peak Serum: 1.5 to 6 hours (Midha 1984)

Pregnancy Considerations Adverse events have not been observed in animal reproduction studies, except when using doses that were also maternally toxic. Prolonged jaundice, extrapyramidal signs, or hyporeflexia have been reported in newborn infants following maternal use of phenothiazines. Antipsychotic use during the third trimester of pregnancy has a risk for extrapyramidal and/or withdrawal symptoms in newborns following delivery. Symptoms in the newborn may include agitation, feeding disorder, hypertonia, hypotonia, respiratory distress, somnolence, and tremor; these effects may be self-limiting or require hospitalization.

◆ **Trifluoperazine HCl** *see* Trifluoperazine *on page 1496*

◆ **Trifluoperazine Hydrochloride** *see* Trifluoperazine *on page 1496*

◆ **Trifluorothymidine** *see* Trifluridine *on page 1497*

Trifluridine (trye FLURE i deen)

Related Information

Systemic Viral Diseases *on page 1709*

Brand Names: US Viroptic [DSC]

Brand Names: Canada APO-Trifluridine; SANDOZ Trifluridine [DSC]; Viroptic

Pharmacologic Category Antiviral Agent, Ophthalmic

Use Herpes keratoconjunctivitis, keratitis: Treatment of primary keratoconjunctivitis and recurrent epithelial keratitis due to herpes simplex virus, types 1 and 2

Local Anesthetic/Vasoconstrictor Precautions
No information available to require special precautions

Effects on Dental Treatment No significant effects or complications reported

Effects on Bleeding No information available to require special precautions

Adverse Reactions

1% to 10%:

Ophthalmic: Burning sensation of eyes (≤5%), stinging of eyes (≤5%), eyelid edema (3%)

Frequency not defined:

Hypersensitivity: Local ocular hypersensitivity reaction

Ophthalmic: Epithelial keratopathy, eye irritation, hyperemia, increased intraocular pressure, keratoconjunctivitis sicca, ocular stromal edema, superficial punctate keratitis

Mechanism of Action Interferes with viral replication by inhibiting thymidylate synthetase and incorporating into viral DNA in place of thymidine (Carmine 1982).

Pharmacodynamics/Kinetics

Half-life Elimination ~12 minutes

Pregnancy Considerations

Adverse effects have not been observed during animal reproduction studies of the ophthalmic solution. Systemic absorption following ophthalmic application is limited. If ophthalmic agents are needed during pregnancy, the minimum effective dose should be used in combination with punctal occlusion to decrease potential exposure to the fetus (Samples 1988).

Trifluridine and Tipiracil
(trye FLURE i deen & tye PIR a sil)

Brand Names: US Lonsurf

Brand Names: Canada Lonsurf

Pharmacologic Category Antineoplastic Agent, Antimetabolite; Antineoplastic Agent, Antimetabolite (Pyrimidine Analog); Thymidine Phosphorylase Inhibitor

Use

Colorectal cancer, metastatic: Treatment of metastatic colorectal cancer in adults previously treated with fluoropyrimidine-, oxaliplatin- and irinotecan-based chemotherapy, an anti-VEGF biological therapy, and if RAS wild-type, an anti-EGFR therapy.

Gastric cancer, metastatic: Treatment of metastatic gastric or gastroesophageal junction adenocarcinoma in adults previously treated with at least two prior lines of chemotherapy which included a fluoropyrimidine, a platinum, either a taxane or irinotecan, and if appropriate, HER2/neu-targeted therapy.

Local Anesthetic/Vasoconstrictor Precautions
No information available to require special precautions

Effects on Dental Treatment Key adverse event(s) related to dental treatment: Stomatitis

Effects on Bleeding Thrombocytopenia, neutropenia and anemia can occur during systemic therapy

Adverse Reactions

>10%:

Central nervous system: Fatigue (≤52%)

Gastrointestinal: Nausea (37% to 48%), decreased appetite (34% to 39%), diarrhea (23% to 32%), vomiting (25% to 28%), abdominal pain (21%)

Hematologic & oncologic: Anemia (63% to 77%; grades 3/4: 18% to 19%), neutropenia (66% to 67%; grades 3/4: 38%;), thrombocytopenia (34% to 42%; grades 3/4: 5% to 6%), febrile neutropenia (grades 3/4: 3%)

Infection: Infection (23% to 27%)

Neuromuscular & skeletal: Asthenia (≤52%)

Miscellaneous: Fever (19%)

1% to 10%:

Cardiovascular: Pulmonary embolism (2% to 3%)

Dermatologic: Alopecia (7%)

Gastrointestinal: Stomatitis (8%; grades 3/4: <1%), dysgeusia (7%)

<1%, postmarketing, and/or case reports: Interstitial pulmonary disease

Mechanism of Action Trifluridine, the active cytotoxic component of trifluridine/tipiracil, is a thymidine-based nucleic acid analogue; the triphosphate form of trifluridine is incorporated into DNA which interferes with DNA synthesis and inhibits cell proliferation. Tipiracil is a potent thymidine phosphorylase inhibitor which prevents the rapid degradation of trifluridine, allowing for increased trifluridine exposure (Mayer 2015).

Pharmacodynamics/Kinetics

Half-life Elimination Trifluridine: 2.1 hours; Tipiracil: 2.4 hours

Time to Peak Plasma: ~2 hours

Reproductive Considerations

Verify pregnancy status in females of reproductive potential prior to therapy initiation. Females of reproductive potential should use effective contraception during therapy and for at least 6 months after the final trifluridine and tipiracil dose. Males who have female partners of reproductive potential should use condoms during therapy and for at least 3 months following the final dose.

Pregnancy Considerations

Based on the mechanism of action and data from animal reproduction studies, in utero exposure to trifluridine/tipiracil may cause fetal harm.

◆ **Trifluridine and Tipiracil Hydrochloride** *see* Trifluridine and Tipiracil *on page 1497*

◆ **Trifluridine/Tipiracil HCl** *see* Trifluridine and Tipiracil *on page 1497*

- **Triglide** *see* Fenofibrate and Derivatives *on page 640*
- **Triglycerides, Medium Chain** *see* Medium Chain Triglycerides *on page 953*

Triheptanoin (trye HEP ta noyn)

Brand Names: US Dojolvi

Pharmacologic Category Anaplerotic Agent; Nutritional Supplement

Use Long-chain fatty acid oxidation disorders: As a source of calories and fatty acids for the treatment of molecularly confirmed long-chain fatty acid oxidation disorders in adults and pediatric patients.

Local Anesthetic/Vasoconstrictor Precautions No information available to require special precautions.

Effects on Dental Treatment No significant effects or complications reported.

Effects on Bleeding No information available to require special precautions.

Adverse Reactions

>10%: Gastrointestinal: Abdominal pain (60%; including abdominal distention, abdominal distress, gastrointestinal pain, upper abdominal pain), diarrhea (44%), nausea (14%), vomiting (44%)

Mechanism of Action Triheptanoin is a medium-chain triglyceride consisting of 3 odd-chain 7-carbon length fatty acids (heptanoate) that provide a source of calories and fatty acids to bypass the long-chain fatty acid oxidation disorder enzyme deficiencies for energy production and replacement.

Pharmacodynamics/Kinetics

Time to Peak Heptanoate: Multiple peak concentrations are observed following oral administration.

Pregnancy Considerations

Information from animal reproduction studies was not considered relevant to maternal use.

Data collection to monitor pregnancy and infant outcomes following exposure to triheptanoin is ongoing. Females exposed to triheptanoin during pregnancy are encouraged to contact the manufacturer (1-888-756-8657).

Product Availability Dojolvi: FDA approved June 2020; anticipated availability July 2020.

Trihexyphenidyl (trye heks ee FEN i dil)

Brand Names: Canada PMS-Trihexyphenidyl

Pharmacologic Category Anti-Parkinson Agent, Anticholinergic; Anticholinergic Agent

Use

Drug-induced extrapyramidal symptoms (treatment): Aid in the control of extrapyramidal symptoms caused by CNS drugs (eg, dibenzoxazepines, phenothiazines, thioxanthenes, butyrophenones)

Parkinsonism: Treatment of all forms of parkinsonism (postencephalitic, arteriosclerotic, and idiopathic) as adjunctive therapy

Local Anesthetic/Vasoconstrictor Precautions No information available to require special precautions

Effects on Dental Treatment Key adverse event(s) related to dental treatment: Xerostomia, dry throat (normal salivary flow resumes upon discontinuation). Prolonged xerostomia may contribute to discomfort and dental disease (ie, caries, periodontal disease, and oral candidiasis).

Effects on Bleeding No information available to require special precautions

Adverse Reactions Frequency not defined.

Cardiovascular: Tachycardia

Central nervous system: Agitation, confusion, delusions, dizziness, drowsiness, euphoria, hallucination, headache, nervousness, paranoia, psychiatric disturbance

Dermatologic: Skin rash

Gastrointestinal: Constipation, intestinal obstruction, nausea, parotitis, toxic megacolon, vomiting, xerostomia

Genitourinary: Urinary retention

Neuromuscular & skeletal: Weakness

Ophthalmic: Blurred vision, glaucoma, increased intraocular pressure, mydriasis

Mechanism of Action Exerts a direct inhibitory effect on the parasympathetic nervous system. It also has a relaxing effect on smooth musculature; exerted both directly on the muscle itself and indirectly through parasympathetic nervous system (inhibitory effect)

Pharmacodynamics/Kinetics

Half-life Elimination 33 hours (Brocks 1999)

Time to Peak Serum: 1.3 hours (Brocks 1999)

Pregnancy Risk Factor C

Pregnancy Considerations Animal reproduction studies have not been conducted. One case report did not show evidence of adverse events after trihexyphenidyl administration during pregnancy (Robottom 2011).

- **Trihexyphenidyl HCl** *see* Trihexyphenidyl *on page 1498*
- **Trihexyphenidyl Hydrochloride** *see* Trihexyphenidyl *on page 1498*
- **Trijardy XR** *see* Empagliflozin, Linagliptin, and Metformin *on page 555*
- **Trijardy XR** *see* Empagliflozin, Linagliptin, and Metformin *on page 555*
- **Triklo [DSC]** *see* Omega-3 Fatty Acids *on page 1137*
- **Trilafon** *see* Perphenazine *on page 1219*
- **Tri-Legest Fe** *see* Ethinyl Estradiol and Norethindrone *on page 614*
- **Trileptal** *see* OXcarbazepine *on page 1154*
- **Tri-Linyah** *see* Ethinyl Estradiol and Norgestimate *on page 616*
- **Trilipix** *see* Fenofibrate and Derivatives *on page 640*
- **Tri-Lo-Estarylla** *see* Ethinyl Estradiol and Norgestimate *on page 616*
- **Tri-Lo-Marzia** *see* Ethinyl Estradiol and Norgestimate *on page 616*
- **Tri-Lo-Mili** *see* Ethinyl Estradiol and Norgestimate *on page 616*
- **Tri-Lo-Sprintec** *see* Ethinyl Estradiol and Norgestimate *on page 616*
- **Triluron** *see* Hyaluronate and Derivatives *on page 761*

Trimethoprim (trye METH oh prim)

Brand Names: US Primsol; Trimpex [DSC]

Pharmacologic Category Antibiotic, Miscellaneous

Use

Cystitis, acute uncomplicated, treatment (tablets, oral solution): Treatment of initial episodes of uncomplicated urinary tract infections due to susceptible strains of *Escherichia coli*, *Proteus mirabilis*, *Klebsiella pneumoniae*, *Enterobacter* species and coagulase-negative *Staphylococcus* species, including *S. saprophyticus*.

Otitis media, acute (oral solution): Treatment of acute otitis media in pediatric patients due to susceptible strains of *Streptococcus pneumoniae* and *Haemophilus influenzae*.

Local Anesthetic/Vasoconstrictor Precautions No information available to require special precautions

Effects on Dental Treatment Key adverse event(s) related to dental treatment: Glossitis.

Effects on Bleeding Trimethoprim has been shown to induce acute thrombocytopenic purpura, as a consequence of immune-mediated platelet destruction. Platelet numbers as low as <5 x 10^9/L have been observed with normal white blood cell counts. A review of clinical case reports indicates the thrombocytopenic purpura risk typically occurs when trimethoprim is coadministered with sulfamethoxazole. Clinicians should be aware of this adverse effect and closely observe patients for cutaneous manifestations and bleeding attributable to thrombocytopenia in order to withdraw the drug promptly.

Adverse Reactions Frequency not always defined.

Dermatologic: Maculopapular rash (200 mg/day: 3% to 7%; incidence higher with larger daily doses), phototoxicity, pruritus (common)

Endocrine & metabolic: Hyperkalemia, hyponatremia

Gastrointestinal: Epigastric distress, glossitis, nausea, vomiting

Hematologic & oncologic: Leukopenia, megaloblastic anemia, methemoglobinemia, neutropenia, thrombocytopenia

Hepatic: Increased liver enzymes

Hypersensitivity: Anaphylaxis, hypersensitivity reaction

Renal: Increased blood urea nitrogen, increased serum creatinine

Miscellaneous: Fever

1%, postmarketing, and/or case reports: Aseptic meningitis, cholestatic jaundice, erythema multiforme, exfoliative dermatitis, Stevens-Johnson syndrome, toxic epidermal necrolysis

Mechanism of Action Inhibits folic acid reduction to tetrahydrofolate by reversible inhibition of dihydrofolate reductase, inhibiting bacterial synthesis of nucleic acids and proteins

Pharmacodynamics/Kinetics

Half-life Elimination

Prolonged with renal impairment

Newborns: 19 hours; range: 11 to 27 hours (Springer 1982)

Infants 2 months to 1 year: 4.6 hours; range: 3 to 6 hours (Hoppu 1989)

Children (Hoppu 1987): 1 to 3 years: 3.7 hours; 8 to 10 years: 5.4 hours

Adults, normal renal function: 8 to 10 hours

Time to Peak Serum: 1 to 4 hours

Pregnancy Risk Factor C

Pregnancy Considerations Trimethoprim crosses the placenta. Trimethoprim may affect folic acid metabolism; adverse fetal events may be associated with maternal trimethoprim use immediately prior to or during pregnancy (Andersen 2013a; Andersen 2013b; Mølgaard-Nielsen 2012; Sun 2014).

Studies evaluating the effects of trimethoprim administration in pregnancy have also been conducted with Sulfamethoxazole and Trimethoprim (see sulfamethoxazole/trimethoprim monograph for details).

◆ **Trimethoprim and Sulfamethoxazole** *see* Sulfamethoxazole and Trimethoprim *on page 1391*

◆ **Trimethoprim-Sulfamethoxazole** *see* Sulfamethoxazole and Trimethoprim *on page 1391*

◆ **Tri-Mili** *see* Ethinyl Estradiol and Norgestimate *on page 616*

Trimipramine (trye MI pra meen)

Related Information

Dentin Hypersensitivity, Acid Erosion, High Caries Index, Management of Alveolar Osteitis, and Xerostomia *on page 1762*

Vasoconstrictor Interactions With Antidepressants *on page 1821*

Brand Names: US Surmontil [DSC]

Brand Names: Canada APO-Trimipramine

Pharmacologic Category Antidepressant, Tricyclic (Tertiary Amine)

Use Depression: Treatment of depression.

Local Anesthetic/Vasoconstrictor Precautions Use with caution; epinephrine and levonordefrin have been shown to have an increased pressor response in combination with TCAs. Trimipramine is one of the drugs confirmed to prolong the QT interval and is accepted as having a risk of causing torsade de pointes. The risk of drug-induced torsade de pointes is extremely low when a single QT interval prolonging drug is prescribed. In terms of epinephrine, it is not known what effect vasoconstrictors in the local anesthetic regimen will have in patients with a known history of congenital prolonged QT interval or in patients taking any medication that prolongs the QT interval. Until more information is obtained, it is suggested that the clinician consult with the physician prior to the use of a vasoconstrictor in suspected patients, and that the vasoconstrictor (epinephrine, mepivacaine and levonordefrin [Carbocaine® 2% with Neo-Cobefrin®]) be used with caution.

Effects on Dental Treatment Key adverse event(s) related to dental treatment: Xerostomia (normal salivary flow resumes upon discontinuation) and unpleasant taste. Long-term treatment with TCAs, such as trimipramine, increases the risk of caries by reducing salivation and salivary buffer capacity.

Effects on Bleeding No information available to require special precautions

Adverse Reactions Frequency not defined.

Cardiovascular: Cardiac arrhythmia, cerebrovascular accident, facial edema, flushing, heart block, hypertension, hypotension, myocardial infarction, palpitations, tachycardia

Central nervous system: Abnormal electroencephalogram, agitation, anxiety, ataxia, confusion, delusions, disorientation, dizziness, drowsiness, exacerbation of psychosis, extrapyramidal reaction, fatigue, hallucination, headache, hypomania, insomnia, nightmares, numbness, paresthesia, peripheral neuropathy, restlessness, seizure, tingling sensation, withdrawal syndrome

Dermatologic: Alopecia, diaphoresis, pruritus, skin photosensitivity, skin rash, urticaria

Endocrine & metabolic: Change in libido, galactorrhea, gynecomastia, hyperglycemia, hypoglycemia, SIADH, weight gain, weight loss

Gastrointestinal: Abdominal cramps, anorexia, constipation, diarrhea, epigastric distress, melanoglossia, nausea, paralytic ileus, parotid gland enlargement, stomatitis, unpleasant taste, vomiting, xerostomia

Genitourinary: Breast hypertrophy, difficulty in micturition, impotence, testicular swelling, urinary retention

Hematologic & oncologic: Agranulocytosis, eosinophilia, petechia, purpura, thrombocytopenia

Hepatic: Cholestatic jaundice, increased liver enzymes

Hypersensitivity: Tongue edema

Neuromuscular & skeletal: Tremor, weakness

Ophthalmic: Accommodation disturbance, angle-closure glaucoma, blurred vision, mydriasis

Otic: Tinnitus

Renal: Polyuria

Mechanism of Action Antidepressant effects are proposed to result from postsynaptic sensitization to serotonin (Cournoyer, 1987).

Pharmacodynamics/Kinetics

Onset of Action Depression: Initial effects may be observed within 1 to 2 weeks of treatment, with continued improvements through 4 to 6 weeks (Papakostas 2006; Posternak 2005; Szegedi 2009).

Half-life Elimination 7 to 40 hours (Abernethy 1984; Bougerolle, 1989; Caille, 1980)

Time to Peak 1 to 6 hours (Abernethy, 1984; Bougerolle, 1989; Caille, 1980)

Pregnancy Considerations Tricyclic antidepressants (TCAs) may be associated with irritability, jitteriness, and convulsions (rare) in the neonate (Yonkers 2009).

The American College of Obstetricians and Gynecologists (ACOG) recommends that therapy for depression during pregnancy be individualized; treatment should incorporate the clinical expertise of the mental health clinician, obstetrician, primary health care provider, and pediatrician (ACOG 2008). According to the American Psychiatric Association (APA), the risks of medication treatment should be weighed against other treatment options and untreated depression. For women who discontinue antidepressant medications during pregnancy and who may be at high risk for postpartum depression, the medications can be restarted following delivery (APA 2010). Treatment algorithms have been developed by the ACOG and the APA for the management of depression in women prior to conception and during pregnancy (Yonkers 2009). TCAs are not the preferred therapy for depression in pregnant women; if a TCA is needed, other agents may be preferred (Larsen 2015).

Pregnant women exposed to antidepressants during pregnancy are encouraged to enroll in the National Pregnancy Registry for Antidepressants (NPRAD). Women 18 to 45 years of age or their health care providers may contact the registry by calling 844-405-6185. Enrollment should be done as early in pregnancy as possible.

Dental Health Professional Considerations See Local Anesthetic/Vasoconstrictor Precautions

◆ **Trimipramine Maleate** *see* Trimipramine *on page 1499*

◆ **Trimpex [DSC]** *see* Trimethoprim *on page 1498*

◆ **TriNessa (28) [DSC]** *see* Ethinyl Estradiol and Norgestimate *on page 616*

◆ **TriNessa Lo [DSC]** *see* Ethinyl Estradiol and Norgestimate *on page 616*

◆ **Tri-Norinyl (28) [DSC]** *see* Ethinyl Estradiol and Norethindrone *on page 614*

◆ **Trintellix** *see* Vortioxetine *on page 1555*

◆ **Triostat** *see* Liothyronine *on page 919*

◆ **Triphasil** *see* Ethinyl Estradiol and Levonorgestrel *on page 612*

◆ **Triple Paste AF [OTC]** *see* Miconazole (Topical) *on page 1019*

◆ **Tri-Previfem** *see* Ethinyl Estradiol and Norgestimate *on page 616*

Triprolidine (trye PROE li deen)

Brand Names: US Dr Manzanilla Antihistamine [OTC] [DSC]; Histex PD [OTC]; Histex PDX [OTC] [DSC]; Histex [OTC]; M-Hist PD [OTC]

Pharmacologic Category Alkylamine Derivative; Histamine H_1 Antagonist; Histamine H_1 Antagonist, First Generation

Use Upper respiratory allergies: Temporary relief of symptoms (runny nose; sneezing; eye, nose, or throat itching) associated with hay fever (allergic rhinitis) or other upper respiratory allergies.

Local Anesthetic/Vasoconstrictor Precautions No information available to require special precautions

Effects on Dental Treatment No significant effects or complications reported

Effects on Bleeding No information available to require special precautions

Adverse Reactions There are no adverse reactions listed in the manufacturer's labeling.

Mechanism of Action Triprolidine is an H_1-receptor antagonist, which provides dose-related suppression of histamine-induced wheel and flare reactions (Simons 1986). It is useful for the prevention and suppression of the signs and symptoms of allergic rhinitis and other upper respiratory allergies.

Pharmacodynamics/Kinetics

Half-life Elimination 2.1 ± 0.8 hours (Simons 1986)

Time to Peak 1.7 ± 0.5 hours (Simons 1986)

Pregnancy Considerations

Information related to the use of triprolidine in pregnancy is limited (Aldridge 2014; Gilboa 2009).

Although triprolidine is approved for the treatment of allergic rhinitis, other agents are preferred for use in pregnancy (BSACI [Scadding 2017]).

◆ **Triprolidine HCl** *see* Triprolidine *on page 1500*

◆ **Triprolidine Hydrochloride** *see* Triprolidine *on page 1500*

◆ **Triptodur** *see* Triptorelin *on page 1500*

Triptorelin (trip toe REL in)

Brand Names: US Trelstar Mixject; Trelstar [DSC]; Triptodur

Brand Names: Canada Decapeptyl; Trelstar

Pharmacologic Category Gonadotropin Releasing Hormone Agonist

Use

Central precocious puberty: Triptodur: Treatment of central precocious puberty in patients 2 years and older

Prostate cancer (advanced): Trelstar: Palliative treatment of advanced prostate cancer

Assisted reproductive technologies: Decapeptyl [Canadian product]: Adjunctive therapy in women undergoing controlled ovarian hyperstimulation for assisted reproductive technologies (ART)

Local Anesthetic/Vasoconstrictor Precautions No information available to require special precautions

Effects on Dental Treatment No significant effects or complications reported

Effects on Bleeding Although significant myelosuppression with associated altered hemostasis has been reported for many chemotherapeutic agents, myelosuppression is not common with triptorelin and no specific precautions appear to necessary.

Adverse Reactions

>10%:

Endocrine & metabolic: Hot flash (prostate cancer: 59% to 73%; central precocious puberty: 2% to 5%), increased serum glucose (prostate cancer)

Hematologic & oncologic: Decreased hemoglobin (prostate cancer), decreased red blood cells (prostate cancer)

Hepatic: Increased serum alanine aminotransferase (prostate cancer), increased serum aspartate aminotransferase (prostate cancer), increased serum transaminases (prostate cancer)

Local: Pain at injection site (central precocious puberty: 45%; prostate cancer: 4%), erythema at injection site (central precocious puberty: 14%)

Nervous system: Headache (2% to 14%)

Neuromuscular & skeletal: Skeletal pain (prostate cancer: 12% to 13%)

Renal: Increased blood urea nitrogen (prostate cancer)

Respiratory: Nasopharyngitis (central precocious puberty: 14%)

1% to 10%:

Cardiovascular: Lower extremity edema (prostate cancer: 6%), hypertension (prostate cancer: ≤4%; central precocious puberty), chest pain (prostate cancer: 2%), peripheral edema (prostate cancer: 1%)

Dermatologic: Injection site pruritus (central precocious puberty: 2%), skin rash (prostate cancer: 2%), pruritus (prostate cancer: 1%)

Endocrine & metabolic: Decreased libido (prostate cancer: 2%), dependent edema (prostate cancer: 2%), gynecomastia (prostate cancer: 2%)

Gastrointestinal: Gastroenteritis (central precocious puberty: 7%), nausea (prostate cancer: 3%), anorexia (prostate cancer: 2%), constipation (prostate cancer: 2%), dyspepsia (prostate cancer: 2%), vomiting (prostate cancer: 2%), abdominal pain (prostate cancer: 1%), diarrhea (prostate cancer: 1%)

Genitourinary: Erectile dysfunction (prostate cancer: 10%), menstruation (central precocious puberty: 8%), testicular atrophy (prostate cancer: 8%), impotence (prostate cancer: 2% to 7%), dysuria (prostate cancer: 5%), mastalgia (prostate cancer: 2%), urinary retention (prostate cancer: 1%), urinary tract infection (prostate cancer: 1%)

Hematologic & oncologic: Anemia (prostate cancer: 1%)

Hepatic: Increased serum alkaline phosphatase (≥2%), hepatic insufficiency (prostate cancer: 1%)

Infection: Influenza (central precocious puberty: 5%)

Local: Swelling at injection site (central precocious puberty: 2%)

Nervous system: Pain (prostate cancer: 2% to 3%), dizziness (prostate cancer: 1% to 3%), anxiety (central precocious puberty: 2%), fatigue (prostate cancer: 2%), mood changes (central precocious puberty: 2%), insomnia (prostate cancer: ≤2%), emotional lability (≤1%)

Neuromuscular & skeletal: Lower extremity pain (prostate cancer: 2% to 5%), back pain (prostate cancer: ≤3%), lower limb cramps (prostate cancer: 2%), arthralgia (prostate cancer: ≤2%), asthenia (prostate cancer: 1%), myalgia (prostate cancer: 1%)

Ophthalmic: Conjunctivitis (prostate cancer: 1%), eye pain (prostate cancer: 1%)

Otic: Otitis externa (central precocious puberty: 5%)

Respiratory: Upper respiratory tract infection (central precocious puberty: 9%), cough (central precocious puberty: 7%; prostate cancer: 2%), bronchitis (central precocious puberty: 5%), pharyngitis (central precocious puberty: 5%; prostate cancer: 1%), sinusitis (central precocious puberty: 5%), dyspnea (prostate cancer: 1%)

Miscellaneous: Postoperative pain (reproductive studies: 3% to 4%), missed abortion (reproductive studies: 2%)

Frequency not defined: Endocrine & metabolic: Increased testosterone level

<1%, postmarketing, and/or case reports: Altered gonadal hormone levels (pituitary-gonadal axis suppression), anaphylactic shock, anaphylactoid shock, angioedema, cerebrovascular accident, deep vein thrombosis, hypersensitivity reaction, interstitial pulmonary disease, intracranial hypertension (Tan 2019), limb pain, myocardial infarction, pituitary apoplexy, pulmonary embolism, seizure, thrombophlebitis, transient ischemic attacks, urticaria, visual disturbance, visual impairment

Mechanism of Action Triptorelin is an agonist analog of gonadotropin releasing hormone (GnRH) and causes suppression of ovarian and testicular steroidogenesis due to decreased levels of LH and FSH with subsequent decrease in testosterone (male) and estrogen (female) levels. After chronic and continuous administration, usually 2 to 4 weeks after initiation, a sustained decrease in LH and FSH secretion occurs. When used for assisted reproductive technologies (ART), prevents premature LH surge in women undergoing controlled ovarian hyperstimulation.

Pharmacodynamics/Kinetics

Half-life Elimination 2.8 ± 1.2 hours

Moderate-to-severe renal impairment: 6.6 to 7.7 hours

Hepatic impairment: 7.6 hours

Time to Peak Trelstar: 1 to 3 hours; Triptodur: 4 hours

Reproductive Considerations

When used for assisted reproductive technologies (ART; not an approved use in the US), pregnancy must be ruled out prior to therapy and nonhormonal contraception should be used until menses occurs. Due to the short half-life of triptorelin (formulations used for ART), it is not expected to be present in the maternal serum at the time of embryo transfer.

Based on the mechanism of action, may impair fertility in males of reproductive potential.

Pregnancy Considerations

Based on the mechanism of action and data from animal reproduction studies, in utero exposure to triptorelin may cause fetal harm.

Hormonal changes that occur with therapy may increase the risk of pregnancy loss. Therefore, use is contraindicated in females who are pregnant. Information following inadvertent exposure in early pregnancy is limited (Elefant 1995).

- ◆ **Triptorelin Embonate** *see* Triptorelin *on page 1500*
- ◆ **Triptorelin Pamoate** *see* Triptorelin *on page 1500*
- ◆ **Tris Buffer** *see* Tromethamine *on page 1502*
- ◆ **Tris(hydroxymethyl)aminomethane** *see* Tromethamine *on page 1502*
- ◆ **Tri-Sprintec** *see* Ethinyl Estradiol and Norgestimate *on page 616*
- ◆ **Triumeq** *see* Abacavir, Dolutegravir, and Lamivudine *on page 51*
- ◆ **Tri-Vi-Flor®** *see* Vitamins (Fluoride) *on page 1550*
- ◆ **Tri-Vi-Flor® with Iron** *see* Vitamins (Fluoride) *on page 1550*
- ◆ **Trivora (28)** *see* Ethinyl Estradiol and Levonorgestrel *on page 612*
- ◆ **Tri-VyLibra** *see* Ethinyl Estradiol and Norgestimate *on page 616*
- ◆ **Tri-VyLibra Lo** *see* Ethinyl Estradiol and Norgestimate *on page 616*
- ◆ **Trixaicin [OTC] [DSC]** *see* Capsaicin *on page 284*
- ◆ **Trixaicin HP [OTC]** *see* Capsaicin *on page 284*
- ◆ **Trizivir** *see* Abacavir, Lamivudine, and Zidovudine *on page 52*
- ◆ **TRK Inhibitor LOXO-101** *see* Larotrectinib *on page 879*
- ◆ **Trocaine Throat [OTC] [DSC]** *see* Benzocaine *on page 228*
- ◆ **Trocal Cough Suppressant [OTC] [DSC]** *see* Dextromethorphan *on page 476*
- ◆ **Trodelvy** *see* Sacituzumab Govitecan *on page 1352*
- ◆ **Trogarzo** *see* Ibalizumab *on page 781*
- ◆ **Trokendi XR** *see* Topiramate *on page 1464*

Tromethamine (troe METH a meen)

Brand Names: US Tham

Brand Names: Canada Tham [DSC]

Pharmacologic Category Alkalinizing Agent, Parenteral

Use Metabolic acidosis: Correction of metabolic acidosis associated with cardiac bypass surgery or cardiac arrest; to correct acidity of stored blood that is preserved with acid citrate dextrose; metabolic acidosis associated with respiratory distress syndrome in neonates and infants.

Local Anesthetic/Vasoconstrictor Precautions No information available to require special precautions

Effects on Dental Treatment No significant effects or complications reported

Effects on Bleeding No information available to require special precautions

Adverse Reactions

Frequency not defined:

Cardiovascular: Localized phlebitis, venospasm, venous thrombosis

Endocrine & metabolic: Hyperkalemia, hypervolemia, hypoglycemia

Hepatic: Hepatic necrosis (resulted during delivery via umbilical venous catheter)

Local: Injection site infection, local irritation

Respiratory: Pulmonary edema, respiratory depression

Miscellaneous: Fever

Mechanism of Action Acts as a proton acceptor, which combines with hydrogen ions, liberating bicarbonate buffer, to correct acidosis. It buffers both metabolic and respiratory acids, limiting carbon dioxide generation. Also an osmotic diuretic.

Pregnancy Considerations Animal reproduction studies have not been conducted.

Tropicamide (troe PIK a mide)

Brand Names: US Mydriacyl

Brand Names: Canada Mydriacyl; Odan-Tropicamide

Pharmacologic Category Ophthalmic Agent, Mydriatic

Use Mydriasis/Cycloplegia: For mydriasis and cycloplegia in diagnostic procedures

Local Anesthetic/Vasoconstrictor Precautions No information available to require special precautions

Effects on Dental Treatment Key adverse event(s) related to dental treatment: Dryness of mouth.

Effects on Bleeding No information available to require special precautions

Adverse Reactions Frequency not defined.

Cardiovascular: Central nervous system dysfunction, tachycardia

Central nervous system: Headache

Dermatologic: Pallor

Gastrointestinal: Nausea, vomiting, xerostomia

Hypersensitivity: Hypersensitivity reaction

Neuromuscular & skeletal: Muscle rigidity

Ophthalmic: Blurred vision, photophobia, stinging of eyes (transient), superficial punctate keratitis

Mechanism of Action Prevents the sphincter muscle of the iris and the muscle of the ciliary body from responding to cholinergic stimulation; produces dilation and prevents accommodation.

Pharmacodynamics/Kinetics

Onset of Action Cycloplegic effect: Peak: 20 to 35 minutes; Mydriatic effect: ~20 to 40 minutes

Duration of Action Cycloplegic effect: <6 hour; Mydriatic effect: ~6 to 7 hours

Pregnancy Considerations

Animal reproduction studies have not been conducted. If ophthalmic agents are needed during pregnancy, the minimum effective dose should be used in combination with punctal occlusion to decrease potential exposure to the fetus (Samples 1988).

Trospium (TROSE pee um)

Related Information

Dentin Hypersensitivity, Acid Erosion, High Caries Index, Management of Alveolar Osteitis, and Xerostomia *on page 1762*

Brand Names: Canada MAR-Trospium; Trosec

Pharmacologic Category Anticholinergic Agent

Use Overactive bladder: Treatment of overactive bladder with symptoms of urgency, incontinence, and urinary frequency

Local Anesthetic/Vasoconstrictor Precautions No information available to require special precautions

Effects on Dental Treatment Key adverse event(s) related to dental treatment: Significant xerostomia and changes in salivation (normal salivary flow resumes upon discontinuation).

Effects on Bleeding No information available to require special precautions

Adverse Reactions

>10%: Gastrointestinal: Xerostomia (9% to 22%)

1% to 10%:

Cardiovascular: Tachycardia (<2%)

Central nervous system: Headache (4% to 7%), fatigue (2%)

Dermatologic: Skin rash (<2%), xeroderma

Gastrointestinal: Constipation (9% to 10%), abdominal pain (1% to 3%), dyspepsia (1% to 2%), flatulence (1% to 2%), abdominal distention (<2%), nausea (1%), dysgeusia, vomiting

Genitourinary: Urinary tract infection (1% to 7%), urinary retention (≤1%)

Infection: Influenza (2%)

Ophthalmic: Dry eye syndrome (1% to 2%), blurred vision (1%)

Respiratory: Nasopharyngitis (3%), dry nose (1%)

<1%, postmarketing, and/or case reports: Anaphylaxis, angioedema, back pain, chest pain, confusion, delirium, dizziness, drowsiness, fecal impaction, gastritis, hallucination, heat intolerance, hypertensive crisis, inversion T wave on ECG, palpitations, rhabdomyolysis, Stevens-Johnson syndrome, supraventricular tachycardia, syncope, visual disturbance

Mechanism of Action Trospium antagonizes the effects of acetylcholine on muscarinic receptors in cholinergically innervated organs. It reduces the smooth muscle tone of the bladder.

Pharmacodynamics/Kinetics

Half-life Elimination Immediate release formulation: 20 hours

Severe renal insufficiency (CrCl <30 mL/minute): ~33 hours; extended release formulation: ~35 hours

Time to Peak 5-6 hours

Pregnancy Risk Factor C

Pregnancy Considerations

Adverse events were observed in animal studies.

- ◆ **Trospium Chloride** *see* Trospium *on page* 1502
- ◆ **Trulance** *see* Plecanatide *on page* 1240
- ◆ **Trumenba** *see* Meningococcal Group B Vaccine *on page* 963
- ◆ **Truvada** *see* Emtricitabine and Tenofovir Disoproxil Fumarate *on page* 558
- ◆ **Truxima** *see* RiTUXimab *on page* 1336
- ◆ **Tryptoreline** *see* Triptorelin *on page* 1500
- ◆ **TSH** *see* Thyrotropin Alpha *on page* 1442
- ◆ **TSPA** *see* Thiotepa *on page* 1439
- ◆ **TST** *see* Tuberculin Tests *on page* 1503
- ◆ **Tuberculin Purified Protein Derivative** *see* Tuberculin Tests *on page* 1503
- ◆ **Tuberculin Skin Test** *see* Tuberculin Tests *on page* 1503

Tuberculin Tests (too BER kyoo lin tests)

Brand Names: US Aplisol; Tubersol

Brand Names: Canada Tubersol

Pharmacologic Category Diagnostic Agent

Use Tuberculosis skin test: An aid in the diagnosis of tuberculosis (TB) infection.

Local Anesthetic/Vasoconstrictor Precautions

No information available to require special precautions

Effects on Dental Treatment No significant effects or complications reported

Effects on Bleeding No information available to require special precautions

Adverse Reactions

Frequency not defined:

Cardiovascular: Presyncope, syncope

Dermatologic: Erythematous rash, localized erythema, localized vesiculation, rash at injection site, skin rash, skin ulceration at injection site, urticaria at injection site

Hypersensitivity: Anaphylactoid reaction, anaphylaxis, angioedema, hypersensitivity reaction

Local: Injection site reactions, discomfort at injection site, hematoma at injection site, injection site scarring, local pruritus, localized edema, local tissue necrosis, pain at injection site

Respiratory: Dyspnea, stridor

Miscellaneous: Fever

Mechanism of Action Tuberculosis results in individuals becoming sensitized to certain antigenic components of the *M. tuberculosis* organism. Culture extracts called tuberculins are contained in tuberculin skin test preparations. Upon intracutaneous injection of these culture extracts, a classic delayed (cellular) hypersensitivity reaction occurs. This reaction is characteristic of a delayed course (peak occurs >24 hours after injection, induration of the skin secondary to cell infiltration, and occasional vesiculation and necrosis). Delayed hypersensitivity reactions to tuberculin may indicate infection with a variety of nontuberculosis mycobacteria, or vaccination with the live attenuated mycobacterial strain of *M. bovis* vaccine, BCG, in addition to previous natural infection with *M. tuberculosis*.

Pharmacodynamics/Kinetics

Onset of Action Delayed hypersensitivity reactions: 5-6 hours; Peak effect: 48-72 hours

Duration of Action Reactions subside over a few days

Pregnancy Risk Factor C

Pregnancy Considerations Animal reproduction studies have not been conducted. Pregnancy is not a contraindication to testing (CDC 2005).

- ◆ **Tubersol** *see* Tuberculin Tests *on page* 1503

Tucatinib (too KA ti nib)

Brand Names: US Tukysa

Pharmacologic Category Antineoplastic Agent, Anti-HER2; Antineoplastic Agent, Tyrosine Kinase Inhibitor

Use Breast cancer, human epidermal growth factor receptor 2 positive, advanced unresectable or metastatic: Treatment of advanced unresectable or metastatic human epidermal growth factor receptor 2 (HER2)-positive breast cancer (in combination with trastuzumab and capecitabine) in adults with or without brain metastases who have received ≥1 prior anti-HER2-based regimens in the metastatic setting.

Local Anesthetic/Vasoconstrictor Precautions

No information available to require special precautions.

Effects on Dental Treatment Key adverse event(s) related to dental treatment: Frequent occurrence of stomatitis; frequency not defined: aphthous stomatitis, glossalgia, lip blister, oral discomfort, oral mucosa ulcer, tongue ulcer, oropharyngeal irritation, oropharyngeal pain.

Effects on Bleeding No information available to require special precautions.

Adverse Reactions Incidences reported for combination therapy with trastuzumab and capecitabine. Comparator: Placebo + trastuzumab + capecitabine.

>10%:

Dermatologic: Palmar-plantar erythrodysesthesia (63%), skin rash (20%)

Endocrine & metabolic: Decreased serum magnesium (40%), decreased serum phosphate (57%), decreased serum potassium (36%), decreased serum sodium (28%), weight loss (13%)

Gastrointestinal: Abdominal pain (≥20%), decreased appetite (25%), diarrhea (81% [comparator: 53%]; severe diarrhea: 4%), nausea (58% [comparator: 44%]), stomatitis (32% [comparator: 21%]); grade 3: 3% [comparator: 0.5%]), vomiting (36% [comparator: 25%])

Hematologic & oncologic: Anemia (21%; grade 3: 4%)

Hepatic: Hepatotoxicity (42% [comparator: 24%]), increased serum alanine aminotransferase (46% [comparator: 27%]; severe hepatotoxicity: >5x ULN: 8%), increased serum alkaline phosphatase (26%), increased serum aspartate aminotransferase (43% [comparator: 25%]; severe hepatotoxicity: >5x ULN: 6%), increased serum bilirubin (47% [comparator: 30%])

Nervous system: Fatigue (≥20%), headache (≥20%), peripheral neuropathy (13%; grade 3: <1%)

Neuromuscular & skeletal: Arthralgia (15%)

Renal: Increased serum creatinine (14% to 33%)

Respiratory: Epistaxis (12%)

1% to 10%: Nervous system: Seizure (2%)

Frequency not defined:

Dermatologic: Allergic dermatitis, dermatitis (including acneiform), erythema of skin, erythematous rash, exfoliation of skin, maculopapular rash, pruritic rash, pustular rash, skin toxicity, urticaria

Gastrointestinal: Aphthous stomatitis, glossalgia, lip blister, oral discomfort, oral mucosa ulcer, tongue ulcer

Nervous system: Peripheral motor neuropathy, peripheral sensory neuropathy, sensorimotor neuropathy (peripheral)

Respiratory: Oropharyngeal irritation, oropharyngeal pain

Mechanism of Action Tucatinib is a tyrosine kinase inhibitor that is highly selective for the human epidermal growth factor receptor 2 (HER2) kinase domain, with minimal inhibition of epidermal growth factor receptor (Murthy 2020). Tucatinib inhibits HER2 and HER3 phosphorylation, resulting in downstream inhibition of MAPK and AKT signaling and cell proliferation; tucatinib demonstrated antitumor activity in HER2-expressing tumor cells and inhibited growth of HER2-expressing tumors. The combination of tucatinib plus trastuzumab exhibited increased antitumor activity compared to either medication alone.

Pharmacodynamics/Kinetics

Half-life Elimination ~8.5 hours.

Time to Peak ~2 hours (range: 1 to 4 hours).

Reproductive Considerations

Evaluate pregnancy status prior to use in females of reproductive potential.

Females of reproductive potential should use effective contraception during tucatinib therapy and for ≥1 week after the last tucatinib dose. Males with female partners of reproductive potential should use effective contraception during tucatinib therapy and for ≥1 week after the last tucatinib dose.

Tucatinib is used in combination with trastuzumab and capecitabine.

Pregnancy Considerations

Based on the mechanism of action and data from animal reproduction studies, in utero exposure to tucatinib may cause fetal harm.

Tucatinib is used in combination with trastuzumab and capecitabine.

- ◆ **Tudorza Pressair** *see* Aclidinium *on page* 74
- ◆ **Tukysa** *see* Tucatinib *on page* 1503
- ◆ **Tulana** *see* Norethindrone *on page* 1117
- ◆ **Turoctocog Alfa** *see* Antihemophilic Factor (Recombinant) *on page* 153
- ◆ **Tuxarin ER** *see* Codeine and Chlorpheniramine *on page* 404
- ◆ **Tuzistra XR** *see* Codeine and Chlorpheniramine *on page* 404
- ◆ **T-VEC** *see* Talimogene Laherparepvec *on page* 1403
- ◆ **T-Vites [OTC]** *see* Vitamins (Multiple/Oral) *on page* 1550
- ◆ **TVP-1012** *see* Rasagiline *on page* 1311
- ◆ **Twinrix** *see* Hepatitis A and Hepatitis B Recombinant Vaccine *on page* 754
- ◆ **Twirla** *see* Ethinyl Estradiol and Levonorgestrel *on page* 612
- ◆ **Twynsta** *see* Telmisartan and Amlodipine *on page* 1414
- ◆ **Ty21a Vaccine** *see* Typhoid Vaccine *on page* 1505
- ◆ **Tybost** *see* Cobicistat *on page* 401
- ◆ **Tydemy** *see* Ethinyl Estradiol, Drospirenone, and Levomefolate *on page* 618
- ◆ **Tygacil** *see* Tigecycline *on page* 1447
- ◆ **Tykerb** *see* Lapatinib *on page* 877
- ◆ **Tylenol [OTC]** *see* Acetaminophen *on page* 59
- ◆ **Tylenol #2** *see* Acetaminophen and Codeine *on page* 65
- ◆ **Tylenol #3** *see* Acetaminophen and Codeine *on page* 65
- ◆ **Tylenol 8 HR [OTC] [DSC]** *see* Acetaminophen *on page* 59
- ◆ **Tylenol 8 HR Arthritis Pain [OTC]** *see* Acetaminophen *on page* 59
- ◆ **Tylenol Children's [OTC]** *see* Acetaminophen *on page* 59
- ◆ **Tylenol Codeine** *see* Acetaminophen and Codeine *on page* 65
- ◆ **Tylenol Extra Strength [OTC]** *see* Acetaminophen *on page* 59
- ◆ **Tylenol Infants' [OTC]** *see* Acetaminophen *on page* 59
- ◆ **Tylenol with Codeine #3 [DSC]** *see* Acetaminophen and Codeine *on page* 65

- ◆ **Tylenol with Codeine #4 [DSC]** *see* Acetaminophen and Codeine *on page 65*
- ◆ **Tylox** *see* Oxycodone and Acetaminophen *on page 1164*
- ◆ **Tymlos** *see* Abaloparatide *on page 53*
- ◆ **Typh-1** *see* Typhoid and Hepatitis A Vaccine *on page 1505*
- ◆ **Typhim Vi** *see* Typhoid Vaccine *on page 1505*

Typhoid and Hepatitis A Vaccine

(TYE foid & hep a TYE tis aye vak SEEN)

Brand Names: Canada ViVaxim

Pharmacologic Category Vaccine; Vaccine, Inactivated (Bacterial); Vaccine, Inactivated (Viral)

Use Note: Not approved in the US

***Salmonella typhi* and hepatitis A disease prevention**: Active immunization against typhoid fever caused by *Salmonella typhi* and against disease caused by hepatitis A virus (HAV) in adolescents ≥16 years and adults

National Advisory Committee on Immunizations (NACI) does not recommend use for routine vaccination but does recommend that immunization be considered in the following groups (NACI 2014; NACI 2016):

- Travelers to areas with a prolonged risk (>4 weeks) of exposure to *S. typhi* or travelers to areas with endemic hepatitis A
- Persons with intimate exposure to a *S. typhi* carrier or who are residing in communities with high endemic rates of hepatitis A virus or at risk of outbreaks
- Laboratory technicians with frequent exposure to *S. typhi* or individuals involved in hepatitis A research or production of hepatitis A vaccine
- Travelers with achlorhydria or hypochlorhydria
- Military personnel, relief workers, or others relocated to areas with high rates of hepatitis A infection
- Persons with lifestyle risks for hepatitis A infection (eg, drug abusers, homosexual men), chronic liver disease, receiving hepatotoxic medication or with disease(s) which may necessitate use of hepatotoxic medications
- Persons with hemophilia A or B treated with plasma-derived clotting factors
- Zookeepers, veterinarians, and researchers who handle nonhuman primates

Local Anesthetic/Vasoconstrictor Precautions No information available to require special precautions

Effects on Dental Treatment No significant effects or complications reported

Effects on Bleeding No information available to require special precautions

Adverse Reactions In Canada, adverse reactions may be reported to local provincial/territorial health agencies or to the Vaccine Safety Section at Public Health Agency of Canada (1-866-844-0018).

>10%:

Central nervous system: Headache (15%)

Local: Pain at injection site (90%), induration at injection site (≤28%), swelling at injection site (≤28%), erythema at injection site (10%)

Neuromuscular & skeletal: Weakness (17%), myalgia (16%)

1% to 10%:

Central nervous system: Malaise (3%), dizziness (1%)

Gastrointestinal: Diarrhea (3%), nausea (3%)

Miscellaneous: Fever (5%)

<1%, postmarketing, and/or case reports (reported with ViVAXIM): Arthralgia, pruritus, skin rash

Mechanism of Action Provides active immunization against typhoid fever through production of antibodies (predominantly IgG) and against hepatitis A infection through production of antihepatitis A virus antibodies.

Pharmacodynamics/Kinetics

Onset of Action Seroprotection rate at 14 days: Hepatitis A: ~96%, typhoid: ~89%; Seroprotection at 28 days: Hepatitis A: ~100%, typhoid: ~90%

Duration of Action Kinetic models suggest antihepatitis A antibodies may persist ≥20 years (NACI 2016); Typhoid: 3 years

Pregnancy Considerations Animal reproduction studies have not been conducted. Although the safety of this combination vaccine during pregnancy has not been determined, consider use in high risk situations. Inactivated vaccines have not been shown to cause increased risks to the fetus (NACI 2015).

Product Availability Not available in the US

Typhoid Vaccine (TYE foid vak SEEN)

Brand Names: US Typhim Vi; Vivotif

Brand Names: Canada Typherix; Typhim Vi; Vivotif

Pharmacologic Category Vaccine; Vaccine, Inactivated (Bacterial); Vaccine, Live (Bacterial)

Use

Typhoid fever prevention: Active immunization against typhoid fever caused by *Salmonella typhi*:

Oral: Immunization of adults and children >6 years of age; complete the vaccine regimen at least 1 week before potential exposure to typhoid bacteria.

Parenteral: Immunization of adults and children ≥2 years of age; complete the vaccine regimen at least 2 weeks before potential exposure to typhoid bacteria.

Not for routine vaccination. In the United States (CDC/ACIP [Jackson 2015]) and Canada, use should be limited to:

- Travelers to areas with a recognized risk of exposure to *S. typhi*
- Persons with intimate exposure to a household contact with *S. typhi* fever or a known carrier
- Laboratory technicians with frequent exposure to *S. typhi*

Additional recommendations: May consider administration to travelers with achlorhydria, or receiving acid suppression therapy; anatomic or functional asplenia (Canadian Immunization Guide)

Local Anesthetic/Vasoconstrictor Precautions No information available to require special precautions

Effects on Dental Treatment No significant effects or complications reported

Effects on Bleeding No information available to require special precautions

Adverse Reactions In the US, all serious adverse reactions must be reported to the Department of Health and Human Services (DHHS) Vaccine Adverse Event Reporting System (VAERS) 1-800-822-7967 or online at https://vaers.hhs.gov/esub/index. In Canada, adverse reactions may be reported to local provincial/territorial health agencies or to the Vaccine Safety Section at Public Health Agency of Canada (1-866-844-0018).

Injection (incidence may vary based on age and/or product used):

>10%:

Central nervous system: Malaise (4% to 24%), headache (16% to 20%), generalized ache (1% to 13%)

Local: Tenderness at injection site (97% to 98%), pain at injection site (27% to 41%), induration at injection site (5% to 15%)

Neuromuscular & skeletal: Muscle tenderness (≤16%)

Miscellaneous: Fever (undefined 2% to 32%)

1% to 10%:

Dermatologic: Pruritus (≤8%)

Gastrointestinal: Nausea (≤8%), vomiting (2%)

Local: Injection site: Erythema at injection site (≤5%), swelling at injection site (≤4%)

Neuromuscular & skeletal: Myalgia (3% to 7%)

Miscellaneous: Fever greater than 100 to 101 degrees (2%)

Postmarketing and/or case reports: Abdominal pain, anaphylaxis, angioedema, arthralgia, asthma, diarrhea, dizziness, flu-like symptoms, Guillain-Barré syndrome, hypersensitivity reaction, hypotension, inflammation at injection site (including angioedema and urticaria), intestinal perforation (jejunum), loss of consciousness, lymphadenopathy, malaise, neck pain, serum sickness, skin rash, syncope (with and without convulsions), tremor, urticaria, vasodilation, weakness

Oral:

1% to 10%:

Central nervous system: Headache (5%)

Dermatologic: Skin rash (1%)

Gastrointestinal: Abdominal pain (6%), nausea (6%), diarrhea (3%), vomiting (2%)

Miscellaneous: Fever (3%)

Postmarketing and/or case reports: Anaphylaxis, demyelinating disease, myalgia, pain, rheumatoid arthritis, sepsis, urticaria, weakness

Mechanism of Action Virulent strains of *Salmonella typhi* cause disease by penetrating the intestinal mucosa and entering the systemic circulation via the lymphatic vasculature. One possible mechanism of conferring immunity may be the provocation of a local immune response in the intestinal tract induced by oral ingesting of a live strain with subsequent aborted infection. The ability of *S. typhi* to produce clinical disease (and to elicit an immune response) is dependent on the bacteria having a complete lipopolysaccharide. The live attenuate Ty21a strain lacks the enzyme UDP-4-galactose epimerase so that lipopolysaccharide is only synthesized under conditions that induce bacterial autolysis. Thus, the strain remains avirulent despite the production of sufficient lipopolysaccharide to evoke a protective immune response. Despite low levels of lipopolysaccharide synthesis, cells lyse before gaining a virulent phenotype due to the intracellular accumulation of metabolic intermediates.

Efficacy: Based on a systematic review and meta-analysis, the estimated 2.5 to 3 year cumulative efficacy was 55% (95% confidence interval [CI]: 30% to 70%) for the injectable vaccine and 48% (CI: 34% to 58%) for the oral vaccine (CDC/ACIP [Jackson 2015]).

Pharmacodynamics/Kinetics

Onset of Action Immunity to *Salmonella typhi*: Oral: ~1 week after completing the series; Parenteral: Antibody response develops within 2 weeks after a single dose.

Duration of Action Immunity: Oral: >5 years; Parenteral: Typhim Vi: ~2 years, Typherix [Canadian product]: ~3 years

Pregnancy Considerations Animal reproduction studies have not been conducted. The manufacturer of the Typhim Vi injection suggests delaying vaccination until the second or third trimester if possible. Untreated typhoid fever may lead to miscarriage or vertical intrauterine transmission causing neonatal typhoid (rare).

- ◆ **Typhoid Vaccine Live Oral Ty21a** *see* Typhoid Vaccine *on page 1505*
- ◆ **Tysabri** *see* Natalizumab *on page 1086*
- ◆ **Tyvaso** *see* Treprostinil *on page 1482*
- ◆ **Tyvaso Refill** *see* Treprostinil *on page 1482*
- ◆ **Tyvaso Starter** *see* Treprostinil *on page 1482*
- ◆ **Tyzeka [DSC]** *see* Telbivudine *on page 1412*
- ◆ **Tyzine [DSC]** *see* Tetrahydrozoline (Nasal) *on page 1435*
- ◆ **506U78** *see* Nelarabine *on page 1091*
- ◆ **U-90152S** *see* Delavirdine *on page 451*
- ◆ **UCB-P071** *see* Cetirizine (Systemic) *on page 328*
- ◆ **Uceris** *see* Budesonide (Systemic) *on page 252*
- ◆ **Uceris** *see* Budesonide (Topical) *on page 255*
- ◆ **Udenyca** *see* Pegfilgrastim *on page 1200*
- ◆ **UK-88,525** *see* Darifenacin *on page 441*
- ◆ **UK-427,857** *see* Maraviroc *on page 947*
- ◆ **UK92480** *see* Sildenafil *on page 1369*
- ◆ **UK109496** *see* Voriconazole *on page 1552*

Ulipristal (ue li PRIS tal)

Brand Names: US Ella

Brand Names: Canada Ella; Fibristal

Pharmacologic Category Contraceptive; Progestin Receptor Modulator

Use

Emergency contraception (ella): Prevention of pregnancy following unprotected intercourse or a known or suspected contraceptive failure. Ulipristal is not intended for routine use as a contraceptive.

Uterine fibroids (Fibristal [Canadian product]): Treatment of moderate to severe signs/symptoms of uterine fibroids in adult women of reproductive age who are eligible for surgery; intermittent treatment of moderate to severe signs/symptoms of uterine fibroids in adult women of reproductive age

Local Anesthetic/Vasoconstrictor Precautions No information available to require special precautions

Effects on Dental Treatment No significant effects or complications reported (see Dental Health Professional Considerations)

Effects on Bleeding No information available to require special precautions

Adverse Reactions

Emergency contraception (ella):

>10%:

Central nervous system: Headache (18% to 19%)

Endocrine & metabolic: Suppressed menstruation (≥7 days later than expected: 19%)

Gastrointestinal: Abdominal pain (8% to 15%), nausea (12% to 13%)

Genitourinary: Dysmenorrhea (7% to 13%)

1% to 10%:
Central nervous system: Fatigue (6%), dizziness (5%)
Endocrine & metabolic: Intermenstrual bleeding (9%)
Genitourinary: Early menses (≥7 days earlier than expected: 7%)
Postmarketing and/or case reports: Acne vulgaris

Treatment of moderate-to-severe signs/symptoms of uterine fibroids (Fibristal [Canadian product]):
>10%:
Central nervous system: Headache (1% to 16%)
Endocrine & metabolic: Hot flash (1% to 25%)
1% to 10%:
Cardiovascular: Edema (≤1%), hypotension (≤1%), sinus bradycardia (≤1%)
Central nervous system: Fatigue (≤4%), vertigo (≤4%), insomnia (≤2%), dizziness (1%), aggressive behavior (≤1%), drowsiness (≤1%), emotional lability (≤1%), migraine (≤1%), sleep disorder (≤1%)
Dermatologic: Night sweats (≤2%), acne vulgaris (≤1%), alopecia (≤1%), seborrhea (≤1%), xeroderma (≤1%)
Endocrine & metabolic: Hypercholesterolemia (3%), hypertriglyceridemia (≤3%), hypothyroidism (≤2%), obesity (1%), amenorrhea (≤1%), increased gamma-glutamyl transferase (≤1%), ovarian cyst (≤1%), ovarian hyperstimulation (≤1%), thyroid disease (≤1%)
Gastrointestinal: Nausea (3%), constipation (1%), dyspepsia (≤1%), upper abdominal pain (≤1%)
Genitourinary: Mastalgia (2%), pelvic pain (1% to 2%), endometrial hyperplasia (≤2%), genital bleeding (≤2%), breast swelling (≤1%), breast tenderness (≤1%), genital discharge (≤1%), uterine disease (≤1%), uterine hemorrhage (≤1%), vaginal dryness (≤1%), vulvovaginal candidiasis (≤1%)
Infection: Herpes virus infection (≤1%)
Neuromuscular & skeletal: Arthralgia (2%), muscle spasm (≤2%), back pain (≤1%), limb pain (≤1%)
Respiratory: Dyspnea (≤1%), epistaxis (≤1%), pharyngitis (≤1%)
Miscellaneous: Fever (≤1%)

Mechanism of Action Prevents progestin from binding to the progesterone receptor. Ulipristal postpones follicular rupture when administered prior to ovulation, thereby inhibiting or delaying ovulation. May also alter the normal endometrium, impairing implantation. When used for the treatment of signs and symptoms of uterine fibroids, ulipristal reduces the size of uterine fibroids by inhibiting cellular proliferation and inducing apoptosis.

Pharmacodynamics/Kinetics

Half-life Elimination Ulipristal: ~32 to 38 hours; Monodemethylated metabolite: ~27 hours

Time to Peak Serum: 1 hour (ulipristal and monodemethylated metabolite)

Reproductive Considerations
When used for emergency contraception, exclude pregnancy prior to therapy; ulipristal is not indicated for terminating an existing pregnancy. A rapid return of fertility is expected following use for emergency contraception; routine contraceptive measures should be initiated or continued following use to ensure ongoing prevention of pregnancy. Barrier contraception is recommended immediately following emergency contraception and throughout the same menstrual cycle; efficacy of hormonal contraceptives may be decreased. The manufacturer recommends waiting ≥5 days after taking ulipristal before resuming oral contraceptives. The CDC notes any contraceptive method may be started immediately after taking ulipristal; however, a barrier method should also be used for 14 days following the dose (or until menses occurs, whichever occurs first) (Curtis 2016a). The manufacturer labeling suggests that ulipristal may be less effective in females with BSA >30 kg/m^2.

When ulipristal is used for treatment of uterine fibroids (Canadian labeling; not in US labeling) a nonhormonal method of contraception is recommended.

Pregnancy Considerations
Use is contraindicated during a known or suspected pregnancy.

Isolated cases of major malformations have been reported following inadvertent use during pregnancy; however, data are not sufficient to determine a causal relationship and no pattern of adverse outcomes has been identified.

When used for emergency contraception, exclude pregnancy prior to therapy; ulipristal is not indicated for terminating an existing pregnancy.

Dental Health Professional Considerations Current hormone contraceptives should not be considered a risk factor for gingival or periodontal disease (Preshaw, 2013).

- ◆ **Ulipristal Acetate** *see* Ulipristal *on page 1506*
- ◆ **Uloric** *see* Febuxostat *on page 637*
- ◆ **Ultiva** *see* Remifentanil *on page 1315*
- ◆ **Ultomiris** *see* Ravulizumab *on page 1313*
- ◆ **Ultracet** *see* Acetaminophen and Tramadol *on page 71*
- ◆ **Ultrafoam Sponge 2x6.25x7CM** *see* Collagen Hemostat *on page 410*
- ◆ **Ultrafoam Sponge 8x6.25x1CM** *see* Collagen Hemostat *on page 410*
- ◆ **Ultrafoam Sponge 8x12.5x1CM** *see* Collagen Hemostat *on page 410*
- ◆ **Ultrafoam Sponge 8x12.5x3CM** *see* Collagen Hemostat *on page 410*
- ◆ **Ultrafoam Sponge 8x25x1CM** *see* Collagen Hemostat *on page 410*
- ◆ **Ultra Freeda A-Free [OTC]** *see* Vitamins (Multiple/Oral) *on page 1550*
- ◆ **Ultra Freeda Iron-Free [OTC]** *see* Vitamins (Multiple/Oral) *on page 1550*
- ◆ **Ultra Freeda With Iron [OTC]** *see* Vitamins (Multiple/Oral) *on page 1550*
- ◆ **Ultram** *see* TraMADol *on page 1468*
- ◆ **Ultram ER [DSC]** *see* TraMADol *on page 1468*
- ◆ **Ultra-Rapid Lispro** *see* Insulin Lispro *on page 824*

Umeclidinium (ue me kli DIN ee um)

Brand Names: US Incruse Ellipta
Brand Names: Canada Incruse Ellipta
Pharmacologic Category Anticholinergic Agent; Anticholinergic Agent, Long-Acting
Use Chronic obstructive pulmonary disease: Maintenance treatment of patients with COPD.
Local Anesthetic/Vasoconstrictor Precautions No information available to require special precautions
Effects on Dental Treatment Key adverse event(s) related to dental treatment: Nasopharyngitis, toothache have been reported
Effects on Bleeding No information available to require special precautions

Adverse Reactions

1% to 10%:

Cardiovascular: Tachycardia (1%)

Gastrointestinal: Toothache (1%), upper abdominal pain (1%)

Hematologic & oncologic: Bruise (1%)

Neuromuscular & skeletal: Arthralgia (2%), myalgia (1%)

Respiratory: Nasopharyngitis (8%), upper respiratory tract infection (5%), cough (3%), pharyngitis (1%), viral upper respiratory tract infection (1%)

<1%, postmarketing, and/or case reports: Anaphylaxis, atrial fibrillation, blurred vision, dysgeusia, dysuria, eye pain, glaucoma, hypersensitivity reaction, urinary retention

Mechanism of Action Competitively and reversibly inhibits the action of acetylcholine at type 3 muscarinic (M_3) receptors in bronchial smooth muscle causing bronchodilation.

Pharmacodynamics/Kinetics

Half-life Elimination 11 hours

Time to Peak 5 to 15 minutes

Pregnancy Considerations Adverse events were not observed in animal reproduction studies. Systemic absorption following oral inhalation in negligible.

Umeclidinium and Vilanterol

(ue me kli DIN ee um & VYE lan ter ol)

Brand Names: US Anoro Ellipta

Brand Names: Canada Anoro Ellipta

Pharmacologic Category Anticholinergic Agent; Anticholinergic Agent, Long-Acting; Beta$_2$ Agonist; Beta$_2$-Adrenergic Agonist, Long-Acting

Use Chronic obstructive pulmonary disease: Maintenance treatment of airflow obstruction in patients with chronic obstructive pulmonary disease, including chronic bronchitis and emphysema.

Local Anesthetic/Vasoconstrictor Precautions No information available to require special precautions

Effects on Dental Treatment No significant effects or complications reported

Effects on Bleeding No information available to require special precautions

Adverse Reactions Also see umeclidinium monograph for additional reactions.

1% to 10%:

Cardiovascular: Chest pain (1%)

Central nervous system: Headache (≥1%), vertigo (≥1%)

Endocrine & metabolic: Diabetes mellitus (≥1%)

Gastrointestinal: Diarrhea (2%), abdominal pain (≥1%), nausea (≥1%), toothache (≥1%), constipation (1%)

Genitourinary: Urinary tract infection (≥1%)

Neuromuscular & skeletal: Limb pain (2%), arthralgia (≥1%), back pain (≥1%), muscle spasm (1%), neck pain (1%)

Respiratory: Pharyngitis (2%), cough (≥1%), lower respiratory tract infection (≥1%), pleuritic chest pain (≥1%), sinusitis (≥1%)

<1%, postmarketing, and/or case reports: Atrial fibrillation, anxiety, blurred vision, chest discomfort, conjunctivitis, dysgeusia, dyspepsia, dysuria, gastroesophageal reflux disease, glaucoma, hypersensitivity reaction (including anaphylaxis, angioedema and urticaria), increased intraocular pressure, musculoskeletal chest pain, myocardial infarction, palpitations, paradoxical bronchospasm, pruritus, skin rash, supraventricular extrasystole, urinary retention, tremor, ventricular premature contractions, voice disorder, vomiting, weakness, xerostomia

Mechanism of Action

Umeclidinium: A long-acting anticholinergic, competitively and reversibly inhibits the action of acetylcholine at type 3 muscarinic (M_3) receptors in bronchial smooth muscle causing bronchodilation.

Vilanterol: A long-acting beta$_2$-agonist, relaxes bronchial smooth muscle by selective action on beta$_2$-receptors with little effect on heart rate.

Pharmacodynamics/Kinetics

Half-life Elimination 11 hours

Pregnancy Risk Factor C

Pregnancy Considerations Animal reproduction studies have not been conducted with this combination. Beta-agonists have the potential to affect uterine contractility if administered during labor. See individual monographs.

- ◆ **Umeclidinium Brm/Vilanterol Tr** *see* Umeclidinium and Vilanterol *on page 1508*
- ◆ **Umeclidinium Bromide** *see* Umeclidinium *on page 1507*
- ◆ **Umeclidinium Bromide and Vilanterol** *see* Umeclidinium and Vilanterol *on page 1508*
- ◆ **Unasyn** *see* Ampicillin and Sulbactam *on page 144*
- ◆ **UNII-LIJ4CT1Z3Y** *see* Alectinib *on page 92*
- ◆ **Uniphyl** *see* Theophylline *on page 1437*
- ◆ **Unithroid** *see* Levothyroxine *on page 900*
- ◆ **Unithroid Direct [DSC]** *see* Levothyroxine *on page 900*
- ◆ **Univasc** *see* Moexipril *on page 1044*
- ◆ **UPA** *see* Ulipristal *on page 1506*

Upadacitinib

(ue PAD a SYE ti nib)

Brand Names: US Rinvoq

Brand Names: Canada Rinvoq

Pharmacologic Category Antirheumatic Miscellaneous; Antirheumatic, Disease Modifying; Janus Associated Kinase Inhibitor

Use

Rheumatoid arthritis: Treatment of moderately to severely active rheumatoid arthritis in adults who have had an inadequate response or intolerance to methotrexate

Limitation of use: Use of upadacitinib in combination with other Janus-associated kinase inhibitors, biologic disease-modifying antirheumatic drugs, or with potent immunosuppressants such as azathioprine and cyclosporine, is not recommended.

Local Anesthetic/Vasoconstrictor Precautions No information available to require special precautions

Effects on Dental Treatment Key adverse event(s) related to dental treatment: Esophageal candidiasis (frequency not reported).

Effects on Bleeding Anemia, neutropenia (frequency not reported). Medical consult may be necessary.

Adverse Reactions

>10%: Respiratory: Upper respiratory tract infection (14%)

1% to 10%:

Gastrointestinal: Nausea (4%)

Hematologic & oncologic: Neutropenia (1%)

Hepatic: Increased serum aspartate aminotransferase (2%)

Neuromuscular & skeletal: Increased creatine phosphokinase in blood specimen (1% to 2%)
Respiratory: Cough (2%)
Miscellaneous: Fever (1%)
<1%: Herpes simplex infection, herpes zoster infection, oral candidiasis, pneumonia
Frequency not defined:
Cardiovascular: Deep vein thrombosis, pulmonary embolism, thrombosis
Dermatologic: Cellulitis
Endocrine & metabolic: Increased HDL cholesterol, increased LDL cholesterol, increased serum cholesterol, increased serum triglycerides
Gastrointestinal: Gastrointestinal perforation
Hematologic & oncologic: Malignant neoplasm, skin carcinoma
Infection: Bacterial infection, cryptococcosis, fungal infection, infection, opportunistic infection, reactivation of HBV, viral infection
Respiratory: Tuberculosis

Mechanism of Action Upadacitinib inhibits Janus kinase (JAK) enzymes, which are intracellular enzymes involved in stimulating hematopoiesis and immune cell function through a signaling pathway. JAKs activate signal transducers and activators of transcription (STATs), which regulate gene expression and intracellular activity. The inhibition of JAKs prevents the activation of STATs.

Pharmacodynamics/Kinetics

Half-life Elimination Terminal: 8 to 14 hours

Time to Peak 2 to 4 hours

Reproductive Considerations

Evaluate pregnancy status prior to use in females of reproductive potential. Females of reproductive potential should use adequate contraception during treatment and for 4 weeks following the last dose of upadacitinib.

Pregnancy Considerations

Based on data from animal reproduction studies, in utero exposure to upadacitinib may cause fetal harm.

- ◆ **Uplizna** *see* Inebilizumab *on page 808*
- ◆ **Uptravi** *see* Selexipag *on page 1364*
- ◆ **Uramit MB [DSC]** *see* Methenamine, Sodium Phosphate Monobasic, Phenyl Salicylate, Methylene Blue, and Hyoscyamine *on page 987*
- ◆ **Urate Oxidase** *see* Rasburicase *on page 1312*
- ◆ **Urate Oxidase, Pegylated** *see* Pegloticase *on page 1203*
- ◆ **Urea Peroxide** *see* Carbamide Peroxide *on page 289*
- ◆ **Urecholine [DSC]** *see* Bethanechol *on page 240*
- ◆ **Urelle** *see* Methenamine, Sodium Phosphate Monobasic, Phenyl Salicylate, Methylene Blue, and Hyoscyamine *on page 987*
- ◆ **Uretron D/S** *see* Methenamine, Sodium Phosphate Monobasic, Phenyl Salicylate, Methylene Blue, and Hyoscyamine *on page 987*
- ◆ **Urex** *see* Methenamine *on page 987*
- ◆ **Uribel** *see* Methenamine, Sodium Phosphate Monobasic, Phenyl Salicylate, Methylene Blue, and Hyoscyamine *on page 987*
- ◆ **Urimar-T** *see* Methenamine, Sodium Phosphate Monobasic, Phenyl Salicylate, Methylene Blue, and Hyoscyamine *on page 987*
- ◆ **Urinary Pain Relief [OTC]** *see* Phenazopyridine *on page 1222*
- ◆ **Urin DS** *see* Methenamine, Sodium Phosphate Monobasic, Phenyl Salicylate, Methylene Blue, and Hyoscyamine *on page 987*
- ◆ **Ur N-C [DSC]** *see* Methenamine, Sodium Phosphate Monobasic, Phenyl Salicylate, Methylene Blue, and Hyoscyamine *on page 987*
- ◆ **Uro-L [DSC]** *see* Methenamine, Sodium Phosphate Monobasic, Phenyl Salicylate, Methylene Blue, and Hyoscyamine *on page 987*
- ◆ **Uro-458** *see* Methenamine, Sodium Phosphate Monobasic, Phenyl Salicylate, Methylene Blue, and Hyoscyamine *on page 987*
- ◆ **UroAv-81** *see* Methenamine, Sodium Phosphate Monobasic, Phenyl Salicylate, Methylene Blue, and Hyoscyamine *on page 987*
- ◆ **UroAv-B** *see* Methenamine, Sodium Phosphate Monobasic, Phenyl Salicylate, Methylene Blue, and Hyoscyamine *on page 987*

Urofollitropin (yoor oh fol li TROE pin)

Brand Names: US Bravelle [DSC]

Brand Names: Canada Bravelle [DSC]

Pharmacologic Category Gonadotropin; Ovulation Stimulator

Use

Multifollicular development during Assisted Reproductive Technologies: Development of multiple follicles with Assisted Reproductive Technologies (ART) in women who have previously received pituitary suppression.

Limitations of use: Prior to therapy, perform a complete gynecologic exam and endocrinologic evaluation and diagnose cause of fertility; exclude the possibility of pregnancy; evaluate the fertility status of the male partner; exclude women with primary ovarian failure

Ovulation induction: Ovulation induction in women who previously received GnRH agonist or antagonist for pituitary suppression.

Limitations of use: Prior to therapy, perform a complete gynecologic exam (including demonstration of tubal patency) and endocrinologic evaluation; exclude the possibility of pregnancy; evaluate the fertility status of the male partner; exclude a diagnosis of primary ovarian failure

Local Anesthetic/Vasoconstrictor Precautions No information available to require special precautions

Effects on Dental Treatment No significant effects or complications reported

Effects on Bleeding Medical consult is suggested.

Adverse Reactions Percentage may vary by indication or route of administration.

>10%:
Central nervous system: Headache
Endocrine & metabolic: Ovarian hyperstimulation syndrome, ovary enlargement
Gastrointestinal: Abdominal cramps
1% to 10%:
Cardiovascular: Hypertension
Central nervous system: Depression, emotional lability, pain (including post-retrieval pain)
Dermatologic: Acne vulgaris, exfoliative dermatitis, skin rash
Endocrine & metabolic: Dehydration, hot flash, ovarian disease (cyst, pain), weight gain
Gastrointestinal: Abdominal pain, constipation, diarrhea, enlargement of abdomen, nausea, vomiting

Genitourinary: Breast tenderness, cervix disease, pelvic cramps, pelvic pain, spotting, urinary tract infection, uterine spasm, vaginal discharge, vaginal hemorrhage

Infection: Infection

Local: Injection site reaction

Neuromuscular & skeletal: Neck pain

Respiratory: Respiratory tract disease, sinusitis

Miscellaneous: Fever

Mechanism of Action Urofollitropin is a preparation of highly purified follicle-stimulating hormone (FSH) extracted from the urine of postmenopausal women. Follitropins stimulate ovarian follicular growth in women who do not have primary ovarian failure. FSH is required for normal follicular growth, maturation, gonadal steroid production, and spermatogenesis.

Pharmacodynamics/Kinetics

Half-life Elimination

IM: 37 hours (single dose), 15 hours (multiple doses)

SubQ: 32 hours (single dose), 21 hours (multiple doses)

Time to Peak

IM: 17 hours (single dose), 11 hours (multiple doses)

SubQ: 21 hours (single dose), 10 hours (multiple doses)

Pregnancy Risk Factor X

Pregnancy Considerations

Urofollitropin is used for the induction of ovulation and with assisted reproductive technologies (ART); use is contraindicated in women who are already pregnant. Ectopic pregnancy, congenital abnormalities, spontaneous abortion, and multifetal gestations/births have been reported. The incidence of congenital abnormality may be slightly higher after ART than with spontaneous conception; higher incidence may be related to parental characteristics (maternal age, genetics, sperm characteristics).

- **Uro-MP** *see* Methenamine, Sodium Phosphate Monobasic, Phenyl Salicylate, Methylene Blue, and Hyoscyamine *on page 987*
- **Urophen MB [DSC]** *see* Methenamine, Phenyl Salicylate, Methylene Blue, Benzoic Acid, and Hyoscyamine *on page 987*
- **Uroxatral** *see* Alfuzosin *on page 101*

Ustekinumab (yoo stek in YOO mab)

Brand Names: US Stelara

Brand Names: Canada Stelara

Pharmacologic Category Antipsoriatic Agent; Interleukin-12 Inhibitor; Interleukin-23 Inhibitor; Monoclonal Antibody

Use

Crohn disease: Treatment of moderately to severely active Crohn disease in adults.

Plaque psoriasis: Treatment of moderate to severe plaque psoriasis in patients ≥6 years of age who are candidates for phototherapy or systemic therapy.

Psoriatic arthritis: Treatment of active psoriatic arthritis (as monotherapy or in combination with methotrexate) in adults.

Ulcerative colitis: Treatment of moderately to severely active ulcerative colitis in adults.

Local Anesthetic/Vasoconstrictor Precautions No information available to require special precautions

Effects on Dental Treatment Key adverse event(s) related to dental treatment: A higher incidence of dental infections was observed in Stelara treated patients when compared with placebo treated patients (1% vs 0.6%) in the placebo controlled portions of the psoriatic arthritis clinical studies.

Effects on Bleeding No information available to require special precautions

Adverse Reactions

>10%:

Immunologic: Antibody development (3% to 12%; associated with reduced efficacy in psoriasis patients)

Infection: Infection (psoriasis: 27% to 72%; infection, severe: ≤3%)

Respiratory: Nasopharyngitis (11% to 24%)

1% to 10%:

Dermatologic: Acne vulgaris (Crohn disease: 1%), pruritus (2% to 4%)

Gastrointestinal: Abdominal pain (ulcerative colitis: 7%), dental disease (infection: 1%), diarrhea (ulcerative colitis: 4%), nausea (3%), vomiting (Crohn disease: 4%)

Genitourinary: Urinary tract infection (Crohn disease: 4%), vaginal mycosis (Crohn disease: ≤5%), vulvovaginal candidiasis (Crohn disease: ≤5%)

Hematologic & oncologic: Malignant neoplasm (excluding nonmelanoma: ≤2%), skin carcinoma (nonmelanoma including squamous cell carcinoma; psoriasis: 2%)

Infection: Influenza (ulcerative colitis: 6%)

Local: Erythema at injection site (1% to 5%)

Nervous system: Depression (psoriasis: 1%), dizziness (psoriasis: 2%), fatigue (3% to 4%), headache (5% to 10%)

Neuromuscular & skeletal: Arthralgia (psoriatic arthritis: 3%), asthenia (Crohn disease: 1%), back pain (psoriasis: 2%)

Respiratory: Bronchitis (Crohn disease: 5%), pharyngolaryngeal pain (psoriasis: 2%), sinusitis (3% to 4%)

Miscellaneous: Fever (ulcerative colitis: 5%)

<1%:

Dermatologic: Cellulitis

Gastrointestinal: Diverticulitis of the gastrointestinal tract

Hypersensitivity: Anaphylaxis

Infection: Herpes zoster infection

Local: Bleeding at injection site, bruising at injection site, induration at injection site, irritation at injection site, itching at injection site, pain at injection site, swelling at injection site

Nervous system: Meningitis due to listeria monocytogenes, reversible posterior leukoencephalopathy syndrome

Ophthalmic: Ocular herpes simplex

Frequency not defined:

Gastrointestinal: Appendicitis, cholecystitis, gastroenteritis

Genitourinary: Perirectal abscess

Infection: Sepsis, viral infection

Neuromuscular & skeletal: Osteomyelitis

Respiratory: Pneumonia

Postmarketing:

Dermatologic: Erythrodermic psoriasis, pustular psoriasis, skin rash, urticaria

Hypersensitivity: Angioedema, hypersensitivity reaction

Infection: Bacterial infection, fungal infection (including opportunistic)

Nervous system: Intracranial hypertension (Tan 2020)

Respiratory: Bronchiolitis obliterans organizing pneumonia, eosinophilic pneumonitis, interstitial pneumonitis, lower respiratory tract infection, tuberculosis

Mechanism of Action Ustekinumab is a human monoclonal antibody that binds to and interferes with the proinflammatory cytokines, interleukin (IL)-12 and IL-23. Biological effects of IL-12 and IL-23 include natural killer (NK) cell activation, CD4+ T-cell differentiation and activation. Ustekinumab also interferes with the expression of monocyte chemotactic protein-1 (MCP-1), tumor necrosis factor-alpha (TNF-α), interferon-inducible protein-10 (IP-10), and interleukin-8 (IL-8). Significant clinical improvement in psoriasis and psoriatic arthritis patients is seen in association with reduction of these proinflammatory signalers.

Pharmacodynamics/Kinetics

Half-life Elimination

SubQ:

Crohn disease, ulcerative colitis: Terminal: ~19 days.

Psoriasis: 14.9 ± 4.6 to 45.6 ± 80.2 days.

Time to Peak Psoriasis: SubQ: Plasma: 45 mg: 13.5 days; 90 mg: 7 days.

Reproductive Considerations

The American Academy of Dermatology considers ustekinumab for the treatment of psoriasis to be acceptable for use in male patients planning to father a child (AAD-NPF [Menter 2019]).

Women and men with well-controlled psoriasis who are planning a pregnancy and wish to avoid fetal exposure can consider discontinuing ustekinumab 15 weeks prior to attempting pregnancy (Rademaker 2018).

Treatment algorithms are available for use of biologics in female patients with Crohn disease who are planning a pregnancy (Weizman 2019). When treatment for inflammatory bowel disease is needed, biologic therapy should be optimized prior to conception (Mahadevan 2019).

Pregnancy Considerations

Ustekinumab crosses the placenta (Klenske 2019; Rowan 2018).

Ustekinumab is a humanized monoclonal antibody (IgG_1). Placental transfer of human IgG is dependent upon the IgG subclass, maternal serum concentrations, birth weight, and gestational age, generally increasing as pregnancy progresses. The lowest exposure would be expected during the period of organogenesis (Palmeira 2012; Pentsuk 2009).

Following administration to two pregnant patients with Crohn disease, cord blood concentrations of ustekinumab were ~2 to 4 times higher than maternal trough levels at delivery. In both cases, ustekinumab was administered throughout pregnancy and stopped 4 to 8 weeks prior to delivery (Klenske 2019; Rowan 2018). In one case, maternal trough concentrations remained stable throughout pregnancy (Rowan 2018).

Vaccination with live vaccines (eg, rotavirus vaccine) should be avoided for the first 6 months of life if exposure to a biologic agent occurs during the third trimester of pregnancy (eg, >27 weeks' gestation) (Mahadevan 2019).

The American Academy of Dermatology considers the safety of ustekinumab for the treatment of psoriasis in pregnancy to be uncertain (AAD-NPF [Menter 2019]).

Inflammatory bowel disease is associated with adverse pregnancy outcomes including an increased risk of miscarriage, premature delivery, delivery of a low birth weight infant, and poor maternal weight gain. Management of maternal disease should be optimized prior to pregnancy. Treatment decreases disease flares, disease activity, and the incidence of adverse pregnancy outcomes. Information related to the use of ustekinumab in pregnancy is limited. When treatment for inflammatory bowel disease is needed in pregnant women, appropriate biologic therapy can be continued without interruption. Serum levels should be evaluated prior to conception and optimized to avoid subtherapeutic concentrations or high levels which may increase placental transfer. Dosing can be adjusted so delivery occurs at the lowest serum concentration. For ustekinumab, the final injection can be given 6 to 10 weeks prior to the estimated date of delivery (4 to 5 weeks before delivery if every-4-week dosing), then continued 48 hours' postpartum (Mahadevan 2019).

- ◆ **Ustell** *see* Methenamine, Sodium Phosphate Monobasic, Phenyl Salicylate, Methylene Blue, and Hyoscyamine *on page 987*
- ◆ **Uticap** *see* Methenamine, Sodium Phosphate Monobasic, Phenyl Salicylate, Methylene Blue, and Hyoscyamine *on page 987*
- ◆ **Utira-C** *see* Methenamine, Sodium Phosphate Monobasic, Phenyl Salicylate, Methylene Blue, and Hyoscyamine *on page 987*
- ◆ **Utrona-C** *see* Methenamine, Sodium Phosphate Monobasic, Phenyl Salicylate, Methylene Blue, and Hyoscyamine *on page 987*
- ◆ **UX007** *see* Triheptanoin *on page 1498*
- ◆ **Vabomere** *see* Meropenem and Vaborbactam *on page 980*
- ◆ **Vaborbactam and Meropenem** *see* Meropenem and Vaborbactam *on page 980*

Vaccinia Immune Globulin (Intravenous)

(vax IN ee a i MYUN GLOB yoo lin IN tra VEE nus)

Brand Names: US CNJ-016

Pharmacologic Category Blood Product Derivative; Immune Globulin

Use Vaccinia conditions: Treatment and/or modification of the following conditions:

- Aberrant infections induced by vaccinia virus that include its accidental implantation in eyes (except in cases of isolated keratitis), mouth, or other areas where vaccinia infection would constitute a special hazard.
- Eczema vaccinatum
- Progressive vaccinia
- Severe generalized vaccinia
- Vaccinia infections in individuals who have skin conditions such as burns, impetigo, varicella-zoster, or poison ivy; or in individuals who have eczematous skin lesions because of either the activity or extensiveness of such lesions

The Advisory Committee on Immunization Practices (ACIP) recommends the following (CDC 2009; CDC [Rotz 2001]; CDC [Wharton 2003]):

Use is recommended for:

- Inadvertent inoculation (considering severity, toxicity of affected person, and pain)
- Eczema vaccinatum
- Generalized vaccinia (severe form or if underlying illness is present)
- Progressive vaccinia

Use may be considered for:
- Severe ocular complications except isolated keratitis

Use is not recommended for:
- Inadvertent inoculation that is not severe
- Mild or limited generalized vaccinia
- Nonspecific rashes, erythema multiforme, or Stevens-Johnson syndrome
- Postvaccinial encephalitis or encephalomyelitis

Local Anesthetic/Vasoconstrictor Precautions No information available to require special precautions

Effects on Dental Treatment No significant effects or complications reported

Effects on Bleeding No information available to require special precautions

Adverse Reactions Frequency not defined. Actual frequency varies by dose and rate of infusion.

Cardiovascular: Peripheral edema

Central nervous system: Dizziness, fatigue, feeling hot, headache, pain, paresthesia, rigors, sensation of cold

Dermatologic: Diaphoresis, erythema, pallor

Gastrointestinal: Decreased appetite, nausea, vomiting

Local: Injection site reaction

Neuromuscular & skeletal: Back pain, muscle spasm, tremor, weakness

Miscellaneous: Fever

<1%, postmarketing, and/or case reports: Abdominal pain, acute intravascular hemolysis, acute renal failure, altered blood pressure, anaphylaxis, apnea, acute respiratory distress, arthralgia, aseptic meningitis, bronchospasm, bullous rash, chills, circulatory shock, coma, cyanosis, diarrhea, dyspnea, epidermolysis, erythema multiforme, flushing, hemolysis, hepatic insufficiency, hypersensitivity reaction, hypoxemia, hypotension, leukopenia, loss of consciousness, malaise, myalgia, pancytopenia, positive direct Coombs test, proximal tubular nephropathy, pulmonary edema, renal disease (osmotic nephropathy), renal insufficiency, seizure, Stevens-Johnson syndrome, syncope, tachycardia, thrombocytopenia, thromboembolism, transfusion-related acute lung injury (TRALI), urticaria, wheezing

Mechanism of Action Antibodies obtained from pooled human plasma of individuals immunized with the smallpox vaccine provide passive immunity

Pharmacodynamics/Kinetics

Half-life Elimination 30 days (range: 13 to 67 days)

Time to Peak Plasma: 1.8 to 2.6 hours

Pregnancy Risk Factor C

Pregnancy Considerations Animal reproduction studies have not been conducted. Immune globulins cross the placenta in increased amounts after 30 weeks gestation. There are no adequate and well-controlled studies in pregnant women. Vaccinia immune globulin is currently not recommended for use in persons with contraindications to smallpox vaccine; inadvertent exposure to smallpox vaccine in high risk populations (eg, pregnant women) should be reported to the CDC so that standardized treatment may be provided.

Prescribing and Access Restrictions Vaccinia immune globulin is not available for general public use. All supplies are currently owned by the federal government for inclusion in the Strategic National Stockpile. The CDC Smallpox Adverse Events Clinical Consultation team will coordinate shipment. The State Health Department should be contacted first concerning severe or unexpected adverse events from smallpox vaccination.

◆ **Vagistat-1 [OTC] [DSC]** *see* Tioconazole *on page 1450*

◆ **Vagistat-3 [OTC] [DSC]** *see* Miconazole (Topical) *on page 1019*

ValACYclovir (val ay SYE kloe veer)

Related Information

Acyclovir (Systemic) *on page 75*

Systemic Viral Diseases *on page 1709*

Viral Infections *on page 1754*

Related Sample Prescriptions

Viral Infections - Sample Prescriptions *on page 43*

Brand Names: US Valtrex

Brand Names: Canada APO-Valacyclovir; Auro-Valacyclovir; BIO-Valacyclovir; CO Valacyclovir [DSC]; DOM-Valacyclovir; JAMP-Valacyclovir; Mar-Valacyclovir [DSC]; MYLAN-Valacyclovir; PHL-Valacyclovir [DSC]; PMS-Valacyclovir; Priva-Valacyclovir; PRO-Valacyclovir; RIVA-Valacyclovir; SANDOZ Valacyclovir; TEVA-Valacyclovir; Valtrex

Generic Availability (US) Yes

Pharmacologic Category Antiviral Agent; Antiviral Agent, Oral

Dental Use Treatment of herpes labialis (cold sores)

Use Treatment of herpes zoster (shingles) in immunocompetent patients; treatment of first-episode and recurrent genital herpes in immunocompetent patients; suppression of recurrent genital herpes and reduction of transmission of genital herpes in immunocompetent patients; suppression of genital herpes in patients with HIV; treatment of herpes labialis (cold sores); treatment of chickenpox in immunocompetent children

Local Anesthetic/Vasoconstrictor Precautions No information available to require special precautions

Effects on Dental Treatment No significant effects or complications reported (see Dental Health Professional Considerations)

Effects on Bleeding There have been rare cases of thrombotic thrombocytopenia purpura (TTP) in HIV-infected patients exposed to valacyclovir at both high doses (8 g/day) and low doses (500 mg twice daily) (see Dental Health Professional Considerations). Although the link between the HIV-infected patient's TTP and valacyclovir may be circumstantial, it is suggested to monitor the patient for hematologic effects during exposure to valacyclovir.

Adverse Reactions

>10%:

Central nervous system: Headache (13% to 38%)

Gastrointestinal: Nausea (5% to 15%), abdominal pain (1% to 11%)

Hepatic: Increased serum AST (2% to 16%), increased serum ALT (≤14%)

Respiratory: Nasopharyngitis (≤16%)

1% to 10%:

Central nervous system: Fatigue (≤8%), depression (≤7%), dizziness (2% to 4%)

Dermatologic: Skin rash (≤8%)

Endocrine & metabolic: Dehydration (children: 2%)

Gastrointestinal: Vomiting (≤6%), diarrhea (children: 5%; adults: <1%)

Genitourinary: Dysmenorrhea (≤8%)

Hematologic & oncologic: Thrombocytopenia (≤3%), leukopenia (≤1%; mild)

Hepatic: Increased serum alkaline phosphatase (≤4%)

Infection: Herpes simplex infection (children: 2%)

Neuromuscular & skeletal: Arthralgia (≤6%)

Respiratory: Rhinorrhea (children: 2%)

Miscellaneous: Fever (children: 4%)

<1%, postmarketing, and/or case reports: Aggressive behavior, agitation, alopecia, anemia, aplastic anemia, ataxia, brain disease, coma, confusion, delirium, dysarthria, erythema multiforme, facial edema, hallucination (auditory and visual), hemolytic-uremic syndrome, hepatitis, hypersensitivity reaction (acute; includes anaphylaxis, angioedema, dyspnea, pruritus, skin rash, urticaria), hypertension, hypersensitivity angiitis, increased serum creatinine, loss of consciousness, mania, psychosis, renal failure, renal pain, seizure, skin photosensitivity, tachycardia, thrombotic thrombocytopenic purpura, tremor, urinary urgency, visual disturbance

Dental Usual Dosage

Herpes labialis (cold sores): Adolescents and Adults: Oral: 2 g twice daily for 1 day (separate doses by ~12 hours)

Chronic suppression of recurrent herpes labialis (cold sores) (off-label use): Immunocompetent adults: 500 mg once daily (Baker 2003)

Dosing

Adult & Geriatric

Bell palsy, new onset (adjunctive therapy) (off-label use): Oral: 1 g 3 times daily for 7 days in combination with corticosteroids; begin within 3 days of symptom onset (AAO-HNSF [Baugh 2013]; Axelsson 2003; Engström 2008). **Note:** Antiviral therapy alone is **not** recommended (AAN [Gronseth 2012]; AAO-HNSF [Baugh 2013]); some experts only recommend addition of an antiviral to steroid therapy in patients with severe Bell palsy (de Almeida 2014; Hato 2008).

Cytomegalovirus, prevention in allogeneic hematopoietic cell transplant recipients (alternative agent) (off-label use): High-risk patients (cytomegalovirus [CMV]-seropositive hematopoietic cell transplant [HCT] recipients and CMV-seronegative HCT recipients with a CMV-seropositive donor): Oral: 2 g 3 to 4 times daily, beginning at engraftment and continued to day 100 (ASBMT/IDSA [Tomblyn 2009]) **or** 2 g 3 times daily, started after initial therapy with IV ganciclovir from day −8 to day −2 prior to transplant, and continued until engraftment or longer in patients on glucocorticoids (Milano 2001; Wingard 2020). **Note:** Both strategies should be combined with screening for CMV reactivation (ASBMT/IDSA [Tomblyn 2009]; Wingard 2020).

Herpes simplex virus, mucocutaneous infection:

Genital:

Immunocompetent patients:

Treatment, initial episode: **Oral**: 1 g twice daily for 7 to 10 days; extend duration if lesion has not healed completely after 10 days (CDC [Workowski 2015]).

Treatment, recurrent episode: **Oral:** 500 mg twice daily for 3 days **or** 1 g once daily for 5 days. **Note:** Treatment is most effective when initiated during the prodrome or within 1 day of lesion onset (CDC [Workowski 2015]).

Suppressive therapy (eg, for severe and/or frequent recurrences): **Oral:** 500 mg or 1 g once daily. **Note:** Reassess need periodically (eg, annually). The 500 mg daily dose may be less effective in patients who experience very frequent (≥10) recurrences per year (CDC [Workowski 2015]).

Immunocompromised patients (including patients with HIV):

Treatment, initial or recurrent episode: **Oral:** 1 g twice daily for 5 to 10 days; extend treatment duration if lesions have not healed completely after 10 days. **Note:** Severe disease should be treated with IV acyclovir for the first 2 to 7 days; may switch to valacyclovir when lesions begin to regress and continue for at least 10 days total and until lesions have resolved completely (CDC [Workowski 2015]; HHS [OI adult 2020]).

Suppressive therapy (eg, for severe and/or frequent recurrences): **Oral:** 500 mg twice daily. **Note:** Reassess need periodically (eg, annually) (CDC [Workowski 2015]; HHS [OI adult 2020]).

Pregnant females:

Treatment, initial episode (alternative agent): **Oral:** 1 g twice daily for 7 to 10 days; extend duration if lesion has not healed completely after 10 days (ACOG 2007; Riley 2020).

Treatment, recurrent episode (symptomatic) (alternative agent): **Oral:** 500 mg twice daily for 3 days **or** 1 g once daily for 5 days (ACOG 2007). **Note:** Some experts reserve treatment of recurrent episodes for patients with severe and/or frequent symptoms (Riley 2020).

Suppressive therapy, for patients with a genital HSV lesion anytime during pregnancy (alternative agent): **Oral:** 500 mg twice daily, beginning at 36 weeks' gestation and continued until onset of labor (ACOG 2007; CDC [Workowski 2015]; Riley 2020). **Note:** Some experts offer suppressive therapy earlier than 36 weeks' gestation for women who have a first-episode lesion during the third trimester (Riley 2020).

Orolabial: **Note:** Initiate therapy at earliest symptom.

Immunocompetent patients:

Cold sores (herpes labialis): **Oral:** 2 g twice daily for 1 day (manufacturer's labeling).

Primary infection (eg, gingivostomatitis): **Oral:** 1 g twice daily for 7 to 10 days (Klein 2020).

Suppressive therapy (eg, for severe and/or frequent recurrences): **Oral:** 500 mg or 1 g once daily (Baker 2003; Gilbert 2007). **Note:** Reassess need periodically (eg, annually) (HHS [OI adult 2020]).

Immunocompromised patients (including patients with HIV):

Treatment, initial or recurrent episode: **Oral:** 1 g twice daily for 5 to 10 days and until complete lesion resolution (HHS [OI adult 2020]).

Suppressive therapy (eg, for severe and/or frequent recurrences): **Oral:** 500 mg twice daily. **Note:** Reassess need periodically (eg, annually) (HHS [OI adult 2020]).

Herpes simplex virus, prevention in immunocompromised patients (off-label use):

Seropositive HCT recipients (allogeneic or autologous) or seropositive patients undergoing leukemia induction chemotherapy: **Oral:** 500 mg twice daily (ASBMT/IDSA [Tomblyn 2009]; Wingard 2018). Initiate with the chemotherapeutic or conditioning regimen and continue until recovery of WBC count and resolution of mucositis; duration may be extended in patients with frequent recurrences or graft-vs-host disease (GVHD) (ASBMT/IDSA [Tomblyn 2009]; ASCO/IDSA [Taplitz 2018]).

Solid organ transplant recipients (HSV-seropositive patients who do **not** require CMV prophylaxis): **Oral:** 500 mg twice daily for at least 1 month (Wilck 2013); some experts recommend continuing for 3 to 6 months after transplantation and during periods of lymphodepletion associated with treatment of rejection (Fishman 2020).

Herpes zoster (shingles), treatment:

Immunocompetent patients: **Oral:** 1 g 3 times daily for 7 days. Initiate at earliest sign or symptom; treatment is most effective when initiated ≤72 hours after rash onset, but may initiate treatment >72 hours after rash onset if new lesions are continuing to appear (Cohen 1999).

Immunocompromised patients (including patients with HIV):

Acute localized dermatomal: **Oral:** 1 g 3 times daily for 7 to 10 days; consider longer duration if lesions resolve slowly (AST-IDCOP [Pergam 2019]; HHS [OI adult 2020]).

Extensive cutaneous lesions or visceral involvement: **Oral:** 1 g 3 times daily to complete a 10- to 14-day course. **Note:** Patients should receive initial treatment with IV acyclovir; when formation of new lesions has ceased and signs/symptoms of visceral infection are improving, may then switch to valacyclovir (AST-IDCOP [Pergam 2019]; HHS [OI adult 2020]).

Herpes zoster ophthalmicus (off-label use): Immunocompetent patients: **Oral:** 1 g 3 times daily for 7 days (Colin 2000). **Note:** Immunocompromised patients and patients who require hospitalization for sight-threatening disease should receive IV acyclovir (Albrecht 2020b).

Varicella (chickenpox), uncomplicated, treatment (off-label): Oral: 1 g 3 times daily. **Note:** Ideally initiate therapy within 24 hours of symptom onset, but may start later if patient still has active skin lesions; continue treatment for at least 5 to 7 days and until all lesions have crusted. Immunocompromised patients generally require IV acyclovir; however, for patients with uncomplicated or mild disease (<50 lesions), some experts treat with valacyclovir (Albrecht 2020a; HHS [OI adult 2020]).

Varicella zoster virus, acute retinal necrosis (off-label use): Oral: 1 g 3 times daily for approximately 6 weeks (following initial treatment with IV acyclovir) (Aizman 2007; Albrecht 2020b; Aslanides 2002; HHS [OI adult 2020]); in patients with HIV, duration is ≥14 weeks and intravitreal ganciclovir should be added (HHS [OI adult 2020]).

Varicella zoster virus, prevention in immunocompromised patients (off-label use):

HCT recipients (allogeneic and autologous):

Postexposure prophylaxis: **Oral:** 1 g 3 times daily; initiate within 96 hours (preferably within 48 hours) of exposure and continue until 22 days after exposure. **Note:** Indicated following exposure **if varicella-zoster immune globulin is unavailable** in seronegative HCT recipients who are <24 months after HCT **or** >24 months after HCT and on immunosuppressive therapy or have chronic GVHD (ASBMT/IDSA [Tomblyn 2009]).

Prevention of VZV reactivation in seropositive patients: **Oral:** 500 mg twice daily for 1 year following transplantation; may extend duration in patients requiring ongoing immunosuppression (some experts continue prophylaxis in these patients until 6 months after discontinuation of all systemic immunosuppression) (ASBMT/IDSA [Tomblyn 2009]).

Solid organ transplant recipients (VZV-seropositive patients who do **not** require CMV prophylaxis): **Oral:** 500 mg twice daily for 3 to 6 months after transplantation and during periods of lymphodepletion associated with treatment of rejection (AST-IDCOP [Pergam 2019]; Fishman 2020).

Renal Impairment: Adult

Herpes zoster (shingles), treatment:

CrCl 30 to 49 mL/minute: Oral: 1 g every 12 hours
CrCl 10 to 29 mL/minute: Oral: 1 g every 24 hours
CrCl <10 mL/minute: Oral: 500 mg every 24 hours

Herpes simplex virus, genital:

Initial episode:
CrCl 10 to 29 mL/minute: Oral: 1 g every 24 hours
CrCl <10 mL/minute: Oral: 500 mg every 24 hours

Recurrent episode: CrCl <29 mL/minute: Oral: 500 mg every 24 hours

Suppressive therapy: CrCl <29 mL/minute: Oral:

For usual dose of 1 g every 24 hours or 500 mg every 12 hours, decrease dose to 500 mg every 24 hours

For usual dose of 500 mg every 24 hours, decrease dose to 500 mg every 48 hours

Herpes simplex virus, orolabial (immunocompetent patients):

CrCl 30 to 49 mL/minute: Oral: 1 g every 12 hours for 2 doses

CrCl 10 to 29 mL/minute: Oral: 500 mg every 12 hours for 2 doses

CrCl <10 mL/minute: Oral: 500 mg as a single dose

Hemodialysis: Dialyzable (~33% removed during 4-hour session); administer dose postdialysis

Chronic ambulatory peritoneal dialysis/continuous arteriovenous hemofiltration dialysis: Pharmacokinetic parameters are similar to those in patients with ESRD; supplemental dose not needed following dialysis

Hepatic Impairment: Adult No dosage adjustment necessary.

Pediatric

Herpes labialis (cold sores), treatment:

Immunocompetent: Children ≥12 years and Adolescents: Oral: 2,000 mg every 12 hours for 1 day (2 doses); initiate at earliest symptom onset

HIV-exposed/-positive: Adolescents: Oral: 1,000 mg twice daily for 5 to 10 days (HHS [adult OI 2017])

Herpes simplex virus (HSV), genital infection; *immuncompetent* patients: Limited data available:

First episode; treatment: Children and Adolescents: Oral: 20 **mg/kg**/dose twice daily, maximum dose: 1,000 mg/dose; for 7 to 10 days (Bradley 2017; CDC [Workowski 2015])

Recurrent episodes; treatment: Begin with onset of symptoms (prodrome) or lesion appearance (CDC [Workowski 2015]): Children and Adolescents:

Patient weight <50 kg: Oral: 20 **mg/kg**/dose twice daily; maximum dose: 1,000 mg/dose; for 5 days (Bradley 2017)

Patient weight ≥50 kg: Oral: 1,000 mg once daily for 5 days (CDC [Workowski 2015])

Suppressive therapy: Children and Adolescents: Oral: 20 **mg/kg**/dose once daily; maximum dose: 1,000 mg/dose (Bradley 2017; CDC [Workowski 2015])

Herpes simplex virus (HSV), prophylaxis in *immunocompromised* patients (eg, HSCT or leukopenic oncology patients): Limited data available (Erard 2007; IDSA [Tomblyn 2009]): Children and Adolescents: Oral:

Early reactivation prevention: Begin at initiation of conditioning and continue until engraftment or resolution of mucositis (IDSA [Tomblyn 2009)

Patient weight <40 kg: 250 mg twice daily

Patient weight ≥40 kg: 500 mg once or twice daily; twice daily dosing should be considered in patients who are highly suppressed

Late reactivation prevention: Continue throughout the first year following HSCT (Erard 2007; IDSA [Tomblyn 2009])

Patient weight <40 kg: 250 mg twice daily

Patient weight ≥40 kg: 500 mg once or twice daily; twice daily dosing should be considered in patients who are highly suppressed

Herpes simplex virus (HSV), treatment of acute retinal disease; step-down therapy: Limited data available: Children ≥50 kg or Adolescents: Oral: 1,000 mg 3 times daily for 4 to 6 weeks; begin after completion of a 10 to 14 day intravenous acyclovir course (HHS [adult OI 2017, pediatric OI 2016])

Herpes simplex virus (HSV), treatment of mucocutaneous infection or gingivostomatitis; *immunocompetent* patients: Limited data available: Infants ≥3 months, Children, and Adolescents: Oral: 20 **mg/kg**/dose twice daily for 5 to 7 days; maximum dose: 1,000 mg/dose (Bradley 2017; Kimberlin 2010)

Mononucleosis (Epstein-Barr virus [EBV]); treatment: Limited data available; efficacy results variable: Adolescents: 1,000 mg 3 times daily; a small trial in college-aged students (age ≥18 years) showed a 14-day course of valacyclovir reduced EBV oral excretion (Balfour 2007; Bradley 2017)

Varicella (chickenpox), prophylaxis in *immunocompromised* patients (eg, HSCT or leukopenic oncology): Limited data available: Children and Adolescents:

Weight-directed: Oral: 15 to 30 **mg/kg**/dose 3 times daily (Bomgaars 2008; Nadal 2002)

Fixed dosing:

Patient weight <40 kg: Oral: 250 or 500 mg twice daily (Erard 2007; IDSA [Tomblyn 2009])

Patient weight ≥40 kg: Oral: 500 mg twice daily (Erard 2007; IDSA [Tomblyn 2009])

Post exposure prophylaxis (IDSA [Tomblyn 2009]): **Note:** Continue for 22 days postexposure.

Patient weight <40 kg: Oral: 500 mg 3 times daily

Patient weight ≥40 kg: Oral: 1,000 mg 3 times daily

Varicella (chickenpox), treatment in *immunocompetent* patients: Note: Routine use in otherwise healthy children not generally recommended; treatment of varicella may be considered in individuals at high risk for a possible moderate-severe course (eg, unvaccinated adolescents, individuals with chronic cutaneous or pulmonary conditions, patients on long-term salicylate therapy or receiving short, intermittent, or aerosolized corticosteroids (*Red Book* [AAP 2015]): Infants ≥3 months, Children, and Adolescents <18 years: Limited data available in patients <2 years of age: Oral: 20 **mg/kg**/dose 3 times daily for 5 days; maximum dose: 1,000 mg/dose; initiate within 24 hours of rash onset (Bradley 2017; *Red Book* [AAP 2015]

Renal Impairment: Pediatric

Herpes labialis: Adolescents:

CrCl 30 to 49 mL/minute: 1,000 mg every 12 hours for 2 doses

CrCl 10 to 29 mL/minute: 500 mg every 12 hours for 2 doses

CrCl <10 mL/minute: 500 mg as a single dose

Genital herpes: Adolescents:

Initial episode:

CrCl 10 to 29 mL/minute: 1,000 mg every 24 hours

CrCl <10 mL/minute: 500 mg every 24 hours

Recurrent episode: CrCl ≤29 mL/minute: 500 mg every 24 hours

Suppressive therapy: CrCl ≤29 mL/minute:

For usual dose of 1,000 mg every 24 hours, decrease dose to 500 mg every 24 hours

For usual dose of 500 mg every 24 hours, decrease dose to 500 mg every 48 hours

HIV-infected patients: 500 mg every 24 hours

Hemodialysis: Dialyzable (~33% removed during 4-hour session); administer dose postdialysis

Hepatic Impairment: Pediatric Children ≥2 years and Adolescents: No dosage adjustment necessary.

Mechanism of Action Valacyclovir is rapidly and nearly completely converted to acyclovir by intestinal and hepatic metabolism. Acyclovir is converted to acyclovir monophosphate by virus-specific thymidine kinase then further converted to acyclovir triphosphate by other cellular enzymes. Acyclovir triphosphate inhibits DNA synthesis and viral replication by competing with deoxyguanosine triphosphate for viral DNA polymerase and being incorporated into viral DNA.

Contraindications Hypersensitivity to valacyclovir, acyclovir, or any component of the formulation

Warnings/Precautions Thrombotic microangiopathy has occurred in immunocompromised patients (at doses of 8 g/day). Safety and efficacy have not been established for treatment/suppression of recurrent genital herpes or disseminated herpes in patients with profound immunosuppression (eg, advanced HIV with CD4 <100 cells/mm^3). CNS adverse effects (including agitation, hallucinations, confusion, delirium, seizures, and encephalopathy) have been reported. Use caution in patients with renal impairment, the elderly, and/or those receiving nephrotoxic agents. Acute renal failure has been observed in patients with renal dysfunction; dose adjustment may be required. Precipitation in renal tubules may occur leading to urinary precipitation; adequately hydrate patient. For cold sores, treatment should begin at the earliest symptom (tingling, itching, burning). For genital herpes, treatment should begin as soon as possible after the first signs and symptoms (within 72 hours of onset of first diagnosis or within 24 hours of onset of recurrent episodes). For herpes zoster, treatment should begin within 72 hours of onset of rash. For chickenpox, treatment should begin with earliest sign or symptom. Use with caution in the elderly; CNS effects have been reported.

Warnings: Additional Pediatric Considerations CNS adverse events (eg, agitation, hallucinations, confusion, delirium, seizures, and encephalopathy) have been reported in children with and without renal dysfunction receiving doses exceeding those recommended for current renal function.

Drug Interactions

Metabolism/Transport Effects Inhibits CYP1A2 (weak)

Avoid Concomitant Use

Avoid concomitant use of ValACYclovir with any of the following: Cladribine; Foscarnet; Varicella Virus Vaccine; Zoster Vaccine (Live/Attenuated)

Increased Effect/Toxicity

ValACYclovir may increase the levels/effects of: CloZAPine; Mycophenolate; Tenofovir Products; Theophylline Derivatives; TiZANidine; Zidovudine

The levels/effects of ValACYclovir may be increased by: Foscarnet; Mycophenolate; Tenofovir Products

Decreased Effect

ValACYclovir may decrease the levels/effects of: Cladribine; Talimogene Laherparepvec; Varicella Virus Vaccine; Zoster Vaccine (Live/Attenuated)

Pharmacodynamics/Kinetics

Half-life Elimination Normal renal function: Children: 1.3 to 2.5 hours, slower clearance with increased age; Adults: 2.5 to 3.3 hours (acyclovir), ~30 minutes (valacyclovir); End-stage renal disease: 14 to 20 hours (acyclovir); During hemodialysis: 4 hours

Time to Peak Children: 1.4 to 2.6 hours; Adults: 1.5 hours

Pregnancy Considerations

Valacyclovir is metabolized to acyclovir. In a pharmacokinetic study, maternal acyclovir serum concentrations were higher in pregnant females receiving valacyclovir than those given acyclovir for the suppression of recurrent herpes simplex virus (HSV) infection late in pregnancy. Amniotic fluid concentrations were also higher; however, there was no evidence that fetal exposure differed between the groups (Kimberlin 1998).

Data from an acyclovir pregnancy registry have shown no increased rate of birth defects than that of the general population; however, there are insufficient data regarding miscarriage or adverse maternal or fetal outcomes.

Untreated herpes simplex during pregnancy increases the risk for fetal complications, including (but not limited to) neonatal chorioretinitis, microcephaly, and skin lesions. Rarely, transplacental transmission resulting in congenital infection may occur. In addition, maternal coinfection with HSV increases the risk for perinatal HIV transmission.

Because more data is available for acyclovir, that agent is preferred for the treatment of genital herpes in pregnant females (CDC [Workowski 2015]); however, valacyclovir may be considered for use due to its simplified dosing schedule (HHS [OI adult 2020]). Pregnant females who have a history of genital herpes recurrence, suppressive therapy is recommended starting at 36 weeks' gestation (ACOG 2007; CDC [Workowski 2015]; HHS [OI adult 2020]).

Breastfeeding Considerations

Valacyclovir is rapidly metabolized to acyclovir. Following administration of valacyclovir, acyclovir is present in breast milk; unchanged valacyclovir has not been detected in breast milk.

Peak acyclovir milk concentrations occurred 4 hours (range: 2 to 4 hours) following maternal administration of a single oral dose of valacyclovir 500 mg to five postpartum females; the half-life of acyclovir in breast milk was ~2 hours (range: 1.3 to 12.2 hours). Acyclovir was detected in the urine of breastfeeding infants following 5 days of maternal treatment with valacyclovir 500 mg twice daily (Sheffield 2002).

According to the manufacturer, the decision to continue or discontinue breastfeeding during therapy should consider the risk of infant exposure, the benefits of breastfeeding to the infant, and the benefits of treatment to the mother. Other sources note that females with HSV infection taking valacyclovir may breastfeed as long as there are not lesions on the breast, body lesions are covered, and strict hand hygiene is practiced (ACOG 82 2007; Jaiyeoba 2012).

Dosage Forms: US

Tablet, Oral:

Valtrex: 500 mg, 1 g

Generic: 500 mg, 1 g

Dosage Forms: Canada

Tablet, Oral:

Valtrex: 500 mg, 1 g

Generic: 500 mg, 1000 mg, 1 g

Dental Health Professional Considerations

Although some conflicting data, dental treatment may be a risk factor for asymptomatic viral shedding of herpes simplex virus type-1 (HSV-1) into human saliva in patients with previous exposure to the virus (Hyland 2007).

It is recommended to reappoint the patient if an active lesion is present. If the lesion is already "crusted" over, treatment will not induce spread of the virus but treatment is aimed at patient comfort during the procedure relating to the wound healing on their lip.

Cases of thrombotic thrombocytopenia purpura (TTP) have been reported in patients who are infected with human immunodeficiency virus (HIV). Manifestations resembling TTP have been reported in HIV-infected patients who were treated with high-dose valacyclovir, 8 g/day. The authors reported in this 2000 issue of Archives of a case of TTP in an HIV-infected patient who was treated with a lower dose of valacyclovir. The patient was on antiretroviral therapy and receiving valacyclovir hydrochloride therapy for 1 year (500 mg twice daily) for recurrent ocular herpes simplex virus infection. The patient was diagnosed as having TTP with fever, neurological changes, renal dysfunction, and thrombocytopenia. The authors state that the link between the TTP and valacyclovir therapy in this case may have been circumstantial; HIV may have been the causative agent. Other studies have reported no cases of TTP among more than 700 HIV-infected patients who were treated with valacyclovir 1 g/day; however, this case highlights the importance of monitoring HIV-infected patients for hematologic issues while exposed to drugs such as valacyclovir (Rivaud 2000).

◆ **Valacyclovir HCl** *see* ValACYclovir *on page 1512*

◆ **Valacyclovir Hydrochloride** *see* ValACYclovir *on page 1512*

Valbenazine (val BEN a zeen)

Brand Names: US Ingrezza

Pharmacologic Category Central Monoamine-Depleting Agent; Vesicular Monoamine Transporter 2 (VMAT2) Inhibitor

Use Tardive dyskinesia: Treatment of adults with tardive dyskinesia

Local Anesthetic/Vasoconstrictor Precautions

Valbenazine is one of the drugs confirmed to prolong the QT interval and is accepted as having a risk of causing torsades de pointes. The risk of drug-induced torsades de pointes is extremely low when a single QT interval prolonging drug is prescribed. In terms of epinephrine, it is not known what effect vasoconstrictors in the local anesthetic regimen will have in patients with a known history of congenital prolonged QT interval or in patients taking any medication that prolongs the QT interval. Until more information is obtained, it is suggested that the clinician consult with the physician prior to the use of a vasoconstrictor in suspected patients, and that the vasoconstrictor (epinephrine, levonordefrin [Neo-Cobefrin®]) be used with caution.

Effects on Dental Treatment No significant effects or complications reported

Effects on Bleeding No information available to require special precautions

Adverse Reactions

>10%: Central nervous system: Drowsiness (≤11%), fatigue (≤11%), sedation (≤11%)

1% to 10%:

Central nervous system: Abnormal gait (≤4%), dizziness (≤4%), equilibrium disturbance (≤4%), falling (≤4%), akathisia (≤3%), restlessness (≤3%), anxiety (1% to <2%), drooling (1% to <2%), extrapyramidal reaction (1% to <2%), insomnia (1% to <2%)

Endocrine & metabolic: Increased serum glucose (1% to <2%), weight gain (1% to <2%)

Gastrointestinal: Vomiting (3%)

Neuromuscular & skeletal: Arthralgia (2%), dyskinesia (1% to <2%)

Respiratory: Respiratory tract infection (1% to <2%)

Frequency not defined:

Endocrine & metabolic: Increased serum prolactin

Hepatic: Increased serum alkaline phosphatase, increased serum bilirubin

<1%, postmarketing and/or case reports: Hypersensitivity reaction, skin rash

Mechanism of Action The mechanism of action of valbenazine in the treatment of tardive dyskinesia is unknown, but is thought to be mediated through the reversible inhibition of vesicular monoamine transporter 2 (VMAT2), a transporter that regulates monoamine uptake from the cytoplasm to the synaptic vesicle for storage and release. Valbenazine and its active metabolite have no appreciable binding affinity for VMAT1 or dopaminergic, serotonergic, adrenergic, histaminergic or muscarinic receptors.

Pharmacodynamics/Kinetics

Half-life Elimination 15 to 22 hours (valbenazine and active metabolite)

Time to Peak Valbenazine: 0.5 to 1 hours; Active metabolite: 4 to 8 hours

Pregnancy Considerations Adverse events were observed in some animal reproduction studies

- ◆ **Valbenazine Tosylate** *see* Valbenazine *on page 1516*
- ◆ **Valcyte** *see* ValGANciclovir *on page 1517*
- ◆ **2-Valent HPV** *see* Papillomavirus (Types 16, 18) Vaccine (Human, Recombinant) *on page 1191*
- ◆ **4-Valent HPV** *see* Papillomavirus (Types 6, 11, 16, 18) Vaccine (Human, Recombinant) *on page 1190*
- ◆ **10-Valent Pneumococcal Nontypeable *Haemophilus influenzae* Protein D Conjugate Vaccine** *see* Pneumococcal Conjugate Vaccine (10-Valent) *on page 1241*
- ◆ **10-Valent Pneumococcal Vaccine** *see* Pneumococcal Conjugate Vaccine (10-Valent) *on page 1241*
- ◆ **13-Valent Pneumococcal Vaccine** *see* Pneumococcal Conjugate Vaccine (13-Valent) *on page 1242*

ValGANciclovir (val gan SYE kloh veer)

Related Information

Ganciclovir (Systemic) *on page 728*

Brand Names: US Valcyte

Brand Names: Canada APO-ValGANciclovir; Auro-Valganciclovir; MINT-Valganciclovir; TEVA-ValGANciclovir; Valcyte

Pharmacologic Category Antiviral Agent

Use

Cytomegalovirus, prophylaxis (solid organ transplant recipients):

Prevention of cytomegalovirus (CMV) in high-risk adult patients (donor CMV seropositive/recipient CMV seronegative) undergoing kidney, heart, or kidney/pancreas transplantation

Prevention of CMV in high risk pediatric patients undergoing kidney transplant (age 4 months to 16 years) or heart transplant (age 1 month to 16 years)

CMV retinitis, treatment (AIDS-related): Treatment of cytomegalovirus (CMV) retinitis in patients with acquired immunodeficiency syndrome (AIDS)

Local Anesthetic/Vasoconstrictor Precautions No information available to require special precautions

Effects on Dental Treatment No significant effects or complications reported

Effects on Bleeding Medical consult is suggested.

Adverse Reactions

>10%:

Cardiovascular: Hypertension (12% to 18%)

Central nervous system: Headache (6% to 22%), insomnia (6% to 20%)

Gastrointestinal: Diarrhea (16% to 41%), nausea (8% to 30%), vomiting (3% to 21%), abdominal pain (15%)

Hematologic & oncologic: Anemia (≤31%), thrombocytopenia (≤22%), neutropenia (3% to 19%)

Immunologic: Graft rejection (24%)

Neuromuscular & skeletal: Tremor (12% to 28%)

Ophthalmic: Retinal detachment (15%)

Renal: Increased serum creatinine (S_{cr} >1.5 to 2.5 mg/dL: 12% to 50%; S_{cr} >2.5: 3% to 17%)

Miscellaneous: Fever (9% to 31%)

1% to 10%:

Cardiovascular: Hypotension (≥5%), peripheral edema (≥5%), cardiac arrhythmia (<5%)

Central nervous system: Peripheral neuropathy (9%), paresthesia (≤8%), anxiety (≥5%), chills (≥5%), depression (≥5%), dizziness (≥5%), fatigue (≥5%), malaise (≥5%), pain (≥5%), agitation (<5%), confusion (<5%), hallucination (<5%), psychosis (<5%), seizure (<5%)

Dermatologic: Dermatitis (≥5%), increased wound secretion (≥5%), night sweats (≥5%), pruritus (≥5%), cellulitis (<5%)

Endocrine & metabolic: Hyperkalemia (≥5%), hypophosphatemia (≥5%), weight loss (≥5%)

Gastrointestinal: Abdominal distention (≥5%), constipation (≥5%), decreased appetite (≥5%), dyspepsia (≥5%), oral mucosa ulcer (≥5%), dysgeusia (<5%), pancreatitis (<5%)

Genitourinary: Hematuria (≥5%), urinary tract infection (≥5%)

Hematologic & oncologic: Bone marrow depression (<5%; including aplastic anemia), febrile neutropenia (<5%), hemorrhage (<5%; associated with thrombocytopenia), pancytopenia (<5%)

Hepatic: Hepatic insufficiency (≥5%), increased serum ALT (<5%), increased serum AST (<5%)

Hypersensitivity: Hypersensitivity reaction (<5%)
Immunologic: Organ transplant rejection (6% to 9%)
Infection: Candidiasis (≥5%; including oral candidiasis), influenza (≥5%), wound infection (≥5%), sepsis (<5%)
Neuromuscular & skeletal: Arthralgia (≥5%), back pain (≥5%), muscle spasm (≥5%), myalgia (≥5%), weakness (≥5%), limb pain (<5%)
Ophthalmic: Eye pain (≥5%), macular edema (<5%)
Otic: Deafness (<5%)
Renal: Decreased creatinine clearance (≥5%), renal impairment (≥5%), renal failure (<5%)
Respiratory: Cough (≥5%), dyspnea (≥5%), pharyngitis (≥5%; including nasopharyngitis), upper respiratory tract infection (≥5%)
Miscellaneous: Postoperative complication (≥5%), postoperative pain (<5%), wound dehiscence (<5%)

Frequency not defined: Genitourinary: Reduced fertility <1%, postmarketing and/or case reports: Agranulocytosis, anaphylaxis, granulocytopenia

Mechanism of Action Valganciclovir is rapidly converted to ganciclovir in the body. Ganciclovir is phosphorylated to a substrate which competitively inhibits the binding of deoxyguanosine triphosphate to DNA polymerase resulting in inhibition of viral DNA synthesis.

Pharmacodynamics/Kinetics

Half-life Elimination

Pediatric patients (heart, kidney, or liver transplant): Mean range:
4 months to 2 years: 2.8 to 4.5 hours
2 to 12 years: 2.8 to 3.8 hours
12 to 16 years: 4.9 to 6 hours
Adults:
Ganciclovir: 4.08 hours, prolonged with renal impairment; Severe renal impairment: Up to 68 hours
Heart, kidney, kidney-pancreas, or liver transplant patients: Mean range: 6.18 to 6.77 hours

Time to Peak Ganciclovir: 1.7 to 3 hours

Reproductive Considerations

[US Boxed Warning]: Based on animal data and limited human data, val ganciclovir may cause temporary or permanent inhibition of spermatogenesis in males and suppression of fertility in females.

Female patients should undergo pregnancy testing prior to initiation and use effective contraception during and for at least 30 days after therapy. Male patients should use a barrier contraceptive during and for at least 90 days after therapy.

Pregnancy Considerations

[US Boxed Warning]: Based on animal data, valganciclovir has the potential to cause birth defects in humans.

Valganciclovir is converted to ganciclovir and shares its reproductive toxicity. Ganciclovir crosses the placenta.

Adverse events following congenital cytomegalovirus (CMV) infection may also occur. Hearing loss, mental retardation, microcephaly, seizures, and other medical problems have been observed in infants with congenital CMV infection.

The indications for treating maternal CMV retinitis during pregnancy are the same as in non-pregnant HIV infected women. In general, intravitreous injections for local therapy are preferred for retinal disease to limit systemic exposure during the first trimester when possible. Valganciclovir is the preferred systemic therapy in pregnant women. Close fetal monitoring is recommended. Use of valganciclovir is recommended to treat maternal infection, but not recommended for the treatment of asymptomatic maternal disease for the sole purpose of preventing infant infection (HHS [OI adult 2020]).

- **Valganciclovir HCl** *see* ValGANciclovir *on page 1517*
- **Valganciclovir Hydrochloride** *see* ValGANciclovir *on page 1517*
- **Valium** *see* DiazePAM *on page 477*
- **Valorin [OTC]** *see* Acetaminophen *on page 59*
- **Valorin Extra [OTC]** *see* Acetaminophen *on page 59*
- **Valproate Semisodium** *see* Valproic Acid and Derivatives *on page 1518*
- **Valproate Sodium** *see* Valproic Acid and Derivatives *on page 1518*
- **Valproic Acid** *see* Valproic Acid and Derivatives *on page 1518*
- **Valproic Acid Derivative** *see* Valproic Acid and Derivatives *on page 1518*

Valproic Acid and Derivatives

(val PROE ik AS id & dah RIV ah tives)

Brand Names: US Depacon [DSC]; Depakene [DSC]; Depakote; Depakote ER; Depakote Sprinkles

Brand Names: Canada APO-Divalproex; APO-Valproic; Depakene; DOM-Divalproex; DOM-Valproic Acid; DOM-Valproic Acid EC; Epival; MYL-Divalproex [DSC]; MYLAN-Divalproex; NOVO-Valproic [DSC]; PHL-Divalproex [DSC]; PHL-Valproic Acid EC [DSC]; PHL-Valproic Acid [DSC]; PMS-Divalproex; PMS-Valproic; PMS-Valproic Acid; RATIO-Valproic [DSC]; SANDOZ Valproic [DSC]; TEVA-Divalproex [DSC]

Pharmacologic Category Anticonvulsant, Miscellaneous; Antimanic Agent; Histone Deacetylase Inhibitor

Use

Bipolar disorder: Treatment of manic episodes (delayed release) or acute manic or mixed episodes with or without psychotic features (extended release) associated with bipolar disorder, as monotherapy or in combination with atypical antipsychotics (BAP [Goodwin 2016])

Focal (partial) onset and generalized onset seizures: Monotherapy and adjunctive therapy in the treatment of patients with focal onset seizures with impairment of consciousness or awareness (complex partial) and generalized onset nonmotor seizures (absence), and as adjunctive therapy for multiple seizure types. May be used off-label as monotherapy for other seizure types.

Migraine prophylaxis (excluding IV formulation): Prophylaxis of migraine headaches

Limitation of use: Do not administer to pregnant women, women who plan to become pregnant, or women of childbearing potential for the treatment of epilepsy or bipolar disorder unless essential for the management of her condition.

Local Anesthetic/Vasoconstrictor Precautions No information available to require special precautions

Effects on Dental Treatment Key adverse event(s) related to dental treatment: Infrequent occurrences of facial edema, orthostatic hypotension, speech disturbance, tardive dyskinesia, periodontal abscess, glossitis, stomatitis, xerostomia, gingival hemorrhage, oral mucosa ulcer, dysgeusia, and fungal infections have been reported. Rare occurrences of erythema multiforme and parotid gland enlargement have also been reported.

Effects on Bleeding Has been associated with dose-related thrombocytopenia. Normal coagulation may generally be expected unless thrombocytopenia is present and severe.

Adverse Reactions As reported with oral administration, unless otherwise noted.

>10%:

Central nervous system: Headache (oral: 31%; intravenous: 3% to 4%), drowsiness (oral: 7% to 30%; intravenous: 2% to 11%), dizziness (oral: 12% to 25%; intravenous: 5% to 7%), insomnia (>1% to 15%), pain (oral: 11%; intravenous: 1%), nervousness (oral: 7% to 11%; intravenous: <1%)

Dermatologic: Alopecia (>1% to 24%)

Gastrointestinal: Nausea (oral: 15% to 48%; intravenous: 3% to 6%), vomiting (oral: 7% to 27%; intravenous: 1%), abdominal pain (oral: 7% to 23%; intravenous: 1%), diarrhea (oral: 7% to 23%; intravenous: <1%), dyspepsia (7% to 23%), anorexia (>1% to 12%)

Hematologic & oncologic: Thrombocytopenia (1% to 27%; dose related)

Infection: Infection (≤20%)

Neuromuscular & skeletal: Tremor (≤57%), asthenia (6% to 27%; intravenous: 7%)

Ophthalmic: Diplopia (>1% to 16%), visual disturbance (amblyopia, blurred vision ≤1% to 12%)

Respiratory: Flu-like symptoms (>1% to 12%)

Miscellaneous: Accidental injury (>1% to 11%)

1% to 10%:

Cardiovascular: Peripheral edema (>1% to 8%), edema (>1% to 5%), facial edema (>1% to 5%), hypertension (>1% to 5%), hypotension (1% to 5%), orthostatic hypotension (1% to 5%), palpitations (>1% to 5%), vasodilation (oral: >1% to 5%; intravenous: <1%), tachycardia (>1% to <5%), chest pain (2%)

Central nervous system: Ataxia (>1% to 8%), amnesia (>1% to 7%), paresthesia (≤7%), abnormality in thinking (>1% to 6%), emotional lability (>1% to 6%), abnormal dreams (>1% to 5%), abnormal gait (>1% to 5%), confusion (>1% to 5%), depression (>1% to 5%), hallucination (>1% to 5%), hypertonia (>1% to 5%), speech disturbance (>1% to 5%), tardive dyskinesia (>1% to 5%), agitation (1% to 5%), catatonia (1% to 5%), chills (1% to 5%), hyperreflexia (1% to 5%), vertigo (1% to 5%), anxiety (>1% to <5%), malaise (>1% to <5%), myasthenia (>1% to <5%), personality disorder (>1% to <5%), twitching (>1% to <5%), sleep disorder (>1%)

Dermatologic: Skin rash (>1% to 6%), maculopapular rash (>1% to 5%), pruritus (>1% to 5%), xeroderma (>1% to 5%), diaphoresis (oral: >1%; intravenous: <1%), erythema nodosum (>1%), vesiculobullous dermatitis (>1%), furunculosis (1% to 5%), seborrhea (1% to 5%)

Endocrine & metabolic: Weight gain (>1% to 9%), weight loss (6%), amenorrhea (>1% to <5%), menstrual disease (>1%)

Gastrointestinal: Increased appetite (>1% to 6%), constipation (>1% to 5%), flatulence (>1% to 5%), periodontal abscess (>1% to 5%), fecal incontinence (1% to 5%), gastroenteritis (1% to 5%), glossitis (1% to 5%), stomatitis (1% to 5%), xerostomia (1% to 5%), eructation (>1% to <5%), hematemesis (>1% to <5%), pancreatitis (>1% to <5%), dysgeusia (2%), dysphagia (>1%), gingival hemorrhage (>1%), hiccups (>1%), oral mucosa ulcer (>1%)

Genitourinary: Cystitis (>1% to 5%), dysmenorrhea (>1% to 5%), dysuria (>1% to 5%), urinary incontinence (>1% to 5%), vaginal hemorrhage (>1% to 5%), urinary frequency (>1% to <5%), vaginitis (>1% to <5%)

Hematologic & oncologic: Ecchymoses (>1% to 5%), petechia (>1% to <5%), hypoproteinemia (>1%), prolonged bleeding time (>1%)

Hepatic: Increased serum alanine aminotransferase (>1% to <5%), increased serum aspartate aminotransferase (>1% to <5%)

Infection: Viral infection (>1% to 5%), fungal infection (>1%)

Local: Pain at injection site (intravenous: 3%), injection site reaction (intravenous: 2%)

Neuromuscular & skeletal: Back pain (>1% to 8%), arthralgia (>1% to 5%), discoid lupus erythematosus (>1% to 5%), lower limb cramps (>1% to 5%), hypokinesia (1% to 5%), neck pain (1% to 5%), neck stiffness (1% to 5%), osteoarthritis (1% to 5%), dysarthria (>1% to <5%), myalgia (>1% to <5%)

Ophthalmic: Nystagmus disorder (1% to 8%), conjunctivitis (1% to 5%), dry eye syndrome (1% to 5%), eye pain (1% to 5%), photophobia (>1%)

Otic: Tinnitus (1% to 7%), deafness (>1% to 5%), otitis media (>1% to <5%)

Respiratory: Pharyngitis (oral: 2% to 8%; intravenous: <1%), bronchitis (5%), rhinitis (>1% to 5%), dyspnea (1% to 5%), cough (>1% to <5%), epistaxis (>1% to <5%), pneumonia (>1% to <5%), sinusitis (>1% to <5%)

Miscellaneous: Fever (>1% to 6%)

<1%, postmarketing, and/or case reports: Abnormal behavior, abnormal thyroid function tests, acute intermittent porphyria, aggressive behavior, agranulocytosis, anaphylaxis, anemia, aplastic anemia, asthenospermia, azoospermia, bone fracture, bone marrow depression, bradycardia, brain disease (rare), breast hypertrophy, cerebral atrophy (reversible or irreversible), change in prothrombin time, changes of hair (color, texture), coma (rare), decreased bone mineral density, decreased plasma carnitine concentrations, decreased platelet aggregation, decreased spermatozoa motility, dementia, developmental delay (learning disorder), disturbance in attention, drug reaction with eosinophilia and systemic symptoms, emotional disturbance, eosinophilia, erythema multiforme, euphoria, Fanconi-like syndrome (rare, in children), female hyperandrogenism, galactorrhea not associated with childbirth, hemorrhage, hepatic failure, hepatotoxicity, hirsutism, hostility, hyperactive behavior, hyperammonemia, hyperammonemic encephalopathy (in patients with UCD), hyperglycinemia, hypersensitivity angiitis, hypersensitivity reaction, hypoesthesia, hypofibrinogenemia, hyponatremia, hypothermia, increased testosterone level, injection site inflammation, leukopenia, lymphocytosis, macrocytosis, male infertility, myelatelia, nail bed changes, nail disease, oligospermia, ostealgia, osteopenia, osteoporosis, pancytopenia, parkinsonism (Easterford 2004), parotid gland enlargement, polycystic ovary syndrome (rare), psychomotor disturbance, psychosis, seizure (paradoxical), severe hypersensitivity reaction (with multiorgan dysfunction), SIADH, skin photosensitivity, sleep disturbance, spermatozoa disorder (abnormal morphology), Stevens-Johnson syndrome, suicidal ideation, suicidal tendencies, toxic epidermal necrolysis (rare), urinary incontinence, urinary tract infection

Mechanism of Action Causes increased availability of gamma-aminobutyric acid (GABA), an inhibitory neurotransmitter, to brain neurons or may enhance the action of GABA or mimic its action at postsynaptic receptor sites. Also blocks voltage-dependent sodium channels, which results in suppression of high-frequency repetitive neuronal firing (Bourin 2009). Divalproex sodium is a compound of sodium valproate and valproic acid; divalproex dissociates to valproate in the GI tract.

Pharmacodynamics/Kinetics

Half-life Elimination Increased in neonates, elderly, and patients with liver impairment

Newborns (exposed to VPA in utero): 30 to 60 hours
Neonates first week of life: 40 to 45 hours
Neonates <10 days: 10 to 67 hours
Infants and Children >2 months: 7 to 13 hours
Children and Adolescents 2 to 14 years: 9 hours (range: 3.5 to 20 hours) (Cloyd 1993)
Adults: 9 to 16 hours

Time to Peak

Oral:
Divalproex sodium:
Delayed release: tablet and sprinkle capsules: ~4 hours
Extended release: 4 to 17 hours
Immediate release enteric-coated tablet [Canadian product]: 4 hours
Valproic acid delayed release capsule: 2 hours
Rectal (off-label route): 1 to 3 hours (Graves 1987)

Reproductive Considerations

[US Boxed Warning]: Due to the risks of adverse fetal events, valproate is contraindicated for prophylaxis of migraine headaches in women of childbearing potential who are not using effective contraception. Valproate should not be used to treat women with epilepsy or bipolar disorder who plan to become pregnant unless other medications have failed to provide adequate symptom control or are otherwise unacceptable. Valproate should not be administered to a woman of childbearing potential unless other medications have failed to provide adequate symptom control or are otherwise unacceptable. In such situations, effective contraception should be used.

Algorithms are available for the management of females of reproductive potential who are taking valproic acid for bipolar disorder. Nonpregnant women who are stable on monotherapy and are planning a pregnancy should undergo a slow taper (>4 weeks); alternative treatment and a faster taper should be introduced in unstable patients during this time. Additional details are available for women planning a pregnancy who are on multiple medications (Anmella 2019).

When pregnancy is being planned in women with epilepsy, consider tapering off of therapy prior to conception if appropriate (Anmella 2019; Harden 2009a); abrupt discontinuation of therapy may cause status epilepticus and lead to maternal and fetal hypoxia.

Counsel women planning a pregnancy and girls at the onset of puberty regarding benefits and risk of valproate use during pregnancy. Folic acid decreases the risk of neural tube defects in the general population; supplementation with folic acid should be used prior to conception and during pregnancy in all females, including those taking valproate.

Cases of male infertility have been reported following valproate use.

Pregnancy Considerations Valproate crosses the placenta (Harden 2009b).

[US Boxed Warning]: Valproate can cause major congenital malformations, particularly neural tube defects (eg, spina bifida). In addition, valproate can cause decreased IQ scores and neurodevelopmental disorders following in utero exposure. Neural tube defects, craniofacial defects (eg, oral clefts, craniosynostosis), cardiovascular malformations, hypospadias, and limb malformations (eg, clubfoot, polydactyly) have been reported. Information from the North American Antiepileptic Drug Pregnancy Registry notes the rate of major malformations to be 9% to 11% following an average exposure to valproate monotherapy 1,000 mg/day; this is an increase in congenital malformations when compared with monotherapy with other antiepileptic drugs (AED). Based on data from the CDC National Birth Defects Prevention Network, the risk of spinal bifida is approximately 1% to 2% following valproate exposure (general population risk estimated to be 0.06% to 0.07%).

Nonteratogenic adverse effects have also been reported. Decreased IQ scores have been noted in children exposed to valproate in utero when compared to children exposed to other antiepileptic medications or no antiepileptic medications; the risk of autism spectrum disorders may also be increased. Hearing loss or impairment may occur following in utero exposure. Fatal hepatic failure and hypoglycemia in infants have been noted in case reports following in utero exposure to valproate.

The pharmacokinetic properties of valproate in pregnancy are highly variable. If use is needed, monitoring of total and unbound serum concentrations should be done prior to and during pregnancy (Johannessen 2018). Clotting factor abnormalities (hypofibrinogenemia, thrombocytopenia, or decrease in other coagulation factors) may develop in the mother following valproate use during pregnancy; close monitoring of coagulation factors is recommended.

[US Boxed Warning]: Due to the risks of adverse fetal events, **valproate is contraindicated for prophylaxis of migraine headaches in pregnant women. Valproate should not be used to treat women with epilepsy or bipolar disorder who are pregnant unless other medications have failed to provide adequate symptom control or are otherwise unacceptable.** Current guidelines recommend complete avoidance of valproate for the treatment of epilepsy in pregnant women whenever possible (Harden 2009a).

A pregnancy registry is available for women who have been exposed to valproic acid. Patients may enroll themselves in the North American Antiepileptic Drug (NAAED) Pregnancy Registry by calling (888) 233-2334. Additional information is available at www.aedpregnancyregistry.org.

Valrubicin (val ROO bi sin)

Brand Names: US Valstar

Brand Names: Canada Valtaxin [DSC]

Pharmacologic Category Antineoplastic Agent, Anthracycline; Antineoplastic Agent, Topoisomerase II Inhibitor

Use Bladder cancer: Intravesical treatment of BCG-refractory bladder carcinoma in situ of the urinary bladder when cystectomy would be associated with unacceptable morbidity or mortality.

Local Anesthetic/Vasoconstrictor Precautions No information available to require special precautions

Effects on Dental Treatment No significant effects or complications reported

Effects on Bleeding This chemotherapy is administered locally and hematologic toxicity is not experienced.

Adverse Reactions In general, local adverse reactions occur during or shortly after instillation and resolve within 1 to 7 days.

>10%: Genitourinary: Irritable bladder (88%), urinary frequency (61%), urinary urgency (57%), dysuria (56%), bladder spasm (31%), hematuria (29%; microscopic: 3%; gross hematuria: 1%), bladder pain (28%), urinary incontinence (22%), cystitis (15%), urinary tract infection (15%), red urine discoloration

1% to 10%:

Cardiovascular: Chest pain (3%), vasodilation (2%), peripheral edema (1%)

Central nervous system: Localized burning (5%), headache (4%), malaise (4%), dizziness (3%)

Dermatologic: Skin rash (3%)

Endocrine & metabolic: Hyperglycemia (1%)

Gastrointestinal: Abdominal pain (5%), nausea (5%), diarrhea (3%), vomiting (2%), flatulence (1%)

Genitourinary: Nocturia (7%), urinary retention (4%), urethral pain (3%), pelvic pain (1%)

Hematologic & oncologic: Anemia (2%)

Neuromuscular & skeletal: Weakness (4%), back pain (3%), myalgia (1%)

Respiratory: Pneumonia (1%)

Miscellaneous: Fever (2%)

<1%, postmarketing, and/or case reports: Ageusia, increased nonprotein nitrogen, pruritus, reduced urine flow, skin irritation (local), tenesmus, urethritis

Mechanism of Action Valrubicin blocks function of DNA topoisomerase II; it inhibits DNA synthesis, causes extensive chromosomal damage, and arrests cell development (G2 phase). Unlike other anthracyclines, valrubicin does not appear to intercalate DNA.

Reproductive Considerations

Females of reproductive potential should use effective contraception during treatment and for 6 months after the final valrubicin dose. Males with female partners of reproductive potential should use effective contraception during treatment and for 3 months after the last valrubicin dose.

Pregnancy Risk Factor C

Pregnancy Considerations

Based on the mechanism of action and data from animal reproduction studies, in utero exposure to valrubicin may cause fetal harm.

Systemic exposure (eg, with bladder perforation) during human pregnancy may result in fetal harm.

Valsartan (val SAR tan)

Related Information

Cardiovascular Diseases *on page 1654*

Brand Names: US Diovan

Brand Names: Canada ACT Valsartan [DSC]; APO-Valsartan; Auro-Valsartan; Diovan; DOM-Valsartan [DSC]; MYLAN-Valsartan [DSC]; PMS-Valsartan [DSC]; RIVA-Valsartan [DSC]; SANDOZ Valsartan; TARO-Valsartan; TEVA-Valsartan

Pharmacologic Category Angiotensin II Receptor Blocker; Antihypertensive

Use

Heart failure with reduced ejection fraction: Treatment of heart failure (NYHA class II to IV).

Hypertension: Management of hypertension.

Post-myocardial infarction: Reduction of cardiovascular mortality in patients with left ventricular dysfunction or failure following myocardial infarction (MI) (eg, acute coronary syndromes such as ST-elevation MI or non-ST-elevation MI).

Local Anesthetic/Vasoconstrictor Precautions No information available to require special precautions

Effects on Dental Treatment Key adverse event(s) related to dental treatment: Patients may experience orthostatic hypotension as they stand up after treatment; especially if lying in dental chair for extended periods of time. Use caution with sudden changes in position during and after dental treatment.

Effects on Bleeding No information available to require special precautions

Adverse Reactions Adverse reactions occurred with heart failure or post-MI unless otherwise indicated.

>10%:

Central nervous system: Dizziness (17%; hypertension: 2% to 8%)

Renal: Increased blood urea nitrogen (>50% increase: 17%)

1% to 10%:

Cardiovascular: Hypotension (6% to 7%; hypertension: <1%), orthostatic hypotension (2%), syncope (>1%; hypertension: <1%)

Central nervous system: Fatigue (2% to 3%), orthostatic dizziness (≤2%), headache (>1%), vertigo (>1%)

Endocrine & metabolic: Hyperkalemia (2%)

Gastrointestinal: Diarrhea (5%), abdominal pain (hypertension: 2%), nausea (>1%), upper abdominal pain (>1%)

Hematologic & oncologic: Neutropenia (2%)

Infection: Viral infection (hypertension: 3%)

Neuromuscular & skeletal: Arthralgia (3%), back pain (3%; hypertension: <1%)

Ophthalmic: Blurred vision (>1%)

Renal: Increased serum creatinine (≤4%), renal insufficiency (>1%)

Respiratory: Dry cough (hypertension: 3%)

<1%, postmarketing, and/or case reports: Alopecia, angioedema, anorexia, anxiety, asthenia, bullous dermatitis, chest pain, constipation, drowsiness, dyspepsia, dyspnea, flatulence, hepatitis, hypersensitivity reaction, impotence, increased liver enzymes, insomnia, muscle cramps, myalgia, palpitation, paresthesia, pruritus, renal failure syndrome, rhabdomyolysis, skin rash, thrombocytopenia, vasculitis, vomiting, xerostomia

Mechanism of Action Valsartan produces direct antagonism of the angiotensin II (AT2) receptors, unlike the ACE inhibitors. It displaces angiotensin II from the AT1 receptor and produces its blood pressure-lowering effects by antagonizing AT1-induced vasoconstriction, aldosterone release, catecholamine release, arginine vasopressin release, water intake, and hypertrophic responses. This action results in more efficient blockade of the cardiovascular effects of angiotensin II and fewer side effects than the ACE inhibitors.

Pharmacodynamics/Kinetics

Onset of Action ~2 hours

Duration of Action 24 hours

Half-life Elimination

Children 1 to 5 years: ~4 hours (Blumer 2009)

Children and Adolescents 6 to 16 years: ~5 hours (Blumer 2009)

Adults: ~6 hours; ~35% longer in elderly patients

Time to Peak Serum:

Children and Adolescents 1 to 16 years: Oral suspension: 2 hours (Blumer 2009)

Adults: Tablets: 2 to 4 hours; Oral solution: 0.7 to 3.7 hours (high-fat, high-calorie meal decreased C_{max} ~44%)

Reproductive Considerations

The use of angiotensin II receptor blockers should generally be avoided in women planning a pregnancy (ACOG 203 2019).

Pregnancy Considerations

[US Boxed Warning]: Drugs that act on the renin-angiotensin system can cause injury and death to the developing fetus. When pregnancy is detected, discontinue as soon as possible. The use of drugs that act on the renin-angiotensin system are associated with oligohydramnios. Oligohydramnios, due to decreased fetal renal function, may lead to fetal lung hypoplasia and skeletal malformations. Oligohydramnios may not appear until after irreversible fetal injury has occurred. Use in pregnancy is also associated with anuria, hypotension, renal failure, skull hypoplasia, and death in the fetus/neonate. The exposed fetus should be monitored for fetal growth, amniotic fluid volume, and organ formation. Infants exposed in utero should be monitored for hyperkalemia, hypotension, and oliguria (exchange transfusions or dialysis may be needed). These adverse events are generally associated with maternal use in the second and third trimesters.

Chronic maternal hypertension may increase the risk of birth defects, low birth weight, preterm delivery, stillbirth, and neonatal death. Actual fetal/neonatal risks may be related to duration and severity of maternal hypertension. Untreated hypertension may also increase the risk of adverse maternal outcomes, including gestational diabetes, myocardial infarction, preeclampsia, stroke, and delivery complications (ACOG 203 2019).

The use of angiotensin II receptor blockers is generally not recommended to treat chronic hypertension in pregnant women (ACOG 203 2019).

Product Availability Prexxartan (valsartan): FDA approved December 2017; anticipated availability currently unknown.

◆ **Valsartan and Sacubitril** *see* Sacubitril and Valsartan *on page 1353*

◆ **Valsartan/Sacubitril** *see* Sacubitril and Valsartan *on page 1353*

◆ **Valstar** *see* Valrubicin *on page 1520*

◆ **Valtoco 5 MG Dose** *see* DiazePAM *on page 477*

◆ **Valtoco 10 MG Dose** *see* DiazePAM *on page 477*

◆ **Valtoco 15 MG Dose** *see* DiazePAM *on page 477*

◆ **Valtoco 20 MG Dose** *see* DiazePAM *on page 477*

◆ **Valtrex** *see* ValACYclovir *on page 1512*

◆ **Vanadom** *see* Carisoprodol *on page 293*

◆ **Vancenase AQ** *see* Beclomethasone (Nasal) *on page 217*

◆ **Vanceril** *see* Beclomethasone (Oral Inhalation) *on page 218*

◆ **Vancocin** *see* Vancomycin *on page 1522*

◆ **Vancocin HCl** *see* Vancomycin *on page 1522*

Vancomycin (van koe MYE sin)

Brand Names: US Firvanq; Vancocin; Vancocin HCl; Vancosol Pack [DSC]

Brand Names: Canada JAMP-Vancomycin; PMS-Vancomycin; Vancocin; Vancomycin HCl

Generic Availability (US) Yes

Pharmacologic Category Glycopeptide

Use

***Clostridioides* (formerly *Clostridium*) *difficile* infection (oral):** Treatment of *C. difficile* infection (CDI)

Endocarditis (injection):

Corynebacteria (diphtheroids): Treatment of diphtheroid endocarditis in combination with either rifampin, an aminoglycoside, or both in early-onset prosthetic valve endocarditis caused by diphtheroids

Enterococcal: Treatment of endocarditis caused by enterococci (eg, *Enterococcus faecalis*), in combination with an aminoglycoside

Staphylococcal: Treatment of staphylococcal endocarditis

Streptococcal: Treatment of endocarditis due to *Streptococcus viridans* or *Streptococcus bovis,* as monotherapy or in combination with an aminoglycoside

Enterocolitis (oral): Treatment of enterocolitis caused by *Staphylococcus aureus* (including methicillin-resistant strains). **Note:** Staphylococcal enterocolitis is uncommon; the disease and treatment are not well described in the literature (Iwata 2014; Lin 2010).

Staphylococcal infections (injection): Treatment of serious or severe infections (eg, bloodstream infections, bone infections, lower respiratory tract infections, skin and skin structure infections) caused by susceptible strains of methicillin-resistant (beta-lactam-resistant) staphylococci; empiric therapy of infections when methicillin-resistant staphylococci are suspected

Local Anesthetic/Vasoconstrictor Precautions

No information available to require special precautions

Effects on Dental Treatment Key adverse event(s) related to dental treatment: Bitter taste. "Red man syndrome", characterized by skin rash and hypotension, is not an allergic reaction but rather is associated with too rapid infusion of the drug. To alleviate or prevent the reaction, infuse vancomycin at a rate of ≥30 minutes for each 500 mg of drug being administered (eg, 1 g over ≥60 minutes); 1.5 g over ≥90 minutes.

Effects on Bleeding Vancomycin has been demonstrated to induce immune thrombocytopenia, causing a significant drop in platelet count following a short (ie, 12-15 hours) period of time after treatment. Both IgG and IgM vancomycin-dependent platelets have been identified post vancomycin administration. Discontinuation has shown to be an effective remedy, as platelet levels return to the pre-exposure counts within 4 days of drug withdrawal.

Adverse Reactions

IV:

Frequency not defined:

Cardiovascular: Chest pain, flushing, hypotension, shock, vasculitis

Dermatologic: Bullous dermatitis, erythema of skin, exfoliative dermatitis (Forrence 1990), pruritus, Stevens-Johnson syndrome (Lin 2014), toxic epidermal necrolysis (Changela 2013)

Gastrointestinal: *Clostridioides difficile* colitis (Hecht 1989)

Hematologic & oncologic: Agranulocytosis (di Fonzo 2018), eosinophilia, leukopenia, neutropenia (reversible) (Black 2011), pancytopenia (Carmichael 1986), thrombocytopenia
Hypersensitivity: Anaphylaxis (Anne 1994), hypersensitivity reaction (Kupstaite 2010), red man syndrome (Symons 1985)
Local: Injection site phlebitis, irritation at injection site, pain at injection site
Nervous system: Chills, dizziness, malaise, vertigo
Neuromuscular & skeletal: Myalgia
Otic: Hearing loss (Klibanov 2003), ototoxicity (Forouzesh 2009), tinnitus (Traber 1981)
Renal: Increased blood urea nitrogen (Bergman 1988), increased serum creatinine, interstitial nephritis (Bergman 1988), renal tubular necrosis (Shah-Khan 2011)
Respiratory: Dyspnea, wheezing
Miscellaneous: Fever (Smith 1999)

Postmarketing:
Cardiovascular: Hypersensitivity angiitis (Pingili 2017)
Dermatologic: Acute generalized exanthematous pustulosis (Mawri 2015), dermatologic disorder (linear IgA bullous dermatosis) (Tashima 2014), erythema multiforme (Khicher 2019), maculopapular rash (Marik 1997)
Gastrointestinal: *Clostridioides difficile* associated diarrhea (Hecht 1989), peritonitis (following intraperitoneal administration during CAPD) (Freiman 1992)
Hematologic & oncologic: Henoch-Schonlein purpura (Min 2017), immune thrombocytopenia (Al Jafar 2015)
Hypersensitivity: Fixed drug eruption (Gilmore 2004)
Immunologic: Drug reaction with eosinophilia and systemic symptoms (Cacoub 2011)
Renal: Acute renal failure (Sawada 2018), nephrotoxicity (Lodise 2009)

Oral:

>10%:
Endocrine & metabolic: Hypokalemia (13%)
Gastrointestinal: Abdominal pain (15%), nausea (17%)

1% to 10%:
Cardiovascular: Peripheral edema (6%)
Gastrointestinal: Diarrhea (9%), flatulence (8%), vomiting (9%)
Genitourinary: Urinary tract infection (8%)
Nervous system: Fatigue (5%), headache (7%)
Neuromuscular & skeletal: Back pain (6%)
Renal: Nephrotoxicity (5%)
Miscellaneous: Fever (9%)

Frequency not defined:
Cardiovascular: Flushing, hypotension
Gastrointestinal: Constipation
Hematologic & oncologic: Anemia
Nervous system: Depression, insomnia
Renal: Increased serum creatinine, renal failure syndrome, renal insufficiency

Postmarketing:
Cardiovascular: Vasculitis
Dermatologic: Exfoliative dermatitis, pruritus, skin rash, Stevens-Johnson syndrome, toxic epidermal necrolysis, urticaria
Hematologic & oncologic: Eosinophilia, thrombocytopenia
Hypersensitivity: Anaphylaxis, nonimmune anaphylaxis, red man syndrome (Arroyo-Mercado 2019)
Nervous system: Chills, drug fever, pain, vertigo
Neuromuscular & skeletal: Muscle spasm (chest and back)
Otic: Tinnitus
Respiratory: Dyspnea, wheezing

Dental Usual Dosage Prophylaxis against infective endocarditis: IV:

Infants >1 month and Children:
Dental, oral, or upper respiratory tract surgery: 20 mg/kg 1 hour prior to the procedure. **Note:** American Heart Association (AHA) guidelines now recommend prophylaxis only in patients undergoing invasive procedures and in whom underlying cardiac conditions may predispose to a higher risk of adverse outcomes should infection occur.
GI/GU procedure: 20 mg/kg plus gentamicin 2 mg/kg 1 hour prior to surgery. **Note:** As of April 2007, routine prophylaxis no longer recommended by the AHA.

Adults:
Dental, oral, or upper respiratory tract surgery: 1 g 1 hour before surgery. **Note:** AHA guidelines now recommend prophylaxis only in patients undergoing invasive procedures and in whom underlying cardiac conditions may predispose to a higher risk of adverse outcomes should infection occur
GI/GU procedure: 1 g plus 1.5 mg/kg gentamicin 1 hour prior to surgery. **Note:** As of April 2007, routine prophylaxis no longer recommended by the AHA.

Dosing

Adult & Geriatric

Usual dosage range: Note: Initial IV dosing in nonobese patients should be based on actual body weight; subsequent dosing should generally be adjusted based on therapeutic monitoring. Trough monitoring has traditionally been used for therapeutic monitoring; however, for serious methicillin-resistant *S. aureus* (MRSA) infections (eg, bacteremia, infective endocarditis, meningitis, osteomyelitis, pneumonia, sepsis), AUC monitoring is preferred (ASHP/IDSA/PIDS/SIDP [Rybak 2020]). For patients with uncomplicated skin and soft tissue infections who are not obese and have normal renal function, therapeutic monitoring is generally not needed (IDSA [Liu 2011]). Risk of toxicity (eg, acute kidney injury) increases as a function of trough concentration, especially when trough is maintained above 15 to 20 mg/L; recent data suggest risk increases along the vancomycin AUC continuum, especially when daily AUC exceeds 650 to 1,300 mg•h/L (ASHP/IDSA/PIDS/SIDP [Rybak 2020]).

Oral: Note: Ineffective for treating systemic infections: 125 to 500 mg 4 times daily.

IV: Note: Ineffective for treating *C. difficile* infections.
Intermittent infusion: 15 to 20 mg/kg/dose (rounded to the nearest 250 mg) every 8 to 12 hours initially to achieve a target AUC/minimum inhibitory concentration determined by broth microdilution (MIC_{BMD}) ratio of 400 to 600 (assuming a vancomycin MIC_{BMD} of 1 mg/L) in patients with serious MRSA infections (eg, bacteremia, infective endocarditis, meningitis, osteomyelitis, pneumonia, sepsis). Trough-only monitoring (target trough: 15 to 20 mg/L) is no longer recommended in patients with serious MRSA infections (ASHP/IDSA/PIDS/SIDP [Rybak 2020]), but may be needed in nonserious MRSA or non-MRSA infections. Early and frequent monitoring for dosage adjustments is recommended, especially when empiric doses exceed 4 g/day (ASHP/IDSA/PIDS/SIDP [Rybak 2020]).

Loading dose: Critically ill patients with documented/suspected MRSA infection: A loading dose of 20 to 35 mg/kg (based on actual body weight; maximum: 3 g/dose) may be considered to rapidly achieve target concentrations (ASHP/IDSA/PIDS/SIDP [Rybak 2020]).

Continuous infusion: **Note:** May be considered for critically ill patients who are unable to achieve AUC target with intermittent infusion dosing. Loading dose: 15 to 20 mg/kg, followed by a maintenance continuous infusion dose of 30 to 40 mg/kg/day (up to 60 mg/kg/day) to achieve a target steady state concentration of 20 to 25 mg/L (ASHP/IDSA/PIDS/SIDP [Rybak 2020]).

Indication-specific dosing:

Bloodstream infection:

Empiric therapy or pathogen-specific therapy for methicillin-resistant S. aureus: **IV:** 15 to 20 mg/kg/dose every 8 to 12 hours initially; adjust based on therapeutic monitoring (ASHP/IDSA/PIDS/SIDP [Rybak 2020]). A loading dose may be considered in seriously ill patients (ASHP/IDSA/PIDS/SIDP [Rybak 2020]; IDSA [Liu 2011]). Treat uncomplicated *S. aureus* infection for ≥14 days from first negative blood culture, with longer courses warranted for endocarditis or metastatic sites of infection (IDSA [Liu 2011]; IDSA [Mermel 2009]).

Empiric therapy or pathogen-specific therapy for methicillin-resistant coagulase-negative staphylococci: **IV:** 15 mg/kg/dose every 12 hours initially; adjust based on therapeutic monitoring (IDSA [Mermel 2009]). Treat uncomplicated bacteremia for 5 to 7 days from day of first negative blood culture, with longer courses warranted for endocarditis or metastatic sites of infection (IDSA [Mermel 2009]; Tufariello 2019). For catheter-related bloodstream infections, consider antibiotic lock therapy for catheter salvage, in addition to systemic therapy (IDSA [Mermel 2009]).

Antibiotic lock technique (catheter-salvage strategy) (off-label use): **Note:** For infections caused by susceptible organisms when the catheter cannot be removed; use in addition to systemic antibiotics. Catheter salvage is **not** recommended for *S. aureus* (Girand 2019; IDSA [Mermel 2009]).

Intracatheter: Prepare lock solution to final concentration of vancomycin 5 mg/mL; may be combined with heparin. Instill into each lumen of the catheter access port using a volume sufficient to fill the catheter (2 to 5 mL) with a dwell time of up to 72 hours, depending on frequency of catheter use. Withdraw lock solution prior to catheter use; replace with fresh vancomycin lock solution after catheter use. Antibiotic lock therapy is given for the same duration as systemic antibiotics (IDSA [Mermel 2009]; LaPlante 2007).

Cerebrospinal fluid shunt infection (off-label use): As a component of empiric therapy or pathogen-specific therapy (eg, methicillin-resistant *S. aureus* or coagulase-negative staphylococci):

IV: 15 to 20 mg/kg/dose every 8 to 12 hours initially; adjust based on therapeutic monitoring (IDSA [Tunkel 2017]). A loading dose may be considered in seriously ill patients (ASHP/IDSA/PIDS/SIDP [Rybak 2020]).

Intraventricular (adjunct to systemic therapy; use a preservative-free preparation): 5 to 20 mg/day; some experts recommend adjusting dosage and administration interval based on cerebrospinal fluid (CSF) vancomycin concentrations (goal: 10 to 20 times MIC of causative organism), ventricular size, and daily output from ventricular drain (IDSA [Tunkel 2017]); data for monitoring are limited (Smetana 2018). When intraventricular vancomycin is administered via a ventricular drain, clamp drain for 15 to 60 minutes after administration (allows solution to equilibrate in CSF) (IDSA [Tunkel 2004]; IDSA [Tunkel 2017]). **Note:** Intraventricular administration is generally reserved for use in patients who fail parenteral therapy despite removal of CSF shunt or when CSF shunt cannot be removed (Baddour 2019).

***Clostridioides* (formerly *Clostridium*) *difficile* infection: Note:** Criteria for disease severity is based on expert opinion and should not replace clinical judgment (IDSA/SHEA [McDonald 2018]).

Oral:

Nonsevere *C. difficile* infection (supportive clinical data: WBC ≤15,000 cells/mm^3 and serum creatinine <1.5 mg/dL):

Initial episode: 125 mg 4 times daily for 10 days (IDSA/SHEA [McDonald 2018]).

First recurrence:

If vancomycin was used for initial episode: Pulsed-tapered regimen: 125 mg 4 times daily for 10 to 14 days, then 125 mg twice daily for 7 days, then 125 mg once daily for 7 days, then 125 mg every 2 or 3 days for 2 to 8 weeks (IDSA/SHEA [McDonald 2018]).

If metronidazole or fidaxomicin was used for initial episode: 125 mg 4 times daily for 10 days (IDSA/SHEA [McDonald 2018]).

Second or subsequent recurrence: Pulsed-tapered regimen as above **or** 125 mg 4 times daily for 10 days followed by rifaximin (SHEA/IDSA [McDonald 2018]).

Severe *C. difficile* infection (supportive clinical data: WBC >15,000 cells/mm^3 and/or serum creatinine ≥1.5 mg/dL): 125 mg 4 times daily (IDSA/SHEA [McDonald 2018]).

Fulminant *C. difficile* infection (supportive clinical data: ileus, megacolon, and/or hypotension/shock): Oral or via nasogastric tube: 500 mg 4 times daily with IV metronidazole; if ileus present, may consider vancomycin retention enema (IDSA/SHEA [McDonald 2018]).

Rectal:

Fulminant *C. difficile* infection with ileus: Retention enema (off-label route): 500 mg in 100 mL NS; retained for as long as possible and administered every 6 hours. Use in combination with oral vancomycin (if the ileus is partial) or in place of oral vancomycin (if the ileus is complete) **plus** IV metronidazole. **Note:** Optimal regimen not established (IDSA/SHEA [McDonald 2018]). Use of rectal vancomycin should be reserved for patients who have not responded to standard therapy and performed by individuals with expertise in administration, as there is risk of colonic perforation (Kelly 2019).

Cystic fibrosis, acute pulmonary exacerbation, moderate to severe (off-label use): Empiric or pathogen-directed therapy for methicillin-resistant *S. aureus*: **IV:** 15 to 20 mg/kg/dose every 8 hours initially; adjust based on therapeutic monitoring (Pettit 2017; Simon 2019). Duration is usually 10 days to 3 weeks or longer based on clinical response (Flume 2009; Simon 2019).

Diabetic foot infection, moderate to severe (off-label use): Empiric or pathogen-directed therapy for methicillin-resistant *S. aureus*: **IV:** 15 to 20 mg/kg/dose every 8 to 12 hours initially; adjust based on therapeutic monitoring (ASHP/IDSA/PIDS/SIDP [Rybak 2020]). Duration (which may include appropriate oral step-down therapy) is usually 2 to 4 weeks in the absence of osteomyelitis (IDSA [Lipsky 2012]; Weintrob 2019).

Endocarditis, treatment:

Enterococcus (native or prosthetic valve) (penicillin-resistant strains or patients unable to tolerate beta-lactams): **IV:** 15 mg/kg/dose every 12 hours initially; adjust to obtain a trough concentration of 10 to 20 mg/L (AHA [Baddour 2015]); some experts favor a trough of 15 to 20 mg/L (BSAC [Gould 2012]; ESC [Habib 2015]). Administer in combination with gentamicin for 6 weeks (AHA [Baddour 2015]).

S. aureus, methicillin-resistant or methicillin-susceptible (severe-beta lactam hypersensitivity) (alternative agent): **IV:**

Native valve: 15 to 20 mg/kg/dose every 8 to 12 hours initially; adjust based on therapeutic monitoring (AHA [Baddour 2015]; ASHP/IDSA/PIDS/SIDP [Rybak 2020]). Duration of therapy is 6 weeks (AHA [Baddour 2015]).

Prosthetic valve: 15 to 20 mg/kg/dose every 8 to 12 hours initially; adjust based on therapeutic monitoring (AHA [Baddour 2015]; ASHP/IDSA/PIDS/SIDP [Rybak 2020]). Duration of therapy: At least 6 weeks (combine with rifampin for the entire duration of therapy and gentamicin for the first 2 weeks) (AHA [Baddour 2015]; IDSA [Liu 2011]).

Viridans group streptococci and S. bovis (native or prosthetic valve) (penicillin or ceftriaxone intolerance): **IV:** 15 mg/kg/dose every 12 hours initially; adjust based on therapeutic monitoring. Duration of therapy is 4 weeks (native valve) or 6 weeks (prosthetic valve) (AHA [Baddour 2015]).

Endophthalmitis, treatment (off-label use): Intravitreal: Usual dose: 1 mg per 0.1 mL NS or sterile water injected into vitreum, usually in combination with ceftazidime (Durand 2020; Endophthalmitis Vitrectomy Study Group 1995). A repeat dose(s) may be considered at 24 to 48 hours based on culture result, severity of the infection, and response to treatment (Durand 2020).

Intra-abdominal infection (off-label use): As a component of empiric therapy or pathogen-specific therapy (eg, methicillin-resistant *S. aureus*): IV: 15 to 20 mg/kg/dose every 8 to 12 hours initially; adjust based on therapeutic monitoring (ASHP/IDSA/PIDS/SIDP [Rybak 2020]; IDSA [Solomkin 2010]).

Intracranial abscess (brain abscess, intracranial epidural abscess) or spinal epidural abscess (off-label use): As a component of empiric therapy or pathogen-specific therapy for methicillin-resistant *S. aureus* : IV: 15 to 20 mg/kg/dose every 8 to 12 hours initially; adjust based on therapeutic monitoring. A loading dose may be considered in seriously ill patients (ASHP/IDSA/PIDS/SIDP [Rybak 2020]; IDSA [Liu 2011]). Duration generally ranges from 4 to 8 weeks for brain abscess and spinal epidural abscess and 6 to 8 weeks for intracranial epidural abscess (Bodilsen 2018; Sexton 2019a; Sexton 2019b; Southwick 2020).

Meningitis, bacterial (off-label use): As a component of empiric therapy or pathogen-specific therapy (eg, methicillin-resistant *S. aureus* or penicillin- and cephalosporin-resistant *S. pneumoniae*): IV: 15 to 20 mg/kg/dose every 8 to 12 hours initially; adjust based on therapeutic monitoring (ASHP/IDSA/PIDS/SIDP [Rybak 2020]; IDSA [Tunkel 2004]; IDSA [Tunkel 2017]). A loading dose may be considered in seriously ill patients (ASHP/IDSA/PIDS/SIDP [Rybak 2020]; IDSA [Liu 2011]).

Osteomyelitis: As a component of empiric therapy or pathogen-specific therapy (eg, methicillin-resistant *S. aureus*): IV: 15 to 20 mg/kg/dose every 8 to 12 hours initially (IDSA [Berbari 2015]; IDSA [Liu 2011]); adjust based on therapeutic monitoring. A loading dose may be considered in seriously ill patients (ASHP/IDSA/PIDS/SIDP [Rybak 2020]). Duration is generally ≥6 weeks; shorter courses are appropriate if the affected bone is completely resected (IDSA [Berbari 2015]; Osmon 2019).

Peritonitis, treatment (peritoneal dialysis patients) (off-label use): Note: Intraperitoneal administration is preferred to IV administration. Adjust to obtain a trough concentration between 15 and 20 mg/L (ISPD [Li 2016]). Consider a 25% dose increase in patients with significant residual renal function (urine output >100 mL/day) (ISPD [Li 2010]; ISPD [Li 2016]; Mancini 2018; Szeto 2018).

Intermittent (preferred): **Intraperitoneal:** 15 to 30 mg/kg added to one exchange of dialysate every 5 to 7 days (allow to dwell for ≥6 hours); supplemental doses and more frequent monitoring of serum levels may be needed for patients receiving automated peritoneal dialysis (ISPD [Li 2016]).

Continuous (with every exchange): **Intraperitoneal:** Loading dose: 30 mg/kg added to first exchange of dialysate; maintenance dose: 1.5 mg/kg/bag for each subsequent exchange of dialysate (Bunke 1983; ISPD [Li 2016]).

Pneumonia, as a component of empiric therapy or pathogen-specific therapy for methicillin-resistant *S. aureus*: IV: 15 to 20 mg/kg/dose every 8 to 12 hours initially; adjust based on therapeutic monitoring (ASHP/IDSA/PIDS/SIDP [Rybak 2020]; IDSA [Liu 2011]; ATS/IDSA [Metlay 2019]). A loading dose may be considered in seriously ill patients (ASHP/IDSA/PIDS/SIDP [Rybak 2009]; IDSA [Liu 2011]). **Note:** Duration of definitive therapy is for ≥7 days and varies based on disease severity and response to therapy (ATS/IDSA [Metlay 2019]; IDSA/ATS [Kalil 2016]; IDSA [Liu 2011]).

Prosthetic joint infection (off-label use): IV:

Pathogen-specific therapy for methicillin-resistant or susceptible S. aureus (alternative agent in beta-lactam intolerance): 15 to 20 mg/kg/dose every 8 to 12 hours initially (Berbari 2019; IDSA [Liu 2011]; IDSA [Osmon 2013]); adjust based on therapeutic monitoring based on therapeutic monitoring. Duration ranges from 2 to 6 weeks depending on prosthesis management, use of rifampin, and other patient-specific factors (IDSA [Osmon 2013]).

Pathogen-specific therapy for Enterococcus spp (penicillin susceptible [alternative agent] or penicillin resistant): 15 mg/kg/dose every 12 hours initially; adjust based on therapeutic monitoring.

Duration: 4 to 6 weeks (Berbari 2019; IDSA [Osmon 2013]).

Note: In select cases (eg, debridement and retention of prosthesis or one-stage arthroplasty), give oral suppressive antibiotic therapy with an appropriate regimen following completion of initial treatment (Berbari 2019; IDSA [Osmon 2013]).

Sepsis/septic shock: As a component of empiric therapy or pathogen-specific therapy for methicillin-resistant *S. aureus*: IV: 15 to 20 mg/kg/dose every 8 to 12 hours initially; adjust based on therapeutic monitoring (ASHP/IDSA/PIDS/SIDP [Rybak 2020]). Administer within 1 hour of identifying sepsis (SCCM [Rhodes 2017]). A loading dose should be considered in seriously ill patients (ASHP/IDSA/PIDS/SIDP [Rybak 2020]; SCCM [Rhodes 2017]). Usual duration of therapy is dependent on underlying source, but is typically 7 to 10 days or longer, depending on clinical response (SCCM [Rhodes 2017]).

Septic arthritis, without prosthetic material: As a component of empiric therapy or pathogen-specific therapy for methicillin-resistant *S. aureus* or coagulase-negative staphylococci: IV: 15 to 20 mg/kg/dose every 8 to 12 hours initially; adjust dose on therapeutic monitoring (ASHP/IDSA/PIDS/SIDP [Rybak 2020]). Total treatment duration is 3 to 4 weeks (in the absence of osteomyelitis), including appropriate oral step-down therapy (Goldenberg 2020; IDSA [Liu 2011]); some experts recommend 4 weeks of parenteral therapy for patients with concomitant bacteremia (Goldenberg 2020).

Skin and soft tissue infection (hospitalized patient): As a component of empiric therapy or pathogen-specific therapy for methicillin-resistant *S. aureus*: IV: 15 mg/kg/dose every 12 hours initially (IDSA [Stevens 2014]); adjust based on therapeutic monitoring (IDSA [Liu 2011]; IDSA [Stevens 2014]). **Note:** For empiric therapy of necrotizing infection, must be used in combination with other agents (IDSA [Stevens 2014]).

Streptococcus (group B), maternal prophylaxis for prevention of neonatal disease (alternative agent) (off-label use): Note: Prophylaxis is reserved for pregnant women with a positive group B streptococcus (GBS) vaginal or rectal screening in late gestation or GBS bacteriuria during the current pregnancy, history of birth of an infant with early-onset GBS disease, and unknown GBS culture status with any of the following: birth <37 0/7 weeks' gestation, intrapartum fever, prolonged rupture of membranes, known GBS positive in a previous pregnancy, or intrapartum nucleic acid amplification testing positive for GBS (ACOG 782 2019).

IV: 20 mg/kg at the onset of labor or prelabor rupture of membranes, then every 8 hours until delivery; maximum single dose: 2 g (ACOG 782 2019). Some experts prefer vancomycin 2 g initially and then 1 g every 12 hours thereafter until delivery (Baker 2019). **Note:** Vancomycin is reserved for use in penicillin-allergic patients at high risk for anaphylaxis, isolates with resistance to clindamycin, or in the absence of susceptibility data (ACOG 782 2019).

Surgical prophylaxis (in combination with other appropriate agents when coverage for methicillin-resistant *S. aureus* is indicated or for gram-positive coverage in patients unable to tolerate beta-lactams) (off-label use): IV: 15 mg/kg (usual maximum: 2 g/dose initially [Anderson 2020]) started within 60 to 120 minutes prior to initial surgical incision. Vancomycin doses may be repeated intraoperatively in 2 half-lives (approximately 8 to 12 hours in patients with normal renal function) if procedure is lengthy or if there is excessive blood loss (ASHP/IDSA/SIS/SHEA [Bratzler 2013]). In cases where an extension of prophylaxis is warranted postoperatively, total duration should be ≤24 hours (Anderson 2014). **Postoperative** prophylaxis is not recommended in clean and clean-contaminated surgeries (CDC [Berrios-Torres 2017]).

Surgical site infection: As a component of empiric therapy or pathogen-specific therapy for methicillin-resistant *S. aureus*: IV: 15 mg/kg/dose every 12 hours initially; adjust based on therapeutic monitoring (ASHP/IDSA/PIDS/SIDP [Rybak 2020]; IDSA [Stevens 2014]).

Toxic shock syndrome, staphylococcal: As a component of empiric therapy or pathogen-specific therapy for methicillin-resistant *S. aureus*: IV: 15 to 20 mg/kg/dose every 8 to 12 hours initially; adjust based on therapeutic monitoring (ASHP/IDSA/PIDS/SIDP [Rybak 2020]; Chu 2019). Duration varies based on underlying etiology; 10 to 14 days of treatment is recommended in the absence of bacteremia or other distinct focus of infection (Chu 2019).

Renal Impairment: Adult

Oral: There are no dosage adjustments provided in the manufacturer's labeling. However, dosage adjustment unlikely due to low systemic absorption.

IV: Note: Vancomycin levels should be monitored in patients with any renal impairment. In critically ill patients with renal insufficiency, the initial loading dose (~25 mg/kg) should not be reduced. However, subsequent dosage adjustments should be made based on renal function and trough serum concentrations (Wang 2001).

Vancomycin Initial Dosage Regimens for Patients With Impaired Renal Function (Golightly 2013)

eGFR (mL/minute per 1.73 m²)	Actual Body Weight			
	<60 kg	60 to 80 kg	81 to 100 kg	>100 kg
>90	750 mg every 8 hours	1,000 mg every 8 hours	1,250 mg every 8 hours	1,500 mg every 8 hours
50 to 90	750 mg every 12 hours	1,000 mg every 12 hours	1,250 mg every 12 hours	1,000 mg every 8 hours
15 to 49	750 mg every 24 hours	1,000 mg every 24 hours	1,250 mg every 24 hours	1,500 mg every 24 hours
<15[a]	750 mg	1,000 mg	1,250 mg	1,500 mg

[a]Check a random vancomycin level in 24 hours after the dose. If random level is ≤20 mg/mL, repeat the dose. If random level is >20 mg/mL, do not redose; repeat random level in 12 hours.

Dialysis: Poorly dialyzable by intermittent hemodialysis; however, use of high-flux membranes and continuous renal replacement therapy (CRRT) increases vancomycin clearance, and generally requires replacement dosing (Launay-Vacher 2002).

End-stage renal disease (ESRD) on intermittent hemodialysis (IHD) (administer after hemodialysis on dialysis days): Following loading dose of 15 to 25 mg/kg, give either 500 to 1,000 mg **or** 5 to 10 mg/kg after each dialysis session (Heintz 2009). **Note:** Dosing dependent on the assumption of 3 times/week, complete IHD sessions.

Redosing based on pre-HD concentrations:
<10 mg/L: Administer 1,000 mg after HD
10 to 25 mg/L: Administer 500 to 750 mg after HD
>25 mg/L: Hold vancomycin
Redosing based on post-HD concentrations: <10 to 15 mg/L: Administer 500 to 1,000 mg
Peritoneal dialysis (PD): 1 g every 4 to 7 days (Aronoff 2007)
Continuous renal replacement therapy (CRRT) (Heintz 2009; Trotman 2005): Drug clearance is highly dependent on the method of renal replacement, filter type, and flow rate. Appropriate dosing requires close monitoring of pharmacologic response, signs of adverse reactions due to drug accumulation, as well as drug concentrations in relation to target trough (if appropriate). The following are general recommendations only (based on dialysate flow/ultrafiltration rates of 1 to 2 L/hour and minimal residual renal function) and should not supersede clinical judgment:
CVVH: Loading dose of 15 to 25 mg/kg, followed by either 1,000 mg every 48 hours **or** 10 to 15 mg/kg every 24 to 48 hours
CVVHD: Loading dose of 15 to 25 mg/kg, followed by either 1,000 mg every 24 hours **or** 10 to 15 mg/kg every 24 hours
CVVHDF: Loading dose of 15 to 25 mg/kg, followed by either 1,000 mg every 24 hours **or** 7.5 to 10 mg/kg every 12 hours
Note: Consider redosing patients receiving CRRT for vancomycin concentrations <10 to 15 mg/L.

Hepatic Impairment: Adult

Oral: There are no dosage adjustments provided in the manufacturer's labeling. However, dosage adjustment unlikely due to low systemic absorption.

IV: There are no dosage adjustments provided in the manufacturer's labeling. However, degrees of hepatic dysfunction do not affect the pharmacokinetics of vancomycin (Marti 1996).

Pediatric

Initial dosage recommendations presented, serum concentrations should be monitored and adjusted accordingly. **Note:** Doses require adjustment in renal impairment. Consider single-dose administration with serum concentration monitoring rather than scheduled dosing in patients with urine output <1 mL/kg/hour or if serum creatinine significantly increases from baseline (eg, doubles). Optimal dose and frequency not established in patients receiving ECMO; available data is very limited and primarily from neonatal experience (Amaker 1996; Buck 1998; Hoie 1990; Mulla 2005). Patient-specific considerations (eg, reason for ECMO) and variability with ECMO procedure itself make extrapolation of pharmacokinetic data and dosing to all patients receiving ECMO difficult; closely monitor serum concentrations and determine individual dosing needs in these patients.

General dosing, susceptible infection: Infants, Children, and Adolescents: IV: 45 to 60 mg/kg/**day** divided every 6 to 8 hours; dose and frequency should be individualized based on serum concentrations (*Red Book* [AAP 2018]). **Note:** Every 6 hour dosing recommended as initial dosage regimen if targeting trough serum concentrations >10 mcg/mL (Benner 2009; Frymoyer 2009) in patients with normal renal function. Close monitoring of serum concentrations and assurance of adequate hydration status is recommended; utilize local antibiogram and protocols for further guidance.

Bacteremia [*S. aureus* (methicillin-resistant)]: Infants, Children, and Adolescents: IV: 15 mg/kg/dose every 6 hours for 2 to 6 weeks depending on severity (IDSA [Liu 2011])

Bone and joint infection:
Osteomyelitis (*S. aureus* [methicillin-resistant]): Infants, Children, and Adolescents: IV: 15 mg/kg/dose every 6 hours for a minimum of 4 to 6 weeks (IDSA [Liu 2011])
Septic arthritis (*S. aureus* [methicillin-resistant]): Infants, Children, and Adolescents: IV: 15 mg/kg/dose every 6 hours for minimum of 3 to 4 weeks (IDSA [Liu 2011])

***C. difficile* infection:**
Manufacturer's labeling: Infants, Children, and Adolescents: Oral: 40 mg/kg/**day** divided every 6 to 8 hours for 7 to 10 days; maximum daily dose: 2,000 mg/day
Guideline recommendations:
Non-severe infection, initial or first recurrence: Children and Adolescents: Oral: 10 mg/kg/dose 4 times daily for 10 days; maximum dose: 125 mg/dose (IDSA/SHEA [McDonald 2018])
Severe/fulminant infection, initial: Children and Adolescents:
Oral: 10 mg/kg/dose 4 times daily for 10 days; maximum dose: 500 mg/dose; may consider adding IV metronidazole in critically ill patients (IDSA/SHEA [McDonald 2018]). If patient is unable to tolerate oral therapy, may use nasogastric administration (ASID [Trubiano 2016]).
Rectal: **Note:** Consider use when ileus is present. Limited data available: Rectal enema: 500 mg in 100 mL NS; dose volume is determined by age (IDSA/SHEA [McDonald 2018]); the optimal doses have not been established in pediatric patients; suggested volumes for children: 1 to 3 years: 50 mL; 4 to 9 years: 75 mL; >10 years: 100 mL (ASID [Trubiano 2016]); administer 4 times daily with or without IV metronidazole (IDSA/SHEA [McDonald 2018])
Second or subsequent recurrence: Children and Adolescents: Pulsed-tapered regimen: Oral: 10 mg/kg/dose 4 times daily for 10 to 14 days; then 10 mg/kg/dose twice daily for 7 days, then 10 mg/kg/dose once daily for 7 days, then 10 mg/kg/dose every 2 or 3 days for 2 to 8 weeks; maximum dose: 125 mg/dose (IDSA/SHEA [McDonald 2018])

CNS infection:
Brain abscess, subdural empyema, spinal epidural abscess [*S. aureus* (methicillin-resistant)]: Infants, Children, and Adolescents: IV: 15 mg/kg/dose every 6 hours for 4 to 6 weeks (some experts combine with rifampin) (IDSA [Liu 2011])
Meningitis: Infants, Children, and Adolescents: IV: 15 mg/kg/dose every 6 hours; **Note:** Maintain trough serum concentrations of 15 to 20 mcg/mL (IDSA [Tunkel 2004]; IDSA [Tunkel 2017])
S. aureus (methicillin-resistant): Infants, Children, and Adolescents: IV: 15 mg/kg/dose every 6 hours for 2 weeks (some experts combine with rifampin) (IDSA [Liu 2011])

VP-shunt infection, ventriculitis: Limited data available: Infants, Children, and Adolescents: Intrathecal/intraventricular **(use a preservative-free preparation)**: 5 to 20 mg/**day**; usual dose: 10 or 20 mg/**day** (IDSA [Tunkel 2004]; IDSA [Tunkel 2017]); due to the smaller CSF volume in infants, some guidelines recommend decreasing the infant dose (IDSA [Tunkel 2017])

Endocarditis, treatment:

Empiric therapy/culture negative: Children and Adolescents: IV 60 mg/kg/**day** divided every 6 hours; maximum daily dose: 2,000 mg/**day**; use in combination with other antibiotics for at least 4 weeks; longer duration may be required if prosthetic material is present; dosage should be adjusted to target trough serum concentrations of 10 to 15 mcg/mL; higher trough concentrations (15 to 20 mcg/mL) may be needed if there is a lack of response or if a resistant organism (MIC >1 mcg/mL) is identified (AHA [Baltimore 2015])

Streptococcus (including enterococcus): Children and Adolescents: IV: 40 mg/kg/**day** divided every 8 to 12 hours for at least 4 to 6 weeks; a longer duration and additional antibiotics may be required depending on organism and presence of prosthetic material; dosage should be adjusted to target trough serum concentrations of 10 to 15 mcg/mL; higher trough concentrations (15 to 20 mcg/mL) may be needed for resistant organisms (MIC >1 mcg/mL) or if there is a lack of response (AHA [Baltimore 2015])

S. aureus:

Non-methicillin resistant: Children and Adolescents: IV: 40 mg/kg/**day** divided every 8 to 12 hours for at least 4 to 6 weeks; a longer duration and additional antibiotics may be required depending on organism and presence of prosthetic material; dosage should be adjusted to target trough serum concentrations of 10 to 15 mcg/mL; higher trough concentrations (15 to 20 mcg/mL) may be needed for resistant organisms (MIC >1 mcg/mL) or if there is a lack of response (AHA [Baltimore 2015])

Methicillin-resistant:

AHA Guidelines: Children and Adolescents: IV: 40 mg/kg/**day** divided every 8 to 12 hours for at least 6 weeks; maximum daily dose: 2,000 mg/**day;** a longer duration may be required depending on the presence of prosthetic material; dosage should be adjusted to target trough serum concentrations of 15 to 20 mcg/mL (AHA [Baltimore 2015])

IDSA Guidelines: Infants, Children, and Adolescents: IV: 60 mg/kg/**day** divided every 6 hours (IDSA [Liu 2011])

Enterocolitis (*S. aureus*): Infants, Children, and Adolescents: Oral: 40 mg/kg/**day** divided every 6 to 8 hours for 7 to 10 days; maximum daily dose: 2,000 mg/**day**

Intra-abdominal infection, complicated (MRSA): Infants, Children, and Adolescents: IV: 40 mg/kg/**day** divided every 6 to 8 hours (IDSA [Solomkin 2010])

Peritonitis (peritoneal dialysis) (ISPD [Warady 2012]):

Prophylaxis: Infants, Children, and Adolescents:

Touch contamination of PD line (if known MRSA colonization): Intraperitoneal: 25 mg per liter

High-risk gastrointestinal procedures: **Note:** Use should be reserved for patients at high risk for MRSA: IV: 10 mg/kg administered 60 to 90 minutes before procedure; maximum dose: 1,000 mg

Treatment: Infants, Children, and Adolescents:

Intermittent: Intraperitoneal: Initial dose: 30 mg/kg in the long dwell; subsequent doses: 15 mg/kg/dose every 3 to 5 days during the long dwell; **Note:** Increased clearance may occur in patients with residual renal function; subsequent doses should be based on serum concentration obtained 2 to 4 days after the previous dose; redosing should occur when serum concentration <15 mcg/mL.

Continuous: Intraperitoneal: Loading dose: 1,000 mg per liter of dialysate; maintenance dose: 25 mg per liter

Pneumonia:

Community-acquired pneumonia (CAP): Infants >3 months, Children, and Adolescents: IV: 40 to 60 mg/kg/**day** every 6 to 8 hours; dosing to achieve AUC/MIC >400 has been recommended for treating moderate to severe MRSA infections (IDSA/PIDS [Bradley 2011])

Alternate dosing: *S. aureus* (methicillin-resistant): Infants, Children, and Adolescents: IV: 60 mg/kg/**day** divided every 6 hours for 7 to 21 days depending on severity (IDSA [Liu 2011])

Health care-associated pneumonia (HAP), S. aureus (methicillin-resistant): Infants, Children, and Adolescents: IV: 60 mg/kg/**day** divided every 6 hours for 7 to 21 days depending on severity (IDSA [Liu 2011])

Septic thrombosis of cavernous or dural venous sinus [*S. aureus* (methicillin-resistant)]: Infants, Children, and Adolescents: IV: 15 mg/kg/dose every 6 hours for 4 to 6 weeks (some experts combine with rifampin) (IDSA [Liu 2011])

Skin and skin structure infections, complicated: [MRSA or *S. aureus* (methicillin sensitive) in penicillin allergic patients]: Infants, Children, and Adolescents (IDSA [Stevens 2014]):

Non-necrotizing infection: IV: 10 mg/kg/dose every 6 hours

Necrotizing infection: IV: 15 mg/kg/dose every 6 hours. Continue until further debridement is not necessary, patient has clinically improved, and patient is afebrile for 48 to 72 hours.

Alternate dosing: *S. aureus* (methicillin-resistant): Infants, Children, and Adolescents: IV: 60 mg/kg/**day** divided every 6 hours for 7 to 14 days (IDSA [Liu 2011])

Surgical (perioperative) prophylaxis: Infants, Children, and Adolescents: IV: 15 mg/kg/dose within 120 minutes prior to surgical incision. May be administered in combination with other antibiotics depending upon the surgical procedure (ASHP/IDSA/SIS/SHEA [Bratzler 2013]).

Renal Impairment: Pediatric

Oral: There are no dosage adjustments provided in manufacturer's labeling; however, dosage adjustment unlikely due to low systemic absorption.

IV: **Note:** Vancomycin levels should be monitored in patients with any renal impairment:

Infants, Children, and Adolescents: The following adjustments have been recommended (Aronoff 2007): **Note:** Renally adjusted dose recommendations are based on doses of 10 mg/kg/dose every 6 hours or 15 mg/kg/dose every 8 hours:

GFR 30 to 50 mL/minute/1.73 m^2: 10 mg/kg/dose every 12 hours

GFR 10 to 29 mL/minute/1.73 m²: 10 mg/kg/dose every 18 to 24 hours

GFR <10 mL/minute/1.73 m²: 10 mg/kg/dose; redose based on serum concentrations

Intermittent hemodialysis: 10 mg/kg/dose; redose based on serum concentrations

Peritoneal dialysis (PD): 10 mg/kg/dose; redose based on serum concentrations

Continuous renal replacement therapy (CRRT): 10 mg/kg/dose every 12 to 24 hours; monitor serum concentrations

Hepatic Impairment: Pediatric

Oral: There are no dosage adjustments provided in the manufacturer's labeling; however, dosage adjustment unlikely due to low systemic absorption.

IV: There are no dosage adjustments provided in the manufacturer's labeling; however, degrees of hepatic dysfunction do not affect the pharmacokinetics of vancomycin (Marti 1996).

Mechanism of Action Inhibits bacterial cell wall synthesis by blocking glycopeptide polymerization through binding tightly to D-alanyl-D-alanine portion of cell wall precursor

Contraindications Hypersensitivity to vancomycin or any component of the formulation

Warnings/Precautions **[US Boxed Warning]: The formulation of vancomycin injection containing the excipients, polyethylene glycol (PEG 400) and N-acetyl D-alanine (NADA), is not recommended for use during pregnancy. PEG 400 and NADA have caused fetal malformations in animal reproduction studies. If use of vancomycin is needed during pregnancy, use other available formulations of vancomycin.**

May cause nephrotoxicity, although limited data suggest direct causal relationship; risk factors include preexisting renal impairment, concomitant nephrotoxic medications (ie, aminoglycosides, loop diuretics, amphotericin B, IV contrast dye, vasopressors, piperacillin/tazobactam, and flucloxacillin), advanced age, increased weight, dehydration, critically ill patients, patients with rapidly changing renal function, sustained high vancomycin serum trough concentrations above 15 to 20 mg/L or daily AUC >650 to 1,300 mg•hour/L, and prolonged exposure (eg, ≥4 days). Studies have defined vancomycin-associated nephrotoxicity as: an increase of 0.5 mg/dL or ≥50% increase from baseline (whichever is greater) in multiple, sequential (≥2) serum creatinine concentrations in the absence of an alternative explanation or an increase in serum creatinine ≥0.3 mg/dL over a 48-hour period (Mehta 2007; Roy 2013; van Hal 2013). Discontinue treatment if signs of nephrotoxicity occur. Nephrotoxicity has also been reported following treatment with oral vancomycin (typically in patients >65 years of age).

May cause neutropenia; prolonged therapy and use of concomitant drugs that cause neutropenia may increase the risk; monitor leukocyte counts periodically in these patients. Prompt reversal of neutropenia is expected after discontinuation of therapy.

Ototoxicity is rarely associated with monotherapy. Ototoxicity manifests as tinnitus, hearing loss, dizziness, or vertigo. It has been most frequently reported in older patients, patients receiving excessive doses, those who have underlying hearing loss, or those receiving concomitant ototoxic drugs (eg, aminoglycosides). Serial auditory function testing may be helpful to minimize risk. Ototoxicity may be transient or permanent; discontinue treatment if signs of ototoxicity occur. Prolonged therapy (>1 week) or total doses exceeding 25 g may increase the risk of neutropenia; prompt reversal of neutropenia is expected after discontinuation of therapy. Prolonged use may result in fungal or bacterial superinfection, including CDI; CDI has been observed >2 months postantibiotic treatment. Use with caution in patients with renal impairment or those receiving other nephrotoxic drugs; dosage modification required and close monitoring is recommended in patients with preexisting renal impairment and those at high risk for renal impairment. Accumulation may occur after multiple oral doses of vancomycin in patients with renal impairment; consider monitoring serum concentrations in this circumstance

IV vancomycin is an irritant and can cause thrombophlebitis; ensure proper needle or catheter placement prior to and during infusion; avoid extravasation. Pain, tenderness, and necrosis may occur with extravasation. If thrombophlebitis occurs, slow infusion rates, dilute solution (eg, 2.5 to 5 g/L) and rotate infusion sites.

Rapid IV administration (eg, over <60 minutes) may result in hypotension, flushing, erythema, urticaria, pruritus, wheezing, dyspnea, and, rarely, cardiac arrest. Reactions usually cease promptly after infusion is stopped. Frequency of infusion reactions may increase with concomitant administration of anesthetics. If used in conjunction with anesthesia, complete the vancomycin infusion prior to anesthesia induction. Hemorrhagic occlusive retinal vasculitis (HORV), including permanent visual loss, has been reported in patients receiving intracameral or intravitreal administration of vancomycin during or after cataract surgery. Safety and efficacy of intraocularly administered vancomycin has not been established; vancomycin is not indicated for prophylaxis of endophthalmitis. Oral vancomycin is only indicated for the treatment of CDI or enterocolitis due to *S. aureus* and is not effective for systemic infections; parenteral vancomycin is not effective for the treatment of enterocolitis. Clinically significant serum concentrations have been reported in patients with inflammatory disorders of the intestinal mucosa who have taken oral vancomycin (multiple doses) for the treatment of CDI. Although use may be warranted, the risk for adverse reactions may be higher in this situation; consider monitoring serum trough concentrations, especially with renal insufficiency, severe colitis, and concurrent enteral vancomycin administration (IDSA/SHEA [McDonald 2018]; Pettit 2015). Use caution when administering intraperitoneally (IP); in some continuous ambulatory peritoneal dialysis (CAPD) patients, chemical peritonitis (cloudy dialysate, fever, severe abdominal pain) has occurred. Symptoms are self-limited and usually clear after vancomycin discontinuation.

Potentially significant interactions may exist, requiring dose or frequency adjustment, additional monitoring, and/or selection of alternative therapy.

Drug Interactions

Metabolism/Transport Effects None known.

Avoid Concomitant Use

Avoid concomitant use of Vancomycin with any of the following: BCG (Intravesical); Cholera Vaccine

Increased Effect/Toxicity

Vancomycin may increase the levels/effects of: Aminoglycosides; Colistimethate; Neuromuscular-Blocking Agents

The levels/effects of Vancomycin may be increased by: Nonsteroidal Anti-Inflammatory Agents; Piperacillin

Decreased Effect

Vancomycin may decrease the levels/effects of: BCG (Intravesical); BCG Vaccine (Immunization); Cholera Vaccine; Lactobacillus and Estriol; Sodium Picosulfate; Typhoid Vaccine

The levels/effects of Vancomycin may be decreased by: Bile Acid Sequestrants

Dietary Considerations May be taken with food.

Pharmacodynamics/Kinetics

Half-life Elimination Biphasic: Terminal:

Newborns: 6 to 10 hours

Neonates receiving ECMO: 6.53 ± 2.1 hours (Buck 1998); others have reported longer: 10.4 ± 6.7 hours (Mulla 2005)

Infants and Children 3 months to 4 years: 4 hours

Children and Adolescents >3 years: 2.2 to 3 hours

Adults: 4 to 6 hours; significantly prolonged with renal impairment

End-stage renal disease (ESRD): 7.5 days

Time to Peak Serum: IV: Immediately after completion of infusion

Reproductive Considerations

Pregnancy status should be evaluated in females of reproductive potential prior to using the IV formulation containing the excipients polyethylene glycol (PEG 400) and N-acetyl D-alanine (NADA).

Pregnancy Considerations

Vancomycin crosses the placenta and can be detected in fetal serum, amniotic fluid, and cord blood (Bourget 1991; Reyes 1989). Adverse fetal effects, including sensorineural hearing loss or nephrotoxicity, have not been reported following maternal use during the second or third trimesters of pregnancy.

The pharmacokinetics of vancomycin may be altered during pregnancy and pregnant patients may need a higher dose of vancomycin. Maternal half-life is unchanged, but the volume of distribution and the total plasma clearance may be increased (Bourget 1991). Individualization of therapy through serum concentration monitoring may be warranted.

Vancomycin is recommended for the treatment of *Clostridioides* (formerly *Clostridium*) *difficile* infections in pregnant women (ACG [Surawicz 2013]). Vancomycin is recommended as an alternative option to prevent the transmission of group B streptococcal (GBS) disease from mothers to newborns in patients at high risk for anaphylaxis to penicillin [or whose risk is unknown], and who do not have GBS susceptible to clindamycin (ACOG 797 2020). In patients colonized with MRSA, vancomycin is recommended as part of the antibiotic regimen for prophylactic use prior to cesarean delivery (ACOG 199 2018).

[US Boxed Warning]: The formulation of vancomycin injection containing the excipients polyethylene glycol (PEG 400) and N-acetyl D-alanine (NADA) is not recommended for use during pregnancy. PEG 400 and NADA have caused fetal malformations in animal reproduction studies. If use of vancomycin is needed during pregnancy, use other available formulations of vancomycin.

Breastfeeding Considerations

Vancomycin is present in breast milk following IV administration.

The relative infant dose (RID) of vancomycin is 4.8% when calculated using the highest breast milk concentration located and compared to an infant therapeutic oral dose of 40 mg/kg/day.

In general, breastfeeding is considered acceptable when the RID is <10% (Anderson 2016; Ito 2000).

Using the highest milk concentration (12.7 mg/mL), the estimated daily infant dose via breast milk is 1.9 mg/kg/day. This milk concentration was obtained 4 hours after maternal administration of IV vancomycin 1 g every 12 hours; therapy had been initiated at least 1 week prior to milk sampling (Reyes 1989).

Vancomycin exhibits minimal oral absorption; therefore, the amount available to pass into the milk would be limited following oral administration.

In general, antibiotics that are present in breast milk may cause non-dose-related modification of bowel flora. Monitor infants for GI disturbances, such as thrush or diarrhea (WHO 2002).

Vancomycin is recommended for the treatment of *Clostridioides* (formerly *Clostridium*) *difficile* infections in breastfeeding women (ACG [Surawicz 2013]). According to the manufacturer, the decision to breastfeed during therapy should consider the risk of infant exposure, the benefits of breastfeeding to the infant, and benefits of treatment to the mother.

Dosage Forms Considerations First-Vancomycin oral solution and Vancomycin+SyrSpend SF oral suspension are compounding kits. Refer to manufacturer's labeling for compounding instructions.

Dosage Forms: US

Capsule, Oral:

Vancocin: 250 mg

Vancocin HCl: 125 mg

Generic: 125 mg, 250 mg

Solution, Intravenous:

Generic: 1000 mg/200 mL (200 mL); 1500 mg/300 mL (300 mL)

Solution, Intravenous [preservative free]:

Generic: 500 mg/100 mL (100 mL); 2000 mg/400 mL (400 mL); 1 g/200 mL in Dextrose 5% (200 mL); 1 g/200 mL in NaCl 0.9% (200 mL); 500 mg/100 mL in Dextrose 5% (100 mL); 750 mg/150 mL in Dextrose 5% (150 mL)

Solution Reconstituted, Intravenous:

Generic: 10 g (1 ea)

Solution Reconstituted, Intravenous [preservative free]:

Generic: 250 mg (1 ea); 500 mg (1 ea); 750 mg (1 ea); 1 g (1 ea); 1.25 g (1 ea); 1.5 g (1 ea); 5 g (1 ea); 10 g (1 ea); 100 g (1 ea)

Solution Reconstituted, Oral:

Firvanq: 25 mg/mL (150 mL, 300 mL); 50 mg/mL (150 mL, 300 mL)

Generic: 250 mg/5 mL (80 mL, 150 mL, 300 mL)

Dosage Forms: Canada

Capsule, Oral:

Vancocin: 125 mg, 250 mg

Generic: 125 mg, 250 mg

Solution Reconstituted, Intravenous:

Generic: 500 mg (1 ea, 10 mL); 1 g (1 ea, 20 mL, 30 mL); 5 g (1 ea); 10 g (1 ea)

◆ **Vancomycin HCl** *see* Vancomycin *on page 1522*

◆ **Vancomycin Hydrochloride** *see* Vancomycin *on page 1522*

◆ **Vancosol Pack [DSC]** *see* Vancomycin *on page 1522*

Vandetanib (van DET a nib)

Related Information

Clinical Risk Related to Drugs Prolonging QT Interval *on page 1675*

Brand Names: US Caprelsa

Brand Names: Canada Caprelsa

Pharmacologic Category Antineoplastic Agent, Epidermal Growth Factor Receptor (EGFR) Inhibitor; Antineoplastic Agent, Tyrosine Kinase Inhibitor; Antineoplastic Agent, Vascular Endothelial Growth Factor (VEGF) Inhibitor

Use

Thyroid cancer, medullary (locally advanced or metastatic): Treatment of metastatic or unresectable locally-advanced medullary thyroid cancer (symptomatic or progressive).

Limitation of use: Use in indolent, asymptomatic, or slowly progressing disease only after careful considerations of vandetanib treatment-related risks.

Local Anesthetic/Vasoconstrictor Precautions Hypertension can occur with the use of this drug, particularly early in the treatment course. Monitor for hypertension prior to using local anesthetic with vasoconstrictor; medical consult if necessary.

Vandetanib is one of the drugs confirmed to prolong the QT interval and is accepted as having a risk of causing torsade de pointes. The risk of drug-induced torsade de pointes is extremely low when a single QT interval prolonging drug is prescribed. In terms of epinephrine, it is not known what effect vasoconstrictors in the local anesthetic regimen will have in patients with a known history of congenital prolonged QT interval or in patients taking any medication that prolongs the QT interval. Until more information is obtained, it is suggested that the clinician consult with the physician prior to the use of a vasoconstrictor in suspected patients, and that the vasoconstrictor (epinephrine, mepivacaine and levonordefrin [Carbocaine® 2% with Neo-Cobefrin®]) be used with caution.

Effects on Dental Treatment Key adverse event(s) related to dental treatment: Xerostomia (normal salivary flow resumes upon discontinuation), mucositis/stomatitis, taste perversion, and oral pain.

Effects on Bleeding Chemotherapy may result in significant myelosuppression, potentially including significant reduction in platelet counts (thrombocytopenia: 9%) and altered hemostasis. In patients who are under active treatment with these agents, medical consult is suggested.

Adverse Reactions

>10%:

Cardiovascular: Hypertension (≤33%), hypertensive crisis (≤33%), prolonged QT interval on ECG (14%)

Central nervous system: Headache (26%), fatigue (24%)

Dermatologic: Skin rash (53%), acneiform eruption (≤35%), acne vulgaris (≤35%), xeroderma (15%), skin photosensitivity (13%), pruritus (11%)

Endocrine & metabolic: Hypocalcemia (11% to 57%), hypoglycemia (24%)

Gastrointestinal: Colitis (≤57%), diarrhea (≤57%), nausea (33%), abdominal pain (21%), decreased appetite (21%), vomiting (15%), dyspepsia (11%)

Hematologic & oncologic: Hemorrhage (grades ≤2: 14%)

Hepatic: Increased serum alanine aminotransferase (51%)

Ophthalmic: Corneal changes (13%)

Renal: Increased serum creatinine (16%)

Respiratory: Upper respiratory tract infection (23%)

1% to 10%:

Cardiovascular: Cerebral ischemia (1%)

Central nervous system: Depression (10%)

Dermatologic: Nail disease (9%), alopecia (8%)

Endocrine & metabolic: Hypomagnesemia (7%), hypothyroidism (6%)

Gastrointestinal: Xerostomia (9%), dysgeusia (8%)

Genitourinary: Proteinuria (10%)

Hematologic & oncologic: Neutropenia (10%), thrombocytopenia (9%)

Neuromuscular & skeletal: Muscle spasm (6%)

Ophthalmic: Blurred vision (9%)

Frequency not defined:

Cardiovascular: Torsades de pointes, ventricular tachycardia

Central nervous system: Reversible posterior leukoencephalopathy syndrome

Dermatologic: Stevens-Johnson syndrome, toxic epidermal necrolysis

Respiratory: Interstitial pulmonary disease, pneumonitis

<1%, postmarketing, and/or case reports: Cardiac failure, intestinal perforation, pancreatitis

Mechanism of Action Vandetanib is a multikinase inhibitor; it inhibits tyrosine kinases including epidermal growth factor reception (EGFR), vascular endothelial growth factor (VEGF), rearranged during transfection (RET), protein tyrosine kinase 6 (BRK), TIE2, EPH kinase receptors and SRC kinase receptors, selectively blocking intracellular signaling, angiogenesis and cellular proliferation

Pharmacodynamics/Kinetics

Half-life Elimination 19 days

Time to Peak 6 hours (range: 4 to 10 hours)

Reproductive Considerations

Pregnancy status should be evaluated prior to vandetanib therapy. Females of childbearing potential should be advised to avoid pregnancy and use effective contraception during and for at least 4 months after the last vandetanib dose.

Pregnancy Considerations

Based on the mechanism of action and data from animal reproduction studies, in utero exposure to vandetanib may cause fetal harm.

Information related to the use of vandetanib in pregnant females is limited (Thomas 2018).

Prescribing and Access Restrictions In Canada, vandetanib is available only through the CAPRELSA Restricted Distribution Program. Prescribers and pharmacies must be certified with the program to prescribe or dispense vandetanib. Further information may be obtained at 1-800-589-6215 or visit www.caprelsa.ca/rdp

Dental Health Professional Considerations See Local Anesthetic/Vasoconstrictor Precautions

- ◆ **Vanos** *see* Fluocinonide *on page 691*
- ◆ **Vantas** *see* Histrelin *on page 759*
- ◆ **Vantin** *see* Cefpodoxime *on page 311*
- ◆ **VAQTA** *see* Hepatitis A Vaccine *on page 755*
- ◆ **VAR** *see* Measles, Mumps, Rubella, and Varicella Virus Vaccine *on page 950*

Vardenafil (var DEN a fil)

Brand Names: US Levitra; Staxyn

Brand Names: Canada APO-Vardenafil; JAMP-Vardenafil; JAMP-Vardenafil ODT; Levitra; MYLAN-VARDENAFIL; Staxyn

Pharmacologic Category Phosphodiesterase-5 Enzyme Inhibitor

Use Erectile dysfunction: Treatment of erectile dysfunction (ED)

Local Anesthetic/Vasoconstrictor Precautions No information available to require special precautions

Effects on Dental Treatment No significant effects or complications reported

Effects on Bleeding No information available to require special precautions

Adverse Reactions

>10%:

Cardiovascular: Flushing (8% to 11%)

Central nervous system: Headache (14% to 15%)

2% to 10%:

Central nervous system: Dizziness (2%)

Gastrointestinal: Dyspepsia (3% to 4%), nausea (2%)

Neuromuscular & skeletal: Back pain (2%), increased creatine phosphokinase (2%)

Respiratory: Rhinitis (9%), flu-like symptoms (3%), nasal congestion (3%), sinusitis (3%)

<2%, postmarketing, and/or case reports: Abdominal pain, abnormal hepatic function tests, allergic edema, anaphylaxis, angina pectoris, angioedema, arthralgia, auditory impairment, basal cell carcinoma (Loeb 2015), blurred vision, chest pain, chromatopsia, conjunctivitis, decreased visual acuity, diaphoresis, diarrhea, drowsiness, dysesthesia, dysphagia, dyspnea, ejaculatory disorder, epistaxis, erythema, esophagitis, eye discomfort, eye pain, facial edema, gastritis, gastroesophageal reflux disease, glaucoma, hearing loss, hypersensitivity reaction, hypertension, hypertonia, hypoesthesia, hypotension, increased gamma-glutamyl transferase, increased intraocular pressure, insomnia, ischemic heart disease, laryngeal edema, malignant melanoma (Loeb 2015), muscle cramps, myalgia, myocardial infarction, neck pain, anterior ischemic optic neuropathy (nonarteritic; NAION), ocular hyperemia, orthostatic hypotension, pain, palpitations, paresthesia, pharyngitis, photophobia, priapism, pruritus, retinal vein occlusion, seizure, skin photosensitivity, skin rash, sleep disorder, syncope, tachycardia, temporary amnesia (global), tinnitus, ventricular tachyarrhythmia, vertigo, vision color changes, vision loss (temporary or permanent), visual disturbance (including dim vision), visual field defect, vomiting, watery eyes, weakness, xerostomia

Mechanism of Action Does not directly cause penile erections, but affects the response to sexual stimulation. The physiologic mechanism of erection of the penis involves release of nitric oxide (NO) in the corpus cavernosum during sexual stimulation. NO then activates the enzyme guanylate cyclase, which results in increased levels of cyclic guanosine monophosphate (cGMP), producing smooth muscle relaxation and inflow of blood to the corpus cavernosum. Vardenafil enhances the effect of NO by inhibiting phosphodiesterase type 5 (PDE-5), which is responsible for degradation of cGMP in the corpus cavernosum; when sexual stimulation causes local release of NO, inhibition of PDE-5 by vardenafil causes increased levels of cGMP in the corpus cavernosum, resulting in smooth muscle relaxation and inflow of blood to the corpus cavernosum; at recommended doses, it has no effect in the absence of sexual stimulation.

Pharmacodynamics/Kinetics

Onset of Action ~60 minutes

Half-life Elimination Terminal: Vardenafil and metabolite: 4 to 6 hours

Time to Peak Plasma: 0.5 to 2 hours

Reproductive Considerations

No effects on sperm motility or morphology were observed in healthy males.

Pregnancy Risk Factor B

Pregnancy Considerations

Adverse events were not observed in animal studies; however, vardenafil is not indicated for use in women.

◆ **Vardenafil HCl** *see* Vardenafil *on page 1532*

◆ **Vardenafil Hydrochloride** *see* Vardenafil *on page 1532*

Varenicline (var e NI kleen)

Brand Names: US Chantix; Chantix Continuing Month Pak; Chantix Starting Month Pak

Brand Names: Canada APO-Varenicline; Champix; Champix Starter Pack; TEVA-Varenicline

Generic Availability (US) No

Pharmacologic Category Partial Nicotine Agonist; Smoking Cessation Aid

Use Smoking cessation: As an aid to smoking cessation treatment.

Local Anesthetic/Vasoconstrictor Precautions

No information available to require special precautions

Effects on Dental Treatment Key adverse event(s) related to dental treatment: Infrequent occurrences of xerostomia (normal salivary flow resumes upon discontinuation) and dysgeusia have been reported. Rare occurrences of Bell palsy, erythema multiforme, oral mucosa ulcer, Stevens-Johnson syndrome, and toothache have also been reported.

Effects on Bleeding No information available to require special precautions

Adverse Reactions

>10%:

Central nervous system: Headache (12% to 19%), insomnia (9% to 19%), abnormal dreams (8% to 13%), irritability (11%), suicidal ideation (11%), depression (4% to 11%)

Gastrointestinal: Nausea (16% to 40%), vomiting (5% to 11%)

1% to 10%:

Cardiovascular: Angina pectoris (4%), chest pain (3%), peripheral edema (2%), myocardial infarction (≤1%)

Central nervous system: Anxiety (8%), malaise (7%), agitation (5% to 7%), sleep disorder (3% to 5%), tension (4%), drowsiness (3%), hostility (2% to 3%), lethargy (1% to 2%), nightmares (1% to 2%)

Dermatologic: Skin rash (3%)

Gastrointestinal: Flatulence (6% to 9%), constipation (5% to 8%), dysgeusia (5% to 8%), abdominal pain (7%), diarrhea (6%), xerostomia (6%), dyspepsia (5%), increased appetite (3% to 4%), anorexia (≤2%), decreased appetite (≤2%), gastroesophageal reflux disease (1%)

Respiratory: Upper respiratory tract infection (5% to 7%), dyspnea (2%), rhinorrhea (≤1%)

<1%, postmarketing, and/or case reports: Abnormal hepatic function tests, abnormality in thinking, abnormal urinalysis, accidental injury, acne vulgaris, acute

coronary syndrome, acute renal failure, aggressive behavior, allergic rhinitis, altered sense of smell, amnesia, anemia, angioedema, arthralgia, asthma, atrial fibrillation, back pain, behavioral changes, Bell palsy, blurred vision, bradycardia, cardiac arrhythmia, cardiac flutter, cataract (subcapsular), cerebrovascular accident, chills, conjunctivitis, cor pulmonale, coronary artery disease, deafness, decreased libido, decreased mental acuity, decreased visual acuity, delusions, diabetes mellitus, difficulty thinking, disorientation, dissociative disorder, dizziness, dysarthria, dysphagia, ECG abnormality, eczema, edema, elevation in serum levels of skeletal-muscle enzymes, emotional disturbance, emotional lability, enterocolitis, epistaxis, equilibrium disturbance, erectile dysfunction, eructation, erythema, erythema multiforme, esophagitis, euphoria, eye irritation, eye pain, fever, flu-like symptoms, flushing, gallbladder disease, gastric ulcer, gastritis, gastrointestinal hemorrhage, hallucination, homicidal ideation, hyperglycemia, hyperhidrosis, hyperlipidemia, hypersensitivity reaction, hypoglycemia, hypokalemia, intestinal obstruction, lack of concentration, leukocytosis, loss of consciousness, lymphadenopathy, mania, Meniere disease, menstrual disease, migraine, multiple sclerosis, muscle cramps, musculoskeletal pain, myalgia, myositis, nephrolithiasis, nocturia, nocturnal amblyopia, nystagmus, ophthalmic vascular disease, oral mucosa ulcer, osteoporosis, palpitations, pancreatitis, panic, paranoia, photophobia, pleurisy, pollakiuria, polyuria, psoriasis, psychomotor agitation, psychomotor retardation, psychosis, pulmonary embolism, respiratory tract disease, restless leg syndrome, seizure, sensory disturbance, sexual difficulty, skin photosensitivity, somnambulism, splenomegaly, Stevens-Johnson syndrome, syncope, tachycardia, thrombocytopenia, thrombosis, thyroid disease, tinnitus, toothache, transient blindness, transient ischemic attacks, tremor, upper respiratory tract inflammation, urethral disease, urinary retention, urine abnormality, urticaria, ventricular premature contractions, vertigo, visual field defect, vitreous opacity, weight gain, xeroderma, xerophthalmia

Dental Usual Dosage Smoking cessation: Oral:

Initial:

Days 1 to 3: 0.5 mg once daily

Days 4 to 7: 0.5 mg twice daily

Maintenance (≥ Day 8): 1 mg twice daily for 11 weeks

Note: Start 1 week before target quit date. Alternatively, patients may consider setting a quit date up to 35 days after initiation of varenicline (some data suggest that an extended pretreatment regimen may result in higher abstinence rates [Hajek, 2011]). If patient successfully quits smoking at the end of the 12 weeks, may continue for another 12 weeks to help maintain success. If not successful in first 12 weeks, then stop medication and reassess factors contributing to failure.

Dosing

Adult & Geriatric

Smoking cessation: Oral:

Initial:

Days 1 to 3: 0.5 mg once daily.

Days 4 to 7: 0.5 mg twice daily.

Maintenance (day 8 and later): 1 mg twice daily; may consider a temporary or permanent dose reduction if usual dose is not tolerated (Tonstad 2006; manufacturer's labeling).

Duration: Continue maintenance dose for 11 weeks (for a total of 12 weeks of treatment); if the patient successfully quits smoking at the end of 12 weeks, an additional 12-week course may increase likelihood of success (Tonstad 2006).

Approaches to selecting a tobacco quit date: May either choose a fixed quit date (ie, start varenicline, then quit on day 8) or a flexible quit date (ie, start varenicline, then quit between days 8 to 35). Alternatively, a gradual quit date (ie, start varenicline and reduce smoking 50% by week 4, reduce an additional 50% by week 8, and continue reducing with a goal of complete abstinence by week 12) is acceptable (Hajek 2011; Rigotti 2020; manufacturer's labeling).

Renal Impairment: Adult

CrCl ≥30 mL/minute: No dosage adjustment necessary.

CrCl <30 mL/minute: Initial: 0.5 mg once daily; maximum maintenance dose: 0.5 mg twice daily

ESRD (receiving hemodialysis): Maximum dose: 0.5 mg once daily

Hepatic Impairment: Adult No dosage adjustment necessary.

Adjustment for Toxicity: Adult Patients who cannot tolerate adverse events may require temporary (or permanent) reduction in dose.

Pediatric

Smoking cessation: Adolescents ≥17 years: **Note:** Efficacy has not been established in patients <17 years of age; a randomized, double-blind, placebo-controlled trial including 216 pediatric patients 12 to 16 years of age showed that varenicline did not improve continuous abstinence rates; use is not recommended in pediatric patients ≤16 years of age. In another double-blind, placebo-controlled trial of 157 adolescents and young adults 14 to 19 years of age (mean age: 19.1 ± 1.5 years), the primary efficacy endpoint of end of treatment (week 12) abstinence was the same in both treatment and placebo groups at 8.9%; significant findings in secondary endpoints were observed, including higher weekly self-reported abstinence rates, and patients who achieved 7-day abstinence reported shorter time to achieve 7 days abstinence (39 days compared to 59 days with placebo) (Gray 2019).

Initial: See "Approaches to selecting a tobacco quit date" for additional information.

Days 1 to 3: Oral: 0.5 mg once daily.

Days 4 to 7: Oral: 0.5 mg twice daily.

Maintenance (≥ Day 8): Oral: 1 mg twice daily for 11 weeks; may consider a temporary or permanent dose reduction if usual dose is not tolerated. If patient successfully quits smoking at the end of the 12 weeks, may continue for another 12 weeks to help maintain success. Patients who are motivated to quit and do not succeed in stopping smoking during prior therapy, or who relapse after treatment, should be encouraged to make another attempt with varenicline once factors contributing to the failed attempt have been identified and addressed.

Approaches to selecting a tobacco quit date: May either choose a fixed quit date (ie, start varenicline, then quit on day 8) or a flexible quit date (ie, start varenicline, then quit between days 8 to 35). Alternatively, a gradual quit date (ie, start varenicline and reduce smoking 50% by week 4, reduce an additional 50% by week 8, and continue reducing with a goal of complete abstinence by week 12) is acceptable.

Dosing adjustment for toxicity: Adolescents ≥17 years: Patients who cannot tolerate adverse events may require temporary (or permanent) reduction in dose.

Renal Impairment: Pediatric

Adolescents ≥17 years:

CrCl ≥30 mL/minute: No dosage adjustment necessary.

CrCl <30 mL/minute: Initial: 0.5 mg once daily; maximum maintenance dose: 0.5 mg twice daily.

End-stage renal disease (ESRD) (receiving hemodialysis): Maximum maintenance dose: 0.5 mg once daily.

Hepatic Impairment: Pediatric Adolescents ≥17 years: No dosage adjustment necessary.

Mechanism of Action Partial neuronal $\alpha_4 \beta_2$ nicotinic receptor agonist; prevents nicotine stimulation of mesolimbic dopamine system associated with nicotine addiction. Also binds to 5-HT_3 receptor (significance not determined) with moderate affinity. Varenicline stimulates dopamine activity but to a much smaller degree than nicotine does, resulting in decreased craving and withdrawal symptoms.

Contraindications Serious hypersensitivity reactions or skin reactions to varenicline or any component of the formulation

Warnings/Precautions Postmarketing cases of serious neuropsychiatric events (including depression, suicidal thoughts, and suicide) have been reported in patients with or without preexisting psychiatric disease; some cases may have been complicated by symptoms of nicotine withdrawal following smoking cessation. Subsequent controlled trials in patients with or without psychiatric disorders, however, have not identified significant differences in neuropsychiatric effects for patients taking varenicline, bupropion, nicotine patches, or placebo (Anthenelli 2013; Anthenelli 2016; Gibbons 2013; Thomas 2015). Monitor all patients for behavioral changes and psychiatric symptoms (eg, agitation, depression, suicidal behavior, suicidal ideation); inform patients to discontinue treatment and contact their health care provider immediately if they experience any behavioral and/or mood changes. Of postmarketing cases, many resolved following therapy discontinuation.

Postmarketing reports of hypersensitivity reactions (including angioedema) and rare cases of serious skin reactions (including Stevens-Johnson syndrome and erythema multiforme) have been reported. Patients should be instructed to discontinue use and contact health care provider if signs/symptoms occur. Treatment may increase risk of cardiovascular events; however, the risk appears lower than nicotine replacement therapy (Benowitz 2018; Carney 2020; Sterling 2016; Ware 2013). Patients should be instructed to contact their health care provider if cardiovascular symptoms occur. Seizures have been reported in patients with or without a history of seizures. Seizures generally occurred within the first month of therapy. Consider the risks against the benefits before initiating in patients with a history of seizures or other factors that can lower the seizure threshold; discontinue use if seizures occur during therapy. Dose-dependent nausea may occur; both transient and persistent nausea has been reported. Dosage reduction may be considered for intolerable nausea. May cause CNS depression, which may impair physical or mental abilities; patients must be cautioned about performing tasks that require mental alertness (eg, operating machinery, driving). There have been postmarketing reports of traffic accidents, near-miss incidents in traffic, or other accidental injuries in patients taking varenicline. Cases of somnambulism, involving harmful behavior to self, others, or property, have been reported. Discontinue treatment if somnambulism occurs.

Use caution in renal dysfunction; dosage adjustment required with severe impairment. Potentially significant drug-drug interactions may exist, requiring dose or frequency adjustment, additional monitoring, and/or selection of alternative therapy.

Warnings: Additional Pediatric Considerations Varenicline has not demonstrated efficacy in patients ≤16 years; the manufacturer conducted a randomized, double-blind, placebo-controlled trial including 216 pediatric patients 12 to 16 years of age as part of the Pediatric Research Equity Act which showed that varenicline did not increase smoking abstinence rates compared to placebo in this age group (FDA 2019).

Drug Interactions

Metabolism/Transport Effects **Substrate** of OCT2

Avoid Concomitant Use There are no known interactions where it is recommended to avoid concomitant use.

Increased Effect/Toxicity

Varenicline may increase the levels/effects of: Alcohol (Ethyl); Nicotine

The levels/effects of Varenicline may be increased by: Erdafitinib; Histamine H2 Receptor Antagonists; Quinolones; Tafenoquine; Trimethoprim

Decreased Effect There are no known significant interactions involving a decrease in effect.

Dietary Considerations Take after eating and with a full glass of water to decrease gastric upset.

Pharmacodynamics/Kinetics

Half-life Elimination ~24 hours

Time to Peak Plasma: ~3 to 4 hours

Pregnancy Considerations

Information related to the use of varenicline in pregnancy is limited (Harrison-Woolrych 2013; Kaplan 2014; Richardson 2017).

Nicotine exposure is associated with adverse events to both the mother and fetus. All pregnant females should be encouraged to stop smoking. However, data is insufficient to recommend varenicline for smoking cessation during pregnancy (ACOG 721 2017).

Breastfeeding Considerations It is not known if varenicline is present in breast milk.

There is insufficient information related to the use of varenicline to recommend use for smoking cessation in breastfeeding women (ACOG 721 2017). Due to the potential for serious adverse reactions in the breastfed infant, the manufacturer recommends a decision be made whether to discontinue breastfeeding or to discontinue the drug, taking into account the importance of treatment to the mother. Infants exposed via breast milk should be monitored for seizures or excessive vomiting.

Dosage Forms: US

Tablet, Oral:

Chantix: 0.5 mg, 1 mg

Chantix Continuing Month Pak: 1 mg

Chantix Starting Month Pak: 0.5 mg x 11 & 1 mg x 42

Dosage Forms: Canada

Miscellaneous, Oral:

Champix Starter Pack: 0.5 MG X 11 & 1 MG X 14 (25 ea)

Generic: 0.5 MG X 11 & 1 MG X 14 (25 ea)

Tablet, Oral:
Champix: 0.5 mg, 1 mg
Generic: 0.5 mg, 1 mg

◆ **Varenicline Tartrate** *see* Varenicline *on page 1532*

◆ **Varicella** *see* Measles, Mumps, Rubella, and Varicella Virus Vaccine *on page 950*

◆ **Varicella, Measles, Mumps, and Rubella Vaccine** *see* Measles, Mumps, Rubella, and Varicella Virus Vaccine *on page 950*

◆ **Varicella Zoster** *see* Varicella-Zoster Immune Globulin (Human) *on page 1535*

Varicella-Zoster Immune Globulin (Human)

(var i SEL a- ZOS ter i MYUN GLOB yoo lin HYU man)

Brand Names: US Varizig

Brand Names: Canada VariZIG

Pharmacologic Category Blood Product Derivative; Immune Globulin

Use

Varicella prophylaxis: Postexposure prophylaxis of varicella in high-risk individuals. High-risk groups include immunocompromised children and adults, newborns of mothers with varicella shortly before or after delivery, premature infants, neonates and infants <1 year, adults without evidence of immunity, and pregnant women.

The Advisory Committee on Immunization Practices (ACIP) recommends varicella-zoster immune globulin (VZIG) to patients who are at high risk for severe varicella infection and complications; and who were exposed to varicella or herpes zoster; and for whom varicella vaccine is contraindicated. The decision to use VZIG should take into consideration if the patient lacks evidence of immunity; if exposure is likely to result in an infection; and if the patient is at greater risk for varicella complications than the general population. The following are patient groups for whom VZIG is recommended (CDC 2013):

- Immunocompromised patients without evidence of immunity (seronegative), including those with neoplastic disease (eg, leukemia or lymphoma); primary or acquired immunodeficiency; immunosuppressive therapy (including steroid therapy equivalent to prednisone ≥2 mg/kg or 20 mg/day)
- Newborn of mother who had onset of varicella (chickenpox) within 5 days before delivery or within 48 hours after delivery
- Hospitalized premature infants (≥28 weeks' gestation) who were exposed during the neonatal period and whose mother has no evidence of immunity
- Hospitalized premature infants (<28 weeks' gestation or ≤1,000 g) regardless of maternal history and who were exposed during the neonatal period
- Pregnant women without evidence of immunity who have been exposed

Local Anesthetic/Vasoconstrictor Precautions
No information available to require special precautions

Effects on Dental Treatment No significant effects or complications reported

Effects on Bleeding No information available to require special precautions

Adverse Reactions

1% to 10%:

Central nervous system: Headache (2% to 4%), chills (≤2%), fatigue (≤2%)
Dermatologic: Skin rash (<2%)
Gastrointestinal: Nausea (<2%)
Local: Pain at injection site (2% to 9%)

<1%, postmarketing, and/or case reports: Deep vein thrombosis, hypersensitivity reaction, serum sickness, thrombosis

Mechanism of Action Antibodies obtained from pooled human plasma of individuals with high titers of varicella-zoster provide passive immunity.

Pharmacodynamics/Kinetics

Duration of Action ≥6 weeks

Half-life Elimination IV: 18 to 24 days; IM: 26.2 ± 4.6 days

Time to Peak IV: <3 hours; IM: 4.5 ± 2.8 days

Pregnancy Risk Factor C

Pregnancy Considerations

Varicella zoster immune globulin (VZIG) is made of purified human IgG. Placental transfer of human IgG is dependent upon the IgG subclass, maternal serum concentrations, birth weight, and gestational age, generally increasing as pregnancy progresses. The lowest exposure would be expected during the period of organogenesis (Palmeira 2012; Pentsuk 2009).

Women who do not have evidence of immunity to varicella may be at increased risk of complications if infected during pregnancy. Varicella infection in the mother can also lead to intrauterine infection in the fetus. VZIG is primarily used to prevent maternal complications, not fetal infection (CDC 2007). The safety of varicella immune globulin during pregnancy has been evaluated (Swamy 2019). VZIG is indicated for postexposure prophylaxis of varicella in high-risk patients, including females who are pregnant (CDC 2013).

◆ **Varizig** *see* Varicella-Zoster Immune Globulin (Human) *on page 1535*

◆ **Varubi [DSC]** *see* Rolapitant *on page 1343*

◆ **Varubi (180 MG Dose)** *see* Rolapitant *on page 1343*

◆ **Vascepa** *see* Omega-3 Fatty Acids *on page 1137*

◆ **Vascular Endothelial Growth Factor Trap** *see* Ziv-Aflibercept (Systemic) *on page 1573*

◆ **Vasodilan** *see* Isoxsuprine *on page 847*

Vasopressin (vay soe PRES in)

Brand Names: US Vasostrict

Pharmacologic Category Antidiuretic Hormone Analog; Hormone, Posterior Pituitary

Use Shock, vasodilatory: To increase blood pressure in adults with vasodilatory shock (eg, postcardiotomy or sepsis) who remain hypotensive despite fluid resuscitation and catecholamines.

Local Anesthetic/Vasoconstrictor Precautions
No information available to require special precautions

Effects on Dental Treatment No significant effects or complications reported

Effects on Bleeding No information available to require special precautions

Adverse Reactions

Frequency not defined:

Cardiovascular: Atrial fibrillation, bradycardia, ischemic heart disease, limb ischemia (distal), low cardiac output, right heart failure, shock (hemorrhagic)
Dermatologic: Skin lesion (ischemic)
Endocrine & metabolic: Hyponatremia
Gastrointestinal: Mesenteric ischemia
Hematologic & oncologic: Decreased platelet count, hemorrhage (intractable)

Hepatic: Increased serum bilirubin
Renal: Renal insufficiency
Postmarketing: Endocrine & metabolic: Diabetes insipidus (reversible)

Mechanism of Action Vasopressin stimulates a family of arginine vasopressin (AVP) receptors, oxytocin receptors, and purinergic receptors (Russell 2011). Vasopressin, at therapeutic doses used for vasodilatory shock, stimulates the AVPR1a (or V1) receptor and increases systemic vascular resistance and mean arterial blood pressure; in response to these effects, a decrease in heart rate and cardiac output may be seen. When the AVPR2 (or V2) receptor is stimulated, cyclic adenosine monophosphate (cAMP) increases which in turn increases water permeability at the renal tubule resulting in decreased urine volume and increased osmolality. Vasopressin, at pressor doses, also causes smooth muscle contraction in the GI tract by stimulating muscular V1 receptors and release of prolactin and ACTH via AVPR1b (or V3) receptors.

Pharmacodynamics/Kinetics

Onset of Action

Antidiuretic: Peak effect: 1 to 2 hours (Murphy-Human 2010).

Vasopressor effect: IV: Rapid with peak effect occurring within 15 minutes of initiation of continuous IV infusion.

Duration of Action SubQ: Antidiuretic: 2 to 8 hours; IV: Vasopressor effect: Within 20 minutes after IV infusion terminated.

Half-life Elimination IV, SubQ: 10 to 20 minutes (apparent half-life: ≤10 minutes).

Pregnancy Risk Factor C

Pregnancy Considerations Animal reproduction studies have not been conducted. Vasopressin may produce tonic uterine contractions; however, doses sufficient for diabetes insipidus are not likely to produce this effect.

◆ **Vasostrict** *see* Vasopressin *on page 1535*
◆ **Vasotec** *see* Enalapril *on page 560*
◆ **Vazculep** *see* Phenylephrine (Systemic) *on page 1227*
◆ **VEC-162** *see* Tasimelteon *on page 1407*
◆ **Vecamyl** *see* Mecamylamine *on page 951*
◆ **Vectibix** *see* Panitumumab *on page 1187*
◆ **Vectical** *see* Calcitriol (Topical) *on page 280*

Vedolizumab (ve doe LIZ ue mab)

Brand Names: US Entyvio

Brand Names: Canada Entyvio

Pharmacologic Category Gastrointestinal Agent, Miscellaneous; Monoclonal Antibody; Monoclonal Antibody, Selective Adhesion-Molecule Inhibitor

Use

Crohn disease: Treatment of Crohn disease in adults.

Ulcerative colitis: Treatment of ulcerative colitis in adults.

Local Anesthetic/Vasoconstrictor Precautions No information available to require special precautions

Effects on Dental Treatment Key adverse event(s) related to dental treatment: Nasopharyngitis (13%), cough (5%), bronchitis (4%), oropharyngeal pain (3%), sinusitis (3%) have all been observed

Effects on Bleeding No information available to require special precautions

Adverse Reactions

>10%:

Immunologic: Antibody development (4% to 13%; neutralizing: 2%)
Nervous system: Headache (12%)
Neuromuscular & skeletal: Arthralgia (12%)
Respiratory: Nasopharyngitis (13%)

1% to 10%:

Dermatologic: Pruritus (3%), skin rash (3%)
Gastrointestinal: Nausea (9%)
Hepatic: Increased serum alanine aminotransferase (≥3 x ULN: <2%), increased serum aspartate aminotransferase (≥3 x ULN: <2%)
Infection: Influenza (4%)
Nervous system: Fatigue (6%)
Neuromuscular & skeletal: Back pain (4%), limb pain (3%)
Respiratory: Bronchitis (4%), cough (5%), oropharyngeal pain (3%), sinusitis (3%), upper respiratory tract infection (7%)
Miscellaneous: Fever (9%), infusion related reaction (4%)

Frequency not defined: Hematologic & oncologic: Malignant neoplasm (excluding dysplasia and basal cell carcinoma)

Postmarketing:

Hepatic: Hepatitis, increased serum bilirubin, increased serum transaminases
Hypersensitivity: Anaphylaxis, bronchospasm, hypersensitivity reaction
Infection: Infection (including anal abscess, sepsis, tuberculosis, salmonella sepsis, meningitis due to *Listeria monocytogenes*, giardiasis, cytomegalovirus disease [colitis])
Nervous system: Progressive multifocal leukoencephalopathy

Mechanism of Action Vedolizumab is a humanized monoclonal antibody that binds to the alpha4beta7 integrin and blocks the interaction of alpha4beta7 integrin with mucosal addressin cell adhesion molecule-1 (MAdCAM-1) and inhibits the migration of memory T-lymphocytes across the endothelium into inflamed gastrointestinal parenchymal tissue. The interaction of the alpha4beta7 integrin with MAdCAM-1 has been implicated as an important contributor to the chronic inflammation that is a hallmark of ulcerative colitis and Crohn disease.

Pharmacodynamics/Kinetics

Half-life Elimination 25 days (serum, at 300 mg dosage)

Reproductive Considerations

Treatment algorithms are available for use of biologics in female patients with Crohn disease who are planning a pregnancy (Weizman 2019). When treatment for inflammatory bowel disease is needed, serum levels of biologic therapy should be optimized prior to conception (Mahadevan 2019).

Pregnancy Considerations Vedolizumab crosses the placenta (Mahadevan 2016).

Vedolizumab is a humanized monoclonal antibody (IgG_1). Placental transfer of human IgG is dependent upon the IgG subclass, maternal serum concentrations, birth weight, and gestational age, generally increasing as pregnancy progresses. The lowest exposure would be expected during the period of organogenesis (Palmeira 2012; Pentsuk 2009).

Information related to the use of vedolizumab in pregnancy is available (Bar-Gil Shitrit 2019; Julsgaard 2017; Mahadevan 2017; Moens 2019; Sheridan 2017). Based on available data, an increased risk of adverse maternal or fetal effects has not been observed following vedolizumab exposure in pregnancy.

The safety of administering live vaccines to infants exposed to vedolizumab in utero is not known. Vaccination with live vaccines (eg, rotavirus vaccine) should be avoided for the first 6 months of life if exposure to a biologic agent occurs during the third trimester of pregnancy (eg, >27 weeks' gestation) (Mahadevan 2019).

Inflammatory bowel disease is associated with adverse pregnancy outcomes including an increased risk of miscarriage, premature delivery, delivery of a low birth weight infant, and poor maternal weight gain. Management of maternal disease should be optimized prior to pregnancy. Treatment decreases disease flares, disease activity, and the incidence of adverse pregnancy outcomes (Mahadevan 2019).

When treatment for inflammatory bowel disease is needed in pregnant women, appropriate biologic therapy can be continued without interruption. Serum levels should be evaluated prior to conception and optimized to avoid subtherapeutic concentrations or high levels which may increase placental transfer. Dosing can be adjusted so delivery occurs at the lowest serum concentration. For vedolizumab, the final injection can be given 6 to 10 weeks prior to the estimated date of delivery (4 to 5 weeks before delivery if every-4-week dosing), then continued 48 hours' postpartum (Mahadevan 2019).

Data collection to monitor pregnancy and infant outcomes following exposure to vedolizumab is ongoing. Health care providers are encouraged to enroll women exposed to vedolizumab during pregnancy in a pregnancy exposure registry. Information about the registry can be obtained by calling 1-877-825-3327.

◆ **VEGF Trap** *see* Ziv-Aflibercept (Systemic) *on page 1573*

◆ **VEGF Trap R1R2** *see* Ziv-Aflibercept (Systemic) *on page 1573*

◆ **Velban** *see* VinBLAStine *on page 1545*

◆ **Velcade** *see* Bortezomib *on page 248*

◆ **Veletri** *see* Epoprostenol *on page 578*

◆ **Velivet** *see* Ethinyl Estradiol and Desogestrel *on page 609*

◆ **Velpatasvir and Sofosbuvir** *see* Sofosbuvir and Velpatasvir *on page 1379*

◆ **Velpatasvir, Voxilaprevir, and Sofosbuvir** *see* Sofosbuvir, Velpatasvir, and Voxilaprevir *on page 1380*

◆ **Vemlidy** *see* Tenofovir Alafenamide *on page 1418*

Vemurafenib (vem ue RAF e nib)

Related Information

Clinical Risk Related to Drugs Prolonging QT Interval *on page 1675*

Brand Names: US Zelboraf

Brand Names: Canada Zelboraf

Pharmacologic Category Antineoplastic Agent, BRAF Kinase Inhibitor

Use

Melanoma, unresectable or metastatic: Treatment of unresectable or metastatic melanoma in patients with a BRAFV600E mutation (as detected by an approved test)

Limitations of use: Not indicated for treatment of wild-type BRAF melanoma

Erdheim-Chester disease: Treatment of Erdheim-Chester disease (ECD) in patients with a BRAF V600 mutation

Local Anesthetic/Vasoconstrictor Precautions Vemurafenib is one of the drugs confirmed to prolong the QT interval and is accepted as having a risk of causing torsade de pointes. The risk of drug-induced torsade de pointes is extremely low when a single QT interval prolonging drug is prescribed. In terms of epinephrine, it is not known what effect vasoconstrictors in the local anesthetic regimen will have in patients with a known history of congenital prolonged QT interval or in patients taking any medication that prolongs the QT interval. Until more information is obtained, it is suggested that the clinician consult with the physician prior to the use of a vasoconstrictor in suspected patients, and that the vasoconstrictor (epinephrine, mepivacaine, and levonordefrin [Carbocaine® 2% with Neo-Cobefrin®]) be used with caution.

Effects on Dental Treatment Key adverse event(s) related to dental treatment: Taste alteration has been reported

Effects on Bleeding Does not cause significant hematologic toxicity.

Adverse Reactions

>10%:

Cardiovascular: Prolonged QT interval on ECG (≤55%), hypertension (≤36%), peripheral edema (17% to 23%)

Central nervous system: Fatigue (38% to ≤55%), peripheral sensory neuropathy (≤36%), headache (23% to 27%)

Dermatologic: Maculopapular rash (9% to ≤59%), alopecia (36% to ≤55%), skin rash (37% to 52%), hyperkeratosis (24% to ≤50%; seborrheic: 10% to ≤41%; pilaris: ≤32%; actinic: 8% to ≤32%), skin photosensitivity (33% to 49%), xeroderma (16% to ≤45%), palmar-plantar erythrodysesthesia (≤41%), pruritus (23% to ≤36%), nevus (≤23%), sunburn (10% to ≤23%), papular rash (5% to ≤23%), erythema (8% to 14%)

Gastrointestinal: Diarrhea (28% to ≤50%), nausea (≤32% to 37%), vomiting (18% to 26%), decreased appetite (18% to 21%), constipation (12% to 16%), dysgeusia (11% to 14%)

Hematologic & oncologic: Cutaneous papilloma (21% to ≤55%), keratoacanthoma (≤41%), squamous cell carcinoma of skin (≤41%; grade 3: 22% to ≤36%)

Hepatic: Increased gamma-glutamyl transferase (5% to 15%)

Neuromuscular & skeletal: Arthralgia (53% to ≤82%), myalgia (13% to 24%), limb pain (9% to 18%), back pain (8% to 11%), musculoskeletal pain (8% to 11%), weakness (2% to 11%)

Renal: Increased serum creatinine (up to 3x ULN: 26% to 86%; greater than 3x ULN: 1% to 9%)

Respiratory: Cough (8% to ≤36%)

Miscellaneous: Fibrosis (Dupuytren contracture) (<20%), fever (17% to 19%)

1% to 10%:

Cardiovascular: Atrial fibrillation, hypotension, vasculitis

Central nervous system: Cranial nerve palsy (facial), dizziness, peripheral neuropathy

Dermatologic: Erythema nodosum, folliculitis, Stevens-Johnson syndrome, toxic epidermal necrolysis

Endocrine & metabolic: Weight loss

Hematologic & oncologic: Basal cell carcinoma, malignant melanoma (new primary), squamous cell carcinoma (oropharyngeal)

Hepatic: Increased serum ALT (≥ grade 3: 3% to ≤9%), increased serum alkaline phosphatase (≥ grade 3: 3% to ≤5%), increased serum bilirubin (≥ grade 3: 2%)

Hypersensitivity: Anaphylaxis, hypersensitivity reaction

Neuromuscular & skeletal: Arthritis, panniculitis

Ophthalmic: Blurred vision, iritis, photophobia, uveitis

Frequency not defined: Hematologic & oncologic: Secondary acute myelocytic leukemia

<1%, postmarketing, and/or case reports: Acute interstitial nephritis, acute tubular necrosis, chronic myelomonocytic leukemia with NRAS mutation (progression of preexisting condition), DRESS syndrome, hepatic injury, increased serum AST, local acneiform eruptions (Ansai 2016), neutropenia, pancreatitis, plantar fasciitis, recall skin sensitization, retinal vein occlusion

Mechanism of Action Vemurafenib is a low molecular weight oral BRAF kinase inhibitor (potent) which inhibits tumor growth in melanomas by inhibiting kinase activity of certain mutated forms of BRAF, including BRAF with V600E mutation, thereby blocking cellular proliferation in melanoma cells with the mutation. Does not have activity against cells with wild-type BRAF. BRAF V600E activating mutations are present in ~50% of melanomas; V600E mutation involves the substitution of glutamic acid for valine at amino acid 600.

Pharmacodynamics/Kinetics

Half-life Elimination 57 hours (range: 30 to 120 hours)

Time to Peak 3 hours.

Reproductive Considerations

Women of reproductive potential should use effective contraception during treatment and for at least 2 weeks after the last dose.

Pregnancy Considerations

Vemurafenib crosses the placenta. Based on the mechanism of action, vemurafenib may cause fetal harm if administered during pregnancy.

Prescribing and Access Restrictions Available through specialty pharmacies. Further information may be obtained from the manufacturer, Genentech, at 1-888-249-4918, or at http://www.zelboraf.com.

Dental Health Professional Considerations See Local Anesthetic/Vasoconstrictor Precautions

◆ **Venclexta** *see* Venetoclax *on page 1538*

◆ **Venclexta Starting Pack** *see* Venetoclax *on page 1538*

Venetoclax (ven ET oh klax)

Brand Names: US Venclexta; Venclexta Starting Pack

Brand Names: Canada Venclexta; Venclexta Starting Pack

Pharmacologic Category Antineoplastic Agent; Antineoplastic Agent, BCL-2 Inhibitor

Use

Acute myeloid leukemia: Treatment of newly-diagnosed acute myeloid leukemia (in combination with azacitidine, decitabine, or low-dose cytarabine) in patients ≥75 years of age, or in patients with comorbidities that preclude use of intensive induction chemotherapy

Chronic lymphocytic leukemia/small lymphocytic lymphoma: Treatment of chronic lymphocytic leukemia or small lymphocytic lymphoma in adults

Local Anesthetic/Vasoconstrictor Precautions No information available to require special precautions

Effects on Dental Treatment No significant effects or complications reported

Effects on Bleeding Chemotherapy may result in significant myelosuppression, potentially including significant reduction in platelet counts (thrombocytopenia grades 3/4:15%) and altered hemostasis. Since there is the potential for bleeding in patients under active treatment with venetoclax, medical consult is suggested.

Adverse Reactions

>10%:

Cardiovascular: Edema (22%)

Central nervous system: Fatigue (32%), headache (18%), dizziness (14%)

Dermatologic: Skin rash (18%)

Endocrine & metabolic: Hypocalcemia (16% to 87%), hyperglycemia (67%), hyperkalemia (17% to 59%), decreased serum albumin (49%), hypophosphatemia (45%), hyponatremia (40%), hyperphosphatemia (14%)

Gastrointestinal: Diarrhea (43%), nausea (42%), abdominal pain (18%), constipation (16%), vomiting (16%), stomatitis (13%)

Hematologic & oncologic: Leukopenia (89%; grades 3/4: 42%; grade 4: 11%), neutropenia (50% to 87%; ≥ grade 3: 45% to 63%; grade 4: 33%), lymphocytopenia (11% to 74%; ≥ grade 3: 7% to 40%; grade 4: 9%), anemia (33% to 71%; ≥ grade 3: 18% to 26%), thrombocytopenia (29% to 64%; ≥ grade 3: 20% to 31%; grade 4: 15%), tumor lysis syndrome (2 to 3 week ramp-up phase: 13%; 5 week ramp-up phase: 2%)

Hepatic: Increased serum aspartate aminotransferase (53%)

Neuromuscular & skeletal: Musculoskeletal pain (29%), arthralgia (12%)

Respiratory: Upper respiratory tract infection (36%), cough (22%), pneumonia (14%), dyspnea (13%), lower respiratory tract infection (11%)

Miscellaneous: Fever (18%)

1% to 10%:

Endocrine & metabolic: Hyperuricemia (10%)

Hematologic & oncologic: Febrile neutropenia (6%; ≥ grade 3: 6%)

Mechanism of Action Venetoclax has cytotoxic activity in tumor cells which overexpress BCL-2. Venetoclax selectively inhibits the anti-apoptotic protein BCL-2, which is overexpressed in chronic lymphocytic leukemia (CLL) cells and acute myeloid leukemia (AML) cells. BCL-2 mediates tumor cell survival and has been associated with chemotherapy resistance. Venetoclax binds directly to the BCL-2 protein, displacing pro-apoptotic proteins and restoring the apoptotic process.

Pharmacodynamics/Kinetics

Half-life Elimination ~26 hours

Time to Peak 5 to 8 hours

Reproductive Considerations

Females of reproductive potential should have a pregnancy test prior to therapy and use effective contraception during treatment and for at least 30 days after the final dose.

Pregnancy Considerations

Based on the mechanism of action and data from animal reproduction studies, venetoclax is expected to cause fetal harm if administered during pregnancy.

Prescribing and Access Restrictions Available through specialty pharmacies and distributors. Further information may be obtained from the manufacturer.

◆ **Venipuncture CPI [DSC]** *see* Lidocaine and Prilocaine *on page 911*

◆ **Venipuncture Px1 Phlebotomy** *see* Lidocaine (Topical) *on page 902*

Venlafaxine (ven la FAX een)

Related Information

Dentin Hypersensitivity, Acid Erosion, High Caries Index, Management of Alveolar Osteitis, and Xerostomia *on page 1762*

Vasoconstrictor Interactions With Antidepressants *on page 1821*

Brand Names: US Effexor XR

Brand Names: Canada ACT Venlafaxine XR; APO-Venlafaxine XR; Auro-Venlafaxine XR; DOM-Venlafaxine XR; Effexor XR; GD-Venlafaxine XR [DSC]; M-Venlafaxine XR; MYLAN-Venlafaxine XR [DSC]; PMS-Venlafaxine XR; RIVA-Venlafaxine XR [DSC]; SANDOZ Venlafaxine XR; TARO-Venlafaxine XR; TEVA-Venlafaxine XR; Venlafaxine XR

Pharmacologic Category Antidepressant, Serotonin/Norepinephrine Reuptake Inhibitor

Use

Generalized anxiety disorder (extended-release capsules only): Treatment of generalized anxiety disorder (GAD)

Major depressive disorder (unipolar): Treatment of unipolar major depressive disorder (MDD)

Panic disorder (extended-release capsules only): Treatment of panic disorder, with or without agoraphobia

Social anxiety disorder (extended-release capsules and tablets only): Treatment of social anxiety disorder, also known as social phobia

Local Anesthetic/Vasoconstrictor Precautions

Although venlafaxine is not a tricyclic antidepressant, it does block norepinephrine reuptake within CNS synapses as part of its mechanisms. It has been suggested that vasoconstrictor be administered with caution and to monitor vital signs in dental patients taking antidepressants that affect norepinephrine in this way. This is particularly important in patients taking venlafaxine, which has been noted to produce a sustained increase in diastolic blood pressure and heart rate as a side effect.

Effects on Dental Treatment Key adverse event(s) related to dental treatment: Significant xerostomia (normal salivary flow resumes upon discontinuation); may contribute to oral discomfort, especially in the elderly; taste perversion. See Effects on Bleeding.

Effects on Bleeding May impair platelet aggregation resulting in increased risk of bleeding events, particularly if used concomitantly with aspirin, NSAIDs, warfarin, or other anticoagulants. Bleeding related to SSRI use has been reported to range from relatively minor bruising and epistaxis to life-threatening hemorrhage. Routine interruption of therapy for most dental procedures is not warranted. In medically complicated patients or extensive oral surgery, the decision to interrupt therapy must be based on the risk to benefit in an individual patient and a medical consult is suggested. If therapy is continued without interruption, the clinician should anticipate the potential for a prolonged bleeding time.

Adverse Reactions Actual frequency may be dependent upon formulation and/or indication. Adverse reactions are reported for the ER tablet and ER capsule formulations.

>10%:

Dermatologic: Diaphoresis (11%)

Endocrine & metabolic: Weight loss (children and adolescents: 18% to 47%; adults: <7%)

Gastrointestinal: Anorexia (8% to 22%), nausea (30%), xerostomia (15%)

Nervous system: Dizziness (16%), drowsiness (15%), insomnia (17% to 24%)

Neuromuscular & skeletal: Asthenia (13%)

1% to 10%:

Cardiovascular: Hypotension (<2%), orthostatic hypotension (<2%), syncope (<2%), tachycardia (<2%), vasodilation (4%)

Dermatologic: Alopecia (<2%), ecchymoses (<2%), pruritus (<2%), skin photosensitivity (<2%), skin rash (<2%), urticaria (<2%)

Endocrine & metabolic: Decreased libido (5% [placebo: 2%]), heavy menstrual bleeding (<2%), hypercholesterolemia (5%), orgasm abnormal (males: ≤10% [placebo: ≤0.5%]), weight gain (<2%)

Gastrointestinal: Bruxism (<2%), constipation (9%), diarrhea (8%), dysgeusia (<2%), gastrointestinal hemorrhage (<2%), vomiting (4%)

Genitourinary: Abnormal uterine bleeding (<2%), ejaculatory disorder (≤10%), impotence (5%), urinary frequency (<2%), urinary incontinence (<2%), urinary retention (<2%), urination disorder (<2%)

Nervous system: Abnormal dreams (3%), agitation (<2%), akathisia (<2%), anorgasmia (2% to 4% [placebo: 0.1% to 0.2%]), apathy (<2%), chills (<2%), confusion (<2%), depersonalization (<2%), hallucination (<2%), hypertonia (<2%), manic reaction (<2%), myoclonus (<2%), nervousness (7% to 10%), paresthesia (2%), seizure (<2%), yawning (4%)

Neuromuscular & skeletal: Tremor (5%)

Ophthalmic: Accommodation disturbance (<2%), mydriasis (<2%), visual disturbance (4%)

Otic: Tinnitus (<2%)

<1%: Nervous system: Hypomania (Chand 2004)

Frequency not defined:

Cardiovascular: Hypertension (Pardal 2001)

Endocrine & metabolic: Increased serum triglycerides

Gastrointestinal: Abdominal pain, dyspepsia

Nervous system: Suicidal ideation, suicidal tendencies, withdrawal syndrome (Sablijic 2011)

Neuromuscular & skeletal: Linear skeletal growth rate below expectation (children and adolescents, most notable for age <12 years), myalgia

Respiratory: Epistaxis

Postmarketing:

Cardiovascular: Cardiomyopathy (takotsubo), hypertensive crisis (Khurana 2003), increased blood pressure (Thase 1998), prolonged QT interval on ECG, sinus tachycardia (Osuagwu 2019), torsades de pointes, ventricular fibrillation, ventricular tachycardia, worsening of heart failure (Colucci 2008)

Dermatologic: Erythema multiforme, Stevens-Johnson syndrome, toxic epidermal necrolysis

Endocrine & metabolic: Hyponatremia (Gupta 1997), increased serum prolactin, SIADH (Romero 2007)

Gastrointestinal: Gingival hemorrhage (Yavasoglu 2008), pancreatitis (Sevastru 2012)

Genitourinary: Erectile dysfunction (Montejo 2001), postpartum hemorrhage (Perotta 2019), priapism (Samuel 2000), sexual disorder (Kennedy 2000), vaginal hemorrhage (Linnebur 2002)

Hematologic & oncologic: Agranulocytosis, aplastic anemia, bruise (Carpenter 2016), mucous membrane bleeding, neutropenia, pancytopenia, prolonged bleeding time, thrombocytopenia

Hepatic: Abnormal hepatic function tests, cholestatic hepatitis (Stadlmann 2012), hepatitis (Horsmans 1999), hepatocellular hepatitis (Liver Tox NIH 2020), hepatotoxicity (Yildirim 2009), increased serum alanine aminotransferase (Liver Tox NIH 2020)

Hypersensitivity: Anaphylaxis, angioedema

Nervous system: Ataxia, balance impairment, delirium, dystonia, extrapyramidal reaction, neuroleptic malignant syndrome, serotonin syndrome (Pan 2003), tardive dyskinesia

Neuromuscular & skeletal: Dyskinesia, rhabdomyolysis

Ophthalmic: Acute angle-closure glaucoma (Ng 2002; Zhao 2018), increased intraocular pressure (open-angle glaucoma) (Botha 2016)

Respiratory: Dyspnea, eosinophilic pneumonitis (Fleisch 2000), interstitial pulmonary disease (Oh 2014), respiratory failure (Fleisch 2000)

Mechanism of Action Venlafaxine and its active metabolite, O-desmethylvenlafaxine (ODV), are potent inhibitors of neuronal serotonin and norepinephrine reuptake and weak inhibitors of dopamine reuptake. Venlafaxine and ODV have no significant activity for muscarinic cholinergic, H_1-histaminergic, or alpha$_2$-adrenergic receptors. Venlafaxine and ODV do not possess MAO-inhibitory activity. Venlafaxine functions like an SSRI in low doses (37.5 mg/day) and as a dual mechanism agent affecting serotonin and norepinephrine at doses above 225 mg/day (Harvey 2000; Kelsey 1996).

Pharmacodynamics/Kinetics

Onset of Action

Anxiety disorders (generalized anxiety, panic, obsessive-compulsive disorder [OCD], posttraumatic stress disorder [PTSD]): Initial effects may be observed within 2 weeks of treatment, with continued improvements through 4 to 6 weeks (WFSBP [Bandelow 2012]); some experts suggest up to 12 weeks of treatment may be necessary for response, particularly in patients with OCD and PTSD (BAP [Baldwin 2014]; Katzman 2014; WFSBP [Bandelow 2012]).

Depression: Initial effects may be observed within 1 to 2 weeks of treatment, with continued improvements through 4 to 6 weeks (Papakostas 2006; Posternak 2005; Szegedi 2009).

Premenstrual dysphoric disorder: Initial effects may be observed within the first few days of treatment, with response at the first menstrual cycle of treatment (ISPMD [Nevatte 2013]).

Half-life Elimination Venlafaxine: 5 ± 2 hours (immediate-release), 10.7 ± 3.2 hours (extended-release); ODV: 11 ± 2 hours (immediate-release), 12.5 ± 3 hours (extended-release); prolonged with cirrhosis (venlafaxine: ~30%, ODV: ~60%), renal impairment (venlafaxine: ~50%, ODV: ~40%), and during dialysis (venlafaxine: ~180%, ODV: ~142%)

Time to Peak

Immediate release: Venlafaxine: 2 hours, ODV: 3 hours

Extended release: Venlafaxine: 6.3 ± 2.3 hours, ODV: 11.6 ± 2.9 hours

Reproductive Considerations

If treatment for major depressive disorder is initiated for the first time in females planning a pregnancy, agents other than venlafaxine are preferred (Larsen 2015).

Pregnancy Risk Factor C

Pregnancy Considerations

Venlafaxine and its active metabolite ODV cross the human placenta (Rampono 2009).

Nonteratogenic adverse events have been observed with venlafaxine or other SNRIs/SSRIs when used during pregnancy. Cyanosis, apnea, respiratory distress, seizures, temperature instability, feeding difficulty, vomiting, hypoglycemia, hypo- or hypertonia, hyperreflexia, jitteriness, irritability, constant crying, and tremor have been reported in the neonate immediately following delivery after exposure to venlafaxine, SSRIs, or other SNRIs late in the third trimester. Prolonged hospitalization, respiratory support, or tube feedings may be required. Some symptoms may be due to the toxicity of the SNRI/SSRIs or a discontinuation syndrome and may be consistent with serotonin syndrome associated with treatment.

Due to pregnancy-induced physiologic changes, some pharmacokinetic parameters of venlafaxine may be altered. Women should be monitored for decreased efficacy (Klier 2007; ter Horst 2014; Westin 2018). The risk of bleeding, including postpartum hemorrhage may be increased following maternal use of venlafaxine (Palmsten Hernández-Díaz 2013; Reis 2010).

Untreated or inadequately treated mental illness may lead to poor compliance with prenatal care. The ACOG recommends that therapy with SSRIs or SNRIs during pregnancy be individualized. Use of a single agent is preferred. According to their recommendations, treatment of depression during pregnancy should incorporate the clinical expertise of the mental health clinician, obstetrician, primary care provider, and pediatrician (ACOG 2008).

If treatment for major depressive disorder is initiated for the first time during pregnancy, agents other than venlafaxine are preferred (Larsen 2015; MacQueen 2016). Women effectively treated with venlafaxine prior to pregnancy may continue treatment (Larsen 2015).

Pregnant women exposed to antidepressants during pregnancy are encouraged to enroll in the National Pregnancy Registry for Antidepressants (NPRAD). Women 18 to 45 years of age or their health care providers may contact the registry by calling 844-405-6185. Enrollment should be done as early in pregnancy as possible.

◆ **Venlafaxine HCl** *see* Venlafaxine *on page* 1539

◆ **Ventolin HFA** *see* Albuterol *on page* 90

◆ **VePesid** *see* Etoposide *on page* 626

◆ **Veramyst [DSC]** *see* Fluticasone (Nasal) *on page* 703

Verapamil (ver AP a mil)

Related Information

Calcium Channel Blockers and Gingival Hyperplasia *on page* 1816

Cardiovascular Diseases *on page* 1654

Brand Names: US Calan SR; Calan [DSC]; Verelan; Verelan PM

Brand Names: Canada APO-Verap; APO-Verap SR; DOM-Verapamil SR; Isoptin SR; MYLAN-Verapamil;

MYLAN-Verapamil SR; NOVO-Veramil SR [DSC]; NOVO-Veramil [DSC]; PMS-Verapamil SR; PRO-Verapamil SR [DSC]; RIVA-Verapamil SR [DSC]; Verelan

Pharmacologic Category Antianginal Agent; Antiarrhythmic Agent, Class IV; Antihypertensive; Calcium Channel Blocker; Calcium Channel Blocker, Nondihydropyridine

Use

Angina: Treatment of angina at rest, including chronic stable angina, vasospastic angina, and unstable angina.

Atrial fibrillation or atrial flutter, rate control:

Oral: IR tablet: Control of ventricular rate at rest and during stress in chronic atrial flutter and/or fibrillation.

IV: Temporary control of rapid ventricular rate in atrial flutter and/or atrial fibrillation (except when the atrial flutter and/or atrial fibrillation are associated with accessory pathways [Wolff-Parkinson-White and Lown-Ganong-Levine syndromes]).

Hypertension: Oral: IR tablet/ER capsule and tablet: Management of hypertension.

Supraventricular tachycardia:

Oral: IR tablet: Prophylaxis of supraventricular tachycardia, such as atrioventricular (AV) nodal reentrant tachycardia, AV reentrant tachycardia, focal atrial tachycardia, or multifocal atrial tachycardia.

IV: Rapid conversion to sinus rhythm.

Local Anesthetic/Vasoconstrictor Precautions No information available to require special precautions

Effects on Dental Treatment Key adverse event(s) related to dental treatment: Frequent occurrence of gingival hyperplasia has been reported. Calcium channel blockers (CCB) have been reported to cause gingival hyperplasia (GH). Verapamil-induced GH has appeared 11 months or more after subjects took daily doses of 240 to 360 mg. The severity of hyperplastic syndrome does not seem to be dose dependent. Gingivectomy is only successful if CCB therapy is discontinued. GH regresses markedly 1 week after CCB discontinuance with all symptoms resolving in 2 months. If a patient must continue CCB therapy, begin a program of professional cleaning and patient plaque control to minimize severity and growth rate of gingival tissue. Infrequent occurrence of erythema multiforme, Stevens-Johnson syndrome, and xerostomia have also been reported.

Effects on Bleeding No information available to require special precautions

Adverse Reactions

>10%:

Central nervous system: Headache (1% to 12%)

Gastrointestinal: Gingival hyperplasia (≤19%), constipation (7% to 12%)

1% to 10%:

Cardiovascular: Peripheral edema (1% to 4%), hypotension (3%), cardiac failure (≤2%), atrioventricular block (1% to 2%), bradycardia (heart rate <50 bpm: 1%), flushing (1%), angina pectoris (oral: ≤1%), atrioventricular dissociation (oral: ≤1%), cerebrovascular accident (oral: ≤1%), chest pain (oral: ≤1%), claudication (oral: ≤1%), ECG abnormality (oral: ≤1%), myocardial infarction (oral: ≤1%), palpitations (oral: ≤1%), syncope (oral: ≤1%)

Central nervous system: Fatigue (2% to 5%), dizziness (1% to 5%), lethargy (3%), pain (2%), paresthesia (1%), sleep disorder (1%), confusion (oral: ≤1%), drowsiness (oral: ≤1%; IV: <1%), equilibrium disturbance (oral: ≤1%), extrapyramidal reaction (oral: ≤1%), insomnia (oral: ≤1%), psychosis (oral: ≤1%), shakiness (oral: ≤1%)

Dermatologic: Skin rash (1% to 2%), alopecia (oral: ≤1%), diaphoresis (oral: ≤1%), erythema multiforme (oral: ≤1%), hyperkeratosis (oral: ≤1%), macular eruption (oral: ≤1%), Stevens-Johnson syndrome (oral: ≤1%), urticaria (oral: ≤1%)

Endocrine & metabolic: Galactorrhea (oral: ≤1%), gynecomastia (oral: ≤1%), hyperprolactinemia (oral: ≤1%), spotty menstruation (oral: ≤1%)

Gastrointestinal: Dyspepsia (3%), nausea (1% to 3%), diarrhea (2%), abdominal distress (oral: ≤1%), gastrointestinal distress (oral: ≤1%), xerostomia (oral: ≤1%)

Genitourinary: Impotence (oral: ≤1%)

Hematologic & oncologic: Bruise (oral: ≤1%), purpuric vasculitis (oral: ≤1%)

Hepatic: Increased liver enzymes (1%)

Neuromuscular & skeletal: Myalgia (1%), arthralgia (oral: ≤1%), muscle cramps (oral: ≤1%), weakness (oral: ≤1%)

Ophthalmic: Blurred vision (oral: ≤1%)

Otic: Tinnitus (oral: ≤1%)

Renal: Polyuria (oral: ≤1%)

Respiratory: Flu-like symptoms (4%), pulmonary edema (≤2%), dyspnea (1%)

<1%, postmarketing, and/or case reports: Asystole, bronchospasm (IV administration), depression (IV administration), diaphoresis (IV administration), drowsiness (IV administration), eosinophilia, exfoliative dermatitis, gastrointestinal obstruction, hair discoloration, laryngospasm (IV administration), muscle fatigue (IV administration), paralytic ileus, Parkinsonian-like syndrome, pruritus (IV administration), respiratory failure (IV administration), rotary nystagmus (IV administration), seizure (IV administration), shock, urticaria (IV administration), vertigo (IV administration), ventricular fibrillation

Mechanism of Action Inhibits calcium ion from entering the "slow channels" or select voltage-sensitive areas of vascular smooth muscle and myocardium during depolarization; produces relaxation of coronary vascular smooth muscle and coronary vasodilation; increases myocardial oxygen delivery in patients with vasospastic angina; slows automaticity and conduction of AV node.

Pharmacodynamics/Kinetics

Onset of Action Peak effect: Oral: Immediate release: 1 to 2 hours (Singh 1978); IV bolus: 3 to 5 minutes.

Duration of Action Oral: Immediate release: 6 to 8 hours; IV: 0.5 to 6 hours (Marik 2011).

Half-life Elimination

Injection: Terminal: 2 to 5 hours.

Oral:

Immediate release: Single dose: 2.8 to 7.4 hours; Multiple doses: 4.5 to 12 hours

Extended release: ~12 hours

Severe hepatic impairment: 14 to 16 hours

Time to Peak Serum: Oral:

Immediate release: 1 to 2 hours

Extended release:

Calan SR: 5.21 hours

Verelan: 7 to 9 hours

Verelan PM: ~11 hours; Drug release delayed ~4 to 5 hours

Pregnancy Considerations Verapamil crosses the placenta.

Chronic maternal hypertension may increase the risk of birth defects, low birth weight, preterm delivery, stillbirth, and neonatal death. Actual fetal/neonatal risks may be related to duration and severity of maternal hypertension. Untreated hypertension may also increase the risks of adverse maternal outcomes, including gestational diabetes, myocardial infarction, preeclampsia, stroke, and delivery complications (ACOG 203 2019).

Calcium channel blockers may be used to treat hypertension in pregnant women; however, agents other than verapamil are more commonly used (ACOG 203 2019; ESC [Regitz-Zagrosek 2018]). Females with preexisting hypertension may continue their medication during pregnancy unless contraindications exist (ESC [Regitz-Zagrosek 2018]).

Women with hypertrophic cardiomyopathy who are controlled with verapamil prior to pregnancy may continue therapy, but increased fetal monitoring is recommended (Gersh 2011). Verapamil may be used IV for the acute treatment of supraventricular tachycardia (SVT) in pregnant women when adenosine or beta-blockers are ineffective or contraindicated. Verapamil may also be used for the ongoing management of SVT in highly symptomatic patients. The lowest effective dose is recommended; avoid use during the first trimester if possible (Page [ACC/AHA/HRS 2016]). Additional guidelines are available for management of cardiovascular diseases during pregnancy (ESC [Regitz-Zagrosek 2018]).

- **Verapamil HCl** *see* Verapamil *on page 1540*
- **Verapamil Hydrochloride** *see* Verapamil *on page 1540*
- **Verdeso** *see* Desonide *on page 461*
- **Verdrocet** *see* Hydrocodone and Acetaminophen *on page 764*
- **Verelan** *see* Verapamil *on page 1540*
- **Verelan PM** *see* Verapamil *on page 1540*
- **Veripred 20 [DSC]** *see* PrednisoLONE (Systemic) *on page 1255*
- **Versacloz** *see* CloZAPine *on page 399*
- **Versed** *see* Midazolam *on page 1020*
- **Vesanoid** *see* Tretinoin (Systemic) *on page 1483*
- **VESIcare** *see* Solifenacin *on page 1380*
- **Vesicare LS** *see* Solifenacin *on page 1380*
- **Vestura [DSC]** *see* Ethinyl Estradiol and Drospirenone *on page 610*
- **Vexol [DSC]** *see* Rimexolone *on page 1330*
- **Vfend** *see* Voriconazole *on page 1552*
- **Vfend IV** *see* Voriconazole *on page 1552*
- **2vHPV** *see* Papillomavirus (Types 16, 18) Vaccine (Human, Recombinant) *on page 1191*
- **4vHPV** *see* Papillomavirus (Types 6, 11, 16, 18) Vaccine (Human, Recombinant) *on page 1190*
- **Viactiv [OTC]** *see* Vitamins (Multiple/Oral) *on page 1550*
- **Viactiv Calcium Flavor Glides [OTC]** *see* Vitamins (Multiple/Oral) *on page 1550*
- **Viactiv Flavor Glides [OTC]** *see* Vitamins (Multiple/Oral) *on page 1550*
- **Viactiv for Teens [OTC]** *see* Vitamins (Multiple/Oral) *on page 1550*
- **Viactiv With Calcium [OTC]** *see* Vitamins (Multiple/Oral) *on page 1550*
- **Viagra** *see* Sildenafil *on page 1369*
- **Vibativ** *see* Telavancin *on page 1411*
- **Vibramycin** *see* Doxycycline *on page 522*
- **Vicks Sinex [OTC] [DSC]** *see* Oxymetazoline (Nasal) *on page 1173*
- **Vicks Sinex 12 Hour Decongest [OTC]** *see* Oxymetazoline (Nasal) *on page 1173*
- **Vicks Sinex Moisturizing [OTC]** *see* Oxymetazoline (Nasal) *on page 1173*
- **Vicks Sinex Severe Decongest [OTC]** *see* Oxymetazoline (Nasal) *on page 1173*
- **Vicodin** *see* Hydrocodone and Acetaminophen *on page 764*
- **Vicodin ES** *see* Hydrocodone and Acetaminophen *on page 764*
- **Vicodin HP** *see* Hydrocodone and Acetaminophen *on page 764*
- **ViCPS** *see* Typhoid Vaccine *on page 1505*
- **Victoza** *see* Liraglutide *on page 920*
- **Vi-Daylin®/F [DSC]** *see* Vitamins (Fluoride) *on page 1550*
- **Vi-Daylin®/F ADC [DSC]** *see* Vitamins (Fluoride) *on page 1550*
- **Vi-Daylin®/F ADC + Iron [DSC]** *see* Vitamins (Fluoride) *on page 1550*
- **Vi-Daylin®/F + Iron [DSC]** *see* Vitamins (Fluoride) *on page 1550*
- **Vidaza** *see* AzaCITIDine *on page 198*
- **Videx [DSC]** *see* Didanosine *on page 492*
- **Videx EC [DSC]** *see* Didanosine *on page 492*
- **Viekira Pak** *see* Ombitasvir, Paritaprevir, Ritonavir, and Dasabuvir *on page 1136*
- **Viekira XR** *see* Ombitasvir, Paritaprevir, Ritonavir, and Dasabuvir *on page 1136*
- **Vienva** *see* Ethinyl Estradiol and Levonorgestrel *on page 612*
- **VIG** *see* Vaccinia Immune Globulin (Intravenous) *on page 1511*

Vigabatrin (vye GA ba trin)

Brand Names: US Sabril; Vigadrone

Brand Names: Canada Sabril

Pharmacologic Category Anticonvulsant, Miscellaneous

Use

Infantile spasms: As monotherapy for pediatric patients 1 month to 2 years of age with infantile spasms for whom the potential benefits outweigh the potential risk of vision loss.

Refractory complex partial seizures: As adjunctive therapy for adults and pediatric patients ≥2 years of age with refractory complex partial seizures who have inadequately responded to several alternative treatments and for whom the potential benefits outweigh the risk of vision loss.

Local Anesthetic/Vasoconstrictor Precautions No information available to require special precautions

Effects on Dental Treatment No significant effects or complications reported

Effects on Bleeding No information available to require special precautions

Adverse Reactions Reported adverse reactions are adjunctive use except in infants for infantile spasms.

>10%:

Dermatologic: Skin rash (infants: 8% to 11%)

Endocrine & metabolic: Weight gain (children and adolescents: 47%; adults: 6% to 17%)
Gastrointestinal: Constipation (infants: 12% to 14%; adults: 8%), diarrhea (10% to 13%), vomiting (infants: 14% to 20%; adults: 7%)
Infection: Viral infection (infants: 19% to 20%)
Nervous system: Dizziness (adults: 24%), drowsiness (infants: 17% to 45%; adults: 22% to 24%; children and adolescents: 6%), fatigue (adults: 23% to 28%; children and adolescents: 10%), headache (adults: 33%), insomnia (infants: 10% to 12%), irritability (infants: 16% to 23%), sedated state (infants: 17% to 19%; adults: 4%)
Neuromuscular & skeletal: Tremor (adults: 15%)
Ophthalmic: Blurred vision (13%), nystagmus disorder (adults: 13%), visual field loss (adults: ≥30%)
Otic: Otic infection (infants: 7% to 14%), otitis media (infants: 10% to 44%)
Respiratory: Bronchitis (infants: 30%), nasal congestion (infants: 4% to 13%), nasopharyngitis (adults: 14%), pneumonia (infants: 11% to 13%), upper respiratory tract infection (infants: 46% to 51%; adults: 7%)
Miscellaneous: Fever (infants: 19% to 29%; adults: 4%)

1% to 10%:
Cardiovascular: Edema (adults: 1%), peripheral edema (adults: 2% to 5%)
Endocrine & metabolic: Increased thirst (adults: 2%)
Gastrointestinal: Abdominal distention (adults: 2%), abdominal pain (adults: 3%), decreased appetite (infants: 7% to 9%), dyspepsia (adults: 4%), nausea (adults: 10%), stomach discomfort (adults: 4%), upper abdominal pain (adults: 5%), viral gastroenteritis (infants: 5% to 6%)
Genitourinary: Dysmenorrhea (adults: 9%), urinary tract infection (4% to 6%)
Hematologic & oncologic: Anemia (adults: 6%), bruise (adults: 3%), decreased hemoglobin (adults: 3%)
Infection: Candidiasis (infants: 3% to 8%), influenza (3% to 5%)
Nervous system: Abnormal behavior (adults: 3%), abnormality in thinking (adults: 3%), abnormal sensory symptoms (adults: 4%), anxiety (adults: 4%), ataxia (adults: 7%), confusion (adults: 4%), depressed mood (adults: 5%), depression (adults: 6%), disturbance in attention (adults: 9%), dysarthria (adults: 2%), hyperreflexia (adults: 4%), hypoesthesia (adults: 4%), hyporeflexia (adults: 4%), hypotonia (≤6%), impaired consciousness (adults: 2%), lethargy (4% to 7%), memory impairment (adults: 7%), paresthesia (adults: 7%), peripheral neuropathy (adults: 1%), seizure (infants: 4% to 7%), status epilepticus (infants: 4% to 6%; adults: 2%), vertigo (adults: 2%)
Neuromuscular & skeletal: Arthralgia (adults: 10%), asthenia (adults: 5%), back pain (adults: 4%), limb pain (adults: 6%), muscle spasm (adults: 3%), myalgia (adults: 3%)
Ophthalmic: Asthenopia (adults: 2%), conjunctivitis (infants: 2% to 5%), diplopia (adults: 7%), strabismus (infants: 5%)
Otic: Tinnitus (adults: 2%)
Respiratory: Cough (infants: 3% to 8%), croup (infants: 1% to 5%), pharyngolaryngeal pain (adults: 7%), sinus headache (adults: 6%), sinusitis (infants: 5% to 9%)

Frequency not defined:
Nervous system: Suicidal ideation, suicidal tendencies
Ophthalmic: Decreased visual acuity, permanent vision loss, tunnel vision, visual field defect (bilateral concentric visual field constriction; may be permanent)

Postmarketing:
Cardiovascular: Facial edema, pulmonary embolism
Dermatologic: Alopecia, maculopapular rash, pruritus, Stevens-Johnson syndrome, toxic epidermal necrolysis
Gastrointestinal: Cholestasis, esophagitis, gastrointestinal hemorrhage
Genitourinary: Sexual disorder (delayed puberty)
Hypersensitivity: Angioedema
Nervous system: Acute psychosis, agitation (neonates), apathy, brain edema (infants: intramyelinic), delirium, developmental delay, dystonia, encephalopathy, hypertonia, hypomania, hypotonia, malignant hyperthermia, myoclonus, psychosis
Neuromuscular & skeletal: Dyskinesia, muscle spasticity
Ophthalmic: Optic neuritis
Otic: Deafness
Respiratory: Laryngeal edema, respiratory failure, stridor
Miscellaneous: Multi-organ failure

Mechanism of Action Irreversibly inhibits gamma-aminobutyric acid transaminase (GABA-T), increasing the levels of the inhibitory compound gamma amino butyric acid (GABA) within the brain. Duration of effect is dependent upon rate of GABA-T resynthesis.

Pharmacodynamics/Kinetics

Duration of Action Resynthesis of GABA-T dependent: Variable (not strictly correlated to serum concentrations)

Half-life Elimination
Terminal: Prolonged in renal impairment.
Pediatric patients:
5 months to 2 years: ~5.7 hours.
3 to 9 years: ~6.8 hours.
10 to 16 years: ~9.5 hours.
Adult patients: ~10.5 hours.

Time to Peak Infants and Children 5 months to 2 years: 2.5 hours; Children and Adolescents 3 to 16 years and Adults: 1 hour (2 hours with food).

Pregnancy Considerations Vigabatrin crosses the placenta (Tran 1998).

Birth defects have been reported following use in pregnancy and include: cardiac defects, limb defects, male genital malformations, fetal anticonvulsant syndrome, renal and ear abnormalities. Time of exposure or maternal dosage was not reported and information is not available relating to the incidence or types of these outcomes in comparison to the general epilepsy population. Visual field examinations have been conducted following in utero exposure in a limited number of children tested at ≥6 years of age; no visual field loss was observed in 4 children and results were inconclusive in 2 others (Lawthom 2009; Sorri 2005).

Data collection to monitor pregnancy and infant outcomes following exposure to vigabatrin is ongoing. Healthcare providers are encouraged to enroll women exposed to vigabatrin during pregnancy in the North American Antiepileptic Drug (NAAED) Pregnancy Registry by calling 1-888-233-2334. Additional information is available at www.aedpregnancyregistry.org.

◆ **Vigadrone** *see* Vigabatrin *on page 1542*

◆ **VIGIV** *see* Vaccinia Immune Globulin (Intravenous) *on page 1511*

◆ **Viibryd** *see* Vilazodone *on page 1544*

◆ **Viibryd Starter Pack** *see* Vilazodone *on page 1544*

◆ **Vilamit MB** *see* Methenamine, Sodium Phosphate Monobasic, Phenyl Salicylate, Methylene Blue, and Hyoscyamine *on page 987*

◆ **Vilanterol and Fluticasone** *see* Fluticasone and Vilanterol *on page 706*

◆ **Vilanterol and Fluticasone Furoate** *see* Fluticasone and Vilanterol *on page 706*

◆ **Vilanterol and Umeclidinium** *see* Umeclidinium and Vilanterol *on page 1508*

Vilazodone (vil AZ oh done)

Related Information

Vasoconstrictor Interactions With Antidepressants *on page 1821*

Brand Names: US Viibryd; Viibryd Starter Pack

Brand Names: Canada Viibryd; Viibryd Starter Pack

Pharmacologic Category Antidepressant, Selective Serotonin Reuptake Inhibitor/5-HT_{1A} Receptor Partial Agonist

Use Major depressive disorder: Treatment of major depressive disorder in adults.

Local Anesthetic/Vasoconstrictor Precautions Although caution should be used in patients taking tricyclic antidepressants, no interactions have been reported with vasoconstrictors and vilazodone, a nontricyclic antidepressant which acts to increase serotonin; no precautions appear to be needed

Effects on Dental Treatment Key adverse event(s) related to dental treatment: Xerostomia (normal salivary flow resumes upon discontinuation) and abnormal taste (see Effects on Bleeding and Dental Health Professional Considerations)

Effects on Bleeding May impair platelet aggregation resulting in increased risk of bleeding events, particularly if used concomitantly with aspirin, NSAIDs, warfarin, or other anticoagulants. Bleeding related to SSRI use has been reported to range from relatively minor bruising and epistaxis to life-threatening hemorrhage. Routine interruption of therapy for most dental procedures is not warranted. In medically complicated patients or extensive oral surgery, the decision to interrupt therapy must be based on the risk to benefit in an individual patient and a medical consult is suggested. If therapy is continued without interruption, the clinician should anticipate the potential for a prolonged bleeding time.

Adverse Reactions

>10%:

Central nervous system: Headache (15%)

Gastrointestinal: Diarrhea (26% to 29%), nausea (22% to 24%)

1% to 10%:

Cardiovascular: Palpitations (1% to 2%)

Central nervous system: Dizziness (6% to 8%), insomnia (6% to 7%), drowsiness (4% to 5%), fatigue (4%), abnormal dreams (3%), restlessness (2% to 3%), paresthesia (2%), delayed ejaculation (1% to 2%), migraine (≥1%), sedation (>1%), panic attack (≤1%), ventricular premature contractions (≤1%)

Dermatologic: Hyperhidrosis (≤1%), night sweats (≤1%)

Endocrine & metabolic: Decreased libido (2% to 4%), weight gain (2%)

Gastrointestinal: Xerostomia (7% to 8%), abdominal pain (4% to 7%), vomiting (4% to 5%), dyspepsia (3%), flatulence (3%), increased appetite (3%), abdominal distension (2%), gastroenteritis (2%)

Genitourinary: Erectile dysfunction (≤3%), orgasm disturbance (1% to 2%)

Neuromuscular & skeletal: Arthralgia (2%), tremor (>1%)

Ophthalmic: Blurred vision (≤1%), xerophthalmia (≤1%)

<1%, postmarketing, and/or case reports: Acute pancreatitis, angle-closure glaucoma, cataract, hallucination, hyponatremia, irritability, mania, seizure, serotonin syndrome, skin rash, sleep paralysis, suicidal ideation, suicidal tendencies, urticaria

Mechanism of Action Vilazodone inhibits CNS neuron serotonin uptake; minimal or no effect on reuptake of norepinephrine or dopamine. It also binds selectively with high affinity to 5-HT_{1A} receptors and is a 5-HT_{1A} receptor partial agonist. 5-HT_{1A} receptor activity may be altered in depression and anxiety.

Pharmacodynamics/Kinetics

Onset of Action Depression: Initial effects may be observed within 1 to 2 weeks of treatment, with continued improvements through 4 to 6 weeks (Papakostas 2006; Posternak 2005; Szegedi 2009; Taylor 2006).

Half-life Elimination Terminal: ~25 hours

Time to Peak Serum: 4 to 5 hours

Pregnancy Considerations Nonteratogenic effects in the newborn following selective serotonin reuptake inhibitor (SSRI)/serotonin and norepinephrine reuptake inhibitor (SNRI) exposure late in the third trimester include respiratory distress, cyanosis, apnea, seizures, temperature instability, feeding difficulty, vomiting, hypoglycemia, hypo- or hypertonia, hyper-reflexia, jitteriness, irritability, constant crying, and tremor. Symptoms may be due to the toxicity of the SSRIs/SNRIs or a discontinuation syndrome and may be consistent with serotonin syndrome associated with SSRI treatment. Persistent pulmonary hypertension of the newborn has also been reported with SSRI exposure. The long-term effects of *in utero* SSRI exposure on infant development and behavior are not known.

The American College of Obstetricians and Gynecologists (ACOG) recommends that therapy with SSRIs or SNRIs during pregnancy be individualized; treatment of depression during pregnancy should incorporate the clinical expertise of the mental health clinician, obstetrician, primary health care provider, and pediatrician. According to the American Psychiatric Association (APA), the risks of medication treatment should be weighed against other treatment options and untreated depression. For women who discontinue antidepressant medications during pregnancy and who may be at high risk for postpartum depression, the medications can be restarted following delivery. Treatment algorithms have been developed by the ACOG and the APA for the management of depression in women prior to conception and during pregnancy. Consideration should be given to using an agent with some safety information in pregnant women (ACOG 2008; APA 2010; Yonkers 2009).

Pregnant women exposed to antidepressants during pregnancy are encouraged to enroll in the National Pregnancy Registry for Antidepressants (NPRAD). Women 18 to 45 years of age or their health care providers may contact the registry by calling 1-844-405-6185. Enrollment should be done as early in pregnancy as possible.

Dental Health Professional Considerations Problems with SSRI-induced bruxism have been reported and may preclude their use; clinicians attempting to evaluate any patient with bruxism or involuntary muscle movement, who is simultaneously being treated with an SSRI drug, should be aware of the potential association.

- ◆ **Vilazodone HCl** *see* Vilazodone *on page 1544*
- ◆ **Vilazodone Hydrochloride** *see* Vilazodone *on page 1544*
- ◆ **Vilevev MB** *see* Methenamine, Sodium Phosphate Monobasic, Phenyl Salicylate, Methylene Blue, and Hyoscyamine *on page 987*
- ◆ **Vimizim** *see* Elosulfase Alfa *on page 550*
- ◆ **Vimovo** *see* Naproxen and Esomeprazole *on page 1084*
- ◆ **Vimpat** *see* Lacosamide *on page 868*

VinBLAStine (vin BLAS teen)

Pharmacologic Category Antineoplastic Agent, Antimicrotubular; Antineoplastic Agent, Vinca Alkaloid

Use

Hodgkin Lymphoma: Treatment of Hodgkin lymphoma

Kaposi sarcoma: Treatment of Kaposi sarcoma

Langerhans cell histiocytosis: Treatment of histiocytosis X (Letterer-Siwe disease)

Non-Hodgkin lymphomas: Treatment of lymphocytic lymphoma, histiocytic lymphoma, and advanced mycosis fungoides

Testicular cancer: Treatment of testicular cancer

Has also been used in the treatment of resistant choriocarcinoma

Local Anesthetic/Vasoconstrictor Precautions No information available to require special precautions

Effects on Dental Treatment Key adverse event(s) related to dental treatment: Stomatitis, metallic taste, and jaw pain.

Effects on Bleeding Chemotherapy may result in significant myelosuppression, potentially including significant reduction in platelet counts and altered hemostasis. In patients who are under active treatment with these agents, medical consult is suggested.

Adverse Reactions Frequency not defined.

Cardiovascular: Angina pectoris, cerebrovascular accident, ECG abnormality, hypertension (common), ischemic heart disease, limb ischemia, myocardial infarction, Raynaud's phenomenon

Central nervous system: Decreased deep tendon reflex, depression, dizziness, headache, malaise (common), metallic taste, neurotoxicity (duration: >24 hours), paresthesia, peripheral neuritis, seizure, tumor pain (common), vertigo

Dermatologic: Alopecia (common), dermatitis, skin blister, skin photosensitivity (rare), skin rash

Endocrine & metabolic: Hyperuricemia, SIADH (syndrome of inappropriate antidiuretic hormone secretion)

Gastrointestinal: Abdominal pain, anorexia, constipation (common), diarrhea, enterocolitis (hemorrhagic), gastrointestinal hemorrhage, intestinal obstruction, nausea (mild), paralytic ileus, stomatitis, toxic megacolon, vomiting (mild)

Genitourinary: Azoospermia, urinary retention

Hematologic & oncologic: Anemia, bone marrow depression (common), granulocytopenia (common; nadir: 5 to 10 days; recovery: 7 to 14 days; dose-limiting toxicity), hemolytic uremic syndrome, leukopenia (common; nadir: 5 to 10 days; recovery: 7 to 14 days; dose-limiting toxicity), rectal hemorrhage, thrombocytopenia (recovery within a few days), thrombotic thrombocytopenic purpura

Local: Local irritation

Neuromuscular & skeletal: Jaw pain (common), myalgia, ostealgia (common), weakness

Ophthalmic: Nystagmus

Otic: Auditory disturbance, deafness, vestibular disturbance

Respiratory: Bronchospasm, dyspnea, pharyngitis

Miscellaneous: Radiation recall phenomenon

Mechanism of Action Vinblastine binds to tubulin and inhibits microtubule formation, therefore, arresting the cell at metaphase by disrupting the formation of the mitotic spindle; it is specific for the M and S phases. Vinblastine may also interfere with nucleic acid and protein synthesis by blocking glutamic acid utilization.

Pharmacodynamics/Kinetics

Half-life Elimination Terminal: ~25 hours

Reproductive Considerations

Females of reproductive potential should avoid becoming pregnant during vinblastine treatment. Reversible amenorrhea may occur when vinblastine is used in some combination regimens (dose related). Aspermia has been reported in males who have received treatment with vinblastine.

Pregnancy Considerations

Based on placental perfusion studies, vinblastine is expected to cross the placenta (Sudhakaran 2008). Outcome information following maternal use of vinblastine as a single agent or as part of combination therapy during pregnancy is available (Avilés 2018; Eyre 2015).

The European Society for Medical Oncology (ESMO) has published guidelines for diagnosis, treatment, and follow-up of cancer during pregnancy. The ESMO guidelines recommend referral to a facility with expertise in cancer during pregnancy and encourage a multidisciplinary team (obstetrician, neonatologist, oncology team). In general, if chemotherapy is indicated, it should be avoided during in the first trimester, there should be a 3-week time period between the last chemotherapy dose and anticipated delivery, and chemotherapy should not be administered beyond week 33 of gestation (Peccatori 2013). An international consensus panel has published guidelines for hematologic malignancies during pregnancy. Vinblastine is a component of the ABVD regimen, which is used for the treatment of Hodgkin lymphoma. If treatment cannot be deferred until after delivery in patients with early stage Hodgkin lymphoma, ABVD may be administered safely and effectively in the latter phase of pregnancy (based on limited data); for patients with advanced-stage disease, ABVD can be administered in the second and third trimesters (Lishner 2016).

A pregnancy registry is available for all cancers diagnosed during pregnancy at Cooper Health (877-635-4499).

◆ **Vinblastine Sulfate** *see* VinBLAStine *on page 1545*
◆ **Vincaleukoblastine** *see* VinBLAStine *on page 1545*
◆ **Vincasar PFS [DSC]** *see* VinCRIStine *on page 1546*

VinCRIStine (vin KRIS teen)

Brand Names: US Vincasar PFS [DSC]

Pharmacologic Category Antineoplastic Agent, Antimicrotubular; Antineoplastic Agent, Vinca Alkaloid

Use

Acute lymphocytic leukemia: Treatment of acute lymphocytic leukemia (ALL)

Hodgkin lymphoma: Treatment of Hodgkin lymphoma

Neuroblastoma: Treatment of neuroblastoma

Non-Hodgkin lymphomas: Treatment of non-Hodgkin lymphomas

Rhabdomyosarcoma: Treatment of rhabdomyosarcoma

Wilms tumor: Treatment of Wilms tumor

Local Anesthetic/Vasoconstrictor Precautions No information available to require special precautions

Effects on Dental Treatment Key adverse event(s) related to dental treatment: Oral ulceration, metallic taste, orthostatic hypotension or hypertension.

Effects on Bleeding Although significant myelosuppression with associated altered hemostasis has been reported for many chemotherapeutic agents, myelosuppression is not common with vincristine and no specific precautions appear to necessary.

Adverse Reactions Frequency not defined.

Cardiovascular: Edema, hypertension, hypotension, ischemic heart disease, myocardial infarction, phlebitis

Central nervous system: Abnormal gait, ataxia, coma, cranial nerve dysfunction (auditory impairment, extraocular muscle impairment, laryngeal muscle impairment, motor dysfunction, paralysis, paresis, vestibular damage, vocal cord paralysis), decreased deep tendon reflex, dizziness, headache, neuralgia (common), neurotoxicity (dose-related), paralysis, paresthesia, parotid pain, peripheral neuropathy (common), seizure, sensorimotor neuropathy, sensory disturbance, vertigo

Dermatologic: Alopecia (common), skin rash

Endocrine & metabolic: Hyperuricemia, uric acid nephropathy (acute), weight loss

Gastrointestinal: Abdominal cramps, abdominal pain, anorexia, constipation (common), diarrhea, intestinal necrosis, intestinal perforation, nausea, oral mucosa ulcer, paralytic ileus, sore throat, vomiting

Genitourinary: Bladder dysfunction (atony), dysuria, urinary retention

Hematologic & oncologic: Anemia (mild), hemolytic uremic syndrome, leukopenia (mild), thrombocytopenia (mild), thrombotic thrombocytopenic purpura

Hepatic: Hepatic sinusoidal obstruction syndrome (formerly known as hepatic veno-occlusive disease)

Local: Local irritation (if infiltrated)

Neuromuscular & skeletal: Amyotrophy, back pain, footdrop, jaw pain, limb pain, myalgia, ostealgia

Ophthalmic: Cortical blindness (transient), nystagmus, optic atrophy with blindness

Otic: Deafness

Renal: Polyuria

Respiratory: Bronchospasm, dyspnea

Miscellaneous: Fever, tissue necrosis (if infiltrated)

<1%, postmarketing, and/or case reports: Anaphylaxis, hypersensitivity reaction, SIADH (syndrome of inappropriate antidiuretic hormone secretion)

Mechanism of Action Vincristine binds to tubulin and inhibits microtubule formation, therefore, arresting the cell at metaphase by disrupting the formation of the mitotic spindle; it is specific for the M and S phases. Vincristine may also interfere with nucleic acid and protein synthesis by blocking glutamic acid utilization.

Pharmacodynamics/Kinetics

Half-life Elimination Terminal: 85 hours (range: 19 to 155 hours)

Reproductive Considerations Females of reproductive potential should avoid becoming pregnant during vincristine treatment.

The effect of vincristine alone on male and female fertility is not known; available information is from use in combination with other agents. Recommendations are available for fertility preservation of male and female adult patients treated with anticancer agents (ASCO [Oktay 2018]).

Pregnancy Considerations

Based on data from animal reproduction studies, in utero exposure to vincristine may cause fetal harm. However, use in pregnancy has been described (NTP 2013).

The European Society for Medical Oncology has published guidelines for diagnosis, treatment, and follow-up of cancer during pregnancy; the guidelines recommend referral to a facility with expertise in cancer during pregnancy and encourage a multidisciplinary team (obstetrician, neonatologist, oncology team). In general, if chemotherapy is indicated, it should be avoided in the first trimester and there should be a 3-week time period between the last chemotherapy dose and anticipated delivery, and chemotherapy should not be administered beyond week 33 of gestation (ESMO [Peccatori 2013]).

When multiagent therapy is needed to treat aggressive non-Hodgkin lymphomas during pregnancy, vincristine (as a component of the CHOP [cyclophosphamide, doxorubicin, vincristine, and prednisone] regimen) may be used when indicated (ESMO [Peccatori 2013]; Lishner 2016).

A pregnancy registry is available for all cancers diagnosed during pregnancy at Cooper Health (1-877-635-4499).

VinCRIStine (Liposomal)

(vin KRIS teen lye po SO mal)

Brand Names: US Marqibo

Pharmacologic Category Antineoplastic Agent, Antimicrotubular; Antineoplastic Agent, Vinca Alkaloid

Use Acute lymphoblastic leukemia (relapsed): Treatment of relapsed Philadelphia chromosome-negative (Ph-) acute lymphoblastic leukemia (ALL) in adults in second or greater relapse or whose disease has progressed after 2 or more antileukemic therapies.

Local Anesthetic/Vasoconstrictor Precautions No information available to require special precautions

Effects on Dental Treatment No significant effects or complications reported

Effects on Bleeding Although significant myelosuppression with associated altered hemostasis has been reported for many chemotherapeutic agents, myelosuppression is not common with vincristine and no specific precautions appear to necessary.

Adverse Reactions

>10%:

Central nervous system: Fatigue (41%), peripheral neuropathy (39%; grades 3/4: 17%), insomnia (32%)

Gastrointestinal: Constipation (57%), nausea (52%), diarrhea (37%), decreased appetite (33%)

Hematologic & oncologic: Febrile neutropenia (38%; grades 3/4: 31%), anemia (34%; grades 3/4: 17%), neutropenia (grades 3/4: 18%), thrombocytopenia (grades 3/4: 17%)

Hepatic: Increased serum AST (grades 3/4: 6% to 11%)

Miscellaneous: Fever (43%)

1% to 10%:

Cardiovascular: Hypotension (grades 3/4: 6%), septic shock (grades 3/4: 6%)

Central nervous system: Pain (grades 3/4: 8%), mental status changes (grades 3/4: 4%), myasthenia (grades 3/4: 1%)

Gastrointestinal: Abdominal pain (grades 3/4: 8%), intestinal obstruction (grades 3/4: 6%)

Infection: Staphylococcal bacteremia (grades 3/4: 6%)

Neuromuscular & skeletal: Weakness (grades 3/4: 5%)

Respiratory: Pneumonia (grades 3/4: 8%), respiratory distress (grades 3/4: 6%), respiratory failure (grades 3/4: 5%)

Mechanism of Action The vincristine liposomal formulation increases the half-life, allowing for enhanced cytotoxic activity in tumor cells. The liposomal formulation of vincristine consists of vincristine encapsulated in sphingosomes, which are composed of sphingomyelin and cholesterol (Bedikian 2006).

Pharmacodynamics/Kinetics

Half-life Elimination 45 hours (urinary half-life); dependent on rate of vincristine release from sphingosome (Bedikian 2006)

Reproductive Considerations Verify pregnancy status prior to treatment initiation in females of reproductive potential. Females of reproductive potential should use effective contraception during therapy and for 6 months after the last vincristine (liposomal) dose. Males with female partners of reproductive potential should use effective contraception during therapy and for 3 months after the last vincristine (liposomal) dose.

Pregnancy Considerations

Based on the mechanism of action and data from animal reproduction studies, in utero exposure to vincristine (liposomal) may cause fetal harm.

◆ **Vincristine (Conventional)** *see* VinCRIStine *on page 1546*

◆ **Vincristine Liposomal Sulfate** *see* VinCRIStine (Liposomal) *on page 1546*

◆ **Vincristine Liposome** *see* VinCRIStine (Liposomal) *on page 1546*

◆ **Vincristine Sulfate** *see* VinCRIStine *on page 1546*

◆ **Vincristine Sulfate Liposome** *see* VinCRIStine (Liposomal) *on page 1546*

Vinorelbine (vi NOR el been)

Brand Names: US Navelbine

Pharmacologic Category Antineoplastic Agent, Antimicrotubular; Antineoplastic Agent, Vinca Alkaloid

Use Non-small cell lung cancer: Treatment (first-line; in combination with cisplatin) of locally advanced or metastatic non-small cell lung cancer (NSCLC); single-agent treatment of metastatic NSCLC.

Local Anesthetic/Vasoconstrictor Precautions

No information available to require special precautions

Effects on Dental Treatment No significant effects or complications reported

Effects on Bleeding Chemotherapy may result in significant myelosuppression, potentially including significant reduction in platelet counts and altered hemostasis. In patients who are under active treatment with these agents, medical consult is suggested.

Adverse Reactions

>10%:

Central nervous system: Neurotoxicity (44%), peripheral neuropathy (20%; grades 3/4: 1%)

Dermatologic: Alopecia (12% to 30%)

Gastrointestinal: Nausea (≤34%), vomiting (≤31%), constipation (29%), diarrhea (12% to 13%)

Hematologic & oncologic: Neutropenia (80% to 85%; grades 3/4: 29% to 69%), leukopenia (81% to 83%; grades 3/4: 12% to 32%), anemia (77%; grades 3/4: 1% to 9%)

Hepatic: Increased serum aspartate aminotransferase (54%)

Local: Injection site reaction (22% to 38%; includes erythema at injection site, vein discoloration), pain at injection site (13%)

Neuromuscular & skeletal: Asthenia (27%)

Renal: Increased serum creatinine (13%)

1% to 10%:

Cardiovascular: Localized phlebitis (10%), chest pain (5%)

Central nervous system: Neuropathy (grades 3/4: 1%)

Hematologic & oncologic: Febrile neutropenia (≤8%), thrombocytopenia (3% to 4%; grades 3/4: 1%)

Hepatic: Increased serum bilirubin (9%)

Infection: Sepsis (≤8%)

Otic: Ototoxicity (1%)

Respiratory: Dyspnea (3%)

Frequency not defined:

Gastrointestinal: Intestinal necrosis, intestinal obstruction, intestinal perforation, paralytic ileus

Hematologic & oncologic: Bone marrow depression

Hepatic: Hepatotoxicity

Respiratory: Interstitial pulmonary disease, pulmonary toxicity (including acute respiratory distress syndrome, interstitial pneumonitis, severe acute bronchospasm)

<1%, postmarketing, and/or case reports: Abdominal pain, abnormal gait, anaphylaxis, angioedema, arthralgia, auditory impairment, back pain, decreased deep tendon reflex, deep vein thrombosis, dermatitis, dysphagia, electrolyte disorder, esophagitis, exfoliation of skin, flushing, headache, hemorrhagic cystitis, hypertension, hyponatremia, hypotension, jaw pain, localized rash, mucositis, myalgia, myasthenia, myocardial infarction, palmar-plantar erythrodysesthesia, pancreatitis, pneumonia, pruritus, pulmonary edema, pulmonary embolism, radiation recall phenomenon, SIADH, skin blister, skin rash, tachycardia, tumor pain, urticaria, urticaria at injection site, vasodilation, vestibular disturbance

Mechanism of Action Vinorelbine is a semisynthetic vinca alkaloid which binds to tubulin and inhibits microtubule formation, therefore, arresting the cell at metaphase by disrupting the formation of the mitotic spindle; it is specific for the M and S phases. Vinorelbine may also interfere with nucleic acid and protein synthesis by blocking glutamic acid utilization.

Pharmacodynamics/Kinetics

Half-life Elimination Triphasic:

Children and Adolescents 2 to 17 years: Terminal: 16.5 ± 9.7 hours (Johansen 2006)

Adults: Terminal: ~28 to 44 hours

Reproductive Considerations

Females of reproductive potential should use effective contraception during vinorelbine treatment and for 6 months after the final vinorelbine dose. Males with female partners of reproductive potential should use effective contraception during treatment and for 3 months following the last vinorelbine dose.

Vinorelbine may damage spermatozoa and may cause decreased fertility in male patients.

Pregnancy Considerations

Based on the mechanism and on findings in animal reproduction studies, vinorelbine may cause fetal harm if administered to a pregnant female.

- ◆ **Vinorelbine, inj** *see* Vinorelbine *on page 1547*
- ◆ **Vinorelbine Tartrate** *see* Vinorelbine *on page 1547*
- ◆ **Viorele** *see* Ethinyl Estradiol and Desogestrel *on page 609*
- ◆ **Viosterol** *see* Ergocalciferol *on page 582*
- ◆ **Viracept** *see* Nelfinavir *on page 1092*
- ◆ **Viramune** *see* Nevirapine *on page 1096*
- ◆ **Viramune XR** *see* Nevirapine *on page 1096*
- ◆ **Virazole** *see* Ribavirin (Oral Inhalation) *on page 1321*
- ◆ **Viread** *see* Tenofovir Disoproxil Fumarate *on page 1419*
- ◆ **Viroptic [DSC]** *see* Trifluridine *on page 1497*
- ◆ **Virt-FeFA Plus** *see* Vitamins (Multiple/Oral) *on page 1550*
- ◆ **Visbiome [OTC]** *see Lactobacillus on page 869*
- ◆ **Viscous Lidocaine** *see* Lidocaine (Topical) *on page 902*
- ◆ **Visine [OTC]** *see* Naphazoline and Pheniramine *on page 1079*
- ◆ **Visine-A [OTC]** *see* Naphazoline and Pheniramine *on page 1079*

Vismodegib (vis moe DEG ib)

Brand Names: US Erivedge

Brand Names: Canada Erivedge

Pharmacologic Category Antineoplastic Agent, Hedgehog Pathway Inhibitor

Use Basal cell carcinoma, metastatic or locally advanced: Treatment of metastatic basal cell carcinoma, or locally-advanced basal cell carcinoma that has recurred following surgery or in adult patients who are not candidates for surgery and not candidates for radiation therapy

Local Anesthetic/Vasoconstrictor Precautions

No information available to require special precautions

Effects on Dental Treatment Key adverse event(s) related to dental treatment: Abnormal taste and loss of taste perception have been reported (see Dental Health Professional Considerations)

Effects on Bleeding No information available to require special precautions

Adverse Reactions

>10%:

Cardiovascular: Increased serum creatine phosphokinase (38%)

Central nervous system: Fatigue (40%)

Dermatologic: Alopecia (64%)

Endocrine & metabolic: Amenorrhea (30%)

Gastrointestinal: Dysgeusia (55%), weight loss (45%), nausea (30%), diarrhea (29%), decreased appetite (25%), constipation (21%), vomiting (14%), ageusia (11%)

Neuromuscular & skeletal: Muscle spasm (72%), arthralgia (16%)

1% to 10%:

Endocrine & metabolic: Hyponatremia (grade 3: 4%), hypokalemia (grade 3: 1%)

Genitourinary: Azotemia (grade 3: 2%)

<1%, postmarketing, and/or case reports: Hepatic injury

Mechanism of Action Basal cell cancer is associated with mutations in Hedgehog pathway components. Hedgehog regulates cell growth and differentiation in embryogenesis; while generally not active in adult tissue, Hedgehog mutations associated with basal cell cancer can activate the pathway resulting in unrestricted proliferation of skin basal cells. Vismodegib is a selective Hedgehog pathway inhibitor which binds to and inhibits Smoothened homologue (SMO), the transmembrane protein involved in Hedgehog signal transduction.

Pharmacodynamics/Kinetics

Half-life Elimination Continuous daily dosing: ~4 days; Single dose: ~12 days

Time to Peak ~2.4 days (Graham 2011)

Reproductive Considerations

[US Boxed Warning]: Verify pregnancy status of females of reproductive potential within 7 days prior to initiating vismodegib. Advise females of reproductive potential to use effective contraception during and after vismodegib. After a negative pregnancy test, initiate highly effective contraception prior to the first vismodegib dose and continue during treatment and for 24 months after the final vismodegib dose.

Amenorrhea may occur in females.

[US Boxed Warning]: Advise males of the potential risk of vismodegib exposure through semen and to use condoms with a pregnant partner or a female partner of reproductive potential. It is not known if the presence of vismodegib in semen can cause embryotoxicity and/or fetotoxicity.

Male patients should not donate sperm during vismodegib treatment and for 3 months after the last vismodegib dose.

Male patients with female partners of childbearing potential should use condoms (even after vasectomy) during vismodegib treatment and for 3 months after the last vismodegib dose.

Pregnancy Considerations

[US Boxed Warning]: Vismodegib can cause embryofetal death or severe birth defects when administered to a pregnant woman. Vismodegib is embryotoxic, fetotoxic, and teratogenic in animals. Teratogenic effects included severe midline defects, missing digits, and other irreversible malformations. Advise pregnant women of the potential risks to a fetus.

Women exposed to vismodegib during pregnancy (directly or via seminal fluid) are encouraged to contact the Pregnancy Exposure Registry (1-888-835-2555).

Prescribing and Access Restrictions

US: Available at specialty pharmacies through the Erivedge Access Solutions program. Further information may be obtained from the manufacturer, Genentech, at 1-888-249-4918, or at www.Erivedge-AccessSolutions.com

Canada: Available through a controlled distribution program called Erivedge Pregnancy Prevention Program (EPPP). Registration with the program is required for participating prescribers and pharmacies. Patients must also be registered with the program and meet all necessary requirements to receive vismodegib. Consult product monograph for detailed information regarding program requirements. Further information may also be obtained at 1-888-748-8926.

Dental Health Professional Considerations Review head and neck exam for changes since previous visit; Refer patient back to dermatologist/physician if changes are noted.

- **Vistaril** *see* HydrOXYzine *on page 780*
- **Vitafol** *see* Vitamins (Multiple/Oral) *on page 1550*
- **Vitamin D_3 and Alendronate** *see* Alendronate and Cholecalciferol *on page 100*
- **Vitamin D and Calcium Carbonate** *see* Calcium and Vitamin D *on page 280*

Vitamin A (VYE ta min aye)

Brand Names: US A-25 [OTC]; Aquasol A; Gordons-Vite A [OTC]; Vitamin A Fish [OTC]

Pharmacologic Category Vitamin, Fat Soluble

Use Treatment and prevention of vitamin A deficiency; parenteral (IM) route is indicated when oral administration is not feasible or when absorption is insufficient (malabsorption syndrome); dietary supplement (OTC)

Local Anesthetic/Vasoconstrictor Precautions No information available to require special precautions

Effects on Dental Treatment No significant effects or complications reported

Effects on Bleeding No information available to require special precautions

Adverse Reactions Frequency not defined: Hypersensitivity: Anaphylactic shock (following IV administration), hypersensitivity reaction (rare), intracranial hypertension (Tan 2019)

Mechanism of Action Vitamin A is a fat soluble vitamin needed for visual adaptation to darkness, maintenance of epithelial cells, immune function and embryonic development.

Reproductive Considerations

Doses greater than the RDA are contraindicated in women who may become pregnant. High doses are used in some areas of the world for supplementation where deficiency is a public health problem (eg, to prevent night blindness); however, single doses >25,000 units should be avoided within 60 days of conception. High-dose supplementation is otherwise not recommended as part of routine antenatal care (WHO 2011c).

Pregnancy Considerations

Excess vitamin A during pregnancy may cause craniofacial malformations, as well as CNS, heart, and thymus abnormalities. Maternal vitamin A deficiency also causes adverse effects in the fetus, and vitamin A requirements are increased in pregnant women (IOM 2000). The manufacturer notes that the safety of doses >6,000 units/day in pregnant women has not been established and doses greater than the RDA are contraindicated in pregnant women.

- **Vitamin A Acetate** *see* Vitamin A *on page 1549*
- **Vitamin A Acid** *see* Tretinoin (Topical) *on page 1484*
- **Vitamin A Fish [OTC]** *see* Vitamin A *on page 1549*
- **Vitamin B_2** *see* Riboflavin *on page 1323*
- **Vitamin B_3** *see* Niacin *on page 1097*
- **Vitamin B_3** *see* Niacinamide *on page 1100*
- **Vitamin B_6** *see* Pyridoxine *on page 1294*
- **Vitamin B9** *see* Folic Acid *on page 709*
- **Vitamin B_{12}** *see* Cyanocobalamin *on page 417*
- **Vitamin B_{12a}** *see* Hydroxocobalamin *on page 778*

Vitamin B Complex Combinations

(VYE ta min bee KOM pleks kom bi NAY shuns)

Pharmacologic Category Vitamin

Use Dietary supplement

Local Anesthetic/Vasoconstrictor Precautions No information available to require special precautions

Effects on Dental Treatment No significant effects or complications reported

Effects on Bleeding No information available to require special precautions

Pregnancy Considerations Water soluble vitamins cross the placenta (IOM, 1998). Refer to individual vitamins for additional information and specific requirements during pregnancy.

- **Vitamin D2** *see* Ergocalciferol *on page 582*
- **Vitamin D3 Super Strength [OTC]** *see* Cholecalciferol *on page 344*
- **Vitamin D3 Ultra Potency [OTC]** *see* Cholecalciferol *on page 344*
- **Vitamin Deficiency System-B12** *see* Cyanocobalamin *on page 417*

Vitamin E (Systemic) (VYE ta min ee)

Brand Names: US Alph-E [OTC]; Alph-E-Mixed 1000 [OTC]; Alph-E-Mixed [OTC]; Aqueous Vitamin E [OTC]; E-400 [OTC] [DSC]; E-400-Clear [OTC]; E-400-Mixed [OTC]; E-Max-1000 [OTC]; E-Pherol [OTC] [DSC]; Formula E 400 [OTC]; Natural Vitamin E [OTC]; Nutr-E-Sol [OTC]; SoluVita E [OTC]; Vita-Plus E [OTC] [DSC]

Pharmacologic Category Vitamin, Fat Soluble

Use Dietary supplement

Note: According to the 2014 USPSTF recommendations for the primary prevention of cardiovascular disease and cancer, the use of vitamin E supplements are not recommended (Moyer 2014).

Local Anesthetic/Vasoconstrictor Precautions No information available to require special precautions

Effects on Dental Treatment No significant effects or complications reported

Effects on Bleeding High doses of vitamin E (800 to 1,200 int. units/day) may increase the overall risk of bleeding. Although the mechanism is unknown, it may affect the coagulation cascade and has the potential to enhance the anticoagulant effects of various anticoagulants.

Adverse Reactions There are no adverse reactions listed in the manufacturer's labeling.

Mechanism of Action Prevents oxidation of vitamin A and C; protects polyunsaturated fatty acids in membranes from attack by free radicals and protects red blood cells against hemolysis

Pregnancy Considerations Vitamin E crosses the placenta. Maternal serum concentrations of α tocopherol increase with lipid concentrations as pregnancy progresses; however, placental transfer remains constant. Additional supplementation is not needed in pregnant women without deficiency (IOM 2000).

◆ **Vitamin G** *see* Riboflavin *on page 1323*

◆ **Vitamin K** *see* Phytonadione *on page 1230*

◆ **Vitamin K$_1$** *see* Phytonadione *on page 1230*

Vitamins (Fluoride) (VYE ta mins, FLOOR ide)

Brand Names: US Poly-Vi-Flor®; Poly-Vi-Flor® With Iron; Soluvite-F; Tri-Vi-Flor®; Tri-Vi-Flor® with Iron; Vi-Daylin®/F + Iron [DSC]; Vi-Daylin®/F ADC [DSC]; Vi-Daylin®/F ADC + Iron [DSC]; Vi-Daylin®/F [DSC]

Pharmacologic Category Vitamin

Use Prevention/treatment of vitamin deficiency; products containing fluoride are used to prevent dental caries; labeled for OTC use as a dietary supplement

Local Anesthetic/Vasoconstrictor Precautions No information available to require special precautions

Effects on Dental Treatment No significant effects or complications reported

Contraindications Hypersensitivity to any component of the formulation; preexisting hypervitaminosis

Warnings/Precautions Not all products can be used in children of all age groups; consult specific product labeling prior to use. Do not exceed recommended doses. Use caution with severe renal or hepatic dysfunction or failure. **[U.S. Boxed Warning]: Products may contain iron. Severe iron toxicity may occur in overdose, particularly when ingested by children; iron is a leading cause of fatal poisoning in children; store out of children's reach and in child-resistant containers.**

Dietary Considerations May take with food to decrease stomach upset.

Dosage Forms: US Content varies depending on product used. For more detailed information on ingredients in these and other multivitamins, please refer to package labeling.

Dental Health Professional Considerations Chronic overdose of fluoride may result in mottling of tooth enamel and osseous changes.

Vitamins (Multiple/Oral)

(VYE ta mins, MUL ti pul/OR al)

Brand Names: US ABDEK [OTC]; Androvite [OTC]; CalciFol; CalciFolic-D; Centamin [OTC]; Centrum Cardio [OTC]; Centrum Flavor Burst [OTC]; Centrum MultiGummies [OTC]; Centrum Performance [OTC]; Centrum Silver Ultra Men's [OTC]; Centrum Silver Ultra Women's [OTC]; Centrum Silver [OTC]; Centrum Ultra Men's [OTC]; Centrum Ultra Women's [OTC]; Centrum [OTC]; Corvite 150; CyFolex; Diatx Zn; Drinkables Fruits and Vegetables [OTC]; Drinkables MultiVitamins [OTC]; Encora; FeRiva; FeRiva 21/7; FeRivaFA; Ferralet 90; Foltrin; Freedavite [OTC]; Fusion Plus; Fusion [OTC]; Genicin Vita-Q; Geri-Freeda [OTC]; Geriation [OTC]; Geritol Complete [OTC]; Geritol Extend [OTC]; Geritol Tonic [OTC]; Glutofac-MX; Gynovite Plus [OTC]; Hemocyte Plus; Hi-Kovite [OTC]; Iberet-500 [OTC] [DSC]; K-Tan Plus; Monocaps [OTC]; Multilex [OTC]; Multilex-T&M [OTC]; Myadec [OTC]; NeoMultivite; Nicadan; NicAzel Forte; NuFera; Nutrimin-Plus [OTC]; Ocuvel; Ocuvite Adult 50+ [OTC]; Ocuvite Extra [OTC]; Ocuvite Lutein [OTC]; Ocuvite [OTC]; One A Day Cholesterol Plus [OTC]; One A Day Energy [OTC]; One A Day Essential [OTC]; One A Day Maximum [OTC]; One A Day Men's 50+ Advantage [OTC]; One A Day Men's Health Formula [OTC]; One A Day Teen Advantage for Her [OTC]; One A Day Teen Advantage for Him [OTC]; One A Day Weight Smart Advanced [OTC]; One A Day Women's Active Mind & Body [OTC]; One A Day Women's [OTC]; One A Day® Women's 50+ Advantage [OTC]; One-Daily/Iron [OTC]; Optivite P.M.T. [OTC]; PreserVision AREDS 2 Formula + Multivitamin [OTC]; PreserVision AREDS [OTC]; PreserVision Lutein [OTC]; Quflora FE; Quintabs [OTC]; Quintabs-M Iron-Free [OTC]; Quintabs-M [OTC]; Replace Without Iron [OTC]; Replace [OTC]; Repliva 21/7; Strovite; Strovite Forte; Strovite Plus [DSC]; T-Vites [OTC]; Thera-Tabs M [OTC]; Theramill Forte [OTC]; TL-HEM 150; Ultra Freeda A-Free [OTC]; Ultra Freeda Iron-Free [OTC]; Ultra Freeda With Iron [OTC]; Viactiv Calcium Flavor Glides [OTC]; Viactiv Flavor Glides [OTC]; Viactiv for Teens [OTC]; Viactiv With Calcium [OTC]; Viactiv [OTC]; Virt-FeFA Plus; Vitafol; Xtramins [OTC]; Yelets [OTC]

Pharmacologic Category Vitamin

Use Prevention/treatment of vitamin and mineral deficiencies; labeled for OTC use as a dietary supplement

Local Anesthetic/Vasoconstrictor Precautions No information available to require special precautions

Effects on Dental Treatment No significant effects or complications reported (see Dental Health Professional Considerations)

Effects on Bleeding No information available to require special precautions

Adverse Reactions See individual vitamin monographs.

Pregnancy Considerations Refer to individual vitamin monographs for requirements during pregnancy.

Dental Health Professional Considerations Dentists may encourage good nutritional habits and may detect signs/symptoms of vitamin deficiency through the intraoral examination. Refer patient back to physician if exam suggests poor nutrition or possible vitamin deficiency.

◆ **Vitamins, Multiple (Oral)** *see* Vitamins (Multiple/Oral) *on page 1550*

◆ **Vitamins, Multiple (Therapeutic)** *see* Vitamins (Multiple/Oral) *on page 1550*

◆ **Vitamins, Multiple With Iron** *see* Vitamins (Multiple/Oral) *on page 1550*

◆ **Vita-Plus E [OTC] [DSC]** *see* Vitamin E (Systemic) *on page 1549*

◆ **Vitekta [DSC]** *see* Elvitegravir *on page 552*

◆ **Vitrakvi** *see* Larotrectinib *on page 879*

◆ **Vi Vaccine** *see* Typhoid Vaccine *on page 1505*

◆ **Vivactil** *see* Protriptyline *on page 1290*

- **Vivarin [OTC]** *see* Caffeine *on page 277*
- **Vivelle Dot** *see* Estradiol (Systemic) *on page 596*
- **Vivelle-Dot** *see* Estradiol (Systemic) *on page 596*
- **Vivitrol** *see* Naltrexone *on page 1077*
- **Vivlodex** *see* Meloxicam *on page 957*
- **Vivotif** *see* Typhoid Vaccine *on page 1505*
- **Vizimpro** *see* Dacomitinib *on page 429*
- **VLB** *see* VinBLAStine *on page 1545*
- **VM-26** *see* Teniposide *on page 1417*
- **Vogelxo** *see* Testosterone *on page 1425*
- **Vogelxo Pump** *see* Testosterone *on page 1425*
- **Volmax** *see* Albuterol *on page 90*
- **Volnea** *see* Ethinyl Estradiol and Desogestrel *on page 609*
- **Voltaren** *see* Diclofenac (Systemic) *on page 484*
- **Voltaren** *see* Diclofenac (Topical) *on page 489*
- **Voltaren Arthritis Pain OTC 1% Gel** *see* Diclofenac (Topical) *on page 489*
- **Vonvendi** *see* von Willebrand Factor (Recombinant) *on page 1551*
- **von Willebrand Factor/Factor VIII Complex** *see* Antihemophilic Factor/von Willebrand Factor Complex (Human) *on page 154*

von Willebrand Factor (Recombinant)

(von WILL le brand FAK tor ree KOM be nant)

Brand Names: US Vonvendi

Pharmacologic Category Antihemophilic Agent

Use von Willebrand disease: Treatment (on demand) and control of bleeding episodes and perioperative management of bleeding in adults with von Willebrand disease (VWD).

Local Anesthetic/Vasoconstrictor Precautions
No information available to require special precautions

Effects on Dental Treatment No significant effects or complications reported

Effects on Bleeding Due to underlying hemophilia, medical consultation is warranted

Adverse Reactions

1% to 10%:

Cardiovascular: Chest discomfort (1%), deep vein thrombosis (1%), hypertension (1%), inversion T wave on ECG (1%), tachycardia (1%)

Central nervous system: Dizziness (4%), vertigo (3%)

Dermatologic: Pruritus (3%)

Endocrine & metabolic: Hot flash (1%)

Gastrointestinal: Nausea (4%), vomiting (4%), dysgeusia (1%)

Immunologic: Antibody development (1%)

Local: Infusion site reaction (paresthesia; 1%)

Neuromuscular & skeletal: Tremor (1%)

Frequency not defined: Hypersensitivity: Hypersensitivity reaction

<1%, postmarketing, and/or case reports: Anaphylaxis, angioedema, infusion related reaction

Mechanism of Action von Willebrand Factor (recombinant) promotes platelet aggregation and adhesion to damaged vascular endothelium and acts as a stabilizing carrier protein for factor VIII.

Pharmacodynamics/Kinetics

Half-life Elimination 19.1 to 22.6 hours

Pregnancy Considerations Pregnant patients with von Willebrand disease may have an increased risk of bleeding following abortion, antenatal procedures, delivery, and miscarriage; close surveillance is recommended. Clotting factors should be monitored at the first antenatal visit, once or twice during the third trimester, at delivery, and prior to surgical or invasive procedures. Changes in von Willebrand factor levels may vary during pregnancy, depending on type. Factor replacement may be required during pregnancy if concentrations are <0.5 IU/mL to prevent maternal bleeding during procedures (including delivery) or if a spontaneous miscarriage occurs. Hemostatic concentrations should be maintained for at least 3 to 5 days following procedures or postpartum. Other agents may be preferred for the treatment of von Willebrand disease in pregnancy; however, when replacement therapy is needed, a recombinant product or a product made from a safe plasma source with viral testing that contains both factor VIII and von Willebrand factor is recommended (AGOG 580 2013; NHF 2018; RCOG [Pavord 2017]).

- **Vopac MDS [DSC]** *see* Diclofenac (Topical) *on page 489*

Vorapaxar (vor a PAX ar)

Related Information

Antiplatelet and Anticoagulation Considerations in Dentistry *on page 1666*

Brand Names: US Zontivity

Pharmacologic Category Antiplatelet Agent; Protease-Activated Receptor-1 (PAR-1) Antagonist

Use History of MI or established peripheral arterial disease: To reduce thrombotic cardiovascular events (cardiovascular death, MI, stroke, urgent coronary revascularization) in patients with a history of MI or with peripheral arterial disease (PAD)

Local Anesthetic/Vasoconstrictor Precautions
No information available to require special precautions

Effects on Dental Treatment Key adverse event(s) related to dental treatment: Vorapaxar increases the risk of bleeding. The risk of bleeding is proportional to the patient's underlying bleeding risk. Older age is an underlying risk factor. The clinician is reminded that the dosing of vorapaxar is usually taken in combination with aspirin and/or clopidogrel. See Dosage. Significant bleeding after invasive dental procedures should be expected. NSAIDs for postoperative pain control should be avoided if possible since NSAIDs may further enhance bleeding in combination with these antiplatelet agents.

Effects on Bleeding Vorapaxar is an antiplatetet agent that works through antagonism of the protease-activated receptor-1 (PAR-1) expressed on platelets, resulting in reduced platelet aggregation and enhanced bleeding. Greater than 10% incidence: Hemorrhage (any GUSTO [Global Utilization of Streptokinase and Tissue Plasminogen Activator for Occluded Arteries] bleeding [severe, moderate, mild]): 25%), major hemorrhage, life-threatening (13%; clinically significant bleeding, including any bleeding requiring medical attention such as intracranial hemorrhage, or clinically significant overt signs of hemorrhage associated with a drop in hemoglobin of ≥3 g/dL). One to 10% incidence: Major hemorrhage (GUSTO bleeding category "moderate or severe": 3%; GUSTO bleeding category "severe": 1%)

Adverse Reactions

>10%:

Hematologic and oncologic: Hemorrhage (any GUSTO [Global Utilization of Streptokinase and Tissue Plasminogen Activator for Occluded Arteries] bleeding [severe, moderate, mild]): 25%), major hemorrhage, life-threatening (13%; clinically significant bleeding, including any bleeding requiring medical attention such as intracranial hemorrhage, or clinically significant overt signs of hemorrhage associated with a drop in hemoglobin of ≥3 g/dL [or when hemoglobin is unavailable, an absolute drop in hematocrit of ≥15% or a fall in hematocrit of 9% to <15%])

1% to 10%:

Central nervous system: Depression (2%)

Dermatologic: Skin rash (2%, includes cutaneous eruptions and exanthemas)

Endocrine & metabolic: Iron deficiency (<2%)

Gastrointestinal: Gastrointestinal hemorrhage (4%)

Hematologic and oncologic: Anemia (5%), major hemorrhage (GUSTO bleeding category "moderate or severe": 3%; GUSTO bleeding category "severe": 1%)

Ophthalmic: Retinopathy (<2%)

<1%, postmarketing, and/or case reports: Diplopia (or oculomotor disturbance), hemorrhagic death, intracranial hemorrhage

Mechanism of Action Vorapaxar, an antagonist of the protease-activated receptor-1 (PAR-1) expressed on platelets, inhibits thrombin-induced and thrombin receptor agonist peptide (TRAP)-induced platelet aggregation. Due to the very long half-life, vorapaxar is effectively irreversible. Vorapaxar reversibly binds to the PAR-1 receptor with a long receptor dissociation half-life of approximately 20 hours; additionally, vorapaxar displays significant inhibition of platelet aggregation that remains for up to 4 weeks after discontinuation due to the very long elimination half-life (Ueno 2010).

Pharmacodynamics/Kinetics

Onset of Action ≥80% inhibition of TRAP-induced platelet aggregation within one week

Duration of Action Dose and concentration dependent; with the recommended dosing, inhibition of TRAP-induced platelet aggregation at a level of 50% can be expected 4 weeks after discontinuation

Half-life Elimination Effective half-life: 3 to 4 days; Terminal elimination half-life (vorapaxar and active metabolite): ~8 days (range: 5 to 13 days)

Time to Peak 1 to 2 hours

Pregnancy Considerations Due to the potential for serious adverse events (eg, maternal bleeding, hemorrhage) and the long half-life of vorapaxar, alternate agents may be preferred in pregnant women. Discontinue use if pregnancy is detected.

◆ **Vorapaxar Sulfate** *see* Vorapaxar *on page 1551*

Voriconazole (vor i KOE na zole)

Related Information

Clinical Risk Related to Drugs Prolonging QT Interval *on page 1675*

Fungal Infections *on page 1752*

Brand Names: US Vfend; Vfend IV

Brand Names: Canada APO-Voriconazole; SANDOZ Voriconazole; TEVA-Voriconazole; Vfend

Pharmacologic Category Antifungal Agent, Oral; Antifungal Agent, Parenteral

Use Treatment of fungal infections in patients ≥2 years of age: Treatment of invasive aspergillosis; treatment of esophageal candidiasis; treatment of candidemia (in non-neutropenic patients); treatment of disseminated *Candida* infections of the skin and abdomen, kidney, bladder wall, and wounds; treatment of serious fungal infections caused by *Scedosporium apiospermum* and *Fusarium* spp. (including *Fusarium solani*) in patients intolerant of, or refractory to, other therapy

Local Anesthetic/Vasoconstrictor Precautions Voriconazole is one of the drugs confirmed to prolong the QT interval and is accepted as having a risk of causing torsade de pointes. The risk of drug-induced torsade de pointes is extremely low when a single QT interval prolonging drug is prescribed. In terms of epinephrine, it is not known what effect vasoconstrictors in the local anesthetic regimen will have in patients with a known history of congenital prolonged QT interval or in patients taking any medication that prolongs the QT interval. Until more information is obtained, it is suggested that the clinician consult with the physician prior to the use of a vasoconstrictor in suspected patients, and that the vasoconstrictor (epinephrine, mepivacaine and levonordefrin [Carbocaine® 2% with Neo-Cobefrin®]) be used with caution.

Effects on Dental Treatment Key adverse event(s) related to dental treatment: Xerostomia (normal salivary flow resumes upon discontinuation).

Effects on Bleeding No information available to require special precautions

Adverse Reactions

>10%:

Cardiovascular: Hypertension (children and adolescents: 11%; adults: <2%)

Dermatologic: Skin rash (children and adolescents: 13%; adults: 2% to 4%)

Endocrine & metabolic: Hyperkalemia (adults: ≤17%), hypokalemia (children and adolescents: 11%; adults: <1%)

Gastrointestinal: Vomiting (children and adolescents: 20%; adults: 1% to 3%), nausea (children and adolescents: 13%; adults: 1% to 4%), abdominal pain (children and adolescents: 12%; adults: <2%), diarrhea (children and adolescents: 11%; adults: <2%)

Hepatic: Increased serum alkaline phosphatase (adults: 4% to 23%; children and adolescents: 8%), increased serum alanine aminotransferase (2% to 23%), increased liver enzymes (2% to 22%), increased serum aspartate aminotransferase (2% to 20%), hyperbilirubinemia (≤19%)

Ophthalmic: Visual disturbance (14% to 26%; likely serum concentration dependent [Imhof 2006; Pascual 2008; Tan 2006])

Renal: Increased serum creatinine (adults: ≤21%; children and adolescents: <5%)

Respiratory: Epistaxis (children and adolescents: 16%; adults: <2%)

Miscellaneous: Fever (children and adolescents: 25%; adults: 2%)

1% to 10%:

Cardiovascular: Hypotension (children and adolescents: 9%; adults: <2%), peripheral edema (≤9%), tachycardia (children and adolescents: 7%; adults: 1%), bradycardia (<5%), flushing (children and adolescents: <5%), palpitations (<5%), phlebitis (<5%), supraventricular tachycardia (<5%), syncope (<5%), acute myocardial infarction (adults: <2%), atrial arrhythmia (adults: <2%), atrial fibrillation (adults: <2%), atrioventricular block (adults: <2%), bigeminy (adults: <2%), bundle branch block (adults: <2%), cardiac failure (adults: <2%), cardiomegaly (adults: <2%), cardiomyopathy (adults: <2%), cerebral ischemia (adults: <2%), cerebrovascular accident (adults: <2%), chest pain (adults: <2%), deep vein thrombophlebitis (adults: <2%), edema (adults: <2%), endocarditis (adults: <2%), extrasystoles (adults: <2%), facial edema (adults: <2%), nodal arrhythmia (adults: <2%), orthostatic hypotension (adults: <2%), prolonged bleeding time (adults: <2%), prolonged QT interval on ECG (adults: <2%), pulmonary embolism (adults: <2%), substernal pain (adults: <2%), supraventricular extrasystole (adults: <2%), thrombophlebitis (adults: <2%), torsades de pointes (adults: <2%), vasodilation (adults: <2%), ventricular arrhythmia (adults: <2%), ventricular fibrillation (adults: <2%), ventricular tachycardia (adults: <2%)

Central nervous system: Headache (children and adolescents: 10%; adults: 2%), hallucination (3% to 5%; likely serum concentration dependent [Imhof 2006; Pascual 2008; Tan 2006]), dizziness (≤5%), agitation (<5%), anxiety (<5%), ataxia (<5%), chills (children and adolescents: <5%; adults: <1%), depression (<5%), emotional lability (children and adolescents: <5%), hypothermia (children and adolescents: <5%), insomnia (<5%), lethargy (children and adolescents: <5%), paresthesia (<5%), seizure (<5%), vertigo (<5%), abnormal dreams (adults: <2%), akathisia (adults: <2%), amnesia (adults: <2%), cerebral edema (adults: <2%), cerebral hemorrhage (adults: <2%), coma (adults: <2%), confusion (adults: <2%), delirium (adults: <2%), dementia (adults: <2%), depersonalization (adults: <2%), drowsiness (adults: <2%), encephalitis (adults: <2%), encephalopathy (adults: <2%), euphoria (adults: <2%), extrapyramidal reaction (adults: <2%), flank pain (adults: <2%), Guillain-Barre syndrome (adults: <2%), hypertonia (adults: <2%), hypoesthesia (adults: <2%), intracranial hypertension (adults: <2%), myasthenia (adults: <2%), neuralgia (adults: <2%), neuropathy (adults: <2%), pain (adults: <2%), psychosis (adults: <2%), suicidal ideation (adults: <2%), tonic clonic epilepsy (adults: <2%), voice disorder (adults: <2%)

Dermatologic: Allergic dermatitis (<5%), alopecia (<5%), contact dermatitis (<5%), dermatitis (children and adolescents: <5%), exfoliative dermatitis (<5%), pruritus (<5%), urticaria (<5%), cellulitis (adults: <2%), cheilitis (adults: <2%), diaphoresis (adults: <2%), ecchymoses (adults: <2%), eczema (adults: <2%), erythema multiforme (adults: <2%), furunculosis (adults: <2%), maculopapular rash (adults: <2%), psoriasis (adults: <2%), skin discoloration (adults: <2%), skin photosensitivity (adults: <2%), Stevens-Johnson syndrome (adults: <2%), toxic epidermal necrolysis (adults: <2%), xeroderma (adults: <2%)

Endocrine & metabolic: Hyperglycemia (children and adolescents: 7%; adults: <2%), hypocalcemia (children and adolescents: 6%; adults: <2%), hypophosphatemia (children and adolescents: 6%; adults: <2%), hypoalbuminemia (children and adolescents: 5%), hypomagnesemia (≤5%), hypercalcemia (<5%), hypermagnesemia (<5%), hyperphosphatemia (children and adolescents: <5%), hypoglycemia (<5%), increased gamma-glutamyl transferase (<5%), adrenocortical insufficiency (adults: <2%), albuminuria (adults: <2%), decreased glucose tolerance (adults: <2%), decreased libido (adults: <2%), diabetes insipidus (adults: <2%), glycosuria (adults: <2%), hypercholesterolemia (adults: <2%), hypernatremia (adults: <2%), hyperthyroidism (adults: <2%), hyperuricemia (adults: <2%), hypervolemia (adults: <2%), hyponatremia (adults: <2%), hypothyroidism (adults: <2%), increased lactate dehydrogenase (adults: <2%), pseudoporphyria (adults: <2%)

Gastrointestinal: Oral inflammation (children and adolescents: 6%), abdominal distention (≤5%), constipation (≤5%), abdominal tenderness (children and adolescents: <5%), cholestasis (<5%), dyspepsia (<5%), ageusia (adults: <2%), anorexia (adults: <2%), cholecystitis (adults: <2%), cholelithiasis (adults: <2%), *Clostridioides difficile* colitis (adults: <2%), duodenitis (adults: <2%), dysgeusia (adults: <2%), dysphagia (adults: <2%), esophageal ulcer (adults: <2%), esophagitis (adults: <2%), flatulence (adults: <2%), gastric ulcer (adults: <2%), gastroenteritis (adults: <2%), gastrointestinal hemorrhage (adults: <2%), gingival hemorrhage (adults: <2%), gingival hyperplasia (adults: <2%), gingivitis (adults: <2%), glossitis (adults: <2%), hematemesis (adults: <2%), intestinal perforation (adults: <2%), melanosis (adults: <2%), melena (adults: <2%), mucous membrane disease (adults: <2%), oral mucosa ulcer (adults: <2%), pancreatitis (adults: <2%), parotid gland enlargement (adults: <2%), perforated duodenal ulcer (adults: <2%), peritonitis (adults: <2%), proctitis (adults: <2%), rectal disease (adults: <2%), stomatitis (adults: <2%), ulcerative bowel lesion (adults: <2%), xerostomia (adults: <2%)

Genitourinary: Abnormal uterine bleeding (adults: <2%), anuria (adults: <2%), blighted ovum (adults: <2%), dysmenorrhea (adults: <2%), dysuria (adults: <2%), epididymitis (adults: <2%), hematuria (adults: <2%), hemorrhagic cystitis (adults: <2%), impotence (adults: <2%), nephrosis (adults: <2%), oliguria (adults: <2%), pelvic pain (adults: <2%), scrotal edema (adults: <2%), uremia (adults: <2%), urinary incontinence (adults: <2%), urinary retention (adults: <2%), urinary tract infection (adults: <2%), uterine hemorrhage (adults: <2%), vaginal hemorrhage (adults: <2%)

Hematologic & oncologic: Thrombocytopenia (children and adolescents: 10%; adults: <2%), anemia (<5%), leukopenia (<5%), pancytopenia (<5%), agranulocytosis (adults: <2%), aplastic anemia (adults: <2%), bone marrow depression (adults: <2%), disseminated intravascular coagulation (adults: <2%), eosinophilia (adults: <2%), granuloma (adults: <2%), hemolytic anemia (adults: <2%), lymphadenopathy (adults: <2%), lymphangitis (adults: <2%), macrocytic anemia (adults: <2%), malignant melanoma (adults: <2%), megaloblastic anemia (adults: <2%), microcytic anemia (adults: <2%), petechia (adults: <2%), purpuric disease (adults: <2%), rectal hemorrhage (adults: <2%), splenomegaly (adults: <2%), squamous cell carcinoma (adults: <2%), thrombotic thrombocytopenic purpura (adults: <2%)

Hepatic: Abnormal hepatic function tests (3% to 6%), jaundice (<5%), cholestatic jaundice (adults: 2%), ascites (adults: <2%), hepatic coma (adults: <2%), hepatic failure (adults: <2%), hepatitis (adults: <2%), hepatomegaly (adults: <2%)

Hypersensitivity: Hypersensitivity reaction (<5%), angioedema (adults: <2%), fixed drug eruption (adults: <2%), nonimmune anaphylaxis (adults: <2%), tongue edema (adults: <2%)

Immunologic: Graft versus host disease (adults: <2%)

Infection: Bacterial infection (adults: <2%), fungal infection (adults: <2%), herpes simplex infection (adults: <2%), infection (adults: <2%), sepsis (adults: <2%)

Local: Catheter pain (children and adolescents: <5%), injection site infection (adults: <2%), inflammation at injection site (adults: <2%), pain at injection site (adults: <2%)

Neuromuscular & skeletal: Arthralgia (<5%), asthenia (<5%), myalgia (<5%), arthritis (adults: <2%), back pain (adults: <2%), discoid lupus erythematosus (adults: <2%), increased creatine phosphokinase blood specimen (adults: <2%), lower limb cramp (adults: <2%), myopathy (adults: <2%), ostealgia (adults: <2%), osteomalacia (adults: <2%), osteonecrosis (adults: <2%), osteoporosis (adults: <2%), tremor (adults: <2%)

Ophthalmic: Photophobia (2% to 6%), conjunctivitis (<5%), dry eye syndrome (<5%), keratitis (<5%), nystagmus disorder (<5%), accommodation disturbance (adults: <2%), blepharitis (adults: <2%), color blindness (adults: <2%), corneal opacity (adults: <2%), diplopia (adults: <2%), eye pain (adults: <2%), keratoconjunctivitis (adults: <2%), mydriasis (adults: <2%), night blindness (adults: <2%), oculogyric crisis (adults: <2%), optic atrophy (adults: <2%), optic neuritis (adults: <2%), papilledema (adults: <2%), retinal hemorrhage (adults: <2%), retinitis (adults: <2%), scleritis (adults: <2%), subconjunctival hemorrhage (adults: <2%), uveitis (adults: <2%), visual field defect (adults: <2%), chromatopsia (adults: ≤1%)

Otic: Tinnitus (<5%), deafness (adults: <2%), otalgia (adults: <2%), otitis externa (adults: <2%), hypoacusis (adults: <2%)

Renal: Renal insufficiency (children and adolescents: 5%; adults: ≤1%), decreased serum creatinine (adults: <2%), hydronephrosis (adults: <2%), increased blood urea nitrogen (adults: <2%), nephritis (adults: <2%), renal pain (adults: <2%), renal tubular necrosis (adults: <2%)

Respiratory: Cough (children and adolescents: 10%; adults: <2%), dyspnea (children and adolescents: 6%; adults: <2%), upper respiratory tract infection (children and adolescents: 5%), hemoptysis (≤5%), bronchospasm (children and adolescents: <5%), nasal congestion (children and adolescents: <5%), respiratory failure (children and adolescents: <5%), tachypnea (children and adolescents: <5%), cyanosis (adults: <2%), flu-like symptoms (adults: <2%), hypoxia (adults: <2%), pharyngitis (adults: <2%), pleural effusion (adults: <2%), pneumonia (adults: <2%), pulmonary edema (adults: <2%), respiratory distress syndrome (adults: <2%), respiratory system disorder (adults: <2%), respiratory tract infection (adults: <2%), rhinitis (adults: <2%), sinusitis (adults: <2%)

Miscellaneous: Multiorgan failure (adults: <2%)

Frequency not defined:

Dermatologic: Cutaneous lupus erythematosus

Hepatic: Fulminant hepatitis

Ophthalmic: Vision color changes

<1%, postmarketing, and/or case reports: Acute renal failure, changes in nails (Malani 2014), periosteal disease (Cormican 2018; Hussain 2018), phototoxicity (Kim 2018), skeletal fluorosis (Cormican 2018; Hussain 2018)

Mechanism of Action Interferes with fungal cytochrome P450 activity (selectively inhibits 14-alpha-lanosterol demethylation), decreasing ergosterol synthesis (principal sterol in fungal cell membrane) and inhibiting fungal cell membrane formation.

Pharmacodynamics/Kinetics

Half-life Elimination Variable, dose-dependent. Steady-state is achieved by day 3 when an IV loading dose is administered and between days 5 and 8 if no loading dose is used (Purkins 2003).

Time to Peak Oral:

Children 2 to <12 years: Median: 1.1 hours (range: 0.73 to 8.03 hours) (Driscoll 2011)

Adults: 1 to 2 hours

Reproductive Considerations

Women of childbearing potential should use effective contraception during treatment.

Pregnancy Considerations

Adverse events were observed in animal reproduction studies. Voriconazole can cause fetal harm when administered to a pregnant woman.

Dental Health Professional Considerations See Local Anesthetic/Vasoconstrictor Precautions

Vorinostat (vor IN oh stat)

Brand Names: US Zolinza

Brand Names: Canada Zolinza

Pharmacologic Category Antineoplastic Agent, Histone Deacetylase (HDAC) Inhibitor

Use Cutaneous T-cell lymphoma: Treatment of cutaneous manifestations of cutaneous T-cell lymphoma (CTCL) in patients with progressive, persistent, or recurrent disease on or following two systemic treatments.

Local Anesthetic/Vasoconstrictor Precautions

Vorinostat is one of the drugs confirmed to prolong the QT interval and is accepted as having a risk of causing torsade de pointes. The risk of drug-induced torsade de pointes is extremely low when a single QT interval prolonging drug is prescribed. In terms of epinephrine, it is not known what effect vasoconstrictors in the local anesthetic regimen will have in patients with a known history of congenital prolonged QT interval or in patients taking any medication that prolongs the QT interval. Until more information is obtained, it is suggested that the clinician consult with the physician prior to the use of a vasoconstrictor in suspected patients, and that the vasoconstrictor (epinephrine, mepivacaine and levonordefrin [Carbocaine® 2% with Neo-Cobefrin®]) be used with caution.

Effects on Dental Treatment Key adverse event(s) related to dental treatment: High incidence of xerostomia (normal salivary flow resumes upon discontinuation) and taste perversion (see Dental Health Professional Considerations)

Effects on Bleeding Chemotherapy may result in significant myelosuppression, potentially including significant reduction in platelet counts (thrombocytopenia grades 3/4: 6%) and altered hemostasis. In patients who are under active treatment with these agents, medical consult is suggested.

Adverse Reactions

>10%:

Cardiovascular: Peripheral edema (13%)

Central nervous system: Fatigue (52%), chills (16%), dizziness (15%), headache (12%)

Dermatologic: Alopecia (19%), pruritus (12%)

Endocrine & metabolic: Hyperglycemia (8% to 69%; grade 3: 5%), weight loss (21%), dehydration (1% to 16%)

Gastrointestinal: Diarrhea (52%), nausea (41%), dysgeusia (28%), anorexia (24%), xerostomia (16%), constipation (15%), vomiting (15%), decreased appetite (14%)

Genitourinary: Proteinuria (51%)

Hematologic & oncologic: Thrombocytopenia (26%; grades 3/4: 6%), anemia (14%; grades 3/4: 2%)

Neuromuscular & skeletal: Muscle spasm (20%)

Renal: Increased serum creatinine (16% to 47%)

Respiratory: Cough (11%), upper respiratory tract infection (11%)

Miscellaneous: Fever (11%)

1% to 10%:

Cardiovascular: Pulmonary embolism (5%), prolonged QT interval on ECG (3% to 4%)

Hematologic & oncologic: Squamous cell carcinoma of skin (4%)

<1%, postmarketing, and/or case reports: Abdominal pain, acute ischemic stroke, angioedema, bacteremia (streptococcal), blurred vision, chest pain, cholecystitis, deafness, deep vein thrombosis, diverticulitis, dysphagia, exfoliative dermatitis, gastrointestinal hemorrhage, Guillain-Barre syndrome, hemoptysis, hypertension, hypokalemia, hyponatremia, infection, infection due to enterococcus, lethargy, leukopenia, myocardial infarction, neutropenia, pneumonia, renal failure, sepsis, spinal cord injury, syncope, T-cell lymphoma, tumor hemorrhage, ureteral obstruction, obstructive uropathy (ureteropelvic junction), urinary retention, vasculitis, weakness

Mechanism of Action Vorinostat inhibits histone deacetylase enzymes, HDAC1, HDAC2, HDAC3, and HDAC6, which catalyze acetyl group removal from protein lysine residues (including histones and transcription factors). Histone deacetylase inhibition results in accumulation of acetyl groups, which alters chromatin structure and transcription factor activation; cell growth is terminated and apoptosis occurs.

Pharmacodynamics/Kinetics

Half-life Elimination ~2 hours

Time to Peak Plasma: With high-fat meal: 4 hours (range: 2 to 10 hours)

Reproductive Considerations

Evaluate pregnancy status prior to treatment. Pregnancy testing should be conducted within 7 days prior to treatment in females of reproductive potential. Females of reproductive potential should avoid pregnancy and use an effective contraceptive during therapy and for at least 6 months after the last vorinostat dose. Males with female partners of reproductive potential should use effective contraception during therapy and for at least 3 months after the last vorinostat dose.

Pregnancy Considerations

Based on the mechanism of action and data from animal reproduction studies, vorinostat may cause fetal harm if administered during pregnancy. Inform patient of potential hazard if used during pregnancy or if pregnancy occurs during treatment.

Dental Health Professional Considerations This drug is known to prolong the QT interval (see Local Anesthetic/Vasoconstrictor Precautions)

Vortioxetine (vor tye OX e teen)

Brand Names: US Trintellix

Brand Names: Canada Trintellix

Pharmacologic Category Antidepressant, Selective Serotonin Reuptake Inhibitor; Serotonin 5-HT_{1A} Receptor Agonist; Serotonin 5-HT_3 Receptor Antagonist

Use Major depressive disorder: Treatment of major depressive disorder (MDD).

Local Anesthetic/Vasoconstrictor Precautions Although caution should be used in patients taking tricyclic antidepressants, no interactions have been reported with vasoconstrictors and vortioxetine, a nontricyclic antidepressant which acts to increase serotonin; no precautions appear to be needed.

Effects on Dental Treatment Key adverse event(s) related to dental treatment: Xerostomia (normal salivary flow resumes upon discontinuation) (see Dental Health Professional Considerations)

Effects on Bleeding Bleeding risk: SSRIs have been reported to impair platelet aggregation resulting in increased risk of bleeding events, particularly if used concomitantly with aspirin, NSAIDs, warfarin, or other anticoagulants. Bleeding related to antidepressant use has been reported to range from relatively minor bruising and epistaxis to life-threatening hemorrhage.

Adverse Reactions

>10%:

Central nervous system: Female sexual disorder (1% to 2%; Arizona Sexual Experiences Scale: 22% to 34%), male sexual disorder (3% to 5%; Arizona Sexual Experiences Scale: 16% to 29%)

Gastrointestinal: Nausea (21% to 32%)

1% to 10%:

Central nervous system: Dizziness (8% to 9%), abnormal dreams (2% to 3%)

Dermatologic: Pruritus (2% to 3%)

Gastrointestinal: Diarrhea (7% to 10%), xerostomia (7% to 8%), constipation (5% to 6%), vomiting (3% to 6%), flatulence (2% to 3%)

Frequency not defined:

Cardiovascular: Flushing

Central nervous system: Suicidal ideation, suicidal tendencies, vertigo

Gastrointestinal: Dysgeusia, dyspepsia

<1%, postmarketing, and/or case reports: Acute pancreatitis, anaphylaxis, angle-closure glaucoma, hypersensitivity reaction, hypomania, hyponatremia, mania, seizure, serotonin syndrome, skin rash, urticaria, weight gain, withdrawal syndrome

Mechanism of Action Inhibits reuptake of serotonin (5-HT); also has agonist activity at the 5-HT_{1A} receptor and antagonist activity at the 5-HT_3 receptor.

Pharmacodynamics/Kinetics

Onset of Action Depression: Initial effects may be observed within 1 to 2 weeks of treatment, with continued improvements through 4 to 6 weeks (Papakostas 2006; Posternak 2005; Szegedi 2009; Taylor 2006).

Half-life Elimination ~66 hours

Time to Peak 7 to 11 hours

Pregnancy Considerations Nonteratogenic effects in the newborn following SSRI/SNRI exposure late in the third trimester include respiratory distress, cyanosis, apnea, seizures, temperature instability, feeding difficulty, vomiting, hypoglycemia, hypo- or hypertonia, hyper-reflexia, jitteriness, irritability, constant crying, and tremor. Symptoms may be due to the toxicity of the SSRIs/SNRIs or a discontinuation syndrome and may be consistent with serotonin syndrome associated with SSRI treatment. Persistent pulmonary hypertension of the newborn (PPHN) has also been reported with SSRI exposure.

The ACOG recommends that therapy with SSRIs or SNRIs during pregnancy be individualized; treatment of depression during pregnancy should incorporate the clinical expertise of the mental health clinician, obstetrician, primary health care provider, and pediatrician (ACOG 2008). According to the American Psychiatric Association (APA), the risks of medication treatment should be weighed against other treatment options and untreated depression. For women who discontinue antidepressant medications during pregnancy and who may be at high risk for postpartum depression, the medications can be restarted following delivery (APA 2010). Treatment algorithms have been developed by the ACOG and the APA for the management of depression in women prior to conception and during pregnancy (Yonkers 2009).

Pregnant women exposed to antidepressants during pregnancy are encouraged to enroll in the National Pregnancy Registry for Antidepressants (NPRAD). Women 18 to 45 years of age or their health care providers may contact the registry by calling 844-405-6185. Enrollment should be done as early in pregnancy as possible.

Dental Health Professional Considerations Problems with SSRI-induced bruxism have been reported and may preclude their use; clinicians attempting to evaluate any patient with bruxism or involuntary muscle movement, who is simultaneously being treated with an SSRI drug, should be aware of the potential association.

◆ **Vortioxetine Hydrobromide** *see* Vortioxetine *on page 1555*

◆ **Vosevi** *see* Sofosbuvir, Velpatasvir, and Voxilaprevir *on page 1380*

◆ **VoSpire ER [DSC]** *see* Albuterol *on page 90*

◆ **Votrient** *see* PAZOPanib *on page 1196*

Voxelotor (vox EL oh tor)

Brand Names: US Oxbryta

Pharmacologic Category Hemoglobin S (HbS) Polymerization Inhibitor

Use Sickle cell disease: Treatment of sickle cell disease in adults and pediatric patients ≥12 years of age.

Local Anesthetic/Vasoconstrictor Precautions No information available to require special precautions.

Effects on Dental Treatment No significant effects or complications reported.

Effects on Bleeding No information available to require special precautions.

Adverse Reactions

>10%:

Central nervous system: Headache (26%), fatigue (14%)

Dermatologic: Skin rash (14%)

Gastrointestinal: Diarrhea (20%), abdominal pain (19%), nausea (17%)

Miscellaneous: Fever (12%)

1% to 10%:

Cardiovascular: Pulmonary embolism (1%)

Hypersensitivity: Hypersensitivity reaction (<10%)

<1%: Severe hypersensitivity reaction

Mechanism of Action Voxelotor is an HbS polymerization inhibitor that reversibly binds to Hb and stabilizes the oxygenated Hb state. Through the increased Hb affinity for oxygen, voxelotor demonstrates dose-dependent inhibition of HbS polymerization, and may inhibit RBC sickling, improve RBC deformability, and reduce whole blood viscosity. Voxelotor may also extend RBC half-life and reduce anemia and hemolysis (Vichinsky 2019).

Pharmacodynamics/Kinetics

Half-life Elimination 35.5 hours.

Time to Peak Median: 2 hours.

Pregnancy Considerations

Adverse events were not observed in animal reproduction studies.

Sickle cell disease increases the risk of adverse maternal and fetal outcomes, including an increased risk for vaso-occlusive crises, preeclampsia, eclampsia, intrauterine growth restriction, preterm delivery, low birth weight, and maternal and perinatal mortality.

◆ **Voxilaprevir, Velpatasvir, and Sofosbuvir** *see* Sofosbuvir, Velpatasvir, and Voxilaprevir *on page 1380*

◆ **VP-16** *see* Etoposide *on page 626*

◆ **VP-16-213** *see* Etoposide *on page 626*

◆ **Vraylar** *see* Cariprazine *on page 293*

◆ **VSL #3 [OTC]** *see Lactobacillus on page 869*

◆ **VSL #3-DS** *see Lactobacillus on page 869*

◆ **VSLI** *see* VinCRIStine (Liposomal) *on page 1546*

◆ **Vumerity** *see* Diroximel Fumarate *on page 504*

◆ **VWF/FVIII Concentrate** *see* Antihemophilic Factor/von Willebrand Factor Complex (Human) *on page 154*

◆ **VWF:RCo** *see* Antihemophilic Factor/von Willebrand Factor Complex (Human) *on page 154*

◆ **vWF:RCof** *see* Antihemophilic Factor/von Willebrand Factor Complex (Human) *on page 154*

◆ **Vyepti** *see* Eptinezumab *on page 580*

◆ **Vyfemla** *see* Ethinyl Estradiol and Norethindrone *on page 614*

◆ **VyLibra** *see* Ethinyl Estradiol and Norgestimate *on page 616*

◆ **Vyondys 53** *see* Golodirsen *on page 745*

◆ **Vytone** *see* Iodoquinol and Hydrocortisone *on page 836*

◆ **Vytorin** *see* Ezetimibe and Simvastatin *on page 634*

◆ **Vyvanse** *see* Lisdexamfetamine *on page 921*

◆ **Vyxeos** *see* Daunorubicin and Cytarabine (Liposomal) *on page 445*

◆ **Vyzulta** *see* Latanoprostene Bunod *on page 881*

◆ **VZIG** *see* Varicella-Zoster Immune Globulin (Human) *on page 1535*

◆ **VZV Vaccine (Varicella)** *see* Measles, Mumps, Rubella, and Varicella Virus Vaccine *on page 950*

◆ **VZV Vaccine (Zoster)** *see* Zoster Vaccine (Live/Attenuated) *on page 1585*

◆ **Wakix** *see* Pitolisant *on page 1239*

Warfarin (WAR far in)

Related Information

Antiplatelet and Anticoagulation Considerations in Dentistry *on page 1666*

Cardiovascular Diseases *on page 1654*

Brand Names: US Coumadin [DSC]; Jantoven

Brand Names: Canada APO-Warfarin; Coumadin; MYLAN-Warfarin [DSC]; TARO-Warfarin

Generic Availability (US) Yes

Pharmacologic Category Anticoagulant; Anticoagulant, Vitamin K Antagonist

Use

Myocardial infarction: Adjunct to reduce risk of systemic embolism (eg, recurrent myocardial infarction, stroke) after myocardial infarction.

Thromboembolic complications: Prophylaxis and treatment of thromboembolic disorders (eg, venous, pulmonary) and embolic complications arising from atrial fibrillation or cardiac valve replacement.

Limitations of use: Warfarin has no direct effect on an established thrombus and does not reverse ischemic tissue damage. The goal of anticoagulant therapy is to prevent further extension of an already formed thrombus and to prevent secondary thromboembolic complications that may result in serious and potentially fatal sequelae.

Local Anesthetic/Vasoconstrictor Precautions
No information available to require special precautions

Effects on Dental Treatment Key adverse event(s) related to dental treatment: Increased risk of bleeding, mouth ulcers, and taste disturbance.

Signs of warfarin overdose may first appear as bleeding from gingival tissue (see Effects on Bleeding and Dental Health Professional Considerations)

For stroke patients undergoing dental procedures (see Effects on Bleeding and Dental Health Professional Considerations)

Effects on Bleeding As with all anticoagulants, bleeding is a potential adverse effect of warfarin during dental surgery; risk is dependent on multiple variables, including the intensity of anticoagulation and patient susceptibility. Consultation with prescribing physician is advisable prior to surgery to determine if temporary dose reduction or withdrawal of medication is indicated. Stroke patients maintained on warfarin should continue therapy during dental procedures as warfarin is unlikely to increase bleeding risk (Armstrong 2013)

Tooth extraction: A recent study assessed the amount of bleeding during a single tooth extraction in patients who remained on warfarin during the procedure versus those who discontinued warfarin (Karsli 2011). All patients had coronary artery disease. There was no significant difference in bleeding with or without warfarin. The mean blood loss was 2486 ± 1408 g in the warfarin group, compared to 1736 ± 876 g in the patients who stopped warfarin. The mean INR value in the warfarin group was 2.6 ± 0.7. Hemostasis was successfully established locally by packing the extraction sockets with oxidized cellulose (Surgicel) and suturing with 3-0 silk sutures.

Concurrent antibiotic use: A retrospective study evaluating over 38,000 patients ≥65 years of age showed exposure to any antibiotic agent was associated with at least a 2-fold increased risk of bleeding that required hospitalization among continuous warfarin users (Baillargeon 2012). All five antibiotic drug classes examined (macrolides, quinolones, cotrimoxazole, penicillins, and cephalosporins) were associated with an increased risk of bleeding. Exposure to an azole antifungal (fluconazole, ketoconazole, or miconazole) while on warfarin was associated with a 4-fold increased risk of bleeding.

Adverse Reactions Bleeding is the major adverse effect of warfarin. Hemorrhage may occur at virtually any site. Risk is dependent on multiple variables, including the intensity of anticoagulation and patient susceptibility.

1% to 10%:

Hematologic & oncologic: Major hemorrhage (≤5%; INR 2.5 to 4.0 generally associated with more bleeding)

Frequency not defined:

Cardiovascular: Purple-toe syndrome, systemic cholesterol micro-embolism, vasculitis

Central nervous system: Chills

Dermatologic: Alopecia, bullous rash, dermatitis, pruritus, skin necrosis, urticaria

Gastrointestinal: Abdominal pain, bloating, diarrhea, dysgeusia, flatulence, nausea, vomiting

Hematologic & oncologic: Minor hemorrhage

Hepatic: Hepatitis

Hypersensitivity: Anaphylaxis, hypersensitivity reaction

Renal: Acute renal failure (in patients with altered glomerular integrity or with a history of kidney disease)

Respiratory: Tracheobronchial calcification

<1%, postmarketing, and/or case reports: Gangrene of skin or other tissue, skin necrosis, vascular calcification (calcium uremic arteriolopathy and calciphylaxis)

Dosing

Adult

The adult dosing recommendations are based upon the best available evidence and clinical expertise. Senior Editor: Edith A Nutescu, PharmD, MS, FCCP.

Note: Dosing must be individualized and use of an institutional protocol is recommended (ACCP [Holbrook 2012]; Nutescu 2013). Response to warfarin is influenced by numerous factors (eg, age, organ function) as described below. Genetic variations in metabolism (eg, CYP2C9 and/or VKORC1 genes) can impact warfarin sensitivity; however, routine genetic testing is not recommended (ACCP [Holbrook 2012]; CPIC [Johnson 2017]).

Oral:

Initial: 5 mg once daily for most patients. A lower or higher starting dose may be used depending upon patient-specific factors (see example warfarin initiation nomogram below). Although an elevation in INR can be seen as soon as 24 to 48 hours after the first dose due to depletion of factor VII, this does not represent therapeutic anticoagulation because other vitamin K–dependent clotting factors with longer half-lives (eg, factors II, IX, and X) must also be depleted. Accordingly, in patients at high risk for thromboembolism, overlap ("bridging") with a parenteral anticoagulant may be necessary during initiation of warfarin until a stable therapeutic INR is attained (Wittkowsky 2018).

Example Warfarin Initiation Nomogram Targeting an INR Range of 2 to 3 (for Outpatients or Clinically Stable Inpatients) (Adapted From Wittkowsky 2018)[a]

	Standard dosing for patients who are *not* expected to be sensitive to warfarin[b]	Reduced dosing for patients expected to be more sensitive to warfarin[c]
Initial dose	5 mg daily for 3 days[d]	2.5 mg daily for 3 days
Check INR the morning of day 4		
<1.5	7.5 to 10 mg daily for 2 to 3 days	5 to 7.5 mg daily for 2 to 3 days
1.5 to 1.9	5 mg daily for 2 to 3 days	2.5 mg daily for 2 to 3 days
2 to 3	2.5 mg daily for 2 to 3 days	1.25 mg daily for 2 to 3 days
3.1 to 4	1.25 mg daily for 2 to 3 days	0.5 mg daily for 2 to 3 days
>4	Hold until INR <3	Hold until INR <3

[a]Dosing nomograms offer a reasonable starting point for estimating an initial warfarin dose and subsequent adjustments but should not serve as a substitute for clinical judgment. If the patient received warfarin previously, history of prior dose requirement is useful for guiding reinitiation of therapy.

[b]Patients who are generally started using "standard dosing" include otherwise healthy adults who are not receiving interacting medications.

[c]Patients expected to be more sensitive to warfarin include adults who are frail, elderly, or undernourished; have liver disease, kidney disease, heart failure, or acute illness; or are receiving a medication known to decrease warfarin metabolism.

[d]Some experts suggest starting select younger, otherwise healthy patients at 7.5 or 10 mg for the first 2 days (ACCP [Holbrook 2012]). A higher initial dose may also be appropriate in a patient who was previously treated with warfarin and required high doses or is receiving a medication that increases warfarin metabolism. However, this nomogram has not been validated for starting doses >5 mg/day.

Maintenance: Usual maintenance dose: 2 to 10 mg once daily. Once INR is therapeutic and stable following initiation, subsequent dosage requirements may be guided with the use of a maintenance dosing nomogram (see example warfarin maintenance dosing nomogram below). INR should be checked at least weekly when it is out of range and approximately every 4 weeks once therapeutic and stable. In chronic therapy, INR values are most affected by the doses administered 2 to 3 days prior to INR measurement.

Example Warfarin Maintenance Dosing Nomogram[a] (Adapted From Hadlock 2018)

Regular-intensity anticoagulation: INR goal 2 to 3	High-intensity anticoagulation: INR goal 2.5 to 3.5	Suggested adjustment(s) to warfarin dose
Adjustment(s) for subtherapeutic (low) INR – Note: If the factor causing subtherapeutic INR is transient (eg, missed warfarin dose or temporary change in vitamin K intake), consider resumption of prior maintenance dose following a one-time supplemental dose, if indicated.		
INR <1.5	INR <2	• Increase weekly maintenance dose by 10% to 20%[b] • Consider a one-time supplemental dose of 1.5 to 2 times the daily maintenance dose[b]
INR 1.5 to 1.7	INR 2 to 2.2	• Increase weekly maintenance dose by 5% to 15% • Consider a one-time supplemental dose of 1.5 to 2 times the daily maintenance dose
INR 1.8 to 1.9	INR 2.3 to 2.4	• No dosage adjustment may be necessary if the last 2 INRs were in range, if there is no clear explanation for the INR to be out of range, and, if in the judgment of the clinician, the INR does not represent an increased risk of thromboembolism for the patient; additional monitoring may be warranted • If dosage adjustment needed, increase weekly maintenance dose by 5% to 10% • Consider a one-time supplemental dose of 1.5 to 2 times the daily maintenance dose
INR within therapeutic range		
INR 2 to 3	INR 2.5 to 3.5	Desired range; no adjustment needed
Adjustment(s) for supratherapeutic (high) INR – Note: If the factor causing elevated INR is transient (eg, temporary change in vitamin K intake, acute illness, acute alcohol ingestion), consider resumption of prior maintenance dose following dose(s) held and low-dose oral vitamin K, if indicated.		
INR 3.1 to 3.2	INR 3.6 to 3.7	• No dosage adjustment may be necessary if the last 2 INRs were in range, if there is no clear explanation for the INR to be out of range, and, if in the judgment of the clinician, the INR does not represent an increased risk of hemorrhage to patient; additional monitoring may be warranted • If dosage adjustment needed, decrease weekly maintenance dose by 5% to 10%
INR 3.3 to 3.4	INR 3.8 to 3.9	• Decrease weekly maintenance dose by 5% to 10%
INR 3.5 to 3.9	INR 4 to 4.4	• Consider holding 1 dose • Decrease weekly maintenance dose by 5% to 15%

(continued)

Example Warfarin Maintenance Dosing Nomogram[a] (Adapted From Hadlock 2018) *(continued)*

INR ≥4 but ≤10 and no bleeding	INR ≥4.5 but ≤10 and no bleeding	• Hold until INR below upper limit of therapeutic range • Decrease weekly maintenance dose by 5% to 20% • If patient considered to be at significant risk for bleeding, consider low-dose oral vitamin K
INR >10 and no bleeding	INR >10 and no bleeding	• Hold until INR below upper limit of therapeutic range • Administer vitamin K orally • Decrease weekly maintenance dose by 5% to 20%

[a]As with initiation therapy nomograms, maintenance therapy nomograms must be used in conjunction with clinical judgment.
[b]As an example, a patient with an INR goal of 2 to 3 and receiving 30 mg of warfarin per week (eg, administered as 5 mg on 5 days and 2.5 mg on 2 days) has an INR result of 1.4. The weekly dose should be increased by 10% to 20% (eg, increase to 35 mg per week by administering 5 mg once daily). A one-time supplemental dose of 7.5 mg may be considered on the day INR was checked, then start new maintenance dose (eg, 5 mg daily) the following day.

Adult Target INR Ranges Based Upon Indication

Indication	Targeted INR range	Treatment duration
Cardiac		
Myocardial infarction with left ventricular thrombus or high risk for left ventricular thrombus (eg, ejection fraction <40% and severe anteroapical wall motion abnormality on imaging 48 hours after reperfusion) (ACCF/AHA [O'Gara 2013]; ACCP [Vandvik 2012]). **Note:** Antiplatelet selection and duration of therapy for treatment of myocardial infarction may vary when used in combination with anticoagulation; consider risks of bleeding and thrombotic events when choosing antithrombotic therapy (ACCP [Vandvik 2012]; Lip 2019).	2 to 3	3 months after myocardial infarction
Atrial fibrillation or atrial flutter (AHA/ACC/HRS [January 2014, January 2019]). **Note:** For eligible patients with *nonvalvular* atrial fibrillation, a direct oral anticoagulant is recommended over warfarin (AHA/ACC/HRS [January 2014, January 2019]).	2 to 3	Indefinite
Stress (takotsubo) cardiomyopathy with acute left ventricular thrombus (ACCP [Vandvik 2012])	2 to 3	3 months
Valvular – Note: For mechanical valves, aspirin in combination with warfarin is recommended indefinitely. For surgically placed bioprosthetic valves, aspirin therapy is recommended indefinitely and concurrent warfarin is suggested for the first 3 to 6 months. When choosing antithrombotic therapy, additional risk factors for thromboembolism (eg, atrial fibrillation, previous thromboembolism, left ventricular systolic dysfunction, hypercoagulable conditions) should be considered. The goal INR is generally the central value in the indicated acceptable range, especially for patients with a mechanical valve (AHA/ACC [Nishimura 2014, Nishimura 2017]).		
On-X mechanical bileaflet aortic valve with no additional risk factors for thromboembolism (AHA/ACC [Nishimura 2017]; Puskas 2014)	Months 1 to 3: 2 to 3 Month 4 and after: 1.5 to 2	Indefinite
Mechanical bileaflet aortic valve (other than On-X) or current-generation single-tilting disc aortic valve with no additional risk factors for thromboembolism (AHA/ACC [Nishimura 2014, Nishimura 2017])	2 to 3	Indefinite

Adult Target INR Ranges Based Upon Indication *(continued)*

Indication	Targeted INR range	Treatment duration
Mechanical aortic valve with additional risk factors for thromboembolism or an older-generation mechanical aortic valve or mechanical mitral valve (including On-X valve) (AHA/ACC [Nishimura 2014, Nishimura 2017])	2.5 to 3.5	Indefinite
Surgically placed bioprosthetic aortic or mitral valve at low risk of bleeding (AHA/ACC [Nishimura 2014, Nishimura 2017])	2 to 3	3 to 6 months
Rheumatic mitral stenosis with atrial fibrillation, previous systemic embolism, or left atrial thrombus (AHA/ACC [Nishimura 2014])	2 to 3	Indefinite
Acute venous thromboembolism treatment – Note: For eligible patients, a direct oral anticoagulant is recommended over warfarin. When warfarin is selected for long-term treatment, a parenteral anticoagulant must be used initially as a bridge until INR measurements are therapeutic and stable. Start warfarin on the first or second day of parenteral anticoagulation and overlap until INR is ≥2 for at least 2 days. Duration of overlap is usually 4 to 5 days (ACCP [Ageno 2012]). The optimal duration of warfarin therapy is dependent on several factors, such as presence of provoking events, patient risk factors for recurrence or bleeding, and patient preferences. If indefinite treatment is suggested, reassess need for anticoagulation at periodic intervals (ACCP [Kearon 2012, Kearon 2016]).		
Venous thromboembolism, provoked (ACCP [Kearon 2012, Kearon 2016])	2 to 3	Minimum of 3 months
Venous thromboembolism, unprovoked (ACCP [Kearon 2012, Kearon 2016]; ISTH [Baglin 2012])	2 to 3	Minimum of 3 months and up to indefinite
Thromboprophylaxis		
Idiopathic or inherited pulmonary artery hypertension (ACCF/AHA [McLaughlin 2009]; ACCP [Klinger 2019]; ESC/ERS [Galiè 2016]; Olsson 2014) – **Note:** Anticoagulation should be considered on an individual basis for patients with idiopathic or inherited pulmonary arterial hypertension after considering risks and benefits. Avoid anticoagulation in patients with scleroderma-associated pulmonary arterial hypertension (Hopkins 2019; Khan 2018; Olsson 2014).	1.5 to 2.5	Indefinite
Chronic thromboembolic pulmonary arterial hypertension (ACCF/AHA [McLaughlin 2009]; ESC/ERS [Galiè 2016])	2 to 3	Indefinite
Antiphospholipid syndrome (ACCP [Holbrook 2012]; Erkan 2019) – **Note:** Antiphospholipid syndrome is an autoimmune syndrome characterized by venous or arterial thrombosis and/or pregnancy loss in the presence of persistent antiphospholipid antibodies. Patients with antiphospholipid antibodies alone, without a history of thromboembolism, should **not** receive anticoagulation unless another indication exists. The PT/INR may be prolonged at baseline, in the absence of anticoagulation, in a small percentage of patients due to the presence of antiphospholipid antibodies. This should **not** be considered a therapeutic effect. An alternative method for monitoring warfarin may be necessary (Erkan 2019).	2 to 3	Indefinite

(continued)

Adult Target INR Ranges Based Upon Indication *(continued)*

Indication	Targeted INR range	Treatment duration
***Total hip arthroplasty or hip fracture surgery* – Note:** May be used as an alternative to low-molecular-weight heparin or low-dose SubQ heparin (ACCP [Falck-Ytter 2012]).	2 to 3	Minimum of 10 to 14 days and up to 35 days
***Total knee arthroplasty* – Note:** May be used as an alternative to low-molecular-weight heparin or low-dose SubQ heparin (ACCP [Falck-Ytter 2012]).	2 to 3	Typically, 10 to 14 days, but consider up to 35 days if there are multiple or persistent risk factors
Heparin-induced thrombocytopenia – Note: If a patient is taking warfarin at the time of diagnosis, it should be discontinued, and vitamin K should be administered to reverse its effect. Initial therapy should be with a parenteral nonheparin anticoagulant. Warfarin may be initiated after the patient has been stably anticoagulated with a parenteral nonheparin anticoagulant and the platelet count has recovered (eg, ≥150 × 10^9/L or at the patient's baseline). Starting dose should be ≤5 mg once daily. Overlap the parenteral nonheparin anticoagulant with warfarin for ≥5 days and until INR is therapeutic. Some nonheparin anticoagulants may elevate INR, complicating interpretation. Recheck INR after effects of the nonheparin anticoagulant have worn off to ensure INR remains therapeutic (ACCP [Linkins 2012]; ASH [Cuker 2018]).		
Heparin-induced thrombocytopenia **without** thrombosis (ACCP [Linkins 2012]; ASH [Cuker 2018])	2 to 3	4 weeks to 3 months (ACCP [Linkins 2012]). Some experts allow for discontinuation of anticoagulation after platelet count recovery, potentially resulting in a shorter duration (ASH [Cuker 2018]).
Heparin-induced thrombocytopenia **with** thrombosis (ACCP [Linkins 2012]; ASH [Cuker 2018])	2 to 3	Optimal duration not well established. Typically, 3 to 6 months (ACCP [Linkins 2012]; ASH [Cuker 2018]).

Transitioning between anticoagulants:

Transitioning from another anticoagulant to warfarin: Note: Apixaban, dabigatran, edoxaban, and rivaroxaban can elevate INR, complicating interpretation if overlapped with warfarin. To minimize interference, check INR near end of direct oral anticoagulant dosing interval.

Transitioning from apixaban to warfarin: Some experts suggest overlapping apixaban with warfarin for ≥2 days until INR is therapeutic. An alternative is to stop apixaban, start warfarin the same day, and bridge with a parenteral anticoagulant until the desired INR is reached (Leung 2019).

Transitioning from dabigatran to warfarin: One option is to stop dabigatran, start warfarin the same day, and bridge with a parenteral anticoagulant until the desired INR is reached (Leung 2019). An alternative option is to overlap the 2 agents. If this is done, the timing of warfarin initiation is based on CrCl as outlined below:

CrCl >50 mL/minute: Initiate warfarin 3 days before discontinuing dabigatran.

CrCl 30 to 50 mL/minute: Initiate warfarin 2 days before discontinuing dabigatran.

CrCl 15 to 30 mL/minute: Initiate warfarin 1 day before discontinuing dabigatran.

CrCl <15 mL/minute: Dosing recommendations cannot be provided. Dabigatran is not recommended for use in patients with severe renal impairment.

Transitioning from edoxaban to warfarin:

Oral option: For patients taking edoxaban 60 mg once daily, reduce the dose to 30 mg once daily and begin warfarin concomitantly. For patients taking edoxaban 30 mg once daily, reduce the dose to 15 mg once daily and begin warfarin concomitantly. Discontinue edoxaban once a stable INR ≥2 is achieved; continue warfarin (Leung 2019).

Parenteral option: Discontinue edoxaban and initiate a parenteral anticoagulant and warfarin at the time of the next scheduled edoxaban dose. Discontinue the parenteral anticoagulant once a stable INR ≥2 is achieved; continue warfarin.

Transitioning from rivaroxaban to warfarin: Some experts suggest overlapping rivaroxaban with warfarin for ≥2 days until INR is therapeutic. An alternative is to stop rivaroxaban, start warfarin the same day, and bridge with a parenteral anticoagulant until the desired INR is reached (Leung 2019).

Transitioning from therapeutic-dose parenteral anticoagulant to warfarin: Start warfarin and continue parenteral anticoagulant until INR is within therapeutic range (Hull 2019a; Wittkowsky 2018). **Note:** For the treatment of venous thromboembolism, overlap parenteral anticoagulant with warfarin until INR is ≥2 for at least 2 days (duration of overlap is usually 4 to 5 days) (ACCP [Ageno 2012]; Hull 2019b).

Transitioning from warfarin to another anticoagulant:

Note: In general, it is reasonable to discontinue warfarin and initiate another anticoagulant as soon as INR is ≤2 depending on the indication and risks of thrombosis and bleeding (Leung 2019). Specific recommendations from manufacturers include:

Transitioning from warfarin to apixaban: Discontinue warfarin and initiate apixaban as soon as INR falls to <2 (US labeling).

Transitioning from warfarin to dabigatran: Discontinue warfarin and initiate dabigatran as soon as INR falls to <2 (US labeling).

Transitioning from warfarin to edoxaban: Discontinue warfarin and initiate edoxaban as soon as INR falls to ≤2.5 (US labeling).

Transitioning from warfarin to rivaroxaban: Discontinue warfarin and initiate rivaroxaban as soon as INR falls to <3 (US labeling) or ≤2.5 (Canadian labeling).

Transitioning from warfarin to parenteral anticoagulation: Stop warfarin and start the parenteral anticoagulant when INR is as close as possible to the lower end of the targeted INR range (Wittkowsky 2018).

Geriatric Patients >60 years of age tend to require lower dosages to produce a therapeutic level of anticoagulation (due to changes in the pattern of warfarin metabolism).

Renal Impairment: Adult

No dosage adjustment necessary. However, patients with renal impairment have an increased risk for bleeding diathesis; monitor INR closely.

Hemodialysis: Not dialyzable (NCS/SCCM [Frontera 2016]).

Hepatic Impairment: Adult There are no dosage adjustments provided in the manufacturer's labeling. However, the response to oral anticoagulants may be markedly enhanced in obstructive jaundice, hepatitis, and cirrhosis. INR should be closely monitored.

Pediatric Note: Labeling identifies genetic factors which may increase patient sensitivity to warfarin based on experience in adult patients. Specifically, genetic variations in the proteins CYP2C9 and VKORC1, responsible for warfarin's primary metabolism and pharmacodynamic activity, respectively, have been identified as predisposing factors associated with decreased dose requirement and increased bleeding risk. Genotyping tests are available, and may provide guidance on initiation of anticoagulant therapy. The American College of Chest Physicians recommends against the use of routine pharmacogenomic testing to guide dosing (Guyatt 2012). For management of elevated INRs as a result of warfarin therapy, see phytonadione monograph or ACCP Guidelines for additional information (ACCP [Monagle 2012]).

Thromboembolic complications; prophylaxis and treatment: Limited data available (ACCP [Monagle 2012]): Individualize dose to achieve target INR based on indication; INRs are primarily extrapolated from adult experience; although there may be some exceptions, for most indications the therapeutic target INR is 2.5 (range: 2 to 3), and for low-dose prophylaxis, a target INR is 1.7 (range: 1.5 to 1.9). Infants, Children, and Adolescents: Oral:

Target International Normalized Ratio (INR) between 2 to 3 (eg, treatment):

Day 1: Initial loading dose (if baseline INR is 1 to 1.3): 0.2 mg/kg/day once daily; maximum dose: 10 mg/dose; use a reduced initial loading dose of 0.1 mg/kg if patient has undergone a Fontan procedure (AHA [Giglia 2013]) or has liver dysfunction (Streif 1999)

Days 2 to 4: Additional loading doses are dependent upon patient's INR:

INR 1.1 to 1.3: Repeat the initial loading dose

INR 1.4 to 1.9: Dose is 50% of the initial loading dose

INR 2 to 3: Dose is 50% of the initial loading dose

INR 3.1 to 3.5: Dose is 25% of the initial loading dose

INR >3.5: Hold the drug until INR <3.5, then restart at 50% of previous dose

Days ≥5: Maintenance doses are dependent upon patient's INR

INR 1.1 to 1.4: Increase dose by 20% of previous dose

INR 1.5 to 1.9: Increase dose by 10% of previous dose

INR 2 to 3: No change

INR 3.1 to 3.5: Decrease dose by 10% of previous dose

INR >3.5: Hold the drug until INR <3.5, then restart at 20% less than the previous dose

Usual maintenance dose: ~0.1 mg/kg/day once daily; range: 0.05 to 0.34 mg/kg/day; the dose in mg/kg/day is inversely related to age. In the largest pediatric study (n=319) (Streif 1999), infants <12 months required a mean dose of 0.33 mg/kg/day, but children 13 to 18 years required a mean dose of 0.09 mg/kg/day; a target INR of 2 to 3 was used for a majority of these patients (75% of warfarin courses). Overall, children required a mean dose of 0.16 mg/kg/day to achieve a target INR of 2 to 3. In another study (Andrew 1994), to attain an INR of 1.3 to 1.8, infants <12 months (n=2) required 0.24 and 0.27 mg/kg/day, but children >1 year required a mean of 0.08 mg/kg/day (range: 0.03 to 0.17 mg/kg/day). Consistent anticoagulation may be difficult to maintain in children <5 years. Children receiving phenobarbital, carbamazepine, or enteral nutrition may require higher maintenance doses (Streif 1999).

Renal Impairment: Pediatric No adjustment required; however, patients with renal failure have an increased risk of bleeding complications. Monitor closely.

Hepatic Impairment: Pediatric There are no dosage adjustments provided in the manufacturer's labeling. However, the response to oral anticoagulants may be markedly enhanced in obstructive jaundice (due to reduced vitamin K absorption) and also in hepatitis and cirrhosis (due to decreased production of vitamin K-dependent clotting factors); INR should be closely monitored.

Mechanism of Action Hepatic synthesis of coagulation factors II (half-life 42 to 72 hours), VII (half-life 4 to 6 hours), IX, and X (half-life 27 to 48 hours), as well as proteins C and S, requires the presence of vitamin K. These clotting factors are biologically activated by the addition of carboxyl groups to key glutamic acid residues within the proteins' structure. In the process, "active" vitamin K is oxidatively converted to an "inactive" form, which is then subsequently reactivated by vitamin K epoxide reductase complex 1 (VKORC1). Warfarin competitively inhibits the subunit 1 of the multi-unit VKOR complex, thus depleting functional vitamin K reserves and hence reduces synthesis of active clotting factors.

Contraindications Hypersensitivity to warfarin or any component of the formulation; hemorrhagic tendencies (eg, active GI ulceration, patients bleeding from the GI, respiratory, or GU tract; cerebral aneurysm; CNS hemorrhage; dissecting aortic aneurysm; spinal puncture and other diagnostic or therapeutic procedures with potential for significant bleeding); recent or potential surgery of the eye or CNS; major regional lumbar block anesthesia or traumatic surgery resulting in large, open surfaces; blood dyscrasias; malignant hypertension; pericarditis or pericardial effusion; bacterial endocarditis; unsupervised patients with conditions associated with a high potential for noncompliance; eclampsia/preeclampsia, threatened abortion, pregnancy (except in women with mechanical heart valves at high risk for thromboembolism)

Warnings/Precautions Use care in the selection of patients appropriate for this treatment. Ensure patient cooperation especially from the alcoholic, illicit drug user, demented, or psychotic patient; ability to comply with routine laboratory monitoring is essential. Use with caution in trauma, acute infection, prolonged dietary insufficiencies, moderate-severe hypertension, polycythemia vera, vasculitis, open wound, active TB, any disruption in normal GI flora, history of PUD, anaphylactic disorders, indwelling catheters, severe diabetes, and menstruating and postpartum women. Use with caution in patients with thyroid disease; warfarin responsiveness may increase (ACCP [Ageno 2012]). Use with caution in protein C deficiency. Use with caution in patients with heparin-induced thrombocytopenia and venous thromboembolism. Warfarin monotherapy is contraindicated in the initial treatment of heparin-induced thrombocytopenia. Reduced liver function, regardless of etiology, may impair synthesis of coagulation factors leading to increased warfarin sensitivity. Use with caution in patients with renal impairment; these patients are at an increased risk for bleeding diathesis; frequent INR monitoring is recommended. Acute kidney injury, possibly as a result of episodes of excessive anticoagulation and hematuria, may occur in patients with a history of kidney disease or in patients with altered glomerular integrity.

[US Boxed Warning]: May cause major or fatal bleeding. Perform regular INR monitoring in all treated patients. INR levels achieved with warfarin therapy may be affected by concomitant

medication, dietary modifications and/or other factors (eg, smoking). Risk factors for bleeding include high intensity anticoagulation (INR >4), age (>65 years), variable INRs, history of GI bleeding, hypertension, cerebrovascular disease, serious heart disease, anemia, malignancy, trauma, renal insufficiency, drug-drug interactions, long duration of therapy, or known genetic deficiency in CYP2C9 activity. Patient must be instructed to report bleeding, accidents, or falls. Unrecognized bleeding sites (eg, colon cancer) may be uncovered by anticoagulation. Patient must also report any new or discontinued medications, herbal or alternative products used, or significant changes in smoking or dietary habits. Necrosis or gangrene of the skin and other tissue can occur, usually in conjunction with protein C or S deficiency. Consider alternative therapies if anticoagulation is necessary. Warfarin therapy may release atheromatous plaque emboli; symptoms depend on site of embolization, most commonly kidneys, pancreas, liver, and spleen. In some cases may lead to necrosis or death. "Purple toes syndrome," due to cholesterol microembolization, may rarely occur. The elderly may be more sensitive to anticoagulant therapy.

Fatal and serious calciphylaxis (calcium uremic arteriolopathy) has been reported in patients with and without end-stage renal disease. If calciphylaxis is diagnosed, discontinue therapy and treat calciphylaxis as appropriate. Consider alternative anticoagulation therapy. Avoid warfarin therapy immediately after bariatric surgery if possible; risk of hemorrhage is increased. When reinitiated, warfarin dose may be reduced but return to preoperative doses 6 to 12 months postoperatively. Monitor INR closely in the early postoperative period and up to 1 year after surgery or when significant nutritional or supplementation changes occur.

Presence of the CYP2C9*2 or *3 allele and/or polymorphism of the vitamin K oxidoreductase (VKORC1) gene may have increased sensitivity to warfarin (eg, lower doses needed to achieve therapeutic anticoagulation). The *2 allele is reported to occur with a frequency of 4% to 11% in African-Americans and Caucasians, respectively, while the *3 allele frequencies are 2% to 7% respectively. Other variant 2C9 alleles (eg, *5, *6, *9, and *11) are also associated with reduced warfarin metabolism and thus may increase sensitivity to warfarin, but are much less common. Lower doses may be required in these patients. Genetic testing may help determine appropriate dosing.

Potentially significant drug-drug interactions may exist, requiring dose or frequency adjustment, additional monitoring, and/or selection of alternative therapy.

When temporary interruption is necessary before surgery, discontinue for approximately 5 days before surgery; when there is adequate hemostasis, may reinstitute warfarin therapy ~12 to 24 hours after surgery. Decision to safely continue warfarin therapy through the procedure and whether or not bridging of anticoagulation is necessary is dependent upon risk of perioperative bleeding and risk of thromboembolism. If risk of thromboembolism is elevated, consider bridging warfarin therapy with an alternative anticoagulant (eg, unfractionated heparin or low-molecular-weight heparin) (ACCP [Ageno 2012]).

Warnings: Additional Pediatric Considerations

Vitamin K-antagonist (VKA) (eg, warfarin) therapy is usually avoided in neonates and infants <4 months due to pharmacodynamic and administration issues which result in a greater risk of bleeding and necessitate more frequent monitoring and dose adjustment in these patients. Pharmacodynamic issues which create problematic dosing and monitoring include: Physiologically decreased neonatal plasma levels of vitamin K-dependent clotting factors (comparable to an adult with an INR 2 to 3 on VKA therapy), and a lower concentration of vitamin K in breast milk relative to infant formula (which is supplemented) making breast-fed infants very sensitive to VKA therapy (eg, much lower doses required to achieve target INR). Administration is problematic since no oral liquid formulation of warfarin is available; although some centers dissolve the appropriate tablet/dose in water, data which verifies stability and full assessment of practice is lacking (ACCP [Monagle 2012]).

Rare hair loss has been reported with warfarin use (ACCP [Monagle 2012]); pediatric cases include two case reports occurring with accidental ingestions in a 2 year old and 6 year old (Watras 2016). Tracheal calcification has been reported in young children and initially was considered a rare observation (ACCP [Monagle 2012]). However, newer data suggests it occurs more frequently; an incidence of 35% (6 out of 17 subjects) was reported in a retrospective analysis evaluating patients ≤10 years of age who underwent cardiac valve replacement and were receiving long-term anticoagulation with warfarin (Golding 2013).

Decreased bone mineral density has been reported in children and adolescents receiving long-term warfarin therapy; a case control study reported a significant reduction in lumbar spinal bone mineral apparent density (BMAD) scores in pediatric patients on warfarin therapy (n=17) compared to age-matched controls (n=321); the mean age of the 17 case subjects was 14.7 years (range: 8 to 18 years) and the mean duration of warfarin treatment was 8.2 years (range: 1 to 14 years) (Barnes 2005). Another cohort study evaluated bone-mineral density in 26 subjects with single ventricle physiology (age range: 5 to 12 years; treatment group [warfarin], n=16) and reported significant reductions of spinal BMD z-score than controls; they also reported lower total body less head BMD z-score (Bendaly 2015). Some centers include bone density monitoring (eg, DXA) as part of routine management for long-term warfarin therapy (Barnes 2005).

Drug Interactions

Metabolism/Transport Effects

Substrate of CYP1A2 (minor), CYP2C19 (minor), CYP2C9 (major), CYP3A4 (minor); **Note:** Assignment of Major/Minor substrate status based on clinically relevant drug interaction potential

Avoid Concomitant Use

Avoid concomitant use of Warfarin with any of the following: Hemin; MiFEPRIStone; Omacetaxine; Oxatomide; Streptokinase; Tamoxifen; Urokinase; Vorapaxar

Increased Effect/Toxicity

Warfarin may increase the levels/effects of: Collagenase (Systemic); Deferasirox; Deoxycholic Acid; Desirudin; Ethotoin; Fosphenytoin; Ibritumomab Tiuxetan; MetFORMIN; Nintedanib; Obinutuzumab; Omacetaxine; Phenytoin; Regorafenib; Sulfonylureas

The levels/effects of Warfarin may be increased by: Acalabrutinib; Acetaminophen; Agents with Antiplatelet Properties; Alemtuzumab; Allopurinol; Amiodarone; Amitriptyline; Androgens; Anticoagulants; Atazanavir; Bicalutamide; Bifonazole; Bromperidol; Cannabinoid-Containing Products; Caplacizumab; Carbimazole; Cephalosporins; Chenodiol; Chloral Betaine; Chloral

Hydrate; Chondroitin Sulfate; Cimetidine; Clopidogrel; Cloxacillin; Cobicistat; Coenzyme Q-10; Corticosteroids (Systemic); Cranberry; CYP2C9 Inhibitors (Moderate); CYP2C9 Inhibitors (Weak); Darunavir; Dasatinib; Desvenlafaxine; Dexmethylphenidate; Disulfiram; Dronabinol; Dronedarone; Econazole; Efavirenz; Elexacaftor, Tezacaftor, and Ivacaftor; Erlotinib; Erythromycin (Ophthalmic); Esomeprazole; Ethacrynic Acid; Ethotoin; Etoposide; Etoposide Phosphate; Exenatide; Fat Emulsion (Fish Oil Based); Fenofibrate and Derivatives; Fenugreek; Fibric Acid Derivatives; Fluconazole; Fluorouracil (Topical); Fluorouracil Products; Fosamprenavir; Fosphenytoin; Frankincense, Indian; Fusidic Acid (Systemic); Gefitinib; Gemcitabine; Ginkgo Biloba; Glucagon; Glucosamine; Green Tea; Hemin; Herbs (Anticoagulant/Antiplatelet Properties); HMG-CoA Reductase Inhibitors (Statins); Ibrutinib; Ifosfamide; Imatinib; Inotersen; Interferons (Alfa); Itraconazole; Ivermectin (Systemic); Ketoconazole (Systemic); Lactulose; Lansoprazole; Leflunomide; LevOCARNitine; Levomilnacipran; Limaprost; Lomitapide; Lumacaftor and Ivacaftor; Macrolide Antibiotics; Maitake; Mesoglycan; Methylphenidate; Metreleptin; MetroNIDAZOLE (Systemic); Miconazole (Oral); Miconazole (Topical); MiFEPRIStone; Milnacipran; Mirtazapine; Multivitamins/Fluoride (with ADE); Multivitamins/Minerals (with ADEK, Folate, Iron); Multivitamins/Minerals (with AE, No Iron); Nelfinavir; Neomycin; Nonsteroidal Anti-Inflammatory Agents (COX-2 Selective); Nonsteroidal Anti-Inflammatory Agents (Nonselective); Omega-3 Fatty Acids; Omeprazole; Oritavancin; Orlistat; Oxatomide; Penicillins; Pentosan Polysulfate Sodium; Pentoxifylline; Phenytoin; Posaconazole; Proguanil; Propacetamol; Propafenone; Prostacyclin Analogues; QuiNIDine; QuiNINE; Quinolones; RaNITIdine (Withdrawn from US Market); RomiDEPsin; Roxithromycin; Salicylates; Salicylates (Topical); Saquinavir; Selective Serotonin Reuptake Inhibitors; Selumetinib; Sodium Zirconium Cyclosilicate; SORAfenib; Streptokinase; Sugammadex; Sulfinpyrazone; Sulfonamide Antibiotics; Sulfonylureas; Sulodexide; Tamoxifen; Tetracyclines; Tezacaftor and Ivacaftor; Thrombolytic Agents; Thyroid Products; Tibolone; Tigecycline; Tipranavir; Tolterodine; Toremifene; Torsemide; TraMADol; Tranilast (Systemic); Urokinase; Valproate Products; Vemurafenib; Venetoclax; Venlafaxine; Vitamin E (Systemic); Vorapaxar; Vorinostat; Zanubrutinib; Zileuton

Decreased Effect

The levels/effects of Warfarin may be decreased by: Adalimumab; Alcohol (Ethyl); Alpelisib; Antithyroid Agents; Apalutamide; Aprepitant; AzaTHIOprine; Barbiturates; Bosentan; CarBAMazepine; Cholestyramine Resin; Cloxacillin; Coenzyme Q-10; Colesevelam; CYP2C9 Inducers (Weak); Darunavir; Dicloxacillin; Direct Acting Antiviral Agents (HCV); Efavirenz; Enzalutamide; Eslicarbazepine; Estrogen Derivatives; Estrogen Derivatives (Contraceptive); Fat Emulsion (Fish Oil and Plant Based); Flucloxacillin; Fosaprepitant; Ginseng (American); Glutethimide; Green Tea; Griseofulvin; Leflunomide; Letermovir; Lopinavir; Lumacaftor and Ivacaftor; Menadiol Diphosphate; Menatetrenone; Mercaptopurine; MetFORMIN; Metreleptin; Multivitamins/Minerals (with ADEK, Folate, Iron); Nafcillin; Nelfinavir; Nevirapine; Obeticholic Acid; Oritavancin; Phytonadione; Progestins; Progestins (Contraceptive); Revaprazan; Ribavirin (Systemic); Rifamycin Derivatives; Ritonavir; St John's Wort; Sucralfate; Telavancin; Teriflunomide; Tobacco (Smoked); Tranilast (Systemic); TraZODone

Food Interactions

Ethanol: Acute ethanol ingestion (binge drinking) decreases the metabolism of oral anticoagulants and increases PT/INR. Chronic daily ethanol use increases the metabolism of oral anticoagulants and decreases PT/INR. Management: Limit alcohol consumption; monitor INR closely.

Food: The anticoagulant effects of warfarin may be decreased if taken with foods rich in vitamin K. Vitamin E may increase warfarin effect. Cranberry juice may increase warfarin effect. Management: Maintain a consistent diet; consult prescriber before making changes in diet. Take warfarin at the same time each day.

Dietary Considerations Foods high in vitamin K (eg, leafy green vegetables) inhibit anticoagulant effect. The list of usual foods with high vitamin K content is well known, however, some unique ones include green tea (*Camellia sinensis*), chewing tobacco, a variety of oils (canola, corn, olive, peanut, safflower, sesame seed, soybean, and sunflower) (Booth 1999; Kuykendall 2004; Nutescu 2011). Snack foods containing Olestra have 80 mcg of vitamin K added to each ounce (Harrell 1999). Some natural products may contain hidden sources of vitamin K (Nutescu 2006). Avoid drastic changes in diet (eg, intake of large amounts of alfalfa, asparagus, broccoli, Brussels sprouts, cabbage, cauliflower, green teas, kale, lettuce, spinach, turnip greens, watercress) which decrease efficacy of warfarin. A balanced diet with a consistent intake of vitamin K is essential. The recommended dietary allowance for vitamin K in adults is 75 to 120 mcg/day (USDA Dietary Reference Intake).

Pharmacodynamics/Kinetics

Onset of Action

Initial anticoagulant effect on INR may be seen as soon as 24 to 72 hours (Harrison 1997; O'Reilly 1968).

Note: Full therapeutic effect generally seen between 5 and 7 days after initiation; dependent on reduction in vitamin K-dependent coagulation factors, especially prothrombin (factor II), which has a half-life of 60 to 72 hours (ACCP [Ageno 2012]; Crowther 1999; Kovacs 2003; manufacturer's labeling).

Duration of Action 2 to 5 days

Half-life Elimination 20-60 hours; Mean: 40 hours; highly variable among individuals

Time to Peak ~4 hours

Reproductive Considerations

Evaluate pregnancy status prior to use in females of reproductive potential. Females of reproductive potential should use effective contraception during therapy and for 1 month after the last dose.

Women who require long-term anticoagulation with warfarin and who are considering pregnancy, low molecular weight heparin (LMWH) substitution should be done prior to conception when possible (AHA/ACC [Nishimura 2014]).

Pregnancy Considerations

Warfarin crosses the placenta; concentrations in the fetal plasma are similar to maternal values. Teratogenic effects have been reported following first trimester exposure and may include coumarin embryopathy (nasal hypoplasia and/or stippled epiphyses; limb hypoplasia may also be present). Adverse CNS events to the fetus have also been observed following exposure during any trimester and may include CNS abnormalities (including ventral midline dysplasia, dorsal midline dysplasia). Spontaneous abortion, fetal hemorrhage, and fetal death may also occur. Use is contraindicated during pregnancy except in women with mechanical heart valves who are at high risk for thromboembolism; use is also contraindicated in women with threatened abortion, eclampsia, or preeclampsia. Frequent pregnancy tests are recommended for women who are planning to become pregnant and adjusted-dose heparin or low molecular weight heparin (LMWH) should be substituted as soon as pregnancy is confirmed or adjusted-dose heparin or LMWH should be used instead of warfarin prior to conception.

In pregnant women with high-risk mechanical heart valves, the benefits of warfarin therapy should be discussed with the risks of available treatments (ACCP [Bates 2012]; AHA/ACC [Nishimura 2014]); when possible avoid warfarin use during the first trimester (ACCP [Bates 2012]) and close to delivery (ACCP [Bates 2012]; AHA/ACC [Nishimura 2014]). Use of warfarin during the first trimester may be considered if the therapeutic INR can be achieved with a dose ≤5 mg/day (AHA/ACC [Nishimura 2014]). Adjusted-dose LMWH or adjusted-dose heparin may be used throughout pregnancy or until week 13 of gestation when therapy can be changed to warfarin. LMWH or heparin should be resumed close to delivery. In women who are at a very high risk for thromboembolism (older generation mechanical prosthesis in mitral position or history of thromboembolism), warfarin can be used throughout pregnancy and replaced with LMWH or heparin near term; the use of low-dose aspirin is also recommended (ACCP [Bates 2012] AHA/ACC [Nishimura 2014]). Women who require long-term anticoagulation with warfarin and who are considering pregnancy, LMWH substitution should be done prior to conception when possible. If anti-Xa monitoring cannot be done, do not use LMWH therapy in pregnant patients with a mechanical prosthetic valve (AHA/ACC [Nishimura 2014]). When choosing therapy, fetal outcomes (ie, pregnancy loss, malformations), maternal outcomes (ie, VTE, hemorrhage), burden of therapy, and maternal preference should be considered (ACCP [Bates 2012]).

Breastfeeding Considerations

Based on available data, warfarin is not present in breast milk.

Breastfeeding women may be treated with warfarin. According to the American College of Chest Physicians (ACCP), warfarin may be used in lactating women who wish to breastfeed their infants (ACCP [Bates 2012]). The manufacturer recommends monitoring of breastfeeding infants for bruising or bleeding.

Dosage Forms: US

Tablet, Oral:

Jantoven: 1 mg, 2 mg, 2.5 mg, 3 mg, 4 mg, 5 mg, 6 mg, 7.5 mg, 10 mg

Generic: 1 mg, 2 mg, 2.5 mg, 3 mg, 4 mg, 5 mg, 6 mg, 7.5 mg, 10 mg

Dosage Forms: Canada

Tablet, Oral:

Coumadin: 1 mg, 2 mg, 2.5 mg, 3 mg, 5 mg

Generic: 1 mg, 2 mg, 2.5 mg, 3 mg, 4 mg, 5 mg, 6 mg, 7.5 mg, 10 mg

Dental Health Professional Considerations It is important to discuss patient with physician or to ask for recent INR result to ensure that patient is within a reasonable range prior to an invasive dental procedure. One clue to determine how stable a patient is on warfarin therapy is to assess how often the patient gets INRs drawn. Recent frequent blood draws may suggest poor control on the patient's warfarin regimen. Surgery is generally acceptable for patients on warfarin with an INR between 2 to 3. Assess potential interactions when prescribing an antibiotic in patients on warfarin. Educate patients, who may require significant acetaminophen doses for multiple consecutive days to control dental pain, on the effects on warfarin (increased INR). NSAIDs do not have effects on INR but may increase the risk of bleeding while on warfarin.

- ◆ **Warfarin Sodium** *see* Warfarin *on page 1557*
- ◆ **WAY-CMA-676** *see* Gemtuzumab Ozogamicin *on page 734*
- ◆ **Weekly-D [OTC]** *see* Cholecalciferol *on page 344*
- ◆ **Welchol** *see* Colesevelam *on page 406*
- ◆ **Wellbutrin XL** *see* BuPROPion *on page 271*
- ◆ **Wellbutrin SR** *see* BuPROPion *on page 271*
- ◆ **Wera** *see* Ethinyl Estradiol and Norethindrone *on page 614*
- ◆ **Westcort [DSC]** *see* Hydrocortisone (Topical) *on page 775*
- ◆ **Westhroid** *see* Thyroid, Desiccated *on page 1442*
- ◆ **Wilate** *see* Antihemophilic Factor/von Willebrand Factor Complex (Human) *on page 154*
- ◆ **WIN-17757** *see* Danazol *on page 433*
- ◆ **Wixela Inhub** *see* Fluticasone and Salmeterol *on page 705*
- ◆ **WP Thyroid** *see* Thyroid, Desiccated *on page 1442*
- ◆ **WR-139007** *see* Dacarbazine *on page 427*
- ◆ **WR-139013** *see* Chlorambucil *on page 332*
- ◆ **Wycillin** *see* Penicillin G Procaine *on page 1210*
- ◆ **Wymzya Fe** *see* Ethinyl Estradiol and Norethindrone *on page 614*
- ◆ **Xadago** *see* Safinamide *on page 1353*
- ◆ **Xalatan** *see* Latanoprost *on page 880*
- ◆ **Xalkori** *see* Crizotinib *on page 415*
- ◆ **Xanax** *see* ALPRAZolam *on page 106*
- ◆ **Xanax XR** *see* ALPRAZolam *on page 106*
- ◆ **Xarelto** *see* Rivaroxaban *on page 1340*
- ◆ **Xarelto Starter Pack** *see* Rivaroxaban *on page 1340*
- ◆ **Xartemis XR** *see* Oxycodone and Acetaminophen *on page 1164*
- ◆ **Xatmep** *see* Methotrexate *on page 990*
- ◆ **Xcopri** *see* Cenobamate *on page 321*
- ◆ **Xcopri (250 MG Daily Dose)** *see* Cenobamate *on page 321*
- ◆ **Xcopri (350 MG Daily Dose)** *see* Cenobamate *on page 321*
- ◆ **Xeljanz** *see* Tofacitinib *on page 1459*
- ◆ **Xeljanz XR** *see* Tofacitinib *on page 1459*
- ◆ **Xelpros** *see* Latanoprost *on page 880*
- ◆ **Xembify** *see* Immune Globulin *on page 803*
- ◆ **Xenical** *see* Orlistat *on page 1145*
- ◆ **Xenleta** *see* Lefamulin *on page 881*
- ◆ **Xenleta** *see* Lefamulin *on page 881*
- ◆ **Xeomin** *see* IncobotulinumtoxinA *on page 806*
- ◆ **Xepi** *see* Ozenoxacin *on page 1178*
- ◆ **Xerava** *see* Eravacycline *on page 581*

Zafirlukast (za FIR loo kast)

Related Information

Respiratory Diseases *on page 1680*

Brand Names: US Accolate

Brand Names: Canada Accolate [DSC]

Pharmacologic Category Leukotriene-Receptor Antagonist

Use Asthma: Prophylaxis and chronic treatment of asthma in adults and children ≥5 years of age. **Note:** The Global Initiative for Asthma recommends zafirlukast in patients with concomitant allergic rhinitis or those who cannot take inhaled corticosteroids (GINA 2020).

Local Anesthetic/Vasoconstrictor Precautions No information available to require special precautions

Effects on Dental Treatment No significant effects or complications reported

Effects on Bleeding No information available to require special precautions

Adverse Reactions Incidences reported in children ≥12 years and adults unless otherwise specified.

>10%: Central nervous system: Headache (13%; children 5 to 11 years: 5%)

1% to 10%:

Central nervous system: Dizziness (2%), pain (2%)

Gastrointestinal: Nausea (3%), diarrhea (3%), abdominal pain (2%; children 5 to 11 years: 3%), vomiting (2%), dyspepsia (1%)

Hepatic: Increased serum ALT (2%)

Infection: Infection (4%)

Neuromuscular & skeletal: Back pain (2%), myalgia (2%), weakness (2%)

Miscellaneous: Fever (2%)

<1%, postmarketing, and/or case reports: Agranulocytosis, angioedema, arthralgia, bruise, depression, edema, eosinophilia (systemic), eosinophilic pneumonitis, hemorrhage, hepatic failure, hepatitis, hyperbilirubinemia, hypersensitivity reaction, insomnia, malaise, pruritus, skin rash, urticaria, vasculitis (with

clinical features of eosinophilic granulomatosis with polyangiitis [formerly known as Churg-Strauss]; rare)

Mechanism of Action Zafirlukast is a selectively and competitive leukotriene-receptor antagonist (LTRA) of leukotriene D4 and E4 (LTD4 and LTE4), components of slow-reacting substance of anaphylaxis (SRSA). Cysteinyl leukotriene production and receptor occupation have been correlated with the pathophysiology of asthma, including airway edema, smooth muscle constriction, and altered cellular activity associated with the inflammatory process, which contribute to the signs and symptoms of asthma.

Pharmacodynamics/Kinetics

Onset of Action Asthma symptom improvement: Peak effect: 2 to 6 weeks

Duration of Action Asthma symptom improvement: 12 hours

Half-life Elimination ~10 hours (range: 8 to 16 hours)

Time to Peak Serum:

Children: 2 to 2.5 hours

Adults: 3 hours

Pregnancy Risk Factor B

Pregnancy Considerations

Information related to the use of zafirlukast in pregnancy is limited (Bakhireva 2007).

Uncontrolled asthma is associated with adverse events in pregnancy (increased risk of perinatal mortality, preeclampsia, preterm birth, low birth weight infants, cesarean delivery, and the development of gestational diabetes). Poorly controlled asthma or asthma exacerbations may have a greater fetal/maternal risk than what is associated with appropriately used asthma medications. Maternal treatment improves pregnancy outcomes by reducing the risk of some adverse events (eg, preterm birth, gestational diabetes) (ERS/TSANZ [Middleton 2020]; GINA 2020).

Agents other than zafirlukast are preferred for the treatment of asthma in pregnancy (ERS/TSANZ [Middleton 2020]; GINA 2020).

Data collection to monitor pregnancy and infant outcomes associated with asthma and the medications used to treat asthma in pregnancy is ongoing. Health care providers are encouraged to enroll exposed pregnant females in the MotherToBaby Pregnancy Studies conducted by the Organization of Teratology Information Specialists (1-877-311-8972 or https://mothertobaby.org). Patients may also enroll themselves.

Zaleplon (ZAL e plon)

Brand Names: US Sonata [DSC]

Pharmacologic Category Hypnotic, Miscellaneous

Use Insomnia: Short-term treatment of insomnia (ie, up to 30 days).

Local Anesthetic/Vasoconstrictor Precautions
No information available to require special precautions

Effects on Dental Treatment Key adverse event(s) related to dental treatment: Xerostomia (normal salivary flow resumes upon discontinuation) (see Dental Health Professional Considerations)

Effects on Bleeding No information available to require special precautions

Adverse Reactions

>10%: Central nervous system: Headache (42%)

1% to 10%:

Cardiovascular: Chest pain (≥1%), peripheral edema (≤1%)

Central nervous system: Dizziness (9%), drowsiness (5% to 6%), amnesia (2% to 4%), paresthesia (3%), altered sense of smell (2%), depersonalization (2%), hypoesthesia (2%), malaise (2%), hyperacusis (1% to 2%), abnormality in thinking (≥1%), anxiety (≥1%), depression (≥1%), migraine (≥1%), nervousness (≥1%), hallucination (1%), hypertonia (1%), vertigo (1%)

Dermatologic: Pruritus (≥1%), skin rash (≥1%), skin photosensitivity (1%)

Gastrointestinal: Nausea (8%), abdominal pain (6%), anorexia (2%), constipation (≥1%), dysgeusia (≥1%), dyspepsia (≥1%), xerostomia (≥1%), colitis (1%)

Genitourinary: Dysmenorrhea (3% to 4%)

Neuromuscular & skeletal: Asthenia (7%), tremor (2%), arthralgia (≥1%), arthritis (≥1%), back pain (≥1%), myalgia (≥1%)

Ophthalmic: Eye pain (3% to 4%), visual disturbance (2%), conjunctivitis (≥1%)

Otic: Otalgia (≤1%)

Respiratory: Bronchitis (≥1%), epistaxis (1%)

Miscellaneous: Fever (≥1%)

<1%: Abnormal gait, abnormal hepatic function tests, abnormal uterine bleeding, accommodation disturbance, acne vulgaris, ageusia, agitation, albuminuria, alopecia, anaphylaxis, anemia, angina pectoris, apathy, aphthous stomatitis, apnea, arthropathy, asthma, ataxia, bigeminy, biliary colic, bladder pain, blepharitis, blepharoptosis, bruxism, bundle branch block, bursitis, cataract, central nervous system stimulation, cerebral ischemia, cheilitis, chills, cholelithiasis, confusion, conjunctival hyperemia (subconjunctival hemorrhage), contact dermatitis, corneal erosion, cyanosis, cystitis, deafness, decreased libido, delusions, diabetes mellitus, diaphoresis, diplopia, dry eye syndrome, duodenal ulcer, dysarthria, dysphagia, dyspnea, dystonia, dysuria, ecchymoses, eczema, edema, emotional lability, enteritis, eosinophilia, eructation, esophageal achalasia, esophagitis, euphoria, facial edema, facial paralysis, flatulence, gastritis, gastroenteritis, gingival hemorrhage, gingivitis, glaucoma, glossitis, goiter, gout, hangover effect, heavy menstrual bleeding, hematuria, hemorrhage (eye), hiccups, hostility, hyperbilirubinemia, hypercholesterolemia, hyperesthesia, hyperglycemia, hyperkinetic muscle activity, hyperreflexia, hypertension, hyperuricemia, hyperventilation, hypoglycemia, hypokinesia, hyporeflexia, hypotension, hypothyroidism, hypotonia, impaired consciousness, impotence, increased appetite, increased bronchial secretions, increased serum alanine aminotransferase, increased serum aspartate aminotransferase, increased thirst, insomnia, intestinal obstruction, irregular menses, ketosis, labyrinthitis, laryngitis, leukocytosis, leukorrhea, lymphadenopathy, lymphocytosis, maculopapular rash, mastalgia, melanosis, melena, menopause, menstrual disease, myasthenia, myoclonus, myositis, neck stiffness, nephrolithiasis, neuralgia, neuropathy, nightmares, nystagmus disorder, oral mucosa ulcer, oral paresthesia, orthostatic hypotension, osteoporosis, palpitations, paradoxical central nervous system stimulation, peptic ulcer, pericardial effusion, photophobia, pleural effusion, pneumonia, psoriasis, psychomotor retardation, pulmonary embolism, purpuric disease, pustular rash, rectal hemorrhage, renal pain, reduced urine flow, retinal detachment, sialorrhea, sinus bradycardia, skin discoloration, skin hypertrophy, slurred speech, snoring, stomatitis, stupor, substernal pain, syncope, tachycardia, tenosynovitis, thrombophlebitis, tinnitus, tongue discoloration,

tongue edema, trismus, urethritis, urinary frequency, urinary incontinence, urinary retention, urinary urgency, urticaria, vaginal hemorrhage, vaginitis, vasodilatation, ventricular premature contractions, ventricular tachycardia, visual field defect, voice disorder, watery eyes, weight gain, weight loss, xeroderma

Frequency not defined:

Central nervous system: Central nervous system depression, complex sleep-related disorder

Hypersensitivity: Angioedema, hypersensitivity condition

Postmarketing: Anaphylaxis, nightmares, nonimmune anaphylaxis

Mechanism of Action Zaleplon is unrelated to benzodiazepines, barbiturates, or other hypnotics. However, it interacts with the benzodiazepine GABA receptor complex. Nonclinical studies have shown that it binds selectively to the brain omega-1 receptor situated on the alpha subunit of the GABA-A receptor complex.

Pharmacodynamics/Kinetics

Onset of Action Rapid

Half-life Elimination ~1 hour

Time to Peak Serum: ~1 hour

Pregnancy Considerations

Adverse events were observed in some animal reproduction studies. A small study of pregnant women did not show an increased risk of teratogenic effects when used early in pregnancy (Wikner 2011). Use during pregnancy is not recommended by the manufacturer.

Controlled Substance C-IV

Dental Health Professional Considerations An adult companion should accompany the patient to and from dental office.

◆ **Zaltrap** *see* Ziv-Aflibercept (Systemic) *on page 1573*

◆ **Zamicet [DSC]** *see* Hydrocodone and Acetaminophen *on page 764*

◆ **Zanaflex** *see* TiZANidine *on page 1455*

Zanamivir (za NA mi veer)

Related Information

Systemic Viral Diseases *on page 1709*

Brand Names: US Relenza Diskhaler

Brand Names: Canada Relenza Diskhaler

Pharmacologic Category Antiviral Agent; Neuraminidase Inhibitor

Use Influenza:

Prophylaxis: Prophylaxis of influenza in adults and pediatric patients 5 years and older.

Treatment: Treatment of uncomplicated acute illness caused by influenza A and B virus in adults and pediatric patients 7 years and older who have been symptomatic for no more than 2 days.

The Advisory Committee on Immunization Practices (ACIP) recommends that **treatment** be considered for the following:

- Persons with severe, complicated or progressive illness
- Hospitalized persons
- Persons at higher risk for influenza complications:
  - Children <2 years of age (highest risk in children <6 months of age)
  - Adults ≥65 years of age
  - Persons with chronic disorders of the pulmonary (including asthma) or cardiovascular systems (except hypertension)
  - Persons with chronic metabolic diseases (including diabetes mellitus), hepatic disease, renal dysfunction, hematologic disorders (including sickle cell disease), or immunosuppression (including immunosuppression caused by medications or HIV)
  - Persons with neurologic/neuromuscular conditions (including conditions such as spinal cord injuries, seizure disorders, cerebral palsy, stroke, mental retardation, moderate to severe developmental delay, or muscular dystrophy) which may compromise respiratory function, the handling of respiratory secretions, or that can increase the risk of aspiration
  - Pregnant or postpartum women (≤2 weeks after delivery)
  - Persons <19 years of age on long-term aspirin therapy
  - American Indians and Alaskan Natives
  - Persons who are morbidly obese (BMI ≥40)
  - Residents of nursing homes or other chronic care facilities
- Use may also be considered for previously healthy, nonhigh-risk outpatients with confirmed or suspected influenza based on clinical judgment when treatment can be started within 48 hours of illness onset.

The ACIP recommends that **prophylaxis** be considered for the following:

- Postexposure prophylaxis may be considered for family or close contacts of suspected or confirmed cases, who are at higher risk of influenza complications, and who have not been vaccinated against the circulating strain at the time of the exposure.
- Postexposure prophylaxis may be considered for unvaccinated healthcare workers who had occupational exposure without protective equipment.
- Pre-exposure prophylaxis should only be used for persons at very high risk of influenza complications who cannot be otherwise protected at times of high risk for exposure.
- Prophylaxis should also be administered to all eligible residents of institutions that house patients at high risk when needed to control outbreaks.

Local Anesthetic/Vasoconstrictor Precautions No information available to require special precautions

Effects on Dental Treatment No significant effects or complications reported

Effects on Bleeding No information available to require special precautions

Adverse Reactions

>10%:

Gastrointestinal: Sore throat (or discomfort; prophylaxis, children: 11%)

Respiratory: Cough (prophylaxis, children: 16%), nasal signs and symptoms (prophylaxis, children: 20%), tonsil disease (discomfort or pain; prophylaxis, children: 11%)

1% to 10%:

Dermatologic: Urticaria (treatment, adolescents and adults: <2%)

Gastrointestinal: Abdominal pain (treatment, adolescents and adults: <2%)

Nervous system: Dizziness (treatment, adolescents and adults: 2%)

Neuromuscular & skeletal: Arthralgia (≤2%), rheumatism (prophylaxis: 2%)

Respiratory: Sinusitis (treatment, adolescents and adults: 3%)

Postmarketing:

Cardiovascular: Cardiac arrhythmia, syncope

Dermatologic: Erythema multiforme, skin rash, Stevens-Johnson syndrome, toxic epidermal necrolysis
Hypersensitivity: Anaphylaxis, facial edema, hypersensitivity reaction (or hypersensitivity-like reaction), oropharyngeal edema
Nervous system: Abnormal behavior, agitation, anxiety, confusion, delirium, delusions, hallucination, impaired consciousness, nightmares, seizure
Respiratory: Bronchospasm, dyspnea

Mechanism of Action Zanamivir inhibits influenza virus neuraminidase enzymes, potentially altering virus particle aggregation and release.

Pharmacodynamics/Kinetics

Half-life Elimination Serum: 2.5 to 5.1 hours

Time to Peak 1-2 hours

Pregnancy Considerations

An increased risk of adverse neonatal or maternal outcomes has not been observed following use of zanamivir during pregnancy (CDC 60[1] 2011).

Untreated influenza infection is associated with an increased risk of adverse events to the fetus and an increased risk of complications or death to the mother. Although neuraminidase inhibitors are currently recommended for the treatment or prophylaxis of influenza in pregnant women and women up to 2 weeks' postpartum, zanamivir is not the preferred agent (ACOG 2018; CDC 60[1] 2011).

◆ **Zanosar** *see* Streptozocin *on page 1389*

Zanubrutinib (ZAN ue BROO ti nib)

Brand Names: US Brukinsa

Pharmacologic Category Antineoplastic Agent; Antineoplastic Agent, Bruton Tyrosine Kinase Inhibitor; Antineoplastic Agent, Tyrosine Kinase Inhibitor

Use Mantle cell lymphoma (relapsed or refractory): Treatment of mantle cell lymphoma in adults who have received at least 1 prior therapy.

Local Anesthetic/Vasoconstrictor Precautions
No information available to require special precautions

Effects on Dental Treatment No significant effects or complications reported

Effects on Bleeding Numerous hematologic toxicities (see adverse reactions section) including thrombocytopenia, neutropenia, leukopenia, and hemorrhage reported. Medical consult suggested prior to invasive dental procedures.

Adverse Reactions

>10%:
Cardiovascular: Hypertension (12%)
Central nervous system: Fatigue (11%)
Dermatologic: Skin rash (25% to 36%)
Endocrine & metabolic: Increased uric acid (29%), hypokalemia (14%)
Gastrointestinal: Diarrhea (20% to 23%), constipation (11% to 13%)
Genitourinary: Urinary tract infection (11% to 13%), hematuria (12%; grades ≥3%: 2%)
Hematologic & oncologic: Petechia (50%), purpuric disease (50%), lymphocytosis (41%, grades 3/4: 16%), neutropenia (38%, grades ≥3: 15% to 27%), thrombocytopenia (27%, grades 3/4: 5% to 10%), leukopenia (25%, grades ≥3%: 5%), bruise (14% to 23%), anemia (14%, grades ≥3: 8%), hemorrhage (10% to 11%, grades ≥3%: 3%)
Hepatic: Increased serum alanine aminotransferase (29%), increased serum bilirubin (24%)
Infection: Bacterial infection (grades ≥3: ≤23%), fungal infection (grades ≥3: ≤23%), opportunistic infection (grades ≥3: ≤23%), serious infection (grades ≥3: ≤23%), viral infection (grades ≥3: ≤23%)
Neuromuscular & skeletal: Musculoskeletal pain (14% to 19%)
Respiratory: Upper respiratory tract infection (38% to 39%), cough (12% to 20%), pneumonia (15% to 18%)

1% to 10%:
Cardiovascular: Atrial fibrillation (2%), atrial flutter (2%)
Central nervous system: Intracranial hemorrhage (5%), headache (4%)
Endocrine & metabolic: Hyperuricemia (6%)
Gastrointestinal: Gastrointestinal hemorrhage (grades ≥3%: 2%)
Hematologic & oncologic: Second primary malignant neoplasm (9%), skin carcinoma (6%), basal cell carcinoma of skin (≤6%), squamous cell carcinoma of skin (≤6%)
Respiratory: Hemothorax (grades ≥3%: 2%)

Frequency not defined:
Hematologic & oncologic: Hematoma
Hepatic: Exacerbation of hepatitis B

Mechanism of Action Zanubrutinib is a highly selective Bruton tyrosine kinase (BTK) inhibitor (Tam 2019). Zanubrutinib forms a covalent bond with a cysteine residue in the BTK active site to inhibit BTK activity. BTK is a signaling molecule of the B-cell antigen receptor and cytokine receptor pathways. BTK signals activation of pathways necessary for B-cell proliferation, trafficking, chemotaxis, and adhesion. Zanubrutinib inhibits malignant B-cell proliferation and reduces tumor growth.

Pharmacodynamics/Kinetics

Half-life Elimination ~2 to 4 hours.

Time to Peak 2 hours.

Reproductive Considerations

Evaluate pregnancy status prior to use in females of reproductive potential. Females of reproductive potential should use effective contraception during therapy and for ≥1 week after the last zanubrutinib dose. Males with female partners of reproductive potential should use effective contraception during therapy and for ≥1 week after the last zanubrutinib dose.

Pregnancy Considerations

Based on data from animal reproduction studies, in utero exposure to zanubrutinib may cause fetal harm.

Prescribing and Access Restrictions Available through specialty pharmacies and distributors. Information regarding distribution is available from the manufacturer at https://www.brukinsa.com/ordering-information-and-distribution-sheet.pdf.

◆ **Zarah** *see* Ethinyl Estradiol and Drospirenone *on page 610*

◆ **Zarontin** *see* Ethosuximide *on page 619*

◆ **Zaroxolyn** *see* MetOLazone *on page 1008*

◆ **Zarxio** *see* Filgrastim *on page 668*

◆ **Zazole [DSC]** *see* Terconazole *on page 1423*

◆ **ZD1033** *see* Anastrozole *on page 150*

◆ **ZD1839** *see* Gefitinib *on page 730*

◆ **ZD6474** *see* Vandetanib *on page 1531*

◆ **ZD9238** *see* Fulvestrant *on page 721*

◆ **ZDV** *see* Zidovudine *on page 1569*

◆ **ZDV, Abacavir, and Lamivudine** *see* Abacavir, Lamivudine, and Zidovudine *on page 52*

Ziconotide (zi KOE no tide)

Brand Names: US Prialt

Pharmacologic Category Analgesic, Nonopioid; Calcium Channel Blocker, N-Type

Use Management of severe chronic pain in patients requiring intrathecal therapy and who are intolerant or refractory to other therapies (eg, systemic analgesics, adjunctive therapies, intrathecal morphine)

Local Anesthetic/Vasoconstrictor Precautions No information available to require special precautions

Effects on Dental Treatment Key adverse event(s) related to dental treatment: Xerostomia (normal salivary flow resumes upon discontinuation) and taste perversion.

Effects on Bleeding No information available to require special precautions

Adverse Reactions

>10%:

Central nervous system: Dizziness (46%), confusion (15% to 33%), memory impairment (7% to 22%), drowsiness (17%), abnormal gait (14%), ataxia (14%), speech disorder (14%), headache (13%), aphasia (12%), hallucination (12%; including auditory and visual)

Gastrointestinal: Nausea (40%), diarrhea (18%), vomiting (16%)

Neuromuscular & skeletal: Increased creatine phosphokinase (40%; ≥3 x ULN: 11%), weakness (18%)

Ophthalmic: Blurred vision (12%)

2% to 10%:

Cardiovascular: Hypotension, orthostatic hypotension, peripheral edema

Central nervous system: Abnormality in thinking (8%), amnesia (8%), anxiety (8%), dysarthria (7%), paresthesia (7%), rigors (7%), vertigo (7%), insomnia (6%), paranoia (3%), delirium (2%), hostility (2%), stupor (2%), absent reflexes, agitation, burning sensation, decreased mental acuity, depression, disorientation, disturbance in attention, fatigue, hypoesthesia, irritability, lethargy, loss of balance, mood disorder, myasthenia, nervousness, pain, sedation

Dermatologic: Pruritus (7%), diaphoresis (5%)

Gastrointestinal: Anorexia (6%), dysgeusia (5%), abdominal pain, constipation, decreased appetite, xerostomia

Genitourinary: Urinary retention (9%), dysuria, urinary hesitancy

Neuromuscular & skeletal: Tremor (7%), muscle spasm (6%), limb pain (5%), muscle cramps, myalgia

Ophthalmic: Nystagmus (8%), diplopia, visual disturbance

Respiratory: Sinusitis (5%)

Miscellaneous: Fever (5%)

<2%, postmarketing, and/or case reports: Acute renal failure, aspiration pneumonia (<1%), atrial fibrillation, attempted suicide (<1%), cerebrovascular accident, ECG abnormality, incoherence, loss of consciousness, mania, meningitis, myoclonus, psychosis (1%), respiratory distress, rhabdomyolysis, seizure (clonic and grand mal), sepsis, suicidal ideation

Mechanism of Action Ziconotide selectively binds to N-type voltage-sensitive calcium channels located on the nociceptive afferent nerves of the dorsal horn in the spinal cord. This binding is thought to block N-type calcium channels, leading to a blockade of excitatory neurotransmitter release and reducing sensitivity to painful stimuli.

Pharmacodynamics/Kinetics

Half-life Elimination IV: 1 to 1.6 hours (plasma); Intrathecal: 2.9 to 6.5 hours (CSF)

Pregnancy Risk Factor C

Pregnancy Considerations Adverse events and maternal toxicity were observed in animal reproduction studies.

Zidovudine (zye DOE vyoo deen)

Related Information

HIV Infection and AIDS *on page 1690*

Brand Names: US Retrovir

Brand Names: Canada ALTI-Zidovudine; APO-Zidovudine; Retrovir (AZT)

Pharmacologic Category Antiretroviral, Reverse Transcriptase Inhibitor, Nucleoside (Anti-HIV)

Use

HIV-1 infection, treatment: Treatment of HIV-1 infection in combination with other antiretroviral agents

Perinatal HIV-1 transmission, prevention: Prevention of mother to fetus HIV-1 transmission

Local Anesthetic/Vasoconstrictor Precautions No information available to require special precautions

Effects on Dental Treatment Key adverse event(s) related to dental treatment: Taste perversion, oral mucosa pigmentation, dysphagia, and mouth ulcer.

Effects on Bleeding No information available to require special precautions relative to hemostasis.

Adverse Reactions Percentages noted with oral administration in adults unless otherwise stated. Pediatric adverse event incidences occurred with combination therapy.

>10%:

Central nervous system: Headache (63%), malaise (53%)

Dermatologic: Skin rash (infants, children, & adolescents: 12%)

Gastrointestinal: Nausea (adults: 51%; infants, children, & adolescents: 8%), anorexia (20%), vomiting (adults: 17%; infants, children, & adolescents: 8%)

Hematologic & oncologic: Macrocytosis (infants, children, & adolescents: >50%), anemia (neonates: 22%; infants, children, & adolescents: 4%; adults, grades 3/4: 1%)

Hepatic: Hepatomegaly (infants, children, & adolescents: 11%)

Respiratory: Cough (infants, children, & adolescents: 15%)

Miscellaneous: Fever (infants, children, & adolescents: 25%)

1% to 10%:

Cardiovascular: Cardiac failure (infants, children, & adolescents: <6%), ECG abnormality (infants, children, & adolescents: <6%), edema (infants, children, & adolescents: <6%), left ventricular dilation (infants, children, & adolescents: <6%)

Central nervous system: Hyporeflexia (infants, children, & adolescents: <6%), irritability (infants, children, & adolescents: <6%), nervousness (infants, children, & adolescents: <6%), chills (≥5%), fatigue (≥5%), insomnia (≥5%), neuropathy (≥5%)

Endocrine & metabolic: Weight loss (infants, children, & adolescents: <6%), increased amylase (infants, children, & adolescents, grades 3/4: 3%)

Gastrointestinal: Diarrhea (infants, children, & adolescents: 8%), constipation (6%), stomatitis (infants, children, & adolescents: 6%), abdominal cramps (≥5%), abdominal pain (≥5%), dyspepsia (≥5%), increased serum lipase (infants, children, & adolescents, grades 3/4: 3%)

Genitourinary: Hematuria (infants, children, & adolescents: <6%)

Hematologic & oncologic: Lymphadenopathy (infants, children, & adolescents: 9%), neutropenia (infants, children, & adolescents, grades 3/4: 8%), splenomegaly (infants, children, & adolescents: 5%), thrombocytopenia (infants, children, & adolescents, grades 3/4: 1%)

Hepatic: Increased serum aspartate aminotransferase (infants, children, & adolescents, grades 3/4: 2%), increased serum alanine aminotransferase (infants, children, & adolescents, grades 3/4: 1%),

Neuromuscular & skeletal: Asthenia (9%), arthralgia (≥5%), musculoskeletal pain (≥5%), myalgia (≥5%)

Otic: Ear sign or symptom (infants, children, & adolescents: 7%)

Respiratory: Nasal congestion (infants, children, & adolescents: ≤8%), rhinorrhea (infants, children, & adolescents: ≤8%), abnormal breath sounds (infants, children, & adolescents: ≤7%), wheezing (infants, children, & adolescents: ≤7%)

Frequency not defined:

Local: Injection site reaction (IV), irritation at injection site (IV), pain at injection site (IV)

<1%, postmarketing and/or case reports: Amblyopia, anaphylaxis, angioedema, anxiety, aplastic anemia, autoimmune disease, back pain, cardiomyopathy, chest pain, confusion, decreased mental acuity, depression, diaphoresis, dizziness, drowsiness, dyschromia, dysgeusia, dysphagia, dyspnea, flatulence, flu-like symptoms, Graves disease, Guillain-Barré syndrome, gynecomastia, hearing loss, hemolytic anemia, hepatitis, hepatomegaly with steatosis, hyperbilirubinemia, hypersensitivity reaction, immune reconstitution syndrome, increased creatine phosphokinase, increased lactate dehydrogenase, jaundice, lactic acidosis, leukopenia, lipotrophy, macular edema, mania, muscle spasm, myopathy, myositis, oral mucosa hyperpigmentation, oral mucosa ulcer, pain, pancreatitis, pancytopenia, paresthesia, photophobia, polymyositis, pruritus, pure red cell aplasia, redistribution of body fat, rhabdomyolysis, rhinitis, seizure, sinusitis, Stevens-Johnson syndrome, syncope, toxic epidermal necrolysis, tremor, urinary frequency, urinary hesitancy, urticaria, vasculitis, vertigo

Mechanism of Action Zidovudine is a thymidine analog which interferes with the HIV viral RNA-dependent DNA polymerase resulting in inhibition of viral replication; nucleoside reverse transcriptase inhibitor

Pharmacodynamics/Kinetics

Half-life Elimination Terminal:

Premature neonate: 6.3 hours

Full-term neonates: 3.1 hours

Infants 14 days to 3 months: 1.9 hours

Infants 3 months to Children 12 years: 1.5 hours

Adults: 0.5 to 3 hours (mean 1.1 hours)

Time to Peak Serum: 30 to 90 minutes

Reproductive Considerations

The Health and Human Services (HHS) perinatal HIV guidelines consider zidovudine an alternative nucleoside reverse transcriptase inhibitor for females living with HIV who are not yet pregnant but are trying to conceive.

For males and females living with HIV and planning a pregnancy, maximum viral suppression below the limits of detection with antiretroviral therapy (ART), modification of therapy (if needed), optimization of the woman's health, and a discussion of the potential risks and benefits of ART therapy during pregnancy is recommended prior to conception (HHS [perinatal] 2019).

Pregnancy Considerations

Zidovudine has a high level of transfer across the human placenta; the placenta also metabolizes zidovudine to the active metabolite.

No increased risk of overall birth defects has been observed following first trimester exposure according to data collected by the antiretroviral pregnancy registry. Maternal antiretroviral therapy (ART) may be associated with adverse pregnancy outcomes including preterm delivery, stillbirth, low birth weight, and small for gestational age infants. Actual risks may be influenced by maternal factors, such as disease severity, gestational age at initiation of therapy, and specific ART regimen, therefore close fetal monitoring is recommended. Because there is clear benefit to appropriate treatment, maternal ART should not be withheld due to concerns for adverse neonatal outcomes. Long-term follow-up is recommended for all infants exposed to antiretroviral medications; children without HIV but who were exposed to ART in utero and develop significant organ system abnormalities of unknown etiology (particularly of the CNS or heart) should be evaluated for potential mitochondrial dysfunction. Cases of lactic acidosis and hepatic steatosis have been reported in pregnant women with use of nucleoside reverse transcriptase inhibitors (NRTIs).

The Health and Human Services (HHS) perinatal HIV guidelines consider zidovudine an alternative NRTI for pregnant females living with HIV who are antiretroviral-naive, who have had ART therapy in the past but are restarting, or who require a new ART regimen (due to poor tolerance or poor virologic response of current regimen). In addition, females who become pregnant while taking zidovudine may continue if viral suppression is effective and the regimen is well tolerated. The pharmacokinetics of zidovudine are not significantly altered in pregnancy and dosing adjustment is not needed.

The HHS perinatal HIV guidelines consider zidovudine in combination with lamivudine as an alternative NRTI backbone for initial therapy in antiretroviral-naive pregnant females. Zidovudine should be administered IV near delivery regardless of antepartum regimen or mode of delivery in females with known or suspected HIV RNA >1,000 copies/mL or unknown HIV RNA status (even in cases of documented zidovudine resistance) and may be considered in females with HIV RNA between 50 to 999 copies/mL, unless there is a history of hypersensitivity.

In general, ART is recommended for all pregnant females living with HIV to keep the viral load below the limit of detection and reduce the risk of perinatal transmission. Therapy should be individualized following a discussion of the potential risks and benefits of treatment during pregnancy. Monitoring of pregnant females is more frequent than in nonpregnant adults. ART should be continued postpartum for all females living with HIV and can be modified after delivery.

Health care providers are encouraged to enroll pregnant females exposed to antiretroviral medications as early in pregnancy as possible in the Antiretroviral Pregnancy Registry (1-800-258-4263 or http://www.APRegistry.com). Health care providers caring for pregnant females living with HIV and their infants may contact the National Perinatal HIV Hotline (1-888-448-8765) for clinical consultation (HHS [perinatal] 2019).

- **Zidovudine, Abacavir, and Lamivudine** *see* Abacavir, Lamivudine, and Zidovudine *on page 52*
- **Zidovudine and Lamivudine** *see* Lamivudine and Zidovudine *on page 874*
- **Ziextenzo** *see* Pegfilgrastim *on page 1200*
- **Zilactin Baby [OTC]** *see* Benzocaine *on page 228*

Zileuton (zye LOO ton)

Related Information

Respiratory Diseases *on page 1680*

Brand Names: US Zyflo; Zyflo CR [DSC]

Pharmacologic Category 5-Lipoxygenase Inhibitor

Use

Asthma: Prophylaxis and chronic treatment of asthma in adults and children ≥12 years of age

Limitations of use: Not indicated for relief of acute bronchospasm

Local Anesthetic/Vasoconstrictor Precautions

No information available to require special precautions

Effects on Dental Treatment No significant effects or complications reported

Effects on Bleeding No information available to require special precautions

Adverse Reactions

>10%: Central nervous system: Headache (23% to 25%)

1% to 10%:

Cardiovascular: Chest pain

Central nervous system: Pain (8%), dizziness, drowsiness, hypertonia, insomnia, malaise, nervousness

Dermatologic: Pruritus, skin rash

Gastrointestinal: Dyspepsia (8%), nausea (5% to 6%), abdominal pain (5%), diarrhea (5%), constipation, flatulence, vomiting

Genitourinary: Urinary tract infection, vaginitis

Hematologic & oncologic: Leukopenia (1% to 3%), lymphadenopathy

Hepatic: Increased serum ALT (≥3 x ULN: 2% to 5%), hepatotoxicity

Hypersensitivity: Hypersensitivity reaction

Neuromuscular & skeletal: Myalgia (7%), weakness (4%), arthralgia, neck pain, neck stiffness

Ophthalmic: Conjunctivitis

Respiratory: Upper respiratory tract infection (9%), sinusitis (7%), pharyngolaryngeal pain (5%)

Miscellaneous: Fever

<1%, postmarketing, and/or case reports: Behavioral changes, hepatic failure, hepatitis, hyperbilirubinemia, jaundice, mood changes, sleep disorder, suicidal tendencies, urticaria

Mechanism of Action Specific 5-lipoxygenase inhibitor which inhibits leukotriene formation. Leukotrienes augment neutrophil and eosinophil migration, neutrophil and monocyte aggregation, leukocyte adhesion, increased capillary permeability, and smooth muscle contraction (which contribute to inflammation, edema, mucous secretion, and bronchoconstriction in the airway of the asthmatic).

Pharmacodynamics/Kinetics

Half-life Elimination ~3 hours

Time to Peak Immediate release: 1.7 hours

Pregnancy Considerations

Uncontrolled asthma is associated with adverse events in pregnancy (increased risk of perinatal mortality, preeclampsia, preterm birth, low birth weight infants, cesarean delivery, and the development of gestational diabetes). Poorly controlled asthma or asthma exacerbations may have a greater fetal/maternal risk than what is associated with appropriately used asthma medications. Maternal treatment improves pregnancy outcomes by reducing the risk of some adverse events (eg, preterm birth, gestational diabetes).

Agents other than zileuton may be preferred for the treatment of asthma during pregnancy (ERS/TSANZ [Middleton 2020]; GINA 2020).

Data collection to monitor pregnancy and infant outcomes associated with asthma and the medications used to treat asthma in pregnancy is ongoing. Health care providers are encouraged to enroll exposed pregnant females in the MotherToBaby Pregnancy Studies conducted by the Organization of Teratology

Information Specialists (1-877-311-8972 or https://mothertobaby.org). Patients may also enroll themselves.

- **Zilretta** *see* Triamcinolone (Systemic) *on page 1485*
- **Zilxi** *see* Minocycline (Topical) *on page 1036*
- **Zinacef [DSC]** *see* Cefuroxime *on page 317*
- **Zinacef in Sterile Water [DSC]** *see* Cefuroxime *on page 317*
- **Zinbryta [DSC]** *see* Daclizumab *on page 428*
- **Zingo** *see* Lidocaine (Topical) *on page 902*
- **Zionodil** *see* Lidocaine (Topical) *on page 902*
- **Zionodil 100** *see* Lidocaine (Topical) *on page 902*

Ziprasidone (zi PRAS i done)

Related Information

Clinical Risk Related to Drugs Prolonging QT Interval *on page 1675*

Brand Names: US Geodon

Brand Names: Canada Auro-Ziprasidone; Zeldox

Pharmacologic Category Second Generation (Atypical) Antipsychotic

Use

Agitation, acute associated with psychiatric disorders (IM only): Treatment of acute agitation in patients with schizophrenia for whom treatment with ziprasidone is appropriate and who need IM antipsychotic medication for rapid control of agitation. May be used off-label for the treatment of acute agitation associated with bipolar disorder (CANMAT [Yatham 2018]).

Bipolar disorder: Monotherapy for the acute treatment of manic or mixed episodes associated with bipolar disorder; for the maintenance treatment of bipolar disorder (manic or mixed episodes) as an adjunct to lithium or valproate.

Schizophrenia: Treatment of schizophrenia.

Local Anesthetic/Vasoconstrictor Precautions Ziprasidone is one of the drugs confirmed to prolong the QT interval and is accepted as having a risk of causing torsade de pointes. The risk of drug-induced torsade de pointes is extremely low when a single QT interval prolonging drug is prescribed. In terms of epinephrine, it is not known what effect vasoconstrictors in the local anesthetic regimen will have in patients with a known history of congenital prolonged QT interval or in patients taking any medication that prolongs the QT interval. Until more information is obtained, it is suggested that the clinician consult with the physician prior to the use of a vasoconstrictor in suspected patients, and that the vasoconstrictor (epinephrine, mepivacaine and levonordefrin [Carbocaine® 2% with Neo-Cobefrin®]) be used with caution.

Effects on Dental Treatment Key adverse event(s) related to dental treatment: Xerostomia and changes in salivation (normal salivary flow resumes upon discontinuation), orthostatic hypotension, tongue edema, and dysphagia.

Effects on Bleeding No information available to require special precautions

Adverse Reactions Frequencies represent oral administration unless otherwise indicated. **Note:** Although minor QTc prolongation (mean: 10 msec at 160 mg/day) may occur more frequently (incidence not specified), clinically relevant prolongation (>500 msec) was rare (0.06%) and less than placebo (0.23%).

>10%:

Central nervous system: Drowsiness (oral and IM: 8% to 31%; may be dose-related), extrapyramidal reaction (oral: 1% to 31%), headache (oral and IM: 5% to 18%), dizziness (oral and IM: 3% to 16%; includes lightheadedness; may be dose-related)

Gastrointestinal: Nausea (oral and IM: 8% to 12%)

1% to 10%:

Cardiovascular: Orthostatic hypotension (IM: ≤5%, oral: ≥1%; may be dose-related), chest pain (3%), hypertension (oral and IM: 1% to 3%), tachycardia (1% to 2%), bradycardia (oral and IM: ≤2%), facial edema (≥1%), angina pectoris (≤1%), peripheral edema (≤1%)

Central nervous system: Akathisia (oral: 8% to 10%; IM: ≤2%), anxiety (oral: 5%; may be dose-related), hypoesthesia (1% to 2%), agitation (oral: ≥1%, IM: ≤2%), personality disorder (IM: ≤2%), speech disturbance (oral and IM: ≤2%), amnesia (≥1%), ataxia (≥1%), chills (≥1%), confusion (≥1%), delirium (≥1%), dystonia (≥1%; may be dose-related), falling (≥1%), flank pain (≥1%), hostility (≥1%), hypothermia (≥1%), vertigo (≥1%), withdrawal syndrome (≥1%), anorgasmia (≤1%), atrial fibrillation (≤1%), male sexual disorder (≤1%), paralysis (≤1%), insomnia

Dermatologic: Skin rash (1% to 5%; may be dose-related), fungal dermatitis (1% to 2%), diaphoresis (IM: ≤2%), furunculosis (IM: ≤2%), skin photosensitivity (≥1%), alopecia (≤1%), contact dermatitis (≤1%), ecchymoses (≤1%), eczema (≤1%), exfoliative dermatitis (≤1%), maculopapular rash (≤1%), urticaria (≤1%), vesiculobullous dermatitis (≤1%)

Endocrine & metabolic: Weight gain (4% to 16%), albuminuria (≤1%), amenorrhea (≤1%), dehydration (≤1%), glycosuria (≤1%), hypercholesterolemia (≤1%), hyperglycemia (≤1%), hypermenorrhea (≤1%), hypokalemia (≤1%), increased lactate dehydrogenase (≤1%), increased thirst (≤1%)

Gastrointestinal: Constipation (oral: 9%, IM: ≤2%), dyspepsia (oral: 8%, IM: 2% to 3%), vomiting (oral and IM: 1% to 5%), xerostomia (oral: 4% to 5%; may be dose-related), diarrhea (oral and IM: ≤5%), sialorrhea (4%; may be dose-related), abdominal pain (oral and IM: ≤2%), anorexia (oral and IM: ≤2%; may be dose-related), dysmenorrhea (IM: ≤2%), dysphagia (≤2%), buccoglossal syndrome (≥1%)

Genitourinary: Hematuria (≤1%), impotence (≤1%), lactation (female: ≤1%), priapism (IM: ≤1%), urinary retention (≤1%)

Hematologic & oncologic: Rectal hemorrhage (oral and IM: ≤2%), anemia (≤1%), eosinophilia (≤1%), leukocytosis (≤1%), leukopenia (≤1%), lymphadenopathy (≤1%)

Hepatic: Increased serum alkaline phosphatase (≤1%), increased serum transaminases (≤1%)

Hypersensitivity: Tongue edema (≤3%)

Local: Pain at injection site (IM: 7% to 8%)

Neuromuscular & skeletal: Weakness (oral: 5% to 6%; may be dose-related), myalgia (1% to 2%), paresthesia (oral and IM: ≤2%), abnormal gait (≥1%), akinesia (≥1%), choreoathetosis (≥1%), dysarthria (≥1%), dyskinesia (≥1%), hyperkinesia (≥1%), hypokinesia (≥1%), hypotonia (≥1%), neuropathy (≥1%), tremor (≥1%; may be dose-related), twitching (≥1%), cogwheel rigidity (oral: ≥1%), hypertonia (≥1%), increased creatine phosphokinase (≤1%), tenosynovitis (≤1%)

Ophthalmic: Visual disturbance (3% to 6%; may be dose-related), diplopia (≥1%), oculogyric crisis (≥1%), blepharitis (≤1%), cataract (≤1%), conjunctivitis (≤1%), photophobia (≤1%), xerophthalmia (≤1%)
Otic: Tinnitus (≤1%)
Renal: Polyuria (≤1%)
Respiratory: Respiratory tract infection (8%), rhinitis (oral: 4%), cough (3%), pharyngitis (3%), dyspnea (1% to 2%), flu-like symptoms (oral: ≥1%), epistaxis (≤1%), pneumonia (≤1%)
Miscellaneous: Accidental injury (4%), fever (≥1%), motor vehicle accident (≥1%)

<1%, postmarketing, and/or case reports: Agranulocytosis, angioedema, arthralgia, basophilia, bundle branch block, cardiomegaly, cerebral infarction, cerebrovascular accident, cholestatic jaundice, decreased glucose tolerance, deep vein thrombophlebitis, diabetic coma, DRESS syndrome, ejaculatory disorder, facial droop, fecal impaction, female sexual disorder, first degree atrioventricular block, galactorrhea, gingival hemorrhage, gout, granulocytopenia, gynecomastia, hematemesis, hemophthalmos, hemoptysis, hepatitis, hepatomegaly, hyperchloremia, hyperkalemia, hyperreflexia, hypersensitivity reaction (including allergic dermatitis, orofacial edema), hyperthyroidism, hyperuricemia, hypocalcemia, hypochloremia, hypocholesterolemia, hypochromic anemia, hypoglycemia, hypomagnesemia, hypomania, hyponatremia, hypoproteinemia, hypothyroidism, increased blood urea nitrogen, increased gamma-glutamyl transferase, increased monocytes, increased serum creatinine, increased serum prolactin, jaundice, keratitis, keratoconjunctivitis, ketosis, laryngismus, liver steatosis, lymphedema, lymphocytosis, mania, melena, myocarditis, myoclonus, myopathy, neuroleptic malignant syndrome, neutropenia, nocturia, nystagmus, oliguria, opisthotonos, oral leukoplakia, oral paresthesia, phlebitis, polycythemia, prolonged QT interval on ECG, pulmonary embolism, respiratory alkalosis, seizure, serotonin syndrome (with or without serotonergic medications), sleep apnea syndrome (obstructive) (Health Canada 2016, Shirani 2011), Stevens-Johnson syndrome, swollen tongue, syncope, tardive dyskinesia, thrombocythemia, thrombocytopenia, thrombophlebitis, thyroiditis, torsades de pointes, torticollis, trismus, urinary incontinence, vaginal hemorrhage, venous thromboembolism, visual field defect

Mechanism of Action Ziprasidone is a benzylisothiazolylpiperazine antipsychotic. The exact mechanism of action is unknown. However, *in vitro* radioligand studies show that ziprasidone has high affinity for D_2, D_3, 5-HT_{2A}, 5-HT_{1A}, 5-HT_{2C}, 5-HT_{1D}, and alpha$_1$-adrenergic; moderate affinity for histamine H_1 receptors; and no appreciable affinity for alpha$_2$-adrenergic receptors, beta-adrenergic, 5-HT_3, 5-HT_4, cholinergic, mu, sigma, or benzodiazepine receptors. Ziprasidone functions as an antagonist at the D_2, 5-HT_{2A}, and 5-HT_{1D} receptors and as an agonist at the 5-HT_{1A} receptor. Ziprasidone moderately inhibits the reuptake of serotonin and norepinephrine.

Pharmacodynamics/Kinetics

Half-life Elimination

Oral: Mean terminal half-life:
Children: Mean: 3.3 to 4.1 hours (Sallee 2006)
Adults: 7 hours
IM: Mean half-life: 2 to 5 hours

Time to Peak

Oral: Children: Mean: 5 to 5.5 hours (Sallee 2006); Adults: 6 to 8 hours
IM: ≤60 minutes

Reproductive Considerations

Ziprasidone may cause hyperprolactinemia, which may cause a reversible reduction of reproductive function in females.

If treatment is needed in a woman planning a pregnancy, use of an agent other than ziprasidone may be preferred (Grunze 2018; Larsen 2015).

Pregnancy Considerations

Antipsychotic use during the third trimester of pregnancy has a risk for abnormal muscle movements (extrapyramidal symptoms [EPS]) and/or withdrawal symptoms in newborns following delivery. Symptoms in the newborn may include agitation, feeding disorder, hypertonia, hypotonia, respiratory distress, somnolence, and tremor; these effects may be self-limiting or require hospitalization.

The American College of Obstetricians and Gynecologists recommends that therapy during pregnancy be individualized; treatment with psychiatric medications during pregnancy should incorporate the clinical expertise of the mental health clinician, obstetrician, primary health care provider, and pediatrician. Safety data related to atypical antipsychotics during pregnancy are limited and routine use is not recommended. However, if a woman is inadvertently exposed to an atypical antipsychotic while pregnant, continuing therapy may be preferable to switching to a typical antipsychotic that the fetus has not yet been exposed to; consider risk: benefit (ACOG 2008). If treatment is initiated during pregnancy, use of an agent other than ziprasidone may be preferred (Grunze 2018; Larsen 2015).

Health care providers are encouraged to enroll women 18 to 45 years of age exposed to ziprasidone during pregnancy in the Atypical Antipsychotics Pregnancy Registry (1-866-961-2388 or https://www.womensmentalhealth.org/pregnancyregistry).

Dental Health Professional Considerations See Local Anesthetic/Vasoconstrictor Precautions

- **Ziprasidone HCl** *see* Ziprasidone *on page 1572*
- **Ziprasidone Hydrochloride** *see* Ziprasidone *on page 1572*
- **Ziprasidone Mesylate** *see* Ziprasidone *on page 1572*
- **Zipsor** *see* Diclofenac (Systemic) *on page 484*
- **Zirabev** *see* Bevacizumab *on page 242*
- **Zithromax** *see* Azithromycin (Systemic) *on page 203*
- **Zithromax TRI-PAK** *see* Azithromycin (Systemic) *on page 203*
- **Zithromax Tri-Pak** *see* Azithromycin (Systemic) *on page 203*
- **Zithromax Z-PAK** *see* Azithromycin (Systemic) *on page 203*
- **Zithromax Z-Pak** *see* Azithromycin (Systemic) *on page 203*

Ziv-Aflibercept (Systemic) (ziv a FLIB er sept)

Brand Names: US Zaltrap

Brand Names: Canada Zaltrap [DSC]

Pharmacologic Category Antineoplastic Agent, Vascular Endothelial Growth Factor (VEGF) Inhibitor; Vascular Endothelial Growth Factor (VEGF) Inhibitor

Use Colorectal cancer, metastatic: Treatment of metastatic colorectal cancer (in combination with fluorouracil, leucovorin, and irinotecan [FOLFIRI]) that is resistant to or has progressed on an oxaliplatin-based regimen.

Local Anesthetic/Vasoconstrictor Precautions Use vasoconstrictor with caution; patients may experience significant hypertension when taking Ziv-Aflibercept (Systemic)

Effects on Dental Treatment Key adverse event(s) related to dental treatment: Stomatitis has been reported in ≤50% of patients

Effects on Bleeding The risk of hemorrhage is increased; GI tract bleeding has been reported

Adverse Reactions Note: Reactions reported in combination therapy with fluorouracil, leucovorin, and irinotecan (FOLFIRI).

>10%:

Cardiovascular: Hypertension (41%)

Dermatologic: Palmar-plantar erythrodysesthesia (11%)

Endocrine & metabolic: Weight loss (32%)

Gastrointestinal: Diarrhea (69%), stomatitis (50%; grades 3/4: 13%), decreased appetite (32%), abdominal pain (27%), severe diarrhea (19%), upper abdominal pain (11%)

Genitourinary: Proteinuria (62%)

Hematologic & oncologic: Leukopenia (78%; grades 3/4: 16%), neutropenia (67%; grades 3/4: 37%), thrombocytopenia (48%; grades 3/4: 3%), hemorrhage (38%; grades 3/4: 3%)

Hepatic: Increased serum aspartate aminotransferase (62%), increased serum alanine aminotransferase (50%)

Immunologic: Antibody development (3%; neutralizing: 35%)

Infection: Infection (46%)

Nervous system: Fatigue (48%), voice disorder (25%), headache (22%)

Neuromuscular & skeletal: Asthenia (18%)

Renal: Increased serum creatinine (23%)

Respiratory: Epistaxis (28%), dyspnea (12%)

1% to 10%:

Cardiovascular: Venous thromboembolism (9%), pulmonary embolism (5%), arterial thromboembolism (3%)

Dermatologic: Hyperpigmentation (8%)

Endocrine & metabolic: Dehydration (9%)

Gastrointestinal: Hemorrhoids (6%), rectal hemorrhage (5%), rectal pain (5%), gastrointestinal hemorrhage (grades 3/4: ≤3%)

Genitourinary: Urinary tract infection (9%), hematuria (grades 3/4: ≤3%)

Hematologic & oncologic: Febrile neutropenia (grades 3/4: 4%), postprocedural hemorrhage (grades 3/4: ≤3%)

Infection: Neutropenic sepsis (grades 3/4: 2%)

Respiratory: Oropharyngeal pain (8%), rhinorrhea (6%)

Miscellaneous: Fistula formation (2%)

Frequency not defined:

Cardiovascular: Angina pectoris, cerebrovascular accident, deep vein thrombosis, transient ischemic attacks

Gastrointestinal: Tooth infection

Hematologic & oncologic: Pulmonary hemorrhage

Local: Catheter infection

Nervous system: Intracranial hemorrhage

Respiratory: Hemoptysis, nasopharyngitis, pneumonia, upper respiratory tract infection

<1%, postmarketing, and/or case reports: Cardiac failure, gastrointestinal perforation, nephrotic syndrome, osteonecrosis of the jaw, reduced ejection fraction, reversible posterior leukoencephalopathy syndrome, thrombotic microangiopathy, wound healing impairment

Mechanism of Action Ziv-aflibercept is a recombinant fusion protein which is comprised of portions of binding domains for vascular endothelial growth factor (VEGF) receptors 1 and 2, attached to the Fc portion of human IgG1. Ziv-aflibercept acts as a decoy receptor for VEGF-A, VEGF-B, and placental growth factor (PlGF) which prevent VEGF receptor binding/activation to their receptors (an action critical to angiogenesis), thus leading to antiangiogenesis and tumor regression.

Pharmacodynamics/Kinetics

Half-life Elimination ~6 days (range: 4 to 7 days)

Reproductive Considerations

Verify pregnancy status in females of reproductive potential prior to initiating ziv-aflibercept. Females of reproductive potential should use effective contraception during therapy and for 1 month following the last ziv-aflibercept dose. Ziv-aflibercept may impair reproductive function in males and females of reproductive potential.

Pregnancy Considerations

Based on the mechanism of action and data from animal reproduction studies, in utero exposure to ziv-aflibercept may cause fetal harm. Aflibercept is a vascular endothelial growth factor (VEGF) inhibitor; VEGF is required to achieve and maintain normal pregnancies (Peracha 2016).

◆ **Zmax [DSC]** *see* Azithromycin (Systemic) *on page 203*

◆ **Zocor** *see* Simvastatin *on page 1372*

◆ **Zodex 6-Day [DSC]** *see* DexAMETHasone (Systemic) *on page 463*

◆ **Zodex 12-Day [DSC]** *see* DexAMETHasone (Systemic) *on page 463*

◆ **Zofran** *see* Ondansetron *on page 1143*

◆ **Zofran ODT [DSC]** *see* Ondansetron *on page 1143*

◆ **Zol 446** *see* Zoledronic Acid *on page 1574*

◆ **Zoladex** *see* Goserelin *on page 746*

◆ **Zoledronate** *see* Zoledronic Acid *on page 1574*

Zoledronic Acid (zoe le DRON ik AS id)

Related Information

Osteonecrosis of the Jaw *on page 1699*

Rheumatoid Arthritis, Osteoarthritis, and Osteoporosis *on page 1697*

Brand Names: US Reclast; Zometa [DSC]

Brand Names: Canada Aclasta; JAMP-Zoledronic Acid; PMS-Zoledronic Acid [DSC]; TARO-Zoledronic Acid; Zoledronic Acid - Z; Zometa

Generic Availability (US) Yes

Pharmacologic Category Bisphosphonate Derivative

Use

Bone metastases, solid tumors: *Zometa*: Treatment of documented bone metastases from solid tumors (in conjunction with standard antineoplastic therapy). Prostate cancer should have progressed following treatment with at least one hormonal therapy.

Hypercalcemia of malignancy: *Zometa*: Treatment of hypercalcemia (albumin-corrected serum calcium ≥12 mg/dL) of malignancy.

Limitations of use: Safety and efficacy for treatment of hypercalcemia associated with hyperparathyroidism or with other non-tumor-related conditions have not been established.

Multiple myeloma: *Zometa*: Treatment of multiple myeloma.

Osteoporosis: *Reclast, Aclasta [Canadian product]*: Treatment and prevention of osteoporosis in postmenopausal females; treatment to increase bone mass in males with osteoporosis; treatment and prevention of glucocorticoid-induced osteoporosis in males and females.

Paget disease: *Reclast, Aclasta [Canadian product]*: Treatment of Paget disease of bone in males and females. **Note:** Zoledronic acid is considered the most efficacious bisphosphonate with respect to treating bone pain as well as suppressing metabolic bone activity. In patients without contraindications, Endocrine Society guidelines as well as some international guidelines recommend zoledronic acid as the treatment of choice (ES [Singer 2014]; Ralston 2019).

Local Anesthetic/Vasoconstrictor Precautions
No information available to require special precautions

Effects on Dental Treatment Key adverse event(s) related to dental treatment: Frequent occurrence of Candidiasis has been observed. Infrequent occurrence of mucositis, dysphagia, stomatitis, and sore throat. Rare occurrences of Stevens-Johnson syndrome and xerostomia (normal salivary flow resumes upon discontinuance) have also been reported.

Medication related osteonecrosis of the jaw (MRONJ) has been reported ranging from infrequent to rare occurrence depending on oncology versus non-oncology applications of the drug. MRONJ is generally associated with local infection and/or tooth extraction and often with delayed healing; has been reported in patients taking bisphosphonates. Symptoms included nonhealing extraction socket or an exposed jawbone. Most reported cases of bisphosphonate-associated osteonecrosis have been in cancer patients treated with intravenous bisphosphonates. However, some have occurred in patients with postmenopausal osteoporosis taking oral bisphosphonates or other antiresorptive therapies. Dental surgery, particularly tooth extraction, may increase the risk for MRONJ. Patients who develop MRONJ while on bisphosphonate therapy should receive care by an oral surgeon. See Dental Health Professional Considerations.

Effects on Bleeding Zoledronic acid has been shown to induce thrombotic thrombocytopenia purpura-hemolytic uremic syndrome (TTP-HUS). In a clinical report, zoledronic acid therapy caused acute anemia and thrombocytopenia, with reticulocyte count at 6% and bilirubin at 1.6 mg/dL, with few fragmented erythrocytes. Treatment for this thrombocytopenia complication is discontinuation of the drug and plasma exchange therapy to increase platelet count.

Adverse Reactions

Oncology indications:

>10%:

Cardiovascular: Lower extremity edema (5% to 21%), hypotension (11%)

Central nervous system: Fatigue (39%), headache (5% to 19%), dizziness (18%), insomnia (15% to 16%), depression (14%), anxiety (11% to 14%), agitation (13%), confusion (7% to 13%), hypoesthesia (12%), rigors (11%)

Dermatologic: Alopecia (12%), dermatitis (11%)

Endocrine & metabolic: Dehydration (5% to 14%), hypophosphatemia (13%), hypokalemia (12%), hypomagnesemia (11%)

Gastrointestinal: Nausea (29% to 46%), vomiting (14% to 32%), constipation (27% to 31%), diarrhea (17% to 24%), anorexia (9% to 22%), weight loss (16%), abdominal pain (14% to 16%), decreased appetite (13%)

Genitourinary: Urinary tract infection (12% to 14%)

Hematologic & oncologic: Anemia (22% to 33%), progression of cancer (16% to 20%), neutropenia (12%)

Infection: Candidiasis (12%)

Neuromuscular & skeletal: Ostealgia (55%), weakness (5% to 24%), myalgia (23%), arthralgia (5% to 21%), back pain (15%), paresthesia (15%), limb pain (14%), skeletal pain (12%)

Renal: Renal insufficiency (8% to 17%; up to 40% in patients with abnormal baseline creatinine)

Respiratory: Dyspnea (22% to 27%), cough (12% to 22%)

Miscellaneous: Fever (32% to 44%; most common symptom of acute phase reaction)

1% to 10%:

Cardiovascular: Chest pain (5% to 10%)

Central nervous system: Somnolence (5% to 10%)

Endocrine & metabolic: Hypocalcemia (5% to 10%; grades 3/4: ≤1%), hypermagnesemia (grade 3: 2%)

Gastrointestinal: Dyspepsia (10%), dysphagia (5% to 10%), mucositis (5% to 10%), sore throat (8%), stomatitis (8%)

Hematologic & oncologic: Granulocytopenia (5% to 10%), pancytopenia (5% to 10%), thrombocytopenia (5% to 10%)

Infection: Infection (nonspecific; 5% to 10%)

Renal: Increased serum creatinine (grades 3/4: ≤2%)

Respiratory: Upper respiratory tract infection (10%)

Nononcology indications:

>10%:

Cardiovascular: Hypertension (5% to 13%)

Central nervous system: Pain (2% to 24%), fever (9% to 22%), headache (4% to 20%), chills (2% to 18%), fatigue (2% to 18%), flank pain (≤2%)

Endocrine & metabolic: Hypocalcemia (≤3%; Paget disease 21%), dehydration (3%)

Gastrointestinal: Nausea (5% to 18%), upper abdominal pain (5%), abdominal distension (≤2%)

Immunologic: Infusion-related reaction (4% to 25%)

Neuromuscular & skeletal: Arthralgia (9% to 27%), myalgia (5% to 23%), back pain (4% to 18%), limb pain (3% to 16%), musculoskeletal pain (≤12%), osteoarthritis (6%)

Respiratory: Flu-like symptoms (1% to 11%)

1% to 10%:

Cardiovascular: Chest pain (1% to 8%), peripheral edema (3% to 6%), atrial fibrillation (1% to 3%), palpitations (≤3%)

Central nervous system: Dizziness (2% to 9%), rigors (8%), malaise (1% to 7%), hypoesthesia (≤6%), lethargy (3% to 5%), vertigo (1% to 4%), paresthesia (2%), hyperthermia (≤2%)

Dermatologic: Skin rash (2% to 3%), hyperhidrosis (≤3%)

Gastrointestinal: Abdominal pain (1% to 9%), diarrhea (5% to 8%), vomiting (2% to 8%), constipation (6% to 7%), dyspepsia (2% to 7%), abdominal discomfort (1% to 2%), anorexia (1% to 2%)

Hematologic & oncologic: Change in serum protein (C-reactive protein increased; ≤5%)

Neuromuscular & skeletal: Ostealgia (3% to 9%), arthritis (2% to 9%), neck pain (1% to 7%), shoulder pain (≤7%), muscle spasm (2% to 6%), weakness (2% to 6%), stiffness (1% to 5%), jaw pain (2% to 4%), joint swelling (≤3%)

Ophthalmic: Eye pain (≤2%)

Renal: Increased serum creatinine (2%)

Respiratory: Dyspnea (5% to 7%)

All indications: <1%, postmarketing, and/or case reports: Acute phase reaction-like symptoms (including pyrexia, fatigue, bone pain, arthralgia, myalgia, chills, influenza-like illness; usually resolves within 3 to 4 days of onset, although may take up to 14 days to resolve), acute renal failure (requiring hospitalization/dialysis), acute renal tubular necrosis (toxic), anaphylactic shock, anaphylaxis, angioedema, arthralgia (sometimes severe and/or incapacitating), blurred vision, bradycardia, bronchoconstriction, bronchospasm, cardiac arrhythmia, cerebrovascular accident, conjunctivitis, diaphoresis, drowsiness, dysgeusia, episcleritis, exacerbation of asthma, Fanconi syndrome (acquired), femur fracture (diaphyseal or subtrochanteric), hematuria, hyperesthesia, hyperkalemia, hypernatremia, hyperparathyroidism, hypersensitivity reaction, hypertension, injection site reaction (eg, itching, pain, redness), interstitial pulmonary disease, iridocyclitis, iritis, muscle cramps, myalgia (sometimes severe and/or incapacitating), numbness, osteonecrosis (including external auditory canal, femur, and hip), osteonecrosis of the jaw, periorbital edema, periorbital swelling, prolonged QT interval on ECG, proteinuria, pruritus, renal insufficiency, scleritis, seizure, skin rash, Stevens-Johnson syndrome, tetany, toxic epidermal necrolysis, tremor, urticaria, uveitis, weight gain, xerostomia

Dosing

Adult & Geriatric Note: Acetaminophen administration after the infusion may reduce symptoms of acute-phase (influenza-like) reactions. Establish adequate calcium and vitamin D intake (diet and/or supplement) prior to infusion when appropriate. Consider delaying therapy initiation until dental health is optimized to reduce the risk of osteonecrosis of the jaw (AAOMS [Ruggiero 2014]).

Oncology uses:

Bone metastases, solid tumors (Zometa):

IV: 4 mg once every 3 to 4 weeks.

Breast cancer or castration-resistant prostate cancer, extended dosing interval (off-label dosing): **IV:** 4 mg once every 12 weeks; dosing once every 12 weeks (versus every 4 weeks) did not result in an increased risk of skeletal events within 2 years in patients with at least 1 site of bone involvement (Himelstein 2017; Hortobagyi 2017). May consider 4 mg once every 4 weeks until bone disease is stabilized, then transition to 4 mg once every 12 weeks (Van Poznak 2020b).

Duration of therapy: May continue indefinitely in patients with breast cancer, although the optimal duration of therapy has not been established in breast cancer or prostate cancer (ASCO [Saylor 2020]; ASCO/CCO [Van Poznak 2017]).

Breast cancer, bone loss associated with aromatase inhibitor therapy in postmenopausal females (off-label use):

Note: May be used in females at elevated risk of bone loss and/or fracture (eg, T-score −2.5 or lower, prior fragility fracture, or T-score between −1 and −2.5 at high fracture risk according to a risk assessment tool (ASCO [Shapiro 2019]).

IV: 4 mg once every 6 months (ASCO [Shapiro 2019]; Brufsky 2012) **or** 5 mg once every 12 months (ASCO [Shapiro 2019]). The optimal duration of therapy has not been established; therapy is typically continued for 3 to 5 years (Brufsky 2012; Gnant 2008).

Breast cancer, early stage, adjuvant therapy in postmenopausal females (off-label use):

Note: May be considered in females with a moderate to high risk of distant recurrence (≥10%) receiving adjuvant systemic therapy (ASCO [Dhesy-Thind 2017]; Hadji 2016; Van Poznak 2020a).

IV: 4 mg once every 6 months for 3 to 5 years (ASCO [Dhesy-Thind 2017]).

Hypercalcemia of malignancy (albumin-corrected serum calcium ≥12 mg/dL) (Zometa):

Note: Asymptomatic or mildly symptomatic patients with chronic hypercalcemia may not require immediate treatment unless albumin-corrected serum calcium level is >14 mg/dL (Shane 2020).

IV: 4 mg (maximum) given as a single dose. May repeat dose after 7 days if hypercalcemia persists.

Multiple myeloma (Zometa):

Note: For use in conjunction with standard multiple myeloma therapy (ASCO [Anderson 2018]; Mhaskar 2017). May consider zoledronic acid for any patient with active multiple myeloma requiring treatment (ASCO [Anderson 2018]), although some reserve zoledronic acid for only those with osteolytic lesions, osteoporosis, or osteopenia (Berenson 2020; Lacy 2006).

IV: 4 mg once every 3 to 4 weeks (ASCO [Anderson 2018]; Rosen 2001; Rosen 2003).

Extended dosing interval (off-label dosing): **IV:** 4 mg once every 12 weeks may be considered in patients with stable/responsive disease (ASCO [Anderson 2018]; Himelstein 2017).

Duration of therapy: Continue for up to 2 years, then reassess risks and benefits; resume therapy upon relapse (ASCO [Anderson 2018]).

Prostate cancer, bone loss associated with androgen deprivation therapy (alternative agent) (off-label use):

Note: For use in males **without** bone metastases treated long-term with androgen deprivation therapy who are at elevated risk of osteoporotic fractures (eg, T-score −2.5 or lower, prior fragility fracture, or T-score between −1 and −2.5 at high fracture risk according to a risk assessment tool) (ASCO [Saylor 2020]; ASCO [Shapiro 2019]).

IV: 5 mg once every 12 months (ASCO [Shapiro 2019]; CCO [Alibhai 2017]) **or** 4 mg once every 6 to 12 months (ASCO [Shapiro 2019]; Michaelson 2007). The optimal duration of therapy has not been established; current studies provide results for up to 36 months of therapy (ASCO [Saylor 2020]; CCO [Alibhai 2017).

Nononcology uses:

Osteoporosis, prevention of fractures (alternative agent): Note: Prior to use, evaluate and treat any potential causes of secondary osteoporosis (eg, hypogonadism in males) (ES [Watts 2012]).

Males and postmenopausal females:

High fracture risk patients, including those with a history of fragility fracture ***or*** *males ≥50 years of age and postmenopausal females with a T-score −2.5 or lower or a T-score between −1 and −2.5 at high fracture risk according to a risk assessment tool* (ES [Watts 2012]; Finkelstein 2020; NOF [Cosman 2014]):

Treatment: IV: 5 mg once every 12 months (Reclast, Aclasta [Canadian product]).

Patients with T-scores between −1 and −2.5 and ***not*** *at high fracture risk according to a risk assessment tool but who desire pharmacologic therapy for prevention of bone loss and/or fracture* (Lewiecki 2020; NOF [Cosman 2014]):

Prevention: IV: 5 mg once every 2 years (Reclast) **or** 5 mg as a single (one-time) dose (Aclasta [Canadian product]).

Duration of therapy: The optimal duration of treatment has not been established. Consider discontinuing after 3 years if bone mineral density (BMD) is stable, there have been no previous fragility fractures, and short-term fracture risk is low. If fracture risk remains high (eg, fragility fracture before or during therapy), consider extending treatment for up to 6 years or switching to alternative therapy. If discontinued, the decision to resume treatment is based on multiple factors, including decline in BMD, duration of discontinuation, and risk factors for fracture (Adler 2016; ES [Eastell 2019]; Watts 2010).

Glucocorticoid-induced:

Note: For use in males ≥50 years of age and postmenopausal females with low bone mineral density (T-scores between −1 and −2.5 in either group) and expected to receive systemic glucocorticoid therapy for at least 3 months at a prednisone dose of ≥7.5 mg/day (or its equivalent) **or** in any patient whose baseline risk of fracture is high and who is receiving a glucocorticoid at any dose or duration (ACR [Buckley 2017]). In younger males and premenopausal females, patient selection must be individualized (Rosen 2020). Avoid use in females who are pregnant, who plan on becoming pregnant, or who are not using effective birth control (ACR [Buckley 2017]).

IV: 5 mg once every 12 months (Reclast, Aclasta [Canadian product]).

Duration of therapy: The optimal duration of treatment has not been established; duration should be individualized based on continuation of glucocorticoid therapy and fracture risk (ACR [Buckley 2017]; NOGG [Compston 2017]).

Paget disease (Reclast, Aclasta [Canadian product]):

Note: For symptomatic patients with active disease and select patients with asymptomatic disease at risk of future complications, or 1 to 3 months prior to planned surgery at an active pagetic site (Charles 2020; ES [Singer 2014]).

Initial: **IV:** 5 mg as a single dose.

Re-treatment: **IV:** A repeat 5 mg dose may be considered after 12 months in patients with biochemical relapse (eg, increase in alkaline phosphatase), radiographic progression of disease, or recurrent pain. Intensive re-treatment based on increased biochemical markers alone is not routinely recommended (Ralston 2019; Tan 2017).

Renal Impairment: Adult Note: Prior to each dose, obtain serum creatinine and calculate the creatinine clearance using the Cockcroft-Gault formula.

Nononcology uses: **Note:** Use actual body weight in the Cockcroft-Gault formula when calculating clearance for nononcology uses.

CrCl 35 to 80 mL/minute: No dosage adjustment is necessary; use with caution.

CrCl <35 mL/minute: Use is contraindicated.

Oncology uses:

Dosage adjustment for renal impairment *prior to* initiating zoledronic acid treatment:

Multiple myeloma and bone metastases from solid tumors:

CrCl >60 mL/minute: 4 mg (no dosage adjustment is necessary).

CrCl 50 to 60 mL/minute: Reduce dose to 3.5 mg.

CrCl 40 to 49 mL/minute: Reduce dose to 3.3 mg.

CrCl 30 to 39 mL/minute: Reduce dose to 3 mg.

CrCl <30 mL/minute: Use is not recommended.

Hypercalcemia of malignancy:

Mild to moderate impairment: No dosage adjustment is necessary.

Severe impairment (serum creatinine >4.5 mg/dL): Evaluate risk versus benefit.

Dosage adjustment for renal toxicity *during* zoledronic acid treatment:

Hypercalcemia of malignancy: Evidence of renal deterioration: Evaluate risk versus benefit.

Multiple myeloma: In patients with bone metastases, treatment should be withheld for deterioration in renal function (increase of serum creatinine ≥0.5 mg/dL in patients with normal baseline serum creatinine, or increase of ≥1 mg/dL in patients with abnormal baseline serum creatinine). Reinitiate therapy (at the same dose) when serum creatinine returns to within 10% of baseline.

American Society of Clinical Oncology (ASCO) guidelines (ASCO [Anderson 2018]) :

Renal deterioration without an apparent cause: Withhold therapy; may resume at the prior dose when renal function returns to within 10% of baseline.

Albuminuria >500 mg/24 hours (unexplained): Withhold dose until return to baseline, then reevaluate every 3 to 4 weeks; consider reinitiating with a longer infusion time of 30 minutes or longer.

Hepatic Impairment: Adult There are no dosage adjustments provided in the manufacturer's labeling (has not been studied); however, zoledronic acid is not metabolized hepatically.

Pediatric

Osteoporosis, primary or secondary: Limited data available: **Note:** Acetaminophen or ibuprofen 30 minutes prior to infusion and 6 hours after is recommended to reduce acute phase reactions (eg, flu-like symptoms including low-grade fever, nausea, myalgias, and fatigue).

Children <2 years (Bowden 2017):

First dose: IV: 0.0125 mg/kg/dose.

Maintenance (to begin 3 months after first dose): IV: 0.025 mg/kg/dose every 3 months.

Children ≥2 years and Adolescents (Bowden 2017; Munns 2007; Trejo 2016):

First dose: IV: 0.0125 mg/kg/dose.

Second dose (3 months after first dose): IV: 0.025 mg/kg/dose.

Maintenance (to begin 6 months after first dose): IV: 0.05 mg/kg/dose every 6 months; maximum dose: 4 mg/dose.

Dose adjustment based on lumbar spine bone mineral density (BMD) Z score: Children ≥2 years and Adolescents:

BMD Z score >−2: Decrease dose to 0.025 mg/kg/dose every 6 months.

BMD Z score >0: Decrease dose to 0.025 mg/kg/dose every 12 months.

Renal Impairment: Pediatric There are no pediatric dosage adjustments provided in the manufacturer's labeling; based on adult experience, dosage adjustment may be needed for mild renal impairment (ie, CrCl 35 to 60 mL/minute) and use avoided in moderate and severe impairment (ie, CrCl <35 mL/minute) and acute renal insufficiency (Bowden 2017).

Hepatic Impairment: Pediatric There are no dosage adjustments provided in the manufacturer's labeling (has not been studied); however, zoledronic acid is not metabolized hepatically.

Mechanism of Action Zoledronic acid is a bisphosphonate which inhibits bone resorption via actions on osteoclasts or on osteoclast precursors; it inhibits osteoclastic activity and skeletal calcium release induced by tumors. Decreases serum calcium and phosphorus, and increases their elimination. In osteoporosis, zoledronic acid inhibits osteoclast-mediated resorption, therefore reducing bone turnover.

Contraindications

US labeling:

Hypersensitivity to zoledronic acid or any component of the formulation; hypocalcemia (Reclast only); CrCl <35 mL/minute and in those with evidence of acute renal impairment (Reclast only).

Canadian labeling:

All indications: Hypersensitivity to zoledronic acid or other bisphosphonates, or any component of the formulation; uncorrected hypocalcemia at the time of infusion; pregnancy, breastfeeding

Nononcology uses: Additional contraindications: Use in patients with CrCl <35 mL/minute and use in patients with evidence of acute renal impairment due to an increased risk of renal failure

Documentation of allergenic cross-reactivity for bisphosphonates is limited. However, because of similarities in chemical structure and/or pharmacologic actions, the possibility of cross-sensitivity cannot be ruled out with certainty.

Warnings/Precautions Osteonecrosis of the jaw (ONJ), also referred to as medication-related osteonecrosis of the jaw (MRONJ), has been reported in patients receiving bisphosphonates. Known risk factors for MRONJ include invasive dental procedures (eg, tooth extraction, dental implants, bony surgery), cancer diagnosis, concomitant therapy (eg, chemotherapy, corticosteroids, angiogenesis inhibitors), poor oral hygiene, ill-fitting dentures, and comorbid disorders (anemia, coagulopathy, infection, preexisting dental disease). Risk may increase with duration of bisphosphonate use and/or may be reported at a greater frequency based on tumor type (eg, advanced breast cancer or multiple myeloma). According to a position paper by the American Association of Maxillofacial Surgeons (AAOMS), MRONJ has been associated with bisphosphonates and other antiresorptive agents (denosumab), and antiangiogenic agents (eg, bevacizumab, sunitinib) used for the treatment of osteoporosis or malignancy; risk is significantly higher in cancer patients receiving antiresorptive therapy compared to patients receiving osteoporosis treatment (regardless of medication used or dosing schedule). MRONJ risk is also increased with monthly IV antiresorptive therapy compared to the minimal risk associated with oral bisphosphonate use, although risk appears to increase with oral bisphosphonates when duration of therapy exceeds 4 years. The manufacturer's labeling states that there are no data to suggest whether discontinuing bisphosphonates in patients requiring invasive dental procedures reduces the risk of ONJ. The manufacturer recommends a dental exam and preventive dentistry be performed prior to placing patients with risk factors on chronic bisphosphonate therapy and that during therapy, invasive dental procedures be avoided, if possible. The AAOMS suggests that if medically permissible, initiation of IV bisphosphonates for cancer therapy should be delayed until optimal dental health is attained (if extractions are required, antiresorptive therapy should delayed until the extraction site has mucosalized or until after adequate osseous healing). Once IV bisphosphonate therapy is initiated for oncologic disease, procedures that involve direct osseous injury and placement of dental implants be avoided. Patients developing ONJ during therapy should receive care by an oral surgeon (AAOMS [Ruggiero 2014]).

Atypical femur fractures (AFF) have been reported in patients receiving bisphosphonates. The fractures include subtrochanteric femur (bone just below the hip joint) and diaphyseal femur (long segment of the thigh bone). Some patients experience prodromal pain weeks or months before the fracture occurs. It is unclear if bisphosphonate therapy is the cause for these fractures; AFFs have also been reported in patients not taking bisphosphonates, and in patients receiving glucocorticoids. Patients receiving long-term (>3 years) IV bisphosphonate therapy may be at an increased risk (Adler 2016; NOF [Cosman 2014]); however, benefits of therapy (when used for osteoporosis) generally outweigh absolute risk of AFF within the first 3 years of treatment, especially in patients with high fracture risk (Adler 2016; ES [Eastell 2019]). Patients presenting with thigh or groin pain with a history of receiving bisphosphonates should be evaluated for femur fracture. Consider interrupting bisphosphonate therapy in patients who develop a femoral shaft fracture; assess for fracture in the contralateral limb.

Severe (and occasionally debilitating) musculoskeletal (bone, joint, and/or muscle) pain have been reported during bisphosphonate treatment. The onset of pain ranged from a single day to several months. Consider discontinuing therapy in patients who experience severe symptoms; symptoms usually resolve upon discontinuation. Some patients experienced recurrence when rechallenged with the same drug or another bisphosphonate; avoid use in patients with a history of these symptoms in association with bisphosphonate therapy.

Hypocalcemia (including severe and life-threatening cases) has been reported with use; patients with Paget disease may be at significant risk for hypocalcemia after treatment with zoledronic acid (because pretreatment rate of bone turnover may be elevated); severe and life-threatening hypocalcemia has also been reported with oncology-related uses. Measure serum calcium prior to treatment initiation. Correct preexisting hypocalcemia before initiation of therapy in patients with Paget disease, osteoporosis, or oncology indications. Use with caution with other medications known to cause hypocalcemia (severe hypocalcemia may develop). Ensure adequate calcium and vitamin D supplementation during therapy. Use caution in patients with disturbances of calcium and mineral metabolism (eg, hypoparathyroidism, thyroid/parathyroid, surgery, malabsorption syndromes, excision of small intestine).

A transient acute phase reaction (eg, fever, chills, pain/myalgia, other influenza-like symptoms) may occur, typically within 3 days following the initial infusion; resolution is usually observed ~3 days after symptom onset but can take up to 14 days. Prophylactic use of acetaminophen may reduce symptoms. The incidence of symptoms may decrease with subsequent infusions.

Nononcology indications: Use is contraindicated in patients with CrCl <35 mL/minute and in patients with evidence of acute renal impairment due to an increased risk of renal failure. Do not use single doses >5 mg and do not infuse over less than 15 minutes. Obtain serum creatinine and calculate creatinine clearance (using actual body weight) with the Cockcroft-Gault formula prior to each administration.

Oncology indications: Use caution in mild to moderate renal dysfunction; dosage adjustment required. In cancer patients, do not use single doses >4 mg and do not infuse over less than 15 minutes (renal toxicity has been reported with doses >4 mg or infusions administered over less than 15 minutes). Risk factors for renal deterioration include preexisting renal insufficiency and repeated doses of zoledronic acid and other bisphosphonates. Dehydration and the use of other nephrotoxic drugs which may contribute to renal deterioration should be identified and managed. Use is not recommended in patients with severe renal impairment (serum creatinine >3 mg/dL or CrCl <30 mL/minute) and bone metastases (limited data); use in patients with hypercalcemia of malignancy and severe renal impairment (serum creatinine >4.5 mg/dL for hypercalcemia of malignancy) should only be done if the benefits outweigh the risks. Diuretics should not be used before correcting hypovolemia. Renal deterioration, resulting in renal failure and dialysis has occurred in patients treated with zoledronic acid after single and multiple infusions at recommended doses of 4 mg over 15 minutes. Assess renal function (eg, serum creatinine) prior to each dose and withhold for renal deterioration [increase in serum creatinine of 0.5 mg/dL (if baseline level normal) or increase of 1 mg/dL (if baseline level abnormal)]; treatment should be withheld until renal function returns to within 10% of baseline.

Adequate hydration is required during treatment (urine output ~2 L/day); avoid overhydration, especially in patients with heart failure. Preexisting renal compromise, severe dehydration, and concurrent use with diuretics or other nephrotoxic drugs may increase the risk for renal impairment. Single and multiple infusions in patients with both normal and impaired renal function have been associated with renal deterioration, resulting in renal failure and dialysis or death (rare). Patients with underlying moderate to severe renal impairment, increased age, concurrent use of nephrotoxic or diuretic medications, or severe dehydration prior to or after zoledronic acid administration may have an increased risk of acute renal impairment or renal failure. Others with increased risk include patients with renal impairment or dehydration secondary to fever, sepsis, gastrointestinal losses, or diuretic use. If history or physical exam suggests dehydration, treatment should not be given until the patient is normovolemic. Transient increases in serum creatinine may be more pronounced in patients with impaired renal function; consider monitoring creatinine clearance in at-risk patients taking other renally eliminated drugs.

Conjunctivitis, uveitis, episcleritis, iritis, scleritis, and orbital inflammation have been reported with zoledronic acid; patients presenting with signs of ocular inflammation may require further ophthalmologic evaluation. Ocular symptoms resolved with topical steroids in some cases. Use caution in patients with aspirin-sensitive asthma (may cause bronchoconstriction) and elderly patients (because decreased renal function occurs more commonly in elderly patients). Rare cases of urticaria and angioedema and very rare cases of anaphylactic reactions/shock have been reported. Do not administer Zometa and Reclast (Aclasta [Canadian product]) to the same patient for different indications.

Breast cancer (metastatic): The American Society of Clinical Oncology (ASCO)/Cancer Care Ontario (CCO) has updated guidelines on the role of bone-modifying agents (BMAs) in metastatic breast cancer patients (ASCO/CCO [Van Poznak 2017]). The guidelines recommend initiating a BMA (denosumab, pamidronate, zoledronic acid) in patients with metastatic breast cancer to the bone. One BMA is not recommended over another (evidence supporting one BMA over another is insufficient). The optimal duration of BMA therapy is not defined; however, the guidelines recommend continuing BMA therapy indefinitely. The analgesic effect of BMAs are modest and BMAs should not be used alone for pain management; supportive care, analgesics, adjunctive therapies, radiation therapy, surgery, and/or systemic anticancer therapy should be utilized. The ASCO/CCO guidelines are in alignment with prescribing information for dosing, renal dose adjustments, infusion times, prevention and management of osteonecrosis of the jaw, and monitoring of laboratory parameter recommendations. BMAs are not the first-line therapy for pain.

Multiple myeloma: The American Society of Clinical Oncology (ASCO) has updated guidelines on bone-modifying agents in multiple myeloma (ASCO [Anderson 2018]). Bisphosphonate (pamidronate or zoledronic acid) therapy should be initiated in patients with radiographic or imaging evidence of lytic bone disease. Bisphosphonates may also be considered in patients with pain secondary to osteolytic disease and as adjunct therapy in patients receiving other interventions for fractures or impending fractures. The guidelines support utilizing IV bisphosphonates in patients with multiple myeloma and osteopenia (osteoporosis) but no radiographic evidence of lytic bone disease. Bisphosphonates are not recommended in patients with solitary plasmacytoma, smoldering (asymptomatic) or indolent myeloma with osteopenia in the absence of lytic bone disease. Bisphosphonates are also not recommended in monoclonal gammopathy of undetermined significance unless osteopenia (osteoporosis) also is present. The guidelines recommend monthly treatment for a period of up to 2 years (less frequent dosing may be considered in patients with stable/responsive disease). After 2 years, consider discontinuing in responsive and stable patients, and reinitiate upon relapse if a new-onset skeletal-related event occurs. The ASCO guidelines are in alignment with prescribing information for dosing, renal dose adjustments, infusion times, prevention and management of osteonecrosis of the jaw, and monitoring of laboratory parameter recommendations. According to the guidelines, in patients with a serum creatinine >3 mg/dL or CrCl <30 mL/minute or extensive bone disease, an alternative bisphosphonate (pamidronate) should be used. Monitor for albuminuria every 3 to 6 months; in patients with unexplained albuminuria >500 mg/24 hours, withhold the dose until level returns to baseline, then recheck every 3 to 4 weeks. Upon reinitiation, the guidelines recommend considering increasing the zoledronic acid infusion time to at least 30 minutes; however, one study has demonstrated that extending the infusion to 30 minutes did not change the safety profile (Berenson 2011).

Survivors of adult cancers with nonmetastatic disease who have osteoporosis (T score of -2.5 or lower in femoral neck, total hip, or lumbar spine) or who are at increased risk of osteoporotic fractures, should be offered bone-modifying agents (utilizing the osteoporosis-indicated dose) to reduce the risk of fracture. For patients without hormonal responsive cancers, when clinically appropriate, estrogens may be administered along with other bone-modifying agents (ASCO [Shapiro 2019]). The choice of bone-modifying agent (eg, oral or IV bisphosphonates or subcutaneous denosumab) should be based on several factors (eg, patient preference, potential adverse effects, quality of life considerations, availability, adherence, cost). Adequate calcium and vitamin D intake, exercise (using a combination of exercise types), as well as lifestyle modifications (if indicated) should also be encouraged. According to guidelines, denosumab is preferred over bisphosphonates in men with nonmetastatic prostate cancer receiving androgen deprivation therapy; however, bisphosphonates may be considered in situations where denosumab is unavailable or contraindicated. Bisphosphonates are not recommended to reduce the risk of first bone metastasis in men with high-risk localized prostate cancer. For preventing or delaying skeletal-related events in men with metastatic castrate-resistant prostate cancer (mCRPC), either zoledronic acid (minimally symptomatic or asymptomatic disease) or denosumab (independent of symptoms) is recommended (both at bone metastasis-indicated dosages). There is not enough evidence to make a recommendation for men with castrate-sensitive prostate cancer and bone metastases. IV bisphosphonates may be considered for palliation in men with mCRPC and bone pain. Adequate calcium and vitamin D intake, exercise (using a combination of exercise types), as well as lifestyle modifications (if indicated) are also recommended (ASCO [Saylor 2020]; CCO [Alibhai 2017]).

Warnings: Additional Pediatric Considerations

Influenza-like reactions have been reported, most commonly after the first dose occurring at 12 to 48 hours after the first infusion, and may include fever, nausea and/or vomiting, myalgia, and bone pain; treatment with standard antipyretic therapy is recommended; symptoms usually do not return with subsequent doses (Bowden 2017; Högler 2004; Munns 2007).

May cause hypocalcemia; administration of a lower initial dose helps to reduce the risk and severity of hypocalcemia (Bowden 2017; Högler 2004; Munns 2007).

Drug Interactions

Metabolism/Transport Effects None known.

Avoid Concomitant Use There are no known interactions where it is recommended to avoid concomitant use.

Increased Effect/Toxicity

Zoledronic Acid may increase the levels/effects of: Deferasirox

The levels/effects of Zoledronic Acid may be increased by: Aminoglycosides; Angiogenesis Inhibitors (Systemic); Calcitonin; Nonsteroidal Anti-Inflammatory Agents; Thalidomide

Decreased Effect

The levels/effects of Zoledronic Acid may be decreased by: Proton Pump Inhibitors

Dietary Considerations

Multiple myeloma or metastatic bone lesions from solid tumors: Take daily calcium supplement (500 mg) and daily multivitamin (with 400 units vitamin D).

Osteoporosis: Ensure adequate calcium and vitamin D intake; if dietary intake is inadequate, dietary supplementation is recommended. Males and females should consume:

Calcium: 1,000 mg/day (males: 50 to 70 years) **or** 1,200 mg/day (females ≥51 years and males ≥71 years) (IOM 2011; NOF [Cosman 2014]).

Vitamin D: 800 to 1,000 int. units/day (males and females ≥50 years) (NOF 2014). Recommended Dietary Allowance (RDA): 600 int. units/day (males and females ≤70 years) **or** 800 int. units/day (males and females ≥71 years) (IOM 2011).

Paget disease: Take elemental calcium 1,500 mg/day (750 mg twice daily or 500 mg 3 times/day) and vitamin D 800 units/day, particularly during the first 2 weeks after administration.

Pharmacodynamics/Kinetics

Half-life Elimination Triphasic; Terminal: 146 hours

Reproductive Considerations

Evaluate pregnancy status prior to use. Females of reproductive potential should use effective contraception during and after treatment with zoledronic acid.

Underlying causes of osteoporosis should be evaluated and treated prior to considering bisphosphonate therapy in premenopausal women; effective contraception is recommended when bisphosphonate therapy is required (Pepe 2020). Bisphosphonates are incorporated into the bone matrix and gradually released over time. Because exposure prior to pregnancy may theoretically increase the risk of fetal harm, most sources recommend discontinuing bisphosphonate therapy in females of reproductive potential as early as possible prior to a planned pregnancy. Use in premenopausal females should be reserved for special circumstances when rapid bone loss is occurring; a bisphosphonate with the shortest half-life should be then used (Bhalla 2010; Pereira 2012; Stathopoulos 2011).

Oral bisphosphonates can be considered for the prevention of glucocorticoid-induced osteoporosis in premenopausal females with moderate to high risk of fracture who do not plan to become pregnant during the treatment period and are using effective birth control (or are not sexually active); intravenous therapy should be reserved for high risk patients only (ACR [Buckley 2017]).

Pregnancy Considerations

It is not known if bisphosphonates cross the placenta, but fetal exposure is expected (Djokanovic 2008; Stathopoulos 2011).

Information specific to zoledronic acid exposure during pregnancy is limited (Djokanovic 2008; Richa 2018). Bisphosphonates are incorporated into the bone matrix and gradually released over time. The amount available in the systemic circulation varies by dose and duration of therapy. Theoretically, there may be a risk of fetal harm when pregnancy follows the completion of therapy; however, available data have not shown that exposure to bisphosphonates during pregnancy significantly increases the risk of adverse fetal events (Djokanovic 2008; Green 2014; Levy 2009; Machairiotis 2019; Sokol 2019; Stathopoulos 2011). Because hypocalcemia has been described following in utero bisphosphonate exposure, exposed infants should be monitored for hypocalcemia after birth (Djokanovic 2008; Stathopoulos 2011).

Breastfeeding Considerations

It is not known if zoledronic acid is present in breast milk.

According to the manufacturer, the decision to breastfeed during therapy should consider the risk of infant exposure, the benefits of breastfeeding to the infant, and the benefits of treatment to the mother.

Dosage Forms: US

Concentrate, Intravenous:
Generic: 4 mg/5 mL (5 mL)

Concentrate, Intravenous [preservative free]:
Generic: 4 mg/5 mL (5 mL)

Solution, Intravenous:
Generic: 4 mg/100 mL (100 mL)

Solution, Intravenous [preservative free]:
Reclast: 5 mg/100 mL (100 mL)
Generic: 4 mg/100 mL (100 mL); 5 mg/100 mL (100 mL)

Dosage Forms: Canada

Concentrate, Intravenous:
Zometa: 4 mg/5 mL (5 mL)
Generic: 4 mg/5 mL (5 mL)

Solution, Intravenous:
Aclasta: 5 mg/100 mL (100 mL)
Generic: 5 mg/100 mL (100 mL)

Dental Health Professional Considerations Zoledronic acid (Reclast) is administered once annually for the treatment of osteoporosis. A single, large prospective, placebo-controlled study established its efficacy for this indication through 3 years of treatment (Black 2007). Two cases of ONJ were reported, one each in the treatment and control groups, suggesting a low risk of ONJ with this treatment protocol through 3 years.

The American Association of Oral and Maxillofacial Surgeons position paper on bisphosphonate-related osteonecrosis of the jaws, 2009 update, stated that IV bisphosphonate exposure in the setting of managing malignancy remains the major risk factor for the development of ONJ. After reviewing case series, case-controlled studies, and cohort studies, the estimates of the cumulative incidence of IV bisphosphonate-associated ONJ ranges from 0.8% to 12%.

Two reports have attempted to assess more accurately the percent of cancer patients developing ONJ after bisphosphonate treatment. Maerevoet et al, reported that among 194 patients treated with Zometa every 3 to 4 weeks, nine developed ONJ. Before receiving Zometa, six had received Aredia 90 mg every 3 to 4 weeks. The median duration of treatment with Aredia was 39 months and for Zometa 18 months. The incidence of ONJ in these patients was calculated to be 4.6%. Durie et al, described the results of a survey by the International Myeloma Foundation in 2004 to assess the risk factors of ONJ. Out of 1,203 respondents, 904 had myeloma and 299 had breast cancer. Of the myeloma patients, 62 developed ONJ and 54 had suspicious findings. Of the breast cancer patients, 13 had ONJ and 23 had suspicious findings. The total number of cases of either ONJ or suspicious findings was 152. ONJ developed in 10% of 211 patients receiving Zometa compared to 4% of 413 receiving Aredia. The mean time to onset of ONJ among patients taking Zometa was 18 months; the mean time to onset after Aredia was 6 years. It should be noted that an early report by authors from Novartis Pharmaceuticals Corporation stressed that Aredia and Zometa had been used in 2.5 million patients world wide and reports of ONJ during their extensive use had been rare (Tarassoff 2003). In addition, these authors stated that review of the reported cases revealed multiple risk factors for avascular necrosis. McMahon et al, followed up with a report that, along with other factors, bisphosphonates are additional stressors of bone health that can tip the balance to osteonecrosis. They suggested that the prevention of ONJ should be stressed such as the elimination of chronic dental infections prior to chemotherapy and bisphosphonate use in cancer patients.

The most comprehensive review to date on osteonecrosis of the jaw bone (ONJ) has been published in the *Journal of Bone and Mineral Research* (Khan 2015), and written by an International Task Force of authors, totaling 34, from academe; industry; clinical medical and dental practice; oral and maxillofacial surgery; bone and mineral research; epidemiology; medical and dental oncology; orthopedic surgery; osteoporosis research; muscle and bone research; endocrinology and diagnostic sciences. The work provides a systematic review of the literature and international consensus on the classification, incidence, pathophysiology, diagnosis, and management of ONJ in both oncology and osteoporosis patient populations. This review of the literature from January 2003 to April 2014, with 299 references, offers recommendations for management of ONJ based on multidisciplinary international consensus.

Incidence of ONJ in oncology patients from the Task Force report:

The incidence of ONJ ranges from 1% to 15% in the oncology patient population where high doses of BPs are used at frequent intervals. The oncology patient with bone metastasis is exposed to more osteoclastic inhibition than those with osteoporosis, thus the incidence of ONJ is much higher.

◆ **Zolinza** *see* Vorinostat *on page* 1554

ZOLMitriptan (zohl mi TRIP tan)

Related Information

Temporomandibular Dysfunction (TMD), Chronic Pain, and Fibromyalgia *on page* 1773

Brand Names: US Zomig; Zomig ZMT

Brand Names: Canada AG-Zolmitriptan; APO-Zolmitriptan; APO-Zolmitriptan Rapid; AURO-Zolmitriptan; CCP-Zolmitriptan; DOM-Zolmitriptan; JAMP Zolmitriptan; JAMP-Zolmitriptan; JAMP-Zolmitriptan ODT; Mar-Zolmitriptan; MINT-Zolmitriptan; MINT-Zolmitriptan ODT [DSC]; MYLAN-Zolmitriptan ODT [DSC]; MYLAN-Zolmitriptan [DSC]; NAT-Zolmitriptan; PMS-Zolmitriptan; PMS-Zolmitriptan ODT; RIVA-Zolmitriptan [DSC]; SANDOZ Zolmitriptan; SANDOZ Zolmitriptan ODT; Septa Zolmitriptan-ODT; TEVA-Zolmitriptan; TEVA-Zolmitriptan OD; VAN-Zolmitriptan ODT [DSC]; Zomig; Zomig Rapimelt

Pharmacologic Category Antimigraine Agent; Serotonin 5-$HT_{1B, 1D}$ Receptor Agonist

Use Migraines:

Nasal inhalation: Acute treatment of migraine with or without aura in adults and pediatric patients ≥12 years.

Oral: Acute treatment of migraine with or without aura in adults.

Local Anesthetic/Vasoconstrictor Precautions No information available to require special precautions

Effects on Dental Treatment Key adverse event(s) related to dental treatment: Xerostomia (normal salivary flow resumes upon discontinuation) and dysphagia.

Effects on Bleeding No information available to require special precautions

Adverse Reactions

>10%: Gastrointestinal: Unpleasant taste (nasal: adults: 17% to 21%; children & adolescents: 6% to 10%)

1% to 10%:

Cardiovascular: Chest pain (oral: 2% to 4%), chest pressure (nasal: 1% to <2%), facial edema (nasal: 1% to <2%), palpitations (nasal: 1% to <2%), cardiac arrhythmia (≤1%), hypertension (≤1%), syncope (≤1%), tachycardia (≤1%)

Central nervous system: Dizziness (adults: 6% to 10%; children & adolescents: 2%), paresthesia (5% to 10%), drowsiness (4% to 8%), local alterations in temperature sensations (oral: 5% to 7%), sensation of pressure (oral: 2% to 5%), hyperesthesia (nasal: 1% to 5%), (1% to 5%), flushing sensation (nasal: 4%), pain (nasal: 2% to 4%), vertigo (oral: 2%), chills (nasal: 1% to <2%), depersonalization (nasal: 1% to <2%), headache (1% to <2%), agitation (≤1%), amnesia (≤1%), anxiety (≤1%), depression (≤1%), emotional lability (oral: ≤1%), insomnia (≤1%), nervousness (nasal: ≤1%)

Dermatologic: Diaphoresis (oral: 2% to 3%), pruritus (≤1%), skin rash (≤1%), urticaria (≤1%)

Gastrointestinal: Nausea (adults: 4% to 9%; children & adolescents: 2%), xerostomia (2% to 5%), dyspepsia (oral: 2% to 3%), dysphagia (1% to 2%), abdominal pain (nasal: 1% to <2%), vomiting (1% to <2%)

Genitourinary: Urinary frequency (oral: ≤1%), urinary urgency (≤1%)

Hypersensitivity: Hypersensitivity reaction (≤1%)

Local: Local pain (4% to 10%; neck/throat/jaw), application site irritation (nasal: 3%)

Neuromuscular & skeletal: Weakness (oral: 5% to 9%; nasal: 3%), arthralgia (nasal: 1% to <2%), myalgia (nasal: 1% to <2%)

Otic: Tinnitus (≤1%)

Renal: Polyuria (≤1%)

Respiratory: Nasal discomfort (nasal: 3%), constriction of the pharynx (nasal: 2%), pressure on pharynx (nasal: 1% to <2%), bronchitis (nasal: ≤1%), cough (nasal: ≤1%), dyspnea (nasal: ≤1%), epistaxis (nasal: ≤1%), laryngeal edema (nasal: ≤1%), pharyngitis (nasal: ≤1%), rhinitis (nasal: ≤1%), sinusitis (nasal: ≤1%)

<1%, postmarketing, and/or case reports: Abnormal dreams, abnormality in thinking, altered sense of smell, amblyopia, anaphylactoid reaction, anaphylaxis, angina pectoris, angioedema, apathy, ataxia, atrial fibrillation, back pain, bradycardia, breast carcinoma, breast neoplasm, bruise, cellulitis, cerebral ischemia, colitis, confusion, conjunctivitis, constipation, convulsions, coronary artery vasospasm, cyanosis, cyst, cystitis, diarrhea, dry eye syndrome, dysmenorrhea, eczema, eructation, erythema, erythema multiforme, euphoria, eye pain, fever, fibrocystic breast disease, flu-like symptoms, gastritis, gastrointestinal carcinoma, gastrointestinal infarction, gastrointestinal necrosis, genitourinary neoplasm, gingivitis, hallucination, hepatic neoplasm, hiccups, hypertensive crisis, hyperthyroidism, hypertonia, hyperventilation, increased appetite, increased bronchial secretions, increased thirst, infection, intestinal obstruction, irritability, ischemic colitis, ischemic heart disease, lacrimation, laryngitis, leukopenia, mania, menorrhagia, myocardial infarction, neoplasm, neuropathy, otalgia, photophobia, pneumonia, psychosis, pyelonephritis, renal pain, salivation, seizure, serotonin syndrome, sialadenitis, skin neoplasm, splenic infarction, stomatitis, tardive dyskinesia, tenosynovitis, thrombophlebitis, thyroid edema, tongue edema, tremor, twitching, urinary tract infection, uterine fibroid enlargement, uterine hemorrhage, vaginitis, vasodilation, ventricular fibrillation, ventricular tachycardia, visual field defect, voice disorder, yawning

Mechanism of Action Selective agonist for serotonin (5-HT_{1B} and 5-HT_{1D} receptors) in cranial arteries and sensory nerves of the trigeminal system; causes vasoconstriction and reduces inflammation associated with antidromic neuronal transmission correlating with relief of migraine

Pharmacodynamics/Kinetics

Half-life Elimination 3 hours

Time to Peak Serum: Tablet: 1.5 hours; Orally-disintegrating tablet and nasal spray: 3 hours

Pregnancy Considerations

Information related to zolmitriptan use in pregnancy is limited in comparison to other medications in this class (Källén 2011; Nezvalová-Henriksen 2010; Nezvalová-Henriksen 2012; Nezvalová-Henriksen 2013; Spielmann 2018).

Until additional information is available, other agents are preferred for the initial treatment of migraine in pregnancy (MacGregor 2014; Worthington 2013).

◆ **Zoloft** *see* Sertraline *on page 1367*

◆ **Zolpak** *see* Econazole *on page 542*

Zolpidem (zole PI dem)

Brand Names: US Ambien; Ambien CR; Edluar; Intermezzo; Zolpimist

Brand Names: Canada APO-Zolpidem ODT; PMS-Zolpidem ODT; Sublinox

Pharmacologic Category Hypnotic, Miscellaneous

Use Insomnia:

IR and sublingual tablets (Edluar only) and oral spray: Short-term treatment of insomnia with difficulty of sleep onset.

ER tablet: Treatment of insomnia with difficulty of sleep onset and/or sleep maintenance.

Sublingual tablet (Intermezzo only): As-needed treatment of insomnia when middle-of-the-night awakening is followed by difficulty returning to sleep and the patient has ≥4 hours of sleep time remaining.

Sublingual tablet (Sublinox only [Canadian product]): Short-term treatment of insomnia (with difficulty of sleep onset, frequent awakenings, and/or early awakenings).

Local Anesthetic/Vasoconstrictor Precautions No information available to require special precautions

Effects on Dental Treatment Key adverse event(s) related to dental treatment: Xerostomia (normal salivary flow resumes upon discontinuation) (see Dental Health Professional Considerations)

Effects on Bleeding No information available to require special precautions

Adverse Reactions As reported with oral administration, unless otherwise noted.

>10%: Central nervous system: Headache (oral: 7% to 19%; sublingual: 3%), drowsiness (2% to 15%), dizziness (1% to 12%)

1% to 10%:

Cardiovascular: Palpitations (2%), chest discomfort (1%), chest pain (1%), increased blood pressure (1%), edema (≤1%), hypertension (≤1%), orthostatic hypotension (≤1%), syncope (≤1%), tachycardia (≤1%)

Central nervous system: Anxiety (2% to 6%), hallucination (4%), disorientation (3%), fatigue (oral: 3%; sublingual: 1%), intoxicated feeling (3%), lethargy (3%), memory impairment (3%), balance impairment (2%), depression (2%), disturbance in attention (2%), hypoesthesia (2%), psychomotor retardation (2%), vertigo (2%), confusion (>1%), euphoria (>1%), insomnia (>1%), abnormal dreams (1%), amnesia (1%), ataxia (1%), depersonalization (1%), disinhibition (1%), eating disorder (1%; binge eating), increased body temperature (1%), paresthesia (1%), sleep disorder (1%), stress (1%), agitation (≤1%), cerebrovascular disease (≤1%), cognitive dysfunction (≤1%), dysarthria (≤1%), emotional lability (≤1%), falling (≤1%), illusion (≤1%), malaise (≤1%), migraine (≤1%), nervousness (≤1%), speech disturbance (≤1%), stupor (≤1%)

Dermatologic: Skin rash (1% to 2%), diaphoresis (≤1%), pallor (≤1%), pruritus (≤1%), urticaria (≤1%), wrinkling of skin (1%)

Endocrine & metabolic: Heavy menstrual bleeding (1%), hyperglycemia (≤1%), increased thirst (≤1%), menstrual disease (≤1%)

Gastrointestinal: Nausea (7%), xerostomia (3%), diarrhea (1% to 3%), constipation (2%), dyspepsia (>1%), hiccups (>1%), abdominal distress (1%), abdominal tenderness (1%), change in appetite (1%), frequent bowel movements (1%), gastroenteritis (1%), gastroesophageal reflux disease (1%), vomiting (1%), anorexia (≤1%), dysgeusia (≤1%), dysphagia (≤1%), flatulence (≤1%)

Genitourinary: Urinary tract infection (>1%), cystitis (≤1%), urinary incontinence (≤1%), vaginitis (≤1%)

Hematologic & oncologic: Bruise (1%)

Hepatic: Abnormal hepatic function tests (≤1%), increased serum alanine aminotransferase (≤1%)

Hypersensitivity: Hypersensitivity reaction (4%)

Infection: Influenza (3%), infection (≤1%)

Neuromuscular & skeletal: Myalgia (4%), back pain (3% to 4%), arthralgia (>1%), asthenia (1%), neck pain (1%), arthritis (≤1%), lower limb cramp (≤1%), tremor (≤1%)

Ophthalmic: Visual disturbance (1% to 3%; including altered depth perception), blurred vision (2%), eye redness (2%), diplopia (>1%), asthenopia (1%), eye irritation (≤1%), eye pain (≤1%), scleritis (≤1%)

Otic: Labyrinthitis (1%), tinnitus (1%)

Respiratory: Sinusitis (4%), pharyngitis (3%), flu-like symptoms (1% to 2%), lower respiratory tract infection (>1%), upper respiratory tract infection (>1%), throat irritation (1%), bronchitis (≤1%), cough (≤1%), dyspnea (≤1%), rhinitis (≤1%)

Miscellaneous: Fever (≤1%), trauma (≤1%)

<1%, postmarketing, and/or case reports: Abnormal gait, abnormal lacrimation, abnormality in thinking, abscess, accommodation disturbance, acne vulgaris, acute myocardial infarction, acute renal failure, aggressive behavior, alteration of saliva, altered sense of smell, anaphylactic shock, anaphylaxis, anemia, angina pectoris, angioedema, apathy, arteritis, behavioral changes, breast fibroadenosis, breast neoplasm, bronchospasm, bullous rash, cardiac arrhythmia, central nervous system depression, cholestatic hepatitis, circulatory shock, complex sleep-related disorder, conjunctivitis, corneal ulcer, decreased libido, delusion, dementia, dental caries, dermatitis, drug tolerance, drug withdrawal, dysphasia, dysuria, enteritis, epistaxis, eructation, esophageal spasm, exacerbation of hypertension, extrasystoles, facial edema, flushing, furunculosis, gastritis, glaucoma, gout, hemorrhoids, hepatic injury, hepatocellular hepatitis, herpes simplex infection, herpes zoster infection, hot flash, hyperbilirubinemia, hypercholesteremia, hyperhemoglobinemia, hyperlipidemia, hypokinesia, hypotension, hypotonia, hypoxia, hysteria, impotence, increased appetite, increased blood urea nitrogen, increased erythrocyte sedimentation rate, increased serum alkaline phosphatase, increased serum aspartate aminotransferase, intestinal obstruction, laryngitis, leukopenia, lymphadenopathy, macrocytic anemia, manic reaction, mastalgia, myasthenia, neuralgia, neuritis, neuropathy, neurosis, nocturia, numbness of tongue, osteoarthritis, otitis externa, otitis media, pain, panic disorder, paresis, periorbital edema, personality disorder, phlebitis, photopsia, pneumonia, polyuria, pulmonary edema, pulmonary embolism, purpuric disease, pyelonephritis, rectal hemorrhage, renal pain, respiratory depression, restless leg syndrome, rigors, sciatica, sialorrhea, skin photosensitivity, strange feeling, suicidal ideation, suicidal tendencies, tendonitis, tenesmus, tetany, thrombosis, urinary frequency, urinary retention, varicose veins, ventricular tachycardia, weight loss, yawning

Mechanism of Action Zolpidem, an imidazopyridine hypnotic that is structurally dissimilar to benzodiazepines, enhances the activity of the inhibitory neurotransmitter, γ-aminobutyric acid (GABA), via selective agonism at the benzodiazepine-1 (BZ_1) receptor; the result is increased chloride conductance, neuronal hyperpolarization, inhibition of the action potential, and a decrease in neuronal excitability leading to sedative and hypnotic effects. Because of its selectivity for the BZ_1 receptor site over the BZ_2 receptor site, zolpidem exhibits minimal anxiolytic, myorelaxant, and anticonvulsant properties (effects largely attributed to agonism at the BZ_2 receptor site).

Pharmacodynamics/Kinetics

Onset of Action Immediate release: 30 minutes.

Duration of Action Immediate release: 6 to 8 hours.

Half-life Elimination

Children 2 to 6 years: Immediate release: 1.8 hours (Blumer 2008).

Children >6 years and Adolescents: Immediate release: 2.3 hours (Blumer 2008).

Adults:

Immediate release, Extended release: ~2.5 hours (range: 1.4 to 4.5 hours); Cirrhosis: Up to 9.9 hours; Elderly: Prolonged up to 32%.

Spray: ~3 hours (range: 1.7 to 8.4).

Sublingual tablet: ~3 hours (range: 1.4 to 6.7 hours).

Time to Peak

Children 2 to 6 years: Immediate release: 0.9 hours (Blumer 2008).

Children >6 to 12 years: Immediate release: 1.1 hours (Blumer 2008).

Adolescents: Immediate release: 1.3 hours (Blumer 2008).

Adults:

Immediate release: 1.6 hours; 2.2 hours with food.

Extended release: 1.5 hours; 4 hours with food.

Spray: ~0.9 hours.

Sublingual tablet: Edluar: ~1.4 hours, ~1.8 hours with food; Intermezzo: 0.6 to 1.3 hours, ~3 hours with food.

Pregnancy Considerations Zolpidem crosses the placenta (Juric 2009).

Severe neonatal respiratory depression and sedation have been reported when zolpidem was used at the end of pregnancy, especially when used concurrently with other CNS depressants. Children born of mothers taking sedative/hypnotics may be at risk for withdrawal; neonatal flaccidity has been reported in infants following maternal use of sedative/hypnotics during pregnancy. Additional adverse effects to the fetus/newborn have been noted in some studies (Sharma 2011; Wang 2010; Wikner 2011). Exposed neonates should be monitored for excess sedation, hypotonia, and respiratory depression.

Controlled Substance C-IV

Dental Health Professional Considerations An adult companion should accompany the patient to and from dental office.

◆ **Zolpidem Tartrate** *see* Zolpidem *on page 1582*

◆ **Zolpimist** *see* Zolpidem *on page 1582*

◆ **Zomacton** *see* Somatropin *on page 1381*

◆ **Zomacton (for Zoma-Jet 10)** *see* Somatropin *on page 1381*

◆ **Zometa [DSC]** *see* Zoledronic Acid *on page 1574*

◆ **Zomig** *see* ZOLMitriptan *on page 1581*

◆ **Zomig ZMT** *see* ZOLMitriptan *on page 1581*

◆ **ZonaCort 7 Day [DSC]** *see* DexAMETHasone (Systemic) *on page 463*

◆ **ZonaCort 11 Day [DSC]** *see* DexAMETHasone (Systemic) *on page 463*

◆ **Zonalon** *see* Doxepin (Topical) *on page 519*

◆ **Zonegran** *see* Zonisamide *on page 1584*

Zonisamide (zoe NIS a mide)

Brand Names: US Zonegran

Pharmacologic Category Anticonvulsant, Miscellaneous

Use Focal (partial) onset seizures: Adjunctive therapy in the treatment of focal onset seizures in adolescents >16 years of age and adults.

Local Anesthetic/Vasoconstrictor Precautions No information available to require special precautions

Effects on Dental Treatment Key adverse event(s) related to dental treatment: Xerostomia (normal salivary flow resumes upon discontinuation) and abnormal taste.

Effects on Bleeding No information available to require special precautions

Adverse Reactions Frequency not always defined. Frequencies noted in patients receiving other anticonvulsants:

>10%:

Central nervous system: Drowsiness (17%), dizziness (13%)

Gastrointestinal: Anorexia (13%)

1% to 10%:

Cardiovascular: Facial edema (1%)

Central nervous system: Headache (10%), agitation (9%), irritability (9%), fatigue (7% to 8%), tiredness (7%), confusion (6%), depression (6%), insomnia (6%), lack of concentration (6%), memory impairment (6%), speech disturbance (2% to 5%), ataxia (≥1% to 6%), decreased mental acuity (4%), anxiety (3%), nervousness (2%), schizophreniform disorder (2%),convulsions (≥1%), hyperesthesia (≥1%), seizure (1%), status epilepticus (1%), hypotonia (≤1%), hyperthermia

Dermatologic: Skin rash (1% to 3%), bruising (2%), pruritus (≥1%), hypohidrosis (children), Stevens-Johnson syndrome, toxic epidermal necrolysis

Endocrine & metabolic: Metabolic acidosis

Gastrointestinal: Nausea (9%), abdominal pain (6%), diarrhea (5%), dyspepsia (3%), weight loss (3%), constipation (2%), dysgeusia (2%), xerostomia (2%), vomiting (≥1%)

Hematologic & oncologic: Agranulocytosis, aplastic anemia

Neuromuscular & skeletal: Paresthesia (4%), abnormal gait (≥1%), tremor (≥1%), weakness (≥1%)

Ophthalmic: Diplopia (6%), nystagmus (4%), amblyopia (≥1%)

Otic: Tinnitus (≥1%)

Renal: Nephrolithiasis (4%, children 3% to 8%), increased blood urea nitrogen

Respiratory: Rhinitis (2%), increased cough (≥1%), pharyngitis (≥1%)

Miscellaneous: Flu-like syndrome (4%), accidental injury (≥1%)

<1%, postmarketing, and/or case reports: Abnormal dreams, acne vulgaris, albuminuria, alopecia, altered sense of smell, amenorrhea, anemia, aphthous stomatitis, apnea, arthralgia, arthritis, atrial fibrillation, bladder calculus, bladder pain, bradycardia, brain disease, cardiac failure, cerebrovascular accident, chest pain, cholangitis, cholecystitis, cholelithiasis, cholestatic jaundice, colitis, conjunctivitis, deafness, decreased libido, dehydration, diaphoresis, DRESS syndrome, duodenitis, dysarthria, dyskinesia, dysphagia, dyspnea, dystonia, dysuria, eczema, edema, esophagitis, euphoria, facial paralysis, fecal incontinence, flank pain, flatulence, gastritis, gastroenteritis, gastrointestinal ulcer, gingival hemorrhage, gingival hyperplasia, gingivitis, glaucoma, glossitis, gynecomastia, hematemesis, hematuria, hemoptysis, hirsutism, hyperkinesia, hypermenorrhea, hyperreflexia, hypersensitivity reaction, hypertension, hypertonia, hypoglycemia, hypokinesia, hyponatremia, hypotension, immunodeficiency, impotence, increased creatine phosphokinase, increased lactic dehydrogenase, increased serum alkaline phosphatase, increased serum ALT, increased serum creatinine, increased thirst, iritis, leg cramps, leukopenia, lupus erythematosus, lymphadenopathy, maculopapular rash, malaise, mastitis, melena, microcytic anemia, movement disorder, myalgia, myasthenia, myoclonus, neck stiffness, neuropathy, nocturia, oculogyric crisis, oral mucosa ulcer, palpitation, pancreatitis, peripheral edema, peripheral neuritis, petechia, photophobia, polyuria, psychomotor disturbance, pulmonary embolism, pustular rash, rectal hemorrhage, rhabdomyolysis, stomatitis, suicidal behavior, suicidal ideation, syncope, tachycardia, thrombocytopenia, thrombophlebitis, twitching, urinary frequency, urinary incontinence, urinary incontinence, urinary retention, urinary urgency, urticaria, vascular insufficiency,

ventricular premature contractions, vertigo, vesiculobullous dermatitis, visual field defect, weight gain, xeroderma

Mechanism of Action Stabilizes neuronal membranes and suppresses neuronal hypersynchronization through action at sodium and calcium channels; does not affect GABA activity.

Pharmacodynamics/Kinetics

Half-life Elimination Plasma: ~63 hours (range: 50 to 68 hours)

Time to Peak 2 to 6 hours

Reproductive Considerations

Women of childbearing potential are advised to use effective contraception during therapy.

Pregnancy Considerations

Zonisamide crosses the placenta and can be detected in the newborn following delivery (Kawada 2002; Shimoyama 1999). Information related to pregnancy outcomes following maternal use of zonisamide is limited (Hernández-Díaz 2014; Kanemoto 2007; Kondo 1996; Ohtahara 2007). Metabolic acidosis is an adverse effect of zonisamide therapy; newborns exposed to zonisamide in utero should be monitored for transient metabolic acidosis after birth and pregnant women taking zonisamide should be monitored and treated as nonpregnant patients. In general, maternal polytherapy with antiepileptic drugs may increase the risk of congenital malformations; monotherapy with the lowest effective dose is recommended. Newborns of women taking antiepileptic medications may be at an increased risk of adverse events (Harden and Meader 2009).

Zonisamide clearance may increase during pregnancy, requiring dosage adjustment (Oles 2008; Reisinger 2013). Until additional data is available, other agents may be preferred for the treatment of epilepsy in pregnant women (Ohtahara 2007).

Patients exposed to zonisamide during pregnancy are encouraged to enroll themselves into the NAAED Pregnancy Registry by calling 1-888-233-2334. Additional information is available at http://www.aedpregnancyregistry.org.

◆ **Zontivity** *see* Vorapaxar *on page 1551*

Zopiclone (ZOE pi clone)

Brand Names: Canada ACT Zopiclone; AG-Zopiclone; APO-Zopiclone; BIO-Zopiclone; DOM-Zopiclone; Imovane; JAMP-Zopiclone; M-Zopiclone; Mar-Zopiclone; MINT-Zopiclone; MYLAN-Zopiclone [DSC]; NRA-Zopiclone; PHL-Zopiclone [DSC]; PMS-Zopiclone; Priva-Zopiclone; PRO-Zopiclone; RATIO-Zopiclone; RIVA-Zopiclone; SANDOZ Zopiclone; Septa-Zopiclone; TARO-Zopiclone

Pharmacologic Category Hypnotic, Miscellaneous

Use Note: Not approved in the US

Insomnia: Short-term and symptomatic relief of insomnia (typically treatment should not exceed 7 to 10 consecutive days).

Local Anesthetic/Vasoconstrictor Precautions No information available to require special precautions

Effects on Dental Treatment Key adverse event(s) related to dental treatment: Coated tongue, dry mouth, halitosis, taste alteration (bitter taste, common).

Effects on Bleeding No information available to require special precautions

Adverse Reactions Frequency not defined. Some incidences tend to be higher in geriatric patients.

Cardiovascular: Palpitations

Central nervous system: Aggressiveness behavior, anxiety, bitter taste, confusion, daytime sedation, depression, dizziness, drowsiness, dysgeusia, euphoria, hypotonia, intoxicated feeling, memory impairment, nervousness, speech disturbance

Dermatological: Diaphoresis

Gastrointestinal: Anorexia, constipation, coated tongue, halitosis, increased appetite, sialorrhea, xerostomia

Neuromuscular & skeletal: Asthenia, tremor

<1%, postmarketing, and/or case reports: Abnormal behavior, abnormality in thinking, agitation, anaphylactoid reaction, anaphylaxis, angioedema, anterograde amnesia, ataxia, delusions, depersonalization, diplopia, disinhibition, disturbance in attention, drug dependence, dyspepsia, hallucination, hostility, increased serum alkaline phosphatase, increased serum transaminases, irritability, lack of concentration, myasthenia, nightmares, paresthesia, psychotic symptoms, rebound insomnia, respiratory depression, restlessness, sleep disorder (complex sleep-related behaviors, usually without recall of the event; includes sleep driving, sleep eating, preparing food, and making telephone calls while not fully awake), somnambulism, withdrawal syndrome

Mechanism of Action Zopiclone is a cyclopyrrolone derivative and has a pharmacological profile similar to benzodiazepines. Zopiclone reduces sleep latency, increases duration of sleep, and decreases the number of nocturnal awakenings.

Pharmacodynamics/Kinetics

Half-life Elimination ~5 hours; Elderly: ~7 hours; Hepatic impairment: ~12 hours

Time to Peak Serum: <2 hours; Hepatic impairment: 3.5 hours

Pregnancy Considerations Use is not recommended during pregnancy. Benzodiazepines may cause congenital malformations during the first trimester and neonatal CNS depression during the last few weeks of pregnancy; it is expected zopiclone may do the same.

Product Availability Not available in the US

◆ **Zorbtive** *see* Somatropin *on page 1381*

◆ **Zorcaine** *see* Articaine and Epinephrine *on page 170*

◆ **Zortress** *see* Everolimus *on page 628*

◆ **Zorvolex** *see* Diclofenac (Systemic) *on page 484*

◆ **Zostavax [DSC]** *see* Zoster Vaccine (Live/Attenuated) *on page 1585*

◆ **Zoster Vaccine Live** *see* Zoster Vaccine (Live/Attenuated) *on page 1585*

Zoster Vaccine (Live/Attenuated)

(ZOS ter vak SEEN)

Related Information

Systemic Viral Diseases *on page 1709*

Brand Names: US Zostavax [DSC]

Brand Names: Canada Zostavax II

Pharmacologic Category Vaccine; Vaccine, Live (Viral)

Use

Herpes zoster prevention: Prevention of herpes zoster (shingles) in patients ≥50 years of age

The Advisory Committee on Immunization Practices (ACIP) recommends zoster vaccine for the prevention of herpes zoster and related complications in immunocompetent adults. Recombinant zoster vaccine (RZV) is preferred for adults ≥50 years. However, zoster vaccine live (ZVL) remains an option for immunocompetent adults ≥60 years (CDC/ACIP [Dooling 2018]).

Limitations of use: Not indicated for treatment of active herpes zoster infection or postherpetic neuralgia (PHN); not indicated for prophylaxis of primary varicella infection (chickenpox).

Local Anesthetic/Vasoconstrictor Precautions
No information available to require special precautions

Effects on Dental Treatment No significant effects or complications reported

Effects on Bleeding No information available to require special precautions

Adverse Reactions

>10%: Local: Pain at injection site (≤54%), erythema at injection site (36% to 48%), swelling at injection site (26% to 40%), localized tenderness (≤34%), injection site pruritus (7% to 11%)

1% to 10%:

Cardiovascular: Cardiac failure (≤2%)

Central nervous system: Headache (1% to 9%)

Gastrointestinal: Diarrhea (2%)

Local: Warm sensation at injection site (2% to 4%), hematoma at injection site (2%), induration at injection site (1%)

Neuromuscular & skeletal: Asthenia (1%), limb pain (1%)

Respiratory: Pulmonary edema (≤2%), respiratory tract disease (1%)

<1%, postmarketing, and/or case reports: Anaphylaxis, arthralgia, exacerbation of asthma, facial nerve paralysis, fever, Guillain-Barre syndrome, herpes zoster infection, hypersensitivity reaction, lymphadenopathy (transient), myalgia, nausea, necrotizing retinitis (patients on immunosuppressive therapy), polymyalgia rheumatica, rash at injection site, skin rash, urticaria at injection site, varicella zoster infection (in immunocompromised patients)

Mechanism of Action

A decline in VZV-specific immunity increases the risk of developing zoster infection. As a live, attenuated vaccine (Oka/Merck strain of varicella-zoster virus), zoster virus vaccine stimulates active immunity to disease caused by the varicella-zoster virus. Administration has been demonstrated to protect against the development of herpes zoster. It may also reduce the severity of complications, including postherpetic neuralgia, in patients who develop zoster following vaccination.

Zoster vaccine live reduced the incidence of zoster by ~70% in those 50 to 59 years of age, 64% in those 60-69 years of age, and 38% in those ≥70 years of age (CDC/ACIP [Dooling 2018]). Additional benefit was afforded to vaccine recipients who developed zoster by reduction in the incidence of PHN: 5% for those 60-69 years of age, 55% for those 70-79 years of age, and 26% for those 80 years and older. Other prespecified zoster-related complications were reported less frequently in subjects who received zoster vaccine compared with subjects who received placebo.

Pharmacodynamics/Kinetics

Onset of Action Seroconversion: ~6 weeks (CDC/ACIP [Harpaz, 2008])

Duration of Action Duration of protection decreases over time with substantial decrease after 1 year. Effectiveness of ZVL in preventing herpes zoster decreased to 32% after 8 years in individuals ≥50 years (Baxter 2017; CDC/ACIP [Dooling 2018]).

Reproductive Considerations

Per the manufacturer, women should avoid becoming pregnant for 3 months after vaccination (4 weeks per CDC) (CDC/ACIP [Harpaz 2008]).

Pregnancy Considerations Use during pregnancy is contraindicated.

Risk to the fetus following exposure to wild-type varicella zoster virus is small, and risk following exposure from the attenuated vaccine is probably even less (CDC/ACIP [Harpaz 2008]). Based on information collected from the manufacturer's pregnancy registry, of women who received a varicella-containing vaccine within 3 months of pregnancy or any time during pregnancy and who were available for analysis, there were no infants born with abnormalities consistent with congenital varicella syndrome. Information specific to exposure following zoster vaccine live was limited. Due to the rare incidence of congenital varicella syndrome and the low rates of varicella vaccine exposure in women of reproductive potential, the pregnancy registry has been closed. Although zoster vaccine live is not licensed for use in women within traditional reproductive ages, inadvertent exposures will still be monitored (Marin 2014).

Any exposures to the vaccine during pregnancy or within 3 months prior to pregnancy should continue to be reported to the manufacturer (Merck & Co, 877-888-4231) or to VAERS (800-822-7967) as suspected adverse reactions (Marin 2014).

Product Availability

Merck will no longer sell Zostavax in the United States, effective July 1, 2020. All remaining product has an expiry date of November 2020. Further information is available at https://www.merckvaccines.com/wp-content/uploads/sites/8/2020/06/US-CIN-00033.pdf.

Zoster Vaccine (Recombinant)

(ZOS ter vak SEEN ree KOM be nant)

Brand Names: US Shingrix

Brand Names: Canada Shingrix

Pharmacologic Category Vaccine; Vaccine, Recombinant

Use

Herpes zoster prevention: Prevention of herpes zoster (shingles) in patients ≥50 years of age

The Advisory Committee on Immunization Practices (ACIP) recommends:

Routine vaccination of immunocompetent patients ≥50 years of age, including those who previously received varicella vaccine or zoster vaccine (live) or who report a previous episode of zoster; and patients with chronic medical conditions (eg, chronic renal failure, diabetes, rheumatoid arthritis, chronic pulmonary disease). Recombinant zoster vaccine is preferred over zoster vaccine (live) in immunocompetent patients (CDC/ACIP [Dooling 2018]).

Limitations of use: Not indicated for prevention of primary varicella infection (chickenpox) or for the treatment of zoster or postherpetic neuralgia (PHN) (CDC/ACIP [Dooling 2018]).

Local Anesthetic/Vasoconstrictor Precautions No information available to require special precautions

Effects on Dental Treatment No significant effects or complications reported

Effects on Bleeding No information available to require special precautions

Adverse Reactions

>10%:

Central nervous system: Fatigue (37% to 57%), headache (29% to 51%), shivering (20% to 36%)

Gastrointestinal: Gastrointestinal adverse effects (14% to 24%)

Local: Pain at injection site (69% to 88%), erythema at injection site (38% to 39%), swelling at injection site (23% to 31%)

Neuromuscular & skeletal: Myalgia (35% to 57%)

Miscellaneous: Fever (14% to 28%)

1% to 10%:

Central nervous system: Chills (4%), malaise (2%), dizziness (1%)

Dermatologic: Injection site pruritus (2%)

Gastrointestinal: Nausea (1%)

Neuromuscular & skeletal: Arthralgia (2%)

<1%, postmarketing, and/or case reports: Gout, high fever, lymphadenitis, optic neuropathy

Mechanism of Action

Stimulates active immunity to disease caused by reactivation of the varicella-zoster virus, thereby protecting against zoster disease (shingles) and associated complications (eg, postherpetic neuralgia [PHN]).

Zoster vaccine (recombinant) reduced the incidence of zoster by ~97% in those 50 to <70 years of age and ~91% in those ≥70 years of age. Additional benefit was afforded to vaccine recipients who developed zoster by reduction in the incidence of PHN: ~89% for those ≥70 years of age.

Pharmacodynamics/Kinetics

Duration of Action ~85% to 93% vaccine efficacy after 4 years

Pregnancy Considerations Based on the lack of data in pregnant women, the ACIP recommends that consideration be given to delaying vaccination with zoster vaccine (recombinant) during pregnancy (CDC/ACIP [Dooling 2018]).

◆ **Zostrix HP [OTC]** *see* Capsaicin *on page 284*

◆ **Zostrix Natural Pain Relief [OTC]** *see* Capsaicin *on page 284*

◆ **Zosyn** *see* Piperacillin and Tazobactam *on page 1236*

◆ **Zovia 1/35E (28)** *see* Ethinyl Estradiol and Ethynodiol Diacetate *on page 611*

◆ **Zovia 1/50E (28) [DSC]** *see* Ethinyl Estradiol and Ethynodiol Diacetate *on page 611*

◆ **Zovirax** *see* Acyclovir (Systemic) *on page 75*

◆ **Zovirax** *see* Acyclovir (Topical) *on page 82*

◆ **ZP10A Peptide** *see* Lixisenatide *on page 925*

◆ **Z-Pak** *see* Azithromycin (Systemic) *on page 203*

◆ **ZTlido** *see* Lidocaine (Topical) *on page 902*

◆ **Z-Tuss AC [OTC]** *see* Codeine and Chlorpheniramine *on page 404*

◆ **Zubsolv** *see* Buprenorphine and Naloxone *on page 270*

Zucapsaicin (zu kap SAY sin)

Brand Names: Canada Zuacta [DSC]

Pharmacologic Category Analgesic, Topical; Topical Skin Product; Transient Receptor Potential Vanilloid 1 (TRPV1) Agonist

Use Note: Not approved in the US

Osteoarthritis of the knee: In conjunction with an oral NSAID or COX-2 inhibitor for short-term (≤3 months) treatment of severe pain associated with osteoarthritis of the knee that is not controlled by NSAID or COX-2 inhibitor monotherapy

Local Anesthetic/Vasoconstrictor Precautions No information available to require special precautions

Effects on Dental Treatment The safety and efficacy of zucapsaicin have only been assessed in treating pain associated with osteoarthritis of the knee; its use as a topical application in treating pain of the temporomandibular joint in the patient with temporomandibular dysfunction has not been studied and is not recommended

Effects on Bleeding No information available to require special precautions

Adverse Reactions

>10%: Local: Application site burning (22% to 35%)

1% to 10%:

Central nervous system: Localized warm feeling (4% to 6%), localized numbness (3%)

Dermatologic: Burning sensation of skin (2%)

Local: Application site reaction (4%; includes application site edema, application site erythema, application site pain, cold sensation, dryness), application site irritation (1%), application-site pruritus (1%), application site rash (1%)

Neuromuscular & skeletal: Arthralgia (1%)

Ophthalmic: Eye irritation (1%)

Respiratory: Cough (2%), sneezing (1%)

<1%, postmarketing, and/or case reports: Arthropathy, dyspnea, flushing, headache, limb pain, nasal congestion, nasal mucosa irritation, osteoarthritis (aggravated), skin photosensitivity, skin rash, skin blister, skin discoloration, throat irritation

Mechanism of Action Actions are thought to be similar to other capsaicinoids, such as capsaicin, which is a transient receptor potential vanilloid 1 receptor (TRPV1) agonist, that activates TRPV1 ligand-gated cation channels on nociceptive nerve fibers, resulting in depolarization, initiation of action potential, and pain signal transmission to the spinal cord; capsaicin exposure results in subsequent desensitization of the sensory axons, depletion of proinflammatory neuropeptides (eg, calcitonin gene-related peptide, substance P) and inhibition of pain transmission initiation. In arthritis, capsaicin induces release of substance P, the principal chemomediator of pain impulses from the periphery to the CNS, from peripheral sensory neurons; after repeated application, capsaicin depletes the neuron of substance P and prevents reaccumulation. The functional link between substance P and the capsaicin receptor, TRPV1, is not well understood.

Pregnancy Considerations Adverse events have not been observed in animal reproduction studies. Zucapsaicin is not absorbed systemically following topical administration. Use during pregnancy is not expected to result in significant exposure to the fetus.

Product Availability Not available in the US

- **Zumandimine** *see* Ethinyl Estradiol and Drospirenone *on page 610*
- **Zuplenz** *see* Ondansetron *on page 1143*
- **Zurampic** *see* Lesinurad *on page 887*
- **ZVL** *see* Zoster Vaccine (Live/Attenuated) *on page 1585*
- **Zyban [DSC]** *see* BuPROPion *on page 271*
- **Zyclara** *see* Imiquimod *on page 802*
- **Zyclara Pump** *see* Imiquimod *on page 802*
- **Zydelig** *see* Idelalisib *on page 795*
- **Zyflo** *see* Zileuton *on page 1571*
- **Zyflo CR [DSC]** *see* Zileuton *on page 1571*
- **Zykadia** *see* Ceritinib *on page 326*
- **Zyloprim** *see* Allopurinol *on page 103*
- **Zymaxid** *see* Gatifloxacin *on page 729*
- **Zypitamag** *see* Pitavastatin *on page 1238*
- **ZyPREXA** *see* OLANZapine *on page 1127*
- **ZyPREXA Relprevv** *see* OLANZapine *on page 1127*
- **Zyprexa Zydis** *see* OLANZapine *on page 1127*
- **ZyPREXA Zydis** *see* OLANZapine *on page 1127*
- **ZyrTEC Allergy [OTC]** *see* Cetirizine (Systemic) *on page 328*
- **ZyrTEC Allergy Childrens [OTC]** *see* Cetirizine (Systemic) *on page 328*
- **ZyrTEC Childrens Allergy [OTC]** *see* Cetirizine (Systemic) *on page 328*
- **Zytiga** *see* Abiraterone Acetate *on page 54*
- **Zyvox** *see* Linezolid *on page 918*
- **ZzzQuil [OTC]** *see* DiphenhydrAMINE (Systemic) *on page 502*

ALPHABETICAL LISTING OF NATURAL PRODUCTS

Acacia Gum

Clinical Overview

Uses

Acacia gum has been used in pharmaceuticals as a demulcent. It has been used topically in wound-healing preparations. Antioxidant, anti-inflammatory, antibacterial (ie, in periodontal disease), and lipidemic effects have been studied; however, robust clinical trials are lacking to support a definitive place in therapy.

Dosing

Clinical trials are generally lacking to provide dosing recommendations. Several trials used gum arabic 30 g orally daily for 6 to 12 weeks for various indications.

Contraindications

Contraindications have not been identified.

Pregnancy/Lactation

Avoid use. Information regarding safety and efficacy in pregnancy and lactation is lacking.

Interactions

None well documented.

Adverse Reactions

Allergic reactions have been reported. Adverse effects reported in clinical trials included unfavorable sensation in the mouth, early morning nausea, mild diarrhea, and bloating.

Toxicology

Acacia is essentially nontoxic when ingested and is generally recognized as safe (GRAS).

Local Anesthetic/Vasoconstrictor Precautions

No information available to require special precautions

Effects on Bleeding None reported

Acai

Clinical Overview

Uses

Antioxidant and anti-inflammatory activity of acai has been documented. Potential exists for use in treating cancer and metabolic syndrome; however, clinical information is limited.

Dosing

Clinical evidence on which to base dosing guidelines is lacking. A pilot study used acai pulp 100 g daily for 1 month.

Contraindications

Hypersensitivity to acai palm or any of its components.

Pregnancy/Lactation

Avoid use. Information regarding safety and efficacy in pregnancy and lactation is lacking.

Interactions

None well documented.

Adverse Reactions

Limited clinical studies exist; however, no adverse events have been reported.

Toxicology

One study reported mutagenicity in the Salmonella typhimurium TA97 assay and clastogenicity when using highly concentrated pulp.

Local Anesthetic/Vasoconstrictor Precautions

No information available to require special precautions

Effects on Bleeding None reported

Agrimony

Clinical Overview

Uses

Agrimony is used as a tea and gargle for sore throat, and externally as a mild antiseptic and astringent.

Dosing

There is no published clinical evidence for a safe or effective dose; however, the German Komission E recommended a daily dose of 3 g of the herb for internal use. Agrimony also is used as a poultice from a 10% decoction of the herb.

Contraindications

Contraindications have not yet been identified.

Pregnancy/Lactation

Information regarding safety and efficacy in pregnancy and lactation is lacking.

Interactions

None well documented.

Adverse Reactions

Agrimony reportedly can produce photodermatitis.

Toxicology

No data.

Local Anesthetic/Vasoconstrictor Precautions

No information available to require special precautions

Effects on Bleeding None reported

Alfalfa

Clinical Overview

Uses

Alfalfa may be useful in lowering cholesterol and treating menopausal symptoms. It also may have hypoglycemic and anti-inflammatory effects; however, clinical information supporting these indications is limited.

Dosing

A general dosing regimen is 5 to 10 g of the dried herb taken 3 times daily. For the treatment of high cholesterol, the seeds may be taken at a dose of 40 g 3 times daily.

Contraindications

The US Food and Drug Administration (FDA) issued an advisory indicating that children, the elderly, and people with compromised immune systems should not consume alfalfa sprouts because they are frequently contaminated with bacteria. Use should be avoided in people with a personal or family history of systemic lupus erythematous (SLE) because of possible effects on immunoregulatory cells by canavanine, a component of alfalfa.

Pregnancy/Lactation

Avoid use. Documented adverse effects of alfalfa during pregnancy include possible uterine stimulation. Although alfalfa has been anecdotally recommended to stimulate milk production, evidence is lacking.

Interactions

Because of its high vitamin K content, alfalfa may antagonize and therefore reduce the effects of warfarin. Alfalfa may interact with immunosuppressant agents, such as cyclosporine, because of its immunostimulatory effects.

Adverse Reactions

Alfalfa seeds and fresh sprouts can be contaminated with bacteria, such as Salmonella enterica and Escherichia coli. The FDA issued an advisory indicating that children, the elderly, and people with compromised immune systems should avoid eating alfalfa sprouts. Ingestion of dried alfalfa preparations is generally safe in healthy adults. Because of its high potassium content, alfalfa may cause hyperkalemia.

Toxicology

Alfalfa tablets have been associated with the reactivation of SLE in at least 2 patients.

Local Anesthetic/Vasoconstrictor Precautions

No information available to require special precautions

Effects on Bleeding As a single agent, alfalfa has no effect on bleeding. Due to the vitamin K content found in alfalfa, it has the potential to reduce the anticoagulant effect of warfarin.

Almond

Clinical Overview

Uses

Almonds are used as a dietary source of protein, unsaturated fats, minerals, micronutrients, phytochemicals, alpha-tocopheral, and fiber, as well as in confectioneries. The efficacy of almonds in altering the lipid profile is weakly supported by the literature; larger, more robust clinical trials of longer duration are required. The almond derivative laetrile/amygdalin has been used as an alternative cancer treatment, but there is no clinical evidence to support this use. Laetrile is banned by the US Food and Drug Administration (FDA) and in Europe for use in cancer therapy.

Dosing

Trials of almond dietary supplementation in adults have used 25 to 168 g of almonds per day. The American Heart Association (AHA) recommends the daily intake of nuts (28.35 to 56.7 g) as part of a healthy diet. There is no widely accepted standard for laetrile/amygdalin dosing due to the potential for toxicity and no evidence for efficacy.

Contraindications

Allergy to almonds or its products.

Pregnancy/Lactation

Consumption of bitter almond or laetrile is not recommended in pregnant or breastfeeding women because of insufficient data and a theoretical risk of birth defects. Consumption of sweet almond has generally recognized as safe (GRAS) status when used as food. Avoid dosages above those found in food because safety is unproven.

Interactions

None well documented.

Adverse Reactions

Adverse reactions similar to those of cyanide poisoning have been reported.

Toxicology

Cyanide poisoning and death have resulted from laetrile and bitter almond consumption.

Local Anesthetic/Vasoconstrictor Precautions

No information available to require special precautions

Effects on Bleeding None reported

Aloe

Clinical Overview

Uses

Topical aloe appears to inhibit infection and promote healing of minor burns and wounds, frostbite, as well as in skin affected by diseases such as psoriasis and seborrheic dermatitis, although studies have had conflicting results. Dried aloe latex should be ingested with caution as a drastic cathartic, but its use is not recommended. In 2002, the US Food and Drug Administration required all over-the-counter aloe laxative products to be removed from the US market or reformulated because manufacturers have not provided the necessary safety data.

Dosing

As a gel, A. vera may be applied externally. The resin product is cathartic and not recommended for internal use.

Contraindications

Ingestion is contraindicated in pregnant and breastfeeding women, children younger than 12 years of age, patients with inflammatory bowel disease, and elderly patients with suspected intestinal obstruction.

Pregnancy/Lactation

Documented adverse effects with ingestion; do not use. Cathartic, reputed abortifacient.

Interactions

Potential interactions between ingested aloe resin and the following medications have been identified: digoxin, furosemide, thiazide diuretics, sevoflurane stimulant laxatives, and antidiabetic agents.

Adverse Reactions

There has been 1 report that aloe gel as standard wound therapy delayed healing. The gel may cause burning sensations in dermabraded skin, and redness and itching also can occur. Use caution with cosmetic products containing A. vera gel. A case of acute hepatitis induced by aloe vera ingestion has been reported.

Toxicology

The resin product is cathartic at doses of 250 mg and is not recommended for internal use.

Local Anesthetic/Vasoconstrictor Precautions

No information available to require special precautions.

Effects on Bleeding None reported

Alpha-Lipoic Acid

Clinical Overview

Uses

Alpha-lipoic acid (ALA) has been used as an antioxidant for the treatment of diabetes and HIV. It also has been used for cancer, liver ailments, and various other conditions.

Dosing

Oral dosage of alpha-lipoic acid given in numerous clinical studies ranges from 300 to 1,800 mg daily. It also is given intravenously at similar daily dosages.

Contraindications

Contraindications have not yet been determined.

Pregnancy/Lactation

Information regarding safety and efficacy in pregnancy and lactation is lacking.

Interactions

None well documented.

Adverse Reactions

No adverse reactions have been reported.

Toxicology

No data.

Local Anesthetic/Vasoconstrictor Precautions

No information available to require special precautions

Effects on Bleeding None reported

Andrographis

Clinical Overview

Uses

Traditionally, andrographis has been used for liver complaints and fever, and as an anti-inflammatory and immunostimulant. In clinical trials, andrographis extract has been studied for use as an immunostimulant in upper respiratory tract infections and HIV infection. The potential for use of andrographolide as an anticancer agent as well as for its immune and anti-inflammatory effects is being investigated. However, limited clinical studies have been published to support any of these uses.

Dosing

The usual daily dose of andrographolides for common cold, sinusitis, and tonsillitis is 60 mg. A clinical trial in children with upper respiratory tract infection reported the use of andrographolide 30 mg daily for 10 days.

Contraindications

Contraindications have not been identified.

Pregnancy/Lactation

Avoid use. Adverse effects, including abortifacient effects, have been documented.

Interactions

None well documented.

Adverse Reactions

In a clinical trial, headache, fatigue, rash, bitter/metallic taste, diarrhea, pruritus, and decreased sex drive were reported with andrographis 10 mg/kg body weight. One HIV-positive participant experienced an anaphylactic reaction.

Toxicology

No data.

Local Anesthetic/Vasoconstrictor Precautions

No information available to require special precautions

Effects on Bleeding None reported

Angelica

Clinical Overview

Uses

Animal studies suggest anticonvulsant, antidepressant/antianxiety, and antioxidant effects of angelica or its constituents; however, clinical trials are lacking to support therapeutic applications or recommend use for any indication. The possibility of increased formation of amyloid-beta peptides exists with use of angelica.

Dosing

Clinical trials are lacking regarding dosage recommendations. Traditional doses of angelica dried root and rhizome range from 3 to 6 g/day (in divided doses).

Contraindications

Contraindications have not been identified.

Pregnancy/Lactation

Avoid use. Adverse effects and emmenagogue effects have been documented.

Interactions

The related Angelica sinensis exhibits antiplatelet aggregating activity.

Adverse Reactions

Limited clinical trials provide information regarding adverse effects. A small clinical trial found no increase in blood pressure or heart rate during 8 weeks of leaf extract use. Allergic dermatitis has been reported, and photosensitization is possible.

Toxicology

Poisoning has been reported with high doses of angelica oils.

Local Anesthetic/Vasoconstrictor Precautions

No information available to require special precautions

Effects on Bleeding Angelica root has the potential to increase the risk of bleeding or potentiate the effects of warfarin.

Anise

Clinical Overview

Uses

Clinical data are lacking to support the wide-ranging traditional uses for anise; limited studies have been conducted in disorders of the GI tract and in menopause. Studies in rodents suggest effects on the CNS. The oil has been used to treat lice, scabies, and psoriasis.

Dosing

GI disorders: In limited clinical studies, anise 3 g powder taken after each meal (3 times per day) for 4 weeks has been studied for treatment of dyspepsia. *Menopausal symptoms:* Capsules containing P. anisum 330 mg taken 3 times daily for 4 weeks has been used for treatment of menopausal symptoms.

Contraindications

Anise is not recommended for use in pregnancy in amounts exceeding those found in food.

Pregnancy/Lactation

Aniseed is a reputed abortifacient. Use in amounts exceeding those found in food is not recommended in pregnancy.

Interactions

None well documented.

Adverse Reactions

Anise may cause allergic reactions of the skin, respiratory tract, and GI tract.

Toxicology

Ingestion of the oil may result in pulmonary edema, vomiting, and seizures.

Local Anesthetic/Vasoconstrictor Precautions

No information available to require special precautions

Effects on Bleeding None reported

Arnica

Clinical Overview

Uses

Arnica and its extracts have been widely used in folk and homeopathic medicine as a treatment for acne, boils, bruises, rashes, sprains, pains, and wounds. There does not appear to be sufficient evidence to support the use of arnica as an anti-inflammatory or analgesic agent or in the prevention of bruising. Heterogeneity of doses, delivery forms, and indications in available clinical studies also makes generalization difficult.

Dosing

Arnica is classified as an unsafe herb by the US Food and Drug Administration (FDA) because of its toxicity and should not be administered orally or applied to broken skin where absorption can occur. No consensus exists on topical dosing, and evidence from clinical trials is lacking to support therapeutic dosing. In homeopathic use, less concentrated strengths, such as 12C, 200C, 1M (1,000C), and 10M (10,000C) (C = centisimal dilution [1 part in 100]; M = millesimal dilution [1 part in 1,000]), are recommended for use before and after surgery.

Contraindications

Contraindications have not been identified.

Pregnancy/Lactation

Avoid use. Uterine stimulation has been documented.

Interactions

None well documented.

Adverse Reactions

Homeopathic doses of arnica are unlikely to result in any adverse reactions because of the small amount ingested. Arnica irritates mucous membranes and causes stomach pain, diarrhea, and vomiting. Allergy and contact dermatitis have been reported.

Toxicology

The plant is poisonous and ingestion can cause gastroenteritis, dyspnea, cardiac arrest, and death. The flowers and roots of the plant have caused vomiting, drowsiness, and coma when eaten by children.

Local Anesthetic/Vasoconstrictor Precautions

May cause serious interactions with anesthetic drugs

Effects on Bleeding May see increased bleeding due to inhibition of platelet aggregation

Artichoke

Clinical Overview

Uses

Artichoke has demonstrated antioxidant, antimicrobial, and anti-inflammatory activities and has been investigated for use in the treatment of cardiovascular disease risk factors (ie, cholesterol), diabetes, GI disease, and liver diseases. However, clinical data are lacking to support use of artichoke for any indication.

Dosing

In clinical trials, dosages of 600 mg/day and 2,700 mg/day of artichoke leaf extract (in divided doses) for 2 months have been studied in patients with liver diseases.

Contraindications

Allergy to plants in the Asteraceae family (eg, daisy, chrysanthemum, marigold, Echinacea, ragweed); bile duct obstruction; gallstones.

Pregnancy/Lactation

Artichoke heads are generally recognized as safe (GRAS) when used as food. Information regarding safety and efficacy of artichoke leaf extract in pregnancy and lactation is lacking; caution is warranted.

Interactions

Cytochrome P450 (CYP-450) 3A4/2C9/2C19/2E1/2-D6/1A2/2B6 substrates: Artichoke may inhibit various CYP-450 isoenzymes, although the mechanism is not fully understood. Therefore, caution is warranted in patients receiving other medications that are substrates for these isoenzymes.

Adverse Reactions

Mild, transient, and infrequent adverse reactions, generally limited to GI complaints such as bloating and flatulence, have been reported. Allergic reactions including anaphylaxis, bronchial asthma, and irritant contact dermatitis, as well as a case of hepatotoxicity, have been reported.

Toxicology

No data.

Local Anesthetic/Vasoconstrictor Precautions

No information available to require special precautions

Effects on Bleeding None reported

Ashwagandha

Clinical Overview

Uses

Ashwagandha has been used as an adaptogen, diuretic, and sedative and is available in the United States as a dietary supplement. Trials supporting its clinical use are limited; however, many in vitro and animal experiments suggest effects on the immune and CNS systems, as well as in the pathogenesis of cancer and inflammatory conditions.

Dosing

Dosing information is limited. W. somnifera root powder has generally been used at dosages of 450 mg to 2 g in combination with other preparations.

Contraindications

Contraindications have not been identified.

Pregnancy/Lactation

Abortifacient properties have been reported for ashwagandha. Avoid use.

Interactions

None well documented.

Adverse Reactions

Limited clinical trials are available and case reports are lacking.

Toxicology

Acute toxicity of W. somnifera is modest; at reasonable doses, ashwagandha is nontoxic.

Local Anesthetic/Vasoconstrictor Precautions

No information available to require special precautions

Effects on Bleeding None reported

Asparagus

Clinical Overview

Uses

Asparagus stalks are commonly consumed as a vegetable. Asparagus has been studied for its diuretic, hypoglycemic, antihypertensive, hypocholesterolemic, CNS, and antioxidant effects; however; there is little to no clinical evidence to support these uses. Other species, such as Asparagus racemosus, have been used in traditional Chinese and Ayurvedic medicine but are not reviewed in this monograph.

Dosing

There is insufficient clinical evidence to provide dosing recommendations for asparagus. A maximum dosage of 2,400 mg daily of dried asparagus root (in divided doses) as part of a combination preparation with parsley (Asparagus-P) has been evaluated for its antihypertensive effects; however, adverse reactions led to participant withdrawal from the study.

Contraindications

Contraindications have not been identified.

Pregnancy/Lactation

Asparagus has "generally recognized as safe" (GRAS) status when used as food. Avoid dosages above those found in food because safety and efficacy have not been established.

Interactions

None well documented.

Adverse Reactions

Symptoms of allergy to asparagus, including rhinitis, occupational asthma, oral allergic syndrome, allergic contact dermatitis, and anaphylaxis, are well documented. Exacerbation of gout has been reported with excessive consumption.

Toxicology

No data.

Local Anesthetic/Vasoconstrictor Precautions

No information available to require special precautions

Effects on Bleeding None reported

Astragalus

Clinical Overview

Uses

Most evidence suggests that astragalus root may modulate immune function and reported benefits are derived from this action, although studies are older and of limited quality. Evidence in the literature for other purported therapeutic uses is lacking.

Dosing

There is no recent clinical evidence to guide dosage of astragalus products; however, recommendations of 2 to 6 g daily of the powdered root are typical.

Contraindications

Contraindications have not yet been identified.

Pregnancy/Lactation

Information regarding safety and efficacy in pregnancy and lactation is lacking.

Interactions

None well documented.

Adverse Reactions

Allergy has been reported. A case report exists of increased carbohydrate antigen 19-9 and induction of reversible liver and kidney cysts in a woman consuming A. membranaceus daily for 1 month.

Toxicology

Evidence is equivocal; however, mutagenicity has been shown in the Ames test.

Local Anesthetic/Vasoconstrictor Precautions

No information available to require special precautions

Effects on Bleeding Astragalus may increase the risk of bleeding.

Barberry

Clinical Overview

Uses

Clinical applications may include use in treating diabetes and dyslipidemia, although clinical trials are limited and are often of poor quality. Other activity includes antimicrobial, antioxidant, and anti-inflammatory effects. No clinical trials exist to support uses related to effects on the cardiovascular and central nervous systems or treating cancer.

Dosing

Daily doses of 2 g of the berries and 1.5 to 3 g daily of dry bark have been used; however, there are limited clinical studies to substantiate barberry's varied uses.

Contraindications

Caution is warranted in the presence of cardiac arrhythmia. Use in children has not been validated.

Pregnancy/Lactation

Avoid use. There are documented adverse effects, including uterine stimulant effects.

Interactions

Case reports are lacking; however, barberry exhibits anti-cytochrome P450 3A4 (CYP3A4) activity similar to that of grapefruit. Caution is warranted with coadministration of potentially toxic medicines such as cyclosporine.

Adverse Reactions

GI symptoms (eg, nausea, vomiting, diarrhea), dizziness, and fainting have been reported. Effects on the cardiovascular system (eg, hypotension, decreased heart rate) and decreased respiration may occur with high dosages. The German Commission E reports that lower doses of berberine are well tolerated. Hypersensitivity has been documented.

Toxicology

Symptoms of poisoning are characterized by lethargy, stupor and daze, vomiting and diarrhea, and nephritis. A median lethal dose (LD_{50}) for berberine was noted as 27.5 mg/kg in humans. Berberine showed mutagenicity in yeast cells and Ames test, while a phototoxic reaction between berberine alkaloid and ultraviolet A (UVA) light has been described.

Local Anesthetic/Vasoconstrictor Precautions

No information available to require special precautions

Effects on Bleeding None reported

Beta Sitosterol

Clinical Overview

Uses

Beta sitosterol has been used to lower low-density lipoprotein (LDL) cholesterol and improve symptoms in mild-to-moderate benign prostatic hypertrophy (BPH). Beta-sitosterol has also been investigated for its immunomodulatory and anticancer effects.

Dosing

Beta sitosterol is incorporated in margarine, yogurt, or other foods to give a daily intake of 1.5-3 g.

Contraindications

Avoid plant sterols such as beta sitosterol in patients with sitosterolemia, a condition in which high plasma concentrations of plant sterols can lead to tendon xanthomas, premature atherosclerosis, and hemolytic anemia.

Pregnancy/Lactation

Beta sitosterol should be avoided in pregnant women due to demonstrated uterine stimulant effects.

Interactions

Plant sterols reduce the absorption of the fat-soluble vitamins beta-carotene, alpha-carotene, and vitamin E. No effects on vitamins A and K have been noted. Beta sitosterol levels may decrease in patients receiving ezetimibe through its inhibition of intestinal absorption of plant sterols.

Adverse Reactions

A review of the literature suggests that beta sitosterol may cause GI adverse effects as well as impotence. In one study, adverse reactions deemed related to beta-sitosterol use were flatulence, discoloration of the feces, appetite changes, dyspepsia, leg cramps, skin rash, and leukopenia. A 1-year study in healthy patients consuming 1.6 g/day of plant sterols contained in a dietary spread demonstrated cholesterol-lowering effects as well as general tolerability with long-term consumption.

Toxicology

Clinical data are lacking.

Local Anesthetic/Vasoconstrictor Precautions

No information available to require special precautions

Effects on Bleeding None reported

Bilberry

Clinical Overview

Uses

Clinical studies are limited. Interest has focused on antioxidant potential in cancer and cardiovascular conditions, and other applications may exist in diabetes, as well as in inflammatory bowel and ocular conditions.

Dosing

Typical bilberry products are standardized to 25% anthocyanoside content, and 100 g of fresh fruit contains anthocyanin content 300 to 700 mg. Limited clinical studies have evaluated supplemental bilberry 100 to 400 g over 4 to 8 weeks' duration.

Contraindications

Contraindications have not yet been identified.

Pregnancy/Lactation

Generally recognized as safe (GRAS) when used as food. Avoid doses above those found in food because safety and efficacy are unproven.

Interactions

None well documented.

Adverse Reactions

Information is lacking.

Toxicology

Information is lacking. Long-term use of bilberry leaves is suspected to lead to adverse effects.

Local Anesthetic/Vasoconstrictor Precautions

No information available to require special precautions

Effects on Bleeding May increase risk of bleeding by inhibiting platelet aggregation

Bitter Melon

Clinical Overview

Uses

Medical literature documents numerous studies of bitter melon use, primarily for its antidiabetic activity, but results are conflicting and inconclusive. There is insufficient evidence to recommend the use of bitter melon as a therapeutic option in type 2 diabetes.

Dosing

Diabetes: Bitter melon juice has been administered for type 2 diabetes at daily doses of 50 to 100 mL; 5 g of dried fruit given 3 times/day has also been used. There is insufficient clinical evidence to substantiate these doses.

Contraindications

Patients deficient in glucose-6-phosphate dehydrogenase should avoid consumption of bitter melon preparations due to the presence of vicine in the seeds.

Pregnancy/Lactation

Avoid use. Documentation of emmenagogue and abortifacient effects exists.

Interactions

None well documented.

Adverse Reactions

Bitter melon generally causes few adverse reactions. GI effects (eg, abdominal pain, diarrhea) and headache have been reported. Case reports of hypoglycemic coma and atrial fibrillation associated with bitter melon intake exist. Bitter melon should be used with caution in patients with impaired hepatic function.

Toxicology

Toxicity resulting in death has been reported in one case report of a child ingesting the red arils around bitter melon seeds.

Local Anesthetic/Vasoconstrictor Precautions

No information available to require special precautions

Effects on Bleeding None reported

Bitter Orange

Clinical Overview

Uses

Pharmacological actions for C. aurantium include antispasmodic, sedative, demulcent, digestive, tonic, and vascular stimulant; as an anti-inflammatory, antibacterial, and antifungal agent; and for reducing cholesterol. Clinical data are limited. Most medical literature focuses on the plant's safety and efficacy in OTC weight loss supplement formulations, with studies using small sample sizes and often focusing on combination products. Therefore, no recommendations for any indication can be made.

Dosing

Follow manufacturer's dosage guidelines because synephrine content may vary in supplement formulations.

Contraindications

Because of potentially additive effects, avoid synephrine use in patients with hypertension, tachyarrhythmia, hyperthyroidism, or narrow-angle glaucoma.

Pregnancy/Lactation

Avoid use. Information regarding safety and efficacy in pregnancy and lactation is lacking.

Interactions

C. aurantium inhibits intestinal CYP3A4 and intestinal efflux in the small intestine and may interact with numerous drugs, including amiodarone, anxiolytics, antidepressants, antiviral agents, calcium channel blockers, dextromethorphan, GI prokinetic agents, vasoconstrictors, and weight loss formulas.

Adverse Reactions

Bitter orange may cause photosensitization, particularly in people with fair skin. There are numerous case reports of adverse cardiac reactions associated with C. aurantium extract use.

Toxicology

Bitter orange is considered generally recognized as safe (GRAS) by the US Food and Drug Administration (FDA) when consumed in amounts found in foods. Medical literature primarily documents cardiovascular toxicity, especially due to the stimulant amines synephrine, octopamine, and N-methyltyramine, which may cause vasoconstriction as well as increased heart rate and blood pressure.

Local Anesthetic/Vasoconstrictor Precautions

Synephrine, the main chemical constituent in the fruit, is a sympathomimetic amine having properties of vasoconstriction and tachycardia. Use vasoconstrictor with caution; synephrine may interact with epinephrine and levonordefrin to cause a pressor response.

Effects on Bleeding None reported

Bittersweet Nightshade

Clinical Overview

Uses

Bittersweet nightshade has been used as a traditional external remedy for skin abrasions and inflammation. The stems were approved by the German Commission E for external use as supportive therapy in chronic eczema (see Toxicology).

Dosing

Traditional use of the stem has been at a dosage of 1 to 3 g/day, usually given as a decoction or infusion in 250 mL of water.

Contraindications

Contraindications have not yet been identified.

Pregnancy/Lactation

Documented teratogenic effects of the glycoalkaloids in animals. Avoid use.

Interactions

None well documented.

Adverse Reactions

No data.

Toxicology

The plant is toxic. Ingestion of unripened berries should be considered a medical emergency. Symptoms may be delayed for several hours.

Local Anesthetic/Vasoconstrictor Precautions

No information available to require special precautions

Effects on Bleeding None reported

Black Cohosh

Clinical Overview

Uses

There is a lack of consensus regarding whether black cohosh is useful for managing some symptoms of menopause. Some official groups state black cohosh can be considered as an alternative nonhormonal therapy for vasomotor symptoms, whereas others state there is a lack of consistent evidence of benefit.

Dosing

Black cohosh extract is generally standardized to 2.5% of triterpene glycosides (ie, 1 mg/dose). Based on clinical use of commercial products, the current recommended black cohosh dose for management of symptoms of menopause is 40 to 80 mg/day, often in divided doses. Therapeutic effects generally begin after 2 weeks of treatment, with maximum effects usually occurring within 8 weeks.

Contraindications

Contraindicated in individuals with aspirin sensitivity because black cohosh contains salicylic acids.

Pregnancy/Lactation

Avoid use in pregnancy and lactation. Black cohosh has been used to improve pregnancy rates following in vitro fertilization and in women with polycystic ovarian syndrome (PCOS). Premature birth may occur with large doses. Concerns regarding labor-inducing, hormonal, emmenagogic, and anovulatory effects exist, based on low-level evidence and expert opinion.

Interactions

None well documented.

Adverse Reactions

Black cohosh is associated with a low incidence of adverse reactions. There are concerns regarding rare, but serious, hepatotoxicity.

Toxicology

Overdose of black cohosh may cause nausea, vomiting, dizziness, nervous system and visual disturbances, reduced pulse rate, and increased perspiration. Case reports primarily document hepatic toxicity; however, cardiovascular and circulatory disorders and 1 case of convulsions have been documented.

Local Anesthetic/Vasoconstrictor Precautions

No information available to require special precautions

Effects on Bleeding None reported

Black Currant

Clinical Overview

Uses

Evidence is conflicting regarding the benefits of black currant as an antioxidant source and in night- and fatigue-related visual impairment. Two small published trials showed some benefit in rheumatoid arthritis, but black currant was not compared to a gold standard. Long-term safety and efficacy have not been studied for any of the above potential uses. Oil and juice extracts have also exhibited limited antimicrobial and prebiotic activities, as well as potential benefit in preventing infant atopic dermatitis, reducing cardiovascular risk, and improving certain exercise performance measures.

Dosing

Limited clinical trial data exist to provide dosage recommendations. Standardization of commercial products has usually been related to anthocyanin and/or vitamin C content. A tea made from 2 to 4 g of chopped leaves can be administered several times per day. Commercial extract products have been used at daily doses ranging from 300 mg to 6 g for 1 to 2 weeks for improvements in exercise performance and recovery. Black currant juice drinks with low (6.4%) and high (20%) juice concentrations have been administered at 250 mL/day for 6 weeks to improve cardiovascular risk parameters.

Contraindications

Contraindications have not been identified.

Pregnancy/Lactation

Information regarding safety and efficacy in pregnancy and lactation is lacking.

Interactions

None well documented.

Adverse Reactions
Self-limiting adverse reactions have been reported, including indigestion, loose bowels, and increased urinary frequency. Although no direct evidence is available, black currant should be used with caution in epileptic patients because lowered seizure threshold has been reported with evening primrose oil.

Toxicology
No data.

Local Anesthetic/Vasoconstrictor Precautions
No information available to require special precautions

Effects on Bleeding None reported

Black Walnut

Clinical Overview

Uses
Black walnut has many traditional uses; however, there are no human trials to support these effects. Black walnuts are a good dietary source of essential fatty acids.

Dosing
No clinical trials are available to support dosage recommendations.

Contraindications
None well documented.

Pregnancy/Lactation
Avoid use. Documented adverse reactions (mutagenic properties).

Interactions
None well documented.

Adverse Reactions
Allergic reactions have occurred.

Toxicology
The quinones juglone and plumbagin found in black walnut are regarded as toxins.

Local Anesthetic/Vasoconstrictor Precautions
No information available to require special precautions

Effects on Bleeding None reported

Blessed Thistle

Clinical Overview

Uses
Blessed thistle has been traditionally used to stimulate secretion of gastric juices and saliva, to increase appetite and facilitate digestion, and to stimulate the flow of bile. It is a common ingredient in combination formulas for gastric health. Anti-inflammatory, antimicrobial, and cytotoxic activities have been reported and thought to be due to the chemical constituent cnicin. However, there are no clinical trials to support these potential uses.

Dosing
No clinical studies exist to provide dosing recommendations for blessed thistle. Doses of 4 to 6 g daily have been traditionally used.

Contraindications
Blessed thistle is contraindicated in patients with gastric ulcers or other inflammatory bowel conditions, such as Crohn disease.

Pregnancy/Lactation
Avoid use. Blessed thistle should not be used in pregnancy. Information regarding safety and efficacy in lactation is lacking.

Interactions
None well documented.

Adverse Reactions
Allergy and cross sensitization have been reported with other members of the Asteraceae family. Stimulation of gastric acid secretion has been reported. Emesis is likely with high dosages.

Toxicology
Clinical information is limited. Emesis is likely with high dosages (5 g or more).

Local Anesthetic/Vasoconstrictor Precautions
No information available to require special precautions

Effects on Bleeding None reported

Blue Cohosh

Clinical Overview

Uses
Blue cohosh has been used to induce uterine contractions in labor; however, there are no quality clinical trials to support any therapeutic application for blue cohosh, and concerns of toxicity outweigh any potential clinical benefit.

Dosing
Despite widespread knowledge or use of blue cohosh, there are no clinical trials on which to base dosage recommendations.

Contraindications
Contraindications have not yet been identified.

Pregnancy/Lactation
Avoid use. Adverse effects have been documented.

Interactions
None well documented.

Adverse Reactions
Information is limited; clinical trials are lacking. Potential for toxicity appears to outweigh any medical benefit.

Toxicology
Blue cohosh root is potentially toxic to humans and to a developing fetus.

Local Anesthetic/Vasoconstrictor Precautions
No information available to require special precautions

Effects on Bleeding None reported

Boldo

Clinical Overview

Uses
In vitro and animal studies suggest that boldo leaf extract and its constituent boldine have antioxidant, anti-inflammatory, and antimicrobial effects and have investigated potential applications in diabetes, GI disorders, cancer, sun protection, osteoporosis, renoprotection, and atopic dermatitis. However, clinical trial data are lacking to recommend use for any indication.

Dosing
No quality clinical trials exist to provide dosing recommendations for boldo leaf extract. Traditional doses include 1 to 2 teaspoons (2 to 3 g) of dry leaf per 240 mL of water; and 0.1 to 0.3 mL of liquid extract (1:1 in 45% alcohol) 3 times a day. Commercial preparations may contain ascaridole, a toxic constituent.

Contraindications
Contraindicated in liver disease and diseases of the bile duct, including gallstones.

Pregnancy/Lactation
Avoid use. Adverse effects have been noted in animal studies.

Interactions

Boldo ingestion may enhance the anticoagulant effect of warfarin; caution is warranted. Boldo may also decrease therapeutic tacrolimus levels; caution is warranted.

Adverse Reactions

Boldo-related adverse events described in case reports include anaphylaxis, prolonged QT interval, ventricular tachycardia, and hepatotoxicity.

Toxicology

No data.

Local Anesthetic/Vasoconstrictor Precautions
No information available to require special precautions

Effects on Bleeding As a single agent, boldo has no effect on bleeding. Boldo may enhance the anticoagulant effects of warfarin when taken simultaneously. This effect has not been confirmed.

Boneset

Clinical Overview

Uses

Boneset has chiefly been used to treat fevers.

Dosing

There is no recent clinical evidence to guide dosage of boneset. Traditional use was at a dose of 2 g of leaves and flowers. Internal use should be tempered by the occurrence of hepatotoxic pyrrolizidine alkaloids in this plant.

Contraindications

Contraindications have not yet been identified.

Pregnancy/Lactation

Documented adverse effects, including cytotoxic constituents. Avoid use.

Interactions

None well documented.

Adverse Reactions

The FDA has classified boneset as an "Herb of Undefined Safety."

Toxicology

The ingestion of large amounts of teas or extracts may result in severe diarrhea. The identification of pyrrolizidine alkaloids in related Eupatorium species is cause for concern until detailed phytochemical investigations are carried out on boneset. This class of alkaloids is known to cause hepatic impairment after long-term ingestion. While direct evidence for a hepatotoxic effect from boneset does not exist, there is sufficient evidence to indicate that any plant containing unsaturated pyrrolizidine alkaloids should not be ingested.

Local Anesthetic/Vasoconstrictor Precautions
No information available to require special precautions

Effects on Bleeding None reported

Borage

Clinical Overview

Uses

Borage has been used in European herbal medicine since the Middle Ages, alone and in combination with fish oil in rheumatoid arthritis, atopic eczema, and osteoporosis, although limited clinical evidence is available to support these uses.

Dosing

Borage seed oil 1 to 3 g/day has been given in clinical trials (1 g/day has been used in children and up to 3 g/day in adults). The content of gamma-linolenic acid is between 20% and 26% of the oil.

Contraindications

Contraindications have not been identified.

Pregnancy/Lactation

Documented adverse effects (pyrrolizidine alkaloids). Avoid use.

Interactions

None well documented.

Adverse Reactions

No adverse effects have been reported. Although no direct evidence is available, caution is advised in patients with epilepsy because of reports of lowered seizure threshold with evening primrose oil.

Toxicology

The presence of unsaturated pyrrolizidine alkaloids in leaves, flowers, and seeds of borage suggests a potential for hepatotoxicity, although the total plant alkaloid content is low.

Local Anesthetic/Vasoconstrictor Precautions
No information available to require special precautions

Effects on Bleeding None reported

Boron

Clinical Overview

Uses

Boric acid is a topical astringent, mild disinfectant and eye wash. Sprinkled in crevices and corners, boric acid powder controls rodents and insects. Sodium borate is used in cold creams, eye washes and mouth rinses. Boron compounds are used to enhance the cell selectivity of radiation therapy.

Dosing

Boron has been studied in several clinical studies at a wide range of doses. Daily dosage of 2.5 to 6 mg as boron has been administered for osteoarthritis and strength conditioning. Intravaginal boric acid (600 mg daily) was administered for vulvovaginal candidiasis. A single dose of 102.6 mg sodium tetraborate was studied for its effects on factor VIIa.

Contraindications

Contraindications have not yet been identified.

Pregnancy/Lactation

Information regarding safety and efficacy in pregnancy and lactation is lacking.

Interactions

None well documented.

Adverse Reactions

There is little or no clinical data about the adverse effects of boron; boron compounds can be toxic to humans.

Toxicology

While boric acid, borates, and other compounds containing boron are used medicinally, they are potentially toxic if ingested or absorbed through nonintact skin.

Local Anesthetic/Vasoconstrictor Precautions
No information available to require special precautions

Effects on Bleeding None reported

Bovine Colostrum

Clinical Overview

Uses

Bovine colostrum may have a role in the management of HIV-associated diarrhea. There is increasing evidence of efficacy in boosting the immune system, preventing upper respiratory tract infection, reducing GI permeability, and enhancing athletic performance, although data are conflicting and are based on small sample sizes and studies of limited quality.

Dosing

Standardization of commercial bovine colostrum products is difficult because antibody content varies widely. Dosages up to 60 g/day for up to 12 weeks have been used in clinical trials evaluating use for athletic enhancement. In trials using bovine colostrum for exercise-induced GI permeability, dosages of 20 g/day for 14 days, or 1 g/day for 20 days have been used; in one trial, a dosage of 1.7 g/kg/day for 7 days prior to an exercise protocol was used.

Contraindications

Contraindications other than milk allergy have not been identified.

Pregnancy/Lactation

Avoid use. Information regarding safety and efficacy in pregnancy and lactation is lacking.

Interactions

None well documented.

Adverse Reactions

Bovine colostrum is well tolerated, with minor GI complaints (eg, nausea, flatulence, diarrhea), unpleasant taste, and skin rash occurring infrequently.

Toxicology

The US Food and Drug Administration (FDA) has accepted the safety of hyperimmune milks on the basis that no adverse health effects have been shown in clinical studies. Past concerns regarding transmission of bovine spongiform encephalopathy (BSE), a feed-borne infection in cattle, have been resolved.

Local Anesthetic/Vasoconstrictor Precautions

No information available to require special precautions

Effects on Bleeding None reported

Brahmi

Clinical Overview

Uses

Brahmi is used for its antioxidant activity. It has been investigated for use in improving cognition.

Dosing

Numerous dosage forms and commercial products are available and marketed for improved short- and long-term memory. A typical commercially available regimen is 2 oral capsules (500 mg; herbal extract of brahmi ratio, 10:1) twice a day with water after meals. Each capsule contains 500 mg (herbal extract of brahmi ratio is 10:1). Brahmi extracts have been used in clinical trials at dosages of 300 to 450 mg per day.

Contraindications

Avoid use with hypersensitivity to any of the components of brahmi.

Pregnancy/Lactation

Avoid use. Information regarding safety and efficacy in pregnancy and lactation is lacking.

Interactions

None well documented.

Adverse Reactions

Commonly reported adverse effects are flu-like symptoms, GI irritation, nausea, increased intestinal motility, and muscle fatigue.

Toxicology

No clinical data are available regarding toxicity.

Local Anesthetic/Vasoconstrictor Precautions

No information available to require special precautions

Effects on Bleeding None reported

Brewer's Yeast

Clinical Overview

Uses

Brewer's yeast is traditionally used as a source of vitamin B, selenium, and chromium, especially by vegetarians. Clinical trials have evaluated yeast for a role in immunomodulation, respiratory infections, prevention of postsurgical infections (as beta-glucan), and as a source of dietary fiber to improve the lipid profile. However, there is a lack of quality trials.

Dosing

Upper respiratory tract infections: S. cerevisiae 500 mg daily has been used in clinical trials over 12 weeks to treat respiratory infections and allergic rhinitis.

Laxative: 6 to 50 g of fresh baker's yeast over 3 days was used in a study for the treatment of cancer-related constipation.

Acute diarrhea: 500 mg daily of brewer's yeast is recommended in the German Commission E Monographs.

Contraindications

Crohn disease; concomitant monoamine oxidase inhibitor (MAOI) therapy.

Pregnancy/Lactation

Information regarding safety and efficacy in pregnancy and lactation is lacking.

Interactions

Brewer's yeast contains tyramine. Avoid concurrent use with MAOIs.

Adverse Reactions

Mild GI symptoms, including flatulence.

Toxicology

Information is limited. Baker's yeast has Food and Drug Administration (FDA) GRAS (generally recognized as safe) status.

Local Anesthetic/Vasoconstrictor Precautions

No information available to require special precautions

Effects on Bleeding None reported

Buchu

Clinical Overview

Uses

Buchu has been used to treat inflammation and kidney and urinary tract infections; as a diuretic and as a stomach tonic. Other uses include carminative action and treatment of cystitis, urethritis, prostatitis and gout. It has also been used for leukorrhea and yeast infections.

Dosing

There is no recent clinical evidence to guide dosage of buchu. Classical doses were from 1 to 2 g of the leaves daily.

Contraindications

Contraindications have not yet been identified.

Pregnancy/Lactation

Documented adverse effects, including uterine stimulant effects. Avoid use.

Interactions

None well documented.

Adverse Reactions

Buchu can cause stomach and kidney irritation and can be an abortifacient. It can also induce increased menstrual flow. Buchu is not recommended during pregnancy.

Toxicology

Poisoning has not been reported. Buchu contains the hepatotoxin pulegone, also known to be present in pennyroyal.

Local Anesthetic/Vasoconstrictor Precautions No information available to require special precautions

Effects on Bleeding None reported

Bupleurum

Clinical Overview

Uses

Bupleurum is being investigated for its antipyretic, immunomodulatory, GI tract, and hepatoprotective effects, as well as its potential in the prevention and treatment of cancers. Clinical trials are generally lacking.

Dosing

No clinical trials exist.

Contraindications

Contraindications have not been identified.

Pregnancy/Lactation

Information regarding safety and efficacy in pregnancy and lactation is lacking.

Interactions

None well documented.

Adverse Reactions

Mild lassitude, sedation, and drowsiness. Large doses may increase flatulence and bowel movements. Allergy to injected bupleurum has been reported.

Toxicology

The toxicity profile appears to be low; however, information is limited.

Local Anesthetic/Vasoconstrictor Precautions No information available to require special precautions

Effects on Bleeding None reported

Bur Marigold

Clinical Overview

Uses

Several Bidens spp. have been used extensively in traditional medicine. Bur marigold may possess anti-inflammatory, antimicrobial, cardiovascular, and cytotoxic activity; however, clinical studies are lacking to support recommendations for use. A B. pilosa extract has been investigated for use in the management of diabetes.

Dosing

Clinical studies are lacking to provide dosing recommendations.

Contraindications

Contraindications have not been identified.

Pregnancy/Lactation

Avoid use. Information regarding safety and efficacy during pregnancy and lactation is lacking.

Interactions

None well documented.

Adverse Reactions

Clinical data regarding adverse effects of bur marigold are lacking; however, a small clinical study reported no adverse effects following administration of a B. pilosa formulation for 90 days. Cross-sensitivity to other members of the Asteraceae family may exist.

Toxicology

Clinical data are limited, especially regarding long-term toxicity.

Local Anesthetic/Vasoconstrictor Precautions No information available to require special precautions

Effects on Bleeding None reported

Butcher's Broom

Clinical Overview

Uses

Butcher's broom has been used in many forms as a laxative, diuretic, treatment for circulatory disease, and cytotoxic agent, although limited results from clinical trials are available.

Dosing

Butchers broom has been used in clinical trials for chronic venous insufficiency standardized to 7 to 11 mg of ruscogenin. Hesperidin methyl chalcone has also been used as a marker for standardization in the product Cyclo 3 Fort. Extracts have been dosed at 16 mg daily for chronic phlebopathy, while a topical cream formulation was used to apply 64 to 96 mg of extract daily.

Contraindications

Contraindications have not yet been identified.

Pregnancy/Lactation

Information regarding safety and efficacy in pregnancy and lactation is lacking. Avoid use.

Interactions

None well documented.

Adverse Reactions

No adverse reactions have been reported.

Toxicology

Not known to be toxic.

Local Anesthetic/Vasoconstrictor Precautions No information available to require special precautions

Effects on Bleeding None reported

Calendula

Clinical Overview

Uses

Limited clinical studies have focused on use of calendula in wound healing, including radiation-induced dermatitis, venous leg ulceration, and burns/acute wounds. Antioxidant, anti-inflammatory, and antimicrobial effects, including in periodontal disease, are also documented. However, quality clinical trial data are lacking to recommend calendula for any indication.

Dosing

Commercial topical preparations are available. Various topical dosage forms and preparations have been evaluated in clinical studies; however, data are lacking regarding specific strengths/concentrations used, and trials are associated with methodological limitations, making dosing recommendations difficult. See specific indications in Uses section.

Contraindications

Contraindications have not been identified.

Pregnancy/Lactation

Avoid use. Information regarding safety and efficacy in pregnancy and lactation is lacking. A study in rats demonstrated a reduction in maternal weight gain when calendula was administered during pregnancy.

Interactions

None well documented.

Adverse Reactions

Allergic reactions, contact sensitization, and one case of anaphylaxis have been reported.

Toxicology

No data.

Local Anesthetic/Vasoconstrictor Precautions
No information available to require special precautions

Effects on Bleeding None reported

Cannabis

Clinical Overview

Uses

The efficacy of cannabis for the management of chemotherapy-induced nausea, spasticity in multiple sclerosis (MS), treatment-resistant seizures, and neuropathic pain has been clinically demonstrated to some extent. A bias towards reporting positive findings exists, both within individual clinical studies as well as within systematic reviews evaluating the role of cannabis in pain management. Undesirable adverse reactions, lack of data regarding long-term effects, and a general lack of comparison to standard treatments limit applications of cannabis; therapeutic use may be limited to either concomitant therapy or alternative therapy when conventional therapy has failed. Clinical studies in the United States have been limited by legal factors.

Dosing

Clinical studies use a wide range of preparations and usually allow dosage titration for effect. For more information regarding dosage recommendations for CBD alone, see the Cannabidiol monograph.

Contraindications

Contraindications have not been identified. There is a risk of hypersensitivity to marijuana or other constituents of the plant. The benefits versus risks of cannabis use should be carefully weighed in individuals with psychosocial disorders.

Pregnancy/Lactation

Avoid use. Information regarding safety and efficacy in pregnancy and lactation is limited. In retrospective studies, cannabis had a modest effect on fetal growth. THC crosses the placental barrier and is excreted in breast milk.

Interactions

Few case reports exist of interactions in which cannabis is solely implicated. Cannabis may interact with the following: alcohol, anticholinergic agents, CNS depressants, cocaine, cytochrome P450 (CYP-450) 1A2 substrates, CYP2C9 inhibitors, CYP3A4 inducers and inhibitors, St. John's wort, and sympathomimetics.

Adverse Reactions

Use of medical cannabis or cannabis preparations is generally considered safe and is devoid of common major adverse reactions, although rare cardiovascular adverse effects and stroke have been noted. Tolerance and dependence have been documented. Major adverse reactions with recreational cannabis use occur more with increasing dosages and include cardiovascular effects, cannabinoid hyperemesis syndrome, psychosis, and others. When recreational use starts at an early age (ie, adolescence), brain development of functional connectivity can be impaired, resulting in declines in intelligence quotient (IQ). The risk of impairments in cognitive and motor function may limit applications of cannabis.

Toxicology

There is a lack of consensus regarding the risk of lung cancer from smoked cannabis or the risk of psychotic events from consumption of oral cannabis preparations. All risk factors should be considered in the context of applications for medical cannabis in intractable diseases. Toxicities due to long-term nonmedical (recreational) cannabis use include increased incidence of psychotic, respiratory, and cardiovascular events, as well as cancers of the lung, head and neck, brain, cervix, prostate, and testis.

Local Anesthetic/Vasoconstrictor Precautions
No information available to require special precautions

Effects on Bleeding None reported

Capsicum Peppers

Clinical Overview

Uses

Many varieties are eaten as vegetables, condiments, and spices. The component capsaicin is an irritant and analgesic used in self-defense sprays, and in a variety of conditions associated with pain. Other studies have evaluated a role in weight loss, GI conditions, postoperative nausea, and rhinitis, although limited information is available.

Dosing

For external uses, capsaicin and Capsicum creams are available in several strengths, from 0.025% to 0.075% capsaicin. Clinical trials are lacking to guide dosage for other uses.

Contraindications

None clearly established.

Pregnancy/Lactation

Generally recognized as safe (GRAS) when used as food. Safety and efficacy for dosages above those in foods are unproven and should be avoided. Studies in animals have shown both positive and negative effects.

Interactions

Use of capsaicin by patients receiving captopril or other angiotensin-converting enzyme (ACE) inhibitors may cause or exacerbate ACE inhibitor-induced cough. Nonheme iron absorption may be inhibited by concomitant chili consumption.

Adverse Reactions

Topical, mucosal, and GI irritations are common. Allergies and cross-sensitization to other allergens have been reported.

Toxicology

Toxicity is evidenced in animal experiments in higher dosages. Controversy exists regarding capsaicin's mutagenicity and tumorigenicity. Toxicity from long-term exposure to chili powder has not been found, and the use of defense sprays likewise has not resulted in reports of toxicity.

Local Anesthetic/Vasoconstrictor Precautions
No information available to require special precautions

Effects on Bleeding May have some antiplatelet effects

Cascara

Clinical Overview

Uses

Clinical studies of cascara have focused on its laxative effects, although cascara is no longer considered safe for this use. Attention has shifted to cascara's constituent emodin and its possible therapeutic applications in the treatment of various conditions, based on animal and in vitro data.

Dosing

Cascara sagrada nonprescription laxative products were declared no longer safe or effective by the US Food and Drug Administration (FDA) in 2002. Typical doses of cascara are 1 g of the bark, 2 to 6 mL as a fluid extract, or 100 to 300 mg of dried bark extract.

Contraindications

Cascara is contraindicated in children younger than 10 years; in ileus of any origin; and in inflammatory diseases of the colon, including ulcerative colitis, irritable bowel syndrome (IBS), and Crohn disease.

Pregnancy/Lactation

Avoid use. Emmenagogue and abortifacient effects have been documented. Anthranoid metabolites may be excreted in breast milk.

Interactions

None well documented.

Adverse Reactions

Extended use may cause chronic diarrhea and consequent electrolyte imbalance. Cases of benign and reversible melanosis coli have been reported.

Toxicology

Overdose of anthraquinone laxatives results in intestinal pain and severe diarrhea, with consequent electrolyte imbalance and dehydration. No causal relationship between long-term use of cascara and colorectal cancer has been established.

Local Anesthetic/Vasoconstrictor Precautions

No information available to require special precautions

Effects on Bleeding None reported

Catnip

Clinical Overview

Uses

There are little clinical data to support any use of catnip in humans, except as an insect repellant. Animal and in vitro studies provide limited data of N. cataria use as an antimicrobial agent or antidepressant.

Dosing

There is no clinical evidence to guide dosage of catnip. A 15% lotion of the essential oil has been used as an insect repellant.

Contraindications

Contraindications have not been identified.

Pregnancy/Lactation

Avoid use. Adverse effects (eg, emmenagogue and abortifacient effects) have been documented.

Interactions

None well documented.

Adverse Reactions

Headache, malaise, conjunctival irritation, and erythema have occurred.

Toxicology

Information is lacking.

Local Anesthetic/Vasoconstrictor Precautions

No information available to require special precautions

Effects on Bleeding None reported

Cat's Claw

Clinical Overview

Uses

Despite multiple purported effects, controlled clinical trials are lacking. Suggested anti-inflammatory, anticancer, and immunostimulant properties are largely based on in vitro and limited animal studies.

Dosing

One gram of root bark given 2 to 3 times daily is a typical dose, while 20 to 30 mg of a root bark extract has been recommended. Clinical trials are generally lacking to support appropriate dosages. A standardized extract containing 8% to 10% carboxy alkyl esters and less than 0.5% oxindole alkaloids has been used in clinical studies in doses of 250 to 300 mg.

Contraindications

Cat's claw products should be avoided before and after surgery, as well as by those using immunosuppressant therapy and in children due to lack of safety data.

Pregnancy/Lactation

Information regarding safety and efficacy during pregnancy and lactation is lacking.

Interactions

Case reports are generally lacking; however, there is a reported interaction with protease inhibitors.

Adverse Reactions

Although reports of adverse effects are rare, GI complaints (nausea, diarrhea, stomach discomfort), renal effects, neuropathy, and an increased risk of bleeding with anticoagulant therapy are possible.

Toxicology

Historical ethnomedicinal evidence and current use by consumers suggest low toxicity; however, toxicological studies are limited.

Local Anesthetic/Vasoconstrictor Precautions

No information available to require special precautions

Effects on Bleeding May cause increased bleeding due to inhibition of platelet aggregation

Chamomile

Clinical Overview

Uses

Chamomile is used topically in skin and mucous membrane inflammations and skin diseases. It can be inhaled for respiratory tract inflammations or irritations; used in baths as irrigation for anogenital inflammation; and used internally for GI spasms and inflammatory diseases. However, clinical trials supporting any use of chamomile are limited.

Dosing

Chamomile has been used as a tea for various conditions and as a topical cream. Typical oral doses are 9 to 15 g/day. Gargles made from 8 g chamomile flowers in 1,000 mL of water have been used in clinical trials.

Contraindications

The use of chamomile-containing preparations is contraindicated in persons with hypersensitivity to ragweed pollens.

Pregnancy/Lactation

Unreferenced adverse reactions have been cited. Avoid use during pregnancy. No clinical data are available on use during lactation.

Interactions

Possible interactions have been reported with warfarin or cyclosporine. Because warfarin and cyclosporine have a narrow therapeutic index, patients taking either of these medications in other than modest amounts should avoid concurrent use of chamomile.

Adverse Reactions

Use of the tea and essential oil has resulted in anaphylaxis, contact dermatitis, and other severe hypersensitivity reactions. Cross-reactivity to asters, chrysanthemums, ragweed, and other members of the Asteraceae family exists.

Toxicology

Animal studies report low toxicity with oral ingestion of chamomile.

Local Anesthetic/Vasoconstrictor Precautions
No information available to require special precautions

Effects on Bleeding None reported

Chaparral

Clinical Overview

Uses

Chaparral has been traditionally used for the treatment of cancer, acne, rheumatism, and diabetes. It has also been promoted for its antioxidant effects by inhibiting free radicals. Chaparral has also been used as a blood purifier and a weight loss agent. However, clinical trials are lacking to support any of these uses.

Dosing

Because chaparral has been documented as hepatotoxic at doses of crude herb from 1.5 to 3.5 g/day, its use is discouraged.

Contraindications

Chaparral was removed from the US Food and Drug Administration's Generally Recognized as Safe (GRAS) list in 1968. Increased risk for hepatotoxicity is expected in patients with hepatic dysfunction. Chaparral is not recommended for use in patients with renal dysfunction due to a risk for accumulation of chaparral and toxicity.

Pregnancy/Lactation

Documented adverse effects (uterine activity, hepatotoxic). Avoid use.

Interactions

None well documented.

Adverse Reactions

The creosote bush can induce contact dermatitis.

Toxicology

Chaparral may cause liver damage, stimulate some malignancies, and cause contact dermatitis.

Local Anesthetic/Vasoconstrictor Precautions
No information available to require special precautions

Effects on Bleeding Nordihydroguaiaretic acid (NDGA), believed to be responsible for the biological activity of chaparral, is a platelet aggregation inhibitor; there is potential for an increased risk of bleeding in patients undergoing invasive dental procedures, particularly in patients taking concomitant anticoagulants, antiplatelet drugs, or any drugs or herbals with antiplatelet properties.

Chaste Tree

Clinical Overview

Uses

Chaste tree extract has been used to manage symptoms related to premenstrual syndrome (PMS) and cyclic mastalgia and may be a suitable alternative to standard pharmacological management. Although the Complete German Commission E Monographs supports its use for PMS and cyclic mastalgia, there are limited clinical trials to support these uses. Limited evidence exists for its use in menopause.

Dosing

Daily doses of chaste tree fruit extract are typically 20 to 40 mg.

Contraindications

Patients who have an allergy to or are hypersensitive to V. agnus-castus or patients who are pregnant or breastfeeding should avoid use. Safe use in children has not been established.

Pregnancy/Lactation

Information regarding safety and efficacy in pregnancy and lactation is lacking. However, chaste tree may have estrogenic, progesterogenic, and/or uterine stimulant activity and should be avoided in pregnancy and while breastfeeding.

Interactions

None well documented.

Adverse Reactions

Generally regarded as safe; mild and reversible adverse effects include GI reactions, itching, rash, headache, fatigue, acne, and menstrual disturbances.

Toxicology

Information is limited and safety has not been determined in children.

Local Anesthetic/Vasoconstrictor Precautions
No information available to require special precautions

Effects on Bleeding None reported

Chinese Cucumber

Clinical Overview

Uses

Chinese cucumber has been studied, primarily in animal and in vitro studies, for its cardiovascular, immune system, antioxidant, antidiabetic, expectorant, and gastroprotective effects. Antiviral activity and potential application in cancer therapy is being investigated. However, a lack of clinical trials and toxicity of the plant's root limit use for any indication.

Dosing

Clinical studies are lacking to provide dosing guidance. In traditional Chinese medicine, Chinese cucumber has most commonly been administered as part of a polyherbal preparation. Seeds of the plant have been used as a dietary source of conjugated linolenic acid (20.8 g of seed kernels per day for 28 days).

Contraindications

Use is contraindicated in pregnancy.

Pregnancy/Lactation

Use is contraindicated. Extracts of the root possess abortifacient activity and are toxic to the fetus.

Interactions

None well documented.

Adverse Reactions

Available published clinical studies are limited. However, one trial in HIV subjects reported myalgia, fever, elevated liver function tests, and mild to moderate anaphylactic reactions.

Toxicology

Extracts of Chinese cucumber are extremely toxic (death has occurred), particularly if administered parenterally.

Local Anesthetic/Vasoconstrictor Precautions
No information available to require special precautions

Effects on Bleeding None reported

Chinese Foxglove

Clinical Overview

Uses

Rehmannia rhizome extracts have been used extensively in traditional Chinese medicine. Because the preparation is often used in combination with other agents, it is difficult to attribute any benefits to R. glutinosa. Efficacy of R. glutinosa acteoside in the management of primary chronic glomerulonephritis has been suggested; however, clinical trials are lacking to support any use.

Dosing

Clinical studies are lacking to inform dosage. Common nonprescription polyherbal products contain varying amounts of Rehmannia root extract.

Contraindications

Chronic liver disease and GI disorders, including diarrhea.

Pregnancy/Lactation

Avoid use. Rehmannia has traditionally been used as an emmenagogue.

Interactions

None well documented.

Adverse Reactions

Minor and transient adverse reactions have been reported and include GI reactions (eg, diarrhea, abdominal pain), edema, heart palpitations, fatigue, and vertigo.

Toxicology

No data.

Local Anesthetic/Vasoconstrictor Precautions

No information available to require special precautions

Effects on Bleeding None reported

Chitosan

Clinical Overview

Uses

There is some evidence of the effect of chitosan on lowering cholesterol and body weight, but the effect is unlikely to be of clinical importance. To some extent, chitosan is used in the emergency setting to control bleeding. Chitosan has been used in various drug delivery systems. Antimicrobial and other effects are being evaluated for use in dentistry.

Dosing

Chitosan has been administered at wide-ranging doses in clinical studies. In studies evaluating weight loss, 2.4 g/day is commonly used.

Contraindications

None well established.

Pregnancy/Lactation

Information regarding safety and efficacy in pregnancy and lactation is lacking.

Interactions

Data are limited. Potentiation of the anticoagulant effect of warfarin was reported in a patient receiving chitosan 2.4 g/day.

Adverse Reactions

The potential for allergy exists in individuals allergic to shellfish. Clinical trials report few adverse events, generally limited to flatulence and constipation.

Toxicology

Chitosan's toxicity profile is relatively low.

Local Anesthetic/Vasoconstrictor Precautions

No information available to require special precautions

Effects on Bleeding None reported

Chondroitin

Clinical Overview

Uses

Chondroitin sulfate has been studied for the treatment of arthritis; however, information on its effectiveness is conflicting. It is commonly given in combination with other agents, such as glucosamine sulfate or glucosamine hydrochloride. It has also been studied for use in drug delivery, antithrombotic and extravasation therapy, and treatment of dry eyes and interstitial cystitis.

Dosing

Chondroitin sulfate has been administered orally for treatment of arthritis at a dosage of 800 to 1,200 mg/day. Positive results often require several months to manifest, and a posttreatment effect has been observed. Animal studies have suggested that the bioavailability of chondroitin sulfate may be increased when given multiple times a day.

Contraindications

Contraindications have not been identified.

Pregnancy/Lactation

Information regarding safety and efficacy in pregnancy and lactation is lacking.

Interactions

An increase in the international normalized ratio (INR) may occur in patients taking anticoagulants, such as warfarin (eg, Coumadin), with either chondroitin alone or in combination with glucosamine.

Adverse Reactions

Potential adverse reactions associated with chondroitin sulfate include alopecia, constipation, diarrhea, epigastralgia, extrasystoles, eyelid edema, lower limb edema, and skin symptoms. Chondroitin sulfate may also exacerbate asthma.

Toxicology

There is little information regarding the long-term effects of chondroitin. Most reports conclude that it is safe.

Local Anesthetic/Vasoconstrictor Precautions

No information available to require special precautions

Effects on Bleeding None reported

Chromium

Clinical Overview

Uses

Chromium supplementation has been studied for a variety of indications, especially diabetes and weight loss, but clinical studies have shown inconsistent results. The role of supplemental chromium remains controversial.

Dosing

The currently accepted value for chromium dietary intake is 25 mcg/day for women and 35 mcg/day for men. Daily dosages used in clinical trials for periods of up to 9 months range as follows: brewer's yeast up to 400 mcg/day; chromium chloride 50 to 600 mcg/day; chromium nicotinate 200 to 800 mcg/day; chromium picolinate 60 to 1,000 mcg/day. The potential for genotoxic effects exists at higher dosages.

Contraindications

None well documented. Renal failure may be considered a relative contraindication.

Pregnancy/Lactation

Information regarding safety and efficacy in pregnancy and lactation is lacking. Limited animal experimentation showed skeletal and neurological defects in the offspring of mice fed chromium picolinate.

Interactions

None well documented.

Adverse Reactions

Ingestion or exposure to certain forms of chromium may cause or contribute to GI irritation and ulcers, dermatitis, hemorrhage, circulatory shock, and renal tubule damage.

Toxicology

No risk of genotoxicity at low dosages over the short-term exists for chromium as a dietary supplement. However, at higher dosages, such as those used in trials evaluating the efficacy of chromium in glycemic control, concern exists for potential genotoxic effects.

Local Anesthetic/Vasoconstrictor Precautions
No information available to require special precautions

Effects on Bleeding None reported

Cinnamon

Clinical Overview

Uses

Cinnamon is used as a spice and aromatic. Traditionally, the bark or oil has been used to combat microorganisms, diarrhea, and other GI disorders, and dysmenorrhea, although there is limited data to support these uses. Evidence is lacking to support the use of cinnamon in the management of diabetes. Research has focused on anti-inflammatory, antioxidant, and antimicrobial activity.

Dosing

Ground cinnamon is generally given at dosages of 1 to 1.5 g/day in studies of diabetes without reported adverse reactions.

Contraindications

Contraindicated in people who are allergic to cinnamon or Peru balsam. Further contraindications have not yet been identified.

Pregnancy/Lactation

Data are insufficient for adequate risk-to-benefit analysis. Cinnamon is generally recognized as safe when used in food.

Interactions

None well documented.

Adverse Reactions

Heavy exposure may cause skin irritation and allergic reactions.

Toxicology

Information is lacking.

Local Anesthetic/Vasoconstrictor Precautions
No information available to require special precautions

Effects on Bleeding None reported

Clove

Clinical Overview

Uses

Clove has historically been used for its antiseptic and analgesic effects. Clove and clove oils are used safely in foods, beverages, and toothpastes. Clove oil cream has been used in the treatment of anal fissures and an extract has exhibited aphrodisiac action in rats; however, there are limited studies supporting clinical applications for clove oil.

Dosing

There are limited studies to support therapeutic dosing for clove oil.

Contraindications

Contraindications have not been identified.

Pregnancy/Lactation

Information regarding safety and efficacy in pregnancy and lactation is lacking.

Interactions

None well documented.

Adverse Reactions

Contact dermatitis has been noted.

Toxicology

Toxicity has been observed following ingestion of the oil, but is rare and poorly documented.

Local Anesthetic/Vasoconstrictor Precautions
No information available to require special precautions

Effects on Bleeding Clove has been reported to have antiplatelet effects; however, case reports and clinical data are lacking. Presently, there is no information available to require special precautions.

Cocoa

Clinical Overview

Uses

Cocoa solid, cocoa butter, and chocolate are all rich sources of antioxidants. Epidemiological studies show an inverse association between the consumption of cocoa and the risk of cardiovascular disease. The likely mechanisms are antioxidant activity; improvement in endothelial function, vascular function, and insulin sensitivity; as well as attenuation of platelet reactivity and reduction in blood pressure.

Dosing

No specific dosing recommendations can be made. Further studies characterizing the polyphenol content of cocoa products and method of measurement are needed. In one study, an inverse relationship was demonstrated between cocoa intake and blood pressure, as well as a 15-year cardiovascular and all-cause mortality; the median cocoa intake among users was 2.11 g/day.

Contraindications

None known.

Pregnancy/Lactation

Generally recognized as safe (GRAS) when used in moderate amounts or in amounts used in foods. Avoid dosages greater than those found in food because safety and efficacy are unproven. Caffeine content should be restricted during pregnancy.

Interactions

None well documented.

Adverse Reactions

Children consuming large amounts of chocolate and caffeinated beverages may exhibit tics or restlessness. Ingredients in chocolate may precipitate migraine headaches, and cocoa products may be allergenic.

Toxicology

Cocoa is nontoxic when ingested in typical confectionery amounts.

Local Anesthetic/Vasoconstrictor Precautions
No information available to require special precautions

Effects on Bleeding None reported

Comfrey

Clinical Overview

Uses

Therapeutic use of comfrey is limited because of its toxicity. A limited number of clinical trials show short-term efficacy of topically applied, alkaloid-free comfrey preparations in skin abrasions and inflammatory conditions. Although not examined in clinical trials, comfrey may possess antifungal and anticancer activity.

Dosing

Oral use of comfrey is not supported because of potential hepatotoxicity. Additionally, because externally applied alkaloids are well absorbed and detected in the urine, topical use of comfrey should not exceed an alkaloid exposure of 100 mcg/day. Limited trials have evaluated the efficacy of alkaloid-free preparations for topical use; however, these studies do not report on hepatic laboratory indices of study participants.

Contraindications

Comfrey is not recommended for internal use because of the hepatotoxic pyrrolizidine alkaloid content. Patients with hypersensitivity or allergic reactions to the plant should avoid external use. Use is contraindicated during pregnancy and lactation, in infants, and in patients with liver or kidney disease.

Pregnancy/Lactation

Contraindicated because of documented adverse effects. Pyrrolizidine alkaloids have abortifacient effects and increase the risk of fatal hepatic veno-occlusive disease. Animal experiments have detected alkaloids in breast milk.

Interactions

None well documented.

Adverse Reactions

Neither internal nor extensive topical use of comfrey is recommended because of numerous reports of liver toxicity (see Toxicology). Case reports show hepatic veno-occlusive disease and pulmonary hypertension related to comfrey use. Infants are more susceptible to pyrrolizidine-related, veno-occlusive disease; therefore, the use of comfrey in this population is contraindicated.

Toxicology

The Food and Drug Administration (FDA) released an advisory in July 2001 recommending that comfrey products be removed from the market because of cases of hepatic veno-occlusive disease. Comfrey is generally considered unsafe, with numerous toxicological effects in animals and humans.

Local Anesthetic/Vasoconstrictor Precautions

No information available to require special precautions

Effects on Bleeding None reported

Cordyceps

Clinical Overview

Uses

Well-controlled clinical trials are lacking.

Dosing

Dosing supported by product quality data is unavailable, and many herbal supplements on the market contain varying undefined levels of this product. Cordyceps 3 to 6 g/day has been used in patients with chronic renal failure for periods ranging from days to years.

Contraindications

Contraindications have not been identified.

Pregnancy/Lactation

Information regarding safety and efficacy in pregnancy and lactation is lacking.

Interactions

None well documented.

Adverse Reactions

Mild GI discomfort, including diarrhea, dry mouth, and nausea, has been reported.

Toxicology

Cordyceps is generally considered safe.

Local Anesthetic/Vasoconstrictor Precautions

No information available to require special precautions

Effects on Bleeding Cordyceps has been reported to have antiplatelet effects; however, case reports and clinical data are lacking. Presently, there is no information available to require special precautions.

Cranberry

Clinical Overview

Uses

Some evidence exists for the use of cranberry in preventing, but not treating, urinary tract infections (UTIs). Other possible uses for cranberry, with limited evidence, include reduction of the risk of cardiovascular disease and cancer.

Dosing

Cranberry juice, juice concentrate, and dried extract have been studied in UTIs; however, consistency in dosage regimens is lacking. Doses of juice cocktail (25% pure cranberry juice) have ranged from 120 to 1,000 mL/day in divided doses. Concentrated cranberry extract in the form of tablets and capsules is available and 600 to more than 1,200 mg/day in divided doses have been used in studies in UTIs.

Contraindications

Predisposition to or history of nephrolithiasis (kidney stones).

Pregnancy/Lactation

Information is limited; however, when ingested at normal food consumption amounts, cranberry is considered relatively safe in pregnancy. Safety during lactation is unknown.

Interactions

An interaction between cranberry and warfarin has been suggested based on case reports; however, evidence for a causal relationship is lacking from clinical trials.

Adverse Reactions

The berries and juice have few adverse reactions associated with their consumption. Large daily doses may produce GI symptoms, such as diarrhea. Concentrated cranberry tablets may predispose patients to nephrolithiasis. Cranberry juice should not be used to clear enteral feeding tubes.

Toxicology

Information is lacking.

Local Anesthetic/Vasoconstrictor Precautions

No information available to require special precautions

Effects on Bleeding None reported

Creatine

Clinical Overview

Uses

Creatine has enhanced performance in short-duration, high-intensity exercise in limited trials. Creatine supplementation has been extensively studied in myopathies and neurodegenerative disorders, but with limited efficacy. Further trials are ongoing.

Dosing

Dosage regimens in clinical trials vary from 2 to 20 g daily, and from 1 to 6 weeks and longer.

Contraindications

Patients with a history of renal impairment or those taking nephrotoxic agents should avoid concomitant creatine supplementation or be monitored closely if supplementation is necessary.

Pregnancy/Lactation

Information regarding safety and efficacy in pregnancy and lactation is lacking.

Interactions

None well documented.

Adverse Reactions

Few adverse reactions have been reported in clinical studies among patients with neurological or muscle disorders, or in healthy individuals

Concerns regarding renal and hepatic toxicity exist; unequivocal proof of safety is lacking and caution is warranted.

Case reports of adverse reactions among athletes include dehydration, electrolyte imbalance, and muscle cramping. Minor GI upset (diarrhea, GI pain, nausea), dizziness, and short-term loss in body mass have also been reported. The safety of creatine in children has not been established.

Toxicology

Information is limited; however, the French Agency for Food, Environmental and Occupational Health & Safety (ANSES) has warned of the potential for production of cytotoxic compounds, especially at high dosages.

Local Anesthetic/Vasoconstrictor Precautions
No information available to require special precautions

Effects on Bleeding None reported

Cumin

Clinical Overview

Uses

Cumin seeds are used in cooking and the oil is used to flavor food and scent cosmetics. Components may have antioxidant, anticancer, hypoglycemic, antiepileptic, antiosteoporotic, ophthalmic, antibacterial, and larvicidal effects; however, there is no clinical evidence to support these claims. Cumin is generally recognized as safe for human consumption as a spice and flavoring.

Dosing

There are no recent clinical studies of cumin that provide a basis for dosage recommendations.

Contraindications

Contraindications have not yet been identified.

Pregnancy/Lactation

Information regarding safety and efficacy in pregnancy and lactation is lacking.

Interactions

None well documented.

Adverse Reactions

The oil may have photosensitizing effects. Cumin may also cause hypoglycemia.

Toxicology

No data are available.

Local Anesthetic/Vasoconstrictor Precautions
No information available to require special precautions

Effects on Bleeding A study published in 1989 showed that cumin inhibits human platelet aggregation in *in vitro* testing; the clinical significance of this effect is unknown at this time.

Damiana

Clinical Overview

Uses

Clinical studies evaluating the effect of T. diffusa are lacking. Studies in rodents suggest damiana has aphrodisiac and anxiolytic effects.

Dosing

There are no recent clinical studies of damiana to provide dosage recommendations. Traditionally, damiana extract British Pharmaceutical Codex (BPC) has been used at a dosage of 0.3 to 0.6 g.

Contraindications

Contraindications have not been identified.

Pregnancy/Lactation

Avoid use. Documented adverse effects include cyanogenic glycosides and risk of cyanide toxicity with high doses of damiana.

Interactions

None well documented.

Adverse Reactions

There is limited clinical information regarding adverse reactions associated with damiana use. The possibility of convulsions, especially in relation to excess alcohol consumption, exists. Damiana-induced hallucinations are unlikely.

Toxicology

Research reveals little or no information regarding toxicity with damiana use. T. diffusa contains potentially toxic chemicals including arbutin, tannins, and cyanogenic glycosides.

Local Anesthetic/Vasoconstrictor Precautions
No information available to require special precautions

Effects on Bleeding None reported

Dandelion

Clinical Overview

Uses

Dandelion has been used for its nutritional value. Other traditional uses include regulation of blood glucose, treatment of liver and gallbladder disorders, appetite stimulation, treatment of dyspeptic complaints, and as a diuretic. However, limited clinical studies are available to provide evidence to support such claims.

Dosing

Clinical trials on which to base dosing are limited. Fresh roots and leaves are often consumed in salads. The *German Commission E Monographs* recommends 3 to 4 g of the root or 10 to 15 drops of root tincture twice a day, or 4 to 10 g of the leaves or 2 to 5 mL of leaf tincture 3 times a day.

Contraindications

Contraindications have not yet been identified.

Pregnancy/Lactation

Generally recognized as safe (GRAS) by the US Food and Drug Administration or used as food. Avoid dosages above those in foods; safety and efficacy of such dosages are unproven.

Interactions

None well documented.

Adverse Reactions

Allergy and mild gastric discomfort have been reported.

Toxicology

The acute toxicity of dandelion is considered low. Decreased fertility in male rats has been observed.

Local Anesthetic/Vasoconstrictor Precautions No information available to require special precautions

Effects on Bleeding None reported

Danshen

Clinical Overview

Uses

Danshen has been used extensively in traditional Chinese medicine as a single herb and in multiherb formulations. Limited clinical studies have shown efficacy in coronary artery disease and acute ischemic stroke, but the quality of methodology limits the validity and extrapolation of these findings.

Dosing

Active components in commercially available preparations of danshen vary greatly. Doses include danshen 20 mg/kg capsules. Dosages of danshen root extract 5 g twice daily for 60 days have been used in diabetic patients with coronary heart disease.

Contraindications

Contraindications have not been identified.

Pregnancy/Lactation

Avoid use. Information regarding safety and efficacy in pregnancy and lactation is lacking.

Interactions

Danshen may interfere with laboratory digoxin plasma levels and increase the anticoagulant effect of warfarin. It may reduce the plasma concentration and therefore pharmacologic effects of midazolam. Danshen inhibits numerous cytochrome P450 (CYP-450) enzymes in vitro.

Adverse Reactions

Adverse reactions include allergy, dizziness, headache, mild GI symptoms, and reversible thrombocytopenia.

Toxicology

No data.

Local Anesthetic/Vasoconstrictor Precautions No information available to require special precautions

Effects on Bleeding Danshen has been shown to inhibit platelet aggregation *in vitro* in animals and is suggested to inhibit platelet aggregation in humans; the clinical significance of this effect is unknown at this time. Case reports described increased anticoagulation in patients taking warfarin, but this appears to be a result of a pharmacokinetic/pharmacodynamic interaction rather than any anticoagulation activity on the part of danshen.

Dehydroepiandrosterone

Clinical Overview

Uses

Adequately powered, long-term clinical trials are lacking to support therapeutic use of dehydroepiandrosterone (DHEA) and dehydroepiandrosterone sulfate (DHEAS) supplementation (hereafter jointly referred to as DHEA/S). Reviews of clinical trials found no convincing evidence to support a place in therapy for DHEA in improving cognitive function or physical strength in elderly patients, or in treating postmenopausal symptoms in women, hyperlipidemia or insulin resistance, schizophrenia, or cancer. Some evidence exists to support the use of DHEA/S supplementation in women with diminished ovarian reserves, in subpopulations of elderly women with osteoporosis, and in mild systemic lupus erythematosus. DHEA is recommended as third-line monotherapy or adjunctive therapy for treatment of major depressive disorder (MDD) by Canadian Network for Mood and Anxiety Treatments (CANMAT) clinical guidelines, and limited data suggest a potential role for DHEA as an anxiolytic.

Dosing

Adrenal insufficiency: 50 mg/day for 3 months is considered a replacement dose, while 200 mg/day achieves supraphysiological circulating levels and is considered a pharmacological dose.

Anorexia nervosa: 100 mg/day for 6 months was used in a pilot study.

Diminished ovarian reserve: DHEA 50 to 75 mg/day (in divided doses) has been used in clinical studies of assisted reproduction.

Exercise training–induced muscle damage: 100 mg/day of DHEA supplementation was administered over 5 days in a study in young men undergoing exercise training.

Major depressive disorder: DHEA doses ranging from 30 to 450 mg/day for 6 to 8 weeks have been used in clinical studies.

Metabolic syndrome: DHEAS 100 mg/day for 3 months has been used in a study evaluating effects against metabolic syndrome in pre- and postmenopausal women.

Postmenopausal women: DHEA 25 mg/day has been suggested because this dose minimizes androgenic adverse effects; however, only studies in which at least 50 mg/day was used demonstrated positive outcomes as hormonal replacement therapy.

Contraindications

Use of DHEA or DHEAS is not recommended in breast or prostate cancer.

Pregnancy/Lactation

Information regarding safety and efficacy in pregnancy and lactation is lacking. DHEA supplementation has been evaluated for use in improving oocyte production in infertility.

Interactions

Supraphysiologic serum DHEAS levels due to DHEA supplementation have been documented to interfere with commercially available progesterone assays, yielding false-positive increases in serum progesterone.

Adverse Reactions

Studies in adrenal insufficiency suggest DHEA is generally well tolerated. However, data from long-term studies are lacking. Observed adverse effects include mania and hypomania, acne, hirsutism, gynecomastia, testicular changes, increased blood pressure, and decreased high-density lipoprotein (HDL) levels.

Use caution in individuals with psychiatric disorders; agitation, confusion, anxiety, paranoia, and suicidal thoughts have been reported. Use of hormones like DHEA may cause erythrocytosis. Use caution in individuals with diabetes, as DHEA may increase insulin resistance or sensitivity. Use caution in individuals with liver dysfunction, as DHEA may exacerbate this condition. Use caution in individuals with polycystic ovarian syndrome, as DHEA may worsen this condition.

Toxicology
No data.

Local Anesthetic/Vasoconstrictor Precautions
No information available to require special precautions

Effects on Bleeding None reported

Devil's Claw

Clinical Overview

Uses
Devil's claw is a folk remedy used for an extensive range of diseases, including arthritis and rheumatism. Clinical trials are generally supportive of its use as an anti-inflammatory and analgesic in low back pain and osteoarthritis.

Dosing
Devil's claw has been studied for low back pain, muscle pain, and osteoarthritis using daily doses of crude tuber up to 9 g, 1 to 3 g of extract, or harpagoside 50 to 100 mg.

Contraindications
Because of the bitterness of the preparation and consequent increase in gastric secretion, devil's claw is contraindicated in patients with gastric or duodenal ulcers.

Pregnancy/Lactation
Documented oxytoxic adverse effects. Avoid use.

Interactions
None well documented.

Adverse Reactions
Rare, generally consisting of headache, tinnitus, or anorexia.

Toxicology
Clinically important toxicity has not been observed in limited, short-term use.

Local Anesthetic/Vasoconstrictor Precautions
No information available to require special precautions

Effects on Bleeding Purpura has occurred in a patient taking warfarin and Devil's Claw concurrently, suggesting over anticoagulation.

Dong Quai

Clinical Overview

Uses
Dong quai is used in combination with other plant extracts in Chinese traditional medicine as an analgesic for rheumatism, an allergy suppressant, and in the treatment of menstrual disorders. Dong quai and its chemical constituents possess antiasthmatic, antispasmodic, anti-inflammatory, and anticoagulant properties. Clinical trials supporting traditional uses are limited. It has also been used to flavor liqueurs and confections.

Dosing
Several forms of the plant exist and dosages vary widely: crude root extract by decoction ranges from 3 to 15 g/day; while in combination, preparations 75 mg to 500 mg may be taken up to 6 times a day.

Contraindications
Relative contraindications in patients receiving warfarin, heparin, or other anticoagulant/antiplatelet therapy, in those with breast cancer, or in the first trimester of pregnancy.

Pregnancy/Lactation
Avoid use. Uterine stimulant and relaxant activity have been reported with A. sinensis, while a related species, Angelica archangelica L., was a reported abortifacient and affected the menstrual cycle.

Interactions
Warfarin, heparin, and other antiplatelet therapy due to anticoagulant/antiplatelet action of A. sinensis.

Adverse Reactions
Case reports exist of fever, gynaecomastia, and bleeding with concurrent warfarin use. A risk of photosensitization exists.

Toxicology
Data are limited. Chemical constituents have demonstrated cytotoxic properties.

Local Anesthetic/Vasoconstrictor Precautions
No information available to require special precautions

Effects on Bleeding May inhibit platelet aggregation and therefore increase bleeding

Du Zhong

Clinical Overview

Uses
The medical literature includes numerous studies on the use of *Eucommia ulmoides* (du zhong) for treating diabetes, inflammation, and obesity. One clinical study exists for its use in treating hypertension.

Dosing
E. ulmoides is commercially available as a combination product or alone as a capsule, tablet, powder, or tea, primarily for treating hypertension. *Tablets*: 3 to 5 (100 mg) tablets 3 times per day with warm water after meals. One clinical study used a 500 mg standardized extract 3 times daily for 8 weeks.

Contraindications
Avoid use in patients who are hypersensitive to any components of *E. ulmoides*. The herb may be contraindicated in patients diagnosed with estrogen-dependent cancers.

Pregnancy/Lactation
Information regarding safety and efficacy in pregnancy and lactation is lacking.

Interactions
None well documented.

Adverse Reactions
One clinical study of *E. ulmoides* documented moderately severe headache, dizziness, edema, and onset of a cold.

Toxicology
No information in humans is available.

Local Anesthetic/Vasoconstrictor Precautions
No information available to require special precautions

Effects on Bleeding
No information available to require special precautions

Echinacea

Clinical Overview

Uses
Although evidence of efficacy in the treatment of infections is limited, use of echinacea as prophylaxis for upper respiratory tract infections has been reported. Use of echinacea for the treatment of anxiety and cancer has been investigated. Specific recommendations for use are unreliable due to variations in the composition of commercial products and inconsistent clinical trial results.

Dosing
A major limitation of available dosing information is the lack of standardization of echinacea preparations. Commercial preparations contain echinacea components derived from different plant parts, species, and varieties. Recommended dosing includes the

following: 300 mg of dry powdered extract (standardized to echinacoside 3.5%), 0.25 to 1.25 mL of liquid extract (1:1 in alcohol 45%), 1 to 2 mL of tincture (1:5 in alcohol 45%), 2 to 3 mL of expressed juice of E. purpurea, and 0.5 to 1 g of dried root or tea (all administered 3 times daily). Long-term use of echinacea or use for longer than 10 days in acute infections in otherwise healthy individuals is not recommended. Parenteral use is not recommended.

Contraindications

Avoid use with known hypersensitivity to plants of the Asteraceae/Compositae family. Echinacea is also contraindicated in patients with rheumatoid arthritis, systemic lupus erythematosus, leukosis, multiple sclerosis, tuberculosis, and HIV infection.

Pregnancy/Lactation

Information regarding safety and efficacy in pregnancy and lactation is lacking. Limited clinical evidence, expert opinion, and long-term traditional use suggest that oral echinacea use is safe during pregnancy at normal dosages. Echinacea should be used with caution during lactation.

Interactions

Specific case reports of interactions are limited, although one report describes an interaction with etoposide. Data regarding echinacea effects on the cytochrome P450 (CYP-450) enzyme system are conflicting.

Adverse Reactions

Adverse reactions with echinacea are rare. The most commonly reported reactions were allergy, GI upset, and rash. A case report of leukopenia, possibly caused by long-term echinacea use, has been published. Due to conflicting data, echinacea should not be used in any condition potentially affected by immune stimulation or suppression such as HIV, tuberculosis, multiple sclerosis, and immunosuppressive therapy.

Toxicology

There is little evidence regarding toxicity with echinacea, despite its widespread use. Echinacea has not been associated with acute or chronic toxic effects. Patients with hepatic impairment should use echinacea with caution, as case reports of hepatotoxicity exist.

Local Anesthetic/Vasoconstrictor Precautions

No information available to require special precautions

Effects on Bleeding None reported

Elderberry

Clinical Overview

Uses

Limited clinical trials have been conducted. Elderberry extracts may have some value in the treatment of influenza and appear to have antioxidant potential.

Dosing

The bioavailability of active constituents in elderberry extracts is considered to be poor. Trials are lacking to provide dosing information. For the treatment of influenza, 15 mL of syrup taken 4 times per day for 5 days has been used in clinical trials.

Contraindications

Contraindications have not been identified.

Pregnancy/Lactation

Information regarding safety and efficacy in pregnancy and lactation is lacking.

Interactions

None well documented.

Adverse Reactions

Consumption of uncooked berries may result in vomiting and diarrhea. Commercial preparations generally do not cause adverse reactions at the recommended dosage. Type 1 allergy to elderberry (positive skin prick tests) has been recorded.

Toxicology

Poisonous alkaloids, lectins, and cyanogenic glycosides are present in some plant parts. Short-term use of elderberry extract preparations appears to be relatively safe; however, long-term toxicological studies are lacking.

Local Anesthetic/Vasoconstrictor Precautions

No information available to require special precautions

Effects on Bleeding None reported

Ephedra

Clinical Overview

Uses

The whole Ephedra sinica plant has traditionally been used to treat symptoms of bronchial asthma, colds, influenza, allergies, and hives in teas or tinctures. Because of adverse events and lack of efficacy, use is not recommended for weight loss or increased athletic performance. Ephedra-containing supplements are banned for sale in the United States.

Dosing

Ephedra-containing dietary supplements are currently banned in the United States. Dosages of ephedra more than 32 mg/day have resulted in adverse reactions.

Contraindications

Cardiovascular and cerebrovascular adverse events have been documented in case reports.

Pregnancy/Lactation

Documented adverse reactions. Avoid use.

Interactions

Interactions are likely to be similar to those established for synthetic ephedrine and include monoamine oxidase inhibitors (MAOIs), the anesthetic propofol, cholinergic agents such as tricyclic antidepressants, caffeine, theophylline, and steroids such as dexamethasone.

Adverse Reactions

Reported adverse reactions include arrhythmia and sudden death, myocardial infarction, stroke, psychiatric symptoms, autonomic hyperactivity, seizures, and ischemic colitis and gastric mucosal injury.

Toxicology

Toxicological data are limited. Periconceptional use of ephedra-containing products has been associated with an increased adjusted odds ratio for anencephaly.

Local Anesthetic/Vasoconstrictor Precautions

Use vasoconstrictor with caution since ephedrine may enhance cardiostimulation and vasopressor effects of sympathomimetics such as epinephrine and levonordefrin.

Effects on Bleeding None reported

Evening Primrose Oil

Clinical Overview

Uses

Evidence suggests that evening primrose oil may be effective for treating rheumatoid arthritis and diabetic neuropathy, but is lacking to support its place in the treatment of atopic dermatitis, menopausal vasomotor symptoms, mastalgia, or multiple sclerosis.

Dosing

Evening primrose oil has been administered orally in clinical trials at doses between 6 and 8 g/day in adults and 2 and 4 g/day in children. The typical content of gamma-linolenic acid (GLA) in the oil is 8% to 10%.

Contraindications

No contraindications have been identified.

Pregnancy/Lactation

Information regarding safety and efficacy in pregnancy and lactation is lacking. A case report exists of transient petechiae in a newborn following oral and intravaginal use of evening primrose oil for cervical ripening for a week prior to the infant's birth. Both linoleic and GLA are normally present in breast milk, and it is reasonable to assume that evening primrose oil may be taken while breastfeeding.

Interactions

A case report exists of an interaction between evening primrose oil and lopinavir in which lopinavir plasma concentrations were elevated to toxic levels.

Adverse Reactions

Evening primrose oil was previously suspected to lower the seizure threshold in schizophrenic patients; however, this is now disputed.

Toxicology

No toxicity, carcinogenicity, or teratogenicity have been reported.

Local Anesthetic/Vasoconstrictor Precautions
No information available to require special precautions

Effects on Bleeding Contains gamma-linolenic acid which can inhibit platelet aggregation and prolong bleeding.

Eyebright

Clinical Overview

Uses

Eyebright preparations have been used to treat a variety of conditions, specifically inflammatory eye disease; however, clinical trial data are lacking to recommend use for any indication.

Dosing

Clinical studies are lacking to provide dosing guidance. Tinctures and extracts of the herb have been used; an orally administered homeopathic product was used in 1 study evaluating effects in preventing conjunctivitis. Various homeopathic eye drops and oral formulations are available commercially.

Contraindications

Contraindications have not been identified.

Pregnancy/Lactation

Avoid use. Information regarding safety and efficacy in pregnancy and lactation is lacking.

Interactions

None well documented.

Adverse Reactions

Multiple adverse effects, including nausea and constipation, confusion, weakness, sneezing, rhinitis, cough, dyspnea, insomnia, polyuria, and diaphoresis, may occur with 10 to 60 drops of eyebright tincture. Homeopathic doses are unlikely to cause adverse reactions because of the minimal amounts ingested. Only sterile ophthalmic preparations should be used.

Toxicology

Information regarding toxicology is limited.

Local Anesthetic/Vasoconstrictor Precautions
No information available to require special precautions

Effects on Bleeding None reported

Fennel

Clinical Overview

Uses

Fennel has been used as a flavoring agent, a scent, and an insect repellent, as well as an herbal remedy for poisoning and GI conditions. It has also been used as a stimulant to promote lactation and menstruation. However, clinical evidence to support the use of fennel for any indication is lacking.

Dosing

Fennel seed and fennel seed oil have been used as stimulant and carminative agents in doses of 5 to 7 g and 0.1 to 0.6 mL, respectively.

Contraindications

Contraindications have not been identified.

Pregnancy/Lactation

There are documented adverse reactions and emmenagogue effects. Avoid use.

Interactions

One study suggested that the fennel constituent 5-methoxypsoralen has the ability to inhibit cytochrome P450 3A4. Therefore, fennel should be used cautiously with medications requiring this isoenzyme as a substrate.

Adverse Reactions

Fennel may cause photodermatitis, contact dermatitis, and cross reactions. The oil may induce reactions, such as hallucinations and seizures. Four case reports of premature thelarche (breast development) in girls have been reported with the use of fennel. Poison hemlock may be mistaken for fennel.

Toxicology

Fennel oil is genotoxic in the Bacillus subtilis DNA repair test. Estragole, present in the volatile oil, has caused tumors in animals.

Local Anesthetic/Vasoconstrictor Precautions
No information available to require special precautions

Effects on Bleeding May see increased bleeding

Fenugreek

Clinical Overview

Uses

Limited clinical trial data suggest fenugreek extracts may have a role in the therapy of dyslipidemia, diabetes, and Parkinson disease; however, studies were limited and provided inconsistent dosing information, making it difficult to provide recommendations. Anti-inflammatory, antioxidant, and cytotoxic properties have yet to be fully explored.

Dosing

Wide-ranging dosages and differing preparations have been used in clinical studies. A standardized hydroalcoholic extract of fenugreek seeds is available, and a trial evaluated its use in patients with Parkinson disease at 300 mg twice daily for a period of 6 months. Studies in patients with type 2 diabetes and hypercholesterolemia have used 5 g/day of seeds or 1 g/day of a hydroalcoholic extract of fenugreek.

Contraindications

Contraindications have not yet been identified. Avoid if an allergy to any member of the Fabaceae family exists. Cross-reactivity to chickpea, peanut, or coriander allergy is possible.

Pregnancy/Lactation

Avoid use in pregnancy. Fenugreek has documented uterine stimulant effects and has been used in traditional medicine to induce childbirth. Studies in pregnant mice have shown intrauterine growth retardation and fetal malformations related to fenugreek seed consumption. Fenugreek has been used to stimulate milk production in breastfeeding mothers; however, the extent of transmission of fenugreek-derived constituents into breast milk is unknown.

Interactions

Interactions with anticoagulant and hypoglycemic agents are possible; monitor therapy.

Adverse Reactions

Dyspepsia and mild abdominal distention have been reported in studies using large doses of the seeds. When ingested in culinary quantities, fenugreek is usually devoid of adverse reactions. Allergy to fenugreek is recognized.

Toxicology

The acute toxicity from large doses of fenugreek has not been characterized, although hypoglycemia is possible.

Local Anesthetic/Vasoconstrictor Precautions

No information available to require special precautions

Effects on Bleeding As a single agent, fenugreek has no effect on bleeding. Fenugreek may enhance the anticoagulant effects of warfarin when taken simultaneously. This effect has not been confirmed.

Feverfew

Clinical Overview

Uses

Feverfew is primarily known for use in prophylactic treatment of migraine headaches and associated nausea and vomiting; however, evidence to support this use is inconclusive. Feverfew has numerous other pharmacological actions, including inhibition of prostaglandin synthesis, blockage of platelet granule secretion, effects on smooth muscle, antitumor activity, inhibition of serotonin release, inhibition of histamine release, and mast cell inhibition, but information from clinical trials is limited.

Dosing

Feverfew is generally given for migraine headaches at a daily dosage of 50 to 150 mg of dried leaves, 2.5 fresh leaves with or after food, or 5 to 20 drops of a 1:5, 25% ethanol tincture. Though optimal doses of feverfew have not been established, an adult dosage of parentholide 0.2 to 0.6 mg/day is recommended for the prevention of migraine. However, parthenolide has not been confirmed as a major active principle for migraine. Numerous feverfew products are commercially available; most are standardized to parthenolide 0.7% in tablet or capsule dosage forms.

Contraindications

Feverfew is contraindicated in patients allergic to other members of the Asteraceae family, such as aster, chamomile, chrysanthemum, ragweed, sunflower, tansy, and yarrow. Due to its potential antiplatelet effects, it is not recommended for use in patients undergoing surgery. Patients with blood-clotting disorders should consult their health care provider prior to using products containing feverfew.

Pregnancy/Lactation

Avoid use because of documented adverse effects. Pregnant women should not use the plant because the leaves possess emmenagogue activity (ejection of the placenta and fetal membranes) and may induce abortion. It is not recommended for breastfeeding mothers or for use in children younger than 2 years of age.

Interactions

None well documented.

Adverse Reactions

Patients withdrawn from feverfew may experience ill effects often known as "postfeverfew" syndrome. Handling fresh feverfew leaves may cause allergic contact dermatitis. Swelling of the lips, tongue, and oral mucosa, in addition to mouth ulceration, have been reported with feverfew use. GI effects, such as abdominal pain, nausea, vomiting, diarrhea, indigestion, and flatulence, may also occur.

Toxicology

No studies of chronic toxicity have been performed on the plant. The safety of long-term use has not been established.

Local Anesthetic/Vasoconstrictor Precautions

No information available to require special precautions

Effects on Bleeding May see increased bleeding due to inhibition of platelet aggregation

Flax

Clinical Overview

Uses

Flaxseed and flaxseed oil contain various essential fatty acids but are particularly rich in alpha linolenic acid (ALA). Flaxseed (but not flaxseed oil) also has a high fiber content that may have health benefits similar to those of other high-fiber products and phytoestrogens. Historically, linseed oil, derived from flaxseed, has been used as a topical demulcent and emollient, as a laxative, and as a treatment for coughs, colds, and urinary tract infections. Interest in flaxseed centers on atherosclerosis, cancer, diabetes, and to a lesser extent, menopause, attention deficit hyperactivity disorder, bipolar disorder, and systemic lupus erythematosus (SLE).

Dosing

Flaxseed (whole or ground) has been used in clinical trials at doses from 5 to 50 g/day or 60 mL flaxseed oil daily, and has been used in children at doses equivalent to 400 mg of ALA in divided doses.

Eight grams of ground flaxseed (or 2.5 g of flaxseed oil) per day provides a daily intake of 1.1 g of ALA for women and 1.6 g for men.

Contraindications

Contraindicated in patients with known hypersensitivity to flaxseed.

Pregnancy/Lactation

The use of flaxseed and flaxseed oil during pregnancy and lactation is not recommended.

Interactions

None well documented.

Adverse Reactions

Flaxseed and flaxseed oil appear to be well tolerated, with few adverse reactions reported except allergy.

Toxicology

The US Food and Drug Administration has not granted GRAS (Generally Recognized as Safe) status to flaxseed or flaxseed oil. The safety of ingested amounts greater than 50 g/day of flaxseed is not established.

Local Anesthetic/Vasoconstrictor Precautions

No information available to require special precautions

Effects on Bleeding None reported

Forskolin

Clinical Overview

Uses

Forskolin has multiple sites of action and should be used with caution. Forskolin derivatives have been developed for use in cardiovascular conditions. Quality clinical trials are lacking to substantiate claims made of the weight loss properties of forskolin, and clinical studies conducted with oral and inhaled forskolin in patients with asthma are limited.

Dosing

Asthma: Oral forskolin has been studied using 10 mg daily over 2 to 6 months.

Obesity: 250 mg of a 10% forskolin extract twice daily for 12 weeks has been studied.

Contraindications

Case reports are lacking.

Pregnancy/Lactation

Information regarding safety and efficacy in pregnancy and lactation is lacking. P. barbatus has been traditionally used as an emmenagogue and oral contraceptive.

Interactions

None well documented.

Adverse Reactions

Clinical trial data are generally lacking. Adverse events reported with the use of colforsin (a forskolin derivative) include tachycardia and arrhythmias. Forskolin should be avoided in patients with polycystic kidney disease.

Toxicology

Information is limited. Embryo-related toxicity has been reported.

Local Anesthetic/Vasoconstrictor Precautions

No information available to require special precautions

Effects on Bleeding Forskolin has been shown *in vitro* to inhibit platelet aggregation. Clinical relevance of this effect is unknown. There are no current published reports of any anticoagulant effect in patients taking Forskolin.

Forsythia

Clinical Overview

Uses

Forsythia has been used for treatment of bacterial infections and upper respiratory tract infections, although the clinical evidence supporting its use is limited.

Dosing

There are no recent clinical studies of forsythia to provide a basis for dosage recommendations.

Contraindications

Contraindications have not yet been identified.

Pregnancy/Lactation

Documented adverse effects. Uterine stimulant, emmenagogue. Avoid use.

Interactions

None well documented.

Adverse Reactions

Forsythia is contraindicated in pregnancy.

Toxicology

Forsythia has minimal potential for toxicity.

Local Anesthetic/Vasoconstrictor Precautions

No information available to require special precautions

Effects on Bleeding None reported

Frankincense, Indian

Clinical Overview

Uses

The oleoresin gum from B. serrata has traditionally been used for its anti-inflammatory effects in conditions such as asthma, osteoarthritis, rheumatoid arthritis, colitis, and irritable bowel syndrome. It has also been used for the management of diabetes, urinary conditions, dermatological ailments, and renal impairment. Boswellic acids have demonstrated immunomodulatory, antiproliferative, cytotoxic, and antimicrobial effects; however, there are no adequate clinical trials to support any of the uses.

Dosing

Administration with high-fat foods may enhance plasma levels of B. serrata. **Asthma:** 300 to 400 mg of an extract (containing 60% boswellic acids) 3 times daily. In one trial, 300 mg 3 times daily of powdered gum resin capsules (S-Compound), or 400 mg 3 times daily of an extract (standardized to 37.5% boswellic acids per dose) was used. **Inflammatory conditions:** 300 to 400 mg of a B. serrata extract (containing 60% boswellic acids) 3 times daily was used in a clinical trial of patients with knee osteoarthritis. Two capsules of Articulin-F (contains B. serrata, Withania somnifera, Curcuma longa, zinc complex) 3 times daily; or supplementation with Casperome (150 mg of boswellic acids) 3 times daily has been used for inflammatory conditions such as osteoarthritis and rheumatoid arthritis. **Ulcerative colitis:** 350 to 400 mg 3 times daily.

Contraindications

Hypersensitivity to B. serrata.

Pregnancy/Lactation

Avoid use. Information regarding safety and efficacy in pregnancy and lactation is lacking.

Interactions

Substrates of cytochrome P450 (CYP-450) 1A2, 2C8, 2C9, 2C19, 2D6, and 3A4: Upon liquid chromatography mass spectrometry analysis, frankincense derived from B. serrata demonstrated inhibition of CYP1A2, 2C8, 2C9, 2C19, 2D6, and 3A4. Therefore, caution is warranted when using B. serrata with medications that are substrates for these isoenzymes. **Substrates for P-glycoprotein (P-gp):** Data suggest that B. serrata extract and the major boswellic acids may be potent inhibitors of P-gp via modulation of transport activity at the GI level, but not at the blood-brain barrier. Therefore, medications that depend on P-gp transport across the GI membrane may be impacted with coadministration of B. serrata. **Warfarin:** According to 2 case reports, coadministration of warfarin and B. serrata may increase international normalized ratio (INR) levels. The interaction may be attributed to inhibition of lipoxygenase and interference with COX-1 by B. serrata. In addition, B. serrata might inhibit CYP2C19, 3A4, and 2C9, which are involved in the metabolism of warfarin. Use of B. serrata in patients receiving warfarin is not recommended.

Adverse Reactions

Diarrhea, abdominal pain, and nausea have been reported.

Toxicology

No data.

Local Anesthetic/Vasoconstrictor Precautions

No information available to require special precautions

Effects on Bleeding None reported

Fruit Acids

Clinical Overview

Uses

Fruit acids have been used to treat a range of dermatological conditions, including acne, photoaging, dry skin, psoriasis, actinic keratosis, and melasma. Additionally, they have been investigated as a treatment for fibromyalgia, dental scaling, and dry mouth, and for prevention and treatment of urinary tract stones. However, apart from topical application, clinical trials are lacking to support any additional indications.

Dosing

Chemical peels: Dosing for chemical peels involving glycolic acid may depend on a variety of factors, including the condition being treated, patient expectations, patient age, cumulative sun exposure, skin type, area being treated, peeling agent used, concentration of peel agent, frequency of application, quantity applied, and length of time applied. Typically, on the first visit, glycolic acid is applied for approximately 2 to 3 minutes to determine sensitivity and provide guidance for future length of exposure. Intervals between peels are generally 2 to 4 weeks; 6 to 8 peels are required for most patients.

Dry skin disorders: Alpha hydroxy acid 8% to 10% cream or lotion applied 2 to 3 times daily to affected area(s). If dry skin persists after 2 weeks, the concentration can be increased by 2% to 4%. Once the skin appears healthy, the frequency can be reduced to every 2 to 3 days.

Fibromyalgia: 3 Super Malic tablets (each containing malic acid 200 mg) twice daily.

Contraindications

Hypersensitive individuals and those with irritated skin should use alpha hydroxy acids cautiously. Patients who have undergone recent cosmetic surgeries, have open wounds, or have used isotretinoin therapy within the last 6 to 12 months should not receive alpha hydroxy acid peels. In patients with a history of recurrent or active herpes simplex lesions, treatment with an oral antiviral agent should occur before undergoing chemical peels.

Pregnancy/Lactation

Information regarding safety and efficacy in pregnancy and lactation is lacking.

Adverse Reactions

Dryness, scaling, burning, erythema, and similar effects may occur in sensitive individuals or with prolonged use.

Toxicology

No data.

Local Anesthetic/Vasoconstrictor Precautions
No information available to require special precautions

Effects on Bleeding None reported

Garcinia (hydroxycitric acid)

Clinical Overview

Uses

The medical literature primarily documents weight loss and lipid-lowering activity for Garcinia cambogia, although trials supporting its use are limited. In short-term clinical trials lasting 12 weeks or less, G. cambogia was ineffective or moderately effective for weight loss in overweight subjects. Results have been inconsistent in studies evaluating the effect of G. cambogia on lipids.

Dosing

The dosages of G. cambogia extract used in clinical trials ranged from 1,500 to 4,667 mg/day (25 to 78 mg/kg/day). The equivalent HCA dosage in the trials ranged from 900 to 2,800 mg/day (15 to 47 mg/kg/day). G. cambogia is available in capsule or tablet form with a maximum dosage of 1,500 mg/day.

Contraindications

Avoid use if there is a known allergy or hypersensitivity to any components of G. cambogia.

Pregnancy/Lactation

Avoid use during pregnancy and lactation. Information regarding safety and efficacy in pregnancy and lactation is lacking.

Interactions

The herb has documented drug interactions.

Adverse Reactions

Fifteen clinical studies involving approximately 900 patients documented very mild adverse reactions, with the most common adverse reactions including headache, dizziness, dry mouth, and GI complaints such as nausea and diarrhea. Hydroxycut dietary supplements for weight loss were voluntarily recalled from the US market in 2009 because of concerns about hepatotoxicity. Although G. cambogia was an ingredient in some formulations of Hydroxycut, its role in cases of hepatotoxicity associated with Hydroxycut is unclear.

Toxicology

Toxicology studies showed no toxicity or deaths in animals given dosages of HCA 5,000 mg/kg, equivalent to HCA 350 g in humans, or 233 times the maximum recommended human dosage of HCA 1.5 g/day.

Local Anesthetic/Vasoconstrictor Precautions
No information available to require special precautions

Effects on Bleeding None reported

Garlic

Clinical Overview

Uses

Garlic has been investigated for its effects in cancer, diabetes, dyslipidemia, hypertension, ischemic heart disease, heart failure, liver disease, osteoarthritis, and peripheral vascular disease, among other conditions. Additionally, garlic's antimicrobial and antiplatelet effects have been evaluated. Most evidence supporting the use of garlic is for dyslipidemia and hypertension, although evidence shows equivocal or mixed results, partially due to the difficulty in developing a true placebo, as well as poor methodology and a lack of standardization of preparation.

Dosing

Suggested average daily doses include 2 to 5 g of fresh raw garlic; 0.4 to 1.2 g of dried garlic powder; 2 to 5 mg of garlic oil; 300 to 1,000 mg of garlic extract (as solid material); and 2,400 mg/day of aged garlic extract (liquid).

In a meta-analysis evaluating effects of garlic on blood pressure, doses of garlic powder ranged from 300 to 2,400 mg/day for 2 to 24 weeks.

Contraindications

Garlic is contraindicated in individuals with known allergy to garlic and its constituents.

Pregnancy/Lactation

Garlic may be used in pregnancy and lactation with caution. Consumption by breastfeeding mothers may impact the infant's behavior during breastfeeding, causing prolonged attachment to the breast and increased sucking. Anecdotal evidence suggests that maternal consumption of garlic may result in colic; however, evidence is conflicting.

Interactions

Conflicting evidence exists regarding garlic's impact on the CYP-450 system, namely CYP1A2, 2D6, and 3A4. Garlic's interactions are likely mediated through its impact on P-glycoprotein rather than the CYP-450 systems.

Garlic may enhance the adverse effects of antiplatelet agents, anticoagulants, and thrombolytics, increasing the risk for bleeding. Garlic may enhance the effects of antidiabetes drugs such as metformin, resulting in lowered blood glucose levels. Additionally, garlic may decrease the concentrations of protease inhibitors, reducing their efficacy.

Adverse Reactions

Body odor and malodorous breath are the most common complaints after garlic ingestion. Mild GI adverse reactions (eg, bloating, flatulence, nausea) have been commonly reported with use. Burns have been documented with topical use. Ingestion of large amounts may increase the risk of postoperative and spontaneous bleeding. Allergy, asthma, pneumonia, contact dermatitis, and anaphylaxis have been reported.

Toxicology

No data.

Local Anesthetic/Vasoconstrictor Precautions
No information available to require special precautions

Effects on Bleeding Causes platelet dysfunction and prolonged bleeding time

Gelsemium

Clinical Overview

Uses

Gelsemium has traditionally been used for its analgesic effects and for the treatment of respiratory conditions. Studies (primarily animal and in vitro) have evaluated the analgesic and anxiolytic effects of gelsemium. However, no clinical trial data support use of gelsemium for any indication; use is not advised due to known toxicity of the plant parts.

Dosing

Current use of gelsemium is primarily homeopathic. However, clinical trials are lacking to provide gelsemium dosing recommendations; use of gelsemium for any indication is not recommended due to toxicity concerns.

Contraindications

Gelsemium is highly toxic; ultralow doses have been evaluated. Gelsemium is rarely used because of toxicity concerns.

Pregnancy/Lactation

Although gelsemium has traditionally been used as a homeopathic treatment around labor and delivery, use should be avoided in pregnancy and lactation due to the potential for toxicity.

Interactions

None well documented.

Adverse Reactions

Toxic symptoms associated with gelsemium include sweating, dizziness, nausea, vomiting, muscle weakness, dilated pupils, paralysis, blurry vision, difficulty breathing, seizures, coma, and death.

Toxicology

All parts of the gelsemium are toxic and can cause death when ingested.

Local Anesthetic/Vasoconstrictor Precautions
No information available to require special precautions

Effects on Bleeding None reported

Ginger

Clinical Overview

Uses

There are many traditional uses for ginger, but recent interest centers on the prevention and management of nausea. However, information to support ginger's use for nausea, especially in pregnancy, is lacking. Ginger may possess anti-inflammatory and analgesic effects, and has been effective in dysmenorrhea in limited studies.

Dosing

Ginger has been used in clinical trials in dosages of 250 mg to 1 g 3 to 4 times daily.

Contraindications

Contraindications have not been identified.

Pregnancy/Lactation

Avoid use. Despite trials conducted to determine its effectiveness in pregnancy-related nausea, data on fetal outcomes are lacking.

Interactions

Anticoagulants (eg, warfarin), agents with antiplatelet properties, nonsteroidal anti-inflammatory agents, salicylates or thrombolytic agents, antihypertensives, and hypoglycemic agents interact with ginger.

Adverse Reactions

The US Food and Drug Administration (FDA) lists ginger as generally recognized as safe (GRAS), but large doses carry the potential for adverse reactions. Mild GI effects (eg, heartburn, diarrhea, mouth irritation) have been reported, and case reports of arrhythmia and immunoglobulin E (IgE) allergic reaction are documented.

Toxicology

Toxicological information regarding the use of ginger in humans is limited, and mutagenicity is contested.

Local Anesthetic/Vasoconstrictor Precautions
No information available to require special precautions

Effects on Bleeding No information available to require special precautions

Ginkgo biloba

Clinical Overview

Uses

Ginkgo has been studied extensively in diverse medical conditions. Findings from large trials have been pivotal in evaluating the efficacy of G. biloba extracts; however, there is not enough quality evidence to support the use of ginkgo for any indication. Evidence is lacking to support a protective role in cardiovascular conditions and stroke. Ginkgo's place in therapy for dementia seems limited, and a role in schizophrenia has not been established. Additionally, data do not support enhanced cognitive function resulting from G. biloba use in healthy individuals. Although interest exists in chemotherapeutic applications, safety concerns persist.

Dosing

Standardized ginkgo leaf extracts have been used in clinical trials for cognitive and cardiovascular disorders at daily doses of 120 to 240 mg.

Contraindications

Contraindications have not been established.

Pregnancy/Lactation

Information regarding safety and efficacy in pregnancy and lactation is lacking. Ginkgo should be used with caution during pregnancy, particularly around labor due to risk of prolonged bleeding time, and should be avoided during lactation.

Interactions

At recommended doses, standardized preparations of ginkgo leaf extract are unlikely to exhibit any clinically important interactions.

Adverse Reactions

Severe adverse reactions are rare; possible reactions include headache, dizziness, heart palpitations, and GI and dermatologic reactions. Ginkgo pollen can be strongly allergenic. Contact with the fleshy fruit pulp may cause allergic dermatitis similar to that caused by poison ivy.

Toxicology

Concerns persist regarding the safety of ginkgo leaf extract, based on studies in rodents that suggested increased mitosis and proliferation of tumor cells, as well as the large Ginkgo Evaluation of Memory (GEM) study in which the potential for an increased risk of certain cancers was noted. Consumption of the seeds may induce a toxic syndrome.

Local Anesthetic/Vasoconstrictor Precautions

No information available to require special precautions

Effects on Bleeding Spontaneous bleeding is a concerning side effect. Significant peri- and postoperative bleeding have been reported. Chronic use inhibits platelet aggregation and prolongs bleeding.

Ginseng

Clinical Overview

Uses

Ginseng root is widely used for its adaptogenic, immunomodulatory, antineoplastic, cardiovascular, CNS, endocrine, and ergogenic effects, but these uses have not been confirmed by clinical trials.

Dosing

According to the Complete German Commission E Monographs, crude preparations of dried root powder 1 to 2 g can be taken daily for up to 3 months. In numerous clinical trials, the dosage of crude root has ranged from 0.5 to 3 g/day and the dose of extracts has generally ranged from 100 to 400 mg.

Contraindications

Contraindications have not been established aside from known hypersensitivity.

Pregnancy/Lactation

Information regarding safety and efficacy in pregnancy and lactation is lacking.

Interactions

Limited evidence exists for any established interactions, with most data derived from laboratory studies and healthy volunteers. Very few case reports exist; however, exercise caution when using the following medicines: antidiabetic drugs/insulin, antipsychotic drugs, caffeine and other stimulants, furosemide, imatinib, monoamine oxidase inhibitors (MAOIs), and nifedipine. Interactions with warfarin and antiviral drugs are conflicting.

Adverse Reactions

It is estimated that more than 6 million people ingest ginseng regularly in the United States. There have been few reports of severe reactions and a very low incidence of adverse events has been reported in clinical trials. Hypersensitivity and anaphylaxis have been reported. Inappropriate use of P. ginseng or ginseng abuse syndrome includes symptoms such as hypertension, diarrhea, sleeplessness, mastalgia, skin rash, confusion, and depression.

Toxicology

None known.

Local Anesthetic/Vasoconstrictor Precautions

Has potential to interact with epinephrine and levonordefrin to result in increased BP; use vasoconstrictor with caution

Effects on Bleeding May prolong thrombin time (TT) and activated partial thromboplastin time (aPTT).

Glucosamine

Clinical Overview

Uses

Glucosamine sulfate and glucosamine hydrochloride have been extensively evaluated in multiple large comparative trials for effects in osteoarthritis, with mixed findings regarding efficacy. Associated guidelines do not recommend the routine use of glucosamine for osteoarthritis. Other potential uses for glucosamine salts include atopic dermatitis, cancer, and osteoporosis.

Dosing

In clinical studies of osteoarthritis, the typical glucosamine dosage (for both sulfate and hydrochloride salt forms) has been 1.5 g/day as a single dose or in divided doses of up to 3 times per day (treatment duration of up to 3 years).

Contraindications

Caution should be used in patients with a shellfish allergy, as glucosamine is derived from the exoskeletons of shellfish.

Pregnancy/Lactation

Information regarding safety and efficacy in pregnancy and lactation is lacking.

Interactions

Agents with antiplatelet properties: Glucosamine may enhance the antiplatelet effect of agents with antiplatelet properties. Monitor therapy.

Warfarin: Glucosamine may enhance the anticoagulant effect of warfarin. Monitor therapy.

Adverse Reactions

Glucosamine is generally considered safe. The majority of reported adverse reactions have been mild, including itching and gastric discomfort (eg, diarrhea, heartburn, nausea, vomiting), which may be alleviated by taking with food. Use caution when administering to individuals with poorly controlled diabetes or liver disease. Use with caution in individuals with allergy to shellfish or with asthma.

Toxicology

No data.

Local Anesthetic/Vasoconstrictor Precautions

No information available to require special precautions

Effects on Bleeding None reported

Goat's Rue

Clinical Overview

Uses

Goat's rue and its derivatives have been used in the management of diabetes mellitus to reduce blood sugar levels. Goat's rue has also been used for its lactogenic effects to increase milk production. It has tonic, liver protectant, and platelet aggregation inhibitory effects, and has been evaluated for its diuretic and weight loss effects. However, limited clinical trials exist to support these uses.

Dosing

Diabetes: Information is lacking to provide dosing recommendations for goat's rue in diabetes. Clinical dosing information focuses on metformin, which is derived from goat's rue.

Galactorrhea: 1 teaspoon (5 mL) of dried herb steeped in 1 cup (240 mL) of water administered twice daily or 1 to 2 mL of tincture administered 3 times daily.

Contraindications

Use caution if administering goat's rue during surgical procedures due to a potential increased risk of bleeding.

Pregnancy/Lactation

Avoid use. Information regarding safety and efficacy in pregnancy is lacking. Silymarin in combination with galega enhances milk production in breastfeeding mothers.

Interactions

Hypoglycemic medications: Additive blood glucose–lowering effects may occur if using goat's rue concomitantly with other hypoglycemic medications such as insulin and sulfonylureas.

Antiplatelet/Anticoagulant medications: Because goat's rue inhibits platelet aggregation, the risk of bleeding may be increased when given concomitantly with other antiplatelet medications or anticoagulants.

Adverse Reactions

Headache, jitteriness, or weakness may occur. Because of its ability to inhibit platelet aggregation, there may be an increased risk of bleeding and bruising with administration of goat's rue.

Toxicology

Toxicity has been observed with other guanidine derivatives.

Local Anesthetic/Vasoconstrictor Precautions

No information available to require special precautions

Effects on Bleeding None reported

Goji Berry

Clinical Overview

Uses

Limited quality clinical trials exist to support therapeutic claims. In vitro and animal experiments suggest antioxidant, hypoglycemic, immune-enhancing, and neuro-, hepato-, and ophthalmic-protective effects.

Dosing

Data are lacking to guide dosage in the clinical setting.

Contraindications

Contraindications have not been identified.

Pregnancy/Lactation

Information regarding safety and efficacy in pregnancy and lactation is lacking.

Interactions

Case reports of interactions with warfarin exist.

Adverse Reactions

Clinical trials report few or no adverse reactions. Information is limited.

Toxicology

Information is lacking.

Local Anesthetic/Vasoconstrictor Precautions

No information available to require special precautions

Effects on Bleeding None reported

Goldenseal

Clinical Overview

Uses

Traditional uses of goldenseal are not validated by clinical studies, although it may be of use in diabetes, dyslipidemia, cardiovascular conditions, and cancer.

Dosing

Clinical evidence is lacking; few well-controlled clinical trials are available to guide dosage for goldenseal root extract.

Recommended dosages vary considerably, from 250 mg to 1 g 3 times daily. Some product labeling suggests higher dosages.

Traditional dosages include 0.5 to 1 g dried rhizomes 3 times daily, and 0.3 to 1 mL 1:1 liquid extract in 60% ethanol 3 times daily.

Contraindications

None well defined.

Pregnancy/Lactation

Avoid use; activity as a uterine stimulant has been documented. Safety in lactation has not been established.

Interactions

Goldenseal may affect the cytochrome CYP-450 (CYP450) system. The clinical importance of this interaction has not been established.

Adverse Reactions

Information from clinical studies is lacking, but adverse reactions with common doses are rare. Very high doses of goldenseal may rarely induce nausea, anxiety, depression, seizures, or paralysis.

Toxicology

Toxicological concerns have been reported, with some evidence of carcinogenicity in rodents.

Local Anesthetic/Vasoconstrictor Precautions

No information available to require special precautions

Effects on Bleeding None reported

Gossypol

Clinical Overview

Uses

According to Chinese studies, gossypol is effective as a nonhormonal male contraceptive; however, it has been documented to have irreversible effects on male fertility and is not recommended for this use. Gossypol is being studied for clinical applications in cancer therapy with equivocal results.

Dosing

Antifertility: There are no dosing recommendations for gossypol due to its potential irreversible effects on male fertility. *Cancer*: Maximum tolerated dosage appears to be 40 mg/day of gossypol (as AT-101).

Contraindications

None well documented.

Pregnancy/Lactation

Avoid use. Documented abortifacient effects.

Interactions

None well documented.

Adverse Reactions

Nausea, emesis, anorexia, diarrhea, altered taste sensation, small intestine obstruction, and fatigue have been reported in clinical trials. The irreversible effects of gossypol on male fertility have been well documented, as has the incidence of hypokalemia. Dose-limiting elevations in liver enzymes have been noted at total doses of 60 mg/day for AT-101, and an increased incidence of hematological toxicities has been observed when AT-101 is combined with cancer chemotherapy, depending on the regimen.

Toxicology

No data.

Local Anesthetic/Vasoconstrictor Precautions

No information available to require special precautions

Effects on Bleeding None reported

Gotu Kola

Clinical Overview

Uses

Gotu kola has potential cardiovascular and dermatological (eg, wound healing) effects. Clinical data are limited.

Dosing

The recommended daily dose of titrated extracts of C. asiatica standardized for asiaticoside, asiatic acid, and madecassic acid is 60 to 120 mg.

Contraindications

Hypersensitivity to C. asiatica or any of its components.

Pregnancy/Lactation

Avoid use during pregnancy and lactation; gotu kola may have emmenagogue effects.

Interactions

Gotu kola extract has been shown to inhibit cytochrome P450 (CYP-450) 3A4, 2C19, and 2B6, but the clinical significance is unknown. Gotu kola may have additive effects when coadministered with antiplatelet agents.

Adverse Reactions

Contact dermatitis has been documented in some clinical trials.

Toxicology

Three cases of hepatotoxicity have been reported with C. asiatica administration for 20 to 60 days.

Local Anesthetic/Vasoconstrictor Precautions

No information available to require special precautions

Effects on Bleeding None reported

Grapefruit and Grapefruit Juice

Clinical Overview

Uses

High-quality clinical trials are lacking to support therapeutic applications of grapefruit and grapefruit juice. Limited data suggest potential benefit for certain patient populations in reducing the risk of renal stones and type 2 diabetes, as well as some cardiovascular risk factors (including improvement in systolic blood pressure, high-density lipoprotein [HDL] cholesterol, and arterial stiffness). Some trials also demonstrate reductions in body fat and waist circumference but data regarding use for weight loss are equivocal. Antimicrobial effects have been reported. Consumption of whole grapefruit has been shown in several analyses to provide improved benefits compared to the juice.

Dosing

Quality clinical trials upon which to base therapeutic dosing recommendations for grapefruit are limited.

Cardiovascular risk factors: 1 grapefruit daily for 30 days has been used in a clinical trial to improve lipid profiles. Fresh grapefruit, grapefruit juice, and grapefruit capsules for 6 or 12 weeks, with naringin doses of the formulations ranging from 81 to 142 mg/day, have been used in randomized controlled trials evaluating effects on cardiovascular risk factors in obese adults. In a trial of healthy postmenopausal women, 340 mL/day (providing 201 mg/day of naringenin) of grapefruit juice was administered for 6 months to evaluate effects on arterial stiffness.

Diabetes risk: Pooled results from 3 prospective longitudinal cohort studies (N=187,382; 3,464,641 person-years of follow-up) reported consumption of 2 to 4 servings per week of grapefruit to reduce the risk of type 2 diabetes. In one cohort of women, 2 to 4 servings per week or 5 or more servings per week of grapefruit (1 serving of grapefruit was one-half of a grapefruit) also reduced risk.

Periodontitis: 2 grapefruits per day for 2 weeks were consumed in a trial evaluating effects on vitamin C status of patients with periodontitis.

Weight and related parameters: 8 oz (237 mL) of grapefruit juice, or half of a fresh grapefruit, 3 times a day before each meal for 12 weeks was used in a clinical trial evaluating effects on body weight and metabolic syndrome. In a meta-analysis evaluating effects on body weight, fresh grapefruit, grapefruit juice, or grapefruit capsules (with naringin dosages of the formulations ranging from 81 to 142 mg) were administered for 6 or 12 weeks in the included randomized controlled trials.

Contraindications

None well defined. In patients with major myocardial structural disorders, pink grapefruit should be avoided due to proarrhythmic effects. The potential for drug interactions with grapefruit should be considered in cases in which an increase or decrease of the coadministered drug is clinically important.

Pregnancy/Lactation

Grapefruit has "generally recognized as safe" (GRAS) status when used as food, according to the US Food and Drug Administration. Safety of amounts greater than those in foods are unproven. Consumption of grapefruit juice increases naringenin levels in breast milk.

Interactions

Grapefruit juice has been reported to interact with numerous drugs; however, case reports of clinically important interactions are rare.

Adverse Reactions

Reports of adverse reactions associated with grapefruit consumption are limited and largely related to drug interactions. Case reports exist of allergy to pectin (a component of grapefruit) and pectin-induced asthma. Constipation and diarrhea have also been reported.

Toxicology

Toxicological studies on whole grapefruit are lacking. A meta-analysis of 3 landmark studies evaluating associations between grapefruit consumption and risk of breast cancer found no increased risk. The grapefruit constituent d-limonene has GRAS status. Grapefruit seed extract has been shown to be toxic to human skin fibroblast cells.

Local Anesthetic/Vasoconstrictor Precautions

No information available to require special precautions

Effects on Bleeding None reported

Grape Seed

Clinical Overview

Uses

Grape seed is known for its antioxidant properties. Limited studies suggest possible cardiovascular, chemopreventive, and cytoprotective effects.

Dosing

Extracts of grape seeds containing mostly proanthocyanidin have been studied for antioxidant and cardiovascular properties, as well as for venous insufficiency and ophthalmologic disorders at doses of 50 to 300 mg/day. A maximum of 900 mg/day has been used.

Contraindications

Contraindicated in patients with known hypersensitivity to grape seed.

Pregnancy/Lactation

Information regarding safety and efficacy in pregnancy and lactation is lacking.

Interactions

Caution is advised when administering supplements containing grape seed polyphenols concomitantly with vitamin C to hypertensive patients because increases in blood pressure may occur.

Adverse Reactions

None well documented. It is contraindicated in patients with known hypersensitivity to grape seed. Gastralgia, headache, and an allergic reaction have been reported in the literature. Additional clinical studies are recommended.

Toxicology

No toxicity in humans has been reported.

Local Anesthetic/Vasoconstrictor Precautions

No information available to require special precautions

Effects on Bleeding None reported

Green Tea

Clinical Overview

Uses

Tea is traditionally consumed as a beverage. Evidence from clinical trials suggests that green tea plays a role in metabolic syndrome because it may have an impact on body weight, glucose homeostasis, and other cardiovascular risk factors. There has been interest in green tea as an agent in cancer prevention. A role in the prevention of stroke and chronic obstructive pulmonary disease (COPD) has also been suggested. Topical as well as oral formulations have been studied for protection from ultraviolet (UV) damage, and a commercial preparation has been approved by the US Food and Drug Administration (FDA) for use in the treatment of anogenital warts.

Dosing

Daily intake of 3 to 5 cups/day (720 to 1,200 mL) of green tea provides at least 180 mg of catechins and at least 60 mg of theanine. Green tea extract should not be taken on an empty stomach due to the potential for hepatotoxicity from excessive levels of epigallocatechin gallate (EGCG).

Anogenital warts: Topical application of sinecatechins (polyphenon E 10% or 15%) was used for up to 16 weeks in a clinical study.

Cardiovascular risks: Green tea catechins or extract (160 to 2,488 mg/day) have been used in trials, often in divided dosages (treatment duration, 2 weeks to 3 months).

Cognitive impairment: Two 430 mg capsules (each capsule containing green tea extract 360 mg and L-theanine 60 mg) administered twice daily, 30 minutes after meals, for 16 weeks (total daily green tea extract dose, 1,440 mg; total daily L-theanine dose, 240 mg).

Depression: 2 to 4 or more cups/day of green tea has been used to lower the prevalence of depressive symptoms.

Diabetes: An EGCG dosage range of 84 to 386 mg/day may be adequate to support glucose homeostasis, based on available literature.

Obesity: ECGC 400 mg twice daily for 8 weeks was used in one clinical trial; green tea extract tablets (containing 125 mg of catechins) and a daily green tea catechin beverage (containing 625 mg of catechins) have also been used in studies of overweight and obese adults.

Contraindications

Contraindications have not been identified; however, use caution in cases of hepatic failure.

Pregnancy/Lactation

Information regarding safety and efficacy in pregnancy and lactation is lacking. Green tea contains caffeine. The FDA advises those who are or may become pregnant to avoid caffeine.

Adverse Reactions

There are no reports of clinical toxicity from daily tea consumption as a beverage. Adverse events associated with tea extracts (including green tea extract) include headache, dizziness, and GI symptoms. Hepatotoxicity, including 1 fatality, has been associated with high plasma levels of EGCG or its metabolites.

Toxicology

No data.

Local Anesthetic/Vasoconstrictor Precautions

No information available to require special precautions

Effects on Bleeding Caffeine in green tea may have antiplatelet effects

Guggul

Clinical Overview

Uses

Guggul has been used in the traditional Ayurvedic medical system for centuries and has been studied extensively in India. Commercial products are promoted for use in hyperlipidemia; however, clinical studies do not substantiate this claim. Anti-inflammatory and cardiovascular effects are being evaluated, as well as use in cancer, obesity, and diabetes.

Dosing

Clinical trials are lacking to provide dosage guidelines; however, in a US clinical trial of hyperlipidemia, 75 to 150 mg of standardized guggulsterones were administered daily. In a study evaluating the anti-inflammatory effect of guggul, 500 mg of gum guggul was taken 3 times per day.

Contraindications

None identified. Caution may be warranted in patients previously experiencing adverse effects to statins.

Pregnancy/Lactation

Information regarding safety and efficacy in pregnancy and lactation is lacking.

Interactions

None well documented.

Adverse Reactions

Although generally accepted as relatively safe, case reports of adverse events exist. Moderate to severe generalized acute eczematous reactions to oral guggul have been reported, and caution may be warranted. A case report exists of rhabdomyolysis possibly caused by guggul consumption.

Toxicology

Research reveals little information regarding toxicology with the use of guggul.

Local Anesthetic/Vasoconstrictor Precautions
No information available to require special precautions

Effects on Bleeding None reported

Gymnema

Clinical Overview

Uses

The plant has been used in traditional medicine, most notably to control blood glucose. Use as a lipid-lowering agent, for weight loss, and for the inhibition of caries have also been investigated, primarily in rodent studies. However, little to no clinical information is available to support the use of gymnema for any indication.

Dosing

Limited controlled studies exist. Clinical studies investigating antidiabetic effects have typically used 200 or 400 mg extract daily standardized to contain 25% gymnemic acids.

Contraindications

None established.

Pregnancy/Lactation

Information regarding safety and efficacy in pregnancy and lactation is lacking.

Interactions

None well documented.

Adverse Reactions

A case report of hepatotoxicity exists.

Toxicology

Information is lacking.

Local Anesthetic/Vasoconstrictor Precautions
No information available to require special precautions

Effects on Bleeding None reported

Hawthorn

Clinical Overview

Uses

Hawthorn may have a role as adjunctive therapy in mild heart failure and exhibits some advantages over digoxin. In more severe cases of congestive heart failure (CHF), its place in therapy is less clear. Studies in animals suggest that hawthorn extracts exert effects on the CNS, including anxiolytic and analgesic action; however, clinical studies are limited. Although limited clinical studies have shown improvement in hyperlipidemia with hawthorn extracts, specific, well-designed trials are needed before hawthorn extracts can be recommended.

Dosing

Trials have evaluated dosages ranging from 160 to 1,800 mg/day standardized extracts (mostly WS 1442) in divided doses over 3 to 24 weeks. A minimum effective dose for adjunctive therapy in mild CHF is suggested to be standardized extract 300 mg daily, and maximum benefit appears after 6 to 8 weeks of therapy. Clinical trials conducted in patients with class II and III CHF found hawthorn extract 900 mg daily to be safe, but not superior to placebo.

Contraindications

Known allergy to members of the rose family.

Pregnancy/Lactation

In the absence of clear data, hawthorn extracts should be avoided in pregnancy and during lactation. Animal studies, however, have not shown any adverse effect on embryonic development.

Interactions

None well documented.

Adverse Reactions

Serious adverse reactions are rarely reported. Mild to moderate dizziness, headache, rash, palpitations, and nausea and other GI symptoms have been reported.

Toxicology

Hawthorn is reportedly toxic in high doses; low doses of hawthorn usually lack adverse effects. No increase in the frequency of fetal malformations or teratogenicity has been found in animal studies.

Local Anesthetic/Vasoconstrictor Precautions
No information available to require special precautions

Effects on Bleeding None reported

Holy Basil

Clinical Overview

Uses

Limited evidence suggests potential applications in treating stress, anxiety disorders, diabetes, and cancer. Anti-inflammatory and antimicrobial activities have also been demonstrated. However, few clinical trials have been conducted to support these uses.

Dosing

Limited clinical trials are available to provide dosing recommendations for holy basil.

CNS disorders: 300 mg/day of an ethanolic leaf extract for 30 days was used in a study evaluating use of holy basil for enhancement of cognition. Dosages of 1,000 mg/day for 8 weeks or 1,200 mg/day for 6 weeks were used in studies evaluating the effects of holy basil extract on stress disorders.

Diabetes/Metabolic syndrome: One clinical trial used 2.5 g of the leaves as a dried powder mixed in 200 mL of water daily for 2 months to produce a hypoglycemic effect.

Contraindications

Contraindications have not been identified.

Pregnancy/Lactation

Avoid use. Information regarding safety and efficacy in pregnancy and lactation is lacking. Emmenagogue and abortifacient effects have been reported for the related species Ocimum basilicum.

Interactions

None well documented.

Adverse Reactions

Clinical information is lacking.

Toxicology

No data.

Local Anesthetic/Vasoconstrictor Precautions
No information available to require special precautions

Effects on Bleeding None reported

Honeybee Products

Clinical Overview

Uses

Honeybee products have been used topically and internally for hundreds of years worldwide as remedies for a variety of illnesses; however, clinical trials are lacking for most uses. Honey and royal jelly exhibit antibacterial properties, and there is some evidence that honey might have a role in wound healing. Discrepancies among studies evaluating honey for wounds may be due to variations in the source and preparation of the honey. Bee pollen is most often used for its nutritional properties, and although it is nutritionally rich, claims that it enhances everyday and athletic performance have not been reliably verified. Data supporting the use of honeybee products for other indications are not well substantiated.

Dosing

Honey is a common food and there are no dose restrictions on its use. It has been ingested and used topically.

The ideal dose of bee pollen is unknown, with doses varying among products because tablets contain differing amounts. Manufacturers' recommendations on product labeling may provide more guidance.

Clinical trials are generally lacking to recommend dosage for royal jelly. Small clinical trials have used royal jelly 6 to 10 g/day for 14 to 28 days when evaluating the effect on hyperlipidemia.

Contraindications

Honey should be used with caution in infant formulations. Allergy to bee venom is considered a relative contraindication to royal jelly. Other contraindications have not been identified for honey, bee pollen, or royal jelly.

Pregnancy/Lactation

Clinical data regarding safety and efficacy of these products in pregnancy and lactation are lacking. Honey is generally recognized as safe (GRAS) during pregnancy and lactation when used as food.

Interactions

None well documented for honey or bee pollen. Case reports of hematuria due to potentiation of warfarin have been documented with royal jelly.

Adverse Reactions

Allergic reactions may occur to pollen in honey when ingested. Attempts to hyposensitize patients by administering bee pollen may produce severe anaphylaxis and other acute or chronic responses. Although rare, bee pollen can cause serious, sometimes fatal, adverse reactions. Some case reports of acute hepatitis and photosensitivity following ingestion of bee pollen have been reported. In many allergic patients, skin tests are positive for royal jelly. Case reports exist of allergy, acute exacerbation of asthma, anaphylaxis, and death.

Toxicology

Contaminated honey containing botulism spores can poison infants. The American Academy of Pediatrics and the World Health Organization recommend that honey should not be given to an infant younger than 12 months due to the potential for botulism. Honey made from the nectar of poisonous plants can be poisonous. Information on the toxicology of bee pollen or royal jelly is lacking.

Local Anesthetic/Vasoconstrictor Precautions

No information available to require special precautions

Effects on Bleeding None reported

Hops

Clinical Overview

Uses

Hops have been used for flavoring; hops and lupulin have been used as a digestive aid, for mild sedation, diuresis, and treating menstrual problems, but no clinical studies are available to confirm these uses.

Dosing

Hops has been used as a mild sedative or sleep aid, with the dried strobile given in doses of 1.5 to 2 g. An extract combination with valerian, Ze 91019 (ReDormin, Ivel) has been studied at a hops dose of 60 mg for insomnia.

Contraindications

Contraindications have not yet been identified.

Pregnancy/Lactation

Information regarding safety and efficacy in pregnancy and lactation is lacking.

Interactions

None well documented.

Adverse Reactions

There are no reported side effects when used in moderation.

Toxicology

Malignant hyperthermic reactions have been observed in dogs that consumed boiled hops residues. A wide safety margin for humans has been extrapolated from animal experiments.

Local Anesthetic/Vasoconstrictor Precautions

No information available to require special precautions

Effects on Bleeding None reported

Horehound

Clinical Overview

Uses

Clinical studies regarding therapeutic uses of horehound are limited. Research has centered on the potential for use in cardiovascular disease, diabetes, and pain and inflammation; however, no clinical evidence supports the use of horehound in these roles or in cough preparations.

Dosing

Clinical trials are lacking to provide dosing guidance. One clinical study evaluating the effect of horehound in type 2 diabetes used horehound infusions prepared with the leaves of M. vulgare and administered in 1 g envelopes, 3 times a day for 21 days.

Dosages of 4.5 g daily as the crude herb and 30 to 60 mL as pressed juice from the herb have been traditionally used.

Contraindications

Use in pregnancy is contraindicated.

Pregnancy/Lactation

Avoid use. Horehound reportedly has emmenagogue and abortifacient effects.

Interactions

None well documented.

Adverse Reactions

In a small clinical study, nausea, dry mouth, excessive salivation, dizziness, and anorexia were reported by some patients drinking a prepared infusion solution of dry leaves of the plant.

Toxicology

Marrubiin, one of the main constituents of *M. vulgare*, has a median lethal dose (LD_{50}) of 370 mg/kg when administered orally to rats and an LD_{50} of 100 mg/kg when injected in mice; marrubiin was not cytotoxic to any of 66 cell lines tested. *M. vulgare* was given to rats at increasing doses of up to 1,000 mg/kg daily for 3 weeks, with no signs of toxicity. As a flavoring agent and essential oil, horehound has been granted generally recognized as safe (GRAS) status by the US Food and Drug Administration (FDA).

Local Anesthetic/Vasoconstrictor Precautions
No information available to require special precautions

Effects on Bleeding None reported

Horse Chestnut

Clinical Overview

Uses

Oral horse chestnut seed extract is effective in the short-term treatment of mild to moderate long-term venous insufficiency. Other investigations focus on the role of the major component aescin in antiobesity and anti-inflammatory effects, as well as potential cancer treatment. Aescin gel has been evaluated for use in bruising.

Dosing

Aescin 20 to 120 mg taken orally has been used for venous insufficiency and is available in tablet form. Oral tinctures and topical gels containing aescin 2% are also available.

Contraindications

Renal or hepatic impairment may be relative contraindications to the use of aescin or horse chestnut derivatives.

Pregnancy/Lactation

Avoid use. Information regarding safety and efficacy in pregnancy and lactation is lacking.

Interactions

None well documented.

Adverse Reactions

The most commonly cited adverse effects include nausea and stomach discomfort, which may be minimized by the use of film-coated tablets. Other mild and infrequent complaints include headache, dizziness, and pruritus. Rare cases of allergy and anaphylaxis have been reported.

Toxicology

All parts of plants in the Aesculus family are potentially toxic, especially the seeds (nuts). Horse chestnut has been classified by the Food and Drug Administration (FDA) as an unsafe herb.

Local Anesthetic/Vasoconstrictor Precautions
No information available to require special precautions

Effects on Bleeding Contains esculin which has antithrombotic effects and may increase the risk of bleeding or bruising.

Horseradish

Clinical Overview

Uses

Horseradish has been used internally as a condiment, GI stimulant, diuretic, and a vermifuge, and externally for sciatica and facial neuralgia. However, there are no clinical trials to support any therapeutic use for horseradish. Animal data suggest potential antibacterial and hypotensive effects.

Dosing

Traditional use for colds and respiratory infections was 20 g/day of fresh root. Externally, preparations with 2% mustard oil have been used.

Contraindications

Contraindicated in patients with GI ulcers and in those with kidney impairment. Not recommended for children younger than 4 years of age.

Pregnancy/Lactation

Documented adverse effects. Avoid use. Use should be avoided during pregnancy and lactation because the allylisothiocyanates are toxic mucosal irritants. Horseradish has abortifacient effects.

Interactions

None well documented.

Adverse Reactions

Irritant effects on GI mucosa. External use may cause erythematous rash. Horseradish is part of the cabbage and mustard family; therefore, it may suppress thyroid function. The isothiocyanates may irritate mucous membranes on contact or if inhaled.

Toxicology

Ingestion of large amounts can cause bloody vomiting and diarrhea.

Local Anesthetic/Vasoconstrictor Precautions
No information available to require special precautions

Effects on Bleeding None reported

Horsetail

Clinical Overview

Uses

Horsetail has traditionally been used as a diuretic, as an astringent to stop bleeding and stimulate healing of wounds and burns, and as a cosmetic component, as well as for treatment of tuberculosis and of kidney and bladder ailments (eg, urethritis, cystitis with hematuria); however, clinical trials are lacking to support these uses. Clinical data demonstrate a hypoglycemic effect with use of E. myriochaetum and efficacy in treating brittle nails with use of E. arvense.

Dosing

Equisetum palustre products are contraindicated for use in humans. **Brittle nails:** A formulation containing E. arvense applied topically every night for 28 days or every other day for 14 days has been used to strengthen fingernails in clinical trials. **Diuretic:** A dry extract of the aerial parts of E. arvense containing 0.026% total flavonoids has been administered as 300 mg orally 3 times daily. **Type 2 diabetes:** A water extract of a related species of horsetail (E. myriochaetum) as a single oral dose of 0.33 g/kg has been used in a clinical study. **Wound healing:** An E. arvense 3% ointment applied topically every 12 hours for 10 days has been used following episiotomy in postpartum mothers.

Contraindications

Horsetail has been listed as an herb of undefined safety by the US Food and Drug Administration (FDA). Horsetail remedies prepared from E. arvense are generally considered safe when used properly. However, another species of horsetail, E. palustre, is poisonous to horses; contraindicated for use in humans.

Pregnancy/Lactation

Avoid use. Information regarding safety and efficacy in pregnancy and lactation is lacking.

Interactions

None well documented.

Adverse Reactions

Documented adverse effects possibly associated with horsetail include acute pancreatitis and an isolated incident of headache.

Toxicology

Horsetail has been listed as an herb of undefined safety by the FDA. Horsetail remedies prepared from E. arvense are generally considered safe when used properly. However, another species of horsetail, E. palustre, is poisonous to horses; contraindicated for use in humans. E. arvense may be toxic, especially in cases of underlying liver disease. There have been reports of children being poisoned by using the stems as blowguns or whistles.

Local Anesthetic/Vasoconstrictor Precautions

No information available to require special precautions

Effects on Bleeding None reported

5-HTP

Clinical Overview

Uses

Clinical trials of 5-HTP conducted in various conditions have resulted in limited evidence suggesting a place in therapy for anxiety, depression, and neurological conditions in which a serotonin deficiency is a contributory factor. 5-HTP may also be an effective appetite suppressant, but further clinical trials are needed.

Dosing

Recent clinical trials do not provide adequate dosing guidelines. Studies in depression have used 5-HTP 200 to 300 mg/day given in 3 to 4 divided doses to prevent possible nausea.

Contraindications

The potential for serotonin syndrome exists with concomitant use of selective serotonin reuptake inhibitors (SSRIs) or monoamine oxidase inhibitors (MAOIs).

Pregnancy/Lactation

Information regarding safety and efficacy in pregnancy and lactation is lacking.

Interactions

The potential for serotonin syndrome exists with concomitant use of SSRIs or MAOIs. 5-HTP augments the effect of citalopram and clomipramine, while carbidopa increases the bioavailability of 5-HTP.

Adverse Reactions

Nausea and vomiting are the most common dose-related adverse events. Diarrhea, abdominal pain, mild headache, and sleepiness have also been reported.

Toxicology

There is little information on the toxicology of 5-HTP. A possible association with fatal eosinophilia-myalgia syndrome in the 1980s and 1990s has now been attributed to contaminated L-tryptophan.

Local Anesthetic/Vasoconstrictor Precautions

No information available to require special precautions

Effects on Bleeding None reported

Human Chorionic Gonadotropin

Clinical Overview

Uses

Existing evidence does not support the use of human chorionic gonadotropin (hCG) in weight reduction, and the use of hCG for this purpose is not supported by the American Medical Association (AMA) or the American Society of Bariatric Physicians. Homeopathic preparations of hCG do not contain significant amount of the active ingredient, and clinical trials have not been conducted to provide evidence for effect.

Dosing

Recommendations for dosing for indications other than those approved for hCG cannot be made because evidence to support efficacy is lacking.

Contraindications

Precocious puberty, prostatic carcinoma or other androgen-dependent neoplasia, prior allergic reaction to chorionic gonadotropin, and pregnancy.

Pregnancy/Lactation

hCG is contraindicated in pregnant women. Avoid use in lactation.

Interactions

None well documented.

Adverse Reactions

Arterial thromboembolism, headache, irritability and other CNS symptoms, genitourinary effects, and hypersensitivity have been reported.

Toxicology

Defects of forelimbs and the CNS, as well as alterations in sex ratio, have been reported in mice on combined gonadotropin and hCG regimens. No mutagenic effect has been clearly established in humans.

Local Anesthetic/Vasoconstrictor Precautions

No information available to require special precautions

Effects on Bleeding None reported

Huperzine A

Clinical Overview

Uses

Historically, club moss has been used for the treatment of bruises, strains, swelling, rheumatism, and colds, to relax muscles and tendons, and to improve blood circulation. Because of its anticholinesterase activity, huperzine A, a constituent of the whole plant, has been studied for potential use in treating Alzheimer disease and other CNS disorders; however, there is still insufficient evidence to support its routine use.

Dosing

Huperzine A has been studied at oral dosages of 0.2 to 0.4 mg/day for Alzheimer disease.

Contraindications

Contraindications have not been identified.

Pregnancy/Lactation

Information regarding safety and efficacy in pregnancy and lactation is lacking.

Interactions

None well documented.

Adverse Reactions

In clinical trials, cholinergic adverse reactions have been noted, including hyperactivity, nasal obstruction, nausea, vomiting, diarrhea, insomnia, anxiety, dizziness, thirst, and constipation. One trial reported abnormalities in electrocardiogram (ECG) patterns (cardiac ischemia and arrhythmia).

Toxicology

Symptoms of acute toxicity are similar to those of other cholinergic inhibitors and include muscular tremor, drooling, tears, increased bronchial secretions, and incontinence. No mutagenicity or teratogenicity were found in rodent studies.

Local Anesthetic/Vasoconstrictor Precautions

No information available to require special precautions

Effects on Bleeding None reported

Hyssop

Clinical Overview

Uses

Toxic effects of hyssop essential oil limit therapeutic applications. Although no clinical evidence supports use, animal research indicates the potential for use of hyssop extract in diabetes and for its antimicrobial and CNS effects.

Dosing

No clinical evidence is available to determine hyssop dosing recommendations.

Contraindications

Contraindications have not been identified.

Pregnancy/Lactation

Avoid use. Documented adverse effects.

Interactions

None well documented.

Adverse Reactions

Information is limited; however, case reports of seizures exist.

Toxicology

Convulsant toxic effects of the essential oil have been established in rodents.

Local Anesthetic/Vasoconstrictor Precautions

No information available to require special precautions

Effects on Bleeding None reported

Iboga

Clinical Overview

Uses

Studies suggest that ibogaine, one of the iboga alkaloids, has potential application in the treatment of addiction to several substances. The US Drug Enforcement Agency (DEA) has designated ibogaine a Schedule I substance under the Controlled Substances Act (CSA).

Dosing

Strict medical supervision is necessary with use. Single oral doses of ibogaine ranging from 500 to 1,000 mg have been used in clinical trials for the treatment of opioid addiction. In patients with drug dependence in a Brazilian drug dependency clinic, an average single dose of 17 mg/kg in combination with psychotherapy was used under close medical supervision. Some literature suggests that based on limited animal data, and applying appropriate safety factors, a maximum initial oral dosage limit of less than 1 mg/kg for the treatment of drug dependence should be adhered to.

Contraindications

Fatalities have been associated with the use of ibogaine; concomitant opioid use and comorbidities (eg, cardiovascular disease, depression, posttraumatic stress disorder, anxiety, stress, schizophrenia, epilepsy, or other imbalances in the autonomic nervous system) increase the risk of life-threatening complications, including sudden cardiac death. Ibogaine should only be used under the supervision of an experienced health care provider.

Pregnancy/Lactation

Avoid use. Information regarding the safety and efficacy in pregnancy and lactation is lacking.

Interactions

None well documented.

Adverse Reactions

Mild acute effects occur frequently and include nausea, vomiting, ataxia, tremors, headaches, and mental confusion. Manic episodes lasting 1 to 2 weeks have also been reported and manifested as sleeplessness, irritability, impulsivity, emotional lability, grandiose delusions, rapid tangential speech, aggressive behavior, and suicidal ideation.

Toxicology

Large doses of iboga can induce agitation, hallucinations, vomiting, ataxia, muscle spasms, weakness, seizures, paralysis, arrhythmias, urinary retention, respiratory insufficiency, and cardiac arrest.

Local Anesthetic/Vasoconstrictor Precautions

No information available to require special precautions

Effects on Bleeding None reported

Ipecac

Clinical Overview

Uses

Ipecac has been used as an emetic and treatment for dysentery. It has amebicidal components. It currently is not recommended as an emetic for childhood poisonings. Activated charcoal now is the treatment of choice. Always consult a health care professional or poison control center when an accidental poisoning occurs.

Dosing

Ipecac syrup, which contains total alkaloids123 to 157 mg per 100 mL, has been used to induce vomiting. The usual dose range for the syrup is 10 to 30 mL, yielding a dose of alkaloids of 12 to 48 mg. Do not confuse the syrup with the fluid extract of ipecac, which is 14 times stronger. Cumulative toxicity requires administration of emetine for amebic dysentery in low doses for a short time with intervals of several weeks before further treatment.

Contraindications

Do not administer ipecac when a patient has a decreased level of consciousness or has ingested either a corrosive substance or hydrocarbon with a high aspiration potential.

Pregnancy/Lactation

Documented adverse effects include uterine stimulation. Avoid use.

Interactions

None well documented.

Adverse Reactions

Repeated exposure to powdered ipecac may cause rhinitis or asthma. Emetine can irritate skin if applied topically. Diarrhea, lethargy, drowsiness, and prolonged vomiting may occur.

Toxicology

Ipecac extracts may be highly toxic; do not confuse with syrup of ipecac. Emetine is a cardiotoxin and has been associated with serious cardiotoxicity.

Local Anesthetic/Vasoconstrictor Precautions

No information available to require special precautions

Effects on Bleeding None reported

Jiaogulan

Clinical Overview

Uses

Limited clinical studies have been conducted to support therapeutic applications. Jiaogulan may have a role in the management of type 2 diabetes, fatty liver disease, immune response (such as asthma), and cancer. *G. pentaphyllum* extracts may also have a place in beneficial antioxidant therapy.

Dosing

Clinical information is lacking. Jiaogulan tea (aqueous extract) 6 g/day, in divided doses twice a day 30 minutes before meals, has been studied in 2 clinical trials in patients with type 2 diabetes.

Contraindications

Contraindications have not yet been identified.

Pregnancy/Lactation

Information regarding safety and efficacy in pregnancy and lactation is lacking.

Interactions

None well documented.

Adverse Reactions

Severe nausea and increased bowel movements are possible.

Toxicology

No data available for human toxicity.

Local Anesthetic/Vasoconstrictor Precautions

No information available to require special precautions

Effects on Bleeding None reported

Jojoba

Clinical Overview

Uses

The toxicity of the constituent simmondsin in jojoba seed meal and some oil components limits the likelihood of clinical applications. Jojoba oil is commonly used in dermatological preparations.

Dosing

There is no clinical evidence to guide dosage of jojoba or its oil; it is primarily used as a vehicle for oxidation-sensitive substances in ointments.

Contraindications

Although absolute contraindications have not been identified, jojoba should not be ingested by humans due to potential toxicity.

Pregnancy/Lactation

Information regarding safety and efficacy in pregnancy and lactation is lacking. Adverse toxicological studies in rodents and birds exist.

Interactions

None well documented.

Adverse Reactions

Case reports of contact dermatitis, confirmed by skin patch tests, exist for jojoba oil.

Toxicology

Constituents of jojoba are toxic. Studies demonstrate hematological toxicity, histological abnormalities, and other adverse effects.

Local Anesthetic/Vasoconstrictor Precautions

No information available to require special precautions

Effects on Bleeding None reported

Juniper

Clinical Overview

Uses

Juniper berries have been used as a flavoring component in alcoholic beverages (eg, gin) and as a seasoning in food; juniper has also been used in traditional medicine for various purposes. Limited animal and in vitro evidence suggests potential antimicrobial, antioxidant, cytotoxic, neuroprotective, hepatoprotective, and hypoglycemic effects; however, no clinical data exist to support use of juniper for any indication.

Dosing

Generally, 2 to 10 g/day of the whole, crushed, or powdered fruit (corresponding to 20 to 100 mg of essential oil) has been used for dyspepsia.

Essential oil: 0.02 to 0.1 mL 3 times daily.

Fluid extract: 1:1 (g/mL); 2 to 3 mL 3 times daily.

Infusion: 2 to 3 g steeped in 150 mL of boiled water for 20 minutes 3 times daily.

Contraindications

Avoid in renal impairment due to potential irritant activity.

Pregnancy/Lactation

Avoid use. Juniper possibly possesses anti-implantation and abortifacient activities. Antiprostaglandin and antiprogestational activities leading to antifertility effects have been suggested.

Interactions

None well documented.

Adverse Reactions

Allergic reactions may occur. Kidney damage and inflammation may result from excessive use of juniper. Juniper berries may increase blood glucose in patients with diabetes.

Toxicology

Large doses of juniper berries may cause catharsis and convulsions. The juniper volatile oil may be nephrotoxic.

Local Anesthetic/Vasoconstrictor Precautions

No information available to require special precautions

Effects on Bleeding None reported

Kava

Clinical Overview

Uses

A number of meta-analyses and systematic reviews of kava use in anxiety have found in favor of kava over placebo, but results are not consistent. Kava has also been studied for effects on cognitive function and for potential cancer applications. However, concerns over hepatotoxicity have limited clinical studies.

Dosing

A maximum daily dose of kavalactones 250 mg is suggested to avoid potential hepatotoxicity. Studies in children are lacking, and use is not recommended.

Contraindications

Kava and kava-containing products are not recommended for use in children or in patients with hepatic disease. Kava should be used cautiously in patients with renal or liver disease, blood disorders, Parkinson disease, or depression.

Pregnancy/Lactation

Documented adverse effects. Avoid use.

Interactions

Kava extracts have been shown to interfere with cytochrome P450 (CYP-450) enzymes; however, specific reports on the metabolism of pharmaceuticals are sparse. Case reports exist on interactions with alprazolam, alcohol, barbiturates, and levodopa. Concomitant administration of kava with haloperidol, risperidone, and metoclopramide, among other drugs, may be associated with adverse reactions.

Adverse Reactions

Heavy kava use may cause a scaly skin rash. A variety of adverse reactions, including visual disturbances, urinary retention, GI discomfort, exacerbation of Parkinson disease, extrapyramidal effects, and rhabdomyolysis, have been reported.

Toxicology

Rare cases of severe liver toxicity have been reported.

Local Anesthetic/Vasoconstrictor Precautions

No information available to require special precautions

Effects on Bleeding None reported

Kudzu

Clinical Overview

Uses

Kudzu is being investigated for its potential use as a therapy for alcoholism; however, sufficient and consistent clinical trials are lacking. The estrogenic activity of kudzu and the cardioprotective effects of its constituent puerarin are also under investigation, but clinical trials are limited.

Dosing

Alcohol abuse: 3 g daily of kudzu extract (25% isoflavone content) has been studied in adults diagnosed with alcohol abuse/dependence. In another study, 2.4 g of kudzu root was given daily. **Unstable angina:** Intravenous (IV) puerarin has been used in studies of unstable angina at dosages of 200 to 500 mg daily for up to 28 days.

Contraindications

Contraindications have not been identified.

Pregnancy/Lactation

Avoid use. Information regarding safety and efficacy in pregnancy and lactation is lacking.

Interactions

None well documented. Because kudzu may decrease blood glucose, additive effects are possible with use of antihyperglycemic agents.

Adverse Reactions

A few case reports of hypersensitivity reactions (ie, maculopapular drug eruption, Stevens-Johnson syndrome-type reaction) exist.

Toxicology

No data.

Local Anesthetic/Vasoconstrictor Precautions

No information available to require special precautions

Effects on Bleeding None reported

Lady's Mantle

Clinical Overview

Uses

Lady's mantle has been traditionally used both topically and internally as a treatment for wounds, GI complaints, and female ailments (eg, menstrual or menopausal complaints); however, clinical studies are lacking to support these uses. Animal studies do not support the use of lady's mantle in diabetes, and limited studies of use in wound healing have been conducted.

Dosing

Clinical studies are lacking to support specific dosing recommendations for lady's mantle. A gel made from the leaves has been used topically for mouth ulcers. Oral dosages of 5 to 10 g of the herb in 1 L of water daily, or of 2 to 4 mL of the liquid herb extract have been traditionally used for the treatment of diarrhea.

Contraindications

Contraindications have not been identified.

Pregnancy/Lactation

Avoid use. Information regarding safety and efficacy in pregnancy and lactation is lacking.

Interactions

None well documented.

Adverse Reactions

None known with use at low doses.

Toxicology

No data.

Local Anesthetic/Vasoconstrictor Precautions

No information available to require special precautions

Effects on Bleeding None reported

Laminaria

Clinical Overview

Uses

Laminaria has been used traditionally as a hygroscopic cervical dilator and inducer of labor, and commercial products are available for this purpose. The basal parts of the blades of Laminaria japonica and Laminaria angustata have been used as a hypotensive agent (ne-kombu) in Japanese folk medicine.

Dosing

Clinical trials are lacking to provide dosing information for uses other than mechanical cervical dilation.

Contraindications

Use is contraindicated during pregnancy.

Pregnancy/Lactation

Laminaria dilators have been used to dilate the cervix and to induce labor in abortions. Information on the use of laminaria for other purposes during pregnancy is lacking. Avoid use.

Interactions

None well documented.

Adverse Reactions

There is a risk of laminaria dilators becoming trapped and fragmenting.

Toxicology

Information is lacking.

Local Anesthetic/Vasoconstrictor Precautions

No information available to require special precautions

Effects on Bleeding None reported

L-arginine

Clinical Overview

Uses

L-arginine is classified as a nonessential amino acid, but it may be considered essential or semiessential under conditions of stress, during which L-arginine synthesis becomes compromised. L-arginine has been evaluated for use in cardiovascular disease because of its antiatherogenic, anti-ischemic, antiplatelet, and antithrombotic properties, and for use in renal disease, diabetes, cystic fibrosis, sickle cell disease, and erectile dysfunction. Its immunostimulatory effects and potential benefits in ophthalmic conditions and preeclampsia have also been evaluated.

Dosing

L-arginine has been studied for a variety of conditions using various dosages and treatment durations; current daily dosage trends range from 6 to 30 g orally in 3 divided doses. Oral and intravenous (IV) formulations have been the most commonly studied.

Contraindications

Contraindications have not been identified. However, L-arginine is not recommended following acute myocardial infarction.

Pregnancy/Lactation

L-arginine supplementation has shown beneficial effects in women with hypertension and in those at risk for preeclampsia. However, due to minimal data regarding safety and efficacy in pregnancy and lactation, L-arginine should only be used in these populations if recommended by and under the supervision of a health care provider.

Interactions

Nitrates: Caution is warranted in patients concomitantly using L-arginine supplementation and nitrates. L-arginine may potentiate the effects of isosorbide mononitrate and other nitric oxide donors, such as glyceryl trinitrate (ie, nitroglycerin) and sodium nitroprusside. *Insulin:* Caution is warranted in patients using insulin concomitantly with L-arginine; effects on insulin are unpredictable. *Cholesterol-lowering drugs:* Caution is warranted in patients using cholesterol-lowering drugs concomitantly with L-arginine; effects on cholesterol-lowering drugs are unpredictable.

Adverse Reactions

Nausea, diarrhea, dyspepsia, palpitations, headache, and numbness have been reported with L-arginine use. Bitter taste may occur with higher doses. Because of L-arginine's vasodilatory effects, hypotension may occur. IV preparations containing L-arginine hydrochloride have a high chloride content that may increase the risk for metabolic acidosis in patients with electrolyte imbalances. Hyperkalemia and elevations in serum urea nitrogen (BUN) levels may occur in patients with renal and/or hepatic impairment.

Toxicology

High concentrations of nitric oxide are considered toxic to brain tissue.

Local Anesthetic/Vasoconstrictor Precautions
No information available to require special precautions

Effects on Bleeding None reported

Lavender

Clinical Overview

Uses

Lavender has been used for anxiety and anxiety-related conditions such as restlessness, insomnia, anxiety, and GI distress. However, trials often included healthy volunteers, and most were considered to be of poor quality and displayed inconsistent results. Limited clinical trials support therapeutic use of lavender for pain, hot flushes, and postnatal perineal discomfort.

Dosing

A single to several drops of lavender essential oil (20 mg to 120 mg) diluted in a base or carrier oil, or added to hot water in a diffuser or humidifier, infiltrated on a cotton pad, or dripped in a jar for inhalation has been described for aromatherapy. For consumption as a tea, 1 to 2 tsp (5 to 10 mL) of lavender herb can be steeped in 1 cup of boiling water. A proprietary oral product, Silexan, is usually dosed at 80 or 160 mg/day for use in anxiety.

Contraindications

Contraindications have not been identified. Cautious use or avoidance is warranted in patients with known allergy/hypersensitivity to lavender.

Pregnancy/Lactation

Information regarding safety and efficacy in pregnancy and lactation is limited. Lavender may possess emmenagogic properties, and excessive internal use should be avoided in pregnancy. Lavender aromatherapy has been used in limited studies during and after labor, with no reported adverse effects.

Interactions

CNS depressants and anticonvulsants may increase or potentiate narcotic and sedative effects when given in combination with lavender-containing products. Anticoagulants may increase the risk of bleeding when given concomitantly with lavender. Lavender may also cause additive cholesterol-lowering effects when given with other drugs that lower cholesterol (eg, statins, nicotinic acid, fibric acid derivatives).

Adverse Reactions

Lavender may cause allergic contact dermatitis and photosensitization. Additionally, several case reports suggest a possible association between topical application of lavender and tea tree oils and prepubertal gynecomastia. GI complaints have been reported with oral use.

Toxicology

A case report describes an accidental ingestion of lavandin resulting in CNS depression in an 18-month-old child. The child's neurological state normalized within 6 hours of ingestion. Consumption of tea made from L. stoechas resulted in supraventricular tachycardia in a 46-year-old woman.

Local Anesthetic/Vasoconstrictor Precautions
No information available to require special precautions

Effects on Bleeding None reported

Lecithin

Clinical Overview

Uses

Lecithin is used for its emulsifying properties in the food, pharmaceutical, and cosmetic industries. Proposed pharmacological use of lecithin includes treatment for hypercholesterolemia, neurologic disorders, manic disorders, and liver ailments. It has also been used to modify the immune system by activating specific and nonspecific defense systems. However, no quality clinical trials exist to support lecithin's use for these indications.

Dosing

Studies of lecithin in cognitive impairment have used a wide range of dosages, from 1 to 35 g daily. In a study of patients with bipolar disorder, 10 mg given 3 times daily was found to improve symptoms of mania.

Contraindications

Contraindications have not yet been identified.

Pregnancy/Lactation

Information regarding safety and efficacy in pregnancy and lactation is lacking.

Interactions

None well documented.

Adverse Reactions

Adverse effects are usually not associated with lecithin. However, there have been reports of anorexia, nausea, sweating, increased salivation, other GI effects, and hepatitis.

Toxicology
Information regarding toxicology with the use of this lecithin is limited.

Local Anesthetic/Vasoconstrictor Precautions
No information available to require special precautions

Effects on Bleeding None reported

Lemon Balm

Clinical Overview

Uses
Primary interest in lemon balm surrounds its effects on the central nervous system. One small study demonstrated decreased stress and agitation in patients with dementia and Alzheimer disease. Lemon balm cream has shown some efficacy in herpes virus lesions in a few small placebo-controlled trials.

Dosing
Crude lemon balm herb is typically dosed at 1.5 to 4.5 g/day. Doses of 600 to 1,600 mg extract have been studied in trials. A standardized preparation of lemon balm (80 mg) and valerian extract (160 mg) has been given 2 or 3 times/day as a sleep aid, and has also been studied in children. A 1% extract cream has been studied as a topical agent for treatment of herpes virus lesions.

Contraindications
Contraindications have not yet been identified.

Pregnancy/Lactation
Information regarding safety and efficacy in pregnancy and lactation is lacking.

Interactions
None well documented.

Adverse Reactions
Clinical trials generally report no adverse reactions.

Toxicology
Research reveals little or no information regarding toxicology with the use of this product.

Local Anesthetic/Vasoconstrictor Precautions
No information available to require special precautions

Effects on Bleeding None reported

Lemongrass

Clinical Overview

Uses
Lemongrass has traditionally been used as a fragrance and flavoring, and for a wide variety of medical conditions. However, clinical trials are lacking to support any uses. Limited clinical or experimental studies have shown antifungal and insecticidal activity, as well as potential anticarcinogenic activity, while suggested hypotensive and hypoglycemic actions have not been confirmed.

Dosing
Information from clinical trials is lacking to provide dosing recommendations. Dose and time-dependent adverse effects of C. citratus leaves on renal function have been reported.

Contraindications
Contraindications have not been identified.

Pregnancy/Lactation
Avoid use. Information regarding safety and efficacy in pregnancy and lactation is lacking.

Interactions
None well documented.

Adverse Reactions
Rare cases of hypersensitivity have been reported. Toxic alveolitis has been associated with inhalation of lemongrass oil. Dose and time-dependent adverse effects of C. citratus leaves on renal function have been reported.

Toxicology
No data. Lemongrass is considered to be of low toxicity at low doses.

Local Anesthetic/Vasoconstrictor Precautions
No information available to require special precautions

Effects on Bleeding None reported

Licorice

Clinical Overview

Uses
Used historically for GI complaints, licorice is primarily used as a flavoring agent in the tobacco and candy industries and to some extent in the pharmaceutical and beverage industries today. The chemical compounds found in licorice have been investigated as cancer therapy as well as for their antiviral activity.

Dosing
Licorice root has been used in daily doses from 2 to 15 g for ulcer and gastritis. Higher doses given for extended periods of time may pose a risk of hyperkalemia. The acceptable daily intake (ADI) for glycyrrhizin is suggested to be 0.2 mg/kg/day.

Contraindications
Contraindications have not yet been identified.

Pregnancy/Lactation
Use during pregnancy should be avoided. Licorice exhibits estrogenic activity and has reputed abortifacient effects. There is no clinical evidence to support the use of licorice tea as a galactogogue.

Interactions
Glycyrrhizin in licorice may alter prednisolone plasma concentrations and may increase the risk of digitalis toxicity.

Adverse Reactions
At lower dosages or normal consumption levels, few adverse reactions are evident. Ocular effects and hypersensitivity have been described. Hypertension and hypokalemia are recognized effects of excessive licorice consumption.

Toxicology
Toxicity from excessive licorice ingestion is well established. Mutagenicity and teratogenicity studies have generally shown no ill effects.

Local Anesthetic/Vasoconstrictor Precautions
No information available to require special precautions

Effects on Bleeding None reported

Lobelia

Clinical Overview

Uses
L. inflata and its major alkaloid, lobeline, have been used in smoking cessation programs and proposed for treatment of other drug dependencies. The sale of over-the-counter (OTC) lobeline products for smoking cessation was prohibited by the US Food and Drug Administration (FDA) in 1993. Lobeline has traditionally been used to treat asthma and bronchitis. However, clinical trial data are lacking to recommend use for any indication.

Dosing
Clinical trials are lacking to support the use of lobelia or provide dosing recommendations. Traditional use of the leaf (ie, as an expectorant) suggests 100 mg of dry herb up to 3 times a day. Doses of 0.6 to 1 g of the leaf are considered toxic, while 4 g of the leaf is considered to be fatal.

Contraindications
Contraindications have not been clearly defined; however, the sale of lobelia OTC products for smoking cessation is prohibited by the FDA due to a lack of efficacy and safety evidence.

Pregnancy/Lactation
Avoid use. Evidence of safety is lacking. Adverse effects have been documented, including loss of uterine tone.

Interactions
None well documented.

Adverse Reactions
Lobelia and lobeline are capable of inducing nausea, vomiting, tremors, and dizziness at high doses. Lobelia alkaloids are cardioactive; cardiotoxicities (ie, hypotension, tachycardia, convulsion) have been reported.

Toxicology
Toxic dosages of the plant have been described: 1 g of leaf is toxic, while 4 g of leaf is considered a fatal dose.

Local Anesthetic/Vasoconstrictor Precautions
No information available to require special precautions

Effects on Bleeding None reported

Lycopene

Clinical Overview

Uses
Scientific literature documents lycopene's antioxidant activity and its use in cancer prevention (breast and prostate), as well as its use in the prevention of cardiovascular disease.

Dosing
Lycopene administered as a pure compound has been studied in clinical trials at dosages of 8 to 75 mg/day. Lycopene is primarily available in capsule and softgel form, with dosage guidelines from manufacturers ranging from 10 to 30 mg taken twice daily with meals. Lycopene is also incorporated in multivitamin and multimineral products.

Contraindications
Avoid with hypersensitivity to lycopene or to any of its food sources, especially tomatoes. Tomato-based products are acidic and may irritate stomach ulcers.

Pregnancy/Lactation
Information regarding safety and efficacy in pregnancy and lactation is lacking. The amount of lycopene in food is assumed to be safe. Tomato consumption increases lycopene concentration in the breast milk and plasma of lactating women.

Interactions
None well documented.

Adverse Reactions
In general, tomato-based products and lycopene supplements are well tolerated. Some GI complaints (eg, diarrhea, dyspepsia, gas, nausea, vomiting) are documented. One trial reported a cancer-related hemorrhage in a patient taking lycopene, but causality was unclear.

Toxicology
None known.

Local Anesthetic/Vasoconstrictor Precautions
No information available to require special precautions

Effects on Bleeding None reported

Maitake

Clinical Overview

Uses
Maitake has been studied for potential therapeutic applications in cancer and in mitigating cardiovascular risk factors and diabetes. CNS, immune-stimulant, and antiviral activities have been demonstrated. However, clinical studies are lacking to support maitake for any use.

Dosing
Clinical studies are lacking to provide dosing guidance. For commercial preparations, manufacturer-recommended disease-preventive daily doses range from 12 to 25 mg of the extract and up to 2,500 mg of the whole powder.

Contraindications
Contraindications have not been identified.

Pregnancy/Lactation
Information regarding safety and efficacy during pregnancy and lactation is lacking.

Interactions
None well documented.

Adverse Reactions
Information is limited.

Toxicology
No data.

Local Anesthetic/Vasoconstrictor Precautions
No information available to require special precautions

Effects on Bleeding None reported

Maritime Pine

Clinical Overview

Uses
Pine bark extract demonstrates antioxidant and anti-inflammatory actions and has been studied for a wide range of clinical conditions, including chronic venous insufficiency, cardiovascular conditions, and erectile dysfunction. However, many clinical studies have been limited in size, with nonrandomized or open-label designs conducted by a limited pool of researchers.

Dosing
Doses of pine bark extract have been studied in clinical trials, most commonly at 150 mg of Pycnogenol per day.

Contraindications
Contraindications have not been identified.

Pregnancy/Lactation
Information regarding safety and efficacy during pregnancy and lactation is lacking.

Interactions
None well documented.

Adverse Reactions
Pine bark extract is generally well tolerated, with minor gastric discomfort, dizziness, nausea, and headache occasionally noted. Clinical studies using Pycnogenol report no clinically important adverse events.

Toxicology
Pine bark extract is generally recognized as safe (GRAS), based on data from clinical trials. Limited toxicological data are available.

Local Anesthetic/Vasoconstrictor Precautions No information available to require special precautions

Effects on Bleeding May see increased bleeding due to inhibition of platelet aggregation

Marshmallow

Clinical Overview

Uses

A. officinalis has been traditionally used for cough, inflammation of the mouth and stomach, and peptic ulcers. It appears to have antimicrobial and anti-inflammatory properties and may be used topically to increase epithelialization of wounds. However, there are no recent clinical trials to support these uses.

Dosing

Root: 6 g/day.

Leaf: 10 g/day.

Marshmallow syrup: 10 g/day.

Topical: 5 to 10 g in an ointment or cream base or 5% powdered marshmallow leaf applied 3 times daily.

Gargle: 2 g soaked in 240 mL of cold water for 2 hours then gargled. Hot water should not be used.

Contraindications

Contraindications have not been identified.

Pregnancy/Lactation

Avoid use. Information regarding safety and efficacy in pregnancy and lactation is lacking.

Interactions

Oral medications: When taken with other oral medications, marshmallow may delay the absorption of the other medications.

Oral hypoglycemic agents/Insulin: Due to potential additive hypoglycemic effects, marshmallow should be used cautiously in patients receiving oral hypoglycemic agents and insulin.

Topical corticosteroids: Marshmallow may enhance the effects of topical corticosteroids. Use caution.

Aminoglycosides: Use caution or avoid use of marshmallow in patients receiving aminoglycosides such as gentamicin.

Adverse Reactions

Anecdotal evidence suggests potential allergic reactions and hypoglycemia.

Toxicology

The acute median lethal dose (LD_{50}) of A. officinalis in mice was greater than 5,000 mg/kg.

Local Anesthetic/Vasoconstrictor Precautions No information available to require special precautions

Effects on Bleeding None reported

Mastic

Clinical Overview

Uses

The purported uses of mastic are diverse. The resin has been used in cancer, infection, surgical wound adhesion, and benign gastric ulcers. Other traditional uses include as an antioxidant and as an insecticide, and for treatment of high cholesterol, Crohn disease, diabetes, and hypertension. However, clinical trials are lacking to support these uses.

Dosing

Mastic resin at a dosage of 1 g daily has been studied for the treatment of duodenal ulcer. Various commercial products are available to help eliminate H. pylori bacterium in the stomach (implicated in a number of GI complaints), including Mastika, which contains mastic gum 250 mg in capsule form. Manufacturer dosage guidelines recommend 4 capsules orally before bed for 2 weeks, followed by a maintenance dosage of 2 capsules daily.

Contraindications

Avoid use in individuals with hypersensitivity to pollen or to any of the ingredients of mastic gum.

Pregnancy/Lactation

Information regarding safety and efficacy in pregnancy and lactation is lacking.

Interactions

None well documented.

Adverse Reactions

Most adverse reactions are associated with hypersensitivity to the plant species or with allergic reactions.

Toxicology

Most toxic effects involve allergic reactions.

Local Anesthetic/Vasoconstrictor Precautions No information available to require special precautions

Effects on Bleeding None reported

Meadowsweet

Clinical Overview

Uses

Meadowsweet has been used for colds, respiratory problems, acid indigestion, peptic ulcers, arthritis and rheumatism, skin diseases, and diarrhea.

Dosing

Doses of 2.5 to 3.5 g/day of flower and 4 to 5 g of herb are considered conventional; however, no clinical trials support the safety or efficacy of these dosages. A tea may be prepared from 4 to 6 g of the dried herb and taken 3 times daily.

Contraindications

Patients with salicylate or sulfite sensitivity. Use with caution in patients with asthma.

Pregnancy/Lactation

Documented adverse effects. Uteroactivity from meadowsweet has been observed in vitro; avoid administration during pregnancy and lactation.

Interactions

Because meadowsweet contains salicylates, it may increase the risk of bleeding when given concomitantly with antiplatelet or anticoagulant drugs, with nonsteroidal anti-inflammatory drugs (NSAIDs), or with any alternative medicines with antiplatelet properties.

Adverse Reactions

Meadowsweet may cause GI bleeding.

Toxicology

Few toxic events have been reported.

Local Anesthetic/Vasoconstrictor Precautions No information available to require special precautions

Effects on Bleeding Limited evidence suggests an anticoagulant effect *in vitro* and *in vivo* by meadowsweet flowers and seeds. Clinical relevance of this effect is unknown. There are no current published reports of any anticoagulant effect in patients taking meadowsweet.

Melatonin

Clinical Overview

Uses

Exogenous melatonin has been extensively studied for its impact on sleep. A beneficial effect on sleep-onset latency and other sleep parameters in special populations (eg, autism spectrum disorder, shift workers, jet lag) is well supported.

In contrast, limited or equivocal data are available regarding use of melatonin to affect atopic dermatitis, bone density, cardiovascular conditions, constipation-predominant irritable bowel syndrome (IBS), infections (eg, periodontal disease), multiple sclerosis (MS), various reproductive problems (ie, in vitro fertilization rates, dysmenorrhea), tardive dyskinesia, or tinnitus. Limited data suggest a potential role for adjunctive use of melatonin in certain patient populations to reduce hepatic and other adverse effects and/or doses of pharmaceutical agents, such as analgesics, antipsychotics, anxiolytics, sedatives, and statins. No data support a role for melatonin in managing dementia- and/or delirium-related cognitive impairment, epilepsy, mood disorders, or organ transplantation graft rejection.

Dosing

Analgesia: Dosages ranging from 3 to 10 mg/day orally for various durations have been used in various pain conditions.

Insomnia: 3 to 5 mg daily in the evening over 4 weeks. Immediate-release melatonin 1 to 2 mg given 1 hour prior to bedtime may be useful in elderly patients. Controlled-release formulations should be avoided in elderly patients due to concerns for prolonged concentrations. American Academy of Sleep Medicine clinical practice guidelines recommend use of strategically timed melatonin in children and adolescents for the treatment of delayed sleep-wake phase disorder and irregular sleep-wake rhythm disorder in those with and without comorbid neurological or psychiatric disorders, based on short-term studies.

Jet lag: In general, lower doses (0.5 to 2 mg orally) preflight, and higher doses (5 mg orally) postflight over a period of up to 4 days has been recommended.

Contraindications

Because melatonin may exacerbate some autoimmune conditions while alleviating others, melatonin should be avoided in patients with autoimmune diseases.

Pregnancy/Lactation

Melatonin was beneficial in delaying early-onset preeclampsia. Although no adverse effects were noted in mothers, fetuses, or newborns, babies born to women receiving melatonin had birthweights less than the 10th percentile for gestation.

Given the minimal information available regarding safety and efficacy, melatonin supplementation in pregnancy and lactation is questionable and should be avoided until further research has been conducted.

Interactions

Melatonin's metabolism involves the CYP-450 system, and therefore has the propensity for numerous drug-drug interactions. Specifically, melatonin is metabolized by CYP1A2 to 6-hydroxymelatonin. Additionally, it is metabolized by CYP2C9 and CYP2C19 to metabolites such as N-acetylserotonin, 5-methoxytryptamine, and 5-methoxylated kynuramines. Additionally, melatonin may result in excessive drowsiness when given with, among others, benzodiazepines, anticholinergics, and alcohol, which all have sedating properties.

Adverse Reactions

Minor adverse reactions associated with melatonin include headache, transient depression, enuresis, dizziness, nausea, stomach cramps, irritability, insomnia, nightmares, hypothermia, and excessive daytime somnolence. Drowsiness may be experienced within 30 minutes after taking melatonin and may persist for approximately 1 hour; as a result, melatonin may affect driving ability.

Toxicology

Studies are limited. There is little or no evidence of major toxicities with melatonin, even at high doses.

Local Anesthetic/Vasoconstrictor Precautions
No information available to require special precautions

Effects on Bleeding None reported

Methylsulfonylmethane (MSM)

Clinical Overview

Uses

MSM is commonly used for osteoarthritis, but may also benefit in alleviating GI upset, musculoskeletal pain, and allergies; boosting the immune system; and fighting antimicrobial infection. Clinical trials are needed to verify these potential uses.

Dosing

MSM commonly is given as 2 to 6 g/day in 2 to 3 divided doses for arthritis and other joint conditions.

Contraindications

Contraindications have not been identified.

Pregnancy/Lactation

Information regarding safety and efficacy in pregnancy and lactation in humans is lacking.

Interactions

None well documented.

Adverse Reactions

No conclusive data on adverse reactions with MSM have been reported.

Toxicology

No toxicity was noted in animal studies.

Local Anesthetic/Vasoconstrictor Precautions
No information available to require special precautions

Effects on Bleeding None reported

Milk Thistle

Clinical Overview

Uses

Milk thistle has been investigated for its anti-inflammatory, antimicrobial, and CNS effects. It has been studied for use in allergic rhinitis, asthma, cancer treatment-related adverse effects, rheumatoid arthritis, type 2 diabetes, drug-induced hepatotoxicity, drug-induced nephrotoxicity, dyslipidemia, and thalassemia; however clinical trials supporting these uses are limited. Milk thistle is most commonly evaluated for use in the management of liver diseases (alcohol-induced and viral hepatitis) but the majority of clinical trials show equivocal results.

Dosing

Milk thistle is considered safe in dosages of 420 mg/day orally in divided doses for up to 41 months. One source suggests daily doses of 12 to 15 g of dry fruits for dyspepsia and disorders of the biliary system, while an extract containing 200 to 400 mg/day of silymarin is considered effective in various liver disorders.

Contraindications

Milk thistle is contraindicated in patients with allergy to any plant in the Asteraceae family. Avoid use of the aboveground parts of the plant in women with hormone-sensitive conditions (eg, breast, uterine, and ovarian cancers; endometriosis; uterine fibroids) unless under the supervision of a physician, due to the extract's possible estrogenic effects. The more commonly used milk thistle seed extracts are not known to have estrogenic effects.

Pregnancy/Lactation

Milk thistle has traditionally been used in pregnancy. Limited clinical studies in pregnancy demonstrate use without apparent adverse effects; however, further data are needed to confirm safety. Caution should be used in pregnant and breastfeeding women.

Interactions

There are mixed data regarding milk thistle's ability to exert inhibitory or inductive activity on cytochrome P450 (CYP-450) 1A2, 2C19, 2D6, 2E1, and 3A4, as well as P-glycoprotein. Therefore, close monitoring is warranted when drugs metabolized by these enzymes are given concomitantly with milk thistle.

Adverse Reactions

Silymarin is well tolerated; the most common adverse effects after oral ingestion were brief GI disturbances (eg, abdominal bloating, abdominal fullness or pain, anorexia, changes in bowel habits, diarrhea, dyspepsia, flatulence, nausea). Headache and pruritus have also been reported.

Toxicology

Toxic effects of silymarin have not been noted clinically at a dosage of 1,200 mg/day; however, mild allergies have been reported with dosages greater than 1,500 mg/day.

Local Anesthetic/Vasoconstrictor Precautions

No information available to require special precautions

Effects on Bleeding None reported

Mistletoe

Clinical Overview

Uses

Mistletoe has been used to treat cancer, although there is a lack of quality clinical trials and no evidence of an effect. Further study is needed. In folk medicine, it has been used for its cardiovascular properties. Clinical efficacy has not been established. Injectable mistletoe extract is widely used in Europe but is not licensed for use in the United States.

Dosing

Crude mistletoe fruit or herb is used to make a tea to treat hypertension at a dosage of 10 g/day. There are a number of proprietary extracts containing low levels of mistletoe lectin-I (ML-I) used as adjuvant cancer therapies. These extracts usually are given by intravenous (IV) or subcutaneous injection at dosages of 0.1 to 30 mg several times per week. Mistletoe preparations, produced according to anthroposophical methods, are given in incrementally increasing dosages depending on the patient's general condition and response to the injection. Use in pediatric patients has been reported. The pharmacokinetics in healthy adults has been determined.

Contraindications

Data are limited. Use of mistletoe extracts in patients with primary or secondary brain tumors, leukemia, or malignant lymphoma is contraindicated.

Pregnancy/Lactation

Mistletoe contains toxic constituents. Avoid use during pregnancy or lactation.

Interactions

None well documented.

Adverse Reactions

Local reactions following injection include redness, itching, inflammation, and induration at the injection site. Systemic reactions include mild fever or flu-like symptoms. Anaphylaxis has been reported.

Toxicology

Poison centers report toxicity of the whole plant, but especially mistletoe berries. The use of preparations standardized to small doses of ML-I or depleted of lectins may reduce toxicity.

Local Anesthetic/Vasoconstrictor Precautions

No information available to require special precautions

Effects on Bleeding None reported

Muira Puama

Clinical Overview

Uses

P. olacoides has been evaluated both alone and as part of a combination product for use in sexual dysfunction; clinical evidence is lacking to support use of P. olacoides alone. Potential use in Alzheimer disease or conditions of cognitive decline has been examined, with studies of P. olacoides in rodents demonstrating improved memory and reversal of cognitive impairment. However, clinical trial data are lacking to recommend use for any indication.

Dosing

There are no quality clinical trials to provide dosing guidance.

Contraindications

Contraindications have not been identified.

Pregnancy/Lactation

Avoid use. Information regarding safety and efficacy in pregnancy and lactation is lacking.

Interactions

None well documented.

Adverse Reactions

Information regarding adverse reactions to muira puama is lacking. Mild adverse reactions (often reported with a combination product) might include stomach bloating, discomfort, dyspepsia, nausea, burping, migraine, headache, nervousness, and agitation.

Toxicology

Robust clinical studies are lacking. In a toxicity study in healthy volunteers taking a 25 mL dose of the combination preparation Catuama (containing 0.875 mL of P. olacoides) twice daily for 28 days, no severe adverse reactions or hematological and biochemical changes were reported. In a pilot study, Revactin (each capsule containing 125 mg of muira puama, as well as other active pharmaceutical ingredients) was taken at a dosage of 2 capsules twice a day for 3 months; a total daily muira puama dose of 500 mg did not result in any severe adverse reactions.

Local Anesthetic/Vasoconstrictor Precautions

No information available to require special precautions

Effects on Bleeding None reported

Mullein

Clinical Overview

Uses

Mullein has traditionally been used to treat various ailments, including cold and cough. Animal and/or in vitro data suggest anti-inflammatory, antimicrobial/anthelmintic, and antioxidant activities of various Verbascum species. Reliable clinical data describing the therapeutic effects (eg, decreased platelet aggregation) of verbascoside, a major active component of mullein, are limited and controversial. Clinical trial data are lacking to recommend use for any indication.

Dosing

Clinical data are lacking to provide dosing recommendations for mullein.

Contraindications

Contraindications have not been identified.

Pregnancy/Lactation

Avoid use. Information regarding safety and efficacy in pregnancy and lactation is lacking.

Interactions

None well documented.

Adverse Reactions

Information is limited. Occupational airborne dermatitis and contact dermatitis have been reported.

Toxicology

No data.

Local Anesthetic/Vasoconstrictor Precautions
No information available to require special precautions

Effects on Bleeding None reported

Nettles

Clinical Overview

Uses

Nettles are primarily used in the management of benign prostatic hyperplasia (BPH), diabetes, and arthritis. However, clinical trials are limited.

Dosing

Clinical trials for BPH have used aqueous extracts of U. dioica root in dosages of 360 mg daily over 6 months and methanol root extract in dosages of 600 to 1,200 mg daily for 6 to 9 weeks. Dosages of 600 mg of freeze-dried nettle leaf have been used in a clinical trial for allergic rhinitis. Standardization of commercial preparations is lacking.

Contraindications

Due to the effects on androgen and estrogen metabolism, nettle preparations are contraindicated in pregnancy and lactation and should not be used in children younger than 12 years.

Pregnancy/Lactation

Avoid use. Adverse effects have been documented.

Interactions

None well documented.

Adverse Reactions

Nettles are primarily known for their ability to induce acute urticaria following contact with exposed skin. Radix urticae extracts and other nettle preparations are generally well tolerated; minor and transient gastric effects, including diarrhea, gastric pain, and nausea, have been reported.

Toxicology

The possibility of oral toxicity with nettle preparations is considered low. Mutagenicity and carcinogenicity studies using the aqueous extract have been negative.

Local Anesthetic/Vasoconstrictor Precautions
No information available to require special precautions

Effects on Bleeding None reported

Nutmeg

Clinical Overview

Uses

Nutmeg and mace, widely accepted as flavoring agents, have been used in higher doses for their aphrodisiac and psychoactive properties.

Dosing

There are no clinical trials to support therapeutic dosing. Consumption of nutmeg at 1 to 2 mg/kg body weight was reported to induce CNS effects. Toxic overdose occurred at a 5 g dose.

Contraindications

Contraindications have not been identified. The excessive use of nutmeg or mace is not recommended in people with psychiatric conditions.

Pregnancy/Lactation

Generally recognized as safe when used in food as a flavoring agent. Safety for doses above those found in foods is unproven; avoid because of possible abortifacient effects.

Interactions

None well documented.

Adverse Reactions

Allergy, contact dermatitis, and asthma have been reported.

Toxicology

CNS excitation with anxiety/fear, cutaneous flushing, decreased salivation, GI symptoms, and tachycardia. Acute psychosis and anticholinergic-like episodes have been documented; death has rarely been reported following the ingestion of large doses of nutmeg.

Local Anesthetic/Vasoconstrictor Precautions
No information available to require special precautions

Effects on Bleeding None reported

Octacosanol

Clinical Overview

Uses

Octacosanol, which has been studied mainly as a constituent of policosanol, may have a role to play in the management of dyslipidemia and may achieve antiplatelet effects similar to those of aspirin. Although octacosanol has been protective in rats with induced parkinsonism, clinical studies in humans have not documented these effects. Clinical trials are lacking to support claims of enhanced athletic performance due to supplemental octacosanol.

Dosing

Limited clinical trials have been conducted with octacosanol. In one pharmacokinetic study, octacosanol 30 mg daily for 4 weeks did not result in measurable serum concentration changes, whereas octacosanol 50 mg was detected in the serum within 8 hours.

Contraindications

Contraindications have not been identified.

Pregnancy/Lactation

Information regarding safety and efficacy in pregnancy and lactation is lacking.

Interactions

None well documented.

Adverse Reactions

Limited clinical trials have been conducted with octacosanol; however, one surveillance study found long-term tolerability with policosanol supplementation.

Toxicology
No data.

Local Anesthetic/Vasoconstrictor Precautions
No information available to require special precautions

Effects on Bleeding None reported

Oleander

Clinical Overview

Uses
Oleander has traditionally been used in the treatment of cardiac illness, asthma, diabetes mellitus, corns, scabies, cancer, and epilepsy, and in wound healing as an antibacterial/antimicrobial. However, limited quality clinical trials are available to support these uses.

Dosing
There is no clinical evidence to support specific doses of oleander. Extreme caution should be used because of its acute cardiotoxicity, hepatotoxicity, and nephrotoxicity.

Contraindications
Oleander is no longer considered safe due to extreme toxicity.

Pregnancy/Lactation
Avoid use. Information regarding safety and efficacy in pregnancy and lactation is lacking.

Interactions
None well documented.

Adverse Reactions
Phytodermatitis caused by contact with oleander has been reported frequently. Oleander ingestion can lead to headache, nausea, vomiting, bradycardia, lethargy, and hyperkalemia. Most symptoms appear 4 hours postingestion.

Toxicology
Oleander is extremely toxic and potentially fatal. Major toxicity reports include disturbances in heart rhythm and death. Signs of toxicity include severe nausea, emesis, abdominal pain, cramping, diarrhea, hyperkalemia, hypertension, lethargy, hepatotoxicity, and nephrotoxicity. Oleander intoxication can negatively impact the lungs, kidneys, spleen, and muscle tissue. Intoxication can occur from ingestion, or from inhalation of smoke from burned plants.

Local Anesthetic/Vasoconstrictor Precautions
No information available to require special precautions

Effects on Bleeding None reported

Olive Leaf

Clinical Overview

Uses
Interest in olive leaf use centers on antioxidant and antiviral activity, as well as its possible role in diabetes and cardiovascular conditions. However, clinical trials do not support its use for any indication.

Dosing
Traditional dosages of olive leaf include 7 to 8 g of dry leaf in 150 mL water. In 1 clinical trial, patients with stage 1 hypertension were administered 500 mg of olive leaf extract twice daily for 8 weeks. A clinical trial in overweight men used oleuropein 51.1 mg and hydroxytyrosol 9.7 mg daily for 12 weeks.

Contraindications
Contraindications have not been identified. Caution may be warranted in hepatic disease.

Pregnancy/Lactation
Information regarding safety and efficacy during pregnancy and lactation is lacking.

Interactions
None well documented.

Adverse Reactions
None well documented. Diabetic patients should be supervised carefully because of potential hypoglycemic effects.

Toxicology
Information is limited.

Local Anesthetic/Vasoconstrictor Precautions
No information available to require special precautions

Effects on Bleeding None reported

Onion

Clinical Overview

Uses
Onion has potential in treating cardiovascular disease (eg, atherosclerosis), osteoporosis, and certain cancers; however, few quality clinical trials are available to support these uses. Topical preparations have been evaluated for the prevention of surgical scarring with varying results.

Dosing
Onion-based quercetin 100 to 500 mg per day has been used in limited clinical studies. Average daily doses of 50 g of fresh onion, or 20 g of dried onion have been suggested. Topical onion extract gels have been used in studies evaluating effects on scarring and are generally applied 3 times daily.

Contraindications
Contraindications have not been identified.

Pregnancy/Lactation
Onion has "generally recognized as safe" (GRAS) status when used as food. Avoid amounts greater than those found in foods because safety has not been established.

Interactions
None well documented.

Adverse Reactions
Few reported.

Toxicology
No data.

Local Anesthetic/Vasoconstrictor Precautions
No information available to require special precautions

Effects on Bleeding None reported

Pantothenic Acid

Clinical Overview

Uses
Clinical studies are limited. Pantothenic acid and its derivatives may have a role in the management of dyslipidemia and in wound healing.

Dosing
The US recommended dietary allowance (RDA) for pantothenic acid in nutritional supplements and foods is age dependent and ranges from 0.2 mg/kg in infants to 5 mg in adults. The RDA during pregnancy and lactation is slightly higher, at 6 and 7 mg daily, respectively.

Clinical studies have used pantethine 600 to 1200 mg/day for dyslipidemia.

Contraindications
Avoid use if hypersensitivity to pantothenic acid exists.

Pregnancy/Lactation

Pantothenic acid has been assigned US Food and Drug Administration (FDA) Pregnancy Category A (studies have failed to demonstrate risk). When dosed above the recommended dietary allowance (6 to 7 mg/day), pantothenic acid is designated Category C.

Interactions

None well documented. Caution may be warranted with concomitant use of biotin.

Adverse Reactions

In high doses, pantothenic acid may inhibit the absorption of biotin produced by the microflora in the large intestine. Diarrhea may occur with large doses of pantothenic acid. Allergic contact dermatitis has been reported with topical use of dexpanthenol.

Toxicology

A tolerable upper intake level for pantothenic acid has not been set because reports of adverse effects are lacking. An oral median lethal dose of 10 g/kg for mice has been reported.

Local Anesthetic/Vasoconstrictor Precautions
No information available to require special precautions

Effects on Bleeding None reported

Papaya

Clinical Overview

Uses

Traditional uses of papaya in some developing countries are being investigated; papaya may provide an alternative to standard treatments for a variety of ailments. C. papaya has a wide range of purported medicinal properties, including antiseptic, antimicrobial, antiparasitic, anti-inflammatory, antihypertensive, diuretic, antihyperlipidemic, antidiabetic, and contraceptive activity. While there are limited data to support most of these uses, there is some clinical evidence for use in treating decubitus ulcers, wounds, and intestinal worms. There is increasing interest in investigating fermented papaya preparations (FPPs) as a nutraceutical.

Dosing

Various topical applications of papaya have been used for wound healing, particularly in developing countries. There are very little data available to make specific recommendations regarding systemic doses of papaya.

One study used 20 mL of an elixir containing air-dried papaya seeds in honey (prepared by mixing 500 g of air-dried, machine-blended seeds with honey, for a total preparation volume of 1,000 mL [ie, 0.2 g of dried C. papaya seeds per milliliter]) to treat helminthiasis in children.

In clinical studies, FPPs have been used at 6 to 9 g per day in divided doses to evaluate effects in patients with diabetes or hypothyroidism.

A commercial papaya preparation (Caricol; 20 mL) has been used for 40 days in a trial evaluating effects in GI disorders.

In the United States, the papaya fruit has "generally recognized as safe" (GRAS) status when used as a food.

Contraindications

Papaya is contraindicated in patients with known hypersensitivity to any of its components (eg, papain). Papaya may induce severe allergic responses in sensitive people. Papaya may cause severe allergic reactions and is therefore contraindicated in sensitive people.

Pregnancy/Lactation

Avoid use. Papaya may be unsafe depending on the part of the plant being used and dose administered.

Interactions

None documented.

Adverse Reactions

Papaya may cause severe allergic reactions in sensitive people. Topically, papaya latex can be a severe irritant and vesicant. Papaya juice and papaya seeds are unlikely to cause adverse effects when taken orally; however, papaya leaves at high doses may cause gastric irritation.

Toxicology

No data.

Local Anesthetic/Vasoconstrictor Precautions
No information available to require special precautions

Effects on Bleeding None reported

Parsley

Clinical Overview

Uses

Parsley, in addition to being a source of certain vitamins and minerals, has been used in the treatment of prostate, liver and spleen diseases, as well as anemia, arthritis, and microbial infections. It has also been found useful as a diuretic and laxative. However, there have been no clinical trials to confirm these uses.

Dosing

Parsley has been used at daily doses of 6 g, however, no clinical studies have been found that support this dose. The essential oil should not be used because of toxicity.

Contraindications

Contraindications have not yet been identified.

Pregnancy/Lactation

Generally recognized as safe or used as food. Safety and efficacy for dosages above those in foods are unproven and should be avoided. Emmenagogue and abortifacient effects in higher doses.

Interactions

None well documented.

Adverse Reactions

Adverse effects from the ingestion of parsley oil include headache, giddiness, loss of balance, convulsions, and renal damage.

Toxicology

While no major toxicities have been reported with the use of parsley, pregnant women should not take parsley because of possible uterotonic effects.

Local Anesthetic/Vasoconstrictor Precautions
No information available to require special precautions

Effects on Bleeding None reported

Passion Flower

Clinical Overview

Uses

Passion flower has been used to treat sleep disorders and historically in homeopathic medicine to treat pain, insomnia related to neurasthenia or hysteria, and nervous exhaustion.

Dosing

No clinical trials of passion flower as a single agent have been reported; however, a daily dose of 4 to 8 g is typical.

Contraindications

Contraindications have not yet been identified.

Pregnancy/Lactation

Documented adverse effects. Avoid use. Passion flower is a known uterine stimulant.

Interactions

None well documented.

Adverse Reactions

Though no adverse effects of passion flower have been reported, large doses may result in CNS depression.

Toxicology

No major clinical trials have been conducted to assess the plant's toxicity.

Local Anesthetic/Vasoconstrictor Precautions

No information available to require special precautions

Effects on Bleeding None reported

Pectin

Clinical Overview

Uses

Pectin has been used in antidiarrheal products and to lower blood lipoprotein levels. Pectin also has been investigated for its effects on cancer, diabetes, and gastroesophageal reflux disease/gastric ulceration. However, quality clinical trials are lacking.

Dosing

Pectin and/or modified pectin have been used in clinical studies in doses of 10 to 20 g daily.

Contraindications

Contraindications have not yet been identified.

Pregnancy/Lactation

Information regarding safety and efficacy in pregnancy and lactation is lacking.

Interactions

Coadministration of pectin with beta-carotene–containing foods or supplements can reduce blood levels of beta-carotene by more than 50%.

Adverse Reactions

Pectin is generally well tolerated when ingested. Occupational asthma has been associated with the inhalation of pectin dust. A cross-sensitivity to cashew and pistachio nuts may exist.

Toxicology

No major toxicities have been reported with the use of pectin.

Local Anesthetic/Vasoconstrictor Precautions

No information available to require special precautions

Effects on Bleeding None reported

Peppermint

Clinical Overview

Uses

Peppermint, peppermint oil, and its menthol extract have been evaluated for use in GI conditions, including nonserious constipation or diarrhea associated with irritable bowel syndrome (IBS) to reduce global symptoms of pain, and bloating; antispasmodic properties of the oil and menthol extract has led to use in endoscopic GI procedures. Quality clinical trials are lacking to recommend use for treatment of dyspepsia. Menthol, a component of peppermint oil, is often added to respiratory products to provide subjective decongestant action and is used as a vasodilatory agent to aid in penetration of topically applied anesthetic drugs. Limited or equivocal data are available for other uses.

Dosing

Up to 1,200 mg daily (180 to 400 mg 3 times daily) of peppermint oil in enteric-coated capsules has been used to treat nonserious constipation and diarrhea associated with IBS.

Contraindications

Peppermint oil should not be administered to patients with gastroesophageal reflux or active gastric ulcers because the oil decreases esophageal sphincter pressure. Peppermint oil should not be applied to the face, especially under the nose of a child or infant. Enteric-coated preparations are not recommended for use in children younger than 8 years.

Pregnancy/Lactation

Adverse reactions, particularly with higher doses, have been documented with use of peppermint. Avoid internal use because of emmenagogue effects.

Interactions

Peppermint oil may inhibit cytochrome P450 (CYP-450) 3A4; use caution when administering with drugs metabolized by this enzyme.

Adverse Reactions

Peppermint oil may cause allergic reactions characterized by contact dermatitis, cutaneous burning, flushing, lacrimation, and headache, and may worsen the symptoms of heartburn, hiatus hernias, and stomach ulcers. Cutaneous and mucosal burns and skin necrosis have been reported with topical formulations.

Toxicology

Peppermint has generally recognized as safe (GRAS) status in amounts used in seasoning or flavoring, but medicinal use of the plant can cause adverse reactions. (See Adverse Reactions.)

Local Anesthetic/Vasoconstrictor Precautions

No information available to require special precautions

Effects on Bleeding None reported

Periwinkle

Clinical Overview

Uses

Periwinkle alkaloids have been used to treat certain cancers; however, use of the plant for this purpose is not recommended without consulting a health care provider.

Periwinkle has been studied for potential antimicrobial and antiprotozoal applications, as well as for use in diabetes and wound healing; however, there is not enough reliable information to recommend the plant for these uses.

Dosing

There is no recent clinical evidence to support specific doses of periwinkle for medicinal use. Traditional doses have included 10 leaves and 10 flowers boiled in water as a tea, or 9 pink flowers in 0.5 L of water for 3 hours ("solar tea") sipped throughout the day. Therapeutic doses for preparations of the pure alkaloids vincristine and vinblastine are available.

Contraindications

Contraindications have not been identified.

Pregnancy/Lactation

Avoid use. Abortifacient effects have been documented.

Interactions

None well documented.

Adverse Reactions

Clinical information is lacking.

Toxicology

Severe, systemic adverse events are associated with the use of the alkaloids vincristine and vinblastine.

Local Anesthetic/Vasoconstrictor Precautions

No information available to require special precautions

Effects on Bleeding None reported

Peru Balsam

Clinical Overview

Uses

Peru balsam has been used in the treatment of dry socket in dentistry, topically as a treatment for wounds and ulcers, and in suppositories for hemorrhoids. However, there are only older, small case studies to support this use. The material is not used internally.

Dosing

Peru balsam has been used topically in 5% to 20% formulations for wounds and burns. Case reports and small clinical studies report the efficacy of balsam combined with other ingredients in the management of certain wounds; however, there are no recent, well-controlled clinical studies to support appropriate dosing.

Contraindications

Contraindications have not been identified.

Pregnancy/Lactation

Information regarding safety and efficacy in pregnancy and lactation is lacking. Systemic toxicity following application of Peru balsam to the nipples of breast-feeding mothers has been reported.

Interactions

None well documented.

Adverse Reactions

Peru balsam is an allergen.

Toxicology

Information is lacking.

Local Anesthetic/Vasoconstrictor Precautions

No information available to require special precautions

Effects on Bleeding None reported

Pineapple

Clinical Overview

Uses

Few well-controlled clinical trials have been published to support the wide range of therapeutic claims for bromelain, a crude, aqueous extract of pineapple. Evidence exists primarily for the use of bromelain in debridement of burns and as an anti-inflammatory agent.

Dosing

Two slices of pineapple contain approximately 100 mg of ascorbic acid (vitamin C). The usual dosage of bromelain is 40 mg taken 3 or 4 times daily. Pineapple products are available commercially in liquid, tablet, and capsule doseforms. Most products contain bromelain 500 mg; manufacturers suggest a dose of 500 to 1,000 mg daily.

Contraindications

Hypersensitivity to any of the components in pineapple. Cross-reaction with honeybee venom, olive tree pollen, celery, cypress pollen, bromelain, and papain have been reported.

Pregnancy/Lactation

Information regarding safety and efficacy in pregnancy and lactation is lacking. Data is lacking to support the historical use of pineapple as an emmenagogue and abortifacient.

Interactions

Potentiation of amoxicillin and tetracycline because of increased volume of distribution by bromelain has been documented.

Adverse Reactions

The juice from unripe pineapples can act as a violent purgative. Bromelain ingestion is associated with a low incidence of adverse reactions, including diarrhea, menorrhagia, nausea, skin rash, and vomiting. Angular stomatitis/cheilitis can result from eating large amounts of the fruit.

Toxicology

Bromelain has very low toxicity.

Local Anesthetic/Vasoconstrictor Precautions

No information available to require special precautions

Effects on Bleeding May cause increased bleeding due to inhibition of platelet aggregation

Plantain

Clinical Overview

Uses

The psyllium in plantain has been used as GI therapy, to treat hyperlipidemia for anticancer effects, respiratory treatment, and other uses.

Dosing

Plantain leaves have been given as a tea for cold and cough at 3 to 6 g/day.

Contraindications

Contraindications have not yet been identified.

Pregnancy/Lactation

Documented adverse effects. Avoid use. Uterine activity, laxative.

Interactions

Patients taking lithium or carbamazepine should avoid coadministration of plantain. Caution patients receiving lithium or carbamazepine to consult their health care provider before using herbal products.

Adverse Reactions

Adverse events include anaphylaxis, chest congestion, sneezing and watery eyes, occupational asthma, and a situation involving the occurrence of a giant phytobezoar composed of psyllium seed husks.

Toxicology

The pollen contains allergenic glycoproteins that react with concanavalin A, as well as components that bind IgE. IgE antibodies have been demonstrated. The IgE-mediated sensitization has contributes to seasonal allergy.

Local Anesthetic/Vasoconstrictor Precautions

No information available to require special precautions

Effects on Bleeding None reported

Poinsettia

Clinical Overview

Uses

Poinsettias are used primarily as Christmas ornamentation but have been used traditionally to treat skin conditions, warts, and toothaches; however, clinical studies are lacking to support these uses.

Dosing

No recent clinical evidence exists to support specific dosing of poinsettia in a therapeutic context.

Contraindications

Contraindications have not been identified.

Pregnancy/Lactation

Avoid use. Information regarding safety and efficacy in pregnancy and lactation is lacking.

Interactions
None well documented.

Adverse Reactions
Allergy and contact dermatitis have been reported. Minor GI irritation following ingestion is possible requiring only supportive therapy.

Toxicology
Although many published reports have warned of the plant's toxicity, there is little clinical evidence to support this claim.

Local Anesthetic/Vasoconstrictor Precautions No information available to require special precautions

Effects on Bleeding None reported

Pokeweed

Clinical Overview

Uses
Young pokeweed leaves and berries may be eaten as food, but only after being cooked properly by boiling in several changes of water.

Dosing
At doses of 1 g, dried pokeweed root is emetic and purgative. At lower doses of 60 to 100 mg/day, the root and berries have been used to treat rheumatism and for immune stimulation; however, there are no clinical trials that support these uses or doses.

Contraindications
Contraindications have not yet been identified.

Pregnancy/Lactation
Documented adverse effects. Avoid use. Uterine stimulant with toxic constituents; is reputed to affect menstrual cycle.

Interactions
None well documented.

Adverse Reactions
GI distress, possibly leading to severe toxicities (see Toxicology).

Toxicology
Ingestion of poisonous parts of the plant may cause severe stomach cramping, nausea with persistent diarrhea and vomiting, slow and difficult breathing, weakness, spasms, hypotension, severe convulsions, and death.

Local Anesthetic/Vasoconstrictor Precautions No information available to require special precautions

Effects on Bleeding None reported

Policosanol

Clinical Overview

Uses
Cholesterol-lowering effects previously attributed to policosanol have not been validated by more recent trials. Policosanol has been studied in platelet aggregation and intermittent claudication, but data are insufficient to support this use.

Dosing
Policosanol is typically initiated at 5 mg/day and titrated up to 20 mg/day for hypercholesterolemia.

Contraindications
Contraindications have not been identified.

Pregnancy/Lactation
Information regarding safety and efficacy in pregnancy and lactation is lacking. Studies in rats and mice demonstrated no adverse effects on fertility, reproduction, teratogenesis, or development at doses equivalent to 1,500 times the normal human dose of 20 mg/kg/day.

Interactions
Because of policosanol's possible effects on platelet aggregation, caution is warranted if policosanol is used concurrently with anticoagulants (eg, warfarin) or antiplatelet agents (eg, aspirin, clopidogrel, prasugrel). In a study in healthy men, policosanol did not affect the pharmacokinetics of warfarin.

Adverse Reactions
Animal and human studies have demonstrated few adverse reactions from policosanol.

Toxicology
Limited animal and human studies have found policosanol to be safe.

Local Anesthetic/Vasoconstrictor Precautions No information available to require special precautions

Effects on Bleeding May see increased bleeding due to inhibition of platelet aggregation

Prickly Pear

Clinical Overview

Uses
Prickly pear is widely cultivated and commercially used in juices, jellies, candies, teas, and alcoholic drinks. American Indians used prickly pear juice to treat burns, and prickly pear has a long history in traditional Mexican folk medicine for treating diabetes. Its use in treating diabetes, lipid disorders, inflammation, and ulcers, as well as its other pharmacologic effects, have been documented. However, there is limited clinical information to support these uses.

Dosing
Prickly pear is commercially available in numerous doseforms, including capsules, tablets, powders, and juices, and as food. Follow manufacturers' suggested guidelines if using commercial products. Typical dosage regimens are two 250 mg capsules by mouth 3 times a day or every 8 hours.

Contraindications
Hypersensitivity to any components of prickly pear.

Pregnancy/Lactation
Avoid use during pregnancy and lactation because of the lack of clinical studies.

Interactions
None well documented.

Adverse Reactions
Dermatitis is the most common adverse reaction to prickly pear.

Toxicology
Little information is available.

Local Anesthetic/Vasoconstrictor Precautions No information available to require special precautions

Effects on Bleeding None reported

Pygeum

Clinical Overview

Uses
Pygeum has been used to improve symptoms of benign prostatic hyperplasia (BPH) and to improve sexual function. However, only studies comparing pygeum to placebo are available.

Dosing
Benign prostatic hyperplasia: 25 to 200 mg/day of P. africana extract standardized to 14% total sterols. The usual dosage is 100 mg/day in 6- to 8-week cycles.

Contraindications
Contraindications have not been identified.

Pregnancy/Lactation

Avoid use. Information regarding safety and efficacy in pregnancy and lactation is lacking.

Interactions

None well documented.

Adverse Reactions

GI irritation and headache have been reported.

Toxicology

A low incidence of toxicity has been demonstrated.

Local Anesthetic/Vasoconstrictor Precautions

No information available to require special precautions

Effects on Bleeding None reported

Quassia

Clinical Overview

Uses

Quassia has a variety of uses, including treatment for measles, diarrhea, fever, and lice. Quassia has antibacterial, antifungal, antifertility, antitumor, antileukemic, and insecticidal actions as well. However, efficacy in clinical trials has not been proven.

Dosing

Quassia wood has been used as a bitter tonic, with a typical oral dose of 500 mg. No studies have been performed to support this dose. Several recent studies of topical quassia tincture for head lice have been reported.

Contraindications

Contraindications have not yet been identified.

Pregnancy/Lactation

Documented adverse reactions. Avoid use.

Interactions

None well documented.

Adverse Reactions

Quassia is used in a number of food products and is considered safe by the FDA. If taken in large doses, this product can irritate the GI tract and cause vomiting. It is not recommended for pregnant women.

Toxicology

Quassia is listed as generally regarded as safe (GRAS) by the FDA. Parenteral administration of quassin is toxic, leading to cardiac irregularities, tremors, and paralysis.

Local Anesthetic/Vasoconstrictor Precautions

No information available to require special precautions

Effects on Bleeding None reported

Queen's Delight

Clinical Overview

Uses

With the exception of prostratin, the other Stillingia factors are likely to be tumor promoters and to possess the typical pleiotropic effects possessed by most other phorbol esters.

Dosing

There is no clinical evidence to support specific dosage recommendations for queen's delight. Classical use of queen's delight called for 2 g of the root, however the documented presence of irritant and tumor-promoting phorbol esters in this plant contraindicates therapeutic use.

Contraindications

No longer considered safe.

Pregnancy/Lactation

Documented adverse effects. Not to be used while nursing. Avoid use.

Interactions

None well documented.

Adverse Reactions

Do not ingest or use topically in human medicine. Observe particular caution with the fresh root, which appears to be more toxic than the dried product. Stillingia root is a purgative and irritant product that should be avoided because of a high likelihood of tumor promotion and documented severe irritancy to skin.

Toxicology

There are reports of sheep poisoned by Stillingia in Florida. Because of the reported phorbol esters, this plant should not be ingested or used topically in human medicine. Observe particular caution with the fresh root, which appears to be more toxic than the dried product.

Local Anesthetic/Vasoconstrictor Precautions

No information available to require special precautions

Effects on Bleeding None reported

Raspberry

Clinical Overview

Uses

There is little pharmacologic evidence to support the use of raspberry leaf in pregnancy, menstruation, or during childbirth. Raspberry fruit and leaf extracts have shown activity on cancer cell lines, possibly due to an antioxidant effect; however, no clinical trials exist.

Dosing

Traditional dosages include 5-10 mg (1-2 tsp) crushed leaf per 240 mL of water up to 6 times per day, or up to 12 g dry leaf. Substantiated clinical applications for dosage recommendations are lacking.

Contraindications

Contraindications have not yet been identified.

Pregnancy/Lactation

Avoid use during pregnancy; adverse effects have been documented. Information regarding safety during lactation is lacking.

Use of raspberry leaf preparations has been promoted by nurse-midwives for strengthening the uterus and shortening the duration of labor. However, there are too few studies upon which to substantiate either the efficacy or the safety of this practice.

Interactions

None well documented.

Adverse Reactions

Information regarding adverse reactions with the use of raspberry fruit is limited. No adverse events were reported in a clinical study evaluating the effect of raspberry tea during pregnancy.

Toxicology

Information is generally lacking for raspberry leaf; raspberry fruit is considered nontoxic.

Local Anesthetic/Vasoconstrictor Precautions

No information available to require special precautions

Effects on Bleeding None reported

Red Clover

Clinical Overview

Uses

Red clover flowers have been used traditionally as a sedative, to purify the blood, and to treat respiratory conditions; topical preparations have been used for psoriasis, eczema, and rashes, and to accelerate wound healing. However, there is no clinical evidence to support any of these uses or for use in menopause-related conditions. Safety of use in treating breast cancer has not been determined, and the epidemiological association of isoflavone consumption in protecting against prostate cancer has not yet been confirmed by clinical trials.

Dosing

Red clover blossoms for sedation were formerly used at doses of 4 g, but is now used primarily as a source of isoflavones. The usual dose is 40 to 80 mg/day of standardized isoflavones, typically containing biochanin A, formononetin, genistein, and daidzein. Several commercial preparations are available.

Contraindications

Red clover is contraindicated in patients with hormonal disorders, estrogen-dependent breast cancer (or risk of), and during pregnancy or lactation. Red clover supplementation is not advised in children younger than 12 years.

Pregnancy/Lactation

Avoid use; red clover has estrogenic activity.

Interactions

Isoflavonoids may interfere with hormonal agents; avoid use with oral contraceptives, estrogen, or progesterone therapies. Case reports are lacking; however, caution is warranted with concomitant use of tamoxifen or letrozole.

Adverse Reactions

Few adverse reactions have been reported in doses used in clinical trials. High doses of isoflavones have been associated with loss of appetite, pedal edema, and abdominal tenderness.

Toxicology

The phytoestrogens in red clover may be expected to act through estrogenic mechanisms, with the associated risk of estrogen-like adverse effects, including increased incidence of endometrial, ovarian, and breast cancers.

Local Anesthetic/Vasoconstrictor Precautions

No information available to require special precautions

Effects on Bleeding Red clover contains coumarins; it may enhance the anticoagulant effects of warfarin when taken simultaneously. This effect has not been confirmed.

Red Yeast Rice

Clinical Overview

Uses

M. purpureus is a natural source of mevinolin, the active ingredient of the drug lovastatin, therefore, having beneficial effects in the treatment of hyperlipidemia. However, red yeast rice should not be used in place of lovastatin and regular medical care because no studies directly compare its use with a statin. Evidence also exists for its antibacterial and anticancer effects, as well as its activity on glycemic metabolism.

Dosing

Red yeast rice is available commercially, primarily as a 600 mg capsule. Most manufacturers suggest an oral dosage of 2 capsules twice a day for a total dose of 2,400 mg/day. Commercial over-the-counter products often contain coenzyme Q_{10} to supplement low levels of this enzyme in patients with statin myopathy. Clinical trials have used dosages of 2,400 mg/day.

Contraindications

Hypersensitivity to any components of red yeast rice. Anaphylactic reactions in certain populations are documented. Because red yeast rice depletes tissue of coenzyme Q_{10}, which may increase the risk of statin-induced myopathy, patients with muscle damage caused by statins should avoid its use.

Pregnancy/Lactation

Avoid use during pregnancy and lactation. The major ingredient in red yeast rice is monacolin K, which is also known as mevinolin or lovastatin and has statin-like activity. Statins are potential teratogens based on theoretical considerations and in small case studies. CNS and limb defects have been reported in newborns exposed to statins in utero.

Interactions

There are many possible drug interactions associated with red yeast rice. Consult a health care provider before using any dietary supplement.

Adverse Reactions

Meta-analysis of the efficacy of 3 red yeast rice preparations (Cholestin, Xuezhikang, and Zhibituo) from 93 randomized trials (9,625 patients) documented no serious adverse reactions. The most common adverse reactions included dizziness, decreased appetite, nausea, stomachache, abdominal distension, and diarrhea. A small number of patients experienced increased serum blood urea nitrogen (BUN) and ALT levels.

Toxicology

The nephrotoxic mycotoxin citrinin has been isolated from some strains of M. purpureus and Monascus ruber. No severe toxicities at high doses have been reported. Not recommended for use in patients with liver or kidney disease.

Local Anesthetic/Vasoconstrictor Precautions

No information available to require special precautions

Effects on Bleeding None reported

Reishi Mushroom

Clinical Overview

Uses

The polysaccharide content of reishi mushroom is responsible for possible anticancer and immunostimulatory effects. Reishi may also provide hepatoprotective action, antiviral activity, and beneficial effect on the cardiovascular system, rheumatoid arthritis, chronic fatigue syndrome, and diabetes. Few clinical trials have been conducted.

Dosing

The Pharmacopoeia of the People's Republic of China recommends 6 to 12 g reishi extract daily. Ganopoly (a Ganoderma lucidum polysaccharide extract) in doses up to 5.4 g daily (equivalent to 81 g of the fruiting body) for 12 weeks has been used in a few clinical trials.

Contraindications

Contraindications have not been identified.

Pregnancy/Lactation

Information regarding safety and efficacy in pregnancy and lactation is lacking.

Interactions

None well documented.

Adverse Reactions

Adverse reactions are mild and may include dizziness, GI upset, and skin irritation.

Toxicology

There are few reports of toxicity with the use of reishi mushroom.

Local Anesthetic/Vasoconstrictor Precautions No information available to require special precautions

Effects on Bleeding Reishi mushroom may have an antiplatelet effect. Clinical significance of this property is unknown.

Rhubarb

Clinical Overview

Uses

Rhubarb is extensively used in traditional Chinese medicine. Rhubarb has been studied for the management of GI and renal function disorders, and for the treatment of hyperlipidemia and cancer. However, sound clinical evidence for its use is lacking.

Dosing

Dried rhubarb extract 20 to 50 mg/kg daily has been used in clinical trials.

Contraindications

Contraindications have not been identified.

Pregnancy/Lactation

Avoid dosages higher than those found in food because safety and efficacy are unproven.

Interactions

Interaction with cardiac glycosides (digoxin) and a reduction in the absorption of orally administered drugs have been noted when rhubarb is taken in large quantities.

Adverse Reactions

A few reactions, primarily GI effects, have been reported in clinical trials.

Toxicology

The leaf blades (but not the stalks) of rhubarb contain enough oxalic acid to cause poisoning. Acute renal failure has been associated with long-term anthraquinone use.

Local Anesthetic/Vasoconstrictor Precautions No information available to require special precautions

Effects on Bleeding None reported

Rose Hips

Clinical Overview

Uses

Rose hips provide vitamin C supplements. Rose hips have been used for diuretic actions, to reduce thirst, to alleviate gastric inflammation, and to flavor teas and jams.

Dosing

There is no recent clinical evidence upon which dosage recommandations can be based. Classical use of rose petals was 3 to 6 g daily.

Contraindications

Contraindications have not yet been identified.

Pregnancy/Lactation

Information regarding safety and efficacy in pregnancy and lactation is lacking.

Interactions

None well documented.

Adverse Reactions

There have been no reported side effects except in those exposed to rose hips dust who have developed severe respiratory allergies.

Toxicology

No data.

Local Anesthetic/Vasoconstrictor Precautions No information available to require special precautions

Effects on Bleeding None reported

Rue

Clinical Overview

Uses

Rue extract is potentially useful as a potassium channel blocker. It has been used to treat many neuromuscular problems and to stimulate the onset of menstruation. Because rue has an antispasmodic effect at relatively low doses, it should be taken with caution. However, considering rue's potential for severe adverse effects, clinical trials are limited.

Dosing

There is no recent clinical evidence to support dosing recommendations for rue. Traditional use calls for 0.5 to 1 g of the herb daily or 65 mg of the essential oil. In larger doses, rue is an emmenagogue, an aphrodisiac, and an abortifacient, and should be considered dangerous.

Contraindications

Contraindications have not yet been identified.

Pregnancy/Lactation

Documented adverse effects, including emmenagogue and abortifacient effects. Avoid use.

Interactions

None well documented.

Adverse Reactions

Rue extracts are mutagenic and furocoumarins have been associated with photosensitization. If ingested, rue oil may result in kidney damage and hepatic degeneration. Large doses can cause violent gastric pain, vomiting, and systemic complications, including death. Because of possible abortifacient effects, the plant should never be ingested by women of childbearing potential. Toxic hepatitis due to Ruta has been reported.

Toxicology

Rue should only be taken with extreme caution. A case report describes multiorgan toxicity in a 78-year-old woman ingesting R. graveolens for cardiovascular protection. After 3 days of use, the patient entered the emergency department with bradycardia, acute renal failure with hyperkalemia necessitating hemodialysis, and coagulopathy.

Local Anesthetic/Vasoconstrictor Precautions No information available to require special precautions

Effects on Bleeding None reported

Safflower

Clinical Overview

Uses

Safflower has demonstrated antioxidant and anti-inflammatory activities and has been investigated for use (though often as a control or comparator agent) in cardiovascular conditions, diabetes, obesity, and pruritus. Animal studies also suggest reproductive, hair growth-promoting, and lung and tendon injury-attenuating effects. However, clinical trial data are lacking to recommend use of safflower for any indication.

Dosing

Safflower oil dosages of 6 g/day and 8 g/day (in divided doses) were used in 2 small studies of obese women to evaluate effects on weight and glycemic indices.

Contraindications

Safflower is contraindicated in pregnancy.

Pregnancy/Lactation

Use is contraindicated in pregnancy; abortifacient and emmenagogue effects have been suggested.

Interactions

None well documented.

Adverse Reactions

Allergy to the flowers has been reported. Safflower oil was generally well tolerated when used as a control in clinical trials. A few cases of acute liver disease have been associated with use of safflower oil supplements.

Toxicology

No data.

Local Anesthetic/Vasoconstrictor Precautions

No information available to require special precautions

Effects on Bleeding None reported

Salvia divinorum

Clinical Overview

Uses

Salvia divinorum is a hallucinogen and is illegal in some jurisdictions. Check individual state legislation.

Dosing

200 to 500 mcg of salvinorin A, or several leaves, smoked or absorbed perorally, is sufficient to cause hallucinations.

Contraindications

S. divinorum should not be used in people with any mental disease.

Pregnancy/Lactation

Use during pregnancy or lactation is not recommended.

Interactions

None well documented.

Adverse Reactions

None systematically reported.

Toxicology

No toxicity was observed in a 2-week study in mice.

Local Anesthetic/Vasoconstrictor Precautions

No information available to require special precautions

Effects on Bleeding None reported

SAMe

Clinical Overview

Uses

SAMe has been studied for the treatment of depressive disorders. Although it has been shown to be equivalent to tricyclics, it has not been compared with newer agents. Information regarding its use in osteoarthritis is conflicting and information regarding its use in liver disorders and hepatitis is limited.

Dosing

Depression: 200 to 1,600 mg/day. *Liver disease:* 800 to 1,000 mg/day. *Osteoarthritis:* 1,200 mg/day initially; then maintenance 400 mg/day.

Contraindications

SAMe should not be used in patients with bipolar depression because of reports of increased anxiety and mania.

Pregnancy/Lactation

Trials conducted in pregnant women documented no harmful effects.

Interactions

None well documented.

Adverse Reactions

Available data indicate nausea, diarrhea, constipation, mild insomnia, dizziness, irritability, anxiety, and sweating to be the most commonly reported adverse reactions associated with the use of SAMe. Data from long-term use are lacking.

Toxicology

Toxicological studies concluded that SAMe is safe even at the highest doses.

Local Anesthetic/Vasoconstrictor Precautions

No information available to require special precautions

Effects on Bleeding None reported

Sarsaparilla

Clinical Overview

Uses

Various smilax extracts have demonstrated anti-inflammatory and antimicrobial properties, as well as effects on cardiovascular risk factors and metabolic syndrome; however, evidence is based largely on animal and in vitro studies, and clinical trials are limited. Sarsaparilla has been traditionally used for treating syphilis, leprosy, and psoriasis; however, clinical evidence to support these uses is lacking. Evidence is also lacking for purported ergogenic/adaptogenic effects. Due to limited clinical study data, use of sarsaparilla cannot be recommended for any indication.

Dosing

Clinical trials are lacking to provide guidance on therapeutic dosages.

Contraindications

Contraindications have not been identified.

Pregnancy/Lactation

Avoid use. Information regarding safety and efficacy in pregnancy and lactation is lacking. Estrogenic and antiestrogenic activities have been described for extracts of at least one of the species.

Interactions

None well documented.

Adverse Reactions

Clinical studies are lacking. GI irritation and increased diuresis have been reported. Occupational asthma caused by sarsaparilla root dust has been reported.

Toxicology

No data.

Local Anesthetic/Vasoconstrictor Precautions

No information available to require special precautions

Effects on Bleeding None reported

Sassafras

Clinical Overview

Uses

Animal and in vitro studies have investigated the potential antifungal, anti-inflammatory, and cardiovascular effects of sassafras and its components. However, clinical trials are lacking, and sassafras is not considered safe for use. Safrole, the main constituent of sassafras root bark and oil, has been banned by the US Food and Drug Administration (FDA), including for use as a flavoring or fragrance, and should not be used internally or externally, as it is potentially carcinogenic. Safrole has been used in the illegal production of 3,4-methylene-dioxymethamphetamine (MDMA), also known by the street names "ecstasy" or "Molly," and the sale of safrole and sassafras oil is monitored by the US Drug Enforcement Administration (DEA).

Dosing

Clinical trials are lacking. External or internal use should be avoided; sassafras oil and the main constituent safrole are potentially carcinogenic. Sassafras oil is toxic in doses as low as 5 mL in adults.

Contraindications

Not considered safe for use.

Pregnancy/Lactation

Avoid use. Emmenagogue and abortifacient effects have been documented. Information regarding use during breastfeeding is lacking.

Interactions

None well documented.

Adverse Reactions

Diaphoresis, hot flashes, and dermatitis have been reported.

Toxicology

Sassafras oil and safrole have demonstrated carcinogenic and hepatotoxic potential in animal studies. Symptoms of sassafras oil poisoning in humans include vomiting, stupor, lowering of body temperature, exhaustion, tachycardia, spasms, hallucinations, and paralysis; effects may be fatal.

Local Anesthetic/Vasoconstrictor Precautions
No information available to require special precautions

Effects on Bleeding None reported

Saw Palmetto

Clinical Overview

Uses

Saw palmetto has been used to treat symptoms of benign prostatic hyperplasia (BPH), but evidence from quality clinical trials and a meta-analysis does not support this use. Data suggesting a positive effect on erectile dysfunction are limited, and results from studies evaluating the effect of saw palmetto on outcomes of transurethral resection of the prostate surgery are equivocal. Some effects on in vitro prostate cancer cells have been described; however, clinical trials are lacking.

Dosing

Benign prostatic hyperplasia: 320 mg/day standardized extract.

Contraindications

Contraindications have not been identified. Use in children younger than 12 years is not recommended.

Pregnancy/Lactation

Information regarding safety and efficacy in pregnancy and lactation is lacking. Effects on androgen and estrogen metabolism have been identified, as well as a lack of rationale for its use in pregnancy, and suggest that saw palmetto should not be used.

Interactions

Case reports of interactions are lacking. Caution may be warranted with concomitant coagulation therapy.

Adverse Reactions

Results from clinical trials note that saw palmetto products are generally well tolerated, with occasional reports of adverse GI effects and headache.

Toxicology

Information is limited.

Local Anesthetic/Vasoconstrictor Precautions
No information available to require special precautions

Effects on Bleeding None reported

Schisandra

Clinical Overview

Uses

Schisandra has been used as a tonic and restorative, and as a treatment for respiratory and GI disorders. Schisandra has also demonstrated liver protectant, nervous system stimulant, and adaptogenic effects. However, clinical trials to support these uses are limited.

Dosing

Schisandra fruit is used as an adaptogen at dosages of 1.5 to 6 g/day of powdered product. In a clinical study, schizandra tablets containing 91.1 mg of extract per tablet (extract standardized for schizandrin and gamma-schizandrin at a level of 3.1 mg/tablet) was used to improve athletic performance. Examples of various doses of schizandra preparations used in official medicine in Russia include the following: Tinctura Fructum Schizandrae prepared with air-dried fruits and 95% ethanol given as 20 to 30 drops twice daily. Tinctura Seminum Schizandrae prepared with dried seeds and 95% ethanol, given as 20 to 30 drops twice daily. Infusion Fructum Schizandrae prepared with air-dried fruits and water (1:20 w/v), given as 150 mL twice daily. Fructum Schizandrae contains air-dried fruits, given at a dose of 0.5 to 1.5 g twice daily. Schizandra seed powder 0.5 to 1.5 g administered twice daily before lunch and the evening meal for 20 to 30 days. Schizandra seed extract prepared by extracting air-dried seeds with 95% ethanol, given as a single dose of 0.05 or 0.2 mL/kg.

Contraindications

Contraindications have not been identified.

Pregnancy/Lactation

Information regarding safety and efficacy in pregnancy and lactation is lacking. Various compounds from the stem of Schisandra propinqua were cytotoxic against rat luteal cells and human decidual cells in vitro.

Interactions

Because of its documented effects on hepatic and gastric enzyme activity, particularly cytochrome P450 (CYP-450) 3A, it is possible that schisandra may interfere with the metabolism of coadministered drugs (eg, midazolam). Findings from a study of healthy volunteers suggest that dosage adjustment may be needed in individuals concomitantly taking P-glycoprotein (P-gp) substrates (eg, tacrolimus).

Adverse Reactions

Research reveals little information regarding adverse reactions with use of schisandra.

Toxicology

No data.

Local Anesthetic/Vasoconstrictor Precautions
No information available to require special precautions

Effects on Bleeding None reported

Scullcap

Clinical Overview

Uses

Scullcap traditionally has been used as a sedative for nervousness and anxiety, although there is little to no data to support any of these uses.

Dosing Limit doses of American skullcap to no more than the package recommendation. Typical doses (see individual product information):

Dried herb: 1 to 2 grams 3 times/day.

Tea: 240 mL 3 times/day (Pour 250 mL of boiling water over 5 to 10 mL of the dried herb and steep for 10 to 15 minutes).

Tincture: 2 to 4 mL 3 times/day.

Contraindications

Contraindications have not yet been identified.

Pregnancy/Lactation

Documented adverse effects in pregnancy. Avoid use. May inhibit pituitary and chorionic gonadotropins, as well as prolactin.

Interactions

None well documented, though it may exaggerate the effects of other drugs that cause drowsiness.

Adverse Reactions

If taken according to the manufacturer's directions, scullcap does not seem to exhibit any adverse effects.

Toxicology

An overdose of the tincture causes giddiness, stupor, confusion, twitching of the limbs, intermission of the pulse, and other symptoms similar to epilepsy.

Local Anesthetic/Vasoconstrictor Precautions

No information available to require special precautions

Effects on Bleeding None reported

Sea Buckthorn

Clinical Overview

Uses

Numerous pharmacological effects of sea buckthorn have been documented in the scientific literature, including antimicrobial, antiulcerogenic, antioxidant, anticancer, radioprotective, and antiplatelet activities, as well as liver and cardiovascular protectant effects. It also has beneficial effects on skin and mucosa. Although sea buckthorn has been used in Asian medicine for thousands of years, there are limited quality clinical trials to support any of these uses.

Dosing

Empirical healers have recommended approximately 20 g/day of fruit. In clinical trials, dosages of 5 to 45 g of freeze-dried sea buckthorn berries, puree, and seed or pulp oil have been used; sea buckthorn juice has been administered in volumes up to 300 mL daily over 8 weeks. **Antimicrobial:** 28 g/day for 90 days. **Atopic dermatitis:** 5 g/day of seed or pulp oil for 4 months. **Cardiovascular risk factors:** Oil or air-dried berries (equivalent to approximately 100 g/day fresh berries); or 300 mL of juice over 8 weeks. **Dry eye:** 1 g twice daily for 3 months. **Liver disease:** 15 g 3 times daily of sea buckthorn extract for 6 months. **Platelet aggregation:** 5 g/day of oil for 4 weeks. **Postmenopausal symptoms:** 1.5 g twice daily for 3 months. **Renal disease:** 350 mg of extract twice daily for 12 weeks; or 2 g/day of oil extract for 8 weeks.

Contraindications

None well documented.

Pregnancy/Lactation

Avoid use. Information regarding safety and efficacy during pregnancy and lactation is lacking.

Interactions

None well documented.

Adverse Reactions

Carotenodermia, a nontoxic accumulation of carotenoids in the skin that manifests as a yellow to orange discoloration of the skin, can result from excessive consumption of sea buckthorn.

Toxicology

No data.

Local Anesthetic/Vasoconstrictor Precautions

No information available to require special precautions

Effects on Bleeding Sea buckthorn inhibits platelet aggregation *in vitro*. One clinical report showed an inhibition of platelet aggregation in 12 healthy volunteers with daily ingestion of sea buckthorn berry oil. The clinician should anticipate that ingestion of sea buckthorn may pose some increased risk of bleeding.

Seaweed

Clinical Overview

Uses

Clinical trials are generally lacking to support definitive therapeutic recommendations for seaweeds. However, seaweeds are an important nutritional source of minerals and elements and are low in sodium. Applications may exist for use in cardiovascular conditions due to potential in cholesterol reduction and appetite suppression. Alginates extracted from seaweed have been used in wound dressings.

Dosing

Clinical trials have used an oral dosage range of 4 to 12 g seaweed daily for up to 2 months.

Contraindications

Contraindications have not been identified.

Pregnancy/Lactation

Information regarding safety and efficacy in pregnancy and lactation is lacking.

Interactions

Patients taking warfarin and consuming a large quantity of food containing seaweed may experience a change in international normalized ratio (INR) because of seaweed's high vitamin K content.

Adverse Reactions

Contact dermatitis, goiter, and, occasionally, GI effects may occur.

Toxicology

Excessive intake of dried seaweed may result in increased serum thyroid-stimulating hormone (TSH). There have been case reports of carotenodermia (yellowing of the skin) with excessive seaweed consumption.

Local Anesthetic/Vasoconstrictor Precautions

No information available to require special precautions

Effects on Bleeding May see increased bleeding due to anticoagulant effects.

Shark Derivatives

Clinical Overview

Uses

Shark cartilage has been investigated for use in treating cancer; however, data are mixed and conflicting. Shark cartilage has been used to treat psoriasis and for its anti-inflammatory effects in conditions such as rheumatoid arthritis.

Dosing

General: Commercial doses range from 0.5 to 4.5 g/day, given in 2 to 6 divided doses. Oral shark cartilage preparations should be taken on an empty stomach, and acidic fruit juices should be avoided for 15 to 30 minutes before and after administration.

Cancer: 80 to 100 g/day or 1 to 1.3 g/kg/day of ground extract in 2 to 4 divided doses. Doses of the shark cartilage derivative AE-941 (Nevostat), used in clinical trials, have ranged from 30 to 240 mL/day or 20 mg/kg twice daily. In one trial, a liquid shark cartilage extract was dosed at 7 and 21 mL daily. In patients with incurable breast and colorectal cancer, a powder formulation (BeneFin) was initially dosed at 24 g/day and titrated upward every 3 days to a target dose of 96 g/day, administered in divided doses 3 to 4 times a day.

Joint diseases: 0.2 to 2 g/kg/day in 2 to 3 divided doses.

Psoriasis: 0.4 to 0.5 g/kg/day for 4 weeks, with dosage reduced to 0.2 to 0.3 g/kg/day for 4 additional weeks if skin lesions improve. Topical preparations containing shark cartilage 5% to 30% are also available.

Contraindications

Use with caution, if at all, in patients with coronary artery disease and peripheral artery disease because of the anti-angiogenic effects of shark cartilage. Due to concerns regarding hypercalcemia, use caution in patients with renal disease, cardiac arrhythmias, or cancer; monitoring is recommended.

Pregnancy/Lactation

Avoid use. Information regarding safety and efficacy in pregnancy and lactation is lacking.

Interactions

Coadministration of shark cartilage with other drugs (eg, calcium supplements, thiazide diuretics) may increase calcium levels.

Adverse Reactions

The most commonly reported adverse effects are mild to moderate and include GI distress, nausea, and taste alterations. Cases of allergic occupational asthma from shark cartilage dust have been reported, and hypercalcemia has occurred in cancer patients. A case of hepatitis has also been reported.

Toxicology

In an analysis of calcium supplements in Korea, shark cartilage-containing calcium supplements were among the highest in mercury and cadmium content, with levels that could be toxic in pediatric and elderly populations. In another study testing 16 shark cartilage products, 15 of the 16 contained beta-*N*-methyl-amino-L-alanine (BMAA), a neurotoxin found in the fins of several species of shark and potentially linked to degenerative brain disease; mercury content was low in these shark fin products. Caution should be used.

Local Anesthetic/Vasoconstrictor Precautions
No information available to require special precautions

Effects on Bleeding None reported

Shark Liver Oil

Clinical Overview

Uses

Shark liver oil (SLO) has been used to help treat cancer, skin conditions, and respiratory ailments, as well as to reduce recurrent aphthous stomatitis and prevent radiation sickness. However, limited clinical data are available. Alkylglycerols have been studied as an immune system stimulant. Animal data suggest SLO may improve fertility.

Dosing

SLO marketed under the name isolutrol has been studied in a clinical trial of acne at a topical concentration of 0.15 g per 100 mL.

Contraindications

Contraindications have not been identified.

Pregnancy/Lactation

Information regarding safety and efficacy in pregnancy and lactation is lacking.

Interactions

None well documented.

Adverse Reactions

Few toxic effects have been reported. SLO supplements may have an unpleasant taste and/or odor. There have been reports of SLO-induced pneumonia in humans and pigs.

Toxicology

No adverse reactions or effects on mortality were noted in rats receiving short- and long-term doses of a supercritical fluid extract of SLO at doses 100 to 200 times that of normal human consumption. In Sweden, a SLO product (Ecomer) was prohibited for use by the National Board of Health and Welfare because of suspected adverse effects.

Local Anesthetic/Vasoconstrictor Precautions
No information available to require special precautions

Effects on Bleeding None reported

Slippery Elm

Clinical Overview

Uses

The mucilaginous property of slippery elm has been used in traditional medicine to treat multiple conditions; however, no clinical studies exist to support these applications. Although limited studies have investigated the antioxidant and anti-inflammatory potential of slippery elm, the information from these studies does not provide any recommendations for use.

Dosing

No clinical studies exist to support dosage guidelines. Traditional use suggests a dosage of 1 to 3 tsp of slippery elm powder in 240 mL of water, up to 3 times a day.

Contraindications

Contraindications have not been identified.

Pregnancy/Lactation

Avoid use in pregnancy. Abortifacient effects have been described, although they may be related to vaginal use of whole bark pieces to induce abortion. Information regarding safety and efficacy in pregnancy and lactation is lacking.

Interactions

None well documented. Because the mucilaginous property of slippery elm may decrease absorption rates of other medicines, it may be beneficial to separate slippery elm doses from those of other medicines by 2 to 3 hours.

Adverse Reactions

Oleoresins from several Ulmus species have been reported to cause contact dermatitis, and the pollen of slippery elm is a known allergen.

Toxicology

Research regarding the toxicity of slippery elm is limited.

Local Anesthetic/Vasoconstrictor Precautions No information available to require special precautions

Effects on Bleeding None reported

Soy

Clinical Overview

Uses

Soy is commonly used as a source of fiber, protein, and minerals. Several meta-analyses evaluating soy use for various indications are available; however, evidence is lacking to support use in the treatment of asthma, menopausal symptoms, obesity, osteoporosis, diabetes, or heart disease. Limited benefit has been demonstrated for irritable bowel disease, polycystic ovary syndrome, and chronic kidney disease. Negative effects of soy consumption have also been noted.

The Italian Society of Diabetology (ISD) and the Italian Society for the Study of Arteriosclerosis (ISSA) state that soy supplementation for cholesterol-lowering purposes may be advised, though with some level of uncertainty and based on low-level evidence, in the general population and in patients with mild hypercholesterolemia who have low to moderate cardiovascular risk.

Dosing

Dosages of various forms of soy in clinical studies evaluating various uses have included 22.7 to 300 mg/day of soy isoflavones, up to 40 g/day of isolated soy protein, 120 g/day of dietary soy foods, 50 to 150 g/day of unfermented soy foods, up to 450 mg/day of genistein, up to 300 mg/day of daidzein, or 70 g/day of whole soy nuts.

Contraindications

Contraindications have not been identified. Women with current or a history of estrogen-dependent tumors, including breast cancer, should consult their physician prior to consuming soy in amounts higher than those typically found in food. An increased risk of some cancers has been documented in men consuming soy.

Pregnancy/Lactation

Soy has "generally recognized as safe" (GRAS) status when used as food. Avoid dosages above those found in food; safety and efficacy have not been established. Soy isoflavones are passed into breast milk. Because of nutritional disadvantages of soy-based infant formulas, the European Society of Pediatric Gastroenterology, Hepatology, and Nutrition (ESPGHAN) and the American Academy of Pediatrics (AAP) recommend amino acid-based and extensively hydrolyzed infant formulas over infant soy formula in nonbreastfed infants with cow's milk protein allergy; a soy formula may be considered in infants on a vegan diet.

Interactions

None well documented; use caution when administering with estrogen derivatives.

Adverse Reactions

Soybeans and their products are generally well tolerated. Minor GI disturbances have been reported. Cross-sensitivity between poly-gamma-glutamic acid (PGA) of fermented soybeans and PGA from jellyfish has been documented in several case reports. Soybeans contain natural goitrogens and can cause hypothyroidism in susceptible patients.

Toxicology

No data.

Local Anesthetic/Vasoconstrictor Precautions No information available to require special precautions

Effects on Bleeding None reported

Spirulina

Clinical Overview

Uses

Spirulina is available in the United States as a health food or supplement. Claims of immunostimulatory, anti-inflammatory, anticoagulant, antihypertensive, antioxidant, antiobesity, hypolipidemic, hypoglycemic, antiviral, and chelating effects exist; however, evidence supporting these claims is limited, and spirulina cannot be recommended for any specific use.

Dosing

Clinical data are insufficient to guide therapeutic dosing of spirulina. Dosages in clinical studies have ranged from 1 to 10 g/day, usually in divided doses, given for up to 12 months.

Contraindications

Phenylketonuria has occurred; however, an association with spirulina has not been substantiated.

Pregnancy/Lactation

Information regarding safety and efficacy in pregnancy and lactation is lacking. Because of the possible presence of mercury and other heavy metal contaminants in spirulina, use should be avoided during pregnancy.

Interactions

None well documented.

Adverse Reactions

Few reports of adverse reactions are available. Cases of anaphylaxis and spirulina-associated hepatotoxicity have been reported, and reactions from heavy metal contamination are possible.

Toxicology

Spirulina is considered nontoxic to humans at usual levels of consumption and has "generally recognized as safe" (GRAS) status according to the US Food and Drug Administration (FDA); however, information is limited.

Local Anesthetic/Vasoconstrictor Precautions No information available to require special precautions

Effects on Bleeding None reported

Stevia

Clinical Overview

Uses

Stevia and its extracts contain sweetening constituents known as steviol glycosides that have been evaluated for their antioxidant, antidiabetic, antimicrobial, and antihypertensive effects. However, clinical trials are lacking to support any uses of stevia, except as a sweetening agent.

Dosing

The acceptable daily intake of stevia is 4 mg/kg.

Note: 1/4 tsp of ground stevia leaves is equal to 1 tsp of sugar.

A standard stevia leaf infusion (1 cup taken 2 to 3 times daily) has been used as a natural aid for diabetes and hypertension. Stevioside 250 to 500 mg capsules administered 3 times daily for 1 to 2 years has been used in clinical studies evaluating antihypertensive effects. A dosage of 1 g of stevia leaf powder for 60 days was used in a small study of patients with type 2 diabetes to reduce postprandial glucose levels.

Contraindications

Contraindications have not been identified.

Pregnancy/Lactation

Information regarding safety and efficacy in pregnancy and lactation is lacking.

Interactions

Coadministration of stevia with drugs that inhibit organic anion transporter 3 (OAT3) uptake of stevia (eg, diclofenac, quercetin, telmisartan, mulberrin) may alter the renal clearance of stevia.

Adverse Reactions

No major adverse reactions have been documented.

Toxicology

Steviol glycosides have "generally recognized as safe" (GRAS) status according to the US Food and Drug Administration (FDA). However, stevia leaf and crude stevia extracts do not have GRAS status and are not FDA-approved for use in food.

Local Anesthetic/Vasoconstrictor Precautions

No information available to require special precautions

Effects on Bleeding None reported

St. John's Wort

Clinical Overview

Uses

Meta-analyses of quality clinical trials support a place for St. John's wort in the treatment of depression as mono- or adjunctive therapy. Effectiveness is comparable with standard antidepressants, while St. John's wort is associated with fewer and milder adverse reactions compared with conventional antidepressants. Benefit in reducing some climacteric symptoms in women with natural menopause has also been demonstrated. Unintended interactions with other drugs and quality control issues need to be considered prior to use. Limited data are available for several other areas of therapeutic use.

Dosing

Preparations vary greatly in chemical content and quality, and may be standardized regarding quantity of hyperforin (commonly 3% to 5%) or hypericin (commonly 0.3%) constituents. Clinical trials evaluating the efficacy of St. John's wort in depression have commonly used 900 mg of extract daily in 3 divided doses for up to 12 weeks (range, 200 to 1,800 mg/day).

Contraindications

Use with various antineoplastics, anticoagulants, and anti-infectives (including antivirals), as well as boceprevir, cobicistat, telaprevir, and voriconazole is contraindicated.

Pregnancy/Lactation

Avoid use. Hypericin and hyperforin have been detected in breast milk. St. John's wort should be avoided during pregnancy and lactation until further long-term studies demonstrate a lack of toxicity in the developing fetus and breastfeeding infants.

Interactions

St. John's wort has been reported to interact with numerous drugs. Drugs with a narrow therapeutic window should be monitored closely. Patients should be cautioned on the potential for interactions and consult their health care provider before taking St. John's wort with prescription or nonprescription drugs.

Adverse Reactions

Adverse reactions are usually mild. Potential adverse reactions include GI symptoms (eg, dry mouth, dizziness, constipation) and confusion. Photosensitization may also occur. In clinical trials, adverse reactions and discontinuations due to adverse effects were usually less with St. John's wort than with standard antidepressants. Other possible rare adverse reactions include induction of mania and effects on male and female reproductive capabilities. Impaired glucose tolerance has been documented in healthy volunteers.

Toxicology

Information is lacking.

Local Anesthetic/Vasoconstrictor Precautions

No information available to require special precautions

Effects on Bleeding None reported

Syrian Rue

Clinical Overview

Uses

In several countries the plant has been traditionally used as an hallucinogen in ceremonies, and has found its way into modern day recreational use. Although in vitro and animal experiments suggest a role as an antimicrobial, vasorelaxant, antidepressant, analgesic, or cytotoxic agent, clinical studies are lacking to support any therapeutic application.

Dosing

Clinical applications are lacking to provide therapeutic dosages. Consumption of decoctions made from 100 to 150 g of seeds has resulted in toxic effects.

Contraindications

Harmala alkaloids (specifically harmine and harmaline) are reversible monoamine oxidase inhibitors (MAOI), thus concomitant use with MAOI medicines and tyramine-containing foods is not advised.

Pregnancy/Lactation

Documented adverse reactions. Avoid use.

Interactions

None well documented.

Adverse Reactions

Case reports of toxicity include nausea and vomiting, visual and auditory hallucinations, confusion, agitation, locomotor ataxia, tremors and convulsions, and life-threatening respiratory depression and coma. Severe gastrointestinal distress, vomiting blood, gastric ulceration, and convulsions have also been reported, as well as bradycardia and low blood pressure. Symptoms are generally of short duration (a few hours) and supportive therapy is recommended.

Toxicology

Information is limited. Elevated renal and liver function tests have been reported.

Local Anesthetic/Vasoconstrictor Precautions

Long-term use of syrian rue has been associated with hypertension, tachycardia, tachypnea, and heart block. Use vasoconstrictor with caution in order to minimize risk of hypertension or tachycardia.

Effects on Bleeding None reported

Tea Tree Oil

Clinical Overview

Uses

Despite an abundance of commercial preparations promoted for antimicrobial use, sound clinical trials are limited. Trials have been conducted in conditions including nail infections, athlete's foot, fungal skin infections, acne, and methicillin-resistant Staphylococcus aureus. Case reports exist for use in other conditions.

Dosing

Decolonization of methicillin-resistant S. aureus: Tea tree oil as a nasal cream (4% to 10%) applied 3 times a day for 5 days and 5% body wash for 5 days. Acne vulgaris: 5% tea tree oil gel applied for 20 minutes twice daily, then washed off. Onchomycosis (fungal nail infections): 100% tea tree oil applied for 6 months. Tinea pedis (athlete's foot): 25% to 50% tea tree oil for 4 weeks.

Contraindications

Oral ingestion is contraindicated.

Pregnancy/Lactation

Information regarding safety and efficacy in pregnancy and lactation is lacking.

Interactions

None well documented.

Adverse Reactions

Case reports exist of dermatitis associated with topical tea tree oil.

Toxicology

Tea tree oil is toxic when ingested orally. Some case studies of accidental and intentional poisoning exist; however, no deaths have been reported to the American Association of Poison Control Centers through 2006. Mutagenicity of tea tree oil appears to be low; however, chemical constituents have been shown to be cytotoxic and embryotoxic.

Local Anesthetic/Vasoconstrictor Precautions

No information available to require special precautions

Effects on Bleeding None reported

Thunder God Vine

Clinical Overview

Uses

Thunder god vine has primarily been evaluated for use in rheumatoid arthritis (RA) and ankylosing spondylitis; however, its adverse event profile and limited quality trials restrict any recommendations for clinical use. Antifertility properties in men have been described, while amenorrhea was observed in women.

Dosing

Clinical trials have evaluated lower (60 mg daily) to higher doses (180 to 350 mg daily) of T. wilfordii for the treatment of RA.

Doses of 20 to 30 mg/day of a refined extract of T. wilfordii (one-third the usual recommended dose for RA) for 1.5 to 5 months has produced antifertility effects in men.

Contraindications

Contraindications have not been identified. Due to immune suppression, thunder god vine preparations should not be used in immunocompromised patients.

Pregnancy/Lactation

Avoid use. Embryotoxicity has been demonstrated in mice.

Interactions

None well documented.

Adverse Reactions

Clinically important adverse events have been reported in clinical trials. GI upset, male and female infertility, and immune suppression are common adverse effects of thunder god vine.

Toxicology

Information is limited.

Local Anesthetic/Vasoconstrictor Precautions

No information available to require special precautions

Effects on Bleeding None reported

Thyme

Clinical Overview

Uses

Thyme has primarily culinary uses. Thyme extracts and thymol have been used in cough mixtures and mouthwashes, as well as for skin conditions, especially fungal infections. Clinical trials are lacking to support these uses.

Dosing

Studies are lacking to guide clinical dosages.

Contraindications

Information is lacking.

Pregnancy/Lactation

Information regarding safety and efficacy in pregnancy and lactation is lacking.

Interactions

None well documented.

Adverse Reactions

Contact dermatitis and systemic allergy have been reported.

Toxicology

Information is lacking.

Local Anesthetic/Vasoconstrictor Precautions

No information available to require special precautions

Effects on Bleeding An extract from thyme has been shown to have antiplatelet aggregating activity. The clinical significance of this effect is unknown.

Tolu Balsam

Clinical Overview

Uses

Tolu balsam is best known for its fragrance and use as flavoring in pharmaceutical products, although it also has mild antiseptic and expectorant properties. There are no clinical data to support its use in any condition.

Dosing

There is no recent clinical evidence to support specific dosing of tolu balsam. Traditional dosage of the herb for colds has been 0.6 g daily.

Contraindications

Contraindications have not yet been determined.

Pregnancy/Lactation

Information regarding safety and efficacy in pregnancy and lactation is lacking.

Interactions

None well documented.

Adverse Reactions

Allergic reactions have been reported.

Toxicology

Information is lacking.

Local Anesthetic/Vasoconstrictor Precautions

No information available to require special precautions

Effects on Bleeding None reported

Turmeric

Clinical Overview

Uses

Limited evidence from meta-analyses suggests that curcumin, the most commonly studied constituent of turmeric, and/or curcuminoids have analgesic, anti-inflammatory, and antioxidant effects and may improve biomarkers and symptoms in patients with osteoarthritis, major depression, cardiovascular risk, obesity, and metabolic syndrome. Data are equivocal in dysglycemic/diabetic populations, and are insufficient to identify a role for curcumin in patients with chronic pruritic skin lesions, cognitive decline, inflammatory bowel disease, nonalcoholic fatty liver disease, oral mucocutaneous conditions, psoriasis, or uveitis.

Dosing

Generally, standardized curcuminoid dosages of 200 mg/day to 6 g/day (treatment durations of up to 8 months) have been used in clinical trials evaluating anti-inflammatory and antioxidant effects of curcumin in a variety of conditions. Lipid-based formulations have shown improved bioavailability over micronized and unformulated curcumin preparations, with greater improvements observed in women compared to men.

Contraindications

Use is contraindicated if hypersensitive to any of the components of curcumin. Avoid use during pregnancy and lactation because of emmenagogue and uterine stimulant effects. Turmeric should not be used in patients with gallstones or bile duct or passage obstruction.

Pregnancy/Lactation

Avoid use. Emmenagogue and abortifacient effects have been documented.

Interactions

C. longa potentially interacts with CYP2D6 and CYP3A substrates, antiplatelet agents, anticoagulants, cladribine, nonsteroidal anti-inflammatory agents, salicylates, and thrombolytic agents.

Adverse Reactions

Clinical trials report few adverse reactions (eg, dyspepsia, pruritus). Rare cases of contact dermatitis and anaphylaxis have also been reported.

Toxicology

No data.

Local Anesthetic/Vasoconstrictor Precautions

No information available to require special precautions

Effects on Bleeding May see increased bleeding due to inhibition of platelet aggregation

Ubiquinone

Clinical Overview

Uses

Ubiquinone may have applications in cardiovascular disease, especially congestive heart failure (CHF), although there is a lack of consensus. Studies in neurological disorders are less promising. Limited clinical trials have been conducted to support its widespread use for other conditions.

Dosing

Cardiovascular and neurologic trials predominantly use ubiquinone dosages of 300 mg/day or idebenone dosages of 5 mg/kg/day. Higher dosages of ubiquinone (up to 3,000 mg/day) have been used. Pharmacokinetic studies suggest split dosing is superior to single daily dosing.

Contraindications

Absolute contraindications have not been identified.

Pregnancy/Lactation

Information regarding safety and efficacy in pregnancy and lactation is lacking.

Interactions

Findings are conflicting. Case reports show ubiquinone decreases the anticoagulant effect of warfarin; however, a randomized clinical trial found no effect on the international normalized ratio (INR).

Adverse Reactions

Adverse effects are rare and include diarrhea, GI discomfort, headache, loss of appetite, and nausea. Allergic reactions have been reported.

Toxicology

An observed intake safety level of 1,200 mg/day is based on clinical data; however, dosages exceeding this amount have been used with no apparent adverse effect. No accumulation in plasma or tissue following cessation of coenzyme Q10 consumption has been noted.

Local Anesthetic/Vasoconstrictor Precautions

No information available to require special precautions

Effects on Bleeding May increase the risk of bleeding

Uva Ursi

Clinical Overview

Uses

Uva ursi has been traditionally used to treat symptoms of mild urinary tract infections. However, there are no clinical trials demonstrating the safety, efficacy, or toxicity of its use. In vitro research supports its use as a urinary antiseptic.

Dosing

Dosing and formulations of uva ursi products available in the United States vary. Doses of arbutin 400 to 840 mg have been used.

Contraindications

Uva ursi is contraindicated during pregnancy and lactation.

Pregnancy/Lactation

Avoid use. Uva ursi is contraindicated during pregnancy and lactation.

Interactions

Uva ursi should not be administered with foods or drugs that acidify the urine.

Adverse Reactions

Ingestion of the dried leaves of uva ursi may cause a greenish-brown discoloration of the urine. Ingestion of uva ursi leaves may cause nausea and vomiting due to its high tannin content. Bull's eye maculopathy has been reported with long-term ingestion (3 years).Topical application has caused leukoderma, erythema, and allergic contact dermatitis.

Toxicology

While uva ursi leaves are not carcinogenic, hydroquinone, a primary constituent of the plant, may be carcinogenic. A recommended therapeutic human daily dose of bearberry leaf extract (420 mg of hydroquinone derivatives calculated as anhydrous arbutin) liberates free hydroquinone in urine at a maximum exposure level of 11 mcg/kg of body weight per day. However, the daily exposure dose, below which there is negligible risk to humans, is 100 mcg/kg.

Local Anesthetic/Vasoconstrictor Precautions

No information available to require special precautions

Effects on Bleeding None reported

Valerian

Clinical Overview

Uses

The evidence to support the common use of valerian in insomnia remains weak. However, as valerian preparations seem to have a wide margin of safety, further trials for insomnia and anxiety may be warranted.

Dosing

Anxiety: Valeprotriates 150 mg/day in 3 divided doses for 4 weeks has been used in a clinical trial. Other trials used the dried herb 0.5 to 2 g, extract 0.5 to 2 mL, and valerian tincture 2 to 4 mL for anxiety. Insomnia: Valerian extract 400 to 600 mg/day taken 1 hour before bedtime for 2 to 4 weeks has been used in clinical trials. Single-dose studies have consistently found no effect for single doses of valerian in insomnia.

Contraindications

Contraindications have not been identified.

Pregnancy/Lactation

Information regarding safety and efficacy in pregnancy and lactation is lacking.

Interactions

None well documented.

Adverse Reactions

In general, clinical studies have found valerian to have a wide margin of safety, be devoid of adverse effects, and have fewer adverse reactions than positive control drugs, such as diazepam. Headache and diarrhea have been reported in clinical trials, but hangover is seldom reported.

Toxicology

Valerian has been classified as GRAS (generally recognized as safe) in the United States for food use; extracts and the root oil are used as flavorings in foods and beverages. The observed in vitro cytotoxicity of valepotriate compounds may not be relevant in vivo because of limited absorption.

Local Anesthetic/Vasoconstrictor Precautions

No information available to require special precautions

Effects on Bleeding None reported

Vinpocetine

Clinical Overview

Uses

Vinpocetine is used to enhance memory and increase brain metabolism. It has also been used for ischemia and reperfusion injury, and is considered a neuroprotective agent. However, there are few robust clinical studies to support the use of vinpocetine in stroke, dementia, or other diseases of the CNS.

Dosing

Most clinical studies have used between 5 and 20 mg vinpocetine, given 3 times daily due to a short half-life (2 to 4 hours).

Contraindications

V. minor whole plant or extract is potentially contraindicated in constipation and hypotension.

Pregnancy/Lactation

Avoid use. Information regarding safety and efficacy in pregnancy and lactation is lacking. Traditional uses for lesser periwinkle include antilactagogue and emmenagogue effects.

Interactions

Caution is warranted in patients on anticoagulant medications.

Adverse Reactions

Vinpocetine is well tolerated. Minor adverse reactions include facial flushing, dry mouth, drowsiness, headache, insomnia, anxiety, dizziness, nausea, and indigestion.

Toxicology

None well documented.

Local Anesthetic/Vasoconstrictor Precautions

No information available to require special precautions

Effects on Bleeding Vinpocetine has the potential to increase the risk of bleeding or potentiate the effects of warfarin. Clinical relevance of this effect is unknown.

Vitamin D

Clinical Overview

Uses

Vitamin D, long recognized as playing a role in bone and calcium homeostasis, is being investigated for use in cardiovascular disease, cancer, diabetes, infections, multiple sclerosis, psoriasis, respiratory health, and other conditions. More clinical trials are needed.

Dosing

The American Academy of Pediatrics recommends 400 units/day of vitamin D in infants and adolescents. Clinical data are not yet sufficiently robust to make definitive recommendations for therapeutic dosages of vitamin D; however, in the elderly, 700 to 1,000 units/day have been shown to reduce the risk of falls.

Contraindications

Contraindications have not been identified.

Pregnancy/Lactation

Routine use of supplemental vitamin D during pregnancy is not supported by safety evidence. However, adequate maternal intake of vitamin D-containing foods during lactation ensures that breast-fed infants receive sufficient vitamin D.

Interactions

The use of statins has been shown to increase serum vitamin D levels. Corticosteriods decrease the metabolism of vitamin D and orlistat reduces its absorption; phenobarbital and phenytoin increase the hepatic metabolism of vitamin D.

Adverse Reactions

High doses of vitamin D have rarely produced adverse events in clinical trials.

Toxicology

Toxicity due to vitamin D is considered to manifest at serum levels greater than 150 ng/mL of 25-hydroxyvitamin D. Symptoms of hypervitaminosis D include fatigue, nausea, vomiting, and weakness associated with hypercalcemia.

Local Anesthetic/Vasoconstrictor Precautions

No information available to require special precautions

Effects on Bleeding None reported

Wild Yam

Clinical Overview

Uses

Clinical trials are generally lacking for topical formulations of Dioscorea for menopausal symptoms. Chinese yam polysaccharides have been evaluated in laboratory studies for potential as prebiotics, with varying results. Dioscorea oppositifolia tubers have been used as a saliva substitute.

Dosing

There are inadequate clinical trials on which to base dosing guidelines.

Contraindications

Contraindications have not been identified.

Pregnancy/Lactation

Information regarding safety and efficacy in pregnancy and lactation is lacking.

Interactions

None well documented.

Adverse Reactions

A clinical study evaluating the daily consumption of wild yam reported no adverse events. Topical preparations of wild yam extract are relatively free from adverse effects. Based on a single study in rats, oral D. villosa should be avoided in people with compromised renal function.

Toxicology

Topical D. villosa (with an upper limit of 3.5% diosgenin) was not found to be systemically toxic or genotoxic.

Local Anesthetic/Vasoconstrictor Precautions

No information available to require special precautions

Effects on Bleeding None reported

Willow Bark

Clinical Overview

Uses

Willow bark can be an effective analgesic if the salicylate content is adequate. Anticancer, antioxidant, and anti-inflammatory activity has been documented in limited trials. Clinical trials have shown that willow has moderate efficacy in treating lower back pain but very little efficacy in treating arthritic conditions.

Dosing

Willow is available in several dosage forms, including tablets, capsules, powder, and liquid. Willow bark has been used for analgesia at daily doses of 1 to 3 g of bark, corresponding to salicin 60 to 120 mg. A clinical study of patients with lower back pain used willow bark at a dose of salicin 120 to 240 mg/day. A proprietary extract of willow bark, Assalix, was standardized to contain 15% salicin. The pharmacokinetics of salicylic acid delivered from willow bark have been studied, and plasma half-life is approximately 2.5 hours. Another pharmacokinetic study of salicylic acid from salicin found peak levels within 2 hours after oral administration.

Contraindications

Patients with known hypersensitivity to aspirin should avoid any willow-containing product. This caution also applies to patients with asthma, impaired thrombocyte function, vitamin K antagonistic treatment, diabetes, gout, kidney or liver conditions, peptic ulcer disease, and in any other medical conditions in which aspirin is contraindicated.

Pregnancy/Lactation

Avoid use because of the lack of information regarding safety and efficacy during pregnancy and lactation.

Interactions

In general, drug interactions associated with salicylates may apply to willow-containing products. Therefore, avoid use with alcohol, barbiturates, sedatives, and other salicylate-containing products because of additive irritant effects and adverse reactions on the GI tract and blood platelets. Willow may also interact with oral anticoagulants (eg, warfarin), seizure medications (eg, phenytoin, valproate acid), and other medications (eg, methotrexate).

Adverse Reactions

Reports from clinical trials primarily document GI discomfort, such as nausea and stomachache, as well as dizziness and rash. An anaphylactic reaction to willow bark has been reported.

Toxicology

There is little or no toxicity information on the use of willow bark. However, the same toxicity associated with salicylates applies to willow. Patients should monitor for blood in stools, tinnitus, nausea or vomiting, and stomach or kidney irritation.

Local Anesthetic/Vasoconstrictor Precautions

No information available to require special precautions

Effects on Bleeding Salicylate derivatives of willow bark had little effect on platelet aggregation when compared with a daily cardioprotective dose of acetylsalicylate 100 mg. The total serum salicylate concentration of salicin, one of the principle salicylates of willow, was bioequivalent to acetylsalicylate 50 mg. There are no reports of bleeding caused by willow bark.

Wormwood

Clinical Overview

Uses

Wormwood was traditionally used to treat worm infestations, although no clinical data support this use. Anti-inflammatory, antipyretic, and chemotherapeutic activity are documented in nonhuman studies. Initial studies suggest that wormwood may improve Crohn disease symptoms, but information regarding the plant's use in immunoglobulin A (IgA) nephropathy is limited. In Germany, woodworm is used to treat loss of appetite, dyspepsia, and biliary dyskinesia. Wormwood is also used as a flavoring agent.

Dosing

Wormwood is commercially available as an essential oil, as well as in capsule, tablet, tincture, and aqueous extract dosage forms. However, no recent clinical evidence supports dosing recommendations. Traditional use of the herb for treating dyspepsia was dosed as an infusion of 2 to 3 g daily.

Contraindications

Avoid use with hypersensitivity to any of the components of wormwood, particularly the essential oil. It may be contraindicated in patients with an underlying defect of hepatic heme synthesis, because thujone is a porphyrogenic terpenoid.

Pregnancy/Lactation

Avoid use. Documented abortifacient and emmenagogue effects.

Interactions

A single case report suggests that wormwood may increase the international normalized ratio (INR) with warfarin.

Adverse Reactions

The volatile oil thujone in wormwood produces a state of excitement and is a powerful convulsant. Repeated ingestion of wormwood may result in absinthism, a syndrome characterized by digestive disorders, thirst, restlessness, vertigo, trembling of the limbs, numbness of the extremities, loss of intellect, delirium, paralysis, and death.

Toxicology

Wormwood is classified as an unsafe herb by the US Food and Drug Administration (FDA) because of the neurotoxic potential of thujone and its derivatives; it is generally regarded as safe if it is thujone free. The safety of wormwood is poorly documented despite its long history as a food additive. Convulsions, dermatitis, and renal failure have been reported.

Local Anesthetic/Vasoconstrictor Precautions

No information available to require special precautions

Effects on Bleeding None reported

Xylitol

Clinical Overview

Uses

Medical literature documents the use of xylitol in medical conditions and applications, including acute otitis media, dental caries, intravenous (IV) nutrition, and osteoporosis, although limited clinical trials exist.

Dosing

Dosage regimens vary. In one study to prevent ear infections in children, the daily dose varied from 8.4 g in chewing gum to 10 g in syrup. Xylitol oral solution at dosages of 5 g orally 3 times a day and 7.5 g orally once a day was well tolerated in young children. Xylitol chewing gum was effective in reducing dental caries when divided into at least 3 consumption periods per day for a total dose of 6 to 10 g. For adults 21 years and older at high risk of caries, consideration may be given for daily use of five 1 gram xylitol lozenges.

Contraindications

Avoid use if allergic to xylitol. Hypersensitivity reactions are documented.

Pregnancy/Lactation

Pregnancy: Category B. Xylitol is considered safe in pregnancy and during breastfeeding, according to the US Food and Drug Administration (FDA). The use of xylitol chewing gum in mothers lowered maternal oral bacterial load and reduced transmission of mutans streptococci to infants late in pregnancy and during the postpartum period.

Interactions

None well documented.

Adverse Reactions

The main adverse effects reported from oral xylitol use at a dosage exceeding 40 to 50 g/day included nausea, bloating, borborygmi (rumbling sounds of gas moving through the intestine), colic, diarrhea, and increased total bowel movement frequency.

Toxicology

Xylitol is generally nontoxic based on various clinical studies and its historical use in foods, pharmaceuticals, and nutraceuticals. Animal studies also confirm its overall safety profile. Renocerebral oxalosis with renal failure is documented with large doses of IV administered xylitol.

Local Anesthetic/Vasoconstrictor Precautions
No information available to require special precautions

Effects on Bleeding None reported

Yarrow

Clinical Overview

Uses

Clinical studies are limited.

Dosing

Traditionally, yarrow herb 4.5 g/day has been used for various conditions. However, there are no quality clinical studies to validate this dosing.

Contraindications

Yarrow use is contraindicated in known allergies to any members of the Aster family. Data for reported contraindications in epilepsy are lacking.

Pregnancy/Lactation

Avoid use. Documented adverse effects.

Interactions

None well documented.

Adverse Reactions

Contact dermatitis is the most commonly reported adverse reaction, but high doses may be associated with anticholinergic effects.

Toxicology

Yarrow is not generally considered toxic; however, an antispermatogenic effect has been reported, and safety data are insufficient to support use of the herb in cosmetic products.

Local Anesthetic/Vasoconstrictor Precautions
No information available to require special precautions

Effects on Bleeding None reported

Yohimbe

Clinical Overview

Uses

Yohimbine has been used primarily in the treatment of sexual dysfunction, weight (body fat) loss, and xerostomia (dry mouth). It has also been used in studies investigating autonomic failure and orthostatic hypotension.

Dosing

Yohimbine 6 mg given 3 times a day has been used in xerostomia trials. A mean dose of 0.4 mg/kg body weight or 30 mg daily, and a maximum of 50 mg, has been used in erectile dysfunction studies. In studies investigating effects on body mass, yohimbine 20 mg daily has been used.

Contraindications

This drug should not be used in the presence of renal or hepatic function impairment.

Pregnancy/Lactation

Do not use during pregnancy or lactation.

Interactions

None well documented.

Adverse Reactions

Clinical trials report few serious adverse reactions. There are case reports of rash, lupus-like syndrome, bronchospasm, severe hypotension, dysrhythmia, heart failure, and death. Increased anxiety, irritability, and excitability have also been reported. Animal studies suggest yohimbine may increase motor activity and seizures at higher dosages. Yohimbe may precipitate psychoses in predisposed individuals.

Toxicology

No data.

Local Anesthetic/Vasoconstrictor Precautions
Has potential to interact with epinephrine and levonordefrin to result in increased BP; use vasoconstrictor with caution

Effects on Bleeding None reported

ORAL MEDICINE TOPICS

PART I:

DENTAL MANAGEMENT AND THERAPEUTIC CONSIDERATIONS IN MEDICALLY COMPROMISED PATIENTS

This first part of the chapter focuses on common medical conditions and their associated drug therapies with which the dentist must be familiar. Patient profiles with commonly associated drug regimens are described.

TABLE OF CONTENTS

CARDIOVASCULAR DISEASES

Cardiovascular disease is the most prevalent human disease affecting over 60 million Americans, accounting for >50% of all deaths in the United States. Surgical and pharmacological therapies have resulted in many cardiovascular patients living healthy and profitable lives. Consequently, patients presenting to the dental office may require treatment planning modifications related to the medical management of their cardiovascular disease. For the purposes of this text, we will cover coronary artery disease (CAD) including angina pectoris, myocardial infarction, cardiac arrhythmias, heart failure, and hypertension.

CARDIOVASCULAR DRUGS: DENTAL CONSIDERATIONS

Some of the drug listings are redundant because the drugs are used to treat more than one cardiovascular disorder. As a convenience to the reader, each table has been constructed as a stand alone listing of drugs for the given disorder.

CORONARY ARTERY DISEASE (CAD)

Any long-term decrease in the delivery of oxygen to the heart muscle can lead to the condition ischemic heart disease. Often arteriosclerosis and atherosclerosis result in a narrowing of the coronary vessels' lumina and are the most common causes of vascular ischemic heart disease. Other causes such as previous infarct, mitral valve regurgitation, and ruptured septa may also lead to ischemia in the heart muscle. The two most common major conditions that result from ischemic heart disease are angina pectoris and myocardial infarction. Sudden death can likewise result from ischemia.

To the physician, the most common presenting sign or symptom of ischemic heart disease is chest pain. This chest pain can be of a transient nature as in angina pectoris or the result of a myocardial infarction. This pain pattern is the more typical presentation in men; women may have more subtle signs of fatigue and general malaise. It is now believed that sudden death represents a separate occurrence that essentially involves the development of a lethal cardiac arrhythmia or coronary artery spasm leading to an acute shutdown of the heart muscle blood supply. Risk factors in patients for coronary atherosclerosis include age (males ≥45, females ≥55 years), family history of premature development, hypertension, hypercholesterolemia, low HDL, cigarette smoking, and diabetes mellitus.

CAD is the cause of about half of all deaths in the United States. CAD has been shown to be correlated with the levels of plasma cholesterol and/or triacylglycerol-containing lipoprotein particles. Primary prevention focuses on averting the development of CAD. In contrast, secondary prevention of CAD focuses on therapies to reduce morbidity and mortality in patients with clinically documented CAD.

Lipid-lowering and cardioprotective drugs provide significant risk-reducing benefits in the secondary prevention of CAD. By reducing the levels of total and low density cholesterol through the inhibition of hydroxymethylglutaryl-coenzyme A (HMG-CoA) reductase, statin drugs significantly improve survival. Cardioprotective drug therapy includes antiplatelet/ anticoagulant agents to inhibit platelet adhesion; aggregation and blood coagulation; beta-blockers to lower heart rate, contractility and blood pressure; and the angiotensin-converting enzyme (ACE) inhibitors to lower peripheral resistance and workload. For a listing of lipid lowering drugs, see Table 1.

Table 1. Drugs Used in the Treatment of Hyperlipidemia

Reduction of Total and Low-Density Cholesterol Levels

HMG-CoA Reductase Inhibitors

Fluvastatin on page 706
Lovastatin on page 940
Pitavastatin on page 1238
Pravastatin on page 1253
Rosuvastatin on page 1348
Simvastatin on page 1372
AtorvaSTATin on page 191

Fibrate Group

Fenofibrate and Derivatives on page 640
Gemfibrozil on page 733

Bile Acid Sequestrants

Cholestyramine Resin on page 345
Colesevelam on page 406
Colestipol

Nicotinic Acid

Niacin on page 1097

Cholesterol Absorption Inhibitor

Ezetimibe on page 633

Antilipemic Agent, Microsomal Triglyceride Transfer Protein (MTP) Inhibitor

Lomitapide on page 927

Table 1. Drugs Used in the Treatment of Hyperlipidemia *(continued)*

PCSK9 Inhibitor

Alirocumab on page 101

Evolocumab on page 631

Miscellaneous

Omega-3-Acid Ethyl Esters

ANGINA PECTORIS (Emphasis on Unstable Angina)

Numerous physiologic triggers can initiate the rupture of plaque in coronary blood vessels. Rupture leads to the activation, adhesion and aggregation of platelets, and the activation of the clotting cascade, resulting in the formation of occlusive thrombus. If this process leads to the complete occlusion of the artery, acute myocardial infarction with ST-segment elevation occurs. Alternatively, if the process leads to severe stenosis but the artery remains partially patent, unstable angina can occur. Triggers which induce unstable angina include physical exertion, mechanical stress due to an increase in cardiac contractility, pulse rate, blood pressure, and vasoconstriction.

Recently, the non-ST-elevation Acute Coronary Syndrome guidelines have been updated by the American Heart Association and the American College of Cardiology Foundation (Amsterdam 2014). These guidelines may be helpful in outlining treatment strategies.

Pharmacologic therapy to treat unstable angina includes antiplatelet drugs, antithrombin therapy, and conventional antianginal therapy with beta-blockers (or non-dihydropyridine calcium channel blockers [eg, diltiazem]) and nitrates. These drug groups and selected agents are listed in Table 2 and see Antiplatelet and Anticoagulation Considerations in Dentistry on page 1666.

Conventional Antianginal Therapy: Beta-Blockers, Nitrates, Calcium Channel Blockers

The pharmacotherapeutic strategy in treating angina is directed at improving myocardial oxygen supply and/or decreasing myocardial oxygen demand. Myocardial oxygen supply can be increased through enhancing coronary blood flow. Myocardial oxygen demand can be reduced by decreasing heart rate, contractility, and myocardial wall tension. Preload, afterload, and myocardial wall thickness are determinants of myocardial wall tension.

Organic Nitrates

Organic nitrates benefit angina by enhancing coronary blood flow via vasodilation of both large epicardial vessels and neighboring collateral vessels and decreasing myocardial oxygen demand by dilating veins and reducing preload. In order to be effective for the chronic prevention of angina, organic nitrates need to be dosed in a manner that does not induce nitrate tolerance.

Beta-Blockers

Beta-blockers are beneficial in treating angina since they decrease heart rate and contractility. Beta-blockers without intrinsic sympathomimetic activity (ISA) are preferred and those with ISA generally should be avoided when treating angina (such beta-blockers may actually increase myocardial workload). Beta-blockers are useful in the treatment of stable and unstable angina; but, since they can induce coronary vasospasm, they should be avoided in patients with vasospastic angina (aka, Prinzmetal's or variant angina).

Beta-blockers are the preferred initial choice, often used in conjunction with an organic nitrate to more positively address the hemodynamic imbalances causing the angina. If the patient cannot tolerate the beta-blocker or if the beta-blocker therapy is contraindicated, a non-dihydropyridine calcium channel blocker (eg, diltiazem) with or without an organic nitrate can be considered. If combination therapy (ie, beta-blocker with an organic nitrate) is ineffective, a calcium channel blocker may be added. Type of calcium channel blocker chosen becomes important when combining with a beta-blocker. Since the combination of a beta-blocker and either of the non-dihydropyridine calcium channel blockers, verapamil or diltiazem, frequently induces undesirable bradycardia, a dihydropyridine calcium channel blocker is often selected in combination with a beta-blocker, unless the patient is experiencing unstable angina. Caution should be used when using beta-blockers in patients with difficult-to-control diabetes mellitus, bronchospastic disease, or peripheral vascular disease. The medications may be dosed as high as possible without inducing symptomatic bradycardia, hypotension, and/or heart blocks. Some patients on beta-blockers will experience fatigue and other adverse effects related to the central nervous system. Abrupt withdrawal of beta-blockers in patients with angina has been known to cause excessive tachycardia, ischemia, and cardiac arrhythmias.

Calcium Channel Blockers

Two categories of agents comprise the calcium channel blockers: Non-dihydropyridines (eg, diltiazem and verapamil) and the dihydropyridine family (eg, nifedipine). These agents are useful in treating stable and unstable angina and are the drugs of choice in treating variant angina. All three agents increase coronary blood flow. Verapamil and diltiazem reduce contractility, heart rate, and, to some extent, afterload (thus reducing wall tension). Dihydropyridines (eg, nifedipine) are potent afterload reducers and have no impact on reducing heart rate. In fact, dihydropyridines may actually increase heart rate in patients not on a beta-blocker and may increase ischemia in patients experiencing unstable angina.

Stable and Unstable Angina

Since stable and unstable angina are nearly always related to CAD, patients should be placed on aspirin and an angiotensin-converting enzyme inhibitor (especially if the patient has heart failure) in addition to antianginal therapy. Clopidogrel or prasugrel may be considered if the patient is allergic to aspirin. If applicable, weight reduction, smoking cessation, and following an appropriate low-cholesterol, low-fat diet should be encouraged as well as an effort to reduce other CAD risk factors. In addition to these lifestyle changes, the patient should be placed on a moderate or high dose statin if no contraindications exist. Titrating statins to LDL-C or non-HDL-C goals as primary or secondary prevention is no longer recommended by the ACC/AHA Blood Cholesterol Guidelines due to insufficient supporting evidence (Stone 2013).

Patients with cardiac stents who have not completed their full course of dual antiplatelet therapy should not have their antiplatelet agents discontinued even if only briefly. Premature interruption of therapy may result in stent thrombosis with subsequent MI. Discussion with the patient's cardiologist is required especially if urgent dental procedures are necessary.

Dental Management

The dental management of the patient with angina pectoris may include sedation techniques for complicated procedures (see the Sedation section in Management of the Patient With Anxiety or Depression on page 1778), to limit the extent of procedures, and to limit the use of local anesthesia containing 1:100,000 epinephrine to two carpules. Anesthesia without a vasoconstrictor might also be selected. The appropriate use of a vasoconstrictor in anesthesia, however, should be weighed against the necessity to maximize anesthesia and control bleeding. Complete history, appropriate referral, and consultation with the patient's physician should be done for patients who are known to be at risk for angina pectoris.

MYOCARDIAL INFARCTION

Myocardial infarction is the leading cause of death in the United States. It is an acute irreversible ischemic event that produces an area of myocardial necrosis in the heart tissue. If a patient has a previous history of myocardial infarction, he/she may be taking a variety of drugs (ie, antihypertensives, lipid lowering drugs, ACE inhibitors or angiotensin receptor blockers, and antianginal medications) to not only prevent a second infarct, but to treat the long-term effects associated ischemic heart disease. Postmyocardial infarction patients are often taking anticoagulants, such as warfarin, or antiplatelet agents, such as aspirin, clopidogrel, or prasugrel. Consultation with the prescribing physician by the dentist is necessary prior to invasive procedures. Temporary dose reduction may allow the dentist to proceed with very invasive procedures. Most procedures, however, can be accomplished without changing the anticoagulant or antiplatelet therapy at all, using local hemostasis techniques and thereby keeping the thromboembolic risk to a minimum.

Aspirin on page 177
Warfarin on page 1557

Thrombolytic drugs, which might dissolve hemostatic plugs, may also be given on a short-term basis immediately following a myocardial infarction and include:

Alteplase on page 111
Reteplase on page 1318
Tenecteplase

Following myocardial infarction and rehabilitation, outpatients may be placed on antiplatelet agents, beta-adrenergic blockers, ACE inhibitors or angiotensin receptor blockers, lipid-lowering therapies, and possibly aldosterone inhibitors and diuretics, if significant heart failure is associated with the MI, or even anticoagulants (such as warfarin) when significant thromboembolic risk coexists. Depending on the presence or absence of continued angina pectoris, patients may also be taking nitrates, beta-blockers, or calcium channel blockers as indicated for treatment of angina.

Beta-Adrenergic Blocking Agents Categorized According to Specific Properties

Alpha-Adrenergic Blocking Activity

Carvedilol on page 294
Labetalol on page 867

Intrinsic Sympathomimetic Activity

Acebutolol on page 58
Pindolol on page 1234

Long Duration of Action and Fewer CNS Effects

Atenolol on page 189
Betaxolol (Systemic) on page 240
Nadolol on page 1070

Beta-1 Receptor Selectivity

Atenolol on page 189
Betaxolol (Systemic) on page 240
Metoprolol on page 1009
Nebivolol on page 1088

Nonselective (blocks both beta-1 and beta-2 receptors)

Nadolol on page 1070
Propranolol on page 1287
Timolol (Systemic)

ARRHYTHMIAS

Abnormal cardiac rhythm can develop spontaneously and survivors of a myocardial infarction are often left with an arrhythmia. An arrhythmia is any alteration or disturbance in the normal rate, rhythm, or conduction through the cardiac tissue. Abnormalities in rhythm can occur in either the atria or the ventricles. Various valvular deformities, drug effects, and chemical derangements can initiate arrhythmias. These arrhythmias can be a slowing of the heart rate (<60 beats/minute) as defined in bradycardia or tachycardia resulting in a rapid heart beat (usually >150 beats/minute). The dentist will encounter a variety of treatments for management of arrhythmias. Usually, underlying causes such as reduced cardiac output, hypertension, and irregular ventricular beats will require treatment. Pacemaker therapy is also sometimes used. Indwelling pacemakers may require supplementation with antibiotics, and consultation with the physician is certainly appropriate.

Beta-blockers are often used to slow cardiac rate and diazepam may be helpful when anxiety is a contributing factor in arrhythmia. When atrial flutter and atrial fibrillation are diagnosed, drug therapy is usually required.

Atrial fibrillation (AF) is an arrhythmia characterized by multiple electrical activations in the atria resulting in scattered and disorganized depolarization and repolarization of the myocardium. Atrial contraction can lead to an irregular and rapid rate of ventricular contraction. The prevalence of AF within the US population ranges between 1% and 4%, with the incidence increasing with age. It is often associated with rheumatic valvular disease and nonvalvular conditions including CAD, heart failure, and hypertension. CAD is present in about one-half of the patients with AF. Atrial fibrillation is a major risk factor for cerebral embolism. It is thought that thrombi develop as a result of stasis in the dilated left atrium and are dislodged by sudden changes in cardiac rhythm. About 10% of all strokes in patients >60 years of age are caused by AF.

The cornerstones of drug therapy for atrial fibrillation are the restoration and maintenance of a normal sinus rhythm through the use of antiarrhythmic drugs, ventricular rate control through the use of beta-blockers, digoxin, or calcium channel blockers, and stroke prevention through the use of anticoagulants.

Antiarrhythmic Drugs

Cardiac rhythm is conducted through the sinoatrial (SA) and atrioventricular (AV) nodes, bundle branches, and Purkinje fibers. Electrical impulses are transmitted within this system by the opening and closing of sodium and potassium channels. Antiarrhythmic drugs are classified by which primary channel they act upon, a classification known as Vaughan Williams. The Class I agents act primarily on sodium channels, and the Class III agents act on potassium channels. In addition, there are subclassifications within the Class I agents according to effects of the drug on conduction and refractoriness within the Purkinje and ventricular tissues. Class IA agents show moderate depression of conduction and prolongation of repolarization.

Atrial Fibrillation: Restoring and Maintaining Normal Sinus Rhythm

Pharmacologic cardioversion may be attempted in hemodynamically stable patients whose ventricular rate is controlled. If a patient has been in atrial fibrillation for ≥48 hours, anticoagulation with warfarin should be considered prior to cardioversion and for at least 4 weeks after cardioversion. Drugs recommended for pharmacologic cardioversion include amiodarone, dofetilide (must be initiated within the hospital), flecainide, or propafenone, depending upon patient's specific characteristics (eg, heart failure).

Ventricular Rate Control

It is accepted practice to treat patients with medication when the resting ventricular rate is >110 beats/minute. Non-dihydropyridine calcium channel blockers and beta-adrenergic blockers are recommended to regulate ventricular rate. Although commonly used, digoxin should be reserved for patients with concurrent heart failure. Digoxin increases the vagal tone to the AV node, non-dihydropyridine calcium channel blockers slow the AV nodal conduction, and the beta-adrenergic blocking drugs decrease the sympathetic activation of AV nodal conduction.

Anticoagulants Useful in Arrhythmias

Warfarin (Coumadin) elicits its anticoagulant effect by interfering with the hepatic synthesis of vitamin K-dependent coagulation factors II, VII, IX, and X. Although warfarin appears to be somewhat effective after myocardial infarction in preventing death or recurrent myocardial infarction, its effectiveness in the treatment of acute coronary syndrome is questionable. Combination therapy with aspirin and heparin, followed by warfarin, has resulted in reduced incidence of recurrent angina, myocardial infarction, death, or all three at 14 days, compared to aspirin alone. In contrast, another study failed to show any additional benefit in the treatment of acute coronary syndrome using a combination of aspirin and warfarin, compared to aspirin alone (Douketis 2012).

Recently, the FDA approved dabigatran (Pradaxa), rivaroxaban (Xarelto), apixaban (Eliquis), and edoxaban (Savavsa) for the prevention of stroke and systemic embolism in patients with atrial fibrillation. Dabigatran was the first FDA-approved replacement available for warfarin. Dabigatran is an anticoagulant that acts by inhibiting thrombin, an enzyme in the blood that is involved in blood clotting. Thrombin (serine protease) enables the conversion of fibrinogen to fibrin during the coagulation cascade, preventing the development of thrombus. Caution is required for patients with mild renal impairment (creatinine clearance 50 to 80 mL/minute), dosage adjustments are required for patients with moderate to severe renal impairment (creatinine clearance 15 to 50 mL/minute), and use is considered contraindicated in patients with a creatinine clearance of <15 mL/minute or those on hemodialysis. Until recently, there have been no direct reversal agents for the novel oral anticoagulant drugs. Idarucizumab (Praxbind) has been approved by the Food and Drug Administration for reversing the anticoagulant effects of dabigatran. Specifically, idarucizumab is intended for use in patients who, while taking dabigatran, require reversal of anticoagulation for emergency surgery/urgent procedures, or those experiencing life-threatening or uncontrolled bleeding. Reversal agents have their own risks and should not be considered for most, if not all planned dental procedures, and consultation with the patient's managing physician is always prudent. The other novel oral anticoagulants which inhibit Factor X (ie, apixaban, edoxaban, and rivaroxaban) do not currently have approved reversal agents available.

Dental clinicians should consider consultation with the patient's health care provider prior to invasive therapies. However, recent reviews have argued that inappropriate adjustments in anticoagulation therapy places the patient at far greater risk of stroke than hemorrhage during most dental procedures (Armstrong 2013; Douketis 2012; Jeske 2003). Therefore, scientific evidence does not support changing regimens of anticoagulation therapy in most instances.

Table 2. Antithrombotic Drugs Used to Manage Unstable Angina

Antiplatelet Drugs

Aspirin on page 177
Clopidogrel on page 390
Prasugrel on page 1252
Ticagrelor on page 1444
Ticlopidine on page 1446

Glycoprotein IIb/IIIa Receptor Antagonists:

Abciximab

Eptifibatide on page 580
Tirofiban on page 1453

Antithrombin Drugs

Indirect Thrombin Inhibitors

Heparin (unfractionated) on page 753

Low molecular weight heparins

Dalteparin on page 431
Enoxaparin on page 566
Nadroparin on page 1071

Direct Thrombin Inhibitors

Bivalirudin on page 246

Factor Xa Inhibitors

Fondaparinux on page 710

REFERENCES

Albert NM. Use of novel oral anticoagulants for patients with atrial fibrillation: systematic review and clinical implications. *Heart Lung.* 2014;43(1):48-59.

American Diabetes Association. Standards of medical care in diabetes − 2013. *Diabetes Care.* 2013;36(Suppl 1):11-66.

Amin H, Nowak RJ, Schindler JL. Cardioembolic stroke: practical considerations for patient risk management and secondary prevention. *Postgrad Med.* 2014;126(1):55-65.

Amsterdam EA, Wenger NK, Brindis RG, et al; ACC/AHA Task Force Members. 2014 AHA/ACC guideline for the management of patients with non-ST-elevation acute coronary syndromes: a report of the American College of Cardiology/American Heart Association Task Force on Practice Guidelines. *Circulation.* 2014; 130(25):e344-426.

Armstrong MJ, Gronseth G, Anderson DC, et al. Summary of evidence-based guideline: periprocedural management of antithrombotic medications in patients with ischemic cerebrovascular disease: report of the Guideline Development Subcommittee of the American Academy of Neurology. Neurology. 2013;80(22):2065-2069.

Aspirin may prevent blood clots in the legs from recurring. *Harvard Heart Lett.* 2013;23(6):8.

Brunzell JD, Davidson M, Furberg CD, et al. Lipoprotein management in patients with cardiometabolic risk: consensus statement from the American Diabetes Association and the American College of Cardiology Foundation. *Diabetes Care.* 2008;31(4):811-822.

Douketis JD. Contra: "bridging anticoagulation is needed during warfarin interruption when patients require elective surgery." *Thromb Haemost.* 2012;108(2):210-212.

Fihn SD, Blankenship JC, Alexander KP, et al. 2014 ACC/AHA/AATS/PCNA/SCAI/STS focused update of the guideline for the diagnosis and management of patients with stable ischemic heart disease: a report of the American College of Cardiology/American Heart Association Task Force on Practice Guidelines, and the American Association for Thoracic Surgery, Preventive Cardiovascular Nurses Association, Society for Cardiovascular Angiography and Interventions, and Society of Thoracic Surgeons. *Circulation.* 2014;130(19):1749-1767.

Fihn SD, Gardin JM, Abrams J, et al. 2012 ACCF/AHA/ACP/AATS/PCNA/SCAI/STS guideline for the diagnosis and management of patients with stable ischemic heart disease: a report of the American College of Cardiology Foundation/American Heart Association Task Force on Practice Guidelines, and the American College of Physicians, American Association for Thoracic Surgery, Preventive Cardiovascular Nurses Association, Society for Cardiovascular Angiography and Interventions, and Society of Thoracic Surgeons. *Circulation.* 2012;126(25):e354-e471.

Gaziano M, Ridker PM, Libby P. Primary and secondary prevention of coronary heart disease. In: Bonow RO, Mann DL, Zipes DP, Libby P, eds. *Braunwald'sHeart Disease: A Textbook of Cardiovascular Medicine.* 9th ed. Saunders; 2011:chap 49.

Heart Failure Society of America, Lindenfeld J, Albert NM, et al. HFSA 2010 comprehensive heart failure practice guideline. *J Card Fail.* 2010;16(6): e1-e194.

Jeske AH, Suchko GD; ADA Council on Scientific Affairs and Division of Science; Journal of the American Dental Association. Lack of a scientific basis for routine discontinuation of oral anticoagulation therapy before dental treatment. *J Am Dent Assoc.* 2003;134(11):1492-1497.

Lee TH, Lee RT. Ask the doctors. There is a long list of drugs and substances that interact with Coumadin (warfarin). Does this mean they make Coumadin more effective, or less effective? *Harvard Heart Lett.* 2013;24(1):2.

New alternatives to warfarin. New drugs may be best when starting treatment for atrial fibrillation, but don't switch if warfarin works for you. *Harvard Heart Lett.* 2013;24(1):4-5.

O'Gara PT, Kushner FG, Ascheim DD, et al. 2013 ACCF/AHA guideline for the management of ST-elevation myocardial infarction: a report of the American College of Cardiology Foundation/American Heart Association Task Force on Practice Guidelines. *Circulation.* 2013;127(4):e362-e425.

Skanes AC, Healey JS, Cairns JA, et al. Focused 2012 update of the Canadian Cardiovascular Society atrial fibrillation guidelines: recommendations for stroke prevention and rate/rhythm control. *Can J Cardiol.* 2012;28(2):125-136.
Smith SC Jr, Benjamin EJ, Bonow RO, et al. AHA/ACCF secondary prevention and risk reduction therapy for patients with coronary and other atherosclerotic vascular sisease: 2011 update: a guideline from the American Heart Association and American College of Cardiology Foundation. *Circulation.* 2011;124(22):2458-2473.
Stone NJ, Robinson J, Lichtenstein AH, et al. 2013 ACC/AHA guideline on the treatment of blood cholesterol to reduce atherosclerotic cardiovascular risk in adults: a report of the American College of Cardiology/American Heart Association Task Force on Practice Guidelines. *Circulation.* 2014; 129 (25 Suppl 2):S1-45.
Vandvik PO, Lincoff AM, Gore JM, et al. Primary and secondary prevention of cardiovascular disease: Antithrombotic Therapy and Prevention of Thrombosis, 9th ed: American College of Chest Physicians Evidence-Based Clinical Practice Guidelines. *Chest.* 2012;141(2 Suppl):e637S-68S.
Wann LS, Curtis AB, January CT, et al. 2011 ACCF/AHA/HRS focused update on the management of patients with atrial fibrillation (updating the 2006 guideline): a report of the American College of Cardiology Foundation/American Heart Association Task Force on Practice Guidelines. *Circulation.* 2011;123(1):104-123.
Yancy CW. ACC/AHA task force on practice guidelines. Circulation. 2013;128(16):e240e327.

HEART FAILURE

Heart failure is a condition in which the heart is unable to pump sufficient blood to meet the metabolic demand of the body. It is caused by impairment of cardiac muscle contraction or ventricular filling. Most frequently, the underlying cause of heart failure is ischemic heart disease. Other major contributory causes include hypertension, idiopathic dilated cardiomyopathy, and valvular heart disease. It is estimated that heart failure affects approximately 5 million Americans. The New York Heart Association functional classification is regarded as the standard measure to describe the severity of a patient's symptom. Class I is characterized by having no limitation of physical activity. There is no dyspnea, fatigue, palpitations, or angina with ordinary physical activity. There is no objective evidence of cardiovascular dysfunction. Class II includes those patients having slight limitation of physical activity. These patients experience fatigue, palpitations, dyspnea, or angina with ordinary physical activity, but are comfortable at rest. There is evidence of minimal cardiovascular dysfunction. Class III is characterized by marked limitation of activity. Less-than-ordinary physical activity causes fatigue, palpitations, dyspnea, or angina, but patients are comfortable at rest. There is objective evidence of moderately severe cardiovascular dysfunction. Class IV is characterized by the inability to carry out any physical activity without discomfort. Symptoms of heart failure may be present even at rest, and any physical activity undertaken increases discomfort. There is objective evidence of severe cardiovascular dysfunction. Drug classes and the specific agents used to treat heart failure are listed in Table 3.

Table 3. Drugs Used in the Treatment of Heart Failure

Angiotensin-Converting Enzyme (ACE) Inhibitors[a]

Benazepril on page 225
Captopril on page 286
Enalapril on page 560
Fosinopril on page 715
Lisinopril on page 922
Moexipril on page 1044
Perindopril Erbumine on page 1218
Quinapril on page 1298
Ramipril on page 1307
Trandolapril on page 1476

Angiotensin II Receptor Blockers

Candesartan on page 282
Losartan on page 938
Valsartan on page 1521

Diuretics

Thiazides

HydroCHLOROthiazide on page 762
Chlorothiazide on page 339

Thiazide-related

Chlorthalidone on page 343
Indapamide
MetOLazone on page 1008

Loop Diuretics

Bumetanide on page 256
Furosemide on page 721
Torsemide on page 1467

Potassium Sparing

Amiloride on page 116
Eplerenone on page 576
Spironolactone on page 1386
Triamterene on page 1493

Table 3. Drugs Used in the Treatment of Heart Failure *(continued)*

Digitalis Glycosides

Digoxin on page 498

Beta-Adrenergic Receptor Blockers

Bisoprolol on page 245

Carvedilol/Carvedilol CR on page 294

Metoprolol succinate (extended release) on page 1009

Supplemental Agents

Direct-Acting Vasodilators

HydrALAZINE

Isosorbide Dinitrate on page 845

Isosorbide Mononitrate on page 845

Nitroglycerin on page 1112

[a]Regarded as the cornerstone of heart failure treatment and should be used routinely and early in all patients.

Drug Classes and Specific Agents Used to Treat Heart Failure

Angiotensin-converting enzyme (ACE) inhibitors reduce left ventricular volume and filling pressure while decreasing total peripheral resistance. They improve cardiac output (modestly) and natriuresis. ACE inhibitors are usually used in all patients with heart failure if no contraindication or intolerance exists. This group of drugs is considered the cornerstone of treatment and is used routinely and early if pharmacologic treatment is indicated. Angiotensin receptor blockers may be used if a patient cannot tolerate an ACE inhibitor or in rare instances used with an ACE inhibitor when persistent symptoms or progressive worsening occurs despite optimal ACE inhibitor and beta-blocker therapy.

Beta-adrenergic receptor blocking drugs (beta-blockers), specifically carvedilol, bisoprolol, and metoprolol extended release, are used in the treatment of heart failure because of their beneficial effect in reducing mortality.

Diuretics increase sodium chloride and water excretion resulting in reduction of preload, thus relieving the symptoms of pulmonary congestion associated with heart failure. They may also reduce myocardial oxygen demand. The thiazides, loop diuretics, and potassium-sparing agents are all useful in reducing preload by way of their diuretic actions.

Digitalis glycosides have been used in the treatment of heart failure for >200 years. Digitalis drugs increase cardiac output by a direct positive inotropic action on the myocardium. This increased cardiac output results in decreased venous pressure, reduced heart size, and diminished compensatory tachycardia.

Other drugs used in the treatment of heart failure include aldosterone blockers and direct-acting vasodilators. Direct-acting vasodilators (hydralazine, isosorbide) may be used in place of an ACE inhibitor or angiotensin receptor blocker. The direct-acting vasodilators reduce excessive vasoconstriction and reduce workload of the failing heart. Aldosterone blockers may be used in severe forms of heart failure to enhance survival; close attention to introduction and monitoring is essential to prevent hyperkalemia.

HYPERTENSION

In the United States, almost 50 million adults 25 to 74 years of age have hypertension. Hypertension is defined as systolic blood pressure ≥140 mm Hg, and/or diastolic pressure >90 mm Hg. People with blood pressure above normal are considered at increased risk of developing damage to the heart, kidney, brain, and eyes, resulting in premature morbidity and mortality.

Hypertension is one of the most common systemic conditions seen in primary care medicine and can lead to myocardial infarction, stroke, renal failure, and death if not detected early and treated appropriately. The Eighth Joint National Committee (JNC 8) Report on Prevention, Detection, Evaluation and Treatment of High Blood Pressure convened in 2008 to begin work on revisions of the JNC 7 which had been in place since 2003. The committee used evidence based principles to determine suggested changes in how HBP is managed. Other international organizations may have slightly different guidelines but the overreaching goals are the same, ie, to recommend lifestyle modifications and pharmacologic regimens that reduce BP to levels that lower these risks. The definitions of high blood pressure have not changed.

The latest guidelines for diagnosis and intervention protocols for hypertension were released November 2017 and simplify the considerations of disease categories. The recommendations remain very detailed into nine specifics and for practicing dentists the primary changes over the JNC 7 and 8 reports relate to relaxing the treatment targets for otherwise healthy patients >60 years of age and suggesting other drugs such as angiotensin-converting enzyme inhibitors, angiotensin receptor blockers and calcium channel blockers as alternative first line therapy as alternatives in addition to thiazide-type diuretics.

The suggested initial goals of drug therapy are the maintenance of an arterial pressure of ≤140/90 mm Hg with concurrent control of other modifiable cardiovascular risk factors. Further reduction to 130/85 mm Hg should be pursued if cardiovascular and cerebrovascular function is not compromised. The Hypertension Optimal Treatment (HOT) randomized trial using patients 50 to 80 years of age found that the lowest incidence of major cardiovascular events and the lowest risk of cardiovascular mortality occurred at a mean diastolic blood pressure of 82.6 and 86.5 mm Hg, respectively. The target blood pressure for patients with diabetes or chronic kidney disease is <130/90 mm Hg.

Table 4. Classification of Blood Pressure for Adults ≥18 Years of Age

BP Classification	Systolic BP (mm Hg)		Diastolic BP (mm Hg)
Normotensive	<120	**and**	<80
Elevated[a]	120 to 129	**and**	≤80
Stage 1 hypertension[b]	130 to 139	**or**	80 to 89
Stage 2 hypertension[c]	≥140	**or**	≥90

[a]Not taking antihypertensive drugs and not acutely ill. When systolic and diastolic blood pressures fall into different categories, the higher category should be selected to classify the individual's blood pressure status. In addition to classifying stages of hypertension on the basis of average blood pressure levels, clinicians should specify presence or absence of target organ disease and additional risk factors. The specificity is important for risk classification and treatment.

[b]Optimal blood pressure with respect to cardiovascular risk is below 120/80 mm Hg. However, unusually low readings should be evaluated for clinical significance.

[c]Based on the average of two or more readings taken at each of two or more visits after an initial screening.

Table 4 adapted from: Whelton PK, Carey RM, Aronow WS, et al. 2017 ACC/AHA/AAPA/ABC/ACPM/AGS/APhA/ASH/ASPC/NMA/PCNA Guideline for the Prevention, Detection, Evaluation, and Management of High Blood Pressure in Adults: A Report of the American College of Cardiology/American Heart Association Task Force on Clinical Practice Guidelines. *J Am Coll Cardiol.* 2017;S0735-1097(17):41519-1.

Original guidelines adapted from: Weber MA, Schiffrin EL, White WB, et al. Clinical practice guidelines for the management of hypertension in the community: a statement by the American Society of Hypertension and the International Society of Hypertension. *J Clin Hypertens (Greenwich).* 2014;16 (1):14-26.

James PA, Oparil S, Carter BL, et al, 2014 evidence-based guideline for the management of high blood pressure in adults. Report from the panel members appointed to the eighth joint national committee (JNC8). *JAMA.* Published online December 18, 2013.

Hypertensive crisis: Systolic over 180 and/or diastolic over 120, with patients needing prompt changes in medication if there are no other indications of problems, or immediate hospitalization if there are signs of organ damage.

Table 5. Lifestyle Modifications to Manage Hypertension[a,b,c,j]

Modification	Recommendation	Approximate Systolic Reduction (Range)
Weight reduction	Maintain normal body weight (body mass index 18.5 to 24.9 kg/m^2)	5 to 20 mm of Hg/10 kg weight loss[d]
Adopt DASH[e] eating plan	Consume a diet rich in fruits, vegetables, and low-fat dairy products with a reduced content of saturated and total fat	8 to 14 mm Hg[f]
Dietary sodium reduction	Reduce dietary sodium intake to ≤100 mmol/day (2.4 g sodium or 6 g sodium chloride)	2 to 8 mm Hg[g]
Physical activity	Engage in regular aerobic physical activity such as brisk walking (≥30 minutes/day, most days of the week)	4 to 9 mm Hg[h]
Moderation of alcohol consumption	Limit consumption to ≤2 drinks (1 oz or 30 mL ethanol); (eg, 24 oz beer, 10 oz wine, or 3 oz 80-proof whiskey) per day in most men and to ≤1 drink/day in women and lighter weight people	2 to 4 mm Hg[i]

[a]Adapted from: US Department of Health and Human Services; National Institutes of Health; National Heart, Lung, and Blood Institute; National High Blood Pressure Education Program

[b]Overall cardiovascular risk education can be achieved by cessation of smoking

[c]The effects of implementing these modifications are dose- and time-dependent and could be greater for some people.

[d]The trials of Hypertension Prevention Collaborative Research Group; He and colleagues

[e]DASH: Dietary Approaches to Stop Hypertension

[f]Sacks and colleagues; Vollmer and colleagues

[g]Sacks and colleagues; Vollmer and colleagues; Chobanian and Hill

[h]Kelley and Kelley; Whelton and colleagues

[i]Xin and colleagues

[j]Eckel RH, Jakicic JM, Ard JD, et al. 2013 AHA/ACC guideline on lifestyle management to reduce cardiovascular risk: a report of the American College of Cardiology/American Heart Association task force on practice guidelines. *Circulation.* 2013.

Table 6. Drug Categories and Representative Agents Used in the Treatment of Hypertension[a]

Diuretics

Thiazide Types

Chlorothiazide on page 339

Chlorthalidone on page 343

HydroCHLOROthiazide on page 762

Indapamide

Methyclothiazide

MetOLazone on page 1008

Table 6. Drug Categories and Representative Agents Used in the Treatment of Hypertension[a] *(continued)*

Loops

Bumetanide on page 256
Furosemide on page 721
Torsemide on page 1467

Potassium-Sparing

AMILoride on page 116
Eplerenone on page 576
Spironolactone on page 1386
Triamterene on page 1493

Beta-Blockers

Cardioselective

Atenolol on page 189
Betaxolol (Systemic) on page 240
Bisoprolol on page 245
Metoprolol on page 1009
Nebivolol on page 1088

Noncardioselective

Nadolol on page 1070
Propranolol on page 1287
Timolol (Systemic)

Alpha-1 Blocker

Doxazosin on page 517
Prazosin on page 1254
Terazosin on page 1421

Alpha-/Beta-Blocker

Carvedilol on page 294
Labetalol on page 867

Angiotensin-Converting Enzyme (ACE) Inhibitors

Benazepril on page 225
Captopril on page 286
Enalapril on page 560
Fosinopril on page 715
Lisinopril on page 922
Moexipril on page 1044
Perindopril Erbumine on page 1218
Quinapril on page 1298
Ramipril on page 1307
Trandolapril on page 1476

Angiotensin II Receptor Blockers

Azilsartan on page 202
Candesartan on page 282
Eprosartan on page 579
Irbesartan on page 840
Losartan on page 938
Olmesartan on page 1131
Telmisartan on page 1413
Valsartan on page 1521

Renin Inhibitor

Aliskiren on page 102

Calcium Channel Blockers

AmLODIPine on page 121
DiltiaZEM on page 499
Felodipine on page 639
Isradipine on page 848
NiCARdipine on page 1100
NIFEdipine on page 1104
Nisoldipine on page 1109
Verapamil on page 1540

Table 6. Drug Categories and Representative Agents Used in the Treatment of Hypertension[a] *(continued)*

Supplemental Agents

Centrally-acting Alpha-2 Agonist

CloNIDine on page 389

GuanFACINE on page 749

Methyldopa on page 995

Direct-Acting Peripheral Vasodilator

HydrALAZINE

Minoxidil (Systemic) on page 1037

Current Thinking Regarding Antihypertensive Drug Selection

Medications in the first eight categories in Table 6 were held to be equally effective in two large-scale studies reported in the *New England Journal of Medicine* and the *Journal of the American Medical Association*, and that any of the medications could be used initially for monotherapy. The JNC 8 panel determined that there is strong evidence to support treating hypertensive persons ≥60 years of age to a BP goal of <150/90 mm Hg and hypertensive persons 30 to 59 years of age to a diastolic goal of <90 mm Hg. However, there is insufficient evidence in hypertensive persons <60 years of age for a systolic goal, or in those <30 years of age for a diastolic goal, so the panel recommends a BP of <140/90 mm Hg for those groups based on expert opinion. The same thresholds and goals are recommended for hypertensive adults with diabetes or nondiabetic chronic kidney disease (CKD) as for the general hypertensive population <60 years of age. There is moderate evidence to support initiating drug treatment with an angiotensin-converting enzyme inhibitor, angiotensin receptor blocker, calcium channel blocker, or thiazide-type diuretic in the nonblack hypertensive population, including those with diabetes. In the black hypertensive population, including those with diabetes, a calcium channel blocker or thiazide-type diuretic is recommended as initial therapy. There is moderate evidence to support initial or add-on antihypertensive therapy with an angiotensin-converting enzyme inhibitor or angiotensin receptor blocker in persons with CKD to improve kidney outcomes.

These guidelines provide evidence-based recommendations for the management of high BP and should meet the clinical needs of most patients. They are not a substitute for clinical judgment, and all clinicians' decisions about care should incorporate the clinical characteristics and co-morbidities of each individual patient.

Beta-blockers are the agents of choice in patients with coronary artery disease or supraventricular arrhythmia, and in young patients with hyperdynamic circulation. Beta-blockers are alternatives for initial therapy and are more effective in white patients than in black patients. Beta-blockers are not considered first choice drugs in elderly patients with uncomplicated hypertension. The beta-blocking drug carvedilol also selectively blocks alpha-1 receptors.

Alpha-1 adrenergic blocking agents (eg, prazosin) can be used as initial therapy in patients with benign prostatic hypertrophy (BPH).

ACE inhibitors are the preferred drugs for patients with coexisting heart failure. They are useful as initial therapy in hypertensive patients with kidney damage or diabetes mellitus with proteinuria, and in non-black patients. No clinically relevant differences have been found among the available ACE inhibitors. The ACE inhibitors are well-tolerated by young, physically active patients and elderly patients. The most common adverse effect of the ACE inhibitors is dry cough. Angiotensin II receptor blockers produce hemodynamic effects similar to ACE inhibitors while avoiding dry cough. These agents are similar to the ACE inhibitors in potency and are useful for initial therapy.

Calcium channel blocking agents are effective as initial therapy in both black and non-black patients, and are well-tolerated by elderly patients. These agents inhibit entry of calcium ion into cardiac cells and smooth muscle cells of the coronary and systemic vasculature. The dihydropyridine calcium channel blockers, nifedipine (Procardia) and amlodipine (Norvasc), are more potent as peripheral vasodilators than diltiazem (Cardizem).

Supplemental antihypertensive agents include the centrally-acting alpha-2 agonists and direct-acting vasodilators. These agents are less commonly prescribed for initial therapy because of the impressive effectiveness of the other drug groups. Clonidine (Catapres) lowers blood pressure by activating inhibitory alpha-2 receptors in the CNS, thus reducing sympathetic outflow. It lowers both supine and standing blood pressure by reducing total peripheral resistance.

The most common oral side effects of the management of the hypertensive patient are related to the antihypertensive drug therapy. A dry, sore mouth can be caused by diuretics and centrally-acting adrenergic inhibitors. Occasionally, lichenoid reactions can occur in patients taking methyldopa. The thiazides are occasionally also implicated. Lupus-like face rashes can be seen in patients taking calcium channel blockers as well.

REFERENCES

American Diabetes Association. Standards of medical care in diabetes — 2013. *Diabetes Care.* 2013;36(suppl 1):S11-S66.

Benavente OR, Coffey CS, Conwit R, et al; SPS3 Study Group. Blood-pressure targets in patients with recent lacunar stroke: the SPS3 randomised trial. *Lancet.* 2013;382(9891):507-515.

Cushman WC, Evans GW, Byington RP, et al; ACCORD Study Group. Effects of intensive blood-pressure control in type 2 diabetes mellitus. *N Engl J Med.* 2010;362(17):1575-1585.

Eckel RH, Jakicic JM, Ard JD, et al. AHA/ACC guideline on lifestyle management to reduce cardiovascular risk: a report of the American College of Cardiology/American Heart Association task force on practice guidelines. *Circulation.* 2013.

Flack JM, Sica DA, Bakris G, et al; International Society on Hypertension in Blacks. Management of high blood pressure in blacks: an update of the International Society on hypertension in blacks consensus statement. *Hypertension.* 2010;56(5):780-800.

Gibbons GH, Harold JG, Jessup M, Robertson RM, OetgenWJ. The next steps in developing clinical practice guidelines for prevention. *J AmColl Cardiol.* 2013;62(15):1399-1400.

Gibbons GH, Shurin SB, Mensah GA, Lauer MS. Refocusing the agenda on cardiovascular guidelines: an announcement from the National Heart, Lung, and Blood Institute. *Circulation.* 2013;128(15):1713-1715.

Hypertension without compelling indications: 2013 CHEP recommendations. Hypertension Canada website. http://www.hypertension.ca/hypertension-without-compelling-indications. Accessed October 30, 2013.

Institute of Medicine. Clinical Practice Guidelines We Can Trust.Washington, DC: National Academies Press; 2011. http://www.iom.edu/Reports/2011/Clinical-Practice-Guidelines-We-Can-Trust.aspx.
James PA, Oparil S, Carter BL, et al. MPH 2014 Evidence-based guideline for the management of high blood pressure in adults report from the panel members appointed to the eighth Joint National Committee (JNC 8). *JAMA*. Published online December 18, 2013.
Kidney Disease; Improving Global Outcomes (KDIGO) Blood Pressure Work Group. KDIGO clinical practice guideline for the management of blood pressure in chronic kidney disease. *Kidney Int Suppl*. 2012;2(5):337-414.
Lindenfeld J, Albert NM, Boehmer JP, et al. HFSA 2010 comprehensive heart failure practice guideline. *J Card Fail*. 2010;16(6):e1-e194.
Mancia G, Fagard R, Narkiewicz K, et al. 2013 ESH/ESC guidelines for the management of arterial hypertension: the task force for the management of arterial hypertension of the european society of hypertension (ESH) and of the european society of cardiology (ESC). *Eur Heart J*. 2013;34 (28):2159-2219.
Pickering TG, Hall JE, Appel LJ, et al. Recommendations for blood pressure measurement in humans and experimental animals: part 1: blood pressure measurement in humans: a statement for professionals from the Subcommittee of Professional and Public Education of the American Heart Association Council on High Blood Pressure Research. *Circulation*. 2005;111(5):697-716.
Verdecchia P, Staessen JA, Angeli F, et al. Cardio-Sis investigators. Usual versus tight control of systolic blood pressure in non-diabetic patients with hypertension (Cardio-Sis): an open-label randomised trial. *Lancet*. 2009;374(9689): 525-533.
Weber MA, Schiffrin EL, White WB, et al. Clinical practice guidelines for the management of hypertension in the community: a statement by the American Society of Hypertension and the International Society of Hypertension. *J Clin Hypertens (Greenwich)*. 2014;16(1):14-26.
Yancy CW, Jessup M, Bozkurt B, et al; American College of Cardiology Foundation/American Heart Association Task Force on Practice Guidelines. 2013 ACCF/AHA guideline for the management of heart failure: a report of the American College of Cardiology Foundation/American Heart Association Task Force on practice guidelines. *Circulation*. 2013;128(16):e240-e327.

CARDIOVASCULAR DISEASE IN WOMEN

American Heart Association Guidelines for Reducing Cardiovascular Risk in Women

Most cardiovascular disease (CVD) in women is preventable, according to the American Heart Association (AHA). In 1999, the AHA published a set of guidelines based on a 1997 review of the literature that described risk factor management and occurrence of CVD in women. The American College of Cardiology has a new guideline for the prevention of cardiovascular disease in women (Mosca 2011).

Cardiovascular disease is the largest single cause of death among women worldwide and accounts for one-third of all deaths. New reports have shown that in the United States, more women than men die every year of CVD.

In general the women who are at risk of CVD are those that have more than one major risk factor for CVD including:

- Cigarette smoking
- Poor diet
- Physical inactivity
- Obesity
- Family history of CVD at <55 years of age in male relative and <65 years of age in female relative
- Hypertension
- Dyslipidemia
- Evidence of subclinical vascular disease (eg, coronary calcification)
- Metabolic syndrome
- Poor exercise capacity on treadmill test
- Abnormal heart rate recovery after stopping exercise

Specific Recommendations

Aspirin:

Aspirin use in high-risk women

As a preventive drug intervention in women, aspirin therapy at a dose of 75 to 162 mg/day should be used in high-risk women unless contraindicated. High-risk women were defined as those with established coronary artery disease, cerebrovascular disease, or peripheral artery disease.

Aspirin use for other at-risk or healthy women

In women ≥65 years of age, consider aspirin therapy 81 mg/day if blood pressure is controlled and benefit for ischemic stroke and myocardial infarction (MI) prevention is likely to outweigh the risk of gastrointestinal bleeding and hemorrhagic stroke. However, the new guidelines suggested that the routine use of aspirin in healthy women <65 years of age is not recommended to prevent MI. It was noted in these new guidelines that previous guidelines by the AHA did not recommend aspirin at all in lower-risk or healthy women.

Smoking Cessation: The guidelines suggest smokers try behavioral modification programs, counseling, nicotine replacement therapy, or prescription smoking cessation medications such as bupropion (Zyban). Also, women should avoid environmental tobacco smoke.

Exercise: Women should accumulate a minimum of 30 minutes of moderate-intensity physical activity on most, and preferably all, days of the week.

Obesity and Exercise: Women who need to lose weight or sustain weight loss should accumulate a minimum of 60 to 90 minutes of moderate-intensity physical activity, such as brisk walking, on most days of the week.

Dietary Intake: Consume a diet rich in fruits and vegetables. Choose whole grain, high fiber foods. Consume fish, especially oily fish such as mackerel or salmon, at least twice a week. Limit intake of dietary saturated fat to <10% of caloric intake, cholesterol intake to <300 mg/day, sodium intake to no more than 1 teaspoonful daily, and consumption of trans-fatty acids to <1% of caloric intake.

Alcohol Consumption: Limit to no more than one drink per day. A drink is equivalent to a 12 ounce bottle of beer, a 5 ounce glass of wine, or a 1.5 ounce shot of 80 proof spirit. It does not matter what form of alcohol is consumed. In contrast to the recommendations by the AHA for moderate alcohol intake as part of the updated guidelines for heart disease prevention in women, a recent report showed that alcohol consumption increases the risk of breast cancer. One to two drinks per day increased the risk of breast cancer by 10% and excessive drinking defined as three or more drinks per day increased the risk by 30%. The researchers examined data from 70,033 women who gave health information during medical examinations during 1978 to 1985. In 2004, follow ups indicated that 2,829 of the women in the study were diagnosed with breast cancer. The study examined alcohol preferences, frequency of drinking one type of alcohol, and overall alcohol consumption. High consumption of any alcohol was linked with a significant increased risk of being diagnosed with breast cancer.

Omega-3 Fatty Acids: As an adjunct to diet, omega-3 fatty acids in capsule form (~850 to 1,000 mg of EPA [eicosapentaenoic acid] and DHA [docosahexaenoic acid] should be considered in those with coronary heart disease and for treatment of women with high triglyceride levels.

In addition, the new guidelines suggested that the following interventions were not useful and may be harmful for CVD or MI in women.

Menopausal Therapy: Hormone replacement therapy, such as Premarin and Prempro, and selective estrogen-receptor modulators (SERMs), such as raloxifene (Evista), should not be used for the primary prevention or secondary prevention of CVD.

Antioxidant Supplements: Antioxidant vitamin supplements such as vitamin E, C, or beta-carotene should not be used for the primary or secondary prevention of CVD.

Folic Acid: Folic acid, with or without vitamin B_6 and B_{12} supplementation, should not be used for the primary or secondary prevention of CVD.

REFERENCES

Bushnell C, McCullough LD, Awad IA, et al. American Heart Association Stroke Council; Council on Cardiovascular and Stroke Nursing; Council on Clinical Cardiology; Council on Epidemiology and Prevention; Council for High Blood Pressure Research. Guidelines for the prevention of stroke in women: a statement for healthcare professionals from the American Heart Association/American Stroke Association. *Stroke*. 2014; 45 (5):1545-1588.

Mehta LS, Beckie TM, DeVon HA, et al. American Heart Association Cardiovascular Disease in Women and Special Populations Committee of the Council on Clinical Cardiology, Council on Epidemiology and Prevention, Council on Cardiovascular and Stroke Nursing, and Council on Quality of Care and Outcomes Research. Acute myocardial infarction in women: a scientific statement from the American Heart Association. *Circulation*. 2016; 133(9):916-947.

Mosca L, Benjamin EJ, Berra K, et al. Effectiveness-based guidelines for the prevention of cardiovascular disease in women – 2011 update: a guideline from the American Heart Association. *J Am Coll Cardiol*. 2011;57(12):1404-1423. Available at http://circ.ahajournals.org/content/123/11/1243.full.pdf

Mosca L, Linfante AH, Benjamin EJ, et al. National study of physician awareness and adherence to cardiovascular disease prevention guidelines. *Circulation*. 2005;111(4):499-510.

ANTIPLATELET AND ANTICOAGULATION CONSIDERATIONS IN DENTISTRY

Over the last 30 years, there has been an increasing use of drugs that relate to the clotting mechanisms in patients, providing a greater number of agents for prevention and management of thromboembolic disease. These drugs have included the widespread use of aspirin, as well as an increasing use of anticoagulants found in warfarin and synthetic drugs that also have anticoagulation effects. Many patients with ischemic heart disease, atherosclerosis, atrial fibrillation, cerebrovascular disease, and in patients at high risk for stroke, we find the increased use of these anticoagulants. Large numbers of these patients are receiving oral anticoagulation therapy as outpatients. In clinical routine, the number of patients receiving antiplatelet therapy and new oral anticoagulants (NOACs) therapy is increasing. Data suggest that NOACs offer benefit in ischemic events when used concomitantly with a single antiplatelet regimen. The dental clinician is often faced with the decision as to how to manage these patients prior to dental procedures. Key factors regarding the patient receiving any form of anticoagulation therapy include:

- Is the surgery urgent or elective?
- Can the procedure be done safely without discontinuing the drug?
- Does the patient understand the nature of the dental procedure and the risks associated with continuing or discontinuing the drug?
- What degree of risk are the patient and the provider willing to accept?
- Is the patient on a single antiplatelet drug or on combination therapy with another drug?
- What is the thromboembolic risk for this patient?
- What is the bleeding risk of the dental procedure planned?
- If an invasive procedure is planned in the face of a high thromboembolic risk, what is the managing physician's opinion on altering the dosage of anticoagulation therapy?

Often, in order to determine these factors, consultation with a patient's physician is necessary. However, recent reviews have argued that inappropriate adjustments in anticoagulation therapy create far greater risk for the patient than the risk of hemorrhage during most dental procedures (Jeske 2003 and others in the reference list). Therefore, the scientific evidence does not support changing regimens of anticoagulation therapy in most instances. This decision can only be determined by weighing the factors described above and discussing the situation with the patient's physician.

Antiplatelet Drugs Used in Cardiovascular Diseases

Aspirin reduces platelet aggregation by blocking platelet cyclo-oxygenase through irreversible acetylation. This action prevents the formation of thromboxane A_2. A number of studies have confirmed that aspirin reduces the risk of death from cardiac causes and fatal and nonfatal myocardial infarction by ~50% to 70% in patients presenting with unstable angina (see Aspirin Alert Update for Dentistry at the end of this chapter).

Clopidogrel (Plavix) inhibits platelet aggregation by affecting the ADP-dependent activation of the glycoprotein IIb/IIIa complex. Clopidogrel is chemically related to ticlopidine but has fewer side effects.

Prasugrel is a prodrug and has no biological activity but is metabolized in the body to an active molecule exhibiting antiplatelet action. The active compound irreversibly blocks P2Y12 component of adenosine diphosphate (ADP) receptors on the platelet for their lifespan, inhibiting activation and decreasing subsequent platelet aggregation. Normal platelet aggregation returns only when new platelets are produced (5 to 9 days after discontinuation of prasugrel).

Ticagrelor (Brilinta) is also a newly released platelet aggregation inhibitor similar to clopidogrel produced by AstraZeneca. Ticagrelor is used along with low-dose aspirin to help prevent myocardial infarction and stroke in people with unstable angina or previous heart attack. It may also be used to prevent heart attack or stroke after certain cardiac surgeries (eg, stent placement, coronary artery bypass graft-CABG, or angioplasty). Trade names include Brilinta, Brilique, Possia. Ticagrelor and its major metabolite reversibly interacts with the platelet $P2Y_{12}$ ADP-receptor to prevent signal transduction and platelet activation.

Platelet Glycoprotein IIb / IIIa Receptor Antagonists

Antagonists of glycoprotein IIb/IIIa, a receptor on the platelet for adhesive proteins, inhibit the final common pathway involved in adhesion, activation, and aggregation. Presently, there exist three classes of inhibitors. One class is murine-human chimeric antibodies of which abciximab is the prototype. The other two classes are the synthetic peptide forms (eg, eptifibatide) and the synthetic nonpeptide forms (eg, tirofiban). These agents, in combination with heparin and aspirin, have been used to treat unstable angina, significantly reducing the incidence of death or myocardial infarction.

Antithrombin Drugs

Unfractionated heparin, in combination with aspirin, has often been used to treat unstable angina. Unfractionated heparin consists of polysaccharide chains which bind to antithrombin III, causing a conformational change that accelerates the inhibition of thrombin and factor Xa. Unfractionated heparin is therefore an indirect thrombin inhibitor. Unfractionated heparin can only be administered intravenously. Low-molecular-weight heparins (LMWH) have a more predictable pharmacokinetic profile than unfractionated heparin and can be administered subcutaneously. These heparins have a mechanism of action and use similar to unfractionated heparin.

The direct thrombin inhibitors decrease thrombin activity in a manner independent of any actions on antithrombin III. Argatroban is a direct antithrombin that is highly specific. It binds directly to thrombin (circulating and clot bound) and inhibits thrombogenic activity.

Until recently there have been no direct reversal agents for the novel new anticoagulation drugs. Idarucizumab has been approved by the Food and Drug Administration for reversing the effects of dabigatran, a novel oral anticoagulant. Specifically, idarucizumab (Praxbind) is intended for use in patients who are taking dabigatran (Pradaxa) during emergency situations when there is a need to reverse its blood-thinning effects. Both drugs are marketed by Boehringer Ingelheim. The other novel anticoagulants are edoxaban (Lixiana, Savaysa), rivaroxaban (Xarelto), betrixaban (Bevyxxa), and apixaban (Eliquis), that inhibit factor Xa (see table below), but there are very few reversal agents available for the direct oral anticoagulants (DOACs). In general most dental procedures do not warrant the use of reversal agents and clinicians are advised to consult with the prescribing physician prior to these considerations. Terminology regarding these agents can be confusing and includes DOACs, target-specific oral anticoagulants, oral direct inhibitors, and NOACs, which stands for "novel oral anticoagulants," "new(er) oral anticoagulants," and "non-vitamin K antagonist oral anti-coagulants". All of these are excreted, at least in part renally, and can be problematic in patients with renal impairment.

A variety of anticoagulant strategies targeting other steps in coagulation are in development for prophylaxis or treatment of venous thromboembolism.

Factor XIa inhibitors:

Osocimab - Osocimab is a monoclonal antibody that binds adjacent to the active site of factor XIa and prevents it from activating factor IX (allosteric inhibition).

Antisense – A factor XI antisense oligonucleotide has been developed to reduce factor XI to undetectable levels.

Synthetic heparin-like small molecule – Sulfated chiro-inositol (SCI) is a synthetic molecule similar to heparin that binds to and alters the conformation of factor XIa, reducing its enzymatic activity (allosteric inhibition). Preclinical testing suggests that this molecule could be effective as an anticoagulant and could be reversed by protamine sulfate.

Tissue factor pathway inhibitors – The recombinant form of tissue factor pathway inhibitor, the physiologic inhibitor of the TF/FVIIa complex, is being tested; specific TF/FVIIa and factor VIIa inhibitors (eg, nematode anticoagulant protein) are also in development.

Factor VIII inhibitor – TB-402 is a human IgG4 monoclonal antibody that partially inhibits factor VIII. As a result of its long half-life (approximately three weeks), this agent may provide a prolonged antithrombotic effect after a single dose.

Thrombomodulin – When thrombin binds to thrombomodulin on the endothelial cell surface, it is converted from a procoagulant enzyme into an anticoagulant enzyme by its ability to activate protein C.

Factor IXa inhibitor – REG1 consists of pegnivacogin (RB006), an injectable RNA aptamer that specifically binds and inhibits factor IXa, and anivamersen (RB007), the complementary oligonucleotide that neutralizes its anti-IXa activity if and when needed (ie, as an antidote). Initial tests of this agent combined with antiplatelet therapy in patients with coronary artery disease appeared promising [133,134]. However, a randomized trial comparing REG1 with bivalirudin in patients undergoing percutaneous coronary intervention was terminated early, after enrollment of 3,232 patients, due to severe allergic reactions with REG1 in 10 of 1,616 patients (1%), compared with 1 of 1,616 patients (0.1%) given bivalirudin [135]. REG1 was associated with reduced stent thrombosis and increased bleeding relative to bivalirudin, but a primary composite endpoint of death, myocardial infarction, stroke, and unplanned revascularization was similar between the two groups.

Factor XIIa inhibitor – The selective factor XIIa inhibitor rHA-Infestin-4 (recombinant human albumin fused to the factor XIIa inhibitor Infestin-4) is highly active in human plasma and profoundly protects mice and rats from pathologic thrombus formation while not affecting hemostasis. This agent is being considered for the prevention and treatment of acute ischemic cardiovascular and cerebrovascular events in humans.

Protein disulfide isomerase inhibitors – Protein disulfide isomerase is an oxidoreductase enzyme that catalyzes redox protein folding in newly synthesized proteins in the endoplasmic reticulum, including coagulation factor XI and tissue factor.

Polyphosphate inhibitors – Polyphosphate (released from platelets upon their activation or from a microbial source) may initiate and/or accelerate coagulation via intrinsic pathway clotting factors. A variety of compounds that inhibit polyphosphate and reduce thrombosis in preclinical models are under investigation.

Warfarin (Coumadin) elicits its anticoagulant effect by interfering with the hepatic synthesis of vitamin K-dependent coagulation factors II, VII, IX, and X. Although warfarin appears to be somewhat effective after myocardial infarction in preventing death or recurrent myocardial infarction, its effectiveness in the treatment of acute coronary syndrome is questionable. Combination therapy with aspirin and heparin, followed by warfarin, has resulted in reduced incidence of recurrent angina, myocardial infarction, death, or all three at 14 days as compared with aspirin alone. In contrast, another study failed to show any additional benefit in the treatment of acute coronary syndrome using a combination of aspirin and warfarin compared to aspirin alone.

Recently, the FDA approved Dabigatran (Pradaxa) for the prevention of stroke and systemic embolism in patients with atrial fibrillation. Dabigatran is the first FDA-approved replacement available for warfarin. Dabigatran is an anticoagulant that acts by inhibiting thrombin, an enzyme in the blood that is involved in blood clotting. Thrombin (serine protease) enables the conversion of fibrinogen to fibrin during the coagulation cascade preventing the development of thrombus. The recommended oral dose is 150 mg twice daily for patients with a creatinine clearance >30 mL/minute. For patients with a creatinine clearance 15 to 30 mL/minute, the recommended oral dose is 75 mg twice daily.

It is quite common for a patient to be taking both warfarin and low-molecular-weight heparins, such as Dalteparin (Fragmin) or Enoxaparin (Lovenox). Low-molecular-weight heparins begin working right away, while warfarin does not. In fact, in the short period of time when a patient first begins taking warfarin, the drug may actually increase the risk of clots. Therefore, warfarin and low-molecular-weight heparins are often taken together. The low-molecular-weight heparins prevent clots while the warfarin begins working. The low-molecular-weight heparins can be stopped once the INR is in the appropriate range.

A similar situation sometimes occurs in patients who have been taking warfarin for a while. If a PT/INR test shows that the patient is at a high risk for clots, a health care provider may recommend using low-molecular-weight heparins as a "bridge therapy" while the warfarin dose is being adjusted. The aPTT is the appropriate test to evaluate the effects of heparin. Bridging guidelines and their application in dental surgery must be discussed with the health care provider on a case-by-case basis.

Dental clinicians should consider consultation with patient's health care provider prior to invasive therapies. However, adjustments in anticoagulation therapy may place the patient at greater risk of stroke than hemorrhage during most dental procedures (Douketis 2012; Jeske 2003). Therefore, scientific evidence does not support changing regimens of anticoagulation therapy in most instances. Given the minimal bleeding risks, stroke patients undergoing dental procedures should routinely continue warfarin (Armstrong 2013).

Evaluating Antiplatelet Response

Partial thromboplastin time and bleeding time (IVY) are appropriate measures for platelet dysfunction. Aspirin, clopidogrel (Plavix), ticagrelor (Brilinta), prasugrel (Effient), and other drugs, such as ticlopidine (Ticlid) are considered antiplatelet drugs, whereas oral Coumadin is considered an oral anticoagulant. Aspirin works by inhibiting cyclo-oxygenase which is an enzyme involved in the platelet system associated with clot formation. As little as one aspirin (300 mg dose) can result in an alteration in this enzyme pathway. Although aspirin is cleared from the circulation very quickly (within 15 to 30 minutes), the effect on the life of the platelet may last up to 7 to 10 days. Most routine dental procedures can be accomplished with no change in these medications using aggressive local hemostasis efforts and prudent treatment planning. The benefit of stroke prevention outweighs the risk of bleeding during most dental treatment. Specifically, the American Academy of Neurology recommends that patients taking aspirin for ischemic stroke prevention continue the aspirin therapy when undergoing any dental procedure (Armstrong 2013).

Evaluating Coumadin Response

The effects of Coumadin on the coagulation within patients occur by way of the vitamin K-dependent clotting mechanism and are generally monitored by measuring the prothrombin time known as the PT. Often, to prevent venous thrombosis, a patient will be maintained at ~2.5 times their normal prothrombin time. Other anticoagulant goals, such as prevention of arterial thromboembolism as in patients with artificial heart valves, may require 2.5 to 3.5 times the normal prothrombin time. It is important for the clinician to obtain the International Normalized Ratio (INR) for the patient. This ratio is calculated by dividing the patient's PT by the mean normal PT for the laboratory, which is determined by using the International Sensitivity Index (ISI) to adjust for the lab's reagents.

The response to oral anticoagulants varies greatly in patients and should be monitored regularly. The dental clinician planning an invasive procedure should consider not only what the patient can tell them from a historical point-of-view, but also when the last monitoring test was performed. In general, all dental procedures can be performed in patients that are 3 times normal or less. Most researchers further suggest that even less than 4 times normal pose little risk in most dental patients and procedures, but these values may be misleading unless the INR is also determined at a time close to the actual planned dental procedure. When in doubt, the prudent dental clinician will consult with the patient's physician and obtain current prothrombin time and INR in order to evaluate fully and plan for his patients.

At recommended therapeutic doses, dabigatran (Pradaxa) prolongs the activated partial thromboplastin time (aPTT). For an oral dose of 150 mg twice daily, the median peak aPTT is approximately twice that of control values. Twelve hours after the last dose, the median aPTT is 1.5 times the control values. The INR test is relatively insensitive to the activity of dabigatran and may not be elevated in patients on this medication.

Regarding dental management patients that are already taking warfarin, the use of analgesics is implicated as a potential source of drug interaction. Hayek, in *JAMA*, found that patients taking warfarin had dangerously elevated INRs and were taking acetaminophen (not necessarily with their physician's recommendation). Additional factors independently influence the INR, as well as a potential interaction with acetaminophen. Effects on the INR are greatest in patients taking acetaminophen at high doses over a protracted time period. Short-term pain management with acetaminophen poses little risk. Other factors influencing INR include advanced malignancy, patients who did not take their warfarin properly (therefore, took more than was necessary), changes in oral intake of liquids or solids, acute diarrhea leading to dehydration, alcohol consumption, and vitamin K intake.

The mechanisms of these augmenting factors for enhancement of the INR are that the cytochrome P450 system is also affected by changes in metabolism associated with these factors. For instance, the metabolism of alcohol in the liver alters its ability to manage the CYP450 enzyme system necessary for warfarin; therefore, enhancing its presence and potentially increasing the half-life of warfarin As oral intake of nutrients declines in patients with either diarrhea or reduced intake of liquids and/or solids, absorption of vitamin K is reduced and the vitamin K-dependent system of metabolism of warfarin changes, therefore increases warfarin blood levels. These factors, along with the liver metabolism of acetaminophen, have resulted in the increased concern that patients, who may be taking acetaminophen as an analgesic or for other reasons, may be at risk for enhancing or elevating, inadvertently, their anticoagulation effect of warfarin. The dentist should be aware of these potential interactions in prescribing any drug containing acetaminophen or in recommending that a patient use an analgesic for relief of even mild pain on a prolonged basis.

Acetaminophen on page 59

It should also be noted that as we learn more about herbal and nutritional supplements, we will find that some of these products have effects on coagulation. Patients sometimes do not include this information in their normal history and it is important for the practitioner to delve into all types of over-the-counter, as well as prescription drugs, that the patient may be taking.

Although not used specifically for this purpose, numerous herbal medicines and natural dietary supplements have been associated with inhibition of platelet aggregation or other anticoagulation effects, and therefore may lead to increased bleeding during invasive dental procedures. Current reports include bilberry, bromelain, cat's claw, devil's claw, dong quai, evening primrose, feverfew, garlic (irreversible inhibition), ginger (only at very high doses), ginkgo biloba, ginseng, grape seed, green tea, horse chestnut, and turmeric.

ASPIRIN ALERT UPDATE FOR DENTISTRY

There are three special alerts provided by the FDA of clinical importance relative to the aspirin patient:

Special Alert 1: Sudden aspirin discontinuation may elevate the risk of myocardial infarction

It was reported in 2004 by Collett et al, that patients with acute coronary syndrome (ACS) who discontinued aspirin use had worse short-term outcomes than individuals not previously on aspirin therapy. Fischer et al, have also reported similar findings and have suggested that discontinuation of aspirin by daily aspirin users may increase the risk of myocardial infarction. A Harvard Health Letter in 2005 also stated that quitting aspirin "cold turkey" could be dangerous and studies have linked aspirin withdrawal to heart attacks.

A more recent review updated the risks associated with discontinuing aspirin antiplatelet therapy and the bleeding risks associated with continuing aspirin during surgical procedures (Lordkipanidze 2009). The article review confirmed the possibility of a pharmacological rebound phenomenon which could lead to adverse ischemic events and supports the warning against premature discontinuation of aspirin issued previously. An analysis of data obtained from 50,279 patients, reported that the increased risk of major adverse cardiac events attributed to aspirin withdrawal/nonadherence was approximately threefold (Biondi-Zoccai 2006).

Special Alert 2: Ibuprofen may interfere with aspirin's cardioprotection

In a statement released on September 8, 2006, the Food and Drug Administration (FDA) notified consumers and health care professionals that the administration of ibuprofen for pain relief to patients taking aspirin for cardioprotection may interfere with aspirin's cardiovascular benefits. The report stated that ibuprofen can interfere with the antiplatelet effect of low-dose aspirin (81 mg daily). This could result in diminished effectiveness of aspirin as used for cardioprotection and stroke prevention. The FDA added that although ibuprofen and aspirin can be taken together, it is recommended that consumers talk with their health care providers for additional information.

Special Alert 3: Strong advisory warning against the discontinuation of dual aspirin and clopidogrel (Plavix) antiplatelet therapy in patients with coronary artery stents

Aspirin and clopidogrel (Plavix) in combination is the primary prevention strategy against stent thrombosis after placement of drug-eluting metal stents in coronary patients (Grines 2007). Premature discontinuation of this drug combination strongly increases the risk of a catastrophic event of stent thrombosis leading to myocardial infarction and/or death (Grines 2007). Discontinuation of Brilinta will increase the risk of MI, stroke, and death. When possible, interrupt therapy with Brilinta for 5 days prior to surgery that has a major risk of bleeding. If Brilinta must be temporarily discontinued, restart as soon as possible.

The AHA stresses a 12-month therapy of aspirin and Plavix combination after placement of a drug-eluting stent in order to prevent thrombosis at the stent site. The AHA also stresses educating both the patient and the health care provider about the hazards of premature antiplatelet drug discontinuation. Any elective surgery should be postponed for 1 year after stent implantation, and if surgery must be performed, consideration should be given to continuing the antiplatelet therapy during the perioperative period in high risk patients with drug-eluting stents.

The recommendations from the AHA advisory panel were summarized for the dental professional according to the following:

> Dental professionals and other health care providers who perform invasive or surgical procedures and are concerned about periprocedural and postoperative bleeding must be made aware of the potential catastrophic risks of premature discontinuation of dual antiplatelet (aspirin, Plavix, or drugs like Brilinta) therapy. The dental professional should contact the patient's cardiologist if issues regarding the patient's antiplatelet therapy are unclear, in order to discuss optimal patient management strategy.
>
> Elective procedures for which there is significant risk of perioperative or postoperative bleeding should be deferred until patients have completed an appropriate course of dual antiplatelet therapy. The course of this therapy is suggested as 12 months after drug-eluting stent implantation if patient is not at high risk of bleeding.

Agents Useful to Aid in Hemostasis During or Prior to Perioperative Bleeding

Aluminum Chloride
Aminocaproic Acid on page 116
Cellulose (Oxidized Regenerated) on page 320
Collagen (Absorbable/Dental) on page 408
Collagen Hemostat on page 410
Fibrin Sealant on page 667
Gelatin (Absorbable) on page 731
Thrombin (Topical) on page 1440
Tranexamic Acid on page 1478

Hemostatic agents inhibit the activation of plasminogen to plasmin, producing antifibrinolytic activity. These agents have been used systemically and locally for treatment and prevention of various bleeding disorders. The oral mucosa tissues are rich in plasminogen activators, making hemostatic agents potentially effective for controlling oral bleeding. Although many hemostatic agents are available, only tranexamic acid and epsilon aminocaproic acid can be prepared and used as mouthwashes. Tranexamic acid is available as an intravenous injection (100 mg/mL). Aminocaproic acid is available as a 500 mg tablet, an injectable solution (250 mg/mL), and a raspberry-flavored oral syrup (250 mg/mL). A potentially critical difference between these drugs is that tranexamic acid is 6 to 10 times more potent that aminocaproic acid, as show in both in vitro and in vivo assays. Neither agent is commercially available as a mouthwash. The EACA oral syrup is most readily usable as a mouthwash; however, due to cost the tablet is usually compounded to form a mouthwash. In addition, the solution for injection may be diluted with sterile water and used as a mouthwash. To ensure stability and sterility, this is commonly prepared the day of surgery. The adverse effects of these agents are dose dependent and generally manifest as nausea, vomiting, abdominal pain, and diarrhea. Theoretically, adverse effects are more likely to occur with systemic use than with local use.

Clinicians managing antithrombotic medications periprocedurally must weigh bleeding risks from drug continuation against thromboembolic risks from discontinuation or interruption in therapy. Data suggesting specific stopping and restarting times are based on drug metabolism, half-life, and excretion rates and may apply to extensive surgical procedures, but most dental manipulations are not in this category. There is a lack of scientific basis for routine discontinuation of oral anticoagulation or antiplatelet therapy before dental treatment. Dental therapy for patients with medical conditions requiring anticoagulation or antiplatelet therapy must provide for potential excess bleeding with local measures and/or appropriate reversal agents as described. Routine discontinuation of these drugs before dental care, however, can place patients at unnecessary medical risk for thromboembolic events and therefore, any changes in anticoagulant therapy must be undertaken in collaboration with the patient's prescribing physician.

Oral Anticoagulant Comparison Chart

Medication	Mechanism of Action	Metabolism	Monitoring Parameters	Pharmacotherapy Pearls	Reversal Strategies[a]
Warfarin	Inhibits formation of vitamin K-dependent clotting factors II, VII, IX, X, and proteins C and S	CYP2C9 CYP1A2 CYP3A4 CYP2C19	PT/INR (individualized; depends on INR stability)	CYP1A2, 3A4, 2C9, and 2C19 drug interactions and vitamin K-containing food interactions Full therapeutic effect usually seen within 5 to 7 days Half-life is ~40 hours	Vitamin K (route and dose will depend on clinical situation and INR) For major bleeding at any INR: Consider inactivated 4-factor PCC + IV vitamin K; if inactivated 4-factor PCC not available, consider 3-factor PCC + IV vitamin K ± FFP
Dabigatran Etexilate (Pradaxa)	Directly inhibits thrombin	Hepatic glucuronidation P-gp substrate	Renal function Routine lab monitoring for extent of anticoagulation not required aPTT, ECA, ECT (if available), TT (most sensitive) may be used to detect the presence of dabigatran	Compliance (BID dosing) Do not open capsules Renal dosing adjustment required; per ACCP guideline, contraindicated with CrCl ≤30 mL/minute Use with caution in patients ≥80 years of age Dose reduction or avoidance required if used with P-gp inhibitors Avoid concurrent use of P-gp inducers when possible Specific conversions to/from warfarin, parenteral anticoagulants Half-life is 12 to 17 hours; prolonged with severe renal impairment	For major bleeding: IdaruCIZUmab If idarucizumab is not available, may consider activated 4-Factor PCC (eg, FEIBA) Always use supportive measures (eg, activated charcoal [if ingestion is within 2 hours], antifibrinolytic agent) ~60% dialyzable – hemodialysis may be considered in addition to other supportive measures
Apixaban (Eliquis)	Directly inhibits factor Xa	CYP3A4 P-gp substrate	Renal and hepatic function Routine lab monitoring for extent of anticoagulation not required Antifactor Xa assay is ideal for excluding the presence of apixaban. Prolonged PT suggests presence of apixaban, but normal PT and aPTT values cannot exclude presence of apixaban.	Compliance (BID dosing) Renal dosing adjustment required for NVAF if 2 of the 3 criteria are met: Age >80 years old, weight <60 kg, SCr >1.5 mg/dL Not recommended in patients with severe hepatic impairment CYP3A4 and P-gp drug interactions Specific conversions to/from warfarin, parenteral anticoagulants Half-life is ~8 to 15 hours; slightly prolonged with renal impairment	For major bleeding: Andexanet alfa[b] If andexanet alfa is not available, may consider inactivated 4-factor PCC or activated 4-factor PCC (ie, FEIBA) Always use supportive measures (eg, activated charcoal [if ingestion is within 2 hours], antifibrinolytic agent) **Not** dialyzable
Betrixaban (Bevyxxa)	Directly inhibits factor Xa	Minimal CYP-independent hydrolysis P-gp substrate	Renal and hepatic function Routine lab monitoring for extent of anticoagulation not required	Administer with food Renal dosing adjustment required Avoid use in moderate and severe hepatic impairment P-gp drug interactions; dose reduction required if used with P-gp inhibitors. Avoid use with P-gp inducers.	For major bleeding: Andexanet alfa[b] If andexanet alfa is not available, may consider inactivated 4-factor PCC or activated 4-factor PCC (ie, FEIBA) Always use supportive measures (eg, activated charcoal [if ingestion is within 2 hours], antifibrinolytic agent)

Oral Anticoagulant Comparison Chart *(continued)*

Medication	Mechanism of Action	Metabolism	Monitoring Parameters	Pharmacotherapy Pearls	Reversal Strategies[a]
Edoxaban (Savaysa)	Directly inhibits factor Xa	CYP3A4 (minor) Hydrolysis (minimal) P-gp substrate	Renal and hepatic function Routine lab monitoring for extent of anticoagulation not required Antifactor Xa assay is ideal for excluding the presence of edoxaban. Prolonged PT suggests presence of edoxaban, but normal PT and aPTT values cannot exclude presence of edoxaban, unless highly sensitive reagents are used.	DVT/PE: Dose reduction necessary for patients <60 kg, concomitant P-gp inhibitor, or if CrCl 15 to 50 mL/minute. Not recommended if CrCl <15 mL/minute NVAF: **Do not use if CrCl >95 mL/minute.** Dose reduction necessary if CrCl 15 to 50 mL/minute. Not recommended if CrCl <15 mL/minute Avoid use in moderate and severe hepatic impairment CYP3A4 and P-gp drug interactions Specific conversions to/from warfarin, parenteral anticoagulants	For major bleeding: Andexanet alfa[b] If andexanet alfa is not available, may consider inactivated 4-factor PCC or activated 4-factor PCC (ie, FEIBA) Always use supportive measures (eg, activated charcoal [if ingestion is within 2 hours], antifibrinolytic agent) **Not** dialyzable
Rivaroxaban (Xarelto)	Directly inhibits factor Xa	CYP3A4 CYP3A5 CYP2J2 P-gp substrate	Renal and hepatic function Routine lab monitoring for extent of anticoagulation not required; Antifactor Xa assay is ideal for excluding the presence of rivaroxaban. Prolonged PT suggests presence of rivaroxaban, but normal PT and aPTT values cannot exclude presence of rivaroxaban, unless highly sensitive reagents are used.	Administer doses ≥15 mg/day with food Dosing frequency depends on indication Renal dosing adjustment required Avoid in moderate or severe hepatic impairment CYP3A4 and P-gp drug interactions Specific conversions to/from warfarin, parenteral anticoagulants Half-life is 5 to 9 hours; slightly prolonged with renal impairment	For major bleeding: Andexanet alfa If andexanet alfa is not available, may consider inactivated 4-factor PCC or activated 4-factor PCC (ie, FEIBA) Always use supportive measures (eg, activated charcoal [if ingestion is within 2 hours], antifibrinolytic agent) **Not** dialyzable

Abbreviations: ACCP = American College of Chest Physicians, AHA/ASA = American Heart Association/American Stroke Association, aPTT = activated partial thromboplastin time, BID = twice daily, DVT = deep venous thrombosis, ECA = ecarin chromogenic assay, ECT = ecarin clotting time, FFP = fresh frozen plasma, INR = international normalized ratio, NVAF = nonvalvular atrial fibrillation, PCC = prothrombin complex concentrate, PE = pulmonary embolism, P-gp = P-glycoprotein, PT = prothrombin time, TT = thrombin time

[a]Management of anticoagulant-associated bleeding requires careful consideration of the indication for anticoagulant therapy and extent of bleeding (eg, epistaxis vs intracranial hemorrhage); minor bleeding may only require local hemostasis.

[b]Andexanet has not been demonstrated to reverse the anticoagulant effects of betrixaban or edoxaban in humans; however, since both are factor-Xa inhibitors similar to apixaban and rivaroxaban, it is likely that andexanet will be effective for betrixaban and edoxaban.

Armstrong MJ, Gronseth G, Anderson DC, et al. Summary of evidence-based guideline: periprocedural management of antithrombotic medications in patients with ischemic cerebrovascular disease: report of the Guideline Development Subcommittee of the American Academy of Neurology. *Neurology.* 2013;80(22):2065-2069. doi:10.1212/WNL.0b013e318294b32d

Cuker A, Burnett A, Triller D, et al. Reversal of direct oral anticoagulants: Guidance from the Anticoagulation Forum. *Am J Hematol.* 2019;94(6):697-709. doi:10.1002/ajh.25475

Doherty JU, Gluckman TJ, Hucker WJ, et al. 2017 ACC expert consensus decision pathway for periprocedural management of anticoagulation in patients with nonvalvular atrial fibrillation: a report of the American College of Cardiology Clinical Expert Consensus Document Task Force. *J Am Coll Cardiol.* 2017;69(7):871-898. doi:10.1016/j.jacc.2016.11.024

Furie KL, Goldstein LB, Albers GW, et al. Oral antithrombotic agents for the prevention of stroke in nonvalvular atrial fibrillation: a science advisory for health care professionals from the American Heart Association/American Stroke Association. *Stroke.* 2012;43(12):3442-3453.

Guyatt GH, Akl EA, Crowther M, et al. Executive summary: antithrombotic therapy and prevention of thrombosis, 9th ed: American College of Chest Physicians evidence-based clinical practice guidelines. *Chest.* 2012;141(2 Suppl):7S-47S.

Tomaselli GF, Mahaffey KW, Cuker A, et al. 2017 ACC expert consensus decision pathway on management of bleeding in patients on oral anticoagulants: a report of the American College of Cardiology Task Force on Expert Consensus Decision Pathways. *J Am Coll Cardiol.* 2017;70(24):3042-3067.

Content adapted from Lexi-Drugs monographs

Oral Antiplatelet Comparison Chart

Medication	Mechanism of Action	Reversible Platelet Inhibition	Prodrug	Metabolism	Pharmacotherapy Pearls	Reversal Strategies[a]
Aspirin	Inhibits cyclooxygenase-1 and 2	No	No	CYP2C9	Chronic NSAID use can compromise antiplatelet effects Monitor for GI ulceration	No specific antidote Consider platelet transfusion ± DDAVP Normal platelet function returns within 7 to 10 days after discontinuation
Cilostazol (Pletal)	Inhibits platelet phosphodiesterase III	Yes	No	CYP3A4 CYP2C19 CYP1A2 CYP2D6	Administer before or 2 hours after meals Contraindicated in patients with heart failure of any severity CYP3A4 and 2C19 drug interactions	No specific antidote Normal platelet function returns within 4 days after discontinuation
Clopidogrel (Plavix)	Inhibits $P2Y_{12}$ component of ADP receptors	No	Yes	CYP2C19 CYP3A4	CYP2C19 inhibitors may reduce concentrations of active metabolite CYP2C19 polymorphisms may affect clopidogrel efficacy	No specific antidote Consider platelet transfusion ± DDAVP Normal platelet function returns within 7 to 10 days after discontinuation
Prasugrel (Effient)	Inhibits $P2Y_{12}$ component of ADP receptors	No	Yes	CYP3A4 CYP2B6	Reduce maintenance dose to 5 mg in patients <60 kg Contraindicated in patients with history of stroke, TIA Not recommended in patients ≥75 years of age	No specific antidote Consider platelet transfusion ± DDAVP Normal platelet function returns within 5 to 9 days after discontinuation
Ticagrelor (Brilinta)	Inhibits $P2Y_{12}$ component of ADP receptors	Yes	No	CYP3A4 CYP3A5	Used in combination with aspirin; daily maintenance aspirin dose should not exceed 81 mg CYP3A4 drug interactions BID dosing Monitor closely for dyspnea, bradyarrhythmia (including ventricular pauses)	No specific antidote Consider aminocaproic acid, tranexamic acid, recombinant factor VIIa Normal platelet function returns within 3 to 5 days after discontinuation
Ticlopidine	Inhibits $P2Y_{12}$ component of ADP receptors	No	Yes	CYP3A4	Black Box warning on hematologic toxicities (aplastic anemia, TTP) Frequent CBC monitoring required BID dosing	No specific antidote Consider platelet transfusion ± DDAVP Normal platelet function returns within 5 to 10 days after discontinuation
Vorapaxar	Inhibits PAR-1	Yes[b]	No	CYP3A4 CYP2J2	Use in combination with aspirin and/or clopidogrel Contraindicated in patients with history of stroke, TIA, or ICH Extremely long effective half-life of 3 to 5 days	No specific antidote Significant inhibition of platelet aggregation remains 4 weeks after discontinuation

[a]Management of antiplatelet-associated bleeding requires careful consideration of the indication for antiplatelet therapy and bleeding extent (eg, epistaxis vs intracranial hemorrhage); minor bleeding may only require local hemostasis.

[b]Due to the very long half-life, vorapaxar is effectively irreversible.

Armstrong MJ, Gronseth G, Anderson DC, et al. Summary of evidence-based guideline: periprocedural management of antithrombotic medications in patients with ischemic cerebrovascular disease: report of the Guideline Development Subcommittee of the American Academy of Neurology. *Neurology*. 2013;80(22):2065-2069.

Hillis LD, Smith PK, Anderson JL, et al. 2011 ACCF/AHA guideline for coronary artery bypass graft surgery: executive summary: a report of the American College of Cardiology Foundation/American Heart Association task force on practice guidelines. *Circulation*. 2011;124(23):2610-2642.

Levi M, Eerenberg E, Kamphuisen PW. Bleeding risk and reversal strategies for old and new anticoagulants and antiplatelet agents. *J Thromb Haemost*. 2011;9(9):1705-1712.

Patrono C, Andreotti F, Arnesen H, et al. Antiplatelet agents for the treatment and prevention of atherothrombosis. *Eur Heart J*. 2011;32(23):2922-2932.

Content adapted from Lexi-Drugs monographs

REFERENCES

Alaali Y, Barnes GD, Froehlich JB, Kaatz S. Management of oral anticoagulation in patients undergoing minor dental procedures. *J Mich Dent Assoc.* 2012;94(8):36-41.

American College of Chest Physicians Evidence-Based Clinical Practice Guidelines (8th Edition). Perioperative Management of Antithrombotic Therapy. *CHEST.* 2008;133:299–339S.

Armstrong MJ, Gronseth G, Anderson DC, et al. Summary of evidence-based guideline: Periprocedural management of antithrombotic medications in patients with ischemic cerebrovascular disease: Report of the Guideline Development Subcommittee of the American Academy of Neurology. *Neurology.* 2013;80(22):2065-2069.

Benjamin EJ, Blaha MJ, Chiuve SE, et al. Heart disease and stroke statistics—2017 Update: a report from the American Heart Association. *Circulation.* 2017.

Breik O, Cheng A, Sambrook P, Goss A. Protocol in managing oral surgical patients taking dabigatran. *Aust Dent J.* 2014;59(3):296-301.

Daniels PR. Peri-procedural management of patients taking oral anticoagulants. *BMJ.* 2015;351:h2391.

Douketis JD, Berger PB, Dunn AS, et al. The perioperative management of antithrombotic therapy: American college of chest physicians evidence-based clinical practice guidelines (8th edition). *Chest.* 2008;133(6_suppl):299S-339S.

Douketis JD, Spyropoulos AC, Spencer FA, et al. Perioperative management of antithrombotic therapy: antithrombotic therapy and prevention of thrombosis, 9th ed: American College of Chest Physicians evidence-based clinical practice guidelines. *Chest.* 2012;141(2 Suppl):e326S-e350S.

Eisenberg MJ, Richard PR, Libersan D, Filion KB. Safety of short-term discontinuation of antiplatelet therapy in patients with drug-eluting stents. *Circulation.* 2009;119(12):1634-1642.

Elad S, Marshall J, Meyerowitz C, Connolly G. Novel anticoagulants: general overview and practical considerations for dental practitioners. *Oral Dis.* 2016;22(1):23-32.

FDA. Ibuprofen and aspirin taken together. http://www.fda.gov/Safety/MedWatch/SafetyInformation/SafetyAlertsforHumanMedicalProducts/ucm150611.htm

Firriolo FJ, Hupp WS. Beyond warfarin: the new generation of oral anticoagulants and their implications for the management of dental patients. *Oral Surg Oral Med Oral Pathol Oral Radiol.* 2012;113(4):431-441.

Friedlander AH, Yoshikawa TT, Chang DS, Feliciano Z, Scully C. Atrial fibrillation: Pathogenesis, medical-surgical management and dental implications. *J Am Dent Assoc.* 2009;140(2):167-177.

Grines CL, Bonow RO, Casey DE, Jr., et al. Prevention of premature discontinuation of dual antiplatelet therapy in patients with coronary artery stents: a science advisory from the American Heart Association, American College of Cardiology, Society for Cardiovascular Angiography and Interventions, American College of Surgeons, and American Dental Association, with representation from the American College of Physicians. *J Am Dent Assoc.* 2007;138(5):652-655.

Grines CL, Bonow RO, Casey DE, Jr., et al. Prevention of premature discontinuation of dual antiplatelet therapy in patients with coronary artery stents: a science advisory from the American Heart Association, American College of Cardiology, Society for Cardiovascular Angiography and Interventions, American College of Surgeons, and American Dental Association, with representation from the American College of Physicians. *Circulation.* 2007;115(6):813-818.

Heidbuchel H, Verhamme P, Alings M, et al. Updated European Heart Rhythm Association Practical Guide on the use of non-vitamin K antagonist anticoagulants in patients with non-valvular atrial fibrillation. *Europace.* 2015.

Heidbuchel H, Verhamme P, Alings M, et al. European Heart Rhythm Association Practical Guide on the use of new oral anticoagulants in patients with non-valvular atrial fibrillation. *Europace.* 2013;15(5):625-651.

Hupp WS. Cardiovascular Diseases. *The ADA Practical Guide to Patients with Medical Conditions.* 2nd ed. Hoboken, NJ: John Wiley & Sons, Inc.; 2016;25-42.

Jeske AH, Suchko GD, ADA Council on Scientific Affairs and Division of Science, Journal of the American Dental Association. Lack of a scientific basis for routine discontinuation of oral anticoagulation therapy before dental treatment. *J Am Dent Assoc.* 2003;134(11):1492-1497.

Lordkipanidzé M, Diodati JG, Pharand C. Possibility of a rebound phenomenon following antiplatelet therapy withdrawal: a look at the clinical and pharmacological evidence. *Pharmacol Ther.* 2009;123(2):178-186.

Managing anticoagulation in the perioperative period: ACCP guidelines. 9th ed; 2012.

Napenas JJ, Oost FC, DeGroot A, et al. Review of postoperative bleeding risk in dental patients on antiplatelet therapy. *Oral Surg Oral Med Oral Pathol Oral Radiol.* 2013;115(4):491-499.

Nematullah A, Alabousi A, Blanas N, Douketis JD, Sutherland SE. Dental surgery for patients on anticoagulant therapy with warfarin: a systematic review and meta-analysis. *J Can Dent Assoc.* 2009;75(1):41.

Perry DJ, Noakes TJC, Helliwell PS. Guidelines for the management of patients on oral anticoagulants requiring dental surgery. *Br Dent J.* 2007;203(7):389-393.

Thean D, Alberghini M. Anticoagulant therapy and its impact on dental patients: a review. *Aust Dent J.* 2015.

United Kingdom National Health Service. Surgical management of the primary care dental patient on antiplatelet medication. National Electronic Library of Medicines: 2007. Accessed October 5 2015.

van Diermen DE, Aartman IH, Baart JA, Hoogstraten J, van der Waal I. Dental management of patients using antithrombotic drugs: critical appraisal of existing guidelines. *Oral Surg Oral Med Oral Pathol Oral Radiol Endod.* 2009;107(5):616-624.

van Diermen DE, van der Waal I, Hoogstraten J. Management recommendations for invasive dental treatment in patients using oral antithrombotic medication, including novel oral anticoagulants. *Oral Surg Oral Med Oral Pathol Oral Radiol.* 2013;116(6):709-716.

Weltman NJ, Al-Attar Y, Cheung J, et al. Management of dental extractions in patients taking warfarin as anticoagulant treatment: A systematic review. *J Can Dent Assoc.* 2015;81:f20.

CLINICAL RISK RELATED TO DRUGS PROLONGING QT INTERVAL

The QT interval is measured as the time and distance between the Q point of the QRS complex and the end of the T wave in the ECG tracing. After adjustment for heart rate, the QT interval is defined as prolonged if it is more than 450 msec in men and 460 msec in women. A long QT syndrome was first described in the 1950s and 60s as a congenital syndrome involving QT interval prolongation, syncope, and sudden death. Some of the congenital long QT syndromes were characterized by a peculiar electrocardiographic appearance of the QRS complex involving a premature atria beat, followed by a pause, then a subsequent sinus beat showing marked QT prolongation and deformity. This type of cardiac arrhythmia was originally termed "torsade de pointes" (translated from the French as "twisting of the points"). In addition to some genetic predisposition to risk of arrhythmic events, numerous studies have also associated prolongation of the QT interval with antidepressant drug therapy and particularly selective serotonin reuptake inhibitors. Asymptomatic individuals with QT alterations usually do not require special care. However, a cardiologist or a cardiac electrophysiologist should evaluate and be consulted regarding such patients on a regular basis.

Prolongation of the QT interval is thought to result from delayed ventricular repolarization. The repolarization process within the myocardial cell is due to the efflux of intracellular potassium. The channels associated with this current can be blocked by many drugs and predispose the electrical propagation cycle to torsade de pointes. In fact there is a wide array of drugs that have been implicated in the prolongation of the QT interval. Some of these drugs have either been restricted or withdrawn from the market due to the increased incidence of fatal polymorphic ventricular tachycardia. The list of drugs that cause QT prolongation continues to grow, and an updated list of specific drugs that prolong the QT interval can be found at www.qtdrugs.org.

Erythromycin, a drug often associated as a dental antibiotic, is considered to have a risk of causing torsade de pointes. Drug-induced torsade de pointes, a specific type of ventricular arrhythmia associated with prolongation of the QT interval, is a well understood form of drug toxicity. The evidence for risk of this event varies among the many drugs associated with torsade de pointes and with the patients' characteristics. The risk of drug-induced torsade de pointes is extremely low when a single QT interval prolonging drug is prescribed. It is not known what effect vasoconstrictors in the local anesthetic regimen will have in patients with a known history of congenital prolonged QT interval or in patients taking any medication that prolongs the QT interval. Until more information is obtained, it is suggested that the clinician consult with the physician prior to the use of a vasoconstrictor in suspected patients, and that the vasoconstrictor (epinephrine, levonordefrin [Neo-Cobefrin]) be used with caution. Other drugs commonly used in oral diseases that have been associated with significant QT interval changes include fluconazole, azithromycin, and levofloxacin, each having variable risk. In May 2012, the FDA notified health care providers that it is aware of the study published in the *New England Journal of Medicine* (May 17) reporting a small increase in cardiovascular deaths and in the risk of death from any cause in patients treated with a 5 day course of azithromycin (Zithromax) compared to patients treated with amoxicillin, ciprofloxacin, or no drug. The FDA is reviewing the results from this study and will communicate any new information on azithromycin and this study or the potential risk of QT interval prolongation after the agency has completed its review.

Patients taking azithromycin should not stop taking their medicine without talking to their health care provider. Health care providers should be aware of the potential for QT interval prolongation and heart arrhythmias when prescribing or administering any macrolide antibiotic.

Thioridazine is another drug confirmed to prolong the QT interval and is accepted as having a risk of causing torsade de pointes. The risk of drug-induced torsade de pointes is extremely low when a single QT interval prolonging drug is prescribed. In terms of epinephrine, it is not known what effect vasoconstrictors in the local anesthetic regimen will have in patients with a known history of congenital prolonged QT interval or in patients taking any medication that prolongs the QT interval. Until more information is obtained, it is suggested that the clinician consult with the physician prior to the use of a vasoconstrictor in suspected patients, and that the vasoconstrictor (epinephrine, levonordefrin [Neo-Cobefrin]) be used with caution.

Drugs Generally Accepted as Having a Risk of Causing Torsade de Pointes

Generic Name	Brand Name	Use
Alfuzosin	Uroxatral	Alpha-1 Blocker
Amiodarone	Cordarone	Antiarrhythmic
Arsenic Trioxide	Trisenox	Antileukemic agent
Artemether and Lumefantrine	Coartem	Antimalarial Agent
Asenapine	Saphris	Antipsychotic
Azithromycin (Systemic)	**Zithromax**	**Antibiotic**
Bedaquiline	-	Antitubercular Agent
Chloroquine	Aralen	Antimalarial
ChlorproMAZINE	-	Antipsychotic
Citalopram	CeleXA	Antidepressant
Clarithromycin	**Biaxin**	**Antibiotic**

Drugs Generally Accepted as Having a Risk of Causing Torsade de Pointes *(continued)*

Generic Name	Brand Name	Use
Crizotinib	Xalkori	Antineoplastic
Disopyramide	Norpace	Antiarrhythmic
Dofetilide	Tikosyn	Antiarrhythmic
Dolasetron	Anzemet	Antiemetic
Dronedarone	Multaq	Antiarrhythmic
Droperidol	-	Antiemetic
Erythromycin (Systemic)	**Various brand names available**	**Antibiotic**
Escitalopram	Lexapro	Antidepressant
Flecainide	Tambocor	Antiarrhythmic
Fluconazole	**Diflucan**	**Antifungal**
FLUoxetine	PROzac	Antidepressant
Gemifloxacin	Factive	Antibiotic
Granisetron	Granisol, Sancuso	Antiemetic
Haloperidol	Haldol	Antipsychotic
Ibutilide	Corvert	Antiarrhythmic
Iloperidone	Fanapt	Antipsychotic
Lapatinib	Tykerb	Antineoplastic
LevoFLOXacin (Systemic)	**Levaquin**	**Antibiotic**
Methadone	Various brand names available	Analgesic, Opioid
MiFEPRIStone	Korlym, Mifeprex	Abortifacient, Cortisol Receptor Blocker
Moxifloxacin (Systemic)	**Avelox**	**Antibiotic**
Nilotinib	Tasigna	Antineoplastic
Ofloxacin (Systemic)	-	Antibiotic
Ondansetron	Zofran, Zofran ODT, Zuplenz	Antiemetic
Paliperidone	Invega, Invega Sustenna	Antipsychotic
Pasireotide	Signifor	Somatostatin Analog
PAZOPanib	Votrient	Antineoplastic Agent, Tyrosine Kinase Inhibitor
Pentamidine	NebuPent	Antibiotic
Pimozide	Orap	Antipsychotic
Procainamide	Procanbid	Antiarrhythmic
Propafenone	Rythmol, Rythmol SR	Antiarrhythmic
Rilpivirine	Edurant	Antiretroviral Agent
QUEtiapine	SEROquel	Antipsychotic
QuiNIDine	-	Antiarrhythmic
QuiNINE	Qualaquin	Antimalarial Agent
Ranolazine	Ranexa	Antianginal
RisperiDONE	RisperDAL	Antipsychotic
RomiDEPsin	Istodax	Antineoplastic Agent, Histone Deacetylase Inhibitor
Saquinavir	Invirase	Antiretroviral Agent
Sotalol	Betapace	Antiarrhythmic
SUNItinib	Sutent	Antineoplastic
Telithromycin	**Ketek**	**Antibiotic**
Tetrabenazine	Xenazine	Huntington's Disease
Thioridazine	-	Antipsychotic
Toremifene	Fareston	Antineoplastic
TraZODone	Oleptro	Antidepressant
Vandetanib	-	Medullary thyroid cancer (symptomatic or progressive)

Drugs Generally Accepted as Having a Risk of Causing Torsade de Pointes *(continued)*

Generic Name	Brand Name	Use
Vemurafenib	Zelboraf	Antineoplastic
Voriconazole	**VFEND**	**Antifungal**
Ziprasidone	Geodon	Antipsychotic
Zuclopenthixol	Clopixol	Antipsychotic

Note: Dental drugs are identified by bold print. This is not a comprehensive list; additional resources should be consulted.

REFERENCES

Barsheshet A, Peterson DR, Moss AJ, et al. Genotype-specific QT correction for heart rate and the risk of life-threatening cardiac events in adolescents with congenital long-QT syndrome. *Heart Rhythm.* 2011;8(8):1207-1213.

Fazio G, Vernuccio F, Grutta G, and Re GL. Drugs to be avoided in patients with long QT syndrome: Focus on the anaesthesiological management. *World J Cardiol.* 2013; 5(4):87–93.

Hedley PL, Jorgensen P, Schlamowitz S, Wangari R, Moolman-Smook J, Brink PA, Kanters JK, et al. The genetic basis of long QT and short QT syndromes: a mutation update. *Hum Mutat.* 2009;30(11): 1486–1511.

Long QT syndrome. *National Heart, Lung, and Blood Institute.* http://www.nhlbi.nih.gov/health/dci/Diseases/qt/qt_. Feb. 10, 2012.

Madias C, Fitzgibbons TP, Alsheikh-Ali AA, et al. Acquired long QT syndrome from stress cardiomyopathy is associated with ventricular arrhythmias and *torsades de pointes. Heart Rhythm.* 2011;8(4):555-561.

Mauriello DA, Johnson JN, Ackerman MJ. Holter monitoring in the evaluation of congenital long QT syndrome. *Pacing Clin Electrophysiol.* 2011;34 (9):1100-1104.

Morita H, Wu J, Zipes DP. The QT syndromes: long and short. *Lancet.* 2008;372(9640):750–763.

Nachimuthu S, Assar MD, Schussler JM. Drug-induced QT interval prolongation: mechanisms and clinical management. *Ther Adv Drug Saf.* 2012; 3 (5):241–253.

Torekov SS, Iepsen E, Christiansen M, Linneberg A, Pedersen O, Holst JJ, Kanters JK, et al. KCNQ1 long QT syndrome patients have hyperinsulinemia and symptomatic hypoglycemia. *Diabetes.* 2014;63(4):1315-1325.

GASTROINTESTINAL DISORDERS

The oral cavity and related structures comprise the first part of the gastrointestinal tract. Diseases affecting the oral cavity are often reflected in GI disturbances. In addition, the oral cavity may indeed reflect diseases of the GI tract, including ulcers, polyps, and liver and gallbladder diseases. The first oral condition that may reflect or be reflected in GI disturbances is taste. Typically, complaints of taste abnormalities are presented to the dentist. The sweet, saline, sour, and bitter taste sensations all vary in quality and intensity and are affected by the olfactory system. Often, anemic conditions are reflected in changes in the tongue, also resulting in potential taste aberrations.

Gastric and duodenal ulcers represent the primary diseases that can be reflected in the oral cavity. Gastroesophageal reflux disease (GERD), also known as gastroesophageal reflux disease (GORD), gastric reflux disease, or acid reflux disease, is a chronic symptom of mucosal damage caused by stomach acid coming up from the stomach into the esophagus. GERD is caused by changes in the barrier between the stomach and the esophagus, including abnormal relaxation of the lower esophageal sphincter, which normally holds the top of the stomach closed, impaired expulsion of gastric reflux from the esophagus, or a hiatal hernia. These changes may be permanent or temporary. When attempting diagnosis of oral diseases, such as taste aberrations, halitosis, and Burning Mouth Syndrome, GERD should be considered as a potential complicating or causative factor.

Another kind of acid reflux, which can cause respiratory and laryngeal signs and symptoms, is called extraesophageal reflux disease (EERD). Unlike GERD, EERD is unlikely to produce heartburn, and is sometimes called "silent reflux." Crohn's disease and ulcerative colitis have also been associated with these conditions and should be ruled out in a differential diagnostic work-up. Chronic recurring oral ulcerations are sometimes associated with Crohn's disease and this association should be considered in patients with a history of both conditions.

Gastric reflux and problems with food metabolism often present as acid erosions to the teeth and occasionally as changes in the mucosal surface as well, resulting in chronic oral ulcerations. In some studies, this has also been associated with burning mouth syndrome. Patients may be identified, upon diagnosis, as harboring the organism *Helicobacter pylori.* Treatment with antibiotics can oftentimes aid in correcting the ulcerative disease.

Celiac disease is a permanent intolerance to certain proteins (collectively called 'gluten') that are present in wheat, rye, and barley and related grains. Ingestion of gluten causes damage to the small intestine through an autoimmune mechanism in genetically susceptible individuals. It can develop at any age when gluten is present in the diet, but if it develops in children while the permanent teeth are developing, abnormalities in the structure of the dental enamel can occur. Common oral and dental manifestations of celiac disease may include the following:

- Enamel defects
- Delayed eruption
- Recurrent aphthous ulcers

Both hypoplasia and hypomineralization of the enamel can occur. A band of hypoplastic enamel is common, often with intact cusps. A break in the enamel and dentine formation can occur at a developmental stage which corresponds with the onset of gastrointestinal symptoms. Specific enamel defects can include pitting and grooving. Sometimes there is complete loss of enamel.

PROTON PUMP AND GASTRIC ACID SECRETION INHIBITORS

Dexlansoprazole on page 471
Esomeprazole on page 594
Lansoprazole on page 876
Lansoprazole, Amoxicillin, and Clarithromycin on page 877
Omeprazole on page 1139
Omeprazole and Sodium Bicarbonate
Pantoprazole on page 1189
RABEprazole on page 1302

HISTAMINE H_2 ANTAGONIST

Cimetidine
Famotidine on page 635
Nizatidine on page 1116
RaNITIdine (Withdrawn from US Market)

The oral aspects of gastrointestinal disease are often nonspecific and are related to the patient's gastric reflux problems. Intestinal polyps occasionally present as part of the "Peutz-Jeghers Syndrome," resulting in pigmented areas of the perioral region that resemble freckles. The astute dentist will need to differentiate these from melanin pigmentation, while at the same time encouraging the patient to seek evaluation for an intestinal disorder.

Diseases of the liver and gallbladder system are complex. Most of the disorders of interest to the dentist are covered in the section on Systemic Viral Diseases on page 1709. All of the new drugs, including interferons, are mentioned in this section.

Multiple Drug Regimens for the Treatment of *H. pylori* Infection in Adult Patients

Medication Regimen	Dosages	Duration of Therapy
	First-Line Therapy (Option 1)	
H_2-Receptor antagonist (H_2RA) **or** proton pump inhibitor (PPI)	Standard dose of H_2RA or PPI[a]	10 to 14 days
	plus	
Bismuth subsalicylate	525 mg 4 times/day	10 to 14 days
	plus	
MetroNIDAZOLE on page 1011	250 mg 4 times/day	10 to 14 days
	plus	
Tetracycline (Systemic) on page 1431	500 mg 4 times/day	10 to 14 days
	First-Line Therapy (Option 2)	
PPI	Standard dose[a]	10 to 14 days
	plus	
Clarithromycin on page 361	500 mg 2 times/day	10 to 14 days
	plus	
Amoxicillin on page 124	1,000 mg 2 times/day	10 to 14 days
	First-Line Therapy (Option 3)	
PPI	Standard dose[a]	10 to 14 days
	plus	
Clarithromycin on page 361	500 mg 2 times/day	10 to 14 days
	plus	
MetroNIDAZOLE on page 1011	500 mg 2 times/day	10 to 14 days
	Salvage Therapy for Persistent Infection (Option 1)	
	PPI (once daily), bismuth, metroNIDAZOLE, and tetracycline (4 times/day) for 7 to 14 days	
	Salvage Therapy for Persistent Infection (Option 2)	
	PPI (standard dose[a]), levofloxacin 500 mg (once daily), and amoxicillin 1,000 mg (2 times/day) for 10 days	

[a]Standard proton pump inhibitor dose: Esomeprazole = 40 mg once daily, lansoprazole = 30 mg 2 times/day, omeprazole = 20 mg 2 times/day, RABEprazole = 20 mg 2 times/day

REFERENCES

Cheng J, Malahias T, Brar P, Minaya MT, Green PH.The association between celiac disease, dental enamel defects, and aphthous ulcers in a United States cohort. *J Clin Gastroenterol.* 2010:44(3):191-194.

Chey WD, Wong BC, Practice Parameters Committee of the American College of Gastroenterology. American College of Gastroenterology guideline on the management of *Helicobacter pylori* infection. *Am J Gastroenterol.* 2007;102(8):1808-1825.

Cobrin GM, Abreu MT. Defects in mucosal immunity leading to Crohn disease. *Immunol Rev.* 2005;206:277-295.

Daley TD, Armstrong JE. Oral manifestations of gastrointestinal diseases. *Can J Gastroenterol.* 2007;21(4):241-244.

Franch AM, Jimenez-Soriano Y, Sarrion-Pérez MG. Dental management of patients with inflammatory bowel disease. *J Clin Exp Dent.* 2010;2(4): e191-195.

Karthik R, Karthik KS, David C, Ameerunnisa, Keerthi G. Oral adverse effects of gastrointestinal drugs and considerations for dental management in patients with gastrointestinal disorders. *J Pharm Bioallied Sci.* 2012;4(Suppl 2):S239–S241.

Padmavathi BN, Sharma S, Astekar M, Rajan Y, Sowmya G. Oral Crohn's disease. *J Oral Maxillofac Pathol.* 2014; 18(Suppl 1):S139–S142.

Pastore L, Carroccio A, Compilato D, Panzarella V, Serpico R, Lo Muzio L. Oral manifestations of celiac disease. *J Clin Gastroenterol.* 2008;42 (3):224-232.

Permin H, Andersen LP. Inflammation, immunity, and vaccines for *Helicobacter* infection. *Helicobacter.* 2005;10(Suppl 1):21-25.

Rashid M, Zarkadas M, Anca A, Limeback H. Oral manifestations of celiac disease: A clinical guide for dentists. *J Can Dent Assoc.* 2011;77:b39.

Saad RJ, Schoenfeld P, Kim HM, Chey WD. Levofloxacin-based triple therapy versus bismuth-based quadruple therapy for persistent *Helicobacter pylori* infection: a meta-analysis. *Am J Gastroenterol.* 2006;101(3):488-496.

Schreiber S, Rosenstiel P, Albrecht M, Hampe J, Krawczak M. Genetics of Crohn disease, an archetypal inflammatory barrier disease. *Nat Rev Genet.* 2005;6(5):376-388.

Tummala S, Keates S, Kelly CP. Update on the immunologic basis of *Helicobacter pylori* gastritis. *Curr Opin Gastroenterol.* 2004;20(6):592-597.

Yuan Y, Padol IT, Hunt RH. Peptic ulcer disease today. *Nat Clin Pract Gastroenterol Hepatol.* 2006;3(2):80-89.

RESPIRATORY DISEASES

Diseases of the respiratory system put dental patients at increased risk in the dental office because of their decreased pulmonary reserve, the medications they may be taking, drug interactions between these medications, medications the dentist may prescribe, and in some patients with infectious respiratory diseases, a risk of disease transmission.

The respiratory system consists of the nasal cavity, the nasopharynx, the trachea, and the components of the lung, including the bronchi, the bronchioles, and the alveoli. The diseases that affect the lungs and the respiratory system can be separated by location of affected tissue. Diseases that affect the lower respiratory tract are often chronic, although infections can also occur. Three major diseases that affect the lower respiratory tract are often encountered in the medical history for dental patients. These include chronic bronchitis, emphysema, and asthma. Diseases that affect the upper respiratory tract are usually of the infectious nature and include sinusitis and the common cold. The upper respiratory tract infections may also include a wide variety of nonspecific infections, most of which are also caused by viruses. Influenza produces upper respiratory type symptoms and is often caused by orthomyxoviruses. Herpangina is caused by the Coxsackie type viruses and results in upper respiratory infections in addition to pharyngitis or sore throat. One serious condition, known as croup, has been associated with *Haemophilus influenzae* infections. Other more serious infections might include respiratory syncytial virus, adenoviruses, and parainfluenza viruses.

The respiratory symptoms that are often encountered in both upper respiratory and lower respiratory disorders include cough, dyspnea (difficulty in breathing), the production of sputum, hemoptysis (coughing up blood), a wheeze, and occasionally chest pain. One additional symptom, orthopnea (difficulty in breathing when lying down), is often used by the dentist to assist in evaluating the patient with the condition pulmonary edema. This condition results from either respiratory disease or congestive heart failure.

No effective drug treatments are available for the management of many of the upper respiratory tract viral infections. However, amantadine (Symmetrel) is a synthetic drug given orally (200 mg/day) and has been found to be effective against some strains of influenza. Treatment other than for influenza includes supportive care products, available over-the-counter. These might include antihistamines for symptomatic relief of the upper respiratory congestion, antibiotics to combat secondary bacterial infections, and in severe cases, fluids, when patients have become dehydrated during the illness (see Pharmacologic Category Index for selection).

SINUSITIS

Sinusitis represents an upper respiratory condition that often comes under the purview of the practicing dentist. Acute sinusitis is characterized by nasal obstruction, fever, chills, and midface head pain. Oftentimes there is only evidence of inflammation rather than true infection. This condition may be discovered as part of a differential workup for other facial or dental pain since the symptoms are often referred to teeth adjacent to the affected sinus. Chronic sinusitis may likewise produce similar dental symptoms. Dental drugs of choice may include ephedrine or nasal drops, antihistamines, and analgesics. When infection accompanies the inflammation of sinusitis, antibiotics may be required. Most commonly, broad spectrum antibiotics such as amoxicillin (often supplemented with clavulanate acid as Augmentin) are prescribed. Levofloxacin (Levoquin) has been specifically approved for sinusitis and has become popular. Antibiotic therapies are often combined with antral lavage to re-establish drainage from the sinus area. Surgical intervention, such as a Caldwell-Luc procedure opening into the sinus, is rarely necessary and many of the second generation antibiotics, such as cephalosporins, are used successfully in treating the acute and chronic sinusitis patient (see Antibiotic Prophylaxis on page 1715).

LOWER RESPIRATORY DISEASES

Lower respiratory tract diseases, including asthma, chronic bronchitis, and emphysema are often identified in dental patients. Asthma is an intermittent respiratory disorder that produces recurrent bronchial smooth muscle spasm, inflammation of the bronchial mucosa, and hypersecretion of mucus. The incidence of childhood asthma appears to be increasing and may be related to the presence of pollutants such as sulfur dioxide and indoor cigarette smoke. The end result is widespread narrowing of the airways and decreased ventilation with increased airway resistance, especially to expiration. Asthmatic patients often suffer asthmatic attacks when stimulated by respiratory tract infections, exercise, and cold air. Medications such as aspirin and some NSAIDs, as well as cholinergic and beta-adrenergic blocking drugs, can also trigger asthmatic attacks in addition to chemicals, smoke, and emotional anxiety.

The classic chronic obstructive pulmonary diseases (COPD) of chronic bronchitis and emphysema are both characterized by chronic airflow obstructions during normal ventilation efforts. They often occur in combination in the same patient and their treatment is similar. One common finding is that the patient is often a smoker. The dentist can play a role in reinforcement of smoking cessation in patients with chronic respiratory diseases.

Treatments include a variety of drugs depending on the severity of the symptoms and the respiratory compromise upon full respiratory evaluation. Patients who are having acute and chronic obstructive pulmonary attacks may be susceptible to infection and antibiotics such as penicillin, ampicillin, tetracycline, or sulfamethoxazole-trimethoprim are often used to eradicate susceptible infective organisms. Corticosteroids, as well as a wide variety of respiratory stimulants, are available in inhalant and/or oral forms. In patients using inhalant medication, oral candidiasis is occasionally encountered. Aclidinium bromide (Tudorza Pressair) has been approved for the long-term maintenance treatment of bronchospasm (narrowing of the airways in the lung) associated with chronic obstructive pulmonary disease (COPD), including chronic bronchitis and emphysema. Aclidinium bromide is a long-acting anticholinergic and, as such, becomes the second approved inhaled long-acting muscarinic antagonist (LAMA), along with tiotropium. Both drugs produce bronchodilation by inhibiting acetylcholine's effect on the muscarinic M3 receptor in the airway smooth muscle. Both drugs are inhaled as dry powders.

Analgesics
Antibiotics
Antihistamines
Decongestants

SPECIFIC DRUGS USED IN THE TREATMENT OF CHRONIC RESPIRATORY CONDITIONS

Beta-2-Selective Agonists

Albuterol on page 90
Arformoterol on page 163
Formoterol on page 711
Indacaterol on page 807
Levalbuterol on page 892
Metaproterenol on page 982
Pirbuterol
Salmeterol on page 1355

Methylxanthines

Aminophylline on page 117
Theophylline on page 1437

Mast Cell Stabilizer

Cromolyn (Systemic) on page 416
Cromolyn (Oral Inhalation) on page 416
Ketotifen (Systemic) on page 866

Corticosteroids

Beclomethasone (Oral Inhalation) on page 218
Budesonide (Systemic) on page 252
Budesonide (Oral Inhalation) on page 254
Ciclesonide (Oral Inhalation) on page 346
Dexamethasone (Systemic) on page 463
Flunisolide (Oral Inhalation) on page 688
Fluticasone (Oral Inhalation) on page 703
MethylPREDNISolone on page 999
Mometasone (Oral Inhalation) on page 1046
PredniSONE on page 1260

Anticholinergics

Aclidinium on page 74
Ipratropium (Oral Inhalation) on page 838
Tiotropium on page 1450

Leukotriene Receptor Antagonists

Montelukast on page 1048
Zafirlukast on page 1565

5-Lipoxygenase Inhibitors

Zileuton on page 1571

Monoclonal Antibody, Antiasthmatic

Omalizumab on page 1134

OBSTRUCTIVE SLEEP APNEA

Obstructive sleep apnea is a condition in which the flow of air pauses or decreases during breathing while you are asleep because the airway has become narrowed, blocked, or floppy. A pause in breathing is called an apnea episode. A decrease in airflow during breathing is called a hypopnea episode. Almost everyone has brief apnea episodes while they sleep. Normally, the upper throat still remains open enough during sleep to let air pass by. However, some people have a narrower throat area. When the muscles in their upper throat relax during sleep, their breathing can stop for a period of time (often more than 10 seconds). This is called apnea. Snoring in people with obstructive sleep apnea is caused by the air trying to squeeze through the narrowed or blocked airway. However, everyone who snores does not have sleep apnea.

Other factors that may also increase your risk include:

- A lower jaw that is short compared to the upper jaw (retrognathia)
- Certain shapes of the palate or airway that cause the airway to be narrower or collapse more easily
- Large neck or collar size (≥17 inches in men and ≥16 inches in women)
- Large tongue, which may fall back and block the airway
- Obesity
- Large tonsils and adenoids in children that can block the airway

At this time, the most effective treatments for sleep apnea are devices that deliver slightly pressurized air to keep the throat open during the night. There are a number of such devices available.

Continuous Positive Airflow Pressure (CPAP)

The best treatment for obstructive sleep apnea is a system known as continuous positive airflow pressure (CPAP). It is safe and effective for people of all ages, including children. Patients with obstructive sleep apnea who use CPAP feel better rested, have less daytime sleepiness, and have improved concentration and memory. In addition, CPAP may potentially reduce the risks for heart problems such as high blood pressure. For maximum benefit, CPAP should be used for at least 6 to 7 hours each night.

CPAP works in the following way:

- The device itself is a machine weighing about 3 pounds that fits on a bedside table.
- A mask containing a tube connects to the device and fits over just the nose.
- The machine supplies a steady stream of air through a tube and applies sufficient air pressure to prevent the tissues from collapsing during sleep.

The standard CPAP machine delivers a fixed, constant flow of air. Variations on CPAP include:

- Autotitrating positive airway pressure (APAP) devices automatically respond to changes in the sleeper's breathing patterns by adjusting and varying the air pressure flow throughout the night. Some patients find this makes CPAP easier to tolerate.
- Bilevel positive airway pressure (BPAP) systems deliver two different pressures, a higher one for inhalation (breathing in) and a lower one for exhalation (breathing out).

OTHER RESPIRATORY DISEASES

Other respiratory diseases include tuberculosis and sarcoidosis which are considered to be restrictive granulomatous respiratory diseases. Sarcoidosis is a relatively rare acquired systemic granulomatous disease affecting multiple organs and tissues. The respiratory system is most commonly affected, with approximately 90% of patients presenting pulmonary findings during the course of their disease. Cutaneous manifestations occur in ~25% of cases but are more common in chronic forms. Head and neck lesions of sarcoidosis are manifested in 10% to 15% of patients. In the maxillofacial region, the salivary glands are frequently involved, with xerostomia and bilateral parotid swelling present. Lesions that occur in the soft tissues of the oral cavity and/or in the jaws are not common but may be the initial presenting findings of sarcoidosis. The diagnosis of sarcoidosis is established by biopsy and the histopathological evidence of typical noncaseating granulomas. These findings are usually supported by elevated serum angiotensin converting enzyme (ACE) levels. Any patient with cutaneous sarcoidosis should be evaluated for the possibility of systemic disease. Testing should include a complete physical exam, chest x-ray, pulmonary function test, electrocardiogram, tuberculin skin testing, a urinalysis, and several blood studies.

Sarcoidosis is a condition that at one time was thought to be similar to tuberculosis; however, it is a multisystem disorder of unknown origin which has a characteristic lymphocytic and mononuclear phagocytic accumulation in epithelioid granulomas within the lung. It occurs worldwide but shows a slight increased prevalence in temperate climates. The treatment of sarcoidosis is usually one that corresponds to its usually benign course; however, many patients are placed on corticosteroids at the level of 40 to 60 mg of prednisone daily. This treatment is continued for a protracted period of time. As in any disease requiring steroid therapy, consideration of adrenal suppression is necessary. Alteration of steroid dosage prior to stressful dental procedures may be necessary, usually increasing the steroid dosage prior to and during the stressful procedures and then gradually returning the patient to the original dosage over several days. Many dentists prefer to use the Medrol Dosepak; however, consultation with the patient's physician regarding dose selection is always advised. Even in the absence of evidence of adrenal suppression, consultation with the prescribing physician for appropriate dosing and timing of procedures is advisable.

PredniSONE on page 1260

Relative Potency of Endogenous and Synthetic Corticosteroids

Agent	Equivalent Dose (mg)
Short-Acting (8 to 12 hours)	
Cortisol	20
Cortisone acetate	25
Intermediate-Acting (18 to 36 hours)	
PrednisoLONE	5
PredniSONE	5
MethylPREDNISolone	4
Triamcinolone	4
Long-Acting (36 to 54 hours)	
Betamethasone	0.75
Dexamethasone	0.75

Potential drug interactions for the respiratory disease patient exist. Check a patient's medical regimen to identify any potential interactions that may affect dental prescribing or a planned dental procedure. An acute sensitivity to aspirin-containing drugs and some of the nonsteroidal anti-inflammatory drugs is a threat for the asthmatic patient. Benzodiazepines may require adjustments, especially if respiratory reserve is limited. Patients that are taking steroid preparations as part of their respiratory therapy may require alteration in dosing prior to stressful dental procedures.

E-Cigarettes

Electronic cigarettes have been available for many years. In the last 5 years, however, these devices have been advocated as a highly recommended alternative to conventional cigarette smoking and have been marketed to adolescents and young adults as an option opposed to conventional smoking products. The safety of E-cigarettes has come into question in the last few years because of concern over the excessive nicotine that is provided through the device. The devices are generally supplied with flavorings and refillable cartridges, making them potentially desirable for adolescent use as well as adult use. There is very little reliable data available regarding the long-term risks of E-cigarettes, regarding their addictive potential and as a potential inducer of premalignant changes in the oral mucosa and the respiratory tract due to chronic exposure to the E-cigarette vapors. Some E-cigarettes also incorporate a concentration of formaldehyde, which by some estimates could deliver exceedingly high concentrations to the user, further increasing the cancer risk. As more information comes available the dentist should be aware of this potential risk and as always be concerned regarding any oral mucosal changes that could indicate premalignancy. More evidence-based risk assessment will be available in the future.

REFERENCES AND SELECTED READINGS

Aurora RN, Casey KR, Kristo D, et al. Practice parameters for the surgical modifications of the upper airway for obstructive sleep apnea in adults. *Sleep*. 2010;33:1408-1413.

de Almeida FR, Lowe AA, Tsuiki S, et al. Long-term compliance and side effects of oral appliances used for the treatment of snoring and obstructive sleep apnea syndrome. *J Clin Sleep Med*. 2005;1(2):143-152.

Dincer HE, O'Neill W. Deleterious effects of sleep-disordered breathing on the heart and vascular system. *Respiration*. 2006;73(1):124-130.

Epstein LJ, Kristo D, Strollo PJ Jr, et al. Adult Obstructive Sleep Apnea Task Force of the American Academy of Sleep Medicine: clinical guideline for the evaluation, management, and long-term care of obstructive sleep apnea in adults. *J Clin Sleep Med*. 2009;5(3):263-276.

Ferguson KA, Cartwright R, Rogers R, Schmidt-Nowara W. Oral appliances for snoring and obstructive sleep apnea: a review. *Sleep*. 2006;29 (2):244-262.

Gay P, Weaver T, Loube D, et al. Evaluation of positive airway pressure treatment for sleep related breathing disorders in adults. *Sleep*. 2006;29 (3):381-401.

Global Initiative for COPD Science Committee. Global strategy for diagnosis, management, and prevention of COPD. 2011. Available at http://www.goldcopd.org/guidelines-global-strategy-for-diagnosis-management.html

Global Initiative for COPD Science Committee. Global strategy for diagnosis, management, and prevention of COPD. 2013. Available at http://www.goldcopd.org/guidelines-global-strategy-for-diagnosis-management.html

Goniewicz ML, Knysak J, Gawron M, et al. Levels of selected carcinogens and toxicants in vapour from electronic cigarettes. *Tob Control*. 2014; 23 (2):133-139.

Goniewicz ML, Kuma T, Gawron M, Knysak J, Kosmider L. Nicotine levels in electronic cigarettes. *Nicotine Tob Res*. 2013; 15(1):158-166.

Hu S, Pallonen U, McAlister AL, et al. Knowing how to help tobacco users. Dentists' familiarity and compliance with the clinical practice guideline. *J Am Dent Assoc*. 2006;137(2):170-179.

Kasai T, Bradley TD. Obstructive sleep apnea and heart failure: pathophysiologic and therapeutic implications. *J Am Coll Cardiol*. 2011;57 (2):119-127.

Kowalczyk JP, Ricotti CA, de Araujo T, Drosou A, Nousari CH. "Strawberry gums" in sarcoidosis. *J Am Acad Dermatol*. 2008;59(5 Suppl):S118-S120.

Lodha S, Sanchez M, Prystowsky S. Sarcoidosis of the skin: a review for the pulmonologist. *Chest*. 2009;136(2):583-596.

McArdle N, Singh B, Murphy M, et al. Continuous positive airway pressure titration for obstructive sleep apnoea: automatic versus manual titration. *Thorax*. 2010;65(7):606-611.

Patil SP, Schneider H, Schwartz AR, Smith PL. Adult obstructive sleep apnea: pathophysiology and diagnosis. *Chest*. 2007;132:325-337.

Popova L, Ling PM. Alternative tobacco product use and smoking cessation: a national study. *Am J Public Health*. 2013; 103(5):923-930.

Schwab R, Kuna S, Remmers JE. Anatomy and physiology of upper airway obstruction. *Principles and Practice of Sleep Medicine*. 4th ed. Kryger MH, Roth T, Dement WC. Philadelphia, PA: Elsevier; 2005;983-1000.

Suresh L, Radfar L. Oral sarcoidosis: a review of literature. *Oral Dis*. 2005;11(3):138-145.

The International Classification of Sleep Disorders: Diagnostic and Coding Manual. 2nd ed. Westchester, IL: American Academy of Sleep Medicine; 2005.

Tomfohr LM, Ancoli-Israel S, Loredo JS, Dimsdale JE. Effects of continuous positive airway pressure on fatigue and sleepiness in patients with obstructive sleep apnea: data from a randomized controlled trila. *Sleep*. 2011;34(1):121-126.

ENDOCRINE DISORDERS AND PREGNANCY

The human endocrine system manages metabolism and homeostasis. Numerous glandular tissues produce hormones that act in broad reactions with tissues throughout the body. Cells in various organ systems may be sensitive to the hormone, or they release, in reaction to the hormone, a second hormone that acts directly on another organ. Diseases of the endocrine system may have importance in dentistry. For the purposes of this section, we will limit our discussion to diseases of the thyroid tissues, diabetes mellitus, management of osteoporosis, conditions requiring the administration of synthetic hormones, and pregnancy.

THYROID

Thyroid diseases can be classified into conditions that cause the thyroid to be overactive (hyperthyroidism) and those that cause the thyroid to be underactive (hypothyroidism). Clinical signs and symptoms associated with hyperthyroidism may include goiter, heat intolerance, tremor, weight loss, diarrhea, and hyperactivity. Thyroid hormone production can be tested by TSH levels and additional screens may include radioactive iodine uptake or a pre-T_4 (tetraiodothyronine, thyroxine) assay or iodine index or total serum T_3 (triiodothyronine). The results of thyroid function tests may be altered by ingestion of antithyroid drugs such as propylthiouracil, estrogen-containing drugs, and organic and inorganic iodides. When a diagnosis of hyperthyroidism has been made, treatment usually begins with antithyroid drugs which may include propranolol coupled with radioactive iodides, as well as surgical procedures, to reduce thyroid tissue. Generally, the beta-blockers are used to control cardiovascular effects of excessive T_4. Propylthiouracil or methimazole are the most common antithyroid drugs used. The dentist should be aware that epinephrine is definitely contraindicated in patients with uncontrolled hyperthyroidism.

Diseases and conditions associated with hypothyroidism may include bradycardia, drowsiness, cold intolerance, thick dry skin, and constipation. Generally, hypothyroidism is treated with replacement thyroid hormone until a euthyroid state is achieved. Various preparations are available, the most common of which is levothyroxine and is generally the drug of choice for thyroid replacement therapy.

Drugs to Treat Hypothyroidism

Levothyroxine on page 900
Liothyronine on page 919
Liotrix on page 919
Thyroid, Desiccated on page 1442

Drugs to Treat Hyperthyroidism

MethIMAzole on page 988
Potassium Iodide
Propranolol on page 1287
Propylthiouracil on page 1289
Sodium Iodide I^{131}

DIABETES

Diabetes mellitus (or diabetes) is a chronic, lifelong condition that affects your body's ability to use the energy found in food. There are three major types of diabetes: Type 1 diabetes, type 2 diabetes, and gestational diabetes. Type 1 diabetes, insulin-dependent diabetes (IDDM), is a condition where there are absent or deficient levels of circulating insulin therefore triggering tissue reactions associated with prolonged hyperglycemia. The kidney's attempt to excrete the excess glucose and the organs that do not receive adequate glucose essentially are damaged. Small vessels and arterial vessels in the eye, kidney, and brain are usually at the greatest risk. Generally, fasting blood sugar levels between 70 to 120 mg/dL are considered to be normal although blood sugar levels greater than 100 mg/dL are considered to be prediabetic and nonpharmacologic interventions are usually recommended at the very least. Inadequate insulin levels allow glucose to rise to greater than the renal threshold which is 180 mg/dL, and such elevations prolonged lead to organ damage.

The goals of treatment of the diabetic are to maintain metabolic control of the blood glucose levels and to reduce the morbid effects of periodic hyperglycemia. Insulin therapy is the primary mechanism to attain management of consistent insulin levels. Insulin preparations are categorized according to their duration of action. Generally, intermediate-acting insulin and long-acting insulin can be used in combination with short-acting or rapid-acting insulins to maintain levels consistent throughout the day.

In Type 2 or noninsulin-dependent diabetes (NIDDM), the receptor for insulin in the tissues is generally down regulated; therefore, the glucose is not utilized at an appropriate rate. There is perhaps a stronger genetic basis for noninsulin-dependent diabetes than for Type 1. Treatment of the diabetes Type 2 patient is generally directed toward early nonpharmacologic intervention, mainly weight reduction, moderate exercise, and lower plasma-glucose concentrations. Oral hypoglycemic agents as seen in the following list are often used to maintain blood sugar levels. Thirty percent of Type 2 diabetics require insulin, as well as oral hypoglycemics, in order to manage their diabetes. Generally, the two classes of oral hypoglycemics are the sulfonylureas and the biguanides. The sulfonylureas are prescribed more frequently. They stimulate beta cell production of insulin, increase glucose utilization, and tend to normalize glucose metabolism in the liver. The uncontrolled diabetic may represent a challenge to the dental practitioner.

Glycosylated hemoglobin or glycol-hemoglobin assays have emerged as a "gold standard" by which glycemic control is measured in diabetic patients. The test does not rely on the patient's ability to monitor their daily blood glucose levels and is not influenced by acute changes in blood glucose or by the interval since the last meal. Glycohemoglobin is formed when glucose reacts with hemoglobin A in the blood and is composed of several fractions. Numerous assay methods have been developed, however, they vary in their precision. Dental clinicians are advised to be aware of the laboratory's particular standardization procedures when requesting glycosylated hemoglobin values. One major advantage of the glycosylated hemoglobin assay is that it provides an overview of the level of glucose in the life span of the red blood cell population in the patient, and therefore is a measure of overall glycemic control for the previous six to twelve weeks. Thus, clinicians use glycosylated hemoglobin values to determine whether their patient is under good control, on average. These assays have less value in medication dosing decisions. Blood glucose monitoring methods are actually better in that respect. The values of glycosylated hemoglobin are expressed as a percentage of the total hemoglobin in the red blood cell population and a normal value is considered to be <6%. The goal is generally for diabetic patients to remain at <7% with a treatment goal of <6%. Values >8% constitute a worrisome signal. Medical conditions such as anemias or any red blood cell disease, numerous levels of myelosuppression, or pregnancy can artificially lower glycosylated hemoglobin values.

Over the last decade there has been a tremendous surge in the development of new drugs to provide primary treatment of diabetes or to provide supplemental therapy to insulin or established drugs such as metformin. Many drugs, therefore, are now recommended in combination therapies. The effects of better control of patients' daily blood sugar levels and glycosylated hemoglobin levels on oral complications of uncontrolled diabetes, such as oral infections and periodontal disease, are under study but the results remain to be proven. Monitoring blood sugar using laser technology (Raman spectroscopy) may eventually eliminate the need for direct blood testing.

Rapid-Acting Insulins

Insulin Lispro (HumaLOG) on page 824
Insulin Aspart (NovoLOG) on page 817
Insulin Glulisine (Apidra) on page 823

Short-Acting Insulin

Insulin Regular on page 829

Intermediate-Acting Insulin

Insulin NPH on page 827

Intermediate- to Long-Acting Insulin

Insulin Detemir on page 820

Long-Acting Insulin

Insulin Glargine on page 822 (various formulations Toujeo Max SoloStar, Toujeo SoloStar, Lantus; and Soliqua [with lixisenatide])

Oral Hypoglycemic Agents

Acarbose on page 57
Albiglutide on page 89
Alogliptin on page 105
Canagliflozin on page 281
ChlorproPAMIDE on page 343
Dapagliflozin on page 435
Dulaglutide
Exenatide on page 633
Empagliflozin on page 555
Glimepiride on page 740
GlipiZIDE on page 740
GlyBURIDE on page 741
LinaGLIPtin on page 917
Liraglutide on page 920
MetFORMIN on page 983
Miglitol on page 1030
Nateglinide on page 1087
Pioglitazone on page 1234
Pramlintide on page 1251
Repaglinide on page 1317
Rosiglitazone on page 1347
SAXagliptin on page 1360
SITagliptin on page 1376
TOLAZamide on page 1460
TOLBUTamide on page 1460

Neuropathic pain can be a significant problem in the management of diabetes. Recently, Tapentadol (Nucynta ER) received approval for use in the management of neuropathic pain in patients with diabetic peripheral neuropathy (DPN). Tapentadol is a dual-acting agent that combines a strong opioid agonist action together with inhibition of norepinephrine and serotonin reuptake. Essentially, it functions in a similar way to combining a schedule II opioid (ie, morphine, oxycodone) with a tricyclic or SNRI antidepressant. Serotonin and especially norepinephrine are important for reducing pain signal transmission in the spinal cord as part of the descending pathways for pain modulation. Opioids also produce spinal analgesia, directly on spinal cord neurons, but also by stimulating the activity of the descending pathways (primarily serotonin). Neuropathic pain is a complex disorder that usually affects ascending pathways initially, but, over time, descending pain pathways can also become damaged or less efficient in pain modulation. Other approved drugs for diabetic neuropathy include pregabalin (Lyrica) and duloxetine (Cymbalta). Unlabeled use of gabapentin (Neurontin) has also shown some efficacy.

Other oral manifestations of uncontrolled diabetes require aggressive dental management and might include abnormal neutrophil function, resulting in a poor response to periodontal pathogens. Increased risk of gingivitis and periodontitis in these patients is common. Candidiasis is also a frequent occurrence. Denture-sore mouth may be more common. Poor wound-healing following extractions may be one of the complications encountered.

OSTEOPOROSIS MANAGEMENT

Prevalence

Osteoporosis effects 25 million Americans of which 80% are women; 27% of American women >80 years of age have osteopenia and 70% of American women >80 years of age have osteoporosis.

Consequences of Osteoporosis

1.3 million bone fractures annually (low impact/nontraumatic) and pain, pulmonary insufficiency, decreased quality of life, and economic costs; >250,000 hip fractures per year with a 20% mortality rate.

Risk Factors of Osteoporosis

Advanced age, female gender, chronic renal disease, hyperparathyroidism, Cushing disease, hypogonadism/anorexia, hyperprolactinemia, cancer, large and prolonged dose heparin or glucocorticoids, anticonvulsants, hyperthyroidism (current or history, or excessive thyroid supplements), sedentary lifestyle, excessive exercise, early menopause, oophorectomy without hormone replacement, excessive aluminum-containing antacids, smoking, and methotrexate have all been at some time associated with risk of osteoporosis.

Diagnosis/Monitoring of Osteoporosis

DXA bone density, history of fracture (low impact or nontraumatic), compressed vertebrae, decreased height, hump-back appearance. Osteomark urine assay measures bone breakdown fragments and may help assess therapy response earlier than DXA but diagnostic value is uncertain as Osteomark does not reveal extent of bone loss. The clinician is referred to Osteonecrosis of the Jaw since the bisphosphonates are associated with this adverse event and its incidence associated with bisphosphonates for osteoporosis management is greater than previously estimated.

Prevention of Osteoporosis

1. Adequate dietary calcium (eg, dairy products)
2. Vitamin D (eg, fortified dairy products, cod, fatty fish)
3. Weight-bearing exercise (eg, walking) as tolerated
4. Fall prevention (eg, visual/hearing checks, minimizing pharmacologic agents that contribute to fall risk, checking environment for safety hazards)
5. Avoidance of tobacco use and excessive alcohol intake
6. Calcium: Adequate intake of at least 1,200 mg **elemental** calcium daily in the form of dietary calcium or calcium supplementation, particularly women ≥50 years of age. Intakes exceeding 1,200 to 1,500 mg offer limited additional benefit and may increase the risk for cardiovascular disease or kidney stones. To minimize constipation, add fiber and start with 500 mg/day for several months, then increase to 500 mg twice daily taken at different times than fiber. Chewable and liquid products are available. Calcium carbonate is given with food to enhance bioavailability. Calcium citrate may be given without regards to meals.
   a. Contraindications: Hypercalcemia, ventricular fibrillation
   b. Side effects: Constipation, anorexia
   c. Drug interactions: Fiber, tetracycline, iron supplement, minerals
7. Vitamin D Supplement: Adequate intake of at least 800 to 1,000 int. units of vitamin D for adults ≥50 years of age. Measuring serum vitamin D concentrations may be warranted, particularly in those at greatest risk for deficiency, to allow for the administration of vitamin D replacement. **Note:** Certain patients at risk for vitamin D deficiency (eg, elderly patients, diseases associated with malabsorption, chronic renal insufficiency) may require higher intakes. Some elderly patients, especially with significant renal or liver disease cannot metabolize (activate) vitamin D and require calcitriol 0.25 mcg orally twice daily or adjusted per serum calcium level, the active form of vitamin D.
   a. Contraindications: Hypercalcemia (weakness, headache, drowsiness, nausea, diarrhea), hypercalciuria, and renal stones
   b. Side effects (uncommon): Hypercalcemia (see above)
   c. Monitor 24-hour urine and serum calcium if using >1,000 units/day

8. Bisphosphonates: Osteoporosis prevention: Postmenopausal Females: See also the chapter on risk of medication related osteonecrosis of the jaw [MRONJ]
   a. Alendronate: Oral: 5 mg once daily **or** 35 mg once weekly
   b. Ibandronate: Oral: 2.5 mg once daily **or** 150 mg once per month
   c. Risedronate: Oral: 5 mg once daily **or** 35 mg once weekly **or** one 75 mg tablet once daily on two consecutive days per month (total: 2 tablets/month) or 150 mg once per month
   d. Zoledronic acid (Reclast): IV: 5 mg infused over at least 15 minutes every 2 years
9. Glucocorticoid-induced osteoporosis prevention: Males and Females:
   a. Alendronate: Oral: 5 to 10 mg once daily
   b. Risedronate: Oral: 5 mg once daily
   c. Zoledronic acid (Reclast): IV: 5 mg every 12 months
10. Estrogen agonist/antagonist (previously known as selective estrogen receptor modulators):
    a. Postmenopausal Females: Raloxifene: Oral: 60 mg once daily; may be taken any time of the day without regard to meals but should be stopped 72 hours prior to or during immobilization due to risk of thromboembolic events.
11. Parathyroid hormone: Initial administration of teriparatide should occur under circumstances in which the patient may sit or lie down, in the event of orthostasis
    a. Glucocorticoid-induced osteoporosis prevention: Males and Females: Teriparatide: SubQ: 20 mcg once daily
12. Estrogens/hormone therapy: Should not be considered first agents for preventing osteoporosis due to increased risk of breast cancer, heart disease, stroke, and deep-vein thrombosis (DVT) found in the Women's Health Initiative study. Estrogens, as well as various combination therapies, including ethinyl estradiol and norethindrone (femhrt) and estradiol and norgestimate (Prefest), have been approved for the prevention of osteoporosis. The FDA recommends that approved nonestrogen treatments should be considered before the use of estrogen/hormone therapy for the sole purpose of prevention of osteoporosis. **Note:** In women with an intact uterus, administer estrogen with oral progesterone; unopposed estrogen can cause endometrial cancer.
13. Bone-modifying agent: Osteoporosis in postmenopausal female: Denosumab: SubQ: 60 mg once every 6 months. Also used to treat bone loss caused by specific cancers or treatments of specific cancers (See chapter on risk of medication related osteonecrosis of the jaw [MRONJ]).

Treatment of Osteoporosis

1. Calcium: Adequate intake of at least 1,200 mg **elemental** calcium daily in the form of dietary calcium or calcium supplementation, particularly women ≥50 years of age. Intakes exceeding 1,200 to 1,500 mg offer limited additional benefit and may increase the risk for cardiovascular disease or kidney stones. To minimize constipation, add fiber and start with 500 mg/day for several months, then increase to 500 mg twice daily taken at different times than fiber. Chewable and liquid products are available. Calcium carbonate is given with food to enhance bioavailability. Calcium citrate may be given without regards to meals.
   a. Contraindications: Hypercalcemia, ventricular fibrillation
   b. Side effects: Constipation, anorexia
   c. Drug interactions: Fiber, tetracycline, iron supplement, minerals
2. Vitamin D Supplement: Adequate intake of at least 800 to 1,000 int. units of vitamin D for adults ≥50 years of age. Measuring serum vitamin D concentrations may be warranted, particularly in those at greatest risk for deficiency, to allow for the administration of vitamin D replacement. **Note:** Certain patients at risk for vitamin D deficiency (eg, elderly patients, diseases associated with malabsorption, chronic renal insufficiency) may require higher intakes. Some elderly patients, especially with significant renal or liver disease cannot metabolize (activate) vitamin D and require calcitriol 0.25 mcg orally twice daily or adjusted per serum calcium level, the active form of vitamin D.
   a. Contraindications: Hypercalcemia (weakness, headache, drowsiness, nausea, diarrhea), hypercalciuria, and renal stones
   b. Side effects (uncommon): Hypercalcemia (see above)
   c. Monitor 24-hour urine and serum calcium if using >1,000 units/day
3. Weight-bearing exercise (eg, walking) as tolerated

4. Estrogens/hormone therapy: Should not be considered first agents for preventing osteoporosis due to increased risk of breast cancer, heart disease, stroke, and deep-vein thrombosis (DVT) found in the Women's Health Initiative study. Estrogens, as well as various combination therapies, including ethinyl estradiol and norethindrone (femhrt) and estradiol and norgestimate (Prefest), have been approved for the prevention of osteoporosis. The FDA recommends that approved nonestrogen treatments should be considered before the use of estrogen/hormone therapy for the sole purpose of prevention of osteoporosis. **Note:** In women with an intact uterus, administer estrogen with oral progesterone; unopposed estrogen can cause endometrial cancer.

5. Bisphosphonates: Oral bisphosphonates should be administered ≥30 minutes before first food or drink (except water) with 6 to 8 ounces tap water (**not** mineral water) and patients should remain upright (or raise head of bed to at least a 30° angle) to avoid ulcerative esophagitis. Consult individual monographs for details regarding use, precautions, dosing, and administration (See chapter on risk of medication related osteonecrosis of the jaw [MRONJ]).

6. Fall prevention: Minimize psychoactive and cardiovascular drugs (monitor BP for orthostasis), give diuretics early in the day, environmental safety check.

	% Elemental Calcium	Elemental Calcium
Calcium gluconate (various)	9	500 mg = 45 mg
Calcium glubionate (Calcionate)	6.5	1.8 g = 115 g per 5 mL
Calcium lactate (various)	13	325 mg = 42.25 mg
Calcium citrate (Citracal)	21	950 mg = 200 mg
Effervescent tabs (Citracal Liquitab)		2,376 mg = 500 mg
Calcium acetate (Phos-Lo)		667 mg = 169 mg
Calcium phosphate, tribasic (Posture)	39	1,565.2 mg = 600 mg
Calcium carbonate		
Tums	40	1.2 g = 500 mg
Oral suspension		1.25 g per 5 mL = 500 mg
Caltrate 600		1.5 g = 600 mg

REFERENCES AND SELECTED READINGS

National Osteoporosis Foundation. Clinician's guide to prevention and treatment of osteoporosis. Washington, DC; 2010. Available at http://www.nof.org/files/nof/public/content/file/344/upload/159.pdf

HORMONAL THERAPY

Two uses of hormonal supplementation include oral contraceptives and estrogen replacement therapy. Drugs used for contraception interfere with fertility by inhibiting release of follicle stimulating hormone, luteinizing hormone, and by preventing ovulation. There are few oral side effects; however, moderate gingivitis, similar to that seen during pregnancy, has been reported.

Drugs commonly encountered include:

Estradiol and Dienogest on page 597
Estradiol and Norethindrone on page 598
Estradiol and Norgestimate on page 599
Ethinyl Estradiol and Drospirenone on page 610
Ethinyl Estradiol and Ethynodiol Diacetate on page 611
Ethinyl Estradiol and Etonogestrel on page 612
Ethinyl Estradiol and Levonorgestrel on page 612
Ethinyl Estradiol and Norethindrone on page 614
Ethinyl Estradiol and Norgestimate on page 616
Ethinyl Estradiol and Norgestrel on page 617
Ethinyl Estradiol, Drospirenone, and Levomefolate on page 618
MedroxyPROGESTERone on page 953
Norethindrone on page 1117
Norethindrone and Mestranol

Estrogens or derivatives are usually prescribed as replacement therapy following menopause or cyclic irregularities and to inhibit osteoporosis. The following list of drugs may interact with antidepressants and barbiturates. New tissue-specific estrogens like Evista may help with the problem of osteoporosis.

Estradiol (Systemic) on page 596
Estradiol and Levonorgestrol on page 598
Estrogens (Conjugated/Equine, Systemic) on page 601
Estrogens (Conjugated A/Synthetic)
Estrogens (Conjugated B/Synthetic) on page 601
Estrogens (Esterified) on page 604
Estrogens (Conjugated/Equine) and Medroxyprogesterone on page 603
Estrogens (Esterified) and Methyltestosterone on page 605
Estropipate on page 605
Raloxifene on page 1304

PREGNANCY

Normal endocrine and physiologic functions are altered during pregnancy. Endogenous estrogens and progesterone increase and placental hormones are secreted. Thyroid stimulating hormone and growth hormone also increase. Cardiovascular changes can result and increased blood volume can lead to blood pressure elevations and transient heart murmurs. Generally, in a normal pregnancy, oral gingival changes will be limited to gingivitis. Alteration of treatment plans might include limiting administration of all drugs to emergency procedures only during the first and third trimesters and medical consultation regarding the patients' status for all elective procedures. Limiting dental care throughout pregnancy to preventive procedures is reasonable. The effects on dental treatment of the "morning after pill" (Plan B and PREVEN) and the abortifacient, mifepristone on page 1028, have not been documented at this time. Consultation with the patient's internist and obstetrician for evaluation of medication safety in pregnancy is advised.

Hypertensive Disorders and Pregnancy

Hypertensive disorders, including chronic or preexisting hypertension and the development of hypertension during pregnancy, occur in 12% to 22% of pregnant women. Oral health professionals should consult with patient's prenatal care provider before initiating dental procedures due to increased bleeding with uncontrolled severe hypertension (blood pressure values ≥160/110 mm Hg).

Diabetes and Pregnancy

Gestational diabetes occurs in 2% to 5% of pregnant women in the US. It is usually diagnosed after 24 weeks of gestation. Any inflammatory process, including acute and chronic periodontal infection, may make diabetes control more difficult. Poorly controlled diabetes is associated with adverse pregnancy outcomes, such as pre-eclampsia, congenital anomalies, and large-for-gestational-age newborns. Meticulous control to avoid or minimize dental infection is important for pregnant women with diabetes. Regulating all sources of acute or chronic inflammation helps manage diabetes.

REFERENCES AND SELECTED READINGS

American Diabetes Association. Standards of medical care in diabetes - 2013. *Diabetes Care*. 2013;36(Suppl 1):S11-S66.

Bertagna X, Guignat L, Groussin L, Bertherat J. Cushing's disease. *Best Pract Res Clin Endocrinol Metab*. 2009;23:607-623.

Carlos-Fabue L, Jimenez-Soriano Y, Sarrion-Perez MG. Dental management of patients with endocrine disorders. *J Clin Exp Dent*. 2010;2(4)e:196–203.

De Groot L, Abalovich M, Alexander EK, et al. Management of thyroid dysfunction during pregnancy and postpartum: an Endocrine Society clinical practice guideline. *J Clin Endocrinol Metab*. 2012;97(8):2543-2565.

Gibson N, Ferguson JW. Steroid cover for dental patients on longterm steroid medication: proposed clinical guidelines based upon a critical review of the literature. *Br Dent J*. 2004;197(11):681-685.

Handelsman Y, Mechanick JI, Blonde L, et al. American Association of Clinical Endocrinologists medical guidelines for clinical practice for developing a diabetes mellitus comprehensive care plan. *Endocr Pract*. 2011;17(Suppl 2):1-53.

Huber MA, Terézhalmy GT. Risk stratification and dental management of the patient with thyroid dysfunction. *Quintessence Int*. 2008;39(2):139-150.

Kelly A, Pomarico L, de Souza IP. Cessation of dental development. in a child with idiopathic hypoparathyroidism: a 5-year follow-up. *Oral Surg Oral Med Oral Pathol Oral Radiol Endod*. 2009;107(5):673-677.

Michalowicz BS, DiAngelis AJ, Novak MJ, et al. Examining the safety of dental treatment in pregnant women. *J Am Dent Assoc*. 2008;139 (6):685-695.

Michalowicz BS, Hodges JS, DiAngelis AJ, et al. Treatment of periodontal disease and the risk of preterm birth. *N Engl J Med*. 2006;355 (18):1885-1894.

Nathan DM, Buse JB, Davidson MB. Medical management of hyperglycemia in type 2 diabetes: a consensus algorithm for the initiation and adjustment of therapy: a consensus statement of the American Diabetes Association and the European Association for the Study of Diabetes. *Diabetes Care*. 2009;32(1):193-203.

Rodbard HW, Jellinger PS, Davidson JA. Statement by an American Association of Clinical Endocrinologists/American College of Endocrinology consensus panel on type 2 diabetes mellitus: an algorithm for glycemic control. *Endocr Pract*. 2009;15(6):540-559.

Stagnaro-Green A, Abalovich M, Alexander E. Guidelines of the American Thyroid Association for the diagnosis and management of thyroid disease during pregnancy and postpartum. *Thyroid*. 2011;21(10):1081-1125.

HIV INFECTION AND AIDS

Human immunodeficiency virus (HIV) represents agents HIV-1 and HIV-2 that produce a devastating systemic disease. The virus causes disease by leading to elevated risk of infections in patients and, from our experience over the last 37 years, there clearly are oral manifestations associated with these patients. Also, there has been a revolution in infection control in our dental offices over the last two decades due to our expanding knowledge of this infectious agent. Infection control practices have been elevated to include all of the infectious agents with which dentists often come into contact. These might include, in addition to HIV, hepatitis viruses (of which the serotypes include A, B, C, D, E, F, and G); the herpes viruses (see Systemic Viral Diseases on page 1709); and STDs such as syphilis, gonorrhea, and papillomavirus (see Sexually-Transmitted Diseases on page 1707).

Acquired immunodeficiency syndrome (AIDS) has been recognized since early 1981 as a unique clinical syndrome manifest by opportunistic infections or by neoplasms complicating the underlying defect in the cellular immune system. These defects are brought on by infection and pathogenesis with human immunodeficiency virus 1 or 2 (HIV-1 is the predominant serotype identified). The major cellular defect brought on by infection with HIV is a depletion of T-cells, primarily the subtype, T-helper cells, known as CD4+ cells. When the CD4 cell count falls below 200 cells/µL, patients are at high risk for life-threatening AIDS-defining opportunistic infections (eg, *Pneumocystis jirovecii* pneumonia, *Toxoplasma gondii* encephalitis, disseminated *Mycobacterium avium* complex disease, tuberculosis, bacterial pneumonia, and oralpharyngeal candidiasis). Over these years, our knowledge regarding HIV infection and the oral manifestations often associated with patients with HIV or AIDS, has increased dramatically. Populations of individuals known to be at high risk of HIV transmission include homosexuals, intravenous drug abuse patients, transfusion recipients, patients with other sexually transmitted diseases, and patients practicing promiscuous sex.

The definitions of AIDS have also evolved over this period of time. The natural history of HIV infection along with some of the oral manifestations can be reviewed in Table 1. The risk of developing these opportunistic infections increases as the patient progresses to AIDS.

Table 1. Natural History of HIV Infection/Oral Manifestations

Time From Transmission (Average)	Observation	CD4 Cell Count
0	Viral transmissions	Normal: 1,000 (±500/mm^3)
2 to 4 weeks	Self-limited infectious mononucleosis-like illness with fever, rash, leukopenia, mucocutaneous ulcerations (mouth, genitals, etc), thrush	Transient decrease
6 to 12 weeks	Seroconversion (rarely requires ≥3 months for seroconversion)	Normal
0 to 8 years	Healthy/asymptomatic HIV infection; peripheral/persistent generalized lymphadenopathy; HPV, thrush, OHL; RAU, periodontal diseases, salivary gland diseases; dermatitis	≥500/mm^3 gradual reduction with average decrease of 50 to 80/mm^3/year
4 to 8 years	Early symptomatic HIV infection previously called (AIDS-related complex): Thrush, vaginal candidiasis (persistent, frequent and/or severe), cervical dysplasia/CA Hodgkin lymphoma, B-cell lymphoma, oral hairy leukoplakia, salivary gland diseases, ITP, xerostomia, dermatitis, shingles; RAU, herpes simplex, HPV, bacterial infections, periodontal diseases, molluscum contagiosum, other physical symptoms: fever, weight loss, fatigue	≥300 to 500/mm^3
6 to 10 years	AIDS: Wasting syndrome, *Candida* esophagitis, Kaposi's sarcoma, HIV-associated dementia, disseminated *M. avium*, Hodgkin's or B-cell lymphoma, herpes simplex >30 days; PCP; cryptococcal meningitis, other systemic fungal infections; CMV	<200/mm^3

Natural history indicates course of HIV infection in absence of antiretroviral treatment. Adapted from: Bartlett JG. A guide to HIV care from the AIDS Care Program of the Johns Hopkins Medical Institutions. 2nd ed.

PCP = *Pneumocystis carinii* pneumonia, ITP = immune thrombocytopenia (formerly known as idiopathic thrombocytopenic purpura), HPV = human papilloma virus, OHL = oral hairy leukoplakia, RAU = recurrent aphthous ulcer

Patients with HIV infection and/or AIDS are seen in dental offices throughout the country. In general, it is the dentist's obligation to treat HIV individuals including patients of record and other patients who may seek treatment when the office is accepting new patients. These patients are protected under the Americans with Disabilities Act and the dentist has an obligation as described. Two excellent publications, one by the American Dental Association and the other by the American Academy of Oral Medicine, outline the dentist's responsibility as well as a very detailed explanation of dental management protocols for HIV patients. These protocols, however, are evolving just as our knowledge of HIV has evolved. New drugs and their interactions present the dentist with continuous need for updates regarding the appropriate management of HIV patients. Diagnostic tests, including determining viral load in combination with the CD4 status, now are used to modify a patient's treatment in ways that allow them to remain relatively illness-free for longer periods of time. This places more of a responsibility on the dental practice team to be aware of drug changes, of new drugs, and of the appropriate oral management in such patients.

Our knowledge of AIDS allows us to properly treat these patients while protecting ourselves, our staff, and other patients in the office. All types of infectious disease require consistent practices in our dental offices known as Standard/Universal Precautions. These agents include sexually transmitted disease agents, the highly virulent hepatitis viruses, and the less virulent but always worrisome HIV. In general, an office that is practicing standard/universal precautions is one that is considered safe for patients and staff. Throughout this spectrum, HIV is placed somewhere in the middle, in terms of infection risk in the dental office. Other sexually transmitted diseases and infectious diseases such as tuberculosis represent a greater threat to the dentist than HIV itself. However, due to the grave danger of HIV infection, many of our precautions have been instituted to assist the dentist in protecting himself, his staff, and other patients in situations where the office may be involved in treating a patient that is HIV positive.

As in the management of all medically compromised patients, the appropriate care of HIV patients begins with a complete and thorough history. This history must allow the dentist to identify risk factors in the development of HIV as well as identify those patients known to be HIV positive. Knowledge of all medications prescribed to patients at risk is also important.

The current antiretroviral therapy used to treat patients with HIV infection and/or AIDS includes three primary classifications of drugs. These are the nucleoside analogs, protease inhibitors, and the non-nucleoside/nucleotide analogs (analogs refers to chemicals that can substitute competitively for naturally produced cell components such as found in DNA, RNA, or proteins). The newest drugs include several nucleoside analogs, abacavir (Ziagen), sub protease inhibitors, amprenavir, several non-nucleoside analogs, efavirenz (Sustiva), and adefovir, as well as the latest combination drugs, such as elvitegravir, cobicistat, emtricitabine, and tenofovir disoproxil fumarate (Stribild; formerly Quad). Finding the perfect "cocktail" of anti-HIV medications still eludes clinicians. This is partly due to the fact that therapies are still too novel and the patient's years too few to study. Numerous studies have indicated that combinations of drugs are far better than individual drug therapy. Several of these studies have looked at two drug combinations, particularly between nucleoside analogs in combination with protease inhibitors. The newer drugs (non-nucleoside analogs) have added the possibility of a triple "cocktail". Recently several studies indicated that this three-drug combination may be the best in managing HIV infection.

When HIV was first discovered, the efforts for monitoring HIV infection focused on the CD4 blood levels and the ratios between the helper cells, suppressor cells within the patient's immune system. These markers were used to indicate success or failure of drug therapies as patients moved through HIV pathogenesis toward AIDS. More recently, however, the advent of protease inhibitors has allowed clinicians to monitor the actual presence of viral RNA within the patient and the term viral load has become the focus of therapy monitoring. The availability of better therapies and our rapidly expanding knowledge of molecular biology of the HIV virus have created new opportunities to control the AIDS epidemic. Cases can be monitored closely looking at the number of copy units or virions within the patient's bloodstream as an indication in combination with other infections and/or declining or increasing CD4 numbers to establish prognostic values for the patient's success. Long-term survival of patients infected with HIV has been accomplished by monitoring and adjusting therapy to these numbers.

Comprehensive coordinated approaches, that have been advocated by researchers, have sought to establish national standards for HIV reporting, greater access to effective newly approved medications, improved access to individual physicians treating HIV patients, and continued protection of patient's privacy. These goals allow the reporting of studies that suggest that combination therapies, some of which have been tried in less controlled individual patient treatments, may prove useful in larger populations of HIV-infected individuals. As these studies are reported, the dental clinician should be aware that patients' drug therapies change rapidly, various combinations may be tried, and the side effects and interactions as described in the chapter on drug interactions and the CYP system will also emerge. The dentist must be aware of these potential interactions with seemingly innocuous drugs such as clarithromycin, erythromycin, and some of the sedative drugs that a dentist may utilize in their practice as well as some of the analgesics. These drug interactions may be the most important part of monitoring that the dentist provides in helping to manage a situation. Some of the antiviral drugs more commonly used for HIV, AIDS, Asymptomatic, CD4 <500, and the newer drugs (ie, protease inhibitors, nucleoside analogs, and non-nucleoside nucleotide analogs) are listed in Table 2.

Table 2. Examples of Drugs

Nucleoside Analogs	Protease Inhibitors	Non-nucleoside Analogs	Nucleotide Analogs	Fusion Protein Inhibitor	CCR5 Antagonist	Integrase Inhibitor
Zidovudine (Retrovir, AZT, SDV)	**Saquinavir** (Invirase)	**Nevirapine** (Viramune)	**Tenofovir disoproxil fumarate** (Viread)	**Enfuvirtide** (Fuzeon)	**Maraviroc** (Selzentry)	**Raltegravir** (Isentress)
Didanosine (Videx, ddi)	**Ritonavir** (Norvir)	**Delavirdine** (Rescriptor)				**Dolutegravir** (Tivicay)
Entecavir (Baraclude)	**Indinavir** (Crixivan)	**Efavirenz** (Sustiva)				
Stavudine (Zerit, d4T)	**Nelfinavir** (Viracept)	**Etravirine** (Intelence)				
LamiVUDine (Epivir)	**Fosamprenavir** (Lexiva)	**Rilpivirine** (Edurant)				
Abacavir (Ziagen)	**Atazanavir** (Reyataz)					
Emtricitabine (Emtriva)	**Darunavir** (Prezista)					
	Tipranavir (Aptivus)					

The presence of other infections is an important part of the health history. Appropriate medical consultation may be mandated after a health history in order to accomplish a complete evaluation of the patients at risk. Uniformity in the taking of a history from a patient is the dentist's best plan for all patients so that no selectivity or discrimination can be implicated.

An appropriate review of symptoms may also identify oral and systemic conditions that may be present in aggressive HIV disease. Medical physical examination may reveal preexisting or developing intra- or extra-oral signs/symptoms of progressive disease. Aggressive herpes simplex, herpes zoster, papillomavirus, Kaposi's sarcoma or lymphoma are among the disorders that might be identified. In addition to these, intra-oral examination may raise suspicion regarding fungal infections, angular cheilitis, squamous cell carcinoma, and recurrent aphthous ulcers. The dentist should be vigilant in all patients regardless of HIV risk.

It will always be up to the dental practitioner to determine whether testing for HIV should be recommended following the history and physical examination of a new patient. Because of the severe psychological implications of learning of HIV positivity for a patient, the dentist should be aware that there are appropriate referral sites where psychological counseling and appropriate discrete testing for the patient is available. The dentist's office should have these sites available for referral should the patient be interested. Candid discussions, however, with the patient regarding risk factors and/or other signs or symptoms in their history and physical condition that may indicate a higher HIV risk than the normal population, should be an area the dentist feels comfortable in broaching with any new patient. Oftentimes, it is appropriate to recommend testing for other infectious diseases should risk factors be present. For example, testing for hepatitis B and hepatitis C may be appropriate for the patient and along with this the dentist could recommend that the patient consider HIV testing. Because of the legal issues involved, anonymity for HIV testing may be appropriate and it is always up to the patient to follow the doctor's recommendations. Currently there are national projects underway to expand HIV disease awareness and included in these initiatives are increased training for dental professionals and in-office screening for HIV. HIV-related oral conditions occur in a large proportion of patients, and frequently are misdiagnosed or inadequately treated. Dental expertise is necessary for appropriate management of oral manifestations of HIV infection or AIDS, but many patients do not receive adequate dental care. Notable HIV-related oral conditions include xerostomia, candidiasis, oral hairy leukoplakia, periodontal diseases such as linear gingival erythema and necrotizing ulcerative periodontitis, Kaposi's sarcoma, human papilloma virus-associated warts, and ulcerative conditions including herpes simplex virus lesions, recurrent aphthous ulcers, and neutropenic ulcers. As therapies have improved and earlier recognition, diagnosis and treatment have been instituted, many of these conditions, including oral hairy leukoplakia and Kaposi's sarcoma, have nearly disappeared in the US and developed countries. Continued vigilance on the part of the dental team however is crucial for identification of other life-threatening complications, such as lymphoma, oral squamous cell carcinoma, and papillomavirus-related diseases remains paramount.

Early Dental Consultation Responsibilities

When a patient has either given a positive history of knowing that they are HIV positive or it has been determined after referral for consultation, the dentist should be aware of the AIDS-defining illnesses. Of course, current medical status and drug therapy that the patient may be undergoing is of equal importance. The dentist, through medical consultation and regular follow-up with the patient's physician, should be made aware of the CD4 count (Table 3), the viral load, and the drugs that the patient is taking. The presence of other AIDS-defining illnesses as well as complications, such as higher risk of endocarditis and the risk of other systemic infections such as tuberculosis, are extremely important for the dentist. These may make an impact on the dental treatment plan in terms of the selection of preprocedural antibiotics or the use of oral medications to treat opportunistic infections in or around the oral cavity.

Table 3. CD4+ Lymphocyte Count and Percentage as Related to the Risk of Opportunistic Infection

CD4+ Cells/mm^3	CD4+ Percentage[a]	Risk of Opportunistic Infection
>600	32 to 60	No increased risk
400 to 500	<29	Initial immune suppression
200 to 400	14 to 28	Appearance of opportunistic infections, some may be major
<200	<14	Severe immune suppression. AIDS diagnosis. Major opportunistic infections. Although variable, prognosis for surviving >3 years is poor
<50	—	Although variable, prognosis for surviving >1 year is poor

[a]Several studies have suggested that the CD4+ percentage demonstrates less variability between measurements, as compared to the absolute CD4+ cell count. CD4+ percentages may therefore give a clearer impression of the course of disease.

Adapted from: Glick M, Silverman S. Dental management of HIV-infected patients. *J Am Dent Assoc* (supplement to reviewers). 1995.

AIDS-defining illnesses, such as oral-pharyngeal candidiasis, herpes infections lasting >30 days, recurrent pneumonia, or lymphoma are clearly important to the dentist. Chemotherapy that might be being given to the patient for treatment for any or all of these disorders can have implications in terms of the patient's response to simple dental procedures.

Drug therapies have become complex in the treatment of HIV/AIDS. Because of the moderate successes with protease inhibitors and the drug combination therapies, more patients are living longer and receiving more dental care throughout their lives. Drug therapies are often tailored to the current CD4 count in combination with the viral load. In general, patients with high CD4 counts are usually at lower risk for complications in the dental office than patients with low CD4 counts. However, the presence of a high viral load with or without a stable CD4 count may be indicative or a more rapid progression of the HIV/AIDS disease process than had previously been thought. Patients with a high viral load and a declining CD4 count are considered to have the greatest risk and the poorest prognosis of all the groups.

In HIV infections, a new drug known as raltegravir is an integrase inhibitor which works by interrupting HIV integration into the host cell DNA. In addition, in 2007, a new class of anti-HIV drugs was introduced, these are the chemokine receptor 5 antagonists or the CCR5 receptor blockers. The drug of interest for this class is maraviroc. This antiviral drug has shown great promise as an adjuvant therapy along with other anti-HIV drugs.

Other organ damage, such as liver compromise potentially leading to bleeding disorders, can be found as the disease progresses to AIDS. Liver dysfunction may be related to preexisting hepatic diseases due to previous infection with a hepatitis virus such as hepatitis B or other drug toxicities associated with the treatment of AIDS. The dentist must have available current prothrombin and partial thromboplastin times (PT and PTT) in order to accurately evaluate any risk of bleeding abnormality. Platelet count and liver function studies are also important. Potential drug interactions include some antibiotics, as well as any anticoagulating drugs, which may be contraindicated in such patients. It may be necessary to avoid NSAIDs, as well as aspirin. (See Drug Interactions: Metabolism/Transport Effects on page 1807).

The use of preprocedural antibiotics is another issue in the HIV patient. As the absolute neutrophil count declines during the progression of AIDS, the use of antibiotics as a preprocedural step prior to dental care may be necessary. If protracted treatment plans are necessary, the dentist should receive updated information as the patient receives such from their physician. It is always important that the dentist have current CD4 counts, viral load assay, as well as liver function studies, AST and ALT, and bleeding indicators including platelet count, PT, and PTT. If any other existing conditions such as cardiac involvement or joint prostheses are involved, antibiotic coverage may also be necessary. However, these determinations are no different than in the non-HIV population and this subject is covered in Antibiotic Prophylaxis - Preprocedural Guidelines for Dental Patients on page 1715. See Laboratory Values/Body Measurements on page 1809 as a general guideline for provision of dental care.

The consideration of current blood values is important in long-term care of any medically compromised patient and in particular the HIV-positive patient. Preventive dental care is likewise valuable in these patients, however, the dentist's approach should be no different than as with all patients. See Table 4 for oral lesions commonly associated with HIV disease and a brief description of their usual treatment (see Part II of this Oral Medicine chapter for more detailed descriptions of these common oral lesions).

The clinician should be aware that several of the protease inhibitors have now been associated with drug interactions. Some of these drug interactions include therapies that the dentist may be utilizing. The basis for these drug interactions with protease inhibitors is the inhibition of cytochrome P450 isoforms, which are important in normal liver function and metabolism of drugs. A detailed description of the mechanisms of inhibition can be found in Drug Interactions: Metabolism/Transport Effects on page 1807, as well as a table illustrating some known drug interactions with antiviral therapy and drugs commonly prescribed in the dental office. The metabolism of these drugs could be affected by the patient's antiviral therapy.

Every dental office should have in place protocols for standard/universal precautions during patient care and for emergency procedures in case of occupational exposure to blood-borne pathogens.

Table 4. Oral Lesions Commonly Seen in HIV/AIDS

Condition	Management
Oral candidiasis	See Fungal Infections on page 1752
Angular cheilitis	
Oral hairy leukoplakia	See Systemic Viral Diseases on page 1709
Periodontal diseases Linear gingivitis Ulcerative periodontitis	See Bacterial Infections on page 1739
Herpes simplex	See Systemic Viral Diseases on page 1709
Herpes zoster	
Chronic aphthous ulceration	Palliation/Thalidomide (Thalomid)
Salivary gland disease	Referral
Human papillomavirus	Laser/Surgical excision
Kaposi's sarcoma	See Antibiotic Prophylaxis on page 1715; Biopsy/Laser
Non-Hodgkin's lymphoma	Biopsy/Referral
Tuberculosis	Referral

Abacavir on page 50
Abacavir and Lamivudine on page 51
Abacavir, Lamivudine, and Zidovudine on page 52
Atazanavir on page 186
Dapsone (Systemic) on page 436
Darunavir on page 441
Delavirdine on page 451
Didanosine on page 492
Dolutegravir on page 511
Efavirenz on page 543
Efavirenz, Emtricitabine, and Tenofovir Disoproxil Fumarate on page 545
Elvitegravir, Cobicistat, Emtricitabine, and Tenofovir Disoproxil Fumarate on page 553
Emtricitabine on page 556
Emtricitabine and Tenofovir Disoproxil Fumarate on page 558
Emtricitabine, Rilpivirine, and Tenofovir Disoproxil Fumarate on page 559
Enfuvirtide on page 564
Entecavir on page 567
Etravirine on page 627
Fosamprenavir on page 712
Indinavir on page 807
LamiVUDine on page 872

Lamivudine and Zidovudine on page 874
Lopinavir and Ritonavir on page 929
Maraviroc on page 947
Nelfinavir on page 1092
Nevirapine on page 1096
Raltegravir on page 1306
Rilpivirine on page 1327
Ritonavir on page 1335
Saquinavir on page 1357
Stavudine on page 1387
Tenofovir Disoproxil Fumarate on page 1419
Thalidomide on page 1435
Tipranavir on page 1452
Zidovudine on page 1569

Several new classes of drugs have been developed as antiretroviral drug classifications in the management of HIV infection. These are fusion inhibitors, CCR5 receptor blockers, integrase inhibitors, post-attachment inhibitors, and pharmacokinetic enhancers. The prototype fusion inhibitor is enfuvirtide (Fuzeon). There are no significant drug interactions; however, there are numerous side effects and toxicities including Guillain-Barré syndrome, as well as taste aberrations with this drug. The prototype CCR5 receptor blocker is maraviroc (Selzentry), the integrase inhibitors are dolutegravir and raltegravir (Isentress) both with no specific oral side effects, post-attachment inhibitor is ibalizumab-uiyk, and pharmacokinetic enhancer is cobicistat. More than 23 combination drugs involving 2, 3, or 4 of these drug classes have been introduced to enhance compliance and long-term control.

First FDA-Approved Medication to Reduce HIV Risk

The FDA has approved a new indication for the existing drug emtricitabine and tenofovir disoproxil fumarate (Truvada) as a once daily dose used in combination with safer sex practices to reduce the risk of sexually-acquired HIV infection in high-risk adults not currently infected with HIV. The drug, first approved for treating HIV infection in 2004, is a combination of the cytosine analogue nucleoside reverse transcriptase inhibitor emtricitabine and the nucleotide reverse transcriptase inhibitor tenofovir disoproxil fumarate, an analog of adenosine 5'-monophosphate. Each drug interferes with HIV viral RNA-dependent DNA polymerase, resulting in inhibition of viral replication. In two large clinical trials, daily use of Truvada was shown to significantly reduce the risk of contracting HIV. In a study sponsored by the National Institutes of Health (NIH) of about 2,500 HIV-negative gay and bisexual men and transgender women, Truvada reduced the risk of infection by ~42%. In a study sponsored by the University of Washington, risk was reduced by 75% in about 4,800 heterosexual couples in which one partner was HIV-positive and the other was not.

It is important that patients recognize that Truvada is not a substitute for safer sex practices. The drug is meant to be used as an adjunct to a comprehensive HIV prevention plan that includes consistent and correct condom use, risk reduction counseling, regular HIV testing, and treatment of any other sexually-transmitted infections. Health care providers must stress that healthy patients adhere to the pill's daily-dose regimen, which is necessary for it to work, and not discontinue other prevention measures, such as condom use. Truvada must be taken every day in order to help prevent HIV infection. One fear is that high-risk patients will not take this medication correctly, become infected, and develop a drug-resistant strain of HIV infection that may be more difficult to treat. These patients may then spread the infection to others, believing they are still HIV-negative.

Common side effects of Truvada include gastrointestinal problems (eg, nausea, abdominal pain, decreased appetite, weight loss, cramping, diarrhea). Joint or muscle pain, pain or tingling in the hands or feet, headache, dizziness, and fatigue are also possible. Obviously, such side effects can compromise daily compliance. Serious side effects may include fatal lactic acidosis and liver disease, as well as muscle weakness, blood disorders, renal failure, and pancreatitis.

The approval of this new indication is not without controversy. The AIDS Healthcare Foundation, a global AIDS organization that provides medical care and services to HIV-infected people, called the FDA's approval of Truvada for HIV prevention "reckless" and criticized the agency for not requiring proof of a negative HIV test in users. In March, the group had filed a petition with the agency urging it to reject Truvada's application, citing concerns about drug side effects, the nearly $14,000 annual cost of the drug and the difficulty of sticking with a daily pill regimen.

FDA Approves HIV Home Test Kit

With the CDC estimating that of the 1.2 million people living with HIV in this country, one-fifth or ~240,000 are unaware of their status. Furthermore, there are ~50,000 new cases of HIV infection added to that number annually. Because of these statistics, many people are unaware they are HIV positive may be transmitting the virus unknowingly. Testing helps slow new infections. In that regard, the FDA approved the first over-the-counter HIV test kit that allows people to test for HIV infection in the privacy of their own homes. The OraQuick In-Home HIV Test detects the presence of antibodies to human immunodeficiency virus type 1 (HIV-1) and type 2 (HIV-2). In essence, the kit is an OTC version of a test used in the clinical setting that was approved by the FDA in 2004. The idea is not for the home test kit to replace medical testing but to provide another route for people to find out their HIV status. In this test, the user takes an oral swab and places it in a specially prepared vial that comes with the kit. The result is ready in 20 to 40 minutes. However, the newly approved OTC kit is not as reliable as being tested by a trained clinician.

The FDA stressed in its approval announcement that the test is not 100% accurate in identifying people with the virus. A trial conducted by test maker OraSure showed OraQuick detected HIV in those carrying the virus only 92% of the time, though it was 99.9% accurate in ruling out HIV in patients not carrying the virus. That means the test could miss one in 12 HIV-infected people (false-negative) who use it but would incorrectly identify only one patient as having HIV for every

5,000 HIV-negative people tested (false-positive). As with other HIV tests performed by trained personnel, a positive result does not necessarily mean that the user is definitely infected with HIV, but that they should then go and be tested in a medical setting to confirm the result. Similarly, a negative result does not necessarily mean the user is definitely not infected, particularly if they may have picked up the virus in the previous 2 to 3 months and have not yet seroconverted. In many areas of the country, Dental and Dental Hygiene students are being trained and certified in using and interpreting these screening tests.

Trends in current HIV treatment approach include preventative and therapeutic vaccine development, gene therapy, immunotherapy, and long acting (easily compliant) treatments. Identification and characterization of naturally immune individuals has shown promise for future success in these efforts.

Updated US Public Health Service Guidelines for the Management of Occupational Exposures to Human Immunodeficiency Virus and Recommendations for Postexposure Prophylaxis

The US Public Health Service has updated its recommendations for the management of health care personnel (HCP) who experience occupational exposure to blood and/or other body fluids that might contain human immunodeficiency virus (HIV). Although the principles of exposure management remain unchanged, recommended HIV postexposure prophylaxis (PEP) regimens and the duration of HIV followup testing for exposed personnel have been updated. This report emphasizes the importance of primary prevention strategies, the prompt reporting and management of occupational exposures, adherence to recommended HIV PEP regimens when indicated for an exposure, expert consultation in management of exposures, follow-up of exposed HCP to improve adherence to PEP, and careful monitoring for adverse events related to treatment, as well as for virologic, immunologic, and serologic signs of infection. To ensure timely postexposure management and administration of HIV PEP, clinicians should consider occupational exposures as urgent medical concerns, and institutions should take steps to ensure that staff are aware of both the importance of and the institutional mechanisms available for reporting and seeking care for such exposures. Summary of recommendations: (1) PEP is recommended when occupational exposures to HIV occur; (2) the HIV status of the exposure source patient should be determined, if possible, to guide need for HIV PEP; (3) PEP medication regimens should be started as soon as possible after occupational exposure to HIV, and they should be continued for a 4-week duration; (4) new recommendation—PEP medication regimens should contain 3 (or more) antiretroviral drugs for all occupational exposures to HIV; (5) expert consultation is recommended for any occupational exposures to HIV and at a minimum for situations described in Box 1; (6) close follow-up for exposed personnel (Box 2) should be provided that includes counseling, baseline and follow-up HIV testing, and monitoring for drug toxicity; follow-up appointments should begin within 72 hours of an HIV exposure; and (7) new recommendation—if a newer fourth-generation combination HIV p24 antigen–HIV antibody test is utilized for follow-up HIV testing of exposed HCP, HIV testing may be concluded 4 months after exposure (Box 2); if a newer testing platform is not available, follow-up HIV testing is typically concluded 6 months after an HIV exposure.

FREQUENTLY ASKED QUESTIONS

How does one get AIDS, aside from having unprotected sex?

Our current knowledge about the immunodeficiency virus is that it is carried via semen, contaminated needles, blood products, transfusion products not tested, and potentially in other fluids of the body. Patients at highest risk include IV drug-abusers, those receiving multiple transfusions with blood that has not been screened for HIV, or patients practicing unprotected sex with multiple partners, where the history of the partner may not be as clear as the patient would like.

Are patients safe from AIDS or HIV infection when they present to the dentist office?

Our current knowledge indicates that the answer is an unequivocal "yes". The patient is protected because dental offices are practicing standard/universal precautions, using antimicrobial handwashing agents, gloves, face masks, eye protection, special clothing, aerosol control, and instrument soaking and autoclaving. All of these procedures stop potential transmission to a new patient, as well as, allow for easy disposal of contaminated office supplies for elimination of microbes by an antimicrobial technique, should they be contaminated through treatment of another patient. These precautions are mandated by OSHA requirements.

What is the most common opportunistic infection that HIV-positive patients suffer that may be important in dentistry?

The most common opportunistic infection important to dentistry is oral candidiasis. This disease can present as white plaques, red areas, or angular cheilitis occurring at the corners of the mouth. Management of such lesions is appropriate by the dentist and is described in this handbook (see Fungal Infections on page 1752). Other oral complications include HIV-associated periodontal disease, as well as the other conditions outlined in Table 4. Of great concern to the dentist is the risk of tuberculosis. In many HIV-positive patients, tuberculosis has become a serious, life-threatening opportunistic infection. The dentist should be aware that appropriate referral for anyone showing such respiratory signs and symptoms would be prudent.

Can one patient infect another through unprotected sex if the other patient has tested negative for HIV?

Yes, there is always the possibility that a sexual partner may be in the early window of time when plasma viremia is not at a detectable level. The antibody response to plasma viremia may be slightly delayed and diagnostic testing may not indicate HIV positivity. This window of time represents a period when the patient may be infectious but not show up yet on normal diagnostic testing.

Can HIV be passed by oral fluids?

As our knowledge about HIV has evolved, we have thought that HIV is inactivated in saliva by an agent possibly associated with secretory leukocyte protease inhibitors known as SLPI. There is, however, a current resurgence in our interest in oral transmission because some research indicates that in moderate to advanced periodontal lesions or other oral lesions where there is tissue damage, the presence of a serous exudate may increase the risk of transmission. The dentist should be aware of this ongoing research and attempt to renew knowledge regularly so that any future breakthroughs will be noted.

REFERENCES AND SELECTED READINGS

Barouch DH, Baden LR, Dolin R. Human immunodeficiency virus vaccines. *Principles and Practice of Infectious Disease.* 6th ed. Mandell GL, Bennett JE, Dolin R, eds. Philadelphia, PA: Churchhill Livingstone; 2005;1707-1717.

Bodhade AS, Ganvir SM, Hazarey VK. Oral manifestations of HIV infection and their correlation with CD4 count. *J Oral Sci.* 2011;53(2):203–211.

DHHS Panel on Antiretroviral Guidelines for Adults and Adolescents. Guidelines for the use of antiretroviral agents in HIV-1-infected adults and adolescents, Department of Health and Human Services. 2013;1-267. Available at http://aidsinfo.nih.gov/contentfiles/lvguidelines/adultandadolescentgl.pdf

DHHS Panel on Antiretroviral Therapy and Medical Management of HIV-Infected Children. Guidelines for the use of antiretroviral agents in pediatric HIV infection, Department of Health and Human Services. 2011;1-268. Available at http://www.aidsinfo.nih.gov

DHHS Panel on Treatment of HIV-Infected Pregnant Women and Prevention of Perinatal Transmission. Recommendations for use of antiretroviral drugs in pregnant HIV-1-infected women for maternal health and interventions to reduce perinatal HIV transmission in the United States. 2012. Available at http://aidsinfo.nih.gov/contentfiles/lvguidelines/perinatalgl.pdf

Ghallab NA. Diagnostic potential and future directions of biomarkers in gingival crevicular fluid and saliva of periodontal diseases: review of the current evidence. *Arch Oral Biol.* 2018;87:115-124.

Kuhar DT, Henderson DK, Struble KA, et al. Updated US Public Health Service guidelines for the management of occupational exposures to human immunodeficiency virus and recommendations for postexposure prophylaxis. *Infect Control Hosp Epidemiol.* 2013; 34(9):875-892.

Merson MH. The HIV-AIDS pandemic at 25-The Global Response. *N Engl J Med.* 2006;354(23):2414-2417.

Petersen PE. Policy for prevention of oral manifestations in HIV/AIDS - The approach of the WHO Global Oral Health Programme. *Adv Dent Res.* 2006;19:17-20.

Petersen PE. World Health Organization global policy for improvement of oral health – World Health Assembly 2007. *Int Dent J.* 2008;58(3):115-121.

Sax PE, Walker BD. Immunology related to AIDS. *Cecil Textbook of Medicine.* 22nd ed. Goldman L, Ausiello D, eds. Philadelphia, PA: Saunders; 2004;2137-2138.

Workowski KA, Berman S, Centers for Disease Control and Prevention (CDC). Sexually transmitted diseases treatment guidelines, 2010. *MMWR Recomm Rep.* 2010;59(RR-12):1-110. Available at http://www.cdc.gov/std/treatment/2010/STD-Treatment-2010-RR5912.pdf

RHEUMATOID ARTHRITIS, OSTEOARTHRITIS, AND OSTEOPOROSIS

RA AND OSTEOARTHRITIS MANAGEMENT

Arthritis and its variations represent the most common chronic musculoskeletal disorders of man. The conditions can essentially be divided into rheumatoid, osteoarthritic, and polyarthritic presentations. Differences in age of onset and joint involvement exist and it is now currently believed that the diagnosis of each may be less clear than previously thought. These degenerative and autoinflammatory diseases have now been shown to affect young and old alike. Criteria for a diagnosis of rheumatoid arthritis include a positive serologic test for rheumatoid factor, subcutaneous nodules, affected joints on opposite sides of the body, and clear radiographic changes. The hematologic picture includes moderate normocytic hypochromic anemia, mild leukocytosis, and mild thrombocytopenia. During acute inflammatory periods, C-reactive protein and tumor-necrosis-factor alpha (TNF-alpha) are elevated and IgG and IgM (rheumatoid factors) can be detected. Osteoarthritis is a degenerative joint disease and lacks these diagnostic features.

Other systemic conditions, such as gout, psoriasis, systemic lupus erythematosus, and Sjögren's syndrome, are often found simultaneously with some of the arthritic conditions.

The goals of rheumatoid arthritis (RA) treatment are to:

- Stop inflammation (put disease in remission)
- Relieve symptoms
- Prevent joint and organ damage
- Improve physical function and overall well-being
- Reduce long-term complications

Some drugs modify the symptoms of RA and are primarily the nonsteroidal antiinflammatory drugs (NSAIDs). Long-term treatment of arthritis includes the use of slow-acting and rapid-acting anti-inflammatory agents ranging from the gold salts to aspirin (see following listings). Long-term usage of these drugs can lead to numerous adverse effects including bone marrow suppression, platelet suppression, and oral ulcerations. The dentist should be aware that steroids (usually prednisone) are the primary drugs that slow the progression of the disease and are often prescribed together with the listed drugs and are often used in dosages sufficient to induce adrenal suppression. Adjustment of dosing prior to invasive dental procedures may be indicated along with consultation with the managing physician. Alteration of steroid dosage, usually increasing the steroid dosage prior to and during the stressful procedures and then gradually returning the patient to the original dosage over several days. Even in the absence of evidence of adrenal suppression, consultation with the prescribing physician for appropriate dosing and timing of procedures is advisable.

Antirheumatic, Disease Modifying Antirheumatic Drugs (DMARDS) including biologic response modifiers

DMARDs, or disease-modifying antirheumatic drugs, are long-term medications meant to slow or alter the progression of rheumatoid arthritis by stopping the immune system from attacking healthy tissue. These drugs protect joints and tissues from permanent damage and gradually reduce daily pain. DMARDs can be taken concurrently or with other pain relievers. A subset of DMARDs are called **biologic response modifiers**. These drugs target specific parts of the immune system that trigger inflammation. One might target and block TNF inhibitors or the activation of T cells, which all plays a role in causing inflammation in the joints. A new subcategory of DMARDs known as "JAK inhibitors" block the Janus kinase, or JAK, pathways, which are involved in the body's immune response. Tofacitinib belongs to this class. Unlike biologics, it can be taken by mouth. These drugs belonging to this class of DMARDS can have significant immunosuppressive properties. Consider a medical consult prior to any invasive treatment for patients under such active treatment. Delayed wound healing due to the immunosuppressive effects and increased potential for postsurgical infection may be of concern.

Abatacept on page 53
Adalimumab on page 83
Anakinra on page 149
Certolizumab Pegol on page 326
Etanercept on page 607
Golimumab on page 744
InFLIXimab on page 809
Tocilizumab on page 1457
Tofacitinib on page 1459

Gold Salts

Auranofin

Metabolic Inhibitor

Leflunomide on page 882
Methotrexate on page 990

Nonsteroidal Anti-inflammatory Agents

Diclofenac (Systemic) on page 484
Diflunisal on page 495
Etodolac on page 622
Fenoprofen on page 642
Floctafenine on page 673
Flurbiprofen (Systemic) on page 701
Ibuprofen on page 786
Indomethacin
Ketoprofen on page 860
Ketorolac (Systemic) on page 861
Meclofenamate on page 952
Mefenamic Acid on page 954
Meloxicam on page 957
Nabumetone on page 1069
Naproxen on page 1080
Oxaprozin on page 1152
Piroxicam on page 1237
Sulindac on page 1394
Tiaprofenic Acid
Tofacitinib on page 1459
Tolmetin

COX-2 Inhibitor NSAID

Celecoxib on page 318

Combination NSAID Product to Prevent GI Distress

Diclofenac and Misoprostol on page 490
Naproxen and Esomeprazole on page 1084

Acetylated Salicylates

Aspirin on page 177

Other

Hydroxychloroquine on page 778
PredniSONE on page 1260

REFERENCES AND SELECTED READINGS

Singh JA, Furst DE, Bharat A, et al. 2012 update of the 2008 American College of Rheumatology recommendations for the use of disease-modifying antirheumatic drugs and biologic agents in the treatment of rheumatoid arthritis. *Arthritis Care Res (Hoboken)*. 2012;64(5):625-639.

OSTEONECROSIS OF THE JAW

Osteonecrosis of the jaw (ONJ), is relevant to the discussion of osteoporosis as well as Perioral Premalignant Lesions and Management of Patients Undergoing Cancer Therapy on page 1781. It is an uncommon condition that results in exposure of bone in the oral cavity. Other signs and symptoms may be associated with changes in bone metabolism and/or poor wound healing, but the ONJ defined condition can also develop spontaneously, such as along the mylohyoid ridge, away from teeth, or any site where acute or chronic trauma could have occurred. It is defined as an area of exposed bone in the maxillofacial region that does not heal within 8 weeks after identification by a health care provider in a patient who is receiving (or been exposed to) a bisphosphonate or other antiresorptive therapy and has not received radiation therapy (Ruggiero 2009; Ruggiero 2013). As this adverse reaction became more familiar in the dental and oncology communities, it became known as bisphosphonate-related ONJ (BRONJ).

Nonbisphosphonate antiresorptive agents denosumab (Prolia and Xgeva) and bevacizumab (Avastin) have also been associated with ONJ. Many researchers are using the term antiresorptive osteonecrosis of the jaw (ARONJ) or medication-related osteonecrosis of the jaw (MRONJ) to refer to ONJ in order to include all putative causal agents other than bisphosphonates. Despite the various terms used, the clinical finding of exposed and necrotic bone of the jaw is accepted as the consistent hallmark in diagnosis (Ruggiero 2013). The American Dental Association recently updated and clarified its guidelines (Hellstein 2011). In this handbook, the acronym ONJ will continue to be used regardless of the etiology.

Cases of ONJ began to emerge in approximately 2003 and were linked primarily with patients with cancer and those receiving the intravenous bisphosphonate drugs such as zoledronic acid (Zometa) and/or pamidronate (Aredia). Patients receiving clodronate (Bonefos) appeared initially to develop this adverse reaction less frequently. Data has continued to emerge related to oral bisphosphonates and the risk of ONJ in patients who are receiving a significantly lower dosage of bisphosphonate via the oral route. Also refer to Perioral Premalignant Lesions and Management of Patients Undergoing Cancer Therapy on page 1781.

Bone disease occurs in many patients with cancer, particularly those with multiple myeloma and metastatic lesions associated with breast cancer, prostate cancer, and other cancers. These changes are often associated with pain and pathologic fractures. This bone destruction often results from changes in the osteoclast and osteoblast activities related to bone remodeling and healing following trauma. Bisphosphonates act at sites of active bone remodeling, changing the activity of the cells necessary for osteoclastic activity. There are no data that indicate that bisphosphonates directly change mineralization of the bone; however, these drugs do result in changes in the vascularity of the bone and cell activity.

Of the 2,408 cases of bisphosphonate-associated ONJ published since 2003, bisphosphonate therapy was used to treat malignancies in 89% and nonmalignant conditions in 11% (Filleul 2010). Tooth extraction preceded 67% of the reported cases and 35% of these patients' cases resolved. The specific bisphosphonate drug used was provided in 1,694 of the cases. Eighty-eight percent of the patients received intravenous therapy, primarily zoledronic acid, and 12% received oral treatment, primarily alendronate (Fosamax) (Filleul 2010). The most recent report by the International Task Force on ONJ suggests that since 2003 the frequency of ONJ in oncology patients receiving oncology doses of bisphosphonate (BP) or denosumab is estimated at 1% to 15%, and the frequency in the osteoporosis patient population receiving much lower doses of BP or denosumab is estimated at 0.001% to 0.01%. In one small but recent study by Voss et al, patients that had transitioned from bisphosphonate therapy to anti RANKL drugs, such as denosumab (Prolia or Xgeva), appeared to have a greater risk of severe ONJ as compared to those on either drug class alone.

Bisphosphonates

Alendronate (Fosamax) on page 95
Clodronate (Clasteon) (Canada only) on page 380
Etidronate (Didronel) on page 620
Ibandronate (Boniva) on page 782
Pamidronate on page 1185
Risedronate (Actonel) on page 1331
Zoledronic acid (Aclasta, Zometa) on page 1574

Antiangiogenic drugs

Bevacizumab (Avastin) on page 242
Cabozantinib (Cometriq)
Everolimus (Afinitor, Zortress) on page 628
SORAfenib (NexAVAR) on page 1383
SUNItinib (Sutent) on page 1396

Nonbisphosphonate antiresorptive drug (Anti-RANKL drug)

Denosumab (Prolia, Xgeva) on page 453
Bevacizumab (Avastin) on page 242

The most comprehensive review to date on osteonecrosis of the jaw bone (ONJ) has been published in the Journal of Bone and Mineral Research and written by an International Task Force of authors (Khan 2015). The American Association of Oral and Maxillofacial Surgeons also has published a position paper in October of 2014 that essentially agrees with the report (Salvatore 2014).

ONJ continues to be defined by the Task Force as (1) exposed bone in the maxillofacial region that does not heal within 8 weeks after identification by a health care provider, (2) exposure to an antiresorptive agent, and (3) no history of radiation therapy to the craniofacial region. Antiresorptive agents include bisphosphonate drugs (BPs), the monoclonal antibody denosumab (Prolia, Xgeva) and antiangiogenic agents such as bevacizumab (Avastin). The clinical staging system currently being used was developed by Ruggiero 2006. The Task Force concurs with this description. Patients with Stage 1 disease have exposed bone but are asymptomatic with no evidence of significant adjacent or regional soft tissue inflammation or infection. Stage 2 disease is characterized by exposed bone with associated pain, adjacent or regional soft tissue inflammatory swelling, or secondary infection. Stage 3 disease is characterized by exposed bone associated with pain, adjacent or regional soft tissue inflammatory swelling, or secondary infection, in addition to a pathologic fracture, an extraoral fistula or oral-antral fistula, or radiographic evidence of osteolysis extending to the inferior border of the mandible or the floor of the maxillary sinus.

After reviewing all literature reports on this subject, the Task Force concluded that the prevalence of ONJ in patients prescribed oral BPs for the treatment of osteoporosis ranges from 0% to to 0.04% with the majority being below 0.001%. However, the Task Force does cite the study of Lo 2010 that evaluated the Kaiser Permanente database and found the prevalence of ONJ in those receiving BPs for >2 years to range from 0.05% to 0.21% and appeared to be related to duration of exposure. The American Dental Association has previously reported that the prevalence of ONJ in osteoporosis patients using oral BPs to be 1 out of 1,000 or 0.1% (Hellstein 2011).

From currently available data, the incidence of ONJ in the osteoporosis patient population appears to be low, ranging from 0.15% to <0.001% person-years drug exposure. In terms of the osteoporosis patient population taking oral BPs, the incidence ranges from 1.04 to 69 per 100,000 patient years of drug exposure. In a trial evaluating the BP known as Reclast (IV zoledronic acid) involving 7,765 patients receiving either zoledronic acid 5 mg or placebo over 3 years, one case of ONJ was identified in each arm.

The incidence of ONJ ranges from 1% to 15% in the oncology patient population in which high doses of BPs are used at frequent intervals. The oncology patient with bone metastasis is exposed to more osteoclastic inhibition than those with osteoporosis, thus the incidence of ONJ is much higher. Clinical studies comparing zoledronic acid 4 mg with denosumab 120 mg dosed monthly for the management of bone metastasis described the incidence of ONJ as ~1% to 2%.

In the osteoporosis patient population, the significant risk factors for the development of ONJ in declining order of importance include local suppuration, BP use, dental extractions and anemia. In the oncology patient population, the significant risk factors for the development of ONJ in declining order of importance are exposure to intravenous zoledronic acid (Zometa), exposure to intravenous pamidronate (Aredia), exposure to denosumab, radiation therapy, dental extraction, chemotherapy, periodontal disease, oral BP use, osteoporosis, local suppuration, glucocorticoid therapy, diabetes, denture use, erythropoietin therapy, tobacco use, hyperthyroidism, renal dialysis, cyclophosphamide therapy, and increasing age.

Management of those at risk

- **General dentistry:** Inform patients of the risk of developing ONJ, but treatment should continue as planned.
- **Oral and maxillofacial surgery:** Inform patients of the risk of developing ONJ and discuss alternative treatment plans, including endodontic treatment, followed by removal of the clinical crown, allowing the roots to exfoliate rather than tooth extraction. Before and after any surgical procedures involving bone, patients should rinse with chlorhexidine twice daily for 4 to 8 weeks after surgery. In addition, antibiotic prophylaxis starting one day before the procedure and for 3 to 7 days after may be effective in preventing ONJ.
- **Restorative dentistry and prosthodontics:** There is no evidence that malocclusion or masticatory forces increase the risk of developing ONJ. Treatment should continue as planned.
- **Orthodontics:** Reports have shown an increase in tooth movement in patients taking bisphosphonates; patients should be advised of this potential complication; the duration of orthodontic treatment may be prolonged and uniform tooth movement may be compromised.
- **Implant placement and maintenance:** Bisphosphonate treatment does not impact implant placement or maintenance, except in extensive cases; treatment should continue as planned.
- **Management of periodontal disease:** Patients who have active periodontal disease should receive appropriate forms of nonsurgical therapy. There is no evidence that periodontal procedures, such as guided tissue regeneration or bone replacement grafts, increase the risk of developing ONJ.
- **Endodontics:** Endodontic treatment is preferable to surgical manipulation if the tooth is salvageable. Limited evidence shows that periapical healing after endodontic therapy is similar regardless of bisphosphonate use.

FREQUENTLY ASKED QUESTIONS

According to the latest literature, what is the incidence of ONJ in oral bisphosphonates users?

Presently, the current estimates of the frequency of occurrence of ONJ in oral bisphosphonate users are the following: Merck drug company, the manufacturer of Fosamax calculated the incidence of ONJ to be 0.7 cases per 100,000 person-years of exposure to oral bisphosphonates. The Medical Consultants of Consumer Reports On-Health Bulletin reported an incidence of one case for every 20,000 users of oral bisphosphonates (0.005%). A recent report from Australia estimated that the frequency of ONJ in osteoporotic patients mainly on weekly oral alendronate (Fosamax) ranged from a minimum of 1 in 8,470 to a maximum of 1 in 2,260 (0.01% to 0.04%) patients. If extractions were performed, the frequency increased to 0.09% to 0.34%. The risk of developing ONJ in patients taking bisphosphonates or denosumab remains low with a prevalence of ~0.1% (1:1,000) (Hellstein 2011).

What numbers can practitioners use to tell the dental patient their risk of developing ONJ with oral bisphosphonates?

The recommendations from the Expert Panel of the American Dental Association suggest that the patient be informed that there is a very low risk of developing ONJ. The true risk posed by oral bisphosphonates remains uncertain but appears to be very small. All the data seem to point to a risk of ~0.1% of total users and that the risk increases with dental extractions to ~0.3%. The risks of developing ONJ can be minimized but never totally eliminated. Good oral hygiene along with regular dental care is the best way to lower the risk of developing ONJ. The current data on incidence of ONJ in patients taking oral bisphosphonates is retrospective information derived primarily from surveys and the number of reported cases in patients taking the drugs. More meaningful assessment of incidence of ONJ in the population at risk must come from prospective cohort investigations.

Is the risk of acquiring osteonecrosis of the jaw bone diminished with the use of other oral bisphosphonates compared to Fosamax?

In addition to alendronate (Fosamax), cases of ONJ, albeit rare, have been reported in patients taking either risedronate (Actonel) or ibandronate (Boniva). Among the class of oral bisphosphonates, more cases have been associated with Fosamax than with Actonel or Boniva. Also, there is no evidence to suggest that the risk of ONJ is less when taking monthly doses of Boniva. Zoledronic acid under the band name of Reclast has recently been approved as a once-annual, 15-minute intravenous infusion of a dose of 5 mg to prevent osteoporosis. This dosing was associated with a significant improvement in bone mineral density and bone metabolism markers. It is unknown whether this dosing schedule places the patient at risk for ONJ; however, data do show a higher risk of serious atrial fibrillation in patients receiving Reclast compared to patients receiving placebo.

Will Fosamax or the other oral bisphosphonates continue to be the standard treatment for osteoporosis?

Yes. The oral bisphosphonates continue to be the most effective class of drugs in reducing the risk of osteoporotic fractures and are the first-line therapy in the treatment of osteoporosis. Fosamax has been shown to prevent bone loss at the spine and hip in postmenopausal women and to reduce fractures by ~50%. Risedronate (Actonel) produced a 30% reduction in hip fractures. Fosamax continues to be in the top 50 of the most widely prescribed drugs in the US.

Do we know the pathogenesis of ONJ?

This question has not been answered and information is only speculative at this time. Osteoporosis can occur due to age-related changes in the number of osteoclasts and bone resorption sites. This overwhelms the production of new bone by osteoblasts and a decrease in bone mass occurs. By inhibiting osteoclastic activity, the oral bisphosphonates seemingly arrest the osteoporotic syndrome. In the process, however, the maxilla and mandible, upon continued exposure to the bisphosphonates, exhibit delayed wound healing following injury from mechanical forces or invasive surgery, such as tooth extraction. This coupled with the antiangiogenic effect (ie, a reduction in bone blood supply by the bisphosphonates) may contribute to jaw bone necrosis. Ruggiero and Drew have suggested that a preferential deposition of the bisphosphonates in the mandible and maxilla may contribute to the necrosis appearing within the jaw rather than within bones outside the craniofacial skeleton.

What are the factors that increase the risk of ONJ in oral bisphosphonate users?

Patients with a history of periodontal disease and dental abscesses are at increased risk of developing ONJ if taking oral bisphosphonates. Also, dentoalveolar trauma will increase the risk. The use of chronic steroids such as prednisone has been identified as a risk factor. Other factors are periodontitis, smoking, wearing dentures, diabetes, and the duration of exposure and age, with longer treatment regimens and age >65 years associated with a greater risk of developing the disease (Hellstein 2011). Patients identified with jaw bone necrosis typically were exposed to oral bisphosphonates for 2 years or longer.

What are the symptoms that an oral bisphosphonates patient would experience which could indicate necrotic jaw bone?

Tooth mobility, mucosal swelling, and/or ulceration. Clinical symptoms would include a nonhealing extraction site, exposed bone surrounded by inflamed soft tissue, and purulent discharge at site of exposed bone. Exposed bone is usually more prevalent in areas such as the tori and the mylohyoid ridge.

What kind of dental procedures can be performed in oral bisphosphonate users with no increase in risk for ONJ?

According to the American Dental Association, all routine procedures can be carried out. Routine dental treatment should not be modified on the basis of oral bisphosphonate use. However, the presence of risk factors, such as steroid use, >65 years of age, or prolonged exposure to oral bisphosphonates, may require consultation with an expert in metabolic bone disease prior to routine dental treatment.

Is dentoalveolar surgery contraindicated in Fosamax users?

According to both Ruggiero et al and Marx et al, no alteration or delay in planned surgery is typically necessary in patients taking an oral bisphosphonate for <3 years and having no other risk factors for ONJ. In asymptomatic patients receiving oral bisphosphonate therapy, dentoalveolar surgery is not contraindicated. Also surgery common to periodontists and other dental providers need not be delayed.

In addition, Marx suggested that if dental implants are placed, informed consent should be obtained related to the potential for implant failure and possible ONJ if the patient continues to take an oral bisphosphonate.

Is a so-called "drug holiday" an effective way to reduce the risks of ONJ?

Although a "drug holiday" would seem logical and has been suggested by some groups, there is no statistically significant evidence indicating in the cancer patient population that this is beneficial in reducing ONJ risk and in fact may be detrimental if the chance of a skeletal-related event increases. The data in oral bisphosphonates use are even less compelling since the incidence is so low to begin with that subjective drug holidays cannot be documented with any degree of confidence. As mentioned earlier, for individuals who have taken a bisphosphonate for <3 years and have no other risk factors for ONJ, no alteration or delay in the planned surgery is recommended, but the caveat is that the risk remains unknown.

In patients about to begin oral bisphosphonate therapy, should the bisphosphonate be delayed until dental health is optimized?

No. It does not appear necessary for patients to initiate prophylactic dental treatment prior to initiating oral bisphosphonate therapy for osteoporosis. It would be prudent, however, to encourage these patients to maintain an optimal level of dental health.

Is diagnostic imaging useful in assessing oral bisphosphonate individuals at risk for ONJ?

Imaging modalities have proved helpful in determining the extent of existing necrotic process, but have not been able to demonstrate any efficacy in assessing patients at risk for ONJ. It has been reported that panoramic and periapical radiographs probably will not reveal significant changes in early stages of osteonecrosis and they are poor screening tools for prediction. Computerized tomography (CT) scan also has not proved helpful with early identification of osteonecrosis in asymptomatic patients.

Do the Fosamax-type drugs increase the risk of ONJ in patients receiving dental implants?

A conclusive cause and effect relationship between bisphosphonate therapy and ONJ still has not been established. Evidence does suggest, however, that such an association may exist, particularly with intravenous bisphosphonate use in cancer patients. Oral bisphosphonates are widely used for the treatment of osteoporosis. It is estimated that 22 to 30 million prescriptions were written for alendronate (Fosamax), the most widely used oral bisphosphonate in the United States, between May 2003 and April 2004. For many years, dental implants have been placed in many patients taking oral bisphosphonates. Prior to the reports on the risk of bisphosphonate-associated ONJ, these patients were treated without any modification of the surgically placed implant procedure. Recently, however, guidelines from the American Dental Association (ADA) and the American Association of Oral and Maxillofacial Surgeons (AAOMS) have suggested a cautious approach to implant surgery and extractions for patients receiving bisphosphonate therapy.

Regarding dental implants, the ADA report cautions practitioners that patients may be at increased risk of developing osteonecrosis of the jaw bone when extensive implant placement or guided bone regeneration is necessary.

If dental implants are to be placed, the AAOMS Task Force suggested contacting the physician who prescribed the oral bisphosphonate prior to surgery to suggest an alternate dosing schedule, a drug holiday (discontinuance of the drug for a short time period), or an alternative to bisphosphonate therapy. It is important to remember that any beneficial or detrimental effects of these drug holidays have not been prospectively studied.

In addition, Marx has suggested the following precautions. Dental implant, if elected, can be placed in the patient about to begin oral bisphosphonate therapy. However, informed consent concerning the potential for implant loss and/or exposed bone related to the bisphosphonates should be obtained as the patient continues bisphosphonate therapy and exceeds 3 years of continuous use. For individuals who have taken an oral bisphosphonate for <3 years and have no clinical or radiographic risk factors, no alteration or delay is necessary for planned dental surgeries. If dental implants are placed, informed consent should be obtained related to the potential for implant failure and possible ONJ if the patient continues to take the bisphosphonate.

For patients who have taken an oral bisphosphonates for >3 years, it is advised that the prescribing physician be contacted and a recommendation made to discontinue the oral bisphosphonate for 3 months prior to the procedure and refrain from reinstating use until 3 months after the procedure.

One report from the UK suggested an even more conservative approach. Scully et al, suggested that when possible, extractions should be avoided in patients receiving oral bisphosphonates and it is best to avoid all elective surgery in these patients, including endosseous implant placement, or treatment should be performed well in advance prior to bisphosphonate therapy. If surgery is performed on patients taking bisphosphonates, they must be counseled about the risk.

A new report showed that implant surgery on patients receiving Fosamax-type drugs did not result in bisphosphonate-associated ONJ. This study, out of the Dentistry/Oral Surgery Group at Montefiore Medical Center, Albert Einstein College of Medicine, reported that of 115 patients taking oral bisphosphonates, none showed evidence or had symptoms of osteonecrosis after implant placement. This report had findings similar to a previous report by Dr Jeffcoat, who showed success in implant placement and no signs of necrosis in patients taking oral bisphosphonates.

The Montefiore study, by Grant et al, used a survey to collect information from patients who had received dental implants and were taking oral bisphosphonates. The study, reported in the *Journal of Oral and Maxillofacial Surgery*, identified 1,319 female patients >40 years of age who had implant surgery between January 1998 and December 2006. A survey was mailed to each of these individuals asking about current and past use of oral bisphosphonates. Of the 1,319 surveys mailed out, 458 (35%) were returned. From those returned, 115 individuals reported taking oral bisphosphonates before or after implant surgery. None reported receiving intravenous bisphosphonates. In this population, it was then determined that a total of 468 implants had been placed in the 115 individuals. This population that responded to the survey was then compared to a random sample of individuals who did not respond with regard to age and number of implants. It was found that only five among 100 nonresponders to the survey had a history of bisphosphonate use compared to the 115 of the 458 responders. The remaining 343 patients indicated that they had not received bisphosphonate therapy. From the pool of 458 responders, there were 1,450 implants placed in these patients and 1,436 had integrated successfully. Implant success was defined using criteria which included the absence of symptoms, such as pain, infection, paresthesia, or neuropathies, and that the dental implant should provide functional service for 5 years in 75% of the cases.

The results were the following:

1. None of the 458 responders to the survey reported symptoms of bisphosphonate-associated ONJ.
2. Since 115 of the 458 responders indicated they were treated with bisphosphonates, it was assumed that none of the 115 responders treated with bisphosphonates had ONJ.
3. Out of the pool of 115 patients, there was a total of 468 implants placed. It was found that 466 of those implants were in function and were considered successful. Only two implants failed. In one case of failure, the patient had taken oral bisphosphonates for 3 years prior to implant placement but no longer was taking any drug at the time of implant placement or thereafter. The investigators removed and replaced the implant and it was still in function for >4 years. In the second case, the patient had been taking bisphosphonates for >8 years and the failure occurred in one implant out of a total of 13 in place. The failed implant was removed, not replaced, and the area healed uneventfully.
4. There were no reports of ONJ from any of the 861 patients who did not return the survey.

This report from Montefiore is consistent with that of the findings of Jeffcoat. She also reported success in implant placement and no signs of necrosis in patients taking oral bisphosphonates. Her method was a single blind controlled study using 50 postmenopausal female dental implant patients. Twenty-five had taken oral bisphosphonates for 1-4 years and the other 25 patients did not take oral bisphosphonates prior to or during the study. In the bisphosphonate group, there was a total of 102 implants that were placed and in the nondrug group, there were 108 implants that were placed. After 3 years, there was 100% success rate with no evidence of infection, pain, or necrosis in patients receiving bisphosphonates. There was 99.2% success rate in the group not taking oral bisphosphonates.

A further review of the literature found only two cases of dental implant failure associated with oral bisphosphonate use. One was a case report from 1995 that suggested that failure of five implants was caused by bisphosphonate therapy. In that case, five implants were placed and successfully integrated in the mandible. The patient then began bisphosphonate therapy 28 months after implant placement and after 4 months, a panoramic radiograph revealed osteolysis around all implants and all five were removed one month later.

In the report by Wang et al, a patient developed a significant bone defect with necrosis after proper implant placement. The patient was a 65-year-old female who had taken Fosamax for 10 years. She received five implants in the mandible. Ten days after surgery, healing appeared to be progressing uneventfully. Four weeks later, upon evaluation, bone defects were observed and noted around two of the implants. The defects were repaired with mineralized human cancellous bone mixed with tetracycline and covered with collagen membrane. Eventually after some further antibiotics and chlorhexidine daily rinsing, complete uneventful healing occurred.

Is the CTX bone marker useful to assess the risk of ONJ in oral bisphosphonate users?

CTX is an acronym for C-terminal telopeptide. During bone resorption, the dominant type 1 collagen is degraded and, during this collagen breakdown, the telopeptide (CTX) is released. Thus, serum levels of CTX can be used as an indicator of bone breakdown/resorption. The CTX blood test, as a risk marker for ONJ, first proposed by Marx in 2007, was used in an Australian study to determine its effectiveness in the prevention and management of ONJ in patients taking bisphosphonates. Essentially, this test was found to be able to identify groups of those individuals in the "risk zone" for developing ONJ, which was defined as a blood level of 150 picograms/mL (pg/mL) to 200 picograms/mL (pg/mL). It was, however, not found to be predictive of the development of ONJ in any individual patient. The CTX test requires a 1 mL sample of whole blood drawn in the morning in fasted individuals. Marx used Quest Diagnostics Nichols East Lab in San Juan Capistrano California to perform the analysis on the samples. Values lower than 100 pg/mL were correlated with a high risk of ONJ; values between 100 pg/mL and 150 pg/mL correlated to a moderate risk and values >150 pg/mL associated with minimal or no risk. According to Ruggiero and Drew, low bone turnover in the jaw due to osteoclastic inhibition by bisphosphonates results in the inability of the bone to repair local microdamage from normal mechanical loading or injury. This ultimately results in bone necrosis. Thus, individuals with low CTX values while taking bisphosphonates are assumed to have jaw bones which may not be able to normally repair themselves and these individuals would have a relatively higher risk of developing ONJ compared to individuals having higher CTX serum values.

Rigorous prospective studies on greater numbers of individuals are required before the use of the CTX serum test could be suggested with any confidence. In 2011, the American Dental Association (ADA) reaffirmed its earlier position that CTX cannot be recommended as a predictive tool for ONJ risk assessment.

Are there other bone markers that may be useful?

Researchers have been seeking screening tools to predict and allow prevention of ONJ. A recent study by the Memorial Sloan-Kettering Cancer Center of New York investigated specific bone turnover markers as predictive models to assess risks of ONJ in patients exposed to bisphosphonates (Morris 2012). This retrospective study showed that N-telopeptide of type-I collagen (NTX) and bone-specific alkaline phosphatase (BAP) did not predict for the development of ONJ. No significant trend for either biomarker was detected. Thus, to date, there is insufficient evidence to recommend the use of serum tests as predictors of ONJ.

Do the new anti-RANK-L drugs such as denosumab (Prolia, Xgeva) increase the risk of ONJ?

ONJ has been reported in clinical studies in patients receiving denosumab at FDA-approved doses for osteoporosis. In clinical studies, patients with advanced cancer treated with 120 mg denosumab administered monthly, have reported a 2% incidence of ONJ. Known risk factors for ONJ include a diagnosis of cancer with bone lesions, concomitant therapies (eg, chemotherapy, antiangiogenic biologics, corticosteroids, radiotherapy to the head and neck), poor oral hygiene, dental extractions, comorbid disorders (eg, preexisting dental disease, anaemia, coagulopathy, infection) and previous treatment with bisphosphonates.

A dental examination with appropriate preventive dentistry should be considered prior to initiating denosumab treatment in patients with concomitant risk factors. These patients should avoid invasive dental procedures if possible during treatment with denosumab. Patients should maintain good oral hygiene during treatment. For patients who develop ONJ while on denosumab therapy, dental surgery may exacerbate the condition. Use clinical judgement and guide the management plan of each patient based on individual risk:benefit evaluation.

Denosumab on page 453

CLINICAL DENTAL MANAGEMENT CONSIDERATIONS

Suggested Preventive Dentistry Before Initiating Chemotherapy, Immunotherapy, or Antiresorptive Therapy

- Remove abscessed and nonrestorable teeth and teeth with severe periodontal disease involvement
- Remove teeth with poor long-term prognosis
- Functionally rehabilitate salvageable dentition, including endodontic therapy
- Perform dental prophylaxis, caries control, and stabilizing restorative dental care
- Examine dentures to ensure proper fit (dentures should be removed at night)
- Educate patients on oral self-care hygiene

Patients at Risk of ONJ Due to Antiresorptive Therapy (Without Any Signs of ONJ):

Invasive dental procedures should be avoided in patients receiving intravenous bisphosphonate therapy. These procedures should also be performed ideally prior to a patient starting bisphosphonate IV therapy. The treating physician should guide the management plan of each patient based on individual benefit:risk assessment and communication with the dentist. For patients requiring dental procedures, there are no prospective data available to suggest whether discontinuation of bisphosphonate treatment reduces the risk of ONJ.

There are five primary actions in this management plan:

1. Patients should be educated on maintaining excellent oral hygiene to reduce the risk of need for invasive procedures in the future.
2. Patients should check and adjust removable appliances such as prostheses to avoid soft tissue injury.
3. Routine cleaning should be performed with care, attempting to reduce any soft tissue injury; however, since hygiene is important, the normal recall planning and treatment should continue.
4. Dental infection should be managed aggressively and nonsurgically when possible. Alternatives such as endodontic therapy over extraction may be advisable.
5. Endodontic therapy is preferable to extractions; treatment with endodontics followed by coronal amputation and root canal therapy on the retained roots may be necessary.

If a Patient Develops Osteonecrosis of the Jaw: Consultations between oral surgeons/dental oncologists and the treating physician are strongly recommended:

- A nonsurgical approach is recommended to prevent further osseous injury.
- Only minimal bony debridement to reduce sharp and rough surfaces to prevent further trauma to adjacent or opposing tissues is recommended.
- A removable appliance or protective stent may be used to protect exposed bone or adjacent tissues.
- Before discontinuing bisphosphonate therapy, patient should be evaluated for potential risk of further osteonecrosis versus the risk of skeletal complications.
- Hyperbaric oxygen therapy is not recommended.
- Biopsy is not recommended unless metastasis to the jaw is suspected.
- Cultures should be taken for directed antimicrobial therapy.
- Prophylactic antibiotic therapy may be considered for pain and disease control.

SAMPLE PRESCRIPTIONS FOR PROPHYLACTIC ANTIBIOTIC THERAPY IF AN INVASIVE PROCEDURE IS PLANNED IN A PATIENT AT HIGH RISK FOR ONJ OR ALREADY HAS A DEFINED ONJ LESION

Rx:

Amoxicillin 875 mg tablets
Disp: 60 tablets
Sig: Take 1 tablet twice daily

Note: Alternatively, 500 mg tablet 3 times daily can be prescribed and may be continued for >1 month. Patients should be cautioned regarding gastrointestinal side effects with long-term use of any antibiotic. Probiotics may help, but evidence is conflicted on true efficacy.

Rx:

Clindamycin (Systemic) 300 mg capsules
Disp: 40 capsules
Sig: Take 1 capsule 3 or 4 times/day for 7 to 10 days

Note: Prescription usually selected for patients allergic to penicillin; may be prescribed for 3 or 4 times/day. This prescription can be continued for >1 month; however, risk of *Clostridioides* (formerly *Clostridium*) *difficile* colitis increases. Patients should be cautioned to take clindamycin with food and monitor for gastrointestinal side effects with long-term use. Probiotics may help, but evidence is conflicted on true efficacy.

Rx:

Chlorhexidine Oral Rinse
Disp: 1 bottle
Sig: Rinse with 20 mL twice daily for 30 seconds and expectorate

ONJ Diagnosis and Definition

- Intraoral pain is variable
- Complaint of roughness along the teeth or ridge
- History of dental procedures (eg, extractions) but may occur on tissues
- Complaint of ill-fitting denture(s)
- Diagnosis of ONJ made clinically with presence of exposed bone in maxillofacial region (>8 weeks duration [with no history of radiation therapy])
- If the presence of exposed bone in maxillofacial region is noted but is <8 weeks duration (with no history of radiation therapy), the clinician must consider other differential diagnoses of:
  - Spontaneous lingual mandibular sequestration with ulceration
  - Trauma
  - Advanced periodontal disease with dehiscence
  - Local malignancy
  - Metastatic cancer

REFERENCES AND SELECTED READINGS

Aljohani S, Gaudin R, Weiser J, et al. Osteonecrosis of the jaw in patients treated with denosumab: a multicenter case series. *J Craniomaxillofac Surg*. 2018;46(9):1515-1525.

Almubarak H, Jones A, Chaisuparat R, et al. Zoledronic acid directly suppresses cell proliferation and induces apoptosis in highly tumorigenic prostate and breast cancers. *J Carcinog*. 2011;10:2.

American Dental Association Council on Scientific Affairs. Dental management of patients receiving oral bisphosphonate therapy: expert panel recommendations. *J Am Dent Assoc*. 2006;137(8):1144-1150.

Badros A, Weikel D, Salama A, et al. Osteonecrosis of the jaw in multiple myeloma patients: clinical features and risk factors. *J Clin Oncol*. 2006;24 (6):945-952.

Filleul O, Crompot E, Saussez S. Bisphosphonate-induced osteonecrosis of the jaw: a review of 2,400 patient cases. *J Cancer Res Clin Oncol*. 2010;136(8):1117-1124.

Grant BT, Amenedo C, Freeman K, Kraut RA. Outcomes of placing dental implants in patients taking oral bisphosphonates: a review of 115 cases. *J Oral Maxillofac Surg*. 2008;66(2):223-230.

Hellstein JW, Adler RA, Edwards B, et al. Managing the care of patients receiving antiresorptive therapy for prevention and treatment of osteoporosis: executive summary of recommendations from the American Dental Association Council on Scientific Affairs. *J Am Dent Assoc*. 2011;142 (11):1243-1251. Available at http://www.ada.org/sections/professionalResources/pdfs/topics_ARONJ_report.pdf. Accessed November 25, 2011.

Hinchy NV et al. Osteonecrosis of the jaw – prevention and treatment strategies for oral health professionals. *Oral Oncology*. 2013;49:878-886.

Katsarelis H, Shah NP, Dhariwal DK, Pazianas M. Infection and medication-related osteonecrosis of the jaw. *J Dent Res*. 2015;94(4):534-539.

Khan AA, Morrison A, Hanley DA, et al. Diagnosis and management of osteonecrosis of the jaw: a systematic review and international consensus. *J Bone Miner Res*. 2015; 30(1):3-23.

Khan AA, Morrison A, Kendler DL, et al. International task force on osteonecrosis of the jaw. case-based review of osteonecrosis of the jaw (ONJ) and application of the international recommendations for management from the international task force on ONJ. *J Clin Densitom*. 2017;20(1):8-24.

Kyrgidis A, Toulis KA. Denosumab-related osteonecrosis of the jaws. *Osteoporos Int*. 2011;22(1):369-370.

Marx RE, Cillo JE Jr, Ulloa JJ. Oral bisphosphonate-induced osteonecrosis: risk factors, prediction of risk using serum CTX testing, prevention, and treatment. *J Oral Maxillofac Surg*. 2007;65(12):2397-2410.

Marx RE. *Oral and Intravenous Bisphosphonate-Induced Osteonecrosis of the Jaws: History, Etiology, Prevention and Treatment*. Chicago, IL: Quintessence Publishing Company; 2007;87-91.

Marx RE, Sawatari Y, Fortin M, Broumand V. Bisphosphonate-induced exposed bone (osteonecrosis/osteopetrosis) of the jaws: risk factors, recognition, prevention, and treatment. *J Oral Maxillofac Surg*. 2005;63(11):1567-1575.

Mavrokokki T, Cheng A, Stein B, Goss A. Nature and frequency of bisphosphonate-associated osteonecrosis of the jaws in Australia. *J Oral Maxillofac Surg*. 2007;65(3):415-423.
Migliorati CA, Casiglia J, Epstein J, Jacobsen PL, Siegel MA, Woo SB. Managing the care of patients with bisphosphonate-associated osteonecrosis: an American Academy of Oral Medicine position paper. *J Am Dent Assoc*. 2005;136(12):1658-1668.
Morris PG, Fazio M, Farooki A, et al. Serum N-telopeptide and bone-specific alkaline phosphatase levels in patients with osteonecrosis of the jaw receiving bisphosphonates for bone metastases. *J Oral Maxillofac Surg*. 2012;70(12):2768-2775.
Mücke T, Deppe H, Hein J, et al. Prevention of bisphosphonate-related osteonecrosis of the jaws in patients with prostate cancer treated with zoledronic acid - a prospective study over 6 years. *J Craniomaxillofac Surg*. 2016;44(10):1689-1693.
Ruggiero SL. Diagnosis and management of antiresorptive-related osteonecrosis of the jaw. *Gen Dent*. 2013;61(7):24-29.
Ruggiero SL, Dodson TB, Fantasia J, et al. American Association of Oral and Maxillofacial Surgeons position paper on medication-related osteonecrosis of the jaw–2014 update. *J Oral Maxillofac Surg*. 2014;72(10):1938-1956.
Ruggiero SL, Dodson TB, Assael LA, et al. American Association of Oral and Maxillofacial Surgeons position paper on bisphosphonate-related osteonecrosis of the jaw − 2009 update. *Aust Endod J*. 2009;35(3):119-130.
Ruggiero SL, Drew SJ. Osteonecrosis of the jaws and bisphosphonate therapy. *J Dent Res*. 2007;86(11):1013-1021.
Ruggiero S, Gralow J, Marx RE. Practical guidelines for the prevention, diagnosis, and treatment of osteonecrosis of the jaw in patients with cancer. *J Oncol Pract*. 2006;2(1):7-14.
Ruggiero SL, Fantasia J, Carlson E. Bisphosphonate-related osteonecrosis of the jaw: background and guidelines for diagnosis, staging and management. *Oral Surg Oral Med Oral Pathol Oral Radiol Endod*. 2006;102(4):433-441.
Ruggiero SL, Mehrotra B, Rosenberg TJ, et al. Osteonecrosis of the jaws associated with the use of bisphosphonates: a review of 63 cases. *J Oral Maxillofac Surg*. 2004;62(5):527-534.
Scheper MA, Badros A, Chaisuparat R, et al. Effect of zoledronic acid on oral fibroblasts and epithelial cells: a potential mechanism of bisphosphonate-associated osteonecrosis. *Br J Haematol*. 2009;144(5):667-676.
Scheper MA, Badros A, Salama AR, et al. A novel bioassay model to determine clinically significant bisphosphonate levels. *Support Care Cancer*. 2009;17(12):1553-1557.
Scheper M, Chaisuparat R, Cullen K, et al. A novel soft-tissue in vitro model for bisphosphonate-associated osteonecrosis. *Fibrogenesis Tissue Repair*. 2010;3:6.
Scully C, Madrid C, Bagan J. Dental endosseous implants in patients on bisphosphonate therapy. *Implant Dent*. 2006;15(3):212-218.
Taylor KH, Middlefell LS, Mizen KD. Osteonecrosis of the jaws induced by anti-RANK ligand therapy. *Br J Oral Maxillofac Surg*. 2010;48(3):221-223.
Voss PJ, Steybe D, Poxleitner P, et al. Osteonecrosis of the jaw in patients transitioning from bisphosphonates to denosumab treatment for osteoporosis. *Odontology*. 2018;106(4):469-480.
Wang HL, Weber D, McCauley LK. Effect of long-term oral bisphosphonates on implant wound healing: literature review and a case report. *J Periodontol*. 2007;78(3):584-594.

SEXUALLY-TRANSMITTED DISEASES

Sexually transmitted diseases (STDs) represent a group of infectious diseases that include bacterial, fungal, and viral etiologies. Several related infections are covered elsewhere. Several viral STDs can be effectively prevented through vaccination with widely available vaccines, including hepatitis A, hepatitis B, and human papilloma virus vaccines.

Human papilloma virus is widespread and serotypes 16 and 18 have been associated with cervical cancer. Although most types that cause oral HPV lesions are not of these serotypes, the clinician should recommend appropriate surgical removal of all such lesions. Lesions in the posterior oral pharyngeal region are of particular concern. Pre-exposure vaccination is one of the most effective methods for preventing transmission of some STDs. Quadrivalent HPV vaccine (Gardasil) and the bivalent HPV vaccine (Cervarix) are available.

GARDASIL 9 is a vaccine indicated in females 9 through 26 years of age for the prevention of cervical, vulvar, vaginal, and anal cancers caused by human papillomavirus (HPV) Types 16, 18, 31, 33, 45, 52, and 58; precancerous or dysplastic lesions caused by HPV Types 6, 11, 16, 18, 31, 33, 45, 52, and 58; and genital warts caused by HPV Types 6 and 11.

GARDASIL 9 is indicated in males 9 through 26 years of age for the prevention of anal cancer caused by HPV Types 16, 18, 31, 33, 45, 52, and 58; precancerous or dysplastic lesions caused by HPV Types 6, 11, 16, 18, 31, 33, 45, 52, and 58; and genital warts caused by HPV Types 6 and 11.

GARDASIL 9 (Human Papillomavirus 9-valent Vaccine, Recombinant) does not eliminate the necessity for girls to continue to undergo recommended cervical cancer screening later in life. Recipients of GARDASIL 9 should not discontinue anal cancer screening if it has been recommended by a health care professional. GARDASIL 9 has not been demonstrated to provide protection against diseases from vaccine HPV types to which a person has previously been exposed through sexual activity.

Cervarix is a bivalent vaccine indicated for the prevention of the following diseases caused by oncogenic human papillomavirus (HPV) types 16 and 18:

- Cervical cancer
- Cervical intraepithelial neoplasia (CIN) grade 2 or worse and adenocarcinoma *in situ*
- Cervical intraepithelial neoplasia (CIN) grade 1

Cervarix is currently no longer available in the US.

Recently, the FDA expanded the approval the HPV 9-valent vaccine, recombinant to include women and men aged 27 to 45 years for the prevention of certain cancers and diseases caused by HPV. Therefore, the HPV 9-valent vaccine (Gardasil 9, Merck) is now approved for males and females aged 9 through 45 years.

Details regarding HPV vaccination are available at www.cdc.gov/std/hpv. Vaccines for other STDs (eg, HIV and herpes simplex virus) are under development or undergoing clinical trials. Vaccines are not available for bacterial or fungal STDs.

The management of a patient with an STD begins with identification. Paramount to the correct management of patients with a history of gonorrhea or syphilis is when the condition was diagnosed, how and with what agent it was treated, did the condition recur, and are there any residual signs and symptoms potentially indicating active or recurrent disease. With standard/universal precautions, the patient with *Neisseria gonorrhoea* or *Treponema pallidum* infection poses little threat to the dentist; however, diagnosis of oral lesions may be problematic. Gonococcal pharyngitis, primary syphilitic lesions (chancre), secondary syphilitic lesions (mucous patch), and tertiary lesions (gumma) may be identified by the dentist. All patients who have gonorrhea should also be tested for other STDs, including chlamydia, syphilis, and HIV. Most gonococcal infections of the pharynx are asymptomatic and can be relatively common in some populations. Gonococcal infections of the pharynx are more difficult to eradicate than urogenital and anorectal infections. Few antimicrobial regimens, including those involving oral cephalosporins, can reliably cure >90% of gonococcal pharyngeal infections. Chlamydial coinfection of the pharynx is unusual; however, because coinfection at genital sites sometimes occurs, treatment for both gonorrhea and chlamydia is recommended.

Gonorrhea is the second most commonly reported bacterial STD. The majority of urethral infections caused by *N. gonorrhoeae* among men produce symptoms that cause them to seek curative treatment soon enough to prevent serious sequelae, but treatment may not be soon enough to prevent transmission to others. Among women, gonococcal infections may not produce recognizable symptoms until complications (eg, pelvic inflammatory disease [PID]) have occurred. PID can result in tubal scarring that can lead to infertility or ectopic pregnancy. Treatment of uncomplicated gonococcal infections of the cervix, urethra, and rectum include ceftriaxone, cefixime, azithromycin, and doxycycline.

Chlamydial genital infection is the most frequently reported infectious disease in the United States and is found more commonly in patients ≤25 years of age. Several important sequelae can result from *C. trachomatous* infection in women including PID, infertility, and ectopic pregnancy. Chlamydia treatment should be provided promptly for all patients testing positive for infection. Coinfection with *C. trachomatous* frequently occurs among patients who have gonococcal infection; therefore, concurrent treatment for both infections is recommended. Chlamydial infections can be treated with azithromycin or doxycycline. Alternative treatments include erythromycin, levofloxacin, or ofloxacin (systemic). If treating gonorrhea concurrently, would not consider use of a fluoroquinolone as resistance is high.

DRUGS USED IN TREATMENT OF CHLAMYDIA, GONORRHEA/SYPHILIS INCLUDE:

Azithromycin (Systemic) on page 203
Cefixime on page 308
CefTRIAXone on page 316
Doxycycline on page 522
Penicillin G Benzathine on page 1208
Penicillin G (Parenteral/Aqueous) on page 1209

The drugs listed above are often used alone or in stepped regimens, particularly when there is concomitant *Chlamydia* infection or when there is evidence of disseminated disease. The proper treatment for syphilis depends on the state of the disease.

HPV PREVENTION:

Papillomavirus (Types 6, 11, 16, 18) Vaccine (Human, Recombinant) (Gardasil) on page 1190
Papillomavirus (Types 16, 18) Vaccine (Human, Recombinant) (Cervarix) on page 1191

REFERENCES AND SELECTED READINGS

Centers for Disease Control and Prevention (CDC). Update to CDC's sexually transmitted diseases treatment guidelines, 2006: fluoroquinolones no longer recommended for treatment of gonococcal infections. *MMWR Morb Mortal Wkly Rep.* 2007;56(14):332-336.

Centers for Disease Control and Prevention (CDC). Update to CDC's sexually transmitted diseases treatment guidelines, 2010: oral cephalosporins no longer a recommended treatment for gonococcal infections. *MMWR Morb Mortal Wkly Rep.* 2012;61(31):590-594.

Corstjens PL, Abrams WR, Malamud D. Detecting viruses by using salivary diagnostics. *J Am Dent Assoc.* 2012;143(10 Suppl):12S-8S.

Little JW. Syphilis: an update. *Oral Surg Oral Med Oral Pathol Oral Radiol Endod.* 2005;100(1):3-9.

Miller WC, Zenilman JM. Epidemiology of chlamydial infection, gonorrhea, and trichomoniasis in the United States – 2005. *Infect Dis Clin North Am.* 2005;19(2):281-296.

Workowski KA, Berman S, Centers for Disease Control and Prevention (CDC). Sexually transmitted diseases treatment guidelines, 2010. *MMWR Recomm Rep.* 2010;59(RR-12):1-110. Available at http://www.cdc.gov/std/treatment/2010/STD-Treatment-2010-RR5912.pdf

SYSTEMIC VIRAL DISEASES

HEPATITIS

The hepatitis viruses are a group of DNA and RNA viruses that produce symptoms associated with inflammation of the liver. Currently, hepatitis A through G have been identified by immunological testing; however, hepatitis A through E have received most attention in terms of disease identification. Recently, there has been increased interest in hepatitis viruses F and G, particularly as related to health care professionals. Our knowledge is expanding rapidly in this area and the clinician should be alert to changes in the literature that might update their knowledge. Hepatitis F, for instance, remains a diagnosis of exclusion, effectively being non-A, B, C, D, E, or G. Hepatitis G has serologic testing available; however, it is not commercially at this time. Research evaluations of various antibody and RT-PCR tests for hepatitis G are under development at this time.

Signs and symptoms of viral hepatitis in general are quite variable. Patients infected may range from asymptomatic to experiencing flu-like symptoms only. In addition, fever, nausea, joint muscle pain, jaundice, and hepatomegaly along with abdominal pain can result from infection with one of the hepatitis viruses. The virus also can create an acute or chronic infection. Usually following these early symptoms or the asymptomatic period, the patient may recover or may go on to develop chronic liver dysfunction. Liver dysfunction may be represented primarily by changes in liver function tests known as LFTs and these primarily include aspartate aminotransferase known as AST and alanine aminotransferase known as ALT. In addition, for A, B, C, D, and E, there are serologic tests for either antigen, antibody, or both. Of hepatitis A through G, five forms have both acute and chronic forms whereas A and E appear to only create acute disease. There are differences in the way clinicians may approach a known postexposure to one of the hepatitis viruses. In many instances, gamma globulin may be used; however, the indications for gamma globulin as a drug limit their use to several of the viruses only. The dental clinician should be aware that the gastroenterologist may choose to give gamma globulin off-label.

Hepatitis A

Hepatitis A virus is an enteric virus that is a member of the Picornavirus family along with Coxsackie viruses and poliovirus. Previously known as infectious hepatitis, hepatitis A has been detected in humans for centuries. It causes acute hepatitis, often transmitted by oral-fecal contamination and having an incubation period of approximately 30 days. Typically, constitutional symptoms are present and jaundice may occur. Drug therapy that the dentist may encounter in a patient being treated for hepatitis A would primarily include immunoglobulin. Hepatitis A vaccine (inactivated) is an FDA-approved vaccine indicated in the prevention of contracting hepatitis A in exposed or high-risk individuals. Candidates at high-risk for HAV infection include persons traveling internationally to highly endemic areas, individuals with chronic liver disease, individuals engaging in high-risk sexual behavior, illicit drug users, persons with high-risk occupational exposure, hemophiliacs or other persons receiving blood products, and pediatric populations. Hepatitis A, caused by infection with HAV, has an incubation period of ~28 days (range: 15 to 50 days). HAV replicates in the liver and is shed in high concentrations in feces from 2 weeks before to 1 week after the onset of clinical illness. HAV infection produces a self-limited disease that does not result in chronic infection or chronic liver disease; however, 10% to 15% of patients experience relapse symptoms during the 6 months after acute illness. Patients with acute hepatitis A usually require only supportive care with no restrictions in diet or activity. Hospitalization may be necessary for patients who become dehydrated due to nausea and vomiting, but is critical for patients with signs or symptoms of acute liver failure. Medications that may cause liver damage or are metabolized by the liver should be used with caution among patients with hepatitis A.

Two products are available for the prevention of HAV infection: Hepatitis A vaccine and immune globulin (IG) for IM administration. Patients recently exposed (within 14 days and prior to development of illness) to HAV and have not received a hepatitis A vaccine should be administered a single dose of the vaccine or IG ([GamaSTAN S/D] 0.02 mL/kg) as soon as possible.

Hepatitis B

Hepatitis B virus is previously known as serum hepatitis and has particular trophism for liver cells. Hepatitis B virus causes both acute and chronic disease in susceptible patients. The incubation period is often long and the diagnosis might be made by serologic markers even in the absence of symptoms.

Hepatitis B is caused by infection with the hepatitis B virus (HBV). The incubation period from the time of exposure to onset of symptoms is 6 weeks to 6 months. The highest concentrations of HBV are found in blood with lower concentrations found in other body fluids.

HBV infection can be self-limited or chronic. In adults, only ~1/2 of newly acquired HBV infections are symptomatic and ~1% of reported cases result in acute liver failure. HBV is efficiently transmitted by percutaneous or mucous membrane exposure to blood or body fluids that contain blood. Preventing disease after exposure in a person without previous hepatitis B vaccine protection is important. Passive-active postexposure prophylaxis (PEP) occurs with administration of hepatitis B immune globulin and hepatitis B vaccine.

Hepatitis C

In the United States, an estimated 4.1 million persons have been infected with hepatitis C virus (HCV), of whom an estimated 3.2 million are living with the infection. The hepatitis C virus (HCV) is an RNA virus. HCV is a major cause of both acute and chronic hepatitis. Persons become infected mainly through parenteral exposure to infected material by blood transfusions or injections with nonsterile needles. Persons who inject illegal drugs and health care workers who are at risk for needlestick and other exposures are at highest risk for HCV infection. Another major risk factor for HCV is high-risk sexual behavior. Cutaneous symptoms or findings relevant to HCV infection manifest in 20% to 40% of patients presenting to dermatologists and in a significant percentage (15% to 20%) of general patients. HCV is suggested and must appear in the differential diagnosis of these patients to avoid missing this important but occult factor in clinical disease in the appropriate setting. HCV has been considered in the differential diagnosis for the causes of oral lichen planus; however, no concrete relationship has been established.

Extrahepatic manifestations of hepatitis C virus are numerous. The most prevalent and most closely linked with HCV is essential mixed cryoglobulins with dermatologic, neurologic, renal, and rheumatologic complications. A less definite relationship to HCV is observed with systemic vasculitis, porphyria cutanea tarda, and the sicca syndromes, which could also affect the oral cavity. HCV is a major public health problem because it causes chronic hepatitis, cirrhosis, and hepatocellular carcinoma (HCC).

Treatment of acute hepatitis C infection has been primarily supportive up to now with monitoring to assess the need for antiviral therapy. Treatment regimens are typically based upon hepatitis C genome, whether the patient is treatment-naïve, has cirrhosis, or has other comorbid conditions, such as HIV. Individuals with Genotype-1 of Hepatitis-C are less likely to respond to standard-of-care HepC medications. Standard-of-care is pegylated interferon (PegIFN) with or without ribavirin. About 50% with genotype-1 and about 80% with genotype-2 or genotype-3 can be virologically cured, but for the others the options to now have been limited. The remaining nonresponders are left with no other treatment options to cure their infection. CDC recommends that all baby boomers (defined as born between 1945 and 1965) be tested for HCV based on the current data that ~2.7 to 3.9 million are infected and most do not know they carry the virus. Recently, Sofosbuvir (Solvaldi) has been approved for the treatment of genotype 1, 2, 3, or 4 chronic hepatitis C in combination with ribavirin or with peginterferon alfa and ribavirin. It is a nucleotide analog polymerase inhibitor, which stops the HCV virus from replicating. Also Sofosbuvir, in combination with ledipasvir (Harvoni), claims a 90% to 99% cure of Hepatitis C.

No vaccine is available for hepatitis C and prophylaxis with immune globulin is not effective in preventing HCV infection after exposure. The OraQuick HCV Rapid Antibody Test (OraSure Technologies) is a rapid assay for the presumptive detection of HCV antibody in fingerstick capillary blood and venipuncture whole blood. Its sensitivity and specificity are similar to those of FDA-approved, laboratory-conducted HCV antibody assays. The Chiron RIBA HCV 3.0 Strip Immunoblot Assay (Novartis Vaccines and Diagnostics) that was recommended for supplemental testing of blood samples after initial HCV antibody testing is no longer available. Testing to determine whether HCV infection has developed is recommended for health care workers after percutaneous or perimucosal exposure to HCV-positive blood.

Historically, HCV treatment was less effective for African Americans than for Caucasians. Researchers identified a gene that was linked with response to pegylated interferon-based treatment, called IL-28B. However, clinical trials of new generation of HCV drugs did not find any difference in cure rates between black and non-black study participants. Hepatitis C also seemed to progress more rapidly in Latinos than in people from other racial and ethnic groups. However, in the clinical trials of several new HCV antivirals, there was no apparent difference in success rates with the drug among Latinos than among non-Latinos.

Hepatitis C, with at least 6 genotypes, is a complex disease also in part because often other liver compromising issues such as cirrhosis and even previous treatments can inhibit the success of newly emerging therapies. Development and approval of a wide variety of drugs to treat selected groups of patients over the last decade has been nothing short of remarkable. In June of 2016 the FDA approved a new combination medicine, the first therapy approved to treat all HCV genotypes (1, 2, 3, 4, 5, or 6). It is also the first single tablet regimen approved for the treatment of patients with HCV genotype 2 and 3, without the need for ribavirin. **EPCLUSA (sofosbuvir 400 mg/velpatasvir 100 mg)** is a once-daily, fixed-dose combination tablet approved for the treatment of adults with chronic HCV genotype 1 to 6. Epclusa for 12 weeks was approved in patients without cirrhosis or with compensated cirrhosis, and in combination with ribavirin for patients with decompensated (advanced) cirrhosis.

Clinicians are advised to refer to liver disease sources such as AASLD-IDSA. See recommendations for testing, managing, and treating hepatitis C at www.hcvguidelines.org in order to assess the data on emerging therapies important in HCV.

Hepatitis D

Hepatitis D, previously known as the delta agent, is a virus that is incomplete in that it requires previous infection with hepatitis B in order to be manifested. Antiviral therapy is not indicated for an acute infection.

Hepatitis E

Hepatitis E virus is an RNA virus that represents a proportion of the previously classified non-A/non-B diagnoses. There is currently no antiviral therapy against hepatitis E.

Hepatitis F

Hepatitis F remains a diagnosis of exclusion. There are no known immunological tests available for identification of hepatitis F at present and currently the Centers for Disease Control have not come out with specific guidelines or recommendations. It is thought that hepatitis F is a blood-borne virus and it has been used as a diagnosis in several cases of post-transfusion hepatitis.

Hepatitis G

Hepatitis G virus (HGV) is the newest hepatitis and is also assumed to be a blood-borne virus. Similar in family to hepatitis C, it is thought to occur concomitantly with hepatitis C and appears to be even more prevalent in some blood donors than hepatitis C. Occupational transmission of HGV is currently under study (see the references for updated information) and currently there are no specific CDC recommendations for postexposure to an HGV individual as the testing for identification remains experimental.

For further information, refer to the following:

Adefovir on page 86
Entecavir on page 567
Hepatitis A Vaccine on page 755
Hepatitis A and Hepatitis B Recombinant Vaccine on page 754
Hepatitis B Immune Globulin (Human) on page 756
Hepatitis B Vaccine (Recombinant) on page 757
Immune Globulin on page 803
Interferon Alfa-2b on page 831
LamiVUDine on page 872
Peginterferon Alfa-2a on page 1201
Peginterferon Alfa-2b on page 1202
Ribavirin (Systemic) on page 1320
Simeprevir on page 1372
Sofosbuvir on page 1378
Telbivudine on page 1412
Tenofovir Disoproxil Fumarate on page 1419

Types of Hepatitis Virus

Features	A	B	C	D	E	F	G
Incubation Period	2 to 6 weeks	8 to 24 weeks	2 to 52 weeks	3 to 13 weeks	3 to 6 weeks	Unknown	Unknown
Onset	Abrupt	Insidious	Insidious	Abrupt	Abrupt	Insidious	Insidious
Symptoms							
Jaundice	Adults: 70% to 80% Children: 10%	25%	25%	Varies	Unknown	Unknown	Unknown
Asymptomatic patients	Adults: 50% Children: Most	~75%	~75%	Rare	Rare	Common	Common
Routes of Transmission							
Fecal/Oral	Yes	No	No	No	Yes	Unknown	Unknown
Parenteral	Rare	Yes	Yes	Yes	No		
Sexual	No	Yes	Possible	Yes	No		
Perinatal	No	Yes	Possible	Possible	No		
Water/Food	Yes	No	No	No	Yes		
Sequelae (% of patients)							
Chronic state	No	Adults: 6% to 10% Children: 25% to 50% Infants: 70% to 90%	>75%	10% to 15%	No	Unknown	Likely
Case-Fatality Rate	0.6%	1.4%	1% to 2%	30%	1% to 2% Pregnant women: 20%	Unknown	Unknown

Preexposure Risk Factors for Hepatitis B

Health care factors:
Health care workers[a]
Special patient groups (eg, adolescents, infants born to HBsAg–positive mothers, military personnel, etc)
Hemodialysis patients[b]
Recipients of certain blood products[c]
Lifestyle factors:
Homosexual and bisexual men
IV drug-abusers
Heterosexually active persons with multiple sexual partners or recently acquired sexually transmitted diseases
Environmental factors:
Household and sexual contacts of HBV carriers
Prison inmates
Clients and staff of institutions for the mentally handicapped
Residents, immigrants, and refugees from areas with endemic HBV infection
International travelers at increased risk of acquiring HBV infection

[a]The risk of hepatitis B virus (HBV) infection for health care workers varies both between hospitals and within hospitals. Hepatitis B vaccination is recommended for all health care workers with blood exposure.

[b]Hemodialysis patients often respond poorly to hepatitis B vaccination; higher vaccine doses or increased number of doses are required. A special formulation of one vaccine is now available for such persons (Recombivax HB, 40 mcg/mL). The anti-HBs (antibody to hepatitis B surface antigen) response of such persons should be tested after they are vaccinated, and those who have not responded should be revaccinated with 1 to 3 additional doses.

Patients with chronic renal disease should be vaccinated as early as possible, ideally before they require hemodialysis. In addition, their anti-HBs levels should be monitored at 6- to 12-month intervals to assess the need for revaccination.

[c]Patients with hemophilia should be immunized SubQ, not IM

PREEXPOSURE VACCINATION

Preexposure vaccination is one of the most effective methods for preventing transmission of some STDs. Human papilloma virus is widespread and serotypes 16 and 18 have been associated with cervical cancer. Although most types that cause oral HPV lesions are not of these serotypes, the clinician should recommend appropriate surgical removal of all such lesions. Lesions in the posterior oral pharyngeal region are of particular concern. Preexposure vaccination is one of the most effective methods for preventing transmission of some STDs. Gardasil 9 is now available.

GARDASIL 9 is a vaccine indicated in females 9 through 26 years of age for the prevention of cervical, vulvar, vaginal, and anal cancers caused by human papillomavirus (HPV) Types 16, 18, 31, 33, 45, 52, and 58; precancerous or dysplastic lesions caused by HPV Types 6, 11, 16, 18, 31, 33, 45, 52, and 58; and genital warts caused by HPV Types 6 and 11.

GARDASIL 9 is indicated in males 9 through 26 years of age for the prevention of anal cancer caused by HPV Types 16, 18, 31, 33, 45, 52, and 58; precancerous or dysplastic lesions caused by HPV Types 6, 11, 16, 18, 31, 33, 45, 52, and 58; and genital warts caused by HPV Types 6 and 11.

GARDASIL 9 (Human Papillomavirus 9-valent Vaccine, Recombinant) does not eliminate the necessity for girls to continue to undergo recommended cervical cancer screening later in life. Recipients of GARDASIL 9 should not discontinue anal cancer screening if it has been recommended by a health care professional. It has not been demonstrated to provide protection against diseases from vaccine HPV types to which a person has previously been exposed through sexual activity. It is not a treatment for external genital lesions; cervical, vulvar, vaginal, and anal cancers; or cervical intraepithelial neoplasia (CIN), vulvar intraepithelial neoplasia (VIN), vaginal intraepithelial neoplasia (VaIN), or anal intraepithelial neoplasia (AIN). Not all vulvar, vaginal, and anal cancers are caused by HPV, and GARDASIL 9 protects only against those vulvar, vaginal, and anal cancers caused by HPV Types 16, 18, 31, 33, 45, 52, and 58. The vaccine is contraindicated in individuals with hypersensitivity, including severe allergic reactions to yeast, or after a previous dose of GARDASIL 9 or if the subject had received the previously available Human Papillomavirus Quadrivalent vaccine (Types 6, 11, 16, and 18). GARDASIL 9 is administered intramuscularly in the deltoid region of the upper arm or in the higher anterolateral area of the thigh. For individuals 9 through 14 years of age, it is administered using a 2-dose or 3-dose schedule. For individuals 15 through 26 years of age, GARDASIL 9 is administered using a 3-dose schedule at 0, 2 months, and 6 months.

Cervarix, an early bivalent vaccine, is no longer marketed in the US.
Recently, the FDA expanded the approval the HPV 9-valent vaccine, recombinant to include women and men aged 27 to 45 years for the prevention of certain cancers and diseases caused by HPV. Therefore, the HPV 9-valent vaccine (Gardasil 9, Merck) is now approved for males and females aged 9 through 45 years.
Details regarding HPV vaccination are available at www.cdc.gov/std/hpv. Vaccines for other STDs (eg, HIV and herpes simplex virus) are under development or undergoing clinical trials. Vaccines are not available for bacterial or fungal STDs.

Hepatitis B vaccination is recommended for all unvaccinated and uninfected patients being evaluated for an STD. In addition, hepatitis A and B vaccines are recommended for men who have sex with men and injection drug users; each of these vaccines should also be administered to HIV-infected patients not yet infected with one or both types of hepatitis virus. Details regarding hepatitis A and B vaccination are available at http://www.cdc.gov/hepatitis.

HPV PREVENTION:

GARDASIL 9 is a vaccine indicated in females 9 through 26 years of age for the prevention of cervical, vulvar, vaginal, and anal cancers caused by human papillomavirus (HPV) Types 16, 18, 31, 33, 45, 52, and 58; precancerous or dysplastic lesions caused by HPV Types 6, 11, 16, 18, 31, 33, 45, 52, and 58; and genital warts caused by HPV Types 6 and 11.

HERPES

The herpes viruses not only represent a topic of specific interest to the dentist due to oral manifestations, but are widespread as systemic infections. Herpes simplex virus is also of interest because of its central nervous system infections and its relationship as one of the viral infections commonly found in AIDS patients. Oral herpes infections will be covered elsewhere. Current recommended drug therapy includes acyclovir, valacyclovir, or famciclovir. Epstein-Barr virus is a member of the herpesvirus family and produces syndromes important in dentistry, including infectious mononucleosis with the commonly found oral pharyngitis and petechial hemorrhages, as well as being the causative agent of Burkitt's lymphoma. The relationship between Epstein-Barr virus to oral hairy leukoplakia in AIDS patients has not been shown to be one of cause and effect; however, the presence of Epstein-Barr in these lesions is consistent. Currently, there is no accepted treatment for Epstein-Barr virus, although acyclovir has been shown in in vitro studies to have some efficacy.

Varicella-zoster virus is another member of the herpesvirus family and is the causative agent of two clinical entities, chickenpox and shingles, or herpes zoster. Oral manifestations of both chickenpox and herpes zoster include vesicular eruptions often leading to confluent mucosal ulcerations. Although the thoracic region is a common site for shingles, the face and/or oral cavity are not rare areas affected. The dentist should be concerned if lesions are confined to one side of the face or oral cavity. Rapid intervention can result in significant reduction in the pain and eruptions of an adult zoster infection. Acyclovir, valacyclovir, or famciclovir are the drugs of choice for treatment of herpes zoster infections.

The vaccine for shingles (Zostavax) is recommended for use in persons ≥60 years of age to prevent shingles. The older a person is, the more severe the effects of shingles typically are. The shingles vaccine is specifically designed to protect people against shingles and will **not** protect people against other forms of herpes, such as genital herpes. The shingles vaccine is **not** recommended to treat active shingles or postherpetic neuralgia (pain after the rash is gone) once it develops. At this time, the CDC does recommend that health care providers within the recommended age group (≥50 years of age) receive the zoster vaccine.

There are other herpes viruses that produce disease in man and animals. These viruses have no specific treatment; therefore, incidence is thought to be less common than those mentioned and the specific treatment is not determined at present. The role of some of these viruses in concomitant infection with the HIV and other coinfection viruses is still under study.

Acyclovir (Systemic) on page 75
Acyclovir (Topical) on page 82
Amantadine on page 112
Atovaquone on page 192
Cidofovir on page 347
Famciclovir on page 635
Foscarnet on page 713
Ganciclovir (Systemic) on page 728
Hepatitis B Immune Globulin (Human) on page 756
Imiquimod on page 802
Immune Globulin on page 803
Interferon Alfa-2b on page 831
Interferon Alfa-n3 on page 833
Oseltamivir on page 1147
Peginterferon Alfa-2a on page 1201
Peginterferon Alfa-2b on page 1202
Penciclovir on page 1207
Ribavirin (Systemic) on page 1320
Rifabutin on page 1323
RiMANTAdine on page 1329
Trifluridine on page 1497
ValACYclovir on page 1512
Zanamivir on page 1567
Zoster Vaccine on page 1585

REFERENCES

AASLD-IDSA HCV Guidance Panel. Hepatitis C guidance: AASLD-IDSA recommendations for testing, managing, and treating adults infected with hepatitis C virus. *Hepatology.* 2015;62(3):932-954. www.hcvguidelines.org.

ACIP Adult Immunization Work Group, Bridges CB, Woods L, Coyne-Beasley T; Centers for Disease Control and Prevention (CDC). Advisory Committee on Immunization Practices (ACIP) recommended immunization schedule for adults aged 19 years and older - United States, 2013. *MMWR Surveill Summ.* 2013;62(Suppl 1):9-19.

Advisory Committee on Immunization Practices (ACIP) Centers for Disease Control and Prevention (CDC). Update: prevention of hepatitis A after exposure to hepatitis A virus and in international travelers. Updated recommendations of the Advisory Committee on Immunization Practices (ACIP). *MMWR Morb Mortal Wkly Rep.* 2007;56(41):1080-1084.

Advisory Committee on Immunization Practices (ACIP). Prevention of hepatitis A through active or passive immunization: recommendations of the Advisory Committee on Immunization Practices (ACIP). *MMWR Recomm Rep.* 2006;55(RR-7):1-23.

Centers for Disease Control and Prevention (CDC). Recommendations of the Advisory Committee on Immunization Practices (ACIP): general recommendations on immunization. *MMWR Recomm Rep.* 2011;60(2):1-64.

Centers for Disease Control and Prevention (CDC). Update on herpes zoster vaccine: licensure for persons aged 50 through 59 years. *MMWR Morb Mortal Wkly Rep.* 2011;60(44):1528.
Cooper C, Lester R, Thorlund K, et al. Direct-acting antiviral therapies for hepatitis C genotype 1 infection: a multiple treatment comparison meta-analysis. *QJM.* 2013;106:153–163.
Corey L, Wald A, Patel R, et al. Once-daily valacyclovir to reduce the risk of transmission of genital herpes. *N Engl J Med.* 2004;350(1):11-20.
Corstjens PL, Abrams WR, Malamud D. Detecting viruses by using salivary diagnostics. *J Am Dent Assoc.* 2012;143(10 Suppl):12S-8S.
Ghany MG, Nelson DR, Strader DB, Thomas DL, Seeff LB; American Association for Study of Liver Diseases. An update on treatment of genotype 1 chronic hepatitis C virus infection: 2011 practice guideline by the American Association for the Study of Liver Diseases. *Hepatology.* 2011;54 (4):1433-1444.
Ghany MG, Strader DB, Thomas DL, Seeff LB; American Association for the Study of Liver Diseases. Diagnosis, management, and treatment of hepatitis C: an update. *Hepatology.* 2009;49(4):1335-1374.
Kaplan JE, Benson C, Holmes KH, et al. Guidelines for prevention and treatment of opportunistic infections in HIV-infected adults and adolescents: recommendations from CDC, the National Institutes of Health, and the HIV Medicine Association of the Infectious Diseases Society of America. *MMWR Recomm Rep.* 2009;58(RR-4):1-207.
Mast EE, Margolis HS, Fiore AE, et al. A comprehensive immunization strategy to eliminate transmission of hepatitis B virus infection in the United States: recommendations of the Advisory Committee on Immunization Practices (ACIP) part 1: immunization of infants, children, and adolescents. *MMWR Recomm Rep.* 2005;54(RR-16):1-31.
Miller CS, Avdiushko SA, Kryscio RJ, Danaher RJ, Jacob RJ. Effect of prophylactic valacyclovir on the presence of human herpesvirus DNA in saliva of healthy individuals after dental treatment. *J Clin Microbiol* . 2005;43(5):2173-2180.
Mofenson LM, Brady MT, Danner SP, et al. Guidelines for the prevention and treatment of opportunistic infections among HIV-exposed and HIV-infected children: recommendations from CDC, the National Institutes of Health, the HIV Medicine Association of The Infectious Diseases Society of America, the Pediatric Infectious Diseases Society, and the American Academy of Pediatrics. *MMWR Recomm Rep.* 2009;58(RR-11):1-166.
Morgan RL, Baack B, Smith BD, Yartel A, Pitasi M, Falck-Ytter Y. Eradication of hepatitis C virus infection and the development of hepatocellular carcinoma. A meta-analysis of observational studies. *Ann Intern Med.* 2013;158:329–337.
Niro GA, Gioffreda D, Fontana R. Hepatitis delta virus infection: open issues. *Dig Liver Dis.* 2011;43(Suppl 1):S19-S24.
Pascarella S, Negro F. Hepatitis D virus: an update. *Liver Int.* 2011;31(1):7-21.
Sherman KE. Hepatitis E virus infection: more common than previously realized? *Gastroenterol Hepatol (N Y).* 2011;7(11):759-761.
Shivkumar S, Peeling R, Jafari Y, Joseph L, Pant Pai N. Accuracy of rapid and point-of-care screening tests for hepatitis C: a systematic review and meta-analysis. *Ann Intern Med.* 2012;157:558–566.
Teshale EH, Hu DJ. Hepatitis E: epidemiology and prevention. *World J Hepatol.* 2011;3(12):285-291.
Triantos C, Kalafateli M, Nikolopoulou V, Burroughs A. Meta-analysis: antiviral treatment for hepatitis D. *Aliment Pharmacol Ther.* 2012;35 (6):663-673.
Workowski KA, Berman S, Centers for Disease Control and Prevention (CDC). Sexually transmitted diseases treatment guidelines, 2010. *MMWR Recomm Rep.* 2010;59(RR-12):1-110. Available at http://www.cdc.gov/std/treatment/2010/STD-Treatment-2010-RR5912.pdf

ANTIBIOTIC PROPHYLAXIS

PREPROCEDURAL GUIDELINES FOR DENTAL PATIENTS

INTRODUCTION

Historically, in dental practice, antibiotic prophylaxis has been mandated for certain at-risk patients to prevent infective endocarditis, orthopedic implant late infection, or contamination through any oral surgical site. Clinical practice guidelines are generally provided through a joint effort of medical and dental organizations and are reviewed and rewritten periodically based upon clinical and scientific evidence. In this section, these guidelines are reviewed. In general, compared with all previous recommendations, there are currently relatively few patient subpopulations for whom antibiotic prophylaxis may be indicated prior to certain dental procedures.

ANTIMICROBIAL STEWARDSHIP

Antimicrobial stewardship refers to coordinated interventions designed to improve and measure the appropriate use of antimicrobials by promoting the selection of the optimal antimicrobial drug regimen, dose, duration of therapy, and route of administration. Antimicrobial stewards seek to achieve optimal clinical outcomes related to antimicrobial use, minimize toxicity and other adverse events, reduce the costs of health care for infections, and limit the selection for antimicrobial resistant strains. Currently, there are no national or coordinated legislative or regulatory mandates designed to optimize use of antimicrobial therapy through antimicrobial stewardship. Given the societal value of antimicrobials and their diminishing effectiveness due to antimicrobial resistance, groups like the ADA support broad implementation of antimicrobial stewardship programs across all health care settings (eg, hospitals, long-term care facilities, long-term acute care facilities, ambulatory surgical centers, dialysis centers, and private practices).

The American Dental Association (ADA) supports the responsible use of antibiotics. As part of this effort toward antibiotic stewardship, the ADA has adopted an evidence-based approach to guideline development, which has resulted in recommendations for decreased indications for, and use of prophylactic antibiotics in people with heart conditions and those who have had joint replacements. Although there are some studies evaluating the appropriateness of antibiotic prescribing in dentistry, a recent paper in *JADA* suggests that it is likely that there are opportunities to improve prescribing practices.

PREVENTION OF INFECTIVE ENDOCARDITIS

In 2007, the American Heart Association (AHA), in conjunction with the American Dental Association (ADA) and other experts in both medicine and dentistry, performed an extensive evidence-based literature review and provided the most recent guidelines regarding the use of antibiotic prophylaxis to prevent infective endocarditis (IE) related to dental procedures. Since the mid-1950s, it has been recommended that patients at risk for IE from a variety of medical conditions should be premedicated with antibiotics prior to dental and other procedures. Earlier changes in the guidelines (1984, 1990, 1997) focused on the recommended antibiotics, dose, and dosing frequency. While indicating a minor modification of recommended antibiotics, the most recent change (2007) focused primarily on the patients for whom prophylaxis is recommended.

Infective endocarditis is the consequence of a sequence of events. This sequence is initiated by the formation of nonbacterial thrombotic endocarditis (NBTE) on the surface of a cardiac valve or elsewhere that endothelial damage occurs within the heart. Turbulent blood flow produced by congenital or acquired heart disease, including flow from high- to low-flow chambers and flow across a narrowed orifice, traumatizes the endothelium. This predisposes for deposition of platelets and fibrin on the endothelial surface and results in NBTE. If bacteremia then occurs following invasion of the bloodstream with a microbial species that has the pathogenic potential to colonize this site, IE can occur. Mucosal surfaces are populated by dense endogenous microflora. Trauma to a mucosal surface releases many different microbial species transiently into the blood stream. Transient bacteremia caused by oral microflora occurs commonly with dental extractions or other dental procedures or with routine daily activities. The frequency and intensity of the resulting bacteremia are related to the nature and magnitude of the trauma, density of the microbial flora, and degree of inflammation or infection at the site. The microbial species entering circulation depends on the unique endogenous microflora that colonize the traumatized site. The ability of the bacteria in the blood stream to adhere to specific NBTE sites determines the anatomic localization of the infection. Mediators of bacterial adherence serve as virulence factors. Common oral flora, including viridans group Streptococci and Staphylococci have cellular components that serve as adhesions to the NBTE and these adhesions are immunogenic. Microorganisms adherent to the vegetation stimulate further deposition of fibrin and platelets on their surface. The buried microorganisms multiply as rapidly as bacteria in broth cultures to reach maximal densities within a short time on the left side of the heart, apparently uninhibited by host defenses in left-sided lesions. Right-sided vegetations have lower bacterial densities due to host defense, such as PMN activity or platelet-derived antibacterial proteins. More than 90% of microorganisms in mature valvular vegetations are metabolically inactive and are therefore less responsive to the bacterial effects of antibiotics.

Viridans group Streptococci are normal oral tract flora and cause more than 50% of cases of community-acquired native valve IE that is not associated with IV drug use. As early as 1935, a report indicated that 11% of patients with poor oral hygiene had positive blood cultures, yet 61% of patients experienced bacteremia with dental extractions. Historically, the additional assumptions associated with antibiotic prophylaxis for IE are that these microorganisms are susceptible to antibiotics recommended for prophylaxis, that antibiotic prophylaxis prevents experimental endocarditis in animals, that a temporal relationship exists between dental procedures and the onset of symptoms of IE, that the risk of adverse drugs reactions is low, and that morbidity and mortality of IE are high.

A primary determinant of the changes for the 2007 guidelines are that the estimated absolute risk for IE from a dental procedure in patients with underlying cardiac conditions increases from 1:1.1 million for mitral valve prolapsed (MVP) to 1:475,000 for congenital heart disease (CHD). The absolute risk increases further for rheumatic heart disease (RHD) (1:142,000), prosthetic valve (1:114,000), and previous IE (1:95,000). Cardiac conditions with predisposition for IE show similar trends. Additionally, mortality associated with prosthetic valve endocarditis (PVE) is >20% and PVE increases the risk of heart failure.

As a result, antibiotic prophylaxis with certain dental procedures is recommended for patients at highest risk of IE due to specific cardiac conditions:

- Prosthetic cardiac valve
- A prior incidence of IE
- Heart transplant patients who develop cardiac valvulopathy
- Patients with CHD are required prophylaxis with the following conditions:
  - Unrepaired cyanotic CHD, including palliative shunts and conduits
  - Completely repaired CHD with prosthetic material or device during the first 6 months after the surgical or catheter intervention procedure
  - Repaired CHD with residual defects at the site or adjacent to the site of a prosthetic patch (which inhibits endothelialization)

These patients with high-risk cardiac conditions are recommended for prophylaxis for all dental procedures involving manipulation of gingival tissue or the periapical region of teeth or perforation of the oral mucosa.

Common dental procedures that **do not** require prophylaxis but do require sound clinical judgement include:

- Routine anesthetic injection into noninfected tissue
- Taking dental radiographs
- Placement of removable prosthodontic or orthodontic appliances
- Adjustment of orthodontic appliances
- Placement of orthodontic brackets
- Shedding of deciduous teeth
- Bleeding from trauma to the lips or oral mucosa

ANTIBIOTIC SELECTION

For examples of sample prescriptions see Prevention of Endocarditis and to Reduce the Risk of Late Infections of Joint Prostheses - Sample Prescriptions on page 40. Dentists should be vigilant in reviewing all current literature for updates.

Table 1 provides the recommended antibiotics and doses. Specific dosage forms available for each antibiotic can be found in the drug monographs. Extended or delayed release dosage formulations should not be used for antibiotic prophylaxis because they will not produce high immediate peak concentrations.

For those patients able to take oral antibiotics and those not allergic to beta-lactam antibiotics (penicillins, cephalosporins, monobactams, and carbapenems), the antibiotic of choice is amoxicillin, an amino penicillin. Aminopenicillins have an extended spectrum of antibacterial action compared to penicillin VK-treating gram-positive aerobes, such as staph and strep, but also some gram-aerobes, such as *Haemophilus influenza*. Aminopenicillins are more stable in the gastro-intestinal tract, allowing them to be taken with food or beverages, providing higher plasma concentrations following oral administration.

For individuals unable to take oral medications and not allergic to beta-lactam antibiotics, intramuscular (IM) or intravenous (IV) ampicillin, also an aminopenicillin, is recommended.

Table 1. Prophylactic Regimens for Infective Endocarditis for Dental Procedures

Situation	Drug	Single Dosage 30 to 60 minutes prior to procedure
Oral	Amoxicillin on page 124	Children: 50 mg/kg Adults: 2 g
Unable to take oral medications	Ampicillin on page 140 **or**	Children: 50 mg/kg IM or IV Adults: 2 g IM or IV
	CeFAZolin on page 301 **or** CefTRIAXone on page 316	Children: 50 mg/kg IM or IV Adults: 1 g IM or IV

(continued)

Table 1. Prophylactic Regimens for Infective Endocarditis for Dental Procedures *(continued)*

Situation	Drug	Single Dosage 30 to 60 minutes prior to procedure
Allergic to penicillins or ampicillin (oral)	Cephalexin on page 322[a,b] **or**	Children: 50 mg/kg Adults: 2 g
	Clindamycin (Systemic) on page 368 **or**	Children: 20 mg/kg Adults: 600 mg
	Azithromycin (Systemic) on page 203 **or** Clarithromycin on page 361	Children: 15 mg/kg Adults: 500 mg
Allergic to penicillins or ampicillin and unable to take oral medications	CeFAZolin on page 301 **or** CefTRIAXone on page 316[b]	Children: 50 mg/kg IM or IV Adults: 1 g IM or IV
	Clindamycin (Systemic) on page 368	Children: 20 mg/kg IM or IV Adults: 600 mg IM or IV

Note: Intramuscular injections should be avoided in patients receiving anticoagulant therapy.

[a]Can use first or second generation oral cephalosporins in equivalent doses.

[b]Cephalosporins should not be used in individuals with immediate-type hypersensitivity reaction (urticaria, angioedema, or anaphylaxis) to penicillins.

Individuals who are allergic to the penicillins, such as amoxicillin or ampicillin, should be treated with an alternate antibiotic. The 2007 guidelines suggest a number of alternate agents, including clindamycin, cephalosporins, azithromycin, and clarithromycin. Patients who do not have a Type I (immediate) allergic (hypersensitivity) reaction to penicillins (urticaria, bronchospasm, angioedema, anaphylaxis) may receive a first or second generation cephalosporin. Oral first generation cephalosporins include cephalexin (Keflex) and cefadroxil (Duricef). First generation cephalosporins have an antibacterial spectrum of activity similar to amoxicillin and ampicillin. Oral second generation cephalosporins include cefaclor (Ceclor), cefprozil, or cefuroxime axetil (Ceftin). Second generation cephalosporins have an antibacterial spectrum of activity broader than aminopenicillins and first generation cephalosporins and similar to amoxicillin with clavulanic acid. For patients unable to take oral cephalosporins, the first generation cephalosporin cefazolin (Ancef) is recommended for IM or IV administration. A third generation cephalosporin, ceftriaxone (Rocephin), is also listed as a parenteral option. Third generation cephalosporins have a broader antibacterial spectrum of activity than first and second generation cephalosporins and should generally be reserved for more serious gram infections or for gram-positive infections not responsive to first-line therapy.

Penicillin and cephalosporin antibiotics have a bactericidal mechanism of action by inhibiting synthesis of the bacterial cell wall. They are most effective in bacteria that are actively growing and reproducing. The most common adverse reaction is a Type I or immediate hypersensitivity reaction which generally produces urticaria, bronchospasm, angioedema, or anaphylaxis. Because both penicillins and cephalosporins are beta-lactam antibiotics, patients with Type I immediate hypersensitivity reactions can be cross-allergic.

Clindamycin (Cleocin) is a lincosamide antibiotic effective against gram-positive aerobes and many anaerobic bacteria. Clindamycin is an option both orally or IM or IV for patients with any penicillin allergy. Clindamycin is a bacteriostatic antibiotic that inhibits bacterial protein synthesis. Adverse effects of clindamycin after a single dose are rare. Although it is estimated that 1% of patients taking clindamycin will develop symptoms of pseudomembranous colitis, these symptoms usually develop after 9 to 14 days of clindamycin therapy. These symptoms are rare and only one case has been reported in a patient taking an acute dose for the prevention of endocarditis.

Azithromycin (Zithromax) and clarithromycin (Biaxin) are members of the class of antibiotics known as macrolides. The pharmacology of these drugs has been reviewed previously in *General Dentistry*. Erythromycins have been available for use in dentistry and medicine since the mid-1950s. Azithromycin and clarithromycin represent the first additions to this class in more than 40 years. The adult prophylactic dose for either drug is 500 mg 30 to 60 minutes before the procedure with no follow-up dose. The pediatric prophylactic dose of azithromycin and clarithromycin is 15 mg/kg orally 30 to 60 minutes before the procedure. Although the erythromycin family of drugs is known to inhibit the hepatic metabolism of theophylline and carbamazepine to enhance their effects, azithromycin has not been shown to affect the liver metabolism of these drugs.

Azithromycin is well-absorbed from the gastrointestinal tract and is extensively taken up from circulation into tissues with a slow release from those tissues. It reaches peak serum levels in 2 to 4 hours and serum half-life is 68 hours. Zithromax is supplied as 250 mg, 500 mg, and 600 mg tablets. It is also available for oral suspension at concentrations of 100 mg per 5 mL, 200 mg per 5 mL, and single-dose packets containing 1 g. In May 2012, the FDA notified health care providers that they are reviewing the results of an azithromycin study published in the *New England Journal of Medicine*. This study reported a small increase in cardiovascular deaths and in the risk of death from any cause in persons treated with a 5-day course of azithromycin (Zithromax) compared to persons treated with amoxicillin, ciprofloxacin, or no medication. The FDA will communicate any new information on azithromycin and this study or the potential risk of QT interval prolongation after the agency has completed its review. Patients taking azithromycin should not stop taking their medicine without talking to their health care provider. Health care providers should be aware of the potential for QT interval prolongation and heart arrhythmias when prescribing or administering any macrolide antibiotic.

Clarithromycin (Biaxin) achieves peak plasma concentrations in 3 hours and maintains effective serum concentrations over a 12-hour period. Reports indicate that it probably interacts with theophylline and carbamazepine by elevating the plasma concentrations of the two drugs. Biaxin is supplied as 250 mg and 500 mg tablets and 500 mg extended release tablets. It is also available as granules for oral suspension at concentrations of 125 mg per 5 mL and 250 mg per 5 mL.

Clinical Considerations for Dentistry

See Figure 1.

Figure 1
Preprocedural Dental Action Plan for Patients With a History Indicative of Elevated Endocarditis Risk

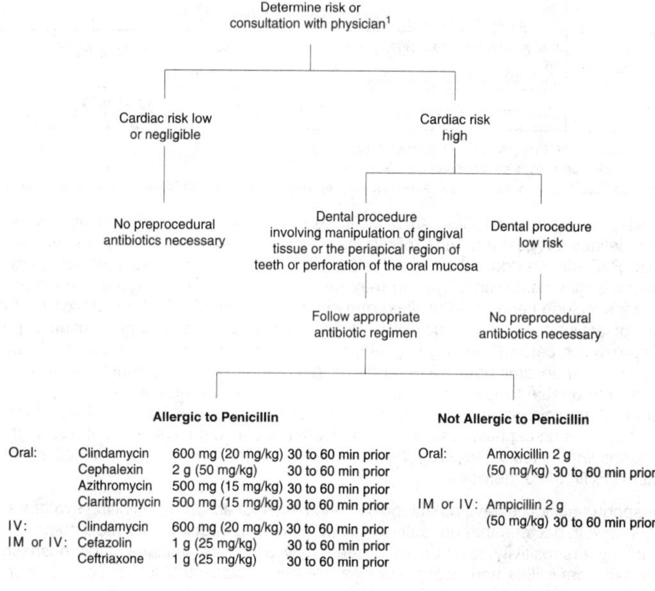

Dosages for children are in parentheses and should never exceed adult dose. Cephalosporins should be avoided in patients with previous Type I hypersensitivity reactions to penicillin due to some evidence of cross-allergenicity.

[1]For Emergency Dental Care, the clinician should attempt phone consultation. If unable to contact patient's physician or determine risk, the patient should be treated as though there is a high risk of cardiac complication and follow the algorithm.

An antibiotic for prophylaxis should be administered in a single dose before the procedure. If the dosage of antibiotic is inadvertently not administered before the procedure, the dosage may be administered up to 2 hours after the procedure. However, administration of the dosage after the procedure should be considered only when the patient did not receive the preprocedural dose.

PREPROCEDURAL ANTIBIOTICS FOR PROSTHETIC IMPLANTS

A significant number of dental patients have had total joint replacements or other implanted prosthetic devices. Prior to performing dental procedures that might induce bacteremia, the dentist has historically been advised to consider the use of antibiotic prophylaxis in these patients. In December 2012, the American Academy of Orthopedic Surgeons (AAOS) and the ADA released an Evidence-Based Guideline and Evidence Report entitled "Prevention of Orthopaedic Implant Infection in Patients Undergoing Dental Procedures". The report concludes that the groups found insufficient evidence to recommend the routine use of antibiotics for joint replacement patients. They advised that there is no direct evidence that routine dental procedures cause prosthetic joint infections. **After 2012, the CPG stated that most patients no longer needed antibiotic prophylaxis, but based on a patient's medical history, consultation with the individuals' health care providers was often recommended.** According to the ADA Chairside Guide, for patients with a history of complications associated with their joint replacement surgery who are undergoing dental procedures that include gingival manipulation or mucosal incision, prophylactic antibiotics should only be considered after consultation with the patient and orthopedic surgeon; in cases where antibiotics are deemed necessary, it is most appropriate that the orthopedic surgeon recommend the appropriate antibiotic regimen and, when reasonable, write the prescription.

Recently the American Dental Association Council on Scientific Affairs convened a panel of experts to provide clarification of Clinical Practice Guidelines (CPG) for dental practitioners, related to the subject of prophylactic antibiotics prior to dental procedures in patients with prosthetic joints. This panel reviewed and supported all of the previous CPG implemented in 2012, related to evidence-based guidelines.

The goal of the new 2014 CPG is to provide additional information and they are published in the Journal of the American Dental Association (Sollecito 2015). The CPG state that in general, there is little or no evidence to support the use of preprocedural antibiotics in prosthetic joint replacement patients. These CPG were developed after an exhaustive re-review and update of those previous 2012 guidelines. Hence, prophylactic antibiotics are not routinely recommended prior to dental procedures in order to prevent prosthetic joint infection.

Regarding clinical conditions that might elevate the risk of late joint infections in this patient population, the panel evaluated the existing evidence related to preoperative conditions and peri/postoperative history of the joint replacement. Berbari EF, et al, published the most significant data in this evidence-based review, which evaluated those preoperative and postoperative factors that have been associated epidemiologically with late prosthetic joint infection. The most clinically relevant of these factors were postoperative problems, especially evidence of multiple joint surgeries, as well as wound drainage, hematoma, or infection postoperatively. History of any of these complications mandate discussion with the orthopedist to determine if antibiotics may be appropriate prior to dental procedures that produce bacteremia.

Other conditions that might be identified preoperatively, such as the comorbidities of diabetes mellitus, rheumatoid arthritis, levels of immune compromise, chronic kidney disease, or evidence of malignancy, were also considered in the risk assessment. These conditions, although extremely important in the overall risk of the subject, do not associate significantly with the risk of prosthetic joint infection but obviously warrant consultation and discussion with the patient's orthopedic and primary care physicians.

In conclusion, the 2014 panel concluded that patients with prosthetic joint implants do not in general require prophylactic antibiotics prior to dental procedures in order to prevent prosthetic joint infections. Dental practitioners must always use their best clinical judgment and all available current scientific knowledge to assess each patient. Therefore, as a general rule, in patients who report preoperative conditions or postoperative complications following the joint implant, open communication/consultation with our medical colleagues to determine an appropriate plan related to possible use of prophylactic antibiotics is advised.

The recommendations from these 2014 CPG increase the importance for dentists when planning invasive oral procedures to consult with the patient's orthopedic surgeon to determine the risk associated with infection and the need for antibiotics.

Table 2. Patients With Medical Conditions Suggesting a Need for Medical Consultation to Determine Potential Risk of Joint Infection

All patients with prosthetic joint replacement who by history report postoperative complications following the joint surgery
Immunocompromised/immunosuppressed patients
Inflammatory arthropathies (eg, rheumatoid arthritis, systemic lupus erythematosus)
Drug-induced immunosuppression (eg, chemotherapy or biologics for autoimmune diseases)
Radiation-induced immunosuppression
Patients with comorbidity (eg, diabetes, obesity, HIV, and smoking)
Previous prosthetic infections
Malnourishment
Hemophilia
HIV infection
Type 1 diabetes mellitus (insulin dependent, IDDM)
Malignancy
Megaprosthesis

Source: January 2013 AAOS Information Statement. Available at http://www.aaos.org/about/papers/advistmt/1033.asp. Original source: American Dental Association; American Academy of Orthopedic Surgeons. Antibiotic prophylaxis for dental patients with total joint replacements. *J Am Dent Assoc.* 2003;134(7):895-899.

Even in these patients, the new 2014 CPG stating that preprocedural antibiotics are not generally necessary should be seriously considered and a medical consultation with the physician will ultimately determine whether or not to use antibiotics. Late infections of implanted prosthetic devices have rarely been associated with microbial organisms of oral origin. Also, since late infections in such patients are often not reported, data is lacking to substantiate or refute this potential.

ANTIBIOTIC REGIMENS

The 2014 CPG should be carefully reviewed for any patient with a prosthetic joint. Clinical judgement decisions can always be made on a case-by-case basis. If using preprocedural antibiotics is found to be appropriate after careful consideration, the antibiotic prophylaxis regimens, as suggested by the advisory panel, are listed in Table 3. These regimens are not exactly the same as those listed in Table 1 (for prevention of endocarditis) and must be reviewed carefully to avoid confusion.

Please review the new Clinical Practice Guidelines (CPG), December 2014, for assessing the need for preprocedural antibiotics to prevent prosthetic joint late infections. The current CPG state that there is no direct evidence linking dental procedures to prostheses infections and that antibiotic prophylaxis is not warranted in most patients. Decisions must be made on a case-by-case basis. If after careful consideration, and/or consultation with the orthopedist, preprocedural antibiotics are found to be appropriate, the following example prescriptions apply. Prescription dispensing amounts are for three visits. These numbers can be adjusted for each patient treatment plan. Clinicians will be advised if and when any more specific guidelines are forthcoming.

The American Association of Orthopedic Surgeons (AAOS) has also developed Appropriate Use Criteria (AUC) for thirteen selected situations encountered by orthopedists, including, "Management of patients with orthopedic implants undergoing dental procedures". This was added as of November 2016.

Regarding antibiotic selection, when after consultation preprocedural antibiotics are deemed necessary, one important change occurred. In the latest release from the AAOS, clindamycin is no longer recommended as the suggested alternative in patients allergic to penicillins. The AAOS now recommends, in allergic patients still able to take oral medication, 2 g cephalexin, or 500 mg of azithromycin or clarithromycin in that order of selection. Since this release the ADA and the AHA have not taken any steps to alter their endocarditis recommendations. Terico AT, Gallagher JC. Beta-lactam hypersensitivity and cross-reactivity. *J Pharm Pract.* 2014; 27(6):530-544 is cited as the reference for considerations of cross allergenicity of cephalosporins and penicillins.

Cephalexin or amoxicillin may be used in patients not allergic to penicillin. The selected antibiotic is given as a single 2 g dose 30 to 60 minutes before the procedure. A follow-up dose is not recommended. Cephalexin (Keflex) and amoxicillin were described earlier in this section.

Parenteral ceftriaxone or ampicillin is the recommended antibiotic for patients unable to take oral medications (see Table 3 for doses). Ceftriaxone is a third generation cephalosporin, effective against anaerobes and aerobic gram-positive bacteria. Ampicillin is an aminopenicillin (described earlier). For patients allergic to penicillin, cephalexin is the recommended antibiotic of choice.

Table 3. Antibiotic Regimens for Patients With Prosthetic Implants

Patients not allergic to penicillin:	Cephalexin or amoxicillin:	2 g orally 1 hour prior to the procedure
Patients not allergic to penicillin and unable to take oral medications:	CefTRIAXone: or Ampicillin:	1 g IM or IV 1 hour prior to the procedure 2 g IM or IV 1 hour prior to the procedure
Patients allergic to penicillin:	Cephalexin:	2 g orally 1 hour prior to the procedure
Second choice:	or Azithromycin (Systemic)	500 mg 1 hour prior to the procedure
Third choice:	or Clarithromycin	500 mg 1 hour prior to the procedure
Patients allergic to penicillin and unable to take oral medications:	CefTRIAXone:	1 g IM or IV 1 hour prior to procedure

Please review the new guidelines for prevention of prosthetic joint late infections. Decisions must be made on a case-by-case basis. If using preprocedural antibiotics is found to be appropriate after careful consideration, the example prescriptions in the section entitled **Prevention of Endocarditis and to Reduce the Risk of Late Infections of Joint Protheses on page 40** apply.

Cephalexin on page 322

As more evidence and data are collected, these recommendations may be revised; however, it is thought to be prudent for the dental clinician to fully evaluate all patients with respect to history and/or physical findings and a medical consultation prior to determining the risk.

In patients in whom concern exists over joint complications and a medical consultation cannot be immediately obtained, the patient should be treated as though antibiotic coverage is necessary until such time that an appropriate consultation can be completed.

Clinical Considerations for Dentistry

See Figure 2.

Figure 2
Preprocedural Dental Action Plan for Patients With Prosthetic Implants

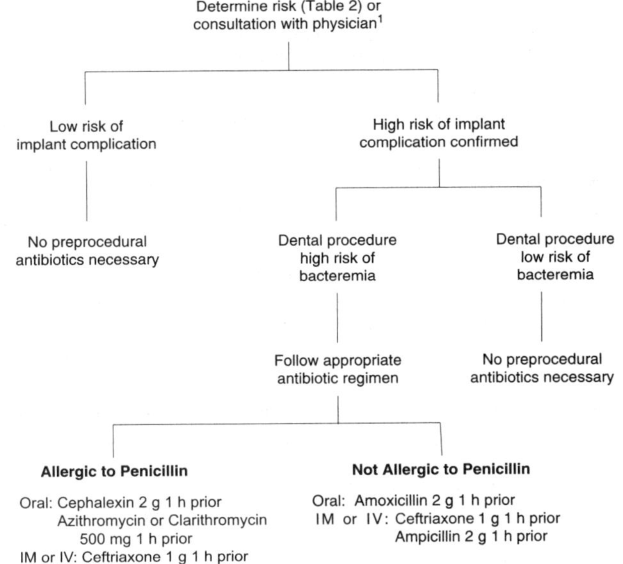

Cephalosporins should be avoided in patients with previous Type I hypersensitivity reactions to penicillin due to some evidence of cross allergenicity. Other risk of cross allergenicity ~1% to 5% (Terico 2014).

[1]For Emergency Dental Care the clinician should attempt phone consultation. If unable to contact patient's physician or determine risk, the patient should be treated as though there is high risk of implant complication and follow the algorithm.

SUMMARY

Compared with previous recommendations, there are currently relatively few patient subpopulations for whom antibiotic prophylaxis may be indicated prior to certain dental procedures.

In patients with prosthetic joint implants, a January 2015 ADA clinical practice guideline, based on a 2014 systematic review states, "In general, for patients with prosthetic joint implants, prophylactic antibiotics are not recommended prior to dental procedures to prevent prosthetic joint infection."

According to the ADA Chairside Guide, for patients with a history of complications associated with their joint replacement surgery who are undergoing dental procedures that include gingival manipulation or mucosal incision, prophylactic antibiotics should only be considered after consultation with the patient and orthopedic surgeon.

For infective endocarditis prophylaxis, current guidelines support premedication for a relatively small subset of patients. Infective endocarditis prophylaxis for dental procedures should be recommended only for patients with underlying cardiac conditions associated with the highest risk of adverse outcome from infective endocarditis (see Figure 1). For patients with these underlying cardiac conditions, prophylaxis is recommended for all dental procedures that involve manipulation of gingival tissue or the periapical region of teeth or perforation of the oral mucosa.

FREQUENTLY ASKED QUESTIONS FOR INFECTIVE ENDOCARDITIS (IE) AND PROSTHETIC IMPLANTS

When should we start following the new prevention of IE and Prosthetic Joint guidelines?

Immediately, since the previous update was from June 2010 for IE and 2014 for Prosthetic Joints.

What should we do for patients who have been premedicated for IE in the past but are no longer recommended for prophylaxis?

If the patient does not fall into one of the highest risk groups, premedication should not be used unless an updated medical consultation suggests additional risks based on previously undisclosed comorbitities.

Should I just premedicate to be safe?

No, the new guidelines are based on evidence which documents that the risk of adverse side effects from the antibiotics (allergy, GI upset, development of microbial resistance, etc) outweigh the benefits in many patients who previously received SBE/IE prophylaxis. The new guidelines clearly recommend the use of prophylactic antibiotics only for those at the highest risk after consultation.

What if a patient did not meet the new high-risk criteria outlined in the new Guidelines and the patient's physician still recommends IE prophylaxis?

Please contact the physician to see if there are compelling medical reasons for continuing IE prophylaxis.

What if a patient who has received IE prophylaxis in the past for a condition that is now deemed as ***not*** *being high risk for IE prophylaxis still insists on being premedicated?*

Recommend that the patient contacts the physician to see if there are compelling medical reasons for continuing IE prophylaxis.

If the patient is presently taking antibiotics for some other ailment, is prophylaxis still necessary?

If a patient is already taking antibiotics for another condition, prophylaxis (when deemed necessary under the new guidelines) should be accomplished with a drug recommendation from another class. For example, in the patient who is not allergic to penicillin and is taking a macrolide antibiotic for a medical condition, amoxicillin would be the drug of choice for prophylaxis. Also, in the penicillin-allergic patient taking clindamycin, prophylaxis would best be accomplished with azithromycin or clarithromycin.

What should I do if medical consultation results in a recommendation that differs from the published guidelines endorsed by the American Dental Association?

The dentist is ultimately responsible for treatment recommendations. Ideally, by communicating with the physician, a consensus can be achieved that is either in agreement with the guidelines or is based on other established medical reasoning.

Is there cross-allergenicity between the cephalosporins and penicillin?

According to a recent study by Terico, the incidence of cross-allergenicity is 5% for first generation drugs and 1% for third generation drugs in the overall population. If a patient has demonstrated a Type I hypersensitivity reaction to penicillin, including urticaria, bronchospasm, angioedema, or anaphylaxis, then this incidence increases to 20%.

Is there definitely an interaction between contraceptive agents and antibiotics?

There are well-founded interactions between contraceptives and antibiotics. The best instructions that a patient could be given by his/her dentist are that should an antibiotic be necessary and the dentist is aware that the patient is on contraceptives, and if the patient is using chemical contraceptives, the patient should seriously consider additional means of contraception during the antibiotic management.

Are PROBIOTICS important in patients receiving long-term or repeated care with antibiotics?

There is always concern regarding disruption of healthy microflora of the gastrointestinal system when antibiotics are prescribed for an extended period of time or on closely repeated occasions. GI symptoms often occur and do not represent any direct drug allergy or toxicity but rather are the effects of this gut flora alteration.

Cultures of direct-fed microorganisms or probiotics are able to multiply in the intestinal tract to create a balance of microflora. Some lactobacillus species used in probiotic applications include *L. acidophilus, L. casei, L. reuteri, L. rhamnosus,* and *Bifidobacterium bifidum*. These and other organisms form a symbiotic or mutual relationship with their host. Each species develops a resistance to the disease-causing potential of such organisms and form mutual beneficial relationships with these organisms. The familiar *L. acidophilus* produces lactic acid, reduces gut pH, and acts as a colonizer. Some forms of antibiotics, such as cephalosporins, clindamycin, or fluoroquinolones, induce colitis, an inflammation of the large intestine, in some individuals. This type of colitis is caused by a toxin produced by the bacteria *Clostridioides* (formerly *Clostridium*) *difficile*, which is resistant to many antibiotics and proliferates in the intestines when other normal bacterial flora in the intestine are altered by the antibiotics.

It is usually recommended to take probiotics at least 3 hours apart from antibiotics. Taking both at the same time defeats the purpose as the friendly bacteria will be totally destroyed by the drug. During antibiotic therapy, a good dose of viable probiotic cells is 6 to 25 billion colony-forming units per day. Probiotics are also being studied as adjunctive therapy to periodontal treatment and treatment of other bacterial infections.

Has there been any change in the guidelines for prophylaxis for patients with prosthetic joint replacements?

Yes, the 2012 Clinical Practice Guidelines and the 2014 panel concluded that patients with prosthetic joint implants do not in general require prophylactic antibiotics prior to dental procedures in order to prevent prosthetic joint infections. Dental practitioners must always use their best clinical judgment and all available current scientific knowledge to assess each patient. Therefore, as a general rule, in patients who report preoperative conditions or postoperative complications following the joint implant, open communication/consultation with our medical colleagues to determine an appropriate plan related to possible use of prophylactic antibiotics is advised. If concern over joint complications exists and a medical consultation cannot be immediately obtained, the dentist should treat the patient as though antibiotic coverage is necessary until an appropriate consultation can be completed.

REFERENCES

American Academy of Orthopaedic Surgeons and American Association of Orthopaedic Surgeons. Statement release for new 2012 clinical practice guideline – new guideline includes shared decision-making tool, implications for practice. 2013. Available at http://www6.aaos.org/news/PDFopen/PDFopen.cfm?page_url=http://www.aaos.org/news/aaosnow/jan13/cover1.asp

American Academy of Orthopaedic Surgeons; American Dental Association. Prevention of orthopaedic implant infection in patients undergoing dental procedures: Evidence-based guideline and evidence report. Rosemont, IL: American Academy of Orthopaedic Surgeons; 2012. Available at www.aaos.org/research/guidelines/PUDP/PUDP_guideline.pdf.

American Dental Association-Appointed Members of the Expert Writing and Voting Panels Contributing to the Development of American Academy of Orthopedic Surgeons Appropriate Use Criteria. American Dental Association guidance for utilizing appropriate use criteria in the management of the care of patients with orthopedic implants undergoing dental procedures. *J Am Dent Assoc.* 2017;148(2):57-59.

Berbari EF, Osmon DR, Carr A, et al. Dental procedures as risk factors for prosthetic hip or knee infection: A hospital-based prospective case-control study (published correction appears in *Clin Infect Dis.* 2010;50(6):944). *Clin Infect Dis.* 2010;50(1):8-16.

Centers for Disease Control and Prevention. Antibiotic/antimicrobial resistance: Threat report 2013. Atlanta: Centers for Disease Control and Prevention; 2013:6,51. Available at: https://www.cdc.gov/drugresistance/threat-report-2013/. Accessed September 21, 2014.

Centers for Disease Control and Prevention. Antibiotic/antimicrobial resistance. U.S. Department of Health & Human Services. Accessed May 20, 2016.

Fluent MT, Jacobsen PL, Hicks LA, OSAP. Considerations for responsible antibiotic use in dentistry. *J Am Dent Assoc.* 2016;147(8):683-686.

Legout L, Beltrand E, Migaud H, Senneville E. Antibiotic prophylaxis to reduce the risk of joint implant contamination during dental surgery seems unnecessary. *Orthop Traumatol Surg Res.* 2012;98(8):910-914.

Lockhart PB, Blizzard J, Maslow AL, Brennan MT, Sasser H, Carew J. Drug cost implications for antibiotic prophylaxis for dental procedures. *Oral Surg Oral Med Oral Pathol Oral Radiol.* 2013;115(3):345-353.

Meurman JH, Stamatova I. Probiotics: contributions to oral health. *Oral Dis.* 2007;13(5):443-445.

Meyer DM. Providing clarity on evidence-based prophylactic guidelines for prosthetic joint infections. *J Am Dent Assoc.* 2015;146(1):3-5.

Nishimura RA, Otto CM, Bonow RO, et al. 2017 AHA/ACC Focused update of the 2014 AHA/ACC Guideline for the management of patients with valvular heart disease: a report of the American College of Cardiology/American Heart Association Task Force on Clinical Practice Guidelines. *Circulation.* 2017;135:e1159-e1195. Accessed June 19, 2017.

Palmer C. ADA News: ADA supports responsible antibiotic use. American Dental Association. June 15, 2015.

Quinn RH, Murray JN, Pezold R, Sevarino KS. The American Academy of Orthopaedic Surgeons Appropriate Use Criteria for the Management of Patients with Orthopaedic Implants Undergoing Dental Procedures. *J Bone Joint Surg Am.* 2017;99(2):161-63.

Rethman MP, Watters W 3rd, Abt E, et al; American Academy of Orthopaedic Surgeons; American Dental Association. The American Academy of Orthopaedic Surgeons and the American Dental Association clinical practice guideline on the prevention of orthopaedic implant infection in patients undergoing dental procedures. *J Bone Joint Surg Am.* 2013;95(8):745-747.

Sollecito TP, Abt E, Lockhart PB, et al. The use of prophylactic antibiotics prior to dental procedures in patients with prosthetic joints: Evidence-based clinical practice guideline for dental practitioners-a report of the American Dental Association Council on Scientific Affairs. *J Am Dent Assoc.* 2015;146(1):11-16.

Swan J, Dowsey M, Babazadeh S, Mandaleson A, Choong PF. Significance of sentinel infective events in haematogenous prosthetic knee infections. *ANZ J Surg.* 2011;81(1-2):40-45.

Terico AT, Gallagher JC. Beta-lactam hypersensitivity and cross-reactivity. *J Pharm Pract.* 2014; 27(6):530-544.

Teughels W, Van Essche M, Sliepen I, Quirynen M. Probiotics and oral healthcare. *Periodontol 2000.* 2008;48:111-147.

Watters W 3rd. Rethman MP, Hanson NB, et al; American Academy of Orthopaedic Surgeons; American Dental Association. Prevention of orthopaedic implant infection in patients undergoing dental procedures. *J Am Acad Orthop Surg.* 2013;21(3):180-189.

Wilson W, Chair, Taubert KA, Gewitz M, et al. Prevention of infective endocarditis: guidelines from the American Heart Association: a guideline from the American Heart Association Rheumatic Fever, Endocarditis, and Kawasaki Disease Committee, Council on Cardiovascular Disease in the Young, and the Council on Clinical Cardiology, Council on Cardiovascular Surgery and Anesthesia, and the Quality of Care and Outcomes Research Interdisciplinary Working Group. *Circulation.* 2007;116:1736-1754.

Wilson W, Taubert KA, Gewitz M, et al. Prevention of infective endocarditis: guidelines from the American Heart Association: a guideline from the American Heart Association Rheumatic Fever, Endocarditis and Kawasaki Disease Committee, Council on Cardiovascular Disease in the Young, and the Council on Clinical Cardiology, Council on Cardiovascular Surgery and Anesthesia, and the Quality of Care and Outcomes Research Interdisciplinary Working Group. *J Am Dent Assoc.* 2008;139 Suppl:3S-24S.

MANAGEMENT OF THE CHEMICALLY DEPENDENT PATIENT

INTRODUCTION

As long as history has been recorded, man has used drugs to alter mood, thought, and feeling. The financial and emotional cost to society due to the abuse and addiction of these substances is staggering. Some reports place the cost to society of alcoholism and alcohol abuse as high as $185 billion dollars annually. Increased on-the-job accidents, absenteeism, welfare costs, and alcohol-related auto fatalities contribute to this cost.

In 1986, the American Dental Association (ADA) passed a policy statement recognizing chemical dependency as a disease. In recognizing this disease, the Association mandated that dentists have a responsibility to include questions relating to a history of chemical dependency, or more broadly, substance abuse in their health history questionnaire. This policy statement included patients who are actively abusing drugs as well as patients who are in recovery. An affirmative response was an alert to the dentist and dental team to use caution with certain medications and that the treatment plan may have to be altered. This policy statement was revised in 1989 and 1991 with minor changes. In October 2005 at the annual ADA session, the House of Delegates passed several resolutions encompassing the use of opioids in management of dental pain, alcohol, and other substance use by pregnant and postpartum patients, and guidelines related to alcohol, nicotine, and/or drug use by child or adolescent patients. The House of Delegates in 2005 reaffirmed the disease concept of alcoholism and other substance use disorders and provided a more current statement on provision of dental treatment for patients with substance use disorders. For an in-depth review of these resolutions, refer to www.ada.org. At the minimum, the patient's past medical history questionnaire should include a question asking if there is a history of chemical dependency and if so, how long they have been in recovery. The ADA recommends that the dental office should have a list available of local resources for drug counseling in the event the patient admits drug use and seeks some help.

This chapter reviews common substances of abuse, where they come from, signs and symptoms of the substance abuser, and some of the dental implications of treating patients actively using or in recovery from these substances. There are many books and articles devoted to this topic that provide greater detail. The reader is referred to several comprehensive texts on this disease. The intent of this chapter is to provide an overview of some of the most prevalent drugs, how abuse of these substances by patients may influence dental treatment, and how to recognize some signs and symptoms of substance abuse and withdrawal.

Substances of abuse originate from many sources. They may be naturally occurring, semisynthetic, synthetic, over-the-counter, or prescription drugs. There is a paucity of information in the dental literature correlating substance abuse with dental manifestations for a simple reason. Most substance abusers do not seek routine dental care because obtaining their drug of choice is their top priority. Most often they will be episodic patients. In fact, that is one of the cardinal signs of addiction, a preoccupation with obtaining the drug or sex or gambling or whatever the addiction. Patients presenting to the dental office solely to obtain opiates or other controlled substances are referred to as "doctor shoppers" because they literally go from doctors' office to office seeking these medications. It can be difficult to distinguish between these drug seekers or the patient that is truly in need of pain medication. Most often these patients have multiple areas of decay and would appear to be in pain, but their main goal is to obtain the opiate medication.

What are some of the warning signs of a "doctor shopper"?

- They can name the medication or may ask for a brand name opiate.
- The patient may be very knowledgeable about contraindications of medications and health problems in order to direct the dentist to prescribe the opiate, for example, the patient may state they have an ulcer and cannot take NSAIDs limiting the prescription choice to opiates.
- The patient may request a prescription over the phone and is not willing to come into the office. Good dental practice dictates that prescriptions for medication never be prescribed over the phone unless the patient has been seen in the office to determine the problem.
- The patient may request to come into the office after hours when the dentist is alone and threaten the dentist to provide the prescription.
- The patient may call and say they are from out of town and need just enough medication to hold them over until they can get to their own dentist.
- The patient may exhibit cutaneous indications of prior drug use.

What can the dentist do to identify a "doctor shopper"?

- Evaluate for signs of drug use. Take the patient's blood pressure, giving you an opportunity to examine the bare arm.
- Check your state's **Prescription Drug Monitoring Program** (PDMP) data base: This information can be accessed to review prescription abuse trends, identify diversion locations, and identify patients who go from doctor to doctor to obtain these prescriptions. These programs are supported mostly by state funds and therefore vary widely in their effectiveness and reliability. However, several states now require the prescriber to consult the PDMP before initially prescribing an opiate or benzodiazepine. In some states, failure to consult the PDMP by the prescriber can result in suspension of their license or a fine. In a PDMP, the dentist is provided with a password which allows them to check the name of a patient whom they suspect as a "doctor shopper" and to see how many prescriptions, and

quantity of controlled substance, the patient has received within a certain period. If the dentist finds that the patient has visited other doctors within a short period of time, the dentist can refuse prescribing the controlled substance. Some states will have a telephone number to alert authorities to have the patient removed from the office.

How to manage the "doctor shopper"

- Perform a thorough examination.
- Document all that you see.
- Prescribe NSAIDs.
  An NSAID in combination with acetaminophen will be much more effective than an opiate analgesic because of the inflammatory nature of dental pain. Opiates are **not** anti-inflammatory. If you must prescribe an opioid analgesic do so in limited amounts and at the lowest possible strength. Routine dental pain (eg, extraction) only requires a two-day supply of medication. If the patient requests a refill by phone, schedule an appointment for follow-up examination. If a dental cause of the pain cannot be identified, the patient should be referred to a pain management center.

As a rule, the central nervous system (CNS) stimulant (uppers) abusing dental patient most likely will not be going to the dentist while under the influence of the drug because the stimulant will amplify their already existing anxiety. It is more likely that a patient will use or abuse a CNS depressant (downer) substance to self-medicate their anxiety. This is important to the dentist because stimulants such as cocaine, methamphetamine, and ecstacy are sympathomimetics and in combination with vasoconstrictor could result in a hypertensive crisis (stroke). **Plain local anesthetic without vasoconstrictor is not contraindicated in that patient.** Patients who self-medicate with depressant drugs such as alcohol, opioids, barbiturates, or marijuana are generally more compliant while in the dental chair, and the drug combination does not pose a serious threat unless the practitioner is using oral or intravenous sedation.

ALCOHOL

Ethyl alcohol (referred to as alcohol) is the most abused drug in the United States today and the most abused drug by dentists. As mentioned above, the cost to society for the treatment of alcoholism and alcohol abuse is billions of dollars annually. Alcohol is a CNS depressant and not a stimulant as many people (particularly the adolescent population) believe. Its effect on the central nervous system is dose-dependent and correlated with the rising blood alcohol concentration rather than the falling concentration. Cognitive ability, reaction time, memory, psychomotor, and perceptual ability are impaired to varying degrees.

Most of the consumed alcohol is absorbed from the small intestine and is, therefore, affected by the gastric emptying time and the consumption of food. Alcohol is metabolized by the liver via acetaldehyde and eventually to carbon dioxide and water. Excess consumption of alcohol can result in hepatic damage that may affect the patient's ability to metabolize medications. Doses of medications that are metabolized by the liver, such as acetaminophen, may have to be reduced when treating a patient with confirmed hepatic damage from alcohol or other substance abuse. Alcohol readily crosses the placental barrier and has the potential of producing fetal alcohol syndrome (FAS), the most severe form of the fetal alcohol spectrum disorders (FASD). It is estimated that the prevalence of FASD in the US ranges from 3.1% to 9.9%. Those who do suffer from some form of FASD exhibit varying degrees of mental retardation, supernumerary teeth, and facial deformities to name a few. These effects are not limited to physical changes but can influence social interactions, and the propensity for substance abuse later in life as well. The two classic signs of FAS in children are the absence of a philtrum and a thin upper lip. The American Dental Association addresses this problem with their resolution passed in 2005 entitled **Statement on Alcohol and Other Substance Use by Pregnant and Postpartum Patients**. There are many other resources that provide greater detail about this preventable syndrome and the reader is referred to those sources as well.

Excessive alcohol use has been associated with an increased incidence of periodontal disease, poor wound healing, chronic orofacial infections, iatrogenic injury, and an increased incidence of oral cancer. Since alcohol is a CNS depressant, any medication that causes respiratory depression should be prescribed or administered with caution or not at all for patients suspected of alcohol abuse. Patients who present to the dental office and are obviously intoxicated should not be provided dental treatment. The major concern with the intoxicated patient is a failure to follow directions while in the chair, and the inability to follow postoperative instructions. An additional concern is the aggressive, combative behavior exhibited by some that are intoxicated.

Signs and Symptoms of Alcohol Use or Abuse	
Lethargic, slow to respond	Odor on breath and/or clothes
Slurred speech	Inability to respond to commands
Telangiectasia	Psychomotor impairment

CANNABIS (MARIJUANA)

The most abused illegal drug by high school students today is marijuana. Marijuana is a plant that grows throughout the world, but is particularly suited for a warm, humid environment. There are three species of plants but the two most frequently cited are *Cannabis sativa* and *Cannabis indica*. All species possess a female and male plant. Approximately 450 chemicals have been isolated of which approximately 85 are described as cannabinoids. Of these, 23 are thought to be psychoactive. The major psychoactive cannabinoid is delta-9-tetrahydrocannabinol and the most abundant. The highest concentration of THC is found in hashish which is derived from the bud of the female plant. The concentration of THC varies according to growing conditions and the part of the plant but has increased from ~2% to 3% in marijuana sold in the 1950s to ~90% sold on the streets today. The term sinsemilla (Hispanic for "without seed") is used to describe marijuana from the unpollinated tops of the female flowers and is associated with a higher concentration of THC. Marijuana can be smoked in cigarettes (joints, spliffs), pipes, water pipes (bongs), or baked in brownies, cakes, candies, etc, and then ingested. However, smoking or inhaling vapers (vaping) marijuana is more efficient, with a faster onset but shorter duration than oral forms. There are new street terms and forms of marijuana that are now used to describe the more potent forms of marijuana such "scat", "dab", "wax", and "shatter", and the use of these forms such as "scatting", "dabbing", etc. Descriptions of these new forms are beyond the scope of this chapter and the reader is directed to current literature. Marijuana is a Schedule I controlled substance but has been promoted as medicinal for the treatment of glaucoma (according to the Glaucoma Research Foundation, "the number of significant side effects generated by long-term oral use of marijuana or long-term inhalation of marijuana smoke make marijuana a poor choice in the treatment of glaucoma, a chronic disease requiring proven and effective treatment"), for increasing appetite in patients who have HIV disease, to prevent the nausea associated with cancer chemotherapy, and as an analgesic for chronic pain. In response to this request, the FDA approved two forms of synthetic THC dronabinol (Marinol, Syndros) and a THC analog nabilone (Cesamet) and placed these medications in Schedule III to be prescribed by physicians for the indicated medical conditions. These synthetic THCs are not psychotropic and in fact are not well-absorbed from the gastrointestinal tract. Thirty-three states have passed legislation to allow marijuana for medical purposes. The laws passed or pending by these states differ in the allowable quantity of usable marijuana, as well as the quantity of plants possessed, and the cannabinoid allowed. For instance, the cannabinoid cannabidiol (CBD) has been approved for treating medication-resistant types of epilepsy but does not produce a psychoactive effect. In June 2018, the FDA approved the first cannabis-derived medication for severe forms of epilepsy, Epidiolex (cannabidiol). The reader should be cautioned when buying commercially available CBD because not all CBD is regulated and much of it is derived from Hemp. Recently, in those states where cannabis is approved for medical, the medical indications for the use of marijuana have been expanded to include multiple sclerosis-induced spasticity, including the neuropathic pain associated with this condition. It is important to remember that none of these indications have been approved by the US Food and Drug Administration (FDA). Eleven states, Alaska, California, Colorado, Illinois, Maine, Massachusetts, Michigan, Nevada, Oregon, Vermont, Washington state, and the District of Columbia, have passed legislation to allow marijuana use for recreational purposes despite the DEA classification as a Schedule I Controlled Substance. Drugs in Schedule I have the highest potential for abuse/addiction and have no accepted medical use in the United States today. This apparent conflict must be resolved as more states approve marijuana for recreational or medicinal use. On August 29, 2013, the Department of Justice issued a statement stating that it would not prosecute any person on the federal level if they abided by state law.

An individual under the influence of marijuana may exhibit no signs or symptoms of intoxication. The pharmacologic effects are dose-dependent and depend to a large extent on the set and setting of the intoxicated individual. As the dose of THC increases, the person experiences euphoria or a state of well-being, often referred to as "mellowing out". Everything becomes comical, problems disappear, and their appetite for snack foods increases. This is called the "munchies". Additionally, marijuana produces time and spatial distortion, which contribute, as the dose increases, to a dysphoria characterized by paranoia, fear, and anxiety. Although there has never been a death reported from marijuana overdose, certainly the higher doses may produce such bizarre circumstances as to increase the chances of accidental death. Since THC is fat soluble, daily consumption of marijuana may result in THC being stored in body fat which will result in detectable amounts of THC being found in the urine for as long as 60 days in some cases. According to the National Institute of Drug Abuse, it is estimated that 9% of marijuana users will become dependent on it and this percentage increases to 17% when marijuana smokers began using in the teenage years. The CDC has reported similar but higher percentages. Recent research suggests that heavy marijuana smokers function at a lower intellectual level compared to nonsmokers, affecting attention span, memory, cognitive ability, and psychomotor skills. These cannabis-induced effects are controversial and the reader should consult additional references. Additional research is needed to ascertain a causal relationship as well as the impact on the dental practice. Studies have indicated that the psychomotor impairment associated with marijuana can extend for up to 24 hours after smoking marijuana.

An endogenous cannabinoid system has been identified in the human, and receptors have been located. This system is referred to as the endocannabinoid system, with endogenous cannabinoids identified as anandamide and 2-arachidonoylglycerol (2-AG). A detailed description, and its medical implications and potential, is not within the scope of this chapter and the reader is referred elsewhere for more detailed descriptions and current research regarding this innate system.

Because of anxiety associated with dental visits, marijuana would be the most likely drug, after alcohol, to be used when coming to the dental office. But, unlike alcohol, marijuana may not produce any detectable odor on the breath nor signs of intoxication. Fortunately, local anesthetics, analgesics, and antibiotics used by the general dentist do not interact with marijuana. The major concern with the marijuana-intoxicated patient, like the alcohol-intoxicated patient, is a failure to follow directions while in the chair, and the inability to follow postoperative instructions. Since marijuana is a CNS depressant, caution with oral and intravenous is advised. Patients under the influence of marijuana exhibit short-term memory impairment which could be a problem following post-op instructions. It is critical that the patient suspected of marijuana intoxication be provided with written post-op instructions and have a witness present for any signed consent.

Signs and Symptoms of Marijuana Use	
Blood shot eyes	Odor on breath and clothes
Lethargic, slow to respond	Inability to respond to commands
Slurred speech	Memory impairment

Synthetic Cannabinoids: These chemicals are illegal (NOT FDA approved) synthetic versions of delta 9-tetrahydrocannabinol (THC), the major psychoactive ingredient in marijuana. They are reported to be 200 to 800 times more potent than THC. The effects of these chemicals are like marijuana: Increased heart rate, increased blood pressure, paranoia, agitation, giddiness, and increased appetite. Synthetic cannabinoids are advertised as being undetectable in urine drug tests for THC; however, this is untrue. The chemicals can be detected by urinalysis, but it takes a very sophisticated system for detection, testing is expensive, and most laboratories do not routinely test for synthetic cannabinoids.

Internet sales of the chemicals have been connected to sources in China, Pakistan, and India. Once the chemicals have been purchased, the final product can be assembled in the United States. It is sold in small packets labeled as herbal incense or potpourri, which contain dried herbal materials that are sprayed with the synthetic cannabinoids. The product is typically smoked and has various street names such as "Spice Diamond," "Dream," "Essence," and "K-2." Packets vary in cost from $20 to $50 and weigh 100 to 300 mg. Liquid synthetic cannabinoids can be vaporized in e-cigarettes.

These "designer" drugs are intended to circumvent the Controlled Substances Act of 1970. The problem for law enforcement is that underground chemists continue to modify chemicals into new ones that are not illegal to possess or use. According to the US Drug Enforcement Administration (DEA) there are 22 of these chemicals that have been placed on the Controlled Substances list and possibly another 75 that have been identified as being sold on the streets in the US but have not been placed on the Controlled Substances list. These synthetic cannabinoids have been implicated as the causative agent in renal and liver failure among our population. And yet they can be purchased over the internet or hand to hand sales on the streets. According to the DEA, a 15-state raid early 2016 seized approximately 16,000 pounds of these packaged synthetic cannabinoids for distribution to the streets. Go to www.DEA.gov for more information about these deadly chemicals.

OPIOIDS

The opioids are often called narcotics and include a variety of commonly prescribed drugs including morphine, oxycodone, and hydrocodone. Illicit opioids available on the street include heroin and fentanyl. Over 70% of people who abuse prescription pain relievers acquire them from friends or relatives. Nearly 1/3 of people ≥12 years of age who abuse these drugs began by using a prescription drug for nonmedical purposes. Numerous studies have reported that approximately 75% of the heroin addicts reported their first misuse of opioids was prescription opioids. From 1999 to 2010, the number of people in the United States dying annually from prescription opioid related overdoses quadrupled, from 4,030 to 16,651 (*JAMA* 2013).

According to the American Society for Addiction Medicine, 94% of people who were being treated for opioid addiction claimed they switched to heroin because of the cost and difficulty obtaining prescription opioids. It is estimated that 134 Americans die evey day from an opioid overdose. According to the Center for Disease Control and Prevention (CDC) from 2000 to 2015 more than half a million people died from drug overdoses. In 2018 the CDC reported that approximately 72,000 people in the United Stated died of a drug overdose in the previous year. Influencing this increased overdose rate is the introduction of newer synthetics such as fentanyl (50 to 100 times more potent than morphine) and carfentanil (referred to as elephant tranquilizer on the street and is 10,000 times more potent than morphine) in the heroin sold on the street. Again, according to the CDC, more people die from opioid overdose every day than die from automobile accidents. The American Medical Association (AMA), the American Dental Association (ADA), the American Pharmaceutical Association (APhA), and the Food and Drug Association (FDA) have called for greater restrictions on opioid prescribing and approval of new opioid entities.

As noted previously in the dental office opioids should be the last choice to relieve postoperative pain. The nature of dental pain is a dull, aching, inflammatory pain and is best controlled by the NSAIDs with acetaminophen as a rescue analgesic. Opioids are **not** anti-inflammatory. Four hundred to 600 mg of ibuprofen every 6 hours by itself or alternating with acetaminophen 500 mg will control 90% of dental pain. Do not exceed 3,000 mg of acetaminophen or 3,200 mg of ibuprofen in 24 hours.

Many patients who have been abusing opioids will exhibit multiple carious lesions, particularly class V lesions. This increased caries rate is probably a result of xerostomia, high intake of sweets, and lack of daily oral hygiene. Patients who are recovering from heroin or other opioid addiction should not be prescribed any kind of opioid analgesic because of the increased chance of relapse. Nonsteroidal anti-inflammatory drugs (NSAIDs) should be used to control any postoperative discomfort in these patients. Patients with a history of intravenous drug abuse may be at higher risk of subacute bacterial endocarditis (SBE), HIV disease, hepatitis, and certainly increased infection postoperatively. The clinician might consider or at least be aware of the increased possibility of postoperative infection in these patients.

Signs and Symptoms of Opioid Use	
Pin point pupils	Glazed eyes
Lethargic, slow to respond	Inability to respond to commands
Slurred speech	Xerostomia

METHAMPHETAMINE

Methamphetamine has been available clinically for 60 years as a medication to curb appetite. Today it is one of the most widely abused drugs on the street. Methamphetamine can be smoked in the form of "ice" (crystal meth), snorted, injected, or consumed orally. The onset of action varies with the route of administration, smoking providing the most rapid onset of action. Clandestine methamphetamine is usually synthesized from pseudoephedrine or ephedrine. Because of this avenue to produce methamphetamine, Congress enacted the Combat Methamphetamine Epidemic Act of 2005 (CMEA) which placed restrictions on the sale of pseudoephedrine. Some states require a prescription for pseudoephedrine and others require identification and limits how much can be purchased over the counter without a prescription. According to the DEA, the majority of methamphetamine is imported to the US from Mexico with very little produced by small clandestine labs within the US According to the most recent surveys from the Monitoring the Future Study for 2018, the abuse of methamphetamine in the last year, the last 30 days, or lifetime in the 8th, 10th, and 12th grades has dramatically decreased.

The methamphetamine molecule can exist in either the "D" isomer or the "L" isomer. The latter isomer has its greatest effect on the cardiovascular system and, in fact, is available commercially over-the-counter as a nasal decongestant. The "D" isomer has its principle effects on the central nervous system as a stimulant (upper) and cannot be converted from the "L" form. It is a sympathomimetic and as such raises blood pressure. This effect on the autonomic nervous system results in increased basal metabolic rate (BMR) and increased body temperature, resulting in the "sweats". Methamphetamine users crave sweets possibly as a source of energy to fuel the increased BMR. Because of the increased sweating the individual becomes dehydrated and thirsty. The sympathetic stimulation produces thick, ropey saliva. This lack of saliva, increased consumption of sweets in the form of soda pop, and lack of routine dental care no doubt is the primary cause of "meth mouth". Initially the meth user experiences a feeling of exhilaration, alertness, and incredible energy. With successive uses, tolerance occurs and the user abuses increasing amounts of methamphetamine looking for the same high they experienced on the first time. They never quite attain it. This has been referred to on the street as "chasing the monkey". As a substitute, the user continues their high for several hours or days in some cases. This is called bingeing. A binge may last for 5 or 6 days. The user becomes very paranoid, develops psychotic episodes, and has the potential of becoming violent. stereotypical behavior develops such as rocking back and forth in a chair, picking their fingernails, or other behavior. During this stage the user begins "tweaking", using small amounts to stay high, and begins to hallucinate. Characteristically, they will describe the feeling that bugs are crawling under their skin and they scratch their arms, face, and any other exposed part of their body. The street term for this hallucination is called "coke bugs". Usually, the user will collapse from the physical exhaustion. Withdrawal can take weeks after the last use. As mentioned above, vasoconstrictor is contraindicated if there has been methamphetamine use within the last 24 hours.

Methamphetamine Signs and Symptoms in the Dental Office	
Dilated pupils	Jittery, irritable behavior
Rapid speech	Unable to sit still, twitching
Tremendous anxiety	Difficult to anesthetize

BENZODIAZEPINES AND OTHER NONALCOHOL SEDATIVES

These drugs are used mainly for treatment of anxiety disorders and, in some instances, insomnia. These drugs are commonly abused, either by themselves or as adjunct to the opioids. They can produce a strong physical dependency on the use of the medication. As tolerance builds up to the drug, the physical dependency increases dramatically. Unlike street drugs, where addiction is a primary consideration, the overuse of benzodiazepine lies in their ability to induce physical dependency. When these drugs are taken for several weeks, there is relatively little tolerance induced. However, after several months, the proportion of patients who become tolerant increases and reducing the dose or stopping the medication produces severe withdrawal symptoms which may result in death.

It is extremely difficult for the physician to distinguish between the withdrawal symptoms and the reappearance of the myriad anxiety symptoms that cause the drug to be prescribed initially. Many patients increase their dose over time because tolerance develops to at least the sedative effects of the drug. The antianxiety benefits of the benzodiazepines continue to occur long after tolerance to the sedating effects. Patients often take these drugs for many years with relatively few ill effects other than the risk of withdrawal. The dentist should be keenly aware of the signs and symptoms and the historical pattern in patients taking benzodiazepines. On the street, the abuser will often mix a benzodiazepine with an opioid to enhance the opioid-induced euphoria. The benzodiazepines are used with methadone to induce a heroin-like high. The dentist should be aware of "doctor shoppers" asking for the benzodiazepines who will then use these medications in conjunction with their opiates or other drugs of abuse. On the street this is referred to as a "benzo boost". The benzodiazepines are also taken along with ecstacy or MDMA to mitigate the crash or coming down from the MDMA. This is referred to as "parachuting" on the street. The most common dental side effect of the benzodiazepines is xerostomia occurring in approximately 10% of the patients who consume these either therapeutically or abusers.

NICOTINE

Cigarette (nicotine) addiction is influenced by multiple variables. Nicotine itself produces reinforcement; users compare nicotine to stimulants such as cocaine or amphetamine, although its effects are of lower magnitude.

Nicotine is absorbed readily through the skin, mucous membranes, and of course, through the lungs. The pulmonary route produces discernible central nervous system effects in as little as 7 seconds. Thus, each puff produces some discrete reinforcement. With 10 puffs per cigarette, the 1 pack per day smoker reinforces the habit 200 times daily. The timing, setting, situation, and preparation all become associated repetitively with the effects of nicotine.

Nicotine has both stimulant and depressant actions. The smoker feels alert, yet there is some muscle relaxation. Nicotine activates the nucleus accumbens reward system in the brain. Increased extracellular dopamine has been found in this region after nicotine injections in rats. Nicotine affects other systems as well, including the release of endogenous opioids and glucocorticoids.

Nicotine Withdrawal Syndrome Signs and Symptoms	
Irritability, impatience, hostility	Restlessness
Anxiety	Decreased heart rate
Dysphoric or depressed mood	Increased appetite or weight gain
Difficulty concentrating	

SMOKING CESSATION PRODUCTS

Several years ago, the journal, *Science* stated that ~80% of smokers say they want to quit, but each year <1 in 10 succeed. Nicotine transdermal delivery preparations (or nicotine patches) were approved by the US Food and Drug Administration in 1992 as aids to smoking cessation for the relief of nicotine withdrawal symptoms. Four preparations were approved simultaneously: Habitrol, Nicoderm, Nicotrol, and ProStep. These products differ in how much nicotine is released and whether they provide a 24- or 16-hour release time.

Studies are still being reported on the effectiveness of nicotine patches on tobacco cessation. Most previous studies had good entry criteria including definition of the Fagerstrom score. Dr Fred Cowan of Oregon Health Sciences University described these Fagerstrom criteria in a previous report on nicotine substitutes in AGD *Impact*. Abstinence of smoking cessation has usually been assessed by self-report, measurement of carbon monoxide in breath, and plasma or urine nicotine products.

In numerous protocols, percentages of study subjects who abstained from smoking after 3 to 10 weeks of patch treatment with nicotine compared to placebo, have never exceeded 40%. After the initial assessment, six studies continued to follow the study subjects through 24 to 52 weeks of patch treatment. The results were even poorer with <25% sustained success. A review of these and additional studies, reveals some general conclusions regarding the effectiveness of nicotine patches in tobacco cessation. In every study, many smokers abstained after treatment with placebo patches; nicotine treatment was initially more effective than placebo; and improved abstinence rates were more marked in the short term (10 weeks) than in the long term (52 weeks). Subjects undergoing tobacco cessation trials tended to gain weight irrespective of whether placebo or nicotine patches were worn. Patients often favor the nicotine polacrilex gum (Nicorette) which releases nicotine into the blood stream via the oral mucosa.

Data are now available from tobacco cessation studies carried out in general medical practices. The effectiveness of nicotine patch substitution under these conditions is like the results described previous. Most patch systems and gum are now available as over-the-counter products; only Habitrol remains prescription. Bupropion (Zyban) is another approach to the treatment of tobacco cessation. This drug is a norepinephrine/serotonin/dopamine reuptake inhibitor and its action directly affects the craving for tobacco. Another new product just introduced is varenicline (Chantix). This product targets certain nicotine receptors to prevent nicotine access and diminishes the mesolimbic dopamine reward associated with nicotine use. The reader is referred to more comprehensive information about these products and the treatment of tobacco cessation. In addition, the reader should familiarize themselves with the supportive ADA posture on the role of the dental team in tobacco cessation treatment.

Many patients have tried traditional therapies to quit smoking. Battery operated E-cigarettes are gaining in popularity, allowing the user to inhale vapors containing nicotine without the tar and carbon monoxide found in cigarettes. A new study indicates that subjects, with no immediate intention of quitting who switched to e-cigarettes demonstrated quitting behavior. They found 10.7% of the subjects who switched to nicotine containing e-cigarettes had completely quit smoking at week 12 and 8.7% were still not smoking 1 year later. Although the US Food and Drug Administration has not approved e-cigarettes for smoking cessation treatment, it is worth considering for patients who want to reduce the harmful effects of smoking but have failed in previous efforts to quit.

Therefore, in patients who smoke but do not intend to quit, the use of e-cigarettes, with or without nicotine (but more successfully with nicotine), decreased cigarette consumption with lasting results, reducing the harmful side effects of smoking (Caponnetto 2013).

The most recent statistics from the 2018 Monitoring the Future Study indicate that 8th, 10th, and 12th graders prefer and more heavily abuse e-cigarettes compared to traditional tobacco products. These e-cigarettes cause a heated source to vaporize the nicotine-containing material giving the perception that they are safer than tobacco products. The reader should be reminded that these e-cigarettes can be used to vaporize other drugs as well such as "crack", methamphetamine, etc. and are not as innocent as they are portrayed. And lastly, nicotine is a very addictive substance regardless of how it is consumed.

COCAINE

Cocaine, referred to on the street as "snow", "nose candy", "girl", and many other euphemisms, has created an epidemic. This drug is like no other local anesthetic. Known for about the last 2,000 years, cocaine has been used and abused by politicians, scientists, farmers, warriors, and of course, on the street. Cocaine is derived from the leaves of a plant called *Erythroxylon* coca which grows in South America. Ninety percent of the world's supply of cocaine originates in Peru, Bolivia, and Colombia. At last estimate, the United States consumes 37% of the world's supply (United Nations Office on Drugs and Crime). The plant grows to a height of ~4 feet and produces a red berry. Farmers go through the fields stripping the leaves from the plant three times a year. During the working day, the farmers chew the coca leaves to suppress appetite and fight the fatigue of working the fields. The leaves are transported to a laboratory site where the cocaine is extracted by a process called maceration. It takes ~7 to 8 pounds of leaves to produce 1 ounce of cocaine.

On the streets of the United States, cocaine can be found in two forms - one is the hydrochloride salt which can be "snorted" or dissolved in water and injected intravenously, the other is the free base form which can be smoked and is sometimes referred to as "crack", "rock", or "free base". It is called crack because it cracks or pops when large pieces are smoked. It is called rock because it is hard and difficult to break into smaller pieces. The most popular method of administration of cocaine is "snorting" in which small amounts of cocaine hydrochloride are divided into segments or "lines" and any straw-like device can be used to inhale one or more lines of the cocaine into the nose. Although cocaine does not reach the lungs, enough cocaine is absorbed through nasal mucosa to provide a "high" within 3 to 5 minutes. Rock or crack, on the other hand, is heated and inhaled from any device available. This form of cocaine does reach the lungs and provides a much faster onset of action as well as a more intense stimulation. There are dangers to the user with any form of cocaine. Undoubtedly, the most dangerous form is the intravenous route.

Signs and Symptoms of Cocaine Use	
Dilated pupils	Tremors
Jitteriness	Talkative
Irritability	Increased blood pressure

The cocaine user, regardless of how the cocaine was administered, presents a potential life-threatening situation in the dental operatory. The patient under the influence of cocaine could be compared to a car going 100 miles per hour. Blood pressure is elevated and heart rate is likely increased. Use of a local anesthetic with epinephrine in such a patient may result in a medical emergency. Such patients can be identified by jitteriness, irritability, talkativeness, tremors, and short abrupt speech patterns. These same signs and symptoms may also be seen in a normal dental patient with preoperative dental anxiety; therefore, the dentist must be particularly alert to identify the potential cocaine abuser. If a patient is suspected, they should never be given a local anesthetic with vasoconstrictor for fear of exacerbating cocaine-induced sympathetic response. Life-threatening episodes of cardiac arrhythmias and hypertensive crises have been reported when local anesthetic with vasoconstrictor was administered to a patient under the influence of cocaine. No local anesthetic used by any dentist can interfere with, nor test positive for cocaine in any urine testing screen. Therefore, the dentist need not be concerned with any false drug use accusations associated with dental anesthesia.

CLUB DRUGS

Perceptual distortions that include hallucinations, illusions, and disorders of thinking such as paranoia can be produced by toxic doses of many drugs. These phenomena also may be seen during toxic withdrawal from sedatives such as alcohol. There are, however, certain drugs that have as their primary effect the production of perception, thought, or mood disturbances at low doses with minimal effects on memory and orientation. These are commonly called *hallucinogenic drugs*, but their use does not always result in frank hallucinations.

Ecstasy (MDMA) and Phenylethylamines (MDA): MDA and MDMA have stimulant, as well as, psychedelic effects and produce degeneration of serotonergic nerve cells and axons. While nerve degeneration has not been well-demonstrated in human beings, the potential remains. Thus, there is possible neurotoxicity with overuse of these drugs. Ecstasy became popular during the 1980s on college campuses and was used by some psychotherapists as an aid to the process of therapy, although very little controlled data is available. These drugs are now classified as Schedule I Controlled Substances and are no longer prescribed. They are, however, a popular street drug of abuse. Acute effects are dose-dependent and include dry mouth, jaw clinching, muscle aches, and tachycardia. At higher doses, effects include agitation, hyperthermia, panic attacks, and visual hallucinations. Frequent, repeated use of psychedelic drugs is unusual and, therefore, tolerance is not commonly seen. However, tolerance does develop to the behavioral effects of various psychedelic drugs, and after numerous doses, the tendency towards behavioral tolerance can be observed. Pure MDMA is referred to as "molly" on the street. Folk lore claims this name comes from "molecule" because of the purity of the drug. These drugs are sympathomimetics and therefore might amplify the effects of vasoconstrictor. Patients who admit to using these drugs within the last 24 hours should not be administered vasoconstrictor. Plain local anesthetic is acceptable.

Lysergic Acid Diethylamide (LSD): LSD is the most potent hallucinogenic drug and produces significant psychedelic effects with a total dose of as little as 25 to 50 mcg. This drug is over 3,000 times more potent than mescaline. It is sold on the illicit market in a variety of forms, as a tablet, capsule, sugar cube, or on blotting paper, a popular contemporary system involving postage stamp-sized papers impregnated with varying doses of LSD (50 to 300 mcg). Most street samples sold as LSD actually do contain LSD, while mushrooms and other botanicals sold as sources of psilocybin and other psychedelics have a low probability of containing the advertised hallucinogenics. Adverse effects which may affect treatment include visual and auditory hallucinations, tachycardia, psychosis, fear, tremors, delirium, hyperglycemia, fever, sweating, flushing, euphoria, hypertonia, nausea, vomiting, coma, seizures, tachypnea, and respiratory arrest.

Bath Salts (synthetic cathinones): These potentially deadly street drugs acquired the name bath salts, because they were packaged in containers that resemble the scented soaps that can be added to bath water. The term "bath salt" is a generic term which originally described three distinct synthetic chemicals: Mephedrone; 3,4-methylenedioxypyrovalerone (MDPV); and methylone. As of October 21, 2011, these substances were designated as Schedule I Controlled Substances by the US Drug Enforcement Administration (DEA). This action makes possession or selling of these chemicals illegal in the United States. These chemicals are synthetic forms of cathinone which is derived from the shrub Catha edulis (khat). There are several street terms for these crystalline chemicals; some of the more popular are "Ivory Wave," "Red Dove," "Vanilla Sky," and "White Lightning." The packages are usually labeled "Not Intended for Human Consumption," to protect the manufacturer, but users will snort, swallow, or inject the contents. A package may weigh from 300 to 500 mg and can cost ~$25 to $40 on the street.

The effects of the chemicals in "bath salts" have been described as a combination of cocaine, ecstasy, and methamphetamine. Psychological effects include insomnia, suicidal ideation, paranoia, agitation, and seizures. The user describes heightened awareness, euphoria, and enhanced sexual ability. Since these medications are sympathomimetics, vasoconstrictors should **not** be used in individuals suspected to be under the influence of "bath salts." Newer drugs have emerged on the street that resemble the synthetic cathinones and are considered more potent, more unpredictable, and therefore more dangerous to the user and law enforcement. These newer drugs are referred to as "flakka", "gravel", etc.

INHALANTS

Anesthetic gases such as nitrous oxide or halothane are sometimes used as intoxicants by medical personnel. Nitrous oxide also is abused by food service employees because it is supplied for use as a propellant in disposable aluminum mini tanks for whipping cream canisters. Nitrous oxide produces euphoria and analgesia and then loss of consciousness. Compulsive use and chronic toxicity rarely are reported, but there are obvious risks of overdose associated with the abuse of this anesthetic. Chronic use has been reported to cause peripheral neuropathy. Glue, correction fluid, gasoline, aerosol key board cleaners, model paint, in fact, any volatile substance has the potential to cause a "high" and like all of the above can become very addictive and deadly.

According to the Monitoring the Future Surveys, abuse of inhalants peaks in the 8th grade and less so in the 10th or 12th grades. Inhalants are CNS depressants and can cause respiratory failure, long-term use results in liver failure, and suffocation.

The dental team should be alert to the signs and symptoms of drug abuse and withdrawal. Further reading is recommended.

REFERENCES AND SELECTED READINGS

American Medical Association. *JAMA*. 2013;309.

Caponnetto P, Campagna D, Cibella F, et al. Efficiency and safety of an electronic cigarette (ECLAT) as tobacco cigarettes substitute: a prospective 12-month randomized control design study. *PLoS One*. 2013;8(6):e66317.

Okie S. A flood of opioids, a rising tide of deaths. *New Engl J Med*. 2010;363(21):1981-1985.

ORAL MEDICINE TOPICS

PART II:

DENTAL MANAGEMENT AND THERAPEUTIC CONSIDERATIONS IN PATIENTS WITH SPECIFIC ORAL CONDITIONS AND OTHER MEDICINE TOPICS

The second part of the chapter focuses on therapies the dentist may choose to prescribe for patients suffering from oral disease or who are in need of special care. Some overlap between these sections has resulted from systemic conditions that have oral manifestations and vice-versa. Cross-references to the descriptions and the monographs for individual drugs described elsewhere in this handbook allow for easy retrieval of information. Example prescriptions of selected drug therapies for each condition are presented so that the clinician can evaluate alternate approaches to treatment, since there is seldom a single drug of choice.

Drug prescriptions shown represent prototype drugs and popular prescriptions and are examples only. The pharmacologic category index is available for cross-referencing if alternatives and additional drugs are sought.

TABLE OF CONTENTS

ORAL PAIN

PAIN PREVENTION

For the dental patient, the prevention of pain aids in relieving anxiety and reduces the probability of stress during dental care. For the practitioner, dental procedures can be accomplished more efficiently in a "painless" situation. Appropriate selection and use of local anesthetics is one of the foundations for success in this arena. Local anesthetics listed below include drugs for the most commonly confronted dental procedures. Ester anesthetics are no longer available in dose form for dental injections, and historically had a higher incidence of allergic manifestations due to the formation of the metabolic byproduct, para-aminobenzoic acid. Articaine, which has an ester side chain, is rapidly metabolized to a non-PABA acid and functions as an amide and has a low allergic potential. The amides, in general, have a nearly negligible incidence of true allergic reactions, and only one well-documented case of amide allergy has been reported by Seng, et al. Although injectable diphenhydramine (Benadryl) has been used in an attempt to provide anesthesia in patients allergic to all the local anesthetics, it is no longer recommended in this context. The vehicle for injectable diphenhydramine can cause tissue necrosis.

Local Anesthetics

Articaine and Epinephrine on page 170
Bupivacaine on page 256
Bupivacaine and Epinephrine on page 257
Chloroprocaine on page 337
Lidocaine and Epinephrine on page 908
Lidocaine (Systemic) on page 901
Mepivacaine on page 972
Mepivacaine and Levonordefrin on page 975
Prilocaine on page 1274
Prilocaine and Epinephrine
Ropivacaine on page 1346
Tetracaine (Topical) on page 1428

The selection of a vasoconstrictor with the local anesthetic must be based on the length of the procedure to be performed, the patient's medical status (epinephrine is contraindicated in patients with uncontrolled hyperthyroidism), and the need for hemorrhage control. The following table lists some of the common drugs with their duration of action. The long-acting amide injectable, Ropivacaine (Naropin) may be useful for postoperative pain management.

Dental Anesthetics (Average Duration by Route)

Product	Infiltration	Inferior Alveolar Block
Articaine HCl 4% and epinephrine 1:100,000	60 minutes	~60 minutes
Articaine HCl 4% and epinephrine 1:200,000	40 minutes	50 minutes
Carbocaine HCl 2% with Neo-Cobefrin 1:20,000 (mepivacaine HCl and levonordefrin)	50 minutes	60 to 75 minutes
Carbocaine Plain 3%	20 minutes	40 minutes
Citanest Plain 4% (prilocaine)	20 minutes	2.5 hours
Citanest Forte with epinephrine 1:200,000 (prilocaine with epinephrine)	2.25 hours	3 hours
Lidocaine HCl 2% and epinephrine 1:100,000	60 minutes	90 minutes
Marcaine HCl 0.5% with epinephrine 1:200,000 (bupivacaine and epinephrine)	60 minutes	5 to 7 hours
Vivacaine 0.5% with epinephrine 1:200,000 (bupivacaine and epinephrine)	60 minutes	5 to 7 hours

The use of articaine 4% with epinephrine 1:100,000 solution for mandibular blocks has been associated occasionally with paresthesia (*J Am Dent Assoc*, 2001, 132(2):177-85).

The use of preinjection topical anesthetics can assist in pain prevention (see also Viral Infections on page 1754 and Ulcerative, Erosive, and Painful Oral Mucosal Disorders on page 1758). It should be noted that the FDA recently warned health care professionals regarding potential risks associated with unsupervised patient cutaneous use of topical anesthetic products. Life-threatening adverse events such as arrhythmias, seizures, coma, and respiratory complications have been reported. Thus, health care professionals are advised to prescribe FDA-approved topical anesthetics in the lowest concentration consistent with pain relief goals. It is not known if oral mucosa misuse may pose the same risk factors.

Clinicians are also using a eutectic mixture of 2.5% lidocaine with 2.5% prilocaine in a periodontal gel form in adults who require localized anesthesia in periodontal pockets during scaling and/or root planing. However, the same mixture available as a skin patch (EMLA) from Astra is not currently approved for oral use.

OraVerse (phentolamine mesylate) injection is a local anesthetic reversal agent that accelerates the return to normal sensation and function following restorative and periodontal maintenance procedures. OraVerse is indicated for the reversal of soft tissue anesthesia (ie, anesthesia of the lip, tongue, and the associated functional deficits resulting from an intraoral submucosal injection of a local anesthetic containing a vasoconstrictor. OraVerse is not recommended for use in children <6 years of age or weighing <15 kg (33 lbs).

Phentolamine (OraVerse), as used in its original context as a medical hypotensive agent, could be expected to cause significant hypotension and reflex tachycardia when used as the anesthetic reversal agent in children. Studies have shown, however, that neither of these reactions occurred in the children receiving the drug. According to the authors of the study, there was an impressive benefit:risk ratio suggesting a safe approach in accelerating recovery from soft tissue anesthesia in children (Tavares, et al. *JADA*. 2008;139(8):1095-1104). There were no serious adverse events observed. The adverse reactions were observed from study populations of 484 adults and 152 children. It should be anticipated that more adverse effects could occur as OraVerse is used in a larger number of patients. The clinical studies used a maximum of 2 cartridges of OraVerse (0.8 mg phentolamine). There is no information published on effects that occur with higher doses of OraVerse. Phentolamine is a very powerful alpha-adrenergic receptor blocker which can cause cardiovascular effects if inadvertently injected in high doses. The manufacturer advises to adhere to the recommended dosing for the OraVerse formulation. The dosing for OraVerse is based on the number of cartridges of local anesthetic with vasoconstrictor administered, with 1 cartridge of OraVerse containing 0.4 mg of phentolamine and 2 cartridges containing 0.8 mg phentolamine. Dosing is as a 1:1 cartridge ratio to local anesthetic using the same injection site and administration technique as that used for the local anesthetic.

Benzocaine on page 228
Lidocaine (Systemic) on page 901
Phentolamine on page 1226
Tetracaine (Topical) on page 1428

PAIN MANAGEMENT

The patient with existing acute or chronic oral pain requires appropriate treatment and sensitivity on the part of the dentist, all for the purpose of achieving relief from the oral source of pain. Pain can be divided into mild, moderate, and severe levels and requires a subjective assessment by the dentist based on knowledge of the dental procedures to be performed, the presenting signs and symptoms of the patient, and the realization that most dental procedures are invasive often leading to pain once the patient has left the dental office. The practitioner must be aware that the treatment of the source of the pain is usually the best management. If infection is present, treatment of the infection will directly alleviate the patient's discomfort. However, a patient who is not in pain tends to heal better and it is wise to adequately cover the patient for any residual or recurrent discomfort suffered. Likewise, many of the procedures that the dentist performs have pain associated with them. Much of this pain occurs after leaving the dentist office due to an inflammatory process or a healing process that has been initiated. It is difficult to assign specific pain levels (mild, moderate, or severe) for specific procedures; however, the dentist should use his or her prescribing capacity judiciously so that overmedication is avoided.

The potential interaction between acetaminophen and warfarin has been recently raised in the literature. The cytochrome P450 system of drug metabolism for these vitamin K-dependent metabolic pathways has raised the possibility that prolonged use of acetaminophen may inadvertently enhance, to dangerous levels, the anticoagulation effect of warfarin. As monitored by the INR, the effects of these drugs may be one and one-half to two times greater than as expected from the warfarin dosage alone. This potential interaction could be of importance in selecting an analgesic/antipyretic drug for the dental patient.

The following categories of drugs and appropriate example prescriptions for each can be found in the Oral Pain - Sample Prescriptions chart. These include management of mild pain with aspirin products, acetaminophen, and some of the nonsteroidal noninflammatory agents (eg, ibuprofen). Management of moderate pain includes codeine, Toradol, Vicodin, Vicodin ES, Opana; and Motrin in the 800 mg dosage. Etodolac is approved as an NSAID for mild-to-moderate acute and chronic pain, as well as, for pain of osteo and rheumatoid arthritis. Severe pain may require treatment with Percodan or Percocet. A new drug, tapentadol is similar to tramadol in its actions and was approved in November 2008 for moderate to severe acute pain. Tapentadol is classified as an opioid analgesic having a unique ability to bind to μ-opiate receptors and inhibit the reuptake of norepinephrine. It shares many properties of traditional opioid drugs including addiction liability. A report by Kleinert et al, showed that a single dose of tapentadol ≥75 mg effectively reduced moderate to severe postoperative dental pain in a dose related fashion and was well tolerated compared to 60 mg morphine. Their study showed that tapentadol was a highly effective, central-acting analgesic with a favorable side effect profile with rapid onset of action (Kleinert 2008). All prescription pain preparations should be closely monitored for efficacy and discontinued if the pain persists or requires a higher level formulation. Combination drugs such as the recently released Combunox containing 5 mg of oxycodone and 400 mg of ibuprofen have proven usefulness in acute moderately severe to severe pain management.

The chronic pain patient represents a particular challenge for the practitioner. Some additional drugs that may be useful in managing the patient with chronic pain of neuropathic origin are covered in the temporomandibular dysfunction section and in the section on Burning Mouth Syndrome within Ulcerative, Erosive, and Painful Oral Mucosal Disorders on page 1758. It is always incumbent on the practitioner to reevaluate the diagnosis, source of pain, and treatment, whenever prolonged use of analgesics is contemplated. Drugs such as Dilaudid are not recommended for management of dental pain in most states. Fibromyalgia, postherpetic and diabetic neuropathies may also require consideration when dealing with the patient with chronic pain although direct oral involvement is uncommon. The dentist may also be confronted with patients being managed at pain centers offering nonsurgical management of acute and chronic pain conditions.

The FDA has formally requested manufacturers to limit the amount of acetaminophen in prescription combination products to no more than 325 mg in each tablet or capsule. Manufacturers had until January 2014 to limit the amount of acetaminophen in their oral prescription drug products. The FDA is also requiring manufacturers to update labeling of all prescription combination acetaminophen products to warn of the potential risk for severe liver injury. The over-the-counter acetaminophen products are not affected by this ruling. Some manufacturers have already reduced acetaminophen amounts to 300 to 325 mg per tablet in combination prescription products.

Examples include the very popular hydrocodone and acetaminophen products such as Norco, Vicodin, and Xodol.

Effective August 18, 2014, Tramadol was classified as a Schedule IV controlled dangerous substance (CDS) under federal regulation. If you dispense Tramadol to your patients, you are required to report this to the Prescription Drug Monitoring Program (PDMP). If you write a prescription for Tramadol, but do **not** dispense this medication, you are not required to report to the PDMP. The Division of Drug Control (DDC) has posted the following information on its web site: USDOJ/DEA, 21 CFR (Federal Register) Part 1308: Schedules of Controlled Dangerous Substances: Placement of Tramadol Into Schedule IV (Final Rule). The link is: DEA (CFR Final Rule) Tramadol Schedule IV Placement (Effective: 8/18/14) (http://dhmh.maryland.gov/laboratories/drugcont/docs/DEA%20%28CFR%20Final%20Rule%29%20Tramadol%20Schedule%20IV%20Placement%20%28Eff.8-18-2014%29.pdf).

Overdose from prescription combination products containing acetaminophen account for nearly half of all cases of acetaminophen-related liver failure in the United States. Many cases result in liver transplant or death. There is no immediate danger to patients taking these combination pain medications. Patients should continue to take them as directed by health care provider. The risk of liver injury primarily occurs when patients take multiple products containing acetaminophen at one time and exceed the current maximum adult dose of 4,000 mg within a 24-hour period. For more information and a complete list of affected products see www.fda.gov/Drugs/DrugSafety/InformationbyDrugClass/ucm239874.htm

Opioid analgesics can be used on a short-term basis or intermittently in combination with non-opioid therapy in the chronic pain patient. Judicious prescribing, monitoring, and maintenance by the practitioner are imperative, particularly whenever considering the use of an opioid analgesic due to the abuse and addiction liabilities. For all prescribers of extended release and long-acting opioid analgesics, patient information as noted below is required. The CDC has released guidelines for opioid prescriptions. Numerous states have adopted prescription monitoring programs particularly targeting opioids and benzodiazapines; refer to your home state guidelines for specific regulations and reporting requirements. In general opioids should not be the first line therapy choice for chronic pain except for active cancer, palliative therapy or end of life care. Please visit www.cdc.gov/drugoverdose/prescribing/guideline.html for more specific details. The FDA also has a required Opioid Analgesic Risk Evaluation and Mitigation Strategy (REMS) for opioid analgesic drug products used in the outpatient setting, see www.opioidanalgesicrems.com.

DOs and DON'Ts of Extended Release/Long-Acting Opioid Analgesics

DO:

- Read the **Medication Guide**
- Take your medicine exactly as prescribed
- Store your medicine away from children and in a safe place
- Check with pharmacy about disposal of unused medicine.
- Call your health care provider for medical advice about side effects. You may report side effects to the FDA at (800) FDA-1088

Call 911 or your local emergency service right away if:

- You take too much medicine
- You have trouble breathing or shortness of breath
- A child has taken this medicine

Talk to your health care provider:

- If the dose you are taking does not control your pain
- About any side effects you may be having
- About all the medicines you take, including over-the-counter medicines, vitamins, and dietary supplements

DON'T:

- **Do not** give your medicine to others
- **Do not** take medicine unless it was prescribed for you
- **Do not** stop taking your medicine without talking to your health care provider
- **Do not** break, chew, crush, dissolve, or inject your medicine. If you cannot swallow your medicine whole, talk to your health care provider
- **Do not** drink alcohol while taking this medicine

MILD PAIN

Acetaminophen on page 59
Aspirin (various products) on page 177
Diflunisal on page 495
Etodolac on page 622
Ibuprofen on page 786
Ketoprofen on page 860
Naproxen on page 1080

MODERATE/MODERATELY SEVERE PAIN

Dihydrocodeine, Aspirin, and Caffeine
HYDROcodone
Hydrocodone and Acetaminophen on page 764
Hydrocodone and Ibuprofen on page 769
Acetaminophen and Tramadol on page 71
Ibuprofen (various products) on page 786
Ketorolac (Systemic) on page 861
OxyMORphone on page 1176
Tapentadol on page 1406

An additional class of NSAIDs has been approved and indicated in the treatment of arthritis, COX-2 inhibitors. Celecoxib (Celebrex) has been approved for use in oral pain management.

The following is a guideline to use when prescribing codeine with either aspirin or acetaminophen (Tylenol):

Codeine No. 2 = codeine 15 mg
Codeine No. 3 = codeine 30 mg
Codeine No. 4 = codeine 60 mg

Example: ASA No. 3 = aspirin 325 mg + codeine 30 mg

HYDROCODONE PRODUCTS

Available hydrocodone oral products are listed in the following table and are scheduled as C-II controlled substances, indicating that prescriptions may either be oral or written. Thus, the prescriber may call in a prescription to the pharmacy for any of these hydrocodone products. All the formulations are combined with acetaminophen except for Vicoprofen, which contains ibuprofen. Most of these brand name drugs are available generically and the pharmacist will dispense the generic equivalent if available, unless the prescriber indicates otherwise.

Hydrocodone Analgesic Combination Oral Products (All Products DEA Schedule C-II)

HYDROcodone is available under numerous brand names with varying dosages and in combination with aspirin or ibuprofen.					
HYDROcodone Bitartrate	**Acetaminophen (APAP[a])**	**Other**	**Brand Name**	**Generic Available**	**Form**
5 mg	300 mg	–	Vicodin	Yes	Tablet
7.5 mg	300 mg	–	Vicodin ES	Yes	Tablet
7.5 mg	325 mg	–	Norco	Yes	Tablet
10 mg	325 mg	–	Norco	Yes	Tablet
10 mg	300 mg	–	Vicodin HP	Yes	Tablet
7.5 mg per 15 mL	325 mg per 15 mL	–	–	Yes	Elixir
7.5 mg	–	Ibuprofen 200 mg	Vicoprofen	Yes	Tablet
5 mg	–	Ibuprofen 200 mg	Ibudone; Reprexain	Yes	Tablet

Note: Although there are products still available with >325 mg of acetaminophen per dosage form, the deadline for reduction of acetaminophen was January 2014. The FDA will institute proceedings to withdraw approval of prescription combinations with >325 mg of acetaminophen.

[a]APAP is the common acronym for acetaminophen and is the abbreviation of the chemical name N-acetyl-para-aminophenol.

SEVERE PAIN

HYDROmorphone on page 776
OxyCODONE on page 1157
Oxycodone and Acetaminophen on page 1164
Oxycodone and Aspirin
Oxycodone and Ibuprofen

Oxycodone is available in a variety of dosages and combinations under numerous brand names.

SAMPLE PRESCRIPTIONS

Rx:
Ibuprofen 800 mg tablets
Disp: 16 tablets
Sig: Take 1 tablet 3 times/day as needed for pain

Note: For severe pain, can be given up to 4 times/day. Also available as 600 mg tablets

Rx:
Norco 10 mg hydrocodone/325 mg acetaminophen
Disp: 16 tablets
Sig: Take 1 or 2 tablets every 4 hours as needed for pain; not to exceed 8 tablets in 24 hours

Note: Restrictions: C-II; no refills
Ingredients: Hydrocodone 10 mg and acetaminophen 325 mg; available as generic equivalent

For additional sample prescriptions see Oral Pain - Sample Prescriptions on page 30

BACTERIAL INFECTIONS

Dental infection can occur for any number of reasons, primarily involving pulpal and periodontal infections. Secondary infections of the soft tissues as well as sinus infections pose special treatment challenges. The drugs of choice in treating most oral infections have been selected because of their efficacy in providing adequate blood levels for delivery to the oral tissues and their proven usefulness in managing dental infections. Penicillin remains the primary drug for treatment of dental infections of pulpal origin. The management of soft tissue infections may require the use of additional drugs.

ANTIMICROBIAL STEWARDSHIP

Antimicrobial stewardship refers to coordinated interventions designed to improve and measure the appropriate use of antimicrobials by promoting the selection of the optimal antimicrobial drug regimen, dose, duration of therapy, and route of administration. Antimicrobial stewards seek to achieve optimal clinical outcomes related to antimicrobial use, minimize toxicity and other adverse events, reduce the costs of health care for infections, and limit the selection for antimicrobial resistant strains. Currently, there are no national or coordinated legislative or regulatory mandates designed to optimize use of antimicrobial therapy through antimicrobial stewardship. Given the societal value of antimicrobials and their diminishing effectiveness due to antimicrobial resistance, groups like the ADA support broad implementation of antimicrobial stewardship programs across all health care settings (eg, hospitals, long-term care facilities, long-term acute care facilities, ambulatory surgical centers, dialysis centers, and private practices).

The American Dental Association (ADA) supports the responsible use of antibiotics. As part of this effort toward antibiotic stewardship, the ADA has adopted an evidence-based approach to guideline development, which has resulted in recommendations for decreased indications for and use of prophylactic antibiotics in people with heart conditions and those who have had joint replacements. Although there are some studies evaluating the appropriateness of antibiotic prescribing in dentistry, a recent paper in *JADA* suggests that it is likely that there are opportunities to improve prescribing practices.

OROFACIAL INFECTIONS

The basis of all infections is the successful multiplication of a microbial pathogen on or within a host. The pathogen is usually defined as any microorganism that has the capacity to cause disease. If the pathogen is bacterial in nature, antibiotic therapy is often indicated.

DIFFERENTIAL DIAGNOSIS OF ODONTOGENIC INFECTIONS

In choosing the appropriate antibiotic for therapy of a given infection, a number of important factors must be considered. First, the identity of the organism must be known. In odontogenic infections involving dental or periodontal structures, this is seldom the case. Secondly, accurate information regarding antibiotic susceptibility is required. Again, unless the organism has been identified, this is not possible. And thirdly, host factors must be taken into account, in terms of ability to absorb an antibiotic, to achieve appropriate host response. When clinical evidence of cellulitis or odontogenic infection has been found and the cardinal signs of swelling, inflammation, pain, and perhaps fever are present, the selection by the clinician of the appropriate antibiotic agent may lead to eradication.

CAUSES OF ODONTOGENIC INFECTIONS

Most acute orofacial infections are of odontogenic origin. Dental caries, resulting in infection of dental pulp, is the leading cause of odontogenic infection.

The major causative organisms involved in dental caries have been identified as members of the viridans (alpha-hemolytic) streptococci and include *Streptococcus mutans, Streptococcus sobrinus,* and *Streptococcus milleri.* Once the bacteria have breached the enamel they invade the dentin and eventually the dental pulp. An inflammatory reaction occurs in the pulp tissue resulting in necrosis and a lower tissue oxidation-reduction potential. At this point, the bacterial flora changes from predominantly aerobic to a more obligate anaerobic flora. The anaerobic gram-positive cocci *(Peptostreptococcus* species), and the anaerobic gram-negative rods, including *Bacteroides, Prevotella, Porphyromonas,* and *Fusobacterium* are most frequently present. An abscess usually forms at the apex of the involved tooth resulting in destruction of bone. Depending on the effectiveness of the host resistance and the virulence of the bacteria, the infection may spread through the marrow spaces, perforate the cortical plate, and enter the surrounding soft tissues.

The other major source of odontogenic infection arises from the anaerobic bacterial flora that inhabits the periodontal and supporting structures of the teeth. The most important potential pathogenic anaerobes within these structures are *Actinobacillus actinomycetemcomitans, Prevotella intermedius, Porphyromonas gingivalis, Fusobacterium nucleatum,* and *Eikenella corrodens.*

Most odontogenic infections (70%) have mixed aerobic and anaerobic flora. Pure aerobic infections are much less common and comprise ~5% incidence. Pure anaerobic infections make up the remaining 25% of odontogenic infections. Clinical correlates suggest that early odontogenic infections are characterized by rapid spreading and cellulitis with the absence of abscess formation. The bacteria are predominantly aerobic with gram-positive, alpha-hemolytic streptococci *(S. viridans)* the predominant pathogen. As the infection matures and becomes more severe, the microbial flora becomes a mix of aerobes and anaerobes. The anaerobes present are determined by the characteristic flora associated with the site of origin, whether it is pulpal or periodontal. Finally, as the infectious process becomes controlled by host defenses, the flora becomes primarily anaerobic. For example, Lewis and MacFarlane found a predominance of facultative oral streptococci in the early infections (<3 days of symptoms) with the later predominance of obligate anaerobes.

In a review of severe odontogenic infections, it was reported that Brook, et al, observed that 50% of odontogenic deep facial space infections yielded anaerobic bacteria only. Also, 44% of these infections yielded a mix of aerobic and anaerobic flora. The results of a study published in 1998 by Sakamoto, et al, were also described in the review. The study confirmed that odontogenic infections usually result from a synergistic interaction among several bacterial species and usually consist of an oral streptococcus and an oral anaerobic gram-negative rod. Sakamoto and his group reported a high level of the *Streptococcus milleri* group of aerobic gram-positive cocci, and high levels of oral anaerobes, including the *Peptostreptococcus* species and the *Prevotella, Porphyromonas,* and *Fusobacterium* species.

Oral streptococci, especially of the *Streptococcus milleri* group, can invade soft tissues initially, thus preparing an environment conducive to growth of anaerobic bacteria. Obligate oral anaerobes are dependent on nutrients synthesized by the aerobes. Thus the anaerobes appear ~3 days after onset of symptoms. Early infections are thus caused primarily by the aerobic streptococci (exquisitely sensitive to penicillin) and late infections are caused by the anaerobes (frequently resistant to penicillin).

It appears logical, as Flynn has noted, to separate infections presenting early in their course from those presenting later when selecting empiric antibiotics of choice for odontogenic infections.

If the patient is not allergic to penicillin, penicillin VK still remains the empiric antibiotic of first choice to treat mild or early odontogenic infections (see Table 1). In patients allergic to penicillin, clindamycin clearly remains the alternative antibiotic for treatment of mild or early infections. Secondary alternative antibiotics still recognized as useful in these conditions are cephalexin (Keflex), or other first generation cephalosporins available in oral dose forms. The first generation cephalosporins can be used in both penicillin-allergic and nonallergic patients, providing that the penicillin allergy is not the anaphylactoid type. Citing concerns over risk of pseudomembranous colitis the American Association of Endodontists has recently altered their recommendations for use of antibiotics to now recommend azithromycin as the alternative to penicillin in allergic individuals and also as a better choice in cases where response to penicillin is inadequate.

PENICILLIN VK

The spectrum of antibacterial action of penicillin VK is consistent with most of the organisms identified in odontogenic infections (see Table 2). Penicillin VK is a beta-lactam antibiotic, as are all the penicillins and cephalosporins, and is bactericidal against gram-positive cocci and the major pathogens of mixed anaerobic infections. It elicits virtually no adverse effects in the absence of allergy and is relatively low in cost. Adverse drug reactions occurring in >10% of patients include mild diarrhea, nausea, and oral candidiasis. To treat odontogenic infections and other orofacial infections, the usual dose for adults and children >12 years of age is 500 mg every 6 hours for at least 7 days (see Table 4). The daily dose for children ≤12 years of age is 25 to 50 mg/kg of body weight in divided doses every 6 to 8 hours (see Table 4). The patient must be instructed to take the penicillin continuously for the duration of therapy.

After oral dosing, penicillin VK achieves peak serum levels within 1 hour. Penicillin VK may be given with meals; however, blood concentrations may be slightly higher when penicillin is given on an empty stomach. The preferred dosing is 1 hour before meals or 2 hours after meals to ensure maximum serum levels. Penicillin VK diffuses into most body tissues, including oral tissues, soon after dosing. Hepatic metabolism accounts for <30% of the elimination of penicillins. Elimination is primarily renal. The nonmetabolized penicillin is excreted largely unchanged in the urine by glomerular filtration and active tubular secretion. Penicillins cross the placenta and are distributed in breast milk. Penicillin VK, like all beta-lactam antibiotics, causes death of bacteria by inhibiting synthesis of the bacterial cell wall during cell division. This action is dependent on the ability of penicillins to reach and bind to penicillin-binding proteins (PBPs) located on the inner membrane of the bacterial cell wall. PBPs (which include transpeptidases, carboxypeptidases, and endopeptidases) are enzymes that are involved in the terminal stages of assembling and reshaping the bacterial cell wall during growth. Penicillins and beta-lactams bind to and inactivate PBPs resulting in lysis of the cell due to weakening of the cell wall.

Penicillin VK is considered a "narrow spectrum" antibiotic. This class of antibiotics produces less alteration of normal microflora thereby reducing the incidence of superinfection. Also, its bactericidal action will reduce the numbers of microorganisms resulting in less reliance on host-phagocyte mechanisms for eradication of the pathogen.

Among patients, 0.7% to 10% are allergic to penicillins. There is no evidence that any single penicillin derivative differs from others in terms of incidence or severity when administered orally. About 85% of allergic reactions associated with penicillin VK are delayed and take >2 days to develop. This allergic response manifests as skin rashes characterized as erythema and bullous eruptions. This type of allergic reaction is mild, reversible, and usually responds to concurrent antihistamine therapy, such as diphenhydramine (Benadryl). Severe reactions of angioedema have occurred, characterized by marked swelling of the lips, tongue, face, and periorbital tissues. Patients with a history of penicillin allergy must never be given penicillin VK for treatment of infections. The alternative antibiotic is clindamycin. If the allergy is the delayed type and not the anaphylactoid type, a first generation cephalosporin may be used as an alternate antibiotic.

CLINDAMYCIN

In the event of penicillin allergy, clindamycin is clearly an alternative of choice in treating mild or early odontogenic infections (see Table 1). It is highly effective against almost all oral pathogens. Clindamycin is active against most aerobic gram-positive cocci, including staphylococci, *S. pneumoniae*, other streptococci, and anaerobic gram-negative and gram-positive organisms, including bacteroides (see Table 3). Clindamycin is not effective against mycoplasma or gram-negative aerobes. It inhibits protein synthesis in bacteria through binding to the 50 S subunit of bacterial ribosomes. Clindamycin has bacteriostatic actions at low concentrations, but is known to elicit bactericidal effects against susceptible bacteria at higher concentrations of drug at the site of infection.

The usual adult oral dose of clindamycin to treat orofacial infections of odontogenic origin is 150 to 450 mg every 6 hours for 7 to 10 days. The usual daily oral dose for children is 8 to 25 mg/kg in 3 to 4 equally divided doses (see Table 4).

Following oral administration of a 150 mg or a 300 mg dose on an empty stomach, 90% of the dose is rapidly absorbed into the bloodstream and peak serum concentrations are attained in 45 to 60 minutes. Administration with food does not markedly impair absorption into the bloodstream. Clindamycin serum levels exceed the minimum inhibitory concentration for bacterial growth for at least 6 hours after the recommended doses. The serum half-life is 2 to 3 hours. Clindamycin is distributed effectively to most body tissues, including saliva and bone. Its small molecular weight enables it to more readily enter bacterial cytoplasm and to penetrate bone. It is partially metabolized in the liver to active and inactive metabolites and is excreted in the urine, bile, and feces.

Adverse effects caused by clindamycin can include abdominal pain, nausea, vomiting, and diarrhea. Hypersensitivity reactions are rare, but have resulted in skin rash. Approximately 1% of clindamycin users develop pseudomembranous colitis characterized by severe diarrhea, abdominal cramps, and excretion of blood or mucus in the stools. The mechanism is disruption of normal bacterial flora of the colon, which leads to colonization of the bacterium *Clostridioides* (formerly *Clostridium*) *difficile*. This bacterium releases endotoxins that cause mucosal damage and inflammation. Symptoms usually develop 2 to 9 days after initiation of therapy, but may not occur until several weeks after taking the drug. If significant diarrhea develops, clindamycin therapy should be discontinued immediately. Theoretically, any antibiotic can cause antibiotic-associated colitis and clindamycin probably has an undeserved reputation associated with this condition. Based on these concerns; however, practitioners should review the updated recommendations of the American Association of Endodontists.

Sandor, et al, also notes that odontogenic infections are typically polymicrobial and that anaerobes outnumber aerobes by at least four-fold. The penicillins have historically been used as the first-line therapy in these cases, but increasing rates of resistance have lowered their usefulness. Bacterial resistance to penicillins is predominantly achieved through production of beta-lactamases. Clindamycin, because of its relatively broad spectrum of activity and resistance to beta-lactamase degradation, is an attractive first-line therapy in treatment of odontogenic infections. Recently, researchers have established a causal link between exposure to antibiotics and antibiotic resistance and they also have established evidence that the development of resistance to one class of antibiotic may confer persistent increased resistance to other antibiotic classes.

FIRST GENERATION CEPHALOSPORINS

Antibiotics of this class, which are available in oral dosage forms, include cefadroxil (Duricef) and cephalexin (Keflex). The first generation cephalosporins are alternates to penicillin VK in the treatment of odontogenic infections based on bactericidal effectiveness against the oral streptococci. These drugs are most active against gram-positive cocci, but are not very active against many anaerobes. First generation cephalosporins are indicated as alternatives in early infections because they are effective in killing the aerobes. First generation cephalosporins are active against gram-positive staphylococci and streptococci, but not enterococci. They are active against many gram-negative aerobic bacilli, including *E. coli, Klebsiella,* and *Proteus mirabilis*. They are inactive against methicillin-resistant *S. aureus* and penicillin-resistant *S. pneumoniae*. The gram-negative aerobic cocci, *Moraxella catarrhalis*, portrays variable sensitivity to first generation cephalosporins.

Cephalexin (Keflex) is the first generation cephalosporin often used to treat odontogenic infections. The usual adult dose is 250 to 1,000 mg every 6 hours with a maximum of 4 g/day. Children's dose is 25 to 50 mg/kg/day in divided doses every 6 hours; for severe infections: 50 to 100 mg/kg/day in divided doses every 6 hours with a maximum dose of 3 g/day (see Table 4).

Cephalexin (Keflex) causes diarrhea in about 1% to 10% of patients. About 90% of the cephalexin is excreted unchanged in urine.

SECOND GENERATION CEPHALOSPORINS

The second generation cephalosporins such as cefaclor (Ceclor) have better activity against some of the anaerobes including some *Bacteroides, Peptococcus,* and *Peptostreptococcus* species. Cefaclor (Ceclor) and cefuroxime (Ceftin) have been used to treat early stage infections. These antibiotics have the advantage of twice-a-day dosing. The usual oral adult dose of cefaclor is 250 to 500 mg every 8 hours (or daily dose can be given in 2 divided doses) for at least 7 days. Children's dose is 20 to 40 mg/kg/day divided every 8 to 12 hours with a maximum dose of 2 g/day. The usual adult oral dose of cefuroxime is 250 to 500 mg twice daily. Children's dose is 20 mg/kg/day (maximum: 500 mg/day) in 2 divided doses.

The cephalosporins inhibit bacterial cell wall synthesis by binding to one or more of the penicillin-binding proteins (PBPs), which in turn inhibit the final transpeptidation step of peptidoglycan synthesis in bacterial cell walls, thus inhibiting cell wall biosynthesis. Bacteria eventually lyse due to ongoing activity of cell wall autolytic enzymes while cell wall assembly is arrested.

BACTERIAL RESISTANCE TO ANTIBIOTICS

If a patient with an early stage odontogenic infection does not respond to penicillin VK within 24 to 36 hours, it is evidence of the presence of resistant bacteria. Bacterial resistance to the penicillins is predominantly achieved through the production of beta-lactamase. A switch to beta-lactamase-stable antibiotics should be made. For example, Kuriyama, et al, reported that past beta-lactam administration increases the emergence of beta-lactamase-producing bacteria and that beta-lactamase-stable antibiotics should be prescribed to patients with unresolved infections who have received beta-lactams. These include either clindamycin or amoxicillin/clavulanic acid (Augmentin). Doses are listed in Table 4.

In the past, all *S. viridans* species were uniformly susceptible to beta-lactam antibiotics. However, over the years, there has been a significant increase in resistant strains. Resistance may also be due to alteration of penicillin-binding proteins. Consequently, drugs which combine a beta-lactam antibiotic with a beta-lactamase inhibitor, such as amoxicillin/clavulanic acid (Augmentin), may no longer be more effective than the penicillin VK alone. In these situations, clindamycin is the recommended alternate antibiotic.

Evidence suggests that empirical use of penicillin VK as the first-line drug in treating early odontogenic infections is still the best way to ensure the minimal production of resistant bacteria to other classes of antibiotics, since any overuse of clindamycin or amoxicillin/clavulanic acid (Augmentin) is minimized in these situations. There is concern that overuse of clindamycin could contribute to development of clindamycin-resistant pathogens.

In late odontogenic infections, it is suggested that clindamycin be considered the first-line antibiotic to treat these infections. The dose of clindamycin would be the same as that used to treat early infections (see Table 4). In these infections, anaerobic bacteria usually predominate. Since penicillin spectrum includes anaerobes, penicillin VK is also useful as an empiric drug of first choice in these infections. It has been reported, however, that the penicillin resistance rate among patients with serious and late infections is in the 35% to 50% range. Therefore, if penicillin is the drug of first choice and the patient does not respond within 24 to 36 hours, a resistant pathogen should be suspected and a switch to clindamycin be made. Clindamycin, because of its relatively broad spectrum of activity and resistance to beta-lactamase degradation, is an attractive first-line therapy in the treatment of these infections. Another alternative is to add a second drug to the penicillin (eg, metronidazole [Flagyl]). Consequently, for those infections not responding to treatment with penicillin, the addition of a second drug (eg, metronidazole), not a beta-lactam or macrolide, is likely to be more effective. Bacterial resistance to metronidazole is very rare. The metronidazole dose is listed in Table 4.

Nonionized metronidazole is readily taken up by anaerobic organisms. Its selectivity for anaerobic bacteria is a result of the ability of these organisms to reduce metronidazole to its active form within the bacterial cell. The electron transport proteins necessary for this reaction are found only in anaerobic bacteria. Reduced metronidazole then disrupts DNA's helical structure, thereby inhibiting bacterial nucleic acid synthesis leading to death of the organism. Consequently, metronidazole is not effective against gram-positive aerobic cocci and most *Actinomyces, Lactobacillus,* and *Cutibacterium* species. Since most odontogenic infections are mixed aerobic and anaerobic, metronidazole should rarely be used as a single agent but it can be useful when combined with penicillins. Alternatively, one can switch to a beta-lactamase resistant drug (eg, amoxicillin/clavulanic acid [Augmentin]). The beta-lactamase resistant penicillins including methicillin, oxacillin, cloxacillin, dicloxacillin, and nafcillin, are only effective against gram-positive cocci and have no activity against anaerobes, hence, should not be used to treat the late stage odontogenic infections.

RESISTANCE IN ODONTOGENIC INFECTIONS

Recently, there has been an alarming increase in the incidence of resistant bacterial isolates in odontogenic infections. Many anaerobic bacteria have developed resistance to beta-lactam antibiotics via production of beta-lactamase enzymes. These include several species of *Prevotella, Porphyromonas, Fusobacterium nucleatum,* and *Campylobacter gracilis. Fusobacterium*, especially in combination with *S. viridans* species, has been associated with severe odontogenic infections. Often, they are resistant to macrolides. Clindamycin is the empiric drug of first choice in these patients.

SEVERE INFECTIONS

In patients hospitalized for severe odontogenic infections, IV antibiotics are indicated and clindamycin is the clear empiric antibiotic of choice. Alternative antibiotics include an IV combination of penicillin and metronidazole or IV ampicillin-sulbactam (Unasyn). Clindamycin, IV cephalosporins (if penicillin allergy is not the anaphylactoid type), and ciprofloxacin have been used in patients allergic to penicillins. Flynn notes that *Eikenella corrodens*, an occasional oral pathogen, is resistant to clindamycin. Ciprofloxacin is an excellent antibiotic for this organism.

Recently approved telavancin (Vibativ) has been approved for severe antibiotic resistant infections. Brand new mechanism of antibacterial effect:

1. Works like vancomycin and penicillins to block bacterial cell wall synthesis at D-alanine-D-alanine portion of cell wall.
2. Disrupts bacterial cell membrane potential due to presence of a lipophilic side chain of telavancin molecule.

Scheduled for use in complicated skin and skin structure infections caused by MRSA, and vancomycin-susceptible enterococcus, strept pyogenes, and strept anginosus.

ERYTHROMYCIN, CLARITHROMYCIN, AND AZITHROMYCIN

In the past, erythromycins were considered highly effective antibiotics for treating odontogenic infections, especially in penicillin allergy. At the present time, however, the current high resistance rates of both oral streptococci and oral anaerobes have rendered the entire macrolide family of antibiotics obsolete for odontogenic infections. Montgomery has noted that resistance develops rapidly to macrolides and there may be cross-resistance between erythromycin and newer macrolides, particularly among streptococci and staphylococci. Hardee has stated that erythromycin is no longer very useful because of resistant pathogens. The antibacterial spectrum of the erythromycin family is similar to penicillin VK. Erythromycins are effective against streptococcus, staphylococcus, and gram-negative aerobes, such as *H. influenzae, M. catarrhalis, N. gonorrhoeae, Bordetella pertussis,* and *Legionella pneumophilia*. Erythromycins are considered narrow spectrum antibiotics.

Both azithromycin and clarithromycin have been used to treat acute odontogenic infections. This is because of the following spectrum of actions: Clarithromycin shows good activity against many gram-positive and gram-negative aerobic and anaerobic organisms. It is active against methicillin-sensitive *S. aureus* and most streptococcus species. *S. aureus* strains resistant to erythromycin are resistant to clarithromycin. Clarithromycin is active against *H. influenzae*. It is similar to erythromycin in effectiveness against anaerobic gram-positive cocci and *Bacteroides sp*. Clarithromycin has been suggested as an alternative antibiotic if the prescriber wants to give an antibiotic from the macrolide family (see Table 3). The recommended oral adult dose is 500 mg twice daily for 7 days.

Azithromycin is active against staphylococci, including *S. aureus* and *S. epidermitis*, as well as streptococci, such as *S. pyogenes* and *S. pneumoniae*. Erythromycin-resistant strains of staphylococcus, enterococcus, and streptococcus, including methicillin-resistant *S. aureus*, are also resistant to azithromycin. It has excellent activity against *H. influenzae*. Inhibition of anaerobes, such as *Clostridium perfringens*, is better with azithromycin than with erythromycin. Inhibition of *Bacteroides fragilis* and other bacteroides species by azithromycin is comparable to erythromycin. Both azithromycin and clarithromycin are presently recommended as alternatives in the prophylactic regimen for prevention of bacterial endocarditis. This past May, the FDA notified health care professionals that it is aware of the study published in the *New England Journal of Medicine* (Ray 2012) reporting a small increase in cardiovascular deaths and in the risk of death from any cause in persons treated with a 5-day course of azithromycin (Zithromax) compared to persons treated with amoxicillin, ciprofloxacin, or no drug. The FDA is reviewing the results from this study and will communicate any new information on azithromycin and this study or the potential risk of QT interval prolongation after the agency has completed its review.

Patients taking azithromycin should not stop taking their medicine without talking to their health care provider. Health care providers should be aware of the potential for QT interval prolongation and heart arrhythmias when prescribing or administering any macrolide antibiotic.

AMOXICILLIN

Some clinicians select amoxicillin over penicillin VK as the penicillin of choice to empirically treat odontogenic infections. Except for coverage of *Haemophilus influenzae* in acute sinus and otitis media infections, amoxicillin does not offer any advantage over penicillin VK for treatment of odontogenic infections. It is less effective than penicillin VK for aerobic gram-positive cocci, and similar to penicillin for coverage of anaerobes. Although it does provide coverage against gram-negative enteric bacteria, this is not needed to treat odontogenic infections, except in immunosuppressed patients where these organisms may be present. If one adheres to the principle of using the most effective narrow spectrum antibiotic, amoxicillin should not be favored over penicillin VK.

Note: The ADA Council on Scientific Affairs has published a review on the subject of antibiotic interaction with oral contraceptives in which a clear statement of the dental professional's responsibility was made. In essence, it was concluded that in any situation where a dentist is planning to prescribe a course of antibiotics, alternative/additional means of contraception should be recommended to the oral contraceptive users. Specifically, patients should be told about the potential for antibiotics to lower the usefulness of oral contraceptives and advised to consult their physician about nonhormonal contraceptive techniques while continuing their oral contraceptive regimen. Even though there is minimal scientific data supporting this position, the risk of possible unwanted pregnancies warrants this simple approach for professionals licensed to prescribe antibiotics (*JADA*. 2002;133:880).

For pretreatment antibiotics and active infections, numerous reviews of antibiotic preferences have been published. Antibiotics used in dentistry by approximate percentage include: Amoxicillin 57%, Clindamycin 15%, Penicillin VK 12%, Azithromycin 5%, Cephalexin 4%, Amoxicillin/Clavulanate 3%, Doxycycline 2%, and others 2% (Durkin 2017).

The following tables have been adapted from Wynn RL, Bergman SA, Meiller TF, Crossley HL. Antibiotics in treating orofacial infections of odontogenic origin. *Gen Dent*. 2001;47(3):238-252.

Amoxicillin on page 124
Amoxicillin and Clavulanate on page 130
Cephalexin on page 322
Cefditoren on page 306
Ceftibuten on page 314
Chlorhexidine Gluconate (Oral) on page 334
Chlorpheniramine on page 361
Clarithromycin on page 361
Clindamycin (Systemic) on page 368
Dicloxacillin on page 491
Erythromycin (Systemic) on page 588
Gemifloxacin on page 733
Loratadine and Pseudoephedrine on page 931
MetroNIDAZOLE (Systemic) on page 1011
Mouthwash (Antiseptic) on page 1062
Moxifloxacin (Systemic) on page 1064
Oxymetazoline (Nasal) on page 1173
Penicillin V Potassium on page 1211
Pseudoephedrine on page 1291
Tetracycline (Systemic) on page 1431

Table 1. Empiric Antibiotics of Choice for Odontogenic Infections

Type of Infection	Antibiotic of Choice
Early (first 3 days of symptoms)	Penicillin VK, amoxicillin Clindamycin Cephalexin (or other first generation cephalosporin)[a]
No improvement in 48 to 72 hours	Consider adding metronidazole or beta-lactamase-stable antibiotic: Clindamycin or amoxicillin/clavulanic acid
Penicillin allergy	Clindamycin Cephalexin (if penicillin allergy is not anaphylactoid type) Clarithromycin (Biaxin)[b]
Late (>3 days)	Clindamycin Penicillin VK-metroNIDAZOLE, amoxicillin-metroNIDAZOLE
Penicillin allergy	Clindamycin (Please see the American Association of Endodontists current recommendations)

[a]For better patient compliance, second generation cephalosporins (cefaclor; cefuroxime) at twice daily dosing have been used; see text.

[b]A macrolide useful in patients allergic to penicillin, given as twice daily dosing for better patient compliance; see text.

If there is no improvement after 48 to 72 hours for a moderately severe oral infection, consider adding metronidazole to the penicillin regimen or discontinue the penicillin and resume therapy with a lactamase-stable antibiotic, such as clindamycin or amoxicillin/clavulanic acid (Augmentin).

- Metronidazole dose = 500 mg tid for 7 to 10 days
- Penicillin VK (or amoxicillin) 500 mg tid for 7 to 10 days
- **Note**: Bacterial resistance to metronidazole is extremely rare

Table 2. Penicillin VK: Antibacterial Spectrum

Gram-Positive Cocci	**Oral Anaerobes**
Streptococci	*Bacteroides*
Nonresistant staphylococci[a]	*Porphyromonas*
Pneumococci	*Prevotella*
	Peptococci
Gram-Negative Cocci	Peptostreptococci
Neisseria meningitides	*Actinomyces*
Neisseria gonorrhoeae	*Veillonella*
	Eubacterium
Gram-Positive Rods	*Eikenella*
Bacillus	*Capnocytophaga*
Corynebacterium	*Campylobacter*
Clostridium	*Fusobacterium*
	Others

[a]Nonresistant staphylococcus represents a small portion of community-acquired strains of *S. aureus* (5% to 15%). Most strains of *S. aureus* and *S. epidermitis* produce beta-lactamases, which destroy penicillins.

Table 3. Clindamycin: Antibacterial Spectrum[a]

Gram-Positive Cocci	Anaerobes[b]
Streptococci[c]	**Gram-Negative Bacilli**
S. aureus[d]	*Bacteroides* species including *B. fragilis*
Penicillinase and nonpenicillinase-producing staphylococcus	*B. melaninogenicus* *Fusobacterium species*
S. epidermitis	**Gram-Positive Nonspore-Forming Bacilli**
Pneumococci	*Cutibacterium* *Eubacterium* *Actinomyces* species
	Gram-Positive Cocci
	Peptococcus Peptostreptococcus Microaerophilic streptococci

[a]In vitro activity against isolates; information from manufacturer's package insert

[b] *Clostridia* are more resistant than most anaerobes to clindamycin. Most *Clostridium perfringens* are susceptible but *C. sporogens* and *C. tertium* are frequently resistant.

[c]Except *S. faecalis*

[d]Some staph strains originally resistant to erythromycin rapidly develop resistance to clindamycin.

Table 4. Oral Dose Ranges of Antibiotics Useful in Treating Odontogenic Infections[a]

Antibiotic	Clinicians must select specific dose and regimen from ranges available to be prescribed based on clinical judgment — Dosage	
	Children	Adults
Penicillin VK	≤12 years: 25 to 50 mg/kg body weight in equally divided doses every 6 to 8 hours for at least 7 days; maximum dose: 3 g/day	>12 years: 500 mg q6h for at least 7 days
Clindamycin	8 to 25 mg/kg in 3 to 4 equally divided doses	150 to 450 mg q6h for at least 7 days; maximum dose: 1.8 g/day
Cephalexin (Keflex)	25 to 50 mg/kg/day in divided doses q6h Severe infection: 50 to 100 mg/kg/day in divided doses q6h; maximum dose: 3 g per 24 hours	250 to 1,000 mg q6h; maximum dose: 4 g/day
Amoxicillin	<40 kg: 20 to 40 mg (amoxicillin)/kg/day in divided doses q8h >40 kg: 250 to 500 mg q8h or 875 mg q12h for at least 7 days; maximum dose 2 g/day	>40 kg: 250 to 500 mg q8h or 875 mg q12h for at least 7 days; maximum dose: 2 g/day
Amoxicillin/clavulanic acid (Augmentin)	<40 kg: 20 to 40 mg (amoxicillin)/kg/day in divided doses q8h >40 kg: 250 to 500 mg q8h or 875 mg q12h for at least 7 days; maximum dose 2 g/day	>40 kg: 250 to 500 mg q8h or 875 mg q12h for at least 7 days; maximum dose: 2 g/day
MetroNIDAZOLE (Flagyl)		500 mg every 6 to 8 hours for 7 to 10 days; maximum dose: 4 g/day

[a]For doses of other antibiotics, see monographs

SAMPLE PRESCRIPTIONS

Rx:

Penicillin V potassium 500 mg
Disp: 40 tablets
Sig: Take 1 tablet 4 times/day for 7 to 10 days (consider a loading dose of 1 g for acute infection)

Rx:

Clindamycin 300 mg
Disp: 40 capsules
Sig: Take 1 capsule 4 times/day for 7 to 10 days

Note: Prescription usually selected for patients allergic to penicillin; may be prescribed for 3 or 4 times/day. This prescription can be continued for treatment of some infections >1 month; however, risk of *Clostridioides* (formerly *Clostridium*) *difficile* infection increases with long-term clindamycin use. Patient should be cautioned to take clindamycin with food and contact health care provider if diarrhea develops even after antibiotic course is completed. Probiotics may help but evidence is conflicted on true efficacy.

Rx:

Amoxicillin 500 mg
Disp: 30 capsules or tablets
Sig: Take 1 capsule or tablet 3 times/day for 7 to 10 days

For additional sample prescriptions see Bacterial Infections and Periodontal Diseases - Sample Prescriptions on page 35

SINUSITIS TREATMENT

Sinusitis represents a common condition which may present with confounding dental complaints. Sinusitis (or rhinosinusitis) is an inflammation of the mucous membrane that lines the paranasal sinuses. It is classified into several categories:

- Acute rhinosinusitis: A new episode that may last ≤4 weeks
- Recurrent acute rhinosinusitis: ≥4 separate episodes of acute sinusitis that occur within 1 year
- Chronic rhinosinusitis: Signs and symptoms last for >12 weeks

All of these types of sinusitis have similar symptoms and are often difficult to distinguish. Acute sinusitis is very common. It has been estimated that 90% of adults have had sinusitis at some point in their lives.

Treatment is sometimes instituted by the dentist, but due to the often chronic and recurrent nature of sinusitis, early involvement of an otolaryngologist is advised. Most sinusitis is brought on by a nasopharyngeal viral infection best treated by sinus lavage, but some infections may require antibiotics of varying spectrum as well as requiring the management of sinus congestion. Although amoxicillin is usually adequate, many otolaryngologists initially prescribe Augmentin. Second-generation cephalosporins and clarithromycin are sometimes used, depending on the chronicity of the problem. Although not the ideal drug for general dental and/or periodontal infections, levofloxacin (Levoquin) is approved for treatment of acute bacterial rhinosinusitis.

For examples of sample prescriptions see Sinus Infection Treatment - Sample Prescriptions on page 41

LYME DISEASE

Lyme disease is a challenging infectious, toxic disease that may exhibit many different symptoms. The clinical picture of Lyme disease can be similar to fibromyalgia, including chronic fatigue, joint pain (arthralgia), or muscle, fibrous tissue, and tendon pain. Lyme disease can also manifest primarily as a neurological disorder, including fatigue and other neurological symptoms. Early, aggressive, and comprehensive treatment improves the prognosis tremendously.

Chronic Persistent Infection

Some symptoms and signs of Lyme disease may not appear until weeks, months, or years after a tick bite. This typically involves intermittent episodes of joint pain or numerous neurological symptoms such as meningitis, Bell's palsy, dysfunction of cardiac rhythm, and migratory pain to joints, tendons, muscle, and bone. Arthritis is most likely to appear as brief bouts of pain and swelling, usually in one or more large joints; however, any combination of symptoms can be present.

In a minority of individuals (~11%), development of chronic Lyme arthritis may lead to erosion of cartilage and/or bone. Other clinical manifestations associated with chronic Lyme arthritis include neurologic complications, such as disturbances in memory, mood, or sleep patterns, and sensations of numbness and tingling.

Oral symptoms can occur as a mimic to atypical facial pain, burning mouth, or other orofacial symptoms with little or no organic basis identified. Although symptoms similar to fibromyalgia are common, the two conditions are not currently thought to be directly connected.

Diagnosis of Lyme Disease

Lyme disease is diagnosed based on history, clinical symptoms, and response to therapy. No test can conclusively rule out lyme disease since routine laboratory tests are usually normal. Liver enzymes may be slightly elevated. The erythrocyte sediment rate (ESR) is most often normal, distinguishing Lyme disease from some of the purely inflammatory disorders such as rheumatoid arthritis or lupus; however, overlap between Lyme disease and autoimmune diseases frequently occurs. A prompt biopsy of the erythema migrans rash can confirm *Borrelia burgdorferi* in the culture. Serological (blood) tests currently available for Lyme disease caused by *B. burgdorferi* include, the immunologically based ELISA and Western blot assays. Clinically, over 75% of patients with Lyme disease are negative by ELISA but positive by Western blot, adding to the complexity of diagnosis (Honegr 2001).

Treatment

Antibiotics are the foundation of Lyme disease therapy. Oral therapy with doxycycline, cefuroxime, or amoxicillin is appropriate for early cases of Lyme disease. Parenteral therapy, usually IV administration, may be used for patients with neurologic involvement, severe arthritis, or any life-threatening manifestation of Lyme disease, such as complete heart block.

Treatment of 2 to 4 weeks is usually effective if initiated at the first appearance of a erythema migrans rash. In patients with symptoms present for more than 6 months, the treatment course may need to be more prolonged or a retreatment course of varying length may be needed. Consult the American Lyme Disease Foundation for treatment suggestions (available at http://www.aldf.com/raad.shtml).

FREQUENTLY ASKED QUESTIONS

What is the best antibiotic modality for treating dental infections?

Penicillin is still the drug of choice for treatment of infections in and around the oral cavity. Phenoxymethyl penicillin (Pen VK) long has been the most commonly selected antibiotic. In penicillin-allergic individuals, clindamycin may be an appropriate consideration, prescribing 300 mg as a loading dose followed by 150 mg 4 times/day would be an appropriate regimen for a dental infection. In general, if there is no response to Pen VK, then Augmentin may be a good alternative in the nonpenicillin-allergic patient because of its slightly altered spectrum. Recommendations would include that the patient should take the drug with food.

Is there cross allergenicity between the cephalosporins and penicillin?

The incidence of cross-allergenicity is 5% to 8% in the overall population. If a patient has demonstrated a Type I hypersensitivity reaction to penicillin, namely urticaria or anaphylaxis, then this incidence would increase to 20%.

Is there definitely an interaction between contraception agents and antibiotics?

There are well founded interactions between contraceptives and antibiotics. The best instructions that a patient could be given by their dentist are that should an antibiotic be necessary and the dentist is aware that the patient is on contraceptives, and if the patient is using chemical contraceptives, the patient should seriously consider additional means of contraception during the antibiotic management.

Are antibiotics necessary in diabetic mellitus patients?

In the management of diabetes, control of the diabetic status is the key factor relative to all morbidity issues. If a patient is well controlled, then antibiotics will likely not be necessary. However, in patients where the control is questionable or where they have recently been given a different drug regimen for their diabetes or if they are being titrated to an appropriate level of either insulin or oral hypoglycemic agents during these periods of time, the dentist might consider preprocedural antibiotics to be efficacious.

Do nonsteroidal anti-inflammatory drugs interfere with blood pressure medication?

At the current time there is no clear evidence that NSAIDs interfere with any of the blood pressure medications that are currently in usage.

REFERENCES AND SELECTED READINGS

ADA Council on Scientific Affairs. Antibiotic interference with oral contraceptives. *JADA*. 2002;133(7):880.

American Dental Association-Appointed Members of the Expert Writing and Voting Panels Contributing to the Development of American Academy of Orthopedic Surgeons Appropriate Use Criteria. American Dental Association guidance for utilizing appropriate use criteria in the management of the care of patients with orthopedic implants undergoing dental procedures. *J Am Dent Assoc*. 2017;148(2):57-59.

Centers for Disease Control and Prevention. Antibiotic/Antimicrobial Resistance U.S. Department of Health & Human Services. Accessed May 20, 2016.

Durkin MJ, Hsueh K, Sallah YH, et al. An evaluation of dental antibiotic prescribing practices in the United States. *JADA*. 2017;148(12):878-886.

Fluent MT, Jacobsen PL, Hicks LA, OSAP. Considerations for responsible antibiotic use in dentistry. *J Am Dent Assoc*. 2016;147(8):683-686

Flynn TR. What are the antibiotics of choice for odontogenic infections, and how long should the treatment course last? *Oral Maxillofac Surg Clin North Am*. 2011;23(4):519-536.

Hayward G, Heneghan C, Perera R, Thompson M. Intranasal corticosteroids in management of acute sinusitis: a systematic review and meta-analysis. *Ann Fam Med*. 2012;10(3):241-249.

Honegr K, Hulínská D, Dostál V, et al. Persistence of *Borrelia burgdorferi* sensu lato in patients with *Lyme borreliosis*. *Epidemiol Mikrobiol Imunol*. 2001;50(1):10-16.

Mayer G. Antibiotics – protein synthesis, nucleic acid synthesis and metabolism. *Medical Microbiology*. 6th ed. Murray PR, Rosenthal KS, Pfaller MA, eds. Elseiver; 2010;Chapter 20.

McDonald LC, Gerding DN, Johnson S, et al. Clinical practice guidelines for clostridium difficile infection in adults and children: 2017 update by the infectious diseases society of america (IDSA) and society for healthcare epidemiology of america (SHEA). *Clin Infect Dis*. 2018;66(7):987-994.

Palmer C. ADA News: ADA supports responsible antibiotic use. American Dental Association. June 15, 2015. Accessed May 20, 2016.

Quinn RH, Murray JN, Pezold R, Sevarino KS. The American Academy of Orthopaedic Surgeons Appropriate Use Criteria for the Management of Patients with Orthopaedic Implants Undergoing Dental Procedures. *J Bone Joint Surg Am*. 2017;99(2):161-163.

Ray WA, Murray KT, Hall K, et al. Azithromycin and the risk of cardiovascular death. *N Engl J Med*. 2012;366:1881-1890.

Rosenfeld RM, Andes D, Bhattacharyya N, et al. Clinical practice guideline: adult sinusitis. *Otolaryngol Head Neck Surg*. 2007;137(3 Suppl):S1-S31.

Smith SR, Montgomery LG, Williams JW Jr. Treatment of mild to moderate sinusitis. *Arch Intern Med*. 2012;172(6):510-513.

Sollecito TP, Abt E, Lockhart PB, et al. The use of prophylactic antibiotics prior to dental procedures in patients with prosthetic joints: Evidence-based clinical practice guideline for dental practitioners–a report of the American Dental Association Council on Scientific Affairs. *J Am Dent Assoc*. 2015;146(1):11-16 e8.

Wilson W, Taubert KA, Gewitz M, et al. Prevention of infective endocarditis: guidelines from the American Heart Association: a guideline from the American Heart Association Rheumatic Fever, Endocarditis and Kawasaki Disease Committee, Council on Cardiovascular Disease in the Young, and the Council on Clinical Cardiology, Council on Cardiovascular Surgery and Anesthesia, and the Quality of Care and Outcomes Research Interdisciplinary Working Group. *J Am Dent Assoc*. 2008;139 Suppl:3S-24S.

Wormser GP, Dattwyler RJ, Shapiro ED, et al. The clinical assessment, treatment, and prevention of lyme disease, human granulocytic anaplasmosis, and babesiosis: clinical practice guidelines by the Infectious Diseases Society of America. *Clin Infect Dis*. 2006;43(9):1089-1134.

Zalmanovici A, Yaphe J. Intranasal steroids for acute sinusitis. *Cochrane Database Syst Rev*. 2009;(4):CD005149.

PERIODONTAL DISEASES

Periodontal diseases are common to mankind affecting, according to some epidemiologic studies, greater than 80% of the worldwide population. The conditions refer primarily to diseases that are caused by accumulations of dental plaque and the subsequent immune response of the host to the bacteria and toxins present in this plaque. Although most of the organisms that have been implicated in advanced periodontal diseases are anaerobic in nature, some aerobes contribute by either coaggregation with the anaerobic species or direct involvement with specific disease types.

As a group of diseases, the soft tissues are affected, supporting the teeth (ie, gingiva) leading to the term gingivitis or inflammation of gingival structures and those conditions that affect the bone and ligament supporting the teeth (ie, periodontitis) result from the infection and/or inflammation of these structures. Diseases of the periodontia can be further subdivided into various types including chronic periodontitis (localized and generalized, mainly in adults), aggressive periodontitis (localized and generalized, including previously classified), early onset periodontitis, prepubertal periodontitis, and rapidly progressing periodontitis. In addition, periodontitis as a manifestation of systemic diseases (hematologic, genetic disorders, not otherwise specified) as well as a necrotizing type due to specific conditions associated with predisposing immunodeficiency disease, such as those found in HIV-infected patients, create further subclassifications of the periodontal diseases, some of which are covered in those chapters associated with those conditions.

Recently, a committee representing both the American Academy of Periodontology (AAP) and the European Federation of Periodontology (EFP) met in November 2017 with the charge of updating the 1999 classification of periodontal disease and conditions. (1) The *Proceedings of the World Workshop on the Classification of Periodontal and Peri-Implant Diseases and Conditions* consists of 19 review papers and four consensus reports.

Periodontal disease and conditions can be broken down into three major categories:

1. **Periodontal health and gingival diseases**
   a. Periodontal and gingival health
   b. Gingivitis caused by biofilm (bacteria)
   c. Gingivitis not caused by biofilm
2. **Periodontitis**
   a. Necrotizing diseases
   b. Periodontitis as a manifestation of systemic disease
   c. Periodontitis (more detailed explanation below)
3. **Other conditions affecting the periodontium**
   a. Systemic diseases affecting the periodontium
   b. Periodontal abscess or periodontal/endodontic lesions
   c. Mucogingival deformities and conditions
   d. Traumatic occlusal forces
   e. Tooth- and prosthesis-related factors

Peri-implant diseases and conditions can be broken down into four major categories:

1. **Peri-implant health**
2. **Peri-implant mucositis**
3. **Peri-implantitis**
4. **Peri-implant soft- and hard-tissue deficiencies**

According to the new classification, when describing periodontitis, we now have to clarify the ***stage, extent, and progression*** with anticipated treatment response. The staging of periodontitis is based on both severity and complexity of management.

Staging of periodontitis:

1. Stage I (initial)
2. Stage II (moderate)
3. Stage III (severe with potential for additional tooth loss)
4. Stage IV (severe with potential for loss of dentition)

Extent and distribution of periodontitis:

1. Localized - BL is around less than 30% of teeth in mouth
2. Generalized - BL is around more than 30% of teeth in mouth
3. Molar-incisor - BL is found around molar (usually first) and anterior incisors

Grading of periodontitis (assessing rate of progression and anticipated response to treatment):

1. Grade A (slow progression)
2. Grade B (moderate progression)
3. Grade C (rapid progression)

This scheme also utilizes the role that diseases, such as diabetes, play in periodontal progression by associating glycosylated hemoglobin levels >7% to grading assignment and likely with treatment outcome expectations. It is well accepted that control of most periodontal diseases requires, at the very minimum, appropriate mechanical cleansing of the dentition and the supporting structures by the patient. These efforts include brushing, some type of interdental cleaning, preferably with either floss or other aids, as well as appropriate sulcular cleaning usually with a brush.

Following appropriate dental treatment by the general dental practitioner and/or the periodontist, aids to these efforts by the patient might include the use of chemical agents to assist in the control of the periodontal diseases, or to prevent periodontal diseases. There are many available chemical agents on the market, only some of which are approved by the American Dental Association (ADA). Several have been tested utilizing guidelines published in 1986 by the ADA for assessment of agents that claim efficacy in the management of periodontal diseases. These chemical agents, including chlorhexidine (Peridex, PerioGard), a quaternary compound, are bisbiguanides. Chlorhexidine, in various concentrations, has shown efficacy in reducing plaque and gingivitis in patients with short-term utilization. Some side effects include staining of the dentition, which is reversible by dental prophylaxis. Chlorhexidine demonstrates the concept of substantivity, indicating that after its use, it has a continued effect in reducing the ability of plaque to form. It has been shown to be useful in a variety of periodontal conditions including acute necrotizing ulcerative gingivitis and healing studies. Some disturbances in taste and accumulation of calculus have been reported; however, chlorhexidine is the most applicable chemical agent of the bisbiguanides that has been studied to date.

Other chemical agents available as mouthwashes include the phenol compound Listerine Antiseptic. These compounds are primarily restricted to prototype agents; the first to be approved by the ADA being Listerine Antiseptic. Listerine Antiseptic has been shown to be effective against plaque and gingivitis in long-term studies and comparable to chlorhexidine in these long-term investigations. However, chlorhexidine performs better than Listerine Antiseptic in short-term investigations. Triclosan, the chemical agent found in the toothpaste Total, has been recently approved by the FDA and is an aid in the prevention of gingivitis. Antiplaque activity of triclosan is enhanced with the addition of zinc citrate and there are no serious side effects to the use of triclosan in the dose found in the dentifrice. Sanguinarine is a principle herbal extract used for antiplaque activity. It is an alkaloid from the plant *Sanguinaria canadensis* and has some antimicrobial properties perhaps due to its enzyme activity although a relationship was found between epithelial mucosa premalignant changes and sanguinarine use in mouth rinse. Zinc citrate and zinc chloride have often been added to toothpastes as well as enzymes such as mucinase, mutanase, and dextrinase which have demonstrated varying results in studies. Some commercial anionic surfactants are available on the market, which include amino alcohols and the agent Plax which essentially is comprised of sodium thiosulfate as a surfactant. Recent studies have shown Plax to have some efficacy when it is added to triclosan.

Long-term use of prescription medications, including antibiotics, is seldom recommended and is not in any way a substitute for general dental/periodontal therapies. As adjunctive therapy, however, benefit has been shown and the new formulations of doxycycline (Periostat [available in Canada] and Atridox), are recommended for long-term or repetitive treatments. It should be noted that the manufacturer's claims indicate that Periostat functions as a collagenase inhibitor not as an antibiotic at recommended low doses for long-term therapy. Atridox functions as an antibiotic and is not recommended for constant long-term therapy, but rather in repetitive applications as necessary. Prescription medications used in efforts to treat periodontal diseases have historically included the use of antibiotics such as tetracycline although complications with use with young patients (ie, teeth intrinsic staining) have often precluded their prescription. Doxycycline is often preferred to tetracycline in low doses. This broad-spectrum bacteriostatic agent has shown efficacy against a wide variety of bacterial organisms found in periodontal disease. Minocycline slow-release (Arestin) has recently been approved.

The drug metronidazole is a nitroimidazole, an agent that was originally used in treatment of protozoan infections and some anaerobic bacteria. It is bactericidal and has a good absorption and distribution throughout the body. The studies using metronidazole have suggested that it has a variety of uses in periodontal treatment and can be used as adjunct in both acute necrotizing ulcerative gingivitis and has specific efficacy against spirochetes, bacteria, and some *Porphyromonas* species. Metronidazole has also been useful alone or with clavulanic acid when combined with amoxicillin for management of acute periodontal infections and in cases of gingival hyperplasia. Recently, it has been used in combination with amoxicillin alone or with clavulanic acid in the management of osteomyelitis associated with bisphosphonate use.

Clindamycin is a derivative of vancomycin and has been useful in treatment of suppurative periodontal lesions. Long-term use is precluded by its complicating toxicities associated with colitis and gastrointestinal problems; however, recent studies have shown that a variety of antibiotics can result in colitis, thus, clindamycin should not be singled out as the sole or main culprit of this reported complication.

When severe gingival inflammation appears to be refractory to routine periodontal therapies the clinician should consider a biopsy since autoimmune conditions that comprise desquamative gingivitis diseases must be considered.

Research has also shown that various combination therapies of metronidazole and tetracycline for localized aggressive periodontitis and metronidazole with amoxicillin for rapidly progressive disease can be useful. The use of other prescription drugs including nonsteroidal anti-inflammatory, as well as other antibacterial agents, have been under study. Effects on prostaglandins of NSAIDs may indirectly slow periodontal disease progression. New research is currently underway in this regard. Perhaps, in combination therapy with some of the antibiotics, these drugs may assist in reducing the patient's immune response or inflammatory response to the presence of disease-causing bacteria.

Of greatest interest has been the improvement in technology for delivery of chemical agents to the periodontally-diseased site. These systems include biodegradable gelatins and biodegradable chips that can be placed under the gingiva and deliver antibacterial agents directly to the site as an adjunct to periodontal treatment. The initial therapy of mechanical debridement by the periodontal therapist is essential prior to using any chemical agent, and the dentist should be aware that the development of newer agents does not substitute for appropriate periodontal therapy and maintenance. The trade names of the gelatin chips and subgingival delivery systems include Periochip, Atridox, and Periostat (available in Canada).

In addition to the periodontal therapy, consideration of the patient's preexisting or developing medical conditions are important in the management of the periodontal patient. Several diseases illustrate these points most acutely. The reader is referred to the chapters on Diabetes, Cardiovascular Disease, Pregnancy, Respiratory Disease, HIV, and Cancer Chemotherapy. It has long been accepted that uncontrolled diabetes mellitus may predispose to periodontal lesions. Now, under current investigation is the hypothesis that preexisting periodontal diseases may make it more difficult for a diabetic patient to come under control. In addition, the inflammatory response and immune challenge that is ongoing in periodontal disease appears to be implicated in the development of coronary artery disease as well as an increased risk of myocardial infarction and/or stroke. The accumulation of intra-arterial plaques appears enhanced by the presence of the inflammatory response often seen systemically in patients suffering with periodontal disease. In addition, the clinician is referred to the section on preprocedural antibiotics in the text for a consideration of antibiotic usage in patients that may be at risk for infective endocarditis. Other conditions including pregnancy and respiratory diseases such as COPD, HIV, and cancer therapy must be considered in the overall view of periodontal diseases. The reader is referred to the sections within the text.

TISSUE REGENERATION

Periodontal therapies rely on disease control and the success of surgery followed by medicinal therapeutics to stabilize and manage patients with advanced periodontal diseases. Efforts in tissue regeneration have largely consisted of free gingival graft procedures, transplanting host tissue from one site to another, or placing lyophilized bone into defects. Recently, the FDA approved a new living cell construct, called GINTUIT, that is made up of an allogeneic cellularized scaffold (McGuire 2011). GINTUIT is intended for use as keratinized tissue to be added to surgical sites to enhance the success and stability of attached gingival surgery and implant placement. Use of this product would not require a donor site surgery, such as a free gingival graft procedure, which may reduce pain and the risk of postoperative infection. It is not known if this product offers long-term improvement in outcomes of periodontal surgery over conventional techniques and materials.

Stem cell research offers a particularly effective potential method for cell transplantation and tissue regeneration (Nguyen 2013). Conventional tissue transplantation solutions are limited by factors, such as insufficient donor tissue and graft rejection and failure. In contrast, stem cells may be able to regenerate new tissue and restore function. A tissue engineering approach to periodontal therapy has been proposed, whereby periodontal tissue would be constructed in the laboratory and then surgically implanted into defects. A promising technique involves harvesting stem cells from the PDL, culturing periodontal cell sheets in vitro and transplanting the tissue into periodontal defects. This has resulted in PDL tissue regeneration in animal models.

REFERENCES

Armitage GC. Development of a classification system for periodontal diseases and conditions. *Ann Periodontol.* 1999;4(1):1-6.

Bulgin D, Hodzic E, Komljenovic-Blitva D. Advanced and prospective technologies for potential use in craniofacial tissues regeneration by stem cells and growth factors. *J Craniofac Surg.* 2011; 22(1):342-348.

Caton G, Armitage G, Berglundh T, et al. A new classification scheme for periodontal and peri-implant diseases and conditions – introduction and key changes from the 1999 classification. *J Clin Periodontol.* 2018;45(suppl 20):S1-S8.

McGuire MK, Scheyer ET, Nevins ML, et al. Living cellular construct for increasing the width of keratinized gingiva: results from a randomized, within-patient, controlled trial. *J Periodontol.* 2011;82(10):1414-1423.

Nguyen TT, Mui B, Mehrabzadeh M, et al. Regeneration of tissues of the oral complex: current clinical trends and research advances. *J Can Dent Assoc.* 2013; 79.

Trounson A, Thakar RG, Lomax G, Gibbons D. Clinical trials for stem cell therapies. *BMC Med.* 2011; 9:52.

NECROTIZING ULCERATING PERIODONTITIS (HIV Periodontal Disease)

Initial Treatment *(In-Office)*

Gentle debridement

Note: Ensure patient has no iodine allergies

Betadine rinse on page 1249

At-Home Treatment

Listerine antiseptic rinse (20 mL for 30 seconds twice daily)

Peridex rinse on page 334

MetroNIDAZOLE (Systemic) (Flagyl) 7 to 10 days on page 1011

Follow-Up Therapy

Proper dental cleaning, including scaling and root planing (repeat as needed)
Continue Peridex and Listerine rinse (indefinitely)

Amoxicillin on page 124
Chlorhexidine Gluconate (Oral) on page 334
Clindamycin (Systemic) on page 368
Doxycycline Hyclate Periodontal Extended-Release Liquid on page 530
Listerine Antiseptic on page 1062
MetroNIDAZOLE (Systemic) on page 1011
Minocycline Hydrochloride (Periodontal) on page 1036
NSAIDs see Oral Pain section on page 1734
Tetracycline (Systemic) on page 1431
Triclosan and Fluoride

For examples of sample prescriptions see Bacterial Infections and Periodontal Diseases on page 35

Pharmacologic Management of Periodontal Diseases

Antibiotic	Adult Dosage
Azithromycin	500 mg once daily for 4 to 7 days
Clindamycin (Systemic)	300 mg tid for 8 days
Doxycycline or minocycline	100 to 200 mg once daily for 21 days
MetroNIDAZOLE (Systemic)	500 mg tid for 8 days
Metronidazole + amoxicillin	250 mg tid for 8 days of each drug

Adapted from: Recommendations from the American Academy of Periodontology. Available at: www.perio.org.

FUNGAL INFECTIONS

Oral fungal infections can result from alteration in oral flora, immunosuppression, and underlying systemic diseases that may allow the overgrowth of these otherwise common but highly opportunistic organisms. These systemic conditions might include infection with the human immunodeficiency virus (and its treatments), diabetes mellitus, long-term xerostomia, adrenal suppression, anemia, and chemotherapy-induced myelosuppression for the management of cancer. Long-term administration of antibiotics such as doripenem used to treat advanced systemic infections, has been implicated in elevating the risk of fungal infections. Also, the use of oral inhalers that include steroids, such as Advair Diskus, have been implicated in the enhancing of the risk of fungal overgrowth. Clinical presentation might include pseudomembranous, erythematous, and hyperkeratotic forms.

Fungus has also been implicated in denture stomatitis, angular cheilitis, and symptomatic geographic tongue (erythema migrans). Patients being treated for fungal skin infections or common oral conditions (eg, angular cheilitis) may also be using topical antifungal preparations coupled with a steroid, such as triamcinolone. *Candida albicans* is the fungal species most commonly isolated from the oral cavity, but other species can be found, some of which are azole resistant, such as *Candida glabrata*.

Nystatin (Mycostatin) is effective topically in the treatment of candidal infections of the skin and mucous membrane. The drug is extremely well tolerated and appears to be nonsensitizing although gastrointestinal upset and nausea are fairly common side effects. Clotrimazole troches are also useful as a topical therapy. Due to the significant sucrose content in nystatin suspension, patients with salivary gland hypofunction may be prescribed an alternative medication, such as clotrimazole troches which do contain dextrose, in order to lessen the caries risk. Clotrimazole is also available as vaginal suppository/troche formulations which do not contain any sugars.

In persons with denture stomatitis in which *Candida albicans* plays at least a contributory role, it is important to soak the prosthesis (laden with organisms) overnight in a nystatin liquid suspension besides treatment of the affected oral mucosa. Nystatin ointment can be placed in the denture during the daytime much like a denture adhesive. Antifungal medication should be continued for at least 14 days in order to prevent relapse and the patient must be reevaluated. Predisposing systemic factors must be reconsidered if the oral fungal infection persists and remake of any prosthesis may be necessary.

Topical applications rely on contact of the drug with the organism within the lesions; therefore, 4 to 5 times daily with a dissolving troche or a nystatin rinse is appropriate. Chronically recurring oral mucosal fungal infections are often seen in patients who use systemic steroids or steroid inhalers for respiratory disease, such as asthma or COPD. Dental prosthesis wearers also often experience recurrent fungal colonization coupled with denture stomatitis. These predisposing conditions may be more resistant to antifungal therapy, possibly requiring a combination of topical and systemic drugs.

Several drugs of different classes can be used in treating systemic and localized fungal infections including, amphotericin B, anidulafungin, caspofungin, ciclopirox olamine, clotrimazole, fluconazole, itraconazole, ketoconazole, micafungin, miconazole, naftifine hydrochloride, nystatin, oxiconazole, posaconazole, and voriconazole. Many of these drugs however are not commonly utilized as topical oral therapies. Clotrimazole, fluconazole, and nystatin are the most commonly prescribed oral topical treatments.

MANAGEMENT OF FUNGAL INFECTIONS REQUIRING SYSTEMIC MEDICATION

If the patient is refractory to topical treatment, consideration of a systemic route usually includes fluconazole (Diflucan) or ketoconazole. Also, when the patient cannot tolerate topical therapy, these choices are effective, well-tolerated, systematic drugs for mucocutaneous candidiasis. Concern over liver function and possible drug interactions must be considered.

In patients who appear to be refractory to ketoconazole, itraconazole, or fluconazole related to the treatment of oropharyngeal candidiasis, posaconazole has been approved for usage. Anidulafungin (Eraxis), caspofungin (Cancidas), micafungin (Mycamine), or voriconazole (VFEND) are also indicated for treatment of serious fungal infections in patients intolerant of, or refractory to, other therapy.

Amphotericin B (Conventional) on page 137
Anidulafungin on page 152
Caspofungin on page 296
Clotrimazole (Oral) on page 396
Fluconazole on page 674
Ketoconazole (Systemic) on page 856
Micafungin on page 1018
Nystatin (Oral) on page 1121
Nystatin (Topical) on page 1122
Nystatin and Triamcinolone on page 1123
Posaconazole on page 1248
Voriconazole on page 1552

Note: Consider Peridex oral rinse or Listerine antiseptic oral rinse for long-term control in immunosuppressed patients.

SAMPLE PRESCRIPTIONS FOR SYSTEMIC TREATMENT

Rx:
Diflucan 100 mg tablets
Disp: 16 tablets
Sig: Take 2 tablets day 1, then 1 tablet/day until gone

Note: Sometimes a shorter course is adequate; however, oral infections commonly are more difficult to eradicate. Often a 21-day (3-week) course, or and even a second course, may be necessary.

Ingredient: Fluconazole

Rx:
Ketoconazole (Systemic) 200 mg
Disp: 14 tablets
Sig: Take 1 tablet daily, with a meal, for 2 weeks

Note: May cause irreversible liver damage; liver function should be monitored with long-term use (ie, >3 weeks)

Ingredient: Ketoconazole

SAMPLE PRESCRIPTIONS FOR TOPICAL TREATMENT

Rx:
Nystatin 100,000 units/mL oral suspension
Disp: 300 mL
Sig: Rinse with 1 teaspoon (5 mL) for 2 minutes 4 to 5 times/day and expectorate

Rx:
Mycelex 10 mg troches
Disp: 70 troches
Sig: Dissolve 1 troche in mouth 4 to 5 times/day until gone; leave any prostheses out during treatment and soak prosthesis in nystatin liquid suspension overnight

Ingredient: Clotrimazole (Oral)

For additional sample prescriptions see Fungal Infections on page 38

MANAGEMENT OF ANGULAR CHEILITIS

Angular cheilitis may represent the clinical manifestation of a multitude of etiologic factors. Cheilitis-like lesions may result from local habits, from a decrease in the intermaxillary space, or from nutritional deficiency. More commonly, angular cheilitis represents a mixed infection coupled with an inflammatory response involving *Candida albicans* and other organisms (most frequently *Staphylococcus aureus*).

The drug of choice is now formulated to contain nystatin and triamcinolone (formerly known as Mycolog and Mycolog II) and the effect is excellent. In addition, an off-label use of iodoquinol and hydrocortisone has also been reported to be effective in the treatment of angular cheilitis.

VIRAL INFECTIONS

Infections of the oropharynx and upper respiratory infections are commonly caused by the Coxsackie group A viruses. Oral cavity proper soft tissue viral infections are most often caused by the herpes simplex viruses. Herpes zoster or varicella-zoster virus, which is one of the herpes family of viruses, can likewise cause similar viral eruptions involving the oral mucosa. Oral manifestations of mononucleosis caused by Epstein-Barr virus (another Herpes family virus) can lead to petechiae on the soft palate during mononucleosis but usually do not require direct therapy and resolve as the systemic condition improves. When EBV causes hairy leukoplakia in HIV/AIDS patients, the lesions usually respond to the anti-retroviral therapies.

Human *Papillomavirus* is causative in a number of oral lesions, the most common of which are *Condyloma acuminatum* and Verruca vulgaris. Within the past few years, certain subtypes of human *Papillomavirus* already proven to cause uterine cervical carcinoma are also responsible for some posterior oral cavity squamous cell carcinomas. Human papillomavirus (HPV) is the broad term for a large group of viruses comprised of more than 150 serotypes. Certain serotypes of HPV cause warts on the skin and others cause warts in the genital region. Some types of HPV are known to cause cervical cancers, as well as cancers of the anus, penis, vulva, vagina, and ***head and neck***.

Disease	HPV type
Common warts	2, 7
Plantar warts	1, 2, 4, 63
Flat warts	3, 10, 8
Anogenital warts	6, 11, 42, 44, and others
Anal lesions	6, 16, 18, 31, 53, 58
Genital cancers	Highest risk: 16, 18, 31, 45 Other high-risk: 33, 35, 39, 51, 52, 56, 58, 59 Probably high-risk: 26, 53, 66, 68, 73, 82
Epidermodysplasia verruciformis	More than 15 types
Focal epithelial hyperplasia (oral)	13, 32
Oral papillomas	6, 7, 11, 16, 32
Oropharyngeal cancer	16
Verrucous cyst	60
Laryngeal papillomatosis	6, 11

HPV-related head and neck cancers occur primarily in the oropharynx (posterior to the tonsillar pillars and on the base of the tongue). Oropharyngeal cancers are more common in white men. Most head and neck cancers are caused by tobacco and alcohol use, but researchers believe that up to 80% of oropharyngeal cancers in the US may be related to long term infection with the HPV virus. HPV-related head and neck cancer occurs in both people who smoke and those who do not smoke.

Salivary diagnostic tests are available for HPV, and involve the use of Polymerase Chain Reaction PCR tests; thus, they are not point of care tests. Kits containing a salivary collector are placed in transport media and sent to a central laboratory for analysis. Investigators in the field have used oral swabs, expectorated saliva or an expectorated oral rinse with mouthwash (OraRisk HPV test, OralDNA Labs, Brentwood, TN, which, to our knowledge, is the only salivary diagnostic test for HPV commercially available in the United States). The latter collection technique probably has the highest sensitivity, because it samples the entire oral cavity and the swishing of the solution dislodges mucosal cells. Investigators in the laboratory use a variety of primers to detect as many HPV types as possible. Early diagnosis is critical for survival of patients with oral squamous cell carcinoma (OSCC), and, thus, it is likely that use of salivary HPV analyses will continue to increase.

Human papilloma virus is widespread and serotypes 16 and 18 have been associated with cervical cancer. Although most types that cause oral HPV lesions are not of these serotypes, the clinician should recommend appropriate surgical removal of all such lesions. Lesions in the posterior oral pharyngeal region are of particular concern. Long-term infection with HPV is still being studied and data regarding oral risk of malignancy is improving. All suspicious lesions should be removed and serotyping performed if counseling the patient seems appropriate. Preexposure vaccination is one of the most effective methods for preventing transmission of some serotypes of HPV. Gardasil 9 is now available.

GARDASIL 9 is a vaccine indicated in females 9 through 26 years of age for the prevention of cervical, vulvar, vaginal, and anal cancers caused by human papillomavirus (HPV) Types 16, 18, 31, 33, 45, 52, and 58; precancerous or dysplastic lesions caused by HPV Types 6, 11, 16, 18, 31, 33, 45, 52, and 58; and genital warts caused by HPV Types 6 and 11.

GARDASIL 9 is indicated in males 9 through 26 years of age for the prevention of anal cancer caused by HPV Types 16, 18, 31, 33, 45, 52, and 58; precancerous or dysplastic lesions caused by HPV Types 6, 11, 16, 18, 31, 33, 45, 52, and 58; and genital warts caused by HPV Types 6 and 11.

GARDASIL 9 (Human Papillomavirus 9-valent Vaccine, Recombinant) does not eliminate the necessity for girls to continue to undergo recommended cervical cancer screening later in life. Recipients of GARDASIL 9 should not discontinue anal cancer screening if it has been recommended by a health care professional. It has not been demonstrated to provide protection against diseases from vaccine HPV types to which a person has previously been exposed through sexual activity. It is not a treatment for external genital lesions; cervical, vulvar, vaginal, and anal cancers;

or cervical intraepithelial neoplasia (CIN), vulvar intraepithelial neoplasia (VIN), vaginal intraepithelial neoplasia (VaIN), or anal intraepithelial neoplasia (AIN). Not all vulvar, vaginal, and anal cancers are caused by HPV, and GARDASIL 9 protects only against those vulvar, vaginal, and anal cancers caused by HPV Types 16, 18, 31, 33, 45, 52, and 58. The vaccine is contraindicated in individuals with hypersensitivity, including severe allergic reactions to yeast, or after a previous dose of GARDASIL 9 or if the subject had received the previously available Human Papillomavirus Quadrivalent vaccine (Types 6, 11, 16, and 18). GARDASIL 9 is administered intramuscularly in the deltoid region of the upper arm or in the higher anterolateral area of the thigh. For individuals 9 through 14 years of age, it is administered using a 2-dose or 3-dose schedule. For individuals 15 through 26 years of age, GARDASIL 9 is administered using a 3-dose schedule at 0, 2 months, and 6 months.

Cervarix is no longer marketed in the US.

Details regarding HPV vaccination are available at www.cdc.gov/std/hpv. Vaccines for other STDs (eg, HIV and herpes simplex virus) are under development or undergoing clinical trials. Vaccines are not available for bacterial or fungal STDs.

The diagnosis of an acute viral infection begins by ruling out bacterial etiology and having an awareness of the presenting signs and symptoms associated with viral infection. Acute onset and vesicular eruption on the soft tissues generally favors a diagnosis of viral infection. Unfortunately, vesicles do not remain for a great length of time in the oral cavity; therefore, the short-lived vesicles rupture leaving ulcerated bases as the only indication of their presence. These ulcers are generally small in size and only when left unmanaged, coalesce to form larger, irregular ulcerations. Distinction must be made between the commonly recurring intraoral atraumatic ulcers (aphthous ulcerations) which do not have a viral etiology and the lesions associated with intraoral recurrent herpes since their effective treatment is distinctly different.

The management of an oral viral infection may be palliative for the most part; however, with the advent of improved antiviral prescription medications there now exists a family of drugs that can assist in managing primary and secondary infection. Aldara has been approved for treatment of genital warts (superficial basal cell carcinomas and actinic keratosis); oral mucosa use is still under study.

It should be noted that herpes can present as a primary infection (gingivostomatitis or pharyngo stomatitis), recurrent lip lesions (herpes labialis of the skin and adjacent vermilion border), and intraoral ulcers (recurrent intraoral herpes), involving the oral and perioral tissues. Primary infection is a systemic infection that leads to acute gingivostomatitis that may involve all moveable and nonmovable sites of the oral cavity (buccal mucosa, lips, tongue, floor of the mouth, palate, and the gingiva). Treatment of primary infections utilizes prescription antivirals such as acyclovir in combination with supportive care. Topical anesthetics, such as lidocaine 1% or dyclonine HCl 1%, used in combination with Benadryl 0.5% in a saline vehicle was found to be an effective oral rinse in the symptomatic treatment of primary herpetic gingivostomatitis. Other agents for symptomatic and supportive treatment include commercially available elixir of Benadryl, Xylocaine viscous, Orajel (OTC), and antibiotics to prevent secondary infections. Systemic supportive therapy should include forced fluids, high concentration protein, vitamin and mineral food supplements, and rest.

Antivirals

Abreva (OTC) on page 508
Acyclovir (Systemic) on page 75
Acyclovir (Topical) on page 82
Famciclovir on page 635
Imiquimod on page 802
L-Lysine on page 925
Nelfinavir on page 1092
Penciclovir on page 1207
ValACYclovir on page 1512

HPV Prevention

GARDASIL 9 is a vaccine indicated in females 9 through 26 years of age for the prevention of cervical, vulvar, vaginal, and anal cancers caused by human papillomavirus (HPV) Types 16, 18, 31, 33, 45, 52, and 58; precancerous or dysplastic lesions caused by HPV Types 6, 11, 16, 18, 31, 33, 45, 52, and 58; and genital warts caused by HPV Types 6 and 11.

Supportive Therapy

DiphenhydrAMINE (Systemic) on page 502
Lidocaine (Topical) on page 902

Prevention of Secondary Bacterial Infection

Penicillin V Potassium on page 1211

SUPPORTIVE CARE FOR PAIN AND PREVENTION OF SECONDARY INFECTION

Primary infections often become secondarily infected with bacteria, requiring antibiotics. Dietary supplement may be necessary. Options are presented due to variability in patient compliance and response.

RECURRENT HERPETIC INFECTIONS

Following the primary herpetic infection, the herpesvirus remains latent until such time as it has the opportunity to recur. The etiology of this latent period and the degree of viral shedding present during latency is currently under study; however, it is thought that some trigger in the mucosa or the skin causes the virus to begin to replicate. This process may involve Langerhans cells which are immunocompetent antigen-presenting cells resident in all epidermal and epithelial surfaces.

The virus replication then leads to physical movement of the virus along the sensory axon leading to eruptions in innervated tissues surrounding the mouth or within. The most common form of recurrence is the lip lesion or herpes labialis; however, intraoral recurrent herpes also occurs with some frequency (attached gingival and hard palate preferentially).

Prevention of recurrences has been attempted with lysine (OTC) 500 to 1,000 mg/day and acyclovir but response has been variable. Herpes zoster outbreaks can also involve the oral and facial tissues, although this is less common. The zoster vaccine (Zostavax) is approved for individuals >50 years of age and may protect against VZV outbreaks. Valacyclovir or famciclovir are the drugs of choice in the event of a shingles outbreak. Of the two medications, famciclovir is reported to be more effective against postherpetic neuralgia. Valacyclovir HCl in 500 mg and 1 g tablets has recently been approved by the FDA for first time generic formulations.

Water-soluble bioflavonoid-ascorbic acid complex, now available as Peridin-C, may be helpful in reducing the signs and symptoms associated with recurrent herpes simplex virus infections. As with all agents used, the therapy is more effective when instituted in the early prodromal stage of the disease process.

PREVENTATIVE SAMPLE PRESCRIPTIONS

Rx:
L-Lysine (OTC) 500 mg
Sig: Take 2 tablets/day as preventive; increase to 4 tablets/day if prodrome or recurrence begins

Rx:
Citrus bioflavonoids and ascorbic acid tablets 400 mg (Peridin-C)
Disp: 10 tablets
Sig: Take 2 tablets at once, then 1 tablet 3 times/day for 3 days

Where a recurrence is usually precipitated by exposure to sunlight, the lesion may be prevented by the application to the area of a sunscreen, with a high skin protection factor (SPF) in the range of ≥25.

SUPPORTIVE CARE FOR PAIN AND MAINTENANCE OF NUTRITION DURING ORAL VIRAL INFECTIONS

Rx:
Benadryl liquid 12.5 mg per 5 mL
Disp: 4 oz bottle
Sig: Rinse with 1 to 2 teaspoonfuls every 2 hours and expectorate

Note: Benadryl is available as a generic diphenhydramine liquid.

Rx:
Benadryl liquid 12.5 mg per 5 mL (mix 50/50) with Kaopectate
Disp: 8 oz total
Sig: Rinse with 1 to 2 teaspoonfuls every 2 hours and expectorate.

Note: Maalox can be used in place of Kaopectate if constipation is a problem. Benadryl is available as a generic diphenhydramine liquid.

Rx:
Xylocaine viscous 2%
Disp: 450 mL bottle
Sig: Swish with 1 tablespoon 4 times/day and spit out

Ingredient: Lidocaine (Topical)

Rx:
Meritene
Disp: 1 lb can (plain, chocolate, eggnog flavors)
Sig: Take 3 servings daily; prepare as indicated on can

Ingredient: Protein-vitamin-mineral food supplement

PRESCRIPTIVE TREATMENT

Acyclovir (Zovirax) possesses antiviral activity against herpes simplex types 1 and 2. Historically, ophthalmic ointments were used topically to treat recurrent mucosal and skin lesions. These do not penetrate well on the skin lesions, thereby providing questionable relief of symptoms. If recommended, use should be closely monitored. Penciclovir, an active metabolite of famciclovir, has been specifically approved in a cream for treatment of recurrent herpes lesions. Valacyclovir and famciclovir have also been approved for treatment of recurrent herpes labialis (see monograph for dosing).

The FDA has also approved acyclovir cream 5% for treatment of herpes labialis in adults and adolescents. Other over-the-counter preparations include 2% tetracaine gel and L-lysine 500 mg tablets.

For sample prescriptions see Viral Infections - Sample Prescriptions on page 43

REFERENCES

ADA Council on Scientific Affairs. Statement on Human Papillomavirus and Squamous Cell Cancers of the Oropharynx (adopted November 2012). Available at: http://www.ada.org/1749.aspx.
Andrews E, Seaman WT, Webster-Cyriaque J. Oropharyngeal carcinoma in nonsmokers and nondrinkers: a role for HPV. *Oral Oncol.* 2009;45 (6):486-491.
Chaturvedi AK, Engels EA, Pfeiffer RM, et al. Human papillomavirus and rising oropharyngeal cancer incidence in the United States. *J Clin Oncol.* 2011;29(32):4294-4301.
Cleveland JL, Junger ML, Saraiya M, Markowitz LE, Dunne EF, Epstein JB. The connection between human papillomavirus and oropharyngeal squamous cell carcinomas in the United States: implications for dentistry. *J Am Dent Assoc.* 2011;142(8):915-924.
Corstjens PL, Abrams WR, Malamud D. Detecting viruses by using salivary diagnostics. *J Am Dent Assoc.* 2012;143(10 Suppl):12S-18S.
Gillison ML, Broutian T, Pickard RK, et al. Prevalence of oral HPV infection in the United States, 2009-2010. *JAMA.* 2012;307(7):693-703.
Jemal A, Simard EP, Dorell C, et al. Annual Report to the Nation on the Status of Cancer, 1975-2009, featuring the burden and trends in human papillomavirus (HPV)-associated cancers and HPV vaccination coverage levels. *J Natl Cancer Inst.* 2013;105(3):175-201. http://jnci.oxfordjournals.org/content/early/2013/01/03/jnci.djs491.full.pdf+html
Kulkarni SS1, Kulkarni SS, Vastrad PP, et al. Prevalence and distribution of high risk human papillomavirus (HPV) Types 16 and 18 in carcinoma of cervix, saliva of patients with oral squamous cell carcinoma and in the general population in Karnataka, India. *Asian Pac J Cancer Prev.* 2011;12 (3):645-648.
Marur S, D'Souza G, Westra WH, Forastiere AA. HPV-associated head and neck cancer: a virus-related cancer epidemic. *Lancet Oncol.* 2010;11 (8):781-789.
Pfister DG and Fury MG. New chapter in our understanding of human papillomavirus-related head and neck cancer. *J Clin Oncol.* 2014;32 (30):3349-3352.

ULCERATIVE, EROSIVE, AND PAINFUL ORAL MUCOSAL DISORDERS

RECURRENT APHTHOUS STOMATITIS - MINOR, MAJOR, AND HERPETIFORM TYPES

Recurrent aphthous stomatitis is an extremely common mucosal disease. Although it is not considered a classic autoimmune disorder, the conditions that have been termed minor, major, and herpetiform types have in common a cellular-mediated event with underlying T-cells activation. This cytotoxicity leads to a destruction of the mucosal surface and is mediated by inflammatory cytokines throughout the oral tissues. The term herpetiform ulcerations is a misnomer and implies a herpes-type appearance to the ulcers when they are present. This is as far as the connection goes since there has never been a viral or bacterial etiology cited for any of the aphthous forms of ulcerations. The different subsets of patients have different triggering factors (eg, stress, hormonal, fluctuations and minor chemical irritations) and thus no one product or treatment technique is universally effective in all patients.

For minor or major aphthous ulcers that severely affect daily living and quality of life, corticosteroids seem to be the mainstay drug. It is believed that the immunomodulating effect of a short-term regimen of corticosteroids in an immunocompetent sufferer is effective without creating the well-known side effects of long-term or high-dose corticosteroid therapy. Sufferers of the herpetiform type of aphthae, in which as many as a hundred small ulcers appear per outbreak, may also obtain relief from an oral suspension corticosteroid (eg, dexamethasone) although management may be more protracted.

Triamcinolone dental paste (Oralone) is indicated for the temporary relief of minor symptoms associated with infrequent recurrences of minor aphthous lesions and ulcerative lesions resulting from trauma. Some clinicians prescribe a soothing rinse containing corticosteroid (eg, dexamethasone), an antifungal agent (eg, nystatin), a topical anesthetic (eg, viscous lidocaine), an antihistamine (eg, diphenhydramine), an antimicrobial/antibiotic (chlorhexidine), and/or coating agent such as attapulgite creating a so-called "magic elixir." The most popular combination contains 1.5 g tetracycline; 60 mg hydrocortisone; nystatin 6 million international units and an equal volume elixir of Benadryl and has been called Mary's Magic potion. Numerous other "Magic Mouthwash" mixtures have been formulated by clinicians, but there are insufficient data to provide evidence for selection of any of these combinations over others. All of the combinations do, however, have reasonable anecdotal evidence of palliative effects.

More severe forms of recurrent aphthous stomatitis may be treated with topical corticosteroids of higher strength (eg, fluocinonide, clobetasol) alone or mixed with Orabase. An oral suspension of tetracycline may be prescribed for avoidance of secondary infection. Tetracycline use is contraindicated during pregnancy, infancy, and childhood to the age of 8 years due to intrinsic staining of teeth. *Lactobacillus acidophilus* preparations (Bacid, Lactinex) are occasionally effective for reducing the frequency and severity of the minor lesions.

With professional oversight, a cauterizing agent, such as Debacterol may markedly decrease the pain associated with the aphthous ulcer. Clinician and patient must be extremely careful in using cauterizing agents within the oral cavity. Patients with long-standing history of recurrent aphthous stomatitis should be evaluated for iron, folic acid, and vitamin B_{12} deficiencies as well as hematological assessments for anemia. One subset of recurrent aphthous stomatitis sufferers markedly improve when tooth dentifrices lacking sodium lauryl sulfate are used.

In patients with medical contraindications for corticosteroid use, alternatives (eg, colchicine, dapsone, immune globulin [intravenous], methotrexate, misoprostol, mycophenolate mofetil, pentoxifylline, tacrolimus, and tretinoin) have had anecdotal reports of effectiveness. These alternative drugs should only be considered in consultation with the patient's physician.

Regular use of Listerine antiseptic has been shown in clinical trials to reduce the severity, duration, and frequency of aphthous stomatitis. An antimicrobial such as chlorhexidine oral rinses (20 mL for 30 seconds 2 to 3 times/day) has also demonstrated efficacy in reducing the duration of aphthae. These effects have generally been attributed to reduction in secondary infection of the open ulcerative lesion. With these products, however, patient intolerance of the burning from the alcohol content is of concern. The newer alcohol-free antimicrobial rinses have not been evaluated. Immunocompromised patients, such as those with AIDS, may have severe ulcer recurrences and thalidomide has been approved for these patients on an FDA orphan drug approved basis. See Periodontal Diseases on page 1748 for HIV-related periodontal considerations.

Two other conditions should be mentioned here since their diagnosis and management requires consideration of all of the ulcerative, erosive, and painful oral mucosal disorders. Necrotizing ulcerative gingivitis (NUG) is a condition that has been recognized for many years. The name historically included the term "acute"; however, most investigators have discontinued this because there is not a chronic form of the disease and it is unnecessary to consider it as anything other than necrotizing gingivitis. The organism *Fusobacterium nucleatum* has been implicated with several other organisms particularly Spirochetes in this condition. The infections seem to occur primarily following periods of psychological stress and this is the most common unifying factor in patients who suffer with NUG. In addition, immunosuppression, smoking, and local trauma have also been implicated. Generally, the classical appearance of NUG includes punched-out interdental papillae that are inflamed and appear blunted, somewhat necrotic at their tips. A pseudomembrane often is present and a strong fetor oris is usually present. The patient sometimes has fever and malaise as well. The treatment is generally conservative using gentle debridement. There is some benefit in using antibiotics such metronidazole, tetracycline, or amoxicillin. Historically, some clinicians have also chosen to add a vitamin supplement, generally a vitamin B complex with vitamin C, to help with the mucosal healing.

Another condition occasionally encountered is plasma cell gingivitis, a diffuse but intense erythema of the gingival complex, including a rapid onset and soreness to the oral gingival tissues. The implicated etiologies in plasma cell gingivitis include various chewing gums, toothpastes with herbal additives, as well as spicy candies, mints, peppers, and other potential allergens. The treatment of plasma cell gingivitis is local use of topical steroids; although by removing the dietary stimulant, generally the condition will resolve spontaneously. If plasma cell gingivitis is being considered as a diagnosis, the autoimmune desquamative gingival diseases must also be considered, including lichen planus, mucous membrane pemphigoid, and pemphigus. A biopsy is usually necessary to determine a diagnosis.

MILD TO MODERATE FORMS OF ULCERATIONS AND EROSIONS

There are several over-the-counter preparations that may give the patient some or total relief, including Ulcerease, BetaCell oral rinse, Cankermelts-GX, Gelclair Bioadherent Oral Gel, Orabase Sooth-N-Seal, OraMoist Dry Mouth Patch, OraPatch, Ricinol P.R.N., Zilactin gel, Canker Cover, Avamin Melts, Benzoin tincture saturated swabsticks, and Orajel Protective Mouth Sore Discs.

Aloclair (Ameseal) is now available as a spray. It is marketed by OMNI Preventive Care as an oral lesion pain relief spray, useful for indications related to aphthous ulcerations and other mild-to-moderate oral erosions. Its prescription companion preparation Gelclair has been suggested for use in the management of mucositis. Oralone is a new formulation of triamcinolone acetonide dental paste which had previously been available as Kenalog in Orabase.

A prescription viscous, mucoadhesive polymer rinse, MuGard, provides a protective coating to the oral mucosa and can help protect against oral mucositis.

SYMPTOMATIC GEOGRAPHIC TONGUE (BENIGN MIGRATORY GLOSSITIS, ERYTHEMA MIGRANS)

Geographic tongue is a localized, transitory loss of the tongue's filiform papillae. Although disconcerting in appearance, it usually is asymptomatic; however, occasionally patients will report a burning sensation. Fungal colonization has been implicated in symptomatic geographic tongue and this condition needs to be ruled out as a contributing factor (see Fungal Infections on page 1752).

After infection has been ruled out, palliation for symptomatic geographic tongue can sometimes be achieved with an approach similar to managing minor oral ulcerations. Benadryl elixir, a potent antihistamine, is used in the oral cavity primarily as a mild topical anesthetic agent for the symptomatic relief of certain allergic deficiencies which should be ruled out as possible etiologies for the oral condition under treatment. It is often used alone as well as in 50:50 solutions with agents such as Kaopectate or Maalox to assist in coating the oral mucosa. Benadryl can also be used systemically in capsule form although the elixir mixed with a coating agent as above provides excellent palliation prior to meals. Frequently, Benadryl alone or in combination with the above agents will be very effective in the relief of symptomatic geographic tongue.

Attapulgite
Chlorhexidine Gluconate (Oral) on page 334
Clobetasol on page 377
Debacterol
Dexamethasone (Systemic) on page 463
DiphenhydrAMINE (Systemic) on page 502
Fluocinonide ointment with Orabase on page 691
Lactobacillus on page 869
MetroNIDAZOLE (Systemic) on page 1011
Mouthwash (Antiseptic) on page 1062
PredniSONE on page 1260
Tetracaine (Topical) on page 1428
Tetracycline (Systemic) on page 1431
Thalidomide on page 1435
Triamcinolone (Topical) on page 1490

EROSIVE LICHEN PLANUS AND OTHER VESICULOEROSIVE DISEASES

Lichen planus is a chronic dermatologic disease that often affects the oral tissues. The name was first selected in 1869 because of the flat appearance of the white lesions on the oral mucosa. The etiology of lichen planus is unknown but significant associations have been made with Hepatitis C and the drug induced form called lichenoid mucositis. Clinically the lesions are identical to the dermatologic form of lichen planus but significant treatment response may be more difficult to achieve.

Lichen planus ranges from being totally asymptomatic to severely painful when present in its erosive forms. Reticular forms of lichen planus with no erosions show a white lacy pattern that has become pathognomic for the condition. The lesions on the skin often have a purplish hue and form slightly raised, pruritic papules, with an occasional white lacy or silvery appearance to the borders of the lesions. Patients do not need to have the skin lesions in order to suffer with oral lichen planus. The diagnosis of lichen planus is best performed by histopathology; however, often the pathognomic appearance and distribution of the lesions allows a presumptive diagnosis to be made from the clinical appearance. Generally, the erosive forms of lichen planus require treatment based on the extent, severity, and pain level of the patient in question. Autoimmune desquamative gingival diseases, including pemphigoid and pemphigus, must also be considered. A biopsy is necessary to determine a diagnosis and systemic work-up for related disease effects must be completed in consultation with patient's physicians. Because of the clinical similarities of these vesiculoerosive diseases, an additional biopsy specimen is needed for diagnostic confirmation; the specimen is placed in Michel's transport media and then direct immunofluorescent studies are performed.

Elixir of dexamethasone, a potent steroidal anti-inflammatory agent, is used topically (as a 5-minute rinse and expectorate) in the management of acute episodes of erosive lichen planus and other vesiculo-erosive disease processes such as benign mucous membrane pemphigoid and pemphigus vulgaris. Some patients will not achieve relief from topical agents and systemic delivery either by swish and swallow or tablets may be necessary. Prednisone corticosteroid tablets are a popular and often effective starting point with a regimen consisting of burst therapy (eg, as high as 60 mg) for several days followed by 7 to 10 days of a maintenance tapering dose. Prescription of a Medrol Dose Pack (which includes a tapering dose over 6 days of 4 mg methylprednisolone), followed by a selected dose, such as 10 mg of prednisone daily and an oral steroid rinse such as dexamethasone can achieve the same effect. Due to the chronicity of these lesions long-term maintenance steroids are usually necessary to achieve control. Historically there has always been a concern that oral erosive lichen planus (ELP) has an association with oral cancer (OC). There has never been a direct relationship established, but because of the clinical similarity in appearance of ELP and OC the clinician must follow patients closely, and any area that does not improve with the above appropriate therapies must be considered suspect and should be rebiopsied to rule out premalignant changes.

Immunosuppressant agents, such as tacrolimus (Protopic), hydroxychloroquine (Plaquenil), and pimecrolimus (Elidel), have shown some efficacy in off-label applications for severe cases. Prolonged use should be carried out in consult with the patient's physician and with a periodical Plaquenil-related ophthalmologic examination. Continued supervision of the patient during treatment is essential and the dentist must be aware that treatment of any secondary infections such as fungal overgrowth may be essential in gaining control of the erosive lesions. Also, patients should be counseled that maximum benefit of the medication will be achieved when oral hygiene is maintained at excellent levels.

For examples of sample prescriptions see Ulcerative and Erosive Disorders - Sample Prescriptions on page 46

BURNING MOUTH SYNDROME

Burning mouth syndrome (BMS) is a relatively common condition, of unknown etiology, and is a significant problem when it occurs, both in diagnosis and in management. Individuals often experience a burning or a scalding pain on the lips, tongue, and sometimes other parts of the oral cavity (eg, anterior hard palate). There are often no visible signs of irritation that the clinician can identify. The etiology of burning mouth syndrome remains unknown. The syndrome has been associated with many systemic conditions, ranging from vitamin deficiencies to the onset of menopause. It is estimated that nearly 5% of the population around the age of 60 may suffer with this condition. The symptoms often include burning mouth, dry mouth, a bitter or metallic taste, other taste alterations, changes in the patient's ability to eat, and onset of pain while attempting to sleep. Systemic conditions associated with BMS are abnormal hormonal fluctuations, diabetes, deficiencies in iron, zinc, and vitamins such as thiamine, B_{12}, niacin, complications associated with cancer therapy, and some patients report that the burning mouth syndrome symptoms occur after dental procedures. Three patterns of pain are reported:

- Type 1: pain absent on waking and developing during the day
- Type 2: pain present day and night
- Type 3: intermittent pain, with pain-free days

Abnormal taste (dysgeusia, parageusia) is either a metallic or bitter taste in the mouth or altered perception of taste particularly of salty or sweet/sour foods. Although the patient may perceive a dryness of the mouth, reduced saliva production is not confirmed on testing.

The evaluation of a patient complaining of burning mouth begins with a detailed history/process of elimination and may lead to a biopsy to determine if any organic reason for the condition is identifiable. Dry mouth often accompanies burning mouth. The clinician should culture the tongue or oral mucosa to rule out oral fungal colonization. A normal hematologic work up will ensure that there is no developing diabetes, allergy, or abnormal liver or thyroid condition. The clinician should carefully examine all of the surfaces of the tissues to see if there are any abrasive components caused by rough teeth or prostheses. It is often necessary to have the patient evaluated by their primary care physician because of the common association of BMS with high stress situations, common in the process of aging. The condition has the features of a neuropathy and could be related to the production of toxic radicals that may be released at the cellular level during times of stress.

These widely divergent hypotheses related to the etiology of BMS have led to equally broad therapeutic suggestions. A variety of drugs have been suggested, including: Topical rinses and anesthetics for palliative management, clonazepam 0.25 to 3 mg/day, amitriptyline 25 to 100 mg/day, nortriptyline 10 to 50 mg/day, gabapentin 900 to 1,500 mg/day, and doxepin cream, applied to the areas affected. Various studies indicate that alpha-lipoic acid in an initial dose of 600 mg may be used with a dose reduction to 200 mg after the initial 20 days. The rationale for attempting alpha-lipoic acid is the relationship between its antioxidant effects and the levels of glutathione and reduction of free radicals cellularly. In addition to alpha-lipoic acid, capsaicin has been used with some success. Capsaicin has been a prescription drug useful in arthritis care as a topical skin product. It has also been prescribed to assist with patients who have had shingles, post herpetic pain neuropathies associated with diabetes and other neuralgias. Its applications in oral use have been studied in very limited trials; however, it has recently been reevaluated in a 0.75% topical application for use in BMS and oral mucositis. Curcumin, the active agent in turmeric, has been recommended to treat BMS, although placebo-controlled trials have not been completed to suggest any consistent response to these products. All of the medications suggested for managing burning mouth are off-label uses and there are limited data from placebo controlled clinical trials.

During a Cochrane analysis, nine clinical trials were reviewed. Of the nine trials, three interventions demonstrated reduction in BMS and all of these included varying effects of clonazepam and alpha-lipoic acid. Although the other trials considered randomized double-blind trials, study designs were small and lacked power to draw and define conclusions. There is little evidence to provide a clear standard of care for treating patients with burning mouth syndrome to date. The clinician must always be aware of this lack of conclusive evidence. These drugs should be selected and managed in collaboration with the patient's physician, particularly since many of these patients suffering with burning mouth syndrome have complicated medical histories including the use of additional medications that could be affected.

REFERENCES AND SELECTED READINGS

Aggarwal BB, Sundaram C, Malani N, Ichikawa H. Curcumin: the Indian solid gold. *Adv Exp Med Biol.* 2007;595:1-75.

Baud CM, Colon LE, Gerberich J, et al. Protection from radiation-induced oral mucositis by MuGard oral rinse a clinical study and *in silico* analysis. Poster presentation at the 18th International MASCC/ISOO supportive care in cancer symposium. 2006. Available at http://www.accesspharma.com/downloads/product-programs/MuGard-Poster.pdf

Buchanan J, Zakrzewska J. Burning mouth syndrome. *Clin Evid (online).* 2008. Available at http://www.ncbi.nlm.nih.gov/pmc/articles/PMC2907957/pdf/2008-1301.pdf.

Carrozzo M, Thorpe R. Oral lichen planus: a review. *Minerva Stomatol.* 2009;58(10):519-537.

Chakrabarty AK, Mraz S, Geisse JK, Anderson NJ. Aphthous ulcers associated with imiquimod and the treatment of actinic cheilitis. *J Am Acad Dermatol.* 2005;52(2 Suppl 1):35-37.

Donovan JC, Hayes RC, Burgess K, Leong IT, Rosen CF. Refractory erosive oral lichen planus associated with hepatitis C: response to topical tacrolimus ointment. *J Cutan Med Surg.* 2005;9(2):43-46.

Femiano F, Gombos F, Scully C. Burning mouth syndrome: open trial of psychotherapy alone, medication with alpha-lipoic acid (thioctic acid), and combination therapy. *Med Oral.* 2004;9(1):8-13.

Goel A, Kunnumakkara AB, Aggarwal BB. Curcumin as "Curecumin": from kitchen to clinic. *Biochem Pharmacol.* 2008;75(4):787-809.

Gremeau-Richard C, Woda A, Navez ML, et al. Topical clonazepam in stomatodynia: a randomised placebo-controlled study. *Pain.* 2004;108 (1-2):51-57.

Hatcher H, Planalp R, Cho J, Torti FM, Torti SV. Curcumin: from ancient medicine to current clinical trials. *Cell Mol Life Sci.* 2008;65(11):1631-1652.

Heckmann SM, Heckmann JG, Ungethüm A, Hujoel P, Hummel T. Gabapentin has little or no effect in the treatment of burning mouth syndrome – results of an open-label pilot study. *Eur J Neurol.* 2006;13(7):e6-e7.

Hens MJ, Alonso-Ferreira V, Villaverde-Hueso A, Abaitua I, Posada de la Paz M. Cost-effectiveness analysis of burning mouth syndrome therapy. *Community Dent Oral Epidemiol.* 2012;40(2):185-192.

Kutluay SB, Doroghazi J, Roemer ME, Triezenberg SJ. Curcumin inhibits herpes simplex virus immediate-early gene expression by a mechanism independent of p300/CBP histone acetyltransferase activity. *Virology.* 2008;373(2):239-247.

Lodi G, Pellicano R, Carrozzo M. Hepatitis C virus infection and lichen planus: a systematic review with meta-analysis. *Oral Dis.* 2010;16(7):601-612.

Mínguez Serra MP, Salort Llorca C, Silvestre Donat FJ. Pharmacological treatment of burning mouth syndrome: a review and update. *Med Oral Patol Oral Cir Bucal.* 2007;12(4):E299-E304.

Olivier V, Lacour JP, Mousnier A, Garraffo R, Monteil RA, Ortonne JP. Treatment of chronic erosive oral lichen planus with low concentrations of topical tacrolimus: an open prospective study. *Arch Dermatol.* 2002;138(10):1335-1338.

Patton LL, Siegel MA, Benoliel R, De Laat A. Management of burning mouth syndrome: systematic review and management recommendations. *Oral Surg Oral Med Oral Pathol Oral Radiol Endod.* 2007;103(Suppl S39):e1-e13.

Petruzzi M, Lauritano D, De Benedittis M, Baldoni M, Serpico R. Systemic capsaicin for burning mouth syndrome: short-term results of a pilot study. *J Oral Pathol Med.* 2004;33(2):111-114.

Petti S, Rabiei M, De Luca M, Scully C. The magnitude of the association between hepatitis C virus infection and oral lichen planus: meta-analysis and case control study. *Odontology.* 2011;99(2):168-178.

Thomson MA, Hamburger J, Stewart DG, Lewis HM. Treatment of erosive oral lichen planus with topical tacrolimus. *J Dermatolog Treat.* 2004;15 (5):308-314.

Vidal MA, Martinez-Fernandez E, Martinez-Vazquez de Castro J, et al. Diabetic neuropathy: effectiveness of amitriptyline and gabapentin. *Rev Soc Esp Dolor.* 2004;11(8):38-52.

White TL, Kent PF, Kurtz DB, Emko P. Effectiveness of gabapentin for treatment of burning mouth syndrome. *Arch Otolaryngol Head Neck Surg.* 2004;130(6):786-788.

Yeon KY, Kim SA, Kim YH, et al. Curcumin produces an antihyperalgesic effect via antagonism of TRPV1. *J Dent Res.* 2010;89(2):170-174.

Zakrzewska JM, Forssell H, Glenny AM. Interventions for the treatment of burning mouth syndrome. *Cochrane Database Syst Rev.* 2005.

DENTIN HYPERSENSITIVITY, ACID EROSION, HIGH CARIES INDEX, MANAGEMENT OF ALVEOLAR OSTEITIS, AND XEROSTOMIA

DENTIN HYPERSENSITIVITY

Dentinal hypersensitivity is one of the most commonly encountered clinical problems. It is an exaggerated response to application of a stimulus to exposed dentine, regardless of its location. True hypersensitivity can develop due to pulpal inflammation and can present the clinical features of irreversible pulpitis, ie, severe and persistent pain, as compared with typical short sharp pain of dentinal hypersensitivity. Suggested steps in resolving dentin hypersensitivity when a thorough exam has ruled-out any other source for the problem:

Treatment Steps

- Home treatment with a desensitizing toothpaste containing potassium nitrate (used to brush teeth as well as a thin layer applied, each night for 2 weeks)
- If needed, in office potassium oxalate (Protect by Butler) and/or in office fluoride iontophoresis
- If sensitivity is still not tolerable to the patient, consider pumice then dentin adhesive and unfilled resin or composite restoration overlaying a glass ionomer base
- The use of 5% sodium fluoride varnishes (Duraflor and Duraphat) have been encouraged for the prevention of decay in persons of high-risk populations and also show some efficacy for reducing sensitivity following multiple applications.
- Gluma is a brand name desensitizer used in dentistry to treat sensitivity. The product is manufactured by Heraeus Kulzer. Its formula of 5% glutaraldehyde and 35% HEMA (hydroxyethyl methacrylate) in water is used to help control both hypersensitive dentin and reduce the incidence of postoperative sensitivity in restorative dentistry procedures.
- Crest Sensi-Stop Strips (Procter & Gamble, Cincinnati, OH) are a patented strip technology layered with an oxalate-containing gel, shown to provide immediate relief from hypersensitivity pain after a single use.

Home Products (all contain nitrate as active ingredient):

Promise
Denquel
Sensodyne
THERADENT

Other major brand name companies have added ingredients to their dentifrice product lines that also make hypersensitivity claims.

REFERENCE

Addy M. Dentine hypersensitivity: new perspectives on an old problem. *Int Dent J.* 2002;52(5)(suppl 1):367-375.
Carey C. Tooth whitening: what we now know. *J Evid Based Dent Pract.* 2014;14(suppl):70-76.
Kassab M, Cohen R. The etiology and prevalence of gingival recession. *JADA.* 2003;134(2):220-225.
Lussi A, ed. *Dental erosion: from diagnosis to therapy. Monogr Oral Sci.* Vol. 20. New York, NY: Karger Publishers; 2006;9-16.
Marvin KL. Bright, white, and sensitive: an overview of tooth whitening and dentin hypersensitivity. http://www.dentistrytoday.com/oral-medicine/1521–sp-1526021429. Published 2008. Accessed July 12, 2017.
Miglani S, Aggarwal V, Ahuja B. Dentin hypersensitivity: Recent trends in management. *J Conserv Dent.* 2010;13(4):218-224.
Saylor C and Overman P. Dentinal hypersensitivity: a review. https://www.dentalacademyofce.com/courses/2573%2FPDF%2F1402cei_saylor_web.-pdf. Published 2011. Accessed July 12, 2017.

ACID EROSION

Acid erosion is the loss of tooth enamel through prolonged exposure to acid rich foods, beverages, and even fruits. The problem has been raised primarily in pediatric patients and can be significant. Several oral care products claim surface remineralization efficacy and should be coupled with dietary counseling to achieve a desirable reduction in tooth damage.

ReNew Remineralizing and Desensitizing Paste
Sensodyne ProNamel for Children
Recaldent, found in GC America's Prospec MI Paste with Recaldent and Trident XTRA CARE chewing gum
Amorphous calcium phosphate (ACP) found in Arm & Hammer Enamel Care Toothpaste
Premier Dental's Enamel Pro polishing paste
SensiStat, found in Ortek Therapeutic's ProClude and DenClude products
NovaMin, a synthetic mineral composed of calcium, sodium, phosphorus, and silica

ANTICARIES AGENTS

Fluoride (Gel 0.4%, Rinse 0.05%) on page 693

Toothpastes with triclosan such as Colgate Total show promise for combined treatment/prevention of caries, plaque, and gingivitis. The use of 5% sodium fluoride varnishes (Duraflor and Duraphat) have been encouraged for the prevention of decay in persons of high-risk populations.

FLUORIDES

Used for the prevention of demineralization of the tooth structure secondary to xerostomia. For patients with long-term or permanent xerostomia, daily application is accomplished using custom applicator trays, such as omnivac. Patients with porcelain crowns should use a neutral pH fluoride (see Fluoride monograph on page 693). Final selection of a fluoride product and/or saliva replacement/stimulant product must be based on patient comfort, taste, and ultimately, compliance. Experience has demonstrated that, often times, patients must try various combinations to achieve the greatest effect and their highest comfort levels. The presence of mucositis during cancer management complicates the clinician's selection of products.

Over-the-Counter (OTC) Products

Form	Brand Name	Strength/Size
Gel, topical (stannous fluoride)	Gel-Kam (cinnamon, fruit and berry, mint flavors)	0.4% (129 g)
Rinse, topical (as sodium)	ACT	0.05% [0.02%] (500 mL, 532 mL)

Adapted from: Wynn RL, Meiller TF, Crossley HL. *Drug Information Handbook for Dentistry*, 25th ed. Hudson, OH: Lexi-Comp, Inc; 2019.

Prescription Only (Rx) Products

Form	Brand Name	Strength/Size
Drops, oral (as sodium)	Fluor-A-Day	0.278 mg/drop [0.125 mg/drop] (30 mL)
	Flura-Drops	0.55 mg/drop [0.25 mg/drop] (24 mL)
Gel, topical (as sodium)	PreviDent (mint, berry flavors)	1.1% (56 g)
Lozenge (as sodium)	Lozi-Flur	2.21 mg [1 mg]
Rinse, topical (as sodium)	Fluorinse	0.2% (480 mL)
Solution, oral (as sodium)	Phos-Flur (bubblegum, grape, mint flavors)	0.044% (473 mL, 500 mL)
Tablet (as sodium)		0.55 mg [0.25 mg]; 1.1 mg [0.5 mg]; 2.2 mg [1 mg]
	Fluor-A-Day	0.55 mg [0.25 mg]
Chewable	Fluor-A-Day, Fluoritab	1.1 mg [0.5 mg]
	Fluor-A-Day, Fluoritab	2.2 mg [1 mg]
Varnish	Duraflor (bubblegum flavor)	5% (1 mL/dose) (10 mL)

Adapted from: Wynn RL, Meiller TF, Crossley HL. *Drug Information Handbook for Dentistry*, 25th ed. Hudson, OH: Lexi-Comp, Inc; 2019.

In-Office-Only Products

Form	Brand Name	Strength/Size
Gel, topical (as acidulated phosphate)	60 Second Taste Gel (bubblegum, chocolate and vanilla, groovy grape, marshmallow, mint, orange twist, strawberry flavors)	1.23% (16 oz bottle) [equivalent to 1.23% F ion]
	Denti-Care 60 Second Fluoride Gel (bubblegum, cherry, grape, mint, orange, strawberry, raspberry flavors)	1.23% (16 oz bottle) [equivalent to 1.23% F ion]
	Iris 60-second (orange smoothie, bubblegum, summer strawberry, California grape, fresh mint flavors)	1.23% (16 oz bottle) [equivalent to 1.23% F ion]
	Kolorz Sixty Second Fluoride Gel (blue raspberry, cherry cheesecake, cotton candy, pina colada, triple mint flavors)	1.23% (16 oz bottle) [equivalent to 1.23% F ion]
	Nupro Fluoride Gel (bubblegum, wild cherry flavors)	1.23% (12 oz bottle) [equivalent to 1.23% F ion]
	PCxx (banana berry, Bazooka bubblegum, grape explosion, mocha cappuccino, marshmallow float, crème de menthe, pina colada, cool peppermint, rootbeer float, raspberry blast, screamin' strawberry, vanilla orange, watermelon splash, wild cherry flavors)	1.23% (16.6 oz bottle) [equivalent 1.23% F ion]
	PediaGel (bubblegum, goofy grape, super strawberry flavors)	1.23% (12 oz bottle) [equivalent to 1.23% F ion]
	Perfect Choice One Minute APF Gel (creamy marshmallow, juicy grape, peppermint stick, pink bubblegum, strawberry delight, vanilla orange, way out watermelon flavors)	1.23% (17½ oz bottle) [equivalent to 1.23% F ion]
	Topex 00:60 APF Second Gel (bubble fun, cherry, mint, orange cream, pina colada flavors)	1.23% (16 oz bottle) [equivalent to 1.23% F ion]
	Zap Gel (bubblegum, cotton candy, grape, marshmallow, orange vanilla, strawberry, watermelon, dye-free mint flavors)	1.23% with xylitol (gluten free) (16 oz bottle) [equivalent to 1.23% F ion]
Gel, topical (as neutral sodium)	Denti-Care Neutral Sodium Fluoride Gel (mint, strawberry, raspberry flavors)	2% (16 oz bottle) [equivalent to 0.9% F ion]
	Nupro (apple cinnamon, mandarin orange, mint flavors)	2% (12 oz bottle) [equivalent to 0.9% F ion]
	PCxx (Bazooka bubblegum, mocha cappuccino, crème de menthe, cool peppermint, raspberry blast, vanilla orange, watermelon splash flavors)	2% (16.6 oz bottle) [equivalent 0.9% F ion]
	PediaGel (apple cinnamon, orange vanilla, way cool spearmint flavors)	2% (12 oz bottle) [equivalent to 0.9% F Ion]
	pH 7 Neutral Fluoride Gel (mint flavor)	2% (16 oz bottle) [equivalent to 0.9% F ion]
	Topex Neutral pH (clearly strawberry [dye-free], mint, pina colada flavors)	2% (16 oz bottle) [equivalent 0.9% F ion]
	Zap Gel (mint flavor)	2% (16 oz bottle) [equivalent to 0.9% F ion]
Foam, topical (as acidulated phosphate)	Denti-Care Denti-Foam (bubblegum, grape, mint, orange, strawberry flavors)	1.23% APF [equivalent to 1.23% F ion]
	Kolorz Sixty Second (blue raspberry, cherry cheesecake, cotton candy, triple mint flavors)	1.23% (125 g) [equivalent to 1.23% F ion]
	Nupro (bubblegum, orange vanilla, spearmint, strawberry flavors)	1.23% (125 g) [equivalent to 1.23% F ion]
	Oral B Minute-Foam (banana splitz, bubblegum, grape punch, mellow mint, orange-A Tangy, strawberry flavors)	1.23% (165 g) [equivalent to 1.23% F]
	PCxx (wild cherry, Bazooka bubblegum, cool peppermint, screamin' strawberry, grape explosion, luscious lime, mocha cappuccino, raspberry blast, vanilla orange flavors)	1.23% [equivalent 1.23% F ion]
	P.U.F.F Fluoride Foam (cotton candy, peppy mint, tropical blast, very berry, wild strawberry flavors)	1.23% (210 g) [equivalent to 1.23% F ion]
	Topex 00:60 Second Foam (bubble fun, grape, orange dream, spearmint, strawberry flavors)	1.23% (125 g) [equivalent to 1.23% F]
	Waterpik UltraControl (bubblegum, melon, mint, strawberry flavors)	1.23% (125 g) [equivalent to 1.23% F]

In-Office-Only Products *(continued)*

Form	Brand Name	Strength/Size
Foam, topical (as sodium)	DentiCare Pro-Foam Neutral (mint, raspberry flavors)	2% (125 g) [equivalent to 0.9% F]
	Kolorz Neutral (triple mint flavor)	2% (125 g) [equivalent to 0.9% F]
	Oral B Neutra-Foam (mint flavor)	2% (165 g) [equivalent to 0.9% F]
	PCxx (Bazooka bubblegum, cool peppermint, vanilla orange, screamin' strawberry, neutral [no flavor] flavors)	2% (210 g) [equivalent to 0.9% F]
	Topex Neutral (mixed berry flavor)	2% (125 g) [equivalent to 0.9% F]
Varnish, topical (as sodium)	Butler (bubblegum, melon madness flavors)	5% (0.5 mL/dose) (36/pkg) [equivalent to 2.26% F]
	CavityShield (bubblegum flavor)	5% (0.25 mL/dose) (32/pkg, 200/pkg) [equivalent to 2.26% F]
	CavityShield (bubblegum flavor)	5% (0.4 mL/dose) (32/pkg, 200/pkg) [equivalent to 2.26% F]
	Colgate Duraphat	5% (1 mL/dose) (10 mL/tube) [equivalent to 2.26% F]
	Colgate PreviDent (mint, raspberry flavors)	5% (0.40 mL/dose) (50/pkg) [equivalent to 2.26% F]
	Duraflor (bubblegum flavor)	5% (1 mL/dose) (10 mL/tube) [equivalent to 2.26% F]
	Duraflor (bubblegum flavor)	5% (0.25 mL/dose) (32/pkg, 200/pkg) [equivalent to 2.26% F]
	Duraflor (rasberry flavor)	5% (0.40 mL/dose) (32/pkg, 200/pkg) [equivalent to 2.26% F]
	Duraflor Halo (spearment, wildberry flavors)	5% (0.50 mL/dose) (32/pkg, 250/pkg) [equivalent to 2.26% F]
	DuraShield Clear (strawberry, watermelon flavors)	5% (0.40 mL/dose) (50/pkg, 200/pkg) [equivalent to 2.26% F]
	Embrace (bubblegum flavor)	5% (0.40 mL/dose) (50/pkg, 200/pkg) [equivalent to 2.26% F]
	Enamel Pro (bubblegum, strawberries n cream, vanilla mint flavors	5% (0.40 mL/dose) (35/pkg, 200/pkg) [equivalent to 2.26% F]
	Enamel Pro Clear (bubblegum flavor)	5% (0.25 mL/dose) (35/pkg) [equivalent to 2.26% F]
	FluoroDose (bubblegum, cherry, melon, mint flavors)	5% (0.30 mL/dose) (120/pkg, 600/pkg, 1200/pkg) [equivalent to 2.26% F]
	Flor-Opal (bubblegum, white mint flavors)	5% (0.50 mL/dose) (40/pkg) [equivalent to 2.26% F]
	Iris (bubblegum, mint, raspberry flavors)	5% sodium fluoride (0.40 mL/dose) [equivalent to 2.26% F]
	Kolorz ClearShield (bubblegum, mint, watermelon flavors)	5% (0.40 mL/dose) (35/pkg, 200/pkg) [equivalent to 2.26% F]
	MI Varnish with RECALDENT (fresh strawberry flavor)	5% (0.50 mL/dose) (50/pkg) [equivalent to 2.26% F]
	Nupro (raspberry flavor)	5% (0.25 mL/dose) [equivalent to 2.26% F]
	Nupro White Varnish (grape, raspberry flavors)	5% (0.40 mL/dose) (50/pkg,100/pkg, 500/pkg) [equivalent to 2.26% F]
	Profluorid (caramel, cherry, melon, mint flavors)	5% (1 mL/dose) (10 mL/tube) [equivalent to 2.26% F]
	Profluorid (caramel, cherry, melon, mint, mixed flavors)	5% (0.40 mL/dose) (48/pkg, 50/pkg, 200/pkg) [equivalent to 2.26% F]
	Profluorid (melon flavor)	5% (0.25 mL) (kids) (50/pkg) [equivalent to 2.26% F]
	Sparkle V (bubblegum, mint flavors)	5% (0.40 mL/dose) (120/pkg) [equivalent to 2.26% F]
	Ultra Thin (bubblegum, melon, mint, strawberry, mixed flavors)	5% (0.40 mL/dose) (25/pkg, 30/pkg, 100/pkg) [equivalent to 2.26% F]
	Vanish (cherry, melon, mint, mixed flavors)	5% Sodium Fluoride White Varnish with TCP (0.50 mL/dose) (50/pkg, 100/pkg, 1000/pkg) [equivalent to 2.26% F]
	Vella (bubblegum, melon, mint, strawberry flavors)	5% Sodium Fluoride Varnish with Xylitol (0.5 mL/dose) (35/pkg, 100/pkg) [equivalent to 2.26% F]
Other fluoride varnishes	Fluor Protector	1% (0.9% difluorsilane) (0.4 mL/dose) (20/pkg) [equivalent to 0.10% F]

ANTIMICROBIAL ORAL RINSE

Chlorhexidine Gluconate (Oral) (Peridex) on page 334
Chlorhexidine Gluconate (Oral) alcohol-free (CHX) on page 334
Mouthwash (Antiseptic) (Listerine) on page 1062

For examples of sample prescriptions see Antimicrobial Oral Rinse on page 34

MANAGEMENT OF ALVEOLAR OSTEITIS

Alveolar osteitis, as compared to simple postoperative pain, occurs in about 2% to 5% of extractions. Factors affecting risk include the complexity of the extraction and other factors, such as smoking, excessive spitting, or poor wound care in the first 5 to 7 days after extraction. Wound healing is a complex process and can be affected by many factors. Alveolar osteitis is the most common healing disturbance of extraction sockets.

Several types of alveolar osteitis can result from disturbances in the healing process. The type that is commonly referred to as dry socket occurs when the initial blood clot that forms after tooth extraction is disturbed or lost during early healing. The healing tissue that normally replaces the blood clot (granulation tissue) fails to grow or is disrupted after beginning to grow, leading to alveolar osteitis. Alveolar osteitis is characterized by grayish slough, moderate to severe pain, and foul odor. The foul odor is a result of a breakdown of the blood clot by putrefaction, rather than by orderly retraction, leaving bare bone visible in the socket. Suppurative osteitis results when the disturbance of extraction socket wound healing is later (usually after day 14), results in infection, and exhibits a purulence in the extraction socket. Disruption of the clot can also result in necrotizing osteitis with bony sequestra.

Signs and Symptoms of Dry Socket or Postop Infection

1. Moderate to severe pain beginning 2 to 5 days after tooth extraction
2. Loss of the blood clot or visible bone in extraction site
3. Foul odor or unpleasant taste in mouth
4. Tenderness or swelling of lymph nodes around jaw
5. At the first signs of suppurative osteitis, antibiotics must be considered.

Treatments of Dry Socket

Irrigation and medicated dressings are primary ways to treat dry socket. Active ingredients in these sedative dressings usually include substances like soluble aspirin, zinc oxide, and eugenol made from oil of cloves. It is usually necessary to repeat treatment for 2 to 5 consecutive days, although it may take longer.

Resorbable dry socket products in the market include:

- Eugenol-soaked Gelfoam can be a one-time treatment with as needed follow-up if necessary
- Alvogyl by Septodont is resorbable but cannot be used on patients having a history of allergic reactions to procaine-type anesthetics or iodine

Nonresorbable dry socket products: **Note:** Must be removed and some have radiopaque markers; thus, patient compliance to return daily must be considered.

- Sultan Dry Socket Paste or Dry Socket Remedy is placed on a gauze strip and packed into the socket, follow-up and removal is needed (guaiacol, balsam peru, eugenol, 1.6% chlorobutanol); used to treat alveolitis and provides instant pain relief. Paste is introduced into socket with flat-bladed instrument, tamped down to cover exposed bone, and allowed to remain in the socket for 3 to 5 days. This is nonresorbable but is claimed to wash out gradually as socket heals.
- Dressol-X by Rainbow is another nonresorbable packing material with radiopaque marker; it contains aspirin and must not be used on patients with ASA allergy or G6PD deficiency.

REFERENCES

Benko P. Emergency dental procedures. Roberts J, et al, eds. *Clinical Procedures in Emergency Medicine*. 5th ed. Philadelphia, Pa.: Saunders Elsevier; 2009.

Cardoso CL, Rodrigues MT, Ferreira Júnior O, Garlet GP, de Carvalho PS. Clinical concepts of dry socket. *J Oral Maxillofac Surg*. 2010;68 (8):1922-1932.

Noroozi AR, Philbert RF. Modern concepts in understanding and management of the "dry socket" syndrome: comprehensive review of the literature. *Oral Surg Oral Med Oral Pathol Oral Radiol Endod*. 2009;107(1):30-35.

MANAGEMENT OF SIALORRHEA

In patients suffering with medical conditions that result in hypersalivation, the dentist may determine that it is appropriate to use an atropine sulfate medication to achieve a dry field for dental procedures or to reduce excessive drooling. Currently there is one ADA approved medication sold under the name of Sal-Tropine. Pro-Banthine (propantheline bromide), an antimuscarinic used for excessive stomach acid production is advocated by some for off-label use. See Atropine (Systemic)

XEROSTOMIA

Xerostomia refers to the subjective sensation of a dry mouth while salivary gland hypofunction can be objectively measured. Numerous factors can play a role in the patient's perception of xerostomia. Changes in salivary function caused by drugs, surgical intervention, or treatment of cancer are among the leading causes of xerostomia. Other factors including aging, smoking, mouth breathing, and autoimmune disorders such as Sjögren syndrome, can also be implicated in a patient's perception of xerostomia. Human immunodeficiency virus (HIV) may produce xerostomia when viral changes in salivary glands are present. Xerostomia often occurs in patients taking antianxiety and antidepressant medication and often accompanies burning mouth syndrome. Xerostomia affects women more frequently than men and is also more common in older individuals. Some alteration in salivary function naturally occurs with age, but it is extremely difficult to quantify the effects. Xerostomia and salivary gland hypofunction in the elderly population are contributory to deterioration in the quality of life.

Once a diagnosis of xerostomia or salivary gland hypofunction is made and possible causes confirmed, treatment for the condition usually involves management of the underlying disease and avoidance of unnecessary medications. In addition, good hydration is essential and water is the drink of choice. Also, the use of artificial saliva substitutes, selected chewing gums, and/or toothpastes formulated to treat xerostomia, is often warranted. In more difficult cases, such as patients receiving radiotherapy for cancer of the head and neck regions or patients with Sjögren syndrome, systemic cholinergic stimulants may be administered if no contraindications exist. The clinician must also rule out and treat concomitant conditions such as fungal colonization and overgrowth which often occur subsequent to xerostomia.

XEROSTOMIA TREATMENTS

Because of the complex nature of xerostomia, management by the dental clinician is difficult. Treatment success is also difficult to assess and is often unsatisfactory. The salivary stimulants, pilocarpine and cevimeline, may aid in some conditions but are only approved for use as sialogogues in patients receiving radiotherapy and in Sjögren patients, specifically as described above. Artificial salivas are available as over-the-counter products and represent the potential for continuous application by the patient to achieve comfort for their xerostomic condition. Coenzyme Q_{10} (ubiquinone) has recently been proven successful with increasing saliva (100 mg daily) (Ryo 2011).

The role of the clinician in attempting treatment of dry mouth is to first achieve a differential diagnosis and to ensure that other conditions are not simultaneously present. For example, many patients suffer burning mouth syndrome or painful oral tissues with no obvious etiology accompanying dry mouth. Also, higher caries incidence may be associated with changes in salivary flow. As previously mentioned, Sjögren syndrome represents an immune complex of disorders that can affect the eyes, oral tissues, and other organ systems. The reader is referred to current oral pathology or oral medicine textbooks for review of signs and symptoms of Sjögren syndrome.

Treatment of cancer often leads to dry mouth. Surgical intervention removing salivary tissue due to the presence of a salivary gland tumor results in loss of salivary function. Also, many of the chemotherapeutic agents produce transitory changes in salivary flow, such that the patient may perceive a dry mouth during chemotherapy. Most notably related to salivary dysfunction is the use of radiation regimens to head and neck tissues. Tumors in or about salivary gland tissue, the oral cavity, and oropharynx are most notably sensitive to radiation therapy and subsequent dry mouth. In the head and neck, therapeutic radiation is commonly used in treatment of squamous cell carcinomas and lymphomas. The radiation level necessary to destroy malignant cells ranges from 40 to 70 Gy. Salivary tissue is extremely sensitive to radiation changes. Radiation dosages >30 Gy are sufficient to permanently change salivary function. In addition to the mucositis and subsequent secondary infection by fungal colonization or viral exacerbation, oral tissues can become exceptionally dry due to the effects of radiation on salivary glands. In fact, permanent damage to salivary gland tissue within the beam path produces significant levels of xerostomia in most patients. Some recovery may be noted by the patient. Most often, the effects are permanent and even progressive as the radiation dosage increases.

Artificial salivas do not produce any protectant or stimulation of the salivary gland. The use of pilocarpine and cevimeline as salivary stimulants in pre-emptive treatment, as well as postradiation treatment, have been shown to have some efficacy in management of dry mouth. The success rate, however, still is often unsatisfactory and post-treatment management by the dentist usually requires fluoride supplements to prevent radiation-induced caries due to dry mouth. Also, management of dry mouth through patient use of the artificial salivary gel, solutions and sprays, or other over-the-counter products for dry mouth (eg, chewing gum, toothpaste, mouthwash, swabsticks, sugar-free candy) is highly recommended. The use of pilocarpine or cevimeline should only be considered by the dentist in consultation with the managing physician. The oftentimes severe and widespread cholinergic side effects of pilocarpine and cevimeline mandate close monitoring of the patient and certain medical conditions contraindicated their use.

The use of artificial salivary substitutes is less problematic for the dentist. The dentist should, in considering selection of a drug, base his or her decision on patient compliance and comfort. Salivary substitutes presently on the market may have some benefit in terms of electrolyte balance and salivary consistency. However, the ultimate decision needs to be based on patients' taste, their willingness to use the medication ad libitum, and improvement in their comfort related to dry mouth. Many of the drugs are pH balanced to reduce additional risk of dental demineralization or caries. Oftentimes, the dentist must try numerous medications, one at a time, prior to finding one which gives the patient some comfort. Another gauge of acceptability is to investigate whether the artificial saliva substitute has the American Dental Association's seal of approval. Most of the currently accepted saliva substitute products have been evaluated by the ADA.

In general, considerations that the clinician might use in a prescribed regimen would be that saliva substitutes are meant to be used regularly throughout the day by the patient to achieve comfort during meals, reduce tissue abrasion, and prevent salivary stagnation on teeth. Other than these, there are no specific recommendations for patients. Recommendations by the dentist need to be tailored to the patient's acceptance. Salivary substitutes may provide an allergic potential in patients who are sensitive to some of the preservatives present in artificial saliva products. In addition to this allergic potential, there is a risk of microbial contamination by placement of the salivary substitute container in close contact with the oral cavity.

Patient education regarding the use of saliva substitutes is also part of the clinical approach. The patient with chronic xerostomia should be educated about regular professional care, high performance in dental hygiene, the need to reevaluate oral soft tissue pathology, and any changes that might occur long term. In patients with severe xerostomia, artificial salivary medications should be given in combination with topical fluoride treatment programs designed by the dentist to reduce caries (see Saliva Substitute monograph on page 1354).

REFERENCE

Ryo K, Ito A, Takatori R, et al. Effects of coenzyme Q_{10} on salivary secretion. *Clin Biochem*. 2011;44(8-9):669-674.

Products and Drugs to Treat Dry Mouth

Medication	Manufacturer and Phone Number	Product Type	Manufacturer's Description	Indication	Ingredients	Directions for Use	Form and Availability
Artificial Salivas (OTC)							
Biotene OralBalance Mouth Moisturizing Gel	Laclede Professional Products, Inc (800) 922-5856	Gel	Sugar-free oral lubricant; relieves dry mouth symptoms up to 8 hours; soothes and protects oral tissue to promote healing; helps to inhibit harmful bacteria; improves retention under dentures	Relieves symptoms of dry mouth: burning, itching, cotton palate, sore tissue swallowing difficulties	Contains the "Biotene" protective salivary enzyme system Active: Glucose oxidase (2,000 units), lactoperoxidase (3,000 units), lysozyme (5 mg), lactoferrin (5 mg) Other: Hydrogenated starch, xylitol, hydroxyethyl cellulose, glycerate polyhydrate, aloe vera	Using a clean fingertip, apply a 1" ribbon of gel on tongue; add additional amount of gel on other dry; use as needed	1.4 oz tube; available at mass merchandise stores, food stores, and drugstores
BreathTech Plaque Fighter Mouth Spray	Omnii Oral Pharmaceuticals (800) 445-3386	Pump dispenser	Plaque inhibitor in vanilla-mint flavor for breath malodor or reduced salivary flow	Treats the discomfort of oral dryness	Microdent patented plaque-inhibitor formula	Spray directly into mouth; spread over teeth and tissue with tongue	18 mL pump dispenser; order directly from manufacturer
Moi-Stir Moistening Solution	Kingswood Laboratories, Inc (800) 968-7772	Pump spray	Saliva supplement for moistening of mouth and mucosal area	Nontherapeutic treatment of dry mouth; intended for comfort only	Water, sorbitol, sodium carboxymethylcellulose, methylparaben, propylparaben, potassium chloride, sodium chloride, flavoring	Spray directly into mouth as necessary to treat drying conditions	4 oz spray bottle; order directly from manufacturer or various distributors
MouthKote Oral Moisturizer	Parnell Pharmaceuticals, Inc (800) 457-4276	Aqueous solution	Pleasant lemon-lime-flavored oral moisturizer to lubricate and protect oral tissue	Treats the discomfort of oral dryness caused by medications, disease, surgery, irradiation, aging	Water, xylitol, sorbitol, yerba santa, citric acid, ascorbic acid, flavor, sodium benzoate, sodium saccharin	Swirl 1 or 2 teaspoonfuls in mouth for 8 to 10 seconds; swallow or spit out; shake well before using	2 oz and 8 oz bottles; available at drugstores or order directly from manufacturer
Oasis Moisturizing Mouthwash	GlaxoSmithKline (800) 777-2500	Oral moisturizer, aqueous solution	Moisturizing mouthwash for a dry mouth indication	Moisturizes mouth and helps it from drying out	Active: Glycerin Other: Water, sorbitol, poloxamer 338, PEG-60 hydrogenated castor oil, cellulose gum, cetylpyridinium chloride, copovidone, disodium phosphate, flavor, methylparaben, propylparaben, sodium benzoate, sodium phosphate, sodium saccharin, xanthan gum, FD&C blue #1	Rinse for 30 seconds with 1 ounce of mouthwash first thing in the morning and before going to bed or as needed; do not swallow; use as part of an effective oral hygiene program	16 oz bottle
Optimoist Oral Moisturizer	Colgate Oral Pharmaceuticals (800) 225-3756	Oral moisturizer, aqueous solution	Pleasant tasting saliva substitute for instant relief of dry mouth and throat without demineralizing tooth enamel	Treats the discomfort of oral dryness	Deionized water, xylitol, calcium phosphate monobasic, citric acid, sodium hydroxide, sodium benzoate, flavoring, acesulfame potassium, hydroxyethylcellulose, polysorbate 20 and sodium monofluorophosphate (fluoride concentration is 2 parts per million)	Spray directly into mouth to relieve dry mouth discomfort; may be swallowed or expectorated; use as needed	2 oz and 12 oz bottles; available at mass merchandise stores, food stores, and drugstores
Salivart Synthetic Saliva, Aqueous Solution	Gebauer Co (800) 321-9348	Aerosol aqueous spray	Oral moisturizer for patients with reduced salivary flow	Replacement therapy for patients complaining of xerostomia	Sodium carboxymethylcellulose, sorbitol, sodium chloride, potassium chloride, calcium chloride dihydrate, magnesium chloride hexahydrate, potassium phosphate dibasic, purified water, nitrogen (propellant)	Spray directly into mouth or throat for 1 to 2 seconds; use as needed	2.48 fl oz (75 g); available at most drugstores or directly from manufacturer

Products and Drugs to Treat Dry Mouth *(continued)*

Medication	Manufacturer and Phone Number	Product Type	Manufacturer's Description	Indication	Ingredients	Directions for Use	Form and Availability
Other Dry Mouth Products (OTC)							
Biotene Dry Mouth Gum	Laclede Professional Products, Inc (800) 922-9348	Chewing gum	Sugar-free; helps stimulate saliva flow; fights cause/effect of bad breath; reduces plaque	Treats oral dryness	Active: Lactoperoxidase (0.11 Units), glucose oxidase (0.15 Units) Other: Sorbitol, gum base, xylitol, hydrogenated glucose, potassium thiocyanate	Chew 1 or 2 pieces; use as needed	Each package contains 17 pieces; available at drugstores or directly from manufacturer
Biotene Dry Mouth Toothpaste	Laclede Professional Products, Inc (800) 922-9348	Toothpaste	Reduces harmful bacteria which cause cavities, periodontal disease, and oral infections	Use in place of regular toothpaste for dry mouth	Active: Lactoperoxidase (15,000 Units), glucose oxidase (10,000 Units), lysozyme (16 mg), sodium monofluorophosphate Other: Sorbitol, glycerin, calcium pyrophosphate, hydrated silica, xylitol, isoceteth-20, cellulose gum, flavoring, sodium benzoate, beta-d-glucose, potassium thiocyanate	Use in place of regular toothpaste; rinse toothbrush before applying; brush for 2 minutes; rinse lightly	4.5 oz tube; available at drugstores or directly from manufacturer
Biotene Gentle Mouthwash	Laclede Professional Products, Inc (800) 922-9348	Mouthwash	Alcohol-free; strong antibacterial formula neutralizes mouth odors; soothes as it cleans to protect teeth and oral tissue	Treats dry mouth or oral irritations	Lysozyme, lactoferrin, glucose oxidase, lactoperoxidase	Use 15 mL (1 tablespoonful); swish thoroughly for 30 seconds and spit out; for dry throat, sip 1 tablespoonful of mouthwash 2 to 3 times/day	Available at drugstores or directly from manufacturer
Moi-Stir Oral Swabsticks	Kingswood Laboratories, Inc (800) 968-7772	Swabsticks	Lubricates and moistens mouth and mucosal area	Lubricates and moistens mouth and mucosal area	Water, sorbitol, sodium carboxymethylcellulose, methylparaben, propylparaben, potassium chloride, sodium chloride, flavoring	Gently swab all intraoral surfaces of mouth, gums, tongue, palate, buccal mucosa, gingival, teeth, and lips where uncomfortable dryness exists	3 swabsticks/packet, 100 packets/case; order directly from manufacturer or from various distributors.
Oasis Moisturizing Mouth Spray	GlaxoSmithKline (800) 777-2500	Oral moisturizer	Moisturizing mouth spray for a dry mouth indication	Moisturizes mouth and helps it from drying out	Active: Glycerin 35% (prediluted) Other: Cetylpyridinium chloride, copovidone, flavor, methylparaben, PEG-60 hydrogenated castor oil propylparaben, sodium benzoate, sodium saccharin, water, xanthan gum, xylitol	Use as required up to a maximum of 30 times or 60 sprays a day; spray 1 to 2 times into the affected area of mouth; do not rinse out	1 oz bottle
XyliMelts Discs	OraHealth (877) 672-6541	Time-release adhering discs	Lubricant	Treats dry mouth, reduces plaque	Xylitol 500 mg, cellulose gum	Use 2 discs as needed	120 tablets

Products and Drugs to Treat Dry Mouth *(continued)*

Medication	Manufacturer and Phone Number	Product Type	Manufacturer's Description	Indication	Ingredients	Directions for Use	Form and Availability
Saliva Substitute (Rx)							
Aquoral	Auriga Laboratories (877) 287-4428	Pump spray	Lipid-based solution designed to moisten and lubricate the oral cavity and oropharynx by formation of lipid film which limits loss of water and restores the viscoelasticity of the oral mucosa	Chronic and temporary xerostomia which may be the result of Sjögren's syndrome, oral inflammation, medication, chemo- or radiotherapy, and stress or aging. **Note:** Contraindicated if patient has a known history of hypersensitivity to any of its ingredients. No known interactions with medicinal or other products.	Oxidized glycerol triesters (TGO), silicon dioxide, aspartame, and artificial flavoring	Shake gently; 1 dose (2 sprays) into the mouth 3-4 times/day; spread product onto inflamed and/or dry areas of the mouth with the tongue.	1 bottle (40 mL = 400 sprays)
Cholinergic Salivary Stimulants (Rx)							
Cevimeline (Evoxac)	Snow Brand Pharmaceuticals (800) 475-6473			Treats symptoms of dry mouth in patients with Sjögren's syndrome	Active: Cevimeline 30 mg Other: Lactose monohydrate, hydroxypropyl cellulose, magnesium stearate	1 capsule (30 mg) 3 times/day	30 mg capsules
Pilocarpine (Salagen)	MGI Pharmaceuticals, Inc (800) 562-5580			Treats xerostomia caused by radiation therapy in patients with head/neck cancer, Sjögren's syndrome	Active: Pilocarpine 5 mg Other: Carnauba wax, hydroxypropyl methylcellulose, iron oxide, microcrystalline cellulose, stearic acid, titanium dioxide	1 to 2 tablets (5 mg) 3 to 4 times/day, not to exceed 30 mg/day	5 mg tablets

CHOLINERGIC SALIVARY STIMULANTS (PRESCRIPTION ONLY)

Pilocarpine (Systemic) (Salagen on page 1230) and cevimeline (Evoxac on page 330) are cholinergic drugs which stimulate salivary flow. They stimulate muscarinic-type acetylcholine receptors in salivary glands within the parasympathetic division of the autonomic nervous system, causing an increase in serous-type saliva. Thus, they are considered cholinergic, muscarinic-type (parasympathomimetic) drugs. Due to significant side effects caused by these drugs, they are available by prescription only.

Pilocarpine (Salagen) is indicated for the treatment of xerostomia caused by radiation therapy in patients with head and neck cancer and xerostomia in patients suffering from Sjögren syndrome. The usual adult dosage is 1 to 2 tablets (5 mg or 7.5 mg/tablet) 3 to 4 times/day, not to exceed 30 mg/day. Patients should be treated for a minimum of 90 days for optimum effect. The most frequent adverse side effect is perspiration, which occurs in about 30% of patients who use 5 mg 3 times/day. Other adverse effects (in about 10% of patients) are nausea, rhinitis, chills, frequent urination, dizziness, headache, lacrimation, and pharyngitis. Salagen is contraindicated for patients with uncontrolled asthma and narrow-angle glaucoma.

Pilocarpine has been documented to overcome xerostomia from different causes. More recent studies confirm its effectiveness in improving salivary flow in patients undergoing irradiation therapy for head and neck cancer. A capstone study by Johnson, et al, reported the effects of pilocarpine in 208 irradiation patients at 39 different treatment sites. Salagen, at a dose of 5 mg 3 times/day, improved salivation in 44% of patients, compared with 25% in the placebo group. They concluded that treatment with pilocarpine (Salagen) produced the best overall outcome with respect to saliva production and relief of symptoms of xerostomia in patients undergoing irradiation therapy.

Additional studies have been published showing the effectiveness of pilocarpine (Salagen) in stimulating salivary flow in patients suffering from Sjögren's syndrome and the FDA has approved the use of Salagen for this indication.

Recent reports suggest that pre-emptive use of pilocarpine may be effective in protecting salivary glands during therapeutic irradiation; further studies are needed to confirm this. As of this publication date, the use of pilocarpine has not been approved to treat xerostomia induced by chronic medication. Pilocarpine could be used as a sialagogue for individuals with xerostomia induced by antidepressants and other medications. However, the potential for serious drug interactions is a concern and more studies are needed to clarify the safety and effectiveness of pilocarpine when given in the presence of other medications.

Cevimeline (Evoxac) is indicated for treatment of symptoms of dry mouth in patients with Sjögren syndrome. The usual dosage in adults is 1 capsule (30 mg) 3 times/day. Cevimeline (Evoxac) is supplied in 30 mg capsules. Some adverse effects reported for Evoxac include increased sweating (19%), nausea (14%), rhinitis (11%), sinusitis (12%), and upper respiratory infection (11%). Evoxac is contraindicated for patients with uncontrolled asthma, narrow-angle glaucoma, acute iritis, and other conditions where miosis is undesirable. Cevimeline's half-life elimination is significantly slower than pilocarpine (0.76 hours versus 5 hours).

Other Drugs Implicated in Xerostomia

>10%	1% to 10%
ALPRAZolam	Acrivastine and Pseudoephedrine
Amoxapine	Albuterol
AtoMOXetine	Almotriptan
BuPROPion	Amantadine
ClomiPRAMINE	Anastrozole
CloNIDine	Armodafinil
Cyclobenzaprine	Bendamustine
Desvenlafaxine	Bevacizumab
Dicyclomine	Chlorpheniramine
DULoxetine	CloZAPine
Disopyramide	Doxazosin
Everolimus	Escitalopram
FluvoxaMINE	Estazolam
GuanFACINE	Flumazenil
IncobotulinumtoxinA	Gabapentin
Interferon alfa-2b	Interferon alfa-2a
Maprotiline	Ipratropium (Oral Inhalation)
Nabilone	Iloperidone
Nefazodone	Isoetharine
Oxybutynin	LamoTRIgine
PARoxetine	Levodopa and Carbidopa
RimabotulinumtoxinB	Loratadine

Other Drugs Implicated in Xerostomia *(continued)*

>10%	1% to 10%
Sertraline	Milnacipran
Tiotropium	Morphine (Systemic)
TiZANidine	OxyCODONE and Acetaminophen
Trospium	Prazosin
Venlafaxine	Propafenone
Zuclopenthixol	Quazepam
	RisperiDONE
	ROPINIRole
	Selegiline
	Tapentadol
	Terbutaline
	Varenicline

TEMPOROMANDIBULAR DYSFUNCTION (TMD), CHRONIC PAIN, AND FIBROMYALGIA

Temporomandibular dysfunction comprises a broad spectrum of signs and symptoms and is the most common cause of chronic nondental facial pain. TMD usually involves the muscles of mastication uni- or bilaterally. Although TMD presents in patterns, diagnosis is often difficult. Evaluation and treatment is time-intensive and no single therapy or drug regimen has been shown to be universally beneficial.

The thorough diagnostician should perform a screening examination for temporomandibular dysfunction on all patients. Ideally, a baseline maximum mandibular opening along with lateral and protrusive movement evaluation should be performed. Secondly, the joint area should be palpated and an adequate exam of the muscles of mastication and the muscles of the neck and shoulders should be made. These muscles include the elevators of the mandible (masseter, internal pterygoid, and temporalis); the depressors of the mandible (including the external pterygoid and digastric); extrusive muscles (including the temporalis and digastric), and protrusive muscles (including the external and internal pterygoids). These muscles also account for lateral movement of the mandible.

The clinician should also be alert to indicators of dysfunction, primarily a history of pain with jaw function, chronic history of joint noise (although this can often be misinterpreted), pain in the muscles of the neck, limited jaw movement, pain in the actual muscles of mastication, and headache or even earache. The signs and symptoms are extremely variable and the clinician should be alert for any or all of these areas of interest. Because of the complexity of both evaluation and diagnosis, the general dentist often finds it too time consuming to spend the countless hours evaluating and treating the temporomandibular dysfunction patient. Therefore, oral medicine specialists trained in temporomandibular evaluation and treatment often accept referrals for the management of these complicated patients. Effective treatment therapies are listed in Tables 1 and 2.

TMD often accompanies other chronic pain conditions, such as facial neuralgia, fibromyalgia, chronic headache, and even Burning Mouth Syndrome. Neuropathic pain is usually unilateral with on and off episodes. A common example of neuropathic pain is trigeminal neuralgia. This presents as pain described as an electric shock often in response to a light touch. Finding the underlying cause of chronic facial pain can be challenging for the diagnostician. Other diagnostic pearls including, giant cell arteritis must be ruled out, especially in patients >50 years of age. Cancer may be the underlying cause of progressive neuropathic pain. While rarely recognized as a neuropathic pain, burning mouth syndrome is most common in perimenopausal women.

Chronic Headache

The lifetime prevalence of headache is >90% for chronic headache patients. Most patients who present with headache have one of three main headache syndromes: Migraine, cluster headache, or tension headache. However, headache and facial pain can have numerous other etiologies that are important for the clinician to consider (eg, pain associated with chronic sinusitis). Two main idiopathic disorders that cause headache and facial pain are midfacial segment pain and atypical facial pain. Midfacial segment pain is a form of tension-type headache of the midface. This pain consists of a symmetric pressure sensation in the nasion, nasal dorsum, periorbital, or malar region. Hyperesthesia of the skin and soft tissues is also found. Treatment consists of low-dose amitriptyline at 10 mg for 6 months and may take up to 6 weeks to show effect. Atypical facial pain is also known as persistent idiopathic facial pain and is constant, deep, and ill-defined, usually crossing recognized dermatomes. The distribution is often unilateral. It occurs most commonly in women older than 40 years of age. The pain may alter in location and psychological factors may play a role. The treatment is similar to that for midfacial segment pain.

Fibromyalgia (Fibromyositis; Fibrositis)

Fibromyalgia is a common syndrome in which a patient has long-term, body-wide pain and tenderness in the joints, muscles, tendons, and other soft tissues. Fibromyalgia has also been linked to fatigue, sleep problems, headaches, depression, and anxiety. The cause of fibromyalgia is unknown; however, suggested causes or triggers include physical or emotional trauma, abnormal pain response, sleep disturbances, or infection (ie, unidentified virus). Fibromyalgia is most common among women 20 to 50 years of age.

Conditions that have been associated with fibromyalgia or mimic its symptoms include chronic neck or back pain, systemic exertion intolerance disease (formerly known as chronic fatigue syndrome), depression, hypothyroidism, Lyme disease, sleep disorders, and atypical facial pain. Patients with fibromyalgia tend to wake up with body aches and stiffness. For some patients, pain improves during the day and gets worse at night, while others experience pain all day long. The pain may get worse with activity, cold or damp weather, anxiety, and stress. Fatigue, depressed mood, and sleep problems (sleep interruption is often reported) are seen in almost all patients with fibromyalgia.

A patient must have at least 3 months of widespread pain and tenderness in at least 11 of 18 areas to be diagnosed with fibromyalgia. These areas may include arms (elbows), buttocks, chest, knees, lower back, neck, rib cage, shoulders, or thighs. Blood and urine tests are usually normal; however, tests may be done to rule out other conditions that may have similar symptoms.

Treatment:

While acute facial pain may be more easily treated by one practitioner, patients with chronic facial pain are best managed by a multidisciplinary team of health professionals (Zakrzewska 2013).

The goal of treatment is to help relieve pain and other symptoms and to help the patient cope with symptoms. The first type of treatment may involve physical therapy, exercise and fitness programs, or stress-relief methods (eg, light massage and relaxation techniques). If these treatments fail, an antidepressant or muscle relaxant may be prescribed. The goal of medication is to improve sleep and pain tolerance. All medications should be used along with exercise and behavior therapy. Duloxetine, pregabalin, and milnacipran are medications that are approved specifically for treating fibromyalgia. People with fibromyalgia are typically treated with pain medicines, antidepressants, muscle relaxants, and sleep medicines. In June 2007, Lyrica (pregabalin) became the first FDA-approved drug for specifically treating fibromyalgia; a year later, in June 2008, Cymbalta (duloxetine) became the second; and in January 2009, Savella (milnacipran) became the third.

Lyrica, Cymbalta, and Savella reduce pain and improve function in some people with fibromyalgia. While those with fibromyalgia have been shown to experience pain differently from other people, the mechanism by which these drugs produce their effects is unknown. There is data suggesting that these drugs affect the release of neurotransmitters in the brain. Lyrica, marketed by Pfizer Inc, was previously approved to treat seizures, as well as pain in people with diabetes (diabetic peripheral neuropathy) and in those who develop pain associated with post-herpetic neuropathy. Side effects of Lyrica including sleepiness, dizziness, blurry vision, weight gain, trouble concentrating, swelling of the hands and feet, and dry mouth. Allergic reactions, although rare, can occur. Cymbalta, marketed by Eli Lilly and Co, was previously approved to treat depression, anxiety, and diabetic peripheral neuropathy. Cymbalta's side effects include nausea, dry mouth, sleepiness, constipation, decreased appetite, and increased sweating. Like some other antidepressants, Cymbalta may increase the risk of suicidal thinking and behavior in people who take the drug for depression. Some people with fibromyalgia also experience depression. Savella, marketed by Forest Pharmaceuticals, Inc, is the first drug introduced primarily for treating fibromyalgia. Savella is not used to treat depression in the United States, but acts like medicines that are used to treat depression. Antidepressants may increase suicidal thoughts or actions in some people. Side effects include nausea, constipation, dizziness, insomnia, excessive sweating, vomiting, palpitations or increased heart rate, dry mouth, and high blood pressure.

Other medications that have been suggested to treat this condition include antiseizure drugs, other antidepressants, muscle relaxants, pain relievers, or sleeping aids. Severe cases of fibromyalgia may require a referral to a pain management clinic.

Some health care providers may recommend an injection in the temporomandibular joint to help alleviate TMJ problems. It is important to note that these treatments have NOT been approved by the Food and Drug Administration (FDA) for treating TMJ disorders.

Botulinum toxin type A (Botox) is a drug made from the same bacterium that causes food poisoning. Used in small dosages, Botox injections can actually help alleviate some health problems and are approved by the Food and Drug Administration (FDA) for certain disorders. However, Botox is currently not approved by the FDA for use in TMJ disorders. Results from recent clinical studies are inconclusive regarding the effectiveness of Botox for treatment of chronic TMJ disorders. Additional research is needed to learn how Botox specifically affects jaw muscles and their nerves and specifically if it has possible efficacy in sleep-related bruxism. Potential adverse effects related to facial expression have been reported.

Steroid injection can be of help in reducing inflammation in cases of an acute flair-up of degenerative joint disease or rheumatoid arthritis. However, it is only a temporary palliative measure and does not address the cause of the problem. Controversy still exists regarding steroid injections as a TMJ treatment.

Hyaluronan (Hyaluronic acid/Hyaluronate) is sometimes used to treat osteoarthritis in the knees or hips; however, there is not enough evidence to judge whether it is helpful for people with TMJ problems. According to the FDA, hyaluronic acid has not been approved to treat TMJ disorders.

Local anesthetics are sometimes injected into the TM joint or jaw muscles for diagnostic purposes to determine the source of the pain. They are also used therapeutically to inject trigger points in the muscles. Such procedures do not need FDA approval as long as the anesthetic agent is an approved drug.

Ozone therapy involves the injection of ozone gas into the temporomandibular joint. Its use is based on the false theory that ozone can kill such bacteria, viruses, and fungi, as well as reduce inflammation and stimulate cartilage growth. Thus, there is no scientific basis for its use in the TM joint and ozone therapy is not approved by the FDA.

Prolotherapy (Sclerotherapy) is a technique in which an irritating solution is injected into a ligament or muscle tendon near a painful area with the intent of inducing the proliferation of new cells and thus strengthening these structures, supporting the weakened muscles, and eliminating the pain. Although it has been used mainly to treat chronic low back pain, it has also been recommended for patients with temporomandibular disorders. However, there is no scientific evidence to show that weakened ligaments and tendons are the cause of pain in TMD patients, or to substantiate the effectiveness of this procedure in eliminating the pain. Moreover, there are no studies to elucidate the risks of collateral tissue effects and prolotherapy should be avoided for TMJ treatments.

Studies are currently being performed to determine the efficacy of chronic pain medications in the specific management of TMD.

The oral medicine specialist in TMD management, the physical therapist interested in head and neck pain, and the oral and maxillofacial surgeon will all work together with the referring general dentist to accomplish successful patient treatment. Table 1 lists the wide variety of treatment alternatives available to the team. Depending on the diagnosis, one or more of the therapies might be selected. For organic diseases of the joint not responding to nonsurgical approaches, a wide variety of surgical techniques are available (Table 2).

ACUTE TMD

Acute TMD oftentimes presents alone or as an episode during a chronic pattern of signs and symptoms. Trauma, such as a blow to the chin or the side of the face, can result in acute TMD. Occasionally, similar symptoms will follow a lengthy wide open mouth dental procedure.

The condition usually presents as continuous deep pain in the TMJ. If edema is present in the joint, the condyle sometimes can be displaced which will cause abnormal occlusion of the posterior teeth on the affected side. The diagnosis is usually based on the history and clinical presentation. Management of the patient includes:

1. Explaining the problem and reassuring the patient
2. Restriction of all mandibular movement to function in a pain-free range of motion
3. Recommending a soft diet (eg, eggs, yogurt, casseroles, soup, ground meat). Avoid chewing gum or eating salads, large sandwiches or fruit that is hard or not sliced into small bites.
4. NSAIDs (eg, Anaprox DS 1 tablet every 12 hours for 7 to 10 days)
5. Moist heat applications to the affected area for 15 to 20 minutes, 4 to 6 times/day
6. Consideration of a muscle relaxant, such as Methocarbamol (Robaxin) on page 988, adult patient of average height/weight, two (500 mg) tablets at bedtime; daytime dose can be tailored to patient

Additional therapies could include referral to a physical therapist for ultrasound therapy 2 to 4 times/week and a single injection of steroid in the joint space. A team approach with an oral maxillofacial surgeon for this procedure may be helpful.

CHRONIC TMD

The most common therapeutic modalities include:

- As with acute TMD: Reassuring the patient, soft diet, applying moist heat, and consideration of muscle relaxants are useful.
- Reducing stress; a monitored exercise program will be beneficial. Usually, working with a physical therapist is ideal.
- Medications include analgesics, anti-inflammatories, and tranquilizers

MEDICATION OPTIONS

Most commonly used medication (NSAIDs)

Choline Magnesium Trisalicylate
Diclofenac (Systemic) on page 484
Diflunisal on page 495
Etodolac on page 622
Fenoprofen on page 642
Flurbiprofen (Systemic) on page 701
Ibuprofen on page 786
Indomethacin
Ketoprofen on page 860
Ketorolac (Systemic) on page 861
Magnesium Salicylate
Meclofenamate on page 952
Mefenamic Acid on page 954
Nabumetone on page 1069
Naproxen on page 1080
Oxaprozin on page 1152
Piroxicam on page 1237
Salsalate on page 1356
Sulindac on page 1394
Tolmetin

Tranquilizers and muscle relaxants, when used appropriately, can provide excellent adjunctive therapy. These drugs should be primarily used for a short period of time to manage acute pain. In low dosages, amitriptyline is often used to treat chronic pain and occasionally migraine headache. Two drugs similar to the prototype drug, amitriptyline, have been approved for use in adults only, for treatment of acute migraine with or without aura: Almotriptan malate (Axert [tablets]; Pharmacia Corp) and frovatriptan succinate (Frova [tablets]; Endo Pharmaceuticals). Other approved abortive (but not preventative) antimigraine triptan drugs include eletriptan (Relpax), naratriptan (Amerge), rizatriptan (Maxalt), sumatriptan (Imitrex), and zolmitriptan (Zomig). Selective serotonin reuptake inhibitors (SSRIs) are sometimes used in the management of chronic neuropathic pain, particularly in patients not responding to amitriptyline. Gabapentin (Neurontin) has been approved for chronic pain. Problems of inducing bruxism with SSRIs, however, have been reported and may preclude their use. Clinicians attempting to evaluate any patient with bruxism or involuntary muscle movement, who is simultaneously being treated with an SSRI, should be aware of this potential association.

Botox (botulinum toxin type A) is a drug made from the same bacterium that causes food poisoning. Used in small doses, Botox injections can actually help alleviate some health problems and have been approved by the Food and Drug Administration (FDA) for certain disorders. However, Botox is currently not approved by the FDA for use in TMJ disorders.

Results from recent clinical studies are inconclusive regarding the effectiveness of Botox for treatment of chronic TMJ disorders. Additional research is under way to learn how Botox specifically affects jaw muscles and their nerves. The findings will help determine if this drug may be useful in treating TMJ disorders.

See individual monographs for dosing instructions.

Common minor tranquilizers include:

ALPRAZolam on page 106
DiazePAM on page 477
LORazepam on page 931

Chronic neuropathic pain management:

Effective treatment usually involves medications. If the patient is unresponsive to medical management then a neurosurgery consultation may be necessary.

Amitriptyline on page 120
CarBAMazepine on page 288
Gabapentin on page 722
OXcarbazepine on page 1154

Acute migraine management:

Almotriptan on page 104
Eletriptan on page 549
Frovatriptan on page 720
Naratriptan on page 1085
Rizatriptan on page 1342
SUMAtriptan on page 1394
ZOLMitriptan on page 1581

Fibromyalgia management:

DULoxetine on page 536
Milnacipran on page 1031
Pregabalin on page 1268

Other non-FDA approved options:

AbobotulinumtoxinA on page 55
Hyaluronate and Derivatives on page 761

Common muscle relaxants include:

Chlorzoxazone on page 344
Cyclobenzaprine on page 418
Methocarbamol on page 988
Orphenadrine on page 1146

Note: Muscle relaxants and tranquilizers should generally be prescribed with an analgesic or NSAID to relieve pain as well.

Opioid analgesics can be used on a short-term basis or intermittently in combination with non-opioid therapy in the chronic pain patient. Judicious prescribing, monitoring, and maintenance by the practitioner is imperative whenever considering the use of opioid analgesics due to the abuse and addiction liabilities.

Table 1. TMD – Nonsurgical Therapies

1. Moist heat and cold spray
2. Injections in muscle trigger areas (procaine)
3. Exercises (passive, active)
4. Medications
   a. Muscle relaxants
   b. Minerals (magnesium, glucosamine, chondroitin)
   c. Multiple vitamins (Ca, B_6, B_{12})
   d. NSAIDs, opioid combinations, antidepressants
5. Orthopedic craniomandibular repositioning appliance (splints)
6. Biofeedback, acupuncture
7. Physiotherapy: TMJ muscle therapy
8. Myofunctional therapy (occasionally)

9. TENS (transcutaneous electrical neural stimulation), Myo-Monitor (occasionally)
10. Dental therapy
    a. Equilibration (coronoplasty) (occasionally)
    b. Restoring occlusion to proper vertical dimension of maxilla to mandible by orthodontics, dental restorative procedures, orthognathic surgery, permanent splint, or any combination of these

Table 2. TMD – Surgical Therapies

1. Cortisone injection into joint (with local anesthetic)
2. Bony and/or fibrous ankylosis: Requires surgery (osteoarthrotomy with prosthetic appliance)
3. Chronic subluxation: Requires surgery, depending on problem (possibly eminectomy and/or prosthetic implant)
4. Osteoarthritis: Requires surgery (arthroscopy), depending on problem
    a. Arthroplasty
    b. Meniscectomy
    c. Arthroplasty with repair of disc
    d. Arthrocentesis
5. Rheumatoid arthritis
    a. Arthroplasty
    b. "Total" TMJ replacement
6. Tumors: Require osteoarthrotomy – removal of tumor and restoring of joint when possible
7. Chronic disc displacement: Arthroscopy with arthrocentesis; possible removal of bone from condyle

REFERENCES

Abeles M, Solitar BM, Pillinger MH, Abeles AM. Update on fibromyalgia therapy. *Am J Med.* 2008;121(7):555-561.

Ernberg M, Hedenberg-Magnusson B, List T, Svensson P. Efficacy of botulinum toxin type A for treatment of persistent myofascial TMD pain: a randomized, controlled, double-blind multicenter study. *Pain.* 2011;152(9):1988-1996.

Fedorowicz Z, van Zuuren EJ, Schoones J. Botulinum toxin for masseter hypertrophy. *Cochrane Database of Systematic Reviews 2013.* Issue 9. Art. No: CD007510.

Gauer RL, Semidey MJ. Diagnosis and treatment of temporomandibular disorders. *Am Fam Physician.* 2015;91(6):378-386.

Häuser W, Bernardy K, Uçeyler N, Sommer C. Treatment of fibromyalgia syndrome with antidepressants: a meta-analysis. *JAMA.* 2009;301 (2):198-209.

Stoustrup P, Kristensen KD, Verna C, Küseler A, Pedersen TK, Herlin T. Intra-articular steroid injection for temporomandibular joint arthritis in juvenile idiopathic arthritis: a systematic review on efficacy and safety. *Semin Arthritis Rheum.* 2013;43(1):63-70.

Wolfe F, Rasker JJ. Fibromyalgia. *Kelley's Textbook of Rheumatology.* 8th ed. Chapter 38. Firestein GS, Budd RC, Harris ED Jr, et al, eds. Philadelphia, PA: Saunders Elsevier; 2008.

Wolfe F, Clauw DJ, Fitzcharles MA, et al. The American College of Rheumatology preliminary diagnostic criteria for fibromyalgia and measurement of symptom severity. *Arthritis Care Res (Hoboken).* 2010;62(5):600-610.

Wright EF, North SL. Management and treatment of temporomandibular disorders: a clinical perspective. *J Man Manip Ther.* 2009;17(4): 247–254.

Zakrzewska JM. Differential diagnosis of facial pain and guidelines for management. *Br J Anaesth.* 2013;111(1):95-104.

MANAGEMENT OF THE PATIENT WITH ANXIETY OR DEPRESSION

ANXIETY AND DEPRESSION

Over the past two decades, there has been a gradual, but steady, increase in the number of patients who are taking antianxiety and antidepressant medications. Much of this is driven by the emergence of new medications for management of these conditions and an increasing awareness on the part of medical clinicians in recognizing signs and symptoms of depression and anxiety. In addition, society has now accepted that the quality of life for these patients can be improved on an outpatient basis.

Anxiety is characterized by apprehension or fear of impending actual or imagined danger, vulnerability, or uncertainty and may be accompanied by restlessness, tension, tachycardia, and dyspnea unattached to a clearly identifiable stimulus. (ICD 10 code F41.1, F41.9, and F43.23)

Depression is an unpleasant, but not necessarily irrational or pathological, mood state characterized by sadness, despair, or discouragement; it may also involve low self-esteem, social withdrawal, and somatic symptoms such as eating and sleep disturbance. (ICD 10 code F32.9 and F33.1)

Oral Manifestations and Considerations

Oral

- Neglect of oral hygiene leading to increased risk of dental caries and periodontal disease, this is a particularly vicious circle: poor oral health leads to painful dentistry, which leads to dental avoidance and even worse oral health.
- Poor nutrition
- Drug-induced xerostomia (chronic xerostomia is associated with fungal overgrowth, burning mouth syndrome, caries, and mucosal irritations and is difficult to manage when it is drug induced)
- Some studies report a positive correlation with temporomandibular disorders and atypical facial pain

Other Potential Disorders/Concerns

- Mitral valve prolapse and GERD
- Children with depression are at increased risk for engaging in high-risk behaviors (promiscuity, smoking, alcohol and drug abuse)

Oral Side Effects of Commonly Prescribed Medications

Depression: SSRIs, Atypical Antidepressants: Xerostomia, dysphagia, sialadenitis; Tricyclic Antidepressants (TCA's): Dysgeusia, stomatitis, gingivitis, glossitis, tongue edema, discolored tongue, and bruxism

Anxiety: SSRIs, Atypical Antidepressants: Xerostomia, dysphagia, sialadenitis; Benzodiazepines: Dysgeusia, stomatitis, gingivitis, glossitis, tongue edema

The dentist often encounters patients taking medications that have the potential to induce mild to moderate adverse oral side effects and may create additional risk based on the types of medication used in the dental practice. In addition to a wide variety of depression-indicated signs and symptoms, antidepressant medications are prescribed for psychiatric disorders, pain control, sleep deprivation, smoking cessation, substance abuse, and eating disorders.

The side effects of these drugs primarily fall into several categories. Xerostomia or altered salivary flow has long been known as a side effect of tricyclic antidepressants. Newer antidepressants, although the effects may be lessened, also have similar side effects. Coupled with xerostomia is an increased risk of fungal infections and a significant association with burning mouth syndrome (BMS). The reader is referred to Fungal Infections on page 1752 and Ulcerative, Erosive, and Painful Oral Mucosal Disorders on page 1758 for management if an infection is suspected. In addition, some drugs, including the selective serotonin reuptake inhibitors (SSRIs), have effects on orthostatic hypotension and there have been rare reports of increased bruxism with chronic use of the drugs. Many of the antianxiety and antidepressant medications have shown some efficacy in the management of chronic pain and some have approval for use in atypical facial pain and temporomandibular dysfunction (TMD). Generally, the dosing for these chronic pain conditions is lower than the dosing for the management of depression or anxiety, but the approved dosing should always be verified before prescribing.

Another potential adverse reaction is cardiotoxicity associated with the use of combination drugs, including the antidepressant medication classes, and the use of a vasoconstrictor in local anesthetics. The reader is referred to Vasoconstrictor Interactions With Antidepressants on page 1821 in the appendix which discusses the classes of antidepressant and antianxiety medications and the potential risk of interactions with local anesthetics.

In reviewing the epidemiology of antidepressant and antianxiety medications, female subjects outnumber males by ~2.3:1 ratio with selective serotonin reuptake inhibitors being the most commonly prescribed medications. Tricyclic antidepressants, atypical third-generation antidepressants, and monoamine oxidase inhibitors are also used. Some of the drugs used for smoking cessation also fall into this atypical antidepressant class.

BIPOLAR DISORDER

Many advances have occurred in the treatment of bipolar illness and a number of drugs have been FDA-approved for use, including some of the atypical antipsychotics (eg, aripiprazole, olanzapine, risperidone, ziprasidone). Treatment options include mood stabilizers (eg, lithium, valproic acid, carbamazepine, oxcarbazepine), antidepressants, electroconvulsive therapy, and antipsychotics (adjunctive therapy). Most people with bipolar disorder take combinations of lithium, valproate, and carbamazepine to manage symptoms and prevent recurrence of bipolar episodes. These medications are often called mood stabilizers, to even out emotional highs and lows. These patients may also be prescribed other medications to treat the agitation, anxiety, and sleep disturbances that may accompany their illness. In patients with concomitant depression, antidepressants can help manage the feelings of sadness, guilt, worthlessness, or hopelessness. Dry mouth, constipation, and nausea are the most common side effects.

SEDATION

Anxiety constitutes the most frequently found psychiatric problem in the general population. Anxiety can range from a simple phobia to a severe debilitating disorder. Functional results of this anxiety can, therefore, range from simple avoidance of dental procedures to panic attacks when confronting stressful situations, such as seen in some patients regarding dental visits. Many patients claim to be anxious over dental care, when in reality, they simply have not been managed with modern techniques of local anesthesia, the availability of sedation, or the caring dental practitioner.

The dentist may detect anxiety in patients during the treatment planning and evaluation phases of care. The anxious person may appear overly alert, may lean forward in the dental chair during conversation, or may appear concerned over time, possibly using this as a guise to cut short the dental visit. Anxious persons may also show signs of being nervous by demonstrating sweating; muscle tension, including their temporomandibular musculature; or they may complain of being tired due to an inability to obtain an adequate night's sleep.

The management of these patients requires a methodical approach to relaxation, discussing their dental needs, and then planning, along with the patient, the best way to accomplish dental treatment in the presence of their fears, either real or imagined. Consideration may be given to sedation. This sedation can be oral or parenteral, or inhalation in the case of nitrous oxide. The dentist must be adequately trained in administering the sedative of choice, as well as in monitoring the patient during the sedated procedures. Numerous medications are available to achieve the level of sedation usually necessary in the dental office: Valium, Ativan, Xanax, Vistaril, Serax, and BuSpar represent a few. These oral sedatives can be given prior to dental visits as outlined in the following prescriptions. They have the advantage of allowing the patient a good night's sleep prior to the day of the procedure and provide on-the-spot sedation during the procedure. Nitrous oxide is an in-the-office administered sedative that is relatively safe, but requires additional training and carefully planned monitoring protocols of auxiliary personnel during inhalation. Both oral and inhalation techniques can be used to manage the anxious patient in the dental office.

It is recommended that patients not drive themselves to or from dental appointments following use of these medications. Also, these medications should not be prescribed during pregnancy. For pediatric patients, oral preprocedural sedatives include primarily hydroxyzine and liquid meperidine. Dosing suggestions are described in each of the respective monographs.

Dental anxiety is linked to poor oral health outcomes, and can be a strain on provider-patient relationships. Fortunately, dentists can help allay patient anxiety by communicating effectively, giving patients control, scheduling appropriately, building a relaxing office with calming distractions, and considering the patient experience before and after the visit. Behavior modification is based on the principles of learning, both in terms of classical conditioning or operant conditioning and of social learning. It aims to change undesirable behavior in certain situations through learning. The strategies involve relaxation along with guided imagery and adjuvant use of physiological monitoring using biofeedback, hypnosis, acupuncture, distraction, positive reinforcement, stop-signaling, and exposure-based treatments, such as systematic desensitization, "tell-show-do", and modeling.

ALPRAZolam on page 106
BusPIRone on page 273
DiazePAM on page 477
HydrOXYzine on page 780
LORazepam on page 931
Meperidine on page 966
Nitrous Oxide on page 1113
Prochlorperazine on page 1279
Triazolam on page 1493

Note: Although various antidepressants have been used for preprocedure sedation, no specific regimens or protocols have been established. Guidelines for use are still under study.

Doxepin (Systemic) on page 518
FLUoxetine on page 697
FluvoxaMINE on page 708
PARoxetine on page 1194
Sertraline on page 1367
TraZODone on page 1481

For examples of sample prescriptions see Sedation (Prior to Dental Treatment) - Sample Prescriptions on page 45

REFERENCES

Anttila S, Knuuttila M, Ylöstalo P, Joukamaa M. Symptoms of depression and anxiety in relation to dental health behavior and self-perceived dental treatment need. *Eur J Oral Sci.* 2006;114(2):109-114.

Armfield JM, Heaton LJ. Management of fear and anxiety in the dental clinic: a review. *Aust Dent J.* 2013;58(4):390-407.

Armfield JM, Stewart JF, Spencer AJ. The vicious cycle of dental fear: exploring the interplay between oral health, service utilization and dental fear. *BMC Oral Health.* 2007;14;7:1.

Brahm CO, Lundgren J, Carlsson SG, Nilsson P, Corbeil J, Hägglin C. Dentists' views on fearful patients. Problems and promises. *Swed Dent J.* 2012;36(2):79-89.

Brodine AH, Hartshorn MA. Recognition and management of somatoform disorders. *J Prosthet Dent.* 2004;91(3):268-273.

Carter AE, Carter G, Boschen M, AlShwaimi E, George R. Pathways of fear and anxiety in dentistry: a review. *World J Clin Cases.* 2014;2(11):642–653.

Cermak SA, Stein Duker LI, Williams ME, et al. Feasibility of a sensory-adapted dental environment for children with autism. *Am J Occup Ther.* 2015;69(3):1–10.

Coulson NS, Buchanan H. Self-reported efficacy of an online dental anxiety support group: a pilot study. *Community Dent Oral Epidemiol.* 2008;36(1):43-46.

Dumitrache MA, Neacsu V, Sfeatcu IR. Efficiency of cognitive technique in reducing dental anxiety. *Procedia Soc Behav Sci.* 2014;149:302–306.

Heaton LJ. Behavioral interventions may reduce dental anxiety and increase acceptance of dental treatment in dentally fearful adults. *J Evid Based Dent Pract.* 2013;13(4):160–162.

Intercollegiate Advisory Committee for Sedation in Dentistry. Standards for Conscious Sedation in the Provision of Dental Care. London: RCS Publications; 2015. Available from: https://www.rcseng.ac.uk/fds/Documents/dental-sedation-report-2015-web-v2.pdf.

Keene JJ Jr, Galasko GT, Land MF. Antidepressant use in psychiatry and medicine: importance for dental practice. *J Am Dent Assoc.* 2003;134(1):71-79.

Klingberg G, Broberg AG. Dental fear/anxiety and dental behaviour management problems in children and adolescents: a review of prevalence and concomitant psychological factors. *Int J Paediatr Dent.* 2007;17(6):391-406.

Lundgren J, Carlsson SG, Berggren U. Relaxation versus cognitive therapies for dental fear – a psychophysiological approach. *Health Psychol.* 2006;25(3):267-273.

Ma R, Xu SJ, Wen XY, et al. Acupuncture for generalized anxiety disorder: a systematic review. *J Psychol Psychother.* 2014;4(5):1000155.

Merry SN, Hetrick SE, Cox GR, et al. Cochrane review: psychological and educational interventions for preventing depression in children and adolescents. *Cochrane Database Syst Rev.* 2012;7(5):1409-1685.

Stenebrand A, Boman UW, Hakeberg M. Dental anxiety and symptoms of general anxiety and depression in 15-year-olds. *Int J Dent Hyg.* 2012.

PERIORAL PREMALIGNANT LESIONS AND MANAGEMENT OF PATIENTS UNDERGOING CANCER THERAPY

PERIORAL PREMALIGNANT LESIONS

Oral mucosal abnormalities present to the dentist in 5% to 15% of patients. The vast majority of these mucosal changes are benign; however, many oral lesions have similar clinical characteristics often making differentiation of relatively benign lesions or reactive conditions from premalignancy difficult. It is very challenging to discriminate between progressive or nonprogressive lesions. Some precancerous lesions may be hidden within mucosa and yet appear normal clinically.

Oral squamous cell carcinoma (OSCC) is the most common oral cancer. The 5-year survival rate is 81% (early stages), 30% (late-stage), and 52% of all patients die within 5 years. The overall 5-year survival rate in whites in US and Europe has increased from 40%, in the 1950's, to 59%, but in black patients, only from 36% to 39%. These survival rates have not significantly changed in many decades. Recognition and diagnosis of oral pathologies other than dental and periodontal diseases is one of the broad-reaching responsibilities of all dental providers, regardless of specialty. The current gold standard for initial detection of oral lesions is through visual and manual inspection of the oral cavity by the dental or medical professional. Unfortunately, the examination process is seldom standardized, hence subjective and not always accurate. These shortcomings have often been blamed for the delay in diagnosis of many pathologies, including common oral diseases but particularly oral cancer. Once noted the dental provider usually recommends other diagnostics or a biopsy if a suspicious region is identified. The ability to accurately detect the disease in a premalignant and earlier stage by minimally invasive means will have significant impact on overall outcome, likely within the next decade with salivary diagnostics to identify disease related biomarkers at the forefront.

Dentists are often the first to recognize early changes in the skin, lips, or oral mucosal tissues that could represent potential premalignancies. The general dentist may refer such patients to an oral and maxillofacial surgeon, oral pathology/oral medicine specialist, or otolaryngologist for biopsy. There are numerous drugs under study to manage premalignancies by preventing the progression of lesions from dysplasia to frank cancer. The condition actinic keratosis on the skin, and the equivalent condition of the lips, actinic cheilitis, create a diagnostic and management challenge for clinicians. Until now 5-fluorouracil preparations have been used with mixed success, but recently, imiquimod (Zyclara) has been approved for actinic keratosis.

For lesions that do not fit these criteria, additional diagnostic steps are often necessary. New approaches are available to aid the dentist in the proper timely management of patients with premalignant lesions or at risk for human papillomas virus infection.

ESTABLISHING A DIFFERENTIAL DIAGNOSIS

For many oral mucosal lesions, a precise diagnosis can be made based solely on patient history and clinical presentation and no additional diagnostic procedures are necessary; however, many lesions share similar clinical features. In order to determine the final diagnosis, additional diagnostic procedures are usually necessary. These procedures most often require removal of some or all of the lesion for microscopic/histologic examination. Diagnostic procedures readily available to the dental team include conventional biopsy, brush biopsy, and exfoliative cytology.

DIAGNOSTIC PROCEDURES

Conventional Biopsy: The microscopic examination of tissue removed from an area of suspected disease. The purpose is to establish an accurate diagnosis so that the disease can be appropriately treated. A conventional biopsy is indicated when:

- Clinical examination fails to lead to a precise diagnosis.
- A lesion fails to respond to conservative therapy within a reasonable period of time.
- A lesion is thought to be premalignant.
- A lesion exhibits clinical features of malignancy.

Incisional Biopsy: The surgical removal of only a sample of the lesion for the purpose of microscopic examination. Once a microscopic diagnosis has been made, it may be necessary to remove the remainder of the lesion.

Excisional Biopsy: The removal of the entire lesion with a margin of clinically uninvolved tissue. The procedure is meant to be both diagnostic and therapeutic. If microscopic examination shows that some of the lesion remains, additional surgery may be necessary.

Punch Biopsy for Oral Mucosal Lesions: Punch biopsy is a convenient method for performing incisional biopsies of oral mucosal lesions. This technique employs a disposable instrument called a biopsy punch that makes a circular incision. A disposable biopsy punch with a diameter of 4 or 6 mm is an excellent choice for many incisional biopsies of oral mucosal lesions. Accessible location of the lesion is a primary consideration for choosing this instrument.

Considerations for selection of the biopsy site:

- The biopsy site should be representative of the disease.
- Important anatomic structures in the submucosa (eg, salivary gland ducts and large blood vessels), should be avoided.
- Tissue that appears to be necrotic should not be included in the biopsy specimen.
- It is usually beneficial to include a margin of clinically uninvolved tissue in the biopsy specimen.

Oral Brush Biopsy: The removal of all layers of the epithelium (including the basal cell layer) using a biopsy brush (a small brush with very firm bristles). Oral CDX is a service available to assess brush samples. In contrast to conventional exfoliative cytology which only provides cells from the surface of the lesion, properly applied brush biopsy generates a transepithelial specimen. If abnormal epithelial cells are detected, a conventional biopsy is indicated.

Indications for oral brush biopsy:

- Brush biopsy is especially suited for the early detection of precancerous and cancerous oral mucosal lesions.

Advantages of oral brush biopsy:

- Requires only a few instruments and supplies
- Easy to perform
- Well tolerated by patient
- Associated with little or no morbidity

Limitations of oral brush biopsy:

- Since only individual cells are examined, the cells cannot be evaluated in their proper tissue relationships.
- If atypical epithelial cells are detected, a conventional biopsy is indicated to confirm the diagnosis.

ORAL EXFOLIATIVE CYTOLOGY

Oral exfoliative cytology is the microscopic examination of cells from the surface of an oral mucosal lesion. Oral exfoliative cytology is a useful adjunct in the diagnosis of surface lesion of oral mucosa.

Indications for oral exfoliative cytology:

- Premalignant / malignant lesions (dysplasia, carcinoma *in situ*)
- Vesiculoulcerative diseases (herpes simplex virus, varicella-zoster virus)
- Superficial fungal infections (candidiasis, geotrichosis)

Advantages of oral exfoliative cytology:

- Requires only a few instruments and supplies
- Easy to perform
- Well tolerated by the patient
- Associated with no morbidity

Limitations of oral exfoliative cytology:

- Because only surface cells are examined, the disease process must involve the mucosal surface.
- Since only individual cells are examined, the cells cannot be evaluated in their proper tissue relationships.
- If atypical epithelial cells are detected, a conventional biopsy is indicated to confirm the diagnosis.

DIRECT OPTICAL FLUORESCENCE VISUALIZATION

Direct optical fluorescence visualization is the process of examining tissue directly with the human eye to assess its autofluorescence properties. In order to detect the fluorescent pattern of the tissue, it must be exposed to a light of specific wavelength and intensity that excites the cells and viewed through special filters that remove all unwanted light normally reflected from the tissue. The fluorescent pattern produced by the cells enables the clinician to differentiate between tissues composed of normal cells and abnormal tissue, specifically premalignant and malignant epithelial neoplasms.

In the oral cavity, direct optical fluorescence visualization is accomplished using the VELscope, a handheld, field-of- view device that provides the clinician with an easy-to-use, adjunctive, screening instrument for early clinical detection of oral premalignant and malignant lesions. The device emits a safe blue light into the oral cavity which excites cells beneath the epithelial surface causing them to fluoresce. Tissue composed of normal cells emits an apple-green fluorescence, while abnormal tissue exhibits a loss of fluorescence and appears dark.

Indications for Use of the Direct Optical Fluorescence Visualization (VELscope):

- Adjunct to routine oral mucosal examination procedures.
- Aid in early clinical detection of oral premalignant and malignant lesions.

Advantages of direct optical fluorescence visualization (VELscope):

- Simple and easy to use.
- Field-of-view technology facilitates efficient screening of oral mucosa and requires the addition of only a few minutes to the examination procedure.
- Noninvasive.

Limitations of direct optical fluorescence visualization (VELscope):

- When viewed through the VELscope, normal tissue exhibits apple-green fluorescence, while abnormal tissue exhibits loss of fluorescence and appears dark.
- If an area of concern is noted, a conventional biopsy is necessary to confirm the diagnosis of premalignancy or malignancy.

HPV AND HEAD & NECK CANCER

Human papillomavirus (HPV) is the broad term for a large group of viruses comprised of more than 200 serotypes. Certain serotypes of HPV cause warts on the skin and others cause warts in the genital region. Some types of HPV are known to cause cervical cancers, as well as cancers of the anus, penis, vulva, vagina and the *head and neck*.

HPV-related head and neck cancers occur primarily in the oropharynx (posterior to the tonsillar pillars and on the base of the tongue). Oropharyngeal cancers are more common in white men. Most head and neck cancers have been shown to be clearly associated with tobacco and alcohol use, but researchers believe more than 80% of oropharyngeal cancers in the US may be related to long-term infection with the HPV virus. HPV-related head and neck cancer occurs in both people who smoke and those who do not smoke and it is assumed that smoking and alcohol use only increase the chances of cancer transformation.

Salivary diagnostic tests are available for HPV, and involve the use of Polymerase Chain Reaction PCR tests; thus, they are not point of care tests. Kits containing a salivary collector are placed in transport media and sent to a central laboratory for analysis. Various investigators have used oral swabs, expectorated saliva, or an expectorated oral rinse with mouthwash, to collect virions and cells for analysis (OraRisk HPV test, OralDNA Labs, Brentwood, TN, is the only salivary diagnostic test for HPV commercially available in the United States). The expectorated oral rinse with mouthwash collection technique has the highest sensitivity, because it samples the entire oral cavity and the swishing of the solution dislodges mucosal cells. Investigators in the laboratory use a variety of primers to detect as many HPV types as possible. Early diagnosis is critical for survival of patients with OSCC and use of salivary HPV analyses is likely to increase.

Human papilloma virus is widespread and serotypes 16 and 18 have clearly been associated with cervical cancer and are also the serotypes associated with the oropharyngeal cancers described above. Although most serotypes that cause commonly encountered oral HPV lesions in the anterior oral cavity are not 16 or 18, the clinician should recommend appropriate surgical removal of all such lesions. Lesions in the posterior oral pharyngeal region are, however, of the greatest concern.

Pre-exposure vaccination is one of the most effective methods for preventing transmission of some serotypes of HPV. Quadravalent (4vHPV) (Gardasil) and the new 9 valent HPV vaccine (9vHPV) (Gardasil) is available in the US and the bivalent HPV vaccine (2vHPV) (Cervarix) is available in numerous other countries but was recently discontinued in the US.

2vHPV, 4vHPV, and 9vHPV all protect against HPV 16 and 18, types that cause about 66% of cervical cancers and the majority of other HPV-attributable cancers in the United States (*1,12*). 9vHPV targets five additional cancer causing types, 9vHPV contains HPV 31, 33, 45, 52, and 58 which account for about 15% of cervical cancers. 4vHPV and 9vHPV also protect against HPV 6 and 11, types that cause anogenital warts.

Gardasil is a vaccine indicated in girls and women 9 to 26 years of age for the prevention of the following diseases caused by Human Papillomavirus (HPV) types included in the vaccine:

- Cervical, vulvar, vaginal, and anal cancer caused by HPV types 16 and 18
- Genital warts (condyloma acuminata) caused by HPV types 6 and 11

And the following precancerous or dysplastic lesions caused by HPV types 6, 11, 16, 18 and HPV 31, 33, 45, 52, and 58:

- Cervical intraepithelial neoplasia (CIN) grade 2/3 and Cervical adenocarcinoma *in situ* (AIS)
- Cervical intraepithelial neoplasia (CIN) grade 1
- Vulvar intraepithelial neoplasia (VIN) grade 2 and grade 3
- Vaginal intraepithelial neoplasia (VaIN) grade 2 and grade 3
- Anal intraepithelial neoplasia (AIN) grades 1, 2, and 3

Gardasil is also indicated in boys and men 9 to 26 years of age for the prevention of the following diseases caused by HPV types included in the vaccine:

- Anal cancer caused by HPV types 16 and 18
- Genital warts (condyloma acuminata) caused by HPV types 6 and 11

And the following precancerous or dysplastic lesions caused by HPV types 6, 11, 16, 18 and HPV 31, 33, 45, 52, and 58:

- Anal intraepithelial neoplasia (AIN) grades 1, 2, and 3

The FDA recently expanded the approval the HPV 9-valent vaccine, recombinant to include women and men aged 27 to 45 years for the prevention of certain cancers and diseases caused by HPV. Therefore, the HPV 9-valent vaccine (Gardasil 9, Merck) is now approved for males and females aged 9 through 45 years.

Details regarding HPV vaccination are available at www.cdc.gov/std/hpv. Vaccines for other STDs (eg, HIV and herpes simplex virus) are under development or undergoing clinical trials. Vaccines are not available for bacterial or fungal STDs.

CANCER PATIENT DENTAL PROTOCOL

As in OSCC, the objective in treatment of any patient with cancer is eradication of the disease. In addition to surgery many cancer patients receive other modalities of treatment including chemotherapy, targeted molecular therapies, and radiation treatment. These treatments often lead to oral complications, such as mucosal ulceration, xerostomia, bleeding, and infections which can cause significant morbidity and may compromise systemic cancer treatment of the patient. With proper oral evaluation before systemic treatment, many of the complications can be minimized or prevented.

MUCOSITIS

Normal oral mucosa acts as a barrier against chemical and food irritants and oral micro-organisms. Disruption of the mucosal barrier can lead to secondary infection, increased pain, delayed healing, and decreased nutritional intake. Mucositis is an inflammation of the mucous membranes; however, its pathogenesis is more complicated, resulting from cytokine signals that lead to surface cell necrosis and delayed new cell proliferation. It is a common reaction to chemotherapy and radiation therapy. It is first seen as an erythematous patch. The mucosal epithelium becomes thin as a result of the killing of the rapidly dividing basal layer mucosal cells. Seven to ten days after cytoreduction chemotherapy and between 1,000 cGy and 3,000 cGy of radiation to the head and neck, mucosal tissues begin to desquamate and eventually develop into frank ulcerations. The mucosal integrity is broken and is often secondarily infected by normal oral flora. The resultant ulcerations can also act as a portal of entry for pathogenic organisms into the patient's bloodstream and may lead to systemic infections. These ulcerations often force interruption of therapy. A specific type of ulcerative stomatitis is encountered in patients treated for cancer with mTOR inhibitors such as everolimus (Afinitor). These ulcers resemble aphthous ulcers and occur on tissues that are freely movable (most commonly the tongue and lips). The lesions are self-limiting but can interrupt chemotherapy. The pathogenesis of the lesions is not well understood, but they appear to respond to steroid rinses.

Prevention of radiation mucositis is difficult. Stents can be constructed to prevent irradiation of uninvolved tissues. Most recently, intensity-modulated radiotherapy has been used as an advanced approach to 3D conformal radiotherapy; it optimizes the delivery of irradiation to irregularly shaped volumes and thus spares normal tissue while delivering an adequate dose to the tumor volumes. The use of multiple ports and fractionation of therapy into smaller doses over a longer period of time can also reduce the severity. Fractured restorations, sharp teeth, and ill-fitted prostheses can damage soft tissues and lead to additional interruption of mucosal barriers. Correction of these problems before radiation therapy can diminish these complications.

CHEMOTHERAPY

Chemotherapy for neoplasia also frequently results in oral complications. Infections and mucositis are the most common complications seen in patients receiving chemotherapy. Also occurring frequently are pain, altered nutrition, and xerostomia, which can significantly affect the quality of life.

Certain chemotherapeutic agents, such as melphalan, 5-fluorouracil, methotrexate, and doxorubicin, are more commonly associated with the development of oral mucositis. Treatment of oral mucositis is mainly palliative, but steps should be taken to minimize secondary pathogenic infections. Culture and sensitivity data should be obtained to select appropriate therapy for the bacterial, viral, or fungal organisms found.

RADIATION CARIES

Dental caries that sometimes follow radiation therapy is called radiation caries. It usually develops in the cervical smooth surface region of the teeth adjacent to the gingiva, often affecting many teeth. It is secondary to the irreversible damage done to the salivary glands and is initiated by dental plaque, but its rapid progress is due to changes in saliva. In addition to the diminution in the amount of saliva, both the salivary pH and buffering capacity are diminished, which decreases anticaries activity of saliva. Oral bacterial flora also change with xerostomia leading to the increase in caries activity. Typically patients that receive a cumulative radiation dose of 30 Gy or more will suffer significant loss of saliva production, some of which will be irreversible.

Osteonecrosis of the jaw (ONJ) is pertinent to cancer patient management and patients with osteoporosis, as well as antiresorptive agents used secondary to multiple myeloma and breast cancer to prevent metastases to the skeleton (see chapter on Osteonecrosis of the Jaw on page 1699 [ONJ, BRONJ, ARONJ, MRONJ]).

SALIVARY CHANGES

Chemotherapy is not thought to directly alter salivary flow, but alterations in taste and subjective sensations of dry mouth are relatively common complaints. Patients with mucositis and graft-vs-host disease following bone marrow or stem cell transplantation often demonstrate signs and symptoms of xerostomia. Radiation does directly affect salivary production. Radiation to the salivary glands produces fibrosis and alters the production of saliva. If all the major salivary glands are in the field, the decrease in saliva can be dramatic and the serous portion of the glands seems to be most severely affected. The saliva produced is increased in viscosity, which contributes to food retention, increased plaque formation, and difficulty swallowing. These xerostomia patients have difficulty in managing a normal diet. Normal saliva also has bacteriostatic properties that are diminished in these patients.

The dental management recommendations for patients undergoing chemotherapy, bone marrow transplantation, and/or radiation therapy for the treatment of cancer are based primarily on clinical observations. The following protocols will provide a conservative, consistent approach to the dental management of patients undergoing chemotherapy or bone marrow transplantation. Many of the cancer chemotherapy drugs produce oral side effects including mucositis, oral ulceration, dry mouth, acute infections, and taste aberrations. Cancer drugs include antibiotics, alkylating agents, antimetabolites, DNA inhibitors, hormones, and cytokines.

All patients undergoing chemotherapy or bone marrow transplantation for malignant disease should have the following baseline:

A. Panoramic radiograph

B. Dental consultation and examination

C. Dental prophylaxis and cleaning (if the neutrophil count is >1,500/mm^3 and the platelet count is >50,000/mm^3)

   – Prophylaxis and cleaning will be deferred if the patient's neutrophil count is <1,500 and the platelet count is <50,000. Oral hygiene recommendations will be made. These levels are arbitrary guidelines and the dentist should consider the patient's oral condition and planned procedure relative to hemorrhage and level of bacteremia.

D. Oral Hygiene: Patients should be encouraged to follow normal hygiene procedures. Addition of a chlorhexidine mouth rinse such as Peridex or PerioGard on page 334 is usually helpful. If the patient develops oral mucositis, tolerance of such alcohol-based products may be limited. A nonalcohol-containing chlorhexidine mouth rinse CHX is also available. Biotène products including Oralbalance are also useful since many patients report alteration of quality and quantity of saliva.

PREVENTION AND TREATMENT OF MUCOSITIS

A. If the patient develops mucositis, bacterial, viral, and fungal cultures should be obtained. There are no standard of care recommendations for prevention of oral mucositis. The intravenous biologic product keratinocyte growth factor, palifermin (Kepivance) is approved to help reduce the chance that certain cancer patients, those with blood cancers undergoing chemotherapy, would develop mucositis. Most therapies are palliative only or help in reducing secondary infection. Sucralfate suspension in a pharmacy-prepared form or Carafate suspension, as well as Benadryl on page 502 or Xylocaine viscous on page 902 solution can assist in helping the patient to tolerate food. In addition to the mucosal-coating drugs described below, various emollients and lubricants can be tried. A cost-effective approach is to rinse with a solution of 1/2 teaspoon of baking soda (and/or 1/2 teaspoon of table salt) in 1 cup of lukewarm water several times a day. Lastly, multiple studies have indicated that lower-level laser therapy can reduce the severity of chemotherapy and radiation-induced oral mucositis.

B. Aloclair is now available as an oral lesion relief spray. It indicated for aphthous ulcerations and other mild to moderate oral erosions.

C. The oral barrier Gelclair and the mucositis treatment aid Caphosol are FDA approved for mucositis. Gargle and spit Gelclair mixture of one single-use packet (15 mL) and water 3 times/day or as needed; follow mixing and administration instructions on packet.

D. Mix contents of 1 blue (A) and 1 clear (B) Caphosol ampul in clean container, swish thoroughly with 1/2 of mixture (15 mL) for 1 minute and spit; repeat. Use immediately after mixing ampuls. Use 4 doses/day from the onset of high dose chemotherapy or radiation treatment. Patients may also require systemic and topical analgesics for pain relief depending on the presence of mucositis. Systemic treatments currently being used with variable success include antioxidants, immunomodulatory drugs, anticholinergic drugs, pentoxifylline, cytokines antiviral drugs, and glutamic acid; a topical analgesic commonly used is lidocaine. Positive fungal cultures may require a nystatin swish-and-swallow prescription or the selection of another antifungal agent (see Fungal Infections on page 1752).

E. The determination of performing dental procedures must be based on the goal of preventing infection during periods of neutropenia and reducing the risk of bleeding when platelet counts are low. Timing of procedures must be coordinated with the patient's hematologic status.

F. If oral surgery is required, at least 7 to 10 days of healing should be allowed before the anticipated date of bone marrow suppression (eg, ANC <1,000/mm^3 and/or platelet count of ≥50,000/mm^3).

G. Daily use of topical fluorides is recommended for those who have received radiation therapy to the head and neck region involving salivary glands. Any patients with prolonged xerostomia subsequent to graft-vs-host disease and/or chemotherapy can also be considered for fluoride supplement. Use the fluoride-containing mouthwashes (Act, Fluorigard, etc) each night before going to sleep; swish, hold 1 to 2 minutes, spit out or use prescription fluorides (gels or rinses); apply daily for 1 to 4 minutes as directed; if mouth is sore (mucositis), use flavorless/colorless gels (Thera-Flur, Gel-Kam, or Prevident). Custom trays for fluoride applications can be produced by the clinician for the patient's home use using heat-formed materials such as omnivac. Patients with porcelain crowns, resin, or glass ionomer restorations should use a neutral pH fluoride. Improvement in salivary flow following radiation therapy to the head and neck has been noted with prescription sialogogue Salagen on page 1230 or Evoxac on page 330. Salagen, containing the nonselective analogue cholinergic agonist, pilocarpine, is currently the sole sialogogic agent approved by the FDA for radiation-induced xerostomia. Evoxac, containing the quinuclidine analogue of acetylcholine, cevimeline, has been found safe and effective in treating xerostomia in patients with Sjögren syndrome and may have merit for the treatment of radiation-induced xerostomia.

Benzonatate on page 231
Cevimeline on page 330
Chlorhexidine Gluconate (Oral) on page 334
DiphenhydrAMINE (Systemic) on page 502
Gelclair Bioadherent Oral Gel on page 1066
Lidocaine (Topical) on page 902
MuGard on page 1066
Pilocarpine (Systemic) on page 1230
Povidone-Iodine (Topical) on page 1249
Sucralfate on page 1389

ORAL CARE PRODUCTS

Bacterial Plaque Control

Patients should use an extra soft bristle toothbrush and dental floss for removal of plaque. Sponge/foam sticks and lemon-glycerine swabs do not adequately remove bacterial plaque.

Cholinergic Agents

See Products for Xerostomia on page 1762

Used for the treatment of xerostomia caused by radiation therapy in patients with head and neck cancer and from Sjögren's syndrome

Cevimeline on page 330
Pilocarpine (Systemic) on page 1230

Fluorides

See Fluorides in the Dentin Hypersensitivity, High Caries Index, and Xerostomia section.

Used for the prevention of demineralization of the tooth structure secondary to xerostomia. For patients with long-term or permanent xerostomia, daily application is accomplished using custom gel applicator trays, such as omnivac. Patients with porcelain crowns should use a neutral pH fluoride (see Fluoride monograph on page 693). Final selection of a fluoride product and/or saliva replacement/stimulant product must be based on patient comfort, taste, and ultimately, compliance. Experience has demonstrated that, often times, patients must try various combinations to achieve the greatest effect and their highest comfort levels. The presence of mucositis during cancer management complicates the clinician's selection of products.

Saliva Substitutes

See Products for Xerostomia on page 1762
Saliva Substitute on page 1354

Oral and Lip Moisturizers/Lubricants

Note: Water-based gels should first be used to provide moisture to dry oral tissues.

Surgilube
K-Y Jelly
Oralbalance
Mouth Moisturizer
Caphosol

PALLIATION OF PAIN

Note: Palliative pain preparations should be monitored for efficacy.

- For relief of pain associated with isolated mucositis or ulcerations, topical anesthetic and protective preparations may be used.
  - Orabase-B with 20% benzocaine on page 228
  - Zilactin-B gel with 10% benzocaine
- For generalized oral pain:
  - Chloraseptic Spray (OTC) anesthetic spray without alcohol
  - Ulcer-Ease anesthetic/analgesic mouthrinse
  - BetaCell oral rinse
  - Xylocaine 2% viscous on page 902

    Note: May anesthetize swallowing mechanism and cause aspiration of food; caution patient against using too close to eating; lack of sensation may also allow patient to damage intact mucosa
  - Tantum Mouthrinse (benzydamine hydrochloride); may be diluted as required

    Note: Available only in Canada and Europe

Patient-Prepared Palliative Mixtures

Coating agents:

Maalox
Mylanta
Kaopectate

These products can be mixed with Benadryl elixir (50:50):

DiphenhydrAMINE (Systemic) (Benadryl) on page 502

Topical anesthetics (diphenhydrAMINE chloride):

Benadryl elixir or Benylin cough syrup on page 502
Note: Choose product with lowest alcohol and sucrose content; ask pharmacist for assistance
Mucotrol gel wafer

Pharmacy Preparations

A pharmacist may also prepare the following solutions for relief of generalized oral pain:

Benadryl-Lidocaine Solution

DiphenhydrAMINE injectable 1.5 mL (50 mg/mL) on page 502
Xylocaine viscous 2% (45 mL) on page 902
Magnesium aluminum hydroxide solution (45 mL)

Swish and hold 1 teaspoonful in mouth for 30 seconds; do not use too close to eating

REFERENCES

ADA Council on Scientific Affairs. Statement on Human Papillomavirus and Squamous Cell Cancers of the Oropharynx (adopted November 2012). Available at: http://www.ada.org/1749.aspx.

Andrews E, Seaman WT, Webster-Cyriaque J. Oropharyngeal carcinoma in nonsmokers and nondrinkers: a role for HPV. *Oral Oncol.* 2009;45(6):486-491.

California-Catalonia Program for Engineering Innovation. Oral cancer detection using optical coherence tomography. 2007-2008 Progress Report.

CDC. Human papillomavirus (HPV)-associated cancers. Atlanta, GA: US Department of Health and Human Services, CDC; 2015. Available at http://www.cdc.gov/cancer/hpv/statistics/cases.htm.

Chaturvedi AK, Engels EA, Pfeiffer RM, et al. Human papillomavirus and rising oropharyngeal cancer incidence in the United States. *J Clin Oncol.* 2011;29(32):4294-4301.

Cleveland JL, Junger ML, Saraiya M, Markowitz LE, Dunne EF, Epstein JB. The connection between human papillomavirus and oropharyngeal squamous cell carcinomas in the United States: implications for dentistry. *J Am Dent Assoc.* 2011;142(8):915-924.

Corstjens PL, Abrams WR, Malamud D. Detecting viruses by using salivary diagnostics. *J Am Dent Assoc.* 2012;143(10 Suppl):12S-18S.

Eisen T, Sternberg CN, Robert C, et al. Targeted therapies for renal cell carcinoma: review of adverse event management strategies. *J Natl Cancer Inst.* 2012;104(2):93-113.

Food and Drug Administration. Highlights of prescribing information. Gardasil 9 (human papillomavirus 9-valent vaccine, recombinant). Silver Spring, MD: US Department of Health and Human Services, Food and Drug Administration; 2014. Available at http://www.fda.gov/downloads/BiologicsBloodVaccines/Vaccines/ApprovedProducts/UCM426457.pdf.

Food and Drug Administration. December 10, 2014 Approval letter—GARDASIL 9. Silver Spring, MD: US Department of Health and Human Services, Food and Drug Administration; 2014. Available at http://www.fda.gov/BiologicsBloodVaccines/Vaccines/ApprovedProducts/ucm426520.htm.

Gillison ML, Broutian T, Pickard RK, et al. Prevalence of oral HPV infection in the United States, 2009-2010. *JAMA.* 2012;307(7):693-703.

Hariri S, Unger ER, Schafer S, et al.; HPV-IMPACT Working Group. HPV type attribution in high-grade cervical lesions: assessing the potential benefits of vaccines in a population-based evaluation in the United States. *Cancer Epidemiol Biomarkers Prev.* 2015;24:393–399.

Jaitley S, Agarwal P, Upadhyay R. Role of oral exfoliative cytology in predicting premalignant potential of oral submucous fibrosis: a short study. *J Cancer Res Ther.* 2015;11(2):471-474.

Jemal A, Simard EP, Dorell C, et al. Annual Report to the Nation on the Status of Cancer, 1975-2009, featuring the burden and trends in human papillomavirus (HPV)-associated cancers and HPV vaccination coverage levels. *J Natl Cancer Inst.* 2013;105(3):175-201. http://jnci.oxfordjournals.org/content/early/2013/01/03/jnci.djs491.full.pdf+html

Kulkarni SS1, Kulkarni SS, Vastrad PP, et al. Prevalence and distribution of high risk human papillomavirus (HPV) Types 16 and 18 in Carcinoma of cervix, saliva of patients with oral squamous cell carcinoma and in the general population in Karnataka, India. *Asian Pac J Cancer Prev.* 2011;12(3):645-648.

Luxembourg A. Program summary and new 9-valent HPV vaccine trial data. Presentation before the Advisory Committee on Immunization Practices (ACIP), October 30, 2014. Atlanta, GA: US Department of Health and Human Services, CDC; 2014. Available at http://www.cdc.gov/vaccines/acip/meetings/downloads/min-archive/min-2014-10.pdf.

Markowitz LE, Dunne EF, Saraiya M, et al. Centers for Disease Control and Prevention (CDC). Human papillomavirus vaccination: recommendations of the Advisory Committee on Immunization Practices (ACIP). MMWR Recomm Rep 2014;63(No. RR-05):1–30.

Marur S, D'Souza G, Westra WH, Forastiere AA. HPV-associated head and neck cancer: a virus-related cancer epidemic. *Lancet Oncol.* 2010;11 (8):781-789.

Mehrotra R, Gupta A, Singh M, Ibrahim R. Application of cytology and molecular biology in diagnosing premalignant or malignant oral lesions. *Mol Cancer.* 2006;5:11.

Messada, D. Diagnostic aids for detection of oral precancerous conditions. *Int J Oral Sci.* 2013;5(2):59-65.

Patton LL, Epstein JB, Kerr AR. Adjunctive techniques for oral cancer examination and lesion diagnosis. *JADA.* 2008;139:1-10.

Pilotte AP, Hohos MB, Polson KM, et al. Managing stomatitis in patients treated with mammalian target of rapamycin inhibitors. *Clin J Oncol Nurs.* 2011;15(5):E83-E89.

Poh CF, MacAulay CE, Laronde DM, Williams PM. Squamous cell carcinoma and precursor lesions: Diagnosis and screening in a technical era. *Periodontol 2000.* 2011; 57(1): 73–88.

Porta C, Osanto S, Ravaud A, et al. Management of adverse events associated with the use of everolimus in patients with advanced renal cell carcinoma. *Eur J Cancer.* 2011;47(9):1287-1298.

Sonis S, Treister N, Chawla S, et al. Preliminary characterization of oral lesions associated with inhibitors of mammalian target of rapamycin in cancer patients. *Cancer.* 2010;116(1):210-215.

Warnakulasuriya S, Ariyawardana A. Malignant transformation of oral leukoplakia: a systematic review of observational studies. *J Oral Pathol Med.* 2015.

DENTIST'S ROLE IN RECOGNIZING DOMESTIC VIOLENCE, ABUSE, AND NEGLECT

Recognition of the signs and symptoms of domestic violence is an important topic for dental and medical professionals throughout the world. Unfortunately, statistics related to domestic abuse and/or neglect of women, children, and elderly patients appear to be on the rise, perhaps, in part, due to increased recognition.

Statistics are indeed staggering; one in four women will experience domestic violence in her lifetime (CDC 2008). In the United States, a woman, child, or elder is physically abused every 5 to 15 seconds. In fact, violence is cited as one of the common causes of emergency room admissions for women 15 to 44 years of age. Furthermore, 50,000 deaths occur annually, which are attributable to violence in the form of homicide or suicide.

The dentist's responsibilities and professional role in this arena are not clear in all states. The literature, however, is clear regarding how each professional has the responsibility to understand current state laws regarding the reporting of domestic violence, abuse of children or elderly patients, and/or neglect. Many states have existing codes defining the role of the professional in these regards. There is a model known as the "ask, validate, document, and refer/report if required by law" model for inquiring about domestic violence.

Many other states, such as Maryland, have adopted continuing education requirements specific to the subject. The overall problem of domestic violence, including child abuse, neglect, and other forms of abuse, are indeed public health issues. Likewise, the costs (eg, medical, dental, psychiatric, hospital, and emergency care fees) are borne to a great extent by the community as well as the individual.

Domestic abuse is defined as "controlling behavior." It is also further defined by the U.S. Centers for Disease Control and Prevention as "physical, sexual or psychological harm by a current or former partner or spouse which can occur among heterosexual or same-sex couples and does not require sexual intimacy." Domestic violence, also known as intimate partner violence, is a serious yet preventable public health issue.

Neglect can take on a myriad of presentations. Although this often includes physical injury, the primary focus of domestic abuse is one person being in control of another person, making that person do something against his/her will. Women are often abused both physically and mentally in relationships that have existed for many years. Children are often the focus of domestic violence; however, the pattern for an entire family's abuse may be present. Abuse comes in many forms and many victims do not even realize that abuse is occurring. Some victims simply "chalk it up" to things that happen within families. Abuse may include battery and physical assault, such as throwing objects, pushing, hitting, slapping, kicking, or attacking with a weapon; sexual assault including the abuser forcing sexual activities upon another; and psychological abuse, such as forcing a victim to perform degrading or humiliating acts, threatening harm to a female or male partner or child, or destroying valued possessions of another. Verbal abuse can also be included; however, psychological forms of abuse are very difficult to ascertain and signs and symptoms may be difficult to separate from other psychological traits. Abuse tends to have a cyclic pattern, often where a partner or the controlling individual is extremely friendly, intimate, and a good household member; however, due to unknown reasons, as tension develops, family violence often erupts. Once battering has begun, it often increases in frequency and in severity with time. Early recognition can often prevent serious effects; however, until physical violence becomes part of the domestic abuse situation, recognition is usually difficult.

It is estimated that nearly 65% of abuse cases (where physical injury is involved) include injury to the head, neck, or mouth; therefore, dental professionals are in a unique position to detect and perhaps, if appropriate in that state, report suspected abuse. In children, these percentages are even higher. Being wards of adults, children are vulnerable. Child abuse includes any act that is not accidental, endangering or impairing a child's safety or emotional health. Types of child abuse may include physical abuse, emotional abuse and neglect, including neglect of proper health care. Any child suspected of suffering from an emotional injury, including sexual abuse or neglect, should be brought to the attention of the social welfare system. Occasionally, "Munchausen syndrome," which is defined as the guardians fabricating or inducing illness in the child, may be observed. Intentional poisoning and safety neglect are also included in this syndrome.

From a medical point-of-view, neglect is much more difficult to determine than abuse. The role of the dentist may be to define the state of normal and customary pediatric or elderly patient health within a locality; however, due to parents and families moving about the country, sometimes one standard may not be appropriate for all locations.

Several key behavioral indicators:

- Child, adult, or elderly patient:
  - Avoids eye contact
  - Is wary of a guardian or spouse
  - Demonstrates fear when touched
  - Exhibits dramatic mood changes (eg, hostile or aggressive behavior)
- History or reports of suicide attempts or running away
- Unexplained injuries or injuries inconsistent with explanation or delay in seeking treatment
- Inappropriate use of prescription drugs (ie, responsible adult controls compliance of a child or elderly patient)
- Individual decides to change practitioner when questioned too intensely

DENTIST'S ROLE IN RECOGNIZING DOMESTIC VIOLENCE, ABUSE, AND NEGLECT

For the dentist, head-neck examination is important and includes gathering an overall visual impression of general cleanliness, dress, and stature and examining for any specific physical indicators such as bruises, welts, bite marks, abrasions, lacerations, or other injuries to the head or neck. Contusions or bruises represent the highest percentage of abuse injuries to the young child. The extremely young child or infant often suffers fractures, which fall to second place in terms of incidence as the child matures. In the adult, fractures are much less common. The dentist needs to document the location since this often represents the characteristic that may be difficult for the person to explain. Common areas for injuries include the bony eminences over the knees, shins, and elbows but could also be on the face, including the zygomatic arch and the chin. Burns are rarer, but represent one of the most serious types of injuries. Intraoral injuries, including trauma to the oral mucosa, tooth fractures, palatal lesions, ecchymoses, and fractures, represent serious evidence of domestic or child abuse. Physical indicators of sexual abuse may not be obvious to the dentist; however, bruising of the hard palate or other evidence of sexual dysfunction may sometimes be found.

The dentist has the responsibility to document, from a forensic point-of-view, the characteristics of abuse that are observed. As with all diagnostic considerations, the dentist must form a differential diagnosis to rule in or out oral and dental pathologies before suspecting abuse or neglect. History and probability are key to making these determinations. If necessary, evidence including impressions for bite marks or photographs to document unexplained injuries to the head, neck, and face may be necessary. The legal liability for the dentist is determined by the state laws governing the dental practice. The dental practitioner's failure to diagnose child abuse and neglect is another consideration which goes along with ethical and legal considerations. States are generally much clearer in the area of child abuse than they are regarding spousal or elderly abuse or overall domestic violence. The dentist has a responsibility to refer a patient for a second opinion, such as to their primary care pediatrician or internist, if there are concerns of abuse.

Under the Federal Child Abuse Prevention and Treatment Act (CAPTA) passed in 1974, all 50 states have passed laws mandating the reporting of child abuse and neglect. CAPTA provides a foundation for states by identifying a minimum set of acts or behaviors that characterize physical abuse, neglect, and sexual abuse. These laws vary from state to state. Each states responsible for the following:

- Providing its own definition of child abuse and neglect
- Describing the circumstances and conditions that obligate mandated individuals to report known or suspected child abuse
- Providing definitions for juvenile/family courts when to take custody of the child
- Specifying the forms of maltreatment that are criminally punishable

Unfortunately, there is little uniformity in the state laws regarding either the responsibility for reporting adult domestic violence or abuse or in protecting the health care professional by reporting, in good faith, abuse situations. When spousal or elderly abuse or other domestic violence is suspected, the definitions become even less clear. They are very similar in ambiguity to those that are faced by the professional regarding neglect as opposed to direct physical or mental abuse. The American Dental Association code is clear on principles and ethics regarding professional conduct regarding the responsibility for recognition of child abuse. They are much less clear on spousal or other abuse and it is likely that in the future, as some consistency is noted between and among the various state laws, the ADA Council will undoubtedly take a stronger position.

It is clearly up to the individual states to take the lead in establishing strict guidelines for recognition and reporting of domestic abuse, including protection under the "good faith" statutes for the practitioner. Rules and regulations regarding malicious reporting should also be better defined. The national position is difficult to define because of the extreme variation among states. Dentists are encouraged to use their best judgment in proceeding in any situation of suspected domestic abuse or neglect. They should primarily know their state laws and join in the discussion of the topic so that appropriate state actions and formation of legal codes can be undertaken. The current move by some states toward requiring continuing education on these subjects is an excellent sign that there is movement in a constructive direction.

RESOURCES

The National Health Resource Center on Domestic Violence, a project of the FVPF, provides support to thousands of health care professionals, policy makers and domestic violence advocates through its four main program areas: Model training strategies, practical tools, technical assistance, and public policy. **Contact information:** 383 Rhode Island St., Suite 304, San Francisco, CA 94103-5133; Phone: (888) Rx-ABUSE; TTY: (800) 595-4889; Fax: (415) 252-8991; email: health@endabuse.org; website: www.endabuse.org/health.

The **American Dental Association (ADA)** has developed a code of ethics and position statements on addressing adult domestic violence and child abuse in the dental health setting. **Contact information:** Phone: (312) 440-2500; website: www.ada.org/

Dental Professionals Against Violence (California Dental Association Foundation) DPAV's training program and print materials are designed to assist dental professionals and their teams to recognize and respond to child abuse/neglect, domestic/intimate partner violence, and elder abuse/neglect. The goal of DPAV is to raise the dental community's awareness of family violence using the most current information regarding patient risk assessment, clinical signs and symptoms, and dental professional's legal obligation to identify and report family violence situations. Dentists, registered dental hygienists, and registered dental assistants are mandated reporters in the state of California. The program includes definitive action steps for dental professionals to use within their practices and communities. **Contact information:** 1201 K Street, Suite 1511, Sacramento, CA 95814; Toll-free: (866) 232-6362 ext. 4921; Phone: (916) 554-4921; Fax: (916) 498-6182; email: foundationinfo@cda.org; website: www.cda.org/public/dpav.

Prevent Abuse and Neglect through Dental Awareness (PANDA) coalition educates dentists about how to effectively intervene in cases of child abuse and neglect and other forms of family violence, including intimate partner violence (domestic violence) and elder abuse and neglect. **Contact information:** Lynn Douglas Mouden, DDS, MPH Director, Office of Oral Health Arkansas Department of Health 4815 W. Markham Street, Slot 41, Little Rock, Arkansas 72205; Phone: (501) 661-2595; Fax: (501) 661-2055; email: Lmouden@healthyarkansas.com.

REFERENCES

American Academy of Pediatric Dentistry. Clinical guideline on oral and dental aspects of child abuse and neglect. *Pediatr Dent.* 2004;26(7 Suppl):63-66.

American Dental Association Council on Ethics, Bylaws and Judicial Affairs. American Dental Association principles of ethics and code of professional conduct, with official advisory opinions. 2012. Available at http://www.ada.org/sections/about/pdfs/code_of_ethics_2012.pdf

Centers for Disease Control and Prevention (CDC). Adverse health conditions and health risk behaviors associated with intimate partner violence – United States, 2005. *MMWR Morb Mortal Wkly Rep.* 2008;57(5):113-117.

Centers for Disease Control and Prevention. Intimate partner violence: definitions. Available at: http://www.cdc.gov/violenceprevention/intimatepartnerviolence/definitions.html.

Dubowitz H, Kim J, Black MM, Weisbart C, Semiatin J, Magder LS. Identifying children at high risk for a child maltreatment report. *Child Abuse Negl.* 2011;35(2):96-104.

Family Violence Prevention Fund. Compendium of State Statutes and Policies on Domestic Violence and Health Care. Available at: https://www.futureswithoutviolence.org/.

Katner DR, Brown CE. Mandatory reporting of oral injuries indicating possible child abuse. *J Am Dent Assoc.* 2012;143(10):1087-1092.

Kellogg ND, American Academy of Pediatrics Committee on Child Abuse and Neglect. Evaluation of suspected child physical abuse. *Pediatrics.* 2007;119(6):1232-1241.

Kenney JP. Domestic violence: a complex health care issue for dentistry today. *Forensic Sci Int.* 2006;159(Suppl 1):S121–S125.

Manea S, Favero GA, Stellini E, Romoli L, Mazzucato M, Facchin P. Dentists' perceptions, attitudes, knowledge, and experience about child abuse and neglect in Northeast Italy. *J Clin Pediatr Dent.* 2007;32(1):19-25.

McAndrew M, Marin MZ. Role of dental professional identification and referral of victims of domestic violence. *N Y State Dent J.* 2012;78(1):16-20.

Nelms AP, Gutmann ME, Solomon ES, Dewald JP, Campbell PR. What victims of domestic violence need from the dental profession. *J Dent Educ.* 2009;73(4):490-498.

Stechey F. P.A.N.D.A. A dentist's introduction to recognizing child abuse. *Dental Practice Management.* 2001. Available at http://www.rcdso.org/life/ll_learning_pdf/DPM_PANDA.pdf

US Department of Health and Human Services, Administration for Children and Families, Child Welfare Information Gateway. Mandatory reporters of child abuse and neglect. 2012. Available at https://www.childwelfare.gov/systemwide/laws_policies/statutes/manda.pdf

Wiseman M. The role of the dentist in recognizing elder abuse. *J Can Dent Assoc.* 2008;74(8):715-720.

APPENDIX TABLE OF CONTENTS

ABBREVIATIONS, ACRONYMS, AND SYMBOLS

Abbreviations Which May Be Used in This Reference

Note: Abbreviations in italics may not be defined within content text.

Abbreviation	Meaning
1/2NS	0.45% sodium chloride
5-HT	5-hydroxytryptamine
AACT	American Academy of Clinical Toxicology
AAP	American Academy of Pediatrics
AAPC	antibiotic-associated pseudomembranous colitis
ABCB1	ATP-binding cassette sub-family B member 1 (also known as P-gP or MDR1)
ABCC2	ATP-binding cassette sub-family C member 2 (also known as MRP2)
ABCG2	ATP-binding cassette sub-family G member 2 (also known as BCRP)
ABG	arterial blood gases
ABMT	autologous bone marrow transplant
ABW	actual body weight
ACC	American College of Cardiology
ACE	angiotensin-converting enzyme
ACLS	advanced cardiac life support
ACOG	American College of Obstetricians and Gynecologists
ACT	activated clotting time
ACTH	adrenocorticotrophic hormone
ADH	antidiuretic hormone
ADHD	attention-deficit/hyperactivity disorder
ADI	adequate daily intake
AdjBW	adjusted body weight
ADLs	activities of daily living
ADT	androgen deprivation therapy
AED	antiepileptic drug
AHA	American Heart Association
AHCPR	Agency for Health Care Policy and Research
AIDS	acquired immunodeficiency syndrome
AIMS	Abnormal Involuntary Movement Scale
ALL	acute lymphoblastic leukemia
ALS	amyotrophic lateral sclerosis
ALT	alanine aminotransferase (formerly called SGPT)
AMA	American Medical Association
AML	acute myeloblastic leukemia
ANA	antinuclear antibodies
ANC	absolute neutrophil count
ANLL	acute nonlymphoblastic leukemia
APL	acute promyelocytic leukemia
aPTT	activated partial thromboplastin time
ARB	angiotensin receptor blocker
ARDS	acute respiratory distress syndrome
ASA-PS	American Society of Anesthesiologists – Physical Status (ASA-PS) I: Normal, healthy patient II: Patient having mild systemic disease III: Patient having severe systemic disease IV: Patient having severe systemic disease which is a constant threat to life V: Moribund patient; not expected to survive without the procedure VI: Patient declared brain-dead; organs being removed for donor purposes
AST	aspartate aminotransferase (formerly called SGOT)
ATP	adenosine triphosphate
AUC	area under the curve (area under the serum concentration-time curve)
A-V	atrial-ventricular
AVNRT	atrioventricular nodal reentrant tachycardia
AVRT	atrioventricular reentrant tachycardia
BCRP	breast cancer resistance protein

Abbreviations Which May Be Used in This Reference *(continued)*

Abbreviation	Meaning
Note: Abbreviations in italics may not be defined within content text.	
BDI	Beck Depression Inventory
BEC	blood ethanol concentration
BLS	basic life support
BMI	body mass index
BMT	bone marrow transplant
BP	blood pressure
BPD	bronchopulmonary disease or dysplasia
BPH	benign prostatic hyperplasia
BPRS	Brief Psychiatric Rating Scale
BSA	body surface area
BSEP	bile salt export pump
BUN	blood urea nitrogen
CABG	coronary artery bypass graft
CAD	coronary artery disease
CADD	computer ambulatory drug delivery
cAMP	cyclic adenosine monophosphate
CAN	Canadian
CAPD	continuous ambulatory peritoneal dialysis
CAS	chemical abstract service
CBC	complete blood cell count
CBT	cognitive behavioral therapy
CDC	Centers for Disease Control and Prevention
CF	cystic fibrosis
CFC	chlorofluorocarbons
CGI	Clinical Global Impression
CHD	coronary heart disease
CHF	congestive heart failure; chronic heart failure
CI	cardiac index
CIE	chemotherapy-induced emesis
C-II	schedule two controlled substance
C-III	schedule three controlled substance
C-IV	schedule four controlled substance
C-V	schedule five controlled substance
CIV	continuous IV infusion
CKD-EPI	chronic kidney disease epidemiology collaboration
CLL	chronic lymphocytic leukemia
C_{max}	maximum plasma concentration
C_{min}	minimum plasma concentration
CML	chronic myelogenous leukemia
CMV	cytomegalovirus
CNS	central nervous system or coagulase negative staphylococcus
COLD	chronic obstructive lung disease
COMT	Catechol-*O*-methyltransferase
COPD	chronic obstructive pulmonary disease
COX	cyclooxygenase
CPK	creatine phosphokinase
CPR	cardiopulmonary resuscitation
CrCl	creatinine clearance
CRF	chronic renal failure
CRP	C-reactive protein
CRRT	continuous renal replacement therapy
CSF	cerebrospinal fluid
CSII	continuous subcutaneous insulin infusion
CT	computed tomography
CVA	cerebrovascular accident
CVP	central venous pressure

Abbreviations Which May Be Used in This Reference *(continued)*

Abbreviation	Meaning
Note: Abbreviations in italics may not be defined within content text.	
CVVH	continuous venovenous hemofiltration
CVVHD	continuous venovenous hemodialysis
CVVHDF	continuous venovenous hemodiafiltration
CYP (CYP-450, CYP3A4, etc.)	cytochrome
D5¼NS	dextrose 5% in sodium chloride 0.2%
D5½NS	dextrose 5% in sodium chloride 0.45%
D5LR	dextrose 5% in lactated Ringer's
D5NS	dextrose 5% in sodium chloride 0.9%
D5W	dextrose 5% in water
D10W	dextrose 10% in water
DBP	diastolic blood pressure
DEHP	di(3-ethylhexyl)phthalate
DIC	disseminated intravascular coagulation
DL_{co}	pulmonary diffusion capacity for carbon monoxide
DM	diabetes mellitus
DMARD	disease modifying antirheumatic drug
DNA	deoxyribonucleic acid
DSC	discontinued
DSM-IV	Diagnostic and Statistical Manual
DVT	deep vein thrombosis
EBV	Epstein-Barr virus
ECG	electrocardiogram
ECHO	echocardiogram
ECMO	extracorporeal membrane oxygenation
ECT	electroconvulsive therapy
ED	emergency department
EEG	electroencephalogram
EF	ejection fraction
EG	ethylene glycol
EGA	estimated gestational age
eGFR	estimated glomerular filtration rate
EIA	enzyme immunoassay
ELBW	extremely low birth weight
ELISA	enzyme-linked immunosorbent assay
EPS	extrapyramidal side effects
ER	extended release
ESA	erythropoiesis-stimulating agent
ESR	erythrocyte sedimentation rate
ESRD	end stage renal disease
E.T.	endotracheal
EtOH	alcohol
FDA	Food and Drug Administration (United States)
FEV_1	forced expiratory volume exhaled after 1 second
FMO	Flavin-containing monooxygenase
FSH	follicle-stimulating hormone
FTT	failure to thrive
FVC	forced vital capacity
G-6-PD	glucose-6-phosphate dehydrogenase
GA	gestational age
GABA	gamma-aminobutyric acid
GAD	generalized anxiety disorder
GE	gastroesophageal
GERD	gastroesophageal reflux disease
GFR	glomerular filtration rate
GGT	gamma-glutamyltransferase
GI	gastrointestinal

Abbreviations Which May Be Used in This Reference *(continued)*

Abbreviation	Meaning
Note: Abbreviations in italics may not be defined within content text.	
GIST	gastrointestinal stromal tumor
GU	genitourinary
GVHD	graft versus host disease
HAM-A	Hamilton Anxiety Scale
HAM-D	Hamilton Depression Scale
HARS	HIV-associated adipose redistribution syndrome
Hb	hemoglobin
HbA_{1c}	hemoglobin A_{1c}
HCAHPS	Hospital Consumer Assessment of Healthcare Providers and Systems
HCM	hypertrophic cardiomyopathy
Hct	hematocrit
HCV	hepatitis C virus
HDL	high-density lipoprotein
HDL-C	high density lipoprotein cholesterol
HER2	human epidermal growth factor receptor 2
HF	heart failure
HFA	hydrofluoroalkane
HFSA	Heart Failure Society of America
HIV	human immunodeficiency virus
HMG-CoA	3-hydroxy-3-methylglutaryl-coenzyme A
HOCM	hypertrophic obstructive cardiomyopathy
HPA	hypothalamic-pituitary-adrenal
HPLC	high performance liquid chromatography
HSV	herpes simplex virus
HTC	hematopoietic cell transplantation
HTN	hypertension
IBD	inflammatory bowel disease
IBS	irritable bowel syndrome
IBW	ideal body weight
ICD	implantable cardioverter defibrillator
ICH	intracranial hemorrhage
ICP	intracranial pressure
ICU	intensive care unit
IDDM	insulin-dependent diabetes mellitus
IDSA	Infectious Diseases Society of America
Ig	immunoglobulin
IgG	immune globulin G
ILCOR	International Liaison Committee on Resuscitation
IM	intramuscular
INR	international normalized ratio
Int. unit	international unit
I.O.	intraosseous
I & O	input and output
IOP	intraocular pressure
IQ	intelligence quotient
IR	immediate release
ITP	immune thrombocytopenia (formerly known as idiopathic thrombocytopenic purpura)
IUGR	intrauterine growth retardation
IV	intravenous
IVH	intraventricular hemorrhage
IVP	intravenous push
IVPB	intravenous piggyback
JIA	juvenile idiopathic arthritis
JNC	Joint National Committee
JRA	juvenile rheumatoid arthritis
kg	kilogram

Abbreviations Which May Be Used in This Reference *(continued)*

Abbreviation	Meaning
Note: Abbreviations in italics may not be defined within content text.	
KIU	kallikrein inhibitor unit
KOH	potassium hydroxide
LAMM	L-α-acetyl methadol
LDH	lactate dehydrogenase
LDL	low-density lipoprotein
LDL-C	low density lipoprotein cholesterol
LE	lupus erythematosus
LFT	liver function test
LGA	large for gestational age
LH	luteinizing hormone
LP	lumbar posture
LR	lactated Ringer's
LV	left ventricular
LVEF	left ventricular ejection fraction
LVH	left ventricular hypertrophy
MAC	*Mycobacterium avium* complex
MADRS	Montgomery Asbery Depression Rating Scale
MAO	monoamine oxidase
MAOI	monamine oxidase inhibitor
MAP	mean arterial pressure
MDD	major depressive disorder
MDR1	multidrug resistence protein 1
MDRD	modification of diet in renal disease
MDRSP	multidrug resistant *streptococcus pneumoniae*
MI	myocardial infarction
MMSE	mini mental status examination
MOPP	mustargen (mechlorethamine), Oncovin (vinCRIStine), procarbazine, and prednisone
M/P	milk to plasma ratio
MPS I	mucopolysaccharidosis I
MRHD	maximum recommended human dose
MRI	magnetic resonance imaging
MRP2	multidrug resistance-associated protein 2
MRSA	methicillin-resistant *Staphylococcus aureus*
MUGA	multiple gated acquisition scan
NAAED	North American Antiepileptic Drug
NAEPP	National Asthma Education and Prevention Program
NAS	neonatal abstinence syndrome
NCI	National Cancer Institute
ND	nasoduodenal
NF	National Formulary
NFD	nephrogenic fibrosing dermopathy
NG	nasogastric
NHL	Non-Hodgkin lymphoma
NIDDM	noninsulin-dependent diabetes mellitus
NIH	National Institute of Health
NIOSH	National Institute for Occupational Safety and Health
NKA	no known allergies
NKDA	no known drug allergies
NMDA	n-methyl-d-aspartate
NMS	neuroleptic malignant syndrome
NNRTI	non-nucleoside reverse transcriptase inhibitor
NPH insulin	neutral protamine Hagedorn insulin
NRTI	nucleoside reverse transcriptase inhibitor
NS	normal saline (0.9% sodium chloride)
NSAID	nonsteroidal anti-inflammatory drug
NSCLC	non-small cell lung cancer

Abbreviations Which May Be Used in This Reference *(continued)*

Abbreviation	Meaning
Note: Abbreviations in italics may not be defined within content text.	
NSF	nephrogenic systemic fibrosis
NSTEMI	Non-ST-elevation myocardial infarction
NYHA	New York Heart Association
OA	osteoarthritis
OAT1/OAT2	organic anion transporter
OCD	obsessive-compulsive disorder
OCT	Organic cation transporter
OCT2	Organic cation transporter 2
OHSS	ovarian hyperstimulation syndrome
O.R.	operating room
OTC	over-the-counter (nonprescription)
PABA	para-aminobenzoic acid
PACTG	Pediatric AIDS Clinical Trials Group
PALS	pediatric advanced life support
PAT	paroxysmal atrial tachycardia
PCA	patient-controlled analgesia
PCI	percutaneous coronary intervention
PCP	*Pneumocystis jirovecii* pneumonia (also called *Pneumocystis carinii* pneumonia)
PCWP	pulmonary capillary wedge pressure
PD	Parkinson's disease; peritoneal dialysis
PDA	patent ductus arteriosus
PDE-5	phosphodiesterase-5
PE	pulmonary embolism
PEG tube	percutaneous endoscopic gastrostomy tube
P-gP	P-glycoprotein
PHN	post-herpetic neuralgia
PICU	Pediatric Intensive Care Unit
PID	pelvic inflammatory disease
PIP	peak inspiratory pressure
PIRRT	prolonged intermittent renal replacement therapy
PMA	postmenstrual age
PMDD	premenstrual dysphoric disorder
PNA	postnatal age
PONV	postoperative nausea and vomiting
PPHN	persistent pulmonary hypertension of the neonate
PPN	peripheral parenteral nutrition
PR interval	–
PROM	premature rupture of membranes
PSVT	paroxysmal supraventricular tachycardia
PT	prothrombin time
PTH	parathyroid hormone
PTSD	post-traumatic stress disorder
PTT	partial thromboplastin time
PUD	peptic ulcer disease
PVB	premature ventricular beats
PVC	polyvinyl chloride
PVD	peripheral vascular disease
PVR	peripheral vascular resistance
P wave	–
QRS complex	–
QTc	corrected QT interval
QTcF	corrected QT interval by Fridericia's formula
QTcI	individual-based corrected QT interval
QT interval	QT interval of the cardiac cycle
Q wave	–
R	Ringer's injection

Abbreviations Which May Be Used in This Reference *(continued)*

Note: Abbreviations in italics may not be defined within content text.

Abbreviation	Meaning
RA	rheumatoid arthritis
RAP	right arterial pressure
RBC	red blood cell [count]
RDA	recommended daily allowance
REM	rapid eye movement
REMS	risk evaluation and mitigation strategies
RIA	radioimmunoassay
RNA	ribonucleic acid
RPLS	reversible posterior leukoencephalopathy syndrome
RSV	respiratory syncytial virus
SA	sinoatrial
SAD	seasonal affective disorder
SAH	subarachnoid hemorrhage
SBE	subacute bacterial endocarditis
SBP	systolic blood pressure
SCLC	small cell lung cancer
SCr	serum creatinine
SERM	selective estrogen receptor modulator
SGA	small for gestational age
SGOT	serum glutamic oxaloacetic aminotransferase
SGPT	serum glutamic pyruvate transaminase
SI	International System of Units or Systeme international d'Unites
SIADH	syndrome of inappropriate antidiuretic hormone secretion
SIDS	sudden infant death syndrome
SL	sodium lactate
SLCO1B1	Solute carrier organic anion transporter family member 1B1
SLE	systemic lupus erythematosus
SLEDD	sustained low-efficiency daily diafiltration
SNRI	serotonin norepinephrine reuptake inhibitor
SRI	serotonin reuptake inhibitor
SSKI	saturated solution of potassium iodide
SSRIs	selective serotonin reuptake inhibitors
STD	sexually transmitted disease
STEM I	ST-elevation myocardial infarction
STI	sexually transmitted infection
ST segment	–
ST-T wave	–
SubQ	subcutaneous
SVR	systemic vascular resistance
SVT	supraventricular tachycardia
SWFI	sterile water for injection
SWI	sterile water for injection
$T_{1/2}$	half-life
T_3	triiodothyronine
T_4	thyroxine
TB	tuberculosis
TC	total cholesterol
TCA	tricyclic antidepressant
TD	tardive dyskinesia
TG	triglyceride
TIA	transient ischemic attack
TIBC	total iron binding capacity
TMA	thrombotic microangiopathy
T_{max}	time to maximum observed concentration, plasma
TNF	tumor necrosis factor
TPN	total parenteral nutrition

Abbreviations Which May Be Used in This Reference *(continued)*

Abbreviation	Meaning
Note: Abbreviations in italics may not be defined within content text.	
TSH	thyroid stimulating hormone
TT	thrombin time
TTP	thrombotic microangiopathy
T wave	–
UA	urine analysis
UC	ulcerative colitis
UGT	UDP-glucuronosyltransferase
ULN	upper limits of normal
URI	upper respiratory infection
USAN	United States Adopted Names
USP	United States Pharmacopeia
UTI	urinary tract infection
UV	ultraviolet
U wave	–
V_d	volume of distribution
V_{dss}	volume of distribution at steady-state
VEGF	vascular endothelial growth factor
VF	ventricular fibrillation
VLBW	very low birth weight
VMA	vanillylmandelic acid
VT	ventricular tachycardia
VTE	venous thromboembolism
vWD	von Willebrand disease
VZV	varicella zoster virus
WBC	white blood cell [count]
WHO	World Health Organization
w/v	weight in volume
w/w	weight in weight
YBOC	Yale Brown Obsessive-Compulsive Scale
YMRS	Young Mania Rating Scale

Common Weights, Measures, or Apothecary Abbreviations

Abbreviation	Meaning
< [a]	less than
>[a]	greater than
≤	less than or equal to
≥	greater than or equal to
ac	before meals or food
ad	to, up to
ad lib	at pleasure
AM	morning
AMA	against medical advice
amp	ampul
amt	amount
aq	water
aq. dest.	distilled water
ASAP	as soon as possible
a.u.[a]	each ear
bid	twice daily
bm	bowel movement
C	Celsius, centigrade
cal	calorie
cap	capsule
cc[a]	cubic centimeter

Common Weights, Measures, or Apothecary Abbreviations *(continued)*

Abbreviation	Meaning
cm	centimeter
comp	compound
cont	continue
d	day
d/c[a]	discharge
dil	dilute
disp	dispense
div	divide
dtd	give of such a dose
Dx	diagnosis
elix, el	elixir
emp	as directed
et	and
ex aq	in water
F	Fahrenheit
g	gram
gr	grain
gtt	a drop
h	hour
hs[a]	at bedtime
kcal	kilocalorie
kg	kilogram
L	liter
liq	a liquor, solution
M	molar
mcg	microgram
m. dict	as directed
mEq	milliequivalent
mg	milligram
microL	microliter
min	minute
mL	milliliter
mm	millimeter
mM	millimole
mm Hg	millimeters of mercury
mo	month
mOsm	milliosmoles
ng	nanogram
nmol	nanomole
no.	number
noc	in the night
non rep	do not repeat, no refills
NPO	nothing by mouth
NV	nausea and vomiting
O, Oct	a pint
o.d.[a]	right eye
o.l.	left eye
o.s.[a]	left eye
o.u.[a]	each eye
pc, post cib	after meals
PM	afternoon or evening
PO	by mouth
P.R.	rectally
prn	as needed
pulv	a powder
q	every
qad	every other day

Common Weights, Measures, or Apothecary Abbreviations *(continued)*

Abbreviation	Meaning
qh	every hour
qid	four times a day
qs	a sufficient quantity
qs ad	a sufficient quantity to make
Rx	prescription drug
S.L.	sublingual
stat	at once, immediately
SubQ	subcutaneous
supp	suppository
syr	syrup
tab	tablet
tal	such
tid	three times a day
tr, tinct	tincture
trit	triturate
tsp	teaspoon
u.d.	as directed
ung	ointment
v.o.	verbal order
w.a.	while awake
x3	3 times
x4	4 times
y	year

[a]ISMP error-prone abbreviation

Additional abbreviations used and defined within a specific monograph or text piece may only apply to that text.

REFERENCE

The Institute for Safe Medication Practices (ISMP) list of Error-Prone Abbreviations, Symbols, and Dose Designations. Available at http://www.ismp.org/Tools/errorproneabbreviations.pdf

AVERAGE WEIGHTS AND SURFACE AREAS

Average Height, Weight, and Surface Area by Age and Gender

Age	Girls			Boys		
	Height (cm)	Weight (kg)	BSA (m^2)	Height (cm)	Weight (kg)	BSA (m^2)
Birth	49.5	3.4	0.22	50	3.6	0.22
3 months	59	5.6	0.3	61	6	0.32
6 months	65	7.2	0.36	67	7.9	0.38
9 months	70	8.3	0.4	72	9.3	0.43
12 months	74.5	9.5	0.44	75.5	10.3	0.46
15 months	77	10.3	0.47	79	11.1	0.49
18 months	80	11	0.49	82	11.7	0.52
21 months	83	11.6	0.52	85	12.2	0.54
2 years	86	12	0.54	87.5	12.6	0.55
2.5 years	91	13	0.57	92	13.5	0.59
3 years	94.5	13.8	0.6	96	14.3	0.62
3.5 years	97	15	0.64	98	15	0.64
4 years	101	16	0.67	102	16	0.67
4.5 years	104	17	0.7	105	17	0.7
5 years	107.5	18	0.73	109	18.5	0.75
6 years	115	20	0.8	115	21	0.82
7 years	121.5	23	0.88	122	23	0.88
8 years	127.5	25.5	0.95	127.5	26	0.96
9 years	133	29	1.04	133.5	28.5	1.03
10 years	138	33	1.12	138.5	32	1.1
11 years	144	37	1.22	143.5	36	1.2
12 years	151	41.5	1.32	149	40.5	1.29
13 years	157	46	1.42	156	45.5	1.4
14 years	160.5	49.5	1.49	163.5	51	1.52
15 years	162	52	1.53	170	56	1.63
16 years	162.5	54	1.56	173.5	61	1.71
17 years	163	55	1.58	175	64.5	1.77
Adult[a]	163.5	58	1.62	177	83.5	2.03

Data extracted from the CDC growth charts based on the 50th percentile height and weight for a given age[b]

Body surface area calculation[c]: Square root of [(Ht x Wt) / 3,600]

[a]McDowell MA, Fryar CD, Hirsch R, Ogden CL. Anthropometric reference data for children and adults: US population, 1999-2002. *Adv Data*. 2005;(361):1-5.

[b]Centers for Disease Control and Prevention (CDC). 2000 CDC growth charts: United States. Available at http://www.cdc.gov/growthcharts. Accessed November 16, 2007.

[c]Mosteller RD. Simplified calculation of body-surface area *N Engl J Med*. 1987;317(17):1098.

BODY SURFACE AREA OF CHILDREN AND ADULTS

Calculating Body Surface Area in Children

In a child of average size, find weight and corresponding surface area on the boxed scale to the left or use the nomogram to the right. Lay a straightedge on the correct height and weight points for the child, then read the intersecting point on the surface area scale. (**Note:** 2.2 lb = 1 kg)

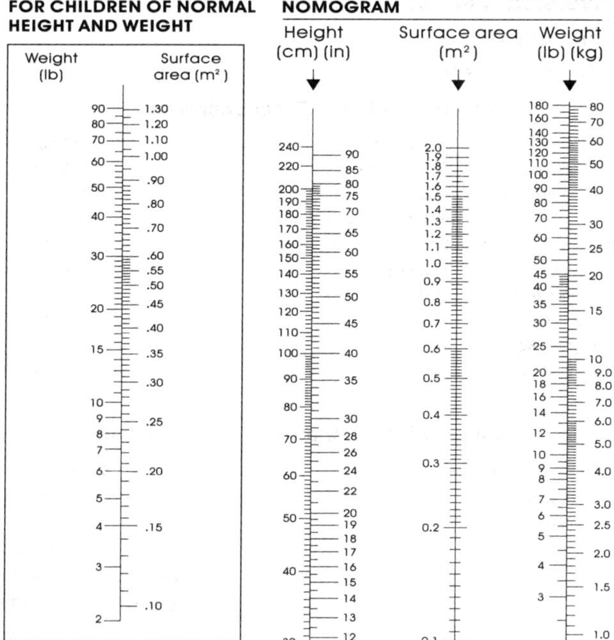

BODY SURFACE AREA FORMULA
(Adult and Pediatric)

$$\text{BSA (m}^2\text{)} = \sqrt{\frac{\text{ht (in)} \times \text{wt (lb)}}{3131}} \quad \text{or, in metric: BSA (m}^2\text{)} = \sqrt{\frac{\text{ht (cm)} \times \text{wt (kg)}}{3600}}$$

References

Lam TK and Leung DT, "More on Simplified Calculation of Body Surface Area," *N Engl J Med*, 1988, 318(17):1130 (letter).

Mosteller RD, "Simplified Calculation of Body Surface Area," *N Engl J Med*, 1987, 317(17):1098 (letter).

METRIC CONVERSIONS

Weight Conversion: Pounds/Kilograms

1 pound = 0.45359 kilograms

1 kilogram = 2.2 pounds

Temperature Conversion: Fahrenheit/Celsius

Fahrenheit to Celsius = (°F - 32) x 5/9 = °C

Celsius to Fahrenheit = (°C x 9/5) + 32 = °F

Apothecary-Metric Exact Equivalents

1 gram (g)	=	15.43 grains (gr)	0.1 mg	=	1/600 gr
1 milliliter (mL)	=	16.23 minims	0.12 mg	=	1/500 gr
1 minim	=	0.06 mL	0.15 mg	=	1/400 gr
1 gr	=	64.8 milligrams (mg)	0.2 mg	=	1/300 gr
1 fluid ounce (fl oz)	=	29.57 mL	0.3 mg	=	1/200 gr
1 pint (pt)	=	473.2 mL	0.4 mg	=	1/150 gr
1 ounce (oz)	=	28.35 g	0.5 mg	=	1/120 gr
1 pound (lb)	=	453.6 g	0.6 mg	=	1/100 gr
1 kilogram (kg)	=	2.2 lb	0.8 mg	=	1/80 gr
1 quart (qt)	=	946.4 mL	1 mg	=	1/65 gr

Apothecary-Metric Approximate Equivalents[a]

Liquids			Solids		
1 teaspoonful	=	5 mL	1/4 grain	=	15 mg
1 tablespoonful	=	15 mL	1/2 grain	=	30 mg
			1 grain	=	60 mg
			1 1/2 grain	=	100 mg
			5 grains	=	300 mg
			10 grains	=	600 mg

[a]Use exact equivalents for compounding and calculations requiring a high degree of accuracy.

DRUG INTERACTIONS: METABOLISM/TRANSPORT EFFECTS

Most drugs are eliminated from the body, at least in part, by being chemically altered to less lipid-soluble products (ie, metabolized), and thus are more likely to be excreted via the kidneys or the bile. Phase I metabolism includes drug hydrolysis, oxidation, and reduction, and results in drugs that are more polar in their chemical structure, while Phase II metabolism involves the attachment of an additional molecule onto the drug (or partially metabolized drug) in order to create an inactive and/or more water soluble compound. Phase II processes include (primarily) glucuronidation, sulfation, glutathione conjugation, acetylation, and methylation.

Virtually any of the Phase I and II enzymes can be inhibited by some xenobiotic or drug. Some of the Phase I and II enzymes can be induced. Inhibition of the activity of metabolic enzymes will result in increased concentrations of the substrate (drug), whereas induction of the activity of metabolic enzymes will result in decreased concentrations of the substrate. For example, the well-documented enzyme-inducing effects of phenobarbital may include a combination of Phase I and II enzymes. Phase II glucuronidation may be increased via induced UDP-glucuronosyltransferase (UGT) activity, whereas Phase I oxidation may be increased via induced cytochrome P450 (CYP) activity. However, for most drugs, the primary route of metabolism (and the primary focus of drug-drug interaction) is Phase I oxidation, and specifically, metabolism.

CYP enzymes may be responsible for the metabolism (at least partial metabolism) of ~75% of all drugs, with the CYP3A subfamily responsible for nearly half of this activity. Found throughout plant, animal, and bacterial species, CYP enzymes represent a superfamily of xenobiotic metabolizing proteins. There have been several hundred CYP enzymes identified in nature, each of which has been assigned to a family (1, 2, 3, etc), subfamily (A, B, C, etc), and given a specific enzyme number (1, 2, 3, etc) according to the similarity in amino acid sequence that it shares with other enzymes. Of these many enzymes, only a few are found in humans, and even fewer appear to be involved in the metabolism of xenobiotics (eg, drugs). The key human enzyme subfamilies include CYP1A, CYP2A, CYP1B, CYP2B, CYP2C, CYP2D, CYP2E, and CYP3A.

CYP enzymes are found in the endoplasmic reticulum of cells in a variety of human tissues (eg, skin, kidneys, brain, lungs), but their predominant sites of concentration and activity are the liver and intestine. Though the abundance of CYP enzymes throughout the body is relatively equally distributed among the various subfamilies, the relative contribution to drug metabolism is (in decreasing order of magnitude) CYP3A4/5 (nearly 50%), CYP2D6 (nearly 25%), CYP2C8/9 (nearly 15%), then CYP1A1/2, CYP2C19, CYP2A6, CYP2E1, CYP1B1, and CYP2B6. Owing to their potential for numerous drug-drug interactions, those drugs that are identified in preclinical studies as substrates of CYP3A enzymes are often given a lower priority for continued research and development in favor of drugs that appear to be less affected by (or less likely to affect) this enzyme subfamily.

Each enzyme subfamily possesses unique selectivity toward potential substrates. For example, CYP1A1/2 preferentially binds medium-sized, planar, lipophilic molecules, while CYP2D6 preferentially binds molecules that possess a basic nitrogen atom. Some CYP subfamilies exhibit polymorphism (ie, multiple allelic variants that manifest differing catalytic properties). The best described polymorphisms involve CYP2C8/9, CYP2C19, and CYP2D6. Individuals possessing "wild type" gene alleles exhibit normal functioning CYP capacity. Others, however, possess allelic variants that leave the person with a subnormal level of catalytic potential (so called "poor metabolizers"). Poor metabolizers would be more likely to experience toxicity from drugs metabolized by the affected enzymes (or less effects if the enzyme is responsible for converting a prodrug to it's active form as in the case of codeine). The percentage of people classified as poor metabolizers varies by enzyme and population group. As an example, ~7% of white patients and only about 1% of Asian patients appear to be CYP2D6 poor metabolizers.

CYP enzymes can be both inhibited and induced by other drugs, leading to increased or decreased serum concentrations (along with the associated effects), respectively. Induction occurs when a drug causes an increase in the amount of smooth endoplasmic reticulum, secondary to increasing the amount of the affected CYP enzymes in the tissues. This "revving up" of the CYP enzyme system may take several days to reach peak activity, and likewise, may take several days, even months, to return to normal following discontinuation of the inducing agent.

CYP inhibition occurs via several potential mechanisms. Most commonly, a CYP inhibitor competitively (and reversibly) binds to the active site on the enzyme, thus preventing the substrate from binding to the same site, and preventing the substrate from being metabolized. The affinity of an inhibitor for an enzyme may be expressed by an inhibition constant (Ki) or IC50 (defined as the concentration of the inhibitor required to cause 50% inhibition under a given set of conditions). In addition to reversible competition for an enzyme site, drugs may inhibit enzyme activity by binding to sites on the enzyme other than that to which the substrate would bind, and thereby cause a change in the functionality or physical structure of the enzyme. A drug may also bind to the enzyme in an irreversible (ie, "suicide") fashion. In such a case, it is not the concentration of drug at the enzyme site that is important (constantly binding and releasing), but the number of molecules available for binding (once bound, always bound).

Although an inhibitor or inducer may be known to affect a variety of CYP subfamilies, it may only inhibit one or two in a clinically important fashion. Likewise, although a substrate is known to be at least partially metabolized by a variety of CYP enzymes, only one or two enzymes may contribute significantly enough to its overall metabolism to warrant concern when used with potential inducers or inhibitors. Therefore, when attempting to predict the level of risk of using two drugs that may affect each other via altered CYP function, it is important to identify the relative effectiveness of the inhibiting/inducing drug on the CYP subfamilies that significantly contribute to the metabolism of the substrate. The contribution of a specific CYP pathway to substrate metabolism should be considered not only in light of other known CYP pathways, but also other nonoxidative pathways for substrate metabolism (eg, glucuronidation) and transporter proteins (eg, P-glycoprotein) that may affect the presentation of a substrate to a metabolic pathway.

SMOKING AND DRUG METABOLISM

A nonpharmaceutical interaction may be equally important because of its constant occurrence in users (tobacco). Smoking induces CYP1A2 activity, possibly causing a reduced effect of its substrates (eg, estradiol). Among post-menopausal women receiving 1 or 2 mg daily of oral estrogen, it has been found that the serum estradiol level in smokers was half that in nonsmokers. The effect was manifested by about a 50% reduction in breast tenderness in smokers. Thus, smoking may affect drugs metabolized by CYP1A2, with various consequences on target organs. A review of the literature suggests that at least a dozen drugs interact with cigarette smoke in a clinically significant manner. Polycyclic aromatic hydrocarbons (PAHs) are largely responsible for enhancing drug metabolism. Cigarette smoke induces an increase in the concentration of CYP1A2, the isoenzyme responsible for metabolism of theophylline. Theophylline is, therefore, eliminated more quickly in smokers than in nonsmokers. As a result of hepatic induction of CYP1A2, serum concentrations of theophylline have been shown to be reduced in smokers. Cigarette smoking may substantially reduce tacrine plasma concentrations. The manufacturer states that mean plasma tacrine concentrations in smokers are about one-third of the concentration in nonsmokers (presumably after multiple doses of tacrine).

Patients with insulin-dependent diabetes who smoke heavily may require a higher dosage of insulin than nonsmokers. Cigarette smoking may also reduce serum concentrations of flecainide. Although the mechanism of this interaction is unknown, enhanced hepatic metabolism is possible. Propoxyphene, a pain reliever, has been found to be less effective in smokers than in nonsmokers. The mechanism for the inefficacy of propoxyphene in smokers compared with nonsmokers may be enhanced biotransformation.

The norepinephrine and serotonin reuptake inhibitors, as a new class of smoking cessation drugs, have also received attention relative to metabolic interactions. In vitro studies indicate that bupropion (Zyban) is primarily metabolized to hydroxybupropion by the CYP2B6 isoenzyme. Therefore, the potential exists for a drug interaction between Zyban and drugs that affect the CYP2B6 isoenzyme metabolism [eg, orphenadrine (Norflex) and cyclophosphamide (Cytoxan)]. The hydroxybupropion metabolite of bupropion does not appear to be metabolized by the cytochrome P450 isoenzymes. No systemic data have been collected on the metabolism of Zyban following concomitant administration with other drugs, or alternatively, the effect of concomitant administration of Zyban on the metabolism of other drugs.

SUMMARY

Once a drug has been metabolized in the liver, it is eliminated through several different mechanisms. One is directly through bile, into the intestine, and eventually excreted in feces. More commonly, the metabolites and the original drug pass back into the liver from the general circulation and are carried to other organs and tissues. Eventually, these metabolites are excreted through the kidney. In the kidney, the drug and its metabolites may be filtered by the glomerulus or secreted by the renal tubules into the urine. From the kidney, some of the drug may be reabsorbed and pass back into the blood. The drug may also be carried to the lung. If the drug or its metabolite is volatile, it can pass from the blood into the alveolar air and be eliminated in the breath. To a minor extent, drugs and metabolites can be excreted by sweat and saliva. In nursing mothers, drugs are also excreted in mother's milk.

The clinical considerations of drug metabolism may affect which other drugs can and should be administered. Drug tolerance may be a consideration, in that larger doses of a drug may be necessary to obtain effect in patients in which the metabolism is extremely rapid. These interactions, via cytochrome P450 or its isoforms, can occasionally be used beneficially to increase/maintain blood levels of one drug by administering a second drug. Dental clinicians should attempt to stay current on this topic of drug interactions as knowledge evolves.

SELECTED READINGS

Bjarnason NH, Christiansen C. The influence of thinness and smoking on bone loss and response to hormone replacement therapy in early postmenopausal women. *J Clin Endocrinol Metab.* 2000;85(2):590-596.

Bjarnason NH, Jørgensen C, Kremmer H, Alexandersen P, Christiansen C. Smoking reduces breast tenderness during oral estrogen-progestogen therapy. *Climacteric.* 2004;7(4):390-396.

Bjornsson TD, Callaghan JT, Einolf HJ, et al. The conduct of in vitro and in vivo drug-drug interaction studies: a PhRMA perspective. *J Clin Pharmacol.* 2003;43(5):443-469.

Drug-Drug Interactions. Rodrigues AD, ed. New York, NY: Marcel Dekker, Inc; 2002.

Hersh EV, Moore PA. Drug interactions in dentistry: the importance of knowing your CYP's. *J Am Dent Assoc.* 2004;135(3):298-311.

Metabolic Drug Interactions. Levy RH, Thummel KE, Trager WF, et al, eds. Philadelphia, PA: Lippincott Williams & Wilkins; 2000.

Wilkinson GR. Drug metabolism and variability among patients in drug response. *N Engl J Med.* 2005;352(21):2211-2221.

Wynn RL, Meiller TF. CYP enzymes and adverse drug reactions. *Gen Dent.* 1998;46(5):436-438.

Zhang Y, Benet LZ. The gut as a barrier to drug absorption: combined role of cytochrome P450 3A and P-glycoprotein. *Clin Pharmacokinet.* 2001;40 (3):159-168.

SELECTED WEBSITES

http://www.bdbiosciences.com/
http://www.cypalleles.ki.se/
http://medicine.iupui.edu/clinpharm/ddis/
http://mhc.com/Cytochromes/

LABORATORY VALUES/BODY MEASUREMENTS

In the following laboratory tests, normal reference values for commonly requested laboratory tests are listed in traditional units and in SI units. The tables are a guideline only. Values are method-dependent and "normal values" may vary between laboratories.

Reference Values for Blood, Plasma, or Serum Laboratory Tests

Determination	Reference Value	
	Conventional Units	SI Units
Alpha-fetoprotein:		
Adult	<15 ng/mL	<15 mcg/L
Pregnant (16 to 18 weeks)	38 to 45 ng/mL	38 to 45 mcg/L
Ammonia (NH_3) - diffusion	20 to 120 mcg/dL	12 to 70 mcmol/L
Ammonia Nitrogen	15 to 45 µg/dL	11 to 32 µmol/L
Amylase	35 to 118 IU/L	0.58 to 1.97 mckat/L
Anion gap (Na^+-\[Cl^- + HCO_3^-]) (P)	7 to 16 mEq/L	7 to 16 mmol/L
Antithrombin III (AT III)	80 to 120 U/dL	800 to 1,200 U/L
Bicarbonate:		
Arterial	21 to 28 mEq/L	21 to 28 mmol/L
Venous	22 to 29 mEq/L	22 to 29 mmol/L
Bilirubin:		
Conjugated (direct)	≤0.2 mg/dL	≤4 mcmol/L
Total	0.1 to 1 mg/dL	2 to 18 mcmol/L
Calcitonin	<100 pg/mL	<100 ng/L
Calcium:		
Total	8.6 to 10.3 mg/dL	2.2 to 2.74 mmol/L
Ionized	4.4 to 5.1 mg/dL	1 to 1.3 mmol/L
Carbon dioxide content (plasma)	21 to 32 mmol/L	21 to 32 mmol/L
Carcinoembryonic antigen	<3 ng/mL	<3 mcg/L
Chloride	95 to 110 mEq/L	95 to 110 mmol/L
Coagulation screen:		
Bleeding time	3 to 9.5 minutes	180 to 570 seconds
Prothrombin time	10 to 13 seconds	10 to 13 seconds
Partial thromboplastin time (activated)	22 to 37 seconds	22 to 37 seconds
Protein C	0.7 to 1.4 µ/mL	700 to 1,400 U/mL
Protein S	0.7 to 1.4 µ/mL	700 to 1,400 U/mL
Copper, total	70 to 160 mcg/dL	11 to 25 mcmol/L
Corticotropin (ACTH) - 0800 h	<60 pg/mL	<13.2 pmol/L
Cortisol:		
800 hours	5 to 30 mcg/dL	138 to 810 nmol/L
1,800 hours	2 to 15 mcg/dL	50 to 410 nmol/L
2,000 hours	≤50% of 0800 hours	≤50% of 0800 hours
Creatine kinase:		
Female	20 to 170 IU/L	0.33 to 2.83 mckat/L
Male	30 to 220 IU/L	0.5 to 3.67 mckat/L
Creatinine kinase isoenzymes, MB fraction	0 to 12 IU/L	0 to 0.2 mckat/L
Creatinine	0.5 to 1.7 mg/dL	44 to 150 mcmol/L
Fibrinogen (coagulation factor I)	150 to 360 mg/dL	1.5 to 3.6 g/L

Reference Values for Blood, Plasma, or Serum Laboratory Tests *(continued)*

Determination	Reference Value			
	Conventional Units		SI Units	
Follicle-stimulating hormone (FSH):				
Female	2 to 13 mIU/mL		2 to 13 IU/L	
Midcycle	5 to 22 mIU/mL		5 to 22 IU/L	
Male	1 to 8 mIU/mL		1 to 8 IU/L	
Glucose, fasting	65 to 115 mg/dL		3.6 to 6.3 mmol/L	
Glucose Tolerance Test (Oral):				
Fasting	*Normal*: 70 to 105 mg/dL	*Diabetic*: ≥140 mg/dL	*Normal*: 3.9 to 5.8 mmol/L	*Diabetic*: ≥7.8 mmol/L
60 minutes	*Normal*: 120 to 170 mg/dL	*Diabetic*: ≥200 mg/dL	*Normal*: 6.7 to 9.4 mmol/L	*Diabetic*: ≥11.1 mmol/L
90 minutes	*Normal*: 100 to 140 mg/dL	*Diabetic*: ≥200 mg/dL	*Normal*: 5.6 to 7.8 mmol/L	*Diabetic*: ≥11.1 mmol/L
120 minutes	*Normal*: 70 to 120 mg/dL	*Diabetic*: ≥140 mg/dL	*Normal*: 3.9 to 6.7 mmol/L	*Diabetic*: ≥7.8 mmol/L
(γ) -Glutamyltransferase (GGT):				
Male	9 to 50 units/L		9 to 50 units/L	
Female	8 to 40 units/L		8 to 40 units/L	
Haptoglobin	44 to 303 mg/dL		0.44 to 3.03 g/L	
Hematologic tests:				
Fibrinogen	200 to 400 mg/dL		2 to 4 g/L	
Hematocrit (Hct):				
Female	36% to 44.6%		0.36 to 0.446 fraction of 1	
Male	40.7% to 50.3%		0.4 to 0.503 fraction of 1	
Hemoglobin A_{1c}	5.3% to 7.5% of total Hgb		0.053 to 0.075	
Hemoglobin (Hb):				
Female	12.1 to 15.3 g/dL		121 to 153 g/L	
Male	13.8 to 17.5 g/dL		138 to 175 g/L	
Leukocyte count (WBC):	3,800 to 9,800/mcl		3.8 to 9.8 × 10^9/L	
Erythrocyte count (RBC)				
Female	3.5 to 5 × 10^6/mcl		3.5 to 5 × 10^{12}/L	
Male	4.3 to 5.9 × 10^6/mcl		4.3 to 5.9 × 10^{12}/L	
Mean corpuscular volume (MCV)	80 to 97.6 mcm^3		80 to 97.6 fl	
Mean corpuscular hemoglobin (MCH)	27 to 33 pg/cell		1.66 to 2.09 fmol/cell	
Mean corpuscular hemoglobin concentrate (MCHC)	33 to 36 g/dL		20.3 to 22 mmol/L	
Erythrocyte sedimentation rate (sedrate, ESR)	≤30 mm/hour		≤30 mm/hour	
Erythrocyte enzymes:				
Glucose-6-phosphate dehydrogenase (G-6-PD)	250 to 5,000 units per 10^6 cells		250 to 5,000 mcunits/cell	
Ferritin	10 to 383 ng/mL		23 to 862 pmol/L	
Folic acid: normal	>3.1 to 12.4 ng/mL		7 to 28.1 nmol/L	
Platelet count	150 to 450 × 10^3/mcl		150 to 450 × 10^9/L	
Reticulocytes	0.5% to 1.5% of erythrocytes		0.005 to 0.015	
Vitamin B_{12}	223 to 1,132 pg/mL		165 to 835 pmol/L	
Iron:				
Female	30 to 160 mcg/dL		5.4 to 31.3 mcmol/L	
Male	45 to 160 mcg/dL		8.1 to 31.3 mcmol/L	
Iron binding capacity	220 to 420 mcg/dL		39.4 to 75.2 mcmol/L	
Isocitrate dehydrogenase	1.2 to 7 units/L		1.2 to 7 units/L	

Reference Values for Blood, Plasma, or Serum Laboratory Tests *(continued)*

Determination	Reference Value	
	Conventional Units	**SI Units**
Isoenzymes:		
Fraction 1	14% to 26% of total	0.14 to 0.26 fraction of total
Fraction 2	29% to 39% of total	0.29 to 0.39 fraction of total
Fraction 3	20% to 26% of total	0.20 to 0.26 fraction of total
Fraction 4	8% to 16% of total	0.08 to 0.16 fraction of total
Fraction 5	6% to 16% of total	0.06 to 0.16 fraction of total
Lactate dehydrogenase	100 to 250 IU/L	1.67 to 4.17 mckat/L
Lactic acid (lactate)	6 to 19 mg/dL	0.7 to 2.1 mmol/L
Lead	≤50 mcg/dL	≤2.41 mcmol/L
Lipase	10 to 150 units/L	10 to 150 units/L
Lipids:		
Total Cholesterol:		
Desirable	<200 mg/dL	<5.2 mmol/L
Borderline-high	200 to 239 mg/dL	<5.2 to 6.2 mmol/L
High	>239 mg/dL	>6.2 mmol/L
LDL:		
Desirable	<130 mg/dL	<3.36 mmol/L
Borderline-high	130 to 159 mg/dL	3.36 to 4.11 mmol/L
High	>159 mg/dL	>4.11 mmol/L
HDL:		
Low	<40 mg/dL	
Desirable	≥60 mg/dL	
Triglycerides:		
Desirable	<150 mg/dL	
Borderline-high	150 to 199 mg/dL	
High	200 to 499 mg/dL	
Very high	≥500 mg/dL	
Magnesium	1.3 to 2.2 mEq/L	0.65 to 1.1 mmol/L
Osmolality	280 to 300 mOsm/kg	280 to 300 mmol/kg
Oxygen saturation (arterial)	94% to 100%	0.94 - fraction of 1
PCO_2, arterial	35 to 45 mm Hg	4.7 to 6 kPa
pH, arterial	7.35 to 7.45	7.35 to 7.45
PO_2, arterial:		
Breathing room air[a]	80 to 105 mm Hg	10.6 to 14 kPa
On 100% O_2	>500 mm Hg	
Phosphatase (acid), total at 37°C	0.13 to 0.63 IU/L	2.2 to 10.5 IU/L or 2.2 to 10.5 mckat/L
Phosphatase alkaline[b]	20 to 130 IU/L	20 to 130 IU/L or 0.33 to 2.17 mckat/L
Phosphorus, inorganic[c] (phosphate)	2.5 to 5 mg/dL	0.8 to 1.6 mmol/L
Potassium	3.5 to 5 mEq/L	3.5 to 5 mmol/L
Progesterone:		
Female:	0.1 to 1.5 ng/mL	0.32 to 4.8 nmol/L
Follicular phase	0.1 to 1.5 ng/mL	0.32 to 4.8 nmol/L
Luteal phase	2.5 to 28 ng/mL	8 to 89 nmol/L
Male	<0.5 ng/mL	<1.6 nmol/L
Prolactin	1.4 to 24.2 ng/mL	1.4 to 24.2 mcg/L

Reference Values for Blood, Plasma, or Serum Laboratory Tests *(continued)*

Determination	Reference Value	
	Conventional Units	**SI Units**
Prostate-specific antigen:	0 to 4 ng/mL	0 to 4 ng/mL
Protein: Total	6 to 8 g/dL	60 to 80 g/L
Albumin	3.6 to 5 g/dL	36 to 50 g/L
Globulin	2.3 to 3.5 g/dL	23 to 35 g/L
Rheumatoid factor	<60 IU/mL	<60 kIU/L
Sodium	135 to 147 mEq/L	135 to 147 mmol/L
Testosterone:		
Female	6 to 86 ng/dL	0.21 to 3 nmol/L
Male	270 to 1,070 ng/dL	9.3 to 37 nmol/L
Thyroid Hormone Function Tests:		
Thyroid-stimulating hormone (TSH)	0.35 to 6.2 mcU/mL	0.35 to 6.2 mU/L
Thyroxine-binding globulin capacity	10 to 26 mcg/dL	100 to 260 mcg/L
Total triiodothyronine (T_3)	75 to 220 ng/dL	1.2 to 3.4 nmol/L
Total thyroxine by RIA (T_4)	4 to 11 mcg/dL	51 to 142 nmol/L
T_3 resin uptake	25% to 38%	0.25 to 0.38 fraction of 1
Transaminase, AST (aspartate aminotransferase, SGOT)	11 to 47 IU/L	0.18 to 0.78 mckat/L
Transaminase, ALT (alanine aminotransferase, SGPT)	7 to 53 IU/L	0.12 to 0.88 mckat/L
Transferrin	220 to 400 mg/dL	2.2 to 4 g/L
Urea nitrogen (BUN)	8 to 25 mg/dL	2.9 to 8.9 mmol/L
Uric acid	3 to 8 mg/dL	179 to 476 mcmol/L
Vitamin A (retinol)	15 to 60 mcg/dL	0.52 to 2.09 mcmol/L
Zinc	50 to 150 mcg/dL	7.7 to 23 mcmol/L

[a]Age-dependent

[b]Infants and adolescents up to 104 U/L

[c]Infants in the first year up to 6 mg/dL

Reference Values for Urine Laboratory Tests

Determination	Reference Value	
	Conventional Units	**SI Units**
Calcium[a]	50 to 250 mcg/day	1.25 to 6.25 mmol/day
Catecholamines:		
EPINEPHrine	<20 mcg/day	<109 nmol/day
Norepinephrine	<100 mcg/day	<590 nmol/day
Catecholamines, 24-hour	<110 μg	<650 nmol
Copper[a]	15 to 60 mcg/day	0.24 to 0.95 mcmol/day
Creatinine:		
Child	8 to 22 mg/kg	71 to 195 μmol/kg
Adolescent	8 to 30 mg/kg	71 to 265 μmol/kg
Female	0.6 to 1.5 g/day	5.3 to 13.3 mmol/day
Male	0.8 to 1.8 g/day	7.1 to 15.9 mmol/day
pH	4.5 to 8	4.5 to 8
Phosphate[a]	0.9 to 1.3 g/day	29 to 42 mmol/day
Potassium[a]	25 to 100 mEq/day	25 to 100 mmol/day
Protein:		
Total	1 to 14 mg/dL	10 to 140 mg/L
At rest	50 to 80 mg/day	50 to 80 mg/day
Protein, quantitative	<150 mg/day	<0.15 g/day

Reference Values for Urine Laboratory Tests *(continued)*

Determination	Reference Value	
	Conventional Units	SI Units
Sodium[a]	100 to 250 mEq/day	100 to 250 mmol/day
Specific gravity, random	1.002 to 1.03	1.002 to 1.03
Uric acid, 24-hour	250 to 750 mg	1.48 to 4.43 mmol

[a]Diet-dependent

Drug Levels[a]

Drug Determination		Reference Value	
		Conventional Units	SI Units
Aminoglycosides	Amikacin:		
	Trough	1 to 8 mcg/mL	1.7 to 13.7 mcmol/L
	Peak	20 to 30 mcg/mL	34 to 51 mcmol/L
	Gentamicin:		
	Trough	0.5 to 2 mcg/mL	1 to 4.2 mcmol/L
	Peak	6 to 10 mcg/mL	12.5 to 20.9 mcmol/L
	Kanamycin:		
	Trough	5 to 10 mcg/mL	nd[b]
	Peak	20 to 25 mcg/mL	nd
	Netilmicin:		
	Trough	0.5 to 2 mcg/mL	nd
	Peak	6 to 10 mcg/mL	nd
	Streptomycin:		
	Trough	<5 mcg/mL	nd
	Peak	5 to 20 mcg/mL	nd
	Tobramycin:		
	Trough	0.5 to 2 mcg/mL	1.1 to 4.3 mcmol/L
	Peak	5 to 20 mcg/mL	12.8 to 21.8 mcmol/L
Antiarrhythmics	Amiodarone	0.5 to 2.5 mcg/mL	1.5 to 4 mcmol/L
	Bretylium	0.5 to 1.5 mcg/mL	nd
	Digitoxin	9 to 25 mcg/L	11.8 to 32.8 nmol/L
	Digoxin	0.8 to 2 ng/mL	0.9 to 2.5 nmol/L
	Disopyramide	2 to 8 mcg/mL	6 to 18 mcmol/L
	Flecainide	0.2 to 1 mcg/mL	nd
	Lidocaine	1.5 to 6 mcg/mL	4.5 to 21.5 mcmol/L
	Mexiletine	0.5 to 2 mcg/mL	nd
	Procainamide	4 to 8 mcg/mL	17 to 34 mcmol/mL
	Propranolol	50 to 200 ng/mL	190 to 770 nmol/L
	QuiNIDine	2 to 6 mcg/mL	4.6 to 9.2 mcmol/L
	Tocainide	4 to 10 mcg/mL	nd
	Verapamil	0.08 to 0.3 mcg/mL	nd
Anticonvulsants	CarBAMazepine	4 to 12 mcg/mL	17 to 51 mcmol/L
	PHENobarbital	10 to 40 mcg/mL	43 to 172 mcmol/L
	Phenytoin	10 to 20 mcg/mL	40 to 80 mcmol/L
	Primidone	4 to 12 mcg/mL	18 to 55 mcmol/L
	Valproic Acid	40 to 100 mcg/mL	280 to 700 mcmol/L

Drug Levels[a] *(continued)*

Drug Determination		Reference Value	
		Conventional Units	SI Units
Antidepressants	Amitriptyline	110 to 250 ng/mL[c]	500 to 900 nmol/L
	Amoxapine	200 to 500 ng/mL	nd
	BuPROPion	25 to 100 ng/mL	nd
	ClomiPRAMINE	80 to 100 ng/mL	nd
	Desipramine	115 to 300 ng/mL	nd
	Doxepin	110 to 250 ng/mL[c]	nd
	Imipramine	225 to 350 ng/mL[c]	nd
	Maprotiline	200 to 300 ng/mL	nd
	Nortriptyline	50 to 150 ng/mL	nd
	Protriptyline	70 to 250 ng/mL	nd
	TraZODone	800 to 1,600 ng/mL	nd
Antipsychotics	ChlorproMAZINE	50 to 300 ng/mL	150 to 950 nmol/L
	FluPHENAZine	0.13 to 2.8 ng/mL	nd
	Haloperidol	5 to 20 ng/mL	nd
	Perphenazine	0.8 to 1.2 ng/mL	nd
	Thiothixene	2 to 57 ng/mL	nd
Miscellaneous	Amantadine	300 ng/mL	nd
	Amrinone	3.7 mcg/mL	nd
	Chloramphenicol	10 to 20 mcg/mL	31 to 62 mcmol/L
	CycloSPORINE[d]	250 to 800 ng/mL (whole blood, RIA) 50 to 300 ng/mL (plasma, RIA)	nd nd
	Ethanol[e]	0 mg/dL	0 mmol/L
	HydrALAZINE	100 ng/mL	nd
	Lithium	0.6 to 1.2 mEq/L	0.6 to 1.2 mmol/L
	Salicylate	100 to 300 mg/L	724 to 2,172 mcmol/L
	Sulfonamide	5 to 15 mg/dL	nd
	Terbutaline	0.5 to 4.1 ng/mL	nd
	Theophylline	10 to 20 mcg/mL	55 to 110 mcmol/L
	Vancomycin:		
	Trough	10 to 20 mcg/mL	nd
	Peak	20 to 40 mcg/mL	nd

[a]The values given are generally accepted as desirable for treatment without toxicity for most patients. However, exceptions are not uncommon.
[b]nd = No data available
[c]Parent drug plus N-desmethyl metabolite
[d]24-hour trough values
[e]Toxic: 50 to 100 mg/dL (10.9 to 21.7 mmol/L)

Average Height, Weight, and Surface Area by Age and Gender

Age	Girls[a]			Boys[a]		
	Height (cm)	Weight (kg)	BSA[b] (m^2)	Height (cm)	Weight (kg)	BSA[b] (m^2)
Birth	49.5	3.4	0.22	50	3.6	0.22
3 months	59	5.6	0.3	61	6	0.32
6 months	65	7.2	0.36	67	7.9	0.38
9 months	70	8.3	0.4	72	9.3	0.43
12 months	74.5	9.5	0.44	75.5	10.3	0.46
15 months	77	10.3	0.47	79	11.1	0.49
18 months	80	11	0.49	82	11.7	0.52

Average Height, Weight, and Surface Area by Age and Gender *(continued)*

Age	Girls[a]			Boys[a]		
	Height (cm)	Weight (kg)	BSA[b] (m^2)	Height (cm)	Weight (kg)	BSA[b] (m^2)
21 months	83	11.6	0.52	85	12.2	0.54
2 years	86	12	0.54	87.5	12.6	0.55
2.5 years	91	13	0.57	92	13.5	0.59
3 years	94.5	13.8	0.6	96	14.3	0.62
3.5 years	97	15	0.64	98	15	0.64
4 years	101	16	0.67	102	16	0.67
4.5 years	104	17	0.7	105	17	0.7
5 years	107.5	18	0.73	109	18.5	0.75
6 years	115	20	0.8	115	21	0.82
7 years	121.5	23	0.88	122	23	0.88
8 years	127.5	25.5	0.95	127.5	26	0.96
9 years	133	29	1.04	133.5	28.5	1.03
10 years	138	33	1.12	138.5	32	1.1
11 years	144	37	1.22	143.5	36	1.2
12 years	151	41.5	1.32	149	40.5	1.29
13 years	157	46	1.42	156	45.5	1.4
14 years	160.5	49.5	1.49	163.5	51	1.52
15 years	162	52	1.53	170	56	1.63
16 years	162.5	54	1.56	173.5	61	1.71
17 years	163	55	1.58	175	64.5	1.77
Adult1	163.5	58	1.62	177	83.5	2.03

[a]Data extracted from the CDC growth charts based on the 50th percentile height and weight for a given age

[b]Body surface area calculation: Square root of [(height (cm) × weight (kg)) / 3,600].

REFERENCES

Centers for Disease Control and Prevention. 2000 CDC growth charts for the United States: Methods and Development. http://www.cdc.gov/growthcharts/2000growthchart-us.pdf. Published May 2002. Accessed November 16, 2007.

McDowell MA, Fryar CD, Hirsch R, Ogden CL. Anthropometric reference data for children and adults: U.S. population, 1999-2002. *Adv Data*. 2005;(361):1-5.

Mosteller RD. Simplified calculation of body-surface area. *N Engl J Med*. 1987;317(17):1098.

CALCIUM CHANNEL BLOCKERS AND GINGIVAL HYPERPLASIA

The last published report on calcium channel blocker-induced gingival hyperplasia (GH) by this author was in 2009 (Wynn 2009). This present update reviews the reports up through 2019, relative to the incidence of GH in patients taking calcium channel blockers (CCBs) and the mechanisms by which these drugs cause GH.

The first reported cases of gingival hyperplasia induced by nifedipine were reported by Ramon et al, in 1984 (Ramon 1984). Since that report, additional reports and case studies have been published describing gingival hyperplasia caused by nifedipine and other calcium channel blockers. The following table lists the number of reported cases with the specific drug involved and the number of cases from 1996 to the present.

FDA Approval	General Preparation	Cases of Gingival Hyperplasia in Clinical Literature Through 1995	Cases Reported in Literature 1996 to Present	Total Reported Cases
1982	Verapamil	7	9	16
1982	DiltiaZEM	20	33	53
1982	NIFEdipine	120	194	314
1989	NiCARdipine	0	0	0
1989	NiMODipine	0	0	0
1991	Isradipine	0	0	0
1992	AmLODIPine	0	58	58
1992	Felodipine	1	8	9
1993	Nisoldipine	0	0	0
2008	Nitrendipine[1]	1	0	1
	Clevidipine	0	0	0
	Pinaverium[a]	0	0	0

[a]Not approved in the United States

Calcium channel blockers are so named because of their effects on calcium at the cellular level. Contractile cells of the myocardium and smooth muscle cells of coronary and systemic arteries are influenced by the movement of calcium across their membranes. Part of this influence is in the regulation of contractile processes in these cells by way of movement of calcium ions through specific membrane channels. By blocking this channel movement of calcium, these drugs cause depression of the mechanical contraction of the myocardial cells, depression of electrical impulse formation and conduction velocity within the myocardium, and depression of smooth muscle contraction in coronary and systemic arteries. Thus, these drugs are useful in cardiovascular diseases, such as angina and hypertension, in which relaxation of these cells to cause vasodilatation is desired. These agents are sometimes referred to as calcium antagonists.

CLINICAL FINDINGS

Typical clinical findings of CCB-induced GH are hyperplastic gingiva around the maxillary and mandibular anterior teeth (Lederman 1984). The hyperplastic gingiva usually originates in the interdental papilla, and in many areas, bleeding upon probing and small ulcerations are present. False periodontal pockets may be present with no evidence of bone loss. Histopathological analysis usually shows a thick layer of stratified squamous epithelium with parakeratosis and elongated rete pegs (Lederman 1984; Lucas 1985). In the submucosa, a proliferation of collagen fibers together with lymphocytic and plasma cell infiltration can be noticed (Lucas 1985). The connective tissue usually shows large bundles of dense collagenous fibers with a moderate increase in fibroblasts. In addition, signs of inflammation are present with lymphocytes and plasma cells located perivascularly (Lucas 1985).

MECHANISMS

Theories abound on the mechanism of CCB-induced gingival hyperplasia, but none have been proven. An early report using cell culture showed that the CCBs may lead to proliferation of selected fibroblasts, leading to an imbalance between regeneration and degeneration of those cells (Pernu 1989). Brown et al, proposed that CCBs influence calcium/sodium flux in gingival fibroblast to result in decreased uptake of folic acid (Brown 1990). The lack of intracellular folic acid then sets off a chain of events resulting in lack of production of active collagenases with no resultant catabolism of interstitial ground substance. The overabundance of ground substance manifests as gingival enlargement. To further the theory on fibroblast proliferation, amlodipine was shown to have direct effects on extracellular matrix of gingival fibroblasts after incubation with fibroblast cell culture (Lauritano 2019). Another theory suggests that these drugs elicit their effects indirectly through mediators which simulate proliferation and/or collagen synthesis by gingival fibroblasts (Giustiniani 1987). Two of the mediators are reported to be Interleukin-2 from T cells and the testosterone metabolite 5-dihydrotestosterone (Nishikawa 1991; Sooriyamoorthy 1990). The report by Sooriyamoorthy et al, showed convincing evidence in controlled experiments that increased levels of 5-dihydrotestosterone occurred in gingival hyperplasia induced by nifedipine (Sooriyamoorthy 1990). Their earlier work also showed that this testosterone metabolite had a stimulatory effect on the synthetic activity of fibroblasts (Sooriyamoorthy 1988). In another theory, Nishikawa et al, suggests that alteration of the intracellular calcium level in gingival cells by nifedipine in combination with some local inflammatory factors is important in eliciting gingival hyperplasia (Nishikawa 1991). Preexisting gingival inflammation may be essential for onset of drug-induced gingival hyperplasia and that strict plaque control would be effective for preventing onset (Nishikawa 1991). A more recent study using rats suggests that CCBs induce epithelial hyperplasia in gingival overgrowth not by an increase in keratinocyte proliferation, but by prolongation of cell life through reduction of apoptosis (controlled cell death) before epithelial hyperplasia is detected (Shimizu 2002). Harel-Raviv et al, have argued that CCB-induced GH must be a calcium-dependent process because drugs, such as phenytoin and cyclosporin, which cause GH, also affect calcium ion cellular flux (Harel-Raviv 1995). For example, phenytoin increases total intracellular calcium accumulation in gingival fibroblasts (Harel-Raviv 1995).

INCIDENCE AND TREATMENT

The frequency and incidence of gingival hyperplasia caused by calcium channel blockers is difficult to assess. Literature numbers tell us that the effect by the calcium blockers is most prevalent with nifedipine (See table). The incidence of nifedipine-induced GH as currently reported are 28 cases out of 442 patients (6.3%), 11 cases out 29 patients (38%), and 79 cases out of 181 patients (44%) (Ellis 1999; Nery 1995; Steele 1994). The other agents are diltiazem, 7 cases out of 33 patients (21%) and 4 cases out of 186 patients (2.2%), and amlodipine, 5 cases out of 150 patients (3.3%) and 3 cases out of 181 patients (1.7%) (Ellis 1999; Jorgensen 1997; Steele 1994). For verapamil, the incidence has been reported as 5 cases out of 26 patients (19%) (Steele 1994). A report from the Mayo clinic described the incidence of verapamil-induced GH as ranging between 4% to 19% (Meraw 1998). Thus to summarize these values, nifedipine incidence ranged from 6.3% to 44%; diltiazem incidence ranged from 2.2% to 21%; amlodipine incidence ranged from 1.7% to 3.3%; and verapamil incidence ranged from 4% to 19%. In a more recent report, 20,636 patients taking a CCB or a non-CCB for treatment of various cardiovascular conditions were evaluated for incidence of gingival hyperplasia (Kaur 2010). The report identified 103 patients with definite CCB-induced gingival hyperplasia. The number of CCB-identified cases included amlodipine (12), nifedipine (13), felodipine (1), verapamil (4), and diltiazem (8). In a report of 2018, Vidal et al evaluated 162 patients with severe refractory hypertension and taking calcium channel blockers. Gingival overgrowth was observed in 55 patients (34.0%). With nifedipine users, 22 had GH and 35 had no GH. With amlodipine users, 15 had GH and 18 had no GH. With felodipine, 7 had GH and 8 had no GH. Eleven of the GH patients were not taking a calcium channel blocker. Three cases of GH associated with amlodipine were reported by Srivastava in 2010. Sharma and Sharma reported one case of amlodipine-associated enlargement in 2012. Sanz 2012, reported that the current use of calcium channel blockers compared to no use of calcium channel blockers doubles the risk of gingival hyperplasia. Nifedipine use alone was shown to nearly triple the risk of gingival hyperplasia. Umeizudike et al (2017) reported that the risk of gingival hyperplasia was nearly three times in calcium channel blocker users than that of non-calcium channel blocker users, and twice higher in amlodipine than nifedipine users in Nigeria. Joshi and Bansal reported a case of amlodipine-induced gingival enlargement in a 45-year old hypertensive patient taking a low dose of 5 mg. According to these authors, there are few reports of gingival enlargement at the dose of 5 mg. Brochet (2017) reported a case of nifedipine-induced gingival hyperplasia in a pregnant patient after 9 months drug exposure. Upon discontinuation of drug, after 48 hours, the gingival hyperplasia improved.

Treatment of CCB-induced GH includes the reinforcement and maintenance of good oral hygiene, along with frequent professional plaque removal (Camargo 2000). The ideal treatment of choice; however, is the discontinuation of the suspected medication. Regression of GH has been demonstrated after discontinuation of the offending CCB (Meraw 1998). In some situations, the use of another drug in the same class of medications has provided similar medical outcomes with reduced incidence of GH (Westbrook 1997). If the nonsurgical approach is ineffective, then gingivectomy or periodontal flap procedures can reduce the enlarged gingival tissues (Camargo 2000).

The following case report is an example of a three-step treatment approach to nifedipine-induced gingival overgrowth (Alandia-Roman 2012). A 61-year old man had severe gingival overgrowth associated with nifedipine use for the management of hypertension. For step one, the treatment protocol was based on a consistent oral health hygiene program and nonsurgical techniques to reduce inflammation. Professional prophylaxis occurred over multiple visits. The patient also received printed and verbal information about oral hygiene and periodontal disease and was given toothbrushes, dental floss, therapeutic dentifrices, and mouthwashes formulated with 0.5% chloramine-T. Chlorhexidine was not used because of its tooth-staining properties. For the second step, the health care provider changed to a different antihypertension medication, in this case an angiotensin-converting enzyme inhibitor. The change in medication controlled the hypertension and the gingival overgrowth showed an expressive but not complete reduction in 4 weeks. Finally, surgical correction of the gingival overgrowth was still necessary and scalpel gingivectomy was conducted at six sites with one site treated per month for 6 months. Per the authors, the measures used to achieve a successful resolution were based on the most commonly cited and discussed techniques found in the literature.

REFERENCES

Alandia-Roman CC, Tirapelli C, Ribas P, Panzeri H. Drug-induced gingival overgrowth: a case report. *Gen Dent.* 2012;60(4):312-315.

Aral CA, Dilber E, Aral K, Sarica Y, Sivrikoz ON. Management of cyclosporine and nifedipine-induced gingival hypeplasia. *J Clin Diagn Res.* 2015; 9 (12):ZD12-15.

Brochet MS, Harry M, Morin F. Nifedipine induced gingival hyperplasia in pregnancy: a case report. *Curr Drug Saf.* 2017;12(1):3-6.

Brown RS, Sein P, Corio R, Bottomley WK. Nitrendipine-induced gingival hyperplasia. First case report. *Oral Surg Oral Med Oral Pathol.* 1990;70 (5):593-596.

Camargo PM, Melnick PR, Pirih FQ, Lagos R, Takei HH. Treatment of drug-induced gingival enlargement: aesthetic and functional considerations. *Periodontol 2000.* 2001;27:131-138.

Carty O, Walsh E, Abdelsalem A, MaCarthy D. Case report: drug-induced gingival overgrowth associated with the use of a calcium channel blocker (amlodipine). *J Ir Dent Assoc.* 2015; 61(5):248-251.

Ellis JS, Seymour RA, Steele JG, Robertson P, Butler TJ, Thomason JM. Prevalence of gingival overgrowth induced by calcium channel blockers: a community-based study. *J Periodontol.* 1999;70(1):63-67.

Giustiniani S, Robustelli della Cuna F, Marieni M. Hyperplastic gingivitis during diltiazem therapy. *Int J Cardiol.* 1987;15(2):247-249.

Harel-Raviv M, Eckler M, Lalani K, Raviv E, Gornitsky M. Nifedipine-induced gingival hyperplasia. A comprehensive review and analysis. *Oral Surg Oral Med Oral Pathol Oral Radiol Endod.* 1995;79(6):715-722.

Jorgensen MG. Prevalence of amlodipine-related gingival hyperplasia. *J Periodontol.* 1997;68(7):676-678.

Joshi S, Bansal S. A rare case report of amlodipine-induced gingival enlargement and review of its pathogenesis. *Case Rep Dent 2013.* 2013:138248.doi:10.1155/2013/138248.

Kaur G, Verhamme KM, Dieleman JP, et al. Association between calcium channel blockers and gingival hyperplasia. *J Clin Periodontol.* 2010;37(7):625-630.

Lauritano D, Luccheses A, DiStasio D, et al. Molecular aspects of drug-induced gingival overgrowth: an in-vitro study on amlodipine and gingival fibroblasts. *Int J Mol Sci.* 2019;20(8). doi: 10.3390/ijms20082047.

Lederman D, Lumerman H, Reuben S, Freedman PD. Gingival hyperplasia associated with nifedipine therapy. Report of a case. *Oral Surg Oral Med Oral Pathol.* 1984;57(6):620-622.

Livada R, Shiloah J. Calcium channel blocker-induced gingival enlargement. *J Hum Hypertens.* 2014;28(1):10-14.

Lucas RM, Howell LP, Wall BA. Nifedipine-induced gingival hyperplasia. A histochemical and ultrastructural study. *J Periodontol.* 1985;56(4):211-215.

Madi M, Shetty SR, Babu SG, Achalli S. Amlodipine-induced gingival hyperplasia – a case report and review. *West Indian Med J.* 2015;64(3):279-282.

Meraw SJ, Sheridan PJ. Medically induced gingival hyperplasia. *Mayo Clin Proc.* 1998;73(12):1196-1199.

Nery EB, Edson RG, Lee KK, Pruthi VK, Watson J. Prevalence of nifedipine-induced gingival hyperplasia. *J Periodontol.* 1995;66(7):572-578.

Nishikawa S, Tada H, Hamasaki A, et al. Nifedipine-induced gingival hyperplasia: a clinical and in vitro study. *J Periodontol.* 1991;62(1):30-35.

Pavlic V, Zubovic N, Ilic S, Adamovic T. Untypical amlodipine-induced gingival hyperplasia. *Case Rep Dent.* 2015; 20215:756976.

Pernu HE, Oikarinen K, Hietanen J, Knuuttila M. Verapamil-induced gingival overgrowth: a clinical, histologic, and biochemic approach. *J Oral Pathol Med.* 1989;18(7):422-425.

Ramon Y, Behar S, Kishon Y, Engelberg IS. Gingival hyperplasia caused by nifedipine – a preliminary report. *Int J Cardiol.* 1984;5(2):195-206.

Sanz M. Current ise of calcium channel blockers (CCBs) is associated with an increased risk of gingival hyperplasia. *J Evid Based Dent Pract.* 2012;12(3 Suppl):147-148.

Sharma S, Sharma A. Amlodipine-induced gingival; enlargement – a clinical report. *Compend Contin Educ Dent.* 2012;33(5):e78-82.

Shimizu Y, Kataoka M, Seto H, Kido J, Nagata T. Nifedipine induces gingival epithelial hyperplasia in rats through inhibition of apoptosis. *J Periodontol.* 2002;73(8):861-867.

Sooriyamoorthy M, Gower DB, Eley BM. Androgen metabolism in gingival hyperplasia induced by nifedipine and cyclosporin. *J Periodontal Res.* 1990;25(1):25-30.

Sooriyamoorthy M, Harvey W, Gower DB. The use of human gingival fibroblasts in culture for studying the effects of phenytoin on testosterone metabolism. *Arch Oral Biol.* 1988;33(5):353-359.

Srivastava AK, Kundu D, Bandyopadhyay P, Pal AK. Management of amlodipine-induced gingival enlargement: series of three cases. *J Indian Soc Periodontol.* 2010;14(4):279-281.

Steele RM, Schuna AA, Schreiber RT. Calcium antagonist-induced gingival hyperplasia. *Ann Intern Med.* 1994;120(8):663-664.

Tejnani A, Mani A, Sodhi NK, et al. Incidence of amlodipine-induced gingival overgrowth in the rural population of Loni. *J Indian Soc Peridontol.* 2014;18(2):226-228.

Umeizuodike KA, Olawuyi AB,Umeizudike TI, Olusequn-Joseph AD, Bello NT. Effect of calcium channel blockers on gingival tissue in hypertensive patients in Lagos, Nigeria: a pilot study. *Contemp Clin Dent.* 2017;8(4):565-570.

Vidal F, deSouza RC, Ferreira DC, Fischer RG, Goncalves LS. Influence of 3 calcium channel blockers on gingival overgrowth in a population of severe refractory hypertensive patients. *J Periodontal Res.* 2018;53(5):721-726.

Westbrook P, Bednarczyk EM, Carlson M, Sheehan H, Bissada NF. Regression of nifedipine-induced gingival hyperplasia following switch to a same class calcium channel blocker, isradipine. *J Periodontol.* 1997;68(7):645-650.

Wynn RL. Calcium channel blockers and gingival hyperplasia – an update. *Gen Dent.* 2009;57(2):105-107.

DENTIFRICES WITHOUT SODIUM LAURYL SULFATE (SLS)A

Brand Name	Ingredients
Arm & Hammer Advance White for Sensitive Teeth	Sodium fluoride 0.24%, triclosan 0.3%
Auromere Herbal Toothpaste	Cardamom, fennel, fine chalk as cleanser, glycerine, Neem with 23 other barks, tooth-whitening Peelu fiber, pomegranite, persian walnut, almond, bedda nut, gluten-free
Orajel Tooth and Gum Cleanser (4 to 18 months of age)	Fluoride-, dairy-, and gluten-free
Burt's Bees Clean and Fresh with & without Fluoride	Sodium monofluorophosphate 0.77% (0.14% w/v fluoride ion)[b]
Biotene Sensitive	Potassium nitrate[c] 5%, sodium monofluorophosphate 0.14% w/v fluoride ion, anticavity
CloSYS	With fluoride 0.24%, and without; water hydrated silica, Clorastan, *naturally activated* chlorine dioxide, coconut derived sarkoysl, peppermint oil
CTx 3 Gel, Grape	Glycerin, hydrogenated starch hydrolysate, grape flavor, hydroxyapatite, xylitol[d]
Desert Essence Natural Tea Oil Toothpaste	Calcium carbonate, glycerin (vegetable-derived), water, fluoride, gluten-free
Dr. Collins Natural	Xylitol 25%[d]
Earthpaste	Purified water, Redmond clay, xylitol, lemon & tangerine essential oils, vegan, gluten-free
hello	Aloe vera, erythritol, fluoride, no dyes or artificial sweeteners
Himalays Botanique	Neem, pomegranite, Triphala, "certified organic ingredients", gluten and saccharin free
Kiss My Face Triple Action Gel	Sorbitol, glycerin, hydrated silica, water, xylitol among other natural ingredients, gluten-free
Life Extensions Toothpaste, Mint	CoQ10, green tea, hydrogen peroxide, aloe vera, xylitol, folic acid, lactoferrin
Lumineux Mineral Rich Toothpaste	Mint, aloe, sea minerals, therapeutic essential oils
Lush USA Toothy Tabs	Baking soda
Miessence Mint Toothpaste[e]	High percent organic ingredients, aloe vera, sodium bicarbonate, mint, sea salt, cinnamon, clove
Mint Sweet Orange Toothpaste	High percent organic ingredients, virgin coconut, sesame, water, organic oils, potassium hydroxide, citric acid
MyntSmile Cosmetic Dental Tooth Cream, formulated for veneers, crowns, and bonding	Sodium monofluorophosphate 0.83%, xylitol, sorbitol, gluten-free
NATIVE, Charcoal, Wild Mint Fluoride and Fluoride Free	Glycerin, water, hydrated silica, xylitol, sodium corcoyl glutamate, xanthan gum, peppermint oil, cocamidopropyl betaine, stevia extract, charcoal powder, carrageenan, titanium dioxide
Oral Essentials	Purified water, Dead Sea Salt, aloe vera, xylitol, essential oils; Whitening formula infused with coconut lemon, and sage oils.
Radius Organic	High percent organic ingredients, tea tree, aloe, Neem, coconut oil, salt, no fluoride
Sensodyne[f], Daily Care Original and Fresh Mint, Fresh Impact, Cool Gel, Tartar Control plus Whitening, Full Protection plus Whitening	Potassium nitrate 5%, sodium fluoride 0.13% w/v fluoride ion, anticavity, gluten-free
Sensodyne ProNamel Mint Essence, Gentle Whitening, Fresh Breath Fresh Wave, Multi-Action	Potassium nitrate 5%, sodium fluoride 0.15% w/v fluoride ion, anticavity, gluten-free
Squigle Tooth Builder	Xylitol 36%, calcium, water, glycerin, gluten-free
Siberian Rose Hips	Siberian juniper and sage extract, red clay
Tom's of Maine Clean and Gentle, SLS Free	Sodium monofluorophosphate 0.76% (0.13% w/v fluoride ion)
Tom's of Maine Fluoride-Free Botanically Bright Whitening	Naturally derived ingredients
The Natural Dentist Whitening The Natural Dentist Cavity Zapper Groovy Grape - Berry Blast	Sodium fluoride 0.24%, gluten-free
The Natural Dentist Fluoride Free	Peppermint oil (0.10%), Sage oil (0.02%), gluten-free

(continued)

Brand Name	Ingredients
Spry	Xylitol, sorbitol, sodium fluoride, all natural ingredients
Uncle Harry's Toothpaste, Jar Formula (peppermint, cinnamon, spearmint, anise)	Natural ingredients, gluten-free
Verve Ultra	Sodium fluoride 0.24%
Vita-Myr	Xylitol, CoQ10, vegan, gluten and sugar-free
Xyliwhite platinum mint	Xylitol 25%, sodium bicarbonate (baking soda, whitening) 9%, papain (whitening), gluten-free

[a]**Note:** Studies have suggested that SLS may have a desquamative effect on oral mucosa and demonstrate an increased incidence of recurrent aphthous ulcers and perioral irritation. http://www.ncbi.nim.nih.gov

[b]Percent Weight/Volume (% w/v) = the weight in grams of a solute per 100 mL of a solution. Hampton Research, Aliso Viejo, CA

[c]Potassium nitrate is used as an antihypersensitivity agent.

[d]Recent studies indicate that xylitol can induce remineralization of tooth enamel. https://www.ncbi.nlm.nih.gov/pubmed/14700079

[e]Cornucopia institute a natural food, Non-Profit Watchdog Organization, whose primary goal is to uphold the integrity of organic products. They produce a toothpaste scorecard based on the percentage of organic ingredients (https:www.cornucopia.org)

[f]All Sensodyne products without SLS have potassium nitrate as a desensitizing agent.

This chart represents a recent list of products that have been researched, updated, and available in the marketplace. It may not be inclusive of all products that do not contain Sodium Lauryl Sulfate. Most products listed are available online.

VASOCONSTRICTOR INTERACTIONS WITH ANTIDEPRESSANTS

Antidepressant	Effects with EPINEPHrine, Levonordefrin	Contraindicated	Recommendation
	Tricyclics		
Amitriptyline (Elavil [DSC])	EPINEPHrine = increased pressor response; cardiac dysrhythmias Levonordefrin = increased pressor response	No	Potentially dangerous; use minimal amounts with caution in local anesthetics
Amitriptyline and Chlordiazepoxide			
Amitriptyline and Perphenazine			
Amoxapine			
ClomiPRAMINE (Anafranil)			
Desipramine (Norpramin)			
Doxepin (Systemic) (Silenor)			
Imipramine (Tofranil [DSC])			
Nortriptyline (Pamelor)			
Protriptyline			
Trimipramine (Surmontil [DSC])			
	Serotonin/Norepinephrine Reuptake Inhibitor		
Desvenlafaxine (Khedezla [DSC], Pristiq)	No adverse interactions reported	No	Suggest caution since serotonin/norepinephrine reuptake inhibitors block norepinephrine reuptake in CNS
Duloxetine (Cymbalta, Drizalma Sprinkle)			
Levomilnacipran (Fetzima, Fetzima Titration)			
Milnacipran (Savella, Savella Titration Pack)			
Venlafaxine (Effexor XR)			
	Serotonin-Only Reuptake Inhibitors		
Citalopram (CeleXA)	No adverse interactions reported	No	No precautions appear to be necessary
Escitalopram (Lexapro)			
FLUoxetine (PROzac, PROzac Weekly [DSC], Sarafem)			
FluvoxaMINE			
Olanzapine and Fluoxetine (Symbyax)			
PARoxetine (Brisdelle, Paxil CR, Paxil, Pexeva)			
Sertraline (Zoloft)			
Vilazodone (Viibryd, Viibryd Starter Pack)			
Vortioxetine (Brintellix [DSC], Trintellix)			
	Central Alpha-2 Antagonist		
Mirtazapine (Remeron SolTab, Remeron)	No adverse interactions reported	No	Suggest caution since mirtazapine increases release of norepinephrine
	DOPamine Reuptake Inhibitor		
BuPROPion (Aplenzin, Buproban [DSC], Forfivo XL, Wellbutrin SR, Wellbutrin XL, Wellbutrin [DSC], Zyban [DSC])	No adverse interactions reported	No	Part of the mechanism of bupropion is to block norepinephrine reuptake within CNS; it has been suggested that vasoconstrictor be administered with caution
Naltrexone and Bupropion (Contrave)			

(continued)

Antidepressant	Effects with EPINEPHrine, Levonordefrin	Contraindicated	Recommendation
	Others		
DULoxetine (Cymbalta, Drizalma Sprinkle)	No adverse interactions reported	No	Part of the mechanism of duloxetine is to block norepinephrine reuptake within CNS; it has been suggested that vasoconstrictor be administered with caution
Maprotiline	Potential for increased pressor response	No	Blocks norepinephrine synaptic reuptake in the CNS; potentially dangerous; use minimal amounts with caution in local anesthetics
	MAO Inhibitors		
Isocarboxazid (Marplan)	No effects on blood pressure or heart rate reported; however, potential exists for slight increase in pressor response	No	Use vasoconstrictor with caution
Moclobemide			
Phenelzine (Nardil)			
Tranylcypromine (Parnate)			
	Serotonin Reuptake Inhibitor/Serotonin Antagonist		
Nefazodone	No adverse interactions reported	No	No precautions appear to be necessary
TraZODone			
	Serotonin Reuptake Inhibitor/5-HT_{1A} Receptor Partial Agonist		
Vilazodone (Viibryd, Viibryd Starter Pack)	No adverse interactions reported	No	No precautions appear to be necessary
	Serotonin Reuptake Inhibitor/5-HT_{1A} Receptor Agonist/5-HT_3 Receptor Antagonist		
Vortioxetine (Brintellix [DSC], Trintellix)	No adverse interactions reported	No	No precautions appear to be necessary

REFERENCES

Becker DE. Review: Adverse drug interactions. *Anesth Prog*. 2011;58(1):31-41.
Becker DE, Reed KL. Local anesthetics: review of pharmacologic considerations. *Anesth Prog*. 2012; 59(2):90-102.
Boakes AL, Laurence DR, Teoh PC, Barar FS, Benedikter LT, Prichard BN. Interactions between sympathomimetic amines and antidepressant agents in man. *Br Med J*. 1973;1(5849):311-315.
Moore PA. Adverse drug interactions associated with local anesthetics, sedatives and anxiolytics. *JADA*. 1999; 130(4):541-554.
Naftalin LW, Yagiela JA. Vasoconstrictors: indications and precautions. *Dent Clin North Am*. 2002;46(4):733-746.
Saraghi M, Golden LR, Hersch EV. Anesthetic considerations for patients on antidepressant therapy-Part I. *Anesth Prog*. 2017;64(4):253-261.
Saraghi M, Golden LT, Hersch EV. Anesthetic considerations for patients on antidepressant therapy-Part II. *Anesth Prog*. 2018;65(1):60-65.
Sisk AL. Vasocondtrictors in local anesthesia for dentistry. *Anesth Prog*. 1992;39(6):187-193.
Svedmyr N. The influence of a tricyclic antidepressive agent (protriptyline) on some of the circulatory effects or noradrenalin and adrenalin in man. *Life Sci*. 1968;7(1):77-84.
Wahl MJ, Brown RS. Dentistry's wonder drugs: Local anesthetics and vasoconstrictors. *Gen Dent*. 2010; 58(2):114-23.
Waits J, Cretton-Scott E, Childers NK, Sims PJ. Pediatric pyschopharmacology and local anesthesia: potential adverse drug reactions with vasoconstrictor use in dental practice. *Pediatr Dent*. 2014; 36(1):18-23.
Yagiela JA. Adverse drug interactions in dental practice: interactions associated with vasoconstrictors. Part V of a series. *J Am Dent Assoc*. 1999;130 (5):701-709.
Yagiela JA. Chapter 1. Injectable and topical anesthetics. *ADA/PDR Guide to Dental Therapeutics*. 5th ed. ADA American Dental Association: Chicago. 2009; 1-23.
Yagiela JA. Local anesthetics. In Yagiela JA, Dowd FJ, Neidle EA, eds. *Pharmacology and Therapeutics for Dentistry*. 5th ed. St Louis: Mosby; 2004.
Yagiela JA, Duffin SR, Hunt LM. Drug interactions and vasoconstrictors used in local anesthetic solutions. *Oral Surg Oral Med Oral Pathol*. 1985;59 (6):565-571.

PHARMACOLOGIC CATEGORY INDEX

Other Offerings from Lexicomp

Clinician's Endodontic Handbook

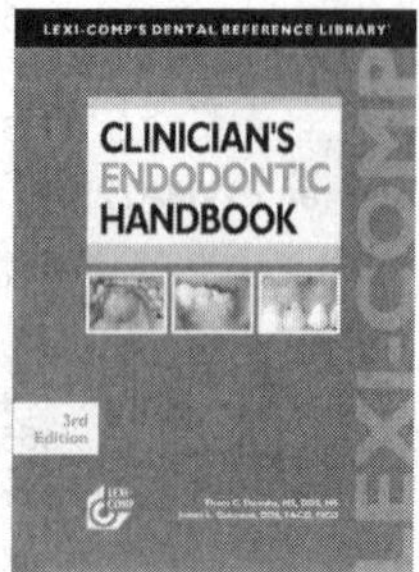

by Thom C. Dumsha, MS, DDS, MS, and James L. Gutmann, DDS, FACD, FICD

The *Clinician's Endodontic Handbook* is a fully illustrated guide to key issues in endodontic therapy. Here, the latest techniques, procedures, and materials are presented, reducing the need for multiple textbooks. This is a valuable reference for all dental practitioners with an interest in endodontics.

Dental Office Medical Emergencies

by Timothy F. Meiller, DDS, PhD; Richard L. Wynn, BSPharm, PhD; Ann Marie McMullin, MD; Cynthia Biron Leiseca, RDH, EMT, MA; Harold L. Crossley, DDS, PhD

The *Dental Office Medical Emergencies* manual facilitates dental office emergency treatment and assists the dentist in addressing any developing situation by reinforcing basic life support techniques. This handy reference is intended for use by the entire dental office staff for preparedness training as well as during times of crisis.

Manual of Clinical Periodontics

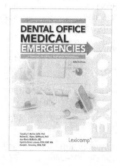

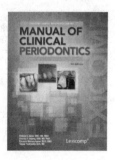

by Francis G. Serio, DMD, MS, MBA; Charles E. Hawley, DDS, MS, PhD; Eduardo Marcuschamer, BDS, DMD; Teppei Tsukiyama, DDS, MS.

The *Manual of Clinical Periodontics* is a quick reference for general dentists, dental hygienists, and students. The manual is a practical resource for both clinical and educational settings, stressing patient-centered, evidence-based diagnosis; treatment planning; and accepted modalities of periodontic therapy.

Manual of Dental Implants

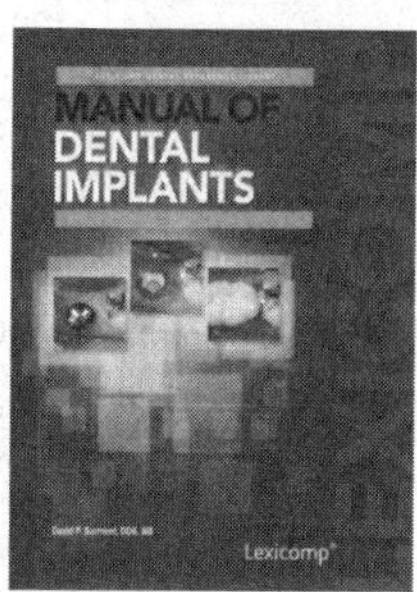

by David P. Sarment, DDS, MS; Beth Peshman, RDH; and Robert F. Faulkner, DDS

The *Manual of Dental Implants* introduces dental professionals to the world of restorative implant dentistry. More than 280 color photographs, diagrams and decision trees help illustrate the diagnosis, treatment, and maintenance of implants. This reference is valuable for increasing levels of knowledge and training, so the user can continue to benefit as he or she gains implant experience.

Other Offerings from Lexicomp

Oral Hard Tissue Diseases

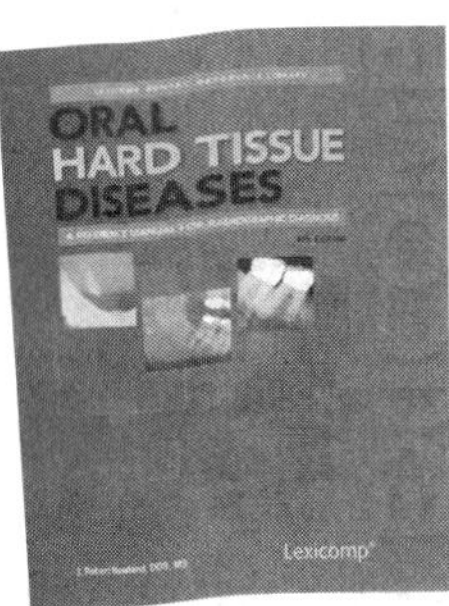

by J. Robert Newland, DDS, MS

Oral Hard Tissue Diseases is a handy reference for visual recognition and diagnosis of common bone lesions. Each section of this manual is devoted to a specific diagnostic category and illustrated with high-quality black-and-white photographs. Recommendations for treatment and follow-up and an alphabetical index are included.

Oral Soft Tissue Diseases

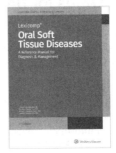

by J. Robert Newland, DDS, MS; Timothy F. Meiller, DDS, PhD; Richard L. Wynn, BSPharm, PhD; Harold L.Crossley, DDS, MS, PhD

In this visually cued manual, each lesion associated with soft tissue disease is illustrated by one or more color photographs depicting typical clinical features and common variations. Recommendations for treatment and follow-up, including sample prescriptions and concise drug monographs, are presented.

The Little Dental Drug Booklet

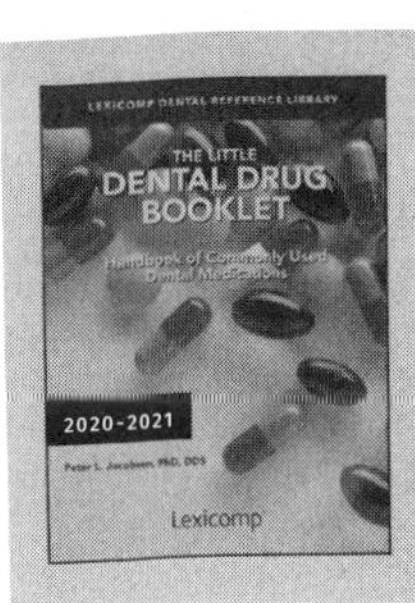

by Peter L. Jacobsen, PhD, DDS

The Little Dental Drug Booklet is a pocket-sized reference to the drugs most commonly used in dental practice. The information provided in this booklet includes practical, practice-oriented suggestions made by dental professionals. A section on prescription writing and prescription requirements is included.